Daniel T. T. Chua, MD
Associate Professor
Department of Clinical Oncology
The University of Hong Kong
Honorary Clinical Consultant
Department of Clinical Oncology
Queen Mary Hospital
Hong Kong

Hans T. Chung, MD
Clinical GU Fellow
Department of Radiation Oncology
UCSF Comprehensive Cancer Center
San Francisco, California

Reiner Class, PhD
Associate Professor
Department of Radiation Oncology
Drexel University College of Medicine
Philadelphia, Pennsylvania

John J. Coen, MD
Department of Radiation Oncology
Massachusetts General Hospital Cancer Center
Boston, Massachusetts

Jay S. Cooper, MD
Director
Maimonides Cancer Center
Brooklyn, New York

Louis S. Constine, MD
Professor and Vice Chair
Department of Radiation Oncology and
   Pediatrics
University of Rochester Medical Center,
   James P. Wilmot Cancer Center
Attending Physician
Department of Radiation Oncology and
   Pediatrics
Strong Memorial Hospital
Rochester, New York

Nils Cordes, MD, PhD
Head, Molecular Targeting Group
OncoRay Center for Radiation Research in Oncology
Medical Faculty Carl Gustav Carus
University of Technology Dresden
Dresden, Germany

Bernard Cummings, MB
Professor
Department of Radiation Oncology
University of Toronto
Staff
Department of Radiation Oncology
Princess Margaret Hospital
Toronto, Ontario, Canada

Walter J. Curran, Jr., MD
Professor and Chairman
Department of Radiation Oncology
Jefferson Medical College of Thomas Jefferson
   University
Clinical Director
Kimmel Cancer at Jefferson
Bodine Center for Cancer Treatment
Philadelphia, Pennsylvania

Brian G. Czito, MD
Associate Professor
Department of Radiation Oncology
Duke University Medical Center
Durham, North Carolina

Rupak Das, PhD
Associate Professor
Department of Human Oncology
University of Wisconsin
Madison, Wisconsin

M. Dolores de la Mata, MD
Radiation Oncology Unit
Clinica La Luz
Madrid, Spain

Thomas F. DeLaney, MD
Associate Professor
Harvard Medical School
Medical Director
Department of Radiation Oncology
Francis H. Burr Proton Therapy Center
Massachusetts General Hospital
Boston, Massachusetts

Gary Deng, MD, PhD
Memorial Sloan-Kettering Cancer Center
New York, New York

Albert S. DeNittis, MD
Chief
Department of Radiation Oncology
Lankenau Hospital
Wynnewood, Pennsylvania

V. Rao Devineni, MD
Department of Radiation Oncology
Washington University/St. Louis
St. Louis, Missouri

Mark W. Dewhirst, MD
Gustavo S. Montana Professor of Radiation
   Oncology
Department of Radiation Oncology
Duke University Medical Center
Durham, North Carolina

Bernadine R. Donahue, MD
Clinical Associate Professor
Department of Radiation Oncology
New York University School of Medicine
Clinical Director
Department of Radiation Oncology
Maimonides Cancer Center
New York, New York

Sarah S. Donaldson, MD
Professor
Department of Radiation Oncology
Stanford University School of Medicine
Associate Chair and Chief of Radiation
   Oncology Services
Department of Radiation Oncology
Stanford University Hospital and Children's
   Hospital at Stanford
Stanford, California

Lei Dong, PhD
Assistant Professor
Department of Radiation Physics
University of Texas MD Anderson Cancer
    Center
Houston, Texas

Tony Y. Eng, MD
Associate Professor
Department of Radiation Oncology
University of Texas Health Science Center at
    San Antonio
Staff
Department of Radiation Oncology
Cancer Therapy and Research Center
San Antonio, Texas

Jean-Pierre Farmer, MD
Associate Professor
Departments of Neurosurgery and Oncology
Pediatric Neurosurgon
The Montreal Children's Hospital
Montreal, Quebec, Canada

Mario Federico, MD
Resident
Residency Program in Radiotherapy
University of Palermo Medical School
Palermo, Italy
Research Fellow
Sbarro Institute for Cancer Research and Molecular
    Medicine
Temple University
Philadelphia, Pennsylvania

John C. Flickinger, MD
Professor
Department of Radiation Oncology
University of Pittsburgh School of Medicine
Attending Radiation Oncologist
Department of Radiation Oncology
UPMC-Presbyterian Hospital
Pittsburgh, Pennsylvania

Silvia C. Formenti, MD
The Sandra and Edward H. Meyer Professor of
    Radiation Oncology
Departments of Radiation Oncology and Medicine
New York University School of Medicine
New York, New York

Carolyn R. Freeman, MB, BS, FRCPC
Michael Rosenbloom Chair in Radiation
    Oncology
Department of Radiation Oncology
The McGill University Health Centre
Professor of Oncology and Pediatrics
McGill University
Montreal, Quebec, Canada

Jorge E. Freire, MD
Assistant Professor
Department of Radiation Oncology
Drexel University College of Medicine
Philadelphia, Pennsylvania

Debra Friedman, MD
Fred Hutchison Cancer Research Center
Seattle, Washington

C. Dave Fuller, MD
Resident
Department of Radiation Oncology
University of Texas Health Science Center at
    San Antonio
San Antonio, Texas

Mirian Gálvez, MD
Medical Physics
Radiation Oncology Unit
Clinica La Luz
Madrid, Spain

Laurie E. Gasper, MD, MBA
Professor and Chair
Department of Radiation Oncology
Grohne Chair in Clinical Oncology
University of Colorado at Denver and
    Health Sciences Center
Aurora, Colorado

Paola A. Gehrig, MD
Associate Professor
Division of Gynecologic Oncology
Department of Obstetrics and Gynecology
University of North Carolina School of Medicine
Chapel Hill, North Carolina

Mark R. Gilbert, MD
Professor and Deputy Chair
Department of Neuro-Oncology
University of Texas MD Anderson
    Cancer Center
Houston, Texas

Ramaswamy Govindan, MD
Associate Professor
Division of Medical Oncology
Department of Internal Medicine
Washington University School of Medicine
St. Louis, Missouri

Perry W. Grigsby, MD, MBA
Professor
Department of Radiation Oncology
Washington University School of Medicine
Radiation Oncologist
Department of Radiation Oncology
Barnes-Jewish Hospital
St. Louis, Missouri

Patrizia Guerrieri, MD
Senior Attending Physician
Department of Radiation Oncology
Regional Cancer Center "M.Ascoli"
Palerno, Italy

Amitabh Gulati, MD
Division of Pain Management
Emory University School of Medicine
Atlanta, Georgia

Leonard L. Gunderson, MD
Getz Family Professor and Chair
Department of Radiation Oncology
Mayo Clinic College of Medicine and Mayo
    Clinic Arizona
Deputy Director for Clinical Affairs
Mayo Clinic Cancer Center-Arizona
Scottsdale, Arizona

Michael Haase, MD
Medford Clinic
Medford, Wisconsin

Bruce G. Haffty, MD
Professor and Chairman
Department of Radiation Oncology
UMDNJ-Robert Wood Johnson Medical School
The Cancer Institute of New Jersey
Chairman
Department of Radiation Oncology
Robert Wood Johnson University Hospital
New Brunswick, New Jersey

Edward C. Halperin, MD
Dean of the School of Medicine
Ford Foundation Professor of Medicine Education
Professor of Radiation Oncology, Pediatrics, and History
University of Louisville
Louisville, Kentucky

Timothy P. Hanna, MD
Resident
Division of Radiation Oncology
Queen's University
Resident
Division of Radiation Oncology
Cancer Centre of Southeastern Ontario
    and Kingston General Hospital
Kingston, Ontario, Canada

Paul M. Harari, MD
Jack Fowler Professor and Chairman
Department of Human Oncology
University of Wisconsin School of Medicine
Madison, Wisconsin

William F. Hartsell, MD
Medical Director
Department of Radiation Oncology
Good Samaritan Hospital
Downer's Grove, Illinois

Curt Heese, MD
Resident
Department of Radiation Oncology
Drexel University College of Medicine
Philadelphia, Pennsylvania

Benjamin J. Heijmen, PhD
Clinical Physicist
Department of Radiation Oncology
Erasmus Medical Center
The Netherlands

Russell W. Hinerman, MD
Associate Professor
Department of Radiation Oncology
University of Florida
Gainesville, Florida

David C. Hodgson, BSc, MD, MPH
Clinical Studies Resource Center Member
Ontario Cancer Institute
Princess Margaret Hospital
Toronto, Ontario, Canada

Henry T. Hoffman, MD, MS
Director of Head and Neck Oncology
Department of Otolaryngology
University of Iowa
Iowa City, Iowa

Kenneth R. Hogstrom, PhD
Professor
Department of Radiation Physics
The University of Texas MD Anderson
    Cancer Center
Houston, Texas

Richard Hoppe, MD
Henry S. Kaplan-Harry Lebeson Professor in
    Cancer Biology
Chairman
Department of Radiation Oncology
Stanford University
Stanford, California

Andrew T. Huang, MD
Professor
Department of Medicine
Duke University
Durham, North Carolina
Professor and CEO
Koo Foundation Sun Yat-Sen Cancer Center
Taipei, Taiwan

Melissa M. Hudson, MD
Member
Department of Hematology-Oncology
St. Jude's Children's Research Hospital
Memphis, Tennessee

Arthur Y. Hung, MD
Department of Radiation Oncology
The University of Texas MD Anderson
    Cancer Center
Department of Medicine/Radiation Oncology
Oregon Health and Science University
Portland, Oregon

Margie Hunt, MS
Department of Medical Physics
Memorial Sloan-Kettering Cancer Center
New York, New York

Rakesh K. Jain, PhD
Andrew Werk Cook Professor
Department of Radiation Oncology
Harvard Medical School
Director, Edwin L. Steele Laboratory
Department of Radiation Oncology
Massachusetts General Hospital
Boston, Massachusetts

Steve B. Jiang, MD
Director of Research
Department of Radiation Oncology
Rebecca and John Moores Comprehensive
   Cancer Center
La Jolla, California

Peter A. S. Johnstone, MD
Professor
Department of Radiation Oncology
Emory University School of Medicine
Department of Radiation Oncology
The Emory Clinic
Atlanta, Georgia

Ellen L. Jones, MD, PhD
Butter Harris Endowed Assistant Professor
Department of Radiation Oncology
Duke University Medical Center
Durham, North Carolina

Monika Jost, PhD
Assistant Professor
Department of Radiation Oncology
Drexel University College of Medicine
Philadelphia, Pennsylvania

Gabor Jozsef, MD
Associate Professor
Department of Radiation Oncology
University of Southern California
Keck School of Medicine
Los Angeles, California

John A. Kalapurakal, MD
Associate Professor
Department of Radiation Oncology
Northwestern University
Associate Professor
Department of Radiation Oncology
Northwestern Memorial Hospital
Chicago, Illinois

Song K. Kang, MD
Resident
Department of Radiation Oncology
Duke University Medical Center
Durham, North Carolina

Brian D. Kavanagh, MD
Professor and Vice-Chair
Department of Radiation Oncology
University of Colorado Comprehensive Cancer Center
Aurora, Colorado
Associate Professor
Department of Radiation Oncology
University of Colorado at Denver and
   Health Sciences Center
Denver, Colorado

Chris R. Kelsey, MD
Assistant Professor
Department of Radiation Oncology
Duke University Medical Center
Durham, North Carolina

Deepak Khuntia, MD
Assistant Professor
Department of Human Oncology
University of Wisconsin-Madison
Madison, Wisconsin

Eric E. Klein, MS, PhD
Associate Professor
Department of Radiation Oncology
Washington University School of Medicine
Chief
Clinical Physics Section
Department of Radiation Oncology
Barnes-Jewish Hospital
St. Louis, Missouri

Michelle M. Kolton, MD
Resident
Department of Radiation Oncology
Drexel University College of Medicine
Philadelphia, Pennsylvania

Ritsuko Komaki, MD
Professor
Department of Radiation Oncology
Gloria Lupton Tennison Distinguished
   Professor of Lung Cancer Research
MD Anderson Cancer Center
Houston, Texas

Kevin R. Kozak, MD, PhD
Holman Research Fellow
Edwin L. Steele Laboratory
Department of Radiation Oncology
Massachusetts General Hospital
Resident
Harvard Radiation Oncology Program
Harvard Medical School
Boston, Massachusetts

Abraham Kuten, MD
Assistant Professor
Department of Radiation and Medical Oncology
The Bruce Rappaport Faculty of Medicine,
   Technion
Chief of Radiation and Medical Oncology
Department of Oncology
Rambam Medical Center
Haifa, Israel

Young Kwok, MD
Assistant Professor
Department of Radiation Oncology
University of Maryland School of Medicine
Assistant Professor
Department of Radiation Oncology
University of Maryland Medical Center
Baltimore, Maryland

George E. Laramore, MD, PhD
Professor and Chair
Department of Radiation Oncology
University of Washington
Director
Department of Radiation Oncology
University of Washington Cancer and Medical Center
Seattle, Washington

Nicole A. Larrier, MD, MSc
Associate
Department of Radiation Oncology
Duke University Medical Center
Durham, North Carolina

Stephen C. K. Law, MD
Honorary Associate Professor
Department of Clinical Oncology
The University of Hong Kong
Chief of Service
Department of Clinical Oncology
Queen Elizabeth Hospital
Hong Kong

Brian D. Lawenda, MD
Assistant Professor
Department of Radiology/Radiological Services
Uniformed Services University of the
    Health Sciences
Bethesda, Maryland
Staff
Department of Radiation Oncology
Naval Medical Center San Diego
San Diego, California

Anne W. M. Lee, MD
Honorary Associate Professor
Department of Clinical Oncology
The University of Hong Kong
Cluster Chief of Service
Department of Clinical Oncology
Pamela Youde Nethersole Eastern Hospital
Hong Kong

Nancy A. Lee, MD
Department of Biochemistry/Molecular Biology
Mayo Clinic
Scottsdale, Arizona

Peter C. Levendag, MD, PhD
Professor and Chairman
Department of Radiation Oncology
Erasmus Medical Center
The Netherlands

Ray Lin, MD
Radiation Oncologist
Scripps Clinic
La Jolla, California

Ruth Lininger, MD
Associate Professor
Attending Radiation Oncologist
21st Century Oncology
Woodbury, New Jersey

Katherine Look, MD
Department of Obstetrics and Gynecology
Indiana University School of Medicine
Indianapolis, Indiana

Daniel Low, PhD
Department of Radiation Oncology
Washington University/St. Louis
St. Louis, Missouri

Laurie Lyckholm, MD
Associate Professor
Department of Internal Medicine, Hematology/
    Oncology
Virginia Commonwealth University School of
    Medicine
Richmond, Virginia

Roger M. Macklis, MD
Professor of Medicine
Department of Radiation Oncology
Cleveland Clinic Lerner College of Medicine
Staff Physician
Department of Radiation Oncology
The Cleveland Clinic
Cleveland, Ohio

Rob MacRae, MD
Assistant Professor
University of Ottawa
Radiation Oncologist
The Ottawa Hospital Regional Cancer Centre
Ottawa, Ontario, Canada

Anthony Mancuso, MD
Professor and Chairman
Department of Radiology
University of Florida
Gainesville, Florida

Rafael R. Mañon, MD
Department of Radiation Oncology
University of Texas MD Anderson Cancer Center
Houston, Texas

David B. Mansur, MD
Assistant Professor
Department of Radiation Oncology
Washington University School of Medicine
Associate Radiation Oncologist
Department of Radiation Oncology
Barnes-Jewish Hospital
St. Louis, Missouri

Robert B. Marcus, Jr., MD
Professor
Department of Radiation Oncology
Emory University
Atlanta, Georgia

Lawrence B. Marks, MD
Professor
Department of Radiation Oncology-Clinical
    Support
Duke University Medical Center
Durham, North Carolina

William H. McBride, D.Sc
Professor
Department of Radiation Oncology
David Geffen School of Medicine at UCLA
Los Angeles, California

Cornelius J. McGinn, MD
Department of Radiation Oncology
Maine Medical Center
Portland, Maine

Minesh P. Mehta, MD
Professor and Chairman
Department of Human Oncology
University of Wisconsin School of Medicine and
    Public Health
Professor and Chairman
Department of Human Oncology
University of Wisconsin Hospitals and Clinics
Madison, Wisconsin

Rosa M. Meirino, MD
Radiation Oncology Unit
Clinica La Luz
Madrid, Spain

Loren K. Mell, MD
Department of Radiation and Cellular Oncology
University of Chicago
Chicago, Illinois

William M. Mendenhall, MD
Professor
Department of Radiation Oncology
University of Florida
Physician
Department of Radiation Oncology
University of Florida Shands Cancer Center
Gainesville, Florida

Helen Michael, MD
Department of Pathology
Indiana University School of Medicine
Indianapolis, Indiana

Jeff M. Michalski, MD, MBA
Professor
Department of Radiation Oncology
Washington University School of Medicine
Clinical Director
Department of Radiation Oncology
Siteman Cancer Center/Barnes-Jewish Hospital
St. Louis, Missouri

Joseph Mikhael, MD
Princess Margaret Hospital
Toronto, Ontario, Canada

Michael T. Milano, MD, PhD
Assistant Professor
Department of Radiation Oncology
University of Rochester
Rochester, New York

Radhe Mohan, PhD
Professor and Chairman
Department of Radiation Physics
The University of Texas MD Anderson Cancer
    Center
Houston, Texas

Mohammed Mohiuddin, MD
Geisinger Henry Cancer Center
Wilkes Barre, Pennsylvania

Gustavo S. Montana, MD
Professor
Department of Radiation Oncology
Duke University Medical Center
Durham, North Carolina

Paolo Montemaggi, MD
Professor of Radiotherapy
University of Palerno Medical School
Head
Department of Radiation Oncology
Regional Cancer Center "M.Ascoli"
Palerno, Italy

Monica Morris, MD
Assistant Professor
Department of Radiation Oncology
Virginia Commonwealth University
Radiation Oncologist
Department of Radiation Oncology
Medical College of Virginia Hospitals
Richmond, Virginia

Gianluca Mortellaro, MD
Resident
Residency Program in Radiotherapy
University of Palerno Medical School
Palerno, Italy

Gerard C. Morton, MD, MRCPI
Assistant Professor
Department of Radiation Oncology
University of Toronto
Radiation Oncologist
Toronto-Sunnybrook Regional Cancer Center
Toronto, Ontario, Canada

Stephan Mose, MD
Head of Department
Department of Radiotherapy and Radiooncology
Schwarzwald-Baar-Klinikum
Villingen-Schwenningen, Germany

Arno J. Mundt, MD
Professor and Chair
Department of Radiation Oncology
University of California, San Diego
Rebecca and John Moores Comprehensive
    Cancer Center
La Jolla, California

Jeffrey N. Myers, MD, PhD
Professor and Director of Research
Deputy Chair for Academic Programs
Department of Head and Neck Surgery
The University of Texas MD Anderson Cancer
    Center
Houston, Texas

Subir Nag, MD
Director of Brachytherapy Services
Department of Radiation Oncology
Kaiser Permanente
Santa Clara, California

Andrea Ng, MD, MPH
Associate Professor
Department of Radiation Oncology
Brigham and Women's Hospital
Dana-Farber Cancer Institute
Harvard Medical School
Boston, Massachusetts

Ajay Niranjan, MD
Associate Professor
Department of Neurosurgery
University of Pittsburgh
Director, Radiosurgery Research
Department of Neurosurgery
UPMC Health System
Pittsburgh, Pennsylvania

Paul Okunieff, MD
Professor
Department of Radiation Oncology
University of Rochester
Chairman
Department of Radiation Oncology
Strong Memorial Hospital
Rochester, New York

Javad Parvizi, MD
Associate Professor of Orthopedic Surgery
Department of Orthopedic Surgery
Surgeon
Department of Orthopedic Surgery
The Rothman Institute
Philadelphia, Pennsylvania

Roy A. Patchell, MD
Professor of Surgery
Division of Neurosurgery
University of Kentucky
Lexington, Kentucky

Todd Pawlicki, MD
Associate Professor
Director
Medical Physics and Clinical Operations
University of California, San Diego
Moores USCD Radiation Oncology
La Jolla, California

Carlos A. Perez, MD
Professor Emeritus
Department of Radiation Oncology
Washington University
St. Louis, Missouri

Zbigniew Petrovich, MD
Department of Radiation Oncology
USC/Norris Comprehensive Cancer Center
Los Angeles, California
(Retired)

Mark H. Phillips, PhD
Professor of Radiation Oncology and
    Neurological Surgery
Department of Radiation Oncology
Washington Medical Center
Seattle, Washington

Leonard R. Prosnitz, MD
Professor of Radiation Oncology
Department of Radiation Oncology
Duke University School of Medicine
Duke University Medical Center
Durham, North Carolina

James A. Purdy, PhD
Professor and Vice Chairman
Department of Radiation Oncology
UC Davis Medical Center
Sacramento, California

Michael E. Ray, MD
Assistant Professor
Department of Radiation Oncology
University of Michigan
Ann Arbor, Michigan

William F. Regine, MD
Professor and Chair
Department of Radiation Oncology
Greenebaum Cancer Center
University of Maryland Medical Center
Baltimore, Maryland

Mack Roach, III, MD
Professor and Chairman
Department of Radiation Oncology
University of California, San Francisco
San Francisco, California

David Roberge, MD
Assistant Professor
Department of Radiation Oncology
McGill University
McGill University Health Centre
Montreal, Quebec, Canada

Kenneth B. Roberts, MD
Associate Professor
Department of Therapeutic Radiology
Yale University School of Medicine
Attending Physician
Department of Therapeutic Radiology
Yale-New Haven Hospital
New Haven, Connecticut

Philip Rubin, MD
Professor Emeritus
Department of Radiation Oncology
University of Rochester School of Medicine
Rochester, New York

Shari B. Rudoler, MD
Assistant Professor
Department of Radiation Oncology
Bodine Center for Cancer Treatment
Thomas Jefferson University
Department of Radiation Oncology
Frankford Hospital-Torresdale Division
Philadelphia, Pennsylvania

Thaddeus V. Samulski, MD
Associate Professor
Department of Radiation Oncology
Director
Division of Physics Department
Duke University
Durham, North Carolina

Todd J. Scarbrough, MD
Medical Director
Department of Radiation Oncology
MIMA Cancer Center
Melbourne, Florida

Paul J. Schilling, MD
Community Cancer Center of North Florida
Gainesville, Florida

Granger R. Scruggs, MD
Clinical Instructor
Department of Radiation Medicine
Ohio State University Medical Center
Columbus, Ohio

Michael Heinrich Seegenschmidt, MD
Clinic for Radiotherapy
Radiotherapy and Nuclear Medicine
Alfried-Krupp von Bohlen and
    Halbach-Krankenhous gGmbH
Essen, Germany

Stuart Seropian, MD
Associate Professor
Department of Internal Medicine (Medical
    Oncology)
Yale Cancer Center, Member
Yale University School of Medicine
New Haven, Connecticut

F. Javier Serrano, MD
Radiation Oncology Service
University Hospital Gregorio Maranon
Madrid, Spain

Hiral K. Shah, MD
Pinellas Radiation Oncology Associates
Clearwater, Florida

George Shenouda, MD, PhD
Associate Professor
Departments of Oncology/Otolaryngology
Department of Radiation
McGill University
Montreal General Hospital
Montreal, Quebec, Canada

Carol L. Shields, MD
Associate Professor
Department of Ophthalmology
Thomas Jefferson University
Department of Ocular Oncology
Wills Eye Hospital
Philadelphia, Pennsylvania

Jerry A. Shields, MD
Professor
Department of Ophthalmology
Thomas Jefferson University
Director
Department of Ocular Oncology
Wills Eye Hospital
Philadelphia, Pennsylvania

Claudio H. Sibata, PhD
Professor and Vice Chairman and
    Director of Physics
Department of Radiation Oncology
Brody School of Medicine/East Carolina
    University
Chief
Department of Radiation Oncology
Pitt County Memorial Hospital
Greenville, North Carolina

Malika L. Siker, MD
Research Assistant
Department of Human Oncology
University of Wisconsin School of Medicine and
    Public Health
Research Associate
Department of Human Oncology
University of Wisconsin Hospital and Clinics
Madison, Wisconsin

Merrill J. Solan, MD
Assistant Professor
Department of Radiation Oncology
Thomas Jefferson University
Philadelphia, Pennsylvania
Medical Director
Jefferson Radiation Oncology at Riddle
Riddle Memorial Hospital
Media, Pennsylvania

Luis Souhami, MD
Division of Oncology/Radiation Oncology
McGill University
Montreal, Quebec, Canada

Joycelyn L. Speight, MD, PhD
Assistant Clinical Professor
Department of Radiation Oncology
Assistant Professor
Department of Urology
UCSF Comprehensive Cancer Center
San Francisco, California

Michael D. Stambaugh, MD
Director
Department of Radiation Oncology
South Jersey Cancer Center
Medical Director
Department of Radiation Oncology
West Jersey Cancer Center
Voorhees, New Jersey

John P. Stein, MD
Associate Professor
Department of Urology
Keck School of Medicine of USC
Los Angeles, California

Michael Story, PhD
Associate Professor and Deputy Director
Department of Radiation Oncology
Director
Simmons Comprehensive Cancer
    Center Genomics Core Facility
University of Texas, Southwestern Medical Center
Dallas, Texas

Jeremy Sugarman, MD, MPH, MA
Harvey M. Meyerhoff Professor of Bioethics and Medicine
Berman Institute of Bioethics and Department of
    Medicine
Johns Hopkins University
Baltimore, Maryland

Roger Taylor, MD
Professor
Department of Radiation Oncology
South West Wales Cancer Center
Singleton Hospital
Swansea, United Kingdom

David N. Teguh, MD
Fellow
Department of Radiation Oncology
Erasmus Medical Center
The Netherlands

Rahul D. Tendulkar, MD
Chief Resident
Department of Radiation Oncology
The Cleveland Clinic
Cleveland, Ohio

Chris H. J. Terhaard, MD, PhD
Associate Professor
Department of Radiotherapy
UMC Utracht
Heidelberg, The Netherlands

Bruce Thomadsen, PhD
Associate Professor
Departments of Medical Physics, Human
    Oncology, Biomedical Engineering, and
    Engineering Physics
University of Wisconsin
Madison, Wisconsin

Charles R. Thomas, Jr., MD
Associate Professor and Vice-Chairman
Department of Radiation Oncology
Adjunct Associate Professor
Department of Medicine
University of Texas Health Science Center at
    San Antonio
Member
Thoracic Oncology Program
San Antonio Cancer Institute
San Antonio, Texas

Gillian M. Thomas, MD
Professor
Department of Radiation Oncology/Obstetrics/
    Gynecology
University of Toronto
Consultant Radiation Oncologist
Department of Oncology
Toronto-Sunnybrook Regional Cancer Center
Toronto, Ontario, Canada

Patrick R. M. Thomas, MD, BS
Former Professor and Chair
Department of Radiation Oncology
Temple University School of Medicine
Radiation Oncologist
Bayfront Cancer Care
Bayfront Medical Center
St. Petersburg, Florida

Wade L. Thorstad, MD
Chief of Head and Neck Service
Assistant Professor
Department of Radiation Oncology
Washington University Medical Center
Siteman Cancer Center
St. Louis, Missouri

Robert D. Timmerman, MD
Professor and Vice-Chair
Department of Radiation Oncology
University of Texas-Southwestern
Dallas, Texas

Wolfgang A. Tome, PhD
Associate Professor
Departments of Human Oncology and Medical
    Physics
University of Wisconsin School of Medicine and
    Public Health
Madison, Wisconsin

Prabhakar Tripuraneni, MD
Chief of Staff
Scripps Green Hospital
Head, Radiation Oncology
Scripps Clinic
La Jolla, California

Richard W. Tsang, MD
Clinical Studies Resource Center Member
Ontario Cancer Institute
Princess Margaret Hospital
Toronto, Ontario, Canada

Richard K. Valicenti, MD
Associate Professor and Clinical Director
Department of Radiation Oncology
Thomas Jefferson University
Philadelphia, Pennsylvania

Mahesh Varia, MD
Professor and Associate Chair
Department of Radiation Oncology
North Carolina Clinical Cancer Center
Chapel Hill, North Carolina

Douglas B. Villaret, MD
Professor
Department of Otolaryngology
University of Florida
Gainesville, Florida

Michael A. Vogelbaum, MD, PhD
Associate Director
Brain Tumor and Neuro-Oncology Center
Director, Center for Translational Therapeutics
Cleveland Clinic/Neurological Institute
Cleveland, Ohio

Eric C. Vonderheid, MD
Professor
Department of Dermatology
Johns Hopkins University Hospital
Baltimore, Maryland

Zeljko Vujaskovic, MD, PhD
Associate Research Professor
Department of Radiation Oncology
Duke University Medical Center
Durham, North Carolina

David E. Wazer, MD
Professor and Chairman
Combined Departments of Radiation Oncology
Tufts-New England Medical Center
Tufts University School of Medicine
Boston, Massachusetts
Radiation Oncologist in Chief
Rhode Island Hospital
Brown University School of Medicine
Providence, Rhode Island

Hans Walter-Weber, MSc
Biologist
Department of Molecular Endocrinology and Bone
   Biology
Merck Research Laboratories
West Point, Pennsylvania

William I. Wei, MD
Professor
Department of Surgery
The University of Hong Kong
Chief of Service
Department of ENT
Queen Mary Hospital
Hong Kong

Tamara E. Weiss, MD
Clinical Associate Professor of Radiation
   Oncology
State University of New York at Stony Brook
Stony Brook, NY

John W. Werning, MD
Professor
Department of Otolaryngology
University of Florida
Gainesville, Florida

Christopher G. Willet, MD
Professor and Chair
Department of Radiation Oncology
Duke University Medical Center
Durham, North Carolina

Jacqueline P. Williams, PhD
Associate Professor
Department of Radiation Oncology
University of Rochester School of Medicine
Rochester, New York

Jeffrey F. Williamson, PhD
Professor and Chair, Division of Medical
   Physics
Department of Radiation Oncology
Virginia Commonwealth University
Chair, Division of Medical Physics
Department of Radiation Oncology
Virginia Commonwealth University Health
   System
Richmond, Virginia

Kathryn Winter, MS
Senior Biostatistician
American College of Radiology
Philadelphia, Pennsylvania

H. Rodney Withers, MD, D.Sc
Professor and Chair
Department of Radiation Oncology
David Geffen School of Medicine at UCLA
Los Angeles, California

Qiuwen, Wu, PhD
Associate Professor
Department of Radiation Oncology
Virginia Commonwealth University
Richmond, Virginia

Santosh Yajnik, MD
Radiation Oncologist
Department of Radiation Oncology
The Cancer Institute at Alexian
   Brothers
Elk Grove Village, Illinois

Michael J. Zelefsky, MD
Professor
Department of Radiation Oncology
Chief
Brachytherapy Service
Memorial Sloan-Kettering Cancer Center
New York, New York

Daniel Zips, MD
Department of Radiotherapy and Radiooncology
Medical Faculty
University Clinic Carl Gustov Carus
Technical University Dresden
Dresden, Germany

Preface

Radiation oncology is the discipline of human medicine which addresses the causes, prevention, and treatment of human cancer with special emphasis on the role of ionizing radiation. Approximately 60% of all cancer patients receive radiation therapy as a component of their treatment. According to American Cancer Society estimates, in 2007 1.44 million new cases of invasive cancer will be diagnosed in the United States. In Europe the incidence of all forms of cancer is 3.2 million. There will be about 560,000 cancer deaths in the United States in 2007 and about 1.7 million cancer deaths in Europe. In the United States cancer accounted for 23% of all deaths, ranking second to heart disease as the nation's leading cause of mortality.

Fortunately, mortality rates for some cancers are on the decline in the economically developed world. This is the result of reductions in smoking, improvement in cancer screening rates (particularly for colorectal cancer), and better treatment. Unfortunately, 60% of the patients who die of, or with cancer, have persistent locoregional tumors. A substantial portion of the resources in cancer care are devoted to control of the locoregional tumor, and we should optimize use of radiation therapy in these patients. The management of the cancer patient involves a complex and close integration of biological and physical sciences in conjunction with sound clinical principles to obtain the best possible therapeutic results. The fifth edition of *Principles and Practice of Radiation Oncology* is designed to provide the reader with a definitive, authoritative, and comprehensive review of the subject.

The addition of two new editors to the fourth edition of the book, Rupert K. Schmidt-Ullrich, M.D., and Edward C. Halperin, M.D., M.A., engendered a review of the mission and vision of the text. A thorough restructuring of the chapters, their subject matter, and their authorship was undertaken and appeared to meet with the approval of our worldwide readership. It is with great sorrow that we report the untimely death of Dr. Schmidt-Ullrich in 2005. A meticulous physician-scientist, and a valued colleague, he is deeply missed.

As we began work on the fifth edition of *Principles and Practice of Radiation Oncology* we quickly realized that, as a result of rapid changes in cancer biology and therapy, the book again required new chapters, new content, and a redesigned format while, at the same time, remaining true to the honorable tradition that has made this book so widely accepted in the discipline. Drs. Perez, Brady, and Halperin agreed that Dr. Halperin would take a lead role in guiding the fifth edition and that three Associate Editors, Drs. Carolyn Freeman, Leonard

Prosnitz, and David Wazer would be added to the team as Associate Editors.

There has been a general evolution of our basic biologic understanding of ionizing radiation and its interactions with living tissue. Increasingly, the discipline of radiation biology has become embedded into a more catholic view of the role of radiation within the field of fundamental cancer biology. The fifth edition addresses the basic science of oncology with updated chapters on molecular cancer biology, radiation biology, and the pathophysiology of solid tumors.

Changes in the technology of radiation therapy have prompted us to expand our sections on medical radiation physics. In addition to updated treatments of the standard topics of photon and electron beam dosimetry and treatment planning, new material has been added which comprehensively addresses three-dimensional conformal therapy, intensity modulated radiation therapy treatment planning, image-guided radiation therapy, brachytherapy, and radiation modifiers.

We have called upon our team of authors to thoroughly update the chapters concerning techniques, modalities, and modifiers in radiation oncology. We have also added entirely new treatments of stereotactic irradiation outside the central nervous system, photodynamic therapy, and oncologic imaging along with updated chapters on particle therapy, intraoperative radiation therapy, and hyperthermia.

The consistent evolution of clinical radiation oncology, abetted by multiple clinical trials, has prompted us to provide the fifth edition with a totally revised treatment of clinical radiation oncology. The chapters discussing disease by anatomic site cover relevant background information on each tumor, including epidemiology, pathology, diagnostic workup, prognostic factors, treatment techniques, applications of surgery and chemotherapy, end results of treatment, and pertinent clinical trials. This edition was extensively revised to include updated reports on new treatment techniques and results. There is a great deal of individuality in the techniques of irradiation. We have attempted to include descriptions of various technical approaches, leaving to the reader the critical task of selecting the most appropriate one for the particular patient under consideration. The comprehensive and rigorous assessment of each tumor site set forth in this text provides the foundation for proper application of radiation therapy techniques and multimodal programs in the treatment of patients with cancer. The old chapters on breast cancer have been replaced with a more complete treatment in three chapters with new authors. Similarly, prostate cancer is addressed in two chapters with new authors. The treatment of head and neck cancer is covered by a combination of new and previous contributors. A fine new chapter on radiotherapy of benign disease has been provided by contributors from Germany.

The constantly evolving treatment of lymphoma, hematologic malignancies, and pediatric cancers has received particular attention. An outstanding revised chapter on Hodgkin's disease compliments this edition of the book as well as an exhaustive revised chapter on non-Hodgkin's lymphoma. New to the fifth edition are a series of chapters on palliative and supportive care and quality of life assessment.

Consistent evolution of our field called for other chapters which have not appeared in prior editions. We have added

chapters on the economics of radiation oncology and radiation oncology in developing countries.

We sincerely hope that the new edition of *Principles and Practice of Radiation Oncology* will continue to advance clinical care, research, and teaching in our discipline. We pray that this new edition will contribute to the amelioration and control of cancer—a disease which causes suffering for many and engenders fear among even more.

Edward C. Halperin, MD, MA

Carlos A. Perez, MD

Luther W. Brady, MD

Preface to the First Edition

Radiation oncology is a discipline of human medicine which addresses the causes, prevention, and treatment of human cancer with special emphasis on the role of ionizing radiation. Approximately 60% of all cancer patients receive radiation therapy as a component of their treatment. According to American Cancer Society estimates, 1.4 million new cases of invasive cancer, 50,000 new cases of carcinoma *in situ* of the uterine cervix, 35,000 new cases of carcinoma *in situ* of the female breast, and 900,000 new cases of nonmelanomatous skin cancer were diagnosed in the United States. Approximately 70% of patients with invasive cancer present with disease limited to the local region and 30% have metastases at the time of initial presentation. Of those who present with locoregional disease, 56% will be cured and 44% will develop recurrent cancer. Unfortunately, at the present time, 60% of the patients who die of or with cancer have persistent locoregional tumors. A substantial portion of the resources in cancer care are devoted to control of the locoregional tumor, and we should optimize use of radiation therapy in these patients. The management of the cancer patient involves a complex and close integration of biological and physical sciences in conjunction with sound clinical principles to obtain the best possible therapeutic results. The fourth edition of *Principles and Practice of Radiation Oncology* is designed to provide the reader with a definitive, authoritative, and comprehensive review of the subject.

The addition of two new editors to the book engendered a thoughtful review of the mission and vision of the text. A thorough restructuring of the chapters, their subject matter, and their authorship will, we hope, meet with the approval of our worldwide readership.

There has been a general evolution of our basic biologic understanding of ionizing radiation and its interactions with living tissue. Increasingly, the discipline of radiation biology has become embedded into a more catholic view of the role of radiation within the field of fundamental cancer biology. The fourth edition addresses the basic science of oncology with new chapters on molecular cancer biology, radiation biology, and the pathophysiology of solid tumors.

Changes in the technology of radiation therapy have prompted us to expand our treatment of medical radiation physics. In addition to updated treatments of the standard topics of photon and electron beam dosimetry and treatment planning, new material has been added which comprehensively addresses three-dimensional conformal therapy and intensity modulated radiation therapy treatment planning.

We have also called upon our team of authors to thoroughly update the chapters concerning techniques, modalities, and modifiers in radiation oncology. The reader will find a brand new chapter on the methodology of clinical trials—essential to the clinician's ability to appreciate evidence-based medicine. We have also added entirely new treatments of intraoperative radiation therapy and hyperthermia.

The consistent evolution of clinical radiation oncology, abetted by multiple clinical trials, has prompted us to provide the fourth edition with a totally revised treatment of clinical radiation oncology. The chapters discussing disease by anatomic site cover relevant background information on each tumor, including epidemiology, pathology, diagnostic workup, prognostic factors, treatment techniques, applications of surgery and chemotherapy, end results of treatment, and pertinent clinical trials. This edition was extensively revised to include updated reports on new treatment techniques and results. There is a great deal of individuality in the techniques of irradiation. We have attempted to include descriptions of various technical approaches, leaving to the reader the critical task of selecting the most appropriate one for the particular patient under consideration. The comprehensive and rigorous assessment of each tumor site set forth in this text provides the foundation for proper application of radiation therapy techniques and multimodal programs in the treatment of patients with cancer. The old chapter on Kaposi's sarcoma in the setting of Acquired Immune Deficiency Syndrome (AIDS) has been replaced with a more complete treatment of malignant neoplasms associated with AIDS. We have also added an entirely new chapter on the role of combined radiotherapy and chemotherapy in the management of locally advanced squamous cell carcinoma of the head and neck. The treatment of breast cancer has been divided into three chapters which now provides adequate space to address the complexities of treatment of Tis tumors, T1-T2 tumors, and locally advanced malignancies. A fine new chapter on tumors of the liver and hepatobiliary tract has been provided by contributors from Taiwan.

The constantly evolving treatment of lymphoma, hematologic malignancies, and pediatric cancers has received particular attention. An outstanding revised chapter on Hodgkin's disease compliments the fourth edition of this book as well as an exhaustive new chapter on non-Hodgkin's lymphoma. New to the fourth edition is a chapter on the role of radiation therapy in the treatment of adult and childhood leukemias.

Consistent evolution of our field called for other chapters which have not appeared in prior editions, Endovascular brachytherapy receives its own chapter. We have also added chapters on technology assessment and cost benefit analysis as well as an overview of ethics and legal considerations in radiation oncology.

We sincerely hope that the new edition of *Principles and Practice of Radiation Oncology* will continue to advance clinical care, research, and teaching in our discipline. We pray that this new edition will contribute to the amelioration and control of cancer—a disease which causes suffering for many and engenders fear among even more.

Carlos A. Perez, MD
Luther W. Brady, MD

Acknowledgments

We are deeply appreciative of the efforts of the Associate Editors and contributors whose expertise, lucid presentations, and promptness eased the task of preparing this edition. An expression of thanks is due to our families who endured our efforts in the preparation of this volume; to the faculty and residents in our departments who were supportive and supplied continued intellectual stimulation, valuable suggestions, and materials toward the completion of the volume; to the editorial and secretarial staff who took on the Herculean task of preparing the manuscript; and to our mentors, who set the standards by which we practice and pursue our profession.

Our special recognition to Ruth M. Aultman, Mary Lou Chin, Gloria Hicken, Lilyan Maitin, Heidi Oehme, and Devon Murphy, who tirelessly and diligently worked on the preparation of materials for the volume. Debbie Habberfield and Susan F. Stone helped manage the considerable flow of paper and mail.

Without the uncompromising devotion of each of these people to the project, it would not have been completed. To every one of them, we owe our everlasting gratitude.

Edward C. Halperin, MD, MA
Carlos A. Perez, MD
Luther W. Brady, MD

Contents

Contributors   *vii*
Preface   *xix*
Preface to the First Edition   *xxi*
Acknowledgments   *xxiii*

Section I   Overview and Basic Science of Radiation Oncology

Chapter 1   **The Discipline of Radiation Oncology**   2
Edward C. Halperin, Carlos A. Perez, and Luther W. Brady

PART A: CANCER BIOLOGY   76

Chapter 2   **Biologic Basis of Radiation Therapy**   76
William H. McBride and H. Rodney Withers

Chapter 3   **Molecular Cancer and Radiation Biology**   109
Michael Baumann, Nils Cordes, Michael Haase, and Daniel Zips

Chapter 4   **Molecular Pathophysiology of Tumors**   126
Rakesh K. Jain and Kevin R. Kozak

PART B: MEDICAL RADIATION PHYSICS   142

Chapter 5   **Principles of Radiologic Physics, Dosimetry, and Treatment Planning**   142
James A. Purdy

Chapter 6   **Photon External-Beam Dosimetry and Treatment Planning**   166
James A. Purdy and Eric E. Klein

Chapter 7   **Electron-Beam Therapy: Dosimetry, Planning, and Techniques**   190
Eric E. Klein

Chapter 8   Three-Dimensional Conformal Radiation Therapy: Physics, Treatment
                   Planning, and Clinical Aspects   218
                   James A. Purdy

Chapter 9   Intensity-Modulated Radiation Treatment Techniques and Clinical
                   Applications   239
                   K. S. Clifford Chao, Radhe Mohan, Nancy A. Lee, Gregory Chronowski, Daniel Low,
                   Qiuwen Wu, and Lei Dong

Chapter 10   Image-Guided Radiation Therapy   263
                   Loren K. Mell, Todd Pawlicki, Steve B. Jiang, and Arno J. Mundt

Section II Techniques, Modalities, and Modifiers in Radiation Oncology

Chapter 11   Altered Fractionation Schedules   300
                   Anesa Ahamad

Chapter 12   Late Effects of Cancer Treatment on Normal Tissues   320
                   Louis S. Constine, Michael T. Milano, Debra Friedman, Monica Morris, Jacqueline P. Williams,
                   Philip Rubin, and Paul Okunieff

Chapter 13   Methodology of Clinical Trials   356
                   Shari B. Rudoler, Kathryn Winter, and Walter J. Curran, Jr.

Chapter 14   Total-Body and Hemibody Irradiation   364
                   Kenneth B. Roberts, Zhe Chen, and Stuart Seropian

Chapter 15   Stereotactic Radiosurgery and Radiotherapy   378
                   John C. Flickinger and Ajay Niranjan

Chapter 16   Stereotactic Irradiation of Tumors Outside the Central Nervous System   389
                   Brian D. Kavanagh, Jeffrey D. Bradley, and Robert D. Timmerman

Chapter 17   Intraoperative Radiotherapy   397
                   Felipe A. Calvo, Rosa M. Meirino, M. Dolores de la Mata, F. Javier Serrano, and Mirian Gálvez

Chapter 18   Particle Beam Radiotherapy   407
                   George E. Laramore, Mark H. Phillips, and Thomas F. DeLaney

Chapter 19   Physics and Biology of Brachytherapy   423
                   Jeffrey F. Williamson and David J. Brenner

Chapter 20   Clinical Applications of Brachytherapy: Low–Dose-Rate and
                   Pulse–Dose-Rate   476
                   Paolo Montemaggi, Patrizia Guerrieri, Mario Federico, and Gianluca Mortellaro

Chapter 21   The Physics and Dosimetry of High–Dose-Rate Brachytherapy   540
                   Bruce Thomadsen and Rupak Das

| Chapter 22 | **Clinical Aspects and Applications of High–Dose-Rate Brachytherapy** | 560 |
| | *Subir Nag and Granger R. Scruggs* | |

| Chapter 23 | **Radioimmunoglobulins and Nonsealed Radionuclide Therapy** | 583 |
| | *Reiner Class, Monika Jost, Stephan Mose, Hans-Walter Weber, and Luther W. Brady* | |

| Chapter 24 | **Photodynamic Therapy** | 599 |
| | *Ron R. Allison and Claudio H. Sibata* | |

| Chapter 25 | **Radiation Oncology in the Developing World** | 604 |
| | *Timothy P. Hanna* | |

| Chapter 26 | **Chemical Modifiers of Radiation Response** | 611 |
| | *David M. Brizel* | |

| Chapter 27 | **Oncologic Imaging/Oncologic Anatomy** | 620 |
| | *Chris R. Kelsey and Lawrence B. Marks* | |

| Chapter 28 | **Hyperthermia** | 637 |
| | *Ellen L. Jones, Thaddeus V. Samulski, Zeljko Vujaskovic, Leonard R. Prosnitz, and Mark W. Dewhirst* | |

| Chapter 29 | **Basic Concepts of Chemotherapy and Irradiation Interaction** | 669 |
| | *Hak Choy, Rob MacRae, and Michael Story* | |

Section III Clinical Radiation Oncology

PART A: SKIN CANCER   690

| Chapter 30 | **Skin** | 690 |
| | *Merrill J. Solan and Luther W. Brady* | |

PART B: AIDS-RELATED MALIGNANCIES   702

| Chapter 31 | **Malignant Neoplasms Associated with the Acquired Immunodeficiency Syndrome** | 702 |
| | *Bernadine R. Donahue and Jay S. Cooper* | |

PART C: CENTRAL NERVOUS SYSTEM TUMORS   717

| Chapter 32 | **Primary Intracranial Neoplasms** | 717 |
| | *Malika L. Siker, Bernadine R. Donahue, Michael A. Vogelbaum, Wolfgang A. Tome, Mark R. Gilbert, and Minesh P. Mehta* | |

Chapter 33   **Pituitary**   751

David Roberge, George Shenouda, and Luis Souhami

Chapter 34   **Spinal Canal**   765

Jeff M. Michalski

PART D: HEAD AND NECK TUMORS   778

Chapter 35   **Eye and Orbit**   778

Jorge E. Freire, Michelle M. Kolton, Luther W. Brady, Jerry A. Shields, and Carol L. Shields

Chapter 36   **Ear**   800

K. S. Clifford Chao and V. Rao Devineni

Chapter 37   **The Role of Combined Radiotherapy and Chemotherapy in the Management of Locally Advanced Squamous Carcinoma of the Head and Neck**   807

David M. Brizel

Chapter 38   **Nasopharynx**   820

Anne W. M. Lee, Carlos A. Perez, Stephen C. K. Law, Daniel T. T. Chua, William I. Wei, and Vincent Chong

Chapter 39   **Nasal Cavity and Paranasal Sinuses**   858

Anesa Ahamad and K. Kian Ang

Chapter 40   **Salivary Glands**   874

Chris H. J. Terhaard

Chapter 41   **Oral Cavity Cancer**   891

Rafael R. Mañon, Jeffrey N. Myers, Deepak Khuntia, and Paul M. Harari

Chapter 42   **Oropharynx**   913

Peter C. Levendag, David N. Teguh, and Ben J. Heijmen

Chapter 43   **Hypopharynx Cancer**   958

Hiral K. Shah, Deepak Khuntia, Henry T. Hoffman, and Paul M. Harari

Chapter 44   **Larynx**   975

William M. Mendenhall, Russell W. Hinerman, Robert J. Amdur, Anthony A. Mancuso, Douglas B. Villaret, and John W. Werning

Chapter 45   **Unusual Nonepithelial Tumors of the Head and Neck**   996

Carlos A. Perez and Wade L. Thorstad

Chapter 46   **Management of the Neck Including Unknown Primary Tumor**   1035

William M. Mendenhall, Robert J. Amdur, Russell W. Hinerman, Anthony A. Mancuso, Douglas B. Villaret, and John W. Werning

Chapter 47   **Thyroid**   1055

Tamara E. Weiss and Perry W. Grigsby

PART E: THORACIC TUMORS   1076

| Chapter 48 | **Lung** | 1076 |

Joe Y. Chang, Jeffrey D. Bradley, Ramaswamy Govindan, and Ritsuko Komaki

| Chapter 49 | **Mediastinum and Trachea** | 1109 |

Arthur Y. Hung, Tony Y. Eng, Todd J. Scarbrough, C. Dave Fuller, and Charles R. Thomas, Jr.

| Chapter 50 | **Esophageal Cancer** | 1131 |

Brian G. Czito, Albert S. Denittis, and Christopher G. Willett

| Chapter 51 | **Tumors of the Heart and Great Vessels** | 1154 |

Rahul D. Tendulkar, Mark A. Chidel, and Roger M. Macklis

PART F: BREAST TUMORS   1162

| Chapter 52 | **Breast: Stage Tis** | 1162 |

David E. Wazer and Douglas W. Arthur

| Chapter 53 | **Early Stage Breast Cancer** | 1175 |

Bruce G. Haffty, Thomas A. Buchholz, and Carlos A. Perez

| Chapter 54 | **Breast Cancer: Locally Advanced and Recurrent Disease, Postmastectomy Radiation, and Systemic Therapies** | 1292 |

Thomas A. Buchholz and Bruce G. Haffty

PART G: GASTROINTESTINAL TUMORS   1318

| Chapter 55 | **Stomach** | 1318 |

Christopher G. Willett and Leonard L. Gunderson

| Chapter 56 | **Cancer of the Pancreas** | 1336 |

Christopher G. Willett, Brian G. Czito, and Johanna C. Bendell

| Chapter 57 | **Liver and Hepatobiliary Tract** | 1349 |

Skye H. Cheng and Andrew T. Huang

| Chapter 58 | **Colon and Rectum** | 1366 |

Mohammed Mohiuddin and Christopher G. Willett

| Chapter 59 | **Anal Cancer** | 1383 |

Bernard J. Cummings and James D. Brierley

PART H: URINARY TRACT TUMORS   1397

| Chapter 60 | **Kidney, Renal Pelvis, and Ureter** | 1397 |

Jeff M. Michalski

Chapter 61   **Bladder**   1412

Zbigniew Petrovich, John P. Stein, Gabor Jozsef, and Silvia C. Formenti

PART I: MALE GENITOURINARY TUMORS   1439

Chapter 62   **Low-Risk Prostate Cancer**   1439

Michael J. Zelefsky, Richard K. Valicenti, Margie Hunt, and Carlos A. Perez

Chapter 63   **Intermediate- and High-Risk Prostate Cancer**   1483

Hans T. Chung, Joycelyn L. Speight, and Mack Roach, III

Chapter 64   **Testis**   1503

Gerard C. Morton and Gillian M. Thomas

Chapter 65   **Penis and Male Urethra**   1519

David B. Mansur and K. S. Clifford Chao

PART J: GYNECOLOGIC TUMORS   1532

Chapter 66   **Uterine Cervix**   1532

Carlos A. Perez and Brian D. Kavanagh

Chapter 67   **Endometrium**   1610

Higinia R. Cardenes, Katherine Look, Helen Michael, and Laura Cerezo

Chapter 68   **Ovary**   1629

Paola A. Gehrig, Mahesh Varia, Smith Apisarnthanarax, Ruth Lininger, and
Michael D. Stambaugh

Chapter 69   **Fallopian Tube**   1650

Patrizia Guerrieri and Luther W. Brady

Chapter 70   **Vagina**   1657

Higinia R. Cardenes and Carlos A. Perez

Chapter 71   **Female Urethra**   1682

Tony Y. Eng

Chapter 72   **Carcinoma of the Vulva**   1692

Gustavo S. Montana and Song K. Kang

PART K: ADRENAL AND RETROPERITONEAL TUMORS   1708

Chapter 73   **Retroperitoneum**   1708

Brian D. Lawenda and Peter A. S. Johnstone

Chapter 74   **Adrenal Gland**   1717

John J. Coen

PART L: LYMPHOMA AND HEMATOLOGIC TUMORS   1721

Chapter 75	**Hodgkin Lymphoma**	1721
	Richard T. Hoppe	
Chapter 76	**Non-Hodgkin's Lymphoma**	1739
	Leonard R. Prosnitz and Andrea Ng	
Chapter 77	**Cutaneous T-Cell Lymphoma**	1766
	Curt Heese, Sushil Beriwal, Luther W. Brady, and Eric C. Vonderheid	
Chapter 78	**Leukemia**	1777
	Kenneth B. Roberts and Stuart Seropian	
Chapter 79	**Plasma Cell Myeloma and Plasmacytoma**	1790
	David C. Hodgson, Joseph Mikhael, and Richard W. Tsang	

PART M: SARCOMAS OF BONE AND SOFT TISSUE   1801

Chapter 80	**Osteosarcoma**	1801
	Nicole A. Larrier	
Chapter 81	**Soft Tissue Sarcomas (Excluding Retroperitoneum)**	1808
	Michael E. Ray and Cornelius J. McGinn	

PART N: PEDIATRIC TUMORS   1822

Chapter 82	**Central Nervous System Tumors in Children**	1822
	Carolyn R. Freeman, Jean-Pierre Farmer, and Roger E. Taylor	
Chapter 83	**Wilms' Tumor**	1850
	John A. Kalapurakal and Patrick R. M. Thomas	
Chapter 84	**Neuroblastoma**	1859
	David B. Mansur and Jeff M. Michalski	
Chapter 85	**Rhabdomyosarcoma**	1872
	John C. Breneman and Sarah S. Donaldson	
Chapter 86	**Ewing Tumor**	1886
	Robert B. Marcus, Jr.	
Chapter 87	**Lymphomas in Children**	1892
	Melissa M. Hudson, Barbara L. Asselin, and Louis S. Constine	
Chapter 88	**Unusual Tumors in Childhood**	1913
	Christian Carrie and Abraham Kuten	

PART 0: BENIGN DISEASES   1933

Chapter 89   **Radiotherapy of Non-Malignant Diseases**   1933
                  Michael Heinrich Seegenschmiedt

Chapter 90   **Endovascular Brachytherapy**   1959
                  Ray Lin and Prabhakar Tripuraneni

Section IV Palliative and Supportive Care

Chapter 91   **Palliation of Brain and Spinal Cord Metastases**   1994
                  Young Kwok, Roy A. Patchell, and William F. Regine

Chapter 92   **Palliation of Bone Metastases**   1986
                  William F. Hartsell and Santosh Yajnik

Chapter 93   **Palliation of Visceral Recurrences and Metastases**   2000
                  Laurie E. Gaspar

Chapter 94   **Pain Management**   2005
                  Gary Deng, Amitabh Gulati, and Barrie R. Cassileth

Chapter 95   **Supportive Care and Quality of Life**   2011
                  Gary Deng and Barrie R. Cassileth

Section V Economics, Ethics, and Technology Assessment

Chapter 96   **Technology Assessment, Cost Benefit, Outcome Analysis Research and
                  Evidence-Based Radiation Oncology**   2022
                  Carlos A. Perez and Edward C. Halperin

Chapter 97   **Ethics, Professional Values, and Legal Considerations in
                  Radiation Oncology**   2035
                  Brian D. Kavanagh, Laurie Lyckholm, and Jeremy Sugarman

Chapter 98   **The Economics of Radiation Oncology**   2043
                  Paul J. Schilling

INDEX   2051

Section I | Overview and Basic Science of Radiation Oncology

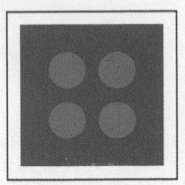

Chapter 1
The Discipline of Radiation Oncology

Edward C. Halperin, Carlos A. Perez, Luther W. Brady

Historical Perspective

On March 27, 1845, in Lennep, Germany, a son, Wilhelm Conrad, was born to the merchant, Friedrich Conrad Röntgen and his wife, Charlotte Constanze (Fig. 1.1). Röntgen's father was a textile merchant and, when Wilhelm was three, the family moved from Prussia to Apeldoorn in the Netherlands, about 100 miles to the northwest, where Wilhelm's maternal grandparents had made their home. Wilhelm was enrolled in the Utrecht Technical School in December 1862. A fellow student caricatured a teacher on the fire screen of the schoolroom. The schoolmaster demanded the name of the unflattering artist, but Wilhelm refused to betray his classmate and was expelled. It seemed that his education would come to an end after this episode. Fortunately, however, the Polytechnical School in Zurich, Switzerland, accepted students based on stiff entrance examinations. The black mark of expulsion from Holland served as no impediment. Röntgen began classes in 1865 and received his diploma in mechanical engineering in 1868 (171,182).

Röntgen's considerable skill in designing and constructing precision instruments for measuring physical phenomena attracted the attention of Dr. August Kundt, a theoretical physicist. Röntgen became Kundt's assistant at the University of Zurich. When Kundt moved, in turn, to the University of Würzburg and then to the University of Strasbourg, Röntgen followed. In 1879, Rontgen struck out on his own as a professor at the University of Giessen.

In 1888, Rontgen accepted a professorship of theoretical physics at the University of Würzburg. On November 8, 1895, Röntgen saw the effects of an unusual phenomenon while doing laboratory experiments. He presented his results to the president of the Physical Society at Würzberg on December 28, 1895 (182,183,353).

There are various accounts of Röntgen's discovery. Among the multitude of reporters who rushed to interview Röntgen was H. J. W. Dam, an Englishman who was a correspondent for the Canadian *McClure's Magazine*. Dam had a letter of introduction from the Royal Institution of Great Britain but, like all other reporters, when he arrived in Würzberg he was turned away. Dam, however, was persistent and wrote a letter in French to Röntgen insisting upon an interview. "You are very difficult, much more difficult than Berthlot, Pasteur, Dewar, and other men of science about whose discoveries I have written." Apparently taken by Dam's audacity and, perhaps, willing to have a sensible article written by a knowledgeable reporter, Röntgen granted Dam an exclusive interview. Dam's lead story in the April 1896 *McClure's* is generally regarded as an accurate depiction (101). Dam told his readers that "in all the history of scientific discovery there has never been, perhaps, so general, rapid, and dramatic an effect wrought on the scientific centers of Europe as has followed, in the past four weeks, upon an announcement made to the Wurzburg Physio-Medical Society, at their December meeting, by Professor William Konrad Röntgen, professor of physics at the Royal University of Wurzberg ... Röntgen's own report arrived, so cool, so business-like, and so truly scientific in character, that it left no doubt either of the truth or of the great importance of the preceding [newspaper] reports" (353). Dam, who was able to converse with Röntgen in English, French, and German, conducted an on-site interview in Röntgen's laboratories and had him describe the circumstances related to the discovery. Dam's charming description, excerpted here, gives an excellent insight into Röntgen the man and the nature of his scientific inquiry.

"Now, Professor," said I, "will you tell me the history of the discovery?"

"There is no history," he said. "I have been for a long time interested in the problems of the cathode rays from a vacuum tube as studied by Hertz and Lenard. I had followed theirs and other researches with great interest, and determined as soon as I had time to make some researches of my own. This time I found at the close of last October. I had been at work for some days when I discovered something new."

"What was the date?"

"The eighth of November."

"And what was the discovery?"

"I was working with a Crookes' tube covered with a shield of black cardboard. A piece of barium platinocyanoide paper lay on the bench there. I had been passing a current through the tube and I noticed a peculiar black line across the paper."

"What of that?"

"The effect was one which could only be produced, in ordinary parlance, by the passage of light. No light could come from the tube, because the shield which covered it was impervious to any light known, even that of the electric arc."

"And what did you think?"

"I did not think; I investigated. I assumed that the effect must have come from the tube, since its character indicated that it could come from nowhere else. I tested it. In a few minutes there was no doubt about it. Rays were coming from the tube which had a luminescent effect on the paper. I tried it successfully at greater and greater distances, even at two metres. It seemed at first a new kind of invisible light. It was clearly something new, something unrecorded."

"Is it light?"

"No."

"Is it electricity?"

"Not in any known form."

"What is it?"

"I don't know. Having discovered the existence of a new kind of rays, I of course began to investigate what they would do. It soon appeared from the tests that the rays had penetrative power to a degree hitherto unknown. They penetrated paper, wood and cloth with ease, and the thickness of the substance made no perceptible difference within reasonable limits. The rays passed through all the metals tested with the facility varying, roughly speaking, with the density of the metal. These phenomena I have discussed carefully in my report to the Würzburg Society and you will find all the technical results therein stated. Since the rays had this great penetrative power, it seemed natural that they should penetrate flesh, and so it proved in photographing the hand I showed you."

"What of the future?"

"I am not a prophet, and I am opposed to prophesying. I am pursuing my investigations, and as fast as my results are verified I shall make them public."

"Do you think the rays can be so modified as to photograph the organs of the human body?"

In answer he took up the photograph of the box of weights. "Here are already modifications," he said, indicating the various

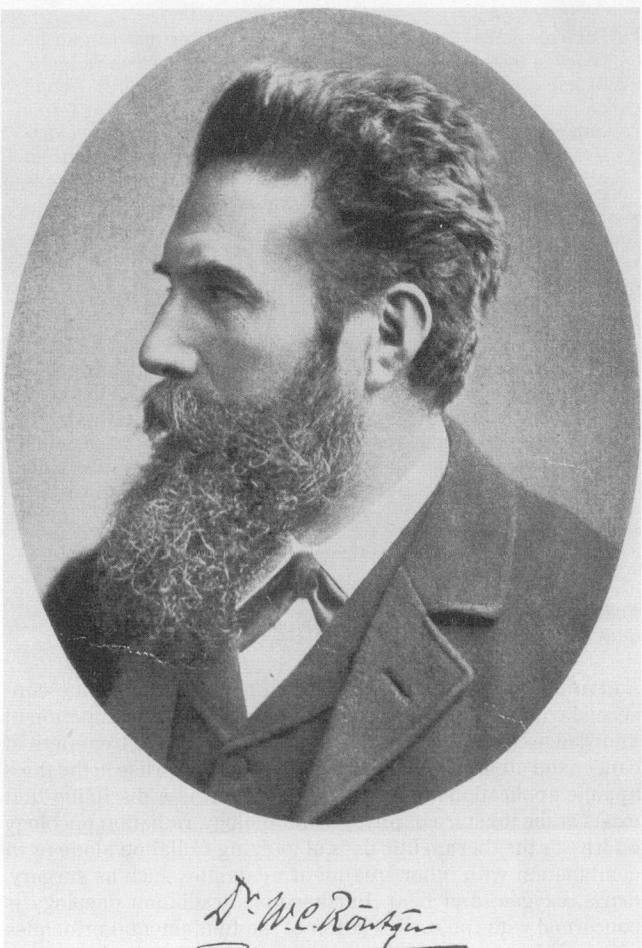

FIGURE 1.1. Wilhelm Conrad von Röntgen was born in Lennep, Germany, in 1845. He studied under Kundt in Zurich and was appointed professor of physics at Giessen in 1879 and at Würzberg in 1888. In 1895, while investigating cathode rays, he noted a new ray of greater penetrating power coming from the cathode tube. Röntgen announced his findings concerning the x-ray before the Würzberg Society in 1895. He received the first Nobel Prize for Physics in 1901. Röntgen died in 1923. (From Glasser O. *Wilhelm Conrad Röntgen and the early history of the Roentgen rays.* Springfield: Charles C. Thomas, 1934, with permission.)

degrees of shadow produced by the aluminum, platinum, and brass weights, the brass hinges, and even the metallic stamped lettering on the cover of the box, which was faintly perceptible.

"But, Professor Neusser has already announced that the photographing of the various organs is possible."

"We shall see what we shall see," he said; "we have the start now; the developments will follow in time."

"When I have done it, I will tell you," he said, smiling resolute in abiding by results. "There is much to do and I am busy, very busy."

"He shook hands with me but his eyes already wandered back to his work in the laboratory." (101)

Kaiser Wilhelm II invited Röntgen to the imperial court at Potsdam in January 1896, less than 2 weeks after the scientist had mailed out reprints to prominent physicists. Röntgen demonstrated his findings and was decorated with the Prussian Order of the Crown, Second Class. On January 23, he gave a lecture to the Würzburg Physical-Medical Society and was startled and overwhelmed by the cheers of the audience. At the end of the talk, Röntgen invited Albert von Killiker, one of Germany's most distinguished anatomists, to come to the podium and have his hand x-rayed. When the audience saw the bones of his hand, it erupted in thunderous applause. This was one of Röntgen's last formal lectures on x-rays. He became flustered before large groups and, to small groups of students, was generally regarded as lusterless and dull.

Röntgen received the Nobel Prize in Physics in 1901 from the Swedish king. He thanked him but gave no speech. He willed the prize money to the University of Würzburg (171). In the presentation speech, the president of the Royal Swedish Academy of Sciences, C. T. Odhner, commented on the enormous potential of Röntgen's discovery for diagnosis and therapy.

The Academy awarded the Nobel Prize in Physics to Wilhelm Conrad Röntgen, Professor in the University of Wurzburg, for the discovery with which his name is linked for all time: the discovery of the so-called Röntgen rays, or, as he himself called them, x-rays. These are, as we know, a new form of energy and have received the name "rays" on account of their property of propagating themselves in straight lines as light does. The actual constitution of this radiation of energy is still unknown. Several of its characteristic properties, however, have been discovered first by Röntgen himself and then by other physicists who have directed their research into this field. And there is no doubt that much success will be gained in physical science when this strange energy form is sufficiently investigated and its wide field has been thoroughly explored. Let us remind ourselves of one of the properties that has been found in Röntgen rays—the basis of the extensive use of x-rays in medical practice. Many bodies, just as they allow light to pass through them in varying degrees, behave likewise with x-rays but with the difference that some that are totally impenetrable to light can be penetrated easily by x-rays, whereas other bodies stop them. Thus, for example, metals are impenetrable to them; wood, leather, cardboard, and other materials are penetrable as are the muscular tissues of animal organisms. Now, when a foreign body impenetrable to x-rays (e. g., a bullet or a needle) has entered these tissues, its location can be determined by illuminating the appropriate part of the body with x-rays and taking a shadowgraph of it on a photographic plate, whereupon the impenetrable body is detected immediately. The importance of this for practical surgery and how many operations have been made possible and facilitated by it is well known to all. If we add that in many cases severe skin diseases (e. g., lupus) have been treated successfully with Röntgen rays, we can say at once that Röntgen's discovery already has brought so much benefit to mankind that to reward it with the Nobel Prize fulfills the intention of the testator to a very high degree. (354)

Following Röntgen's discovery, clinical and technologic advances accumulated more rapidly than did basic biologic knowledge. Several scientists began investigating whether or not rays similar to x-rays might be produced by ordinary fluorescent or phosphorescent substances. Henri Becquerel placed fluorescent mineral crusts on photographic plates wrapped in light-tight black paper, exposed them to sunlight, and observed an image on the plates. In February 1896, when poor weather prevented exposing his plates to sunlight, Becquerel put the prepared plates and minerals away in a drawer. On March 1, 1896, he removed them and, for an unknown reason, developed them before any exposure to sunlight. He saw images of the crust shapes on the developed plates and concluded that neither sunlight, fluorescence, nor phosphorescence was necessary to produce the effect. This form of radiation, initially called Becquerel rays, could penetrate thin strips of aluminum and copper. The next day, he presented his findings at the French Academy of Sciences. He later collaborated with the Curies and shared the Nobel Prize for Physics with them in 1903 (504).

Marie Sklodowoska Curie and Pierre Curie showed that Becquerel radiations could be measured using ionization techniques, and that radiation intensity was proportional to the amount of uranium in a substance. They also discovered polonium (named after Marie Curie's country of birth) and, in December 1898, radium (100,504).

External beam radiation therapy quickly showed itself to be a useful form of cancer treatment. Only 8 years after Röntgen's discovery, Dr. Charles L. Leonard, in 1903, observed that

in spite of the most diligent study, there is nothing known of the etiology and histology of malignant disease that aids its treatment. Its development and fatal termination cannot be retarded, if the diseased tissue be permitted to remain in the body. Total extirpation by surgical intervention has been the only chance of cure. Leonard, however, discerned some promise in a new form of treatment. The results obtained by the use of the Röntgen rays seems to ... have demonstrated their power to alter the character of malignant cells, to prevent their spread and development, and to produce retrograde changes that result in fatty and cystic degeneration or absorption, and often terminate in a restoration of the affected part to a nearly normal state .... The Röntgen treatment applied as a palliative in many hopeless, operatively impossible cases, has resulted frequently in cures, that, if not permanent, have at least restored the patient to health and given months and even years of usefulness .... The results so far obtained are, therefore, very encouraging. An agent has been found which has a greater influence in retarding the growth of malignant tumors than any heretofore known. Many remarkable and apparently permanent cures have been obtained. (281)

At the International Congress of Oncology in Paris in 1922, Coutard (94) and Hautant presented evidence that advanced laryngeal cancer could be cured without disastrous, treatment-induced sequelae. By 1934, Coutard (95) had developed a protracted, fractionated scheme that remains the basis for current radiation therapy and, in 1936, Paterson (377) published results on the treatment of cancer with x-rays.

The use of brachytherapy, starting with radium-226 (^{226}Ra) needles and tubes, has increased steadily in the treatment of malignant tumors in many anatomic locations. Isotopes such as caesium, iridium-192 (^{192}Ir), iodine-125 (^{125}I), and palladium-103 (^{103}Pd) were generated from nuclear reactors, and the use of afterloading techniques, including remote afterloading devices and high–dose-rate brachytherapy, brought a revival of this important treatment modality. With time ionizing radiation became more precise, high-energy photons, electrons, protons, and neutrons became available, and treatment planning and delivery became more accurate and reproducible. Advances in computer and electronic technology fostered the development of more sophisticated treatment planning and delivery techniques, leading to the development and eventually broad implementation of three-dimensional conformal (3DCRT) and intensity-modulated radiation therapy (IMRT).

∷ | A Call to Arms

An Institute on Cancer study was conducted at the University of Wisconsin in Madison in 1936. Among the prominent scientists in attendance were James Ewing, professor of oncology at Cornell University Medical College, after whom Ewing sarcoma is named, Gioacchino Failla, the famous radiation physicist of the Memorial Hospital for Cancer and Allied Diseases of New York, and Henri Coutard, pioneer radiation therapist of the Curie Institute of Paris. Glenn Frank, president of the University of Wisconsin, addressed the scientists on the first day of the meeting. Seventy years later, Frank's opening address remains a moving call to arms for basic science, translational, and clinical researchers, physicists, and clinicians (268).

> Down the ages, cancer has been the most hideously persistent and the most persistently hideous enemy of mankind, the suffering it lays upon men intolerably horrible, its toll of life progressively devastating, its blows falling so often just when men have reached the years of ripest usefulness to family and state. But not all these tragic consequences together are the worse evil wrought by cancer. For every *body* that is *killed* by the *fact* of cancer, multiplied thousands of *minds* are *unnerved* by the *fear* of cancer. What cancer, as an unsolved mystery, does to the morale of millions who may never know its ravages

is incalculable. This is an incidence of cancer that cannot be reached by the physician's medicaments, the surgeon's knife, or any organized advice against panic. Nothing but the actual conquest of cancer itself will remove this sword that today hangs over every head. I can remember, as a boy in rural Missouri, that death from cancer was rarely mentioned and then only with bated breath. I realize now that this reaction was born of a feeling of utter helplessness and awe in the presence of a mysterious enemy. That almost primitive reaction to cancer has happily vanished. We have not penetrated the mystery, but, thanks to you and your colleagues the world over, we have made notable rents in the veil surrounding the mystery. The world is determined to conquer this thing that steals upon men like a thief in the night and without warning strikes down the strong and weak alike. By one thing alone can this conquest come, and that is by the tireless, painstaking, and self-sacrificing genius of scientists who, like yourselves, go to their laboratory tables as to an altar and sink their lives in the great adventure of emancipating mankind from the fact and fear of this plague. Surely, if anywhere in the secular activities of men, there is a spark or divinity in lives do dedicated! (268)

∷ | A Definition of Radiation Oncology

Radiation oncology is that discipline of human medicine concerned with the generation, conservation, and dissemination of knowledge concerning the causes, prevention, and treatment of cancer and other diseases involving special expertise in the therapeutic applications of ionizing radiation. As a discipline that exists at the juncture of physics and biology, radiation oncology addresses the therapeutic uses of ionizing radiation alone or in combination with other treatment modalities such as surgery, drugs, oxygen, and heat. Furthermore, radiation oncology is concerned with the investigation of the fundamental principles of cancer biology, the biologic interaction of radiation with normal and malignant tissue, and the physical basis of therapeutic radiation. As a learned profession, radiation oncology is concerned with clinical care, scientific research, and the education of professionals within the discipline.

Radiation therapy is a clinical modality dealing with the use of ionizing radiations in the treatment of patients with malignant neoplasias (and occasionally benign diseases). The aim of radiation therapy is to deliver a precisely measured dose of irradiation to a defined tumor volume with as minimal damage as possible to surrounding healthy tissue, resulting in eradication of the tumor, a high quality of life, and prolongation of survival at competitive cost. In addition to curative efforts, radiation therapy plays a major role in cancer management in the effective palliation or prevention of symptoms of the disease: pain can be alleviated, luminal patency can be restored, skeletal integrity can be preserved, and organ function can be reestablished with minimal morbidity (89).

In 1962, Buschke (63) defined a radiotherapist as a physician whose practice is limited to radiation therapy. He emphasized the active role of the radiation oncologist:

> While the patient is under our care we take full and exclusive responsibility, exactly as does the surgeon who takes care of a patient with cancer. This means that we examine the patient personally, review the microscopic material, perform examinations and take a biopsy if necessary. On the basis of this thorough clinical investigation we consider the plan of treatment and suggest it to the referring physician and to the patient. We reserve for ourselves the right to an independent opinion regarding diagnosis and advisable therapy and if necessary, the right of disagreement with the referring physician.... During the course of treatment, we ourselves direct any additional medication that may be necessary... and are ready to be called in an emergency at any time.

To integrate the various disciplines and provide better care to patients, it is extremely important for the radiation oncologist to cooperate closely with specialists in other fields (64,394).

The Etymology of *Radiate*

The defining verb of the discipline of radiation oncology, *radiate*, is derived from the Latin verb *radiatus*. *Radiatus* is the participial stem. Some dictionaries cite the origin of the word *radiate* as being from other tenses of the verb such as the present infinitive *radiarae* or the first person singular present indicative *radio*. Radiate is defined as "to spread from the common center" or "to diverge or spread from the common point" or "to issue and raise." Radiate shares a common root and related meanings with other English words such as *ray*, *radius*, and *radial*. The verb *radiate* is more distantly related to other words. For example, if one proceeds along the ray from the political center to the extreme, then one is called *radical*.

The verb *irradiate* means "to direct rays upon" or "to cause rays to fall upon something." In Latin, the prefix *in* conveys the meaning of in, within, on, upon, or against. When the prefix *in* is used with the word that begins with the letter *r*, the letter *r* is substituted for the letter *n* in the prefix to assimilate the initial sound of the verb. Thus, the verb that indicates the placement of water within or on the ground changed from *inrigate* to *irrigate*. Similarly, *inradiate* was changed to *irradiate*.

An object may be said to radiate something or to emit a ray. For example, "The block of cobalt 60 radiates all who come near." The verb that indicates directing rays on or into an object is *irradiate*. An example of proper usage would be "I recommend that we irradiate the tumor to a total dose of 45 Gy." Incorrect usage would be "I think the primary tumor should be radiated to a dose of 45 Gy" (213).

The Planning and Conduct of a Course of Radiation Therapy

When a physician proposes administering radiation therapy to a patient, five fundamental questions must be answered. Once these questions have been answered, an appropriate first step has been taken toward the development of a comprehensive justification and plan for the conduct of a course of radiation therapy. The five questions are:

1. What is the *indication* for radiation therapy?
2. What is the *goal* of radiation therapy?
3. What is the planned treatment *volume*?
4. What is the planned treatment *technique*?
5. What is the planned treatment *dose*?

The *indication* for radiation therapy is that body of data that can be brought to bear showing that radiation therapy would be efficacious for the patient's condition. Such data might exist in the form of retrospective single institution reviews of the specific malignancy, which provide evidence favoring the role of radiotherapy. Phase I and II studies demonstrating safety and possible efficacy could be invoked to justify a course of radiation therapy. The gold standard, however, is a prospective, randomized, phase III trial that demonstrates the value of radiation therapy.

Radiation therapy can be justified either because it improves local tumor control, ameliorates a specific symptom, improves the quality of life, or increases the probability of cure. Any data used to justify a course of radiation therapy must have a clearly defined end point, appropriate data analysis, and accepted statistical methodology. It is incumbent on the skilled radiation oncologist to know how to critically evaluate the scientific literature and synthesize it in the best interest of the patient.

There remains a role for sound personal clinical experience. Although there is increasing reliance on published trials, and special deference is given to prospective randomized phase III trials, it is still appropriate for a physician to rely firmly on his or her clinical experience in the context of an intimate knowledge of the patient's problems. A sound scientific basis and an extensive knowledge of clinical research augment the essential nature of the physician–patient relationship, but they do not substitute for it.

There are two possible *goals* of radiation therapy. *Curative* radiation therapy is used for the purpose of curing the patient where one is willing to engender a small risk of significant side effects in return for the possibility of cure. An example is the use of radiation therapy for the treatment of early stage breast cancer. In return for a high probability of cure, one is willing to engender a small risk of pneumonitis, for example. *Palliative* radiation therapy is designed to ameliorate a specific symptom such as pain, obstruction, or bleeding. In palliative radiation therapy used in the context of an incurable malignancy, one is not willing to engender a significant risk of side effects to achieve a palliative goal. Thus, if one wishes to relieve pain from lung cancer metastatic to a bone, one would pick a dose and technique of radiation therapy sufficient to achieve the relief of pain but not enough to run a risk of radiation osteonecrosis.

The questions of *indication* and *goal* are generic. They should be answered irrespective of the modality of therapy being used for the treatment of malignancy. It is reasonable to ask for indications and goal if one is planning on using chemotherapy, surgery, hyperthermia, biologic therapy, or radiation therapy. Oncologists are, in general, better at formulating indications for curative therapy than for palliative therapy. It must be borne in mind that it is not good palliative medicine to make the patient ill from therapy while making asymptomatic metastatic masses smaller. In palliative treatment of cancer, one must treat the patient and his or her symptoms and not treat the mass devoid of its context.

The remaining three of the five major questions, *volume*, *dose*, and *technique*, are not generic—they are specific to the discipline of radiation oncology. First, the radiation oncologist must consider *volume* (Fig. 1.2). What is the appropriate volume of tissue that needs to be irradiated for the purpose of achieving the desired curative or palliative goal in the context of the justification? Does one need to treat strictly the visualized or

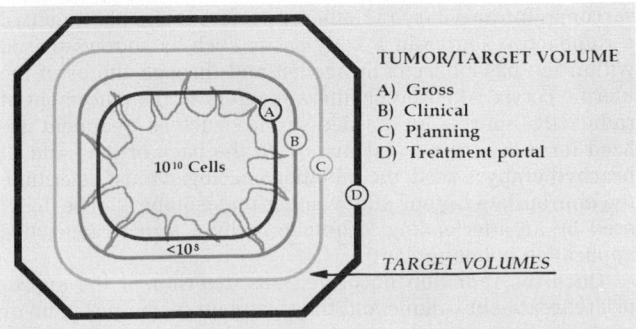

FIGURE 1.2. Schematic representation of "volumes" in radiation therapy. The treatment portal volume includes the tumor volume, potential areas of local and regional microscopic disease around the tumor, and a margin of surrounding normal tissue. (Modified from Perez CA, Purdy JA. Rationale for treatment planning in radiation therapy. In: Levitt SH, Khan FM, Potish RA, eds. *Levitt and Tapley's technological basis of radiation therapy: practical clinical applications*, 2nd ed. Philadelphia: Lea & Febiger, 1992; with permission.)

palpable tumor mass? Is it also appropriate to treat the mass and surrounding lymphatic drainage? Does one have to worry about the routes of spread of microscopic disease? All of these are crucial questions in formulating a plan for a course of radiation therapy. If radiation oncologists only needed to treat visible or palpable masses, then radiation oncology would be more of a physics exercise than an exercise in human medicine. Understanding a cancer's routes of spread and the tolerance of organs surrounding the cancer requires honed clinical judgment.

An example of the problem of volume in the radiation therapy of cancer is medulloblastoma. Medulloblastoma is a tumor that arises in the posterior fossa of the human brain. If, however, one treats with resection alone, patients almost uniformly relapse both locally and by leptomeningeal dissemination via the cerebrospinal fluid. Thus, the treatment volume for radiation therapy of medulloblastoma, in children >3 years old, is the posterior fossa wherein the tumor arises and the entire craniospinal axis. Another example of the problem of treatment volume would be in head and neck cancer. Many of these tumors, by physical examination and by diagnostic imaging, appear to be localized at their site of origin. For many of these squamous cell cancers there is, however, a high incidence of dissemination to the lymph nodes of the neck. Thus, the appropriate radiation therapy treatment volume would include both the primary tumor site and the neck.

The next question that the radiation oncologist must face is what is the appropriate *technique*? Radiation oncologists, in general, have two techniques at their disposal. The first, *teletherapy*, has a similar etymology to telephone, telegraph, and telepathy. It refers to the projection of radiation through space. Teletherapy is administered with external beam sources such as a cobalt-60 (^{60}Co) machine or a linear accelerator. If one elects to treat a patient with teletherapy, one must derive appropriate external beam treatment plans. These plans include considerations such as whether the patient should be treated with photons or electrons; with parallel opposed fields, four fields, or multiple oblique fields; with IMRT; with or without wedges; with or without compensators, and the like. There has been an explosion of interest in new techniques of external beam radiation therapy (EBRT) related to improvements in diagnostic imaging and the increasing power of computers to allow manipulation of vast amounts of data.

Another technique of radiation therapy is *brachytherapy*. The word brachytherapy shares an etymology with words such as brachycephaly and brachydactyly. It refers to short or slow therapy (i.e., a radioactive implant). There are several broad categories of brachytherapy. These include interstitial brachytherapy, intracavitary brachytherapy, and mold therapy. Interstitial brachytherapy refers to the placement of radioactive sources directly into tissue. An example might be the implantation of the tumor bed for breast cancer or soft-tissue sarcoma. Intracavitary radiotherapy refers to the placement of a radioactive source in a body cavity such as sources placed within the nasopharynx or against and through the os of the uterine cervix. Mold brachytherapy refers to the placement of radioactive sources on the skin surface, such as treatment utilized for a superficial malignancy on the back of the hand. If brachytherapy is used, the radiation oncologist must determine the appropriate isotope and whether that isotope is to be delivered by an afterloading technique or by a direct radioactive application (a hot implant).

Once the radiation oncologist has determined the appropriate treatment volume and the treatment technique(s), he or she must determine the appropriate radiation *dose*. Radiation dose selection is a complex issue. One must determine the correct number of fractions of radiation per day, the correct dose per fraction, and the proposed total dose of irradiation. Furthermore, in certain situations, the dose rate (i.e., the number of cGy per minute) matters, such as in total body irradiation

for bone marrow transplantation and brachytherapy. Decisions concerning dose will, in part, be driven by decisions concerning treatment volume and technique. Paramount in the physician's mind will be the goal of treatment. The physician must determine what the correct dose is to achieve the proposed curative or palliative goal. In broad terms, the radiation oncologist has two factors that will guide his or her selection of dose. The first factor concerns what is known about the dose–response relationship for tumor control in a particular clinical situation. This subject, addressed in detail elsewhere in this chapter, concerns the probability of tumor control within a radiation therapy field as a function of the dose administered. Second, the radiation oncologist must consider normal tissue tolerance. In general terms, the probability of acute and late ill effects of radiation is a function of dose. Ultimately, the prescription of a dose requires the radiation oncologist to engage in a balancing act between a sufficient dose of radiation to achieve the desired treatment goal while not giving so much dose as to engender an unacceptable risk of side effects.

The five fundamental questions of radiation therapy—*indication*, *goal*, *volume*, *dose*, and *technique*—are not questions for the physician alone. A patient has the right to be apprised of the physician's views on these questions. This information should be presented to the patient in an appropriate intellectual, social, and cultural context (i.e., in a manner in which the patient can understand) because the patient is a full partner in his or her care.

External-Beam Radiation Treatment Planning

Treatment Volume

Tumor cell killing by ionizing radiation is an exponential function of dose. The dose required for a certain level of tumor control probability (TCP, or local control) is proportional to the logarithm of the number of clonogenic cells in the tumor. Subclinical extensions of tumor (also called microscopic disease or disease below the level of ready clinical detection) should be controlled, in general, by a lower dose of external beam radiation than is required for a palpable tumor mass. Microscopic tumor extensions may be less likely than bulky tumors to contain hypoxic cells. This also means that they may be more readily controlled by radiation.

Insofar as the dose tolerated by normal tissue is inversely related to the volume of normal tissue irradiated, delivering a uniform physical dose of radiation requires that one choose between the risks of marginal recurrence around small volumes of high dose, central recurrences in large volumes of low dose, or excessive normal tissue damage and large volumes of high dose. We may conclude that different doses of radiation are required for a given probability of tumor control, depending on the type and initial number of clonogenic cells present.

A shrinking field technique is a rational approach to the problem of heterogeneous tumor distribution (Fig. 1.3). Withers et al. (603) have argued that "in the ideal case, the doses would be graded to provide a homogeneous TCP throughout the treatment volume rather than a homogeneous physical dose distribution." We are entering an era of "dose painting" where a heterogenous dose will be layered on a tumor as determined by sophisticated imaging tools (33). The radiation oncologist delivers varying radiation doses to certain portions of the tumor (periphery versus central portion or metabolically active versus inactive on CT/PET) or may vary the dose in cases in which gross tumor has been surgically removed.

The International Commission on Radiation Units and Measurements (ICRU) report 50 has recommended definitions of

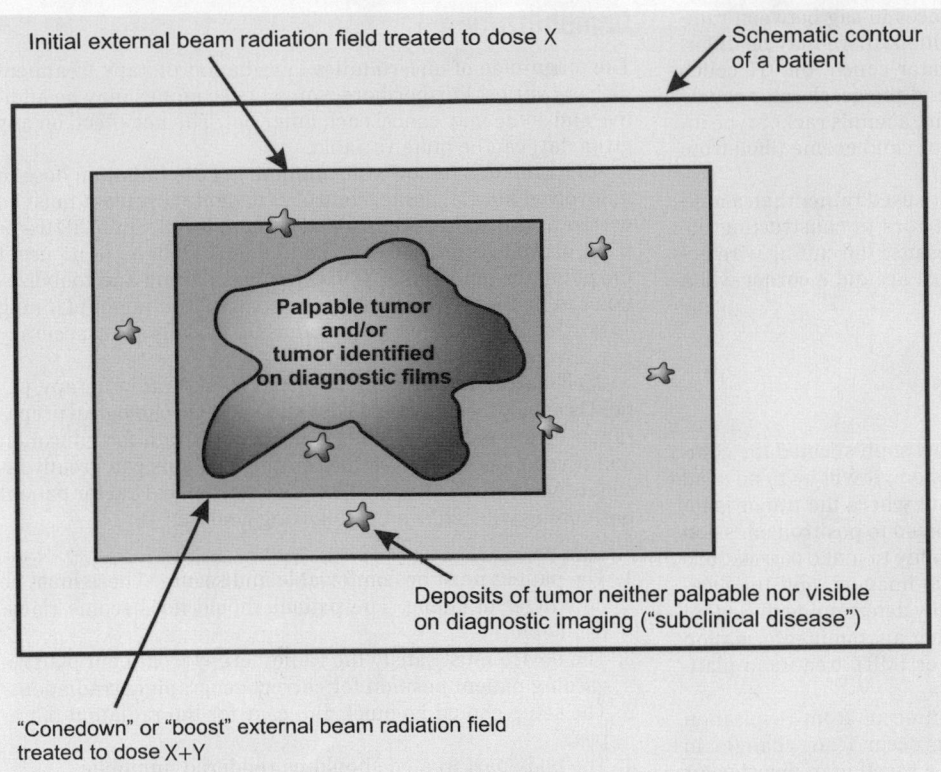

Initial external beam radiation field treated to dose X

Schematic contour of a patient

Palpable tumor and/or tumor identified on diagnostic films

Deposits of tumor neither palpable nor visible on diagnostic imaging ("subclinical disease")

"Conedown" or "boost" external beam radiation field treated to dose X+Y

FIGURE 1.3. Cell killing by ionizing radiation is an exponential function of dose. It follows that the dose required for a certain level of tumor control probability (TCP) is directly proportional to the logarithm of the number of clonogenic cells in the tumor deposit. It would be reasonable to expect that subclinical extensions of disease could be controlled by a lower dose of irradiation than what is required for a bulky palpable tumor mass. It has been argued by some researchers that microscopic tumor extensions are less likely to contain hypoxic foci that will minimize the requirement for reoxygenation for their control—but this is controversial. Insofar as the dose tolerated by a tissue is inversely related to the volume of tissue irradiated, delivering a uniform physical dose requires that one choose between the risk of marginal recurrences around small volumes of high dose, central occurrences in large volumes of low dose, or excessive normal tissue damage in large volumes of high dose. A reasonable approach is to use a shrinking-field technique in which one delivers an initial external-beam field that is treated to dose X and then "cones down" to a smaller field to treat to dose X + Y. In the ideal case, doses are graded to provide a homogeneous TCP throughout the treatment volume rather than a homogeneous physical dose distribution. (This diagram was prepared based on a concept articulated by Withers HR, Peters LJ. Biologic aspects of radiotherapy. In: Fletcher GH, ed. *Textbook of radiotherapy,* 3rd ed. Philadelphia: Lea & Febiger, 1980;142.)

terms and concepts for radiation therapy treatment volumes and margins (246):

- The gross tumor volume (GTV) denotes demonstrable tumor. It includes all known gross disease including abnormally enlarged regional lymph nodes. In the determination of GTV, it is important to use the appropriate computed tomography (CT) and/or magnetic resonance imaging (MRI) settings and, if appropriate, PET scan to give the maximum dimension of what is considered potential gross disease.
- The clinical target volume (CTV) denotes the GTV and subclinical disease (i.e., volumes of tissue with suspected tumor).
- The planning target volume (PTV) denotes the CTV and includes margins for geometric uncertainties. One also should account for variation in treatment setup and other anatomic motion during treatment such as respiration.

Because the PTV does not account for treatment machine characteristics, the actual treated volume is that volume enclosed by an isodose surface that is selected and specified by the radiation oncologist as being appropriate to achieve the goal of treatment. It is impossible to design a radiation therapy treatment plan that limits the prescribed dose to the PTV only. Some tissues en route to the target or near the target also will be irradiated to the same dose as the target. The treated volume is, therefore, almost always larger than the PTV and usually has a somewhat simpler shape.

- The irradiated volume is that volume of tissue that receives a dose considered significant in relationship to tissue tolerance. This would include tissues in the exit region of unopposed photon beams or in the penumbra region of a beam.
- The planning organ at risk volume refers to the definition of margins around organs at risk for injury by radiation. For example, one might define a 0.5-cm margin around the optic chiasm to avoid the risk of blindness.

Uncertainties

There are, inevitably, uncertainties in the planning and delivery of a course of radiation therapy. These were well characterized by the esteemed dosimetrist Gunilla Bentel (32) (1936–2000), to whom we are grateful for the following discussion.

We may, in broad terms, divide uncertainties into two general categories:. First, there are uncertainties related to the delivery of dose. These include inhomogeneities in the beam, problems related to dose calculations, variables in the output of treatment machines, instability of the beam monitoring technique, and problems related to beam flatness. Spatial uncertainties in the delivery of radiation therapy may be divided into those related to mechanical inaccuracies in the equipment and those related to the patient.

Mechanical Uncertainties

- *Field size settings.* There can be errors related either to mechanical dials or digital settings in which the field size set on the machine is not precisely the same as that delivered.
- *Rotational settings.* Mechanical or digital settings that display the degree of angulation of the gantry or the collimator may be in error.
- *Cross hairs.* Wires in the linear accelerator designed to show the central axis or the field edges may become displaced.
- *Isocenter.* Deviations in the position of the isocenter may occur as a result of sagging of the gantry head.
- *Light-beam congruence.* The light beam within the linear accelerator may be in error. These misalignments may be caused by small shifts in the mirror or the light bulb.
- *Alignment systems.* The laser beam systems used for alignment may be in error. They may not intersect exactly at the isocenter, they may not be perpendicular, and some systems may display relatively thick lines allowing for errors in judgment.

- *Couch top.* There can be differences in sag between radiation treatment couches. In addition, there may be differences in sag between the simulator couch, the CT couch used for 3D or IMRT planning, and the accelerator couch. Sometimes, in the treatment room, a tennis racket-type insert is used. Over time, couch tops can become tilted from side-to-side or from end-to-end.
- *Beam-shaping blocks.* If blocks are used rather than a multileaf collimator, there may be errors in constructing the blocks related to user error or because the cutting wire becomes too hot or is moved too fast around a corner when the Styrofoam mold is cut.

Patient-Related Uncertainties

- *Target delineation.* No matter how sophisticated the computerized treatment planning system, it will be to no avail if the physician is uncertain about where the tumor is located. The inherent problems related to positron emission tomography, MRI, CT, and our ability to make correlations between anatomic and functional imaging, and the location of tumor may result in difficulty determining the extent of tumor as well as in transferring anatomic information from imaging studies to the 3D or IMRT treatment planning system.
- *Organ motion.* Organ motion can occur from respiration or heartbeat. In addition, it can occur from changes in the size or shape of an organ as a function of digestive or excretory function (i.e., changes in the size and position of the stomach, intestines, bladder, rectum, and, in the last case, its influence on prostate position) (Fig. 1.4).
- *Skin marks.* Skin marks can shift relative to deeper tissues. This can change as a result of alterations in patient weight, patient positioning, or the use of steroids during a course of radiation therapy. A particular problem is related to the width of setup lines drawn by therapists on the patient's skin. Variation in the width of the lines drawn and variation in the position of the light fields in relationship to the lines can cause uncertainty in treatment delivery.
- *Repositioning.* Day-to-day problems in reproducing the position may occur.
- *Patient motion.* Some patients simply will not hold still during radiation therapy. Whether this is related to the patient being in pain, demented, or subject to a neurologic disorder, it can lead to uncertainties in radiation therapy treatment delivery.

Immobilization

The magnitude of uncertainties in radiation therapy treatment delivery varies. Furthermore, some uncertainties may be additive and some may cancel each other out. The net effect, on any given day, can be quite variable.

To irradiate a tumor while minimizing the radiation dose to uninvolved normal tissue, control of patient movement must be precise and absolute. Sophisticated tumor localization, 3D treatment planning, radiosurgery, and/or IMRT will be of no use if the patient is not holding still. Often, positioning and mobilization can be the weakest link in the chain of treatment planning (204). Quality radiotherapy demands that a daily setup accuracy of a few millimeters be ensured.

Mechanical immobilization of the awake radiotherapy patient is an adjunct to patient education and psychological preparation of the patient. Although not a substitute for education and psychological preparation, mechanical aids can greatly facilitate accurate treatment. The ideal mechanical aid for patient positioning will achieve the following goals (214):

1. The patient must be comfortable and secure. There must be no danger of falling. The patient should not become claustrophobic.
2. The device must satisfy the radiotherapy treatment plan regarding patient position for correct geographic irradiation.
3. The setup should be quick and easy for the radiation therapist.
4. The body part treated should be rendered immobile.
5. Position of the body part should be reproducible for daily treatment.
6. Construction of the device should be reasonably quick. It should not be difficult to train therapists, dosimetrists, and physicians in the construction procedure.
7. The stabilization device should not adversely affect beam buildup and backscatter characteristics.
8. This system should be economical.
9. If anesthesia is being used in pediatric cases, the device must not interfere with the establishment of a secure airway, intravenous access, or the use of monitoring equipment.

A variety of immobilization devices meet these stated criteria to varying degrees. There is no perfect system. Techniques will vary among institutions. It is reasonable to expect, however, that the radiation oncologist should be knowledgeable in several techniques that can be brought to bear as the situation demands.

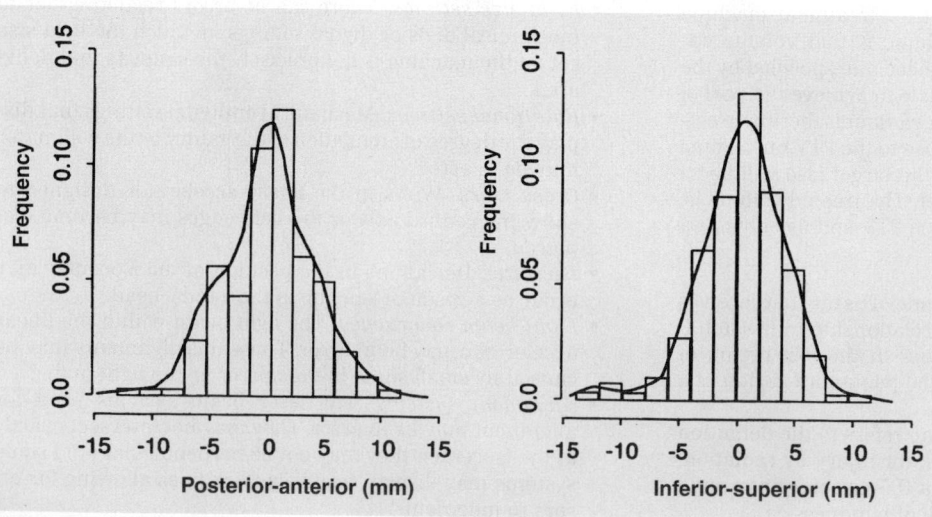

FIGURE 1.4. Precision radiotherapy treatment planning must take physiologic target motion into account. Wu et al. evaluated the treatment errors from setup and interfraction prostatic motion with port films and implanted prostate fiducial markers during conformal radiotherapy for localized prostate cancer. These histograms show the frequency distribution of prostate motion in the anteroposterior and superoinferior planes. Prostate motion can contribute to setup and treatment error in external-beam radiotherapy. (From Wu J, Haycocks T, Alasti H, et al. Position errors and prostate motion during conformal prostate radiotherapy using on-line isocentre set-up verification and implanted prostate markers. *Radiother Oncol* 2001;61:127–133, with permission.)

There are a variety of stabilization devices. These include commercially available accessories such as plastic headholders and sponges, bite blocks, thermoplastics, plaster of Paris, vacuum-molded thermoplastics, polyurethane foams, vacuum bags, intrarectal balloons to stabilize the prostate and rectal wall during prostate radiotherapy, gated radiotherapy and therapy while breath holding to minimize respiratory excursion, and mechanical devices to compensate for patient movement by compensatory couch movement or collimator leaf movement.

Accuracy of external beam placement is assessed periodically with portal (localization) films, online imaging verification (electronic portal imaging) devices, or online CT, fluoroscopy, or ultrasound (322,511,530). Portal localization errors may be systematic or occur at random. Online electronic portal imaging has been used to document inter- or intratreatment portal displacement (511) (see Fig. 1.4).

Patient movement clearly adversely influences the quality of external beam radiotherapy. In a review of 48 patients on whom multiple digital portal verification images were obtained, Bissett et al. (40) noted that displacements of the field were 2.9 mm in the transverse and 3.4 mm in the craniocaudal dimensions. Mean rotational displacement was 2 degrees. The mean treatment field coverage was 95%. There were some variations in the assessment of the translational errors when observations of several radiation oncologists were analyzed. Rabinowitz et al. (415), in a comparison of simulator and portal films of 71 patients, noted some discrepancies between the simulator and the localization (treatment) portal films. With an average value of 3-mm standard deviation of the variations, the mean worst case discrepancy averaged 3.5 mm in the head and neck region, 9.2 mm in the thorax, 5.1 mm in the abdomen, 8.4 mm in the pelvis, and 6.9 mm in the extremities. Other investigators have documented similar localization errors on the basis of portal film review analysis (307,415). Hendrickson (231) reported a 3.5% error frequency in multiple parameters (setting of field size, timer, gantry and collimator angles, and patient positioning) with one technologist working. The error rate declined to 0.82% when two technologists worked together.

Doss (119), in a study of patients with upper airway carcinoma, showed that in 21/28 patients (75%) with treatments in which 30% or more portals exhibited a blocking error, a recurrence developed, whereas tumor failure was noted in only 2/12 patients (17%) without such errors. Perez et al. (384) also reported a higher incidence of failures in patients with carcinoma of the nasopharynx on whom shielding of the ear inadvertently caused some blocking of tumor volume.

A growing body of evidence supports the benefit of stabilization devices in reducing patient motion. Marks et al. (306,307) demonstrated, by systematic use of verification films, a high frequency of localization errors in patients irradiated for head and neck cancer or malignant lymphomas. These errors were corrected with improved patient immobilization; with the use of a bite block in patients with head and neck tumors localization errors were reduced from 16% to 1% (307) (Table 1.1). The growing popularity of 3DCRT and IMRT, as well as the emphasis on stereotactic body radiosurgery, has led to several excellent contributions to the literature assessing the value of stabilization devices. Such devices are particularly important in the treatment of lung, liver, and paraspinal tumors. Often, these devices include a combination of a thermoplastic body cast, vacuum pillow, arm and leg support, wooden backing and/or sides, or a carbon plate. It has been demonstrated that such devices can achieve setup errors and deviations in the 1 to 3 mm range (295, 457). Some institutions, particularly in the United Kingdom, rely on vacuum molded plastic shells. These devices, similarly, will achieve displacements on the order of 1 to 3 mm (243).

One of the most unique recent studies was performed by a research team at the Karolinska University Hospital in Stockholm, Sweden. In this randomized trial, patients with head and neck

Table 1.1	THE IMPACT OF STABILIZATION DEVICES ON EXTERNAL-BEAM SETUP REPRODUCIBILITY	
	Number of Position Adjustments Per Number of Times Tested (%)	*p*
Hodgkin's disease (n = 56)[a]		
Short cradle stabilization device	48/237 (20)	0.009
Whole-torso cradle stabilization device	21/213 (10)	—
Head and neck cancer (n = 71)[b]		
Three casting strip stabilization device	55/307 (18)	0.23
Customized mask device	40/291 (14)	—
Lung cancer (n = 60)[c]		
No stabilization device	17/119 (14)	0.139
Cradle	14/171 (8)	—

[a]Bentel GC, Marks LB, Krishnamurthy R, et al. Comparison of two repositioning devices used during radiation therapy for Hodgkin's disease. *Int J Radiat Oncol Biol Phys* 1997; 38(4):791–795.
[b]Bentel GC, Marks LB, Hendren K, et al. Comparison of two head and neck immobilization systems. *Int J Radiat Oncol Biol Phys* 1997;38(4):867–873.
[c]Bentel GC, Marks LB, Krishnamurthy R. Impact of cradle immobilization on setup reproducibility during external beam radiation therapy for lung cancer. *Int J Radiat Oncol Biol Phys* 1997;38(4):527–531.

cancer were randomly assigned to be stabilized with a thermoplastic head mask or a thermoplastic head and shoulder mask. Reproducibility was assessed by comparing port films in these three dimensionally planned patients with simulator films. This was done twice during treatment and by comparing the actual treatment table positions weekly. Patient tolerance and skin reactions were also assessed. A total of 241 patients were evaluated. There were no statistically significant differences between the head mask stabilization device or the head and shoulder mask stabilization device in terms of reproducibility. It was of note, however, that patients with the thermoplastic mask extending over the head and shoulders experienced significantly more claustrophobic reactions and greater skin reactions. This study has been criticized for its reliance on thermoplastic devices rather than the vacuum formed clear polyethylene masks (428).

Because different stabilization devices are utilized in different clinical situations, there is no simple way to know which is the best stabilization device. An excellent comparative study done at the Northeast Proton Therapy Center of the Harvard Medical School analyzed the length for which there is a 95% probability that the total displacement will be smaller as a result of intrafractional patient motion. It is reasonable to expect that customized closely fitting molds should achieve intrafractional stabilization of 2 to 7 mm, with the best stabilization being obtained in precision treatment of the brain utilizing a rigid halo and bite block (Table 1.2) (142).

We may expect further benefits from research on stabilization. For example, air-filled rectal balloons have been shown to decrease prostate motion during prostate radiotherapy. The perturbation of the radiation dose near the air–tissue interface appears to produce some sparing of the rectal mucosa without incremental detriment to the dose to the prostate (499). Active breathing control, gated radiotherapy, and compensatory motion of the treatment couch to account for patient motion are also all under active investigation (114,123).

Respiratory-Dampened, Respiratory-Gated, and Respiration-Synchronized Radiotherapy

The movement associated with respiration affects the position of multiple organs. If the radiation oncologist wishes to administer highly conformal fractionated or single-fraction treatment(s)

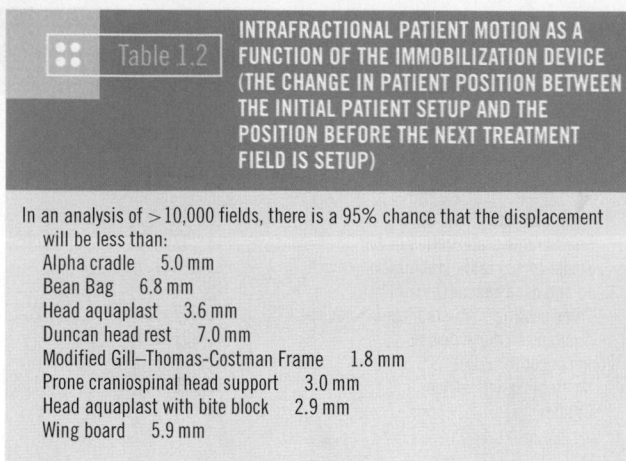

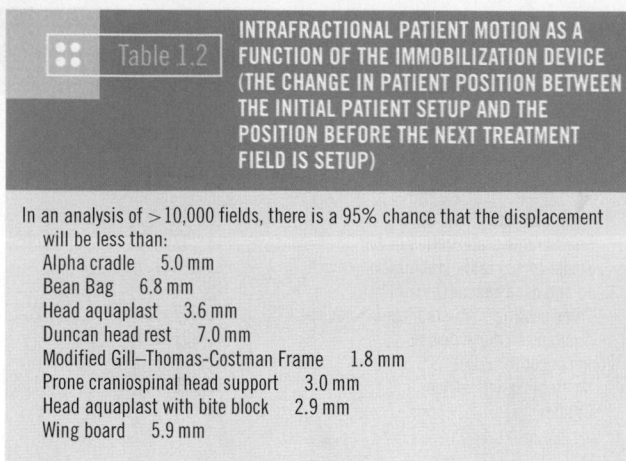 Table 1.2	INTRAFRACTIONAL PATIENT MOTION AS A FUNCTION OF THE IMMOBILIZATION DEVICE (THE CHANGE IN PATIENT POSITION BETWEEN THE INITIAL PATIENT SETUP AND THE POSITION BEFORE THE NEXT TREATMENT FIELD IS SETUP)

In an analysis of >10,000 fields, there is a 95% chance that the displacement will be less than:

Alpha cradle   5.0 mm
Bean Bag   6.8 mm
Head aquaplast   3.6 mm
Duncan head rest   7.0 mm
Modified Gill–Thomas-Costman Frame   1.8 mm
Prone craniospinal head support   3.0 mm
Head aquaplast with bite block   2.9 mm
Wing board   5.9 mm

Modified from Engelsman M, Rosenthal SJ, Michaud SL, et al. Intra and Interfractional patient motion for a variety of immobilization devices. *Med Phys* 2005;32:3468–3474.

Table 1.3	AVERAGE DIAPHRAGM MOTION DURING ACTIVE BREATHING CONTROL (ABC) (MEAN, RANGE)	
By Fluoroscopy at Simulation	By Fluoroscopy during Treatment	Beam's Eye View During Treatment
1.4 mm (0–3.4 mm)	1.2 mm (0.4–2.5 mm)	0.5 mm (0–4.2 mm)

From References 103,129,611.

to tumors of the liver, lung, pancreas, kidney, retroperitoneum, thoracic wall, mediastinal region, and adjacent structures, it will be necessary to either account for respiration-induced movement by putting a larger margin around the tumor or use an intervention to reduce this movement.

One method for limiting respiratory motion during radiotherapy is the *abdominal compression method*. This involves placing a plate or some other restrictive device above or around the abdomen and chest, sometimes in association with supplemental oxygen, in an effort to minimize the amount of diaphragmatic motion during radiotherapy (30). This is also referred to as *respiratory-dampened radiotherapy* (510). Another technique involves general anesthesia and high-frequency jet ventilation to minimize diaphragm motion during liver radiosurgery (173).

Respiratory-gated radiotherapy involves turning the beam on only during portions of the respiratory cycle. One such method calls for the patient to hold his or her breath during the irradiation. A device called the Active Breathing Coordinator (ABC, Elekta, Norcross, GA) attempts to standardize breath holding. The patient is coached to hold his or her breath at a certain consistent depth of inspiration by watching a monitor. The ABC device uses a mouth piece, nose plug, bacterial filter, tubing, and a balloon valve that, when triggered to inflate by the caregiver, will prevent airflow to and from the patient. The patient controls the switch, which must be enabled to allow the operation of the device. Using the ABC system, the caregiver can initiate a patient's breath hold at a predetermined title volume. At the time of simulation, the patient practices in-exhale breath hold under guidance of the radiation therapist. At the moment of fixed inspiration, a valve device engages to prevent additional inspiration or expiration. The beam-on time is coordinated with breath holding (103,129,611).

Investigation of the ABC system has focused on treatment of lung and liver. As seen in Table 1.3, the system can be used to minimize diaphragmatic motion and, therefore, reduce the amount of hepatic excursion during precision radiation therapy.

DNA Damage by Ionizing Radiation

The biologic effects of ionizing radiation are largely the result of DNA damage, which is caused directly by ionization within the DNA molecule or indirectly from the action of chemical radicals formed as a result of local ionizations in water. The general forms of DNA damage are base damage, DNA-protein cross-

links, single-strand breaks, double-strand breaks, and complex combinations of all of these (Fig. 1.5).

Normal mammalian cells repair a significant proportion of radiation-induced DNA damage. Long-term biologic consequences are the result of those injuries, which are irreparable or misrepaired. The cell will attempt to repair DNA injury induced by radiation via several pathways. Key genes affecting these radiation-repair pathways include ATM (associated with ataxia telangiectasia), Ku (involved in repair of double-strand DNA breaks), and XRCC2.

There is some evidence that clustered local damage to DNA, such as a double-strand break accompanied by additional breaks, base damage, or DNA-protein cross-links, are especially difficult for cells to repair. Even lesions that are potentially repairable may be repaired incorrectly (misrepaired) if lesions are accumulating very rapidly because of high–dose-rate or dose-rate radiation or if the cell enters M phase and attempts DNA synthesis while repair is in progress. Conversely, radiation, which is given at a low dose rate or is highly fractionated, provides the best opportunity for repair of radiation-induced lesions and recovery from injury. DNA damage that is not repaired may cause cell death, prevent cell division, or permanently give rise to heritable lesions such as point mutations, small and large deletions and translocations of DNA sequences, and a wide variety of DNA aberrations (291) (Tables 1.4 and 1.5).

Relevance of Radiobiologic Concepts in Clinical Radiation Therapy

Radiation and Cancer Biology's Contributions to the Clinical Practice of Radiation Oncology

Generations of radiation oncologists have grappled with the question of radiation and cancer biology's contribution to the clinical practice of radiation oncology. The question was posed and addressed by Stanford's Henry S. Kaplan (258), in his 1970 Failla lecture to the Radiation Research Society as well as by Harvard's Herman D. Suit (486) in his 1983 Failla lecture. Treading on the ground prepared for us by Kaplan and Suit, we will reconsider the question in the context of the explosion of knowledge concerning the molecular and cellular basis of cancer at the start of the 21st century.

One can look at the history of cancer biology's contribution to the clinical practice of radiation oncology in terms of two debates: *empiricism versus research-based radiation oncology* and *biology versus physics*.

Empiricism versus Research-Based Radiation Oncology

Empiricism harkens to the views of David Hume (1711–1776) and other British philosophers of the 17th and 18th centuries

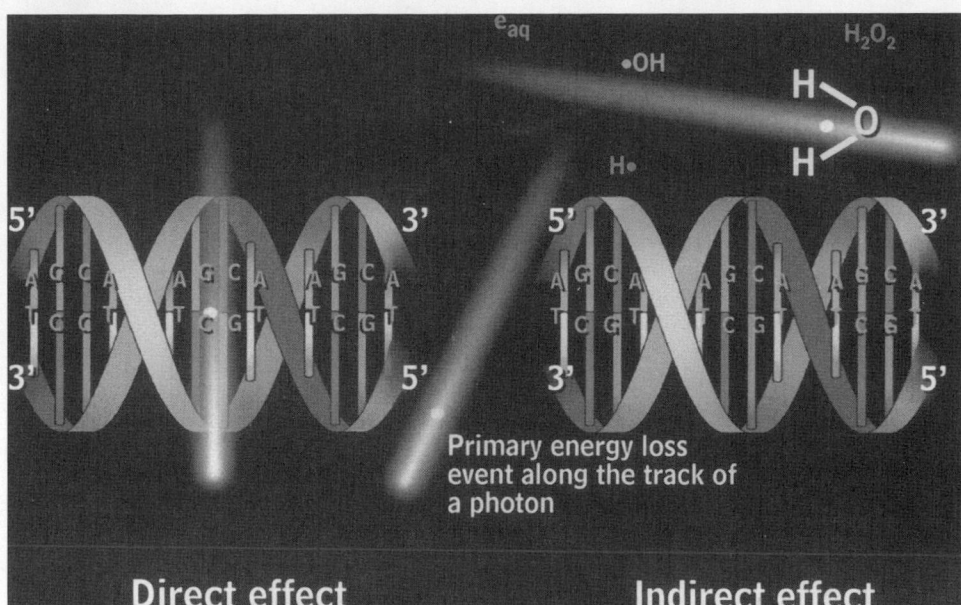

FIGURE 1.5. The direct effect of ionizing radiation occurs when a photon interacts directly with the DNA helix. The indirect effect occurs via an interaction of ionizing radiation with water. Free radicals are generated that, in turn, interact with DNA. The most common lethal injurious effect of ionizing radiation is the production of DNA double-strand breaks. (From Dutton JJ, Haik BG. *Thyroid eye disease.* New York: Marcel Dekker Inc, 2002, with permission.)

and their distrust of the power of unaided reason. In the philosopher's view of empiricism, the best contact between one's understanding of knowledge and the world is not the point at which a mathematical proof crystallizes, but the point at which you see and touch a familiar object. Their paradigm was knowledge by sensory experience rather than by reason alone (42,344,474).

Empirical radiation oncologists rely on accumulated clinical experience, also known as "what has worked in the past." They are suspicious of therapies based on theories and laboratory

research and feel safest when treading the pathway of tested experience. One can find very strong signs of empiricism in the radiation oncology literature: case reports; single-institution retrospective clinical series; and a marked concern with retrospective clinical analyses of radiation therapy that mine clinical experience to aid the selection of radiation treatment volume, dose, and treatment techniques.

There can be no doubt that the development of radiation oncology has been extensively based on empiricism. As Fowler wrote: "If therapists had waited for a fully scientific basis for

---

Table 1.4   THE MICROENVIRONMENT AND THE RADIATION RESPONSE

A. Issues and problems
    Tumor and its interaction with normal tissue and stroma
       Identifying tumor from normal tissue
       Abnormal physiology; stress response and epigenetic changes
       Normal tissue and stromal component—cytokines, growth factors, cell–cell contact
       Immunologic response
       Inflammatory processes
       Interstitial pressure—a barrier to therapy?
       Drug distribution—depends on size, charge, solubility
       Heterogeneity—very complex and hard to replicate in the lab
       Instability—genetic, environmental; inherent cellular genetic instability also is subject to dynamic changes (e.g., ischemia-reperfusion)

B. New opportunities
    Laser-capture microscopy—analyze heterogeneity
    cDNA microarray—molecular phenotype and identification of families of genes and genes that modify the impact of mutated genes
    Protein function depends on conformation such that a normal gene product may function abnormally in the tumor microenvironment
    Tumor progression may be the result of a combination of tumor and stromal cell factors
    Normal tissues within the tumor may become therapeutic target (e.g., endothelial cells)
    Immunologic response—adoptive immunotherapy, enhancing immunogenicity with costimulatory molecules and factors and possibly with radiation to increase antigen
       expression
    Heterogeneity of radiation dose-intensity within tumor—intensity-modulated radiation therapy, brachytherapy, radiolabeled molecules (antibodies, ligands, peptides)
    Inflammatory processes and inflammatory molecules and their role in tumor resistance to therapy
    Late effects; these may be a continuous/continual "chronic active" process
    Interstitial space analysis—microdialysis, pharmacokinetics
    Drug/nutrient distribution—target abnormal tumor physiology with hypoxia activation of drugs and genes
    Instability—genetic, environmental
    Need to understand selection pressure based on environment; successful treatment or prevention strategies may require abrogating the tumor cell's ability to evolve a more
       malignant phenotype

From Coleman CN. International Conference on Translational Research and Preclinical Strategies in Radio-Oncology (ICTR): conference summary. *Int J Radiat Oncol Biol Phys* 2001;49:301–309, with permission.

Table 1.5	THE NANO-TO-PICO ENVIRONMENT AND THE RADIATION RESPONSE

A. Issues and problems
  Where the real action is
    Subcellular dosimetry—heterogeneity at nano-level where dense ionizations occur
    Multiple molecular target beyond DNA
    Molecular pharmacology—cell is highly compartmentalized
    For effective cancer treatment both drug and radiation therapy-induced radical or other biochemical perturbation—must be
      at right concentration, right place at the right time

B. New opportunities
  Subcellular dosimetry—understanding of molecular dosimetry, tracks, and impact of dense ionization on non-DNA processes
  Fractionation effects—low-dose hypersensitivity, adaptive response, and bystander effect—what is impact on normal tissue
    and tumors
  Molecular targets beyond DNA
  New drug discovery
    Designer molecules synthesized using specific target and structural biology
    Combinatorial molecules can create many molecules and then one sorts out activity
  Imaging—functional and molecular of tumor and normal-tissue positron emission tomography, magnetic resonance, electron
    paramagnetic resonance, etc. (e.g., image oxygen)
  Nanotechnology—biomolecular sensors/probes (e.g., imaging biochemical processes)
  Targeting radioisotopes—select isotope (α, β, or γ) by desired path length
  Ultimate planning of biology plus physics *Nano Inverse planning*
  Radiation oncology more than technology; we need to convey the concept of "focused biology" to colleagues

From Coleman CN. International Conference on Translational Research and Preclinical Strategies in Radio-Oncology (ICTR): conference summary. *Int J Radiat Oncol Biol Phys* 2001;49:301–309, with permission.

treating the first patient, radiotherapy would not have started yet" (258,259). We must note, however, that radiation biologists worked closely with the early radiation oncologists. It would be erroneous to suggest that the early history of radiation oncology was completely devoid of reliance on radiation biology.

The theme of hostility to empiricism and support for finding a firm basis for clinical radiation oncology in radiation and cancer biology research is also easily identified in the development of the specialty. "Some people do the same thing wrong for 30 years and then call it accumulated clinical experience," said one critic; or it has been said, "If radiation oncologists were put in charge of the war against polio, they certainly would have perfected the iron lung by now." Knowledge of the genome, proteomics, secondary messengers, solid tumor biology, angiogenesis, oxygenation, and cell-cycle control are changing the present and future of medicine. If clinical radiation oncologists have a future, these individuals say, then they must actively participate in the investigation of the molecular and cellular basis of cancer and in translational research.

Physics versus Biology

One also may formulate the debate over the role of basic biology in clinical radiation oncology as a pull and tug between physics and biology. Medical radiation physics has dominated the thinking of clinical radiation oncologists. Among the major achievements of this discipline are the following:

- The identification and characterization of physical units of radiation dose.
- Significant improvement in radiation therapy apparatus (initially, kilovoltage and later ^{60}Co, and high-energy linear accelerators, the Gamma Knife (Elekta Corp, Stockholm), and the CyberKnife (Accuray, Sunnyvale, CA).
- The development of 3D treatment planning for identification of tumor volume and characterization of irradiated normal tissue.
- IMRT for improved conformality of treatment beams.
- Particle therapy including neutrons, protons, pions, and stripped nuclei.

- Improved stabilization devices to aid the reproducibility of treatment.
- Advances in brachytherapy technology including new isotopes, the afterloading technique, and remote high–dose-rate machines.
- The apparatus for intraoperative radiation therapy (IORT).
- Equipment for heat deposition in tumors leading to the clinical applications of hyperthermia.

At present, a considerable effort in clinical radiation oncology is focused on the tools and techniques provided to the physician by the physicist. Radiation oncology meetings are dominated by discussions of 3D treatment planning, IMRT, radiosurgery/conformal radiation, and innovations in equipment. Simply put, these techniques all offer better radiation dose distributions, which, one hopes, will lead to an increase in local control of tumors and a decrease in normal tissue toxicity. At present, a better dose distribution is the solution physics offers to the problems of oxygenation, monitoring of tumor blood flow, tumor pH, secondary messengers, tumor-suppressor genes, oncogenes, the biology of metastasis, normal tissue radioprotectors, and tumor radiosensitizers. Could it be that "if all you have is a hammer, than everything looks like a nail"?

What has cancer biology ever done for the clinical radiation oncologist? It is, we think, a generally fair question, although it might be characterized as somewhat narcissistic, along the lines of "What have you done for me lately?" (258,259,486). Among the areas one should consider on the list of laboratory contributions to the clinic are the following:

- As early as 1906, Bergonie and Tribondeau (35) enunciated a series of famous laws of radiosensitivity. This was followed by the work of the French investigator Regaud and Ferroux (418), who demonstrated that whereas a single dose of radiation to the testes always produced maximal damage to the scrotal skin, fractionated exposure spared the skin but destroyed spermatogenesis. They speculated that this same technique of fractionation might be differentially advantageous in the treatment of tumors. This led to Coutard's (94) study that culminated in the fractionated EBRT techniques of today.

- The identification of the relationship between radiation dose and cell kill led to the characterization of the radiation cell survival curve. This contributed mightily to our understanding of radiation therapy dose and fractionation and, consequently, contributed to our understanding of radiation repair. This development placed our understanding of radiation fractionation on sound footing and led to investigations of alternative fractionation schemes. This has contributed to improved tumor control as well as limitation of normal tissue toxicity. Ultimately, the radiation cell survival curve also provided the underpinnings for our understanding of elements of the dose–response relationship for tumor control and normal tissue toxicity.

- In 1909, Schwarz (452) demonstrated that compression of the skin to diminish capillary blood flow reduces severity of cutaneous radiation reactions. This may have been the first demonstration of the "oxygen effect" (364). L. H. Gray (194) pointed out the relevance of the "oxygen effect" to radiation oncology by identifying the fact that human neoplasms contain a significant subpopulation of hypoxic cells (507). A series of important developments has driven home the centrality of hypoxia to our understanding of radiation's effects on tumors. Clearly, histopathologic studies and invasive measurements of intratumoral partial oxygen pressure have shown that many human tumors contain regions with low oxygen tension (54). We now believe that there are at least two different mechanisms, called *diffusion-limited* and *perfusion-limited* hypoxia, behind this observation. Some have called these *permanent* and *transient* hypoxia (364). Diffusion-limited hypoxia results from inadequate angiogenesis, whereas perfusion-limited hypoxia is associated with intermittent closure of tumor vessels, leading to acute hypoxic conditions for tumor cells downstream from the obstruction. In addition, we now understand how hypoxia activates genes and may produce tumor differentiation and increase a tumor's metastatic potential. Clinical studies have associated the prognostic value of hemoglobin level with tumor local control (235,364). The characterization of the hypoxia problem has led to a variety of strategies to overcome it. One has been to have the patient breathe high–oxygen-content gas mixtures or to irradiate patients in hyperbaric oxygen chambers. Another option involves the use of oxygen-mimetic chemicals. Other treatment strategies include blood transfusions or the specific use of hypoxic-specific cytotoxins such as mitomycin-C.

- There has been considerable growth in our understanding of cell proliferation, the cell cycle, and cell-repair mechanisms. We now understand that cells are more sensitive to radiation in M phase and more sensitive to hyperthermia in S phase. Our understanding of the differential sensitivity of cells to radiation during the cell cycle helps provide a rational basis for the use of radiation and chemotherapy. Furthermore, our understanding of the influence of the cell cycle on sensitivity has led to work on the halogenated pyrimidine analogs, which appear to sensitize cells to radiation's lethal effects by increasing the yield of nonrepairable double-strand breaks (278). A large number of clinical trials have resulted. Although this line of research has not, to date, borne major clinical fruit, it has been a rationally based area of investigation that may yet prove itself.

- As an extension of the knowledge associated with the radiation cell-survival curve, clinicians obviously need to have a good understanding of the radiation dose and response for both normal and malignant tissue. The development of research involving the lethal dose 50% (LD50), local control rates, and normal tissue toxicity in animal models has led to an improved understanding of the radiation

dose–response relationship. Correlates of this understanding have included the use of the progressive shrinking-field technique; IORT; brachytherapy as "boost"; the use of increasingly conformal beams associated with our improved understanding of how radiation dose should be associated with tumor volume and dose painting. One expects, in the future, to see increasing work in intentional dose heterogeneity as a technique for improving local control.

In his 1983 Failla lecture, Herman Suit (486) considered the evolution of the principles of clinical radiation therapy. He prepared a table in which he attempted to articulate the principles of radiation therapy invoked in the United States in 1956 and 1982. This is reproduced in the first two columns of Table 1.6. The authors of this chapter have added a third column identifying the appropriate principles for 2007. One can see, by scanning across the table, the significant changes that have taken place in our discipline. It is clear that the future holds a role both for empiricism and for research-based radiation oncology as well as a role for improvements in physics and biology. Through cooperation and constructive dialogue, all may contribute to the future of cancer care.

:: | Logarithmic Cell Kill

Among the simplest exercises a radiation oncologist–in-training can undertake is the creation of a table of logarithmic cell kill. At first, such an exercise seems trivial. The effort expended on this somewhat tedious exercise, will, however be repaid many times over.

Let us assume that we have a tumor that follows a typical cell-survival curve. These tumor cells have a 50% probability of cell survival after a radiation dose of 2 Gy. If we assume, for the purpose of this exercise, that there are no changes in the probability of cell kill wrought by changes in tumor oxygenation, pH, or other factors during the course of treatment; that there is no accelerated repopulation; and that only the simplest conditions apply (i.e., that there is 50% kill for each dose), then we can create a table showing the number of cells killed and the number of cells remaining after each dose (Table 1.7).

Let us assume that we begin with a relatively small tumor (i.e., a spherical tumor a bit more than 1 cm in diameter containing, say, 10^9 cells). At each dose of 2 Gy, 50% of the cells are killed. Thus, after the first dose, 500 million cells are killed and 500 million cells remain. At each successive dose 50% of the cells are killed. Therefore, by the end of the course of radiation, very few cells are killed with each individual dose.

One can see, from going through the exercise, that even for a very small tumor the number of initial cells is very large and the marginal killing of the absolute number of cells, with the last few doses, is small. It is not surprising, therefore, that for a tumor of average radiation sensitivity, quite a high dose of radiation is required.

Obviously, the exercise would change if we were to use a different radiation dose per fraction, producing a different probability of survival, or if the intrinsic radiosensitivity of the tumor cell line were different and the probability of survival were different. (Based on Suit HD. Radiation biology: a basis for radiotherapy. In Fletcher GH, ed. *Textbook of radiotherapy*. Philadelphia: Lea & Febiger, 1966.)

Coleman (86), in a summary of the International Conference on Translational Research in Radiation Oncology, emphasized the importance of radiation oncologists remaining current with newer scientific findings that will be critical in the development of improved therapeutic strategies. Approaches that alter the

Table 1.6	PRINCIPLES OF RADIATION ONCOLOGY DERIVED FROM THE INITIAL WORK OF SUIT	
1956	**1982**	**2007**
1. Aim for uniform dose throughout the treatment volume. Treatment volume is constant for entire treatment (i.e., no shrinking field).	1. Use shrinking-field technique (i.e., a nonuniform dose distribution related to number of tumor cells).	1. Moderate and conform the external-beam or brachytherapy dose distribution in accordance with the viable tumor-cell distribution.
2. Initial large treatment volume is carried to tolerance.	2. Dose to the initial volume is usually less than tolerance. Only the final treatment volume is carried to tolerance dose level.	2. Dose to the initial volume is less than tolerance and may be moderated because of the specific host and treatment factors affecting tolerance.
3. No special emphasis to push dose to higher levels for larger tumors.	3. Dose aim is planned on the basis of tumor size or estimated tumor cell number. a. Maximum doses (with higher risk of morbidity) for large tumors. b. Modest well-tolerated dose levels for subclinical disease. c. For combination of radiation and surgery use less than radical dose level.	3. Dose aim is planned on the basis of tumor size or estimated tumor cell number, and biologic predictors of tumor aggressiveness. a. Maximum doses (with higher risk of morbidity) for large and more aggressive tumors. b. Modest well-tolerated dose levels for subclinical disease. c. For combinations of radiation and surgery, chemotherapy, and/or biologic therapy one might use less than radical dose level in certain situations. d. For combinations of external-beam radiation therapy and brachytherapy or radiation therapy and hyperthermia, the dose of each modality is modified as a function of the other modalities used.
4. Little priority given to planned combination of radiation and surgery.	4. Major emphasis on planned combinations of radiation and surgery.	4. Major emphasis on planned combinations of radiation, surgery, chemotherapy, hormonal therapy, and biologic therapy.
5. Treatment fields are square or rectangular.	5. Secondary collimation is utilized on virtually all fields to reduce irradiation of tissues not suspected of involvement by tumor.	5. Multileaf collimators and intensity modulation are used on virtually all fields in an attempt to improve conformality of the radiation and reduce irradiation of tissue not suspected of being involved with tumor. Radiation dose distribution is often based on sophisticated imaging technologies.
6. Radiation alone is the general rule.	6. Multidisciplinary approach accepted as most effective for most tumor problems.	6. The radiation oncologist is expected to be trained in and make use of pathology for tumor subtyping and grading; anatomic and molecular staging; diagnostic imaging; and the therapeutic role of chemotherapy, hormonal therapy, biologic therapy, and surgical therapy.
7. Results of treatment described almost exclusively in terms of absolute survival at a fixed period (e.g., 5 years).	7. Results analyzed on basis of detailed assessment of causes of failure (e.g., local persistence or regrowth, local complication, marginal miss, regional spread, distant metastases, intercurrent disease).	7. The phase III randomized prospective trial is the gold standard for clinical decision making. Decisions based on properly planned and conducted cancer trials concerning radiation therapy dose, volume, and technique are most appropriate. If such trials are not available or are inadequate, then phase II trials or retrospective reviews involving survival, local control, patterns of failure, and multivariate analysis of outcome are often useful. The future will depend on basic and translational research in cancer biology and medical physics being brought to the clinic.

content of cyclins or activation of cyclin p34 may overcome cellular resistance. By exploitation of cellular mechanisms related to apoptosis, it may be possible to kill cells with irradiation by inducing changes other than unrepaired DNA damage. With understanding of the tumor microenvironment and new techniques such as cDNA microarrays, as well as an understanding of how growth factors may alter cellular processes, innovative bioinformatics and improved combined-modality strategies may emerge. The ability to study many genes simultaneously will provide information beyond the era when biologic effects were attributed to a single gene. Better understanding of hypoxia may improve clinical outcome with antihypoxia strategies, including hypoxic cell radiosensitizers and hypoxic cytotoxic agents. Cyclins and growth factors may be useful as clinical radiation modifiers.

There is a critical need to balance the investment in technical aspects of radiation therapy with concepts and innovative approaches derived from better understanding of cancer biology. Coleman (86) has presented a complex model of the biologic factors influencing radiation oncology (Figs. 1.6–1.8). These scientific developments will greatly alter the way in which we practice our discipline.

Radiosensitivity and Radiocurability

In 1906, Bergonie and Tribondeau (35) formulated a law relating radiosensitivity to reproductive capacity of cells, based on their experiments on rat testis in which they were able to destroy the germinal cells while the interstitial tissue and Sertoli syncytium remained unimpaired. They wrote that "X-rays are more effective on cells which have a greater reproductive activity; the effectiveness is greater on those cells which have a longer dividing future ahead.... From this law, it is easy to understand

⋮⋮ Table 1.7	VARIOUS LEVELS OF IRRADIATION WILL YIELD DIFFERENT PROBABILITIES OF TUMOR CONTROL, DEPENDING ON THE SIZE OF THE LESION		
Cumulative Dose (Gy)	**Initial Cell Number**	**Probability of Survival**	**Remaining Cell Number**
2	1,000,000,000	× 0.5 =	500,000,000
4	500,000,000	× 0.5 =	250,000,000
6	250,000,000	× 0.5 =	125,000,000
8	125,000,000	× 0.5 =	62,500,000
10	67,500,000	× 0.5 =	31,250,000
12	33,750,000	× 0.5 =	15,625,000
14	15,625,000	× 0.5 =	7,812,500
16	7,823,500	× 0.5 =	3,906,250
18	3,906,250	× 0.5 =	1,953,125
20	1,953,125	× 0.5 =	976,562
22	976,562	× 0.5 =	488,281
24	488,281	× 0.5 =	244,140
26	244,140	× 0.5 =	122,070
28	122,070	× 0.5 =	61,035
30	61,035	× 0.5 =	30,517
32	30,517	× 0.5 =	15,258
34	15,258	× 0.5 =	7,629
36	7,629	× 0.5 =	3,814
38	3,814	× 0.5 =	1,907
40	1,907	× 0.5 =	953
42	953	× 0.5 =	476
44	476	× 0.5 =	238
46	238	× 0.5 =	119
48	119	× 0.5 =	59
50	59	× 0.5 =	29
52	29	× 0.5 =	15
54	15	× 0.5 =	7
56	7	× 0.5 =	4
58	4	× 0.5 =	2
60	2	× 0.5 =	1
62	1	× 0.5 =	<1

that roentgen radiation destroys tumors without destroying healthy tissues." Fletcher (153) felt that this observation, which was interpreted to indicate that radiosensitivity of tumors was linked to that of the mother organ, did much harm to clinical radiation therapy, leading to the erroneous concept that undifferentiated tumors with mitotic activity were radiosensitive and that more differentiated tumors were radioresistant.

In 1914, Schwarz (451) introduced the concept of fractionation by postulating that it was inefficient to deliver the total radiation dose in one treatment because cells were in different states of radiosensitivity and because there was a better chance that multiple exposures could hit the cells in a radiosensitive phase (e.g., mitosis). Fractionation was assumed to create a favorable therapeutic ratio because the tolerance of normal tissues increased relative to that of tumors and because malignant cells had a greater reproductive capacity and were, therefore, more likely to be in a radiosensitive phase.

Based on these and other observations, the term *radiocurability* was coined. It refers to the eradication of tumor at the primary or regional site and reflects a direct effect of the irradiation; this does not necessarily equate with the patient's cure from cancer. In contrast, *radiosensitivity* is a measure of tumor–radiation response, thus describing the degree and speed of regression during and immediately after radiotherapy. However, for most malignant tumors no significant correlation exists between the responsiveness of a tumor to irradiation and its radiocurability.

The response of human tumors to irradiation is a key issue for radiation oncologists and has been addressed by many leading radiobiologists. At least four explanations have been considered that could alone or in combination account for the different radiosensitivities of tumors (209,513):

1. *Hypoxia.* To explain the spectrum of clinical radioresponsiveness on this basis, it is likely that the less-responsive tumors either have a high hypoxic fraction, have failed to reoxygenate during fractionated treatment, or both (478). Direct oxygen electrode measurements have shown that cervical cancer, breast cancer, and squamous cell cancers are human tumors reported to have mean oxygen pressures below those of the surrounding tissue (236,356,529). Despite a wide range of values, the oxygen pressure in tumors tends to decrease with increasing tumor size (528). Although it is not possible to prove that hypoxia is unimportant in conventional radiation therapy, some doubts about its importance have been expressed based on the limited success of neutron therapy or hypoxic cell radiosensitizers (111,125). Recent studies have shown that hypoxia can act as an important determinant of selecting for tumor cells of a more malignant phenotype that is likely to adversely affect treatment outcome (107,238).

2. *Proportion of clonogenic cells.* Proliferating cells are more radiosensitive and have a greater turnover (cell-loss) rate. Tumor regression during irradiation may be proportional to the total number of proliferating cells (growth fraction) or the proliferative rate, which may accelerate for certain tumor cells as a result of adaptive processes (accelerated repopulation) during fractionated irradiation.

3. *Inherent radiosensitivity of tumor cells.* Fertil and Malaise (148) and Deacon et al. (105) established a positive correlation between the steepness of the initial slope of the oxic cell survival curve for human tumor cells and their response to radiation. The magnitude of differences between cell lines at low doses is sufficient to explain the range of curability observed clinically. Steel and Peacock (478) analyzed human

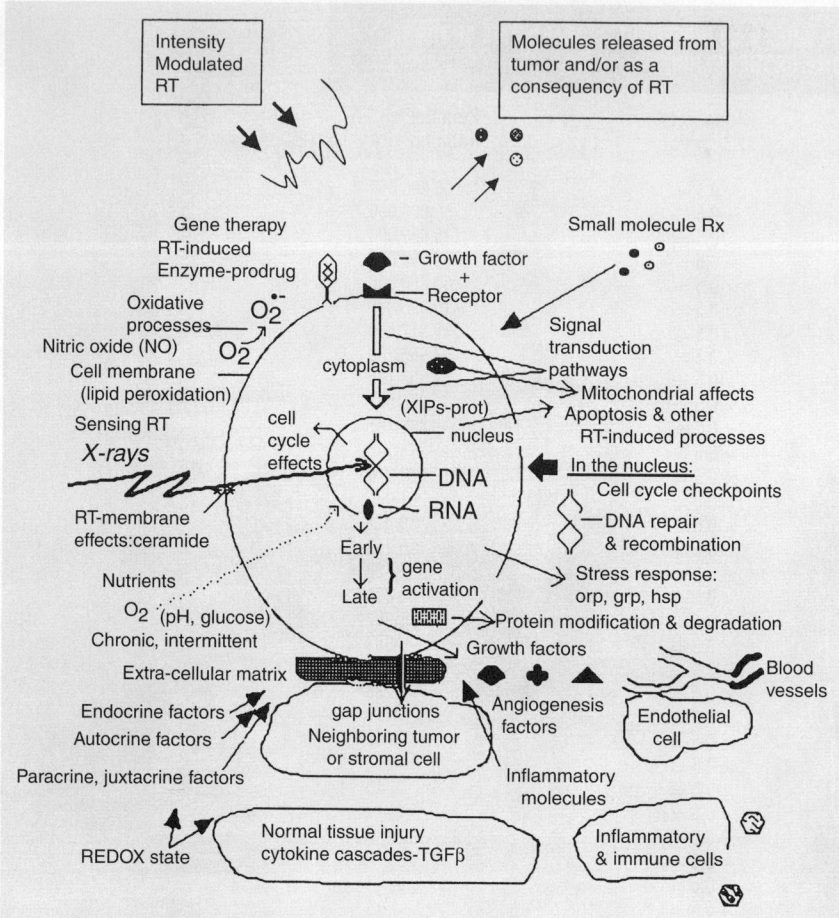

FIGURE 1.6. Radiation oncology sciences: focused biology. This figure includes the many targets for modifying the radiation response. In addition to the biologic targets within the tumor, this figure includes the concept of intensity-modulated radiation therapy (RT) with the radiation being deliverable by external beam, brachytherapy, or radiolabeled molecules. Also included is the so-called abscopal effect of radiation and the tumor, in that tumor-derived products may produce systemic symptoms, conceivably including immune alteration. (From Coleman CN. International Conference on Translational Research and Preclinical Strategies in Radio-Oncology (ICTR): conference summary. *Int J Radiat Oncol Biol Phys* 2001;49:301–309, with permission.)

tumor radiosensitivity in light of existing concepts of cell killing based on the linear-quadratic (LQ) equation. However, despite encouraging correlations in some studies, these radiobiological parameters have not been accepted for routine clinical use.

4. *Repair of radiation damage.* Repair of sublethal damage (split-dose effect) is observed in almost all tumor cell lines (132). Potentially lethal damage repair after a single dose varies considerably from one cell line to another and has been reported by Weichselbaum and Little (549) to correlate with clinical radiocurability, with less curable tumors showing the greatest degree of potentially lethal damage recovery. To date, these repair parameters have not been confirmed in larger clinical experiences to justify their use as predictors of radiotherapy outcomes (see later in this chapter).

Some investigators have reported a correlation between the clinical or pathological response of a tumor after the completion of irradiation with ultimate probability of local tumor control (491). For this analysis to be valid, it is necessary to compare patients with the same initial stage because, in general, more advanced lesions have a greater probability of tumor persistence at the completion of radiation therapy, and local recurrence may be more frequent. Barkley and Fletcher (23) reported 82% tumor control in 88 patients with tumors of the oropharynx that had regressed completely at the end of therapy, in contrast to 41% in 237 patients with persistent tumor at completion of therapy. Sobel et al. (473) concluded that local tumor control in head and neck carcinomas could be predicted with the greatest accuracy and consistency 1 to 3 months after completion of radiotherapy. They noted that the prediction was 80% accurate in favorable tumors (T1 and T2) but decreased

to 50% to 60% in more advanced primary lesions; complete tumor clearance was a more accurate predictor of tumor control. This was confirmed for the radiotherapeutic management of N2 (>3 cm) neck disease, where complete clinical resolution of tumor within 8 weeks of completion of irradiation correlated with a >90% freedom from neck failures (254,303). As an example of considerable variation with different tumors and clinical experiences, a good correlation between the probability of local tumor control and complete or partial regression of tumor after radiotherapy has been reported for carcinoma of the uterine cancer (252,302). Such a correlation was not found in patients with localized carcinoma of the prostate treated with irradiation (391).

Tumor Radiosensitivity and Predictive Assays

Since the inception of the use of ionizing radiation, many investigators have categorized the response of tumors according to their sensitivity to irradiation. Wetterer (554) in 1913 characterized tumor radiosensitivity based on histologic types, and Paterson (375) divided tumors into three groups: radiosensitive, intermediate, and radioresistant. The first category included germ cell tumors and reticuloses; the second included squamous cell and adenocarcinomas; and the third group included soft-tissue and bone sarcomas and melanomas (440). However, depending on variation in proliferative rates and cell loss, end points for response assessment may vary substantially, as has been pointed out for malignant melanoma (446). Attempts have been made to predict the response of tumors to radiation depending on several parameters, such as the assay proposed by Glucksmann

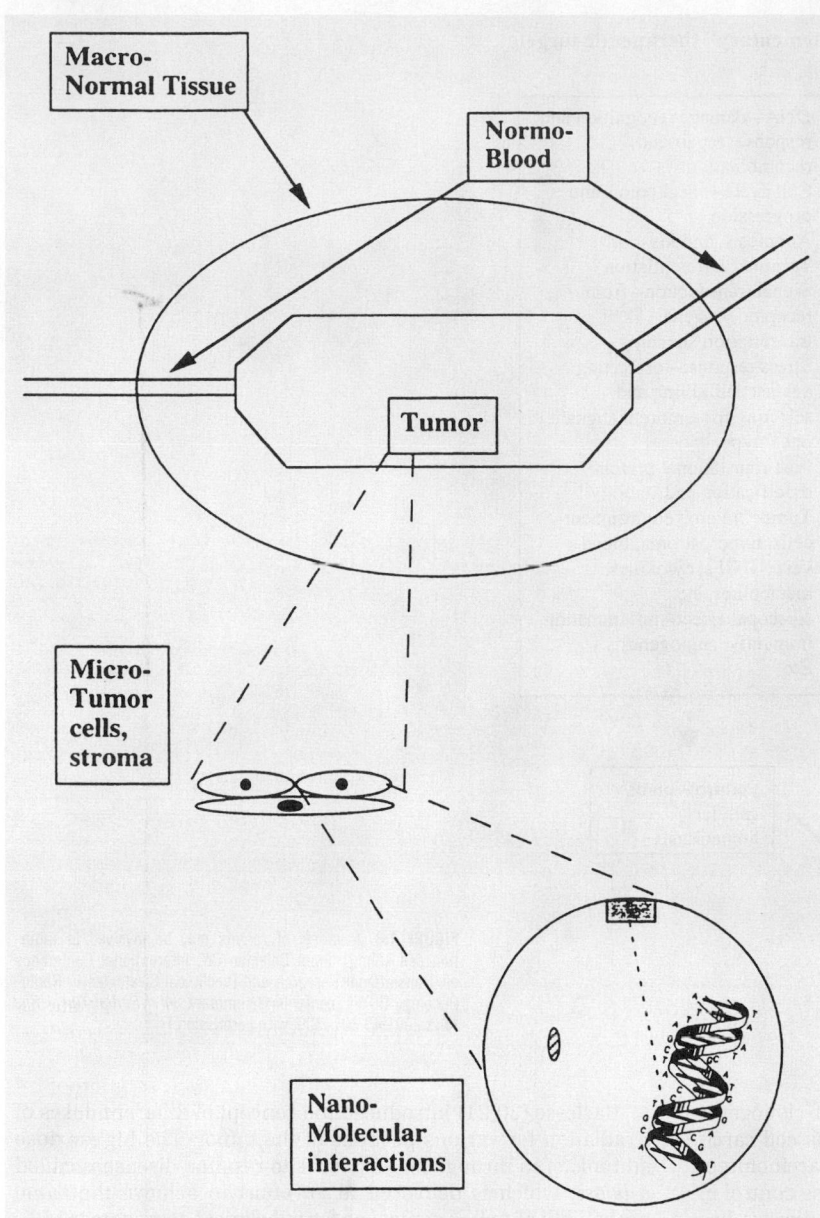

FIGURE 1.7. Radiation research address the normal tissue macroenvironment, the microenvironment of tumor cell and surrounding stroma, and molecular processes involved in the radiation response. (From Coleman CN. International Conference on Translational Research and Preclinical Strategies in Radio-Oncology (ICTR): conference summary. *Int J Radiat Oncol Biol Phys* 2001;49: 301–309, with permission.)

(185) consisting of differential cell counts of mitotic, resting, and degenerating cells in biopsy samples from the growing edge of the tumor before and after initiation of radiotherapy. It is generally accepted that tumors contain mixed-cell populations of stem cells with differing sensitivity to antineoplastic agents and that therapy can be selected for resistant cell populations or, in the case of certain cytotoxic agents, to induce cellular resistance (66). Peters et al. (397,398) described a predictive assay to assess tumor response *in vitro* and the difficulties in predicting the probability of tumor control by irradiation in a given patient. Unfortunately, despite promising correlations between radiosensitivity *in vitro* and radioresponsiveness of normal tissues and tumors (34,517), sufficiently powered predictive assays have not been identified. Given the inherent intertumor variability of predictive parameters, such as SF_2 (41,299) or T_{POT} (143,424), a single predictive assay is unlikely to carry sufficient predictive power. The incorporation of multiple radiobiologic tumor–cell parameters (e. g., markers for radiosensitivity and proliferation potential) into TCP (see later in this chapter) models appears more promising but awaits broader validation in clinical trials (59).

Probability of Tumor Control

For many histological types of cancer, higher radiation doses produce better tumor control. Numerous dose–response curves for a variety of tumors have been published. The first dose–response data were reported for skin cancer by Miescher (323) in 1934; 10 years later Strandqvist (484) published a dose–response curve for skin cancer. The Strandqvist plots were refined by von Essen (534), who demonstrated from a large skin carcinoma experience that the slopes for 97% tumor control and 3% skin necrosis differed and permitted, through appropriate fractionation schedules also considering the volume of disease, a dissociation of the two end points. As Fletcher (153) pointed out, meaningful dose–response curves can be generated only when a group of homogeneous tumors is given a range of radiation doses, indicating that tumor control is a probabilistic event. For every increment of radiation dose, a certain fraction of cells will be killed; therefore, the total number of surviving clonogenic cells will be proportional to the initial number present and the fraction killed with each dose (136). Thus, various levels of irradiation will yield different probabilities of tumor control,

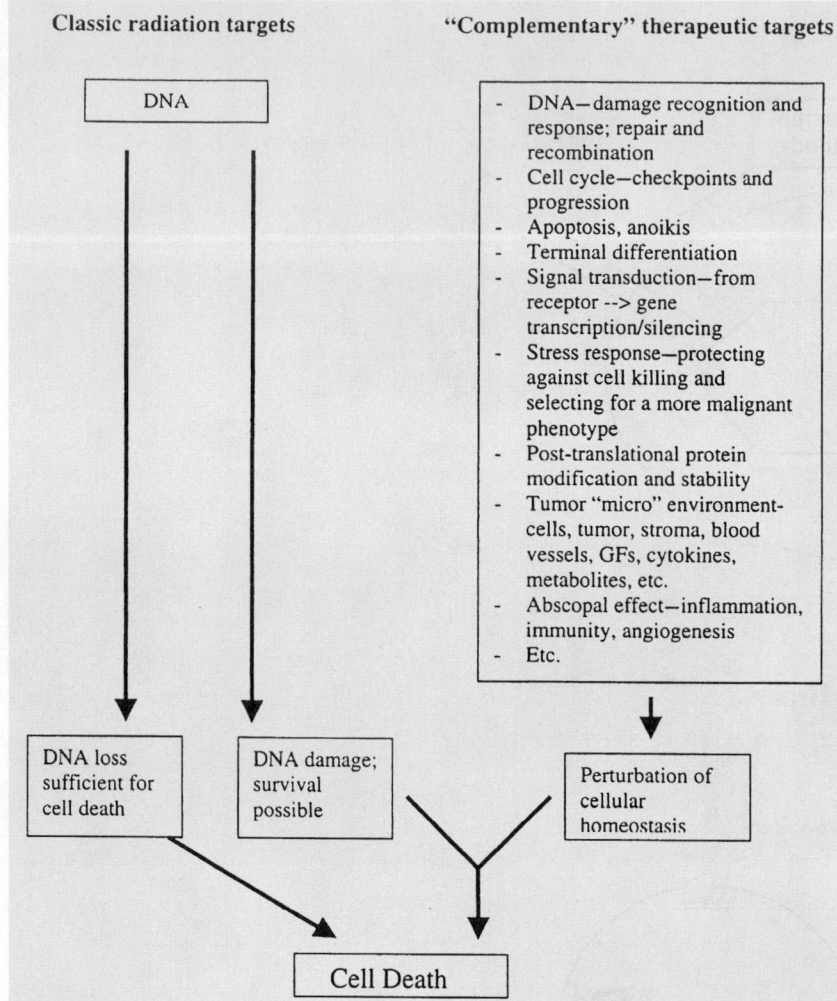

FIGURE 1.8. A variety of targets may be involved in radiation cell killing. (From Coleman CN. International Conference on Translational Research and Preclinical Strategies in Radio-Oncology (ICTR): conference summary. *Int J Radiat Oncol Biol Phys* 2001;49:301–309, with permission.)

depending on the extent of the lesion (number of clonogenic cells present). For subclinical disease in squamous cell carcinoma of the upper-respiratory tract or for adenocarcinoma of the breast, doses of 45 to 50 Gy will result in disease control in more than 90% of patients (154,320). Subclinical disease has been referred to as deposits of tumor cells that are too small to be detected clinically and even microscopically but, if left untreated, subsequently may evolve to clinically apparent tumor (374). It must be emphasized that microscopic evidence of tumor, such as at the surgical margin, should not be regarded as subclinical disease; cell aggregates $\geq 10^6/cm^3$ are required for the pathologist to detect them. Therefore, these volumes must receive higher doses of irradiation, in the range of 60 to 65 Gy in 6 to 7 weeks for epithelial tumors. This distinction of disease extent is re-emphasized by clinical results, demonstrating the need of irradiating patients with likely subclinical carcinoma to postoperative doses near 60 Gy (399,602).

For clinically palpable head and neck tumors, doses of 65 (for T1) to 75 to 80 Gy or higher (for T4 tumors) are required at 2 Gy/day using five fractions weekly. This dose range and probability of tumor control have been documented for squamous cell carcinoma and adenocarcinoma (153,154,321,460). Even with preoperative irradiation, the dose effect on probability of tumor control can be documented. At Memorial Hospital, with doses of 20 Gy (4 Gy/day for 1 week) to the neck combined with radical neck dissection, the failure rate was 22%, whereas it was only 7% when 50 Gy in 5 weeks was given postoperatively (532).

Baclesse (20,21) introduced the concept of different doses of irradiation for various portions of the tumor. The higher dose administered through small portals to residual disease is called a *boost*, which is delivered in an effort to achieve the same probability of tumor control as for subclinical aggregates (153). One consequence of the concepts discussed earlier is use of portals that are progressively reduced in size. This *shrinking field* technique administers higher radiation doses to the entire gross tumor where more clonogenic cells (including hypoxic cells) reside, relative to lower doses to tissues in the immediate proximity of the clinically apparent (gross) tumor. The tissues comprising the "tumor margin" contain a lower number of tumor clonogens that are better oxygenated (see Fig. 1.3).

Normal Tissue Effects

A variety of normal tissue changes are induced by ionizing radiation, depending on the total dose, fractionation schedule (daily dose and overall treatment time), and volume treated. These factors are closely interrelated (Fig. 1.9).

It has been postulated that for many normal tissues the radiation dose necessary to produce a particular sequela increases as the irradiated fraction of volume of the organ decreases. This concept was demonstrated for skin by Paterson (377), who plotted doses delivered with orthovoltage x-rays that would produce moist desquamation (Fig. 1.10). The same phenomenon later was reported for supervoltage irradiation of other organs (476) and for brachytherapy.

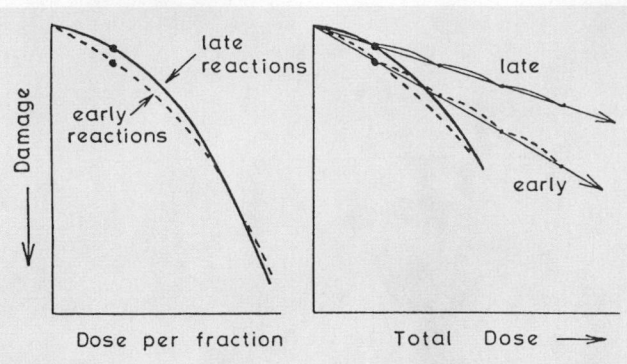

FIGURE 1.9. Difference in cell-survival curves for acute- and late-radiation effects with single or multifractionated doses of irradiation. (From Fowler JF. Fractionation and therapeutic gain. In: Steel GG, Adams GE, Peckham MT, eds. *Biological basis of radiotherapy.* Amsterdam: Elsevier Science, 1983;181–194, with permission.)

Several authors have observed higher tolerance doses (TD) than initially reported for a variety of organs (305,315, 333,382,406,407), which stresses the importance of updating this information in light of more precise treatment planning and delivery of irradiation and more accurate evaluation and recording of sequelae. Excellent examples are radiation dose escalation studies, using conformal radiotherapy delivery techniques, for prostate (218) and lung carcinomas (Radiation Therapy Oncology Group [RTOG] trial 93–11). A compilation from the literature of data on tolerance doses for whole or partial organ irradiation was published by Emami et al. (138) but requires refinement as has recently been demonstrated for preservation of parotid gland function using IMRT (131). Estimates from data of Emami et al. (138) were used by Burman et al. (62) to develop a series of tolerance curves for multiple organs.

In studying late radiation effects, an organ can be considered to be made up of multiple functional subunits (FSUs) that are arranged serially or in parallel (449,604). For serially structured organs, such as gastrointestinal tract or nervous tissue, damage to one portion of the organ may render the entire organ dysfunctional. In contrast, in organs with parallel structure, FSU damage may not impair the entire organ function because the remaining FSUs operate independently from the damaged group, and clinical injury occurs only when a critical volume of the organ (or proportion of FSUs) is damaged and the surviving FSUs are unable to maintain organ function. Therefore, the sensitivity of an organ depends on the number of FSUs. Marks (308) discussed the importance of organ structure in determining late radiation effects and pointed out that conventional dose–volume histograms (DVHs) and normal tissue complication probability (NTCP) models are frequently inadequate because they ignore functional and structural heterogeneities. Such considerations will be particularly important for partial irradiation of lung, liver, and kidney to doses that approach the tolerance of the organs' functional units. Yorke et al. (621) developed a biologically based model for NTCP as a function of dose and irradiation volume fractions for kidney and lung in which the organ was assumed to be composed of FSUs arranged in a parallel architecture. Jackson et al. (248) presented a thorough discussion of the subject, including its mathematical basis, and addressed the problem of calculating NTCP for inhomogeneously irradiated organs with parallel architecture. They showed that variations in FSUs and functional reserve in a patient population may produce NTCP dose–response curves, the widths of which are comparable with those observed clinically.

Structural alterations without anatomic or functional impairment may be noted, whereas in other instances substantial injuries with tissue destruction, severe dysfunction, or even death may occur (141). Normal tissues have a substantial capacity to recover from sublethal or potentially lethal damage induced by radiation (at tolerable dose levels). Injury to normal tissues may be caused by the radiation effect on the microvasculature or the support tissues (stromal or parenchymal cells) (513).

Rubin et al. (439) indicated the usefulness of assigning a certain percentage of risk of complication, depending on the dose of the radiation. The minimal tolerance dose is defined as $TD_{5/5}$, which represents the dose of radiation that could cause no more than a 5% severe complication rate within 5 years after treatment. (Some authors use the equivalent terms "tissue tolerance dose," or $TTD_{5/5}$. Both the $TD_{5/5}$ and the $TTD_{5/5}$ are based on treatment at 2 Gy per fraction, five fractions per week.) An acceptable complication rate for severe injury is 5% in most curative clinical situations. Moderate sequelae are noted in varying proportions (10% to 25% of patients), depending on the dose of irradiation given and the organs at risk.

Chronologically, the effects of irradiation are subdivided into acute (first 3 months) and late effects (more than 3 months after irradiation), according to the National Cancer Institute Common Toxicity Criteria. The gross manifestations depend on the kinetic properties of the cells (slow or rapid renewal) and the total radiation dose given (436).

Early applications of time–dose considerations were applied by Baclesse (20) based on observations by Coutard (96) that various degrees of mucositis and moist desquamation were repaired by re-epithelialization of the mucosa and skin from the periphery of the irradiated field and from cells surviving in the center of the field. Protracted fractionation schedules for carcinoma of the breast with lower daily doses over 10 to 12 weeks were successful in avoiding acute moist desquamation (20), but the higher radiation doses caused severe tissue damage in a large number of patients (64).

No correlation has been established between the incidence and severity of acute reactions and the occurrence of late effects. In 286 patients irradiated for head and neck carcinomas, Geara et al. (179) observed no significant difference in local tumor failure rates in patients with maximum grade 1 or 2 versus grade 3 or 4 acute mucositis (28% and 18%, respectively) (p =. 17). Also, no correlation was found between severity of late reactions and local tumor control. Withers et al. (608) compiled data depicting isoeffect lines for acute or late effects in several organs. The slopes for late reactions were steeper than for acute effects, and there was a lack of correlation between the doses producing similar severities of acute or late effects (503).

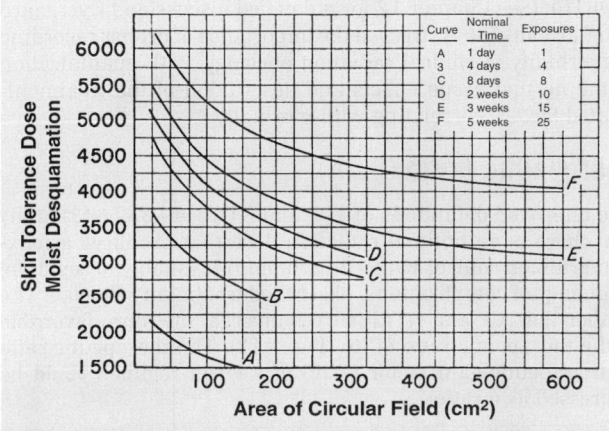

Curve	Nominal Time	Exposures
A	1 day	1
B	4 days	4
C	8 days	8
D	2 weeks	10
E	3 weeks	15
F	5 weeks	25

FIGURE 1.10. Graph showing the relationship between dose and size of area irradiated (healthy skin in an "average" site) to produce moist desquamation for various overall treatment times (daily irradiation at about 50 R/min for each exposure with radiation of half-value layer 1.5 mm Cu). (From Paterson R. *The treatment of malignant disease by radium and x-rays.* Baltimore: Williams & Wilkins, 1949;39, with permission.)

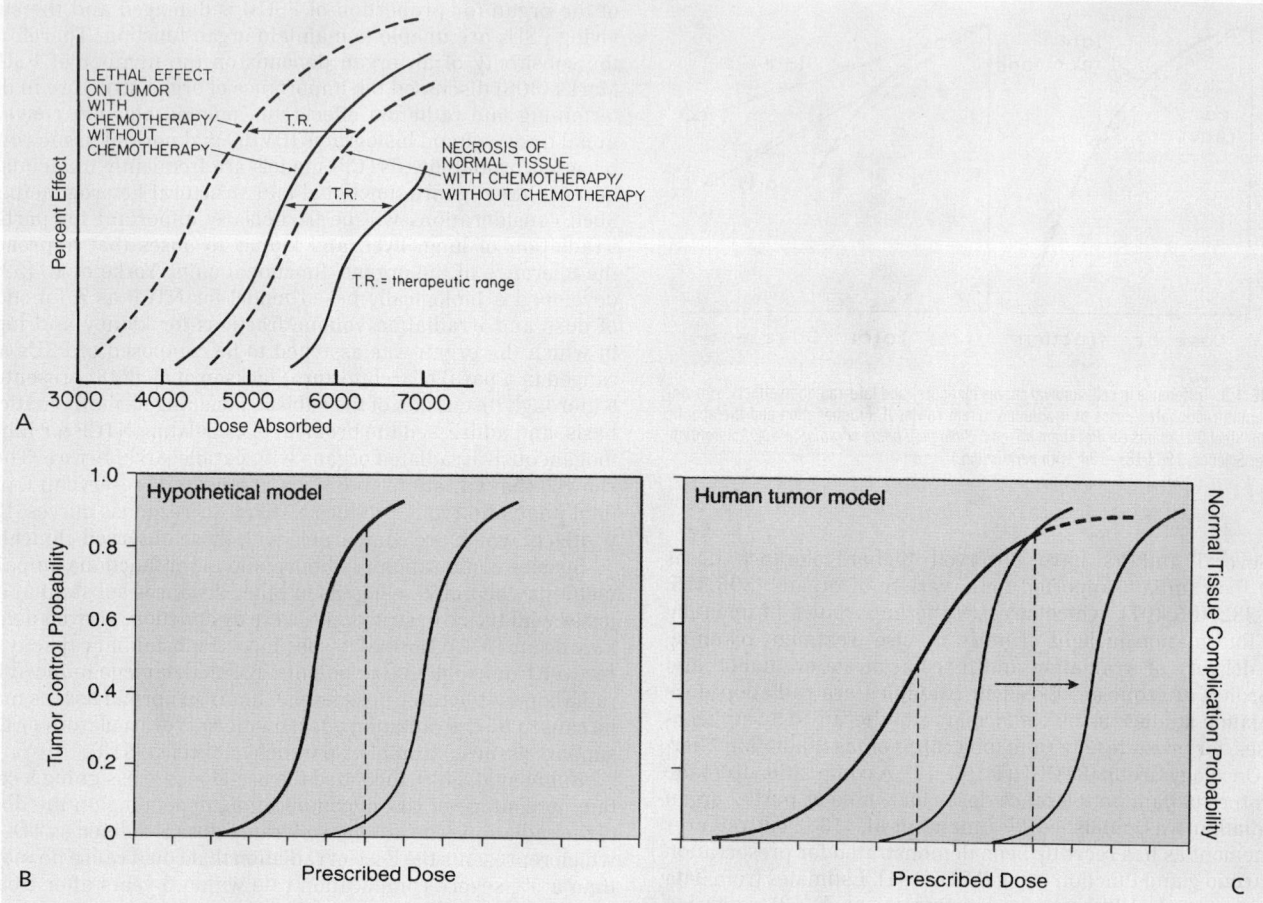

FIGURE 1.11. A: Theoretical curves for tumor control and complications as a function of radiation dose with and without chemotherapy. *TR* is the therapeutic ratio, or the difference between tumor control and complication frequency. (Perez CA, Thomas PRM. Radiation therapy: basic concepts and clinical implications. In: Sutow WW, Fernbach DJ, Vietti TJ, eds. *Clinical pediatric oncology*, 3rd ed. St. Louis, MO: CV Mosby, 1984;167–209.) **B:** Hypothetical dose–response curves for tumor control and for normal tissue injury. Because the tumor control and the normal tissue complication curves are approximately parallel in shape and are sufficiently separated, the dose levels necessary to cure a high percentage of patients can be administered without producing excessive normal tissue damage (indicated by the *vertical dotted line*). **C:** Human tumor model. The slope of the tumor-control curve is less steep than the normal tissue-complication curve; thus, for an acceptable level of normal tissue injury, the probability of tumor control is decreased compared to the hypothetical model. Because of the volume effect, reducing the volume of normal tissues shifts the curve to the higher dose region, thereby effectively increasing the separation of the dose–response curves. Consequently, a higher dose can be given to the tumor, improving the probability of tumor control without increasing the probability of normal tissue injury. (From Leibel SA, Fuks Z, Zelefsky MJ, et al. Intensity-modulated radiotherapy. *Cancer J* 2002;8[2];60–166, with permission.)

This may result from the difference in the slopes of cell-survival curves for acute or late-reacting tissues (162) (Fig. 1.11).

Combining irradiation with surgery or cytotoxic agents frequently modifies the tolerance of normal tissues to a given dose of irradiation, which may necessitate adjustments in treatment planning and dose prescription (395). The lack of correlation between acute and late-reacting tissues represents one rationale for combining radiotherapy with chemotherapy. As long as the enhanced acute toxicities of combined treatment can be managed, no significant increased damage in late-reacting tissues is expected (503).

▐ Quantitation of Treatment Toxicity

There is a critical need to accurately assess and record morbidity of treatment because this, in addition to therapeutic efficacy, is a crucial parameter in the evaluation of new regimens and in the selection of therapy for an individual patient. Multiple schemata have been developed, although a complete consensus has not been reached as to ideal grading scores. Toxicity grading systems for various organs were developed by RTOG and the

European Organisation for Research and Treatment of Cancer (EORTC). (See Chapter 12 for a detailed discussion.) Overgaard and Bartelink (365) stressed the importance of proper recording of morbidity in clinical radiation oncology, with quantification of the normal tissue effects and description of the treatment-related factors correlating with morbidity.

Therapeutic Ratio (Gain)

The improved definitions of TCP and NTCP (49,332,613) imply that there is an optimal radiation dose that produces a maximum tumor control with a minimum (reasonably acceptable) frequency of complications, also called treatment sequelae. The farther the TCP and NTCP curves diverge, the more favorable is the therapeutic ratio (436) (Fig. 1.12). The therapeutic ratio or therapeutic gain factor (TGF) of a given regimen could be expressed as a ratio:

$$\text{TGF} = \frac{\%\,\text{tumor control with therapy A versus therapy B}}{\%\,\text{complications with therapy A versus therapy B}}$$

The higher the TGF, the more efficient a particular therapy is. Such a quantitative expression could be used to compare

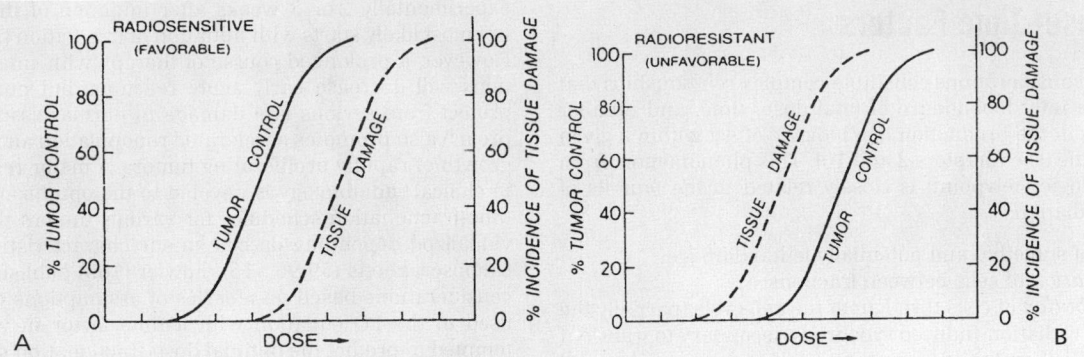

FIGURE 1.12. Different therapeutic ratios exist in different clinical circumstances depending on the radiosensitivity (dose–response curves) for the tumor versus critical normal tissue in the treatment field. **A:** Favorable. **B:** Unfavorable. (From Rubin P. *Clinical oncology: a multidisciplinary approach for physicians and students,* 7th ed. Philadelphia: W.B. Saunders, 1993, with permission.)

different therapeutic strategies. Mendelsohn (319) expressed this concept in terms of "uncomplicated tumor ablation" (Fig. 1.13). The selection of a dose must weigh the probability of major complications for any potential enhancement of tumor control. Models for decision making, using Bayesian theory, incorporate values assigned to positive or negative outcomes (318). Positive outcome is considered tumor cure without complication, whereas negative outcomes include tumor cure with significant complications or tumor recurrence with or without complications.

Impact of Local Tumor Control on Survival

Over the past two decades, the importance of systemic chemotherapy was emphasized as the dominant therapeutic modality that could improve survival of cancer through control of systemic metastatic disease. Significant but modest improvements in patients' survival rates for carcinoma of the breast (150,151), for example, have firmly established cytotoxic chemotherapy as a component of breast cancer treatment. However, attempts of further enhancing the benefits of chemotherapy with high-dose (HDCT), marrow-ablative regimens were disappointing and did not provide a benefit over standard chemotherapy. The effect of locoregional tumor control on patient survival has been emphasized repeatedly (226,227,488). Clinical experiences and randomized trials (446) demonstrate for cancers with high metastatic potential, such as breast, prostate, and lung, that improved locoregional control by radiotherapy with or without chemotherapy enhances overall survival. This has revived the interest in locoregional radiotherapy as a survival-prolonging treatment modality, also confirming earlier clinical experiences in patients with carcinoma of the lung (381), prostate (391), and uterine cervix (387).

Because of the emphasis on control of systemic disease, assessment of the importance of locoregional tumor control in patients with malignant tumors has been relatively underemphasized (108). In a large proportion of patients with cancer seen in the United States, locoregional recurrence is just as prevalent (69% of patients dying with locoregional disease) as distant metastases. A large proportion of patients (50%) have both locoregional recurrence and distant metastases (see Table 1.6).

Clinical data have matured over the past decade, demonstrating that tumor persistence after initial therapy does, because of tumor progression, carry as poor a prognosis as treatment of a more advanced cancer. In addition, radiotherapy has been shown for tumor with high metastatic potential, such as breast, prostate, and lung, to prolong overall survival if higher radiation doses are delivered and achieve improved local control rates (87,218,369,381,391,446).

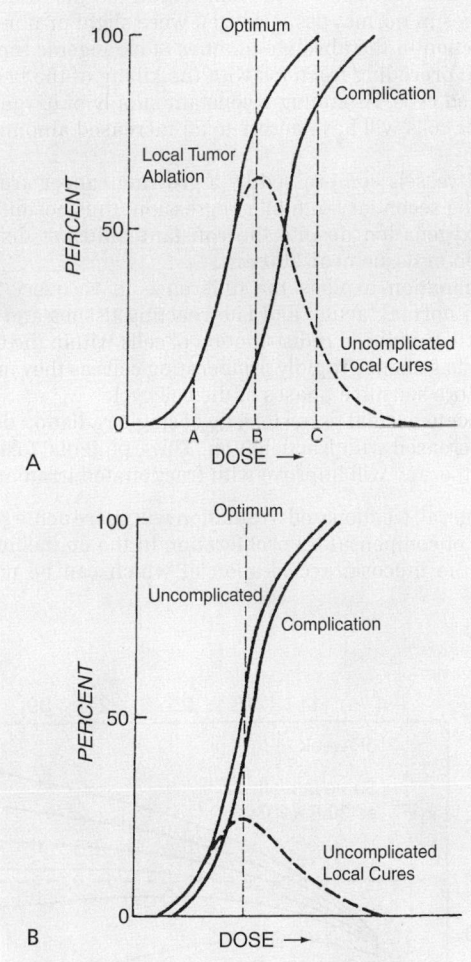

FIGURE 1.13. Treatment outcomes. Uncomplicated curves *(dashed line)* are the desired results of treatment. This is illustrated as a function of the therapeutic ratio; that is, the greater the separation of the tumor-control curve and the normal tissue-complication curve, the greater the number of uncomplicated cures that will result. The letters *A, B,* and *C* represent three different dose levels, which, if chosen, would lead to three different outcomes: *A* would result in few tumor cures but no complications; *C* would lead to complete cure in many cases, but virtually all patients would suffer complications. The optimal choice in this group of dose levels is *B,* which would result in the greatest number of cured patients without complications. (From Mendelsohn ML. The biology of dose-limiting tissues. In: *Time and dose relationships in radiation biology as applied to radiotherapy.* Brookhaven National Laboratory [BNL] Report 5023 [C-57]. Upton, NY: Brookhaven National Laboratory, 1969;154–173, with permission.)

Dose–Time Factors

Dose–time considerations constitute complex relationships that express the interdependence of total dose, time, and number of fractions in the production of a biologic effect within a given tissue volume (see Chapters 2 and 10). This phenomenon, from a radiobiologic viewpoint, is closely related to the four Rs of ionizing radiation:

1. *Repair* of sublethal and potentially lethal damage;
2. *Repopulation* of cells between fractions;
3. *Redistribution* of cells throughout the cell cycle (partially the result of radiation-induced synchrony secondary to transient arrest at cell-cycle checkpoints and cell-cycle–dependent cell killing); and
4. *Reoxygenation* occurring during repeated radiation exposures.

The advantages of dose fractionation include (339):

1. Reduction in the number of hypoxic cells through cell killing and reoxygenation. Cater and Silver (72) demonstrated increased oxygenation in the tumor after irradiation, whereas changes in normal tissue oxygen were slight or nonexistent.
2. Reduction in the absolute number of clonogenic tumor cells by the preceding fractions with the killing of the better oxygenated cells. Assuming a constant supply of oxygen, fewer cancer cells will have access to an increased amount of oxygen.
3. Blood vessels compressed by a growing cancer are decompressed secondary to tumor regression, thus permitting better oxygenation despite the constant diffusion distance of oxygen in tissue near 200 μm.
4. Fractionation exploits the difference in recovery rate between normal, acute, and late-reacting tissues and tumors. Radiation-induced redistribution of cells within the cell cycle tends to sensitize rapidly proliferating cells as they move into the more sensitive phases of the cell cycle.
5. The acute normal tissue toxicity of single radiation doses can be decreased with fractionation. Thus, patients' tolerance of radiotherapy will improve with fractionated irradiation.

In general, fractionated irradiation will spare acute reactions because of compensatory proliferation in the epithelium of the skin or the mucosa, acceleration of which can be measured experimentally 2 or 3 weeks after initiation of therapy (106), but most likely starts with initiation of irradiation (33,165,447). However, a prolonged course of therapy with small daily fractions will decrease early acute reactions but not necessarily protect from serious late damage to normal tissues. This approach also promotes accelerated repopulation and permits the growth of rapidly proliferating tumors. A major research effort in clinical radiobiology is devoted to the optimization of dose–time-fractionation schedules for various tumors that are individualized depending on cell kinetic characteristics and clinical observations (59,96,515). Fowler (163) published theoretic considerations based on a series of assumptions of the values used in the LQ equation with a time factor in which he attempted to predict the optimal dose-fractionation schedules for tumors with various cell-doubling times. He concluded that optimal overall times depend primarily on the doubling time of the tumor cells and intrinsic radiosensitivity, alpha (assumed to be proportional to α/β). Short overall treatment times are required for tumors with a low α/β ratio or fast proliferation. For median potential doubling times of 5 days and intermediate radiosensitivity, overall times of 2.5 to 4 weeks would be optimal. More slowly proliferating tumors should be treated with longer overall times (Fig. 1.14). *In vitro* techniques to assess tumor radiosensitivity in biopsy specimens ultimately may be helpful as predictive assays.

Altered Fractionation

Without a solid biologic basis and out of empiricism and convenience, the "standard fractionation" for radiation therapy has evolved into five fractions weekly. Other fractionation schedules have been proposed that deliver multiple fractions daily or six fractions weekly or use a hyperfractionation split-course regimen (Fig. 1.15). The characteristics for hyperfractionation, accelerated fractionation, or split-course schedules as well as potential advantages or disadvantages are summarized in Table 1.8. Based on the narrow window between improvements in tumor control and enhanced normal tissue toxicities (396), any altered fractionation schedule is potentially harmful and must be approached with great caution. However, the improved quality of clinical trials by national study groups and by individual institutions has generated a growing body of clinical outcome data, that, together with improved biological modeling, allows relatively accurate predictions of clinical outcomes based on

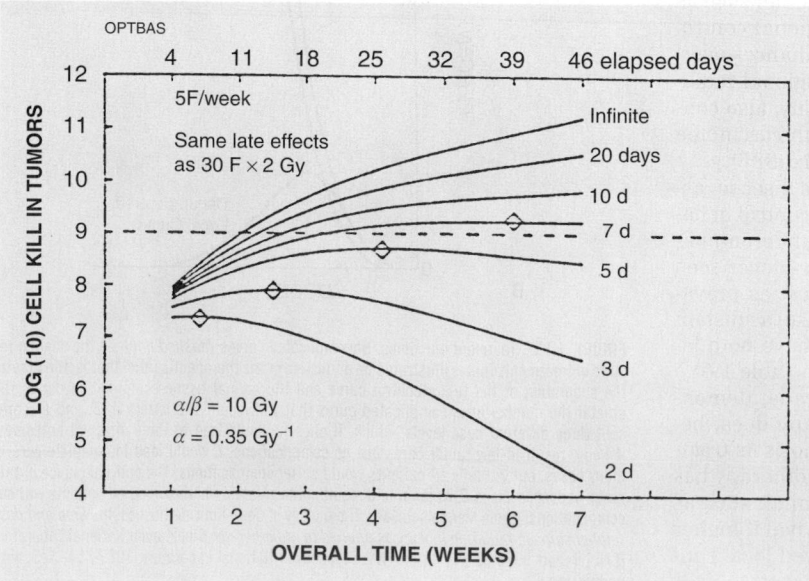

FIGURE 1.14. Log cell kill in tumors as a function of overall time, for schedules using five fractions per week to a total dose that gives the same late effects as 30 fractions of 2 Gy (assuming $\alpha/\beta = 3$ Gy for late effects). Each curve is for the stated proliferation doubling time (average over the overall time). The diamond-shaped symbols show the maximum cell kill for that doubling time, at the optimum overall time for that number of fractions per week. If there is no diamond, the optimum overall time is longer than 7 weeks. The dotted line is drawn arbitrarily at 9 logs of cell kill. (From Fowler JF. How worthwhile are short schedules in radiotherapy? A series of exploratory calculations. *Radiother Oncol* 1990;18:165–181, with permission.)

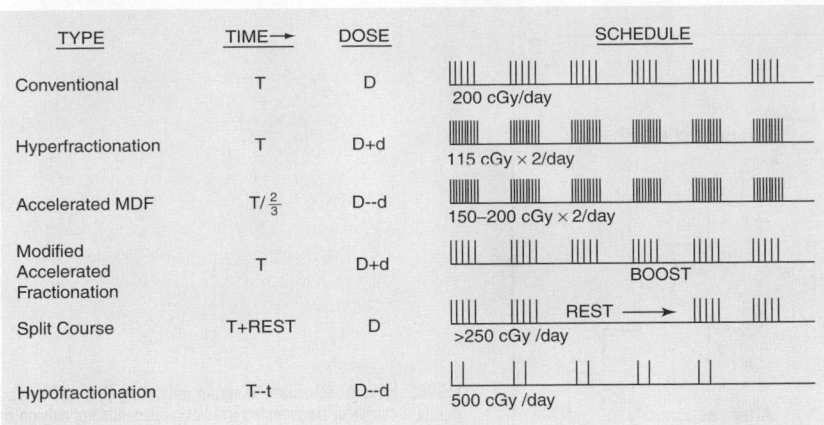

FIGURE 1.15. Various types of fractionation used in radiation therapy.

relative biological effectiveness (RBE) calculations (331). Thus, an increasing number of clinical trials have demonstrated that altered fractionation schedules permit dose escalation to tumors with increased late normal tissue toxicity (175,337,338) or similar tumor-control rates with reduced late normal tissue sequelae in children with rhabdomyosarcoma (117).

Multiple daily fractions are likely to be more effective in rapidly growing tumors with a high growth fraction. Normal tissues behave as actively proliferating cells for expression of acute reactions but as slowly proliferating cells in the manifestation of late injury (606). As suggested by several biologic studies (167), clinical trial results conducted by EORTC and RTOG demonstrated that a minimum of 6 hours interfraction interval should be allowed when multiple daily fractions are used to allow maximum repair of normal tissues. This is supported by reduced complication rates in patients irradiated for carcinoma of the lung and a highly uniform cohort of patients with tonsillar squamous cell carcinomas (164,602).

Accelerated fractionation aims at shortening the overall treatment time. Schedules may use larger than standard size fractions five times weekly or more than five fractions per week of 2 Gy (366). In addition, multiple fractions of radiation may be given daily exclusively or in combination with standard fractions of 2 Gy. Some reduction in the total dose delivered may have to be used for fractions >2 Gy for normal tissue sparing. These schedules may be preferable with hypoxic cell sensitizers or other chemical modifiers of radiation response that require the presence of a high concentration of the compound in the tumor at the time of the radiation exposure.

With hyperfractionation, a larger number of smaller-than-conventional dose fractions are given daily; the total daily dose is usually 10% to 20% greater than with standard fractionation; the total period of time is minimally changed; and the total dose needs to be escalated to achieve tumor toxicity similar to that of standard fractionation. The aim of hyperfractionation is to achieve the same incidence of late effects on normal tissue as observed with a comparable conventional regimen while increasing the probability of tumor control through dose escalation (603).

Accelerated Repopulation

Withers and Taylor (604) described experimental observations documenting accelerated repopulation of tumor cells during fractionated radiotherapy and provided convincing evidence that this phenomenon occurs in clinical situations (Figs. 1.16–1.18). Although Withers and Taylor's analyses suggested that accelerated repopulation occurs preferentially after the 4th week of radiotherapy, reanalysis of the same data by Bentzen (33) and Thames et al. (502) and independent derivations by Fowler (165) suggested that repopulation starts early during fractionated irradiation. The latter is supported by experimental data of Schmidt-Ullrich et al. (447), showing that molecular processes of accelerated repopulation, mediated through radiation-induced receptor activation and cellular growth stimulation, occur after a single radiation exposure of 2 Gy. The effectiveness of a course of fractionated irradiation depends in part on the killing by individual fractions as well as on the rate of proliferation of surviving cells between irradiation fractions. Neoadjuvant chemotherapy also may lead to increased proliferation of surviving tumor cells after partial regression of the

Table 1.8	COMPARISON OF VARIOUS FRACTIONATION SCHEDULES			
	Conventional	**Split-Course**	**Accelerated Fractionation**	**Hyperfractionation**
Indication, in tumors, of growth rate	Average	Average or slow	Rapid	Slow (with large cell-loss factors)
Normal tissue effects, acute	Standard	Standard or greater	Greater	Standard or greater
Normal tissue effects, late	Standard	Greater	Standard (if complete repair of sublethal damage occurs) or greater	Lower
Advantages	—	Shorter actual treatment time (fewer fractions)	Destroys more tumor cells; prevents tumor cell repopulation; less overall treatment time	Lower OER with small doses; spares late damage, allows reoxygenation; allows stem cell repopulation
Disadvantages	—	May permit tumor repopulation	—	More fractions

OER, oxygen enhancement ratio.

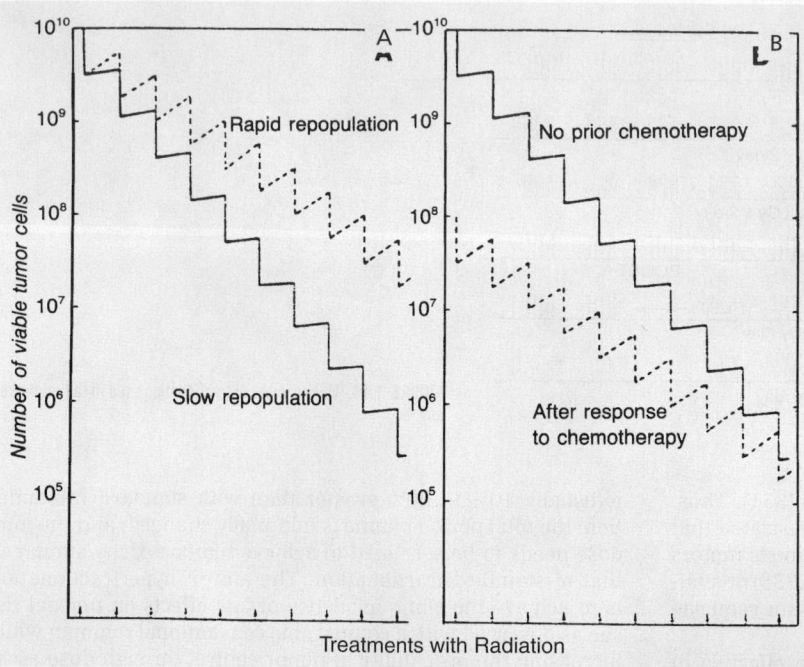

FIGURE 1.16. A: Schematic diagram indicating that cell survival during a course of fractionated irradiation depends not only on the proportion of cells killed with each dose (equal for the two curves shown) but also on the rate of proliferation of surviving cells between dose fractions, which differs for the two curves. **B:** Hypothetical diagram to illustrate the number of surviving cells in a tumor during treatment with irradiation alone (*solid line*) or during radiation therapy delivered to a tumor that has responded to chemotherapy (i.e., cell number reduced to 1% at start of irradiation) but where proliferation has been stimulated (*dashed line*). Note that cell survival is similar after fractionated irradiation, despite the initial response to drugs. (From Tannock IF. Combined modality treatment with radiotherapy and chemotherapy. *Radiother Oncol* 1989;16:83–101, with permission.)

lesion, which could result in decreased cell killing by subsequent fractionated irradiation.

Isoeffect Graphs

To express an equal biologic effect produced by various fractionation schedules, isoeffect lines have been generated. Kronig and Friedrich (269) first published the observation that a specific physical dose of irradiation is less biologically effective if given in multiple fractions, which embodies the original concept of recovery between fractions. Later, MacComb and Quimby (297) and Reisner (419) established the rate of recovery in experimentally produced skin reactions in patients.

In 1944, Strandqvist (484) published a monograph describing the results of treatment of 280 patients with skin cancer

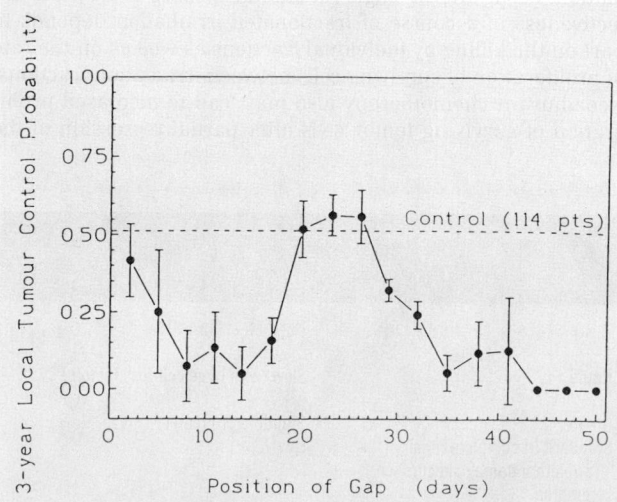

FIGURE 1.17. Dependence of tumor control probability (TCP) on the position of a single treatment gap in 533 patients. Gap duration ranged from 3 to 20 days. Position of a gap is defined by its starting point. Each point shows the TCP averaged over 3 consecutive days (± SD). (From Skladowski K, Law MG, Maciejewski B, et al. Planned and unplanned gaps in radiotherapy: The importance of gap position and gap duration. *Radiother Oncol* 1994;30:109–120, with permission.)

(squamous cell and basal cell carcinoma); most tumors were treated within 14 and 29 days, and only one was treated within 45 days. An isoeffect line was drawn, with a slope of 0.22. He fitted the recovery factors of MacComb and Quimby and Reisner using an extrapolated value of 0.35 per day as the time for a single dose. He also produced a graph for various degrees of radiation reaction on the skin, ranging from erythema to necrosis (Fig. 1.19). It should be emphasized that in these curves, the vertical coordinate represents the total dose given, and the abscissa represents the total duration in days after the first irradiation. However, some authors have plotted similar graphs representing the number of fractions in the horizontal coordinate. It is critical to identify these two parameters because one could deliver 60 Gy in 6 weeks in 30 fractions given five times weekly or the same dose delivered in 18 fractions given three times weekly. The effects on normal tissues certainly would be different. Von Essen (534), using the Strandqvist data as well as his own, pointed out the importance of the volume irradiated when isoeffect parameters are studied and generated a 3D display of these data.

Dutreix et al. (128) published observations on the influence of fraction size in patients with cancer of the lung, on whom one of the supraclavicular areas received a single exposure and the other area received two exposures separated by 6 hours. They noticed that two fractions of 1 Gy produced the same skin reaction as one fraction of 2 Gy. As the fraction size increased, however, it took a higher dose in the two-fraction schedule to produce the same reaction as with the single-fraction schedule. With mucositis of the faucial arch used as an end point, researchers at M.D. Anderson Cancer Center observed that 10 Gy per week given in five fractions of 2 Gy is equivalent to 11 Gy given in 10 fractions, twice a day, separated by 3 hours (153).

The slopes for reactions for various normal tissues differ, as do slopes of tumor curability and normal tissue late effects. In general, the slope for tumor curability is less steep than that for normal tissue reactions (84). Isoeffect lines for various squamous cell carcinomas of the head and neck, different stages, have slopes varying from 0.33 to 0.38 (156,180,476,501). Furthermore, as stated earlier, tolerance of normal tissues is strongly related to the volume irradiated. Whereas 60 Gy could be given safely in 5 weeks for a small glottic tumor with a 5-cm

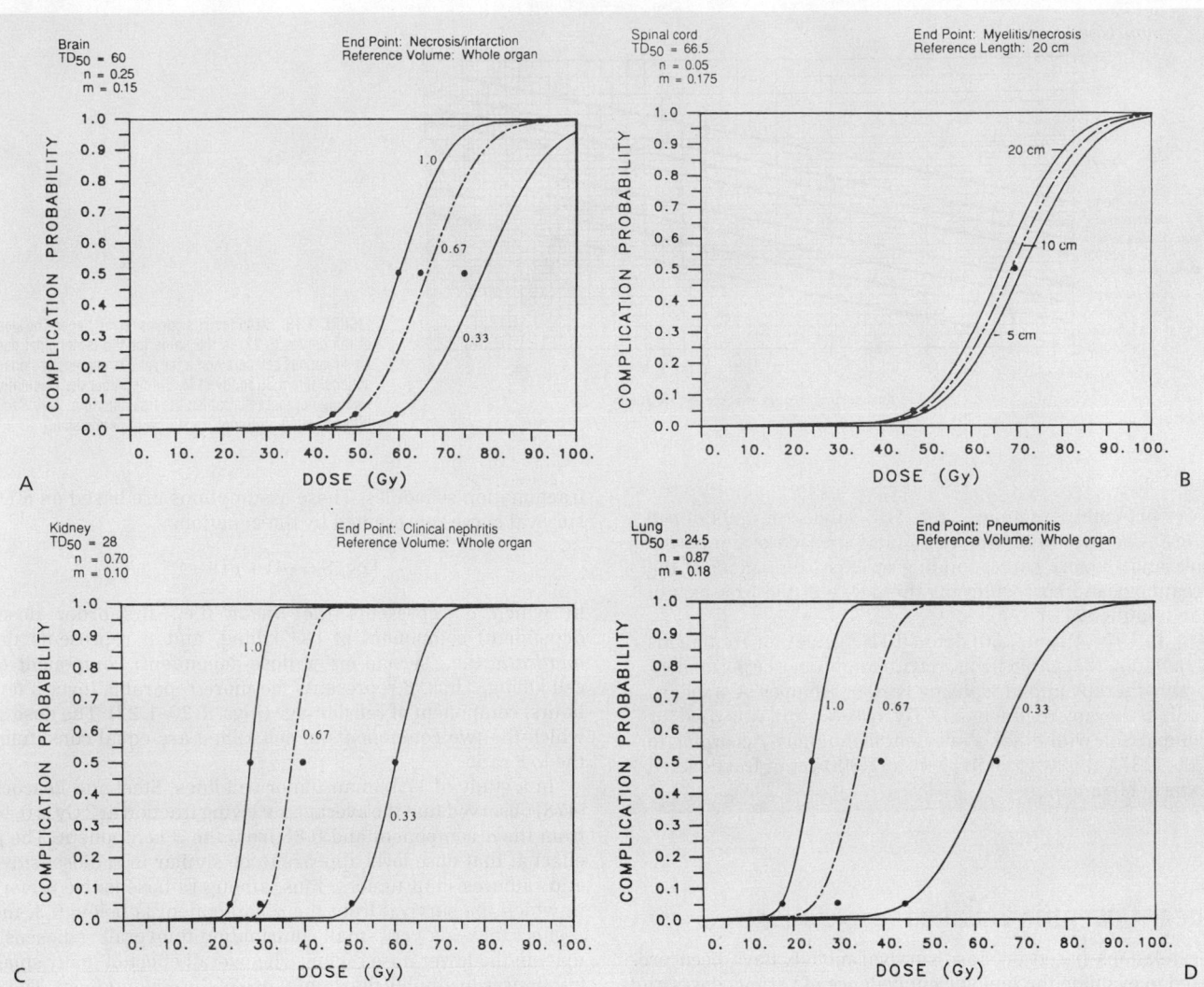

FIGURE 1.18. Complication probability correlated with irradiation dose for (**A**) brain, (**B**) spinal cord, (**C**) kidney, and (**D**) lung. (From Burman C, Kutcher GJ, Emami B, et al. Fitting of normal tissue tolerance data to an analytic function. *Int J Radiat Oncol Biol Phys* 1991;21:123–135, with permission.)

by 4-cm portal, the same dose delivered in the same period for a supraglottic carcinoma, with a larger portal covering the entire larynx, would result in more severe acute and late sequelae (156).

Nominal Standard Dose and Time–Dose Factor

The nominal standard dose (NSD) concept is of historic interest. For 20 years NSD was used frequently to express equivalency of clinical doses of irradiation based on human skin tolerance and curability of squamous cell carcinoma. Cohen (85) pointed out that the regression coefficient for squamous cell carcinoma was different from that of normal skin (0.24). In 1969, Ellis (135) suggested that if one number could be used to represent the dose of irradiation that reached normal tissue tolerance, this would be advantageous in comparing different techniques. This figure should represent the normal connective tissue tolerance because this was, in his thinking, the limiting factor in most tumor therapies.

The unit for NSD expression was the *ret*. It could never be assumed that the NSD value represented a "single equivalent dose" because the isoeffect time calculated by Ellis used data from four to 30 fractions. Another flaw of the NSD calculation was that it did not allow for the effect of variations in volume treated or for interruptions of therapy (split-course therapy). Orton (358) estimated that NSD calculations were misused about 50% of the time by unaware clinicians comparing different radiation therapy regimens. The NSD formula did not predict isoeffect in pig skin irradiation with ^{60}Co using two to five fractions per week (557). Moreover, early reactions did not predict the magnitude of late damage when dose fractionation was altered from conventional daily schedules.

In 1973, Orton and Ellis (362) published a simplification of the NSD concept more applicable to clinical radiation therapy, stating that when a treatment did not result in normal connective tissue tolerance, treatment effectiveness should be described in terms of partial tolerance. Although there was no definite basis for the application of the time–dose factor (TDF) concept to clinical radiation therapy, equivalency of various dose schedules is sought constantly.

(Continued)

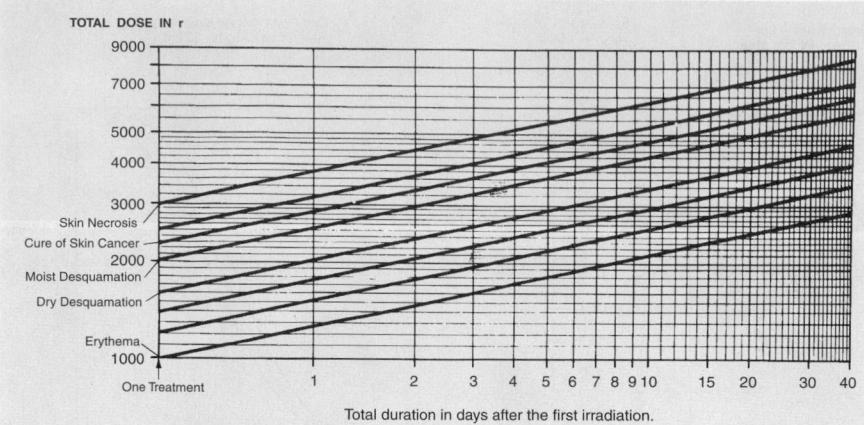

FIGURE 1.19. Strandqvist's curves on log paper. The slope of the curves (0.22) is the same for the tumoricidal dose for squamous cell carcinoma for various degrees of skin reactions. (From Strandqvist M. Sutdien uber die kumulative wirkung der rontgenstrahlen bie frakionierung. *Acta Radiol* [Stockh] 1944;55[Suppl]:1–300, with permission.)

For split-course regimens, the TDF values (in units of ret) were used by adding the TDF value for each of the partial tolerance factors corresponding to each component of the treatment and correcting for the decay of the first part of the treatment TDF.

In 1974, Orton (360) defined TDF values for continuous irradiation that could be used with temporary or permanent brachytherapy implants, using various isotopes. A standard radium therapy regimen of 60 Gy in 168 hours was used for comparison with other equivalent techniques. According to Ellis (137), this was equivalent to 1,800 ret of fractionated external irradiation.

Linear-Quadratic Equation (α/β Ratio)

Formulations based on dose survival models have been proposed to evaluate the biologic equivalence of various doses and fractionation schedules. These assumptions are based on a LQ survival curve represented by the equation:

$$\text{Log}_e S = \alpha D + \beta D^2,$$

in which α represents the *linear* (i.e., first-order dose-dependent) component of cell killing, and β represents the *quadratic* (i.e., second-order dose-dependent) component of cell killing. Thus, β represents the more reparable (over a few hours) component of cell damage (Figs. 1.20–1.22). The dose at which the two components of cell killing are equal constitutes the α/β ratio.

In a study of 17 human tumor cell lines, Steel and Peacock (478) observed that the average surviving fraction at 2 Gy is 0.44 from the α component and 0.88 from the β component. The β effect at that dose level appears to be similar in radiosensitive and radioresistant tumors; thus, among radiosensitive tumors in which the survival from the α component is below 0.3, the β effect makes a very small contribution to overall radiosensitivity in the lower dose region. The overall effect of many small fractions is to amplify the dominance of the α component. The β

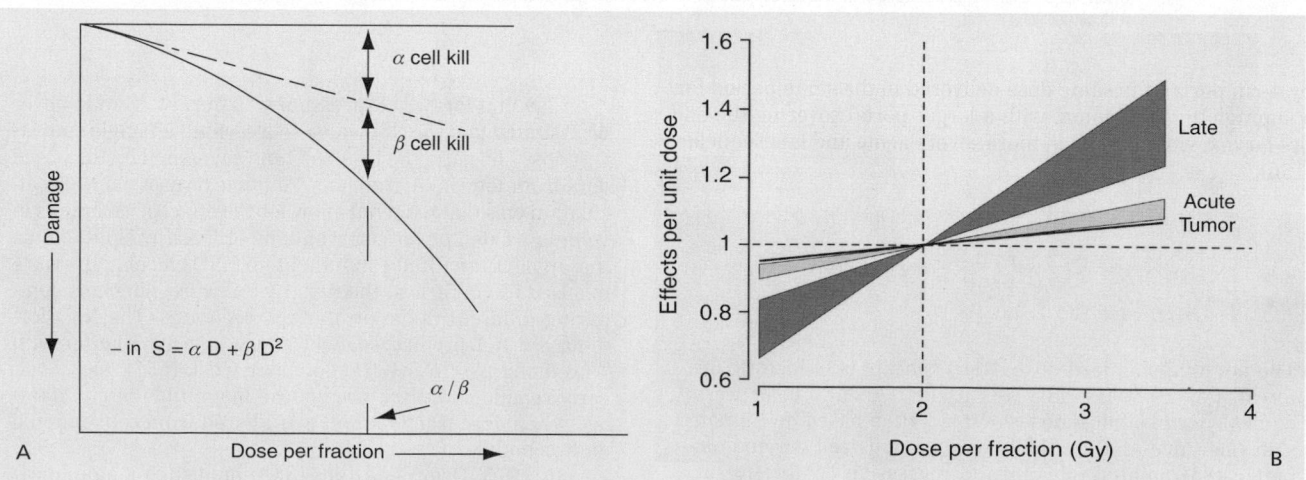

FIGURE 1.20. A: At a dose equal to the α/β ratio, the log cell kill due to the α-process (nonreparable) is equal to that due to the β-process (reparable injury); α/β is thus a measure of how soon the survival curve begins to bend over significantly. The α/β ratio for late effects on normal tissue generates a "curvier curve" than the α/β ratio for radiation's effects on acutely reacting normal tissue and tumor cells. Thus, the relative effect of dose per fraction is higher for late-responding tissue than for acutely responding tissues. In particular, for the central nervous system, high dose per fraction radiation therapy is associated with an increased risk of late effects. An α/β ratio of 2 to 3 commonly is used in calculations of radiation effects on late-reacting tissue, whereas the ratio of 10 is used more commonly for acute-responding tissues or tumor. (From Fowler JR. Fractionation and therapeutic gain. In: Steel GG, Adams GE, Peckham MJ, eds. *The biological basis of radiotherapy*. Amsterdam: Elsevier Science, 1983;181–194, with permission.) **B:** A schematic representation of biologic data relating dose per fraction to effect on tumors, early reacting, and late-reacting normal tissues. (From Saunders MI. Programming of radiotherapy in the treatment of non-small-cell lung cancer—a way to advance cure. *Lancet Oncol* 2001;2[7]:401–408, with permission.)

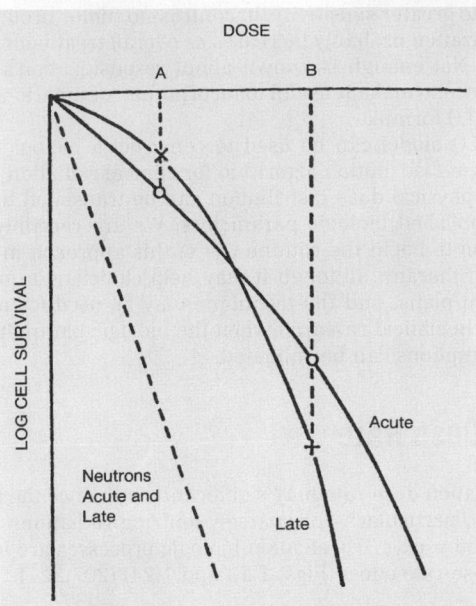

FIGURE 1.21. Hypothetical survival curves for the target cells for acute and late effects in normal tissues exposed to x-rays or neutrons. The α/β ratio in the equation for surviving fractions (SF = $e^{-\alpha D + \beta D_2}$) is higher for late effects than for acute effects in x-irradiated tissues, resulting in a greater rate of change in effect in late-responding tissues with change in dose. At dose A, survival of target cells is higher in late-effects than in acute-effects tissues, whereas at dose B, the reverse is true. Therefore, increasing the dose per fraction from A to B results in a relatively greater increase in late rather than acute injury. In the case of neutrons, the α/β ratio is low, with no detectable influence on the quadratic function ($e\beta D \pm D2$) over the first two decades of reduction in cell survival, implying that accumulation of sublethal injury plays a negligible role in cell killing by doses of neutrons of clinical interest. At these doses, the relative biologic effectiveness is higher for late effects than it is for acute effects. (From Fowler JR. Fractionation and therapeutic gain. In: Steel GG, Adams GE, Peckham MJ, eds. *The biological basis of radiotherapy.* Amsterdam: Elsevier Science, 1983;181–194, with permission.)

effect is unimportant because repair will be almost complete. In the more radiocurable tumors, cell killing by the α component represents the predominant fraction of tumor cell killing.

The shape of the dose-survival curve with photons differs for acutely and slowly responding normal tissues. This difference in shape is not observed with neutrons. The severity of late effects changes more rapidly with a variation in the size of dose per fraction when a total dose is selected to yield equivalent acute effects. With a decreasing size of dose per fraction, the total dose required to achieve a certain isoeffect increases more for late-responding tissues than for acutely responding tissues. Thus, in hyperfractionated regimens, the tolerable dose would be increased more for late effects than for acute effects. Conversely, if large doses per fraction are used, the total dose required to achieve isoeffects in late-responding tissues would be reduced more for late effects than for acute effects. In general, tumors and acutely reacting tissues have a high α/β ratio (8 to 15 Gy), whereas tissues involved in late effects have a low α/β ratio (1 to 5 Gy). Some values obtained in animal experiments and clinical studies are summarized in Table 1.9.

The values for α and β can be obtained from graphs in which the reciprocal of the total dose (Gy^{-1}) and the dose per fraction (Gy) are plotted. A straight line is obtained. The intercept of this line with the zero dose-per-fraction axis is proportional to α and equal to $\alpha/\ln S$, wherein S is the natural logarithm of survival. The slope is proportional to β and equal to $\beta/\ln S$ (126,507).

The algebraic functions to derive the straight line from the reciprocal total dose per fraction plot are provided as follows. Tumor cell survival following n fractions, each of dose d:

$$-\ln S = n(\alpha d + \beta d)^2$$
$$= \alpha nd + \beta nd^2$$
$$= nd(\alpha + \beta d).$$

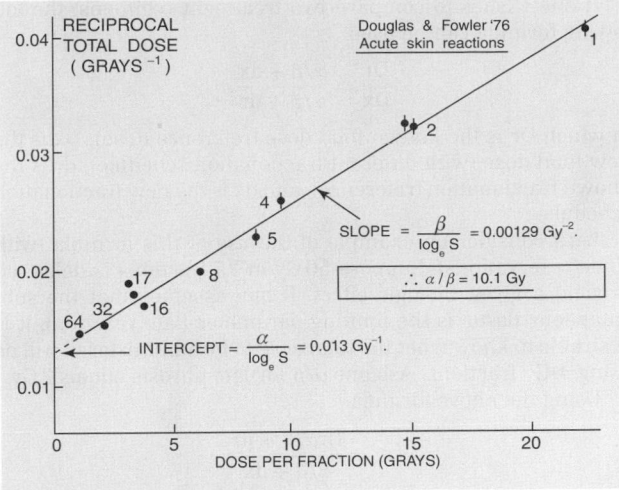

FIGURE 1.22. Values of α and β. If the reciprocal of total dose (for several multifraction schedules) is plotted against dose per fraction, a straight line will be obtained. The intercept of this line with the zero dose-per-fraction axis is proportional to α ($\alpha/\ln S$). The slope is proportional to β ($\beta/\ln S$). The α/β ratio is readily determined. For absolute values of α and β, clonogenic assay is necessary for the end point. (From Fowler JR. Fractionation and therapeutic gain. In: Steel GG, Adams GE, Peckham MJ, eds. *The biological basis of radiotherapy.* Amsterdam: Elsevier Science, 1983;181–194, with permission.)

Dividing both sides by total dose nd:

$$\frac{-\ln S}{nd} = \alpha + \beta d$$
$$\uparrow \qquad \uparrow .$$
$$\text{Intercept} \quad \text{Slope}$$

Withers et al. (606) proposed a method for using these survival-curve parameters for calculating the change in total dose necessary to achieve an equal response in tissue when the dose per fraction is varied, using the α/β ratios. This calculation accounts only for the effect of repair of cellular injury. The iso-effect curves vary for different tissues. A biologically equivalent dose (BED) can be obtained using this formula:

$$BED = \frac{\ln S}{\alpha}.$$
$$BED = nd[1 + d/(\alpha/\beta)]$$

Table 1.9	RATIO OF LINEAR (α) TO QUADRATIC (β) TERMS FROM MULTIFRACTION EXPERIMENTS AND CLINICAL DATA	
	α/β Ratio (Gy)	
Tissue	**Experimental**	**Clinical**
Early reactions		
Skin/subcutaneous tissues	9–12	5–10
Jejunum	6–10	2.2–8
Colon	10–11	—
Testis	12–13	—
Callus	9–10	—
Late reactions		
Spinal cord	1.0–4.9	3.3
Kidney	1.5–2.4	—
Lung	2.4–6.3	4.2–4.7
Bladder	3.1–7.0	3.4–4.5

Modified from Fowler JF. Fractionation and therapeutic gain. In: Steel GG, Adams GE, Peckham MJ, eds. *The biological basis of radiotherapy.* Amsterdam, The Netherlands: Elsevier Science, 1983;181–194.

If one wishes to compare two treatment regimens, the following formula can be used:

$$\frac{Dr}{Dx} = \frac{\alpha/\beta + dx}{\alpha/\beta + dr},$$

in which Dr is the known total dose (reference dose), Dx is the new total dose (with different fractionation schedule), dr is the known fractionation (reference), and dx is the new fractionation schedule.

Let's consider an example of the use of this formula (with some reservations). Suppose 50 Gy in 25 fractions is delivered to yield a given biologic effect. If one assumes that the subcutaneous tissue is the limiting parameter (late reaction), it is desirable to know what the total dose to be administered will be using 4-Gy fractions. Assume α/β for late fibrosis equals 2 Gy.

Using the above formula:

$$Dx = \frac{Dr\alpha/\beta + dr}{\alpha/\beta + dx}.$$

Thus

$$Dx = 500\,Gy\left(\frac{5+2}{5+4}\right) = 39\,Gy.$$

The basic LQ equation addresses the inactivation of a homogeneous population of cells. One should be wary, however, of accepting the basic equation as being complete. Because it is likely that accelerated repopulation of tumor clonogens occurs during the course of radiotherapy, and that cell cycle redistribution and reoxygenation also occur, we should consider how these factors can be accounted for in the formula (52,207,618).

Repopulation may be accounted for, in broad approximation, by describing the number of clonogens (N) at time t as being related to the initial number of clonogens (No).

Then,

$$N = No^{e\lambda t}.$$

The parameter λ determines the speed of cell repopulation and is given by

$$\lambda = \frac{loge^2}{Tpot} = \frac{0.693}{Tpot},$$

where Tpot is the effective doubling time of cells in the tumor. If we ignore spontaneous cell loss, then Tpot is approximately the same as the measurable *in vitro* doubling time of tumor cells. Reported values of Tpot are 2 to 25 days with a median value of approximately 5 days. For late-responding tissues, Tpot is so large that λ is effectively zero.

Incorporating the allowance for tumor proliferation, with t representing time, the LQ equation becomes

$$E = nd\left(1 + \frac{d}{\alpha/\beta}\right) - \frac{0.693t}{\alpha Tpot}.$$

Let's assume an α/β for an acutely reacting tissue, such as a tumor, of 10, and an α of 0.3 with a Tpot of 5. The BED of 70 Gy of 2 Gy/fraction, 5 fractions per week, in 46 days, is

$$BED = 70(1 + 0.2) = 84\,Gy_{10}.$$

Now let's add the correction for tumor repopulation during the course of treatment:

$$\frac{E}{\alpha} = 70\left(1 + \frac{2}{10}\right) - \frac{0.693}{0.3} \times \frac{46}{5}$$
$$BED = 84 - 21 = 63\,Gy_{10}.$$

The decrease in clonogens by radiotherapy is attenuated, in part, by the repopulation of the surviving clonogens.

In the LQ equation, redistribution in the cell cycle and reoxygenation may be modeled by a single term called *resensitization*. Immediately after a dose of radiation, the average radiosensitivity of the cell population falls and then gradually returns to greater sensitivity. In contrast to tumor proliferation, resensitization probably increases as overall treatment time increases. Not enough is known about resensitization's clinical importance to make it useful to incorporate a numeric value for it in the LQ formula.

The LQ model can be used to construct a biologically oriented dose-distribution algorithm for clinical radiation therapy (280). A physical dose distribution can be translated to a BED using published biologic parameters. We are certainly not in a position to begin the routine use of this approach in clinical radiation therapy, although it may help clinicians to optimize treatment plans, and the technique may be used for outcome analysis in clinical research when the biologic parameters and the assumptions can be validated.

:: | Dose Rate

The radiation dose rate may significantly influence the biologic response, particularly for sparsely ionizing radiations such as x-rays and γ-rays. Three main biologic processes are involved in the dose-rate effect (Figs. 1.23 and 1.24) (207,227).

1. Repair of sublethal damage occurs when radiation is delivered at a low dose rate, and the treatment time is extended to a point where it is comparable to the repair half-time. As the dose rate is reduced, more sublethal damage is repaired because the radiation injury is spread over a longer period. The cell survival curves become progressively less steep, and at the same time the extrapolation number approaches unity.
2. Cell proliferation occurs during protracted radiation exposure if the dose rate is low enough or the cell cycle time is short enough.

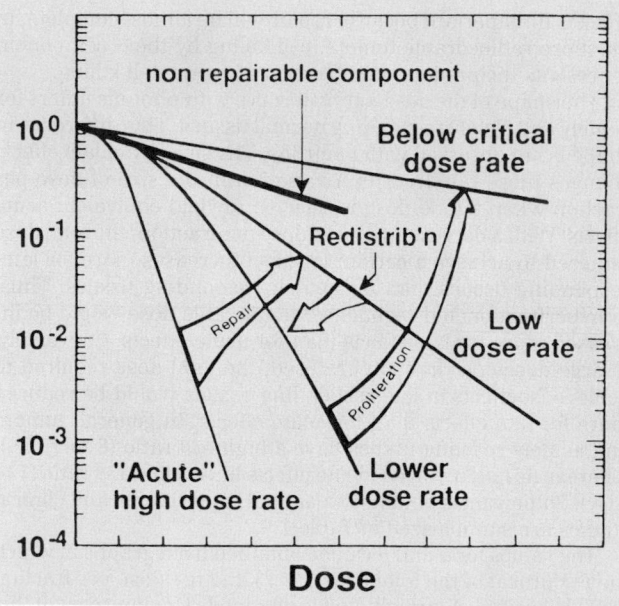

FIGURE 1.23. The dose-rate effect as a result of repair of sublethal damage, redistribution in the cycle, and cell proliferation. The dose–response curve for acute exposures is characterized by a broad initial shoulder. As the dose rate is reduced, the survival curve becomes progressively shallower as more and more sublethal damage is repaired, but cells are "frozen" in their positions in the cycle and do not progress. As the dose rate is lowered further and for a limited range of dose rates, the survival curve steepens again because cells can progress through the cycle to pile up at a block in G2, a radiosensitive phase, but still cannot divide. A further lowering of dose rate allows cells to escape the G2 block and divide; cell proliferation then may occur during the protracted exposure, and survival curves become shallower as cell birth from mitosis offsets cell killing from the irradiation. (Based on the ideas of Dr. Joel Bedford, and from Hall EJ. *Radiobiology for the radiologist*, 4th ed. Philadelphia: J.B. Lippincott, 1994, with permission.)

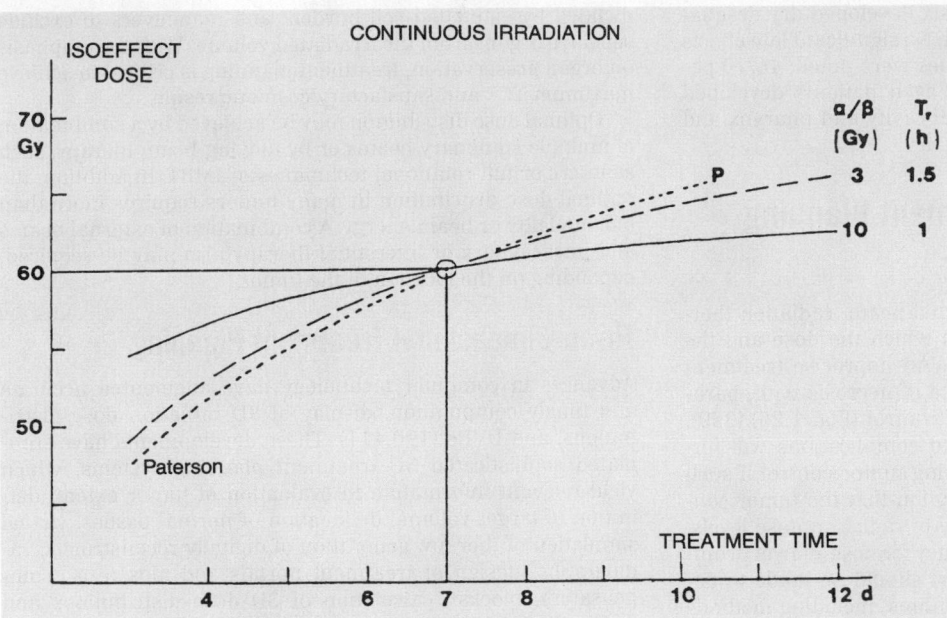

FIGURE 1.24. Low–dose-rate irradiation. Isoeffect dose equivalent to 60 Gy in 7 days. Two sets of parameters have been considered for the computation, which would presumably correspond to skin and mucosa early reactions and to the effect on the epithelioma ($\alpha/\beta = 10$ Gy, Tr = 1 hour) and to late reactions ($\alpha/\beta = 3$ Gy, Tr = 1.5 hour). (From Dutreix J. Expression of the dose rate effect in clinical curietherapy. *Radiother Oncol* 1989;15:25–37, with permission.)

3. Redistribution and accumulation of cells throughout the cell cycle occur with a low dose rate in which proliferation is decreased because cells are arrested and accumulate in G_2. This phase of the cycle is relatively radiosensitive. As a result, cell killing may be greater for a lower dose rate. This effect occurs over a narrow dose-rate range and is known as the inverse dose-rate effect.

With the advent of moderate– and high–dose-rate remote control afterloading devices, increased emphasis has been placed on the biologic effects of dose rate. Many *in vitro* and *in vivo* experimental observations indicate variations in cell killing and repair of sublethal or potentially lethal damage with varying dose rates. The so-called dose-rate effect is most dramatic between 1 cGy/minute and 1 Gy/minute (204). The biologic effect achieved by a given irradiation dose decreases as the dose rate diminishes, chiefly as a result of the increase in cell repair that occurs during continuous prolonged irradiation, because cell proliferation is virtually negligible in the range of treatment times used in low–dose-rate brachytherapy (127).

In some experiments, a bending of the cell-survival curve at very low dose rates has been noted, instead of the expected exponential result, possibly because of cell redistribution (625) or a decline in the repair capacity with large doses (525). At a very low dose rate, because the cell killing is caused only by direct lethal events that are considered independent of the dose rate, cell repair is also negligible. The induction of sublethal injury is relatively slow compared with the rate of repair, and cell killing, by accumulation of sublethal injury, remains minimal. Variation of the isoeffect dose occurs mainly in the range of medium dose rates (1 to 10 Gy/hour), and it vanishes at very high dose rates because the cell repair is negligible during the short treatment time (127).

The dose-rate effect in clinical brachytherapy was described initially by Green and Paterson (136,360,376). The historic isoeffect curve showed a significant increase in dose when time was increased from 2 to 7 days. However, the validity of Paterson's curve was questioned by Pierquin et al. (402), who used the same dose of 70 Gy with treatment times ranging from 3 to 8 days for the treatment of head and neck tumors with ^{192}Ir implants and did not observe any difference in the control rate or incidence of necrosis. The agreement with Paterson's curve

is acceptable when the α/β value equals 3 Gy and repair half-time (T_r) equals 1.5 hours, but the curve is shallower when α/β equals 10 Gy and T_r equals 1 hour. One should expect Paterson's curve to correspond to late reactions and to overestimate the variation for early reactions and control of squamous cell carcinoma.

Several important concepts should be considered regarding the clinical relevance of dose rate (51,205):

1. At ultra-high doses and instantaneous dose rates (i.e., 10 Gy pulsed in nanoseconds), the rapid deposition of energy consumes oxygen too quickly for diffusion to maintain an adequate level of oxygenation, and dose–response curves are characteristic of hypoxia. There is little interest in clinical application of this approach.
2. Based on laboratory data, it may be possible to design schedules with a pulse width of several minutes and a pulse interval of about 1 hour to achieve cell killing equivalent to that obtained with a continuous 30 Gy in 60 hours (0.5 Gy/hour).
3. Using the LQ equation, it is possible to estimate the equivalency of high–dose-rate (HDR) and low–dose-rate (LDR) exposures with a variety of fractionation schedules (remembering that a lower number of fractions may result in enhanced late effects).

Special consideration should be given to the effect of HDR brachytherapy on normal tissues. The tumor dose must be decreased 30% to 50% in comparison with that delivered with conventional low dose rates (361,363). (For further discussion, see Chapters 20–22.)

In the past, there was some interest in continuous LDR irradiation with external cobalt units (601). Pierquin et al. (401) used a modified ^{60}Co unit with a small industrial source (activity 45 Ci). Radiation was delivered at 1 to 1.39 Gy/hour to administer daily tumor doses of 8 to 10 Gy in 7 to 8 hours. A minimum of five treatments was given per week, although occasionally weekends and holidays caused schedule modifications. Patients were given short rest periods every 1 or 2 hours. Tumor doses of approximately 63 Gy were delivered in eight to 11 fractions, with the volume reduced to 8 by 10 cm after 45 Gy. Nineteen patients with advanced tumors of the mouth and pharynx were treated; 15 had no evidence of tumor 3 months after treatment. Only three patients developed recurrences. Of 19 patients, two developed moist desquamation and six developed dry desquamation; the others had only erythema. No significant late effects on the skin or the subcutaneous tissues were noted; 16/19 patients developed severe mucositis. Seven patients developed necrosis, six in large areas of the oral cavity and pharynx and in several instances at the tumor site.

Importance of Treatment Planning in Radiation Therapy

The predicted consequences of external-beam, radiation therapy are based on the precision with which the dose and the irradiated volume are defined (253). An imprecise treatment system could lead to a high incidence of necrosis with, paradoxically, a low probability of tumor control (Fig. 1.25) (359). Decreasing irradiation doses to avoid complications will further reduce the probability of achieving tumor control if such action is based on the wrong assumption that the tumor control/complication ratio is related only to radiation dose levels. The ICRU recommends a ± 5% accuracy for dose-delivery computations (245). However, every effort should be made to develop accurate dose-calculation algorithms, including methods to correct for inhomogeneities in tissue density and the shape of the patient's body, and to develop practical treatment planning capabilities to obtain the highest possible dose optimization in the irradiated volume (tumor and normal tissues). There are benefits of reducing the treatment volume in an effort to deliver higher doses of irradiation. This may improve the quality of tumor control without excessively irradiating surrounding normal tissues, thereby decreasing treatment-related morbidity.

Various steps can be taken to decrease toxicity in normal tissues, including precise treatment planning and irradiation techniques, selective decreased volume receiving higher doses

dictated by estimated cell burden, and maneuvers to exclude sensitive organs from the irradiated volume. With the emphasis on organ preservation, treatment planning is critical to achieve maximum TCP and satisfactory cosmetic results.

Optimal dose distribution may be achieved by a combination of multiple stationary beams or by moving-beam therapy, such as in arc or full-rotational techniques or IMRT. In addition, the optimal dose distribution in many tumors requires more than one modality or beam energy. A combination of external beams and intracavitary or interstitial therapy also may be required, depending on the location of the tumor.

Three-Dimensional Treatment Planning

Advances in computer technology have augmented accurate and timely computation, display of 3D radiation dose distributions, and DVHs (190,411). These developments have stimulated sophisticated 3D treatment planning systems, which yield relevant information in evaluation of tumor extent, definition of target volume, delineation of normal tissues, virtual simulation of therapy, generation of digitally reconstructed radiographs, design of treatment portals and aids (e. g., compensators, blocks), calculation of 3D dose distributions and dose optimization, and critical evaluation of the treatment plan (188,389,413).

The potential benefits of 3D planning and delivery systems are great. It is, however, not clear which specific disease sites and treatment situations will be benefited by 3D planning (412). With advanced computerized and display technologies, contiguous CT slices are used to define anatomic structures and target volumes. External radiation beams of any possible orientation are simulated. A significant feature of these systems is the so-called beam's eye view, in which patient contours are viewed as if the observer's eye is placed at the source of radiation looking out along the axis of the radiation beam (317). These systems allow simulation of the geometric setup; evaluation of the plan for dose optimization still is made on the merits of volumetric dose distributions.

Quantitative treatment planning evaluation is crucial in selection of the best portals and radiation beams to deliver an optimal dose to the tumor with relative sparing of normal tissues (232). The ICRU report 50 and its supplement G2 define 3D volumes for the prescription and reporting of EBRT (246). The GTV is defined as the gross demonstrable extent and location of malignant growth; the CTV allows a margin around the GTV for subclinical disease; the PTV allows margins on the CTV for variation in position, size, and shape so that the prescribed dose is received by the CTV; and the treated volume is that area receiving a dose considered appropriate to the purpose of treatment such as tumor eradication or palliation (Fig. 1.2).

The DVH is useful as a means of dose display, particularly in assessing several treatment plan dose distributions (79). A DVH provides a complete summary of the entire 3D dose matrix, showing the amount of target volume or critical structure receiving more than a specified dose level. Because a DVH does not provide spatial dose information, it cannot replace the other methods of dose display; it can only complement them.

Models for optimization of 3D dose distribution using biologic models of tumor and normal tissue responses correlated with physical radiation doses have been described (384). Mohan et al. (330), in a theoretical analysis, concluded that for certain clinical situations it is not sufficient to specify objectives of optimization purely on the basis of pattern of irradiation dose and that dose-volume effects and biologic indices also must be incorporated into the formulation.

Niemierko et al. (352) described a technique for optimization of 3D conformal radiation therapy plans with biologic models of tumor and normal tissue response to irradiation as well as with scores based on physical dose. Optimization programs attempted to minimize dose gradient across the target volume,

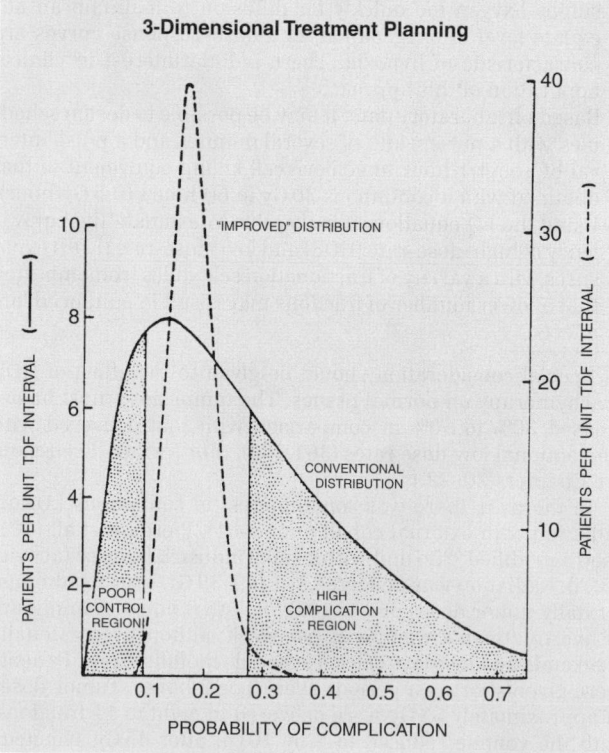

FIGURE 1.25. Frequency distribution of patients treated to different probabilities of complication. (From Orton CG. Other considerations in three-dimensional treatment planning. In: Bagne F, ed. *Computerized treatment planning systems.* HHS Publications FDA 84–8223, 1984;136–141, with permission.)

match specified isodose contours to the target and critical organs, match specified dose-volume constraints, minimize integral dose to the entire volume of patient treated, minimize maximum dose to critical organs, and constrain dose to specified normal tissues below a tolerance-dose level. The solutions were based on TCP, NTCP, various dose levels given to specified volumes of the patient, discrete or continuous values of beam parameters, number of beams, and logical combination of any constraints.

Intensity-Modulated Radiation Therapy

An increasingly popular approach to 3D treatment planning and conformal therapy optimizes the delivery of irradiation to irregularly shaped volumes through a process of complex inverse treatment planning and dynamic delivery of irradiation that results in modulated fluence of photon beam profiles (49).

Treatment planning begins with the determination of the GTV and the CTV, which contains the GTV, and an estimate of where the tumor may spread. CT, MRI, and fluorodeoxyglucose positron emission tomography (FDG-PET) imaging along with image fusion have enhanced the possibilities for determining the target more accurately. The PTV accounts for inaccuracies in positioning patients' and organ motion.

In "forward" planning, software calculates the dose distribution, displays it with a 3D anatomical model, and provides analytical and graphical metrics for assessing the adequacy of tumor treatment and normal tissue avoidance. The physician decides if the plan is acceptable. If not, an alteration is made in the beam arrangement, and the process is repeated.

Computerized optimization techniques have lead to "inverse" planning. Goals of an acceptable treatment plan are delineated, and the inverse planning algorithm searches through many thousands of possibilities to find a plan that best satisfies the goals. In IMRT, the beams are broken up into "beamlets" (on the order of 0.5 by 0.5 or 1 by 1 cm) that can each have different intensity. IMRT may improve the ability to treat with a high radiation dose while minimizing dose to nearby critical structures.

There are a variety of forms in which IMRT can be administered:

1. The North American Scientific (NOMOS) Corporation (Chatsworth, CA) Peacock system: an array of individual beamlets, each consisting of a narrow incident arc photon beam that exposes the target. The radiation fluence is modulated with a small dynamic multileaf collimator (MLC) (MIMiC) activated by a preprogrammed controller.
2. A linear accelerator and multileaf collimation, with a variety of portals at various angles, may be used; the MLC determines the portal shape of each of the portals. Photon modulated fluency may be obtained (a step-and-shoot method).
3. Dynamic computer-controlled IMRT is delivered when the configuration of the portals with the MLC is changing at the same time that the gantry or the accelerator is changing positions around the patient.
4. In helical tomotherapy, the photon fan beam continually rotates around the patient as the couch transports the patient longitudinally through the ring gantry (273). The verification processes for helical tomotherapy are enabled by the use of the ring gantry; the geometry of a CT scanner allows tomographic processes to be reliably performed. Dose reconstruction is a key process of tomography; the treatment detector sinogram computes the actual dose deposited in the patient. The length of the beam is 40 cm at the central axis and has a width that can vary between 0.5 and 5 cm. Like the NOMOS MIMiC MLC, the lengths of the MLC in helical tomography are temporarily modulated or binary in the sense that they are rapidly driven either in or out by air system actuators rather than beam slowly pushed by motors driving lead screws as in the conventional MLC.
5. The robotic arm IMRT system consists of a miniaturized 6-MV photon linear accelerator mounted on a highly mobile arm and a set of ceiling-mounted x-ray cameras to provide near real-time information on patient position and target exposure during treatment.

The majority of the IMRT systems use 6-MV x-rays, but energies of 8 to 10 MV may be more desirable in some anatomic sites (to decrease skin and superficial subcutaneous tissue dose). The dose-distribution and field-shaping parameters are based on inverse 3D planning using specially defined minimal dose to target and dose constraints for surrounding normal tissues (46,49,70,621). Inverse planning starts with an ideal dose distribution and finds through trial and error or multiple iterations (simulated annealing) the beam characteristics (fluence profiles), then produces the best approximation to the ideal dose defined in a 3D array of dose voxels organized in a stack of 2D arrays (365,547).

A back-projection technique through careful choice of filters, beam placement, and shaping of the portals conforms the irradiation dose to the shape of the tumor, minimizing dose to critical adjacent structures. When this technique is used, it is critical to adhere to basic concepts of treatment planning and evaluation of the pathobiology of malignant disease. Well-designed treatment plans based on radiographic imaging (CT or MRI), which in most instances demonstrates gross disease, are necessary to minimize the risk of missing or underirradiating adjacent microscopic or subclinical tumor.

Given the added time and labor involved in IMRT, numerous issues require study:

1. Can the tumor be localized with sufficient accuracy to take advantage of the improved dose localization?
2. Treatment plans that produce a rapid drop in dose between the edge of the tumor and the normal tissue require more exact patient positioning; otherwise, there is a high risk of under-dosing the tumor or overdosing normal tissue.
3. Some IMRT plans treat the center of the tumor with a very high dose to achieve an acceptable dose at the edge. This may not be optimal.
4. Many IMRT techniques spread a low dose over a larger volume or normal tissue. This may increase the risk of secondary malignancies years later (253,336).

Heavy Particle Beams

The vast majority of radiation therapy is administered with photon or electron external beams or photon-generating brachytherapy sources. Physicians and physicists have explored the possibility that alternative forms of ionizing radiation might be clinically useful.

One can imagine two possible mechanisms by which one could improve on therapeutic x-rays with an alternative particle. First, the alternative particle could have energy deposition characteristics that lead to a superior dose distribution. A beam, conceivably, could have more skin sparing than x-rays, better stopping characteristics, and/or less side scatter. This might allow a more conformal therapy. Second, the alternative particle could have advantageous radiobiologic properties. It might be more toxic than x-rays to hypoxic cells or cells in the late S phase of the mitotic cell cycle. Such a particle would have, perhaps, a lower oxygen enhancement ratio (OER) and a higher RBE than x-rays. These two possible mechanisms of improving on x-rays are not mutually exclusive. A particle could have both superior physical dose distribution and radiobiologic properties.

The effort to identify improved alternatives to x-rays has focused on the group of particles called hadrons. These are particles constituted of strongly interacting particles called quarks and gluons. The hadrons include the mesons and the baryons. The latter include protons, neutrons, negative pions, and the nuclei of heavier atoms such as He^2 (helium), C^6 (carbon), O^8 (oxygen), Ne^{10} (neon), and Ar^{18} (argon). All of these forms of radiation are distinguished from x-rays and electrons by their greater masses. These alternative radiation modalities are relatively difficult to produce, are expensive, and are considerably more difficult to control.

Proton beams have attracted radiation oncologists because they offer interesting and potentially beneficial dose distribution characteristics. Radiobiologically, their properties are not significantly different from x-rays. When a proton beam traverses tissue, the dose is deposited in an approximately constant rate. The rate of energy loss (also called the "stopping power") of a heavy charged particle is proportional to the square of the particle charge and inversely proportional to the square of its velocity. As a proton slows down, its rate of energy loss increases and so does the ionization or absorbed dose to the tissue. Near the end of the proton's range, the deposition of energy rises very sharply before dropping to almost zero. This peaking of dose near the end of the particle range is called the Bragg peak. As a result of the Bragg peak effect and minimal scattering, the proton offers the potential advantage and the ability to concentrate dose inside and immediately adjacent to the tumor volume and minimize dose to surrounding normal tissues. There are proton treatment facilities operational and under construction throughout the economically developed world. The technology has been evaluated most extensively in the management of choroidal melanoma, base of skull tumors, soft-tissue sarcomas, and prostate cancer.

A Glossary of Terms Pertinent to Heavy Particle Beam Radiation Therapy

baryon: A hadron made from three quarks. The proton and the neutron are both baryons. They also may contain additional quark–antiquark pairs.

Bragg, William Henry (1862–1942): He was born at Westward, Cumberland, and educated at King William's College, Isle of Mann; Trinity College, Cambridge; and the Cavendish Laboratory. In collaboration with his son (*vide infra*), he developed techniques of systematically analyzing crystal structures using x-rays. This was recognized by the award of the Nobel Prize in Physics jointly to father and son in 1915.

Bragg, William Lawrence (1890–1971): He was born in Adelaide, South Australia, where his father was a professor. He came to England with his father (*vide supra*) and entered Trinity College, Cambridge. He and his father published *X-rays and Crystal Structure* in 1915. Later in his career, he used x-ray analysis to investigate the structure of proteins. Having been awarded the Nobel Prize with his father, he was, at 25 years of age, the youngest-ever Laureate.

Bragg peak: The region of high dose at the end of the range of a heavy charged particle.

charge: A quantum number carried by a particle. Determines whether the particle can participate in an interaction process. A particle with electric charge has electrical interactions; one with strong charge has strong interactions, and so forth.

electric charge: The quantum number that determines participation in electromagnetic interactions.

electromagnetic interaction: The interaction resulting from electric charge; this includes magnetic effects that have to do with moving electric charges.

electron: The least massive electrically charged particle, hence absolutely stable. It is the most common lepton, with electric charge –1.

fermion: Any particle that has odd-half-integer (1/2, 3/2, . . .) intrinsic angular momentum (spin). As a consequence of this peculiar angular momentum, fermions obey the Pauli exclusion principle, which states that no two fermions can exist in the same state at the same place and time. Many of the properties of ordinary matter arise because of this rule. Electrons, protons, and neutrons are all fermions, as are all the fundamental matter particles, both quarks and leptons.

gluon: The carrier particle of strong interactions.

hadron: A particle made of strongly interacting constituents (quarks and/or gluons). These include the mesons and baryons. Such particles participate in residual strong interactions.

lepton: A fundamental fermion that does not participate in strong interactions. The electrically charged leptons are the electron, the muon, the tau, and their antiparticles. Electrically neutral leptons are called neutrinos.

meson: A hadron made from an even number of quark constituents. The basic structure of most mesons is one quark and one antiquark.

neutron: A baryon with electric charge zero; it is a fermion with a basic structure of two down quarks and one up quark (held together by gluons). The neutral component of an atomic nucleus is made from neutrons. Different isotopes of the same element are distinguished by having different numbers of neutrons in their nucleus.

nucleon: A proton or a neutron; that is, one of the particles that makes up a nucleus.

nucleus: A collection of neutrons and protons that forms the core of an atom.

particle: A subatomic object with a definite mass and charge.

photon: The carrier particle of electromagnetic interactions.

pion: The least massive type of meson, pions can have electric charges + 1 or 0.

proton: The most common hadron, a baryon with electric charge (+1) equal and opposite to that of the electron (–1). Protons have a basic structure of two up quarks and one down quark (bound together by gluons). The nucleus of a hydrogen atom is a proton. A nucleus with electric charge Z contains Z protons; therefore, the number of protons is what distinguishes the different chemical elements.

quark: A fundamental fermion that has strong interactions. Quarks have electric charge of either 2/3 (*up, charm, top*) or –1/3 (*down, strange, bottom*) in units where the proton charge is 1.

strong interaction: The interaction responsible for binding quarks, antiquarks, and gluons to make hadrons. Residual strong interactions provide the nuclear binding force.

subatomic particle: Any particle that is small compared to the size of the atom.

These definitions are derived from Welsh JS. Quarks, leptons, fermions, bosons: the subatomic pharmacology of radiation therapy. *Science Med* 2005;10:124–136, 2005; The Nobel Museum (www.nobel.se/physics/laureates); The Atlas Experiment (http://atlasexperiment.org/glossary.html); and Khan FM. *The physics of radiation therapy*, 3rd ed. Philadelphia: Lippincott Williams & Wilkins, 2003.

This section of Chapter 1 offers only the briefest overview of proton and neutron therapy. For a thorough discussion of these two forms of radiation, as well as a consideration of pi meson therapy and charged nuclei therapy such as helium ions and neon ions, the reader is referred to Chapter 18 of this volume.

Boron Neutron Capture Therapy

The fundamental concept of boron neutron capture therapy is the production of high–linear energy transfer (LET) particles ($^7Li^{3+}$ and $^4He^{2+}$) when one "tags" or "labels" a tumor cell with a compound having a large cross-section capable of capturing a "slow" (thermal) neutron. After the compound captures the neutron, it goes into an excited state. The excited fission of the ^{11}B nucleus will release energy, which drives the heavy ion products over short distances comparable to the dimensions of one cell. A 0.48 MeV photon is also produced in 94% of the fission events. This is useful for monitoring the reaction but is of little consequence for cell killing (Fig. 1.26).

The neutron has a mass of 0.782 MeV, more than that of the proton. Neutrons were identified in 1932 by Chadwick (74) at Cambridge University's Cavendish Laboratory. Subsequently, Fermi (147) discovered that neutrons react most efficiently with a number of elements after they are slowed by passage through a hydrogen-rich substance such as paraffin. Chadwick and Goldhaber (75), Taylor and Goldhaber (497), and Burcham and Goldhaber (60) showed that slow neutron bombardment of specific stable isotopes of boron, lithium, and nitrogen yield charged particle tracts in photographic plates. The tracts from boron's interaction with neutrons were short and straight and were consistent with the formation of two particles traveling in opposite trajectories. In photographic gelatin, their average travel distance was 7.6 μm. The boron neutron capture process is highly localized. In principle, one could kill a tumor cell containing boron while sparing an adjacent normal cell that does not contain boron.

A Glossary of Terms Pertinent to Neutron Capture Therapy

Epithermal neutrons: Energetic neutrons pass through an intermediate energy range on the way to becoming slow or thermal neutrons. This intermediate energy range is called epithermal.

Fast neutrons: Fast neutrons are highly energetic and travel quickly.

Moderation: Neutrons generated from the fission process or from particle bombardment of materials have significant energy. They lose that energy by colliding with atoms in their environment and create energetic recoil atoms. After a sufficient number of collisions, the neutrons lose essentially all of their energy and become thermal. This process of energy loss is called moderation. The material that provides the atoms the fast neutrons collide with is called a moderator. Water is the usual moderator.

Slow neutrons: Slow neutrons have little energy. They also are referred to as thermal neutrons because they have the same average kinetic energy as gas molecules in their environment.

Thermalize: Epithermal neutron beams, as they penetrate tissue, become additionally moderated. This is called becoming thermalized.

From Yanch JC, Shefer RE, Busse PM. Boron neutron capture therapy. *Science Med* 1999;January/February:18–27.

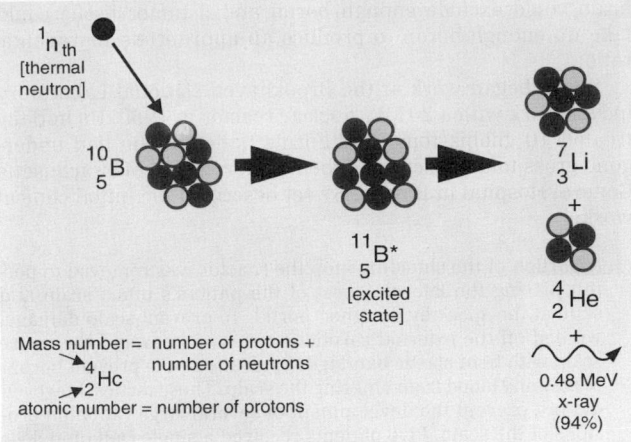

FIGURE 1.26. The bombardment of stable Bo^{10} by a thermal neutron results in a nuclear reaction. This reaction yields Li^7 nuclei and α-particles. These fission products have short path links and a high linear energy transfer (LET). This high-LET radiation, over a short path length, offers the possibility of a lethal effect highly localized within a cell.

The complete chemical reaction is as follows:

$$^{10}B + {}^1n \rightarrow {}^7Li + {}^4He + \gamma + 2.4\,MeV.$$

The attraction of boron neutron capture therapy (BNCT), for many clinicians, has been the notion of the "magic bullet." The idea that one could specifically label tumor cells with a compound with an enlarged cross-sectional area, not label surrounding normal tissue, and therefore deposit radiation only in the tumor is most attractive. Unfortunately, reality is far different from the ideal.

Fast neutrons differ from x-rays in the mode of their interaction with tissue. Whereas x-ray photons interact with the orbital electrons of atoms via the Compton or photoelectric process and set fast electrons in motion, neutrons interact with the nuclei of the atoms of the absorbing tissue. Neutrons put fast recoil protons, α-particles, and heavier nuclear fragments in motion. At energies above about 6 MeV, inelastic scattering by neutrons takes place. A neutron may interact, for example, with a carbon or an oxygen nucleus to produce α-particles. These lead to nuclear fragments called spallation products. The LET is considerably higher for neutrons than for x-rays. Because the LET of neutron radiation is higher, the slope of the cell-survival curve becomes steeper and the size of the initial shoulder gets smaller. This produces a beam with a lower OER than x-rays—neutrons are considerably more toxic to hypoxic cells than x-rays. Also, neutrons are more toxic to cells in phases of the cell cycle that are relatively radioresistant to x-rays. Thus, the RBE of neutrons is higher than x-rays.

In 1936, Locher (294) published a theoretical account of the possible biologic effects and therapeutic possibilities of boron neutron capture. In a prescient comment, he wrote:

> The possibility of destroying or weakening cancerous cells, by the general or selective absorption of neutrons by themselves and particularly there is the possibility of introducing small quantities of neutron absorbers into the regions where it is desired to liberate ionizing energy. A simple illustration would be the injection of a soluble non-toxic compound of boron, lithium, or gold into a superficial cancer followed by bombardment with slow neutrons.

In a 1950 paper by Conger and Giles (90) from Oakridge National Laboratories, they reported that the trace amounts of boron normally present in lily bulbs were responsible for most of the radiation changes in the plants following exposure to slow neutrons. This demonstrated the biologic fact clearly and led William H. Sweet (492) and others to see if the normal brain could exclude enough boron and if tumor tissue could take up enough boron to produce an appropriate therapeutic ratio.

Sweet began work at the Brookhaven National Laboratory in New York with a 20 MW nuclear reactor in 1950. He initially treated 10 glioblastoma multiforme patients who had undergone gross total resection of their tumors at the Massachusetts General Hospital in Boston. Sweet described the initial clinical work:

A portion of the shielding atop the reactor was removed to permit placing the lateral aspect of the patient's intact scalp and skull at the specially designed portal. To prevent scalp damage, we tied off the external carotid arteries and covered the entire scalp with tight elastic bandages in an attempt to prevent boron-containing blood from entering the scalp. These tactics, however, did not prevent the development of several large radiation erosions of the scalp. Five patients received a single radiation dose and the remaining 5 were given the treatment in 2 to 4 fractions. Although there were no life threatening complications of therapy, all of the patients died from 6 to 21 weeks after the first session of neutron capture therapy, which was usually the case in the 1950s for glioblastoma patients treated by any means. Postmortem studies done in 6 of the patients showed abundant viable tumor. Their painful scalp lesions together with the inadequacy of the radiation dose lead us to attempt to deliver the thermal neutron beam directly to the grossly normal but microscopically tumor-infiltrated brain. The Rockefeller Foundation made this approach possible with a $500,000 gift to the Massachusetts Institute of Technology [MIT] to provide additional features to a nuclear reactor that was then being constructed. Included was a surgical operating room immediately beneath the reactor core. This permitted us to turn down the scalp, bone, and dural flap used in the prior removal of gross tumor. At reopening the cerebrospinal fluid replacing tumor was also drained away to give maximally unimpeded access of the thermal neutrons through sterile air to the tumor-infiltrated brain. (492)

Sweet treated 18 patients at MIT. They died from 10 days to 11.5 months after radiation. In every patient the cause of death was cerebral, and extensive irradiation necrosis of the brain was induced in nine cases. In two cases only recurrent tumor was seen, and in one patient there was extensive radiation necrosis and tumor.

Some of the initial work with BNCT was highly controversial and, decades later, led to investigations concerning the nature of informed consent for these human experiments. President William J. Clinton created, by executive order, a commission to study the ethics of cold war–era medical experimentation using radiation. One of the collateral effects of this commission's report was that Sweet and his colleagues were sued for malpractice 40 years after the BNCT experiments. Although the plaintiffs were awarded substantial damages at trial, the decision was eventually overturned on appeal (212).

Clinical trials, largely in Japan, have argued that there is benefit to BNCT of glioblastoma multiforme. However, to date, no randomized clinical trials of BNCT have been performed. Although Japanese investigators have reported a survival rate for grade 3 and 4 malignant glioma patients as high as 58% with BNCT, this has been called into question by Laramore et al. (276). They investigated 14 U.S. patients who were treated with BNCT for glioblastoma multiforme in Japan. A comparison of the survival of these patients with a matched set of conventionally treated patients using the prognostic factors of the RTOG showed no statistical difference compared to the BNCT patients. This is almost certainly the result of patients with relatively favorable characteristics being selected for boron neutron capture therapy such as lower histologic grade, young age, good functional status, and superficial location. Because neutron beams have a significant normal tissue toxicity, and because their depth-dose characteristics are not superior to

x-rays, their applicability has been limited, and clinical results, to date, have been quite mixed. Clinical studies have been reported concerning the use of neutrons in salivary gland and other head and neck tumors, soft-tissue sarcomas, and prostate cancer.

Lack of progress in BNCT may be attributed to two primary factors: inadequate tumor specificity of the boron compounds used to localize in the tumor and poor penetration into tissue of the thermal neutrons. In addition, the thermal and antithermal neutron beams produced by nuclear reactors have considerable contamination with γ-rays and fast neutrons. These can cause normal tissue damage even in the absence of boron concentration in tissues. In addition, there are a number of compounds in normal tissue that can interact with thermal neutrons and have capture events of their own, producing biologic damage even to non–boron-containing tissue.

The development of suitable boron-carrying agents remains a stumbling block to clinical programs. The ideal agent will be nontoxic, will have a high tumor to normal tissue ratio, and will have a high absolute boron concentration. Three classifications are helpful for defining boron agents:

1. *Global agents* have little selectivity for tumor cells. The clinician is relying on a conformal neutron beam to achieve selectivity rather than selective accretion of boron.
2. *Tumor selective agents* accumulate selectivity in tumors. L-4-dihydroxyborylphenylanine has been used as a boron-carrying agent (Fig. 1.27). This compound is a dopamine analog in the melanin synthetic pathway and concentrates in pigmented tumors. It has been thought to be of potential use in the treatment of melanoma, and initial clinical trials are under way. Tumor-selective agents include, in addition to borylphenylalanine compounds, investigations of boronated porphyrins, amino acids, and nucleic acids that are borinated. Melanin is an intracellular protein synthesized from the amino acid tyrosine. Incorporating boronic acid into the paraposition of phenylalanine, producing p-borophenylallanine, would result in a molecule that behaved like tyrosine and might be able to selectively put boron-10 into melanoma cells. These compounds are capable of achieving a tumor-to-normal-tissue ratio of 3 or 4 to 1. It is not, however, because they are a substrate for tyrosinase, the first enzyme in the pathway to melanin. Nonetheless, they are capable of producing high levels of boron-10 in tumors (611).
3. *Tumor-targeted agents* have a structural feature that binds to a specific portion of the cancer cell. Tumor-targeted agents include the use of polycomplex peptides, known as starburst dendrimers, which may allow boron to be attached to an antibody without causing a loss of specificity, and carry boron in low-density lipoprotein vesicles.

Investigations of improved ways of delivering thermal neutrons have centered on two areas: the use of nuclear reactors

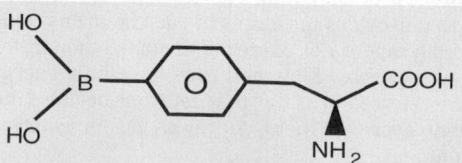

FIGURE 1.27. P-borophenylallanine (BPA) was synthesized in the late 1950s for use in boron neutron capture therapy. It has been shown to accumulate selectively in B16 melanoma cells both *in vivo* and *in vitro*. Clinical trials have been performed of BPA-mediated boron neutron capture therapy for cutaneous melanoma. The compound also has been studied in brain tumor therapy.

and useful alternatives to reactors. For reasons of safety, reactors generally use a low enriched fuel with uranium. However, one would have considerable doubts about the political and social feasibility of the placement of such units in major medical centers in populated areas. Therefore, some investigators have been pursuing nonreactive sources of thermal and epithermal neutrons with a sufficiently high flux to be used for BNCT.

The most intense way to generate a neutron beam is with a nuclear reactor. Despite the high neutron intensities available from these reactors, it is widely recognized that alternative neutron sources will be necessary for BNCT to be performed. First of all, there are few suitable nuclear reactors in operation. A patient would have to travel a long distance for treatment. Second, nuclear reactors, for political and social reasons, are not likely to be sited near major population centers in the future. A major reactor facility located far from a population center would have to be provided with its own clinical infrastructure, and it is not obvious that the target patient population would be large enough to support the operation of more than a few medical reactors (611). Therefore, some investigators have been pursuing nonreactive sources of thermal and epithermal neutrons with a sufficiently high flux to be used for boron neutron capture therapy (83,274,492,545).

An alternative to the reactor would be a neutron source from radioactive decay such as californium-252 (^{252}Cf). However, production of a neutron beam with sufficient intensity for BNCT would require more than the entire present annual supply of ^{252}Cf. Another alternative source is a particle accelerator. Accelerator-based neutron beams are created when light ions such as protons or deuterons are accelerated in an electric field and are made to bombard target materials. Several accelerator techniques now exist that may be capable of producing intense beams for boron neutron capture theory.

Several current clinical protocols are under way, or have recently been completed, concerning BNCT. These trials attempt to evaluate patients with advanced-stage melanoma of the extremities and are designed to determine the maximally tolerated dose of boron neutron capture theory to the skin and overlying connective tissue. Other studies are evaluating treatment with BNCT of glioblastoma multiforme or brain metastasis from malignant melanoma. Animal studies have been initiated on BNCT synovectomy for treatment of rheumatoid arthritis (221,545).

Effects of Irradiation on Cells

The radiation-induced lesion most detrimental to cell survival involves damage to the DNA. This may result in either mitotic cell death or apoptosis (Fig. 1.28). If the cell survives and repairs the damage, it may achieve a normal status. If there is misrepair, it may be associated with permanent mutations and induction of carcinogenesis. The physical interaction of ionizing radiation with the molecular infrastructure of the cell results in chemical reactions that occur within 10^{-18} to 10^{-3} seconds (541). Absorption of the photon energy destabilizes the target molecule, resulting in molecular breaks or release of energetic electrons and secondary energy-attenuated photons, which may interact with other cellular molecules, leading to a chain reaction that produces a variety of short-lived ions and chemically unstable free radicals (542,543). The most common radicals are produced from the radiolysis of cellular water and include hydroxyl radicals ($^{\bullet}$OH), hydrated electrons (e_{aq}), hydrogen atoms ($H^{\bullet}$), and hydrogen peroxide (H_2O_2). Free radicals are extremely unstable and interact nearly instantaneously with neighboring molecules to produce chemically stable lesions. This process can be modified by free radical scavengers or by oxygen, which have opposing effects on the number of stable lesions and on the level of cellular radiosensitivity (460). However, if all factors

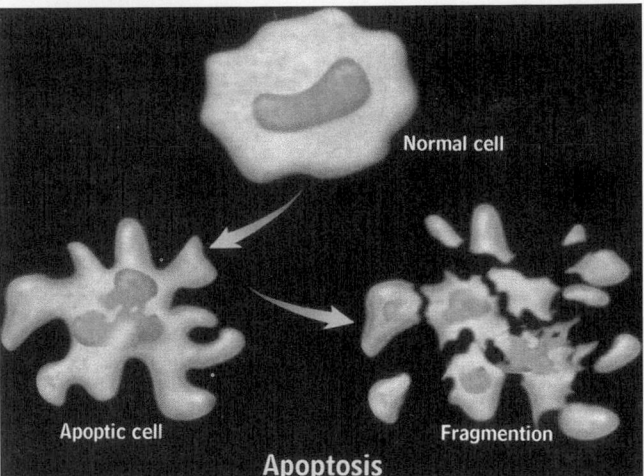

FIGURE 1.28. Programmed cell deaths or apoptosis results in DNA laddering and cell fragmentation. (From Dutton JJ, Haik BG. *Thyroid eye disease.* New York: Marcel Dekker Inc, 2002, with permission.)

remain constant, the permanent damage is linear with dose. Experiments in which the cell nucleus and the cytoplasm were selectively irradiated show that the dose required in the cytoplasm to kill a cell is larger than doses required in the nucleus (86,341). It is generally accepted that most target molecules for radiation-induced cell killing are located in the nucleus and involve damage to the DNA (114). However, other targets such as the cell membrane and the membrane of mitochondria have been proposed as the origin of apoptotic cascades that follow irradiation also contributing to cell death.

In many cells, radiation-induced lethality is not instantaneous because cells continue to function and even undergo several divisions before final mitotic death occurs (466). Noncycling lymphocytes, thymocytes, and hematopoietic cells were shown to undergo an interphase cell death without progressing through the mitotic phase of the cell cycle (6,610). Two patterns of morphologic changes are associated with cell death in mammalian cells (177). Cell necrosis, which is degenerative, is the most usual type of cell damage. Necrotic cell death results from collapse of cellular metabolism and depletion of its adenosine triphosphate storage (604). The final events of necrosis involve membrane rupture, loss of lysosomal enzymes, degradation of nuclear chromatin, and karyolysis (177). The other process of radiation-induced cell death is apoptosis. Programmed cell death, or apoptosis, is a physiologic process that involves a series of characteristic, genetically controlled steps. These include chromatin condensation and segmentation, fragmentation of the nucleus into apoptotic bodies, cell shrinkage, and loss of cellular contact with neighboring cells (18,258,262,614). Apoptosis culminates in the engulfment of the cell by neighboring cells, such as macrophages, without a concomitant inflammatory response (309). Apoptosis occurs spontaneously in various solid tumors (272,605) and contributes to the balance between tumor cell gain and cell loss.

Within minutes after irradiation, signal transduction pathways mediated by protein kinase C and tyrosine kinase are stimulated (76). Genes and enzymes involved in genetic control of radiation damage repair are activated, stress genes are induced, and growth factors and cytokines that modulate response of mammalian cells to ionizing radiation are activated (177). Radiation-induced stimulation is probably critical to induction of many genes and proteins, including early response genes, which, in turn, activate other genes, including those for tumor necrosis factor, fibroblast growth factor, and transforming

Table 1.10	APPLICATION OF RADIOBIOLOGIC CONCEPTS TO RADIATION THERAPY	
Process	**Potential Manipulation**	**Examples of Therapy**[a]
DNA damage	Increase damage in tumor cells	Hypoxic-cell sensitizers, thymidine analogs
DNA repair	Decrease repair in tumor cells	Fluoropyrimidines, hydroxyurea, cisplatin
Signal transduction	Inhibit protective signaling cascades in tumor cells	Protein kinase C inhibitors (?), phosphotyrosine kinase inhibitors (?)
Radiation-induced gene expression	Use gene therapy	Tumor necrosis factor linked to radiation-responsive promoter (?)
Growth-factor expression	Administer or increase expression of protective factors	Interleukin-1, granulocyte colony-stimulating factor, granulocyte-macrophage colony-stimulating factor, basic fibroblast growth factor (?)
	Block expression of factors producing long-term toxicity	Antibodies or antisense RNA against epidermal growth factor, transforming growth factor β (?)
Apoptosis	Force tumor cells to undergo apoptosis	Transfection of wild-type p53 (?)
Cell cycle	Synchronize tumor cells in sensitive phase of cycle (early S or M phase)	Antimetabolites (early S phase), paclitaxel phase (M), cyclin inhibitors (G_1 to S phase) (?)
	Prevent G_2 arrest in tumor cells	Cyclin inhibitors (G_2 to M phase) (?)

[a]A question mark indicates potential therapy.
From Lichter AS, Lawrence TS. Recent advances in radiation oncology. *N Engl J Med* 1995;332:371–379, with permission.

growth factor (86). In addition, new proteins, such as tissue plasminogen activator, are synthesized (161). This cascade of gene activation and transcription and protein synthesis is related to key cellular functions that the cell invokes in an attempt to survive a dose of radiation (161) (Table 1.10).

Modifiers of Radiation Response

Several approaches have been used to enhance the therapeutic ratio in radiation therapy:

1. *Physical modifiers of low-LET radiations.* IMRT, three-dimensional treatment planning, improvements in anatomic and functional imaging, the increasing power of computer hardware and software, and linear accelerator improvements have led to better photon and electron dose distributions; less side scatter; less differential absorption in bone and normal tissues; and, with charged particles, selective energy deposition at specific depths.
2. *High-LET radiations.* The importance of tumor hypoxia and cells residing in relatively resistant phases of the mitotic cycle are factors that are less likely to cause unsatisfactory results with neutrons, pi-mesons, and heavy ions than with standard radiation doses delivered with low-LET beams (166).
3. *Hyperbaric oxygen or tourniquet techniques.* These techniques involve use of increased oxygen tension to improve the effects of irradiation on the tumor (112) or use of a tourniquet to produce severe hypoxia in the surrounding normal tissues so that higher irradiation doses can be delivered (491). Theoretically, these approaches yield better tumor control without damaging normal tissues. Interest in the tourniquet technique waned years ago. Some investigators continue to evaluate hyperbaric oxygen. The logistics often are formidable, and clinical trials have not been conclusive (82,112,232,253,524).
4. *Hypoxic sensitizers.* Compounds with electron affinity, from the nitroimidazole group, theoretically produce free radicals in a manner similar to that of oxygen, selectively sensitizing hypoxic cells to radiation. Misonidazole (RO-07–0582) was evaluated in numerous clinical trials by the RTOG, with no evidence of clinical efficacy (544); however, in the Danish Head and Neck Cancer trial there was a highly significant survival benefit in the subgroup of patients with pharynx tu-

mors (367). New compounds, such as SR-2508, have been tested in phase I and II studies without clearly positive results.
5. *Perfluorocarbons.* These agents are administered in emulsion (they are insoluble in water) in sufficient concentrations coupled with inhalation of 95% to 100% oxygen to enhance oxygen transport and release in the presence of low oxygen tension (192,429). Their potential application in the treatment of patients with cancer is under evaluation (155,429).
6. *Cytotoxic agents.* Actinomycin-D, doxorubicin, 5-fluorouracil, cyclophosphamide, cisplatin, methotrexate, bleomycin, and others have been shown to interact with radiation in several forms to maximize tumor cell killing. In some instances, increased normal tissue reactions have been observed.
7. *Radioprotectors.* Sulfhydryl-containing compounds, such as cystine and cysteamine, have been used in animals to protect normal tissues against irradiation. Amifostine (WR-2721), a thiophosphate derivative of cysteamine, has been shown to selectively protect normal tissues, including bone marrow, salivary glands, and intestinal mucosa in animals, with little effect on tumor response to irradiation (522). This compound is being widely investigated in phase II and III clinical trials (53,498).
8. *Hyperthermia.* Heat at temperatures of more than 42.5 °C kills cells by itself or enhances the effects of irradiation and numerous cytotoxic agents. Heat selectively kills cells that are chronically hypoxic, acidotic, and nutritionally deficient—characteristics shared by tumor cells in comparison with the better oxygenated and better nourished normal cells. Furthermore, heat preferentially kills cells in the S phase of the proliferative cycle, which are known to be relatively resistant to irradiation (106,500).

A complete review of these topics will be found in Chapters 30, 32, and 33.

Genes and the Biology of Cancer

The infectious nature of some cancers was demonstrated by Francis Peyton Rous (1879–1970) in a 1910 experiment showing that defined, submicroscopic, filterable agents (viruses) isolated from a chicken sarcoma could induce new sarcomas in healthy chickens. Rous and his work languished in obscurity before being rediscovered and recognized with the Nobel Prize in Physiology or Medicine in 1966 (482). In his Nobel Lecture, "The Challenge to Man of the Neoplastic Cell," Rous considered the possible existence of growth-promoting genes—what he called oncogens and what are now called oncogenes.

> Tumors destroy man in a unique and appalling way, as flesh of his own flesh which has somehow been rendered proliferative, rampant, predatory and ungovernable. They are the most concrete and formidable of human maladies, yet despite more than 70 years of experimental study they remain the least understood. This is the more remarkable because they can be evoked at will for scrutiny by any one of a myriad chemical and physical means which are left behind as tumors grow. These had acted merely as initiation. Few situations are more exasperating to the inquirer than to watch a tiny nodule form on a rabbit's skin at a spot from which the chemical agent inducing it has long since been gone, and to follow the nodule as it grows, and only too often becomes a destructive epidermal cancer. What can be the why for these happenings?
>
> Every tumor is made up of cells that have been so singularly changed as to no longer obey the fundamental law whereby the cellular constituents of an organism exist in harmony and act together to maintain it. Instead the changed cells multiply at its expense and inflict damage that can be mortal. We term the lawless cells neoplastic because they form new tissue, and the growth itself is a neoplasm; but on looking into medical dictionaries, hoping for more information, we are told, in effect, that *neoplastic* means "of or pertaining to a neoplasm," and turning to *neoplasm* learn that it is "a growth which consists of neoplastic cells." Ignorance could scarcely be more stark.
>
> The chemical and physical initiators ordinarily are called *carcinogens;* but this is a misleading term because they not only induce the malignant epithelial growths known as carcinomas but also other neoplasms of widely various kinds. In this chapter the less often used term oncogenes will be used, meaning "thereby capable of producing a tumor." It hews precisely to the fact . . . .
>
> What can be the nature of the generality of neoplastic changes, the reason for their persistence; for their irreversibility; and for the discontinuous, steplike alterations that they frequently undergo? A favorite explanation has been that oncogenes cause alterations in the genes of the body—somatic mutations as these are termed. But numerous facts, when taken together, decisively exclude this supposition. (354)

Rous, it turned out, was unequivocally wrong about oncogenes. Theodor Boveri (46) was right. In 1914 he used his studies of normal mitosis in sea urchins and worms as a platform for suggesting that cancer might be caused by the abnormal gain or loss of chromosomes and their function (38). In a 1929 English translation of his 1926 book, *The Origin of Malignant Tumors*, Boveri wrote:

> The unlimited tendency to rapid proliferation in malignant tumor cells [could result] from a permanent predominance of the chromosomes that promote division. . . . Another possibility [to explain cancer] is the presence of definite chromosomes which inhibit division . . . . Cells of tumors with unlimited growth would arise if those "inhibiting chromosomes" were eliminated . . . [since] each kind of chromosome is represented twice in the normal cell, the depression of only one of these two might pass unnoticed. (46)

Boveri predicted that the genetic abnormalities leading to the development of cancer are of two sorts: growth-promoting genes and growth-suppressing genes. If the growth-promoting genes are excessive in number or activity, they lead to cell proliferation. If, however, the growth-suppressing genes are defective in amount or activity, they fail to halt cell proliferation and lead to unbridled cell replication (Fig. 1.29). These growth-promoting genes are called *oncogenes*. The growth-suppressing genes are called *tumor-suppressor genes*.

We may think of oncogenes and tumor-suppressor genes as analogous to the accelerator pedal and the brake pedal of an

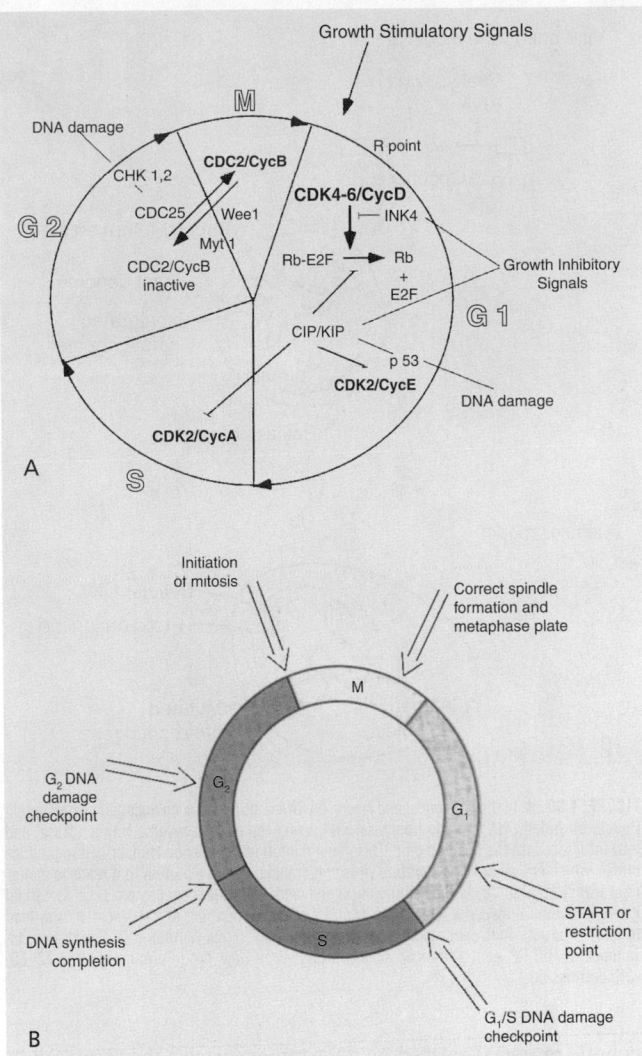

FIGURE 1.29. Schematic representation of cell cycle and checkpoints. **A:** Schematic representation of the eukaryotic cell cycle. The major regulatory kinases are indicated at their approximate points of action in the cell cycle. **B:** Schematic illustration of the two major checkpoints in the cell cycles: arrest after DNA damage at the G2/M border and arrest at metaphase of mitosis/meiosis. (From Murakami MS, Strobel LMC, Vande Woude GF. Cell cycle regulation, oncogenes, and antineoplastic drugs. In: Mendelsohn J, Howled PM, Israel MA, et al., eds. *The molecular basis of cancer.* Philadelphia: W.B. Saunders, 1995;3–17, with permission.)

automobile. The car can move forward when it is idling with the transmission in drive either by pushing on the accelerator pedal, by taking pressure off the brake pedal, or by doing both simultaneously. Similarly, cell growth and proliferation, leading to cancer, can occur either by the activity of the oncogenes or inactivity of the suppressor genes.

There are clearly a wide variety of physiologic conditions that call for the effective use of growth-promoting and growth-suppressing genes. There must be a mechanism to cause the fetus to grow and then, at the appropriate time, to restrain growth. There must be a way of causing fibroblasts to proliferate to heal a wound and then, at the appropriate time, halt the fibroblasts (except in the case of keloid formation). Uncontrolled cell growth, or cancer, may be thought of as a set of physiologic controls of cell growth gone awry.

Oncogenes

The experiments that initially identified oncogenes were based largely on transformed retroviruses in transplantable tumors in chickens, mice, and rats (273). Oncogenes were described as the

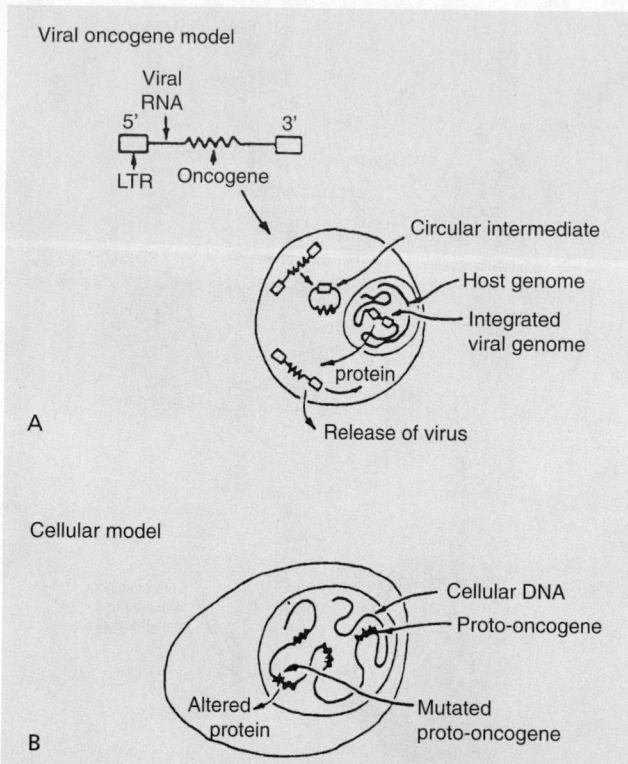

FIGURE 1.30. A: In the viral oncogene model, an RNA virus carrying an oncogene enters a cell. Double-stranded DNA is made from viral RNA, using the enzyme reverse transcriptase, and may integrate into the host genome. This genetic information may be transcribed to produce mRNA, which is packaged as a mature virus or is translated into a protein that leads to malignant transformation. **B:** In the cellular oncogene model, proto-oncogenes are seen as normal genes in mammalian cells. Alterations by mutation, amplification, or translocation may lead to gene products that cause malignant transformation. (From Minden MD. Oncogenes. In: Tannock IF, Hill RP, eds. *The basic science of oncology.* New York: Pergamon, 1987;72–88, with permission.)

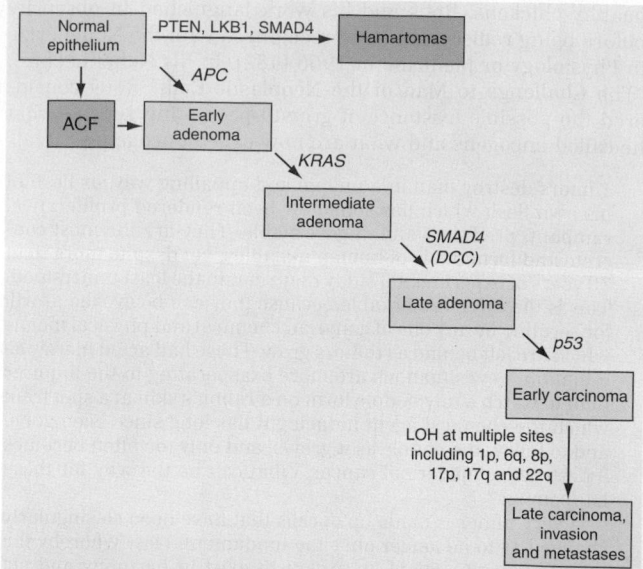

FIGURE 1.31. A variety of oncogenes and tumor-suppressor genes are responsible for cancer carcinogenesis. The archetype for the process of multistaged carcinogenesis is the conversion of normal epithelium of the colon to increasingly more severe degrees of adenomatous dysplasia until the development of frank adenocarcinoma. This diagram shows the associated oncogenes and tumor-suppressor genes, in the sequence, that are now known to be responsible for this transformation. (From MacDonald F, et al. *Molecular biology of cancer,* 2nd ed. London: BIOS Scientific Publishers, 2004, with permission.)

genetic material carried by RNA tumor viruses that resulted in rapid malignant transformation of target cells. The name oncogene was given to virus-encoded single genes that alone or in combination with other genes induced a transformed phenotype in affected cells (38) (Figs. 1.30 and 1.31).

The definition of an oncogene (from the Greek *onkos*, a mass or tumor) is still under debate. Duesberg (124) pointed out that the only "true" oncogenes are those found in retroviruses. However, not all cellular genes capable of transforming cells have been identified within the genome of known retroviruses. It is accepted that an oncogene is a gene capable of contributing directly to the conversion of a normal cell to a tumorigenic one and that a proto-oncogene is a cellular gene convertible to an oncogene by various molecular mechanisms: sequence mutations, gene amplification, chromosomal translocation, viral transduction, and insertional mutagenesis. In general, these perturbations result in two net effects: altered regulation or augmented expression of an oncogene through mutation or rearrangement of the nucleotide sequences that constitute signals for control of transcription, mRNA processing, and stability via insertion of a strong foreign promoter or by increased gene dosage; and altered biochemical function or ectopic expression of a protein product as a result of a mutation or translocation within the protein-coding region of the oncogene (187). Proto-oncogene products are involved in the regulation of normal cellular growth and differentiation (431).

A large number of viral oncogenes have been identified. In addition, oncogenes have been identified that are not associated with RNA tumor viruses but are recognized either by their activity in transformation or by their association with chromosome

translocations (326). When DNA-probing techniques were used, it was found that sequences homologous to the oncogene region of the virus were present in the DNA of all tissues of virus-free chickens. The normal cellular sequences are proto-oncogenes (37,483). The oncogene carried by a virus is referred to as *v-onc*, whereas the proto-oncogene is referred to as *c-onc*. In the normal cell the expression of proto-oncogene is well controlled and appears to play a role in the growth and development of the organism. The function of some of these genes has been determined, whereas for others a close association between cell proliferation and gene expression has been established (326) (Fig. 1.32).

Stimulation of a nonmalignant cell into a proliferative state often depends on an external signal, which is received by a receptor on the cell membrane and transferred through the membrane into the cytoplasm and ultimately to the nucleus where DNA synthesis is initiated. Proto-oncogenes have been found that function at each step of this pathway. The *erb*-B oncogene is homologous to the gene encoding for cell membrane receptor of epidermal growth factor (EGF). The interaction of EGF with this receptor reduces the proliferation of epidermal cells such as breast epithelium.

Strong evidence suggests that malignancy induction may be associated with genetic changes in the cell. Examples of this are the finding of specific chromosome abnormalities in malignant cells, association of tumor development with DNA-damaging agents such as ionizing irradiation and chemical carcinogens, and increasing incidence of cancer in hereditary diseases such as xeroderma pigmentosum (326). It is recognized that oncogenes are normal cellular genes that may contribute to the development of the malignant cell if their expression is altered through mutation, translocation, amplification, or some other mechanism. Evidence suggests that several genetic changes are needed to produce a cancer cell, and oncogene studies support this concept (326).

Chromosome translocations occur at a high frequency in some types of tumors, suggesting that they may play a role in their development. Examples of translocations are the t(9;22)

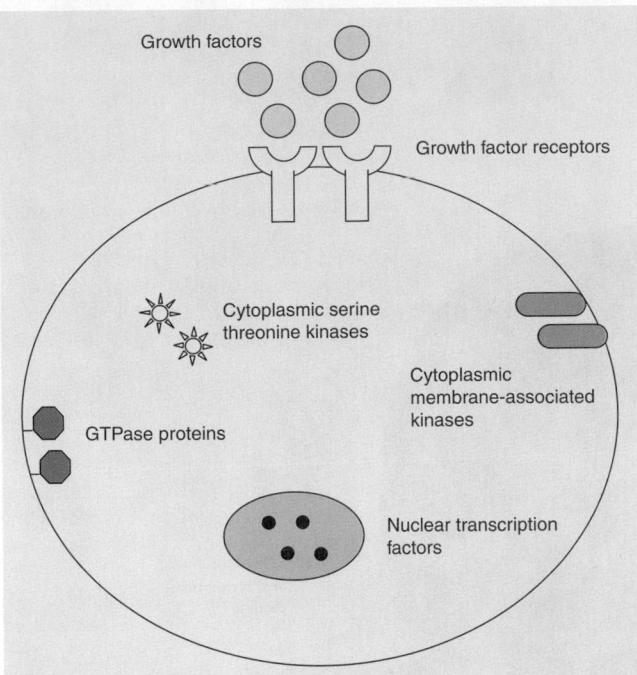

FIGURE 1.32. Cellular functions of proto-oncogene products are demonstrated in this schematic. (From MacDonald F, et al. *Molecular biology of cancer*, 2nd ed. London: BIOS Scientific Publishers, 2004, with permission.)

Philadelphia chromosome in chronic myelogenous leukemia (CML), the t(15;17) in promyelocytic leukemia, and several translocations involving chromosome 8 seen in lymphatic malignancies. Common sites of translocations in malignant cells are frequently near an oncogene (435). Those translocations such as the t(9;22) in CML can result in the formation of a new protein that is intimately involved in the tumorigenic transformation of the cell. In the CML example, the *ber*-gene is translocated next to the *abl*-oncogene, forming the new *bcr-abl* gene. The proteinaceous product of this newly formed gene is a hyperactive protein kinase that provides permanent growth signals to the cell (Figs. 1.33 and 1.34).

Role of Proto-Oncogenes in Normal and Transformed Cells

Proto-oncogenes are genes with apparent oncogenic potential, and because they are apparently present in all animals, it is speculated that some kind of activation of proto-oncogenes could be associated with the initiation and progression of neoplasia. Activated oncogenes are detected in a large percentage of human tumors, suggesting a prominent role of these genes in their development; association between activated oncogenes and neoplastic diseases must have some kind of specificity for both the oncogene and the tumor (187).

Oncogene protein products can be grouped into several classes depending on their location and reactivity: nuclear, cytoplasmic, and membrane protein kinases; cytoplasmic guanosine triphosphate-binding proteins; growth factors; and others. The protein products of the proto-oncogenes *src*, *abl*, and *ras* are cytoplasmic in location. The proto-oncogene products of *myc*, *fos*, *ski*, and *myb* are nuclear in location and are believed

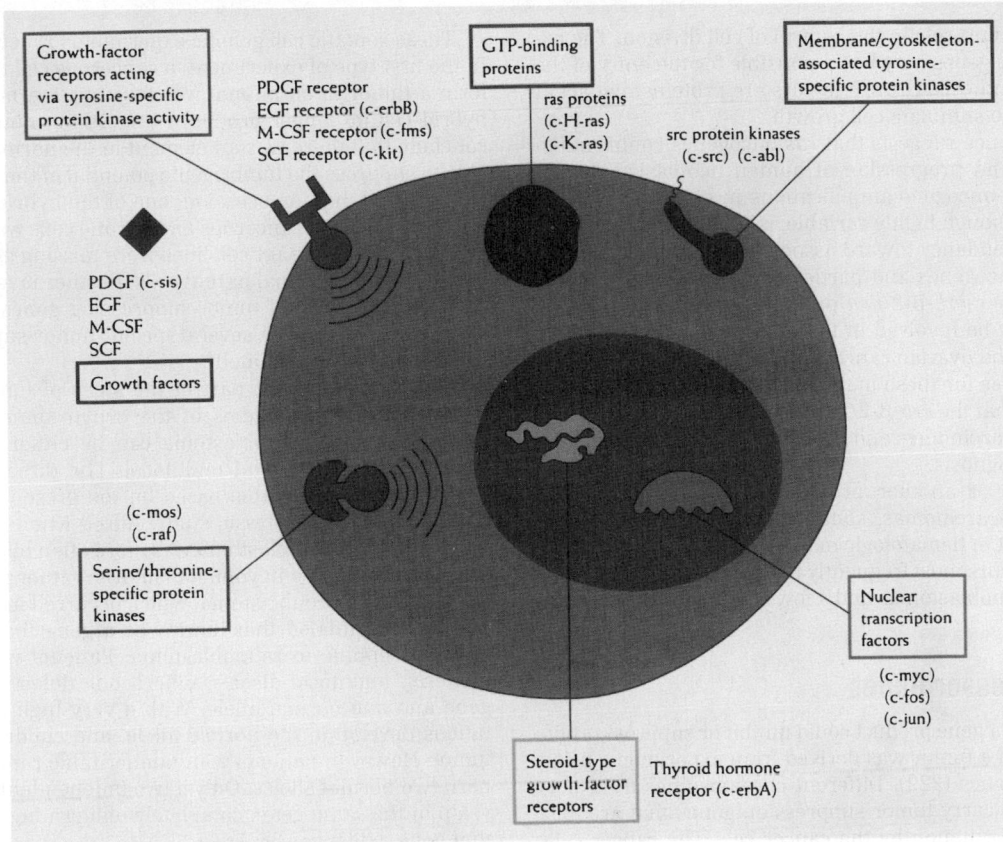

FIGURE 1.33. Proto-oncogenes generate protein products that act within and outside the cell. EGF,; GTP,; M-CFS,; PDGF,; SCF, (From Varmus H, Weinberg RA. *Genes and the biology of cancer*. New York: Scientific American Library, 1993, with permission.)

Overview and Basic Science of Radiation Oncology

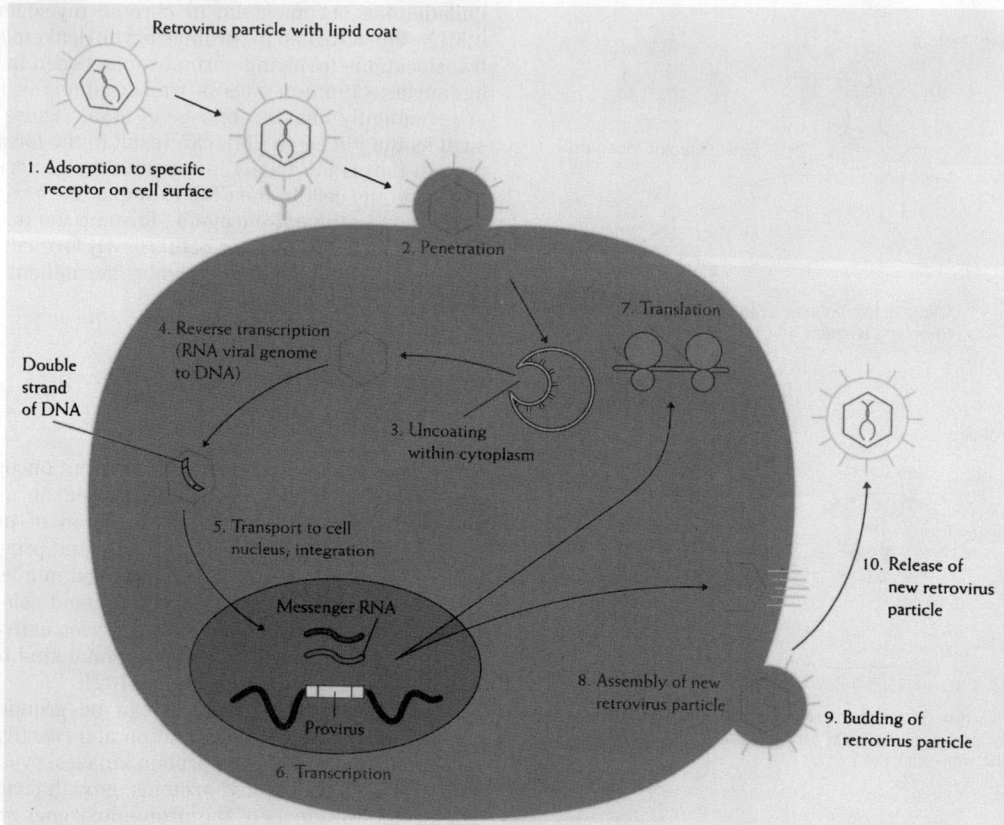

FIGURE 1.34. The retrovirus life cycle occurs within the cell. (From Varmus H, Weinberg RA. *Genes and the biology of cancer.* New York: Scientific American Library, 1993, with permission.)

to play an important role in the control of cell division. The expression of these genes may be responsible for the entry of the cell into DNA synthesis. Growth factors are proteins that act at the cell surface to stimulate cell growth.

Current evidence suggests that *ras* oncogenes contribute to both initiation and progression of human neoplasia. The incidence of proto-oncogene amplifications in biopsy specimens from tumors, although highly variable, is usually low. However, there may be a tendency toward association of amplification of specific proto-oncogenes and particular types of tumors. Amplifications of the c-*erb*-B-2/*neu* proto-oncogene (also referred to as *her*-2) may be involved in the etiology of human breast, salivary gland, and ovarian cancers and might serve as a useful prognostic marker for these malignancies (466). Slamon et al. (467) observed that the *erb*-B-2/*neu* locus is amplified in 30% of primary breast carcinomas and that amplification is associated with a worse prognosis.

Amplification of another proto-oncogene, C-*myc*, occurs mainly in adenocarcinomas, squamous cell carcinomas, and sarcomas but not in hematologic malignancies, whereas N-*myc* amplification occurs most frequently in neuroblastomas and occasionally in retinoblastomas and a few small-cell lung carcinomas (171).

Tumor-Suppressor Genes

The concept that a gene product could inhibit or suppress proliferation of cells in a tumor was derived from experiments using somatic cell genetics (222). Different chromosomes from normal human cells carry tumor suppression genes that are able to block tumor formation by the cancer cell. The cancer cells must sustain mutation in both alleles of these genes to develop the ability to produce tumors (282).

These somatic cell genetic experiments relied on cell fusion. In the first type of experiment, a cancerous cell that was able to form a tumor in an animal was fused with a normal cell. The hybrid cell no longer produced tumors in animals. One could conclude that there was an element in the normal cell that was able to suppress the tumorigenic potential of the cancerous cell. It was found that, on occasion, one of the hybrid cell lines produced by fusion of cancerous and normal cells was tumorigenic. Why? These malignant cell lines were missing genetic material supplied by the normal parent cells. Further investigation identified the presence of tumor-suppressing genes from the normal parent. Eventually, several specific tumor-suppressor genes were identified and named.

The next important part of the story of tumor-suppressor genes comes from studies of the ocular tumor of infancy—retinoblastoma. Retinoblastoma can be either unilateral and unifocal or bilateral and multifocal. The disease also can be heritable or nonheritable based on the presence of a positive family history. In a classic study, Alfred Knudson (264) noted that heritable retinoblastoma was more often bilateral and multifocal and occurred in younger children rather than nonheritable unilateral retinoblastoma, which occurred in older children. Knudson postulated that there was a gene that renders children susceptible to retinoblastoma. Patients with early onset bilateral, multifocal disease inherit one defective copy of this gene and one normal allele. With a very high frequency, mutations develop in the normal allele, and children develop the tumor. However, patients with nonheritable retinoblastoma inherit two normal alleles. Only if two independent mutations develop in the same gene, completely obliterating the function of that gene, will a cancer arise.

Knudson concluded that it requires two genetic injuries in two alleles to produce retinoblastoma. This is called the

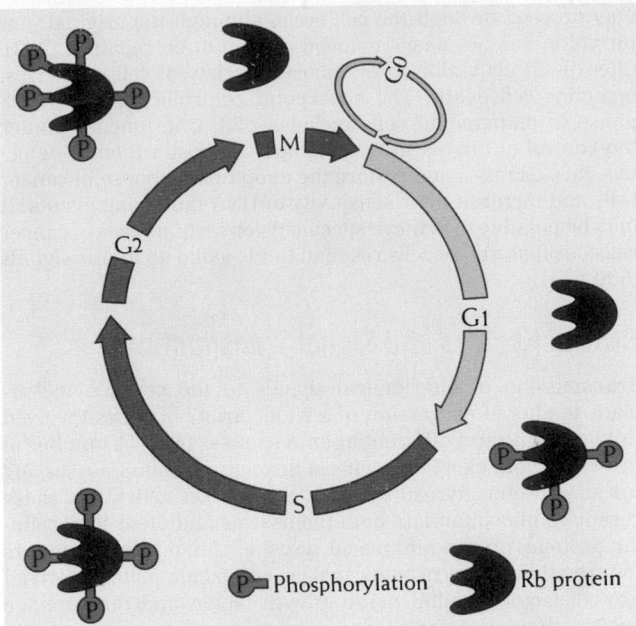

FIGURE 1.35. The retinoblastoma gene product (pRb) is increasingly phosphorylated as the cell moves toward G2. All the phosphate groups are stripped of M. pRb loses its ability to stop cell growth when it becomes phosphorylated. (From Varmus H, Weinberg RA. *Genes and the biology of cancer.* New York: Scientific American Library, 1993, with permission.)

"Knudson two hit" hypothesis. The hypothesis predicts that if only one of the two gene copies remains active, there is sufficient growth-suppression activity to keep the cell normal. Only if both copies are inactivated is there sufficient loss of genetic activity to allow unbridled cell proliferation. The retinoblastoma gene, *Rb*, was isolated on the long arm of chromosome 13. Because the short arm of chromosomes is abbreviated as p and the long arm as q, the deletion of the *Rb* gene is abbreviated as 13q- (Fig. 1.35).

A number of distinctions separate the oncogenes from the tumor-suppressor genes (Table 1.11). It is almost certain that, in most human cancers, there is a multistep pathway to tumor development, which involves the accumulation of mutations in a series of oncogenes and suppressor genes (282).

Many tumor-suppressor genes have been cloned (APC, BRCA, DCC, MLM, NF1, NF2, Rb, p53, VHL, and WT1). The suppressor p53 gene resides in 20 kb of DNA located in chromosome 17p13.1 (24). The gene is a nuclear phosphoprotein composed of 393 amino acid residues in humans (282). p53 mutations have been detected in a wide variety of malignant human tumors. The p53 gene encompasses 16 to 20 kilobase (kb) of DNA on the short arm of human chromosome 17. Loss of normal p53 function is associated with cell transformation *in vitro* and development of neoplasms *in vivo*. Abrogation of the normal p53 pathway is a common feature in human cancers, and it appears to be critical in the pathogenesis and progression of these tumors (73). In some cases, candidate tumor-suppressor genes have been identified based on an association between loss or inactivation and tumor development, the causal connection being only inferred.

Cell-Cycle Control

The cell cycle, which consists of four phases (G1, S, G2, and M), regulates the duplication of genetic information and distribution of duplicated chromosomes to daughter cells. The Nobel Prize in Physiology or Medicine for 2001 was awarded to Leland H. Hartwell, R. Timothy Hunt, and Sir Paul M. Nurse for their discoveries regarding the control of the cell cycle. The Nobel presentation speech by Professor Anders Zetterberg succinctly describes the important controls of cell replication elucidated by these three scientists.

Cell division is a fundamental process of life. All living organism on earth are descended from an ancestral cell that appeared about 3 billion years ago, and which has undergone an unbroken series of cell divisions since then. Each human being also began life as one single cell—a cell that divided repeatedly to give rise to all one hundred thousand billion cells that we consist of .... Every second millions of cells divide in our body.

The cycle of events that a cell completes from one division to the next is called the cell cycle. During the cell cycle the cell grows in size, duplicates its hereditary material—that is, it copies the DNA molecules in the chromosomes—and divides into two daughter cells.

This year's Nobel Laureates have discovered the key regulators of the cell cycle—cyclin dependent kinase (CDK) and cyclin. Together these two components form an enzyme, in which CDK is comparable to a "molecular engine" that drives the cell through the cell cycle by altering the structure and function of other proteins in the cell. Cyclin is the main switch that turns the "CDK engine" on and off. This cell-cycle engine operates in the same way in such widely disparate organisms as yeast cells, plants, animals, and humans.

How were the key regulators CDK and cyclin discovered? Lee Hartwell realized the great potential of genetic methods for cell-cycle studies. He chose baker's yeast as a model organism. In the microscope he could identify genetically altered cells—mutated cells—that stopped in the cell cycle when they were cultured at an elevated temperature. Using this method Hartwell discovered, in the early 1970s, dozens of genes specific to the cell-division cycle, which he named CDC genes. One of these genes, CDC28, controls the initiation of each cell cycle, the "start"

:: Table 1.11	**PROPERTIES OF PROTO-ONCOGENES AND TUMOR-SUPPRESSOR GENES**	

Property	Proto-Oncogenes	Tumor-Suppressor Genes
Number of mutational events required to contribute to the cancer	One	Two
Function of the mutant allele	Gain of function, acts in a dominant fashion	Loss of function, acts in a recessive fashion
Mutant allele may be inherited through the germ line	No examples at this time	Frequently has an inherited form
Somatic mutation contributes to cancer	Yes	Yes
Tissue specificity of mutational event	Some, but can act in many tissues	Inherited form commonly has a tissue preference

From Levine AJ. Tumor suppressor genes. In: Mendelsohn J, Howley PM, Israel MA, et al., eds. *The molecular basis of cancer.* Philadelphia: W.B. Saunders, 1995;89, with permission.

function. Hartwell also formulated the concept of "checkpoints," which ensure that cell-cycle events occur in the correct order. Checkpoints are comparable to the program in a washing machine that checks if one step has been properly completed before the next can start. Checkpoint defects are considered to be one of the reasons behind the transformation of normal cells into cancer cells.

Paul Nurse also used the genetic approach in his cell-cycle studies but in a different kind of yeast. In the late 1970s and early 1980s he discovered the gene CDC2, which could be mutated in two different ways. Either the cells did not divide, or they divided too early. From this he correctly concluded that CDC2 controls cell division. He later discovered that CDC2 not only controls cell division, the final event of the cell cycle; it also has a key regulatory function for the whole cell cycle, including that described for CDC28 in baker's yeast. This key function was shown to be that of CDK in the cell-cycle engine. By moving human genes into yeast cells, in 1987 Nurse isolated a human CDC2 gene. This human CDC2 gene functioned perfectly in yeast cells. Thus, the CDK function in the cell-cycle engine had been conserved through more than 1 billion years of evolution—from yeast to man.

Tim Hunt discovered the other key component of the cell-cycle engine, the protein cyclin, which regulates the function of the CDK molecule. Working with sea urchin eggs as a model organism, in 1982 he discovered a specific protein that increased in amount before cell division but disappeared abruptly when the cells divided. Because of these cyclic variations, he named the protein cyclin. These experiments not only led to the discovery of cyclin, but also demonstrated the existence of periodic protein degradation in the cell cycle—a fundamental control mechanism. Hunt also showed the existence of cyclins in other, unrelated species. Thus cyclins, like CDK, had been conserved during evolution.

It is now almost 50 years since the structure of the DNA molecule—the double helix—was discovered, leading to a molecular explanation of how a gene can make a copy of itself. With the discoveries of CDK and cyclin we are now beginning to understand, at the molecular level, how the cell can make a copy of itself. (354)

To ensure that the daughter cells possess a full complement of genetic information, checkpoints exist to ensure fidelity of DNA duplication and accuracy of chromosome segregation (341). Checkpoint pauses permit editing and repair of genetic information so that each daughter cell receives a full complement of genetic information identical to the parent cell (see Fig. 1.29). In some cells, there are checkpoints for initiation of mitosis. Mutation of the checkpoint genes allows the cell to enter mitosis after x-irradiation (342). For example, the rad-9 gene is a G2/M checkpoint gene because it responds to two different types of signals (344). Experimental observations suggest that the p53 gene, shown to be a transcriptional activator (409), may be critical for G1 checkpoint control. p53 has been shown to induce transcription of p21, which in turn inhibits the association of CDK 4,6 with PCNA and cyclin D. As a consequence, the retinoblastoma protein cannot be phosphorylated and stays in complex with the transcription factor E2 F, effectively blocking the transcription of cell–cycle-promoting proteins and causing a cell-cycle arrest.

Checkpoints are signal-transduction systems that must receive a signal, amplify it, and transmit it to other components that regulate the cell cycle. Double-strand DNA breaks, unexcised ultraviolet light-induced dimers in DNA, and centromeres not engaged by the spindle are potential signals (29,223,257). Checkpoints ensure the fidelity of genomic replication and segregation. Biologically significant levels of spontaneous damage require checkpoint control for cells to maintain a high fidelity of chromosome transmission. Therefore, restoration of compromised checkpoints could slow cancer cell evolution even in the absence of exogenous sources of DNA damage (223). Many signal-transduction systems, including checkpoint controls, exhibit adaptation; that is, in the presence of a constant stimulus, the response diminishes with time. As a consequence, the cell

may proceed through the cell cycle, although the original perturbation has not been removed or cannot be repaired (223). Checkpoint activation may induce a variety of cell responses, including cell death. The checkpoint controlling entry into S phase in mammalian cells includes p53. One function under the control of this pathway is apoptosis. Restoration of defective checkpoints could restore the apoptotic response of cancer cells and increase their sensitivity to DNA-damaging agents. It may be possible to achieve specificity for certain types of cancer cells because not all cells respond to the same apoptotic signals (600,614).

Growth Factors and Signal Transduction

Transmission of biochemical signals to the cellular nucleus leads to altered expression of a wide variety of genes involved in microgenic and differentiation responses (472). A number of growth factors exert their effects through receptors possessing intrinsic protein tyrosine kinase activity. On activation, these receptors phosphorylate both themselves and other intracellular proteins on the aminoacid tyrosine. Among the receptors for growth factors are epidermal growth factor, platelet derived growth factor, insulin, nerve growth factor, and macrophage colony stimulatory factor. The mitogenic signaling pathway activated by protein-tyrosine-kinase receptors involves the activation of ras proteins. Ras undergoes conformational change and interacts with additional down stream targets. A protein kinase cascade is activated, which conveys the growth factor–initiated signal to the nucleus via the raf, mek, map kinase, and other proteins (346) (Fig. 1.36).

Telomeres

Human chromosomes are linear. At each end of the chromosome are structures known as telomeres from the Greek *telo* for end and *mere* for structure. Telomeres are composed of specialized DNA and DNA-binding proteins. As chromosomes are replicated, telomeres shorten each time during the process of cell division. Continued cycles of cell division result in shortened telomeres. The telomeres, for example, in the fibroblasts of older adults are shorter than those in children. Normal human cells senesce when the telomeres shorten to a critical length.

Stem cells and cancer cells must maintain their telomere lengths to prevent senescence. Two mechanisms of telomere maintenance have been identified: expression of the telomerase enzyme, and the recombination of telomeres.

The telomere hypothesis states that critical telomere shortening prevents somatic cells from dividing. In contrast, the maintenance of telomere length allows cancer cells to continue to divide. An increasing body of experimental evidence supports the telomere hypothesis and its association with cancer (476).

The capacity of cells to respond to ionizing radiation is determined by multiple factors. There are a variety of syndromes associated with molecular defects that are characterized by

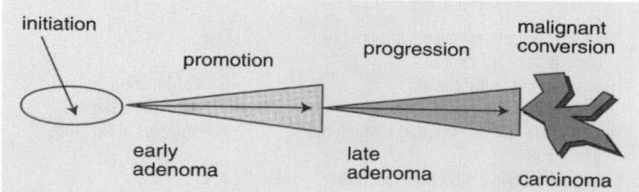

FIGURE 1.36. Carcinogenesis is a multistage process that begins with the genetic event of initiation. Initiation is followed by the selective proliferation of altered cells during the process of tumor promotion. The example here is schematic of the conversion of normal colonic epithelium to early and late adenomas and then frank carcinoma. (From Perantoni AO. Carcinogenesis. In: McKinnell RG, et al. *The biological basis of cancer.* New York: Cambridge University Press, 1998; with permission.)

clinical radiosensitivity. These include ataxia, telangiectasia, Nijmegen breakage syndrome, and ataxia telangiectasia-like disorder. These syndromes all have defective telomere maintenance in common. It has been hypothesized, therefore, that the radiosensitivity phenotype and the telomere dysfunction phenotype may be linked. A variety of experimental models suggest that telomere maintenance and radiosensitivity are associated, and this may offer the opportunity for a therapeutic target (431).

Apoptosis

Apoptosis or programmed cell death, a phenomenon distinct from necrosis, was described in 1972 by Kerr et al. (263). Apoptosis is programmed by specific signals in the cell that cause an endonuclease to cleave DNA at internucleosomal sites.

Apoptosis is detected by histologic evaluation of membrane blebbing and chromatin condensation, by flow cytometry using fluorescent nucleotides and terminal transferase to detect fragmented DNA, by detecting apoptotic cells that are usually very small with characteristic profiles of right angle and forward light scattering, or by using DNA fluorochrome to detect a decrease in fluorescence as small DNA fragments diffuse from the cell that is undergoing apoptosis (80,616). An early change in apoptosis, the flip-flop of the phospholipid phosphatidylserine (PS) from the inner to the outer leaflet of the bilayer membrane, also can be detected using a fluorescently labeled annexin V protein that has a high binding affinity to PS. Several oncogenes, cytokines, and growth factors have been reported to play a role in promoting or reducing radiation-induced apoptosis (110).

Most radiation-induced cell lethality (loss of reproductive integrity) for dividing cells appears to be caused by mitotic-linked death resulting in loss of genetic information as cells with chromosomal aberrations divide. Apoptosis, frequently seen within 4 to 6 hours after irradiation, occurs spontaneously and is enhanced by radiation as observed *in vivo* in the intestinal crypt and salivary and lacrimal glands with nondividing cells and nondividing lymphocytes. Apoptotic cells are eliminated rapidly *in vivo*, making it difficult to quantify. In contrast, this cell death mechanism is easy to quantify *in vitro* because apoptotic cells persist in culture for many hours. However, cell division of nonapoptotic cells complicates quantification (110). In cell lines susceptible to apoptosis, this process sometimes occurs early before cells enter mitosis or later after the cells divide. Late apoptosis may be associated with mitotically linked death and, in fact, may be triggered by chromosomal aberrations. Apoptosis may be quite important for clinically relevant doses of fractionated irradiation, even if it causes a relatively small reduction in clonogenic survival. However, this requires that cells be recruited into the apoptotic-susceptible fraction after each dose fraction.

It appears that with progression of certain tumors, spontaneous and therapy-related apoptosis occurs less frequently. The apoptotic response to irradiation can be modified by cytokines to protect normal tissues (176) or to induce tumor cell killing (210,230). Tumor necrosis factor increases apoptosis after irradiation in some tumors while protecting the hematopoietic compartment, possibly by blocking apoptosis (349). Irradiation prevents extensive cellular proliferation by increasing differentiation in both tumors and normal tissues. Also, irradiation appears to increase the aging of normal cells. Another mechanism of reversible loss of proliferative capacity induced by irradiation is necrosis, which occurs with high doses of irradiation and is a major mechanism seen with large dose fractions such as in stereotactic irradiation (Figs. 1.37 and 1.38).

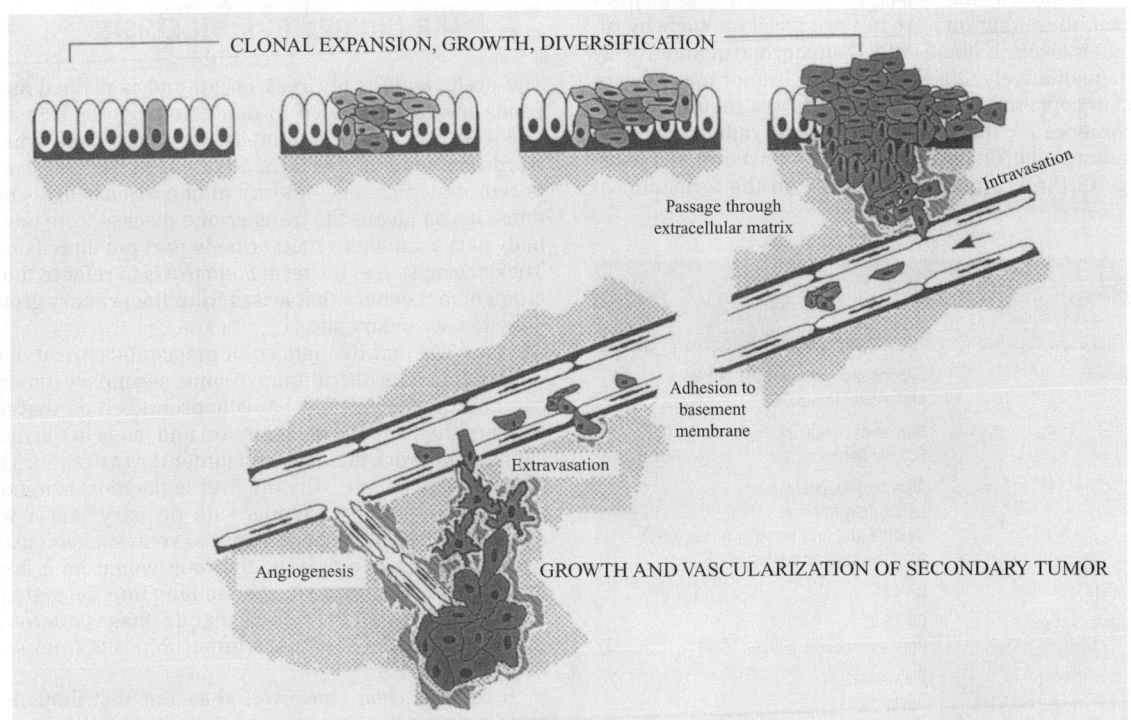

FIGURE 1.37. A transformed cell will give rise to progeny that compose the primary tumor. Tumors are heterogeneous. Some tumor cells are able to give rise to metastatic colonies. These subclones of metastatic-prone cells bind and disrupt the basement membrane upon which they rest and then invade the extracellular matrix. Eventually, they make their way to the basement membrane of a blood vessel and engage in intravasation. This ability to migrate requires cell motility and cell detachment. The cells must have the ability to penetrate the vascular lymphatic system, circulate, survive the assault of the immune system during transit in the blood system, and eventually adhere at a distant site. (From Cotran RS, et al. *Pathologic basis of cancer*, 5th ed. Philadelphia: W.B. Saunders, with permission.)

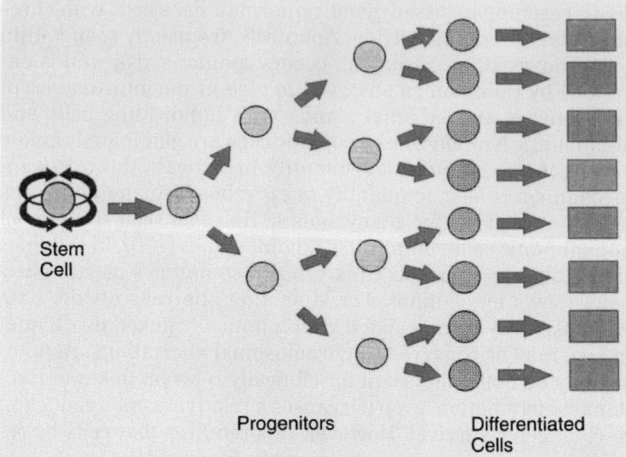

FIGURE 1.38. The renewal of human tissue is the result of a balance between the production of new differentiated cells and the loss of older cells. These older cells are lost either through sloughing or apoptosis. New, specialized cells, which are represented as squares, are produced via the differentiation of immature precursor cells, which are represented by the dense stipple pattern. These, in turn, were produced via the proliferation and maturation of progenitor cells shown as the stippled circles. Stem cells, while usually quiescent, enter the cell cycle periodically to produce progenitor cells and reproduce the stem cell population as needed. When a cancer develops, the system is perturbed and cell production and differentiation become disconnected and cell production and cell loss are no longer in balance. (From Parchment RE. Biotherapy. In McKinnell RG, et al. *The biological basis of cancer.* New York: Cambridge University Press, 1998; with permission.)

Tumor Markers

Tumor markers may be detected in body fluids, are produced by or associated with a variety of tumors, and may be used to aid in tumor diagnosis and prognosis, to assess tumor cell burden, and to detect early recurrent tumors after therapy. They also may be helpful in the selection and scheduling of therapy. However, these markers are not produced uniquely by tumors, and their levels in blood differ from normal quantitatively rather than qualitatively (304) (Table 1.12). Tumor markers are present in low concentrations in the plasma and require sophisticated techniques for their detection such as radioimmunoassay, immunoradiometric assay, or enzyme-linked immunosorbent assay. All three procedures depend on the formation of antigen-antibody complexes, in which a purified preparation of a particular marker is used initially to prepare the specific antibodies (usually monoclonal); these antibodies are attached to a solid support such as Sephadex beads (Sigma-Aldrich Inc, St. Louis, MO).

Sensitivity of a marker refers to the proportion of patients with a particular tumor who have elevated plasma levels of the marker. Specificity is indicated by the proportion of patients who do not have this particular pathologic process who exhibit normal plasma levels of the marker. Ideally a marker will have a high sensitivity and specificity.

Oncofetal proteins are present during a variable period of normal embryonic or fetal life, do not disappear entirely in the adult, and may reappear with certain malignancies. Classic examples are carcinoembryonic antigen (CEA) and α-fetoprotein (AFP).

Elevated CEA blood levels have been identified in some nonmalignant diseases, such as cirrhosis and chronic obstructive pulmonary disease, and modest elevations may occur in smokers. Increased levels of the protein, seen in a variety of epithelial tumors, such as colorectal, breast, lung, and pancreatic cancer, have led to the suggestion that "de-repression" may be a characteristic of malignant growth or, alternatively, that stem cells or other primitive progenitor cells populate the tumor (303). The half-life of CEA in plasma is about 6 to 8 days.

AFP is an α_1-globulin product of the fetal liver, gastrointestinal tract, and yolk sac and is normally present in fetal circulation. Marked increases in plasma AFP levels are noted in 80% of patients with hepatocellular carcinoma and about 60% of patients with nonseminomatous testis tumors. AFP also may be elevated in the presence of nonmalignant liver disease, especially cirrhosis. AFP has a half-life in plasma of about 5.5 days.

Tumor-associated antigens have been described in a variety of tumors as a result of the widespread availability of techniques for production of monoclonal antibodies, including prostate-specific antigen (PSA), ovarian antigen CA125, and others.

The Biology of Metastasis

The prefix *meta* is of Greek origin and is defined as after, beyond, or over. It is used to denote change or transformation. The word *stasis* means stand or stationary. Thus, when the two words are combined to form *metastasis*, the new word is used to represent a change in location of a disease or its manifestations. It also means the transfer of a disease from one organ or body part to another organ or body part not directly connected. The oncologist uses the term *metastasis* to refer to the manifestation of malignancy that arises from the primary growth but is now in a secondary site.

It is clear that the pattern of metastatic spread of cancer is not random. The distribution of some secondary tumor deposits can be explained on mechanistic grounds (i.e., that the tumor cells are shed into the bloodstream and lodge in the first narrow capillary network that they encounter downstream). This would explain, for example, why the liver is the most common site for secondary tumors in patients with primary cancer within the catchment area of the hepatic portal vein, such as gastrointestinal malignancies. Similarly, the lung would be a favored site in patients with primary tumor spilling into the systemic veins. There can be no doubt that vascular drainage patterns influence the distribution of secondary tumor deposits from some types of primary cancer.

It is also clear, however, that the distribution of some metastatic tumors cannot be explained solely by patterns of encountering and lodging in the nearest narrow capillary bed. The seminal paper addressing this problem was by Stephen Paget (1855–1926). Paget was the fourth and youngest son of the famous British physician Sir James Paget. Stephen Paget worked

Table 1.12	CLASSIFICATION OF TUMOR MARKERS SHOWING SELECTED EXAMPLES
Oncofetal proteins	Carcinoembryonic antigen (CEA)
	Alpha-fetoprotein (AFP)
Hormones	Human chorionic gonadotropin (hCG)
	Ectopic hormones
Enzymes	Alkaline phosphatase
	Lactic dehydrogenase
	Gamma glutamyl transpeptidase (GGT)
	Neurone-specific enolase (NSE)
Immunoglobulins	CA-125
Tumor-associated antigens	CA 15.3
	Prostate-specific antigen (PSA)
Miscellaneous markers	Polyamines
	Nucleosides
	Tissue polypeptide antigen (TPA)
	Acute phase proteins

From Malkin A. Tumor markers. In: Tannock IF, Hill RP, eds. *The basic science of oncology,* 2nd ed. New York: McGraw-Hill, 1992;196–206, with permission.

as an assistant surgeon at the West London and Metropolitan Hospitals in England. Later in life, he devoted himself to public health issues and became a highly regarded biographer and essayist (370). Writing in the *Lancet* on March 23, 1889, on "The distribution of secondary growth in cancer of the breast," Paget wondered:

> The question ought to be asked, and if possible answered: "What is it that decides what organs shall suffer in a case of disseminated cancer?" If the remote organs in such a case are all alike passive and, so to speak, helpless—all equally ready to receive and nourish any particle of the primary growth which may "slip through the lungs," and so be brought to them—then the distribution of cancer throughout the body must be a matter of chance. But if we can trace any sort of rule or sequence in the distribution of cancer, any relation between the character of the primary growth and the situation of the secondary growths derived from it, then the remote organs cannot be altogether passive or indifferent as regards embolism.... Every single cancer cell must be regarded as an organism, alive and capable of development. When a plant goes to seed, its seeds are carried in all directions; but they can only live and grow if they fall on congenial soil. (371)

Paget observed, in a large number of autopsies of women with breast cancer, that the lymph nodes, liver, lung, bone, and brain commonly were involved. However, he found that the kidney and spleen rarely were involved despite receiving a significant amount of cardiac output. He was struck by the discrepancy between the relative blood supplies and the relative frequencies of metastatic tumors in various organs. From his data, Paget expounded his "seed and soil hypothesis." He argued that metastasis required both a willing seed (intrinsic cellular factors) and hospitable soil (host organ). There must be intrinsic cellular factors that lead to a satisfactory interaction between the tumor cell and the host organ resulting in successful metastasis. In contemporary terms, we understand this to mean that the tumor cell must have favorable adhesion molecules, and the host organ must be accepting receptors on its endothelial cells, which results in appropriate sites for the circulating tumor cells to bind, migrate into the organ, and subsequently grow.

Metastasis formation is an inefficient process. Fidler and Zeidman injected melanoma cells into the peripheral vein of a mouse whose DNA had been labeled with radioactive iodine. They found that, shortly after the injection, most of the injected cells rested in the lung (i.e., the nearest narrow capillary bed). Most of the tumor cells, however, went on to die in the lung. Only a few live cells continued to circulate. Within a day, only 1% of the injected cells were alive, and after 2 weeks, no known metastasis could be seen in the lungs. Only 0.1% of the cells originally injected were still alive (351). Bloodborne metastasis must be a highly selective process. Only a very small proportion of malignant cells that enter into the bloodstream are able to survive and grow.

There are three major pathways of metastasis. They are:

- Across body cavities such as the peritoneal cavity or within the cerebrospinal fluid. This is the way, for example, that medulloblastoma disseminates via the leptomeninges or that ovarian tumors form on the peritoneal surface of the intestine.
- Via the lymphatic system. Axillary masses following breast cancer, that are easily palpable, would be a common example.
- Hematogenously, usually via veins rather than arteries. The spread of a limb sarcoma to the lungs would be an example (Fig. 1.39)

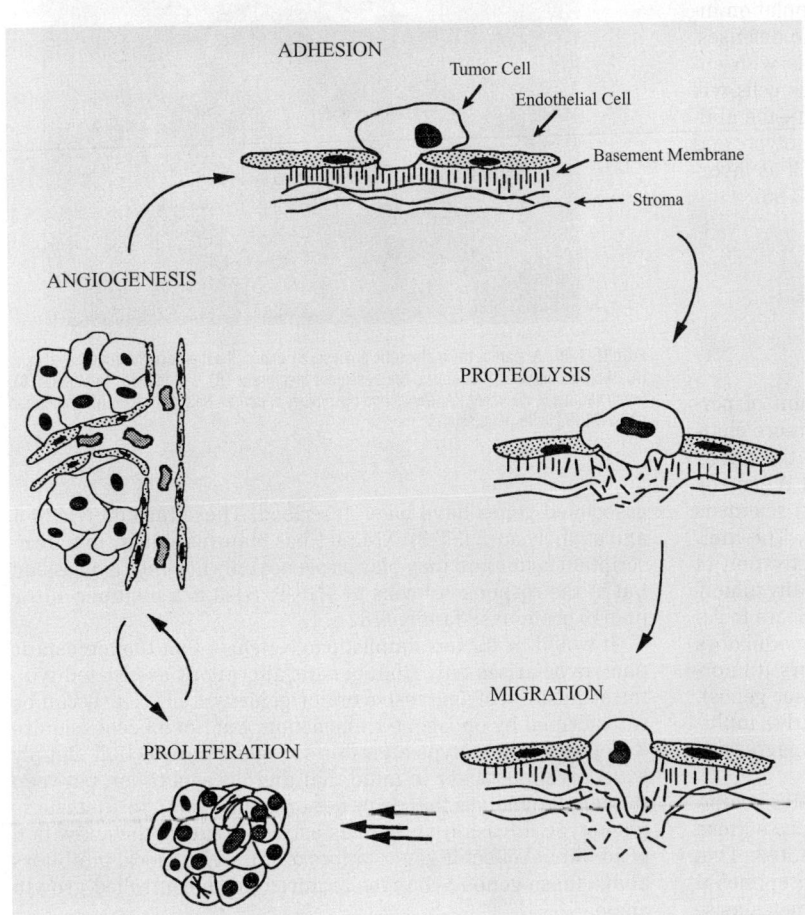

FIGURE 1.39. The metastatic cascade, which involves primary tumor growth, angiogenesis, and the three components of invasion: adhesion, proteolysis, and migration. (From Alessandro R, Bicher A, Kohn E. Tumor invasion and metastases. In: Hoskins WJ, Perez CA, Young RC, eds. *Principles and practice of gynecologic oncology*, 2nd ed. Philadelphia: Lippincott-Raven, 1997; with permission.)

The molecular mechanism of tumor metastasis is a multistep process involving many tumor cells—host cell interactions as well as cell-matrix associations (483). The crucial processes are as follows:

- Tumor cell adhesion to other tumor cells at the site of the primary malignancy, host cells, or components of the extracellular matrix;
- Proteolysis of the extracellular matrix during invasion;
- Tumor cell motility through the extracellular matrix to reach the vascular or lymphatic endothelium;
- Embolism into the lymphatic system and/or the blood circulation;
- Tumor cell survival despite both the mechanical trauma endured by the cell in-transit in the vascular system as well as the body's immunologic assault directed against the circulating tumor cell;
- Adherence to the endothelium when the tumor cell comes to rest at the metastatic site in the secondary organ;
- Dissolution of the cell–cell junction and the basement membrane of the blood vessel into the organ parenchyma;
- Satisfactory response of microenvironment in the host organ to permit growth of the tumor deposit; and
- Tumor cell proliferation in the new organ and angiogenesis (Fig. 1.40).

Only if all of these steps can be negotiated successfully can the tumor cell ultimately "setup shop" as a metastatic focus. The fact that only a small fraction of tumor cells survive and successfully establish a metastasis would suggest that the ultimately successful cells must be quite unusual. It would be reasonable to believe that they represent a subpopulation of tumor cells that are endowed with particular characteristics that make for successful metastasis. As the population of tumor cells evolves, it is likely that aggressive subpopulations, having diverse properties, will arise and that their frequency in the population increases under selective pressure of the host immune defenses. This will lead, ultimately, to the emergence of cells with enhanced malignancy (483). The successful metastatic cells will possess characteristics of neoplastic transformation—the ability to turn on an angiogenic switch, an invasive phenotype, and the capacity to evade the immune response—as well as favorable cell adhesion and motility characteristics (158–160).

The Molecular Biology of the Metastatic Phenotype and Angiogenesis

Foulds defined tumor progression as the acquisition of permanent, irreversible, qualitative changes in one or more characteristics of neoplasm that ultimately will lead to the tumor becoming more autonomous and malignant (482). A genetic analysis of the stages of tumor progression has led scientists to formulate the multistep theory of tumorigenesis. The multistep theory involves activation of oncogenes, inactivation of tumor suppression genes, and the identification of many tumor-associated molecules. The metastatic phenotype appears to require cells to have the additive effect of positive modulators (oncogenes) as well as the loss of negative effectors (tumor-suppressor genes, invasion and metastasis suppressor genes). Thus, the molecular biology of a metastatic cell is clearly a multistep process of diversification and clonal selection for aggressive cells.

The mutated *ras* oncogene sequences, when transfected into mouse embryo-derived fibroblasts (NIH 3T3 cells), cause those transfected cells to produce numerous metastases (509). This finding has been confirmed in both fibroblasts and epithelial cells of human and rodent origin. A number of other metastasis-

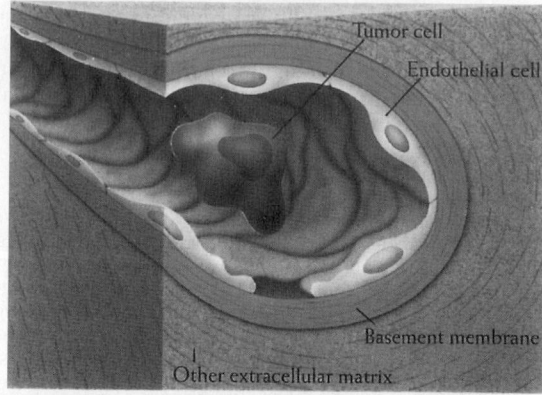

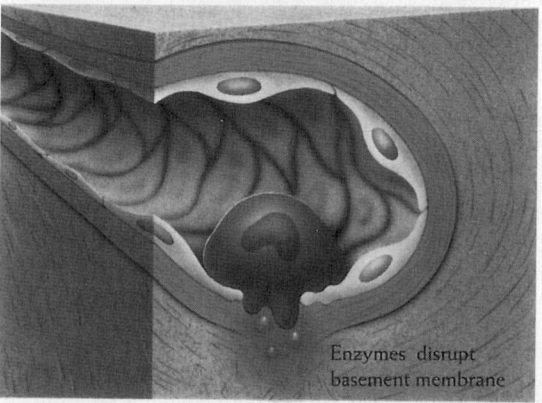

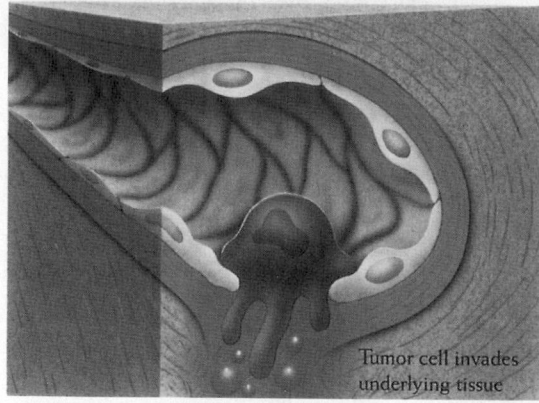

FIGURE 1.40. As part of the metastatic process, a tumor cell adheres to the endothelial cells **(A)**, secretes enzymes that cleave the basement membrane **(B)**, and invades the tissue **(C)**. (From Varmus H, Weinberg RA. *Genes and the biology of cancer.* New York: Scientific American Library, 1993, with permission.)

associated genes have been described. These include NM23-1 and stomelysm-3 (ST-3). NM23-1 has features similar to a transcription factor and may play a role not only in *c-myc* expression but in the response of cells to TGF-B. ST-3 is a member of the matrix proteinase family (482).

It would be far too simplistic to conclude that the metastatic phenotype arises only from genetic alterations associated with the acquisition of aggressive tumorigenicity. Cells clearly can be transformed by oncogene transfection, but not all cells acquire a metastatic phenotype after this oncogene transfection. Simply stated, we must bear in mind that there is separation between the genetic changes that drive tumorigenicity and the metastatic phenotype. Invasion and metastasis will require the activation of additional effector genes or loss of suppressor local inhibitors above those genetic changes required for uncontrolled growth alone.

The successful development of a metastatic focus requires new blood vessel growth. Recent evidence has identified angiogenesis promoters and inhibitors that may be modified or removed during the tumor-induced angiogenic response. Tumor angiogenesis in the nascent metastasis is a tightly regulated process in a delicate balance between the pro- and antiangiogenic factors (283).

Angiogenesis

The success of growth of a tumor is, in part, governed by a complex interplay between the tumor cells and the surrounding normal tissue. A dramatic example of this interplay is the process of tumor angiogenesis (also called tumor neovascularization).

The growth of the tumor depends on the tumor's access to nutrients and oxygen as well as its ability to eliminate metabolic waste and carbon dioxide. In very small tumors, these requirements are addressed by diffusion. As the tumor enlarges, however, diffusion is inadequate. The growing tumor requires direct access to the circulatory system.

Tumor access to the circulatory system is secured through angiogenesis, through which the tumor cells encourage the ingrowth of capillaries and larger vessels from the adjacent normal tissue. The tumor cells recruit these vessels through the release of angiogenic factors. These cause the proliferation of endothelial growth factor and, almost certainly, tissue growth factor–β. The generation of tumor vessels is the result of a delicate balance between angiogenesis-promoting factors and angiogenesis-inhibiting factors. These factors have now provided a growing body of therapeutic targets in the treatment of cancer.

Some authorities encourage us to think about the tumor as a structure composed of varied compartments including the actual clonogenic cells, a connective structure, and the blood vessels. Utilizing this way of thinking about tumors, we envision cancer treatment as striking at different components of the tumor (i.e., antiangiogenesis agents directed against the vasculature and anticlonogenic agents directed against proliferating cells). Experimental evidence suggests that, in certain tumor systems, combination of radiation and antiangiogenic agents are a fruitful way of treating cancer. We may expect to see an increasing body of evidence for the use of combinations of radiation, chemotherapy, hormonal therapy, and antiangiogenesis agents in the coming years.

The hallmark of an invasive cancer is its ability to disrupt the epithelial basement membrane and the presence of cancer cells in the stromal compartment. It makes sense, therefore, that two broad classes of molecules have been implicated repeatedly in contributing to the metastatic ability: cell–cell adhesion molecules and motility molecules play a crucial role in the development of metastatic potential (48). The ability of tumor cells to adhere to other tumor cells, cells of the host, or components of the extracellular matrix affect multiple components of the metastatic cascade. These interactions depend on several classes of molecules expressed on the cell surface. Cadherins are calcium-dependent molecules that mediate homophilic cell–cell adherence. Integrins are heterodimeric transmemory proteins that are formed by the noncovalent association of α- and β-subunits. The binding of the extracellular matrix ligands to integrins is known to initiate similar transduction pathways (181). These pathways lead to cell proliferation, differentiation, migration, or cell death.

Selectins act through a terminal calcium-dependent lexon domain. They are prominently involved in heterotypic cell–cell adhesion between blood cells and endothelial cells (58).

Tumor adherence to the extracellular matrix and cell motility is the next crucial component of the metastatic cascade. Tumor cells are able to attach to a specific lipoprotein of the extracellular matrix such as fibronectin, collagen, and laminin. These adherences are formed either through integrin or non-integrin cell-surface receptors. CD44 is a crucial transmembrane glycoprotein with a large echo domain and a single cytoplasm domain. CD44 is involved in cell adhesion to hyaluronan (471).

Antiangiogenesis Therapy of Cancer

Tumor vessels are fundamentally different from normal blood vessels insofar as they are usually irregular and disorganized. In vessels that are leaky, hemorrhagic, torturous, and those containing poorly oxygenated blood that may flow backward and forward in the same vessel, tumor vasculature may provide an interesting therapeutic target. The general public and the scientific community have recently experienced a wave of considerable excitement associated with the possibility that antiangiogenesis agents may be employed clinically to disrupt tumor angiogenesis. This form of therapy may complement existing cancer treatments. Some of the drugs in the therapeutic pipeline include:

- *Angiostatin* appears to be able to inhibit endothelial cell migration, tubule formation, and endothelial cell proliferation in response to growth factors. Angiostatin may also induce apoptosis in endothelial cells (216).
- *Bevacizumab* is a recombinant humanized monoclonal IgG1 antibody that binds to and inhibits the biologic activity of human vascular endothelial growth factor (VEGF) in *in vitro* and *in vivo* assay systems. Bevacizumab binds VEGF and prevents the interaction of VEGF with its receptors (Flt-1 and KDR) on the surface of endothelial cells. The interaction of VEGF with its receptors leads to endothelial cell proliferation and new blood vessel formation in *in vitro* models of angiogenesis. Administration of bevacizumab to xenotransplant models of colon cancer in nude (athymic) mice caused reduction of microvascular growth and inhibition of metastatic disease progression. This drug appears effective in metastatic colorectal cancer.
- *Endostatin* is a potent natural inhibitor of angiogenesis. It is a C-terminal fragment of collagen XVIII, which is mainly localized in the basement membrane zones of the vessels, particularly in newly formed, tumor-associated blood vessel. Elevated serum levels of Endostatin (Sigma-Aldrich Inc, St. Louis, MO) have been found in metastatic cancer patients.
- *Thrombospondin-1* is a potent inhibitor of angiogenesis and inhibits a wide variety of angiogenic stimuli, including VEGF, proteins that act via tyrosine kinase receptors, G proteins, serine/threonine kinase receptors, and lipids.
- *Tumstatin* is a M(r) 28,000 C-terminal NC1 fragment of type alpha3 (IV) collagen that inhibits angiogenesis and suppresses proliferation of endothelial cells and growth of tumors.

For further reading, see Jain RK. Normalization of tumor vasculature: an emerging concept in antiangiogenic therapy. *Science* 2005;307:58–62; Denekamp J. Angiogenesis, neovascular proliferation and vascular pathophysiology as targets for cancer therapy. *Br J Radiol* 1993;66: 181–196; and Hurwitz H et al. Bevacizumab plus irinotecan, fluorouracil, and leucovorin for metastatic colorectal cancer. *N Engl J Med* 2004;350:2334–2342.

Overview and Basic Science of Radiation Oncology

The potentially metastatic cell must overcome a series of tissue barriers. These include the basement membrane and connective tissue. These must be traversed by the tumor cells during the metastatic process. Five classes of naturally occurring proteinases have been associated with aggressive tumor cells and implicated in metastases. These include members of the gene family of matrix metalloproteinases. These enzymes, each of which is secreted by a proenzyme that subsequently requires activation, may be divided into three general subclasses: interstitial collagenase, type-4 collagenase (gelatinases), and stromelysins. Once having dissolved barriers, active tumor cell motility is required for the penetration of the basement membrane and the interstitial stoma. Successful migration of metastatic cells requires transition of propulsive force from the extracellular matrix to the cytoskeleton. Tumor cells exhibit amoeboid movement, which is characterized by pseudopod extension. For the protrusion and retraction of pseudopods, the network of intracellular polymerized cross-linked filaments must be disassembled and then reassembled (483).

Management of the Patient with Cancer

The optimal care of cancer patients is a multidisciplinary effort that may combine two or more disciplines: surgery, radiation therapy, and chemotherapy. Many professionals, including physicians, physicists, laboratory scientists, nurses, rehabilitation staff, sociologists, and social workers, are intimately involved. Pathologists, radiologists, clinical laboratory physicians, and immunologists are integral members of the team that renders the correct diagnosis. Biology, biochemistry, and pharmacology have contributed greatly to the advancement of methods used to evaluate and treat cancer patients (e.g., biomarkers, cell kinetics indicators, oncogenes).

The radiation oncologist, like any other physician, must assess all conditions relative to the patient and the tumor under consideration for treatment and systematically review the need for diagnostic and staging procedures as well as the best therapeutic strategy. This has been well illustrated in a series of "decision trees" designed by the Patterns of Care Study Group for radiation therapy (241). In several instances, a clear relationship existed between compliance with guidelines for diagnostic or therapeutic procedures (best current management consensus) and therapy outcome, as defined by survival, recurrence patterns, or complications of treatment.

Emphasis on screening and early diagnosis of cancer, as well as improvements in therapeutic strategies, have had a significant positive impact on the survival of patients with cancer. In the United States, results of the Surveillance Epidemiology and End Results program (169) have shown a small but steady improvement in survival for a variety of tumor sites. Relative survival of patients with cancer at various times after diagnosis has improved substantially since 1960.

Combination of Therapeutic Modalities

Irradiation and Surgery

The rationale for preoperative radiation therapy relates to its potential ability to eradicate subclinical or microscopic disease beyond the margins of the surgical resection, to diminish tumor implantation by decreasing the number of viable cells within the operative field, to sterilize lymph node metastases outside the operative field, to decrease the potential for dissemination of clonogenic tumor cells that might produce distant metastases, and to increase the possibility of resectability. The disadvantages of preoperative irradiation are that it may interfere with normal healing of the tissues affected by the radiation, it delays

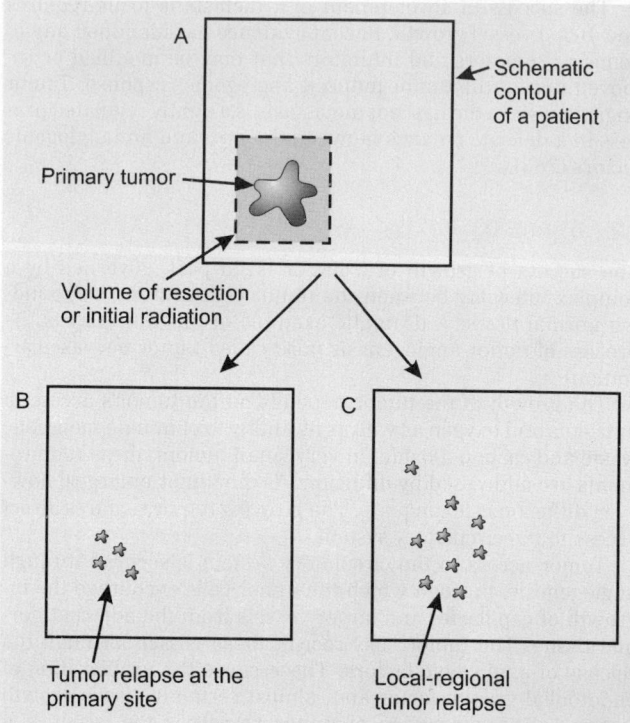

FIGURE 1.41. A: A pattern of failure analysis is useful to improve treatment of malignancies. **B:** If the tumor after surgery and/or radiotherapy tends to relapse at the primary site within the volume treated, it would suggest that the local therapy is insufficiently intense. **C:** If, however, there is a local-regional tumor relapse, it would suggest that the initial surgery or radiotherapy field size is insufficient to cover microscopic extension of disease that has the potential to be controlled. A pattern of failure as shown in panel (C) is not, by itself, sufficient to make the case for extended field radiation. One must have a pattern of failure such as that which is seen in panel (C) and also be able to show that intervention with large field irradiation can alter that pattern in a favorable manner.

surgery, and it may disrupt surgical staging of the tumor and/or the expression of histologic or immunohistochemical prognostic factors.

The rationale for postoperative irradiation is based on the fact that it is possible to eliminate subclinical foci of tumor cells in the tumor bed (including lymph node metastases). By delivering higher doses to the volume of high-risk or known residual disease than can be achieved with preoperative irradiation, a greater tumor control may be obtained. For example, Vikram and Farr (531) and Fletcher (153) reported improved survival rates in patients with head and neck tumors treated with combined therapy in comparison with surgery alone.

The potential disadvantages of postoperative irradiation are related to the delay in initiation of radiation therapy until wound healing is completed. Theoretic and experimental evidence suggests that the radiation effect may be impaired by vascular changes produced in the tumor bed by surgery. Experimental data suggest that preoperative irradiation may be more effective than postoperative irradiation (392) (Fig. 1.41).

Irradiation and Chemotherapy

Tumor or *normal tissue enhancement* describes any increase in effect greater than that observed with either chemotherapy or irradiation alone (400). Agents used in chemoirradiation include those with cytotoxic activity against the tumor, which may show additive, subadditive, or supra-additive effects, such as 5-fluorouracil or mitomycin-C in anal carcinoma; agents with minimal or no significant activity against a specific tumor, which may, however, enhance the irradiation effect; radiation hypoxic cell cytotoxins or bioreductive agents; and radioprotectors (Fig. 1.42).

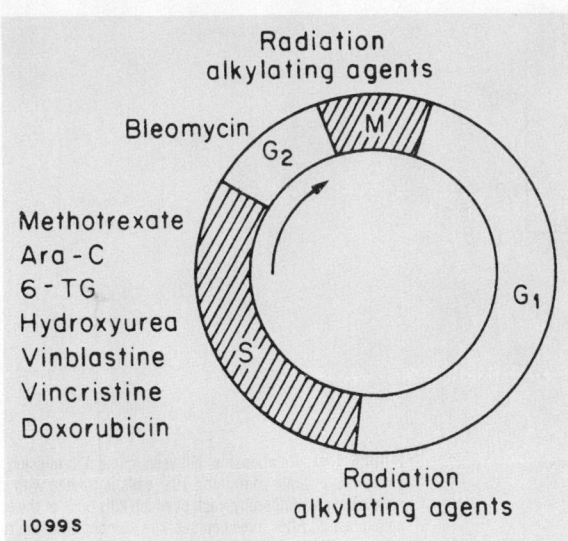

FIGURE 1.42. The position in the cell cycle at which anticancer drugs and radiation most often exert their maximum lethal toxicity. Drugs and radiation also may act to delay progression around the cycle (e.g., vinblastine and vincristine induce mitotic arrest). (From Tannock IF. Principles of cell proliferation: cell kinetics. In: DeVita VT Jr, Hellman S, Rosenberg SA, eds. *Cancer: principles and practice of oncology,* 3rd ed. Philadelphia: J.B. Lippincott, 1989;3–13, with permission.)

Chemotherapy alone or combined with irradiation may be used in several settings (494). *Primary chemotherapy* is used as part of the primary lesion treatment (even if later followed by other local therapy) and when the primary tumor response to the initial treatment is the key identifier of systemic effects (340). *Adjuvant chemotherapy* is used as an adjunct to other local modalities as part of the initial curative treatment. Frei (170) proposed the term *neoadjuvant chemotherapy* when this modality is used in the initial treatment of patients with localized tumors, before surgery or irradiation.

The effects of combined radiation therapy–chemotherapy can be independent, additive, or interactive. Chemotherapy and irradiation can be administered sequentially or concomitantly. Sequencing of treatment at the appropriate time is significantly related to the residual tumor cell burden at the point of introduction of each new treatment program (612).

Administration of chemotherapy before irradiation may produce cell killing and reduce the number of cells to be eliminated by the irradiation. Use of chemotherapy concurrently with radiation therapy has a strong rationale because it could interact with the local treatment (additive and even supra-additive action) and also could affect subclinical disease early in treatment. However, the combination of modalities may enhance normal tissue toxicity. When agents with added toxicity are used, lower tumor control may result because the added morbidity requires lowering the doses of the effective agents or prolonging overall irradiation treatment time. When fatal toxicity from chemotherapy occurs, it prevents some dying patients from demonstrating tumor response that could have been observed had they survived. Overall patient survival may be compromised as well.

Biologic Considerations in Combinations of Chemotherapy and Irradiation

Many experimental animal studies have shown therapeutic benefit from a combination of irradiation and drugs, but most are phenomenologic. Therapeutic benefit requires differential properties on tumor and normal tissues, which may be exploited for therapeutic gain. These include genetic instability of tumors compared with normal tissues, differences in cell proliferation (particularly cell repopulation during fractionated ra-

diation therapy), and environmental factors such as hypoxia and acidity (which usually are confined to tumors). There are variations in sensitivity or resistance to irradiation or drugs. The mechanisms for resistance to these agents may be shared in some tumors and different in other tumors. Resistance to anticancer drugs may have implications for resistance to radiation therapy; many drug mechanisms for resistance are multifactorial, such as in cisplatin, in which this phenomenon may be the result of decreased drug uptake, increased repair of DNA, increased expression of sulfhydryl compounds such as glutathione and metallothionein, and increased expression of glutathione-S-transferase. Combined treatment with radiation and drugs might result in an improved therapeutic index if mechanisms of resistance are independent (496).

Oxygen, pH, and nutrient supply can play an important role in the combined effects of chemotherapy and irradiation on tumor cells (126). Hypoxic cells are less radiosensitive and chemosensitive to many drugs, and chronic hypoxia can alter cell-cycle age distribution and proliferation rate—both important modifiers of cellular response to ionizing radiation and drugs. In addition, chronic hypoxia can affect cellular ability to repair radiation- and drug-induced DNA damage. Bioreductive drugs such as mitomycin-C are activated to toxic species and affect solid animal tumors under hypoxic conditions (416). DNA repair, cell-cycle age distribution, and the activity and stability of some chemotherapeutic drugs may be pH dependent; thus, this factor plays a role in the sensitivity of cells to irradiation and cytotoxic agents.

It is possible that hypoxic conditions, which commonly exist in tumors, may lead to amplification of genes. Activation and increased expression of certain oncogenes, such as *ras*, c-*myc*, and c-*raf*-1, have been associated with increased radioresistance in some malignant and normal human cell lines *in vitro* (77,465). Although this has been demonstrated in several mouse tumor cell lines, it was not observed in three human cell lines studied by Tannock (493). Investigation of the role and mechanisms of action of cytotoxic agents, as well as further studies on factors that modulate the activation and expression of genes encoding these substances, may enhance our understanding of the molecular basis of genetic regulation of cellular sensitivity or resistance to irradiation and chemotherapy (175).

Some cytokines such as tumor necrosis factor-α or interleukin (610) and growth factors such as platelet-derived and fibroblast growth factors are seen in malignant and normal human cells after irradiation (608). These cytokines and growth factors enhance the cytotoxic effects of irradiation and chemotherapy in tumor cells (271) or offer radioprotection in normal cells (350).

Possible molecular or cellular mechanisms of interaction of chemotherapy and irradiation include:

1. Modification of the slope of the dose–response curves, such as has been shown with actinomycin D, cisplatin, doxorubicin, mitomycin-C, 5-fluorouracil, and other agents.
2. Decreased accumulation or inhibition of repair of sublethal damage, as induced by actinomycin D, cisplatin, bleomycin, hydroxyurea, and nitrosoureas (69,261,463). Doxorubicin and other DNA intercalators decrease the shoulder widths but do not decrease the slope or suppress the repair of lethal damage in *in vitro* studies (118).
3. Inhibition of repair of potentially lethal damage, as has been shown with actinomycin D, doxorubicin, and cisplatin (121,538).
4. Perturbation of cell kinetics, for example, after treatment with hydroxyurea, which kills cells in the S phase, when cells may become partially synchronized and blocked at the G1/S phase of the cell cycle. If irradiation is delivered during this sensitive phase, as the cells subsequently emerge from the block, an enhanced cytotoxic effect may be expected.

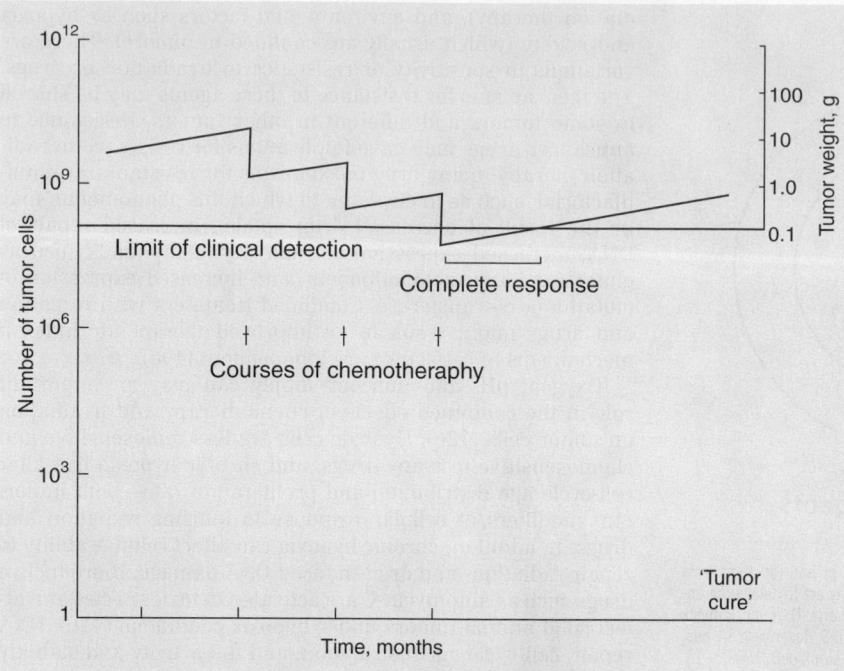

FIGURE 1.43. Relationship between clinical remission and cure. A 10-g tumor containing 10^{10} cells is treated with three courses of chemotherapy, each of which kills 90% of the tumor cells present. After three courses, the number of viable tumor cells is $<10^8$ (<0.1 g) and the patient is judged to be in clinical and radiologic complete remission. Note that this is a small step toward tumor cure. Moreover, additional chemotherapy may not be helpful if drug-resistant cells have been selected after three courses of chemotherapy. (From Tannock IF. Combined modality treatment with radiotherapy and chemotherapy. *Radiother Oncol* 1989;16:83–101, with permission.)

5. Selective cytotoxicity and radiosensitization of hypoxic cells, which have been reported with mitomycin-C and cisplatin (267,294,416).
6. Inhibition of cell repopulation.
7. Decrease in tumor bulk leading to improved blood supply, reoxygenation, and cell-cycle recruitment, resulting in increased radiosensitivity and chemosensitivity.

A possible danger in the administration of cytotoxic drugs before radiation therapy is accelerated cell proliferation or repopulation. Because some tumor regression is induced by the cytotoxic agent (drugs or irradiation), the distance between the tumor cells, and adjacent functional capillaries decreases, this may induce tumor cell proliferation so that higher doses of irradiation would be required to produce a given tumor control. In fact, neoadjuvant chemotherapy has been reported to induce significant regression of malignant tumors in the head and neck, without improvement in survival (480). This may occur because, during radiation therapy, tumor cells surviving neoadjuvant chemotherapy may be stimulated to repopulate at a faster rate. Because of this effect, the initial advantage in cell killing by drugs is lost, and the survival curves for fractionated radiation therapy may come together or even cross over. As pointed out by Tannock (496), although this mechanism is hypothetical, it suggests caution in the use of induction chemotherapy and explains why an initial tumor response may not necessarily translate to a therapeutic advantage with combined-modality treatment given in this fashion. In the example in Fig. 1.43, three courses of induction chemotherapy reduced tumor cell numbers from 10^{10} to 10^8 (from 10 g to about 0.1 g), which is considered a complete clinical tumor regression. Even a pathologic complete response has limited long-term implications; a complete pathologic regression is consistent with the presence of about 106 tumor cells per gram, a substantial biologic cell burden.

Integrated Multimodality Cancer Management and Organ Preservation

Combinations of two or all three of the classic modalities frequently are used to improve tumor control and patient survival.

Steel and Peckham (477,479) postulated the biologic basis of cancer therapy as spatial cooperation, in which an agent is active against tumor cells spatially missed by another agent, addition of antitumor effects by two or more agents, and nonoverlapping toxicity and protection of normal tissues (388). Large primary tumors or metastatic lymph nodes must be removed surgically or treated with definitive radiation therapy. Regional microextensions are eliminated effectively by irradiation without the anatomic and at times physiologic deficit produced by equivalent medical surgery. Chemotherapy is applied mainly to control disseminated subclinical disease, although it also has an effect on some larger tumors.

Organ preservation is being vigorously promoted because it enhances the quality of life and psychoemotional feelings of patients with excellent tumor control and survival, as has been demonstrated in many tumors (107,142,196,263,324,383, 385,496). In some types and stages of head and neck tumors, breast cancer, gastrointestinal malignancies, genitourinary tumors, soft-tissue sarcomas, and pediatric tumors, studies have shown that less radical surgical procedures combined with chemotherapy and radiation therapy yield the same local tumor control at the primary site and survival as did radical procedures. Advances in reconstructive surgery have greatly improved our ability to repair defects of radical surgery.

Cancer Prevention

Cancer is a largely preventable disease. Epidemiologic studies have identified the causative agents for a significant proportion of adult cancers (Figs 1.44–1.46) (Tables 1.13 and 1.14). Approximately 30% to 35% of cases of cancer in the United States are associated with tobacco use. Another 30% to 35% of cases are associated with excessive dietary fat and obesity. Approximately 5% of cancer is related to alcohol use. Another 5% is associated with exposure to viral agents (115). Among the other causative factors of cancer, each responsible for a small percentage of malignancies, are occupational exposures, a family history of cancer, environmental pollution, ionizing and

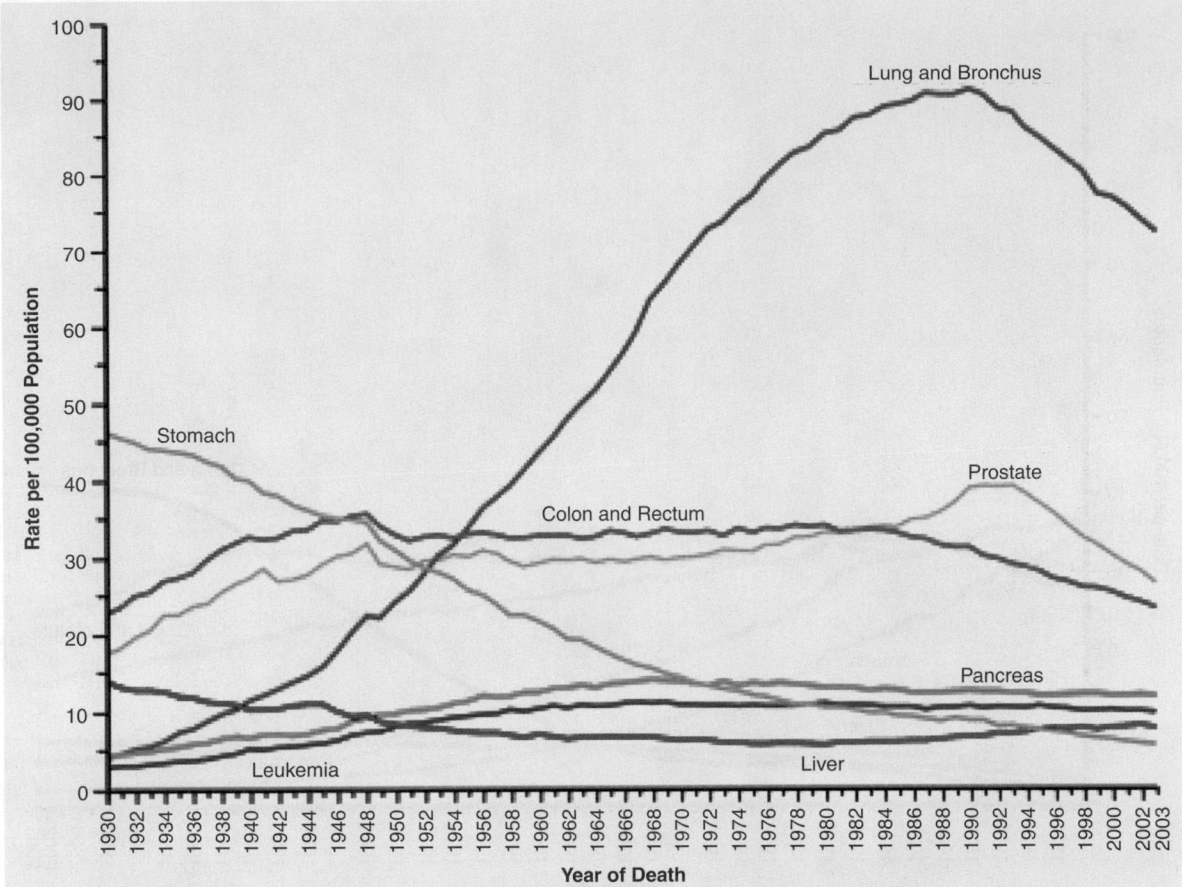

FIGURE 1.44. Annual age-adjusted cancer death rates among males, United States, 1930–2002. (From Jemal A, et al. Cancer statistics 2006. *CA Cancer J Clin* 2006;56:106 130, with permission.)

ultraviolet irradiation, prescription drugs, and medical procedures (91,470).

There are two general approaches to cancer prevention. They are referred to as *primary prevention strategies* and *secondary prevention strategies.* A primary preventive strategy may be invoked when there is an explicit and indisputable behavior that should be avoided or adopted because of its association with a predictable and certain reduction in cancer risk for an individual. A secondary prevention is distinguished from primary prevention in that it is an intervention focused on altering the natural history of a disease and thus avoiding disease-related adverse outcomes (92). The most commonly used secondary prevention strategy is broad-based or targeted population screening.

The principal primary prevention strategies are directed against cancers that have been associated with certain behaviors. They begin, first and foremost, with avoidance of tobacco. Tobacco use, either in the form of cigarette, pipe, or cigar smoking or the use of snuff or chewing tobacco, is strongly associated with carcinoma of the lung, larynx, pharynx, oral cavity, and esophagus. Tobacco also appears to be an important contributing factor in cancer of the pancreas, bladder, kidney, stomach, colon, and uterine cervix. In addition to its role in the etiology of cancer, tobacco also is associated with coronary heart disease, chronic lung disease, stroke, and other maladies. Tobacco is the single largest preventable cause of death in the Western world today.

In recent years, we have come to understand the role of excessive fat consumption and obesity in the etiology of cancer.

Studies suggest a direct correlation between average dietary fat intake in various countries and the incidence of breast cancer. Classic studies have shown that the incidence of stomach cancer among Japanese decreases when Japanese individuals migrate to Hawaii. Second-generation Japanese residents of Hawaii have an incidence of stomach cancer equivalent to that of the white population (316). Clearly, a more healthy diet could reduce the incidence of cancer (312).

Excessive alcohol consumption also is associated with cancer. Alcohol consumption is particularly harmful among cigarette smokers. It appears that smoking acts as an initiator, producing injurious mutations, and alcohol acts as a promoter in cancer of the oral cavity, oropharynx, pharynx, larynx, and esophagus.

A variety of occupational exposures also are associated with specific cancers. These include cancer in asbestos miners and workers, various forms of cancer in workers in the chemical industry, cancers associated with pesticide exposure in agricultural workers, and radiation-associated cancers in uranium miners. An obvious preventive strategy is to minimize or eliminate such harmful exposures in the workplace.

In recent years, scientists have become increasingly aware of various genetic syndromes associated with the etiology of cancer. These include the multiple endocrine neoplasia syndromes and their association with medullary cancer of the thyroid, susceptibility genes that increase the risk of colon cancer, and the association of the BRCA1 and BRCA2 genes with carcinoma of the breast and ovary (456). For some of these genetic-susceptibility traits, the best that the physician can offer

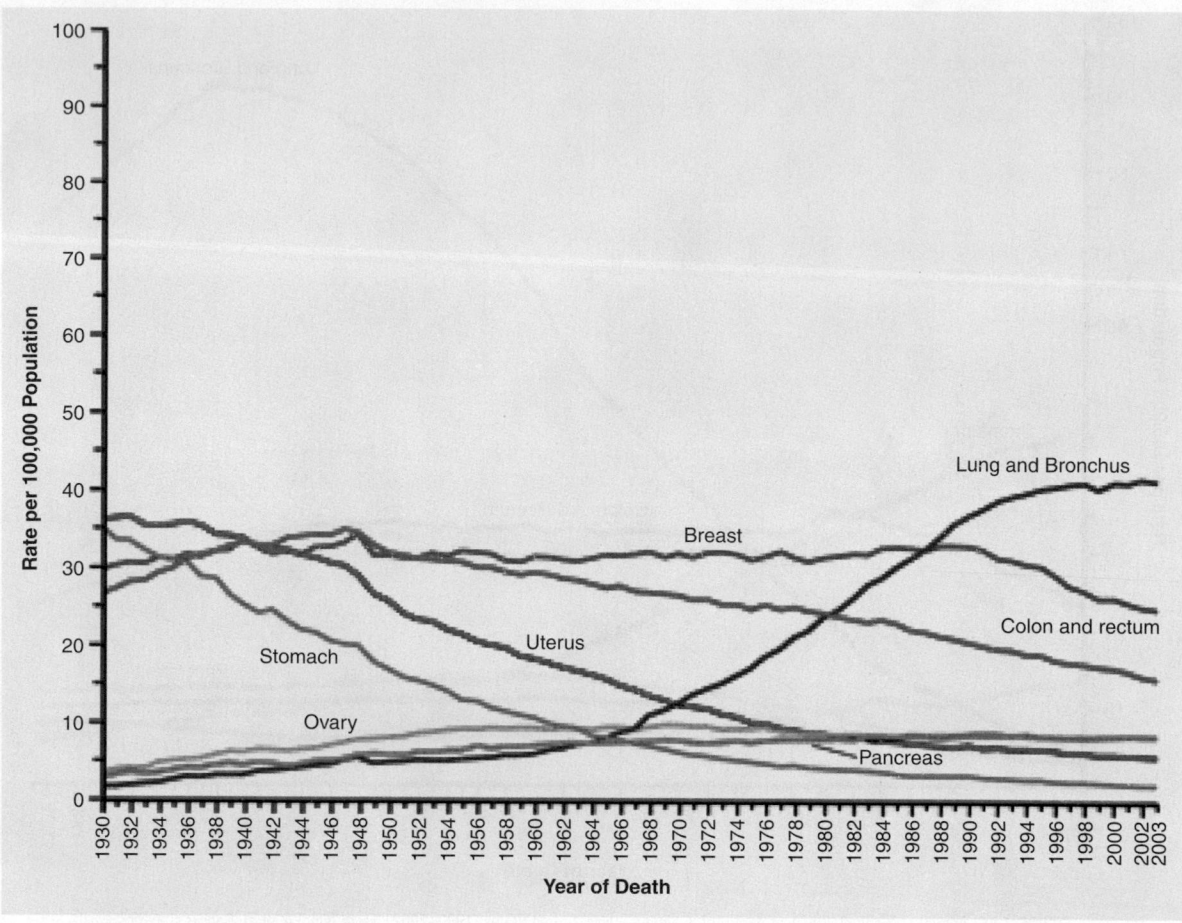

FIGURE 1.45. Annual age-adjusted cancer death rates among females, United States, 1930–2001. (From Jemal A, et al. Cancer statistics 2006. *CA Cancer J Clin* 2006;56:106–130, with permission.)

is close follow-up. There are certain situations where the avoidance of a potentially lethal cancer may lead an individual to consider prophylactic surgery. For example, consider the problem of a woman who is treated for breast-conserving surgery followed by radiotherapy for breast cancer. She subsequently is found to have a deleterious mutation of BRCA1 or BRCA2. The patient has a risk of relapse in the treated breast, development of a tumor in the contralateral breast, and development of ovarian cancer (201). Is the patient best handled by close follow-up? Should bilateral mastectomies be offered (345)? At present, the answer is unclear. In a study reported in 2002, investigators found that prophylactic salpingo-oophorectomy in women with BRCA1 and BRCA2 mutations significantly reduced their risk of not only ovarian cancer but also of breast cancer (3,313). This effect, presumably, is the result of decreasing endogenous estrogen exposure in the setting of BRCA genes, rendering the breast susceptible to estrogen-induced DNA damage (47).

Since the publication of the previous edition of this textbook, the most exciting development in cancer prevention is the successful clinical trial of a vaccine capable of reducing, by about 70%, the incidence of HPV-associated cervical cancer. The U.S. Food and Drug Administration approved this vaccine for clinical use in summer 2006. This vaccine, along with the use of routine Pap testing, has the potential to make invasive cervical cancer an exceedingly rare event.

Cancer screening is the most frequently considered secondary preventive strategy. A cancer screening procedure

should lead to the early detection of an asymptomatic or unrecognized disease by the application of simple, inexpensive tests or examinations in a targeted population. For cancer screening to be appropriate and successful, several criteria should be met. These include the following:

1. The cancer for which one is screening should have a substantial morbidity and/or mortality rate that warrants the screening procedure.
2. The cancer for which one is screening should have a sufficiently high prevalence in a detectable, preclinical state to warrant screening.
3. Once the cancer is detected by a screening procedure, there should be an effective treatment related to early detection. This criteria is quite important because there is little value in screening for an untreatable malignancy.
4. The screening test should have a high sensitivity and specificity.
5. The screening test should be of low cost such that the expense of screening a large population would be more than offset by the reduced cost to society of treating early rather than advanced malignancy.
6. Individuals screened should suffer little inconvenience and discomfort.

There is no perfect screening test. Those tests currently used generally meet most, but not all, of the aforementioned criteria (92,422).

There are several examples of currently used screening tests. For breast cancer, these include self-examination, examination

Estimated New Cases

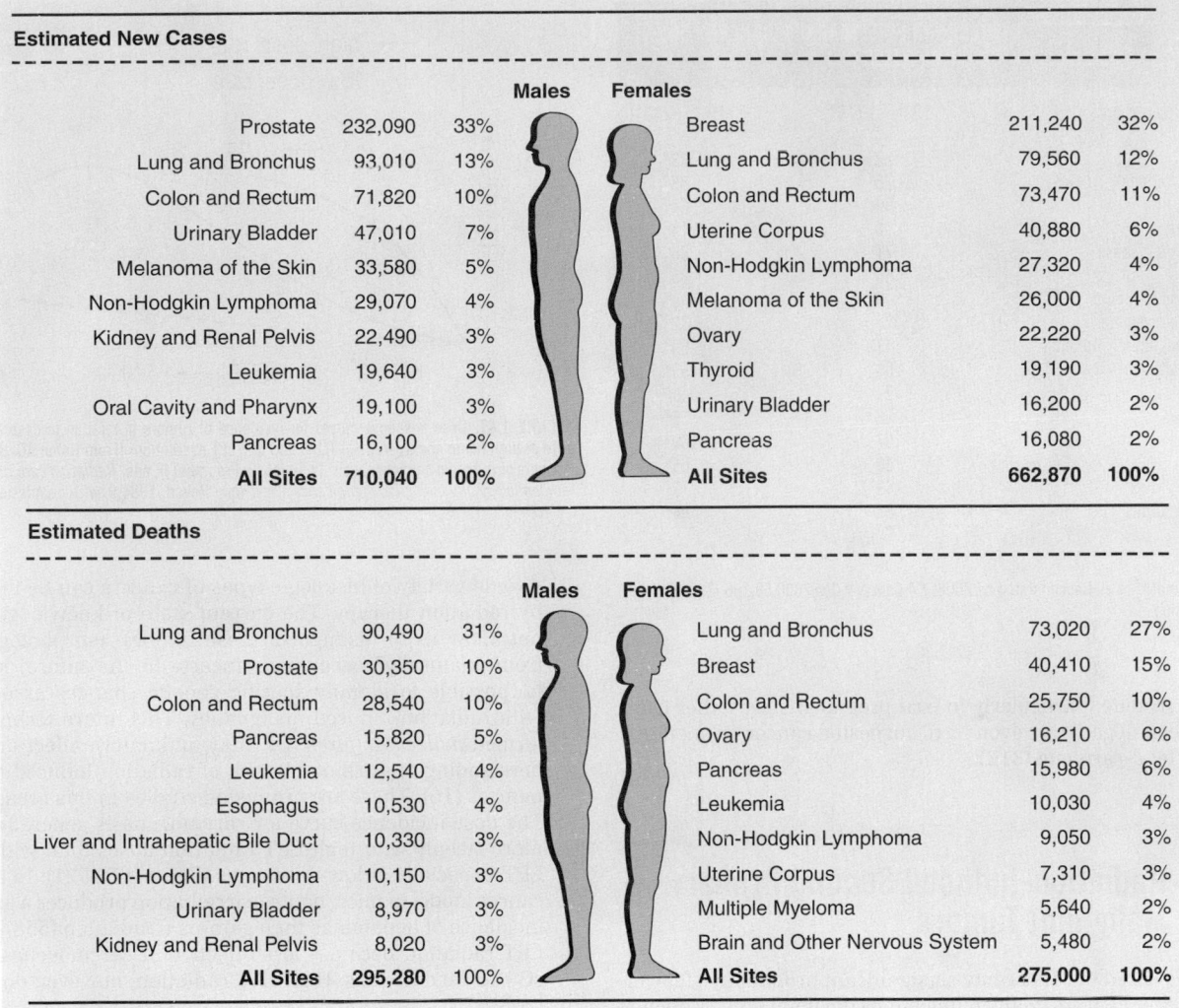

	Males			Females		
Prostate	232,090	33%		Breast	211,240	32%
Lung and Bronchus	93,010	13%		Lung and Bronchus	79,560	12%
Colon and Rectum	71,820	10%		Colon and Rectum	73,470	11%
Urinary Bladder	47,010	7%		Uterine Corpus	40,880	6%
Melanoma of the Skin	33,580	5%		Non-Hodgkin Lymphoma	27,320	4%
Non-Hodgkin Lymphoma	29,070	4%		Melanoma of the Skin	26,000	4%
Kidney and Renal Pelvis	22,490	3%		Ovary	22,220	3%
Leukemia	19,640	3%		Thyroid	19,190	3%
Oral Cavity and Pharynx	19,100	3%		Urinary Bladder	16,200	2%
Pancreas	16,100	2%		Pancreas	16,080	2%
All Sites	**710,040**	**100%**		**All Sites**	**662,870**	**100%**

Estimated Deaths

	Males			Females		
Lung and Bronchus	90,490	31%		Lung and Bronchus	73,020	27%
Prostate	30,350	10%		Breast	40,410	15%
Colon and Rectum	28,540	10%		Colon and Rectum	25,750	10%
Pancreas	15,820	5%		Ovary	16,210	6%
Leukemia	12,540	4%		Pancreas	15,980	6%
Esophagus	10,530	4%		Leukemia	10,030	4%
Liver and Intrahepatic Bile Duct	10,330	3%		Non-Hodgkin Lymphoma	9,050	3%
Non-Hodgkin Lymphoma	10,150	3%		Uterine Corpus	7,310	3%
Urinary Bladder	8,970	3%		Multiple Myeloma	5,640	2%
Kidney and Renal Pelvis	8,020	3%		Brain and Other Nervous System	5,480	2%
All Sites	**295,280**	**100%**		**All Sites**	**275,000**	**100%**

FIGURE 1.46. Ten leading cancer types and cancer deaths, by sex, United States, 2005 (excludes basal and squamous skin cancers and *in situ* cancer except for bladder). (From Jemal A, et al. Cancer statistics 2006. *CA Cancer J Clin* 2006;56:106–130, with permission.)

by a trained health practitioner, and mammography, augmented, when appropriate, by ultrasound and MRI. The value of these tests in various populations of women is currently highly disputed. In screening for colorectal cancer, the tools available to the clinician include testing for fecal occult blood, sigmoidoscopy, colonoscopy, and barium enema studies, and the developing field of virtual colonoscopy. There is a general consensus that screening for fecal occult blood and, in the appropriate aged population, screening colonoscopy are worthwhile. Among the most controversial areas for cancer screening is the role of screening in the detection of early prostate cancer. There was rapid general acceptance of the use of physical examination and PSA testing to ascertain the presence of early prostate cancer. On further consideration, however, many investigators fear that we have, as a society, successfully identified large numbers of men who would never have been diagnosed with symptomatic prostate cancer in their remaining lifetime or required treatment. The appropriate role of screening for prostate cancer has generated as much controversy as the debate over mammography in breast cancer. A considerable amount of anxiety has been generated in asymptomatic men compulsively watching their PSA levels. Far less controversial, however, has been the use of the Pap test for early detection of carcinoma of the cervix. Where properly used, the test

appears to have resulted in a decrease of mortality from this malignancy.

Cancer chemoprevention is defined as a pharmacologic intervention with specific nutrients or other chemicals intended to suppress or reverse carcinogenesis and to prevent the development of invasive cancer. Trials involving chemopreventive therapy require large numbers of individuals who are at high risk for malignancy because of family history, carcinogenic exposure, or the presence of a mutated gene. The ideal chemopreventive agent would have minimal side effects because it would be given to a considerable number of people, none of whom have cancer. Chemoprevention trials differ from other types of cancer prevention studies and from therapeutic studies in important ways. The participants are healthy volunteers, and one seeks to measure a reduction in morbidity and mortality in the long run. Chemoprevention trials are, by definition, large. There are strict enrollment criteria that reflect the group of interest. These studies are often long term and expensive. To date, the best-studied agents in human preventive trials are retinoids (the natural derivatives and synthetic analogs of vitamin A) and one member of the carotenoid class, β-carotene. A number of randomized cancer prevention trials involving carotenoids and retinoids have been completed. Some of these trials have reported chemopreventive effects for various retinoids and

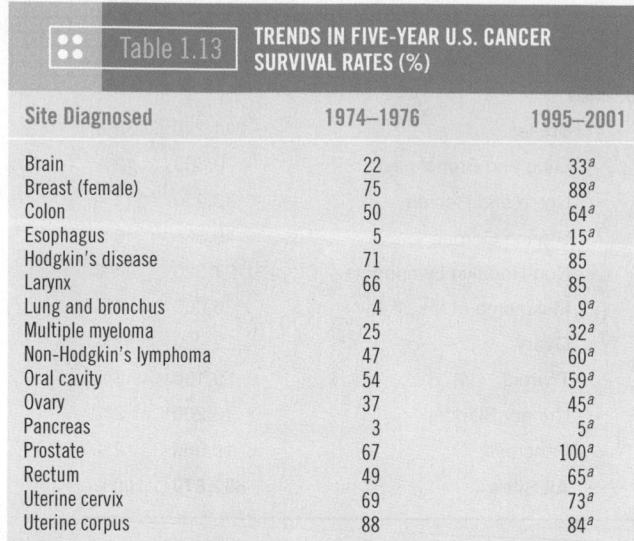

Table 1.13	TRENDS IN FIVE-YEAR U.S. CANCER SURVIVAL RATES (%)	
Site Diagnosed	**1974–1976**	**1995–2001**
Brain	22	33[a]
Breast (female)	75	88[a]
Colon	50	64[a]
Esophagus	5	15[a]
Hodgkin's disease	71	85
Larynx	66	85
Lung and bronchus	4	9[a]
Multiple myeloma	25	32[a]
Non-Hodgkin's lymphoma	47	60[a]
Oral cavity	54	59[a]
Ovary	37	45[a]
Pancreas	3	5[a]
Prostate	67	100[a]
Rectum	49	65[a]
Uterine cervix	69	73[a]
Uterine corpus	88	84[a]

[a]p <.05.
From Jemal A, et al. Cancer statistics 2006. *CA Cancer J Clin* 2006;56:106–130, with permission.

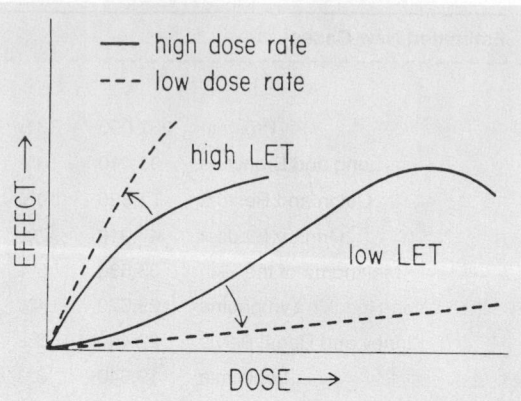

FIGURE 1.47. Dose–response curves for incidence of tumors in relation to dose and dose rate of high linear energy transfer (LET) and low-LET irradiation. (From Upton AC. Biological aspects of radiation carcinogenesis. In: Boice JD, Fraumeni JF, eds. *Radiation carcinogenesis: epidemiology and biological significance.* New York: Raven, 1984;9, with permission.)

for β-carotene, particularly in oral premalignancy. Other trials have been negative or even have suggested cancer promotional effects by β-carotene (312).

Radiation-Induced Second Primary Malignant Tumors

Patients cured of cancer have a significant probability of developing other cancers. Many publications document the frequency of second malignant neoplasms, associated with radiation therapy, in cancer survivors (214). Several principles characterize radiation-induced cancers:

Table 1.14	ESTIMATED NEW U.S. CANCER CASES AND DEATHS, 2006	
	New Cases	**Deaths**
All sites	1,399,790	564,830
Oral cavity and pharynx	30,990	7,430
Digestive system	263,060	136,180
Respiratory system	186,370	167,050
Bones and joint	2,760	1,260
Soft tissue (excluding heart)	9,530	3,500
Skin (excluding basal and squamous)	68,780	10,710
Breast	214,640	41,430
Genital system	321,490	56,060
Urinary system	102,740	26,670
Eye and orbit	2,360	230
Brain and other nervous system	18,820	12,820
Endocrine system	32,260	2,290
Lymphoma	66,670	20,330
Multiple myeloma	16,570	11,310
Leukemia	35,070	22,280
Other and unspecified primary sites	27,680	45,280

Data from Jemal A, et al. Cancer statistics 2006. *CA Cancer J Clin* 2006;56:106–130, with permission.

1. A wide variety of histologic types of cancers can be induced by radiation therapy. The current state of knowledge does not allow us to distinguish these tumors, morphologically, from "naturally" occurring cancers. In the future, it may be possible to identify specific genetic changes associated with radiation-induced malignancy. This future technology, termed *molecular forensics*, may, ultimately, affect our understanding of attributable risk of radiation-induced malignancies (16). There are promising studies in this areas (45).

2. The dose incidence curve for carcinogenesis generally rises more steeply with high-LET radiation doses than with low-LET, especially at low-dose rates (Fig. 1.47) (521). In a liver cancer model in mice, neutron irradiation produces a greater incidence of hepatomas than gamma irradiation (558). Low-LET radiation becomes less effective at carcinogenesis per cGy as the dose falls. High-LET radiation, however, does not (265).

3. When one compares the frequency of second malignant neoplasms over time, it appears that orthovoltage radiation therapy is more likely to be carcinogenic than megavoltage therapy. This may be a dose-related phenomenon insofar as orthovoltage irradiation gives a higher dose to bone. It is also possible that the longer term follow-up available for survivors of orthovoltage irradiation may, somewhat artifactually, lead to a higher reported incidence of tumors (224,312,405).

4. The sensitivity of tissues to radiation-induced malignancies is not uniform. Current evidence indicates that the thyroid gland and the breast are sensitive to cancer induction at relatively low doses of radiation; lymphoid tissue, lung, and liver require moderate doses; and bone requires the highest dose. It also seems likely that the relationship between dose and response may vary according to the type of induced tumor. One can estimate the cancer risk from radiation either per unit dose measured in Gy or per unit dose equivalent measured in sievert. When one measures in sieverts, a quality factor (Q) is used to take account of the varying biologic effectiveness of the different forms of radiation. For example, for a conventional γ-ray or x-ray, Q = 1. For neutron irradiation, Q = 20. A review of the available literature indicates that the lifetime cancer mortality risk for a working population of both sexes is 0.008 per Sv for high doses and 0.004 per Sv for low doses (209). The cancer mortality risk for the general population after whole body exposure is 0.0001 to 0.0004 per cGy per person.

5. One of the most puzzling aspects of radiation-induced cancer concerns the issue of the relation of low radiation dose to carcinogenesis. Most of the data we have concerns relatively

high doses. Much of the public debate, however, concerns exposure to relatively low doses. Because we have few exact data regarding low doses, extrapolation is, for the most part, used to predict risk at low doses. This can be a particularly vexing problem in litigation where a plaintiff sues for an alleged radiation-induced malignancy following relatively low-dose exposure to radiation.

6. Any assessment of the radiation–dose-response curve for the production of second malignant neoplasms has to take into account the fact that neoplasms also can be induced by agents other than radiation. These include chemotherapy, environmental exposures, and hereditary disposition.

7. Because the risk of radiation-induced carcinogenesis is very small, a large denominator of radiated patients followed for a long period with thorough follow-up would be necessary to calculate risk with any reliability.

8. Latent periods for the production of radiation-induced tumor vary according to the type of induced tumor. One type of latency is exemplified by the risk of leukemia in survivors of the atomic bomb. This consisted of an early pulse of increased risk followed by a gradual decline to baseline levels. The second pattern of occurrence, more typical of solid tumors, is an increase in the relative risk of second malignant neoplasms over many years that remains constant over time thereafter. It is important to remember, therefore, that the duration of follow-up for any study population is very likely to influence the frequency of tumors seen.

9. Age is a critical factor in determining radiation risk. In children, second cancers would be more likely to occur in tissues undergoing rapid proliferation such as bone and thyroid tissue.

There are several classically cited episodes of human radiation carcinogenesis. These include:

1. Individuals who are treated with radiation for ankylosing spondylitis suffered from an increase in leukemia. Mortality from colon cancer, which is associated with spondylitis through a common association with ulcerative colitis, was increased in irradiated patients. Mortality for patients with cancers other than leukemia or colon cancer also rose (102).

2. Diagnostic x-rays of the abdomen and pelvis taken of a pregnant woman to ascertain the size of the pelvic outlet before delivery are associated with an increased risk of malignancy in the offspring.

3. A large number of immigrants entered the State of Israel following its founding in 1948. X-ray epilation was used to treat tinea capitis. There was an increased incidence of brain and nervous system tumors (1.8 excess risk per 10,000 persons per year) in 10,834 children irradiated for tinea capitis compared with the same number of nonirradiated matched controls and 5,392 siblings. There were 12 malignant brain tumors in the irradiated patients versus five and one suspected in nonirradiated people. The average dose received was 4 Gy in 5 consecutive days. Irradiation doses of 1 to 2 Gy significantly increased the risk of neurologic tumors (427).

4. The United States dropped atomic bombs on Hiroshima and Nagasaki in Japan in August 1945. Radiation-related risks among bomb survivors show that the incidence of leukemia rose. The increased risk appeared 1 to 3 years after the bombing and peaked at 6 to 7 years. In solid tumors, excess tumor risk was manifest only after exposed individuals reached the age at which the cancer was normally prone to develop.

5. Uranium miners suffered an increase of lung cancer as a result of inhalation of radon gas. Workers who painted luminous radium dials on watch faces developed bone sarcomas because of the habit of shaping the paintbrush in the mouth and ingesting bone-seeking radium (174).

6. In the past, thorotrast was used as a contrast medium in diagnostic radiology. This material is a colloidal suspension of the α-emitter thorium dioxide. The compound was associated with the late development of angiosarcoma (5).

7. Canadian studies of women with tuberculosis who were fluoroscoped repeatedly for monitoring of an induced pneumothorax demonstrated an increased incidence of breast cancer.

8. The Chernobyl Nuclear Power Plant accident of April 26, 1986, appears to be associated with an increased risk of thyroid cancer in Belarus and Ukraine.

An important review of radiation-induced sarcomas was published by Cahan et al. (65) in 1948. Cahan's criteria, which were used to define a radiation-induced sarcoma, have wide applicability and are used, by some investigators, as the standard for demonstration of any alleged radiation-induced malignancy. The Cahan Criteria, modified from his original definition, are:

(a) A radiation-induced malignancy must have arisen in an irradiated field.

(b) A sufficient latent period, preferably longer than 4 years, must have elapsed between the initial irradiation and the alleged induced malignancy.

(c) The treated tumor must have been biopsied. The alleged induced tumor must have been biopsied. The two tumors must be of different histologies.

(d) The tissue in which the alleged induced tumor arose must have been normal (i.e., metabolically and genetically normal) prior to radiation exposure.

Quality Assurance in Radiation Oncology

Quality assurance (QA) in radiation oncology is a set of processes and procedures designed to improve the practice of radiation therapy by confirming that radiation therapy will be or was administered appropriately and safely and documented properly.

Clinical Quality Assurance for External-Beam Radiation Therapy

Clinical QA for EBRT is based on regular chart audits seeking to demonstrate the existence of specific elements of the medical record and assess the quality of these elements. The chart should have an electronic, computer-printed, typewritten, or legibly handwritten clinical evaluation of the patient, containing a complete medical history, physical examination, and recommendations for therapy. In some teaching institutions, the initial history and physical note is augmented by a separate attending physician note that documents the faculty member's recommendations for radiotherapy. If a course of EBRT is recommended, there should be documentation in the chart of a discussion with the patient and his or her family of issues related to informed consent. This should be supplemented by a signed consent form. Chart audits also should identify a treatment planning note and/or simulation note indicating the course of radiation therapy proposed and documenting the physician's thinking process as regards the treatment volume and technique selected for simulation. For patients undergoing or having completed treatment, there should be a series of progress notes (also called "on treatment notes") documenting the conduct of the course of EBRT. After completion of treatment, there should be follow-up notes. A pathology or cytology report documenting the existence of cancer, x-ray and other diagnostic imaging reports, and laboratory results also should be present.

The chart audit also should be able to identify, in every case, an EBRT prescription page that clearly shows the physician's prescription for the body site to be irradiated, the body position during treatment, the stabilization device to be used (if any), the energy and direction of beams specified, radiation dose per fraction, number of fractions per day, number of fractions per week, and total dose of radiation proposed. There should be a clear indication of whether the patient is enrolled on a specific protocol and whether the intent of treatment is curative or palliative. When IMRT is employed many insurance carriers expect to see a note indicating that an IMRT plan was compared to alternatives and was judged preferable *for this particular patient*.

It is also reasonable to expect, during a QA chart audit, that the reviewer can identify a page documenting the parameters for treatment established during the simulation, such as field size, use of blocks, beam energy, and documentation of the daily administered EBRT treatments. There should be a section of the chart containing documentation of dosimetry, treatment plans, isodose curves, and DVHs. One should be able to find a record of the patient's vital signs, documentation of the patient's weight, and pertinent hematologic studies such as complete blood counts and PSA (for men). Charts also include listings of the patient's medications and drug allergies. It has become increasingly popular, in recent years, to have a section of the chart devoted to the documentation of the level of a patient's pain as the "fifth" vital sign.

During a QA chart audit, it is customary for the reviewer to have a checklist or form on which he or she indicates that the aforementioned elements are present and satisfactory. The mere presence of the appropriate material is not sufficient. When one reviews the chart, one should be persuaded that the therapy is indicated; that it is appropriate in its intent; and that the radiation dose, treatment volume, and technique are appropriate.

The chart audit for EBRT should be accompanied by a review of the simulation and port films. The reviewer should feel that the beams are appropriate, that blocks are appropriately designed and placed, and that the therapy was implemented correctly.

The External-Beam Quality Assurance Conference Chart Rounds

In many radiation oncology departments, it is customary to conduct the routine chart audit in the context of a weekly conference referred to either as a QA conference or chart rounds. This conference generally serves as the mainstay of the external-beam QA process.

Chart rounds should be attended by all of the department's physicians. It is essential that physicians not "check themselves" during chart rounds. Rather, differing perspectives and the give and take of discussion and debate should characterize this time. Physicians should be willing to question each other and probe the proposed treatment plan. Junior physicians should not be hesitant at questioning their senior counterparts. In some radiation oncology departments, chart rounds are only conducted on patients just starting treatment. In other departments, all patients are reviewed on a weekly basis while under treatment.

In addition to the departmental physicians, chart rounds also should be attended by representatives of medical physics, dosimetry, nursing, and radiation therapy. In some departments, members of the social work staff and secretaries also attend. Telemedicine may be used to allow distant departments to participate. The conference room should have suitable light boxes or x-ray projection equipment so that simulator and port films can be readily displayed and critiqued. The conference room should be free from distractions such as pagers, cell phones, and outside phone calls. The serious nature of chart rounds should be emphasized by the demeanor of the presiding physician, and appropriate minutes should be taken.

In general, chart rounds for a QA program should include broad efforts in the following areas:

1. *Statistics on patient-related activities.* Statistics should include the total number of new patients seen and treated per year, number of retreated patients, anatomic site of tumors treated, and number of procedures performed (consultations, treatment visits, fields treated, simulations, treatment plans done, brachytherapy procedures, and follow-up visits).
2. *Patient records and forms.* Radiation oncology records ideally should be kept separate from the hospital records to ensure ready access to both types of records in different areas of the hospital when required. Copies of appropriate sections of the radiation therapy record should be sent to the referring physician as well as to the hospital record room or made available in the electronic medical record.

   Every patient must have a complete consultation note, with a history and physical examination, description of pertinent physical findings required for staging, and laboratory and radiographic studies that may be helpful in the selection of therapy. Histologic or cytologic documentation of cancer (or a compelling reason for lack of verification) should be an integral part of the record. Drawings or photographs illustrating the extent, character, location, and stage of the tumor always should be included.

   The details of treatment planning, volume treated (portals), dose prescription, calculations, simulator and periodic portal localization films, and dose distribution (isodose curves) must be documented. The record should indicate the position of the patient; any special immobilization, shielding, or beam-modifying devices; doses of irradiation given, monitoring units, exposure time of daily treatment (when applicable); and daily and cumulative tumor doses delivered. Following is a checklist for completion of treatment chart review, suggested by the American College of Radiology (8):

   - Diagnosis stated
   - Stage of disease recorded
   - Pertinent histopathology report in chart
   - Relevant history of the disease stated in consult note
   - Physical findings relevant to the disease stated
   - Treatment plan or prescription dated and signed by responsible physician at beginning of treatment
   - Planned dose and method of delivery planned
   - Treatment site or treatment volume specified
   - Fields documented by actual or electronic portal films
   - Dosimetry calculations in chart and checked by physicist
   - Isodose calculations in chart and checked by physicist
   - Treatment record checked weekly by physician
   - Treatment record checked weekly by physicist or dosimetrist
   - Evidence of weekly evaluation of patient by responsible physician
   - Summary or completion of therapy report prepared
   - Follow-up plan stated
   - Other comments
   - Name of person completing review and date

   Every radiation oncology center should develop or adopt appropriate forms for patient registration, tumor staging, dose prescription and recording (including brachytherapy procedures), and follow-up information. Pathology reports and laboratory data can be copied from the hospital chart, obtained from the respective departments, or shared electronically for inclusion in the radiation oncology record. Forms are available for staging purposes in each anatomic site; many of them were designed following suggestions of the American Joint Committee on Cancer (195).
3. *Treatment planning/dosimetry procedures.* To verify the validity of administration of the radiation therapy, data

concerning the planned treatment techniques, technical factors, and dose prescription should be reviewed by both the radiation oncologist directing the treatment and the physics or dosimetry staff. Electronic or conventional simulation and localization films and photographs are required to document the appropriateness of the irradiation portals. The dosimetry review includes initial and periodic verification of the maximum doses and tumor doses delivered to the tumor, draining lymphatics, and critical normal structures throughout the course of irradiation.

4. *Equipment evaluation and calibration procedures.* Each radiation oncology facility should have a formal equipment QA program, developed by the chief radiation physicist in close cooperation with the medical director. QA procedures and results from periodic performance tests and calibration of all therapy machines must be documented accurately (85). It is strongly recommended that an electronic or paper log book be kept at each therapy machine console to allow the machine operator (therapy technologist) to document immediate problems related to machine performance that could affect radiation and mechanical safety. QA requirements in each of these areas are outlined elsewhere (247).

Three-Dimensional External-Beam Radiation Therapy Chart Rounds

The proliferation of 3D treatment planning, conformal field irradiation, IMRT, and related technologies creates special opportunities and challenges for QA. In many radiation oncology departments, special QA chart rounds are conducted specifically for patients treated with 3D treatment planning and IMRT techniques. These chart rounds share many essential elements with conventional EBRT chart rounds. To wit: the selection of radiation dose, treatment volume, technique, treatment goals, and indications are reviewed carefully for each case.

The unique aspect of 3D radiotherapy and IMRT QA chart rounds is the review, in a group setting, of the treatment plan. These plans often involve noncoplanar fields, unconventional angles, and the use of multileaf collimators.

Considerable attention must be given to the technology utilized to display the treatment plan in a group setting. In some departments, the staff gathers around a computer screen to view the 3D or IMRT plan. In other departments, special technology is used to project the plan on multiple television monitors or a large screen. As technology evolves for treatment planning, QA rounds serve both the expected purpose of documenting the proper and safe administration of radiotherapy as well as the additional purpose of group learning.

•• | Clinical Quality Assurance •• | for Brachytherapy

Elements of Brachytherapy Quality Assurance

As for a patient receiving EBRT, the radiation therapy chart of a patient treated with brachytherapy must contain certain elements. These include a history and physical examination note, a discussion of the indications for brachytherapy, goals of treatment, and proposed technique. A brachytherapy summary should describe the procedure used for brachytherapy, the isotope used, the dose distribution selected, the duration of the radioactive implant, and the dose administered. Such notes should be accompanied by a description of the procedure, analogous to an operative note, which documents the findings at the time of the brachytherapy procedure and any complications encountered.

There also should be documentation of the work of the participating physicist and dosimetrist, including, if appropriate, the receipt of the radioactive isotope from an outside supplier or the logging out and logging in of the isotope from the department's radioactive material storage facility. The activity of the isotope should be specified as well as the calculation of its decay during the course of the radioactive implant, if appropriate. Multiple dose distributions should be presented in the chart to indicate the dose distribution of the radioactive application in multiple planes. Diagnostic quality radiographs showing the placement of the afterloading catheters, generally with dummy seeds in place, are important to have along with photographs of the implant.

Documentation of radiation safety procedures during brachytherapy are also necessary. These might include documentation of room surveys with the scintillation counter before and after placement and removal of the brachytherapy sources and an accounting of the number of seeds or sources.

Brachytherapy Quality Assurance Conference/Chart Rounds

In some departments, brachytherapy chart rounds are combined with EBRT chart rounds. In other departments, a separate brachytherapy chart round is conducted every week, every 2 weeks, or every month—depending on the volume of brachytherapy procedures. The obvious difference between EBRT chart rounds and brachytherapy chart rounds is that, in the case of EBRT, chart rounds are conducted for patients beginning or undergoing treatment. In brachytherapy chart rounds, however, charts are reviewed *after* the brachytherapy application. Thus, in the case of brachytherapy, chart rounds serve as a monitoring technique, for reporting of complications, and, most importantly, as a method of continuous quality improvement.

During a brachytherapy QA conference, each case is presented briefly and the appropriate x-rays and photographs are shown to document the brachytherapy application. In addition, the dose distribution is either passed around the room or projected on a screen for all to view. A give-and-take discussion follows in which the audience probes the indications, nature of the procedure, and complications in an effort to glean every possible bit of information from the procedure and its outcome.

Complications and unanticipated events deserve special emphasis. In an active brachytherapy practice, events such as uterine perforation, "lost seeds," hemorrhage, unanticipated "hot spots," and device failures inevitably will occur. Such events should not be "swept under the rug"; they should be discussed and serve as an opportunity for learning and improvement.

Quality Assurance for Hyperthermia

As an evolving technique of cancer treatment, hyperthermia presents new problems and opportunities for QA. In those departments performing hyperthermia, chart rounds should be conducted on a regular basis. The indications for hyperthermia should be discussed in each case, and specific protocol accrual for investigative studies should be discussed. Temperature distributions, equipment problems, and complications should be reviewed. A hyperthermia QA checklist should be developed, depending on the equipment used and the protocols open, for each department.

Quality Assurance for Protocol Compliance in Radiation Oncology

The essential element of a phase I, II, or III protocol for cancer treatment is a clearly written protocol. The protocol must specify the goals of the study, eligible patients, nature and specifics of the treatment plan, data to be accrued, statistical methods, and the requirements for informed consent. When protocols are conducted by multiple physicians, at multiple locations, often in several countries and on several continents, the data will be meaningless unless there is assurance that all patients are treated to protocol specifications. This includes assurance that EBRT machines or brachytherapy sources are calibrated appropriately; that the dose of radiation administered is within protocol guidelines; that the radiation therapy fields used are those specified by the protocol; and, in the case of EBRT, that the daily dose and total dose are appropriate.

To fulfill the aforementioned goals, protocols generally call for data concerning radiation oncology treatment to be sent to a centralized QA office in paper or electronic form. At this office, the specifics of the radiation therapy administered are reviewed and checked for compliance with the protocol. Often, there is a "rapid turnaround" procedure in which the radiation therapy treatment plan is reviewed within a few days of starting the course of treatment. Any discrepancy from the protocol guidelines can be noted and the treating physician is contacted for possible correction. After the course of radiation therapy is completed, the treatment course is reviewed again at the central QA office and is judged as to its level of appropriateness. In cases in which there is serious deviation from the protocol guidelines, the patient may be judged "unevaluable" and, in this manner, the quality of the clinical data for the study is defended.

QA for radiation oncology in cancer protocols is expensive. It is, therefore, often an area targeted for attempted cost savings. This tendency is to be discouraged. QA is essential to obtaining valid data in clinical research. The clinical literature in radiation oncology abounds with examples of studies that would have obtained entirely different answers were it not for the modifications wrought by appropriate QA procedures (215).

The Department Quality Assurance Committee

Every radiation oncology department should have a QA committee that meets on a regular basis. There should be representation from the physician staff, medical physics, nursing, dosimetry, radiation therapy, and, often, social work and administration.

The essential elements of the regular QA meeting should include a review of departmental statistics concerning the number of external-beam treatments and brachytherapy procedures. This should be followed by a report from the designated physician representative concerning problems identified in clinical care and corrective action taken. Similarly, there should be a report from medical physics concerning machine calibrations, problems identified, and corrective actions. Dosimetry and therapy should report any errors that occurred during the reporting period and corrective actions taken. On a regular basis, there should be a targeted area for quality improvement. In many departments, a specific disease site is reviewed every 6 months to 1 year as a venue for quality improvement.

Every QA committee should have regular minutes kept that should be, on request, available for review by appropriate oversight bodies. Of particular importance in these minutes should be the notation of problems identified and, in subsequent minutes, the corrective action taken.

The External Practice Audit

Radiation oncology departments may, from time to time, be subject to a practice audit. Practice audits are performed for the reassurance that the department is delivering state-of-the-art radiation therapy. They also may be performed for the purpose of certification by an external governing body, a university medical center with whom the practice wishes to affiliate, or an accreditation organization. In addition, practice audits sometimes are performed when a problem in a practice has been alleged and one wishes to obtain objective data to assess the existence, nature, and severity of the alleged problem.

In a practice audit, the reviewing team generally consists of a physician and medical physicist. They either will review a series of charts of patients treated during a specified time period or request a random pull of charts. Some reviewers will review charts based on disease sites such as five cases of lung cancer, five cases of breast cancer, three cases of lymphoma, and so on. The reviewing team will go through each chart and appropriate port films, or films documenting the brachytherapy application, and review them in accordance with a prearranged checklist. At the end of the chart audit, a verbal and written report are given to the audited physicians and/or hospital and an opinion is rendered concerning the state of the practice.

The performance of a practice audit calls for, on the part of the auditors, not only expertise in radiation oncology and medial physics but a high level of diplomacy and tact. Having one's charts reviewed by a colleague is obviously anxiety-producing. The auditor must make clear that the goals of the practice audit are quality assurance, quality improvement, and information gathering rather than a punitive exercise.

●● Documentation of Acute and Late Ill ●● Effects of Radiation Therapy

Radiation therapy is a powerful and potentially dangerous treatment for cancer. Almost every course of treatment has some risk of acute and late ill effects. When these occur, they must be properly documented.

There are various techniques for documenting untoward effects of treatment. Although many physicians rely on a simple narrative or conventional clinic note, there is much to be said for using standardized reporting systems relying on scales or grading systems. This is particularly common in cancer protocols, and a variety of such scales are available. Using an established scale and returning to it over time allows one to more fully appreciate the onset and time course of an ill effect.

●● How Many Linear Accelerators, Gamma Knifes, CyberKnifes, Intraoperative Radiotherapy Machines, Proton Units, Neutron Units, and Staff Does a Department Need?

The practicing radiation oncologist often faces a decision as to when to buy a new linear accelerator or when to replace an existing machine, what sort of radiosurgery equipment to buy, and whether to buy more exotic equipment such as high–dose-rate remote afterloaders, Gamma Knifes or CyberKnifes, or particle therapy units. We will consider these questions in this section of the chapter.

How many patients can be treated on a single linear accelerator? At what point do the demands on a piece of equipment become so high that it justifies a second machine? In those states in the United States, provinces in Canada, or national health authorities in other countries that control linear accelerators through a certificate of need process or its equivalent, what guidelines should be used for issuing permits to acquire linear accelerators? These are all practical and important questions that deserve reasonable answers.

Government regulatory bodies in the economically developed world have often sought to curb the rise in health care costs by capping purchases of new equipment. They hope that

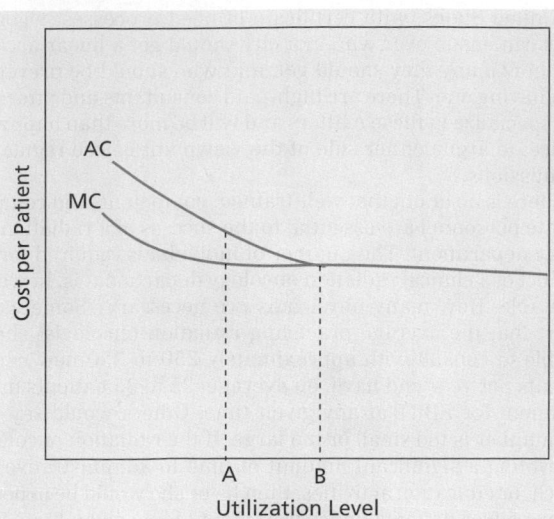

FIGURE 1.48. The theoretical relation between the cost per patient and rate of use of a linear accelerator for cancer therapy. As the rate of use of a linear accelerator increases, the average cost (AC) of treatment per patient declines until all economies of scale have been achieved (*point B*). The average cost of a radiotherapy treatment will fall as long as any additional patients can be treated at a marginal cost (MC) lower than the AC. It is important to remember that point B represents only the minimized cost of operating the linear accelerator. If you add in costs such as the travel time for a patient to go a considerable distance to reach the linear accelerator, the lost time from work for the patient and anyone traveling with them, child care costs, and stress, then the total societal expenditure for a linear accelerator will not be minimized at point B. It will, instead, be reached at point A. We are, however, quite poor at accounting for costs such as travel, loss of work time, and stress so it is difficult to determine point B and, in turn, the need for a new linear accelerator. If you wish to persuade a government regulatory agency to grant a certificate of need for a piece of radiotherapy equipment at a moderate distance from an existing facility, then you will have an economic incentive to inflate the importance of travel and inconvenience. In the United States, this behavior is increasing as institutions try to justify the need for linear accelerators, radiosurgery, and proton therapy units. The corporations that manufacture and market these units have a vested interest in contributing to this exaggeration of need. (Modified from Suit HD, Urie M. Proton beams in radiation therapy. *J Natl Cancer Inst* 1992;84:155–164, with permission.)

by reducing large capital expenses, consolidating clinical services so that economies of scale are achieved, and eliminating duplication health care costs will be reduced without compromising the quality of care (Fig. 1.48). In the increasingly competitive global marketplace, large corporations find themselves competing with companies throughout the world. If a U.S. automobile manufacturer provides expensive and comprehensive health care benefits to its workforce, and if these workers avail themselves of expensive high technology medical care, then the price of the automobile will have to rise in order to generate sufficient profit margin to pay, not only for the steel, plastic, aluminum, and other materials necessary to build the car, but also for the health care insurance of the workers. If an Asian competitor pays far less for health care for its workers, then they will be able to undercut the American manufacturer's price and they will, over time, increase their market share. This series-of-events has not been lost on U.S. industry, and we now see increasing pressure from the business world to reduce health care costs. Recently, for example, the St. Louis Business Coalition successfully lobbied to force two St. Louis hospitals to cooperate to get a single Gamma Knife unit rather than allow each to purchase its own (334).

Starting in 1986, the Intersociety Council for Radiation Oncology published a set of guidelines in a small pamphlet titled "Radiation Oncology in Integrated Cancer Management." This subsequently has been updated. The work is a joint effort of the American Association of Physicists in Medicine, American College of Radiology, American Radium Society, American Society for Therapeutic Radiology and Oncology, Radiation Research Society, Radiological Society of North America, and the Society

of Chairman of Academic Radiation Oncology Programs. The organization has offered guidelines for equipment utilization and a mechanism for determining a "realistic load for a megavoltage [linear accelerator] unit."

The methodology used in the guidelines was relatively straightforward: assume that a linear accelerator can treat, on average, one patient every 15 minutes. Thus, one can treat four patients per hour. If one assumes an 8-hour workday with 1 hour for the radiation therapists' QA procedures, warm-up, room preparation, lunch, and clean-up, then this offers 7 hours for treatment, or $7 \times 4 = 28$ treatments per day. Twenty-eight treatments per day multiplied by 5 days per week and 52 weeks per year converts to 7,280 standard treatments per accelerator per year. From this number, the authors of the guidelines subtracted an allowance for the extra time required for the first day of treatment for patients, the need for additional time for port films and verifications, and machine down time and holidays. They offer an estimate that the average linear accelerator should be able to administer roughly 6,000 standard treatments (single patient visit equivalents) per year.

Critical evaluation of the recommended 6,000 single patient visit equivalents immediately raises many questions and problems. For example, are all patient treatments equivalent? Is it reasonable to assert that treating a child with retinoblastoma under anesthesia with IMRT is an "equivalent treatment" to using parallel opposed anterior and posterior fields to treat a metastasis from lung cancer to the humerus in an adult? Is it reasonable to assert that total body irradiation is more complex than palliative bone irradiation? Is it reasonable to assert that a craniospinal field for medulloblastoma is more complex than a palliative whole-brain field, or that a IMRT treatment plan setup is more complex to implement than a conventionally simulated setup?

It would seem reasonable to accept the assertion that some forms of external radiotherapy are more complex than others. This would lead one to think that there should be some multiples in which one could convert the complexity of one type of radiotherapy to a numeric value. Perhaps one would assert that a complex planned treatment for the child with retinoblastoma under anesthesia is two-, three-, or fourfold more complicated that the "standard patient equivalent treatment," and perhaps not.

One also could question the recommendation for 6,000 standard treatments (single patient visit equivalents) per year on other grounds. Is it reasonable to assume an 8-hour workday? Perhaps the linear accelerator should, as a matter of course, be operated from 7:00 AM to 7:00 PM each day with overlapping shifts of radiation therapists so that the machine is operated through the lunch hour rather than taking a break. Perhaps it is reasonable to assert that one can, in some circumstances, treat five patients per hour rather than four. However, some institutions may only be able to treat two or three patients per hour. It rapidly becomes clear that, as one carefully explores the assumptions that underlie the single patient visit equivalent/standard treatment methodology, one can get enormously different answers. We are aware, for example, that in one state in the United States, the number of treatments per linear accelerator using this methodology ranges from 4,000 to 14,000.

All of these issues would be simply intellectual matters, providing an interesting focus for discussion, were it not for a single factor: *money*. The type of methodology used to determine the need for linear accelerators can be manipulated in a machiavellian manner to advantage some hospitals or practices in obtaining linear accelerators and prevent others from obtaining them. In a competitive medical marketplace, such as the United States, a tremendous amount is at stake in the manipulation of the methodology for equipment utilization. This methodology can be used to financially advantage some practices and drive competitors from the market.

It is easy to think of simple examples as to how the methodology can be manipulated to be an advantage for some institutions and not others. An academic health center might want to assert, for example, that the techniques more often used at that center require inflated multiples to make it more likely that they will get approval for more linear accelerators. They also might assert, for example, that all pediatric radiotherapy cases are, by definition, fivefold more complicated than standard radiotherapy treatments or that total body irradiation or the treatment of severely immunocompromised patients is vastly more complicated. However, a private practice that recently has purchased IMRT software might demand that multiples be used to show that all IMRT setups are, by definition, more complicated and deserve a high multiplier.

Pitched battles will ensue before state health care commissions as these matters are played out. Some practices will assert that they are entitled to a new linear accelerator simply because they are in a relatively geographically isolated area, and that an accelerator is necessary to "reduce patient's driving time." The reader readily can imagine that we have only touched the tip of the iceberg in this heated and somewhat unseemly debate. The issues become additionally complex when the argument is expanded into intraoperative radiotherapy units, proton machines, and dedicated radiosurgery units.

Another highly nuanced question is how many linear accelerators are required to serve a given population. Assume, for example, that you wish to serve a city of 100,000 people. The incidence of cancer is on the order of three to four newly diagnosed cases of cancer per year per 1,000 people. Thus, we would expect the city to encounter 300 to 400 new cases of cancer per year. If, on average, 60% of all patients with cancer received radiation therapy as some part of their treatment, then the city would expect to have between 180 and 240 new radiotherapy patients per year.

To see how the number of new cancer patients seen in a city per year converts to demand for linear accelerators, let's return to our hypothetical example of the linear accelerator that is supposed to provide roughly 6,000 standard treatments (single patient visit equivalents) per year. If half of the patients are seen for palliation and half for cure, then we can engage in some simple multiplication. Let's begin with 250 patients. The 125 patients who were treated for cure will receive on average, say, 35 treatments each. This results in a need for 4,375 standard treatments (single patient visit equivalents) during the course of the year. The 125 patients treated for palliation will require, on average, say, 10 treatments each. This results in 1,250 standard treatments (single patient visit equivalents) per year. Thus, to treat 250 patients, we would need a total of 5,625 standard treatments (single patient visit equivalents) per year, and we might conclude that one accelerator could serve about 250 new radiation oncology consultations per year. By this calculation, therefore, one linear accelerator should be more than adequate for our hypothetical city of 100,000 people.

As with the problem of the 6,000 standard treatments (single patient visit equivalents) per year, the assertion that one linear accelerator should be able to serve a population of 100,000 to 120,000 people can break down with a critical look at the methodology. For example, in some states in the United States, the frequency of newly diagnosed cancers is more on the order of four to five cases per thousand. In other states, it is decidedly less than three newly diagnosed cases per thousand. The presence or absence of Veterans Administration treatment facilities, state cancer hospitals, and dedicated special purpose treatment units only used for total body irradiation or radiosurgery; the need for specialized procedures; the use of single versus multiple fraction treatment of bone metastases; and patient travel and access all can create wide variation in the alleged needs for new linear accelerator units. And, of course, as in the problem of 6,000 treatments per year, money comes into play. In

the United States, with certificate of need processes, vigorous fights can ensue over who in a city should get a linear accelerator, how many they should get, and who should be prevented from having one. There are high-paid consultants and attorneys who specialize in these matters and will be more than happy, for a price, to argue either side of the viewpoint before regulatory commissions.

There is no doubt that well-trained, competent, and compassionate personnel are essential to the success of a radiation oncology department. The number of individuals required for the conduct of a clinical radiation oncology department is, however, debatable. How many physicians are necessary? Some would assert that the average practicing radiation oncologist should be able to consult with approximately 250 to 350 new cancer patients per year and have, on average, 25 to 35 patients under treatment for EBRT at any given time. Others would say that this number is too small or too large. If the radiation oncologist is devoting a significant amount of time to administrative, research, or education activities, then he or she would be expected to have fewer patients under treatment at any given time. Similarly, a medical radiation physicist is thought, by some authorities, to serve approximately 400 patients annually. Depending, however, on the considerable demands on a physicist's time engendered by an IMRT program, brachytherapy, or electron units, this may be a gross overstatement.

There clearly is a large number of other personnel required for the successful operation of a clinical radiation oncology service. These include a radiation therapist-in-chief, staff radiation therapists, nurses, transporters, dietitians, social workers, maintenance engineers, information technology specialists, receptionists, billing clerks, business managers, and secretaries. The Intersociety Council for Radiation Oncology issued guidelines in this regard (247) (Table 1.15).

The dated guidelines offered by the Intersociety Council are, as we have previously shown, highly fungible. Let's consider the case of a hospital-based radiation oncology practice in which the physician bills for professional services and the hospital collects for technical services. It is, in such arrangements, generally customary that the hospital serves as the employer of the radiation therapists, physicists, nurses, and other support personnel. It would be in the financial best interest of the physician to insist that the hospital provide large numbers of personnel. It is in the hospital's financial interest to keep the number of personnel as small as possible. To either end, the guidelines suggested above can be manipulated to either be an advantage to the position of the physician or to the position of the hospital. Discussions over staffing, therefore, become a mixture of high road considerations of QA and patient care and a more sordid discussion of money.

The extraordinary cost of some radiation therapy equipment, particularly Gamma Knifes, CyberKnifes, and particle therapy units, has prompted some creative physicians, their business managers and attorneys, and equipment manufacturers to promote the concept of "regional units." In this technique, the organizers argue that they are not building a high-technology radiotherapy unit for their own benefit. Rather, they say, they will open the unit to practitioners over a wide geographic area—as long as these practitioners meet "accreditation and qualification" standards which are, of course, established by the owner of the unit (24). Thus, the government regulatory agency can assert that it is helping to provide high-technology radiotherapy over a broad geographic area and forcing a consolidation of services (334). In practice, such arrangements sometimes work and sometimes are a carefully constructed shell game designed to allow major health care providers to buy what they want.

In some Certificate of Need decisions, the government regulatory agency is hopelessly outgunned by the lobbying of physicians and their allies in the equipment manufacturing sector. If

Table 1.15	**SUGGESTED PERSONNEL REQUIREMENTS FOR CLINICAL RADIATION THERAPY**[a]
Category	Staffing
Radiation oncologist-in-chief	One per program
Staff radiation oncologist	One additional for each 250–300 patients treated annually
Radiation physicist	One per center additional in ratio of 1 per 400 patients treated annually
Treatment planning staff Dosimetrist Physics technologist Radiation therapy technologist	One per 300 patients treated annually
Supervisor	One per center
Staff (treatment)	Two to three per megavoltage unit up to 40 patients treated daily per unit Four to six per megavoltage unit up to 60 patients treated daily per unit
Staff (simulation)	One to two per simulator
Staff (brachytherapy)	As needed
Maintenance engineer or electronics technician	One per two megavoltage units
Treatment aid	As needed
Nurse	One per center
Additional RN, LPN	One per 300 patients treated annually
Social worker	As needed
Dietitian	As needed
Physical therapist	As needed

[a]Additional personnel are required for research and education programs.
Modified from *Inter-Society Council for Radiation Oncology: Radiation oncology in integrated cancer management.* Philadelphia: American College of Radiology, 1991.

there already is a linear accelerator–based radiotherapy unit in a city, is there a need for a Gamma Knife? On the one hand, the proponents of the linear accelerator will assert its relatively low cost and the benefit that the linear accelerator is serving more than one purpose. On the other hand, the proponents of the Gamma Knife will allege that it is somehow better.

This debate will next be stretched into the debate over how many proton therapy units are needed in a country, state, region, or city. One could make an entirely plausible argument that a very few proton units are needed, in the foreseeable future, for the treatment of exotic pediatric, ocular, and CNS tumors while appropriate randomized, prospective trials are performed to see if this technology is of any value in more common tumors. The salesmen for proton units, however, will be more than happy to see a unit installed on every street corner in the absence of clinical trials and will assert, along with some physicians, that clinical trials are unnecessary in a technology that is "self-evidently" better. If the proton unit is financed by venture capitalists, and the physicians have a financial incentive to treat patients with protons, then the chance of an objective assessment of the technology declines.

It will be important, as we debate the need for new equipment in radiotherapy, to measure a variety of outcomes. It is nearly impossible to prove the benefits of simulation versus not simulating, linear accelerator versus cobalt-60, conventional treatment planning versus IMRT, or any other new technology if one focuses only on survival. In many diseases, the marginal benefit of the new technology and the relatively short duration of survival make it unlikely that one could ever show a survival benefit in a sufficiently powered study. If, on the other hand, one focuses on quality of survival (i.e., survival following treatment of lung cancer without the morbidity and societal cost of radiation-induced transverse myelitis), then it may be possible

to show the benefit of certain forms of technological innovation in specific disease (122).

In this section, we have aimed at demonstrating the principles and methodology used in determining needs for radiotherapy equipment and personnel. One hopes that, in the future, these discussions become increasingly data driven and based on time–motion studies by management engineers that are carefully conducted, carefully reviewed, and published. We fear, however, that there will be an equal amount of debate, in this venue, driven by money and power.

Legal Principles Concerning Malpractice in Radiation Oncology

A plaintiff initiates a radiation oncology malpractice lawsuit by filing papers with the court claiming that he or she was harmed by the radiation oncologist and is entitled to legal redress. The claim of malpractice must be set out in the plaintiff's *prima facie* case. This will include a statement of the facts and legal theories that establish that the plaintiff believes he or she is legally entitled to enforceable claims against the physician. There are four essential elements to a *prima facie* case of medical malpractice. They are the establishment of duty, breach, causation, and damages. To demonstrate medical malpractice, a plaintiff–patient must show that the radiation oncologist had a duty to provide nonnegligent care to the patient, that the provider breached that duty by providing negligent care, and that this breech caused the patient injury or damage (421).

To establish a *duty*, the plaintiff must have facts that demonstrate a legal relationship between the radiation oncologist and the patient. It is a basic rule of Anglo-American law that there is no duty to another person unless there is a legally recognized relationship with that person. The plaintiff–patient must demonstrate the existence of a physician–patient relationship (421).

To establish a *breach*, the patient–plaintiff must demonstrate facts that illustrate the radiation oncologist breached the legal duties implied in the physician–patient relationship or duties that would be generally imposed on members of society. The plaintiff must establish that the appropriate standard of care was violated. Although, in theory, the establishment of the standard of care and the breach of that standard are legally separate, in reality, unless there is a factual question about what the radiation oncologist actually did, the proof of the standard of care also would demonstrate the defendant's breach. Most commonly, in law, the definition of *standard of care* is how similarly qualified radiation oncologists would have managed the patient's care under the same or similar circumstances. In most medical malpractice cases, both the standard of care and the breach are established through the testimony of expert witnesses (284).

Negligence is defined as "the omission to do something which a reasonable man guided by those ordinary considerations which ordinarily regulate human affairs would do, or the doing of something which a reasonable and prudent man would not do." The person who brings a malpractice claim is asserting that he or she is owed some duty by the defendant physician and that the violation of that duty by the physician must have caused some injury. The court will make a determination concerning the propriety or impropriety of the defendant physician's performance on the basis of "the reasonable man" had he or she been in the same situation as the individual being judged. Negligence may derive from the physician's lack of training or experience. It may also result from the physician's carelessness or inadvertence (43).

To understand the concept of an expert witness, we must consider the legal doctrines of the *school of practice*, the *locality rule*, and the concept of the *qualifications of an expert*. The legal doctrine of the school of practice is designed to deal with the historic problem of the competing interests of physicians. Physicians generally do not want to testify against their colleagues, but they often are tempted to try to run their competitors out of business. Allopathic physicians were happy to label homeopathic physicians as quacks, and many medical doctors would be happy to dispute the competence of a chiropractor. To deal with the problem, the courts use the legal doctrine of the *school of practice* in which they refuse to allow physician experts to question a different school based on philosophic or psychologic beliefs (421). The school of practice rule now generally is used to differentiate physicians in the self-designated specialties (we use the term *self-designated* because few state licensing boards recognize specialties or limit physician's rights to practice the specialties in which they have been trained). The *locality rule* refers to the concept that a physician's competence should be determined by comparison with other physicians in the community or in similar neighboring communities (421). However, with the development of national standards for the practice of radiation oncology, there is no justification for rules that shelter substandard medical decision making by using an excuse that it is the norm for a given community. A radiation oncologist, for example, could not be held at fault for failing to treat a patient with an unusual or exotic technology if that technology were not available in his or her local community. However, physicians are required to inform the patients of the limitations of the available facilities and recommend prompt transfer if indicated. Failure to refer patients when a provider lacks the experience to appropriately treat may create malpractice liability. Furthermore, if a radiation oncologist does not give a patient information about the potential result associated with not seeing a subspecialist able to use a specific technology, then the initial radiation oncologist may be held liable. Physicians must recognize when a particular medical problem is beyond their capacity for diagnosis or treatment. They are responsible for obtaining timely and adequate consultations when indicated and to refer the patient to an appropriate specialist or facility whenever the requirements for the appropriate or specialized care could not be satisfied at the available facilities. The continued expansion of knowledge in radiation oncology and the increasingly specialized training of physicians make it essential that the radiation oncologist be able to recognize any limitations in their capabilities or on their ability to treat a given patient with what is perceived to be standard of care. Failure to obtain an appropriate consultation or make an appropriate referral may denote negligence (13,14,277).

Qualified experts sometimes disagree as to the standard of care. When alternative schools of thought exist, the physician defendant is entitled to be judged by the tenants of the school he or she follows. In such states, this is called the *minority practice doctrine*. With this doctrine, also called the *respectable minority rule*, the physician may show that although the course of therapy followed was not the same as other practitioners would have followed, it was one that was accepted by a respectable minority group of practitioners (421).

A problem that is increasingly facing physicians in the United States, and has evolved considerably since the previous edition of this book, has been the pressure radiation oncologists face from health maintenance organizations (HMO) and insurance companies to conform their proposed care to a predetermined regimen. Despite legislative initiatives to hold managed care organizations accountable, the radiation oncologist will, for the most part, carry a significant portion of the risk of liability in cases where the patient asserts that he or she was unable to obtain the most accurate and appropriate diagnostic and therapeutic measures. It is essential that the radiation oncologist come to his or her own conclusions about the standard of care irrespective of any pressures applied by an HMO or an insurance company. In litigation, the radiation oncologist's best defense against a claim of malpractice is if he or she can demonstrate action only in the interest of the patient, regardless of any financial consideration or bureaucratic restraint imposed by an insurance company, HMO, or any other financial consideration. If a conflict arises between the radiation oncologists recommendations for the best course of treatment and the level of care authorized by the HMO, the physician must give the best care to the patient even it if means the physician will not ultimately be compensated (242).

Radiation oncologists will, on occasion, be called on to serve as expert witnesses in malpractice cases. Physicians, trained to give opinions, may find the give and take of the court room off-putting. For an expert witness, the foremost qualifications are effective presentation and teaching ability. The radiation oncologist, serving as an expert witness, must educate the attorneys, the judge, and jury. Once there is a perception of understanding, the radiation oncologist may be able to convince the judge and jury that they can make an independent decision that his or her testimony is correct.

Both the plaintiff's attorney and the defense attorney will retain expert witnesses who will be persuaded to "take sides." The expert witness will be asked to swear, under oath, what influence the radiation dose, volume, or technique had on the risk of an ill effect of radiation therapy on normal tissue or alleged failure to control the tumor. This expert witness system troubles many physicians who feel that they can bring a dispassionate and scientific view to such cases and come to a reasonable conclusion about whether or not malpractice occurred outside the process of litigation (242). Whatever the wishes of the physician, a trial is an adversarial process. The physician is best advised, therefore, to state his or her opinion about the case frankly and not attempt to predict or handicap how a trial will turn out. The physician should do his or her best to provide an opinion and then step aside to let a system, in which he or she has little expertise or experience, run its course in the hands of the attorneys and judge. Although often frustrating and distressing, the physicians will find themselves out of their league if they attempt to act as attorney or judge.

Each physician must make a determination as to whether he or she feels comfortable participating in the legal process as an expert witness. Some radiation oncologists accept employment as expert witnesses in both plaintiffs' actions and in defense. Some only choose to participate as expert witnesses for the defendant physicians or simply wash their hands in the matter and will have nothing to do with the process. The lure of money is strong and serving as an expert witness can be quite lucrative. Each physician must, however, determine for him- or herself whether the financial compensation for serving as an expert witness outweighs the considerable difficulties and troubling aspects of the process.

It is important that radiation oncologists understand the concept in malpractice law of *res ipsa loquitur* (421). The doctrine of *res ipsa loquitur*, roughly translated as "the thing speaks for itself," is used to deal with cases in which the actual negligent act may not be proved, but it is clear that the injury was caused by negligence. In law, this doctrine was first recognized in the case of a man who was injured when a barrel rolled out of a second story window of a warehouse. The defense attorney argued that the plaintiff did not know what events preceded the barrel rolling out of the window and, therefore, it could not be proven that an employee of the warehouse was negligent. The plaintiff, however, countered that barrels do not normally fall out of second story warehouse windows. The simple fact that the barrel fell from the window and caused an injury "spoke for itself" and demonstrated that someone must have been negligent.

In medical malpractice law, *res ipsa loquitur* is used to shift the burden of proof to the defendant's position regarding causation. *Res ipsa loquitur* can be invoked if the patient suffers an injury that is not an expected complication of medical care, the injury does not normally occur unless someone has been negligent, and the defendant was responsible for the patient's well-being at the time of the injury. Examples in which this concept has been invoked include the dislocation of a patient's shoulder while aligning it for a chest x-ray, knocking out a patient's tooth while the patient was under anesthesia for a tonsillectomy, nerve injury due to a hypodermic injection, leaving a sponge in the abdomen during an operation, or fracturing a patient's jaw while extracting a tooth (421).

An *intentional tort* is an action that can result in harm to the plaintiff. The classic intentional tort in medical malpractice law is forcing unwanted medical care on a patient. Even if care clearly would benefit a patient, if that care were refused and the radiation oncologist had no state mandate to force care on the patient, but did so anyway, the patient might sue for intentional tort. The most common intentional tort is *battery*. The legal standard for a battery is "an intentional unconsented touching" (283).

Battery is not the same, in law, as *assault*. Assault is the act of putting a person in fear of bodily harm. Most battery claims against physicians are based on real attacks. However, battery claims also can be created by the circumstances of the medical treatment. The legal standard of care is that male health care providers do not examine female patients without a female attendant present. Although the standard frequently is ignored, it should not be. An attorney representing a plaintiff–patient may attempt to demonstrate that allowing an unattended examination of a female patient by a male radiation oncologist is concrete evidence that, at the very least, the physician has very poor judgment.

Of particular concern to radiation oncologists, in the realm of malpractice, is the concept of *loss of chance*. This usually is evoked in circumstances where physicians failed to diagnose a terminal illness. The loss of chance stems from the failure to diagnose in time for the patient to have a chance of cure. Not all states recognize this standard. In those states that do, however, the patient must show that the loss of chance is statistically significant (421).

It is generally viewed that any patient injured by exposure to a defective x-ray machine will be compensated as a matter of law (43). If, however, the radiation oncologists did not know or could not have reasonably been expected to know that a machine was defective they will generally not be held liable if the radiation oncologist used the machine properly (15). Radiation oncologists are bound by the usual standards of skill, knowledge, and appropriate diligence that apply to the specialists within the field.

If a patient is hypersensitive to radiation therapy, and in the absence of any reasonable way to predict this, the radiation oncologist will not be expected to predict or prevent it (17,441,559). There is, however, the possibility that the plaintiff's attorney will invoke *res ipsa loquitur* in certain circumstances (91). For example, in a patient who received radiation therapy for a benign condition and suffered a severe radiation cutaneous reaction that required bilateral amputation, the radiation oncologist was found to be negligent (536). In the employment of diagnostic radiation, minimal exposure is involved, but it is not expected that a skin reaction will be produced. Thus, if a skin reaction does ensue, many courts would infer negligence (28). If a part of the body is unintentionally irradiated and injured, liability will generally follow. For example, a patient who is undergoing radiation therapy to the head and neck was compensated when he suffered severe injury to the arms (310). A patient given radiation therapy to the ear suffered reaction of the head, face, and neck. Liability was also imposed (143). It is reasonable to expect that patients give informed consent for radiation therapy and will accept a certain risk of ill effects. This does not mean that the patient assumes a risk of negligent care (199,239).

In a case where a patient with carcinoma of the rectum was given radiation therapy at a dose above that recognized as proper and suffered severe ill effects, the radiation oncologist offered a defense that such dosage had been given in accordance with the recommendation of a recently delivered scientific paper. The court rejected this claim. In the court's view, this was not a generally accepted course or program of therapy, and the patient's specific consent to the variance in therapy had not been obtained (2).

One must be particularly cautious in dealing with women of childbearing age concerning the possibility of pregnancy before exposing her to radiation therapy. Since the fetus might be injured, producing birth defects or necessitating an abortion, the patient has a right to refuse or at least should be given the full chance of providing informed consent (443).

One must also be wary of injury through other forms of negligence involving radiation therapy. Injuries of this type include allowing the patient to fall, unstrapped, off the couch of a linear accelerator as it is being moved into the correct position, being struck by a fluoroscopic screen or other equipment from a treatment machine or a simulator, being shocked or burned, or being permitted to come in contact with high-tension electrical wires (356).

There are some data specifically concerning the types of malpractice claims brought in radiation oncology. From 1975 through 1994, a total of 18,860 malpractice suits were brought in Cook County, Illinois, naming at least one codefendant physician; 8% named a radiation oncologist as one of the defendants. The number of suits directed against radiation oncologists fell sharply in Cook County after 1982. At that time allegations that thyroid cancer in adults developed from tonsillar irradiation administered in childhood for benign disease halted when such suits proved unsuccessful. The most common complaints initiating radiation oncology suits in recent years relate to:

(a) Alleged complications of radiotherapy,
(b) Alleged administration of radiotherapy for inappropriate indications, and
(c) Alleged inappropriate withholding of radiotherapy (378).

An interesting survey of 107 radiation oncology lawsuits conducted by the Fletcher Society found that 59% of the plaintiff patients were female. The four most common organ sites involved in the suits were gynecologic (17%), breast (16%), head and neck (14%), and urologic (12%). The actuarial probability of a radiation oncologist remaining free of a lawsuit after 30 years in practice was 35% (455).

The National Association for Insurance Commissioners conducted an extensive study of medical liability claims and insurance indemnity. It was published yearly between 1977 and 1980. The final report was based on data collected from over 70,000 medical liability claims arising from over 62,000 alleged injuries or incidences that were closed with payments to the plaintiffs by insurers. These data show that 4% of paid claims were related to external-beam radiation therapy (346).

Brachytherapy as the origin of a malpractice action poses particular problems for the radiation oncologist. Brachytherapy procedures are relatively rare. Therefore, expertise is often limited and the individual experience of the practicing radiation oncologist may be minimal. The existence of postimplant films, which document the location of the radioactive material, can be used to challenge the quality of the implant procedure. Brachytherapy complications can take years to occur and, because brachytherapy is often employed in treatment of carcinoma of the prostate, cervix, and uterus, the development of fistulas in long-term survivors can often be the cause of a malpractice action.

Radiation oncologists conduct their practice with the assistance of others: physicists, dosimetrists, nurses, and therapists. It is necessary, therefore, for radiation oncologists to understand *vicarious liability*. In general, employers are responsible for the actions of their employees. This is called *respondent superior*—also called the master–servant relationship (284). The fundamental issue that determines whether a person is legally treated as an employee is the extent to which the person hiring the worker may control the details of that work. Nurses, physician assistants, radiation therapists, and other physician extenders are professionals, but in most states in which they are licensed, they generally have a limited license. The extent to which they make medical decisions is determined by state law, but they usually must work under the supervision of a practicing physician. The physician's license, however, is unlimited. The physician, for example, may perform nursing tasks without violating nursing practice laws. Injury caused by extenders may, ultimately, lead to a malpractice claim against the physician. Physician liability for the actions of hospital employees is particularly problematic for radiation oncologists. Many radiation oncologists practice in hospital-based clinics. In general, the *doctrine of the borrowed-servant* or the *captain of the ship doctrine* states that all actions of hospital employees are attributable to the patient's attending physician. Under such a doctrine, the radiation oncologist may be found liable for the actions of a nurse, dosimetrist, or radiation therapist who the physician can neither hire, fire, nor otherwise directly control (284).

When radiation oncologists are directors of clinical services, they also should be aware of the fact that they may be vicariously liable for the behavior of employees if they tolerate inappropriate activity or do not properly screen employees for dangerous tendencies. If, for example, a radiation therapist has assaulted persons in the past and the radiation oncologist was negligent in discovering this, the radiation oncologist could be held liable under the theory of negligent hiring. The radiation oncologist also could be held liable for negligent retention if there were complaints about the behavior of the radiation therapist and the physician failed to act on them (421).

The captain of the ship doctrine means that physicians may have responsibility for the mistakes of their radiation therapists, dosimetrists, physicists, nurses, and fellow practicing physicians allegedly under their supervision or control. It is, therefore, incumbent upon the responsible radiation oncologist to take care in staff selection, training, and supervision. There is a risk in delegating such matters to an office manager. Ultimately, the physician must maintain an active role in ascertaining that he or she can fully trust the person selected to assist in all aspects of patient care. This means that the radiation oncologist must protect against allegations of sexual misconduct or abuse, alcohol or drug impairment, or mental illness potentially affecting patient care since the physician is ultimately liable for the care given to a patient, the radiation oncologist must play an active role in ongoing training and professional development of his or her staff (266).

If an accident or allegation of misconduct occurs, the radiation oncologist must have a thorough, efficient, and adequate means of investigation of the matter and, if necessary, discipline or dismissal. Adequate employment records must be maintained (242).

One of the most vexing problems now facing the practicing radiation oncologist is the matter of substance and alcohol abuse in the workplace and potential criminal records of employees. Some practices are instituting mandatory preemployment screening for alcohol and drug abuse and criminal background checks. These issues, however, are extremely complicated, and it is not yet clear which drugs should be tested for, when the testing should occur, who should be evaluated for a potential criminal background, which positive criminal background checks merit a decision not to employ an individual or to dismiss the person, under what circumstances a person can be felt to have paid his or her debt to society in a way that allows the individual to practice in a health care environment, and to what extent a radiation oncologist can be held liable for failure to exercise due caution in this process. Obtaining sound advice from an expert in personnel relations and legal counsel is advisable (36).

It is well recognized that no radiation oncologist can be available at all times and in all circumstances. A physician may arrange, during his or her absence for vacation or ill health, for practice coverage by another physician. When one radiation oncologist "covers" for another, there are risks to patient safety, and possible susceptibility to malpractice claims, if clinical care "falls through the cracks." To minimize the risk of malpractice claims, the following guidelines should be followed:

- When you are away from your practice, you should select a covering radiation oncologist who possesses knowledge and skill at least equal to yours.
- Inform and obtain consent from those patients who will be affected.
- Apprise your covering physician of any important clinical information pertaining to patients he or she will see in your absence.
- The covering physician is expected to do more than just "fill in." He or she must apply the same degree of medical skill and care as the regular radiation oncologist.
- When the regular radiation oncologist returns, he or she should receive a report of any noteworthy patient care events, laboratory tests or diagnostic imaging results that deserve follow-up, and any other "loose-ends" (31).

It cannot be overemphasized that well-maintained medical records are crucial to a satisfactory legal defense in malpractice claims in radiation oncology. In law, the concept of spoliation refers to the destruction of evidence of significance or a meaningful alteration of a document. In medical malpractice cases, this would refer to the absence or disappearance of medical records. One radiation oncologist wisely counseled:

> Now and then pick up an old chart, see if you can trace all of your steps in making decisions and executing treatments. Would this chart be sufficient to defend yourself against a malpractice claim? (455)

The Nature of Grievances and Malpractice Claims in Radiation Oncology

Dissatisfied patients act in various ways. Some ignore their physician's advice, and others seek a new physician. Assertive patients may confront their physician. It is also commonplace for patients to discuss their complaints about physicians with friends and relatives.

In Anglo American law and custom, patients whose dissatisfaction prompts formal action have several options. These include bringing a malpractice claim and seeking redress in courts. Other options include filing a complaint with a government medical board; filing a complaint with the "patient relations office" of a hospital or group practice; directing a complaint to a hospital's chief of medical staff or credentials office; or submitting a grievance to the local, state, district, or national medical society. Why some dissatisfied patients do nothing and others take formal action is not well studied. The general nature of patient grievances against physicians, however, has been evaluated by several authors (211). Complaints fall into several broad categories:

- Alleged failure of physicians to fulfill the patient's expectations for examination and treatment (i.e., inadequate therapy, failure to obtain informed consent prior to a procedure, inadequate physical examination, or lack of prompt attention following hospitalization);
- Alleged failure to make a prompt diagnosis;
- Alleged rude or discourteous behavior;
- Alleged unacceptable practice behavior, such as producing excessive pain or practicing outside an area of expertise;
- Alleged inappropriate behavior related to billings and collections;
- Alleged physician's use of alcohol or drugs;
- Alleged sexual misconduct;
- Alleged errors in prescribing; and
- Alleged insurance fraud.

Formal complaints, including malpractice suits, represent only the tip of the iceberg of patient dissatisfaction. Patients far more often deal with their dissatisfaction by complaining to family and friends or switching doctors than by submitting a written complaint. A study by the Harvard Medical Practice Study Group, for example, found that <2% of patients who had adverse events because of medical malpractice ever filed malpractice claims (293). Patients pursued medical malpractice claims for a variety of reasons. The four most common include an attempt to hold the offending caregiver accountable, to seek a more complete or satisfying explanation for the adverse event, to stop similar events from occurring to other patients, and to obtain financial compensation (533).

Two episodes in the United Kingdom remind us of the problem of systematic overdose and underdose in radiation oncology. It was discovered at Exeter, in 1998, that 207 patients were given a radiation dose >25% than that generally deemed appropriate for the treatment of breast cancer. Some patients had more marked radiation reactions than appropriate. When this became known, adverse publicity appeared in the press. At Stafford ~1,000 patients received ~25% underdosing over a 20-year period. An investigation concluded that in ~500 patients there was a real possibility that underdosage may have affected the outcome of treatment and, in a small number of patients, produced a cancer recurrence higher rate than that expected (373).

The causes of these two incidents were analyzed in great detail and may have been related to inadequate medical physics staffing. A Royal College of Radiologists' survey showed that radiation oncologists in many U.K. radiotherapy departments were seeing ≥600 new patients per year as compared to the usual 250 to 300 patients seen in France, Germany, and the United States.

⠿ The RAGE Campaign

In 1991, a group of women formed an organization in the United Kingdom called RAGE (Radiation in Action Group Exposure). The campaign began when a patient developed serious brachial plexus damage following surgery and radiotherapy for breast cancer. The patient wrote a letter to several newspapers describing these events and criticizing the medical and legal processes. This produced an outpouring of concern from other patients who claimed to have suffered from the same side effects. RAGE called for significant changes in the use of radiotherapy for the treatment of breast cancer (373). The group successfully applied to the legal aid board for funds to undertake research toward a group legal action and, in 1995, constituted a group of plaintiffs in a group malpractice case. Publicity associated with the litigation prompted the Royal College of Radiology

to establish a multidisciplinary working party that made recommendations to ensure that patients with symptoms that might be due to radiation-associated brachial plexus injury had access to a network of health care professionals and cancer centers with the necessary skills for diagnosis, functional assessment, and treatment. The case highlighted the risks of high-dose per fraction radiation therapy used in the 1970s and 1980s. When the case eventually came to judgment, Justice Ebsworth concluded that there was no negligence and costs were directed against the plaintiffs. The justice commented that "it was unfortunate that litigation in turns of medical negligence was felt to be the only mechanism available," particularly in view of the fact that the cost of litigation exceeded £4 million. The case is instructive on several grounds:

1. The ill effects of radiation therapy may take a long time to become manifest.
2. Communication with patients concerning the causes and treatment of the disability is crucial.
3. The cost of litigation is quite high, and one would certainly hope that in the future society can derive alternative mechanisms to costly malpractice actions to allow patients to understand how and why injuries occur (113,270,324).

A disagreement between a patient and his or her radiation oncologist may cause the patient to have diminished trust in the physician, to be dissatisfied with the clinical results, to change physicians or health plans, to file a complaint, or to undertake litigation. For physicians, however, disagreements with patients may result in frustration, anger, a feeling of loss of control, and career dissatisfaction.

It is important to document your explanation of the risks and benefits of radiation therapy and to obtain the patient's written authorization to proceed, with a full understanding of those risks. In discussing any procedure or treatment with the patient or his or her guardian, the radiation oncologist should endeavor to explain all of the risks in sufficient detail to permit the patient to make a well-educated decision. Written informed consent should be obtained. But simply having the patient sign a standard form is not the end of the matter. The forms need to be easily understood and written in clear language. It is unwise for a physician to adopt standard printed forms without giving them proper scrutiny. Radiation oncologists must also be sure that the consent form is properly filled out. If, for example, there are blanks for explanations of particular risks involved for the procedure, they should be properly filled in (242).

It is essential that radiation oncologists use fundamental communication skills to avoid grievances and malpractice claims, understand the patient's worries and concerns, express empathy, actively discuss care options, negotiate differences of opinion, and allow time for adequate conversation. The challenge for radiation oncologists is to recognize patients' unfulfilled expectations and to engage patients in a discussion with the goal of identifying and avoiding dissatisfaction while building a trusting therapeutic relationship.

⠿ Health Insurance Portability and Accountability Act

Since the Health Insurance Portability and Accountability Act of 1996 (HIPPA) has come fully into effect, considerable changes have occurred in the area of health care fraud and abuse. This marks a change since the previous edition of this textbook. HIPPA created new criminal offenses and brought civil remedies while strengthening existing ones. More important for the practicing radiation oncologist, however, HIPPA is part of a larger political initiative in which health care fraud and abuse became a top law enforcement priority. Large numbers of civil investigations have been brought regarding alleged abuses of Medicare and Medicaid. Many physicians and organizations have been excluded from federally funded health care programs, and there have been criminal convictions and collection of large amounts of money in criminal fines (242).

Risk Management in Radiation Oncology

In an era of increasing litigation and, unfortunately, a growth in adversarial situations between physicians and patients, it is critical for the radiation oncologist and staff to make every effort to decrease professional liability risks.

The origins of medical malpractice suits include (434):

- Medical accidents that may not be adequately understood by the patient or explained by the treating physician.
- Less than successful or unexpected adverse results of treatment.
- Poor results from previous treatment elsewhere and ill-advised comments by other physicians or health care personnel.
- Rejection of a plan of therapy without appropriate documentation that the physician has advised the patient of the consequences of declining treatment. Some physicians document this discussion in the chart and send a certified letter advising the patient of the consequences of rejection of treatment.
- Complaint of experimentation when the patient has not been appropriately informed of the nature of the therapy to be administered.
- An angry patient who may find this a way to vent anger or frustration about any events surrounding treatment, including lack of communication, discourteous treatment by the physician or staff, or the amount of the medical bill.

The best prevention against a lawsuit is good rapport with the patient and relatives, effective communication and QA programs in all activities related to patient management, and clear and accurate records with documentation of all procedures, discussions, and events that take place before, during, and after treatment.

After appropriate clinical assessment, the histologic diagnosis of the patient must be confirmed at the treating institution; this includes review of outside pathologic slides. Rationale of therapy and any changes in treatment plan should be duly explained and documented in the record. All procedures performed on the patient should be recorded in the chart, including details of daily treatments, such as use of special treatment aids (i.e., wedges, immobilization devices), and any problems related to equipment operation. All treatment parameters and calculations should be accurately recorded and verified by a physicist or dosimetrist, in addition to the radiation oncologist. We should remember that, as professional liability attorneys say, "If it is not recorded on the chart, we may assume it never happened."

The physician and staff may help in their own professional liability defense in case a lawsuit occurs. It is extremely important for the physician to understand and, at an appropriate time, identify early warning signs of an impending malpractice suit. The physician should promptly contact his or her attorney, risk management office, and insurance carrier.

The physician should prepare an incident report in anticipation of potential litigation, describing all details regarding potential liability, including dates when events took place and actors and witnesses to be identified by name, affiliation, and status. Incident reports are confidential information between the physician and the attorney, risk manager, or insurance carrier. The report should be prepared while the facts are still fresh when it is likely that documentation will be optimal.

Clear and well-kept records with notes documenting every discussion and procedure that is performed on the patient should help in case of a lawsuit. A full discussion with the patient and relatives regarding planned therapy, particularly side effects of irradiation, and a well-documented informed consent form are valuable in risk management.

Informed Consent

The need to obtain informed consent for treatment is based on the patient's right to self-determination and the fiduciary relationship between the patient and physician (420). The law requires that the treating physician adequately apprise every patient of the nature of the disease requiring treatment, recommended course of therapy and details regarding it, alternative treatments available, benefits of recommended treatment, and all minor and major risks (acute and late effects) associated with the recommended therapy (Table 1.16). If the plan of therapy is modified, this should be discussed with the patient, and, if warranted, a second informed consent may be required. It is advisable to discuss the informed consent contents in the presence of a witness and have that person sign an informed consent form or the chart verifying that the information was discussed with the patient.

Informed consent is a process, not a form. A consent form documents and codifies the process but does not substitute for clear and appropriate provision of information to the patient with adequate time for questions, answers, and free discussion and exchange. Ultimately, the competent adult patient or a legal representative must agree to the treatment and give approval. For unemancipated minors or legally incompetent adults, informed consent must be signed by the parents, adult brothers or sisters, or a responsible near-relative or legal guardian. For incompetent adults, spouses may be allowed by the state to sign. Emancipated minors may provide their own consent. It is extremely important for the radiation oncologist and the staff to spend as much time as is needed to ensure that the patient and, if necessary, relatives understand all aspects of the radiation therapy, particularly the specific description of the various potential deleterious effects of this modality. Many physicians indicate which situations may require surgery to treat a complication and, specifically, when a gastrostomy, colostomy, ileal bladder, or other organ-substituting operation may be necessary to correct sequelae of therapy.

The radiation oncologist is always balancing a full disclosure of risks and options without overwhelming the patient with data and causing distress. It is reasonable to expect the patient to come away from a meeting with the treating radiation oncologist with a general realistic hope regarding the proposed course of treatment and honest understanding of the side effects, and a sense of trust for the physician and the organization (242). Good documentation is crucial and, if a malpractice action were to occur, liability may hinge on who said what to whom at what point of the treatment process. Absent or lost records will reflect extremely poorly on the radiation oncologist (242).

It must be stressed that in dealing with children or mentally incompetent adults, a thorough discussion of the plan of therapy and sequelae should be held with the parents, relatives, or legal guardian of the patient. Also, they must sign the informed consent.

Although, in case of a lawsuit, having a properly executed informed consent form in the record is helpful, more important is the incontrovertible documentation in the chart of the pertinent discussion held with the patient. Table 1.16 describes

Table 1.16	POSSIBLE SPECIFIC SEQUELAE OF THERAPY DISCUSSED IN INFORMED CONSENT	

Anatomic Site	Acute Sequelae	Late Sequelae
Brain	Earache, headache, dizziness, hair loss, erythema	Hearing loss Damage to middle or inner ear Pituitary gland dysfunction Cataract formation Brain necrosis
Head and neck	Odynophagia, dysphagia, hoarseness, xerostomia, dysgeusia, weight loss	Subcutaneous fibrosis, skin ulceration, necrosis Thyroid dysfunction Persistent hoarseness, dysphonia, xerostomia, dysgeusia Cartilage necrosis Osteoradionecrosis of mandible Delayed wound healing, fistulae Dental decay Damage to middle and inner ear Apical pulmonary fibrosis Rare: myelopathy
Lung and mediastinum or esophagus	Odynophagia, dysphagia, hoarseness, cough Pneumonitis Carditis	Progressive fibrosis of lung, dyspnea, chronic cough Esophageal stricture Rare: chronic pericarditis, myelopathy
Breast or chest wall	Odynophagia, dysphagia, hoarseness, cough Pneumonitis (asymptomatic) Carditis Cytopenia	Fibrosis, retraction of breast Lung fibrosis Arm edema Chronic endocarditis, myocardial infarction Rare: osteonecrosis of ribs
Abdomen or pelvis	Nausea, vomiting Abdominal pain, diarrhea Urinary frequency, dysuria, nocturia Cytopenia	Proctitis, sigmoiditis Rectal or sigmoid stricture Colonic perforation or obstruction Contracted bladder, urinary incontinence, hematuria (chronic cystitis) Vesicovaginal fistula Rectovaginal fistula Leg edema Scrotal edema, sexual impotency Vaginal retraction or scarring Sterilization Sexual impotence Damage to liver or kidneys
Extremities	Erythema, dry/moist desquamation	Subcutaneous fibrosis Ankylosis, edema Bone/soft-tissue necrosis

many of the specific sequelae in several anatomic sites that should be included in the informed consent. Radiation oncologists, and physicians in general, also should be aware of the recent court decisions that place a greater burden on the physician to disclose statistical life-expectancy information to critically ill patients as part of the informed consent and as an affirmation of patient-centered decision making (regarding treatment) in the context of a physician–patient relationship based on trust (12).

Smart Radiation Oncology Is Coming

Sequencing of the human genome is now complete. There are now vigorous efforts under way by government, academia, and industry to catalog specific genes and to identify the protein makeup of cells—disciplines called genomics and proteomics.

What do genomics and proteomics mean for the future of radiation oncology? Engaging in predictions is a highly risky endeavor. We think it is reasonable, however, to expect that the next 10 years will demonstrate trends toward the development of a new, more informed, smarter radiation oncology.

First, we think that there will continue to be a movement away from anatomic staging of cancer toward molecular staging. When cancer staging was first developed, it was based on whether tumors could be labeled "operable" or "inoperable." Our discipline then moved toward anatomic staging, in which an assessment of the status of the tumor was made by inspection and palpation. Typical examples of this were the Jewett system for prostate cancer or the League of Nations system for cervical cancer. Staging now has developed into a system based on physical examination, radiographic studies, and, in some cases, pathologic assessment. The most widely used system includes an assessment of tumor status (T), nodal status (N), and the presence or absence of distant metastasis (M).

There is a trend toward a more molecular-based staging of cancer in which one assesses the genetic component of an individual tumor as a predictor of outcome and as a guide toward treatment. We already are seeing evidence of this trend in the use of DNA ploidy, presence or absence of n-*myc,* the presence

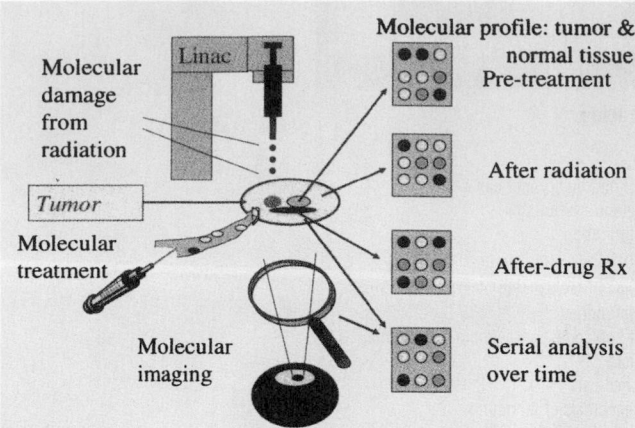

FIGURE 1.49. New developments in biotechnology will permit an analysis of how the genome or proteome of a tumor changes with treatment. This may allow researchers to identify novel therapeutic targets or find predictors of treatment outcome. The interaction between ionizing radiation and a biologic system may be thought of as a molecular event. Before, during, and after radiation gene expression profiles using microarrays may be generated. (From Coleman CN. Radiation oncology–linking technology and biology in the treatment of cancer. *Acta Oncolog* 2002;41:6–13, with permission.)

or absence of H-erb-2B, and study of subtypes of gene rearrangements in the staging of leukemias and solid tumors. With more detailed molecular staging, one will be able to more finely tailor therapy to the specific needs of the patient (555).

There will be an increasing trend toward the use of genomics and proteomics to identify high-risk patients for development of cancer. There are many cancers that have an obvious genetic basis. Population screening tests based on the presence or absence of a gene could change significantly the stage distribution of malignancies the clinician faces (145). It is hoped that screening will allow us to identify earlier cases that would be more amenable to treatment. It certainly will be preferable to have a clear-cut genetic test for the early detection of colorectal cancer, for example, rather than the cumbersome, uncomfortable, and relatively expensive use of colonoscopy.

Developments in genetics and proteomics are highly likely to modify the clinician's use of drugs and radiation (Fig. 1.49). Currently, physicians treat individuals as a statistically average person. Medications are prescribed because they are thought, on average, to bring about a certain affect in the average patient and have a known risk of side effects. It would be preferable to understand the genetic profile of the individual patient and to more precisely predict whether he or she will respond to a drug and whether he or she would be more or less likely to have side effects from the medication. Genomics offers the possibility of developing a personalized medicine in which one would match medication-prescribing practices to the specific DNA profile of an individual patient. This evolving discipline is called pharmacogenomics (145).

Predictive assays for tumor control and the risk of normal tissue complications are under active investigation. Among the hypotheses being explored are the possible correlation of gene activity promoting or inhibiting apoptosis with tumor response to radiation, the correlation of the presence or absence of tumor markers for hypoxia with the chance of local tumor control with radiation, whether skin fibroblast radiosensitivity correlates with normal tissue complication risk from radiotherapy, the possible association of transforming growth factor β-1 polymorphisms with the risk of radiation-induced normal tissue damage, the possible correlation between *in vitro* chromosomal radiosensitivity of lymphocytes and normal tissue damage following external-beam radiotherapy, the pretreatment predictive power of microarray technology for gene expression in tu-

mors, and protein expression profiling (proteomics) of tumors and normal tissue. This latter two technologies, because of their ability to measure many thousands of genes or proteins quickly, may allow the clinician of the future to obtain profiles of the tumor before, during, and after treatment, predict outcome, and, perhaps, tailor treatment according to the molecular response of the tumor (22,97,202,281,282,420,442).

Finally, we may hope to see a fine tuning of the individual patient's and his or her tumor's genome to affect therapy. Overproduction of oncogenes or inadequate production of tumor-suppressor genes might be genetically modified to place tumors into remission. Such activities are, almost certainly, far off in the future and will be enormously complex. One biotechnology executive artfully characterized the problem, as it regards the p53 tumor-suppressor gene, as follows:

> This is a gene that produces a tumor suppressor protein.... If it is under expressed [the cell] becomes cancerous. So when your p53 is lowered, the whole intelligence network of the cell is altered, and that's where cancer begins.
>
> However, researchers now have identified that if p53 is too high, that same gene produces osteoporosis, wrinkled skin, and shriveled organs—results that are linked to premature aging and a number of other diseases. A healthy human being, then, has an exact regulation of the p53 gene. There appears only to be a fine line between premature old age and cancer. It's obviously a very important gene, but we don't know much about how it works yet. (555)

One of the evolving areas in external beam radiotherapy will, undoubtedly, be the attempt to develop *dose painting* or *biologically based optimization*. These techniques strive to marry diagnostic imaging, which identifies the tumor location with metabolic imaging to show tumor activity (PET and PET/CT), along with calculations of tumor control probability, normal tissue complication probability, and uncomplicated tumor control probability. The software packages for these techniques strive to conform the radiation dose not only to the anatomic location of the tumor but to the most metabolically active areas of the tumor while, at the same time, minimizing the dose to those areas of normal tissue most likely to produce complications (379).

A new, smart form of radiation oncology offers enormous promise to the practicing clinician. An exciting age of medicine is before us. Obviously, developments in biotechnology pose formidable ethical problems that will vex the clinician. How much will be known about each individual patient's genetic makeup? How will that information be shared with the patient's family, insurance company, and employer? What protection will be built into a system in which enormous amounts of very private information will exist in electronic form? One only can hope that ethics and law will keep up with scientific progress.

References

1. Adami HO, Sparen P, Bergstrom R, et al. Increasing survival trend after cancer diagnosis in Sweden: 1960–1984. *J Natl Cancer Inst* 1989;81:1640–1674.
2. Ahern v. Veterans' Administration, 537 F 2d 1098, CCA 10 NM, 1976.
3. Ahmad K. Oopherectomy reduces cancer risk. *Lancet Oncol* 2002;3:393.
4. Alessandro R, Bicher A, Kohn E. Tumor invasion and metastases. In: Hoskins WJ, Perez CA, Young RC, eds. *Principles and practice of gynecologic oncology*, 2nd ed. Philadelphia: Lippincott-Raven, 1996.
5. Alison M, Sarraf M. *Understanding cancer: from basic science to clinical practice.* Cambridge: Cambridge University Press, 1997:37–57.
6. Allan DJ. Radiation-induced apoptosis: its role in a MADCaT (mitosis-apoptosis-differentiation-calcium toxicity) scheme of cytotoxicity mechanisms. *Int J Radiat Biol* 1992;62:145.
7. Amdur RJ, Parsons JT, Fitzgerald LT, et al. The effect of overall treatment time on local control in patients with adenocarcinoma of the prostate treated with radiation therapy. *Int J Radiat Oncol Biol Phys* 1990;19:1377–1382.
8. American College of Radiology. *Draft standards for radiation oncology, April 11, 1990.* Philadelphia: American College of Radiology, 1990.
9. American Medical Association. Report of the Council on Ethical and Judicial Affairs of the American Medical Association. Updated June 1994.
10. Andrews JR. Benefit, risk and optimization by ROC analysis in cancer radiotherapy. *Int J Radiat Oncol Biol Phys* 1985;11:1557–1562.

11. Ang KK. Accelerated fractionation: what is the price for speeding? *Radiother Oncol* 1997;44:97–99.
12. Annas GJ. Informed consent, cancer, and truth in prognosis. *N Engl J Med* 1994;330:223–225.
13. Anonymous. Duty to consult. *JAMA* 1973;226:111.
14. Anonymous. Duty to refer patient to medical specialist. *JAMA* 1968;204:281.
15. Anonymous. Radiation therapy. *JAMA* 1972;220:1807.
16. Anonymous. Report on a workshop to examine methods to arrive at risk estimates for radiation-induced cancer in the human based on laboratory data. *Radiat Res* 1993;135:434–437.
17. Antowill v. Friedman N, 188 NYS 777 NY 1921.
18. Arends MJ, Morris RG, Wyllie AH. Apoptosis: the role of the endonuclease. *Am J Pathol* 1990;136:593.
19. Auffray C, Strominger JL. Molecular genetics of the human major histocompatibility complex. *Adv Hum Genet* 1986;15:197.
20. Baclesse F. Carcinoma of the larynx. *Br J Radiol* 1949;3:1–62.
21. Baclesse F. Roentgentherapy alone in the cancer of the breast. *Acta Unio Int Contra Cancrum* 1959;15:1023–1026.
22. Barber JB, Burrill W, Spreadborough AR, et al. Relationship between in vitro chromosomal radiosensitivity of peripheral blood lymphocytes and the expression of normal tissue damage following radiotherapy for breast cancer. *Radiother Oncol* 2002;55:179–186.
23. Barkley HT, Fletcher GH. The significance of residual disease after external irradiation of squamous cell carcinoma of the oropharynx. *Radiology* 1977;124:493–495.
24. Barnett GH. Evolution and organization of a regional Gamma Knife center. *Stereotactic Funct Neurosurg* 1996;66[Suppl 1]:365–369.
25. Barsky SH, Rao CN, Williams JE, et al. Laminin molecular domains which alter metastasis in a murine model. *J Clin Invest* 1984;74:843–848.
26. Begg AC, Stewart FA, Dewit L, et al. Interactions between cisplatin and radiation in experimental rodent tumors and normal tissues. In: Hill BT, Bellamy AS, eds. *Antitumor drug-radiation interactions*. Boca Raton, FL: CRC Press, 1990;153–190.
27. Benchimol S, Lamb P, Crawford LC, et al. Transformation associated p53 protein is encoded by a gene on human chromosome 17. *Somat Cell Mol Genet* 1985;11:505.
28. Benedict SH. Immobilization, localization, and repositioning methods in stereotactic body radiation therapy. In: Kavanagh BD, Timmerman RD, eds. *Stereotactic body radiation therapy*. Philadelphia: Lippincott Williams & Wilkins, 2005;51–56.
29. Bennett CB, Lewis AL, Baldwin KK, et al. Lethality induced by a single site-specific double-strand break in a dispensable yeast plasmid. *Proc Natl Acad Sci U S A* 1993;90:5613–5617.
30. Bennett v. Los Angeles Tumor Institute 227 P 2d 473 Cal, 1951.
31. Bentel GC. *Patient positioning and immobilization in radiation oncology*. New York: McGraw-Hill, 1999.
32. Bentel GC. *Radiation therapy planning*, 2nd ed. New York: McGraw-Hill, 1996.
33. Bentzen SM. Dose-plainting by numbers. Theranostic imaging for radiation oncology. *Lancet Oncol* 2005;6:112–117.
34. Bentzen SM. Potential clinical impact of normal-tissue intrinsic radiosensitivity testing. *Radiother Oncol* 1997;43:121–131.
35. Bergonie J, Tribondeau L. Interpretation of some results of radiotherapy and an attempt at determining a logical technique of treatment. *Radiat Res* 1959;11:587–588. [Translation of original article in CR Acad Sci 1906;143:983.]
36. Berlin L. Malpractice issues in radiology: liability when covering for another radiation oncologist. *Am J Roent* 1999;172:1189–1192.
37. Bishop JM. Cellular oncogenes and retroviruses. *Ann Rev Biochem* 1983;52:301–354.
38. Bishop JM. The molecular genetics of cancer. *Science* 1987;235:305–311.
39. Bishop JM, Weinberg RA. Introduction. In: Bishop JM, Weinberg RA, eds. *Scicntific American: molecular oncology*. New York: Scientific American, 1996;1–12.
40. Bissett R, Leszczynski K, Loose S, et al. Quantitative vs. subjective portal verification using digital portal images. *Int J Radiat Oncol Biol Phys* 1996;34:489–495.
41. Bjork-Erikson T, West C, Karlsson E, et al. Tumor radiosensitivity (SF2) is a prognostic factor for local control in head and neck cancers. *Int J Radiat Oncol Biol Phys* 2000;46:13–19.
42. Blackburn S. *Think: a compelling introduction to philosophy*. Oxford: Oxford University Press, 1999.
43. Blackman NS, Bailey CP. *Liability in medical practice: A reference for physicians*. Chur, Switzerland: Harwood Academic Publishers, 1990.
44. Boente PM, Beckman M, Bast RCA. Immunology and immunotherapy of gynecologic cancers. In: Hoskins WJ, Perez CA, Young RC, eds. *Principles and practice of gynecologic oncology*, 2nd ed. Philadelphia: Lippincott-Raven, 1996.
45. Bogni A, Cheng C, Liu W, et al. Genome-wide approach to identify risk factors for therapy-related myeloid leukemia. *Leukemia* 2006;20:239–246.
46. Boveri T. *The origin of malignant tumors*. Baltimore: Williams & Wilkins, 1929.
47. Boyer TG, Lee WH. Breast cancer susceptibility genes. *Sci Med* 2002;8:138–149.
48. Bracke, ME, van Roy FM, Mareel MM. The E-cadherin/catenin complex in invasion and metastasis. *Curr Top Microbiol Immunol* 1996;213(pt 1):123.
49. Brahme A. Optimization of stationary and moving beam radiation therapy techniques. *Radiother Oncol* 1988;12:129–140.
50. Brahme A. Optimized radiation therapy based on radiobiological objectives. *Semin Radiat Oncol* 1999;9:35–47.
51. Brenner DJ, Dale R, Orton C, et al. Radiobiology of high dose-rate, low dose-rate, and pulsed dose-rate brachytherapy. In: Joslin CAF, Flynn A, Hall EJ, eds. *Principles and practice of brachytherapy: using afterloading systems*. London: Arnold, 2001:189–204.
52. Brenner DJ, Hlatky LR, Hahnfeldt PJ, et al. A convenient extension of the linear-quadratic model to include redistribution and reoxygenation. *Int J Radiat Oncol Biol Phys* 1995;32:379–390.
53. Brizel DM. Does amifostine have a role in chemoradiation treatment? *Lancet Oncol* 2003;4:378–81.
54. Brizel DM, Rosner GL, Harrelson J, et al. Pretreatment oxygenation profiles of human soft tissue sarcomas. *Int J Radiat Oncol Biol Phys* 1994;30(3):635–642.
55. Brizel DM, Scully SP, Harrelson JM, et al. Radiation therapy and hyperthermia improve the oxygenation of human soft tissue sarcomas. *Cancer Res* 1996;56:5347–5350.
56. Brizel DM, Sibley GS, Prosnitz LR, et al. Tumor hypoxia adversely affects the prognosis of carcinoma of the head and neck. *Int J Radiat Oncol Biol Phys* 1997;38(2):285–289.
57. Brown JM, Siim BG. Hypoxia-specific cytotoxins in cancer therapy. *Semin Radiat Oncol* 1996;6:22–36.
58. Buck A. Adhesion mechanisms controlling cell-cell and cell-matrix interactions during the metastatic process. In: Mendelsohn J, Howley P, Israel M, eds. *The molecular basis of cancer*. Philadelphia: W.B. Saunders Company, 1995.
59. Buffa FM, Davidson SE, Hunter RD, et al. Incorporating biologic measurements (SF(2), CFE) into a TCP model increases their prognostic significance: a study in cervical carcinoma treated with radiation therapy. *Int J Radiat Oncol Biol Phys* 2001;50:1113–1122.
60. Burcham WE, Goldhaber M. The disintegration of nitrogen by slow neutrons. *Proc Cambridge Philosophl Soc* 1936;32:632–636.
61. Burck KB, Liu ET, Larrick JW. *Oncogenes: an introduction to the concept of cancer genes*. New York: Springer-Verlag, 1988.
62. Burman C, Kutcher GJ, Emami B, et al. Fitting of normal tissue tolerance data to an analytic function. *Int J Radiat Oncol Biol Phys* 1991;21:123–135.
63. Buschke F. What is a radiotherapist?[editorial]. *Radiology* 1962;79:319–321.
64. Bush RS. The complete oncologist: the Buschke lecture. *Int J Radiat Oncol Biol Phys* 1982;8:1019–1027.
65. Cahan WG, Woodard HQ, Higinbotham ND, et al. Sarcoma arising in irradiated bone: report of eleven cases. *Cancer* 1948;1:3–29.
66. Calabresi P, Dexter DL, Heppner GA. Clinical and pharmacological implications of cancer cell differentiation and heterogeneity. *Biochem Pharmacol* 1979;28:1933–1941.
67. Calle R, Fletcher GH, Pierquin B. Le bases de la radiotherapie curative des eipthe-liomas mammaires. *J Radiol Electrol* 1973;54:929–938.
68. Cao Y. Tumor angiogenesis in therapy. *Biomed Pharmaco Ther* 2005;59[Suppl 2]:S340–S343.
69. Carde PL. Effects of cis-dichlorodiammineplatinum (II) and x-rays on mammalian cell survival. *Int J Radiat Oncol Biol Phys* 1981;7:929–933.
70. Carol MP, Targovnik H. Importance of the user in creating optimized treatment plans with Peacock. *Med Phys* 1994;21:913.
71. Castro JR, Collier JM, Potti PL, et al. Charged particle radiotherapy for lesions encircling the brain stem or spinal cord. *Int J Radiat Oncol Biol Phys* 1989;17:477–484.
72. Cater DB, Silver IA. Quantitative measurements of oxygen tension in normal tissues and in the tumours of patients before and after radiotherapy. *Acta Radiol* 1960;53:233–256.
73. Catterall M. Neutron therapy at Hammersmith Hospital 1970 to 1985: a re-examination of results. *Strahlenther Onkol* 1989;165:298–301.
74. Chadwick J. The existence of a neutron. *Proc Roy Soc London* 1932;136:692–708.
75. Chadwick J, Goldhaber M. Disintegration by slow neutrons. *Nature* 1935;135:65.
76. Chae HP, Jarvis LJ, Uckum FM. Role of tyrosine phosphorylation in radiation-induced activation of c-jun proto-oncogene in human lymphohematopoietic precursor cells. *Cancer Res* 1993;53:447–451.
77. Chang EH, Pirollo KF, Zou ZQ, et al. Oncogenes in radioresistant non-cancerous skin fibroblasts from a cancer prone family. *Science* 1987;237:1036–1039.
78. Chang F, Syrjönen S, Syrjönen K. Implications of the p53 tumor-suppressor gene in clinical oncology. *J Clin Oncol* 1995;13:1009–1022.
79. Chen GTY, Austin Seymour M, Castro JR, et al. Dose volume histograms in treatment planning evaluation of carcinoma of the pancreas. In: *International Conference on Computers in Radiation Therapy: proceedings of 8th International Conference*. IEEE Computer Press, 1984.
80. Chrest FJ, Buchholz MA, Kim YH, et al. Identification and quantitation of apoptotic cells following anti-CD3 activation of murine G0 T-cells. *Cytometry* 1993;14:883–890.
81. Chung CK, Stryker JA, O'Neill M Jr. , et al. Evaluation of adjuvant postoperative radiotherapy for lung cancer. *Int J Radiat Oncol Biol Phys* 1982;8:1877–1880.
82. Churchill Davidson I. Oxygen effect on radiosensitivity. In: *Proceedings of the Conference on Research of the Radiotherapy of Cancer*. New York: American Cancer Society, 1961.
83. Coderre JA, Morris GM. The radiation biology of boron neutron capture therapy. *Radiol Res* 1999;151:1–18.
84. Cohen L. Clinical radiation dosage. II. Interrelation of time, area and therapeutic ratio. *Br J Radiol* 1949;22:706–713.
85. Cohen L. Theoretical "iso-survival" formulae for fractionated radiation therapy. *Br J Radiol* 1968;41:522–528.
86. Coleman CN. International Conference on Translational Research and Preclinical Strategies in Radio-Oncology (ICTR): conference summary. *Int J Radiat Oncol Biol Phys* 2001;49:301–309.
87. Coleman CN, Stevenson MA. The hallmark of modern radiation oncology. *Int J Radiat Oncol Biol Phys* 1994;30:1247–1249.
88. Coleman CN. *Understanding cancer: a patient's guide to diagnosis, prognosis, and treatment*, 2nd ed. Baltimore: Johns Hopkins University Press, 2006.
89. Committee for Radiation Oncology Studies. *Criteria for radiation oncology in multidisciplinary cancer management: report to the director of the National Cancer Institute, National Institutes of Health*. Philadelphia: American College of Radiology, 1986.
90. Conger AD, Giles NH Jr. Cytogenic effect of slow neutrons. *Genetics* 1950;35:397–419.
91. Costa v. Regents of the University of California, 254 P 2d 85 Cal, 1953.
92. Costanza ME, Li FP, Finn LM, et al. Cancer prevention: strategies for practice. In: Lenhard RE Jr., Osteen RT, Gansler T, eds. *Clinical oncology*. Atlanta: American Cancer Society, 2001;75–122.
93. Coutard H. Cancer of the larynx: results of roentgen therapy after five and ten years of control. *Am J Roentgenol* 1938;40:509.
94. Coutard H. Principles of x-ray therapy of malignant diseases. *Lancet* 1934;2:1–8.
95. Coutard H. Roentgentherapy of epitheliomas of the tonsillar region, hypopharynx and larynx from 1920 to 1926. *Am J Roentgenol* 1932;28:313–331.
96. Cox JD. Fractionation: a paradigm for clinical research in radiation oncology. *Int J Radiat Oncol Biol Phys* 1987;13:1271–1281.
97. Cuddihy AR, Bristow RG. The p53 protein family and radiation sensitivity: yes of no? *Cancer Metastasis Rev* 2004;23:237–257.
98. Cunningham JR. Development of computer algorithms for radiation treatment planning. *Int J Radiat Oncol Biol Phys* 1989;16:1367–1376.
99. Cummings BJ, Keane TJ, O'Sullivan B, et al. Epidermoid anal cancer: treatment by radiation alone or by radiation and 5-fluorouracil with and without mitomycin C. *Int J Radiat Oncol Biol Phys* 1991;21:1115–1125.
100. Curie P, Curie MP, Bemont G. Sur une nouvelle substance fortement radioactive

contenue dans la pechblende (note presented by M. Becquerel). *Compt Rend Acad Sci (Paris)* 1898;127:1215–1217.
101. Dam HJW. The new marvel in photography. *McClure's Magazine* 1896;6:403.
102. Darby SC, Dall R, Gill SK, et al. Long-term mortality after a single treatment course with x-rays in patients treated for ankylosing spondylitis. *Br J Cancer* 1987;55:179–190.
103. Dawson LA, Brock KK, Kazanjania S, et al. The reproducibility of organ position using active breathing control (ABC) during liver radiotherapy. *Int J Radiat Oncol Biol Phys* 2001;51:1410–1421.
104. Dawson LA, Eccles C, Bissonnettee JP, et al. Accuracy of daily image guidance for hypofractionated liver radiotherapy with active breathing control. *Int J Rad Oncol Bio Phys* 2005;62:1247–1252.
105. Deacon J, Peckham MJ, Steel GG. The radioresponsiveness of human tumours and the initial slope of the cell survival curve. *Radiother Oncol* 1984;2:317–323.
106. Denekamp J. Changes in the rate of repopulation during multifraction irradiation of mouse skin. *Br J Radiol* 1973;46:381–387.
107. Denko NC, Giaccia AJ. Tumor hypoxia, the physiological link between Trousseau's syndrome (carcinoma-induced coagulopathy) and metastasis. *Cancer Res* 2001;61:795–798.
108. DeVita VT, Lippman M, Hubbard SM, et al. The effect of combined modality therapy on local control and survival. *Int J Radiat Oncol Biol Phys* 1986;12:487–501.
109. Dewey WC, Hopwood LE, Sapareto SA, et al. Cellular responses to combinations of hyperthermia and radiation. *Radiology* 1977;123:463–474.
110. Dewey WC, Ling CC, Meyn RE. Radiation-induced apoptosis: relevance to radiotherapy. *Int J Radiat Oncol Biol Phys* 1995;33:781–796.
111. Dische S. Chemical sensitizers for hypoxic cells: a decade of experience in clinical radiotherapy. *Radiother Oncol* 1985;3:97–115.
112. Dische S. Hyperbaric oxygen: the Medical Research Council trials and their clinical significance. *Br J Radiol* 1979;51:888–894.
113. Dische S, Joslin CA, Miller S. The RAGE litigation. *Lancet* 1998;351:1967–1968.
114. Dizdaroglu M. Measurement of radiation-induced damage in DNA at the molecular level. *Int J Radiat Biol* 1992;61:175.
115. Doll R, Peto R. *The causes of cancer: quantitative estimates of avoidable risks of cancer in the United States.* Oxford: Oxford University Press, 1981.
116. Donaldson S. Lessons from our children. *Int J Radiat Oncol Biol Phys* 1993;26:739–749.
117. Donaldson SS, Meza J, Breneman JC, et al. Results from the IRS-IV randomized trial of hyperfractionated radiotherapy in children with rhabdomyosarcoma—a report from the IRSGI. *Int J Radiat Oncol Biol Phys* 2001;51:718–728.
118. Donaldson SS, Moskowitz PS, Canty EL, et al. Combination radiation-adriamycin therapy: renoprival growth, functional and structural effects in the immature mouse. *Int J Radiat Oncol Biol Phys* 1980;6:851–859.
119. Doss LL. Localization error and local recurrence in upper airway carcinoma. *Proceedings of the Workshop on Quality Control in the Radiotherapy Department of the Cancer and Leukemia Group B (CALGB).* New York; May 31, 1979.
120. Douglas BG, Fowler JF. The effect of multiple small doses of x-rays on skin reactions in the mouse and a basic interpretation. *Radiat Res* 1976;66:401–426.
121. Dritschilo A, Piro AJ, Kelman AD. The effect of cisplatinum on the repair of radiation damage in plateau phase Chinese hamster (V-79) cells. *Int J Radiat Oncol Biol Phys* 1979;5:1345–1349.
122. Dritschilo A, Sherman D, Emami B, et al. The cost effectiveness of a radiation therapy simulator: a model for the determination of need. *Int J Rad Oncol Biol Phys* 1979;5:243–247.
123. D'Souza WD, Naqvi SA, Yu CX. Real-time intra-fraction-mation tracking using the treatment couch: a feasibility study. *Phys Med Biol* 2005;50:4021–4033.
124. Duesberg PH. Activated proto-oncogenes: Sufficient or necessary for cancer? *Science* 1985;228:669–677.
125. Duncan W. A clinical evaluation of fast neutron therapy. In: Steel GG, Adams GE, Peckham MJ, eds. *The biological basis of radiotherapy.* Amsterdam, The Netherlands: Elsevier Science BV, 1983;277–286.
126. Durand RE. The influence of microenvironmental factors on the activity of radiation and drugs. *Int J Radiat Oncol Biol Phys* 1991;20:253–258.
127. Dutreix J. Expression of the dose rate effect in clinical curietherapy. *Radiother Oncol* 1989;15:25–37.
128. Dutreix J, Wambersie A, Bounik C. Cellular recovery in human skin reactions: application to dose fraction number overall time relationship in radiotherapy. *Eur J Cancer* 1973;9:159–167.
129. Eccles C, Brock KK, Bissonette J-P, et al. Reproducibility of liver position using active breathing coordinator for live cancer radiotherapy. *Int J Radiat Oncol Biol Phys* 2006;63:751–759.
130. Eichhorn H-J, Lessel A. Four years' experiences with combined neutron-telecobalt therapy: investigations on tumor reaction of lung cancer. *Int J Radiat Oncol Biol Phys* 1977;3:277–280.
131. Eisbruch A, Kim HM, Terrell JE, et al. A. Xerostomia and its predictors following parotid-sparing irradiation of head-and-neck cancer. *Int J Radiat Oncol Biol Phys* 2001;50:695–704.
132. Elkind MM. DNA damage and cell killing: cause and effect. *Cancer* 1985;45:2123–2127.
133. Elkind MM, Sutton H. Radiation response of mammalian cells grown in culture. I. Repair of x-ray damage in surviving Chinese hamster cells. *Radiat Res* 1960;13:556–593.
134. Elliott K, Walner K, Merrick G, et al. Medical malpractice of prostate brachytherapy. *Brachytherapy* 2004;3:231–236.
135. Ellis F. Dose, time and fractionation: a clinical hypothesis. *Clin Radiol* 1969;20:1–7.
136. Ellis F. Time and dose relationships in radiation biology as applied to radiotherapy. Brookhaven National Laboratory. *BNL* 1969;50203(C-57):313.
137. Ellis F. Time, fractionation, and dose rate in radiotherapy. In: Vaeth JM, ed. *Frontiers of radiation therapy and oncology*, vol. 3. Basel, Switzerland: Karger, 1968;131–140.
138. Emami B, Lyman J, Brown A, et al. Tolerance of normal tissue to therapeutic irradiation. *Int J Radiat Oncol Biol Phys* 1991;21:109–122.
139. Emami B, Myerson RJ, Scott C, et al. Phase I/II study combination of radiotherapy and hyperthermia in patients with deep-seated malignant tumors: report of a pilot study by the Radiation Therapy Oncology Group. *Int J Radiat Oncol Biol Phys* 1991;20:73–79.
140. Emrie v. Tice, 258 P Td 332, Kans, 1953.
141. Engleman MA, Woloschak G, Small W, Jr., Radiation induced skeletal injury. *Cancer Treat Res* 2006;128:155–169.
142. Engelsman M, Rosenthal SJ, Michaud SL, et al. Intra and interfractional patient motion for a variety of immobilization devices. *Med Phys* 2005;32:3468–3474.
143. Eschwege F, Bourhis J, Girinski T, et al. Predictive assays of radiation response in patients with head and neck squamous cell carcinoma: a review of the Institute Gustave Roussy experience. *Int J Radiat Oncol Biol Phys* 1997;39:849–853.
144. Ettinghausen SE, Lipford EH III, Mule JJ, et al. Recombinant interleukin-2 stimulates in vivo proliferation of adoptively transferred lymphokine activated killer (LAK) cells. *J Immunol* 1985;135:3623–3635.
145. Ezzell C. Proteins rule. *Sci Am* 2002;286:40–47.
146. Fayos JV, Lampe I. Radiation therapy of carcinoma of the tonsillar region. *Am J Roentgenol Radium Ther Nucl Med* 1971;111:85–94.
147. Fermi E. Artificial radioactivity produced by neutron bombardment. In: Holberg MA, ed. *Les Prix Nobel in 1939.* Stockholm: Norstedt and Söner, 1939; .
148. Fertil B, Malaise EP. Inherent cellular radiosensitivity as a basic concept for human tumor radiotherapy. *Int J Radiat Oncol Biol Phys* 1981;7:621–629.
149. Fidler IJ, Hart IR. Biological diversity in metastatic neoplasms: origins and implications. *Science* 1982;217:998–1003.
150. Fisher B, Anderson S. Conservative surgery for the management of invasive and noninvasive carcinoma of the breast: NSABP trials. National Surgical Adjuvant Breast and Bowel Project. *World J Surg* 1994;18:63–69.
151. Fisher B, Redmond C, Poisson R, et al. Eight year results of a randomized clinical trial comparing total mastectomy and lumpectomy with or without irradiation in the treatment of breast cancer. *N Engl J Med* 1989;320:822–828.
152. Fletcher GH. Clinical dose-response curve of human malignant epithelial tumors. *Br J Radiol* 1973;46:1–12.
153. Fletcher GH, ed. *Textbook of radiotherapy*, 3rd ed. Philadelphia: Lea & Febiger, 1980.
154. Fletcher GH. Keynote address: the scientific basis of the present and future practice of clinical radiotherapy. *Int J Radiat Oncol Biol Phys* 1983;9:1073–1082.
155. Fletcher GH. Local results of irradiation in the primary management of localized breast cancer. *Cancer* 1972;29:545–551.
156. Fletcher GH, Shukovsky LJ. The interplay of radiocurability and tolerance in the irradiation of human cancers. *J Radiol Electrol* 1975;56:383–400.
157. Folkman J, Klagsbrun M. Angiogenic factors. *Science* 1987;235:442.
158. Folkman J, Shing Y. Angiogenesis. *J Biol Chem* 1992;267:10931–10934.
159. Folkman J. Tumor angiogenesis: therapeutic implications. *N Engl J Med* 1971;285:1182.
160. Folkman J, Watson K, Ingber D, et al. Induction of angiogenesis during the transition from hyperplasia to neoplasia. *Nature* 1989;339:58.
161. Fornace AJ Jr. Mammalian genes induced by radiation: activation of genes associated with growth control. *Annu Rev Genet* 1992;26:507–526.
162. Fowler JF. Fractionation and therapeutic gain. In: Steel GE, Adams GE, Peckham MT, eds. *Biological basis of radiotherapy.* Amsterdam, The Netherlands: Elsevier Science, 1983;181–194.
163. Fowler JF. How worthwhile are short schedules in radiotherapy? A series of exploratory calculations. *Radiother Oncol* 1990;18:165–181.
164. Fowler JF. Late normal tissue complications: new insights. *Int J Radiat Oncol Biol Phys* 1995;33:759–760.
165. Fowler JF. Rapid repopulation in radiotherapy: a debate on mechanism. The phantom of tumor treatment—continually rapid proliferation unmasked. *Radiother Oncol* 1991;22:156–158.
166. Fowler JF. Rationale for high linear energy transfer radiotherapy. In: Steel GG, Adams GE, Peckham JM, eds. *The biological basis of radiotherapy.* Amsterdam, The Netherlands: Elsevier Science, 1983;261–268.
167. Fowler JF. The linear quadratic formula and progress in fractionated radiotherapy: a review. *Br J Radiol* 1989;62:679–694.
168. Fowler JF, Denekamp J, Page AL, et al. Fractionation with x-rays and neutrons in mice: response of skin and C3H mammary tumours. *Br J Radiol* 1972;45:237–249.
169. Fraumeni JF Jr., Hoover RN, Devesą SS, et al. Epidemiology of cancer. In: DeVita VT Jr., Hellman S, Rosenberg SA, eds. *Cancer: principles and practice of oncology*, 3rd ed. Philadelphia: J.B. Lippincott, 1989;196–235.
170. Frei E III. What's in a name: neoadjuvant. *J Natl Cancer Inst* 1989;80:1088–1089.
171. Friedman M, Friedland GW. *Medicine's 10 greatest discoveries.* New Haven, CT: Yale University Press, 1998.
172. Friend SH, Dryja TP, Weinberg RA. Oncogenes and tumor-suppressing genes. *N Engl J Med* 1988;318:618–622.
173. Fritz P, Kraus HJ, Dolken W, et al. Technical note: gold marker implants and high-frequency jet ventilation for stereotactic, single-dose irradiation of liver tumors. *Technol Cancer Res Treat* 2006;5:9–14.
174. Fry SA. Studies of US radium dial workers: an epidemiological classic. *Radiat Res* 1998;150:521–529.
175. Fu KK. Interactions of chemotherapeutic agents and radiation. In: Meyer JL, Vaeth JM, eds. *Frontiers of radiation therapy and oncology, radiotherapy/chemotherapy interactions in cancer therapy*, vol. 26. Basel, Switzerland: Karger, 1992;16–30.
176. Fuks Z, Alfieri A, Haimovitz-Friedman A, et al. Intravenous basic fibroblast growth factor protects the lung but not mediastinal organs against radiation-induced apoptosis. *Cancer J Sci Am* 1995;1:62–72.
177. Fuks Z, Weischselbaum RR. Radiation therapy. In: Mendelsohn J, Howley PM, Israel MA, et al., eds. *The molecular basis of cancer.* Philadelphia: W.B. Saunders, 1995;404–431.
178. Galvin JM, Chen X-G, Smith RM. Combining multileaf fields to modulate fluence distributions. *Int J Radiat Oncol Biol Phys* 1993;27:697–705.
179. Geara FB, Peters LJ, Ang KK. Comparison between normal tissue reactions and local tumor control in head and neck cancer patients treated by definitive radiotherapy. *Int J Radiat Oncol Biol Phys* 1996;35:455–462.
180. Ghossein A, Bataini JP, Ennuyer A, et al. Local control and site of failure in radically irradiated supraglottic laryngeal cancer. *Radiol* 1974;112:187–192.
181. Giancotti FG, Ruoslahti E. Integrin signaling. *Science* 1999;285:1028.
182. Glasser O. *Dr. W.C. Röntgen.* Springfield: Charles C. Thomas, 1945.
183. Glasser O. *Wilhelm Conrad Röntgen and the early history of the Roentgen rays.* Springfield: Charles C. Thomas, 1934.
184. Glatstein E. Dr. Strange (high) tech or how I learned to stop worrying and love my MLC/3D treatment planning, stereotactic LINAC. *Int J Radiat Oncol Biol Phys* 1999;45:1097–1101.
185. Glucksmann A. Preliminary observations on the quantitative examination of human biopsy material taken from irradiated carcinomata. *Br J Radiol* 1941;14:187–198.

186. Glicksman AS, Chu FCH. Organ and functional preservation in the management of cancer: editorial introduction. *Cancer Invest* 1995;13:55–56.
187. Godwin AK, Schultz DC, Hamilton TC, et al. Oncogenes. In: Hoskins WJ, Perez CA, Young RC, eds. *Principles and practice of gynecologic oncology*, 2nd ed. Philadelphia: Lippincott-Raven, 1996; .
188. Goitein M, Abrams M. Multi-dimensional treatment planning. I. Delineation of anatomy. *Int J Radiat Oncol Biol Phys* 1983;9:777–787.
189. Goitein M. Computed tomography in planning radiation therapy. *Int J Radiat Oncol Biol Phys* 1979;5:445–447.
190. Goitein M. The comparison of treatment plans. *Semin Radiat Oncol* 1992;2:246–256.
191. Gore v. Brockman, 119 SW 1082, Mo 1909.
192. Graham ML, Cheng AY, Geer LY, et al. A method to analyze 2-dimensional daily radiotherapy portal images from an on-line imaging system. *Int J Radiat Oncol Biol Phys* 1991;20:613–619.
193. Graham ML, Purdy JA, Emami B, et al. Preliminary results of a prospective trial using three-dimensional radiotherapy for lung cancer. *Int J Radiat Oncol Biol Phys* 1995;33:993–1000.
194. Gray LH. Oxygenation in radiotherapy. I. radiobiological considerations. *Br J Radiol* 1957;30:403–406.
195. Greene FL, Page DL, Fleming ID. *AJCC cancer staging manual*, 6th ed. New York: Springer-Verlag, 2002.
196. Greenwald P, Nixon DW, Malone WF, et al. Concepts in cancer chemoprevention research. *Cancer* 1990;65:1483–1490.
197. Griffin TW, Pajak TF, Laramore GE, et al. Neutron vs. photon irradiation of inoperable salivary gland tumors: results of an RTOG-MRC cooperative study. *Int J Radiat Oncol Biol Phys* 1988;15:1085–1090.
198. Griffin TW, Pajak TF, Maor MH, et al. Mixed neutron/photon irradiation of unresectable squamous cell carcinomas of the head and neck: the final report of a randomized cooperative trial. *Int J Radiat Oncol Biol Phys* 1989;17:959–965.
199. Gross v. Robinson, 218 SW 924, Mo, 1920.
200. Gunderson LL. Combined treatment approaches in the management of rectal cancer. *Rec Results Cancer Res* 1988;110:119–129.
201. Haffty BG, Harrold E, Khan AJ, et al. Outcome of conservatively managed early-onset breast cancer by BRCA 1/2 status. *Lancet* 2002;359:1471–1477.
202. Haikonen J, Rantanen V, Pekkola K, et al. Does skin fibroblast radiosensitivity predict squamous cancer cell radiosensitivity of the same individual? *Int J Cancer* 2003;103:784–788.
203. Hall EJ. ASTRO Gold Medal: the function of a radiologist is to make the clinician think. *Int J Radiat Oncol Biol Phys* 1994;30:891–892.
204. Hall EJ. Dose-rate considerations. In: Hilaris BS, Batata MA, eds. *Brachytherapy oncology—1983*. New York: Memorial Sloan-Kettering Cancer Center, 1983;33–39.
205. Hall EJ. Intensity modulated radiation therapy, protons, and the risk of second cancers. *Int J Rad Oncol Biol Phys* 2006.
206. Hall EJ. Molecular biology in radiation therapy: the potential impact of recombinant technology on clinical practice. *Int J Radiat Oncol Biol Phys* 1994;30:1019–1028.
207. Hall EJ. *Radiobiology for the radiologist*, 5th ed. Philadelphia: Lippincott Williams & Wilkins, 2000.
208. Hall EJ, Brenner DJ. The dose-rate effect revisited: radiobiological considerations of the importance in radiotherapy. *Int J Radiat Oncol Biol Phys* 1991;21:1403–1414.
209. Hall EJ, Wuu CS. Radiation-induced second cancers: the impact of 3D-CRT and IMRT. *Int J Radiat Oncol Biol Phys* 2003;56:83–88.
210. Hallahan DE, Beckett MA, Kufe DW, et al. The interaction between recombinant human tumor necrosis factor and radiation in 13 human tumor cell lines. *Int J Radiat Oncol Biol Phys* 1990;19:69–74.
211. Halperin EC. Formal grievances directed against physicians. *Western Med J* 2000;173:235–238.
212. Halperin EC. Historical review: particle therapy for cancer. *Lancet Oncol* 2006;7:676–685.
213. Halperin EC. The right verb. *Int J Radiat Oncol Biol Phys* 1987;13:143.
214. Halperin EC, Constine LS, Kun LE, et al. Chapter 22. *Pediatric radiation oncology*, 4th ed. Philadelphia: Lippincott Williams & Wilkins, 2004.
215. Halperin EC, Laurie F, Fitzgerald TJ. An evaluation of the relationship between the quality of prophylactic cranial radiotherapy in childhood acute leukemia and institutional experience: a quality assurance review center-pediatric oncology group study. *Int J Radiat Oncol Biol Phys* 2002;53(4):1001–1004.
216. Hanford HA, Wong CA, Kassan H, et al. Angiostatin 4,5-mediated apoptosis of vascular endothelial cells. *Cancer Res* 2003;63:4275–4280.
217. Hanks GE, Diamond JJ, Krall JM, et al. A ten-year follow-up of 682 patients treated for prostate cancer with radiation therapy in the United States. *Int J Radiat Oncol Biol Phys* 1987;13:499–505.
218. Hanks GE, Hanlon AL, Pinover WH, et al. Survival advantage for prostate cancer patients treated with high-dose three-dimensional conformal radiotherapy. *Cancer J Sci Am* 1999;5:152–158.
219. Hanks GE, Kinzie JJ, White RL, et al. Patterns of Care outcome studies: results of the national practice in Hodgkin's disease. *Cancer* 1983;51:569–573.
220. Hanks GE, Lee WR, Schultheiss TE. Clinical and biochemical evidence of control of prostate cancer at 5 years after external beam radiation. *J Urol* 1995;154:456–459.
221. Harling OK, Zamenhof RG, Yanch JC, et al. Boron neutron capture and radiation synovectomy research at the MIT research reactor. *J Nucl Sci Engin* 1992;110:330.
222. Harris H, Miller OJ, Klein G, et al. Suppression of malignancy by cell fusion. *Nature* 1969;223:363.
223. Hartwell LH, Kastan MB. Cell cycle control and cancer. *Science* 1994;266:1821–1828.
224. Haselow RE, Nesbit M, Dehner LP, et al. Second neoplasms following megavoltage radiation in a pediatric population. *Cancer* 1978;42:1185–1191.
225. Hawthorne MF. New horizons for therapy based on the boron neutron capture reaction. *Molec Med Today* 1998;4:174–181.
226. Hellman S. Reanalysis of a trial comparing total mastectomy with lumpectomy. *N Engl J Med* 1996;334:989.
227. Hellman S. Roentgen Centennial Lecture: discovering the past, inventing the future. *Int J Radiat Oncol Biol Phys* 1996;35:15–20.
228. Hellman S, Vokes EE. Advancing current treatments for cancer. *Sci Am* 1996;275:118–123.
229. Hellman S, Weichselbaum RR. Radiation oncology. *JAMA* 1996;275:1852–1853.
230. Hellman S, Weichselbaum RR. Radiation oncology and the new biology. *Cancer J Sci Am* 1995;1:174–179.
231. Hendrickson FR. Four P's of human error in treatment delivery. *Int J Radiat Oncol Biol Phys* 1978;4:913–914.
232. Henk JM, Smith CW. Radiotherapy and hyperbaric oxygen in head and neck cancer. *Lancet* 1977;1:104–105.
233. Herring DF. The consequences of dose response curves for tumor control and normal tissue injury on the precision necessary in patient management. *Laryngoscope* 1975;85:1112.
234. Hicklin DJ, Ferrone S. HLA class I antigen loss in cancer. *Sci Med* 2002;8:86–95.
235. Hirst DG. Anemia: a problem or an opportunity in radiotherapy. *Int J Radiat Oncol Biol Phys* 1986;12:2009–2017.
236. Höckel M, Knoop C, Schlenger K, et al. Intratumor pO2 predicts survival in advanced cancer of the uterine cervix. *Radiother Oncol* 1993;26:45–50.
237. Höckel M, Schlenger K, Mitze M, et al. Hypoxia and radiation response in human tumors. *Semin Radiat Oncol* 1966;6:3–9.
238. Hoeckel M, Vaupel P. Biological consequences of tumor hypoxia. *Semin Oncol* 2001;28:36–41.
239. Holland v. Sisters of St. Joseph of Peace, 552 P Td 208, Ore 1974.
240. Holmgren J, ed. *Tumor marker antigens*. Goteborg, Sweden: Studentlitteratur, 1985.
241. Hoppe RT, ed. *Patterns of care process study newsletter (Hodgkin's disease), 1990–1991*. Philadelphia: American College of Radiology, 1991.
242. Horn III C, Caldwell DH Jr., Osborn DC. *Law for physicians: an overview of medical legal issues*. Chicago: American Medical Association, 2002.
243. Humphreys M, Guerrero Urbano MT, Mubata C, et al. Assessment of a customized immobilization system for head and neck IMRT using electronic portal imaging. *Radiother Oncol* 2005;77:39–44.
244. Huvos AG, Woodard HQ, Cahan WG, et al. Postradiation osteogenic sarcoma of bone and soft tissue. *Cancer* 1985;55:1244–1255.
245. International Commission of Radiation Units. Determination of absorbed dose in a patient irradiated by beams of x- or gamma rays. In: *Radiotherapy procedures, ICRU Report 24*. Washington, DC: International Commission of Radiation Units and Measurements, 1976.
246. International Commission on Radiation Units and Measurements. Prescribing, recording, and reporting photon beam therapy: ICRU Report 50. Bethesda, MD: International Commission of Radiation Units and Measurements, 1993.
247. Inter-Society Council for Radiation Oncology. *Radiation oncology in integrated cancer management*. Philadelphia: American College of Radiology, December 1991.
248. Jackson A, Kutcher GJ, Yorke ED. Probability of radiation-induced complications for normal tissues with parallel architecture subject to non-uniform irradiation. *Med Phys* 1993;20:613–625.
249. Jacobs AJ, Faris C, Perez CA, et al. Short-term persistence of carcinoma of the uterine cervix following radiation: an indicator of long-term prognosis. *Cancer* 1986;57:944–950.
250. Jain NL, Kahn MG. Ranking radiotherapy treatment plans using decision-analytic and heuristic techniques. *Comp Biochem Res* 1992;25:374–383.
251. Jefford M, Marashovsky E, Cabon J, et al. The use of dendrite cells in cancer therapy. *Lancet Oncol* 2001;2:343–353.
252. Johnson CR, Silverman LN, Clay LB, et al. Radiotherapeutic management of bulky cervical lymphadenopathy in squamous cell carcinoma of the head and neck: is postradiotherapy neck dissection necessary? *Radiat Oncol Invest* 1998;6:52–57.
253. Johnson RJR. Gynecological cancer treated with cobalt under hyperbaric conditions. First Annual San Francisco Cancer Symposium. 1966:185–194.
254. Jung M, Dritschillo A. NF-kappa B signaling pathway as a target for human tumor radiosensitization. *Semin Rad Oncol* 2001;11:346–351.
255. Kaanders JH, Bussink J, van der Kogel AJ. Clinical studies of hypoxia modification in radiotherapy. *Semin Radiat Oncol* 2004;14:233–240.
256. Kaanders JH, Wijffels KI, Marres HA, et al. Pimonidazole binding and tumor vascularity predict for treatment outcome in head and neck cancer. *Cancer Res* 2002;62:7066–7074.
257. Kagan AR. Malpractice in radiation oncology: redefining the role of the medical expert. *IJROBP* 2005;61:638–639.
258. Kaplan HS. Historic milestones in radiobiology and radiation therapy. *Semin Oncol* 1979;6(4).
259. Kaplan HS. Radiobiology's contribution to radiotherapy: promise or mirage? Failla Memorial Lecture. *Radiat Res* 1970;43:460–476.
260. Kaufman DS, Winter KA, Shipley WU, et al. The initial results in muscle-invading bladder cancer of RTOG 95–06: phase I/II trial of transurethral surgery plus radiation therapy with concurrent cisplatin and 5-fluorouracil followed by selective bladder preservation or cystectomy depending on the initial response. *Oncologist* 2000;5:417–476.
261. Kelland LR, Steel GG. Inhibition of recovery from damage induced by ionizing radiation in mammalian cells. *Radiother Oncol* 1988;13:285–299.
262. Kerr JFR, Harmon BV. Definition and incidence of apoptosis: an historical perspective. In: Tomei LD, Cope FO, eds. *Apoptosis: the molecular basis of cell death*. Cold Spring Harbor, NY: Cold Spring Harbor Laboratory Press, 1991;5.
263. Kerr JFR, Wyllie AH, Currie AR. Apoptosis: a basic biological phenomenon with wide-ranging implications in tissue kinetics. *Br J Cancer* 1972;26:239–257.
264. Knudson AG Jr. Mutation and cancer: statistical study of retinoblastoma. *Proc Natl Acad Sci U S A* 1971;68:820–823.
265. Kohn HI, Fry RJM. Radiation carcinogenesis. *N Engl J Med* 1984;310:504–511.
266. Kopf AW. Prevention and early detection of skin cancer: melanoma. *Cancer* 1988;62:1791.
267. Korbelik M, Skov KA. Inactivation of hypoxic cells by cisplatin and radiation at clinically relevant doses. *Radiat Res* 1989;119:145–156.
268. Kreyberg L, et al. *A symposium on cancer given at the Institute on Cancer conducted at the Medical School of the University of Wisconsin*. Madison: University of Wisconsin Press, 1938.
269. Kronig S, Friedrich W. *Physikalische und biologische Grundlagen der Strahlentherapie*. Sonderbtrband der Strahlentherapie, 1918.
270. Kunkler I. Recommendations after the RAGE litigation. *Lancet* 1998;352:657. Breast radiation injury litigation and RAGE *Clin Oncol R Col Radiol* 1999;11:138–139.
271. Kwok TT, Sutherland RM. Enhancement of sensitivity of human squamous carcinoma cells to radiation by epidermal growth factor. *J Natl Cancer Inst* 1989;81:1020–1024.

272. Kyprianou N, English HF, Isaacs JT. Programmed cell death during regression of PC-82 human prostate cancer following androgen ablation. *Cancer Res* 1990;50:3748.
273. Land H, Parada LF, Weinberg RA. Cellular oncogenes and multistep carcinogenesis. *Science* 1983;222:771–778.
274. Laramore GE. The use of neutrons in cancer therapy: a historical perspective through the modern era. *Semin Oncol* 1997;24:672–686.
275. Laramore GE, Krall JM, Griffin TW, et al. Neutron versus photon irradiation for unresectable salivary gland tumors: final report of an RTOG-MRC randomized clinical trial. *Int J Radiat Oncol Biol Phys* 1993;27:235–240.
276. Laramore GE, Krall JM, Thomas FJ, et al. Fast neutron radiotherapy for locally advanced prostate cancer: final report of a Radiation Therapy Oncology Group randomized clinical trial. *Am J Clin Oncol* 1993;16:164–167.
277. Largess v. Tatem, 291 A 2d 398, Vt 1972.
278. Lawrence TS, Maybaum J. Fluoropyrimidines as radiation sensitizers. *Semin Radiat Oncol* 1993;3:20–28.
279. Lawrence TS, Tesser RJ, Ten Haken RK. An application of dose-volume histograms to treatment of intrahepatic malignancies with radiation therapy. *Int J Radiat Oncol Biol Phys* 1990;19:1041–1047.
280. Lee SP, Leu MY, Smathers JB, et al. Biologically effective dose distribution based on the linear quadratic model and its clinical relevance. *Int J Radiat Oncol Biol Phys* 1995;33:372–389.
281. Leonard CL. The röntgen rays as a palliative in the treatment of cancer. *Amer Med* 1903;6:854–855.
282. Levine AJ. Tumor suppressor genes. In: Mendelsohn J, Howley PM, Israel MA, et al., eds. *The molecular basis of cancer.* Philadelphia: W.B. Saunders, 1995;86–104.
283. Li CY, Shan S, Huang Q, et al. Initial stages of tumor cell-induced angiogenesis: evaluation via skin window chambers in rodent models. *J Natl Cancer Inst* 2000;92(2):143–147.
284. Liang BA. *Health law and policy: a survival guide to medicolegal issues for practitioners.* Boston: Butterworth Heinemann, 2000.
285. Lichter AS, Lawrence TS. Recent advances in radiation oncology. *N Engl J Med* 1995;332:371–379.
286. Lindegaard JC, Overgaard J, Bentzen SM, et al. Is there a radiobiological basis for improving the treatment of advanced stage cervical cancer? *J Natl Cancer Inst Monogr* 1996;21:105–112.
287. Liotta LA. Gene products which play a role in cancer invasion and metastasis. *Breast Cancer Res Treat* 1988;11:113–124.
288. Liotta LA. Tumor invasion and metastases: role of the extracellular matrix: Rhoads Memorial Award Lecture. *Cancer Res* 1986;46:1–7.
289. Liotta LA, Mandler R, Murano G, et al. Tumor cell autocrine motility factor. *Proc Natl Acad Sci U S A* 1986;83:3302–3306.
290. Liotta LA, Thorgeirsson UP, Garbisa SL. Role of collagenases in tumor cell invasion.
291. Little MP. Cancer after exposure to radiation in the course of treatment for benign and malignant disease. *Lancet Oncol* 2001;2:212–220.
292. Liu K, Moss D, Persky V. Dietary cholesterol, fat, and fibre, and colon-cancer mortality. *Lancet* 1979;2:782.
293. Localio AR, Lawthers AG, Brennan TA, et al. Relation between malpractice claims and adverse events due to negligence: results of the Harvard Medical Practice study III. *N Engl J Med* 1991;325:245–251.
294. Locher GL. Biologic effects and therapeutic possibilities of neutrons. *Am J Roentgenol* 1936;36:1.
295. Lovelock DM, Hua C, Wang P, et al. Accurate setup of paraspinal patients using a noninvasive patient immobilization cradle and portal imaging. *Med Phys* 2005;32:2606–2614.
296. Lyon JL, Gardner JW, West DW. Cancer incidence in Mormons and non-Mormons in Utah during 1967–75. *J Natl Cancer Inst* 1980;65:1055.
297. MacComb WS, Quimby EH. The rate of recovery of human skin from the effects of hard or soft roentgen rays or gamma rays. *Radiology* 1936;27:196–207.
298. Maciejewski B, Withers HR, Taylor JMG, et al. Dose fractionation and regeneration in radiotherapy for cancer of the oral cavity and oropharynx. II. Normal tissue responses: acute and late effects. *Int J Radiat Oncol Biol Phys* 1990;18:101–111.
299. Mackay RI, Hendry JH. The modelled benefits of individualizing radiotherapy patients' dose using cellular radiosensitivity assays with inherent variability. *Radiother Oncol* 1999;50:67–75.
300. Mackie TR, Balog J, Ruchala K, et al. Homography. *Semin Radiat Oncol* 1999;9:108–117.
301. MacLennen R, Jensen OM, Mosbech J, et al. Diet, transit time, stool weight, and colon cancer in two Scandinavian populations. *Am J Clin Nutr* 1978;31[Suppl]:239.
302. Mak AC, Morrison WH, Garden AS, et al. Base-of-tongue carcinoma: treatment results using concomitant boost radiotherapy. *Int J Radiat Oncol Biol Phys* 1995;33:289–296.
303. Malkin A. Tumor markers. In: Tannock IF, Hill RP, eds. *The basic science of oncology*, 2nd ed. New York: McGraw Hill, 1992;196–206.
304. Malkin D, Li FP, Strong LC, et al. Germ line p53 mutations in a familial syndrome of breast cancer, sarcomas, and other neoplasms. *Science* 1990;250:1233–1238.
305. Marcus RB Jr. , Million RR. The incidence of myelitis after irradiation of the cervical spinal cord. *Int J Radiat Oncol Biol Phys* 1990;19:3–8.
306. Marks JE, Haus AG. The effect of immobilization on localization errors in the radiotherapy of head and neck cancer. *Clin Radiol* 1976;27:175–177.
307. Marks JE, Haus AG, Sutton HG, et al. Localization error in the radiotherapy of Hodgkin's disease and malignant lymphoma with extended mantle fields. *Cancer* 1974;34:83–90.
308. Marks LB. The impact of organ structure on radiation response. *Int J Radiat Oncol Biol Phys* 1996;34:1165–1171.
309. Martin GS. Normal cells and cancer cells In: Bishop JM, Weinberg RA, eds. *Scientific American: molecular oncology.* New York: Scientific American, 1996;13–40.
310. Martin v. Eschelman, 33 SW 2d 827 Tex, 1930.
311. Martin v. Stratton, 515 P 2D 1366, Okla, 1973.
312. Mayne ST, Lippman SM. Cancer prevention; diet and chemopreventive agents: retinoids, carotenoids, and micronutrients. In: DeVita VT Jr., Hellman S, Rosenberg SA, eds. *Cancer: principles and practice of oncology*, 6th ed. Philadelphia: Lippincott Williams & Wilkins, 2001;575–589.
313. McCarthy M. Advances highlighted at US cancer meeting. *Lancet* 2002;359:1835.
314. McCaughan JS Jr. Overview of experience with photodynamic therapy for malignancy in 192 patients. *Photochem Photobiol* 1987;46:903–909.
315. McCunniff AJ, Laing MJ. Radiation tolerance of the cervical spinal cord. *Int J Radiat Oncol Biol Phys* 1989;16:675–678.
316. McLaughlin JR, Boyd NF. Epidemiology of cancer. In: Tannock IF, Hill RP, eds. *The basic science of oncology*, 3rd ed. New York: McGraw-Hill, 1998:6–25.
317. McShan DL, Fraass BA, Lichter AS. Full integration of the beam's eye view concept into computerized treatment planning. *Int J Radiat Oncol Biol Phys* 1990;18:1485–1494.
318. Mendelsohn ML. Radiotherapy and tolerance. In: Vaeth JM, ed. *Frontiers of radiation therapy and oncology.* Baltimore: University Park Press, 1972;512–528.
319. Mendelsohn ML. The biology of dose-limiting tissues. In: *Time and dose relationships in radiation biology as applied to radiotherapy. Brookhaven National Laboratory (BNL) Report 5023 (C-57).* Upton, NY: Brookhaven National Laboratory, 1969;154–173.
320. Mendenhall WM, Million RR, Cassisi NJ. Elective neck irradiation in squamous cell carcinoma of the head and neck. *Head Neck Surg* 1980;3:15–20.
321. Meoz-Mendez RT, Fletcher GH, Guillamondegui OM, et al. Analysis of the results of irradiation in the treatment of squamous cell carcinomas of the pharyngeal walls. *Int J Radiat Oncol Biol Phys* 1978;4:579–585.
322. Michalski JM, Wong JW, Gerber RL, et al. The use of on-line image verification to estimate the variation in radiation therapy dose delivery. *Int J Radiat Oncol Biol Phys* 1978;27:707–716.
323. Miescher G. Erfolge der karzinombehandlung an der Dermatologischen Klinik Zurich. Einzeitige Hochstdosis and Fraktionierte Behandlung. *Strahlentherapie* 1934;49:65–81.
324. Millington J. Breast radiation injury litigation and RAGE. *Clin Oncol (R Col Radiol)* 1999;11:137–138.
325. Million RR. The larynx . . . so to speak: everything I wanted to know about laryngeal cancer I learned in the last 32 years. *Int J Radiat Oncol Biol Phys* 1992;23:691–704.
326. Minden MD. Oncogenes. In: Tannock IF, Hill RP, eds. *The basic science of oncology.* New York: Pergamon, 1987;72–88.
327. Minden MD, Pauson AJ. Oncogenes. In: Tannock IF, Hill RP, eds. *The basic science of oncology*, 2nd ed. New York: McGraw Hill, 1992;61–87.
328. Moench HC, Phillips TL. Carcinoma of the nasopharynx: review of 146 patients with emphasis on radiation dose and time factors. *Am J Surg* 1982;124:515–518.
329. Mohan MJ, Seaton T, Mitchell J, et al. The tumor necrosis factor-alpha converting enzyme (TACE). A unique metalloprotein are with highly defined substrate selectivity. *Biochemistry* 2002;41:9462–9469.
330. Mohan R, Wang Z, Jackson A, et al. The potential and limitations of the inverse radiotherapy technique. *Radiother Oncol* 1994;32:232–248.
331. Mohan R, Wu Q, Manning M, et al. Radiobiological considerations in the design of fractionation strategies for intensity-modulated radiation therapy of head and neck cancers. *Int J Radiat Oncol Biol Phys* 2000;46:619–630.
332. Mohan R, Wu Q, Niemierko A, et al. Optimization of IMRT plans based on biologically equivalent uniform dose. In: Proceedings of Sixth International Conference on Dose, Time and Fractionation in Radiation Oncology. *Biological and physical basis of IMRT and tomotherapy.* Madison, WI: Medical Physics Publishing, 2001.
333. Montana GS, Fowler WC, Varia MA, et al. Carcinoma of the cervix, stage III: results of radiation therapy. *Cancer* 1986;57:148–154.
334. Moore JC Jr. Device truce in St. Louis: hospital must cooperate to get a single Gamma Knife. *Mod Healthc* 1997;27:28–29.
335. Moran JM, Elshaikh MA, Lawrence TS. Radiotherapy: what can be achieved by technical improvements in dose delivery? *Lancet Oncol* 2005;6:51–58.
336. Morris MJ, Reuter VE, Kelly WK, et al. HER-2 profiling and targeting in prostate carcinoma. *Cancer* 2002;94:980–986.
337. Morris MJ, Scher HL. Novel strategies and therapeutics for the treatment of prostate carcinoma. *Cancer* 2000;89:1329–1348.
338. Morris MM, Schmidt-Ullrich R, Johnson CR. Advances in radiotherapy for carcinoma of the head and neck. *Surg Oncol Clin North Am* 2000;9:563–575.
339. Moss WT, Brand WN, Battifora H, eds. *Radiation oncology: rationale, techniques, results*, 5th ed. St. Louis: C.V. Mosby, 1979;24–25.
340. Muggia FM. Primary chemotherapy: concepts and issues. In: Wagedner DJJ, Blijham GH, Smeets JBG, et al., eds. *Primary chemotherapy in cancer medicine.* New York: Alan R Liss, 1985;377–383.
341. Munro TR. The relative radiosensitivity of the nucleus and the cytoplasm of the Chinese hamster fibroblast. *Radiat Res* 1990;42:451.
342. Murakami MS, Strobel LMC, Vande Woude GF. Cell cycle regulation, oncogenes, and antineoplastic drugs. In: Mendelsohn J, Howley PM, Israel MA, et al., eds. *The molecular basis of cancer.* Philadelphia: W.B. Saunders, 1995;3–17.
343. Murray AW. Creative blocks: cell-cycle checkpoints and feedback controls. *Nature* 1992;359:599–604.
344. Nagel T. *What does it all mean? A very short introduction to philosophy.* New York: Oxford University Press, 1987.
345. Narod S. What options for treatment of hereditary breast cancer? *Lancet* 2002;359:1451–1452.
346. National Association for Insurance Commissioners. *NAIC malpractice claims, 1975–79: final compilation*, Vol. 2, No. 2, Brookfield, WI: 1980.
347. Nau MM, Brooks BJ, Battey J, et al. L-*myc*, a new *myc*-related gene amplified and expressed in human small cell lung cancer. *Nature* 1985;317:69–73.
348. Nelson WG, Kastan MB. DNA strand breaks: the DNA template alterations that trigger p53-dependent DNA damage response pathways. *Mol Cell Biol* 1994;14:1815–1823.
349. Neta R, Oppenheim JJ. Radioprotection with cytokines: learning from nature to cope with radiation damage. *Cancer Cells* 1991;3:391–396.
350. Neta R, Oppenheim JJ, Douches SD. Interdependence of the radioprotective effects of human recombinant interleukin 1 alpha, tumor necrosis factor alpha, granulocyte colony stimulating factor, and murine recombinant granulocyte macrophage colony stimulating factor. *J Immunol* 1988;140:108–111.
351. Nicholson G. Cancer metastasis. In: Friedberg EC, ed. *Cancer biology.* New York: W.H. Freeman and Company, 1986;138–148.
352. Niemierko A, Urie M, Goitein M. Optimization of 3D radiation therapy with both physical and biological end points and constraints. *Int J Radiat Oncol Biol Phys* 1992;23:99–108.
353. Nitske WR. *The life of Wilhelm Conrad Röntgen: discoverer of the x ray.* Tucson: University of Arizona Press, 1971.
354. Nobel e-Museum. Available at: http://www.nobel.se.
355. Northrop M, Fletcher GH, Jesse RH, et al. Evolution of neck disease in patients with primary squamous cell carcinoma of the oral tongue, floor of mouth, and

palatine arch, and clinically positive neck nodes neither fixed nor bilateral. *Cancer* 1972;29:23–30.
356. Okunieff M, Hockel EP, Dunphy EP, et al. Oxygen tension distributions are sufficient to explain the local response of human breast tumors treated with radiation alone. *Int J Radiat Oncol Biol Phys* 1993;26:631–636.
357. Order S. Presidential address: systemic radiotherapy: the new frontier. *Int J Radiat Oncol Biol Phys* 1990;18:981–992.
358. Orton CG. Errors in applying the NSD concept. *Radiol* 1975;115:233–235.
359. Orton CG. Other considerations in 3-dimensional treatment planning. In: Bagne F, ed. *Computerized treatment planning systems.* HHS Publication FDA 84–8223. Washington, DC: U.S. Government Printing Office, 1984;136–141.
360. Orton CG. Time-dose factors (TDFs) in brachytherapy. *Br J Radiol* 1974;47:603–607.
361. Orton CG, Cohen L. A unified approach to dose-effect relationships in radiotherapy. I. Modified TDF and linear quadratic equations. *Int J Radiat Oncol Biol Phys* 1988;14:549–556.
362. Orton CG, Ellis F. A simplification in the use of the NSD concept in practical radiotherapy. *Br J Radiol* 1973;46:529–537.
363. Orton CG, Seyedsadr M, Somnay A. Comparison of high and low dose rate remote afterloading for cervix cancer and the importance of fractionation. *Int J Radiat Oncol Biol Phys* 1991;21:1425–1434.
364. Overgaard J. Sensitization of hypoxic tumour cells—clinical experience. *Int J Rad Biol* 1989;56(5):801–811.
365. Overgaard J, Bartelink H. About tolerance and quality: an important notice to all radiation oncologist [editorial]. *Radiother Oncol* 1995;35:1–3.
366. Overgaard J, Hansen HS, Overgaard M, et al. A randomized double-blind phase III study of nimorazole as a hypoxic radiosensitizer of primary radiotherapy in supraglottic larynx and pharynx carcinoma. Results of the Danish head and neck cancer study (DAHANCA) protocol 5–85. *Radiother Oncol* 1998;46:135–146.
367. Overgaard J, Horsman MR. Modification of hypoxia-induced radio-resistance in tumors by the use of oxygen and sensitizers. *Semin Radiat Oncol* 1996;6:10–21.
368. Overgaard J, von der Maase H, Overgaard M. A randomized study comparing two high-dose per fraction radiation schedules in recurrent or metastatic malignant melanoma. *Int J Radiat Oncol Biol Phys* 1985;11:1837–1839.
369. Overgaard M, Jensen MB, Overgaard J, et al. Postoperative radiotherapy in high-risk postmenopausal breast-cancer patients given adjuvant tamoxifen: Danish breast cancer cooperative group DBCG 82c randomized trial. *Lancet* 1999;353:1641–1648.
370. Paget S. A centennial celebration of Dr. Stephen Paget's "Seed and Soil" hypothesis. *Cancer Metastasis Rev* 1989;8:93–97.
371. Paget S. The distribution of secondary growths in cancer of the breast. *Lancet* 1889;1:571–573.
372. Paik S, Hazan R, Fisher ER, et al. Pathologic findings from the National Surgical Adjuvant Breast and Bowel Project: prognostic significance of erbB-2 protein overexpression in primary breast cancer. *J Clin Oncol* 1990;8:103–112.
373. Paine C. Il dissoluto Punito: medicine in the age of blame. *Medical-Legal J* 2002;70:161–175.
374. Parsons JT. Time-dose-volume relationships in radiation therapy. In: Million RR, Casissi NJ, eds. *Management of head and neck cancer: a multidisciplinary approach.* Philadelphia: J.B. Lippincott, 1984;137–172.
375. Paterson R. Studies in optimum dosage. *Br J Radiol* 1952;25:505–516.
376. Paterson R. *The treatment of malignant disease by radium and x-ray: being a practice of radiotherapy.* Baltimore: Williams & Wilkins, 1949.
377. Paterson RP. The radical x-ray treatment of the carcinomata. *Br J Radiol* 1936;9:671–679.
378. Pawson T. The biochemical mechanisms of oncogene action. In: Bishop JM, Weinberg RA, eds. *Scientific American: molecular oncology.* New York: Scientific American, 1996.
379. Penagaricano JA, Papanikolaou N, Wu C, et al. An assessment of biologically-based optimization (BORT) in the IMRT era. *Med Dosim* 2005;30:12–19.
380. Perez CA, Ackerman LV, Mill WB, et al. Malignant tumors of the tonsil: analysis of failures and factors affecting prognosis. *Am J Roentgenol Radium Ther Nucl Med* 1972;114:43–58.
381. Perez CA, Bauer M, Edelstein S, et al. Impact of tumor control on survival in carcinoma of the lung treated with irradiation. *Int J Radiat Oncol Biol Phys* 1986;12:539–547.
382. Perez CA, Breaux S, Bedwinek JM, et al. Radiation therapy alone in the treatment of carcinoma of the uterine cervix. II. Analysis of complications. *Cancer* 1984;54:235–246.
383. Perez CA. Carcinoma of the prostate: a model for management under impending health care system reform. *Radiology* 1995;196:309–322.
384. Perez CA, Devineni VR, Marcial-Vega V, et al. Carcinoma of the nasopharynx: factors affecting prognosis. *Int J Radiat Oncol Biol Phys* 1992;23:271–280.
385. Perez CA, Gardner P, Glasgow GP. Radiotherapy quality assurance in clinical trials. *Int J Radiat Oncol Biol Phys* 1984;10:119–125.
386. Perez CA, Grigsby PW, Galakatos A, et al. Irradiation in management of carcinoma of the vulva with emphasis on conservation therapy. *Cancer* 1993;71:3707–3716.
387. Perez CA, Kuske RR, Camel HM, et al. Analysis of pelvic tumor control and impact on survival in carcinoma of the uterine cervix treated with radiation therapy alone. *Int J Radiat Oncol Biol Phys* 1988;14:613–621.
388. Perez CA, Marks J, Powers WE. Preoperative irradiation in head and neck cancer. *Semin Oncol* 1977;4:387–397.
389. Perez CA, Michalski JM, Purdy JA, et al. Three-dimensional conformal therapy or standard irradiation in localized carcinoma of prostate: preliminary results of a nonrandomized comparison. *Int J Radiat Oncol Biol Phys* 2000;47:629–637.
390. Perez CA, Pajak T, Emami B, et al. Randomized phase III study comparing irradiation and hyperthermia with irradiation alone in superficial measurable tumors: final report by the Radiation Therapy Oncology Group. *Am J Clin Oncol* 1991;14:133–141.
391. Perez CA, Pilepich MV, Zivnuska F. Tumor control in definitive irradiation of localized carcinoma of the prostate. *Int J Radiat Oncol Biol Phys* 1986;12:523–531.
392. Perez CA, Powers WE. Studies on optimal dose of preoperative irradiation and time for surgery in the cure of a mouse lymphosarcoma. *Radiology* 1967;89:116–122.
393. Perez CA, Purdy JA, Harms W, et al. Design of a fully integrated three-dimensional computed tomography simulator and preliminary clinical evaluation. *Int J Radiat Oncol Biol Phys* 1994;30:887–897.
394. Perez CA. Quest for excellence: the ultimate goal of the radiation oncologist. *Int J Radiat Oncol Biol Phys* 1993;6:565–580.
395. Perez CA, Thomas PRM. Radiation therapy: basic concepts and clinical implications. In: Sutow W, Fernbach DJ, Vietti TJ, eds. *Clinical pediatric oncology*, 3rd ed. St. Louis: C.V. Mosby, 1984;167–209.
396. Peschel RE, Fischer JJ. Multiple daily fractionation schedules. *Int J Radiat Oncol Biol Phys* 1982;8:1811–1812.
397. Peters LJ. Inherent radiosensitivity of tumor and normal tissue cells as a predictor of human tumor response. *Radiother Oncol* 1990;17:177–190.
398. Peters LJ, Brock WA, Chapman JD, et al. Predictive assays of tumor radiocurability. *Am J Clin Oncol* 1988;11:275–287.
399. Peters LJ, Goepfert H, Ang KK, et al. Evaluation of the dose for postoperative radiation therapy of head and neck cancer: first report of a prospective randomized trial. *Int J Radiat Oncol Biol Phys* 1993;26:3–11.
400. Phillips TL. Biochemical modifiers: drug-radiation interactions. In: Mauch PM, Loeffler JS, eds. *Radiation oncology: technology and biology.* Philadelphia: W.B. Saunders, 1994;113–151.
401. Pierquin B, Baillet F, Brown CH. Low dose irradiation in advanced tumors of head and neck. *Acta Radiol* 1975;14:497–504.
402. Pierquin B, Chassagne D, Baillet F, et al. Clinical observations on the time factor in interstitial radiotherapy using Iridium 192. *Clin Radiol* 1973;24:506–509.
403. Pitot HC. Principles of cancer biology: chemical carcinogenesis. In: DeVita VT Jr., Hellman S, Rosenberg SA, eds. *Cancer: principles and practice of oncology.* Philadelphia: J.B. Lippincott, 1985;79–100.
404. Pollack A, Zagars GK, Smith LG, et al. Preliminary results of a randomized radiotherapy dose-escalation study comparing 70 Gy with 78 Gy for prostate cancer. *J Clin Oncol* 2000;18:3904–3911.
405. Potish R, Dehner L, Haselow R, et al. The incidence of second neoplasms following megavoltage radiation for pediatric tumors. *Cancer* 1985;56:1534–1537.
406. Pourquier H, Delard R, Achille E, et al. A quantified approach to the analysis and prevention of urinary complications in radiotherapeutic treatment of cancer of the cervix. *Int J Radiat Oncol Biol Phys* 1987;13:1025–1033.
407. Pourquier H, Dubois JB, Delard R. Cancer of the uterine cervix: dosimetric guidelines for prevention of late rectal and rectosigmoid complications as a result of radiotherapeutic treatment. *Int J Radiat Oncol Biol Phys* 1982;8:1887–1895, 559–567.
408. *Prescribing, recording and reporting photon beam therapy (Supplement to ICRU Report 50).* Bethesda, MD: International Commission on Radiation Units and Measurements, 1999.
409. Prives C. Doing the right thing: feedback control and p53. *Curr Opin Cell Biol* 1993;5:214.
410. Puck TT, Marcus PI. Actions of x-rays on mammalian cells. *J Exp Med* 1956;103:653–666.
411. Purdy JA. Photon dose calculations for three-dimensional radiation treatment planning. *Semin Radiat Oncol* 1992;2:235–245
412. Purdy JA, Wong JW, Harms WB, et al. State of the art of high energy photon treatment planning. *Front Radiat Ther Oncol* 1987;21:4–24.
413. Purdy JA, Wong JW, Harms WB, et al. Three dimensional radiation treatment planning system. In: *Proceedings of the 9th International Conference on the Use of Computers in Radiation Therapy.* The Netherlands, North Holland: Scheveningen, 1987.
414. Quarmby S, Fakhoury H, Levine E, et al. Association of transforming growth factor beta-1 single nucleotide polymorphisms with radiation-induced damage to normal tissues in breast cancer patients. *Int J Radiat Biol* 2003;79:137–143.
415. Rabinowitz I, Broomberg J, Goitein M, et al. Accuracy of radiation field alignment in clinical practice. *Int J Radiat Oncol Biol Phys* 1985;11:1857–1867.
416. Rauth AM, Mohindra JK, Tannock IF. Activity of mitomycin C for aerobic and hypoxic cells in vitro and in vivo. *Cancer Res* 1983;43:4154–4158.
417. Rayner AA, Grimm EA, Lotze MT, et al. Lymphokine-activated killer (LAK) cell phenomenon: analysis of factors relevant to the immunotherapy of human cancer. *Cancer* 1985;55:1327–1333.
418. Regaud C, Ferroux R. Discordance des effects de rayons X, d'une part dans le testicule, par le fractionnement de la dose. *CR Soc Biol* 1927;97:431–434.
419. Reisner A. Hauterythem und rotgenstrahlung. *Ergeb Med Strahlenforsch* 1933;6:1.
420. Reuter SR. An overview of informed consent for radiologists. *AJR* 1987;148:219–227.
421. Richards EP, Rathbun KC. *Law and the physician: a practical guide.* Boston: Little, Brown and Company, 1993.
422. Rimer BK, Schildkraut J, Hiatt RA. Cancer screening. In: DeVita VT Jr., Hellman S, Rosenberg SA, eds. *Cancer principles and practice of oncology*, 6th ed. Philadelphia: Lippincott Williams & Wilkins, 2001;575–589.
423. Risch HA, Jain M, Choi NW, et al. Dietary factors and the incidence of cancer of the stomach. *Am J Epidemiol* 1985;122:947–959.
424. Roberts SA, Hendry JH. A realistic closed-form radiobiological model of clinical tumor-control data incorporating intertumor heterogeneity. *Int J Radiat Oncol Biol Phys* 1998;41:689–699.
425. Roberts SA, Hendry JH. Time factors in larynx tumor radiotherapy: lagtimes and intertumor heterogeneity in clinical datasets from four centers. *Int J Radiat Oncol Biol Phys* 1999;45:1247–1257.
426. Roentgen WC. On a new kind of rays (preliminary communication). Translation of a paper read before the Physikalische-medicinischen Gesellschaft of Würzburg on December 28, 1985. *Br J Radiol* 1931;4:32.
427. Ron E, Modan B, Boice JD, et al. Tumors of the brain and nervous system after radiotherapy in childhood. *N Engl J Med* 1988;319:1033–1039.
428. Roques T, Dagless M, Tames J. Randomized trial on two types of the thermoplastic masks for patient immobilization during radiation therapy for head-and-neck cancer: in regard to Sharp et al. *Int J Rad Oncol Biol Phys* 2005;62:942.
429. Rose C, Lustig R, McIntosh N, et al. A clinical trial of fluosol DA 20% in advanced squamous cell carcinoma of the head and neck. *Int J Radiat Oncol Biol Phys* 1988;12:1325–1327.
430. Rosen II. Treatment planning for intensity modulated radiation therapy. Paper presented at the Intensity Modulated Radiation Therapy Workshop. Durango, CO; May 17–18, 1996.
431. Rosen N. Oncogenes. In: Mendelsohn J, Howley PM, Israel MA, et al., eds. *The molecular basis of cancer.* Philadelphia: W.B. Saunders, 1995;105–116.
432. Rosenberg SA, Longo DL, Lotze MT. Principles and applications of biologic therapy.

In: DeVita VT Jr., Hellman S, Rosenberg SA, eds. *Cancer: principles and practice of oncology*, 3rd ed. Philadelphia: J.B. Lippincott, 1989;301–347.
433. Rosenberg SA, Lotze MT, Muul LM, et al. A progress report on the treatment of 157 patients with advanced cancer using lymphokine-activated killer cells and interleukin-2 or high-dose interleukin-2 alone. *N Engl J Med* 1987;316:889–897.
434. Rosenthal RS. Malpractice: cause and its prevention. *Laryngoscope* 1978;88:1–11.
435. Rowley JD. Biological implications of consistent chromosome rearrangements in leukemia and lymphoma. *Cancer Res* 1984;44:3159–3168.
436. Rubin P. *Clinical oncology: a multidisciplinary approach for physicians and students*, 7th ed. Philadelphia: W.B. Saunders, 1993.
437. Rubin P. The emergence of radiation oncology as a distinct medical specialty. *Int J Radiat Oncol Biol Phys* 1985;11:1247–1270.
438. Rubin P, Casarett GW. *Clinical radiation pathology*, vols 1 and 2. Philadelphia: W.B. Saunders, 1968.
439. Rubin P, Cooper R, Phillips TL, eds. *Radiation biology and radiation pathology syllabus* (Set RT 1: Radiation Oncology). Chicago: American College of Radiology, 1975.
440. Rubin P, Siemann DW. Principles of radiation oncology and cancer radiotherapy. In: Rubin P, McDonald S, Qazi R, eds. *Clinical oncology: a multidisciplinary approach for physicians and students*, 7th ed. Philadelphia: W.B. Saunders, 1993.
441. Runyan v. Goodrum, 228 SW 397 Ark 1921.
442. Russell NS, Begg AC. Predictive assays for normal tissue damage. *Radiother Oncol* 2002;64:125–129.
443. Salinetro v. Nystrom, 341 So 2d 1059, Fla, 1977.
444. Saunders MI. Programming of radiotherapy in the treatment of non-small-cell lung cancer—a way to advance cure. *Lancet Oncol* 2001;2(7):401–408.
445. Sause WT, Stewart JR, Plenk HP, et al. Late skin changes following twice-weekly electron beam radiation to post-mastectomy chest wall. *Int J Radiat Oncol Biol Phys* 1981;7:1541–1544.
446. Schmidt-Ullrich RK. Local tumor control and survival: clinical evidence and tumor biologic basis. *Surg Oncol Clin North Am* 2000;9:401–414.
447. Schmidt-Ullrich RK, Contessa JN, Dent P, et al. Molecular mechanisms of radiation-induced accelerated repopulation. *Radiat Oncol Invest* 1999;7:321–330.
448. Schneider JJ, Fletcher GH, Barkley HT Jr. Control by irradiation alone of nonfixed clinically positive lymph nodes from squamous cell carcinoma of the oral cavity, oropharynx, supraglottic larynx, and hypopharynx. *Am J Roentgenol Radium Ther Med* 1975;123:42–48.
449. Schultheiss TE, Stephens LC, Ang KK, et al. Volume effects in rhesus monkey spinal cord. *Int J Radiat Oncol Biol Phys* 1994;29:67–72.
450. Schwartz WB, Joskow PL. Duplicated hospital facilities: how much can we save by consolidating them? *N Eng J Med* 1980;303:1449–1457.
451. Schwarz G. Heilung teifliegender Karzinome durch Rontgen-bestrahlung von der Korperoberflache. *Munch Med Wochenschr* 1914;61:1733.
452. Schwarz G. Ueber desensibilisierung gegen Rontgen—und radiumstrahlen. *Munchener medizinische wochenschrift* 1909;24:1–2.
453. Seeger RC, Broudeur GM, Sather H, et al. Association of multiple copies of the N-myc oncogene in untreated human neuroblastomas. *N Engl J Med* 1985;313:1111–1116.
454. Sharkey RM, Blumenthal RD, Hansen HJ, et al. Biological considerations for radioimmunotherapy. *Cancer Res* 1990;50[Suppl]:964–969.
455. Sherman NE, Rich TA, Peters LJ. Professional liability in radiotherapy: experience of the Fletcher Society. *Int J Radiat Oncol Biol Phys* 1991;20:563–566.
456. Sherry RM. Cancer prevention: role of surgery in cancer prevention. In: DeVita VT Jr., Hellman S, Rosenberg SA, eds. *Cancer: principles and practice of oncology*, 6th ed. Philadelphia: Lippincott Williams & Wilkins, 2001;575–589.
457. Shioyama Y, Nakamura K, Anai S, et al. Stereotactic radiotherapy for lung and liver tumors using a body cast system: setup accuracy and preliminary clinical outcome. *Radiat Med* 2005;23:407–413.
458. Shipley WU, Kaufman DS, Heney NM, et al. An update of combined modality therapy for patients with muscle invading bladder cancer using selective bladder preservation or cystectomy. *J Urol* 1999;162:445–451.
459. Shipley WU, Munzenrider JE, McManus PL, et al. Results of a randomized trial of total radiation dose for stage T3-T4 prostate cancer boosting with photons (to 67.2 CGE) or with conformal protons (to 75.6 CGE). *Int J Radiat Oncol Biol Phys* 1994;30[Suppl 1]:211.
460. Shukovsky LJ. Dose, time, volume relationships in squamous cell carcinoma of the supraglottic larynx. *Am J Roentgenol* 1970;108:27–29.
461. Shukovsky LJ, Baeza MR, Fletcher GH. Results of irradiation of squamous cell carcinomas of the glossopalatine sulcus. *Radiology* 1976;120:405–408.
462. Shukovsky LJ, Fletcher GH. Time-dose and tumor volume relationships in the irradiation of squamous cell carcinoma of the tonsillar fossa. *Radiology* 1973;107:621–626.
463. Siemann DW. Interactions between nitrosoureas and x-irradiation. In: Hill BT, Bellamy AS, eds. *Antitumor drug-radiation interactions*. Boca Raton, FL: CRC Press, 1990;141–151.
464. Sinclair WK. Fifty years of neutrons in biology and medicine: the comparative effects of neutrons in biological systems. In: Booz J, Ebert H, eds. *Proceedings of the Eighth Symposium in Microdosimetry*. Luxembourg: Eur 8395 Commission European Communities, 1983;1.
465. Sklar MD. The ras oncogenes increase the intrinsic resistance of NIH-3T3 cells to ionizing radiation. *Science* 1988;239:645–647.
466. Slamon DJ, Clark GM, Wong SG, et al. Human breast cancer: correlation of relapse and survival with amplification of the HER-2/neu oncogene. *Science* 1987;235:177–182.
467. Slamon DJ, Godolphin W, Jones LA, et al. Studies of the HER-2/neu proto-oncogene in human breast and ovarian cancer. *Science* 1989;244:707–712.
468. Slijepecic P. Commentary: is there a link between telomere maintenance and radiosensitivity? *Rad Res* 2004;161:82–86.
469. Smith AR, Gerber RL, Hughes DB, et al. Treatment planning structure and process in the United States: a "Patterns of Care" study. *Int J Radiat Oncol Biol Phys* 1995;32:255–262.
470. Smith RA, Meltin CJ. Cancer detection. In: Lenhard RE Jr., Osteen RT, Gansler T, eds. *Clinical oncology*. Atlanta: American Cancer Society, 2001;75–122.
471. Sneath RJ, Mangham DC. The normal structure and function of CD44 and its role in neoplasia. *Mol Pathol* 1998;51:191.
472. Sobel ME. Metastasis suppressor genes. *J Natl Cancer Inst* 1990;82(4):267–276.
473. Sobel S, Rubin P, Keller B, et al. Tumor persistence as a predictor of outcome after radiation therapy of head and neck cancers. *Int J Radiat Oncol Biol Phys* 1976;1:873–880.
474. Solomon RC, Higgins KM. *A passion for wisdom: a very brief history of philosophy*. New York: Oxford University Press, 1997.
475. Song CW, Zhang WL, Pence DM, et al. Increased radiosensitivity of tumors by perfluorochemicals and carbogen. *Int J Radiat Oncol Biol Phys* 1985;11:1833–1836.
476. Spanos WJ Jr., Shukovsky LJ, Fletcher GH. Time, dose, and tumor volume relationships in irradiation of squamous cell carcinomas of the base of the tongue. *Cancer* 1976;37:2591–2599.
477. Steel GC. The combination of radiotherapy and chemotherapy. In: Steel GG, Adams GE, Peckham MJ, eds. *The biological basis of radiotherapy.* Amsterdam: Elsevier Science, 1983;239–248.
478. Steel GG, Peacock JH. Why are some human tumours more radiosensitive than others? *Radiother Oncol* 1989;15:63–72.
479. Steel GG, Peckham MJ. Exploitable mechanisms in combined radiotherapy-chemotherapy: the concept of additivity. *Int J Radiat Oncol Biol Phys* 1979;5:85–91.
480. Stell PM, Rawson NSB. Adjuvant chemotherapy in head and neck cancer. *Br J Cancer* 1990;61:779–787.
481. Sterneck ES, ed. *The theory and practice of intensity modulated radiation therapy.* Madison, WI: Advanced Medical Publishing, 1997.
482. Stetler-Stevenson W, Kleiner D. Molecular biology of cancer: invasion and metastases. In: Devita V Jr., Hellman S, Rosenberg S, eds. *Cancer principles and practice of oncology*, 6th ed. Philadelphia: Lippincott Williams & Wilkins, 2001; .
483. Stracke M, Liotta L. *Molecular mechanisms of tumor cell metastasis. The molecular basis of cancer.* Philadelphia: W.B. Saunders, 1995;233–247.
484. Strandqvist M. Sutdien uber die kumulative wirkung der rontgenstrahlen bie frakionierung. *Acta Radiol* (Stockh)1994;55[Suppl]:1–300.
485. Stuschke M, Pottgen C. Localized small-cell lung cancer: which type of thoracic radiotherapy and which time schedule. *Lung Cancer* 2004;45[Suppl 2]:5133–5137.
486. Suit H. Radiation biology: the conceptual and practical impact on radiation therapy. *Radiat Res* 1983;94:10–40.
487. Suit HD. Radiation biology, a basis for radiotherapy. In: Fletcher GH, ed. *Textbook of radiotherapy*, 2nd ed. Philadelphia: Lee and Febiger, 1973;78.
488. Suit HD, Urie M. Proton beams in radiation therapy. *J Natl Cancer Inst* 1992;84:155–164.
489. Suit HD, Westgate SJ. Impact of improved local tumor control on survival. *Int J Radiat Oncol Biol Phys* 1986;12:453–458.
490. Suit HD. Impact of improved local control on survival in patients with soft tissues sarcoma. *Int J Radiat Oncol Biol Phys* 1986;12:699–700.
491. Suit H, Lindberg R. Radiation therapy administered under conditions of tourniquet-induced local tissue hypoxia. *Am J Roentgenol* 1968;2:27–37.
492. Sweet WH. Early history of development of boron neutron capture therapy of tumors. *J Neuro Oncol* 1997;33:19–26.
493. Tannock IF. Eradication of a disease: how we cured symptomless prostate cancer. *Lancet* 2002;359:1341–1342.
494. Tannock IF. New perspectives in combined radiotherapy and chemotherapy treatment. *Lung Cancer* 1994;10[Suppl 1]:29–51.
495. Tannock IF. Population kinetics of carcinoma cells, capillary endothelial cells, and fibroblasts in a transplanted mouse mammary tumor. *Cancer Res* 1970;30:2470–2476.
496. Tannock IF. Potential for therapeutic gain from combined-modality treatment. In: Meyer JL, Vaeth JM, eds. *Frontiers of radiation therapy and oncology, radiotherapy/chemotherapy interactions in cancer therapy*, vol 26. Basel, Switzerland: Karger, 1992;1–15.
497. Taylor JH, Goldhaber M. Detection of nuclear disintegration in a photographic emulsion. *Nature* 1935;135:34.
498. Taylor RE, Bailey CC, Robinson KJ, et al. Impact of radiotherapy parameters on outcome in the International Society of Paediatric Oncology/United Kingdom Children's Cancer Study Group PNET-5 study of preradiotherapy chemotherapy for MO-M1 medulloblastoma. *Int J Radiat Oncol Biol Phys* 2004;58:1184–1193.
499. Teh BS, Dong L, McGary JE, et al. Rectal wall sparing by dosimetric effect of rectal balloon used during intensity-modulated radiation therapy (IMRT) for prostate cancer. *Med Dosim* 2005;30:25–30.
500. Terasima T, Tolmach LJ. Variations in several responses of HeLa cells to x-irradiation during the division cycle. *Biophys J* 1963;3:11–33.
501. Tester W, Caplan R, Heaney J, et al. Neoadjuvant combined modality program with selective organ preservation for invasive bladder cancer: results of Radiation Therapy Oncology Group Phase II trial 8802. *J Clin Oncol* 1996;14:119–126.
502. Thames HD, Withers HR, Mason KA, et al. Dose-survival characteristics of mouse jejunal crypt cells. *Int J Radiat Oncol Biol Phys* 1981;7:1591–1597.
503. Thames HD Jr., Withers HR, Peters LJ, et al. Changes in early and late radiation responses with altered dose fractionation: implications for dose-survival relationships. *Int J Radiat Oncol Biol Phys* 1982;8:219–226.
504. Thomas AMK, ed. *The Röntgen centenary: the invisible light: 100 years of medical radiology*. Oxford: Blackwell Science, 1995.
505. Thomas RJ, Abbott M, Bhathal PS, et al. High dose photoirradiation of esophageal cancer. *Ann Surg* 1987;206:193–199.
506. Thomason JF, Lombard LS, Grahn D, et al. RBE of fission neutrons for life shortening and tumorigenesis. In: Broerse JJ, Gerber GB, eds. *Neutron carcinogenesis.* Luxembourg: Commission of the European Communities, 1982;75.
507. Thomlinson RH, Gray LH. The histological structure of some human lung cancers and the possible implications for radiotherapy. *Br J Cancer* 1955;9:539–549.
508. Thompson LH, Suit HD. Proliferation kinetics of x-irradiated mouse L cells studied with time-lapse photography. II. *Int J Radiat Biol Relat Stud Phys Chem Med* 1969;15:347.
509. Thorgeirsson UP, Turpeenniemi-Hujanen T, Williams JE, et al. NIH/3T3 cells transfected with human tumor DNA containing activated ras oncogenes express the metastatic phenotype in nude mice. *Mol Cell Biol* 1985;5:259.
510. Timmerman RD, Kavangh BD. Stereotactic body radiation therapy. *Curr Probl Cancer* 2005;29:120–157.
511. Tinger A, Michalski JM, Bosch WR, et al. An analysis of intratreatment and intertreatment displacements in pelvic radiotherapy using electronic portal imaging. *Int J Radiat Oncol Biol Phys* 1996;34:683–690.
512. Touchette N. Evolutions: cancer genes. *J NIH Res* 1992;4:92–96.
513. Travis EL. *Primer of medical radiobiology*, 2nd ed. Chicago: Year Book Publishers, 1989.

514. Tronick SR, Aaronson SA. Growth factors and signal transduction. In: Mendelsohn J, Howley PM, Israel MA, et al., eds. *The molecular basis of cancer.* Philadelphia: W.B. Saunders, 1995;117–140.

515. Tubiana M, Richare JM, Malaise E. Kinetics of tumor growth and of cell proliferation in U.R.D.T. cancers: therapeutic implications. *Laryngoscope* 1975;85:1039–1052.

516. Tucker JD, Preton RJ. Chromosome aberrations micronuclei, aneuploidy, sister chromatid exchanges, and cancer risk assessment. *Mut Res* 1996;365:147–159.

517. Tucker SL, Geara FB, Peters LJ, et al. How much could the radiotherapy dose be altered for individual patients based on a predictive assay of normal-tissue radiosensitivity? *Radiother Oncol* 1996;38:103–113.

518. Turesson I, Notter G. The influence of fraction size in radiotherapy on the late normal tissue reaction. I. Comparison of the effects of daily and once-a-week fractionation on human skin. *Int J Radiat Oncol Biol Phys* 1984;10:593–598.

519. Ulaner GA. Review: telomere maintenance in clinical medicine. *Am J Med* 2004;117:262–269.

520. United States Department of Health and Human Services, Centers for Disease Control. Smoking-attributable mortality and years of potential life lost in the United States, 1984. *MMWR* 1987;36:693–697.

521. Upton AC. Biological aspects of radiation carcinogenesis. In: Boice JD, Fraumeni JF, eds. *Radiation carcinogenesis: epidemiology and biological significance.* New York: Raven, 1984;9.

522. Utley JF, Seaver N, Newton GL, et al. Pharmacokinetics of WR-1065 in mouse tissues following treatment with WR-02721. *Int J Radiat Oncol Biol Phys* 1984;10:1525–1528.

523. van de Vijver M, van de Bersselaar R, Devilee P, et al. Amplification of the neu (c-erbB-2) oncogene in human mammary tumors is relatively frequent and is often accompanied by amplification of the linked c-erbA oncogene. *Mol Cell Biol* 1987;7:2019–2023.

524. van den Brenk HAS. Hyperbaric oxygen in radiation therapy. *Am J Roentgenol* 1968;102:8–26.

525. Van Rongen E. Analysis of cell survival after multiple fractions and low dose-rate irradiation of two in vitro cultured rat tumor cell lines. *Radiat Res* 1985;104:28–46.

526. Varmus H, Weinberg RA. *Genes and the biology of cancer.* New York: Scientific American Library, 1993.

527. Varmus HE. The molecular genetics of cellular oncogenes. *Ann Rev Genet* 1984;18:553–612.

528. Vaupel P, Kelleher DK, Hockel M. Oxygen status of malignant tumors: pathogenesis of hypoxia and significance for tumor therapy. Treatment resistance of solid tumors: role of hypoxia and anemia. *Semin Oncol* 2001;28:29–35.

529. Vaupel P, Schlenger K, Knoop C, et al. Oxygenation of human tumors: evaluation of tissue oxygen distribution in breast cancers by computerized tension measurements. *Cancer Res* 1991;51:3316–3322.

530. Verhey LV, Goitein M, McNulty P, et al. Precise positioning of patients for radiation therapy. *Int J Radiat Oncol Biol Phys* 1982;8:289–294.

531. Vikram B, Farr HW. Adjuvant radiation therapy in locally advanced head and neck cancer. *Cancer* 1983;33:134–138.

532. Vikram B, Strong EW, Shah JP, et al. Failure in the neck following multimodality treatment for advanced head and neck cancer. *Head Neck Surg* 1984;6:724–729.

533. Vincent C, Young M, Phillips A. Why do people sue doctors? A study of patients and relative taking legal action. *Lancet* 1974;343:1609–1613.

534. Von Essen CF. A spatial model of time-dose-area relationships in radiation therapy. *Radiology* 1963;81:881–883.

535. Votava C Jr., Fletcher GH, Jesse RH Jr. et al. Management of cervical nodes, either fixed or bilateral, from squamous cell carcinoma of the oral cavity and faucial arch. *Radiology* 1972;105:417–420.

536. Waddle v. Sutherland, 126 SO 201 Miss, 1930.

537. Wallner K, Elliott K. Malpractice in radiation oncology: redefining the role of the medical expert in regard to Kagan. *Int J Radiat Oncol Biol Phys* 2005;62:1254–1255.

538. Wallner KE, Li GC. Effect of cisplatin resistance on cellular radiation response. *Int J Radiat Oncol Biol Phys* 1987;13:587–591.

539. Wang CC. Improved local control for advanced oropharyngeal carcinoma following twice daily radiation therapy. *Am J Clin Oncol* 1985;8:512–516.

540. Wang CC, Blitzer PH, Suit HD. Twice-a-day radiation therapy for cancer of the head and neck. *Cancer* 1985;55:2100–2104.

541. Ward JF. DNA damage produced by ionizing radiation in mammalian cells: identities, mechanisms of formation and repairability. *Prog Nucleic Acids Mol Biol* 1988;35:95.

542. Ward JF. The yield of DNA double-strand breaks produced intracellularly by ionizing radiation: a review. *Int J Radiat Biol* 1990;57:1141.

543. Wasserman TH, Brizel DM. The role of amifostine as a radioprotector. *Oncology* 2001;15:1349–1354; discussion 1357–1360.

544. Wasserman TH. Hypoxic cell radiosensitizers: present and future [editorial]. *Int J Radiat Oncol Biol Phys* 1981;7:849–852.

545. Watson-Clarke RA, et al. Model studies directed toward the application of boron neutron capture theory of rheumatoid arthritis: boron delivery by liposomes to rat collagen-induced arthritis. *PNAS USA* 1998;95:2531–2534.

546. Watson JD. The human genome project: past, present, and future. *Science* 1990;248:44–49.

547. Webb S. *The physics of three-dimensional radiation therapy: conformal radiotherapy, radiosurgery and treatment planning.* Bristol, England: Institute of Physics Publishing, 1993.

548. Weichselbaum RR, Little JB. Radioresistance in some human tumor cells conferred in vitro by repair of potentially lethal x-ray damage. *Radiology* 1982;145:511–513.

549. Weichselbaum RR, Little JB. The differential response of human tumours to frac-

550. tionated radiation may be due to a post-irradiation repair process. *Br J Cancer* 1982;46:532–537.

550. Weinberg RA. Tumor suppressor genes. *Science* 1991;254:1138–1146.

551. Weinberg RA, Hanahan D. The molecular pathogenesis of cancer. In: Bishop JM, Weinberg RA, eds. *Scientific American: molecular oncology.* New York: Scientific American, 1996; .

552. Weiner LM, Holmes M, Adams GP, et al. A human tumor xenograft model of therapy with a bispecific monoclonal antibody targeting c-erbB-2 and CD16. *Cancer Res* 1993;53:94–100.

553. Weinstein B. The origins of human cancer: molecular mechanisms of carcinogenesis and their implications for cancer prevention and treatment. *Cancer Res* 1988;48:4135–4143.

554. Wetterer J. *Handbuch der Rontgen Therapie.* Leipzig i:176, 1913–1914.

555. White T. Smart medicine is coming. *Vital Speeches of the Day* 2002;68:326–331.

556. Wilder RB, McGann JK, Sutherland WR, et al. The hypoxic cytotoxic SR 4233 increases the effectiveness of radioimmunotherapy in mice with human non-Hodgkin's lymphoma xenografts. *Int J Radiat Oncol Biol Phys* 1994;28:119–126.

557. Wile AG, Dahlman A, Burns RG, et al. Laser photoradiation therapy of cancer following hematoporphyrin sensitization. *Lasers Surg Med* 1982;2:163–168.

558. Wiley Al Jr., Vogel HH Jr., Clifton KH. The effect of variations in LET and cell cycle on radiation hepatocarcinogenesis. *Radiat Res* 1973;54:284–293.

559. Wilkinson v. Harrington, 243 A 2d, 745 RI 1968.

600. Williams GT, Smith CA. Molecular regulation of apoptosis: genetic controls of cell death. *Cell* 1993;74:777–779.

601. Wilson JF. Low dose rate teletherapy: review of recent clinical study. In: *Proceedings of 2nd International Dose-Time Conference*, University of Wisconsin, Madison, WI; September 12–14, 1984.

602. Withers HR, Peters LJ, Taylor JM, et al. Late normal tissue sequelae from radiation therapy for carcinoma of the tonsil: patterns of fractionation study of radiobiology. *Int J Radiat Oncol Biol Phys* 1995;33:563–568.

603. Withers HR, Peters LJ, Thames HD, et al. Hyperfractionation. *Int J Radiat Oncol Biol Phys* 1982;8:1807–1809.

604. Withers HR, Taylor JM. Critical volume model. *Int J Radiat Oncol Biol Phys* 1992;25:151–152.

605. Withers HR, Thames HD Jr. , Flow BL, et al. The relationship of acute to late skin injury in 2 and 5 fractions/week x-ray therapy. *Int J Radiat Oncol Biol Phys* 1978;4:595–601.

606. Withers HR, Thames HD, Peters LJ. A new isoeffect curve for change in dose per fraction. *Radiother Oncol* 1983;1:187–191.

607. Withers HR, Thames HD, Peters LJ. Differences in fractionation response of acutely and late responding tissues. In: Karcher KH, Kogelnik HD, Reinartz G, eds. *Progress in radio-oncology II.* New York: Raven, 1982;287–296.

608. Witte L, Fuks Z, Friedman-Himovitz A, et al. Effects of radiation on the release of growth factors from cultured bovine, porcine, and human endothelial cells. *Cancer Res* 1989;49:5066–5072.

609. Wm. Phenomena leading to cell survival values which deviate from linear quadratic models. *Mutual Res* 2004;568:33–39.

610. Woloschak GE, Liu GMC, Jones S, et al. Modulation of gene expression in Syrian hamster embryo cells following ionizing radiation. *Cancer Res* 1990;50:339–344.

611. Wong JW, Sharpe MB, Jaffray DA, et al. The use of active breathing control (ABC) to reduce margin for breathing motion. *Int J Radiat Oncol Biol Phys* 1999;44:911–919.

612. Wrba E. Ubersicht uber 198 maligne pulmonale Erkrankungen im Jahre 1975: Therapie und Erbenisse (Eng Abstr) *Wien Medworkenscher* 1980;103:436–439.

613. Wu J, Haycocks T, Alasti H, et al. Position errors and prostate motion during conformal prostate radiotherapy using on-line isocentre set-up verification and implanted prostate markers. *Radio Oncol* 2001;61:127–133.

614. Wyllie AH. Apoptosis. *Br J Cancer* 1993;67:205–208.

615. Wyllie AH. The biology of cell death in tumours. *Anti Cancer Res* 1985;5:131.

616. Wyllie AH, Kerr JFR, Currie AR. Cell death: the significance of apoptosis. *Int Rev Cytol* 1980;68:251–306.

617. Wynder EL, Graham EA. Tobacco smoking as a possible etiologic factor in bronchogenic carcinoma: a study of 684 proved cases. *JAMA* 1950;143:329–336.

618. Yaes RJ. Linear-quadratic model isoeffect relations for proliferating tumor cells for treatment with multiple fractions per day. *Int J Radiat Oncol Biol Phys* 1989;17:901–905.

619. Yamada T, Ohyama H. Radiation-induced interphase death of rate thymocytes is internally programmed (apoptosis). *Int J Radiat Biol* 1988;53:65.

620. Yanch JC, Shefer RE, Busse PM. Boron neutron capture therapy. *Sci Med* 1999;January/February:18–27.

621. Yorke ED, Kutcher GJ, Jackson A, et al. Probability of radiation-induced complications in normal tissues with parallel architecture under conditions of uniform whole or partial organ irradiation. *Radiother Oncol* 1993;26:226–237.

622. Zagars GK, von Eschenbach AC, Johnson DE, et al. Stage C adenocarcinoma of the prostate: an analysis of 551 patients treated with external beam irradiation. *Cancer* 1987;60:1489–1499.

623. Zelefsky MJ, Cowen D, Zuks Z, et al. Long term tolerance of high dose three-dimensional conformal radiotherapy in patients with localized prostate carcinoma. *Cancer* 1999;85:2460–2468.

624. Zeman EM, Bedford JS. Dose rate effects in mammalian cells. V. Dose fractionation effects in non-cycling C3H 10 T1/2 cells. *Int J Radiat Oncol Biol Phys* 1984;10:2089–2098.

625. Zeman EM, Brown JM. Aerobic radiosensitization by SR 4233 in rodent and human cell lines: mechanistic and therapeutic implications. *Int J Radiat Oncol Biol Phys* 1991;59:117–131.

626. Zhan Q, Bae I, Kastan MB, et al. The p53-dependent gamma-ray response of GADD45. *Cancer Res* 1994;54:2755–2760.

Overview and Basic Science of Radiation Oncology

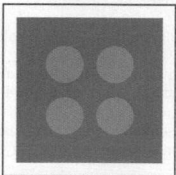

Chapter 2
Biologic Basis of Radiation Therapy

William H. McBride, H. Rodney Withers

Injury to DNA is the primary mechanism by which ionizing radiation kills cells (4,83). Most DNA damage is repaired, but lethal double-strand breaks are thought to persist in the form of locally multiply damaged sites (300) of about 15 to 20 nucleotides in size that cause micronuclei formation, chromosome aberrations, and cell death through loss of the reproductive integrity of the cell's genome (38,66,112,158,235,236). However, many biologic factors affect the relationship between the amount of physical energy deposited, the extent of DNA damage that is caused, the number of cells that are killed, and the severity of the tissue response.

The energy initially deposited by ionizing radiation is largely converted into the generation of free radicals. Since cells are made up largely of water (about 85%), most of the damage to biologic molecules caused by x-rays (perhaps 65% or more) is mediated through free radicals formed by activated water, and in particular, hydroxyl radicals, and most DNA damage is therefore indirect. A chain of physicochemical reactions is initiated that is heavily influenced by the intracellular milieu, which influences the persistence of free radicals and the other chemical species that are formed, and the damage that results. Perhaps the most important molecular presence is that of oxygen (5), although other electron-affinic molecules will also play a role. Oxygen can participate in the free radical-generation chain, fix free radical damage, and limit chemical repair. Conversely, sulfhydryl molecules, which vary in natural abundance, scavenge free radicals and may limit the extent of damage.

In contrast to sparsely ionizing x-rays, densely ionizing high linear energy transfer (LET) radiations (e.g., neutrons, α-particles) deposit their energy so intensely along their tracks that lethality relies more on direct ionization to cause damage in DNA and other molecules than on indirect action through ionization of water. The outcome of the interaction of the physicochemical events initiated by ionizing radiation with the biologic system therefore varies with the nature of the radiation and the intracellular milieu, in addition to obvious factors such as dose and dose rate.

Further complexities are that cells sense and respond to radiation damage and this mechanism varies, depending on their biochemical and genetic make-up. Several molecules have been identified by which cells sense damage to DNA (the DNA damage response), and to other intracellular structures and molecules,

including mitochondria, membrane lipids, and certain growth factor receptors. Recognition of damage leads to activation of signal transduction pathways aimed at making a coherent and appropriate response to injury. The internal molecular signaling network that exists within a cell as well as the external signals they are receiving (e.g., from hypoxia, cytokines, cell-cell contact, and the extracellular matrix) influence the nature of the response. The resultant radiation-induced pathways can promote cell death or survival, cell cycle arrest or progression, and DNA repair or instability. In other words, the way the cell "perceives" radiation damage plays an important role in determining the final response. Since tumorigenesis requires mutations in molecular pathways that govern cell death, cell cycle, and DNA repair, it follows that genetic alterations associated with cancer frequently affect the response to radiation therapy. It should be noted that similar pathways are often activated in response to stresses other than radiation, including chemotherapy, hyperthermia, oxidative agents, and inflammation. However, radiation differs from these in that it causes a relatively large number of large lesions in DNA that are not only frequently lethal but drive a predominance of pathways triggered by DNA double-strand break formation.

Finally, in addition to molecular and cellular factors that determine intrinsic cellular radiosensitivity, tissue-related and clinical features of radiation exposure add several additional layers of complexity. For example, the number of cells in a tissue capable of regenerating function will be important, as will the way the regenerative potential is distributed as functional subunits within the tissue. Tissue responses may not relate directly to radiation's cytotoxic effects. For example, in tumors, although local control requires elimination of tumor clonogens, in some circumstances vascular damage could be important, especially when irradiation is combined with biologics or chemotherapeutic drugs. Also, irradiation modifies the tumor-host relationship, including interactions with infiltrating cells, such as macrophages and lymphocytes, which have been shown to be able to both promote and inhibit tumor growth. Effects have been described, mainly *in vitro*, in which the irradiated cell affects the viability or mutability of surrounding "bystander" cells. Such bystander effects may involve more than one mechanism but are presumably, *in vivo* in normal tissues, a "danger" signaling mechanism for responses to irradiation aimed at tissue healing. Further, some side effects of radiation therapy on normal tissues (13) may result from the release of cytokines and other biologic factors or may be associated with remodeling of the normal tissues, rather than cell death *per se*. For example, late radiation-induced normal tissue fibrosis depends to an extent on cell depletion by radiation, but is more an attempt at a healing response that can be modified by numerous factors, including health status, presence of infection, surgery, injury, and so on.

So, while the initial deposition of energy and subsequent radiochemical events are complete within thousandths of a second following irradiation, a chain of biologic events is initiated that induce programmed cell death or survival, tissue repair and remodeling, all of which depend on the intercellular signaling network, all of which are influenced by systemic and local physiologic conditions. Given the complexity of the biologic condition, it is impossible to predict biologic or clinical outcomes from the amount of physical energy deposited. In other words, biological dose differs from physical dose.

Remarkably, while cells and tissues may respond differently to the same physical dose of radiation, any given tissue appears to respond in a fairly predictable way. The reason for this apparent constancy is that tissue responses are governed largely by cell turnover and the regenerative reserve in the tissue that is generally similar between individuals. Therefore, normal mucosal reactions occur at the same time interval after the start of irradiation and have similar dose-response relationships in most patients. While tumor responses may be more variable than those in normal tissues, certain histologic types of tumors are regarded as more curable by irradiation, and others are not. Reproducible differences in biologic response between tissues are, in fact, exploited for therapeutic benefit. A good example is the use of standard dose fractionation in conventional radiation therapy. This protocol was derived empirically but actually exploits differences in the biologic response between tumor and normal tissues to the same physical dose of radiation. The radiobiologic rationale for the use of dose fractionation in standard radiation therapy has been encapsulated in the 4 "Rs" (reoxygenation, redistribution, repair, and repopulation) (311). This chapter aims to explain how radiobiologic concepts derived from studies dealing with responses within and between normal tissues and tumors are relevant in clinical radiotherapy.

▪▪ | Normal Tissue Radiobiology

Modes of Cell Death after Irradiation

Mitotic Death

Pioneers in radiobiology recognized that cells lethally injured by clinically relevant doses of radiation typically execute one or more divisions before undergoing "mitotic death," the number depending on the size of the radiation dose (273,274). After 2 Gy, two to three attempts may be made. The progeny of these cells may all die or a proportion may survive to contribute to the reproductive pool, and in the case of tumor recurrence.

Interphase Death

The early pioneers also realized that, in contrast to mitotic death, certain cell types, including many lymphocytes, and some oligodendrocytes and serous cells in the salivary gland, thyroid, intestinal crypt, and hair follicles may undergo relatively rapid "interphase death" within about 2 to 6 hours after irradiation. Typically, only low doses of radiation are required; that is, interphase death is a characteristic of "radiosensitive" cells. Importantly, cells that die during interphase cannot contribute to the reproductive pool. While interphase death was a phenomenon recognized by radiobiologists for decades, recognition of the fact that cells could die by more than one pathway has only recently received wider credence as different pathways leading to cell death have become delineated (67,147,191,256). Interphase death is now acknowledged to represent death by rapid apoptosis.

Apoptotic Death

The morphologic characteristics of apoptosis are nuclear condensation, cell shrinkage, membrane blebbing, and nuclear fragmentation with formation of apoptotic bodies. At the biochemical level, endonucleases are activated that fragment DNA into nucleosomal-sized pieces that are multiples of 180 to 200 base pairs (the size of a nucleosome) and that produce a characteristic "ladder" pattern on agarose gel electrophoresis. In tissue sections, apoptosis can be recognized morphologically. Alternatively, fluorescein or other labels can be attached to the 5′-ends of apoptotic DNA strand breaks using terminal deoxynucleotidyl transferase (TUNEL technique) to allow visualization. In apoptosis, neighboring cells phagocytose cell remnants, and inflammation is not induced. Within a few hours, the whole process is complete, leaving no trace, which makes it easy to underestimate the role of apoptosis in cell loss. Radiation-induced apoptosis in normal tissues is often, but not always, dependent on activation of the tumor suppressor gene p53 (144). Importantly, apoptosis is an active form of cell "suicide" since it requires active metabolic processes. Apoptosis is the primary mechanism by which the body creates organ structures during morphogenesis and tissue sculpting. This is why apoptosis is often called *programmed cell death type I*. In the adult, apoptosis is required for normal tissue homeostasis; for example, removal of excess cells at sites of proliferation, self-reactive lymphocytes, some cell types as they age or lose the influence of survival signals, virally infected cells, hypoxic cells, or cells damaged by irradiation. It recycles many cell types and removes potentially harmful cells.

The ability to undergo rapid apoptosis is restricted to particular cell types, and even then only at certain positions within tissues that relate to their developmental stage (144). Only cells that have their internal molecular "rheostat" on a proapoptosis setting appear to undergo rapid apoptosis following irradiation. In other words, irradiation tends to increase the frequency of apoptosis only in tissues and tumors in which the cells already have a proapoptotic tendency. Thus, lymphomas generally have proapoptotic tendencies, whereas glioblastoma multiforme cells do not, with or without irradiation.

Necrotic Death

In contrast to apoptosis, necrosis is, for the most part, a pathologic, rather than a physiologic, process that does not require active metabolic cellular processes. It is involved in tissue healing in response to injury or invasion by pathogens. Necrosis can also be a pathologic response to vascular damage, as well as a "default" death pathway for cells that lack an effective apoptotic apparatus. Membrane integrity is lost, cells increase in size, lysosomal enzymes are released, and inflammatory responses are generated with release of cytokines that link cell death to the development of specific immunity. DNA from cells undergoing necrosis forms a "smear" on agarose gel electrophoresis.

Another alternative death style following irradiation is autophagy, where cells internalize cellular organelles within vacuoles and digest them. This is most often seen in nutrient deprivation but is also another form of "programmed" cell death (type II) involved in morphogenesis and tissue sculpting. Other outcomes may be important in specific cell types.

Radiation-induced differentiation, senescence, or quiescence are possible outcomes that may achieve the same objective as death in removing damaged tumor cells from the reproductive pool and limiting the chances of carcinogenesis. A difference is that in these cases some function is retained for some time. For example, terminal differentiation of fibrocytes gives a cell phenotype that can contribute to radiation-induced fibrosis through enhanced collagen production (121).

While radiation-induced interphase death can easily be ascribed to apoptosis, mitotic death may involve several mechanisms; for example, failure of spindle formation in M phase, loss of the G2 checkpoint leading to "mitotic catastrophe," or improper chromosome segregation due to damage and loss of genetic material, which may be manifested microscopically as chromosome alterations. Furthermore, mechanistically, the molecular machinery that is employed can be apoptotic, necrotic, or any other. Mitotic death, by its very nature, is normally delayed, occurring over a period of days. Unlike "rapid" (interphase) apoptosis, there is no evidence to suggest that cells that die by "delayed" (mitotic) apoptosis are particularly radiosensitive.

The molecular pathways that participate in cell death are described in another chapter, but it is appropriate here to consider specific phenomena that might relate to *in vivo* responses. The presence of "survival" signals appropriate for the cell's environment, such as those provided by growth factors, cell-cell contact, and extracellular matrix, will be important in determining response to irradiation. Their loss leads to a phenomenon known as "anoikis" (97) or homelessness, which is a form of "death by neglect." This is why lymphocytes activated by growth factors are more radioresistant than resting lymphocytes and endothelial cells are more radioresistant in the presence than in the absence of mitogenic basic fibroblast growth factor (98). This may be a broadly applicable concept and explain why blocking receptor tyrosine signaling with cetuximab, Iressa, or similar agents, or NF-κB activation with bBortezomib, may radiosensitize tumor cells.

Survival pathway signaling may also underlie some of the phenomena ascribed to potentially lethal damage repair (PLDR) following irradiation. In PLDR, the cellular microenvironment determines the likelihood of cell death. Classically, PLDR occurs when cells are irradiated and maintained in a contact-inhibited, plateau-phase culture (111,229). If such contact-inhibited cells are trypsinized immediately, or soon after irradiation, survival is compromised, as demonstrated, for example, by lowered clonogenicity. The cells are rendered "homeless" by trypsinization and are more likely to die. It must be noted, however, that PLDR has been invoked as a mechanism that increases survival under diverse sets of experimental conditions and that multiple mechanisms may contribute to the final outcome (282).

As opposed to "death by neglect," certain positive signals can cause death of susceptible cells. Classically, such signals involve members of the tumor necrosis factor (TNF) family of cytokines (e.g. TNF-α, fasL, Trail). Activation of TNF receptor (TNFR) family members that contain a death domain in their cytoplasmic tail can trigger apoptosis. Other members of the same family of receptors that do not have a death domain, as well as soluble receptors and receptor antagonists, can counteract these death threats. Therefore, the type of receptor and related molecules that a cell expresses may determine its response to TNF. TNF-α causes proliferation of some cell types, such as fibroblasts or their CNS equivalent, astrocytes. In contrast, TNF-α can induce growth arrest or apoptosis in many tumors and in some normal cells, such as oligodendrocytes. Since radiation can induce expression of both TNF and TNFR family, these pathways can contribute indirectly to death or survival of some cell types following irradiation (114,115,125). For example, mice lacking TNFR2, which does not have a death domain and drives cell survival, are particularly sensitive to late

effects of irradiation to the brain (61). The cytotoxicity of certain chemotherapeutic agents, such as 5-fluorouacil and cisplatin, can also involve TNF-α (206). Because TNF-α is a primary mediator of inflammation, a proinflammatory cytokine cascade is activated in tissues following irradiation that may also activate bystander cells.

●● Cell Death in Irradiated Normal
●● Tissues

Radiation-induced apoptosis varies with location within a tissue, reflecting the fact that apoptosis is inherently programmed in a position-dependent manner. For understandable reasons, most of the information on radiation-induced apoptosis in normal tissues comes from studies in mice. Radiation-induced rapid apoptosis in the mouse small intestine is maximal around position 4 from the base of the crypt (232), which is the site of the proliferative compartment and of spontaneous apoptosis. In contrast, apoptosis is not so marked in the colon and is not seen in the proliferative region. Indeed, the antiapoptotic molecule Bcl-2 is expressed by cells in this region (184). In lymphoid tissues, small intestine, hair follicles, and ependyma, there is some concordance between the position of apoptotic cells and radiation-induced up-regulated expression of p53 (54,183,184,232). In subpopulations of cells in other tissues, p53 can be up-regulated with little evidence of rapid apoptosis, while most cells in liver, skeletal muscle, and brain show neither p53 nor much apoptosis (144,169,177,206). In the thymus, developing T lymphocytes with the potential to respond to foreign antigens are selected by apoptotic elimination of both self-reacting and nonreacting T cells in the cortex (positive and negative selection). About 98% of the cells that are generated by mitotic division die (about 5×10^7 cells per day in a young adult mouse). After irradiation, massive rapid, p53-dependent apoptosis of T cells is seen in the cortex, but less apoptosis is evident in the medulla, which contains more mature cells.

The role of apoptosis in normal tissue responses to irradiation has yet to be fully evaluated, but inevitably it will depend on the physiologic role of the proapoptotic cells. If the proapoptotic cells are superfluous to needs, radiation-induced cell death in this compartment may have little impact, but if they are critical to tissue function the opposite will be true. For example, in the mouse small intestine, the cells that die by rapid apoptosis may contribute little to the clonogenic crypt stem cell population. Thus, there is little difference between p53 wild type and p53-null mice in their clonogenic responses following gut irradiation (118), although variation with dose and dose rate is evident (117). In the mouse brain, radiation-induced apoptosis is seen in endothelial cells, oligodendrocytes, and the neuroepithelial subventricular zone (122) where it depends on the protein that is mutated in ataxia telengiectasia and p53, both of which are phosphorylated by radiation and act as sensors of DNA damage, as well as TNFR expression. The extreme radiosensitivity of the developing brain is probably due to its high apoptotic index. Although little information is available in humans, acute parotitis can develop in the first 24 hours of treatment of patients receiving head and neck irradiation, and this reflects apoptotic death of serous cells (251). There is no such acute death in the mucous cells; hence, the mouth is dry and the saliva more viscous.

●● Pathobiology and Kinetics of Radiation
●● Injury in Normal Tissues

The time to development of most normal tissue injury depends critically on the turnover time of the tissue, that is, on the kinetics of cell differentiation, loss, and renewal. The terms *acute, subacute,* or *late* are commonly used to describe the time to occurrence of functional inadequacy after irradiation and reflect kinetic differences between tissues while saying little about the underlying pathogenesis of the response. The terms are also often loosely used to describe the tissues in which such effects are seen, as in "acute effects tissue," but this can be misleading since tissues and organs comprise more than one cell type, each with its own turnover rate characteristics. Any one tissue can therefore express both acute and late symptoms of radiation damage, depending on the cell type that is limiting function at that time. Also, a severe acute injury from irradiation can lead to nonspecific late (consequential) changes such as fibrosis, atrophy, or ulceration (35,223,329) (e.g., stenosis consequent to mucosal ulceration of the bowel, or fibrosis or necrosis of skin or oropharyngeal tissues consequent to desquamation and acute ulceration).

Acute Responses

Acute responses to radiation therapy are defined as occurring during a standard 6- to 8-week course of therapy and are seen in tissues with large populations of cells that turn over rapidly (gastrointestinal mucosa, bone marrow, skin, and oropharyngeal and esophageal mucosa). Hierarchical organization exists in such tissues (187–189,303) with a small number of stem cells that proliferate slowly to produce a highly proliferative compartment of progenitor cells that differentiate into mature, nonproliferative, functional cells. Irradiation may deplete the stem and progenitor cell pools, but nonproliferating, differentiated cells maintain tissue function until they are lost through continuing normal cell turnover.

After irradiation, depleted stem and progenitor cell pools may first reconstitute their own numbers before differentiating to restore function, although the extent to which this occurs varies with the tissue. A useful model to consider is that under normal steady-state circumstances (i.e., not growing or involuting), tissues have, by definition, a cell-loss factor (ϕ) of 1. The only requirement for growth of a tissue is a decrease in ϕ to less than 1, which is characteristic of the embryo and fetus, tissue regeneration, and malignancy. After irradiation, some tissues (e.g., jejunal crypts) reduce ϕ to 0 and regenerate quickly; others (e.g., skin) may reduce it to about 0.5 and regenerate less quickly, but continuously produce some functional cells; others (e.g., seminiferous epithelium) show little change in ϕ and mostly continue in steady state, producing sperm in numbers that are reduced for months or years in direct proportion to the extent of stem cell depletion.

Because acute-responding tissues are organized in a hierarchical fashion, the *severity* of radiation injury depends on both the extent of stem/progenitor cell depletion and the length of the delay before new functional cells are released into the differentiated compartment. Severity of injury naturally increases with dose, but providing the proliferative pool does not fall below a critical value symptoms are transient and recovery is complete. Dose fractionation can lessen the severity of acute effects by allowing regeneration from the stem/progenitor cell compartment during the course of therapy. Unlike the *extent* of injury, the *rate* at which acute injury develops and the latent time to the appearance of symptoms is relatively (187), although not completely (175), independent of dose. This is because latency is mainly determined by the rate of loss of differentiated cells.

Because cell turnover kinetics determines the time to a normal tissue effect, latency is not an indicator of radiosensitivity. For example, in hematopoiesis, leukocyte and platelet numbers drop quickly after bone marrow irradiation because they have a fast turnover rate, whereas anemia is not an obvious acute effect because red cells turn over slowly. Similarly, in the testis, each spermatogenic stem cell division ultimately produces more than 1,000 sperm through successive divisions of spermatogo-

nia and spermatocytes—a process that in humans takes more than 60 days. Early differentiating spermatogonia are few in number and are selectively depleted by doses that have little effect on cells in the more mature stages of spermatogenesis. This is why sperm counts remain normal for several weeks after exposure, falling steeply only at the time when the progeny of the irradiated spermatogonia would normally have reached the seminal vesicles. In the mucosa of the small bowel, mitotic activity is confined to the crypts; the cells lining the villus are nonproliferative. Because crypt cells divide rapidly (an average of more than once daily in humans), they are lost within days if sterilized by radiation. The villus shows no immediate effect of irradiation, with shortening becoming evident only as programmed shedding of differentiated cells into the lumen continues in the absence of renewal from the crypts. This is why symptoms take about 2 weeks to appear in patients undergoing standard daily doses of abdominal irradiation.

Subacute Responses

Certain tissues may display subacute reactions several months after irradiation, reflecting failure of a cell population with a longer turnover time. Symptoms are generally reversible, although in some instances they may be associated with severe damage and even death. Examples of transient effects are Lhermitte's syndrome after spinal cord irradiation, somnolence after brain irradiation, and subacute pneumonitis 2 to 3 months after the start of lung irradiation. Subacute effects occur most often during the remodeling phase in irradiated tissues and prior to the onset of late effects that are associated with slowly progressing damage.

Late Responses

Late reactions to radiation therapy in normal tissues can be severe, and recovery is often limited. They are generally considered to be the result of the depletion of slowly proliferating "target" cells that are lost from the tissue at a slow rate, for example, from central (oligodendroglia) or peripheral (Schwann cells) nervous tissue, kidney (tubule epithelium), blood vessels (endothelium), dermis (fibroblasts), and bones (osteoblasts and chondroblasts). However, abortive rounds of attempts at healing may involve different cell types in distinct cellular compartments, and lesions can appear to evolve with time in a dose-dependent manner (278). Some lesions, such as those associated with artherosclerosis and heart disease (238), can take decades to occur after irradiation and are an increasing problem as patients live longer following cancer therapy. Pathologic findings following collapse of late effects tissues can be very variable. For example, late demyelination after brain irradiation may be ascribed to loss of oligodendrocytes and subsequently of neurons (50), but coincident with and preceding any neurologic changes, proliferation of astrocytes and microglial cells can be observed (51), as can vascular lesions with edema, hemorrhage, or inflammatory infiltrates (45). Infiltrating cells may contribute to the pathogenesis of radiation injury, as is illustrated by involvement of infiltrating cells in the pathogenesis of radiation pneumonitis, or recovery from injury as in the slower healing of skin wounds in mice receiving total body irradiation compared with those irradiated only at the local site (293).

Unlike acute responding hierarchical tissues, slowly proliferating, late effects tissues contain cells that are usually both functional and able to proliferate on demand. In an operational sense, such tissues can be regarded as "flexible" (187–189). This does not deny the presence of stem cells with limited function or functional cells that do not proliferate, but the roles of such cells are probably of lesser importance than in hierarchical tissues. The relative inability of late effects tissues to be repopulated from a stem cell pool makes radiation reactions in these tissues more chronic and debilitating, diminishing the quality of life for those afflicted.

As in acute-responding tissues, the *rate* at which radiation injury develops in late effects tissues reflects the turnover rate of proliferative cells, which may be also functional cells in this case (e.g., liver, kidney). Therefore, dose has a greater apparent influence on <u>latency</u>, with late injury developing more quickly with increase in dose. This may be because the greater the dose, the fewer the number of division cycles the cells can successfully negotiate before death (166,177,273). Another reason may be that as cells die, residual (mostly lethally injured) target cells are increasingly recruited to the proliferative pool, causing a cascade or "avalanche" of cell death and functional tissue failure. A third explanation may be that because interactions between cell types tend to be involved in the causation of late effects, the nature of the lesion may vary with time, depending on which cell type is critically limiting at that time (45,284,285). The time course to development of injury can be accelerated and the severity increased by various insults such as surgery, chemotherapy, infection, or physical trauma (105,106). Indeed, such factors may play a major role in precipitating the onset of late effects in humans (e.g., necrotic, nonhealing ulcers after trauma). Conversely, slowing the proliferation process and decreasing stress may reduce their incidence and severity.

Whereas a severe early response in a rapidly proliferating tissue permits adjustment of the dose schedule during the course of standard radiation therapy, this is not the case for late injuries, since they occur after completion of therapy. Tolerance doses for individual patients are therefore based on past experience. Such tolerance doses have not been precisely defined, even though, generally accepted limits to doses considered tolerable by various organs do exist in practice (85,241).

An issue of growing clinical importance is the extent to which late radiation effects can be reversed. It has been shown recently that certain agents given late after radiation can modify injury in tissues. For example, captopril, an angiotensin-converting enzyme inhibitor, slows the development of radiation-induced nephritis (194,196), pneumopathy, and lung fibrosis (192) in rats. Steroids also can prevent death from radiation pneumonitis in animals, although their withdrawal before the end of the usual period of pneumonitis can result in accelerated mortality (109). Pentoxifylline, alone or in combination with vitamin E, protects against radiation-induced late effects in some experimental models (69,151) and in a clinical study, Delanian et al. (63) found that the combination, but neither agent alone, reversed chronic radiation-induced fibrosis. It is not clear how these agents act and whether they promote cellular recovery, but such studies point to ways to improve the future management of late complications of radiation therapy (189).

Functional Subunits

The tolerance of a tissue to irradiation is determined by the number of cells with regenerative potential and the way they are organized, in addition to their intrinsic radiosensitivity. Tissues can be thought of as being composed of functional subunits (FSUs), which is the minimum clonogenic entity required for regeneration of a structure. For example, epilation requires doses lower than those for desquamation. This is not because the cells in the hair follicle differ in their radiosensitivity from those in the basal epithelium, but because there is a smaller number of clonogenic cells in the FSU that produces a hair than in the sheet of basal cells that is capable of regenerating itself. Similarly, hair is depigmented by relatively low doses of radiation (294), but the epidermis loses pigmentation only after higher

doses. This is because each hair follicle contains a small number of melanocytes, sometimes only one, whereas melanocytes are more numerous in the epidermis.

In the kidney, each nephron is an FSU (324). If a tubule is completely de-epithelialized, it is lost permanently because it is not repopulated from adjacent nephrons. Therefore, the tolerance dose for the kidney is determined more by the number of tubule cells per nephron than the number of nephrons. For example, if the kidney contained 10^{11} clonogenic tubule cells distributed as 10^4 cells in each of 10^7 nephrons and any one of these 10^4 cells were capable of regenerating the tubule, then most tubules should regenerate after a dose that reduced survival to 10^{-4} (or an average of one cell per tubule). Because of the random nature of events, some tubules would then contain more than one surviving cell and others would contain none. From Poisson distribution statistics, 37% of FSU nephrons would be eliminated. The "tolerance" dose would be different if the organ were composed of 10^4 nephrons, each containing 10^7 cells: The dose that would eliminate 37% of the nephrons would be that to reduce survival to 10^{-7}. In a multifractionated dose regimen, during which a logarithmic decline in cell number occurs, this is 7/4 (1.75) times that required to reduce survival to 10^{-4}. This is why tolerance doses can vary so much among tissues and organs, even if the target cells have the same intrinsic radiosensitivity.

It is easy to appreciate the structural organization of FSUs for hair and kidney, but not for some other tissues. For example, in mouse skin, the survival of about 10 cells per cm^2, from what is normally approximately 10^6 basal stem cells per cm^2, is required to maintain uninterrupted integrity and prevent overt desquamation (308). Therefore, the FSU would be about 1/10 cm^2. Organs with acinar or alveolar architecture (e.g., salivary glands, pancreas, sweat glands, testis, mammary epithelium, lung, and perhaps liver) may resemble the kidney in having structurally defined FSUs, while the target cells in dermis, CNS, mucosae, gut, and epidermis are less restricted by physical barriers and cellular migration may influence regeneration.

Known tolerance doses are consistent with FSUs being relatively small in tissues such as kidney with structurally well-defined FSUs, are intermediate in the spinal cord, and large in the dermis. Obviously, a primary tumor is just one large FSU in which one surviving clonogen can lead to recurrence. Clonogenic cell number will play a big role in determining local tumor control. For metastatic deposits, regional control will depend not only on the number of clonogenic cells each contains but also the number of metastatic deposits. In general, a larger number of small metastatic deposits will be cured with lower radiation doses than a small number of larger metastases, even if the total cell number is the same in both cases.

Volume Effects

Traditionally, radiation oncologists have reduced the total dose when treating large volumes of normal tissue. In fact, the now widespread reduction in dose per fraction from 2 to 1.8 Gy had its origin in a volume effect; the longer treatment duration enhanced mucosal tolerance in large head and neck treatment fields (93). In the orthovoltage era, a reduction in dose with increase in treatment volume was generally recommended (218), but with the advent of skin-sparing megavoltage beams, the volume effect received less attention, especially as larger tumors (and larger treatment volumes) require higher doses for their control.

In fact, the concept of decreasing dose with increasing treatment volume has little radiobiologic basis, except in specific circumstances. For example, if FSUs are arranged in series, like links in a chain, as they are in nerve tracts, spinal cord, and the cylindrical sheath of peritoneum covering the small intestine,

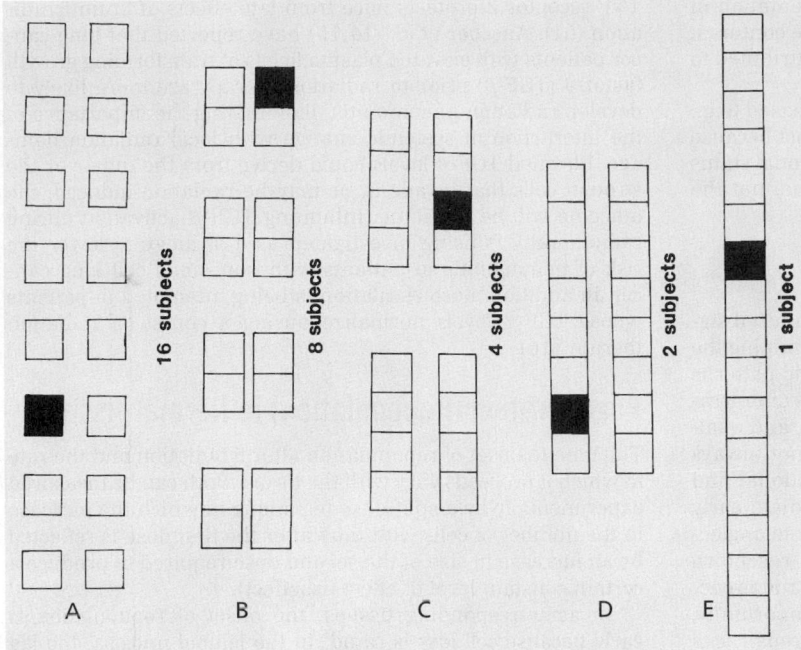

FIGURE 2.1. Diagrammatic representation of the influence on the probability of a complication from increasing the treatment volume in a tissue where functional subunits (FSUs) are arranged serially. The average survival of FSUs was 1 in 16, sterilized FSUs being denoted by the black squares. With the small volumes (**A**), the probability of myelitis was 6% (1/16), whereas it would approach 100% if 16 FSUs in one patient were exposed (**E**). The actual probabilities can be calculated using the equation in the text. (From Withers HR, Taylor JMG, Maciejewski B. Treatment volume and tissue tolerance. *Int J Radiat Oncol Biol Phys* 1988;14:751, with permission.)

the loss of one subunit may result in an overt expression of injury, regardless of the state of the other subunits in the series. The probability of injury increases with volume (number of FSUs exposed) (Fig. 2.1). Such a volume effect has been demonstrated clinically for small bowel obstruction (160,231) and experimentally for myelitis (126,246,286).

The relationship between the number of FSUs irradiated (n) and the probability of a complication (P) is described by the following formula:

$$P = 1 - (1 - p)^n$$

where p is the probability of the loss of one FSU. This relationship is illustrated in Figure 2.2. Increasing the volume (number of FSUs exposed) reduces the dose necessary to produce a complication and increases the steepness of the dose-response curves. The effect would be predicted to occur when the

average number of surviving cells per FSU is reduced to almost one and when the length of serial arrangement of FSUs is small. This may be less true for the small bowel (100,160,319) than for spinal cord.

Nonradiobiologic "volume effects" exist that can result from multiple mechanisms. There are some mechanisms that can be excluded. For example, there is no evidence that cellular radiosensitivity is affected by an increase in treatment volume (332). The radiosensitivity of skin epithelium is constant over a 5,000-fold range of treatment area (308,332). Also, no evidence exists for an increased role for vascular damage as volume increases (326). On the other hand, "volume effects" can be seen when (332):

1. A patient tolerates a small area of injury (such as ulceration) better than a large area of the same severity because pain, exudation, infection are worse, healing is slower, and consequential contraction and scarring are more of a problem. The effect of increasing volume is to make the injury more incapacitating, even though the severity of the radiation response is independent of volume treated.
2. Large gradients in dose distribution and heterogeneity develop as volume increases. Without prudent planning, a tumor dose may be prescribed at the 80% level, leading to a 25% higher dose in the region of D_{max}. Also, with large fields, large variations in contour may exist. These variations could result in a high-dose region where tissue thickness is less than that measured at the midplane; as, for example, in the spinal cord at the thoracic inlet in thoracic irradiation and in tangential fields for treatment of the breast. If the threshold-sigmoid curve of the probability of normal tissue complications against dose is steep, as it is in experimental studies (266), a 25% increase in total dose could produce a marked change in the incidence of complications. This increase in physical dose is further compounded by the biologic effectiveness of each dose per fraction being increased by more than 25%, or the "double trouble" of increased physical and biological dose. The magnitude of the increase in "biological" dose will depend on the dose per fraction and the type of normal tissue, but will be greatest in late-responding normal tissues for reasons that will be explained later in terms of the nonlinear rate of increase in injury with increase in

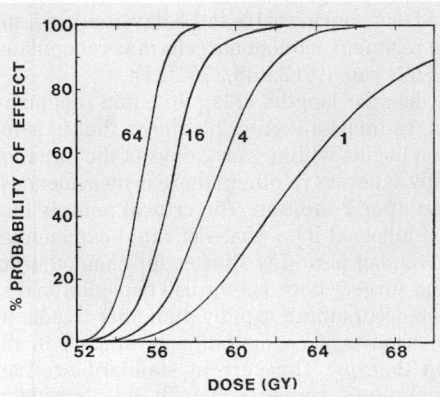

FIGURE 2.2. Curves illustrating how the probability of producing a complication increases with increase in the number of serially arranged functional subunits (FSUs) included in the treatment volume. The curves were positioned by assuming that 58 Gy in 2-Gy fractions sterilized 10% of FSUs and that for a series of 2-Gy fractions the effective D_0 for the target cells was 4 Gy. The curves are shifted to the left and are steeper with increase in number of FSUs exposed, but this effect becomes less obvious once large numbers of subunits are involved. (From Withers HR, Taylor JMG, Maciejewski B. Treatment volume and tissue tolerance. *Int J Radiat Oncol Biol Phys* 1988;14:751, 1988, with permission.)

dose per fraction. Because this additional augmentation of biologic doses is not evident from physical isodose contours, an increased biologic effect may be erroneously attributed to the large volume being treated *per se*.

3. If organ "reserve" is obliterated as volume is increased (e.g., lung, salivary gland), this is not a true volume effect because sequelae are determined by the volume and functional status of the tissue *excluded* from the treatment volume, not the volume irradiated.

Molecular Responses in Normal Tissues

As discussed in the introductory section, radiation-induced signal transduction pathways can be important in determining the cellular response to damage. Cell- and tissue-specific patterns of molecular responses are detected minutes to hours after irradiation that can vary with radiation dose, dose rate, and quality, and with dose-response relationships that are not always linear. The most rapid response includes transcriptional and posttranscriptional activation of members of immediate early gene families, such as c-jun and c-fos, ATM (ataxia telangiectasia), p53, c-abl, EGFR (epidermal growth factor receptor), and other molecules. Phosphorylation/dephosphorylation reactions or other activating mechanisms are invoked. Importantly, these pathways couple molecular damage to DNA repair, cell cycle arrest, phenotypic changes, and cell death. Another part of the early response involves the induction of sets of secreted molecules such as proinflammatory cytokines, proteases and antiproteases, cell adhesion molecules, and extracellular matrix materials that together form a regulated acute tissue reaction (125) to trigger subsequent tissue remodeling. Such "danger" signaling can extend beyond the radiation field and may be responsible for some of the observed "abscopal" effects of irradiation. The overall function of radiation-induced molecular responses is to preserve cell and tissue integrity after irradiation by promoting cell death/survival and tissue recovery and remodeling.

Radiation-induced inflammatory responses, as well as initiating healing responses in tissues, may "prime" cells and tissues for adaptive responses to further radiation doses. For example, radiation-induced basic fibroblast growth factor may act through autocrine pathways to promote survival of endothelial cells (98). *In vivo*, antagonists of radiation-induced interleukin (IL)-1 and TNF-α increase the intrinsic sensitivity of mice to bone marrow death after irradiation (200,201), suggesting that these responses also have adaptive survival value. On the other hand, radiation-induced TNF-α can cause certain cells to apoptose (115) and may trigger clinical symptoms that can not be ascribed to cell death (16,130). Examples are nausea or vomiting that can occur within hours of irradiation of the upper abdomen, acute erythema and edema associated with vascular leakage, fatigue in patients receiving irradiation to a large volume, especially within the abdomen, and somnolence that can develop within a few hours of cranial irradiation. Radiation-induced proliferative responses such as gliosis (51) or certain forms of fibrosis could also cause symptoms unrelated to cell depletion.

Recently, it has been shown that during the latent period leading up to the expression of late effects, waves of molecular responses occur that may reflect repeated attempts at tissue recovery and remodeling (49). As a result, the concept that late effects represent dysregulation of an integrated injury and healing process that involves both parenchymal and vascular elements, as well as inflammatory cells, has gained in prominence. Failure of any of the required elements could give rise to a late effect.

Cytokines and growth factors are thought to play important roles in late effects. For example, signaling through the TNF receptor 2 protects mice from late effects of brain irradiation (61). Anscher et al. (14,15) have reported that lung cancer patients with elevated plasma levels of transforming growth factor-β (TGF-β) prior to radiation therapy are more likely to develop radiation pneumonitis, illuminating the importance of the interaction of systemic change with local radiation damage. Elevated TGF-β levels could derive from the tumor or the stromal cells that invade it, or may be radiation-induced; the outcome will be the same. Inhibiting TGF-β activation during radiotherapy is being investigated as a strategy to lower the risk of pneumonitis in patients with non–small cell lung cancer. In addition, dose escalation is being attempted in patients whose TGF-β levels normalize during a course of radiation therapy (16).

Regeneration (Repopulation) in Normal Tissues

The time to onset of repopulation after irradiation and the rate at which it proceeds vary with the tissue. Both can be measured experimentally by a split-dose technique in which the increase in the number of cells with time after the first dose is reflected by an increase in size of the second dose required to produce a certain constant level of effect (isoeffect).

In acute-responding tissues, the onset of repopulation is early because cell loss is rapid. In the jejunal mucosa, the lag time before the onset of radiation-induced proliferation may be <24 hours. In the colon and stomach, it is slightly longer. In contrast, in renal tubules, there is no histologic evidence of cell depletion for many months after irradiation, and there is a long lag period before the onset of repopulation. In the mouse, it takes more than 12 months to reconstitute a tubule (324). The rate of repopulation has, similarly, not been well quantified in acutely and, especially, in late-responding tissues. In mice, some approximate doubling times for clonogenic cells are 8, 12, and 22 hours for jejunum, colon (310), and skin (309), respectively.

In humans, tissue turnover kinetics are slower than in mice. They have been approximated for oropharyngeal mucosa from consideration of responses to various dose-fractionation regimens. Mucositis begins to appear 14 to 21 days after the start of a regimen of 2 Gy given five times per week, but repopulation begins at about 10 to 12 days (288). High initial doses may shorten the lag period, but only by 1 or 2 days. Repopulation can increase the tolerance of the mucosa to a conventional dose regimen by an *average* of at least 1 Gy/day, which is equivalent to approximately a doubling of clonogenic cell numbers every 2 days, and it may be significantly faster (321). If daily irradiation is suspended (e.g., during a 10- to 14-day break in a split-course accelerated regimen), clonogenic cells may repopulate at two or three times this rate (9,12,288,299,321).

These values for lengths of lag time and repopulation rates are, at best, estimates. Figure 2.3 shows that in some tissues, regeneration begins within 1 or 2 days of the initiation of radiation therapy, whereas in others there is no evidence for regeneration even after 2 months. The critical point is that there is a lag period followed by a phase of rapid exponential growth. In general, the lag period is shorter for chemotherapy, hyperthermia, and surgery because the cell depletion that stimulates regeneration occurs more rapidly than after irradiation.

The importance of repopulation is implicit in the history of radiation therapy. The current standard protracted overall treatment times confer a benefit by allowing regeneration of acute-responding tissues, which reduces toxicity. When attempts are made to deliver curative therapy more quickly, acute responses become more severe and dose-limiting.

Growth factors may be useful in protecting normal tissues from irradiation by shortening the apparent lag phase and accelerating recovery in irradiated tissues. Hematopoietic growth

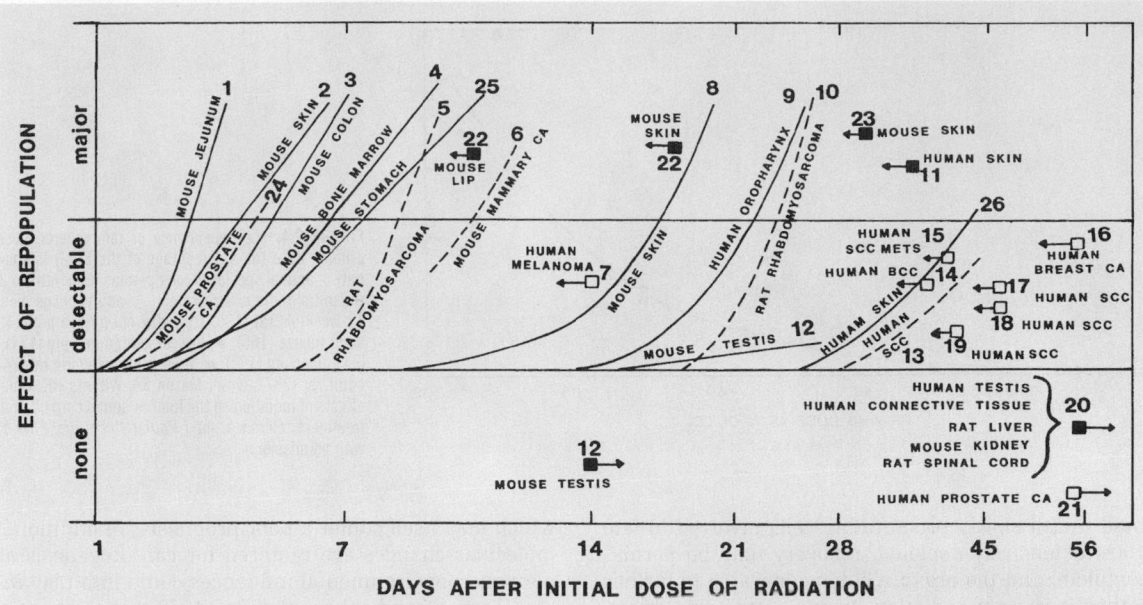

FIGURE 2.3. Representation of the approximate kinetics of regeneration of irradiated normal tissues (*solid lines, solid symbols*) and tumors (*dashed lines, open symbols*). Curves are based on measurements or estimates of regeneration; symbols denote times at which an effect of regeneration has already appeared (◄–■) or has not yet appeared (■–►). The logarithmic abscissa is for convenience of presentation only and has no biologic rationale. In general, the human data are displaced to the right of experimental animal data, reflecting a slower initiation of repopulation because human tissues proliferate more slowly than do their rodent counterparts, they were exposed to protracted dose regimens; and less-sensitive end points were used to detect onset of repopulation in humans. Numbers on the curve and symbols refer to the sources of data. 1, Withers (310); 2, Withers (309); 3, Withers and Mason (322); 4, McCulloch and Till (179); 5, Hermens and Barendsen (120); 6, Suit et al. (259); 7, Choi et al. (53); 8, Denekamp (64); 9, Fletcher (93), Horiot et al. (128), van der Schueren et al. (288), Wang (297,298), and Wang et al. (299); 10, Barendsen and Broerse (21); 11, Arcangeli et al. (17); 12, Withers et al. (320) and Meistrich et al. (180); 13, Maciejewski et al. (168–172); 14, Allen (2); 15, Maciejewski et al. (169); 16, Barker et al. (22); 17, Wang (297,298) and Wang et al. (299); 18, Parsons et al. (216); 19, Maciejewski et al. (168); 20, Pedrick and Hoppe (219), Maciejewski et al. (170), Fisher and Hendry (91), Withers and Mason (324), and van der Kogel (284,285); 21, White and Hornsey (304); and Withers et al. (337); 22, Xu et al. (338) and Ang et al. (12); 23, Ang et al. (9); 24, Kummermehr and Trott (154); 25, Chen and Withers (48); and 26, Turesson and Notter (279).

factors such as G-CSF, GM-CSF, erythropoietin, and IL-11 can accelerate proliferation of hematopoietic cells (199). In doing so, they minimize the danger of infection. In epithelial tissues keratinocyte growth factor, which is specific for epithelial cells, has similar potential. It protects the oral mucosa, small intestine, lung, and hair follicles against chemotherapy or radiation injury (73,87,88,339) in preclinical models and has shown efficacy in clinical bone marrow transplantation trials.

"Remembered" Dose: Tolerance to Retreatment

Conventional teaching in radiation oncology has been that a heavily irradiated tissue will not tolerate retreatment. The postulated reason was that the basis of late effects was vascular damage and was irreversible. While irradiation may limit the tolerance of a tissue to retreatment, in fact, retreatment is often possible and may be better tolerated than previously expected (156). Factors that determine the extent to which residual injury will limit retreatment tolerance include the amount of cell depletion caused by prior treatment, the time elapsed since that treatment and therefore the extent of regeneration, and the tissue at risk. High prior doses, short intervals between treatment courses, and slow regeneration of target cells will reduce retreatment tolerance.

Some data for experimental radiation myelitis are shown in Figure 2.4. The plot shows the effect of size of the first dose on the dose required to produce myelitis in a second regimen. Recovery is complete after low doses, but is progressively compromised as the initial dose approaches tissue tolerance (174). It should be remembered that clinical "tolerance" doses for the spinal cord of 45 to 50 Gy in 1.8- to 2-Gy fractions are low in terms of the injury evaluated in Fig. 2.4 (50% incidence of myelitis). The time to recovery for the spinal cord is not accurately known, but in rats at 100 days it is about half of what it reaches by 200 days (287). In monkeys, there was extensive recovery from 44 Gy in 2.2-Gy fractions by 2 years, but a detailed profile of the time course could not be established (7).

Not all tissues, or elements within tissues, recover at an equal rate or to an equal extent from the effects of irradiation. Acute-responding epithelial and hemopoietic tissues generally recover quickly and demonstrate a high tolerance to retreatment in terms of acute responses. However, the fibrovascular support in skin and mucosa and the stroma in bone marrow are less tolerant to retreatment because they respond more slowly. The kidney shows poor retreatment tolerance as assessed functionally in mice (253). Reirradiation tolerance in this organ is inversely related to the initial dose, but tolerance decreases significantly with increasing interval between treatments, suggesting progression rather than recovery from the initial damage.

Because different tissues show different levels of tolerance to retreatment, caution should be exercised in the application of these concepts to the clinic. Also, the experimental studies deal with well-defined end points within a limited time scale. If different end points in the same tissue are examined or the time is extended, the same guidelines may not apply. It should

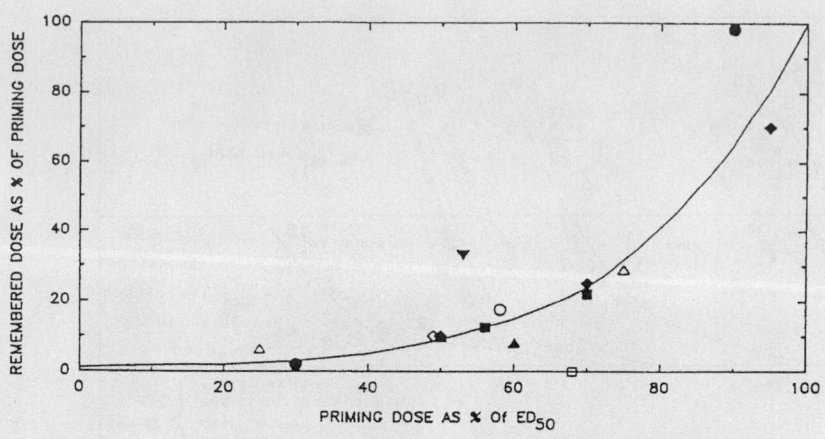

FIGURE 2.4. The dependence of remembered dose on size of priming dose (as a percentage of the ED_{50}) is shown for a variety of animal species at long periods (6 months to 2 years) after the initial radiation treatment: ○, adult rhesus monkey (10); △, 12-week-old rat (130); ▫, 1-day-old guinea pig (149); ●, young adult mouse (165); ▲, 8-week-old guinea pig (174); ▼, 8-week-old guinea pig (198); ■, 3-week-old weanling rat (243); ◆, young adult rat (287). (From Mason KA, Withers HR, Chiang CS. Late effects of radiation on the lumbar spinal cord of guinea pigs: Retreatment tolerance. *Int J Radiat Oncol Biol Phys* 1993;26:643, with permission.)

also be noted that if slowly proliferating cells involved in late responses are extensively depleted, recovery may be permanently incomplete, and the organ will be vulnerable to further injury whether it is from radiation, trauma, cytotoxic drugs, or any other insult. For example, hyperthermia can precipitate myelitis in a patient who has had high, but otherwise tolerable, doses of x-irradiation (161), and trauma from dental intervention frequently precipitates mandibular necrosis.

Tumor Radiobiology

Cell Death in Tumors and Predictive Assays

As is obvious from clinical practice, the doses of irradiation required for a certain control rate vary widely among human tumors. Tumor types that are traditionally radiocurable tend to show greater cellular radiosensitivity *in vitro* (62,89). Although there is a wide spectrum of radiosensitivities within one tumor type (39,225,227,302), these data can be taken as evidence that intrinsic pathways play a role in determining clinical radiation response. Further evidence is that mutations in oncogenes and tumor suppressor genes that affect pathways integral to cell death and proliferation alter intrinsic radiosensitivity (see Chapter 3,4). Therefore, considerable effort has been expended to develop molecular or cellular assays for molecules involved in cell death/survival, proliferation/arrest, and DNA repair so as to predict clinical responses to radiation therapy, and to identify potential targets for tumor radiosensitization.

Apoptotic cells, which are seen in many tumors, have received attention as possible predictors of response. Their clinical relevance is suggested by the fact that tumors of those histologic types that are traditionally radiocurable are also those that have a tendency to apoptose. Lymphocytic tumors generally apoptose more than carcinomas, whereas melanomas, sarcomas, and astrocytomas are relatively resistant (185). Also, experiments in animals have shown that tumors that have a high rate of spontaneous apoptosis exhibit a higher apoptotic index after irradiation and are relatively radiosensitive (191). Importantly, apoptotic cells reappear between fractionated exposures (186). Also, genetic modification of cells to introduce a proapoptotic phenotype frequently, although not always, radiosensitize.

In spite of these encouraging findings, studies specifically designed to find relationships between molecular markers of apoptosis and radiocurability of human tumors have yielded mixed and sometimes contradictory results (220). This may be because the phenotype is not associated with the clonogenic cells or is linked to other features, such as excess proliferation, which may itself confer a poor prognosis. In addition, multiple molecular changes are required for carcinogenesis and complex microenvironmental influences come into play *in vivo*, so many genetic and epigenetic factors affect to the outcome of radiation therapy. Some of these, such as the fraction of tumor cells that are clonogenic, reoxygenation, and regrowth kinetics have already been alluded to. It is therefore unlikely that any single molecular marker will be a useful predictor of individual response. Even molecular screening for expression of thousands of genes using gene microarray technology thus far has not given useful markers, although molecular profiling of tumors will be of future benefit, even if it is only to improve subclassification.

In Vivo Kinetics of Tumor Responses

Most tumors regress during a course of radiation therapy and are considered analogous to acute-responding normal tissues in their radiation dose-fractionation responses, although prostate cancer has recently been suggested to have a low $\alpha\beta$ ratio, like late-responding tissues. As for normal tissues, regression of a tumor after radiation therapy reflects the *rate* of cell loss, which is determined by its turnover kinetics. Thus, tumors with a small cell loss factor can respond slowly after irradiation, even though all their clonogens have been sterilized, as evidenced by their failure to recur.

Cell-Loss Factors in Tumors

A cell-loss factor (ϕ) of less than one is characteristic of tissue growth. In tumors, especially carcinomas, ϕ is actually close to 1 (250), which is why their growth rate is much slower (on average, doubling times of about 60 days) (47) than could be predicted by their proliferative activity. Mitotic count, S-phase count, or labeling index would suggest a potential doubling time of about 3 to 7 days. It follows that a high proliferative index is not necessarily evidence of a rapidly growing tumor. A classic example is the slow-growing basal cell skin carcinoma, in which numerous mitotic figures are commonly visible. They have a high ϕ due to extensive apoptosis (145,146). Necrosis, apoptosis, and exfoliation of cells are the usual mechanisms contributing to ϕ in tumors.

Tumor Regression after Irradiation

Tumors with a high rate of cell loss will regress rapidly during and after irradiation, regardless of pretreatment growth rate, and, providing that the overall treatment duration is not unduly protracted, the prognosis will be good (250,325). Until the cell loss factor decreases, the regressing clonogen pool will contribute little to cell replacement. On the other hand, rapid regression would also be expected in a tumor with a low cell-loss rate if a large proportion of its cells are actively cycling and it is growing quickly, although in this case the prognosis will be poor. Therefore, rapid regression is not a universal prognostic indicator (325) although, in practice, tumors with a high cell-loss rate are more common than those with a low cell-loss rate, and rapid regression is usually a favorable prognostic sign. However, rapid regression may also trigger an accelerated repopulation, and overall treatment durations should not be protracted.

The same arguments can be applied to tumors that regress slowly, such as prostate carcinoma, some cases of nodular sclerosing Hodgkin's disease, teratocarcinomas of testis, some soft tissue sarcomas, choroidal melanomas, meningiomas, pituitary adenomas, chordomas, or glomus tumors. This may reflect slow proliferation, low cell-loss factor, residual stroma, or, sometimes, treatment failure. Slow regression of a tumor type that usually regresses quickly is prognostic of a lower probability of local control, but not necessarily of treatment failure (23).

Repopulation occurs as a homeostatic response to cell depletion caused by treatment. The rate of cell loss slows (the cell loss factor decreases), as in acute-responding normal tissues, to permit rapid repopulation. Tumors with a high rate of cell production and a high cell-loss factor will behave similarly and are likely to regress quickly, but recur early and regrow rapidly after unsuccessful irradiation, chemotherapy, or surgery (2).

A practical implication of the complex reasons for different rates of tumor response to radiation therapy is that it is not a good idea to reduce the total dose just because a tumor regresses rapidly (260). Also, local control of tumors that grow slowly because of high cell-loss factors may initiate an early repopulation response, and local control may be prejudiced by protraction of treatment time beyond normal, just as it is for fast-growing tumors that are initially fast growing (204,331). Well-differentiated tumors (which have a high cell-loss factor) are more prone to an early reduction in cell-loss factor and, consequently, an early repopulation response, which prejudices local control, especially if overall duration of treatment is protracted (72).

:: | Tumor Regeneration after Irradiation

Potential Doubling Time

The potential regeneration rate of tumors after cytotoxic injury is better predicted by preirradiation proliferative activity than by preirradiation tumor growth rate. The *potential doubling time* (T_{pot}) (29,31,250,307), which is the time that would be required for the number of clonogenic cells to double if the cell-loss factor were zero, is a measure of the S-phase (T_s) and the fraction of cells in S-phase, measured by labeling index (LI):

$$T_{pot} = \lambda T_s / LI$$

where λ is a correction factor for the cell-cycle distribution of the population.

T_{pot} is a logical predictor of the kinetics of a regenerative response; attempts were made to use it to predict which tumors would benefit from acceleration of treatment that aims to minimize such repopulation (29,128,307). Early results indicated that it might be of some value, but more recent analyses indicate otherwise (30,133). This may be because the cell cycle time measured in an unperturbed tumor before treatment is differ-

ent from that during or after treatment. The regrowth rate of a tumor could exceed that predicted by T_{pot} or may never reach it. Further, other measures that can reflect the rate of cell loss, such as rate of tumor regression or apoptotic index and the length of the lag period before accelerated regrowth, may need to be taken into account.

Growth Fraction

The *growth fraction* (181) is the fraction of tumor cells that are cycling. In solid tumors, this is usually a small proportion of the total (e.g., 20%). The growth fraction may decrease as tumors enlarge and grow more slowly (see control curve, Figure 2.5). This changing growth rate can be approximated by a Gompertz equation (250). In contrast, after cytoreductive therapy, the growth fraction probably increases and contributes to accelerated regrowth. An analogous response is found in some normal tissues (liver, dermis), which have only a small fraction of cells in cycle, but can regenerate rapidly through recruiting resting, G0-phase cells into cycle.

Regeneration in Experimental Tumors

Hermens and Barendsen (120) showed a rapid exponential increase of surviving clonogenic tumor cells in a rat rhabdomyosarcoma several days after irradiation. Since only 1% of the initial clonogens survived, tumors did not enlarge; rather, the tumor mass was still regressing when repopulation began (Fig. 2.5). Using a mouse mammary carcinoma, Kummermehr and Trott (154) also demonstrated clones of regenerating malignant cells in regressing tumors after irradiation, and the same occurs during regression of many clinical tumors.

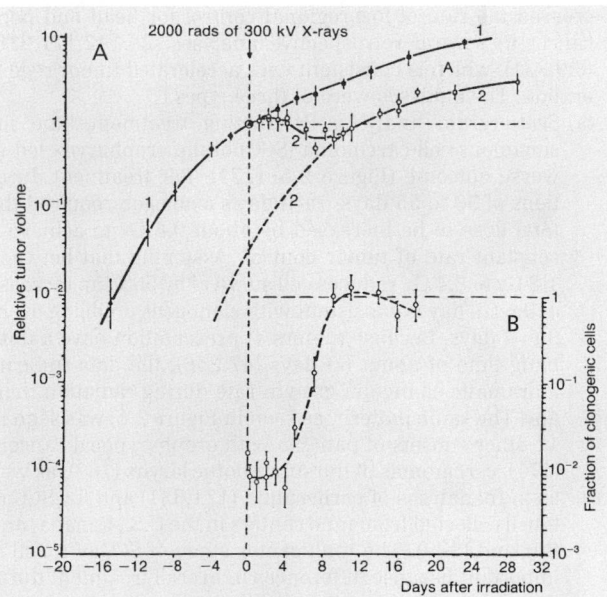

FIGURE 2.5. Growth curves for a rat rhabdomyosarcoma and its constituent clonogenic cells after a dose that reduced survival to 1%. The upper curve (1) shows unperturbed growth of tumors; the middle curve (2) shows regression and regrowth of tumors irradiated on day 0 with a dose that reduced cell survival to 1%; the lower curve (B) traces the repopulation of the tumor by surviving clonogens. Exponential regrowth of the surviving clonogenic cells occurs while the gross tumor is regressing. (From Hermens AF, Barendsen GW. Changes of cell proliferation characteristics in a rat rhabdomyosarcoma before and after x-irradiation. *Eur J Cancer* 1969;5:173, 1969, with permission.. Copyright 1969, Pergamon Press, Ltd.)

Regeneration in Human Tumors

Clonogen regeneration in human tumors can be assessed by an increase in dose required for tumor control as treatment duration is increased (259). Alternatively, if a constant dose has been used, the decrease in tumor control rate as treatment time is extended is a measure of repopulation. These techniques have been used to derive evidence for accelerated regrowth during a standard radiation therapy regimen for head and neck cancer, but it is likely to occur in all tumor sites, although at different times and rates. The magnitude and timing of regeneration will also vary from tumor to tumor of the same type and, for normal tissues, among different types.

The concept of accelerated repopulation by human tumor clonogens during and after a course of fractionated radiation therapy is supported by several observations and is of particular concern when already prolonged delivery times are further prolonged.

1. Time to tumor recurrence: One tumor cell must undergo nearly 30 doublings (to 2^{30} or about 10^9) to become detectable as a recurrence; even 10,000 surviving cells would have to undergo 15 to 17 doublings. Most local recurrences of head and neck cancer are detectable within 12 months after radiation therapy (93,215), which would be consistent with an *average* tumor volume doubling time of about 2 to 3 weeks if 10,000 cells survived. Therefore, since the median volume doubling time for tumors at presentation is about 2 months (47), growth rate of residual clonogens must accelerate following unsuccessful treatment. Similar rapid postirradiation regrowth was seen in pulmonary metastases after subcurative irradiation (290).

2. Split-course treatment: Split-course regimens for head and neck squamous cell carcinomas gave lower local control rates than continuous regimens of the same total dose (215,216), suggesting that tumor growth occurred during the time extension. Prostate cancer, which has an indolent growth pattern, was an exception (217,230).

3. Protracted treatment: Protraction of treatment time decreased the rate of locoregional control for head and neck cancer in several retrospective analyses (24,142,171,210, 329,331), which is consistent with accelerated tumor regeneration. The analyses were of three types.

   (a) Scattergram analysis. Protracting treatment time for squamous cell carcinoma (SCC) of the oropharynx led to worse outcome (Figure 2.6) (171). For treatment durations of 30 to 55 days, each day's extension required the total dose to be increased by about 0.6 Gy to achieve a constant rate of tumor control. Assuming that between 1.8 Gy to 2.4 Gy reduces cell survival by 50%, an increase of 0.6 Gy/day is consistent with clonogens doubling every 3 to 4 days. Because tumors at presentation have a doubling time of about 60 days (47,250), the data indicate a dramatic change in growth rate during radiation therapy. The same pattern, as seen in Figure 2.6, was seen in 11 other subsets of patients with oropharyngeal cancers (171), carcinomas of the supraglottic larynx (169), as well as in reanalyses of earlier data (171,331) and for SCC of tonsil collected from nine centers in the U.S., Canada, and England (329). The multicenter study of SCC of tonsil is important because differences in overall treatment duration predominantly reflect institutional policy; it rules out selection of longer treatments for worse tumors as a factor in the increase of tumor control dose 50 (TCD$_{50}$), with extension of overall treatment time.

   (b) TCD$_{50}$ analysis. Figure 2.7 presents TCD$_{50}$ values for SCC of head and neck calculated from the literature (331). They are independent of treatment duration up to about 28 days, after which they increase rapidly (consistent with 0.6 Gy/day). The suggestion is that, *on average*, head and neck SCCs exhibit a lag period of 3 to 4 weeks before beginning to repopulate with an average doubling time of 3 to 4 days.

   (c) Analysis of primary tumor control rate. When a standard prescription (e.g., 50 Gy in 20 fractions in 4 weeks) is given, but the overall duration of therapy is extended for whatever reason, the control rate decreases, commonly by 1% to 2% per day for head and neck and cervix cancer (Fig. 2.6B) (24,95,99,142).

   It should be noted that a lag period of up to 4 weeks and thereafter a 0.6 Gy/day increase in the "isocontrol" dose are *not* evidence that radiation therapy for head and neck cancer is best given in 4 weeks. Repopulation of mucosa begins at about 10 to 12 days and is more rapid than tumor, requiring thereafter an average daily dose increment of at least 1 Gy for a mucosal isoresponse (331). Thus, a therapeutic gain in mucosal tolerance relative to tumor control is still achieved by extending treatment beyond 4 weeks. It is only late-responding tissues, which do not benefit from repopulation, that lose out. Thus, the overall therapeutic differential will be greatest if the tolerance dose for the critical late-responding tissue is delivered in the shortest overall time consistent with an acceptable acute response (313,331) and without compromising the total dose delivered to the tumor.

4. Accelerated treatment: If accelerated tumor growth contributes to treatment failure, acceleration of standard treatment may benefit some tumors. In nonrandomized studies, shortening the overall duration of treatment improved the local control in inflammatory breast cancer (22), melanoma metastases to brain (53), and head and neck cancer (149,297–299). Randomized studies of accelerated treatment of head and neck cancer validated the benefit; however, not all tumor sites have been evaluated. Exceptions may be cancer of the prostate, which is slow growing (217,230) and Burkitt's lymphoma, which may be growing too rapidly for any acceleration to be detected (204). Dose-intensity studies (134,135,148) suggest that chemotherapy also accelerates tumor regrowth. Furthermore, the lack of benefit from neoadjuvant chemotherapy given for two or three cycles before the start of radiation therapy for head and neck cancer, despite shrinkage of the gross tumor mass, is consistent with accelerated regrowth of the subclinical residual clonogens before, or early in, the course of radiation therapy, compromising its efficacy.

Cell-Cycle Redistribution after Irradiation

Cells change in their radiosensitivity as they traverse the division cycle (249,262). There is enormous variation in initial slope of the survival curve (Fig. 2.8). The difference in radiosensitivity between late S-phase and G$_2$-M cells is greater than that between euoxic and hypoxic cells.

After exposure of an asynchronous population of cells to 2 Gy, the survivors will be partially synchronized in relatively radioresistant cell cycle phases (because of the preferential killing of cells in sensitive phases). When these survivors resume their progression through the division cycle, they move into more sensitive phases. If they were to do so in a synchronized fashion this could be exploited (81). Unfortunately, they do not. However, a greater proportion of the surviving population will be in sensitive phases of the division cycle than immediately after irradiation, which will produce a net "self-sensitization" effect that will not occur in a nonproliferating cell population. Dose fractionation will enhance the therapeutic ratio by permitting

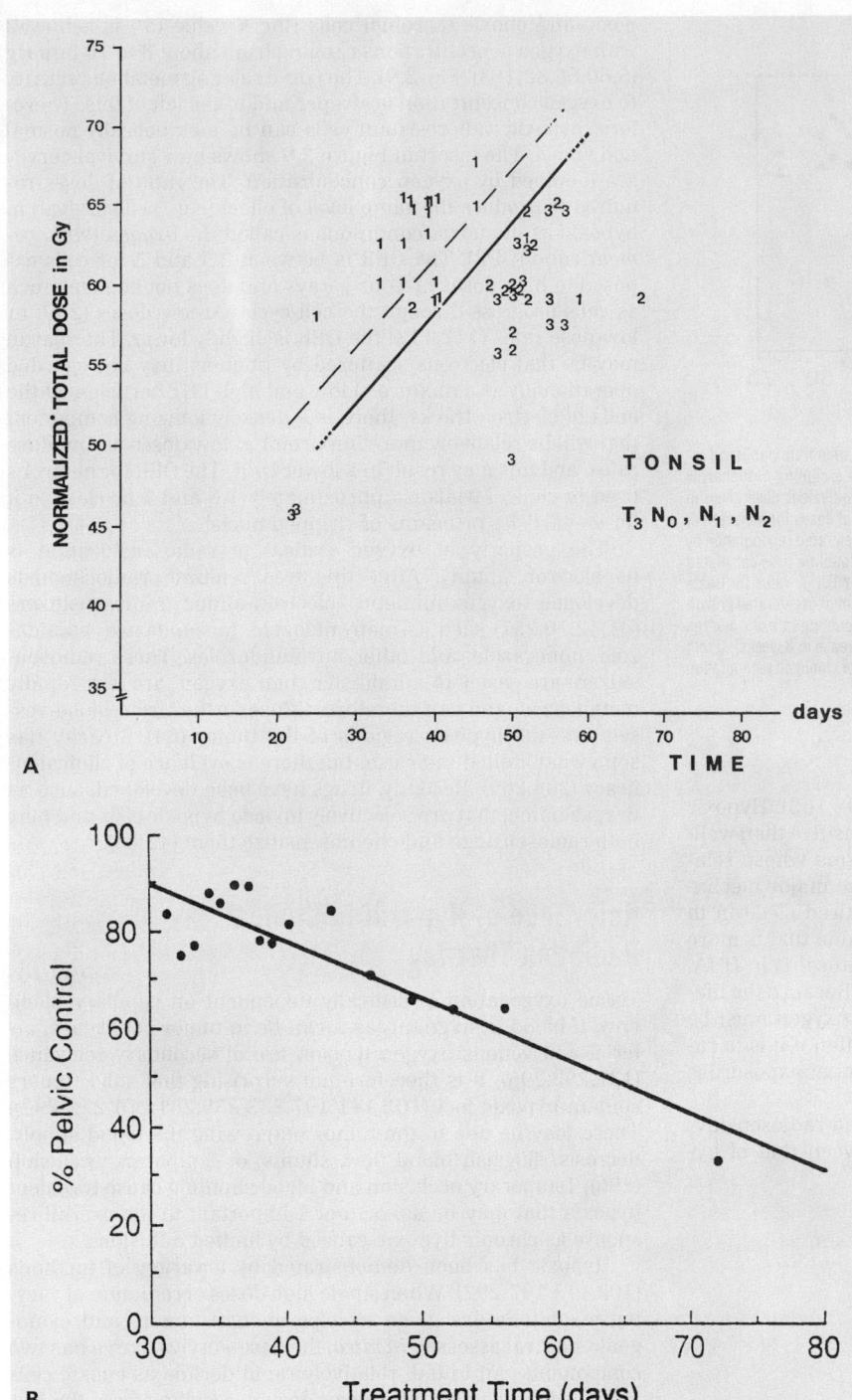

FIGURE 2.6. A: Scattergram with TCD$_{50}$ and TCD$_{90}$ (tumor control dose) curves for 3-year local control of squamous cell carcinoma of the tonsil (1, local control; 2, recurrence; 3, persistence of detectable disease). For a given total dose, local control decreased with protraction of overall treatment time. For a given overall time, local control improved with increase in dose. The total doses were normalized to be equivalent to the total dose in 2.5-Gy fractions using the linear quadratic isoeffect curve (see Fig. 2.22). An α/β value of 2.5 Gy was used, being the best estimate from these and other data. (From Maciejewski B, Withers HR, Taylor JMG. Dose fractionation and regeneration in radiotherapy for cancer of the oral cavity and oropharynx. I. Tumor dose-response and repopulation. *Int J Radiat Oncol Biol Phys* 1989;16:831, with permission.) **B:** Pelvic control as a function of treatment time for 621 patients treated with a total dose of 85 Gy. (From Keane TJ, Fyles A, O'Sullivan B, et al. The effect of treatment duration on local control of squamous carcinoma of the tonsil and carcinoma of the cervix. *Semin Radiat Oncol* 1992;2:27, with permission.)

redistribution among tumor cells but not nonproliferating cells in late-responding normal tissues (312). The differential is greater the smaller the dose per fraction and is amplified as an exponential function of the number of fractions delivered. This amplification of small differentials between cycling tumor cells and the nonredistributing target cells in late-responding normal tissues was the initial rationale for clinical trials of hyperfractionation (312), before important intrinsic differences in response to low dose fractionation between late-responding normal tissues and tumors were appreciated (270,335).

The effect of cell-cycle redistribution on tumor and normal tissue responses to multifraction irradiation is difficult to demonstrate (323). It is probably the cause of spermatogenic stem cell sensitivity to split-dose irradiation (152,320), but in most

circumstances it may be overwhelmed by the effects of repopulation. However, it is difficult to envision that it does not influence multifraction responses in all proliferating tissues and the therapeutic benefit that can be obtained from dose fractionation.

The Oxygen Effect

Many early clinicians and radiobiologists reported that restricting the blood flow to a tissue decreased its radiation response. They thought it was a metabolic effect, but in 1951, Read (235) showed that oxygen sensitized cells through a radiochemical mechanism. Now, oxygen is recognized as the most potent

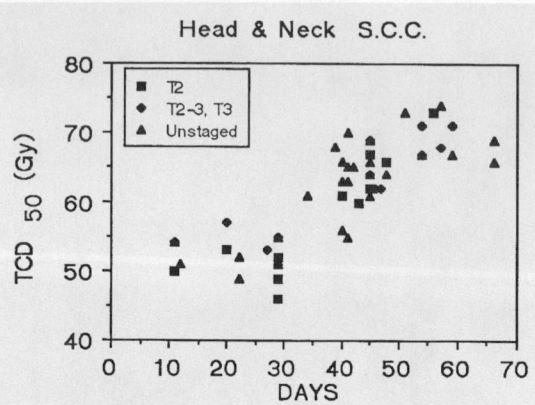

FIGURE 2.7. Estimated TCD_{50} values as a function of treatment duration from published results of radiation therapy for squamous carcinomas of head and neck excluding nasopharynx and true vocal cord. TCD_{50} values are expressed as $LQED_{2Gy}$ (the equivalent dose given in 2-Gy fractions calculated using the linear quadratic [LQ] model). Total doses for an isoeffect increase steeply with protraction of treatment duration, implying accelerated repopulation by surviving tumor clonogens, consistent with the 3- to 4-day average doubling time calculated from scattergrams (171,328) (see Fig. 2.6A). The relatively constant TCD_{50} value for treatments lasting up to 4 weeks is consistent with an average time of onset of accelerated growth at about 4 weeks. Growth of clonogens at the average preirradiation doubling rate of 2 months would have little detectable effect on TCD_{50} values (about 2.5-Gy increase in 8 weeks). (From Withers HR, Taylor JMG, Maciejewski B. The hazard of accelerated tumor clonogen repopulation during radiotherapy. *Acta Oncol* 1988;27:131, with permission.)

chemical modifier of radiosensitivity (66,82,108,163). Hypoxic mammalian cells are 2.5 to 3 times less radiosensitive than well-oxygenated cells, reflecting multiple mechanisms whose relative contributions are not precisely known. The major mechanism may be oxygen combining with an unpaired electron in the outer shell of a free radical to yield a peroxide that is more stable and toxic than the free radical. If the radical is in DNA, damage may be "fixed" and less easy to repair. Because the lifetime of a free radical is in microseconds (34), oxygen must be present close to the DNA at the time of irradiation if it is to radiosensitize. Adding it even 1/100 of a second after exposure is ineffective.

The relationship between oxygen tension and radiosensitivity varies, but a radiosensitivity halfway between that of hy-

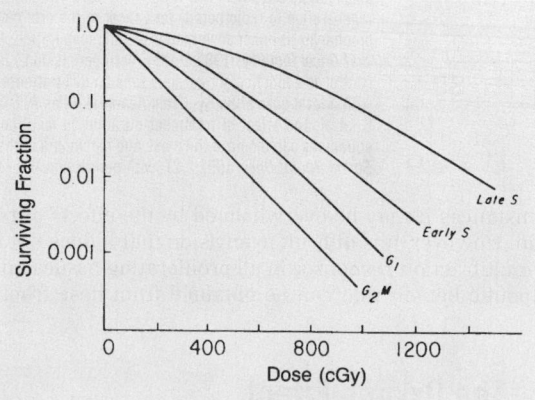

FIGURE 2.8. Radiation dose-survival curves for one line of mammalian cells (V-79 Chinese hamster) synchronized in four positions in the division cycle (249). Significant differences occur in the survival of cells at different ages, with the differences relative to absolute survival being greatest at lower doses. The survival ratio between late S and G_2M cells after 2 Gy is approximately 5. (From Withers HR, Peters LJ. Biological aspects of radiation therapy. In: Fletcher GH, ed. *Textbook of radiotherapy*, 3rd ed. Philadelphia: Lea & Febiger, 1980, with permission.)

poxic and euoxic (aerobic) cells (the k value (5)) is achieved with oxygen concentrations ranging from about 3 to 10 mm Hg (5,60,66,82,163) (Fig. 2.9). The curve relating metabolic activity to oxygen concentration is steeper and to the left of this. Therefore, hypoxic radioresistant cells can be metabolically normal and viable. The insert in Figure 2.9 shows how survival curves are modified by oxygen concentration. The ratio of doses required to produce the same level of effect (e.g., cell survival) in hypoxic as in euoxia conditions is called the *oxygen enhancement ratio* (OER). The OER is between 2.5 and 3 for cells exposed to high doses of x- or γ-rays and does not change much as cells progress through the cell cycle. At low doses (239) or low-dose rates (112,113) the OER is slightly lower. The reason may be that electrons scattered by photons may be regarded operationally as a mixture of low and high LET particles. At the ends of electron tracks, there is a densely ionizing component that will be relatively more important at low doses or low-dose rates, and this may result in a lower OER. The OER for neutrons used in clinical trials is approximately 1.6 and 1 or close to it for α-particles or beams of stripped nuclei.

The property of oxygen critical to radiosensitization is its electron affinity. After this was realized, radiochemists developed oxygen-mimetic, electron-affinic radiosensitizers (41,42,70,257) such as metronidazole, misonidazole, etanidazole, nimorazole, and other nitroimidazoles. These radiosensitizers are easier to administer than oxygen, are less rapidly metabolized, and can therefore diffuse further from blood vessels into the hypoxic regions of the tumor (64). Toxicity has somewhat limited their use, but there is evidence of clinical efficacy (208,209). Recently, drugs have been developed, such as tirapazamine, that are selectively toxic to hypoxic cells and may both radiosensitize and chemosensitize them (42,65).

Relevance of Hypoxia to Clinical Radiation Therapy

Tissue oxygenation is critically dependent on capillary blood flow. If blood is stagnant, as it can be in tumor capillaries, arterial and venous oxygen tension are of secondary relevance (137,292,296). It is therefore not surprising that solid tumors contain hypoxic foci (102,141,197,233,259,261,271,272,292). These may be due to the tumor outgrowing the blood supply, necrosis, sluggish blood flow, shunts, or temporary occlusion (296). Temporary occlusion and blood shunting cause transient hypoxia that may be as, or more, important to the overall response as chronic hypoxia caused by limited diffusion.

Hypoxia has been demonstrated by a variety of methods (102,113,197,292). When single high doses of radiation of varying magnitude are given to experimental tumors and clonogenic survival assessed *in vitro*, the dose-survival curve has two components: An initial, relatively rapid decline as euoxic cells are killed, and a second, slower decline resulting from the less efficient killing of radioresistant hypoxic cells (233). Recently, polarographic oxygen electrodes have been used to measure oxygen tension (pO_2) within human and experimental tumors (46,102,292) as have DNA strand break (Comet) assays (207), detection of binding of the 2-nitroimidazole by immunohistochemistry (EF5) (150,281) or positron emission tomography-imaging, and immunohistochemistry for localized expression of hypoxia–inducible factor-1α, or its downstream effectors (27). It is not clear which of these techniques is the most reliable measure of radiobiologic hypoxia, but hypoxia-related molecular pathways are often activated under nonhypoxic conditions, and oxygen electrodes or nitroimidazole binding seem more robust.

Hypoxia is being increasingly linked with clinical outcome. Hyperbaric oxygen (71,119,283) or correction of anemia (43,71,86) has been reported to improve outcome, and high

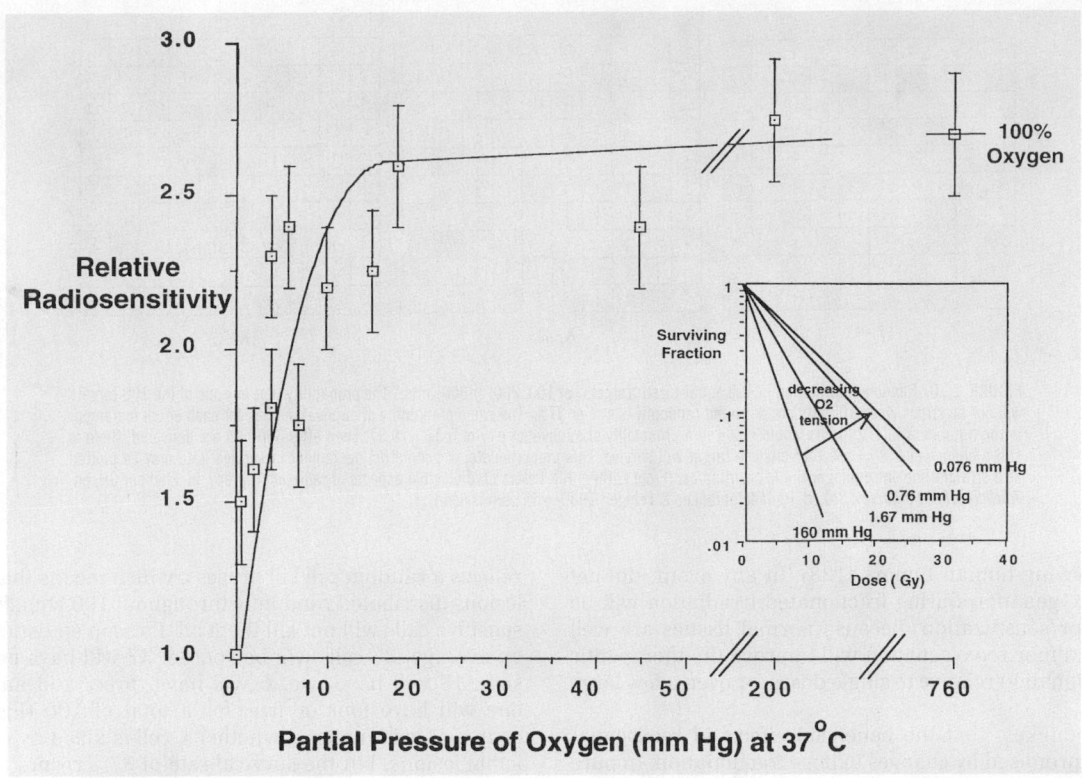

FIGURE 2.9. Curve relating cellular radiation sensitivity to partial pressure of O_2 at the time of irradiation. Data were obtained by scoring anaphase aberrations in Ehrlich ascites tumor cells (66), but similar curves have been obtained for killing of bacteria (4). About 50% of the total sensitization by O_2 is seen at a partial pressure of approximately 4 mm Hg at 37°C. The inset shows survival curves for different levels of oxygenation (82).

hypoxic fraction (102,292) portends poor local control and survival rates in head and neck and cervix cancer treated with radiation therapy (37,242). However, outcome of patients with uterine cervix cancers treated with surgery only also correlated with hypoxia (124). A possible explanation for this comes from studies showing that hypoxia can provide a growth advantage for cells with mutated p53 (107). Hypoxia can therefore select for more aggressive tumors.

Despite the probable existence of hypoxic cells within many, if not all, solid tumors of humans, the importance of hypoxia as a predictor of individual response to radiation therapy has yet to be established. It may not be a constant cause of failure (330). An important issue is whether reoxygenation occurs during a course of fractionated radiotherapy. If hypoxia is simply a marker of tumor aggression, reoxygenation may not be important for outcome, but if hypoxia is radiobiologically relevant, the rate and extent of reoxygenation will be critical.

Tumor Reoxygenation

It is important to know the extent to which tumors become reoxygenated during a fractionated course of radiotherapy. If 30% of tumor clonogens were hypoxic and 70% were euoxic, and no change were to occur in the distribution of oxygenation during a course of 2-Gy fractions, the majority of surviving cells would be hypoxic after the first few fractions, and 70 Gy in 2-Gy fractions would not reduce the fraction of cells surviving to less than 10^{-4}. A general lack of reoxygenation is therefore incompatible with high rates of tumor control in the clinic. Reoxygenation must occur, although incomplete reoxygenation could still be a cause of some treatment failures. The magnitude of the effect of reoxygenation on the response to multiple dose fractions can be appreciated from Table 2.1. For example, the dose to a tumor that repeatedly returns to an 80-to-20 euoxic-to-hypoxic

cell mixture would need to be 15% higher than it would if all tumor cells were oxic.

Reoxygenation may result from reduction in total tumor cells with less loss of blood vessels, decreased interstitial pressure, and better oxygen diffusion as a result of increased vascular density and less temporary occlusions (137,141). It should be noted that free radicals generated during reoxygenation may be particularly toxic to cells, although the importance of this potential mechanism of radiosensitization has yet to be evaluated.

Most studies on the kinetics of reoxygenation in animal tumors have used relatively large dose fractions and indicate considerable variation between tumors. In most cases, reoxygenation occurs rapidly and is completed within 6 to 24 hours (132,271). In human tumors, the kinetics of reoxygenation is still a matter of controversy (167,176). The variation between tumors and tumor sites seems considerable. It is anticipated that reoxygenation would be more effective if multiple small doses than single large doses are given, and that rapidly growing experimental tumors would be poor guides for the behavior

	RATIOS OF DOSE FOR ISOSURVIVAL
Table 2.1	**EQUIVALENT TO THAT FROM 2 GY IN OXIC CONDITIONS**[a]

Ratio of Euoxic to Hypoxic Cells	Dose Modification Factor
100/0	1
90/10	1.07
80/20	1.15
70/30	1.23
60/40	1.35

[a] Assuming a constant oxygen enhancement ratio of 2.5 at all doses.

Overview and Basic Science of Radiation Oncology

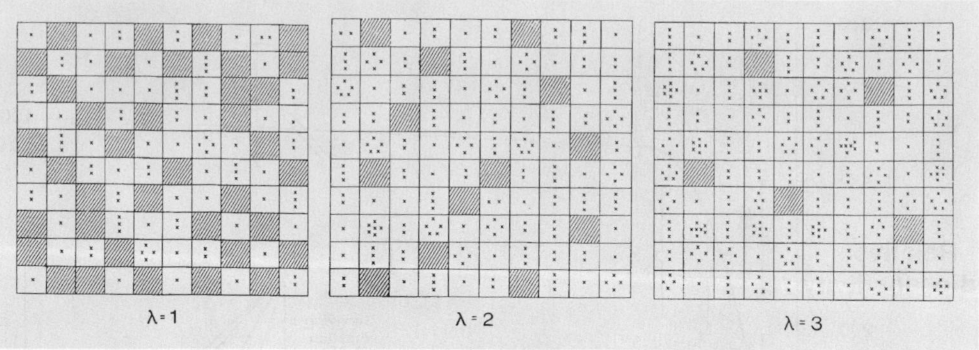

FIGURE 2.10. Random distribution in 100 equal-sized "targets" of 100, 200, or 300 "hits." The probability that any one of the 100 targets will not be struck when 100 hits are delivered randomly is e^{-1} or 37%. The same probability of survival applies for each equal increment in the number of hits: 200 hits would result in a probability of survival of e^{-2} or 0.37×0.37. Even after 300 hits are delivered, there is still a chance of $e^{-3} = 5\%$ that any one target will survive. This proportionate, or geometric, decrement in survival rate may be plotted as a straight line on semilogarithmic coordinates. (From Withers HR, Peters LJ. Biological aspects of radiation therapy. In: Fletcher GH, ed. *Textbook of radiotherapy,* 3rd ed. Philadelphia: Lea & Febiger, 1980, with permission.)

of slowly growing human tumors (123). In any event, the net effect of reoxygenation during fractionated irradiation will be relative tumor sensitization. Because normal tissues are well oxygenated, tumor reoxygenation will improve the therapeutic ratio of fractionation relative to single doses, or even a few large fractions.

It seems unlikely that the beneficial effects of reoxygenation are compromised by changes in dose fractionation. In pure hyperfractionation, where the dose per fraction is small, responses will be little affected by 10% to 20% of the cells being hypoxic, especially because the OER is lowest at low doses of x-rays (213). Also, the overall duration of the course of radiation therapy is not shortened, so the time available for reoxygenation will be the same. In accelerated regimens, the theoretical problem of the proportion of surviving cells that are hypoxic and are increasing with time is of more concern. However, the rapid reoxygenation kinetics observed in experimental tumors as well as high control rates achieved experimentally and clinically with brachytherapy and in centers using 3- or 4-week overall treatment durations suggest that reoxygenation is adequate in most tumors, even with short courses of fractionated or low-dose rate irradiation.

Where large dose fractions are given as a single exposure, as in intraoperative radiation therapy, single-dose stereotactic radiosurgery, and high-dose rate brachytherapy, outcome may be more compromised by hypoxia. However, results show that local control is often achieved, suggesting that advantageous physical factors must outweigh any lack of reoxygenation. Nevertheless, these are situations in which a large dose of a hypoxic cell sensitizer or cytotoxin might have most effect. In chemoradiotherapy or bioradiotherapy protocols that target tumor vasculature or angiogenesis, the extent of reoxygenation might also be an issue.

Quantitative Radiobiology and Dose Fractionation

Random Nature of Cell Killing

Our earliest understanding of dose-response relationships for irradiated cells came from studies with bacteria (4,158). Bacterial cell survival decreases geometrically with dose. In other words, the dose that reduces the survival rate to 50% will, when doubled, reduce it to 25%, and if tripled, to 12.5%, and so forth. When such a relationship is plotted semilogarithmically, a straight line results. Such a dose-survival relationship

reflects a random cell kill process, which means that 100 lethal lesions distributed randomly throughout 100 equally radiation-sensitive cells will not kill them all. Poisson statistics state that, on average, 37 cells will be spared, 37 will have one lethal lesion, 18 will have two, 6 will have three, and an occasional one will have four or five, for a total of 100 (Fig. 2.10). Of course, it is immaterial whether a cell is killed by one or more lethal lesions, but the survival rate of 37% recurs for each additional mean lethal dose, which ensures the semilogarithmic relationship.

The mathematic bent of early radiation biologists, many of whom were also physicists, caused them to describe the slope of survival curves in terms of the mean lethal dose (D_{37} or D_0), which reduces survival by one natural logarithm (e^{-1}), rather than D_{10}, which reduces it by one common logarithm and is an easier term for biologists to think in. It is useful to remember that D_{10} is about 2.3 times D_0.

Mammalian Cell Survival Curves

Puck and Marcus (234) published the first survival curve for mammalian cells in 1956. Logarithmic decreases in cell survival with dose were found that fitted the model described for bacteria, but with two important differences. D_0 values for cells are generally between 0.75 and 2 Gy, which is less than one tenth of values for most bacteria, largely reflecting the latter's smaller target size (less DNA). Also, unlike those for bacteria, mammalian cell survival curves often have a shoulder before the logarithmic decline (Fig. 2.11). The biological basis for the shoulder is not firmly established, but it is simplest to consider it in terms of single-hit and multiple-hit killing. At low doses, the rate of deposition of energy by a charged particle is inversely proportional to its energy. Hence, intratrack ionization events are initially sparse, but as energy is lost through collisions and scattering, they become more densely distributed. The dense ionization at the end of the electron track probably causes most of the irreversible single lethal hits with a predominance of "deletion-type" chromosome lesions. At high doses, there is additional accumulation of ionization injury from other electron tracks (intertrack). This "sublethal" injury can be converted to lethal injury with a relative increase in "exchange-type" chromosome aberrations that form from more than one double-strand break (DSB) lesion. High levels of injury might also reduce the capacity of the cell to repair injury (4,265). Lethal lesions are generally considered to be DNA double-strand breaks with large "locally multiply damaged sites" involving 15 to 20 base pairs (300).

An additional complexity in dose-response curves is that hyperradiosensitivity to very low radiation doses (<10 cGy) has

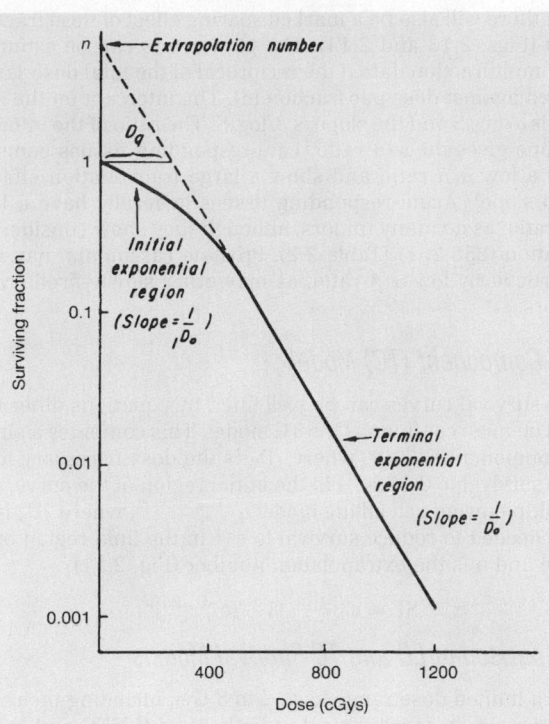

FIGURE 2.11. A two-component survival curve for mammalian cells is characterized by a "shoulder" followed by a terminal exponential region, the slope of which is defined by a D_0 value (slope = $1/D_0$). The position of the curve on the radiation dose axis can be fixed by the intercepts of the terminal exponential region extrapolated back to the zero dose axis (n) or to the 100% survival level (D_q): n is termed the *extrapolation number*, and D_q the *quasithreshold dose*. Although n and D_q are parameters that define the width of the shoulder on the survival curve, they do not indicate its shape, which is of prime importance in radiation therapy. The survival curve shoulder can be considered to consist of an initial exponential region (the slope of which is defined by $_1D_0$), followed by a downward-bending segment that merges asymptotically into the final exponential region of the survival curve. (From Withers HR, Peters LJ. Biological aspects of radiation therapy. In: Fletcher GH, ed. *Textbook of radiotherapy,* 3rd ed. Philadelphia: Lea & Febiger, 1980, with permission.)

expected frequency of postradiation chromosomal aberrations, but in the future they may provide novel opportunities for therapeutic intervention. In any event, they do not significantly impact the mathematical models that have been proposed for radiation cytotoxicity, which were derived to fit existing data within the clinically relevant dose range.

Linear Quadratic (LQ) Formula

Lea (158) and Read (235,236) quantified biologic responses to irradiation in terms of a linear dose coefficient (α) and a coefficient (β) for the square of the dose,

$$\text{Effect is proportional to } \alpha D + \beta D^2.$$

This can be used to fit a continuously bending curve to cell survival data:

$$\text{S.F. (survival fraction)} = e^{-(\alpha D + \beta D^2)}$$

The linear component (αD) of this dose-survival relationship dominates the response at low doses and is of major significance if radiation therapy is delivered in fractions of about 2 Gy (Fig. 2.12). Its importance was largely ignored in the 1960s, but was "rediscovered" in the early 1970s when Dutreix and associates (77) demonstrated that reducing doses per fraction below 3 Gy did not result in additional sparing of acute effects in human skin. Now it is accepted that low-dose brachytherapy or

been shown in some systems. Then, as dose increases above about 30 cGy, radioresistance increases until about 1 Gy, when cell survival begins to follow the usual downward-bending curve with increasing dose (140). This phenomenon is not universal but has been seen in many human cell lines *in vitro* and in experimental studies in mouse skin, kidney, and lung. The precise mechanisms are still unclear; however, the increased radioresistance may be similar to adaptive responses in which small conditioning or "priming" doses increase resistance to higher "challenge" doses given hours later. Clinical attempts are underway to exploit the "hypersensitivity" phenomenon.

Other phenomena also challenge any simple relationship between DNA strand lesions and radiation response. One is radiation-induced genomic instability, in which the rate of genomic alterations increases with increasing number of divisions of irradiated cells, as manifested by chromosomal rearrangements, formation of micronuclei, gene amplification, or cell killing (3,26). Another is the nontargeted radiation effect in which cells that were not irradiated but were bystanders at the time of irradiation are affected. In some, not all, cases, culture medium from irradiated cells is active (164,193). Again, chromosome-related alterations, mutations, gene induction, and cell killing are observed end points. The relevance of low-dose hypersensitivity, adaptive responses, induced genetic instability, and bystander effects to clinical radiotherapy have yet to be fully evaluated. They clearly challenge classic radiobiologic paradigms. They are probably most relevant to radiation-induced carcinogenesis, where they can explain the higher than

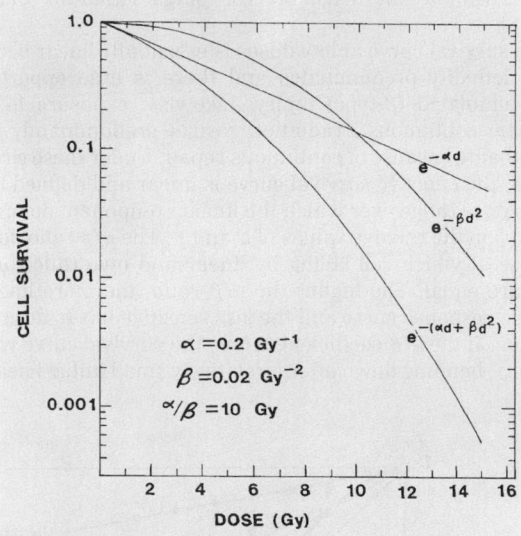

FIGURE 2.12. Model dose-survival curves for mammalian cells showing that the experimentally determined curve for acute exposures (lowest curve) is the product of two mechanisms: Single-hit injury described by an exponential curve ($e^{-\alpha d}$) and multiple-hit, or cumulative, injury described by a continuously bending curve related by a coefficient, β, to the square of the dose. At doses of clinical relevance, cell death from the single-hit mechanism predominates. The rate at which the survival curve bends from an initial, essentially exponential region depends on the ratio (α/β) of the coefficients for single-hit and multiple-hit killing: The lower the value, the sooner and more steeply the curve bends. The value of α/β is the dose at which single- and multiple-hit mechanisms contribute equally to cell killing. In these curves, $\alpha/\beta = 10$ Gy, which is a value characteristic of acutely-responding tissues. Target cells in late-responding normal tissues are characterized by low α/β values; hence, their survival curves are curvier. The flexure dose, D_f, is the dose at which deviation from the initial exponential part of the curve is difficult to detect and, for available biologic assay systems, is about one-tenth of α/β. When doses in a multifraction regimen are less than D_f, further dose fractionation does not produce detectable "sparing" (because cell killing is essentially all the result of single-hit events, the lesions potentially contributing to multievent killing being completely repaired during the fractionation intervals). The lower the α/β value, the lower the dose at which multiple-hit mechanisms cause cell death, the lower the value of D_f, and the lower the dose per fraction below which a sparing effect of dose fractionation is lost. The curve for single-hit killing ($e^{-\alpha d}$) can be measured experimentally using very small dose fractions or a continuous low-dose rate exposure, but the curves for multiple-hit killing ($e^{-\beta d^2}$) can be determined only indirectly from a knowledge of the other two curves.

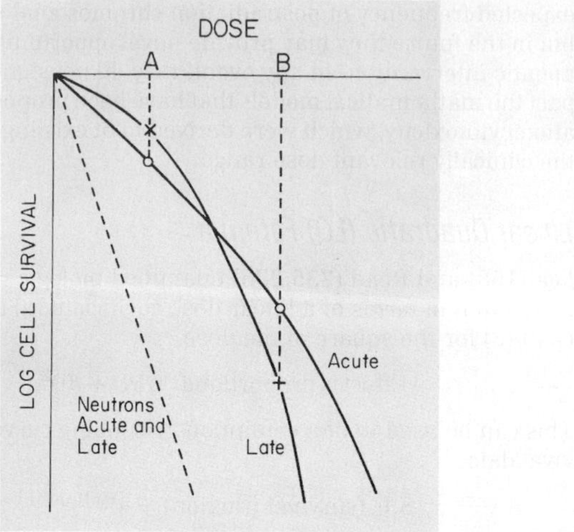

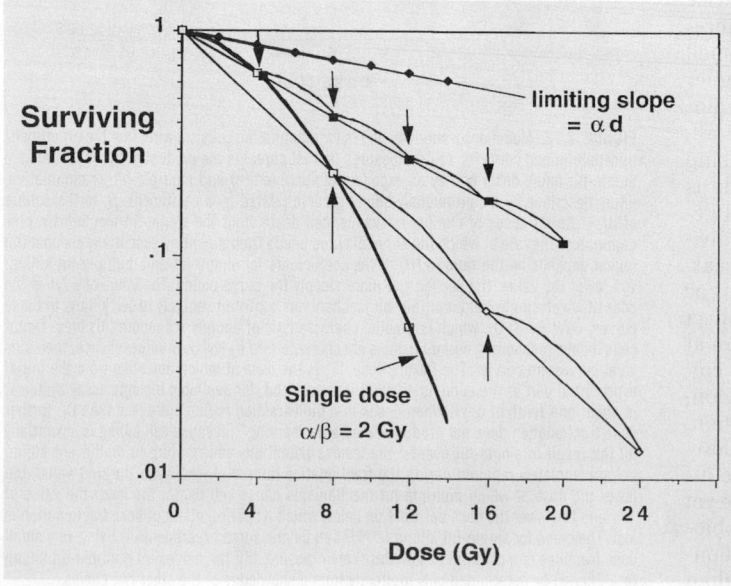

FIGURE 2.13. Hypothetical survival curves for the target cells for acute and late effects in normal tissues exposed to x-rays or neutrons. The α/β ratio is lower for late effects than for acute effects in x-irradiated tissues, resulting in a greater change in effect in late-responding tissues with change in dose. At dose A, survival of target cells is higher in late-effects than in acute-effects tissues; at dose B, the reverse is true. Increasing the dose per fraction from A to B results in a relatively greater increase in late than in acute injury. For neutrons, the α/β ratio is high, with no detectable influence of the quadratic function (βd^2) over the first two decades of reduction in cell survival, implying that accumulation of sublethal injury plays a negligible role in cell killing by doses of neutrons of clinical interest. (From Withers HR, Thames HD, Peters LJ. Biological bases for high RBE values for late effects of neutron irradiation. *Int J Radiat Oncol Biol Phys* 1982;8:2071, with permission.)

standard fractionated radiation therapy could not eradicate cancer without the existence of single-lethal-hit damage (40,318).

The survival curve at low doses is essentially linear because α-type lethality predominates and there is little opportunity for accumulated (β-type) injury. Likewise, exposure to low-dose rate continuous irradiation results predominantly in α-type lethality because of continuous repair. Under these circumstances, the effective survival curve is linear and defined by α.

The dose range over which the linear component dominates depends on the relative values of α and β. The α/β ratio defines the dose at which cell killing by linear and quadratic components are equal. The higher the α/β ratio, the more linear is the dose-response curve and the less sensitive it is to dose fractionation. If the α/β coefficient is low, the survival curve will be "curvier," bending down after a relatively small initial linear re-

gion; there will also be a marked sparing effect of dose fractionation (Figs. 2.13 and 2.14). The parameters can be estimated from multifraction data if the reciprocal of the total dose 1/nd is plotted against dose per fraction (d). The intercept on the ordinate is $\alpha/\log_e S$ and the slope is $\beta/\log_e S$. The ratio of the intercept to slope gives the α/β ratio. Late-responding tissues generally have a low α/β ratio and show a large fractionation effect (a steep slope). Acute-responding tissues generally have a large α/β ratio, as do many tumors, although they show considerable variation (258,261) (Table 2.2). Prostate carcinoma may have a particularly low α/β ratio, as may other slowly-proliferative tumors.

Two-Component (TC) Model

Dose survival curves can be well fitted by equations other than LQ. The most common is the TC model. This combines a single-hit component $e^{-D/_1D_0}$, where $_1D_0$ is the dose necessary to reduce survival to $0.37(e^{-1})$ in the initial region of the curve, with a multiple-event cell killing model $e^{-(1-e^{-D/_nD_0})^n}$, where $_nD_0$ is the dose needed to reduce survival to e^{-1} in the final region of the curve and n is the extrapolation number (Fig. 2.11).

$$SF = e^{-D/_1D} \cdot (1 - [e^{-D_n/D_0}]^n)$$

Comparison of LQ and TC Survival Models

Over a limited dose range (e.g., 2 to 8 Gy), including the region that matters in most clinical radiotherapy, the TC and the LQ models "fit" data indistinguishably (Fig. 2.15). At high doses, the LQ model fits some cell survival curves better as they appear to continue to bend, while the TC model better fits those that seem more linear. Importantly, the models are significantly different at predicting responses to doses below 2 Gy using data from doses above 2 Gy (139). The differences may appear small but would be amplified if a dose of 1.15 Gy, for example, were repeated 70 times or more, as could happen in a hyperfractionated radiation therapy regimen (Fig. 2.16).

The LQ model has gained popularity (20,74,94,143,159, 240,265,270,335,336) because it is simpler and because α/β ratios can be determined from *in vivo* multifraction experiments even though the absolute values of each coefficient are unknown. Adding to the utility of the LQ model is that responses of tissues to change in dose fractionation can be predicted from just the α/β ratio (270). Examples of α/β ratios for different tissue and tumors are given in Table 2.2.

FIGURE 2.14. Multifraction dose-survival curves compared with a single-dose curve. Effective survival curves for multifraction regimens that produce an equal (proportionate) decrement in survival from each dose are linear, with shallower slopes than the single-dose curve at the same dose. Slopes of the multifraction curves become less steep with a decrease in fraction size until the dose per fraction is so low that multiple-hit killing contributes negligibly and the slope is the limiting one determined by single-hit killing (and $_eD_0 = 1/\alpha$). The dose per fraction below which the effective survival curve becomes no shallower is a function of the curviness of the single-dose survival curve and is lower than the α/β value.

Table 2.2 α/β VALUES[a]

Early-Responding Tissues	α/β (Gy)	Late-Responding Tissues	α/β (Gy)
Skin (desquamation)	9.4–21	Spinal cord (paresis)	1.6–5
Skin—pig (desquamation)		—Cervical	2–3.4
—Time ≤16 d	8.7	—Lumbar	4–5
—Time >16 d	0.9	Brain (LD$_{50}$/10 months)	2.1
Lip mucosa (desquamation)	7.9	Kidney (multiple end points)	0.4–5
Jejunal mucosa (clones)	7–13	Lung (pneumonitis)	1.6–4.5
Tongue mucosa (ulceration)	11.6	Lung (fibrosis)	2.3
Colonic mucosa (clones)	7–8.5	Heart failure	3.7
Hair follicles (epilation)		Liver (clones)	2.5
—Anagen	7.5	Bladder (frequency)	7.2
—Telogen	5.5	Bladder (contraction)	5.8–11
Testis (clones)	13.9	Bowel (stricture/perforation)	3.5–5
Spleen (clones)	8.9	Bowel (fistula/obstruction)	10.7
Bone marrow (clones)	9	Bowel (rectal stenosis, <5 d)	6.2
Melanocytes (depigmentation)	6.5	Bowel (rectal stenosis, >5 d)	1.1
		Dermal contraction	1.5–3.5
Tumors (cure)		Dermal wound healing	2.5
		Eye cataracts	1.2
Experimental tumors	10–35	Bone — human fracture	2.2
Most human tumors	6–25	Cartilage and submucosa	1–4.9
Human prostate cancer	1.5	Total-body irradiation (LD$_{50}$/1 yr)	5.1

[a]These values represent a synthesis from many sources. Individual values are means from one study. Where a range is given, it represents mean values from multiple studies. They come from our own data (94,270,306,320—2013;323) and that of others (32,44,90,91,106,110,127,166,171,211,212,245,252,265,279,280,285,289,291,305,322,328). Further references can be obtained in Perez, 4th edition.

Multifraction Survival Curves

In 1959, Elkind and Sutton (81) showed that sublethal damage (SLD) is repaired, given a few hours of normal metabolic activity. The extent and rate of repair of SLD can be estimated by the change in survival fraction with increasing time between two dose fractions or by the increase in total dose necessary to achieve the same level of cell survival (D2-D1) (Fig. 2.17). If two doses are separated by enough time to permit complete repair of SLD, it is as though the survivors of the first dose had not been previously irradiated and harbor no residual injury. Net survival is the product of the survival after each exposure. In other words, if 2 Gy reduces survival to 50% (S.F.$_{2Gy}$ = 0.5), two doses of 2 Gy would reduce it to $(0.5)^2$ and n doses to $(0.5)^n$, that is, there is an equally proportionate decrease in the survival rate with each equal increment in dose. Although this and the absence of regeneration between doses are not universally accurate assumptions, they are sufficiently for modeling purposes. Thus, the dose-survival relationship for a series of equal dose fractions can be considered logarithmic and to give a straight line when plotted on semilogarithmic coordinates (Fig. 2.18). The multifraction survival curve will extrapolate to 1 (n = 1) from any dose level, unlike most single-dose x-ray survival curves. The slope of such a linear multifraction curve is always less than that for the single-dose curve at an equivalent total dose and becomes shallower the smaller the dose per fraction (Fig. 2.14).

The slope of a linear multifraction cell survival curve can be described by an "effective D$_0$" ($_{eff}$D$_0$, or $_e$D$_0$) (325), which is the dose that reduces survival to e^{-1} for that particular fractionation pattern. In clinical radiation therapy where most treatment involves multiple dose fractions, $_{eff}$D$_0$ values for survival curves for a series of 2 Gy fractions are much more relevant than D$_0$ values, and are commonly in the range of 2.5 to 5 Gy. Because the multifraction dose-survival curve is linear, and if S.F.$_{2Gy}$ were 0.5, the corresponding $_e$D$_0$ value for a series of 2 Gy fractions would be 2.9 Gy (S.F. = e$^{-D/effD_0}$). If the S.F.$_{2Gy}$ values ranged from 0.45 to 0.67, the $_{eff}$D$_0$ values would range from 2.5 to 5 Gy. In mice, S.F.$_{2Gy}$ values for jejunal crypt and spermatogenic stem cells are about 0.6 and for colonic cells about 0.65, giving $_{eff}$D$_0$ values for 2 Gy fractions of about 3.9 and 5 Gy, respectively. It can be calculated, in two ways, that 30 fractions of 2 Gy would reduce survival of jejunal crypt cells to 2×10^{-7}:

S.F. after 30×2 Gy = (S.F. 2 Gy)^{30} = $(0.6)^{30}$ = 2×10^{-7} or SF after 60 Gy in 2 Gy fractions = $e^{-60/effD_0}$ = $e^{-60/3.9}$ = 2×10^{-7}

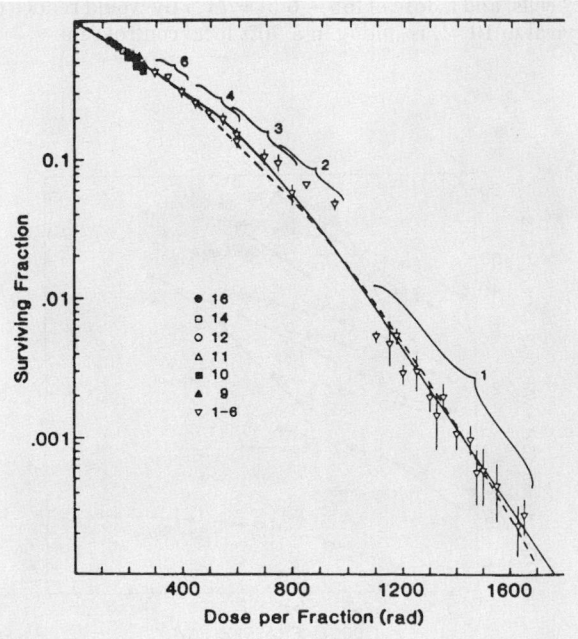

FIGURE 2.15. Effective single-dose survival curves for clonogenic cells of jejunal crypts fitted to multi-fraction data using linear quadratic (LQ) (*broken curves*) and two-component (TC) (*solid lines*) models. Numbered brackets illustrate that the data were from experiments using that number of fractions. Mean survival curve parameters are, for LQ model, $\alpha = 0.23$ Gy, $\beta = 0.018$ Gy^{-2}, and for TC model, $_1$D$_0$ = 3.57 Gy, D$_0$ = 1.43 Gy, $_n$D$_0$ = 2.37 Gy, and n = 20.4. (From Thames HD, Withers HR, Mason KA, et al. Dose-survival characteristics of mouse jejunal crypt cells. *Int J Radiat Oncol Biol Phys* 1981;7:1591, with permission.)

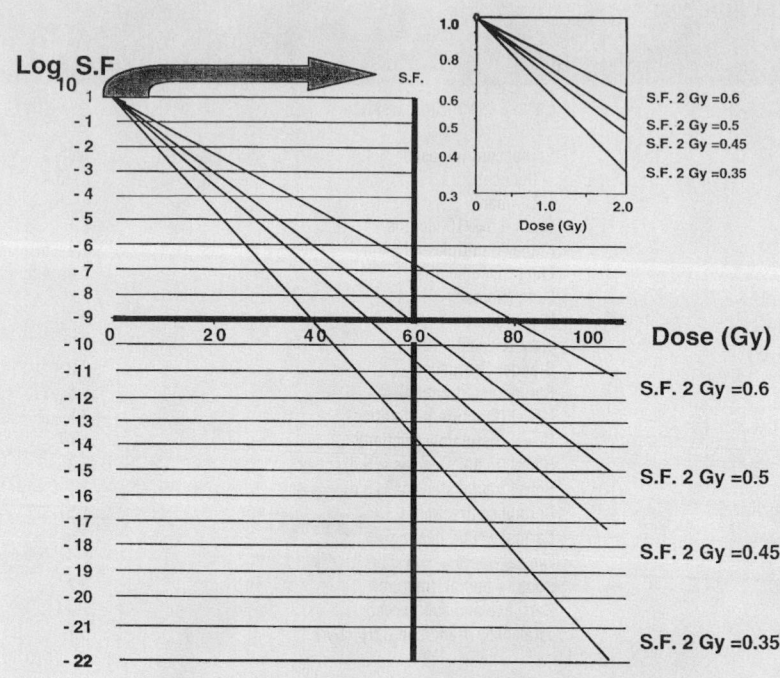

FIGURE 2.16. Effective multifraction dose-survival curves for cell populations, the survival of which from 2 Gy varies from 0.65 to 0.35. When survival from 2 Gy is 0.5, survival from 30 × 2 Gy is (0.5) (30) = approximately 10^{-9}. When this figure was constructed, this survival value was taken as an arbitrary standard against which the relative survival of other populations exposed to 30 × 2 Gy was plotted. The abscissa at the standard survival shows the total doses in 2-Gy fractions necessary to achieve that standard survival level in different cell populations. In all cases, an equal effect per dose fraction was assumed. The ratios of cell survival after a total dose of 60 Gy illustrate the exponential amplification of survival differences with increasing dose. Thus, dose fractionation can transform small differences in response at low doses (2 Gy) to large ultimate differences; measurements must be made accurately after a dose of 2 Gy to predict accurately the ultimate outcome of high-dose multifraction irradiation. (From Withers HR. Predicting late normal tissue responses. *Int J Radiat Oncol Biol Phys* 1986;12:693, with permission.)

Small differences between cell types in their intrinsic radiosensitivity to dose fractions of 2 Gy could amplify into large differences after many fractions, which could have a major influence on the outcome of therapy. For example, if $S.F._{2Gy}$ in one tissue were 0.6 and 0.5 in another, the ratio of cell survival after 30 doses of 2 Gy would be $\left(\frac{0.6}{0.5}\right)^{30}$, or 237-fold. For n = 35, the difference would increase to 590-fold. The effect of differences in $S.F._{2Gy}$ ranging from 0.35 to 0.6 on outcome after 30 fractions is shown in Fig. 2.16 (264). That the differences are very large can be judged from the ratios of cell survival rate (on the ordinate), or the range of total doses needed to achieve the same level of cell survival (approximately 10^{-9}) (abscissa).

Common Logarithms and $_eD_{10}$

The effective survival curve for a multifraction regimen is more easily considered in terms of $_eD_{10}$, which reduces survival to 10% (10^{-1}), than in terms of $_eD_0$. An approximate value for $_eD_{10}$ for 2 Gy fractions is 6.5 to 7 Gy, which corresponds with $S.F._{2Gy}$

of about 0.5. Remembering that about 10^9 tumor cells tightly packed would have a volume of about 1 cm^3 and that 10^{10} cells would form a sphere about 2.2 cm diameter, then an average T_3 tumor would contain about 10^{10} clonogenic cells. Assuming an $_eD_{10}$ of 7 Gy, a T_3 tumor treated with 70 Gy would have its surviving clonogen number reduced by 10^{-10} ($10^{-70/7}$), or to an average of one clonogen per tumor. Because of the random nature of cell survival, 37% of such tumors would contain 0 clonogens and would be locally controlled. If $_eD_{10}$ were 6.5 Gy, 65 Gy would be sufficient to cure 37% of tumors containing 10^{10} cells, and a dose of (65 + 6.5) = 71.5 Gy would reduce cell survival to 10^{-11}, resulting in a 90% local control rate.

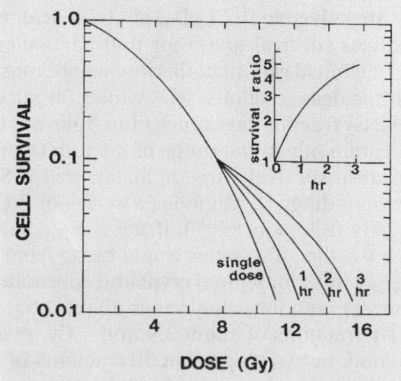

FIGURE 2.17. Recovery curves of the type first described by Elkind and Sutton (81). The repair of sublethal injury begins immediately and can be measured in terms of survival ratio (inset) or the increment in dose to achieve isosurvival.

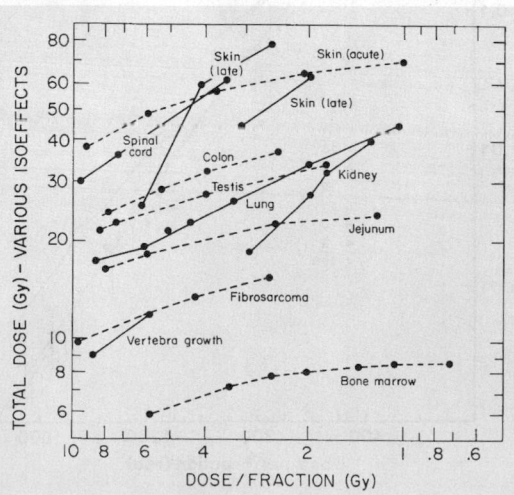

FIGURE 2.18. Isoeffect curves in which the total dose necessary for a certain effect in various tissues is plotted as a function of dose per fraction (late effects, *solid lines*; acute effects, *broken lines*). Data were selected to exclude an influence on the total dose of regeneration during the multifraction experiments. The isodoses for late effects increase more rapidly with decrease in dose per fraction than is the case for acute effects. (From Withers HR. Biologic basis for altered fractionation schemes. *Cancer* 1985;55:2086, with permission.)

Tumor Response and Dose Fractionation

There is a wide spectrum of radiosensitivities within and between tumor types (39,225,227,302) and variation in their α/β ratios (258,261) (Table 2.2). There is also uncertainty in attributing weight to each of the major phenomena affecting survival of tumor cells during a course of radiation therapy; these have been called the four "Rs" of dose fractionation (311): *Repair* of sublethal damage, *repopulation, redistribution* through the division cycle (312,340), and *reoxygenation* (141) of hypoxic tumor clonogens. If the effects of such phenomena on the response to each dose were constant throughout the course of a multifraction regimen, the resulting survival curve would be linear and the slope would depend on the extent to which each phenomenon affected the response. More likely, their influence, and particularly the effect of reoxygenation and regeneration, varies with time as treatment progresses. In some normal tissues (e.g., oropharyngeal mucosa), regeneration of surviving clonogenic cells late in a course of 1.8 to 2 Gy fractions may outstrip the cytocidal effect of treatment and the net survival curve will have a positive slope. The same phenomenon may occasionally happen within a tumor during treatment. In spite of the uncertainties, it is possible to model dose-response relationships for tumors and to use these models to guide treatment.

Tumor Control Probability (TCP)

TCP for Clinically Detectable Disease

The probability of tumor control increases, but not linearly, as radiation dose increases and clonogenic tumor cell survival decreases. Success or failure in controlling a tumor depends on killing the last surviving clonogen. For permanent tumor control (not palliation), if even one clonogen survives, the whole dose is "wasted"; conversely, control is achieved abruptly as the last clonogen is sterilized.

A plot of control versus dose for a single tumor therefore shows no response up to a certain dose and then an immediate increase to 100% response at death of the last clonogen. For a series of patients, even if they have identical tumors, the shape of the tumor control probability curve is different because cell killing is a random process. After a certain dose of irradiation, the numbers of surviving clonogens per tumor will begin to follow a Poisson distribution. For example, if cell survival is reduced to an average of one clonogen per tumor there would be, on average, 37% with no survivors, 37% with one, 18.4% with two, 6.1% with three, and 1.5% with four or more surviving clonogens. Obviously, the local control rate would be 37%, not 0%. Poisson statistics correlate probability of tumor control with cell survival rate by:

$$P_{cure} = e^{-x} = e^{-(SF \cdot M)}$$

where x is the average number of surviving clonogens per tumor, which in turn is the product of S.F. (fraction of cells surviving) and M (initial cell number). For example, if a tumor contains 10^{10} clonogens, doses that reduce survival to 10^{-10} would give an average cell survival of 1 and a P_{cure} to e $- (10^{10} \cdot 10^{-10}) = e^{-1} = 0.37$ or 37%.

If the total dose were increased by two $_{eff}D_0$ values, cell survival would be further reduced by two natural logarithms, from 1 to $1 \times e^{-2}$, that is, to an average of 0.135 cells per tumor, and $P_{cure} = e^{-0.135} = 0.87$, or 87%. It can be calculated that an increase in dose by three $_{eff}D_0$ values is sufficient to increase the probability of cure from 10% to 90%.

If $P_{cure} = 10\% = 0.1 = e^{-x}$ then x = 2.3. In other words, at 10% local control rate there is an average of 2.3 clonogens per tumor. After an increase in dose by three $_{eff}D_0$ values, $P_{cure} = e^{-(2.3 \cdot e^{-3})} = e^{-(0.115)} = 0.89$, or 89%.

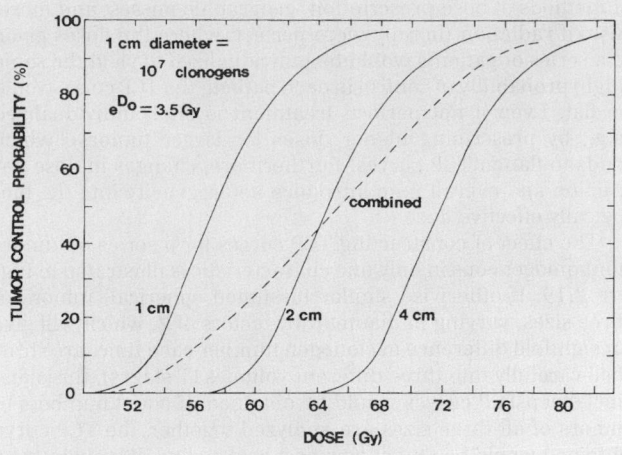

FIGURE 2.19. Theoretic tumor control probability (TCP) curves for three sizes of spherical tumors (*solid lines*) and one that would result from a study incorporating into the dose-response analysis all three tumor sizes in equal proportions (*broken line*). They were calculated on the assumptions that the dose was given in 2-Gy fractions, that the $_eD_0$ value for 2 Gy per fraction was 3.5 Gy, and that a 1-cm diameter spherical tumor contained 10^7 clonogens. As tumor volume increases, so does the dose required for a certain probability of control. The cell number increases by eight times and 64 times as the spherical tumor increases from 1-cm diameter to 2 and 4 cm, respectively. An exponential increase in clonogen number is related to a linear increase in dose for an isoeffect. Heterogeneity of even one factor, initial clonogen number, causes the TCP curve to be shallower (*broken line*). Retrospective clinical studies incorporate a large number of causes for heterogeneity of response.

This relationship between probability of cure and dose, above a certain threshold, is described by a sigmoid curve (Fig. 2.19). It is obvious from the previous equations and calculations that the slope of the curve is a function of the $_{eff}D_0$ values for the last few surviving tumor clonogens. It is steeper for neutrons or for single-dose x-ray treatments than for multifraction x-ray exposures and steeper (by the oxygen-enhancement ratio) for euoxic than for hypoxic cells.

The dose that yields a 50% control rate is known as the tumor control dose 50 (TCD_{50}). A higher rate is usually sought in clinical practice. For experimental studies, the TCD_{50} is useful because it is in a steep part of the TCP curve and is sensitive to small changes in the effectiveness of therapy. (Actually, the curve is steepest at TCD_{37} [i.e., where an average of one clonogenic cell survives per tumor].)

TCP curves from experimental animal data are steep, but those for human tumor control are shallower than would be predicted from estimates of tumor cell radiosensitivity (1,25,92,103,116,182,226,247,248,268). This reflects heterogeneity in various clinical tumor characteristics and treatment prescriptions that give a wider spread of responses to a given (nominal) dose. Originally, a nominal standard dose (NSD) equation was used in an effort to normalize differences resulting from differences between physical and biological isodose contours resulting from differences in dose fractionation patterns and to construct TCP curves (247,248), although it is now known to be inappropriate for these purposes (325). However, even in recent analyses where variation in tumor characteristics and treatment parameters has been minimized or adjusted for, and uniformity facilitated by analyzing a body of data large enough to allow relatively homogeneous stages of disease to be studied independently, the TCP curves have been fairly shallow (32,170,268,328).

Heterogeneity that could give rise to relatively shallow TCP curves from analyses of clinical data may come from differences in initial numbers of clonogens, their intrinsic radiosensitivity, repair of sublethal or potentially lethal injury, redistribution and repopulation kinetics, reoxygenation rates, dose rate, dose calculation, inhomogeneities of dose distribution, inconsistency of methods of dose prescription, geographic misses, and more. Also, if radiation therapy were perfect, where the doses given to a series of patients would be individualized to yield the same (high) probability of control in each patient, the TCP curve would be flat. Even if not perfect, treatment is often individualized (e.g., by prescribing higher doses for larger tumors), which tends to flatten TCP curves. Furthermore, changes in dose per fraction and overall time introduce heterogeneity into the biologically effective dose

The effect of constructing TCP curves for a series of tumors nonhomogeneous in only one characteristic is illustrated in Figure 2.19. If otherwise similar (assumed spherical) tumors of three sizes, varying in diameter by factors of 2, which will give an eightfold difference in clonogen number each time, are stratified carefully into three different volumes (T stages), three distinct steep TCP curves would be obtained. If equal numbers of tumors of all three sizes are analyzed together, the TCP curve obtained would be that shown as a broken line. It would not be appropriate to include tumors with a 64-fold range of volumes in a clinical TCP analysis, but the range in clonogen numbers in human cancers of similar T-stage may be large so that heterogeneity of this magnitude is not impossible. Variations in clonogenic cell content may come not only from the range of volumes included in a given T-stage, but also from differences in the ratio of stem cells to differentiated cells, necrosis, or extent of normal cell infiltration (such as fibrovascular stroma and macrophages). Further variation in the effective number of clonogens would also arise from differences in inherent tumor growth kinetics and in accelerated repopulation potential of surviving cells during radiation therapy.

Normal tissue dose-response curves for the incidence of a certain complication are also sigmoid above a certain threshold. Such curves are used for estimating lethal damage (LD_{50}) or effective dose (ED_{50}) values, the doses that cause in 50% of cases lethality or any specified effect, respectively. Because normal tissues are more homogeneous than tumors in their composition and radiation responses, complication probability curves are steeper than those for tumor control (175,266).

The art of radiation therapy can be quantified in a risk-benefit analysis as a balance between the TCP and the probability of complications, NTCP, (both represented by sigmoid curves illustrated in Fig. 2.20), but with many factors involved. Different points illustrate this:

1. If there is to be therapeutic gain, the biologic effectiveness of radiation therapy must be greater in the tumor than in normal tissues; i.e., normal tissues must be preferentially spared.
2. In the steep midrange of TCP or complication frequency, a small change in the biologic effectiveness of therapy can give a substantial change in clinical outcome. Converely, if a change in treatment produces a modest difference in effect (e.g., in TCP or in frequency of complications), that percentage difference should not be interpreted as being due to a large change in the biologic effectiveness. The change should be expressed more appropriately in terms of change in dose to achieve a certain isoeffect, that is, by quantifying the lateral shift of the TCP or NTCP curve, not the vertical change for a fixed dose. This ratio of isoeffect doses is the dose-modification factor.
3. At incidences of about <10% and about >85%, changes in biologically effective dose will appear less effective than in the midrange. For example, if the TCP is 90%, minor therapeutic gain would be achieved from an increase in dose, and perhaps a therapeutic disadvantage if there was already an associated incidence of severe complications that lay on the steep part of the NTCP curve.
4. Because dose-response curves for normal tissues and most human tumors are close together, it is usually inappropriate to never produce complications. Within the treatment volume, a certain incidence of injury to normal tissues sufficient to be defined as a complication is a prerequisite to good curative radiation therapy under most circumstances where TCP is not close to 100%.
5. If the TCP is predominantly to the right of the normal tissue complications curve, tumor control without a high incidence of complications is unlikely, and other modalities should be used, either independently or as adjuvants. For example, suppose the TCP curves for large tumors lie to the right of those for complications, whereas those for smaller tumors are to the left. In this situation, a therapeutic gain could be derived from excision of the main mass of a large tumor by surgery or some form of chemotherapy that would add to the effect of irradiation without increasing normal tissue toxicity. However, a 50% or even 90% debulking is of modest value. A 90% reduction in tumor volume represents only a one decade decrease in cell number, equivalent to about 6.5 to 7 Gy in 2-Gy fractions, other things being equal.
6. It defies biologic rationale to deny the existence of a potential benefit from maximizing the dose in a patient considered to have some finite chance of tumor control merely because retrospective studies show a shallow TCP curve (1,116).

TCP for Subclinical Disease

The threshold-sigmoid curve for tumor control probability for clinically detectable tumors is inappropriate if applied to subclinical metastases. If 10^n clonogens represent the upper limit of clinical undetectability of metastases and in a group of patients some have overt metastases at presentation (i.e., $>10^n$ metastatic clonogens) and some have no metastatic clonogens, then those who harbor subclinical metastases must have a tumor burden of between 1 and 10^n cells. Given that micrometastases grow exponentially (173), it is reasonable (as a working hypothesis) to assume that there is within a series of patients, an even distribution of the logarithm of metastatic clonogens (between 1 and 10^n cells) (178,327).

If it is further assumed that a reasonable value for n is 9, then 11% of patients with subclinical metastases would have between 1 and 10 metastatic clonogens, another 11% between 10 and 100, another 11% of patients between 10^2 and 10^3, and so forth. Based on this simple model, the dose-response curve would exhibit no threshold and would be shallow. The lack of a

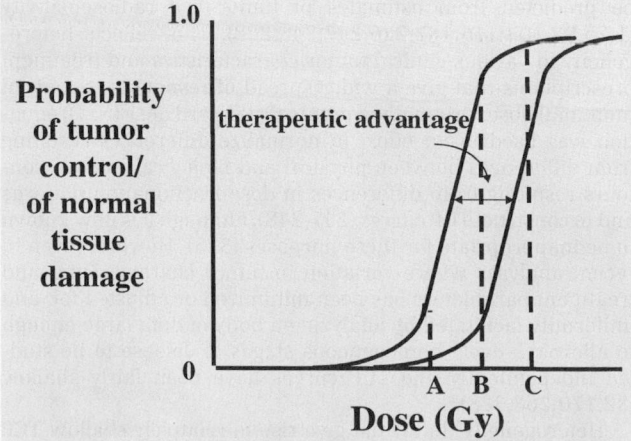

FIGURE 2.20. Theoretical curves showing the probability of tumor control and normal tissue complications. Both curves have a threshold and are log sigmoid in nature. The art of radiotherapy is to increase the distance between these two curves; that is, to derive a therapeutic benefit. If the normal tissue damage curve is to the left of that for TCP, tumor control is unlikely without unacceptable normal tissue complications.

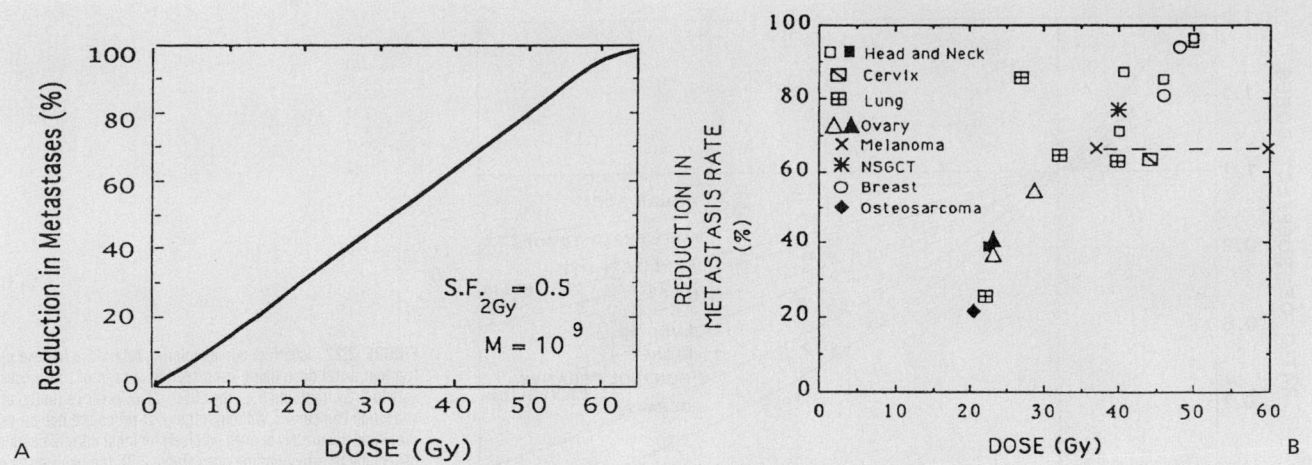

FIGURE 2.21. Percentage control rate as a function of dose for subclinical metastases. **A:** Modeling on the basis of a uniform distribution of the logarithm of numbers of metastatic tumor cells per patient ranging between 1 and 10^9. An SF_{2Gy} value of 0.5 was used. The intercept of this theoretic curve is displaced slightly from zero because of the random statistical chance that any cell will survive any dose of radiation. Also, at high doses, the probability of sterilizing all tumor cells approaches 100% asymptotically for the same reason. **B:** Percentage reductions in recurrence as a function of dose from reports in the literature for various tumor types. Solid symbols represent data from prospective randomized trials. Other data are retrospective comparisons between control rates with and without elective irradiation. (From Withers HR, Peters LJ, Taylor JMG. Dose-response relationship for radiation therapy of subclinical disease. *Int J Radiat Oncol Biol Phys* 1995;31:353, with permission.)

detectable threshold would reflect the existence of a very small number of metastatic cells in some patients, and the shallow slope would reflect the wide variation in cell burden within the population harboring subclinical metastases. The model in Figure 2.21A illustrates these concepts. Although this distribution could be modified by many factors (notably Gompertzian growth of micrometastases), it is generally consistent with results of irradiation of sites of subclinical metastases (Fig. 2.21B).

Time-Dose Isoeffect Formulae and Dose Fractionation

History

Early isoeffect curves related the total dose required to produce certain skin reactions or to achieve a certain TCP to the treatment time over which the dose regimen was delivered (237,255). That work preceded the demonstration by Puck and Marcus (234) in 1956 that mammalian cell survival curves had a shoulder. It also preceded the work of Elkind and Sutton (81) in 1959 demonstrating that sublethal injury could be repaired, and, therefore, that the number of fractions, not just overall time, was important. Fowler and Stern (96) varied the number of fractions (N) and overall time (T) experimentally and showed that they were independent variables. Ellis (84) developed the NSD formula to incorporate these two variables into an isoeffect curve that was thought to be more relevant to radiation therapy than the original Strandqvist curves (255).

More recently, isoeffect curves that are based on parameters of dose-survival curves only (20,55,74,270,336) or that include other biologic parameters, such as regeneration, have been proposed (56,277). We now understand that there can be no single universally applicable isoeffect equation or curve because tissues (and tumors) differ in the characteristics which determine their fractionation responses and repopulation kinetics.

Acute Versus Late-Responding Tissues

The most general biologic phenomenon influencing the fractionation response is repair of sublethal injury (81). This varies among tissues, with slow-responding tissues consistently showing a greater capacity than rapidly responding tissues (20,138,157,270,334–336). This may be because surviving cells in early responding tissues redistribute through the division cycle during the interfraction interval and express unrepaired damage as they do so or they may move into cell cycle phases that are more radiation-sensitive. Alternatively, repair of sublethal injury often seems to continue longer in late-responding than in early responding tissues (8,205,263,265,267). Regardless of the mechanism, late-responding tissues are spared more than acute-responding tissues by dose fractionation; that is, the dose for an isoeffect increases more rapidly in late-responding tissues as dose per fraction is reduced.

The slopes of the isoeffect curves in Figures 2.18 and 2.22 reflect the shape of the dose-survival or dose-function curves for responses in various tissues. Those in Figure 2.22 are constructed using the LQ formula (see later discussion) to correct the total dose (normalized to 1) to that which would be given if the dose per fraction were a standard 2 Gy. Shown for comparison is a plot based on the NSD formula (84) where the correction for time is ignored; i.e., where $D = NSD \times N^{0.24}$.

In terms of the LQ cell survival model, late effects tissues have a low α/β ratio (270,333–335), describing a curvier curve than that for acute-responding tissues (Fig. 2.13). Thus, increasing the dose per fraction produces a relatively larger increment in effect in late-responding than in early-responding tissues. Conversely, decreasing dose per fraction spares late-responding tissues more than acute-responding tissues. Examples of α/β values for tissues are in Table 2.2.

Some specific clinical implications of the differences in fractionation response between acutely and late-responding tissues are:

1. Large dose fractions are relatively more harmful for late-responding tissues. If the same acute reactions are achieved with two different fractionation regimens—one using large, the other small doses per fraction—late responses will be more severe from the large dose per fraction regimen. This has been observed in many clinical studies (6,59,172,212, 270,279,335,336).

2. Since the therapeutic differential between late-responding tissues and tumors increases with decreasing dose per

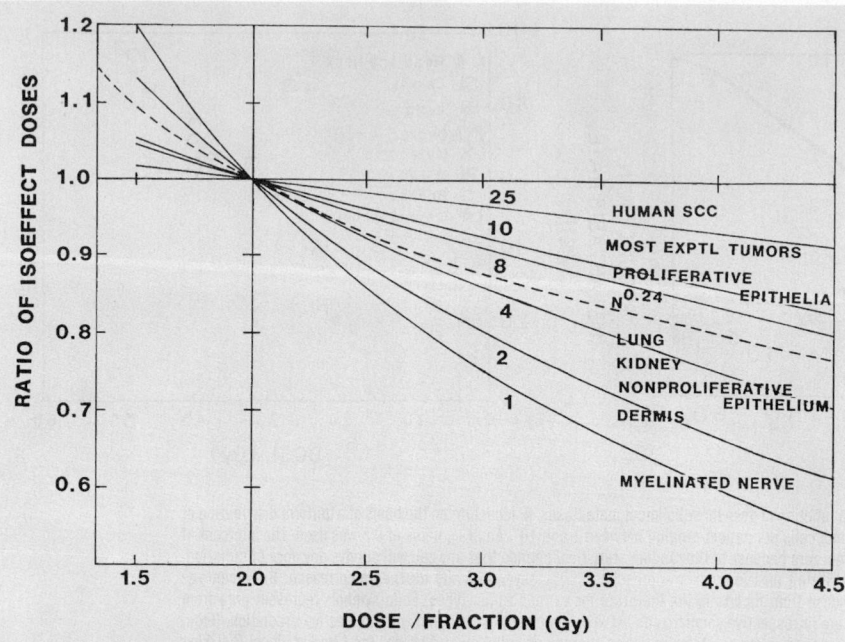

FIGURE 2.22. Isoeffect curves relating total dose to dose per fraction, total dose being expressed as a ratio of that necessary in 2-Gy fractions (i.e., the $LQED_{2Gy}$). α/β ratios (in Gy) are shown on the curves. Although the α/β ratios are not yet established accurately or even precisely for most normal tissues, especially late-responding ones (Table 2.2), the likely order of fractionation sensitivities is as shown. The broken line traces the change in dose as it would have been predicted by a factor $N^{0.24}$ in the nominal standard dose (84) formula. Phenomena other than repair of sublethal injury, specifically repopulation, are not accounted for by these curves. SCC, squamous cell carcinoma. (From Withers HR. Contrarian concepts in the progress of radiotherapy. *Radiat Res* 1989;119:395, with permission.)

fraction, a therapeutic gain may result from use of the smallest practical dose per fraction (129). For example, if two fractions of 1.15 Gy achieve the same effect in a late-responding tissue as one fraction of 2 Gy, but two fractions of only 1.05 Gy achieve the same tumor control rate, the therapeutic gain would be 1.15/1.05 = 1.1. Thus hyperfractionation using two fractions of 1.15 Gy to replace one fraction of 2 Gy would increase the biologically effective tumor dose by 10% with no increase in late complications, although acute-responding normal tissues will also receive an increased biologic dose.

3. To maximize the potential therapeutic gain from hyperfractionation, repair of sublethal damage in late-responding tissues must be complete, implying fractionation intervals of at least 6 hours (8,224,263–265). For the spinal cord, a longer interval may be prudent (8,10,72,244,284).

4. The relative biologic efficiency (RBE) for neutrons (or charged particles such as carbon ions) for late effects is greater at low doses than high doses because the great sparing effect from fractionated x-ray doses is lost, as is illustrated in Figure 2.13 (136,334).

LQ Formula for Calculating Isoeffect Relationships

It is possible to use the LQ response formula to change the size of dose per fraction (within limits) (336):

$$D_{new}/D_{ref} = (\alpha/\beta + d_{ref})/(\alpha/\beta + d_{new})$$

where D_{new} is the new total dose for a change in size of dose per fraction to d_{new}; D_{ref} is the previous total dose in fractions of d_{ref}; and α/β is for the tissue in question, all doses being expressed in Gray. For example, if d_{new} were 4 Gy and d_{ref} were 2 Gy, the ratio of total doses to achieve the same effects in a tissue with an α/β value of 2 Gy would be 0.66. For a tissue with an α/β value of 10 Gy, it would be 0.85. This calculation was used to derive the curves in Figure 2.22.

The following caveats apply to this use of the LQ isoeffect formula:

1. The LQ response model does not apply equally well at all dose levels. It fits experimental data well over a limited dose range (e.g., 2 to 8 Gy), but its validity and precision beyond

that range has yet to be established, especially for such vital structures as the spinal cord (7) and especially at doses per fraction less than about 2 Gy (11,139).

2. Using uncertain values for α/β ratios has more of an effect in late-responding tissues and carries more risk. There is little difference in isoeffect curves for different dose-per-fraction regimens delivered to tissues with α/β values of 10 Gy or more, whereas the difference is much larger for tissues with α/β values of 1 and 2 Gy (Fig. 2.22).

3. Dose corrections are most affected at low doses per fraction, which is also the region where the LQ response model is least validated. Using the isoeffect formula here, or the curves in Fig. 2.22, compare the ratios of isoeffect doses for a tissue characterized by an α/β value of 2 Gy when the dose per fraction is changed from 2 to 1 Gy (a 33% increase) and from 2 to 3 Gy (a 20% decrease). The greatest change in predicted isoeffect doses occurs in the least defined region of the curves (low doses) and for (late effects) tissues, which are most affected by change in dose per fraction.

4. No account is taken of cell regeneration within tissues during multifraction regimens, and repair must be complete (8,263,265,267).

For the previously mentioned reasons, the LQ formula or curve should be used cautiously.

Influence of Regeneration (Repopulation)

Normal Tissues

The influence of overall duration of therapy on fractionation responses comes largely from large differences in the time of onset and kinetics of regeneration (repopulation) among various normal and neoplastic tissues (Fig. 2.3). This is why a constant exponent for overall treatment time in an isoeffect formula (e.g., time in days as used in NSD, cumulative radiation effect, time-dose factor formulas) without regard to tissue is a dangerous simplification with no biologic foundation (325). For example, early regeneration of intestinal mucosa or bone marrow makes a major contribution to the net response if a treatment regimen is spread out over several weeks, whereas it provides little or no benefit to spinal cord, kidney, or dermis. A constant exponent of less than 1 also implies a greater effect on isoeffect dose when values for T are small, whereas the major contribution of regeneration occurs when T values are large (e.g., 10 to 60 days).

Tumors

Like acute-responding normal tissues, tumors accelerate their growth in response to injury. Some clinical implications of tumor regeneration for curative radiation therapy are:

1. Protracting treatment longer than necessary will likely be a disadvantage. For example, using 1.8 Gy rather than 2 Gy fractions given five times per week extends overall treatment time by about 10% and should be reserved for situations in which acute responses are likely to limit the rate of dose accumulation or where there may be substantial inhomogeneities in dose distribution. Inhomogeneity can lead to double trouble, with areas receiving a high total dose areas also receiving high doses per fraction. The increase in physical dose has an added biologic component because of the large dose per fraction that is more of a problem if later-responding tissues are involved (Fig. 2.23).
2. If a break in treatment is necessary because of acute toxicity, it should be kept as short as is tolerable.
3. Planned split-course therapy is inadvisable unless it is part of an accelerated treatment protocol that ultimately shortens the overall treatment duration (discussed later).
4. Breaks in therapy for nonmedical reasons (machine breakdown, holidays) may merit "catch-up" treatments in patients being treated for cure, for example, by treating twice on some remaining days.
5. Obviously, rapidly growing tumors must be treated rapidly. However, it is reasonable to accelerate treatment of tumors with a high proliferative index, regardless of their growth rate, because they are likely to reduce their rate of cell loss

and regenerate earlier and faster during treatment. In fact, treatment should never be unnecessarily protracted (consistent with other considerations) because it is difficult to predict the accelerated repopulation response of individual tumors.

Modification of Dose Fractionation Patterns

Standard radiation therapy regimens, using about 2 Gy per day 5 days per week, have developed empirically over the decades as a good overall pattern of dose fractionation. However, from the preceding discussion, it should be obvious that this may not be the best for all clinical situations and that it is certainly inappropriate in some (e.g., in obviously rapidly growing tumors) (94,95,204,269,313).

Some biologic factors relevant to modification of dose fractionation are:

1. Tissues differ in their response to multiple dose fractions (Figs. 2.14, 2.18, and 2.22), and tissue-related factors have to be taken into account.
2. Acute-responding normal tissues have an enormous capacity for repopulation (Fig. 2.3).
3. Tumors also show accelerated repopulation (Figs. 2.5–2.7). Although there is probably great variability from tumor to tumor, on average, the lag time before its onset is longer and its rate slower than for acute-responding normal tissues.
4. Cell-cycle redistribution to asynchrony between dose fractions produces a net sensitization in proliferative tissues, but not in nonproliferative, late-responding tissues.
5. Hypoxia affects tumor responses to a lesser extent at low doses, but the kinetics of reoxygenation are probably rapid in relation to the duration of most radiation therapy regimens, and it may be a factor only if single or a few large doses are used.
6. Slow-responding tissues repair sublethal damage better than acute-responding tissues.
7. Repopulation in normal tissues, and possibly in tumors, may occur rapidly during any treatment break.
8. The lag time to the onset of repopulation may be shortened (although to a limited extent) by causing injury faster; for example, by increasing dose intensity or by concomitant chemotherapy.

In the following discussion of altered fractionation, two treatments that are most often disadvantageous will be discussed before those that are more often likely to be advantageous.

Hypofractionation

Many clinical and experimental animal studies have shown that increasing the size of dose fractions increases the severity of late responses in relation to acute responses. Since the fractionation response of acute-responding normal tissues is not dissimilar to that of most tumors (171,306) with exceptions (195,258,261) from the viewpoint of differentials in α/β ratios, increasing the size of dose fractions (hypofractionation) usually provides a therapeutic disadvantage.

If we assume α/β ratios of 10 Gy and 3 Gy for tumor and critical late-responding normal tissue, respectively, and change a treatment of 66 Gy in 2 Gy fractions to a 4 Gy regimen, the isoeffective total dose for the late-responding tissue, determined using the LQ isoeffect formula, would be 0.71 of 70 Gy (49.7 Gy). However, to keep tumor control rate constant would require a reduction to only 0.86 of 70 Gy (60.4 Gy). By giving 49.7 Gy, the incidence and severity of late sequelae would remain unchanged, but the tumor would be relatively underdosed,

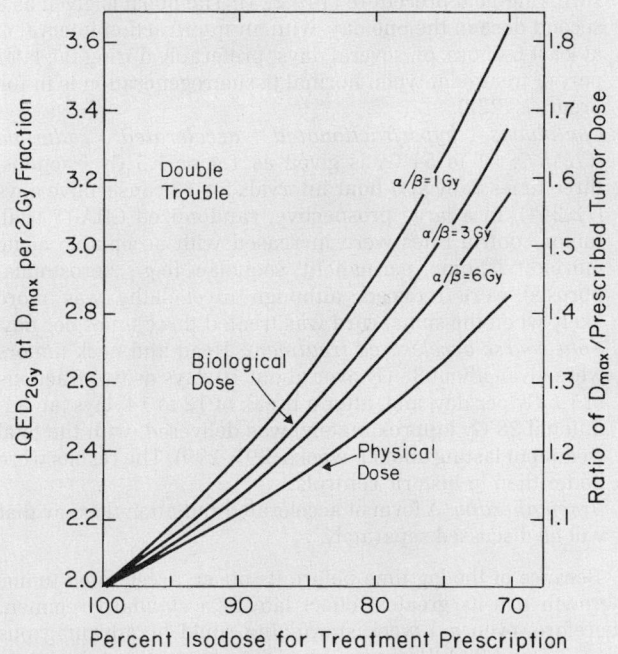

FIGURE 2.23. Influence of dose heterogeneity on physical and biologic doses as a function of the isodose line chosen for defining the tumor dose and of α/β ratio of the tissue located at D_{max}. The divergence of biologic and physical doses reflects the change in biologic dose that results from change in dose per fraction that derives from the heterogeneity of dose distribution. The lower the α/β ratio, the greater the divergence between biologic and physical doses. This "double-trouble" is not reflected in physics isodose distributions and may explain not only a spurious volume effect but also may contribute to low values of tolerance doses that have appeared in the literature from time to time.

receiving only 83% (0.71/0.86) of the dose biologically equivalent to the reference dose of 70 Gy in 2-Gy fractions. For the biologic effect on the tumor to be maintained would require giving a total of 60.4 Gy, and the biologic dose to the late-responding tissues would be 20% (0.86/0.71) too high. Obviously, the therapeutic ratio will be reduced regardless of whether the change in total dose was aimed at an isoeffect for late responses (49.7 Gy) or for an isocontrol rate of the tumor (60.4 Gy). Although logistic advantages in palliative treatment, or physical advantages derived from highly localized dose (e.g., in stereotactic radiosurgery and high-dose-rate afterloading brachytherapy) may outweigh the biologic disadvantage of hypofractionation, in general, hypofractionation should be reserved for when the tumor has an α/β value the same or lower than the normal tissue at risk, as may be the case for prostate cancer (36,76).

Protraction of Overall Treatment Duration

If irradiation were protracted for months, acute-responding tissues could tolerate enormous doses because of repopulation, but late-responding tissues would be dose-limiting. Because many tumors show an accelerated response some time after the start of a multifraction regimen, and some are already growing rapidly before treatment has begun, it is illogical to extend the overall duration of a curative course of radiation therapy for longer than is necessary to limit acute normal tissue toxicity.

Hyperfractionation

Hyperfractionation is defined as the use of smaller-than-standard doses per fraction. It can be achieved without extending the overall treatment duration by treating once a day for 6 or 7 days per week, but is usually achieved by giving two fractions per day for up to 5 days per week. Its aim is to increase the therapeutic differential between late-responding normal tissues and acute-responding tumors. It does this primarily by exploiting differences in their α/β ratios (223,335,337) although, historically, it was introduced to exploit the self-sensitizing effect of cell-cycle redistribution present in the tumor but absent in late-responding normal tissues (312). A third rationale is that the OER is lower at low doses (79,112,113). When two fractions are given per day, the interfraction interval should be as long as possible, but preferably not less than 6 hours (8,11,214,263,265,267,284,287), and longer if CNS tissue is involved, since repair there may continue for more than 12 hours (8,214,263). Hyperfractionation may not be an advantage in the treatment of slowly proliferating tumors because, like slowly proliferating normal tissues, their α/β ratio may be low.

Clinical evidence suggests that to achieve comparable toxicity in fibrovascular tissues, one fraction of 2 Gy/day should be replaced with two fractions of about 1.2 Gy (101,129). For comparison, the dose per fraction necessary for an isoeffect in acute-responding tissues (and most tumors) would be about 1.05 Gy (101,129,328,329). Assuming that the isoeffect dose for late-responding tissues was increased by 20% and that it was increased for tumor by only 5%, the therapeutic differential would be increased by 1.2/1.05 = 1.14. Therefore, if two fractions of 1.2 Gy/day replaced one fraction of 2 Gy/day, the acute responses of normal tissues and cytotoxicity for tumors would be increased as if the dose had been increased by 14% while late responses would be unaltered. Coincidentally, if the overall treatment time were unchanged, the "biologic" rate of treatment of the tumor and acute-responding normal tissues would also be accelerated by 14% (316). Hyperfractionation has improved tumor control rates, but also increases acute toxicity (79,101,129,224,301).

Accelerated Treatment

Accelerated treatment may be defined as a shortening of the overall treatment duration without a comparable reduction in total dose. However, in practice, lower doses (e.g., 50 to 55 Gy in 3 to 4 weeks) are generally given commonly using dose fractions of greater than 2 Gy, although in a clinical trial of an accelerated hyperfractionated regimen (CHART) doses of 1.5 Gy three times per day, 7 days per week were given. The aim of accelerated treatment is to minimize tumor growth or regeneration during therapy. The importance of accelerated repopulation during tumor treatment can be visualized by appreciating that two to three doublings of surviving clonogens should add about the same (four- to eightfold) increment in tumor cell burden as a one-step increase in T stage. The difficulty is to avoid excess toxicity in acute-responding normal tissues by reducing the benefit normally derived from repopulation. Using larger doses per fraction would accelerate treatment, but this is not advised in curative therapy for reasons discussed earlier. In practice, accelerated regimens should use conventional or even reduced doses per fraction given more frequently than usual (i.e., six or more times per week).

There are numerous ways to increase the intensity of dose accumulation from the "standard" of 2 Gy, five times per week (a regimen that is already accelerated 10% in relation to 1.8 Gy fractions)

1. *Multiple standard 2 Gy fractions per day* have been given in a continuous course lasting less than 2 weeks with good local control rates but a high frequency of severe complications (18,104,202,221,239).
2. *Relative hypofractionation*: About 50 Gy given in 15 fractions in 3 weeks (78,254), or 20 fractions in 4 weeks (116,119) are standard in a number of centers.
3. *Concomitant boosting*: The boost dose to a reduced volume is given "concomitantly" with the treatment of the initial larger volume rather than as a sequel, as would be standard in a shrinking-field procedure (149,224). The boost is given as a second dose in the one day, with an interfraction interval of at least 6 hours, on several days, preferably during the later part of treatment when normal tissue regeneration is in full progress (222).
4. *Continuous hyperfractionated accelerated radiation (CHART):* 51 to 54 Gy is given as 1.4 or 1.5 Gy fractions, three times daily at 6-hour intervals for 12 consecutive days (72,244). In a large prospective, randomized CHART trial, tumor control rates were increased with acceptable acute morbidity. Some permanent sequelae (e.g., xerostomia, fibrosis) were reduced, although myelopathy was more likely when the spinal cord was treated three times per day.
5. *Split-course accelerated treatment*: Head and neck tumors were given about 38 Gy over about 10 days as two fractions of 1.6 Gy per day, and, after a break of 12 to 14 days, an additional 28 Gy (approximately) was delivered, with the total treatment lasting about 6 weeks (297–299). The results were better than in historic controls.
6. *Brachytherapy:* A form of accelerated radiation therapy that will be discussed separately.

Because of the lag time before its onset, accelerated tumor regrowth has its greatest effect late in a standard regimen. Therefore, even a 1-week shortening could be advantageous (Figs. 2.5 and 2.6). However, excessive shortening to less than the lag time (e.g., to less than 3 to 4 weeks in head and neck cancer) may not improve tumor control rates, especially if the total dose is reduced to maintain acceptable acute toxicity.

Patients most suited to accelerated regimens are those with tumors that are rapidly growing (204) or have a high potential for rapid regrowth (269); for example, with a high proliferative index or a high cell loss factor. It may become possible to predict which tumors will repopulate early and quickly (31,72,128). One sign may be rapid regression, which could signify a tumor likely to repopulate quickly. In principle, all tumors should be treated in an overall time that is as short as possible consistent with acceptable acute morbidity, but caution should be taken to avoid self-defeating reductions in total dose below standard levels. Likewise, aggressive treatments that result in gaps in treatment due to severe acute toxicity can be counterproductive.

Although modifying and individualizing fractionation patterns may improve the outcome for some patients, accelerated tumor growth, repopulation in acute-responding tissues, and differences in response between late-responding normal tissues and tumors have important implications for everyday conventional treatment (331). For example, radiation therapy, at least for head and neck cancers, should not be completed on a Monday after a weekend break because this is a 3-day extension. Likewise, a course of curative therapy should not start on a Friday. In general, breaks in treatment (such as public holidays, patient demands) should be accounted for by delivering more than five fractions in at least one of the weeks of treatment without resorting to large fractions. Chemotherapy given over several weeks before the start of radiation therapy may also initiate accelerated repopulation and compromise the chance for local tumor control. Such neoadjuvant therapy might be more effective if given during or after radiation therapy, at a time when surviving tumor clonogens are actively proliferating, but, again, the total radiation dose should be maintained and acute toxicity kept tolerable.

Low-Dose Rate Irradiation

Low-dose rate continuous irradiation has the same biologic advantages as hyperfractionation. Additionally:

1. Proliferative cells may be delayed in their progression through the division cycle (28,68,80,112,131,274) in particular in late G2 phase. Such a skewed redistribution could self-sensitize proliferative tissues and tumors, without affecting late-responding normal tissues.
2. The overall duration of therapy is shortened.
3. The high-dose regions near the radioactive sources have a high probability of being completely sterilized of tumor cells. However, when the logarithmic nature of cell killing is considered, this is not as great an advantage as it may seem. For example, radiation "cautery" of 50% of the tumor cells represents a gain that is equivalent to about 2 to 2.5 Gy of a standard multifraction regimen.
4. The volume of normal tissue receiving a high dose is minimized. Not only is the total dose beyond the treatment volume lower, but so is the dose rate, boosting further the sparing of late-responding tissues. This can be considered an inverse double-trouble effect, or a double advantage.
5. A potential biologic disadvantage is that the relatively rapid fall-off in dose beyond the treatment volume, and in unintentional "cold spots," could decrease the probability of tumor cell eradication if the tumor lay beyond the specified minimum tumor isodose (geographic miss).

In contrast to low-dose rate brachytherapy, the advantages of high-dose rate, high-dose-per-fraction brachytherapy come from improved logistics and staff protection, as well as because normal tissues can be tolerably displaced from the high-dose field. Its biologic disadvantages may be loss of therapeutic differential between late effects tissues and tumors, reduced influence of cell-cycle redistribution and delay, and increased influence of tumor hypoxia.

Permanent implants of low dose rate radioisotopes with long half-lives (e.g., ^{125}I) also have radiobiologic disadvantages because late-responding normal tissues may accumulate high doses and, unlike the acute-responding normal tissues, are not spared appreciably by repopulation. Furthermore, if a set total dose is to be delivered over a relatively long time, the initial dose rate may have to be so low as to facilitate "escape" of tumor clonogens. As with high-dose rate brachytherapy, other considerations may overwhelm these radiobiologic disadvantages.

Optimal Dose Rate

A change in dose rate, even between relatively high-dose rates such as 10 Gy/min (600 Gy/h) to 1 Gy/min (60 Gy/h), can affect the response of tissues by allowing concomitant sublethal damage repair. However, sparing is most pronounced with changes among the lower dose rates more characteristic of brachytherapy, especially between about 10 and 0.1 Gy/h. However, in acute-responding tissues, and presumably also in a proportion of tumors, at low-dose rates, repopulation may be more important than repair.

In late-responding tissues, such as rat spinal cord (245) and lung (75), a large-dose rate effect is seen with change from 4 to 2 Gy/h. Technical factors in such experiments make investigation of lower dose rates difficult, but if 2 Gy/h data are compared with multifraction data, potential for substantial sparing with a further decrease in dose rate below 2 Gy/h is indicated (8,263,284,285). Such a large sparing effect of the reduced dose rate is to be expected in late-responding tissues for the same reasons as hyperfractionation spares such tissues.

Low-Dose Rate Total-Body Irradiation

Because proliferative bone marrow populations and leukemia (123) cells are characterized by a high α/β ratio (Table 2.2), it is reasonable to prepare patients for bone marrow transplantation using either multiple small dose fractions or continuous low-dose rate exposure (58,228,276). The low-dose rates between about 1 and 7 Gy/h that have been chosen for various continuous total-body irradiation regimens are where biologic effectiveness changes rapidly and even lower dose rates may provide even better therapeutic differential (75,214,245,276). Because such low-dose rates in a single sitting are often not practical, many transplantation centers give multifraction exposures using low doses per fraction and at a low-dose rate. In general, low doses per fraction and low-dose rates provide the best therapeutic differentials, provided the overall treatment duration is kept short in relation to the growth rate of the leukemia cells and lymphocytic stem cells.

Intensity-Modulated Radiation Therapy

Stereotactic and intensity-modulated radiation therapy can increase the therapeutic index by developing steep dose gradients between the tumor and adjacent normal tissues. They can also facilitate the generation of planned or inadvertent cold or hot spots within the tumor.

Geographic Underdosage of Tumor

The impact of geographic underdosage (cold spots) of areas within tumor on the TCP depends on:

1. Number of clonogens underdosed
2. Magnitude of the underdosage
3. TCP for homogeneous dose distribution
4. Radiosensitivity of the tumor clonogens

The likely decline in TCP can be modeled if it is assumed that the tumor clonogens are distributed uniformly throughout the clinical tumor volume and are of uniform radiosensitivity. The tumor can then be regarded as a large number of "tumorlets" each receiving a specified, although variable, dose. The overall

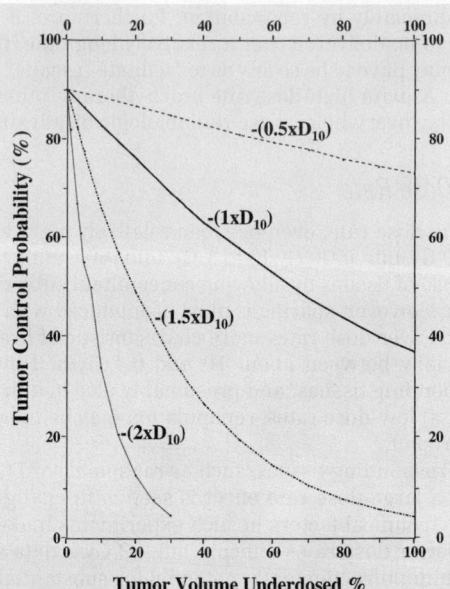

FIGURE 2.24. Effect of varying degrees of underdosage (in terms of D_{10} values) on tumor control probability as a function of tumor volume underdosed. Note that the most important determinant is the magnitude of the underdosage (317).

TCP can be estimated by summing the TCPs for all the tumorlets. As illustrated in Figure 2.24, this TCP will decrease more the greater the number of underdosed tumorlets (volume) and the larger the decrement in dose. In a given patient, the probability of cure if the dose were distributed homogeneously (Fig. 2.26), as well as the radiosensitivity of the tumor clonogens, will be important. (Note that inhomogeneities in dose introduce heterogeneities in dose per fraction, which amplifies inhomogeneity in biologic dose beyond the variation in physical dose to an extent that will depend on the α/β ratio.)

Figure 2.24 traces the decline in TCP as a function of volume of tumor underdosed and the magnitude of the underdosage. The magnitude of the underdose is shown as multiples of D_{10}, the dose that would reduce the number of surviving clonogens to 10% of the initial number: About 7 Gy for a standard regimen of 2-Gy fractions. Thus, from Figure 2.24, it can be seen that a 7 Gy ($1 \times D_{10}$) underdosage to 10% of the tumor would reduce TCP from 90% to 83%, whereas a 14 Gy underdosage to only 5% of the tumor would reduce TCP from 90% to 55%. The extent of underdosage is more important than the volume underdosed.

Dose-Volume Histograms and TCP

Heterogeneity of Dose in Subvolumes

Theoretical dose-volume histograms (DVHs) are presented in Figure 2.25. The smallest deviation from 100% dose to 100% tumor is outlined by a-e, showing 5% of the tumor being underdosed by about 5% ($0.5 \times D_{10}$). Underdosage by 10% ($1 \times D_{10}$), 15% ($1.5 \times D_{10}$), or 20% ($2 \times D_{10}$) in a 70 Gy regimen is shown by b-e, c-e, and d-e, respectively. The impact on TCP of the four levels of underdosage depicted by the DVHs in Figure 2.25 can be read from Fig. 2.24. Assuming that 70 Gy in 2-Gy fractions yields a TCP of 90%, then the effect of underdosing 5% of the tumor by 5% ($0.5 \times D_{10}$), 10% ($1 \times D_{10}$), 15% ($1.5 \times D_{10}$) or 20% ($2 \times D_{10}$) would be a decline in TCP by 1%, 3.5%, 12.5% and 35%, respectively (Fig. 2.24).

It is obvious that most of the DVH is irrelevant to TCP, but that small increments in the indentation along the x-axis in the upper right hand corner may be critical, signifying that moderate-to-large reductions in dose to even small volumes are dangerous.

Heterogeneity of Subvolumes Receiving an Underdose

The DVHs b-e, b-f, and b-g in Figure 2.25 illustrate a 10% underdosage to 5%, 10%, and 20% of the tumor. From Figure 2.24, it can be seen that this 10% underdosage would decrease the calculated TCP by 3.5%, 7%, and 14%, respectively, much less of a loss than associated with the smaller indentations along the x-axis.

Clearly, the extent of underdosage is a more important determinant of TCP than the volume of tumor underdosed. Thus, the indentation along the x-axis of the upper right corner of the tumor DVH in Figure 2.25 is more ominous than the indentation in the y-axis when considering TCP.

Geographic Overdosage (Hot Spots)

Small areas of elevated dose, or hot spots (e.g., in 30% or less of the tumor) produce a negligible change in overall TCP, especially if the TCP from the homogeneous dose is already high (Fig. 2.26). Obviously, the larger the volume of tumor included in the overdosed region, the greater the potential for an increase in TCP, especially if the TCP from the homogeneously lower dose was already low (lower curves, Fig. 2.26). In general, raising the dose to the tumor by "dose-painting" subvolumes, offers little advantage whereas elevating the dose to the whole tumor could be of great value. For example, an escalation of dose to 30% of the tumor by $1 \times D_{10}$ could raise the TCP from 10% to nearly 18%, whereas the same increment to the whole tumor could raise the TCP from 10% to 80%.

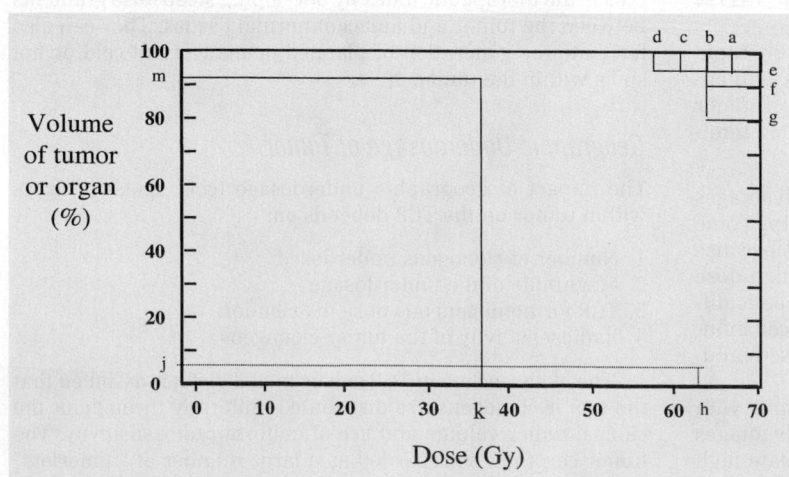

FIGURE 2.25. Multiple theoretical dose volume histograms. By reference to Fig. 2.24, the impact on tumor control probability (TCP) of indentations in the upper right corner of the dose-volume histogram (DVH) can be estimated (see text). The underdosage (a-e, b-e, c-e, d-e) is the most important determinant of TCP. The histogram h-j depicts a dangerous DVH for an organ with serially-arranged functional subunits such as spinal cord, but benign for lung, liver, kidney, and so forth. Histogram k-m depicts danger for liver, lung, kidney, but not for spinal cord.

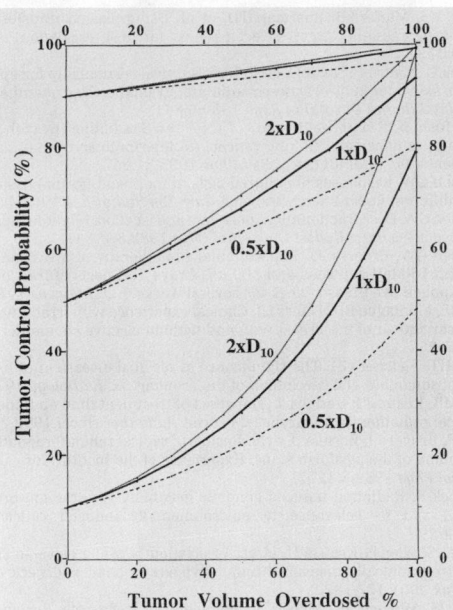

FIGURE 2.26. Modeling of the effect on tumor control probability (TCP) of increasing dose to increasing proportions of the tumor. Small hot spots are not very useful, especially if TCP is already high. The closer to 100% of the tumor being "overdosed" the steeper the TCP curve (317).

A significant advantage would only derive from introducing small "hot spots" in subvolumes within an otherwise homogeneous tumor dose distribution if the hot spots accurately targeted areas of substantially and consistently greater radioresistance (e.g., a nidus of chronically hypoxic cells). A tumor with such a radioresistant nidus would not be cured by a relatively low homogeneous dose. At present, there are no proven ways of localizing tumor foci that are consistently radioresistant. Thus, with current levels of understanding and technical expertise, the largest and most certain benefits are likely to be achieved if the dose to the whole tumor is escalated. This is illustrated by the increasing slope of the curves in Figure 2.26 as the volume receiving the higher dose approaches 100%.

Effective Uniform Dose

The effects of inhomogeneous dose distribution on TCP can be quantified by the equivalent uniform dose (EUD) (203). An EUD produces a constant probability of tumor control for different volumes of tumor under- or overdosed. In Figures 2.24 and 2.26, a horizontal line for any chosen TCP would join EUDs for various volumes exposed to doses differing by various multiples of D_{10}, the relevant EUD value being the homogeneous dose that produced that TCP.

Dose-Volume Histograms for Normal Tissues

The effect of the volume of a normal organ exposed to irradiation is discussed elsewhere. Heterogeneity of dose in the exposed volume will produce different levels of injury, but the net pathophysiologic outcome is dictated by the structure and function of the organ.

An organ such as spinal cord with its functional subunits arranged in series can be injured by a high dose to even a small volume (Fig. 2.25, h-j), but not by a low dose to a large volume (Fig. 2.25, k-m). However, a large dose to a small volume (Fig. 2.25, h-i) is of little consequence in an organ with a large "reserve" volume of functional subunits. Conversely, a relatively low dose to a large volume (e.g., Fig. 2.25, k-m), which may

be of little consequence to spinal cord, could be devastating if applied to lung, liver, or kidney. Thus, DVH configurations must be viewed against an understanding of the structure and physiology of the specific tissue, as discussed earlier.

Alterations in Quality of Radiation

Linear Energy Transfer

The rate at which a charged particle, such as an electron or proton, deposits its energy along its track is described as its linear energy transfer (LET); the heavier the particle, the higher its LET. Thus, electrons have a predominantly low LET, protons a slightly higher LET, neutrons an even higher LET, and heavy charged particles the highest LET of clinically used radiations.

The rate of energy transfer increases as particles slow, which means that LET is only an average value that is little more than a useful guide to the radiation therapist. As the LET of a beam increases, so does its biologic efficiency, although the increase is most rapid and peaks around 100 to 150 kv/μm. This is thought to represent where ionization events are spaced so that they are most likely to hit both strands of DNA. It then decreases per unit of measured physical dose with further increase in LET (an "overkill" phenomenon). As LET increases, OER decreases inversely with biological effectiveness (19), and the impact of variations in cell cycle–related radiosensitivity become less (33). At high LET, single-hit, nonrepairable cell killing increases relative to that from accumulation of sublethal injury, so that the survival curve for neutrons or heavy charged particles is essentially linear over at least the first decade of cell killing, and there is little sparing from dose fractionation, reducing the differential in fractionation response between late-responding and acute-responding tissues (334).

Relative Biologic Efficiency

Relative biologic efficiency is a ratio of doses from two beams to produce the same effect:

$$RBE = dose\,(standard\,beam)\,/dose\,(test\,beam).$$

RBE is usually used to compare high and low LET radiations but it has wider applicability for comparing the effectiveness of treatment approaches such as high- and low-dose-rate x-irradiation. Initially, the standard photon beam was 250 kVp x-rays, but now, at least from the viewpoint of radiation therapy, it is ^{60}Co (250 kVp x-rays are about 15% more efficient than ^{60}Co in killing mammalian cells). It is not widely appreciated that even at relatively high dose rates, photon beam effectiveness varies with dose rate and also that this is an important determinant of RBE. Furthermore, it can only be measured accurately if the same effect is achieved by both radiations. The conditions of RBE measurements must, therefore, be explicitly and precisely stated.

Neutrons

Neutrons deposit energy in a tissue through collisions with nuclei (mainly of hydrogen) rather than with electrons, as occurs with photon beams. Although neutrons are uncharged, they eject protons from the nucleus, and, therefore, the cellular injury they produce is through free radicals formed from ion pairs—the same basic mechanism as that for x-rays. The difference is that the column of ionization produced by the proton ejected from the nucleus by the neutron is much denser than that produced by an electron ejected by a photon. Because of the density of resulting free radicals, neutrons are more likely than x-rays to cause irreparable single-lethal-hit injury to DNA.

The high density of ionization from neutron irradiation also results in a reduced OER. If the OER is 2.6 for x-rays and 1.6 for neutrons, the ratio, which has been called the *hypoxic gain factor*, would be 2.6/1.6 = 1.6. In other words, if a course of neutrons is given that produces normal tissue sequelae equivalent to those from 66 Gy of x-rays given in 2-Gy fractions, the biologic effect of the neutrons on a completely hypoxic tumor would be equivalent to that from (1.6 × 66 Gy) = 106 Gy of x-rays. Of course, not all tumor cells are hypoxic, and so the therapeutic gain factor is lower than 1.6, and will depend on the percentage of hypoxic cells and, in a multifraction regimen, the extent of reoxygenation (315).

The response of cells to neutrons is less influenced by position in the cell cycle than is the case with x-rays (323). Therefore, the RBE is greater for cells in x-ray–resistant than x-ray–sensitive phases of the cell cycle. This may affect the therapeutic gain or loss from using neutrons (314). For example, if a tumor were to consist entirely of cells in an x-ray–resistant phase of the cell cycle, for which the RBE were 5, and if the critical normal tissue were to have an RBE of 3, then the therapeutic gain factor would be 5/3 = 1.66.

Because single-hit nonrepairable events are greater with neutrons, cell survival rate is more nearly exponential over a wider dose range, and steeper, than for x-rays. In terms of the LQ survival curve formula, neutrons have a very high α/β value (e.g., 30 to 100 Gy). Therefore, dose fractionation is of less significance in neutron than in x-ray radiation therapy.

Neutrons may have a therapeutic advantage for poorly reoxygenating, poorly redistributing, intrinsically x-ray–resistant, rapidly growing, and rapidly repopulating tumors. Predictive assays would be needed to identify such tumors prospectively, which would also permit more selective modification of x-ray regimens (315).

Acknowledgments

Jan Haas helped in the preparation of this manuscript.

References

1. Agren CA, Kallman P, Turesson I, et al. Volume and heterogeneity dependence of the dose-response relationship for head and neck tumours. *Acta Oncol* 1995;34:851.
2. Allen EP. A trial of radiation dose prescription based on dose-cell survival formula. *Australas Radiol* 1984;28:156.
3. Almasan A, Linke SP, Paulson TG, et al. Genetic instability as a consequence of inappropriate entry into and progression through S-phase. *Cancer Metastasis Rev* 1995;14:59.
4. Alper T. *Cellular radiobiology*. London: University Press, 1979.
5. Alper T, Howard-Flanders P. The role of oxygen in modifying the radiosensitivity of *E. coli* B. *Nature* 1956;178:978.
6. Andrews JR. Dose-time relationships in cancer radiotherapy: A clinical radiobiology study of extremes of dose and time. *Am J Roentgenol Rad Ther Nucl Med* 1965;93:56.
7. Ang KK, Jiang GL, Feng Y, et al. Extent and kinetics of recovery of occult spinal cord injury. *Int J Radiat Oncol Biol Phys* 2001;50:1013.
8. Ang KK, Jiang GL, Guttenberger R, et al. Impact of spinal cord repair kinetics on the practice of altered fractionation schedules. *Radiother Oncol* 1992;25:287.
9. Ang KK, Landuyt W, Rijnders A, et al. Differences in repopulation kinetics in mouse skin during split-course multiple fractions per day or daily fractionated irradiation. *Int J Radiat Oncol Biol Phys* 1985;10:95.
10. Ang KK, Price RE, Stephens LC, et al. The tolerance of primate spinal cord to re-irradiation. *Int J Radiat Oncol Biol Phys* 1993;25:459.
11. Ang KK, van der Kogel AJ, van der Schueren E. Lack of evidence for increased tolerance of rat spinal cord with decreasing fraction doses below 2 Gy. *Int J Radiat Oncol Biol Phys* 1985;11:105.
12. Ang KK, Xu FX, Vanuytsel L, et al. Repopulation kinetics in irradiated mouse lip mucosa: The relative importance of treatment protraction and time distribution of irradiation. *Radiat Res* 1985;101:162.
13. Anno GH, Baum SJ, Withers HR, et al. Symptomatology of acute radiation effects in humans after exposure to doses of 0.5–30 Gy. *Health Phys* 1989;56:821.
14. Anscher MS, Kong FM, Andrews K, et al. Plasma transforming growth factor beta1 as a predictor of radiation pneumonitis. *Int J Radiat Oncol Biol Phys* 1998;41:1029.
15. Anscher MS, Kong FM, Jirtle RL. The relevance of transforming growth factor beta1 in pulmonary injury after radiation therapy. *Lung Cancer* 1998;19:109.
16. Anscher MS, Marks LB, Shafman TD, et al. Using plasma transforming factor beta1 during radiotherapy to select patients for dose escalation. *J Clin Oncol* 2001;19:3758.
17. Arcangeli G, Mauro F, Nervi C, et al. Dose survival relationship for epithelial cells of human skin after multi-fraction irradiation: Evaluation by a quantitative method in vivo. *Int J Radiat Oncol Biol Phys* 1980;6:841.
18. Ball DL, Bishop JF. A phase III study of accelerated radiotherapy with and without carboplatin in nonsmall cell lung cancer: An interim toxicity analysis of the first 100 patients. *Int J Radiat Oncol Biol Phys* 1995;31:267.
19. Barendsen GW. Responses of cultured cells, tumors and normal tissues to radiations in different linear energy transfer. *Curr Top Radiat Res* 1968;4:295.
20. Barendsen GW. Dose fractionation, dose rate and isoeffect relationships for normal tissue responses. *Int J Radiat Oncol Biol Phys* 1982;8:1981.
21. Barendsen GW, Broerse JJ. Experimental radiotherapy of a rat rhabdomyosarcoma with 15 MeV neutrons and 300 kV X rays. II. Effects of fractionated treatments, applied five times a week for several weeks. *Eur J Cancer* 1970;6:89.
22. Barker JL, Montague ED, Peters LJ. Clinical experience with irradiation of inflammatory carcinoma of the breast with and without elective chemotherapy. *Cancer* 1980;45:625.
23. Barkley HT, Fletcher GH. The significance of residual disease after external irradiation of squamous cell carcinoma of the oropharynx. *Radiology* 1977;124:493.
24. Barton MB, Keane TJ, Gadalla T. The effect of treatment time on tumor control in the radical radiotherapy of laryngeal cancer. *Radiother Oncol* 1992;23:137.
25. Bataini P, Brugere J, Bernier J, et al. Results of radical radiotherapy treatment of carcinoma of the pyriform sinus: Experience of the Institut Curie. *Int J Radiat Oncol Biol Phys* 1982;8:1277.
26. Baverstock K. Radiation-induced genomic instability: a paradigm-breaking phenomenon and its relevance to environmentally induced cancer. *Mut Res* 2000;454:89.
27. Becker A, Stadler P, Krause U, et al. Association between elevated serum VEGF and polarographically measured tumor hypoxia in head and neck carcinomas. *Strahl Onk* 2001;177:182.
28. Bedford JS, Mitchell JB. Mitotic accumulation of HeLa cells during continuous irradiation. *Radiat Res* 1977;70:173.
29. Begg AC. Prediction of repopulation rates and radiosensitivity in human tumours. *Int J Radiat Biol* 1994;65:103.
30. Begg AC, Haustermans K, Hart AA, et al. The value of pretreatment cell kinetic parameters as predictors for radiotherapy outcome in head and neck cancer: a multicenter analysis. *Radiother Oncol* 1999;50:13.
31. Begg AC, McNally NJ, Shrieve DC, et al. A method to measure the duration of DNA synthesis and the potential doubling time from a single sample. *Cytometry* 1985;6:620.
32. Bentzen SM, Christensen JJ, Overgaard J, et al. Some methodological problems in estimating radiobiological data from clinical data. *Acta Oncol* 1988;27:105.
33. Blakely EA, Chang PY, Lommel: Cell-cycle-dependent recovery from heavy-ion damage in G1-phase cells. *Radiat Res* 1985;104[Suppl]:S145.
34. Boag JW. The time scale in radiobiology. In: Nygaard OF, Adler HI, Sinclair WK, eds. *Radiation research, proceedings of 5th International Congress of Radiation Research*. New York: Academic Press, 1975;9–29.
35. Bourne RG, Kearsley J, Groves WD. The relationship of early and late gastrointestinal complications of radiation for carcinoma of the cervix. *Int J Radiat Oncol Biol Phys* 1983;9:1445.
36. Brenner DJ. Toward optimal external-beam fractionation for prostate cancer. *Int J Radiat Oncol Biol Phys* 2000;48:315.
37. Brizel DM, Sibley GS, Prosnitz LR, et al. Tumor hypoxia adversely affects the prognosis of carcinoma of the head and neck. *Int J Radiat Oncol Biol Phys* 1997;38:285.
38. Brock WA. Kinetics of micronucleus expression in synchronized irradiated Chinese hamster ovary cells. *Cell Tissue Kinet* 1985;18:247.
39. Brown WA. Predictive assays. In: Withers HR, Peters LJ, eds. *Innovations in radiation oncology*. Heidelberg: Springer-Verlag, 1988;11–24.
40. Brown BW, Thompson JR, Barkley HT, et al. Theoretical considerations of dose rate factors influencing radiation strategy. *Radiology* 1974;110:197.
41. Brown JM. Sensitizers in radiotherapy. In: Withers HR, Peters LJ, eds. *Innovations in radiation oncology*. Heidelberg: Springer-Verlag, 1988;247–264.
42. Brown JM. SR4233 (Tirapazamine): A new anticancer drug exploiting hypoxia in solid tumors. *Br J Cancer* 1993;67:1163.
43. Bush RS, Jenkin RDT, Alh WEC, et al. Definitive evidence for hypoxic cells influencing cure in cancer therapy. *Br J Cancer* 1978;37[Suppl 3]:302.
44. Caldwell WL. Time dose factors in fatal post-irradiation nephritis. In: Alper T, ed. *Cell survival after low doses of radiation*. Bristol, England: John Wiley & Sons, 1975;328–332.
45. Calvo W, Hopewell JW, Reinhold MS, et al. Time- and dose-related changes in the white matter of the rat brain after single of doses of x-rays. *Br J Radiol* 1988;61:1043.
46. Cater DB, Silver IA. Quantitative measurement of oxygen tension in normal tissues and in the tumours of patients before and after radiotherapy. *Acta Radiol* 1960;53:233.
47. Charbit A, Malaise EP, Tubiana M. Relation between the pathological nature and the growth rate of human tumors. *Eur J Cancer* 1971;7:307.
48. Chen KY, Withers HR. Survival characteristics of stem cells of gastric mucosa exposed to localized gamma irradiation in C3H mice. *Int J Radiat Oncol Biol Phys* 1972;21:521.
49. Chiang CS, Hong JH, Stalder A, et al. Delayed molecular responses to brain irradiation. *Int J Radiat Biol* 1997;72:45.
50. Chiang CS, McBride WH, Withers HR. Myelin-associated changes in mouse brain following irradiation. *Radiother Oncol* 1993;27:229.
51. Chiang CS, McBride WH, Withers HR. Radiation-induced astrocytic and microglial responses in mouse brain. *Radiother Oncol* 1993;29:60.
52. Chiarugi V, Magnelli L, Cinelli M, et al. Dominant oncogenes, tumor suppressors, and radiosensitivity. *Cell Mol Biol Res* 41995;1:161.
53. Choi KN, Withers HR, Rotman M. Metastatic melanoma in brain: Rapid treatment or large dose fractions. *Cancer* 1985;56:10.
54. Clarke AR, Gledhill S, Hooper ML, et al. p53 dependence of early apoptotic and proliferative responses within the mouse intestinal epithelium following gamma-irradiation. *Oncogene* 1994;9:1767.
55. Cohen L. Theoretical "iso-survival" formulae for fractionated radiation therapy. *Br J Radiol* 1968;41:522.

56. Cohen L, Creditor M. Isoeffect tables for tolerance of irradiated normal human tissues. *Int J Radiat Oncol Biol Phys* 1983;9:233.
57. Cori CF, Cori GT. Carbohydrate metabolism of tumors: Changes in sugar, lactic acid, and CO_2-combining power of blood passing through tumor. *J Biol Chem* 1925;65:397.
58. Cosset JM, Baume D, Pico L, et al. Single dose versus hyperfractionationed total body irradiation before allogeneic bone marrow transplantation: A non-randomized comparative study of 54 patients at the Institut Gustave-Roussy. *Radiother Oncol* 1989;15:151.
59. Cosset JM, Henry-Amar M, Girinski T, et al. Late toxicity of radiotherapy in Hodgkin's disease. *Acta Oncol* 1988;27:123.
60. Cullen B, Lansley I. The effect of preirradiation growth conditions on the relative radiosensitivities of mammalian cells at low oxygen concentrations. *Int J Radiat Biol* 1974;26:579.
61. Daigle JL, Hong JH, Chiang CS, et al. The role of tumor necrosis factor signaling pathways in the response of murine brain to irradiation. *Cancer Res* 2001;61:8859.
62. Deacon J, Peckham MJ, Steel GG. The radioresponsiveness of human tumors and the initial slope of the cell survival curve. *Radiother Oncol* 1984;2:317.
63. Delanian S, Balla-Mekias S, Lefaix JL. Striking regression of chronic radiotherapy damage in a clinical trial of combined pentoxifylline and tocopherol. *J Clin Oncol* 1999;17:3283.
64. Denekamp J. Changes in the rate of repopulation during multi-fraction irradiation of mouse skin. *Br J Radiol* 1973;46:381.
65. Denny WA, Wilson WR. Tirapazamine: A bioreductive anticancer drug that exploits tumour hypoxia. *Expert Opin Investig Drugs* 2000;9:2889.
66. Deschner EE, Gray LH. Influence of oxygen tension on x-ray–induced chromosomal damage in Ehrlich ascites tumor cells irradiated in vitro and in vivo. *Radiat Res* 1959;11:115.
67. Dewey WC, Ling CC, Meyn RE. Radiation-induced apoptosis: Relevance to radiotherapy. *Int J Radiat Oncol Biol Phys* 1995;33:781.
68. Dewey WC, Robinette SM. Progression of viable and nonviable synchronized Chinese hamster cells into the S phase after X-irradiation in mitosis or the S phase. *Int J Radiat Biol* 1969;16:495.
69. Dion MW, Hussey DH, Doornbos JF, et al. Preliminary results of a pilot study of pentoxifylline in the treatment of late radiation soft tissue necrosis. *Int J Radiat Oncol Biol Phys* 1990;19:401.
70. Dische S. Review of chemical radiosensitizers: Update to 1988. In: McNally NJ, ed. *The Scientific Basis of Modern Radiotherapy, BIR Report 19,* London: BIR, 1989;91–96.
71. Dische S, Anderson PJ, Sealy R, et al. Carcinoma of the cervix: Anaemia, radiotherapy and hyperbaric oxygen. *Br J Radiol* 1983;56:251.
72. Dische S, Saunders MI. Continuous hyperfractionated accelerated radiotherapy. *Br J Cancer* 1989;59:325. Radiother Oncol 15:19,1989
73. Dorr W, Noack R, Spekl K, et al. Modification of oral mucositis by keratinocyte growth factor: single radiation exposure. *Int J Radiat Biol* 2001;77:341.
74. Douglas BG, Fowler JF. The effect of multiple small doses of x-rays on skin reactions in the mouse and a basic interpretation. *Radiat Res* 1976;66:401.
75. Down JD, Easton DF, Steel GG. Repair in the mouse lung during low dose rate irradiation. *Radiother Oncol* 1986;6:29.
76. Duchesne GM, Peters LJ. What is the alpha/beta ratio for prostate cancer? Rationale for hypofractionated high-dose-rate brachytherapy. *Int. J Radiat Oncol Biol Phys* 1999;44:747.
77. Dutreix J, Wambersie A, Bounik C. Cellular recovery in human skin reactions: Application to dose, fraction number, overall time relationship in radiotherapy. *Eur J Cancer* 1973;9:159.
78. Easson EC, Pointon RCS. *The radiotherapy of malignant disease*. Berlin, Springer-Verlag, 1985
79. Edsmyr F, Anderson L, Esposti PL, et al. Irradiation therapy with multiple small fractions per day in urinary bladder cancer. *Radiother Oncol* 1985;4:197.
80. Elkind MM, Han A, Volz KW. Radiation response of mammalian cells grown in culture. IV. Dose dependence of division delay and postirradiation growth of surviving and nonsurviving Chinese hamster cells. *J Natl Cancer Inst* 1963;30:705.
81. Elkind MM, Sutton H. X-ray damage and recovery in mammalian cells in culture. *Nature* 1959;184:1293.
82. Elkind MM, Swain RW, Alescio T, et al. Oxygen, nitrogen, recovery and radiation therapy. In: Shalek R, ed. *Cellular radiation biology*. Baltimore, MD: Williams & Wilkins, 1965: 442–466.
83. Elkind MM, Whitmore GF. The radiobiology of cultured mammalian cells. New York, Gordon & Breach, 1967.
84. Ellis F. Nominal standard dose and the ret. *Br J Radiol* 1971;44:101.
85. Emami B, Lyman J, Brown A, et al. Tolerance of normal tissue to therapeutic irradiation. *Int J Radiat Oncol Biol Phys* 1991;21:109.
86. Evans JC, Per Bergsjo MD. The influence of anaemia on the results of radiotherapy in carcinoma of the cervix. *Radiology* 1965;84:709.
87. Farrell CL, Bready JV, Rex KL, et al. Keratinocyte growth factor protects mice from chemotherapy and radiation-induced gastrointestinal injury and mortality. *Cancer Res* 1998;58:933.
88. Farrell CL, Rex KL, Kaufman SA, et al. Effects of keratinocyte growth factor in the squamous epithelium of the upper aerodigestive tract of normal and irradiation mice. *Int J Radiat Biol* 1999;75:609.
89. Fertil B, Malaise EP. Intrinsic radiosensitivity of human cell lines is correlated with radioresponsiveness of human tumors. *Int J Radiat Oncol Biol Phys* 1985;11:1699.
90. Field SB, Hornsey S, Kutsutani Y. Effects of fractionated irradiation on mouse lung and a phenomenon of slow repair. *Br J Radiol* 1976;49:700.
91. Fisher DR, Hendry JH. Dose fractionation and hepatocyte clonogens. *Radiat Res* 1988;113:51.
92. Fletcher GH. Clinical dose-response curves of human malignant epithelial tumours. *Br J Radiol* 1973;46:1.
93. Fletcher GH. *Textbook of radiotherapy*, I, II and III eds. Philadelphia, Lea & Febiger, 1966,1973, 1980.
94. Fowler JF. J.F. Kirk Memorial Lecture: What next in fractionated radiotherapy. *Br J Cancer* 1984;49[Suppl 6]:285.
95. Fowler JF, Lindstrom MJ. Loss of local control with prolongation in radiotherapy. *Int J Radiat Oncol Biol Phys* 1992;23:457.
96. Fowler JF, Stern BE. Dose-time relationships in radiotherapy and the validity of cell survival curve models. *Br J Radiol* 1963;36:163.
97. Frisch SM, Francis H. Disruption of epithelial cell-matrix interactions induces apoptosis. *J Cell Biol* 1994;124:619.
98. Fuks Z, Persaud RS, Alfieri A, et al. Basic fibroblast growth factor protects endothelial cells against radiation-induced programmed cell death in vitro and in vivo. *Cancer Res* 1994;54:2582.
99. Fyles A, Keane TJ, Barton M, et al. The effect of treatment duration in the local control of cervix cancer. *Radiother Oncol* 1992;25:273.
100. Gallagher MS, Brereton HD, Rostock RA, et al. A prospective study of treatment techniques to minimize the volume of pelvic small bowel with reduction of acute and late effects associated with pelvic irradiation. *Int J Radiat Oncol Biol Phys* 1986;12:1565.
101. Garden AS, Morrison WH, Ang KK, et al. Hyperfractionated radiation in the treatment of squamous cell carcinomas of the head and neck: A comparison of two fractionation schedules. *Int J Radiat Oncol Biol Phys* 1995;31:493.
102. Gatenby RA, Coia LA. Oxygen distribution in squamous cell carcinoma metastases: Relationship to outcome of radiation therapy. *Am J Clin Oncol* 1987;10:101.
103. Ghossein NA, Bataini JP, Ennuyer A, et al. Local control and site of failure in radically irradiated supraglottic laryngeal cancer. *Radiology* 1974;112:187.
104. Gonzales-Gonzales B, Breur K, van der Schueren E. Preliminary results in advanced head and neck cancer in radiotherapy by multiple fractions per day. *Clin Radiol* 1980;31:417.
105. Gorodetsky R, McBride WH, Withers HR. Assay of radiation effects in mouse skin as expressed in wound healing. *Radiat Res* 1988;116:135.
106. Gorodetsky R, Mou X, Fisher DR, et al. Radiation effect in mouse skin: Dose fractionation and wound healing. *Int J Radiat Oncol Biol Phys* 1990;18:1077.
107. Graeber TG, Osmanian C, Jacks T, et al. Hypoxia-mediated selection of cells with diminished apoptotic potential in solid tumors. *Nature* 1996;379:88.
108. Gray LH, Conger AD, Ebert M, et al. The concentration of oxygen dissolved in tissues at the time of irradiation as a factor in radiotherapy. *Br J Radiol* 1953;26:638.
109. Gross NJ, Narine KR. Experimental radiation pneumonitis: Corticosteroids increase the replicative activity of alveolar type 2 cells. *Radiat Res* 1988;115:543.
110. Habermalz HJ, Valley B, Habermalz E. Radiation myelopathy of the mouse spinal cord in isoeffect correlations after fractionated radiation. *Strahlenther Onkol* 1987;163:626.
111. Hahn GM, Little JB. Plateau-phase cultures of mammalian cells: An in vitro model for human cancer. *Curr Top Radiat Res Q* 1972;8:39.
112. Hall EJ. Radiation dose-rate: A factor of importance in radiobiology and radiotherapy. *Br J Radiol* 1972;45:81.
113. Hall EJ, Bedford JS, Oliver R. Extreme hypoxia, its effect on the survival of mammalian cells irradiated at high and low dose rates. *Br J Radiol* 1966;39:302.
114. Hallahan DE, Haimovitz FA, Kufe DW, et al. The role of cytokines in radiation oncology. *Important Adv Oncol* 1993;71.
115. Hallahan DE, Spriggs DR, Beckett M, et al. Increased tumor necrosis factor α mRNA after cellular exposure to ionizing radiation. *Proc Natl Acad Sci U S A* 1989;86:10104.
116. Harwood AR, Beale FA, Cummings JB, et al. Supraglottic laryngeal carcinoma: An analysis of dose-time-volume factors in 410 patients. *Int J Radiat Oncol Biol Phys* 1983;9:311.
117. Hendry JH, Broadbent DA, Roberts SA, et al. Effects of deficiency in p53 or bcl-2 on the sensitivity of clonogenic cells in the small intestine to low dose-rate irradiation. *Int J Radiat Oncol Biol* 2000;76:559.
118. Hendry JH, Cai WB, Roberts SA, et al. p53 deficiency sensitizes clonogenic cells to irradiation in the large but not the small intestine. *Radiat Res* 1997;148:254.
119. Henk JM, Kunkler PB, Smith CW. Radiotherapy and hyperbaric oxygen in head and neck cancer. *Lancet* 1977;2:101.
120. Hermens AF, Barendsen GW. Changes of cell proliferation characteristics in a rat rhabdomyosarcoma before and after x-irradiation. *Eur J Cancer* 1969;5:173.
121. Herskind C, Rodemann HP. Spontaneous and radiation-induced differentiation of fibroblasts. *Exp Gerontol* 2000;35:747.
122. Herzog KH, Chong MJ, Kapsetaki M, et al. Requirement for Atm in ionizing radiation-induced cell death in the developing central nervous system. *Science* 1998;280:1089.
123. Hewitt HB. Fundamental aspects of the radiotherapy of cancer. In: *The Scientific Basis of Medicine: Annual Review*. London: Athlone Pr Humanities, 1962:305.
124. Hockel M, Schlenger K, Hockel S, et al. Hypoxic cervical cancers with low apoptotic index are highly aggressive. *Cancer Res* 1999;59:4525.
125. Hong J, Chiang C, Campbell IL, et al. Induction of acute phase gene expression by brain irradiation. *Int J Radiat Oncol Biol Phys* 1996;33:619.
126. Hopewell JW, Morris AD, Dixon-Brown A. The influence of field size on the late tolerance of the rat spinal cord to single doses of x-rays. *Br J Radiol* 1987;60:1099.
127. Hopewell JW, Wiernik G. Tolerance of pig kidney to fractionated x-irradiation. In: *Radiobiological research and radiotherapy*, vol 1. Vienna: IAEA, 1977:65–73.
128. Horiot JC, Begg AC, LeFur FR, et al. Present status of EORTC trials of hyperfractionated and accelerated radiotherapy on head and neck carcinoma. *Rec Res Cancer Res* 1994;134:111.
129. Horiot JC, LeFur FR, Nguyen T, et al. Hyperfractionation versus conventional fractionation in oropharyngeal carcinoma: Final analysis of a randomized trail of the EORTC cooperative group of radiotherapy. *Radiother Oncol* 1992;25:231.
130. Hornsey S, Myers R, Warren P. Residual injury in the spinal cord after treatment with x-rays or neutrons. *Br J Radiol* 1982;55:516.
131. Howard A, Pelc SR. Synthesis of deoxyribonucleic acid in normal and irradiated cells and its relation to chromosome breakage. *Heredity* 1952;6[Suppl]:261.
132. Howes AE. An estimation of changes in the proportions and absolute numbers of hypoxic cells after irradiation of transplanted C_3H mammary tumours. *Br J Radiol* 1969;42:441.
133. Hoyer M, Jorgensen K, Bundgaard T, et al. Lack of predictive value of potential doubling time and iododeoxyuridine labelling index in radiotherapy of squamous cell carcioma of the head and neck. *Radiother Oncol* 1998;46:147.
134. Hryniuk WM. The importance of dose intensity in outcome of chemotherapy. In: DeVita VT, Hellman S, Rosenberg SA, eds. *Important advances in oncology 1988*. Philadelphia: JB Lippincott, 1988:121–142.
135. Hryniuk WM. Will increases in dose intensity improve outcome. *Proc Am J Med* 1995;99[Suppl]:69.
136. Hussey DH, Fletcher GH. Clinical features of 16 and 50 $MeV_{d/Be}$ neutrons. *Eur J Cancer* 1974;10:357.
137. Jain RK. Barriers to drug delivery in solid tumors. *Sci Am* 1994;271:58.

138. Jirtle RL, McLain JR, Strom SC, et al. Repair of radiation damage in noncycling parenchymal hepatocytes. *Br J Radiol* 1982;55:847.

139. Joiner MC. The dependence of radiation response on the dose per fraction. In: McNally NJ, ed. *The scientific basis of modern radiotherapy, BIR Report 19,* London: BIR, 1989;20–26.

140. Joiner MC, Marples B, Lambin P, et al. Low-dose hypersensitivity: current status and possible mechanisms. *Int J Radiat Oncol Biol Phys* 2001;49:379.

141. Kallman RF. The phenomenon of reoxygenation and its implication for fractionated radiotherapy. *Radiology* 1972;105:135.

142. Keane TJ, Fyles A, O'Sullivan B, et al. The effect of treatment duration on local control of squamous carcinoma of the tonsil and carcinoma of the cervix. *Semin Radiat Oncol* 1992;2:26.

143. Kellerer AM, Rossi HH. A generalized formulation of dual radiation action. *Radiat Res* 1978;75:471.

144. Kemp CJ, Sun S, Gurley KE. p53 induction and apoptosis in response to radio- and chemotherapy in vivo is tumor-type-dependent. *Cancer Res* 2001;61:327.

145. Kerr JF, Searle J. A suggested explanation for the paradoxically slow growth rate of basal-cell carcinomas that contain numerous mitotic figures. *J Pathol* 1972;107:41.

146. Kerr JF, Winterford CM, Harmon BV. Apoptosis: Its significance in cancer and cancer therapy. *Cancer* 1994;73:2013 [erratum *Cancer* 1994;73:3108.].

147. Kerr JFR, Wyllie AH, Currie AR. Apoptosis: A basic biological phenomenon with wide-ranging implications in tissue kinetics. *Br J Cancer* 1972;26:239.

148. Kim JJ, Tannock IF. Repopulation of cancer cells during therapy: An important cause of treatment failure. *Nat Rev Cancer* 2005;5:516.

149. Knee R, Field RS, Peters LJ. Concomitant boost radiotherapy for advanced squamous cell carcinoma of the head and neck. *Radiother Oncol* 1985;4:1.

150. Koh WJ, Bergman KS, Rasey JS, et al. Evaluation of oxygenation status during fractionated radiotherapy in human nonsmall cell lung cancers using [F-18] fluoromisonidazole positron emission tomography. *Int J Radiat Oncol Biol Phys* 1995;33:391.

151. Koh WJ, Stelzer KJ, Peterson LM, et al. Effect of pentoxifylline on radiation-induced lung and skin toxicity in rats. *Int J Radiat Oncol Biol Phys* 1995;31:71.

152. Kohn HI, Kallman RF. The effect of fractionated x-ray dosage upon the mouse testis. I. Maximum weight loss following 80 to 240 R given in 2 to 5 fractions during 1 to 4 days. *J Natl Cancer Inst* 1995;15:891.

153. Kolstad P. The development of the vascular bed in tumours as seen in squamous cell carcinoma of the cervix uteri. *Br J Radiol* 1965;38:216.

154. Kummermehr J, Trott KR. Rate of repopulation in a slow and a fast growing mouse tumor. In: Karcher KH, Kogelnik HD, Reinartz G, eds. *Progress in radio-oncology II.* New York: Raven, 1982:299.

155. Lane DP, Lu X, Hupp T, et al. The role of the p53 protein in the apoptotic response. *Philos Trans R Soc Lond [Biol]* 1994;345:277.

156. Laramore GE, Griffin TW, Parker RG, et al. The use of electron beams in treating local recurrence of breast cancer in previously irradiated fields. *Cancer* 1978;41:991.

157. Lauk S, Ruth S, Trott KR. The effects of dose-fractionation on radiation-induced heart disease in rats. *Radiother Oncol* 1987;8:363.

158. Lea DE. *Actions of radiation on living cells,* 2nd ed. Cambridge, England: Cambridge University Press, 1955.

159. Leith JT, DeWyngaert JK, Glicksman AS. Radiation myelopathy in the rat: An interpretation of dose effect relationships. *Int J Radiat Oncol Biol Phys* 1981;7:1673.

160. Letschert JG, Lebesque JV, Aleman BM, et al. The volume effect in radiation-related late small bowel complications: Results of a clinical study of the EROTC Radiotherapy Cooperative Group in patients treated for rectal carcinoma. *Radiother Oncol* 1994;32:116.

161. Levin W, Blair RM. Pattigrew technique of inducing whole-body hyperthermia. *NIC Monogr* 1982;61:377.

162. Levine AJ, Perry ME, Chang A, et al. The 1993 Walter Hubert Lecture: The role of the p53 tumour-suppressor gene in tumorigenesis. *Br J Cancer* 1994;69:409.

163. Littbrand B, Revesz L. The effect of oxygen on cellular survival and recovery after radiation. *Br J Radiol* 1969;42:914.

164. Little JB. Repair of potentially lethal radiation damage in mammalian cells: Enhancement by conditioned medium from stationary cultures. *Int J Radiat Biol* 1971;20:87.

165. Lo Y-C, McBride WH, Lavey RS, et al. Remembered radiation dose in mouse spinal cord. Presented at 40th Annual Meeting of Radiation Research Society; March 1992; Salt Lake City, Utah. Abstract P102-2.

166. Lo Y-C, Taylor JMG, McBride WH, et al. The effect of fractionated doses of radiation on mouse spinal cord. *Int J Radiat Oncol Biol Phys* 1993;27:309.

167. Lyng H, Sundfor K, Rofstad EK. Changes in tumor oxygen tension during radiotherapy of uterine cervical cancer: relationships to changes in vascular density, cell density, and frequency of mitosis and apoptosis. [Comment In: *Int J Radiat Oncol Biol Phys* 2001;49:282–289UI:21119560.] *Int J Radiat Oncol Biol Phys* 2000;46:935.

168. Maciejewski B, Majewski S. Dose fractionation and tumour repopulation in radiotherapy for bladder cancer. *Radiother Oncol* 1991;21:163.

169. Maciejewski B, Preuss-Bayer G, Trott KR. The influence of the number of fractions and overall treatment time on the local tumor control of cancer of the larynx. *Int J Radiat Oncol Biol Phys* 1983;9:321.

170. Maciejewski B, Taylor JMG, Withers HR. Alpha/beta value and the importance of size of dose per fraction for late complications in the supraglottic larynx. *Radiother Oncol* 1986;7:323.

171. Maciejewski B, Withers HR, Taylor JMG. Dose fractionation and regeneration in radiotherapy for cancer of the oral cavity and oropharynx. I. Tumor dose-response and repopulation. *Int J Radiat Oncol Biol Phys* 1989;16:831.

172. Maciejewski B, Withers HR, Taylor JMG. Dose fractionation and regeneration in radiotherapy for cancer of the oral cavity and oropharynx. II. Acute and late effects in normal tissues. *Int J Radiat Oncol Biol Phys* 1990;18:101.

173. Mason KA, Withers HR. RBE of neutrons generated by 50 MeV deuterons on beryllium for control of artificial pulmonary metastases of a mouse fibrosarcoma. *Br J Radiol* 1977;50:652.

174. Mason KA, Withers HR, Chiang CS. Late effects of radiation on the lumbar spinal cord of guinea pigs: Re-treatment tolerance. *Int J Radiat Oncol Biol Phys* 1993;26:643.

175. Mason KA, Withers HR, Davis CA. Dose dependent latency of fatal gastrointestinal and bone marrow syndrome. *Int J Radiat Biol* 1989;55:1.

176. Mayr NA, Yuh WT, Oberley LW, et al. Serial changes in tumor oxygenation during the early phase of radiation therapy in cervical cancer—are we quantitating hypoxia change? *Int J Radiat Oncol Biol Phys* 2001;49:282.

177. McBride WH, Withers HR. In vitro studies of ante-mortem proliferation kinetics. *Br J Cancer* 1986;53[Suppl 7]:386.

178. McBride WH, Withers HR. Radiobiology of subclinical disease. *Front Radiat Ther Oncol* 1994;28:46.

179. McCulloch EA, Till JE. Proliferation of hematopoietic colony-forming cells transplanted into irradiated mice. *Radiat Res* 1964;22:383.

180. Meistrich ML, Hunter NR, Suzuki N, et al. Gradual regeneration of mouse testicular stem cells after ionizing radiation. *Radiat Res* 1978;74:349.

181. Mendelsohn ML. The growth fraction: a new concept applied to tumors. *Science* 1960;132:1496.

182. Meoz-Mendez RT, Fletcher GH, Guillamondegui OM, et al. Analysis of the results of irradiation in the treatment of squamous cell carcinomas of the pharyngeal walls. *Int J Radiat Oncol Biol Phys* 1978;4:579.

183. Merritt AJ, Potten CS, Kemp CJ, et al. The role of p53 in spontaneous and radiation-induced apoptosis in the gastrointestinal tract of normal and p53-deficient mice. *Cancer Res* 1994;54:614.

184. Merritt AJ, Potten CS, Watson AJ, et al. Differential expression of bcl-2 in intestinal epithelia: Correlation with attenuation of apoptosis in colonic crypts and the incidence of colonic neoplasia. *J Cell Sci* 1995;108:2261.

185. Meyn RE, Stephens LC, Ang KK, et al. Heterogeneity in the development of apoptosis in irradiated murine tumours of different histologies. *Int J Radiat Biol* 1993;64:583.

186. Meyn RE, Stephens LC, Hunter NR, et al. Reemergence of apoptotic cells between fractionated doses in irradiated murine tumors. *Int J Radiat Oncol Biol Phys* 1994;30:619.

187. Michalowski AS. Effects of radiation on normal tissues: Hypothetical mechanisms and limitations of in situ assays of clonogenicity. *Radiat Environ Biophys* 1981;19:157.

188. Michalowski AS. Post-irradiation modification of normal-tissue injury: Lessons from the clinic. *Br J Radiol* 1992;24[Suppl]:183.

189. Michalowski AS. The pathogenesis and conservative management of radiation injuries. *Neoplasma* 1995;42:289.

190. Midgley CA, Owens B, Briscoe CV, et al. Coupling between gamma irradiation, p53 induction and the apoptotic response depends upon cell type in vivo. *J Cell Sci* 1995;108:1843.

191. Milas L, Stephens LC, Meyn RE. Relation of apoptosis to cancer therapy. *In Vivo* 1994;8:665.

192. Molteni A, Moulder JE, Cohen EF, et al. Control of radiation-induced pneumopathy and lung fibrosis by angiotensin-converting enzyme inhibitors and an angiotensin II type 1 receptor blocker. *Int J Radiat Biol* 2000;76:523.

193. Mothersill C, Seymour C. Radiation-induced bystander effects: past history and future directions. *Radiat Res* 2001;155:759.

194. Moulder JE, Cohen EP, Fish BL, et al. Prophylaxis of bone marrow transplant nephropathy with captopril, an inhibitor of angiotensin-converting enzyme. *Radiat Res* 1993;136:404.

195. Moulder JE, Dutreix J, Rockwell S, et al. Applicability of animal tumor data to cancer therapy in humans. *Int J Radiat Oncol Biol Phys* 1988;14:913.

196. Moulder JE, Fish BL, Cohen EP. Treatment of radiation nephropathy with ACE inhibitors. *Int J Radiat Oncol Biol Phys* 1993;27:93.

197. Moulder JE, Rockwell S. Hypoxic fractions of solid tumors: Experimental techniques, methods of analysis and a survey of existing data. *Int J Radiat Oncol Biol Phys* 1984;10:695.

198. Murray, D, McBride WH. Radioprotective agents. In: Kroschwitz JI, Howe-Grant M, eds. *Encyclopedia of chemical technology,* 4th ed. New York: John Wiley & Sons, 1996:963–1006.

199. Neta R. Modulation of radiation damage by cytokines. *Stem Cells* 1997;15[Suppl 2 2–3]:87.

200. Neta R, Okunieff P. Cytokine-induced radiation protection and sensitization. *Semin Radiat Oncol* 1996;6:306.

201. Neta R, Oppenheim JJ, Schreiber RD, et al. Role of cytokines (interleukin 1, tumor necrosis factor, and transforming growth factor beta) in natural and lipopolysaccharide-enhanced radioresistance. *J Exp Med* 1991;173:1177.

202. Nguyen TD, Panis X, Froissart D, et al. Analysis of late complications after rapid hyperfractionated radiotherapy in advanced head and neck cancers. *Int J Radiat Oncol Biol Phys* 1988;14:23.

203. Niemierko A. Reporting and analyzing dose distributions: A concept of equivalent uniform dose. *Med Phys* 1997;24:103–110.

204. Norin T, Onyango J. Radiotherapy in Burkitt's lymphoma: Conventional or superfractionated regime: Early results. *Int J Radiat Oncol Biol Phys* 1987;2:339.

205. Nyman J, Turesson I. Does the interval between fractions matter in the range of 4–8 h in radiotherapy? A study of acute and late human skin reactions. *Radiother Oncol* 1995;34:171.

206. Okamoto M, Kasetani H, Kaji R, et al. cis-Diamminedichloroplatinum and 5-fluorouracil are potent inducers of the cytokines and natural killer cell activity in vivo and in vitro. *Cancer Immunol Immunother* 1998;47:233.

207. Olive PL, Trotter T, Banath JP, et al. Heterogeneity in human tumour hypoxic fraction using the comet assay. *Br J Cancer* 1996;27:S191.

208. Overgaard J. Clinical evaluation of nitromidazoles as modifiers of hypoxia in solid tumors. *Oncol Res* 1994;6:509.

209. Overgaard, J, Hansen HS, Overgaard M, et al. A randomized double-blind phase III study of nimorazole as a hypoxic radiosensitizer of primary radiotherapy in supraglottic larynx and pharynx carcinoma. Results of the Danish Head and Neck Cancer Study (DAHANCA) Protocol 5-85. *Radiother Oncol* 1998;46:135.

210. Overgaard J, Hjelm-Hansen M, Vendelbo Johansen L, et al. Comparison of conventional and split-course radiotherapy as primary treatment in carcinoma of the larynx. *Acta Oncol* 1988;27:147.

211. Overgaard M. The clinical implication of non-standard fractionation. *Int J Radiat Oncol Biol Phys* 1985;11:1225.

212. Overgaard M. Spontaneous radiation-induced rib fractures in breast cancer patients treated with postmastectomy irradiation: A clinical radiobiological analysis of fraction size and dose response relationship in late bone damage. *Acta Oncol* 1988;27:117.

213. Palcic B, Skarsgard LD. Reduced oxygen enhancement ratio at low doses of ionizing radiation. *Radiat Res* 1984;100:328.

214. Parkins CS, Fowler JF. Repair in mouse lung of multi-fraction X-rays and neutrons. *Br J Radiol* 1985;58:1087.
215. Parsons JT. Time-dose-volume relationships in radiation therapy. In: Million RR, Cassisi NJ, eds. *Management of head and neck cancer*. Philadelphia: JB Lippincott, 1984:137–172.
216. Parsons JT, Bova FJ, Million RR. A reevaluation of split-course technique for squamous cell carcinoma of the head and neck. *Int J Radiat Oncol Biol Phys* 1980;6:1645.
217. Parsons JT, Thar TL, Bova FJ, et al. An evaluation of split-course irradiation for pelvic malignancies. *Int J Radiat Oncol Biol Phys* 1980;6:175.
218. Paterson RP. The treatment of malignant disease by radium and x rays. London: Edward Arnold, 1948.
219. Pedrick TJ, Hoppe RT. Recovery of spermatogenesis following pelvic irradiation for Hodgkin's disease. *Int J Radiat Oncol Biol Phys* 1986;12:117.
220. Peltenburg LT. Radiosensitivity of tumor cells. Oncogenes and apoptosis. *Q J Nuc Med* 2000;44:355.
221. Peracchia G, Salti C. Radiotherapy with thrice-a-day fractionation in a short overall time. *Int J Radiat Oncol Biol Phys* 1981;7:99.
222. Peters LJ. Accelerated fractionation using the concomitant boost: A contribution of radiobiology to radiotherapy. *Br J Radiol* 1992;24[Suppl]:200.
223. Peters LJ, Ang KK, Thames HD. Fractionation in the treatment of head and neck cancer: A critical comparison of different strategies. *Acta Radiol Oncol* 1988;27:185.
224. Peters LJ, Ang KK, Thames HD. Altered fractionation schedules. In: Perez CA, Brady LW, eds. *Principles and practice of radiation oncology*, 2nd ed. Philadelphia: JB Lippincott, 1992:97–113.
225. Peters LJ, Brock WA, Chapman JD, et al. Predictive assays of tumor radiocurability. *Am J Clin Oncol* 1988;11:275.
226. Peters LJ, Thames HD. Dose-response relationship for supraglottic laryngeal carcinoma. *Int J Radiat Oncol Biol Phys* 1983;9:421.
227. Peters LJ, Tofilon PJ, Groepfert H, et al. Radiosensitivity of primary tumor cultures as a determinant of human head and neck cancers. In: McNally NJ, ed. *The scientific basis of modern radiotherapy, BIR Report 19*. London: BIR, 1989:132–135.
228. Peters LJ, Withers HR, Cundiff JH, et al. Radiobiological considerations in the use of total body irradiation for bone marrow transplantation. *Radiology* 1979;131:243.
229. Phillips RA, Tolmach LJ. Repair of potentially lethal damage in x-irradiated HeLa cells. *Radiat Res* 1966;29:413.
230. Pino Y, Torres JL, Lee DJ, et al. Local control and reduced complications in split course irradiation of prostatic cancer. *Int J Radiat Oncol Biol Phys* 1981;7:43.
231. Potish RA. Importance of predisposing factors in the development of enteric damage. *Am J Clin Oncol* 1982;5:189.
232. Potten CS, Merritt A, Hickman J, et al. Characterization of radiation-induced apoptosis in the small intestine and its biological implications. *Int J Radiat Biol* 1994;65:71.
233. Powers WE, Tolmach LJ. A multicomponent x-ray survival curve for mouse lymphosarcoma cells irradiated in vivo. *Nature* 1963;197:710.
234. Puck TT, Marcus PI. Action of x-rays on mammalian cells. *J Exp Med* 1956;103:653.
235. Read J. The effect of ionizing radiation on the broad bean root. *Br J Radiol* 1952;25:89;154.
236. Read J. *Radiation biology of vicia faba in relation to the general problem*. Oxford, England, Blackwell Scientific, 1959
237. Reisner A. Der hauterythemverlauf bei fraktionierter verabfolgung grosser strahlenmengen. *Fortschr Rongtenstrahlen* 1982;45:293.
238. Renner SM, Massel D, Moon BC. Mediastinal irradiation: A risk factor for atherosclerosis of the internal thoracic arteries. *Can J Cardiol* 1999;15:597.
239. Resouly A, Svoboda VHJ. Management of advanced head and neck squamous carcinoma by multiple daily sessions of radiotherapy. In: Karcher KH, ed. *Progress in radio-oncology II*. New York: Raven, 1982. L339–348.
240. Rossi HH. A note on the effects of fractionation of high LET radiations. *Radiat Res* 1976;66:170.
241. Rubin P, Casarett GW. *Clinical radiation pathology*, vols 1 and 2. Philadelphia, WB Saunders, 1968.
242. Rudat V, Stadler P, Becker A, et al. Predictive value of the tumor oxygenation by means of pO2 histography in patients with advanced head and neck cancer. *Strahl Onk* 2001;177:462.
243. Ruifrok ACC, Kleiboer BJ, van der Kogel AJ. Reirradiation tolerance on the immature rat spinal cord. *Radiother Oncol* 1992;23:249.
244. Saunders MI, Dische S, Grosch EJ, et al. Experience with CHART. *Int J Radiat Oncol Biol Phys* 1991;21:871.
245. Scalliet P, Landuyt W, van der Schueren E. Repair kinetics as a determining factor for the late tolerance of central nervous system to low dose rate irradiation. *Radiother Oncol* 14:345,1989
246. Schultheiss TE, Stephens LC, Ang KK. Volume effects in rhesus monkey spinal cord. *Int J Radiat Oncol Biol Phys* 1994;29:67.
247. Shukovsky LJ. Dose, time, volume relationships in squamous cell carcinoma of the supraglottic larynx. *Am J Roentgenol* 1970;108:27.
248. Shukovsky LJ, Fletcher GH. Time-dose and tumor volume relationships in the irradiation of squamous cell carcinoma of the tonsillar fossa. *Radiology* 1973;107:621.
249. Sinclair WK. Dependence of radiosensitivities upon cell age. In: *Time and Dose Relationships in Radiation Biology as Applied to Radiotherapy*. Brookhaven National Lab Report 50203 (C-57), 1969:97.
250. Steel GG. *Growth kinetics of tumours*. New York: Oxford University Press, 1977.
251. Stephens LC, Ang KK, Schultheiss TE, et al: Target cell and mode of radiation injury in rhesus salivary glands. *Radiother Oncol* 1986;7:165.
252. Stewart FA. Late normal tissue damage after combined chemotherapy and radiotherapy. In: McNally NJ, ed: *The scientific basis of modern radiotherapy, BIR Report 19*. London: BIR, 1989:95.
253. Stewart FA, Oussoren Y, van Tinteren H, et al. Loss of reirradiation tolerance in the kidney with increasing time after single or fractionated partial tolerance doses. *Int J Radiat Oncol Biol* 1994;66:169.
254. Stewart JG, Jackson AW. The steepness of the dose response curve for both tumor cure and normal tissue injury. *Laryngoscope* 1975;85:1107.
255. Strandqvist M. Studien uber die kumulative wirking der rontgenstrahlen bei fraktionierung. *Acta Radiol Suppl (Stockh)* 1944;55:1.
256. Strasser A, O'Connor L, Dixit VM. Apoptosis signaling. *Ann Rev Biochemistry* 2000;69:217.
257. Stratford IJ, Sheldon PW, Adams GE. Hypoxic cell radiosensitizers. In: Steel GG, Adams GE, Peckham MJ, eds. *The biological basis of radiotherapy*. Amsterdam: Elsevier, 1983:211–223.
258. Stuschke M, Budach V, Budach W, et al. Repair capacity of human soft tissue sarcomas. In: Karcher KH, ed. *Progress in radio-oncology IV*. New York: Raven, 1988:53–57.
259. Suit HD, Howes AF, Hunter N. Dependence of response of a C3H mammary carcinoma to fractionated irradiation on fractionation number and intertreatment interval. *Radiat Res* 1977;72:440.
260. Suit HD, Lindberg RD, Fletcher GH. Prognostic significance of extent of tumor regression at completion of radiation therapy. *Radiology* 1965;84:1100.
261. Suit HD, Zietman A, Miralbell R, et al. Human tumor xenografts for study of the radiation response of human tumors. In: *Prediction of Radiation Response in Radiation Therapy, AAPM Symposium Proceedings 7*. New York: American Institute of Physics, 1989:251–262.
262. Terasima T, Tolmach LJ. Variations in several responses of HeLa cells to x-irradiation during the division cycle. *Biophys J* 1963;3:11.
263. Thames HD, Ang KK, Stewart FA, et al. Does incomplete repair explain the apparent failure of the basic LQ model to predict spinal cord and kidney responses to low doses per fraction? *Int J Radiat Biol* 1988;54:13.
264. Thames HD, Bentzen SM, et al. Fractionation parameters for human tissues and tumors. *Int J Radiat Biol* 1989;56:701.
265. Thames HD, Hendry JH. *Fractionation in radiotherapy*. London: Taylor & Francis, 1987.
266. Thames HD, Hendry JH, Moore JV, et al. The high steepness of dose-response curves for late-responding tissues. *Radiother Oncol* 1989;15:49.
267. Thames HD, Mason KA, Bentzen SM. Split dose recovery in mouse jejunal crypt cells. In: McNally NJ, ed. *The Scientific basis of modern radiotherapy, BIR Report 19*. London: BIR, 1989:37–42.
268. Thames HD, Peters LJ, Spanos W, et al. Dose response of squamous cell carcinomas of the upper respiratory and digestive tracts. *Br J Cancer* 1980;41[Suppl IV]:35.
269. Thames HD, Peters LJ, Withers HR, et al. Accelerated fractionation vs. hyperfractionation: Rationale for several treatments per day. *Int J Radiat Oncol Biol Phys* 1983;9:127.
270. Thames HD, Withers HR, Peters LJ, et al. Changes in early and late radiation responses with altered dose fractionation: Implications for dose-survival relationships. *Int J Radiat Oncol Biol Phys* 1982;8:219.
271. Thomlinson RH. Reoxygenation as a function of tumor size and histopathological type. In: *Time and dose relationships in radiation biology as applied to radiotherapy*. Upton, NY: Brookhaven National Lab Report 50203 (C-57), 1970:242–254.
272. Thomlinson RH, Gray LH. The histological structure of some human lung cancers and possible implications for radiotherapy. *Br J Cancer* 1955;9:539.
273. Thompson LH, Suit HD. Proliferation kinetics of x-irradiated mouse L cells studied with time-lapse photography. II. *Int J Radiat Biol* 1969;15:347.
274. Tolmach LJ. Growth patterns in irradiated HeLa cells. *Ann NY Acad Sci* 1961;95:743.
275. Travis EL, Parkins CS, Down JD, et al. Repair in mouse lung between multiple small doses of x-rays. *Radiat Res* 1983;94:326.
276. Travis EL, Peters LJ, McNeill J. Effect of dose-rate on total body irradiation: Lethality and pathologic findings. *Radiother Oncol* 1985;4:341.
277. Travis EL, Tucker SL. Isoeffect models and fractionated radiation therapy. *Int J Radiat Oncol Biol Phys* 1987;13:283.
278. Turesson I. The progression rate of late radiation effects in normal tissue and its impact on dose-response relationships. *Radiother Oncol* 1989;15:217.
279. Turesson I, Notter G. The influence of the overall treatment time in radiotherapy on the acute reaction: Comparison of the effects of daily and twice-a-week fractionation on human skin. *Int J Radiat Oncol Biol Phys* 1984;10:599.
280. Turesson I, Notter G. Accelerated versus conventional fractionation. *Acta Oncol* 1988;27:169.
281. Urtusan RC, Chapman JD, Raleigh JA, et al. A novel technique for measuring human tissue hypoxia at the cellular level. *Br J Cancer* 1986;54:453.
282. Utsumi H, Elkind MM. Two forms of potentially lethal damage have similar repair kinetics in plateau- and in log-phase cells. *Int J Radiat Biol Relat Stud Phys Chem Med* 1985;47:569.
283. van den Brenk HAS. The oxygen effect in radiation therapy. *Curr Top Radiat Res* 1969;5:197.
284. van der Kogel AJ. Radiation tolerance of the rat spinal cord: Time-dose relationships. *Radiology* 1977;122:505.
285. van der Kogel AJ. Mechanisms of late radiation injury in the spinal cord. In: Meyn R, Withers HR, eds. *Radiation biology in cancer research*. New York: Raven, 1980:461–470.
286. van der Kogel AJ. Effect of volume and localization on rat spinal cord. In: Fielden EM, Fowler JF, Hendry JH, Scott D, eds. *Proceedings of the 8th International Congress of Radiation Research*. London: Taylor & Francis, 1987:352.
287. van der Kogel AJ. Central nervous system radiation injury in small animal models. In: Gutin PJ, Leibel SA, Sheline GE, eds. *Radiation injury to the nervous system*. New York: Raven, 1991:91.
288. van der Schueren E, van den Bogaert W, Ang KK. Radiotherapy with multiple fractions per day. In: Steel GG, Adams GE, Peckham MJ, eds. *The biological basis of radiotherapy*. Amsterdam: Elsevier, 1983:195.
289. van Dyk J, Mah K, Keane TJ. Radiation-induced lung damage: Dose-time fractionation considerations. *Radiother Oncol* 1989;14:55.
290. van Peperzeel HA. Effects of single doses of radiation on lung metastases in man and experimental animals. *Eur J Cancer* 1972;8:665.
291. van Rongen E, Kuijpers WC, Madhuizen HT, et al. Effects of multi-fraction irradiation on the rat kidney. *Int J Radiat Oncol Biol Phys* 1988;15:1161.
292. Vaupel P, Schlenger K, Hoeckel M. Blood flow and tissue oxygenation of human tumors: An update. *Adv Exp Med Biol* 1992;317:139.
293. Vegesna V, Withers HR, Holly FE, et al. The effect of local and systemic irradiation on impairment of wound healing in mice. *Radiat Res* 1993;135:431.
294. Vegesna V, Withers HR, Taylor JMG. The effect on depigmentation after multi-fraction irradiation of mouse resting hair follicle. *Radiat Res* 1987;111:464.
295. Vegesna V, Withers HR, Taylor JMG. Repair kinetics of mouse lung. *Radiother Oncol* 1989;15:115.
296. Vogel AW. Intratumoral vascular changes with increased size of a mammary adenocarcinoma: A new method and results. *J Natl Cancer Inst* 1965;34:571.

297. Wang CC. Accelerated fractionation. In: Withers HR, Peters LJ, eds. *Innovations in radiation oncology*. Heidelberg, Germany: Springer-Verlag, 1988:239–243.
298. Wang CC. Accelerated hyperfractionation radiation therapy for carcinoma of the nasopharynx. *Cancer* 1989;63:2461.
299. Wang CC, Blitzer PH, Suit HD. Twice-a-day radiation therapy for cancer of the head and neck. *Cancer* 1985;55:2100.
300. Ward JF. DNA damage produced by ionizing radiation in mammalian cells: Identities, mechanisms of formation and repairability. *Prog Nucl Acids Res Mol Biol* 1988;35:96.
301. Wendt CD, Peters LJ, Ang KK, et al. Hyperfractionated radiotherapy in the treatment of squamous cell carcinomas of the supraglottic larynx. *Int J Radiat Oncol Biol Phys* 1989;17:1057.
302. West CM. Intrinsic radiosensitivity as a predictor of patient response to radiotherapy. *Br J Radiol* 1995;68:837.
303. Wheldon TE, Michalowski AS, Kirk J. The effect of irradiation on function in self-renewing normal tissues with differing proliferative organisation. *Br J Radiol* 1982;55:759.
304. White A, Hornsey S. Time-dependent repair of radiation damage in the rat spinal cord after X rays and neutrons. *Eur J Cancer* 1980;16:957.
305. Williams MV, Denekamp J. Radiation induced renal damage in mice: Influence of fraction size. *Int J Radiat Oncol Biol Phys* 1984;10:885.
306. Williams MV, Denekamp J, Fowler JF. A review of $\alpha\beta$ ratios for experimental tumors. *Int J Radiat Oncol Biol Phys* 1985;11:87.
307. Wilson GD, Dische S, Saunders MI. Studies with bromodeoxyuridine in head and neck cancer and accelerated radiotherapy. *Radiother Oncol* 1995;36:189.
308. Withers HR. The dose-survival relationship for irradiation of epithelial cells of mouse skin. *Br J Radiol* 1967;40:187.
309. Withers HR. Recovery and repopulation in vivo by mouse skin epithelial cells during fractionated irradiation. *Radiat Res* 1967;32:227.
310. Withers HR. Regeneration of intestinal mucosa after irradiation. *Cancer* 1971;28:75.
311. Withers HR. The 4 R's of radiotherapy. In: Lett JT, Alder H, eds. *Advances in radiation biology, vol 5*. New York: Academic, 1975:241.
312. Withers HR. Cell cycle redistribution as a factor in multi-fraction irradiation. *Radiology* 1975;114:199.
313. Withers HR. Biologic basis for altered fractionation schemes. *Cancer* 1985;55:2086.
314. Withers HR. Neutron radiobiology and clinical consequences. *Strahlentherapie* 1985;161:739.
315. Withers HR. Neutrons and other clinical trials: Impossible dreams? *Int J Radiat Oncol Biol Phys* 1987;13:1967.
316. Withers HR. Inherent acceleration of tumor dose-rate in hyperfractionated regimens. *Int J Radiat Oncol Biol Phys* 1988;14:400.
317. Withers HR. Biological aspects of conformal therapy. *Acta Oncol* 2000;39:569.
318. Withers HR, Chen KY. Poor man's neutrons? *Br J Radiol* 1971;44:818.
319. Withers HR, Cuasay L, Mason KA, et al. Elective radiation therapy in the curative treatment of cancer of the rectum and rectosigmoid. In: Strohlein JR, Romsdahl JR, eds. *Gastrointestinal cancer*. New York: Raven, 1981:351–361.
320. Withers HR, Hunter N, Barkley HT, et al. Radiation survival and regeneration of characteristics of spermatogenic stem cells of mouse testis. *Radiat Res* 1974;57:88.

321. Withers HR, Maciejewski B, Taylor JMG. Biology of options in dose fractionation. In: McNally NJ, ed. *The scientific basis of modern radiotherapy, BIR Report 19*. London: BIR, 1989:27–36.
322. Withers HR, Mason KA. The kinetics of recovery in irradiated colonic mucosa of the mouse. *Cancer* 1974;34:896.
323. Withers HR, Mason KA, Reid BO, et al. Response of mouse intestine to neutrons and gamma-rays in relation to dose fractionation and division cycle. *Cancer* 1974;34:39.
324. Withers HR, Mason KA, Thames HD. Late radiation response of kidney assayed by tubule cell survival. *Br J Radiol* 1986;59:587.
325. Withers HR, Peters LJ. Biological aspects of radiation therapy. In: Fletcher GH, ed. *Textbook of radiotherapy*, 3rd ed. Philadelphia: Lea & Febiger, 1980:103–180.
326. Withers HR, Peters LJ, Kogelnik HD. The pathobiology of late effects of irradiation. In: Meyn RE, Withers HR, eds. *Radiation biology in cancer research*. New York: Raven, 1980:439–448.
327. Withers HR, Peters LJ, Taylor JMG. Dose-response relationship for radiation therapy of subclinical disease. *Int J Radiat Oncol Biol Phys* 1995;31:353.
328. Withers HR, Peters LJ, Taylor JMG, et al. Local control of carcinoma of the tonsil by radiation therapy: An analysis of patterns of fractionation in nine institutions. *Int J Radiat Oncol Biol Phys* 1995;33:549.
329. Withers HR, Peters LJ, Taylor JMG, et al. Late normal tissue sequelae from radiation therapy for carcinoma of the tonsil: Patterns of fractionation study of radiobiology. *Int J Radiat Oncol Biol Phys* 1995;33:563.
330. Withers HR, Suit HD. Is oxygen important in the radiocurability of human tumors? In: Friedman M, ed. *The biological and clinical basis of radiosensitivity*. Springfield, IL: Charles C Thomas, 1974:548.
331. Withers HR, Taylor JMG, Maciejewski B. The hazard of accelerated tumor clonogen repopulation during radiotherapy. *Acta Oncol* 1988;27:131.
332. Withers HR, Taylor JMG, Maciejewski B. Treatment volume and tissue tolerance. *Int J Radiat Oncol Biol Phys* 1988;14:751.
333. Withers HR, Thames HD. Dose fractionation and volume effects in normal tissues and tumors. *Am J Clin Oncol* 1988;11:313.
334. Withers HR, Thames HD, Peters LJ. Biological bases for high RBE values for late effects of neutron irradiation. *Int J Radiat Oncol Biol Phys* 1982;8:2071.
335. Withers HR, Thames HD, Peters LJ. Differences in the fractionation response of acute and late-responding tissues. In: Karcher KH, Kogelnik HD, Reinartz G, eds. *Progress in radio-oncology II*. New York: Raven, 1982:287–296.
336. Withers HR, Thames HD, Peters LJ. A new isoeffect curve for change in dose per fraction. *Radiother Oncol* 1983;1:187.
337. Withers HR, Thames HD, Peters LJ, et al. Normal tissue radioresistance in clinical radiotherapy. In: Fletcher GH, Nervi C, Withers HR, eds. *Biological bases and clinical implications of tumor radioresistance*. New York:Masson, 1983:139.
338. Xu F, van der Schueren E, Ang KK. Acute reactions of the lip mucosa of mice to fractionated irradiations. *Radiother Oncol* 1984;1:369.
339. Yi ES, Williams ST, Lee H, et al. Keratinocyte growth factor ameliorates radiation-and bleomycin-induced lung injury and mortality. *Am J Pathol* 1996;149:1963.
340. Zeman EM, Bedford JS. Changes in early and late effects with dose-per-fraction: Alpha, beta, redistribution and repair. *Int J Radiat Oncol Biol Phys* 1984;10:1039.

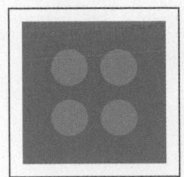

Chapter 3
Molecular Cancer and Radiation Biology

Michael Baumann, Nils Cordes, Michael Haase, Daniel Zips

During the last 3 decades molecular cancer research has become a rapidly growing branch of the biomedical sciences. Many advances in our understanding of cancer are closely related to innovations in biotechnology, for example, techniques to knock out or to knock in a specific gene of interest, experimental maneuvers to manipulate temporal and spatial gene expression, the development of high-throughput methods to study the entire genome and proteome of cancer cells, and a vastly growing methodology to specifically interfere with signal transduction. This chapter provides an introductory overview of molecular cancer and radiation biology (32,116,120,180,304,305).

Cell biology approaches contribute to modern radiobiology and help to better understand effects of ionizing radiation on cells, tumors, and normal tissues. Knowledge in molecular cancer biology is important for clinical decision-making in oncology and the development of novel biology-driven strategies in the multidisciplinary clinical environment (18,59–61,146,207). *Molecular pathology* of tumors increasingly supplements classic histopathology and immunohistochemistry, thereby providing the basis for improved treatment stratification in oncology (69,123). *Molecular pathophysiology* describes mechanisms leading to a characteristic microenvironment of tumors or the mechanisms that eventually lead to the manifestation of radiation sequelae in normal tissues (15,146,295). *Molecular imaging* has not only become important for staging but also for biologic characterization of tumors, and for determination of target volumes in radiation oncology, including new approaches such as dose painting (28,44,58,145,166,247,293,335). *Molecular targeting* in radiotherapy may either increase the tumor response or protect normal tissues, thereby enhancing the therapeutic gain of the treatment (21,38,53,54,93,136, 239,324).

Compared to other fields of oncology, radiotherapy appears to be particularly promising to integrate molecular targeting approaches (21). Firstly, the radiobiologic mechanisms of the response of tumors and normal tissues to radiotherapy are well characterized, and the molecular pathways involved in these responses are increasingly known. Secondly, similar to conventional chemotherapeutic drugs, the novel drugs developed so far are not curative in themselves. In contrast, radiotherapy in itself is extremely efficient in eradicating clonogenic tumor cells, and recurrences often occur from only one or a few surviving cells (181,286). Thus, even if novel drugs have only the potential to kill a limited number of tumor cells, this might be sufficient to increase local control when combined with radiotherapy. The same argument applies when these drugs increase the radiosensitivity of tumor cells or when normal tissues are specifically protected. Thirdly, in contrast to systemic chemotherapy, radiotherapy can be modulated in dose, time, and space. This allows individual tailoring of the effects of combined treatments in consideration of the spatial distribution of clonogenic tumor cell burden as well as with consideration of normal tissues. Preclinical data and early clinical results corroborate these arguments (20,21,39,199) and support further translational research on biologically enhanced radiotherapy.

PRINCIPLES OF MOLECULAR CANCER BIOLOGY

The majority of human cancers arise from single somatic cells as a result of a stepwise evolutionary process of accumulation of multiple genetic and epigenetic aberrations (237,256). Genetic changes include point mutation, deletion, insertion, gene amplification, chromosomal instability, loss of heterozygosity, and translocation. Promoter hypermethylation and thereby silencing of tumor suppressor genes represents an important epigenetic mechanism of tumorigenesis (22). Infection with oncogenic viruses might contribute to the development of human cancer, for example, human papilloma viruses in cervical cancer, hepatitis B viruses in hepatocellular carcinoma, and human immunodeficiency viruses in Kaposi's sarcoma (138). The hostile micromilieu in solid tumors, particularly hypoxia, further promotes progressive genomic alterations and clonal selection (296). Consequently, cells gain advantage in proliferation and survival, which eventually results in malignant transformation, a prerequisite for the development of cancer and metastatic spread.

Conceptually, two classes of cancer genes can be distinguished. Firstly, *oncogenes* are activated in cancer cells by genetic alterations resulting in a gain of function. Mutations in proto-oncogenes acting in a dominant fashion (i.e., a genetic alteration in one of the alleles) are sufficient for gene activation. Typical oncogene functions are stimulation of cell proliferation (e.g., by activation of Ras) and increase in cell survival (e.g., by activation of PI3K/Akt signaling). Disorders in the second class of cancer genes, *tumor suppressor genes*, cause a loss of function. Mutations in one allele of a tumor suppressor gene are recessive because they can be functionally compensated by the second, nonmutated (wild type) allele. While some cancers can be attributed to single genetic alterations, most sporadic solid tumors exhibit a wide range of disorders in numerous cancer genes. Simplified mathematical modeling of the increasing incidence of common cancers as a function of age suggests that four to seven somatic gene alterations are required for carcinogenesis (171,256). A typical example for multistep tumorigenesis is the adenoma-carcinoma sequence in colorectal cancer (105).

Inherited cancer predisposition can be divided into the rare group of inherited cancer syndromes and familial cancers (strong predisposition) and into the more frequent group of predisposition without evident family clustering (weak predisposition) (237). The first group includes syndromes caused by germline mutations affecting DNA repair, genomic stability, and cell cycle control, for example *TP53* (Li Fraumeni syndrome), nucleotid excision repair genes (Xeroderma pigmentosum), *ATM* (ataxia telangietasia), DNA mismatch repair genes (hereditary nonpolyposis colorectal cancer, HNPCC), and *BRCA 1/2* (familial breast cancer) (302). An example of a familial cancer syndrome related to oncogene activation is neurofibromatosis type I, in which the mutated *NF1 gene* results in activation of the oncogene Ras (57). Germline mutational inactivation of in

Table 3.1	THE SIX HALLMARKS OF CANCER WITH INVOLVED ONCOGENIC AND TUMOR SUPPRESSIVE MOLECULES (SELECTION)
Hallmark	**Involved Oncogenic and Tumor Suppressive Molecules (Selection)**
Loss of growth control	
1. Self-sufficiency in growth signals	p53, TGF-β, RTKs, Ras, pRB, cyclin D, cdk4, p16/ARF, p27, Akt, PTEN, cytokine
2. Insensitivity to antigrowth signals	receptors, JAK/STAT, APC, β-catenin, myc
3. Resistance to apoptosis	Caspase 8, FLIP, Bcl-2, Apaf-1, HSPs, IAPs, Akt, PTEN
4. Induction and sustaining angiogenesis	VEGF, PDGF, FGF, TSP-1, angiostatin, endostatin
5. Tissue invasion and metastasis	MMPs, integrins, E-Cadherin
6. Limitless replicative potential	p53, pRB, telomerase

Adapted from Hanahan D, Weinberg RA. The hallmarks of cancer. *Cell* 2000;100:57–70.

the adhesion molecule E-cadherin is a finding in familial diffuse gastric carcinoma (140).

The essential molecular biology of cancer can be summarized by a simplified concept based on a small number of underlying principles. In their seminal article, Hanahan and Weinberg (135) described these principles shared by most human tumor types as the *"six hallmarks of cancer"* (Table 3.1). These six hallmarks are the consequence of specific genetic alterations in important oncogenes and tumor suppressor genes.

The Hallmarks of Cancer

Cancer is characterized by the loss of growth control, due to acquired capabilities of autonomy of growth signaling, deteriorations in the cell cycle regulation, and insensitivity to growth inhibitory signals (135). Normal cell division is tightly regulated by stimulatory and inhibitory growth signals. Growth signaling involves interaction of diffusible growth factors or cytokines with transmembrane receptors, as well as regulation of growth by components of the extracellular matrix and by cell-cell-interactions. Once a resting cell receives a sufficient growth stimulus, it enters the cell cycle by passing the restriction point and four distinct phases of cytokinesis and mitogenesis: Gap-1 (G1), DNA synthesis (S), Gap-2 (G2) and mitosis (M) (253,299). Passage through the restriction point and entry into S and M (G1/S and G2/M checkpoints) are governed by several proto-oncogenes and tumor suppressor genes. Each phase of the cell cycle is regulated by specific complexes of cyclins (cyclin A-E) and their respective partners, the cyclin-dependent kinases (cdk). Important complexes are cyclin D/cdk4 and cyclin D/cdk6 (restriction point, G1), cyclin E/cdk2 (G1/S), cyclin A/cdk2 (S, G2) and cyclinB/cdk1 (M). Cyclins are directly upregulated by growth factors and indirectly via c-myc and Ras. Several cyclin/cdk complexes phosphorylate the retinoblastoma protein (pRB) facilitating the G1/S transition as well as blocking differentiation. The activity of the cdks is regulated by phosphorylation and various inhibitory small molecules, for example, by members of the INK4 (p15, p16, p18 and p19) and Cip1/Kip1 (p21, p27 and p57) families. The proteins p15 and p21 are related to two important tumor suppressors, the antiproliferative factor TGF-β (transforming growth factor-β) and p53, respectively.

Self-Sufficiency in Growth Signals

Mitogenic signals from growth factors, cytokines, extracellular matrix, and cell-cell-adhesion molecules are transferred into the cell by different classes of transmembrane receptors (135). Malignant cells acquire the capability to escape from the tightly regulated dependency from extracellular growth signals. The molecular mechanisms include overexpression of growth factors as well as growth factor receptors (autocrine and paracrine stimulation), receptor mutations leading to constitutive receptor

activation without ligand binding, and molecular aberrations in the intracellular signal transduction pathways.

Receptor tyrosine kinases (RTKs) represent a group of oncogenic, transmembrane receptors consisting of an extracellular ligand-binding domain, a transmembrane part, and an intracellular catalytic domain with tyrosine kinase activity (37). On ligand binding and receptor homo/heterodimerization, the protein kinase is subsequently activated, resulting in phosphorylation of tyrosine residues of the receptor itself (autophosphorylation) or target proteins. Depending on the cellular context, this triggers an intracellular signal cascade that eventually leads to proliferation, survival, differentiation, and migration. Among the known human RTKs are the epidermal growth factor receptors (EGFRs), the platelet-derived growth factor receptors (PDGFs), the vascular endothelial growth factor receptors, the fibroblast growth factor receptors, the ephrin receptors, and tyrosine kinase receptor in endothelial cells. The *EGFR family* consists of four distinct members (EGFR/ErbB-1, HER2/ErbB-2, HER3/ErbB-3, and HER4/ErbB-4) (333). The receptor ligands such as epidermal growth factor, tumor growth factor-α, and neuroregulin-1, as well as their cognate receptors, are abundantly expressed in a large variety of human cancers including lung, breast, head and neck, and gliomas and have been related to poor prognosis leading to the recognition of the EGFRs as important targets for cancer therapy. Mechanisms underlying the increased activation of the EGFR pathway in cancer cells include gene amplification and activating mutations, for example, EGFRvIII, a constitutively ligand-independent EGFR mutant (333).

RTK-Initiated Signal Transduction

The extracellular signals received by the RTKs are translated into a large variety of different cellular responses by a cascade of molecular processes, that is, signal transduction (37). This RTK signaling involves several distinct molecular pathways that are often deregulated in cancer cells, that is, the Ras/RAF/MAPK (mitogen-activated protein kinase) pathway, the PI3K (phosphoinositide 3' kinases)/Akt pathway, the jak/stat molecules, and the protein kinase C. Co-operative cross-talk between the different transduction pathways forms a complex signaling network.

An important signal transduction route that has been extensively studied in EGFR signaling represents the Ras/Raf/MAPK pathway. The *Ras proteins* (H-Ras, K-Ras4A, K-Ras4B, and N-Ras) are GTPases and are attached in their active state (GTP-bound) to the inner surface of the cell membrane. The Ras proto-oncogene, predominantly K-Ras, is mutated in about one third of human cancers. Activating mutations are frequent in adenocarcinomas of the pancreas (up to 90%), colorectum (about 50%), and the lung (about 30%) (68,104,165). The processing and membrane attachment of the functional Ras is governed by farnesyltransferases, which are the molecular target for specific pharmaceutical inhibitors of activated Ras (49,208). EGFR activation channels via the Grb2/SOS complex to the Ras molecule.

Activated Ras binds to *Raf,* facilitating its function as a serine/threonine kinase. Constitutively activated Raf proteins as a result of genetic alterations in the Raf genes have been shown in a large variety of human malignancies (23). Raf associates with MEK1/2 kinases, which in turn activate *MAPKs.* Activated MAPKs are subsequently translocated to the nucleus and initiate transcription by the activation of several transcription factors, for example, Elk-1. Consequently, gene expression is changed and proliferative processes are triggered.

In addition to Raf, activated Ras has an effect on various downstream molecules including *PI3K* (37,117). Following either direct activation by RTKs or indirect Raf-mediated activation, this group of kinases phosphorylates the 3'-OH group of the inositol ring in inositolphopholipids. Signaling mediator molecules of PI3K include phospohoinositide-dependent–kinase 1, Akt, protein kinase C, and subsequently the nuclear transcription factor NFκB. The cellular responses on activation of the PI3K pathway are cell-type specific and include changes in gene expression, cell cycle progression, survival, and apoptosis. The latter has been linked to PKB/Akt negatively controlling apoptosis-regulating molecules, such as Bad, caspase 9, Fas ligand, CREB, and IκB kinase. The tumor suppressor protein *PTEN* negatively regulates the PI3K/Akt pathway. Akt overexpression or hyperactivity, and PTEN mutations, are found in numerous human malignancies (254). Akt phosphorylates mTOR, the molecular target of rapamycin, a compound that exhibits anticancer activity (35).

Cytokine Receptors

A large number of growth-stimulating hormones, growth factors, and cytokines such as the interleukins, erythropoietin, and prolactin bind to the class of cytokine receptors that are structurally different from the previously described RTKs (236). The intracellular signaling in response to cytokine receptor activation includes the *JAK* and *STAT* kinases. In addition to the cytokine receptors, many RTKs can activate the JAK/STAT pathway. In malignant cells the autonomy of growth signaling can be associated with mutations in cytokine receptors (e.g., in the erythropoietin receptor) and constitutively upregulated activity of the JAK/STAT pathway in haematopoetic malignancies. STAT activation may result from transformation of tyrosine kinases such as v-src, v-Abl, and Bcr/Abl by viral oncoproteins from HTLV or EBV (125,274).

Wnt Signaling

Wnt proteins are diffusible growth factors that bind to specific surface receptors (Frizzeled) and trigger distinct intracellular pathways leading to cell growth (24,33,163). Wnt signaling involves the tumor suppressor protein adenomatous polyposis coli (*APC*) and regulates by phosphorylation the steady-state levels of cytosolic β-catenin. An increased level of *β-catenin* facilitates its transit into the nucleus, activation of transcription factors, and subsequently transcription of β-catenin target genes including c-myc, c-jun, and cyclin D1. The aberrant activation of Wnt signaling caused by mutations in the β-catenin and APC genes are typical findings in colon cancer and melanoma but have been identified as well in a large variety of other human cancers.

Cytoplasmic, nonreceptor kinases are often activated in malignant disease. For example, the *Bcr/Abl* fusion protein kinase resulting from the translocation t(9;22) is a typical molecular finding in chronic myelogenous leukemia and represents the molecular target for small molecule inhibitors such as imatinib (169). This drug also inhibits *c-KIT,* a cytoplasmic tyrosine kinase that has been shown to be activated by mutation in gastrointestinal stroma tumors (81).

Transcription factors bind to the DNA and activate the expression of specific genes. Oncogenic transcription factors are overactive in most human cancers and contribute to the au-

tonomy of growth signaling. Based on their mechanism of activation, three groups can be separated (79). First are the *steroid receptors,* which are found in hormone-sensitive breast or prostate cancer. The second group of transcription factors resides in the nucleus, is governed by kinase signals, and consists of various different members including *myc, AP-1 (activator protein 1),* and *E2F.* Myc transcription factors are induced in cancer by different mechanisms including translocation and gene amplification. For example, c-myc is activated by chromosomal translocation t(8;14), which brings the c-myc gene under the control of the IgG enhancer and thereby leads to constitutive expression in 80% of Burkitt lymphomas. N-myc and L-myc amplification are found in neuroblastoma and small cell lung cancer, respectively. AP-1 consisting of JUN, FOS, ATF, and MAF, can exhibit oncogenic or antioncogenic effects depending on the cellular context (99). The third group of oncogenic transcription factors, the latent transcription factors, is activated by ligand-receptor interactions and includes the STATs (see previous discussion), the WNT-β-catenin pathway (see previous discussion), the nuclear factor κB (NFκB), and the molecules Notch (323) and Hedgehog (149). NFκB levels have been shown to be constitutively active in lymphomas, leukemias, and breast and colon cancer (164).

Loss of Cell Cycle Control

Retinoblastoma Tumor Suppressor Protein (pRB)

The retinoblastoma protein is an important regulator of cell cycling and cell differentiation (4,96,219). Loss of pRB function is often found in malignant cells and leads to an uncontrolled G1/S transition, genomic instability, and loss of differentiation. Hypophosphorylated pRB binds to several proteins including the E2F transcription factors and histone deacetylases. These proteins are released on phosphorylation of pRB, for example by cyclin D/cdk4, cyclin E/cdk2 and cyclin A/cdk2, and contribute to cell cycle transition and/or to inhibition of terminal differentiation. As a result, the cell is switched from a quiescent phenotype toward a proliferative state. Released E2F activates transcription of genes required for DNA synthesis such as dihydrofolate reductase, thymidylate reductase, and DNA polymerase. Loss of pRB function can result from mutation or inactivation by oncogenic viral proteins such as HPV E7. Somatic mutations in the RB gene have been detected in a variety of epithelial and mesenchymal malignancies (264). Loss of cell cycle control by impairment of the pRB pathway can also result from overexpression of cyclin D, activating mutations and amplification of cdk4, and loss of p16 (INK4) leading to a constitutive expression of E2F target genes (56). Loss of function in the pRB pathway contributes to genomic instability by E2F-mediated overexpression of MAD2, an important component of the mitotic checkpoint (143). The encoding RB gene was the first characterized tumor suppressor gene that is involved in retinoblastoma, a rare childhood tumor. Retinoblastoma is a typical example for the two-hit model of tumor induction (171). The first hit, that is, mutation in one RB allele, is either a germline (inherited form, often bilateral) or an acquired somatic mutation (sporadic form, mostly unilateral). An acquired somatic mutation in the other RB allele causes the inactivation of the pRB and consequently tumorigenesis.

TP53 tumor suppressor gene is inactivated in the majority of cancers and has been associated with poor prognosis in some cancers (45). Wild type p53 binds to specific DNA sequences and activates transcription of numerous genes including *MDM2, GADD45, p21^{CIP-1}, cyclin D,* and the proapoptotic BAX. On the other hand, p53 also can negatively regulate gene transcription (e.g., for genes such as *myc, cyclin A, MDR1*) and the antiapoptotic *Bcl-2* (307). The role of p53 for radiation response is discussed later in this chapter. Loss of p53 function has numerous biologic consequences including a loss of cell cycle arrest in G1/S phase transition of the cell cycle after genotoxic stress, inhibition of apoptosis, and differentiation (303). Furthermore, loss of p53 function seems to be critical for chromosomal stability as p53 is involved in DNA repair, recombination, and replication. Inactivation of the TP53 gene is the most common genetic alteration in human cancer. More than 80% of the p53 alterations result from missense mutations in the DNA binding domain (309). The obvious predominance of specific missense mutations in human tumors with the presence of a full-length protein suggests an additional role of mutant p53 as an oncogenic protein with gain-of-function and dominant negative properties (276). In addition to mutations, p53 function can be compromised by aberration of its negative regulator MDM2 or by viral proteins HPV E6/E7 (271). While most of the *TP53* mutations are sporadic, a high proportion of patients with Li-Fraumeni syndrome, a rare cancer syndrome with a spectrum of carcinomas and sarcomas at early age, carry germline mutations.

Insensitivity to Growth Inhibitory Signals

TGF-β regulates multiple cell functions such as proliferation, extracellular matrix synthesis, angiogenesis, immune response, apoptosis, and differentiation (150). The TGF-β family (TGF-β1−5) belongs to the superfamily of peptide hormones. The different TGF-β isoforms bind to specific cell surface receptors (TβRI to TβRV) (85). TGF-β–mediated growth inhibition is associated with activation and repression of target gene transcription. Genes of proproliferative kinases such as cdks are repressed, whereas genes of the major cyclin-dependent kinase inhibitors p15 and p21 are transcriptionally activated. Ligand binding to TβRV stimulates serine/threonine-specific phosphatases, which inhibit proliferation by dephosphorylation of pRB. Alteration of TGF-β signaling in tumors, for example, by mutations and transcriptional silencing, leads to insensitivity to the growth inhibitory ligand effects.

Resistance to Apoptosis

Under physiologic conditions, tissue homeostasis results from the balance of cell division and cell loss. This balance is disturbed in most tumors by increased cell division rate due to the molecular mechanisms previously described and by an inappropriate rate of cell death, such as by senescence and apoptosis ([45,261,301]; Compare Table 3.2). While the acquired capability to escape from apoptosis is a prerequisite for tumorigenesis, it does not necessarily correlate with resistance to cancer treat-

ment (45). Apoptosis is a complex, multistep process involving numerous molecules, including adapter proteins, members of the *Bcl-2* family, and *caspases* (cysteine-aspartate proteases) (25,109,244). The latter are divided into initiator caspases (caspases 1, 2, 4, 5, 8, 9, 10, 12) and effector caspases (caspases 3, 6, 7, 11, 13). Caspases activate specific substrates by proteolytic cleavage. The activity of caspases is regulated by heat shock proteins and inhibitor of apoptosis proteins. The executive phase of the apoptotic program includes the release of cytochrome C from mitochondria after membrane depolarization, formation of the apoptosome complex (Apaf-1, pro-caspase 9, cytochrome c), and activation of effector caspases, leading subsequently to morphologic changes (e.g., DNA condensation and fragmentation). Initiator caspases are activated by two major pathways, that is, the extrinsic, receptor-mediated pathway and the intrinsic, mitochondria-mediated pathway (301). The extrinsic apoptotic signaling starts from binding of death ligands, such as Fas, tumor necrosis factor (TNF), and *TRAIL*, to their corresponding cell-surface receptors. Subsequently, a cell-type specific intracellular program is executed, including caspases, and members of the Bcl-2 family (*Bax, Bid, Bak*) eventually trigger the release of cytochrome C (type II) or directly activate effector caspase 3 (type I). The intrinsic, mitochondria-mediated pathway is triggered in response to cellular stress, such as DNA damage, chemotherapy, ionizing radiation, growth factor withdrawal, and kinase inhibition.

An important mediator between the recognition of DNA alterations and apoptosis is the tumor suppressor p53 (307). On DNA damage, p53 is stabilized and induces cell cycle arrest (see previous discussion), senescence, or apoptosis. Promotion of apoptosis by p53 results from transcriptional repression of antiapoptotic proteins (e.g., Bcl-2 and *survivin*), and activation of the proapoptotic proteins, including *Bax, PUMA,* and *NOXA*. Importantly, the apoptotic pathways are closely linked to protein kinase signaling. Thus, protein kinases such as MAPK and PI3K/Akt (see previous discussion) are able to modulate the balance between death and survival stimuli in the cell. Given the complex regulation of apoptosis, it is not surprising that a large variety of molecular alterations can result in an escape of cancer cells from this form of cell death (301). For instance, the extrinsic pathway is affected by down-regulation of caspase 8 activity by promotor methylation, mutation, and up-regulation of the negative regulator *FLIP*. Many tumor cells show a deregulated intrinsic, mitochondria-related apoptotic pathway caused by an imbalance of expression levels of pro- and antiapoptotic proteins of the Bcl-2 family. Abnormal expression levels of Apaf-1, inhibitor of apoptosis proteins, and heat-shock proteins result in an impaired execution phase of apoptosis in cancer cells.

| **Table 3.2** | **TYPES OF RADIATION-INDUCED CELL DEATH AND THEIR CHARACTERISTICS** |

Type of Cell Death	Important Morphologic Characteristics	Important Molecular Mechanisms
Mitotic catastrophe	During or after mitosis, mis-segregation of chromosomes, cell fusion, micronuclei, giant cell formation	Lethal chromosome damage, caspase independent
Apoptosis	Chromatin condensation, nuclear fragmentation, blebbing of cell membrane	Damage to DNA and/or membranes and/or alterations of intracellular signaling, caspase dependent (intrinsic pathway via caspase 9)
Senescence	Metabolically active but nondividing, functionally differentiated cells	Damage to DNA and/or alterations of intracellular signaling, generally p53-dependent terminal growth arrest, increased senescence associated β galactosidase
Autophagy	Partial chromatin condensation, cell membrane blebbing, increased number of autophagic vesicles	Protein degradation characterized by double-membrane vesicles in the cytoplasm, possibly related to DNA protein kinase (DNA-PK) activity
Necrosis	Increased vacuolation, swelling of organelles and cells, rupture of cell membranes, formation of necrotic mass	Unregulated traumatic cell destruction; After irradiation consequence of, e.g., mitotic catastrophe or vascular damage

DNA-PK
Adapted from Brown JM, Wouters BG. Apoptosis, p53, and tumor cell sensitivity to anticancer agents. *Cancer Res* 1999;59:1391–1399, and Okada H, Mak TW. Pathways of apoptotic and non-apoptotic death in tumour cells. *Nat Rev Cancer* 2004;4:592–603.

Moreover, important mediators and regulators of the apoptotic program such as p53, PI3K/Akt, PTEN, and MAPK are often functionally deregulated. While it is well established that the escape from apoptosis represents an important and possibly essential step in tumorigenesis, the importance of this phenomenon for therapy resistance, outcome prediction, and as a potential target to improve conventional cancer therapies remains unclear (45,301).

Limitless Replicative Potential

Loss of growth control and resistance to cell death are not sufficient for the development of macroscopic tumors (135). Normal cells have the capacity for a finite number of cell divisions, that is, a limited replicative potential; Thereafter they stop proliferating and enter the process of senescence. During tumorigenesis, some premalignant cells become immortal by circumventing senescence, that is, acquired capability of limitless replicative potential (139). Importantly, malignant tumors consist of heterogeneous populations differing in their replicative potential. While most cancer cells have a limited replicative potential, a small subpopulation (i.e., cancer stem cells) have an infinite replicative capacity to reconstitute the tumor (6,34,229). Thus, this subpopulation represents the target for curative cancer therapy, that is, all of these stem cells have to be inactivated by therapy to achieve cure.

The molecular mechanisms underlying the escape from senescence and other modes of cell death include loss of tumor suppressor proteins such as p53 and pRB as well as telomere maintenance (135). Telomeres are chromatin segments located at the ends of the chromosomes and protecting these regions from recombination and degradation (36). As telomeres are incompletely replicated they become progressively shorter during each cell division, subsequently resulting in loss of chromosomal protection, which in turn triggers senescence. Cancer cells generally have shorter telomeres than normal cells but are able to perpetuate their replicative potential by expressing telomerase, a complex including DNA polymerase, which reconstitutes the telomeres (36).

Induction and Sustaining Angiogenesis

To grow beyond microscopically sized cell aggregates of 1 to 2 mm, tumors depend on angiogenesis. Proliferating cells require appropriate oxygen and nutrient supply, which is physiologically limited to a distance of 100 to 200 μm from the next blood vessel. Therefore, malignant cells must induce and sustain their own vascular system to form tumors and metastases (13,30,50,95,106,111,134,157,241). The process of the *angiogenic switch* during tumorigenesis (i.e., the transition from the avascular phase to the vascular stage) is governed by different molecular changes in tumor cells and in cells of the surrounding stroma. The major event of the angiogenic switch is that proangiogenic factors—mostly growth factors such as the vascular endothelial growth factors (VEGFs), the fibroblast growth factors, and PDGFs—outbalance antiangiogenic factors, such as thrombospondin (*TSP-1*), *angiostatin*, and *endostatin*. The driving forces toward the imbalance of angiogenic factors in tumors include activation of oncogenes;for example, Ras and myc activation results in VEGF up-regulation (43) and TSP-1 repression (316). The loss of function in tumor suppressor proteins also contributes to the angiogenic switch by transcriptional regulation of angiogenic factors. For example, p53 up-regulates TSP-1 and down-regulates VEGF gene expression (30). Hypoxia promotes tumor angiogenesis via the hypoxia inducible factor 1, which transcriptionally regulates many angiogenic molecules (265). As originally proposed by Folkman (110), effective targeting of molecules and pathways involved in angiogenesis has been shown to exhibit anticancer activity (107).

Tissue Invasion and Metastasis

Locoregional and distant spread of tumor cells requires detachment from the primary tumor, invasion into surrounding tissues, intravasation into blood or lymphatic vessels, adhesion to endothelial cells at distant sites, extravasation, and eventually colonization in distant organs. The acquired capability of cancer cells to grow invasively and to metastasize is associated with multiple genetic and biochemical alterations of the cell-cell and cell-matrix interactions. Tissue invasion and metastasis require, at different steps, contrary capabilities, for example, detachment from the primary tumor versus adhesion at the metastatic site, suggesting that rapid adaptations, genetic instability, and clonal selection play an important role. Gene expression profiling revealed metastatic signatures in primary tumors (292) but also host polymorphisms, resulting in a genetically determined individual disposition to develop metastases (151). The often observed nonrandom pattern of metastasis in different types of cancer led to the "seed and soil" hypothesis describing the complex interplay between cancer cells and environmental factors (108). Recent experimental data suggest that bone marrow-derived endothelial progenitor cells exhibit preconditioning functions for metastases;that is, they reside in tumor-specific metastatic sites before the colonization with tumor cells and prepare the optimal environment for tumor cell homing (162).

Many physiologic functions of the cell such as proliferation, migration, survival, and differentiation are regulated by interactions with neighboring cells and with molecules of the extracellular matrix (ECM). The ECM consists of a large variety of different components including collagens, fibronectins, laminins, tenascin, proteoglycans, matrix proteases, and their specific inhibitors. Altered composition of the ECM is a typical finding in malignant tissues. For example, tenascin overexpression was found in the stroma of breast cancer, colon carcinoma, and glioma (227). It has been suggested that, due to the antiadhesive properties of tenascin, this change in the ECM facilitates detachment of cancer cells and subsequently tissue invasion and metastasis. *Matrix proteases* are important for ECM turnover and enable tumor cells to degrade extracellular barriers, a prerequisite for tissue invasion and metastasis (101). The different classes of matrix proteases include serine proteases (plasminogen activator, plasmin, and elastase), cysteine proteases (cathepsins), and matrix metalloproteinases (collagenases, stromelysins). The latter are released from the cells in an inactive form and activated by binding to zinc ions. The activity of the matrix proteases, and thereby the ECM turnover rate is also determined by inhibitors of the proteases such as tissue inhibitors of metalloproteases or plasminogen activator inhibitor. It has been shown that tissue invasion and metastasis in various types of cancer are associated with increased expression of matrix proteases and decreased activity of their inhibitors compared with normal cells (148,198).

Cell-cell and cell-matrix interactions are mediated by different adhesion molecules including integrins, cadherins, immunoglobulinelike cell adhesion molecules, and the hyaluronan receptor CD44 (51). These molecules exert not only structural functions but are also important modulators of signaling pathways. *Integrins* represent a class of heterodimeric transmembrane ECM receptors (42,153,185). At least 24 integrin receptors are formed by 18 α and 8 β subunits with overlapping binding affinity to ECM components and functions. Further diversity in the integrins results from postranslational modification such as alternative splicing. Intracellular signal transduction on binding of integrins to ECM components includes activation of the focal adhesion kinase and subsequent association with PI3K, which is required for focal adhesion kinase-promoted cell migration and survival. Other signaling partners of integrins include ILK, protein kinase C, Rho family of small

G proteins as well as cytoplasmic kinases (src, Abl), which contribute to activation of MAPK/JNK and subsequently stimulate proliferation and migration.

Besides the ability to bind ECM proteins such as fibronectin, collagen, or laminin, some integrins recognize members of the ADAM (A Disintegrin And Metalloproteinase) family or counter receptors on neighboring cells such as immunoglobulin-type receptors like intercellular cell adhesion molecules or vascular cell adhesion molecules (78). Several cross-talks between integrin signaling, growth factor signaling, and tumor suppressor proteins such as PTEN and p53 have been described. The capability of tissue invasion and metastatic spread has been associated with altered integrin function in tumors (158). In general, cancer cells show a more pronounced variability in integrin combinations, an abnormal expression pattern, and aberrant spatial expression compared with nonmalignant cells facilitating interaction with ECM of different composition and thereby permitting cancer cell survival and proliferation at distant sites. Alternative splicing of the hyaluronan receptor *CD44* results in a complex cell-type specific expression pattern that has been demonstrated to be altered in many tumors and metastasis (144). *E-Cadherin* is a glycoprotein expressed at the cell surface and intracellularly linked to the cytoskeleton via catenin proteins. In addition E-cadherin is connected to multiple intracellular signaling pathways. The function of E-cadherin as a tumor suppressor was established from experimental and clinical observations that a loss of function (e.g., by mutation, promoter methylation, increased proteolytic degradation by matrix metalloproteinases, increased endocytotic degradation induced by phosphorylation) is a frequent finding in human cancers and is associated with an invasive and metastatic phenotype (140). The multifunctional immunoglobulinelike cell adhesion molecules are expressed in a large variety of cell types. Some members of this superfamily such as NCAM, CEA, Mel-CAM,

and L1 are involved in tumorigenesis, metastasis, and invasion (51).

MOLECULAR RADIATION BIOLOGY

Target Molecules of Radiation Damage

Radiation effects may occur as direct ionizations in an organic molecule or indirectly via free-radical processes. As cells consist mostly of water, most ionizations produced by irradiation occur in water molecules. Within only 10^{-10} seconds, radiolysis of water leads, among other entities, to e^-aq, $H\cdot$, and $OH\cdot$. About 60% to 70% of cellular DNA damage produced by ionizing radiation is caused by $OH\cdot$ (310,313). The radiation-induced reactive oxygen species (ROS) will undergo further reactions, for example, production of H_2O_2 from two hydroxyl radicals. Aerobes have evolved antioxidant defenses to protect themselves against the oxygen-derived species generated *in vivo* or from external sources. These defenses include enzymes (such as superoxide dismutases, catalase, and gluthathione peroxidase), low-molecular mass agents (such as α-tocopherol and ascorbic acid) and proteins that bind metal ions in forms unable to catalyse the generation of free radicals. In contrast to those defensive mechanisms, the oxygen molecule has a high affinity to free radicals, which may give rise to further cascades of radical production and thereby to the fixation of free radical damage to important macromolecules of the cell (e.g., DNA). This is one explanation of the oxygen effect of radiation damage, that is, the fact that well-oxygenated cells are more radiosensitive than hypoxic cells (126,328,329).

By far the most important target for the biologic effects of ionizing radiation is the DNA (Fig. 3.1). This is obvious for the

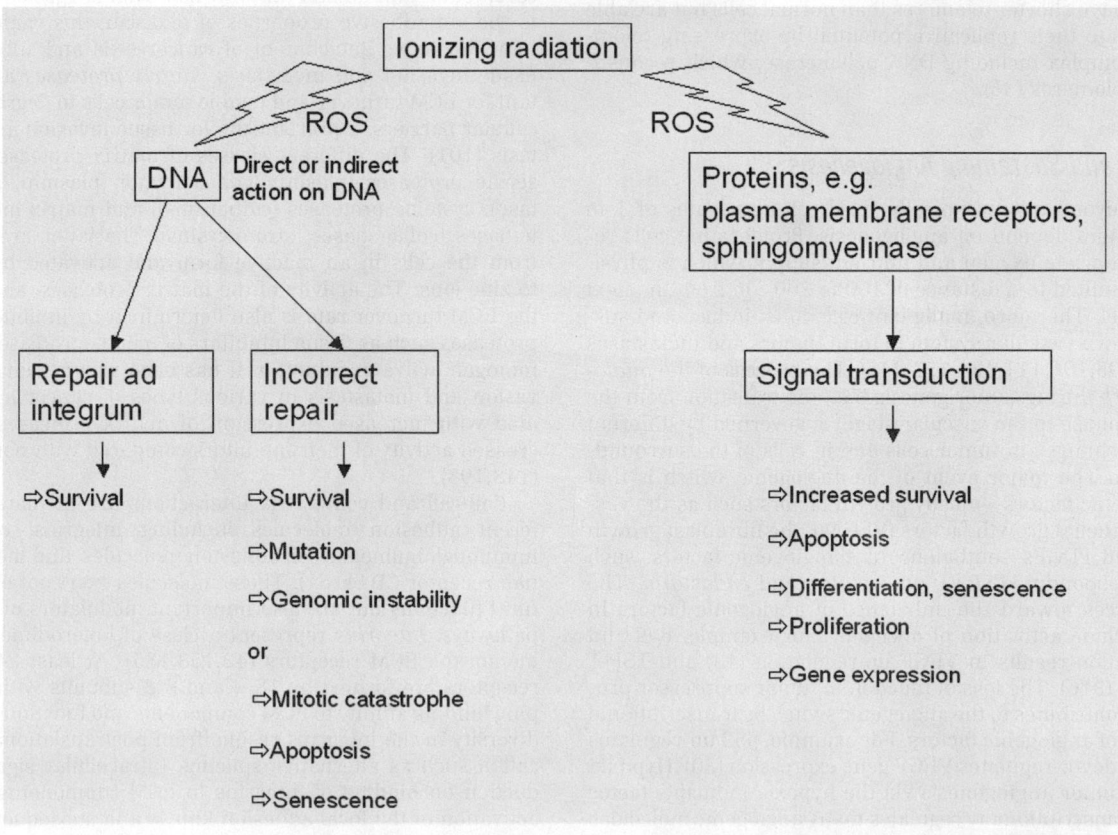

FIGURE 3.1. Simplified illustration of biologic effects of ionizing radiation mediated via DNA and non-DNA target molecules. ROS, reactive oxygen species.

induction of mutations but has also been consistently demonstrated for the killing of cells in a number of different experiments. Irradiation of the cytoplasm of cells with short-range α-particles only leads to cell kill at very high doses, whereas 1,000-fold lower doses to the nucleus are sufficient to kill the cell (218). Radioactive isotopes with short-range emission effectively kill cells when incorporated into the DNA, but not when predominantly incorporated in cell membranes (315). Modification of radiation-induced cell kill by different measures including hypoxia, high linear energy transfer radiation, or hyperthermia is linked closely with a change in the induction and repair of DNA double-strand breaks (113). Exposure of cells to about 1 Gy causes approximately 3,500 DNA injuries, 1,500 to 2,500 of which are damaged bases, 1,000 single-strand breaks (SSB), 40 double-strand breaks (DSB), and an estimated 100 to 200 local multiple-damaged sites (312), where one or several DSBs occur in close proximity to SSBs and base damages (314). It will be discussed later that most radiation-induced DNA damage is recognized and very efficiently repaired by the cell.

Beside effects on DNA, ionizing radiation also evokes biologically important responses on proteins (e.g., transmembrane receptors) and on lipids (e.g., ceramides) (Fig. 3.1). Radiation-induced activation of receptors will be discussed later. Ionizing irradiation induces rapid sphingomyelin hydrolysis by acid sphingomyelinase to generate ceramide, an inductor of apoptosis (130,172,255,317).

Biological Consequences of Irradiation

The effects of ionizing radiation on cellular target molecules may lead to various functional consequences. These functional effects can be broadly categorized into cell death, repair, cell cycle effects, altered gene expression, modification of signal transduction, or mutagenesis and genomic instability (Fig. 3.2). These categories are not exclusive.

Cell Death

Among the functional consequences of ionizing radiation, cell death is the most important for radiation oncology. Cells can die in several ways (45,225), by apoptosis, mitotic catastrophe, senescence, necrosis, and autophagy (Table 3.2). Most important for the effect of radiotherapy of solid tumors is *mitotic catastrophe,* which is caused by lethal chromosome damage. After irradiation, cells can pass through one or few mitotic cycles before mis-segregation of chromosomes or cell fusion leads to the loss of the replicative potential (or clonogenicity)

of cells. Often micronuclei, containing unrepaired chromosome fragments, can be detected. Those micronuclei, and hence essential genetic information, will be lost during the following cell cycle, which results in cell death. Frequent multinucleate giant cells reflect a radiation-induced failure of cytoplasmatic separation on cell division.

Neoplastic hematopoetic or lymphatic cells often die from radiation-induced *apoptosis* via the intrinsic, caspase 9-dependent pathway. Two different forms of radiation-induced apoptosis can be distinguished, early or premitotic versus late or postmitotic (112,273). Early apoptosis is p53-dependent, occurs within few hours after irradiation before the cells enter mitosis, and is primarily a consequence of DNA damage. Early apoptosis represents a distinct mode of radiation-induced cell death. In contrast, secondary apoptosis occurs after mitosis and is one of several possible manifestations of radiation-induced lethal chromosome aberrations. In most cancers, particularly in solid tumors, apoptosis appears not to be the main mechanism of radiation-induced cell death. No clear evidence exists that either apoptotic index or levels of p53, Bcl-2, or other Bcl-2 family members are predictive of the response of solid tumors to radiotherapy (45–47). For example, overexpression of Bcl-2 was shown to decrease significantly apoptotic fraction in response to irradiation. However, this did not translate into a change of clonogenic cell survival after irradiation (327).

Radiation-induced *senescence* plays an important role for development of normal tissue damage, for example, fibrosis (246). Cells survive and are metabolically active but lose their replicative potential. The mechanism of radiation-induced senescence involves p53-mediated cell cycle arrest but apparently not telomere shortening (278). *Necrosis* is an unregulated process of cell destruction by the release of intracellular components. This is usually the consequence of a pathophysiologic conditions such as ischemia and inflammation (225). So far no distinct pathway has been described that directly leads to cellular necrosis after clinical relevant doses of irradiation. However, it is well known that tumors after neoadjuvant radiotherapy or radiochemotherapy often show massive necrosis, which in some tumors correlates with improved prognosis (89,281,297). It is likely that this radiation-induced induction of necrosis is explained by several factors, including mitotic catastrophe of tumor cells and the effects of irradiation on tumor vessels leading to changes in the microenvironment, which consequently causes cell death.

Autophagy is a form of nonapoptotic and non-necrotic cell death that is related to lysosomal degradation of proteins and cell organelles (225). This mode of programmed cell death is triggered by growth factor withdrawal, differentiation, and developmental stimuli. Recent experimental data indicate that ionizing radiation also may induce autophagy (75,228). However, the contribution of autophagy to inactivation of clonogenic cells after clinically relevant radiation doses, its dependency on cell type, and molecular regulation so far are poorly understood.

Recognition of Radiationinduced DNA Damage

DNA damage, in particular DSB, is sensed by different proteins that trigger an ataxia telangiectasia mutated (ATM)-dependent or, in some cases, ataxia telangiectasia and Rad3-related (ATR)–dependent signaling cascade (3,291) (Fig. 3.3). ATM activation requires the telomeric protein TRF2 and the MRN complex consisting of Rad50, Mre11 (meiotic recombination protein 11), and NBS1 (Nijmegen breakage syndrome protein 1), MDC1 (mediator of DNA damage checkpoint protein-1), and 53BP1 (54,183,195,197,242,290). In addition of proper activation of downstream DNA repair proteins, histone H2HAX molecules need to be phosphorylated in the vincinity of the DSB. All of these proteins assemble at the site of the breaks and presumably control the choice for one of several repair pathways. In

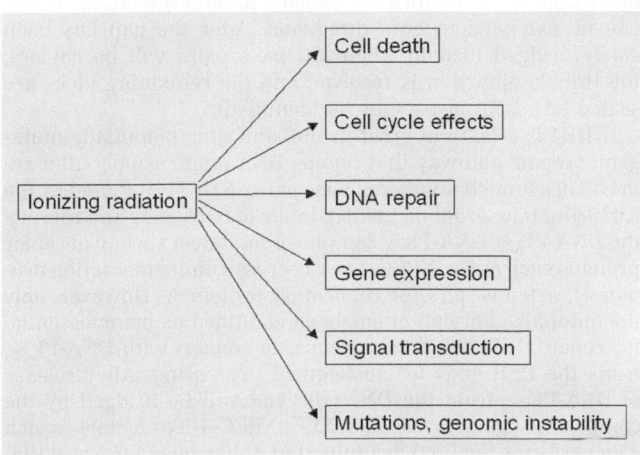

FIGURE 3.2. Functional effects of ionizing radiation on cells. The categories are not exclusive.

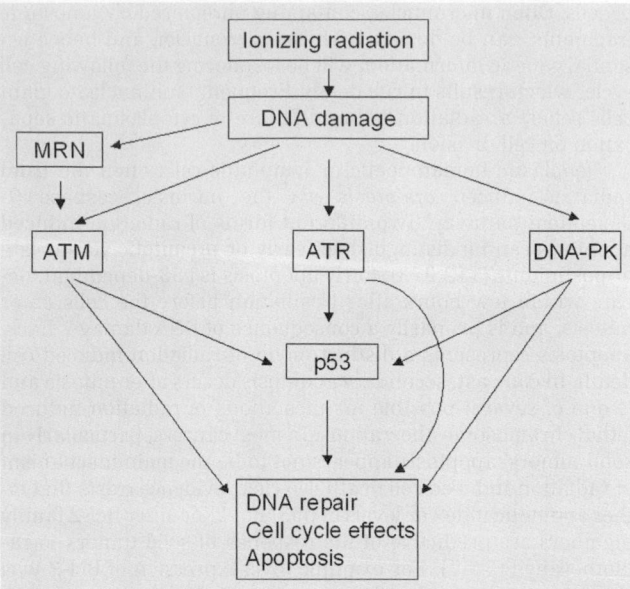

FIGURE 3.3. Simplified pathways of radiation-induced DNA damage recognition. MRN, Mrc 11, Rad50, NB51 complex; ATM, ataxia telengiectasia mutated; ATR, ataxia telangiectasia and Rad3-related; PK, protein kinase.

addition to its role in repair, ATM is involved in the regulation of multiple cell cycle checkpoints (G1/S, S, G2/M) after DNA damage (168). ATM, ATR, and DNA-PK$_{CS}$ (DNA-dependent kinase-catalytic subunit) phoshrpylate p53 and a number of proteins involved in cell cycle delay, apoptosis, and induction of DNA repair (291). ATR appears to be important for sensing ultraviolet and other types of bulky lesions, and damage that induces a replication block, while ATM seems to be the sensor for DSB induced by ionizing radiation (3,291). ATR may serve in some cases as a backup for ATM.

DNA Repair

Genome integrity is essential to the survival of cells and organisms. It is estimated that about 10^4 DNA lesions occur in a single human cell every day (191). Most of the damage is caused by endogenous sources such as oxygen free radicals, replicative errors, and spontaneous desaminations. To cope with the plethora of permanent damage initially, a repair system has developed during evolution that also acts on external challenge such as radiation or chemical DNA damage. To enable repair of massive DNA damage, the cells stop proliferation. This may prevent replication or segregation of damaged genetic material. If repair is not possible, the cells either die or, in case of survival, may propagate mutated DNA (Fig. 3.2). When the DNA replication machinery meets damaged DNA, replication may continue despite the damage by translesion synthesis, which requires DNA polymerase with low fidelity. Different mechanisms are involved in DNA repair (26,55,71,73,97,127,191,194,257,279,291,298).

Base Excision Repair (BER)

The mechanism of BER is responsible for the repair of various kinds of base damage (abasic sites, oxidized bases, deaminated bases, and alkylated bases) and SSB. Base damages and SSB are the most frequent types of DNA damage after irradiation. The major BER pathway is the short-patch pathway, which involves excision of only one base. The minor pathway, the long-patch repair, excises 2 to 10 nucleotides. In the short-patch pathway, DNA glycosylases recognize damaged bases and excise them from DNA. APE1 (apurinic/apyrimidinic endonuclease 1,

synonyms: HAP-1, redox effector factor 1) (330) hydrolyzes the phosphodiester bond 5′ to the abasic site (331). Alternatively, an AP-lyase cleaves the 3′ sugar-phosphate bond. In both cases, the sugar residue is removed by either a 5′or 3′-phosphodiesterase. Polymerase β (Pol-β) incorporates a single nucleotide into the gap and, finally, the nick in the DNA is sealed by DNA ligase III, which interacts with Pol-β. In this process, XRCC1 (x-ray repair cross-complementing protein) interacts with several enzymes in this pathway and regulates their activity (27,178,300). For the long-patch repair, the nick produced by AP-endonuclease or AP-lyase is extended to a gap 2 to 10 nucleotides by either 5′- 3′exonuclease, that is, exonuclease function of polymerase δ or ε (Pol-δ or ε) or by removal of a flap-end by Fen-1 (flap-end endonuclease-1). Pol δ or ε and associated replication factors (proliferating cell nuclear antigen andreplication factor C) will then fill the gap. After the synthesis, DNA ligase I or, less frequently ligase III, seals the nick (55,204,230).

Double Strand Break (DSB) Repair

Spontaneous DSBs occur either on topoisomerase failure during recombination and is forced by replication errors or are due to thermodynamic fluctuation. In germ cells, DSBs are produced during meiotic crossover in T and B lymphocytes during a sik-specific DNA recombination of variable diversity and joining genes (VDJ) on maturation of T-cell receptors and antibodies. Radiation-induced DSBs are, despite their relatively low induction frequency (40 per Gy per cell), biologically much more important than base damage and SSB. Two major pathways, homologous recombination (HR) and non-homologous end-joining (NHEJ), have evolved to repair DSB (55,72,155,222,291,294,322) (Fig. 3.4). Whereas NHEJ occurs in all phases of the cell cycle, HR is particularly important in the S/G2 transition of the cell cycle (248).

HR is a slow, high-fidelity repair pathway. Regions of DNA homology, usually the sister chromatid, are used as the template. During HR, activated ATM recruits endonucleases that process broken ends, which ultimately creates single-stranded 3′ends (195,291). For the processing, the MRN complex is required. In concert with on BRCA1, BRCA2, and Rad51 paralogues (XRCC2, XRCC3, Rad51B, Rad51C, Rad51D, Rad52, Rad54), the Rad51 protein binds to single-stranded DNA with the aid of replication protein A and searches for a homologous sequence on the sister chromatid. On strand invasion, Rad51 enables the formation of a temporary triple helix. Once the complementary strands have paired, the 3′ end of the damaged DNA will be elongated by polymerases (not yet identified) beyond the position of former DSB. When the 3′ single strand of the second end of the DSB also invades the structure, a quadruple-helix is formed called *Holliday-junction*, which can be extended in both directions. After the gap has been safely bridged (usually about 50 base pairs will be copied), the Holliday-junction is resolved and the remaining nicks are sealed by a DNA ligase (not yet identified).

NHEJ is a fast but error-prone, and thus potentially mutagenic, repair pathway that rejoins DNA ends, usually after removal of a limited number of base pairs. NHEJ is initiated by the Ku70/Ku80 heterodimer, which binds to DNA ends and recruits the DNA-PK$_{CS}$. DNA-PK$_{CS}$ can phosphorylate a variety of repair proteins such as Ku, XRCC-4 (x-ray cross-complementation protein 4), artemis, p53, or replication protein A. However, only the autophosphorylation has been identified as being essential for repair (159,200,243). Artemis, in concert with DNA-PK$_{CS}$, trims the DSB ends for subsequent processing. After release of DNA-PK$_{CS}$, from the DNA, the end will be bridged by the complex of ligase IV/XRCC-4/XLF (XRCC-4-like factor), which also performs the final ligations step. It has been observed that NHEJ can, to some extent, occur in the absence of several core proteins. This gave raise to the idea of a backup pathway

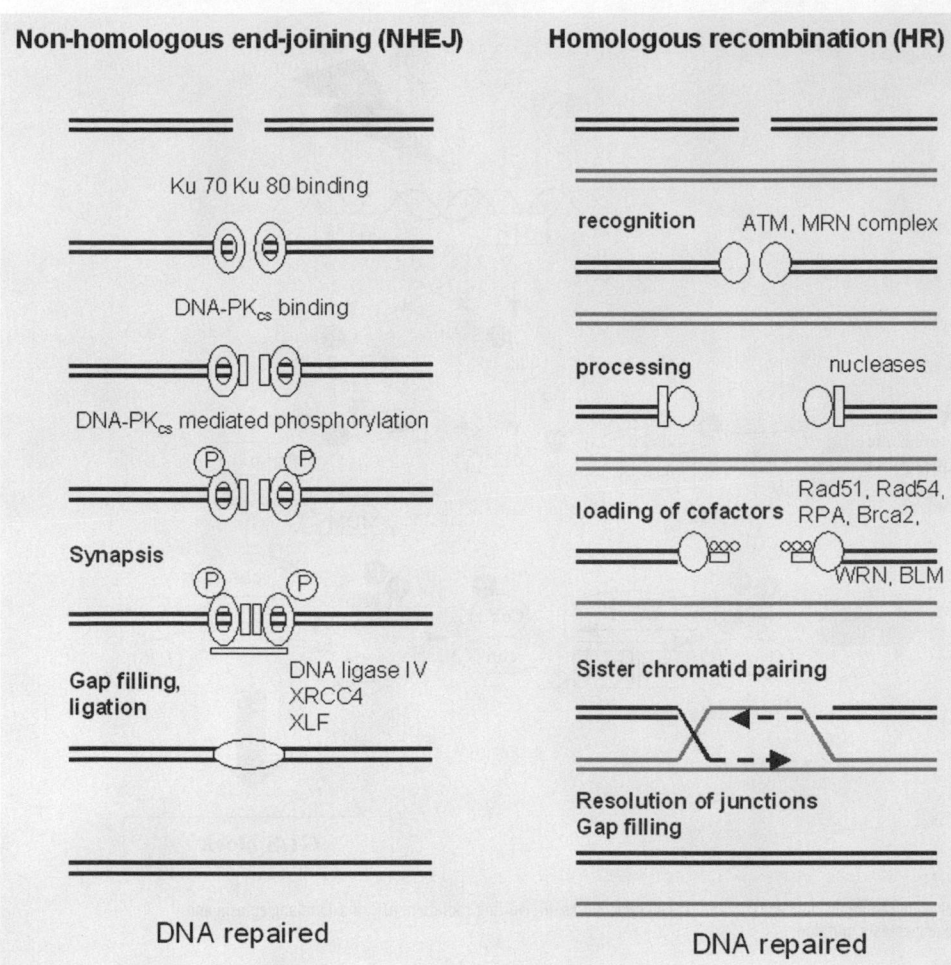

Non-homologous end-joining (NHEJ)

Ku 70 Ku 80 binding

DNA-PK$_{cs}$ binding

DNA-PK$_{cs}$ mediated phosphorylation

Synapsis

Gap filling, ligation

DNA ligase IV
XRCC4
XLF

DNA repaired

Homologous recombination (HR)

recognition   ATM, MRN complex

processing   nucleases

loading of cofactors   Rad51, Rad54, RPA, Brca2, WRN, BLM

Sister chromatid pairing

Resolution of junctions
Gap filling

DNA repaired

FIGURE 3.4. Mechanisms of DNA double-strand break repair in mammalian cells.

that only operates when the DNA-PK–dependent NHEJ fails (233,311). Recent data suggest that, beside the genuine repair proteins, the tumor suppressor p53 is involved in controlling the repair. P53 appears to suppress both HR and NHEJ in case error-free repair is not possible and thereby reduces the mutagenic risk of error-prone repair (5,74,321).

Radiation-Induced Cell Cycle Delay

It has long been recognized that radiation-induced DNA damage is associated with delay in the cell cycle, which has been interpreted as allowing additional time for the cells to repair.

G1 Phase

The G1 cell cycle checkpoint prevents damaged DNA from being replicated and is the best understood checkpoint in mammalian cells (16). Radiation-induced G1 phase cell cycle arrest is regulated by p53 (Fig. 3.5). Loss of p53 function, which is found in the majority of tumors, leads to a lack of G1 phase arrest. Instead, these cells exert a dose-dependent blockage in the G2 and M phase of the cell cycle. Central to the G1 checkpoint is the accumulation and activation of the p53 protein, which is controlled by the ATM and ATR kinases. These kinases together with DNA-PK are activated by and recruited to radiation-induced DNA lesions. Physiologically, p53 expression levels are low due to interaction with its negative regulator MDM2, which targets p53 for nuclear export and proteosome-mediated degradation in the cytoplasm (7). Following radiation-induced DNA damage, ATM activates the downstream cell cycle

checkpoint kinase Chk2 by phosphorylation at position Thr68 (147), which in turn phosphorylates amino acid residue Ser20 of p53. This results in a pronounced tetramerization, activity, and stability. The p53-Ser20 phosphorylation inhibits p53/MDM2 interaction, resulting in p53 accumulation. Moreover, ATM exerts p53 stability by directly phosphorylating MDM2 on Ser395 (206). While allowing maintenance of MDM2/p53 interaction, this event prevents p53 nuclear export to the cytoplasm for degradation. *In vitro* studies showed Ser20 phosphorylation of p53 by the ATR-related cell cycle checkpoint-dependent kinase Chk1 (272). Transcriptional transactivation activity is mediated via Ser15 phosphorylation of p53 (94). Both ATM and ATR are able to directly phosphorylate this residue in response to irradiation. P53 target genes include several genes that are involved in the DNA damage response (e.g., MDM2, GADD45a, p21[Cip1]). Accumulation of the cyclin-dependent kinase inhibitor p21[Cip1] blocks G1/S phase progression by binding to the cyclinE/cdk2 complex, reducing cdk2 activity, which has an important function in phosphorylation of pRB.

S phase

After irradiation, the rate of DNA synthesis is decreased via ATM- and NBS1-dependent pathways (280). Radiation-induced DNA damage activates ATM for Thr68 phosphorylation of Chk2 (103). Activated Chk2 targets CDC25A phosphatase for ubiquitination. As a result of CDC25A degradation, inhibitory phosphorylations of Cdk2 at Thr14 and Tyr15 reside. The Cdk2/Cyclin E and Cdk2/Cyclin A complexes remain inactive, which prevents completion of DNA synthesis and G2 entry.

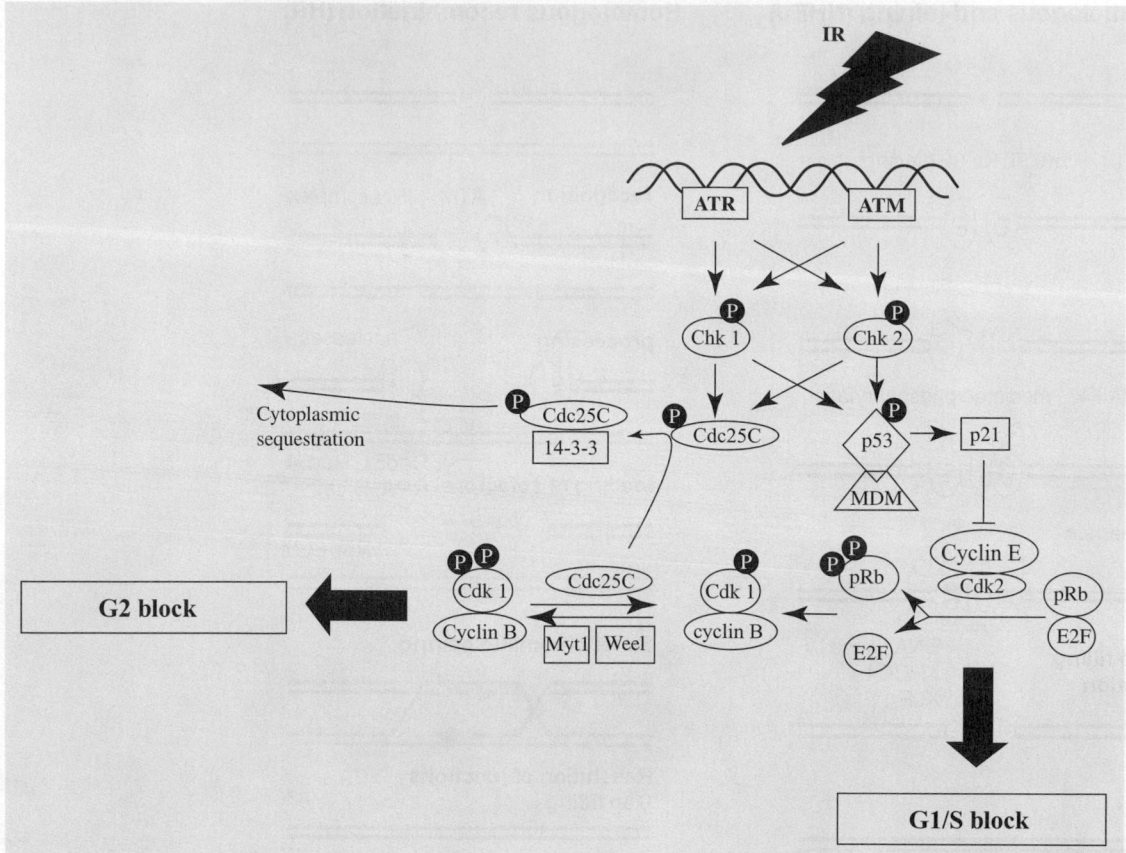

FIGURE 3.5. Pathways involved in radiation-induced G1/S and G2 cell cycle blocks. IR, ionizing radiation; ATR, ataxia telangiectasia and Rad3-related; ATM, ataxia telengiectasia mutated.

Alternatively, radiation-activated ATM phosphorylates several downstream substrates, including BRCA1 at Ser1387, NBS1 at Ser343, and SMC1 at Ser957 and Ser966 (103, 170). ATR phosphorylates the cell cycle checkpoint kinase Chk1 at Ser317 and Ser345. Subsequently, Chk1 phosphorylates CDC25A, which results in cytoplasmic sequestration and thereby in inhibition of S-G2 transition (339).

G2 Phase

In contrast to the G1 checkpoint, all mammalian cells, normal or transformed, undergo cell cycle arrest in G2 after radiation-induced damage (82). The G2 cell cycle checkpoint is the essential final determinator allowing cells to divide. The entry into mitosis is regulated by the activity of the cyclin-dependent kinase Cdk1 (221) (Fig. 3.5). Phosphorylation of Thr14 and Tyr15 of Cdk1 blocks cell cycling into G2. These phosphorylations are removed by the phosphatase CDC25C. After irradiation, ATR and ATM activate the downstream checkpoint kinases Chk1 and Chk2, which phosphorylate CDC25C at Ser216 (232). This results in binding of 14-3-3 proteins. The CDC25C/14-3-3 protein complex is translocated into the cytoplasm for sequestration. As a consequence of this CDC25C degradation, Cdk1 remains phosphorylated, thereby preventing entry into mitosis. ATM appears to be more dominant at the early stage of G2/M checkpoint activation, whereas ATR seems to contribute mainly to sustained checkpoint events (231).

Radiation-Induced Gene Expression

Radiation may modify gene expression (179,193). Many of the transcriptionally activated proteins have been shown to be cen-

trally involved in the pathogenesis of radiation damage or to modulate the effect of radiation on tumor cells. Early responses may occur within hours after irradiation and involve mostly transcription factors such as the proto-oncogenes jun, fos, junB (270), and Egr1 (early growth response gene 1) (133,238). Sustained activation of early radiation response genes such as NFκB may contribute to late radiation damage (128). Other examples for radiation-induced genes that may occur early and/or late after irradiation include TGF-β, TNF-α, bFGF, PDGF, and IL-1 (119,132,173,174,252).

Induction of *jun* is partly mediated by protein kinase C (133) and by reactive oxygen intermediates (80). In addition to transcriptional activation, prolongation of the half-life of jun has also been observed (270). Jun and fos form a heterodimer that represents the transcription factor *AP-1*. This transcription factor is a central regulator of cell proliferation, differentiation and death (10,268,269); For example, activation of AP-1 results in transcriptional suppression of MAPK phosphatases (161). Furthermore, AP-1 appears to be an important regulator of the transcription of other radiation-induced genes, such as in the early transcription of TGF-β (202). Redox-dependent DNA binding activity of AP-1 is regulated by the DNA repair protein Ref-1 (330,331).

Gene expression and DNA binding activity of *NFκB* is induced shortly after ionizing radiation (41). NFκB is a sequence-specific DNA binding protein complex that binds to DNA as a dimer. Five mammalian proteins have been identified that belong to this family: NFκB1 (p50 and its precursor p105), NFκB2 (p52 and its precursor p100), c-Rel, RelA (p65), and RelB (266). The most frequently occuring dimer is p50/p65. In the nonactivated state, this dimer is retained in the cytoplasm by binding to its inhibitor IκB (inhibitor of NFκB). On activation of the NFκB pathway, IκB is phosphorylated by a kinase complex named *IKK* (IκB kinase), consisting of the three subunits α, β, and γ (48,52,87,114,115,212,249,326,332,336,337). According to its multiple functions, NFκB can also be activated by a variety of agents, like membrane receptors as TNFR or Toll-like receptors (129) and oxidative stress (262,282). Radiation-induced activation of NFκB is mediated by IKK (160,188). This response does not depend on a nuclear signal as it also occurs in enucleated cells (86). However, it has been shown that ATM is required for chronic activation of the transcription factor NFκB (235). NFκB acts antiapoptotic and protects the intestinal epithelium from radiation damage (100).

Radiation exposure induces immediate and sustained *TGFβ1* gene expression as well as activation of this cytokine (137,306). On transcriptional activation TGF-β is produced as an inactive latent form and secreted. Latent TGF-β is stored in the extracellular matrix and proteolytically activated in irradiated tissues (14). Active TGF-β1 binds and activates the TGF-β1 type I receptor, resulting in TGF-β1-dependent gene expression inducing, for example, p21, p27, collagen, and TIMP (21,202). This is most likely responsible for the cellular effects of TGF-β, such as modulation of proliferation, differentiation and radiation sensitivity of fibroblasts, and for the biochemical events (e.g., collagene deposition, characteristic of radiation-induced fibrosis) (245). Also TGF-β secreted by tumor cells on irradiation might contribute to the development of radiation-induced fibrosis (11). Intervention into the TGF-β mediated effects (e.g., by TGF-β1 neutralizing antibodies and superoxide dismutase) offer a promising strategy to prevent radiation-induced fibrosis (21,202).

TNF-α belongs to the group of proinflammatory cytokines involved in radiation-induced normal tissue damage, such as pneumonitis and lung fibrosis. Immediately after irradiation, TNF-α is transcriptionally up-regulated and released by the bronchiolar epithelium. TNF-α enhances phagocytosis and cytotoxicity by neutrophilic granulocytes, and modulates the expression of other cytokines such as IL1 and IL6 (250). Experimental data show that also tumor lines, particulary paediatric sarcomas, may produce large quantities of bioactive TNF-α after irradiation. This may be of potential importance for tumor response and for normal tissue reactions after radiotherapy (251).

Induction of genes by ionizing radiation has been experimentally exploited for therapy. For example, the early-response gene Egr1 was inserted upstream to TNF-α, which may act as a radiosensitizer. This provides a strategy for spatial and temporal control of the biologic effect by radiotherapy (179,319,320).

Radiation Effects on Signal Transduction

Ionizing radiation may activate intracellular signaling (258). The general mechanisms of activation involve the dose-dependent production of ROS and reactive nitrogen species (RNS) that stimulate, for example, cytoplasmic protein kinases, phosphatases, cell membrane receptors, or disturb, for example, the lipid and protein metabolism (213). Many signalling pathways are simultaneously activated in a cell type-dependent manner, which may contribute to different radiation responses in different cell types. Cooperative and mutual cross-talk occurs between parallel and up- and downstream signaling routes (224). Examples of important intracellular signaling pathways and their modulation by ionizing radiation are discussed in the following paragraphs.

EGFR-Mediated Signaling

The EGFR family belongs to the group of RTKs and consists of four different single receptors (EGFR/ErbB-1, HER2/ErbB-2, HER3/ErbB-3, and HER4/ErbB-4) that are dimerized after ligand binding to the extracellular domain (152). In ad-

dition to activation through its natural ligands such as EGF, TGF-α, or amphiregulin, ionizing radiation is able to stimulate EGFR (17,259). Radiation doses of 1 to 2 Gy activate the EGFR and its downstream signaling cascades similarly efficient as physiologic EGF concentrations of 0.1 to 1 nM. Recent reports provide evidence that the radiation-dependent production of ROS/RNS plays a critical role in EGFR activation and downstream signaling via MAPK (184,213). It was shown that protein tyrosine phosphatases contain ROS/RNS-sensitive cysteine residues at a site essential for phosphatase activity. Thus, the radiation-dependent activation of EGFR is likely to be controlled by ROS/RNS-regulated protein phosphatases. In addition, paracrine and autocrine activation of the EGFR can also result from radiation-induced release of TGF-α from irradiated cells (83,284).

EGFR signaling via Ras-Raf-MAPK after irradiation has been implicated in increased proliferation (259), which corresponds to observations that EGFR overexpression is associated with repopulation during fractionated irradiation (29,102,175). In addition, EGFR-dependent signaling via PI3K/Akt has been associated with increased cellular survival and cell cycle progression (84,201,210). Another EGFR downstream pathway represents the c-Src-mediated activation of STAT3. STAT3 is involved in the TGF-α-mediated autocrine growth (124) and contributes to the regulation of angiogenesis by production of vascular endothelial growth factor (VEGF) (220). After radiation-induced activation, the EGFR is internalised and may function as a nuclear transcription factor (190,226,318). In addition, internalized EGFR can activate DNA-PK. Pharmacologic inhibitors can block EGFR signaling at different levels and thereby influence several mechanisms of radioresistance such as DNA repair, repopulation, antiapoptotic signaling, and tumor hypoxia (20,90,91,136,176,216,259,260). The specific mutational status of the cells, for example, Ras mutations (283,284), and the class of drugs (19,176) may critically modify effects of EGFR inhibition on radiation reponse. The concept of EGFR inhibition to improve outcome of radiotherapy has been proven recently in a phase III clinical trial (39). An important variant of the EGFR for radiation oncology is the constitutively active, truncated EGFRvIII, which is coexpressed with EGFR in a significant proportion of solid tumors (196). EGFRvIII lacks the ability of EGF binding due to a deletion of the NH(2)-terminal domain but, as wild type EGFR, can be activated by irradiation (182). Current evidence suggests that EGFRvIII has altered signaling properties compared to normal EGF receptor, and represents a cancer cell-specific target (196). Experimental data indicate that activation of EGFRvIII leads to more pronounced cytoprotective responses to radiation than EGFRwt (182).

Ras Signaling

Mutant, constitutively active Ras, an important component of the MAPK pathway, has been found in many types of human cancers. Farnesyltransferase inhibitors (FTIs) can effectively block Ras mediated signal transduction (31,208). Application of FTI renders cells more sensitive to ionizing radiation. Combination of FTI with radiotherapy is currently under preclinical and clinical investigation (49,203).

PDGF-Mediated Signaling

Radiation-induced autocrine and paracrine PDGF signaling plays an important role in fibroblast and endothelial cell activation and proliferation *in vitro* (187). Increased phosphorylation of the PDGFR has been observed after irradiation (187). Combination of irradiation with PGDFR tyrosine kinase inhibitors resulted in decreased clonogenic survival of endothial cells and fibroblasts *in vitro* (187). Recent data suggest that inhibition of PDGFR signaling may attenuate development of radiation-induced pulmonary fibrosis (1).

VEGFR-Mediated Signaling

Transmembrane receptors for VEGF and related ligands include VEGFR-1 (Flt-1), VEGFR-2 (KDR/Flk-1), and VEGFR-3 (Flt-4), neuropilin-1, and neuropilin-2 (70). On irradiation, VEGF is up-regulated via the EGFR/STAT signaling and released by tumor cells and exert, via VEGFR/PI3K/Akt signaling, prosurvival stimuli on tumor and endothial cells (2,122,308,340). Up-regulated VEGFR expression has been found after ionizing irradiation (167,341). Besides normalizing the tumor micromilieu (325), inhibition of radiation-induced VEGF/VEGFR signaling represents the rationale for combining anti-VEGF strategies with radiotherapy, which is currently under preclinical and clinical investigation (223,342).

Cyclo-Oxygenase–Mediated Signaling

The rate-limiting enzyme in the synthesis of prostaglandins is cyclo-oxygenase (COX). Two isoforms, COX-1 and COX-2, exist. COX-2 is typically not expressed or is expressed at relatively low levels in normal tissues, but overexpressed in 40% to 80% of cancers of the lung, colon, head and neck, breast, prostate, brain, and pancreas (215). COX-2 enzyme inhibitors are potential enhancers of tumor radioresponse (214). Among other stimuli, irradiation has been shown to up-regulate expression of COX-2 in tumors and normal tissues (156,277,334). Specific inhibition of COX-2 has been demonstrated to enhance radiation responses of tumor cells in vivo and in vitro (234). Several mechanisms, including reduced angiogenesis, increased apoptosis, and immune responses, have been implicated in the radiosensitizing effects of COX-2 inhibitors. Recent experimental data suggest that inhibition of DNA repair by COX-2 inhibitors via down-regulation of Ku70, and thereby inhibition of DNA-PK$_{CS}$, contributes significantly to the radiosensitizing effects (240). Furthermore, COX-2 inhibitors appear to attenuate radiation gene expression via inihbiton of NFκB (240). Ongoing early clinical trials in combination with radiotherapy indicate feasibility of this approach (189).

Integrin-Mediated Signaling

Interactions between cells and extracellular matrix (ECM) proteins are facilitated mainly by the integrin family of cell adhesion molecules (154). Besides the influence of growth factors and cytokines, these interactions add a further facet to the circuitry of microenvironmental factors that modulate the cellular behavior on exposure to ionizing radiation (Fig. 3.6). Chemotherapeutic compounds as well as ionizing radiation showed less cytotoxic efficacy in cells adherent to ECM compared to cells growing in suspension or on plastic surfaces (65). Resistance-promoting effects by integrin-mediated adhesion to ECM were found in cell lines from solid tumors of the lung (118,267), breast (211), liver (338), colon, pancreas (65,217), ovary (205), prostate (98), brain (289), and leukemia cells (76). Certain integrins seem to communicate increased radiation and drug resistance. For example, α5β1 integrin, the "classic" fibronectin receptor, acts as a major antagonist of cell death induced by doxorubicin or melphalan in multiple myeloma (141), by paclitaxel in breast cancer or small cell and non–small cell lung cancer (NSCLC) (12,62), or by cisplatin or mitomycin C in non–small cell lung cancer (62). Additional studies underscored the important role of β1 integrins in promoting resistance against ionizing radiation on the basis of signaling events via the adapter proteins paxillin and p130Cas to the survival-regulating protein kinase JNK (66,263). Further regulatory cytoplasmic cascades downstream of β1

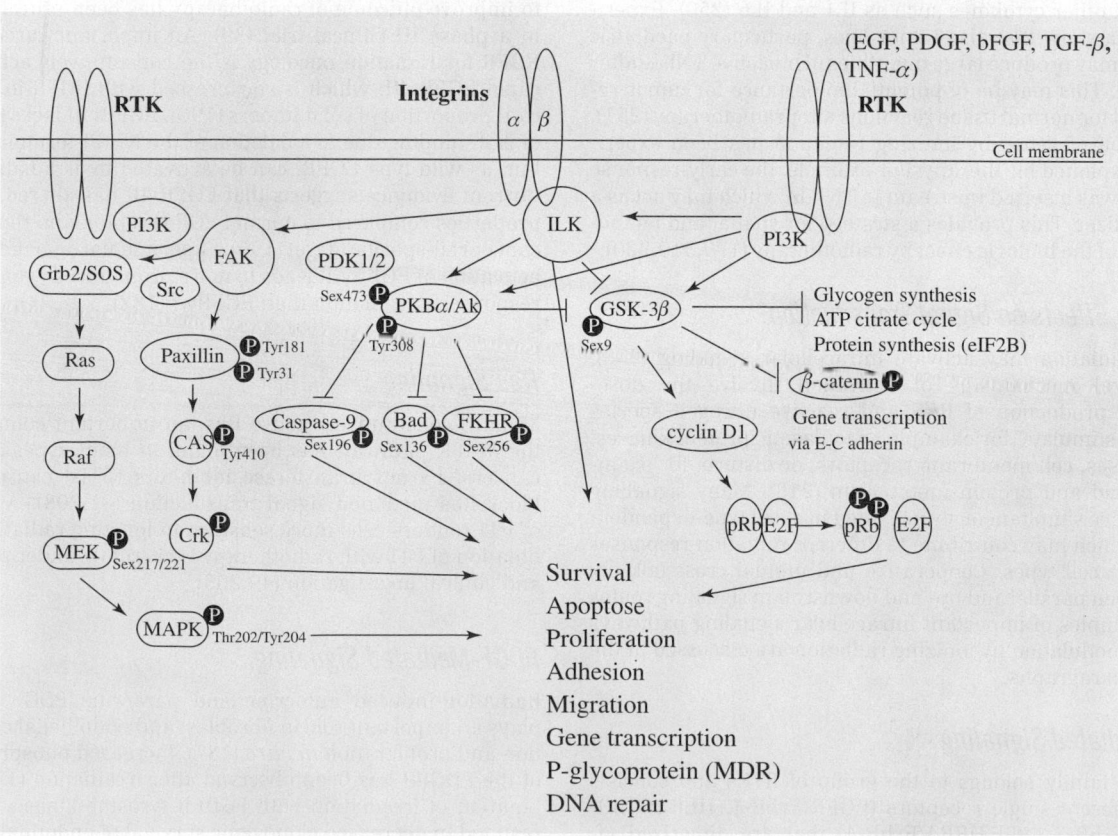

FIGURE 3.6. Cross-talk between receptor tyrosine kinase (RTK) and integrin-mediated signaling.

integrins that exert survival advantage on treatment with geno-toxic agents included regulation of the proapoptotic proteins Bim and Bax (77,142) and the antiapoptotic Bcl-2-like proteins or Bcl-2/Bax ratio (76). In addition to regulating cell survival, cell-matrix interactions impact on radiation-induced cell cycle arrest, that is, adhesion of cells to matrix proteins prolongs the G1- and G2 cell cycle blockage in parallel to enhanced activation of DNA repair pathways involving the checkpoint kinase Chk1 and Chk2, Cdk1, p53, and diverse cyclins (67,88,121,177).

Following radiation exposure, the expression of several integrin subunits including $\beta1$, $\beta3$, $\alpha5$, and αv, is up-regulated in human skin and lung fibroblasts (65), endothelial cells, and keratinocytes (209), as well as in tumor cells of the colon, hematopoetic cells (92), prostate (275), lung (63), brain (64), and melanomas (65). Integrin-mediated adhesion to matrix proteins does not always cause chemo- or radioresistance but, in some tumor lines, also may promote apoptosis (9,186).

Mutagenesis and Genomic Instability

Cells may survive radiation despite unrepaired or misrepaired DNA-damage, that is, with mutations or chromosomal aberrations. These may remain silent or result in radiation-related secondary primary cancers or, as germline mutations, cause hereditary disease (8,40,131,192,285,287). In addition to directly induced mutations, radiation may induce a heritable, genome-wide process of instability (i.e., genomic instability) that leads to an enhanced frequency of genetic changes occurring among the progeny of the original irradiated cell, which is transmissible over many generations of cell replication (192). Whereas most mutations induced directly by radiation involve loss of large parts of the tested gene leading to a loss of heterozygosity, most mutations resulting from radiation-induced genomic instability involve point mutations and small deletions (192,288). While some studies, particularly on thyroid cancer in children after the Chernobyl fallout, suggest a nonrandom pattern of chromosomal damage, generally no fingerprint alterations have been identified that would unequivocally indicate radiation-induced cancer (287).

References

1. Abdollahi A, Li M, Ping G, et al. Inhibition of platelet-derived growth factor signaling attenuates pulmonary fibrosis. *J Exp Med* 2005;201:925–935.
2. Abdollahi A, Lipson KE, Han X, et al. SU5416 and SU6668 attenuate the angiogenic effects of radiation-induced tumor cell growth factor production and amplify the direct anti-endothelial action of radiation in vitro. *Cancer Res* 2003;63:3755–3763.
3. Abraham RT. Cell cycle checkpoint signaling through the ATM and ATR kinases. *Genes Dev* 2001;15:2177–2196.
4. Adams PD. Regulation of the retinoblastoma tumor suppressor protein by cyclin/cdks. *Biochim Biophys Acta* 2001;1471:M123–133.
5. Akyuz N, Boehden GS, Susse S, et al. DNA substrate dependence of p53-mediated regulation of double-strand break repair. *Mol Cell Biol* 2002;22:6306–6317.
6. Al-Hajj M, Wicha MS, Benito-Hernandez A, et al. Prospective identification of tumorigenic breast cancer cells. *Proc Natl Acad Sci U S A* 2003;100:3983–3988.
7. Alarcon-Vargas D, Ronai Z. p53-Mdm2–the affair that never ends. *Carcinogenesis* 2002;23:541–547.
8. Allan JM, Travis LB. Mechanisms of therapy-related carcinogenesis. *Nat Rev Cancer* 2005;5:943–955.
9. Andjilani M, Droz JP, Benahmed M, et al. Alpha6 integrin subunit mediates laminin enhancement of cisplatin-induced apoptosis in testicular tumor germ cells. *Int J Cancer* 2005;117:68–81.
10. Angel P, Karin M. The role of Jun, Fos and the AP-1 complex in cell-proliferation and transformation. *Biochim Biophys Acta* 1991;1072:129–157.
11. Anscher MS, Kong FM, Murase T, et al. Short communication: normal tissue injury after cancer therapy is a local response exacerbated by an endocrine effect of TGF beta. *Br J Radiol* 1995;68:331–333.
12. Aoudjit F, Vuori K. Integrin signaling inhibits paclitaxel-induced apoptosis in breast cancer cells. *Oncogene* 2001;20:4995–5004.
13. Augustin HG. Tubes, branches, and pillars: the many ways of forming a new vasculature. *Circ Res* 2001;89:645–647.
14. Barcellos-Hoff MH. Integrative radiation carcinogenesis: interactions between cell and tissue responses to DNA damage. *Semin Cancer Biol* 2005;15:138–148.
15. Barcellos-Hoff MH, Park C, Wright EG. Radiation and the microenvironment—tumorigenesis and therapy. *Nat Rev Cancer* 2005;5:867–875.
16. Bartek J, Lukas J. Mammalian G1- and S-phase checkpoints in response to DNA damage. *Curr Opin Cell Biol* 2001;13:738–747.
17. Baselga J, Arteaga CL. Critical update and emerging trends in epidermal growth factor receptor targeting in cancer. *J Clin Oncol* 2005;23:2445–2459.
18. Baumann M, Bentzen SM, Doerr W, et al. The translational research chain: is it delivering the goods? *Int J Radiat Oncol Biol Phys* 2001;49:345–351.
19. Baumann M, Dorr W, Petersen C, et al. Repopulation during fractionated radiotherapy: much has been learned, even more is open. *Int J Radiat Biol* 2003;79:465–467.
20. Baumann M, Krause M. Targeting the epidermal growth factor receptor in radiotherapy: radiobiological mechanisms, preclinical and clinical results. *Radiother Oncol* 2004;72:257–266.
21. Baumann M, Krause M, Zips D, et al. Molecular targeting in radiotherapy of lung cancer. *Lung Cancer* 2004;45[Suppl 2]:S187–197.
22. Baylin SB, Ohm JE. Epigenetic gene silencing in cancer—a mechanism for early oncogenic pathway addiction? *Nat Rev Cancer* 2006;6:107–116.
23. Beeram M, Patnaik A, Rowinsky EK. Raf: a strategic target for therapeutic development against cancer. *J Clin Oncol* 2005;23:6771–6790.
24. Behrens J, Lustig B. The Wnt connection to tumorigenesis. *Int J Dev Biol* 2004;48:477–487.
25. Belka C, Budach W. Anti-apoptotic Bcl-2 proteins: structure, function and relevance for radiation biology. *Int J Radiat Biol* 2002;78:643–658.
26. Benhamou S, Sarasin A. Variability in nucleotide excision repair and cancer risk: a review. *Mutat Res* 2000;462:149–158.
27. Bennett RA, Wilson DM, 3rd, Wong D, et al. Interaction of human apurinic endonuclease and DNA polymerase beta in the base excision repair pathway. *Proc Natl Acad Sci U S A* 1997;94:7166–7169.
28. Bentzen SM. Theragnostic imaging for radiation oncology: dose-painting by numbers. *Lancet Oncol* 2005;6:112–117.
29. Bentzen SM, Atasoy BM, Daley FM, et al. Epidermal growth factor receptor expression in pretreatment biopsies from head and neck squamous cell carcinoma as a predictive factor for a benefit from accelerated radiation therapy in a randomized controlled trial. *J Clin Oncol* 2005;23:5560–5567.
30. Bergers G, Benjamin LE. Tumorigenesis and the angiogenic switch. *Nat Rev Cancer* 2003;3:401–410.
31. Bernhard EJ, Kao G, Cox AD, et al. The farnesyltransferase inhibitor FTI-277 radiosensitizes H-ras-transformed rat embryo fibroblasts. *Cancer Res* 1996;56:1727–1730.
32. Bertino J. *Encyclopedia of Cancer*. Academic Press, 2002.
33. Bienz M. The subcellular destinations of APC proteins. *Nat Rev Mol Cell Biol* 2002;3:328–338.
34. Bjerkvig R, Tysnes BB, Aboody KS, et al. Opinion: the origin of the cancer stem cell: current controversies and new insights. *Nat Rev Cancer* 2005;5:899–904.
35. Bjornsti MA, Houghton PJ. The TOR pathway: a target for cancer therapy. *Nat Rev Cancer* 2004;4:335–348.
36. Blasco MA. Telomeres and human disease: ageing, cancer and beyond. *Nat Rev Genet* 2005;6:611–622.
37. Blume-Jensen P, Hunter T. Oncogenic kinase signalling. *Nature* 2001;411:355–365.
38. Bonner JA, De Los Santos J, Waksal HW, et al. Epidermal growth factor receptor as a therapeutic target in head and neck cancer. *Semin Radiat Oncol* 2002;12:11–20.
39. Bonner JA, Harari PM, Giralt J, et al. Radiotherapy plus cetuximab for squamous-cell carcinoma of the head and neck. *N Engl J Med* 2006;354:567–578.
40. Bouffler SD, Bridges BA, Cooper DN, et al. Assessing radiation-associated mutational risk to the germline: repetitive DNA sequences as mutational targets and biomarkers. *Radiat Res* 2006;165:249–268.
41. Brach MA, Hass R, Sherman ML, et al. Ionizing radiation induces expression and binding activity of the nuclear factor kappa B. *J Clin Invest* 1991;88:691–695.
42. Brakebusch C, Fassler R. The integrin-actin connection, an eternal love affair. *Embo J* 2003;22:2324–2333.
43. Breier G, Blum S, Peli J, et al. Transforming growth factor-beta and Ras regulate the VEGF/VEGF-receptor system during tumor angiogenesis. *Int J Cancer* 2002;97:142–148.
44. Bremer C, Ntziachristos V, Weissleder R. Optical-based molecular imaging: contrast agents and potential medical applications. *Eur Radiol* 2003;13:231–243.
45. Brown JM, Attardi LD. The role of apoptosis in cancer development and treatment response. *Nat Rev Cancer* 2005;5:231–237.
46. Brown JM, Wilson G. Apoptosis genes and resistance to cancer therapy: what does the experimental and clinical data tell us? *Cancer Biol Ther* 2003;2:477–490.
47. Brown JM, Wouters BG. Apoptosis, p53, and tumor cell sensitivity to anticancer agents. *Cancer Res* 1999;59:1391–1399.
48. Brown K, Franzoso G, Baldi L, et al. The signal response of IkappaB alpha is regulated by transferable N- and C-terminal domains. *Mol Cell Biol* 1997;17:3021–3027.
49. Brunner TB, Hahn SM, Gupta AK, et al. Farnesyltransferase inhibitors: an overview of the results of preclinical and clinical investigations. *Cancer Res* 2003;63:5656–5668.
50. Carmeliet P. Angiogenesis in health and disease. *Nat Med* 2003;9:653–660.
51. Cavallaro U, Christofori G. Cell adhesion and signalling by cadherins and Ig-CAMs in cancer. *Nat Rev Cancer* 2004;4:118–132.
52. Chariot A, Princen F, Gielen J, et al. IkappaBalpha enhances transactivation by the HOXB7 homeodomain-containing protein. *J Biol Chem* 1999;274:5318–5325.
53. Chinnaiyan P, Allen GW, Harari PM. Radiation and new molecular agents, part II: targeting HDAC, HSP90, IGF-1R, PI3K, and Ras. *Semin Radiat Oncol* 2006;16:59–64.
54. Choudhury A, Cuddihy A, Bristow RG. Radiation and new molecular agents part I: targeting ATM-ATR checkpoints, DNA repair, and the proteasome. *Semin Radiat Oncol* 2006;16:51–58.
55. Christmann M, Tomicic MT, Roos WP, et al. Mechanisms of human DNA repair: an update. *Toxicology* 2003;193:3–34.
56. Chudnovsky Y, Adams AE, Robbins PB, et al. Use of human tissue to assess the oncogenic activity of melanoma-associated mutations. *Nat Genet* 2005;37:745–749.
57. Cichowski K, Jacks T. NF1 tumor suppressor gene function: narrowing the GAP. *Cell* 2001;104:593–604.
58. Coleman CN. Linking radiation oncology and imaging through molecular biology (or now that therapy and diagnosis have separated, it's time to get together again!). *Radiology* 2003;228:29–35.

59. Coleman CN. Molecular biology in radiation oncology. Radiation oncology perspective of BRCA1 and BRCA2. *Acta Oncol* 1999;38[Suppl 13]:55–59.

60. Coleman CN, Stevenson MA. Biologic basis for radiation oncology. *Oncology (Williston Park)* 1996;10:399–411; Discussion: 395–411.

61. Colevas AD, Brown JM, Hahn S, et al. Development of investigational radiation modifiers. *J Natl Cancer Inst* 2003;95:646–651.

62. Cordes N, Beinke C, Plasswilm L, et al. Irradiation and various cytotoxic drugs enhance tyrosine phosphorylation and beta(1)-integrin clustering in human A549 lung cancer cells in a substratum-dependent manner in vitro. *Strahlenther Onkol* 2004;180:157–164.

63. Cordes N, Blaese MA, Meineke V, et al. Ionizing radiation induces up-regulation of functional beta1-integrin in human lung tumour cell lines in vitro. *Int J Radiat Biol* 2002;78:347–357.

64. Cordes N, Hansmeier B, Beinke C, et al. Irradiation differentially affects substratum-dependent survival, adhesion, and invasion of glioblastoma cell lines. *Br J Cancer* 2003;89:2122–2132.

65. Cordes N, Meineke V. Cell adhesion-mediated radioresistance (CAM-RR). Extracellular matrix-dependent improvement of cell survival in human tumor and normal cells in vitro. *Strahlenther Onkol* 2003;179:337–344.

66. Cordes N, Seidler J, Durzok R, et al. Beta1-integrin-mediated signaling essentially contributes to cell survival after radiation-induced genotoxic injury. *Oncogene* 2006;25:1378–1390.

67. Cordes N, van Beuningen D. Arrest of human lung fibroblasts in G2 phase after irradiation is regulated by converging phosphatidylinositol-3 kinase and beta1-integrin signaling in vitro. *Int J Radiat Oncol Biol Phys* 2004;58:453–462.

68. Cowgill SM, Muscarella P. The genetics of pancreatic cancer. *Am J Surg* 2003;186:279–286.

69. Crocker J. Demystified. Molecular pathology in oncology. *Mol Pathol* 2002;55:337–347.

70. Cross MJ, Dixelius J, Matsumoto T, et al. VEGF-receptor signal transduction. *Trends Biochem Sci* 2003;28:488–494.

71. D'Andrea AD, Grompe M. The Fanconi anaemia/BRCA pathway. *Nat Rev Cancer* 2003;3:23–34.

72. Daboussi F, Dumay A, Delacote F, et al. DNA double-strand break repair signalling: the case of RAD51 post-translational regulation. *Cell Signal* 2002;14:969–975.

73. Dahm-Daphi J, Dikomey E, Brammer I. DNA-repair, cell killing and normal tissue damage. *Strahlenther Onkol* 1998;174[Suppl 3]:8–11.

74. Dahm-Daphi J, Hubbe P, Horvath F, et al. Nonhomologous end-joining of site-specific but not of radiation-induced DNA double-strand breaks is reduced in the presence of wild-type p53. *Oncogene* 2005;24:1663–1672.

75. Daido S, Yamamoto A, Fujiwara K, et al. Inhibition of the DNA-dependent protein kinase catalytic subunit radiosensitizes malignant glioma cells by inducing autophagy. *Cancer Res* 2005;65:4368–4375.

76. Damiano JS, Cress AE, Hazlehurst LA, et al. Cell adhesion mediated drug resistance (CAM-DR): role of integrins and resistance to apoptosis in human myeloma cell lines. *Blood* 1999;93:1658–1667.

77. Damiano JS, Hazlehurst LA, Dalton WS. Cell adhesion-mediated drug resistance (CAM-DR) protects the K562 chronic myelogenous leukemia cell line from apoptosis induced by BCR/ABL inhibition, cytotoxic drugs, and gamma-irradiation. *Leukemia* 2001;15:1232–1239.

78. Danen EH. Integrins. regulators of tissue function and cancer progression. *Curr Pharm Des* 2005;11:881–891.

79. Darnell JE Jr. Transcription factors as targets for cancer therapy. *Nat Rev Cancer* 2002;2:740–749.

80. Datta R, Hallahan DE, Kharbanda SM, et al. Involvement of reactive oxygen intermediates in the induction of c-jun gene transcription by ionizing radiation. *Biochemistry* 1992;31:8300–8306.

81. De Giorgi U, Verweij J. Imatinib and gastrointestinal stromal tumors: where do we go from here? *Mol Cancer Ther* 2005;4:495–501.

82. Denekamp J. Cell kinetics and radiation biology. *Int J Radiat Biol Relat Stud Phys Chem Med* 1986;49:357–380.

83. Dent P, Reardon DB, Park JS, et al. Radiation-induced release of transforming growth factor alpha activates the epidermal growth factor receptor and mitogen-activated protein kinase pathway in carcinoma cells, leading to increased proliferation and protection from radiation-induced cell death. *Mol Biol Cell* 1999;10:2493–2506.

84. Dent P, Yacoub A, Fisher PB, et al. MAPK pathways in radiation responses. *Oncogene* 2003;22:5885–5896.

85. Derynck R, Zhang YE. Smad-dependent and Smad-independent pathways in TGF-beta family signalling. *Nature* 2003;425:577–584.

86. Devary Y, Rosette C, DiDonato JA, et al. NF-kappa B activation by ultraviolet light not dependent on a nuclear signal. *Science* 1993;261:1442–1445.

87. DiDonato JA, Hayakawa M, Rothwarf DM, et al. A cytokine-responsive IkappaB kinase that activates the transcription factor NF-kappaB. *Nature* 1997;388:548–554.

88. Dimitrijevic-Bussod M, Balzaretti-Maggi VS, Gadbois DM. Extracellular matrix and radiation G1 cell cycle arrest in human fibroblasts. *Cancer Res* 1999;59:4843–4847.

89. Dincbas FO, Koca S, Mandel NM, et al. The role of preoperative radiotherapy in nonmetastatic high-grade osteosarcoma of the extremities for limb-sparing surgery. *Int J Radiat Oncol Biol Phys* 2005;62:820–828.

90. Dittmann K, Mayer C, Fehrenbacher B, et al. Radiation-induced epidermal growth factor receptor nuclear import is linked to activation of DNA-dependent protein kinase. *J Biol Chem* 2005;280:31182–31189.

91. Dittmann K, Mayer C, Rodemann HP. Inhibition of radiation-induced EGFR nuclear import by C225 (Cetuximab) suppresses DNA-PK activity. *Radiother Oncol* 2005;76:157–161.

92. Dong L, Sun H, Liu W, et al. Effect of ligustrazine on expression of adherent molecule CD49d and cyclin D2 in hematopoietic cells in acute radiation injured mice. *J Tongji Med Univ* 1999;19:99–101.

93. Dorr W, Reichel S, Spekl K. Effects of keratinocyte growth factor (palifermin) administration protocols on oral mucositis (mouse) induced by fractionated irradiation. *Radiother Oncol* 2005;75:99–105.

94. Dumaz N, Meek DW. Serine15 phosphorylation stimulates p53 transactivation but does not directly influence interaction with HDM2. *Embo J* 1999;18:7002–7010.

95. Dvorak HF. Angiogenesis: update 2005. *J Thromb Haemost* 2005;3:1835–1842.

96. Dyson N. The regulation of E2F by pRB-family proteins. *Genes Dev* 1998;12:2245–2262.

97. Eckstein R, Lilley DMJ. *DNA Repair*. Berlin and Heidelberg, Springer, 1998.

98. Edlund M, Miyamoto T, Sikes RA, et al. Integrin expression and usage by prostate cancer cell lines on laminin substrata. *Cell Growth Differ* 2001;12:99–107.

99. Eferl R, Wagner EF. AP-1: a double-edged sword in tumorigenesis. *Nat Rev Cancer* 2003;3:859–868.

100. Egan LJ, Eckmann L, Greten FR, et al. IkappaB-kinasebeta-dependent NF-kappaB activation provides radioprotection to the intestinal epithelium. *Proc Natl Acad Sci U S A* 2004;101:2452–2457.

101. Egeblad M, Werb Z. New functions for the matrix metalloproteinases in cancer progression. *Nat Rev Cancer* 2002;2:161–174.

102. Eriksen JG, Steiniche T, Overgaard J. The influence of epidermal growth factor receptor and tumor differentiation on the response to accelerated radiotherapy of squamous cell carcinomas of the head and neck in the randomized DAHANCA 6 and 7 study. *Radiother Oncol* 2005;74:93–100.

103. Falck J, Mailand N, Syljuasen RG, et al. The ATM-Chk2-Cdc25A checkpoint pathway guards against radioresistant DNA synthesis. *Nature* 2001;410:842–847.

104. Fearon ER, Gruber SB. Molecular Abnormalities in colon and rectal cancer. In: Mendelsohn J, Howley PM, Israel MA, et al., eds. *The molecular basis of cancer*. Philadelphia: Saunders, 2001:289–312.

105. Fearon ER, Vogelstein B. A genetic model for colorectal tumorigenesis. *Cell* 1990;61:759–767.

106. Ferrara N, Gerber HP, LeCouter J. The biology of VEGF and its receptors. *Nat Med* 2003;9:669–676.

107. Ferrara N, Kerbel RS. Angiogenesis as a therapeutic target. *Nature* 2005;438:967–974.

108. Fidler IJ. The pathogenesis of cancer metastasis: the 'seed and soil' hypothesis revisited. *Nat Rev Cancer* 2003;3:453–458.

109. Fischer U, Janicke RU, Schulze-Osthoff K. Many cuts to ruin: a comprehensive update of caspase substrates. *Cell Death Differ* 2003;10:76–100.

110. Folkman J. Tumor angiogenesis: therapeutic implications. *N Engl J Med* 1971;285:1182–1186.

111. Folkman J. Role of angiogenesis in tumor growth and metastasis. *Semin Oncol* 2002;29:15–18.

112. Forrester HB, Vidair CA, Albright N, et al. Using computerized video time lapse for quantifying cell death of X-irradiated rat embryo cells transfected with c-myc or c-Ha-ras. *Cancer Res* 1999;59:931–939.

113. Frankenberg-Schwager M. Review of repair kinetics for DNA damage induced in eukaryotic cells in vitro by ionizing radiation. *Radiother Oncol* 1989;14:307–320.

114. Franzoso G, Biswas P, Poli G, et al. A family of serine proteases expressed exclusively in myelo-monocytic cells specifically processes the nuclear factor-kappa B subunit p65 in vitro and may impair human immunodeficiency virus replication in these cells. *J Exp Med* 1994;180:1445–1456.

115. Franzoso G, Carlson L, Poljak L, et al. Mice deficient in nuclear factor (NF)-kappa B/p52 present with defects in humoral responses, germinal center reactions, and splenic microarchitecture. *J Exp Med* 1998;187:147–159.

116. Freireich EJ, Stass SA. *Molecular basis of oncology*. Blackwell Science, Cambridge, 1995.

117. Fresno Vara JA, Casado E, de Castro J, et al. PI3K/Akt signalling pathway and cancer. *Cancer Treat Rev* 2004;30:193–204.

118. Fridman R, Giaccone G, Kanemoto T, et al. Reconstituted basement membrane (matrigel) and laminin can enhance the tumorigenicity and the drug resistance of small cell lung cancer cell lines. *Proc Natl Acad Sci U S A* 1990;87:6698–6702.

119. Fuks Z, Persaud RS, Alfieri A, et al. Basic fibroblast growth factor protects endothelial cells against radiation-induced programmed cell death in vitro and in vivo. *Cancer Res* 1994;54:2582–2590.

120. Futreal PA, Coin L, Marshall M, et al. A census of human cancer genes. *Nat Rev Cancer* 2004;4:177–183.

121. Gadbois DM, Bradbury EM, Lehnert BE. Control of radiation-induced G1 arrest by cell-substratum interactions. *Cancer Res* 1997;57:1151–1156.

122. Gorski DH, Beckett MA, Jaskowiak NT, et al. Blockage of the vascular endothelial growth factor stress response increases the antitumor effects of ionizing radiation. *Cancer Res* 1999;59:3374–3378.

123. Grade M, Becker H, Ghadimi BM. The impact of molecular pathology in oncology: the clinician's perspective. *Cell Oncol* 2004;26:275–278.

124. Grandis JR, Drenning SD, Chakraborty A, et al. Requirement of Stat3 but not Stat1 activation for epidermal growth factor receptor-mediated cell growth In vitro. *J Clin Invest* 1998;102:1385–1392.

125. Grassmann R, Aboud M, Jeang KT. Molecular mechanisms of cellular transformation by HTLV-1 Tax. *Oncogene* 2005;24:5976–5985.

126. Gray LH, Conger AD, Ebert M, et al. The concentration of oxygen dissolved in tissues at the time of irradiation as a factor in radiotherapy. *Br J Radiol* 1953;26:638–648.

127. Grompe M, D'Andrea A. Fanconi anemia and DNA repair. *Hum Mol Genet* 2001;10:2253–2259.

128. Haase MG, Klawitter A, Geyer P, et al. Sustained elevation of NF-KappaB DNA binding activity in radiation-induced lung damage in rats. *Int J Radiat Biol* 2003;79:863–877.

129. Hacker H, Redecke V, Blagoev B, et al. Specificity in Toll-like receptor signalling through distinct effector functions of TRAF3 and TRAF6. *Nature* 2006;439:204–207.

130. Haimovitz-Friedman A, Kan CC, Ehleiter D, et al. Ionizing radiation acts on cellular membranes to generate ceramide and initiate apoptosis. *J Exp Med* 1994;180:525–535.

131. Hall EJ. Intensity-modulated radiation therapy, protons, and the risk of second cancers. *Int J Radiat Oncol Biol Phys* 2006;65:1–7.

132. Hallahan DE, Spriggs DR, Beckett MA, et al. Increased tumor necrosis factor alpha mRNA after cellular exposure to ionizing radiation. *Proc Natl Acad Sci U S A* 1989;86:10104–10107.

133. Hallahan DE, Sukhatme VP, Sherman ML, et al. Protein kinase C mediates x-ray inducibility of nuclear signal transducers EGR1 and JUN. *Proc Natl Acad Sci U S A* 1991;88:2156–2160.

134. Hanahan D. Signaling vascular morphogenesis and maintenance. *Science* 1997;277:48–50.

135. Hanahan D, Weinberg RA. The hallmarks of cancer. *Cell* 2000;100:57–70.

136. Harari PM, Huang S. Radiation combined with EGFR signal inhibitors: head and neck cancer focus. *Semin Radiat Oncol* 2006;16:38–44.
137. Hauer-Jensen M, Richter KK, Wang J, et al. Changes in transforming growth factor beta1 gene expression and immunoreactivity levels during development of chronic radiation enteropathy. *Radiat Res* 1998;150:673–680.
138. Haverkos HW. Viruses, chemicals and co-carcinogenesis. *Oncogene* 2004;23: 6492–6499.
139. Hayflick L. The illusion of cell immortality. *Br J Cancer* 2000;83:841–846.
140. Hazan RB, Qiao R, Keren R, et al. Cadherin switch in tumor progression. *Ann N Y Acad Sci* 2004;1014:155–163.
141. Hazlehurst LA, Dalton WS. Mechanisms associated with cell adhesion mediated drug resistance (CAM-DR) in hematopoietic malignancies. *Cancer Metastasis Rev* 2001;20:43–50.
142. Hazlehurst LA, Damiano JS, Buyuksal I, et al. Adhesion to fibronectin via beta1 integrins regulates p27kip1 levels and contributes to cell adhesion mediated drug resistance (CAM-DR). *Oncogene* 2000;19:4319–4327.
143. Hernando E, Nahle Z, Juan G, et al. Rb inactivation promotes genomic instability by uncoupling cell cycle progression from mitotic control. *Nature* 2004;430:797–802.
144. Herrlich P, Morrison H, Sleeman J, et al. CD44 acts both as a growth- and invasiveness-promoting molecule and as a tumor-suppressing cofactor. *Ann N Y Acad Sci* 2000;910:106–118; Discussion 118–120.
145. Herschman HR. Non-invasive imaging of reporter genes. *J Cell Biochem Suppl* 2002;39:36–44.
146. Hill RP, Rodemann HP, Hendry JH, et al. Normal tissue radiobiology: from the laboratory to the clinic. *Int J Radiat Oncol Biol Phys* 2001;49:353–365.
147. Hirao A, Kong YY, Matsuoka S, et al. DNA damage-induced activation of p53 by the checkpoint kinase Chk2. *Science* 2000;287:1824–1827.
148. Hojilla CV, Mohammed FF, Khokha R. Matrix metalloproteinases and their tissue inhibitors direct cell fate during cancer development. *Br J Cancer* 2003;89:1817–1821.
149. Hooper JE, Scott MP. Communicating with hedgehogs. *Nat Rev Mol Cell Biol* 2005;6:306–317.
150. Huang SS, Huang JS. TGF-beta control of cell proliferation. *J Cell Biochem* 2005;96:447–462.
151. Hunter K. Host genetics influence tumour metastasis. *Nat Rev Cancer* 2006;6:141–146.
152. Hynes NE, Lane HA. ERBB receptors and cancer: the complexity of targeted inhibitors. *Nat Rev Cancer* 2005;5:341–354.
153. Hynes RO. Integrins: versatility, modulation, and signaling in cell adhesion. *Cell* 1992;69:11–25.
154. Hynes RO. Integrins: bidirectional, allosteric signaling machines. *Cell* 2002;110: 673–687.
155. Iliakis G, Wang H, Perrault AR, et al. Mechanisms of DNA double strand break repair and chromosome aberration formation. *Cytogenet Genome Res* 2004;104:14–20.
156. Jaal J, Dorr W. Radiation induced inflammatory changes in the mouse bladder: the role of cyclooxygenase-2. *J Urol* 2006;175:1529–1533.
157. Jain RK. Molecular regulation of vessel maturation. *Nat Med* 2003;9:685–693.
158. Janes SM, Watt FM. New roles for integrins in squamous-cell carcinoma. *Nat Rev Cancer* 2006;6:175–183.
159. Jeggo PA, Lobrich M. Artemis links ATM to double strand break rejoining. *Cell Cycle* 2005;4:359–362.
160. Jung M, Kondratyev A, Lee SA, et al. ATM gene product phosphorylates I kappa B-alpha. *Cancer Res* 1997;57:24–27.
161. Kamata H, Honda S, Maeda S, et al. Reactive oxygen species promote TNFalpha-induced death and sustained JNK activation by inhibiting MAP kinase phosphatases. *Cell* 2005;120:649–661.
162. Kaplan RN, Riba RD, Zacharoulis S, et al. VEGFR1-positive haematopoietic bone marrow progenitors initiate the pre-metastatic niche. *Nature* 2005;438:820–827.
163. Karim R, Tse G, Putti T, et al. The significance of the Wnt pathway in the pathology of human cancers. *Pathology* 2004;36:120–128.
164. Karin M, Cao Y, Greten FR, et al. NF-kappaB in cancer: from innocent bystander to major culprit. *Nat Rev Cancer* 2002;2:301–310.
165. Kelley MJ, Johnson BE. Molecular biology of lung cancer. In: Mendelsohn J, Howley PM, Israel MA, et al., eds. *The molecular basis of cancer*. Philadelphia: Saunders, 2001:260–287.
166. Kelloff GJ, Krohn KA, Larson SM, et al. The progress and promise of molecular imaging probes in oncologic drug development. *Clin Cancer Res* 2005;11:7967–7985.
167. Kermani P, Leclerc G, Martel R, et al. Effect of ionizing radiation on thymidine uptake, differentiation, and VEGFR2 receptor expression in endothelial cells: the role of VEGF(165). *Int J Radiat Oncol Biol Phys* 2001;50:213–220.
168. Khanna KK, Lavin MF, Jackson SP, et al. ATM, a central controller of cellular responses to DNA damage. *Cell Death Differ* 2001;8:1052–1065.
169. Kharas MG, Fruman DA. ABL oncogenes and phosphoinositide 3-kinase: mechanism of activation and downstream effectors. *Cancer Res* 2005;65: 2047–2053.
170. Kim ST, Xu B, Kastan MB. Involvement of the cohesin protein, Smc1, in Atm-dependent and independent responses to DNA damage. *Genes Dev* 2002;16:560–570.
171. Knudson AG. Two genetic hits (more or less) to cancer. *Nat Rev Cancer* 2001;1:157–162.
172. Kolesnick R, Fuks Z. Radiation and ceramide-induced apoptosis. *Oncogene* 2003;22:5897–5906.
173. Kovacs EJ. Fibrogenic cytokines: the role of immune mediators in the development of scar tissue. *Immunology Today* 1991;12:17–23.
174. Kovacs EJ, DiPietro LA. Fibrogenic cytokines and connective tissue production. *Faseb J* 1994;8:854–861.
175. Krause M, Ostermann G, Petersen C, et al. Decreased repopulation as well as increased reoxygenation contribute to the improvement in local control after targeting of the EGFR by C225 during fractionated irradiation. *Radiother Oncol* 2005.
176. Krause M, Schutze C, Petersen C, et al. Different classes of EGFR inhibitors may have different potential to improve local tumour control after fractionated irradiation: a study on C225 in FaDu hSCC. *Radiother Oncol* 2005;74:109–115.
177. Kremer CL, Schmelz M, Cress AE. Integrin-dependent amplification of the G2 arrest induced by ionizing radiation. *Prostate* 2006;66:88–96.
178. Kubota Y, Nash RA, Klungland A, et al. Reconstitution of DNA base excision-repair with purified human proteins: interaction between DNA polymerase beta and the XRCC1 protein. *Embo J* 1996;15:6662–6670.
179. Kufe D, Weichselbaum R. Radiation therapy: activation for gene transcription and the development of genetic radiotherapy-therapeutic strategies in oncology. *Cancer Biol Ther* 2003;2:326–329.
180. Kufe D, Bast R, Hait W, et al. *Cancer Medicine 7*. BC Becker, Ontario, 2006.
181. Kummermehr J, Trott KR. Tumour stem cells. In: Potten CS, ed. *Stem cells*. London: Academic Press, 1997:363–399.
182. Lammering G, Hewit TH, Valerie K, et al. EGFRvIII-mediated radioresistance through a strong cytoprotective response. *Oncogene* 2003;22:5545–5553.
183. Lavin MF. The Mre11 complex and ATM: a two-way functional interaction in recognising and signaling DNA double strand breaks. *DNA Repair (Amst)* 2004;3:1515–1520.
184. Leach JK, Black SM, Schmidt-Ullrich RK, et al. Activation of constitutive nitric-oxide synthase activity is an early signaling event induced by ionizing radiation. *J Biol Chem* 2002;277:15400–15406.
185. Lee JW, Juliano R. Mitogenic signal transduction by integrin- and growth factor receptor-mediated pathways. *Mol Cells* 2004;17:188–202.
186. Lewis JM, Truong TN, Schwartz MA. Integrins regulate the apoptotic response to DNA damage through modulation of p53. *Proc Natl Acad Sci U S A* 2002;99:3627–3632.
187. Li M, Gong P, Plathow C, et al. Small molecule receptor tyrosine kinase inhibitor of platelet-derived growth factor signaling (SU9518) modifies radiation response in fibroblasts and endothelial cells. *BMC Cancer* 2006;6:79.
188. Li N, Banin S, Ouyang H, et al. ATM is required for IkappaB kinase (IKKk) activation in response to DNA double strand breaks. *J Biol Chem* 2001;276:8898–8903.
189. Liao Z, Komaki R, Milas L, et al. A phase I clinical trial of thoracic radiotherapy and concurrent celecoxib for patients with unfavorable performance status inoperable/unresectable non-small cell lung cancer. *Clin Cancer Res* 2005;11:3342–3348.
190. Lin SY, Makino K, Xia W, et al. Nuclear localization of EGF receptor and its potential new role as a transcription factor. *Nat Cell Biol* 2001;3:802–808.
191. Lindahl T. Instability and decay of the primary structure of DNA. *Nature* 1993;362:709–715.
192. Little JB. Induction of genetic instability by ionizing radiation. *C R Acad Sci III* 1999;322:127–134.
193. Little JW, Mount DW. The SOS regulatory system of Escherichia coli. *Cell* 1982;29:11–22.
194. Ljungman M, Lane DP. Transcription—guarding the genome by sensing DNA damage. *Nat Rev Cancer* 2004;4:727–737.
195. Lobrich M, Jeggo PA. The two edges of the ATM sword: co-operation between repair and checkpoint functions. *Radiother Oncol* 2005;76:112–118.
196. Lorimer IA. Mutant epidermal growth factor receptors as targets for cancer therapy. *Curr Cancer Drug Targets* 2002;2:91–102.
197. Lou Z, Minter-Dykhouse K, Franco S, et al. MDC1 maintains genomic stability by participating in the amplification of ATM-dependent DNA damage signals. *Mol Cell* 2006;21:187–200.
198. Lynch CC, Matrisian LM. Matrix metalloproteinases in tumor-host cell communication. *Differentiation* 2002;70:561–573.
199. Ma BB, Bristow RG, Kim J, et al. Combined-modality treatment of solid tumors using radiotherapy and molecular targeted agents. *J Clin Oncol* 2003;21:2760–2776.
200. Ma Y, Pannicke U, Lu H, et al. The DNA-dependent protein kinase catalytic subunit phosphorylation sites in human Artemis. *J Biol Chem* 2005;280:33839–33846.
201. Marmor MD, Skaria KB, Yarden Y. Signal transduction and oncogenesis by ErbB/HER receptors. *Int J Radiat Oncol Biol Phys* 2004;58:903–913.
202. Martin M, Lefaix J, Delanian S. TGF-beta1 and radiation fibrosis: a master switch and a specific therapeutic target? *Int J Radiat Oncol Biol Phys* 2000;47:277–290.
203. Martin NE, Brunner TB, Kiel KD, et al. A phase I trial of the dual farnesyltransferase and geranylgeranyltransferase inhibitor L-778,123 and radiotherapy for locally advanced pancreatic cancer. *Clin Cancer Res* 2004;10:5447–5454.
204. Matsumoto Y, Kim K, Hurwitz J, et al. Reconstitution of proliferating cell nuclear antigen-dependent repair of apurinic/apyrimidinic sites with purified human proteins. *J Biol Chem* 1999;274:33703–33708.
205. Maubant S, Cruet-Hennequart S, Poulain L, et al. Altered adhesion properties and alphav integrin expression in a cisplatin-resistant human ovarian carcinoma cell line. *Int J Cancer* 2002;97:186–194.
206. Maya R, Balass M, Kim ST, et al. ATM-dependent phosphorylation of Mdm2 on serine 395: role in p53 activation by DNA damage. *Genes Dev* 2001;15:1067–1077.
207. McKenna WG, Muschel RJ. Targeting tumor cells by enhancing radiation sensitivity. *Genes Chromosomes Cancer* 2003;38:330–338.
208. McKenna WG, Muschel RJ, Gupta AK, et al. The RAS signal transduction pathway and its role in radiation sensitivity. *Oncogene* 2003;22:5866–5875.
209. Meineke V, Muller K, Ridi R, et al. Development and evaluation of a skin organ model for the analysis of radiation effects. *Strahlenther Onkol* 2004;180:102–108.
210. Mendelsohn J, Baselga J. The EGF receptor family as targets for cancer therapy. *Oncogene* 2000;19:6550–6565.
211. Menendez JA, Vellon L, Mehmi I, et al. A novel CYR61-triggered 'CYR61-alphavbeta3 integrin loop' regulates breast cancer cell survival and chemosensitivity through activation of ERK1/ERK2 MAPK signaling pathway. *Oncogene* 2005;24:761–779.
212. Mercurio F, Zhu H, Murray BW, et al. IKK-1 and IKK-2: cytokine-activated IkappaB kinases essential for NF-kappaB activation. *Science* 1997;278:860–866.
213. Mikkelsen RB, Wardman P. Biological chemistry of reactive oxygen and nitrogen and radiation-induced signal transduction mechanisms. *Oncogene* 2003;22:5734–5754.
214. Milas L. Cyclooxygenase-2 (COX-2) enzyme inhibitors as potential enhancers of tumor radioresponse. *Semin Radiat Oncol* 2001;11:290–299.
215. Milas L. Cyclooxygenase-2 (COX-2) enzyme inhibitors and radiotherapy: preclinical basis. *Am J Clin Oncol* 2003;26:S66–69.
216. Milas L, Mason KA, Ang KK. Epidermal growth factor receptor and its inhibition in radiotherapy: in vivo findings. *Int J Radiat Biol* 2003;79:539–545.
217. Miyamoto H, Murakami T, Tsuchida K, et al. Tumor-stroma interaction of human pancreatic cancer: acquired resistance to anticancer drugs and proliferation regulation is dependent on extracellular matrix proteins. *Pancreas* 2004;28:38–44.
218. Munro TR. The relative radiosensitivity of the nucleus and cytoplasm of Chinese hamster fibroblasts. *Radiat Res* 1970;42:451–470.

219. Nguyen DX, McCance DJ. Role of the retinoblastoma tumor suppressor protein in cellular differentiation. *J Cell Biochem* 2005;94:870–879.

220. Niu G, Wright KL, Huang M, et al. Constitutive Stat3 activity up-regulates VEGF expression and tumor angiogenesis. *Oncogene* 2002;21:2000–2008.

221. Nurse P. Universal control mechanism regulating onset of M-phase. *Nature* 1990;344:503–508.

222. O'Driscoll M, Jeggo PA. The role of double-strand break repair—insights from human genetics. *Nat Rev Genet* 2006;7:45–54.

223. O'Reilly MS. Radiation combined with antiangiogenic and antivascular agents. *Semin Radiat Oncol* 2006;16:45–50.

224. Oda K, Matsuoka Y, Funahashi A, et al. A comprehensive pathway map of epidermal growth factor receptor signaling. *Mol Syst Biol* 2005;1:E1–E17.

225. Okada H, Mak TW. Pathways of apoptotic and non-apoptotic death in tumour cells. *Nat Rev Cancer* 2004;4:592–603.

226. Oksvold M, Huitfeldt H, Stang E, et al. Localizing the EGF receptor. *Nat Cell Biol* 2002;4:E22; Author reply E22–23.

227. Orend G. Potential oncogenic action of tenascin-C in tumorigenesis. *Int J Biochem Cell Biol* 2005;37:1066–1083.

228. Paglin S, Hollister T, Delohery T, et al. A novel response of cancer cells to radiation involves autophagy and formation of acidic vesicles. *Cancer Res* 2001;61:439–444.

229. Pardal R, Clarke MF, Morrison SJ. Applying the principles of stem-cell biology to cancer. *Nat Rev Cancer* 2003;3:895–902.

230. Pascucci B, Stucki M, Jonsson ZO, et al. Long patch base excision repair with purified human proteins. DNA ligase I as patch size mediator for DNA polymerases delta and epsilon. *J Biol Chem* 1999;274:33696–33702.

231. Peng A, Chen PL. NFBD1/Mdc1 mediates ATR-dependent DNA damage response. *Cancer Res* 2005;65:1158–1163.

232. Peng CY, Graves PR, Thoma RS, et al. Mitotic and G2 checkpoint control: regulation of 14-3-3 protein binding by phosphorylation of Cdc25C on serine-216. *Science* 1997;277:1501–1505.

233. Perrault R, Wang H, Wang M, et al. Backup pathways of NHEJ are suppressed by DNA-PK. *J Cell Biochem* 2004;92:781–794.

234. Petersen C, Baumann M, Petersen S. New targets for the modulation of radiation response—selective inhibition of the enzyme cyclooxygenase 2. *Curr Med Chem Anticancer Agents* 2003;3:354–359.

235. Piret B, Schoonbroodt S, Piette J. The ATM protein is required for sustained activation of NF-kappaB following DNA damage. *Oncogene* 1999;18:2261–2271.

236. Platanias LC. Mechanisms of type-I- and type-II-interferon-mediated signalling. *Nat Rev Immunol* 2005;5:375–386.

237. Ponder BA. Cancer genetics. *Nature* 2001;411:336–341.

238. Prasad AV, Mohan N, Chandrasekar B, et al. Induction of transcription of "immediate early genes" by low-dose ionizing radiation. *Radiat Res* 1995;143:263–272.

239. Raben D, Bianco C, Milas L, et al. Targeted therapies and radiation for the treatment of head and neck cancer: are we making progress? *Semin Radiat Oncol* 2004;14:139–152.

240. Raju U, Ariga H, Dittmann K, et al. Inhibition of DNA repair as a mechanism of enhanced radioresponse of head and neck carcinoma cells by a selective cyclooxygenase-2 inhibitor, celecoxib. *Int J Radiat Oncol Biol Phys* 2005;63:520–528.

241. Rak J, Yu JL, Kerbel RS, et al. What do oncogenic mutations have to do with angiogenesis/vascular dependence of tumors? *Cancer Res* 2002;62:1931–1934.

242. Rappold I, Iwabuchi K, Date T, et al. Tumor suppressor p53 binding protein 1 (53BP1) is involved in DNA damage-signaling pathways. *J Cell Biol* 2001;153:613–620.

243. Riballo E, Kuhne M, Rief N, et al. A pathway of double-strand break rejoining dependent upon ATM, Artemis, and proteins locating to gamma-H2AX foci. *Mol Cell* 2004;16:715–724.

244. Riedl SJ, Shi Y. Molecular mechanisms of caspase regulation during apoptosis. *Nat Rev Mol Cell Biol* 2004;5:897–907.

245. Rodemann HP. Role of radiation-induced signaling proteins in the response of vascular and connective tissues. In: Milas L, Ang KK, Nieder C, eds. *Biological modification of radiation response*. Berlin: Springer, 2003:15–28.

246. Rodemann HP, Bamberg M. Cellular basis of radiation-induced fibrosis. *Radiother Oncol* 1995;35:83–90.

247. Rohren EM, Turkington TG, Coleman RE. Clinical applications of PET in oncology. *Radiology* 2004;231:305–332.

248. Rothkamm K, Kruger I, Thompson LH, et al. Pathways of DNA double-strand break repair during the mammalian cell cycle. *Mol Cell Biol* 2003;23:5706–5715.

249. Rothwarf DM, Zandi E, Natoli G, et al. IKK-gamma is an essential regulatory subunit of the IkappaB kinase complex. *Nature* 1998;395:297–300.

250. Rube CE, Uthe D, Wilfert F, et al. The bronchiolar epithelium as a prominent source of pro-inflammatory cytokines after lung irradiation. *Int J Radiat Oncol Biol Phys* 2005;61:1482–1492.

251. Rube CE, van Valen F, Wilfert F, et al. Ewing's sarcoma and peripheral primitive neuroectodermal tumor cells produce large quantities of bioactive tumor necrosis factor-alpha (TNF-alpha) after radiation exposure. *Int J Radiat Oncol Biol Phys* 2003;56:1414–1425.

252. Rubin P, Johnston CJ, Williams JP, et al. A perpetual cascade of cytokines postirradiation leads to pulmonary fibrosis. *Int J Radiat Oncol Biol Phys* 1995;33:99–109.

253. Sanchez I, Dynlacht BD. New insights into cyclins, CDKs, and cell cycle control. *Semin Cell Dev Biol* 2005;16:311–321.

254. Sansal I, Sellers WR. The biology and clinical relevance of the PTEN tumor suppressor pathway. *J Clin Oncol* 2004;22:2954–2963.

255. Santana P, Pena LA, Haimovitz-Friedman A, et al. Acid sphingomyelinase-deficient human lymphoblasts and mice are defective in radiation-induced apoptosis. *Cell* 1996;86:189–199.

256. Sarasin A. An overview of the mechanisms of mutagenesis and carcinogenesis. *Mutat Res* 2003;544:99–106.

257. Scharer OD. Chemistry and biology of DNA repair. *Angew Chem Int Ed Engl* 2003;42:2946–2974.

258. Schmidt-Ullrich RK, Dent P, Grant S, et al. Signal transduction and cellular radiation responses. *Radiat Res* 2000;153:245–257.

259. Schmidt-Ullrich RK, Mikkelsen RB, Dent P, et al. Radiation-induced proliferation of the human A431 squamous carcinoma cells is dependent on EGFR tyrosine phosphorylation. *Oncogene* 1997;15:1191–1197.

260. Schmidt-Ullrich RK, Valerie K, Fogleman PB, et al. Radiation-induced autophosphorylation of epidermal growth factor receptor in human malignant mammary and squamous epithelial cells. *Radiat Res* 1996;145:81–85.

261. Schmitt CA. Senescence, apoptosis and therapy—cutting the lifelines of cancer. *Nat Rev Cancer* 2003;3:286–295.

262. Schreck R, Rieber P, Baeuerle PA. Reactive oxygen intermediates as apparently widely used messengers in the activation of the NF-kappa B transcription factor and HIV-1. *Embo J* 1991;10:2247–2258.

263. Seidler J, Durzok R, Brakebusch C, et al. Interactions of the integrin subunit beta1A with protein kinase B/Akt, p130Cas and paxillin contribute to regulation of radiation survival. *Radiother Oncol* 2005;76:129–134.

264. Sellers WR, Kaelin WG Jr. Role of the retinoblastoma protein in the pathogenesis of human cancer. *J Clin Oncol* 1997;15:3301–3312.

265. Semenza GL. Targeting HIF-1 for cancer therapy. *Nat Rev Cancer* 2003;3:721–732.

266. Senftleben U, Karin M. The IKK/NF-kappaB pathway. *Crit Care Med* 2002;30:S18–S26.

267. Sethi T, Rintoul RC, Moore SM, et al. Extracellular matrix proteins protect small cell lung cancer cells against apoptosis: a mechanism for small cell lung cancer growth and drug resistance in vivo. *Nat Med* 1999;5:662–668.

268. Shaulian E, Karin M. AP-1 in cell proliferation and survival. *Oncogene* 2001;20:2390–2400.

269. Shaulian E, Karin M. AP-1 as a regulator of cell life and death. *Nat Cell Biol* 2002;4:E131–136.

270. Sherman ML, Datta R, Hallahan DE, et al. Ionizing radiation regulates expression of the c-jun protooncogene. *Proc Natl Acad Sci U S A* 1990;87:5663–5666.

271. Sherr CJ. The INK4a/ARF network in tumour suppression. *Nat Rev Mol Cell Biol* 2001;2:731–737.

272. Shieh SY, Ahn J, Tamai K, et al. The human homologs of checkpoint kinases Chk1 and Cds1 (Chk2) phosphorylate p53 at multiple DNA damage-inducible sites. *Genes Dev* 2000;14:289–300.

273. Shinomiya N, Kuno Y, Yamamoto F, et al. Different mechanisms between premitotic apoptosis and postmitotic apoptosis in X-irradiated U937 cells. *Int J Radiat Oncol Biol Phys* 2000;47:767–777.

274. Silva CM. Role of STATs as downstream signal transducers in Src family kinase-mediated tumorigenesis. *Oncogene* 2004;23:8017–8023.

275. Simon EL, Goel HL, Teider N, et al. High dose fractionated ionizing radiation inhibits prostate cancer cell adhesion and beta(1) integrin expression. *Prostate* 2005;64:83–91.

276. Soussi T, Lozano G. p53 Mutation heterogeneity in cancer. *Biochem Biophys Res Commun* 2005;331:834–842.

277. Steinauer KK, Gibbs I, Ning S, et al. Radiation induces upregulation of cyclooxygenase-2 (COX-2) protein in PC-3 cells. *Int J Radiat Oncol Biol Phys* 2000;48:325–328.

278. Suzuki K, Mori I, Nakayama Y, et al. Radiation-induced senescence-like growth arrest requires TP53 function but not telomere shortening. *Radiat Res* 2001;155:248–253.

279. Svejstrup JQ. Mechanisms of transcription-coupled DNA repair. *Nat Rev Mol Cell Biol* 2002;3:21–29.

280. Taylor AM, Groom A, Byrd PJ. Ataxia-telangiectasia-like disorder (ATLD)-its clinical presentation and molecular basis. *DNA Repair (Amst)* 2004;3:1219–1225.

281. Thomas M, Rube C, Semik M, et al. Impact of preoperative bimodality induction including twice-daily radiation on tumor regression and survival in stage III non-small-cell lung cancer. *J Clin Oncol* 1999;17:1185.

282. Toledano MB, Leonard WJ. Modulation of transcription factor NF-kappa B binding activity by oxidation-reduction in vitro. *Proc Natl Acad Sci U S A* 1991;88:4328–4332.

283. Toulany M, Dittmann K, Baumann M, et al. Radiosensitization of Ras-mutated human tumor cells in vitro by the specific EGF receptor antagonist BIBX1382BS. *Radiother Oncol* 2005;74:117–129.

284. Toulany M, Dittmann K, Kruger M, et al. Radioresistance of K-Ras mutated human tumor cells is mediated through EGFR-dependent activation of PI3K-AKT pathway. *Radiother Oncol* 2005;76:143–150.

285. Travis LB, Rabkin CS, Brown LM, et al. Cancer survivorship–genetic susceptibility and second primary cancers: research strategies and recommendations. *J Natl Cancer Inst* 2006;98:15–25.

286. Trott KR. Tumour stem cells: the biological concept and its application in cancer treatment. *Radiother Oncol* 1994;30:1–5.

287. Trott KR, Rosemann M. Molecular mechanisms of radiation carcinogenesis and the linear, non-threshold dose response model of radiation risk estimation. *Radiat Environ Biophys* 2000;39:79–87.

288. Trott KR, Teibe A. Lack of specificity of chromosome breaks resulting from radiation-induced genomic instability in Chinese hamster cells. *Radiat Environ Biophys* 1998;37:173–176.

289. Uhm JH, Dooley NP, Kyritsis AP, et al. Vitronectin, a glioma-derived extracellular matrix protein, protects tumor cells from apoptotic death. *Clin Cancer Res* 1999;5:1587–1594.

290. Uziel T, Lerenthal Y, Moyal L, et al. Requirement of the MRN complex for ATM activation by DNA damage. *Embo J* 2003;22:5612–5621.

291. Valerie K, Povirk LF. Regulation and mechanisms of mammalian double-strand break repair. *Oncogene* 2003;22:5792–5812.

292. van't Veer LJ, Dai H, van de Vijver MJ, et al. Gene expression profiling predicts clinical outcome of breast cancer. *Nature* 2002;415:530–536.

293. van Baardwijk A, Baumert BG, Bosmans G, et al. The current status of FDG-PET in tumour volume definition in radiotherapy treatment planning. *Cancer Treat Rev* 2006.

294. van Gent DC, Hoeijmakers JH, Kanaar R. Chromosomal stability and the DNA double-stranded break connection. *Nat Rev Genet* 2001;2:196–206.

295. Vaupel P. Tumor microenvironmental physiology and its implications for radiation oncology. *Semin Radiat Oncol* 2004;14:198–206.

296. Vaupel P, Harrison L. Tumor hypoxia: causative factors, compensatory mechanisms, and cellular response. *Oncologist* 2004;9[Suppl 5]:4–9.

297. Vecchio FM, Valentini V, Minsky BD, et al. The relationship of pathologic tumor regression grade (TRG) and outcomes after preoperative therapy in rectal cancer. *Int J Radiat Oncol Biol Phys* 2005;62:752–760.

298. Venkitaraman AR. Tracing the network connecting BRCA and Fanconi anaemia proteins. *Nat Rev Cancer* 2004;4:266–276.

299. Vermeulen K, Van Bockstaele DR, Berneman ZN. The cell cycle: a review of

regulation, deregulation and therapeutic targets in cancer. *Cell Prolif* 2003;36: 131–149.

300. Vidal AE, Boiteux S, Hickson ID, et al. XRCC1 coordinates the initial and late stages of DNA abasic site repair through protein-protein interactions. *Embo J* 2001;20:6530–6539.

301. Viktorsson K, Lewensohn R, Zhivotovsky B. Apoptotic pathways and therapy resistance in human malignancies. *Adv Cancer Res* 2005;94:143–196.

302. Vogelstein B, Kinzler KW. *The genetic basis of cancer.* New York: McGraw-Hill, 1998.

303. Vogelstein B, Lane D, Levine AJ. Surfing the p53 network. *Nature* 2000;408:307–310.

304. Vogelstein B, Kinzler KW. *The genetic basis of human cancer.* New York: McGraw-Hill, 2002.

305. Vogelstein B, Kinzler KW. Cancer genes and the pathways they control. *Nat Med* 2004;10:789–799.

306. Von Pfeil A, Hakenjos L, Herskind C, et al. Irradiated homozygous TGF-beta1 knockout fibroblasts show enhanced clonogenic survival as compared with TGF-beta1 wild-type fibroblasts. *Int J Radiat Biol* 2002;78:331–339.

307. Vousden KH, Lu X. Live or let die: the cell's response to p53. *Nat Rev Cancer* 2002;2:594–604.

308. Wachsberger P, Burd R, Dicker AP. Tumor response to ionizing radiation combined with antiangiogenesis or vascular targeting agents: exploring mechanisms of interaction. *Clin Cancer Res* 2003;9:1957–1971.

309. Walker DR, Bond JP, Tarone RE, et al. Evolutionary conservation and somatic mutation hotspot maps of p53: correlation with p53 protein structural and functional features. *Oncogene* 1999;18:211–218.

310. Wallace SS. Enzymatic processing of radiation-induced free radical damage in DNA. *Radiat Res* 1998;150:S60–79.

311. Wang H, Perrault AR, Takeda Y, et al. Biochemical evidence for Ku-independent backup pathways of NHEJ. *Nucleic Acids Res* 2003;31:5377–5388.

312. Ward JF. Mechanisms of DNA repair and their potential modification for radiotherapy. *Int J Radiat Oncol Biol Phys* 1986;12:1027–1032.

313. Ward JF. DNA damage produced by ionizing radiation in mammalian cells: identities, mechanisms of formation, and reparability. *Prog Nucleic Acid Res Mol Biol* 1988;35:95–125.

314. Ward JF. DNA damage as the cause of ionizing radiation-induced gene activation. *Radiat Res* 1994;138:S85–88.

315. Warters RL, Hofer KG, Harris CR, et al. Radionuclide toxicity in cultured mammalian cells: elucidation of the primary site of radiation damage. *Curr Top Radiat Res Q* 1978;12:389–407.

316. Watnick RS, Cheng YN, Rangarajan A, et al. Ras modulates Myc activity to repress thrombospondin-1 expression and increase tumor angiogenesis. *Cancer Cell* 2003;3:219–231.

317. Watters D. Molecular mechanisms of ionizing radiation-induced apoptosis. *Immunol Cell Biol* 1999;77:263–271.

318. Waugh MG, Hsuan JJ. EGF receptors as transcription factors: ridiculous or sublime? *Nat Cell Biol* 2001;3:E209–211.

319. Weichselbaum RR, Hallahan DE, Beckett MA, et al. Gene therapy targeted by radiation preferentially radiosensitizes tumor cells. *Cancer Res* 1994;54:4266–4269.

320. Weichselbaum RR, Kufe DW, Hellman S, et al. Radiation-induced tumour necrosis factor-alpha expression: clinical application of transcriptional and physical targeting of gene therapy. *Lancet Oncol* 2002;3:665–671.

321. Willers H, McCarthy EE, Wu B, et al. Dissociation of p53-mediated suppression of homologous recombination from G1/S cell cycle checkpoint control. *Oncogene* 2000;19:632–639.

322. Willers H, Dahm-Daphi J, Powell SN. Repair of radiation damage to DNA. *Br J Cancer* 2004;90:1297–1301.

323. Wilson A, Radtke F. Multiple functions of Notch signaling in self-renewing organs and cancer. *FEBS Lett* 2006.

324. Wilson GD, Bentzen SM, Harari PM. Biologic basis for combining drugs with radiation. *Semin Radiat Oncol* 2006;16:2–9.

325. Winkler F, Kozin SV, Tong RT, et al. Kinetics of vascular normalization by VEGFR2 blockade governs brain tumor response to radiation: role of oxygenation, angiopoietin-1, and matrix metalloproteinases. *Cancer Cell* 2004;6: 553–563.

326. Woronicz JD, Gao X, Cao Z, et al. IkappaB kinase-beta: NF-kappaB activation and complex formation with IkappaB kinase-alpha and NIK. *Science* 1997;278:866–869.

327. Wouters BG, Denko NC, Giaccia AJ, et al. A p53 and apoptotic independent role for p21waf1 in tumour response to radiation therapy. *Oncogene* 1999;18: 6540–6545.

328. Wouters BG, Koritzinsky M, Chiu RK, et al. Modulation of cell death in the tumor microenvironment. *Semin Radiat Oncol* 2003;13:31–41.

329. Wright EA, Howard-Flanders P. The influence of oxygen on the radiosensitivity of mammalian tissues. *Acta Radiol* 1957;48:26–32.

330. Xanthoudakis S, Curran T. Identification and characterization of Ref-1, a nuclear protein that facilitates AP-1 DNA-binding activity. *Embo J* 1992;11: 653–665.

331. Xanthoudakis S, Miao G, Wang F, et al. Redox activation of Fos-Jun DNA binding activity is mediated by a DNA repair enzyme. *Embo J* 1992;11:3323–3335.

332. Yamaoka S, Courtois G, Bessia C, et al. Complementation cloning of NEMO, a component of the IkappaB kinase complex essential for NF-kappaB activation. *Cell* 1998;93:1231–1240.

333. Yarden Y, Sliwkowski MX. Untangling the ErbB signalling network. *Nat Rev Mol Cell Biol* 2001;2:127–137.

334. Yeoh AS, Bowen JM, Gibson RJ, et al. Nuclear factor kappaB (NFkappaB) and cyclooxygenase-2 (Cox-2) expression in the irradiated colorectum is associated with subsequent histopathological changes. *Int J Radiat Oncol Biol Phys* 2005;63:1295–1303.

335. Zakian KL, Koutcher JA, Ballon D, et al. Developments in nuclear magnetic resonance imaging and spectroscopy: application to radiation oncology. *Semin Radiat Oncol* 2001;11:3–15.

336. Zandi E, Chen Y, Karin M. Direct phosphorylation of IkappaB by IKKalpha and IKKbeta: discrimination between free and NF-kappaB-bound substrate. *Science* 1998;281:1360–1363.

337. Zandi E, Rothwarf DM, Delhase M, et al. The IkappaB kinase complex (IKK) contains two kinase subunits, IKKalpha and IKKbeta, necessary for IkappaB phosphorylation and NF-kappaB activation. *Cell* 1997;91:243–252.

338. Zhang H, Ozaki I, Mizuta T, et al. Beta 1-integrin protects hepatoma cells from chemotherapy induced apoptosis via a mitogen-activated protein kinase dependent pathway. *Cancer* 2002;95:896–906.

339. Zhou XY, Wang X, Hu B, et al. An ATM-independent S-phase checkpoint response involves CHK1 pathway. *Cancer Res* 2002;62:1598–1603.

340. Zingg D, Riesterer O, Fabbro D, et al. Differential activation of the phosphatidylinositol 3'-kinase/Akt survival pathway by ionizing radiation in tumor and primary endothelial cells. *Cancer Res* 2004;64:5398–5406.

341. Zips D, Eicheler W, Geyer P, et al. Enhanced susceptibility of irradiated tumor vessels to vascular endothelial growth factor receptor tyrosine kinase inhibition. *Cancer Res* 2005;65:5374–5379.

342. Zips D, Hessel F, Krause M, et al. Impact of adjuvant inhibition of vascular endothelial growth factor receptor tyrosine kinases on tumor growth delay and local tumor control after fractionated irradiation in human squamous cell carcinomas in nude mice. *Int J Radiat Oncol Biol Phys* 2005;61:908–914.

Overview and Basic Science of Radiation Oncology

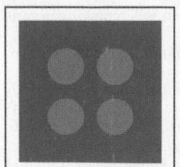

Chapter 4
Molecular Pathophysiology of Tumors

Rakesh K. Jain, Kevin R. Kozak

A solid tumor is an organlike structure containing neoplastic and stromal cells nourished by the tumor vasculature composed of endothelial cells, basement membrane, and perivascular cells. All of these components are embedded in an extracellular matrix (Fig. 4.1). The interactions between these cells, their surrounding matrix, and their local microenvironment influence the expression of various genes. The products encoded by these genes, in turn, control the pathophysiologic characteristics of the tumor. The tumor pathophysiology affects tumor growth, invasion, and metastasis, as well as the response to radiation and other therapies. In this chapter, we will discuss various pathophysiologic parameters that characterize the vascular and extravascular compartments of a tumor as well as the molecular players involved in the formation and function of these compartments. Finally, we will point out some clinical implications of the findings and present a future perspective.

⠶ Vascular Compartment

Neoplastic cells, similar to normal cells, need oxygen and other nutrients for their survival and growth. Every reproductively intact normal cell in our body is located within 100 to 200 μm from a blood capillary so that it can receive adequate levels of oxygen and other nutrients by the process of diffusion. Likewise, cells undergoing neoplastic transformation depend on nearby capillaries for growth. These preneoplastic (i.e., dysplastic or hyperplastic) cells can grow as spherical or ellipsoidal cellular aggregates. However, once the size of the cellular aggregate reaches the diffusion limit for critical nutrients, the aggregate may become dormant. Indeed, human tumors may remain dormant for a number of years despite active cell proliferation because of a balance between proliferation and cell death. However, once they have access to new blood vessels, the tumor may grow and metastasize. What triggers the growth of new vessels? What molecular and cellular players are involved? How do these vessels compare with normal vessels with respect to their structure and function?

Angiogenesis

The fact that the vascular system is associated with tumor growth in animals and humans has been known for nearly a century (92). Ide et al. (115) and Algire and Chalkley (3) provided powerful insight into the neovascularization of transplanted tumors using transparent window techniques (for reviews, see 136,137,141). In 1968 Greenblatt and Shubik (93) and Ehrmann and Knoth (64) suggested the possibility that tumors produce an "angiogenic" substance. In 1971 Folkman (69) proposed the hypothesis that blocking angiogenesis should block tumor growth and metastasis. In 1978 Gullino (97) demonstrated that a tissue acquires angiogenic capacity during neoplastic transformation and proposed that antiangiogenesis approaches be used to prevent cancer. Both of these hypotheses have been validated in a number of preclinical studies (42,130). A wide range of anti- and proangiogenic strategies are being evaluated in the clinic to prevent or treat a large number of diseases, including cancer (40,131). Most importantly, despite testing in patients with advanced or refractory disease, antiangiogenic strategies have yielded overall survival benefits in patients with colorectal cancer, non–small-cell lung cancer, renal cell cancer, and gastrointestinal stromal tumors and have shown progression-free survival benefits in breast cancer (23,114,131, 179,242).

The net balance between pro- and antiangiogenic factors governs both normal and pathologic angiogenic processes (22,101,126). This balance is spatially and temporally regulated under physiologic conditions so that the "angiogenic switch" is "on" when needed (e.g., during embryonic development, wound healing, formation of corpus luteum) and "off" otherwise. During neoplastic transformation and tumor progression, this regulation is deranged, which results in ectopically formed blood vessels to support the growing mass (70,97,100).

Cellular Mechanisms

At least four cellular mechanisms are involved in the vascularization of tumors: co-option, intussusception, sprouting (angiogenesis), and vasculogenesis (Fig. 4.2). Tumor cells can co-opt and grow around the existing vessels to form "perivascular" cuffs. However, as stated earlier, these cuffs cannot grow beyond the diffusion limit of critical nutrients, and they actually may cause the collapse of the vessels as a result of the growth pressure (referred to as "solid stress") (105,225). Alternatively, an existing vessel may enlarge in response to the growth factors released by tumors, and an interstitial tissue column may grow in the enlarged lumen and partition the lumen to form an expanded vascular network. This mode of intussusceptive microvascular growth has been observed during tumor growth, wound healing, and gene therapy (226,228,229).

"Sprouting" angiogenesis is perhaps the most widely studied mechanism of vessel formation. During sprouting angiogenesis, the existing vessels become leaky in response to growth factors released by cancer or stromal cells; the basement membrane and the interstitial matrix dissolve; the pericytes dissociate from the vessel; endothelial cells (EC) migrate and proliferate to form an array/sprout; a lumen is formed in the sprout (referred to as canalization); branches and loops are formed by confluence and anastomoses of sprouts to permit blood flow; and finally, these immature vessels are invested in basement membrane and pericytes. During physiologic angiogenesis, these vessels differentiate into mature arterioles, capillaries, and venules, whereas in tumors they may remain immature (39,126,137).

During embryonic development, a primitive vascular plexus is formed from endothelial precursor cells (EPCs) by a process referred to as vasculogenesis. Isner (118), Lyden et al. (176), and Rafii et al. (234) showed that circulating EPCs mobilized from the bone marrow or peripheral blood also can contribute to postnatal vasculogenesis in tumors and other tissues. The challenge now is to discern the relative contribution of each of the four mechanisms of new vessel formation in tumors to optimize antiangiogenic treatment of cancer (60, 257).

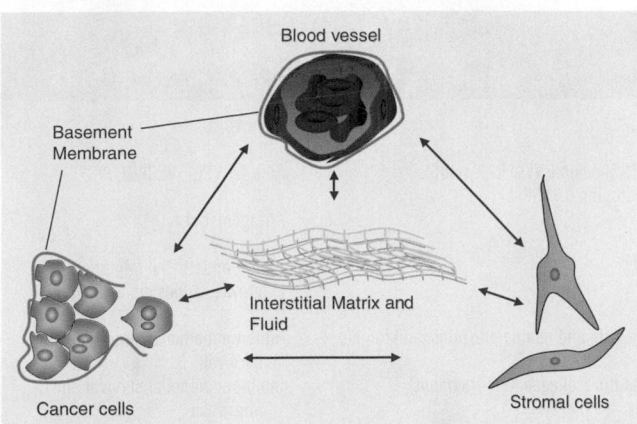

FIGURE 4.1. Schematic representation of a solid tumor. The key components include cancer cells, host cells, and vasculature made of endothelial and perivascular cells—all embedded in a matrix bathed in interstitial fluid. Arrows indicate interactions between the components. [From Jain RK. Vascular and interstitial biology of tumors. In: Abeloff MD, Armitage JO, Niederhuber JE, et al., eds. *Clinical oncology,* 3rd ed. Philadelphia: Elsevier, 2004;153–172, with permission.]

Molecular Mechanisms

Various pro- and antiangiogenic molecules that orchestrate different steps in vessel formation and their functions are listed in Table 4.1. Vascular endothelial growth factor (VEGF) is, perhaps, the most critical angiogenic molecule. Originally discovered in 1983 as the vascular permeability factor by Dvorak and colleagues (61) and cloned in 1989 by Ferrara and colleagues (68), VEGF increases vascular permeability, promotes migration and proliferation of ECs, serves as an EC survival factor, and is known to up-regulate leukocyte adhesion molecules on ECs (61,68,188). During tumor progression, the variety and concentration of angiogenic molecules produced by a tumor can increase. Thus, if VEGF were blocked, tumor growth might continue as a result of the action of other angiogenic molecules (e.g., basic fibroblast growth factor [bFGF], interleukin-8 [IL-8], stromal cell-derived factor 1α [SDF1α]) (10,44,146,198,285). Other positive regulators include angiopoietins that are involved in blood vessel maturation (284); various proteases involved in extracellular matrix remodeling and growth factor release (173); and organ-specific angiogenic stimulators, such as endocrine gland-VEGF (162,163).

Angiogenesis inhibitors include soluble receptors of various proangiogenic ligands as well as molecules that down-regulate stimulator expression (e.g., interferons), interfere with stimu-

lator release, or block binding of stimulators to their receptors (e.g., platelet factor 4). Thrombospondins are among the first and best characterized endogenous inhibitors that interfere with the growth, adhesion, migration, and survival of ECs (22). Other endogenous inhibitors include fragments of various plasma or matrix proteins, for example, angiostatin—fragment of plasminogen (219); endostatin—fragment of collagen XVIII (218); tumstatin—fragment of collagen IV (177). An understanding of the mechanisms of action of these inhibitors is beginning to emerge (150,264).

The generation of pro- and antiangiogenic molecules can be triggered by injury, metabolic stress (e.g., low partial pressure of oxygen [P_{O2}], low pH, or hypoglycemia), mechanical stress (e.g., shear stress, solid stress), immune/inflammatory responses (e.g., immune/inflammatory cells that have infiltrated the tissue), and genetic mutations (e.g., activation of oncogenes or deletion of suppressor genes that control the production of angiogenesis regulators) (22,73,83,101,282). These molecules can emanate from cancer cells, endothelial cells, stromal cells, blood, and extracellular matrix (27,72,104,269) (Fig. 4.3). Because the host cells differ among organs, angiogenesis depends on host–tumor interactions (53,74,91,110,201,270,289). Furthermore, because the tumor microenvironment is likely to change during tumor growth, regression, and relapse after treatment, profiles of pro- and antiangiogenic molecules are likely to change with time and space (10,119,140,278,279). The challenge now is to develop a unified theoretic framework to describe the temporal and spatial profiles of this increasing number of angiogenesis regulators to develop effective therapeutic strategies (236).

Vascular Architecture

In normal tissue, blood flows systematically from an artery to an arteriole to capillaries to venules to a vein. Although the tumor vasculature originates from these host vessels and the mechanisms of angiogenesis are similar, its organization may be completely different depending on the tumor type, its location, and whether it is growing, regressing, or relapsing (8,84). In general, tumor vessels are dilated, saccular, tortuous, and chaotic in their patterns of interconnection (122). For example, whereas the normal vasculature is characterized by dichotomous branching, the tumor vasculature has many trifurcations and branches with uneven diameters (166,167). The fractal dimensions and minimum path lengths of tumor vasculature are different from those of the normal host vasculature (7,8,84).

The molecular mechanisms of this abnormal vascular architecture are not entirely understood, but it seems reasonable

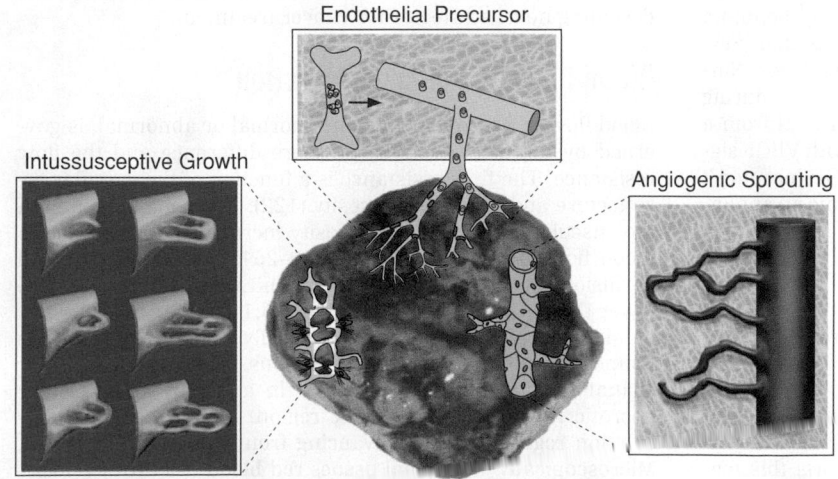

FIGURE 4.2. Cellular mechanisms of vascularization in tumors. At least four mechanisms are involved: intussusception—tumor vessels enlarge and an interstitial tissue column grows in the enlarged lumen, expanding the network; vasculogenesis—endothelial precursor cells mobilized from the bone marrow or peripheral blood contribute to the endothelial lining of tumor vessels, sprouting angiogenesis—the existing vascular network expands by forming sprouts or bridges; and co-option (not shown)—tumor cells grow around existing vessels to form "perivascular" cuffs. (Adapted from Carmeliet P, Jain RK. Angiogenesis in cancer and other diseases. *Nature* 2000;407:249–257, with permission.)

| Table 4.1 | SELECT ANGIOGENESIS ACTIVATORS AND INHIBITORS[a] | | |

Activators	Function	Inhibitors	Function
VEGF family members[c,d]	Stimulate angio-vasculogenesis, permeability, leukocyte adhesion	VEGFR-1; soluble VEGFR-1; soluble neuropilin-1 (NRP-1)	Sink for VEGF, VEGF-B, PIGF
VEGFR[d], NRP-1, NRP-2	Integrate angiogenic and survival signals	Ang2[b,d]	Antagonist of Ang1
EG-VEGF	Stimulate growth of endothelial cells derived from endocrine glands	TSP-1,2	Inhibit endothelial migration, growth, adhesion, and survival
Ang1 and Tie2[c,d]	Stabilize vessels	Angiostatin and related plasminogen kringles	Inhibit endothelial migration and survival
PDGF-BB and receptors	Recruit smooth muscle cells	Endostatin (collagen XVIII fragment)	Inhibit endothelial survival and migration
TGF-$\beta1^b$, endoglin, TGF-β receptors	Stimulate extracellular matrix production	Tumstatin	Inhibit endothelial protein synthesis
FGF, HGF, MCP-1	Stimulate angio-arteriogenesis	Vasostatin; calreticulin	Inhibit endothelial growth
Integrins $\alpha_v\beta_3^b$, α_5, β_5, $\alpha_5\beta_1$	Receptors for matrix macromolecules and proteinases	Platelet factor-4	Inhibit binding of bFGF and VEGF
VE-cadherin; PECAM (CD31)	Endothelial junctional molecules	Tissue-inhibitors of MMP (TIMPs); MMP-inhibitors; PEX	Suppress pathologic angiogenesis
Ephrins[d]	Regulate arterial/venous specification	Meth-1; Meth-2	Inhibitors containing MMP-, TSP- and disintegrin-domains
Plasminogen activators, MMPs	Remodel matrix, release growth factor	IFN -α, -β, -γ; IP-10, IL-4, IL-12, IL-18	Inhibit endothelial migration; down-regulate bFGF and VEGF
PAI-1	Stabilize nascent vessels	Prothrombin kringle-2; anti-thrombin III fragment	Suppress endothelial growth
NOS; COX-2	Stimulate angiogenesis and vasodilation	16 kD-prolactin	Inhibit bFGF/VEGF
AC133	Regulate angioblast differentiation	VEGI	Modulate cell growth
Chemokines[b]	Pleiotropic role in angiogenesis	Fragment of SPARC	Inhibit endothelial binding and activity of VEGF
Id1/Id3	Inhibit differentiation	Osteopontin fragment	Interfere with integrin signaling
		Maspin	Protease inhibitor
		Canstatin, Proliferin-related protein, Restin	Mechanisms unknown
		Netrins	Regulate blood vessel guidance by endothelial cell repulsion
		Slits	Mechanism unknown

bFGF, basic fibroblast growth factor; COX, cyclooxygenase; EG-VEGF, endocrine-gland-derived vascular endothelial growth factor; FGF, fibroblast growth factor; HGF, hepatocyte growth factor; Id, inhibitor differentiation; IFN, interferon; IP, interferon-inducible protein; IL, interleukin; kD, kilodalton; MCP, monocyte chemoattractant protein; Meth, methamphetamine; MMPs, matrix metalloproteinases; NRP, neuropilin; NOS, nitric oxide synthase; PAI, plasminogen activator inhibitor; PDGF, platelet-derived growth factor; PECAM, platelet endothelial cell adhesion molecule; PIGF, placental growth factor; TGF, transforming growth factor; TIMPs, tissue inhibitors of metalloproteinases; TSP, thrombospondin; SPARC, secreted, protein acidic, and rich in cysteine; VE-cadherin, vascular endothelial cadherin; VEGF, vascular endothelial growth factor; VEGI, vascular endothelial growth inhibitor
[a]Selected list updated from Carmeliet P, Jain RK. Angiogenesis in cancer and other diseases. *Nature* 2000;407:249–257 and Carmeliet P, Tessier-Lavigne M. Common mechanisms of nerve and blood vessel wiring. *Nature* 2005;436:193–200. For complete function and references, see supplementary information (http://steele.mgh.harvard.edu).
[b]Opposite effect in some contexts.
[c]Also present in or affecting nonendothelial cells
[d]See reference (284).

to hypothesize that an imbalance of pro- and antiangiogenic molecules is a key contributor (126,127,135). By extension, modulation of this angiogenic imbalance may allow for the correction of the tumor vascular abnormalities, leaving behind a more structurally and functionally normal vascular bed. Several observations support this "normalization" hypothesis. Normalization of tumor xenograft vasculature is observed during therapies that lower VEGF (e.g., hormone withdrawal from a hormone-dependent tumor [140]), that interfere with VEGF signaling (e.g., treatment with anti-VEGF or anti-VEGF receptor-2 antibody [148,267,280,286]) (Fig. 4.4), or that mimic an antiangiogenic cocktail (e.g., trastuzumab treatment of a her2 overexpressing tumor [119]). Emerging clinical data from cancer patients treated with bevacizumab, an anti-VEGF antibody, or AZD2171, a pan-vascular endothelial growth factor receptor (VEGFR) tyrosine kinase inhibitor, lend even more compelling support to this hypothesis (10,131,278,279).

Mechanical stress generated by proliferating tumor cells also may lead to partially compressed or totally collapsed vessels often found in tumors (105,157). Decompression of blood vessels by inducing apoptosis in perivascular cells supports this me-

chanical hypothesis (94,225). Perhaps the combination of both molecular and mechanical factors renders the tumor vasculature abnormal; thus, both must be taken into account when designing novel strategies for cancer treatment.

Blood Flow and Microcirculation

Blood flow in a vascular network, normal or abnormal, is governed by the arteriovenous pressure difference and the flow resistance. The flow resistance is a function of the vascular architecture and the blood viscosity (122). Abnormalities in both the vasculature and blood viscosity increase the resistance to blood flow in tumors (166,167,249–251). As a result, overall perfusion rates (blood flow rate per unit volume) in tumors are lower than in many normal tissues (96,143,273).

Macroscopically and microscopically, tumor blood flow is temporally and spatially heterogeneous. Macroscopically, four spatial regions can be recognized in a tumor: an avascular necrotic region, a seminecrotic region, a stabilized microcirculation region, and an advancing front (67,133) (Fig. 4.5A). Microscopically, in normal tissues red blood cell (RBC) velocity

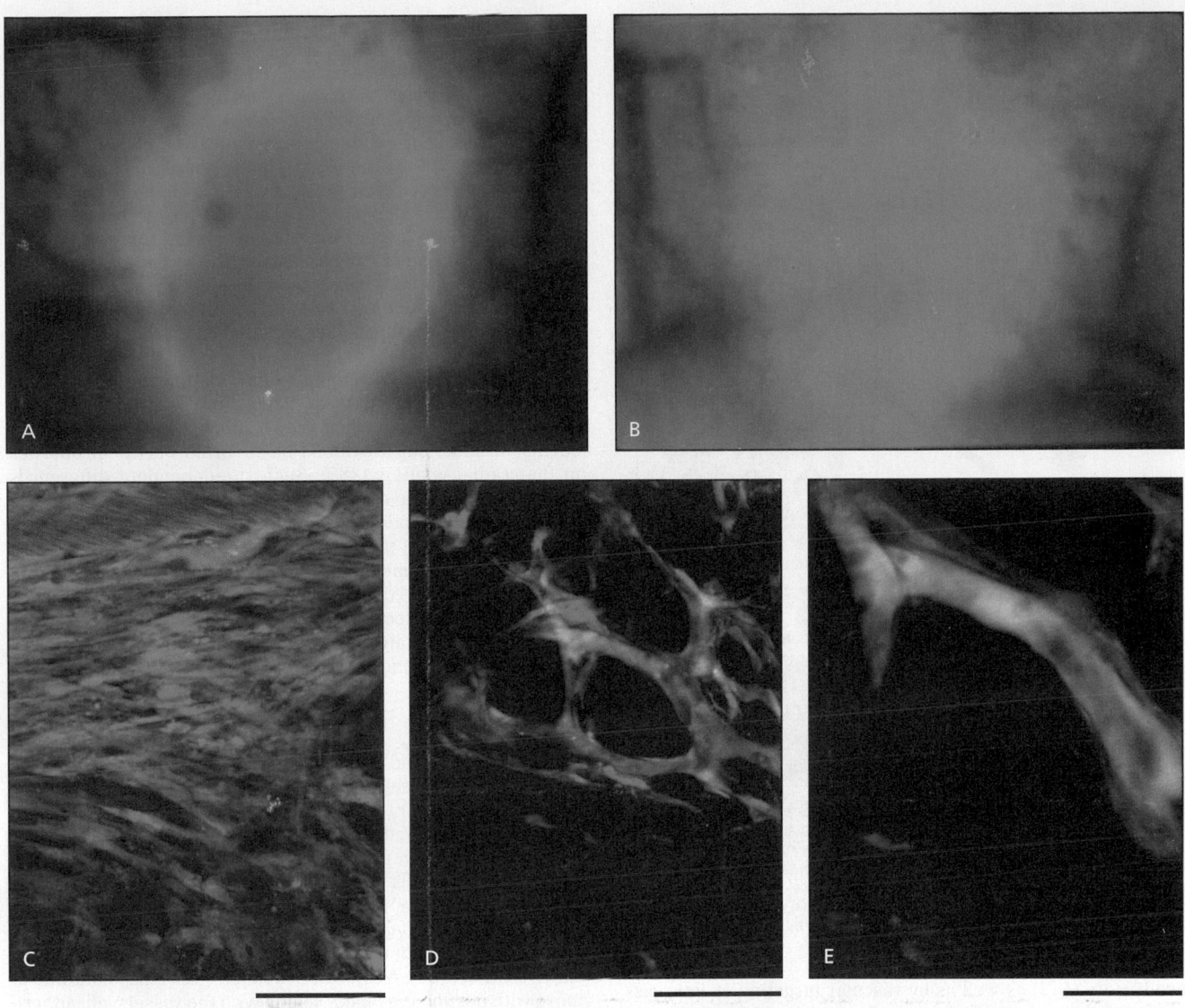

100 μm   100 μm   50 μm

FIGURE 4.3. Tumor induction of host promoter activity in stromal cells. The expression of vascular endothelial growth factor (VEGF) in host cells can be examined using transgenic mice expressing green fluorescent protein (GFP) under the control of the VEGF promoter. **A:** A murine mammary carcinoma xenograft shows host cell VEGF expression mainly at the periphery of the tumor after 1 week. **B:** After 2 weeks, the VEGF expressing host cells have infiltrated the tumor. (From Fukumura D, Xavier R, Sugiura T, et al. Tumor induction of VEGF promoter activity in stromal cells. *Cell* 1998;94:715–725, with permission). **C:** A GFP-expressing layer of host cells can be seen at the tumor-host interface. **D, E:** The VEGF-expressing host cells colocalize with the angiogenic tumor vessels. (From Brown EB, Campbell RB, Tsuzuki Y, et al. *In vivo* measurement of gene expression, angiogenesis and physiological function in tumors using multiphoton laser scanning microscopy. *Nat Med* 2001;7:866–870, with permission.)

is dependent on vessel diameter, but there is no such dependence in most tumors (74,170,289). Furthermore, the average RBC velocity may be an order of magnitude lower in some tumors compared to the host tissue (289). In a given tumor vessel, blood flow fluctuates with time and can even reverse its direction (24,67,170).

In addition to the elevated geometric and viscous (rheologic) resistance, other molecular and mechanical factors contribute to this spatial and temporal heterogeneity. These include imbalance between pro- and antiangiogenic molecules (236), solid stress generated by proliferating cancer cells (94,105,157,225), vascular remodeling by intussusception (227), and coupling between luminal and interstitial fluid pressure via hyperpermeability of tumor vessels (8,9,200,214). As discussed later, this heterogeneity contributes to both acute and chronic hypoxia in

tumors—a potential cause of resistance to radiation and other therapies and increased metastatic potential.

Considerable effort has gone into modulating tumor blood flow to improve cancer treatment. This has been difficult to achieve reproducibly because the tumor vasculature consists of both vessels co-opted from the preexisting host vasculature and vessels resulting from the angiogenic response of host vessels to cancer cells. The former are invested in normal contractile perivascular cells, whereas the latter either lack perivascular cells or are abnormally invested (1,152,203). As a result, efforts to increase tumor blood flow and the delivery of cytotoxins, by pharmacologic or physical agents, have not always been successful (122,143). In contrast, efforts to "starve" tumors by decreasing or shutting down tumor blood flow by "stealing" blood away from the passive component of the tumor vasculature by

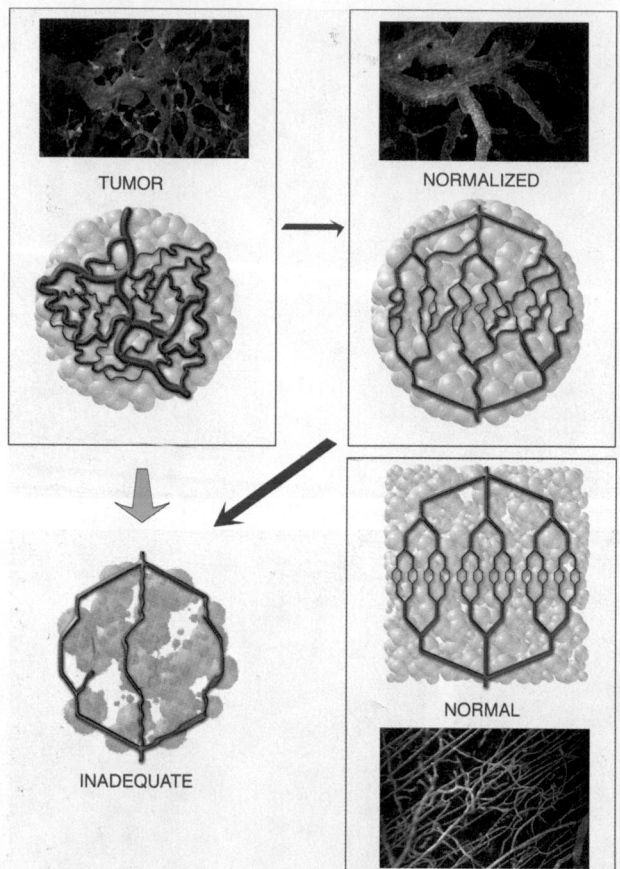

FIGURE 4.4. Normalization of tumor vasculature. **A:** Normal vessels are well organized with even diameters. **B:** In contrast, tumor vessels are tortuous with increased vessel diameter, length, density, and permeability. **C:** Antiangiogenic therapies "normalize" the tumor vascular network and ultimately may reduce the vasculature to the point that it provides inadequate support for tumor growth. (From Jain RK. Normalizing tumor vasculature with anti-angiogenic therapy: a new paradigm for combination therapy. *Nat Med* 2001;7:987–989 and Jain RK, Carmeliet PF. Vessels of death or life. *Sci Am* 2001;285:38–45, with permission.)

vasodilators (143) as well as by vascular targeting or intravascular coagulation have shown promise in experimental systems (59,112,210). It also appears that judiciously applied antiangiogenic therapy may "normalize" the abnormal tumor vasculature and the resulting "normalized" vessels might be more responsive to vasoactive agents (125,127) (Fig. 4.4).

Vascular Permeability

Once a bloodborne molecule has reached an exchange vessel, its extravasation occurs by diffusion, convection, and, to some extent, presumably by transcytosis (62,120). The diffusive permeability of a molecule depends on the size, shape, charge, and flexibility of the molecule as well as the size, shape, charge, and dynamics of the transvascular transport pathway. In normal vessels, these pathways include diffusion through the EC membrane (for lipophilic solutes), trans-EC diffusion, interendothelial junctions (<7 nm), open or closed fenestrations (<10 nm), and transendothelial channels (including vesicles or vesicovacuolar organelles [VVOs]) (62,120). Some of these pathways may be lined with glycocalyx on EC, thus effectively reducing the size of the pathway. A basement membrane may retard further the movement of molecules. Ultrastructural studies show widened interendothelial junctions; an increased number of fenestrations, vesicles, and VVOs in tumor vessels; and a lack of normal basement membrane and pericytes (62,103,110,120,181).

In concert with these ultrastructural findings, both vascular permeability to solutes and water permeability (referred to

as hydraulic conductivity) of tumors, in general, are significantly higher than that of various normal tissues (66,85,172, 252,288,289). Furthermore, unlike normal vessels, tumor vessels lack selectivity for the size of extravasating molecules (287). However, positively charged molecules have a higher affinity for the negatively charged angiogenic tumor vessels (36,54,266). Despite increased overall permeability, not all blood vessels of a tumor are leaky. Even the leaky vessels have a finite pore size that is tumor dependent (110), and ultrastructural studies show that the larger pore size in tumors represents wide interendothelial junctions (103,110). Not only do the vascular permeability and pore size vary from one tumor to the next, but within the same tumor they vary both spatially and temporally as well as during tumor growth, regression, and relapse (110,119,140).

The local microenvironment plays an important role in controlling vascular permeability. For example, a human glioma (HGL21) is fairly leaky when grown subcutaneously in immunodeficient mice, but it exhibits blood–brain barrier properties in the cranial window (289). Such site-dependent differences for other tumors have been observed in other orthotopic sites (74,201,270). One possible explanation is that the host–tumor interactions control the production and secretion of cytokines associated with permeability increase (e.g., VEGF) and decrease (e.g., angiopoietin 1) (126,135,202,284,286). A better understanding of the molecular mechanisms of permeability regulation in tumors is likely to yield strategies for improved delivery of molecular medicine to tumors (276).

Movement of Cells across Vessel Walls

Both cancer cells and immune cells frequently move across the walls of blood vessels—the former in the process of metastasis and the latter during immune response or cell-based immunotherapy. Both transendothelial and periendothelial pathways have been proposed as a route for intravasation and extravasation of cells. Very little is known about intravasation, except that a tumor may shed more than a million cells per gram per day and most of these are not clonogenic (14,95,262). More is known about the molecular and cellular mechanisms of extravasation (134). A cell within a blood vessel may continue to move with the flowing blood, collide with the vessel wall, adhere transiently or stably, and finally extravasate. These interactions are governed by both local hydrodynamic forces and adhesive forces. The former are determined by the vessel diameter and fluid velocity and the latter by the expression, strength, and kinetics of binding between adhesion molecules and by the surface area of contact (134,190,192,195,207,290). Deformability of cells affects both types of forces (189).

Rolling of endogenous leukocytes is generally low in tumor vessels, whereas stable adhesion (≥30 seconds) is comparable between normal and tumor vessels (71). However, both rolling and stable adhesion are nearly zero in angiogenic vessels induced in collagen gels by bFGF or VEGF, two of the most potent angiogenic factors (53). Whether the latter is due to a low flux of leukocytes into angiogenic vessels and/or down regulation of adhesion molecules in these immature vessels is currently not known. Age may also play an important role in leukocyte–endothelial interactions (283).

Further insight into the biology of cells that adhere to tumor vessels comes from studies on the localization of IL-2 activated natural killer (A-NK) cells in normal and tumor tissues in mice using positron emission tomography (183,184). Immediately following systemic injection, these cells localized primarily in the lungs, whereas a nondetectable number of cells arrived in the tumor (183). Increased rigidity caused by IL-2 activation may contribute to the mechanical entrapment of these cells in the lung microcirculation (185,244). Constitutive expression of certain adhesion molecules in the lung vasculature also may

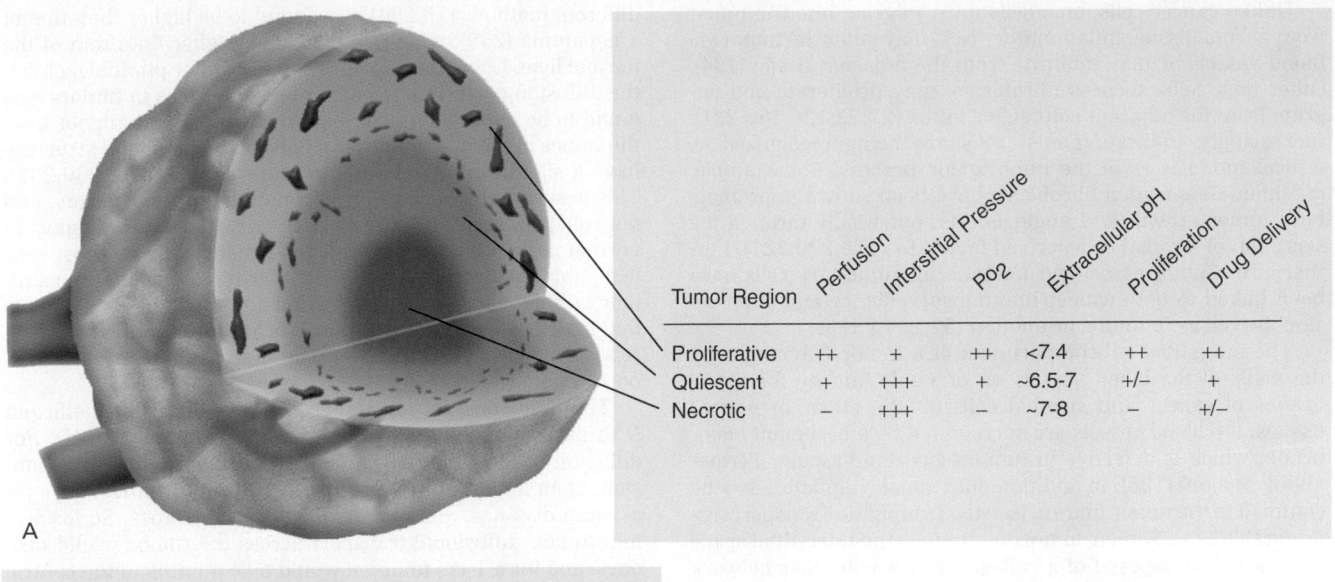

Tumor Region	Perfusion	Interstitial Pressure	Po2	Extracellular pH	Proliferation	Drug Delivery
Proliferative	++	+	++	<7.4	++	++
Quiescent	+	+++	+	~6.5-7	+/−	+
Necrotic	−	+++	−	~7-8	−	+/−

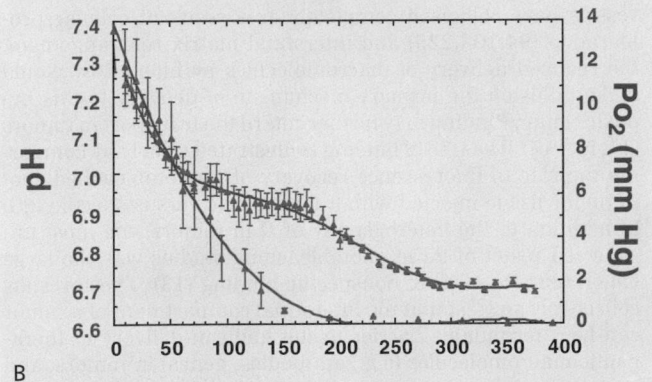

FIGURE 4.5. A: The tumor microenvironment is heterogeneous with proliferative, quiescent, and necrotic regions. These regions can be characterized in terms of various physiologic parameters. Decreasing magnitude of these parameters is indicated as + + +, + +, +, +/−, and − in the adjoining table. (From Jain RK, Forbes NS. Commentary—can engineered bacteria help control cancer? *Proc Natl Acad Sci U S A* 2001;98:14748–14750, with permission.) **B:** pH and Po2 as a function of distance from a blood vessel in a tumor. The tumor environment becomes progressively more hypoxic and acidic farther away from a blood vessel. (From Helmlinger G, Yuan F, Dellian M, et al. Interstitial pH and Po2 gradients in solid tumors in vivo: high-resolution measurements reveal a lack of correlation. *Nat Med* 1997;3:177–182, with permission.)

facilitate their localization in the lungs (134). One approach to reducing lung entrapment is to reduce the rigidity of these cells (186,189). Alternatively, the lung can be circumvented by injecting A-NK cells directly into the blood supply of tumors. In this case, A-NK cells, both xenogeneic and syngeneic, adhered to some blood vessels in three different tumor models (184,191,245) via CD18 and very late antigen-4 (VLA-4) on the A-NK cells and intercellular adhesion molecule-1 (ICAM-1), vascular cell adhesion molecule-1 (VCAM-1), and E-selectin on the activated endothelium of angiogenic vessels (188,205,206).

These molecules can be up-regulated by a number of cytokines, including tumor necrosis factor-α (TNF-α) and a protein of 90kD molecular weight (p90), secreted by some neoplastic cells (144,187,190) and down-regulated by others, for example, transforming growth factor-β (TGF-β) also, presumably, secreted by cancer cells (80–82,91). Surprisingly, the proangiogenic VEGF also can up-regulate these molecules (55,140,148,188,269), presumably via VEGFR1, a VEGF receptor, whereas another proangiogenic molecule, bFGF, can down-regulate these molecules (188). The challenge now is to decrease nonspecific entrapment of immune cells in normal vessels and to increase their delivery to tumor vessels to improve various cell-based therapies, including gene therapy.

Extravascular Compartment

Composition and Origin

The extravascular compartment of a solid tumor consists of neoplastic cells (parenchyma) and host cells (e.g., inflammatory cells, fibroblasts) residing in an interstitial subcompartment bathed by the interstitial fluid (Fig. 4.1). Depending on the tumor type and its stage of differentiation, neoplastic cells may be dispersed in the matrix as individual cells (e.g., lymphomas, melanomas) or as clumps or nests (e.g., carcinomas). More than 80% of tumors are carcinomas arising from epithelial cells. The remaining include sarcomas arising from mesenchymal cells (e.g., bone or muscle cells), lymphomas arising from lymphoid tissue, leukemias arising from hematopoietic cells, and hemangiomas arising from endothelial cells. In a poorly differentiated carcinoma, the cancer cells may be loosely packed in clumps, whereas in a well-differentiated carcinoma, the cells may be connected with intercellular junctions and tightly packed in a nest enveloped by a basement membrane. With tumor progression, cancer cells may invade the basement membrane and spread to other regions (62).

Unlike cancer cells, host cells must migrate into the tumor from normal tissue. Inflammatory cells may enter the tumor via blood vessels or may infiltrate from the adjacent tissue (134). Other host cells, such as fibroblasts, may proliferate and migrate from the adjacent connective tissue (27,72,126,150,231). Increasingly, infiltrating host cells are being recognized as critical modulators of the tumorigenic process. For example, carcinoma-associated fibroblasts have been shown to promote both tumor growth and angiogenesis, potentially through the secretion of stromal cell–derived factor-1α (174,220,221). Furthermore, tumor-associated immune/inflammatory cells have been linked to both cancer immunosurveillance and suppression as well as to tumor promotion (52,204,231).

The interstitial subcompartment of a tumor is bounded by the walls of the blood vessels on one side and by the membranes of cancer and stromal cells on the other. In normal tissues, the blood vessels are surrounded by a basement membrane, which is defective in tumors (see the Vascular Permeability section) (126). In addition, functional lymphatics may be confined to the tumor margin (see the Lymphatic Transport section) (132,223). Similar to normal tissues, the interstitial space of tumors is composed of a collagen and elastin fiber network that provides structural support to the tissue. Interdispersed in this cross-linked structure are the interstitial fluid and macromolecular constituents (polysaccharides hyaluronan and proteoglycans [PG]), which form a hydrophilic gel.

Compared with our understanding of blood vessel formation, our understanding of stroma generation is minimal. Dvorak et al. (62) have proposed that the extravasated plasma protein fibrinogen, a key component of the tumor interstitial fluid (TIF), clots to form fibrin, which serves as a major component of the provisional stroma. This provisional stroma eventually is replaced by more mature connective tissue stroma. The TIF also contains several proteins including fibronectin, vitronectin, osteopontin, thrombospondin, decorin, and tenascin. These proteins are present in both free and bound forms and contain the amino acid sequence arg-gly-asp (RGD). The RGD sequence provides a binding site for adhesion that assists in the migration of various cells, including stromal cells. In addition to extravasating from the leaky tumor vessels, these proteins, along with collagen and various PGs, also are synthesized by the stromal cells, albeit in a form that is different from that in the plasma or normal tissues (62). TIF also may contain various growth factors that facilitate stroma formation. For example, *in vitro* studies suggest that platelet-derived growth factor-β is involved in the recruitment of fibroblasts to tumors, and TGF-β controls the production of collagen and other matrix molecules in tumors (65,126). With the increasing interest in using the fragments of matrix constituents for controlling angiogenesis, our understanding of the molecular and cellular mechanisms of stroma generation in tumors is likely to increase (149).

Interstitial Transport

Once a molecule has extravasated, its movement through the interstitial space occurs by diffusion and convection (121). Diffusion is proportional to the concentration gradient in the interstitium, and convection is proportional to the interstitial fluid velocity, which, in turn, is proportional to the pressure gradient in the interstitium. Just as the interstitial diffusion coefficient, D (cm^2/s), relates the diffusive flux to the concentration gradient, the interstitial hydraulic conductivity, K (cm^2/mm Hg·s), relates the interstitial velocity to the pressure gradient (121). Values of these transport coefficients are governed by the structure and composition of the interstitial compartment as well as by the physicochemical properties of the solute molecule (28,45,51,217,230,259).

The value of K (interstitial hydraulic conductivity) for a human colon carcinoma xenograft (LS174T), measured using two different methods (16,294), was found to be higher than that of a hepatoma (259), which, in turn, was higher than that of the normal liver. Using fluorescence recovery after photobleaching, the diffusion coefficient (D) of various molecules in tumors was found to be about one-third that in water (13) and higher than the values in the host tissue (45). Collagen content and structure have a significant effect on D in tumors (16,51,212,230,237). This is surprising because hyaluronan and proteoglycans, and not collagen, account for most of the resistance to transport in normal tissues. Because collagen is produced by the host cells (e.g., fibroblasts), the penetrability of macromolecules into a tumor will depend on the host–tumor interaction. Thus, agents that interfere with collagen synthesis and/or organization (e.g., relaxin, bacterial collagenase) may increase interstitial transport in tumors (26,182).

The time constant for a molecule with diffusion coefficient D to diffuse across a distance L is approximately $L^2/4D$. For diffusion of IgG (immunoglobulin G) in tumors, this time constant is on the order of 1 hour for a 100-μm distance, days for a 1-mm distance, and months for a 1-cm distance. So for a 1-mm tumor, diffusional transport across the tumor would take days, and for a 1-cm tumor, it would take months. If the central vessels have collapsed completely as a result of cellular proliferation (94,105,225) and interstitial matrix rearrangement, the reduced delivery of macromolecules by blood flow would make diffusion the primary mechanism of delivery to this hypoxic center. Binding may further retard the transport in tumors (11,13,147). The role of binding is illustrated clearly by comparing the rate of fluorescence recovery of a photobleached spot in tumor tissue injected with a nonspecific versus specific IgG. In addition to the heterogeneity of D in tumors, the most unexpected result of these photobleaching studies was the large extent (30% to 40%) of nonspecific binding (13). These results collectively suggest that the interstitial compartment of a tumor can be a formidable barrier to the uniform delivery of therapeutic macromolecules (e.g., antibodies, genes) in tumors, and strategies are needed to overcome this barrier (182).

Lymphatic Transport

In most normal tissues, extravasated plasma and macromolecules are taken up by the lymphatics and returned to the central circulation. Although it is widely accepted that lymphatic vessels are present in the tumor margin and the peritumoral tissue, the hotly debated issue for nearly a century has been whether anatomically defined lymphatic vessels are present within solid tumors (96), and, if so, whether they function (168,223). Currently available immunohistochemical markers stain for structures in some tumors that resemble lymphatic vessels. However, because many of these markers lack specificity (43,132,223), it is not clear whether they stain functional lymphatic vessels, endothelial cells from remnant lymphatic vessels, or some other structures or cell types (e.g., preferential fluid channels (16)). It is likely that the stress induced by proliferating cancer cells compresses and impairs lymphatic vessels that are co-opted or formed in a tumor (105,225) and/or lymphatic valves are impaired by tumor growth (117). The impaired lymphatic vessels, in turn, may contribute to the interstitial hypertension characteristic of animal and human tumors (see the Interstitial Hypertension section). In addition, invasion of the functional peritumoral lymphatics is considered to be a poor prognostic factor for a number of tumors, and lymphatic metastasis is a major cause of morbidity and mortality.

Our understanding of the mechanisms of lymphangiogenesis lags behind our understanding of the mechanisms of angiogenesis. However, considerable progress has recently been made toward identifying molecular players responsible for lymphangiogenesis. VEGF-C, acting through VEGFR-3, appears to play a central role in tumor-associated lymphangiogenesis.

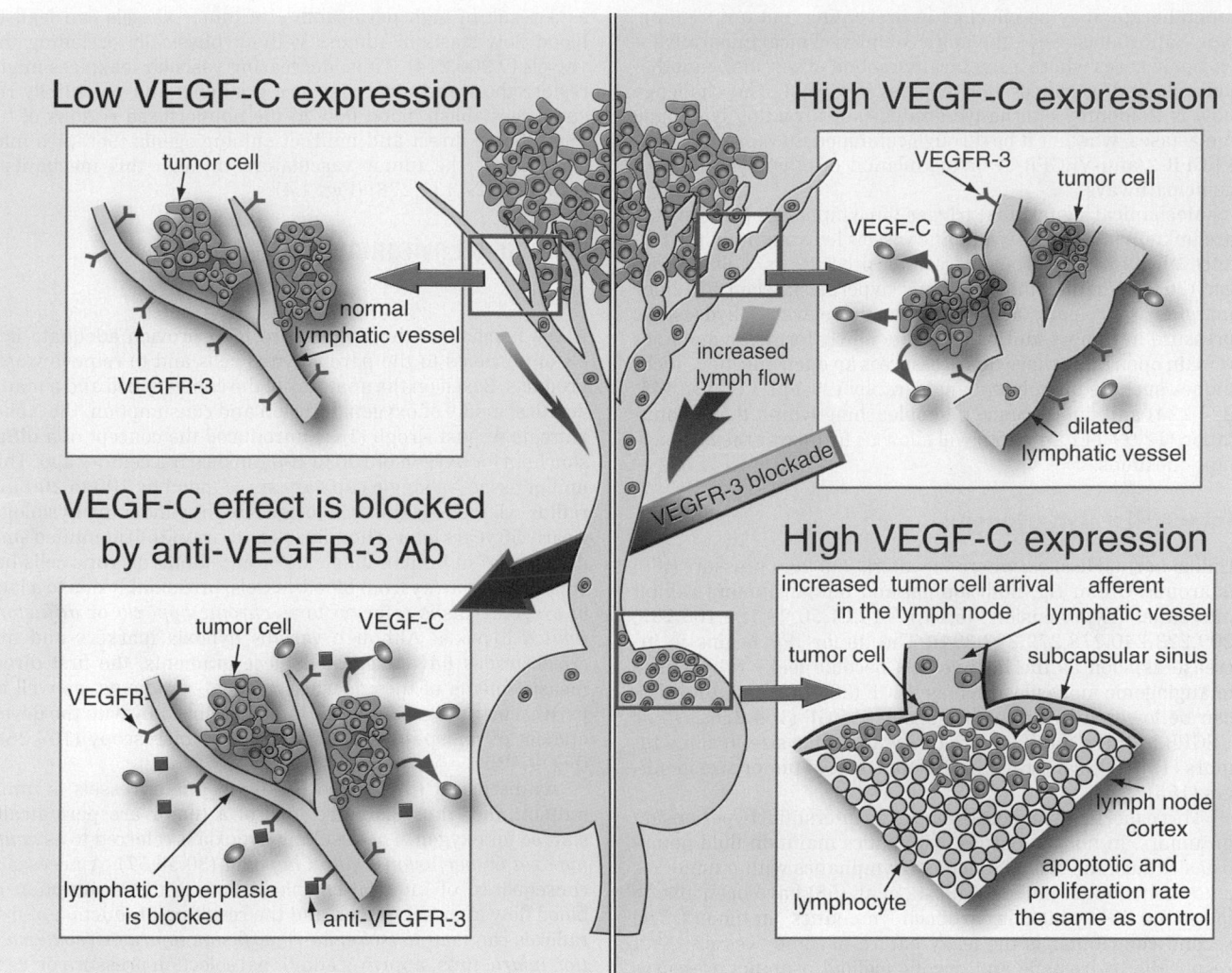

FIGURE 4.6. Schematic of lymphatics in low (*left*) versus high (*right*) VEGF-C expressing tumors. VEGF-C secreted from tumor cells stimulates VEGFR-3 expressed in lymphatic endothelial cells inducing peritumor lymphatic hyperplasia (*top right*). An increase in lymphatic surface area may increase the opportunity for tumor cell entry into lymphatic vessels. Augmented lymph flow enhances tumor cell delivery to draining lymph nodes (*bottom right*). In the absence of VEGF-C overexpression, peritumor lymphatic hyperplasia is less pronounced and fewer tumor cells are delivered to draining lymph nodes (*left*). Anti-VEGF-C/anti-VEGFR-3 treatment inhibits VEGF-C–induced lymphatic hyperplasia and tumor cell delivery to draining lymph nodes (*bottom left*). (From Hoshida T, Isaka N, Hagendoorn J, et al. Imaging steps of lymphatic metastasis reveals that vascular endothelial growth factor-C increases metastasis by increasing delivery of cancer cells to lymph nodes: therapeutic implications. *Cancer Res* 2006;66:8065–8075, with permission.)

Several experimental (111,151,178,222,223,254,281) and clinical (2,215) studies have demonstrated a positive correlation between VEGF-C expression and peritumoral lymphatic vessel density, lymphatic metastasis, and, in some cases, poor clinical outcomes. Like in vascular angiogenesis, other positive and negative regulators, such as VEGF (49,208), VEGF-D (255), hepatocyte growth factor (37), platelet-derived growth factor-BB (38), and angiopoietins (78) are involved in lymphangiogenesis. Furthermore, mechanisms analogous to cooption, intussusception, sprouting, and vasculogenesis may operate in lymphatic growth (42) (see the Angiogenesis: Cellular Mechanisms section). Similar to the recently discovered organ-specific angiogenic molecule (EG-VEGF) (162) and endothelial precursor cells (176,233,234), there may be organ-specific lymphangiogenic molecules and lymphatic endothelial precursor cells that contribute to tumor-associated lymphangiogenesis (238). Moreover, the proteolytic processing of lymphangiogenesis molecules, as well as the phenotype and function of the resulting lymphatics, may depend on the tumor type as well as on the host organ in which the tumor is growing (4,138,139,148).

The precise roles for these lymphangiogenic molecules in the induction of lymphatic metastasis are imperfectly understood. Recent data demonstrate that tumor VEGF-C overexpression induces peritumoral lymphatic hyperplasia through activation of VEGFR-3. Consequently, lymph fluid volumetric flow increases (111). This results in increased tumor cell delivery to lymph nodes and a higher rate of lymphatic metastasis (111) (Fig. 4.6). It remains unclear how VEGF-C overexpression impacts tumor cell entry into lymphatic vessels; however, an attractive hypothesis is that the increased lymphatic surface area simply increases the probability of tumor cell entry and dissemination. Alternatively, VEGF-C may stimulate the release of a chemotactic factor that recruits tumor cells into lymphatic vessels. Of potential clinical importance, VEGFR-3 blockade was shown to inhibit VEGF-C–induced lymphatic hyperplasia, tumor cell delivery to draining lymph nodes, and lymphatic metastasis when treatment was started at the time of tumor initiation. However, lymphatic metastases were not significantly reduced if VEGFR-3 blockade was started after tumor cell seeding of draining lymph nodes (111). These data suggest that anti-VEGFR-3 monotherapy may be effective in preventing, but not treating, lymphatic metastases—the more common clinical imperative—except in cases where a significant fraction of vascular endothelial cells and/or cancer cells express VEGFR-3. The challenge now is to identify alternative strategies for treating lymphatic metastases, whether it be through combined therapy (e.g., anti-VEGFR-2/anti-VEGFR-3) or modulation of other lymphangiogenic pathways.

Mechanical signals that trigger the lymphangiogenic switch are unknown. Because lymphatic vessels help maintain the balance of fluid in tissues, hydrostatic pressure is a likely trigger (261). Whether the lymphatic hyperplasia seen in tumor margins is, in part, a response to the elevated hydrostatic pressure in tumors and whether the newly formed lymphatics remain open and relieve this pressure is an open question. Techniques such as microlymphangiography (99,111,117,137,145, 223,224) and fluorescence photobleaching lymph flow quantitation (12,99,111,169,260) will allow us to answer these important questions.

Interstitial Hypertension

Unlike normal tissues, where the interstitial fluid pressure (IFP) is around 0 mm Hg, both animal and human tumors exhibit interstitial hypertension (6,15,17–19,21,50,98,121,165,197, 209,223,240,278,279,293,294). The tumor IFP begins to increase as soon as the host vessels become leaky in response to angiogenic molecules such as VEGF (20,100), and, thus, IFP can be lowered by antibodies against VEGF (164,278,279) or VEGFR2 (267). The IFP increases with tumor size in some tumors (15,18,98) and remains independent of tumor size in others (165).

Three mechanisms contribute to the interstitial hypertension in tumors. In normal tissues, lymphatics maintain fluid homeostasis; thus, the lack of functional lymphatics within tumors is a key contributor. Indeed, DiResta et al. (58) have been able to lower the IFP by placing "artificial lymphatics" in tumors. The second contributor is the leaky nature of tumor vessels. As a result, the hydrostatic and oncotic (colloid osmotic) pressures become almost equal between the intravascular and extravascular space (17,142,256,267). At least two pieces of evidence support this hypothesis. First, lowering permeability by blocking VEGF signaling lowers IFP (164,267,278,279). Second, IFP goes up and down with the microvascular pressure within seconds (211,213,292). The two mechanisms described so far can only explain hypertension up to 20 to 30 mm Hg—the microvascular pressure of most exchange vessels in our body—but IFPs as high as 94 mm Hg have been measured in human tumors (240). Because the microvascular pressure (MVP) is the driving force for IFP in tumors, these tumors must have a high MVP. Indeed, this is the case (17). There are two possible explanations for the elevated MVP in tumors: (i) the tumor vessels have reduced arterial resistance so that the MVP becomes closer to arterial pressure, and/or (ii) the tumor vessels have increased venous resistance as a result of compression and tortuosity so that the whole vascular network is under hypertension. Indirect evidence for the latter comes from the decrease in IFP following decompression of tumor vessels by drug-induced apoptosis of perivascular cancer cells (94,225).

The elevated pressure can compromise the tumor microcirculation and delivery of therapeutics in three ways. First, reduced transmural pressure gradients resulting from equilibrium between MVP and IFP reduce convection across tumor vessels and thus compromise the transport of macromolecules (17,128,142,213,267). Second, because IFP is nearly uniform throughout a tumor and drops precipitously in the tumor margin, the interstitial fluid "oozes" out of the tumor into the surrounding normal tissue, carrying macromolecules with it (15,35,128). Finally, transmural coupling between IFP and MVP

as a result of high permeability of tumor vessels can lead to blood flow stasis in tumors without physically occluding the vessels (9,200,214). Thus, decreasing vascular leakiness might restore the transmural pressure gradients and potentially resume/reestablish blood flow in the nonperfused regions of tumors. Some direct and indirect antiangiogenic therapies may "normalize" the tumor vasculature through this mechanism (119,125,127,131,278) (Fig. 4.4).

Metabolic Environment

Hypoxia

A key function of the vasculature is to provide adequate levels of nutrients to the parenchymal cells and to remove waste products. Based on the anatomy of the capillary bed and a mathematical model of oxygen diffusion and consumption, the Nobel laureate August Krogh (161) introduced the concept of a diffusion limit for oxygen of 100 to 200 μm nearly a century ago. This unit of tissue—a single capillary surrounded by 100 to 200 μm radius cylinder—is referred to as a Krogh cylinder in physiology. Nearly 50 years later, Thomlinson and Gray (265) identified similar "cords" in human lung cancer and found necrotic cells beyond 180 μm away from blood vessels, presumably due to a lack of oxygen. This is referred to as *chronic hypoxia* or *diffusion-limited* hypoxia. Although various hypoxia markers and microelectrodes have suggested these gradients, the first direct measurements of these perivascular Po_2 gradients, as well as perivascular pH gradients, became possible only with the development of phosphorescence quenching microscopy (107,268) (Fig. 4.5B).

As discussed earlier, blood flow in tumor vessels is intermittent, and, thus, some regions of a tumor are periodically starved for oxygen. The resulting hypoxia is referred to as *acute hypoxia* or *perfusion-limited hypoxia* (30,56,57). A necessary consequence of intermittent blood flow is the resumption of blood flow after shutdown, and the resulting production of free radicals can lead to *ischemia-reperfusion injury* or *reoxygenation injury*; thus, applying additional selection pressure on cancer cells can cause them to become more locally aggressive, metastatic, and resistant to therapy (31,102,232).

Low pH

Another consequence of the abnormal microcirculation of the tumor is low extracellular pH. There are at least two sources of H+ ions in tumors—lactic acid and carbonic acid (106). The former results from glycolysis, and the latter results from conversion of CO_2 and H_2O via carbonic anhydrase. However, the intracellular pH of cancer cells remains neutral or alkaline (≥ 7.2) despite the acidic extracellular pH. Because carbonic anhydrase-9 and various glucose transporters (GLUT-1, -3) and enzymes in the glycolytic pathway are up-regulated by hypoxia (102,232), one would expect low extracellular pH and hypoxia to track each other and to colocalize with regions of low blood flow. It is surprising that there is a lack of spatial correlation among these parameters—a discovery made possible by recent developments in optical techniques that permit the simultaneous high-resolution mapping of multiple physiologic parameters (107). A potential explanation for this lack of concordance is that some perfused tumor vessels carry hypoxic blood (107). Thus, although they may not be able to deliver enough oxygen to the surrounding cells, they may be able to carry away the waste products (e.g., lactic acid).

Therapeutic Consequences

The presence of molecular oxygen during irradiation can "fix" biologic (e.g., DNA) free radicals, making radiation-induced damage irreparable (oxygen fixation hypothesis). Thus, hypoxia reduces the radiation sensitivity of neoplastic and normal cells both *in vitro* and *in vivo* (46). Similarly, hypoxia can compromise the efficacy of some chemotherapeutics (29). Independently, hypoxia can increase the metastatic potential of cancer cells (31,102,232). Therefore, for nearly half a century considerable preclinical and clinical effort has been focused on alleviating hypoxia through a multitude of interventions such as improving tumor perfusion with mild hyperthermia or drugs, increasing oxygen content of the blood via hyperbaric oxygenation, and increasing hemoglobin/hematocrit by transfusion or exogenous erythropoietin (46). Unfortunately, the clinical outcomes have not met expectations. Although early studies suggested a marked benefit of transfusion in anemic cervical cancer patients undergoing definitive radiotherapy (34), careful analysis suggests that these studies are confounded by selection biases that preclude the conclusion that anemia correction by transfusion impacts outcome (32,33,77). Furthermore, erythropoietin (or analog) treatment showed encouraging survival results in anemic cancer patients receiving nonplatinum chemotherapy (175) and in anemic lung cancer patients receiving chemotherapy (271). However, subsequent trials in anemic head and neck cancer patients (108) and mainly nonanemic metastatic breast cancer patients (171) actually suggested outcomes may be impaired by erythropoietic agents. There are multiple possible reasons such interventions have yielded mixed results. These include the inability to increase tumor Po_2 as markedly as systemic Po_2 (153,154,258), the inability to increase Po_2 in all areas of a tumor to optimal levels due to abnormal vasculature (127) and undesired "off-target" effects of interventions (e.g. immunosuppression with transfusion (63,90,243)). Furthermore, tumors may reoxygenate during radiation therapy with standard fractionation, potentially minimizing the impact of providing additional oxygen to the target tissue.

Similarly, low extracellular pH can adversely (or favorably) affect the uptake and cytotoxicity of some therapeutics (47,275). The pH gradient difference between tumor and normal tissue may offer a tumor specific target for weak acid chemotherapeutics for the treatment of cancer (86–89,159). The specific development of drugs that exploit this pH difference and strategies to modulate pH in tumors have not yet reached the clinic but are anticipated (232).

Two broad strategies targeting the unique tumor metabolic environment are emerging: (a) exploit hypoxia to activate drugs or attract tumoricidal anaerobic bacteria and (b) dissect hypoxia-induced pathways to identify novel targets for drug development. The first strategy has led to the development of drugs such as tirapazamine (29) and to rejuvenated interest in bacteriolytic therapy (133); both approaches are in clinical trials. The second strategy has revealed several molecular players in the physiologic and pathophysiologic response to hypoxia (109,232,247). The balance between hypoxia-induced apoptosis/necrosis on one hand and the increased resistance to cell death mediated by various hypoxia-induced pathways on the other determines whether a tumor can survive and even grow under hypoxic conditions. Ultimately, hypoxia selects for tumor cells that are more malignant, more invasive, and genetically unstable, rendering them resistant to various therapies. Therefore, certain players in the hypoxia-induced pathways now are being targeted in the development of diagnostic and therapeutic agents. Hypoxia-induced pathways include genes involved in oxygen delivery, glycolysis and glucose uptake, pH control, stress-response pathways, growth-factor signaling, angiogenesis, transcription, apoptosis, growth inhibition, and invasion and metastasis (Table 4.2) (102,109).

Table 4.2	SELECT GENES IN HYPOXIA-INDUCED PATHWAYS
Oxygen delivery	Erythropoietin
	Heme oxygenase 1
Glycolysis and glucose uptake	Glucose transporter-1, -3 (GLUT1, GLUT3)
	Hexokinase-1, -2
pH control	Carbonic anhydrase-9, -12
Stress-response pathways	Growth arrest- and DNA damage-induced gene (GADD 153)
Growth-factor signaling	Insulinlike growth factor-2 (IGF-2)
	Interleukin-6, -8 (IL-6, IL-8)
	Platelet-derived growth factor-B (PDGF-B)
Angiogenesis	Angiopoietin-2 (Ang-2)
	Cyclooxygenase-2 (COX-2)
	Fibroblast growth factor-3 (FGF-3)
	Hepatocyte growth factor (HGF)
	Nitric oxide synthase (NOS)
	Placental growth factor-B (PDGF-B)
	Tie-2 (an angiopoietin receptor)
	Transforming growth factor-α, -$\beta 1$, -$\beta 2$ (TGF-α, TGF-$\beta 1$, TGF-$\beta 2$)
	Vascular endothelial growth factor-A (VEGF-A)
	VEGF receptor 1 (VEGFR1)
Transcription	FOS
	Hypoxia-inducible factor-1α, -2α (HIF-1α, HIF-2α)
	JUN
	Nuclear factor-$\kappa\beta$ (NF-$\kappa\beta$)
	Apoptosis 19 kilodalton interacting protein-3 (NIP3)
	Annexin V
	BCL-interacting killer (BIK)
	NIP3-like protein X (NIX)
Growth inhibition	Growth arrest- and DNA damage-induced gene (GADD153), p21, p27
Invasion and metastasis	Metalloproteinases (MMP), MMP-13
	Plasminogen activator inhibitor-1 (PAI-1)

Adapted from Harris AL. Hypoxia: a key regulatory factor in tumour growth. *Nat Rev Cancer* 2002;2:38–47.

Overview and Basic Science of Radiation Oncology

Of the various molecular players involved in sensing and responding to hypoxia, hypoxia-inducible factor-1a (HIF-1α) has received the most attention. This transcription factor is up-regulated in a number of human tumors (102,247,263,291). Regulated by proline and asparagine hydroxylases, (HIF-1α) activates genes involved in an array of physiological responses including angiogenesis, vasodilation, glycolysis, and RBC production by binding to the hypoxia-response element (HRE). Although an attractive therapeutic target, the pleiotropic action of HIF-1α may prove to be a major challenge for clinical exploitation. For example, teratomas arising from HIF-1α(−/−) embryonic cells grow more rapidly despite lower levels of VEGF and angiogenesis (41). This counterintuitive finding may be a result of the ability of HIF-1α(−/−) cells to survive under hypoxic conditions, instead of undergoing apoptosis (27). HIF-1α has also been shown to play an important role in determining tumor radioresponsiveness through the regulation of multiple, and sometimes opposing, processes (199). Under some circumstances, HIF-1α inhibition *reduces* tumor cell radiosensitivity by protecting hypoxic cells from radiation-induced apoptosis and enhancing clonogenic survival potentially through reductions in adenosine triphosphate metabolism, cellular proliferation, and p53 activation (199). Furthermore, HIF-1α serves a key function in inflammatory cell energy metabolism, and its inhibition results in profound immunodeficiency (48). Consequently, molecular therapies that target HIF-1α or HRE, as well as more selective therapies that target key downstream effectors of HIF-1α, are under intensive investigation for cancer detection and treatment (193,232,247).

Clinical Implications

Two major problems currently plague the nonsurgical treatment of malignant solid tumors. First, physiologic barriers within tumors impede the delivery of therapeutics and oxygen (a key radiation sensitizer) at effective concentrations to all cancer cells (123,124). Second, inherent or acquired resistance resulting from genetic and epigenetic mechanisms reduces the effectiveness of conventional as well as novel therapies (180). Can we take advantage of the unique pathophysiology of tumors to overcome these problems for better management of cancer? As discussed next, recent clinical data offer some hope.

Prognostic Implications

Multiple indices of tumor pathophysiology have been evaluated as potential predictors of treatment outcome including vessel density (reviewed in [253]), oxygen level (reviewed in [194, 272]), and interstitial pressure (75,76,197,240). Vessel density can be evaluated in biopsies and is measured either in "hot spots" (i.e., regions of most active angiogenesis) or in the tissue as a whole. The former presumably provides a measure of a tumor's aggressiveness, and the latter reflects the status of global oxygenation. Most studies to date show that poor outcome of radiation therapy correlates with high vessel density in "hot spots" and/or low overall microvessel density. There are, however, several studies showing a lack of correlation or an opposite correlation. This discrepancy may be the result of the morphometric techniques used or to differences in tumor types or treatment schedules.

The oxygen level in a tumor also has a potential prognostic value, and it can be directly measured with microelectrodes. Alternatively, immunohistochemical analysis of tumor tissue for endogenous or exogenous hypoxic markers (e.g., HIF-1α, glucose transporter-1, carbonic anhydrase-9, pimonidazole) can be used as a surrogate for tumor oxygenation status. However, immunohistochemical assessments of hypoxia do not necessarily correlate with oxygen status measured directly with microelectrodes (216). Finally, a concerted effort is under way to assess hypoxia using novel, noninvasive imaging techniques (248). Several studies have shown that tumor hypoxia is a predictor of a poor outcome of radiation therapy when used alone or in combination with other therapies. These findings are consistent with *in vitro* and *in vivo* preclinical studies showing the adverse effect of hypoxia on radiation responses.

Finally, because the IFP is a reflection of the global physiology of tumors, a correlation between tumor IFP and the response to radiation therapy has been suggested. One cervical cancer study has shown that elevated tumor IFP can, indeed, independently predict a poor outcome of radiation therapy (75,76). Further studies are needed to evaluate the prognostic significance of IFP in tumors. However, one potential application of the steep rise of pressure at the tumor periphery is improved localization of tumors before their removal (129).

Although each of these approaches has advantages, key disadvantages include their invasiveness as well as their potential for sampling error. With rapid developments in the field of noninvasive imaging, it is likely that the measurement of various physiologic and molecular parameters in tumors will become more refined and convenient for patients. Examples of such imaging approaches include blood-oxygen level-dependent magnetic resonance imaging (BOLD MRI) (160), electron paramagnetic resonance spectroscopy/imaging (79), and [^{18}F]-misonidazole positron emission tomography (FMISO-PET) (235,239,248). The promise of such imaging approaches has just started to be realized. FMISO-PET has been evaluated in a substudy of patients with stage III or IV squamous-cell carcinoma of the head and neck randomized to concurrent radiotherapy with either tirapazamine and cisplatin or infusional fluorouracil and cisplatin. Pretreatment FMISO-PET–detected hypoxia was associated with a higher risk of locoregional recurrence among patients who did not receive the tirapazamine-containing regimen compared to patients who did receive tirapazamine (239). This study suggests that FMISO-PET can provide clinically meaningful information about tumor physiology and simultaneously provides evidence that tirapazamine acts by specifically targeting hypoxic tumor cells. Such progress will continue and physiologic/molecular profiles of patients' tumors will yield improved and better-tailored therapies for individual patients.

Therapeutic Implications

Given the physiologic barriers to the delivery and effectiveness of various therapeutics, a strategy that is gaining increasing interest is targeting the tumor vasculature. This strategy has the advantage of targeting ECs that are easily accessible to a blood-borne drug and are presumably genetically stable. In addition, each EC supports multiple cancer cells, thus providing "therapeutic amplification." However, the inability to target *all* ECs in a tumor can reduce the effectiveness of antivascular therapy. Similarly, the dependence of ECs on multiple angiogenic molecules can limit the effectiveness of various antiangiogenic therapies when used alone (42,119,130). These challenges may explain why currently available antiangiogenic agents, although demonstrating biological activity, are unable to provide durable tumor control when used as monotherapy.

Although of limited utility when used alone, the judicious combination of antiangiogenic therapies with conventional cytotoxic therapies has led to improved tumor control in mice and lengthened survival in certain types of human tumors (5,25,114, 131,155,156,158,246). For example, in two human tumor xenograft models, a VEGFR-2–blocking antibody decreased the dose of fractionated radiation required to control 50% of tumors (TCD50) by 11 to 27 Gy without modifying in-field skin reactions (158). Thus, to maximize clinical gains, these agents must

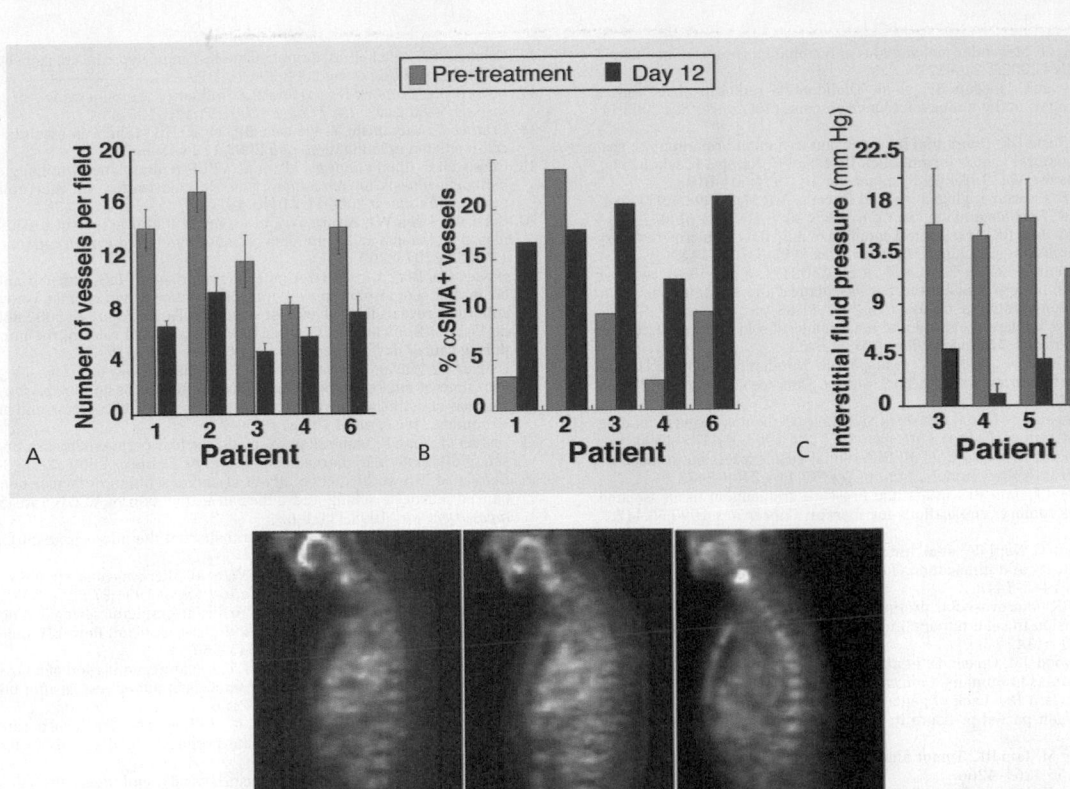

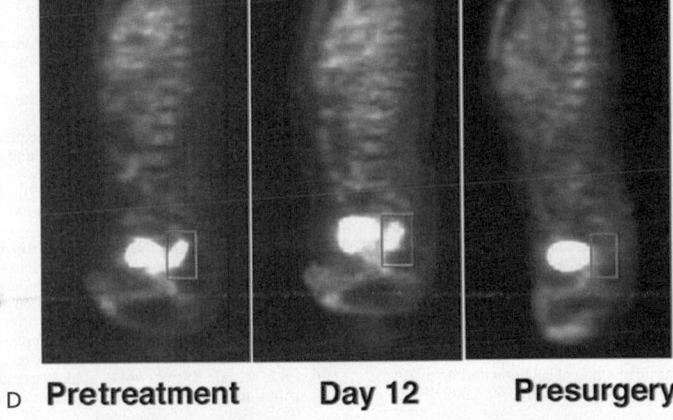

D Pretreatment   Day 12   Presurgery

FIGURE 4.7. Vascular "normalization" in rectal cancer patients following treatment with the anti-VEGF antibody, bevacizumab. Tumor vessel "normalization" following a single injection of bevacizumab is suggested by the **(A)** reduced tumor microvessel density, **(B)** increased fraction of tumor vessels with pericyte coverage and **(C)** reduced interstitial fluid pressure. **D:** Positron emission tomography reveals no change in 18-fluorodeoxyglucose (FDG) uptake after a single dose of bevacizumab and complete resolution of FDG uptake following neoadjuvant chemoradiation (bevacizumab, 5-fluorouracil, pelvic external beam radiation therapy). The stability of FDG uptake following bevacizumab monotherapy, despite marked reductions in microvessel density, suggests the efficiency of persistent tumor blood vessels after bevacizumab treatment is improved. (From Willett CG, Boucher Y, di Tomaso E, et al. Direct evidence that the VEGF-specific antibody bevacizumab has antivascular effects in human rectal cancer. *Nat Med* 2004;145–147, with permission.)

be employed in combination with radiation and chemotherapy. The challenge now is to optimally combine these therapies in patients. Destruction of tumor vasculature by antiangiogenic agents should antagonize chemo- and radiotherapy by compromising the delivery of therapeutics and oxygen, respectively. However, judiciously applied antiangiogenic therapy can prune inefficient tumor vessels and render the remaining vasculature more efficient (Fig. 4.4) (125,127). This "normalization" of tumor vasculature has been demonstrated in various preclinical models (5,113,116,119,140,148,196,241,246,267,274,277, 280,286) and in rectal cancer and glioblastoma patients (10,278) (Fig. 4.7). Vascular "normalization" should result in improved delivery of cytotoxic chemotherapy and radiosensitizing oxygen, thereby improving tumor control. This principle has been rigorously tested in animal models (5,113,241, 246,277,280) and confirmatory data on the impact of vascular "normalization" on patient outcomes await mature results of ongoing and future clinical trials.

Acknowledgments

We thank Kathryn Held, Leo Gerweck, Sergey Kozin, Theodore Hong, Timothy Padera, and Hennng Willers for critically reviewing this chapter. The work summarized here was supported by continuous support from the National Cancer Institute since 1980.

References

1. Abramsson A, Berlin O, Papayan H, et al. Analysis of mural cell recruitment to tumor vessels. *Circulation* 2002;105:112–117.
2. Achen MG, Mann GB, Stacker SA. Targeting lymphangiogenesis to prevent tumour metastasis. *Br J Cancer* 2006;94:1355–1360.
3. Algire GH, Chalkley HW. Vascular reactions of normal and malignant tissues in vivo. I. Vascular reactions of mice to wounds and to normal and neoplastic transplants. *J Natl Cancer Inst* 1945;6:73–85.

4. Alitalo K, Carmeliet P. Molecular mechanisms of lymphangiogenesis in health and disease. *Cancer Cell* 2002;1:219–227.

5. Ansiaux R, Baudelet C, Jordan BF, et al. Thalidomide radiosensitizes tumors through early changes in the tumor microenvironment. *Clin Cancer Res* 2005;11: 743–750.

6. Arbit E, Lee J, DiResta GR. Interstitial hypertension in human brain tumors: possible role in peritumoral edema formulation. In: Nagai H, Kamiya K, Ishi S, eds., *Intracranial pressure*, Vol. 9. Tokyo: Springer-Verlag, 1994;604–619.

7. Baish JW, Jain RK. Cancer, angiogenesis and fractals. *Nat Med* 1998;4:984–984.

8. Baish JW, Jain RK. Fractals and cancer. *Cancer Res* 2000;60:3683–3688.

9. Baish JW, Netti PA, Jain RK. Transmural coupling of fluid flow in microcirculatory network and interstitium in tumors. *Microvasc Res* 1997;53:128–141.

10. Batchelor TT, Sorensen AG, di Tomaso E, et al. AZD2171, a pan-VEGF receptor tyrosine kinase inhibitor, normalizes tumor vasculature and alleviates vasogenic edema in glioblastoma patients. *Cancer Cell* 2007;11:83–95.

11. Baxter LT, Jain RK. Transport of fluid and macromolecules in tumors. III. Role of binding and metabolism. *Microvasc Res* 1991;41:5–23.

12. Berk DA, Swartz MA, Leu AJ, et al. Transport in lymphatic capillaries. II. Microscopic velocity measurement with fluorescence photobleaching. *Am J Physiol* 1996;39:H330–H337.

13. Berk DA, Yuan F, Leunig M, et al. Direct in vivo measurement of targeted binding in a human tumor xenograft. *Proc Natl Acad Sci U S A* 1997;94:1785–1790.

14. Bockhorn M, Roberge S, Sousa C, et al. Differential gene expression in metastasizing cells shed from kidney tumors. *Cancer Res* 2004;64:2469–2473.

15. Boucher Y, Baxter LT, Jain RK. Interstitial pressure gradients in tissue-isolated and subcutaneous tumors: implications for therapy. *Cancer Res* 1990;50:4478–4484.

16. Boucher Y, Brekken C, Netti PA, et al. Intratumoral infusion of fluid: estimation of hydraulic conductivity and implications for the delivery of therapeutic agents. *Br J Cancer* 1998;78:1442–1448.

17. Boucher Y, Jain RK. Microvascular pressure is the principal driving force for interstitial hypertension in solid tumors: implications for vascular collapse. *Cancer Res* 1992;52:5110–5114.

18. Boucher Y, Kirkwood JM, Opacic D, et al. Interstitial hypertension in superficial metastatic melanomas in humans. *Cancer Res* 1991;51:6691–6694.

19. Boucher Y, Lee I, Jain RK. Lack of general correlation between interstitial fluid pressure and oxygen partial-pressure in solid tumors. *Microvasc Res* 1995;50: 175–182.

20. Boucher Y, Leunig M, Jain RK. Tumor angiogenesis and interstitial hypertension. *Cancer Res* 1996;56:4264–4266.

21. Boucher Y, Salehi H, Witwer B, et al. Interstitial fluid pressure in intracranial tumours in patients and in rodents. *Br J Cancer* 1997;75:829–836.

22. Bouck N, Stellmach V, Hsu SC, eds. How tumors become angiogenic. *Adv Cancer Res.* 1996;69:135–174.

23. Branca MA. Multi-kinase inhibitors create buzz at ASCO. *Nat Biotechnol* 2005;23:639.

24. Brizel DM, Klitzman B, Cook JM, et al. A comparison of tumor and normal tissue microvascular hematocrits and red cell fluxes in a rat window chamber model. *Int J Radiat Oncol Biol Phys* 1993;25:269–276.

25. Browder T, Butterfield CE, Kraling BM, et al. Antiangiogenic scheduling of chemotherapy improves efficacy against experimental drug-resistant cancer. *Cancer Res* 2000;60:1878–1886.

26. Brown E, McKee T, diTomaso E, et al. Dynamic imaging of collagen and its modulation in tumors in vivo using second-harmonic generation. *Nat Med* 2003;9:796–800.

27. Brown EB, Campbell RB, Tsuzuki Y, et al. In vivo measurement of gene expression, angiogenesis and physiological function in tumors using multiphoton laser scanning microscopy. *Nat Med* 2001;7:1069–1069.

28. Brown EB, Boucher Y, Nasser S, et al. Measurement of macromolecular diffusion coefficients in human tumors. *Microvasc Res* 2004;67:231–236.

29. Brown JM. The hypoxic cell: a target for selective cancer therapy—eighteenth Bruce F. Cain Memorial Award lecture. *Cancer Res* 1999;59:5863–5870.

30. Brown JM, Giaccia AJ. The unique physiology of solid tumors: opportunities (and problems) for cancer therapy. *Cancer Res* 1998;58:1408–1416.

31. Brown JM, Wilson WR. Exploiting tumour hypoxia in cancer treatment. *Nat Rev Cancer* 2004;4:437–447.

32. Bush RS. Current status and treatment of localized disease and future aspects. *Int J Radiat Oncol Biol Phys* 1984;10:1165–1174.

33. Bush RS. The significance of anemia in clinical radiation therapy. *Int J Radiat Oncol Biol Phys* 1986;12:2047–2050.

34. Bush RS, Jenkin RD, Allt WE, et al. Definitive evidence for hypoxic cells influencing cure in cancer therapy. *Br J Cancer Suppl* 1978;37:302–306.

35. Butler TP, Grantham FH, Gullino PM. Bulk transfer of fluid in interstitial compartment of mammary tumors. *Cancer Res* 1975;35:3084–3088.

36. Campbell RB, Fukumura D, Brown EB, et al. Cationic charge determines the distribution of liposomes between the vascular and extravascular compartments of tumors. *Cancer Res* 2002;62:6831–6836.

37. Cao R, Bjorndahl MA, Gallego MI, et al. Hepatocyte growth factor is a lymphangiogenic factor with an indirect mechanism of action. *Blood* 2006;107:3531–3536.

38. Cao R, Bjorndahl MA, Religa P, et al. PDGF-BB induces intratumoral lymphangiogenesis and promotes lymphatic metastasis. *Cancer Cell* 2004;6:333–345.

39. Carmeliet P. Mechanisms of angiogenesis and arteriogenesis. *Nat Med* 2000;6: 389–395.

40. Carmeliet P. Angiogenesis in life, disease and medicine. *Nature* 2005;438:932–936.

41. Carmeliet P, Dor Y, Herbert JM, et al. Role of HIF-1alpha in hypoxia-mediated apoptosis, cell proliferation and tumour angiogenesis. *Nature* 1998;394:485–490.

42. Carmeliet P, Jain RK. Angiogenesis in cancer and other diseases. *Nature* 2000; 407:249–257.

43. Carreira CM, Nasser SM, di Tomaso E, et al. LYVE-1 is not restricted to the lymph vessels: expression in normal liver blood sinusoids and down-regulation in human liver cancer and cirrhosis. *Cancer Res* 2001;61:8079–8084.

44. Casanovas O, Hicklin DJ, Bergers G, et al. Drug resistance by evasion of antiangiogenic targeting of VEGF signaling in late-stage pancreatic islet tumors. *Cancer Cell* 2005;8:299–309.

45. Chary SR, Jain RK. Direct measurement of interstitial convection and diffusion of albumin in normal and neoplastic tissues by fluorescence photobleaching. *Proc Natl Acad Sci U S A* 1989;86:5385–5389.

46. Coleman CN, Mitchell JB, Camphausen K. Tumor hypoxia: chicken, egg, or a piece of the farm? *J Clin Oncol* 2002;20:610–615.

47. Cowan DS, Tannock IF. Factors that influence the penetration of methotrexate through solid tissue. *Int J Cancer* 2001;91:120–125.

48. Cramer T, Yamanishi Y, Clausen BE, et al. HIF-1alpha is essential for myeloid cell-mediated inflammation. *Cell* 2003;112:645–657.

49. Cursiefen C, Chen L, Borges LP, et al. VEGF-A stimulates lymphangiogenesis and hemangiogenesis in inflammatory neovascularization via macrophage recruitment. *J Clin Invest* 2004;113:1040–1050.

50. Curti BD, Urba WJ, Alvord WG, et al. Interstitial pressure of subcutaneous nodules in melanoma and lymphoma patients: changes during treatment. *Cancer Res* 1993;53:2204–2207.

51. Davies CD, Berk DA, Pluen A, et al. Comparison of IgG diffusion and extracellular matrix composition in rhabdomyosarcomas grown in mice versus in vitro as spheroids reveals the role of host stromal cells. *Br J Cancer* 2002;86:1639–1644.

52. de Visser KE, Eichten A, Coussens LM. Paradoxical roles of the immune system during cancer development. *Nat Rev Cancer* 2006;6:24–37.

53. Dellian M, Witwer BP, Salehi HA, et al. Quantitation and physiological characterization of angiogenic vessels in mice—effect of basic fibroblast growth factor vascular endothelial growth factor vascular permeability factor, and host microenvironment. *Am J Pathol* 1996;149:59–71.

54. Dellian M, Yuan F, Trubetskoy VS, et al. Vascular permeability in a human tumour xenograft: molecular charge dependence. *Br J Cancer* 2000;82:1513–1518.

55. Detmar M, Brown LF, Schon MP, et al. Increased microvascular density and enhanced leukocyte rolling and adhesion in the skin of VEGF transgenic mice. *J Invest Dermatol* 1998;111:1–6.

56. Dewhirst MW. Concepts of oxygen transport at the microcirculatory level. *Semin Radiat Oncol* 1998;8:143–150.

57. Dewhirst MW, Kimura H, Rehmus SW, et al. Microvascular studies on the origins of perfusion-limited hypoxia. *Br J Cancer Suppl* 1996;27:S247–S251.

58. DiResta GR, Lee J, Healey JH, et al. "Artificial lymphatic system": A new approach to reduce interstitial hypertension and increase blood flow, pH and Po$_2$ in solid tumors. *Ann Biomed Eng* 2000;28:543–555.

59. Dolmans D, Kadambi A, Hill JS, et al. Vascular accumulation of a novel photosensitizer, MV6401, causes selective thrombosis in tumor vessels after photodynamic therapy. *Cancer Res* 2002;62:2151–2156.

60. Duda DG, Cohen KS, Kozin SV, et al. Evidence for incorporation of bone marrow-derived endothelial cells into perfused blood vessels in tumors. *Blood* 2006;107:2774–2776.

61. Dvorak HF. Vascular permeability factor/vascular endothelial growth factor: a critical cytokine in tumor angiogenesis and a potential target for diagnosis and therapy. *J Clin Oncol* 2002;20:4368–4380.

62. Dvorak HF, Nagy JA, Feng D, et al. Tumor architecture and targeted delivery. In: Abrams PG, Fritzberg AR, eds., *Radioimmunotherapy of cancer*. New York: Marcel Dekker, Inc., 2000;107–135.

63. Dzik S, Mincheff M, Puppo F. Apoptosis, transforming growth factor-beta, and the immunosuppressive effect of transfusion. *Transfusion* 2002;42:1221–1223.

64. Ehrmann RL, Knoth M. Choriocarcinoma—transfilter stimulation of vasoproliferation in hamster cheek pouch studied by light and electron microscopy. *J Natl Cancer Inst* 1968;41:1329–1341.

65. Elenbaas B, Weinberg RA. Heterotypic signaling between epithelial tumor cells and fibroblasts in carcinoma formation. *Exp Cell Res* 2001;264:169–184.

66. Endo M, Jain RK, Witwer B, et al. Water channel (aquaporin 1) expression and distribution in mammary carcinomas and glioblastomas. *Microvasc Res* 1999;58:89–98.

67. Endrich B, Reinhold HS, Gross JF, et al. Tissue perfusion inhomogeneity during early tumor growth in rats. *J Natl Cancer Inst* 1979;62:387–395.

68. Ferrara N. Role of vascular endothelial growth factor in regulation of physiological angiogenesis. *Am J Physiol Cell Physiol* 2001;280:C1358–C1366.

69. Folkman J. Tumor angiogenesis. In: Holland JF, Frei E III, Bast RC Jr., et al., eds., *Cancer medicine*, 5th ed. Ontario, Canada: B.C. Decker Inc., 2000;132–152.

70. Folkman J, Watson K, Ingber D, et al. Induction of angiogenesis during the transition from hyperplasia to neoplasia. *Nature* 1989;339:58–61.

71. Fukumura D, Salehi HA, Witwer B, et al. Tumor necrosis factor alpha-induced leukocyte adhesion in normal and tumor vessels: effect of tumor type, transplantation site, and host strain. *Cancer Res* 1995;55:4824–4829.

72. Fukumura D, Xavier R, Sugiura T, et al. Tumor induction of VEGF promoter activity in stromal cells. *Cell* 1998;94:715–725.

73. Fukumura D, Xu L, Chen Y, et al. Hypoxia and acidosis independently up-regulate vascular endothelial growth factor transcription in brain tumors in vivo. *Cancer Res* 2001;61:6020–6024.

74. Fukumura D, Yuan F, Monsky WL, et al. Effect of host microenvironment on the microcirculation of human colon adenocarcinoma. *Am J Pathol* 1997;151:679–688.

75. Fyles A, Milosevic M, Hedley D, et al. Tumor hypoxia has independent predictor impact only in patients with node-negative cervix cancer. *J Clin Oncol* 2002;20:680–687.

76. Fyles A, Milosevic M, Pintilie M, et al. Long-term performance of interstitial fluid pressure and hypoxia as prognostic factors in cervix cancer. *Radiother Oncol* 2006;80:132–137.

77. Fyles AW, Milosevic M, Pintilie M, et al. Anemia, hypoxia and transfusion in patients with cervix cancer: a review. *Radiother Oncol* 2000;57:13–19.

78. Gale NW, Thurston G, Hackett SF, et al. Angiopoietin-2 is required for postnatal angiogenesis and lymphatic patterning, and only the latter role is rescued by angiopoietin-1. *Dev Cell* 2002;3:411–423.

79. Gallez B, Baudelet C, Jordan BF. Assessment of tumor oxygenation by electron paramagnetic resonance: principles and applications. *NMR Biomed* 2004;17:240–262.

80. Gamble JR, Khew-Goodall Y, Vadas MA. Transforming growth factor-beta inhibits E-selectin expression on human endothelial cells. *J Immunol* 1993;150:4494–4503.

81. Gamble JR, Vadas MA. Endothelial adhesiveness for blood neutrophils is inhibited by transforming growth factor-beta. *Science* 1988;242:97–99.

82. Gamble JR, Vadas MA. Endothelial cell adhesiveness for human T lymphocytes is inhibited by transforming growth factor-beta 1. *J Immunol* 1991;146:1149–1154.

83. Garkavtsev I, Kozin SV, Chernova O, et al. The candidate tumour suppressor protein ING4 regulates brain tumour growth and angiogenesis. *Nature* 2004;428:328–332.

84. Gazit Y, Baish JW, Safabakhsh N, et al. Fractal characteristics of tumor vascular architecture during tumor growth and regression. *Microcirculation* 1997;4:395–402.
85. Gerlowski LE, Jain RK. Microvascular permeability of normal and neoplastic tissues. *Microvasc Res* 1986;31:288–305.
86. Gerweck LE. Tumor pH: implications for treatment and novel drug design. *Semin Radiat Oncol* 1998;8:176–182.
87. Gerweck LE, Kozin SV, Stocks SJ. The pH partition theory predicts the accumulation and toxicity of doxorubicin in normal and low-pH-adapted cells. *Br J Cancer* 1999;79:838–842.
88. Gerweck LE, Seetharaman K. Cellular pH gradient in tumor versus normal tissue: potential exploitation for the treatment of cancer. *Cancer Res* 1996;56:1194–1198.
89. Gerweck LE, Vijayappa S, Kozin S. Tumor pH controls the in vivo efficacy of weak acid and base chemotherapeutics. *Mol Cancer Ther* 2006;5:1275–1279.
90. Gharehbaghian A, Haque KM, Truman C, et al. Effect of autologous salvaged blood on postoperative natural killer cell precursor frequency. *Lancet* 2004;363:1025–1030.
91. Gohongi T, Fukumura D, Boucher Y, et al. Tumor-host interactions in the gallbladder suppress distal angiogenesis and tumor growth: Involvement of transforming growth factor beta 1. *Nat Med* 1999;5:1203–1208.
92. Goldman E. The growth of malignant disease in man and the lower animals with special reference to the vascular system. *Lancet* 1907;2:1236–1240.
93. Greenblatt M, Shubik P. Tumor angiogenesis: transfilter diffusion studies in the hamster by the transparent chamber technique. *J Natl Cancer Inst* 1968;41:111–124.
94. Griffon-Etienne G, Boucher Y, Brekken C, et al. Taxane-induced apoptosis decompresses blood vessels and lowers interstitial fluid pressure in solid tumors: Clinical implications. *Cancer Res* 1999;59:3776–3782.
95. Gullino PM Techniques in tumor pathophysiology. In: Busch H, ed., *Methods in cancer research*. New York: Academic Press, 1970;45–92.
96. Gullino PM. Extracellular compartments of solid tumors. In: Becker FF, ed., *Cancer*. New York: Plenum, 1975;327–354.
97. Gullino PM. Angiogenesis and oncogenesis. *J Natl Cancer Inst* 1978;61:639–643.
98. Gutmann R, Leunig M, Feyh J, et al. Interstitial hypertension in head and neck tumors in patients: Correlation with tumor size. *Cancer Res* 1992;52:1993–1995.
99. Hagendoorn J, Padera TP, Kashiwagi S, et al. Endothelial nitric oxide synthase regulates microlymphatic flow via collecting lymphatics. *Circ Res* 2004;95:204–209.
100. Hagendoorn J, Tong R, Fukumura D, et al. Onset of abnormal blood and lymphatic vessel function and interstitial hypertension in early stages of carcinogenesis. *Cancer Res* 2006;66:3360–3364.
101. Hanahan D, Weinberg RA. The hallmarks of cancer. *Cell* 2000;100:57–70.
102. Harris AL. Hypoxia: a key regulatory factor in tumour growth. *Nat Rev Cancer* 2002;2:38–47.
103. Hashizume H, Baluk P, Morikawa S, et al. Openings between defective endothelial cells explain tumor vessel leakiness. *Am J Pathol* 2000;156:1363–1380.
104. Helmlinger G, Endo M, Ferrara N, et al. Formation of endothelial cell networks. *Nature* 2000;405:139–141.
105. Helmlinger G, Netti PA, Lichtenbeld HC, et al. Solid stress inhibits the growth of multicellular tumor spheroids. *Nat Biotechnol* 1997;15:778–783.
106. Helmlinger G, Schell A, Dellian M, et al. Acid production in glycolysis-impaired tumors provides new insights into tumor metabolism. *Clin Cancer Res* 2002;8:1284–1291.
107. Helmlinger G, Yuan F, Dellian M, et al. Interstitial pH and Po_2 gradients in solid tumors in vivo: high-resolution measurements reveal a lack of correlation. *Nat Med* 1997;3:177–182.
108. Henke M, Laszig R, Rube C, et al. Erythropoietin to treat head and neck cancer patients with anaemia undergoing radiotherapy: randomised, double-blind, placebo-controlled trial. *Lancet* 2003;362:1255–1260.
109. Hirota K, Semenza GL. Regulation of angiogenesis by hypoxia-inducible factor 1. *Crit Rev Oncol Hematol* 2006;59:15–26.
110. Hobbs SK, Monsky WL, Yuan F, et al. Regulation of transport pathways in tumor vessels: Role of tumor type and microenvironment. *Proc Natl Acad Sci U S A* 1998;95:4607–4612.
111. Hoshida T, Isaka N, Hagendoorn J, et al. Imaging steps of lymphatic metastasis reveals that vascular endothelial growth factor-C increases metastasis by increasing delivery of cancer cells to lymph nodes: therapeutic implications. *Cancer Res* 2006;66:8065–8075.
112. Huang X, Molema G, King S, et al. Tumor infarction in mice by antibody-directed targeting of tissue factor to tumor vasculature. *Science* 1997;275:547–550.
113. Huber PE, Bischof M, Jenne J, et al. Trimodal cancer treatment: beneficial effects of combined antiangiogenesis, radiation, and chemotherapy. *Cancer Res* 2005;65:3643–3655.
114. Hurwitz H, Fehrenbacher L, Novotny W, et al. Bevacizumab plus irinotecan, fluorouracil, and leucovorin for metastatic colorectal cancer. *N Engl J Med* 2004;350:2335–2342.
115. Ide AG, Baker NH, Warren SL. Vascularization of the Brown-Pearce rabbit epithelioma transplant as seen in the transplant ear chamber. *Am J Radiol* 1939;42:891–899.
116. Inai T, Mancuso M, Hashizume H, et al. Inhibition of vascular endothelial growth factor (VEGF) signaling in cancer causes loss of endothelial fenestrations, regression of tumor vessels, and appearance of basement membrane ghosts. *Am J Pathol* 2004;165:35–52.
117. Isaka N, Padera TP, Hagendoorn J, et al. Peritumor lymphatics induced by vascular endothelial growth factor-C exhibit abnormal function. *Cancer Res* 2004;64:4400–4404.
118. Isner JM. Myocardial gene therapy. *Nature* 2002;415:234.
119. Izumi Y, Xu L, di Tomaso E, et al. Tumor biology—Herceptin acts as an anti-angiogenic cocktail. *Nature* 2002;416:279–280.
120. Jain RK. Transport of molecules across tumor vasculature. *Cancer Metastasis Rev* 1987;6:559–593.
121. Jain RK. Transport of molecules in the tumor interstitium: a review. *Cancer Res* 1987;47:3039–3051.
122. Jain RK. Determinants of tumor blood flow: a review. *Cancer Res* 1988;48:2641–2658.
123. Jain RK. Barriers to drug delivery in solid tumors. *Sci Am* 1994;271:58–65.
124. Jain RK. The next frontier of molecular medicine: delivery of therapeutics. *Nat Med* 1998;4:655–657.
125. Jain RK. Normalizing tumor vasculature with anti-angiogenic therapy: a new paradigm for combination therapy. *Nat Med* 2001;7:987–989.
126. Jain RK. Molecular regulation of vessel maturation. *Nat Med* 2003;9:685–693.
127. Jain RK. Normalization of tumor vasculature: an emerging concept in antiangiogenic therapy. *Science* 2005;307:58–62.
128. Jain RK, Baxter LT. Mechanisms of heterogeneous distribution of monoclonal antibodies and other macromolecules in tumors: significance of elevated interstitial pressure. *Cancer Res* 1988;48:7022–7032.
129. Jain RK, Boucher Y, Stacey-Clearm A, et al. Method for locating tumors prior to needle biopsy. Patent 5,396,897. USA, March 14, 1995.
130. Jain RK, Carmeliet PF. Vessels of death or life. *Sci Am* 2001;285:38–45.
131. Jain RK, Duda DG, Clark JW, et al. Lessons from phase III clinical trials on anti-VEGF therapy for cancer. *Nat Clin Pract Oncol* 2006;3:24–40.
132. Jain RK, Fenton BT. Intratumoral lymphatic vessels: a case of mistaken identity or malfunction? *J Natl Cancer Inst* 2002;94:417–421.
133. Jain RK, Forbes NS. Can engineered bacteria help control cancer? *Proc Natl Acad Sci U S A* 2001;98:14748–14750.
134. Jain RK, Koenig GC, Dellian M, et al. Leukocyte-endothelial adhesion and angiogenesis in tumors. *Cancer Metastasis Rev* 1996;15:195–204.
135. Jain RK, Munn LL. Leaky vessels? Call Angl1! *Nat Med* 2000;6:131–132.
136. Jain RK, Munn LL, Fukumura D. Transparent window models and intravital microscopy: imaging gene expression, physiological function and drug delivery in tumors. In: Teicher BA, ed., *Tumor models in cancer research*. Totowa, NJ: Humana Press, Inc., 2001;647–672.
137. Jain RK, Munn LL, Fukumura D. Dissecting tumour pathophysiology using intravital microscopy. *Nat Rev Cancer* 2002;2:266–276.
138. Jain RK, Padera TP. Prevention and treatment of lymphatic metastasis by antilymphangiogenic therapy. *J Natl Cancer Inst* 2002;94:785–787.
139. Jain RK, Padera TP. Development: lymphatics make the break. *Science* 2003;299:209–210.
140. Jain RK, Safabakhsh N, Sckell A, et al. Endothelial cell death, angiogenesis, and microvascular function after castration in an androgen-dependent tumor: role of vascular endothelial growth factor. *Proc Natl Acad Sci U S A* 1998;95:10820–10825.
141. Jain RK, Schlenger K, Hockel M, et al. Quantitative angiogenesis assays: progress and problems. *Nat Med* 1997;3:1203–1208.
142. Jain RK, Tong R, Munn LL. Effect of vascular normalization by anti-angiogenic therapy on interstitial hypertension, peri-tumor edema and lymphatic metastasis: insights from a mathematical model. *Cancer Res* 2007;67:2729–2735.
143. Jain RK, Ward-Hartley K. Tumor blood flow: Characterization, modifications, and role in hyperthermia. *IEEE Trans Son Ultrason* 1984;31:504–526.
144. Jallal B, Powell J, Zachwieja J, et al. Suppression of tumor growth in vivo by local and systemic 90K level increase. *Cancer Res* 1995;55:3223–3227.
145. Jeltsch M, Kaipainen A, Joukov V, et al. Hyperplasia of lymphatic vessels in VEGF-C transgenic mice. *Science* 1997;276:1423–1425.
146. Jin DK, Shido K, Kopp HG, et al. Cytokine-mediated deployment of SDF-1 induces revascularization through recruitment of CXCR4+ hemangiocytes. *Nat Med* 2006;12:557–567.
147. Juweid M, Neumann R, Paik C, et al. Micropharmacology of monoclonal antibodies in solid tumors: direct experimental evidence for a binding site barrier. *Cancer Res* 1992;52:5144–5153.
148. Kadambi A, Carreira CM, Yun C, et al. Vascular endothelial growth factor (VEGF)-C differentially affects tumor vascular function and leukocyte recruitment: Role of VEGF-receptor 2 and host VEGF-A. *Cancer Res* 2001;61:2404–2408.
149. Kalluri R. Basement membranes: structure, assembly and role in tumor angiogenesis. *Nat Rev Cancer* 2003;3:422–433.
150. Kalluri R, Zeisberg M. Fibroblasts in cancer. *Nat Rev Cancer* 2006;6:392–401.
151. Karpanen T, Egeblad M, Karkkainen MJ, et al. Vascular endothelial growth factor C promotes tumor lymphangiogenesis and intralymphatic tumor growth. *Cancer Res* 2001;61:1786–1790.
152. Kashiwagi S, Izumi Y, Gohongi T, et al. NO mediates mural cell recruitment and vessel morphogenesis in murine melanomas and tissue-engineered blood vessels. *J Clin Invest* 2005;115:1816–1827.
153. Kelleher DK, Matthiensen U, Thews O, et al. Tumor oxygenation in anemic rats: effects of erythropoietin treatment versus red blood cell transfusion. *Acta Oncol* 1995;34:379–384.
154. Kelleher DK, Mattheinsen U, Thews O, et al. Blood flow, oxygenation, and bioenergetic status of tumors after erythropoietin treatment in normal and anemic rats. *Cancer Res* 1996;56:4728–4734.
155. Kerbel R, Folkman J. Clinical translation of angiogenesis inhibitors. *Nat Rev Cancer* 2002;2:727–739.
156. Klement G, Baruchel S, Rak J, et al. Continuous low-dose therapy with vinblastine and VEGF receptor-2 antibody induces sustained tumor regression without overt toxicity. *J Clin Invest* 2000;105:R15–R24.
157. Koike C, McKee TD, Pluen A, et al. Solid stress facilitates spheroid formation: potential involvement of hyaluronan. *Br J Cancer* 2002;86:947–953.
158. Kozin SV, Boucher Y, Hicklin DJ, et al. Vascular endothelial growth factor receptor-2-blocking antibody potentiates radiation-induced long-term control of human tumor xenografts. *Cancer Res* 2001;61:39–44.
159. Kozin SV, Shkarin P, Gerweck LE. The cell transmembrane pH gradient in tumors enhances cytotoxicity of specific weak acid chemotherapeutics. *Cancer Res* 2001;61:4740–4743.
160. Krishna MC, Subramanian S, Kuppusamy P, et al. Magnetic resonance imaging for in vivo assessment of tissue oxygen concentration. *Semin Radiat Oncol* 2001;11:58–69.
161. Krogh A. *The anatomy and physiology of capillaries*. New York: Yale University Press, 1922.
162. LeCouter J, Kowalski J, Foster J, et al. Identification of an angiogenic mitogen selective for endocrine gland endothelium. *Nature* 2001;412:877–884.
163. LeCouter J, Lin R, Ferrara N. Endocrine gland-derived VEGF and the emerging hypothesis of organ-specific regulation of angiogenesis. *Nat Med* 2002;8:913–917.
164. Lee CG, Heijn M, di Tomaso E, et al. Anti-vascular endothelial growth factor treatment augments tumor radiation response under normoxic or hypoxic conditions. *Cancer Res* 2000;60:5565–5570.
165. Less JR, Posner MC, Boucher Y, et al. Interstitial hypertension in human breast and colorectal tumors. *Cancer Res* 1992;52:6371–6374.

166. Less JR, Posner MC, Skalak TC, et al. Geometric resistance and microvascular network architecture of human colorectal carcinoma. *Microcirculation* 1997;4:25–33.

167. Less JR, Skalak TC, Sevick EM, et al. Microvascular architecture in a mammary carcinoma: branching patterns and vessel dimensions. *Cancer Res* 1991;51:265–273.

168. Leu AJ, Berk DA, Lymboussaki A, et al. Absence of functional lymphatics within a murine sarcoma: A molecular and functional evaluation. *Cancer Res* 2000;60:4324–4327.

169. Leu AJ, Berk DA, Yuan F, et al. Flow velocity in the superficial lymphatic network of the mouse tail. *Am J Physiol* 1994;267:H1507–H1513.

170. Leunig M, Yuan F, Menger MD, et al. Angiogenesis, microvascular architecture, microhemodynamics, and interstitial fluid pressure during early growth of human adenocarcinoma LS174T in SCID mice. *Cancer Res* 1992;52:6553–6560.

171. Leyland-Jones B, Semiglazov V, Pawlicki M, et al. Maintaining normal hemoglobin levels with epoetin alfa in mainly nonanemic patients with metastatic breast cancer receiving first-line chemotherapy: a survival study. *J Clin Oncol* 2005;23:5960–5972.

172. Lichtenbeld HC, Yuan F, Michel CC, et al. Perfusion of single tumor microvessels: application to vascular permeability measurement. *Microcirculation* 1996;3:349–357.

173. Liotta LA, Kohn EC. The microenvironment of the tumour-host interface. *Nature* 2001;411:375–379.

174. Littlepage LE, Egeblad M, Werb Z. Coevolution of cancer and stromal cellular responses. *Cancer Cell* 2005;7:499–500.

175. Littlewood TJ, Bajetta E, Nortier JW, et al. Effects of epoetin alfa on hematologic parameters and quality of life in cancer patients receiving nonplatinum chemotherapy: results of a randomized, double-blind, placebo-controlled trial. *J Clin Oncol* 2001;19:2865–2874.

176. Lyden D, Hattori K, Dias S, et al. Impaired recruitment of bone-marrow-derived endothelial and hematopoietic precursor cells blocks tumor angiogenesis and growth. *Nat Med* 2001;7:1194–1201.

177. Maeshima Y, Sudhakar A, Lively JC, et al. Tumstatin, an endothelial cell-specific inhibitor of protein synthesis. *Science* 2002;295:140–143.

178. Mandriota SJ, Jussila L, Jeltsch M, et al. Vascular endothelial growth factor-C-mediated lymphangiogenesis promotes tumour metastasis. *EMBO J* 2001;20:672–682.

179. Marx J. Cancer. Encouraging results for second-generation antiangiogenesis drugs. *Science* 2005;308:1248–1249.

180. McCormick F. New-age drug meets resistance. *Nature* 2001;412:281–282.

181. McDonald DM, Choyke PL. Imaging of angiogenesis: from microscope to clinic. *Nat Med* 2003;9:713–725.

182. McKee TD, Grandi P, Mok W, et al. Degradation of fibrillar collagen in a human melanoma xenograft improves the efficacy of an oncolytic herpes simplex virus vector. *Cancer Res* 2006;66:2509–2513.

183. Melder RJ, Brownell AL, Shoup TM, et al. Imaging of activated natural killer cells in mice by positron emission tomography: preferential uptake in tumors. *Cancer Res* 1993;53:5867–5871.

184. Melder RJ, Elmaleh D, Brownell AL, et al. A method for labeling cells for positron emission tomography (PET) studies. *J Immunol Methods* 1994;175:79–87.

185. Melder RJ, Jain RK. Kinetics of interleukin-2 induced changes in rigidity of human natural killer cells. *Cell Biophys* 1992;20:161–176.

186. Melder RJ, Jain RK. Reduction of rigidity in human activated natural-killer-cells by thioglycollate treatment. *J Immunol Methods* 1994;175:69–77.

187. Melder RJ, Koenig GC, Munn LL, et al. Adhesion of activated natural killer cells to tumor necrosis factor-alpha-treated endothelium under physiological flow conditions. *Nat Immunol* 1996;15:154–163.

188. Melder RJ, Koenig GC, Witwer BP, et al. During angiogenesis, vascular endothelial growth factor and basic fibroblast growth factor regulate natural killer cell adhesion to tumor endothelium. *Nat Med* 1996;2:992–997.

189. Melder RJ, Kristensen CA, Munn LL, et al. Modulation of A-NK cell rigidity: in vitro characterization and in vivo implications for cell delivery. *Biorheology* 2001;38:151–159.

190. Melder RJ, Munn LL, Yamada S, et al. Selectin- and integrin-mediated T-lymphocyte rolling and arrest on TNF-alpha-activated endothelium: augmentation by erythrocytes. *Biophys J* 1995;69:2131–2138.

191. Melder RJ, Salehi HA, Jain RK. Interaction of activated natural-killer-cells with normal and tumor vessels in cranial windows in mice. *Microvasc Res* 1995;50:35–44.

192. Melder RJ, Yuan J, Munn LL, et al. Erythrocytes enhance lymphocyte rolling and arrest in vivo. *Microvasc Res* 2000;59:316–322.

193. Melillo G. Inhibiting hypoxia-inducible factor 1 for cancer therapy. *Mol Cancer Res* 2006;4:601–605.

194. Menon C, Fraker DL. Tumor oxygenation status as a prognostic marker. *Cancer Lett* 2005;221:225–235.

195. Migliorini C, Qian Y, Chen H, et al. Red blood cells augment leukocyte rolling in a virtual blood vessel. *Biophys J* 2002;83:1834–1841.

196. Miller DW, Vosseler S, Mirancea N, et al. Rapid vessel regression, protease inhibition, and stromal normalization upon short-term vascular endothelial growth factor receptor 2 inhibition in skin carcinoma heterotransplants. *Am J Pathol* 2005;167:1389–1403.

197. Milosevic M, Fyles A, Hedley D, et al. Interstitial fluid pressure predicts survival in patients with cervix cancer independent of clinical prognostic factors and tumor: oxygen measurements. *Cancer Res* 2001;61:6400–6405.

198. Mizukami Y, Jo WS, Duerr EM, et al. Induction of interleukin-8 preserves the angiogenic response in HIF-1alpha-deficient colon cancer cells. *Nat Med* 2005;11:992–997.

199. Moeller BJ, Dreher MR, Rabbani ZN, et al. Pleiotropic effects of HIF-1 blockade on tumor radiosensitivity. *Cancer Cell* 2005;8:99–110.

200. Mollica F, Jain RK, Netti PA. A model for temporal heterogeneities of tumor blood flow. *Microvasc Res* 2003;65:56–60.

201. Monsky WL, Carreira CM, Tsuzuki Y, et al. Role of host microenvironment in angiogenesis and microvascular functions in human breast cancer xenografts: mammary fat pad versus cranial tumors. *Clin Cancer Res* 2002;8:1008–1013.

202. Monsky WL, Fukumura D, Gohongi T, et al. Augmentation of transvascular transport of macromolecules and nanoparticles in tumors using vascular endothelial growth factor. *Cancer Res* 1999;59:4129–4135.

203. Morikawa S, Baluk P, Kaidoh T, et al. Abnormalities in pericytes on blood vessels and endothelial sprouts in tumors. *Am J Pathol* 2002;160:985–1000.

204. Muller AJ, Scherle PA. Targeting the mechanisms of tumoral immune tolerance with small-molecule inhibitors. *Nat Rev Cancer* 2006;6:613–625.

205. Munn LL, Koenig GC, Jain RK, et al. Kinetics of adhesion molecule expression and spatial organization using targeted sampling fluorometry. *Biotechniques* 1995;19:622–631.

206. Munn LL, Melder RJ, Jain RK. Analysis of cell flux in the parallel-plate flow chamber: implications for cell capture studies. *Biophys J* 1994;67:889–895.

207. Munn LL, Melder RJ, Jain RK. Role of erythrocytes in leukocyte-endothelial interactions: mathematical model and experimental validation. *Biophys J* 1996;71:466–478.

208. Nagy JA, Vasile E, Feng D, et al. Vascular permeability factor/vascular endothelial growth factor induces lymphangiogenesis as well as angiogenesis. *J Exp Med* 2002;196:1497–1506.

209. Nathanson SD, Nelson L. Interstitial fluid pressure in breast cancer, benign breast conditions, and breast parenchyma. *Ann Surg Oncol* 1994;1:333–338.

210. Neri D, Bicknell R. Tumour vascular targeting. *Nat Rev Cancer* 2005;5:436–446.

211. Netti PA, Baxter LT, Boucher Y, et al. Time-dependent behavior of interstitial fluid pressure in solid tumors: implications for drug delivery. *Cancer Res* 1995;55:5451–5458.

212. Netti PA, Berk DA, Swartz MA, et al. Role of extracellular matrix assembly in interstitial transport in solid tumors. *Cancer Res* 2000;60:2497–2503.

213. Netti PA, Hamberg LM, Babich JW, et al. Enhancement of fluid filtration across tumor vessels: Implication for delivery of macromolecules. *Proc Natl Acad Sci U S A* 1999;96:3137–3142.

214. Netti PA, Roberge S, Boucher Y, et al. Effect of transvascular fluid exchange on pressure-flow relationship in tumors: a proposed mechanism for tumor blood flow heterogeneity. *Microvasc Res* 1996;52:27–46.

215. Nisato RE, Tille JC, Pepper MS. Lymphangiogenesis and tumor metastasis. *Thromb Haemost* 2003;90:591–597.

216. Nordsmark M, Loncaster J, Aquino-Parsons C, et al. Measurements of hypoxia using pimonidazole and polarographic oxygen-sensitive electrodes in human cervix carcinomas. *Radiother Oncol* 2003;67:35–44.

217. Nugent LJ, Jain RK. Extravascular diffusion in normal and neoplastic tissues. *Cancer Res* 1984;44:238–244.

218. O'Reilly MS, Boehm T, Shing Y, et al. Endostatin: an endogenous inhibitor of angiogenesis and tumor growth. *Cell* 1997;88:277–285.

219. O'Reilly MS, Holmgren L, Shing Y, et al. Angiostatin: a novel angiogenesis inhibitor that mediates the suppression of metastases by a Lewis lung carcinoma. *Cell* 1994;79:315–328.

220. Orimo A, Gupta PB, Sgroi DC, et al. Stromal fibroblasts present in invasive human breast carcinomas promote tumor growth and angiogenesis through elevated SDF-1/CXCL12 secretion. *Cell* 2005;121:335–348.

221. Orimo A, Weinberg RA. Stromal fibroblasts in cancer: a novel tumor-promoting cell type. *Cell Cycle* 2006;5:1597–1601.

222. Padera TP, Boucher Y, Jain RK. Correspondence re: S. Maula et al., intratumoral lymphatics are essential for the metastatic spread and prognosis in squamous cell carcinoma of the head and neck. *Cancer Res* 2003;63:1920–1926. [Author reply: *Cancer Res* 2003;63:8555–8556.]

223. Padera TP, Kadambi A, di Tomaso E, et al. Lymphatic metastasis in the absence of functional intratumor lymphatics. *Science* 2002;296:1883–1886.

224. Padera TP, Stoll BR, So PT, et al. Conventional and high-speed intravital multi-photon laser scanning microscopy of microvasculature, lymphatics, and leukocyte-endothelial interactions. *Mol Imaging* 2002;1:9–15.

225. Padera TP, Stoll BR, Tooredman JB, et al. Pathology: cancer cells compress intratumour vessels. *Nature* 2004;427:695.

226. Patan S. Vasculogenesis and angiogenesis. *Cancer Treat Res* 2004;117:3–32.

227. Patan S, Alvarez MJ, Schittny JC, et al. Intussusceptive microvascular growth: a common alternative to capillary sprouting. *Arch Histol Cytol* 1992;55[Suppl]:65–75.

228. Patan S, Munn LL, Jain RK. Intussusceptive microvascular growth in a human colon adenocarcinoma xenograft: a novel mechanism of tumor angiogenesis. *Microvasc Res* 1996;51:260–272.

229. Patan S, Tanda S, Roberge S, et al. Vascular morphogenesis and remodeling in a human tumor xenograft: blood vessel formation and growth after ovariectomy and tumor implantation. *Circ Res* 2001;89:732–739.

230. Pluen A, Boucher Y, Ramanujan S, et al. Role of tumor-host interactions in interstitial diffusion of macromolecules: Cranial vs. subcutaneous tumors. *Proc Natl Acad Sci U S A* 2001;98:4628–4633.

231. Pollard JW. Tumour-educated macrophages promote tumour progression and metastasis. *Nat Rev Cancer* 2004;4:71–78.

232. Pouyssegur J, Dayan F, Mazure NM. Hypoxia signalling in cancer and approaches to enforce tumour regression. *Nature* 2006;441:437–443.

233. Rafii S. Circulating endothelial precursors: mystery, reality, and promise. *J Clin Invest* 2000;105:17–19.

234. Rafii S, Lyden D, Benezra R, et al. Vascular and haematopoietic stem cells: novel targets for anti-angiogenesis therapy? *Nat Rev Cancer* 2002;2:826–835.

235. Rajendran JG, Schwartz DL, O'Sullivan J, et al. Tumor hypoxia imaging with [F-18] fluoromisonidazole positron emission tomography in head and neck cancer. *Clin Cancer Res* 2006;12:5435–5441.

236. Ramanujan S, Koenig GC, Padera TP, et al. Local imbalance of proangiogenic and antiangiogenic factors: a potential mechanism of focal necrosis and dormancy in tumors. *Cancer Res* 2000;60:1442–1448.

237. Ramanujan S, Pluen A, McKee TD, et al. Diffusion and convection in collagen gels: implications for transport in the tumor interstitium. *Biophys J* 2002;83:1650–1660.

238. Religa P, Cao R, Bjorndahl M, et al. Presence of bone marrow-derived circulating progenitor endothelial cells in the newly formed lymphatic vessels. *Blood* 2005;106:4184–4190.

239. Rischin D, Hicks RJ, Fisher R, et al. Prognostic significance of [18F]-misonidazole positron emission tomography-detected tumor hypoxia in patients with advanced head and neck cancer randomly assigned to chemoradiation with or without tirapazamine: a substudy of Trans-Tasman Radiation Oncology Group Study 98.02. *J Clin Oncol* 2006;24:2098–2104.

240. Roh HD, Boucher Y, Kalnicki S, et al. Interstitial hypertension in carcinoma of uterine cervix in patients: Possible correlation with tumor oxygenation and radiation response. *Cancer Res* 1991;51:6695–6698.

241. Salnikov AV, Roswall P, Sundberg C, et al. Inhibition of TGF-beta modulates macrophages and vessel maturation in parallel to a lowering of interstitial fluid pressure in experimental carcinoma. *Lab Invest* 2005;85:512–521.

242. Sandler A, Gray R, Perry MC, et al. Paclitaxel-carboplatin alone or with bevacizumab for non–small-cell lung cancer. *N Engl J Med* 2006;355:2542–2550.

243. Santin AD, Bellone S, Palmieri M, et al. Effect of blood transfusion during radiotherapy on the immune function of patients with cancer of the uterine cervix: role of interleukin-10. *Int J Radiat Oncol Biol Phys* 2002;54:1345–1355.

244. Sasaki A, Jain RK, Maghazachi AA, et al. Low deformability of lymphokine-activated killer cells as a possible determinant of in vivo distribution. *Cancer Res* 1989;49:3742–3746.

245. Sasaki A, Melder RJ, Whiteside TL, et al. Preferential localization of human adherent lymphokine-activated killer cells in tumor microcirculation. *J Natl Cancer Inst* 1991;83:433–437.

246. Segers J, Fazio VD, Ansiaux R, et al. Potentiation of cyclophosphamide chemotherapy using the anti-angiogenic drug thalidomide: Importance of optimal scheduling to exploit the 'normalization' window of the tumor vasculature. *Cancer Lett* 2006;244:129–135.

247. Semenza GL. Targeting HIF-1 for cancer therapy. *Nat Rev Cancer* 2003;3:721–732.

248. Serganova I, Humm J, Ling C, et al. Tumor hypoxia imaging. *Clin Cancer Res* 2006;12:5260–5264.

249. Sevick EM, Jain RK. Geometric resistance to blood flow in solid tumors perfused ex vivo: effects of tumor size and perfusion pressure. *Cancer Res* 1989;49:3506–3512.

250. Sevick EM, Jain RK. Viscous resistance to blood flow in solid tumors: effect of hematocrit on intratumor blood viscosity. *Cancer Res* 1989;49:3513–3519.

251. Sevick EM, Jain RK. Effect of red blood cell rigidity on tumor blood flow: increase in viscous resistance during hyperglycemia. *Cancer Res* 1991;51:2727–2730.

252. Sevick EM, Jain RK. Measurement of capillary filtration coefficient in a solid tumor. *Cancer Res* 1991;51:1352–1355.

253. Sharma S, Sharma MC, Sarkar C. Morphology of angiogenesis in human cancer: a conceptual overview, histoprognostic perspective and significance of neoangiogenesis. *Histopathology* 2005;46:481–489.

254. Skobe M, Hawighorst T, Jackson DG, et al. Induction of tumor lymphangiogenesis by VEGF-C promotes breast cancer metastasis. *Nat Med* 2001;7:192–198.

255. Stacker SA, Caesar C, Baldwin ME, et al. VEGF-D promotes the metastatic spread of tumor cells via the lymphatics. *Nat Med* 2001;7:186–191.

256. Stohrer M, Boucher Y, Stangassinger M, et al. Oncotic pressure in solid tumors is elevated. *Cancer Res* 2000;60:4251–4255.

257. Stoll BR, Migliorini C, Kadambi A, et al. A mathematical model of the contribution of endothelial progenitor cells to angiogenesis in tumors: implications for antiangiogenic therapy. *Blood* 2003;102:2555–2561.

258. Sundfor K, Lyng H, Kongsgard UL, et al. Polarographic measurement of Po$_2$ in cervix carcinoma. *Gynecol Oncol* 1997;64:230–236.

259. Swabb EA, Wei J, Gullino PM. Diffusion and convection in normal and neoplastic tissues. *Cancer Res* 1974;34:2814–2822.

260. Swartz MA, Berk DA, Jain RK. Transport in lymphatic capillaries. I. Macroscopic measurements using residence time distribution theory. *Am J Physiol* 1996;39:H324–H329.

261. Swartz MA, Boardman KC Jr. The role of interstitial stress in lymphatic function and lymphangiogenesis. *Ann N Y Acad Sci* 2002;979:197–210; discussion 229–134.

262. Swartz MA, Kristensen CA, Melder RJ, et al. Cells shed from tumours show reduced clonogenicity, resistance to apoptosis, and in vivo tumorigenicity. *Br J Cancer* 1999;81:756–759.

263. Talks KL, Turley H, Gatter KC, et al. The expression and distribution of the hypoxia-inducible factors HIF-1alpha and HIF-2alpha in normal human tissues, cancers, and tumor-associated macrophages. *Am J Pathol* 2000;157:411–421.

264. Teodoro JG, Parker AE, Zhu X, et al. p53-mediated inhibition of angiogenesis through up-regulation of a collagen prolyl hydroxylase. *Science* 2006;313:968–971.

265. Thomlinson RH, Gray LH. The histological structure of some human lung cancers and the possible implications for radiotherapy. *Br J Cancer* 1955;9:539–549.

266. Thurston G, McLean JW, Rizen M, et al. Cationic liposomes target angiogenic endothelial cells in tumors and chronic inflammation in mice. *J Clin Invest* 1998;101:1401–1413.

267. Tong RT, Boucher Y, Kozin SV, et al. Vascular normalization by vascular endothelial growth factor receptor 2 blockade induces a pressure gradient across the vasculature and improves drug penetration in tumors. *Cancer Res* 2004;64:3731–3736.

268. Torres-Filho IP, Leunig M, Yuan F, et al. Noninvasive measurement of microvascular and interstitial oxygen profiles in a human tumor in SCID mice. *Proc Natl Acad Sci U S A* 1994;91:2081–2085.

269. Tsuzuki Y, Fukumura D, Oosthuyse B, et al. Vascular endothelial growth factor (VEGF) modulation by targeting hypoxia-inducible factor-1alpha–> hypoxia response element–> VEGF cascade differentially regulates vascular response and growth rate in tumors. *Cancer Res* 2000;60:6248–6252.

270. Tsuzuki Y, Mouta Carreira C, Bockhorn M, et al. Pancreas microenvironment promotes VEGF expression and tumor growth: novel window models for pancreatic tumor angiogenesis and microcirculation. *Lab Invest* 2001;81:1439–1451.

271. Vansteenkiste J, Pirker R, Massuti B, et al. Double-blind, placebo-controlled, randomized phase III trial of darbepoetin alfa in lung cancer patients receiving chemotherapy. *J Natl Cancer Inst* 2002;94:1211–1220.

272. Varlotto J, Stevenson MA. Anemia, tumor hypoxemia, and the cancer patient. *Int J Radiat Oncol Biol Phys* 2005;63:25–36.

273. Vaupel P, Kallinowski F, Okunieff P. Blood flow, oxygen and nutrient supply, and metabolic microenvironment of human tumors: a review. *Cancer Res* 1989;49:6449–6465.

274. Vosseler S, Mirancea N, Bohlen P, et al. Angiogenesis inhibition by vascular endothelial growth factor receptor-2 blockade reduces stromal matrix metalloproteinase expression, normalizes stromal tissue, and reverts epithelial tumor phenotype in surface heterotransplants. *Cancer Res* 2005;65:1294–1305.

275. Vukovic V, Tannock IF. Influence of low pH on cytotoxicity of paclitaxel, mitoxantrone and topotecan. *Br J Cancer* 1997;75:1167–1172.

276. Weis SM, Cheresh DA. Pathophysiological consequences of VEGF-induced vascular permeability. *Nature* 2005;437:497–504.

277. Wildiers H, Guetens G, De Boeck G, et al. Effect of antivascular endothelial growth factor treatment on the intratumoral uptake of CPT-11. *Br J Cancer* 2003;88:1979–1986.

278. Willett CG, Boucher Y, di Tomaso E, et al. Direct evidence that the VEGF-specific antibody bevacizumab has antivascular effects in human rectal cancer. *Nat Med* 2004;10:145–147.

279. Willett CG, Boucher Y, Duda DG, et al. Surrogate markers for antiangiogenic therapy and dose-limiting toxicities for bevacizumab with radiation and chemotherapy: continued experience of a phase I trial in rectal cancer patients. *J Clin Oncol* 2005;23:8136–8139.

280. Winkler F, Kozin SV, Tong RT, et al. Kinetics of vascular normalization by VEGFR2 blockade governs brain tumor response to radiation: role of oxygenation, angiopoietin-1, and matrix metalloproteinases. *Cancer Cell* 2004;6:553–563.

281. Wong SY, Haack H, Crowley D, et al. Tumor-secreted vascular endothelial growth factor-C is necessary for prostate cancer lymphangiogenesis, but lymphangiogenesis is unnecessary for lymph node metastasis. *Cancer Res* 2005;65:9789–9798.

282. Xu L, Fukumura D, Jain RK. Acidic extracellular pH induces vascular endothelial growth factor (VEGF) in human glioblastoma cells via ERK1/2 MAPK signaling pathway—mechanism of low pH-induced VEGF. *J Biol Chem* 2002;277:11368–11374.

283. Yamada S, Melder RJ, Leunig M, et al. Leukocyte rolling increases with age. *Blood* 1995;86:4707–4708.

284. Yancopoulos GD, Davis S, Gale NW, et al. Vascular-specific growth factors and blood vessel formation. *Nature* 2000;407:242–248.

285. Yoshiji H, Harris SR, Thorgeirsson UP. Vascular endothelial growth factor is essential for initial but not continued in vivo growth of human breast carcinoma cells. *Cancer Res* 1997;57:3924–3928.

286. Yuan F, Chen Y, Dellian M, et al. Time-dependent vascular regression and permeability changes in established human tumor xenografts induced by an anti-vascular endothelial growth factor/vascular permeability factor antibody. *Proc Natl Acad Sci U S A* 1996;93:14765–14770.

287. Yuan F, Dellian M, Fukumura D, et al. Vascular permeability in a human tumor xenograft: molecular size dependence and cutoff size. *Cancer Res* 1995;55:3752–3756.

288. Yuan F, Leunig M, Berk DA, et al. Microvascular permeability of albumin, vascular surface area, and vascular volume measured in human adenocarcinoma LS174T using dorsal chamber in SCID mice. *Microvasc Res* 1993;45:269–289.

289. Yuan F, Salehi HA, Boucher Y, et al. Vascular permeability and microcirculation of gliomas and mammary carcinomas transplanted in rat and mouse cranial windows. *Cancer Res* 1994;54:4564–4568.

290. Yuan J, Melder RJ, Jain RK, et al. Lateral view flow system for studies of cell adhesion and deformation under flow conditions. *Biotechniques* 2001;30:388–394.

291. Zhong H, De Marzo AM, Laughner E, et al. Overexpression of hypoxia-inducible factor 1alpha in common human cancers and their metastases. *Cancer Res* 1999;59:5830–5835.

292. Zlotecki RA, Boucher Y, Lee I, et al. Effect of angiotensin II induced hypertension on tumor blood flow and interstitial fluid pressure. *Cancer Res* 1993;53:2466–2468.

293. Znati CA, Rosenstein M, Boucher Y, et al. Effect of radiation on interstitial fluid pressure and oxygenation in a human tumor xenograft. *Cancer Res* 1996;56:964–968.

294. Znati CA, Rosenstein M, McKee TD, et al. Irradiation reduces interstitial fluid transport and increases the collagen content in tumors. *Clin Cancer Res* 2003;9:5508–5513.

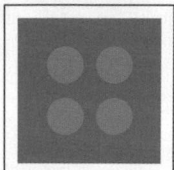

Chapter 5
Principles of Radiologic Physics, Dosimetry, and Treatment Planning

James A. Purdy

A solid foundation in the principles of radiologic physics, dosimetry, and treatment planning is essential for the practice of modern-day radiation oncology. In this chapter, the basic concepts and parameters that provide the basis for the photon external beam treatment planning and dose/monitor unit calculations methods covered in Chapter 6 are discussed. More details on these basic concepts can be found in the medical physics textbooks listed in the references (19,30,63).

Atomic and Nuclear Structure

The *atom* may be thought of as consisting of a centrally located core, the *nucleus,* surrounded by small orbiting particles called *electrons.* The overall dimension of an atom is about 10^{-10} m, and the nucleus is about 10^{-14} m. An electron has a rest mass (m_e) of 9.109×10^{-31} kg and has a negative electrical charge equal to 1.602×10^{-19} coulomb (C). Most of the mass of the atom is contained in the nucleus, making it extremely dense $(10^{15}$ kg/m$^3)$. The nucleus is composed of two kinds of particles, *protons* and *neutrons,* known collectively as *nucleons.* A proton has a rest mass (m_p) of 1.673×10^{-27} kg and has a positive electrical charge equal in magnitude to the charge of the electron $(1.602 \times 10^{-19}$ C). Collectively, the protons constitute the electrical charge of the nucleus. A neutron is slightly more massive than a proton $(m_n = 1.675 \times 10^{-27}$ kg) and has no electrical charge.

Units used to describe atomic processes include the *atomic mass unit (amu)* for mass, *nanometer (nm)* for distance, *electron volt (eV)* for energy, and *electronic charge (e)* for electrical charge. The *amu* is defined as one-twelfth the mass of the neutral carbon 12 atom. Thus, 1 amu $= 1.660 \times 10^{-27}$ kg. In terms of amu, a proton's rest mass is equal to 1.00727 amu, a neutron's rest mass is equal to 1.00866 amu, and an electron's rest mass is equal to 0.000548 amu. The *electron volt (eV)* is defined as the kinetic energy acquired by an electron accelerated through a potential difference (voltage) of 1 volt. One eV is equal to 1.6×10^{-19} Joule of energy. One keV is equal to 10^3 eV, and 1 million electron volts (MeV) $= 10^6$ eV. The nanometer is defined as equal to 10^{-9} meter, and the electronic unit of charge is defined as equal to 1.602×10^{-19} coulomb.

The planetary model of the atom is attributed to Niels Bohr, who in 1913 theorized that the hydrogen atom consisted of an electron orbiting around a nucleus of equal and opposite charge. He extended his theory to multielectron atoms requiring the electrons surrounding a nucleus to be arranged in distinct, concentric shells or energy levels as shown in Figure 5.1. Energy is released when an electron moves to an orbit closer to the nucleus, and energy is required to move an electron into a higher orbit. Historically, the shells are labeled, from innermost outward, by the letters *K, L, M,* and so forth. There are a maximum number of electrons that can be accommodated in each shell: 2 in the first shell, 8 in the second, 18 in the third, and so on. The maximum number of electrons allowed in each shell is given by the relationship $2n^2$, where n is an integer specific to each shell and is called the *principal quantum number.* Other properties of the electron also have discrete values specified by quantum numbers. These include the electron's angular momentum as it orbits the nucleus, denoted by other quantum numbers l $(l = 0, 1 \ldots, n - 1)$; Its spin about its axis, denoted by s $(s = \pm 1/2)$; And its magnetic moment, denoted by m_l $(m_l = 0, \pm 1, \ldots, \pm l)$. Thus, each electron in an atom has an associated set of quantum numbers (n, l, s, m_l). This is the basis of the *Pauli Exclusion Principle,* which states that no two electrons can have the same set of quantum numbers within a particular atom.

Modern physics has replaced the simplistic orbiting electron model of Bohr with an abstract quantum mechanical model of diffuse electron clouds that represent probability functions of the electron's position. However, for an understanding of radiologic physics, the simple Bohr model of a nucleus composed of protons and neutrons and surrounded by orbiting electrons in distinct orbits (energy levels) is sufficient.

The atom of an *element* is specified by its *atomic number,* denoted by the symbol Z, and its *mass number,* denoted by the symbol A. The atomic number is equal to the number of protons in the nucleus, and the mass number is equal to the number of nucleons (protons and neutrons) in the nucleus. Hence, A minus Z is equal to the number of neutrons, denoted by the symbol N, within the nucleus. In addition, each element has an associated chemical symbol (e.g., Co for cobalt). When these definitions are used, the standard notation to specify an atom is $^A_Z X$, as illustrated by $^{60}_{70}$Co, which is a radioactive isotope of the element cobalt that has an atomic number of 27 (i.e., 27 protons) and

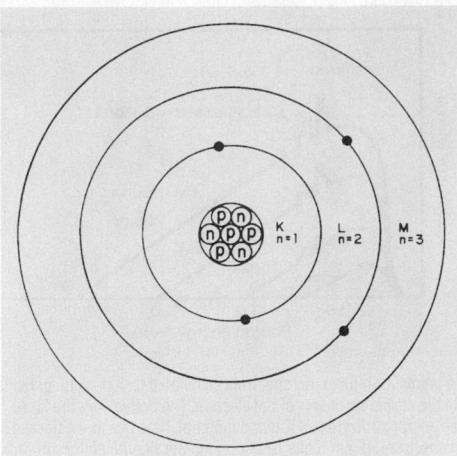

FIGURE 5.1. Schematic drawing of the Bohr model of the atom. The nucleus contains protons (p) and neutrons (n). Electrons revolve around the nucleus in specific orbits having discrete energy levels. By convention, the orbits (energy levels) are assigned either quantum numbers (n = 1, 2, 3...) or letters (K, L, M...).

a mass number of 60 (i.e., 60 nucleons, or 27 protons and 33 neutrons).

Isotopes of an element (e.g., $_{27}^{58}Co$, $_{27}^{59}Co$ and $_{27}^{60}Co$) have the same atomic number but different numbers of neutrons and, therefore, different mass numbers. Isotopes have the same chemical properties but have different physical properties. Atoms such as $_{27}^{60}Co$ and $_{28}^{60}Ni$, which have the same mass number but different numbers of protons and neutrons, are called *isobars*. Atoms such as $_{27}^{57}Co$ and $_{26}^{56}Fe$, which have the same number of neutrons but different atomic and mass numbers, are called *isotones*.

Every atom has a characteristic atomic mass A_m (sometimes referred to as atomic weight). The *gram-atomic mass* of an isotope is the amount of isotope in grams that is numerically equaled to the isotope's atomic mass. For example, 1 g-atomic mass of carbon-12 is 12 g. One gram-atomic mass contains 6.0228×10^{23} atoms, a constant that is called *Avogadro's number (N_A)*. Useful parameters that can be calculated using Avogadro's number are as follows:

Number atoms/g = N_A/A_m
Number electrons/g = $(N_A \, Z)/A_m$
Number g/atom = A_m/N_A

The closer the electrons are to the nucleus, the more tightly bound they are to the nucleus. This results from the attraction between the negatively charged electrons and the positively charged nucleus and is referred to as the *Coulomb* or *electrostatic force*. To move an electron from an inner shell to an outer shell (*excitation*) or to remove it completely from the atom (*ionization*), energy must be supplied. The energy required to remove an electron completely from an atom is called the *binding energy* for the electron. Binding energies are considered negative because energy must be supplied to remove the electron from its orbit. Atomic shells often are described in terms of binding energy, as shown in Figure 5.2 for the tungsten atom. The binding energies for the *K, L,* and *M* shells are −69,500 eV, −11,000 eV, and −2,500 eV, respectively. The electrons in the outermost shells are called *valence electrons* and have a binding energy of only a few electron volts because they are very loosely bound. These electrons determine the atom's chemical properties.

Electromagnetic Radiation

Electromagnetic radiation can be represented by a varying electric and magnetic field that is conveniently described using a sine-wave model. The sine wave is characterized by two parameters: the *frequency*, represented by the Greek letter ν, and the *wavelength*, represented by the Greek letter λ. The wavelength is the distance from one crest of the sine wave to another; the frequency is the number of complete cycles or oscillations per second and is measured in *hertz (Hz)*. The product of the frequency and wavelength is the speed with which the wave is propagated, which in a vacuum is the speed of light (c = 3 × 10^8 m/sec).

Electromagnetic radiation wavelengths extend from approximately 10^7 m to 10^{-13} m. The frequencies associated with these radiations are approximately 10^1 to 10^{21} Hz. the electromagnetic spectrum shown in Figure 5.3 includes the radio and television bands; Radar and microwaves; the infrared, visible, and ultraviolet regions; and x-rays and cosmic rays.

Quantum physics allows electromagnetic radiation to be represented as a wave and also as particles, called *photons*. This is referred to as the *wave-particle duality of nature*. The photon energy is directly proportional to the classic wave frequency and is related to it through a constant of proportionality known as *Planck's constant (h)*, which has a numerical value of 6.625 × 10^{-34} J-sec. The relationship between energy, *E,* and frequency, ν, is given by the following equation:

$$E = h\nu$$

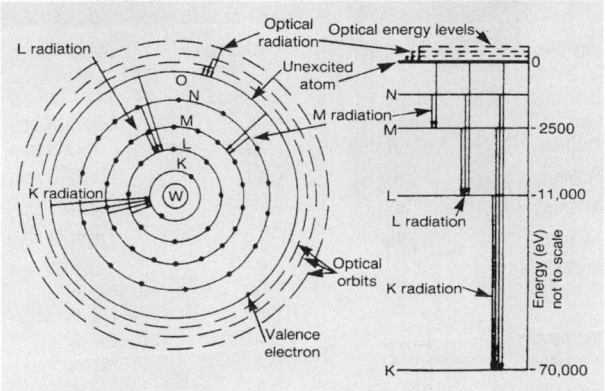

FIGURE 5.2. Schematic drawing of tungsten atom showing electron configuration and energy levels. (From Johns HE, Cunningham JR. *The physics of radiology,* 4th ed. Springfield, IL: Charles C Thomas, 1983, with permission.)

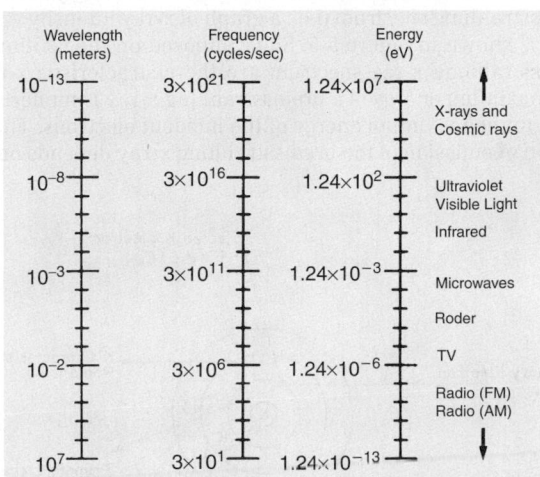

FIGURE 5.3. Electromagnetic spectrum extending over several orders of magnitude listing values of wavelengths, frequency, and identifying values in some of the more common regions of the spectrum.

The relationship between photon energy and photon wavelength is given by the following equation:

$$E = hc/\lambda$$

in which c is the speed of light in a vacuum. These relationships show that as the wavelength becomes shorter or the frequency becomes larger, the energy of the photon becomes greater.

X-Rays

Wilhelm Conrad Röentgen discovered *x-rays* on November 8, 1895 (57). He observed that a paper screen coated with fluorescent material glowed when placed in the vicinity of a tube of gas at low pressure through which electricity was being passed. We now know that the x-rays were produced where the electron beam struck the anode. Energetic electrons that impinge on matter interact with either the orbital electrons or the nuclei of target atoms. The kinetic energy of the electrons then is converted into thermal energy or electromagnetic energy (in the form of x-rays).

The impinging electron's kinetic energy is converted to thermal energy through the interaction with an outer-shell electron of a target atom that raises it to a higher energy level (referred to as *excitation*). The excited electron then returns to the normal energy level with the emission of low-energy electromagnetic radiation (*infrared*).

If the impinging electron's kinetic energy is high enough, the interaction can free an orbital electron (referred to as *ionization*), which then can result in the production of electromagnetic radiation (*characteristic x-rays*) when an outer orbital electron moves to the electron vacancy produced via ionization (Fig. 5.4). The characteristic x-ray energy is equal to the difference in the binding energies of the two orbital electrons involved. Occasionally, this excess energy is transferred directly to another orbital electron, causing it to be emitted from the atom. Such electrons are called *Auger electrons*.

The impinging electron also can lose its kinetic energy via a process called *bremsstrahlung* (braking radiation), which occurs when the incident electron interacts with the electric field of the nucleus (rather than the orbiting electrons) and is deflected and loses energy. This loss of energy reappears in the form of an x-ray photon. The impinging electron can lose any amount of its kinetic energy in the bremsstrahlung process. Thus, the x-radiation produced via the bremsstrahlung process is characterized by having a continuous range of energy values, unlike characteristic x-rays, which have only discrete energy values. A bremsstrahlung spectrum (i.e., a graph of x-ray intensity vs. energy) is shown in Figure 5.5. Superimposed on the continuous bremsstrahlung x-ray spectrum are the characteristic x-rays. The maximum energy of a bremsstrahlung x-ray is numerically equal to the maximum energy of the incident electrons. The direction of emission of the bremsstrahlung x-ray depends on the

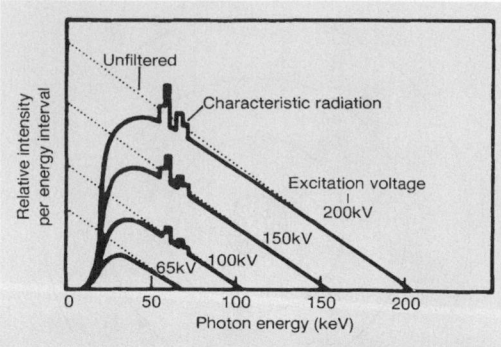

FIGURE 5.5. A bremsstrahlung x-ray spectrum calculated for a thick tungsten target extending from zero to the maximum energy of the electron. The *dotted lines* are for no filtration, and the *solid curves* are for a filtration of 1 mm aluminum. Note the superimposed characteristic x-ray emission spectrum. (From Johns HE, Cunningham JR. *The physics of radiology*, 4th ed. Springfield, IL: Charles C Thomas, 1983, with permission.)

energy of the incident electron, with higher energy electrons producing more forward-directed x-rays.

Radioactivity

In 1896 Henri Becquerel conducted experiments in which he wrapped a photographic plate in black paper to keep out the light and then placed pieces of various elements against the wrapped plate (45). He discovered that the mineral pitchblende emitted x-rays. Other elements—such as thorium, actinium, and two new elements (polonium and radium) discovered by Pierre and Marie Curie—also emitted x-rays. Further experiments showed that the radioactive elements emitted three types of radiation: *α-particles,* having a positive electrical charge; *β-particles,* having a negative charge; and high-energy *γ-rays,* having no charge at all. We now know that an α-particle is a helium nucleus, β-particles are electrons, and *γ-rays* are electromagnetic radiation that is similar to x-rays except that it originates from within the nucleus of the atom.

Many other elementary particles have since been discovered and are important topics of current physics research, but they are not germane to our discussion of radiation oncology physics. Properties of the particles relevant to radiation therapy are listed in Table 5.1.

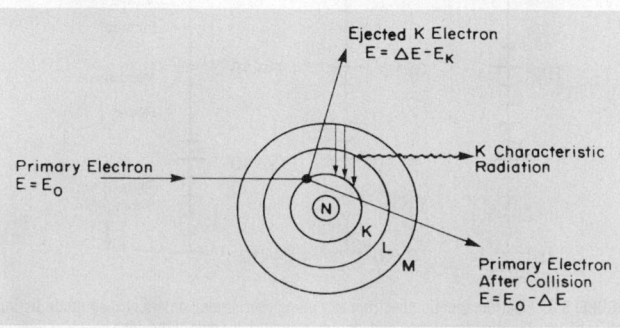

FIGURE 5.4. Schematic diagram illustrating characteristic x-ray production.

Table 5.1 PARTICLES OF INTEREST IN RADIATION THERAPY			
Particle	**Symbol**	**Charge**	**Mass**
Photon	$h\nu, \gamma$	0	0
Electron	e, e^-, β^-	−1	0.000549 amu[a]
Positron	e^+, β^+	+1	0.000549 amu
Proton	$p, {}^1_1H$	+1	1.007277 amu
Neutron	$n, {}^1_0n$	0	1.008665 amu
Alpha	$\alpha, {}^4_2He^{++}$	+2	4.002604 amu
Neutrino	ν	0	$<1/2{,}000\ m_0$[b]
Pi mesons	π^+, π^-	+1, −1	$273\ m_0$
	π°	0	$264\ m_0$
Mu mesons	μ^+, μ^-	+1, −1	$207\ m_0$
K mesons	K^+, K^-	+1, −1	$967\ m_0$
	K^0	0	$973\ m_0$

[a] 1 amu = 1.66043×10^{-27} kg.
[b] m_0 = rest mass of an electron = 9.1091×10^{-31} kg.

The radioactive decay processes are related to the forces involved. Huge electrostatic (coulomb) forces of repulsion exist between the positively charged and closely spaced protons in a nucleus. However, a nuclear force of attraction (called the *strong nuclear force*) exists among the neutrons and protons, binding them together to form the nucleus. The strong nuclear force is much more complicated than the *electrostatic (coulomb) force* and is still not completely understood. However, it is known that the strong nuclear force between nucleons depends on the distance between them and is effective only over a very short distance, whereas the electrostatic force decreases with the square of the distance. The strong nuclear force easily overcomes the repelling electrostatic force as long as the protons are very close together. However, for a large nucleus, the strong nuclear force binding the nucleons together may be weaker on opposite sides of the nucleus than the repelling electrostatic force. Therefore, a large nucleus is not as stable as a smaller nucleus.

Because neutrons interact through the attractive strong nuclear force and not the repelling electrostatic force, they can be considered stabilizing particles for the nucleus. For example, in light nuclei, only an equal number of neutrons and protons are required, but in heavier nuclei, the number of neutrons must be about 1.5 times greater than the number of protons to counteract the repelling electrostatic forces of the protons. A nuclide having too many more protons than neutrons is said to have an unfavorable *N*-to-*Z* ratio and thus undergoes *radioactive decay* to reach a stable configuration.

The *decay constant* of a radioactive nucleus is defined as the fraction of the total number of atoms that decay per unit of time and is denoted by the symbol λ. The decay process can be represented mathematically. If N_0 radioactive nuclei are initially present in a particular sample, the number of radioactive nuclei, N, remaining at a particular time, t, is given by the following equation:

$$N = N_0 e^{-\lambda t}$$

Activity, which describes the radioactivity of a sample and is denoted by the symbol A, is defined as the total number of disintegrations per unit of time interval and is given by the following relationship:

$$A = \frac{\Delta N}{\Delta t} = -\lambda N$$

This decay constant equation can be expressed in terms of activity:

$$A = A_0 e^{-\lambda t}$$

where A is the activity at time t and A_0 is the initial activity. The *curie* (Ci), a unit of activity, is equal to 3.7×10^{10} disintegrations per second, the approximate number of decays per second by one g of ^{226}Ra. The *Becquerel* (Bq), the special name for the SI (international system of units) unit for activity, is equal to one disintegration per second (Table 5.2).

The *half-life* of a radioactive nuclide is the time required for the number of atoms in a particular sample to decrease by one-half. The half-life, $T_{1/2}$, is related to the decay constant by the following equation:

$$T_{1/2} = \frac{0.693}{\lambda}$$

The *average life*, T_a, of a radioactive nuclide is related to the decay constant and the half-life by the following equation:

$$T_a = \frac{1}{\lambda} = 1.44 \, T_{1/2}$$

The average life represents the time period that a hypothetical source would need—if it retained its original activity for that time period and then suddenly decayed to zero activity—to produce the same number of disintegrations as produced over an infinite time period by the source if it decayed exponentially.

Gamma decay occurs when a nucleus undergoes a transition from a higher to a lower energy level. In this process, a high-energy photon, called a γ-*ray*, is emitted. These γ-rays are identical to the x-rays emitted by excited atoms, except that γ-rays originate from within the nucleus and x-rays originate from outside the nucleus. Half-lives for γ decay are usually very short, typically 10^{-15} seconds.

Closely related to gamma decay is the process called *internal conversion*. Instead of emitting a γ-ray, the excess energy from the excited nucleus is transferred to an electron in one of the inner atomic shells, causing ejection of the electron from the atom with emission of characteristic x-rays. The probability of internal conversion occurring increases as the atomic number increases.

In *beta decay*, a neutron within the nucleus is converted into a proton, and an electron and an *antineutrino* are emitted, or a proton is converted into a neutron, and a *positron* and a *neutrino* are emitted.

$$\beta^- \text{ decay} : n \longrightarrow p + \beta^- + \overline{v}$$
$$\beta^+ \text{ decay} : n \longrightarrow p + \beta^+ + v$$

The positron was discovered in cosmic-ray experiments in 1932. It is a positively charged particle with the same mass and spin as the electron and is considered the antiparticle of the electron. The neutrino and its antiparticle, the antineutrino, are massless particles (or at least a very small mass) having no charge that carry opposite spins and account for the conservation of energy and continuous energy spectrum observed for beta decay. Particle–antiparticle pairs interact by annihilating each other, converting all their mass to electromagnetic energy (two γ-ray photons, each of 0.51 MeV). In β decay, the emitted particles may vary in the kinetic energy they possess, which is rarely greater than 3 MeV. Half-lives for beta decay are long compared with gamma decay half-lives, varying from seconds to years. The forces responsible for the beta decay processes are weak compared with both the *strong nuclear force* and the *electrostatic force* among the nucleons. Accordingly, the force responsible for beta decay is referred to as the *weak nuclear force*.

:: Table 5.2	INTERNATIONAL SYSTEM OF UNITS (SI UNITS) FOR RADIATION THERAPY		
Quantity	**SI Unit (Special Name)**	**Non-SI Unit**	**Conversion Factor**
Exposure	C kg^{-1}	Roentgen (R)	1 C kg$^{-1} \approx$ 3876 R
Absorbed dose, kerma	J kg^{-1} (gray [Gy])	Rad	1 Gy = 100 rad
Dose equivalent	J kg^{-1} (sievert [Sv])	Rem	1 Sv = 100 rem
Activity	s^{-1} (becquerel [Bq])	Curie	1 Bq = 2.7 × 10^{-11}Ci

Electron capture is an alternative to *positron decay*. In this process, an electron, usually in the K shell, is captured within the nucleus and combined with a proton to create a neutron. Electron capture most often is followed by γ-decay to release any excess nuclear energy.

Alpha decay occurs in nuclides with atomic numbers above 82 and where the ratio of neutrons to protons is low, thus resulting in the repulsive coulomb force of the protons overcoming the attractive strong nuclear force. The emitted α-particle is a helium nucleus (two protons and two neutrons). The kinetic energy for a particular alpha decay is monoenergetic (i.e., the transition may be to an excited energy state with subsequent γ emission) and often 4 to 5 MeV. Half-lives range from 10^{-3} to 10^{10} years. The radioactive decay of radium to radon is an example of alpha decay, where the Q term represents the total energy release in the transition (called *transition energy*).

$$^{226}_{88}\text{Ra} \longrightarrow {}^{222}_{86}\text{Rn} + {}^{4}_{2}\alpha + \gamma + Q$$

The latest periodic table of the elements shows a grouping of 118 elements. (Note: elements 117 and 118 have not yet been observed, but are included to show their expected positions.) Only the first 92 occur naturally; the remaining have been produced artificially. In general, the elements with high atomic number tend to be radioactive; in fact, all but one of the elements with atomic number above 82 (lead) are radioactive; only $^{209}_{83}\text{Bi}$ is stable.

The naturally occurring radioactive elements have been grouped into three radioactive series called the *uranium series,* the *actinium series,* and the *thorium series,* all of which terminate with a stable isotope of lead. The uranium series provides an example of radioactive nuclides undergoing successive transformations through α and β decay, in which the parent nuclide produces a radioactive product called the *daughter nuclide.*

When the half-life of the parent nuclide is longer than the half-life of the daughter nuclide, an equilibrium condition exists. When this occurs, the ratio of the activity of the daughter nuclide to the activity of the parent nuclide becomes constant and the apparent decay rate of the daughter nuclide is controlled by the parent nuclide's decay rate. Two types of radioactive equilibrium conditions are defined: *transient equilibrium* and *secular equilibrium.* Transient equilibrium is established when the parent nuclide's half-life is not much greater than the daughter nuclide's half-life (Fig. 5.6). In secular equilibrium, the half-life of the parent nuclide is much greater than that of the daughter nuclide (Fig. 5.7). The two types of equilibrium are described mathematically by the following equations, in which

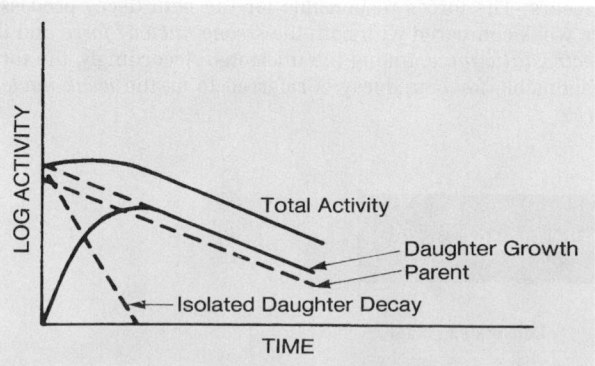

FIGURE 5.6. Transient equilibrium. Shown is a semilog plot of activity versus time for parent and daughter radionuclides illustrating conditions of transient equilibrium that may be achieved when the parent nuclide's half-life is not much greater than the half-life of the daughter nuclide. Once equilibrium is established, the daughter activity exceeds the parent activity, and both decay with the half-life of the parent.

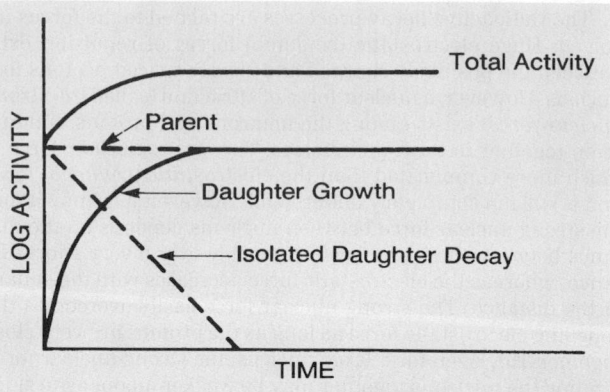

FIGURE 5.7. Secular equilibrium. Shown is a semilog plot of activity versus time for parent and daughter radionuclides illustrating conditions of secular equilibrium that may be achieved when the parent nuclide's half-life is much greater than the half-life of the daughter nuclide. Once secular equilibrium is established, activities of both parent and daughter are equal.

A_P and A_D represent the activity of the parent and daughter nuclides, respectively:

$$\text{Transient equilibrium:} \quad \frac{A_D}{A_P} = \frac{\lambda_D}{\lambda_D - \lambda_P}$$
$$\text{Secular equilibrium:} \quad A_D = A_P$$

Interaction of Photons with Matter

As stated previously, x-rays and γ-rays may be considered as bundles of energy called *photons.* If an x-ray photon enters a thin layer of matter, it is possible that it will pass through without interaction, or it may interact (usually with the atomic electrons, but sometimes with the atomic nuclei) in one of several ways (only the *photoelectric effect, Compton scattering,* and *pair production* interactions are discussed here). The probability that a photon will interact when it traverses through a given thickness of material is the product of the individual interaction probabilities for each of these three processes. The attenuation process can be described mathematically by the following equation:

$$N = N_0\, e^{-\mu x}$$

where N_0 is the number of photons in the beam impinging on an absorber of thickness x, e is the base of the natural logarithm, and μ is the linear attenuation coefficient. The quantity μ is actually the sum of the individual attenuation coefficients for the five processes. Its numerical value depends on the energy of the photon and the type of attenuating material.

There is a variety of tabulated attenuation coefficients, including the *linear attenuation coefficient* (μ), *mass attenuation coefficient* (μ/ρ), *mass energy-transfer coefficient* (μ_t/ρ), and *mass energy-absorption coefficient* (μ_{en}/ρ). Each type of coefficient is intended for use in the solution of different types of attenuation or energy-absorption problems; division by ρ, the physical density of the medium, makes the coefficient medium-independent. Figure 5.8 shows the mass attenuation coefficient for lead and water as a function of incident photon energy. The discontinuities, where the attenuation coefficient suddenly increases, are called absorption edges and occur at photon energies just equal to the binding energy of a specific electron shell.

The thickness of material that reduces the number of photons transmitted to one-half the incident number is termed the

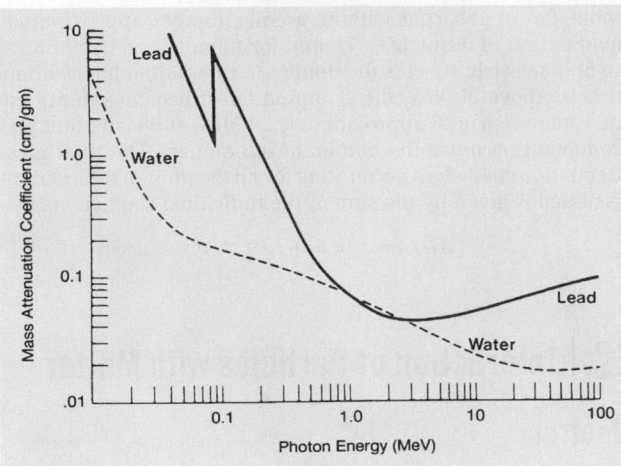

FIGURE 5.8. Mass attenuation coefficient for lead and water. Note sharp discontinuities, which are called *absorption edges.* (From Johns HE, Cunningham JR. *The physics of radiology,* 4th ed. Springfield, IL: Charles C Thomas, 1983, with permission.)

half-value layer (HVL). The HVL is related to the linear attenuation coefficient by the following equation:

$$HVL = \frac{0.693}{\mu}$$

This parameter is used to describe the quality or penetrability of the radiation and is discussed later in this chapter.

Photoelectric Effect

In the *photoelectric effect,* the total energy of the photon is transferred to an orbital electron, usually close to the nucleus, and the photon disappears. The electron then is ejected from the atom with an energy equal to the energy of the photon minus the binding energy of the electron (Fig. 5.9). The direction in which the electron is emitted depends on the energy of the incident photon. For the low-energy photons (e.g., 50 keV) the photoelectron is ejected at a large angle with respect to the incoming photon's direction, increasing in the forward direction as the photon's energy increases. After ejection of the electron, the neutral atom becomes a positively charged ion with a vacancy in an inner shell that must be filled. The atom returns to a stable condition by filling the vacancy with a nearby, less tightly

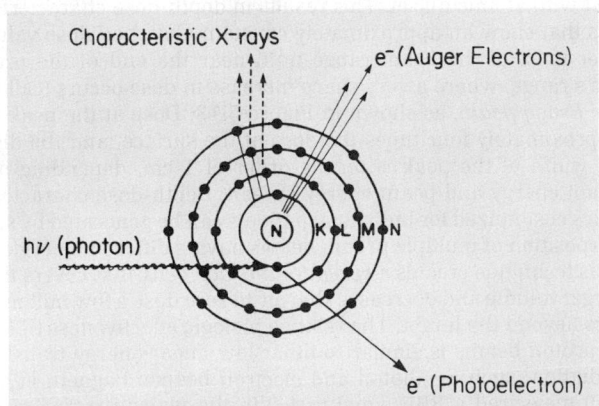

FIGURE 5.9. Photoelectric effect. In this type of photon interaction, the incident photon disappears, and an electron is ejected with kinetic energy equal to the incident photon's energy minus the binding energy of the electron. Characteristic x-rays and Auger electrons are emitted as the atom's electrons cascade to fill the vacancy created by the ejected electron.

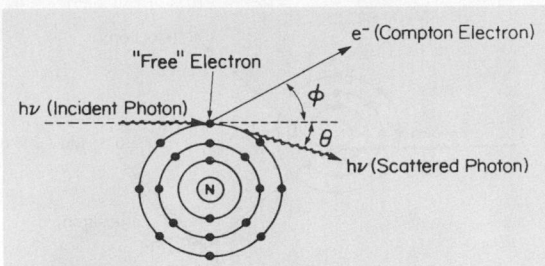

FIGURE 5.10. Compton effect. In this type of photon interaction, the incident photon interacts with one of the atom's outer electrons and the energy is shared between the ejected electron and a scattered photon.

bound electron farther out from the nucleus, and characteristic x-rays or an Auger electron is emitted.

The probability that a given photon will interact by means of the photoelectric process (denoted by τ/ρ) is a function of both the photon's energy and the atomic number of the target atom. For the process to occur, the incident photon must have energy greater than the binding energy of the involved orbital electron. In general, the probability per electron that a photon will undergo a photoelectric interaction is inversely proportional to the third power of the photon's energy and directly proportional to the third power of the atomic number of the target atom.

Compton Effect

The *Compton effect* is the interaction of a photon with a loosely bound orbital electron in which part of the incident photon's energy is transferred to the electron as kinetic energy and the remaining energy is carried away by another photon (Fig. 5.10). The binding energy of the electron is insignificant compared with the incident photon's energy, and thus can be ignored. The energy of the Compton-scattered photon is equal to the difference between the energy of the incident photon and the energy transferred to the electron. If the incoming photon's energy is low (e.g., 100 keV), very little energy is transferred to the electron. As the photon's energy increases, a greater proportion of the energy is transferred to the electron, so the scattered photon necessarily retains a smaller proportion of the incident energy. The photon may be scattered at any angle with respect to the direction of the incident photon, but the Compton electron is confined to angles between zero and 90 degrees with respect to the direction of the incident photon. If the incoming photon's energy is low, the distribution of the scattered photons is isotropic (equal in all directions). The scatter angles decrease for photons and electrons as the incident photon's energy increases (e.g., at megavoltage photon energies, both are scattered predominantly in the forward direction).

As a result of conservation of energy and momentum, the energies of the incident photon, $h\upsilon_0$, the scattered photon, $h\upsilon'$, and the scattered electron, $E,$ are given by the following relationships:

$$E = h\upsilon_0 \frac{\alpha(1 - cos\,\theta)}{1 + \alpha(1 - cos\,\theta)}$$

$$h\upsilon' = h\upsilon_0 \frac{1}{1 + \alpha(1 - cos\,\theta)}$$

$$cot(\phi) = (1 + \alpha)tan(\theta/2)$$

where $\alpha = h\upsilon_0/m_0 c^2$, and $m_0 c^2$ is the rest energy of the electron (0.511 MeV). If $h\upsilon_0$ is expressed in MeV, then $\alpha = h\upsilon_0/0.511$.

The probability that a photon will interact with a target atom via the Compton process (σ_c/ρ) depends on the energy of the incoming photon, generally decreasing as the energy of the photon is increased. The probability of a Compton interaction is

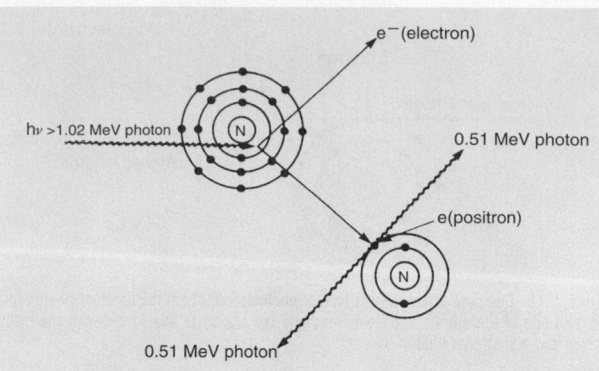

FIGURE 5.11. Pair production. In this type of photon interaction, the incident photon interacts with the electromagnetic field of the nucleus. The incident photon disappears, and two energetic electrons (a positron and a negatron) are produced. Two annihilation photons of energy 0.511 MeV then are produced when the positron interacts with its antiparticle, another electron.

nearly independent of the atomic number of the absorber and is directly proportional to the number of electrons per gram.

Pair Production

Pair production (Fig. 5.11) is possible only with photons having energies greater than 1.02 MeV. When such an energetic photon approaches closely enough to the nucleus of the target atom, the incident photon energy may be converted directly into an electron–positron pair. Energy possessed by the photon in excess of 1.02 MeV appears as kinetic energy, which may be distributed in any proportion between the electron and the positron. When the positron comes to rest, it combines with an electron, and both particles then undergo mutual annihilation, with the appearance of two photons with energy of 0.511 MeV traveling in opposite directions. The probability of pair production (π/ρ) occurring increases rapidly with incident photon energy above the 1.02-MeV threshold and is proportional to Z^2 per atom, Z per electron, and approximately Z per gram.

Relative Importance of Interaction Processes

Figure 5.12 illustrates the relative importance of the photoelectric, Compton, and pair-production processes—the three principal modes of interactions pertinent to radiation therapy—as a function of energy and atomic number of the absorber. For example, for an absorber with an atomic number approximately equal to that of tissue ($Z = 7$), and for monoenergetic photons, the photoelectric effect is the dominant interaction below about 30 keV. Above 30 keV, the Compton effect becomes dominant and remains so until approximately 24 MeV, at which point pair production becomes the dominant interaction. The total mass attenuation coefficient accounting for all the photon interactions discussed is given by the sum of the individual coefficients:

$$\mu_{en}/\rho = \tau/\rho + \sigma_c/\rho + \pi/\rho$$

Interaction of Particles with Matter

Electrons

An electron loses its kinetic energy when traversing matter via interactions that can be either *elastic*, in which no kinetic energy is lost, or *inelastic*, in which some portion of the kinetic energy is changed into some other form of energy. Elastic collisions occur with either atomic electrons or with atomic nuclei and are characterized by a change in direction of the incident electron with no loss of kinetic energy. Inelastic collisions can occur with atomic electrons resulting in *ionizations* and *excitations* of atoms, or inelastic collisions with atomic nuclei, which result in the production of bremsstrahlung x-rays (*radiative losses*). In the case of ionization, it is possible for the ejected electron to acquire enough kinetic energy to cause additional ionizations of its own. These electrons are called *secondary electrons* or *delta rays* and they can go on to produce additional ionizations and excitations. The typical energy loss in tissue for a therapeutic electron beam, averaged over its entire range, is about 2 MeV/cm in water.

The complete description of the energy and depth of penetration of the moving electrons at any point in the medium is complicated by the fact that the electrons are very much lighter than the atomic nuclei. As a result, the electron can lose a very large fraction of its energy in a single process and, thus, can be deflected by very large angles. This means that even if the electron beam is monoenergetic when first impinging on a medium, there will be a large variation among all the moving electrons as to where in the medium each will stop. This is referred to as *range-straggling*.

Protons and Heavy Ions

Protons traverse relatively straight paths through matter, slowing down continuously by interactions with atomic electrons and with atomic nuclei. This results in depth-dose characteristics that show an approximately constant absorbed dose value over most of the beam range until near the end of the proton's range, where a very sharp increase in dose occurs (called the *Bragg peak*), as shown in Figure 5.13. Dose at the peak is approximately four times the dose at the surface, and the distal width of the peak is on the order of 1 cm, depending on beam energy and beam energy spread. Depth-dose characteristics customized for individual patients can be generated by superposition of multiple proton beams having different energies. This technique creates a *spread-out Bragg peak* that covers the target volume and decreases sharply to zero dose a few millimeters beyond the target. The relative biologic effectiveness (RBE) of proton beams is similar to other low linear-energy transfer radiation, such as photon and electron beams; Pagnetti et al. (50) measured a RBE equal to 1.0 in the plateau region, and a RBE equal to 1.1 in the center of the Bragg peak for a 250-MeV beam. Therefore, the clinical response established for photon and electron treatments is considered applicable to proton treatments.

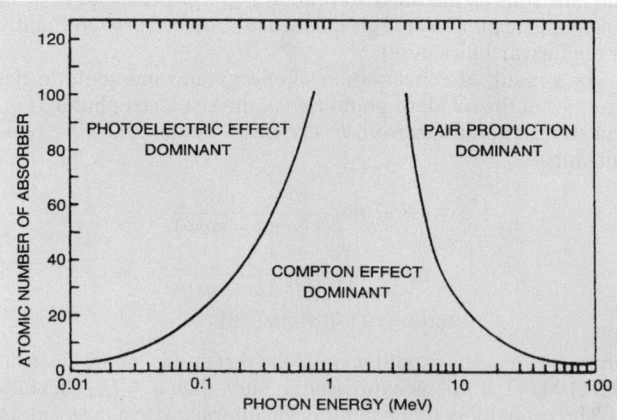

FIGURE 5.12. Relative importance of the three principal modes of interaction as a function of photon energy and atomic number of absorber. (From Hendee WR, Ritenour ER. *Medical imaging physics*, 3rd ed. St. Louis: Mosby-Year Book, 1992, with permission.)

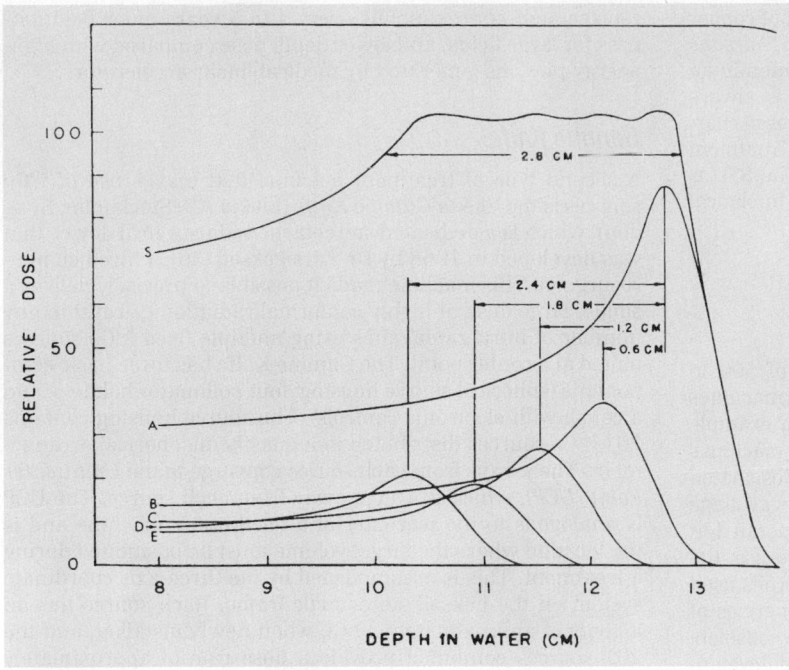

FIGURE 5.13. Drawing illustrating the way in which the Bragg peak for a proton beam can be spread out. Curve A is the depth-dose distribution for the primary beam of 160-MeV protons at the Harvard cyclotron. Beams of lower intensity and shorter range, as illustrated by curves B, C, D, and E, can be added to give a composite curve S, which results in a uniform dose of more than 2.8 cm. (From Hall EJ. *Radiobiology for the radiologist,* 4th ed. Philadelphia: JB Lippincott, 1994, with permission.)

Neutrons

Neutrons, like photons, are uncharged and thus are an indirectly ionizing radiation, which are exponentially attenuated by matter. The interactions are through processes that are primarily nuclear. They include elastic scattering with nuclei that make up the body's tissues (hydrogen, oxygen, carbon, nitrogen, and so forth). Neutron interactions result in recoil protons and charged nuclear fragments that have relatively low energy. The RBEs of these resultant particles are not fully known, thereby complicating the understanding of the relationship between clinical response and absorbed dose.

●● | Radiation Therapy Treatment ●● | Machines

Kilovoltage Units

Before 1951, most radiation-treatment units were kilovoltage x-ray machines capable of producing photon beams having only limited penetrability. Today, many modern radiation oncology clinics still use this type of machine for the treatment of skin cancer. In these machines, the electrons are accelerated by an electric field produced from a high voltage generated in a transformer that is applied directly between the filament (cathode) and the x-ray target (anode). A schematic diagram of a radiation therapy x-ray tube is shown in Figure 5.14. The potential difference (kVp) is variable on these machines, and metal filters can be added to absorb the lower-energy photons preferentially, changing the penetrability of the beam. The combination of variable kVp and different filtration provides the capability of generating multiple x-ray beams. The degree of penetrability is used to categorize the units as *contact, superficial,* and *orthovoltage* (deep-therapy) x-ray machines. A detailed review of these type treatment machines is provided by Biggs et al. (8).

Contact Units

A contact x-ray machine typically operates at potentials of 40 to 50 kVp and at a tube current of 2 to 5 milliamperes (mA). Attached cones are used for a source–skin distance (SSD) of typically 2 cm or less. Filters of 0.5 to 1.0 mm aluminum are used to give a typical HVL of 0.6 mm aluminum. The x-ray tube is rod-shaped with an extremely thin mica-beryllium window, having an inherent filtration of 0.03 mm aluminum equivalency, and the radiation is emitted axially. The primary radiation therapy application of a contact x-ray unit is for endocavitary irradiation of selected rectal carcinomas (55,58).

Superficial Units

A superficial unit is an x-ray machine that operates at potentials of 50 to 150 kVp and 5 to 10 mA. Added thickness of filtration (1 mm Al to 1 mm Al + 0.25 mm Cu) produces HVLs of 1.0 to 8.0 mm of aluminum. Attached cones typically are used; lead masks are used to define irregular fields. The SSD is typically 15 or 20 cm. These machines are used primarily to treat skin lesions and are still in relatively widespread use.

Orthovoltage (Deep-Therapy) Units

Orthovoltage x-ray machines operate at potentials between 150 and 500 kV, with most operating between 200 and 300 kV, and

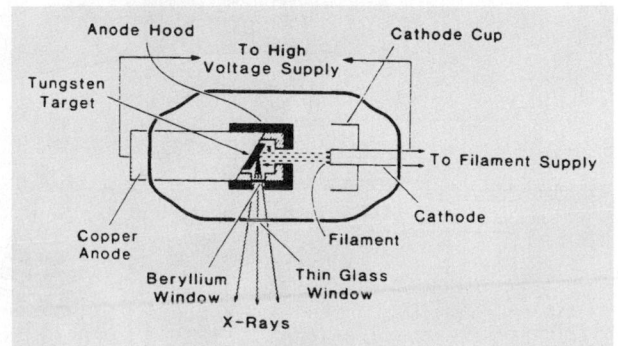

FIGURE 5.14. Schematic diagram of radiation therapy x-ray tube. (From Khan FM. *The physics of radiation therapy,* 3rd ed. Baltimore: Williams & Wilkins, 1994, with permission.)

with tube currents of 10 to 20 mA. HVLs of 1 to 4 mm of copper are common with the use of added filters, such as the *Thoreaus filter,* a combination of thin sheets of tin, copper, and aluminum arranged so that the highest atomic number sheet is always closest to the x-ray target, ensuring that the higher-energy characteristic x-rays are absorbed by the lower Z metal. Treatment fields usually are defined using detachable cones. The SSD is typically 50 cm. Very few of these machines are still in clinical use.

Supervoltage and Megavoltage Photon and Electron Beam Treatment Units

X-ray treatment machines operated in the range of 500 to 1,000 kV were designated as *supervoltage therapy* machines (59). The *resonant transformer x-ray machine* is an example of this type of kilovoltage machine. X-ray treatment machines that can produce beams 1 MV or greater have been designated as *megavoltage therapy* machines. One of the first megavoltage machines was the *Van de Graaff generator,* which operated at 1 to 2 MV. Another early type megavoltage machine was the *betatron,* first developed in 1941 by Kerst (29). Betatrons used in radiation oncology produced x-ray beams with energies of more than 40 MV. All of these early machines are now obsolete and no longer in clinical use. Details on the history and development of these early accelerators used in radiation therapy can be found in the textbook by Karzmark et al. (28).

⁶⁰Co Teletherapy

The first *cobalt-60 teletherapy* machine was loaded with its ⁶⁰Co source in August 1951 in the Saskatoon Cancer Clinic in Canada, and the first patient was treated on November 8 of that year (56). A detailed review of ⁶⁰Co teletherapy machines is provided by Glasgow (17). The advantages of a ⁶⁰Co teletherapy machine are its relative constancy of beam output, predictability of decay because of a well-defined half-life, and lack of day-to-day small-output fluctuations typically found in electrical machines. Modern isocentric ⁶⁰Co teletherapy machines, such as the Theratronics International Ltd. (Kanata, Canada) Theratron-780 and Theratron-1000, have a source-to-axis distance of 80 cm or 100 cm, respectively. Source activities vary from about 5,000 to 13,000 Ci in 1.5- to 2.0-cm diameter sources, and yield exposure rates of 150 to 250 R/min at 1 m. A typical design for the Theratron-780 source head is illustrated in Fig. 5.15. Maximum field sizes of 40 × 40 cm at the machine isocenter now are available on some newer machines. The radiation consists of 1.17- and 1.33-MeV γ-rays having a $d_{1/2}$ in tissue (the depth at which the dose has been reduced to 50% of the maximum dose value) of about 10 cm. Disadvantages of ⁶⁰Co units include the need for source

replacement approximately every 4 to 5 years, poor field flatness for large fields, and lower depth dose compared with high-energy photons generated by medical linear accelerators.

Gamma Knife

A second type of treatment machine that makes use of ⁶⁰Co sources is the Elekta *Gamma Knife* (Elekta AB, Stockholm, Sweden), which is a dedicated stereotactic radiosurgical device that was developed in 1968 by Dr. Lars Leksell (36), a Swedish neurosurgeon. This machine made it possible to precisely deliver a single, large dose of highly conformal radiation (γ-rays) to any number of intracranial sites using multiple fixed ⁶⁰Co sources aimed at a center point. The Gamma Knife has three basic components (spherical source housing, four collimator helmets, and a couch with electronic controls). The source housing contains 201 ⁶⁰Co sources distributed in a quasihemispherical arrangement. The γ-rays from each source converge to the *Unit Center Point (UCP)*, which is 40 cm away from each source. The UCP is analogous to the isocenter of a teletherapy machine and is the location where the target volume must be positioned during a treatment. This is accomplished by the three-axis coordinate system on the Leksell stereotactic frame. Each source has an activity of approximately 30 Ci, when newly installed, and the 201 sources combined provide a dose rate of approximately 300 cGy/min at the UCP. Along the path to the UCP, the radiation beam from each source is collimated twice, once by a primary collimator, and then by one of four secondary collimator helmets. For each helmet, 201 tungsten collimators define specified circular apertures (4, 8, 14, or 18 mm projected at the UCP). In order to conform the radiation dose to the shape of the target in the patent, various combinations of aperture diameters, aperture blocking (*plugging*), irradiation times, and head positions are used. A specific combination of these four parameters defines what is referred to as a *shot* in Gamma Knife terminology. Several 100,000s of patients have been treated using this type of treatment machine.

Linear Accelerators

The first microwave electron linear accelerator (8 MV) for medical use became operational in 1953 at the Radiation Research Center of the Medical Research Council at Hammersmith Hospital in London (43). The design for an isocentric gantry mount for the accelerator first was conceived by P. Howard-Flanders (21). Shortly thereafter, Ginzton et al. (16) at Stanford developed a 6-MV isocentric medical linear accelerator (linac). Since then there have been continued advances in accelerator design and construction, and today medical linear accelerators (referred to as *linacs*) account for most of the operational megavoltage treatment units in clinical use (52).

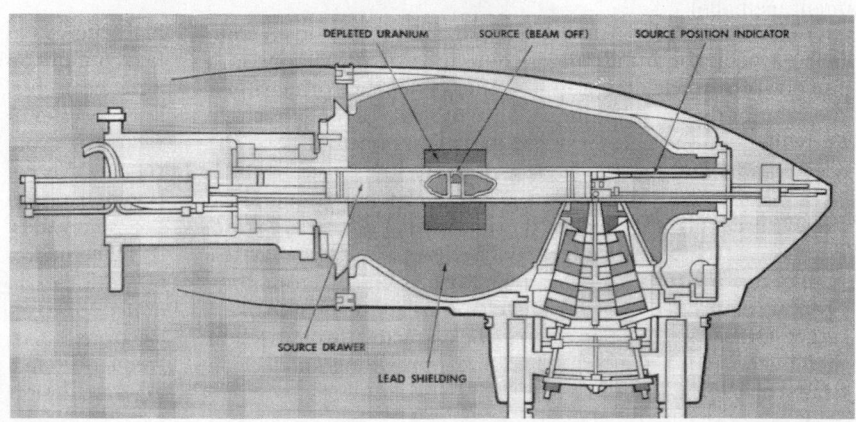

FIGURE 5.15. Schematic cutaway diagram showing Theratron-780 ⁶⁰Co source head. (Courtesy of Theratronics International, Limited.)

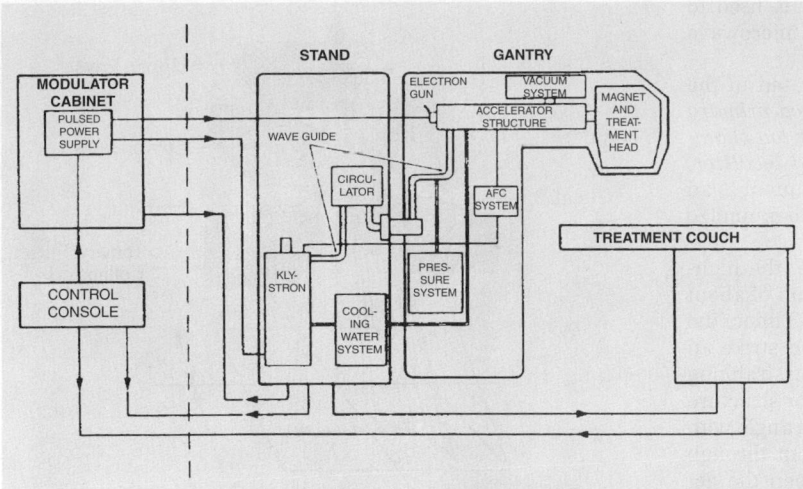

FIGURE 5.16. Schematic block diagram showing major components of high-energy bent-beam medical linear accelerator. (Courtesy of Varian Associates, Palo Alto, CA.)

Figure 5.16 is a block diagram of a high-energy, bent-beam medical linear accelerator showing the major components. The linac uses electromagnetic waves of frequencies in the *S-band* microwave region (2,856 megahertz [MHz]) to generate an electric field. The microwave radiation is propagated through a device called an *accelerator structure* and the electrons injected into the structure are accelerated by the electric field in a straight line. The accelerator structure consists of a stack of cylindrical metal cavities having an axial hole through which the accelerated electrons pass. The accelerator structure's electric field produced by the microwaves can be either a *traveling wave* or *standing wave* design. In a traveling wave design, the electrons travel with the electric field as the field propagates through the structure with time, somewhat in the manner of a surfboarder riding the crest of an ocean wave. In a standing wave accelerator, the reflected microwave power is used to produce a standing wave electric field. In that case, the microwave power is coupled into the accelerator structure by side-coupling cavities, rather than through the accelerator structure's axial cavity apertures.

The accelerator structure in low-energy (4 to 6 MV) linacs most often is mounted vertically in the treatment head collinear

along with the components associated with producing, controlling, and monitoring the x-ray beam (Fig. 5.17, left). High-energy (15 to 18 MV) linacs use a horizontally mounted accelerator structure with a beam-bending magnet system (Fig. 5.17, right). Accelerator structure technology now makes possible multiple high-dose–rate photon beams of widely separated energies.

Other important components of a linac are the modulator, microwave power sources, electron gun, and the beam-handling components. The *modulator* is the source of pulsed DC (direct current) power, which is needed for the production of *microwave power*. Pulsed DC power is also supplied to the *electron gun* (a hot-wire filament that serves as the source of the accelerated electrons). The electrons are bunched before acceleration by a device called a *buncher*. The electron beam thus consists of pulses of bunched electrons in the form of a narrow pencil beam. The *magnetron* is a device that serves as both the source of the microwaves and as a power amplifier. The *klystron* is a device used to amplify the microwave power that is generated from a separate microwave source *(RF Driver)*. The microwave power coming from the magnetron or klystron is transported to the accelerator structure by a metallic pipe

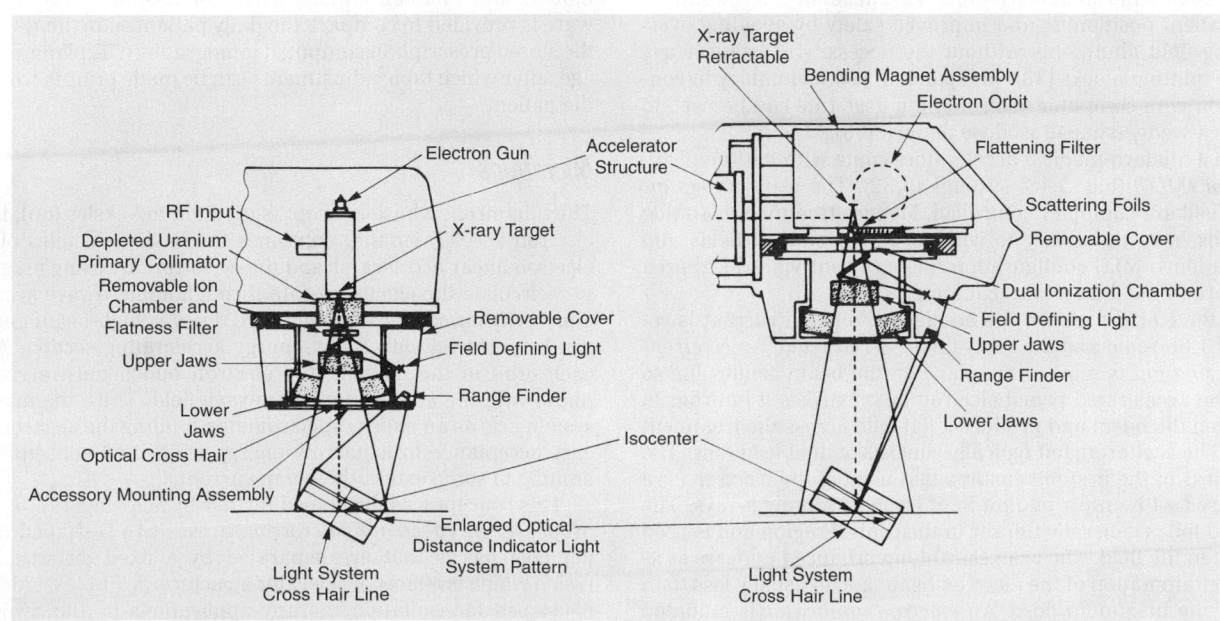

FIGURE 5.17. Schematic cutaway diagram of treatment heads for a low-energy straight-beam (left) and high-energy bent-beam (right) medical linear accelerators. (Courtesy of Varian Associates, Palo Alto, CA.)

called a *waveguide*. A device called the *circulator* is used to isolate the klystron/magnetron from the reflected microwave power.

Other important components in a linac are located in the treatment head. These include the *x-ray target, fixed primary collimator, scattering foils, flattening filter, monitor ion chamber, movable secondary collimator jaws, light field localizer,* and *optical distance indicator.* In addition, the treatment head contains a significant amount of shielding material to minimize leakage radiation.

At the exit window of the accelerator structure, the high-energy electrons emerge in the form of a pencil beam of about 2 to 3 mm in diameter. In a low-energy (4 to 6 MeV) linac, the accelerated electrons proceed in a straight line and strike an x-ray target, when in photon mode, producing bremsstrahlung x-rays. In high-energy linacs, because the accelerator structure is much longer and is placed horizontally or at some angle with respect to the horizontal, the electrons must be bent through a suitable angle, usually 90 or 270 degrees between the accelerator structure and the target. This is enabled by the beam transport system, which consists of an *achromatic focusing and bending magnet*, as well as *steering* and *focusing coils*.

The *primary collimator* is a fixed collimator located just below the x-ray target and used to collimate the x-ray beam in the direction of the patient treatment and reduces the leakage radiation from the x-ray source. The angular distribution of the bremsstrahlung x-rays produced by megavoltage electrons incident on a target is forward-peaked. To make the x-ray beam intensity uniform across the field, a conical metal *flattening filter* is inserted in the beam. Filters have been constructed of lead, tungsten, uranium, steel, and aluminum (or some combination of these), depending on x-ray energy. The flattened x-ray beam then passes through a *monitor ionization chamber*. In most cases, this system consists of several transmission-type parallel-plate ionization chambers, which cover the entire beam. These ion chambers are used to monitor the field symmetry, dose rate, and the integrated dose per monitor unit.

After passing through the monitor chamber, the beam can be further collimated by continuously movable x-ray collimators, consisting of two pairs of lead or tungsten jaws, which provide rectangular field sizes ranging from zero to typically 40 × 40 cm at a distance of 100 cm. The field size is defined by a *light localizer* and a *mirror assembly. Independent jaw* capability is available on modern units. This flexibility allows simplified patient positioning and improved safety by avoiding overlapping field abutments without the necessity of using heavy beam-splitting blocks (33). Independent jaw technology in conjunction with computer control of the dose rate can be used to create a wedge-shaped isodose pattern (35).

Most modern medical accelerators come with *multileaf collimator (MLC)* (Fig. 5.18) systems (5,32). The leaf settings for each field are computer controlled. Modern treatment planning systems have the ability to configure MLC shaped fields and the patient's MLC configuration files are sent via a local area network to the linac's MLC computer.

In the electron mode, the accelerator's beam current is reduced 1,000-fold and the x-ray target is retracted. An *electron-scattering foil* is moved into place on the beam center line so that the accelerated pencil electron beam strikes it in order to broaden the beam and produce a flat field across the treatment field. The scattering foil typically consists of dual lead foils. The thickness of the first foil ensures that most of the electrons are scattered with only a minimum of bremsstrahlung x-rays. The second foil is generally thicker in the central region and is used to flatten the field. The bremsstrahlung produced appears as x-ray contamination of the electron beam and is usually less than 5% of the maximum dose. An *electron applicator* is mounted below the movable collimator jaws to provide the final field collimation. A schematic diagram of all the treatment head sub-

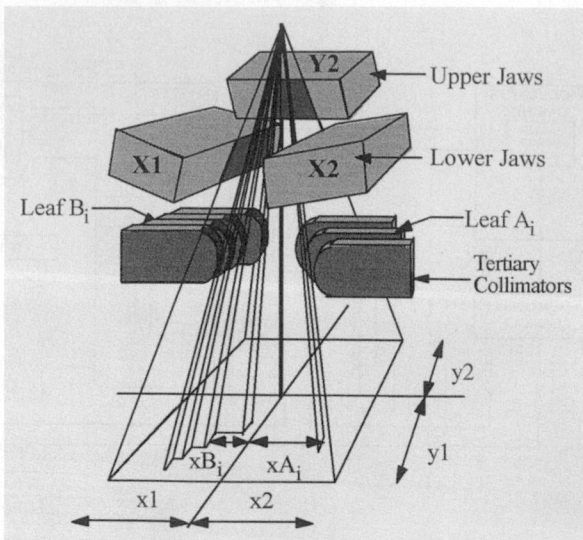

FIGURE 5.18. Schematic illustrating geometry of multileaf collimator for Varian linear accelerators. The *x*-direction is the field width across each leaf pair, and the *y*-direction is the field length. (Courtesy of Varian Associates, Palo Alto, CA.)

systems for both x-ray and electron beams is shown in Fig. 5.19.

The latest development in conventional medical linacs is the addition of advance imaging capabilities having cone beam computed tomography capability. Such linacs are referred to as *image-guided radiation therapy* (IGRT) linacs. The first commercial cone beam computed tomography IGRT linac was the *Elekta Synergy* (Elekta) (24,25); the other medical linac manufacturers have also embraced the IGRT concept and have either produced their own version of an IGRT linac, *Varian Trilogy* (Varian Medical Systems, Palo Alto, CA), or are in the process of such developments, Siemens *ARTISTE* (Siemens Medical Solutions USA, Inc., Malvern, PA). The Synergy IGRT system (referred to as XVI) consists of a retractable kV x-ray source, an amorphous silicon flat panel-imager mounted on the linear accelerator perpendicular to the radiation beam direction, and a software module for processing the data and tools for registering the images (Fig. 5.20). The XVI system provides for planar, motion, and volumetric imaging capabilities. Registration software is provided to compare the daily patient setup image with the stored prescription computed tomography (CT) planning image, after which table adjustments can be made prior to treating the patient.

Microtrons

The microtron, whose concept is credited to Veksler (66), is an electron accelerator that combines the basic principles of the electron linear accelerator and the cyclotron. By using magnets to recirculate the electron beam through a microwave accelerator cavity (or cavities) one or more times, a high-beam energy can be achieved with a low-energy accelerating section. After each orbit in the magnet, the electron bunch must arrive in phase with the accelerator microwave field. Thus, the magnet system acts as an energy spectrometer, limiting the electron energy acceptance to a narrow energy width and consequently limiting to some extent the beam current.

This concept was developed further by Schwinger (60), who proposed the *racetrack microtron*. It uses two D-shaped magnet pole pieces that are separated by a fixed distance, between which is a linac accelerator structure. A 50-MeV unit was developed for radiation therapy applications by the Swedish firm Scanditronics (Uppsala, Sweden), and was one of the first modern intensity-modulated radiation therapy delivery systems

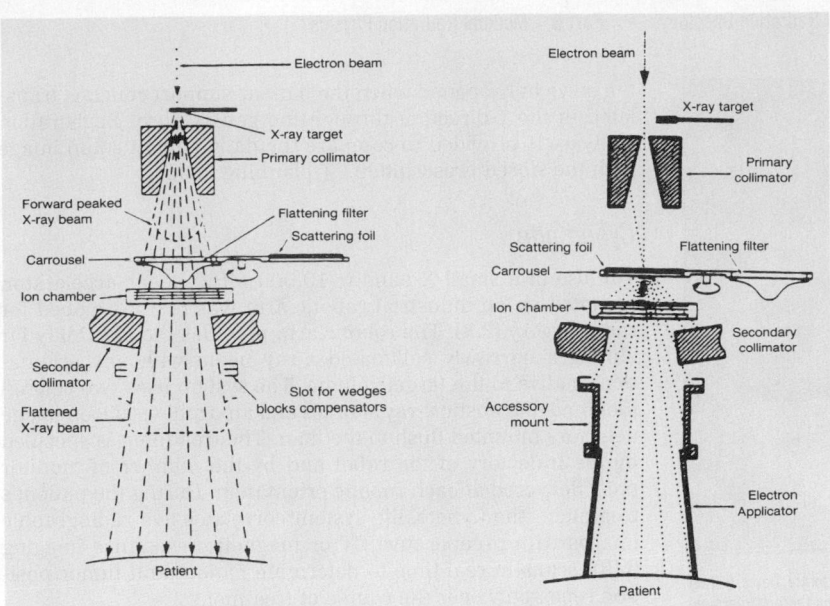

FIGURE 5.19. Schematic diagram of beam subsystems for x-ray beam (**A**) and electron beam therapy (**B**). (From Karzmark CJ, Morton RJ. *A primer on theory and operation of linear accelerators in radiation therapy.* Reprinted with permission of the Department of Health and Human Services, Public Health Service, Food and Drug Administration, Bureau of Radiological Health, Rockville, MD.)

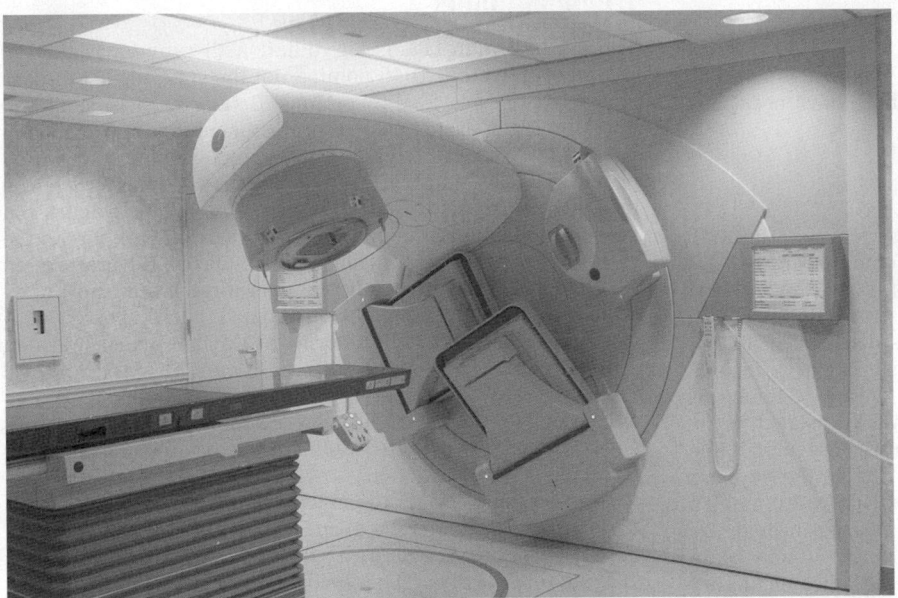

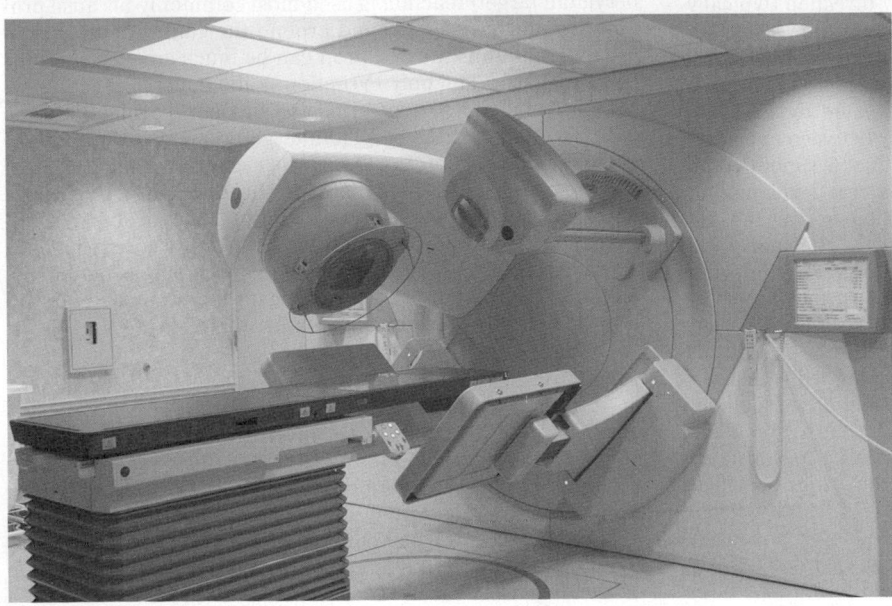

FIGURE 5.20. Elekta Synergy installed at University of California, Davis. Unit consists of a conventional multimodality medical linac with a retractable kV x-ray source, an amorphous silicon flat panel imager mounted on the linear accelerator perpendicular to the radiation beam direction, and a software module (referred to as the XVI system). The upper panel shows the x-ray source, with the amorphous silicon flat panels retracted, and the lower panel shows them extended.

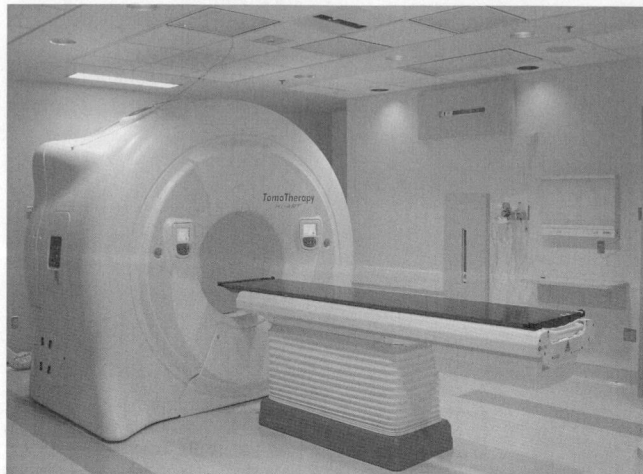

FIGURE 5.21. TomoTherapy HI-ART system installed at University of California, Davis. A short in-line 6-MV linac rotates on a ring-gantry. Intensity-modulated radiation therapy treatment is delivered while the patient-support couch is translated through the gantry bore in the same way as a helical computed tomography study is conducted. The width of the beam in the patient-translated direction is defined by a pair of jaws that is fixed for any particular patient treatment, and laterally the treatment beam is modulated by a 64-leaf binary multileaf collimator.

described in the literature (9). Only two of this type microtrons were installed in the United States, and both have now been replaced.

Tomotherapy

Helical tomotherapy was first proposed by Mackie et al. (38) and is now commercially available as the TomoTherapy HI-ART system (TomoTherapy, Inc., Madison, WI) (26,39,68). A short in-line 6-MV linac (Siemens Oncology Systems, Concord, CA) rotates on a ring gantry, at a source–axis distance of 85 cm. Figure 5.21 shows the unit installed at Univeristy of California, Davis. The intensity-modulated radiation therapy treatment is delivered while the patient-support couch is translated in the y-direction (toward gantry) through the gantry bore in the same way as a helical CT study is conducted. Thus, in the patient's reference frame, the treatment beam is angled inward along a helix, with the midpoint of the fan beam passing through the center of the bore. Similar to helical CT, the treatment beam *pitch* is defined as the distance traveled by the couch per gantry rotation, divided by the field width in the y-direction (typically between 0.2 and 0.5). The width of the beam in the y-direction is defined by a pair of jaws that is fixed for any particular patient treatment to one of three selectable values (1, 2.5, or 5 cm). Laterally, the treatment beam is modulated by a 64 leaf binary MLC, whose leaves transition rapidly between open and closed states. Each leaf has a projected width of 6.25 mm at the bore center for a maximum possible open lateral field length of 40 cm. Intensity modulation is accomplished by varying the fraction of time different leaves are opened. The individual modulation pattern can change with angle (divided into exactly 51 projections over a full revolution). During the treatment, the gantry rotates at a constant velocity with a period ranging between 10 and 60 seconds per rotation. The extent to which a treatment beam projection is modulated is characterized through what is called, the *modulation factor,* defined as the ratio of the maximum leaf open time to the average leaf open time for the projection. Pitch and maximum permissible modulation factor are new parameters needing to be specified by the treatment planner. Highly modulated treatments achieve greater conformality but they inevitably take longer to deliver. A helical MVCT image is acquired using the on-board xenon CT detector system and the 6-MV linac (detuned to 3.6 MV) with

the leave fully opened when the patient-support couch is translated in the y-direction through the gantry bore. Registration software is provided to compare the daily patient setup image with the stored prescription CT planning image.

CyberKnife

The use of a small X-band (~10,000 MHz) linear accelerator, mounted on an industrial robotic arm was first developed for radiosurgery (2,3). The robotic arm provides the capability for aiming a narrowly collimated x-ray beam with any orientation relative to the target volume. The system uses two ceiling-mounted diagnostic x-ray sources and amorphous silicon image detectors mounted flush to the floor. The treatment is specified by the trajectory of the robot and by the number of monitor units delivered at each robotic orientation. During the patient's treatment, the CyberKnife system correlates live radiographic images with preoperative CT or magnetic resonance imaging (MRI) scans in real time to determine patient and tumor position repeatedly over the course of treatment.

Proton, Heavy Particle, Neutron Beam Treatment Units

The use of proton beams for radiation therapy is credited to Wilson (69), who in 1946 pointed out the superior depth-dose characteristics provided by protons. Details on the history and development of proton beam therapy machines are provided in the text by Breuer and Smit (10). In most existing or proposed proton and heavy particle treatment facilities, either a *cyclotron* or a *synchrotron* is used for the accelerator. The synchrotron has the advantage of simple energy variability, whereas the cyclotron is capable of higher beam intensity. Several proton treatment facilities presently are operating within the United States, including but not limited to, Loma Linda University Medical Center, University of California at Davis, Northeast Proton Therapy Center at the Massachusetts General Hospital, and The Proton Therapy Center at The University of Texas M. D. Anderson Cancer Center (12,44). Several more proton beam therapy facilities in the United States are near opening or being planned.

Modern neutron therapy machines use cyclotrons to accelerate protons or deuterons to energies of about 50 MeV, to produce neutron beams with depth-dose characteristics equivalent to about 6-MV x-rays. The p,Be (protons accelerated to strike a beryllium target) reaction is used most commonly because protons are much easier to bend around the gantry of an isocentric unit, and thus the cyclotron can be much smaller and thus less expensive. The only exception is the superconducting cyclotron installed at Harper Hospital in Detroit which uses the d,Be (deuterions strike beryllium target) reaction (41). With superconducting technology, the entire cyclotron is small enough to be rotated around the patient on isocentric rings, thus eliminating the need for bending the deuteron beam around a rotating gantry. In addition, the neutron yield for the d,Be reaction is about five times that for p,Be reaction. More details on the history and development of neutron beam therapy machines are provided in the review by Maughan and Yudelev (42).

Cyclotron

The cyclotron (Fig. 5.22) was invented by Ernest Lawrence of the University of California in 1929. It accelerates heavy charged particles such as protons, deuterons, and heavy ions using a high-frequency, alternating voltage (potential difference) applied across two conducting D-shaped evacuated half-cylinders (Ds). A fixed magnetic field, perpendicular to the top of the two Ds, forces the charged particles to travel in a

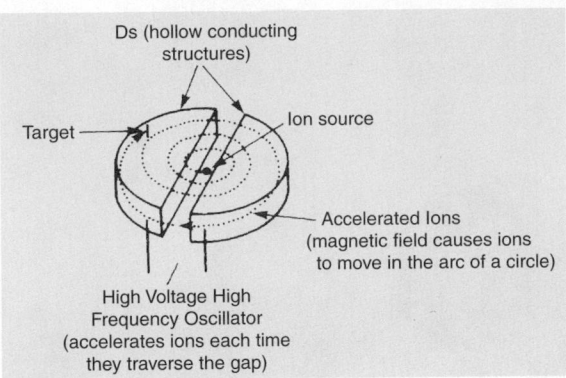

FIGURE 5.22. Schematic drawing showing principles of cyclotron operation. This machine is used for accelerating positive ions and is used clinically to produce proton and neutron beams. Metal half-disks (Ds) have an evacuated center through which the protons can travel. The protons are accelerated by an oscillating electric field operating between the half-disks. A magnetic field perpendicular to the plane of the half-disks confines the charged particles in the half-disks.

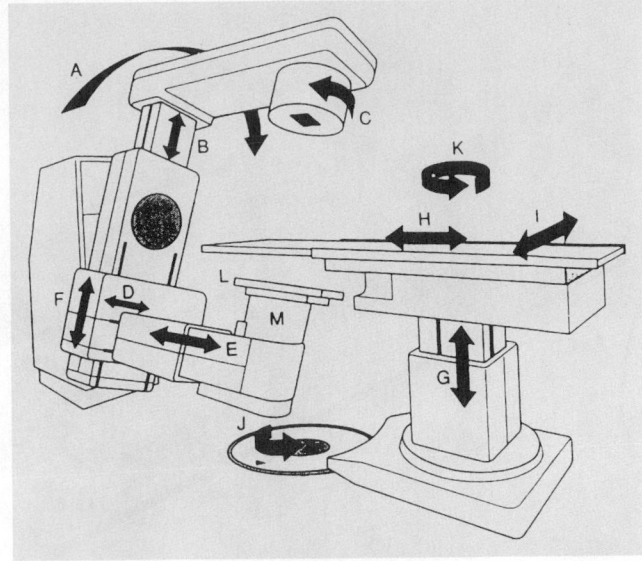

FIGURE 5.23. The basic components and motions of a radiation therapy simulator: **A:** gantry rotation, **B:** source-axis distance, **C:** collimator rotation, **D:** image intensifier (lateral), **E:** image intensifier (longitudinal), **F:** image intensifier (radial), **G:** patient table (vertical), **H:** patient table (longitudinal), **I:** patient table (lateral), **J:** patient table rotation about isocenter, **K:** patient table rotation about pedestal, **L:** film cassette, and **M:** image intensifier. Motions not shown include field size delineation, radiation beam diaphragms, and source—tray distance. (From Van Dyk J, Mah K. Simulators and CT scanners. In: Williams JR, Thwaites DI, eds. *Radiotherapy physics.* New York: Oxford Medical Publications, 1993, with permission.)

circular path. The charged particles accelerate only when passing through the gap between the two Ds. The beam spirals out to the edge of the container as the particles' speeds increase. At this point, the particles' speed approaches the speed of light. Proton beam energies of 200 to 250 MeV is considered adequate for most radiation therapy applications. Beam intensity from the accelerator must be adequate to overcome losses in the beam delivery system and provide tolerable treatment times. Beam spreading is accomplished by passive modulation (scattering foils) or dynamic pencil beam-scanning systems. Hall (18) has recently pointed out that there is significant neutron leakage radiation for those proton treatment machines that use a scattering foil and recommends moving to the pencil beam-scanning systems.

Synchrocyclotron, Synchrotrons

A *synchrocyclotron* varies either the magnetic field or the frequency of the applied electric field; a *synchrotron* varies both. By increasing these parameters appropriately as the particles gain energy, their path can be held constant as they are accelerated. This allows the vacuum container for the particles to be a large, thin torus. In reality it is easier to use some straight sections and some bent sections using multiple bend magnets, thus creating the shape of a rounded cornered polygon. The Loma Linda proton beam facility is an example of this type accelerator (12).

▪▪ | Simulators

Conventional Simulator

Details on the historic development of the *radiation therapy simulator* and the selection, acceptance testing, and quality assurance of radiation therapy simulators is provided in the review article by Van Dyk and Munro (64). The modern conventional simulator mimics the functions and allowed motions of a therapy unit and uses a diagnostic x-ray tube to simulate the radiation properties of the treatment beam (Fig. 5.23). A simulator allows the beam direction and the treatment fields to be determined to encompass the projection of the target volume. Radiographic visualization of internal structures in relation to external landmarks allows special shielding devices (Cerrobend blocks) to be constructed to help minimize the dose to normal critical structures. Gantry arms are rigid enough to

support heavy shielding blocks and simulated electron cones; Couch widths are similar to therapy unit couch widths; and operating consoles feature digital displays of parameters and programmable settings for source-to-axis distance, gantry angles, and field sizes. Conventional simulators are equipped with x-ray fluoroscopy to expedite field setup and beam angulations and have automatic exposure controls for improved radiographic techniques. One of the major changes in the imaging chain design for conventional simulator is the replacement of the image intensifier and video camera system with amorphous silicon detectors (47). The new imagers produce high spatial and contrast-resolution images that approach film quality, facilitating the concept of filmless radiation oncology departments, and provide cone-beam CT capability.

CT Simulators

In the 1980s and early 1990s, research led to the integration of a diagnostic CT scanner with what was essentially a three-dimensional (3-D) treatment planning system which led to the concept of *virtual simulation* (11,46,49,51,62). Such a system is referred to as a *CT simulator* and consists of a CT scanner, a flat tabletop, patient position-alignment system including an orthogonal laser system, virtual simulation workstation, and hardcopy output device (Fig. 5.24). A CT simulator provides many advanced image manipulation and viewing features including *beam's eye view* display, which allows the anatomy to be viewed from the perspective of the radiation beams and allows field shaping to be done electronically at the graphics display station, and the generation of *digitally reconstructed radiographs*. Modern CT simulation systems incorporate large-bore CT scanners especially designed for radiation oncology (15), with multislice capability, high-quality laser patient positioning/marking systems, and sophisticated virtual simulation software features. Details of the virtual simulation process will be discussed in some detail in Chapter 8. More details on CT simulation can be found in he review articles by Van Dyk and Taylor (65) and Mutic et al. (47).

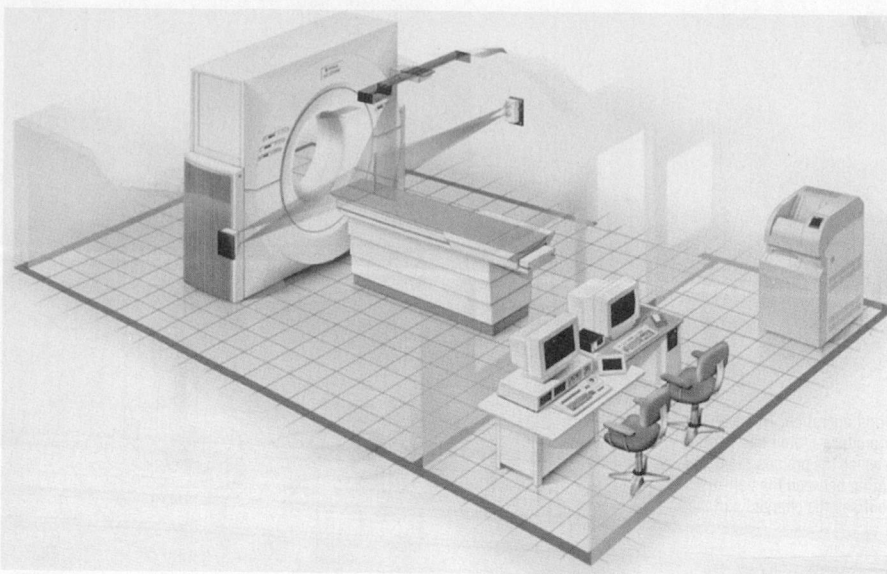

FIGURE 5.24. Typical computed tomography simulation suite showing the scanner, flat tabletop, orthogonal laser system, virtual simulation workstation, and hardcopy output device. (Reproduced with permission of Philips Inc.)

Quality of Radiation

The penetrability of an x-ray beam, referred to as the *quality* of the beam, is completely specified by its spectral distribution curve (i.e., the relative intensities of photons of various energies), which is the result of fluctuations of tube potential, the bremsstrahlung radiation process, characteristic radiation, and multiple interactions of the incident electrons and the x-ray target. The distribution of the photon energies, including the peak photon energy, in the continuous spectrum is governed solely by the x-ray tube potential. However, the energy of the characteristic photons increases with increasing atomic number of the target element. All other factors being equal, the radiation intensity is proportional to the atomic number of the target element.

Spectral distribution of an x-ray beam can be modified by placing absorbing materials of various thicknesses (i.e., filters) in the beam. In general, a filter removes relatively more low-energy photons than high-energy photons, although photons of all energies are removed to some extent. For radiation in the orthovoltage region (except for the absorption edge effect), the lower the energy of the photons, the larger the total mass attenuation coefficient and therefore the greater the likelihood that the photon will be absorbed. Thus, the beam emerges from the filter with a larger percentage of high-energy photons than it had on entering the filter. The beam has a greater penetration power and is said to have been *"hardened"* by the filter. The quality of an x-ray beam improves with increasing tube potential and with increasing thickness and atomic number of the filter.

A specification of beam quality based entirely on a spectral distribution is too cumbersome for radiation therapy. The usual method of specifying beam quality in superficial and orthovoltage therapy is to list the HVL and the accelerating potential. For megavoltage beams, only the maximum energy of the electrons striking the x-ray target typically is used. The *homogeneity coefficient* denotes how homogeneous an x-ray beam is with respect to its photon energies. It is defined as the ratio of the first HVL to the second HVL. As the filtration is increased, the exposure rate decreases; therefore, there is a practical limit of filter thickness in orthovoltage therapy with a given combination of kilovolts, milliamperes, and treatment distance. In certain situations, it is convenient to express the quality of the x-ray beam in terms of

an "equivalent energy," which can be derived from knowledge of the HVL. The type of x-ray beam that is used in radiation therapy is always heterogeneous; however, the x-ray beam can be considered to have an *equivalent energy* of a monoenergetic x-ray beam that has a HVL equal to the measured HVL of the heterogeneous beam.

Radiation Exposure

In 1928 at the Second International Congress of Radiology, the ionization of air, called *exposure*, was adopted as the measurable effect of radiation of a photon beam (45). As the beam passes through a material, it creates ion pairs via the ionization process. In air, these ion pairs have some mobility and may be collected by applying an electric field across the air. The number of ion pairs collected is a measure of the quantity of radiation passing through the air.

The *roentgen* (R), the unit for exposure, also was defined at the 1928 Congress. The definition has been modified slightly by subsequent congresses, but the basic concept remains the same. The roentgen is that amount of x- or γ-radiation that causes the associated corpuscular emission per 0.001293 g of air to produce, in air, ions carrying one electrostatic unit of charge of either sign. The value 0.001293 g is the mass of 1 cm^3 of air at 0°C and 760 mm Hg pressure; "associated corpuscular emission" refers to the Compton and pair-production electrons set in motion by the interactions between the incident photons and the air molecules. By conversion of units, the roentgen can be expressed as follows:

$$1R = 2.58 \times 10^{-4} \, C/kg \, of \, air$$

With the advent of SI units, the roentgen no longer is used as a special name for a radiation unit, and the SI unit for exposure is coulomb per kilogram (C/kg), which is equivalent to approximately 3876 R (Table 5.2).

The condition of electronic equilibrium must exist for the definition of the roentgen to be satisfied (Fig. 5.25). According to the definition, the electrons produced in a specified volume must spend all of their energies by ionization in air and the total charge must be measured. However, because some electrons produced inside the specified volume create ion pairs outside the volume and some electrons produced outside the volume

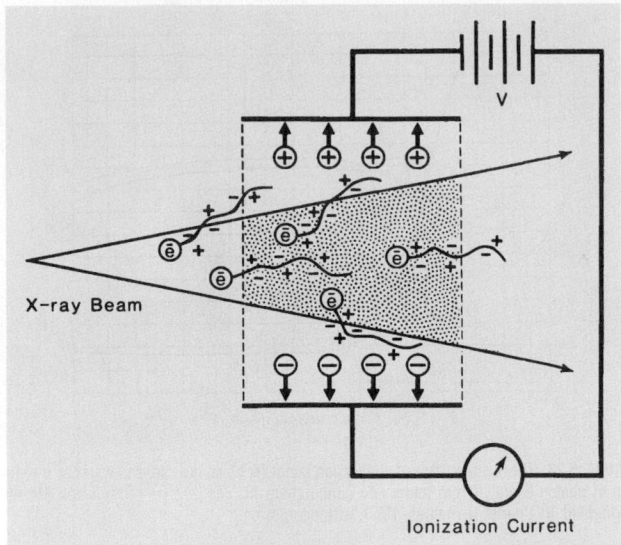

FIGURE 5.25. Schematic illustrating electronic equilibrium. (From Khan FM. *The physics of radiation therapy,* 3rd ed. Baltimore: Williams & Wilkins, 1994, with permission.)

contribute ionization inside the specified volume, the gain and loss of ion pairs must be the same for the definition of the roentgen to be satisfied.

The free-air ionization chamber is used to measure exposure directly in roentgens (30). It is designed to collect all the ions produced in a defined volume by the radiation beam and is used primarily by standards laboratories. Free-air chambers are bulky and too complicated to use for routine measurements. Instead, small ionization chambers called *thimble chambers* are typically used to measure exposure. The chamber gives a measure of the ionization produced, which then is converted to exposure in roentgens by use of an *exposure calibration factor,* N_x, traceable to the National Institute of Standards and Technology. Thimble chambers are designed for use at specific energies; the thickness of the chamber wall is equal to the maximum electron range (electronic equilibrium established). If they are used at higher energies, at which the electron range is greater, an added wall thickness or *buildup cap* must be used.

To determine the exposure rate from an x-ray or γ-ray machine, an exposure-calibrated thimble chamber (with appropriate wall thickness) and connected to an *electrometer*, is placed at beam center, in air, at right angles to the beam's central axis and at the point where the exposure rate is to be specified. The field size for which the exposure rate is to be measured is set, and the radiation machine is turned on for a specified time, T, to achieve a reading, M, on the connected electrometer. The reading is corrected for *temperature and atmospheric pressure, timer error, stem effect,* and *ion-recombination effects.* The therapy machine exposure rate $\dot{X}$, is given in roentgens per minute by the following equation:

$$\dot{X} = \frac{M \cdot N_x \cdot C_{tp} \cdot C_{st} \cdot C_s}{T + \alpha}$$

where M is the raw ionization chamber reading, N_x is the exposure calibration factor obtained from a standards laboratory, C_{tp} is the temperature (t) and pressure (p) correction factor, C_{st} is the stem effect correction factor, C_s is the ion-recombination correction factor, T is timer (min) or monitor unit setting, and α is the timer error. The temperature-pressure correction factor C_{tp} is given by the following equation:

$$C_{tp} = \left(\frac{t + 273.16}{295.16} \right) \left(\frac{760}{p} \right)$$

The timer error α is given by the following equation:

$$\frac{M_1}{T + \alpha} = \frac{M_2}{T + n\alpha}$$

where M_1 is the instrument reading for a single long exposure of T, M_2 is the instrument reading for n short exposures of total time T, and α is the timer error (monitor end effect for linacs) for a single exposure (30).

Beyond 3 MeV, the roentgen cannot be measured accurately, thus, calibrations of radiation therapy machines at these higher energies are performed using an exposure-calibrated ionization chamber as a Bragg-Gray cavity, and the ionization readings are converted to absorbed dose as discussed in the following section.

Absorbed Dose

In 1953 the International Commission on Radiological Units and Measurements introduced the concept of *absorbed dose* and defined its unit, the *rad* (45). Before its definition can be presented, the reader must understand the concept of dose absorption. As a beam of radiation passes through an absorbing medium, it interacts with it in a two-stage process. The first step occurs when energy carried by the photons, the indirectly ionizing particles, is transformed into kinetic energy of high-speed electrons; the second step occurs as these electrons, the directly ionizing particles, are slowed down and deposit their energy in the medium.

Kerma, an acronym for the kinetic energy released in the medium, represents the transfer of energy from the photons to the directly ionizing particles (step 1). The subsequent transfer of energy from the directly ionizing particles to the medium (step 2) is represented by the absorbed dose and is defined in terms of the energy deposited by the radiation beam as it passes through the medium. The relationship between kerma and absorbed dose is illustrated in Figure 5.26.

The *rad* represents the absorption of 0.01 J/kg of the absorbing material (1 rad = 0.01 J/kg). The rad now has been replaced with the *SI unit* for absorbed dose (1 J/kg) given the special name of *gray (Gy)* (Table 5.2). By conversion of units, the gray can be expressed as follows:

$$1\,Gy = 1\,J/kg = 100\,cGy = 100\,rad$$

Determination of Absorbed Dose

It is difficult to measure absorbed dose directly, but two direct methods, *calorimetry* and *Fricke dosimetry*, are available in some laboratories. Neither method is particularly practical nor widely used, and the reader is referred to the literature for more details (34). Instead, a simpler, indirect method using an exposure-calibrated ionization chamber is used to determine absorbed dose.

Absorbed Dose Calculation from Exposure Measurement

For photon energies of ^{60}Co and lower, an ionization chamber having an exposure calibration factor assigned by an appropriate national calibration facility (e.g., National Institute of Standards and Technology or an American Association of Physicists in Medicine [AAPM] accredited dosimetry calibration laboratory) can be used to measure exposure in air as described in the section Radiation Exposure. Absorbed dose then can be calculated from the exposure as explained here. The energy deposited in a fixed mass of air from a known exposure can be calculated because it is known that an exposure of 1 R creates a finite number of ion pairs per unit mass of air (i.e., 1.61×10^{15} ion pairs per kilogram of air) and that the mean energy

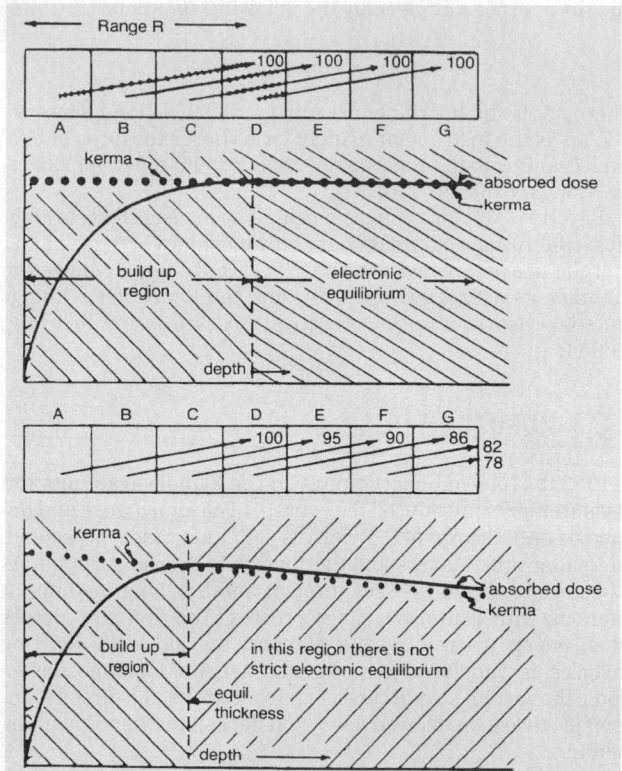

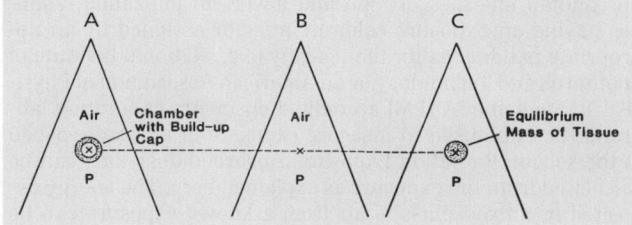

FIGURE 5.26. Graphs showing schematic relationship of kerma and absorbed dose. (From Johns HE, Cunningham JR. *The physics of radiology*, 4th ed. Springfield, IL: Charles C Thomas, 1983, with permission.)

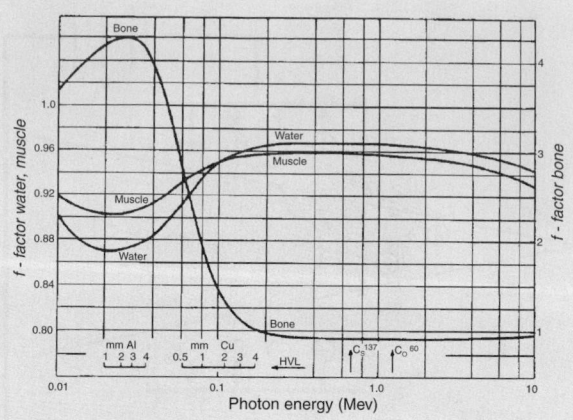

FIGURE 5.28. The roentgen-to-rad conversion factor for bone, muscle, and water as a function of photon energy. (From Johns HE, Cunningham JR. *The physics of radiology*, 4th ed. Springfield, IL: Charles C Thomas, 1983, with permission.)

required to create an ion pair in air (denoted by W) is equal to 33.97 eV per ion pair. When these values are used, the relationship between the exposure, X, and the dose to air, D_{air}, is given by the following expression:

$$D_{air}\,(Gy) = \left(8.76\,\frac{Gy}{R}\right) \cdot X(R)$$

The *dose in free space*, D_{fs} is defined as the dose at the center of a small mass of phantomlike material just large enough to provide electronic equilibrium (Fig. 5.27) and can be derived from D_{air} using the ratio of the mass energy absorption coefficients (u_{en}/ρ) and an attenuation correction factor A_{eq} that accounts for the photon attenuation in the small mass of phantomlike material.

$$D_{fs} = \left(0.873 \cdot \frac{(+\mu_{en}/\rho)_{med}}{(\mu_{en}/\rho)_{air}}\right) \cdot X \cdot A_{eq}$$

The term in brackets is called the *f-factor* or the *roentgen-to-rad conversion factor* and is represented as f_{med}, giving the

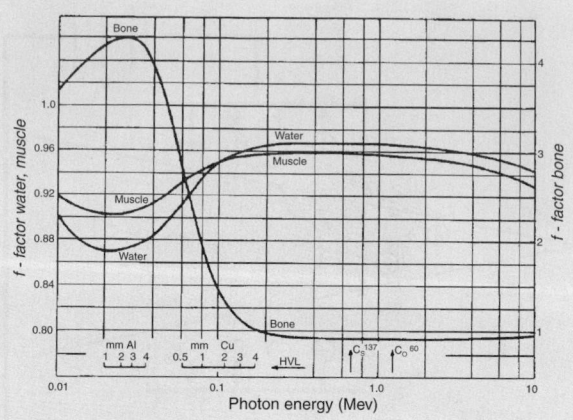

dose in free space as follows:

$$D_{fs} = f_{med} \cdot X \cdot A_{eq}$$

Values of f_{med} are shown in Figure 5.28 over the energy range commonly used in radiation therapy. Notice that f factor is a function of the medium and the energy of the photon beam. Typical values of A_{eq} are 0.989 and 1.00 for ^{60}Co and 250 kV energies, respectively.

An in-air calibration procedure is performed as follows: The calibrated ion chamber (with wall thick enough to ensure electronic equilibrium) is placed in air with its sensitive volume on the central axis of the beam and its stem at right angles to the beam direction. The center of the chamber most often is placed at a distance from the source (or target) equal to the nominal SSD of the machine plus the buildup depth. A standard field size is set, usually 10 × 10 cm, using either movable collimators or the standard treatment applicator. An exposure is made for a known time or number of monitor units. The ionization chamber reading is converted to units of Gy/min at the depth of the maximum dose within a phantom, d$_{med}$, using the following equation:

$$\dot{D}_{med} = \frac{M \cdot N_x \cdot C_{tp} \cdot C_{st} \cdot C_s \cdot A_{eq} \cdot f_{med} \cdot TAR(d_{max})}{(T + \alpha)}$$

where M, N_x, C_{tp}, C_{st}, C_s, A_{eq}, f_{med}, T, and α are used as defined earlier. The term $TAR(d_{max})$ represents the tissue–air ratio at the depth of maximum dose (i.e., the *backscatter* or *peakscatter factor*) and converts the dose in free space to the dose in a phantom at the depth of maximum dose. This parameter is discussed in more detail later. The preceding equation can be rewritten as follows:

$$\dot{D}_{med} = \dot{X} \cdot f_{med} \cdot A_{eq} \cdot TAR(d_{max})$$

And

$$\dot{D}_{med} = \dot{D}_{fs} \cdot TAR(d_{max})$$

This method is also valid when the measurements are made with the exposure-calibrated ion chamber embedded within a medium, such as a water phantom. In that case, the $TAR(d_{max})$ term is not included in the calculation, and the A_{eq} factor is replaced by a displacement factor, A_m. The numerical value of A_m is very close to that of A_{eq}, and for exposure measurements made within a water phantom, the dose rate is given by the following expression:

$$\dot{D}_{med} = \dot{X} \cdot f_{med} \cdot A_m$$

FIGURE 5.27. Schematic illustrating ionization measurement in air to determine dose in free space. (From Khan FM. *The physics of radiation therapy*, 2nd ed. Baltimore: Williams & Wilkins, 1994, with permission.)

Absorbed Dose Calculation from Bragg-Gray Cavity Ionization Measurement

For energies above the level of ^{60}Co, exposure calibration factors are not available from the standards laboratories because of measurement limitations. In 1983, the AAPM introduced a protocol for the calibration of high-energy photon and electron beams that was based on *Bragg-Gray cavity theory* and allowed one to calculate dose directly from ion chamber measurements in a medium for energies above the level of ^{60}Co (7). The protocol updated physical parameters and procedures for calibration and measurement and accounted for the different phantom materials (e.g., plastic and water) used for calibration and differences in ion chamber design and construction. The protocol introduced the *cavity-gas calibration factor* (N_{gas}), which is related to the ion chamber's ^{60}Co exposure-calibration factor N_x and is used in conjunction with restricted stopping-power ratios, $\overline{L}/\rho$, for the radiation beam in question to convert the ionization reading to absorbed dose using to the following expression:

$$D_{med} = M \cdot N_{gas} \cdot (\overline{L}/\rho)_{gas}^{med} \cdot P_{ion} \cdot P_{repl} \cdot P_{wall}$$

where M is the raw ionization chamber reading per monitor unit corrected for temperature and pressure, P_{ion} is the ion recombination correction factor, P_{repl} is a correction factor for replacement of phantom material by the ionization chamber, and P_{wall} is a correction factor to account for ionization chamber wall composition.

In 1999, the AAPM published a new protocol (TG-51) for the calibration of high-energy photon and electron beams (4). This protocol uses ion chambers with absorbed-dose-to-water calibration factors, $N_{D.W}^{Co-60}$, which are traceable to national primary standards via the ^{60}Co standard. The absorbed dose to water D_W^Q, at the point of measurement of the ion chamber placed under reference conditions is given by the following equation:

$$D_W^Q = M \cdot k_Q \cdot N_{D,W}^{Co-60}$$

where Q is the beam quality of the clinical beam, M is the fully corrected ion chamber reading, and k_Q is the *quality conversion factor* that converts the calibration factor for a ^{60}Co beam to that for a beam of quality Q. The protocol is designed to be a simplification of the AAPM's TG-21 protocol in the sense that large tables of stopping-power ratios and mass-energy absorption coefficients are no longer needed and the user does not need to calculate any theoretical dosimetry factors (22,23).

Other Dosimetry Methods

Thermoluminescence Dosimetry

Certain crystalline materials exhibit a phenomenon known as *thermoluminescence*. When a crystal capable of thermoluminescence is irradiated, a small portion of the energy absorbed is stored in the structure of the crystal lattice. If the material is heated, the energy is released in the form of visible light. Several thermoluminescent phosphors are available, but lithium fluoride, with an effective atomic number of 8.2, is the most commonly used.

The physical theory of thermoluminescence dosimetry can be explained as follows (34). In the individual atom, electrons occupy discrete energy levels. However, in the crystal lattice, the electronic energy levels are perturbed by mutual interactions between atoms, giving rise to energy bands, so-called *allowed energy bands* and *forbidden energy bands*. Impurities in the crystal create energy traps in the forbidden bands, allowing metastable states to exist; for example, when the phosphor is irradiated, some of the electrons in the valence band (ground state) receive sufficient energy to be raised to the conduction band. If there is an instantaneous emission of light, the phenomenon is called *fluorescence*. If an electron in the trap requires energy to get out of the trap and return to the valence band, the emission of light is called *phosphorescence*. If the emission of light is slow at room temperature but can be sped up with heating, the process is called *thermoluminescence*.

Thermoluminescence dosimeters must be calibrated before they can be used for measuring an unknown dose. Because the response of the thermoluminescent material is affected by its radiation and thermal histories, the material must be annealed to remove residual effects. The standard preirradiation annealing procedure for lithium fluoride is 1 hour of heating at 400°C and 24 hours at 80°C.

Film Dosimetry

When an x-ray film is exposed to ionizing radiation, the exposed silver bromide crystals form a latent image. In the film development process, the affected crystals cause a darkening of the film, and the unaffected crystals leave the film clear. The degree of blackening of the film is proportional to the energy absorbed and is measured by determining the optical density with a densitometer. The optical density is defined as follows:

$$OD = \log(I_0/I_T)$$

where I_0 is the amount of light detected without the film in place and I_T is the amount of light detected with the film in place. For radiation dosimetry, the net optical density is obtained by subtracting the densitometric reading for the base fog (clear portion of the film) from the measured optical density. Most films are exposed to yield an optical density between 1.3 and 1.7 for optimal viewing.

A plot of net optical density as a function of radiation exposure or dose is called the *sensitometric curve* or the *Hunter-Driffield (H-D) curve*. If the curve is nonlinear, appropriate corrections must be applied to convert net optical density to absorbed dose.

The use of film is a relatively straightforward method of dosimetry for electron beams, but it must be done with extreme care in photon dosimetry. The problem is that the photoelectric effect depends on Z^3 ($Z_{silver} = 47$), and the film emulsion strongly absorbs radiation below 100 kV. A concise review of radiographic film dosimetry can be found in the article by Kron (34).

Radiochromic Film Dosimetry

Recommendations for radiochromic film dosimetry are provided in the AAPM Task Group 55 Report (48). Radiochromic film consists of a thin (7 to 23 mm), radiosensitive colorless leuco dye bonded to a 100-mm thick Mylar base. Radiochromic films are colorless before irradiation and turn deep blue when irradiated without physical, chemical, or thermal processing. The film is approximately tissue equivalent, integrates simultaneously at all measurement points, and has a high spatial resolution (more than 1,200 lines per mm). It shows a stable, reproducible response if protected from ultraviolet light, unstable temperatures, and humidity. Because radiochromic dye is an aromatic hydrocarbon, like plastic scintillator, it has an energy response superior to that of diode and comparable with thermoluminescence dosimetry. Interest in radiochromic film as a quantitative dosimeter has been stimulated by the appearance of a fourfold more sensitive film (model MD-55), which extends its response down to the 5-Gy level. More details on radiochromic film dosimetry are given in the article by Kron (34).

Semiconductor Dosimetry

Semiconductor diodes offer many advantages for clinical dosimetry, including high sensitivity, real-time read-out, robustness, and air pressure independence. Most semiconductor diodes are made from silicon, which is either n type (silicon doped with group V material, such as phosphorus) or p type (silicon doped with group III material, such as boron) (34). To form a diode detector, a p-n junction must be created.

The physical theory of semiconductor dosimetry can be explained as follows. During irradiation, electron-hole pairs are created both within and outside the depletion region in the body of the diode detector. The charge carriers are swept across the depletion region and collected rapidly under the action of the electric field that exists across it. In this way, a current is generated, flowing in the reverse direction to normal diode current flow, which can be measured and related to absorbed dose.

Dosimetry diodes are operated without an external reverse bias voltage and connected via cable to a simple electrometer. Details on their use for *in vivo* dosimetry are provided in AAPM Report 87 (6). Calibration of diodes typically is performed by comparison of readings against an ion chamber in a standard setup to establish a diode calibration factor for absorbed dose to water and the establishment of a series of correction factors to account for calibration differences when measurements are performed under various experimental conditions. Typical concerns are energy dependence, temperature sensitivity, directional dependence, and radiation damage. Each radiation therapy center should establish the responses of their diodes under the various conditions encountered and monitor them as the cumulative dose to the diodes increases. Frequency of checks should be adjusted according to the frequency of use of the diodes and the variability encountered.

Metal oxide semiconductor-field effect transistors are another example of a semiconductor dosimeter. Originally developed for space dosimetry, the operation is based on the buildup of charge in the silicon oxide transistor gate created by ionizing radiation. The reader is referred to the article by Kron (34) for more details on this type dosimeter.

Polymer-Gel Dosimetry

Maryanski et al. (40) reported on a polymer-gel dosimetry using MRI that may provide an innovative solution to the problem of recording 3-D dose distributions from complex radiation fields in a tissue-equivalent material. The method exploits the radiation-induced free-radical chain polymerization of acrylic monomers, dispersed in an aqueous gel. When irradiated, discrete, microscopic regions of cross-linked polymer are formed, the concentration of which is proportional to radiation dose. The water proton nuclear magnetic resonance relaxation rates in the gel are strongly affected by local changes in the polymer molecular structure and dynamics; thus, the distribution of radiation dose may be visualized and quantified with high-resolution using MRI. Because the polymer microparticles scatter light, the dose distribution also can be visualized in the transparent gel as a dose-dependent 3-D optical turbidity. Several publications are now available on the precision and accuracy of dose measurements in photon radiotherapy using gel dosimetry (37,67).

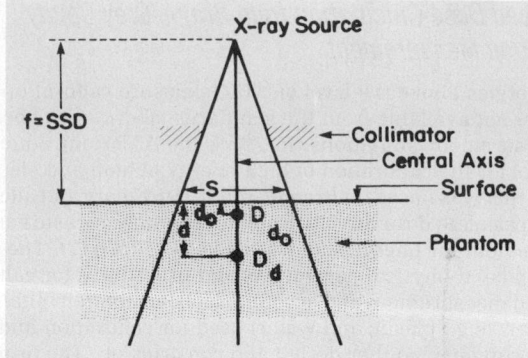

FIGURE 5.29. Schematic drawing illustrating definition of percentage depth dose, where d is any depth and d_0 is the reference depth, usually d_{max}.

Dosimetry Parameters

Percentage Depth Dose

Percentage depth dose (PDD) may be understood by reference to Fig. 5.29. It is the ratio, expressed as a percentage, of the absorbed dose on the central axis at depth d to the absorbed dose at the reference point d_0. Percentage depth dose is given by

$$PDD(d, d_0, S, f, E) = \frac{D_d}{D_{d_0}} \times 100$$

The functional symbols have been inserted in the expression to make it clear that the PDD is affected by a number of parameters, including d, d_0, field dimension S, source-to-surface distance f, and radiation beam energy (or quality) E. S refers to the side length of a square beam at a specified reference depth. Nonsquare beams may be designated by their equivalent square. Field shape and added beam collimation also can affect the central axis depth-dose distribution. Photon beam PDD increases with increasing energy, SSD, and field size. Figure 5.30 shows that the depth of the 50th percentile increases from approximately 14 cm for 4-MV x-rays to nearly 23 cm for 25-MV x-rays. The depth of maximum dose varies from about 1 cm for 4-MV x-rays to more than 3.5 cm for 25-MV x-rays.

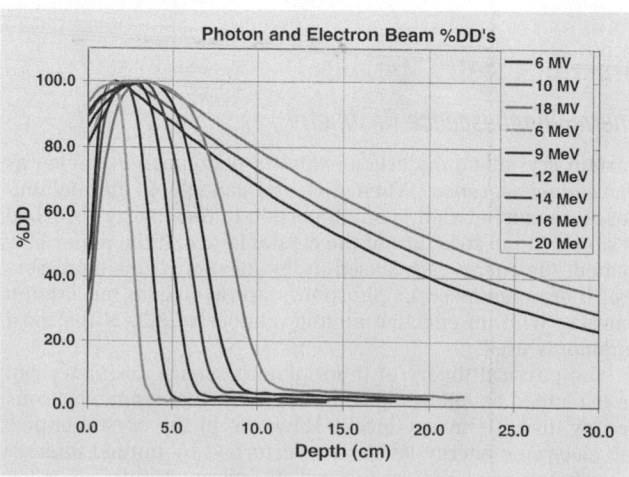

FIGURE 5.30. Examples of central axis percentage depth dose (DD) for megavoltage x-ray beams ranging from ^{60}Co to 18-MV x-rays and 6-MeV to 20-MeV electron beams.

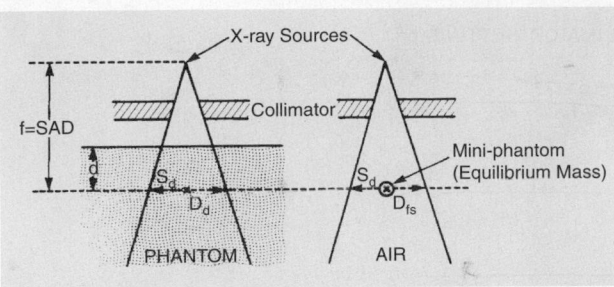

FIGURE 5.31. Schematic drawing illustrating the definition of tissue–air ratio, where d is the thickness of overlying material.

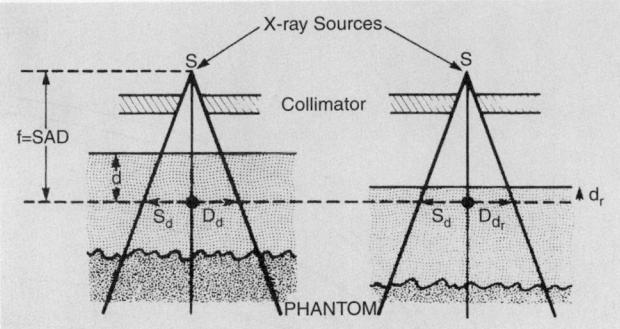

FIGURE 5.33. Schematic drawing illustrating the definition of tissue–phantom ratio and tissue–maximum ratio, where d is the thickness of overlying material and d_r is the reference thickness.

The PDD for one SSD is related to the PDD at a second SSD by the following equation:

$$PDD(d, S, f_2) = PDD(d, S, f_1) \left(\frac{f_1 + d}{f_2 d} \cdot \frac{f_2 + d_{max}}{f_1 + d_{max}} \right)^2$$

The term in the brackets is called the *Mayneord F factor* (51).

Tissue–Air Ratio

The tissue–air ratio (TAR) is defined as the ratio of the absorbed dose D_d at a given point in the phantom by the absorbed dose in free space, D_{fs}, that would be measured at the same point but in the absence of the phantom, if all other conditions of the irradiation (e.g., collimator, distance from the source) are equal (Fig. 5.31). The TAR is expressed as:

$$TAR(d, S_d, E) = \frac{D_d}{D_{fs}}$$

where d is depth, E is radiation beam energy, and S_d is the beam dimension measured at depth d. TAR depends on depth, field size, and beam quality but for all practical purposes it is independent of the distance from the source.

The TAR at the depth of maximum dose is called the *peakscatter factor*. It is perhaps better known as the backscatter factor, but because of the finite depth d_0, this tends to be misleading. Figure 5.32 shows the peakscatter factors for various field sizes and beam qualities.

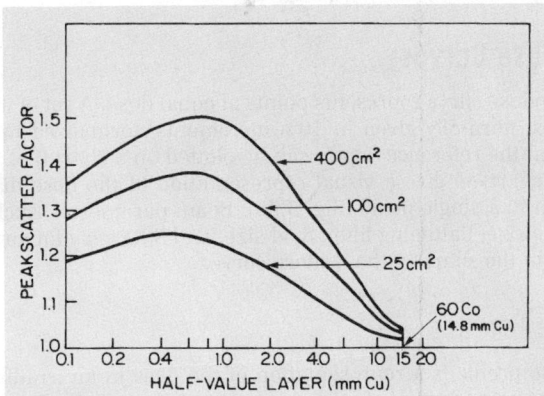

FIGURE 5.32. Variation of peakscatter factor with beam quality (half-value layer). (From Johns HE, Cunningham JR. *The physics of radiology*, 4th ed. Springfield, IL: Charles C Thomas, 1983, with permission.)

Tissue–Phantom Ratio and Tissue–Maximum Ratio

The concepts of tissue–phantom ratio (TPR) and tissue–maximum ratio (TMR) were proposed for high-energy radiation as alternatives to TAR in response to arguments raised against the use of in-air measurement for a photon beam with a maximum energy greater than 3 MeV (20,27). As originally defined, TPR is given by the ratio of two doses:

$$TPR(d, d_r, S_d, E) = \frac{D_d}{D_{d_r}}$$

where D_{dr} is the dose at a specified point on the central axis in a phantom with a fixed reference depth, d_r, of tissue-equivalent material overlying the point; D_d is the dose in phantom at the same spatial point as before but with an arbitrary depth, d, of overlying material; and S_d is the beam width at the level of measurement (Fig. 5.33). In each instance, underlying material is sufficient to provide for full backscatter. There is no general agreement about the magnitude of the reference depth to be used for this quantity, particularly for high energies. The TPR is intended to be analogous to the TAR but has an advantage because the reference dose, D_{d_r}, is directly measurable over the entire range of x-rays and γ-rays in use, eliminating problems in obtaining a value for the dose in free space when the depth for electronic buildup is great.

The original TMR definition is similar to the definition of TPR, except that the reference depth, d_r, is the depth of maximum dose. However, the depth of maximum dose for megavoltage x-ray beams varies significantly with field size and also is a function of SSD. Thus, the definition of TMR creates a measurement problem because a variable d_r is required and the TMR depends on SSD. A modification by Khan et al. (31) proposed that the reference depth, d_r, must be equal to or greater than the largest depth of maximum dose.

Purdy (54) reported on the relationships between the central axis percentage depth dose and the TPR, TMR, or tissue–air ratio. This work suggested that the degree to which the TPR and TMR are independent of distance from the radiation source depends largely on the linac's collimator/flattening-filter scatter component of the beam.

Scatter–Air Ratio and Scatter–Maximum Ratio

The scatter-air ratio (SAR) can be thought of as the scatter component of the TAR (13). It is defined as follows:

$$SAR(d, S_d, E) = TAR(d, S_d, E) = TAR(d, 0, E)$$

SAR is the difference between the TAR for a field of finite area and the TAR for a zero-area field size. The zero-area TAR

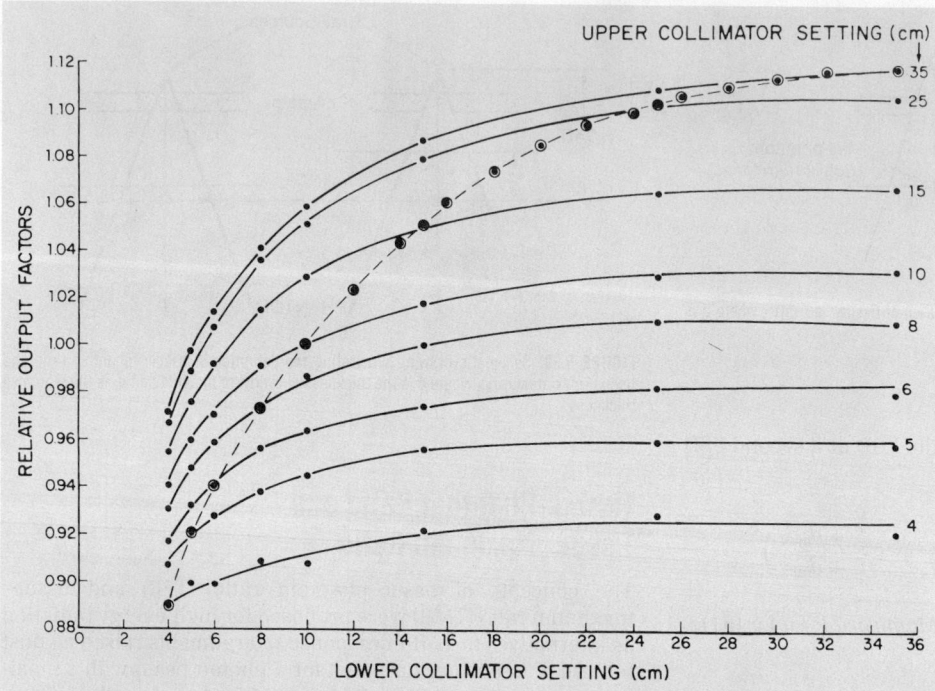

FIGURE 5.34. Example of output factor as a function of lower and upper collimator settings for a medical linear accelerator 18-MV x-ray beam.

is a mathematical abstraction obtained by extrapolation of the TAR values measured for finite field sizes.

Similarly, the scatter-maximum ratio (SMR), the scatter component of the TMR, is defined as follows:

$$SMR(d, S_d, E) = TMR(d, S_d, E) \cdot \frac{S_p(S_d, E)}{S_p(S_0, E)} - TMR(d, 0, E)$$

where S_p is a phantom scatter correction factor, which takes into account changes in scatter radiation originating in the phantom at the reference depth as the field size is changed (31).

Output Factor

The output factor for a given field size is defined as the ratio of the dose rate at the depth of maximum dose for a given field size to that for the reference field size (usually 10×10 cm) at its d_{max}. The output factor varies with field size (Fig. 5.34) as a result of two distinct phenomena. As the collimator jaws are opened, the primary dose, D_p at d_{max} on the central ray per monitor unit increases as a result of a larger number of primary x-ray photons scattered out of the flattening filter. In addition, the scatter dose, $D_s(d_{max}, r)$, at the measurement point per unit D_p increases as the scattering volume irradiated by primary photons increases with increasing collimated field size. These two components can vary independently of one another if nonstandard treatment distances or extensive secondary blocking is used.

Khan et al. (31) described a method for separating the overall output factor, $S_{c,p}$, into two components. One is the collimator scatter factor, $S_c(r_c)$, which is a function only of the collimator opening, r_c, projected to isocenter. The other is the phantom scatter factor, $S_p(r)$, which is a function only of the cross-sectional area or effective field size, r, irradiated at the treatment distance. They demonstrate that:

$$S_{c,p}(r) = S_c(r_c) \cdot S_p(r)$$

In practice, the total and collimator scatter factors both are measured and the phantom scatter factor is calculated using the

relationship listed previously. $S_c(r_c)$ is measured in air using an ion chamber fitted with an equilibrium-thickness buildup cap and given by the ratio of the reading for the given collimator opening to the reading for a reference field (typically 10×10 cm) collimator opening. The overall output factor is measured in-phantom using the standard treatment distance and is given by the reading relative to that for a 10×10 cm field size. By carefully extrapolating this measured ratio to zero-field size, the zero-field size phantom scatter factor, $S_p(0)$, is obtained. If a small ion chamber is positioned axially in the beam, it is possible to measure $S_{c,p}$ for field sizes as small as 1×1 cm. Because of the loss of lateral secondary electron equilibrium encountered near the edges of high-energy photon beams, S_p deviates significantly from unity. Consistent separation of primary and scatter dose components significantly improves the accuracy of dose predictions for irregular field calculations, especially near block edges and the resultant dose falloff resulting from lateral electron disequilibrium, and under blocks, overcoming many of the dose-modeling problems presented by use of extensive customized blocking (31).

Isodose Curves

An isodose curve represents points of equal dose. A set of these curves, normally given in 10% increments normalized to the dose at the reference depth, can be plotted on a chart (i.e., isodose chart) to give a visual representation of the dose distribution in a single plane (Fig. 5.35). Beam parameters, such as source size, flattening filter, field size, and SSD, play important roles in the shape of the isodose curve.

Dose Profiles

A dose profile is a representation of the dose in an irradiated volume as a function of spatial position along a single line (53). Dose profiles are particularly well suited to the description of field flatness and penumbra. The data most often are given as ratios of doses normalized to the dose on the central axis

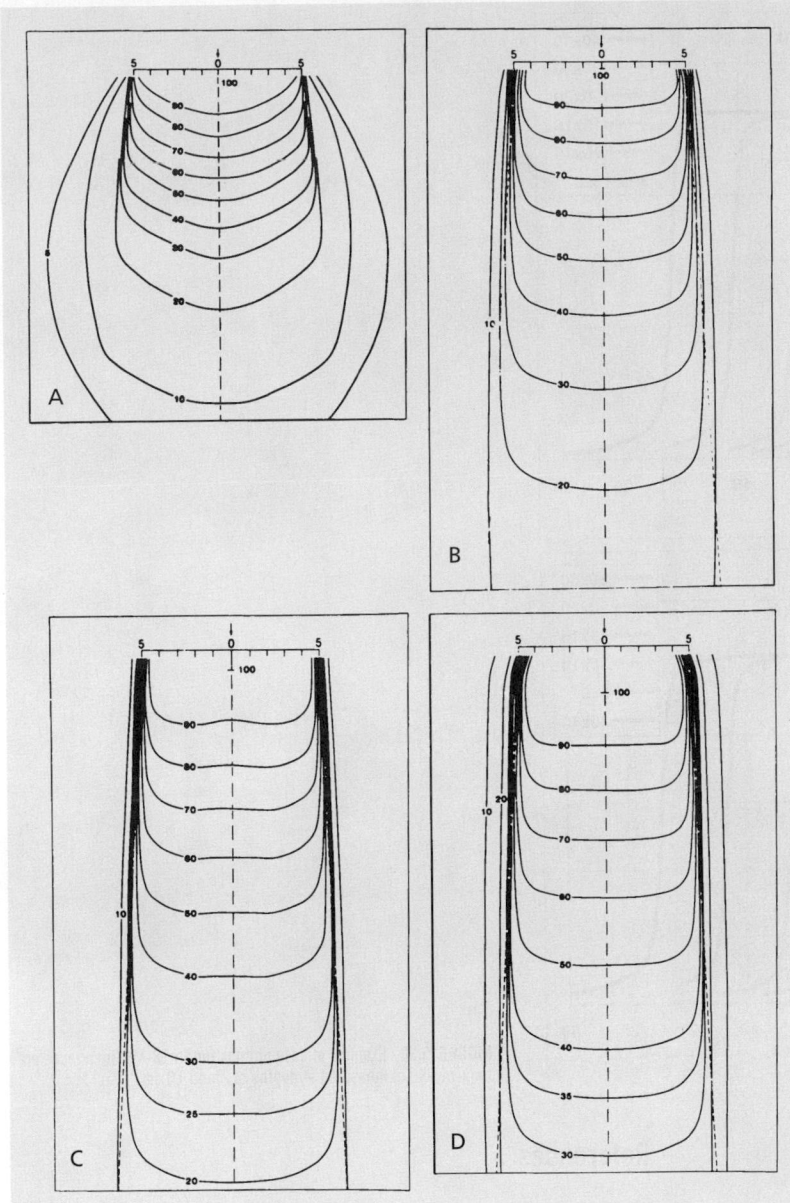

FIGURE 5.35. Isodose distributions for different quality radiations. **A:** 200 kVp, source–skin distance (SSD) = 50 cm, half-value layer (HVL) = 1 mm Cu, field size = 10 × 10 cm. **B:** ^{60}Co, SSD = 80 cm, field size = 10 × 10 cm. **C:** 4-MV x-rays, SSD = 100 cm, field size = 10 × 10 cm. **D:** 10-MV x-rays, SSD = 100 cm, field size = 10 × 10 cm. (From Khan FM. *The physics of radiation therapy,* 3rd ed. Baltimore: Williams & Wilkins, 1994, with permission.)

(Fig. 5.36). The profiles, called *off-axis factors* or *off-center ratios,* may be measured in air (i.e., with only a buildup cap) or in a phantom at selected depths. The in-air off-axis factor gives only the variation in primary beam intensity; the in-phantom off-center ratio shows the added effect of phantom scatter.

Wedge Filter

Wedge filters, first introduced by Ellis and Miller (14), generally are constructed of brass, steel, or lead. When placed in the beam they progressively decrease intensity across the field, causing the isodose distribution to have a planned asymmetry (Fig. 5.37).

The wedge angle is defined as the angle the isodose curve subtends with a line perpendicular to the central axis at a specific depth and for a specified field size. Current practice is to use a depth of 10 cm. Past definitions were based on the 50th percentile isodose curve and, more recently, the 80th percentile isodose curve. The wedge angle is a function of field size and

depth. The wedge factor is defined as the ratio of the dose measured in a tissue-equivalent phantom at the depth of maximum buildup on the central axis with the wedge in place to the dose at the same point with the wedge removed.

Wedge isodose curves can be normalized in different ways as shown in Figure 5.37. The wedged isodose distribution on the left side of the figure has been normalized to 100% at d_{max} on the central axis with the wedge in place; on the right, the normalization is done without the wedge in place. Thus, it is imperative that the normalization and the use of the wedge factor should be clearly understood before wedges are used clinically.

Beam hardening occurs when a wedge is inserted into the radiation beam. The PDD, therefore, can be considerably increased at depth. Differences in PDD of nearly 7% have been reported for a 4-MV x-ray, 60-degree wedge field, compared with the open field at a depth of 12 cm, and there have been reports of as much as a 3% difference between the 60-degree wedge field and the open field for a 25-MV x-ray beam (1,61).

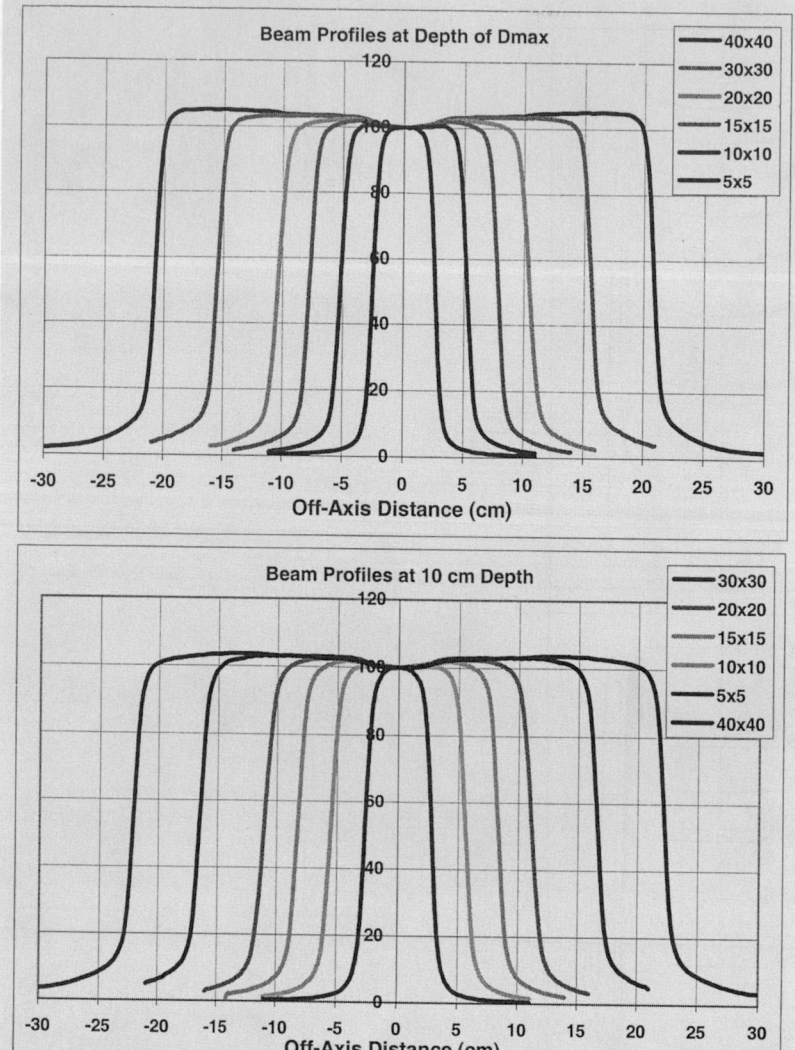

FIGURE 5.36. Example of dose profiles for an 18-MV linear accelerator x-ray beam measured at depths of 3 and 10 cm.

References

1. Abrath FG, Purdy JA. Wedge design and dosimetry for 25-MV x-rays. *Radiology* 1980;136:757–762.
2. Adler JR, Chang SD, Murphy MJ, et al. The CyberKnife: a frameless robotic system for radiosurgery. *Stereotact Funct Neurosurg* 1997;69:124–128.
3. Adler JR, Murphy MJ, Chang SD, et al. Image-guided robotic radiosurgery. *Neurosurgery* 1999;44:1299–1307.
4. Almond PR, Biggs PJ, Coursey BM, et al. AAPM's TG-51 protocol for clinical reference dosimetry of high-energy photon and electron beams. *Med. Phys.* 1999;26:1847–1870.
5. American Association of Physicists in Medicine. Report 72: basic applications of multileaf collimators: report of Task Group 50 of the Radiation Therapy Committee. 2001; 1–48.
6. American Association of Physicists in Medicine. Report 87: diode in vivo dosimetry for patients receiving external beam radiation: report of Task Group 62 of the Radiation *Therapy Committee*. Madison, WI: Medical Physics Publishing, 2005: 1–76.
7. American Association of Physicists in Medicine Task Group 21, Radiation Therapy Committee, American Association of Physicists in Medicine. A protocol for the determination of absorbed dose from high-energy photon and electron beams. *Med Phys* 1983;10:741–771.
8. Biggs P, Ma C-M, Doppke K, et al. Kilovoltage X-rays. In: Van Dyk J, ed. *The Modern technology of radiation oncology*. Madison, WI: Medical Physics Publishing, 1999: 287–312.
9. Brahme A. Design principles and clinical possibilities with a new generation of radiation therapy equipment: a review. *Acta Oncol* 1987;26:403–412.
10. Breuer H, Smit BJ. *Proton therapy and radiosurgery*. Berlin: Springer-Verlag, 2000.
11. Coia LR, Schultheiss TE, Hanks G, ed. *A practical guide to CT simulation*. Madison, WI: Advanced Medical Publishing, 1995.
12. Coutrakon G, Bauman M, Lesyna D, et al. A prototype beam delivery system for the proton medical accelerator at Loma Linda. *Med Phys* 1991;18:1093–1099.

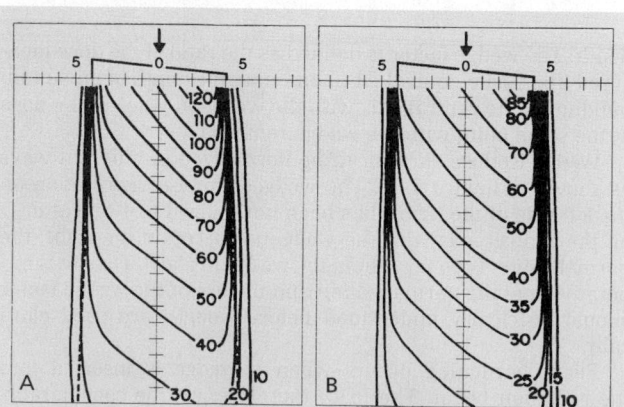

FIGURE 5.37. Isodose curves for a wedge filter. **A:** Normalized to D_{max}. **B:** Normalized to D_{max} without the wedge. ^{60}Co, wedge angle = 45 degrees, field size = 8 × 10 cm, source–skin distance = 80 cm. (From Khan FM. *The physics of radiation therapy*, 3rd ed. Baltimore: Williams & Wilkins, 1994, with permission.)

13. Cunningham JR. Scatter-air ratios. *Phys Med Biol* 1972;17:42–51.
14. Ellis F, Miller H. The use of wedge filters in deep x-ray therapy. *Br J Radiol* 1944;17:90.
15. Garcia-Ramirez JL, Mutic S, Dempsey JF, et al. Performance evaluation of an 85-cm-bore x-ray computed tomography scanner designed for radiation oncology and comparison with current diagnostic CT scanners. *Int J Radiat Oncol Biol Phys* 2002;52:1123–1131.
16. Ginzton EL, Mallory KB, Kaplan HS. The Stanford medical linear accelerator: I. Design and development. *Stanford Med Bull* 1957;15:123–140.
17. Glasgow GP. Cobalt-60 teletherapy. In: Van Dyk J ed. *The modern technology of radiation oncology*. Madison, WI: Medical Physics Publishing 1999:313–348.
18. Hall EJ. Intensity-modulated radiation therapy, protons, and the risk of second cancer. *Int J Radiat Oncol Biol Phys* 2006;65:1–7.
19. Hendee WR, Ibbott GS. *Radiation therapy physics.* St. Louis: Mosby, 1996.
20. Holt JG, Laughlin JS, Moroney JP. The extension of the concept of Tissue-Air Ratios (TAR) to high energy s-ray beams. *Radiology* 1970;96:437–446.
21. Howard-Flanders P. The development of the linear accelerator as a clinical instrument. *Acta Radiol* 1954;116:649–655.
22. Huq MS, Andreo P. Reference dosimetry in clinical high-energy photon beams: comparison of the AAPM TG-51 and AAPM TG-21 dosimetry protocols. *Med Phys* 2001;28:46–54.
23. Huq MS, Song H. Reference dosimetry in clinical high-energy electron beams: comparison of the AAPM TG-51 and AAPM TG-21 dosimetry protocols. *Med Phys* 2001;28:2077–2087.
24. Jaffray DA, Drake DG, Moreau M, et al. A radiographic and tomographic imaging system integrated into a medical linear accelerator for localization of bone and soft-tissue targets. *Int J Radiat. Oncol Biol Phys* 1999;45:773–789.
25. Jaffray DA, Siewerdsen JH, Wong JW, et al. Flat-panel cone-beam computed tomography for image-guided radiation therapy. *Int J Radiat Oncol Biol Phys* 2002;53:1337–1349.
26. Jeraj R, Mackie TR, Balog J, et al. Radiation characteristics of helical tomotherapy. *Med Phys* 2004;31:396–404.
27. Karzmark CJ, Deubert A, Loevinger R. Tissue-phantom ratios: An aid to treatment planning. *Br J Radiol* 1965;38:185.
28. Karzmark CJ, Nunan CS, Tanabe E. *Medical electron accelerators.* New York: McGraw-Hill, 1993.
29. Kerst DW. The betatron. *Radiology* 1943;40:120–127.
30. Khan FM. *The physics of radiation therapy.* Philadelphia: Lippincott Williams & Wilkins, 2003.
31. Khan FM, Sewchand W, Lee J, et al. Revision of tissue-maximum ratio and scatter-maximum ratio concepts for cobalt 60 and higher energy x-ray beams. *Med Phys* 1980;7:230–237.
32. Klein EE, Harms WB, Low DA, et al. Clinical implementation of a commercial multileaf collimator: dosimetry, networking, simulation, and quality assurance. *Int J Radiat Oncol Biol Phys* 1995;33:1195–1208.
33. Klein EE, Taylor M, Michaletz-Lorenz M, et al. A mono-isocentric technique for breast and regional nodal therapy using dual asymmetric jaws. *Int J Radiat Oncol Biol Phys* 1994;28:753–760.
34. Kron T: Dose measuring tools. In: Van Dyk J, ed. *The modern technology of radiation oncology.* Madison, WI: Medical Physics Publishing 1999: 753–821.
35. Leavitt DD, Martin M, Moeller JH, et al. Dynamic wedge field techniques through computer-controlled collimator motion and dose delivery. *Med Phys* 1990;17:87–91.
36. Leksell L. Cerebral radiosurgery: I. Gammathalamotomy in two cases of intractable pain. *Acta Chir Scand* 1968;134:585–595.
37. MacDougall ND, Pitchford WG, Smith MA. A systematic review of the precision and accuracy of dose measurements in photon radiotherapy using polymer and Fricke MRI gel dosimetry. *Phys Med Biol* 2002;47:R107–R121.
38. Mackie TR, Holmes T, Swerdloff S, et al. Tomotherapy: a new concept for the delivery of dynamic conformal radiotherapy. *Med Phys* 1993;20:1709–1719.
39. Mackie TR, Kapatoes J, Ruchala K, et al. Image guidance for precise conformal radiotherapy. *Int J Radiat Oncol Biol Phys* 2003;56:89–105.
40. Maryanski MJ, Ibbott GS, Eastman P, et al. Radiation therapy dosimetry using magnetic resonance imaging of polymer gels. *Med Phys* 1996;23:699–705.
41. Maughan RL, Powers WE. A superconducting cyclotron for neutron radiation therapy. *Med Phys* 1994;21:779–785.
42. Maughan RL, Yudelev M. Neutron therapy. In: Van Dyk J, ed. *The modern technology of radiation oncology*. Madison, WI: Medical Physics Publishing 1999: 871–917.
43. Miller CW. Traveling-wave linear accelerator for x-ray therapy. *Nature* 1953;171:297.
44. Miller D. A review of proton beam radiation therapy. *Med Phys* 1995;22:1943–1954.
45. Mould RF. *A Century of x-rays and radioactivity in medicine.* Bristol: Institute of Physics Publishing, 1993.
46. Mutic S, Palta JR, Butker EK, et al. Quality assurance for computed-tomography simulators and the computed-tomography-simulation process: report of the AAPM Radiation Therapy Committee Task Group No. 68. *Med Phys* 2003;30:2762–2792.
47. Mutic S, Purdy JA, Michalski JM, et al. The simulation process in the determination and definition of the treatment volume and treatment planning. In: Levitt SH, Purdy JA, Perez CA, et al., ed. *Technical basis of radiation therapy.* Berlin: Springer, 2006:107–133.
48. Niroomand-Rad Z, Blackwell CR, Coursey BM, et al. Radiochromic film dosimetry: recommendations of AAPM Radiation Therapy Committee Task Group 55. *Med Phys* 1998;25:2093–2115.
49. Nishidai T, Nagata Y, Takahashi M, et al. CT simulator: A new 3-D planning and simulation system for radiotherapy. I. Description of system. *Int J Radiat Oncol Biol Phys* 1990;18:499–504.
50. Paganetti H, Niemierko A, Ancukiewicz M, et al. Relative biological effectiveness (RBE) values for proton beam therapy. *Int J Radiat Oncol Biol Phys* 2002;53:407–421.
51. Perez CA, Purdy JA, Harms WB, et al. Design of a fully integrated three-dimensional computed tomography simulator and preliminary clinical evaluation. *Int J Radiat Oncol Biol Phys* 1994;30:887–897.
52. Podgorsak EB, Metcalfe P, Van Dyk J. Medical accelerators. In: Van Dyk J, ed. *The modern technology of radiation oncology.* Madison, WI: Medical Physics Publishing 1999: 349–435.
53. Powers WE, Korba A, Purdy JA, et al. Dose profiles in treatment planning. *Radiology* 1976;121:741–742.
54. Purdy JA. Relationship between tissue-phantom ratio and percentage depth dose. *Med Phys* 1977;4:66–67.
55. Purdy JA, Prasad SC, Walz BJ, et al. Radiation protection considerations for endocavitary. *Int J Radiat Oncol Biol Phys* 1985;11:2177–2181.
56. Robison RF. The race for megavoltage. *Acta Oncol* 1995;34:1055–1074.
57. Roentgen WC. A new kind of rays. *Trans Wurzburg Phys Med Soc* 1895;December.
58. Schild SE, Martenson JA, Gunderson LL. Endocavitary radiotherapy of rectal cancer. *Int J Radiat Oncol Biol Phys* 1993;34:677–682.
59. Schulz MD. The supervoltage story. *Am J Roentgenol Radium Ther Nucl Med* 1975;124:541–559.
60. Schwinger J. On the classical radiation of accelerated electrons. *Phys Rev* 1949;75:1912–1925.
61. Sewchand W, Khan FM, Williamson J. Variations in depth-dose data between open and wedge fields for 4-MV x-rays. *Radiology* 1978;127:789–792.
62. Sherouse GW, Mosher CE, Novins K, et al. Virtual simulation: concept and implementation, in the use of computers in radiation therapy. Proceedings of the 9th International Conference on the Use of Computers in Radiation Therapy, June 22–25, 1987; Scheveningen, The Netherlands.
63. Van Dyk J, ed.: *The modern technology of radiation oncology.* Madison, WI: Medical Physics Publishing, 1999.
64. Van Dyk J, Munro PN. Simulators. In: Van Dyk J, ed. *The modern technology of radiation oncology.* Madison, WI: Medical Physics Publishing, 1999:95–129.
65. Van Dyk J, Taylor JS: CT simulators. In: Van Dyk J, ed. *The modern technology of radiation oncology.* Madison, WI: Medical Physics Publishing, 1999:131–168.
66. Veksler VJ. A new method for acceleration of relativistic particles. *Dokl Akad Nauk SSSR* 1944;43:329.
67. Vergote K, De Deene Y, Claus F, et al. Application of monomer/polymer gel dosimetry to study the effects of tissue inhomogeneities on intensity-modulated radiation therapy (IMRT) dose distribution. *Radio Oncol* 2003;67:119–128.
68. Welsh JS, Patel RR, Ritter MA, et al. Helical tomotherapy: an innovative technology and approach to radiation therapy. *Technol Cancer Res Treat* 2002;1:311–6.
69. Wilson RW. Radiological use of fast protons. *Radiology* 1946;47:487–491.

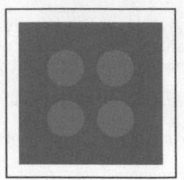

Chapter 6
Photon External-Beam Dosimetry and Treatment Planning

James A. Purdy, Eric E. Klein

The radiation oncologist, when planning the treatment of a patient with cancer, is faced with the problem of prescribing a treatment regimen with a radiation dose that is large enough potentially to cure or control the disease, but does not cause serious normal tissue complications. This task is a difficult one because tumor control and normal tissue effect responses are typically steep functions of radiation dose; that is, a small change in the dose delivered ($+5\%$) can result in a dramatic change in the local response of the tissue ($\pm20\%$) (25,35,80). Moreover, the prescribed curative doses are often, by necessity, very close to the doses tolerated by the normal tissues. Thus, for optimum treatment, the radiation dose must be planned and delivered with a high degree of accuracy.

One can readily compute the dose distribution resulting from photons, electrons, or a mixtures of these radiation beams impinging on a regularly shaped, flat-surface, homogeneous unit-density phantom. However, the patient presents a much more complicated situation because of irregularly shaped topography and having tissues of varying densities and atomic composition (called *heterogeneities*). In addition, beam modifiers, such as wedges, compensating filters, or bolus, are sometimes inserted into the radiation beam, further complicating the dose calculation.

In this chapter, several aspects of photon external beam dosimetry and treatment planning are reviewed, including methods used for dose/monitor unit calculation, correction for the effects of patient topography, and internal heterogeneities on the photon dose distribution, isodose distributions for combined fields, field junctions, field shaping and design of treatment aids, and related quality assurance (QA) issues.

Monitor Unit and Dose Calculation Methods

Monitor unit (MU) calculations relate the dose at any point on the central ray of the treatment beam, regardless of depth, treatment distance, secondary blocking configuration, or collimator opening selected, to the calibrated output of the treatment machine (described in units commonly described as *dose per monitor unit*) (32). This is accomplished by using the various dosimetric quantities described in Chapter 5 to relate the dose corresponding to an arbitrary set of treatment parameters to a single standard treatment setup where the output of the machine is specified in terms of Gy/MU. The reference distance, field size, and depth of output specification are denoted by the symbols SCD, r_{cal}, and d_{cal}, respectively. Usually, but by no means universally, it is assumed that:

$$SCD = SAD\ (source–axis\ distance) + d_{max}$$
$$r_{cal} = 10\,cm \times 10\,cm$$
$$d_{cal} = d_{max}$$

Normal incidence and open-beam geometry (i.e., absence of trays or any beam-modifying filters) are assumed. The previous setup parameters are described as fixed source-to-skin distance (SSD) calibration geometry. Treatment machines often are calibrated isocentrically with the point of MU specification located

at distance SAD rather than at distance SAD + d_{max} as described here. For isocentric calibration, SCD = SAD.

If the machine is a linear accelerator, it is calibrated by adjusting the sensitivity of its internal monitor transmission chamber so that:

$$1Gy/1MU = D(SCD, r_{cal}, d_{cal})/MU$$

MU Calculation for Fixed Fields

When the patient is to be treated isocentrically, the point of dose prescription is located at the isocenter regardless of the target depth. When the notation of Khan et al. (45) is used, the MU needed to deliver a prescribed tumor dose to isocenter (TD_{iso}) for a depth d of overlying tissue on the central ray is given by:

$$MU = \frac{TD_{iso}}{TMR(d, r_d) \cdot S_c(r_c) \cdot S_p(r_d) \cdot TF \cdot WF \left(\frac{SCD}{SAD}\right)^2}$$

where *TF* and *WF* denote the tray and wedge factors, respectively. They are defined as the ratio of the central ray dose with the tray or wedge filter in place relative to the dose in the open beam geometry. The collimated field size is denoted by r_c and is usually described as the square field size equivalent to the rectangular collimator opening projected to isocenter. The effective field size is denoted by r_d and is always specified to the isocenter distance (SAD). The inverse-square law factor accounts for the difference in distances from the source-to-point of dose prescription relative to the point of MU specification. When isocentric calibration is used, this factor is unity. Note that collimator-defined field size is used for lookup of the collimator scatter factor, S_c, whereas effective field size projected to isocenter is used for lookup of tissue-maximum ratio (TMR) and the phantom scatter factor, S_p. By separately accounting for the effect of collimator opening on the primary dose component and the influence of cross-sectional area of tissue irradiated, most of the difficulties in accurately delivering a dose in the presence of extensive blocking are overcome.

When a fixed distance between the target and entry skin surface (SSD) is used to treat the patient, a dose-calculation formalism based on percentage depth dose (PDD) is used rather than one based on isocentric dose ratios. When a dose TD is to be delivered to depth d, MUs are given by:

$$MU = \frac{TD \cdot 100}{PDD(SSD, d, r) \cdot S_c(r_c) \cdot S_p(r) \cdot TF \cdot WF \left(\frac{SCD}{SSD + d_{max}}\right)^2}$$

The field size (or its equivalent square) on the skin surface at central axis is denoted by r and is used for lookup of both *PDD* and S_p. The collimated field size r_c at the isocenter must be used for lookup of S_c. When an extended treatment distance is used, the collimated field size at isocenter differs significantly from that at the skin surface of the patient. Note that PDD is a function of treatment distance, SSD, depth, and effective field size. Collimator scatter factors measured at SAD are valid over a wide range of extended treatment distances (45).

When this dose calculation formalism for highly extended treatment distances such as encountered in administering whole-body irradiation is used, care must be taken to verify the validity of inverse square law at these distances. It is recommended that such setups always be verified by ion chamber measurement. Because of the large scatter contribution to effective primary dose originating from the flattening filter and other components in the treatment head, the virtual source of radiation may be as much as 2 cm proximal to the target of the accelerator.

The tissue-air ratio (TAR) system of dose calculation is a widely used alternative to the Khan formalism. It is simply an extension of the familiar TAR and backscatter factor concepts, as used in ^{60}Co and orthovoltage dosimetry, to the megavoltage photon energy range. The needed dosimetry parameters are determined from ion chamber measurements (both in-phantom and in-air) like those performed for ^{60}Co, but now using a much larger buildup cap (radius thickness = d_{max}). Thus the megavoltage peakscatter factor, $PSF(r)$, for an effective field size r, is simply the ratio of the two ion chamber readings as shown here.

$$PSF(r) = \frac{ionization\ at\ depth\ d_{max}\ in\ phantom}{ionization\ with\ build-up\ cap\ in\ air\ at\ same\ point\ in\ space}$$

And the megavoltage beam dose rate (Gy/MU) in free space, $\dot{D}_{fs}$, is given by:

$$\dot{D}_{fs}(SAD + d_{max}, r_c) = \frac{\dot{D}(SSD, r_c, d_{max})}{PSF(r_c)}$$

where the numerator is the measured d_{max} dose at distance SSD = SAD + d_{max} and collimator setting r_c. Implementation of this system requires a table of, $\dot{D}_{fs}(SAD + d_{max}, r_c)$ values for each collimator opening and a table of PSF versus effective field size. Then, dose at d_{max} per MU for any distance, effective field size, and collimator opening can be calculated easily.

When the patient is to be treated isocentrically, the MU needed to deliver a prescribed isocenter dose (ID) to a depth d on the central axis is given by:

$$MU = \frac{ID}{TAR(d, r_d) \cdot \dot{D}_{fs}(SAD + d_{max}, r_c) \cdot TF \cdot WF \left(\frac{SCD}{SAD}\right)^2}$$

If the treatment is fixed SSD, the MU needed to deliver a prescribed dose (TD) to a depth d on the central ray is given by:

$$MU = \frac{TD \times 100}{PDD(d, r) \cdot \dot{D}_{fs}(SAD + d_{max}, r_c) \cdot PSF(r) \cdot TF \cdot WF \left(\frac{SCD}{SSD + d_{max}}\right)^2}$$

The TAR system, like the Khan scatter analysis, accounts separately for the influence of collimator opening on the primary dose component and the size of the scattering volume on the scatter-to-primary ratio. Unlike the Khan formalism, it does not use extrapolation to zero field size to separate scatter and primary dose components. It is approximately equivalent to assuming that $S_p(0) = S_p(2 \times d_{max})$ in the Khan system (i.e., requiring that the extrapolation stop at the smallest field size for which lateral electron equilibrium exists). By ignoring these effects, the TAR system assigns a larger relative value to the primary dose component. Although both systems give identical results well away from beam edges, the TAR system underestimates dose falloff near sharp primary fluence gradients relative to the Khan model.

All MU calculation formalisms require some means of estimating the square field size, r, that is equivalent, in terms of scattering characteristics, to an arbitrary rectangular field of width a and length b. Such an equivalence is of great practical importance because it reduces the dimensionality of table lookups by one. In addition, those formalisms that distinguish between overall and effective field size require some means of estimating the square or rectangular field size that is equivalent to an arbitrary irregular field. Perhaps the most widely used rectangular equivalency principal is the "A/P" rule. It states that a square and a rectangle are equivalent if they have the same area/perimeter ratio; that is:

$$r = \frac{2(a \times b)}{(a + b)}$$

Another widely used approach to reducing rectangular estimates of effective field size to square field sizes is the equivalent square table published in the *British Journal of Radiology* (9). The problem of estimating the effective field size equivalent to an irregular field is most accurately handled by irregular field calculations (12).

MU Calculations for Asymmetric X-Ray Collimators

Asymmetric x-ray collimators (also referred to as *independent jaws*) allow independent motion of an individual jaw and may be available for one jaw pair or both pairs. Because MU calculations and treatment-planning methods generally rely on symmetric jaw data, the dosimetric effects for asymmetric jaws must be well documented before clinical use. Several investigators have examined the effects of asymmetric jaws on PDD, collimator scatter, and isodose distributions; the reader is referred to the review article by Mellenburg (64) for more details. In general, the only change to MU calculations for asymmetric fields is the need to incorporate an off-axis factor OAR(x) to account for off-axis beam intensity changes. PDD is only minimally affected, but isodose curve shape can be altered and should be investigated for any particular linac.

MU Calculations for Multileaf Collimator

Multileaf collimators (MLCs) are now standard in clinics around the world as a replacement for alloy field shaping. The effects resulting from field area shaped by tertiary MLC systems on PDD and beam output parameters are similar to those resulting from lead alloy field shaping (46). Thus, dose/MU calculation methods as discussed previously apply and one simply uses the equivalent area as defined by the MLC. The collimator scatter factor and the dose in free space are determined using the x-ray collimator jaw settings, with an off-axis factor applied for any asymmetric jaw settings. However, it should be noted that for MLC systems that replace the lower jaws, the MLC field shape can be a determining factor in selecting the appropriate output factor (66). Therefore, because of machine manufacturer MLC design differences and the fact that MLC designs continue to change, each institution is advised to study carefully the impact of the MLC on the basic MU calculation procedure before clinical use.

MU Calculations for Rotation Therapy

MU calculations for rotation therapy can be computed using the following expression:

$$MU = \frac{ID}{TAR_{avg} \cdot \dot{D}_{fs} \left(\frac{SCD}{SAD}\right)^2}$$

and the MU per degree setting is given by:

$$MU/deg = \frac{monitor\ unit\ setting}{degrees\ of\ rotation}$$

where the symbols have the previous meaning and TAR_{avg} is an average TAR (averaged over radii at selected angular intervals, such as 10 or 20 degrees).

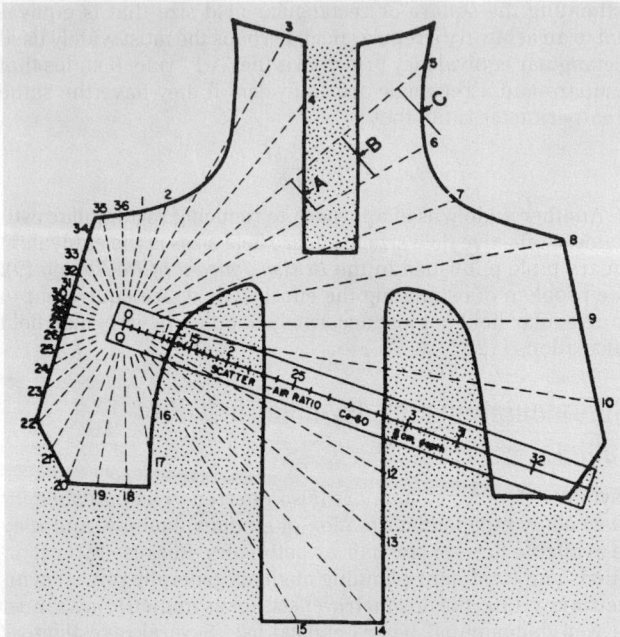

FIGURE 6.1. Outline of mantle field illustrating method of determining scatter-to-air ratio, used for irregular-field dose calculations. (From Cundiff JH, Cunningham JR, Golden R, et al. A method for the calculation of dose in the radiation treatment of Hodgkin's disease. *Am J Roentgenol* 1973;117:30–34, with permission.)

MU Calculations for Irregular Fields

For large, irregularly shaped fields and at points off the central axis, it is necessary to take account of the off-axis change in intensity (relative to the central axis) of the beam, the variation of the SSD within the field of treatment, the influence of the primary collimator on the output factor, and the scatter contribution to the dose. Changes in the beam quality as a function of position in the radiation field also should be considered (33,34).

The general method used for irregular-field calculations consists of summation at each point of interest of the primary and scatter irradiation, with allowance for the off-axis change in intensity (off-axis factor) and SSD (12). The MUs required to deliver a specified tumor dose at an arbitrary point in an irregular field (Fig. 6.1) can be calculated as follows:

$$MU = \frac{TD}{[TAR(d, 0) + \overline{SAR}(d)] \cdot \dot{D}_{fs}(SSD + d_{max}, r_c) \cdot TF \cdot OAF \left(\frac{SSD + d_{max}}{SSD + g + d} \right)^2}$$

where the parameters used are:

TAR(d, 0) = zero-field size TAR at depth d

$\quad$ SAR(d) = average SAR for point in question at depth d
$\qquad\qquad$ determined using the Clarkson technique

$\qquad$ $\dot{D}_{fs}$ = Gy/MU in a small mass of tissue, in air, on the
$\qquad\qquad$ central axis at normal SSD + d_{max} for the
$\qquad\qquad$ collimated field size

$\qquad$ SSD = nominal SSD for treatment constraints

$\qquad$ d_{max} = depth of dose maximum

$\qquad\quad$ TF = blocking tray attenuation factor

$\qquad\quad$ g = vertical distance between skin surface over
$\qquad\qquad$ point in question and nominal

$\qquad$ SSD = (beam vertical)

$\qquad\quad$ d = vertical depth, skin surface to point in question

$\qquad$ OAF = in-air off-axis factor

Computer implementations vary, but typically include using the expanded field size at a depth for the SAR calculation, determining the off-axis factor using the distance from the central axis to the slant projection of the point of calculation to the SSD plane along a ray from the source, and determining the zero-area TAR using the slant depth along a ray going from the source to the point of calculation. It is generally accepted that the off-axis factor should be multiplied by the sum of the zero-area TAR and the SAR as originally proposed.

Beam quality is a function of position in the field for beams generated by linear accelerators (33,34). The TAR_0 may be expressed as a function of position in the beam so that changes in beam quality can be incorporated into calculations, and it can be related to the half-value layer (HVL) of water by the following equation:

$$TAR(d, 0, r) = e \left[\frac{-0.693(d - d_{max})}{HVL(r)} \right]$$

where d is the depth of the point of reference, d_{max} is the depth of maximum dose, r is the radial distance from the central axis of the beam to the point of calculation, e is the base of the natural logarithm, and *HVL(r)* is the beam quality expressed as the HVL measured in water.

One final point about irregular-field or off-axis dose calculations concerns the off-axis factor. In some computerized treatment planning systems, the calculation of dose to points off the central axis is based on the assumption that the off-axis factor can be represented by a separable function given by:

$$OAF(x, y) = OAF(x, 0) \cdot OAF(0, y)$$

where x and y are the symmetry axes perpendicular to the beam axis and the functions *OAF(x, 0)* and *OAF(0, y)* are equal for a square open field. For some accelerator-generated beams, this assumption is invalid because measured values differ from those predicted by the previous equation by as much as 20% (53).

●● | Correction for Varying Patient
●● | Topography (Air Gaps)

Because basic dose distribution data are obtained for idealized geometries (e.g., flat surface, unit density media), corrections are needed to determine the dose distribution in actual patients. Methods have been developed to account for the air gap caused by the patient's varying topography and for internal heterogeneities. In one approach, the dose data calculated for idealized geometry are multiplied by a correction factor (CF) to obtain the revised dose distribution and are reviewed in the following sections (40).

Air Gap CF: Ratio of Tissue-Air Ratio or Tissue-Phantom Ratio Method

In the ratio of TAR or tissue-phantom ratio (TPR) method, the surface (along a ray line) directly above point A is unaltered, so the primary dose distribution at this point is unchanged (Fig. 6.2). For relatively small changes in surface topography, the scatter component is essentially unchanged. Thus, the dose at point A can be considered as unaltered by patient shape. However, for point B, where there are considerable variations in the patient's topography, both the primary and scatter components of the radiation beam are altered. The CF may be determined using two TARs or TPRs as follows:

$$CF = \frac{T(d - h, s_d)}{T(d, s_d)}$$

where h = air gap.

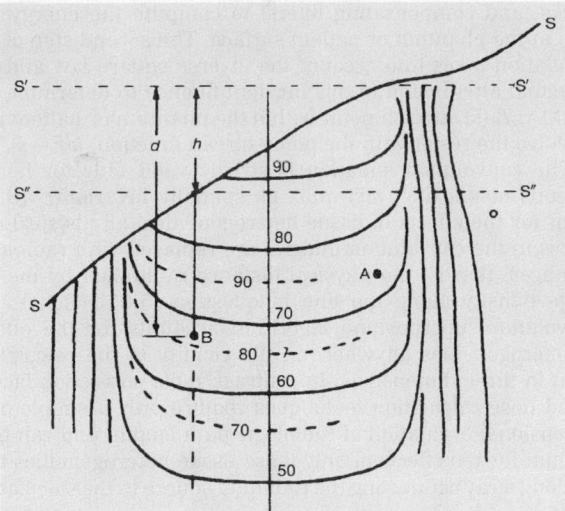

FIGURE 6.2. Schematic drawing illustrating tissue-air ratio and effective source-to-skin distance (SSD) methods for the correction of isodose curves under a sloping surface (*solid lines* for SSD = S'; *dashed lines* for SSD = S''). (From International Commission of Radiation Units and Measurements. *Report 24: Determination of absorbed dose in a patient irradiated by beams of × or gamma rays in radiotherapy procedures.* Washington, DC: International Commission of Radiation Units and Measurements, 1976, with permission.)

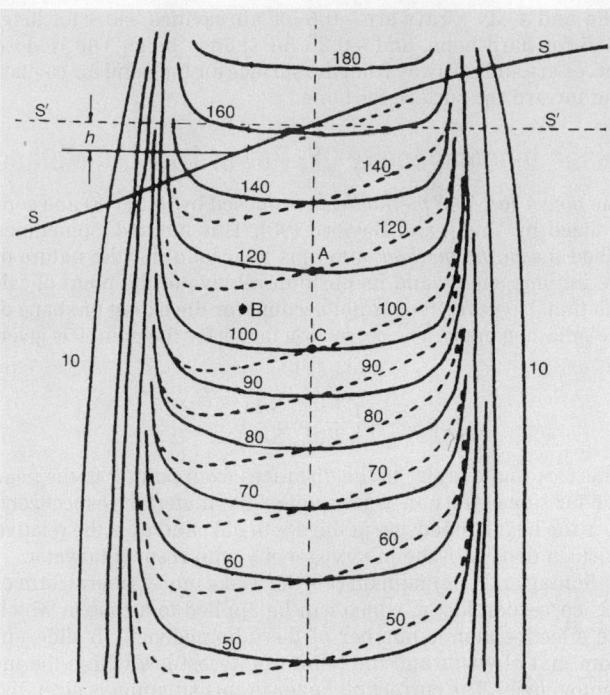

FIGURE 6.3. Schematic diagram illustrating isodose shift method of correcting isodose curves under a sloping surface. *Solid lines*, source-to-skin distance = S'; *dashed lines*, shifted source-to-skin distance. (From International Commission of Radiation Units and Measurements. *Report 24: Determination of absorbed dose in a patient irradiated by beams of × or gamma rays in radiotherapy procedures.* Washington, DC: International Commission of Radiation Units and Measurements, 1976, with permission.)

Air Gap CF: Effective Source-Skin Ratio Method

In the effective SSD method, the isodose chart to be used is placed on the contour representation, positioning the central axis at the distance for which the curve was measured (Fig. 6.2). It then is shifted down along the ray line for the length of the air gap, h. The PDD value at point B is read and modified by an inverse-square calculation to account for the effective change in the peak dose. The CF can be expressed as follows:

$$CF = \frac{P(d - h, d_O, S, f, E)}{P(d, d_O, S, f, E)} \cdot \left(\frac{f + d_O}{f + h + d_O}\right)^2$$

Air Gap CF: Isodose Shift Method

Manual construction of an entire dose distribution for an actual patient with the previous methods would be time-consuming. The isodose shift method (Fig. 6.3), although simplistic, is efficient and gives satisfactory results in most cases. In this method, the isodose chart is moved down along a diverging ray by a fractional amount of the air gap, h. The intersection of the isodose lines with this ray are read off directly. For ^{60}Co radiation, a shift of two-thirds of h is used, and for 25-MV x-rays, a shift of one-half of h is used.

⠿ | Correction for Tissue Inhomogeneities

Current dose calculation algorithms can be broadly classified into correction factor-based and kernel-based models; a detailed review of photon beam dose calculation algorithms is provided by Ahnesjö and Aspradakis (6). Correction factor-based models correct the dose distribution computed for a regularly shaped, homogeneous water phantom for the presence of beam modifiers, surface topography variations, and tissue heterogeneities encountered in treatment planning of real patients. Kernel-based models (also called *superposition/convolution methods*) directly compute the dose in a phantom or patient accounting for lateral transport of radiation, beam energy, geometry, beam modifiers, patient surface topography, and electron density distribution.

Most of the correction factor-based models discussed here rely mainly on "one-dimensional" effective pathlength approaches, some of which were developed before x-ray computed tomography. These models consider the effect of patient structure only along the ray joining the point of computation and the source of radiation and are limited in accuracy under some circumstances.

Tissue Inhomogeneity CF: Ratio of Tissue-Air Ratio Method

The ratio of TAR (RTAR) method of correction for inhomogeneities is given by:

$$CF = \frac{T(d_{eff}, S_d)}{T(d, S_d)}$$

where the numerator is the TAR for the equivalent water thickness, d_{eff}, and the denominator is the TAR for the actual thickness, d, of tissue between the point of calculation and the surface along a ray passing through the point. S_d is the dimension of the beam cross-section at the depth of calculation. The RTAR method accounts for the field size and depth of calculation. It does not account for the position of the point of calculation with respect to the heterogeneity. It also does not take into account the shape of the inhomogeneity; instead, it assumes that it extends the full width of the beam and has a constant thickness (i.e., a slab-type geometry).

Tissue Inhomogeneity CF: Isodose Shift Method

Isodose lines are shifted by an amount equal to a constant times the thickness of the inhomogeneity as measured along a line parallel to the central axis and passing through the calculation point. Values for the shift constant empirically determined for

[60]Co and 4-MV x-rays are −0.6 for air cavities, −0.4 for lung, +0.5 for hard bone, and +0.25 for spongy bone. The isodose curves are shifted away from the surface for lung and air cavities and toward the surface for bone.

Tissue Inhomogeneity CF: Power Law TAR Method

The *power law TAR method* was proposed by Batho (8) and generalized by Young and Gaylord (90). This method, sometimes called the *Batho method*, attempts to account for the nature of the inhomogeneity and its position relative to the point of calculation. However, it does not account for the extent or shape of the inhomogeneity. The correction factor for the point P is given by:

$$CF = \left(\frac{T(d_2, S_d)}{T(d_1, S_d)} \right)^{\rho_2 - 1}$$

where d_1 and d_2 refer to the distances from point P to the near and far side of the non–water-equivalent material, respectively; S_d is the beam dimension at the depth of P; and ρ_2 is the relative electron density of the inhomogeneity with respect to water.

Sontag and Cunningham (79) derived a more general form of this correction factor, which can be applied to a case in which the effective atomic number of the inhomogeneity is different from that of water and the point of interest lies within the inhomogeneity. The correction factor in this situation is given by:

$$CF = \frac{T(d_2, S_d)^{(\rho_b - 1)}}{T(d_1, S_d)^{(\rho_b - \rho_a)}} \times \frac{(\mu_{en}/\rho)_a}{(\mu_{en}/\rho)_b}$$

where ρ_a is the density of the material in which point P lies at a depth d below the surface and ρ_b is the density of an overlying material of thickness $(d_2 - d_1)$; $(\mu_{en}/\rho)_a$ and $(\mu_{en}/\rho)_b$ are the mass energy absorption coefficients for the medium a and b.

Convolution/Superposition Method for Accounting for Tissue Inhomogeneities

The convolution/superposition dose calculation algorithm is based on the following equation (6):

$$D(\vec{r}) = \iiiint T_E(\vec{s}) h(E, \vec{r} - \vec{s}) d^3s\, dE$$

where D represents the dose at some point $\vec{r}$, $T_E(\vec{s})$ represents the total energy released by primary photon interactions per unit mass (or TERMA), and $h(E, \vec{r} - \vec{s})$ is the *point-spread function* (also called *dose spread array*, *differential pencil beam*, and *energy deposition kernal*). The point-spread function represents the fraction of the energy deposited (per unit volume) at point $\vec{s}$ that is subsequently transported to the calculation point, $\vec{r}$. Hence, the dose at point $\vec{r}$ is computed by integrating over all space the contributions from photons and electrons produced at all other points in the phantom or patient.

Ahnesjö et al. (5) showed that the point-spread function, $h(E, \vec{r} - \vec{s})$, changes only slightly as a function of energy, and thus, can be replaced by $h(\vec{r} - \vec{s})$ (defined as the average point-spread function weighted by the spectral components of the beam), reducing the basic convolution four-dimensional integral to a three-dimensional integral over all space. Point-spread functions for monoenergetic photons are generally precomputed using Monte Carlo methods (5). The energy dependence of the TERMA, $T_E(\vec{s})$, can be expressed by applying the inverse-square law and exponential attenuation to the photon fluence at the surface of the phantom or patient.

The three-dimensional integral is typically evaluated in a two-step process. The first step takes into account the properties of the accelerator (including the finite source size, primary collimator, flattening filter, collimator jaws, MLCs and any beam-modifying devices used for the treatment, such as wedges, alloy blocks, and compensating filters) to compute the energy fluence at the phantom or patient surface. The second step of the calculation takes into account the inverse square law and exponential attenuation to this incident fluence to determine the TERMA, $T_E(\vec{s})$, at each point within the phantom or patient and convolve the result with the point-spread function, $h(\vec{r} - \vec{s})$.

The convolution equation is strictly valid only for homogeneous media (i.e., $h(\vec{s})$ must be spatially invariant). To account for the effects of tissue heterogeneities, all physical distances in the convolution integral are replaced with radiologic distances; that is, the physical distance multiplied by the average density along the line in question (5,61). Hence, the convolution/superposition algorithm accounts for the effects of heterogeneities anywhere in the vicinity of the calculation point in three dimensions. In contrast, most correction factor-based dose-calculation techniques require only a simple one-dimensional evaluation of radiologic path length, and can thus account for the effects of only those tissue heterogeneities that lie along a ray connecting the radiation source to the calculation point.

Several investigators have tested the convolution/superposition algorithm against measurements and Monte Carlo–generated data for complex phantom geometries including both homogeneous and heterogeneous phantoms and found that the convolution/superposition model gave accurate results, even in parts of the buildup region and penumbra (4,59).

Monte Carlo Method for Accounting for Tissue Inhomogeneities

Monte Carlo is, in principle, the only method capable of computing the dose distribution accurately for all situations encountered in radiation therapy, including being able to accurately predict the dose near interfaces of materials with very dissimilar atomic number, such as near metal prostheses, or different densities such as tumors in lung tissue (78). The Monte Carlo method uses the known cross-sections for electron and photon interactions in matter and follows individual photons and the associated electrons set in motion through the entire heterogeneous phantom or patient. By calculating the trajectories and interactions of a very large number of photon and electrons, one can accurately model the dose distribution. Recently, several Monte Carlo codes have been developed for radiotherapy treatment planning (13,25,74,87). The reader is referred to the review article by Siebers et al. (78) for more details on Monte Carlo calculation for external beam radiation therapy.

Correcting for Tissue Heterogeneities: Recommendations

In 2004, the American Association of Physicists in Medicine (AAPM) published Report 85 (Task Group 65) on tissue inhomogeneity corrections from megavoltage photon beams (2). The task group recommended an accuracy goal for tissue heterogeneity corrections of 2% in order to achieve an overall 3% accuracy in dose delivery. The AAPM report recommended heterogeneity corrections be applied to plans and prescriptions, with the condition that the algorithm used for calculations be reviewed and rigorously tested by medical physicists. A brief summary of the site specific recommendations is presented here (2). For the head and neck region, a one-dimensional path correction algorithm for point-dose estimations beyond mandible and ear cavities was thought to be reasonable. However, for soft tissue regions and volumes that are adjacent to these heterogeneities, superposition/convolution or Monte Carlo algorithms should be used. For the larynx, specifically, if the target volume was adjacent to the air cavity or severe case of disease in the anterior commissure, then the superposition/convolution or

Monte Carlo algorithms should be used. For treatment of lung cancer, for interest points well beyond the lung interface, one-dimensional path corrections were thought to be reasonable. However, accounting for doses at tumor lung interfaces, the superposition/convolution or Monte Carlo algorithms should be used. Also, the report recommended that photon energies of 12 MV or less should be used for treatment of lung cancer in order to minimize nonequilibrium conditions that exist with higher energies. For breast cancer treatment (particularly if the dose of interest of the target volume is considered to be chest wall), it is recommended that calculations be performed with superposition/convolution or Monte Carlo. However, for simple intact breast planning, one-dimensional algorithms are adequate. For the upper gastrointestinal tract, one-dimensional corrections were adequate. However, one should be leery of barium contrast used that can erroneously call for increased dose due to interpretation of the high atomic number material. In terms of the pelvis and prostate, one-dimensional corrections were quite reasonable except in the presence of high-Z implanted hip prosthesis. (Note: The dosimetric considerations for patients with hip prosthesis undergoing pelvic irradiation are discussed in a latter section). The study by Frank et al. (28) provides a clear method for safely transitioning clinical use from one based on planning that assumes a homogeneous unit-density patient, to one using a heterogeneous patient model.

Clinical Photon Beam Dosimetry

Percent Depth Dose and Single-Field Isodose Charts

As explained in Chapter 5, the central-axis PDD expresses the penetrability of a radiation beam. Table 6.1 summarizes beam characteristics for x-ray and γ-ray beams typically used in radiation therapy and lists the depth at which the dose is maximum (100%) and the 10-cm depth PDD value. Representative PDD curves are shown in Figure 6.4 for conventional SSDs. As a rule of thumb, an 18-MV, 6-MV, and ^{60}Co photon beam loses approximately 2%, 3.5%, and 4.5% per centimeter, respectively, beyond the depth of maximum dose, d_{max} (values are for a 10×10 cm field, 100-cm SSD). There is no agreement as to what is the single optimal x-ray beam energy; instead, institutional bias or radiation oncologist training typically influences its selection, and it is usually treatment site specific. As pointed out in Chapter 5, most modern linacs are multimodality, and provide a range of photon and electron beam energies ranging from 4 to 25 MV, with 6- and 15 or 18-MV x-ray beams the most common.

Isodose charts as discussed in Chapter 5 provide much more information about the radiation beam characteristics than do central axis PDD data alone. However, even isodose charts are limited in that they represent the dose distribution in only one plane (typically the one containing the beam's central axis) and are usually available only for square or rectangular fields. Isodose charts are usually measured in a water phantom with the radiation beam directed perpendicular to the phantom's flat surface. Isodose curves show the relative uniformity of the beams across the field at various depths, and also provide a graphical depiction of the width of the beam's penumbra region. ^{60}Co teletherapy units exhibit a relatively large penumbra, and their isodose distributions are more rounded than those from linac x-ray beams. This is due to the relatively large source size (typically 1 to 2 cm in diameter vs. only a few millimeters for linacs). Linac beam penumbra width does increase slightly as a function of energy and if unfocused MLC leaves are used, but is still much less than that for ^{60}Co units. In addition to the smaller penumbra, linac x-ray isodose distributions have relatively flat isodose curves at depth. However, at shallow

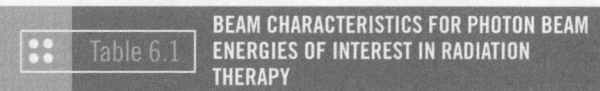

Table 6.1	**BEAM CHARACTERISTICS FOR PHOTON BEAM ENERGIES OF INTEREST IN RADIATION THERAPY**

200 kVp, 2-mm Cu HVL, SSD = 50 cm

- Depth of maximum dose = surface
- Rapid fall-off with depth due to (a) low energy and (b) short SSD
- Sharp beam edge due to small focal spot
- Significant dose outside beam boundaries due to Compton scattered radiation at low energies

^{60}CO, SSD = 80 cm

- Depth of maximum dose = 0.5 cm
- Increased penetration (10 cm PDD = 55%)
- Beam edge not as well defined—penumbra due to source size
- Dose outside beam low because most scattering is in forward direction
- Isodose curvature increases as the field size increases

4-MV x-ray, SSD = 80 cm

- Depth of maximum dose = 1 to 1.2 cm
- Penetration slightly greater than cobalt (10 cm PDD = 61%)
- Penumbra smaller
- "Horns" (beam intensity off-axis) due to flattening filter design ≈14%

6-MV x-ray, SSD = 100 cm

- Depth of maximum dose = 1.5 cm
- Slightly more penetration than ^{60}Co and 4 MV (10 cm PDD = 67%)
- Small penumbra
- Horns (beam intensity off-axis) due to flattening filter design ≈9%

18-MV x-ray, SSD = 100 cm

- Depth of maximum dose = 3—3.5 cm
- Much greater penetration (10 cm PDD = 80%)
- Small penumbra
- Horns (beam intensity off-axis) due to flattening filter design ≈5%
- Exit dose often higher than entrance dose

HVL, half-value layer; SSD, source-to-skin distance; PDD, percentage depth dose.

depths, particularly at d_{max}, linac x-ray beams typically exhibit an increase in beam intensity away from the central axis; this beam characteristic is referred to as the dose profile *horns* and depends on flattening filter design. In general, each treatment unit has unique radiation beam characteristics, and thus, isodose distributions must be measured, or at least verified, for each specific unit.

Another important point to understand is how the radiation field size is defined. The radiation field size dimensions refer to

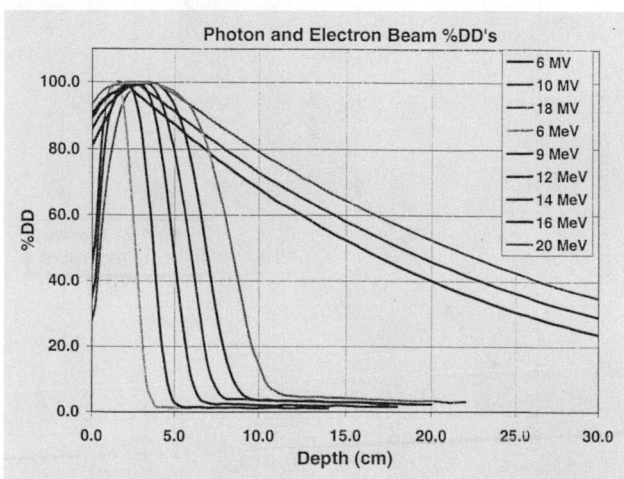

FIGURE 6.4. Typical x-ray or photon beam central-axis percentage depth dose (DD) curves for a 10×10 cm beam for megavoltage x-ray beams ranging from ^{60}Co to 18-MV x-rays and 6- to 20-MeV electron beams.

Overview and Basic Science of Radiation Oncology

Table 6.2	BUILD-UP REGION RELATIVE DEPTH DOSE FOR 6, 10, 18 MV X-RAY BEAMS								
Depth (cm)	6 MV, 5 × 5 cm[a]	10 MV, 5 × 5 cm	18 MV, 5 × 5 cm	6 MV, 15 × 15 cm	10 MV, 15 × 15 cm	18 MV, 15 × 15 cm	6 MV, 25 × 25 cm	10 MV, 25 × 25 cm	18 MV, 25 × 25 cm
0.0000	0.0561	0.0416	0.0509	0.1713	0.1587	0.1994	0.2779	0.2640	0.3193
0.0127	0.1329	0.0883	0.0803	0.2413	0.2080	0.2324	0.3422	0.3120	0.3523
0.0254	0.1854	0.1238	0.1036	0.2912	0.2444	0.2564	0.3883	0.3477	0.3766
0.0508	0.2714	0.1875	0.1442	0.3717	0.3063	0.2982	0.4635	0.4078	0.4188
0.1000	0.3473	0.2434	0.1796	0.4413	0.3608	0.3336	0.5270	0.4583	0.4518
0.2000	0.5160	0.3841	0.2784	0.5970	0.4943	0.4295	0.6694	0.5819	0.5431
0.5000	0.8050	0.6713	0.5152	0.8533	0.7567	0.6489	0.8912	0.8150	0.7411
1.0000	0.9614	0.8790	0.7376	0.9776	0.9295	0.8331	0.9892	0.9557	0.8957
1.5000	1.0000	0.9718	0.8730	1.0000	0.9957	0.9345	1.0000	1.0068	0.9680
2.0000		0.9958	0.9410		1.0032	0.9745		0.9901	0.9908
2.5000		1.0000	0.9786		1.0000	0.9927		1.0000	0.9996
3.0000			1.0000			1.0000			1.0000

[a]Field size

the distance perpendicular to the beam's direction of incidence that corresponds to the 50% isodose at the beam's edge. It is defined at the skin surface for SSD treatments, and at the axis depth for *source-to-axis distances* (SADs) for isocentric treatments. The linac's light field is typically set using this definition (radiation–light field agreement tolerance is typically ± mm).

Depth-Dose Buildup Region

When a photon beam strikes the tissue surface, electrons are set in motion, causing the dose to increase with depth until the maximum dose is achieved at depth d_{max}. Table 6.2 lists the buildup of dose as a function of depth beneath the entry surface for common photon energies. As the energy of the photon beam increases, the depth of the buildup region is increased. The subcutaneous tissue-sparing effects of higher-energy x-rays, combined with their great penetrability, make them well suited for treating deep lesions. For specific x-ray energy, the magnitude of the skin dose generally increases with increasing field size and with the insertion of plastic blocking trays in the beam (Fig. 6.5) (71,86). The blocking trays should be at least

20 cm above the skin surface because skin doses are significantly increased for lesser distances. Copper, lead, or lead glass filters beneath plastic trays can be used to remove the undesired lower-energy electrons that contribute to skin dose, but this is rarely done routinely in the clinic (71).

As the angle of the incident radiation beam becomes more oblique, the surface dose increases, and d_{max} moves toward the surface (Fig. 6.6). This is due to more secondary electrons being ejected along the oblique path of the beam (31).

Depth Dose/Exit Dose Region

The skin and superficial tissue on the side of the patient from which the beam exits receive a reduced dose if there is insufficient backscatter material present. The amount of dose reduction is a function of x-ray beam energy, field size, and the thickness of tissue that the beam has penetrated reaching the exit surface. For a 6-MV beam, Purdy (71) measured a 15% reduction in dose with little dependency on field size. This work was repeated for 18-MV beams by Klein and Purdy (52), who reported an 11% reduction in exit dose. In general, the addition of a thickness of tissue-equivalent material on the exit side equivalent in thickness to approximately two-thirds of the d_{max} depth is sufficient to provide full dose to the build-down region on the exit side. Figure 6.7 shows the effects of various backscattering media when placed directly behind the exit surface.

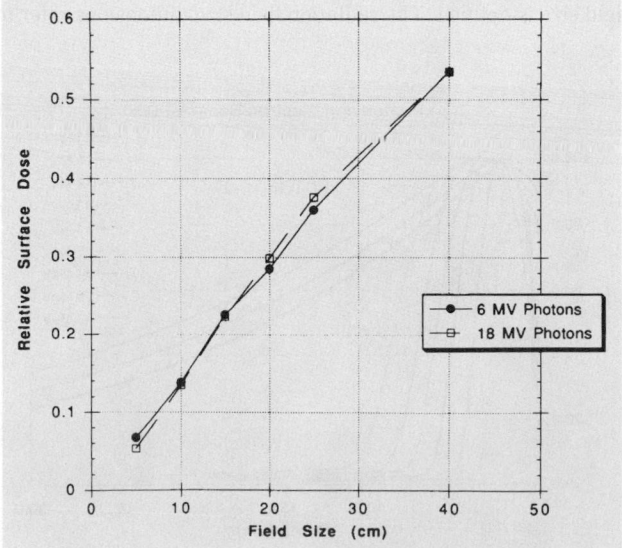

FIGURE 6.5. Relative surface dose versus field size with blocking tray in place for 6- and 18-MV photons. (From Klein EE, Purdy JA. Entrance and exit dose regions for Clinac-2100C. *Int J Radiat Oncol Biol Phys* 1993;27:429–435, with permission.)

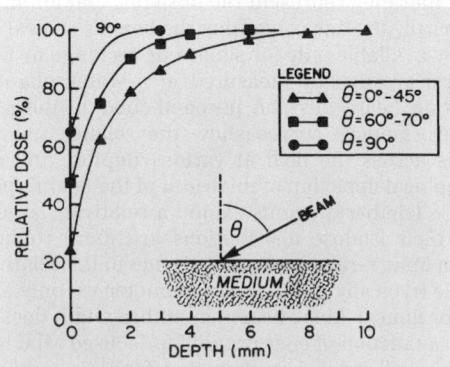

FIGURE 6.6. The variation of surface dose and depth of maximum dose as a function of the angle of incidence of the x-ray beam with the surface (4 MV, 10 × 10 cm).

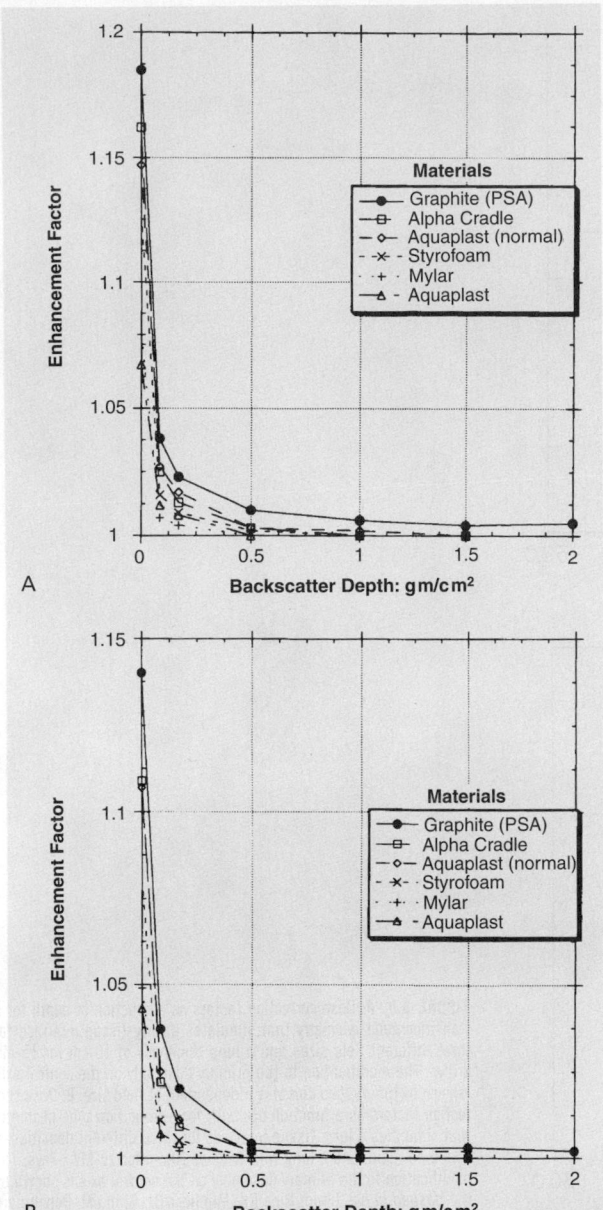

FIGURE 6.7. Enhancement of exit dose for **(A)** 6-MV and **(B)** 18-MV photons for a 15 × 15 cm field at 100 cm source-to-axis distance versus backscatter depth for various backscattering materials. (From Klein EE, Purdy JA. Entrance and exit dose regions for Clinac-2100C. *Int J Radiat Oncol Biol Phys* 1993;27:429–435, with permission.)

Tissue Interface Dosimetry

The dose distribution in the patient in transition zones (interfaces of different media) depends on radiation field size (scatter influence), distance between interfaces (e.g., air cavities), differences between physical densities and atomic number of the interfacing media, and the size and shape of the different media. Interface dose measurements usually are done with parallel-plate ionization chambers. Corrections should be used to account for plate separation, energy (ionization ratio), and guard width (30,86). Thermoluminescent dosimeters and film also have been used for transition zone measurements, but the problems associated with thickness and atomic number (respectively) and the associated QA needed make measurements with these dosimeters more laborious, and the results typically have a greater uncertainty. Several benchmark mea-

surements have been reported for various geometries simulating clinical situations and are discussed briefly in the following sections.

Air Cavities

Epp et al. (22) performed measurements with a parallel-plate ionization chamber for ^{60}Co beams that showed significant losses of ionization on the central axis after traversing air cavities of varying dimensions. The losses, which were due to lack of forward-scattered electrons, were approximately 12% for a typical larynxlike air cavity, but recovered within 5 mm in the new buildup region. Epp et al. (21) reported a 14.5% loss at the distal interface for 10-MV photons with a buildup curve that plateaued within 20 mm behind the interface.

Lung Interfaces

Although the problem of reestablishing equilibrium for lung interfaces is not as severe as with air cavities, a transition zone region at the lung–tissue interface still exists over the range of typical clinical photon beam energies. Rice et al. (75) measured responses in various simulated lung media using a parallel-plate chamber and phantom constructed of simulated lung material (average lung material density, $\rho = 0.31$ g/cm^3). They measured correction factors with a 10-cm layer of lung material versus water and observed minor differences at the interface compared with regions beyond the lung and a small dependence on field size (7% for 4 MV) (Fig. 6.8A). A considerable buildup curve was observed (10% change in correction factor) for a 5×5 cm field for the 15-MV beam, which began in the distal region of the lung and plateaued beyond the lung (Fig. 6.8B). Klein et al. (51) measured the effects of nonequilibrium for tissue-equivalent volumes in lung media and found significant underdosage, especially for small volumes and high-energy beams.

Bone Interfaces

Das et al. (14,15) measured dose perturbation factors (DPFs) proximal and distal for simulated bone–tissue interface regions using a parallel-plate chamber for both 6- and 24-MV x-ray beams. They reported DPFs of 1.1 for the 6-MV beam and 1.07 for the 24-MV beam at the proximal interface. A 7% enhancement (build-down) was measured for the 24-MV beam at the distal interface, whereas the 6-MV beam exhibited a new buildup region distally with a DPF of 0.95 at the interface. Buildup or build-down regions dissipate within a few millimeters and the perturbations are independent of thickness and lateral extent of the bone or radiation field size.

Prostheses (Steel and Silicone)

Das et al. (14) measured forward dose perturbation factors following a 10.5-mm-thick stainless steel layer simulating a hip prosthesis geometry. They measured an enhancement of 19% for 24-MV photons, but only 3% for 6-MV photons. They also measured backscatter dose perturbation factors for various energies for many high-Z materials, including steel, and reported an enhancement of 30% for steel due to backscattered electrons independent of energy, field size, or lateral extent of the steel. These interface effects dissipated within a few millimeters in polystyrene.

The most complete information currently available on hip prosthesis dosimetry is found in AAPM Report 81 (72). The report points out that the complete understanding and method of clinical dosimetry for these situations is still incomplete, but is intended to reflect the current state of scientific understanding and technical methods in clinical dosimetry for radiation

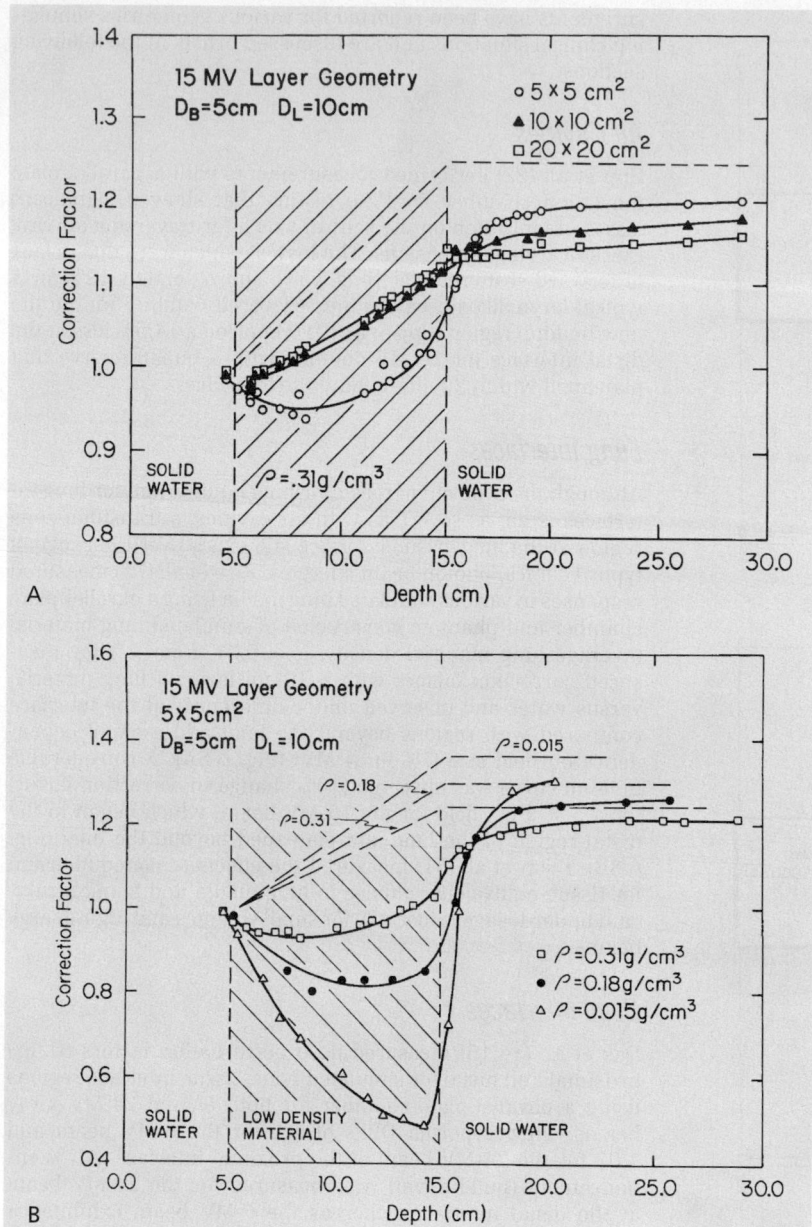

FIGURE 6.8. A: Dose correction factors as a function of depth for a transition zone geometry that simulates a lung-tissue interface for three different field sizes and a lung thickness of 10 cm for 15-MV x-rays. The modification to the primary dose only on the central axis (shown by the *dashed curve*) is independent of field size. **B:** Dose correction factors as a function of depth for a transition zone geometry that simulates a lung-tissue interface for three different densities, a 5 × 5 cm field, and a lung thickness of 10 cm for 15-MV x-rays. The modification to the primary dose only on the central axis is shown by the *dashed curve.* (From Rice RK, Mijnheer BJ, Chin LM. Benchmark measurements for lung dose corrections for x-ray beams. *Int J Radiat Oncol Biol Phys* 1988;15:399–409, with permission.)

oncology patients with high-Z hip prostheses. Beam arrangements that avoid the prosthesis should always be a first consideration. If this cannot be done, valuable information is available in Report 81, including values for different prostheses electron density, approximate attenuation of the beam passing through the prosthesis, and possible dose increase to the hip bone (72). An isodose distribution should be generated using the treatment planning system's most physically rigorous dose-calculation algorithm using the appropriate electron density for the prothesis. During the first fraction, exit dose measurements (with diodes, films, or thermoluminescent dosimeters) should be performed to confirm (and, if necessary), modify the treatment-planning calculations and input characteristics. It should also be noted that some of the data and recommendations are also applicable to patients having other implanted high-Z prosthetic devices such as pins and humeral head replacements.

Klein and Kuske (48) reported on interface perturbations around silicone breast prostheses. Such prostheses have a density similar to breast tissue but have a different atomic number.

They observed a 6% enhancement at the proximal interface and a 9% loss at the distal interface.

Wedge Filter Dosimetry

When a wedge filter is inserted into the beam, the dose distribution is angled at some specified depth to some desired angle relative to the incident beam direction over the entire transverse dimension of the radiation beam (Fig. 6.9). For cobalt units, the depth of the 50% isodose usually is selected for specification of the wedge angle, whereas for high-energy linacs, higher-percentile isodose curves, such as the 80% curve, or the isodose curves at a specific depth (10 cm), are used to define the wedge angle.

Cobalt unit wedges are typically designed for specific field sizes (nonuniversal wedges) to keep the dose rate of the unit within a useful clinical range. Linacs are typically equipped with multiple wedges (*universal wedges*) that may be used with an allowed range of field sizes. Although linac wedges can be

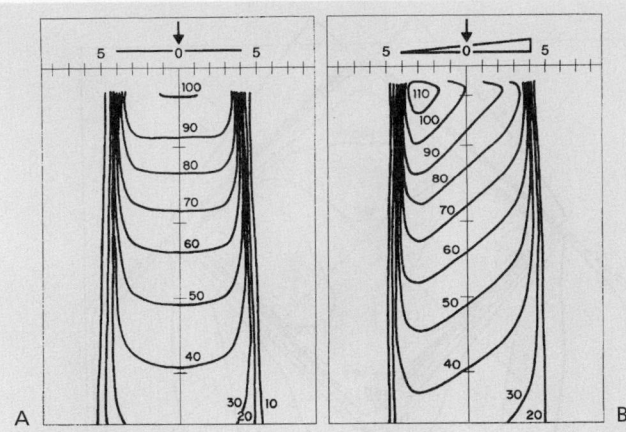

FIGURE 6.9. Isodose distributions for a 6-MV x-ray beam with an 8 × 8 cm field size. **A:** Open field. **B:** Field with a 45-degree wedge. (From Khan FM. *The physics of radiation therapy*, 2nd ed. Baltimore: Williams & Wilkins, 1994, with permission.)

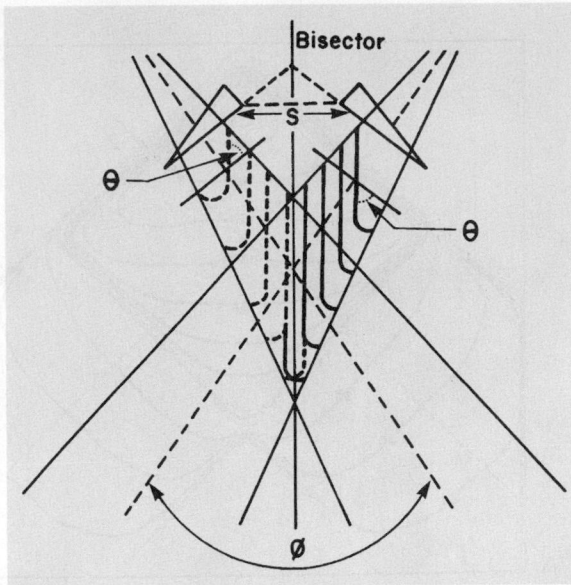

FIGURE 6.10. Parameters of the wedge beams: ϕ is the wedge angle, θ is the hinge angle, and S is separation. Isodose curves for each wedge field are parallel to the bisector. (From Khan FM. *The physics of radiation therapy*, 2nd ed. Baltimore: Williams & Wilkins, 1994, with permission.)

designed for any desired *wedge angle*, 15-, 30-, 45-, and 60-degree wedges are the most common.

Some linacs (Elekta AB, Sweden) feature a single wedge, referred to as a *motorized wedge*, located in the treatment head, and the desired wedged dose distribution is obtained by the proper combination of wedged and unwedged treatment. A simple approximate model for combining open and wedged fields was first proposed by Tatcher (83), in which the effective wedge angle θ_E, resulting by the addition of a wedged and unwedged beam, is equal to the nominal wedge angel θ_W for wedged beam, weighted by the fraction of wedged field, B:

$$B = \theta_E/\theta_W$$

The Philips Medical Systems Division (1) proposed a slightly different method as follows:

$$B = tan(\theta_E)/tan(\theta_W)$$

Petti and Siddon (69) investigated both methods and showed that these are approximations to an exact theoretical solution which is given by:

$$B = f/([tan(\theta_W)/tan(\theta_E)] + f - 1)$$

Most importantly, their investigations showed that Tatcher's approximation is good only for values of θ_W less than 45 degrees, and thus is inadequate for accelerators such as Elekta, which use a 60-degree motorized wedge. They did show that for the field sizes studied (up to 20 × 20 cm), the Philips relationship was valid to within 3 degrees.

The wedged isodose curves can be normalized in two different ways. In some older systems, the wedge dose distributions have the wedge factor (i.e., the ratio of the measured central axis dose rate with and without the wedge in place) incorporated into the wedged isodose distribution. More commonly, the wedge isodose curves are normalized to 100% at d_{max}, and a separate *wedge factor* is used to calculate the actual treatment MUs or time. McCullough et al. (63) noted that wedge factors measured at d_{max} usually are accurate to within 2% for depths up to 10 cm, but at greater depths can be inaccurate to 5% or more. The inclusion (or noninclusion) of the wedge factor is an extremely important point to understand because serious error in dose delivered to the patient can occur if used improperly.

Sewchand et al. (76) and Abrath and Purdy (3) pointed out that beam hardening results when a wedge is inserted into the radiation beam. The PDD, therefore, can be considerably increased at depth. Differences reported were nearly 7% for a 4-MV 60-degree wedge field PDD from the open field PDDs at

12-cm depth, and 3% difference in depth-dose values between the wedge field and the open field for a 60-degree wedge using 25-MV x-rays.

Modern computer-controlled medical linacs now have software features that allow the user to create a wedge-shaped dose distribution by moving one collimator jaw across the field in conjunction with adjustment of the dose rate over the course of the daily single-field treatment (55). This technology provides superior dose distributions and eliminates the previously mentioned beam-hardening problem seen in physical wedges. This feature can deliver a greater number of wedge angles, and over larger field sizes, including asymmetric field sizes (30 cm in the wedge direction, with 20 cm toward the wedge "heel," and 10 cm toward the wedge "toe"). The increased number of angles enhances planning options but also complicates commissioning and QA (49,50).

When the patient's treatment is planned, wedged fields are commonly arranged such that the angle between the beams, the *hinge angle (θ)*, is related to the wedge angle (ϕ) by the following relationship (Fig. 6.10):

$$\theta = 90 \, degrees - \phi/2$$

For example, as shown in Figure 6.11, 45-degree wedge fields orthogonal to one another yield a uniform dose distribution.

Treatment Planning: Combination of Treatment Fields

Parallel-Opposed Fields

When only two unmodified x-ray beams are used in radiation therapy, they usually are parallel-opposed beams (i.e., directed toward each other from opposite sides of the anatomic site with the central axes coinciding). Figure 6.12 presents the normalized relative axis dose profiles from parallel-opposed photon beams for a 10 × 10 cm field at an SSD of 100 cm and for patient diameters of 15 to 30 cm in 5-cm increments. The weight of a beam denotes a numeric value assigned to the beam at some normalization point. For SSD beams, the weight specifies

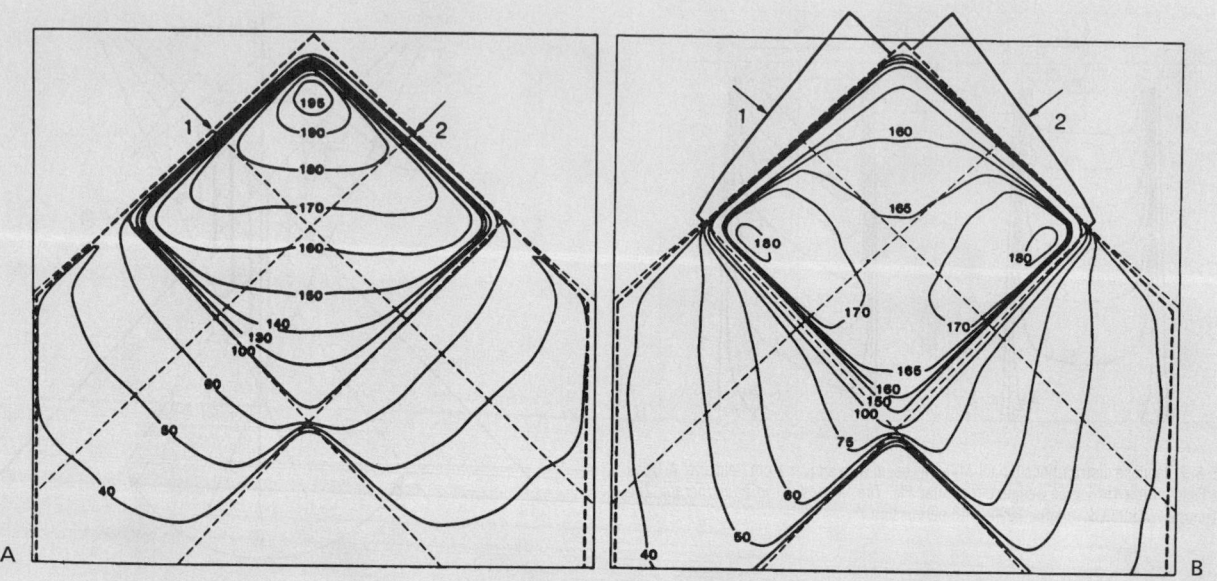

FIGURE 6.11. Isodose distribution for two angled beams. **A:** Without wedges. **B:** With wedges. Both: 4-MV; field size, 10 × 10 cm; source-to-skin distance, 100 cm; wedge angle, 45 degrees. (From Khan FM. *The physics of radiation therapy*, 2nd ed. Baltimore: Williams & Wilkins, 1994, with permission.)

the relative dose assigned to the beam at d_{max}, and for isocentric beams, at isocenter. The beams shown are weighted 1 to 1 (i.e., assigned equal value 100% at d_{max}), and the dose profiles have been normalized to the cumulative midline PDD.

The maximum patient diameter easily treated with parallel-opposed beams for a midplane tumor requiring 50 Gy or less with low-energy megavoltage beams is approximately 18 cm. For "thicker" patients, higher x-ray energies produce improved dose profiles with less dose variation along the central axis without resorting to more complex multibeam arrangements.

For some treatment sites, the underdosing achieved near the skin surface with very–high-energy, parallel-opposed x-ray beams is a highly advantageous feature, but in others it may be desirable to achieve a higher dose nearer to the skin. With very–high-energy x-ray beams traversing small anatomic thicknesses, the exit dose can exceed the entry dose, and the exact dose distribution in the regions beneath the entry and exit surfaces from parallel-opposed high-energy x-ray beams must be carefully evaluated to consider properly the contribution from both entrance and exit components.

Unequal beam weightings are advantageous if the target volume is not midline. Figure 6.13 shows normalized central-axis dose profiles for other weightings, such as 2 to 1 and 3 to 1. The greater the unequal weighting, the greater will be the shift of the higher-dose region toward one surface and away from midline. Although in some anatomic sites unequal weighting may be advantageous, special attention must be directed to the anatomic structures in the high-dose volume.

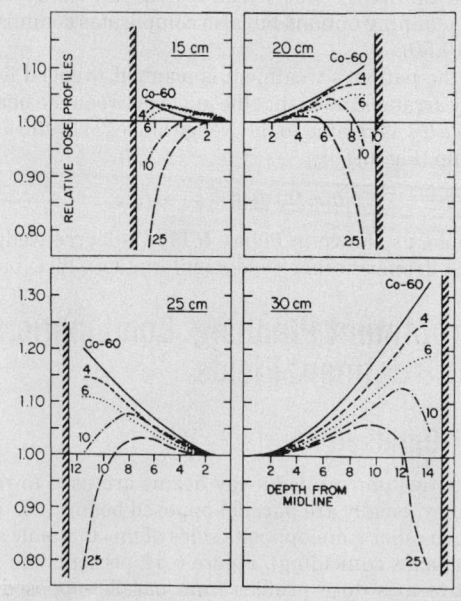

FIGURE 6.12. Relative central-axis dose profiles as a function of x-ray energy (^{60}Co or 4, 6, 10, and 25 MV) and patient thickness (15, 20, 25, and 30 cm). The parallel-opposed beams are equally weighted, and the profiles are normalized to unity at midline. Because of symmetry, only half of each profile is shown.

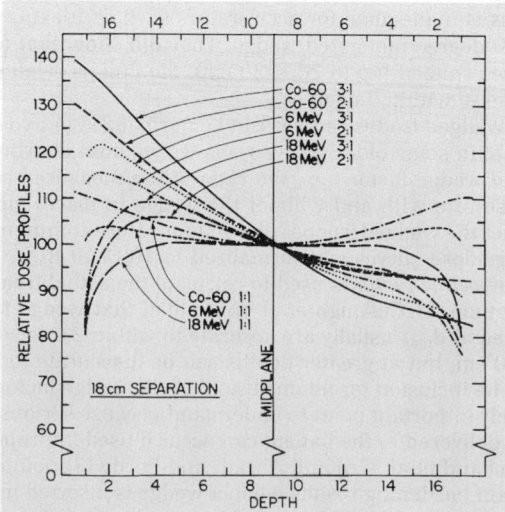

FIGURE 6.13. Dose profiles achieved with unequal weightings of parallel-opposed photon beams; profiles are normalized to unity at midline.

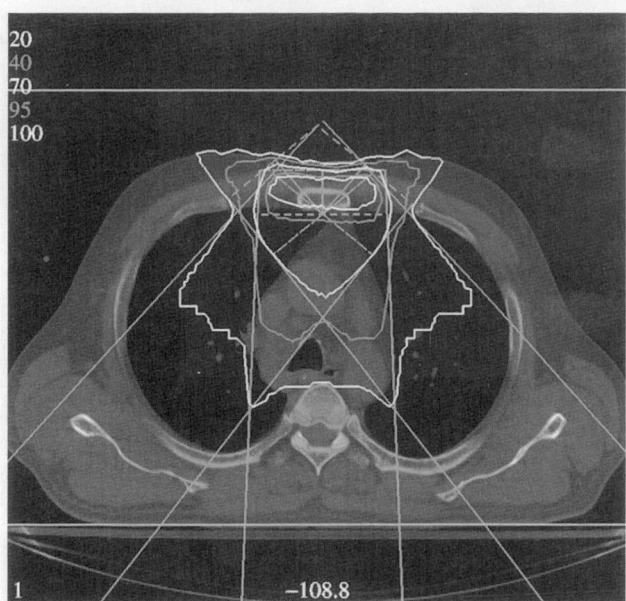
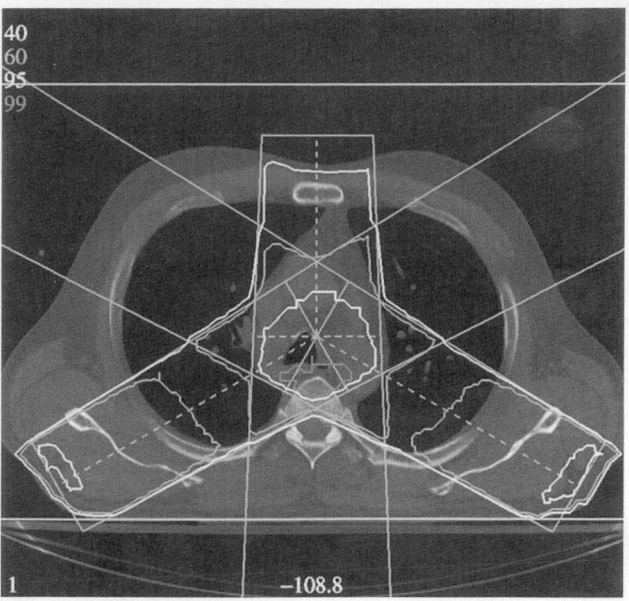

FIGURE 6.14. Three-field coaxial beam arrangements: Dose distribution for two different beam arrangements using 6-MV x-ray beams, 8 × 10 cm field size, 100-cm source-to-skin distance. Isodose curves have been renormalized to show the 100% line almost encompassing the target volume. **A:** Anterior field with two anterior oblique fields at 40 degrees off the midline, all equally weighted. **B:** Anterior field with a weight of 0.8 with two equally weighted (1) posterior oblique fields separated by 120 degrees.

Multiple-Beam Arrangements

Figure 6.14 shows three commonly used coaxial three-field beam arrangements. A direct anterior field with two anterior oblique fields can be used to generate a high-dose region where the three fields overlap, whereas a low-dose region exists beyond this intersection point. For example, if this arrangement is used for treating the mediastinum, the spinal cord might be included in the anterior beam but spared by the anterior oblique beams. Moving the anterior oblique fields laterally to form a parallel-opposed pair yields a rectangular isodose region with a more uniform dose gradient; however, the magnitude of the dose gradient is determined by the relative weighting of the beams and the thickness of tissue traversed. An anterior field with two symmetrically placed posterior oblique beams yields elongated isodose curves. The degree of elongation is determined by the relative thickness of tissue each beam traverses to the point of intersection and by the relative weights of the beams. Three-field arrangements are often useful for treating tumors lateral to the midline of a patient.

Three-field nonaxial (noncoplanar) arrangements are readily achieved with linacs by rotating the table and gantry. A common technique for treating pituitary tumors uses two lateral fields and a vertex field with the beam entering through the top the head. Astrocytomas often are treated with parallel-opposed lateral fields and a frontal field entering through the forehead. A 90-degree couch rotation is used with the gantry rotated laterally for the vertex or frontal fields. The lateral fields are also rotated by collimator to ensure the "heels" of the wedges are in the plane of the vertex/frontal field trajectory.

Four-field techniques typically are used in such sites as the abdomen or the pelvis. In most instances, the arrangements consist of pairs of parallel-opposed fields, with a common intersecting point, which yield a "boxlike" isodose distribution. Figure 6.15 compares the dose distributions achieved with a four-field "box-technique" for 6- and 18-MV x-ray beams. The central dose distribution is similar for all beam energies, but the greater penetrability of the higher-energy beams yields a lower dose to the region outside the box. Variations in the dose

gradient are achieved by differential weighting of each pair of beams. Figure 6.16 shows other possible four-beam arrangements. Angulation of the beams yields a diamond-shaped dose distribution. A butterfly-shaped distribution is achieved if each pair of beams has a point of intersection lying on a common line but separated by a few centimeters.

With the advent of *three-dimensional conformal radiation therapy* and *intensity-modulated radiation therapy* (IMRT), there has been an increase in multiple-field treatments such as the three-dimensional conformal radiation therapy six-field technique used for the treatment of prostate carcinoma (7), and the nine-field commonly used for head and neck cancer IMRT treatments (89).

Rotation Therapy

Rotational (or *arc*) *therapy* techniques, in which the treatment is delivered while the gantry (and thus the radiation beam) rotates around the patient, can be thought of as an infinite extension of the multiple-field techniques already described. This technique is most useful when applied to small, symmetric, deep-seated tumors, and usually is limited to field sizes less than approximately 10 cm in width for the treatment of centrally located lesions (i.e., there is approximately an equal amount of tissue in all directions around the lesion).

Dose distributions generated by rotational techniques are not very sensitive to the energy of the photon beam. Figure 6.17 illustrates this fact, showing the dose distribution achieved using a 6-MV x-ray beam, and also the distribution using an 18-MV x-ray beam. There is a little less elongation in the direction of the shorter dimension of the patient's anatomy for the 18-MV beam, and the dose distribution in the periphery is slightly lower.

In arc therapy techniques, one or more sectors of a 360-degree rotation are skipped to reduce the dose to critical normal structures. When a sector is skipped, the high-dose region is shifted away from the skipped region. Therefore, the isocenter must be moved toward the skipped sector; this technique is referred to as *past-pointing*. Examples are shown in Figure 6.18.

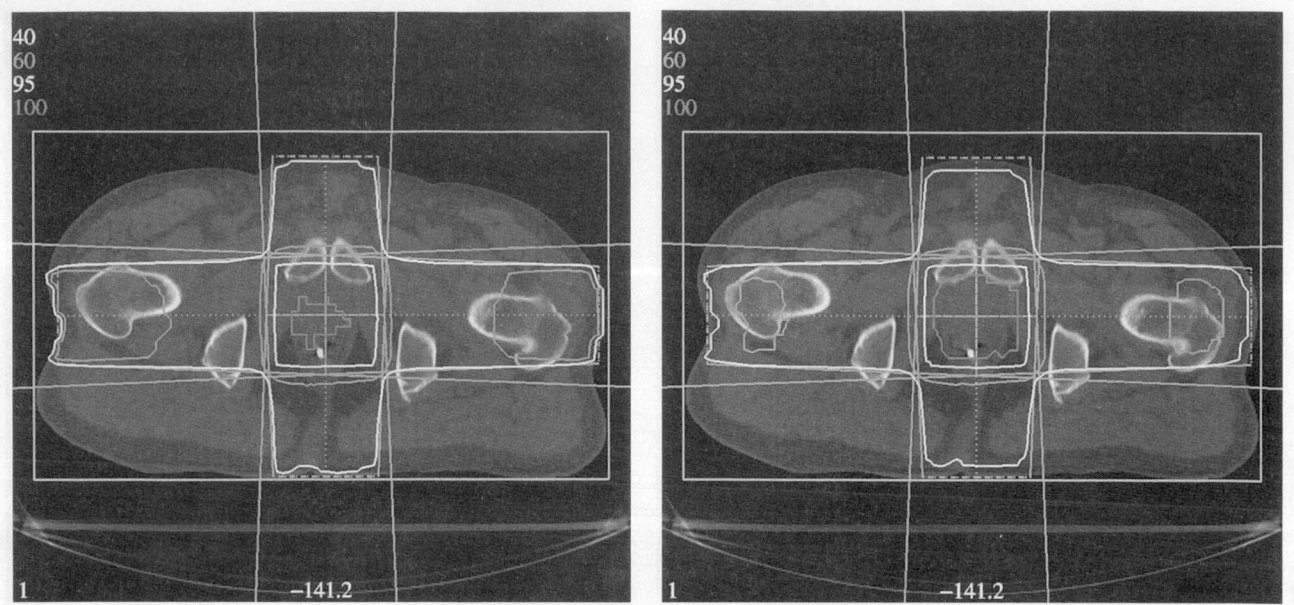

FIGURE 6.15. Four-field "box technique" coaxial beam arrangements (equal beam weightings): **A:** 6-MV x-ray beams. **B:** 18-MV x-ray beams. Note the improved dose distribution with the higher-energy beam technique (more uniform dose in the target region and lower doses near the femoral head region of the lateral fields) as a result of the increased percentage depth for 18-MV x-rays.

The prostate, bladder, cervix, and pituitary are clinical sites that have been treated, either initially or for boost doses, with rotational or arc therapy techniques. Although the dose distributions achieved by rotation or arc therapy yield high target-volume doses, these techniques normally result in a greater volume of normal tissue being irradiated (albeit at low doses) than fixed, multiple-field techniques. The advent of tomotherapy treatment machines, which use a rotational approach to deliver IMRT, has increased the awareness of the radiation oncology community on the effects on the dose distribution due to rotation (11,16).

Field Shaping

A major constraint in the treatment of cancer using radiation is the limitation in the dose that can be delivered to the tumor because of the dose tolerance of the critical normal tissues surrounding or near the target volume. Shielding of normal tissues has allowed the radiation oncologist to increase the dose to the tumor volume while maintaining the dose to critical organs below some tolerance level. The frequently used tolerance doses for these organs are not absolute, and larger doses are

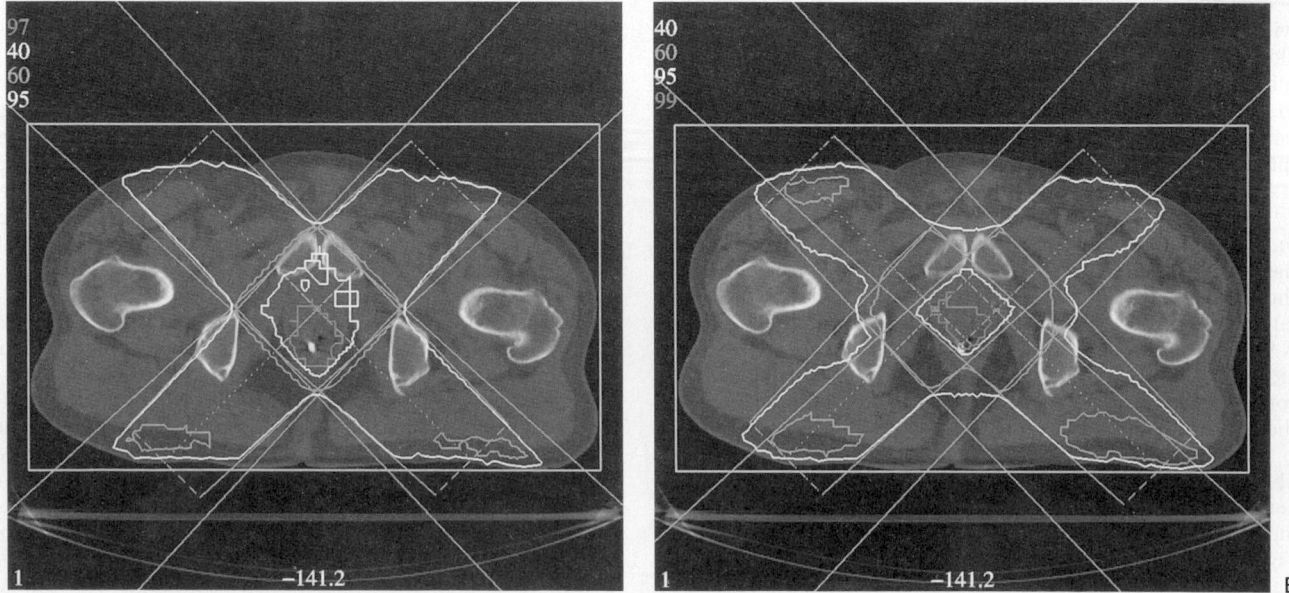

FIGURE 6.16. Four-field "oblique technique" coaxial beam arrangements (6-MV x-rays, equal beam weightings): **A:** With common isocenter resulting in a diamond-shaped dose distribution. **B:** Each beam pair intersecting at two different points on a common line resulting in a butterfly-shaped isodose distribution.

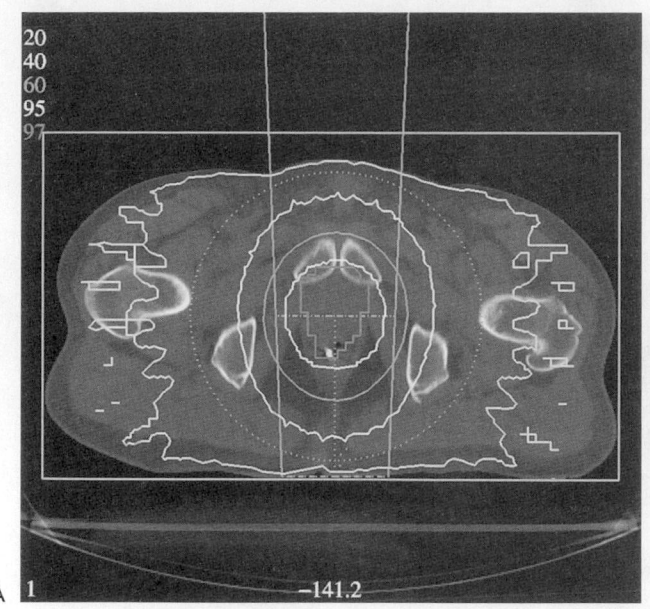 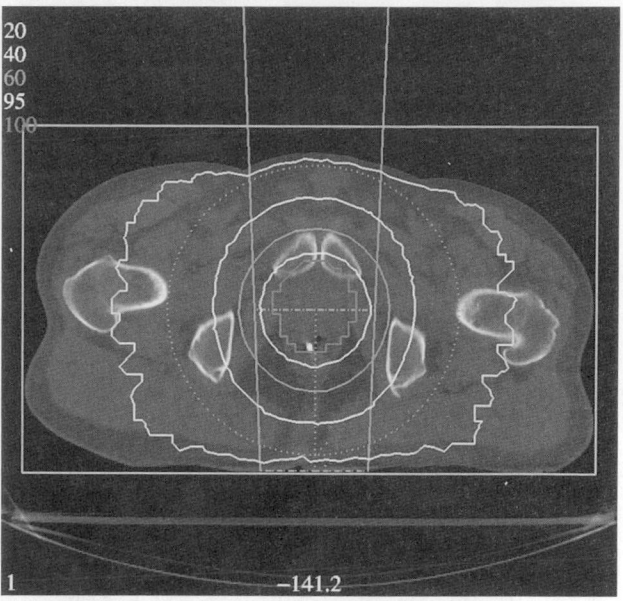

FIGURE 6.17. A 360-degree rotational therapy technique. **A:** 6-MV x-ray beams. **B:** 18-MV x-ray beams. Note that there is little difference in the dose distribution when using a higher-energy beam as a result of the offsetting effects of increased percentage depth versus higher exit dose.

sometimes given to fractional volumes of these organs (20). Shielding is usually accomplished using low–melting-point alloy blocks or MLCs, in which the beam aperture (field shape) is customized for individual patients.

Low-Melting Alloy Blocks

The Lipowitz metal (Cerrobend) shielding block system was introduced by Powers et al. (69). Lipowitz metal consists of 13.3% tin, 50% bismuth, 26.7% lead, and 10% cadmium. The physical density at 20°C is 9.4 g/cm³, compared with 11.3 g/cm³ for lead.

The block fabrication procedure is illustrated in Figure 6.19 and briefly described here. More details on using this form of field shaping can be found in the review article by Leavitt and Gibbs (54). A simulation radiograph is obtained with the patient in the treatment position and the central axis positioned approximately in the center of the treatment field to avoid excessively heavy blocks. The source-to-film distance is marked on the radiograph for future reference when fabricating the block. The desired treatment field aperture is drawn on the radiograph by the radiation oncologist. The marked radiograph is then placed on the illuminated surface of the hot-wire cutting device and aligned such that the central ray image coincides with the axis

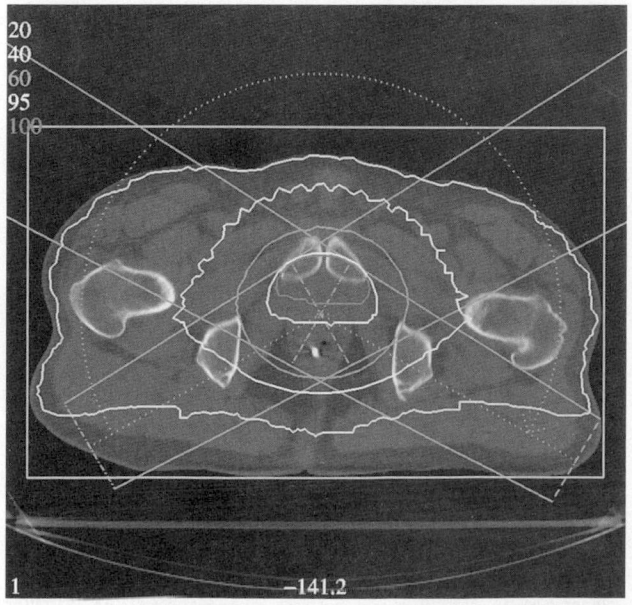 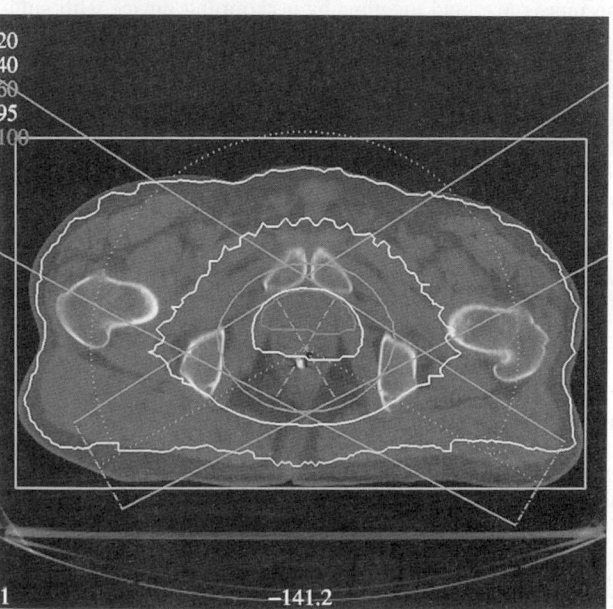

FIGURE 6.18. Arc therapy technique for 6-MV x-rays. **A:** 240-degree arc. Note that when a sector of the full 360-degree rotation is skipped, the high-dose isodose curves are shifted away from the skipped sector. **B:** 240-degree arc, but patient positioned so that isocenter is 2 cm lower toward the skipped sector (this technique is called *past-pointing*). Note high-dose isodose curves now encompass the target volume.

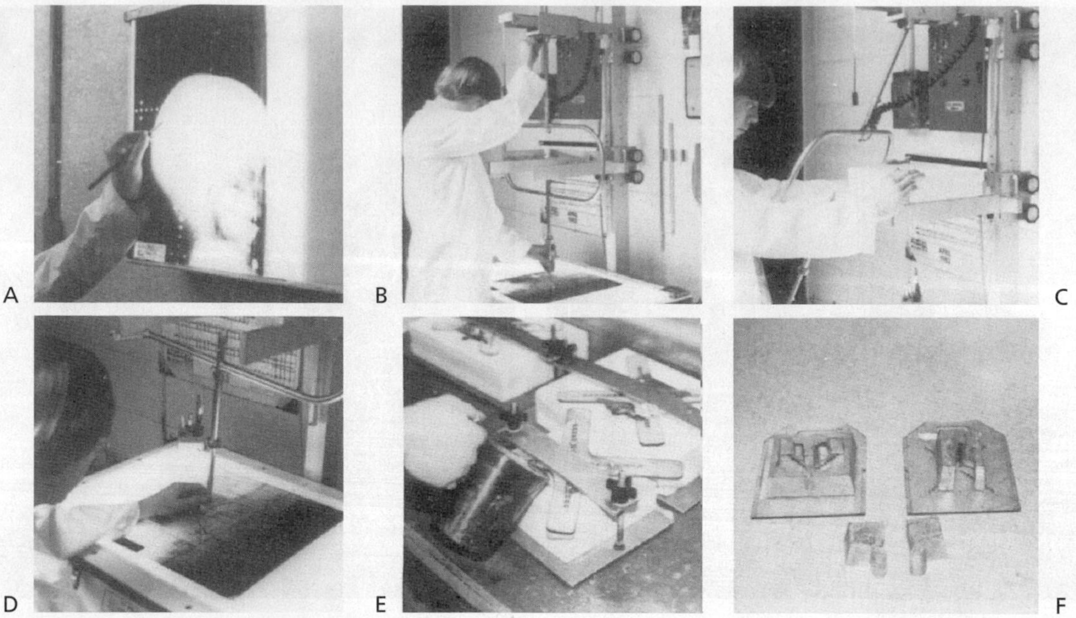

FIGURE 6.19. Composite photographs illustrating the low–melting-point alloy shielding block design and fabrication process. **A:** Physician defining the treatment volume on the x-ray simulator radiograph. **B:** Physics technician adjusting the source-to-skin distance and skin-to-film distance of a hot-wire cutter to emulate simulator geometry. **C:** Proper-thickness foam block aligned to the central axis of the cutter. **D:** Foam mold cut with hot-wire cutter. **E:** Foam pieces aligned and held in place using a special clamping device. Molten alloy is poured into the mold and allowed to harden. **F:** Examples of typical shielding blocks cast using this system. (From Purdy JA. Secondary field shaping. In: Wright AE, Boyer AL, eds. *Advances in radiation therapy treatment planning*. New York: American Institute of Physics, 1983, with permission.)

of the cutting device. The distance between the pivot point of the cutting arm and the film is adjusted to be equal to the simulation source-to-film distance. A foam block of appropriate size and thickness is placed on the hot-wire cutter's block holder and adjusted to the exact source-to-tray distance for the treatment unit. The foam mold is cut with the hot-wire stretched inside a C-arm stylus. The periphery of the treatment field is cut first, and then a rectangular outline slightly larger than the collimator jaw positions is cut. The inner piece of foam, corresponding to the beam aperture, and the outside piece of foam are placed on a flat metal holder and aligned with a plastic blocking tray. The pieces are held together by a clamping device with sufficient pressure to prevent leakage of the molten alloy. The total time required for a block to solidify typically is approximately 45 minutes, after which the pieces of foam mold are removed. The block should then be visually inspected for defects or voids. Rigorous QA checks should be performed to ensure that both the fabrication and the mounting of the block on the plastic tray have been correctly performed.

Alloy Block Dosimetry

Doses to critical organs may be limited by using either a full-thickness block, usually five HVLs (3.125% transmission) or six HVLs (1.562% transmission), or a partial transmission shield, such as a single HVL (50% transmission) of shielding material. The actual dose delivered under the shielded area is usually greater than these stated transmission levels because of scatter radiation beneath the blocks from adjacent unshielded portions of the field. The scatter component of the dose increases with depth as more radiation scatters into the shielded volume beneath the block. Thus, the dose to the blocked area is a function of block material, thickness (and width), field size, and energy. Figure 6.20 shows the attenuation of Lipowitz metal of x-rays produced at 2, 4, 10, and 18 MeV and ^{60}Co γ-rays (38). Alloy blocks made from the standard thickness (7.6 cm) of foam molds

reduce the primary beam intensity to 5% of its unattenuated value. Increasing the block thickness usually is not worthwhile because it makes the block heavier, whereas the scatter radiation contributes an equal or greater share of the dose under the blocks.

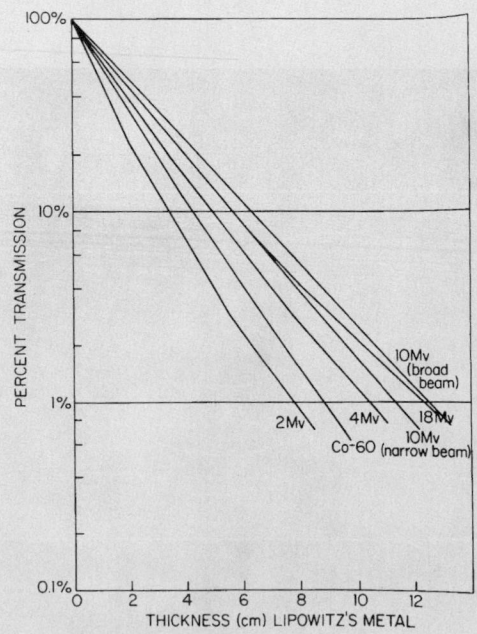

FIGURE 6.20. Attenuation in Lipowitz metal of x-rays produced at 2, 4, 10, and 18 MV and γ-rays from ^{60}Co. (From Huen A, Findley DO, Skov DD. Attenuation in Lipowitz's metal of x-rays produced at 2, 4, 10, and 18 MV and gamma rays from cobalt-60. *Med Phys* 1979;6:147, with permission.)

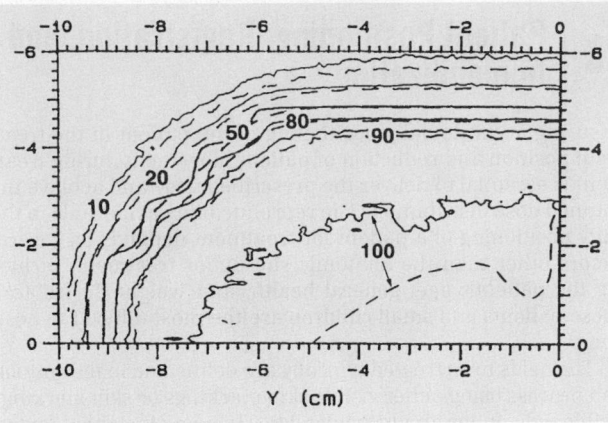

FIGURE 6.21. Comparison of beam's-eye-view isodose curves at 10-cm depth for multileaf collimator (*solid line*) and Cerrobend-shaped (*dashed line*) beam apertures for 18-MV photons. (From Klein EE, Harms WB, Low DA, et al. Clinical implementation of a commercial multileaf collimator: Dosimetry, networking, simulation, and quality assurance. *Int J Radiat Oncol Biol Phys* 1995;33:1195–1208, with permission.)

MLC and Associated Dosimetry

MLC, introduced first in Japan in the 1960s (82), has now gained widespread acceptance and has replaced alloy blocking as the standard of practice for field shaping in modern radiation therapy clinics. The different linac manufacturers' MLC systems vary with respect to field size coverage, leaf design, and MLC location. AAPM Report No. 72 provides a review of basic applications for MLCs (1). The reader is referred to this document for more details on the design configurations for the various commercial systems, MU calculations, accepting testing commissioning and safety, clinical applications, and QA.

Klein et al. (47) reported leaf transmission values of 1.5% to 2% for a Varian 6-MV beam (Varian Oncology Systems, Palo Alto, CA), and 1.5% to 5% for an 18-MV beam. Transmission through the screw attachment plane was 2.5%. These values are lower than those found for alloy blocks (3.5%), but higher than those for collimator jaw transmission (<1%). Transmission through abutted (closed) leaf pairs was as high as 28% for 18-MV photons on the central axis. The abutment transmission decreased as a function of off-axis distance to as low as 12%.

Figure 6.21 shows a comparison of MLC and alloy blocks regarding penumbra. The discrete steps of the MLC systems introduce undulations in the isodose lines. This effect causes an apparent increase in penumbra with wave patterns after the undulations. Some investigators describe this apparent penumbra increase as an "effective" penumbra accounting for the maximum and minimums of the undulations. Single, focused MLC systems have a slightly larger penumbra than do alloy shields and have an even larger difference compared with collimator jaws. Boyer et al. (10) found the penumbra (80% to 20%) generated by leaf ends to be wider than those generated by upper collimator jaws by 1 to 1.5 mm, and 1 to 2.5 mm compared with the lower jaws, depending on energy and field size. Powlis et al. (70) compared MLC and alloy field shaping and found few differences. LoSasso and Kutcher (59) found similar results and concluded that geometric accuracy is even improved with MLC.

The penumbras measured for the leaf sides are comparable with those found for upper jaws because of their divergent nature. The penumbra increase and stair-stepping effect are most prominent at d_{max}. The effects diminish at depth owing to the influence of scattered electrons and photons because the scatter-to-primary ratio increases with depth. Adding an opposed beam leads to further smoothing of the undulations, and penumbra differences become less significant. For multibeam arrangements, the differences in dose distribution between MLC and alloy shields are negligible.

Two methods for designing the optimal MLC configurations to fit the treatment plan's field apertures have evolved:

i. Configuring the MLC using a digitized film image using a dedicated MLC workstation (with or without automated optimization); and
ii. Configuring the MLC using treatment planning system software.

The main limitation in optimizing the MLC leaf settings to conform to the shaped field is the discrete leaf steps. Most field shapes require only minor adjustment of collimator angle to achieve minimal discrepancy between the desired and resultant field shape. The criteria for optimizing the MLC leaf settings are governed by placing the most leaf ends possible tangent to the field and also maintaining the same internal area as originally prescribed. MLC shaping systems typically provide an option to place the leaf ends entirely outside the field (exterior), entirely within the field (interior), or crossing the field at midleaf (leaf-center insertion). The last is the most widely used criterion because the desired field area is more closely maintained. However, this choice leads to regions in which some treatment areas are shielded and some normal tissues are irradiated. Zhu et al. (91) reported on a variable insertion technique in which leaves are placed only far enough into the field to cause the 50% isodose contour to undulate outside and up to the desired contour. LoSasso et al. (58) reported on a method in which each leaf is inserted such that the treatment area covered by the leaf equals the normal tissue area that is not spared. Du et al. (18) reported on a method that defines optimal leaf positioning in combination with optimal collimator angulation. Typically, the optimal direction for the leaf motion is along the narrower axis. For a simple ellipse, the optimal leaf direction is parallel to the short axis.

Klein et al. (47) showed that lunglike heterogeneities tended to increase MLC penumbra (especially for 18-MV photons), and bonelike heterogeneities tended to decrease MLC penumbra. However, when multibeam arrangements were used, the summed dose distribution consistently showed a superior dose distribution for the MLC fields, despite the stair-stepping effects, as opposed to alloy blocks.

Because MLC systems are still evolving, a careful evaluation of the effect of MLC on MU calculations and the resultant dose distributions over the range of field sizes and shapes to be used must be performed before actual clinical use.

Compensating Filters

The compensating filter, introduced by Ellis et al. (19), counteracts the effects caused by variations in patient surface curvature while still preserving the desirable skin-sparing feature of megavoltage photon beams. This is accomplished by placing the custom-designed compensating filter in the beam, sufficiently "upstream" from the patient's surface.

Several different compensator systems are in clinical use (73). They vary in complexity and technologic sophistication from the simple Ellis technique, using an array of stacked aluminum and brass blocks, to the latest imaged-based planning systems. Early methods required the patient's presence for long periods (typically 45 minutes) for acquisition of topographic surface data and actual fabrication of the compensator shape. New approaches separate these two operations and require the patient's presence for only a very brief time. The new methods use computerized milling units to construct the actual filter or filter mold. These systems require limited human interaction during the construction process and provide registration guides that improve filter alignment.

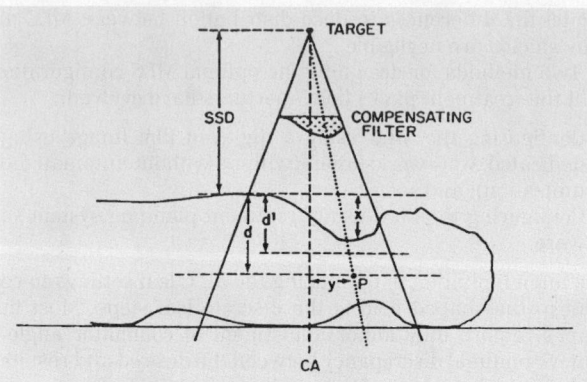

FIGURE 6.22. Schematic illustrating typical geometry used in the design of a compensator filter to account for patient's irregularly shaped surface. SSD, source-to-skin distance; CA, central axis.

A compensating filter system can be separated into several distinct subsystems, including a method to measure the missing tissue deficit, a means to demagnify patient topography, a method for constructing the compensating filter, a method of aligning and holding the filter in the beam, and a means of quality control inherent to it. Figure 6.22 shows a typical situation in which the principles of tissue compensation are illustrated. An air gap or tissue deficit, x, exists over point P. All points at depth d are to receive the same dose as the point P. These points all lie in a plane, each at an effective depth (d – x). Thus, one must determine the tissue deficit, x, and the distance, y, from some reference point (usually the central axis) for all points within the irradiated area. This surface topography must then be demagnified back to the level at which the compensating filter will be placed in the radiation beam.

The appropriate filter thickness depends primarily on the material used. It also depends on the field size, x-ray beam energy, depth of target volume, and distance of compensator from the topographic deficit. Compensators made of material that is nearly tissue-equivalent usually must have a thickness less than the missing tissue deficit to correct adequately for the lack of scatter produced as a result of the missing tissue. Hence, compensators are designed to compensate to a specified depth, for a given geometry and beam energy. Overcompensation (less dose) usually occurs above and under compensation (more dose) below the specified compensator depth.

Bolus

Tissue-equivalent material placed directly on the patient's skin surface to reduce the skin sparing of megavoltage photon beams is referred to as *bolus*. A tissue-equivalent bolus should have electron density, physical density, and atomic number similar to those of tissue or water and be pliable so that it conforms to the skin surface contour. Inexpensive, nearly tissue-equivalent materials used as a bolus in radiation therapy include slabs of paraffin wax, rice bags filled with soda, gauze coated with petrolatum, and synthetic-based substances, such as Super-Flab or Super Stuff (39).

Thin slabs of bolus that follow the surface contour increase the dose to the skin beneath the bolus with a maximum reduction when the bolus thickness is approximately equal to the d_{max} depth for the photon beam. In addition, adding bolus to fill a tissue deficit may smooth an irregular surface. A bolus also can be shaped to alter the dose distribution as well, but normally missing tissue compensators or wedges are used to alter the dose distribution for megavoltage photon beams to retain skin sparing.

Patient Positioning, Registration, and Immobilization

Ensuring accurate daily positioning of the patient in the treatment position and reduction of patient movement during treatment is essential to deliver the prescribed dose and achieve the planned dose distribution. The reproducibility achievable in the daily positioning of a patient for treatment depends on several factors other than the anatomic site under treatment, including the patient's age, general health, and weight. In general, obese patients and small children are the most difficult to position.

The fields to be treated typically are delineated in the simulation process using either visible skin markings or skin markings visible only under an ultraviolet light. In some instances, external tattoos are applied. These markings are used in positioning a patient on the treatment machine using the machine's field localization light and distance indicator and laser alignment lights mounted in the treatment room that project transverse, coronal, and sagittal light lines (or dots) on the patient's skin surface.

Numerous patient restraint and repositioning devices have been designed and used in treating specific anatomic sites. For example, the disposable foam plastic head holder provides stability for the head when the patient is in the supine position. If the patient is treated in the prone position, a face-down stabilizer can be used. This device has a foam rubber lining covered by disposable paper with an opening provided for the patient's eyes, nose, and mouth. It allows comfort and stability as well as air access for the patient during treatment in the prone position.

A vacuum-form body immobilization system is commercially available. This system consists of a vacuum pump and an outer rubber bag filled with plastic minispheres. The rubber bag containing the minispheres is positioned to support the patient's treatment position. A vacuum is then applied, causing the minispheres to come together to form a firm, solid support molded to the patient's shape. The bite block (Fig. 6.23) is another device used as an aid in patient repositioning in the treatment of head and neck cancer. With this device, the patient, in the treatment position, bites into a specially prepared dental impression material layered on a fork that is attached to a supporting device. When the material hardens, the impression of the teeth is recorded. The bite-block fork is connected to a support arm, which is attached to the treatment couch, and may be used either with or without scales for registration.

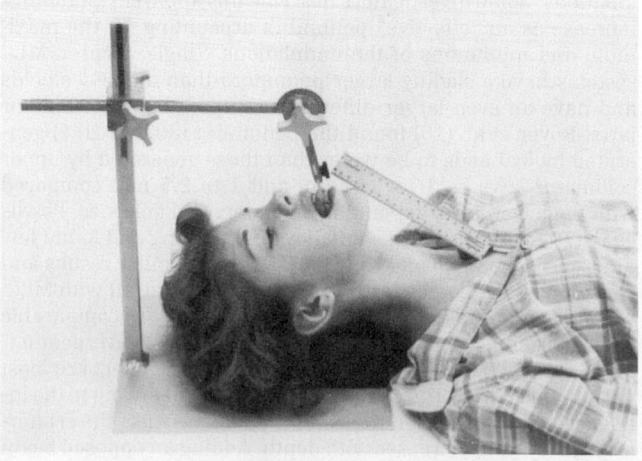

FIGURE 6.23. Example of a bite-block registration and immobilization system used in treatment of head and neck cancer. (Courtesy of Radiation Products Design, Buffalo, MN.)

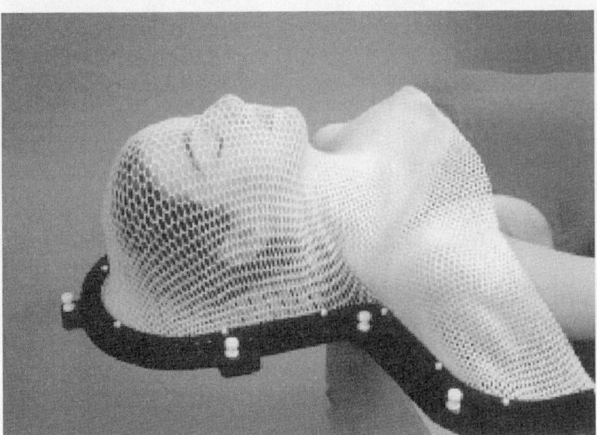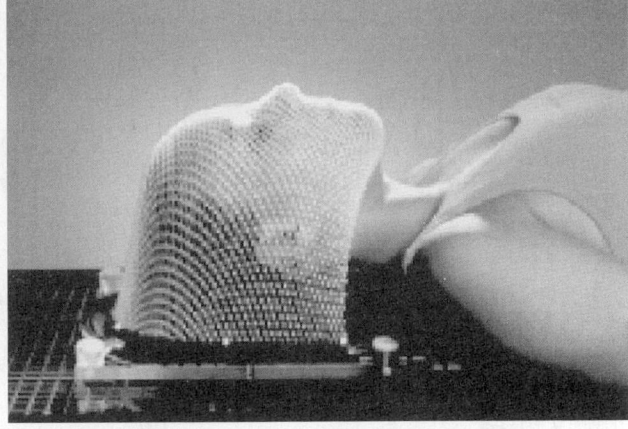

FIGURE 6.24. Example of a registration and immobilization system (thermal plastic mask) used in treatment of head and neck cancer. (Courtesy of MED-TEC, Inc., Orange City, IA.)

The traditional plaster casting technique is still used in some clinics but has not gained widespread use in the United States. Transparent, form-fitting plastic shells that are fabricated using a special vacuum device are also used extensively in Great Britain and Canada, but again have not gained acceptance in the United States. Both methods are described in detail by Watkins (88). Thermal plastic masks are now widely used in the United States (Fig. 6.24). A plastic sheet is placed in warm water and draped over the site, and hardens on cooling (29). The use of thermal plastic masks allows treatments with few skin marks made on the patient because most of the reference lines can be placed on the mask. Treatments can be given through the mask; however, there is some loss of skin sparing. When skin sparing is critical, the mask may be cut out to match the treatment portal, although some of the structural rigidity is lost.

Custom molds constructed from polyurethane formed to patient contours have gained widespread use as aids in immobilization and repositioning (Fig. 6.25). The constituent chemicals

for the polyurethane foam are mixed in liquid form and allowed to expand and harden around the patient while the patient is in the treatment position. These molds are used for treatment of Hodgkin's disease with the mantle irradiation technique, in patients with cancer of the thorax or prostate, and for extremity repositioning/immobilization. Johnson et al. (42) reported on the effect on surface dose caused by the mold for ^{60}Co, 6- and 18-MV photon beams. Also, when concerned about surface dose effects caused by immobilization devices, one should not neglect understanding the effects also caused by carbon fiber couch inserts (36).

In the past, we have used either a bite-block system or a thermal plastic face mask system to immobilize our patients with head and neck tumors. Our experience has shown that patients immobilized with the bite-block system typically require a larger number of adjustments than when more effective systems like the thermal face mask are used. Also, patients prefer the face mask because most of the reference marks are on the mask rather than on the skin; radiation therapists have greater

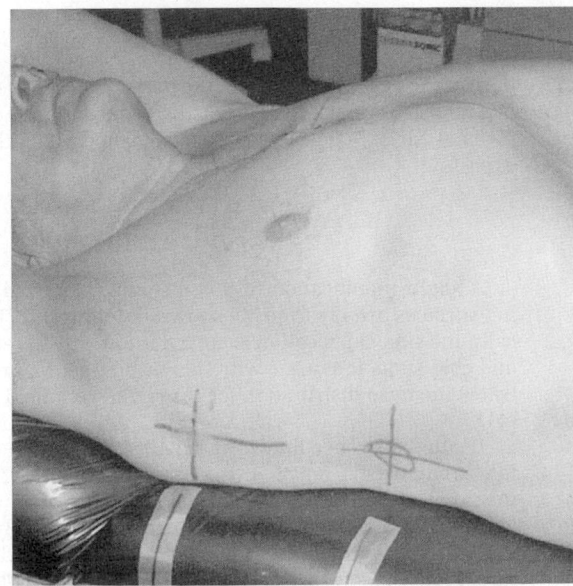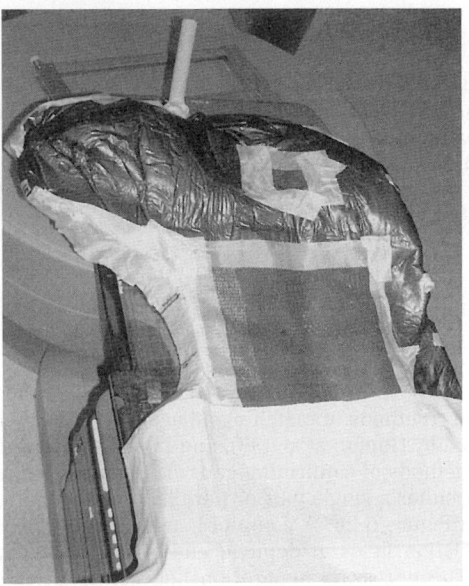

A B

FIGURE 6.25. Examples of registration and immobilization systems (foam mold) used in treatment of the thorax. **A:** Mold is registered to table and the patient is registered to the mold by fiducial markings. **B:** Mold with cutout area to allow clear access to the treatment area, and built-in handgrip.

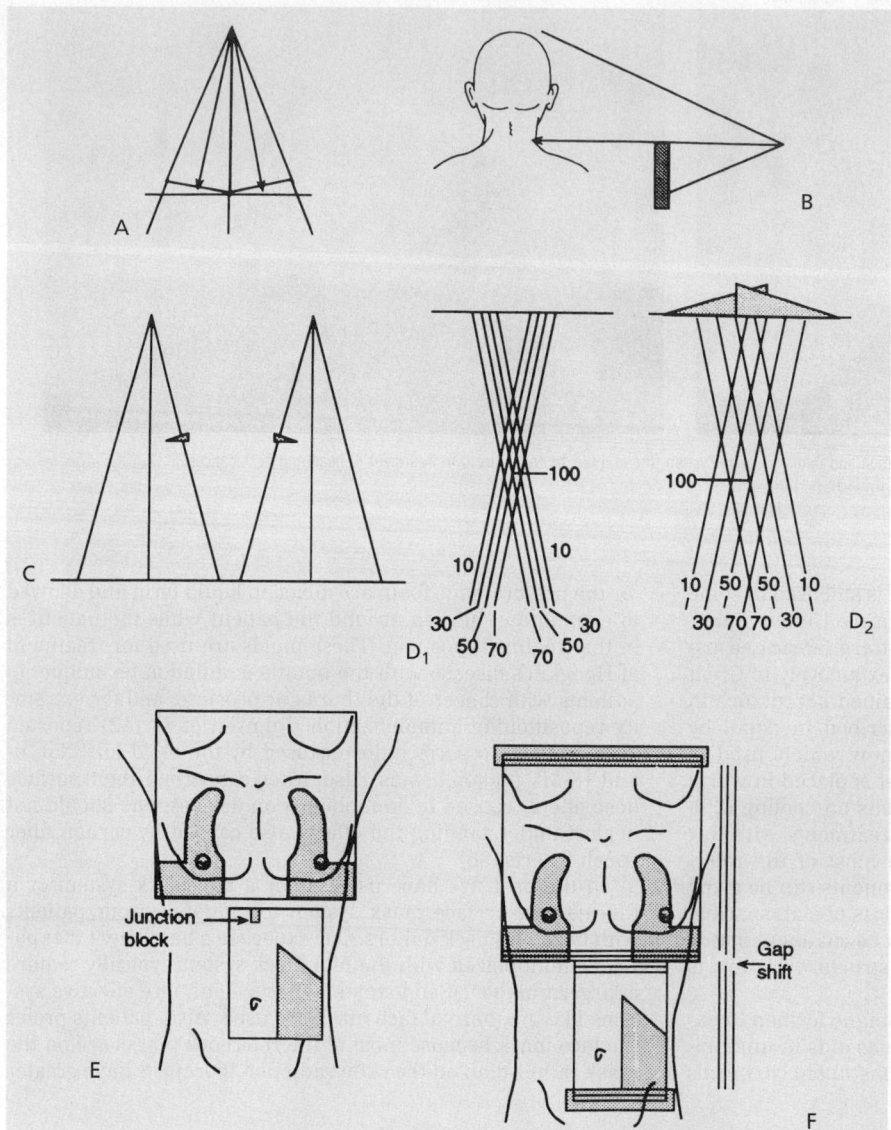

FIGURE 6.26. Different techniques for matching adjacent fields. **A:** Beam's central rays are angled slightly away from one another so that the diverging beams are parallel. **B:** Half-beam block to eliminate divergence. **C:** Penumbra generators (small wedges) to increase width of penumbra, as illustrated in D_1 and D_2. **E:** Junction block over spinal cord. **F:** Moving gap technique. (From Bentel GC, ed. *Radiation therapy planning*, 2nd ed. New York: McGraw-Hill, 1996, with permission.)

confidence in the accuracy of the treatment with the face mask. However, the final assessment of accuracy and reproducibility of the daily treatment is obtained by radiographic imaging of the area treated because there is the possibility of patient movement within the mask, especially if significant tumor shrinkage or weight loss has taken place.

Separation of Adjacent X-Ray Fields

Field Junctions

The numerous methods of matching adjacent x-ray fields have been reviewed by Hopfan et al. (37), and Dea (17) reviewed radiographic methods of confirming gaps. The geometries of adjacent fields, either a single pair or parallel-opposed pairs, are illustrated in Figure 6.26. A commonly used method matches adjacent radiation fields at depth d and is illustrated in Figure 6.27A. The necessary separation between adjacent field edges necessary to produce junction doses similar to central-axis doses follows from the similar triangles formed by the half-field length and SSD in each field. The field edge is defined by the

dose at the edge that is 50% of the dose at d_{max}. For two contiguous fields of lengths L_1 and L_2, the separation, S, of these two fields at the skin surface can be calculated using the following expression:

$$s = \frac{1}{2}L_1\left(\frac{d}{SSD}\right) + \frac{1}{2}L_2\left(\frac{d}{SSD}\right)$$

A slight modification of this formula is needed when sloping surfaces are involved, as shown in Figure 6.27B (44). Typically, the skin gap location is moved frequently to reduce the hot and cold spots that arise with this technique. Figure 6.28 illustrates the dose distribution for three different field separations (41).

Beam divergence may be eliminated by using a "beam splitter," created using a five- or six-HVL block over half of the treatment field. The central axes of the adjacent fields, where there is no divergence, are then matched. As previously discussed, this is a useful method on linacs with the independent jaw feature. Match-line wedges or penumbra generators that generate a broad penumbra for linac beams have been reported but have not found widespread use (26). Here the intent is to broaden the narrow penumbra of the linacs so that it is not so difficult to

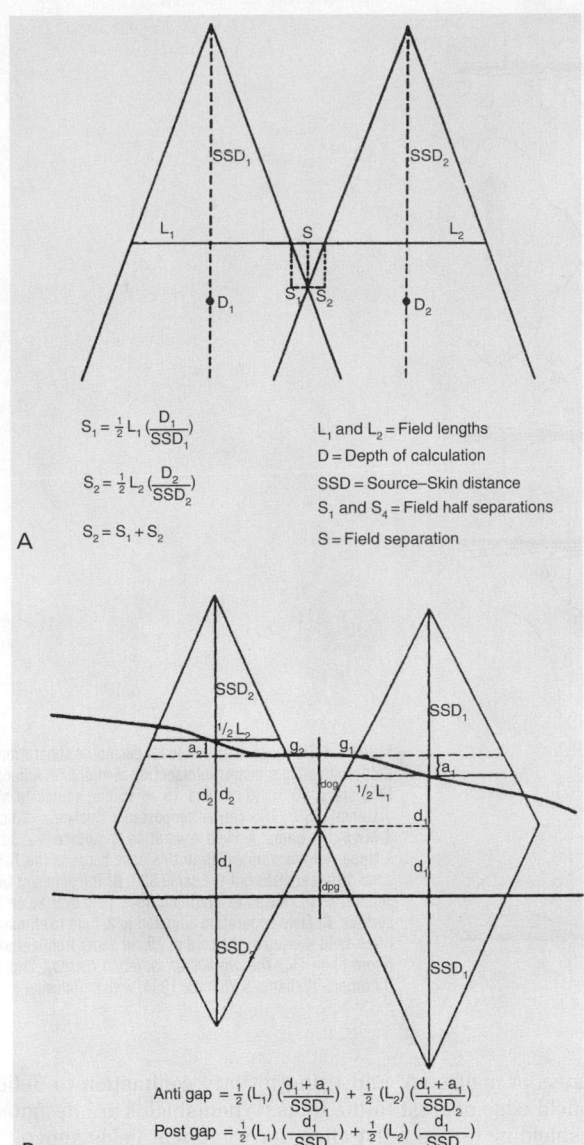

$S_1 = \frac{1}{2}L_1\left(\frac{D_1}{SSD_1}\right)$

$S_2 = \frac{1}{2}L_2\left(\frac{D_2}{SSD_2}\right)$

$S_2 = S_1 + S_2$

L_1 and L_2 = Field lengths
D = Depth of calculation
SSD = Source–Skin distance
S_1 and S_4 = Field half separations
S = Field separation

A

Anti gap $= \frac{1}{2}(L_1)\left(\frac{d_1 + a_1}{SSD_1}\right) + \frac{1}{2}(L_2)\left(\frac{d_1 + a_1}{SSD_2}\right)$

Post gap $= \frac{1}{2}(L_1)\left(\frac{d_1}{SSD_1}\right) + \frac{1}{2}(L_2)\left(\frac{d_1}{SSD_2}\right)$

B

FIGURE 6.27. A: Standard formula for calculating the gap at the skin surface for a given depth using similar triangles. **B:** Modified formula for calculating the gap for matching four fields on a sloping surface. (From Keys RA, Grigsby PW. Gapping fields on sloping surfaces. *Int J Radiat Oncol Biol Phys* 1990;18:1183–1190, with permission.)

match the 50% isodose levels. The resulting dose distributions are similar to those obtained with a moving gap technique.

Orthogonal Field Junctions

Figure 6.29 illustrates the geometry of matching abutting orthogonal photon beams. Such techniques are necessary, particularly in the head and neck region where the spinal cord can be in an area of beam overlap, in the treatment of medulloblastoma with multiple spinal portals (85) and lateral brain portals, as well as in multiple-field treatments of the breast (77). A common method of avoiding overlap is to use a half-block, as previously discussed, so that abutting anterior and lateral field edges are perpendicular to the gantry axis (43). In addition, a notch in the posterior corner of the lateral oral cavity portal is commonly used to ensure overlap avoidance of the spinal cord when midline cord blocks cannot be used on anteroposterior portals irradiating the lower neck and matched to the oral cav-

ity portals. Other techniques rotate the couch about a vertical axis to compensate for the divergence of the lateral field, with the angle of rotation given by:

$$\tan \theta^{-1} = \left(\frac{\frac{1}{2}\text{field width}}{\text{SAD}}\right)$$

Another technique is to leave a gap, *S*, on the anterior neck surface between the posterior field of length *L* and lateral field edges, where *d* is the depth of the spine beneath the posterior field and where

$$s = \frac{1}{2}(L)\left(\frac{d}{\text{SAD}}\right)$$

Craniospinal irradiation is well established as a standard method of treatment of suprasellar dysgerminoma, pineal tumors, medulloblastomas, and other tumors involving the central nervous system. Uniform treatment of the entire craniospinal target volume is possible using separate parallel-opposed lateral cranial portals rotated so that their inferior borders match with the superior border of the spinal portal, which is treated with either one or two fields, depending on the length of the spine to be treated. Lim (56,57) describes the dosimetry of optional methods of treating medulloblastoma with excellent descriptions and diagrams. Two junctional moves are made at one-third and two-thirds of the total dose. The spinal field central axis is shifted away from the brain by 0.5 cm and the field size length reduced by 0.5 cm with corresponding increases in the length of the cranial field, so that a match exists between the inferior border of the brain portal and the superior border of the spine portal. To achieve the match, the whole-brain portals are rotated by an angle given by the following relationship:

$$\tan \theta^{-1} = \left(\frac{\frac{1}{2} \text{ spinal field length}}{SAD}\right)$$

To eliminate the divergence between the cranial portal and spinal portal, the table is rotated through a floor angle:

$$\tan \alpha^{-1} = \left(\frac{\frac{1}{2} \text{ cranial field length}}{SAD}\right)$$

Potential for the occurrence of radiation myelopathy resulting from the potentially excessive dose from misaligned overlapping fields is always a concern when central nervous system tumors are treated at doses greater than 20 Gy.

●● ┃ Radiation Therapy Patients
●● ┃ with Cardiac Pacemakers

To treat patients with cardiac pacemakers safely, it is important to understand the potential effects of radiation therapy on pacemaker operation and to take steps to minimize any actions that could jeopardize the cardiac health of the patient. Potential interactions between a functioning pacemaker and the radiation therapy environment fall into two categories. First, transient malfunctions may be caused by strong high- and low-frequency electromagnetic fields created by the treatment machine in the course of producing high-energy photon and electron beams. Secondly, modern pacemakers are radiosensitive and have a significant probability of failing catastrophically at radiation doses well below normal tissue tolerance and, therefore, should never be irradiated by the direct beam. Table 6.3 provides a list of widely accepted clinical management guidelines based on recommendations by the AAPM (62).

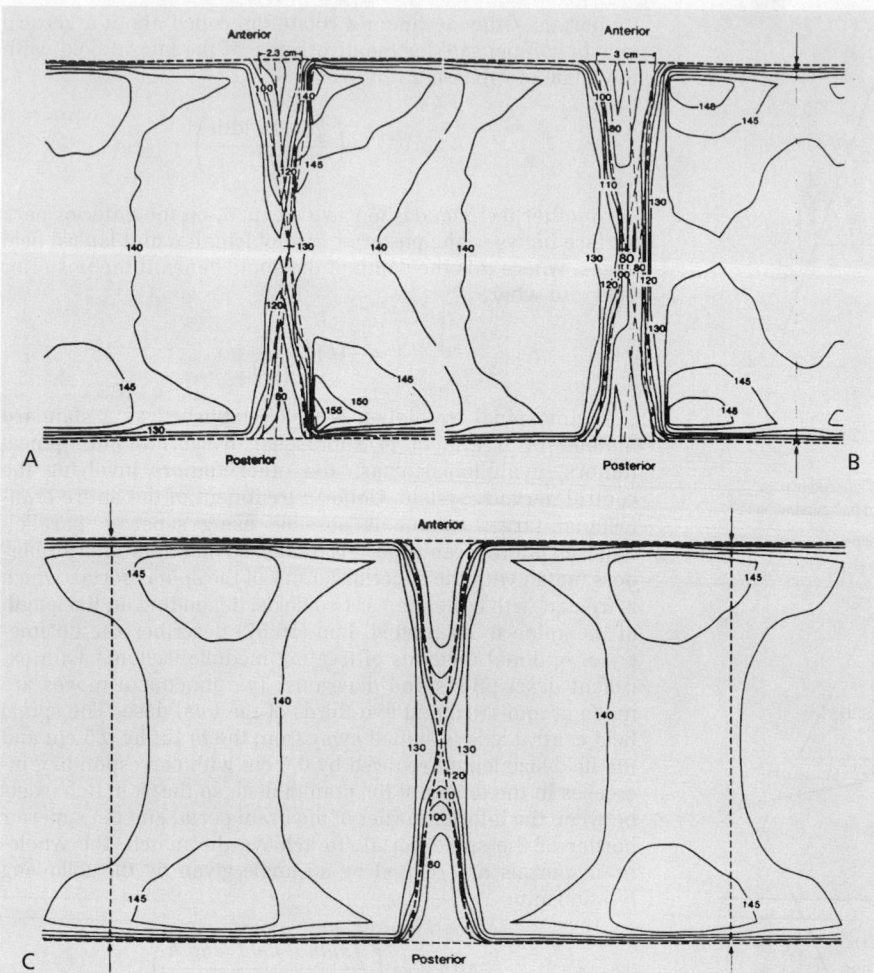

FIGURE 6.28. Dose distribution for geometric separation of fields with all four beams intersecting at midpoint. Adjacent field sizes: 30 × 30 cm and 15 × 15 cm; source-to-skin distance (SSD), 100 cm; anteroposterior thickness, 20 cm; 4-MV x-ray beams. **A:** Field separation at surface is 2.3 cm. A three-field overlap exists in this case because the fields have different sizes but the same SSD. **B:** The adjacent field separation increased to eliminate three-field overlap on the surface. **C:** Field separation adjusted to 2.7 cm to eliminate three-field overlap at the cord at 15 cm depth from anterior. (From Khan FM. *The physics of radiation therapy*, 2nd ed. Baltimore: Williams & Wilkins, 1994, with permission.)

Fetal Dose

Radiation therapy is standard treatment for several malignancies (e.g., Hodgkin's lymphoma, breast cancer) in which the population of women is often of childbearing age. The issues are complex and the patient, along with the radiation oncologist, must evaluate treatment risk to the fetus in such cases. Radiation effects to the fetus are not fully understood and cannot be comfortably predicted for each case. If the decision is to irradiate, the dose levels outside the treatment fields should be quantified, and every effort should be made to lower the dose to the fetus. This may require changes in irradiation technique (i.e., modified mantle fields), elimination of double-exposure portal films, and the addition of special patient shields. An AAPM report provides data and techniques to estimate and reduce radiation dose to the fetus for beam energies ranging from ^{60}Co to 18 MV (81). Before the pregnant patient is treated, the pregnancy stage should be known to estimate the size and location of the fetus throughout the treatment. Dose-estimation points should be selected that allow estimation of dose throughout the fetus (e.g., fundus, symphysis pubis, and umbilicus).

Two methods can be used to reduce the dose to the fetus, namely, modification of treatment techniques and the use of special shields. Modifications include changing field angle (avoiding placement of the gantry close to the fetus, that is, treatment of a posterior field with the patient lying prone on a false table top), reducing field size, choosing a different radiation energy (avoiding ^{60}Co because of high leakage or energies of >10 MV

because of neutrons), and using tertiary collimation to define the field edge nearest to the fetus. When shields are designed, the shielding device must allow for treatment fields above the diaphragm and on the lower extremities. Safety to the patient and personnel is a primary consideration in shield design. As part of the management of a pregnant patient, the treatment planning tasks listed in Table 6.4 should be performed to ensure that the dose to the fetus is kept to a minimum (81).

Gonadal Dose

Many of the same reports used to estimate peripheral dose and fetal dose apply to dose estimations to both testes and ovaries. Estimations by calculated methods (27) and by extrapolated measurements (84) have been reported specific to gonadal dose. Simultaneously, there have been studies to determine the genetically significant dose (GSD) as it applies to peripheral radiotherapy dosage to ovaries and testes. Niroomand-Rad and Cumberlin (65) combined measured data and GSD data to determine the GSD for particular treatment techniques that deliver peripheral dose to ovaries and testes. They summarized that GSDs from conventional therapies are minimal. However, there are circumstances, such as treatment of seminoma, when it is necessary to use a testicular shield to surround the testes to reduce head scatter and leakage, and some internal scatter (24).

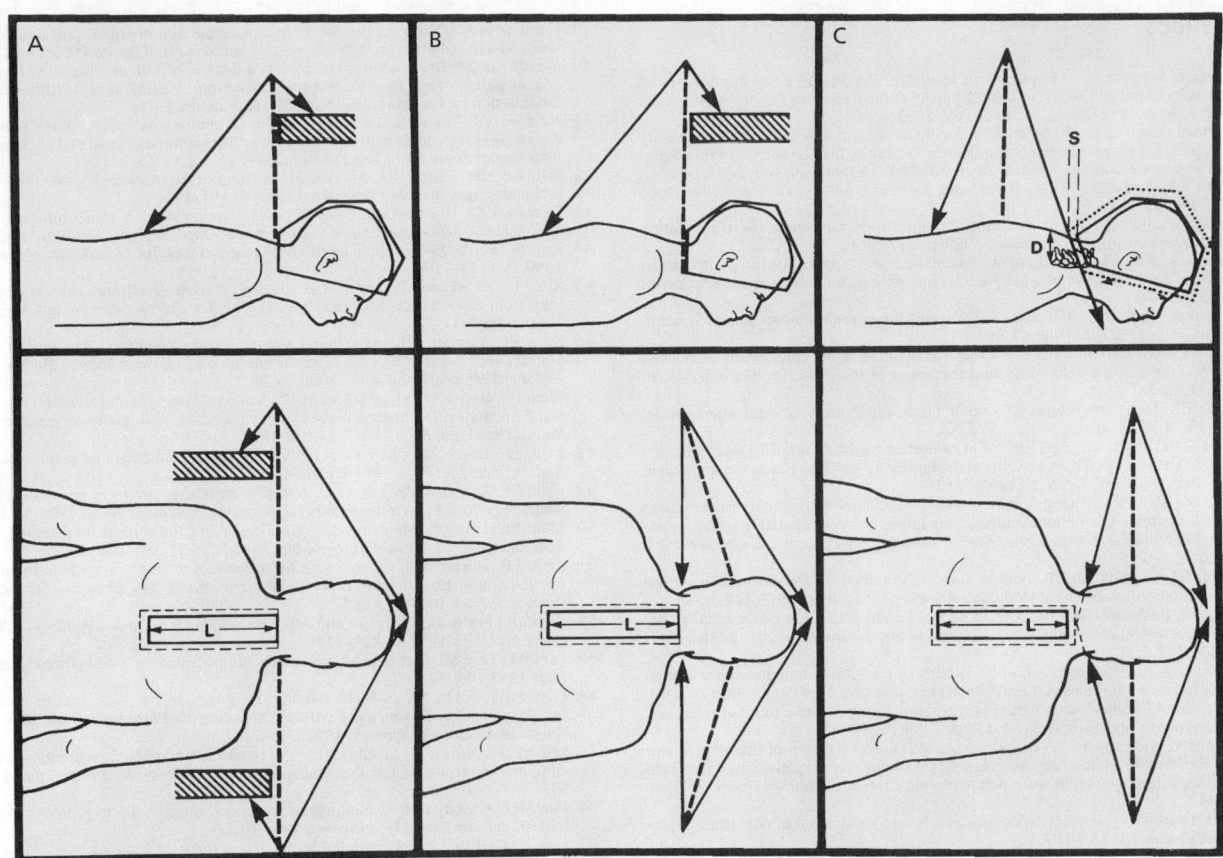

FIGURE 6.29. Some solutions for the problem of overlap for orthogonal fields. **A:** A beam splitter, a shield that blocks half of the field, is used on the lateral and posterior fields and on the spinal cord portal to match the nondivergent edges of the beams. **B:** The divergence in the lateral beams may also be removed by angling the lateral beams so that their caudal edges match. Because most therapy units cannot be angled like this, the couch is rotated through small angles in opposite directions to achieve the same effect. **C:** A gap technique allows the posterior and lateral field to be matched at depth using a gap *S* on the skin surface. The *dashed lines* indicate projected field edges at depth *D*, where the orthogonal fields meet. (From Williamson TJ. A technique for matching orthogonal megavoltage fields. *Int J Radiat Oncol Biol Phys* 1979;5:111, 1979, with permission.)

⋮⋮ Table 6.3	**MANAGEMENT GUIDELINES FOR RADIATION THERAPY PATIENTS WITH CARDIAC PACEMAKERS**

1. Pacemaker-implanted patients should never be treated with a betatron.
2. Have the patient's coronary and pacemaker status evaluated by a cardiologist before and soon after completion of therapy.
3. Always keep the pacemaker outside the machine-collimated radiation beam, both during treatment and when taking portal films.
4. Carefully observe the patient during the first therapy session to verify that no transient malfunctions are occurring and during subsequent treatments if magnetron or klystron misfiring (sparking) occurs.
5. Before treatment, estimate and record the dose (from scatter) to be received by the pacemaker. The total accumulated dose should not exceed approximately 2 Gy.
6. If treatment within these guidelines is not possible, the physician should consider having the pacemaker either temporarily or permanently moved before irradiation.
7. If a patient has an automatic implantable cardioverter–defibrillator (AICD), the physicist should follow the same steps as one would for pacemakers in contacting the manufacturer and simultaneously ascertaining the dose expected to the AICD. If there is no manufacturer information concerning radiation effects to the ACID, a conservative threshold of 100 cGy should be considered.

Modified from Marbach et al. *Med Phys* 1994;21:85–90 (see ref. 62)

⋮⋮ Table 6.4	**TREATMENT-PLANNING TASKS TO ENSURE THAT DOSE TO THE FETUS IS KEPT TO A MINIMUM**

1. Complete all planning as though the patient were not pregnant.
2. Consider modifications of the plan that would minimize the fetal dose (e.g., changing field size and angle, using a different energy).
3. Estimate dose to fetus without shielding using a phantom or data from the AAPM report (2).
4. Design and construct special shielding if necessary; four or five HVLs of lead usually suffice.
5. Measure dose to fetus in a phantom during simulated treatment with shielding in place.
6. Document the treatment plan and discuss the treatment with all personnel involved with the treatment.
7. Check all aspects of safety, including the load-bearing limits of the couch and support and movement of the shields, to ensure that there will be no injury to the patient or to personnel. The setup of each field should be photographed for documentation.
8. Monitor fetal size and location throughout the course of therapy and update estimates of fetal dose if necessary.
9. Document the completion of treatment by estimating the total dose to the fetus due to the radiation therapy.

Modified from Stovall et al. 1995;22:63–82 (see ref. 81)

References

1. American Association of Physicists in Medicine. Report 72: Basic applications of multileaf collimators: Report of Task Group 50 of the Radiation Therapy Committee. Medical Physics Publishing, Madison, WI: 2001:1–48.
2. American Association of Physicists in Medicine. Report 85: Tissue inhomogeneity corrections for megavoltage photon beams: Report of Task Group 65 of the Radiation Therapy Committee. Medical Physics Publishing, Madison, WI: 2004:1–130.
3. Abrath FG, Purdy JA. Wedge design and dosimetry for 25-MV x rays. *Radiology* 1980;136:757–762.
4. Ahnesjö A. Collapsed cone convolution of radiant energy for photon dose calculation in heterogeneous media. *Med Phys* 1989;16:577–592.
5. Ahnesjö A, Andreo P, Brahme A. Calculation and application of point spread functions for treatment planning with high energy photon beams. *Acta Oncol* 1987;26:49–56.
6. Ahnesjö A, Aspradakis MM. Dose calculations for external photon beams in radiotherapy. *Phys Med Biol* 1999;44:R99–R155.
7. Akazawa PF, Roach MI, Pickett B, et al. Three dimensional comparison of blocked arcs vs. four and six field conformal treatment of the prostate. *Radiother Oncol* 1996;41:83–88.
8. Batho, HF. Lung corrections in Cobalt 60 beam therapy. *J Can Assoc Radiol* 1964;15:79–83.
9. Central axis depth dose data for use in radiotherapy. *Br J Radiol* 1996;25[Suppl]:
10. Boyer A, Ochran TG, CE, et al. Clinical dosimetry for implementation of a multileaf collimator. *Med Phys* 1992; 19:1255–1261.
11. Chao KSC, Majhail N, Huang C, et al. Intensity-modulated radiation therapy reduces late salivary toxicity without compromising tumor control in patients with oropharyngeal carcinoma: A comparison with conventional techniques. *Radiother Oncol* 2001;61:275–280.
12. Cundiff JH, Cunningham JR, Golden R, et al. A method for the calculation of dose in the radiation treatment of Hodgkin's disease. *Am J Roentg* 1973;117:30–44.
13. Cygler JE, Daskalov GM, Chan GH, et al. Evaluation of the first commercial Monte Carlo dose calculation engine for electron beam treatment planning. *Med Phys* 2004;31:142–153.
14. Das IJ, Kase KR, Meigooni AS, et al. Validity of transition-zone dosimetry at high atomic number interfaces in megavoltage photon beams. *Med Phys* 1990;17:10–16.
15. Das IJ, Khan FM. Backscatter dose perturbation at high atomic number interfaces in megavoltage photon beams. *Med Phys* 1989;16:367–375.
16. De Neve W, De Gersem W, Derycke S, et al. Clinical delivery of intensity modulated conformal radiotherapy for relapsed or second-primary head and neck cancer using a multileaf collimator with dynamic control. *Radiother Oncol* 1999;50:301–314.
17. Dea D. Dosimetric problems with adjacent fields: Verification of gap size. *Am AssocMed Dosim J* 1985;10:37.
18. Du MN, Yu CX, Symons M, et al. A multi-leaf collimator prescription preparation system for conventional radiotherapy. *Int J Radiat Oncol Biol Phys* 1995;32:513–520.
19. Ellis F, Hall EJ, Oliver R. A compensator for variations in tissue thickness for high energy beams. *Br J Radiol* 1959;32:421–422.
20. Emami B, Lyman J, Brown A, et al. Tolerance of normal tissue to therapeutic irradiation. *Int J Radiat Oncol Biol Phys* 1991;21:109–122.
21. Epp ER, Boyer AL, Doppke KP. Underdosing of lesions resulting from lack of electronic equilibrium in upper respiratory air cavities irradiated by 10 MV x-ray beams. *Int J Radiat Oncol Biol Phys* 1977;2:613.
22. Epp ER, Lougheed MN, McKay JW. Ionization build-up in upper respiratory air passages during teletherapy units with cobalt-60 irradiation. *Br J Radiol* 1958;31:361.
23. Fischer JJ, Moulder JE. The steepness of the dose-response curve in radiation therapy. *Radiology* 1975;117:179–184.
24. Fraass BA, Kinsella TJ, Harrington ES, et al. Peripheral dose to the testes: The design and clinical use of a practical and effective gonadal shield. *Int J Radiat Oncol Biol Phys* 985;11:609–616.
25. Fraass BA, Smathers J, Deye JA. Summary and recommendations of a National Cancer Institute workshop on issues limiting the clinical use of Monte Carlo dose calculation algorithms for megavoltage external beam radiation therapy. *Med Phys* 2003;30:3206–3216.
26. Fraass BA, Tepper JE, Glatstein E, et al. Clinical use of a match line wedge for adjacent megavoltage radiation field matching. *Int J Radiat Oncol Biol Phys* 1983;9:209–216.
27. Francois P, Beurtheret C, Dutreix A. Calculation of the dose delivered to organs outside the radiation beams. *Med Phys* 1988;15:879–883.
28. Frank SJ, Forster KM, Stevens CW, et al. Treatment planning for lung cancer: Traditional homogeneous point-dose prescription compared with heterogeneity-corrected dose-volume prescription. *Int J Radiat Oncol Biol Phys* 2003;56:1308–1318.
29. Gerber RL, Marks JE, Purdy JA. The use of thermal plastics for immobilization of patients during radiotherapy. *Int J Radiat Oncol Biol Phys* 1982;8:1461.
30. Gerbi BJ, Khan FM. Measurement of dose in the buildup region using fixed-separation plane-parallel ionization chambers. *Med Phys* 1990;17:17–26.
31. Gerbi BJ, Meigooni A, Khan FM. Dose buildup for obliquely incident photon beams. *Med Phys* 1987;14:393–399.
32. Gibbons JP, ed. *Monitor unit calculations for external photon and electron beams*. Madison, WI, Advanced Medical Publishing, 2000.
33. Hanson WF, Berkley LW. Calculative technique to correct for the change in linear accelerator beam energy at off-axis points. *Med Phys* 1980;7:147–150.
34. Hanson WF, Berkley LW. Off-Axis beam quality change in linear accelerator x-ray beams. *Med Phys* 1980;7:145–146.
35. Herring DF. The consequences of dose response curves for tumor control and normal tissue injury on the precision necessary in patient management. *Laryngos* 1975;85:119–125.
36. Higgins DM, Whitehurst P, Morgan AM. The effect of carbon fiber couch inserts on surface dose with beam size variation. *Med Dosim* 2001;26:251–254.
37. Hopfan S, Reid A, Simpson L, et al. Clinical complications arising from overlapping of adjacent fields: Physical and technical considerations. *Int J Radiat Oncol Biol Phys* 1977;2:801–808.
38. Huen A, Findley DO, Skov DD. Attenuation in Lipowitz's metal of x-rays produced at 2, 4, 10, and 18 MV and gamma rays from cobalt-60. *Med Phys* 1979;6:147–148.
39. Humphries SM, Boyd K, Cornish P, et al. Comparison of super stuff and paraffin wax bolus in radiation therapy of irregular surfaces. *Med Dosim* 1996;21:155–157.
40. *Report No. 24: Determination of absorbed dose in a patient irradiated by beams of x or gamma rays in radiotherapy procedures*. Washington, DC, International Commission on Radiation Units and Measurements, 1976.
41. Johnson JM, Khan FM. Dosimetric effects of abutting extended source to surface distance electron fields with photon fields in the treatment of head and neck cancers. *Int J Radiat Oncol Biol Phys* 1994;28:741–747.
42. Johnson MW, Griggs MA, Sharma SC. A comparison of surface doses for two immobilizing systems. *Med Dosimetry* 1995;20:191–194.
43. Karzmark CJ, Huisman PA, Palos BB, et al. Overlap at the cord in abutting orthogonal fields: A perceptual anomaly. *Int J Radiat Oncol Biol Phys* 1980;6:1366.
44. Keys R, Grigsby PW. Gapping fields on sloping surfaces. *Int J Radiat Oncol Biol Phys* 1990;18:1183–1190.
45. Khan FM, Sewchand W, Lee J, et al. Revision of tissue-maximum ratio and scatter-maximum ratio concepts for cobalt 60 and higher energy x-ray beams. *Med Phys* 1980;7:230–237.
46. Klein EE. Monitor unit calculations with multileaf collimators. In: Gibbons JP ed. *Monitor unit calculations for external photon and electron beams*. Madison, WI: Advanced Medical Publishing, 2000:75–82.
47. Klein EE, Harms WB, Low DA, et al. Clinical implementation of a commercial multileaf collimator: Dosimetry, networking, simulation, and quality assurance. *Int J Radiat Oncol Biol Phys* 1995;33:1195–1208.
48. Klein EE, Kuske RR. Changes in photon dosimetry due to breast prosthesis. *Int J Radiat Oncol Biol Phys* 1993;25:541–549.
49. Klein EE, Low DA, Maag D, et al. A quality assurance program for ancillary high technology devices on a dual-energy accelerator. *Radiother Oncol* 1996;38:51–60.
50. Klein EE, Low DA, Meigooni AS, et al. Dosimetry for clinical implementation of dynamic wedge. *Int J Radiat Oncol Biol Phys* 1995;31:583–592.
51. Klein EE, Morrison A, Purdy JA, et al. A volumetric study of measurements and calculations of lung density corrections for 6 and 18 MV photons. *Int J Radiat Oncol Biol Phys* 1997;37:1163–1170.
52. Klein EE, Purdy JA. Entrance and exit dose regions for Clinac-2100C. *Int J Radiat Oncol Biol Phys* 1993;27:429–435.
53. Lam WC, Lam KS. Errors in off-axis treatment planning for a 4 MeV machine. *Med Phys* 1983;10:480.
54. Leavitt DD, Gibbs FA Jr. Field shaping. In: Purdy JA ed. *Advances in radiation oncology physics: Dosimetry, treatment planning, and brachytherapy*. New York: American Institute of Physics, 1992:500–523.
55. Leavitt DD, Martin M, Moeller JH, et al. Dynamic wedge field techniques through computer-controlled collimator motion and dose delivery. *Med Phys* 1990;17:87–91.
56. Lim MLF. A study of four methods of junction change in the treatment of medulloblastoma. *Am Assoc Med Dosim J* 1985;10:17–24.
57. Lim MLF. Evolution of medulloblastoma treatment techniques. *Am Assoc Med Dosim J* 1986;11:25–33.
58. LoSasso T, Chui CS, Kutcher GJ. The use of multileaf collimator for conformal radiotherapy of carcinomas of the prostate and nasopharynx. *Int J Radiat Oncol Biol Phys* 1993;25:161–170.
59. LoSasso T, Kutcher GJ. Multi-leaf collimation vs. cerrobend blocks: Analysis of geometric accuracy. *Int J Radiat Oncol Biol Phys* 1995;32:499–506.
60. Lydon JM. Photon dose calculations in homogeneous media for a treatment planning system using a collapsed cone superposition convolution algorithm. *Phys Med Biol* 1998;43:1813–1822.
61. Mackie TR, Scrimger JW, Battista JJ. A convolution method of calculating dose for 15-MV x-rays. *Med Phys* 1985;12:188–196.
62. Marbach JR, Sontag MR, Van Dyk J, et al. Management of radiation oncology patients with implanted cardiac pacemakers: Report of AAPM Task Group No. 34. *Med Phys* 1994;21:85–90.
63. McCullough EC, Gortney J, Blackwell CR. A depth dependence determination of the wedge transmission factor for 4-10 MV photon beams. *Med Phys* 1988;15:621–623.
64. Mellenberg DE. Monitor unit calculations for asymmetric fields. In: Gibbons JP, ed. *Monitor unit calculations for external photon and electron beams*. Madison, WI: Advanced Medical Publishing, 2000:61–73.
65. Niroomand-Rad A, Cumberlin RL. Measured dose to ovaries and testes from Hodgkin's fields and determination of genetically significant dose. *Int J Radiat Oncol Biol Phys* 1993;25:745–751.
66. Palta JR, Yeung DK, Frouhar V. Dosimetric considerations for a multileaf collimator system. *Med Phys* 1996;23:1219–1224.
67. Petti PL, Siddon RL. Effective wedge angles with a universal wedge. *Phys Med Biol* 1985;30:985–991.
68. Philips Medical Systems Division Product Data 764. Eindhoven: The Netherlands, 1983.
69. Powers WE, Kinzie JJ, Demidecki AJ, et al. A new system of field shaping for external-beam radiation therapy. *Radiology* 1973;108:407–411.
70. Powlis WD, Smith AR, Cheng E, et al. Initiation of multileaf collimator conformal radiation therapy. *Int J Radiat Oncol Biol Phys* 1993;25:171–179.
71. Purdy JA. Buildup/surface dose and exit dose measurements for 6-MV linear accelerator. *Med Phys* 1986;13:259–262.
72. Reft C, Alecu R, Das IJ, et al. Dosimetric considerations for patients with HIP prostheses undergoing pelvic irradiation. Report of the AAPM Radiation Therapy Committee Task Group 63. *Med Phys* 2003;30:1162–1182.
73. Reinstein LE. New approaches to tissue compensation in radiation oncology. In: Purdy JA, ed. *Advances in radiation oncology physics: Dosimetry, treatment planning, and brachytherapy*. New York: American Institute of Physics, 1992:535–572.
74. *Report No. 42: Use of computers in external beam radiotherapy procedures with high energy proton and electrons*. Bethesda, MD. International Commission Radiation Units and Measurements, 1987.
75. Rice RK, Mijnheer BJ, Chin LM. Benchmark measurements for lung dose corrections for x-ray beams. *Int J Radiat Oncol Biol Phys* 1988;15:399–409.
76. Sewchand W, Khan FM, Williamson J. Variations in depth-dose data between open and wedge fields for 4-MV x rays. *Radiology* 1978;127:789–792.
77. Siddon RL, Tonnesen GL, Svensson GK. Three-field techniques for breast treatment using a rotatable half-beam block. *Int J Radiat Oncol Biol Phys* 1981;7:1473–1477.
78. Siebers JV, Keall PJ, Kawrakow I. Monte Carlo dose calculations for external beam radiation therapy. In: Dyk JV, ed. *The modern technology of radiation oncology—a*

compendium for medical physicists and radiation oncologists, vol 2. Madison, WI: Medical Physics Publishing, 2005:91–130.

79. Sontag MR, Cunningham JR. Corrections to absorbed dose calculations for tissue inhomogeneities. *Med Phys* 1977;4:431–436.

80. Stewart J, Jackson A. The steepness of the dose response curve for both tumor cure and normal tissue injury. *Laryngoscope* 1975;85:1107–1111.

81. Stovall M, Blackwell CR, Cundiff J, et al. Fetal dose from radiotherapy with photon beams: Report of AAPM Radiation Therapy Committee Task Group No. 36. *Med Phys* 1995;22:63–82.

82. Takahaski S. Conformation radiotherapy-rotation techniques as applied to radiography and radiotherapy of cancer. *Acta Radiol Suppl* 1965;242:1–142.

83. Tatcher M. A method for varying effective angle of wedge filters. *Radiology* 1970;97:132.

84. Van Der Giessen PH. A simple and generally applicable method to estimate the peripheral dose in radiation teletherapy with high energy x-rays or gamma radiation. *Int J Radiat Oncol Biol Phys* 1996;35:1059–1068.

85. Van Dyk J, Jenkin RDT, Leung PMK, et al. Medulloblastoma: Treatment technique and radiation dosimetry. *Int J Radiat Oncol Biol Phys* 1977;2:993–1005.

86. Velkley De, Manson DJ, Purdy JA, et al. Build-up region of megavoltage photon radiation sources. *Med Phys* 1975;2:14–18.

87. Verhaegen F, Seuntjens J. Monte Carlo modeling of external radiotherapy photon beams (topical review). *Phys Med Biol* 2003;48:R107–R164.

88. Watkins DMB. *Radiation therapy mold technology*. Toronto, Canada: Pergamon Press, 1981.

89. Wu Q, Manning M, Schmidt-Ullrich R, et al. The potential for sparing of parotids and escalation of biologically effective dose with intensity-modulated radiation treatments of head and neck cancers: A treatment design study. *Int J Radiat Oncol Biol Phys* 2000;46:195–205.

90. Young MEJ, Gaylord JD. Experimental tests of corrections for tissue inhomogeneities in radiotherapy. *Br J Radiol* 1970;43:349–355.

91. Zhu Y, Boyer AL, Desorby GE. Dose distributions of x-ray fields as shaped with multileaf collimators. *Phys Med Biol* 1992;37:163–173.

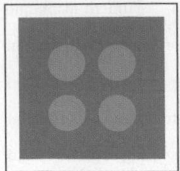

Chapter 7
Electron-Beam Therapy: Dosimetry, Planning, and Techniques

Eric E. Klein

Megavoltage-photon–based radiation therapy treatment of shallow tumor volumes is complicated by the buildup and radiation transport properties of megavoltage beams. These beams are capable of treating both shallow and deep tumors, but when treating shallow tumors, the radiation beams transit through the entire patient, exposing distal normal tissues. Megavoltage electron beams have the property of a finite range and, therefore, do not deliver significant radiation doses to distal depths. Electron-beam therapy is therefore suitable for shallow tumors (<5 cm deep), such as head and neck cancers, skin and lip cancers, chest wall irradiation for breast cancer, and boost dose to nodes. Electrons will typically provide dose uniformity in these target volumes, with minimal dose to distal organs. In fact G.H. Fletcher (21) had gone as far as saying, "there is no alternative treatment to electron-beam therapy." Even the strongest proponents of photon therapy acknowledge electron therapy is necessary to complete any radiotherapy program.

In 1976 Tapley (91) published one of the earlier comprehensive treatises on electron radiation therapy, in which she states, "There is no practical way for every radiation therapy department, either in hospitals or private offices, to be equipped with all modalities of irradiation beams. Ideally, electron beams should be available for those clinical situations where electrons are indispensable or very clearly superior." Electrons are now used at most radiation therapy centers. It still might be advantageous to refer patients to regional centers for special treatment techniques utilizing electrons.

Since the late 1970s, there have been three developments in electron-beam radiation therapy technology that have improved significantly our ability to deliver electron therapy. First, the advent of computed tomography (CT)-based treatment planning allowed for coverage of the planning target volume (PTV) by the therapeutic dose and the dose to normal tissues and structures to be more accurately assessed. Use of CT provides a physical description of the anatomy, which is required for accurate dose calculations (26,34). Second, the development of the electron pencil-beam algorithms (PBAs) and their implementation into treatment planning systems in the early 1980s provided a mechanism for accurately calculating dose (30,31,38). More recently, use of Monte Carlo calculations has moved development to commercial platforms. They have demonstrated high degrees of accuracy, especially with the presence of homogenetics. Third, manufacturers refined the quality of their electron beams (i.e., depth dose, off-axis uniformity, and penumbral width) by improving dual-scattering foil systems and electron applicators. Klein et al. (50) describe dosimetric improvement with the most recent Varian electron-beam delivery system. Presently, the differences in the electron-beam dose characteristics of various radiation therapy machines from different vendors are minimal.

Electron-beam therapy is advantageous because it delivers a reasonably uniform dose from the surface to a specific depth, after which dose falls off rapidly, eventually to a near-zero value. The depth of treatment is controlled by selecting the appropriate energy, and when necessary, the bolus thickness. Using electron beams with energies up to 20 MeV allows disease within approximately 6 cm of the surface to be treated effectively, sparing deeper normal tissues.

Electron-beam therapy is useful in treating cancer of the skin and lips, upper-respiratory and digestive tract, head and neck (20,67), breast, and a variety of other sites (53,91,93). Treatment sites of the skin include the eyelids, nose, ear (70), scalp (91,92), and more widely spread diseases of the limbs (e.g., melanoma and lymphoma) (96), or total skin (e.g., mycosis fungoides) (39,45). Treatment sites of upper respiratory and digestive tract include the floor of mouth, soft palate, retromolar trigone, and salivary glands (20,95). Treatments of the breast include chest-wall irradiation following mastectomy (78,90,91); nodal irradiation, often internal mammary chain and occasionally axillary; and boost to the surgical bed following mastectomy or lumpectomy (81). Current techniques of using tangential photon adjunct fields abutting supraclavicular and posterior axillary fields are difficult enough without the addition of treating a separate medial breast internal mammary field with a mixture of photon and electrons. Other sites of electron-beam therapy include the retina (48), orbit (17), spine (craniospinal irradiation) (13,16,62,63), paraspinal muscles (26,58), pancreas and other abdominal structures (intraoperative therapy) (65), vulva (77), and cervix (intracavitary irradiation) (64).

The purpose of this chapter is to discuss the treatment and treatment-planning techniques necessary to deliver the most effective electron-beam therapy. This requires a basic knowledge of dose distribution in water, dose in the heterogeneous patient, treatment-planning tools and principles, and special techniques using electron beams.

Dose Distribution in Water

To appreciate the clinical use of electron beams, their dose distributions in water must be understood. Understanding the properties of depth dose, off-axis ratios, and two-dimensional (2D) isodose contour plots will clarify the concept of dose distribution in water. As well, an understanding of the dependence of the dose distribution on incident energy, field size, and source-to-surface distance (SSD) is required. It is assumed that the dose distribution for a specified energy, field size, and SSD is machine dependent. Applicator dependence might have a minor influence on dose distributions and more significant influence.

Depth Dose

This section discusses percentage of dose (values are normalized to 100% at the depth of dose maximum, R_{100}) versus depth in water. Central-axis depth dose implies that the electron field is symmetric about the central axis, and the focus initially will be on square fields. Electron depth dose varies with field size; however, once the field reaches a certain size, side-scatter equilibrium is achieved, and further increasing the size has an

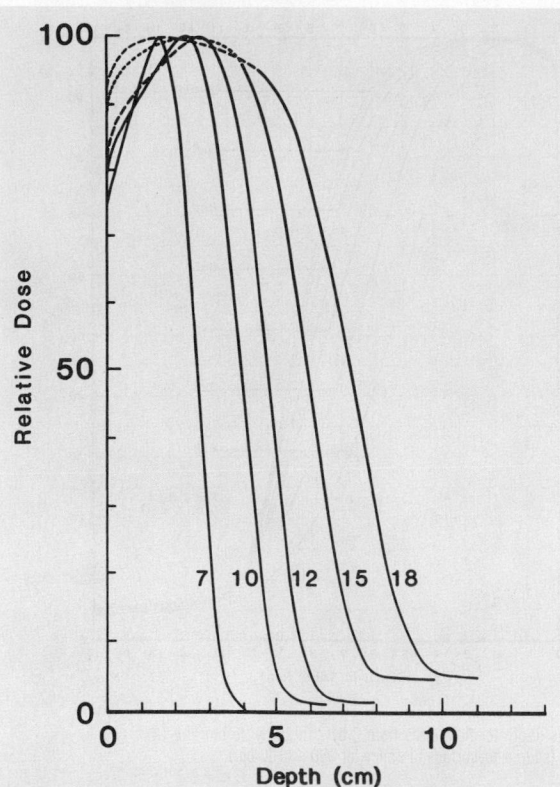

FIGURE 7.1. Energy dependence of depth dose. Plot of relative dose (%) versus depth for a 10 by 10 cm² field size for 7 to 18 MeV beams on a Siemens Mevatron 77 radiation therapy unit (source-to-surface distance, or SSD = 100 cm). (From Meyer JA, Palta JR, Hogstrom KR. Demonstration of relatively new electron dosimetry measurement techniques on the Mevatron 80. *Med Phys* 1984;11:670–677, with permission.)

3. The practical range (R_p) (maximum penetration) of the electrons increases as energy increases.
4. X-ray dose due to bremsstrahlung that lies beyond the electron dose component is characterized by its value (D_x), is taken from the PDD curve 10 cm beyond the practical range (R_p). D_x increases as energy increases.
5. The R_100 depth (dmax) can vary irregularly with depth and model of electron treatment machine; its dependence is insignificant for treatment planning, although it is significant to the medical physicist for constructing percent depth–dose data and in beam calibration.

Table 7.1 gives dosimetric parameters for a modern (0) linear accelerator.

Depth dose has a significant dependence on field size, and the dependence varies with incident electron energy. The primary reason for the field-size dependence is loss of side-scatter equilibrium, which has been discussed in detail by Hogstrom (37) and Kahn et al. (46). Figure 7.2A,B, which show the field-size dependence of percentage depth dose at 9 and 20 MeV, respectively, clearly illustrates that it is a greater issue at higher energies. Loss of side-scatter equilibrium, which begins first at the deeper depths, results in R_90 shifting toward the surface as field size decreases. As the field size gets even smaller, the maximum dose decreases, and when it is normalized to 100%, the relative dose at the surface, D_s, increases. Also, the effects on the distal portion of the depth–dose curve are greater. The most clinically significant effect is the decrease in R_90 with decreasing field size, which can require a greater energy than initially proposed for treatment using very small fields.

Depth–dose variations with SSD are usually minimal. Differences in the depth dose resulting from inverse square effect are small because electrons do not penetrate that deep (6 cm or less in the therapeutic region) and because the significant growth of penumbra width with SSD restricts the SSD in clinical practice to typically 115 cm or less. The primary effect of inverse square is that R_90 penetrates a few millimeters deeper at extended SSD at the higher energies, as illustrated in Figure 7.3. In relatively few cases (e.g., when the electron beam has a large component of collimator-scattered electrons) the variation in depth dose with SSD can become more significant. In such cases the collimator-scattered electrons are scattered out of the beam, resulting in a depth dose with a lower D_s and greater R_90 (87).

For rectangular fields, Hogstrom et al. (30) derived and others have confirmed (66,87) that percentage of depth dose can be calculated by taking the geometric mean of the percentage of depth doses for a square field of length dimension (L) and one of width dimension (W). That is:

$$\%D(d; LxW) = \sqrt{\%D(d; LxL) \cdot \%D(d; WxW)} \qquad (1)$$

If the square field, percentage of depth–dose curves do not have a common R_100, then the result of equation 1 must be

insignificant effect on depth dose (37,46). In the energy range of up to 20 MeV, a 10 by 10 cm² field size typically will achieve side-scatter equilibrium on central axis. The energy dependence of depth dose is illustrated in Figure 7.1, where central-axis depth dose is plotted for a 10 by 10 cm² field for energies in the range of 7 to 18 MeV. The family of curves illustrates how the dosimetric characteristics vary with the incident electron energy:

1. Surface dose (D_s) increases from approximately 75% to 95% as energy increases. The slow increase in dose from the surface to the depth of maximum dose (R_100) occurs as a result of electrons undergoing multiple Coulomb scattering in water (37).
2. Depth of distal 90% (R_90), often the therapeutic prescription depth, increases as energy increases.

Nominal Energy	Measured E_0 (MeV)	Measured E_p (MeV)	R_90: Depth of 90% (cm)	R_50: Depth of 50% (cm)	R_p (cm)	Dx (%)
6	5.55	6.08	1.53	2.38	2.95	0.1
9	8.41	8.84	2.69	3.61	4.33	0.3
12	11.77	12.23	3.85	5.05	6.02	0.9
16	15.63	16.02	5.10	6.71	7.900	1.6
20	19.62	20.78	6.14	8.42	10.25	2.1

Table 7.1 TRILOGY MEASURED ELECTRON DEPTHS (R_p, R_50) AND CALCULATED ENERGIES (E_p, E_0)

E_0: Average energy at the surface, where $E_0 = 2.33 \times R_{50}$.
E_p: Most probable electron energy at the surface, where $E_p = C_1 + C_2 R_p = C_3 R_p^2$; where C1, C2, and C3, are constants, with C1 = 0.22 MeV, C2 = 1.98 MeV cm^1, and C3 = 0.01025 MeV cm^2.

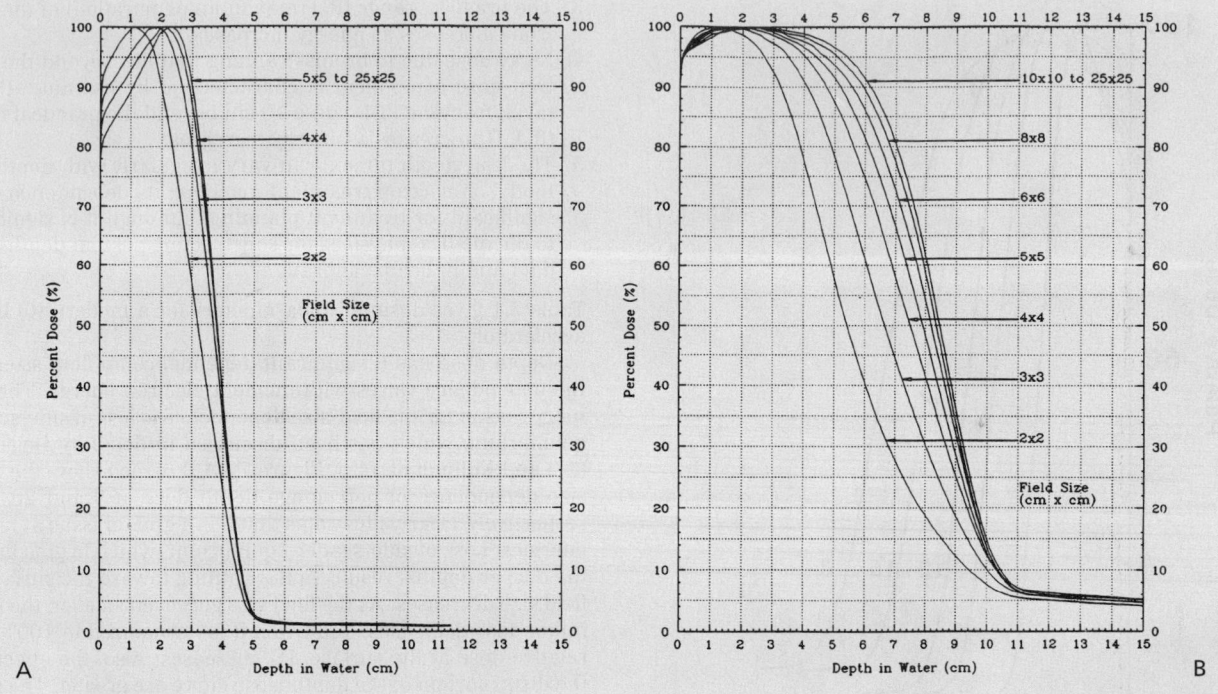

FIGURE 7.2. Field-size dependence of depth dose. Plot of percent dose versus depth for field sizes from 2 by 2 to 25 by 25 cm² for **(A)** 9-MeV and **(B)** 20-MeV beams on a Varian Clinac 2100C radiation therapy unit (source-to-surface distance, or SSD = 100 cm).

normalized such that its maximum equals 100%. This method is referred to as the *square-root method*.

In some instances (e.g., intraoperative, intraoral, or intravaginal cones) circular fields are used. In such cases, it will be necessary to measure their dose distributions independent of those determined for square or rectangular fields.

Usually, a collimating insert is placed inside an electron applicator to form an irregular-shaped field, occasionally blocking the central axis. In such cases, central-axis depth dose makes little sense, and the term *central-field depth dose* should be used, providing that the field has an axis of symmetry. In cases where the insert is irregular, the depth dose can be approximated using a rectangular-shaped field that approximates the irregular-shaped field (36). In highly irregular-shaped fields, the dose dis-

tribution should be calculated using an appropriate dose algorithm in a three-dimensional (3D) treatment-planning system. For very small fields, irregular or otherwise, it is highly recommended that PPD measurements be performed to properly determine prescriptive choices (i.e, R_{90}).

Off-Axis Dose

Dose distributions in the dimensions perpendicular to the central axis can be described by off-axis ratios (OAR). The OAR is defined as the ratio of dose at an off-axis position to that on the central axis at the same depth. Off-axis ratios measured in water are used to assess off-axis beam quality, which is

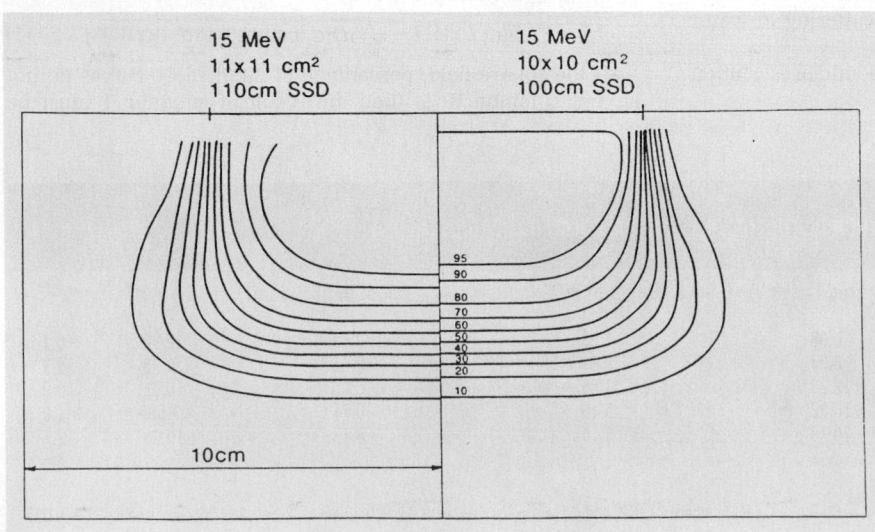

FIGURE 7.3. Source-to-surface distance (SSD) dependence of depth dose. Comparison of isodose plots for 15-MeV beam, 10 by 10 cm² at 100-cm SSD with 11 by 11 cm² field at 110-cm SSD. (From Hogstrom KR. Clinical electron-beam dosimetry: Basic dosimetry data. In: Purdy JA, ed. *Advances in radiation oncology physics: Dosimetry, treatment planning, and brachytherapy.* Woodbury: American Institute of Physics, Inc., 1991;390–429, with permission.)

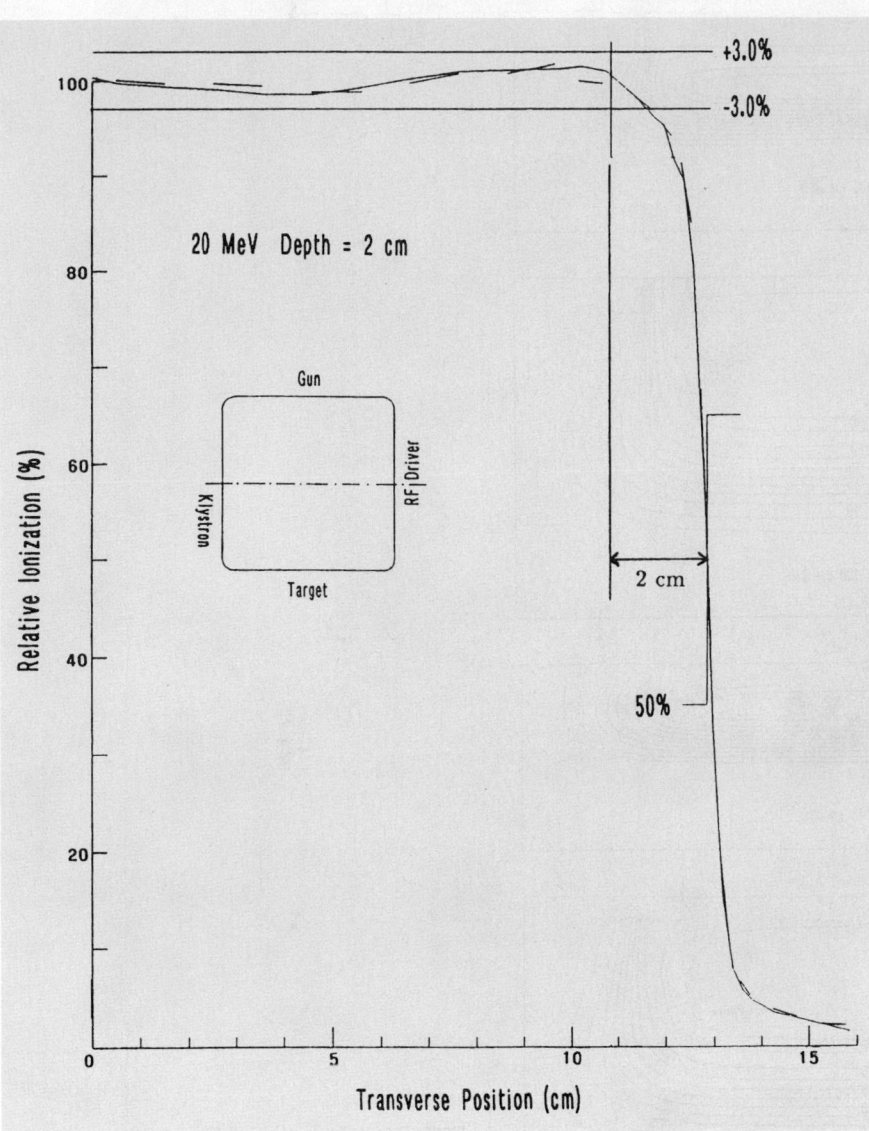

FIGURE 7.4. Beam uniformity verification. Plot of off-axis ratios versus position along a major axis. Data having a negative position (*dashed curve*) is reflected about central axis for comparison with data having a positive position (*solid curve*). Data measured at a depth of 2 cm in water at 100-cm SSD for a 20-MeV beam (Varian Clinac 2100C, 25 by 25 cm² open applicator).

characterized by flatness and symmetry in the uniform portion of the beam and by its falloff in the region of the penumbra (e.g., 90% to 10%, or 80% to 20%, respectively).

Manufacturers should be able to provide electron beams with a symmetry specification of 2% for opposing points in the beam and a flatness specification of ±3% of the *central-axis value* along the major axes (±4% along diagonals). The American Association of Physicists in Medicine (AAPM) Task Group 25 recommended that flatness and symmetry should be evaluated along major axes (lines containing central axis and perpendicular to the collimator edges) and along diagonal axes (46). Task Group 25 also recommended that flatness and symmetry be evaluated at depths near the surface and therapeutic depth. Practically, this is performed at R_{100}.

Flatness and symmetry are evaluated inside the penumbra, which usually is ensured by setting the boundaries of evaluation 2 cm inside the collimating edge $2\sqrt{2}$ cm along diagonals). When physicists acceptance test a treatment machine, and during subsequent annual reviews, they use the AAPM Task Group 40 recommendations of 2% symmetry and 5% flatness. This is usually performed for each energy with an average size applicator, but should be tested for each energy applicator during acceptance. Figure 7.4 shows the result for a typical accelerator performance evaluation (54).

Penumbra of electron beams is predetermined by the design of the beam flattening system, the air gap between the final collimator, and the scatter of electrons in water. Penumbra, a function of depth, is the root mean square addition of two penumbral components, one the result of the air gap and one the result of scatter in the water (30,38). This dependence is complex, but can be appreciated qualitatively by the illustration in Figure 7.5, which compares isodose plots for normal (100 cm) and extended (110 cm) SSD at 6 and 16 MeV, respectively. These data show that penumbra grows in a nonlinear fashion with depth, that air gap is more significant at the lower energies, and that scatter in water dominates at the higher energies. Fortunately, the complex dependence of penumbra can be modeled accurately in treatment-planning systems using the pencil-beam or more sophisticated dose algorithms (27,35–37).

Isodose Plots

Combining depth dose with off-axis ratios results in the 3D dose distribution, and the properties of the 3D dose distribution can

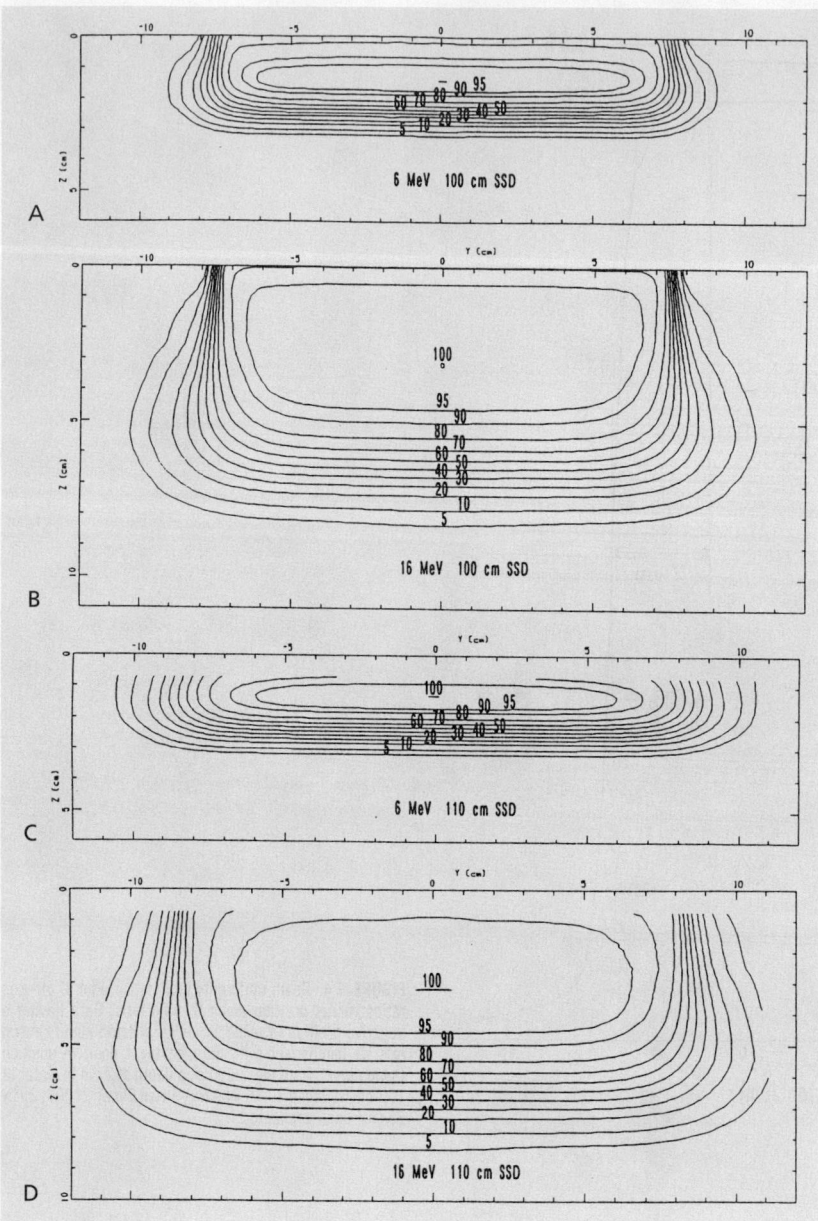

FIGURE 7.5. Variation of dose distribution with energy and SSD. Isodose plots (5% to 100%) in water for open 15 by 15 cm² applicator and for **(A)** 6 MeV, 100-cm SSD, **(B)** 16 MeV, 100-cm SSD, **(C)** 6 MeV, 110-cm SSD, and **(D)** 16 MeV, 110-cm SSD (Varian Clinac 2100C).

be appreciated by viewing 2D isodose contour plots in a plane containing the central axis and a major axis. Examples of these plots for a 15 by 15 cm² field are illustrated in Figure 7.5. As field width decreases or increases, the penumbra shape changes insignificantly, as it is most significantly influenced by air gaps and by collimation type. Collimating on the skin, for example, reduces penumbra significantly.

Data required for isodose contours are acquired for an inclusive spread of field sizes at each energy. Two-dimensional isodose contour plots and data are useful for manual treatment planning, input data required by dose algorithms, verification of dose calculated by a treatment-planning system, and quality assurance standards (22,37,46).

Dose in the Heterogeneous Patient

For most clinical circumstances, the ideal irradiation condition is for the electron beam to be incident normal to a flat surface with underlying homogeneous soft tissues. The dose distribu-

tion for this condition, similar to that for a water phantom described previously, contains a reasonably uniform dose inside the penumbra from the surface to R$_{90}$, and it has the sharpest possible fall-off laterally and with depth. As the angle of incidence deviates from normal, as the surface becomes irregular, and as internal heterogeneous tissues (e.g., air, lung, and bone) become present, the qualities of the dose distribution degrade (33). Internal heterogeneities can change the depth of beam penetration as a result of differences in the rate of energy loss, which can result in PTV underdose and critical structure overdose. Both irregular surfaces and internal heterogeneities create changes in side-scatter equilibrium, producing volumes of increased dose (hot spots) and decreased dose (cold spots), potentially leading to an increased dose to critical structures and decreased dose to the PTV (26,33). These pertubations can be reduced or eliminated by modifying the treatment technique.

Irregular Surfaces

Two geometries that illustrate the effects on the dose distribution caused by an irregular patient surface are the sloped

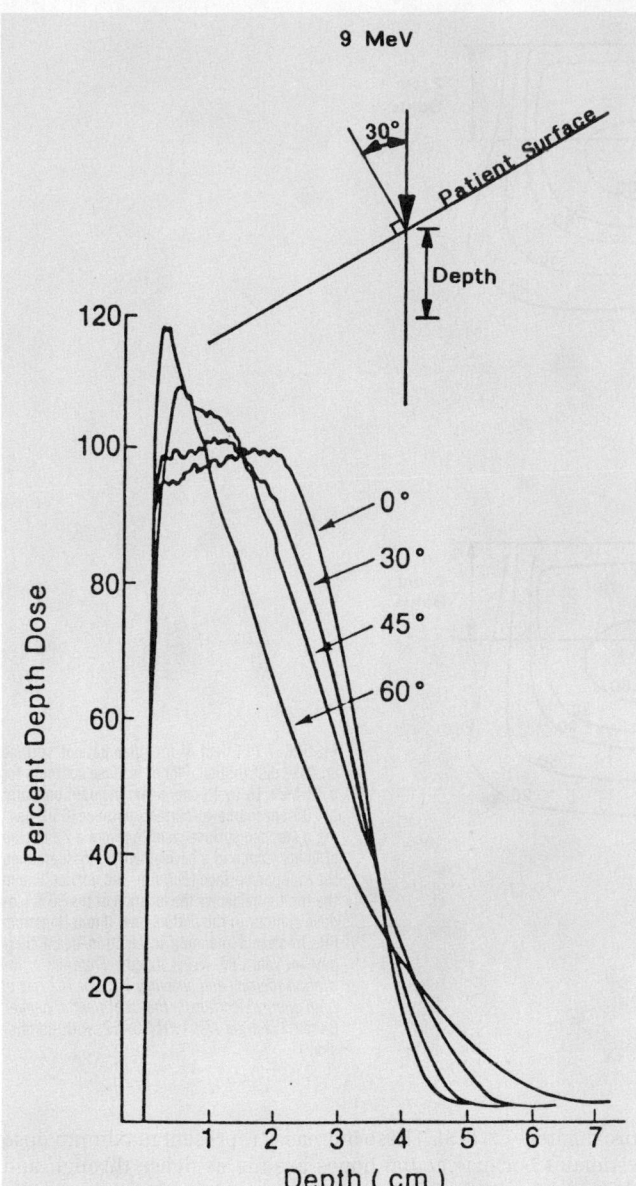

FIGURE 7.6. Effect of angle of incidence on depth dose. Dose versus depth for a 9-MeV beam incident on water angled 0 degrees to 60 degrees from the normal. (From Ekstrand KE, Dixon RL. The problem of obliquely incident beams in electron-beam treatment planning. *Med Phys* 1982;9:276–278, with permission.)

the lateral chest wall cannot be encompassed with a wide anterior beam, as the surface dose would be too great and the penetration would be too little.

Any time a sharp gradient (stepped surface) occurs on the patient's surface, side-scatter equilibrium will be lost, resulting in a cold spot beneath the proximal surface and a hot spot beneath the distal surface (7,33,35,85). This can occur as a result of a bolus edge, surgical defects, or normal anatomy. For example, in the use of uniform thickness bolus that partially covers a field, a 90-degree edge can result in hot or cold spots as great as 20%, as illustrated in Figure 7.7. In such a case, the bolus should be tapered as much as possible; the results of the 45-degree tapered bolus in Figure 7.7 show a reduction in the hot spot but, more significantly, an increased coverage of the 90% isodose contour. The nose is a protrusion that creates a cold spot beneath itself, often the location of the tumor (31,33,35). The ear canal (Fig. 7.8) and surgical voids, which are characterized by a depression in the patient's surface, can result in hot spots in excess of 50%, depending on void dimension and beam energy (71,79). Such depressions normally should be filled with some type of bolus material. Normal anatomy contains many irregular surface depressions and protrusions (e.g., the ear canal and the nose, respectively) and should be accounted for by accurate treatment planning.

Air Cavities

The influence of an internal air cavity is illustrated in Figure 7.9, which compares isodose contours beneath an air cavity to those without the air cavity. Results show that (a) the isodose contours in the shadow of air are shifted distally, (b) the dose beneath the air cavity increases as a result of loss of side-scatter equilibrium, and (c) the influence of the air increases laterally with depth. Internal air cavities of clinical interest primarily occur in treatment of the head and neck (e.g., nasal passages, ethmoid sinuses, maxillary sinuses, larynx, and mastoids) (33,35).

Another significant effect is the reduction in dose in unit density tissue lateral to an air cavity. Electrons scattering from the unit density tissue into the air are not replaced because air is unable to scatter an equal amount back into the unit density tissue. Frequently, nose tumors can spread into the septum, in which case bolus should be used to eliminate or reduce underdosing.

Lung

In lung, electrons can penetrate three to four times farther than in unit density tissue. This is demonstrated in Figure 7.10, where isodose contours from a typical electron chest wall treatment are compared with those in which the lung is assumed unit density. Assuming a given dose of 50 Gy, the 40% isodose contour corresponds to 20 Gy, approximately the threshold for pneumonitis, if significant lung volume is irradiated. Ignoring the low density of lung would grossly underestimate the volume of lung above 20 Gy (35).

This effect increases with energy. For example, increasing the beam energy from 9 to 12 MeV results in an additional 1.5 cm of penetration in waterlike tissue (electrons lose energy at a rate of approximately 2 MeV/cm in water), and this corresponds to as much as 6.0 cm in lung (assuming a lung density of 25%). Consider the patient whose chest wall thickness requires an energy of 10 MeV for treatment and that 12 MeV must be selected. This results in as much as 4 cm in depth of needless irradiation in lung, unless 1 cm of bolus is used to effectively lower the energy incident on the patient to 10 MeV.

skin surface and the stepped skin surface. Figure 7.6 illustrates changes in the depth–dose curve as a result of nonnormal incidence of an electron beam onto a flat surface. Compared with normal incidence, the nonnormal incident, central-axis, depth–dose curve shows: (a) an increased surface dose, (b) an increased dose maximum, (c) a decreased penetration of the therapeutic dose (R_{90}), and (d) an increased range of penetration (18,46). These changes can be clinically significant, particularly at angles of incidence >30 degrees from the normal. Such conditions can occur when irradiating curved patient surfaces with large fields (e.g., chest wall, limbs, neck, and scalp). Also, it should be appreciated that the depth of R_{90} is specified along the central axis of the beam, and if the depth is taken perpendicular to the surface, then the depth is further reduced (approximately) by the factor cos (Ø), where Ø is the deviation of the incident angle from the normal. These data explain why

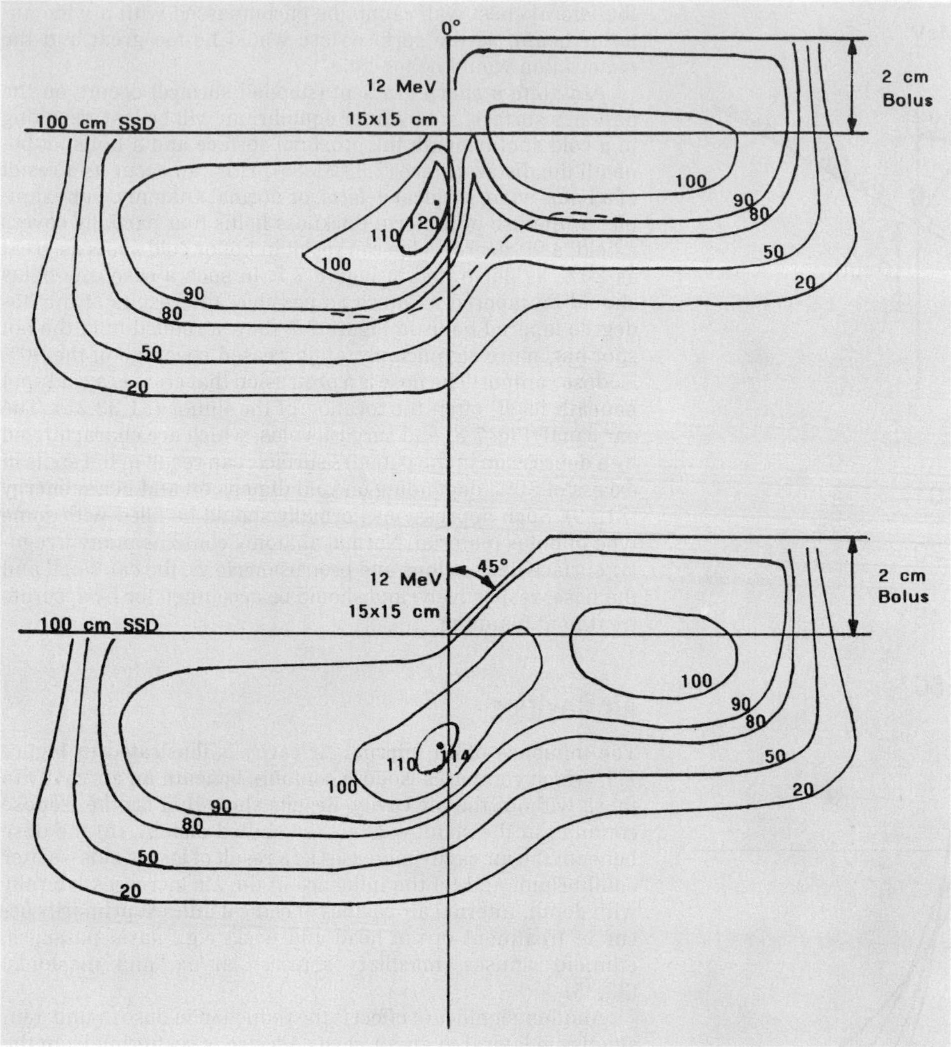

FIGURE 7.7. Effect of irregular patient surface on dose distribution. Plot of isodose contours for a 12-MeV, 15 by 15 cm^2 beam incident on water at 100-cm source-to-surface distance (SSD) having a stepped surface resulting from a 2-cm slab of bolus (*top*) and a beveled edge (45 degree) on the stepped surface (*bottom*). The dashed line in the top figure shows the location of the 90% isodose contour in the bottom one. (From Hogstrom KR. Treatment planning in electron-beam therapy. In: Vaeth JM, Meyer JL, eds. *Frontiers of radiation therapy and oncology Vol. 25: The role of high energy electrons in the treatment of cancer.* Basel: S. Karger AG, 1991;30–52, with permission.)

Bone

The influence of bone is illustrated in Figure 7.11, which compares isodose contours beneath hard bone to those without the bone. The results show that:

1. The isodose contours in the shadow of the bone are shifted proximally,
2. Dose outside (inside) the bone-water interface increases (decreases) by approximately 5% as a result of loss of side-scatter equilibrium, and
3. The lateral dimension of the region having its dose perturbed by the bone increases with depth.

Actual bones are not uniformly dense throughout their cross-section, and in most cases their edges are not parallel to the incident beam. Both differences decrease the influence of bone in generating inhomogeneity in the patient's dose distribution. Dense bones that significantly affect the dose distribution include the mandible, bones of the skull (e.g., frontal bone and zygoma in orbit treatment or temporal bone in treatment of parotid), clavicles, and vertebral processes (e.g., craniospinal irradiation).

Another question that occasionally arises is What is the clinical significance of the increase in dose in or around bone due to increased scatter? The maximum dose increase expected as a result of backscattered electrons is 5%, and the maximum dose increase expected inside bone and in adjacent exit tissues is ap-

proximately 7% (83). These increases represent maximum dose estimates because actual bones are not as dense through and through as are the bone substitute in which these data were taken. These estimates of the increased dose are not expected to be clinically significant. In fact, untoward effects in or around bone that can be attributed to dosimetry have not been observed in patients treated with electron-beam therapy.

Dose Prescription and Calculation of Monitor Units

Dose Prescription

It is recommended that dose be prescribed to given dose or 90% of given dose. Intermediate or lower prescription (95%, 85%, 80%) can be prescribed if the energy (typically stepped in 3 to 4 MeV increments) choices are too course to maintain a single baseline prescription recipe. Given dose is defined as the maximum central-axis dose in a water phantom at the SSD of the patient for the energy, applicator, and field size identical to that used for patient treatment. If the field shape is irregular, then the field size is taken to be a rectangular field representative of the irregular field shape. The most representative rectangular field is not well defined; however, Hogstrom et al.

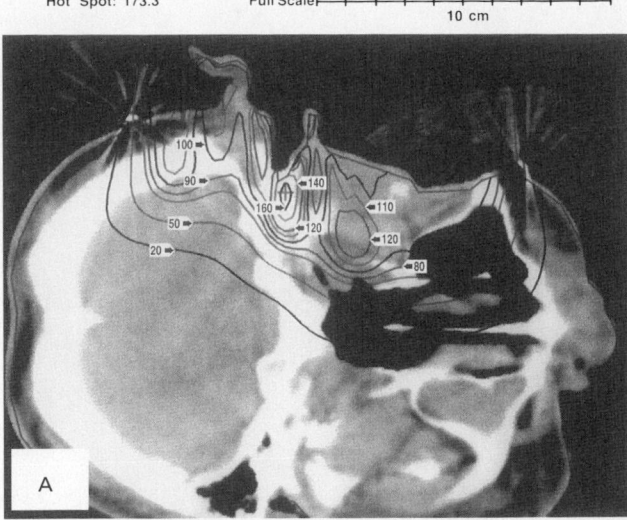

Hot Spot: 173.3   Full Scale

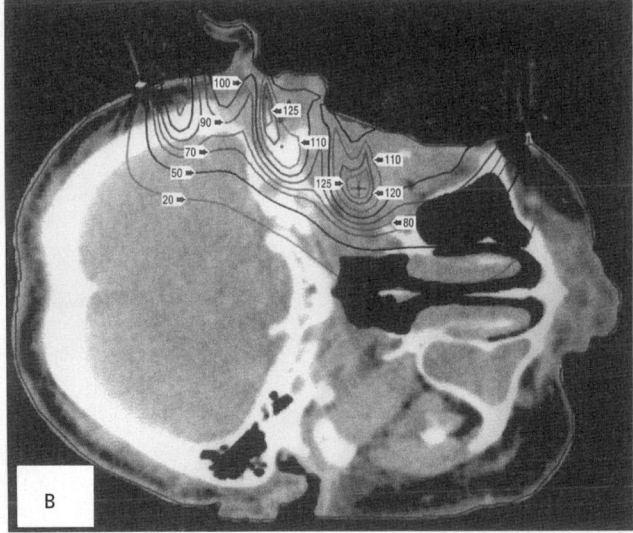

Hot Spot: 130.2   Full Scale

FIGURE 7.8. Impact of irregular surface anatomy on dose distribution. A 15-MeV electron beam irradiates the left side of a patient treated for dermal squamous carcinoma with perineural invasion. A beeswax bolus protects the posterior cranial fossa and the maxillary sinus. Isodose contours, expressed as a percentage of given dose, show **(A)** how the ear canal results in an unacceptable hot spot of 160% to the middle ear and **(B)** how filling the ear canal with bolus (saline solution) eliminates that hot spot. The residual hot spot of 125% is a result of the external ear. (From Morrison WH, Wong PF, Starkschall G, et al. Water bolus for electron irradiation of the ear canal. *Int J Radiat Oncol Biol Phys* 1995;33:479–483, with permission.)

(27) have provided one methodology for determining its estimate.

It is recommended that dose be prescribed to given dose or a percentage of it and not to a point in the patient. It is quite possible that a dose prescription point in the patient could be in a region of increased or decreased dose because of tissue heterogeneity or irregular surface, which could result in PTV underdose or overdose, respectively.

Calculation of Monitor Units

Monitor units can be determined by

$$MU = \frac{D_{prescribed}/\%D}{O(E, C, LxW, SSD)} \qquad (2)$$

where $D_{prescribed}$ is the prescribed dose, $\%D$ is the percentage of given dose to which dose is prescribed (e.g., 90%), and $O(E,$

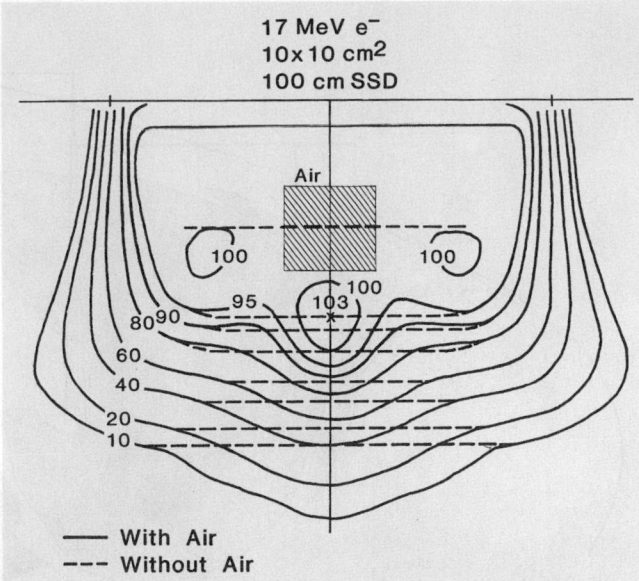

FIGURE 7.9. Effect of internal air cavity on underlying dose distribution. Dose calculated by the pencil-beam algorithm (PBA) for a 2 by 2 cm² cylinder of air located 2 cm below the surface in water is compared to that in its absence. (From Hogstrom KR. Dosimetry of electron heterogeneities. In: Wright AE, Boyer AL, eds. *Advances in radiation therapy treatment planning.* New York: American Institute of Physics, Inc., 1983;223–243, with permission.)

$C, LxW, SSD)$ is the output (dose per monitor unit) for a beam of energy E, applicator C, field size LxW, and SSD. To use this methodology, the medical physicist must measure dose output as a function of square field size and SSD for each energy-applicator combination at the time of commissioning the accelerator. Output for rectangular fields can be determined using the *square-root method* of Mills et al. (69,70) and Shiu et al. (87):

$$O(E,C,LxW,SSD) = [O(E,C,LxL,SSD) \cdot O(E,C,WxW,SSD)]^{1/2} \qquad (3)$$

Output for rectangular fields also can be determined using an equivalent square method (5,46,47,66); however, Biggs et al. (5) recommend limiting this method to an aspect ratio ($L{:}W$) of 2:1. The square-root method is not limited to the aspect ratio, and Shiu et al. (87) have shown it to be more accurate. Figure 7.12 illustrates beam output data at 9 MeV for four common applicators used on the Varian Clinac 2100C (Varian Medical Systems, Palo Alto, CA) at 100 cm SSD.

Output at extended SSD can be determined by either the air-gap method or the effective-source method (46). The effective-source method is covered in detail by Khan (47). The air-gap method has a sounder physical basis. Although both methods give similar answers, only the air-gap method will be covered here (66). Output at extended SSD is given by the product of output at the nominal SSD (SSD_0), the air-gap factor (fair), and an inverse square term,

$$O(E,C,LxW,SSD) = O(E,C,LxW,SSD_0)f_{air}(E,LxW,SSD)$$
$$\times \left(\frac{SSD_o + R_{100}}{SSD + R_{100}}\right) \qquad (4)$$

f_{air} is determined by measuring dose output for square fields at the extended SSD and then solving equation 4. For rectangular fields, the air gap factor is determined using the square-root method (87):

$$f_{air}(E,LxW,SSD) = \sqrt{f_{air}(E,LxL,SSD) \cdot f_{air}(E,WxW,SSD)} \qquad (5)$$

As f_{air} is assumed independent of applicator, the dose output needs to be measured only for the smallest applicator that

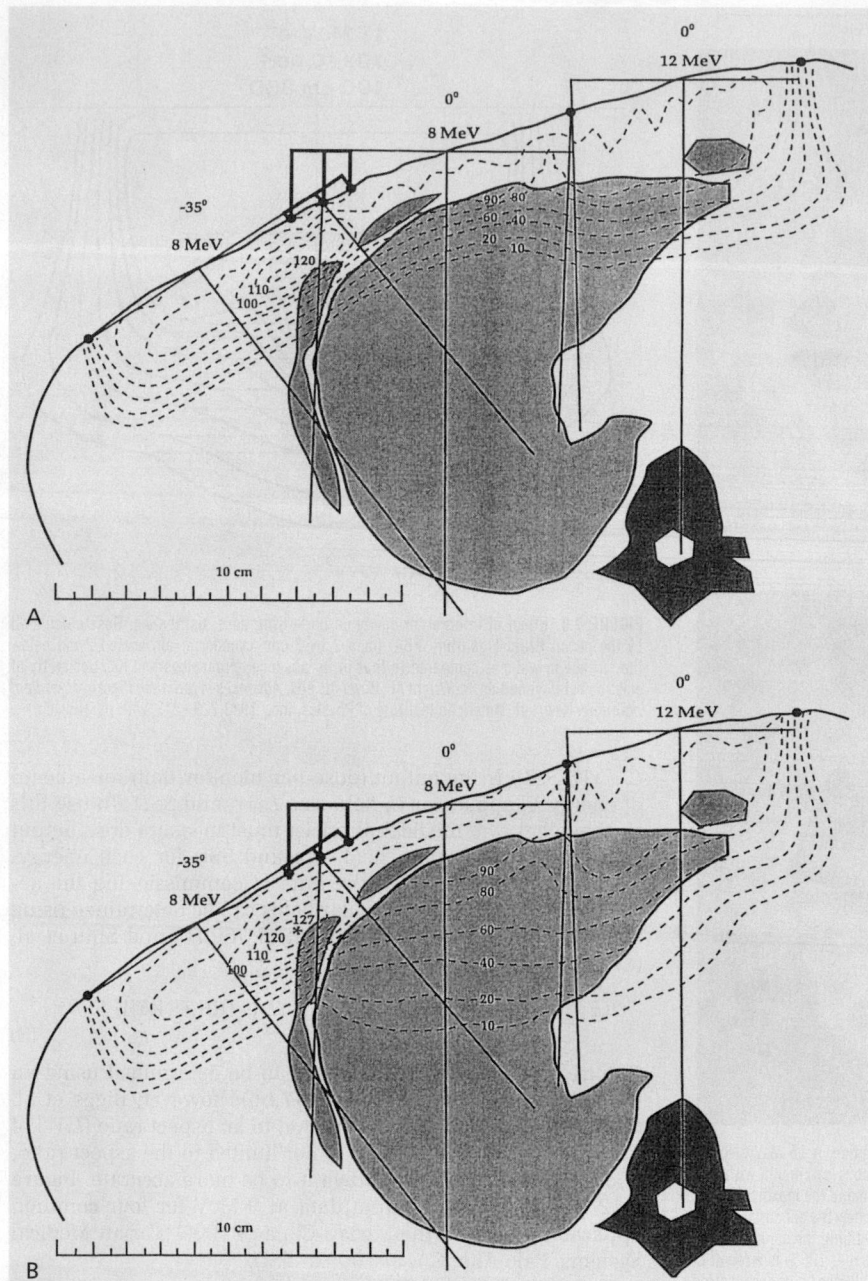

FIGURE 7.10. Effect of lung on dose distribution underlying chest wall. Comparison of dose calculated by the pencil-beam algorithm (PBA) for 8-MeV chest-wall irradiation, assuming **(A)** patient is water and **(B)** heterogeneous anatomy based on computed tomography data.

contains the square field size. Figure 7.13 plots the square field air gap factors for the 9-MeV beam of the Varian Clinac 2100C for SSD from 100 to 120 cm. For a more detailed explanation of dose output and sample calculations of monitor units for electron beams, refer to Hogstrom et al. (36). Another practical option is to fix incremented SSDs to be used clinically (i.e., 100, 105, 110, 115 cm) and establish tabular outputs for each energy/applicator SSD combination.

Calculation of Dose in Patient

Standards for Patient Dose Calculations

Sound treatment-planning decisions require accurate dose calculation in the patient. Therefore, the following recommenda-

tions are made for electron-beam treatment planning. First, dose should be calculated in the full three dimensions to allow for evaluation of dose homogeneity in the PTV, coverage of the PTV by the 90% dose contour, and dose to critical structures. Second, the dose algorithm should account for patient heterogeneity. Failure to properly account for patient heterogeneity can result in failure to appreciate dose heterogeneity, PTV underdose, or normal-tissue overdose (26,33,35). Third, the dose algorithm should be accurate, and those conditions for which this is not the case should be understood to allow proper interpretation of the dose calculations.

To expand on the final recommendation, a dose algorithm must meet certain criteria to be most effective in the clinic (32). First, it should be accurate to within 4% in regions of low-dose gradients or within 2 mm in regions of high-dose gradient (e.g., penumbra or depth-dose falloff region). Second, the dose algorithm should be commissioned easily by a qualified medical

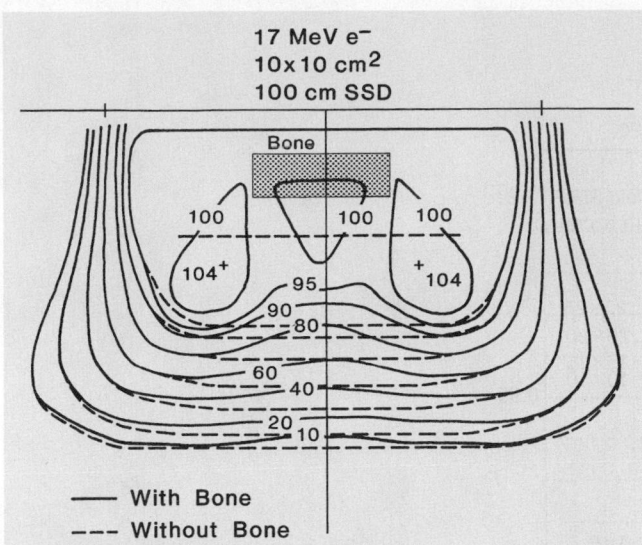

FIGURE 7.11. Effect of hard bone on underlying dose distribution. Dose calculated by the pencil-beam algorithm (PBA) for a 3 by 1 cm² cylinder of hard bone substitute located 1 cm below the surface in water is compared to that in its absence. (From Hogstrom KR. Dosimetry of electron heterogeneities. In: Wright AE, Boyer AL, eds. *Advances in radiation therapy treatment planning.* New York: American Institute of Physics, Inc., 1983;223–243, with permission.)

physicist. Third, the accuracy of the dose algorithm should be well documented. Since 1981, the PBA has best met this requirement. Presently, several new, more accurate algorithms, both analytical and Monte Carlo–based, are being implemented into commercial treatment-planning systems and will replace or supplement the PBA in due time. Regardless of the algorithm, it is the medical physicist's responsibility to commission the algorithm, to understand its accuracy, and to train medical dosimetrists and radiation oncologists in its use.

Dose Algorithms

For the past 20 years, the standard methodology for dose calculation in the patient has been the PBA. Various versions have been implemented into commercial treatment-planning systems and many are based on the Hogstrom algorithm (30,31). As computing power increased, it was possible to implement the algorithms into 3D format (89). Detailed instructions for commissioning the dose algorithm and documentation of its accuracy have been published (31,32,38). The PBA has been shown to be quite accurate in water at standard and extended SSD, correctly predicting the changes in penumbra (35–37). It is also quite accurate in predicting changes in dose resulting from oblique incidence and irregular surfaces (31,32). Regarding internal heterogeneities, it correctly predicts the penetration in lung and the growth of the penumbra width in lung (30,32); however, it tends to underestimate the dose in lung near the mediastinum as a result of its central axis approximation (32). In bone, it correctly predicts the shortening of the dose penetration behind the bone, and it slightly underestimates (<5%) the magnitude of the hot and cold spots under the edge of a thick hard bone such as the mandible (31). The PBA does not predict the increased dose (<5%) resulting from backscatter at the proximal tissue–bone interface, nor does it predict the increased dose (>7%) in bone resulting from increased scatter. The PBA underestimates the hot and cold spots under the air–tissue interfaces (31,32).

New dose algorithms that are accurate to 4% or better are becoming available in commercial treatment-planning systems. Many of these algorithms have been reviewed by Hogstrom and Steadham (32). One of these is the pencil-beam redefinition algorithm (PBRA), whose commissioning is similar to that of the conventional PBA, although its accuracy is significantly improved (8,9,84). Figure 7.14 illustrates the improvement of the PBRA.

Many of the newer algorithms are based on Monte Carlo methods, which allow them to be quite accurate (19,41,61,73,

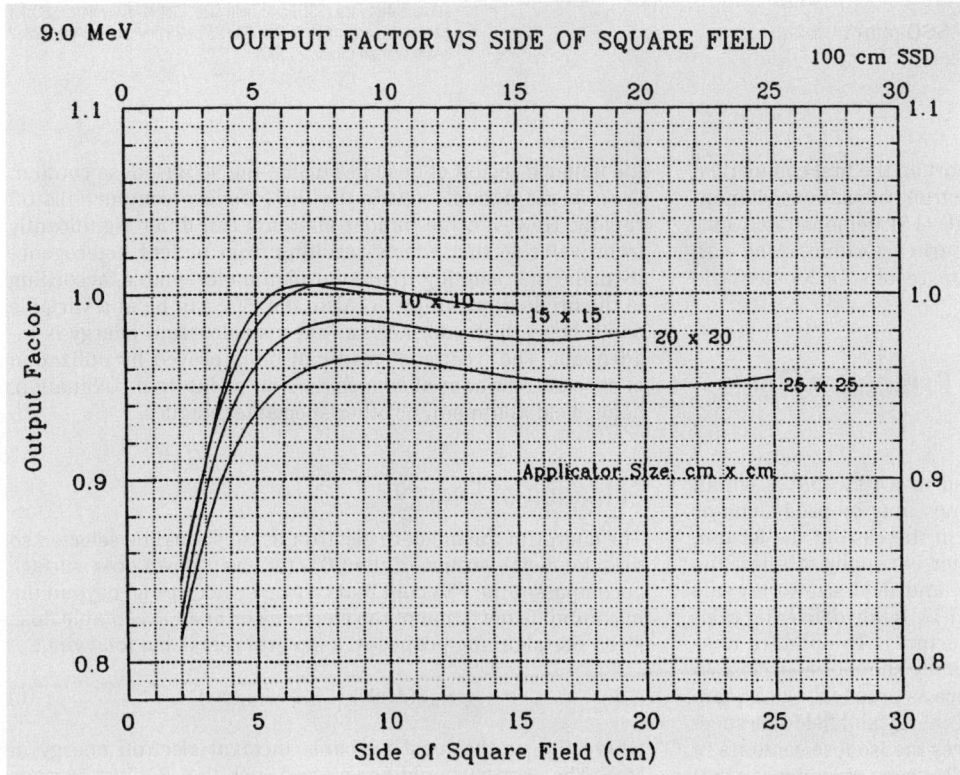

FIGURE 7.12. Field-size dependence of output (dose/monitor unit). Plot of output factor (cGy/MU) versus side of square field from 2 by 2 cm² to the open applicator for four applicators and for the 9-MeV beam of a Varian Clinac 2100C.

Overview and Basic Science of Radiation Oncology

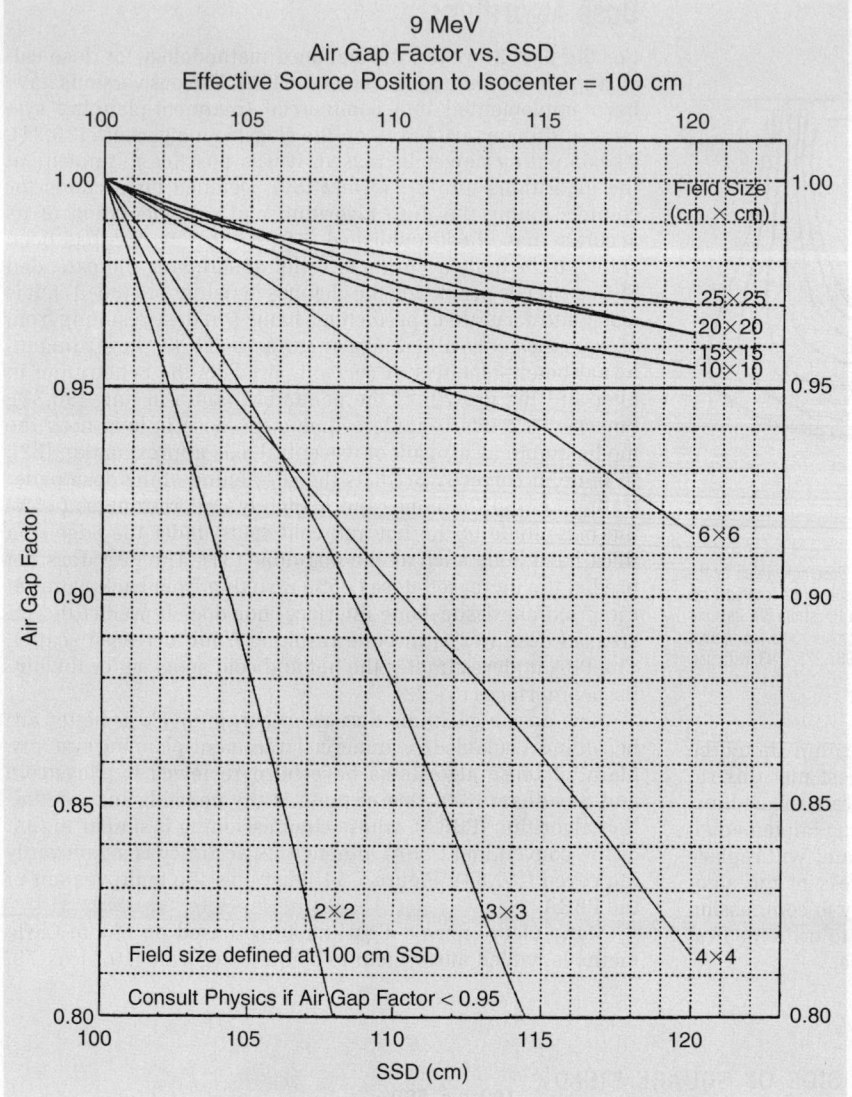

FIGURE 7.13. Dependence of air-gap factors on source-to-surface distance (SSD) and field size. Plot of f_{air} versus SSD for field sizes ranging from 2 by 2 to 25 by 25 cm² and for the 9-MeV beam (Varian Clinac 2100C).

74). Cygler et al. (10) published a report on the first commercial system using Monte Carlo–based electron calculations, demonstrating excellent results. Ding et al. (15) demonstrated outstanding results for a macro–Monte Carlo algorithm, along with a companion report showing superior results for Monte Carlo compared with PBA (14).

Treatment-Planning Principles, Tools, and Methods

Electron therapy usually is restricted to a PTV that is within 6 cm of the patient's surface. Electrons may be used alone or in conjunction with photon beams. In the case of the former, the objective of the treatment planner is usually to select the appropriate beam direction, energy, and field size to provide as uniform a dose as possible to the PTV while delivering minimal dose to normal tissue and structures. To optimize dose homogeneity, the beam direction usually should be as close to normal incidence to the patient surface as practical. Once beam direction is specified, the selection of energy and field size specification follows. Figure 7.15 compares the isodose contours in water with the beam edges and R90. Electrons are unique in that

the uniform region of dose lies inside the 90% isodose contour. Dose in the patient outside the 90% isodose contour falls off rapidly. However, the patient anatomy can differ significantly from water so that effects resulting from patient heterogeneity make the resulting treatment plan unacceptable, according to the original prescription. Also, the PTV can be at a variable depth beneath the surface so that a single beam energy is inadequate. The treatment plan can be improved by utilization of special treatment aids such as skin or internal collimation, bolus, field abutment, or other special techniques.

Selection of Energy

The energy of the incident electron beam should be selected so that the distal surface of the 90% (of given dose) dose surface encompasses the PTV and that critical structures lie beyond the maximum penetration of the electrons or at an acceptable dose level. For planning purposes, a general rule is the following:

$$E_{p,0}(MeV) \sim 3.3 \cdot R_{90}(cm) \tag{6}$$

where $E_{p,0}$ is the most probable incident electron energy in MeV. The energy should be selected such that R_{90} just exceeds

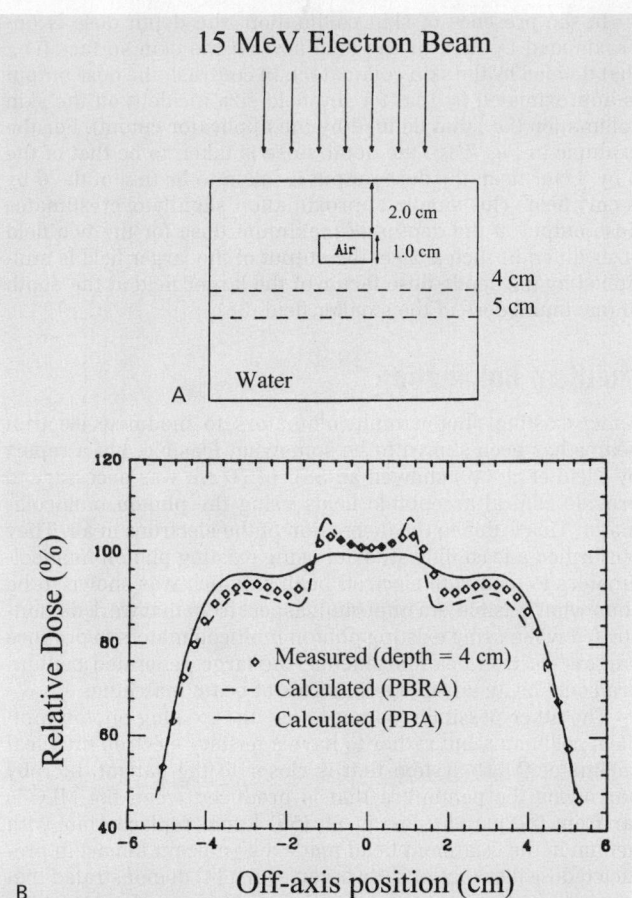

FIGURE 7.14. Evaluation of accuracy of dose algorithms below air cavity. **A:** Dose is measured distal to an internal air cavity. **B:** Measured dose profile at a depth of 4 cm is compared to that calculated by the pencil-beam algorithm and the pencil-beam redefinition algorithm; PBA, pencil-beam algorithm; PRBA, pencil-beam redefinition algorithm. (From Shiu AS, Hogstrom KR. Pencil-beam redefinition algorithm for electron dose distributions. *Med Phys* 1991;18:7–18, with permission.)

the maximum depth of the PTV. This approximation is true in water for field sizes large enough to have side-scatter equilibrium on the central axis. For small field sizes that do not have side-scatter equilibrium, R_{90} will be less, so a higher energy might be required. Also, heterogeneous tissue (e.g., bone or air) can affect the penetration requiring greater or lesser energy, respectively.

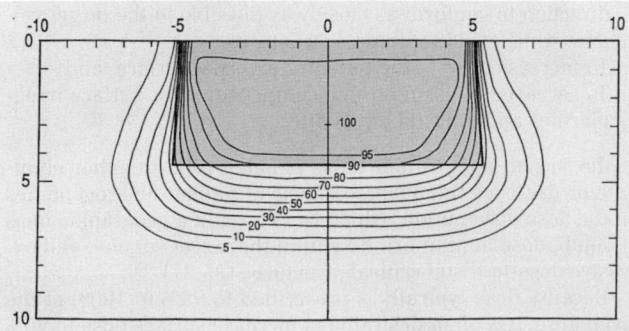

FIGURE 7.15. Plot of isodose curves for a 15-MeV, 10 by 10 cm² electron beam in water (source-to-surface distance, or SSD = 100 cm). Note the shape of the 90% isodose contour with respect to the shaded area, which is framed by the diverging field edges and the R_{90} depth.

Similarly, for planning purposes, a general rule is the following:

$$E_{p,0}(MeV) = 2 \cdot R_p(cm) \qquad (7)$$

where R_p is the practical range in centimeters of the electron beam (35). The treatment planner can select an energy such that R_p is less than the minimal depth of a critical structure. This approximation has no field-size limitation; however, as before, heterogeneous tissue (e.g., bone, lung, or air) can affect the penetration, allowing greater or lesser energy.

As an example of how to use these general rules, consider irradiating the posterior cervical nodes of the neck with electrons to spare the spinal cord because its dose is already near tolerance. If the maximum depth of the nodes is 3 cm and the minimum depth of the spinal cord is 6 cm, then equations 6 and 7 indicate that the minimum energy to cover the PTV is 9.9 MeV and the maximum energy that protects the spinal cord is 12 MeV, respectively. Hence, beam energies in the range of 10 to 12 MeV should be acceptable. In all cases, the energy of the beam should be confirmed by performing a 3D dose calculation for the planned treatment using a CT representation of the patient. Bolus may be strategically used to tune the beam penetration either globally or in discrete areas.

Design of Electron Collimation

Electron collimation consists of multiple collimating components; however, the electron field shape usually is defined by an applicator's collimating insert and/or skin collimation. Custom electron collimators are constructed from lead or low melting-point lead alloy (Lipowitz metal). The lead thickness in millimeters required to stop the primary electrons equals one-half the incident most probable energy of the electron beam in MeV (37,46). To account for small variations in thickness resulting from the lead-sheet manufacturing process, a 1-mm surplus can be added. That is:

$$t_{Pb}(mm) = 0.5 \cdot E_{p,0}(MeV) + 1 \qquad (8)$$

For example, an 18-MeV beam requires 10 mm of lead. Lipowitz metal comprised mostly of lead along with bismuth has a density 20% less than that of lead; therefore, its thickness should be 20% greater. For example, an 18-MeV beam requires 12 mm of Lipowitz metal. Lipowitz metal collimating inserts usually are fabricated at a constant thickness—namely, that sufficient for the greatest energy on the treatment machine. For a machine whose maximum energy is 20 MeV, the Lipowitz metal thickness should be a minimum of 13 mm.

Skin collimation thickness is usually available in units of 0.0625-inch lead sheets and normally is taken to be the minimum thickness necessary to reduce the collimator's weight. The maximum possible dose beneath the skin collimation occurs at the skin surface with no air gap between the two (46,66). The transmitted dose, which is the result of bremsstrahlung photons from the incident beam and those generated by electrons stopping in the lead, is slightly greater than that with no lead present. It is recommended that a table of measured dose under the lead, as a function of lead thickness, is available for each beam energy (37). As the air gap between the lead and the patient increases, the transmitted dose to the patient decreases. These values can be measured at the time of beam commissioning. If not, and for cases where precise determination of dose beneath a block is critical, in vivo dosimetry (e.g., thermoluminescent dosimetry) should be used.

In designing the shape of the aperture of a collimating insert, due consideration is made for the penumbra. Typically, there is approximately a 1-cm margin between the projected edge of the collimator and outer boundary of target volume when both are projected to the isocenter. This margin varies with energy, depth, and air gap, and it only can be appreciated by utilization of isodose curves (see Figs. 7.5 and 7.15). Again, the adequacy of the margin between the aperture and PTV should be confirmed by performing a 3D dose calculation for the planned treatment using a CT representation of the patient.

Skin Collimation

The closer the field-defining collimator is to the patient, the sharper the beam's penumbra; hence, skin collimation provides the sharpest possible penumbra. Because of the significant effort often required to fabricate skin collimation, its use is restricted to applications for which it has the greatest benefit, for example: (a) small-field treatments, (b) providing maximal protection to adjacent critical structures, (c) reducing penumbra beneath a bolus, (d) reducing penumbra when treating at an extended air gap, and (e) reducing penumbra in electron arc therapy. Proper use of skin collimation requires that it be in contact with the skin surface and that it extend sufficiently inwardly and outwardly to intercept the penumbra from upstream collimation (28–30).

The utility of skin collimation for small-field treatments is illustrated in Figure 7.16. A 6-MeV, 3 by 3 cm² field with a 10-cm air gap (collimator to surface) is essentially all penumbra, resulting in an unsatisfactory dose distribution. However, by opening the collimator to 6 by 6 cm² and then forming the 3 by 3-cm² field using skin collimation, the dose distribution becomes clinically satisfactory. This application is used for treatment of the eyelid, nose, and other small target volumes.

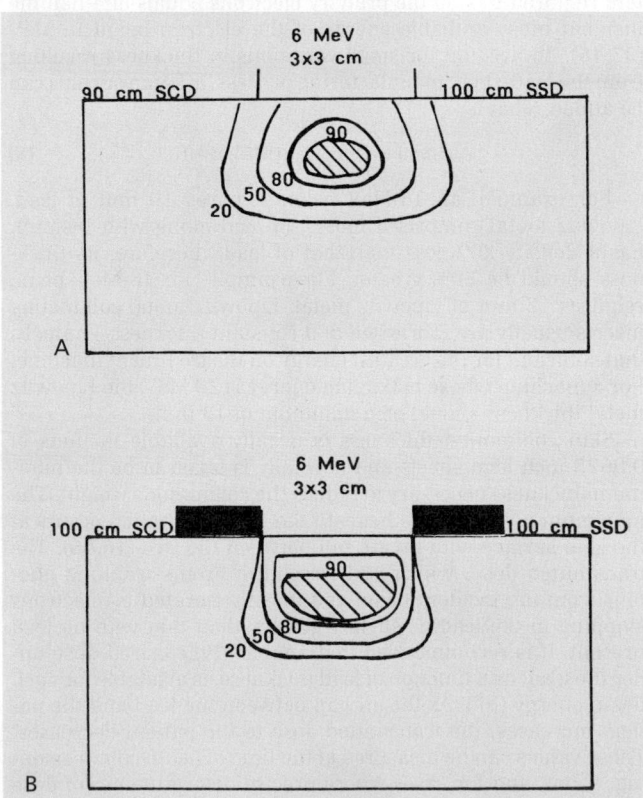

FIGURE 7.16. Impact of skin collimation for small electron fields. Isodose plots are compared for results of a computer simulation of a 6-MeV electron beam in water for **(A)** a 3 by 3 cm² field formed by an applicator insert 10 cm above the patient and **(B)** a 3 by 3 cm² field formed by collimation at the surface with a 6 by 6 cm² applicator insert 10 cm above the patient. (From Hogstrom, KR. Clinical electron-beam dosimetry: Basic dosimetry data. In: Purdy JA, ed. *Advances in radiation oncology physics: Dosimetry, treatment planning, and brachytherapy.* Woodbury: American Institute of Physics, Inc., 1991;390–429, with permission.)

In the presence of skin collimation, the depth dose is approximated by that for the field size on the skin surface (i.e., that defined by the skin collimator). In contrast, the dose output is approximated by that for the field size incident on the skin collimation (i.e., that defined by the applicator cutout). For the example in Fig. 7.16, the depth dose is taken to be that of the 3 by 3 cm² field; the dose output is taken to be that of the 6 by 6 cm² field. This simple approximation slightly overestimates dose output, if the depths of maximum dose for the two field sizes differ. In such a case, the output of the larger field is multiplied by the depth–dose factor of the larger field at the depth of maximum dose of the smaller field (36).

Multileaf Collimation

Using existing photon multicollimators to modulate electron beams has been shown to be somewhat feasible, but a report by Klein et al. (49) showed an SSD of 70 cm was necessary to provide clinical acceptable fields using the photon multicollimator. This is due to the dispersion of the electrons in air. They performed a feasibility study of using existing photon multicollimators to modulate electron beams, which was shown to be somewhat feasible. An important aspect from that work demonstrated when using existing photon multicollimators to produce narrow electron-beam segments, the large generated penumbra could be an advantage in terms of beam matching.

The other possibility is not to use the existing photon multileaf collimator, but rather to have a tertiary electron multileaf collimator (MLC) system that is closer to the patient, thereby narrowing the penumbra that is produced when the MLC is far from the patient. Lee et al. (56) found replacing air with helium in the treatment head made a significant impact in predicted dose distributions. Karlsson et al. (44) demonstrated that penumbra, effective source position, field shape, and matching could be optimized by replacing air with helium in the treatment head below the MLC leaves and by shifting the position of the scattering foils, monitor chamber, and MLC position.

Bolus

Bolus is an essential tool for the delivery of optimal electron radiation therapy. Electron bolus is defined as water- or near water-equivalent material that normally is placed either in direct contact with the patient's skin surface, close to the patient's skin surface, or inside a body cavity. This material is designed to provide extra scattering or energy degradation of the electron beam. Its purpose usually is to shape the dose distribution to conform to the target volume or to provide a more uniform dose inside the target volume (35,37). More specifically, electron bolus has three primary applications:

1. To shape the coverage of the treatment volume in the depth direction to conform as closely as possible to the target volume while avoiding critical structures,
2. To increase dose to the patient's external surface, and
3. To serve as a missing tissue compensator for surface irregularities and internal air cavities.

In the second application, bolus is being used to either eliminate or decrease the adverse effects of patient heterogeneities on the dose distribution, which can result in a geographic miss at depth, dose nonuniformity within the target volume, and excessive dose-to-distal critical structures (35,37).

Because dose typically is prescribed to 90% to 100% of the given dose, it is often desirable to increase surface dose to 90% or higher when treating with low-energy electrons. To accomplish this, a higher energy beam is selected and a uniformly thick bolus is placed on or near the skin surface. The surface dose of the higher energy electron beam is greater, and the bolus

Table 7.2	VALUES OF SURFACE DOSE AND THERAPEUTIC DEPTH FOR VARIOUS ENERGY–BOLUS COMBINATIONS					
Superflab Thickness (cm)	**0.0**	**0.3**	**0.5**	**1.0**	**1.5**	**2.0**
Energy: 6 MeV						
D_s (%)	72	79	83	93	100	–
R_{90} (cm)	2.0	1.7	1.5	1.0	0.5	–
Energy: 9 MeV						
D_s (%)	78	83	85	89	95	99
R_{90} (cm)	3.0	2.7	2.5	2.0	1.5	1.0
Energy: 12 MeV						
D_s (%)	83	88	89	91	94	96
R_{90} (cm)	4.0	3.7	3.5	3.0	2.5	2.0
Energy: 16 MeV						
D_s (%)	87	92	93	96	97	98
R_{90} (cm)	5.0	4.7	4.5	4.0	3.5	3.0
Energy: 20 MeV						
D_s (%)	91	96	97	98	99	100
R_{90} (cm)	6.1	5.8	5.6	5.1	4.6	4.1

places the skin at a deeper depth, further increasing the surface dose. The energy–bolus thickness combination is selected to place R_{90} at the prescription depth while increasing the surface dose (D_s) to near 90%. To assist in usage of this technique, a table that allows selection of the optimal energy–bolus thickness combination is recommended. Table 7.2 illustrates a sample for the five electron-beam energies of a typical radiation therapy machine.

Two bolus methods are used for this function. One places flexible sheet material (e.g., Superflab) directly on the skin surface. This material is approximately water equivalent and comes in thickness increments of 0.3 to 4 cm. It is particularly useful for chest-wall irradiation, both for fixed-beam and arced-beam therapies. In some treatments, the bolus is used for only a portion of the field, in which case care must be taken to ensure the edge of the bolus is tapered to reduce the magnitude of the hot or cold spot created by the surface irregularity (cf. Fig. 7.7) (35,37).

For highly irregular or sensitive skin surfaces, which often are encountered in head and neck or postsurgical irradiations, it is advantageous to have a rigid bolus sheet (often referred to as a scatter plate because it not only degrades the energy of the electron beam but also scatters the beam) close to but not necessarily in direct contact with the patient (35). For such cases standard thicknesses of polymethylmethacrylate (PMMA) (0.125 to 0.25 inches) are placed perpendicular to the beam, as illustrated in Figure 7.17. To restore a sharp penumbra, skin collimation usually is recommended with use of the scatter-plate bolus method. Rules for using skin collimation with the bolus have been discussed by Hogstrom (35). It is important that the bolus be in contact or close to the patient because too large of an air gap can create an exceedingly large penumbra. This is

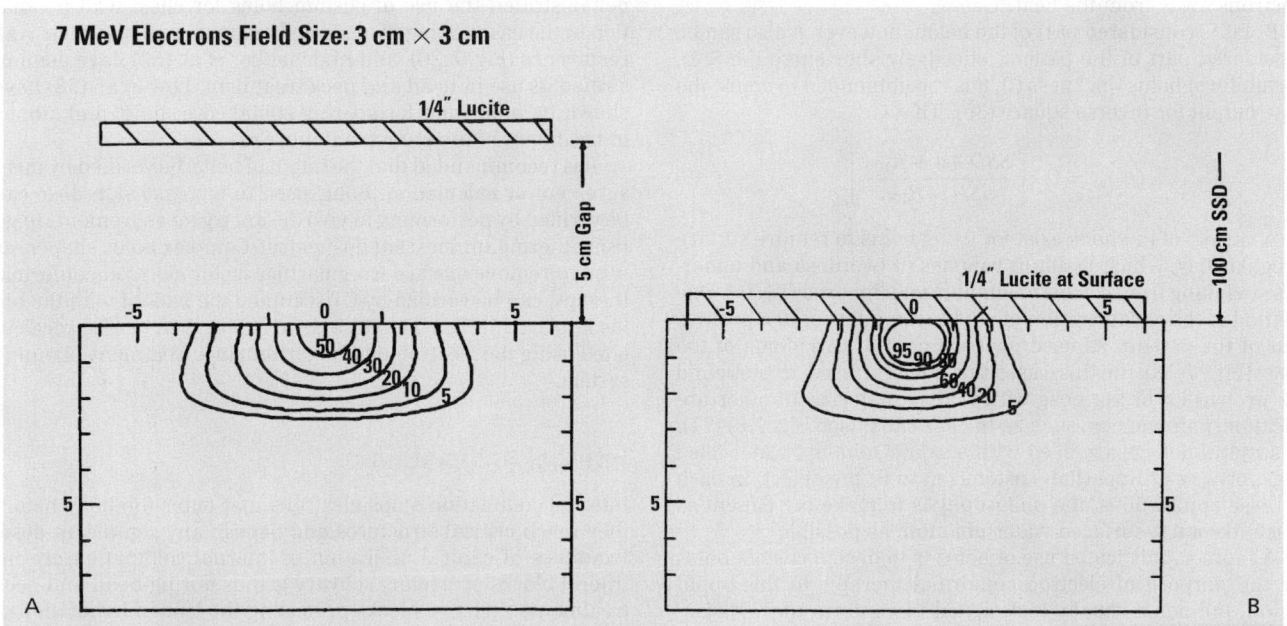

FIGURE 7.17. Proper location of slab bolus. Constant thickness (slab) bolus is used to increase surface dose and to fine tune electron-beam penetration (see Table 7.2). Its location is important for irradiation by a small field (3 by 3 cm^2) and low energy (7 MeV) electron beam. **A:** If a 0.25-inch polymethylmethacrylate (PMMA) plate is located 5 cm above patient, electrons are scattered away from the field resulting in needless broadening of the penumbra and a decrease in given dose of approximately 50% (given dose without the bolus is 100%). **B:** Placing the 0.25-inch PMMA plate on the surface preserves both the given dose and beam penumbra.

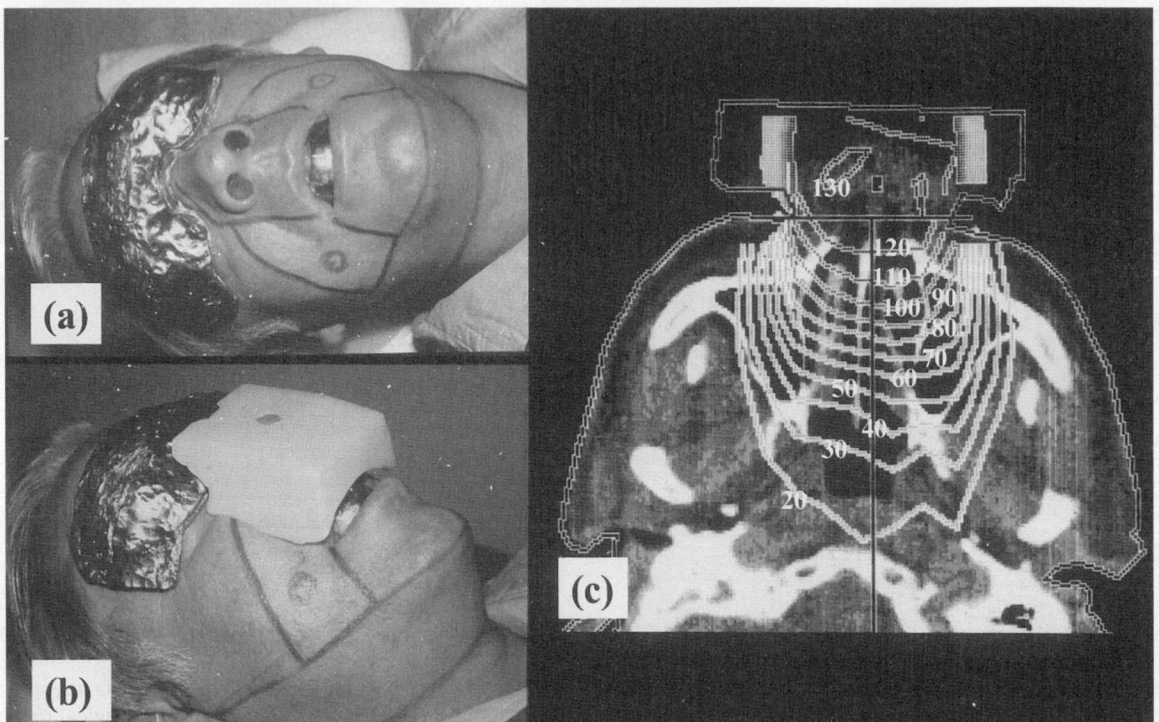

FIGURE 7.18. Utility of bolus to remove dose inhomogeneity caused by surface irregularity of nose. **A:** Bolus in nasal air passages prevents cold spots in the septum. (Also, note the skin collimation used to restore penumbra under nose bolus and the intraoral stent used to protect the tongue.) **B:** Wax bolus surrounding the nose eliminates irregular patient surface. **C:** Isodose curves superimposed on a transverse computed tomography scan illustrate how the bolus makes the patient more like a water phantom, resulting in a homogeneous dose distribution characteristic of that in a water phantom. The patient dose is delivered 12-MeV electrons: ^{60}Co photons = 4:1. (Note that the surface dose is lower than that shown because the treatment-planning system calculated the photon dose assuming the bolus was in place during its delivery, which is not the case.) (From Hogstrom KR. Treatment planning in electron-beam therapy. In: Vaeth JM, Meyer JL, eds. *Frontiers of radiation therapy and oncology Vol. 25: The role of high energy electrons in the treatment of cancer.* Basel: S. Karger AG, 1991;30–52, with permission.)

demonstrated in Figure 7.17, where a 5-cm air gap results in a 50% decrease in the given dose because of the bolus scattering electrons away from the field.

Bolus is considered part of the beam; however, it also can be considered part of the patient, effectively shortening the SSD. For uniform bolus thickness (t), it is recommended to adjust the dose output for inverse square (36). That is:

$$O_{bolus} = O \cdot \left[\frac{SSD + t + R_{100}}{SSD + R_{100}} \right]^2 \qquad (9)$$

A variety of methods exist for using bolus to remove surface irregularities, which result in volumes of overdose and underdose resulting from scatter inequilibrium if ignored (34,35). One method involves fabrication of a beeswax bolus onto a positive cast of the patient, as used for treatment of carcinoma of the nose (Fig. 7.18). In this case, the bolus is used to surround the protrusion of the nose with scatter material. In other applications, air cavities, such as the ear canal (see Fig. 7.8) (71), or surgical defects are filled with a saline solution, water-filled bags, or wax or Superflab customized to fit the defect. In each of these applications, the philosophy is to make the patient as much like a flat-surfaced water phantom as possible.

A more sophisticated use of bolus is to design custom bolus for the purpose of electron conformal therapy. In this application, the bolus usually is designed to conform the 90% isodose line to the PTV while minimizing dose to nearby critical structures and maintaining dose uniformity as much as possible within the 90% dose contour. Proper design of custom bolus requires use of a 3D treatment-planning system (88) that utilizes bolus design operators (57) and a 3D PBA (89). The methodology of bolus design to optimize target coverage and critical structure searing is seen in Figure 7.19. Perkins et al. (78) have demonstrated the use of custom bolus for chest-wall irradiation in the cases of highly distorted anatomy and of a chest wall recurrence (Fig. 7.20), and Kudchadker et al. (52) have demonstrated its use in head and neck treatment. Low et al. (58) have shown its utilization for sparing spinal cord, lung, and kidney in treatment of the paraspinal muscles.

It is recommended that the intent of bolus be verified by measurement or calculation. Bolus used to increase skin dose can be verified by performing in vivo dosimetry measurements (e.g., using thermoluminescent dosimetry). Complex bolus shapes, as used to remove surface irregularities or for electron conformal therapy, can be verified by CT scanning the patient with the bolus in place (58,78). The dose distribution then can be recalculated using the electron dose algorithm in a treatment-planning system.

Internal Collimation

Internal collimation stops electrons that enter the body before they reach critical structures and deposit any significant dose. Examples of clinical utilization of internal collimation are intraoral blocks protecting salivary glands during head and neck treatments (91); eye blocks protecting the lens in irradiation of the eyelid (86), orbit, or retina; and sheets of lead used to protect internal structures during intraoperative therapy.

There are two important concepts to remember in the use of internal collimation. First, the collimator must be sufficiently thick to stop the energy of the electrons in the beam at depth.

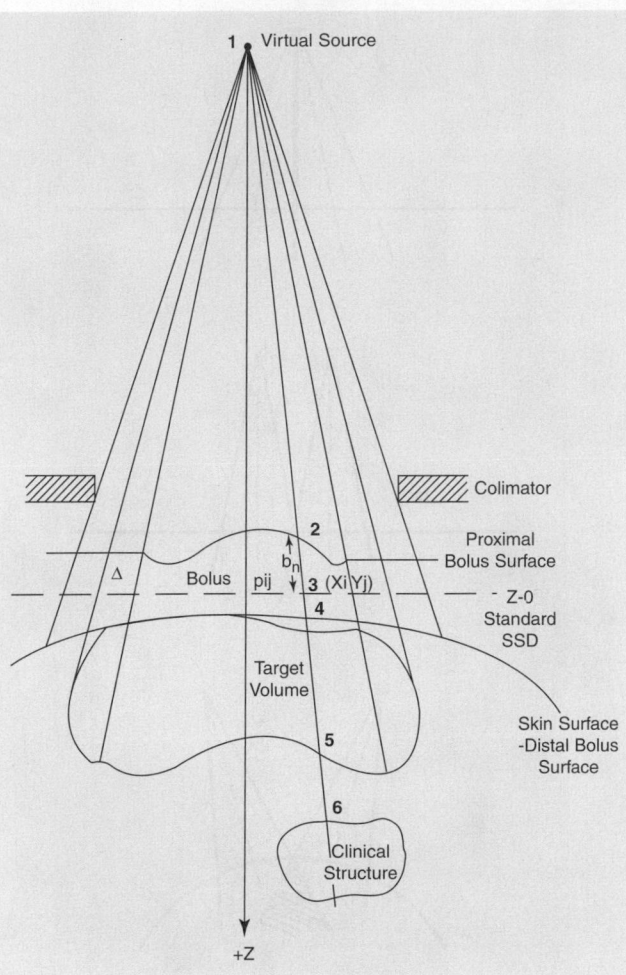

FIGURE 7.19. Schematic representation of the patient contour, target volume, and compensating bolus designed to optimize the coverage of the target while minimizing the dose to the underlying critical structure (From Low DA, Starkschall G, Bujnowski SW, et al. Electron bolus design for radiation therapy treatment planning: Bolus design algorithms. *Med Phys* 1992;19:115–124, with permission.)

Electron-beam energy is reduced by 2 MeV per cm in unit density tissue; hence, the energy of a 12-MeV beam at a depth of 2 cm is 8 MeV. The thickness of lead required to stop 8-MeV electrons is 4 mm (8 MeV · 0.5 mm/MeV).

One application where ensuring that collimation is sufficiently thick that has been sometimes overlooked is the use of internal eye shields. Shiu et al. (86) showed that x-ray eye shields constructed of plastic-coated lead and designed to shield the eyes from kilovoltage x-rays did not stop 6-MeV electrons, resulting in penetration of approximately 50% of the given dose. However, electron eye shields constructed of enamel-coated tungsten can stop electrons with energies as great as 9 MeV (Fig. 7.21). By using higher density tungsten ($\rho = 19.3$) instead of lead ($\rho = 11.5$), the eye shields remain sufficiently thin to fit under the eyelid. If only x-ray eye shields are available, bolus should be placed on top of the eye and eye shield to ensure that the electron energy is reduced sufficiently so that electrons do not penetrate the eye shield.

Second, electrons backscattered from lead at a lead-tissue interface increase dose, the increase ranging from approximately 20% at 20 MeV to 60% at 4 MeV, where the energy is the average energy of electrons incident on the lead (46,51). Das and Bushe (11) published a comprehensive data set demonstrating the range for backscatter electrons as a function of energy, on the order of a few mm, and increases as a function of energy. Inserting two half-value layers of bolus between the lead and the tissue usually reduces the dose to upstream tissue to a clinically acceptable value. The thickness of one half-value layer ranges from approximately 1 cm at 10 MeV to 0.5 cm at 3 MeV (46,55). Intraoral lead stents are coated routinely with acrylic (64), and a material such as dental wax can be applied easily to lead sheets placed between the mucosa and gums. Eye shields, however, only have clearance for 1 to 2 mm of coating; hence, backscatter dose to the eyelids is important in treatment management (86). When determining lead thickness for an internal shielding at a particular depth, one must first determine the energy of the electron beam at that location. The energy of the electron beam on the surface is $E_{o,p}$ typically close to the "console selected" energy. As electrons lose energy by 2 MeV/cm, one can determine the remaining energy of any depth. For example, 12 MeV beams at surface would be approximate 6 MeV after 3 cm.

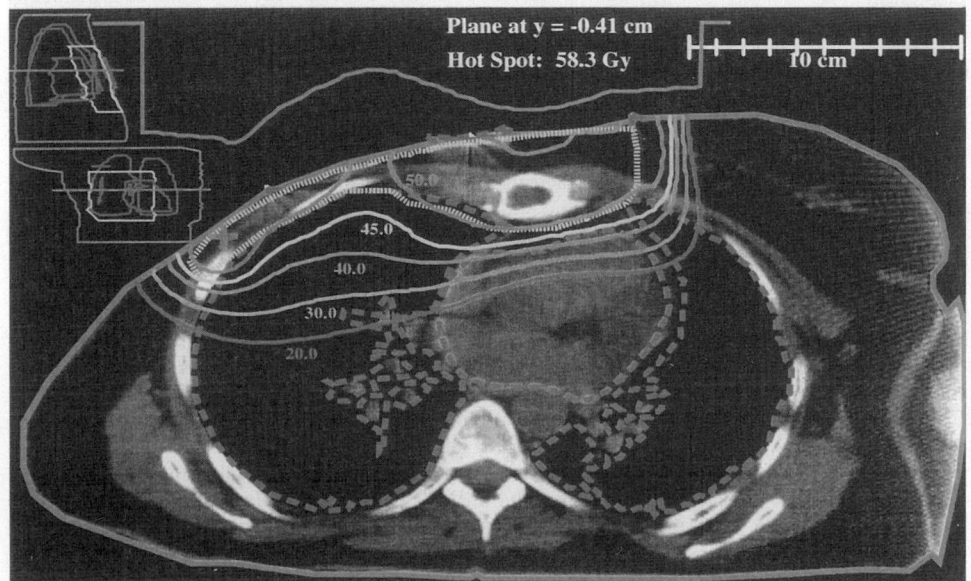

FIGURE 7.20. Conformal electron therapy using variable thickness bolus. Bolus is used to shape the 90% isodose surface (45 Gy) to the distal surface of the chest wall in treating a chest wall occurrence, optimally sparing lung. (From Perkins GH, McNeese MD, Antolak JA, et al. A custom three-dimensional electron bolus technique for optimization of postmastectomy irradiation. *Int J Radiat Oncol Biol Phys* 2001;51:1142–1151, with permission.)

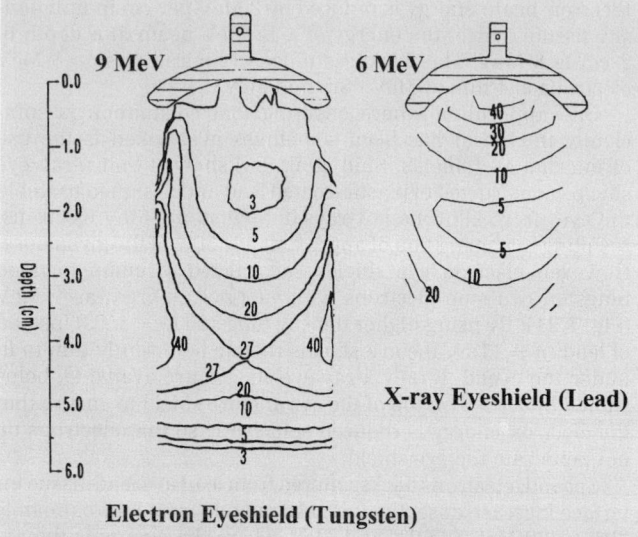

FIGURE 7.21. Electron eye shields. The dose distribution under tungsten electron eye shields demonstrates its ability to stop 9-MeV electrons. The dose distribution under a lead x-ray eye shield shows its inability to stop 6-MeV electrons. (From Shiu AS, Tung SS, Gastorf RJ, et al. Dosimetric evaluation of lead and tungsten eye shields in electron-beam treatment. *Int J Radiat Oncol Biol Phys* 1996;35:599–604, with permission.)

Field Abutment

The purpose of field abutment usually is to enlarge the radiation field or to change the beam energy or modality. In either case, beam uniformity requires that three criteria be met. First, the beams must abut along the entire border (35,37,40,46). If the edges of the two beams coincide exactly (Fig. 7.22A), then the two beams will be equivalent to a single beam and optimal uniformity will be achieved. If the central axes of the two beams are parallel (see Fig. 7.22B), then the diverging beam edges will overlap, creating a cold spot upstream and a hot spot downstream of the region of intersection. This is least significant for narrow fields, as encountered in irradiation of the cervical nodes of the neck or abutting the internal mammary and medial chest-wall fields. If the central axes are converging (see Fig. 7.22C), then there is an even greater amount of overlap. This is the case for abutting lateral and medial chest-wall fields. In such cases, feathering the beam edge ±1 cm can reduce the dose heterogeneity. This is illustrated in Figure 7.23 for a standard postmastectomy chest-wall irradiation using electrons.

The second criterium is that the beam penumbra must be matched. This is the case for the two spinal fields referred to earlier, but it is not the case in general, particularly in abutting electron to photon fields. In such cases, either one or both of the field edges must be feathered. Third, it is best that the penumbra be somewhat broad. This reduces the impact of misalignment on the uniformity of dose in the abutted region. Harms and Purdy (24) demonstrated the influence of SSD energy and match bolus on match-line dosimetry. Figure 7.24 displays dose homogeneity for abutted 12 MeV fields depending on gap. In addition, matching of electron and photo fields is a planning challenge, as two differing penumbra are abutted. Johnson and Khan (43) performed a study of matched electron/photon fields as a function of energy and SSD. Figure 7.25 demonstrates match-line profiles for a typical head and neck field match.

Mixed-Beam Therapy

Electron beams frequently are mixed with photon beams to create an appropriate treatment. The mixed beams can irradiate a

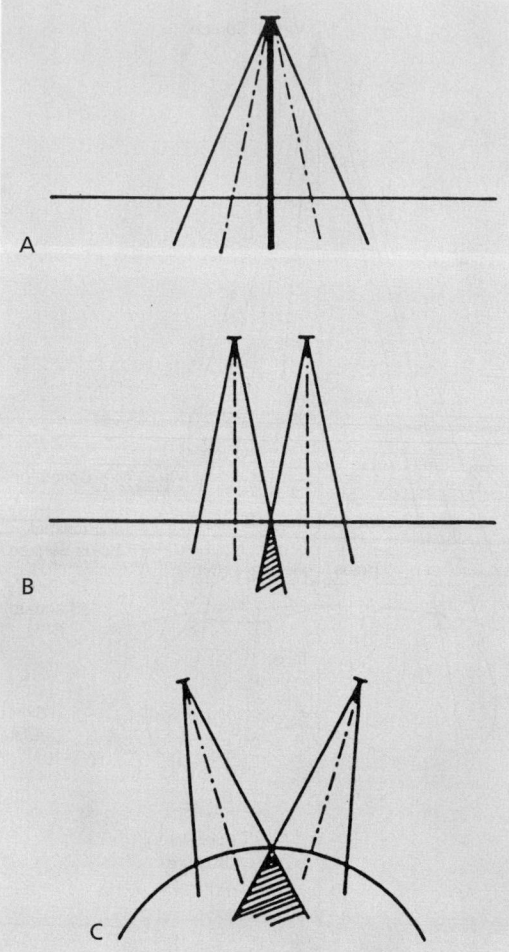

FIGURE 7.22. Comparison of abutment geometries. **A:** Common edge is created by having diverging central axes. **B:** Parallel central axes result in overlapping edges. **C:** Converging central axes result in the greatest overlap. (From ICRU Report 35. *Radiation dosimetry: Electron beams with energies between 1 and 50 MeV.* Bethesda: International Commission on Radiation Units and Measurement, 1984, with permission.)

common volume of tissue, or they can be abutted. In the former case, an electron field may be added to a primarily photon-beam treatment or a photon field may be added to a primarily electron-beam treatment. For example, electron boosts are used to deliver localized dose to the surgical site following photon breast irradiation, to treat the postcervical nodes once spinal cord tolerance is reached, and to reduce spinal cord dose (e.g., in lymphoma treatment) (68). In some head and neck treatments, the photon beam is a surrogate to the electron beam, being used to reduce skin dose and to increase dose penetration while still sparing the contralateral salivary gland (20,91). With the future availability of intensity-modulated photon and modulated electron therapy, the effectiveness of mixed-beam therapy can be expected to increase in breast and head and neck radiation therapy.

Abutted mixed beams are used when separate portions of the anatomy can benefit from the two individually. The most common application of this process is the utilization of electron fields for irradiation of the internal mammary chain, supraclavicular, or axillary lymph nodes as part of breast or chest-wall irradiation (91). Matching of tangential photon fields and internal mammary chain (IMC) electron fields is complex due to surface irregularities and heterogeneities. Careful treatment planning must be performed, especially if prescriptive decisions for electron energy and dosage are predicated on the resultant dose

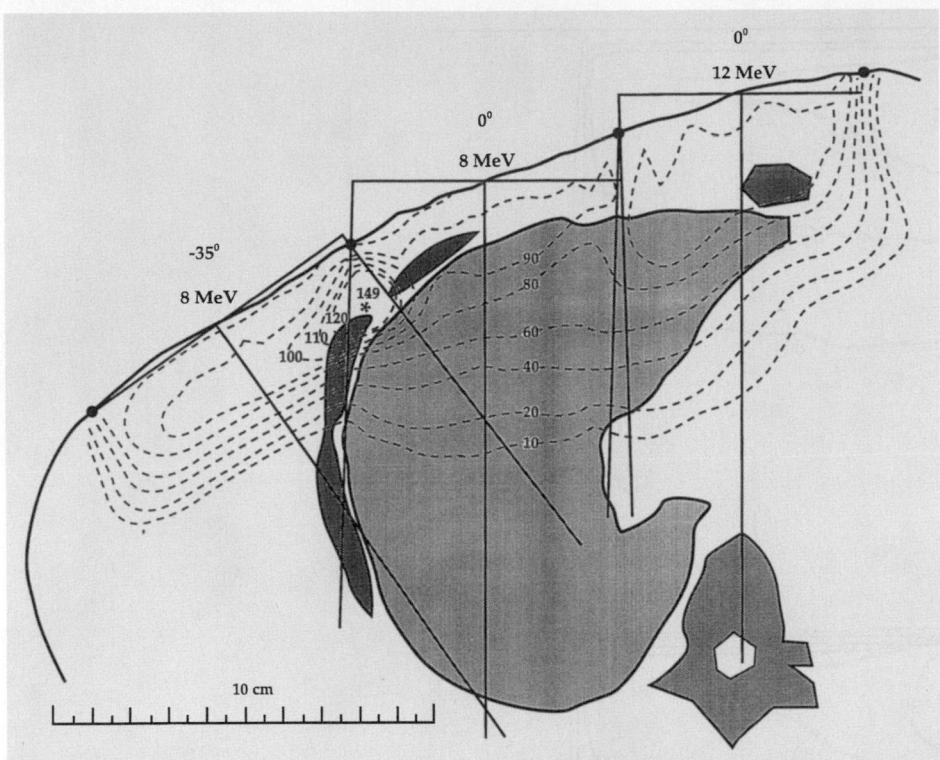

FIGURE 7.23. Clinical example of abutting electron fields in chest wall treatment. Dose homogeneity is acceptable at the border of internal mammary chain (IMC) and medial chest-wall fields because central axes are parallel and field widths are small. Dose homogeneity is unacceptable at the border of medial and lateral chest-wall fields because central axes are converging (see Fig. 7.10B). Dose homogeneity is improved at border of medial and lateral chest-wall fields by delivering equal doses with the match line being moved 1 cm twice during treatment.

distribution. Figure 7.26 displays a tangential photon IMC electron field initial plan with a plan performed with partially wide tangent, a technique suggested to remove the field abutment dilemma (82). This technique is also used for irradiating the total scalp or for craniospinal irradiation, which are described later. The use of combined modulated photon and electron fields has been reported. This has the potential to be an ideal therapy for particular treatment sites. Thus far this combined therapy has been demonstrated with Microtron (helium head) machines. Early publications demonstrated conventional

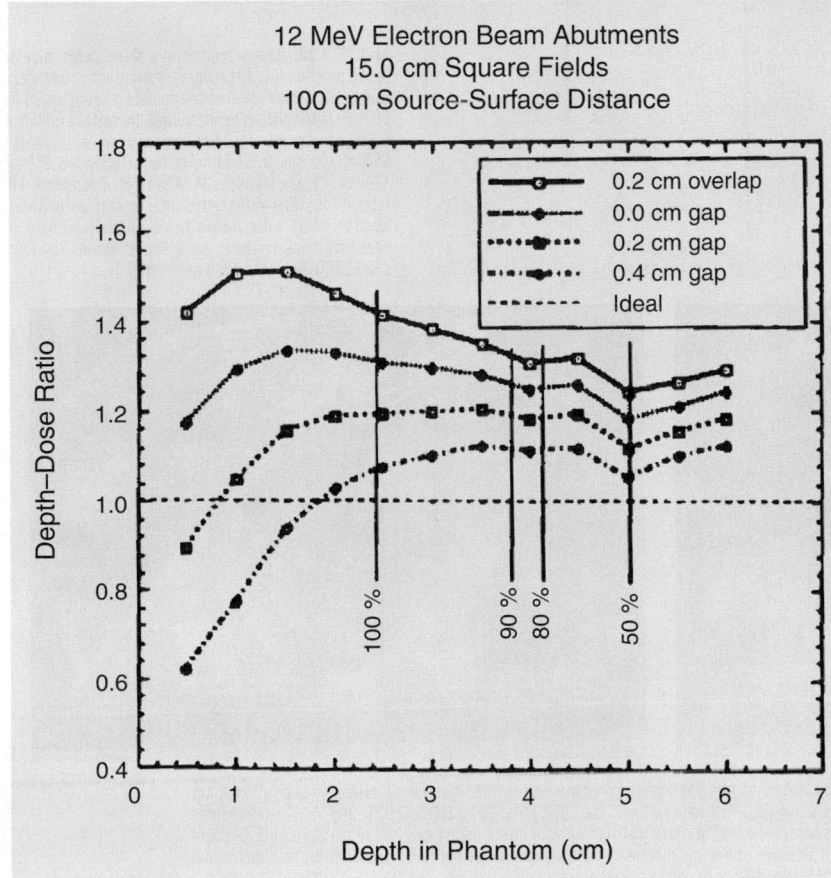

FIGURE 7.24. Graph depicting dose homogeneity for abutted 12 MeV electron fields for a series of gaps. (From Harms WB, Purdy JA. Abutment of high energy electron fields. *Int J Radiat Oncol Biol Phys* 1991;20(4):853–858, with permission.)

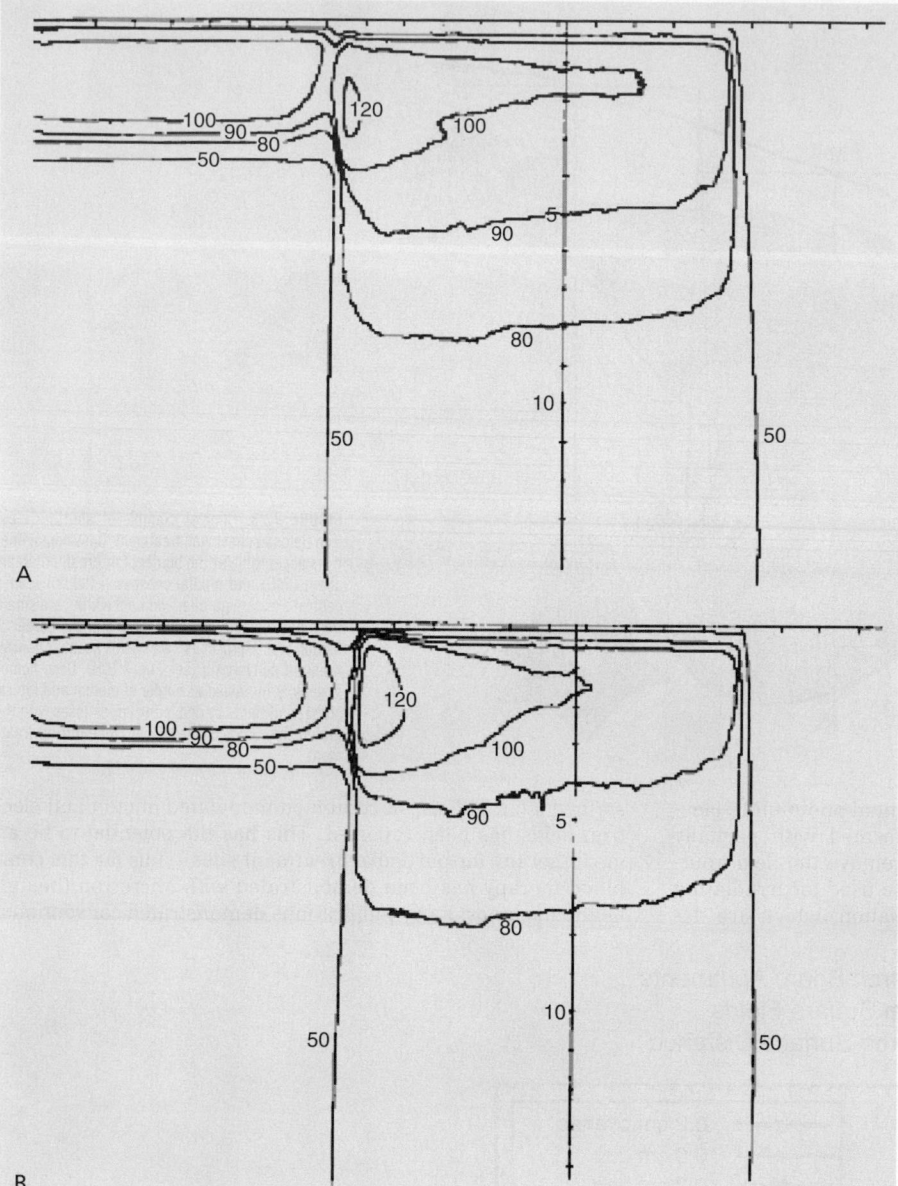

FIGURE 7.25. Isodose curves in a plane perpendicular to the junction line between abutting photon and electron fields. 9-MeV electron beam; field size equals 10 by 10 cm^2; 6-MV photon beam; source-to-surface distance (SSD) equals 100 cm. **A:** Electron beam at standard SSD of 100 cm. **B:** Electron beam at extended SSD of 120 cm. (From Johnson JM, Khan FM. Dosimetric effects of abutting extended source to surface distance electron fields with photon fields in the treatment of head and neck cancers. *Int J Radiat Oncol Biol Phys* 1994;28(3):741–747, with permission.)

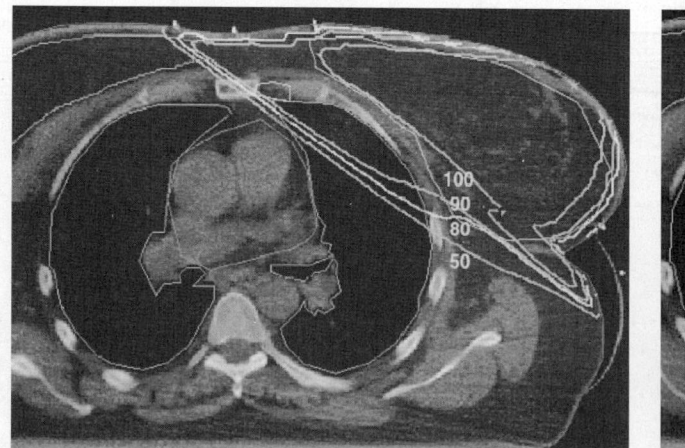

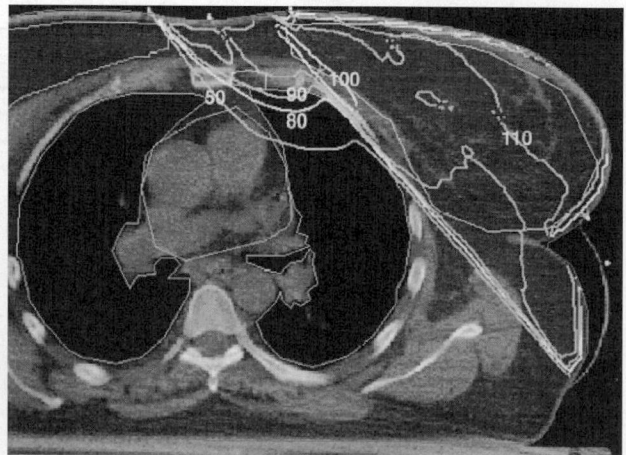

FIGURE 7.26. Dose distribution with partially wide tangentials (PWT) versus photon/electron (P/E) illustrating difference in position of hot spots. Left lung, heart, IMC, left breast or chest, and right breast were outlined. The 50%, 80%, 90%, 100%, 110%, and 120% isodose lines are displayed. **A:** Dose distribution with intact breast and PWT. **B:** Dose distribution with intact breast and P/E. (From Severin D, Connors S, Thompson H, et al. Breast radiotherapy with inclusion of internal mammary nodes: A comparison of techniques with three-dimensional planning. *Int J Radiat Oncol Biol Phys* 2003;55(3):633–644, with permission.)

(nonmodulated) use of photons and electrons as collimated by MLC. Zackrisson and Karlsson (98) described a technique for matching of electron and photon beams for conformal therapy of target volumes at moderate depths. More recent efforts have explored the use of photons and electrons. Mu et al. (72) showed mixed photon and electron was superior in obtaining planning goals versus IMRT alone. One essential aspect was the reduction of integral dose. The same computer-controlled MLC of Microtron model is used for photons and electrons. Das et al. (12) developed an algorithm using automated beam orientation and modality selection for optimal beam arrangement selection in intensity-modulated radiotherapy (IMRT) of mixed photon and electron beams. And finally Ma et al. (59) performed a comparative study on tangential photon beams, IMRT, and modulated electron radiotherapy (MERT) for breast cancer treatment.

:: | Specialized Electron Techniques

Although electron-beam therapy is used less frequently than is photon-beam therapy, it remains an essential modality. To fully use electron-beam therapy, there must be access to comprehensive electron treatment and treatment-planning techniques. This includes specialized electron techniques, which, in the present context, are defined as those that are seldom required and that use a complex treatment geometry, special treatment delivery hardware, or special treatment-planning software. It is not recommended that all radiation therapy facilities offer all techniques, but radiation oncologists should be aware of these techniques and should be able to refer patients to a regional center for those that are impractical in smaller settings. This recommendation is based on the significant time, resources, and costs of implementing, maintaining, and providing some of the more complex special electron procedures. The American College of Medical Physics has reviewed the effort and cost associated with several special procedures, which include electron arc therapy, intraoperative electron therapy, and total-skin electron irradiation (27).

Four types of special techniques are discussed here. First, the treatment of internal tissues is exemplified by intraoperative radiation therapy and intracavitary radiation therapy. Second, the utilization of abutted electron and photon fields is exemplified by craniospinal and total-scalp treatment techniques. Third, the treatment of superficial tissues for a cylindric geometry is exemplified by the total-limb and total-skin treatment techniques. Fourth, an alternative to fixed-beam therapy of the chest wall is exemplified by arc therapy.

Intracavitary Irradiation

Cones of appropriate design can be used for intracavitary electron irradiation, which delivers an improved dose distribution over that traditionally delivered using orthovoltage x-rays. Intracavitary irradiation most frequently is used to boost the primary site while sparing nearby normal tissues. Intracavitary irradiation has been a choice for intraoral, transvaginal, and intraoperative treatments. Wang (95) showed the benefit of intraoral cones for boosting the oral lesions of the floor of the mouth, soft palate, tongue, and retromolar trigone while sparing mandible, teeth, gum, and salivary glands. McGinnis et al. (64) reported using a transvaginal cone to boost carcinoma of the cervix with electrons, reducing bulk tumor to subsequently allow intracavitary brachytherapy. Intraoperative radiation therapy can be used in many sites (93); however, it is used primarily for abdominal sites. Merrick et al. (65) reviewed the experience in the United States of using intraoperative radiotherapy for treatment of pancreatic, biliary, and gastric carcinomas.

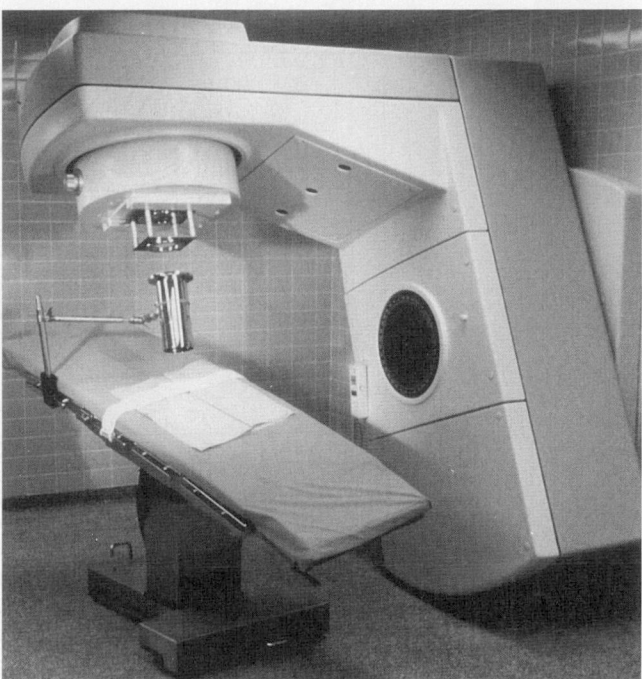

FIGURE 7.27. Intraoperative electron radiation therapy accelerator. View of dedicated Siemens intraoperative radiation therapy unit in operating room. Note the separation between the treatment cone and the radiation therapy treatment head. A laser alignment system provides soft docking between treatment head and the cone. (From Hogstrom KR, Boyer AL, Shiu AS, et al. Design of metallic electron-beam cones for an intraoperative therapy linear accelerator. *Int J Radiat Oncol Biol Phys* 1990;18:1223–1232, with permission.)

The criteria for intracavitary electron irradiation are similar, regardless of site. A treatment cone is necessary in order that healthy tissue can be restrained from intercepting electrons irradiating the tumor. The cone wall must be sufficiently thick to stop electrons from escaping to outside tissue while being thin enough not to interfere with tumor access. Guidelines for accomplishing this for intraoperative cones have been discussed by Hogstrom et al. (25). Another issue is how to ensure accurate alignment while maintaining patient safety with a cone. Appropriate cone positioning requires having a method for looking down the cone to view the tumor. Proper alignment of the cone after inserting it into the patient requires methods for docking it to the machine. For soft docking, the cone is not physically attached to the machine (Fig. 7.27) (25). For hard docking, the cone is physically attached to the machine, and there are methods for its breaking away under stress (6,64). Many of the intraoral and transvaginal cones are x-ray cones converted for use with electrons; however, intraoperative cones are larger and typically designed for that specific purpose.

Treatment planning for intracavitary cones typically is done manually because it is not possible to CT scan the patient in the treatment position or under operating room conditions. The electron energy and cone size are selected to match measured isodose distributions to the dimensions of the clinical target volume. Examples of dose distributions for intraoperative cones are shown in Figure 7.28 (75). These examples show two characteristics of such cones. First, for the larger diameter cones, scatter off the wall of the cone can lead to hot spots near the cone's periphery. Second, ends of the cones often are beveled to make it easy to establish contact when the anatomic plane is not perpendicular to the direction of approach (i.e., the central axis of the beam). Note how the depth of the 90% isodose contour beneath the surface decreases from 3.6 cm at 0-degrees incidence to 3.0 cm at 30-degrees incidence, as a result of the effects described earlier.

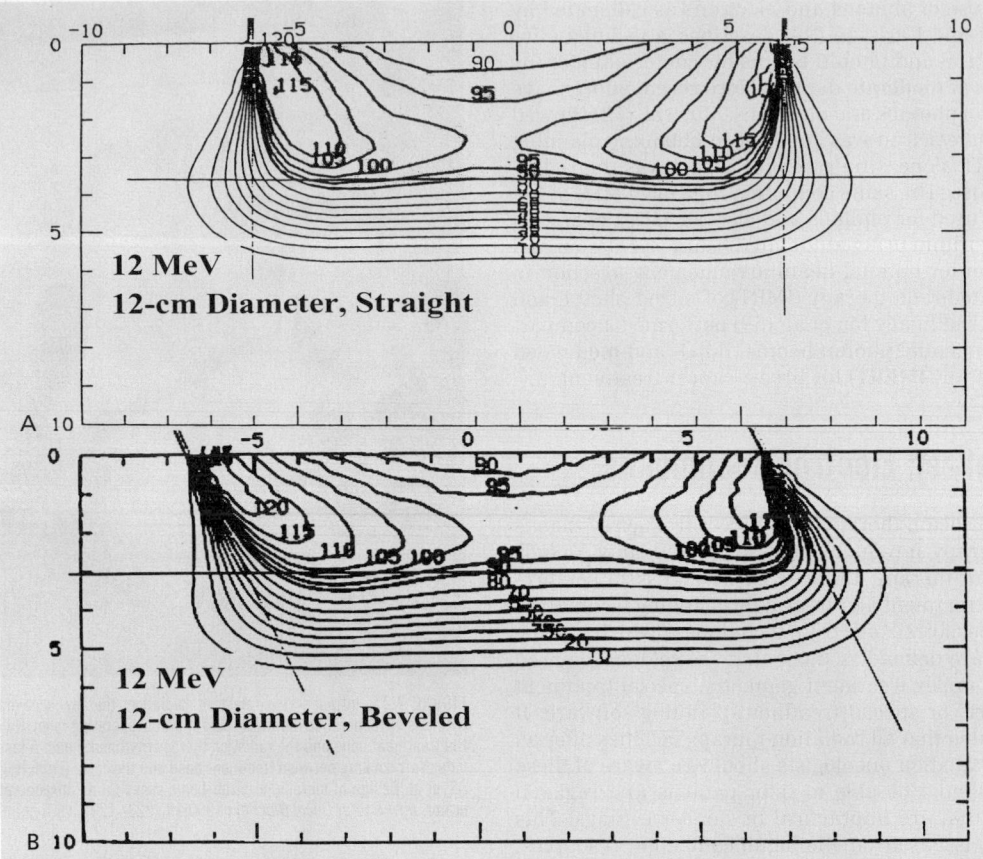

FIGURE 7.28. Isodose plots illustrating typical intraoperative dose distributions at 12 MeV. **A:** 12-cm diameter cone, normal incidence and **(B)** 30-degree beveled, 12-cm diameter cone. Note the decreased depth of the 90% dose beneath the surface for the beam 30 degrees from normal incidence relative to that for normal incidence. (From Nyerick CE, Ochran TG, Boyer AL, et al. Dosimetry characteristics of metallic cones for intraoperative radiation therapy. *Int J Radiat Oncol Biol Phys* 1991;21:501–510, with permission.)

Craniospinal Irradiation

Craniospinal irradiation is important for management of brain tumors that seed along the pathways of the cerebrospinal fluid (e.g., medulloblastoma, malignant ependymoma, germinoma, and infratentorial glioblastoma) (62). Utilization of a high-energy electron beam in lieu of photons to irradiate the spinal cord can reduce dose to the upper aerodigestive and lower gastrointestinal tracts, lymph nodes, and the vertebral bodies. This should result in reduced probability to acute complications and late effects (62,63). Challenges to this technique are

1. Proper selection of energy to account for effect of bone;
2. Abutment scheme in the neck to achieve uniform dose at the abutment of the posterior electron field of the spine with the parallel opposed, lateral photon fields irradiating the brain; and
3. Abutment scheme for the two electron fields usually used to treat the spine.

Two similar techniques for craniospinal techniques are reported by Maor et al. (62,63) at M.D. Anderson Cancer Center and by Dewit et al. (13) at University Hospital in Leuven.

Total-Scalp Irradiation

Total-scalp irradiation is sometimes necessary in the management of malignancies (e.g., cutaneous lymphoma, melanoma, and angiosarcoma) that present with widespread involvement of the scalp and forehead (91,92). Electron-beam therapy is a practical means of achieving the therapeutic goal of delivering a uniform dose to the scalp with minimal dose to underlying brain. For many years, total-scalp irradiation was achieved by patching multiple electron fields (1,91). Although effective, the treatment was tedious as a result of the large number of fields, their requirement for skin collimation, and the need to move the abutment border to improve dose homogeneity (1). Akazawa (2) from the University of California–San Francisco reported a simpler technique that abuts lateral electron fields to parallel opposed photon fields, the latter of which treats the rind of the scalp while avoiding brain tissue. Tung et al. (92) modified the abutment scheme to account for beam divergence and demonstrated improved dose uniformity by comparing 3D dose calculations with in vivo dose measurements.

Figure 7.29 illustrates the abutment scheme. The outer edge of the electron field overlaps the inner edge of the 6 MV x-ray field by 3 mm to account for the divergence of the contralateral 6 MV x-ray field. Because the electron and x-ray penumbras are not matched, their common border is moved 1 cm toward beam center halfway through treatment to improve dose homogeneity. Figure 7.30 shows the dose distribution in a transverse CT plane, which illustrates the dose homogeneity achieved in the region of abutment and the sparing of brain tissue. Initially, the common border is set at approximately 0.5 cm inside the inner table of the skull. Moving the common border further toward the inner table of the skull reduces brain irradiation at the expense of the x-ray beam being replaced by an electron beam that would begin to graze the skull. As discussed earlier, grazing radiation penetrates less deeply, possibly underdosing the scalp in this region. Also noticeable in Figure 7.30 is a 6-mm thick wax bolus, which increases surface dose for both the electron

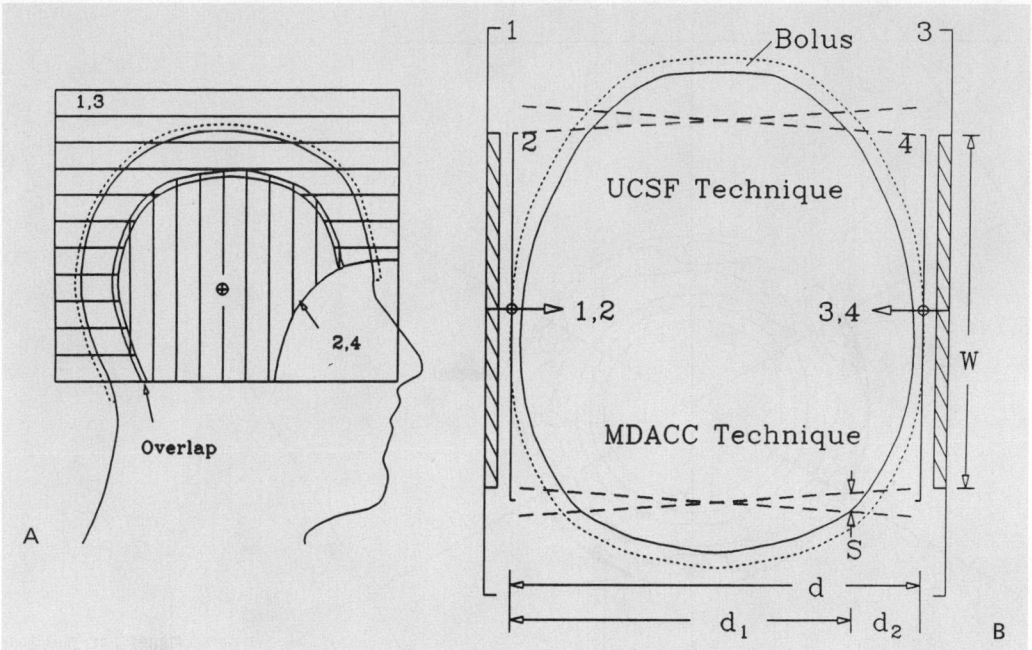

FIGURE 7.29. Abutment scheme for total-scalp irradiation (x-ray fields, 1,3; electron fields, 2,4). **A:** The electron field edge, placed just inside the skull, overlaps the edge of the ipsilateral x-ray field by approximately 3 mm to account for divergence of the edge of the contralateral x-ray field. Halfway through treatment, the field edges are moved 1 cm to improve dose homogeneity in the region of abutment. **B:** The need for the 3-mm overlap (MDACC technique) is better appreciated viewing the divergent edges of all fields in a transverse plane. (From Tung SS, Shiu AS, Starkschall G, et al. Dosimetric evaluation of total scalp irradiation using a lateral electron-photon technique. *Int J Radiat Oncol Biol Phys* 1993;27:153–160, with permission.)

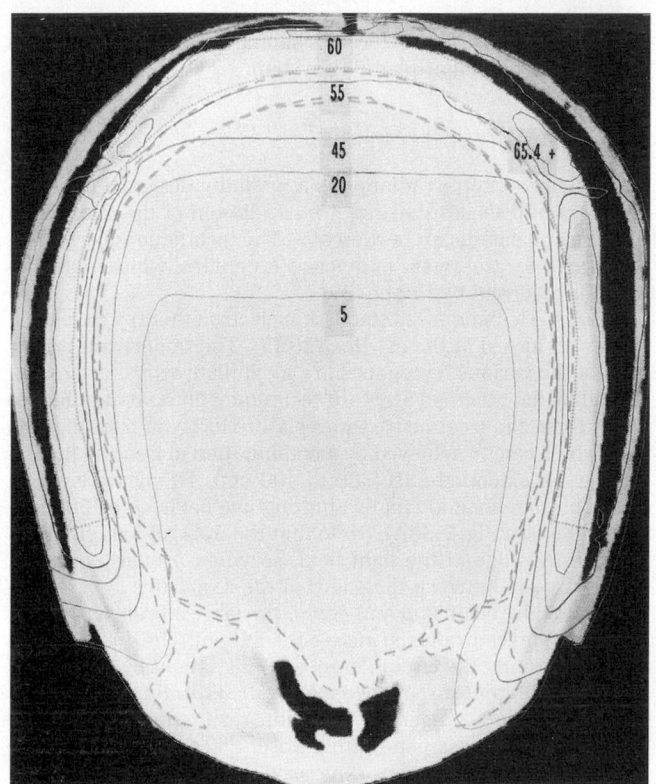

FIGURE 7.30. Dose distribution in a transverse computed tomography plane, illustrating the homogeneity of dose in the abutment region and the degree of brain sparing with this technique. Isodose values in Gy. (From Tung SS, Shiu AS, Starkschall G, et al. Dosimetric evaluation of total scalp irradiation using a lateral electron-photon technique. *Int J Radiat Oncol Biol Phys* 1993;27:153–160, with permission.)

and x-ray fields. Although this technique is straightforward to plan and implement, concern of hot spots along to the midline superior brain tissue along the plane is a concern.

Walker et al. (94) described a six-field electron-beam technique for treatment of mycosis fungoides of the scalp. This technique of overlapping beams was verified with thermoluminescent dosimetry measurements. The dose prescriptions were 20 and 30 Gy for the two patients in this study. Yaparpalvi et al. (97) developed a technique for scalp irradiation that used a single posterior-superior field with concentric circles that varied in electron energy. This interesting technique was not confirmed with anthropomorphic phantom dosimetry studies. Peters (80) described use of an electron reflector to improve dose uniformity to the scalp during total-skin electron therapy.

Total-Limb Irradiation

It may be advantageous to irradiate the superficial anatomy of a limb for management of cancer (e.g., melanoma, lymphoma, Kaposi's sarcoma). If the depth beneath the surface is 2 cm or less, electrons offer a uniform dose while sparing deep tissues and structures. This technique has been described by Wooden et al. (96) for the treatment of the lower calf of a patient with Kaposi's sarcoma. Illustrated in Figure 7.31, six equally spaced 5-MeV electron beams are used to irradiate a 9-cm diameter cylinder. Each beam is sufficiently wide, so that the entire circle falls within the uniform portion of each beam. Tangential radiation to the surface of the cylinder delivers a greater dose as a result of oblique incidence, which is partially offset by the inverse square effect. Also, the tangential radiation penetrates less deeply. The utilization of six or more beams begins to simulate 360-degree arc therapy (which is not feasible due to collisions). The resulting dose distribution illustrates three interesting characteristics. First, the average maximum dose along each radius is approximately 2.5 times the given dose of each

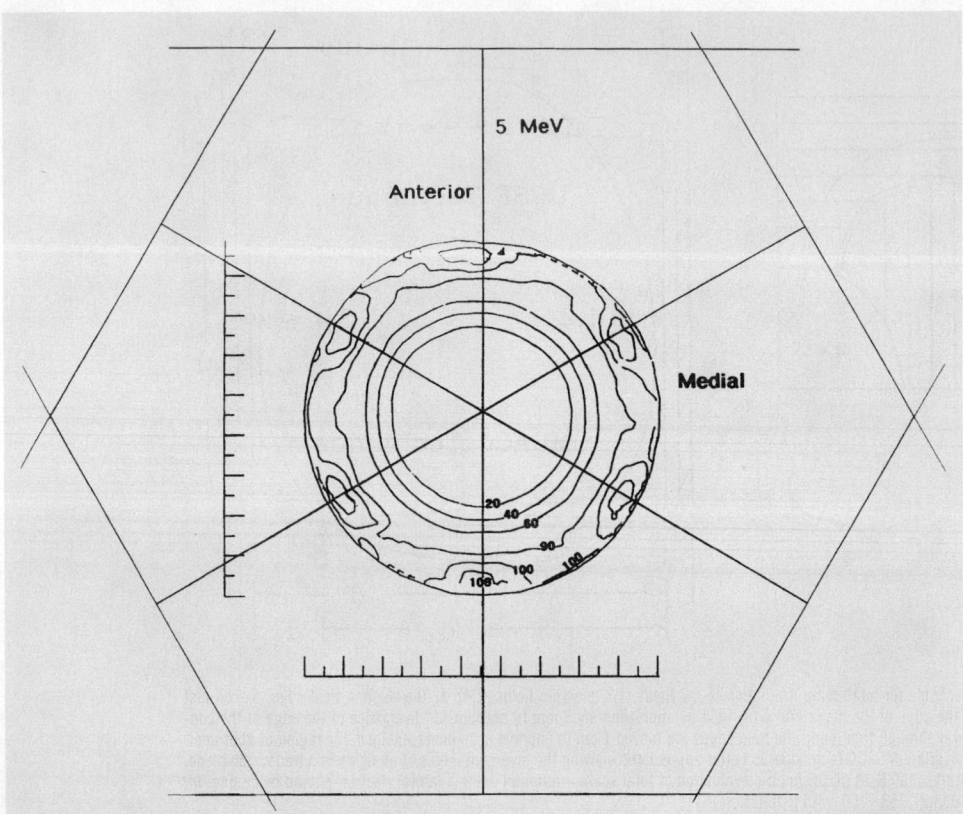

FIGURE 7.31. Dose distribution for total-limb irradiation. Six equally spaced 17-cm wide, 5-MeV electron beams are used to irradiate a 9-cm diameter cylinder. 100% equals 2.55 times the given dose from a single field. (From Wooden KK, Hogstrom KR, Blum P, et al. Whole-limb irradiation of the lower calf using a six-field electron technique. *Med Dosim* 1996;21:211–218, with permission.)

of the six fields. Second, 90% of the average maximum dose penetrates 8 to 10 mm, reduced from the value of 15 mm for a single beam incident normally on a flat surface (Fig. 7.32). Third, the surface dose has increased to 90% or greater of average maximum dose compared with approximately 70% of the given dose for a single beam incident normally on a flat surface. This is the result of the self-bolusing effect of tangential electron radiation.

The dosimetric characteristics should be carefully evaluated using one's treatment-planning system.

Total-Skin Irradiation

Total-skin electron irradiation is a modality designed for management of diseases that require irradiation of the entire skin surface or a significant portion of it. The technique is used most frequently for treatment of mycosis fungoides, whose management is reviewed by Hoppe (39).

Multiple techniques for total-skin electron therapy have been reviewed in AAPM Report No. 23 (45). The underlying principles of the various techniques are all similar, which are exemplified by the modified Stanford technique, illustrated in Figure 7.33. First, the treatment requires a broad beam from right to left, which can be achieved by a combination of treating the patient at an extended SSD (300 to 400 cm). The beam is made uniform from head to foot by abutting two fields at the 50% off-axis ratio (see Fig. 7.33A). (Note that the 50% off-axis ratio lies outside the edge of the light field, so when properly abutted, there is a gap between the edges of the respective light fields.) By aiming the beams up and down, the largest bremsstrahlung contribution (central axis) misses the patient. The dose is made uniform around the circumference of the patient by irradiating from six different directions (see Fig. 7.33B). Similar to total-limb irradiation, tangential radiation results in a higher surface dose and a less penetrating dose. Placed upstream of the patient is a plastic screen that serves as both an energy degrader and a scatterer. Dose homogeneity is also dependent on patient position, and reproducing the positions of the Stanford technique (see Fig. 7.33C) is important. Despite efforts to create a homogeneous dose, there always will be areas that are underdosed (e.g., top of scalp, sole of feet, perineum, and

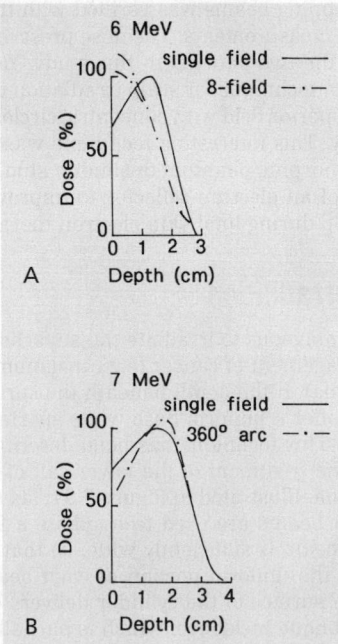

FIGURE 7.32. Treating circular anatomy with multiple beams spaced over 360 degrees. Depth dose along a radial axis depends on the field width. **A:** Depth dose for a broad, 6-MeV beam, resulting from an 8-field technique around a 20-cm diameter water cylinder, is governed by grazing radiation, typical of total-skin and total-limb irradiation. **B:** Depth dose for a narrow, 7-MeV beam, resulting from rotating around a 20-cm diameter water cylinder, is governed by focusing of the radiation toward isocenter, typical of arc electron therapy.

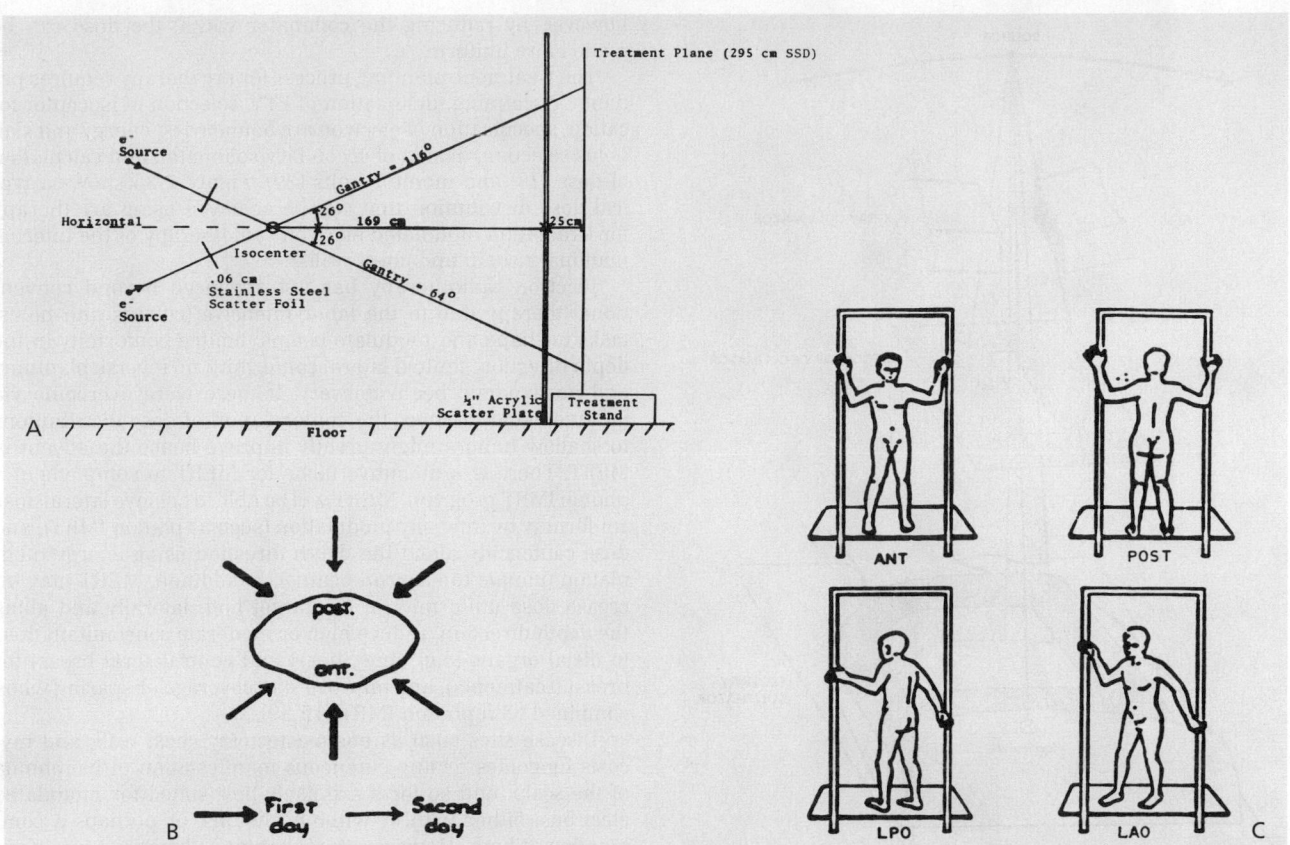

FIGURE 7.33. Schematic of modified Stanford technique. **A:** Side view of setup shows the relative position of patient plane, scatter plate, isocenter, and gantry angles. **B:** Six beam directions are achieved by placing patient in **(C)** six patient positions. (From Almond, PR. Total skin electron irradiation technique and dosimetry. In: Kereiakes JG, Elson HR, Born CG, eds. *Radiation oncology physics 1986.* New York: American Institute of Physics, Inc., 1987;296–332; and Karzmark CJ, Anderson J, Fessenden P, et al. *AAPM Report No. 23, total skin electron therapy: Technique and dosimetry.* New York: American Institute of Physics, Inc., 1987, with permission.)

under the breast or under the panniculus of obese individuals). These areas and sometimes tumorous lesions require separate treatment and boosting, respectively. In contrast, fingers, feet, and toes typically receive excess dose and are shielded for a portion of the treatment. In vivo measurement of patient dose on an individual basis is important when making decisions on prescriptions for supplemental treatments.

Implementation of this technique is complex. It requires an external patient stand with a plastic diffuser, an external scattering foil to broaden the beam, special dosimetry equipment for quality assurance and calibration, special shields for selected parts of the patient, and access to in vivo dosimetry (3). It is also necessary for the radiation therapy accelerator to have a high–dose-rate mode and interlocks for electron energy, gantry angle, and x-ray jaws. Implementation of this technique has been estimated at 105 hours (27). An institution must have a warranted patient population requiring this technique.

Electron Arc Therapy

Electron arc therapy is useful for treating postmastectomy chest wall (29,90). It is used in lieu of parallel-opposed tangential photon irradiation. It is more useful in barrel-chested women, where tangential beams can irradiate too much lung. It is also difficult to achieve homogeneous dose in the region where the medial tangential beam used for the chest wall abuts the anterior beam used for the internal mammary chain. In such cases, treating both areas with only opposed tangent photon beams irradiates too much lung. In such cases electron arc therapy is

a viable option. This can be particularly important in patients with bilateral disease.

The treatment geometry and dosimetry for arc therapy are unique and are discussed in detail by Hogstrom and Leavitt (29). There are three levels of collimation in electron arc therapy: the primary x-ray collimators, a shaped secondary cerrobend insert, and skin collimation (Fig. 7.34). The secondary collimator typically projects a 5- to 6-cm beam width at isocenter. There is typically a large air gap between the secondary collimating insert and the patient, resulting in a large penumbra; also, the finite width of the field results in a broad edge at the end of the arc. The sharpness of the penumbra is restored utilizing skin collimation. This requires that the edge of the field of the secondary collimator extends well beyond the edge of the field defined by skin collimation. In the plane of rotation, this is achieved by rotating approximately 15 degrees beyond the treatment field edge (Fig. 7.35).

As previously discussed, depth dose for an arced beam differs from that for a fixed beam (see Fig 7.27B); the surface dose is significantly less and the dose falloff becomes slightly sharper. Consequently, bolus may be required to deliver adequate dose superficially. Another consequence of arcing is that a constant width of the secondary collimator results in dose inhomogeneity in the cephalocaudal direction. The radius of curvature of the patient with respect to the accelerator isocentric axis is typically less superiorly, as the neck is approached. If the radius of curvature is less, then the skin is farther from the electron source (i.e., a greater SSD). Contrary to fixed-beam therapy, the dose to that region increases rather than decreases as a result of focusing of the electron fluence toward isocenter (29);

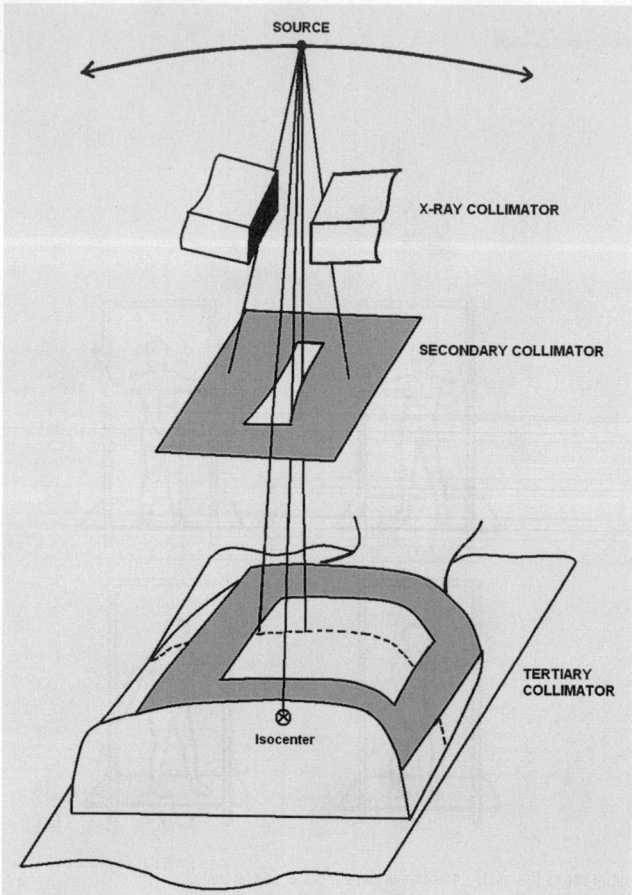

FIGURE 7.34. Schematic of treatment geometry for electron arc therapy. Skin collimation is required because of the large air gap between secondary collimator and patient, which is needed to allow rotation of the gantry around the patient.

however, by reducing the collimator width, the dose can be made more uniform.

The treatment-planning process for arc therapy requires patient CT scanning, delineation of PTV, selection of isocenter location, specification of electron arc boundaries, energy and slab bolus selection, design of secondary collimator, and calculation of dose (28) and monitor units (29). Figure 7.36 shows a typical dose distribution that can be achieved using arc therapy for irradiation modulated electron radiotherapy of the internal mammary chain and chest wall.

Electron radiotherapy has not advanced beyond conventional therapy due to the labor intensive (cutouts and bolus) tasks to shape and modulate beams, limited conformity in the depth direction, limited lateral conformity, no inverse planning, and no dynamic beam delivery. If these were overcome via an automated method, the conformation of dose distributions to shallow tumors might greatly improve hence the advent of MERT. There is a definitive niche for MERT to complement a photon IMRT program. MERT will be able to achieve lateral dose conformity by intensity modulation (such as photon IMRT), and dose conformity along the depth direction using energy modulation (unique to electron beams). In addition, MERT may increase dose uniformity in the target both laterally and along the depth direction, reduce high or moderate concomitant dose to distal organs (e.g., lung, heart and contralateral breast for breast treatments), and improve skin coverage or sparing when combined with photon IMRT (15,59).

Disease sites such as postmastectomy chest wall, and mycosis fungoides or any cutaneous manifestation of lymphoma of the scalp, and so forth are likely best suited for modulated electrons, either with or without photons, or perhaps a combination of both. However, the inherent collimation systems in modern accelerators were optimized for megavoltage photons and are not conducive to electron-beam delivery (in lieu of extended applicators), nor do commercial treatment planning systems model electrons collimated without applicators.

As an example of targeted sites that would be improved with MERT, treatment to the chest wall stands out. Current techniques of using tangential photon adjunct fields abutting

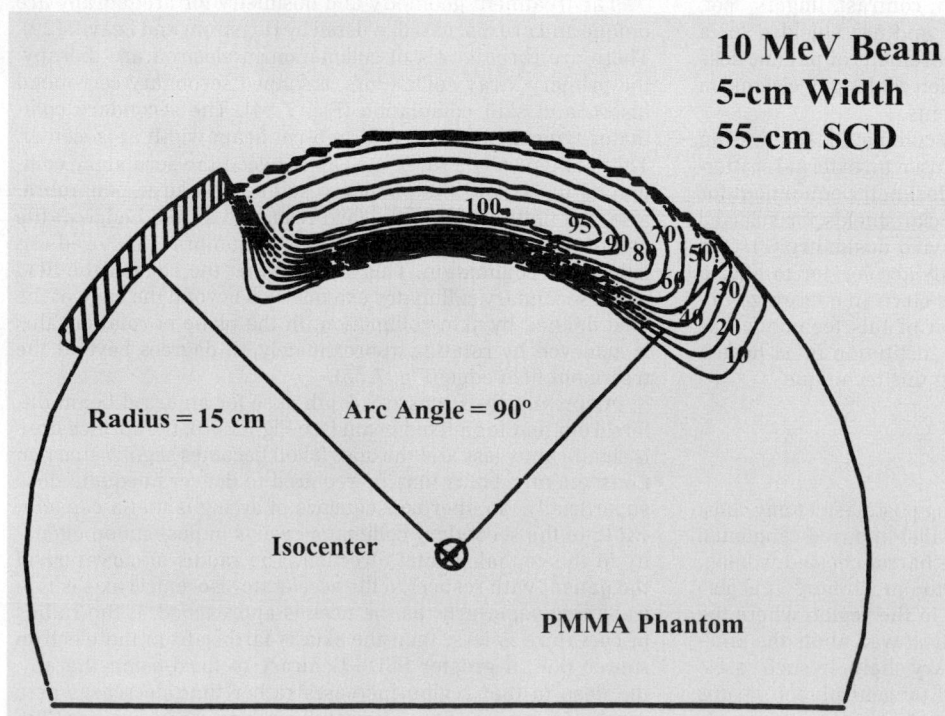

10 MeV Beam
5-cm Width
55-cm SCD

FIGURE 7.35. Comparison of dose distribution with and without skin collimation. The uncollimated edge has a slow dose falloff that is useful for abutting to other arced fields. The skin collimation restores the beam edge but requires rotating the beam 15 degrees beyond the edge of the skin collimator.

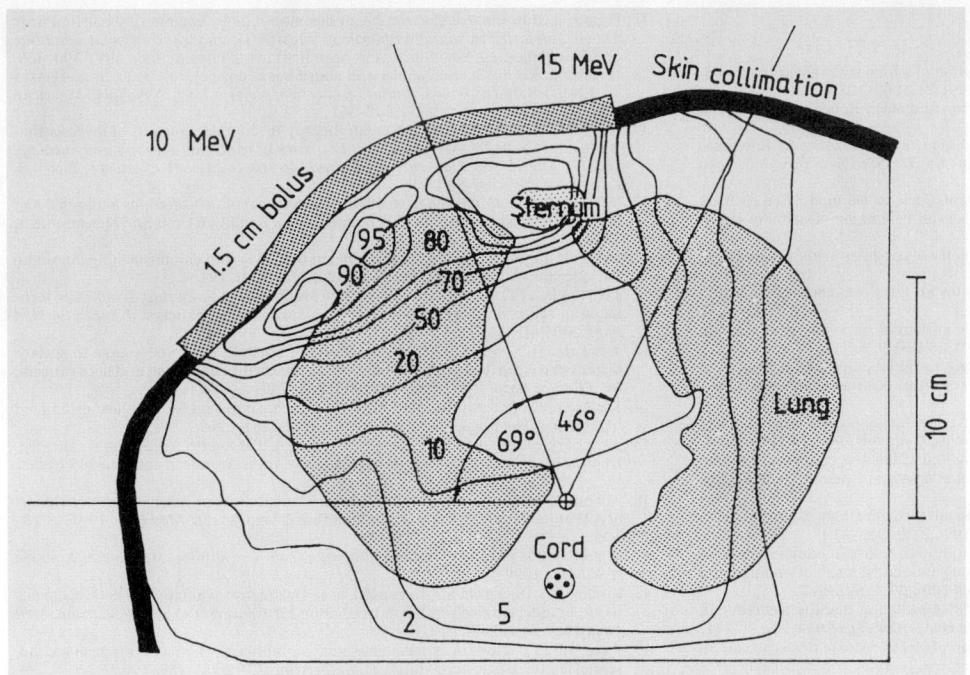

FIGURE 7.36. Typical dose distribution achieved by arc electron therapy. Note the different energies used for the IMC and chest-wall fields, the exact abutment of the internal mammary chain and chest-wall fields, the rotation 15 degrees beyond the skin edges of the skin collimator, and the use of bolus to increase the surface dose. (From Hogstrom KR, Kurup RG, Shiu AS, et al. A two-dimensional pencil-beam algorithm for calculation of arc electron dose distributions. *Phys Med Biol* 1989;34:315–341, with permission.)

supraclavicular and posterior axillary fields are difficult enough without the addition of treating a separate medial breast internal mammary field with a mixture of photon and electrons. Although there has been extensive work to optimize these techniques (42), there are short comings due to match-line problems and delivery of unacceptable doses to volumes of heart, lung, and contralateral breast. The clinical side effects can be edema, fibrosis, heart disease, and pneumonitis. Delivery by tangential photon beams to the chest wall is also not ideal because of the heterogeneous dose delivered in the secondary electron buildup region of the breast. Bolus may be used, but this unfortunately reduces skin sparing. Electron arc therapy was developed in the 1980s to address the limitations of tangential photon-beam treatments (23), but it was extremely time-consuming to implement.

Many centers have used photon IMRT to improve dose conformity, but the fundamental limitations due to megavoltage photon beams, such as excess distal dose and the buildup dose, are still challenges. MERT has been proposed as an alternative, particularly for postmastectomy patients (15,59). The principal advantage is the rapid distal dose falloff. In principle, electron beams are well suited for these shallow targets, as they will spare distal regions, such as lung and heart.

Optimization is another important aspect for a MERT program. Many people have come up with inverse planning techniques for photons and even more recently for electrons. Al-Yahya et al. (4) came up with a method of optimizing electron-beam planning for a few electron-leaf collimators (FELC). Planning was performed via Monte Carlo calculations and optimization using simulated annealing, a powerful mathematical tool that is the basis for inverse planning. FELC consists of four motor-driven trimmer bars at the end of an applicator that creates rectangular shapes. The report claims potential treatment times of 15' or less. Olofsonn et al. (76) devised an algorithm that was based on energy and range selection methods for optimization. Very comprehensive work by Lee et al. (56) described a Monte Carlo optimization scheme for modulated electron-beam radiotherapy based on a stop and shoot technique. One of the most challenging things in both calculating and optimizing is the leaf scatter where distributions could

vary up to 20% depending on leaf positions. Lee et al. performed MLC planning accomplished by calculating composite distributions for electron beamlets as collimated by tertiary electron MLC. Scatter and leakage contributions were included in the final dose calculation. An inverse planning dose optimization engine designed weights for each beamlet. The particle generation and absorption within the MLC leaves created demanding calculations, but were necessary for accurate organ-at-risk calculations. Therefore, modeling of leaf scatter and transmissions is vital for accurate dose calculations. It is key that a multiple source model be developed. And finally, Oloffson et al. (76) studied use of MLC computer optimization to select energies for 1 cm by 1 cm beamlets, depending on depths to treat. They found that simple plans with four segments worked well for postmastectomy patients to reduce dose to lung and heart and cover chest wall tissue. The delivery was to be accomplished with computer controlled MLC of Microtron, which was modeled for electrons.

Summary

Electron-beam therapy remains an important modality to the practice of radiation therapy. As discussed earlier, its effective use requires knowledge of the unique properties of electron-beam dose distributions, the impact of the patient on the dose distribution, and the basic principles for good practice. It requires access to and the proper use of comprehensive treatment planning and delivery tools. It also requires access to special techniques that offer unique treatment solutions for a limited number but broad range of patient conditions.

Electron therapy can be expected to become more sophisticated in the future as the enthusiasm for modulated electron radiation therapy grows. Advances in electron dose calculations, methods for electron-beam optimization, and availability of multileaf collimators for electrons will enable the practice of combined intensity-modulated photon and energy-modulated electron therapy. This will advance both electron conformal and mixed-beam therapy.

References

1. Able CM, Mills MD, McNeese MD, et al. Evaluation of a total scalp electron irradiation technique. *Int J Radiat Oncol Biol Phys* 1991;21:1063–1072.
2. Akazawa C. Treatment of the scalp using photon and electron beams. *Med Dosim* 1989;14:129–131.
3. Almond, PR. Total skin electron irradiation technique and dosimetry. In: Kereiakes JG, Elson HR, Born CG, eds. *Radiation oncology physics 1986*. New York: American Institute of Physics, Inc., 1987;296–332.
4. Al-Yahya K, Hristov D, Verhaegen F, et al. Monte Carlo based modulated electron beam treatment planning using a few-leaf electron collimator—feasibility study. *Phys Med Biol* 2005;50(5):847–857.
5. Biggs PJ, Boyer AL, Doppke KP. Electron dosimetry of irregular fields on Clinac-18. *Int J Radiat Oncol Biol Phys* 1979;5:433–440.
6. Biggs PJ, Wang CC. Breakaway safety feature for an intra-oral cone system. *Int J Radiat Oncol Biol Phys* 1984;10:1117–1119.
7. Boyd RA, Hogstrom KR, Antolak JA, et al. A measured data set for evaluating electron-beam dose algorithms. *Med Phys* 2001;28:950–958.
8. Boyd RA, Hogstrom KR, Rosen II. Effect of using an initial polyenergetic spectrum with the pencil-beam redefinition algorithm for electron-dose calculations in water. *Med Phys* 1998;25:2176–2185.
9. Boyd RA, Hogstrom KR, Starkschall G. Electron pencil-beam redefinition algorithm dose calculations in the presence of heterogeneities. *Med Phys* 2001;28:2096–2104.
10. Cygler JE, Daskalov GM, Chan GH, et al. Evaluation of the first commercial Monte Carlo dose calculation engine for electron beam treatment planning. *Med Phys* 2004;31(1):142–153.
11. Das IJ, Bushe HS. Backscattering and transmission through a high Z interface as a measure of electron beam energy. *Med Phys* 1994;21(2):315–319.
12. Das SK, Bell M, Marks LB, et al. A preliminary study of the role of modulated electron beams in intensity modulated radiotherapy, using automated beam orientation and modality selection. *Int J Radiat Oncol Biol Phys* 2004;59(2):602–617.
13. Dewit L, Van Dam J, Rijnders A, et al. A modified radiation therapy technique in the treatment of medulloblastoma. *Int J Radiat Oncol Biol Phys* 1984;10:231–241.
14. Ding GX, Cygler JE, Yu CW, et al. A comparison of electron beam dose calculation accuracy between treatment planning systems using either a pencil beam or a Monte Carlo algorithm. *Int J Radiat Oncol Biol Phys* 2005;63(2):622–633.
15. Ding GX, Duggan DM, Coffey CW, et al. First macro Monte Carlo based commercial dose calculation module for electron beam treatment planning—new issues for clinical consideration. *Phys Med Biol* 2006;51(11):2781–2799.
16. Dominiak GS. Dose in spinal cord following electron irradiation. The University of Texas Health Science Center at Houston, Graduate School of Biomedical Sciences, 1991.
17. Donaldson SS, Findley DO. Treatment of orbital lymphoid tumors with electron beams. In: Vaeth JM, Meyer JL, eds. *Frontiers of radiation therapy and oncology Vol. 25: The role of high energy electrons in the treatment of cancer*. Basel: S. Karger AG, 1991;187–200.
18. Ekstrand KE, Dixon RL. The problem of obliquely incident beams in electron-beam treatment planning. *Med Phys* 1982;9:276–278.
19. Faddegon B, et al. Clinical considerations of Monte Carlo for electron radiotherapy treatment planning. *Radiat Phys Chem* 1998;53:217–227.
20. Fields RS, Hogstrom KR. Optimization of electron-photon mixed beam planning. In: *Proceedings of the Eighth International Conference on the Use of Computers in Radiation Therapy*. Silver Spring: IEEE Computer Society Press, 1984;248–254.
21. Fletcher GH. Clinical applications of the electron beam. In: Tapley N, ed. New York, Wiley, 1976;1.
22. Fraass B, Doppke K, Hunt M, et al. American Association of Physicists in Medicine Radiation Therapy Committee Task Group 53: Quality assurance for clinical radiotherapy treatment planning [Review]. *Med Phys* 1998;25(10):1773–1829.
23. Gaffney DK, Leavitt DD, Tsodikov A, et al. Electron arc irradiation of the postmastectomy chest wall with CT treatment planning: 20-year experience. *Int J Radiat Oncol Biol Phys* 2001;51(4):994–1001.
24. Harms WB, Purdy JA. Abutment of high energy electron fields. *Int J Radiat Oncol Biol Phys* 1991;20(4):853–858.
25. Hogstrom KR, Boyer AL, Shiu AS, et al. Design of metallic electron beam cones for an intraoperative therapy linear accelerator. *Int J Radiat Oncol Biol Phys* 1990;18:1223–1232.
26. Hogstrom KR, Fields RS. Use of CT in electron beam treatment planning: Current and future development. In: Ling CC, Rogers CC, Morton RJ, eds. *Computed tomography in radiation therapy*. New York: Raven Press, 1983;241–252.
27. Hogstrom KR, Horton JL, Kutcher GJ, et al. *ACMP Task Group Report: Survey of physics resources for radiation oncology special procedures*. Reston: American College of Medical Physics, 1998.
28. Hogstrom KR, Kurup RG, Shiu AS, et al. A two-dimensional pencil-beam algorithm for calculation of arc electron dose distributions. *Phys Med Biol* 1989;34:315–341.
29. Hogstrom KR, Leavitt D. Dosimetry of electron arc therapy. In: Kereiakes JG, Elson HR, Born CG, eds. *Radiation oncology physics 1986*. New York: American Institute of Physics, 1987;265–295.
30. Hogstrom KR, Mills MD, Almond PR. Electron beam dose calculations. *Phys Med Biol* 1981;26:445–459.
31. Hogstrom KR, Mills MD, Meyer JA, et al. Dosimetric evaluation of a pencil-beam algorithm for electrons employing a two-dimensional heterogeneity correction. *Int J Radiat Oncol Biol Phys* 1984;10:561–569.
32. Hogstrom KR, Steadham RE. Electron beam dose computation. In: Palta JR, Mackie TR, eds. *Teletherapy: Present and future*. Madison: Advanced Medical Publishing, 1996;137–174.
33. Hogstrom KR. Dosimetry of electron heterogeneities. In: Wright AE, Boyer AL, eds. *Advances in radiation therapy treatment planning*. New York: American Institute of Physics, Inc., 1983;223–243.
34. Hogstrom KR. Implementation of CT treatment planning. In: Wright AE, Boyer AL, eds. *Advances in radiation therapy treatment planning*. New York: American Institute of Physics, Inc., 1983;268–281.
35. Hogstrom KR. Treatment planning in electron beam therapy. In: Vaeth JM, Meyer JL, eds. *Frontiers of radiation therapy and oncology Vol. 25: The role of high energy electrons in the treatment of cancer*. Basel: S. Karger AG, 1991;30–52.
36. Hogstrom, KR, Steadham RE, Wong PF, et al. Monitor unit calculations for electron beams. In: Gibbons JP, ed. *Monitor unit calculations for external photon and electron beams*. Madison: Advanced Medical Publishing, Inc., 2000;113–126.
37. Hogstrom, KR. Clinical electron beam dosimetry: basic dosimetry data. In: Purdy JA, ed. *Advances in radiation oncology physics: Dosimetry, treatment planning, and brachytherapy*. Woodbury: American Institute of Physics, Inc., 1991;390–429.
38. Hogstrom, KR. Evaluation of electron pencil beam dose calculations. In: Kereiakes JG, Elson HR, Born CG, eds. *Radiation oncology physics 1986*. New York: American Institute of Physics, Inc., 1987;532–557.
39. Hoppe, RT. Total skin electron beam therapy in the management of mycosis fungoides. In: Vaeth JM, Meyer JL, eds. *Frontiers of radiation therapy and oncology Vol. 25: The role of high energy electrons in the treatment of cancer*. Basel: S. Karger AG, 1991;80–89.
40. ICRU Report 35. *Radiation dosimetry: Electron beams with energies between 1 and 50 MeV*. Bethesda: International Commission on Radiation Units and Measurement, 1984.
41. Jiang SB, Kapur A, Ma CM. Electron beam modeling and commissioning for Monte Carlo treatment planning. *Med Phys* 2000;27(1):180–191.
42. Jin JY, Klein EE, Kong FM, et al. An improved internal mammary irradiation technique in radiation treatment of locally advanced breast cancers. *J Appl Clin Med Phys* 2005;6(1):84–93.
43. Johnson JM, Khan FM. Dosimetric effects of abutting extended source to surface distance electron fields with photon fields in the treatment of head and neck cancers. *Int J Radiat Oncol Biol Phys* 1994;28(3):741–747.
44. Karlsson MG, Karlsson M, Ma CM. Treatment head design for multileaf collimated high-energy electrons. *Med Phys* 1999;26(10):2161–2167.
45. Karzmark CJ, Anderson J, Fessenden P, et al. *AAPM Report No. 23, total skin electron therapy: Technique and dosimetry*. New York: American Institute of Physics, Inc., 1987.
46. Khan FM, Doppke KP, Hogstrom KR, et al. Clinical electron-beam dosimetry: Report of AAPM Radiation Therapy Committee Task Group No. 25. *Med Phys* 1991;18:73–109.
47. Khan FM. *The physics of radiation therapy*. 2nd ed. Baltimore: Lippincott Williams & Wilkins, 1994.
48. Kirsner SM, Hogstrom KR, Kurup RG, et al. Dosimetric evaluation in heterogeneous tissue of anterior electron beam irradiation for treatment of retinoblastoma. *Med Phys* 1987;14:772–779.
49. Klein EE, Li Z, Low DA. A feasibility study of multileaf collimated electrons with a scattering foil based accelerator. *Radiother Oncol* 1996;41:189–196.
50. Klein EE, Low DA, Purdy JA. Dosimetric changes with the new scattering foil applicator system on a C12100C. *Int J Radiat Oncol Biol Phys* 1995;32:483–490.
51. Klevenhagen SC, Lambert GD, Arbabi A. Backscattering in electron beam therapy for energies between 3 and 35 MeV. *Phys Med Biol* 1982;27:363–373.
52. Kudchadker RJ, Hogstrom KR, Garden AS, et al. Electron conformal radiation therapy using bolus and intensity modulation. *Int J Radiat Oncol Biol Phys* 2002;53:1023–1037.
53. Kun LE. Electron beam therapy in children. In: Vaeth JM, Meyer JL, eds. *Frontiers of radiation therapy and oncology Vol. 25: the role of high energy electrons in the treatment of cancer*. Basel: S. Karger AG, 1991;201–206.
54. Kutcher GJ, Coia L, Gillin M, et al. Comprehensive QA for radiation oncology: Report of AAPM Radiation Therapy Committee Task Group 40. *Med Phys* 1994;21(4):581–618.
55. Lambert GD, Klevenhagen SC. Penetration of backscattered electrons in polystyrene for energies between 1 and 25 MeV. *Phys Med Biol* 1982;27:721–725.
56. Lee MC, Jiang SB, Ma CM. Monte Carlo and experimental investigations of multileaf collimated electron beams for modulated electron radiation therapy. *Med Phys* 2000;27(12):2708–2718.
57. Low DA, Starkschall G, Bujnowski SW, et al. Electron bolus design for radiation therapy treatment planning: Bolus design algorithms. *Med Phys* 1992;19:115–124.
58. Low DA, Starkschall G, Sherman NE, et al. Computer-aided design and fabrication of an electron bolus for treatment of the paraspinal muscles. *Int J Radiat Oncol Biol Phys* 1995;33:1127–1138.
59. Ma CM, Ding M, Li JS, et al. A comparative dosimetric study on tangential photon beams, intensity-modulated radiation therapy (IMRT) and modulated electron radiotherapy (MERT) for breast cancer treatment. *Phys Med Biol* 2003;48(7):909–924.
60. Ma CM, Faddegon BA, Rogers DW, et al. Accurate characterization of Monte Carlo calculated electron beams for radiotherapy. *Med Phys* 1997;24(3):401–416.
61. Ma CM, Mok E, Kapur A, et al. Clinical implementation of a Monte Carlo treatment planning system. *Med Phys* 1999;26(10):2133–2143.
62. Maor MH, Fields RS, Hogstrom KR, et al. Improving the therapeutic ratio of craniospinal irradiation in medulloblastoma. *Int J Radiat Oncol Biol Phys* 1985;11:687–697.
63. Maor MH, Hogstrom KR, Fields RS, et al. Newer approaches to cerebrospinal irradiation in pediatric brain tumors. In: Brooks BF, ed. *Malignant tumors of childhood*. Austin: University of Texas Press, 1986;245–254.
64. McGinnis WL, Bischof CJ, Latourette HB. Transvaginal cone electron beam technique for a Varian 18 MeV linear accelerator. *Int J Radiat Oncol Biol Phys* 1979;5:123–125.
65. Merrick HW III, Dobelbower RR Jr, Konski AA. Intraoperative radiation therapy for pancreatic, biliary and gastric carcinoma: The US experience. In: Vaeth JM, Meyer JL, eds. *Frontiers of radiation therapy and oncology Vol. 25: The role of high energy electrons in the treatment of cancer*. Basel: S. Karger AG, 1991;246–257.
66. Meyer JA, Palta JR, Hogstrom KR. Demonstration of relatively new electron dosimetry measurement techniques on the Mevatron 80. *Med Phys* 1984;11:670–677.
67. Million RR, Parson JT, Bova FJ, et al. Electron beam: the management of head and neck cancer. In: Vaeth JM, Meyer JL, eds. *Frontiers of radiation therapy and oncology Vol. 25: The role of high energy electrons in the treatment of cancer*. Basel: S. Karger AG, 1991;107–127.
68. Mills MD, Fuller LM, Zagars GK, et al. Spinal cord dose reduction using an anterior 13 MeV electron field situated between a split anterior ^{60}Co supraclavicular field. *Int J Radiat Oncol Biol Phys* 1987;13:1571–1575.
69. Mills MD, Hogstrom KR, Almond PR. Prediction of electron beam output factors. *Med Phys* 1982;9:60–68.
70. Mills MD, Hogstrom KR, Fields RS. Determination of electron beam output factors for a 20-MeV linear accelerator. *Med Phys* 1985;12:473–476.
71. Morrison WH, Wong PF, Starkschall G, et al. Water bolus for electron irradiation of the ear canal. *Int J Radiat Oncol Biol Phys* 1995;33:479–483.
72. Mu X, Olofsson L, Karlsson M, et al. Can photon IMRT be improved by combination with mixed electron and photon techniques? *Acta Oncol* 2004;43(8):727–735.

73. Neuenschwander H, Born EJ. A macro Monte-Carlo method for electron-beam dose calculations. *Phys Med Biol* 1992;37(1):107–125.
74. Neuenschwander H, Mackie TR, Reckwerdt PJ. MMC—a high-performance Monte Carlo code for electron beam treatment planning. *Phys Med Biol* 1995;40(I):543–574.
75. Nyerick CE, Ochran TG, Boyer AL, et al. Dosimetry characteristics of metallic cones for intraoperative radiation therapy. *Int J Radiat Oncol Biol Phys* 1991;21:501–510.
76. Olofsson L, Karlsson MG, Karlsson M. Effects on electron beam penumbra using the photon MLC to reduce bremsstrahlung leakage from an add-on electron MLC. *Phys Med Biol* 2005;50(6):1191–1203.
77. Perez CA. Management of vulvar cancer. In: Vaeth JM, Meyer JL, eds. *Frontiers of radiation therapy and oncology Vol. 25: The role of high energy electrons in the treatment of cancer*. Basel: S. Karger AG, 1991;183–186.
78. Perkins GH, McNeese MD, Antolak JA, et al. A custom three-dimensional electron bolus technique for optimization of postmastectomy irradiation. *Int J Radiat Oncol Biol Phys* 2001;51:1142–1151.
79. Perry DJ, Holt JG. A model for calculating the effects of small inhomogeneities on electron beam dose distributions. *Med Phys* 1980;7:207–215.
80. Peters VG. Use of an electron reflector to improve dose uniformity at the vertex during total skin electron therapy. *Int J Radiat Oncol Biol Phys* 2000;46(4):1065–1069.
81. Recht A, Triedman SA, Harris JR. The "boost" in the treatment of early-stage breast cancer: Electrons versus interstitial implants. In: Vaeth JM, Meyer JL, eds. *Frontiers of radiation therapy and oncology Vol. 25: The role of high energy electrons in the treatment of cancer*. Basel: S. Karger AG, 1991;169–179.
82. Severin D, Connors S, Thompson H, et al. Breast radiotherapy with inclusion of internal mammary nodes: A comparison of techniques with three-dimensional planning. *Int J Radiat Oncol Biol Phys* 2003;55(3):633–644.
83. Shiu AS, Hogstrom KR. Dose in bone and tissue near bone-tissue interface from electron beam. *Int J Radiat Oncol Biol Phys* 1991;21:695–702.
84. Shiu AS, Hogstrom KR. Pencil-beam redefinition algorithm for electron dose distributions. *Med Phys* 1991;18:7–18.
85. Shiu AS, Tung S, Hogstrom KR, et al. Verification data for electron beam dose algorithms. *Med Phys* 1992;19:623–636.
86. Shiu AS, Tung SS, Gastorf RJ, et al. Dosimetric evaluation of lead and tungsten eye shields in electron beam treatment. *Int J Radiat Oncol Biol Phys* 1996;35:599–604.
87. Shiu AS, Tung SS, Nyerick CE, et al. Comprehensive analysis of electron beam central axis dose for a radiation therapy linear accelerator. *Med Phys* 1994;21:559–566.
88. Starkschall G, Antolak JA, Hogstrom KR. Electron beam bolus for 3-D conformal radiation therapy. In: Purdy JA, Emami B, eds. *3-D radiation treatment planning and conformal therapy, proceedings of an international symposium*. Madison, WI: Medical Physics Publishing, 1995;265–282.
89. Starkschall G, Shiu AS, Bujnowski SW, et al. Effect of dimensionality of heterogeneity corrections on the implementation of a three-dimensional electron pencil-beam algorithm. *Phys Med Biol* 1991;36:207–227.
90. Stewart JR, Leavitt DD, Prows J. Electron arc therapy of the chest wall for breast cancer: Rationale, dosimetry, and clinical aspects. In: Vaeth JM, Meyer JL, eds. *Frontiers of radiation therapy and oncology Vol. 25: The role of high energy electrons in the treatment of cancer*. Basel: S. Karger AG, 1991;134–150.
91. Tapley ND, ed. *Clinical applications of the electron beam*. New York: John Wiley & Sons, Inc., 1976.
92. Tung SS, Shiu AS, Starkschall G, et al. Dosimetric evaluation of total scalp irradiation using a lateral electron-photon technique. *Int J Radiat Oncol Biol Phys* 1993;27:153–160.
93. Vaeth JM, Meyer JL, eds. *Frontiers of radiation therapy and oncology Vol. 25: The role of high energy electrons in the treatment of cancer*. Basel: S. Karger AG, 1991.
94. Walker C, Wadd NJ, Lucraft HH. Novel solutions to the problems encountered in electron irradiation to the surface of the head. *Br J Radiol* 1999;72(860):787–791.
95. Wang, CC. Intraoral cone for carcinoma of the oral cavity. In: Vaeth JM, Meyer JL, eds. *Frontiers of radiation therapy and oncology Vol. 25: The role of high energy electrons in the treatment of cancer*. Basel: S. Karger AG, 1991;128–131
96. Wooden KK, Hogstrom KR, Blum P, et al. Whole-limb irradiation of the lower calf using a six-field electron technique. *Med Dosim* 1996;21:211–218.
97. Yaparpalvi R, Fontenla DP, Beitler JJ. Improved dose homogeneity in scalp irradiation using a single set-up point and different energy electron beams. *Br J Radiol* 2002;75(896):670–677.
98. Zackrisson B, Karlsson M. Matching of electron beams for conformal therapy of target volumes at moderate depths. *Radiother Oncol* 1996;39(3):261–270.

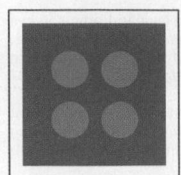

Chapter 8
Three-Dimensional Conformal Radiation Therapy: Physics, Treatment Planning, and Clinical Aspects

James A. Purdy

Modern anatomic imaging technologies, such as x-ray computed tomography (CT) and magnetic resonance imaging (MRI) provide a fully three-dimensional model of the cancer patient's anatomy, which is often complemented with functional imaging, such as positron emission tomography (PET) or magnetic resonance spectroscopy. Such advanced imaging now allows the radiation oncologist to more accurately identify tumor volumes and their relationship with other critical normal organs. Powerful x-ray CT-simulation and three-dimensional treatment planning systems (3DTPS) have been commercially available since the early 1990's and three-dimensional conformal radiation therapy (3DCRT) is now firmly in place as the standard of practice (79,102,113). In addition, advances in radiation treatment-delivery technology continue and medical linear accelerators now come equipped with sophisticated computer-controlled multileaf collimator systems (MLCs) and integrated volumetric imaging systems that provide beam aperture and/or beam-intensity modulation capabilities that allow precise shaping and positioning of the patient's dose distributions (10).

Conformal treatment plans generally use an increased number of radiation beams that are shaped to conform to the target volume. To improve the conformality of the dose distribution, conventional beam modifiers (e.g., wedges, partial transmission blocks, and/or compensating filters) are sometimes used. This *"forward planning"* approach to 3DCRT is rapidly giving way to an *"inverse planning"* approach referred to as *intensity-modulated radiation therapy* (IMRT), which can achieve even greater conformity by optimally modulating the individual beamlets that make up the radiation beams (104,149). IMRT dose distributions can be created to conform much more closely to the target volume, particularly for those volumes having complex/concave shapes, and shaped to avoid critical normal tissues in the irradiated volume. This increased conformality results in IMRT treatments being much more sensitive to geometric uncertainties than the two-dimensional or 3DCRT approaches, and has spurred the development of treatment machines integrated with advanced volumetric imaging capabilities (52), which is again pushing the edge of our frontiers in conformal therapy practice from IMRT to what is now referred to as *image-guided IMRT*, or simply *image-guided radiation therapy* (IGRT) (10,67). Of course, the concept of image guidance is not revolutionary, and really should be viewed as an evolutionary component in the development of conformal therapy. In the past, many systems and/or processes have been developed to help better localize the patient for treatment (and hence conform the dose), including dedicated x-ray simulators, megavoltage radiographic port films, electronic portal imaging devices, implanted radiopaque markers, ultrasound imaging systems, and optical surface tracking systems (24,88). Even the early isocentric cobalt-60 teletherapy machines in the 1960s came equipped with a kilovolt x-ray tube attached to the beam stop.

This chapter will review the critical components that make up the conformal therapy planning and delivery process, focusing mainly on the forward-planned 3DCRT process. However, it should be understood that most of concepts and tasks discussed apply equally well to IMRT and IGRT, particularly with regard to target volume definition. In addition, the reader should understand that the use of the terms *2D* (two-dimensional), *3D* (three-dimensional), and even *4D* (four-dimensional) (55) as descriptors for the conformal therapy planning and delivery process is referring to a process and tools used, and not merely to beam arrangements. For example, 3D treatment planning certainly does not require the use of "noncoplanar" beams, a common misconception, but does require the ability to plan and visualize volumetric dose distributions for such beam arrangements. Even today, newer tools are being developed that allow 4D image-based treatment planning, that is, target volume segmentation and dose calculation in the presence of respiratory motion, that will be used to deliver 3DCRT treatments for lung cancer (121). Thus, the reader will be able to appreciate the conformal therapy approach much more fully, if viewed as a workflow process using appropriate software and technology.

Historical Development of Conformal Therapy and 3-D Treatment-Planning Systems

Conformational treatment methods were pioneered in the 1950s and 1960s by several groups, including Takahashi in Japan (137); Proimos (101), Wright et al. (154), and Trump et al. (140) in the United States; and Green (39) and Green et al. (40) in Great Britain. This work continued into the 1970s, when several groups actually implemented computer-controlled radiation therapy, including the Joint Center in Boston project led by Bjarngard et al. (9) and Kijewski et al. (56), and the Tracking Cobalt Project led by Davy et al. (21–23) at the Royal Free Hospital in London.

Sterling et al. (135,136) are credited with the first 3D approach (dose calculation and display) to treatment planning. They demonstrated a technique by which a computer-generated film loop gave the illusion of a 3D view of the patient's relevant anatomic features and the calculated isodose distribution (2D color washes) throughout a treatment volume. However, this effort did not result in a practical 3DTPS and was viewed as simply a demonstration project. Reinstein et al. (117) and McShan et al. (77) at Rhode Island Hospital, Brown University, made the first real step in implementing a clinically usable 3DTPS based on a new type of display, called *beam's-eye-view* (BEV), which simulates the treatment planner's viewing point from the perspective of the radiation source looking out along the axis of the radiation beam, similar to that obtained when viewing a simulation radiograph.

The advent of CT spurred further development of 3D planning systems. In 1983, Goitein and Abrams (37) and Goitein et al. (38) reported on their system, which took advantage of CT and increased minicomputer capabilities. The system produced high-quality color BEV displays and could display radiographic images computed from the digital CT data; such computed radiographs are now called *digitally reconstructed radiographs* (DRRs). By the latter half of the 1980s, several other groups had developed 3D planning systems having powerful new features such as the real-time *room's-eye-view* (REV) display first

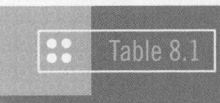

Table 8.1	NATIONAL CANCER INSTITUTE RESEARCH CONTRACTS IN SUPPORT OF THREE-DIMENSIONAL RADIATION THERAPY TREATMENT PLANNING

Evaluation of Treatment Planning for Heavy Particles (1982–1986)
- University of Pennsylvania School of Medicine and Fox Chase Cancer Center
- Lawrence Berkeley Laboratory and University of California
- Massachusetts General Hospital
- M.D. Anderson Cancer Center - University of Texas

Evaluation of Treatment Planning for External-Beam Photons (1984–1987)
- University of Pennsylvania School of Medicine and Fox Chase Cancer Center
- Memorial Sloan-Kettering Cancer Center
- Massachusetts General Hospital
- Washington University in St. Louis

Evaluation of Treatment Planning for External-Beam Electrons (1986–1989)
- University of Michigan
- M.D. Anderson Cancer Center - University of Texas
- Washington University in St. Louis

Development of Radiation Therapy Treatment Planning Software Tools (1989–1994)
- University of North Carolina
- University of Washington
- Washington University in St. Louis

developed at Washington University in 1986 (30,84,110,131). The REV display provides the treatment planner a viewing point simulating any arbitrary location within the treatment room.

In the 1990s, the commercial availability of 3DTPSs led to widespread adoption of 3D planning and conformal therapy as the standard of practice. One of the keys to this development was a series of research contracts funded by the National Cancer Institute (NCI) in the 1980s and 1990s to evaluate the potential of 3D planning and to make recommendations to the NCI for future research in this area (134,162). Each of the research contracts funded a collaborative working group (CWG) (the participating institutions in each CWG are shown in Table 8.1) whose charge was to evaluate various aspects of this new planning process and develop new software tools needed. The CWGs were composed of physicists, clinicians, and computer scientists. Many important developments and/or refinements in 3D planning came from these NCI research CWGs, particularly planning evaluation software tools such as *dose–volume histograms* (DVHs) (25,26), *electronic view-box* (11), and biologic effect models such as *tumor control probability* (TCP) and *normal tissue complication probability* (NTCP) models. Just as important was the CWG efforts that helped stimulate and document the current state of knowledge about 3D planning and conformal therapy. Even IMRT has benefited from the CWG approach, as a consensus statement was developed in 2001 that helped clarify many issues regarding that form of conformal therapy (51). Conformal therapy could perhaps benefit once more from a CWG that focused on newly emerging IGRT.

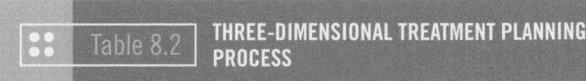

Table 8.2	THREE-DIMENSIONAL TREATMENT PLANNING PROCESS

Step 1: Patient positioning and immobilization
- Construct patient repositioning/immobilization device
- Establish patient reference marks/patient coordinate system

Step 2: Image acquisition and input
- Acquire/input CT (MR or other imaging data) into three-dimensional radiation therapy treatment planning system.

Step 3: Anatomy definition
- Geometrically register all input data (such as CT, MR)
- Define and display contours and surfaces for organs at risk
- Define and display contours and surfaces for target volumes
- Generate electron density representation from CT or from assigned bulk density information

Step 4: Dose prescription
- Specify dose prescription for planning target volume(s)
- Specify dose tolerances for organs at risk

Step 5: Beam technique
- Determine beam arrangements (beam's-eye-view and room's-eye-view displays)
- Design field shape (blocks, multileaf collimator leaf settings)
- Determine beam modifiers (compensators, wedges, partial transmission blocks)
- Determine beam weighting

Step 6: Dose calculations
- Select dose-calculation algorithm and calculation grid
- Input dose prescription
- Perform dose calculations
- Set relative and absolute dose normalizations

Step 7: Plan evaluation/improvement
- Generate two- and three-dimensional isodose displays
- Generate dose–volume histograms
- Perform visual DVH and isodose comparisons
- Use automated optimization tools if available
- Modify plan based on evaluation of the dose distribution

Step 8: Plan review and documentation
- Perform overall review of all aspects of plan and obtain physician approval
- Generate hard copy output including digitally reconstructed radiographs

Step 9: Plan implementation and verification
- Transfer plan parameters into treatment machine record-and-verify system
- Set up (register) the real patient according to plan (verification simulation optional)
- Perform patient treatment QA checks including independent check of monitor units

CT, computed tomography; MR, magnetic resonance; DVH, dose-volume histogram; QA, quality assurance.

Three-Dimensional Treatment Planning

Forward-based 3D planning for conformal therapy typically involves a series of procedures summarized in Table 8.2; these include establishing the patient's treatment position (including constructing a patient repositioning immobilization device when needed), obtaining a volumetric image dataset of the patient in treatment position, contouring target volume(s) and critical normal organs using the volumetric planning image dataset, determining beam orientation and designing beam-block apertures or MLC leaf settings, computing a 3D dose distribution

according to the dose prescription, evaluating the treatment plan, and, if needed, modifying the plan (e.g., beam orientations, apertures, weights, modifiers) until an acceptable plan is approved by the radiation oncologist. The approved plan must then be implemented on the treatment machine and the patient's treatment verified using appropriate quality assurance (QA) procedures. All of these tasks make up the forward-planned conformal therapy process and are discussed in the ensuing sections.

It should be clearly understood that 3D treatment planning and the conformal therapy process represents a radical change in practice for the radiation oncologist still using the 2D approach, which emphasizes the use of a conventional x-ray simulator to visualize bony landmarks on planar radiographs for designing beam portals for standardized beam arrangement techniques. In contrast, the 3D treatment planning/conformal therapy process emphasizes a volumetric image-based virtual simulation approach for defining tumor and critical structure volumes for the individual patient (79,102). This process puts increased demands on the radiation oncologist to specify target volume(s) and critical structure(s) with far greater

Overview and Basic Science of Radiation Oncology

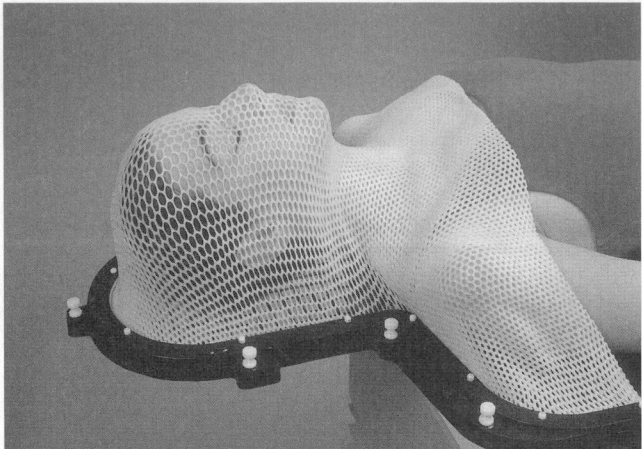

FIGURE 8.1. Example of immobilization repositioning system used for patients undergoing radiation therapy for head and neck cancer. It should be clearly understood that being able to accurately reposition the patient and accounting for internal organ movement, in order to accurately deliver the planned dose distribution, is one of the most important steps in the conformal therapy process. (Reproduced with permission of MEDTEC, Inc., Orange City, IA)

accuracy than previously. Moreover, conformal therapy also places increased demands on the radiation oncology physicist to insure adequate QA measures are in place, such as checks regarding use of multi-modality imaging (including fusion QA), patient setup reproducibility checks, organ motion assessment, and treatment delivery verification.

Patient Treatment Position/Immobilization and Planning CT Scan

In the initial part of the conformal therapy process (preplanning), the proposed treatment position of the patient is determined and the immobilization device to be used during treatment is fabricated. It should be clearly understood that being able to accurately reposition the patients and accounting for internal organ movement, in order to accurately deliver the planned dose distribution, is one of the most important steps in the conformal therapy process. Errors may occur if patients are

inadequately immobilized, with resultant treatment fields inaccurately aligned from treatment to treatment (interfraction). In addition, patients and/or their tumor volume may also move during treatment (intrafraction) because of either inadequate immobilization or physiologic activity.

Determining the treatment position of the patient and construction of the immobilization device can be performed on a conventional radiation therapy simulator, but more preferably, is done in a dedicated radiation therapy CT-simulator facility as described in Chapter 5 (91,97). The CT simulator is used to acquire a volumetric planning CT scan of the patient, which is then used to create a virtual patient model for use with the virtual simulation software that mimics the functions of a conventional radiation therapy simulator. The CT scan must be performed with the patient in the treatment position, as determined in the preplanning step. CT tomograms should be generated first and reviewed prior to acquiring the planning scan to ensure patient alignment is correct; adjustments are made if needed. Radiopaque markers are typically placed on the patient's skin and the immobilization device to serve as fiducial marks to assist in any coordinate transformation needed as a result of 3D planning and eventual plan implementation. An example of a typical immobilization repositioning system used for patients undergoing radiation therapy for head and neck cancer is shown in Figure 8.1. Some complex treatment techniques, such as tangential breast irradiation, are difficult or nearly impossible to set up because of older CT scanner bore-size limitations. However, as shown in Figure 8.2, the large-bore (85-cm) CT scanner developed by Marconi (now part of Philips Inc., Cleveland, OH) designed specifically for radiation oncology applications has largely solved this problem (33). Other aids in radiation treatment planning, such as the use of intravenous contrast to help delineate target volumes, need to be considered during CT simulation.

Planning CT scan protocols are tumor site-dependent and typically range from 2- to 8-mm slice thicknesses and 50 to 200 slices. In general, a 3-mm slice thickness provides adequate quality DRRs (35). The planning CT dataset provides an accurate geometric model of the patient as well as the electron density information needed for the calculation of the 3D dose distribution that takes into account tissue heterogeneities.

The planning CT dataset is typically transferred to a 3DTPS or virtual simulation computer workstation via a computer

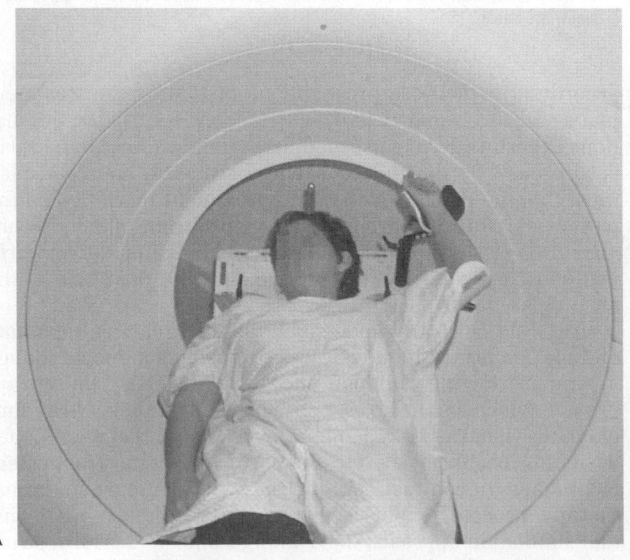
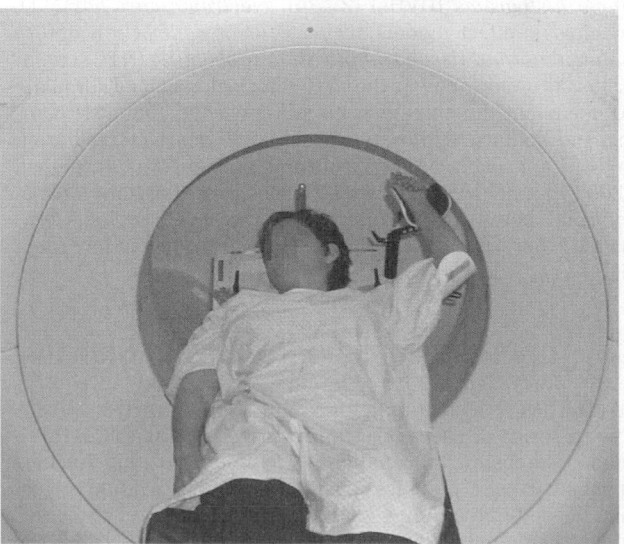

A   B

FIGURE 8.2. Some complex treatment techniques, such as tangential breast irradiation, are difficult or nearly impossible to set up in small-bore computed tomography (CT) scanners. Shown is a comparison of breast CT simulation with a breast board for a 70-cm bore scanner **(A)** and breast CT simulation with a breast board for a 85-cm bore scanner **(B)**.

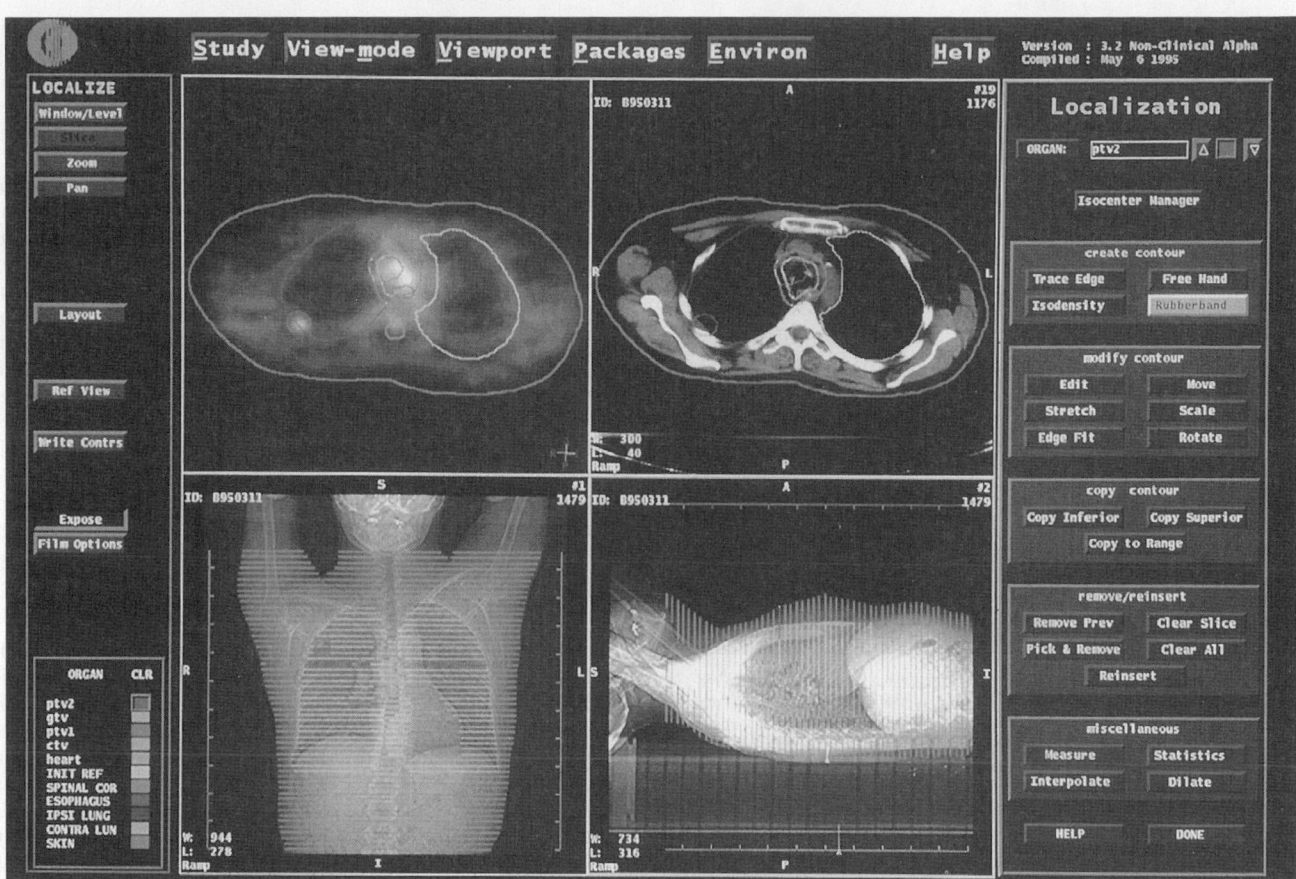

FIGURE 8.3. Image segmentation software provides tools for radiation oncologists and treatment planners to determine critical structures and tumor and target volumes for three-dimensional planning. Computed tomography (CT) data are displayed and contours are drawn by the treatment planner/radiation oncologist around the tumor, target, and normal tissues on a slice-by-slice basis, as seen in upper right panel. At the same time, planar images from both anteroposterior and lateral projections are displayed in bottom right and left panels. Upper left panel shows positron emission tomography scan data with overlying contours after image registration with the CT data.

network. Data transfer issues will be discussed in more detail in a later section.

Tumor, Target Volume, and Critical Structure Delineation and Dose Prescription

Delineation of tumor/target volume and organs at risk contours using the volumetric CT dataset is typically performed by the radiation oncologist and the medical dosimetrist, working as a team. The CT data are displayed and contours are drawn manually using a computer mouse or stylus on a slice-by-slice basis. Some organs at risk with distinct boundaries (e.g., skin, lung) can be contoured automatically, with only minor editing required; others (e.g., brachial plexus, optic chiasm) require the "hands-on" effort of the radiation oncologist. When modern 3DTPS image segmentation software is used (Fig. 8.3), contouring generally takes 1 to 2 hours, depending on disease site. However, for some complex sites, such as head and neck cancer, where many organs at risk and complex tumor/target volumes are often the norm, this task can take up to 4 hours.

No doubt, one of the most important factors that has contributed to the success of the current conformal therapy process has been the standardization of nomenclature and methods for defining the volume of known tumor, suspected microscopic spread, and marginal volumes necessary to account for setup variations and organ and patient motion published in the International Commission on Radiation Units and Measurements (ICRU) Reports 50 (49) and 62 (50). Details on the use of this method are discussed in a separate section.

Designing Beam Arrangement and Field Apertures

Design of the beam arrangement and beam apertures is the next step in the forward-planned conformal therapy process. The planning system must have the capability to simulate each of the treatment machine motion functions, including gantry angle, collimator length, width and angle, MLC leaf settings, couch latitude, longitude, height, and angle. When noncoplanar beam arrangements are used, care must be taken to avoid the selection of a gantry and couch angles that results in table/gantry collisions or other treatment room restrictions.

An essential tool for conformal therapy planning is the BEV display (Fig. 8.4), in which the observer's viewing point is at the source of radiation looking out along the axis of the radiation beam (38,77,117). The BEV display allows the planner to easily view the critical structure volumes and the target volume so that shielding blocks or MLC defined apertures can be defined. The REV display (Fig. 8.5) complements the BEV in the beam design phase of treatment planning, particularly in positioning of beam isocenter depth and in visualizing all, or selected, beams, to better appreciate the beam arrangement geometry (110,114).

Dose Calculation

A rectilinear coordinate system affixed to the patient 3D CT image set is typically assumed for dose calculations. This "patient or CT system" typically has its x-axis along the horizontal axis

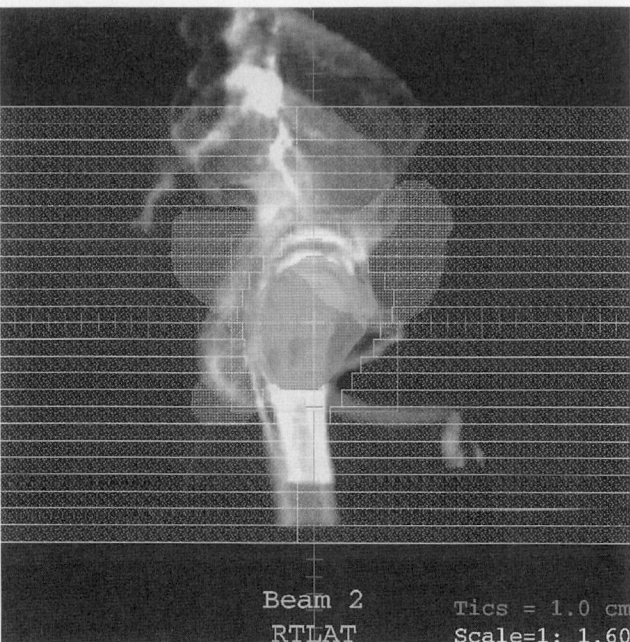

FIGURE 8.4. Beam's-eye-view (BEV) display is the cornerstone of three-dimensional radiation therapy treatment planning. BEV display is useful in identifying best gantry, collimator, and couch angles at which to irradiate target and avoid irradiating adjacent normal structures by interactively moving patient and treatment beam. Critical structures and target volumes are outlined on the patient's serial computed tomography sections. Contours are seen in perspective, as though the observer's eye is at radiation source looking out along the axis of the radiation beam. Outlines of beam-shaping blocks are displayed.

of the transverse CT images, the y-axis along the vertical axis, and the z-axis along the couch motion. Contour points are specified as a sequence of points having x, y, z coordinates in this system. The center of each voxel in the 3D CT image matrix is computed relative to the same coordinate system and is used to look up the relative electron density values. The selection of grid spacing for the 3D dose matrices is an important consideration regarding dose computational accuracy, calculation speed, and computer hardware requirements. Drzymala et al.

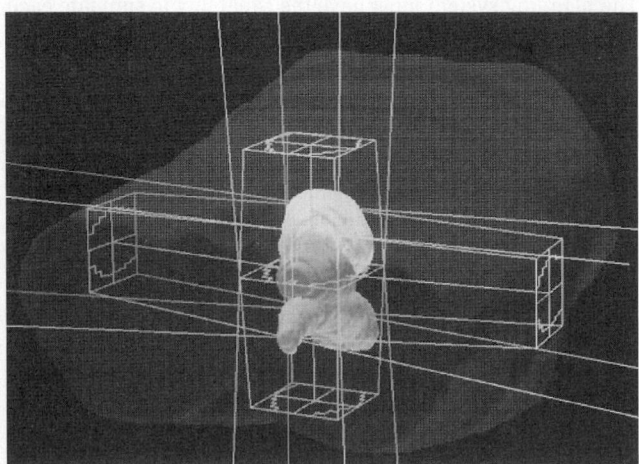

FIGURE 8.5. Real-time interactive room's-eye-view (REV) display for patient with prostate cancer showing multiple beams. All contours except those for the bladder, rectum, and prostate planning target volume have been turned off. The REV display helps the treatment planner better to appreciate the overall treatment technique geometry and placement of the isocenter. (From Purdy JA, Harms WB, Matthews JW, et al. Advances in 3-dimensional radiation treatment planning systems: Room-view display with real time interactivity. *Int J Radiat Oncol Biol Phys* 1993;27:933–944, with permission.)

(26) point out that a 2% dose accuracy or 2-mm isodose positional accuracy can generally be achieved with a grid spacing of 5 mm. However, in regions of high-dose gradients, a finer grid is typically needed, which creates larger computer files and increases the 3DTPS memory and mass storage requirements.

The reader should also understand that CT numbers are not used directly in photon dose calculations. Instead, the CT numbers are correlated with the electron density of the corresponding tissues at each voxel relative to the electron density of water (6,48,100). This is because Compton scattering is the dominant mode of interaction for the type photon beams used in radiation therapy (cobalt-60 through 25 MV x-rays) and the absorption and scattering of photons in tissue depends primarily on the electron density of the tissue. Errors in CT numbers can result in inaccurate dose calculations. Generally, however, errors of 10% or less in electron density (CT numbers) will not result in significant errors in the dose distribution (34,141). Details on specific dose calculation algorithms are discussed in a later section.

Plan Evaluation and Improvement

Plan evaluation and improvement for forward-based conformal planning involves an iterative, interactive approach. The initial beam arrangement is selected based primarily on clinical experience using BEV and REV displays. The beam arrangement can then be modified based on the evaluation of the dose distribution using multilevel 2D displays showing isodose lines superimposed on CT images (Fig. 8.6), or as a spectrum of colors superimposed on the anatomic information represented by modulation of intensity (color wash), and REV 3D dose clouds (Fig. 8.7). However, because of the large amount of dosimetric data that must be analyzed when a 3DCRT plan is evaluated, methods for condensing and presenting the data in easily understandable formats have been developed. The most useful data reduction tool for conformal therapy planning is the DVH, which is discussed in detail in a later section (26).

The planned dose distribution approved by the radiation oncologist is most often one in which a uniform dose is delivered to the target volume (e.g., +7% and −5% of prescribed dose) with doses to critical structures held below some tolerance level that has been specified by the radiation oncologist (27).

Plan Implementation and Treatment Verification

Once the treatment plan has been designed, evaluated, and approved, documentation for plan implementation must be generated. Documentation includes beam parameter settings transferred to the treatment machine record and verify system, hard copy block templates for the block fabrication room or MLC parameters communicated over a network to the computer system that controls the treatment machine's MLC system, DRR generation and printing, or transfer to the electronic medical record database.

QA checks used to confirm the validity and accuracy of the conformal plan include an independent check of the treatment plan and monitor unit calculation by a physicist, isocenter placement check on the treatment machine using orthogonal DRRs compared to similar orthogonal radiographs (Fig. 8.8), field apertures check using portal films or electronic portal images, and diode or metal-oxide semiconductor field-effect transistor (MOSFET) *in vivo* dosimeter checks. A record and verify system is now considered essential to help manage conformal therapy treatments. However, careful scrutiny must be given to ensure that the input data into the record and verify system are correct.

If a clinic is in the initial phases of implementing conformal techniques, a verification simulation procedure is recommended

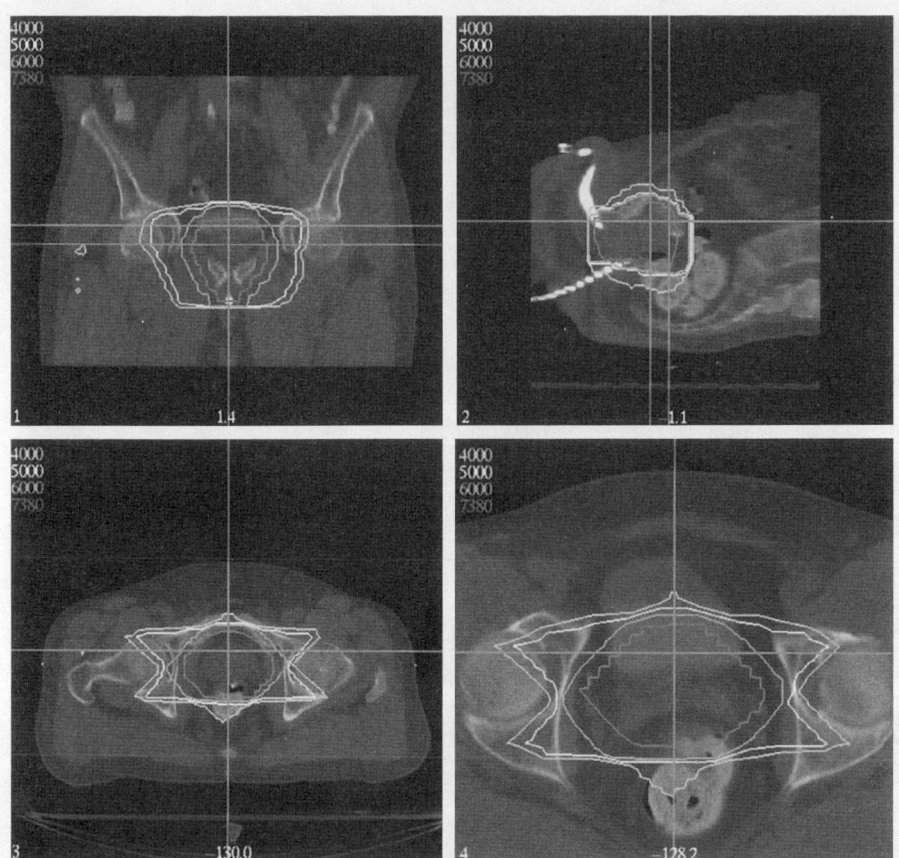

FIGURE 8.6. Dose distribution displays for a patient with prostate cancer showing coronal, sagittal, and two axial computed tomography (CT) sections with superimposed color-coded isodose lines (73.8, 60, 50, and 40 Gy). Vertical and horizontal lines displayed on each CT section indicate the positions of each section. Evaluating volumetric three-dimensional dose distributions using only this type of two-dimensional display is difficult and time-consuming.

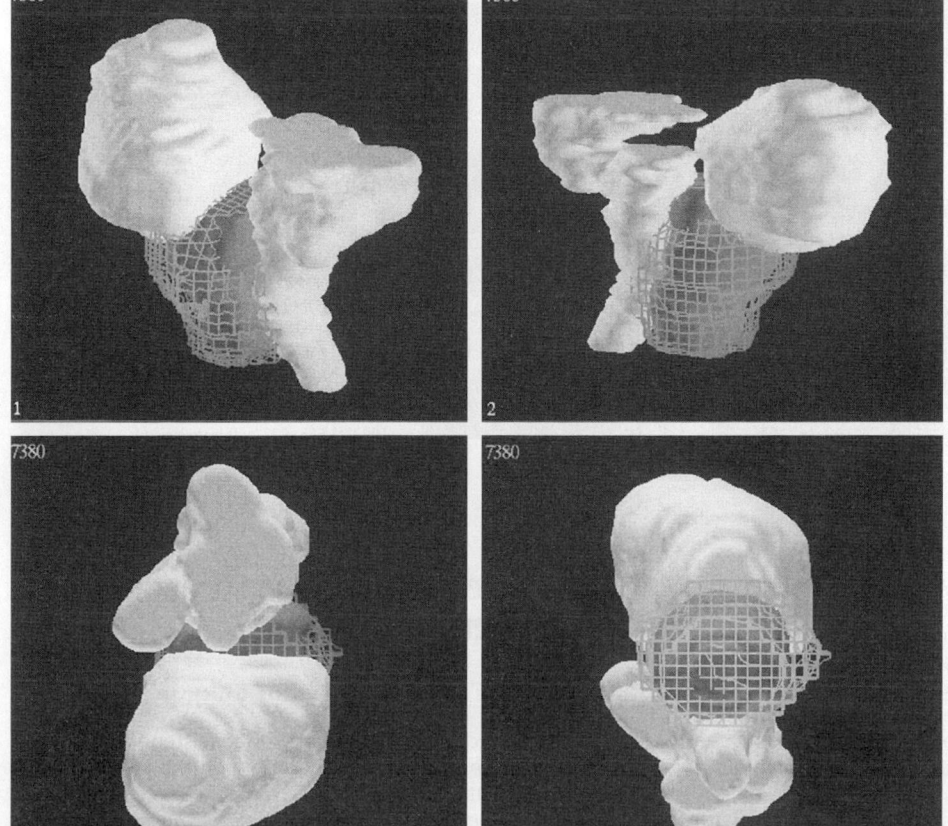

FIGURE 8.7. Room's-eye-view (REV) three-dimensional (3D) isodose surface display with real-time interactivity is a valuable tool for evaluation of 3D dose distributions in terms of adequate coverage of target volumes and sparing of critical structures. The REV display enables radiation oncologists to view target volume or normal tissue volume with superimposed isodose surfaces or "dose clouds" from any arbitrary viewing angle. Shown is a four-panel REV display of the 73.8-Gy isodose volume, the prostate planning target volume (PTV), bladder, and rectum of a patient with prostate cancer treated with a six-field technique. The location of the PTV region not covered by the specified dose level is easily discernible using the REV display. (From Purdy JA. Three-dimensional treatment planning and conformal dose delivery: A physicist's perspective. In: Mittal BB, Purdy JA, Ang KK, eds. *Advances in radiation therapy*. Boston: Kluwer Academic Publishers, 1998:1–33, with permission.)

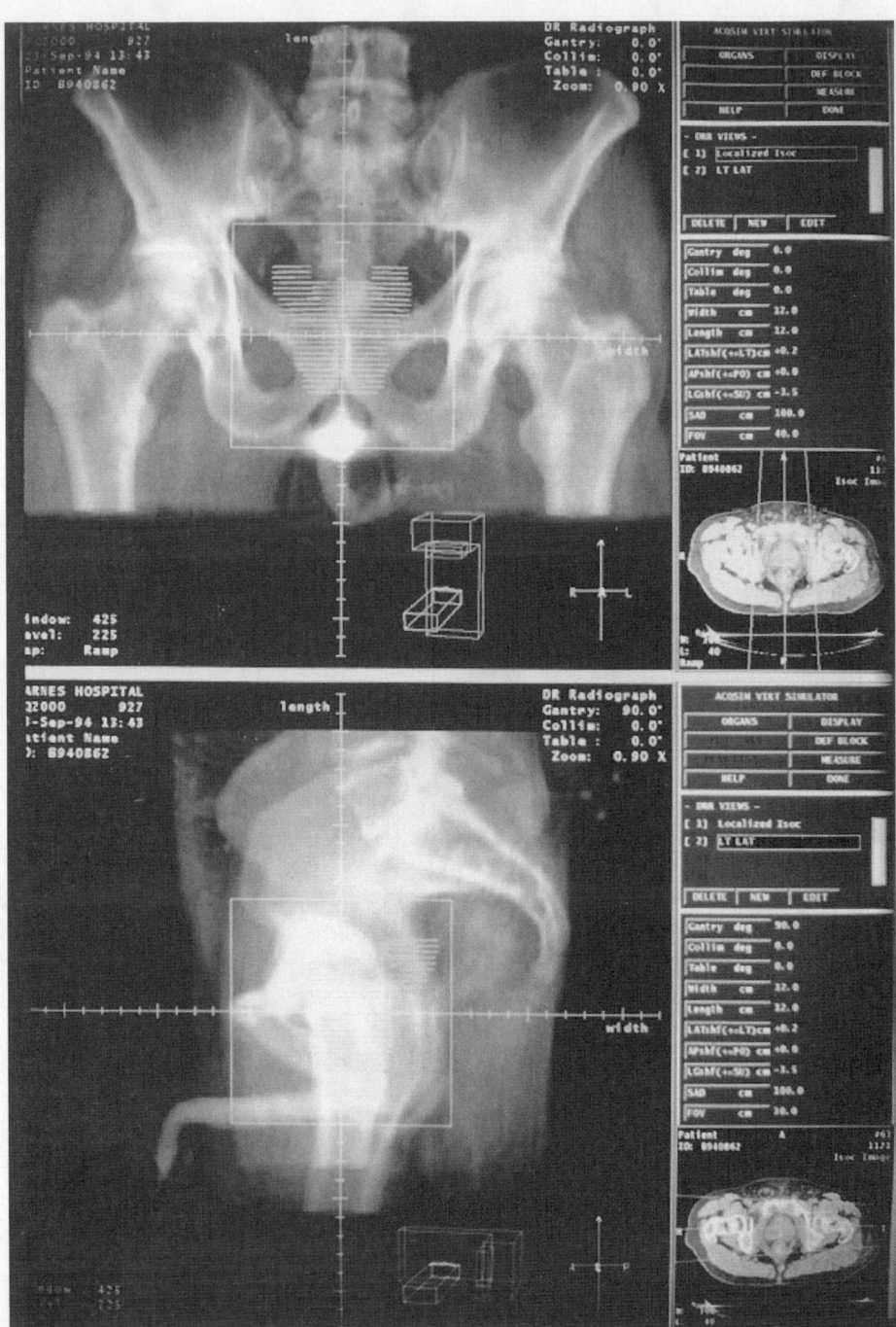

FIGURE 8.8. Digitally reconstructed radiograph (DRR). Illustrated are orthogonal setup DRRs of a patient with prostate cancer showing prostate target volume contours and collimator positions. Icon at lower right depicts gantry and treatment couch position. Icon at far lower right depicts patient orientation. (From Purdy JA. Advances in three-dimensional treatment planning and conformal dose delivery. *Semin Oncol* 1997;24:655–672, with permission.)

to confirm the geometric validity and accuracy of the 3D treatment plan. DRRs are used for comparison with the verification simulation radiographs to confirm the correctness of the beam orientations in the physical implementation. Orthogonal radiographs should always be taken and compared with similar orthogonal DRRs to ensure correct isocenter positioning. The optical distance indicator is also useful in assessing the correctness of the setup of a particular beam. Documentation provides a depth of isocenter below the skin surface on the central ray of the beam, which can then be compared with the isocenter depth measured on the simulator or treatment machine after the beam is set up using the couch and gantry positions specified by the treatment plan.

Volume and Dose Specification for Conformal Therapy

Definition of Tumor and Target Volumes

The ICRU first addressed the issue of consistent volume and dose specification in radiation therapy with the publication of ICRU Report 29 in 1978 (ICRU, 1978 #867). That report defined the *target volume* as *the volume containing those tissues that are to be irradiated to a specified absorbed dose according to a specified time-dose pattern* (Fig. 8.9A). It is interesting to note that this report (even though published in the 2D era) attempted

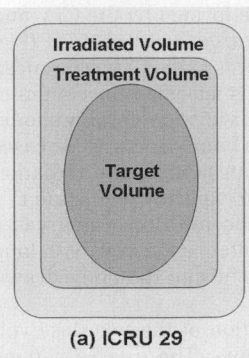
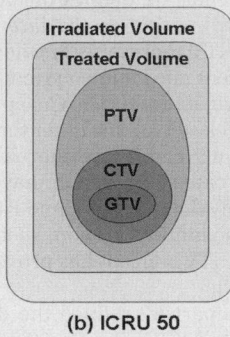
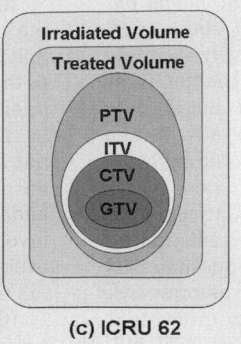

| (a) ICRU 29 | (b) ICRU 50 | (c) ICRU 62 |

FIGURE 8.9. A: Schematic illustration of the boundaries of the volumes defined by International Commission on Radiation Units and Measures (ICRU) Report 29: Target Volume, Treatment Volume, and Irradiated Volume. **B:** Boundaries of the volumes defined by ICRU Report 50: Gross Tumor Volume (GTV), Clinical Target Volume (CTV), Planning Target Volume (PTV), Treated Volume, and Irradiated Volume. **C:** Boundaries of the volumes defined by ICRU Report 62: GTV, CTV, Internal Target Volume (ITV), PTV, Treated Volume, and Irradiated Volume.

to address spatial uncertainties by pointing out that the size and shape of a target volume may change during the course of a treatment and that one should take into account the following parameters when describing the target volume:

a. expected movements (e.g., caused by breathing) of those tissues that contain the target volume relative to anatomic reference points (e.g., skin markings, suprasternal notch),
b. expected variation in shape and size of the target volume during a course of treatment (e.g., urinary bladder, stomach), and
c. inaccuracies or variations in treatment setup during the course of treatment.

However, the report did not address the issues of coordinate systems (e.g., patient vs. treatment machine) and no attempt was made to define and explicitly separate the margins for the different types of uncertainties.

In addition to the target volume, ICRU Report 29 defined two other volumes: (a) the *treatment volume*, and (b) the *irradiated volume*. These volumes were not based on anatomy, but instead were based on the dose distribution. The treatment volume was defined as *the volume enclosed by the isodose surface representing the minimal target dose*, and the irradiated volume was defined as *the volume that receives a dose considered significant in relation to normal tissue tolerance* (e.g., 50% isodose surface).

Report 29 defined *organs at risk* (OAR) as *specially radiosensitive organs in or near the target volume whose presence influences treatment planning and/or prescribed dose*. The report also recognized the importance of tissues outside the target area that received a dose higher than 100% of the specified target dose. This was defined as a *hot spot* and was considered clinically meaningful only if the corresponding isodose curve enclosed an area of at least 2 cm^2 in a section.

In retrospect, ICRU Report 29 recommendations were well suited for the technology of the 1970s and 1980s, that is, using a conventional simulator to generate a planning radiograph for designing beam portals based on bony and soft tissue landmarks for standardized beam arrangement techniques applied to whole classes of comparable patients. Several generations of radiation oncologists were trained using this nomenclature and method, and the ICRU recommendation for reporting dose and volumes helped advance radiation oncology.

In 1993, the ICRU updated its recommendations for specifying dose/volume in Report 50, and were well suited for conformal therapy. The target volume definition was separated into three distinct volumes: (a) visible tumor, that is, *gross tumor volume* (GTV), (b) a volume to account for uncertainties in microscopic tumor spread, that is, *clinical target volume* (CTV), and (3) a volume to account for geometric and other uncertainties, that is, *planning target volume* (PTV) as illustrated in Fig. 8.9B.

The GTV and CTV are anatomic-clinical concepts that should be defined before a choice of treatment modality and technique is made. Labels or subscripts with the GTV nomenclature can be used to distinguish between primary disease and other areas of macroscopic tumor involvement such as involved lymph nodes that are visible on imaging studies (e.g., GTV$_{primary}$ and GTV$_{nodal}$, or GTV-T and GTV-N). Similarly, the GTV together with this surrounding volume of local subclinical involvement that defines the CTV can be denoted as CTV-T. Note that even if the GTV has been removed by radical surgery, the volume can be designated as CTV-T. In specifying the CTV, the physician must not only consider microextensions of the disease near the GTV, but also the natural avenues of spread for the particular disease and site, including lymph node, perivascular, and perineural extensions. These may be designated CTV-N (and, if necessary, CTV-N1, CTV-N2, and so forth).

The *PTV* is defined by specifying the margins that must be added around the CTV to manage the effects of organ, tumor and patient movements, inaccuracies in beam and patient setup, and any other uncertainties. The PTV is a static, geometrical concept used for treatment planning and for specification of dose. Its size and shape depend primarily on that of the GTV/CTV and the effects caused by internal motions of organs and the tumor, technical aspects of treatment technique (e.g., patient fixation). The PTV can be considered a 3D envelope in which the tumor and any microscopic extensions reside and move within this envelope. Once the PTV is defined, appropriate beam sizes to account for penumbra and beam arrangements must be selected to ensure the desired dose coverage of the PTV. Note that multiple PTVs may be defined for a patient's radiation therapy treatment. For example, it is common practice to plan a higher dose to the PTV enclosing the GTV, and a lower dose to the PTV containing the CTV. Such planning volumes are typically subscripted using the dose level prescribed; for example, PTVs for 66 Gy and 54 Gy can be represented as PTV$_{66}$ and PTV$_{54}$.

ICRU Report 50 essentially retained the definition of the two dose volumes defined in ICRU Report 29, changing the treatment volume name to *treated volume*, and refining the definition as *the volume enclosed by an isodose surface, selected and specified by the radiation oncologist as being appropriate to achieve the purpose of treatment* (e.g., tumor eradication, palliation), and the irradiated volume as that *tissue volume that receives a dose that is considered significant in relation to normal tissue tolerance*.

Report 50 refined the definition of organs at risk as *normal tissues whose radiation sensitivity may significantly influence treatment planning and/or prescribed dose*. The report did state that any possible movement of the organ at risk during treatment, as well as uncertainties in the setup during the whole treatment course, must be considered, but did not provide a method to do so.

The hot spot definition was modified to be *a volume outside the PTV that received a dose larger than 100% of the specified PTV dose*. This was considered clinically meaningful only if the minimum diameter exceeded 15 mm (note: previously it had been 2 cm^2). However, if the hot spot occurs in a small organ, such as the optic nerve, a dimension smaller than the recommended 15 mm should be considered.

As previously stated, Report 50 was well suited to conformal therapy and it stimulated broad interest in the radiation oncology community. However, its use raised new questions and prompted numerous publications (3,118). Also, as previously pointed out, irradiation techniques continued to evolve (e.g., IMRT), and advances in imaging procedures (e.g., PET, MRI) provided even more information on functionality, the location, shape, and limits of tumor/target volumes, and organs at risk. In response to these developments, the ICRU in 1999 published Report 62 (50), which expanded on some of the definitions and concepts of Report 50 and took into account the consequences of the technical and clinical progress referred to previously. However, it should be clearly understood that Report 62 is intended to complement the recommendations contained in Report 50, and not to replace it.

ICRU Report 62 refined the definition of PTV by introducing the concept of an *internal margin* to take into account variations in size, shape, and position of the CTV in reference to the patient's coordinate system using anatomic reference points, and also the concept of a *setup margin* to take into account all uncertainties in patient-beam positioning in reference to the treatment machine coordinate system. Identification of these two types of margins is needed as they compensate for different types of uncertainties and refer to different coordinate systems. Internal margin uncertainties are due to physiologic variations (e.g., filling of rectum, movements due to respiration) and are difficult or almost impossible to control from a practical viewpoint. Setup margin uncertainties are related largely to technical factors that can be dealt with by more accurate setup and immobilization of the patient and improved mechanical stability of the machine. However, exactly how these margins should be combined is still not clear. This point will be discussed further in a later section, but for now understand that the selection of an overall margin and delineation of the border of the PTV typically involves a compromise that requires the experience and the judgment of the radiation oncologist and the treatment-planning team.

ICRU Report 62 defines the volume formed by the CTV and the internal margin as the *internal target volume* (ITV) (Fig. 8.9C). The ITV represents the movements of the CTV referenced to the patient coordinate system and is specified in relation to internal and external reference points, which preferably should be rigidly related to each other through bony structures. In cases not involving significant internal organ motion, the radiation oncologist can simply ignore having to explicitly define the ITV and use only the GTV, CTV, and PTV concepts. However, in cases involving significant motion, such as often is the case with lung cancer, the ITV concept has proven useful and should be drawn (53,68,132).

ICRU Report 62 refined the definition of the two dose volumes defined ICRU Report 50 as follows: The *treated volume is the tissue volume that (according to the approved treatment plan) is planned to receive at least a dose selected and specified by radiation oncology team as being appropriate to achieve the purpose of the treatment, e.g., tumor eradication or palliation, within the bounds of acceptable complications*. The irradiated volume is the *tissue volume that receives a dose that is considered significant in relation to normal tissue tolerance*.

Report 62 refined the definition of organs at risk as *normal tissues (e.g., spinal cord) whose radiation sensitivity may significantly influence treatment planning and/or prescribed dose*. The report also included a discussion regarding a system of classifying organs at risk as "serial," "parallel," or "serial-parallel." Report 62 also addressed what was perhaps the most criticized limitation of Report 50, which was that it did not provide a method to account for organ at risk movements and changes in shape and/or size, as well as setup uncertainties. To account for such spatial uncertainties, Report 62 introduced the concept of the *planning organ at risk volume* (PRV), in which a margin is added around the organ at risk to compensate for that organ's geometric uncertainties. The PRV margin around the organ at risk is analogous to the PTV margin around the CTV. The introduction of the PRV concept is timely as its use is even more important for those conformal therapy cases involving IMRT because of the increased sensitivity of this type treatment to geometric uncertainties. For example, it is common practice to add a 0.5-cm rind around the spinal cord contour. Note, that the PTV and the PRV may overlap, and often do so, which implies searching for a compromise in weighting the importance of each in the planning process. A summary of the ICRU volume nomenclature recommendations per report is presented in Table 8.3.

Table 8.3 SUMMARY OF THE INTERNATIONAL COMMISSION ON RADIATION UNITS AND MEASUREMENTS (ICRU) NOMENCLATURE FOR VOLUMES (1970S TO PRESENT)

ICRU Report 29: 1970s–1993	ICRU Report 50: 1993–Present	ICRU Report 62: 1999–Present
• Target volume	• GTV • CTV • PTV	• GTV • CTV • ITV • PTV
• Treatment volume	• Treated volume	• Treated volume
• Irradiated volume	• Irradiated volume	• Irradiated volume
• Organ at risk	• Organ at risk	• Organ at risk • PRV
• Hot spot (area outside target that receives dose larger than 100% of specified target dose) • (at least 2 cm^2 in a section)	• Hot spot (volume outside PTV that receives dose larger than 100% of specified PTV dose) • (>15 mm diameter)	• Hot spot (volume outside PTV that receives dose larger than 100% of specified PTV dose) • (>15 mm diameter)
• Dose heterogeneity (no value given)	• Dose heterogeneity (+7 to −5% of prescribed dose)	• Dose heterogeneity (+7 to −5% of prescribed dose)

GTV, gross tumor volume; CTV, clinical target volume; PTV, planning target volume; ITV, internal target volume; PRV, planning risk volume.

Dose Reporting and Dose Prescription

ICRU Reports 50 and 62 define a series of doses, including the minimum, maximum, mean dose, and *ICRU Reference Dose* (defined at the *ICRU Reference Point*) for reporting dose. The ICRU Reference Point for a particular treatment plan should be chosen based on the following criteria:

a. be clinically relevant and can be defined in an unambiguous way;
b. be located where the dose can be accurately determined; and
c. be located in a region where there are no steep dose gradients.

In general, this point should be in the central part of the PTV. In cases where the treatment beams intersect at a given point, it is recommended that the intersection point be chosen as the ICRU Reference Point.

It should be noted that ICRU Reports 50 and 62 do not make strict recommendations regarding dose prescription; rather ICRU states that "...the radiation oncologist should have the freedom to prescribe the parameters in his/her own way, mainly using what is current practice to produce an expected clinical outcome of the treatment" (49).

With regard to dose homogeneity, ICRU Report 50 does recommend that the dose coverage of the PTV be kept within specific limits, namely +7% and −5% of the prescribed dose (49). This level of dose homogeneity may not be achieved in all cases (particularly for current IMRT techniques), and the reader is reminded that ICRU Report 50 explicitly states that if this degree of homogeneity cannot be achieved, it is the responsibility of the radiation oncologist to decide whether the dose heterogeneity can be accepted or not, pointing out that in those parts of the PTV where the highest malignant cell concentration may be expected (i.e., GTV), a higher dose may even be an advantage.

Using the GTV, CTV, and PTV Concept

From this brief review, the reader should clearly see that there has been a deliberate attempt to keep the definitions of the volumes used for reporting external photon beam radiation therapy similar and consistent over time. Modifications have occurred when advances in the technologies used for planning and delivering radiation therapy suggest further refinement is needed. Although the current recommendations direct the radiation oncologist to specifically account for microscopic disease uncertainty, and patient setup and organ movement uncertainties in defining the PTVs and PRVs, it must be recognized that, with current technology, in reality this is still a judgment call and not an exact science for most cases. In performing this task, the radiation oncologist must rely on his or her experience and judgment drawn from study of the literature, and observation and evaluation of patients treated regarding risk of failure versus normal tissue complications. In other words, when confronted with the problem of defining the volume to receive a prescribed dose, or defining an organ at risk in order to avoid or limit dose, the radiation oncologist must make a series of trade-offs, which are discussed in this section.

Some limitations and practical issues must be clearly understood when the ICRU Report 50 and 62 methods are adopted (103,105,107–109). First, the physical treatment planning process depends on the delineation of the three volumes (GTV, CTV, and PTV) and the prescription of the target dose. The GTV, CTV, and PTV must be specified by the radiation oncologist independent of the dose distribution: The GTV in terms of the patient's anatomy, the CTV in terms of the patient's anatomy or as a quantitative margin to be added to the GTV, and the PTV in terms of a quantitative margin to be added to the CTV to account for positional uncertainties.

The reproducibility and accuracy of GTV delineation for most treatment sites is generally not very well known, as it is based mostly on clinical judgment. It is known that the shape and size of the GTV can depend significantly on the imaging modality (123,150). Leunens et al. (63) reported that they observed a considerable intra- and interobserver variation in GTV delineation for brain tumors. Ten Haken et al. (138) and Rasch et al. (115) compared GTVs defined using both CT and MRI. In both reports, the target volume defined using CT and MRI was different than the volume defined using CT alone. Furthermore, Rasch et al. (116) concluded that MRI-derived target volumes had less interobserver variation than CT only-derived target volumes. In another study, Roach et al. (123) compared the delineated prostate volumes using both CT and MRI for a series of patients and found significant volume differences in approximately one third of the cases, depending on the imaging modality used.

That said, CT is still the principal source of imaging data used for defining the GTV for conformal therapy planning for most sites, but this imaging modality presents several potential pitfalls. First, when contouring the GTV, it is essential that the appropriate CT window and level settings be used in order to determine the maximum dimension of what is considered potential gross disease (Fig. 8.10). Secondly, for those treatment sites in which there is considerable organ motion, such as for tumors in the thorax, CT images do not correctly represent either the time-averaged position of the tumor or its shape (14). This can be understood by reference to Figure 8.11 and appreciating the fact that today's CT-simulation process relies almost exclusively on the use of fast, spiral CT technology, and thus acquires data essentially in 2D. This has the effect of capturing the tumor cross-section images at particular positions in the breathing cycle. Caldwell et al. (14) studied this problem showing that if the tumor motion is large, different, and possibly noncontiguous, transverse sections of the tumor could be imaged at different points of the breathing cycle, leading to volume uncertainties. They pointed out that the interpolation process in spiral CT technology adds further to the uncertainty and concluded that 3D reconstruction of the GTV from temporally variant 2D images will contain distortions that are not only nonrepresentative of the true geometry of the stationary tumor, but also not a good representation of the tumor and its motion. In their study, they further concluded that PET imaging could provide a more accurate representation of the GTV encompassing motion of such tumors, and thus has the potential to provide patient-specific motion volumes for an individualized ITV. Multislice CT technology (so-called *4D CT imaging*) is just now being adopted for CT simulation, and will minimize this problem (120,121). Until that occurs, however, one must be very careful when defining a GTV using helical single-slice CT images in those cases in which the tumor motion is significant.

Unfortunately, in many sites, anatomic-imaging techniques (i.e., CT or MRI) do not always distinguish malignant from normal tissues. Thus, there is growing interest in incorporating the complementary information available from functional imaging, such as PET, when defining the GTV (18,64–66,73,90,130). For example, Caldwell et al. (15) reported high observer variability in CT-based definition of the GTV for non–small cell lung cancer patients when compared with the GTV defined using ^{18}F-flurodeoxyglucose (FDG)-hybrid PET images coregistered with CT. Chao et al. (16) provide another example of the use of functional imaging in target volume definition; they proposed the use of PET employing a hypoxic tumor-specific tracer to define the hypoxic region of the GTV for potentially guiding IMRT treatment delivery. If PET or other modality imaging studies are used to complement the CT planning process, they must be accurately registered to the planning CT dataset (47,89,125). Although significant improvements in 3DTPS fusion software have been made, image registration remains one of the serious pitfalls that can befall the radiation oncologist when defining

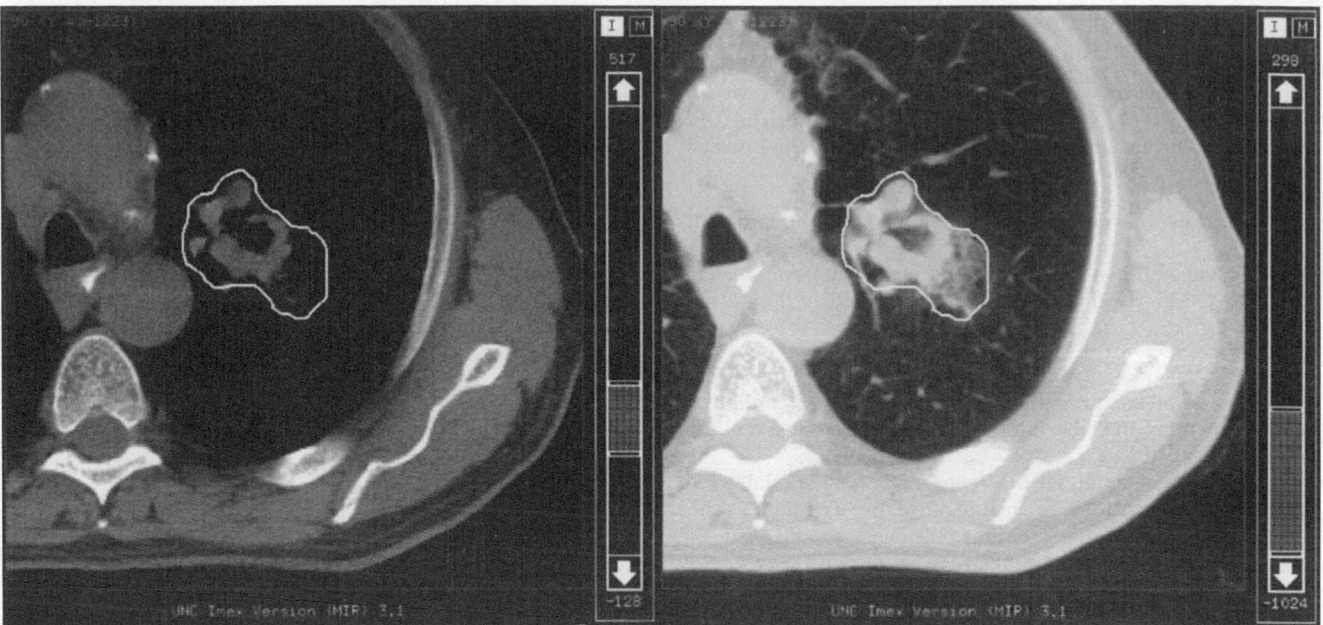

FIGURE 8.10. Computed tomography (CT) slice for patient with lung cancer showing that the appropriate CT window and level settings (right frame) must be used to determine the maximum dimensions of the gross tumor volume (GTV). Note that a much smaller GTV would have been contoured with the settings used in the left frame. (From Purdy JA. Advances in three-dimensional treatment planning and conformal dose delivery. *Semin Oncol* 1997;24:655–672, with permission.)

the GTV (126). The radiation oncologist and treatment planner must be especially vigilant when using multiple imaging studies when defining volumes and be sure that robust QA processes are in place (89).

Delineating the CTV is a much more complicated task than delineating either the GTV or most organs at risk. At this time, it is more an art than a science because current imaging techniques are not capable of detecting subclinical tumor involvement directly. When defining GTV/CTVs and organs at risk on

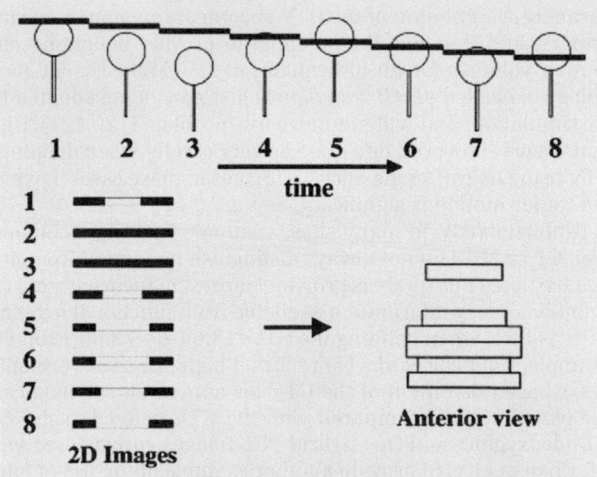

FIGURE 8.11. Schematic illustrating computed tomography (CT) data acquisition of a sphere moving in the longitudinal plane. At each point in time (1 through 8), the sphere is located at a different position in the motion cycle. The x-ray plane (represented by the solid gray rectangle) of the CT scanner moves inferiorly with time. At each time interval, the reconstructed two-dimensional (2D) image (represented by black/white rectangles on the left side) captures a different section of the sphere (white section embedded in black rectangles). An anterior digitally reconstructed radiograph reconstruction from the 2D images displays an object that is non-representative of either the stationary sphere or the volume traced by the moving sphere. Note that the schematic is not to scale. (From Caldwell et al. *Int J Radiat Oncol Biol Phys* 2003;55:1381–1393, with permission.)

axial CT slices, assistance from a diagnostic radiologist is often helpful. Publications and symposiums addressing the problem of establishing a consistent CTV for various clinical sites are now becoming more common (17,41,74). There is no question that image-based cross-sectional anatomy training should be an explicit requirement in radiation oncology residency training programs as the modern-day radiation oncologist needs to become much more expert in image recognition of normal tissue anatomy and gross tumor changes in order to take full advantage of advances in imaging. Research efforts that will allow a more accurate determination of CTV may be the single most important area to further advance conformal therapy.

Specifying the margins around the CTV to create the PTV is also not an exact science. The treating physician should take into account data from published literature and/or any uncertainty studies performed in their clinic. A review by Langen and Jones (61) provides the most comprehensive compilation of organ motion data to date. Interfraction organ motion studies have focused mainly on the treatment of prostate cancer (2,4,122,124,139,143), while intrafraction motion studies have focused on variations caused by respiratory motion (5,43) for disease in the thoracic and upper abdominal regions. However, how to use target organ mobility and setup error data to determine the appropriate margin between the CTV and PTV is still not clearly defined, and is an active area of investigation (3,118,119,144). In fact, there is some inconsistency between Reports 50 and 62 regarding compromising the margins of the PTV if it encroaches on an organ at risk. Current thinking is for those cases in which the PTV encroaches or overlaps another PTV, OAR or PRV, the PTV margins should not be compromised. Instead, additional regions within the PTV corresponding to different prescribed doses should be defined. Similar methods may also be used in case of overlapping PTVs.

The asymmetrical nature of the GTV/CTV geometric uncertainties must also be addressed when defining the PTV (Fig. 8.12). For example, organ motion for the prostate gland has been shown to be anisotropic (4,78,98). Daily setup errors may also be anisotropic as side-to-side or rotational shifts of patients

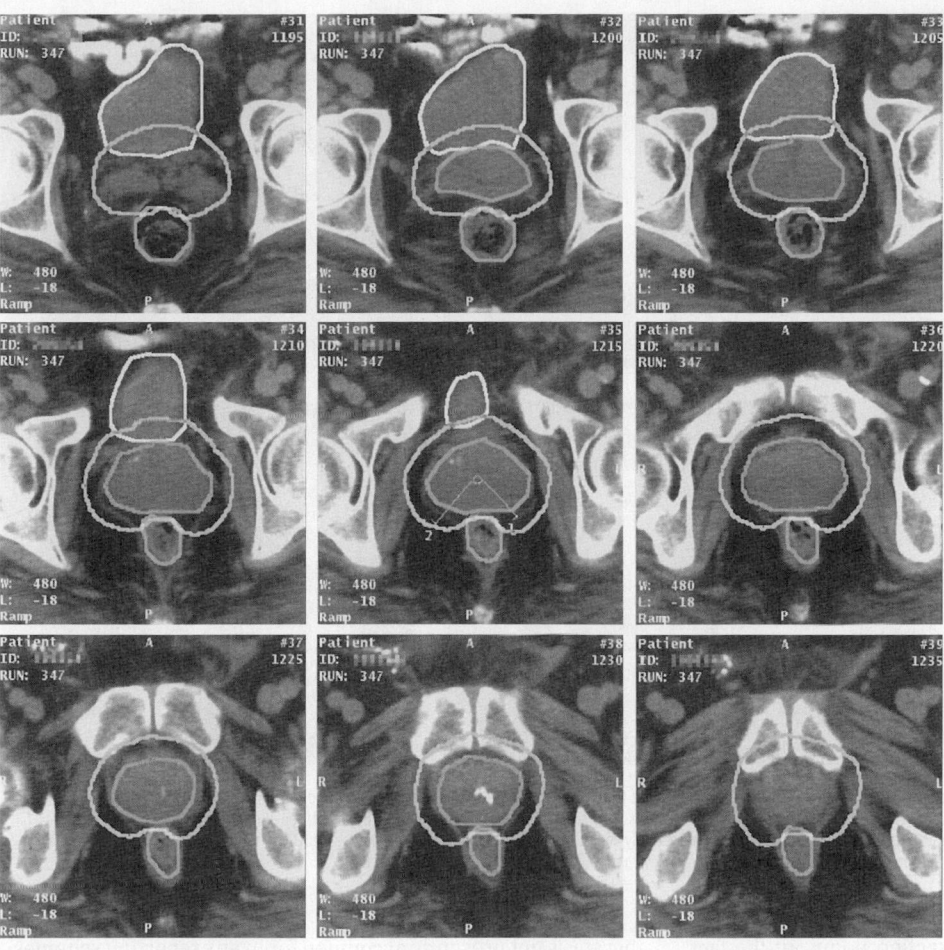

FIGURE 8.12. Computed tomography images of patient with prostate cancer showing the contour outlines for the gross tumor volume (GTV), planning target volume (PTV), bladder, and rectum. The physician made the decision that no additional margin around the prostate for the clinical target volume (CTV) was required (i.e., CTV = GTV). Note that a nonuniform margin around the GTV/CTV was used to define the PTV in the region of the rectum (see middle frame). Also note the additional PTV contours needed to cap the GTV/CTV (upper left and lower right frame). (From Purdy JA. Three-dimensional treatment planning and conformal dose delivery: A physicist's perspective. In: Mittal BB, Purdy JA, Ang KK, eds. *Advances in radiation therapy*. Boston: Kluwer Academic Publishers, 1998:1–33, with permission.)

are likely to be different from setup differences in the antero-posterior direction.

Another point of concern is the fact that some 3DTPSs still do not possess accurate methods for providing a true 3D margin around the GTV/CTV when delineating the PTV. The problem is illustrated in Figure 8.13. For large contour differences in the GTV/CTV in neighboring slices, a margin expansion drawn or specified in 2D around the GTV/CTV contour will result in margins that are too small in the cranial-caudal direction. Bedford and Shentall (7) describe methods to compute 3D target volume margins resolving this problem. The point that must be understood is that physicians must know the method used on the radiation treatment planning (RTP) system; if it is 2D, a larger contour in the adjoining slice should be used and be sure to also cap the GTV/CTV inferiorly and superiorly.

Another potential pitfall occurs in those cases where the PTV extends outside the patient's skin contour (e.g., PTV for tangential irradiation of the breast, or for some head and neck cancer sites). In such cases, part of PTV will have an airlike density, causing an artifact in the dose distribution calculated and displayed. For practical purposes, one must change the density used for that part of the PTV to unity, or require the PTV margin to coincide with the skin surface. Neither method is totally correct, but regardless, it is important that the treating physician be aware of the approximation used when setting or approving field margins and evaluating the dose distribution.

A serious limitation currently present with some planning systems occurs when a PTV overlaps with an organ at risk or its associated PRV. For such systems, the overlapping voxels can be assigned to only one of the volumes, typically the target volume, thus truncating the overlapping organ at risk volume

(e.g., a PTV that overlaps a parotid gland). In such cases, DVH evaluation for the organ at risk is compromised, as is the digital data export of the contour data to the national QA centers (112). Concentric PTVs ($PTV_{HighDose}$ and $PTV_{LowDose}$) present this same type of limitation for these planning systems. Thus, it is essential that the physician and the physicist fully understand the planning system's method (and limitations) used in assigning voxels, both for DVH evaluation and for digital data export.

Returning to the problem of creating the margin between the CTV and PTV using organ motion and setup error data, ICRU Report 62 states that a quadratic approach similar to that recommended by the Bureau International des Poids et Mesures can be used (13,83). Antolak and Rosen (3) concluded that to ensure that every point on the edge of the CTV be within the PTV approximately 95% of the time, the CTV should be expanded using a normalized radius of expansion of 1.65 times the SD in each direction. Craig et al. (19) concluded that a coverage of about 95% is a reasonable goal for PTV design and that geometric uncertainties from different sources should be added in quadrature, unless there are compelling reasons to do otherwise.

van Herk et al. (145) calculated probability distributions of the cumulative dose over a population of patients (which they called *dose-population histograms*) and studied the effects of systematic and random geometrical deviations on the cumulative dose distribution to the CTV. A margin recipe to create the PTV could be obtained from a single point on this type histogram and is given by the following relationship, where Σ is the standard deviation of the systematic errors and σ is the standard deviation of the random errors.

$$PTV\ Margin = 2.5\Sigma + 0.7\sigma$$

Overview and Basic Science of Radiation Oncology

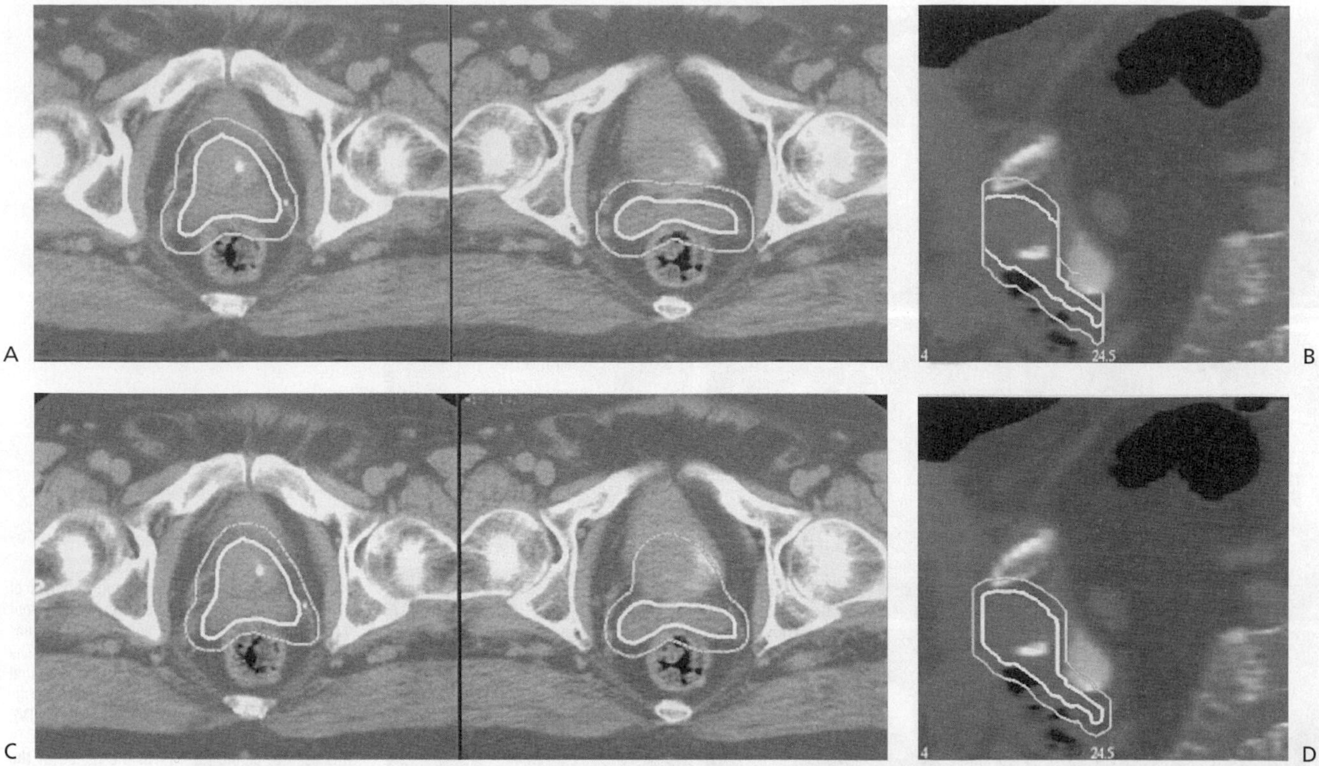

FIGURE 8.13. Multiple two-dimensional margins around a prostate gross tumor volume in a transverse computed tomography (CT) slice **(A)** may yield margins that are too small in the craniocaudal direction, as shown in a sagittal reconstruction **(B)**. The three-dimensional margins may appear too large in a transverse CT slice **(C)**, but are actually correct as shown in a sagittal reconstruction **(D)**. (From Purdy JA. 3D treatment planning and intensity-modulated radiation therapy. *Oncology* 1999;13:155–168, with permission.)

All of the issues discussed in this section point out the fact that the PTV/PRV concept is a useful tool that simplifies accounting for geometric uncertainties. However, its use does give rise to several dilemmas. Particularly important is the loss of actual tumor and normal organ volumes information reported for researchers developing TCP and NTCP models. Although it does not appear possible to totally eliminate the PTV concept at this time, it does appear possible to use smaller margins for some sites if more frequent imaging or other technical innovation is used to reduce geometric uncertainties. For example, for prostate cancer, the use of daily ultrasound imaging or daily electronic portal imaging of implanted radiopaque markers to relocate the target volume in reference to the machine isocenter does allow for a smaller margin for the PTV (4,24,62). However, one must still be prudent in the amount of margin reduction for the prostate PTV when using these technologies. For treatment sites in the thorax, ways to minimize respiratory motion and its effects include the use of ventilatory-based gating, breath-holding, and active breathing control (58,72,127,133,153). The different methods include various tradeoffs ranging from treatment machine control, which is not dependent on the patient, to systems that are completely dependent on the patient. Again, regardless of which technique is used to reduce the overall PTV margin, one must be prudent in the amount of margin reduction.

Yan et al. (157,158) have proposed an individual patient-based approach for determining PTV (called *adaptive radiation therapy*), as opposed to the current situation of using population-based averages of the setup errors or organ motion. In this approach, multiple CT scans and daily portal images are performed during the first week of the patient's treatment to determine the required margins for the patient's later treatments.

Yan and Lockman (156) have pointed out that the temporal dose-volume variation brought on by fractionated radiation therapy is not presently accounted for in any reporting schemes; that is, the location of the organ/tumor/patient varies with respect to the radiation beams during a course or radiation therapy. In other words, the temporal variation of each tissue voxel irradiated is currently not taken into account, causing uncertainties in understanding the tumor and normal tissue dose response, thereby limiting reliable treatment evaluation and optimization. Improved models that account for organ deformation and movements will be needed to address this important issue.

One final practical issue should be clearly understood by the reader. Once the PTV has been defined, additional margin beyond the PTV is needed when designing the beam portal in order to obtain dose coverage because of beam penumbra and treatment technique. Typically, 7 to 9 mm margin (port edge to PTV) is generally a good starting point for 3DCRT techniques, but one should consider the actual characteristics of the beams used to make this starting point determination. Also, in the case of coplanar treatment techniques, the margins required across the axial plane of treatment and the margins orthogonal to this plane will be different. For example, a larger inferior-superior portal margin is always needed for coplanar techniques to ensure that the prescribed isodose surface covers the PTV. Also, in many situations, the lateral and anterior-posterior portal margins for each field can be reduced (providing better organ at risk sparing) by adjusting each beam's relative weighting. It should be clear that making a hard rule about margin sizes is unrealistic and requires some planning iteration to find the best mix of superior-inferior, anterior-posterior, lateral margins, and beam weights. The ability of IMRT to reduce beam margin by increasing fluence at the PTV periphery is a significant advantage of this form of conformal therapy in achieving PTV dose coverage while improving the sparing of adjacent organs at risk.

3D Dose-Calculation Algorithms

In the past, dose calculation methods have traditionally been based on parameterizing dose distributions measured in water phantoms under standard conditions and applying correction factors to the beam representations for the nonuniform surface contour of the patient or the obliquity of the beam, tissue heterogeneities, and beam modifiers such as blocks, wedges, and compensator. However, more advanced models have been developed for 3D planning that compute the dose more from first principles and only use a limited set of measurements to obtain a better fit of the model. Examples of the more advanced type of algorithms include the superposition/convolution method developed by Mackie et al. (71) and the differential pencil beam method developed by Mohan et al. (85). The reader is referred to Chapter 6 and to the review by Ahnesjö and Aspradakis (1) for more details on these advanced dose calculation algorithms.

Briefly, the superposition/convolution method uses energy deposition kernels that describe the distribution of dose about a single primary photon interaction site. The convolution kernels are most often obtained by using Monte Carlo simulations to interact monoenergetic primary photons at the origin in a phantom and to transport the charged particles and scattered and secondary photons that are set in motion. The energy that gets deposited about the primary photon interaction site is tabulated and stored for use in the superposition/convolution method. In addition to describing how scattered photons contribute to dose absorbed at some distance away from the interaction site of primary photons, the kernels take into account charged particle transport.

It is the author's opinion that heterogeneity-corrected 3D treatment plans generated using such advanced algorithms should be standard of practice today. The study by Frank et al. (32) provides a clear method for safely transitioning from a clinical experience based on planning assuming a homogeneous unit density patient to a heterogeneous patient model.

Even the convolution/superposition dose calculation algorithm will eventually be replaced by the Monte Carlo technique (20,31,146). Monte Carlo is, in principle, the only method capable of computing the dose distribution accurately for all situations encountered in radiation therapy, including being able to accurately predict the dose near interfaces of materials with very dissimilar atomic number, such as near metal prostheses, or different densities such as tumors in lung tissue.

Dose-Volume Histograms

The large amount of dosimetric data that must be analyzed when a 3DCRT plan is evaluated has prompted the development of new methods of condensing and presenting the data in more easily understandable formats. One such data reduction tool is the DVH (26); two types, the *differential DVH* and the *cumulative DVH*, are used in conformal therapy planning.

Differential Dose-Volume Histograms

Figures 8.14 and 8.15 illustrate how a differential DVH is generated for a defined volume that is subjected to an inhomogeneous dose distribution. First, the volume under consideration is divided into a 3D grid of volume elements (voxels), the size of which is small enough so that the dose can be assumed to be constant within one voxel. The volume's dose distribution is then divided into dose bins and the voxels grouped according to dose bin without regard to anatomic location. A plot of the number of voxels in each bin (x-axis) versus the bin dose range (y-axis) is by definition a differential DVH. The size of the dose

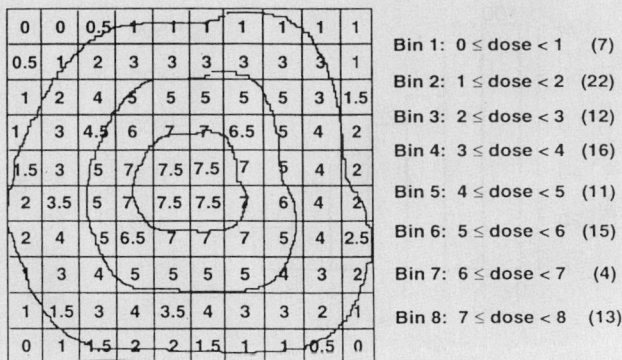

FIGURE 8.14. Dose grid for a hypothetical plan. In this plan, an irradiated organ has been divided into 100 5-cm³ voxels, each of which receives 0 to 7.5 Gy. The number of voxels receiving a given dose range is indicated. For example, 22 voxels received at least 1 Gy but less than 2 Gy. (From Lawrence TS, Kessler ML, Ten Haken RK. Clinical interpretation of dose-volume histograms: The basis for normal tissue preservation and tumor dose escalation. *Front Radiat Ther Oncol* 1996;29:57–66, with permission.)

bins determines the height of each bin of the differential DVH. For example, if the bin widths were increased, the heights of the histogram bins generally would increase because more voxels would fall into any given bin. Thus, it should be clearly understood that the detailed shape of a differential DVH depends on the bin choice, even though the underlying dose-volume data are not different.

Cumulative Dose-Volume Histograms

A cumulative DVH is a plot in which each bin represents the volume, or percentage of volume (y-axis), that receives a dose equal to or greater than an indicated dose (x-axis). An example of a cumulative DVH is shown in Figure 8.16, in which the value at any dose bin is computed by summing the number of voxels of the corresponding differential DVH to the right of that dose bin. Note that the volume value for the first bin (dose origin) is the full volume of the structure because the total volume receives at least zero dose, and the volume for the last bin is that which receives the maximum dose bin.

Dose-Volume Statistics

Explicit values of dose-volume parameters can be extracted from the DVH data and are called *dose-volume statistics* or

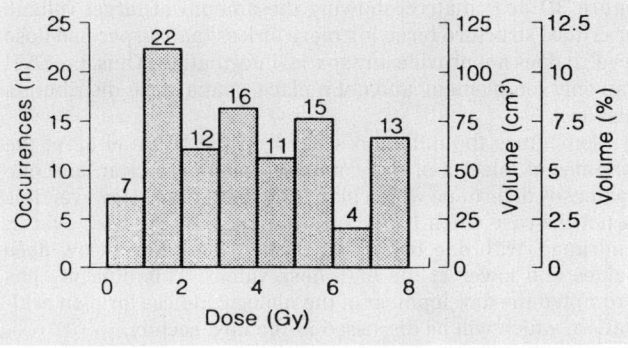

FIGURE 8.15. Differential dose-volume histogram display of the voxels shown in Fig. 8.17. The abscissa shows the 1-Gy bin sizes. The ordinate is expressed in a variety of equally valid units: Number of voxels (directly from Fig. 8.17), volume (cubic centimeters; equal to the voxel number × 5 cm³ per voxel), and volume (percentage; equal to the fraction of the total volume in that bin). For instance, 11 voxels (or 60 cm³ or 11% of the organ) received 2 Gy or more but less than 3 Gy. (From Lawrence TS, Kessler ML, Ten Haken RK. Clinical interpretation of dose-volume histograms: The basis for normal tissue preservation and tumor dose escalation. *Front Radiat Ther Oncol* 1996;29:57–66, with permission.)

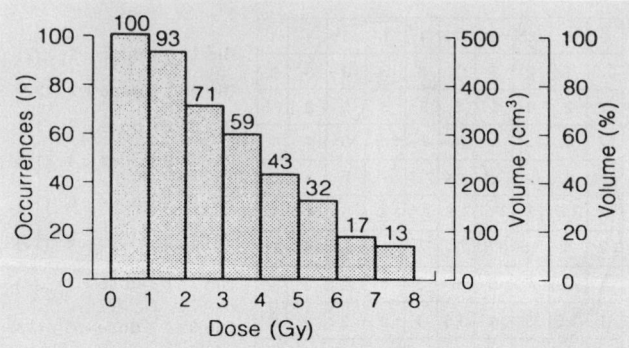

FIGURE 8.16. Cumulative dose–volume histogram (DVH) display of the voxels shown in Fig. 8.15. This figure contains the same data as shown in Fig. 8.15, but now displayed as a cumulative DVH. For instance, 71 voxels (or 350 cm^3 or 71% of the organ) received 2 Gy or more. (From Lawrence TS, Kessler ML, Ten Haken RK. Clinical interpretation of dose-volume histograms: The basis for normal tissue preservation and tumor dose escalation. *Front Radiat Ther Oncol* 1996;29:57–66, with permission.)

simply *dose statistics*. Examples include maximum point dose, minimum point dose, mean dose, percentage volume receiving greater than or equal to the prescription dose for target volumes and maximum point dose, mean dose, and percentage volume receiving greater than or equal to an established tolerance dose for organs at risk. There is some question as to whether a single point in the 3D dose matrix is meaningful clinically; typically, the maximum dose averaged over a small but clinically significant volume is more meaningful.

Plan Evaluation Using DVHs and Dose-Volume Statistics

The DVH is an essential tool used for conformal therapy plan evaluation. The planner can review the DVHs for the PTV and PRVs for the dose distribution under review, or superimpose DVHs for a specific PTV or PRV from several competing plans on one plot and compare them directly. The DVH display effectively points out the PRVs receiving excessive dose as well as any target volume(s) that may be underdosed. It is useful to generate a DVH for what is called "unspecified tissues" (i.e., those voxels within the skin contour that are not contained within contours for which DVHs have been generated). The unspecified tissue DVH helps prevent the radiation oncologist from overlooking high-dose regions that may be clinically significant.

Although a set of DVHs provides a complete summary of the entire 3D dose matrix, showing the amount of target volume or critical structure receiving more or less than a specified dose level, it does not provide any spatial information. Thus, the DVH can only complement, and not replace, spatial dose-distribution displays.

Sometimes the differences between the DVHs of all of the volumes of interest of two compared plans are clear, and one can easily determine which plan is the better one. However, this is not the case when DVHs for a normal tissue crosses over in midrange, with one being higher than the other at low dose values and lower at the high dose values. This difficulty has prompted the development of the biologic indices for plan evaluation, which will be discussed in the next section.

Biologic Models for Plan Evaluation

It is not always clear what degree of dose uniformity in the PTV can be tolerated as dose levels are escalated using conformal therapy or how exactly high a dose can be tolerated by a small portion of a normal structure volume. In the past, class solu-

tions based on clinical experience were used because quantitative 3D dose-volume data were not available. Researchers are now developing biophysical models that attempt to translate the dose-volume information into estimates of biologic impact (i.e., TCP and NTCP models). Today, most agree that the TCP and NTCP models developed thus far are not accurate to the extent that the absolute values can be used to predict response, but most agree that they can be used to compare rival plans. In any case, such biologic models should be used clinically only under protocol conditions until their utility has been firmly established for routine clinical use.

Normal Tissue Complication Probability

Currently there are two different approaches in modeling NTCP: The empiric model introduced by Lyman and Wolbarst (69,70), and the functional models based on the functional subunit concept (54,95,152).

The Lyman model can be expressed by an error function of dose and volume:

$$NTCP = \frac{1}{\sqrt{2\pi}} \int_{-\infty}^{1} \exp(-t^2/2) dt$$

where

$$V = V/V_{ref},$$
$$t = (D - TD_{50}(v))/(m \cdot TD_{50}(v))$$

and

$$TD_{50}(1) = TD_{50}(v) \cdot V^{-n}$$

TD$_{50}$(1) is the tolerance dose for 50% complications for uniform whole-organ irradiation, whereas *TD$_{50}$(v)* is the 50% tolerance dose for uniform partial-organ irradiation to the partial volume V. The arbitrary variables m and n are found by fitting tolerance doses for uniform whole and uniform partial organ irradiation, where m characterizes the gradient (slope) of the dose-response function at TD_{50} and n characterizes the effect of volume. When n is near unity, the volume effect is large; conversely, when n is near zero, the volume effect is small. When NTCP is plotted against dose, the NTCP equation demonstrates a sigmoid shape.

Two methods are currently used to extend this method to nonuniform organ irradiation. The interpolation method, proposed by Lyman and Wolbarst (70), modifies the DVH to one in which the organ receives an effective dose, D$_{eff}$, which is less than or equal to the maximum organ dose. The *effective volume method*, proposed by Kutcher and Burman (59), modifies the DVH to one in which a fraction of the organ, v$_{eff}$, receives the maximum organ dose. In this method, a uniformly irradiated dose equivalent is calculated for each tissue that contains dose heterogeneities (Fig. 8.17). For example, each step in the histogram of height ΔV_i and extension D_i is assumed to satisfy a power-law relationship so that it adjusts to one of smaller volume V$_{eff}$ and extension D$_{max}$ using

$$V_{eff} = \Delta V_{max} + \Delta V_i (D_i/D_{max})^{\frac{1}{n}} + \Delta V_2 (d_2/D_{max})^{\frac{1}{n}} + \cdots$$

where n is a size parameter.

Other NTCP models include the *critical volume model* proposed by Niemierko and Goitein (94), which they applied to the appearance of nephritis. Its form is similar to that of Lyman and Wolbarst (69) but it includes additional terms to account for the radiosensitivity of functional subunit in the kidney. The group at the University of Michigan has proposed a simple phenomenologic model for normal tissue complication, based on the sigmoid relationship derived by Goitein (36). In their model, however, they have nested the sigmoid cell-killing function into another sigmoid relationship describing complication or functional damage of an organ.

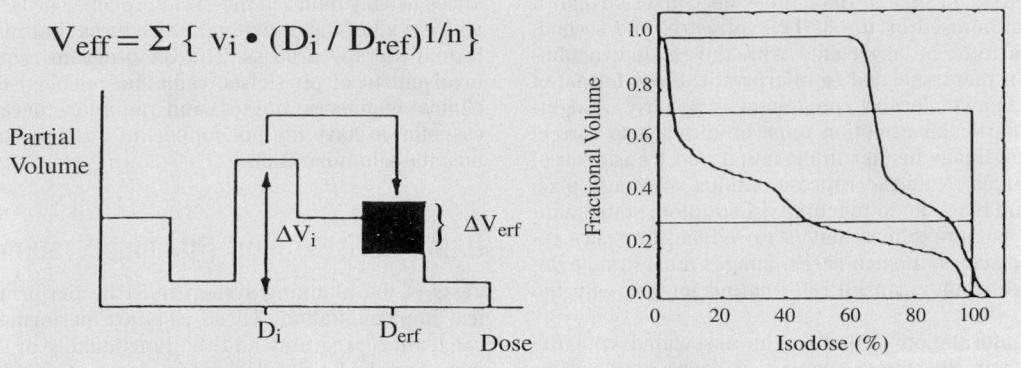

FIGURE 8.17. Illustration of the effective volume dose-volume histogram (DVH) reduction scheme. For a differential DVH (**A**), volume elements at one dose level are transposed to an effective volume at the reference dose level through use of the power-law relationship. This results in the single-step DVH (**B**), predicted to yield normal tissue complication probabilities identical to the original nonuniform irradiation DVHs. (Modified from Kutcher G, Berman C. Calculation of complication probability factors for non-uniform tissue irradiation: The effective volume method. *Int J Radiat Oncol Biol Phys* 1989;16:1623–1630, with permission.)

Tumor Control Probability

Tumor control probabilities have been modeled by Brahme (12) and Goitein (36), who proposed that, for a uniform dose within a tumor volume, TCP may be computed using the following equation:

$$TCP = \frac{1}{\left(1 + \left(\frac{Dose}{D_{50}}\right)^{-K}\right)}$$

where

$$K = 4/\Gamma$$

and Γ is equal to the slope of the dose response curve at 50% cell death.

For a nonuniform dose distribution, the total volume is reduced to smaller volumes having "uniform" doses within. TCPs are computed for each volume element and are then weighted according to their volume-fractions and summed according to the following equation:

$$\ln TCP = \sum \left(\frac{\Delta V}{V_0}\right) \ln TCP(V_0, D(x, y, z))$$

where

$$V_0 = \text{total tumor volume}$$

and

$$\Delta V = \text{volume element of dose D.}$$

When TCP is plotted against dose, the TCP equation demonstrates a sigmoid shape.

Equivalent Uniform Dose

Equivalent uniform dose (EUD) is a concept introduced by Niemierko (92) for use in evaluating and reporting inhomogeneous dose distributions. For tumors, it is generally accepted that the expected number of surviving clonogens determines the probability of local control. Therefore, two different inhomogeneous target dose distributions are equivalent if the corresponding expected numbers of surviving clonogens are equal. Using SF_2, (defined as the surviving fraction of cells irradiated to a dose of 2 Gy), as a measure of cell radiosensitivity, EUD is given by:

$$EUD = 2Gy \frac{\ln\left[\sum_i v_i(SF_2)^{\frac{D_i}{2Gy}}\right]}{\ln(SF_2)}$$

where v_i is the partial volume corresponding to dose D_i and the sum is taken over all bins of the differential DVH for the target volume. It should be noted that McGary et al. (75,76) have pointed out that there are conditions in which EUD is not adequate as a single parameter to report or analyze inhomogeneous dose distributions (e.g., when the minimum dose is significantly lower than the mean dose) (93).

Management of Conformal Therapy Data

To perform the steps involved in conformal therapy, several forms of patient imaging and other data must be acquired, displayed, manipulated, and stored. Typically, patient image data acquired from several imaging subsystems must be communicated to the planning system to permit these images to be used for defining target volumes and organs at risk. Several software components also must be integrated so that the output of one processing step can be made available for use as input to the next step. The issues in data management in all forms of conformal therapy are complex and continue to be somewhat problematic (106).

It is important to understand that nontrivial differences exist in the way various planning systems describe the details of radiation treatment, including units of measure and coordinate systems for specifying the geometric relationship between the patient and treatment beams. The American College of Radiology/National Electrical Manufacturers Association (NEMA) Digital Imaging and Communication in Medicine (DICOM) 3.0 standard for representing and communicating digital medical image and radiation therapy (RT) objects such as contours (RT structures), treatment plan specifications (RT-Plan), and 3D dose distributions (RT-Dose) is rapidly becoming the standard used in radiation oncology (8).

Several protocols have been developed to support the transfer of data files between computers. File transfer protocol (FTP) was developed for data file transport between computers on the Internet and is part of the Transmission Control Protocol/Internet Protocol suite of network protocols. FTP client and server software has been implemented for a wide range of computer hardware and operating systems. Because of its flexibility, FTP has found application both locally (e.g., to transfer data files between a CT scanner computer and the main 3DTPS file server) and between computers at widely separated sites on the Internet (e.g., to exchange 3DTPS data for multi-institutional clinical studies) (111).

Once image data have been acquired and transferred from the imaging system to the planning system, two important steps still remain. First, the image data must be converted into a format that can be used by the 3DTPS software, and second, the image data must be associated with the related, nonimage information that is needed to interpret it. If the format of image files is known, format conversion is a fairly straightforward task. Particular attention must be directed to correct interpretation of image header information and translation of image data values. Numeric representations of image pixel values vary from machine to machine. In addition, some manufacturers use compression schemes to reduce the space required to store images. In such cases, images must first be decompressed before they can be reformatted for use with the 3DTPS.

Nonimage information that must be associated with the image comes from the image acquisition process as well as from the clinical environment. An example of the former is calibration information that permits interpretation of image pixel values, such as the CT values representing air and water and the size of image pixels. Clinical information includes patient identification and demographics, as well as the date and time of acquisition and identification of the image acquisition system.

The amount of digital data transferred/stored (and thus the available information) in a radiation oncology department has drastically increased with the development/implementation of IGRT treatment machines. Daily kilovoltage cone-beam computed tomography (CBCT) images or MV helical CT images are acquired during a patient's treatment course adding several dozen Mbytes to Gbytes of information that need to be stored such that the data can be accessed when needed in an efficient manner. At the same time, the patient's treatment planning data, which often only exists in a system-specific proprietary format, need to be similarly stored and be able to be readily accessed. In addition, cancer biology imaging techniques currently used (or those under development) generate huge digital data files that require storage. But storage is not the only issue; new software tools to effectively use the imaging data (for clinical workflow issues, outcomes research, and basic research) are needed if radiation oncology is to take full advantage of all the new information. IGRT clearly points to the need for a new type picture archive communication system (PACS) specifically designed for radiation oncology (i.e., a RO-PACS) (86). The development of a robust RO-PACS will be one of the most important developments for radiation oncology as the use of information technology will be mission-critical in order to make radiation oncology more effective and efficient.

Another important informatics effort in radiation oncology is that being led by the Image-guided Therapy QA Center as part of the Advanced Technology QA Consortium (http://atc.wustl.edu/) (112). NCI-sponsored advanced technology trials in several sites are now in progress in which the patient's 3D planning and verification digital data are submitted via the Internet. All target volumes and designated critical structures contours superimposed on CT display, first-day portal films on all patients, and the 3D dose distribution are reviewed using web-based tools. The data are stored in a treatment planning-verification database. This database resource is allowing researchers to mine the data so as to better understand the relationship between dose and outcomes of 3DCRT/IMRT, and ultimately develop robust TCP and NTCP models.

Quality Assurance for Conformal Therapy

The precision and accuracy required for the 3D treatment planning and conformal therapy process exceeds accepted toler-

ances usually found in the 2D approach. The QA program must address all of the individual procedures that make up the conformal therapy process. The QA program requires the active involvement of physicists, radiation oncologists, dosimetrists, clinical engineers, nurses, and radiation therapists. It is also essential to have the full support of the department chair and hospital administration.

QA of the Treatment-Planning System

Tests of the planning system must be performed before clinical implementation. These tests are performed to check the calculation programs and the functionality of the system software and the hardware used for data entry and output. American Association of Physicists in Medicine Task Group 53 report, which describes the acceptance testing and commissioning of image-based planning systems, is currently the most extensive QA resource regarding these tests (29).

Software tests should follow the flow of the computer-based portions of the treatment planning process as much as possible: Patient data acquisition (obtaining scans from CT or MRI), patient anatomy definition (contouring of normal critical structures and tumor/target volumes), beam setup, dose computation, beam dose summation and dose display, DVH calculation and display, and hard copy output (e.g., beam settings, dose distributions, patient anatomy, custom portal plots, DRRs). The treatment planner initiates some of these steps, whereas others are the result of the normal flow of the planning system software (e.g., multiple-beam dose distribution summation).

Dose-calculation program and algorithm verification involves the testing of the implementation of the algorithm and includes a review of all input (modeling) data used for such calculations. A suite of tests that can be performed in a reasonable period to ensure that a software release functions predictably and correctly and that any hardware input/output devices used with the system function correctly is mandatory. Examples of such tests can be found in the articles by Harms et al. (44–46). Van Dyk et al. (142) have published recommendations of tolerance criteria for specific hardware and software tests and provide guidelines that can be used to supplement the testing described in the following paragraphs.

Each imaging modality to be used for patient data acquisition must be validated before its clinical use. Typically, a phantom (with documented geometry) is scanned over a range of slices in a fashion identical to scanning patients, and the image data are transferred to the planning system. The transferred images can be compared with the known phantom geometry to ensure correct orientation (anterior, posterior, right, and left) and slice position. If slice position changes are required because of differing coordinate systems on the CT scanner and the planning system (usually opposite signs on the slice position coordinates or left and right), the modifications required should be documented and reviewed for correctness. Because patient orientation on the scanner (prone, supine, head-first, feet-first) can affect the orientation of the transferred images, all orientations to be used for patients to be planned must be validated through this type of testing. The dimensions of the phantom in the image, subsequent to its transfer to the planning system, must be verified and documented. As a minimum, both horizontal and vertical dimensions should be reviewed. If the image pixel size on the scanner is variable, images of two different pixel sizes must be transferred and evaluated to ensure that the correct operation noted in the first test was not dependent on a particular pixel size. In addition, the planning system must be tested to determine if pixel sizes for a set of images (for a single patient) may have varying pixel dimensions from image to image and still be properly handled by the planning system.

If not, the software should explicitly prevent this from occurring.

The results of the conversion of the CT numbers to electron density must be verified, and bulk density assignments (as may be required for MRI-based patient data) also must be evaluated. Contouring software used to provide appropriate information about treatment setup and dose-volume information must be tested.

Defining a beam, setting it up to the proper orientation, and computing doses are so intermingled that it requires a broad definition of the verification tests to be performed. The actual verification of the dose-calculation algorithm is a separate test and is typically performed for single-beam dose computations. Examples of other tests to be performed are changing basic beam parameters such as energy, modality, and setup type (isocentric, arc, source-to-surface distance) to ensure that the change has been properly effected; adding and deleting treatment aids such as wedges, compensating filters, and custom portals to verify that they have been removed or replaced properly and are reflected in the subsequent dose distribution; changing all variable parameters for a beam of fixed energy and modality, using any and all means of manipulation, and ensuring that the changes are properly reflected in the graphic and text displays as well as in the dose display; evaluating the accuracy of digitizers and other methods of entering custom beam portals; and calculating and displaying DRRs for several known geometries and comparing with actual radiographs, BEV anatomy projections, or manual calculations of edge positions.

Although algorithm verification deals with individual beams, the validation process must check for proper summation of multiple-beam dose distributions. A simple manual check of beam summation is typically performed. For example, four single-beam plans are set up with four different gantry angles corresponding to anterior, posterior, right lateral, and left lateral angulations, and several point doses are extracted from each distribution. These point doses are manually summed and compared with point doses extracted from a single plan containing all four beams. To ensure that when beams are deleted from a treatment plan the doses for each beam are properly removed from a distribution, each of the four beams should be deleted from the previously described four-beam plan and the subsequent dose distribution evaluated using the extracted point doses as before.

Arc beam dose distributions are typically computed by simulating the arc with multiple static beams separated by a constant angle from start to stop angle. Therefore, point dose extractions should be performed to ensure that a summation of superimposed static field dose distributions simulating a rotational beam matches the dose distribution for the plan containing the arc beam.

Isodose contour displays can be tested using a single slice of the test phantom with superimposed isodoses for a plan that may be generated and be compared with the measured point doses.

A DVH test should involve a specially constructed phantom with well-defined internal structures and nested target volumes and with an equally well-defined dose distribution. This well-defined geometry and dose distribution then allows for manual generation of the DVHs for comparison with the computer-generated DVHs to ensure that the histograms are calculating and displaying correctly.

Both the hard copy output and the digital transfer of plan parameters to the record and verify and electronic medical record must be tested to ensure that all is correct. Typical outputs to be tested are beam settings (e.g., gantry position, couch positions, collimator positions, isocenter depth), dose distributions, patient anatomy, custom portal contours, DVH plots, DRR films, and any other output that may be available or required physically to implement a treatment plan.

QA of Plan Implementation

Ensuring that the patient is in the proper treatment position and that the numeric setup parameters of the treatment beams in the planning system are correctly transferred to the actual patient treatment is one of the most important steps in treatment plan implementation. It requires coordinate system alignment between the 3D treatment plan and the physical implementation of the treatment. Similar immobilization/registration support devices, modified to account for different couch constructions, are used on the simulator, CT simulator, and treatment machines.

It is possible to define beam orientations that are physically impossible to set up, and this process requires use of clinical judgment by the dosimetrist generating the treatment plan. Thus, the ability physically to set up a particular beam orientation must be reviewed and verified, particularly for beam orientations involving couch rotation, in which experiments may have to be performed to verify clearance between the treatment machine gantry and the patient or the gantry and the treatment couch before finalizing the treatment plan. Also, peer review of critical structure and tumor and target volumes and treatment plans is critical to conformal therapy delivery.

The conformal plan and associated documentation required for implementation and for the patient's chart must be reviewed for correctness and consistency. Documentation typically includes beam-setting parameters, custom MLC leaf settings (or block fabrication templates), DRRs, hard copy of appropriate REVs, which provides an overall view of the beam orientations relative to the patient, and DVHs for all targets and critical structures. Multiple REVs may be required for complex beam orientations or when too many beams are being used to be able to identify clearly the orientation of each beam.

After the treatment planner's initial review and documentation generation are completed, a physicist should evaluate the appropriateness of the plan and the ability physically to implement it on a treatment machine. The physicist should review the dose distribution for atypical or anomalous doses that may flag a previously undetected error in dose calculation, functioning of the planning system, or patient data entry. Finally, the radiation oncologist must perform the final review to assess the acceptability of the plan for both setup and dose, and approve it.

Verification Simulation

If a clinic is in the initial phases of implementing conformal therapy techniques or if experienced users implement nonconventional beam orientations, a verification simulation procedure is recommended to confirm planning systems are used for comparison with the verification simulation radiographs to confirm the correctness of the beam orientations in the physical implementation. When a beam orientation cannot be simulated, orthogonal radiographs may be taken and compared with similar DRRs to ensure correct isocenter positioning.

The optical distance indicator is also useful in assessing the correctness of the setup of a particular beam. Documentation provides a depth of isocenter below the skin surface on the central ray of the beam, which can then be compared with the isocenter depth measured on the simulator or treatment machine after the beam is set up using the couch and gantry positions specified by the treatment plan.

Treatment Verification

After verification that the treatment plan generated has been correctly implemented on the therapy simulator, the patient setup and beam arrangements must be accurately transferred to, and set up, on the treatment machine. This requires that the radiation therapist fully understand the methods of immobilization and beam orientation being used and precisely follow the setup instructions. On-line electronic portal imaging systems and/or cone beam CT systems for daily verification of each treatment are rapidly being implemented and are likely to replace the weekly checks of isocenter placement using orthogonal radiographs, which is commonly used today. Of course, first-day checks of portals apertures and beam orientations should always be performed for conformal therapy techniques. In addition, record-and-verify systems are considered essential components of a conformal therapy QA program. However, careful QA checks must also be in place to ensure that the input data into the record-and-verify system are correct.

Summary

Hypothetical benefits of 3D planning and conformal therapy are improved local tumor control because of better coverage of target volume with a specific dose of irradiation, less acute and late morbidity, capability of carrying out dose-escalation studies if morbidity is held to acceptable levels, and improved survival. Phase I/II and III conformal therapy dose-escalation studies in several disease sites have been conducted (or are underway) by the Radiation Therapy Oncology Group under cooperative agreement with the NCI (128). Particular note should be given to the Radiation Therapy Oncology Group dose-escalation study 94-06 in which a total of more than 1,000 patients were accrued (80–82,129). The latest report continues to show the observed tolerance to 3DCRT with 78 Gy in 2-Gy fractions remains better than expected compared with historical controls (81). In addition, there are many other individual institutional studies that have been published that have shown the benefits of 3D planning and conformal therapy, particularly for prostate cancer, head and neck cancer, and lung cancer (28,42,57,60,87,96,99,147,148,151,155,159–161).

The author strongly believes that the use of 3D treatment planning and conformal therapy has had (and will continue to have) a major impact on the practice of radiation therapy. Patients identified to benefit most from 3D planning and conformal therapy are those with tumors in sites with complex anatomy, irregularly shaped tumor volumes, tumors adjacent to radiation-sensitive normal structures, and small-volume or high-dose treatments. But as with any major technical advance in radiation oncology, its use must be supported with enhanced quality assurance from all members of the treatment team.

References

1. Ahnesjö A, Aspradakis MM. Dose calculations for external photon beams in radiotherapy. *Phys Med Biol* 1999;44:R99–R155.
2. Althof VGM, Hoekstra CJM, te Loo HJ. Variation in prostate position relative to adjacent bony anatomy. *Int J Radiat Oncol Biol Phys* 1996;34:709–715.
3. Antolak JA, Rosen II. Planning target volumes for radiotherapy: How much margin is needed. *Int J Radiat Oncol Biol Phys* 1999;44:1165–1170.
4. Balter JM, Lam K, Sandler HM, et al. Measurement of prostate movement over the course of routine radiotherapy using implanted markers. *Int J Radiat Oncol Biol Phys* 1995;31:113–118.
5. Balter JM, Lam KL, McGinn CJ, et al. Improvement of CT-based treatment-planning models of abdominal targets using static exhale imaging. *Int J Radiat Oncol Biol Phys* 1998 41:939–943.
6. Battista JJ, Rider WD, Van Dyk J. Computed tomography for radiotherapy planning. *Int J Radiat Oncol Biol Phys* 1980;6:99–108.
7. Bedford JL, Shentall GS. A digital method for computing target margins in radiotherapy. *Med Phys* 1998;25:224–231.
8. Bennett B, McIntyre, J: *Understanding DICOM 3.0, Version 1.0.* Kodak Health Imaging Systems, Rochester, NY, 1993.
9. Bjarngard B, Kijewski P, Pashby C. Description of a computer-controlled machine. *Int J Radiat Oncol Biol Phys* 1977;2:142–152.
10. Bortfeld T, Schmidt-Ullrich R, De Neve W, et al. *Image-guided IMRT.* Berlin, Springer, 2006.
11. Bosch WR, Low DA, Gerber RL, et al. The electronic viewbox: A software tool for radiation therapy treatment verification. *Int J Radiat Oncol Biol Phys* 1995;31:135–142.
12. Brahme A. Dosimetric precision requirements in radiation therapy. *Acta Radiol Oncol* 1984;23:379–391.
13. Bureau International des Poids et Mesures. Recommendation R(I)-1 in BIPM Com. Cons. Etalons Mes. Ray. Ionisants (Section I). (Offilib, F-75240 Paris Cedex 05) R(I)15. Paris: Bureau International des Poids et Mesures.
14. Caldwell CB, Mah K, Skinner M, et al. Can PET provide the 3D extent of tumor motion for individualized internal target volumes? A phantom study of the limitations of CT and the promise of PET. *Int J Radiat Oncol Biol Phys* 2003;55:1381–1393.
15. Caldwell CB, Mah K, Ung YC, et al. Observer variation in contouring gross tumor volume in patients with poorly defined non-small cell lung tumors on CT: The impact of 18FDG-Hybrid PET fusion. *Int J Radiat Oncol Biol Phys* 2001;51:923–931.
16. Chao KSC, Bosch WR, Mutic S, et al. A novel approach to overcome hypoxic tumor resistance: Cu-ATSM-guided intensity-modulated radiation therapy. *Int J Radiat Oncol Biol Phys* 2001;49:1171–1182.
17. Chao KSC, Ozyigit G, ed. *Intensity modulated radiation therapy for head and neck cancer.* Philadelphia: Lippincott Williams & Wilkins, 2003
18. Chapman JD, Bradley JD, Eary JF, et al. Molecular (functional) imaging for radiotherapy applications: An RTOG symposium. *Int J Radiat Oncol Biol Phys* 2003;55:294–301.
19. Craig T, Battista J, Moisennko V, et al. Considerations for the implementation of target volume protocols in radiation therapy. *Int J Radiat Oncol Biol Phys* 2001;49:241–250.
20. Cygler JE, Daskalov GM, Chan GH, et al. Evaluation of the first commercial Monte Carlo dose calculation engine for electron beam treatment planning. *Med Phys* 2004;31:142–153.
21. Davy TJ. Physical aspects of conformation therapy using computer-controlled tracking units. In: Orton, CG, ed. *Progress in medical radiation Physics: 2.* New York: Plenum, 1985.
22. Davy TJ, Brace JA. Dynamic 3-D treatment using a computer-controlled cobalt unit. *Br J Radiol* 1979;53:612–616.
23. Davy TJ, Johnson PH, Redford R, et al. Conformation therapy using the tracking cobalt unit. *Br J Radiol* 1975;48:122–130.
24. Dawson LA, Balter JM. Interventions to reduce organ motion effects in radiation delivery. *Semin Radiat Oncol* 2004;14:76–80.
25. Drzymala RE, Holman MD, Yan D, et al. Integrated software tools for the evaluation of radiotherapy treatment plans. *Int J Radiat Oncol Biol Phys* 1994;30:909–919.
26. Drzymala RE, Mohan R, Brewster L, et al. Dose-volume histograms. *Int J Radiat Oncol Biol Phys* 1991;21:71–78.
27. Emami B, Lyman J, Brown A, et al. Tolerance of normal tissue to therapeutic irradiation. *Int J Radiat Oncol Biol Phys* 1991;21:109–122.
28. Fiveash JB, Hanks G, Roach M, et al. 3D conformal radiation therapy (3DCRT) for high grade prostate cancer: A multi-institutional review. *Int J Radiat Oncol Biol Phys* 2000;47:335–342.
29. Fraass B, Doppke K, Hunt M, et al. AAPM Radiation Therapy Committee Task Group 53: Quality assurance for clinical radiotherapy treatment planning. *Med Phys* 1998;25:1773–1829.
30. Fraass BA, McShan DL. 3-D treatment planning. I. Overview of a clinical planning system. Proceedings of the 9th International Conference on the Use of Computers in Radiation Therapy. 1987; June 22–25, 1987. Scheveningen, The Netherlands.
31. Fraass BA, Smathers J, Deye JA. Summary and recommendations of a National Cancer Institute workshop on issues limiting the clinical use of Monte Carlo dose calculation algorithms for megavoltage external beam radiation therapy. *Med Phys* 2003;30:3206–3216.
32. Frank SJ, Forster KM, Stevens CW, et al. Treatment planning for lung cancer: Traditional homogeneous point-dose prescription compared with heterogeneity-corrected dose-volume prescription. *Int J Radiat Oncol Biol Phys* 2003;56:1308–1318.
33. Garcia-Ramirez JL, Mutic S, Dempsey JF, et al. Performance evaluation of an 85-cm-bore x-ray computed tomography scanner designed for radiation oncology and comparison with current diagnostic CT scanners. *Int J Radiat Oncol Biol Phys* 2002;52:1123–1131.
34. Geise RA, McCullough EC. The use of CT scanners in megavoltage photon-beam therapy planning. *Radiology* 1977;124:133–141.
35. Gerber RL, Purdy JA, Harms WB, et al. Introduction to the CT-simulation/3D treatment planning process. In: Purdy JA, Starkschall G, ed. *Practical guide to 3-D planning and conformal radiation therapy.* Madison, WI: Advanced Medical Publishing, Inc., 1999:27–55.
36. Goitein M. The probability of controlling an inhomogeneously irradiated tumor. In: Goitein M, Lyman J, Maor M, et al, ed. *Report of the Working Groups on the Evaluation of Treatment Planning for Particle Beam Radiotherapy.* 1987.
37. Goitein M, Abrams M. Multi-dimensional treatment planning: I. Delineation of anatomy. *Int J Radiat Oncol Biol Phys* 1983;9:777–787.
38. Goitein M, Abrams M, Rowell D, et al. Multi-dimensional treatment planning: II. Beam's eye view, back projection, and projection through CT sections. *Int J Radiat Oncol Biol Phys* 1983;9:789–797.
39. Green A. Tracking cobalt project. *Nature* 1965;207:1311.
40. Green A, Jennings WA, Christie HM. Rotational roentgen therapy in the horizontal plane. *Acta Radiol* 1960;31:275–320.
41. Gregoire V, Coche E, Cosnard G, et al. Selection and delineation of lymph node target volumes in head and neck conformal radiotherapy. Proposal for standardizing terminology and procedure based on the surgical experience. *Radiother Oncol* 2000;56:135–150.
42. Hanks GE, Hanlon AL, Schultheiss TE, et al. Dose escalation with 3D conformal treatment: Five year outcomes, treatment optimization, and future directions. *Int J Radiat Oncol Biol Phys* 1998;41:501–510.
43. Hanley J, Debois MM, Mah D, et al. Deep inspiration breath-hold technique for lung tumors: The potential value of target immobilization and reduced lung density in dose escalation. *Int J Radiat Oncol Biol Phys* 1999;45:603–611.
44. Harms WB Sr, Low DA, Purdy JA. Commissioning a three-dimensional dose-calculation algorithm for clinical use. In: Purdy JA, Fraass BA, ed. *Syllabus: A categorical course in physics.* Oak Brook, IL: Radiological Society of North America, 1994:111–115.
45. Harms WB Sr, Purdy JA. Evaluating commercially available three-dimensional radiotherapy treatment planning systems. *Semin Radiat Oncol* 1997;7:83–94.
46. Harms WB Sr, Purdy JA, Emami B, et al. Quality assurance for three-dimensional treatment planning. In: Purdy JA, Fraass BA, ed. *Syllabus: A categorical course in physics.* Oak Brook, IL: Radiological Society of North America, 1994:161–167.
47. Hill DLG, Batchelor PG, Holden M, et al. Medical image registration. *Phys Med Biol* 2001;46:R1–R45.

48. Hobday P, Hodson JJ, Husband J, et al. Computed tomography applied to radiotherapy treatment planning: Techniques and results. *Radiology* 1979;133:477–482.
49. ICRU Report 50: Prescribing, recording, and reporting photon beam therapy. Bethesda, MD: International Commission on Radiation Units and Measurements, 1993.
50. ICRU Report 62: Prescribing, recording, and reporting photon beam therapy (Supplement to ICRU Report 50). Bethesda, MD: International Commission on Radiation Units and Measurements, 1999.
50a. ICRU Report 29. Dose specification for reporting external beam therapy with photons and electrons. Washington, DC: International Commission on Radiation Units and Measurements, 1978.
51. IMRTCWG. NCI IMRT Collaborative Working Group: Intensity modulated radiation therapy: Current status and issues of interest. *Int J Radiat Oncol Biol Phys* 2001;51:880–914.
52. Jaffray DA, Siewerdsen JH, Wong JW, et al. Flat-panel cone-beam computed tomography for image-guided radiation therapy. *Int J Radiat Oncol Biol Phys* 2002;53:1337–1349.
53. Jin J-Y, Ajlouni M, Chen Q, et al. A technique of using gated-CT images to determine internal target volume (ITV) for fractionated stereotactic lung radiotherapy. *Radiother Oncol* 2006;78:177–184.
54. Källman P, Lind BK, Brahme A. An algorithm for maximizing the probability of complication free tumor control in radiation therapy. *Int J Radiat Oncol Biol Phys* 1992;37:871–890.
55. Keall PJ. 4-dimensional computed tomography Imaging and Treatment Planning. *Semin Radiat Oncol* 2004;14:81–90.
56. Kijewski PK, Chin LM, Bjarngard BE. Wedge-shaped dose distributions by computer-controlled collimator motion. *Med Phys* 1978;5:426–429.
57. Kong F-M, Hayman JA, Griffith KA, et al. Final toxicity results of a radiation-dose escalation study in patients with non-small-cell lung cancer (NSCLC): Predictors for radiation pneumonitis and fibrosis. *Int J Radiat Oncol Biol Phys* 2006;65:1075–1086.
58. Kubo HD, Wang L. Compatibility of Varian 2100C gated operations with enhanced dynamic wedge and IMRT dose delivery. *Med Phys* 2000;27:1732–1737.
59. Kutcher G, Berman C. Calculation of complication probability factors for non-uniform tissue irradiation: The effective volume method. *Int J Radiat Oncol Biol Phys* 1989;16:1623–1630.
60. Lagerwaard FJ, Senan S, van Meerbeeck JP, et al. Has 3-D conformal radiotherapy (3D CRT) improved the local tumour control for stage I non-small cell lung cancer? *Radiother Oncol* 2002;63:151–157.
61. Langen KM, Jones DTL. Organ motion and its management. *Int J Radiat Oncol Biol Phys* 2001;50:265–278.
62. Lattanzi J, McNeeley S, Pinover W, et al. A comparison of daily CT localization to a daily ultrasound-based system in prostate cancer. *Int J Radiat Oncol Biol Phys* 1999;43:719–725.
63. Leunens G, Menten J, Weltens C, et al. Quality assessment of medical decision making in radiation oncology: Variability in target volume delineation for brain tumors. *Radiother Oncol* 1993;29:169–175.
64. Lin LL, Mutic S, Malyapa RS, et al. Sequential FDG-PET brachytherapy treatment planning in carcinoma of the cervix. *Int J Radiat Oncol Biol Phys* 2005;63:1494–1504.
65. Lin LL, Yang Z, Mutic S, et al. FDG-PET imaging for the assessment of physiologic volume response during radiotherapy in cervix cancer. *Int J Radiat Oncol Biol Phys* 2006;65:177–181.
66. Ling CC, Hum68.m J, Larson S, et al. Towards multidimensional radiotherapy (MD-CRT): Biological imaging and biological conformality. *Int J Radiat Oncol Biol Phys* 2000;47:551–560.
67. Ling CC, York E, Fuks Z. From IMRT to IGRT: Frontierland or Neverland? *Radiother Oncol* 2006;78:119–122.
68. Liu HH, Koch N, Starkschall G, et al. Evaluation of internal lung motion for respiratory-gated radiotherapy using MRI: Part II–margin reduction of internal target volume. *Int J Radiat Oncol Biol Phys* 2004;60:1473–1483.
69. Lyman JT, Wolbarst AB. Optimization of radiation therapy. III. A method of assessing complication probabilities from dose-volume histograms. *Int J Radiat Oncol Biol Phys* 1987;13:103–109.
70. Lyman JT, Wolbarst AB. Optimization of radiation therapy. IV: A dose-volume histogram reduction algorithm. *Int J Radiat Oncol Biol Phys* 1989;17:433–436.
71. Mackie TR, Scrimger JW, Battista JJ. A convolution method of calculating dose for 15-MV x-rays. *Med Phys* 1985;12:188–196.
72. Mageras GS, Yorke E. Organ motion in radiation treatment. *Semin Radiat Oncol* 2004;14:65–75.
73. Malyapa RS, Mutic S, Low DA, et al. Physiologic FDG-PET three-dimensional brachytherapy treatment planning for cervical cancer. *Int J Radiat Oncol Biol Phys* 2002;54:1140–1146.
74. Martinez-Monge R, Fernades PS, Gupta N, et al. Cross-sectional nodal atlas: A tool for the definition of clinical target volumes in three-dimensional radiation therapy planning. *Radiology* 1999;211:815–828.
75. McGary JE, Grant W, Woo SY. Applying the equivalent uniform dose formulation based on the linear—quadratic model to inhomogeneous tumor dose distributions: Caution for analyzing and reporting. *J Appl Clin Med Phys* 2000;1:126–137.
76. McGary JE, Grant W, Woo SY, et al. Comment on "Reporting and analyzing dose distributions: A concept of equivalent uniform dose" [Med Phys 1997;24:103–109]. *Med Phys* 1997;24:1323–1324.
77. McShan DL, Silverman A, Lanza D, et al. A computerized three-dimensional treatment planning system utilizing interactive color graphics. *Br J Radiol* 1979;52:478–481.
78. Melian E, Mageras GS, Fuks Z, et al. Variation in prostate position: Quantitation and implications for three dimensional conformal radiation therapy. *Int J Radiat Oncol Biol Phys* 1997;38:73–81.
79. Meyer JL, Purdy JA, ed. *3-D conformal radiotherapy: A new era in the irradiation of cancer*. Basel: Karger, 1996.
80. Michalski JM, Purdy JA, Winter K, et al. Preliminary report of toxicity following: 3D radiation therapy for prostate cancer on 3DOG/RTOG 9406. *Int J Radiat Oncol Biol Phys* 2000;46:391–402.
81. Michalski JM, Winter K, Purdy JA, et al. Toxicity after three-dimensional radiotherapy for prostate cancer on RTOG 9406 dose Level V. *Int J Radiat Oncol Biol Phys* 2005;62:706.
82. Michalski JM, Winter K, Purdy JA, et al. Toxicity after three-dimensional radiotherapy for prostate cancer with RTOG 9406 dose level IV. *Int J Radiat Oncol Biol Phys* 2004;58:735–742.
83. Mijnheer BJ, Battermann JJ, Wambersie A. What degree of accuracy is required and can be achieve in photon and neutron therapy. *Radiother Oncol* 1987;8:237–252.
84. Mohan R, Barest G, Brewster LJ, et al. A comprehensive three-dimensional radiation treatment planning system. *Int J Radiat Oncol Biol Phys* 1988;15:481–495.
85. Mohan R, Chui C, Lidofsky L. Differential pencil beam dose computation model for photons. *Med Phys* 1986;13:64–73.
86. Moore C, Lehmann J, Purdy JA. A prototype radiation therapy picture archive communication system (RT PACS) design for clinics implementing IGRT (abstract). *Med Phys* 2006;33:2060.
87. Morris DE, Emami B, Mauch PM, et al. Evidence-based review of three-dimensional conformal radiotherapy for localized prostate cancer: An ASTRO outcomes initiative. *Int J Radiat Oncol Biol Phys* 2005;62:3–19.
88. Murphy MJ. Tracking moving organs in real time. *Semin Radiat Oncol* 2004;14:91–100.
89. Mutic S, Dempsey JF, Bosch WR, et al. Multimodality image registration quality assurance for conformal three-dimensional treatment planning. *Int J Radiat Oncol Biol Phys* 2001;51:244–260.
90. Mutic S, Grigsby PW, Low DA, et al. PET-guided three-dimensional treatment planning of intracavitary gynecologic implants. *Int J Radiat Oncol Biol Phys* 2002;52:1104.
91. Mutic S, Palta JR, Butker EK, et al. Quality assurance for computed-tomography simulators and the computed-tomography-simulation process: Report of the AAPM Radiation Therapy Committee Task Group No. 68. *Med Phys* 2003;30:2762–2792.
92. Niemierko A. Reporting and analyzing dose distributions: A concept of equivalent uniform dose. *Med Phys* 1997;24:103–110.
93. Niemierko A. Response to "Comment on 'Reporting and analyzing dose distributions: A concept of equivalent uniform dose'" *Med Phys* 1997;24:1323–1324]. *Med Phys* 1997;24:1325–1327.
94. Niemierko A, Goitein M. Calculation of normal tissue complication probability and dose-volume histogram reduction schemes for tissues with a critical element architecture. *Radiother Oncol* 1991;20:166–176.
95. Olsen DR, Kambestad BK, Kristoffersen DT. Calculation of radiation induced complication probabilities for brain, liver and kidney, and the use of a reliability model to estimate critical volume fractions. *Br J Radiol* 1994;67:1218–1225.
96. Perez CA, Michalski JM, Purdy JA, et al. Three-dimensional conformal therapy or standard irradiation in localized carcinoma of prostate: Preliminary results of a nonrandomized comparison. *Int J Radiat Oncol Biol Phys* 2000;47:629–637.
97. Perez CA, Purdy JA, Harms WB, et al. Design of a fully integrated three-dimensional computed tomography simulator and preliminary clinical evaluation. *Init J Radiat Oncol Biol Phys* 1994;30:887–897.
98. Pickett B, Roach M, Verhey L, et al. The value of nonuniform margins for six-field conformal irradiation of localized prostate cancer. *Int J Radiat Oncol Biol Phys* 1995;32:211–218.
99. Pollack A, Zagars GK, Starkschall G, et al. Prostate cancer radiation dose response: Results of the M. D. Anderson phase III randomized trial. *Int J Radiat Oncol Biol Phys* 2002;53:1097–1105.
100. Prasad SC, Glasgow GP, Purdy JA. Dosimetric evaluation of computed tomography treatment planning system. *Radiology* 1979;130:777–781.
101. Proimos BS. Synchronous field shaping in rotational megavoltage therapy. *Radiology*. 1960;74:753–757.
102. Purdy JA. 3-D radiation treatment planning: A new era. In: Meyer JL, Purdy JA, ed. *Frontiers of radiation therapy and oncology. 3-D conformal radiotherapy: A new era in the irradiation of cancer*. Basel: Karger, 1996:1–16.
103. Purdy JA. Defining our goals: Volume and dose specification for 3-D conformal radiation therapy. In: Meyer JL, Purdy JA, ed. *Frontiers of radiation therapy and oncology. 3-D conformal radiotherapy: A new era in the irradiation of cancer*. Basel: Karger, 1996:24–30.
104. Purdy JA. Intensity-modulated radiation therapy. *Int J Radiat Oncol Biol Phys* 1996;35:845–846.
105. Purdy JA. Volume and dose specification, treatment evaluation, and reporting for 3D conformal radiation therapy. In: Palta J, Mackie TR, ed. *Teletherapy: Present and future*. College Park, MD: Advanced Medical Publishing, 1996:235–251.
106. Purdy JA (guest ed). Data management in radiation oncology. *Semin Radiat Oncol* 1997;7:1–94.
107. Purdy JA. Dose-volume specification and reporting. In: Shiu AS, Mellenberg DE, ed. *General practice of radiation oncology physics in the 21st century*. Madison, WI: Medical Physics Publishing, 2000:3–15.
108. Purdy JA. Dose-volume specification: New challenges with intensity-modulated radiation therapy. *Semin Radiat Oncol* 2002;12:199–209.
109. Purdy JA. Current ICRU definitions of volumes: Limitations and future directions. *Semin. Radiat Oncol* 2004;14:27–40.
110. Purdy JA, Harms WB, Matthews JW, et al. Advances in 3-dimensional radiation treatment planning systems: Room-view display with real time interactivity. *Int J Radiat Oncol Biol Phys* 1993;27:933–944.
111. Purdy JA, Harms WB, Michalski J, et al. Multi-institutional clinical trials: 3-D conformal radiotherapy quality assurance. In: Meyer JL, Purdy JA, ed. *Frontiers of radiation therapy and oncology. 3-D conformal radiotherapy: A new era in the irradiation of cancer*. Basel: Karger, 1996:255–263.
112. Purdy JA, Harms WB, Michalski JM, et al. Initial experience with quality assurance of multi-Institutional 3D radiotherapy clinical trials. *Strahlentherapie nd Onkologie* 1998;174:40–42.
113. Purdy JA, Starkschall G. *A practical guide to 3-D planning and conformal radiation therapy*. Madison, WI: Advanced Medical Publishing, 1999.
114. Purdy JA, Wong JW, Harms WB, et al. Three dimensional radiation treatment planning system. Proceedings of the 9th International Conference on the Use of Computers in Radiation Therapy, June 22–25, 1987. Scheveningen, The Netherlands.
115. Rasch C, Barillot I, Remeijer P, et al. Definition of the prostate in CT and MRI: A multi-observer study. *Int J Radiat Oncol Biol Phys* 1999;43:57–66.
116. Rasch C, Keus R, Pameijer FA, et al. The potential impact of CT-MRI matching on tumor volume delineation in advanced head and neck cancer. *Int J Radiat Oncol Biol Phys* 1997;39:841–848.

117. Reinstein LE, McShan D, Webber BM, et al. A computer-assisted three-dimensional treatment planning system. *Radiology* 1978;127:259–264.

118. Remeijer P, Rasch C, Lebesque JV, et al. A general methodology for three-dimensional analysis of variation in target volume delineation. *Med Phys* 1999;26:931–940.

119. Remeijer P, Rasch C, Lebesque JV, et al. Margins for translational and rotational uncertainties: A probability-based approach. *Int J Radiat Oncol Biol Phys* 2002;53:464–474.

120. Rietzel E, Chen GTY, Choi NC, et al. Four-dimensional image-based treatment planning: Target volume segmentation and dose calculation in the presence of respiratory motion. *Int J Radiat Oncol Biol Phys* 2005;61:1535–1550.

121. Rietzel E, Pan T, Chen GT. Four-dimensional computed tomography: Image formation and clinical protocol. *Med Phys* 2005;32:874–889.

122. Roach M, Faillace-Akazawa P, Malfatti C. Prostate volumes and organ movements defined by serial computerized tomographic scans during three-dimensional conformal radiotherapy. *Radiat Oncol Invest* 1997;5:187–194.

123. Roach M, Faillace-Akazawa P, Akazawa C, et al. Prostate volumes defined by magnetic resonance imaging and computerized tomographic scans for three-dimensional conformal radiotherapy. *Int J Radiat Oncol Biol Phys* 1996;35:1011–1018.

124. Roeske JC, Forman J, Mesina CF, et al. Evaluation of changes in the size and location of the prostate, seminal vesicles, bladder, and rectum during a course of external beam radiation therapy. *Int J Radiat Oncol Biol Phys* 1995;33:1321–1329.

125. Rosenman J. Incorporating functional imaging information into radiation treatment. *Semin Radiat Oncol* 2001;11:83–92.

126. Rosenman JG, Miller EP, Tracton G, et al. Image registration: An essential part of radiation therapy treatment planning. *Int J Radiat Oncol Biol Phys* 1998;40:197–205.

127. Rosenzweig KE, Hanley J, Mah D, et al. The deep inspiration breath-hold technique in the treatment of inoperable non-small-cell lung cancer. *Int J Radiat Oncol Biol Phys* 2000;48:81–87.

128. RTOG. Image-Guided Radiation Therapy Committee. *Int J Radiat Oncol Biol Phys* 2001;51:60V.

129. Ryu JK, Winter K, Michalski JM, et al. Interim report of toxicity from 3D conformal radiation therapy (3D-CRT) for prostate cancer on 3DOG/RTOG 9406, Level III (79.2 GY). *Int J Radiat Oncol Biol Phys* 2002;54:1036–1046.

130. Schnall M, Rosen M. Primer on imaging technologies for cancer. *J Clin Oncol* 2006;24:3225–3232.

131. Sherouse GW, Mosher CE, Novins K, et al. Virtual simulation: Concept and implementation, in the use of computers in radiation therapy. Proceedings of the 9th International Conference on the Use of Computers in Radiation Therapy. June 22–25, 1987, Scheveningen, The Netherlands.

132. Shih HA, Jiang SB, Aljarrah KM, et al. Internal target volume determined with expansion margins beyond composite gross tumor volume in three-dimensional conformal radiotherapy for lung cancer. *Int J Radiat Oncol Biol Phys* 2004;60:613–622.

133. Sixel KE, Aznar MC, Ung YC. Deep inspiration breath hold to reduce irradiated heart volume in breast cancer patients. *Int J Radiat Oncol Biol Phys* 2001;49:199–204.

134. Smith AR, Purdy JA, eds. Three-dimensional photon treatment planning: Report of the Collaborative Working Group on the Evaluation of Treatment Planning for External Photon Beam Radiotherapy. *Int J Radiat Oncol Biol Phys* 1991;21:1–266.

135. Sterling TD, Knowlton KC, Weinkam JJ, et al. Dynamic display of radiotherapy plans using computer-produced films. *Radiology* 1973;107:689–691.

136. Sterling TD, Perry H, Katz L. Automation of radiation treatment planning V. Calculation and visualization of the total treatment volume. *Br J Radiol* 1965;38:906–913.

137. Takahaski S. Conformation radiotherapy-rotation techniques as applied to radiography and radiotherapy of cancer. *Acta Radiol Suppl* 1965;242:1–142.

138. Ten Haken RK, Thornton AF, Sandler HM, et al. A quantitative assessment of the addition of MRI to CT-based, 3-D treatment planning of brain tumors. *Radiother Oncol* 1992;25:121–133.

139. Tinger A, Michalski JM, Cheng A, et al. A critical evaluation of the planning target volume for 3-D conformal radiotherapy of prostate cancer. *Int J Radiat Oncol Biol Phys* 1998;42:213–221.

140. Trump JG, Wright KA, Smedal MI, et al. Synchronous field shaping and protection in 2-million-volt rotational therapy. *Radiology* 1961;76:275–283.

141. Urie MM, Goitein M, Doppke K, et al. The role of uncertainty analysis in treatment planning. *Int J Radiat Oncol Biol Phys* 1991;21:91–107.

142. Van Dyk J, Barrett RB, Cygler JE, et al. Commissioning and quality assurance of treatment planning computers. *Int J Radiat Oncol Biol Phys* 1993;26:261–273.

143. van Herk M, Bruce, A, Kroes APG, et al. Quantification of organ motion during conformal radiotherapy of the prostate by three dimensional image registration. *Int J Radiat Oncol Biol Phys* 1995;33:1311–1320.

144. van Herk M, Remeijer P, Lebesque JV. Inclusion of geometric uncertainties in treatment plan evaluations. *Int J Radiat Oncol Biol Phys* 2002;52:1407–1422.

145. van Herk M, Remeijer P, Rasch C, et al. The probability of correct target dosage: Dose-population histograms for deriving treatment margins in radiotherapy. *Int J Radiat Oncol Biol Phys* 2000;47:1121–1135.

146. Verhaegen F, Seuntjens J. Monte Carlo modeling of external radiotherapy photon beams (topical review). *Phys Med Biol* 2003;48:R107–R164.

147. Vicini F, Winter K, Straube W, et al. A phase I/II trial to evaluate three-dimensional conformal radiation therapy confined to the region of the lumpectomy cavity for stage I/II breast carcinoma: Initial report of feasibility and reproducibility of Radiation Therapy Oncology Group (RTOG) study 0319. *Int J Radiat Oncol Biol Phys* 2005;63:1531–1537.

148. Vicini FA, Remouchamps V, Wallace M, et al. Ongoing clinical experience utilizing 3D conformal external beam radiotherapy to deliver partial-breast irradiation in patients with early-stage breast cancer treated with breast-conserving therapy. *Int J Radiat Oncol Biol Phys* 2003;57:1247–1253.

149. Webb S. The physical basis of IMRT and inverse planning. *Br J Radiol* 2003;76:678–689.

150. Weltens C, Menten, J, Feron M, et al. Interobserver variations in gross tumor volume delineation of brain tumors on computed tomography and impact of magnetic resonance imaging. *Radiother Oncol* 2001 60:49–59.

151. Wilson EM, Joy Williams, F, Ethan Lyn, B, Aird, EGA. Comparison of two dimensional and three dimensional radiotherapy treatment planning in locally advanced non-small cell lung cancer treated with continuous hyperfractionated accelerated radiotherapy weekend less. *Radiother Oncol* 2005;74:307–314.

152. Withers HR, Taylor JMG, Maciejewski B. Treatment volume and tissue tolerance. *Int J Radiat Oncol Biol Phys* 1988;14:751–759.

153. Wong J, Sharpe M, Jaffray D, et al. The use of active breathing control (ABC) to reduce margin for breathing control. *Int J Radiat Oncol Biol Phys* 1999;44:911–919.

154. Wright KA, Proimos BS, Trump JG, et al. Field shaping and selective protection in megavoltage therapy. *Radiology* 1959;72:101.

155. Wu K-L, Jiang G-L, Liao Y, et al. Three-dimensional conformal radiation therapy for non-small-cell lung cancer: A Phase I/II dose escalation clinical trial. *Int J Radiat Oncol Biol Phys* 2003;57:1336–1344.

156. Yan D, Lockman D. Organ/patient geometric variation in external beam radiotherapy and its effects. *Med Phys* 2001;28:593–602.

157. Yan D, Lockman D, Brabbins D, et al. An off-line strategy for constructing a patient-specific planning target volume in adaptive treatment process for prostate cancer. *Int J Radiat Oncol Biol Phys* 2000;48:289–302.

158. Yan D, Ziaga E, Jaffray D. The use of adaptive radiation therapy to reduce setup error: A prospective clinical study. *Int J Radiat Oncol Biol Phys* 1998;41:715–720.

159. Zelefsky MJ, Cowen D, Fuks Z. Long-term tolerance of high dose three-dimensional conformal radiotherapy in patients with localized prostate carcinoma. *Cancer* 1999;85:2460–2468.

160. Zelefsky MJ, Leibel SA, Gaudin PB, et al. Dose escalation with three-dimensional conformal radiation therapy affects the outcome in prostate cancer. *Int J Radiat Oncol Biol Phys* 1998;41:491–500.

161. Zheng X-K, Ma J, Chen L-H, et al. Dosimetric and clinical results of three-dimensional conformal radiotherapy for locally recurrent nasopharyngeal carcinoma. *Radiother Oncol* 2005;75:197.

162. Zink S. 3-D radiation treatment planning: NCI perspective. In: Purdy JA, Emami B, ed. *3D radiation treatment planning and conformal therapy*. Madison, WI: Medical Physics Publishing, 1995:1–10.

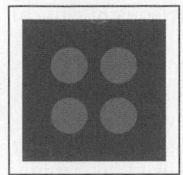

Chapter 9
Intensity-Modulated Radiation Treatment Techniques and Clinical Applications

K. S. Clifford Chao, Radhe Mohan, Nancy A. Lee, Gregory Chronowski, Daniel Low, Qiuwen Wu, Lei Dong

Since its introduction into clinical use (21,76,77), intensity-modulated radiation therapy (IMRT) has generated widespread interest. IMRT optimally assigns nonuniform intensities (i.e., weights) to tiny subdivisions of beams, which have been called rays or "beamlets." The ability to optimally manipulate the intensities of individual rays within each beam permits greatly increased control over the radiation fluence, enabling custom design of optimum dose distributions. These improved dose distributions potentially may lead to improved tumor control and reduced normal tissue toxicity. IMRT requires the settings of the relative intensities of tens of thousands of rays comprising an intensity-modulated treatment plan. This task cannot be accomplished manually and requires the use of specialized computer-aided optimization methods.

The optimum beamlet intensities are determined using a systematic iterative process during which the computer sequentially generates intensity-modulated plans one by one, evaluates each of them according to user-selected criteria ("desired objectives"), and makes incremental changes in the ray intensities based on the deviation from the desired objectives. The quality of an intensity-modulated treatment plan produced in this manner depends on a number of factors. These include the mathematical function and its parameters used by the optimization process to evaluate and compare competing treatment plans; the mathematics and algorithms of optimization; the number, orientation, and energy of radiation beams; margins assigned to the planning target volume (PTV) and to normal structures; dose-calculation algorithms; and so on. We will discuss many of these in detail in this chapter.

The term *IMRT* is used to mean much more than its literal meaning might suggest. Strictly speaking, the use of wedges and conventional compensators to compensate for surface curvature is also intensity modulation. In this chapter, IMRT is a form of three-dimensional (3D) conformal radiation therapy (CRT) in which a *computer-aided optimization process is used to determine customized nonuniform fluence distributions to attain certain specified dosimetric and clinical objectives.*

IMRT Rationale

IMRT has many potential advantages. It can be used to produce dose distributions that are far more conformal than those possible with standard 3D conformal radiation therapy (3DCRT). Dose distributions within the PTV, in theory, can be made more homogeneous and, if so desired, a sharper fall-off of dose at the PTV boundary can be achieved. Experience with current IMRT systems has led to an impression among many that IMRT inherently produces inhomogeneous dose distribution within the target volume. Inhomogeneity commonly observed is the result of the overriding need to partially or wholly protect one or more critical organs. In other words, the dose distributions tend to be more heterogeneous because the homogeneity criterion is made less important than the normal structure avoidance criterion. If all things were equal, the IMRT plan always should produce more homogeneous dose distribution than a plan made with uniform beams. A sharper fall-off of dose at the PTV boundary, in turn, means that the volume of normal tissues exposed to high doses may be reduced significantly. These factors may allow escalation of tumor dose, reduction of normal tissue dose, or both, hopefully leading to an improved outcome. A lower rate of complications also may mean lower cost of patient care following the treatment. In addition, IMRT has the potential to be more efficient with regard to treatment planning and delivery than standard 3DCRT, although gains in this direction are being realized rather slowly. The treatment design process is relatively insensitive to the choice of planning parameters, such as beam directions. There are no secondary field-shaping devices other than the computer-controlled multileaf collimator (MLC). Furthermore, large fields and boosts can be integrated into a single treatment plan, and, in many cases, electrons can be dispensed with, permitting the use of the same integrated boost plan for the entire course of treatment. An integrated boost treatment may offer an additional radiobiologic advantage in terms of lower dose per fraction to normal tissues while delivering higher dose per fraction to the target volume. Higher dose per fraction also reduces the number of fractions and hence lowers the cost of a treatment course.

IMRT Limitations and Risks

We should recognize, however, that IMRT has limitations. There are many dose distributions (or dose-volume combinations) that are simply not physically achievable. Furthermore, our knowledge about what is clinically optimal and achievable and how best to define clinical and dosimetric objectives of IMRT is limited. Moreover, the best solution may elude us because of the limitations of the mathematical formalism used or because of the practical limits of computer speed and the time required for finding it.

Uncertainties of various types (e.g., those related to daily, or interfraction, positioning; displacement and distortions of internal anatomy; intrafraction motion; and changes in physical and radiobiologic characteristics of tumors and normal tissues during the course of treatment) may limit the applicability and efficacy of IMRT. Dosimetry characteristics of a delivery device, such as radiation scattering and transmission through the MLC leaves, introduce some limitations in the accuracy and deliverability of IMRT fluence distributions. In addition, the limited spatial and temporal coverage and overall accuracy of current IMRT dosimetric verification systems (based principally on radiographic film) diminish the confidence in the delivered dose. Furthermore, most current dose-calculation models are limited in their accuracy, especially for the small, complex shapes required for IMRT. It is quite conceivable that inaccuracies in dose calculations may yield a solution different from the one derived if dose calculations were accurate. Perhaps the most important factor that may limit the immediate success of IMRT is the inadequacy of imaging technology to define the true extent of the tumor, its extensions, and radiobiologic characteristics as well as geometric, dose-response, and functional characteristics of normal tissues.

We also should be aware of the risks of IMRT. The effect of large fraction sizes used in integral boost IMRT on tissues embedded within the gross tumor volume (GTV) is uncertain and may present an increased risk of injury (97). There also may be an increased risk that improper use of spatial margins, coupled with the high degree of conformation with IMRT, may lead to geographic misses of the disease and recurrences, especially for disease sites where positioning and motion uncertainties play a large role or where there are significant changes in anatomy and radiobiology during the course of radiotherapy. Similarly, high doses in close proximity to normal critical structures may pose a greater risk of normal tissue injury. In addition, IMRT dose distributions are unusual and highly complex and existing experience is too limited to interpret them properly and evaluate their efficacy. This may lead to unforeseen sequelae.

These limitations and risks point to the need for continued investigations to improve the method and to minimize the uncertainties. Such investigations are essential to exploit the full power of IMRT.

IMRT—An Unconventional Paradigm

The application, process, and dose distributions of IMRT are significantly different from those of conventional two-dimensional (2D) CRT or 3DCRT. This means the traditional methods of specification and fractionation of treatments, evaluation of treatment plans, and reporting of results are limited and new methods need to be introduced.

The traditional 3DCRT process involves "forward planning," in which beam parameters (directions, apertures and their margins, beam weights, beam modifiers) are specified and dose distributions are computed. The treatment plan is evaluated by a human being, and, if necessary, beam parameters are modified to achieve a satisfactory dose distribution. In IMRT, an inverse process ("inverse planning") is used in which the desired dosimetric and clinical objectives are stated mathematically (in the form of an "objective function"). The term *inverse planning* sometimes is confused with matrix inversion of a given dose distribution. In the present context it is used to distinguish it from forward planning for conventional 3DCRT. The IMRT optimization software iteratively adjusts beam parameters with the aim of obtaining the best possible approximation of the desired dose distribution. In each optimization iteration, the optimization software computes the value of the objective function (i.e., the IMRT plan score) to judge the overall quality of each of a large number of plans to choose the optimum one.

IMRT is most conformal and most efficient if all target volumes (gross disease, subclinical extensions, and electively treated nodes) are treated simultaneously using different fraction sizes. Such a treatment strategy has been called the simultaneous integrated boost (SIB) (97). This is in contrast to conventional radiotherapy in which the same fraction size (typically 1.8 or 2 Gy) is used for all target volumes with successive reductions in field sizes to protect critical normal structures and to limit the dose to electively treated and subclinical disease regions.

Alternative IMRT Approaches

During the past 15 years, a variety of techniques have been explored for designing and delivering optimized IMRT (5, 8–10,11,13–16,20,21,27,30,34,35,53,60,76,77,86,91–93,96,97, 115–120,128,131–136,147,148). Many of these are implemented in commercial IMRT systems. The most significant differences among the various approaches are in terms of the mechanisms they use for the delivery of nonuniform fluences. Although the merits of each often are speculated, the superiority of any of the approaches is difficult to assess because there have been no systematic comparisons of clinical treatment plans.

Of the various approaches proposed, two dominant but significantly different methods have emerged. Mackie et al. (85,86) proposed an approach called *tomotherapy* in which intensity-modulated photon therapy is delivered using a rotating slit beam. A temporally modulated slit MLC is used to rapidly move leaves in or out of the slit. Like a computed tomography (CT) unit, the radiation source and the collimator continuously revolve around the patient. Either the patient is translated between successive rotations (serial tomotherapy) or during rotation (helical tomotherapy). For helical tomotherapy, the system looks like a conventional CT scanner and includes a megavoltage portal detector to provide for the tomographic reconstruction of the delivered dose distribution. The first clinical tomotherapy machine is in the process of being implemented.

A commercial slit collimator (called *MIMiC*) of the type proposed by Mackie et al. (85,86) has been designed and built by the NOMOS Corporation (North American Scientific Chatsworth, CA). It has been incorporated into their serial tomotherapy system, known as Peacock (Fig. 9.1), for planning and rotational delivery of intensity-modulated treatments (21).

In the second approach, implemented first into clinical use at Memorial Sloan-Kettering Cancer Center (76,77,91,92, 96,98,131,132), a standard MLC is used to deliver the optimized fluence distribution in either dynamic mode (defined as the leaves moving while the radiation is on) or static mode, i.e., "step-and-shoot" mode (defined as sequential delivery of radiation subportals that combine to deliver the desired fluence distribution), to deliver a set of intensity-modulated fields incident from fixed-gantry angles. These techniques are gaining wide acceptance rapidly. Every major commercial treatment-planning system manufacturer has implemented one or both of these approaches (Fig. 9.2).

A third approach, called *intensity-modulated arc therapy* or IMAT, developed by Yu (147), uses a combination of dynamic multileaf collimation and arc therapy. The shape of the field formed by the MLC changes continuously during gantry rotation. Multiple superimposing arcs are used, and the field shape for a specific gantry angle changes from one arc to the next appropriately so that the cumulative fluence distribution of all arcs is equal to the desired distribution.

In addition to these approaches, the University of Michigan has used the so-called multisegment approach in which each of a number of beams is divided into multiple segments. One segment for each beam frames the entire target while the others spare one or more normal structures. Each segment is uniform in intensity. The weights of segments of all beams are optimized to produce the desired treatment plan. The treatments are delivered as a sequence of multiple uniform field segments. A similar approach previously was proposed by Mohan et al. (94). In almost all of these significantly different treatment-delivery approaches, the underlying principles of optimization are similar, although the specifics may be quite different.

The IMRT Process Overview

As mentioned previously, there are significant differences in 3DCRT and IMRT concepts and processes. However, there are also many similarities. In particular, IMRT relies on many of the same imaging, dose calculations, plan evaluation, quality assurance (QA), and delivery tools as 3DCRT.

The IMRT planning, QA, and delivery phases of the dynamic or static MLC process are shown in Figure 9.3. Figures 9.4–9.6 show the steps in each phase of the IMRT process. The tomotherapy process is similar, except that the fixed-beam angle selection is replaced by selection of the slice thickness and, for serial tomotherapy, the gantry rotation angles.

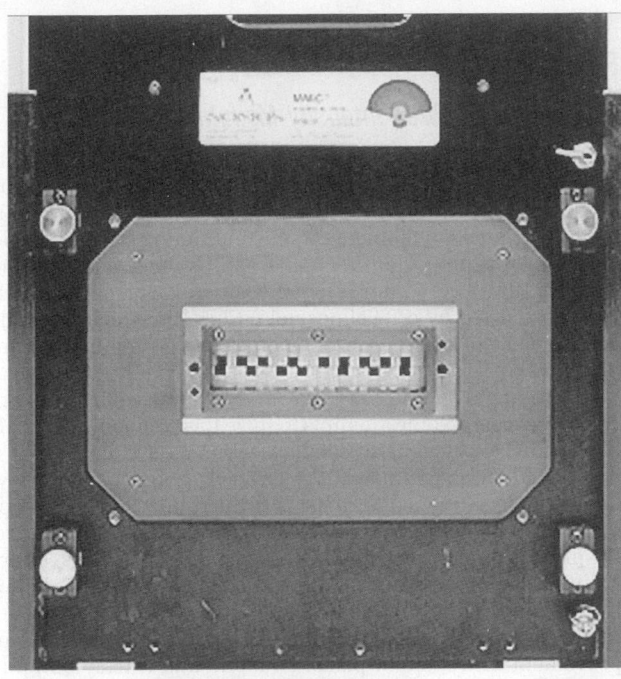
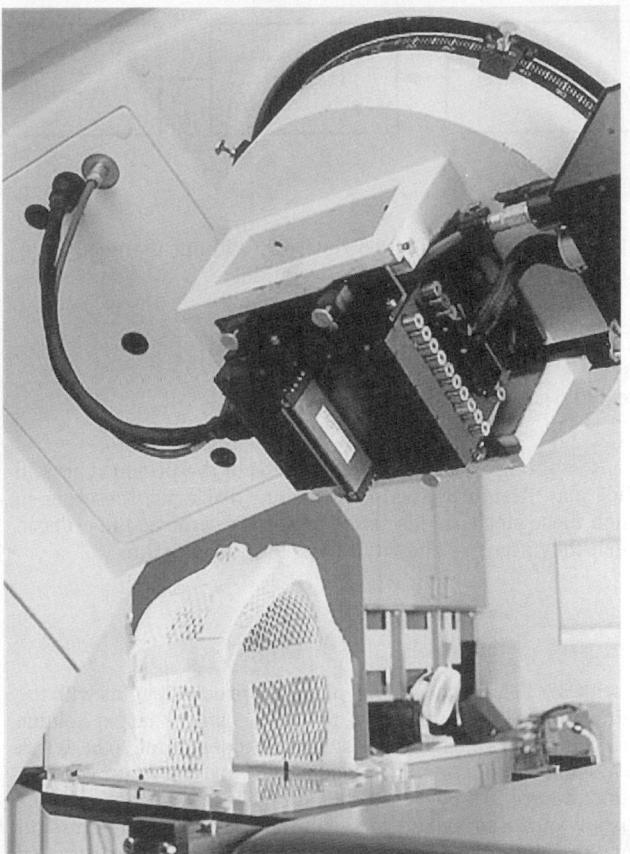

A   B

FIGURE 9.1. Commercial serial tomotherapy delivery hardware mounted on a conventional linear accelerator. **A:** View looking into the collimator toward the radiation source. A leaf pattern is shown that highlights the system's capability for delivering complex fluence patterns. **B:** The multileaf collimator mounted to a conventional linear accelerator.

In the preparatory phase of the IMRT process, volumes of interest (such as tumors and normal organs) are delineated on 3D CT images, often with assistance from other coregistered imaging modalities. Also, the desired objectives in the form

FIGURE 9.2. A typical multileaf collimator used for delivery of intensity-modulated radiation therapy looking toward the radiation source. In the dynamic mode, the leaves move back and forth or sweep across the field continuously to form the sequence of required field shapes while the beam is on. In the static or step-and-shoot mode, the beam is turned off when the leaves move to form the required field shapes. (Photograph courtesy of Varian Medical Systems.)

of an objective function, its parameter values, and the IMRT fractionation strategy are specified, and beam configuration is defined.

In the treatment-plan optimization phase, an iterative process is used to adjust and set the intensities of rays of each beam (or portion of the arc) so that the resulting intensity distributions yield the best approximation of the desired objectives. The IMRT plan then is evaluated to ensure that the trade-offs made by the optimization system are acceptable. If further improvement is deemed necessary and possible, the objective function parameters are modified and the optimization process is repeated until a satisfactory treatment plan is achieved.

In the leaf sequence-generation phase, the intensity distributions are converted into sequences of leaf positions. It is conceivable that certain dose distributions cannot be delivered as a result of the leakage characteristics of the delivery devices. Therefore, in most treatment-planning systems, the leaf sequences are used in a reverse process to calculate the dose distributions they are expected to deliver. These dose distributions, called the *deliverable dose distributions*, are evaluated for clinical adequacy. If necessary, objective function parameters are further adjusted to produce an intensity distribution that leads to a deliverable dose distribution that meets the desired objectives. This is the practice in most systems. However, in some systems, the leaf sequence-generation process is incorporated into the IMRT plan optimization loop so that the optimized and deliverable dose distributions are identical. More details on this are given later in this chapter.

The leaf sequences then are transmitted to the treatment machine and used to verify that the dose distribution that will be delivered to the patient is correct and accurate. The patient then is set up in the usual fashion and treated. In general, the

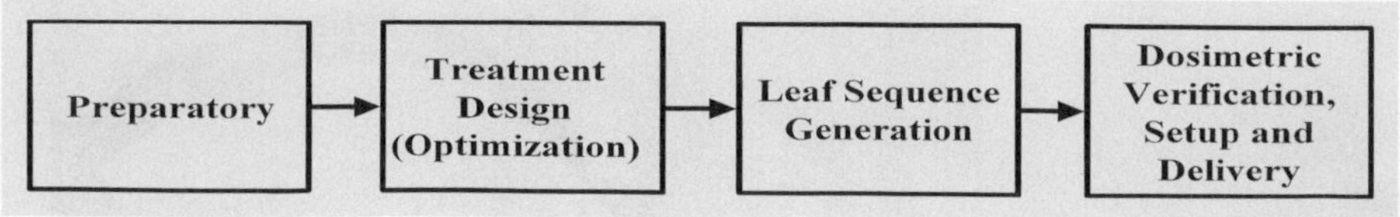

Preparatory → Treatment Design (Optimization) → Leaf Sequence Generation → Dosimetric Verification, Setup and Delivery

FIGURE 9.3. Overview of a typical intensity-modulated radiation therapy planning and delivery process.

entire treatment is delivered remotely without the need to re-enter the treatment room in between fields.

•• Preparatory and IMRT Planning Phases

This section discusses each of the steps of the preparatory and IMRT plan design phases. For reasons of clarity, the order in which these steps are discussed is not the same as the order in which they occur as shown in Figs. 9.4 through 9.6.

Imaging and Volumes of Interest

As with 3DCRT, the treatment-planning process begins with the delineation of the outlines of the GTV, clinical target volume (CTV), and the critical normal structures considered to be at risk on a sequence of CT image sections. In an important contrast with standard 3DCRT, regions of subclinical extension (volume typically enclosed by a 1- to 2-cm margin around the gross tumor) and potential subclinical disease (e.g., electively treated lymph–node-bearing regions) also need to be outlined. The optimization process considers explicitly and simultaneously both the gross disease and the larger volumes of occult or microscopic disease to design an IMRT plan. As will be explained later, this strategy has some distinct advantages. A supplementary margin is added to allow for uncertainties related to the movement of the tumor volume from one day to the next and for intrafraction motion to obtain the PTVs. The number of normal structures that need to be drawn also increases. In conventional radiotherapy, in which the use of large uniform fields is typical and the treatment plans are evaluated manually, a clinician can make a reasonable estimate of dose received by a volume of interest even if it is not explicitly drawn. In IMRT, in which dose is being escalated to unprecedented levels, where dose distributions are highly nonuniform, and where plans are generated and evaluated by the computer during the iterative optimization process, all structures to which the dose must be constrained need to be delineated.

Beam Configurations

Systems Using Fixed Intensity-Modulated Fields

The beam configuration can have a significant impact on the quality of an optimized IMRT plan. It may be argued that, because of the greater control over dose distributions afforded by optimized intensity modulation, the fine-tuning of beam angles may not be as important for IMRT as it is for standard radiotherapy. However, optimization of beam angles may find paths least obstructed by critical normal tissues, thus facilitating the achievement of desired distribution with a minimum of compromise.

Beam-angle optimization, however, is not a trivial problem. There have been some attempts to solve this problem (108,121), but a satisfactory general solution has not yet been found. To appreciate the magnitude of the problem, consider the following example. If the angle range is divided into 5-degree steps, nearly 60,000 combinations would need to be tested for three beams, nearly 14 million combinations for five beams, nearly 1.5 billion combinations for seven beams, and so on. Considering the magnitude of the search space, none of the optimization methods is likely to be able to demonstrate a significant improvement in treatment plans, let alone find a truly optimum combination when the number of beams is five or more. Furthermore, the beam-angle optimization problem is known to have multiple minima, which means that fast gradient-based optimization techniques may fail.

Another question that may be asked is how many beams are optimal. In principle, a larger number of beams would provide a larger number of parameters to adjust and therefore a greater opportunity to achieve desired dose distributions. (Thus, in theory, a rotational beam would be the ultimate.) However, for fixed-beam IMRT, it may be desirable to minimize the number of beams to reduce the time and effort required for planning, QA, dosimetric verification, and delivery of treatments. Fewer intensity-modulated beams would be needed if beam angles were optimized than if the beams were placed at equiangular steps.

Considering the difficulties of optimizing beam angles, beam directions are selected intuitively, based on conventional experience, or placed at equiangular steps. For equiangular beams,

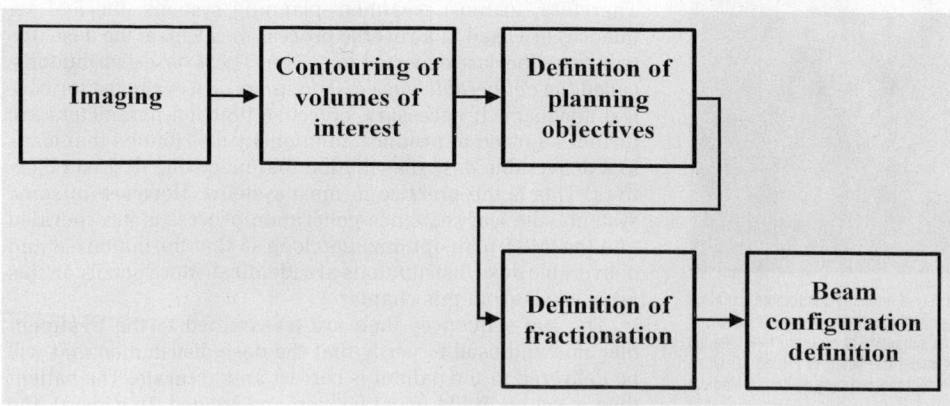

FIGURE 9.4. Intensity-modulated radiation therapy process: Preparatory phase.

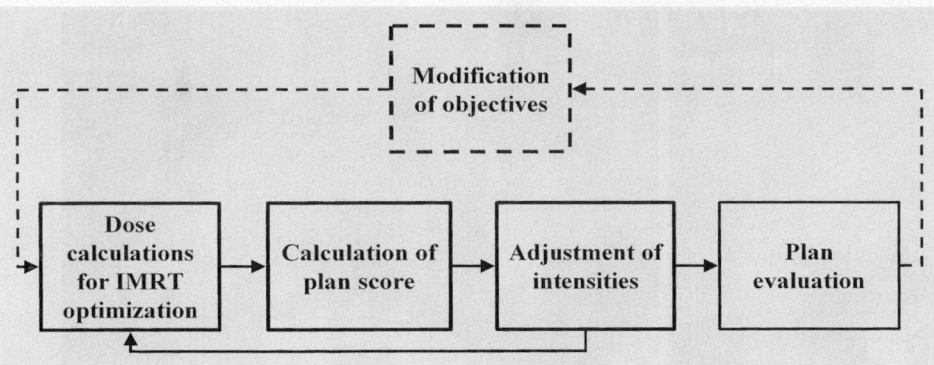

FIGURE 9.5. Intensity-modulated radiation therapy (IMRT) process: Plan optimization phase.

in general, the quality of a plan improves as the number of beams increases; but as the number of beams increases, the additional gain achieved diminishes. It is not evident *a priori* how many intensity-modulated beams would be adequate. The ideal minimum number would depend in a complex manner on a combination of geometric and biologic factors including the size, shape, and location of the target volume; the sizes, shapes, tolerances, tissue architectures, and relative locations of the surrounding normal tissues; and the prescription dose. This number may have to be determined by trial and error for each class of radiotherapy problems.

Figure 9.7 (a) through (d) compare head and neck IMRT plans designed with 5, 7, 9, and 15 equally spaced beams. Consistent with published experience, the plan quality improves but the incremental improvement diminishes with increasing number of beams. Optimum nonuniform placement of beams can further improve dose distribution. Figure 9.8A and B shows another head and neck IMRT case for two different beam angles. The patient, treated with beam configuration shown in Figure 9.8A, developed significant mucositis at the early phase of treatment. This was consistent with the "horn" in dose distribution pointed to by the arrow. Revising beam angle arrangement as shown in Figure 9.8C led to improved dose distribution shown in Figure 9.8D.

In general, it is most advantageous to place beams so that they are maximally avoiding each other and the opposing beams with the stipulation that directions that overlap significant obstructions, such as heavily attenuating bars in the treatment couch, be avoided. For simplicity, beams often are constrained to lie in the same transverse plane. However, noncoplanar beams will provide an additional degree of freedom and potentially an additional gain in the quality of treatments.

Although reducing the number of beams is a desirable goal for IMRT delivered with several fixed-gantry angles and dynamic MLC, it should not be the overriding consideration. IMRT can be planned and delivered automatically in times not significantly different from the times for much simpler conventional treatments. Therefore, the delivery times for 6 to 20 beams may be quite acceptable. Keep in mind, however, that some of the current linear accelerators are limited in their ability to accurately deliver a large number of intensity-modulated beams each with a very small number of monitor units (MUs).

Systems Using Rotating Slit (Tomotherapy) Approach

Tomotherapy delivery has substantial differences from fixed-portal IMRT. The linear accelerator rotates during delivery, and the beam is modulated during rotation. Typically, the modulation is subdivided into small gantry angle ranges (e.g., 5 degrees) and the beam is independently modulated at each gantry angle. Each leaf is used to deliver a single rotating pencil. The pencil-beam modulation is conducted for each leaf by opening that leaf for a fraction of the gantry range consistent with the fractional fluence to be delivered from that gantry angle. For example, for a 5-degree angle range bin, if a leaf is to deliver 50% fluence, the leaf will be open for 2.5 degrees over the 5-degree range. Because of geometric constraints of modulating the radiation fan beams, only one or two thin planes can be treated with each rotation. The Peacock system, for instance, uses two banks of opposing leaves projecting to 1.7 or 3.4 cm, depending on user-selected mechanical stops. This delivers modulated beams to two abutting, independently modulated planes. The helical tomotherapy unit uses a single leaf bank with a backup collimator that allows the radiation field width to be continuously adjusted. Narrower leaf widths provide higher spatial resolution for modulation but require more treatment arcs and consequently more delivery time.

Aperture Margins

IMRT has the inherent capacity to reduce margins attributable to the beam penumbra. When a photon beam traverses the body, it is scattered, depositing dose not only along the path of each ray of the beam but also at points away from it. The electrons knocked out by the incident photons travel laterally to points in the neighborhood of each ray, depositing dose along the way. Near the middle of a uniform beam, outgoing electrons are offset by incoming electrons and equilibrium exists. However, at and just inside the boundaries of the beam, there are no incoming electrons to balance electrons flowing out of the beam. Therefore, a "lateral disequilibrium" exists that leads to a dose deficit inside the boundaries of beams. For lower energy beams and at large depths, scattered photons significantly contribute to this effect also. The conventional approach to overcome this deficiency is to add a margin for the "beam penumbra" to the PTV so that the tumor dose is maintained at the required level.

For IMRT plans, there is another method to counterbalance the dose deficit. The intensity of rays just inside the beam boundary may be increased. Because some of the increased energy must also flow out, a very large increase would be required if the margin for the penumbra were set to zero or to a very small value. Therefore, an increase in boundary fluence alone is not enough. A combination of an increased fluence and the addition of a margin, albeit a much smaller one, is a better solution. This reduction in margin can be exploited quite usefully to reduce the volume of normal tissues exposed to high doses

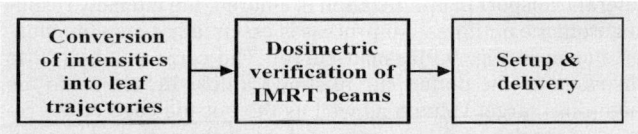

FIGURE 9.6. Intensity-modulated radiation therapy (IMRT) process: Quality assurance and delivery phase.

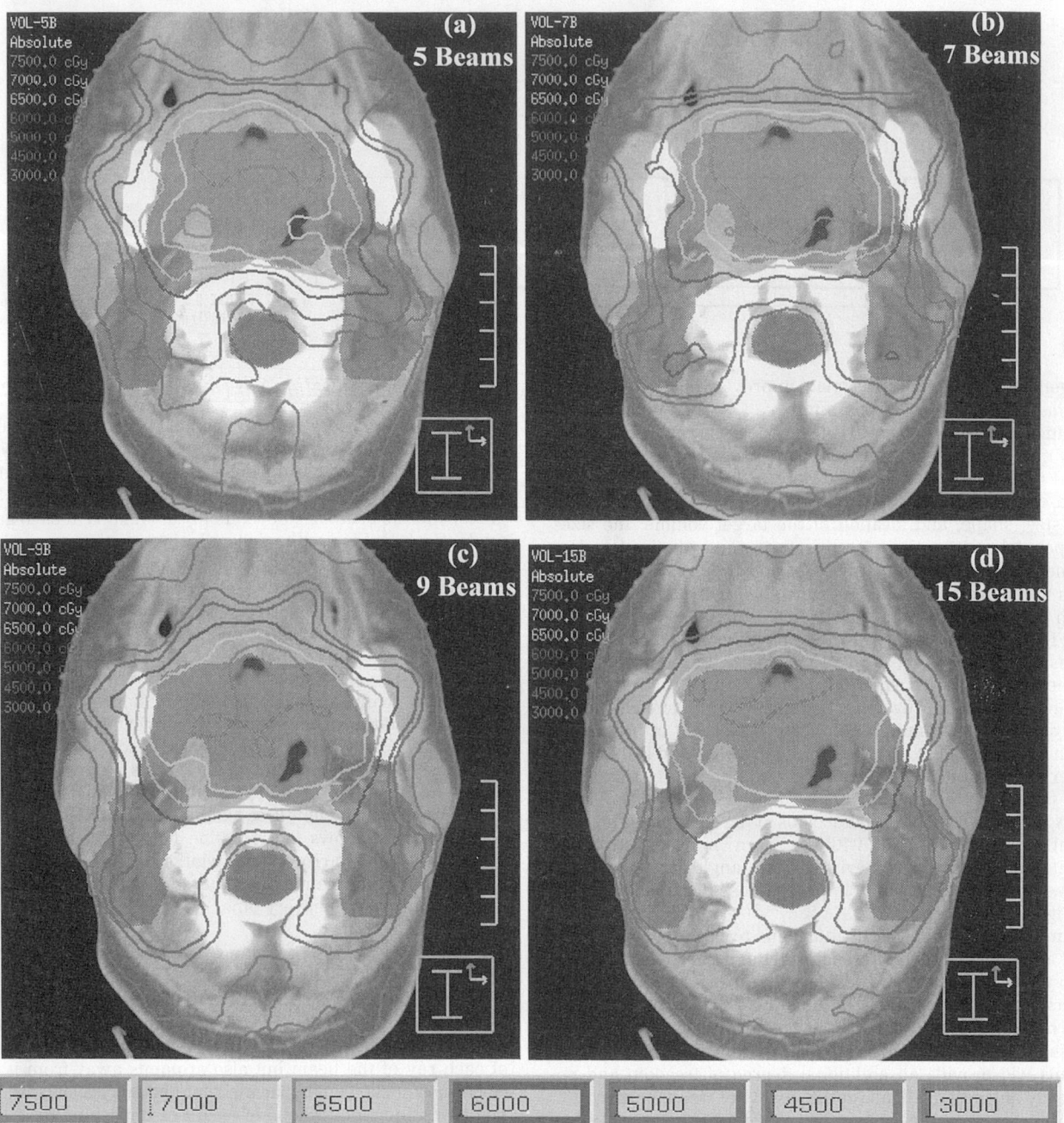

FIGURE 9.7. (*See* Color Figures 9.7 a through d.) Head and neck intensity-modulated radiation therapy (IMRT) plans designed based on dose-volume criteria using **(a)** 5, **(b)** 7, **(c)** 9, and **(d)** 156-MV beams placed at equiangular steps. The quality of IMRT plans improves as the number of beams increases. However, the additional gain above nine beams is clinically negligible.

of radiation with a corresponding reduction in toxicity and a further potential for dose escalation.

The beam–boundary-sharpening and margin-reduction feature of IMRT can be taken advantage of only if the dose-computation method is able to adequately take into account the lateral transport of radiation and if the intensity matrix grid size is sufficiently small. Initially, dose distribution for a given configuration of beams is computed by taking lateral transport into consideration. In each optimization iteration, the intensity distribution first is designed ignoring lateral transport. At the end of the iteration, the dose distribution is recalculated, thereby incorporating the effects of field-shaping devices on lateral transport and revealing the resulting deviations from the anticipated dose distribution. In the next iteration, ray intensities are adjusted further to rectify the deviations, and so on (25,98).

A schematic example shown in Figure 9.9A through C illustrates the issues involved. Figure 9.9A shows a normal organ overlapping the target volume. The target volume is being irradiated by two parallel-opposed beams. It is desired that the dose to the region of overlap be 60% of the target dose. If more dose is delivered, damage to the normal organ may result; but lower than the desired dose may cause local failure. If the role of lateral transport in optimization is ignored, the intensity resulting from the optimization process is essentially a step function, as shown in Fig. 9.9B (solid curve). The corresponding dose distribution (the dotted curve) shows a dose deficit inside the high-dose target volume as well as the outside edge of the region of overlap and an excess of dose in the region of overlap adjacent to the high-dose volume. If lateral transport is incorporated by adjusting fluence, the fluence and dose patterns shown

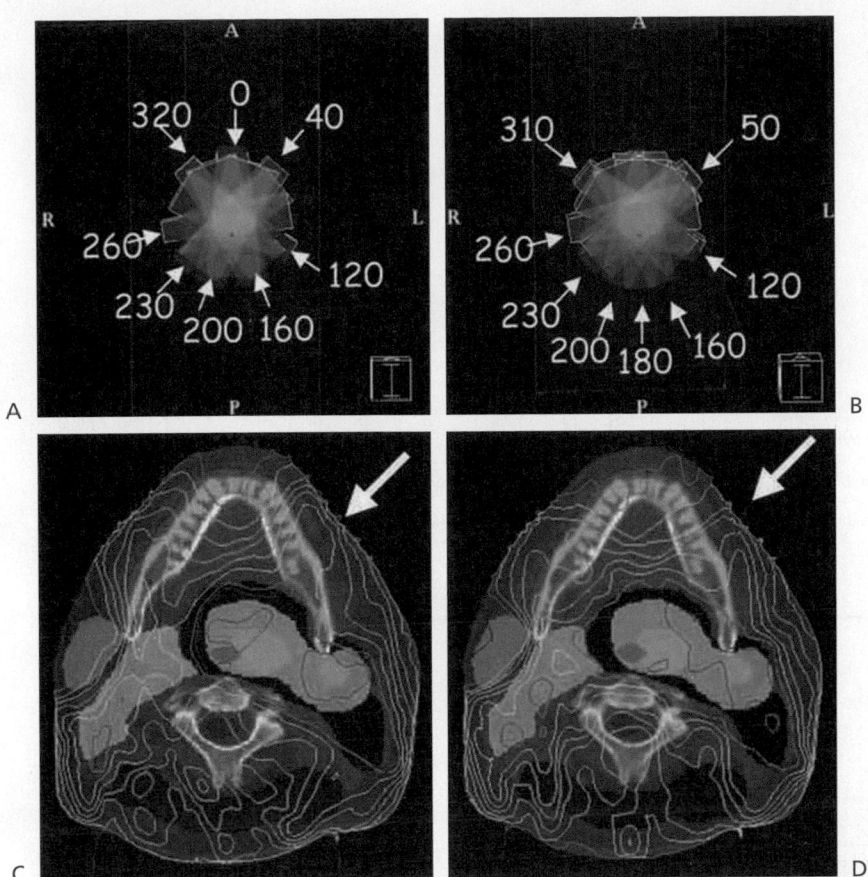

FIGURE 9.8. (*See* Color Figures 9.8A through D.) A patient with carcinoma of the base of tongue was treated with intensity-modulated radiation therapy. **A,B** depict the beam angle arrangement and the resulting isodose distribution. Arrow on (**C**) indicated a "horn" of high dose to the left oral tongue and buccal mucosa. By rearranging anterior beam placement (**B**) lead to improvement of dose distribution to the normal mucosa of left anterior oral cavity (**D**).

in Figure 9.9C result. Fluence is increased at both boundaries. It also is increased in the high-dose side of the interface with the overlap region and decreased on the lower-dose side. The dose is now much closer to the desired dose. Comparing Figures 9.9B and C, it also appears that a modest increase in fluence just inside the boundary does not lead to a perceptible increase in dose outside the beam boundary. This is presumably the result of the fact that the excess dose flowing out of the target periphery is deposited in a much larger volume of tissue. A reduction of margins attributable to penumbra by as much as 8 mm has been found to be feasible for prostate treatments (25,98).

IMRT Fractionation

In principle, conventional fractionation strategies can be used to design IMRT plans as well. For example, in a strategy similar to the conventional 1.8-Gy to 2-Gy/fx schedule, a major portion of the dose could be delivered in the initial phase using uniform fields designed with standard 3D conformal methods followed by an IMRT boost. Alternatively, separate IMRT plans could be designed for both the initial large-field treatment and the boost treatment. It may be intuitively obvious that, if a large portion of the dose already has been delivered using large fields, it may be very difficult, if not impossible, to achieve a high level of dose conformation with the remaining fractions in the IMRT-boost phase (97). As indicated earlier in this chapter, IMRT may be most conformal if all targets volumes (gross disease, subclinical extensions, and electively treated nodes) are treated simultaneously using different fraction sizes (97). Such a treatment strategy has been called the simultaneous integrated boost (SIB) (97). The SIB IMRT strategy not only produces superior dose distributions; it is also an easier, more efficient, and perhaps less error-prone way of planning and delivering IMRT because it involves the use of the same plan for the entire course of treat-

ment. Furthermore, in many cases, there is no need for electron fields and the nodal volumes can be included in the IMRT fields, thus avoiding the perennial problem of field matching encountered in the treatment of many sites.

Because each of the target regions receives different doses per fraction in the SIB IMRT strategy, prescribed nominal (physical) dose and dose per fraction must be adjusted appropriately. The adjusted nominal dose and fraction size for each target region depends on the number of IMRT fractions. The fraction sizes may be estimated using an isoeffect relationship based on the linear-quadratic model and the values of its parameters (such as α/β ratios, tumor doubling time).

The effect of the modified fractionation on acute and late toxicity of normal tissues both outside and within the volumes to be treated also should be considered. Because of the improved conformality of IMRT plans, dose to normal tissues outside the target volume is typically lower than for conventional treatment plans. In addition, if the number of fractions is greater than the number of fractions used to deliver large fields in conventional therapy, the dose per fraction to normal tissues is lower. Therefore, the biologically effective dose would be lower still. However, normal tissues embedded within or adjacent to the target volumes would receive high doses per fraction and may be at higher risk. Isoeffect formulae for normal tissues also may be derived to estimate the effect of a particular fractionation strategy. These formalisms would need to incorporate regeneration and change in sensitivity over the treatment course.

The values of parameters for the computation of altered fractionation may, in theory, be obtained from published studies. Studies by Maciejewski et al. (84) and Withers et al. (138, 139,140), for example, have yielded important information for estimating tumor parameters for head and neck carcinoma. In general, the data available are limited. Furthermore, there is considerable uncertainty in the data, and there are concerns

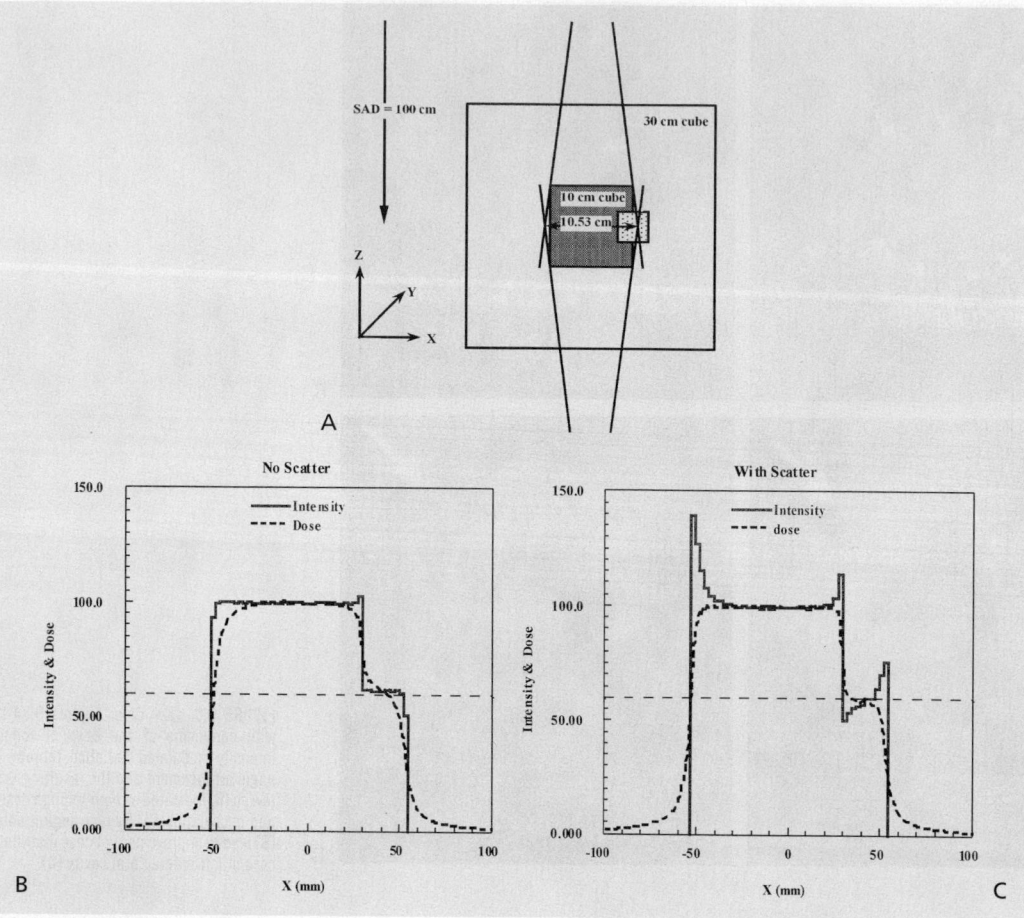

FIGURE 9.9. A schematic example illustrating the sharpening of penumbra with intensity-modulated radiation therapy. See text for details.

about the validity of numerous assumptions in the linear-quadratic model and the isoeffect formalism, especially with regard to normal tissues. Nevertheless, various investigators have carried out the necessary calculations and adopted SIB IMRT fractionation strategies. Continued investigations and clinical trials are needed to develop more reliable time-dose fractionation models, to produce better estimates of their parameters, and to evaluate alternate SIB IMRT fractionation strategies for all sites. The following are some examples of IMRT fractionation strategies currently being used for IMRT of head and neck cancers.

In Radiation Therapy Oncology Group H-0022 protocol, 30 daily fractions are used to simultaneously deliver 66 Gy (2.2 Gy per fraction) to the PTV, 60 Gy (2 Gy per fraction) to the high-risk subclinical disease ("first echelon nodes or dissected neck area containing lymph node metastases"), and 54 Gy (1.8 Gy per fraction) to subclinical disease. These are biologically equivalent to 70, 60, and 50 Gy, respectively, if given in 2 Gy per fraction. For normal structures, brainstem, spinal cord, and mandible are maintained below 54, 45, and 70 Gy, respectively. The mean dose to the parotid glands is maintained below 26 Gy and/or 50% of one of the parotids is maintained below 30 Gy and/or at least 20 mL of the combined volume of both parotids is constrained to receive no more than 20 Gy (43).

The SIB strategy at Virginia Commonwealth University involves a dose-escalation protocol in which primary nominal dose levels of 68.1, 70.8, and 73.8 Gy, given in 30 fractions (biologically equivalent to 74, 79, and 85 Gy, respectively, if given in 2 Gy per fraction) are used (143). Simultaneously, the subclinical disease and electively treated nodes were prescribed 60 and 54 Gy, respectively (biologically equivalent to 60 and 50 Gy, respec-

tively, if given in 2 Gy fractions). Spinal cord and brainstem are maintained below 45 and 55 Gy, respectively, and an attempt is made to allow no more than 50% of at least one parotid to receive higher than 26 Gy.

At the Mallinckrodt Institute of Radiology, the SIB strategy for definitive IMRT prescribes 70 Gy in 35 fractions in 2 Gy per fraction to the volume of gross disease with margins. The adjacent soft tissue and nodal volumes at high risk were treated to 63 Gy in 1.8 Gy per fraction and simultaneously 56 Gy in 1.6 Gy per fraction to the elective nodal regions. This regimen has been shown to be well tolerated when combined with concurrent chemotherapy (25).

Optic nerve and optic chiasm are maintained below 55 Gy, retina below 45 Gy, brainstem below 50 to 55 Gy, spinal cord to below 45 to 48 Gy, parotid glands to below 20 to 30 Gy, and mandible to below 70 Gy.

Optimization of Intensity Maps

The optimization of ray intensities may be carried out using one of several mathematical formalisms and algorithms (also termed *optimization engines*). Each method has its strengths and weaknesses. The choice depends in part on the nature of the objective function and in part on individual preference. Although the details are complex, the basic principles are not difficult to comprehend. As depicted schematically in Figure 9.10, each ray of each beam is traced from the source of radiation through the patient. Only the rays that pass through the target volume need to be traced (plus through a small margin assigned to ensure that the lateral loss of scattered radiation does not compromise the treatment). Others are set to a weight of zero.

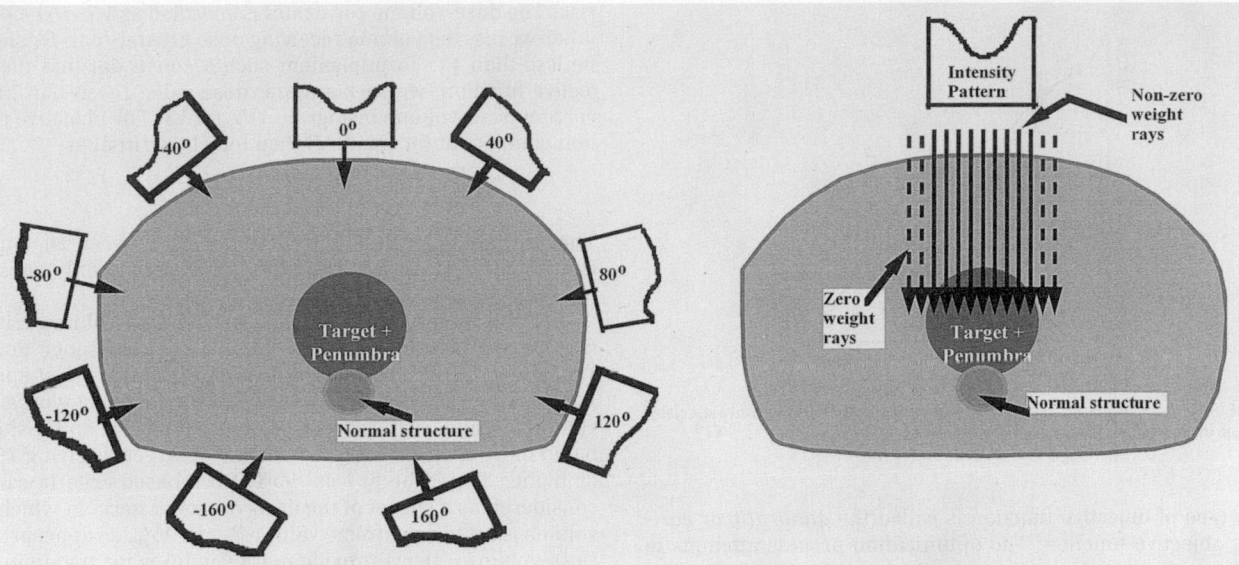

FIGURE 9.10. Each ray of each beam is traced from the source of radiation through the patient. Only the rays that pass through the target volume need to be traced (also through a small margin assigned to ensure that the lateral loss of scattered radiation does not compromise the treatment). Others are set to a weight of zero.

The patient's 3D image is divided into voxels. The dose at every voxel in the patient is calculated for an initial set of ray weights. The resulting dose distribution is used to compute the "score" of the treatment plan (i.e., the value of the objective function that mathematically states the clinical objectives of the intended treatment).

The ray-tracing process identifies the tumor and normal tissue voxels that lie along the path of the ray. The effect of a small change in a ray weight on the score then is calculated. If the increase in ray weight would result in favorable consequences for the patient, the weight is increased, and vice versa. Mathematically speaking, the ray weight is changed by an amount proportional to the gradient of the score with respect to the ray weight. Realizing that the improvement in the plan at each point comes from rays from many beams and that each ray affects many points, only a small change in ray weight may be permitted at a time. This process is repeated for each ray. At the end of each complete cycle (an iteration), a small improvement in the treatment plan results. The new pattern of ray intensities then is used to calculate a new dose distribution and the new score of the plan, which then is used as the basis of further improvement in the next iteration. The iterative process continues until no further improvement takes place, the optimization process is assumed to have converged, and the optimum plan is assumed to have been achieved.

Many current optimization systems use variations of gradient techniques to optimize IMRT plans. Methods of this type are by far the fastest computationally. However, the use of gradient techniques assumes that there is a single extremum (a minimum or a maximum, depending on the form of the objective function). This is indeed the case for objective functions based on variance of dose and when only ray weights are optimized. For other cases, it would be necessary to determine whether multiple extrema exist and whether such multiple extrema have an impact on the quality of the solution found. Multiple extrema have been found to exist when beam directions are optimized or when dose–response-based objective functions are used to optimize weights of uniform beams (88,94,120). One can expect that multiple minima also exist when dose–response-based objective functions are used to optimize IMRT plans. Using simple schematic examples, it also has been shown that multiple minima exist when dose–volume-based objectives are used (40).

Although this may be the case in theory, the existence of multiple minima has not been found to be a serious impediment in dose–volume-based or dose–response-based optimization using gradient techniques. In fact, in a recent study of dose–volume-based IMRT optimization, Wu and Mohan (142) found that, starting from vastly different initial intensities, the solutions converged to nearly the same plans. The reasons for this have been speculated but not conclusively proven and need to be investigated further.

It is possible that multiple minima do become a factor under a specific set of circumstances. These circumstances need to be determined. If multiple minima are discovered to be a factor, then some form of stochastic optimization technique may need to be considered. At the simplest, one may use a random search technique in conjunction with one of the gradient techniques. A more sophisticated stochastic technique is "simulated annealing" or its variation, the "fast simulated annealing" (88,94). These techniques allow the optimization process to escape from the local minima traps. Other forms of stochastic approaches, such as "genetic algorithms," also have been proposed (45). In principle, the simulated annealing technique and other stochastic approaches can find the global minimum, but, practically, there is no guarantee that the absolute optimum has been found, only that the best among the solutions examined has been found. Furthermore, stochastic techniques tend to be extremely slow and should be used in routine work only if it is established that they are necessary. Nevertheless, some commercial systems have implemented the simulated annealing approach for IMRT optimization (21).

Objective Functions

Dose-Based Objective Functions

A simple example of an objective function is the criteria stated in terms of the sum of the squares of the differences of desired dose and computed dose at each point within each of the volume of interest. That is,

$$S = \sum_i (D_{T,0} - D_{Ti})^2 + \sum_n p_n \times \sum_j H(D_{n,0} - D_{n,j}) \quad (9.1)$$
$$\times (D_{n,0} - D_{n,j})^2$$

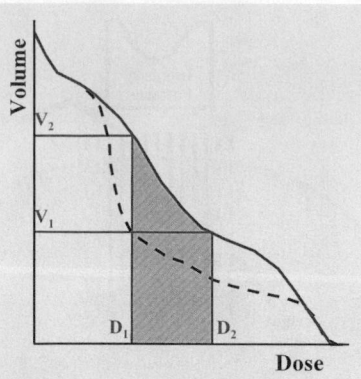

FIGURE 9.11. A method of incorporating dose-volume constraints in intensity-modulated radiation therapy optimization. (Adapted from Wu et al. [141].)

This type of objective function is called the *quadratic* or *variance* objective function. The optimization process attempts to minimize the treatment plan score $S.D_{T,0}$ in expression (Eq. 9.1) is the desired dose to the target volume and $D_{n,0}$ is the tolerance dose of the n'th normal structure. $D_{T,i}$ is the computed dose in the i'th voxel of the target and $D_{n,j}$ is the computed dose at the j'th voxel of the n'th normal structure. For normal organs, the function $H(D_{n,j} - D_{n,0})$ is defined as follows:

$$H(D_{n,j} - D_{n,.0}) = 0 \text{ for } D_{n,j} \leq D_{n,0} \text{ and} \qquad (9.2)$$
$$= 1 \text{ for } D_{n,j} > D_{n,0}.$$

In other words, so long as the dose in a normal tissue voxel does not exceed the tolerance limit, the voxel does not contribute to the score function. The quantity p_n is the "relative penalty" for exceeding the tolerance dose.

Dose–Volume-Based Objective Functions

Purely dose-based criteria, such as the one previously described, are not sufficient. In general, the response of the tumor and normal tissues is a function of not only radiation dose but also (to varying degrees depending on the tissue type) of the volume subjected to each level of dose. Currently, dose–volume-based objective functions are the most widely used clinically. Dose–volume-based objective functions are expressed in terms of the limits on the volumes of each structure that may be allowed to receive a certain dose or higher.

A practical scheme to incorporate dose–volume-based objectives has been suggested by Bortfeld et al. (12). It is explained in Figure 9.11 using a simple schematic example of one organ at

risk. The dose-volume constraint is specified as $V(>D_1) <V_1$. In other words, the volume receiving dose greater than D_1 should be less than V_1. To implement such a constraint into the objective function, we seek another dose value D_2 so that in the current dose–volume histogram $V(D_2) = V_1$. The objective function component for this OAR then may be written as:

$$p_n \cdot \sum_j H(D_2 - D_j) \cdot H(D_j - D_1) \cdot (D_j - D_1)^2 \qquad (9.3)$$

That is, only the points with dose values between D_1 and D_2 contribute to the score. Therefore, they are the only ones penalized.

For the target volumes, two types of dose-volume criteria may be specified to limit both the hot and cold spots. For instance, for the desired target dose of 80 Gy, we may specify $V(>85 \text{ Gy}) \leq 5\%$ and $V(>79 \text{ Gy}) \geq 95\%$. In other words, the volume of the target receiving dose greater than 85 Gy should be no more than 5%, and the volume of target receiving 79 Gy or higher should be at least 95%. Dose-based criteria can be considered as a subset of the dose-volume criteria in which the volume is set to an extreme value (0% or 100%, as appropriate). Dose-volume criteria provide more flexibility for the optimization process and greater control over dose distributions. The reason is that dose-based optimization penalizes all the points above the dose limit, whereas the dose–volume-based optimization penalizes only the subset of points within the lower end of range of dose values above the dose limit. For the example of Figure 9.11, the dose–volume-based optimization process attempts to bring only the points between D_1 and D_2 into compliance with the constraint. In contrast, the dose-based optimization process attempts to constrain all of the points above D_1. Furthermore, dose-volume criteria are highly "degenerate" functions of dose distributions (i.e., there are an infinite number of dose distributions that correspond to the same dose-volume constraint). Therefore, the optimization system has a large solution space to choose from, making it easier to find a better solution.

Limitations of Dose–Volume-Based Objective Functions

Dose–volume-based criteria have been demonstrated to have limitations. To illustrate one such limitation, consider the example in Figure 9.12A of a normal structure for which a constraint has been specified that no more that 25% of the volume is to receive 50 Gy or higher. All three dose–volume histograms (DVHs) shown meet this criteria. However, the DVH represented by the solid curve clearly causes the least damage. One can argue that we can overcome this limitation by specifying multiple dose-volume constraints or even the entire DVH. However, as illustrated in Figure 9.12B, this would be too limiting. Multiple

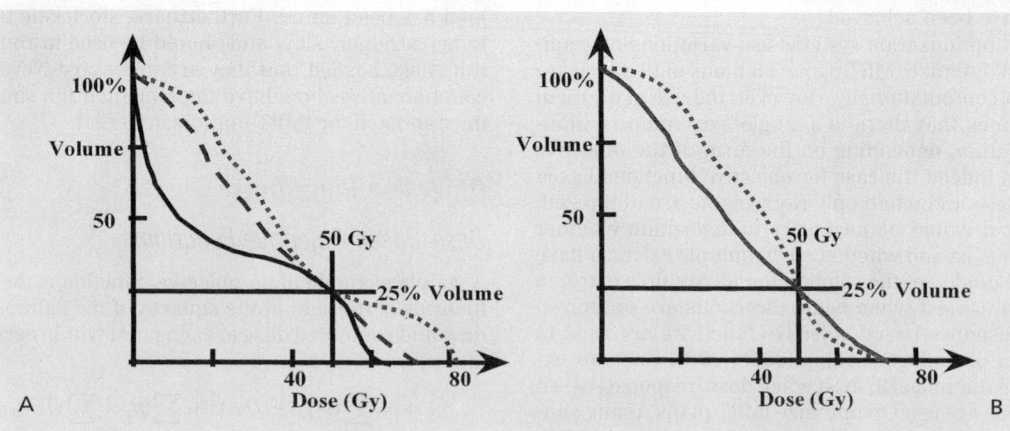

FIGURE 9.12. Limitations of dose–volume-based criteria.

DVHs, in fact an infinite number of them, could lead to an equivalent injury to a particular organ, but each DVH may produce a different effect on other organs and the tumor. When this happens, DVHs usually cross each other, as shown in Figure 9.12B. Only one of them is optimum so far as the tumor and other organs are concerned.

To overcome the limitations of dose–volume-based criteria, they may be supplemented with biologic (or dose–response-based) criteria, for instance, in terms of such indices as tumor control probability (TCP), normal tissue complication probabilities (NTCPs), and equivalent uniform dose (EUD). Dose–response-based objective functions are the subject of ongoing investigations (94,144).

Objective Function Parameters

The desired IMRT dose distributions are specified in terms of parameters of the objective function. In Equation 9.1, for instance, the parameters of the objective function are the desired dose limits $D_{T,0}$ and $D_{n,0}$ for target and normal structures and the relative importance (or penalty) factors p_n for deviating from desired dose limits. Most often, the objective functions are specified in terms of one or more "soft" dose-volume constraints for each volume of interest, one for each constraint. That is, if the computed dose deviates from the desired value, the plan is not rejected, but it is assessed a penalty. The optimization software computes a "subscore" corresponding to each constraint. The subscore value depends on the deviation of dose distribution from the desired dose distributions and the penalty factor. The overall score of an IMRT plan is an accumulation of subscores of individual volumes of interest. The IMRT optimization system uses the IMRT plan score to arrive at the optimum plan according to the specified objective function. The optimized solution involves trade-offs that balance specified normal tissue objectives against each other and against tumor objectives. An IMRT treatment-planning system should provide parameters that allow the treatment planner to adjust the trade-off for each crit-

ical structure in a straightforward manner. An example of this is shown in Figure 9.13, where a head and neck target volume nearly abuts the parotid gland (9). Plans C and F use parameters that emphasize parotid-gland sparing and tumor coverage, respectively. This is an excellent example of the flexibility of moving the steep dose gradient in and out of the target volume.

The plan considered to be the best by the computer may not be the best (or even good enough) by the treatment planner. Parameters are adjusted by trial and error to obtain a satisfactory plan. A confounding factor is that a change in a parameter of one volume of interest affects not only its own subscore and DVH but also the subscores and DVHs of other structures in a complicated manner. For a complex IMRT problem, in which there may be several dozen parameters, their adjustment is an extremely difficult task. The trial-and-error approach used currently is time-consuming and leads to suboptimal results. Future research based on artificial intelligence techniques may provide a systematic means of determining optimum parameter values.

Treatment Plan Evaluation

IMRT dose distributions tend to be highly conformal but complex and unconventional. Traditional methods of evaluation and reporting may be too limited for such dose distributions. In principle, the target dose distributions for IMRT should be more homogeneous than for 3DCRT. In practice, the opposite is the case, due in part to the competing demands of sparing of normal tissues and in part to the inadequacy of objective functions. Dose distributions in normal structures as well are, in general, more nonuniform than for 3DCRT.

In the current practice of radiotherapy, treatment plans are evaluated using dose and dose-volume parameters including such quantities as dose to a point in the volume of interest, minimum dose, maximum dose, minimum dose to a specified fractional volume, or the volume of the structure receiving a specified dose or higher. MUs are set to deliver the prescribed

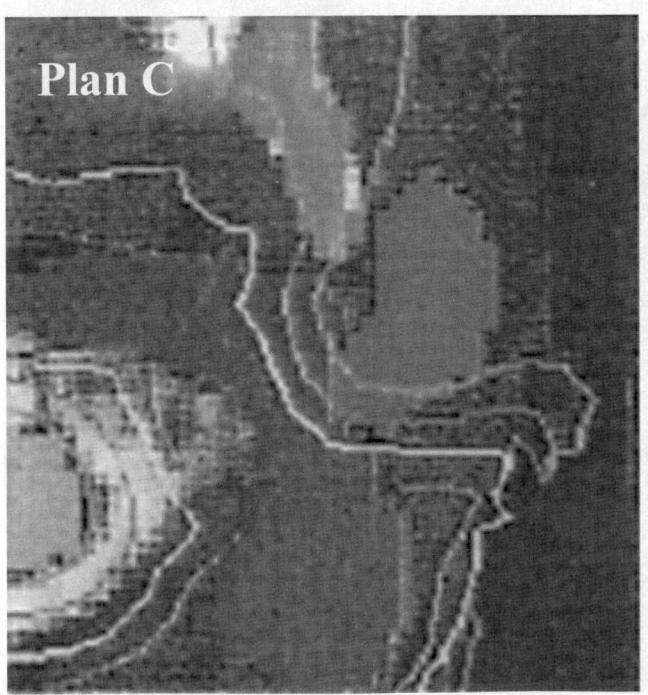
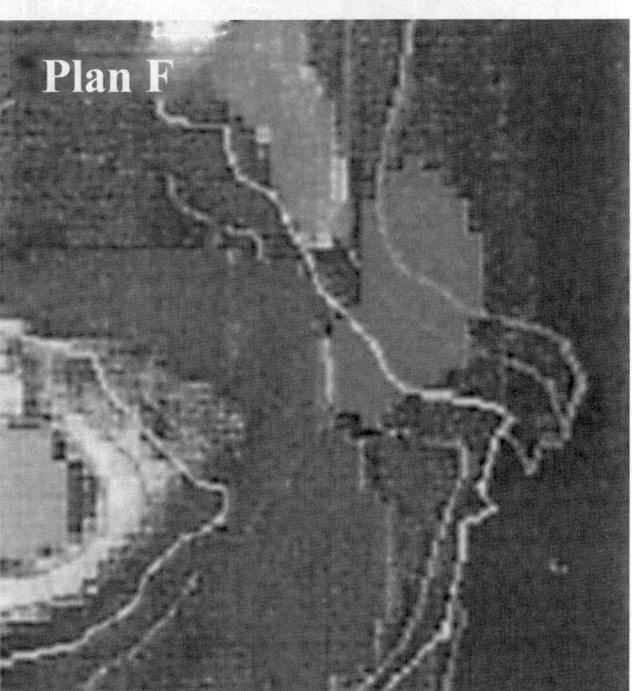

FIGURE 9.13. (*See* Color Figure 9.13.) Effect of adjusting dose-prescription parameters on the resulting treatment plan. The parotid gland and target are shown in green and blue, respectively. Plan C emphasizes parotid sparing, and plan F emphasizes tumor coverage. (From Chao KSC, Low DA, Perez CA, et al. Intensity-modulated radiation therapy in head and neck cancers: The Mallinckrodt experience. *Int J Cancer* 2000;90:92–103, with permission.)

dose to a specified point or to an isodose line (or surface) just enclosing the target volume. For some sites and techniques (e.g., stereotactic radiosurgery of brain tumors), an index of conformality (the ratio of volume occupied by the prescription isodose surface and the volume of the target) is used for plan evaluation. Cumulative dose and dose-volume data are reported as a part of the patient's chart and used for correlation with outcome.

Because of the unconventional nature of IMRT dose distributions, especially the high degree of dose heterogeneity and fluctuations in dose as a function of position in volumes of interest, indices such as dose to a point, minimum dose, or maximum dose may not correlate well with dose response. Instead, dose to a specified fractional volume is more appropriate. For instance, dose to 98% or 99% and to 1% or 2% of the target volume may be more meaningful than minimum and maximum dose, respectively.

Limitations of dose and dose-volume plan evaluation parameters have been articulated in the literature (49). These limitations become more significant for the complex dose distributions of IMRT. It has been argued that biophysical dose-response indices, which summarize complex dose distributions using a single clinically relevant index in each volume of interest, may be more appropriate. Currently, indices such as TCP, NTCPs, and biologically EUD often are computed and recorded, but rarely are used for routine plan evaluation. This is because of the unreliability of published dose-response data and weaknesses of models to compute these indices. This is, in turn, the result of the various sources of uncertainty in both the quantification of response and in doses delivered to the structures. In a recent report, Levegrun et al. (73), from their analysis of patients with prostate cancer treated at Memorial Sloan-Kettering Cancer Center, concluded that the biopsy-based response did

not correlate with minimum tumor dose, EUD, or TCP. Instead, they found the mean dose to be a very good predictor of response. They attributed this observation to large treatment margins for PTV, substantial target motion, and relatively homogeneous dose distributions. There are similar other examples in the literature in which lack of dose response or correlation with mean dose may be attributable to uncertainties in the extent of the disease, target position, normal structure positions, and dose delivered. Such examples highlight the importance of continued efforts to reduce sources of uncertainty.

Generation of Leaf Sequences

Fixed Intensity-Modulated Fields

For the IMRT mode using multiple fixed fields, the plan optimization process produces nonuniform intensity distributions (Fig. 9.14) for each set of fields. In principle, such intensity distributions can be delivered using custom-fabricated compensators made of lead alloys to attenuate the appropriate amount of radiation along each ray of the beam. Such devices would have to be produced using computerized milling machines. In addition, to use them it would be necessary for the operator (radiation therapist) to enter the treatment room to insert the device for each field. This process would be highly labor-intensive and impractical considering that a large number of beams often may be needed for optimum intensity-modulated treatments.

The most efficient means of delivering fixed-field IMRT is the standard MLC in dynamic mode using such methods as "sliding-window" technique or the step-and-shoot technique. In either

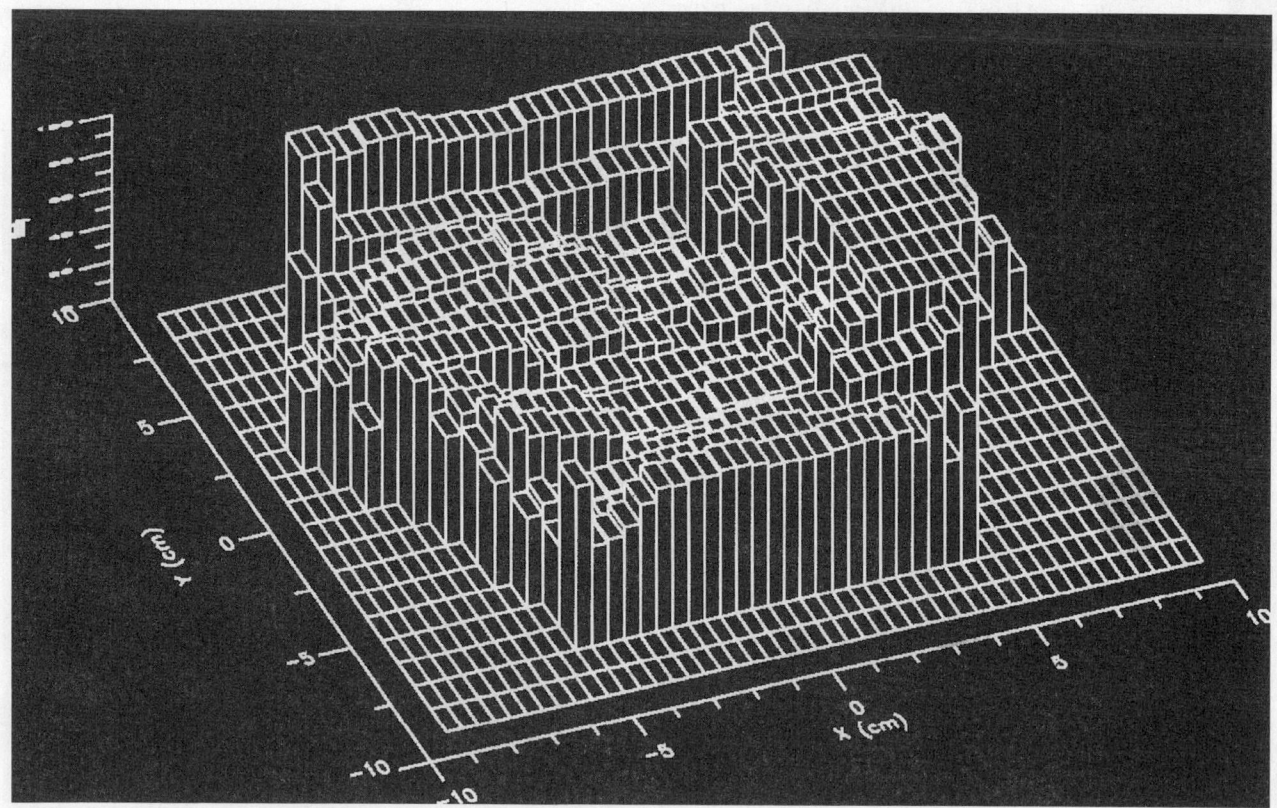

FIGURE 9.14. Intensity profile of the left lateral beam of an intensity-modulated radiation therapy plan designed for the treatment of the cervix. Intensity distribution in a plane through the isocenter and normal to the direction of the beam is plotted. The grid size along the y-axis is 1 cm, corresponding to the width of multileaf collimator leaves. Each intensity curve along the x-axis corresponds to one pair of opposing leaves.

case, leaf position sequences as a function of MUs need to be generated. The MLC leaves are made of approximately 5- or 6-cm thick tungsten and are typically 0.5 or 1 cm wide (projected to isocenter). MLCs with leaves of a width as small as 1 mm have been introduced. Smaller leaf width may be of greater value for IMRT than for standard 3DCRT. For the former, the leaf width affects the dose delivered to the entire slice, whereas for the latter, it affects only the shape of the boundary. A smaller leaf width undoubtedly would produce more conformal dose distributions, but the electromechanical complexity and cost of the device would increase. Because of the smearing caused by finite-sized radiation sources, lateral secondary electron transport, and the use of multiple fields and because of motion and positioning uncertainties, an acceptable leaf width may not need to be very small. The minimum desirable leaf width would depend on numerous factors including shapes and locations of volumes of interest, dose gradients desired, and number and orientations of beams. Although the issue of leaf width has been debated for quite some time, there are no definitive studies to guide the choice of the most suitable width.

MLCs transmit only 0.5% to 2% of incident radiation (except through small interleaf gaps and the rounded ends of some MLCs). However, as discussed later in this chapter, because intensity-modulated treatments require substantially larger number of MUs than do the conventional uniform field treatments, the cumulative effective transmission may be considerably larger.

Leaf Sequence Generation—Sliding-Window Technique

In the sliding-window method, the gap formed by each pair of opposing leaves is swept across the target volume under computer control while the radiation is on. The gap opening and its speed are optimally adjusted. Because the dose rate of the treatment machine might fluctuate slightly, the motion is indexed to MUs rather than time. The basic principle is that as the gap slides across a point, the radiation received by the point is proportional to the number of MUs delivered during the time the tip of the leading leaf goes past the point and exposes it until the tip of the trailing leaf moves in to block it again. (The point also receives additional radiation transmitted through or scattered from the leaves, which must be accounted for. See later discussion in this chapter.) The setting of the gap opening and its speed for each pair at any instant are determined by a technique first introduced by Convery and Rosenbloom (33) and refined and studied further by Bortfeld et al. (10), Spirou and Chui (117) and Spirou et al. (118), Stein et al. (119), Svensson et al. (122), and others (95,99,131). Knowledge of the maximum leaf speed is taken advantage of to maximize the gap between the opposing pair of leaves and, therefore, to minimize the treatment time. The number of leaves participating in the delivery of a beam depends on the projected size of the target volume. The data describing leaf trajectories, produced by the leaf sequence-generation process, are in the form of a table of positions of leaves versus the corresponding MUs (depicted graphically in Fig. 9.15).

Leaf Sequence Generation—Step-and-Shoot and Multisegment Techniques

With the step-and-shoot technique (as well as for multisegment technique) the fixed-gantry radiation beam is composed of multiple static MLC segments, with each segment having its own aperture shape and weight or monitor (MU) settings. The leaf sequence-generation algorithms take the optimized intensity pattern as the input and decompose it into multiple segments, each to be shaped as an aperture formed by the MLC.

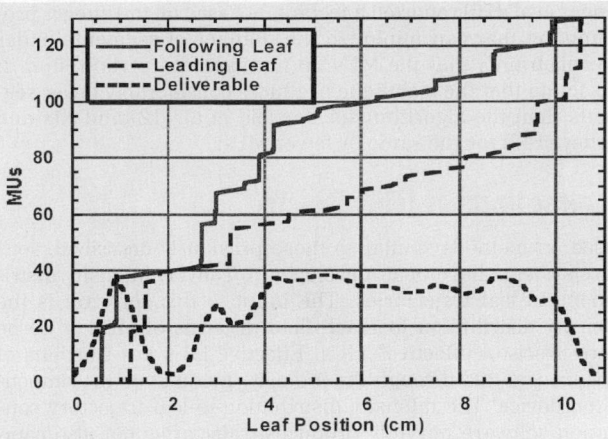

FIGURE 9.15. A typical trajectory of one of the pairs of leaves used to deliver intensity-modulated beam profiles of the type shown in Fig. 9.14. Intensity-modulated radiation therapy optimization based on deliverable dose distributions using the sliding-window technique. Positions of the leading and following leaves are plotted as a function of monitor units (MUs). The gap formed by the pair of leaves moves from left to right. Its width and speed are adjusted by the computer to allow a predetermined amount of radiation to reach each point within the field. Note that the fluence (intensity) is the differences in MUs for the left leaf and the right leaf.

Fluence intensity throughout each MLC segment is relatively uniform. The summation of all static segments yields the required intensity-modulated dose distributions. Ideally, the segments are sorted to minimize the MLC leaf travel time between the segments. Note that such sorting is neither necessary nor possible for the sliding-window technique.

The first step of the leaf sequence-generation process is the discretization of the continuous intensity distribution into a limited number of intensity levels. These intensity levels then are converted into leaf sequences using one of several methods described in the literature. Bortfeld et al. (10), for example, have proposed a method in which each row of intensity is handled separately, similar to the sliding-window algorithm. The advantage is that the total number of MUs is small but at the cost of possibly large numbers of segments. Xia and Verhey (145) proposed the so-called areal algorithm. Instead of dividing the intensities into levels of equal steps, they divided them into levels in powers of 2 to reduce the number of steps and to gain efficiency. Wu et al. (144) proposed a technique called the *K-means clustering* in which the intensity levels are grouped together based on their values and the user-specified error tolerance levels. The intensity levels are not equally spaced and can be arbitrary.

Unlike the sliding-window algorithm, the maximum leaf speed is not important for the step-and-shoot and multisegment techniques. Similarly, while the number of segments is not an issue for the sliding-window techniques, it could affect the step-and-shoot delivery efficiency significantly. For the former, the only penalty of the large number of segments is the size of computer storage, whereas for the latter it leads to inefficiency because the beam is off during the transition between the segments. Furthermore, for some linear accelerators, there is an overhead time associated with each segment.

Que (109) compared several step-and-shoot algorithms and found that the algorithm used by Xia and Verhey (145) frequently, but not always, produces the least number of segments. Other investigators have reported methods to minimize the number of segments as well. The algorithm of Dai and Zhu (38) checks numerous candidates for each segment, and the candidate that would result in a residual intensity matrix with the least complexity selected. If more than one candidate exists with the same complexity, the one with the largest size is chosen.

Langer et al. (70) reported a technique based on the integer programming that can minimize the number of segments under the constraints that the MUs do not exceed a certain limit. It was found that the technique produces considerably fewer segments than the algorithms of Bortfeld et al. (12) and Xia and Verhey (145) for the same or fewer MUs.

Monitor Units of IMRT Beams

Based on methods similar to those previously described, software systems have been developed to convert intensity distributions to leaf trajectories. The input to this software is the intensity distribution for each field in terms of MUs or, to be more precise, "effective" MUs. Effective MUs are fractions of MUs transmitted through the intensity-modulation or compensation device. The intensity distribution-to-leaf trajectory conversion software not only produces trajectories but also computes actual MU settings for each beam as a natural byproduct of the conversion process. Trajectories of leaves and the MUs for each beam are transmitted to the computer-controlled radiation treatment machine for dosimetric verification and the delivery of treatment.

It is important to note that the relationship between the prescribed dose and MUs required for delivering each of the intensity-modulated beams is highly complex and not obvious. There is no practical way to calculate MUs by hand as is done for traditional treatments as an independent check of the predicted MU values. To ensure patient safety and to satisfy the requirements of the independent check, some systems have implemented independent software for a second MU calculation. Others have adopted the policy to measure the dose or dose distribution for each of the beams before the first treatment.

Impact of MLC Characteristics

Adjustments to leaf trajectories are required to account for the various effects associated with MLC characteristics, including the rounded leaf tips, tongue-and-groove leaf design, interleaf and intraleaf transmission, leaf scatter, and collimator scatter upstream from the MLC. The accuracy of dose delivered and the agreement between calculated and measured dose distributions depend on the adequate accounting of these effects. Approximate empirical corrections are applied for these effects by algorithms and software that convert optimized intensity distributions into leaf trajectories.

MLCs have an interlocking tongue-and-groove leaf design to minimize interleaf leakage. However, there is a difference in interleaf leakage and leakage through the leaves. This difference can become significant for beams that require large number of MUs and in portions of the beams that receive large fractions of their dose through leakage. Currently, this effect is ignored, although the use of Monte Carlo techniques to account for it is being investigated (63,113).

In addition, there are circumstances during creation of intensity profiles when a thin strip of the irradiated medium is shielded by the tongue of one leaf pair or the groove of the adjacent leaf pair rather than being completely exposed or completely blocked. van Santvoort and Heijmen (128) have demonstrated that this leads to an underdosage in the thin strip. They, and subsequently Webb et al. (135), also showed that this effect could be removed by the use of leaf motion-synchronizing techniques. However, such techniques result in an increase in the number of MUs. Furthermore, this effect is not considered to be of significant clinical consequence because of the smearing caused by multiple fields and the positioning and motion uncertainties. Using different collimator angles for each field can reduce this effect further.

Depending on the complexity (the frequency and amplitudes of peaks and valleys) of the intensity pattern, points within the field aperture may receive a substantial portion of the dose as a result of radiation transmitted through or scattered from the leaves when the points are in the shadow of the leaves. Points outside the leaf aperture receive their entire dose through these "indirect" sources. The complexity of intensity distributions produced by the IMRT optimization process depends on a combination of several clinical factors including the shapes, sizes, and relative locations of tumor and normal tissues; required tumor dose; dose homogeneity; and dose-volume limits of normal tissues. Intensity distributions for head and neck cases, for example, tend to be considerably more complex than for prostate cases. For beams with highly complex intensity patterns, the average window width to deliver the treatment tends to be small and, for the same dose received by the tumor, the treatment time (i.e., the number of MUs) is long. Consequently, the contribution of radiation transmitted through and scattered from the leaves may form a significant fraction of the total dose delivered. Because these contributions are accounted for approximately, the uncertainty in dose delivered is increased. In addition, the differences between interleaf and intraleaf transmissions may no longer be negligible. Another consequence of complex intensity patterns is that the lower limit of the deliverable intensity is high.

The deliverable dose distributions may be significantly different from the original optimized ones. There are different ways to overcome the difficulties resulting from the differences in desired and deliverable dose distributions. For example, if the deliverable dose to a particular normal structure is higher than the original optimized dose, the planner could modify the objective function to demand an appropriately lower dose. Alternatively, as shown in Figure 9.16, the optimization loop could include a pass through leaf sequence generation and calculation of deliverable dose distributions. The optimizer then adjusts ray weights based on deliverable dose distributions rather than the idealized ones. This scheme has been investigated by Siebers et al. (114).

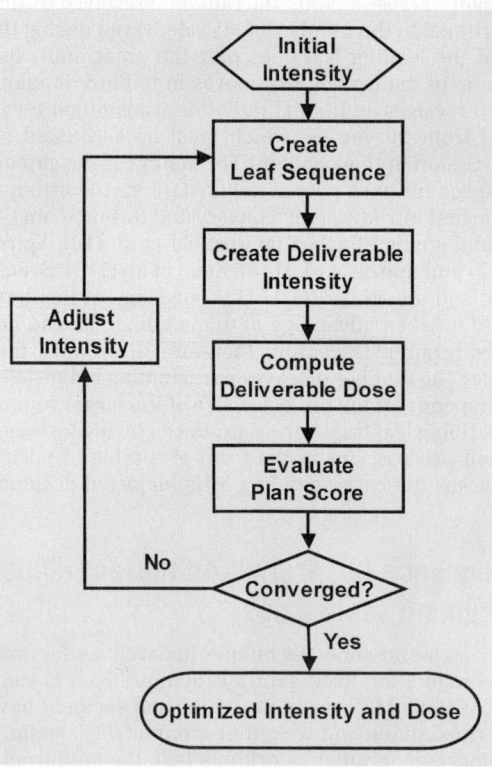

FIGURE 9.16. Intensity-modulated radiation therapy optimization based on deliverable dose distributions.

QA for Intensity-Modulated Treatments

A number of QA steps unique to IMRT are needed to ensure the accuracy and safety of treatments. These include QA of the MLC in dynamic mode, dosimetric verification for each dynamic beam as well as for the composite treatment plans, portal imaging, treatment verification, *in vivo* dosimetry, and reduction in uncertainty associated with daily positioning and internal organ motion during irradiation.

When using conventional 3DCRT, MLC leaf position calibration errors influence the accuracy of the radiation distribution at the portal boundary. Because of PTV and beam penumbra margins, small errors in leaf calibration will have a minimal effect on the target volume dose. The accepted leaf calibration accuracy is 2 mm (1). However, for IMRT the MLCs are used to generate inhomogeneous fluence distributions. In the sliding-window technique, for instance, this is done by adjusting the velocity and width of leaf gaps during radiation delivery. If the MLC calibration is inaccurate, the delivered dose distribution will be in error. The error is a function of the ratio of leaf calibration error to the sliding-window width. For example, a 1-mm imprecision in the gap would result in a 10% error in dose if a uniform field were to be delivered using a sliding window of 1 cm. For step-and-shoot delivery, magnitudes of dose errors are greater (owing to the steep dose gradients near the MLC leaf edges), but they are confined to the subfield edges. Thus, it is important that the manufacturers of MLCs used for IMRT ensure that the leaves can be positioned with accuracy of better than 0.25 mm, and the physicists must ensure through routine QA procedures that such precise positioning is achieved and maintained. It is interesting that integral dose error is similar for both the step-and-shoot and sliding-window techniques, but the distribution of the error is different.

Because MLC leaf calibration and the accuracy of MLC operations influence the delivered dose distribution, new, more rigorous MLC QA procedures have been developed. Chui et al. (31) and LoSasso and Chui C-S, Ling (77), among others, have developed QA procedures specifically for MLCs used in dynamic mode. Periodic QA checks must ensure that the leaves of the MLC do indeed move to their designated positions at the specified values of MUs. Moreover, to ensure safe and accurate delivery of treatments with an MLC, the manufacturers must include redundant and independent sensors for the leaves of the MLC. Furthermore, in the event of treatment field interruption and resumption, there should be no perceptible change in dose delivered.

Another aspect of QA important for IMRT is the daily positioning uncertainty and motion during irradiation. IMRT is a highly conformal and highly precise form of radiotherapy frequently used to escalate dose. Dose distributions may have steep dose gradients between the target and the neighboring normal structures. Furthermore, margins may be much smaller than in conventional treatments. Patient positioning and immobilization requirements are more stringent than ever to ensure that the target volumes are covered adequately and the normal tissues are spared adequately. In fact, special immobilization devices and techniques are being developed to reproducibly and accurately position the target volume and normal anatomy. Many of these devices already are available commercially (e.g., rectal inserts to improve positioning for prostate IMRT).

Similarly, motion during treatment, mainly as a consequence of respiration, also can be a serious problem for IMRT of sites in the thorax and abdomen. Because IMRT is delivered dynamically, the moving target volume may move in and out of the instantaneous field of radiation. Some portions of the target volume may get more than the planned dose, whereas others may get less. A way to minimize effects of respiratory motion would be to use "gated treatments" in which radiation and leaf motion is turned on only during a specific, reproducible portion of the respiratory cycle or in an interval during which the patient's breath is voluntarily, or involuntarily, held (65,141). In any case, it is also important that imaging used for planning of treatments be gated in a similar way.

Dosimetric Verification of Intensity-Modulated Treatments

To implement a new treatment technology into routine clinical use, there are usually three distinct but closely-related phases: *Acceptance tests:* This is the initial set of tests that ensures the hardware and software meet the factory or customer-provided specifications. Usually, but not always, the written specifications contain the necessary instructions or guidelines for these tests (in order to avoid legal ambiguity in the measurements). It is also a good opportunity for the users to establish some performance baselines, especially for the hardware purchased. *Commissioning tests:* The IMRT commissioning is a process to implement IMRT treatments using the customer's hardware and beam data. Various groups have studied the general guidelines for commissioning a treatment planning system. The process usually starts with collection of essential beam data for beam modeling. The parameters of the dose-calculation algorithm are then tuned to provide the best performance for the user's beam. Additional tests should be performed to evaluate the limitations of the treatment-planning system and a solution or a workaround should be found if the problem is clearly identified. Then IMRT phantom measurements should be performed to test the accuracy of the delivery system and data connectivity. If the accuracy is judged to be acceptable, the system can be released to the clinic after the necessary user training and procedural implementations. It is recommended that a small (interdisciplinary) focus group should be assigned to lead the IMRT implementation in the clinic. The "train-the-trainer" approach has proven to be effective in translating new technology into routine clinical practice. *On-going QA:* After the system is released to the clinic, it is important to establish a routine QA program. The performance of various steps involved in performing IMRT treatments needs to be tracked so that the quality of the treatments can be maintained. The ongoing QA program can be separated into patient-specific QA and equipment QA, which will be described in more detail below.

Patient- and Equipment-Specific QA

Because of the complexity of irregular field shapes, small-field dosimetry, and time-dependent deliverable leaf sequences, it is recommended by the American Association of Physicists in Medicine and ASTRO, that patient-specific QA should be performed as a part of the IMRT management process and a requirement for billing for IMRT services. Figure 9.17 shows the general categories of patient- and equipment-specific QA which are detailed in the following.

Patient setup, although not specific to IMRT dosimetry, is considered a key step in ensuring accurate IMRT treatments. A variety of image-guided localization techniques have been proposed for use with IMRT treatments, from simple orthogonal portal films to the beam's eye view portal film with IMRT intensity pattern overlays (79), daily electronic portal imaging of implanted fiducials (48,137), daily ultrasound-guided localization (6,64,82), and to the most integrated tomotherapy solutions (87). The detailed discussion of these specific image-guided procedures is out of the scope of this chapter, but QA in patient positioning remains an important issue for IMRT.

The implementation of patient-specific QA depends highly on each institution. For example, dosimetric measurements of MU

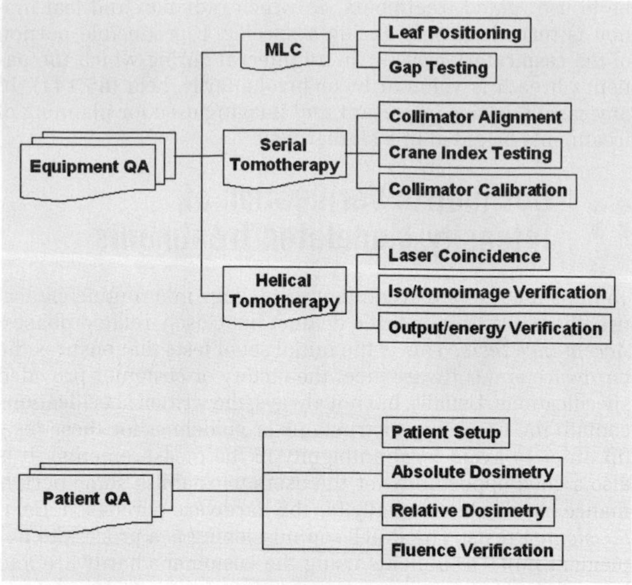

FIGURE 9.17. Overview of intensity-modulated radiation therapy quality assurance (QA) includes patient-specific and equipment-specific procedures. MLC, multileaf collimator.

settings can be verified for each beam individually (usually in a flat [slab] phantom geometry) or for the composite treatment plan (usually in a specially designed phantom, but it is also possible to use the simple slab phantom setup). Unlike single-beam verification in which the single-beam dose distribution can be significantly different from the original patient plan, the advantage of measuring the composite treatment plan in a phantom (regardless of the shape of the phantom) is that the composite dose distribution or the dose "pattern" generated in a phantom is usually similar to those in the original patient plan. This can be useful in selecting the measurement points or in visualizing potential dose errors. Absolute dosimetry is usually referred to as "MU verification" for IMRT. The traditional manual process for MU verification is virtually impossible to perform because of the large number of fields involved and the irregular shape and size of the treatment segments. Attempts have been made to verify MU settings in an IMRT plan using alternative calculation methods (102,112,129). However, these alternative calculation methods cannot predict the uncertainties during the actual delivery at the treatment machines and are also subject to limitations and approximations in their dose-calculation models. The most reliable and practical technique currently for IMRT MU verification is still the ion chamber-based point dose measurement in a phantom. Absolute dose measurement in a phantom is usually performed through a process called the *hybrid phantom plan*. In this plan, all beam angles and deliverable intensity patterns for a patient plan are transferred to the phantom, and doses in the phantom are computed for QA. The basic assumption in this process is that if the dose calculated in the phantom agrees with the measurement in the phantom, then the dose delivered to the patient agrees with the dose calculated in the patient. Relative dosimetry is usually performed using radiographic films or 2D array detectors. The process is similar to absolute dose measurement using the hybrid phantom plan technique. For film dosimetry, it is important to convert film density into relative dose using a film-calibration process. Because of the additional dimensionality, it becomes difficult to define good numerical criteria for evaluating relative 2D/3D measurements. Various numerical indicators (such as the distance to agreement, and gamma, or normalized agreement test) were proposed. In particular, the concept of gamma, combining the dose difference and distance to agreement, is appealing in

evaluating 2D or 3D dose distributions. For clinical applications, the most reliable and practical way to evaluate 2D distribution is to overlay the measurement isodose lines with the calculated ones. Special attention should be made to the low-dose regions near critical structures in the original patient plan. Attention should also be made to the systematic shifts of isodose lines, which may reveal if the isocenter or any reference setup point may be off. The relative dosimetry verification for IMRT should be performed in conjunction with the absolute dose verification for IMRT. It would be useful if the relative dose distribution can be normalized to the absolute dose measurement point, which converts the relative dose measurement into absolute dose distributions (71).

Two-dimensional fluence verification of intensity patterns gained popularity with the invention of 2D array detectors and the necessary software (59,66,146). Fluence verification usually is performed for each IMRT beam at a fixed gantry angle with or without a flat phantom geometry. The purpose of fluence verification is to make sure the intensity patterns created in each IMRT plan can be faithfully delivered under ideal conditions (2D, beam's eye view). Fluence verification should be combined with other patient-specific and equipment QAs to make sure that IMRT treatments are executed accurately.

Figure 9.17 also illustrates equipment-specific QA procedures. In general, IMRT QA is a subset of general equipment QA processes. The technology of IMRT and techniques for QA are also evolving. It is strongly suggested that users of IMRT should attempt to attend national meetings and technology conferences or training courses so that their knowledge about the use of IMRT can be updated regularly.

IMRT has been variously termed as *opaque, unintuitive,* and *nontransparent*, partly because it is delivered using dynamic techniques. Many are skeptical about whether the dose distribution displayed on an IMRT plan is, in fact, delivered. Furthermore, because of the complexity of computations involved, there is no practical way to verify the MU settings by hand calculations as is done for conventional treatments. Moreover, because of the inherent nonuniformity of IMRT fields, it is important to know the dose accurately at every point within the beam. One way to check if the intended dose would be delivered to the patient at the time of the treatment is to conduct dosimetric verification measurements.

Two broad categories of IMRT treatment-plan verification approaches have been developed for MLC-based IMRT. First, the dose distribution from radiation fields are independently measured and evaluated. This often is accomplished by using a flat homogeneous water-equivalent phantom and irradiating each field independently. The film-measured dose distributions are compared against calculations conducted by the treatment-planning system under the same geometric conditions. The process is explained in Figure 9.18. For calculation of dose distributions, each field is transferred to a treatment plan with flat homogeneous phantom. A typical example for a sliding-window intensity-modulated beam dosimetric verification is shown in Figure 9.19. This technique has the advantage that discrepancies between the planned and delivered dose can be attributed to individual radiation portals. However, the total integrated dose distribution is not checked.

The second method uses a phantom that is irradiated by all beam portals, allowing the evaluation of the total dose distribution delivered (80,130). Typically, ionization chambers and radiographic film are the dosimeters used for these measurements. Although ionization chambers can be benchmark-quality dosimeters, they suffer from volume averaging and are inefficient for measuring multiple points. Because of the complexity of the dose distributions being measured, a 2D dosimeter is required for thorough evaluations of nonuniform dose distribution. Quantitative radiographic film measurements require careful dose calibrations using independently measured

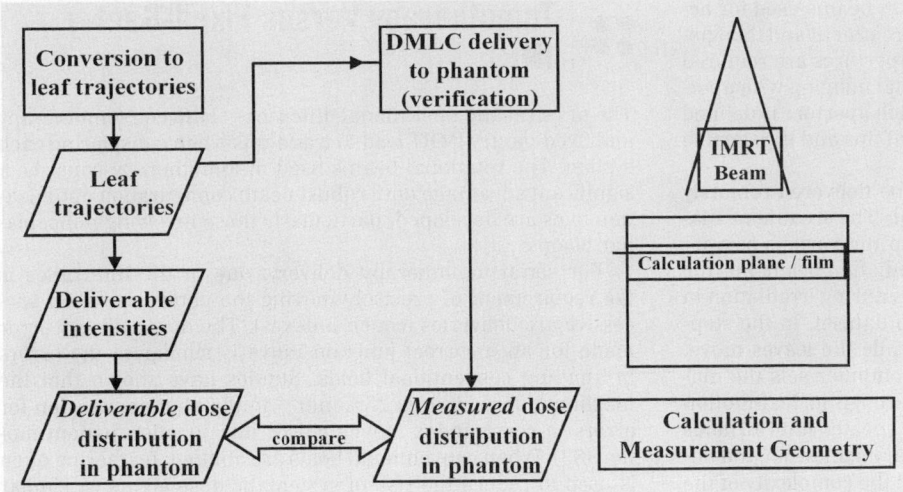

FIGURE 9.18. Diagram illustrating dosimetric verification of individual intensity-modulated radiation therapy fields. DMLC, dynamic multi-leaf collimator; IMRT, intensity-modulated radiation therapy

sensitometric curves. The film optical densities are measured and converted to absolute dose using film-calibration data and compared with the predictions of the treatment-planning system (42).

In vivo dosimetry commonly is used to verify the dose delivered by conformal therapy radiation fields. The complex fluence distribution of IMRT fields makes quantitative use of *in vivo* dosimetry, specifically the use of skin-surface mounted dosimeters, difficult.

Film, thermoluminescent dosimeters, and diodes may not be sufficiently accurate; are laborious to use; and, in the case of thermoluminescent dosimeters and diodes, are incapable of providing detailed information. In the long run, the most efficient way to verify fixed intensity-modulated fields is expected to be with real-time 2D dosimetry systems using appropriately calibrated electronic portal imaging devices. Such devices could be used for dosimetric verification of IMRT beams before treatment delivery and for exit dosimetry using transmitted portal dose images (PDIs). For electronic portal imaging devices to be used for pretreatment dosimetric verification and exit dosimetry, they must operate in the integration mode to capture the transmitted radiation over the entire exposure of each beam. The result is a PDI that can be compared with an intensity-modulated digitally reconstructed PDI. For pretreatment dosimetric verification of a given beam, a PDI may be created using a 3D-treatment-planning system to compute dose deposited in the electronic portal imaging device detector. For exit dosimetry, the PDI may be calculated using the 3D CT image of the patient. In either case, for accurate dosimetric verification, the effect of scattered radiation and the variation in response of the detector with energy must be included. The former effect can be taken into account with dose-spread kernel superposition methods, but both can be accounted for using Monte Carlo techniques.

Treatment Setup and Delivery

Fixed-Gantry Intensity-Modulated Fields

As for conventional radiotherapy, for IMRT techniques using fixed intensity-modulated fields, it is necessary to verify the

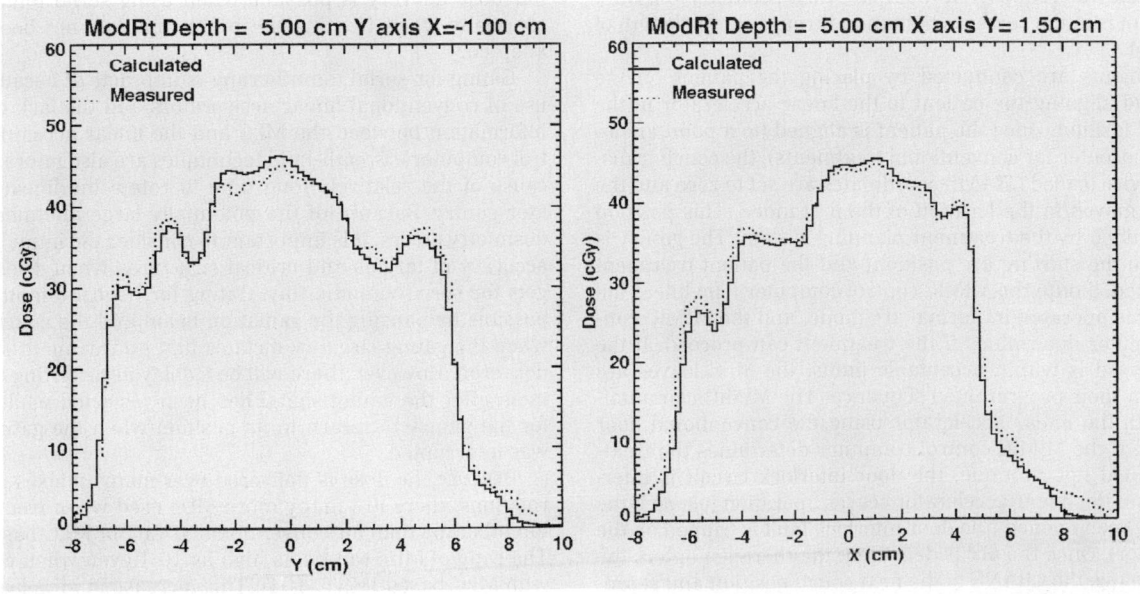

FIGURE 9.19. Dosimetric verification example comparing measured and calculated dose profiles of a right-lateral field generated with sliding-window technique for the intensity-modulated radiation therapy of gynecologic cancer.

patient alignment using portal images with beams used for actual treatment before the delivery of first treatment and then periodically thereafter. However, no beam apertures are required for IMRT. Therefore, special fields for portal imaging with apertures are created in which the shape of each aperture is defined by the terminal positions of the leading leaf tips and the starting positions of the trailing leaf tips.

Intensity-modulated treatments may be delivered remotely or automatically under computer control. The treatment machine computer may automatically set up the various components of the machine and switch on the radiation beam. For the sliding-window technique, it moves leaves during irradiation in the sequence specified in the leaf motion dataset. In the step-and-shoot mode, the radiation pauses while the leaves move. At the completion of the first field, the computer sets the machine for the next field and again goes through its leaf-motion sequence and irradiation. This process is repeated until all fields are delivered. The treatment times may vary somewhat and depend on the number of fields involved and the complexity of the fluence distribution. Current time estimates range from 5 to 20 minutes, excluding patient setup (76,77,131).

Setup and IMRT Delivery with Serial Tomotherapy

Because there are no specific beam directions or portals associated with serial tomotherapy beam delivery, the treatment QA concentrates on patient positioning and immobilization. The add-on multileaf collimator (MIMiC) is relatively heavy and its removal is time consuming, so portal films often are acquired with the MIMiC in place. This limits the portal fields to a roughly 3.4×20 cm^2 field size. Therefore, the imaging of useful, immobile, bony anatomic landmarks is critical for each port film, meaning that the selection of the portal film locations is critical to the accurate determination of patient-positioning accuracy. The positions of the films do not need to coincide with the locations of the treated indices, but the digitally reconstructed radiograph that is used to compare against the portal film must be simulated at the same relative couch position as the portal film is acquired. Typically, anteroposterior and lateral films are acquired, and if the target is longer than 10 cm and is in a location where patient structures are flexible (e.g., in the neck), portal films may be required at multiple couch positions to assure the patient is in the correct orientation throughout the length of treatment.

Treatments are conducted by placing the patient on the couch and aligning the patient to the linear accelerator in the standard fashion. Once the patient is aligned (to a point analogous to isocenter for conventional treatments), the couch translation device (called *CRANE*) coordinates are set to zero and the couch is moved to the location of the first index. This position is determined by the treatment-planning system. The gantry is rotated to the starting arc position, and the patient treatment plan is loaded onto the MIMiC control computer. The linear accelerator is operated in normal arc mode, and the MIMiC control computer determines if the treatment can proceed. If the gantry speed is within acceptable limits, the MLC leaves are opened in their programmed sequence. The MIMiC communicates with the linear accelerator using the conventional door interlock. If the MIMiC control computer determines the treatment should not continue, the door interlock circuit is interrupted and the linear accelerator ceases operation just as if the door had been opened (the door interlock fault is tripped on the accelerator). Once the arc is delivered, the therapist enters the room to move the CRANE to the next couch position and reprograms the MIMiC controlling computer by following the screen prompts.

Tomotherapy Versus Fixed-Gantry IMRT

The physical and operational differences between tomotherapy and fixed-gantry IMRT lead to trade-offs when considering each system. The rotational beams used in tomotherapy could be a significant advantage until robust beam configuration optimization tools are developed, particularly those involving noncoplanar beams.

For serial tomotherapy delivery, one of the difficulties is the requirement of precisely moving the patient between successive arc deliveries (couch indexes). The dose-delivery error made for an incorrect junction move is similar to the errors in abutting conventional fields. Studies have shown that the maximum dose error is 25% mm^{-1} in the abutment region for errors in couch index movement or intrajunction patient motion (83). When conventional fields are abutted, feathering often is used to reduce the risk of systematic dose errors. A similar technique has been suggested for distributing the abutment regions for serial tomotherapy (41) by creating multiple treatment plans with modified target volumes to force a redistribution of indexes.

Even when perfectly abutted, there are dose heterogeneities within the abutment region caused by the divergent radiation fields, especially when arcs of less than 360 degrees are used. Low et al. (83) studied the abutment region dose distributions for arcs ranging from 180 degrees to 340 degrees and determined that the tumor doses can have significant cold spots when short arcs are used. These become more severe when the longer leaf setting (1.7 cm) is used. The accuracy of the treatment-planning system in predicting these heterogeneities was not evaluated, but the system tends to underestimate the severity of the heterogeneities. Although the divergence in the radiation beams is still present in helical tomotherapy, the helical path of the field edge distributes the diverging distribution such that dose errors caused by inaccuracies in couch motion, or by patient movement, are significantly smaller than with serial tomotherapy.

One of the advantages of fixed-gantry IMRT is the availability of noncoplanar directions. The commercial hardware device used to precisely move the couch between successive indexes also is produced in a model that attaches directly to the couch, allowing for couch rotations. Although limited noncoplanar dose delivery is possible when using serial tomotherapy, especially when treating the brain, this has not been widely adopted.

Gating for serial tomotherapy is impractical because of the use of conventional linear accelerators and the lack of shared information between the MLC and the linear accelerator control computers. Breath-hold techniques are also impractical because of the relatively long time to rotate the linear accelerator gantry. Because of the potentially large abutment-region dosimetry errors, it is important to consider the immobilization accuracy of targets and critical structures when selecting targets for serial tomotherapy. Gating for helical tomotherapy is possible by pausing the radiation beam and the couch motion when the gating circuitry dictates that no treatment should be delivered. However, there will be a delay in restarting the treatment after the gating signal has been restarted while waiting for the gantry to return to its position when the gating signal was interrupted.

Because the dose is delivered over many indexes or gantry rotations, there are many more MUs used when treating with tomotherapy than for conventional 3DCRT or MLC-based IMRT. The ratio of MUs can be as high as 10:1 even when compared with MLC-based IMRT (104). This increase in MUs leads to increases in whole-body dose that may yield a significant increase in secondary radiation-induced malignancies. The solution to this is to improve the linear accelerator head shielding, the source of most of the whole-body dose in tomotherapy.

Another limitation of tomotherapy is the lack of electron beams. Electron beams (including energy and intensity-modulated electron beams), by themselves or in combination with intensity-modulated photon beams, are expected to play an important role in the treatment of certain sites (e.g., breast).

A major advantage of helical tomotherapy is that it is a dedicated IMRT device. However, MLC-based IMRT is likely to compete as a delivery mode resulting in part from the limitations of tomotherapy discussed earlier. Furthermore, the large base of MLC-mounted linear accelerators will mean that the adoption of tomotherapy for significant numbers of IMRT patient treatments will take many years.

Special Requirements of Facility Design for IMRT

The room-shielding design characteristics for IMRT delivery are different than those for conventional radiotherapy. Shielding requirements are determined separately for primary and scattered radiation barriers and for tomotherapy and MLC-based IMRT. For MLC-based IMRT, the total integrated radiation fluence remains similar to that used in conformal therapy, so no change in primary barrier thicknesses is expected. However, the increase in MUs of about a factor of 3 is expected to increase the required secondary shielding barrier attenuation, at least until the linear accelerator manufacturers improve the head leakage characteristics. For serial tomotherapy without a beam stopper, the same primary barrier is struck for each couch index, indicating that an increase in primary barrier thickness may be required. However, the use of a rotating beam, and the relatively small angle subtended by the MIMiC, reduces the effective use factor to the point that it almost exactly cancels the number of times the beam strikes the primary barrier. Increases in secondary shielding, however, may be greater than for IMRT because the total number of MUs is significantly greater.

Clinical Experience with IMRT

IMRT of Head and Neck Cancer

The first report of the application of IMRT to head and neck neoplasms was from Baylor College. Kuppersmith et al. (68) reported a decrease in dose to the parotid glands to less than 30 Gy in 28 patients treated with IMRT using serial tomotherapy. They also found the incidence of acute toxicity to be drastically lower than with conventional radiation therapy. Later, Butler et al. (18) implemented the "simultaneous modulated accelerated radiation therapy" (SMART) technique, an equivalent of the SIB technique, and found that 19 out 20 patients treated had complete response with acceptable toxicity. Low et al. (81) have described the application of the serial tomotherapy technique and QA practices for head and neck treatments at Washington University in St. Louis. Preliminary results of the use of these techniques for 17 patients have been reported by Chao et al. (23) and showed that the tumor control is promising with no severe adverse acute side effects. A prospective clinical study conducted by Chao et al. (22) also showed that the sparing of parotid glands translated into objective and subjective improvement of both xerostomia and quality-of-life scores in patients with head and neck cancers treated with IMRT.

In another publication, Chao et al. (24) also reported that the dosimetric advantage of IMRT did translate into significant reduction of late salivary toxicity in patients with oropharyngeal carcinoma and had no adverse impact on tumor control and disease-free survival. In this study, 430 patients with carcinoma of the oropharynx were treated. There were 260 patients with primary tumors of the tonsil and 170 patients with tumors arising from the base of the tongue. Twenty-four (6%) patients had stage I disease, 88 (20%) had stage II, 128 (30%) had stage III, and 190 (44%) had stage IV disease. Patients were divided into five groups. Group I consisted of 109 patients who received preoperative conventional radiation therapy. Group II consisted of 142 patients who received postoperative conventional radiation therapy. Group III consisted of 153 patients who received definitive conventional radiation therapy. Serial tomotherapy IMRT was used to treat 14 patients postoperatively (group IV) and 12 patients definitively without surgery (group V). With a median follow-up of 3.9 years, the 2-year locoregional control values for the five studied groups were 78%, 76%, 68%, 100%, and 88%, respectively. The 2-year disease-free survival values for the five studied groups were 68%, 74%, 58%, 92%, and 80%, respectively. IMRT significantly reduced the incidence of late xerostomia. The benefit of IMRT in nasopharyngeal carcinoma has been reported by Cheng et al. (28), who showed that target coverage of the primary tumor was maintained and nodal coverage was improved with IMRT in 17 nasopharyngeal carcinoma patients, as compared with conventional beam arrangements. Also, the ability of IMRT to spare parotid gland was considerably superior. Hunt et al. (56) reported similar results with 23 primary nasopharyngeal carcinoma patients. Lee et al. (72) reported data for 67 head and neck cancer patients treated with IMRT using three different techniques:

a. Manually cut partial transmission blocks,
b. Computer-controlled auto-sequencing multisegment approach, and
c. Serial tomotherapy (MIMiC).

Fifty patients received concomitant cisplatinum and adjuvant cisplatinum and 5-fluorouracil chemotherapy according to the Intergroup 0099 trial. Twenty-six patients had fractionated high–dose-rate intracavitary brachytherapy boost and one patient had gamma-knife radiosurgery boost after external-beam radiotherapy. With a median follow-up of 31 months, the 4-year estimates of local progression-free, locoregional progression-free, and distant metastases-free rates were 97%, 98%, and 66%, respectively. IMRT provided excellent tumor target coverage and allowed the delivery of a high dose to the target leading to excellent locoregional control for nasopharyngeal carcinoma with significant sparing of the salivary glands and other nearby critical normal tissues.

IMRT also has been found to be suitable for patients with carcinoma of the paranasal sinuses. Claus et al. (32) observed no dry eye or other visual disturbances in 11 ethmoid sinus cancer patients, finding that the optic pathway dose can be reduced selectively by IMRT and that the IMRT has the potential to save binocular vision. In this study, however, no evaluation of retinopathy was done because the follow-up period was short. Similar significant advantages of IMRT were shown for six patients over conventional radiation therapy and 3DCRT for treatment of maxillary sinus carcinoma (2).

The Virginia Commonwealth University group has reported data on a dose-escalation trial of advanced head and neck squamous cell carcinomas (143). In their protocol, IMRT was designed and delivered using the SIB strategy. Primary dose levels of 68.1, 70.8, and 73.8 Gy, given in 30 fractions (biologically equivalent to 74, 79, and 85 Gy, respectively, if given in 2 Gy per fraction), were evaluated. Simultaneously, the subclinical disease and electively treated nodes were prescribed 60 and 54 Gy, respectively (biologically equivalent to 60 and 50 Gy, respectively, if given in 2 Gy fractions). For each prescribed dose level, the required cord and brainstem sparing and a variable degree of parotid gland sparing were achieved. Dose homogeneities for GTV were on average 6.2%, 8.3%, and 8.8% for the three dose levels. An average of 25.8 Gy to the contralateral parotid gland and 40.8 Gy to the ipsilateral parotid gland were achieved.

In patients treated with IMRT, local recurrences have been mainly within the high-dose region. Chao et al. (26) reported the patterns of failure in 126 head and neck IMRT patients treated with serial tomotherapy. Seventeen locoregional failures were detected, and nine of those failures were inside the GTV. Two-year actuarial locoregional control rate was 85%, and 2-year ultimate locoregional control rate after salvage surgery was 89%. Dawson et al. (39) reported the patterns of failure analysis of 58 patients. Patients were treated with forward-planning IMRT and 3DCRT. The actuarial locoregional control rate was 79% with a median follow-up of 27 months. For 14 out 15 patients, the locoregional failures were in the region containing gross disease and in the adjacent soft tissue at risk.

IMRT of Prostate Cancer

Zelefsky et al. (149) reported the results of 171 patients with localized prostate cancer treated with IMRT using fixed-gantry beams and sliding-window techniques. They found that IMRT improved target coverage and significantly reduced the volumes of rectal and bladder walls exposed to high doses. Acute grade 1 to 2 and late grade 2 rectal toxicities were significantly lower in the IMRT group in comparison with the 3DCRT group despite the fact that the latter mostly used lower target doses. In another publication, Zelefsky et al. (150) reported the results of 772 patients with clinically localized prostate cancer treated with IMRT. A total of 698 patients (90%) were treated to 81 Gy, and 74 patients (10%) were treated to 86.4 Gy. The 3-year actuarial prostate-specific antigen relapse-free survival rates for favorable, intermediate, and unfavorable risk group patients were 92%, 86%, and 81%, respectively. Eleven patients (1.5%) developed late grade 2 rectal bleeding. Four patients (0.1%) experienced grade 3 rectal toxicity. No grade 4 rectal complications have been observed. The 3-year actuarial likelihood of late grade 2 rectal toxicity was 4%. Seventy-two patients (9%) experienced late grade 2 urinary toxicity, and five (0.5%) developed grade 3 urinary toxicity (urethral stricture). The 3-year actuarial likelihood of late grade 2 urinary toxicity was 15%. These data represented the largest compilation of patients treated with IMRT and demonstrated the feasibility of high-dose radiation delivery with IMRT for patients with localized prostate cancer. Acute and late rectal toxicities seemed to be significantly reduced compared with what has been observed with conventional 3DCRT. Short-term prostate-specific antigen control rates also seemed to be at least comparable to those achieved with 3DCRT at similar dose levels.

Pollack et al. (106) reported their preliminary results of acute toxicity on 100 patients treated on a randomized trial of 76 Gy in 38 fractions versus 70.2 Gy in 26 fractions. All patients were treated using IMRT. The hypofractionated regimen appeared to be well tolerated but did have slightly higher rates of acute GI toxicity. Kupelian et al. (67) reported the results of a single-arm hypofractionated IMRT protocol using 70 Gy in 28 fractions and found that biochemical relapse free survival was 97%, 88%, and 70%, respectively, for low, intermediate, and high-risk disease. Rates of grade 2 or 3 rectal toxicity at 5 years were 5%.

Other studies of prostate IMRT include one conducted at Royal Marsden Hospital. This study of 10 patients with prostate cancer showed that, when both prostate gland and pelvic lymph nodes are included in the target volume, a reduction in critical pelvic volume irradiated can be achieved with IMRT allowing a modest dose escalation with acceptable complication rates (105). Teh et al. (124) reported acceptable acute genitourinary toxicity with a mean dose of 69 Gy in 40 postprostatectomy patients. Using a rectal balloon for prostate immobiliza-

tion, they further reported the treatment results of 100 patients with prostate cancer with definitive IMRT. They found that there was no grade III or IV acute gastrointestinal (GI) and genitourinary toxicity (125). Morr et al. (100) have evaluated the clinical feasibility of daily computer-assisted transabdominal ultrasonography for target position verification in the setting of IMRT for prostate cancer. Twenty-three patients with clinically localized prostate cancer were treated with serial tomotherapy and transabdominal ultrasonography. They found that this localization technique can be practically implemented as part of a daily setup routine and could be a useful tool in the clinical practice of IMRT for prostate cancers.

IMRT Experience with Other Cancer Sites

In addition to strong data supporting the use of IMRT in head and neck and prostate cancer, there are a number of preliminary studies reporting the feasibility and outcomes of IMRT of other cancers; many of these reports are theoretical dosimetric studies. Theoretically improved dosimetry alone probably does not serve as sufficient justification for the routine use of IMRT in these cases, and in the absence of robust clinical data regarding actual treatment outcomes, IMRT in these settings should be considered investigational.

IMRT of Breast Cancer

Commercial systems are now available that can autocontour the volume of breast tissue within conventionally designed tangential photon portals and then use an inverse planning algorithm to optimize dose homogeneity within these tangential portals (67). However, most commercial inverse planning systems could not handle the "skin flash" appropriately. Due to setup uncertainties and breathing motion, a portion of the breast (target) tissue may move outside the skin line as indicated by the treatment planning CT images of the patient. The traditional IMRT technique to overcome target motion uncertainty is to expand the PTV and optimize the dose coverage to the entire PTV. However, this strategy may not work because a portion of the PTV will be expanded into the air, which does not have the necessary mass to absorb the dose. Some treatment-planning systems ignore the regions outside the skin contour entirely. Therefore, it may be necessary to add "virtual" tissues in the PTV for the inverse planning system. Sometimes it may require users to manually open certain IMRT segments to take care of the skin flash effect.

Nevertheless, there has been interest in using IMRT for left-sided beast cancers in order to spare myocardium from the high-dose region of the radiotherapy fields. No robust data regarding clinical outcomes after IMRT for breast cancer exist; however, a variety of dosimetric studies (29,44,54,75,110,126,127) have suggested reductions in lung and myocardium doses when IMRT is compared to conventional radiotherapeutic techniques. Hurkmans et al. (57) used a normal tissue complication probability (NTCP) model to estimate the NTCP for cardiac and lung complications due to radiotherapy and found that IMRT did decrease the NTCP for late cardiac toxicity compared to more conventional radiotherapy techniques, but had a minimal effect on the NTCP for radiation pneumonitis.

Hong et al. (54) reported a dosimetric study of IMRT in 10 cases of intact breast cancer showing significant reduction of dose to the coronary arteries, ipsilateral lung, and surrounding soft tissues. It simultaneously improved dose homogeneity throughout the target volume. Li et al. (74) described a combined electron and IMRT technique for breast cancer treatment, which led to improvement over the conventional treatment technique using tangential fields with reduced dose to the ipsilateral lung and the heart. Other studies (44,127) also confirmed that IMRT reduces the high-dose volume in tangential breast irradiation significantly and enables more complete cardiac sparing without compromising PTV coverage in some patients. Furthermore, IMRT creates a possibility to improve field matching in case of multiple field irradiations of the breast and lymph nodes (62,69,127). In addition, IMRT for tangential breast radiation therapy was found to be an effective and efficient method to achieve uniform dose throughout the breast. Preliminary findings reveal minimal or no acute skin reactions for patients with different breast sizes in 32 patients with early-stage breast cancer (62).

IMRT of Gynecologic Cancer

In regard to the targeting of pelvic lymphatics, with IMRT, Taylor et al. (123) mapped the pelvic lymphatics of 20 patients using MRI with the administration of iron oxide particles and found that a modified CTV margin of 7 mm around the iliac vessels resulted in adequate coverage of the pelvic lymphatics.

Ahamad et al. (3) analyzed the normal tissue-sparing effects of IMRT in the treatment of the pelvis after hysterectomy in patients with gynecologic cancers and found that although more small bowel, bladder, and rectum could be spared with IMRT compared to conventional radiotherapeutic techniques, these benefits rapidly diminished with even small expansions of the target volumes. D'Souza et al. (37) used the same dataset of patients as Ahamad et al. (3) and found that IMRT may allow higher doses of radiation (54 Gy) to be delivered safely to the node-bearing regions of the pelvis and the vaginal apex compared to conventional techniques that administer 50.4 Gy.

Salema et al. (111) reported 13 patients treated with extended field pelvic and paraaortic radiotherapy using IMRT and found that 2 patients experienced grade 3 or higher toxicity Both of these patients received concurrent cisplatin-based chemotherapy.

Portelance et al. (107) reported dosimetric comparison between 3DCRT and IMRT for 10 patients with cervical cancer. They demonstrated that, with similar target coverage, normal tissue-sparing was superior with IMRT. Mundt et al. (101) reported the clinical experience of 40 patients with gynecologic malignancy who underwent IMRT to the pelvis. Compared with 35 historic control patients who were treated with conventional techniques, patients treated with IMRT experienced fewer acute GI symptoms than those treated with conventional whole-pelvic radiotherapy.

IMRT of Gastrointestinal Cancer

Crane et al. (36) reported the results of a phase I dose-escalation study of radiotherapy with concurrent gemcitabine chemotherapy. The aim of this study was to alternate escalating the radiation dose by 3 Gy and the gemcitabine dose by 50 mg/m^2. The starting dose of gemcitabine was 350 mg/m^2 and 33 Gy per 11 fractions of IMRT to the regional lymphatics and primary disease. All three patients in the first cohort who were treated suffered dose-limiting toxicity, and the trial was ultimately closed because of excessive myelosuppression and upper GI toxicity.

Ben-Josef et al. (7) reported on 15 patients with pancreatic cancer treated with concurrent capecitabine and IMRT (45 to 55 Gy) and reported that only 1 patient had grade 3 GI toxicity, specifically GI ulceration that responded to medical management.

Brown et al. (17) performed a dosimetric analysis of 15 patients with pancreatic cancer and compared 3DCRT, IMRT with sequential boost, and IMRT with integrated boost, and found that IMRT with integrated boost allowed dose escalation up to 64.8 Gy to the primary tumor.

Guerrero-Urbano et al. (51) performed a dosimetric evaluation in five patients with locally advanced rectal cancer and found that IMRT with simultaneous integrated boost theoretically reduced the radiation dose to the small bowel compared to 3D conformal techniques. However, clinical data regarding outcomes of patients treated with IMRT for rectal cancer are lacking at this time.

Milano et al. (90) reported on 17 patients with squamous cell carcinomas of the anal canal treated with IMRT with whole pelvic radiation does of 45 Gy followed by boost to the anal canal. Thirteen patients received concurrent 5-fluorouracil and mitomycin-C chemotherapy. Treatment was well tolerated with no grade 3 or higher nonhematologic toxicity, and no required treatment breaks from skin or GI toxicity. However, one patient receiving mitomycin-C chemotherapy did experience grade 4 hematologic toxicity. Three patients who did not achieve a complete response required abdominoperineal resection and colostomy. With a mean follow-up of 20.3 months, there were no other local failures.

Milano et al. (89) also reported on seven patients with gastric cancer treated with IMRT to a dose of 50.4 Gy. No patient experienced grade 3 toxicity. The treated IMRT plans were compared to conventional AP:PA and three-field plans, and the IMRT plans were found to provide better coverage of the target volumes compared to conventional techniques, with better sparing of the liver and kidneys.

IMRT of Lung Cancer

Because of concerns regarding respiratory motion in radiotherapy of lung cancer, the use of IMRT in lung cancer requires some method to account for tumor and organ motion during treatment planning and delivery; these techniques include both respiratory gating (61) and 4D CT planning (4).

The poor local control rates of conventional radiotherapy doses in the treatment of lung cancer (19) have led to much interest in using IMRT to allow for dose escalation to improve local control. Holloway et al. (52) reported the initial results of five patients with unresectable stage II and III non–small cell carcinoma treated on a phase I dose-escalation trial using induction chemotherapy followed by IMRT to a dose of 84 Gy using 2.4 Gy daily fractions. PET CT was used to define target volumes. One patient developed lethal radiation pneumonitis and the trial was halted.

Murshed et al. (103) performed a dosimetric analysis of 41 patients initially treated with 3DCRT to a dose of 63 Gy. IMRT plans were then generated using these patients' initial planning CTs, and IMRT was found to decrease the volume of lung irradiated to both 10 and 20 Gy (V10 and V20). Target coverage was improved with IMRT, and the volumes of heart and esophagus irradiated were also reduced.

Grills et al. (50) performed a dosimetric comparison of four radiotherapy techniques in 18 patients with stage I-IIB lung cancer. The study compared IMRT, optimized multiple beam 3DCRT, two- to three-beam 3DCRT, and traditional wide-field radiotherapy with elective nodal irradiation. This study found that IMRT and optimized 3DCRT resulted in similar doses of radiotherapy to normal tissues in node-negative patients; however, in node-positive patients, IMRT resulted in a 15% decrease in the volume of lung treated to 20 Gy (V20) and a 30% decrease in the NTCP for radiation pneumonitis.

IMRT of Intracranial Malignancies

Iuchi et al. (58) from Japan published a retrospective report on 25 patients with malignant astrocytomas (World Health Organization grade III and IV) treated with IMRT using a hypofractionated regimen of 48 to 68 Gy in 8 fractions. Thirteen patients were treated to 68 Gy and 12 patients received doses of 48 to 65 Gy. The IMRT group was compared to 60 patients treated with conventional techniques to doses of 40 to 60 Gy using 2 Gy daily fractions. The 2-year overall survival was significantly improved ($p = .043$) in patients treated with hypofractionated IMRT (55.6%) compared to those patient treated with conventional techniques (19.4%).

Floyd et al. (46) reported a pilot study of 20 patients treated with hypofractionated IMRT. Treatment was administered during 2 weeks (10 fractions), and 50 Gy (5 Gy/day) was prescribed to enhance disease or the surgical cavity and 30 Gy (3 Gy/day) was prescribed simultaneously to peritumoral edema. Three patients experienced grade 4 brain necrosis, requiring surgical re-excision. There was no mortality from brain necrosis; in fact, those patients manifesting brain necrosis had longer survival times.

Hwang et al. (55) reported on 15 patients with pediatric medulloblastoma treated with conventional craniospinal radiotherapy followed by a boost to the posterior fossa using IMRT. IMRT delivered much lower doses of radiation to the auditory apparatus while maintaining full doses to the desired target volume. Their findings suggested that, despite receiving higher doses of cisplatin and despite receiving radiotherapy before cisplatin therapy, IMRT can significantly decrease the rate of hearing loss in children treated for medulloblastoma.

In closing, IMRT clearly results in improved radiation dose distributions in a variety of cancers. In some cases, the superior dosimetry of IMRT has resulted in improved clinical outcomes for patients; however, the scientific evidence documenting these clinical improvements lags far behind the data documenting improved dosimetry. It is incumbent on radiation oncologists to continue to document improved clinical outcomes with IMRT in the peer-reviewed literature if we wish to justify the use of this expensive technology to our communities in an era of skyrocketing medical costs.

References

1. 50 A Rortctg Basic applications of multileaf collimators. In: Publishing MP (ed.). Madison, 2001.
2. Adams EJ, Nutting CM, Convery DJ, et al. Potential role of intensity-modulated radiotherapy in the treatment of tumors of the maxillary sinus. *Int J Radiat Oncol Biology Phys* 2001;51:579–588.
3. Ahamad A, D'Souza W, Salehpour M, et al. Intensity-modulated radiation therapy after hysterectomy: Comparison with conventional treatment and sensitivity of the normal-tissue-sparing effect to margin size. *Int J Radiat Oncol Biol Phys* 2005;62:1117–1124.
4. Alasti H, Cho YB, Vandermeer AD, et al. A novel four-dimensional radiotherapy method for lung cancer: Imaging, treatment planning and delivery. *Phys Med Biol* 2006;51:3251–3267.
5. Barth NH. The verification of an inverse problem in radiation Therapy. *Int J Radiat Oncol Biology Phys* 1990;18:425–431.
6. Bednarz G, Saiful Huq M, Rosenow UF. Deconvolution of detector size effect for output factor measurement for narrow Gamma Knife radiosurgery beams. *Phys Med Biol* 2002;47:3643–3649.
7. Ben-Josef E, Shields AF, Vaishampayan U, et al. Intensity-modulated radiotherapy (IMRT) and concurrent capecitabine for pancreatic cancer. *Int J Radiat Oncol Biol Phys* 2004;59:454–459.
8. Bortfeld T, Burkelbach J, Boesecke R, et al. Methods of image reconstruction from projections applied to conformation radiotherapy. *Phys Med Biol* 1990;35:1423–1434.
9. Bortfeld T, Burkelbach J, Boesecke R, et al. Three-dimensional solution of the inverse problem in conformation radiotherapy. In: Breit A, ed. *Advanced radiation therapy: Tumor response monitoring and treatment planning.* Berlin: Springer-Verlag, 1992:503–508.
10. Bortfeld T, Kahler DL, Waldron TJ, et al. X-ray field compensation with multileaf collimators. *Int J Radiat Oncol Biology Phys* 1994;28:723–730.
11. Bortfeld T, Schlegel W, Dykstra C, et al. Physical vs. biological objectives for treatment plan optimization [Letter]. *Radiother Oncol* 1996.
12. Bortfeld T, Stein J, Preiser K. Clinically relevant intensity modulation optimization using physical objectives. In: *XII International Conference on the Use of Computers in Radiotherapy.* Salt Lake City, Utah, 1997:1–4.
13. Bortfeld T, Schlegel W. Optimization of beam orientations in radiation therapy: Some theoretical considerations. *Phys Med Biol* 1993;38:291–304.
14. Brahme A. Optimization of stationary and moving beam radiation therapy techniques. *Radiother Oncol* 1988;12:129–140.
15. Brahme A, Roos J, Lax I. Solution of an integral equation encountered in radiation therapy. *Phys Med Biol* 1982;27:1221–1229.
16. Brown MW, Ning H, Arora B, et al. A dosimetric analysis of dose escalation using two intensity-modulated radiation therapy techniques in locally advanced pancreatic carcinoma. *Int J Radiat Oncol Biol Phys* 2006;65:274–283.
17. Butler EB, Teh BS, Grant WH, et al. SMART (Simultaneous Modulated Accelerated Radiation Thearpy) boost: A new accelerated fractionation schedule for the treatment of headn and neck cancer with intensity modulated radiotherapy. *Int J Radiat Oncol Biology Phys* 1999;45:21–32.
18. Byhardt RW, Scott C, Sause WT, et al. Response, toxicity, failure patterns, and survival in five Radiation Therapy Oncology Group (RTOG) trials of sequential and/or concurrent chemotherapy and radiotherapy for locally advanced non-small-cell carcinoma of the lung. *Int J Radiat Oncol Biol Phys* 1998;42:469–478.
19. Carol MP. Integrated 3-D conformal multi-vane intensity modulation delivery system for radiotherapy. In: XIth International Conference on the Use of Computers in Radiation Therapy. Manchester, UK, 1994:172–173.
20. Carol MP. Peacock: A system for planning and rotational delivery of intensity-modulated fields. *Int J Imag Sys Technol* 1995;6:56–61.
21. Chao KS, Deasy JO, Markman J, et al. A prospective study of salivary function sparing in patients with head-and-neck cancers receiving intensity-modulated or three-dimensional radiation therapy: Initial results. *Int J Radiat Oncol Biol Phys* 2001;49:907–916.
22. Chao KS, Low DA, Perez CA, et al. Intensity-modulated radiation therapy in head and neck cancers: The Mallinckrodt experience. *Int J Cancer* 2000;90:92–103.
23. Chao KS, Majhail N, Huang CJ, et al. Intensity-modulated radiation therapy reduces late salivary toxicity without compromising tumor control in patients with oropharyngeal carcinoma: A comparison with conventional techniques. *Radiother Oncol* 2001;61:275–280.
24. Chao KS, Ozyigit G, Tran BN, et al. Patterns of failure in patients receiving definitive and post-operative IMRT for head and neck cancer. *Int J Radiat Oncol Biol Phys* 2003;55:312–321.
25. Chao KS, Wippold FJ, Ozyigit G, et al. Determination and delineation of nodal target volumes for head-and-neck cancer based on patterns of failure in patients receiving definitive and postoperative IMRT. *Int J Radiat Oncol Biol Phys* 2002;53:1174–1184.
26. Chen Z, Wang X, Bortfeld T, et al. The influence of scatter on the design of the optimized intensity modulators. *Med Phys* 1995;22:1727–1733.
27. Cheng JC, Chao KS, Low DA. Comparison of intensity modulated radiation therapy (IMRT) treatment techniques for nasopharyngeal carcinoma. *Int J Cancer* 2001;96:126–131.
28. Cho BC, Schwarz M, Mijnheer BJ, et al. Simplified intensity-modulated radiotherapy using predefined segments to reduce cardiac complications in left-sided breast cancer. *Radiother Oncol* 2004;70:231–241.
29. Chui CS, LoSasso T, Spirou S. Dose calculations for photon beams with intensity modulation generated by dynamic jaw or multi-leaf collimations. *Med Phys* 1994;21:1237–1243.
30. Chui CS, Spirou S, LoSasso T. Testing of dynamic multileaf collimation. *Med Phys* 1996;23:635–641.
31. Claus F, De Gersem W, De Wagter C, et al. An implementation strategy for IMRT of ethmoid sinus cancer with bilateral sparing of the optic pathways. *Int J Radiat Oncol Biol Phys* 2001;51:318–331.
32. Convery DJ, Rosenbloom ME. The generation of intensity-modulated fields for conformal radiotherapy by dynamic collimation. *Phys Med Biol* 1992;37:1359–1374.
33. Cormack A. A problem in rotation therapy with x-rays. *Int J Radiat Oncol Biology Phys* 1987;13:623–630.
34. Cormack AM, Cormack RA. A problem in rotation therapy with x-rays: Dose distributions with an axis of symmetry. *Int J Radiat Oncol Biology Phys* 1987;13:1921–1925.
35. Crane CH, Antolak JA, Rosen II, et al. Phase I study of concomitant gemcitabine and IMRT for patients with unresectable adenocarcinoma of the pancreatic head. *Int J Gastrointest Cancer* 2001;30:123–132.
36. Dai J, Zhu Y. Minimizing the number of segments in a delivery sequence for intensity-modulated radiation therapy with a multileaf collimator. *Med Phys* 2001;28:2113–2120.
37. Dawson LA, Anzai Y, Marsh L, et al. Patterns of local-regional recurrence following parotid-sparing conformal and segmental intensity-modulated radiotherapy for head and neck cancer. *Int J Radiat Oncol Biol Phys* 2000;46:1117–1126.
38. Deasy JO. Multiple local minima in radiotherapy optimization problems with dose-volume constraints. *Med Phys* 1997;24:1157–1161.
39. Dogan N, Leybovich LB, King S, et al. Improvement of treatment plans developed with intensity-modulated radiation therapy for concave-shaped head and neck tumors. *Radiology* 2002;223:57–67.
40. Dong L, Antolak J, Salehpour M, et al. Patient-specific point dose measurement for IMRT monitor unit verification. *Int J Radiat Oncol Biol Phys* 2003;53:867–877.
41. D'Souza WD, Ahamad A, Iyer R, et al. Feasibility of dose escalation using intensity-modulated radiotherapy in posthysterectomy cervical carcinoma. *Int J Radiat Oncol Biol Phys* 2005;61:1062–1070.
42. Eisbruch A, Chao KSC, Garden A. RTOG 0022 Phase I/II study of conformal and intensity modulated irradiation for oropharyngeal cancer. Active 2002-2006. RTOG Protocol. 2002.
43. Evans PM, Donovan EM, Partridge M, et al. The delivery of intensity modulated radiotherapy to the breast using multiple static fields. *Radiother Oncol* 2000;57:79–89.
44. Ezzell GA. Genetic and geometric optimization of three-dimensional radiation therapy. *Med Phys* 1996;23:293–305.
45. Floyd NS, Woo SY, Teh BS, et al. Hypofractionated intensity-modulated radiotherapy for primary glioblastoma multiforme. *Int J Radiat Oncol Biol Phys* 2004;58:721–726.
46. Frank SJ, McNeese MD, Strom EA, et al. Advances in radiation treatments of breast cancer. *Clin Breast Cancer* 2004;4:401–406.
47. Garcia-Vicente F, Delgado JM, Peraza C. Experimental determination of the convolution kernel for the study of the spatial response of a detector. *Med Phys* 1998;25:202–207.
48. Goitein M. The comparison of treatment plans. *Semin Radiat Oncol* 1992;2:246–256.
49. Grills IS, Yan D, Martinez AA, et al. Potential for reduced toxicity and dose escalation in the treatment of inoperable non-small-cell lung cancer: A comparison of intensity-modulated radiation therapy (IMRT), 3D conformal radiation, and elective nodal irradiation. *Int J Radiat Oncol Biol Phys* 2003;57:875–890.
50. Guerrero-Urbano MT, Henrys AJ, Adams EJ, et al. Intensity-modulated radiotherapy in patients with locally advanced rectal cancer reduces volume of bowel treated to high dose levels. *Int J Radiat Oncol Biol Phys* 2006;65:907–916.

51. Holloway CL, Robinson D, Murray B, et al. Results of a phase I study to dose escalate using intensity modulated radiotherapy guided by combined PET/CT imaging with induction chemotherapy for patients with non-small cell lung cancer. *Radiother Oncol* 2004;73:285–287.

52. Holmes T, Mackie TR. A filtered backprojection dose calculation method for inverse treatment planning. *Med Phys* 1994;21:303–313.

53. Hong L, Hunt M, Chui C, et al. Intensity-modulated tangential beam irradiation of the intact breast. *Int J Radiat Oncol Biol Phys* 1999;44:1155–1164.

54. Huang E, Teh BS, Strother DR, et al. Intensity-modulated radiation therapy for pediatric medulloblastoma: Early report on the reduction of ototoxicity. *Int J Radiat Oncol Biol Phys* 2002;52:599–605.

55. Hunt MA, Zelefsky MJ, Wolden S, et al. Treatment planning and delivery of intensity-modulated radiation therapy for primary nasopharynx cancer. *Int J Radiat Oncol Biol Phys* 2001;49:623–632.

56. Hurkmans CW, Cho BC, Damen E, et al. Reduction of cardiac and lung complication probabilities after breast irradiation using conformal radiotherapy with or without intensity modulation. *Radiother Oncol* 2002;62:163–171.

57. Iuchi T, Hatano K, Narita Y, et al. Hypofractionated high-dose irradiation for the treatment of malignant astrocytomas using simultaneous integrated boost technique by IMRT. *Int J Radiat Oncol Biol Phys* 2006;64:1317–1324.

58. Jursinic PA, Nelms BE. A 2-D diode array and analysis software for verification of intensity modulated radiation therapy delivery. *Med Phys* 2003;30:870–879.

59. Kallman P, Lind B, Eklof A, et al. Shaping of arbitrary dose distributions by dynamic multi-leaf collimation. *Phys Med Biol* 1988;33:1291–1300.

60. Keall P, Vedam S, George R, et al. The clinical implementation of respiratory-gated intensity-modulated radiotherapy. *Med Dosim* 2006;31:152–162.

61. Kestin LL, Sharpe MB, Frazier RC, et al. Intensity modulation to improve dose uniformity with tangential breast radiotherapy: Initial clinical experience. *Int J Radiat Oncol Biol Phys* 2000;48:1559–1568.

62. Kim JO, Siebers JV, Keall P, et al. Characteristics of radiation transmitted and scattered from multi-leaf collimators. *Med Phys* 2001;28:2497–2506.

63. Kitamura K, Shirato H, Shimizu S, et al. Registration accuracy and possible migration of internal fiducial gold marker implanted in prostate and liver treated with real-time tumor-tracking radiation therapy (RTRT). *Radiother Oncol* 2002;62:275–281.

64. Kubo H. Respiration gated radiotherapy treatment: A technical study. *Phys Med Biol* 1996;41:83–91.

65. Kung JH, Chen GT, Kuchnir FK. A monitor unit verification calculation in intensity modulated radiotherapy as a dosimetry quality assurance. *Med Phys* 2000;27:2226–2230.

66. Kupelian PA, Thakkar VV, Khuntia D, et al. Hypofractionated intensity-modulated radiotherapy (70 gy at 2.5 Gy per fraction) for localized prostate cancer: Long-term outcomes. *Int J Radiat Oncol Biol Phys* 2005;63:1463–1468.

67. Kuppersmith RB, Greco SC, Teh BS, et al. Intensity-modulated radiotherapy: First results with this new technology on neoplasms of the head and neck. *Ear Nose Throat J* 1999;78:238–241.

68. Landau D, Adams EJ, Webb S, et al. Cardiac avoidance in breast radiotherapy: A comparison of simple shielding techniques with intensity-modulated radiotherapy. *Radiother Oncol* 2001;60:247–255.

69. Langer M, Thai V, Papiez L. Improved leaf sequencing reduces segments or monitor units needed to deliver IMRT using multileaf collimators. *Med Phys* 2001;28:2450–2458.

70. Lattanzi J, McNeeley S, Hanlon A, et al. Ultrasound-based stereotactic guidance of precision conformal external beam radiation therapy in clinically localized prostate cancer. *Urology.* 2000;55:73–78.

71. Lee N, Xia P, Quivey JM, et al. Intensity-modulated radiotherapy in the treatment of nasopharyngeal carcinoma: An update of the UCSF experience. *Int J Radiat Oncol Biol Phys* 2002;53:12–22.

72. Levegrun S, Jackson A, Zelefsky MJ, et al. Analysis of biopsy outcome after three-dimensional conformal radiation therapy of prostate cancer using dose-distribution variables and tumor control probability models. *Int J Radiat Oncol Biol Phys* 2000;47:1245–1260.

73. Li JG, Williams SS, Goffinet DR, et al. Breast-conserving radiation therapy using combined electron and intensity-modulated radiotherapy technique. *Radiother Oncol* 2000;56:65–71.

74. Li JG, Xing L, Boyer AL, et al. Matching photon and electron fields with dynamic intensity modulation. *Med Phys* 1999;26:2379–2384.

75. Ling CC, Burman C, Chui CS, et al. Conformal radiation treatment of prostate cancer using inversely-planned intensity-modulated photon beams produced with dynamic multileaf collimation. *Int J Radiat Oncol Biol Phys* 1996;35:721–730.

76. Ling CC, Burman C, Chui CS, et al. Implementation of photon IMRT with dynamic MLC for the treatment of prostate cancer. In: Sternick ES, ed. *The theory & practice of intensity-modulated radiation therapy.* Pittsburgh: NOMOS, 1997: 219–228.

77. LoSasso T, Chui C-SLing CC. Physical and dosimetric aspects of a multileaf collimation system used in the dynamic mode for implementing intensity modulated radiotherapy. *Med Phys* 1998;25:1919–1917.

78. Low D, Parikh, P, Dempsey, J, et al. Ionization chamber volume averaging effects in dynamic intensity modulated radiation therapy beams. *Med Phys* 2003;30:1706–1711.

79. Low DA. Quality assurance of intensity-modulated radiothearpy. *Semin Radiother Oncol* 2002;12:219–228.

80. Low DA, Chao KS, Mutic S, et al. Quality assurance of serial tomotherapy for head and neck patient treatments. *Int J Radiat Oncol Biol Phys* 1998;42:681–692.

81. Low DA, Dempsey JF, Markman J, et al. Toward automated quality assurance for intensity-modulated radiation therapy. *Int J Radiat Oncol Biol Phys* 2002;53:443–452.

82. Low DA, Mutic S, Dempsey JF. Abutment region dosimetry for serial tomotherapy. *Int J Radiat Oncol Biol Phys* 1999;45:193–203.

83. Maciejewski B, Withers HR, Taylor JMJ, et al. Dose fractionation and regeneration in radiotherapy for cancer of the oral cavity and oropharynx: Tumor dose-response and repopulation. *Int J Radiat Oncol Biol Phys* 1989;16:831–843.

84. Mackie TR, Holmes TW, Reckwerdt PJ, et al. Tomotherapy: A proposal for a dedicated computer-controlled delivery and verification system for conformal radiotherapy. In: *Proceedings of the XIth International Conference on the use of Computers in Radiation therapy.* 1994:176–177.

85. Mackie TR, Holmes TW, Swerdloff S, et al. Tomotherapy: A new concept for the delivery of conformal radiotherapy. *Med Phys* 1993;20:1709–1719.

86. Mackie TR, Kapatoes J, Ruchala K, et al. Image guidance for precise conformal radiotherapy. *Int J Radiat Oncol Biol Phys* 2003;56:89–105.

87. Mageras GS, Mohan R. Application of fast simulated annealing to optimization of conformal radiation treatments. *Med Phys* 1993;20:639–647.

88. Milano MT, Garofalo MC, Chmura SJ, et al. Intensity-modulated radiation therapy in the treatment of gastric cancer: Early clinical outcome and dosimetric comparison with conventional techniques. *Br J Radiol* 2006;79:497–503.

89. Milano MT, Jani AB, Farrey KJ, et al. Intensity-modulated radiation therapy (IMRT) in the treatment of anal cancer: Toxicity and clinical outcome. *Int J Radiat Oncol Biol Phys* 2005;63:354–361.

90. Mohan R. Intensity modulation in radiotherapy. In: AAPM Summer School. Vancouver, BC, Canada, 1996:761–792.

91. Mohan R, Leibel SA. Intensity modulation of the radiation Beam. In: DeVita VT, Hellman S, Rosenberg SA, eds. *Cancer: Principles and practice of oncology,* 5th ed. Philadelphia: Lippincott-Raven, 1997:3093–3106.

92. Mohan R, Ling CC, Stein J, et al. The number of beams in intensity-modulated treatments: In response to the letter to the editor by Soderstrom and Brahme. *Int J Radiat Oncol Biology Phys* 1996;34:758–759.

93. Mohan R, Mageras GS, Baldwin B, et al. Clinically relevant optimization of 3D conformal treatments. *Med Phys* 1992;19:933–944.

94. Mohan R, Tong S, Arnfield M, et al. The impact of fluctuations in intensity patterns on the number of monitor units and the quality and accuracy of intensity modulated radiotherapy. *Med Phys* 2000;27:1226–1237.

95. Mohan R, Wang X, Jackson A, et al. The potential and limitations of the inverse radiotherapy technique. *Radiother Oncol* 1994;32:232–248.

96. Mohan R, Wu Q, Manning M, et al. Radiobiological considerations in the design of fractionation strategies for intensity-modulated radiation therapy of head and neck cancers. *Int J Radiat Oncol Biol Phys* 2000;46:619–630.

97. Mohan R, Wu Q, Wang X-H, et al. Intensity modulation optimization, lateral transport of radiation and margins. *Med Phys* 1996;23:2011–2022.

98. Mohan R, Wu Y, Wu Q. Delivery of intensity-modulated radiotherapy with dynamic multi-leaf collimators. In: AAPM 2000 Summer School, General Practice of Radiation Oncology Physics in the 21st Century. Northern Illinois University, Dekalb, IL, July 29-August 1, 2000. 2000:113–135.

99. Morr J, DiPetriollo T, Tsai JS, et al. Implementation and utility of a daily ultrasound-based localization system with intensity-modulated radiotherapy for prostate cancer. *Int J Radiat Oncol Biol Phys* 2002;53:1124–1129.

100. Mundt AJ, Lujan AE, Rotmensch J, et al. Intensity-modulated whole pelvic radiotherapy in women with gynecologic malignancies. *Int J Radiat Oncol Biol Phys* 2002;52:1330–1337.

101. Murphy MJ. Fiducial-based targeting accuracy for external-beam radiotherapy. *Med Phys* 2002;29:334–344.

102. Murshed H, Liu HH, Liao Z, et al. Dose and volume reduction for normal lung using intensity-modulated radiotherapy for advanced-stage non-small-cell lung cancer. *Int J Radiat Oncol Biol Phys* 2004;58:1258–1267.

103. Mutic S, Low DA, Klein EE, et al. Room shielding for intensity-modulated radiation therapy treatment facilities. *Int J Radiat Oncol Biol Phys* 2001;50:239–246.

104. Nutting CM, Convery DJ, Cosgrove VP, et al. Reduction of small and large bowel irradiation using an optimized intensity-modulated pelvic radiotherapy technique in patients with prostate cancer. *Int J Radiat Oncol Biol Phys* 2000;48:649–656.

105. Pollack A, Hanlon AL, Horwitz EM, et al. Dosimetry and preliminary acute toxicity in the first 100 men treated for prostate cancer on a randomized hypofractionation dose escalation trial. *Int J Radiat Oncol Biol Phys* 2006;64:518–526.

106. Portelance L, Chao KS, Grigsby PW, et al. Intensity-modulated radiation therapy (IMRT) reduces small bowel, rectum, and bladder doses in patients with cervical cancer receiving pelvic and para-aortic irradiation. *Int J Radiat Oncol Biol Phys* 2001;51:261–266.

107. Pugachev AB, Boyer AL, Xing L. Beam orientation optimization in intensity-modulated radiation treatment planning. *Med Phys* 2000;27:1238–1245.

108. Que W. Comparison of algorithms for multileaf collimator field segmentation. *Med Phys* 1999;26:2390–2396.

109. Remouchamps V, Vicini FA, Sharpe MB, et al. Significant reductions in heart and lung doses using deep inspiration breath hold with active breathing control and intensity-modulated radiation therapy for patients treated with locoregional breast irradiation. *Int J Radiat Oncol Biol Phys* 2003;55:392–406.

110. Salama JK, Mundt AJ, Roeske J, et al. Preliminary outcome and toxicity report of extended-field, intensity-modulated radiation therapy for gynecologic malignancies. *Int J Radiat Oncol Biol Phys* 2006;65:1170–1176.

111. Serago CF, Chungbin SJ, Buskirk SJ, et al. Initial experience with ultrasound localization for positioning prostate cancer patients for external beam radiotherapy. *Int J Radiat Oncol Biology Phys* 2002;53:1130–1138.

112. Siebers JV, Keall PJ, Kim JO, et al. A method for photon beam Monte Carlo multileaf collimator particle transport. *Med Phys* 2003;30:574–582.

113. Siebers JV, Lauterbach M, Keall PJ, et al. Incorporating multi-leaf collimator delivery constraints into iterative IMRT optimization. *Med Phys* 2002;29:952–959.

114. Söderström S, Brahme A. Selection of suitable beam orientations in radiation therapy using entropy and fourier transform measures. *Phys Med Biol* 1992;37:911–924.

115. Söderström S, Gustafsson A, Brahme A. Optimization of the dose delivery in few field techniques using radiobiological objective functions. *Med Phys* 1993;20:1201–1210.

116. Spirou SV, Chui CS. Generation of arbitrary fluence profiles by dynamic jaws or multileaf collimators. *Med Phys* 1994;21:1031–1041.

117. Spirou SV, Stein J, LoSasso T, et al. Incorporation of the source distribution function and rounded leaf edge effects in dynamic multileaf collimation. *Med Phys* 1996;23:1074–1074(abstr).

118. Stein J, Bortfeld T, Doerschel B, et al. Dynamic x-ray compensation for conformal radiotherapy by means of multi-leaf collimation. *Radiother Oncol* 1994;32:163–173.

119. Stein J, Mohan R, Wang X-H, et al. Optimum number and orientations of beams for intensity-modulated treatments. *Med Phys* 1996;23:1063–1063(abstr).

120. Stein J, Mohan R, Wang X-H, et al. Number and orientations of beams in intensity-modulated radiation treatments. *Med Phys* 1997;24:149–160.

121. Svensson R, Kallman P, Brahme A. An analytical solution for the dynamic control of multileaf collimators. *Phys Med Biol* 1994;39:37–61.

122. Taylor A, Rockall AG, Reznek RH, et al. Mapping pelvic lymph nodes: Guidelines for delineation in intensity-modulated radiotherapy. *Int J Radiat Oncol Biol Phys* 2005;63:1604–1612.

123. Teh BS, Mai WY, Augspurger ME, et al. Intensity modulated radiation therapy (IMRT) following prostatectomy: More favorable acute genitourinary toxicity profile compared to primary IMRT for prostate cancer. *Int J Radiat Oncol Biol Phys* 2001;49:465–472.

124. Teh BS, Mai WY, Uhl BM, et al. Intensity-modulated radiation therapy (IMRT) for prostate cancer with the use of a rectal balloon for prostate immobilization: Acute toxicity and dose-volume analysis. *Int J Radiat Oncol Biol Phys* 2001;49:705–712.

125. Thilmann C, Sroka-Perez G, Krempein R, et al. Inversely planned intensity modulated radiotherapy of the breast including the internal mammary chain: A plan comparison study. *Tech Cancer Res Treat* 2004;3:69–75.

126. van Asselen B, Raaijmakers CP, Hofman P, et al. An improved breast irradiation technique using three-dimensional geometrical information and intensity modulation. *Radiother Oncol* 2001;58:341–347.

127. van Santvoort JPC, Heijmen BJM. Dynamic multileaf collimation without "tongue-and-groove" underdosage effects. *Phys Med Biol* 1996;41:2091–2105.

128. Verellen D, Soete G, Linthout N, et al. Quality assurance of a system for improved target localization and patient set-up that combines real-time infrared tracking and stereoscopic X-ray imaging. *Radiother Oncol* 2003;67:129–141.

129. Verhey LJ. Issues in optimization for planning of intensity-modulated radiation therapy. *Semin Radiat Oncol* 2002;12:210–218.

130. Wang X, Spirou S, LoSasso T, et al. Dosimetric verification of an intensity modulated treatment. *Med Phys* 1996;23:317–328.

131. Wang XH, Mohan R, Jackson A, et al. Optimization of intensity modulated 3D conformal treatment plans based on biological indices. *Radiother Oncol* 1995;37:140–152.

132. Webb S. Optimization of conformal radiotherapy dose distributions by simulated annealing. *Phys Med Biol* 1989;34:1349–1370.

133. Webb S. Optimization of conformal radiotherapy dose distributions by simulated annealing: 2. Inclusion of scatter in the 2D technique. *Phys Med Biol* 1991;36:1227–1237.

134. Webb S, Bortfeld T, Stein J, et al. The effect of stair-step leaf transmission on the "tongue-and-groove problem" in dynamic radiotherapy with a multileaf collimator. *Phys Med Biol* 1997;42.

135. Webb S, Convery DJ, Bortfeld T, et al. A general analysis of the "tongue-and-groove" effect in dynamic MLC therapy. In: *XII International Conference on the Use of Computers in Radiotherapy.* Salt Lake City, UT: 1997:342–345.

136. Westermark M, Arndt J, Nilsson B, et al. Comparative dosimetry in narrow high-energy photon beams. *Phys Med Biol* 2000;45:685–702.

137. Withers HR, Peters LJ, Taylor JMG, et al. Late normal tissue sequelae from radiation therapy for carcinoma of the tonsil: Patterns of fractionation study of radiobiology. *Int J Radiat Oncol Biol Phys* 1995;33:563–568.

138. Withers HR, Peters LJ, Taylor JMG, et al. Local control of carcinoma of the tonsil by radiation therapy: An analysis of patterns of fractionation in nine institutions. *Int J Radiat Oncol Biol Phys* 1995;33:549–562.

139. Withers HR, Taylor JMG, Maciejewski B. The hazard of accelerated tumor clogen repopulation during radiotherapy. *Acta Oncologica* 1988;27:131–146.

140. Wong J, Sharpe M, Jaffray D. The use of Active Breathing Control (ABC) to minimize breathing motion in conformal therapy. In: *XIIth International Conference on the Use of Computers in Radiation Therapy.* Salt Lake City, UT: 1997:220–222.

141. Wu Q, Mohan R. Multiple local minima in IMRT optimization based on dose-volume criteria. *Med Phys* 2002;29:1514–1527.

142. Wu Q, Mohan R, Morris M, et al. "Simultaneous integrated boost" IMRT of advanced head and neck squamous cell carcinomas. *Int J Radiat Oncol Biol Phys* 2003;56:573–585.

143. Wu Y, Yan D, Sharpe MB, et al. Implementing multiple static field delivery for intensity modulated beams. *Med Phys* 2001;28:2188–2197.

144. Xia P, Verhey LJ. Multileaf collimator leaf sequencing algorithm for intensity modulated beams with multiple static segments. *Med Phys* 1998;26: 1424–1434.

145. Xing L, Chen Y, Luxton G, et al. Monitor unit calculation for an intensity modulated photon field by a simple scatter-summation algorithm. *Phys Med Biol* 2000;45:N1–7.

146. Yu CX. Intensity-modulated arc therapy with dynamic multileaf collimation: An alternative to tomotherapy. *Phys Med Biol* 1995;40:1435–1449.

147. Yu CX, Jaffray DA, Wong JW. Calculating the effects of intra-treatment organ motion on dynamic intensity modulation. In: *XIIth International Conference on the Use of Computers in Radiation Therapy.* Salt Lake City, UT: 1997:231–233.

148. Zelefsky MJ, Fuks Z, Happersett L, et al. Clinical experience with intensity modulated radiation therapy (IMRT) in prostate cancer. *Radiother Oncol* 2000;55:241–249.

149. Zelefsky MJ, Fuks Z, Hunt M, et al. High-dose intensity modulated radiation therapy for prostate cancer: Early toxicity and biochemical outcome in 772 patients. *Int J Radiat Oncol Biol Phys* 2002;53:1111–1116.

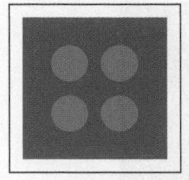

Chapter 10
Image-Guided Radiation Therapy

Loren K. Mell, Todd Pawlicki, Steve B. Jiang, Arno J. Mundt

The field of radiation oncology is amid a period of rapid technological change. Advancements in imaging, treatment planning, and delivery now enable unprecedented sophistication in the approach to radiation therapy (RT). Such advancements enhance the quality of treatment through better target delineation, dose delivery, and normal tissue sparing, which collectively promise to improve the therapeutic ratio. A key element of this technological progress is the use of modern imaging techniques to augment both the initial treatment plan and treatment delivery. The array of techniques implementing these modern imaging approaches has been termed *image-guided RT* (IGRT).

The term *image guided* is relatively noninformative, since radiation oncology has essentially always been guided by images. Moreover, the definition of IGRT is not standardized, remaining open to various interpretations. A global definition might include *any* aspect of RT involving imaging, from fluoroscopic simulation, to computed tomography (CT)-based treatment planning, to weekly port films. For the purposes of this chapter, however, the term *IGRT* is defined as in the contemporary vernacular, namely the use of modern imaging modalities, especially those incorporating functional or biological information, to augment target delineation, and the use of imaging to adjust for target motion or positional uncertainty, and, potentially, to adapt treatment to tumor response.

IGRT as an Oncology Technique

Purpose of IGRT

In the late 1960s, the chair of a well-known radiation oncology department met with a Certificate of Need board to secure approval for a fluoroscopic simulator, a recent and expensive technological development at that time. The chair, emphasizing the importance of imaging to the practice of radiation oncology, asked rhetorically: "When you drove here this evening, how many of you used your headlights? You all did, of course, so you could see where you were going. That's all I'm trying to do" (Hellman S, personal communication, May 1, 2006).

Without accurate targeting, one is, at least figuratively, practicing in the dark. Target identification itself, however, can be a "moving target." Shifting patterns of clinical presentation of cancer and advances in local and systemic therapies altering patterns of failure make optimal target definition a constant, evolving challenge. Modern imaging modalities assist in this regard by improving disease detection and refining target definition, thus optimizing therapeutic results. The role of IGRT will continue to expand as newer imaging modalities are incorporated into routine use.

A key feature of IGRT is the facilitation of four-dimensional (4D) target localization. For example, reproducibly positioning the patient is an important element of fractionated RT delivery. However, both systematic and stochastic errors in patient setup contribute to variation in daily positioning. Reproducibility is also hindered by movement or changes occurring in target and normal tissues between (*inter*fraction) or even during (*intra*fraction) treatment. IGRT incorporates strategies to more accurately localize the target and optimize RT during the treatment course, ideally leading to more effective and less toxic therapy. Adjustments can take place between fractions (offline) or while the patient is in the treatment position (online). Such corrections may allow reductions of planning margins, sparing of normal tissue, or adaptation of treatment plans to optimize dose delivery.

Although targeting accuracy has always been a goal, the impetus to adopt IGRT has taken on greater importance with the growing popularity of intensity-modulated RT (IMRT) (180). Some concerns about IMRT, however, include the prolongation of treatment time and the presence of steep dose gradients. Both factors accentuate uncertainties related to target localization and heighten the need for IGRT to compensate for them.

A second impetus for IGRT is the greater need to decrease toxicity. Concurrent chemoradiotherapy is now standard treatment in many disease sites, but it is generally associated with high rates of acute toxicity. IGRT, especially when combined with IMRT, could reduce such toxicities and/or permit implementation of more aggressive, but isotoxic, regimens. In addition, interest in hypofractionation is increasing, especially in sites where it may have distinct radiobiological and/or logistical advantages (82,220). Use of high fraction sizes requires optimal target definition and stereotaxis, however, to limit complication risk. Finally, as systemic therapies improve prolonging survival, the importance of reducing chronic treatment effects becomes greater. As toxicity is often the major factor limiting the applicability of RT, it is imperative to reduce toxicity so the therapeutic role of RT is both maintained and advanced.

Lastly, the advent of functionally based imaging techniques, including positron emission tomography (PET), has been a key development. The understanding of the relationship between tumor hypoxia and both radioresistance (108) and adverse outcomes (114,198), which may be overcome by altered fractionation or dose escalation, continues to grow. The concept of a "biological target volume" has been promulgated (165), emphasizing the existence of biological heterogeneity within the target and indicating the possibility of tailoring dose and fraction size to inherent biologic characteristics. The potential radiotherapeutic applications of functional imaging are yet to be fully understood, posing one of the exciting challenges for 21st-century radiation oncology.

Image-Guided Target Delineation

An important aspect of IGRT is the incorporation of modern imaging techniques in target delineation. At most centers, CT-based planning is now commonplace, and its impact on improved target delineation is well known. Interest is now focused on incorporation of more sophisticated imaging approaches, particularly those that provide functional and biologic information.

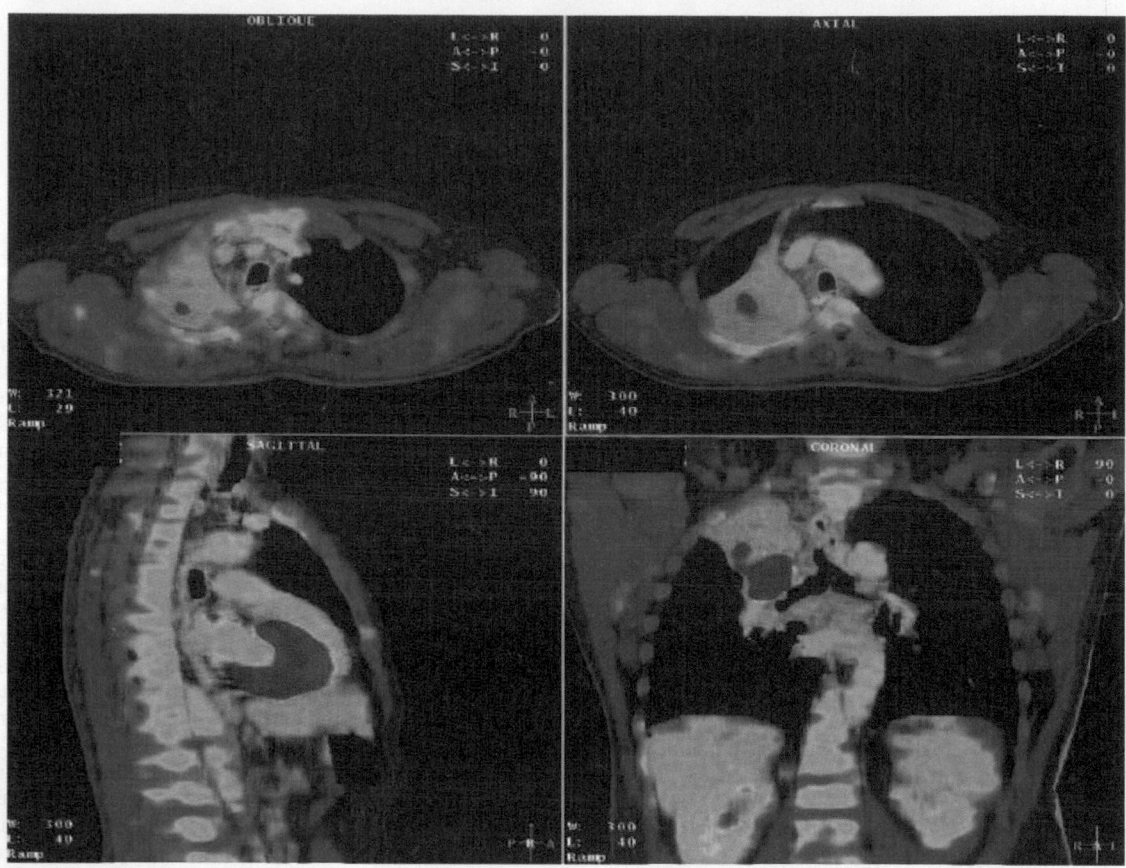

FIGURE 10.1. Fluorodeoxyglucose-positron emission tomography (FDG-PET) imaging was useful in this patient to differentiate between the primary tumor and atelectasis within the right upper lobe of the lung. (From Bradley J, Thorstad WL, Mutic S, et al. Impact of FDG-PET on radiation therapy volume delineation in non-small-cell lung cancer. *Int J Radiat Oncol Biol Phys* 2004;59[1]:78–86, with permission.)

Positron Emission Tomography

PET has made key contributions to the staging and treatment of cancer (172,216,242,243), enabling better selection and design of appropriate therapy for each patient. Most studies have focused on 18-fluorodeoxyglucose ([18]FDG). However, a variety of other radioactive tracers have been used, including ^{11}C-methionine (^{11}C-MET), ^{11}C-acetate, [11]C- or ^{18}F-choline, ^{18}F-thymidine ([18]FLT), ^{18}F-misonidazole (^{18}F-MISO), ^{18}F-azomycin arabinoside (^{18}F-FAZA), and [60]Cu(II)-diacetyl-bis(N[4]-methylosemicarbazone) ([60]Cu-ATSM). [15]O and [13]N—labeled H_2O, CO_2, O_2, or NH_3—molecules have also been used to measure blood flow or identify necrosis with PET (213), and other novel PET tracers are continually being developed and tested.

Multiple studies have investigated the role of [18]FDG-PET in RT planning for non–small cell lung cancer (NSCLC) (9,32,60,287). [18]FDG-PET imaging alters treatment volumes in approximately 40% of patients (103). It is particularly valuable in distinguishing tumor from atelectasis (88,209), which can otherwise be difficult on CT (Fig. 10.1). Vanuytsel et al. (287) found that [18]FDG-PET-CT altered treatment volumes in 45/73 (62%) lymph node positive patients staged by mediastinoscopy; in 16 the volume was enlarged, and in 29 it was contracted. Bradley et al. (32) confirmed the utility of [18]FDG-PET in NSCLC treatment planning, noting significant changes in the gross tumor volume (GTV) and planning target volumes (PTV) in 58% of patients. Interobserver target definition is also improved with PET (9).

Studies of [18]FDG-PET in head and neck cancer have found similar results, with RT volumes frequently altered after incorporating PET imaging (88,103,209,243,244). PET-guided volumes are more often smaller than those based on CT, but may be larger in some cases (209). In a study of 40 head and neck cancer patients, Paulino et al. (209) compared IMRT plans based on [18]FDG-PET to those based on CT. In 25% of patients, CT-based plans were suboptimal in covering the PET-delineated GTV. In a prospective analysis of 20 patients, Schwartz et al. (244) found that IMRT plans could be optimized with the aid of [18]FDG-PET-CT to improve parotid and laryngeal sparing and allow dose escalation up to 81 Gy. Although promising, concern exists regarding the technical aspects of PET-guided RT in head and neck cancer, including difficulties in establishing optimal image registration (98) and large interobserver variability in target definition (228).

[18]FDG-PET also appears useful in RT planning in other sites, notably esophageal (159,290,296) and pelvic (74,190) tumors. For example, Wieder et al. (296) examined changes in tumor [18]FDG avidity in patients undergoing preoperative chemoradiotherapy for esophageal carcinoma (Fig. 10.2). In 27 patients undergoing midtreatment [18]FDG-PET, a decline in standardized uptake value (SUV) >30% was associated with improved 2-year overall survival and histopathologic response. Investigators from Washington University have shown the feasibility of [18]FDG-PET-guided targeting for cervical cancer patients with involved para-aortic lymph nodes (189). With IMRT, doses up to 59.4 Gy can be accomplished with acceptable sparing of normal tissues.

Application of [18]FDG-PET in central nervous system (CNS) tumors is limited by high background uptake of FDG by normal brain cells (100). ^{11}C-MET may overcome this limitation, since its uptake in neural tissue is low. Grosu et al. (106)

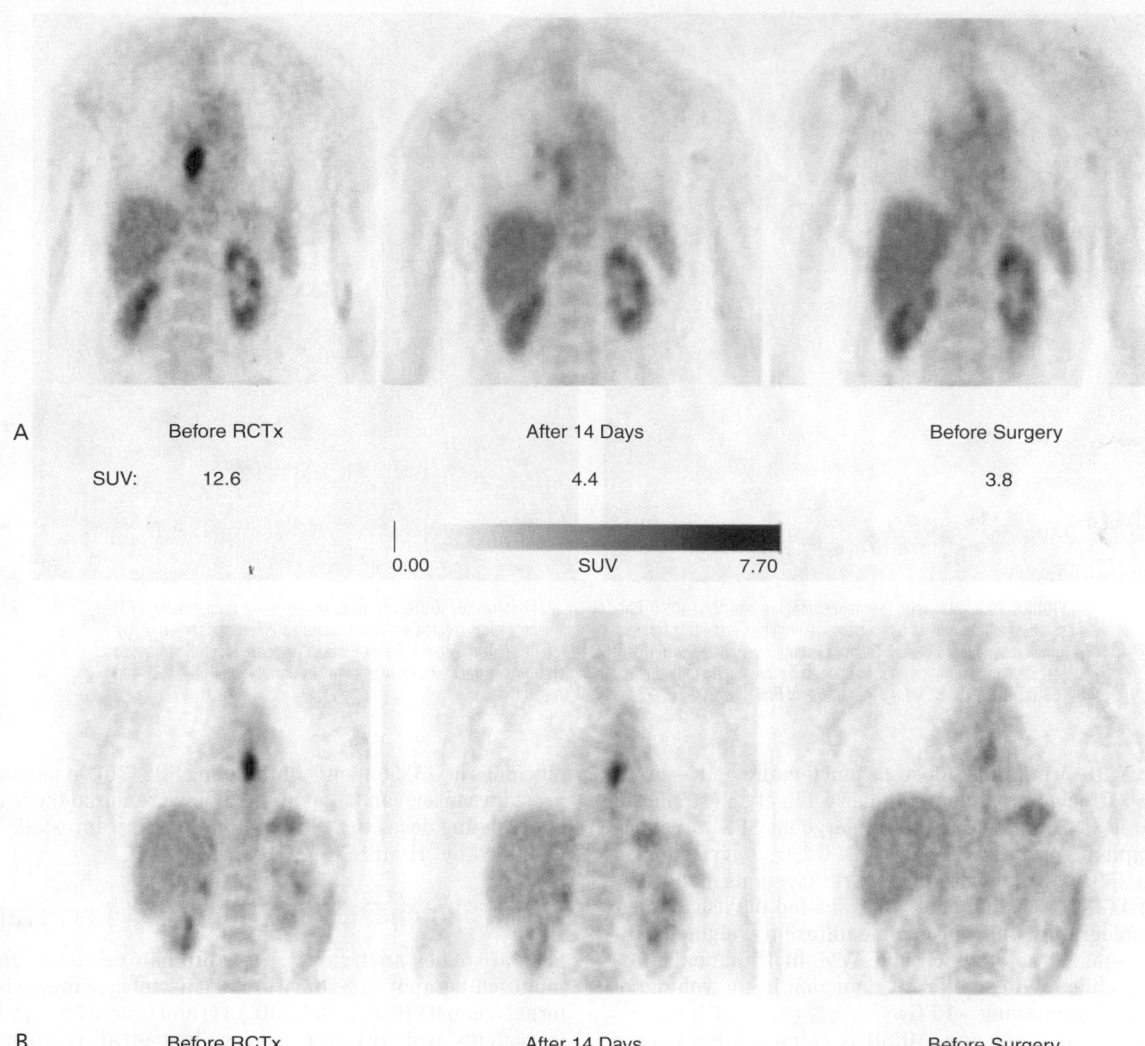

FIGURE 10.2. Coronal slices from fluorodeoxyglucose-positron emission tomography (FDG-PET) scans in patients with histopathologically responding **(A)** and nonresponding **(B)** esophageal cancer. In the responding tumor, FDG uptake decreased to background levels 14 days after beginning chemoradiotherapy. At the same time point in the non-responding tumor, FDG uptake is essentially unchanged. (From Wieder HA, Brucher BL, Zimmermann F, et al. Time course of tumor metabolic activity during chemoradiotherapy of esophageal squamous cell carcinoma and response to treatment. *J Clin Oncol* 2004;22:900–908, with permission.)

analyzed 39 resected glioblastoma multiforme (GBM) patients; in 29 patients (74%), ^{11}C-MET uptake extended (up to 4.5 cm) beyond the tumor identified by magnetic resonance imaging (MRI). ^{11}C-MET may also be useful in the delineation of CNS tumors with high interobserver reproducibility (e.g. meningioma) (105). Both ^{11}C-MET- and [18]FDG-PET have been used in target design for stereotactic radiosurgery (SRS) and fractionated RT (105,262). A limitation of ^{11}C-based PET, however, is the short half-life of [11]C (20 minutes). Milker-Zabel et al. (181) evaluated [68]Ga-(0)-D-Phe (1)-Tyr (221)-octreotide (DOTATOC)-PET in 26 meningiomas patients, a technique that takes advantage of high expression of the somatostatin type 2 receptor that binds DOTATOC. In 19 patients, DOTATOC-PET significantly influenced target design (Fig. 10.3).

Several investigators have explored PET-guided RT using hypoxia radio tracers, including ^{18}F-MISO (227) and ^{18}F-FAZA (102). [60]Cu-ATSM, however, has attracted attention due to its potential biokinetic advantages and better resolution (225). Chao et al. (40) demonstrated the feasibility of dose-escalated IMRT treatment using [60]Cu-ATSM-PET-guided hypoxia imaging in head and neck cancer patients (Fig. 10.4). The Trans-Tasman Radiation Oncology Group correlated hypoxia identified on ^{18}F-MISO-PET with outcomes in 45 stage III or IV head and neck

cancer patients undergoing chemoradiotherapy, with or without the hypoxic cytotoxin tirapazamine (230). Baseline hypoxia and residual hypoxia (detected on ^{18}F-MISO-PET scans at week 4 or 5 of treatment) were correlated with higher rates of locoregional failure. Four of six patients with residual hypoxia recurred locally compared to 4/23 patients without residual hypoxia.

Other applications of [18]FDG-PET relevant to IGRT include automated target delineation techniques (48) and PET-guided intracavitary brachytherapy planning for cervical cancer (189). In summary, an emerging body of literature supports PET as a useful modality for image-guided treatment planning. Future research will hopefully clarify the optimal utilization of this technology to improve cancer treatment.

Magnetic Resonance Imaging

Numerous studies have established the advantages of MRI in defining targets, with the clearest benefits seen in CNS (7), head and neck (69), and prostate cancers (35,206). MR simulators are now becoming increasingly available (35).

In addition to conventional MRI, functional MRI (fMRI) has been used to guide RT planning. Hamilton et al. (109) explored

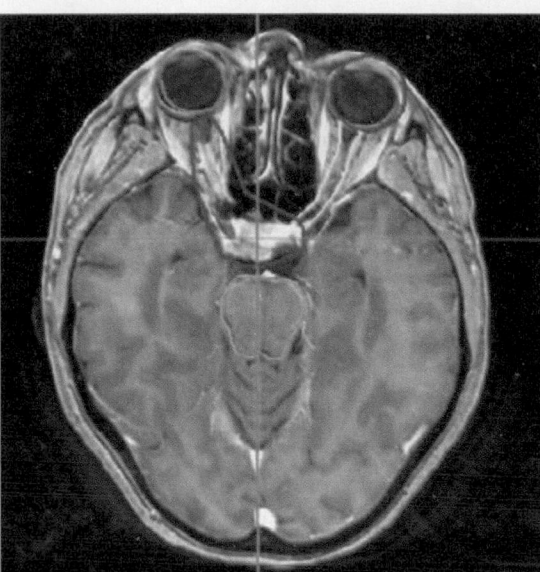
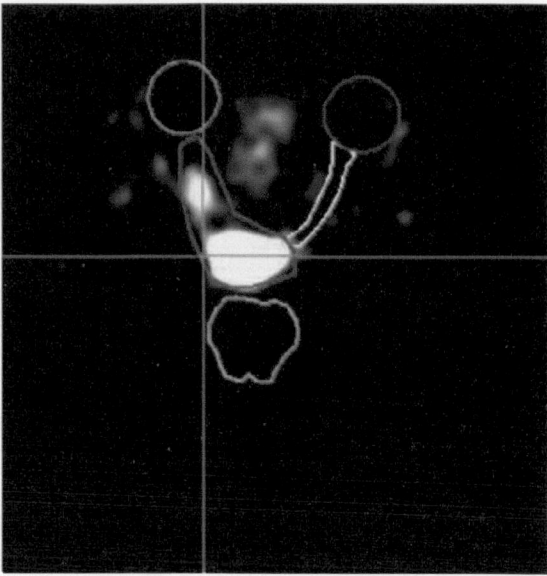

FIGURE 10.3. Magnetic resonance imaging and ^{68}Ga-(0)-D-Phe (1)-Tyr (221)-octreotide (DOTATOC) positron emission tomography (PET) scans of a patient with a recurrent meningioma extending from the right sphenoid wing, treated with fractionated stereotactic radiotherapy. Tumor extension to the orbital apex is better visualized with DOTATOC-PET. (From Milker-Zabel S, Zabel-du Bois A, Henze M, et al. Improved target volume definition for fractionated stereotactic radiotherapy in patients with intracranial meningiomas by correlation of CT, MRI, and [68Ga]-DOTATOC-PET. *Int J Radiat Oncol Biol Phys* 2006;65:222–227, with permission.)

the use of fMRI to minimize dose to functionally active brain areas in an astrocytoma patient. Similarly, Liu et al. (169) used fMRI in three CNS tumor patients undergoing SRS to reduce dose to eloquent cortex by 30% to 40%. Others have reported the utility of fMRI to guide targeting of arteriovenous malformations (AVMs) (239). Aoyama et al. (6) evaluated the use of magnetoencephalography and anisotropic diffusion weighted MRI to plan 20 patients, 15 of which had AVM. In 15 patients, targets were modified with significant reduction in the volume of sensitive regions receiving >15 Gy.

MR-spectroscopic imaging (MRSI) is gaining interest as a technique for image-guided treatment planning. ^{1}H-MRSI has been shown to be useful for planning in low- and high-grade gliomas (217,218). Moreover, exclusion of metabolically active areas identified by ^{1}H-MRSI has been associated with worse

outcomes in GBM patients undergoing SRS (36). In patients with prostate cancer, van Lin et al. (286) have reported the feasibility of escalating doses to 90 Gy to dominant intraprostatic lesions identified by ^{1}H-MRSI (Fig. 10.5).

Single Photon Emission Computed Tomography

Several studies analyzing ^{111}In-capromab pendetide radioimmunoscintigraphy (RIS) have found it useful in planning both external beam RT (EBRT) (87,130,131) and brachytherapy (67,68) in patients with prostate cancer. Jani et al. (130) reported that RIS influenced RT volumes and decision making in a significant proportion of patients undergoing postprostatectomy salvage RT. Of 54 evaluable patients, 18.5% had treatment plans altered by RIS, including four who were not offered RT

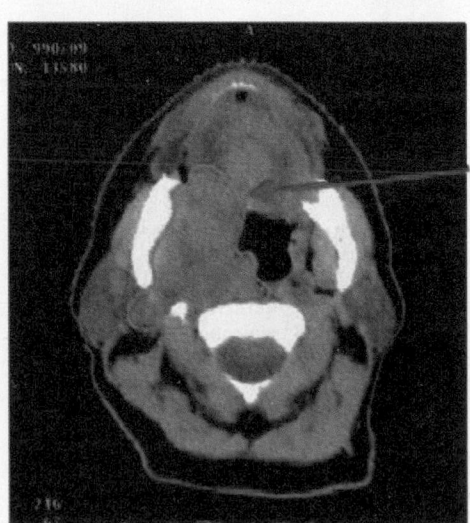

Tumor volume was defined on CT scan

The tumor contour was shown on the corresponding ^{60}Cu-ATSM image after image registration and fusion

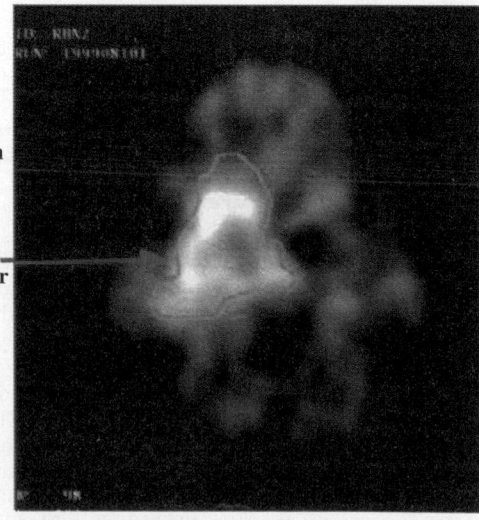

FIGURE 10.4. Comparison of computed tomography and fused ^{60}Cu-ATSM (^{60}Cu[II]-diacetyl-bis[N^4-methylosemicarbazone]) positron emission tomography scans delineating the gross tumor volume and its ATSM-avid fraction. (From Chao KS, Bosch WR, Mutic S, et al. A novel approach to overcome hypoxic tumor resistance: Cu-ATSM-guided intensity-modulated radiation therapy. *Int J Radiat Oncol Biol Phys* 2001;49:1171–1182, with permission.)

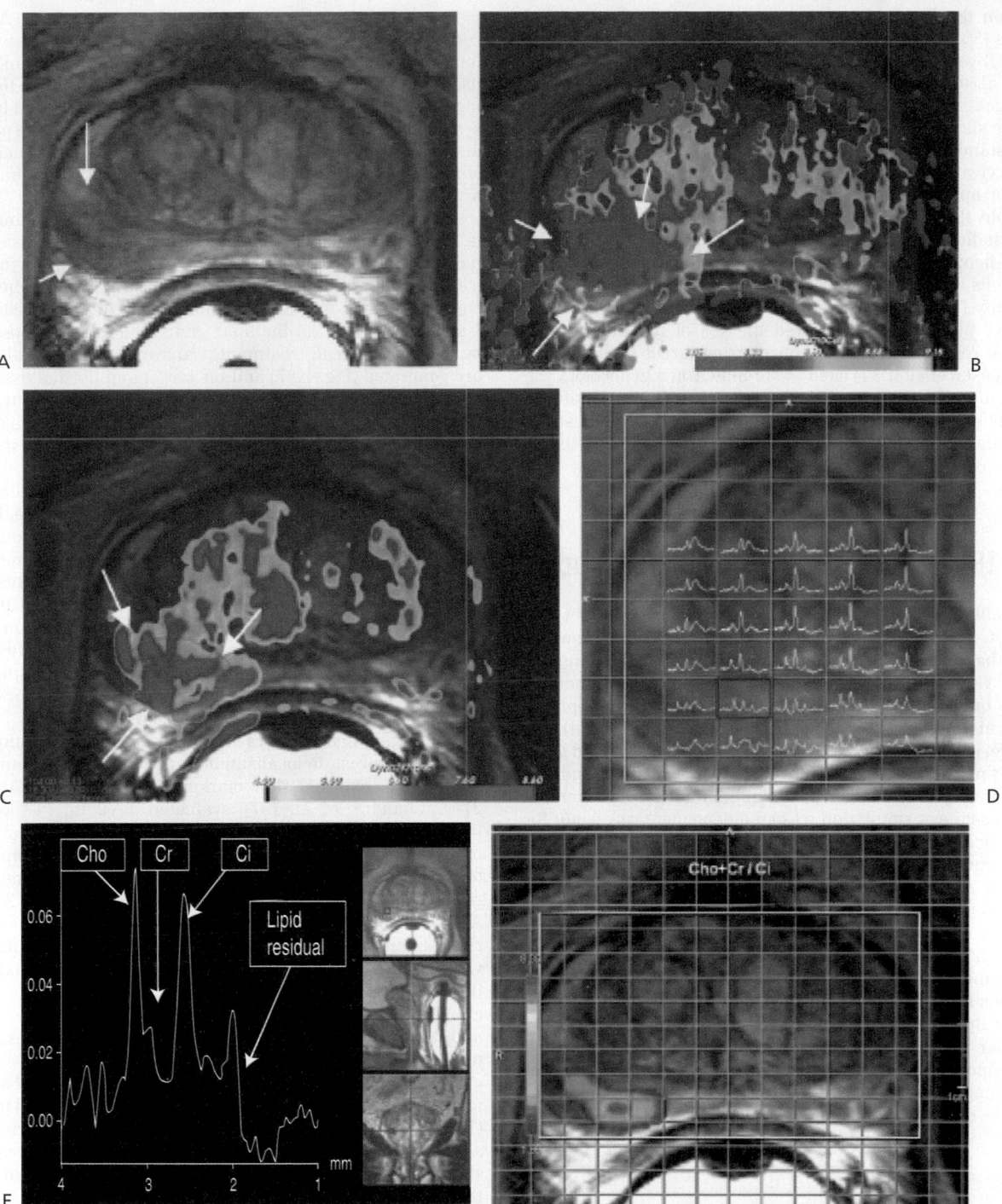

FIGURE 10.5. Dynamic contrast-enhanced (DCE) magnetic resonance imaging (MRI) and ¹H-spectroscopic MR-spectroscopic imaging (MRSI) results for a prostate cancer patient with a dominant intraprostatic lesion. **A:** Axial T_2-weighted image with decreased signal intensity in the right peripheral zone (*arrows*), without evidence of capsular invasion. **B,C:** DCE-MRI results: (B) Start-of-enhancement parameter demonstrated earlier enhancement in part of low-signal-intensity lesion (*arrows*) compared with the left peripheral zone. (C) Volume transfer constant was elevated in low-signal-intensity lesion (*arrows*) indicating tumor tissue. **D:** MRSI detected elevated choline and low citrate peaks in seven voxels. Blue box indicates voxel from which spectrum originated. **E:** ¹H-MRI spectrum from voxel in right peripheral zone. Increased choline (Cho) plus creatinine (Cr)/citrate(Ci) ratio indicated prostate cancer. **F:** Strongly interpolated (choline+creatinine)/citrate map was used to visualize MRSI-based tumor nodule. (From van Lin EN, Futterer JJ, Heijmink SW, et al. IMRT boost dose planning on dominant intraprostatic lesions: gold marker-based three-dimensional fusion of CT with dynamic contrast-enhanced and 1H-spectroscopic MRI. *Int J Radiat Oncol Biol Phys* 2006;65:291–303, with permission.)

based on the RIS findings. In a multivariate analysis of 107 patients (53 planned with RIS), RIS was associated with an improved 3-year biochemical failure-free survival (bFFS) (131). Ellis et al. (68) treated 80 low-intermediate risk prostate cancer patients with RIS-assisted brachytherapy. Regions of the prostate showing increased RIS uptake were prescribed 150% of the standard dose. The overall 4-year biochemical failure-free survival was 97.4%.

Other applications of single photon emission computed tomography (SPECT)-guided treatment planning have been studied, including [123]IMT SPECT for gliomas (101,104) and meta-[123]iodo-benzylguanidine (MIBG) scans for neuroblastoma (77). In patients with NSCLC, Christian et al. (46) used ^{99m}Tc-SPECT to identify functioning regions of lung for avoidance using inverse RT planning, and showed the V_{20} of functioning lung could be reduced without compromising target coverage. Finally, Roeske et al. (231) used ^{99m}Tc-SPECT in a gynecology patient to identify hematopoietically active bone marrow sites in the female pelvis (Fig. 10.6A). IMRT planning could be used to reduce dose to these regions, potentially reducing the risk of hematotoxicity in patients receiving chemoradiotherapy (Fig. 10.6B).

IGRT Technologies and Clinical Studies

The problems created by inter- and intrafraction target and normal tissue motion have long been recognized. Innumerable studies have quantified the magnitude of motion and setup errors for various disease sites (154). The extent of such motions may be quite substantial, leading to inaccurate or suboptimal treatment plans and poorer tumor control (70,93,117,174). For example, in a study of 127 prostate cancer patients treated *without* daily prostate localization, de Crevoisier et al. (56) found that significant rectal distension resulting in anterior displacement of the prostate at simulation was an independent risk factor for biochemical failure.

Strategies to address motion have included wide margins, elaborate immobilization techniques, resimulation and replanning, and portal radiography. IGRT approaches take advantage of more frequent and sophisticated imaging to setup the patient and localize the target with greater accuracy, ostensibly improving treatment delivery and allowing reduction of margins.

In this section, the various IGRT technologies developed to address interfraction and intrafraction motion are reviewed. Particular attention is placed on their clinical applications and data supporting their use. Issues surrounding respiratory motion management (e.g., 4D CT and respiratory gating) are discussed in detail in the following section.

Ultrasound Systems

The use of high-frequency sound waves to produce images of internal anatomy, ultrasound is one of the most common IGRT approaches in current practice. Although three operational modes are available, B (brightness) mode is the primary one used. The ultrasound process involves the emission of high-frequency sound waves by a transducer encased in a probe applied to the skin surface. These waves are partly reflected (as "echoes") when a change in impedance is encountered due to density differences between tissues (e.g., between the prostate and rectum). The time an echo takes to return is used to calculate the depth of the tissue interface. Image information is obtained along the beamline of the probe, with a complete two-dimensional (2D) or three-dimensional (3D) image created by sweeping across the region of interest. Readers interested in a more complete description of the physics of ultrasound are referred elsewhere (110).

Several ultrasound systems are currently available. An issue common to all is the necessity to map the image coordinate system to the linear accelerator (linac) coordinate system, which itself is mapped to the simulation images. This is done by tracking the position of a stereotactic arm or by an infrared imaging system to detect the probe position. The location of the patient's anatomy prior to beam-on is thus determined and the necessary shifts to bring the anatomy back into its position at simulation are calculated.

The most common ultrasound system in current clinical use is the B-mode acquisition and targeting (BAT) transabdominal system (NOMOS Radiation Oncology Division, North American Scientific, Chatsworth, CA), consisting of a probe and a computer-based targeting system. The probe is registered to a stereotactic arm on the linac gantry, allowing its position to be tracked. Prior to treatment, transverse and sagittal images are generated (Fig. 10.7) and the target and normal tissue contours from the planning CT scan are overlaid on the ultrasound images. If the target is displaced, the CT structures are maneuvered on a touch-screen and the necessary 3D couch shifts are calculated.

Another system in use is SonArray (Varian Medical Systems, Palo Alto, CA), which combines ultrasound localization with an optical guidance system to track the position of the probe in the treatment room (29,272). A similar system is available from BrainLAB (Heimstetten, Germany). The I-Beam system (Computerized Medical Systems Inc, St. Louis, MO) uses a machine vision pattern recognition technique to calibrate the probe relative to the gantry. Restitu (Resonant Medical Inc., Montreal, Canada) obtains ultrasound images in both the treatment and simulation rooms, eliminating potential errors inherent in cross-modality image comparisons.

Numerous investigators have compared ultrasound-based systems for prostate localization with conventional setup techniques (i.e., external skin markers) (37,84,155,158,167,245, 274). Chandra et al. (37) evaluated BAT in 147 prostate IMRT patients and reported interfraction standard deviations of prostate position of 4.9, 4.4, and 2.8 mm in the anteroposterior (AP), superior-inferior (SI) and lateral (RL) dimensions, respectively (37). The percentage of shifts >5 mm was 28.6% in AP, 23% in SI, and 9% in RL, respectively. In a review of nine series, Kuban et al. (148) reported that shifts from the initial setup were greatest in the AP direction, where standard deviations in the various studies ranged from 2.7 to 6.4 mm. Standard deviations in the SI and RL directions ranged from 2.8 to 7.3 mm and 2.1 to 4.6 mm, respectively, with maximum values of 30.3 mm and 34.9 mm.

Several investigators have evaluated setup shifts based on ultrasound in prostate patients undergoing daily portal imaging (167,274), removing the impact of patient setup uncertainty. In a study of 35 patients, Little et al. (168) reported mean BAT shifts of −1.3, −1.6, and −0.89 mm in the AP, SI and RL directions, respectively. In contrast, Trichter and Ennis (274) reported larger mean shifts in a cohort of 10 patients, namely 4.3 mm, 3.2 mm, and 3 mm in the AP, SI, and RL directions, respectively. The margins necessary to cover the prostate at the 95% confidence level *without* daily BAT (despite portal imaging) were 9.2, 14.6, and 10.2 mm in the RL, SI, and AP directions, respectively. Organ motion was found to be greater than setup error.

Although ultrasound-based localization accounts for interfraction organ motion, it does not address intrafraction motion. Fortunately, the magnitude of such motion in patients with prostate cancer appears to be small. In a study of 20 patients undergoing pre- and posttherapy BAT, Huang et al. (124) noted mean shifts of 0.01 ± 0.4 mm, 0.2 ± 1.3 mm and 0.1 ± 1 mm in the RL, AP, and SI directions, respectively. However, while Trichter and Ennis (274) similarly noted small mean intrafraction shifts using BAT pre- and posttherapy, large

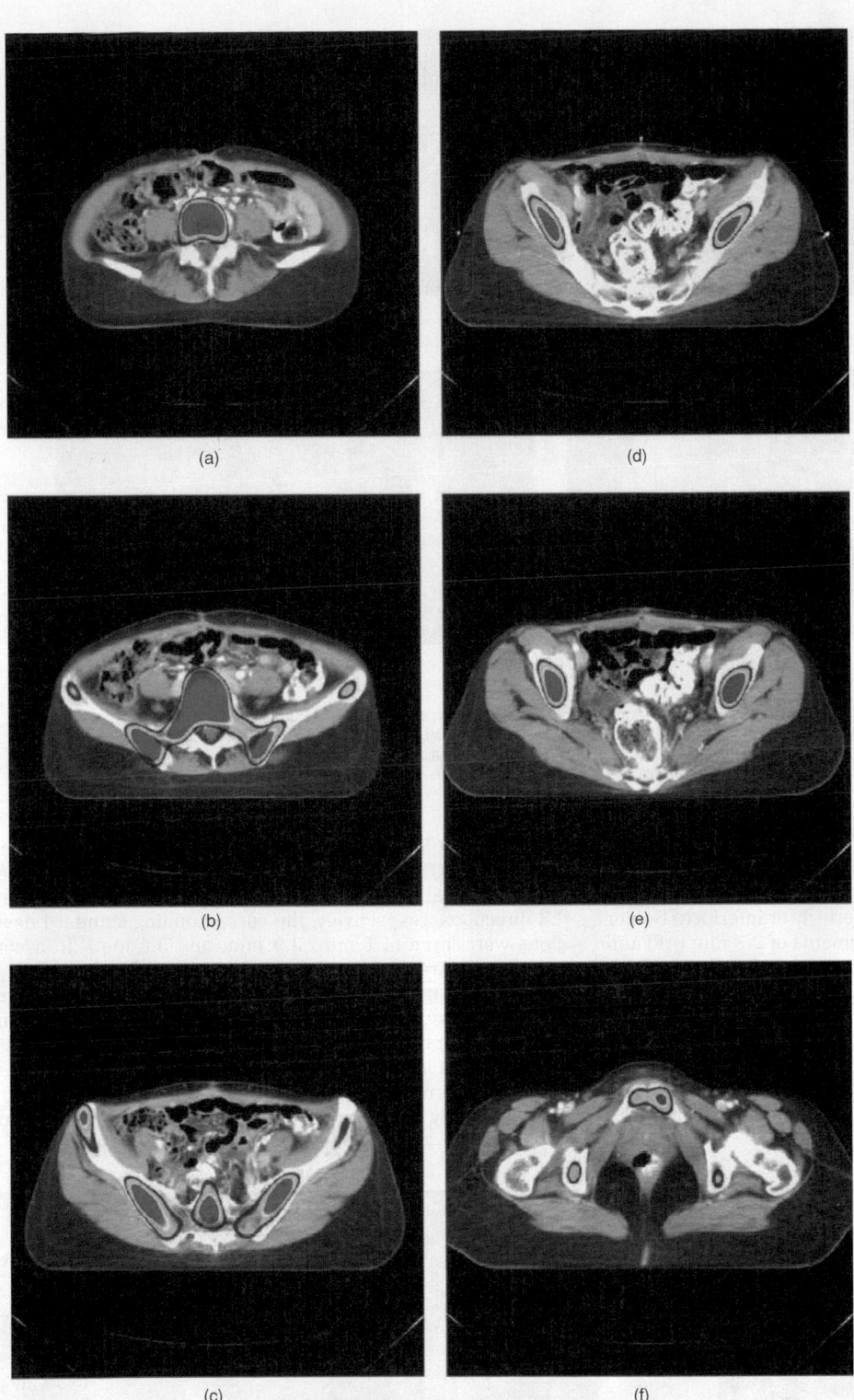

FIGURE 10.6. A: Colorwash overlay of single photon emission computed tomography (SPECT) bone marrow images on planning computed tomography (CT) images of a patient with cervical cancer. *(a)* Lumbar vertebrae; *(b)* Lumbar vertebrae and iliac crests; *(c)* Sacrum and iliac crest; *(d)* Mid-pelvis; *(e)* Hip; *(f)* Pubic symphysis.)

A

maximum shifts were noted: 8.1, 20.4, and 8.3 mm in the AP, SI, and RL directions, respectively.

An important concern is the added time required with ultrasound-based approaches. However, image acquisition and positional adjustments at experienced centers require 5 minutes or less (37,274). Additional time is necessary when the technology is first adopted and if changes are checked online by a physician (84). At most centers, adjustments are made by therapists. Fortunately, major misalignments are infrequent (37).

Other concerns include image quality, interuser variability and reproducibility, and probe-induced organ motion. Although some centers report high rates (95%) of acceptable image quality (37), others note less favorable rates (66% to 83%) (155,245). Poor image quality appears to be correlated with larger skin-to-prostate distances, increased thickness of tissue anterior to the bladder, and less prostate gland present superior to the symphysis (245). Most (85,245,274) but not all (71,155) investigators have reported high rates of reproducibility and low variability using ultrasound-based prostate localization techniques.

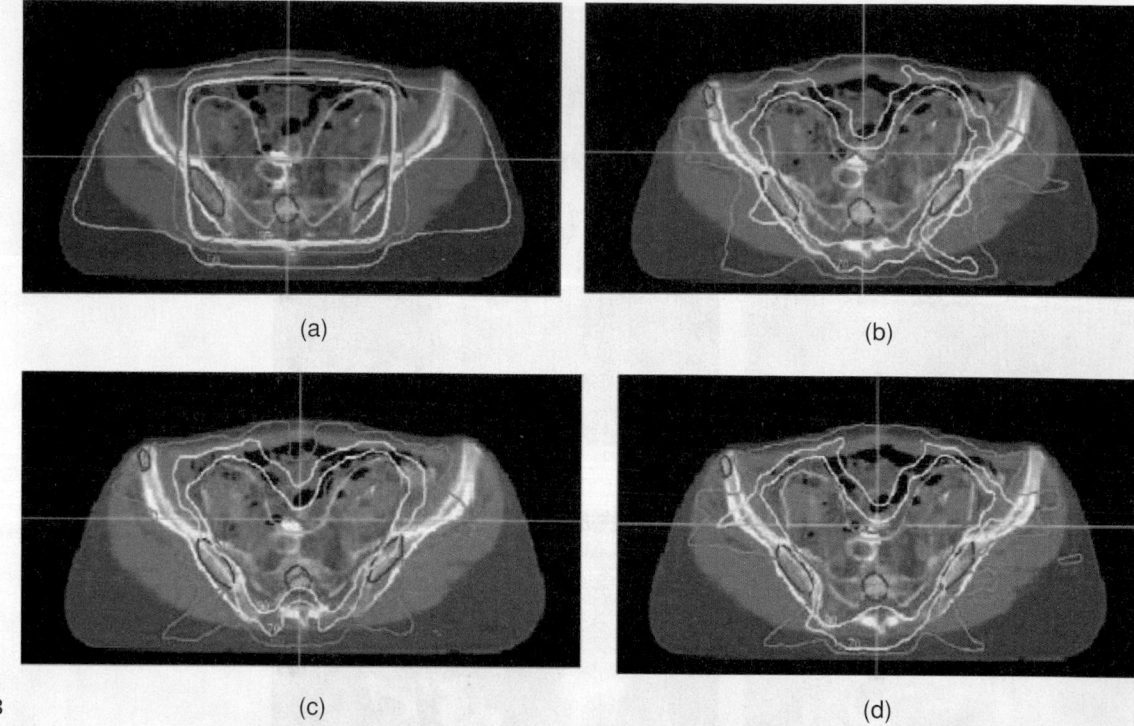

(a)   (b)

B   (c)   (d)

FIGURE 10.6. (Continued) **B:** Isodose curves overlaid on an axial CT slice in a cervical cancer patient for *(a)* four-field pelvic radiation therapy (PRT); *(b)* intensity-modulated (IM)-PRT; *(c)* IM-PRT to spare iliac bone marrow (BM); *(d)* IM-PRT to spare SPECT-identified BM. (Both figures from Roeske JC, Lujan A, Reba RC, et al. Incorporation of SPECT bone marrow imaging into intensity modulated whole-pelvic radiation therapy treatment planning for gynecologic malignancies. *Radiother Oncol* 2005;77:11–17, with permission.)

Potential probe-induced motion has received considerable attention (8,37,63,245,274). Serago et al. (245) noted discernible displacements in 7/16 prostate patients, with average displacements of 3.1 mm, either posteriorly or inferiorly. Dobler et al. (63) reported maximal displacements of 2.3 mm (AP) and 1.9 mm (SI) and 2.5 degrees of rotation in 10 patients. With improper probe handling, displacements up to 1 cm were seen.

Ultrasound prostate localization has been compared with CT (65,148,157,158) and implanted fiducial markers (155,238,285). Lattanzi et al. (158) evaluated CT and BAT in 35 patients. Average disagreements between the modalities was small: −0.09 mm (AP), −0.16 mm (LR), and −0.03 mm (SI).

Dong et al. (65) compared ultrasound and CT in 15 patients treated on a CT-on-rails unit. Although mean differences were relatively small: −0.9, −0.1, and 0.7 mm in the AP, SI, and LR directions, respectively, the corresponding standard deviations were large (4.1 mm, 3.9 mm, and 3.4 mm). In a comparison of ultrasound and fiducial markers, Scarbrough et al. (238) noted significantly different shifts in 40 patients. Ultrasound was associated with significantly greater systematic and random errors than fiducial markers, leading the authors to conclude that larger expansions would be necessary using ultrasound (~9 mm) compared to fiducial markers (~3 mm). In the only study comparing different ultrasound systems, Cury

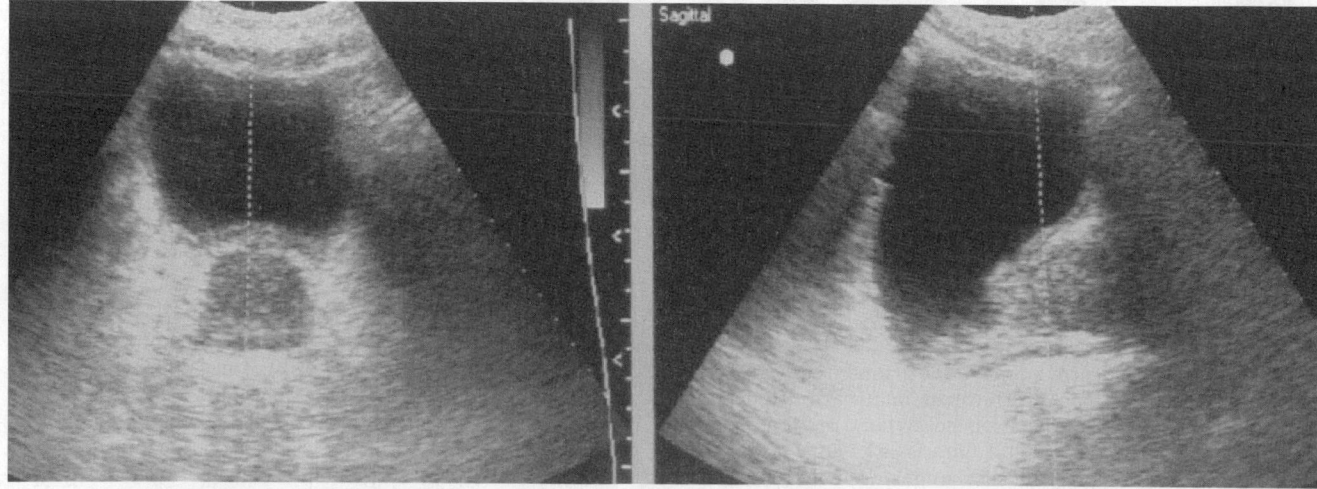

FIGURE 10.7. Example axial and sagittal ultrasound images of a prostate cancer patient performed using the B-mode acquisition and targeting (BAT) system. (From Serago CF, Chungbin SJ, Buskirk SJ, et al. Initial experience with ultrasound localization for positioning prostate cancer patients for external beam radiotherapy. *Int J Radiat Oncol Biol Phys* 2002;53:1130–1138, with permission.)

et al. (52) found significant differences in average prostate displacements up to 6 mm (SI direction) between BAT and Restitu.

Despite its popularity, limited data exist regarding the impact of ultrasound-based IGRT on patient outcome. Indirect support is garnered, however, from the excellent outcome of prostate cancer patients treated using daily ultrasound guidance. In a series of 100 patients undergoing short-course IMRT, BAT was used to allow tight margins around the target: 4 mm posteriorly, 8 mm laterally, and 5 mm in other directions (150). At a median follow-up of 66 months, the 5-year bFFS was 85%, with 5% of patients developing grade 2 or 3 rectal sequelae.

Two case series of prostate cancer patients undergoing IMRT with or without ultrasound guidance have been published (132,133). Jani et al. (132) evaluated acute urinary and rectal toxicity in 50 patients treated with BAT versus 49 patients without BAT. Although no differences were seen in urinary toxicity, BAT patients experienced less rectal toxicity. Moreover, BAT usage was the sole factor correlated with *less* rectal toxicity on multivariate analysis. In a subsequent study, Jani et al. (133) analyzed chronic sequelae in patients treated with or without BAT. Although less toxicity was noted with its use, BAT usage was not statistically significant on multivariate analysis.

Ultrasound-based IGRT approaches may also be useful in the postprostatectomy setting (44,207). Chinnaiyan et al. (44) evaluated the utility of SonArray in 16 prostate cancer patients, six of whom were treated following surgery. In postoperative patients, the average shifts from the initial setup were 5 ± 4 mm, 3 ± 3 mm, and 3 ± 4 mm in the AP, LR, and SI directions, respectively.

Clinical data evaluating ultrasound-based IGRT in other tumor sites are limited. Boda-Heggeman et al. (27) treated a patient with an inoperable liver metastasis with frameless SRS and ultrasound-guided tumor localization, using active breathing control to reduce tumor motion. Fuss et al. (86) evaluated ultrasound-based IGRT in 62 patients with upper abdominal malignancies, predominantly pancreatic cancer. The mean shifts in the x, y, and z directions were 4.9 ± 4.35 mm, 6 ± 5.31 mm, and 6 ± 6.7 mm, respectively. Meeks et al. (177) performed ultrasound-guided extracranial SRS using SonArray. In 16 patients analyzed, single-fraction doses ranging from 12.5 to 24.0 Gy were delivered without significant acute complications. In a series of 10 gallbladder cancer patients treated to a median dose of 59 Gy with daily ultrasound localization (83), all but one experienced grade 2 or less acute toxicity.

Video Systems

Video-based techniques for patient positioning have been used for over 25 years. Connor et al. (50) described a close-circuit television camera and monitor system plus a videodisc recorder that reduced positional errors to <1 mm. The recorder stored a reference image of each treatment setup and was superimposed, in reverse color, on the live camera image. More recently, investigators at the University of Chicago developed an online video "subtraction" setup system, consisting of wall- and ceiling-mounted charge-coupled device cameras linked to a computer equipped with a frame grabber (138,182). After optimal positioning, a reference image is obtained and, on subsequent days, is subtracted in real-time from live video images. Subtraction images are displayed on an in-room monitor and used to interactively realign the patient (Fig. 10.8). Milliken et al. (182) reported high levels of accuracy in both 2D and 3D repositioning using this system.

Johnson et al. (138) performed a clinical study of this system in five head and neck cancer patients undergoing twice daily RT. Conventional setup was used in the morning, with the video used simply to record the final patient position. In the afternoon, patients were first aligned with conventional techniques and then live subtraction images were used for setup

correction. Although the standard deviation of setup error using room lasers was $\sigma = 3.9$ mm, it was reduced by 56% ($\sigma = 1.7$ mm) using video setup. The entire process generally required approximately 1 minute.

Several investigators have evaluated video-based setup techniques in breast cancer patients. Baroni et al. (15) developed a video system based on optoelectronics and close-range photogrammetry that captures in real-time the position of markers on the patient that are used to monitor and adjust the patient position. Bert et al. (24) investigated a commercial stereo-vision surface imaging system (AlignRT, Vision RT Ltd, London, UK) for setup of partial-breast irradiation patients who use close-range photogrammetry to generate a 3D image of the patient's surface. The resultant image is compared to an image generated at simulation or of the patient's external surface generated from a CT data set. Phantom studies found that the system was capable of identifying submillimeter translational shifts and rotations of <0.1 degree.

Investigators at Johns Hopkins University have developed a real-time 3D video-guided IMRT approach in breast cancer patients using a video camera system capable of capturing full-frame 3D surface images through a single video snapshot (62,162). Patient setup parameters are determined semiautomatically, and the IMRT leaf segments are modified in real-time. Unlike other video approaches, this system compensates for changes in surface topology by modifying the treatment plan rather than adjusting the patient position. This system is also being applied to patients undergoing fractionated stereotactic RT (164).

Planar Imaging Systems

Electronic Portal Imaging Devices

Electronic portal imaging devices (EPIDs) provide a means of generating an electronic image of a treatment field with the patient on the treatment table. Similar to conventional portal imaging, EPIDs produce images using the therapeutic (megavoltage) beam. However, EPIDs overcome many of the limitations of conventional port films, including delays due to image processing. Moreover, EPID images can be digitally processed for better visualization of the relevant anatomy and stored for offline review.

Numerous EPID classes have been introduced including video-based, liquid ion chamber, and solid state systems. Most commercial systems in use today are based on flat-panel amorphous silicon (aSi) detectors. With this method, a scintillator first converts x-rays to visible light. A photodiode array then converts the light to electrons, which in turn activate pixels in a layer of aSi. The pixels are then read out in successive rows, processed, and displayed on a computer screen for viewing. Readers interested in an overview of EPID technologies are referred to several excellent reviews (5,30).

Clinical studies illustrating the benefits of EPID-based IGRT approaches initially appeared in the early 1990s (57,94,180). De Neve et al. (57) evaluated EPID as an online setup tool in 21 patients. Of 533 setups, 92 (17.2%) were adjusted. Michalski et al. (180) randomized 32 patients to EPID monitoring versus standard port films. Of the 1,011 fields monitored, 1.4% required an intervention, with the percentage of errors >1 cm decreasing from 11.2% to 6.1% ($p < .01$), primarily in pelvic patients. The value of EPID-based setup techniques in many disease sites, including head and neck (16), lung (54), breast (75), and pelvic (204) cancers, has been reviewed by Herman (121).

Several investigators have reviewed their experience using online EPID IGRT approaches (267,284) (Fig. 10.9). In 16 inoperable lung cancer patients, Van de Steene et al. (284) used the locations of the lung apices and the carina for alignment. In-house software was used to calculate translational and

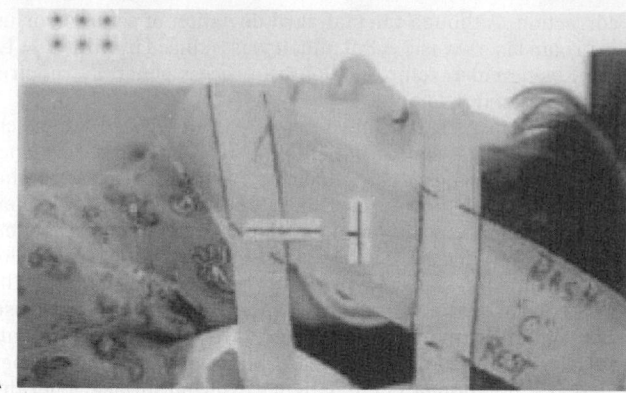

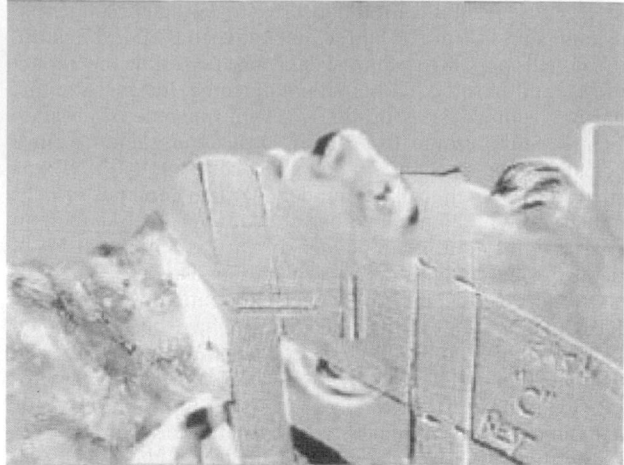

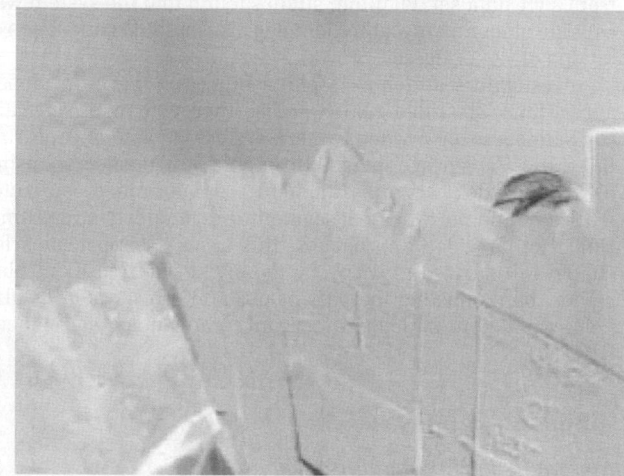

FIGURE 10.8. The video-subtraction positioning system involves the acquisition of a reference image **(A)** on the first day of treatment after positioning based on portal imaging. On subsequent treatment days, reference images are retrieved from the archive and subtracted in real-time from the live video **(B)**. Using a computer monitor in the treatment room, the therapists utilize the live subtraction images to interactively fine tune the patient's position **(C)**. (From Johnson S, Milliken BD, Hadley SW, et al. Initial clinical experience with a video-based patient positioning system. *Int J Radiat Oncol Biol Phys* 1999;45:205–213, with permission.)

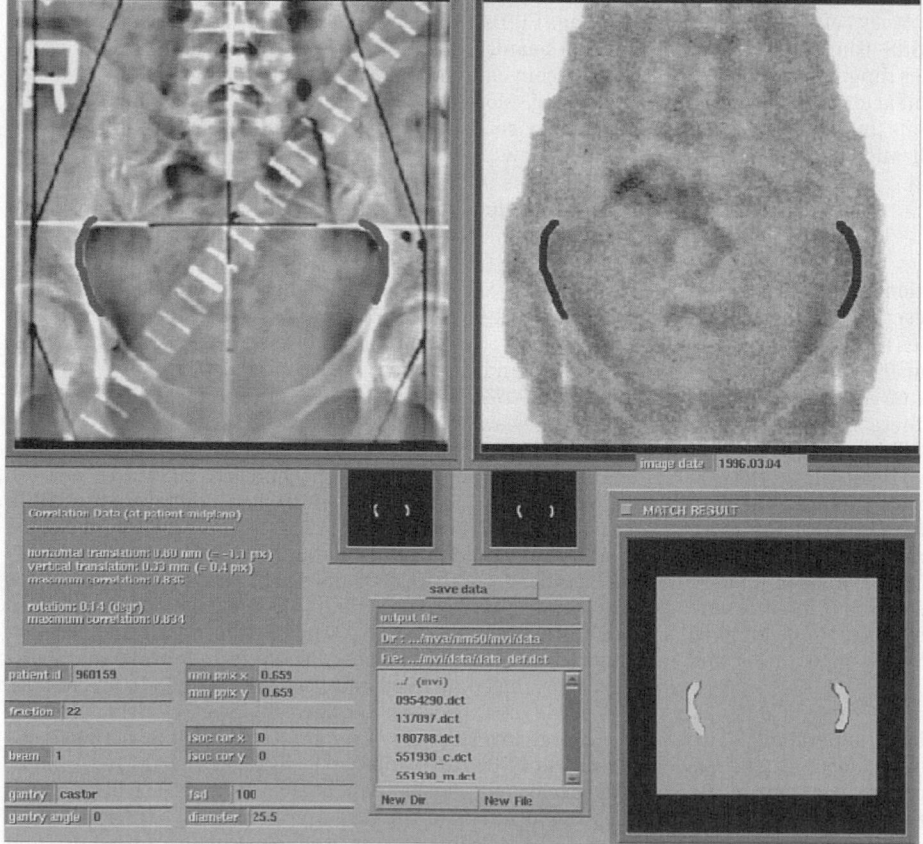

FIGURE 10.9. Illustration of an online positioning approach using electronic portal imaging devices (EPID) in a gynecology patient. The reference image is shown in the left upper image with a manually drawn contour (*gray*). In the upper right image, an EPID image is shown on which a similar structure is contoured (*black*). The two images in the middle depict the binary images used from the cross-correlation match. The match result is visualized in the lower right image; where the black and gray contours overlap, the contours become light gray. Resulting translation values are shown on the bottom left. (From Stroom JC, Olofsen-van Acht MJJ, Quint S, et al. Online setup corrections during radiotherapy of patients with gynecologic tumors. *Int J Radiat Oncol Biol Phys* 2000;46:499–506, with permission.)

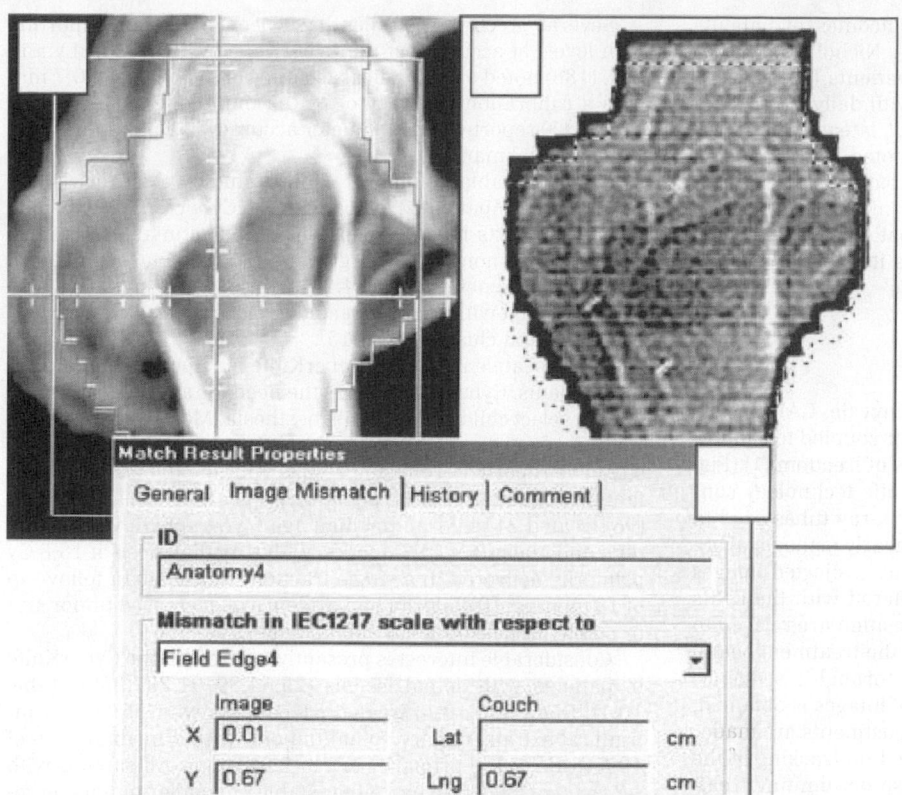

FIGURE 10.10. Electronic portal imaging devices (EPID) as an online setup approach in a prostate cancer patient with implanted fiducial markers. Marker positions on the initial digitally reconstructed radiograph (DRR) obtained at simulation are compared with the online EPID image. A "Mismatch Summary" is obtained describing couch translations required to correct for prostate motion and setup errors. (From Chung PWM, Haycocks T, Brown T, et al. Online aSi portal imaging of implanted fiducial markers for the reduction of interfraction error during conformal radiotherapy of prostate carcinoma. *Int J Radiat Oncol Biol Phys* 2004;60:329–334, with permission.)

rotational errors. If either exceeded 2 mm, a correction was performed, resulting in corrections in 85% of set-ups.

Concerns over increased workload and excess dose have increased interest in offline EPID approaches. One such approach is the so-called *shrinking action level* (SAL) strategy (17). Initially, EPID images are obtained on a given number (N_{max}) of consecutive days. The 3D setup deviation and length of the average vectors of the 3D setup deviation in the x, y, and z directions are then calculated offline and the length of the deviation vector is compared to a predetermined "action level." If exceeded, a setup correction is performed at the next session. The feasibility of this approach was assessed in a multi-institutional prostate cancer trial (18). Prior to its application, the percentage of mean 3D deviations >5 mm was 26% to 36%. After it was applied, accuracy improved, with mean 3D deviations >5 mm ranging from 0% to 1.6%. Favorable results have also been reported using the SAL approach in lung (73) and head and neck (55) cancers.

An alternative approach is the no action level (NAL) strategy, whereby the mean setup error over a fixed number of fractions is calculated and always corrected for. Using a database of 600 prostate cancer patients with measured setup errors, the NAL protocol achieved a higher level of accuracy than the SAL strategy for a similar workload (53).

Considerable attention has also been focused on EPID as a means of prostate localization in conjunction with implanted seed markers (47,120,221,289,293). Pouliot et al. (221) have presented an overview of the prostate seed marker protocol developed at the University of California–San Francisco (UCSF) using EPID. Prior to simulation, three gold markers were inserted (two laterally on each side of the prostate and one in the apex). A planning CT scan was performed, the location of each marker was contoured, and a digitally reconstructed radiograph (DRR) with the location of each marker was generated. Prior to treatment, a left lateral EPID image was obtained to assess SI and

AP shifts, requiring approximately 2 cGy of dose. Comparison of the center of mass of the markers with its expected position on the DRR was used to evaluate the need for repositioning. If shifts were >3 mm, the treatment couch was adjusted. Chung et al. (47) reported their initial experience using EPID and implanted prostate seed markers in 17 patients (Fig. 10.10). Using an action level of 3 mm, 19% of the treatment fractions were adjusted, requiring, on average, 6.1 additional minutes when no adjustments were required and 8.7 minutes when adjustments were made. Although seed marker placement is generally well tolerated, transient symptoms have been reported (59).

A concern with EPID-based marker localization is image quality. However, most investigators report excellent marker visualization (47,120,289), particularly when gold markers are used (293), with a minimum diameter of 0.9 mm (118). At the Princess Margaret Hospital, at least two gold markers were visualized in 99% of EPID images (47). High intra- and interradiation therapist reproducibility has been reported using this approach (279).

Another concern with implanted prostate markers is the potential for migration. However, numerous investigators have reported no or only minimal migration of implanted markers (47,221,240,289,293). Kupelian et al. (151) evaluated seed marker position throughout the course of treatment in 56 prostate cancer patients. Of 2,037 alignments, the average directional variation of all intermarker distances was −0.31 ± 1.41 mm. Only two markers (1%) showed frequent changes in position, most likely caused by prostate deformation. Of note, others have reported marker movement in patients undergoing hormonal therapy as the prostate involutes (198).

Limited data exist using EPID and implanted markers in other tumor sites. Kaatee et al. (139) evaluated EPID in 10 cervical cancer patients with radio-opaque tantalum markers attached to the cervix. Although image quality was very good, nearly half of the markers were lost before the completion of therapy.

Several investigators have reported outcomes of patients treated with EPID-based IGRT techniques. Nichol et al. (196) treated 140 stage T1–2 prostate cancer patients (Gleason ≤8 and PSA ≤20) to a total dose of 75.6 Gy with daily EPID setup corrections based on bony anatomy. Overall, late grade ≥2 gastrointestinal and urinary toxicities were noted in 2% and 1% of patients, respectively. Others have reported favorable results using EPID and the SAL approach (211). Unfortunately, no series has included a comparison group of patients treated without EPID-based IGRT techniques and thus its benefit remains unknown.

CyberKnife

The CyberKnife system (Accuray Inc., Sunnyvale, CA) consists of a compact x-band 6 MV linear accelerator coupled to a multi-jointed robotic manipulator with 6 degrees of freedom (1) (Fig. 10.11). The current generation of CyberKnife technology consists of two precisely calibrated diagnostic x-ray tubes fixed to the ceiling of the treatment vault and two nearly orthogonal aSi flat-panel detectors. After coarse alignment, projected images from the cameras are automatically registered with the DRRs from the planning CT. Changes in target position are relayed to the robotic arm, which adjusts pointing of the treatment beam. During treatment, the robotic arm moves through a sequence of positions (nodes). At each node, a pair of images is obtained, the patient position is determined, and adjustments are made.

CyberKnife treatment was initially based on tracking of the skeletal anatomy of the skull and upper spine, limiting treatment to tumors of the brain, head and neck, and upper spine. Subsequently, the ability to track implanted fiducial markers was introduced, allowing treatment of lower spinal tumors. More recently, software has been developed that obviates the need for implanted fiducials in spine patients and enables respiratory tracking.

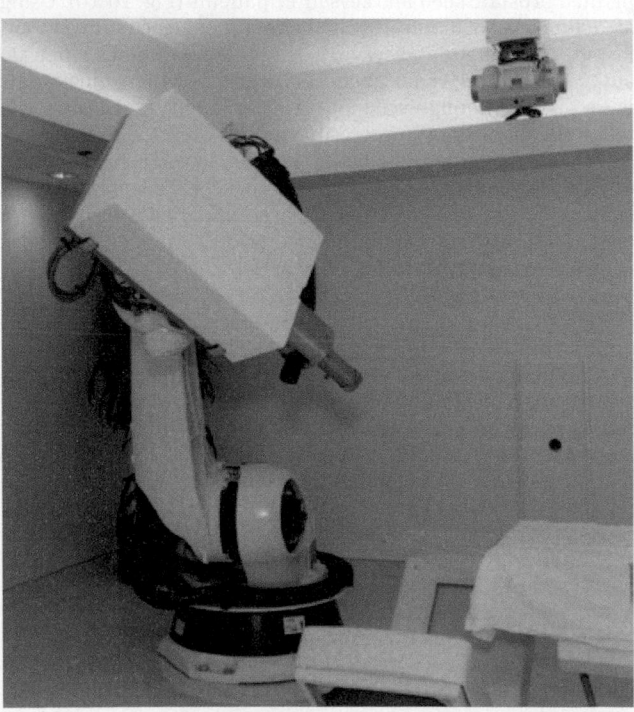

FIGURE 10.11. CyberKnife Radiosurgery System. Two amorphous silicon x-ray detectors are positioned orthogonally to the treatment couch. (From Gerszten PC, Ozhasoglu C, Burton SA, et al. Cyberknife frameless stereotactic radiosurgery for spinal lesions: clinical experience in 125 cases. *Neurosurgery* 2004;55:89–99, with permission.)

Several preclinical studies have been published reporting high levels of accuracy of the CyberKnife system. Murphy and Cox. (186) noted a mechanical accuracy of the beams of 0.7 mm with a calibration accuracy of ± 0.5 mm along each axis. Yu et al. (313) reported submillimeter accuracy in a phantom study using fiducial markers.

A considerable volume of clinical studies exist describing the outcome of patients treated with the CyberKnife. Favorable outcome reports have been published on pituitary adenomas (140), schwannomas (127), gliomas (312), metastases (249), and trigeminal neuralgia (164,232). Excellent results have also been achieved with tumors treated in close proximity to the optic nerves and chiasm (178,215).

A provocative use of the CyberKnife is in pediatric brain tumor patients. CyberKnife avoids the need for a rigid head frame and, in select children, general anesthesia. Moreover, frameless treatment can be fractionated. Investigators at Baylor University have reported promising results with the CyberKnife in infants (95) and the general pediatric population (96). Giller et al. (96) treated 21 children (median age 6 years) with various benign and malignant CNS tumors, with a median dose of 18.8 Gy primarily delivered in a single fraction. At a median follow-up of 18 months, 10 children had evidence of decreased tumor size or stable disease on follow-up imaging.

Considerable interest is presently focused on the CyberKnife in patients with spinal lesions (25,64,89–91,237,259) (Table 10.1). Dodd et al. (64) treated 51 patients with 55 benign intradural extramedullary spinal tumors, with a median dose of 19.6 Gy delivered primarily in 1 or 2 fractions. All patients with >2 years of follow-up had either stable or smaller tumors on repeat imaging. Most patients had stable or improved symptoms. One developed a spinal cord injury 8 months following treatment. Investigators at the University of Pittsburgh reported on 125 primarily malignant spinal lesions (115 patients) treated to a median dose of 14 Gy in 3 to 5 fractions (91) (Fig. 10.12). Total treatment time was 1 to 2 hours. At a median follow-up of 18 months, no patient developed new symptoms or had evidence of RT sequelae, despite the fact that 68% had received prior RT. Of 79 patients presenting with pain, 74 (94%) noted improvement. Others have reported similarly promising results in patients with benign and malignant spinal tumors (25,39,89,90, 259).

Recently, the CyberKnife is being considered in the treatment of extracraniospinal sites, notably the prostate (143) and lung (199). Interest in prostate cancer is not surprising given the growing use of implanted fiducials to localize the prostate on a daily basis with other IGRT approaches. However, outcome data remain limited (112). Nuyttens et al. (199) treated 20 patients with lung tumors in whom fiducial markers had been implanted for tumor tracking. A system of light-emitting diodes placed on the patient's abdomen was used to monitor the location of fiducials with respect to respiratory motion, and provide feedback to the robotic arm of the CyberKnife for tracking. Four-dimensional CT simulation scans were acquired and patients were treated with hypofractionated radiation (36 to 60 Gy in three fractions). With a median follow-up of 4 months, no local failures were observed. Prolonged treatment times are also a concern with using CyberKnife in sites outside the brain and spine. It is likely, therefore, that the role for CyberKnife in such patients will be limited to the delivery of hypofractionated treatment regimens.

Novalis

The Novalis system (BrainLab Inc, Westchester, IL) consists of a 6 MV linear accelerator equipped with a micromultileaf collimator. Infrared camera and stereoscopic kV x-ray imaging technologies are used for patient positioning. Two 80 to 100 kV x-ray tubes mounted in the floor of the treatment room are used

⁞⁞ Table 10.1   OUTCOME OF SPINAL TUMORS TREATED WITH THE CYBERKNIFE

Author	Pts/Lesions	Tumor Histology	Median Dose, Gy (range)	#Fractions	Median Follow-Up, Months	Outcome
Dodd [64]	51/55	Various (all benign)	19.6 (16–30)	1–5	36	100% LC[a] 25–50% improved pain 1 late spinal cord injury
Ryu [237]	16/16	Various (benign and malignant)	11–25	1–5	≥6	100% LC No complications
Sinclair [259]	15/15	AVM	20.5[b] (20–25)	2–5	27.9	86%[c] ↓volume No new symptoms, No hemorrhage
Gerszten [90]	18/18	Sacral tumors (94% malignant)	15 (12–20)	1	6	100% LC No new neurologic symptoms
Gerszten [89]	26/26	Metastases	18 (16–20)	1	16	All patients underwent kyphoplasty 92% improved pain
Gerszten [91]	115/125	108 metastases 17 benign	14 (12–20)	1	18	No new neurologic symptoms 94%[d] improved pain
Bhatnagar [25]	NS/35	Various (all benign)	16 (10–31)	1 (95%)	8	96% LC[e]

LC = local control. AVM = arteriovenous malformation.
[a]Of 28 patients with >2 years of follow-up.
[b]Mean dose.
[c]Of 7 patients with >3 years of follow-up.
[d]Of 79 patients presenting with pain.
[e]Of patients with follow-up imaging (includes non-spinal extracranial tumors).

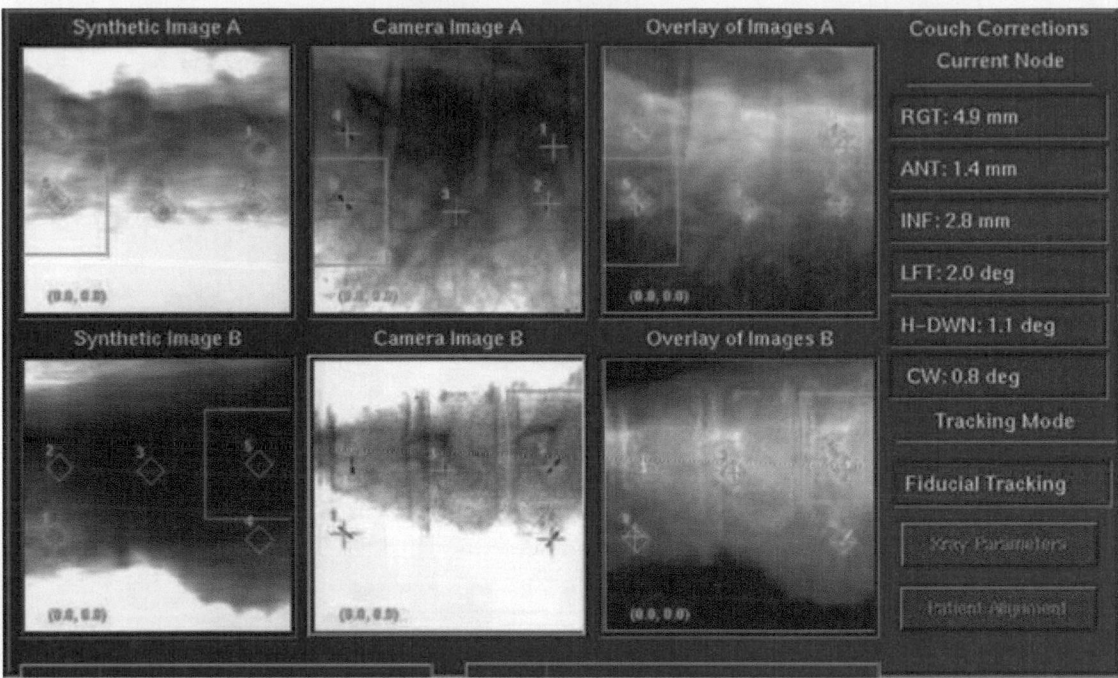

FIGURE 10.12. X-rays illustrating tracking of implanted fiducial markers in a patient with a spinal lesion treated with the CyberKnife system. The measured position of the fiducial markers is communicated to a robotic manipulator, which redirects the beam to the intended target. (From Gerszten PC, Ozhasoglu C, Burton SA, et al. Cyberknife frameless stereotactic radiosurgery for spinal lesions: clinical experience in 125 cases. *Neurosurgery* 2004;55:89–99, with permission.)

to acquire images of internal anatomy (e.g., the vertebral bodies), which are automatically compared with the DRRs from the planning CT scan. The cameras are used to detect the positions of sensors on the patient's skin, which are automatically compared with their position at simulation to determine necessary couch shifts.

In an analysis of the positional accuracy of the Novalis system, simulated infrared marker shifts revealed that positioning errors of the planned isocenter were 0.6 ± 0.3, 0.5 ± 0.2, and 0.7 ± 0.2 mm along the lateral, longitudinal, and vertical axes, respectively (310). Simulated target shifts indicated that positioning errors of the planned isocenter were 0.6 ± 0.3, 0.7 ± 0.2, and 0.5 ± 0.2 mm along the three axes. Others studies have similarly reported submillimeter accuracy with the Novalis system (224).

Various investigators have reported the outcome of patients treated on the Novalis system (42,72,210,295). In a series of 32 trigeminal neuralgia patients, Chen et al. (42) noted good to excellent pain relief in 78%. Pedroso et al. (210) treated 44 cranial AVM patients to a median dose of 15 Gy in a single fraction. The obliteration rate was 52.5%. Three patients (6.8%) bled following treatment; however, none developed significant late sequelae.

Others have reported on the use of Novalis in spinal tumors (20,58,235,236,295). Investigators at Henry Ford Hospital treated 10 spinal metastases with external beam RT (25 Gy in 10 fractions) followed by a 6 to 8 Gy SRS boost on a Novalis unit (236) (Fig. 10.13). All patients presenting with pain experienced significant relief. No acute or chronic sequelae were noted, at a median follow-up of 6 months. These same investigators reported their experience with SRS alone (10 to 16 Gy) in 49 patients with 61 spinal metastases (235). Complete and partial pain relief was noted in 85% of patients. Others have reported similarly promising results in malignant and benign spinal tumors (20,58).

The Novalis system is being increasingly used in other tumor sites. Ryu et al. (234) treated 13 head and neck cancer

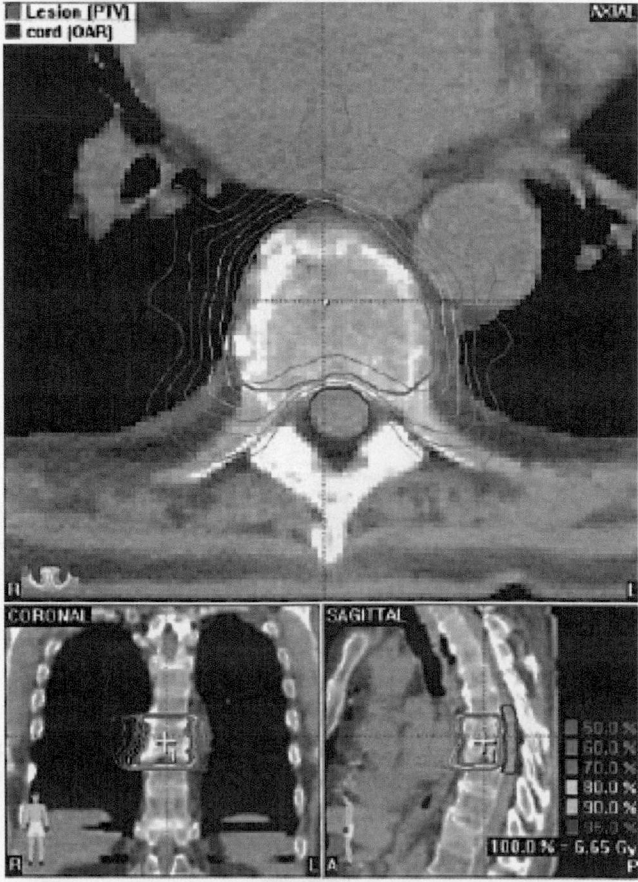

FIGURE 10.13. An intensity-modulated stereotactic spinal radiosurgery plan in a patient treated on a Novalis unit. The patient had multiple myeloma involving the seventh and eighth thoracic vertebral bodies. (From Ryu S, Yin FF, Rock J, et al. Image-guided and intensity-modulated radiosurgery for patients with spinal metastasis. *Cancer* 2003;97:2013–2018, with permission.)

tumors, with either SRS (12 to 18 Gy in one fraction) or hypofractionated RT (30 to 36 Gy in six fractions). Six patients achieved a complete and three a partial response. Soete et al. (260) reported short-term outcome of prostate cancer patients treated with hypofractionated RT (56 Gy in 3.5 Gy daily fractions). Grade 2 rectal and bladder acute toxicities were noted in 12% and 29% of patients, respectively. None experienced grade $\geq$3 toxicity. In a separate study, Soete et al. (261) noted significant improvements in positioning of prostate cancer patients using Novalis compared to conventional setup techniques. Setup errors of $\geq$5 mm occurred in 2% to 14% of patients positioning with Novalis versus 28% to 53% with conventional positioning.

Real-Time Tumor Tracking

The Real-Time Tumor-Tracking (RTRT) system (Mitsubishi Electronics Co. Ltd, Tokyo, Japan) consists of four sets of diagnostic x-ray tubes and imagers (253) (Fig. 10.14). Each x-ray unit is comprised of a 1.5 mega heat unit (MHU) x-ray tube with a fixed collimator mounted in the floor with a corresponding imager mounted in the ceiling. During treatment, two of the four x-ray systems are selected to track an implanted fiducial marker using motion tracking software (113). The treatment beam is gated to irradiate when the position of the marker coincides with its planned position.

Phantom experiments demonstrate that the RTRT system is highly accurate, with geometric accuracy better than 1.5 mm for moving targets up to a speed of 40 mm/sec. Dose due to the diagnostic x-ray monitoring ranges from 0.01% to 1% of the

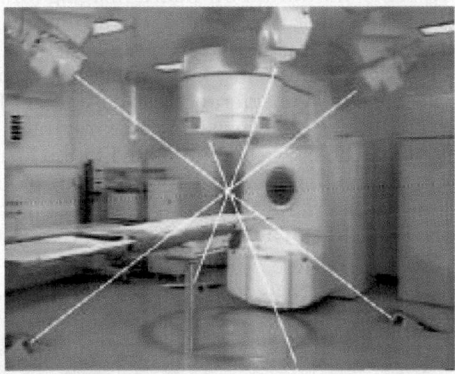

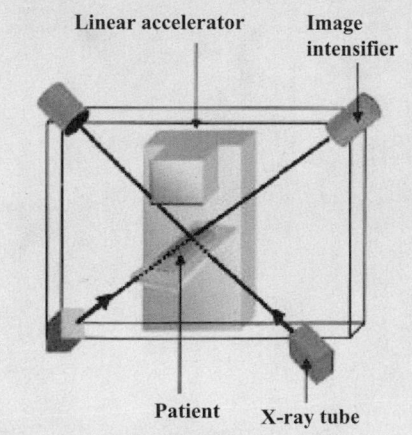

Linear accelerator   Image intensifier

Patient   X-ray tube

FIGURE 10.14. The Real-Time Tumor-Tracking (RTRT) system. (From Harada T, Shirato H, Ogura S, et al. Real-time tumor-tracking radiation therapy for lung carcinoma by the aid of insertion of a gold marker using broncho-fiberoscopy. *Cancer* 2002;95:1720–1727, with permission.)

target dose measured in a chest phantom (253). A 4D RTRT system has also been developed (252).

Investigators at Hokkaido University in Japan have presented a number of clinical studies using the RTRT system (113,115,126,144–146,251,253,254,305). In an early report, Shirato et al. (253) described the treatment of 14 patients with a variety of tumors, including lung, bladder, prostate, liver, and rectal cancers. All patients were treated with tight PTV margins (<10 mm). At a median follow-up of 6 months, no local or marginal recurrences were noted.

These investigators and others have explored the use of the RTRT system in tumors of the lung (113,126,251,254), prostate (144,146), gastrointestinal tract (2,115), and female genital tract (305). In a study of 18 lung cancer patients, Harada et al. (113) placed gold markers via bronchofiberoscopy under video guidance. Markers were shown to be stable in 65% of tumors throughout treatment. All patients received 35 to 40 Gy in four fractions, with "tight" (5 mm) margins around the tumor. At a median follow-up of 9 months, all were locally controlled, with only one patient developing symptomatic pneumonitis.

Kitamura et al. (146) reviewed the outcome of 31 patients on a dose escalation trial, with 12 patients receiving 65 Gy and 19 receiving 70 Gy, both in 2.5 Gy fractions using RTRT. In the 65 Gy group, no patient experienced acute toxicity and 8.3% developed late grade 1 rectal toxicity. In the 70 Gy group, grade 1 acute rectal and grade 1 or 2 acute bladder toxicities were seen in 5.3% and 15% of patients. Three patients developed a biochemical relapse (one 65 Gy and two 70 Gy patients).

Hashimoto et al. (115) treated 20 gastrointestinal tumor patients (14 esophagus, two stomach, and four duodenum) with the RTRT system. Markers were placed either intraoperatively or via endoscopy and tight (5 mm) margins were used. At a median follow-up of 10.2 months, no grade $\geq$3 late toxicities were noted. Ahn et al. (2) used the RTRT system in three unresectable pancreatic cancer patients. All received intraoperative electrons and external beam RT. None developed grade $\geq$2 acute toxicities. At a median follow-up of 3 months, three partial responses and one stable disease were noted. The RTRT system is discussed further in the following section.

University of Michigan System

Investigators at the University of Michigan developed an IGRT system for high-dose irradiation of intrahepatic tumors consisting of a racetrack microtron and diagnostic x-ray tubes mounted on the floor and ceiling of the treatment room (12). An in-room shielded control booth allows direct visual contact of the patient during kV imaging. This system was designed to be used in conjunction with an active breathing control (ABC) apparatus to reduce tumor motion due to respiration (299).

In a feasibility study, daily orthogonal images were obtained under ABC and aligned to the planning CT, using the diaphragm for SI alignment, and the vertebral bodies for LR and AP alignment (12). Overall, 171/262 (65%) fractions required repositioning. Setup errors were reduced from 4.0 mm (LR), 6.7 mm (SI), and 3.8 mm (AP) to 2.1 mm (LR), 3.5 mm (SI), and 2.3 mm (AP). Treatment time was 25 to 30 minutes, with breath holds of up to 35 seconds.

In a review of the 128 patients with unresectable intrahepatic tumors treated with high-dose conformal RT (recent patients with the in-house IGRT system) and hepatic artery floxuridine, Ben-Josef et al. (19) reported a median survival of 15.8 months, significantly improved over historical controls. Grade 3 and 4 toxicities were noted in 21% and 9% of patients, respectively. Unfortunately, the outcomes of patients treated with or without online setup corrections were not compared and thus their effect on patient outcome is not clear. However, indirect support for its use is garnered by the fact that the sole factor correlated with survival was total dose.

Prototype Gantry-Mounted Systems

Investigators at Tohoku University in Japan have modified a commercial linear accelerator to include x-ray generators (mounted of the gantry at ±45 degrees from the beam axis) opposite two sets of aSi flat panel sensors with images obtained at 15 frames per second (270) (Fig. 10.15). Takai et al. (269) used this system to image a gold seed on a rotating disk and a seed implanted in a metastatic lung tumor and reported excellent visualization of both. In a subsequent study (270), this system was combined with a dynamic multileaf collimator approach potentially allowing tracking and continuously irradiating a moving target.

Inter- and intrafractional prostate organ motion have been evaluated using this system in eight patients with implanted gold markers (33). After alignment using skin marks, images were obtained and isocenter shifts were calculated. Images were also obtained prior to every field with corrections of intrafractional displacements >1 mm. The mean magnitudes of interfractional displacements were 1.76, 3.14, and 3.78 mm in the LR, SI, and AP directions, respectively. Corresponding intrafractional displacements were 0.45, 1.08, and 1.45 mm, respectively. Of 214 fractions, 84 (39%) required intrafractional corrections.

An integrated radiotherapy imaging system (IRIS) consisting of two gantry-mounted diagnostic x-ray units on either side of the machine head opposite two aSi flat panel detectors has been developed at Massachusetts General Hospital (MGH) (21) (Fig. 10.16). The system corotates with the gantry, maintaining relative positions between the megavoltage and kilovoltage x-ray beams. It is also integrated with the pulsing of the linac to limit the amount of megavoltage noise during imaging. Each flat panel has an active area of 39.7 by 29.8 cm. To accommodate larger coverage for cone-beam CT acquisition (see "Volumetric Imaging Systems" below), the panels are able to slide 13.2 cm along their long axes from their home position. Un-

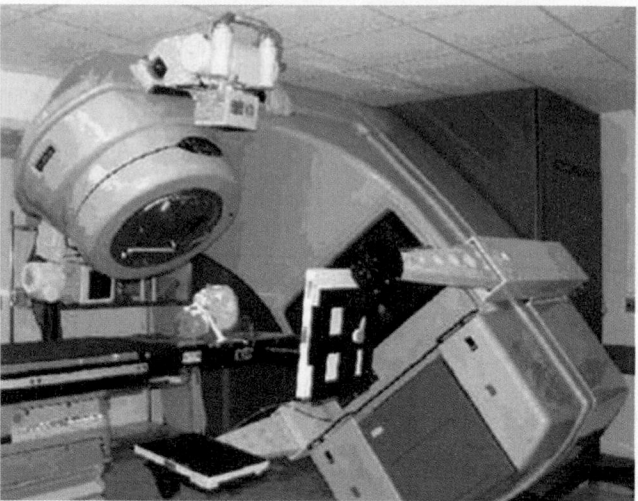

FIGURE 10.16. The integrated radiotherapy imaging system (IRIS) developed at Massachusetts General Hospital. (Photo courtesy of Steve Jiang, Ph.D.)

like commercially available systems, the dual-imager IRIS provides a *stereoscopic* view of the tumor, allowing assessment of the 3D trajectory of tumor motion. To date, no clinical studies have been published using this system. See "Respiratory Motion Management" below for additional information on the IRIS system.

Commercial Gantry-Mounted Systems

Two commercial gantry-mounted planar imaging systems are currently available: the Varian On-Board Imaging (OBI) system (Varian Medical Systems, Palo Alto, CA) and the Elekta Synergy (Elekta Oncology Systems, Norcross, GA). Both produce high-resolution diagnostic quality x-ray images of the patient in treatment position with considerably less dose than EPID.

The Varian OBI system consists of an x-ray tube opposed to an aSi flat panel detector, both mounted to the linac gantry orthogonal to the treatment beam axis. The x-ray tube and aSi detector panel can be retracted from the imaging position via robotic arms (Fig. 10.17). The x-ray tube produces 40 to 150 kV

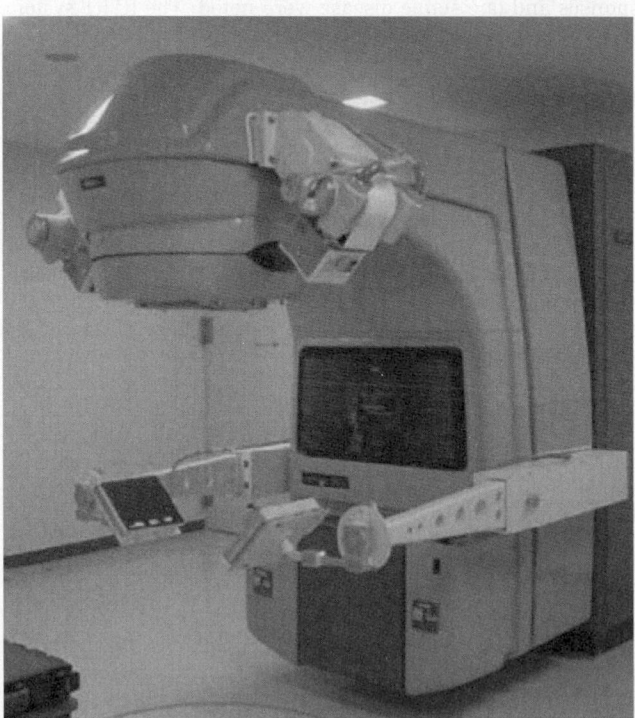

FIGURE 10.15. The prototype gantry-mounted image-guided radiation therapy (IGRT) system developed by Takai et al. at Tohoku University in Japan. (From Takai Y, Mitsuya M, Nemoto K, et al. Development of a new linear accelerator mounted with dual x-ray flouroscopy using amorphous silicon flat panel x-ray sensors to detect a gold seed in a tumor at real treatment position. *Int J Radiat Oncol Biol Phys* 2001;51[Suppl]:381[abstr], with permission.)

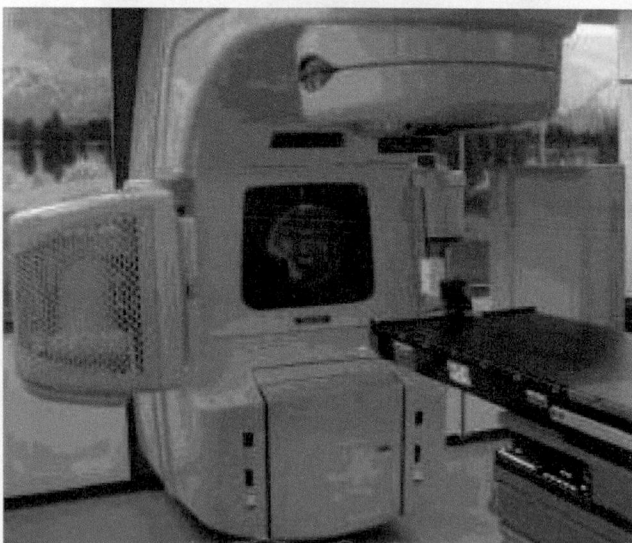

FIGURE 10.17. The Varian On-Board Imaging (OBI) system. (From Fox T, Huntzinger C, Johnstone P, et al. Performance evaluation of an automated image registration algorithm using an integrated kilovoltage imaging and guidance system. *J Appl Clin Med Phys* 2006;7:97–104, with permission.)

x-rays with an image size of 40 by 30 cm^2. Images are acquired at 7.5 frames per second at 0.195 mm per pixel and 15.0 frames per second at 0.390 mm per pixel.

Fox et al. (81) recently presented an overview of the Varian OBI software and hardware, and a performance evaluation of the automated image registration algorithm. In phantom verification tests, the registration algorithm was capable of detecting known translations and rotations with an accuracy of <1.4 mm for a 3D vector offset (0.4 mm, 1.1 mm, and 0.8 mm in the lateral, longitudinal and vertical dimensions, respectively). Earlier work demonstrated that the isocenter stability of the linear accelerator with the OBI arms extended is <1 mm (316).

The Elekta Synergy system consists of an x-ray tube opposed to an aSi flat panel detector, both mounted to the linac gantry orthogonal to the treatment beam axis. Similar to the Varian system, the x-ray tube and aSi detector panel can be retracted via mechanical arms. The x-ray tube produces 60 to 150 kV x-rays with an image size of 41 by 41 cm^2. Modern day linac-based kV imaging systems were originally developed by investigators at the William Beaumont Hospital (Fig. 10.18). A full description of their original in-house system is provided by Jaffray et al. (129).

Given their recent clinical introduction, limited experience is available with commercial gantry-mounted planar x-ray systems. Pisani et al. (219) evaluated the accuracy of online setup errors using a kV and MV dual-beam imaging system mounted on an Elekta SL-20 linear accelerator. Interobserver variability was found to be less with kV imaging and the intraobserver variability was also less for kV for most cases.

Perkins et al. (213) presented the outcome of 13 gastrointestinal tumor patients undergoing IMRT and concomitant chemotherapy with daily online setup corrections based on bony landmarks and/or surgical clips using the Varian OBI system. Of 276 fractions, average isocenter shifts were 0.30 ± 0.42 cm (vertical), 0.33 ± 0.34 cm (longitudinal), and 0.35 ± 0.39 cm (lateral). Maximum corresponding shifts were 4.0, 2.3, and 2.4 cm, respectively. Grade ≥2 acute nausea and diarrhea were noted in five and two patients, respectively. At a median follow-up of 6 months, 21% had disease regression and 71% stable disease.

Investigators at Karolinska University recently presented their initial clinical experience using the Varian OBI system in prostate cancer patients with implanted gold markers (264). Shifts were determined by comparing daily orthogonal films of

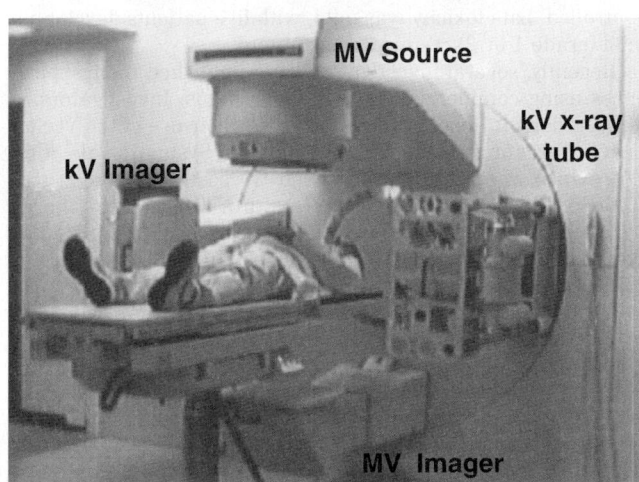

FIGURE 10.18. A modified Elekta linear accelerator (linac) with dual kV and MV imaging capability. From Jaffray SA, Drake DG, Moreau M, et al. A radiographic and tomographic imaging system integrated into a medical linear accelerator for localization of bone and soft-tissue targets. *Int J Radiat Oncol Biol Phys* 1999;45:773–789, with permission.)

the patient on the treatment couch with reference DRRs at simulation, using a 2D matching algorithm with couch movements made remotely. The entire process added ≤1 minute to each patient's treatment. These investigators are also applying the Varian OBI system to patients with gynecologic, lung, head and neck, and brain tumors.

Volumetric Imaging Systems

In-Room CT Systems

FOCAL System

The FOCAL (fusion of computed tomography and linear accelerator) system is comprised of a Mitsubishi EXL-15DP linear accelerator (Mitsubishi Electric, Tokyo, Japan), a high-speed DX/I General Electric CT scanner (GE Yokogawa Medical Systems, Tokyo, Japan), and conventional x-ray simulator (Fig. 10.19). Developed at the National Defense Medical College in Japan, this system was designed primarily for stereotactic irradiation of lung tumors (278). The gantry axes of the linac, CT scanner, and simulator are all coaxial, and the table can be rotated in three directions, allowing imaging of the patient by the CT scanner and simulator and also treatment with the linac. Accuracy of the matching of the linac isocenter with the CT image is ≤0.5 mm.

Uematsu et al. (275–278) have published a series of reports on the utility of the FOCAL unit. Lung cancer patients are immobilized supine and instructed to perform shallow breathing, often with the aid of an oxygen mask. The position and motion of the lung tumor are first evaluated using planar x-rays. The table is then rotated to the CT and serial thin-slice scans are performed at 4 seconds per slice to ensure capturing of the full extent of tumor motion. The target volume is then determined, the plan generated, and the table is then rotated to the linac for treatment. Using this approach, Uematsu et al. (276) treated 50 stage I or II lung cancer patients, primarily with 50 to 60 Gy in five to 10 fractions. At a median follow-up of 36 months, local control was 94%. No adverse sequelae were noted, apart from minor bone fractures and temporary pleural pain in two and six patients, respectively.

In a separate study, the FOCAL unit was used to evaluate intrafraction tumor stability in 38 lung and 12 liver tumor patients (277). Overall, no intrafraction movements >10 mm were noted. In fact, 68% of lesions had clinically negligible changes in position (0 to 5 mm). The percentage of upper lung, lower lung, and liver tumors with ≤5 mm movements were 100%, 50%, and 25%. However, in addition to coaching all patients on shallow breathing, abdominal belts were used in select patients to further reduce motion.

MSKCC System

Investigators at the Memorial Sloan-Kettering Cancer Center (MSKCC) have constructed a specially designed treatment system, consisting of a conventional CT scanner (Phillips Medical Systems, Milpitas, CA) and a Clinac 2100EX linear accelerator (Varian Medical Systems, Palo Alto, CA) (123,302,304,311). The CT scanner couch and linac table are aligned permitting a smooth transfer to the linac after the CT is performed.

In an initial report, Yenice et al. (312) described the treatment of paraspinal patients with this system. Patients were first immobilized in a stereotactic body frame, using pressures points on select skeletal structures. A planning CT scan was then performed and an IMRT plan generated. A CT scan in the treatment room was then obtained and automatically registered using bony landmarks and surgical hardware to the planning CT scan. Prior to treatment, a second registration was performed using fiducial markers on the frame and patient. The entire process required approximately 1 to 1.25 hours for

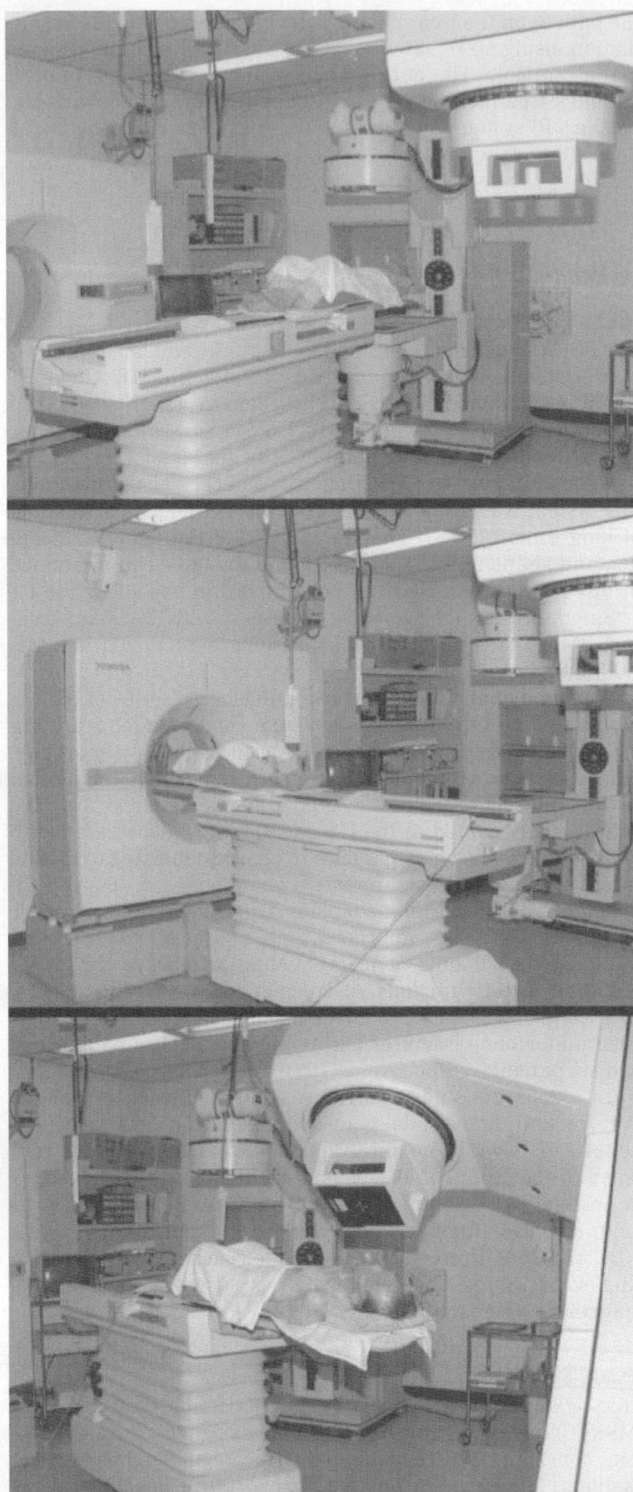

FIGURE 10.19. Fusion of computed tomography (CT) and linear accelerator (linac) (FOCAL) unit (*upper image*). The table is rotated to the x-ray simulator to monitor respiratory motion, then to the CT for scanning (*middle image*), and finally to the linac for treatment (*lower image*). (From Uematsu M, Shioda A, Suda A, et al. Intrafractional tumor position stability during computed tomography (CT)-guided frameless stereotactic radiation therapy for lung or liver cancers with a fusion of CT and linear accelerator (FOCAL) unit. *Int J Radiat Oncol Biol Phys* 2000;48:443–448, with permission.)

the initial fraction. Overall 3D accuracy of the system was 1.3 ± 0.8 mm.

The outcome of 35 paraspinal tumor patients (14 primary, 21 metastatic) undergoing IMRT using the MSKCC system has been presented (305). Overall, 24 (68%) had received prior RT. A planning margin of 10 mm was used, except at the spinal cord interface where 5 mm was used. The median prescribed dose was 2000 cGy in five fractions. At a median follow-up of 11 months, the 2-year actuarial local control rates for primary and metastatic tumors were 75% and 81%, respectively. Of 30 patients with >3 months follow-up, 90% experienced excellent palliation. No patient developed late RT-related sequelae. In their latest report focusing on previously irradiated patients (302), daily CT myelograms were performed to improve localization of the spinal cord and cauda equina.

CT-On-Rails

The initial CT-on-Rails system was developed at the University of Yamanashi in Japan consisting of a linear accelerator, a CT scanner, and a common treatment couch, with the linac and the CT gantries positioned at opposite ends of the patient couch (152). This system minimizes patient movement and displacement by moving the gantry of the CT scanner instead of the couch within the gantry. The basis of this system is the Smart Gantry system (GE-Yokogawa Medical Systems, Tokyo, Japan), which is comprised of two side and one middle rails. The side rails ensure controlled horizontal gantry movement, whereas the middle rail guides the gantry forward and backward in the direction of scanning. Kuriyama et al. (152) reported that the positional accuracy of the common couch was 0.2, 0.18, and 0.39 mm in the lateral, longitudinal, and vertical directions, respectively. The scan-position accuracy of the CT gantry was <0.4 mm in all three axes.

In a series of reports Onishi et al. (204,205) described the utility of the CT-on-Rails system in patients with unresected lung cancer. In a series of 22 stage I to IIIB patients, all were treated using voluntary breath hold and self-directed beam control (i.e., patients were able to turn the beam on or off using a hand-held switch) (204). Using fluoroscopy, a comfortable degree of breath hold was identified, which maintained tumor position. Tumor position was found to be highly reproducible with average positional differences of 2.2 mm, 1.4 mm, and 1.3 mm in the SI, AP, and RL positions, respectively, between the daily and planning CT scans. In a separate report, Onishi et al. (205) treated 35 stage I lung cancer patients with 60 Gy in 10 fractions. At a median follow-up of 13 months, 94% of tumors were locally controlled. Late toxicity was mild, with five patients developing mild (grade 1 or 2) respiratory symptoms.

Recently, several investigators have published their experiences using commercial CT-on-Rails systems. Investigators at M.D. Anderson Hospital have described their use of the Varian ExaCT Targeting system (Varian Medical Systems, Palo Alto, CA), which integrates a high-speed CT scanner on rails (GE Medical Systems, Milwaukee, WI) with a Varian dual-energy linac equipped with a 120 multileaf collimator (MLC) (38,255). The couch base is rotated to position the patient for either treatment or scanning, without the need to transfer onto the CT couch. Court et al. (51) reviewed the accuracy of this system and noted that the largest single uncertainty was the couch position on the CT side after a rotation (0.5 mm in the lateral direction). All other sources of uncertainty, including the difference in couch sag between the CT and linac, were <0.3 mm.

Chang et al. (38) treated 15 patients with spine metastases with IMRT on a nondose escalating phase I clinical trial using the ExaCT Targeting system. All patients were immobilized in a stereotactic body frame and received 30 Gy in five fractions, with a maximum allowed cord dose of 10 Gy. On average, the duration of the daily procedure was 1.5 hours. At a

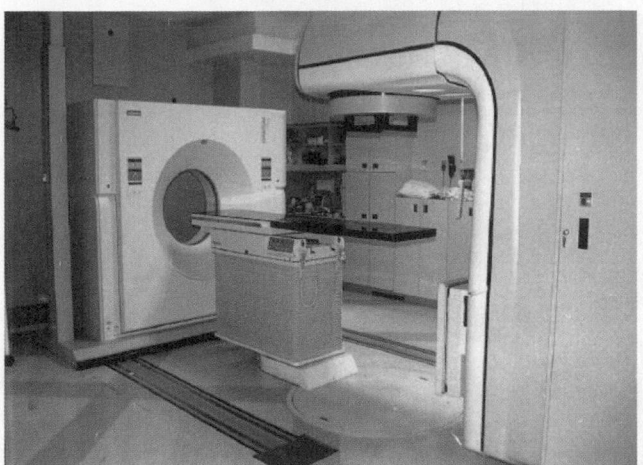

FIGURE 10.20. The Siemens Primatom CT-on-Rails system. (From Wong JR, Grimm L, Uematsu M, et al. Image-guided radiotherapy for prostate cancer by CT-linear accelerator combination: prostate movements and dosimetric considerations. *Int J Radiat Oncol Biol Phys* 2005;61:561–569, with permission.)

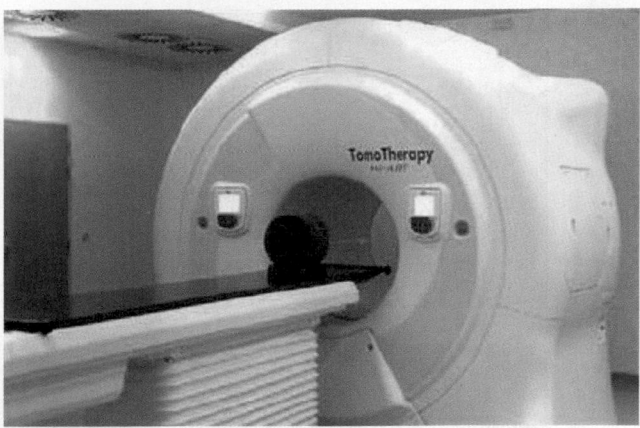

FIGURE 10.21. The helical Tomotherapy system. (From Tomsej M. The Tomotherapy Hi-Art System for sophisticated IMRT and IGRT with helical delivery: recent developments and clinical applications. *Cancer Radiother* 2006;10:288–295.

median follow-up of 9 months, no patient developed significant RT-related sequelae.

Others have reported their experiences using the Siemens Primatom CT-on-Rails system (Siemens Oncology Systems, Concord, CA), which consists of a Somatom CT scanner and a Primus Linear Accelerator in the same vault sharing a common table/couch (43,208,300) (Fig. 10.20). As with other CT-on-Rails systems, the CT scanner is moved on a pair of horizontal rails. Wong et al. (300) utilized the Primatom system in 108 prostate cancer patients undergoing IMRT to deliver the final 10 Gy. Overall, isocenter adjustments were common. The percentage of adjustments in the AP, SI, and LR directions were 54%, 27%, and 34%, respectively. Corresponding shifts of 1 cm or greater were noted in 15%, 4%, and 5% of patients, respectively.

Ma and Paskalev (170) have provided an excellent review of in-room CT systems and techniques. The future of such systems remains unclear given the increasing availability of other commercial volumetric imaging systems, including on-board cone-beam CT and helical tomotherapy. However, the value and possible applications of in-room high-quality conventional CT images remains an interesting area for clinical research.

Megavoltage Systems

Early MCVT Systems

Considerable interest has been focused on the use of the megavoltage (MV) treatment beam to generate volumetric CT images of the patient on the treatment table. The underlying principle of MVCT is analogous to kilovoltage CT, namely an x-ray source and detectors are used to reconstruct 2D images into 3D data sets. The first MVCT system was developed in 1982, consisting of a modified 4 MV linear accelerator with a detector array mounted on the linac gantry (258). In addition to the appeal of using the MV beam for imaging, MVCT has the added benefit of producing images free of the streaking artifacts common in kilovoltage CT, secondary to dental fillings or hip prostheses.

More recently, investigators at the University of Tokyo mounted a small detector on the gantry of a 6 MV linac in order to generate MVCT images in lung tumor patients undergoing SRS (190,191). All patients were instructed to maintain shallow breathing during planning and treatment to minimize organ motion. Moreover, at simulation, tumor motion was assessed by fluoroscopy and, if >1 cm, an oxygen mask and a belt compressing the chest and abdomen were used. Immediately prior

to treatment, a MVCT was obtained on the treatment table and appropriate shifts are made. In a series of 14 patients treated with a median single fraction dose of 20 Gy using this approach, the overall local control was 95%. Moreover, although all patients with >3 months follow-up had interstitial lung changes, only one developed symptomatic pneumonitis.

Helical Tomotherapy

The Tomotherapy system (Tomotherapy Inc., Madison, WI) is comprised of a 6 MV linac and a detector array mounted opposite each other on a ring gantry that continuously rotates while the couch is translated through the gantry (171,273) (Fig. 10.21). MVCT imaging on the Tomotherapy system is performed by reducing the nominal energy of the incident electron beam to 3.5 MeV (134). Three acquisition modes are available (fine, normal, and coarse).

Investigators at the University of Wisconsin evaluated the utility of Tomotherapy MVCT imaging for optimizing setup in eight dogs undergoing RT (79) (Fig. 10.22). Prior to treatment, a MVCT scan was obtained and aligned with the planning kilovoltage CT scan in the transverse and sagittal planes. MVCT images were of sufficient quality for verification of treatment setup in all eight animals, although soft tissue contrast was inferior to that of the kV CT scans. Both the primary tumor and adjacent bony landmarks were used for alignment. The entire process took approximately 5 to 12 minutes, including ~3 minutes for image acquisition.

Mahan et al. (173) reported on the use of the Tomotherapy system for optimizing patient setup in eight patients undergoing reirradiation of spinal metastases. The mean retreatment dose was 28 Gy, with the maximum cord dose of 27% to 56% of the prescribed dose. Prior to treatment, MVCT images were acquired and autofused with the planning CT scan, allowing calculation of couch translations. The range of interfraction displacement was as great as 1.5 cm, with standard deviations of ±4 mm (AP), ±4.1 mm (RL). and ±4.3 mm (SI). At a median follow-up of 15.2 months, all eight patients responded (two partial, six complete). None developed an in-field recurrence or significant late toxicity. Others have reported the value of daily setup verification using the Tomotherapy system in other sites, notably lung cancer (122,294).

A concern with the use of the Tomotherapy system for daily setup verification is image quality. Although less of a concern when bony landmarks are used, this is important when alignment is based solely on soft tissues. Song et al. (263) evaluated the feasibility of using Tomotherapy for daily prostate localization. MVCT images were acquired and compared to the

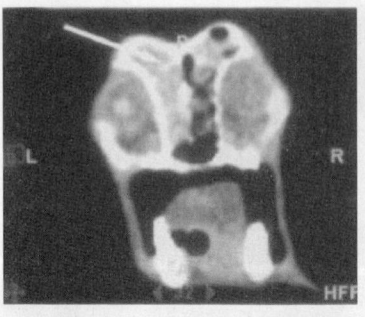

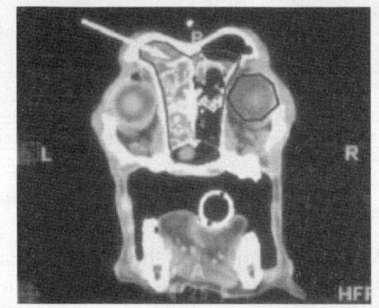

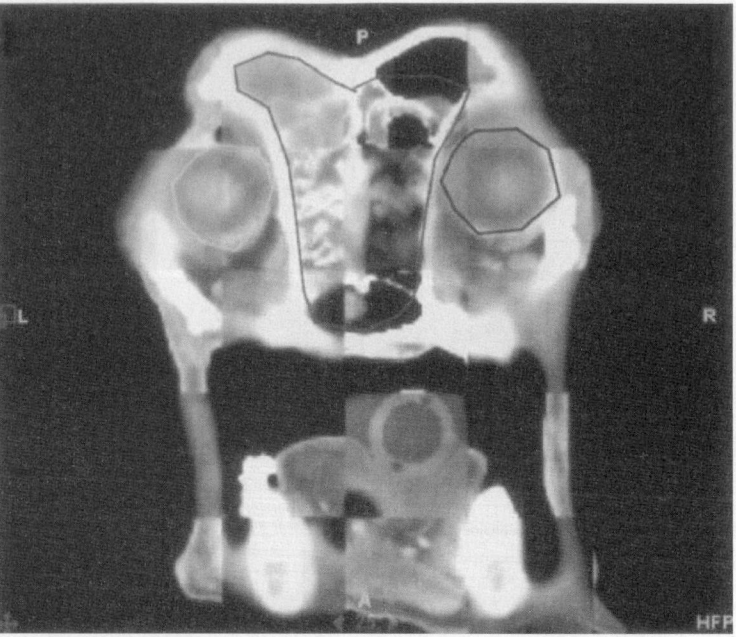

FIGURE 10.22. Megavoltage computed tomography (MVCT) obtained on a Tomotherapy unit **(A)**, kilovoltage computed tomography (CT), **(B)** and aligned images of the nasal cavity **(C)** of a dog with a nasopharyngeal tumor at the level of the eyes. On the aligned image (C), the darker gray, checkerboard regions represent the MVCT image superimposed over the CT image. (From Forrest LJ, Mackie TR, Ruchala K, et al. The utility of megavoltage computed tomography images from a helical tomotherapy system for setup verification purposes. *Int J Radiat Oncol Biol Phys* 2004;60:1639–1644, with permission.)

planning kV CT images in five patients. Of note, prostate volumes were smaller and more consistent on kV CT scans. Moreover, inter- and intraobserver contouring uncertainty was greater for MVCT. Daily alignment can be improved in prostate patients, however, with implanted fiducials, which are well visualized on the Tomotherapy system (156).

Given its relative recent clinical implementation, outcome data of patients treated with Tomotherapy remain limited. This will certainly change in the coming years given the number of dosimetric studies supporting its benefits (125,214,248). Tomotherapy may be particularly beneficial in patients undergoing hypofractionated stereotactic body radiosurgery. Hodge et al. (122) treated nine patients with medically inoperable T1–2 lung cancers with 60 Gy in five fractions using Tomotherapy. To aid in target delineation and treatment delivery, patients underwent a 4D CT scan (see "Respiratory Motion Management" below) and daily pretreatment MVCT image guidance. The average treatment time was 22 minutes. Treatment was well tolerated with no patients developing grade ≥2 pulmonary sequelae.

MV Cone-Beam Systems

Considerable attention has been focused on cone-beam CT (CBCT) imaging generated using the treatment beam (128). Megavoltage CBCT imaging is accomplished by first generating a series of 2D projections around the patient with the MV beam and a detector. A 3D data set is then reconstructed using the Feldkamp et al. (76) algorithm, in a process analogous to conventional CT imaging whereby an x-ray source and a detector are mounted on a rotating gantry. However, whereas a conventional CT system uses a 1D linear detector array, the CBCT system uses a 2D detector array.

Multiple investigators have evaluated the utility of MV CBCT imaging (78,184,185,200,222,256), with the largest published experience from UCSF (184,222). Pouliot et al. (222) described the feasibility of MV CBCT imaging for both patient alignment and dose verification, using a 6-MV Primus linear accelerator (Siemens Oncology Systems, Concord, CA) operating

in arc mode equipped with an aSi flat-panel EPID. MV CBCT scans were generated using an anthropomorphic head phantom, frozen sheep/pig cadaver heads, and head and neck cancer patients, requiring doses of 5 to 15 cGy. Acquisition and processing times were both on the order of 90 seconds. MV CBCT and conventional CT data sets were registered with millimeter and degree accuracy.

Morin et al. (184) evaluated the potential benefits of MV CBCT imaging in head and neck, lung, and pelvic patients treated on a prospective clinical trial (Fig. 10.23). In a locally advanced head and neck cancer patient, MV CBCT detected a misalignment of the vertebral bodies and spinal cord in the neck not seen on portal imaging. MV CBCT has also been found to complement treatment planning in patients with implanted metallic objects (10). No clinical outcome data, however, have been published to date in patients undergoing MV CBCT scanning.

Kilovoltage Systems

Mobile Flouroscopic C-Arm Systems

Several groups have reported the generation of kilovoltage (kV) CBCT scans using a mobile flouoroscopic C-arm imager (166,265). Sorenson et al. (265) and Kriminiski et al. (147) modified a commercial mobile isocentric fluoroscopic C-arm (Power-Mobil, Siemens Medical Solutions, Erlangen, Germany), replacing the standard image intensifier with an aSi flat-panel detector. A projection set of 100 to –1,000 images are obtained while the C-arm rotates around the patient in a 180-degree arc. Similar to MV CBCT imaging, kV CBCT images are reconstructed using the Feldkamp et al. (76) algorithm, modified due to the limited projection arc (257). Similar units have been developed at other centers (223).

The feasibility of using kV CBCT imaging produced by a mobile C-arm system in patients with prostate and head/neck cancer to improve setup and target localization has been presented (265). Patients underwent kV CBCT imaging weekly and the images were assessed offline. Overall, the imaging procedure was performed in <5 minutes with a dose less than

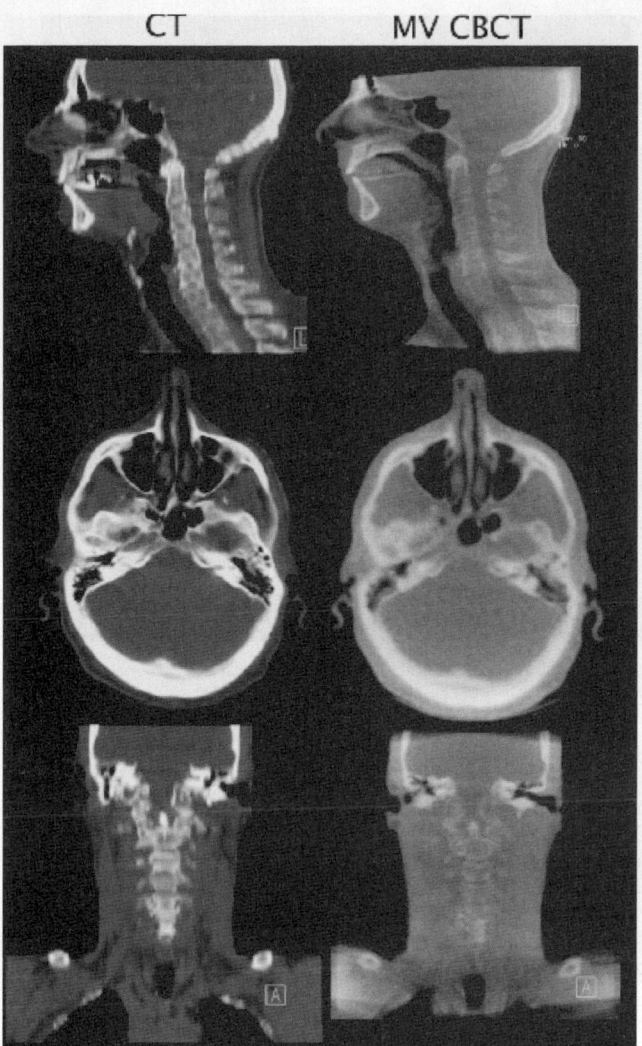

FIGURE 10.23. Comparison of a kilovoltage computed tomography (CT) scan (*left*) with a MV cone-beam CT (*right*) of a head-and-neck cancer patient. The window level of both images was adjusted to provide the best soft-tissue contrast. (From Morin O, Gillis A, Chen J, et al. Megavoltage cone-beam CT: system description and clinical applications. *Med Dosim* 2006;31:51–61, with permission.)

conventional CT. Although spatial resolution was good, image quality was not ideal (e.g. differentiation of the prostate from the rectum in the area of the prostate-rectum interface was poor) (Fig. 10.24). Clearly, if such systems are to become widely used, image quality must be substantially improved. In sites prone to respiratory-induced motion, image quality can be improved by correlating the CBCT acquisition with breathing (147).

Gantry-Mounted CBCT Systems

All major linear accelerator vendors currently offer gantry-mounted kV CBCT solutions or plan to in the near future. The Elekta Synergy (Elekta Oncology Systems, Norcross, GA) and the Varian On-Board Imager (Varian Medical Systems, Palo Alto, CA) systems consist of kilovoltage x-ray tubes mounted opposite flat panel detectors orthogonal to the treatment beam on retractable arms (161,264,268). In collaboration with investigators at the University of Heidelberg, Siemens (Siemens Oncology Systems, Concord, CA) is developing an "in-line" system which places the diagnostic x-ray tube at 180 degrees to the MV source (201,271) (Fig. 10.25). All three systems acquire kV projections during a 360-degree gantry rotation. These images are then reconstructed into a 3D data set (202).

The initial prototype (and its corresponding commercial counterpart) of the Elekta kV CBCT system has been presented in a series of reports from William Beaumont Hospital (160,161,202). In an initial evaluation of its feasibility in prostate cancer (161), kV CBCT was found in a phantom to achieve a setup accuracy of ≤1 mm in the LR, AP, and SI directions. Setup error was reduced in nearly all cases and was generally within ± 1.5 mm. The entire image guided process required 23 to 35 minutes.

Others have recently presented their initial experiences using the Elekta kV CBCT system (107,119,176). In 20 patients with various tumors, McBain et al. (176) noted sufficient image quality in all patients, including those in whom full gantry rotations were not possible (extremity and breast tumor patients). In general, soft tissue delineation was sufficient to allow assessment of the target and normal tissues. However, prostate images were not sufficiently distinct to allow organ contouring, compensation for small (<3 mm) movements, or for verification of small PTV margins.

Guckenberg et al. (107) compared the utility of the Elekta kV CBCT system with EPID in terms of setup accuracy in 24 patients with a variety of tumors. Kilovoltage CBCT was found to add little in the assessment of translational errors. Translational errors detected with either approach differed by <1 mm in 70.7% and <2 mm in 93.2% of measurements. However, CBCT was superior in the detection of rotational errors. Rotational errors >2 degrees were noted in 3.7%, 26.4%, and 12.4% of pelvic, thoracic, and head and neck tumors, respectively. Such rotational errors led to poorer target coverage and increased normal tissue dose in cases with elongated targets in close proximity to normal tissues.

Investigators at Karolinska University have presented their initial experience with the Varian kV CBCT system (264) (Fig. 10.26). Overall, kV CBCT images were generated with low total doses (~45 mGy) and the entire process including acquisition, reconstruction, and 3D registration added only 5 minutes to each patient's treatment. Image quality was felt to be slightly poorer than conventional CT imaging. However, several potential means of improvement were identified including replacing the table top with a homogenous carbon fiber composite, decreasing the field of view, and using the full fan mode.

Thilmann et al. (271) recently evaluated the utility of the in-line kV CBCT system developed in collaboration with Siemens. In a study of various tumor sites, bony landmarks were easily visualized on all images, allowing table shifts to be automatically calculated. Soft tissue contrast was acceptable except in only one morbidly obese patient. Using an action level of 2 mm, setup corrections were performed in four of six patients. Approximately 10 to 12 minutes were required to perform imaging, reconstruction, analysis, and positional corrections.

No clinical outcome studies are yet available in patients treated using kV CBCT for either setup or target localization. However, Groh et al. (99) compared the performance of MV and kV cone-beam CT technologies. MV CBCT was found to offer an advantage in terms of simplicity of mechanical integration with a linear accelerator. In contrast, kV CBCT was found to be superior in terms of imaging of soft tissue structures and the signal-to-noise ratio per unit dose.

In the coming years, numerous advancements are expected in kV CBCT technology. One area of active research is digital tomosynthesis (DTS), a method of reconstructing 3D slices from 2D cone beam x-ray projections data acquired with limited source angulation (e.g., 40 degrees). Unlike conventional kV CBCT approaches, DTS requires less scan time and results in less radiation exposure to the patient. Investigators from Duke University recently illustrated the ability to generate high-quality images using the DTS approach in patients with prostate, head and neck, and liver tumors (97).

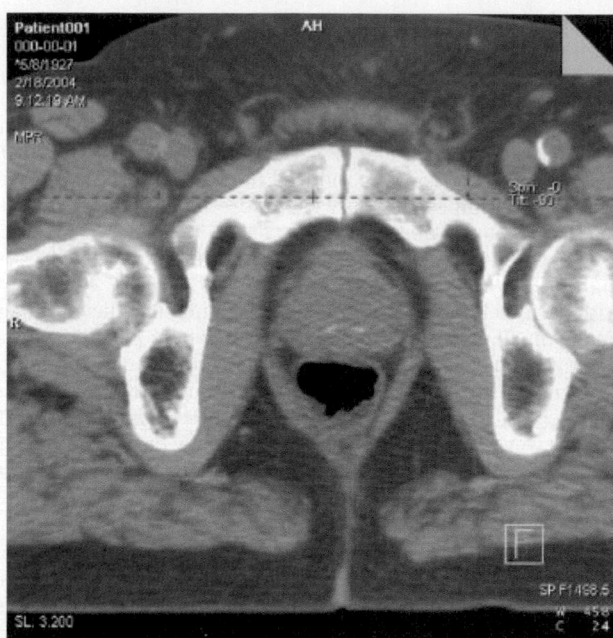 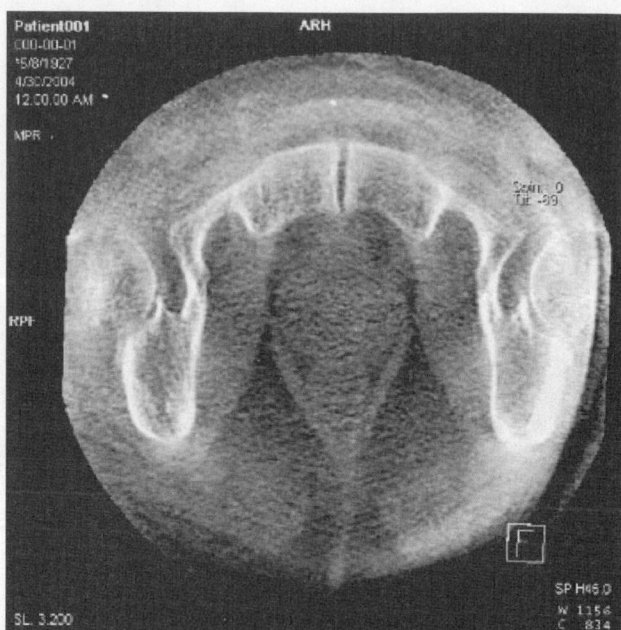

FIGURE 10.24. Comparison of a conventional computed tomography (CT) scan (*left*) with a kilovoltage cone-beam CT scan (*right*) obtained using a mobile fluoroscopic c-arm imager in a patient with prostate cancer. (From Sorensen SP, Chow PE, Kriminiski S, et al. Image-guided radiotherapy using a mobile kilovoltage x-ray device. *Med Dosim* 2006;31:40–50, with permission.)

Respiratory Motion Management

Respiratory-induced organ motion is a major problem in RT, particularly in tumors in the thorax and upper abdomen. Tumors in these sites can move up to 2.5 cm or more during free breathing (66,92,266) (Fig. 10.27). Such motions result in imaging artifacts (41) and positional uncertainty that compromise the accuracy of target delineation and treatment delivery.

A common method to account for uncertainties in targeting has been to use standard, population-based, PTV margins, typically 5 to 15 mm. However, this approach can result in irradiation of large volumes of normal tissues in some patients, while underdosing the target in others (3). Customized margins have been advocated based on the maximum excursion of tu-

mor observed during fluoroscopy (66) or serial free-breathing CT imaging (3,281). Others have explored the use of breath-hold techniques that "freeze" the target in a specific phase of the respiratory cycle, notably ABC (301) and deep inspiration breath hold (DIBH) (233). However, such approaches may not be well tolerated in many patients, particularly those with poor pulmonary function. More sophisticated methods to improve target delineation and treatment of mobile tumors are respiratory gating and 4D imaging.

Respiratory Gating

The two main approaches to respiratory gating are internal and external gating. Internal gating utilizes internal tumor motion surrogates such as implanted fiducial markers, whereas external gating uses external respiratory surrogates such as markers placed on the surface of the patient's abdomen. Other methods for acquiring a respiratory signal have been described including spirometry (315) and thermocoupling (297).

The only internal gating system currently in clinical use is the RTRT system (253). This system and its clinical applications have been described in detail in the previous section (see "Planar Imaging Systems"). Its major strength is precise and real-time localization of the tumor position during the treatment. Implanted markers are often good surrogates for tumor position, and marker migration is usually not an issue, particularly if multiple markers are used. Major weaknesses include its invasiveness and the high imaging dose required for fluoroscopic tracking.

The real-time position management (RPM) system (Varian Medical Systems, Palo Alto, CA) can be viewed as representative of external gating systems (Fig. 10.28). This system consists of a lightweight plastic block with two passive infrared reflective markers placed on the patient's anterior abdominal surface and monitored by a charge-coupled-device video camera mounted on the treatment room wall. The surrogate signal is the abdominal surface motion. Both amplitude and phase gating are allowed. During treatment, a periodicity filter checks the regularity of the breathing waveform and disables the beam when

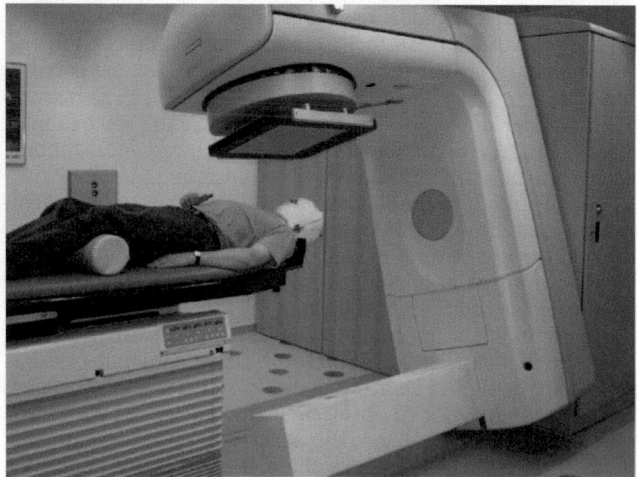

FIGURE 10.25. The Siemens "in-line" system developed in collaboration with the University of Heidelberg. (From Thilmann C, Nill S, Tucking T, et al. Correction of patient positioning errors based on in-line cone beam CTs: clinical implementation and first experiences. *Radiat Oncol* 2006;1:16–21, with permission.)

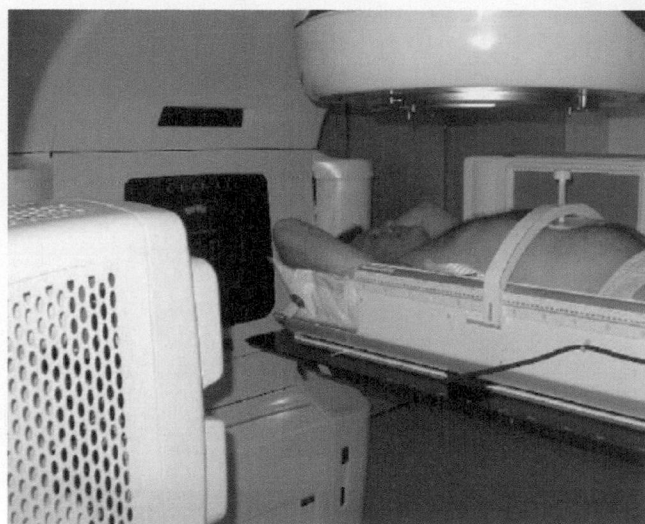
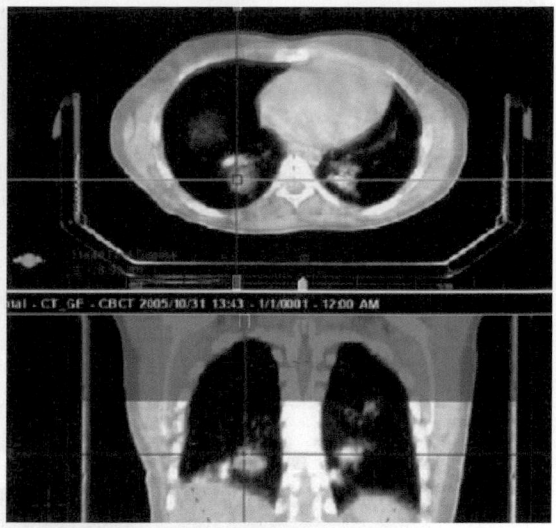

FIGURE 10.26. Kilovoltage cone-beam computed tomography (CBCT) imaging using the Varian On-Board Imaging system in a patient undergoing extracranial stereotactic treatment at Karolinska University (*left*). The kV CBCT of the patient in the stereotactic body frame is shown registered with the planning CT scan (*right*). (From Sorcini B, Tilikidis A. Clinical application of image-guided radiotherapy, IGRT [on the Varian OBI platform]. *Cancer Radiother* 2006;10:252–257.

the waveform becomes irregular, such as with patient motion or coughing, and re-enables the beam after establishing breathing is again regular. The RPM is also used during simulation to acquire the patient's geometry in the gating window and to setup the gating window.

Major strengths of external gating are that it is noninvasive, relatively easy to use, and well tolerated by patients (23). Moreover, it does not require any radiation dose for imaging. However, it should be noted that tracking the external marker is not equivalent to tracking the tumor, thus blindly trusting the exter-

nal surrogate can result in errors. In particular, the relationship between the tumor motion and the surrogate signal may change over time, inter- and intrafractionally.

4D Imaging

4D imaging combines the spatial (e.g., 3D) data with time-dependent changes during respiration. Although 4D PET and MRI techniques have been described (193,250), their application to radiation oncology has not yet been extensively explored;

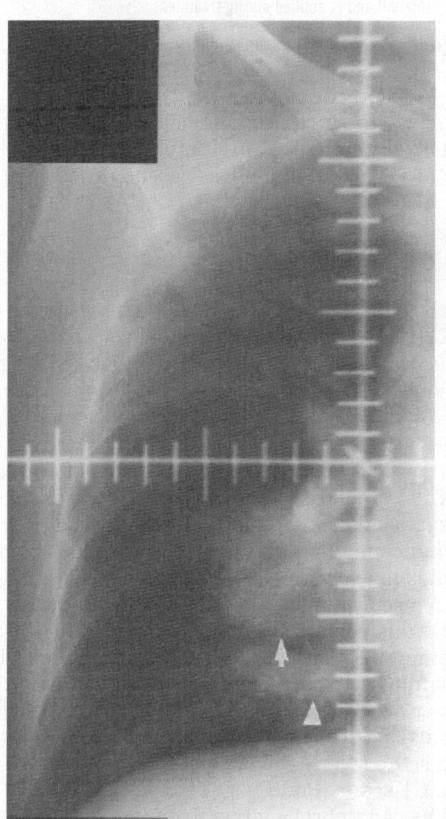
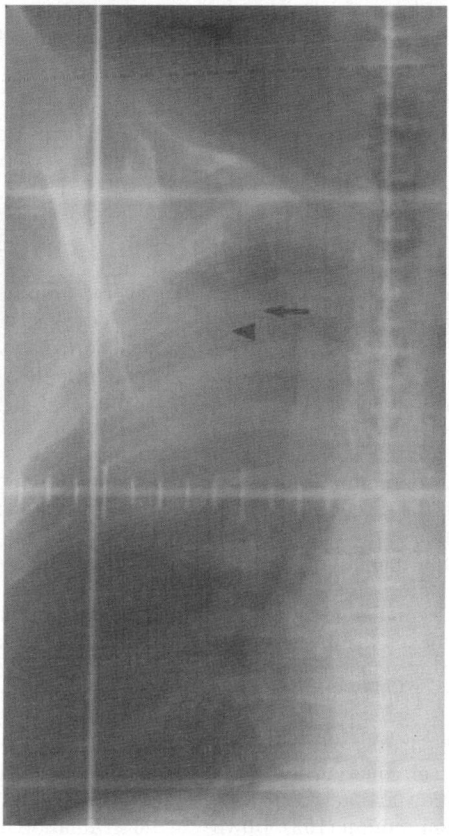

FIGURE 10.27. Double-exposure radiographs from two different patients with lung cancer. **A:** Respiratory-dependent superior-inferior (SI) tumor motion shown in a patient with a 5.5 cm non–small cell lung cancer of the right lower lobe. SI motion of 2.2 cm was noted between expiration (*arrowhead*) and inspiration (*arrow*). **B:** Lateral motion of a lung tumor, illustrated by the change in the medial tumor edge with inspiration (*arrowhead*) and expiration (*arrow*). (From Stevens CW, Munden RF, Forster KM, et al. Respiratory-driven lung tumor motion is independent of tumor size, tumor location, and pulmonary function. *Int J Radiat Oncol Biol Phys* 2001;51:62–68, with permission.)

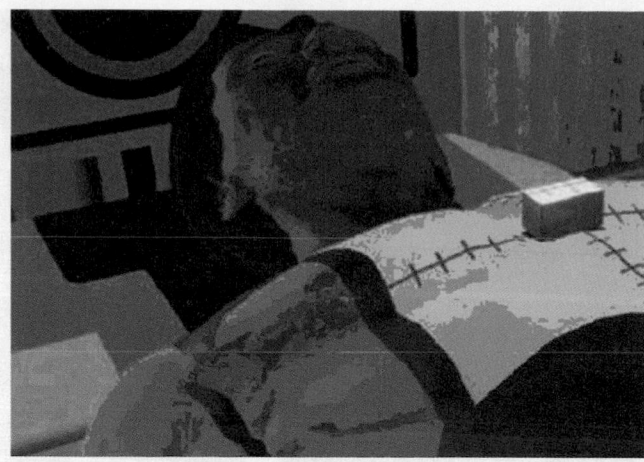

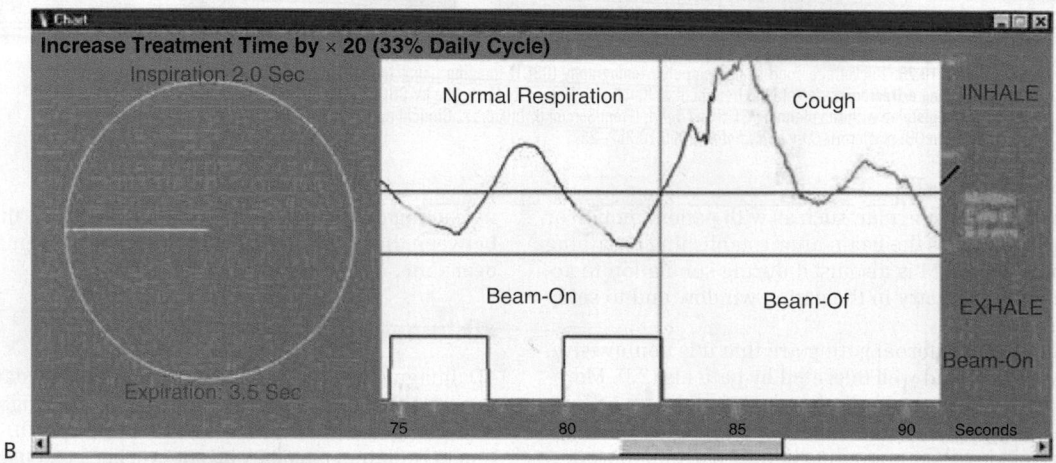

FIGURE 10.28.   The Varian Real-Time Position Management (RPM) system. **A:** A passive infrared reflective marker block is used to track chest (or abdominal) wall motion. **B:** Gating software is used during simulation to optimize the beam-on interval and is applied during treatment delivery with beam gating based on the patient's breathing pattern. (Adapted from Huntzinger C. Image guided radiation therapy. Accessed from varian.mediaroom.com/file.php/mr_varian/spinsite_docfiles/148/IGRT_Full_Paper_Sept1.pdf on December 2, 2006, with permission.)

this section will thus concentrate on 4D CT. Readers interested in potential applications of 4D PET and a more extensive discussion of 4D imaging are referred elsewhere (141,303).

Motion artifacts during CT scanning are due to the fact that the CT scan is performed during free breathing. Depending on the scanning speed relative to the tumor motion speed, artifacts appear in different ways. If the scan speed is much *slower* than the tumor speed, a smeared image is captured. If the scan speed is much *faster*, tumor position and shape are captured at an arbitrary breathing phase. If the scan and tumor speeds are *comparable*, which is the case in most currently available helical CT scanners, the tumor position and shape are heavily distorted. This scenario has been extensively reviewed by Chen et al. (41). Based on an experiment and computer simulations, it was found that distortions along the axis of motion could result in either a lengthening or shortening of the target (Fig. 10.29). In addition to shape distortion, the center of the imaged target can be displaced by as much as the amplitude of the motion.

To overcome these problems, a respiratory-correlated or 4D CT is performed. The idea behind 4D CT is that, at every position of interest along patient's long axis, images are oversampled and each image is tagged with breathing phase information. After the scan is done, images are sorted based on the corresponding breathing phase signals. Many 3D CT sets are thus obtained, each corresponding to a particular breathing phase, and together they constitute a 4D CT set covering the whole breathing cycle. 4D CT decreases motion artifacts and accurately assesses the extent of intrafraction motion (153). Down-

sides to 4D CT include the increased time for image acquisition and increased dose to the patient from multiple CT scans. An excellent review of 4D CT scanning was recently presented by Keall (141).

4D Target Delineation

Several approaches to 4D target delineation have been described (4,153,229,280,298). These approaches enable construction of an *integrated target volume* (ITV) consisting of imaging data acquired in separate phases of respiration into a combined 3D volume containing the probable location of tumor. Allen et al. (4) created a composite volume based on the tumor delineated on maximal inhalation and exhalation scans in 16 patients. This structure was significantly smaller than a 1 cm uniform expansion around the GTV delineated on a free-breathing scan, indicating that a standard approach using a 1-cm expansion leads to overtreatment of normal tissues. Lager-waard et al. (153) used multiple "slow" CT scans to define the CTV, showing that this volume provided better target coverage than a free-breathing CT-derived CTV with isotropic margins. This method is limited to some extent, however, by motion artifacts that hamper accurate target delineation. Wolthaus et al. (298) have used artifact-free mid-ventilation CT scans selected from the 4D data set to reduce the irradiated volume compared to free-breathing CT scans. Underberg et al. (280) showed that individualized ITVs can improve target definition for stereotactic irradiation of stage I NSCLC (Fig. 10.30).

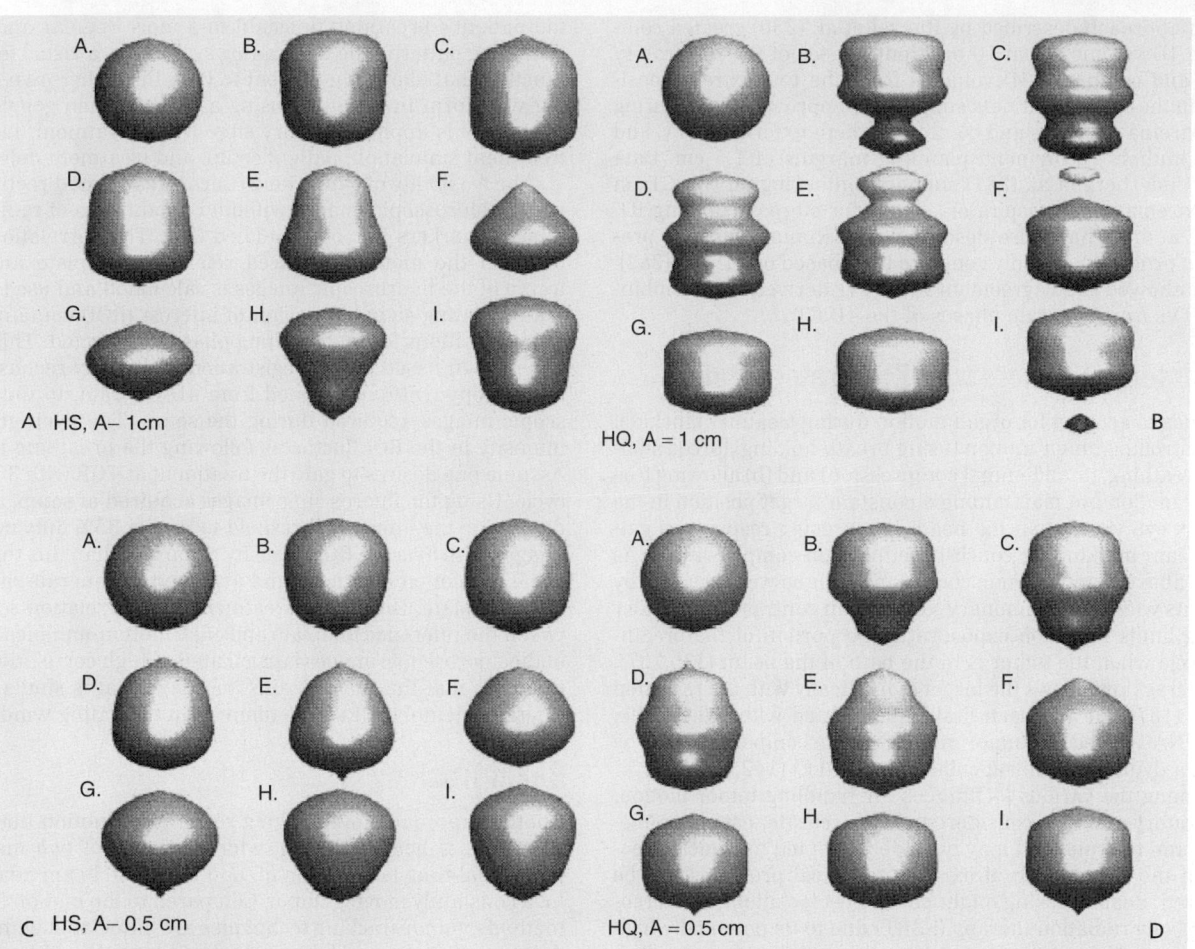

FIGURE 10.29. Simulations of helical scanning of a 3-cm radius sphere under different conditions. Object A in each series is a volumetric representation of the object scanned in static mode. Objects B–I represent the sphere as reconstructed beginning with initial phase (ϕ) = 0, and incremented by $\pi/4$ for each subsequent object. **A:** High speed (HS) mode (slice thickness 3.75 mm, effective speed 0.2 s/slice, pitch 1.5 cm), amplitude 1 cm; **(B)** High quality (HQ) mode (slice thickness 3.75 mm, effective speed 0.4 s/slice, pitch 0.75 cm), amplitude 1 cm; **(C)** HS mode, amplitude 0.5 cm; and **(D)** HQ mode, amplitude 0.5 cm (From Chen GT, Kung JH, Beaudette KP. Artifacts in computed tomography scanning of moving objects. *Semin Radiat Oncol* 2004;14:19–26, with permission.)

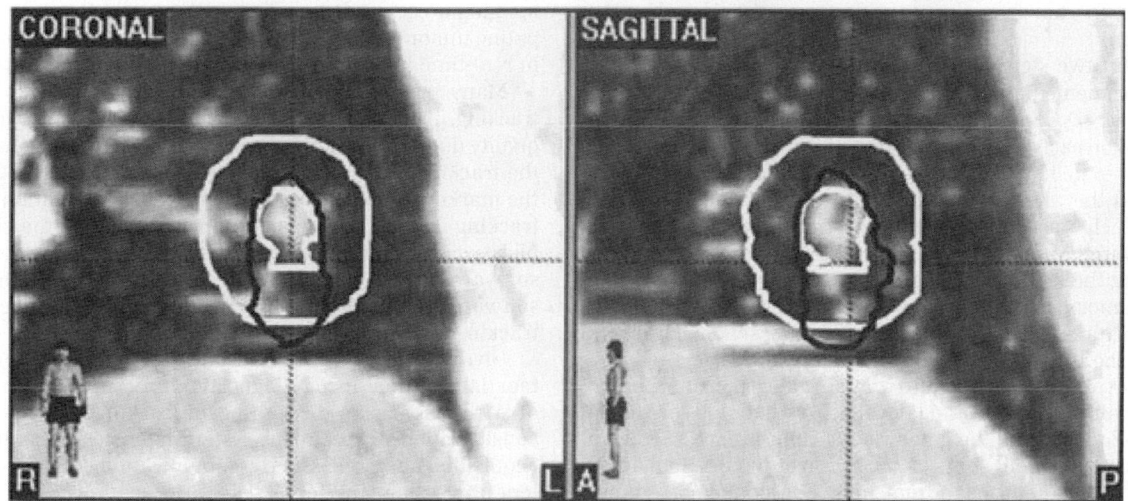

FIGURE 10.30. Internal target volume (ITV) generated from a four-dimensional computed tomography (4D CT) scan (*black*) versus a gross tumor volume (GTV) generated from an image in a "random" portion of the respiratory cycle (*inner white line*). The planning target volume generated by adding a 1 cm margin around the GTV (*outer white line*) fails to cover the ITV from the 4D CT caudally. (From Underberg RW, Lagerwaard FJ, Cuijpers JP, et al. Four-dimensional CT scans for treatment planning in stereotactic radiotherapy for stage I lung cancer. *Int J Radiat Oncol Biol Phys* 2004;60:1283–1290, with permission.)

An approach described by Rietzel et al. (230) created composite 4D volumes from 10 different phases of the respiratory cycle and compared 4D volumes from the two extrema positions in the cycle. Their data support the approach of contouring the extrema positions and combining them to form an ITV, and these authors recommend planning margins of 1.5 cm. Data from Underberg et al. (281) support contouring on two CTs in the extrema of the respiratory phase for stereotactic lung RT. These authors have also described a maximum intensity projection protocol to rapidly generate ITVs based on 4D CTs (282). These showed good agreement with ITVs derived from combining GTVs from separate phases of the 4D CT.

Treatment of Tumors with Respiratory Motion

Methods to account for organ motion during treatment include: (a) controlling tumor motion (using breath holding, forced shallow breathing, or abdominal compression) and (b) allowing free tumor motion but maintaining a constant target position in the beam's eye view when the beam is on (using respiratory gating, beam tracking, or couch-based motion compensation). As noted above, tumor motion control may not be well tolerated by patients with poor pulmonary function. In contrast, respiratory gating limits radiation exposure to the portion of the breathing cycle when the tumor is in the path of the beam (136,137). Beam tracking follows the target dynamically with the radiation beam (187), an approach first implemented with CyberKnife. For LINAC-based RT, tumor motion can be compensated for by using a dynamic multileaf collimator (DMLC) (142,195).

Among the various techniques for handling tumor motion, respiratory gating is considered to be accurate, easy to implement and tolerate, and may be widely adopted in clinical practice in the near future, if existing technical problems can be resolved. Beam tracking might be the best technique for stereotactic body radiation therapy (SBRT) due to its potentially high treatment efficiency and precision, although it is more technically challenging.

To ensure an accurate externally gated treatment, four key steps are required. During treatment simulation, the tumor reference gating position should be accurately measured using techniques such as 4D CT. During planning, the patient and tumor geometry at the gating position should be used. During setup, the tumor gating position at the current fraction should be matched to the reference gating position. Finally, during the treatment delivery, the gating position should be maintained the same (i.e., the tumor is always at the same position when the beam is on).

The first two steps are relatively straightforward and have been implemented at MGH (137). For each patient undergoing gated RT, a 4D CT scan is acquired. The GTV and/or CTV are contoured on each 4D CT data set in the gating window and then combined to define an ITV. The ITV is then fused to the 4D CT data set at the gating position, that is, the end of exhale (EOE) phase, which is used as the planning CT data. Critical structures are contoured on the EOE CT data set. A margin is then added generating the PTV, and a treatment plan is generated.

The tumor gating EOE position, relative to skin tattoos or bony structures, can vary significantly from fraction to fraction. At MGH, the IRIS system (see "Prototype Gantry-Mounted Systems" above), is used to acquire gated radiographs for patient setup. A pair of gated AP and lateral IRIS radiographs are taken at the EOE phase, and the gated radiographs are matched with DRRs to detect patient shifts (137). For liver tumors, implanted fiducial markers are used for matching. For lung tumors, tumor mass or anatomic features near the tumor, such as diaphragm, are used.

The tumor EOE position for a treatment fraction is measured during patient setup. This position can vary after the treatment begins. One means of minimizing this variation is to coach the patient's breathing to establish a more regular and stable breathing pattern. The RPM gating system has a visual feedback function that allows the patient to view his or her own breathing waveform in real-time using a pair of video goggles. The procedure is applied to every step of the treatment, including treatment simulation, patient setup, and treatment delivery.

The feasibility of gating lung cancer treatment directly based on the fluoroscopic images without implantation of radiopaque fiducial markers has been studied (22). The correlation score between the motion-enhanced reference template and each frame of the fluoroscopic images is calculated and used to generate a gating signal. A region of interest (ROI) containing the tumor positions for all breathing phases is selected. This ROI is determined based on the registration of digitally reconstructed fluoroscopy (DRF), generated from 4D CT data, to the fluoroscopic images acquired during the setup. The average image intensity in the ROI fluctuates following the breathing pattern. Assume one desires to gate the treatment at EOE with 35% duty cycle. Using the fluoroscopic images acquired at setup, one can determine the intensity threshold to have a 35% duty cycle. All images with average ROI intensity value less than this threshold are then motion enhanced and averaged to generate the reference template. During the treatment, the correlation score between the reference template and each motion-enhanced frame of the fluoroscopic images is calculated. A high correlation score indicates that the ROI contains an image that is similar to the reference template (i.e., the tumor is in the gating window).

Beam Tracking

Another approach to managing respiratory motion during the treatment is beam tracking, which consists of two major aspects: real-time localization of, and real-time beam adaptation to, a constantly moving tumor. Compared to the motion freezing methods, tumor tracking techniques are associated with higher delivery efficiency and less residual target motion. These factors may be particularly important to SBRT of thoracic and abdominal tumor sites, where a large dose is delivered during a single or a few relatively lengthy treatment sessions. In addition, beam tracking is applicable to regularly fractionated IMRT and three-dimensional conformal radiation therapy (3DCRT) treatment of mobile tumors.

One should note that real-time beam adaptation is not feasible without precise real-time localization of the tumor position in 3D. Owing to system latency and the desire to reduce the imaging dose, predictive filters are usually required for anticipating tumor position. Errors in localization should be identified in real-time in order to avoid irradiating the wrong target.

Many practical challenges exist with fluoroscopic marker tracking, including changes in marker shape and poor image quality due to MV beam interference. There is no guarantee that the tracking algorithm will always be able to correctly localize the marker or tumor position. Accurate identification of system tracking failures thus has an important role in the clinical application of a tumor tracking system (247). When the tracking software fails, the treatment beam must be held off until the software resumes correct tracking. Repeated or unrecoverable tracking failures require human intervention.

Given that one can locate and track the position of a tumor in real-time using diagnostic x-ray imaging, the delivery of a treatment plan through beam tracking requires adequate consideration of treatment system latencies, including image acquisition and processing, communication delays, control system processing, and for DMLC based beam tracking, MLC mechanical latencies. Furthermore, the imaging dose given over long SRS procedures or multiple RT fractions must be considered. Reducing the sampling rate of the imaging system can mitigate the adverse side effects of extended fluoroscopic exposure. Hence, predictive models are needed to reduce tumor localization errors that may result from the larger system latencies and slower imaging rate (246).

Beam tracking by means of a DMLC shaped aperture is an active area of investigation. DMLC has become a standard means of IMRT delivery on some gantry-mounted linacs. The MLC leaf travel speed can safely reach 2.5 cm/sec, which is comparable with respiration-induced tumor motion speed. Since it only moves the beam aperture in 2D, the approach cannot compensate out-of-plane tumor motion. However, the resultant dosimetric error should be small.

Because of its potential for providing high-dose conformity and a high-duty cycle, as well as its technical complexity, real-time beam adaptation methods are suitable for hypofractionated thoracic and abdominal cancer. However, there are a number of technical hurdles before this approach becomes clinically feasible, including treatment planning, and the accurate response of the MLC to tumor positions measured in real-time. The actual tumor movement as well as its relationship to surrounding critical structures during the treatment cannot be known at the time of treatment planning. Therefore, planning can only be done based on some kind of average patient geometry information or at best on 4D CT simulation data, and an adaptive scheme must be used throughout the treatment course.

Synchronized moving aperture radiation therapy (SMART) is a simplified implementation of DMLC based real-time beam adaptation technology (194,195). The basic assumption is that, under breath coaching or other kinds of breath regulation, the tumor motion pattern is stable and reproducible during the whole treatment course; therefore, it can be measured prior to treatment and used to modify the treatment plan. The practical implementation includes: (a) during treatment simulation and planning, tumor motion data are measured and the average tumor trajectory (ATT) is derived; then the IMRT MLC leaf sequence is modified to compensate for tumor motion; (b) during treatment delivery, respiratory surrogates or implanted markers are monitored and used to synchronize the treatment with tumor motion. Treatment can be interrupted and resumed if target motion differs from the average trajectory.

Studies have shown the practicality and effectiveness of breath coaching for improving the regularity and reproducibility of patient breathing (194). A method for deriving the ATT from the measured tumor trajectory has been developed (195). Including tumor motion into an IMRT MLC leaf sequence seems a straightforward superposition process. However, it can be very complicated when considering the hardware constraints of MLC, such as the maximum leaf travel speed, communication time delay, minimum leaf gap, and acceleration constraints.

Instead of modifying an existing leaf sequence to include tumor motion, one can also consider the tumor motion at the leaf sequencing stage, or include the motion at the treatment planning stage, if 4D CT data are available. When 4D CT data are available, it is possible to optimize the SMART treatment plan incorporating the tumor motion present in the images. Jiang et al. (135) have developed an optimization scheme that does not require mapping voxel displacements between image sets at different phases. The optimization results in one intensity map for each breathing phase and field. The leaf sequencing algorithm for SMART is analogous to that for intensity modulated arc therapy (IMAT), with breathing phase corresponding to the gantry angle from 0 to 360 degrees (135). Further studies are needed in order to make this approach clinically useful.

Adaptive Radiotherapy

RT treatment planning has traditionally been a static process, whereby a plan is generated based on a single snapshot of the patient's anatomy and delivered over a number of weeks. However, IGRT approaches will most likely transform this static process into a *dynamic* one, whereby plans are altered throughout the treatment course or perhaps even throughout the treatment fraction. In many ways, altering the treatment plan during treatment is not new, for example, patients are often replanned due to significant weight loss and/or tumor response. What is different is the level of sophistication IGRT offers to this process.

Adaptive RT (ART) is a broad concept. One approach is to use the knowledge of patient setup and organ motion obtained from imaging during treatment to alter the treatment plan. This approach was introduced by investigators at William Beaumont Hospital in patients with prostate cancer. As initially conceived, treatment is initiated with a population-based margin and setup errors are measured daily using EPID imaging (290,291). Systematic and random setup errors and the time-dependent drift of treatment setup are then predicted (307). Yan et al. (309) reported that this strategy could be used to modify treatment margins and the total prescribed dose. Setup errors were estimated at the 95% confidence level with ≤ 9 EPID images. Moreover, a significant percentage of patients could have their dose safely increased due to the use of smaller margins. In a separate report, Yan et al. (307) applied this approach prospectively to a cohort of 20 patients and reported that the average number of treatment days to confidently predict the setup error was 6.

More recently, volumetric imaging has been introduced into the Beaumont adaptive RT process (31) (Fig. 10.31). Based on the planning CT simulation, an initial treatment plan is generated with a 1-cm generic CTV-PTV margin. Each of the first 4 days of therapy, daily EPIs and CT scans are acquired immediately before or after treatment. Confidence-limited PTV (cl-PTV) margins are generated based on each patient's setup inaccuracies and internal organ motion. Rectal and bladder constraints are used to determine the individual patient's total dose, ranging from 70.2 to 79.2 Gy. These investigators earlier demonstrated that five CT scans are enough to meet the criteria of dose reduction by 2% in the CTV due to organ motion in more than 80% of patients (31).

Vargas et al. (288) treated a total of 331 T1–3 prostate patients using the Beaumont adaptive process. At a median follow-up of 1.6 years, grade 2 chronic rectal toxicity was seen in 10% of patients; nine (3%) developed grade 3 chronic rectal toxicity. The 2-year actuarial rate of grade ≥ 2 and ≥ 3 rectal chronic sequelae were 17% and 3%, respectively. No difference was noted between dose levels, supporting the adaptive process. Brabbins et al. (31) evaluated chronic toxicities in 280 patients followed for a minimum of 1 year and noted no differences in toxicity rates between higher and lower doses.

Another adaptive approach is to alter treatment based on *changes* in the tumor and/or normal tissues. Multiple investigators have reported significant morphologic changes in tumors and/or normal tissues in a wide variety of tumor sites during RT, including head and neck cancers (14,111), lung cancer (149,228), and gynecologic tumors (283). Barker et al. (14) noted a mean volume reduction of the GTV of 0.2 cm^3/day in head and neck cancer patients treated on a CT-on-Rails system. Of note, the parotid gland volume decreased by 0.19 cm^3/day and the glands shifted medially, on average, by 3.1 mm. In seven lung cancer patients undergoing daily MV CT imaging, Ramsey et al. (226) reported a mean GTV reduction of 31%. Kupelian et al. (149) treated 10 NSCLC patients with the Tomotherapy system and observed an average decrease in GTV of 1.2% per day; five of six replanned cases demonstrated small increases in tumor dose delivery. Van de Bunt et al. (283) reported an average reduction in the GTV of 46% in 14 cervical cancers reimaged with MRI after the delivery of 30 Gy (Fig. 10.32). In contrast, no significant changes have been reported in other tumor sites, notably prostate cancer (61).

Several investigators have reported that adapting to morphologic changes may improve treatment delivery. Ramsey et al. (226) found that the lung V$_{20}$ would be decreased from 23%

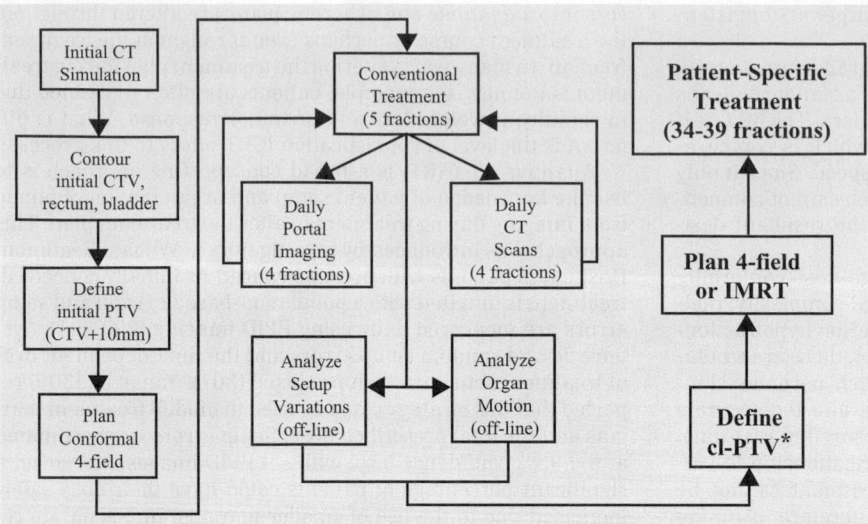

FIGURE 10.31. The Beaumont adaptive radiation therapy process. An offline analysis of setup error and organ motion is performed during the first 5 days of treatment. These characterizations are used to predict variations over the remaining fractions, and the confidence-limited planning target volume (CL-PTV) is designed to provide dosimetric coverage of the nonsystematic components of these variations. CTV, clinical target volume; IMRT, intensity modulated radiation therapy. (From Brabbins D, Martinez A, Yan D, et al. A dose-escalation trial with the adaptive radiotherapy process as a delivery system in localized prostate cancer: analysis of chronic toxicity. *Int J Radiat Oncol Biol Phys* 2005;61:400–408, with permission.)

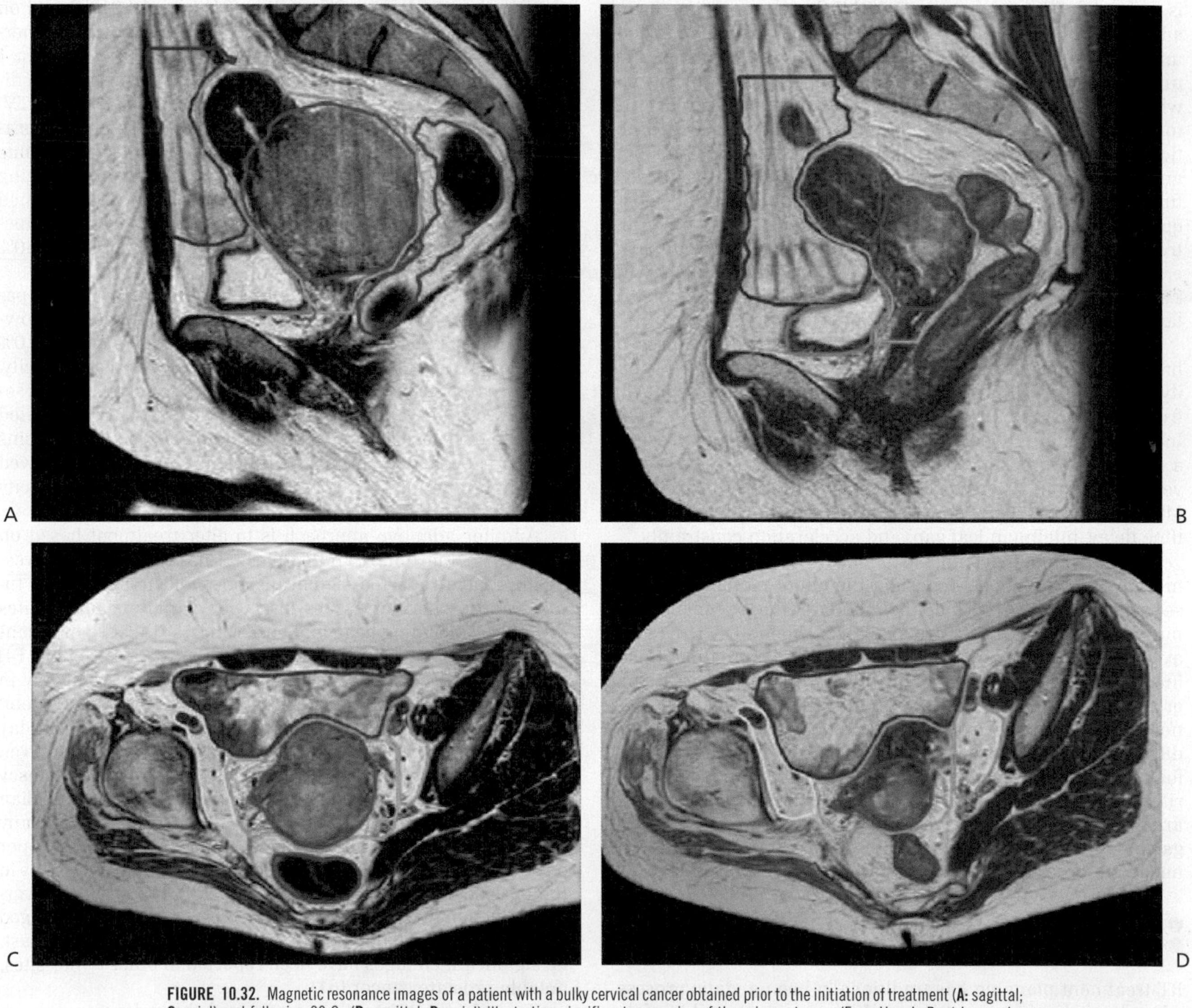

FIGURE 10.32. Magnetic resonance images of a patient with a bulky cervical cancer obtained prior to the initiation of treatment (**A:** sagittal; **C:** axial) and following 30 Gy (**B:** sagittal; **D:** axial) illustrating significant regression of the primary tumor. (From Van de Bunt L, van der Heided UA, Ketelaars M, et al. Conventional, conformal and intensity modulated radiation therapy treatment planning of external beam radiotherapy for cervical cancer: the impact of tumor regression. *Int J Radiat Oncol Biol Phys* 2006;64:189–196, with permission.)

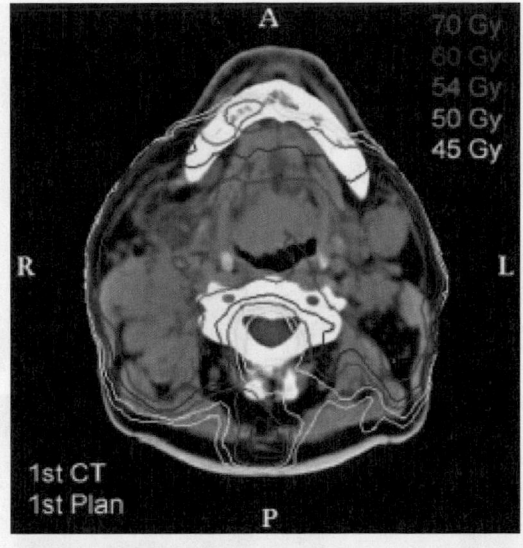

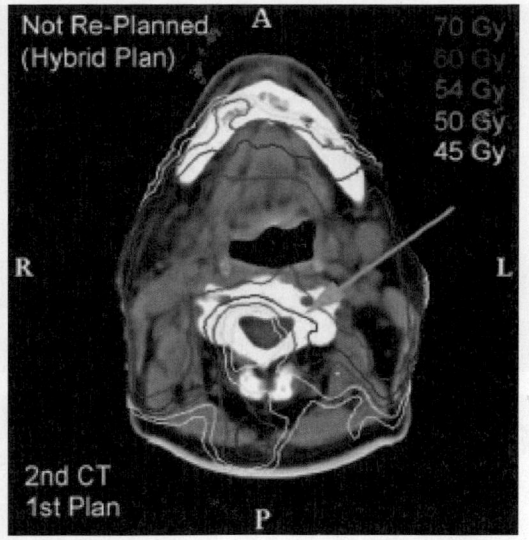

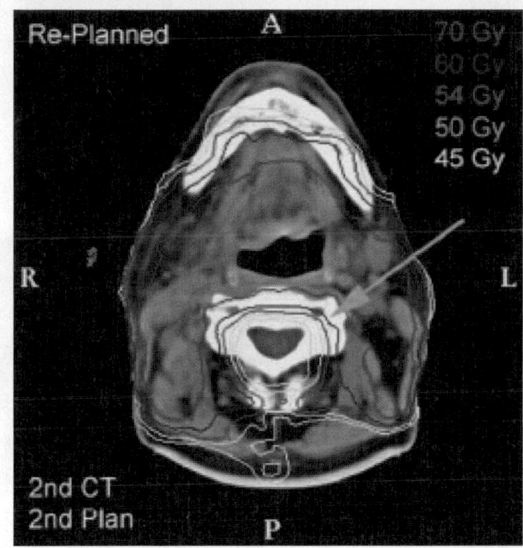

FIGURE 10.33. The benefit of replanning midway through treatment is illustrated in a patient with a T2N2C base of tongue carcinoma. **A:** The initial intensity modulated radiation therapy (IMRT) plan generated from the initial planning computed tomography (CT) scan. **B:** A second CT scan during treatment showing the isodose lines obtained without replanning. **C:** The same slice from the second CT scan, with isodose lines obtained by replanning. The second CT was obtained after 22 fractions and after a 12% weight loss from the start of treatment. The arrow demonstrates the increased spinal cord dose without replanning. (From Hansen EK, Bucci MK, Quivey JM, et al. Repeat CT imaging and re-planning during the course of IMRT for head-and-neck cancer. *Int I Radiat Oncol Biol Phys* 2006;64:355-362, with permission.)

Overview and Basic Science of Radiation Oncology

to 17% by adapting to reductions in the GTV in lung cancer patients, corresponding to 17% less reduction in lung perfusion. Hansen et al. (111) evaluated the impact of re-planning in a cohort of 13 head and neck cancer patients with either significant weight loss and/or tumor response during IMRT (Fig. 10.33). Compared to replanning, not replanning significantly decreased dose to the target volume and increased doses to normal tissues (spinal cord and brainstem). The D_{95} of the PTV_{GTV} and the PTV_{CTV} decreased by up to 6.3 Gy and 7.4 Gy, respectively.

Adaptation could potentially be extended beyond morphologic changes in the tumor. For example, plans could be altered based on normal tissue imaging changes occurring during RT (26). An intriguing idea is to adapt the plan to *functional* changes of the tumor. This approach has received little attention to date, most likely due to the fact that current IGRT technologies do not allow in-room functional imaging. However, increasing data suggest that functional changes in tumors are correlated with outcome (296). Whether adapting the plan (e.g., intensifying treatment in patients with suboptimal metabolic changes) would improve patient outcome remains unclear.

From a technical standpoint, a major concern is *how* to efficiently adapt to changes in the tumor and/or normal tissues during treatment. Although it may be trivial to occasionally

replan a limited number of patients, frequent replanning of many patients requires new software tools and approaches. Recontouring is time consuming, impractical, and prone to variability, even when performed by the same individual. To date, several groups have explored automated segmentation algorithms in a number of disease sites using various imaging technologies (13,28,49,175,192). Automated segmentation in IGRT is particularly problematic since repeat imaging is performed without contrast and may have less than optimal soft tissue contrast.

A challenging problem in adaptive IGRT is the registration of serial images due to changes in the size and shape of the target and normal tissues. Fortunately, several groups have developed deformable registration algorithms to account for such changes (34,45,80,169,241,291,292). Investigators at M.D. Anderson Hospital have developed a deformable registration approach based on the "Demons" algorithm, which iteratively minimizes differences in intensities between the reference and subsequent images (291) (Fig. 10.34). This approach has been shown to be highly accurate in both phantom studies and evaluation of serial CT images in prostate and head and neck cancer patients. Recently, this algorithm has been enhanced, improving its calculation speed and tolerance of large organ deformations (292).

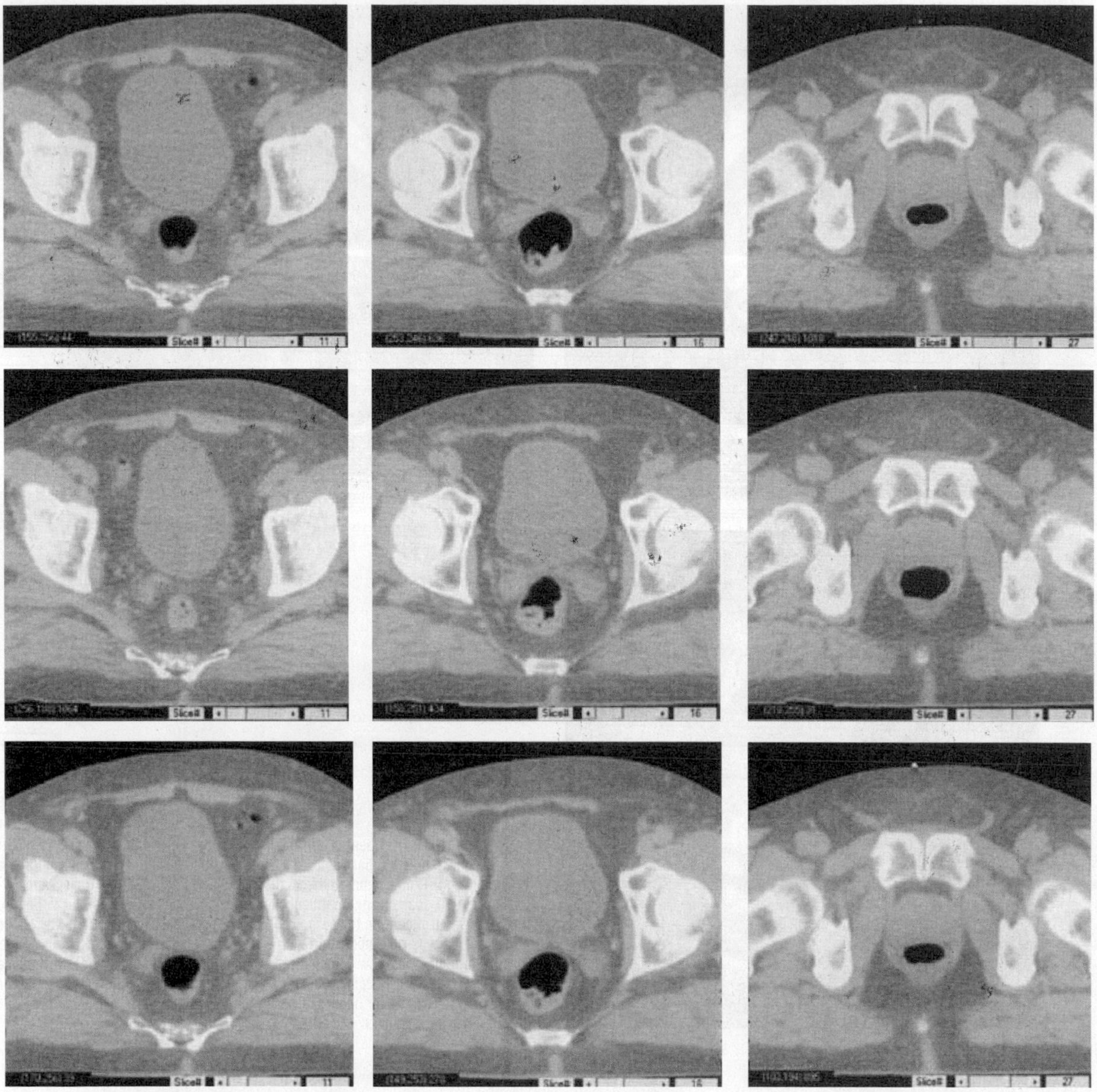

FIGURE 10.34. Deformable image registration of patient computed tomography (CT) sets obtained from two separate CT sessions. The top row includes three slices of the pelvic CT images obtained during session one. The middle images are corresponding CT slices during session two. The bottom row illustrates algorithm deformed session two images to match session one images. (From Wang H, Dong L, Fwu M, et al. Implementation and validation of a three-dimensional deformable registration algorithm for targeted prostate cancer radiotherapy. *Int J Radiat Oncol Biol Phys* 2005;61:725–735, with permission.)

Lu et al. (169) developed a fully automatic voxel similarity based free-form deformable registration algorithm using the calculus of variations. This approach has been shown to produce highly accurate deformations in patients with lung cancer imaged at different phases of the respiratory cycle and in prostate cancer patients imaged on different days. Commercial systems are also being developed that will aid in contouring of large numbers of serial images (11).

Deformable image registration may alter our interpretation of target and tumor tissue dose-volume histograms. Traditionally, a DVH was generated prior to treatment to help guide the selection between various treatment plans. Deformable registration will also alter the generation of actual DVH based on the daily dose distribution, organ position, and shape. Using a thin-plate spline deformable registration technique, Schaly et al. (241) calculated a cumulative dose distribution in a prostate cancer patient undergoing serial CT imaging during RT. Large differences in the dose to the normal tissues were noted. A

smaller difference was noted in terms of the target DVH. Such techniques may help reduce the toxicity in select patients. Moreover, it may allow one to adapt the treatment plan midway through treatment if the actual dose deposition is worse than the predicted DVH.

To improve the efficiency of the adaptive RT process, Mohan et al. (183) have proposed an alternative to full-fledged reoptimization, namely deformation of the IMRT dose distribution based on the deformation of the anatomy in the beam's eye view projection (Fig. 10.35). For select prostate and head-and-neck patient examples, the results of the deformed intensities were found to be a good approximation of full-fledged replanning. In both cases, the results were superior to the use of a single treatment plan used throughout the treatment course. Other approaches to streamline the adaptive IGRT process have also been described (116).

Many questions remain to be answered before true adaptive RT can be introduced into clinical practice. For example, how

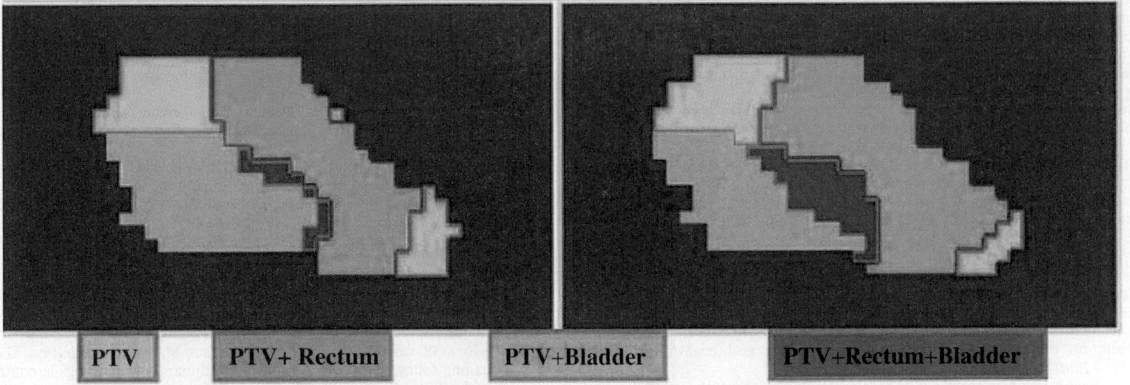

(a) Segmented BEV based on Pre-tx CT   **(a) Segmented BEV based on fx 7 CT**

| PTV | PTV+ Rectum | PTV+Bladder | PTV+Rectum+Bladder |

(c) Initial Intensity Distributions   **(d) Deformably Mapped to Fraction 7**

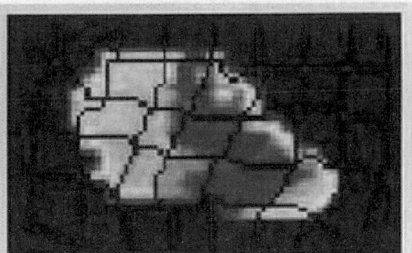

FIGURE 10.35. Illustration of the aperture segment by aperture segment deformation of intensity distributions. The beam's eye view (BEV) apertures for each beam are segmented into regions of overlap of the planning target volume with normal structures. The intensity distributions within each segment from the original pretreatment intensity-modulated radiation therapy (IMRT) plan are then mapped to the corresponding segment with the current treatment's BEV. (From Mohan R, Zhang X, Wang H, et al. Use of deformed intensity distributions for on-line modification of image-guided IMRT to account for interfractional anatomic changes. *Int J Radiat Oncol Biol Phys* 2005;61:1258–1266, with permission.)

often should new plans be generated? Once? Weekly? Daily? Another question is whether altering the target volume would *adversely* impact tumor control. In the Hansen et al. (111) study, attempts were made to "maintain the size of the original GTV in the second plan without extending it beyond the skin contour or into adjacent normal structures," ensuring irradiation of potential microscopic disease spread. Such concerns are quite reasonable in infiltrative tumors such as head and neck cancers. However, such concerns may be less valid in noninfiltrative tumors (e.g., bulky lymphadenopathy). Altering the target volume as the tumor responds in this situation should carry less risk. Moreover, it should reduce the risk of toxicity and allow the delivery of higher, more effective doses. The answer to these and other questions can only be answered by carefully designed clinical trials.

Conclusions

IGRT is a cornerstone of modern radiation oncology that holds considerable promise to improve cancer treatment. However, as discussed in this chapter, most IGRT technologies have not yet been proven to change patients' ultimate outcomes. In addition, IGRT may be associated with significant increases in cost to patients and the medical system, and economic competition is likely to have an important impact on its implementation in general radiation oncology practice. Therefore, continued careful study and quantification of the effects of IGRT on treatment outcomes are needed so that definitive statements may be made about its necessity in everyday radiotherapy.

References

1. Adler JR, Murphy MJ, Chang SD, et al. Image guided robotic radiosurgery. *Neurosurgery* 1999;44:1299–1306.
2. Ahn YC, Shimizu S, Shirato H, et al. Application of real-time tumor-tracking and gated radiotherapy system for unresectable pancreatic cancer. *Yonsei Med J* 2004;45:584–590.
3. Allen AM, Siracuse KM, Hayman JA, et al. Evaluation of the influence of breathing on the movement and modeling of lung tumors. *Int J Radiat Oncol Biol Phys* 2004;58:1251–1257.
4. Allen AM, Siracuse KM, Hayman JA, et al. Evaluation of the influence of breathing on the movement and modeling of lung tumors. *Int J Radiat Oncol Biol Phys* 2004;58:1251–1257.
5. Antonuk L. Electronic portal imaging devices: a review and historical perspective of contemporary technologies and research. *Phys Med Biol* 2002;47:R31–R65.
6. Aoyama H, Kamada K, Shirato H, et al. Integration of functional brain information into stereotactic irradiation treatment planning using magnetoencephalography and magnetic resonance axonography. *Int J Radiat Oncol Biol Phys* 2004;58:1177–1183.
7. Aoyama H, Shirato H, Nishioka T, et al. Magnetic resonance imaging system for three-dimensional conformal radiotherapy and its impact on gross tumor volume delineation of central nervous system tumors. *Int J Radiat Oncol Biol Phys* 2001;50:821–827.
8. Artignan X, Smitsmans MH, Lebesque JV, et al. Online ultrasound image guidance for radiotherapy of prostate cancer: impact of image acquisition on prostate displacement. *Int J Radiat Oncol Biol Phys* 2004;59:595–601.
9. Ashamalla H, Rafla S, Parikh K, et al. The contribution of integrated PET/CT to the evolving definition of treatment volumes in radiation treatment planning in lung cancer. *Int J Radiat Oncol Biol Phys* 2005;63:1016–1023.
10. Aubin M, Morin O, Chen J, et al. The use of megavoltage cone-beam CT to complement CT for target definition in pelvic radiotherapy in the presence of hip replacement. *Br J Radiol* 2006;79:918–921.
11. Available at: http://www.ikoetech.com/. Last accessed November 27, 2006.
12. Balter J, Brock K, Litzenberg DW, et al. Daily targeting of intrahepatic tumors for radiotherapy. *Int J Radiat Oncol Biol Phys* 2002;52:266–271.
13. Barber DC, Hose DR. Automatic segmentation of medical images using image registration diagnostic and simulation applications. *J Med Eng Technol* 2005;29:53–63.
14. Barker JL, Garden AS, Ang KK, et al. Quantification of volumetric and geometric changes during fractionated radiotherapy for head-and-neck cancer using an integrated CT/linear accelerator system. *Int J Radiat Oncol Biol Phys* 2004;59:960–970.
15. Baroni G, Ferrigno G, Orrechia R, et al. Real-time opto-electronic verification of patient position in breast cancer radiotherapy. *Comput Aided Surg* 2000;5:296–306.

16. Bel A, Keus R, Vijlbrief RE, et al. Setup deviations in wedged pair irradiation of parotid gland and tonsillar tumors, measured with an electronic portal imaging device. *Radiother Oncol* 1995;37:153–159.
17. Bel A, van Herk M, Bartelink H, et al. A verification procedure to improve patient setup accuracy using portal images. *Radiother Oncol* 1993;29:253–260.
18. Bel A, Vos PH, Rodrigus PTR, et al. High precision prostate cancer irradiation by clinical application of an offline patient setup verification procedure, using portal imaging. *Int J Radiat Oncol Biol Phys* 1996;35:321–332.
19. Ben-Josef E, Normolle D, Ensminger WD, et al. Phase II trial of high-dose conformal radiation therapy with concurrent hepatic artery floxuridine for unresectable intra-hepatic malignancies. *J Clin Oncol* 2005;23:8739–8747.
20. Benzil DL, Saboori M, Mogilner AY, et al. Safety and efficacy of stereotactic radiosurgery for tumors of the spine. *J Neurosurg* 2004;101[Suppl 3]:413–418.
21. Berbeco RI, Jiang SB, Sharp GC, et al. Integrated radiotherapy imaging system (IRIS): design considerations of tumour tracking with LINAC gantry-mounted diagnostic x-ray systems with flat-panel detectors. *Phys Med Biol* 2004;49:243–255.
22. Berbeco RI, Mostafavi H, Sharp GC, et al. Towards fluoroscopic respiratory gating for lung tumours without radiopaque markers. *Phys Med Biol* 2005;50:4481–4490.
23. Berson AM, Emery R, Rodriguez L, et al. Clinical experience using respiratory gated radiation therapy: comparison of free-breathing and breath-hold techniques. *Int J Radiat Oncol Biol Phys* 2004;60:419–426.
24. Bert C, Metheany KG, Doppke K, et al. A phantom evaluation of a stereo-vision surface imaging system for radiotherapy patient setup. *Med Phys* 2005;32:2753–2762.
25. Bhatnagar AK, Gerszten PC, Ozhasaglu C, et al. Cyberknife frameless radiosurgery for the treatment of extracranial benign tumors. *Technol Cancer Res Treat* 2005;4:571–576.
26. Blomlie V, Rofstad EK, Skjonsberg A, et al. Female pelvic bone marrow: serial MR imaging before, during and after radiation therapy. *Radiology* 1995;194:537–543.
27. Boda-Heggemann J, Walter C, Mai S, et al. Frameless stereotactic radiosurgery of a solitary liver metastasis using active breathing control and stereotactic ultrasound. *Strahlenther Onkol* 2006;182:216–221.
28. Bondiau PY, Malandain G, Chanalet S, et al. Atlas-based automatic segmentation of MR images: validation study on the brainstem in radiotherapy context. *Int J Radiat Oncol Biol Phys* 2005;61:289–298.
29. Bouchet LG, Meeks SL, Goodchild G, et al. Calibration of three-dimensional ultrasound images for image-guided radiation therapy. *Phys Med Biol* 2001;46:559–577.
30. Boyer AL, Antonuk L, Fenster A, et al. A review of electronic portal imaging devices (EPIDs). *Med Phys* 1992;19:1–16.
31. Brabbins D, Martinez A, Yan D, et al. A dose-escalation trial with the adaptive radiotherapy process as a delivery system in localized prostate cancer: analysis of chronic toxicity. *Int J Radiat Oncol Biol Phys* 2005;61:400–408.
32. Bradley J, Thorstad WL, Mutic S, et al. Impact of FDG-PET on radiation therapy volume delineation in non-small-cell lung cancer. *Int J Radiat Oncol Biol Phys* 2004;59(1):78–86.
33. Britton KR, Takai Y, Mitsuya M, et al. Evaluation of inter- and intrafraction organ motion during intensity modulated radiation therapy for localized prostate cancer measured by a newly developed on-board image-guided system. *Rad Med* 2005;23:14–24.
34. Brock KK, Dawson LA, Sharpe MB, et al. Feasibility of a novel deformable image registration technique to facilitate classification, targeting, and monitoring of tumor and normal tissue. *Int J Radiat Oncol Biol Phys* 2006;64:1245–1254.
35. Buyyounouski MK, Horwitz EM, Price RA, et al. Intensity-modulated radiotherapy with MRI simulation to reduce doses received by erectile tissue during prostate cancer treatment. *Int J Radiat Oncol Biol Phys* 2004;58:743–749.
36. Chan AA, Lau A, Pirzkall A, et al. Proton magnetic resonance spectroscopy imaging in the evaluation of patients undergoing gamma knife surgery for grade IV glioma. *J Neurosurg* 2004;101:467–475.
37. Chandra A, Dong L, Huang E, et al. Experience of ultrasound-based daily prostate localization. *Int J Radiat Oncol Biol Phys* 2003;56:436–447.
38. Chang EL, Shiu AS, Lii MF, et al. Phase I clinical evaluation of near-simultaneous computed tomographic image-guided stereotactic body radiotherapy for spinal metastasis. *Int J Radiat Oncol Biol Phys* 2004;59:1288–1294.
39. Chang SD, Martin DP, Lee E, et al. Stereotactic radiosurgery and hypofractionated stereotactic radiotherapy for residual or recurrent cranial base and cervical chordomas. *Neurosurg Focus* 2001;10:E5.
40. Chao KS, Bosch WR, Mutic S, et al. A novel approach to overcome hypoxic tumor resistance: Cu-ATSM-guided intensity-modulated radiation therapy. *Int J Radiat Oncol Biol Phys* 2001;49:1171–1182.
41. Chen GT, Kung JH, Beaudette KP. Artifacts in computed tomography scanning of moving objects. *Semin Radiat Oncol* 2004;14:19–26.
42. Chen JC, Girvigian M, Greathouse H, et al. Treatment of trigeminal neuralgia with linear accelerator radiosurgery: initial results. *J Neurosurg* 2004;101[Suppl 3]:346–350.
43. Cheng CW, Wong J, Grimm L, et al. Commissioning and clinical implementation of a sliding gantry CT scanner installed in an existing treatment room and early clinical experience for precise tumor localization. *Am J Clin Oncol* 2003;26:28–36.
44. Chinnaiyen P, Tomee W, Patel R, et al. 3D-ultrasound guided radiation therapy in the post-prostatectomy setting. *Technol Cancer Res Treat* 2003;2:455–458.
45. Christensen GE, Carlson B, Chao KSC, et al. Image-based dose planning of intracavitary brachytherapy: registration of serial-imaging studies using deformable anatomic templates. *Int J Radiat Oncol Biol Phys* 2001;51:227–243.
46. Christian JA, Partridge M, Nioutsikou E, et al. The incorporation of SPECT functional lung imaging into inverse radiotherapy planning for non-small cell lung cancer. *Radiother Oncol* 2005;77:271–277.
47. Chung PWM, Haycocks T, Brown T, et al. On-line aSi portal imaging of implanted fiducial markers for the reduction of interfraction error during conformal radiotherapy of prostate carcinoma. *Int J Radiat Oncol Biol Phys* 2004;60:329–334.
48. Ciernik IF, Huser M, Burger C, et al. Automated functional image-guided radiation treatment planning for rectal cancer. *Int J Radiat Oncol Biol Phys* 2005;62:893–900.
49. Ciernik IF, Huser M, Burger C, et al. Automated functional image-guided radiation treatment planning for rectal cancer. *Int J Radiat Oncol Biol Phys* 2005;62:893–900.
50. Connor W, Boone M, Veomett R, et al. Patient repositioning and motion detection using a video cancellation system. *Int J Radiat Oncol Biol Phys* 1975;1:147–153.
51. Court L, Rosen I, Mohan R, et al. Evaluation of mechanical precision and alignment uncertainties for an integrated CT/linac system. *Med Phys* 2003;30:1–13.
52. Cury F, Shenouda G, Souhami L, et al. Comparison of BAT system and a new 3D trans-abdominal ultrasound-based image-guided system for prostate daily localization during external beam radiotherapy. *Int J Radiat Oncol Biol Phys* 2004;60:S329.
53. de Boer HCJ, Meijman BJM. A protocol for the reduction of systematic patient setup errors with minimal portal imaging workload. *Int J Radiat Oncol Biol Phys* 2001;50:1350–1365.
54. de Boer HCJ, Sornsen de Koste JR, Senan S, et al. Analysis and reduction of 3D systematic and random setup errors during the simulation and treatment of lung cancer patients with CT-based external beam radiotherapy dose planning. *Int J Radiat Oncol Biol Phys* 2001;49:857–868.
55. de Boer HCJ, van Sornsen de Koste JR, Creutzbeerg CL, et al. Electronic portal image assisted reduction of systematic set-up errors in head and neck irradiation. *Radiother Oncol* 2001;61:299–308.
56. De Crevoisier, Tucker SL, Dong L, et al. Increased risk of biochemical and local failure in patients with distended rectum on the planning CT for prostate cancer radiotherapy. *Int J Radiat Oncol Biol Phys* 2005;62:965–973.
57. De Neve W, van den Heuvel F, de Beukeleer M, et al. Routine clinical on-line portal imaging followed by immediate field adjustment using a tele-controlled patient couch. *Radiother Oncol* 1992;24:45–54.
58. De Salles AA, Pedroso AG, Medin P, et al. Spinal lesions treated with Novalis shaped beam intensity-modulated radiosurgery and stereotactic radiotherapy. *J Neurosurg* 2004;101[Suppl 3]:435–440.
59. Dehnad H, Nederveen AJ, van der Heide UA, et al. Clinical feasibility study for the use of implanted gold seeds in the prostate as reliable positioning markers during megavoltage irradiation. *Radiother Oncol* 2003;67:295–302.
60. Deniaud-Alexandre E, Touboul E, Lerouge D, et al. Impact of computed tomography and ^{18}F-deoxyglucose coincidence detection emission tomography image fusion for optimization of conformal radiotherapy in non-small-cell lung cancer. *Int J Radiat Oncol Biol Phys* 2005;63:1432–1441.
61. Deurloo KE, Steenbakkers RJ, Zijp LJ, et al. Quantification of shape variation of prostate and seminal vesicles during external beam radiotherapy. *Int J Radiat Oncol Biol Phys* 2005;61:228–238.
62. Djajaputra D, Li S. Real-time surface-image-guided beam setup in radiotherapy of breast cancer. *Med Phys* 2005;32:65–75.
63. Dobler B, Mai S, Ross C, et al. Evaluation of possible prostate displacement induced by pressure applied during transabdominal ultrasound image acquisition. *Strahlenther Onkol* 2006;182:240–246.
64. Dodd RL, Ryu MR, Kamnerdsupaphon P, et al. CyberKnife radiosurgery for benign intradural extramedullary spinal tumors. *Neurosurgery* 2006;58:674–685.
65. Dong L, De Crevoisier R, Bonnen M, et al. Evaluation of an ultrasound-based prostate target localization technique with in-room CT-on-rails. *Int J Radiat Oncol Biol Phys* 2004;60:S332(abstr).
66. Ekberg L, Holmberg O, Wittgren L, et al. What margins should be added to the clinical target volume in radiotherapy treatment planning for lung cancer? *Radiother Oncol* 1998;48(1):71–77.
67. Ellis RJ, Sodee DB, Spirnak JP, et al. Feasibility and acute toxicities of radioimmunoguided prostate brachytherapy. *Int J Radiat Oncol Biol Phys* 2000;48:683–687.
68. Ellis RJ, Vertocnik A, Kim E, et al. Four-year biochemical outcome after radioimmunoguided transperineal brachytherapy for patients with prostate adenocarcinoma. *Int J Radiat Oncol Biol Phys* 2003;57:362–370.
69. Emami B, Sethi A, Petruzzelli GJ. Influence of MRI on target volume delineation and IMRT planning in nasopharyngeal carcinoma. *Int J Radiat Oncol Biol Phys* 2003;57:481–488.
70. Engelsman M, Damen EM, De Jaeger K, et al. The effect of breathing and set-up errors on the cumulative dose to a lung tumor. *Radiother Oncol* 2001;60:95–105.
71. Enke CA, Ayyangar KM, Saw CB, et al. Inter-observer variation in prostate localization utilizing BAT. *Int J Radiat Oncol Biol Phys* 2002;54:S269(abstr).
72. Ernst-Stecken A, Lambrecht U, Mueller R, et al. Dose escalation in large anterior skull-base tumors by means of IMRT. First experience with the Novalis system. *Strahlenther Onkol* 2006;182:183–189.
73. Erridge SC, Seppenwoolde Y, Muller SH, et al. Portal imaging to assess setup-errors, tumor motion and tumor shrinkage during conformal radiotherapy of non-small cell lung cancer. *Radiother Oncol* 2003;66:75–85.
74. Esthappan J, Mutic S, Malyapa RS, et al. Treatment planning guidelines regarding the use of CT/PET-guided IMRT for cervical carcinoma with positive para-aortic lymph nodes. *Int J Radiat Oncol Biol Phys* 2004;58:1289–1297.
75. Fein DA, McGee KP, Schultheiss TE, et al. Intra- and inter-fractional reproducibility of tangential breast fields: a prospective on-line portal imaging study. *Int J Radiat Oncol Biol Phys* 1996;34:733–740.
76. Feldkamp LA, Davis LC, Kress JW. Practical cone-beam algorithm. *J Opt Soc Am A* 1984;1:612–619.
77. Fenig E, Mishaeli M, Yerushalmi R, et al. Treatment of neuroblastoma using the fused imaging guided radiotherapy (FIGURA) system. *Clin Nucl Med* 2006;31:256–258.
78. Ford EC, Chang J, Mueller K, et al. Cone-beam CT with megavoltage beams and an amorphous silicon electronic portal imaging device: potential for verification of radiotherapy of lung cancer. *Med Phys* 2002;29:2913–2934.
79. Forrest LJ, Mackie TR, Ruchala K, et al. The utility of megavoltage computed tomography images from a helical tomotherapy system for setup verification purposes. *Int J Radiat Oncol Biol Phys* 2004;60:1639–1644.
80. Foskey M, Davis B, Goyal L, et al. Large deformation three-dimensional image registration in image-guided radiation therapy. *Phys Med Biol* 2005;50:5869–5892.
81. Fox T, Huntzinger C, Johnstone P, et al. Performance evaluation of an automated image registration algorithm using an integrated kilovoltage imaging and guidance system. *J Appl Clin Med Phys* 2006;7:97–104.
82. Fukumoto S, Shirato H, Shimzu S, et al. Small-volume image-guided radiotherapy using hypofractionated, coplanar, and noncoplanar multiple fields for patients with inoperable stage I non–small cell lung carcinomas. *Cancer* 2002;95:1546–1553.
83. Fuller CD, Thomas CR, Wong A, et al. Image-guided intensity-modulated radiation therapy for gallbladder carcinoma. *Radiother Oncol* 2006;81:65–72.

84. Fung AYC, Enke CA, Ayyangar KM, et al. Prostate motion and isocenter adjustment from ultrasound-based localization during delivery of radiation therapy. *Int J Radiat Oncol Biol Phys* 2005;61:984–992.
85. Fuss M, Cavanugh SX, Fuss C, et al. Daily stereotactic ultrasound prostate targeting: inter-user variability. *Technol Cancer Res Treat* 2003;2:161–170.
86. Fuss M, Salter BJ, Cavanagh SX, et al. Daily ultrasound-based image-guided targeting for radiotherapy of upper abdominal malignancies. *Int J Radiat Oncol Biol Phys* 2004;59:1245–1256.
87. Ganswindt U, Paulsen F, Corvin S, et al. Intensity modulated radiotherapy for high risk prostate cancer based on sentinel node SPECT imaging for target volume definition. *BMC Cancer* 2005;5:91.
88. Geets X, Daisne JF, Gregoire V, et al. Role of 11-C-methionine positron emission tomography for the delineation of the tumor volume in pharyngo-laryngeal squamous cell carcinoma: comparison with FDG-PET and CT. *Radiother Oncol* 2004;71:267–273.
89. Gerszten PC, Germanwala A, Burton SA, et al. Combination kyphoplasty and spinal radiosurgery: a new treatment paradigm for pathological fractures. *J Neurosurg Spine* 2005;3:296–301.
90. Gerszten PC, Ozhasoglu C, Burton SA, et al. Cyberknife frameless single-fraction stereotactic radiosurgery for tumors of the sacrum. *Neurosurg Focus* 2003; 15:E7.
91. Gerszten PC, Ozhasoglu C, Burton SA. et al. CyberKnife frameless stereotactic radiosurgery for spinal lesions: clinical experience in 125 cases. *Neurosurgery* 2004;55:89–99.
92. Gierga DP, Brewer J, Sharp GC, et al. The correlation between internal and external markers for abdominal tumors: implications for respiratory gating. *Int J Radiat Oncol Biol Phys* 2005;61:1551–1558.
93. Gierga DP, Chen GT, Kung JH, et al. Quantification of respiration-induced abdominal tumor motion and its impact on IMRT dose distributions. *Int J Radiat Oncol Biol Phys* 2004;58:1584–1595.
94. Gildersleve J, Dearnaley DP, Evans PM, et al. A randomized trial of patient repositioning during radiotherapy using a megavoltage imaging system. *Radiother Oncol* 1994;31:161–168.
95. Giller CA, Berger BD, Gillo JP, et al. Feasibility of radiosurgery for malignant brain tumors in infants by use of image-guided robotic radiosurgery: preliminary report. *Neurosurgery* 2004;55:916–924.
96. Giller CA, Berger BD, Pistenmaa DA, et al. Robotically guided radiosurgery for children. *Pediatr Blood Cancer* 2005;45:304–331.
97. Godfrey DJ, Yin FF, Oldham M, et al. Digital tomosynthesis with an on-board kilovoltage imaging device. *Int J Radiat Oncol Biol Phys* 2006;65:8–15.
98. Gregoire V, Daisne JF, Geets X. Comparison of CT- and FDG-PET-defined GT: in regard to Paulino et al. *Int J Radiat Oncol Biol Phys* 2005;63:308–309.
99. Groh BA, Siewerdsen JH, Drake DG, et al. A performance comparison of flat-panel imager-based MV and KV cone-beam CT. *Med Phys* 2002;29:967–975.
100. Gross MW, Weber WA, Feldmann HJ, et al. The value of F-18-fluorodeoxyglucose PET for the 3-D radiation treatment planning of malignant gliomas. *Int J Radiat Oncol Biol Phys* 1998;41:989–995.
101. Grosu AL, Feldmann H, Dick S, et al. Implications of IMT-SPECT for postoperative radiotherapy planning in patients with gliomas. *Int J Radiat Oncol Biol Phys* 2002;54:842–854.
102. Grosu AL, Molls M, Zimmermann FB, et al. High-precision radiation therapy with integrated biological imaging and tumor monitoring: evolution of the Munich concept and future research options. *Strahlenther Onkol* 2006;182:361–368.
103. Grosu AL, Piert M, Weber WA, et al. Positron emission tomography for radiation treatment planning. *Strahlenther Onkol* 2005;181:483–499.
104. Grosu AL, Weber W, Feldmann HJ, et al. First experience with I-123-alpha-methyl-tyrosine SPECT in the 3-D radiation treatment planning of brain gliomas. *Int J Radiat Oncol Biol Phys* 2000;47:517–526.
105. Grosu AL, Weber WA, Astner ST, et al. 11C-methionine PET improves the target volume delineation of meningiomas treated with stereotactic fractionated radiotherapy. *Int J Radiat Oncol Biol Phys* 2006;66:339–334.
106. Grosu AL, Weber WA, Riedel E, et al. L-(methyl-11C) methionine positron emission tomography for target delineation in resected high-grade gliomas before radiotherapy. *Int J Radiat Oncol Biol Phys* 2005;63:64–74.
107. Guckenberg M, Meyer J, Vordermark D, et al. Magnitude and clinical relevance of translational and rotational patient setup errors: a cone-beam CT study. *Int J Radiat Oncol Biol Phys* 2006;65:934–942.
108. Hall EJ, Giaccia AJ. Oxygen effect and reoxygenation. In: Hall EJ, Giaccia AJ, eds. *Radiobiology for the radiologist*. Philadelphia: Lippincott, 2006;88–91.
109. Hamilton RJ, Sweeney PJ, Pelizzari CA, et al. Functional imaging in treatment planning of brain lesions. *Int J Radiat Oncol Biol Phys* 1997;37:181–188.
110. Hangiandreou NJ. B-mode US: Basic concepts and new technology. *Radiographics* 2003;23:1019–1033.
111. Hansen EK, Bucci MK, Quivey JM, et al. Repeat CT imaging and re-planning during the course of IMRT for head-and-neck cancer. *Int J Radiat Oncol Biol Phys* 2006;64:355–362.
112. Hara W, Patel D, Pawlicki T, et al. Hypofractionated stereotactic radiotherapy for prostate cancer: early results. *Int J Radiat Oncol Biol Phys* 2006;66:S324–325(abstr).
113. Harada T, Shirato H, Ogura S, et al. Real-time tumor-tracking radiation therapy for lung carcinoma by the aid of insertion of a gold marker using broncho-fiberoscopy. *Cancer* 2002;95:1720–1727.
114. Harrison LB, Chadha M, Hill RJ, et al. Impact of tumor hypoxia and anemia on radiation therapy outcomes. *Oncologist* 2002;7:492–508.
115. Hashimoto T, Shirato H, Kato M, et al. Real-time monitoring of a digestive tract marker to reduce adverse effects of moving organs at risk in radiotherapy for thoracic and abdominal tumors. *Int J Radiat Oncol Biol Phys* 2005;61:1559–1564.
116. Haslam JJ, Mundt AJ, Roeske JC. Adaptive treatment planning using position compensated plans. *Int J Radiat Oncol Biol Phys* 2006;66:S123(abstr).
117. Hector CL, Evans PM, Webb S. The dosimetric consequences of inter-fractional patient movement on three classes of intensity-modulated delivery techniques in breast radiotherapy. *Radiother Oncol* 2001;59:281–291.
118. Henry AM, Stratford J, Davies J, et al. An assessment of clinically optimal gold marker length and diameter for pelvic radiotherapy verification using an amorphous silicon flat panel electronic portal imaging device. *Br J Radiol* 2005;78:737–741.
119. Henry AM, Stratford J, McCarthy C, et al. X-ray volume imaging in bladder radiotherapy verification. *Int J Radiat Oncol Biol Phys* 2006;64:1174–1178.
120. Herman MG, Pisnaky TM, Kruse JJ, et al. Technical aspects of daily online positioning of the prostate for three-dimensional conformal radiotherapy using an electronic portal imaging device. *Int J Radiat Oncol Biol Phys* 2003;57:1131–1140.
121. Herman MG. Clinical use of electronic portal imaging. *Sem Radiat Oncol* 2005;15:157–167.
122. Hodge W, Tome WA, Jaradat HA, et al. Feasibility report of image guided stereotactic body radiotherapy (IG-SBRT) with tomotherapy for early stage medically inoperable lung cancer using extreme hypofractation. *Acta Oncol* 2006;45:890–896.
123. Hua C, Lovelock DM, Mageras GS, et al. Development of a semi-automatic alignment tool for accelerated localization of the prostate. *Int J Radiat Oncol Biol Phys* 2003;55:811–824.
124. Huang E, Dong L, Chandra A, et al. Intrafraction prostate motion during IMRT for prostate cancer. *Int J Radiat Oncol Biol Phys* 2002;53:261–268.
125. Hui SK, Kapatoes J, Fowler J, et al. Feasibility study of helical tomotherapy for total body or total marrow irradiation. *Med Phys* 2005;32:3214–3224.
126. Imura M, Yamazaki K, Shirato H, et al. Insertion and fixation of fiducial markers for setup and tracking of lung tumors in radiotherapy. *Int J Radiat Oncol Biol Phys* 2005;63:1442–1447.
127. Ishihara H, Saito K, Nishizaki T, et al. Cyberknife radiosurgery for vestibular schwannoma. *Minim Invasive Neurosurg* 2004;47:290–293.
128. Jaffray DA. Emergent technologies for 3-dimensional image-guided radiation delivery. *Sem Radiat Oncol* 2005;15:208–216.
129. Jaffray SA, Drake DG, Moreau M, et al. A radiographic and tomographic imaging system integrated into a medical linear accelerator for localization of bone and soft-tissue targets. *Int J Radiat Oncol Biol Phys* 1999;45:773–789.
130. Jani AB, Blend MJ, Hamilton R, et al. Influence of radioimmunoscintigraphy on postprostatectomy radiotherapy treatment decision making. *J Nucl Med* 2004;45:571–578.
131. Jani AB, Blend MJ, Hamilton R, et al. Radioimmunoscintigraphy for post-prostatectomy radiotherapy: analysis of toxicity and biochemical control. *J Nucl Med* 2004;45:1315–1322.
132. Jani AB, Gratzle J, Muresan E, et al. Analysis of acute toxicity with the use of transabdominal ultrasonography for prostate positioning during intensity modulated radiotherapy. *Urology* 2005;65:504–508.
133. Jani AB, Gratzle J, Muresan E, et al. Impact on late toxicity of using transabdominal ultrasound for prostate cancer patients treated with intensity modulated radiotherapy. *Technol Cancer Res Treat* 2005;4:115–120.
134. Jeraj R, Mackie TR, Balog J, et al. Radiation characteristics of helical tomotherapy. *Med Phys* 2004;31:396–404.
135. Jiang S, Bortfeld T, Trofimov A, et al. Synchronized moving aperture radiation therapy (SMART): treatment planning using 4D CT data. Paper presented at: The 14th International Conference on the Use of Computers in Radiation Therapy, 2004; Seoul, Korea.
136. Jiang SB. Radiotherapy of mobile tumors. *Semin Radiat Oncol* 2006;16:239–248.
137. Jiang SB. Technical aspects of image-guided respiration-gated radiation therapy. *Med Dosim* 2006;31:141–151.
138. Johnson S, Milliken BD, Hadley SW, et al. Initial clinical experience with a video-based patient positioning system. *Int J Radiat Oncol Biol Phys* 1999;45:205–213.
139. Kaatee RS, Olofesen MJ, Verstraate MB, et al. Detection of organ movement in cervix cancer patients using a fluoroscopic electronic portal imaging device and radiopaque markers. *Int J Radiat Oncol Biol Phys* 2002;54:576–583.
140. Kajiwara K, Saito K, Yoshikawa K, et al. Image-guided radiosurgery with the Cyberknife for pituitary adenomas. *Minim Invasive Neurosurg* 2005;48:91–96.
141. Keall P. 4-Dimensional computed tomography imaging and treatment planning. *Semin Radiat Oncol* 2004;81–90.
142. Keall PJ, Kini VR, Vedam SS, et al. Motion adaptive x-ray therapy: a feasibility study. *Phys Med Biol* 2001;46:1–10.
143. King CR, Lehmann J, Adler JR, et al. Cyberknife radiotherapy for localized prostate cancer: rationale and technical feasibility. *Technol Cancer Res Treat* 2003;2:25–30.
144. Kitamura K, Shirato H, Seppenwoolde Y, et al. Three-dimensional intrafractional movement of the prostate measured during real-time tumor-tracking radiotherapy in supine and prone treatment positions. *Int J Radiat Oncol Biol Phys* 2002;53:1117–1123.
145. Kitamura K, Shirato H, Seppenwoolde Y, et al. Tumor location, cirrhosis and surgical history contribute to tumor movement in the liver, as measured during stereotactic irradiation using a real-time tumor-tracking radiotherapy system. *Int J Radiat Oncol Biol Phys* 2003;56:221–228.
146. Kitamura K, Shirato H, Shinohara N, et al. Reduction in acute morbidity using hypofractionated intensity-modulated radiation therapy assisted with a fluoroscopic real-time tumor-tracking system for prostate cancer: preliminary results of a phase I/II study. *Cancer J* 2003;9:268–276.
147. Kriminiski S, Mitschke M, Sorensen S, et al. Respiratory correlated cone-beam computed tomography on an isocentric c-arm. *Phys Med Biol* 2005;50: 5263–5280.
148. Kuban DA, Dong L, Cheung R, et al. Ultrasound-based localization. *Semin Radiat Oncol* 2005;15:180–191.
149. Kupelian PA, Ramsey C, Meeks SL, et al. Serial megavoltage CT imaging during external beam radiotherapy for non-small-cell lung cancer: observations on tumor regression during treatment. *Int J Radiat Oncol Biol Phys* 2005;63:1024–1028.
150. Kupelian PA, Thakkar VV, Khuntia D, et al. Hypofractionated intensity-modulated radiotherapy (70 Gy at 2.5 Gy per fraction) for localized prostate cancer: long-term outcomes. *Int J Radiat Oncol Biol Phys* 2005;63:1463–1468.
151. Kupelian PA, Willoughby TR, Meeks SL, et al. Intraprostatic fiducials for localization of the prostate gland: monitoring inter-marker distances during radiation therapy to test for marker stability. *Int J Radiat Oncol Biol Phys* 2005;62:1291–1296.
152. Kuriyama K, Onishi H, Sano N, et al. A new irradiation unit constructed of self-moving gantry-CT and LINAC. *Int J Radiat Oncol Biol Phys* 2003;55:428–435.
153. Lagerwaard FJ, Van Sornsen de Koste JR, Nijssen-Visser MR, et al. Multiple "slow" CT scans for incorporating lung tumor mobility in radiotherapy planning. *Int J Radiat Oncol Biol Phys* 2001;51;932–937.
154. Langen KM, Jones DT. Organ motion and its management. *Int J Radiat Oncol Biol Phys* 2001;50:265–278.
155. Langen KM, Pouliot J, Anezinos C, et al. Evaluation of ultrasound-based prostate localization for image-guided radiotherapy. *Int J Radiat Oncol Biol Phys* 2003;57:635–644.

156. Langen KM, Zhang Y, Andrews RD, et al. Initial experience with megavoltage (MV) CT guidance for daily prostate alignments. *Int J Radiat Oncol Biol Phys* 2005;62:1517–1524.
157. Lattanza J, McNeeley S, Donnelly S, et al. Ultrasound-based stereotactic guidance in prostate cancer—quantification of organ motion and set-up errors in external beam radiation therapy. *Comput Aided Surg* 2000;5:289–295.
158. Lattanzi J, McNeeley S, Hanlon A, et al. Ultrasound-based stereotactic guidance of precision conformal external beam radiation therapy in clinical localized prostate cancer. *Urology* 2000;55:73–78.
159. Leong T, Everitt C, Yuen K, et al. A prospective study to evaluate the impact of FDG-PET on CT-based radiotherapy treatment planning for oesophageal cancer. *Radiother Oncol* 2006;78:254–261.
160. Letourneau D, Martinez AA, Lockman D, et al. Assessment of residual error for online cone-beam XT-guided treatment of prostate cancer patients. *Int J Radiat Oncol Biol Phys* 2005;62:1239–1246.
161. Letourneau D, Wong JW, Oldham M, et al. Cone-beam-CT guided radiation therapy: technical implementation. *Radiother Oncol* 2005;75:279–286.
162. Li S, Geng J. Real-time-3D-video-guided IMRT: Emerging technology. In: Mundt AJ, Roeske JC, eds. *Intensity modulated radiation therapy: a clinical perspective.* Toronto: B.C. Decker Inc, 2005;407–413.
163. Li S, Liu D, Yin G, et al. Real-time 3D surface-guided head refixation useful for fractionated stereotactic radiotherapy. *Med Phys* 2006;33:492–503.
164. Lim M, Villavicencio AT, Burneikiene S, et al. Cyberknife radiosurgery for idiopathic trigeminal neuralgia. *Neurosurg Focus* 2005;18:E9.
165. Ling CC, Humm J, Larson S, et al. Towards multidimensional radiotherapy (MD-CRT): biological imaging and biological conformality. *Int J Radiat Oncol Biol Phys* 2000;47:551–560.
166. Linsenmaier U, Rock C, Euler E, et al. Three-dimensional CT with a modified c-arm image intensifier: feasibility. *Radiology* 2002;224:286–292.
167. Little DJ, Dong L, Levy LB, et al. Use of portal images and BAT ultrasonography to measure setup error and organ motion for prostate IMRT: implications for treatment margins. *Int J Radiat Oncol Biol Phys* 2003;56:1218–1224.
168. Liu WC, Schulder M, Narra V, et al. Functional magnetic resonance imaging aided radiation treatment planning. *Med Phys* 2000;27:1563–1572.
169. Lu W, Olivera GH, Chen Q, et al. Deformable registration of the planning image (kVCT) and the daily images (MVCT) for adaptive radiation therapy. *Phys Med Biol* 2006;51:4357–4374.
170. Ma CM, Paskalev K. In-room techniques for image-guided radiation therapy. *Med Dosim* 2006;1:30–39.
171. Mackie TR, Kapatoes J, Ruchala K, et al. Image guidance for precise conformal radiotherapy. *Int J Radiat Oncol Biol Phys* 2003;56:89–105.
172. MacManus MP, Hicks RJ, Matthews JP, et al. High rate of detection of unsuspected distant metastases by PET in apparent stage III non-small-cell lung cancer: implications for radical radiation therapy. *Int J Radiat Oncol Biol Phys* 2001;50:287–293.
173. Mahan SL, Ramsey CR, Scaperoth DD, et al. Evaluation of image-guided helical tomotherapy for the re-treatment of spinal metastasis. *Int J Radiat Oncol Biol Phys* 2005;63:1576–1583.
174. Manning MA, Wu Q, Cardinale RM, et al. The effect of setup uncertainty on normal tissue sparing with IMRT for head-and-neck cancer. *Int J Radiat Oncol Biol Phys* 2001;51:1400–1409.
175. Mazzara GP, Velthuizen RP, Pearlman JL, et al. Brain tumor target volume determination for radiation ttreatment planning through automated MRI segmentation. *Int J Radiat Oncol Biol Phys* 2004;59:300–312.
176. McBain CA, Henry AM, Sykes J, et al. X-ray volumetric imaging in image-guided radiotherapy: the new standard in on-treatment imaging. *Int J Radiat Oncol Biol Phys* 2006;64:625–634.
177. Meeks SL, Buatti JM, Bouchet LG, et al. Ultrasound-guided extracranial radiosurgery: technique and application. *Int J Radiat Oncol Biol Phys* 2003;55:1092–1101.
178. Mehta VK, Lee QT, Chang SD, et al. Image-guided stereotactic radiosurgery for lesions in proximity to the anterior visual pathways: a preliminary report. *Technol Cancer Res Treat* 2002;1:173–180.
179. Mell LK, Mehrotra AK, Mundt AJ. Intensity-modulated radiation therapy use in the United States, 2004. *Cancer* 2005;104:1296–1303.
180. Michalski JM, Graham MV, Bosch WR, et al. Prospective clinical evaluation of a electronic portal imaging device. *Int J Radiat Oncol Biol Phys* 1996;34:943–951.
181. Milker-Zabel S, Zabel-du Bois A, Henze M, et al. Improved target volume definition for fractionated stereotactic radiotherapy in patients with intracranial meningiomas by correlation of CT, MRI, and [68Ga]-DOTATOC-PET. *Int J Radiat Oncol Biol Phys* 2006;65:222–227.
182. Milliken BD, Rubin SJ, Hamilton RJ, et al. Performance of a video-image-subtraction-based patients positioning system. *Int J Radiat Oncol Biol Phys* 1997;38:855–866.
183. Mohan R, Zhang X, Wang H, et al. Use of deformed intensity distributions for on-line modification of image-guided IMRT to account for interfractional anatomic changes. *Int J Radiat Oncol Biol Phys* 2005;61:1258–1266.
184. Morin O, Gillis A, Chen J, et al. Megavoltage cone-beam CT: system description and clinical applications. *Med Dosim* 2006;31:51–61.
185. Mosleh-Shirazi MA, Evans PM, Swindell W, et al. A cone-beam megavoltage CT scanner for treatment verification in conformal radiotherapy. *Radiother Oncol* 1998;48:319–328.
186. Murphy MJ, Cox RS. The accuracy of dose localization for an image-guided frameless radiosurgery system. *Med Phys* 1996;23:2043–2049.
187. Murphy MJ. Tracking moving organs in real time. *Semin Radiat Oncol* 2004;14:91–100.
188. Mutic S, Grigsby PW, Low DA, et al. PET-guided three-dimensional treatment planning of intracavitary gynecologic implants. *Int J Radiat Oncol Biol Phys* 2002;52:1104–1110.
189. Mutic S, Malyapa RS, Grigsby PW, et al. PET-guided IMRT for cervical carcinoma with positive para-aortic lymph nodes-a dose-escalation treatment planning study. *Int J Radiat Oncol Biol Phys* 2003;55:28–35.
190. Nakagawa K, Aoki Y, Akanuma A, et al. Technological features and clinical feasibility of megavoltage CT scanning. *Eur Radiol* 1992;2;184–189.
191. Nakagawa K, Aoki Y, Tago M, et al. Megavoltage CT-assisted stereotactic radiosurgery for thoracic tumors: original research in the treatment of thoracic neoplasms. *Int J Radiat Oncol Biol Phys* 1000;48:449–457.
192. Nanayakkara ND, Samarabandu J, Fenster A. Prostate segmentation by feature enhancement using domain knowledge and adaptive region based operations. *Phys Med Biol* 2006;51:1831–1848.
193. Nehmeh SA, Erdi YE, Pan T, et al. Four-dimensional (4D) PET/CT imaging of the thorax. *Med Phys* 2004;31:3179.
194. Neicu T, Berbeco R, Wolfgang J, et al. Synchronized moving aperture radiation therapy (SMART): improvement of breathing pattern reproducibility using respiratory coaching. *Phys Med Biol* 2006;51:617–636.
195. Neicu T, Shirato H, Seppenwoolde Y, et al. Synchronized moving aperture radiation therapy (SMART): average tumour trajectory for lung patients. *Phys Med Biol* 2003;48:587–598.
196. Nichol A, Chung P, Lockwood G, et al. A phase II study of localized prostate cancer treated to 75.6 Gy with 3D conformal radiotherapy. *Radiother Oncol* 2005;76:11–17.
197. Nichol AM, Rosewall T, Catton CN, et al. Intra-prostatic fiducial markers and concurrent androgen deprivation. *Clin Oncol (R Coll Radiol)* 2005;17:465–468.
198. Nordsmark M, Overgaard J. A confirmatory prognostic study on oxygenation status and loco-regional control in advanced head and neck squamous cell carcinoma treated by radiation therapy. *Radiother Oncol* 2000;57:39–43.
199. Nuyttens JJ, Prevost JB, Praag J, et al. Lung tumor tracking during stereotactic radiotherapy treatment with the CyberKnife: marker placement and early results. *Acta Oncol* 2006;45(7):961–965.
200. Oelfke U, Tucking T, Nill S, et al. LINAC-integrated kv-cone beam CT: technical features and first applications. *Med Dosim* 2006;31:62–70.
201. Oelfke U, Tucking T, Nill S, et al. LINAC-integrated kv-cone beam CT: technical features and first applications. *Med Dosim* 2006;31:62–70.
202. Oldham M, Letourneau D, Watt L, et al. Cone-beam-CT guided radiation therapy: a model for on-line application. *Radiother Oncol* 2005;75:271–278.
203. Olofsen-van Acht M, van den Berg H, Quint S, et al. Reduction of irradiation small bowel volume and accurate patient positioning by use of a bellyboard device in pelvic radiotherapy of gynecological cancer patients. *Radiother Oncol* 2001;59:87–93.
204. Onishi H, Kuriyama K, Komiyama T, et al. A new irradiation system for lung cancer combining linear accelerator, computed-tomography, patient self-breath-holding, and patient-directed beam-control without respiratory monitoring devices. *Int J Radiat Oncol Biol Phys* 2003;56:14–20.
205. Onishi H, Kuriyama K, Komiyama T, et al. Clinical outcomes of stereotactic radiotherapy for stage I non-small cell lung cancer using a novel irradiation technique: patient self-controlled breath-hold and beam switching using a combination linear accelerator and CT scanner. *Lung Cancer* 2004;45:45–55.
206. Parker CC, Damyanovich A, Haycocks T, et al. Magnetic resonance imaging in the radiation treatment planning of localized prostate cancer using intra-prostatic fiducial markers for computed tomography co-registration. *Radiother Oncol* 2003;66:217–224.
207. Paskalev K, Feigenberg S, Jacob R, et al. Target localization for post prostatectomy patients using CT and ultrasound image guidance. *J Appl Clin Med Phys* 2005;6:40–49.
208. Paskalev K, Feigenberg S, Jacob R, et al. Target localization for post-prostatectomy patients using CT and ultrasound image guidance. *J Appl Clin Med Phys* 2005;6:40–49.
209. Paulino AC, Koshy M, Howell R, et al. Comparison of CT- and FDG-PET-defined gross tumor volume in intensity-modulated radiotherapy for head-and-neck cancer. *Int J Radiat Oncol Biol Phys* 2005;61:1385–1392.
210. Pedroso AG, De Salles AA, Tajik K, et al. Novalis shaped beam radiosurgery of arteriovenous malformations. *J Neurosurg* 2004;101[Suppl 3]:425–434.
211. Peeters STH, Heemsbergen WD, van Putten WLJ, et al. Acute and late complications after radiotherapy for prostate cancer: results of a multicenter randomized trial comparing 68 Gy to 78 Gy. *Int J Radiat Oncol Biol Phys* 2005;61:1019–1034.
212. Pelizzari CA, Lujan AE. Imaging and fusion technologies. In: Mundt AJ, Roeske JC, eds. *Intensity modulated radiation therapy: a clinical perspective.* Toronto: B.C. Decker, 2005;102–104.
213. Perkins CL, Fox T, Elder E, et al. Image-guided radiation therapy in gastrointestinal tumors. *J Pancreas* 2006;7:372–381.
214. Pezner RD, Liu A, Han C, et al. Dosimetric comparison of helical tomotherapy treatment and step-and-shoot intensity-modulated radiotherapy of retroperitoneal sarcoma. *Radiother Oncol* 2006;81:81–87.
215. Pham CJ, Chang SD, Gibbs IC, et al. Preliminary visual field preservation after staged Cyberknife radiosurgery for perioptic lesions. *Neurosurgery* 2004;54:799–810.
216. Pieterman RM, van Putten JW, Meuzelaar JJ, et al. Preoperative staging of non-small-cell lung cancer with positron-emission tomography. *N Engl J Med* 2000;343:254–261.
217. Pirzkall A, Li X, Oh J, et al. 3D MRSI for resected high-grade gliomas before RT: tumor extent according to metabolic activity in relation to MRI. *Int J Radiat Oncol Biol Phys* 2004;59:126–137.
218. Pirzkall A, Nelson SJ, McKnight TR, et al. Metabolic imaging of low-grade gliomas with three-dimensional magnetic resonance spectroscopy. *Int J Radiat Oncol Biol Phys* 2002;53(5):1254–1264.
219. Pisani L, Lockman D, Jaffray D et al. Setup error in radiotherapy: on-line correction using electronic kilovoltage and megavoltage radiographs. *Int J Radiat Oncol Biol Phys* 2000;47:825–839.
220. Pollack A, Hanlon AL, Horwitz EM, et al. Dosimetry and preliminary acute toxicity in the first 100 men treated for prostate cancer on a randomized hypofractionation dose escalation trial. *Int J Radiat Oncol Biol Phys* 2006;64:518–526.
221. Pouliot J, Aubin M, Langen KM, et al. (Non)-migration of radiopaque markers used for on-line localization of the prostate with an electronic portal imaging device. *Int J Radiat Oncol Biol Phys* 2003;56:862–866.
222. Pouliot J, Bani-Hashemi A, Chen J, et al. Low-dose megavoltage cone-beam CT for radiation therapy. *Int J Radiat Oncol Biol Phys* 2005;61:552–650.
223. Rafferty MA, Siewerdsen JH, Chan Y, et al. Investigation of C-arm cone-beam CT-guided surgery of the frontal recess. *Laryngoscope* 2005;115:2138–2143.
224. Rahimian J, Chen JC, Rao AA, et al. Geometrical accuracy of the Novalis stereotactic radiosurgery system for trigeminal neuralgia. *J Neurosurg* 2004;101:351–355.
225. Rajendran JG, Hendrickson KR, Spence AM, et al. Hypoxia imaging-directed radiation treatment planning. *Eur J Nucl Med Mol Imaging* 2006;33:44–53.

226. Ramsey CR, Langen KM, Kupelian PA, et al. A technique for adaptive image-guided helical tomotherapy for lung cancer. *Int J Radiat Oncol Biol Phys* 2006;64:1237–1244.
227. Rasey JS, Koh WJ, Evans ML, et al. Quantifying regional hypoxia in human tumors with positron emission tomography of [18F]fluoromisonidazole: a pretherapy study of 37 patients. *Int J Radiat Oncol Biol Phys* 1996;36:417–428.
228. Riegel AC, Berson AM, Destian S, et al. Variability of gross tumor volume delineation in head-and-neck cancer using CT and PET/CT fusion. *Int J Radiat Oncol Biol Phys* 2006;65:726–732.
229. Rietzel E, Liu AK, Doppke KP, et al. Design of 4D treatment planning target volumes. *Int J Radiat Oncol Biol Phys* 2006;66:287–295.
230. Rischin D, Hicks RJ, Fisher R, et al. Prognostic significance of [18F]-misonidazole positron emission tomography-detected tumor hypoxia in patients with advanced head and neck cancer randomly assigned to chemoradiation with or without tirapazamine: a substudy of Trans-Tasman Radiation Oncology Group Study 98.02. *J Clin Oncol* 2006;24:2098–2104.
231. Roeske JC, Lujan A, Reba RC, et al. Incorporation of SPECT bone marrow imaging into intensity modulated whole-pelvic radiation therapy treatment planning for gynecologic malignancies. *Radiother Oncol* 2005;77:11–17.
232. Romanelli P, Heit G, Chang SD, et al. Cyberknife radiosurgery for trigeminal neuralgia. *Stereotact Funct Neurosurg* 2003;81:105–109.
233. Rosenzweig KE, Yorke E, Amols H, et al. Tumor motion control in the treatment of non-small cell lung cancer. *Cancer Invest* 2005;23:129–133.
234. Ryu S, Khan M, Yin FF, et al. Image-guided radiosurgery of head and neck cancers. *Otolaryngol Head Neck Surg* 2004;130:690–697.
235. Ryu S, Rock J, Rosenblum M, et al. Patterns of failure after single-dose radiosurgery for spinal metastasis. *J Neurosurg* 2004;101[Suppl 3]:402–405.
236. Ryu S, Yin FF, Rock J, et al. Image-guided and intensity-modulated radiosurgery for patients with spinal metastasis. *Cancer* 2003;97:2013–2018.
237. Ryu SI, Chang SD, Kim DH, et al. Image-guided hypo-fractionated stereotactic radiosurgery to spinal lesions. *Neurosurgery* 2001;49:838–846.
238. Scarbrough TJ, Golden NM, Ting JY, et al. Comparison of ultrasound and implanted seed marker prostate localization methods: implications for image-guided radiotherapy. *Int J Radiat Oncol Biol Phys* 2006;65:378–387.
239. Schad LR, Bock M, Baudendistel K, et al. Improved target volume definition in radiosurgery of arteriovenous malformations by stereotactic correlation of MRA, MRI, blood bolus tagging, and functional MRI. *Eur Radiol* 1996;6:38–45.
240. Schallenkamp JM, Herman MG, Kruse JJ, et al. Prostate position relative to pelvic bony anatomy based on intraprostatic gold markers and electronic portal imaging. *Int J Radiat Oncol Biol Phys* 2005;63:800–811.
241. Schaly B, Kepe JA, Bauman GS, et al. Tracking the dose distribution in radiation therapy by accounting for variable anatomy. *Phys Med Biol* 2004;49:791–805.
242. Schoder H, Noy A, Gonen M, et al. Intensity of 18-fluorodeoxyglucose uptake in positron emission tomography distinguishes between indolent and aggressive non-Hodgkin's lymphoma. *J Clin Oncol* 2005;23:4643–4651.
243. Schwartz DL, Ford E, Rajendran J, et al. FDG-PET/CT imaging for preradiotherapy staging of head-and-neck squamous cell carcinoma. *Int J Radiat Oncol Biol Phys* 2005;61:129–136.
244. Schwartz DL, Ford EC, Rajendran J, et al. FDG-PET/CT-guided intensity modulated head and neck radiotherapy: a pilot investigation. *Head Neck* 2005;27:478–487.
245. Serago CF, Chungbin SJ, Buskirk SJ, et al. Initial experience with ultrasound localization for positioning prostate cancer patients for external beam radiotherapy. *Int J Radiat Oncol Biol Phys* 2002;53:1130–1138.
246. Sharp GC, Jiang SB, Shimizu S, et al. Prediction of respiratory tumour motion for real-time image-guided radiotherapy. *Phys Med Biol* 2004;49:425–440.
247. Sharp GC, Jiang SB, Shimizu S, et al. Tracking errors in a prototype real-time tumour tracking system. *Phys Med Biol* 2004;49:5347–5356.
248. Sheng K, Molloy JA, Read PW. Intensity-modulated radiation therapy (IMRT) dosimetry of the head and neck: a comparison of treatment plans using linear accelerator-based IMRT and helical tomotherapy. *Int J Radiat Oncol Biol Phys* 2006;65:917–923.
249. Shimamoto S, Inoue T, Shiomi H, et al. Cyberknife stereotactic irradiation for metastatic brain tumors. *Radiat Med* 2002;20:299–304.
250. Shimizu S, Shirato H, Aoyama H, et al. High-speed magnetic resonance imaging for four-dimensional treatment planning of conformal radiotherapy of moving body tumors. *Int J Radiat Oncol Biol Phys* 2000;48:471–474.
251. Shimizu S, Shirato H, Ogura S, et al. Detection of lung tumor movement in real-time tumor-tracking radiotherapy. *Int J Radiat Oncol Biol Phys* 2001;51:304–310.
252. Shirato H, Shimizu S, Kitamura K, et al. Four-dimensional treatment planning and fluoroscopic real-time tumor tracking radiotherapy for moving tumor. *Int J Radiat Oncol Biol Phys* 2000;48:435–442.
253. Shirato H, Shimizu S, Kuneida T, et al. Physical aspects of a real-time tumor-tracking system for gated radiotherapy. *Int J Radiat Oncol Biol Phys* 2000;48:1187–1195.
254. Shirato H, Suzuki K, Sharp GC, et al. Speed and amplitude of lung tumor motion precisely detected in four-dimensional setup and in real-time tumor-tracking radiotherapy. *Int J Radiat Oncol Biol Phys* 2006;64:1229–1236.
255. Shiu AS, Chang EL, Ye JS, et al. Near simultaneous computed tomography image-guided stereotactic spinal radiotherapy: an emerging paradigm for achieving true stereotaxy. *Int J Radiat Oncol Biol Phys* 2003;57:605–613.
256. Sidhu K, Ford EC, Spirou S, et al. Optimization of conformal thoracic radiotherapy using cone-beam CT imaging for treatment verification. *Int J Radiat Oncol Biol Phys* 2003;55:757–767.
257. Siewerdsen JH, Moseley DJ, Burch S, et al. Volume CT with a flat-panel detector on a mobile, isocentric C-arm: pre-clinical investigation in guidance of minimally invasive surgery. *Med Phys* 2005;32:241–254.
258. Simpson RG, Chen CT, Grubbs EA, et al. A 4-MV CT scanner for radiation therapy: the prototype system. *Med Phys* 1982;9:574–579.
259. Sinclair J, Chang SD, Gibbs IC, et al. Multisession Cyberknife radiosurgery for intramedullary spinal cord arteriovenous malformations. *Neurosurgery* 2006;58:1081–1089.
260. Soete G, Arcangeli S, De Meerleer G, et al. Phase II study of a four-week hypofractionated external beam radiotherapy regimen for prostate cancer: report on acute toxicity. *Radiother Oncol* 2006; (in press).
261. Soete G, Verellen D, Michielsen D, et al. Clinical use of stereoscopic x-ray positioning of patients treated with conformal radiotherapy for prostate cancer. *Int J Radiat Oncol Biol Phys* 2002;54:948–952.
262. Solberg TD, Agazaryan N, Goss BW, et al. A feasibility study of 18F-fluorodeoxyglucose positron emission tomography targeting and simultaneous integrated boost for intensity-modulated radiosurgery and radiotherapy. *J Neurosurg* 2004;101:381–389.
263. Song WY, Chiu B, Bauman GS, et al. Prostate contouring uncertainty in megavoltage computed tomography images acquired with a helical tomotherapy unity during image-guided radiation therapy. *Int J Radiat Oncol Biol Phys* 2006;65:595–607.
264. Sorcini B, Tilikidis A. Clinical application of image-guided radiotherapy, IGRT (on the Varian OBI platform). *Cancer Radiother* 2006; (in press).
265. Sorensen SP, Chow PE, Kriminiski S, et al. Image-guided radiotherapy using a mobile kilovoltage x-ray device. *Med Dosim* 2006;31:40–50.
266. Stevens CW, Munden RF, Forster KM, et al. Respiratory-driven lung tumor motion is independent of tumor size, tumor location, and pulmonary function. *Int J Radiat Oncol Biol Phys* 2001;51:62–68.
267. Stroom JC, Olofsen-van Acht MJJ, Quint S, et al. On-line setup corrections during radiotherapy of patients with gynecologic tumors. *Int J Radiat Oncol Biol Phys* 2000;46:499–506.
268. Sykes JR, Amer A, Czjka J, et al. A feasibility study for image guided radiotherapy using low dose, high speed, cone beam x-ray volumetric imaging. *Radiother Oncol* 2005;77:45–52.
269. Takai Y, Mitsuya M, Nemoto K, et al. Development of a new linear accelerator mounted with dual x-ray flouroscopy using amorphous silicon flat panel x-ray sensors to detect a gold seed in a tumor at real treatment position. *Int J Radiat Oncol Biol Phys* 2001;51[Suppl]:381(abstr).
270. Takai Y, Mitsuya M, Nemoto K, et al. Development of a real-time tumor tracking system with dMLC with dual x-ray fluoroscopy and amorphous silicon flat panel on the gantry of a linear accelerator. *Int J Radiat Oncol Biol Phys* 2002;54[Suppl:193–194(abstr).
271. Thilmann C, Nill S, Tucking T, et al. Correction of patient positioning errors based on in-line cone beam CTs: clinical implementation and first experiences. *Radiat Oncol* 2006;1:16–21.
272. Tome WA, Meeks SL, Orton NP, et al. Commissioning and quality assurance of an optically guided three-dimensional ultrasound target localization system for radiotherapy.
273. Tomsej M. The Tomotherapy Hi-Art System for sophisticated IMRT and IGRT with delical delivery: recent developments and clinical applications. *Cancer Radiother* 2006; (in press).
274. Trichter F, Ennis RD. Prostate localization using transabdominal ultrasound imaging. *Int J Radiat Oncol Biol Phys* 2003;56:1225–1233.
275. Uematsu M, Fukui T, Shioda A, et al. A dual computed tomography linear accelerator unit for stereotactic radiation therapy: a new approach without cranially fixated stereotactic frames. *Int J Radiat Oncol Biol Phys* 1996;35:587–592.
276. Uematsu M, Shioda A, Suda A, et al. Computed tomography-guided frameless stereotactic radiotherapy for stage I non-small cell lung cancer: a 5-year experience. *Int J Radiat Oncol Biol Phys* 2001;51:666–670.
277. Uematsu M, Shioda A, Suda A, et al. Intrafractional tumor position stability during computed tomography (CT)-guided frameless stereotactic radiation therapy for lung or liver cancers with a fusion of CT and linear accelerator (FOCAL) unit. *Int J Radiat Oncol Biol Phys* 2000;48:443–448.
278. Uetmatsu M, Shioda A, Tahara K, et al. Focal, high dose and fractionated modified stereotactic radiation therapy for lung carcinoma patients: a preliminary experience. *Cancer* 1998;82:1062–1070.
279. Ullman KL, Ning H, Susil RC, et al. Intra- and inter-radiation therapist reproducibility of daily isocenter verification using prostatic fiducial markers. *Radiation Oncol* 2006;1:2–6.
280. Underberg RW, Lagerwaard FJ, Cuijpers JP, et al. Four-dimensional CT scans for treatment planning in stereotactic radiotherapy for stage I lung cancer. *Int J Radiat Oncol Biol Phys* 2004;60:1283–1290.
281. Underberg RW, Lagerwaard FJ, Slotman BJ, et al. Benefit of respiration-gated stereotactic radiotherapy for stage I lung cancer: an analysis of 4DCT datasets. *Int J Radiat Oncol Biol Phys* 2005;62:554–560.
282. Underberg RW, Lagerwaard FJ, Slotman BJ, et al. Use of maximum intensity projections (MIP) for target volume generation in 4DCT scans for lung cancer. *Int J Radiat Oncol Biol Phys* 2005;63:253–260.
283. Van de Bunt L, van der Heided UA, Ketelaars M, et al. Conventional, conformal and intensity modulated radiation therapy treatment planning of external beam radiotherapy for cervical cancer: the impact of tumor regression. *Int J Radiat Oncol Biol Phys* 2006;64:189–196.
284. Van de Steene J, Van den Heuvel F, Bel A, et al. Electronic portal imaging with on-line correction of setup error in thoracic irradiation: clinical evaluation. *Int J Radiat Oncol Biol Phys* 1998;40:967–976.
285. Van den Heuvel F, Powell T, Seppi E, et al. Independent verification of ultrasound based image-guided radiation treatment, using electronic portal imaging and implanted gold markers. *Med Phys* 2003;30:2878–2887.
286. van Lin EN, Futterer JJ, Heijmink SW, et al. IMRT boost dose planning on dominant intraprostatic lesions: gold marker-based three-dimensional fusion of CT with dynamic contrast-enhanced and 1H-spectroscopic MRI. *Int J Radiat Oncol Biol Phys* 2006;65:291–303.
287. Vanuytsel LJ, Vansteenkiste JF, Stroobants SG, et al. The impact of (18)F-fluoro-2-deoxy-D-glucose positron emission tomography (FDG-PET) lymph node staging on the radiation treatment volumes in patients with non-small cell lung cancer. *Radiother Oncol* 2000;55:317–324.
288. Vargas C, Yan D, Kestin LL, et al. Phase II dose escalation study of image-guided adaptive radiotherapy for prostate cancer: use of dose-volume constraints to achieve rectal isotoxocity. *Int J Radiat Oncol Biol Phys* 2005;62:141–149.
289. Vigneault E, Pouliot J, Laverdiere J, et al. Electronic portal imaging device detection of radiopaque markers for the evaluation of prostate position during megavoltage radiation: a clinical study. *Int J Radiat Oncol Biol Phys* 1997;37:205–212.
290. Vrieze O, Haustermans K, De Wever W, et al. Is there a role for FDG-PET in radiotherapy planning in esophageal carcinoma? *Radiother Oncol* 2004;73:269–275.
291. Wang H, Dong L, Fwu M, et al. Implementation and validation of a three-dimensional deformable registration algorithm for targeted prostate cancer radiotherapy. *Int J Radiat Oncol Biol Phys* 2005;61:725–735.

292. Wang H, Dong L, O'Daniel J, et al. Validation of an accelerated 'demons' algorithm for deformable image registration in radiation therapy. *Phys Med Biol* 2005;50:2887–2905.

293. Welsh JS, Berta C, Borzillary S, et al. Fiducial markers implanted during prostate brachytherapy for guiding conformal external beam radiation therapy. *Technol Cancer Res Treat* 2004;3:359–364.

294. Welsh JS, Bradley K, Ruchala KJ, et al. Megavoltage computed tomography imaging: a potential tool to guide and improve the delivery of thoracic radiation therapy. *Clin Lung Cancer* 2004;5:303–306.

295. Whang CJ, Yee GT, Choi CY, et al. First experience in using Novalis shaped beam radiosurgery in Korea. *J Neurosurg* 2004;101[Suppl 3]:341–345.

296. Wieder HA, Brucher BL, Zimmermann F, et al. Time course of tumor metabolic activity during chemoradiotherapy of esophageal squamous cell carcinoma and response to treatment. *J Clin Oncol* 2004;22:900–908.

297. Wolthaus JW, Schneider C, Sonke JJ, et al. Mid-ventilation CT scan construction from four-dimensional respiration-correlated CT scans for radiotherapy planning of lung cancer patients. *Int J Radiat Oncol Biol Phys* 2006;65:1560–1571.

298. Wolthaus JW, Schneider C, Sonke JJ, et al. Mid-ventilation CT scan construction from four-dimensional respiration-correlated CT scans for radiotherapy planning of lung cancer patients. *Int J Radiat Oncol Biol Phys* 2006;65:1560–1571.

299. Wong J, Sharpe MB, Jaffray DA, et al. The use of active breathing control (ABC) to reduce margin for breathing motion. *Int J Radiat Oncol Biol Phys* 1999;44:911–919.

300. Wong JR, Grimm L, Uematsu M, et al. Image-guided radiotherapy for prostate cancer by CT-linear accelerator combination: prostate movements and dosimetric considerations. *Int J Radiat Oncol Biol Phys* 2005;61:561–569.

301. Wong JW, Sharpe MB, Jaffray DA, et al. The use of active breathing control (ABC) to reduce margin for breathing motion. *Int J Radiat Oncol Biol Phys* 1999;44:911–919.

302. Wright JL, Lovelock DM, Bilsky MH, et al. Clinical outcomes after reirradiation of paraspinal tumors. *Am J Clin Oncol* 2006;29:495–502.

303. Xing L, Thorndyke B, Schreibmann E, et al. Overview of image-guided radiotherapy. *Med Dosim* 2006;31:91–112.

304. Yamada Y, Lovelock DM, Yenice KM, et al. Multifractionated image-guided and stereotactic intensity-modulated radiotherapy of paraspinal tumors: a preliminary report. *Int J Radiat Oncol Biol Phys* 2005;62:53–61.

305. Yamamoto R, Yonesaka A, Watari H, et al. High dose three-dimensional conformal boost (3DCB) using an orthogonal diagnostic x-ray set-up for patients with gynecological malignancy: a new application of real-time tumor-tracking system. *Radiother Oncol* 2004;73:219–222.

306. Yan D, Lockman D, Brabbins D, et al. An off-line strategy for constructing a patient-specific planning target volume in adaptive treatment process for prostate cancer. *Int J Radiat Oncol Biol Phys* 2000;48:289–302.

307. Yan D, Wong J, Gustafson G, et al. A new model for "accept or reject" strategies in off-line and on-line megavoltage treatment evaluation. *Int J Radiat Oncol Biol Phys* 1995;31:943–952.

308. Yan D, Wong J, Vicini F, et al. Adaptive modification of treatment planning to minimize the deleterious effects of treatment setup errors. *Int J Radiat Oncol Biol Phys* 1997;38:197–206.

309. Yan D, Ziaja E, Jaffray D, et al. The use of adaptive radiation therapy to reduce setup errors: a prospective clinical study. *Int J Radiat Oncol Biol Phys* 1998;41:715–720.

310. Yan H, Yin FF, Kim JH. A phantom study on the positioning accuracy of the Novalis body system. *Med Phys* 2003;30:2052–2060.

311. Yenice KM, Lovelock DM, Hunt MA, et al. CT image-guided intensity-modulated therapy for paraspinal tumors using stereotactic immobilization. *Int J Radiat Oncol Biol Phys* 2003;55:583–593.

312. Yoshikawa K, Saito K, Kajiwara K, et al. Cyberknife stereotactic radiotherapy for patients with malignant glioma. *Minim Invasive Neurosurg* 2006;49:110–115.

313. Yu C, Main W, Taylor D, et al. An anthropomorphic phantom study of the accuracy of Cyberknife spine radiosurgery. *Neurosurgery* 2004;55:1138–1149.

314. Yu CX. Intensity-modulated arc therapy with dynamic multileaf collimation: an alternative to tomotherapy. *Phys Med Biol* 1995;40:1435–1449.

315. Zhang T, Keller H, O'Brien MJ, et al. Application of the spirometer in respiratory gated radiotherapy. *Med Phys* 2003;12:3165–3171.

316. Zinniker J, Filiberti R, Huntzinger C. Isocenter stability of Clinac with an on-board imager. *Med Phys* 2004;31:1783(abstr).

Section II

Techniques, Modalities, and Modifiers in Radiation Oncology

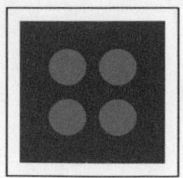

Chapter 11
Altered Fractionation Schedules

Anesa Ahamad

Alternative fractionation schedules discussed in this chapter are contrasted with conventional fractionation in the United States; that is, fractional doses of 1.8 to 2 Gy given once daily, Monday through Friday, to total doses determined by the tumor feature and the tolerance of critical normal tissues. In *hyperfractionation*, the total dose is increased, the size of dose per fraction is significantly reduced, the number of dose fractions is increased, and overall time is relatively unchanged. In *accelerated fractionation*, overall time is significantly reduced, and the number of dose fractions, total dose, and size of dose per fraction are either unchanged or somewhat reduced, depending on the extent of overall time reduction. In this chapter, such regimens are classified as predominantly hyperfractionated or predominantly accelerated, according to which rationale carries the greatest weight.

Background Radiobiology

Perhaps the most important consequence of altering a fractionation schedule is that late effects are more sensitive to changes in size of dose per fraction, and acute reactions are more sensitive to changes in the rate of dose accumulation.

The classic descriptions of early and late reactions are couched in terms of target cell killing. This characterization is on firmer ground with acute effects, where direct connections can be made between depletion of identified cell populations and measurable injury, than with late effects, where such identification is more problematic (147) (see also Chapter 2 of this volume). Despite this shortcoming, the conventional understanding of the potential advantages of alternative fractionation strategies is framed within the target cell concept.

Time–Dose Parameters

The time–dose parameters that determine normal tissue tolerance are total dose, overall duration of treatment, size of dose per fraction, and frequency of dose fractions. The latter two determine the rate of dose accumulation, sometimes referred to as the *weekly dose rate*. The intensity of acute reactions in epithelial and other tissues organized into stem cell, maturation, and functional compartments (e.g., bone marrow) reflects the balance between the rate of cell killing by irradiation and the rate of regeneration of surviving stem cells. This balance depends primarily on the rate of dose accumulation. The fraction size is also a factor in determining the severity of acute reactions (large fractions being more damaging Gray-for-Gray than small ones), but to a lesser extent than is the case for late reactions. After an acute reaction has peaked (e.g., moist desquamation of the skin or confluent mucositis of the mucosa has occurred), further stem-cell killing cannot produce an increase in *intensity* of the acute reaction but manifests as an increased time to heal the reaction. If sufficient stem cells do not survive to repopulate tissues, acute reactions may progress into a *consequential* late injury (118).

The conventional view is that late reactions occur in tissues characterized by slow cellular turnover, such as mature connective tissues and the parenchymal cells of various organs. Because cellular depletion in such tissues does not manifest until after a typical course of radiation therapy is completed, the rate of dose accumulation and overall duration of treatment would be of minor significance in determining the severity of late reactions. Therefore, late reactions would depend primarily on total dose, size of dose per fraction, and interfraction interval.

There are difficulties with this simplified description. For example, there is evidence that the frequency of some late reactions correlates with the level of acute reactions, possibly through an influence of the rate of dose accumulation (49,88, 154). In addition, there is evidence that late effects can be modified by pharmacologic intervention. For example, amifostine administration protects lung tissue and the esophageal mucosa in the treatment of lung cancer (142), and other agents have been shown to affect the development of radiation-induced nephritis (captopril) and fibrosis (pentoxifylline and vitamin E). In this chapter, I describe alternative fractionation in the conventional terms used during the last two decades, with the caveat that future studies may have a significant impact on our description.

Size of Dose Per Fraction and Length of Interfraction Interval

The influence of the dose per fraction on the results of radiation therapy is manifest through the slope of the response to multifractionated doses, and this is a reflection of the *repair capacity* of the target cells. The experimental literature was reviewed (151), and the results shown in Figure 2.18 (Chapter 2) indicate that changes in isoeffect doses for late effects with changing dose per fraction (solid curves) are steeper than for acute effects (dashed curves). The significance of this is that if tumors are similar to acutely responding normal tissues in their sensitivity to changing fraction size, then a gain in the therapeutic ratio can be realized by significantly reducing the fraction sizes and escalating the total dose (hyperfractionation). These results are independent of any mathematical models and rest instead on the data shown in Figure 2.18. It is, however, convenient to be able to quantify the fractionation sensitivity, and this is easiest using the linear-quadratic (LQ) model, assuming that the target cell hypothesis is correct and that the LQ model correctly describes the target-cell survival curves. Given these conditions, the ratio α/β of the parameters of the LQ model is a quantitative measure of this sensitivity to changes in fraction size (151): low ratios signify high fractionation sensitivity, and high ratios signify low fractionation sensitivity. Low ratios imply relatively large changes in isoeffective dose when dose per fraction is changed, and the converse for high values. The implication is that the tolerance dose for late effects can be increased more by the use of smaller fraction sizes than the tolerance dose for tumors and acute effects (hyperfractionation). The α/β ratios for some animal normal tissues are set out in Table 2.1 (Chapter 2), and for human tissues and tumors in Table 11.1.

In general, the estimated values of α/β for early and late reactions in human normal tissues are consistent with results

Table 11.1	**ESTIMATES OF α/β FOR HUMAN TISSUES AND TUMORS**	

Tissue/Tumor	Authors (Reference)	Estimate/Bound of α/β in Gy (95% Confidence Limits)
Acutely Responding		
Skin		
Desquamation (time $\leq$29 d)	Turesson and Thames (154)	11.2 (8.5–17.6)
Erythema	Turesson and Thames (154)	8.8 (6.9–11.6)
	Bentzen et al. (16)	12.3 (2–23)
Mucous membrane—ulcer	Rezvani et al. (127)	15 (0–45.2)
Lung—acute	Cox (45)	>8.8
Late Responding		
Supraglottic larynx—late sequelae	Maciejewski et al. (99)	3.8 (0.8–14)
Larynx—cartilage necrosis	Henk and James (75)	~3.4
	Horiot et al. (80)	$\leq$4.4
	Fletcher et al. (65)	$\leq$4.2
	Stell and Morrison (139)	
Larynx—pharynx	Taylor et al. (143)	7.8 (3–∞)
	Rezvani et al. (127)	3.5 (1.1–5.9)
Oropharynx—late sequelae	Horiot et al. (82)	~4.5
Skin		
Subcutaneous fibrosis	Bentzen et al. (21)	1.9 (0.8–3)
Telangiectasia	Turesson and Thames (154)	3.9 (2.7–4.8)
	Bentzen et al. (21)	3.7 (0.2–4.7)
	Bentzen and Overgaard (17)	2.8 (0–8.1)
Mucosal ulceration (consequential effects)	Withers et al. (166)	21.3 (5.2–∞)
Shoulder—impaired movement	Bentzen et al. (18)	3.5 (0.7–6.2)
Rib—fracture	Overgaard (113)	1.8–2.8
Bone—exposure/necrosis	Withers et al. (166)	0.8 (0–2.4)
Lung		
Pneumonitis	Cox (45)	$\leq$3.8
Computed tomography density	van Dyk et al. (157)	3.3 (0.5–6.5)
Spinal cord—myelopathy	Dische et al. (52)	$\leq$3.3
Brachial plexus—plexopathy	Powell et al. (124)	$\leq$5.3
Bowel—stricture/perforation	Bennett (14), Edsmyr et al. (61)	2.2 $\leq\alpha/\beta\leq$8
Tumors		
Tonsil	Withers et al. (166)	14.7 (4.4–∞)
Vocal cord	Harrison et al. (73)	>9.9
Larynx	Rezvani et al. (128)	12[a]:18 (0–42), T3[a]:13 (3–23)
Oral cavity/oropharynx	Maciejewski et al. (100)	~25
	Byhardt et al. (36)	>6.5
	Cox et al. (46)	~10.3
	Handa et al. (72)	>7
Lung—non–small cell carcinomas	Cox et al. (46)	50–90
Cervix	Watson et al. (162)	>13.9
Skin	Trott et al. (153)	8.5 (4.5–11.3)
Prostate	Brenner et al. (32)	1.2 (0.03–4.1)
	Brenner and Hall (31)	1.5 (0.8–2.2)
	Fowler et al. (66)	1.5 (1.3–1.8)
	King and Fowler (90)	1.8–2.8
Melanoma	Bentzen et al. (18)	0.6 (0–2.5)[b]
Liposarcoma	Thames and Suit (149)	0.4 (0–5.4)[b]

[a]American Joint Committee on Cancer staging system.
[b]Lower confidence limit is negative, but is listed as 0, because a negative α/β has no biologic meaning.
Modified from Thames HD, Hendry JH. *Fractionation in radiotherapy.* London: Taylor & Francis, 1987, with permission.

from experimental animals. With regard to tumors, squamous-cell carcinomas of the head and neck, cervix, and skin, and non–small cell lung cancers (NSCLC) are characterized by high α/β ratios, in agreement with rodent models. However, available data from melanomas and liposarcomas suggest somewhat lower α/β ratios for these tumor types. There is also a hint that the α/β ratio for breast adenocarcinomas may be lower than those for other carcinomas listed in Table 11.1 (110), but the data are insufficient to reach any firm conclusion.

The situation may be different with prostate tumors, which contain unusually small fractions of cycling cells (74). Several groups (28,60) reasoned that prostate tumors might not respond to changes in fractionation in the same way as other cancers, and that prostate tumors might respond to changes in fractionation more like a late-responding normal tissue. In mathematical terms, the suggestion was that the α/β ratio for prostate cancer might be low, comparable to that for late sequelae. If so, much of the rationale for using many fractions, or

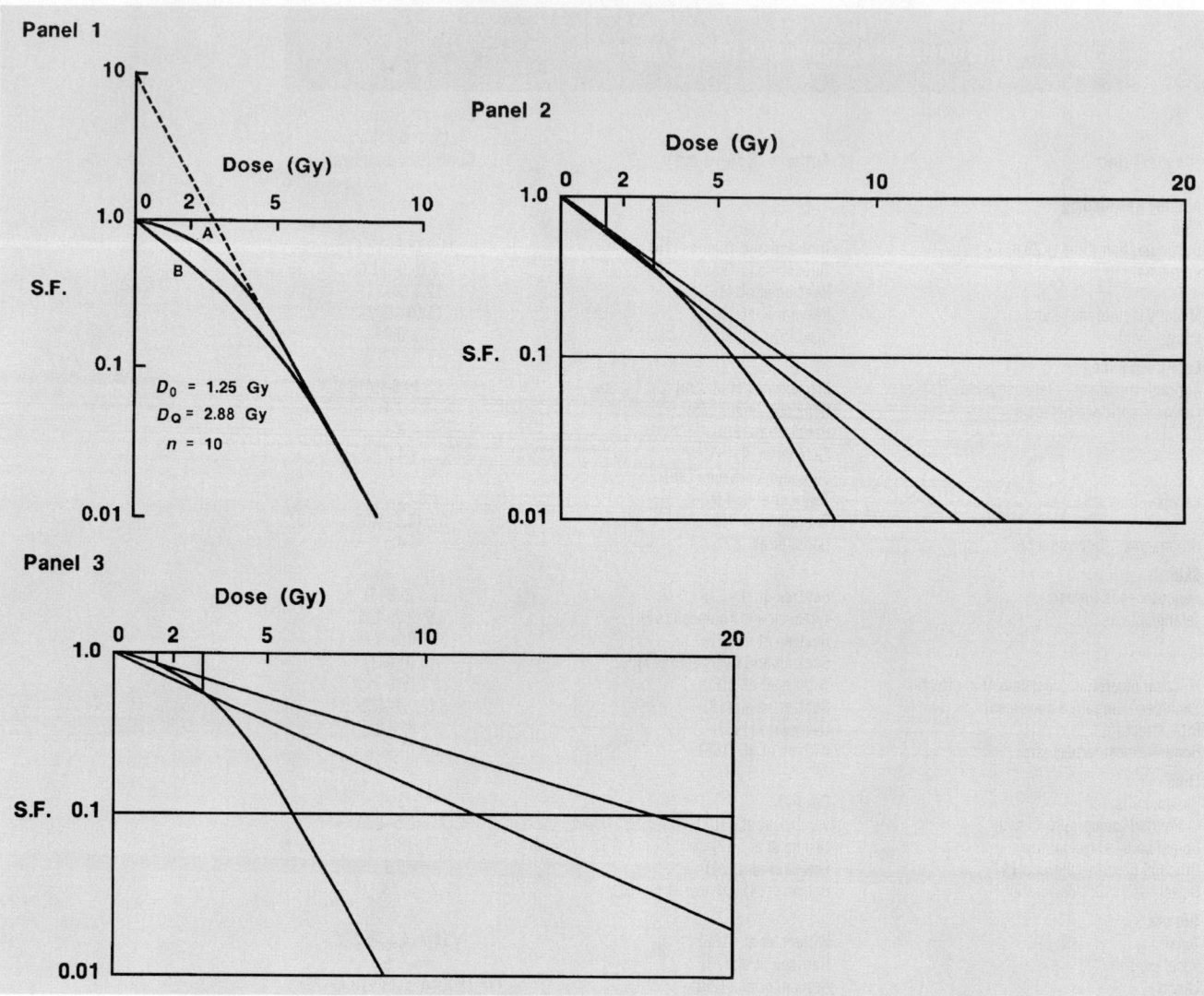

FIGURE 11.1. The importance of survival curve shoulder *shape* rather than width for the response to fractionated irradiation. *Panel I:* Two survival curves with the same D_0, D_q, and n, but with different initial slopes and shoulder curvatures. In terms of the linear quadratic model of cell survival, the α/β ratio is lower for curve A than for curve B. *Panels 2 and 3:* Effect of change in fraction size on the dose required for a given effect. Panel 2 shows that when the shoulder has a steep initial slope and little curvature (high α/β), a change in dose per fraction from 3 to 1.5 Gy would only slightly increase the total dose needed to produce a given survival fraction. Panel 3 shows that when the shoulder has a shallow initial slope and marked curvature (low α/β), a much greater increase in total dose is necessary to produce a given survival fraction when the same change in dose per fraction is made. (From Peters LJ, Brock WA, Travis EL. Radiation biology at clinically relevant fractions. In: DeVita V, Hellman S, Rosenberg SA, eds. *Important advances in oncology.* Philadelphia: J.B. Lippincott, 1991;65–83, with permission.)

using low dose rate, would disappear for prostate radiotherapy. There are now many studies (29,32,95,97) that suggest that the value is low (in the range 1 to 3 Gy), comparable to that for late-responding tissues, opening up the possibility of hypofractionation or HDR (high–dose rate) brachytherapy.

The arguments presented here really relate to the α/β value for prostate cancer *in relation to the α/β value for the relevant late-responding normal tissue.* There is good evidence both from animal (28,51,59,70,144,156) and from human (30,56,88,160) studies that for late rectal sequelae $\alpha/\beta > 4$ Gy is higher than for most other late sequelae. If the α/β value for prostate cancer is actually less than that for the surrounding late-responding normal tissue, hypofractionation (by external beam or HDR) at the appropriate dose, would be expected to yield increased tumor control for a given level of late complications, or decreased late complications for a given level of tumor control.

Hypofractionation in a curative setting, even when the dose is appropriately lowered, is a *prima facie* unsettling idea, par-

ticularly as the literature has many examples of large dose per fraction resulting in unacceptable late effects (44,120). None of these reports are for prostate cancer, however. To the contrary, there is a report of 22 years' experience (1962–84) with 232 prostate cancer patients treated in London with a six fraction 6-Gy protocol (42); even with the much poorer dose distributions than are now routine, minimal long-term urologic or bowel morbidity was reported. There is also extensive early experience from the Christie Hospital, Manchester, of treating prostate cancer with a 15 fraction 3.1 Gy protocol, both before and since the era of conformal therapy, with satisfactory results and without excess late sequelae (97). Clinical trials of prostate cancer hypofractionation have been started in the intensity-modulated radiation therapy (IMRT) era, in the United States, Canada, United Kingdom, Australia, Japan, and Greece. In those studies that have reported on potential late sequelae, there is to date little indication of any unexpected late sequelae after median follow-up periods of 31 months (2), 48 months (96), 66 months (91), 68 months (98), and 97 months (42).

Repair Kinetics

To realize an increase in tolerance of late-responding tissues through dose fractionation, it is essential for the time interval between the dose fractions to be long enough to allow repair to approach completion. If doses are too closely spaced, injury will accumulate between dose fractions, and successive doses will become increasingly more damaging. This emphasizes the importance of *repair kinetics*, which is quantified by the half-time for repair. Of the tissues in experimental models in which repair kinetics have been studied, half-times for repair tend to be longest (1 to several hours) in the skin, kidney, and spinal cord, shortest (approximately half an hour) in the jejunal mucosa, and intermediate in the lung and colon (7,9,57,68,76,84,129,147,150,152,158). The exact values vary according to the experimental protocol, and considerable overlap exists in the confidence limits of repair half-time. The important point is to ensure an adequate interfraction interval during hyperfractionation.

Repair kinetics is of particular importance in determining the response of the spinal cord to fractionation schedules of more than one daily fraction. In rats, experimental data have shown that repair is best described by a biexponential function, in which the slower component has a half-time of 3.8 hours (5). This would imply that any fractionation schedule using more than one fraction per day is associated with some degree of incomplete repair in the spinal cord. A clinical report of radiation myelopathy occurring in four patients whose spinal cords received 45 to 48 Gy in 28 fractions of 1.5 Gy, three times a day with a 6-hour interval over 9 consecutive days, supports this observation (135), although incomplete repair cannot fully account for the observed frequency of injury (71). Two reports from the Radiation Therapy Oncology Group (RTOG) (47,102) have shown an increased rate of other late complications in patients treated on hyperfractionated protocols when the mean interval was <4.5 hours. For clinical practice, it is prudent to account for the potential compounding effect of incomplete repair. Therefore, most protocols now stipulate a minimum 6-hour interval between dose fractions. A review of the clinical data suggests that this is adequate for normal tissues other than the spinal cord (148).

Data on repair kinetics in human normal tissues are extremely sparse, but, as indicated earlier, some evidence suggests that interfraction recovery may be slower in humans than in rodents. More recently, Bentzen et al. (19) have analyzed late complications in the continuous, hyperfractionated, accelerated radiation therapy (CHART) randomized trial, and their findings are in agreement with this picture. Estimated repair half-times, with 95% confidence intervals, were 4.9 hours (3.2, 6.4) for laryngeal edema, 3.8 hours (2.5, 4.6) for skin telangiectasia, and 4.4 hours (3.8, 4.9) for subcutaneous fibrosis. These results were shown to be consistent with observations from two other published trials of altered fractionation, European Organization for Research and Treatment of Cancer (EORTC) 22791 and EORTC 22851. It is clear that 6 hours must be regarded as the absolute minimum interfraction interval for twice-daily fractionation.

Overall Time

The intensity of acute reactions is determined primarily by the rate of dose accumulation (weekly dose rate). Acute reactions represent a deficit in the balance between the rate of cell killing by radiation and cell regeneration from surviving stem cells. After the stem-cell population is depleted the acute reaction peaks, and further depopulation produces no apparent increase in severity of the reaction. This means that the peak intensity of acute reactions is influenced more by the rate of dose accumu-

lation than by the total dose, after a certain threshold of total dose has been reached.

Conversely, the time taken to heal depends on total dose, provided that the weekly dose rate exceeds the regenerative ability of the surviving stem cells. This is because healing is a function of the absolute number of stem cells surviving the course of treatment, and the higher the total dose, the lower the number of stem cells surviving. Although most classic late radiation sequelae (e.g., spinal cord injury) show little or no dependence on overall time (provided full recovery occurs between dose fractions), overall time may be of significance for another set of late effects classed as consequential late effects in which total doses were less than or similar to conventional regimens and in which a higher incidence of late reactions was observed (116,141,155). To explain these results, a distinction needs to be drawn between "true" late effects and "consequential" late reactions (50,118). Many of the late effects seen in these studies can be attributed to severe and prolonged epithelial denudation rather than to direct radiation injury of the mesenchymal tissues normally associated with late reactions.

The cure rates of many cancers (particularly squamous cell carcinomas) are also highly dependent on overall treatment time, and this has been interpreted in terms of accelerated regeneration of tumor clonogens (167). Studies of the increase in tumor control dose with increasing treatment time suggest that after a variable lag period, surviving tumor clonogens regenerate rapidly during fractionated radiation therapy to the extent that each additional day of treatment requires approximately 0.6 Gy, on average, to offset clonogenic cell regeneration, again suggesting a clonogenic cell doubling time of 3.5 to 5 days. This is illustrated in Figure 2.6 (Chapter 2) (20,58,145).

In addition to the results shown in Figure 2.6, other evidence has been adduced for accelerated regeneration of surviving tumor cells after therapeutic intervention (3). The majority of recurrences of squamous cell carcinomas of the head and neck occur within 2 years of treatment (62), and because the recurrences occurred from a population of tumors in which many were controlled, it follows that many recurrences must have arisen from one or a few surviving clonogenic cells. This would have required approximately 30 volume doublings, and the median doubling time of nonsterilized tumor clonogens must have been about 6 days (5). Comparison of split-course treatment with continuous-course treatment suggests that 0.5 Gy per day is required to compensate for treatment interruption. Assuming that 2 to 3 Gy in 2-Gy fractions is necessary to reduce the surviving fractions of clonogenic cells by 50%, four to six doublings must occur during the 3-week treatment split, yielding a clonogenic cell doubling time of 3.5 to 5 days. It appears from all three types of analyses that after initiation of radiotherapy, surviving clonogens in squamous-cell carcinomas of the head and neck are able to regenerate with doubling times as short as 3 to 5 days.

Isoeffect Formulas

The effect of changes of dose fractionation schedule on the total dose required to produce a certain level of biologic effect is approximated by isoeffect curves or formulas. The first clinical isoeffect curve was produced by Strandqvist (140). This was followed by other studies (39–41,67), culminating in the nominal standard dose (NSD) formula of Ellis (64): $D = N^{0.24} \times T^{0.11}$ (D is the dose; N is the number of dose fractions; T is the overall time). None of these explicitly included dose per fraction.

In the early 1980s, it was pointed out that the different exponents for early and late effects could be interpreted in terms of survival curves for different target cell populations (151), in which the curves for late effects were "curvier" than those for acute effects. The consequence of this is that isoeffect doses

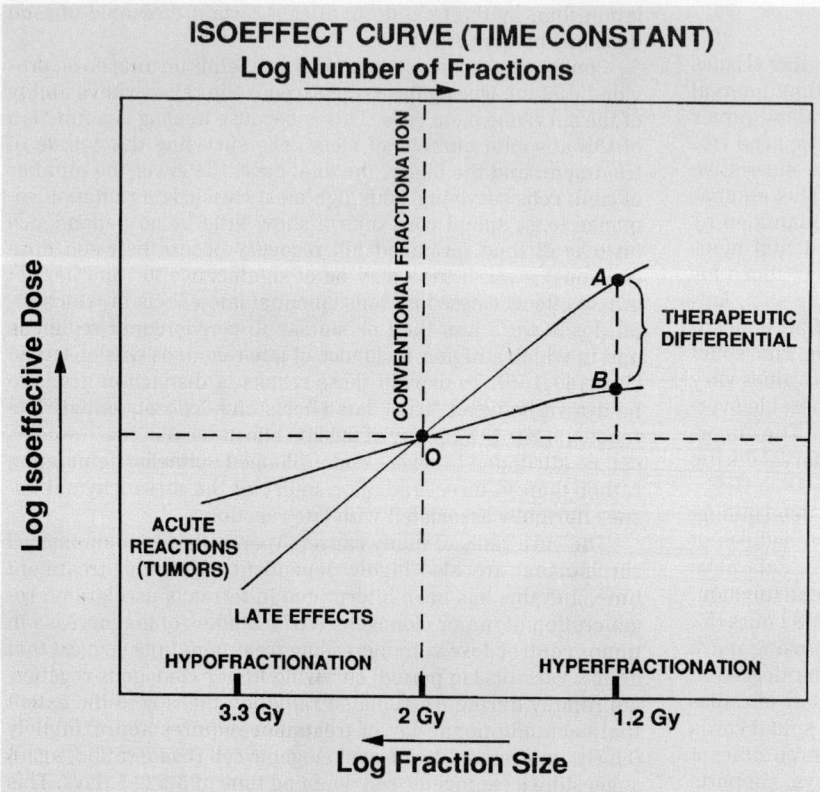

ISOEFFECT CURVE (TIME CONSTANT)
Log Number of Fractions

FIGURE 11.2. Effect of change in size of dose fraction (with overall time held constant) on the total dose necessary to produce a given level of acute and late effects. The curves are normalized to the "conventional" 2 Gy per fraction. Changes in fraction size have a relatively greater effect on the isoeffective doses for late reactions than for acute reactions and for the response of tumors with high α/β ratios. Consequently, by reducing the dose per fraction—for example, from 2 to 1.2 Gy—the total dose for equivalent late effects can be increased from O to A, which is greater than the increase (O to B) required to achieve an equivalent tumor response. The increment in dose from B to A represents the therapeutic differential achieved by hyperfractionation.

for various late effects in normal tissues are more sensitive to changes in dose per fraction than are corresponding doses for acute effects. With the widespread use of the LQ model to quantify the fractionation sensitivity, the following model has gained in popularity:

$$D_1 = D_2 \, (\alpha/\beta + d_2) \, / \, (\alpha/\beta + d_1)$$

where D_2 is the reference total dose given in fractions of size d_2, and it is desired to calculate the total dose D_1 in fractions of size d_1 that would be isoeffective. This basic formula assumes complete repair between dose fractions, and no time factor is incorporated in it (see Chapter 2 for a detailed discussion). Thus, the basic formula may be used only when dose fractions are spaced widely enough apart to ensure complete repair and when the end point is either time independent (as with most late reactions) or the two schedules being compared involve the same overall time–dosing intensity.

Whereas the LQ-based isoeffect model is internally consistent for a wide range of tissue types and end points, clinical application of the model for derivation of new fractionation schedules is limited by at least two factors. First, there is the lack of precision of estimates of α/β. Even in closely controlled animal systems, estimates of α/β show large confidence intervals (Table 2.1, chapter 2). The α/β ratios of available human data are consistent with the experimentally determined α/β ratios, but have very wide confidence bounds (see Table 11.1). Second, as discussed earlier, the severity of complications can be modulated by various agents, including growth factors, radioprotectors, and pharmacologic agents, and current isoeffect concepts will doubtlessly have to be modified as the results of future studies become available. *The bottom line is that no isoeffect formula is sufficiently reliable to preempt clinical judgment, and, in the*

final analysis, each new fractionation schedule must be tested clinically to establish its safety.

Rationale for Hyperfractionation

The basic rationale of hyperfractionation is that the use of small dose fractions allows higher total doses to be administered within the tolerance of late-responding normal tissues, and this translates into a higher biologically effective dose to the tumor. For this rationale to hold, the α/β ratio for tumor cells must be greater than that for the dose-limiting normal tissue. Acutely responding tissues as a class have higher α/β ratios than late-responding normal tissues. Because of the kinetic similarity between tumors and acutely responding normal tissues, it may be predicted that tumors (with possible exceptions, such as the prostate) also tend to have large α/β ratios. Other rationales for hyperfractionation are radiosensitization through redistribution and lesser dependence on oxygen effect. The greater the number of dose fractions, the greater the chance that cells would be in a more radiosensitive phase at the time of the next fraction. With small fractional doses, the influence of tumor cell hypoxia is reduced on two counts. First, the proportion of hypoxic cells needs to be higher to increase significantly the surviving fraction and, second, the oxygen enhancement ratio is lower (114).

Hyperfractionation has been tested in more than 20 randomized trials, and these are summarized in the data presented in Table 11.2.

Rationale for Accelerated Fractionation

The rationale for accelerated fractionation is that reduction in overall treatment time decreases the opportunity for tumor

Table 11.2 DATA OF PHASE III CLINICAL TRIALS ADDRESSING HYPERFRACTIONATION

Tumor Site and Type	No. of Patients	Dose/Fx (Gy)	Fx/d	Total Dose (Gy)	Overall Time	Tumor Response	Side Effects	Authors (Reference)
Head and neck carcinomas								
Oropharynx Stage III–IV	98	1.1 / 2.0	2 / 1	70.4 / 66.0	6.5 / 6.5	Tumor response: 84% vs. 64% ($p = 0.02$). 3.5-y OS: 27% vs. 8% ($p = 0.03$).	Earlier onset of acute reactions with HF. Late complications: no details.	Pinto et al. (122)
Oropharynx. T2-3 N0-1	356	1.15 / 2.0	2 / 1	80.5 / 70.0	7.0 / 7.0	5-y LRC: 59% vs. 40% ($p = 0.02$). Improved local control of T3 tumors.	More acute mucositis with HF. No difference in late complication rate.	Horiot et al. (81); Horiot (78)
Various sites. T3-4 N0 or any TN+	331	1.45 / 2.55	2 / 1	58.0 / 51.0	4.0 / 4.0	5-y LRC: 45% vs. 37% ($p = 0.01$). 5-y OS: 40% vs. 30% ($p = 0.01$).	More acute mucositis with HF. 5-y grade 3–4 late toxicity: 8% vs. 14% ($p = 0.31$).	Cummings et al. (48)
Various sites. Stage III–IV, stage II of tongue base, hypopharynx	1073	1.2 / 1.8* / 1.6 / 2.0	2 / 1–2 / 2 / 1	81.6 / 72.0 / 67.2 / 70.0	6.0 / 7.0 / 6.0 / 7.0	LRC: higher with HF and CB ($p = 0.045$ and 0.05). DFS: trend in favor of HF and CB ($p = 0.067$ and 0.054) but no difference in OS.	More acute mucositis with all altered fractionations. No difference in late complication rate.	Fu et al. (69)
Bladder cancer (TCC)								
T2-4	168	1.0 / 2.0	3 / 1	84.0 / 64.0	8.0 / 8.0	Survival: higher with HF with a RH of 1.52 (95% CI: 1.10–2.09) OS benefit persists at 10 years.	Trend for increase in bowel injury requiring surgical treatment.	Naslund et al. (108)
Non–small cell lung cancer								
Stage II–III (surgically unresectable)	458	1.2 / 2.0	2 / 1	69.6 / 60.0	5.8 / 6.0	No significant difference in median or 5-year survival. (Induction chemotherapy arm yielded better OS.)	Late toxicity not presented in detail.	Sause et al. (136)
Brainstem tumors								
Age: 3–21 y	130	1.17 / 1.80	2 / 1	70.2 / 54.0	6.0 / 6.0	No significant difference in time to disease progression and overall survival.	Morbidity similar in both arms.	Mandell et al. (101)
Cranial radiation for treatment of high-risk all acute lymphoblastic leukemia								
Children treated on two consecutive protocols for high-risk all	369	0.9 / 1.8	2 / 1	18.0 / 18.0	2.0 / 2.0	8-y EFS 72% +/– 3% vs. 80% +/– 3% ($p = 0.06$) OS 78% +/– 3% vs. 85% +/– 3% ($p = 0.06$). CNS HF may compromise antileukemic efficacy.	Provides no benefit in terms of cognitive late effects. No difference in intelligence, academic achievement, visuospatial reasoning, or verbal learning. Children on HF arm exhibited a modest advantage for visual memory ($p \leq 0.05$).	Weber et al. (162); LeClerc et al. (93)
Children with rhabdomyosarcoma								
Children enrolled into the Intergroup RMS Study IV with Group III RMS	490	1.1 / 1.8	2 / 1	59.4 / 50.4	5.5 / 5.5	No difference in 5-y FFS or OS between HF and SF.	Analysis by intention to treat; high noncompliance analysis by actual treatment also shows no difference. Higher acute toxicity with HF.	Donaldson et al. (55)
Unresected brain metastases (hyperfractionation versus accelerated hypofractionation)								
RTOG 9104; patients with measurable brain metastasis and KPS at least 70; AHF versus AF	429	1.6 / 3.0	2 / 1	54.4 / 30.0	3.5 / 2.0	No difference in OS 1-y OS: 19% in AF vs. 16% in AHF.	Grade III or IV toxicity was equivalent in both arms.	Murray et al. (107)

The outcome data are given x% vs. y% implies x is the experimental arm result.

AF, accelerated fractionation; ALL, acute lymphoblastic leukemia; CNS, central nervous system; DFS, disease-free survival; EFS, event-free survival; FFS, failure-free survival; HF, hyperfractionation; LC, local control; LRC, locoregional control; MST, median survival time; NSCLC, non–small cell lung cancer; OS, overall survival; TCC, transitional cell carcinoma; RMS, rhabdomyosarcoma; SF, standard fractionation; TN, .

cell regeneration during treatment and therefore increases the probability of tumor control for a given total dose. Because overall treatment time has little influence on the probability of late normal tissue injury, a therapeutic gain should be realized, provided the size of dose per fraction is not increased and the interval between dose fractions is sufficient for complete repair to take place.

When the overall duration of treatment is markedly reduced, it is necessary to reduce total dose to prevent excessively severe acute reactions. A therapeutic gain is then realized only if the reduction in dose is less than the dose equivalent of blocked regeneration of tumor cells due to shortened time.

Strategies to accelerate radiation can be divided into two categories: (i) *pure accelerated fractionation* regimens, with reduced overall treatment time without concurrent changes in the fraction size or total dose (examples are given in Table 11.3); And (ii) *hybrid accelerated fractionation*, with reduced overall treatment time in conjunction with changes in other parameter(s) such as the fraction size, total dose, and time distribution. Four forms of hybrid accelerated fractionation were designed, and the regimes tested in randomized clinical trials are given in Table 11.4. The categories are further described as type A: drastic reduction of the overall time with substantial decrease in the total dose; type B: duration of treatment is more modestly reduced with total dose kept in the same range and there is a break in treatment; and type C: duration of treatment is more modestly reduced with total dose kept in the same range with a concomitant boost phase.

Clinical Studies

This section will summarize the results of hyperfractioned (HF) radiotherapy trials and accelerated fractionation (AF) radiotherapy trials; the combination of altered fractionation with concurrent chemotherapy; critical fractionation issues to consider when IMRT is used; common clinically practiced fractionation schedules; and future directions in combining molecular targeting with altered fractionation.

Hyperfractioned Radiotherapy Trials

Table 11.2 summarizes 10 reported prospective, randomized trials addressing hyperfractionation for the treatment of patients with head and neck, bladder, lung, brainstem tumors, whole brain radiotherapy for pediatric acute lymphoblastic leukemia, whole brain radiotherapy for brain metastases, and rhabdomyosarcoma. The most striking results are from trials in head and neck squamous-cell carcinoma (HNSCC) where hyperfractionation was accompanied by an increase in dose.

The key findings were:

- HF is better than standard fractionation in locoregional control of intermediate to locally advanced head and neck carcinoma. This was also associated with an improvement in survival in three trials (167).
- Reducing the fraction size from 2 Gy to 1.1 to 1.2 Gy permits a 7% to 17% total radiation dose escalation without increase in late complications. This supports the existence of differential fractionation sensitivity (variable α/β ratios) between human late-responding normal tissues and head and neck carcinomas.

Head and Neck

In all four head and neck trials (48,69,78,81,122) HF allowed a higher total dose to be delivered, which produced improved locoregional control by 8% to 20%. In three of these trials, HF improved overall survival by 10% to 19%. In all four studies, HF

produced more severe acute mucositis but no increase in late morbidity. The Brazilian Group (122) tested HF of 70.4 Gy at 1.1 Gy twice daily and showed improved local response by 20% and 3.5-year overall survival from 8% to 27%. The EORTC tested 80.5 Gy HF at 1.15 Gy per fraction, twice per day in 7 weeks (81). The 10-Gy increase in dose improved locoregional control from 38% to 56% and overall survival (20,78). The Princess Margaret Hospital tested 58 Gy at 1.45 Gy twice per day over 4 weeks versus 51 Gy at 2.55 Gy per fraction once daily (a standard fractionation at that institute) (48). The 7-Gy increase in dose improved locoregional control from 37% to 45% and improved 5-year overall survival from 30% to 40%.

The RTOG 9003 trial (69) tested 81.6 Gy at 1.2 Gy per fraction HF twice per day over 6 weeks versus 70 Gy at 2 Gy per fraction versus two AF regimes (a continuous and a split course accelerated regime), as shown in Tables 11.2 and 11.4. HF improved locoregional control from 46% to 54.4% (similar to the improvement by AF with the concomitant boost arm of the trial). This trial gives strong evidence that total dose and treatment duration are important to outcome. Locoregional control was significantly improved by an increase of the total dose without changing overall time using HF or by accelerated overall treatment time without changing total dose using concomitant boost fractionation.

A recent meta-analysis of hyperfractionated and accelerated radiotherapy in unresected locally advanced squamous-cell carcinoma of the head and neck showed a substantial prolongation of median survival (14.2 months; $p <0.001$) for hyperfractionated compared to conventional radiotherapy (36). They studied four trials (69,81,122) and a trial from Barcelona (130) that has been criticized for questionable quality (26). All four trials studied showed a statistically significant survival benefit. Studies testing HF without dose escalation did not show a survival advantage (12,165). HF is simply the best tool to enable dose escalation without an increase of severe late toxicity.

Bladder Cancer

In the study by Edsmyr et al. (61), T2-4 bladder tumors were randomized to either three 1-Gy daily fractions 4-hour with interfraction intervals to 84 Gy, or a single daily fraction of 2 Gy to total dose of 64 Gy, both given in a split course over 8 weeks. The cystoscopic complete response rate increased from 36% to 65% by HF ($p <0.001$), and the 5-year survival rate also significantly increased. However, severe late complications were higher in the hyperfractionated arm, indicating that the dose chosen might not be equivalent for late normal tissue injury. An updated analysis revealed that the survival benefit persisted for 10 years, and that there was a trend for higher bowel complications requiring surgery in the HF group (108).

Non–Small Cell Lung Cancer

The joint Intergroup trial (136) of the RTOG, Eastern Cooperative Oncology Group (ECOG), and Southwest Oncology Group (SWOG) compared induction chemotherapy (cisplatin and vinblastine) plus 60 Gy in 2-Gy fractions or HF (69.6 Gy in 1.2-Gy fractions) with conventional fractionation (60 Gy in 2-Gy fractions). HF, although slightly better, did not significantly improve survival over the standard fractionation.

Childhood Brainstem Tumor

The trial of the Pediatric Oncology Group (POG) (101) compared the efficacy of 70.2 Gy given in 1.17 Gy per fraction versus 54 Gy in 1.8-Gy fractions, both in combination with 100 mg/m^2 of cisplatin. This study showed no difference in the median time to disease progression, median time to death, or survival rates at 1 and 2 years with no significant difference in toxicity.

Table 11.3 DATA OF PHASE III CLINICAL TRIALS ADDRESSING PURE ACCELERATED FRACTIONATION

Tumor Site and Type	No. of Patients	Dose/Fx (Gy)	Fx/d and Ti (h)	Total Dose (Gy)	Overall Time	Tumor Response	Side Effects	Authors (Reference)
Inoperable non–small cell lung cancer	204	2.0 2.0	2 1	60 ± Carbo 60 ± Carbo	3.0 6.0	No significant difference in median survival time and 2-y OS.	Esophageal toxicity significantly greater in AF.	Ball et al. (11)
Various head and neck carcinomas. Stage III–IV	82	2.0 2.0	2 (≥6) 1	66.0 66.0	3.4 6.8	CR: 35% vs. 29% ($p = 0.18$). No difference in 3-y relapse-free survival.	Grade 3–4 reactions: 27 vs. 8 ($p = 0.00005$). Grade 4 late toxicity: 8 vs. 2 ($p = 0.10$).	Jackson et al. (87)
Various head and neck carcinomas, T2-4 N0-1	100	1.8–2.0 1.8–2.0	1 1	~70.0 ~70.0	5.0 7.0	3-y LC: 82% vs. 37% ($p \leq 0.0001$) and 3-y OS: 78% vs. 32% ($p \leq 0.0001$).	Severe mucositis: 62% vs. 26%. Late complications: 10% vs. 0%.	Skladowski et al. (137)
Various head and neck carcinomas, all stages	1485	2.0 2.0	1 1	~66.0 ~66.0	6.0 7.0	5-y LRC: 66% vs. 57% ($p = 0.01$). 5-y DFS: 72% vs. 65% ($p = 0.04$). No difference in OS.	More acute mucositis with AF. No difference in late complication rate.	Overgaard et al. (112)
Larynx carcinomas, T1-3N0	395	2.0 2.0	1–2 (≥6) 1	66.0 66.0	5.5 6.5	LRC: higher with AF ($p = 0.03$).	More acute reactions with AF. No difference in late complications except for telangiectasia.	Hliniak et al. (77)
Nasopharynx cancer	416	1.8–1.9 1.8–1.9 2.0	1 1 1	74–76 74–76 +Cis/5-FU 70–76	6.0 6.0 7.0	LR 16.7% vs. 13.6% vs. 27.3% ($p \leq 0.05$). 5-y OS 53.6% vs. 57.6% vs. 43.8% ($p \leq 0.05$) Acceleration had a similar improvement as concurrent chemotherapy.	Acute reactions higher with acceleration.	Wang et al. (161)

The outcome data are given x% vs. y% implies x is the experimental arm result.
AF, accelerated fractionation; Carbo, carboplatin; Cis, cisplatin; CR, complete response; DFS, disease-free survival; 5-FU, 5-flourouracil; LC, local control; LR, local recurrence; LRC, local-regional control; OS, overall survival.

Table 11.4 DATA OF PHASE III CLINICAL TRIALS ADDRESSING HYBRID ACCELERATED FRACTIONATION

Tumor Site and Type	No. of Patients	Dose/Fx (Gy)	Fx/d and Ti (h)	Total Dose (Gy)	Overall Time	Tumor Response	Side Effects	Authors (Reference)
Accelerated fractionation with total dose reduction (Type A)								
Various head and neck carcinomas, mainly stage II–IV	918	1.5 / 2.0	3 (6 h) / 1	54.0 / 66.0	2.0 / 6.5	No difference in LRC, disease-free interval, and OS.	More acute mucositis but less epidermis, telangiectasia, mucosal ulceration, and edema with AF.	Dische et al. (53)
Various head and neck carcinomas. Stage III–IV	350	1.8 / 2.0	2 (≥6) / 1	59.4 / 70.0	3.5 / 7.0	5-y LRC: 52% vs. 47% ($p = 0.30$). 5-y DFS: 41% vs. 35% ($p = 0.32$). 5-y DSS: 46% vs. 40% ($p = 0.40$).	More severe acute mucositis ($p = 0.00008$) but reduced incidence of grade ≥2 late soft tissue effects ($p \leq 0.05$) with AF (except for mucosal late effect).	Poulsen et al. (123)
All sites of head and neck carcinomas. Oropharynx 75%; T4 70%	268	2.0 / 2.0	2 / 1	~63.0 / 70.0	3.3 / 7.0	2-y LRC: 58% vs. 34% ($p \leq 0.01$). No difference in OS.	Grade 3–4 mucositis: 83% vs. 28% ($p < 0.01$). Similar late toxicity.	Bourhis et al. (27)
Postoperative head and neck	70	1.4 / 2.0	3 (6 h) / 1	46.2 / 60.0	2.0 / 6.0	3-y LRC: 88 +/− 4% vs. 57% +/− 9% ($p = 0.01$). OS: 60 +/− 10% vs. 46 +/− 9% ($p = 0.29$).	More rapid and more severe mucositis. Fibrosis and edema more frequent after accelerated.	Awwad et al. (10)
Stage IIIA and B unresectable head and neck	141	1.5 / 2.0	3 / 1	57.6 / 60.0	2.5 / 6.5	Trend suggesting a survival advantage MS 20.3 vs. 14.9 mo ($p = 0.28$). 2-y OS 44% vs. 34% 3-y OS 24% vs. 14%	Study included induction CT closed prematurely because concurrent CRT now seems more effective; 388 patients were needed.	Belani et al. (13)
RTOG 9104; patients with measurable brain metastasis and KPS at least 70; AHF versus AF	429	3.0 / 1.6	1 / 2	30.0 / 54.4	2.0 / 3.5	No difference in OS 1-y OS: 19% in AF vs. 16% in AHF.	Grade III or IV toxicity was equivalent in both arms.	Murray et al. (107)
Locally advanced non–small cell lung cancer	563	1.5 / 2.0 Split course	3 (6 h) / 1	54.0 / 60.0	2.0 / 6.0	2-y OS: 29% vs. 20% ($p = 0.008$). Lower risk of local progression ($p = 0.033$).	No difference in short- or long-term morbidity.	Saunders et al. (132)
Split-course (Type B) and concomitant boost (Type C) accelerated fractionation								
Various head and neck carcinomas, T2-4 N0-1	500	1.6 / 2.0 Split course	3 / 1	72.0 / 70.0	5.0 / 7.0	5-y LRC: 59% vs. 46% ($p = 0.02$). Trend for higher 5-y DFS ($p = 0.08$) but no difference in OS ($p = 0.96$).	More severe acute mucositis and higher incidence of severe late morbidity ($p \leq 0.001$) with AF.	Horiot et al. (79)

Table 11.4 DATA OF PHASE III CLINICAL TRIALS ADDRESSING HYBRID ACCELERATED FRACTIONATION

Tumor Site and Type	No. of Patients	Dose/Fx (Gy)	Fx/d and Ti (h)	Total Dose (Gy)	Overall Time	Tumor Response	Side Effects	Authors (Reference)
Various head and neck carcinomas, stage III–IV, stage II of tongue base, hypopharynx	1073	1.8[a] 1.20 1.60 Split course 2.0	1–2 2 2 1	72.0 81.6 67.2 70.0	6.0 7.0 6.0 7.0	LRC: higher with CB and HF ($p = 0.05$ and 0.045). DFS: strong trend in favor of CB and HF ($p = 0.054$ and 0.067) but no difference in OS.	More acute mucositis with all altered fractionations. No difference in late complication rate.	Fu et al. (69)
Unresectable epidermoid tumors of oropharynx.	192	2.0 1.6 Split course 2[b]	1 2 1	66–70 64–67.2 66–70	6.5–7 5.5 6.5–7	No difference in 2-y EFS and OS between SF, AFS, and SF chemo, 2-y DFS higher with SF chemo (42%) than SF 23% or AFS 20% ($p = 0.22$)	SF had less severe mucositis than AFS or SF chemo.	Olmi et al. (111)
T2-3 N0-1 bladder tumors	229	1.8 (a.m.) 2 (p.m.) Split course 2.0	2 1	60.8 64.0	5.0 6.5	No difference in 3- or 5-y DFS and OS 5-y OS 37% vs. 40%.	More acute bowel reactions with AF.	Horwich et al. (83)
Various head and neck carcinomas, high-risk surgical-pathologic features	151	1.8 1.8	1–2 1	63.0 63.0	5.0 7.0	A trend for higher LRC ($p = 0.11$) and OS ($p = 0.08$) with CB. Cumulative time was a significant prognostic factor for LRC ($p = 0.005$) and OS ($p = 0.03$)	More acute mucositis with CB. No difference in late complication rate.	Ang et al. (8)
High-risk features (pT4, + margins, pN >1, perineural/lymphovascular invasion, extracapsular extension, subglottic extension) after surgery	226	1.8 1.8	1–2 1	64.0 60.0	5.0 6.0	No difference in OS and LRC but trend for improved LRC among patients who had delayed RT.	More acute mucositis with CB.	Sanguineti et al. (131)
Accelerated hyperfractionation								
Glioblastoma multiforme	231	1.6 1.8	2 1	70.4 ± DMFO 59.4 ± DMFO	4.4 6.5	No difference in PFS ($p = 0.32$) and OS ($p = 0.48$).	Cerebral necrosis was not observed. Morbidity more common in the DFMO arms.	Prados et al. (125)

The outcome data are given x% vs. y% implies x is the experimental arm result.
Hybrid accelerated of which there are three types: accelerated with dose reduction (A); accelerated with split course (B); accelerated with concomitant boost (C).
[a]Boost dose given in 1.5 Gy fractions.
[b]Third arm with concurrent chemotherapy.

AF, accelerated fractionation; AFS, accelerated hyperfractionated split-course; AHF, accelerated hyperfractionated; CB, concomitant boost; CRT, concurrent chemoradiation; CT, chemoradiation; DFS, disease-free survival; DMFO, difluoromethylornithine; DSS, disease-specific survival; EFS, event-free survival; HF, hyperfractionation; KPS, Karnofsky performance score; LRC, local-regional control; MS, median survival; OS, overall survival; PFS, progression-free survival; RTOG, Radiation Therapy Oncology Group; SF, standard fractionation; SF, chemo, standard fraction plus concomitant chemotherapy.

Cranial Radiation Therapy for High-Risk Acute Lymphoblastic Leukemia

To test whether hyperfractionated (twice daily) therapy can reduce incidence and severity of late toxicities associated with 18-Gy prophylactic cranial radiotherapy, 369 children on two consecutive Dana-Farber Cancer Institute Consortium protocols were randomized to 18 Gy delivered in 10 1.8-Gy fractions, once daily over 2 weeks versus 18 Gy delivered in 20 0.9-Gy fractions. No benefit was seen in terms of cognitive late effects, and the results suggested that HF may compromise antileukemic efficacy (93,163).

Group III Rhabdomyosarcoma

A study of 490 children with group III rhabdomyosarcoma (RMS) who were randomized to hyperfractionated radiotherapy (HFRT) (59.4 Gy in 54 1.1-Gy twice daily fractions) versus conventionally fractionated radiotherapy (CFRT) to 50.4 Gy in the Intergroup RMS Study IV showed that HFRT did not improve local/regional control, failure-free survival, or overall survival compared with CFRT, and that HFRT actually produced more acute toxicity (55). Unlike studies in HNSCC of positive results with dose-escalated HFRT, an escalation of dose by 9.5 Gy did not improve outcome for RMS.

Unresected Brain Metastasis

RTOG 9104 compared 1-year survival and acute toxicity rates between an accelerated hyperfractionated radiotherapy (1.6 Gy twice a day) to a total dose of 54.4 Gy versus an accelerated hypofractionated arm of 30 Gy in 10 daily fractions in patients with unresected brain metastasis. Of 429 analyzable patients, the median survival time was 4.5 months in both arms. The 1-year survival rate was 19% in the hypofractionated arm versus 16% in the hyperfractionated arm. Grade III or IV toxicity was equivalent in both arms. In spite of an escalated dose, HF was of no benefit (107).

Results of Accelerated Radiotherapy Trials

Key findings of AF regimens include the following:

- Modest acceleration by 1 week by delivering six fractions of 2 Gy per week or a concomitant boost regimen without dose reduction or treatment break yields superior locoregional control of head and neck carcinomas without increase in late toxicity but without clear impact on survival. Acceleration by more than 3 weeks with a 10% total dose reduction (<6 to 7 Gy) also improves the locoregional control without demonstrable increase in late complications. However, a further 5% to 8% total dose reduction abrogates the gain in tumor control but appears to reduce the severity of some late normal tissue complications, such as fibrosis and edema.
- Mucositis per se or its consequential late toxicity prevents delivery of more than 12 Gy per week when given in two fractions of 2 Gy per day, 5 days a week or daily fractions throughout weekends to a total dose of 66 to 70 Gy (pure acceleration).
- Acceleration achieves significantly improved local control for well-differentiated tumors and advanced primary mucosal site tumors but may be of little benefit to advanced nodal disease and poorly differentiated tumors. This supports the existence of the accelerated proliferation phenomenon in mucosa-derived tumor cells.

The trials are classified into either pure accelerated, with same total dose or hybrid accelerated of which there are three types: (i) accelerated with dose reduction, (ii) accelerated with split course, and (iii) accelerated with concomitant boost.

Pure Accelerated Fractionation

Table 11.3 summarizes the radiation regimens and outcomes of six reported randomized trials of pure AF for the treatment of patients with NSCLC head and neck carcinoma.

Non–Small Cell Lung Cancer

A study of 204 patients randomized them to 60 Gy in 3 weeks versus 60 Gy in 6 weeks, both with or without concurrent carboplatin (11). The results showed no survival advantage with either AF or concurrent carboplatin. The study showed that 60 Gy in 3 weeks induced a significantly greater esophagitis than 60 Gy in 6 weeks.

Head and Neck Cancer

The first two HNSCC studies shown in Table 11.3 (87,137) induced unacceptable toxicity leading to early termination, and these two fractionations have been abandoned. However, two of the other three trial showed positive results (112,161), while one (77) showed no benefit and similar late toxicity.

The Polish Cooperative Group compared 66 Gy given in 33 fractions over 38 days (two fractions every Thursday) as compared with a conventional regimen of 66 Gy given in 33 fractions over 45 days. In the study 395 patients with T1-3, N0, M0, glottic and supraglottic laryngeal cancer were randomized. There was no difference in terms of locoregional control ($p = 0.37$) (77).

The Danish trial, one of the largest trials of altered fractionation (112), accrued 1,485 patients with larynx, oropharynx, and oral cavity carcinomas of all stages. Six versus 7 weeks' treatment was achieved by giving a sixth fraction each week. Overall 5-year locoregional control rates improved (70% vs. 60%; $p = 0.0005$). The benefit of shortening treatment time was seen for primary tumor control (76% vs. 64%; $p = 0.0001$), but not for neck-node control. Acceleration from 7 to 6 weeks improved voice preservation in laryngeal cancer (80% vs. 68%; $p = 0.007$) and improved disease-specific survival (73% vs. 66%; $p = 0.01$) but not overall survival. Multivariate analysis of 754 larynx cancers showed that AF was beneficial in tumors that were moderately and well differentiated with no benefit for the poorly differentiated. This effect suggests that the mechanism of repopulation in the primary tumor may be similar to the response in the original normal mucosa and in its functional mechanism of regeneration. This capacity to respond to the trauma of irradiation is more likely to exist in well-differentiated tumors, and the process may be facilitated by signaling from the surrounding normal mucosa. Accelerated proliferation may, therefore, be a response of the primary tumor and not the nodal metastases (15).

Nasopharynx

Pure acceleration for nasopharynx cancer was tested in Guangxi, China. In the study, 416 patients were randomized to three arms: all had 7,400 to 7,600 given either as AF six fractions per week versus AF with concurrent cisplatin and 5-fluorouracil (AFC) versus the conventional five (CF) 2-Gy fractions per week. The local recurrence rates were 16.7% in the AF group, 13.6% in the AFC group, and 27.3% in the CF group ($p < 0.05$). The 5-year survival rates were 53.6%, 57.6%, and 43.8% ($p < 0.05$), respectively. The interesting finding was that acceleration had a similar effect as concurrent chemotherapy with acceleration for nasopharynx cancer (161).

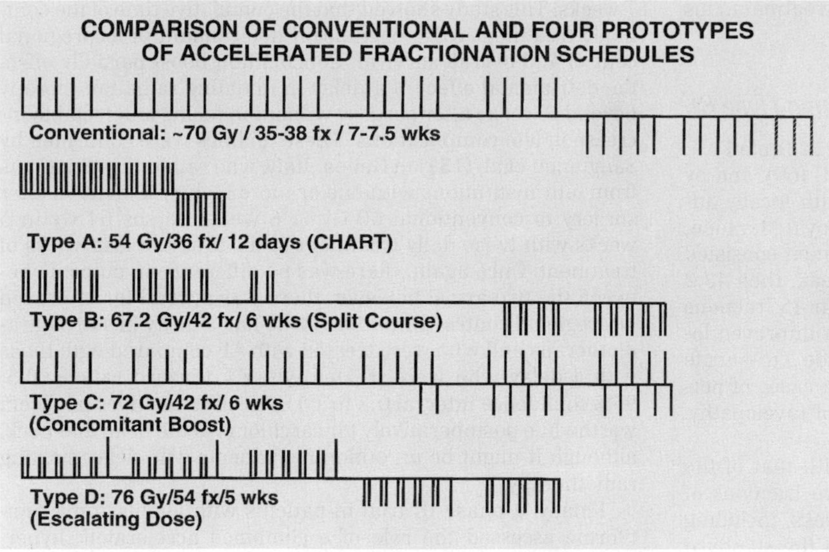

**COMPARISON OF CONVENTIONAL AND FOUR PROTOTYPES
OF ACCELERATED FRACTIONATION SCHEDULES**

Conventional: ~70 Gy / 35-38 fx / 7-7.5 wks

Type A: 54 Gy/36 fx/ 12 days (CHART)

Type B: 67.2 Gy/42 fx/ 6 wks (Split Course)

Type C: 72 Gy/42 fx/ 6 wks
(Concomitant Boost)

Type D: 76 Gy/54 fx/5 wks
(Escalating Dose)

FIGURE 11.3. Conventional and accelerated fractionation schedules. For each regimen, the large-field treatment is depicted by the bars above the horizontal line and the boost-field irradiation by the bars below the line. The dotted bars represent treatment omitted in the lower ranges of total dose. fx, fraction

Techniques, Modalities, and Modifiers in Radiation Oncology

Hybrid Accelerated Fractionation

Table 11.4 summarizes the details of regimens and outcomes of 14 reported prospective, randomized trials addressing the role of types A to C hybrid accelerated fractionation.

Type A

AF regimens (with dose reduction) were addressed in seven trials shown in Table 11.4, including a trial in HNSCC (definitive and postoperative), brain metastases, and NSCLC. It includes trails by the British Medical Research Council (MRC), Trans-Tasman Radiation Oncology Group (TROG), the French Radiotherapy Oncology Group for Head and Neck Cancer (GORTEC), and the Eastern Cooperative Oncology Group (ECOG).

Head and Neck

As shown in Table 11.4, two trials for HNSCC—the British MRC CHART (53) and TROG regimens (123)—did not yield improvement in locoregional control and disease-free and overall survival rates. In contrast, the GORTEC regimen (26) for locally advanced head and neck carcinoma with a 3.5-week acceleration and only 7-Gy (10%) dose reduction significantly improved the locoregional control with no gain in the overall survival rate.

Based on the assumption of accelerated proliferation after surgery, Awwad et al. (10) in Cairo explored acceleration in postoperative radiotherapy of locally advanced HNSCC. The study consisted of 70 patients with (T2/N1-2) or (T3-4/any N) squamous-cell carcinoma of the oral cavity, larynx, and hypopharynx who, following surgery, were randomized to accelerated hyperfractionation 46.2 Gy in 12 days versus conventional 60 Gy per 6 weeks. The 3-year locoregional control rate was better with accelerated treatment (88% +/− 4%) versus (57%+/− 9%) conventional group ($p = 0.01$) with no difference in survival (60% +/− 10% vs. 46% +/− 9%; $p = 0.29$). As expected, acute mucositis was more severe in the accelerated group and fibrosis and edema also tended to be more frequent; this finding contrasts with the results in two postoperative studies of type C (concomitant boost) described later and in Table 11.4 (8,131).

Non-Small Cell Lung Cancer

One randomized controlled trial showed that CHART improves survival over standard radiotherapy of 60 Gy in 30 fractions

in patients with locally advanced unresectable stage III NSCLC. This British MRC trial (132) showed that CHART with a 4-week acceleration and 6-Gy (10%) dose reduction decreased the risk for local progression and improved the overall survival significantly without increasing short- and long-term morbidity. These patients are now routinely given concurrent chemotherapy. However, in some countries, selected patients who are not fit for chemotherapy or patients who prefer radiotherapy only may be considered for CHART. The ECOG tested accelerated radiotherapy after induction chemotherapy (two cycles of carboplatin plus paclitaxel) in stage IIIA and B NSCLC. Acceleration was achieved with 57.6 Gy (1.5 Gy three times a day for 2.5 weeks) versus conventional 64 Gy (2 Gy per day). Of 141 patients enrolled, 83% were randomly assigned, 60 accelerated and 59 conventional. The median survival was 20.3 and 14.9 respectively ($p = 0.28$). With the acceptance that concurrent

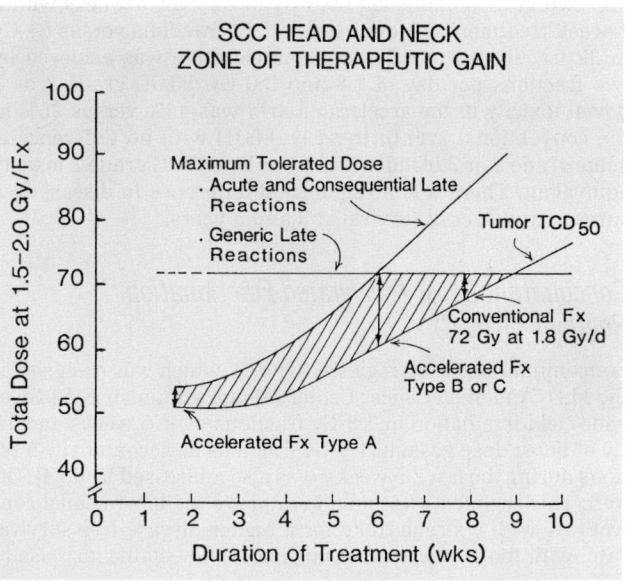

FIGURE 11.4. Zone of therapeutic gain in squamous-cell carcinomas of the head and neck for different accelerated fractionation schedules. Type A is 54 Gy in 36 fractions over 12 days, type B is 67.2 Gy in 42 fractions over 42 days, and type C is 72 Gy in 42 fractions over 40 days. For explanation, see text. (From Peters LJ, Brock WA, Travis EL. Radiation biology at clinically relevant fractions. In: DeVita V, Hellman S, Rosenberg SA, eds. *Important advances in oncology.* Philadelphia: J.B. Lippincott, 1991;65–83, with permission.)

chemoradiation is more effective than sequential treatment, this trial closed early (13).

Split-Course Accelerated Fractionation Regimen (Type B)

Split-Course AF regimens (type B) are also shown in Table 11.4. This was addressed by the EORTC (79) and RTOG (69), and by a study from Firenze, Italy (111), in patients with locally advanced head and neck carcinomas and by the Royal Marsden, London, in bladder cancer (83). The EORTC regimen consisted of 28.8 Gy over 7 days followed by a 2-week break, then 43.2 Gy over 11 days to a cumulative dose of 72 Gy in 45 fractions over 5 weeks. Although the 2-week acceleration improved locoregional control, it produced twice as many grade 3 to 4 acute morbidities, more late toxicity (p <0.001), seven cases of permanent peripheral neuropathy, and two cases of myelopathy. This regimen has been abandoned.

The RTOG split regimen was comparable with that of the Massachusetts General Hospital study (159): two fractions of 1.6 Gy per day to a total dose of 67.2 Gy in 6 weeks, including a 2-week break in treatment after 38.4 Gy with the standard 70 Gy in 7 weeks. This 1-week acceleration with a 3.8-Gy (5%) dose reduction increased the acute mucositis without improving the locoregional control rate (69), with the concomitant boost and hyperfractionation arm being superior. Olmi et al. (111) reported an Italian multicenter randomized trial that treated 192 patients with advanced carcinoma of the oropharynx with conventional radiotherapy (arm A: 66 to 70 Gy in 33 to 35 fractions, 5 days a week over 6.5 to 7 weeks) versus accelerated split course radiotherapy (arm B: 64 to 67.2 Gy, two fractions of 1.6 Gy 5 days a week with 2-week split at 38.4 Gy) concomitant chemoradiation (arm C: same radiotherapy as arm A plus concomitant carboplatin and 5-fluorouracil). Although there was no significant difference in overall survival and event-free survival, the 2-year disease-free survival was superior in arm C (p = 0.022): 42% for arm C versus 23% for arm A and 20% for arm B, but this improvement was associated with a higher incidence of acute morbidity.

The Royal Marsden in London evaluated the efficacy and toxicity of an AF regimen to treat T2 or T3, N0 or N1 muscle invasive bladder cancer. The 229 patients were randomized into two groups and given 60.8 Gy in 32 over 5 weeks with a 1-week treatment gap after the first 12 fractions versus 64 Gy in 32 fractions over 6.5 weeks. Acceleration was achieved by two fractions per day of 1.8 and 2.0 Gy. RTOG grade 2 or 3 bowel toxicity in the accelerated arm was 44% versus 26% in the conventional arm (p trend = 0.001) with no difference is acute grade 2 or 3 bladder toxicity or late RTOG grade 2 toxicity equivalent. There was no significant difference in disease-free survival and overall survival at 3 and 5 years.

Concomitant Boost Accelerated Fractionation Regimen (Type C)

Concomitant boost AF regimen (type C), which was designed at the M.D. Anderson Cancer Center (4) and administers 54 Gy of wide-field irradiation in 1.8-Gy fractions over 6 weeks and 18 Gy of boost dose given in 1.5-Gy fractions as second daily fractions during the last 2.5 weeks, was also addressed by the RTOG (69). This regimen was found to improve the locoregional control rate with a strong trend for a higher disease-free survival rate, with more severe mucositis but no detectable increase in late complications.

Concomitant boost-type fractionation was also tested for postoperative radiation therapy in two phase III trials (6,131). Ang et al. () randomized patients with high-risk pathologic features to 63 Gy given in 35 fractions over either 5 weeks (daily fractions for 3 weeks then two fractions per day for 2 weeks) or

7 weeks. This study showed that the cumulative time of the combined treatment was a significant determinant of locoregional control and overall survival. Concomitant boost partially offset the detrimental effect of a delay in initiating radiation therapy beyond 6 weeks after surgery without inducing a detectable increase in late complications. These findings were confirmed by Sanguineti et al. (131) in Genoa, Italy, who randomized patients from four institutions with one or more high-risk features after surgery to conventional 60 Gy in 6 weeks versus 64 Gy in 5 weeks with twice daily treatment in the first and last weeks of treatment. Once again, there was no difference in outcome between the two arms; however, there was a trend for improved locoregional control for patients who had a delay in starting radiotherapy and who were treated with AF compared with those with a delay who were treated with CF (hazard ratio = 0.5; 95% confidence interval 0.2 to 1.1). Acceleration does not seem worthwhile postoperatively for carcinoma of the head and neck, although it might be an option for patients who delay starting radiotherapy.

Finally, a phase III trial in patients with glioblastoma multiforme assessed the role of a combined accelerated, hyperfractionated regimen with a 2-week reduction of therapy duration and a dose increment of 11 Gy (18%) (125). This radiation regimen, with or without difluoromethylornithine (DMFO), was found to yield no better progression-free and overall survival rates.

The Combination of Altered Fractionation with Concurrent Chemotherapy

In a recent meta-analysis conducted at Villejuif, an absolute benefit of 3% (from 36% to 39%, hazard ratio [HR] 0.92; 95% CI 0.87 to 0.97; p = 0.004) was observed at 5 years in favor of the altered fractionation regimens (25). In light of the data in support of the superiority of altered fractionation to standard radiotherapy alone and findings of improved local control and survival with the addition of concurrent chemotherapy to radiotherapy in several randomized studies (37,103,164) and two recent meta-analyses (63,121), at least 11 studies reported on investigation of addition of chemotherapy to altered fractionation (Table 11.5). These studies did not explore chemotherapy results with varying fractionation regimens, except for one study (1,2), which tested the addition of chemotherapy to radiation in patients with unresectable squamous-cell HNSCC by adding chemotherapy to either standard fractionation or a complicated prolonged split course regime.

Key Findings of Combined Altered Fractionation with Concurrent Chemotherapy

Although the magnitude of its effect was less marked for survival indices than for local-regional control, the addition of chemotherapy to altered fractionation regimens results in a clear improvement compared with hyperfractionated or accelerated regimens alone; however, the effect on normal tissues' late toxicities is not fully known.

In nasopharynx cancer, the benefit of concurrent chemotherapy is similar to that of acceleration without chemotherapy. The potential biological interactions between chemotherapy and radiotherapy by the addition of to radiation have been summarized as follows (22):

1. Shift of cell survival curves toward higher cell killing levels and lower cell surviving fractions for a given dose of irradiation;
2. Cooperation to prevent the emergence of resistant clones;
3. A decrease in tumor mass and reoxygenation;
4. Specific toxicity for hypoxic cells;

Author (Reference)	Tumor Site and Stage	No. of Patients	Therapy Regimens	Tumor Response	Complications
Accelerated fractionation plus chemotherapy					
Dobrowsky & Naude (54)	Various sites T1-4 N0-3	239	V-CHART: 55.3 Gy/17 d (2.5 Gy on d 1, then 1.65 Gy, b.i.d., on d 2–17). V-CHART + MMC 20 mg/m² on day 5. CF: 70 Gy/7 wk.	V-CHART + MMC yielded higher LRC (p <0.05) and survival (p ≤0.03) than V-CHART and CF.	V-CHART induced more mucositis than CF but not intensified by MMC. Late toxicity not reported.
Staar et al. (138)	Stage III–IV unresectable oropharynx and hypopharynx	240	69.9 Gy/5.5 wk + carboplatin (70 mg/m²/d) and 5-FU (600 mg/m²/d) for 5 days × 2. 69.9 Gy/5.5 wk (1.8 Gy every day for 3.5 wk, then b.i.d., 1.8 Gy + 1.5 Gy, for 2 wk).	2-y OS: 48% vs. 39% (p = 0.11). 2-y LRC 51% vs. 45% (p = 0.14). Patients receiving G-CSF had worse LRC (p = 0.007)	Grade 3–4 mucositis: 68% vs. 52% (p = 0.01). Grade 3–4 vomiting: 8.2% vs. 1.6% (p = 0.02). Late swallowing problems and feeding tube dependency: 51% vs. 25% (p = 0.02).
Bourhis et al. (27)	Various sites Advanced-inoperable	109	62–64 Gy/5 wk + cis (100 mg/m² on day 1, 16, 32) and 5-FU (1 g/m²/d on d 1–5, 31–35). 62–64 Gy/3 wk.	Not reported yet.	Early cessation due to higher treatment-related deaths in the combined arm.
Wang et al. (161)	Nasopharynx cancer	416	74–76 Gy in 6 wk (6 fractions per wk) + Cis/5-FU. 74–76 Gy in 6 wk (6 fractions per wk). 70–76 Gy in 7 weeks.	LRC 13.6% 16.7% vs. 27.3% (p <0.05). 5-y OS 57.6% vs. 53.6% vs. 43.8% (p < 0.05). Acceleration had a similar improvement as concurrent chemotherapy.	Acute reactions higher with acceleration.
Alternating chemoradiation versus partly accelerated radiotherapy in locally advanced squamous cell carcinoma of the head and neck					
Corvo et al. (43)	Unfavorable stage II or stage III–IV	136	1 wk Cis (20 mg/m²/d + 5-FU 200 mg/m²)/d for 5 days alternated with three 2-wk courses of 20 Gy 2 Gy/d, 5 d/wk (60Gy) vs. 75 Gy/40 CB in 6 wk	3-y OS: 37% vs. 29%; 3-y PFS: 35% vs. 27%. 3-y LRC: 32% vs. 27%.	Acute skin and late mucosal and skin toxicities significantly less with chemoradiation but radiotherapy dose was 15 Gy or less.
Split-course accelerated fractionation plus chemotherapy					
Denham et al. (49)	Various sites T2-4 N0-3	122	RT: 70 Gy/47 d in 1.25 Gy b.i.d. (7–10/d break after 40 Gy) + Cis and 5-FU wk 1 and 6. RT alone: 75Gy/42 d in 1.25 Gy, b.i.d.	3-y LRC: 70% vs. 44% (p = 0.01). 3-yr RFS: 61% vs. 41% (p = 0.07). 3-y OS: 55% vs. 34% (p = 0.07).	Similar mucositis. Increased internal feeding and sepsis. Similar late complications.
Byhardt et al. (36)	Various sites Stage III–IV	270	70.2 Gy/51 d plus Cis, 5-FU, and leucovorin. 70.2 Gy/51 d (23.4 Gy in 1.8-Gy fractions, b.i.d., for 3 cycles with 10–1 break).	3-y LRC: 36% vs. 17%, (p <0.004). 3-y OS: 48% vs. 24% (p <0.0003).	Grade 3–4 acute mucositis: 38% vs. 16% (p <0.001) Serious late side effects: 10% vs. 6.4% (NS)

Table 11.5 — PHASE III TRIALS ADDRESSING CONCURRENT CHEMOTHERAPY AND ALTERED FRACTIONATION IN PATIENTS WITH HEAD AND NECK CANCER

Author (Reference)	Tumor Site and Stage	No. of Patients	Therapy Regimens	Tumor Response	Complications
Chemoradiation with split-course prolonged radiotherapy					
Adelstein et al. (1)	Stage III or IV unresectable disease	295	30 Gy at 2 Gy/d with concurrent 5-FU and Cis wk 1–3, 5-wk break with chemotherapy followed by 30–40 Gy/wk 8–11 vs. 70 Gy at 2 Gy/d plus Cis on d 1, 22, and 43 vs. (3) 70 Gy at 2 Gy/d alone	3-y projected OS:27 vs. 37 vs. 23%. Median survival: 13.8 vs. 19.1 vs. 12.6 mo. No difference between arm 1 and 3. 3-y DSS 41% vs. 51% vs. 33%. Arm 2 was better ($p = 0.01$).	Grade 3 or worse toxicity: 77% vs. 89% vs. 52% ($p < 0.001$).
Hyperfractionation plus chemotherapy					
Denham et al. (50)	Various sites stage III–IV	130	77 Gy/7 wk + Cis (6 mg/m²/d). 77 Gy/7 wk (1.1 Gy, b.i.d.).	5-y LRPFS: 50% vs. 36% ($p = 0.04$). 5-y PFS: 46% vs. 25% ($p = 0.007$). 5-y DMFS: 86% vs. 57% ($p = 0.001$). 5-y OS: 46% vs. 25%. ($p = 0.008$).	No significant difference in acute morbidity (except for leucopenia, $p = 0.006$) or late toxicity.
Hugeunin et al. (85)	Squamous cell carcinomas of the head and neck	224	74.4 Gy; 1.2 Gy b.i.d. + Cis 20 mg/m² (on 5 d wk 1 and 5). 74.4 Gy; 1.2 Gy b.i.d.	Failure-free rate at 2.5 y was 45% and 33%. LRC was significantly improved log-rank test ($p < 0.039$)	Late toxicity was comparable.
Hyperfractionated accelerated chemoradiation with concurrent chemotherapy versus dose-escalated hyperfractionated accelerated radiation therapy alone in locally advanced head and neck cancer					
Budach et al. (35)	Various sites stage III–IV	384	70.6 Gy in 6 weeks (30 Gy, 2 Gy/d + 40.6 at 1.4 Gy b.i.d.) + 5-FU (600 mg/m²) + mitomycin (10 mg/m². 77.6 Gy (14 Gy at 2 Gy/d + 1.4 Gy b.i.d.): dose-escalated radiotherapy.	5-y LRC 49.9% vs. 37.4% ($p = 0.001$). 5-y OS: 28.6% vs. 23.7% ($p = 0.023$).	Maximum acute mucositis, moist desquamation, and erythema were higher in dose-escalated radiotherapy; no differences in late reactions.

b.i.d., twice-a-day irradiation; CB,concomitant boost; CF, conventional fractionation; Cis, cisplatin; DMFS, distant metastasis-free survival; DSS, disease-specific survival; 5-FU, 5-flourouracil; LC, local control; LRC, locoregional control; LRPFS, locoregional progression-free survival; MMC, mitomycin-C; NS, not significant; OS, overall survival; PFS, progression-free survival; QD, once-a-day irradiation; RFS, relapse-free survival; V-CHART, Vienna variation of continuous hyperfractionated accelerated radiation therapy.

5. Selective toxicity depending on cell-cycle phase;
6. Cytokinetic cooperation;
7. Action on DNA repair;
8. Increased apoptosis.

Table 11.5 summarizes the results of 11 randomized studies investigating the efficacy of concurrent chemotherapy regimens with altered fractionation.

Acceleration versus Chemoradiation or with Chemotherapy

An Austrian three-arm trial tested the addition of mitomycin C (MMC) on day 5 of treatment to Vienna variation of continuous, hyperfractionated, accelerated radiation therapy (V-CHART): 55.3 Gy in 17 days. The three arms were 70 Gy conventional fractionation alone versus V-CHART, versus V-CHART with concurrent MMC on day 5 (V-CHART + MMC) (54). The 239 patients were randomized. Locoregional tumor control was 31% after conventional fractionation, 32% after V-CHART and 48% after V-CHART + MMC, respectively (p <0.05). Overall crude survival was 24% after conventional fractionation, 31% after V-CHART, and 41% after V-CHART + MMC, respectively (p <0.05). Therefore, reducing the treatment time from 7 weeks to 17 consecutive days and dose of radiotherapy from 70 to 55.3 Gy produced identical results, while the addition of MMC on day 5 to the accelerated fractionated treatment produced a significant improvement in local tumor control and survival. This supports an argument for adding chemotherapy to AF.

A German Cooperative Group compared a concomitant boost radiation regimen with or without carboplatin and 5-fluorouracil (138). The addition of chemotherapy produced a trend for better locoregional control and survival rates, but it induced a significantly higher incidence of chronic dysphagia, resulting in feeding-tube dependency (51% vs. 25%). A secondary randomization to receive or not receive granulocyte colony stimulating factor to reduce mucositis produced the startling finding that *the administration of granulocyte colony stimulating factor significantly reduced the probability of locoregional control in both treatment arms*.

The French Cooperative Group, GORTEC, tested the combination of 62 to 64 Gy given in 5 weeks with cisplatin and 5-fluorouracil and terminated the trial prematurely due to unacceptable toxicity (48). The nasopharynx trial from China gave a very interesting finding that accelerated radiotherapy provides the same benefit as adding concurrent chemotherapy and is discussed in the section above on accelerated radiotherapy (160).

Alternating chemoradiotherapy was studied in Italy by Corvo et al. (43) and compared with high-dose accelerated radiotherapy. The 136 patients with unfavorable stage II or stage III to IV head and neck carcinoma were randomized to alternating cisplatin and 5-fluorouracil with three 2-week courses of radiotherapy (20 Gy at 2 Gy per day: 60 Gy vs. 75 Gy at 40 fractions in 6 weeks) using a concomitant boost technique. At 60 months there was no differences in overall survival, progression-free survival, or locoregional control.

Split-course altered fractionation with or without concurrent chemotherapy was tested in two trials. Both added cisplatin and 5-fluorouracil to split-course type AF schedules (70 Gy in 42 to 51 days) (33,164). Both showed that a chemotherapy regime improved locoregional control versus altered fractionation alone. However, a split course accelerated regimen is now known to be no more effective than standard fractionation. The locoregional control improved with an 18% to 26% increase in late effects. The larger trial showed improved overall survival.

Adelstein et al. (1) reported on the Head and Neck Intergroup's trial to test the addition of chemotherapy to radiation in patients with unresectable squamous cell HNSCC by adding chemotherapy to either standard fractionation or a prolonged split-course regime. The 295 patients were randomized into three arms: 70 Gy at 2 Gy per day (RT only) versus the same radiation therapy with concurrent bolus cisplatin (RT + C) versus a third arm: split course radiotherapy with chemotherapy during the break radiotherapy (split RT + C) from week 9. They did not meet the accrual goal. Grade 3 or worse toxicity occurred in 52% of patients in the RT only arm, 89% in RT + C (p <0.0001) and 77% in split RT + C arm (p <0.001). The 3-year projected overall survival for patients RT only arm was 23%, compared with 37% for RT + C arm (p = 0.014) and 27% for split RT + C arm (p = not significant). The addition of concurrent high-dose, single-agent cisplatin to conventional radiation significantly improves survival and increased toxicity; however, multiagent chemotherapy did not offset the loss of efficacy resulting with prolongation by split-course radiation.

Concurrent Chemotherapy in Addition to Hyperfractionated Radiotherapy

A randomized trial by Jeremic et al. (89) tested the addition of low-dose daily cisplatin to 77 Gy at 1.1 Gy per fraction twice daily over 7 weeks. Daily cisplatin improved the results of HF radiation with better locoregional progression-free survival (50% vs. 36%; p = 0.04), 5-year progression-free survival (46% vs. 25%; p = 0.007), 5-year distant metastases-free survival (86% vs. 57%; p = 0.001), and 5-year overall survival (46% vs. 25%; p = 0.008). This was a true therapeutic gain because there was no difference in late side effects.

A study conducted in Zurich also reported similar results (85). The 224 patients with squamous-cell carcinomas were randomized to two cycles of concurrent cisplatin 20 mg/m^2 on 5 days of weeks 1 and 5 with HF radiotherapy (median dose, 74.4 Gy; 1.2 Gy twice daily) versus the same radiotherapy. Locoregional control and distant disease-free survival were significantly improved with cisplatin (log-rank test; p = 0.039 and 0.011, respectively) with no difference in overall survival and similar late toxicity. The therapeutic index of HF radiotherapy was improved by concomitant cisplatin.

A third trial reported by the German Cancer Society with an even greater number of patients confirmed this outcome using a nonplatinum regime with HF accelerated radiation versus dose escalated HF accelerated radiation (34). The 84 patients with stage III (6%) and IV (94%) oropharyngeal (59.4%), hypopharyngeal (32.3%), and oral cavity (8.3%) cancer were randomized to concurrent chemotherapy and HF accelerated radiation therapy to 70.6 Gy in 6 weeks versus HF accelerated radiation therapy alone to 77.6 Gy. Chemotherapy was 5-fluoroucil (600 mg/m^2, 120 hours continuous infusion) days 1 through 5 and mitomycin (10 mg/m^2) on days 5 and 36. At 5 years, the locoregional control was 49.9% versus 37.4% (p = 0.001) and overall survival was 28.6% versus 23.7% (p = 0.023), respectively. Progression-free and freedom from metastases rates were 29.3% and 51.9% versus 26.6% and 54.7%, respectively (p = 0.009 and p = 0.575, respectively). There were no differences in late reactions. They concluded that concurrent chemotherapy with HF accelerated radiotherapy to 70.6 Gy is superior to dose-escalated HF radiotherapy to 77.6 Gy with less acute reactions and equivalent late reactions, indicating an improvement of the therapeutic ratio.

Pending Results of Radiation Therapy Oncology Group Trial of Concurrent Chemotherapy to Select Fractionation Schedules

The RTOG conducted a randomized trial to determine whether altered fractionation improves the outcome of concurrent cisplatin chemotherapy (i.e., whether the benefit of altered fractionation remains true in the setting of concurrent chemotherapy) (126). Patients with stage III or IV squamous-cell carcinoma of the oral cavity, oropharynx, hypopharynx, or larynx were randomized into two arms: *conventional standard radiation* (70 Gy in 35 fractions once daily over 7 weeks) with three cycles of concurrent cisplatin (100 mg/m^2 given every 3 weeks during radiotherapy) versus *concomitant boost* (72 Gy in 42 fractions in 6.5 weeks) with two cycles of the same chemotherapy. This type of study schema, standard radiotherapy plus chemotherapy versus accelerated radiotherapy plus chemotherapy, has not been previously reported. The study has completed accrual and outcome is pending.

Critical Fractionation Issues to Consider When Intensity Modulated Radiation Treatment Is Used

The new era of high-precision radiation therapy brings two major advantages: improved coverage of tumor volumes by the prescribed dose without the use of multiple matched fields, and increased sparing of normal tissues, such as parotid gland, spinal cord, brainstem, brain, and optic using IMRT. However, there are two important fractionation issues to be considered:

- If a single plan is used, all targets are treated in the same overall number of fractions. This may result in treating secondary targets to a lower dose per fraction. This has to be corrected by alteration of the total dose to the secondary targets to avoid the potentially serious disadvantage of delivering a lower biologically effective dose.
- IMRT may allow an increased dose to be delivered if the dose-limiting toxicity can be spared by organ avoidance. This may be delivered as additional fractions with prolongation of the duration of treatment or by giving more than one fraction per day. Alternatively, the dose per fraction may be increased and the total escalated dose delivered in the same or shortened treatment time.

Potential Delivery of Lower Biologically Effective Dose to Targets and Lower Probability of Cure

Classic non-IMRT techniques for HNSCC deliver doses at a fixed dose per fraction to all targets. A large initial field delivers an initial dose to the entire volume, and the field is reduced sequentially to boost additional regions to a higher dose (shrinking field technique). For example, a classic head and neck three-field plan uses opposed lateral photon fields and abutting electron fields to deliver 50 Gy at 2 Gy per fraction to gross disease at the primary site and nodes, elective nodal regions, and regions around the tumor that may contain microscopic tumor cells. Smaller fields are then used to deliver an additional 16 to 20 Gy in eight to 10 fractions to boost the gross tumor and nodal disease to 66 to 70 Gy, depending on the size of the gross tumor. A posterior electron field may be added to bring the dose adjacent to the gross nodal tumor to 56 to 60 Gy. This type of fractionation is used especially with concurrent chemotherapy. This contrasts with IMRT, with which the dose prescribed to various portions of the treatment volume is delivered simultaneously. Each fraction delivers a specific constant dose per fraction throughout the treatment to each target. All targets are treated in the same number of fractions. For example, 70 Gy in 35 fractions prescribed to the gross tumor will deliver 2 Gy per fraction to this volume. The 56 Gy and 50 Gy prescribed to secondary target volumes will also be delivered in 35 fractions in 7 weeks using IMRT at a 1.6 and 1.43 dose per fraction over 7 weeks, respectively. The biologically effective dose to 56 Gy and 50 Gy in 35 fractions in 7 weeks is lower using IMRT because of the effect of the smaller dose per fraction and longer

Dose/Fractionation	GTVs (Gy)	Intermediate (Gy)	Microscopic (Gy)
United States: IMRT[a]			
70/33 f; s.i.d. with chemo	70	60—63	57–60
Concomitant boost			
72 Gy/42 f	72	57–63	54
b.i.d. for 10–12 days			
66/30 f s.i.d.	66	60	54
Without chemotherapy			
Postoperative			
60–66/ 30 f s.i.d.	66	56–57	54
Canada (PMH): IMRT[a]			
70 Gy/35 f s.i.d.	70	63	56
60 Gy/25 f	60	56	50
T2-N0 larynx small T1–2 oropharynx			
64 Gy/40 f; b.i.d.	64	56	46
T3, T4 with low volume nodal disease			
Postop Boost			
66 Gy/33 f; s.i.d.	66	60	56
60 Gy/30 f; s.i.d.	60	60	54
51 Gy/20 f			
T1aN0M0 Glottic cancer			
Manchester (Christie Hospital)			
50–52.5/16 f for small volume(5–6 cm) larynx			
55 in 20 f for modest volumes up to 10 cm long			
Postop 50/20 f with chemo			
50–52.5/20 f without chemo			
Denmark			
70Gy/35 f; 6 f per wk			

The biologically isoeffective dose for tumor control to intermediate and with IMRT takes into consideration the effect of reduced dose per fraction and the effect of prolonged overall treatment time. f, fraction; IMRT, intensity-modulated radiotherapy.
[a]Single phase treatment schedules.

treatment time. This must be compensated for by increasing the total dose to the elective and intermediate dose targets as shown in Table 11.6.

Prospect for Improving the Therapeutic Ratio by Dose Escalations to Targets without Increased Dose to Normal Tissues

The experience and conclusions of altered fractionation studies are based entirely on results of traditional radiotherapy techniques and conventional conformal techniques. These techniques deliver the boost dose to a much larger volume of tissue of normal tissues, which inevitably receive the full boost dose. However, IMRT delivers much reduced doses to normal structures with potential for less toxicity. For example, IMRT produced significant reduction in incidence and severity of xerostomia with parotid-sparing head and neck (94,106,115). However, a further advantage of IMRT may be its potential for dose escalation. Preclinical comparative dosimetry studies have suggested that dose escalation may be feasible using simultaneous boosts to tumor subvolumes (105). Further work is ongoing to try to explore whether the boost volume may be localized using metabolic or hypoxic imaging (38).

Common Standard Clinical Practice

An analysis by the Meta-analysis of Chemotherapy on Head and Neck Cancer Collaborative Group revealed that concurrent chemoradiation yielded a larger survival benefit than that achieved with altered fractionation regimens (121). This benefit is seen predominantly in more locally advanced (i.e., stage IV) HNSCC, and concurrent chemoradiation is often recommended for patients with large T3 or T4 tumors or with N2-3 nodes usually given with standard fractionation.

Since accelerated regimens seem to preferentially benefit local control at the primary site and not nodal control, it is reasonable to choose altered fractionation for patients with T2, exophytic T3 or N0-1 disease who are not routinely given chemotherapy and those with more advanced locoregional tumor who are unfit to receive chemotherapy (109).

In much of the United States and Europe, standard fractionation remains 2 Gy per day. However, there is considerable variation in common practice, and despite the results of randomized studies, institutions tend to adhere to dose fractionation schedules with which they are experienced. Examples of commonly used schedules in Manchester, Canada, Denmark, and the United States are shown in Table 11.6.

Future Directions: Combining the Gains of Molecular Imaging and Molecular Targeting with Altered Fractionation

Advances in the understanding of tumor biology have opened exciting new opportunities to develop specific molecularly targeted strategies to selectively enhance tumor response to radiation. For example, epidermal growth factor receptor (EGFR) overexpression was a strong independent prognostic indicator for overall survival and disease-free survival and a robust predictor for locoregional relapse but not for distant metastasis in a correlative study of the impact on survival and pattern of failure in patients with advanced HNSCCs enrolled in the RTOG 9003 trial (69). There was no correlation between EGFR expression and T stage, N stage, stage grouping, and recursive partitioning analysis classes ($r = -0.07$ to 0.17). The overall and disease-free survival rates of patients with high EGFR-expressing HNSCCs were significantly lower ($p = 0.0006$ and $p = 0.0016$, respectively), and the locoregional relapse rate was significantly higher ($p = 0.0031$) compared with those of patients with low EGFR-expressing HNSCCs. Multivariate analysis showed that EGFR expression was an independent determinant of survival and a robust independent predictor of locoregional relapse. The data suggest that EGFR immunohistochemistry should be considered for selecting patients for more aggressive combined therapies or enrollment into trials targeting EGFR-signaling pathways (4).

Promising preclinical and earlier phase clinical results support the use of EGFR blockade in combination with radiation for advanced HNSCC (104). These results were corroborated by the recently reported phase III multinational trial that demonstrated radiosensitization following molecular inhibition of EGFR signaling. The agent cetuximab, a monoclonal antibody against the EGFR, when added to high-dose radiation in patients with locoregionally advanced HNSCC, produced improved locoregional control and reduced mortality without increasing the common toxic effects. In this study, 424 patients were randomized to receive either radiation alone for 6 to 7 weeks (RT), or radiation plus weekly cetuximab 400 mg/m^2 (RT + C). The median duration of locoregional control was 24.4 months in the RT + C arm versus 14.9 months in the RT only arm (hazard ratio for locoregional progression or death, 0.68; $p = 0.005$). At median follow-up of 54.0 months, the median overall survival was 49.0 months in the RT + C arm versus 29.3 months in the RT only arm (hazard ratio for death, 0.74; $p = 0.03$). Cetuximab significantly prolonged progression-free survival (hazard ratio for disease progression or death, 0.70; $p = 0.006$). With the exception of acneiform rash and infusion reactions, the incidence

of grade 3 or greater toxic effects, including mucositis, did not differ significantly between the two groups (23,24).

Further exploration will be done to test the benefit of adding cetuximab to chemotherapy plus altered fractionation. The RTOG is conducting a randomized trial of concurrent accelerated radiation and cisplatin versus concurrent accelerated radiation, cisplatin, and cetuximab in stage III and IV HNSCC.

References

1. Adelstein DJ, Li Y, Adams GL, et al. An intergroup phase III comparison of standard radiation therapy and two schedules of concurrent chemoradiotherapy in patients with unresectable squamous cell head and neck cancer. *J Clin Onc* 2003;21(1):92–98.
2. Akimoto T, Muramatsu H, Takahashi M, et al. Rectal bleeding after hypofractionated radiotherapy for prostate cancer: correlation between clinical and dosimetric parameters and the incidence of grade 2 or higher rectal bleeding. *Int J Radiat Biol Oncol Phys* 2004.
3. Andrews JR. Dose-time relationships in cancer radiotherapy: a clinical radiobiology study of extremes of dose and time. *AJR Am J Roentgenol* 1965;93:56–74.
4. Ang KK, Berkley BA, Tu X, et al. Impact of epidermal growth factor receptor expression on survival and pattern of relapse in patients with advanced head and neck carcinoma. *Cancer Res* 2002;62:7350–7356.
5. Ang KK, Jiang GL, Guttenberger R, et al. Impact of spinal cord repair kinetics on the practice of altered fractionation schedules. *Radiother Oncol* 1992;25:287–294.
6. Ang KK, Landuyt W, Xu FX. The effect of small radiation doses per fraction on mouse lip mucosa assessed using the concept of partial tolerance. *Radiother Oncol* 1987;8:79–86.
7. Ang KK, Thames HD, van der Kogel AJ, et al. Is the rate of repair of radiation-induced sublethal damage in rat spinal cord dependent on the size of dose per fraction? *Int J Radiat Oncol Biol Phys* 1987;13:557–562.
8. Ang KK, Trotti A, Brown BW, et al. Randomized trial addressing risk features and time factors of surgery plus radiotherapy in advanced head and neck cancer. *Int J Radiat Oncol Biol Phys* 2001;51:571–578.
9. Ang KK, Xu FX, Landuyt W. The kinetics and capacity of repair of sublethal damage in mouse lip mucosa during fractionated irradiations. *Int J Radiat Oncol Biol Phys* 1985;11:1977–1985.
10. Awwad KH, Lotayef M, Shouman T, et al. Accelerated hyperfractionation (AHF) compared to conventional fractionation (CF) in the postoperative radiotherapy of locally advanced head and neck cancer: influence of proliferation. *Br J Cancer* 2002;86(4):517–523.
11. Ball D, Bishop J, Smith J, et al. A randomised phase III study of accelerated or standard fraction radiotherapy with or without concurrent carboplatin in inoperable non-small cell lung cancer: final report of an Australian multi-centre trial. *Radiother Oncol* 1999;52:129–136.
12. Beck-Bornholdt HP, Dubben HH, Liertz-Petersen C, et al. Hyperfractionation: where do we stand? *Radiother Oncol* 1997;43:1–21.
13. Belani CP, Wang W, Johnson DH, et al. Phase III study of the Eastern Cooperative Oncology Group (ECOG 2597): induction chemotherapy followed by either standard thoracic radiotherapy or hyperfractionated accelerated radiotherapy for patients with unresectable stage IIIA and B non–small cell lung cancer. *J Clin Oncol* 2005;23(16):3760–3767.
14. Bennett MR. The treatment of stage III squamous carcinoma of the cervix in air and hyperbaric oxygen. *Br J Radiol* 1978;51:68.
15. Bentzen J, Bastholt L, Hansen O, et al. On behalf of the Danish Head and Neck Cancer Study Group. Five compared with six fractions per week of conventional radiotherapy of squamous-cell carcinoma of head and neck: DAHANCA 6&7 randomized controlled trial. *Lancet* 2003;363:933–940.
16. Bentzen SM, Juul-Christensen J, Overgaard J. Some methodological problems in estimating radiobiological parameters from clinical data: alpha/beta ratios and electron RBE for cutaneous reactions in patients treated with postmastectomy radiotherapy. *Acta Oncol* 1988;27:105–116.
17. Bentzen SM, Overgaard M. Relationship between early and late normal-tissue injury after postmastectomy radiotherapy. *Radiother Oncol* 1991;20:159–165.
18. Bentzen SM, Overgaard M, Thames HD. Fractionation sensitivity of a functional endpoint: impaired shoulder movement after post-mastectomy radiotherapy. *Int J Radiat Oncol Biol Phys* 1989;17:531–537.
19. Bentzen SM, Saunders MI, Dische S. Repair halftimes estimated from observations of treatment-related morbidity after CHART or conventional radiotherapy in head and neck cancer. *Radiother Oncol* 1999;53:219–226.
20. Bentzen SM, Thames HD. Clinical evidence for tumour clonogen regeneration: interpretations of the data. *Radiother Oncol* 1991;22:161–166.
21. Bentzen SM, Thames HD, Overgaard M. Latent-time estimation for late cutaneous and subcutaneous radiation reactions in a single follow-up clinical study. *Radiother Oncol* 1989;15:267–274.
22. Bernier J. Alteration of radiotherapy fractionation and concurrent chemotherapy: a new frontier in head and neck oncology? *Nature* 2005;2(6):305–314.
23. Bonner JA, Harari PM, Giralt J, et al. Cetuximab prolongs survival in patients with locoregionally advanced squamous cell carcinoma of head and neck: a phase III study of high dose radiation therapy with or without cetuximab. *American Society for Clinical Oncology Proceedings* 2004(abstr 5507).
24. Bonner JA, Harari PM, Giralt J, et al. Radiotherapy plus cetuximab for squamous-cell carcinoma of the head and neck. *N Engl J Med* 2006;354(6):634–636.
25. Bourhis J, Audry H, Overgaard J, et al. Meta-analysis of conventional versus altered fractionated radiotherapy: in head and neck squamous cell carcinomas (HNSCC): final analysis. 46th American Society of Therapeutic Radiology and Oncology (ASTRO) meeting, 3–7 October 2004, Atlanta. *Int J Rad Oncol Biol Phys* 60[Suppl]:S190–S191.
26. Bourhis J, Lapeyre M, Tortochaux J, et al. Very accelerated versus conventional radiotherapy in HNSCC: results of the GORTEC 94-02 randomized trial. *Int J Radiat Oncol Biol Phys* 2000;48:S111.
27. Bourhis J, Lapeyre M, Tortochaux J, et al. Preliminary results of the GORTEC 96-01 randomized trial, comparing very accelerated radiotherapy versus

concomitant radio chemotherapy for locally inoperable HNSCC. *Int J Radiat Oncol Biol Physics* 2001;51[Suppl 1]:39.
28. Brenner D, Armour E, Corry P, et al. Sublethal damage repair times for a late responding tissue relevant to brachytherapy (and external-beam radiotherapy): implications for new brachytherapy protocols. *Int J Radiat Oncol Biol Phys* 1998;41:135–138.
29. Brenner DJ. Toward optimal external-beam fractionation for prostate cancer. *Int J Radiat Oncol Biol Phys* 2000;48:315–316.
30. Brenner DJ. Fractionation and late rectal toxicity. *Int J Radiat Oncol Biol Phys* 2004;60:1013–1015.
31. Brenner DJ, Hall EJ. Fractionation and protraction for radiotherapy of prostate carcinoma. *Int J Radiat Oncol Biol Phys* 1999;43:1095–1101.
32. Brenner DJ, Martinez AA, Edmundson GK, et al. Direct evidence that prostate tumors show high sensitivity to fractionation (low alpha/beta ratio), similar to late-responding normal tissue. *Int J Radiat Oncol Biol Phys* 2002;52:6–13.
33. Brizel DM, Albers ME, Fisher SR, et al. Hyperfractionated irradiation with or without concurrent chemotherapy for locally advanced head and neck cancer. *N Engl J Med* 1998;338:1798–1804.
34. Budach V, Stuschke M, Budach W, et al. Hyperfractionated accelerated chemoradiation with concurrent fluorouracil-mitomycin is more effective than dose-escalated hyperfractionated accelerated radiation therapy alone in locally advanced head and neck cancer: final results of the radiotherapy cooperative clinical trials group of the German Cancer Society 95-06 Prospective Randomized Trial. *J Clin Oncol* 2005;23(6):1125–1135.
35. Budach W, Hehr T, Budach V, et al. A meta-analysis of hyperfractionated and accelerated radiotherapy and combined chemotherapy and radiotherapy regimens in unresected locally advanced squamous cell carcinoma of the head and neck. *BMC Cancer* 2006;6:28.
36. Byhardt RW, Greenberg M, Cox JD. Local control of squamous carcinoma of oral cavity and oropharynx with 3 vs 5 treatment fractions per week. *Int J Radiat Oncol Biol Phys* 1977;2:415–420.
37. Calais G, Alfonsi M, Bardet E, et al. Randomized trial of radiation therapy versus concomitant chemotherapy and radiation therapy for advanced stage oropharynx carcinoma. *J Natl Cancer Inst* 1999;91:2081–2086.
38. Chao KS, Bosch WR, Mutic S, et al. A novel approach to overcome hypoxic tumor resistance: Cu ATSM-guided intensity modulated radiation therapy. *Int J Radiat Oncol Biol Phys* 2001;49(4):1171–1182.
39. Cohen L. Clinical radiation dosage: I. *Br J Radiol* 1949;22:160–163.
40. Cohen L. Clinical radiation dosage: II. *Br J Radiol* 1949;22:706–713.
41. Cohen L, Kerrich JE. Estimation of biological dosage factors in clinical radiotherapy. *Br J Cancer* 1951;5:180–193.
42. Collins CD, Lloyd-Davies RW, Swan AV. Radical external beam radiotherapy for localized carcinoma of the prostate using a hypofractionation technique. *Clin Oncol (R Coll Radiol)* 1991;3:127–132.
43. Corvo R, Benasso M, Sanguineti G, et al. Alternating chemoradiotherapy versus partly accelerated radiotherapy in locally advanced squamous cell carcinoma of the head and neck results from a phase III randomized trial. *Cancer* 2001;92(11):2856–2867.
44. Cox JD. Large-dose fractionation (hypofractionation). *Cancer* 1985;55:2105–2111.
45. Cox JD. Presidential address. Fractionation: a paradigm for clinical research in radiation oncology. *Int J Radiat Oncol Biol Phys* 1987;13:1271–1281.
46. Cox JD, Byhardt RW, Komaki R. Reduced fractionation and the potential of hypoxic cell sensitizers in irradiation of malignant epithelial tumors. *Int J Radiat Oncol Biol Phys* 1980;6:37–80.
47. Cox JD, Pajak TF, Marcial VA, et al. ASTRO Plenary. Interfraction interval is a major determinant of late effects, with hyperfractionated radiation therapy of carcinomas of the upper respiratory and digestive tracts: results from Radiation Therapy Oncology Group Protocol 8313. *Int J Radiat Oncol Biol Phys* 1991;20:1191–1195.
48. Cummings B, O'Sullivan B, Keane T, et al. 5-year results of a 4 week/twice daily radiation schedule: the Toronto Trial. *Radiother Oncol* 2000;56:S8.
49. Denham JW, Hauer-Jensen M, Kron T, et al. Treatment-time-dependence models of early and delayed radiation injury in rat small intestine. *Int J Radiat Oncol Biol Phys* 2000;48:871–887.
50. Denham JW, Hauer-Jensen M, Peters LJ. Is it time for a new formalism to categorize normal tissue radiation injury? *Int J Radiat Oncol Biol Phys* 2001;50:1105–1106.
51. Dewit L, Oussoren Y, Bartelink H, et al. The effect of cis-diamminedichloroplatinum (II) on radiation damage in mouse rectum after fractionated irradiation. *Radiother Oncol* 1989;16:121–128.
52. Dische S, Martn WMC, Anderson P. Radiation myelopathy in patients treated for carcinoma of the bronchus using a six fraction regime of radiotherapy. *Br J Radiol* 1981;54:29–35.
53. Dische S, Saunders M, Barrett A, et al. A randomised multicentre trial of CHART versus conventional radiotherapy in head and neck cancer. *Radiother Oncol* 1997;44:123–136.
54. Dobrowsky W, Naude J. Continuous hyperfractionated accelerated radiotherapy with/without mitomycin C in head and neck cancers. *Radiother Oncol* 2000;57:119–124.
55. Donaldson SS, Meza J, Breneman JC, et al. Children's Oncology Group Soft Tissue Sarcoma Committee (formerly Intergroup Rhabdomyosarcoma Group) representing the Children's Oncology Group and the Quality Assurance Review Center. Results from the IRS-IV randomized trial of hyperfractionated radiotherapy in children with rhabdomyosarcoma—a report from the IRSG. *Int J Radiat Oncol Biol Phys* 2002;54(5):1579–1580.
56. Dörr W, Hendry JH. Consequential late effects in normal tissues. *Radiother Oncol* 2001;61:223–231.
57. Down JD, Easton DF, Steel GG. Repair in mouse lung during low dose-rate irradiation. *Radiother Oncol* 1986;6:29–42.
58. Dubben HH. Local control, TCD50 and dose-time prescription habits in radiotherapy of head and neck tumours. *Radiother Oncol* 1994;32:197–200.
59. Dubray BM, Thames HD. Chronic radiation damage in the rat rectum: an analysis of the influences of fractionation, time and volume. *Radiother Oncol* 1994;33:41–47.
60. Duchesne GM, Peters LJ. What is the α/β ratio for prostate cancer? Rationale for hypofractionated high-dose rate brachytherapy. *Int J Radiat Oncol Biol Phys* 1999;44:747–748.
61. Edsmyr F, Andersson L, Esposti PL, et al. Irradiation therapy with multiple small fractions per day in urinary bladder cancer. *Radiother Oncol* 1985;4:197–203.
62. El Badawi SA, Goepfert H, Fletcher GH, et al. Squamous cell carcinoma of the pyriform sinus. *Laryngoscope* 1982;92:357–364.
63. El-Sayed S, Nelson N. Adjuvant and adjunctive chemotherapy in the management of squamous cell carcinoma of the head and neck region. a meta-analysis of prospective and randomized trials. *J Clin Oncol* 1996;14:838–847.
64. Ellis F. Nominal standard dose and the ret. *Br J Radiol* 1971;44:101–108.
65. Fletcher GH, Barkley HT, Shukovsky LJ. Present status of the time factor in clinical radiotherapy: II. The nominal standard dose formula. *J Radiol* 1974;55:745–751.
66. Fowler J, Chappell R, Ritter M. Is α/β for prostate tumors really low? *Int J Radiat Oncol Biol Phys* 2001;50:1021–1031.
67. Fowler JF, Stern BE. Dose-time relationships in radiotherapy and the validity of cell survival curve models. *Br J Radiol* 1963;36:335–353.
68. Fowler JF, Whitred CA, Joiner MD. Repair kinetics in mouse lung: a fast component at 1.1 Gy per fraction. *Int J Radiat Biol* 1989;56:335–353.
69. Fu KK, Pajak TF, Trotti A, et al. A radiation therapy oncology group (RTOG) phase III randomized study to compare hyperfractionation and two variants of accelerated fractionation to standard fractionation radiotherapy for head and neck squamous cell carcinomas: first report of RTOG 9003. *Int J Radiat Oncol Biol Phys* 2000;48:7–16.
70. Gasinska A, Dubray B, Hill SA, et al. Early and late injuries in mouse rectum after fractionated x-ray and neutron irradiation. *Radiother Oncol* 1993;26:244–253.
71. Guttenberger R, Ang KK, Thames HD. Is the experience with CHART compatible with experimental data? New model of repair kinetics and computer simulations. *Radiother Oncol* 1992;25:280–286.
72. Handa K, Edioliya TN, Pandey RK. A radiotherapeutic clinical trial of twice per week vs five times per week in oral cancer. *Stralentherapie* 1980;156:626–631.
73. Harrison D, Crennan E, Cruickshank D. Hypofractionation reduces the therapeutic ratio in early glottic carcinoma. *Int J Radiat Oncol Biol Phys* 1988;15:365–372.
74. Haustermans KM, Hofland I, van Poppel H, et al. Cell kinetic measurements in prostate cancer. *Int J Radiat Oncol Biol Phys* 1997;37:1067–1070.
75. Henk JM, James KW. Comparative trials of large and small fractions in the radiotherapy of head and neck cancer. *Clin Radiol* 1978;29:611–616.
76. Henkleman RM, Lam GKY, Kornelsen RO. Explanation of dose-rate and split-dose effects in mouse foot reaction using the same time factor. *Radiat Res* 1980;84:276–289.
77. Hliniak A, Gwiazdowska B, Szutkowski Z, et al. Radiotherapy of the laryngeal cancer: the estimation of the therapeutic gain and the enhancement of toxicity by the one-week shortening of the treatment time. Results of the randomized phase III multicenter trial. *Radiother Oncol* 2000;56:S5.
78. Horiot JC. Controlled clinical trials of hyperfractionated and accelerated radiotherapy in otorhinolaryngologic cancers. *Bull Acad Natl Med* 1998;182(6):1247–1260; discussion 1261.
79. Horiot JC, Bontemps P, van den Bogaert V, et al. Accelerated fractionation (AF) compared to conventional fractionation (CF) improved head and neck cancers: results of the EROTC 22851 randomized trial. *Radiother Oncol* 1997;44:111–121.
80. Horiot JC, Fletcher GH, Ballantyne AJ. Analysis of failures in early vocal cord cancer. *Radiology* 1972;103:663–665.
81. Horiot JC, LeFur RN, Guyen T, et al. Hyperfractionation versus conventional fractionation in oropharyngeal carcinoma: final analysis of a randomized trial of the EORTC cooperative group of radiotherapy. *Radiother Oncol* 1992;25:231–241.
82. Horiot JC, van den Bogaert W, Ang KK. European Organization of Research on Treatment of Cancer trials using radiotherapy with multiple fractions per day: a 1978–1987 survey. *Front Radiat Ther Oncol* 1988;22:149–161.
83. Horwich A, Dearnaley D, Huddart R, et al. A randomized trial of accelerated radiotherapy for localized invasive bladder cancer. *Radiother Oncol* 2005;75(1):34–43.
84. Huczkowski J, Trott KR. Jejunal crypt stem cell survival after fractionated gamma-irradiation performed at different dose rates. *Int J Radiat Biol* 1987;51:131–137.
85. Hugeunin P, Beer KT, Allal A, et al. Concomitant cisplatin significantly improves locoregional control in advanced head and neck cancers treated with hyperfractionated radiotherapy. *J Clin Oncol* 2004;22(23):4665–4673.
86. Huguenin P, Beer KT, Allal A, et al. Concomitant cisplatin significantly improves locoregional control in advanced head and neck cancers treated with hyperfractionated radiotherapy. *J Clin Oncol* 2005;23(1):248.
87. Jackson SM, Weir LM, Hay JH, et al. A randomised trial of accelerated versus conventional radiotherapy in head and neck cancer. *Radiother Oncol* 1997;43:39–46.
88. Jereczek-Fossa BA, Jassem J, Badzio A. Relationship between acute and late normal tissue injury after postoperative radiotherapy in endometrial cancer. *Int J Radiat Oncol Biol Phys* 2002;52:476–482.
89. Jeremic B, Shibamoto Y, Milicic B, et al. Hyperfractionated radiation therapy with or without concurrent low-dose daily cisplatin in locally advanced squamous cell carcinoma of the head and neck: a prospective randomized trial. *J Clin Oncol* 2000;18:458–464.
90. King CR, Fowler JF. A simple analytic derivation suggests that prostate cancer alpha/beta ratio is low. *Int J Radiat Oncol Biol Phys* 2001;51:213–214.
91. Kupelian PA, Thakkar VV, Khuntia D, et al. Hypofractionated intensity-modulated radiotherapy (70 Gy at 2.5 Gy per fraction) for localized prostate cancer: long-term outcomes. *Int J Radiat Oncol Biol Phys* 2005;63:1463–1468.
92. Lamb D, Spry N, Gray A, et al. Accelerated fractionated radiotherapy for advanced head and neck cancer. *Radiother Oncol* 1990;18:107–116.
93. LeClerc JM, Billett Al, Gelber Rd, et al. Treatment of childhood acute lymphoblastic leukemia: results of Dana-Farber ALL Consortium Protocol 87-01. *J Clin Oncol* 2002;20(1):237–246.
94. Lin A, Kim HM, Terrell JE, et al. Quality of life after parotid-sparing IMRT for head and-neck cancer: a prospective longitudinal study. *Int J Radiat Oncol Biol Physics.* 2003;57(1):61–70.
95. Lindsay PE, Moiseenko VV, Van Dyk J, et al. The influence of brachytherapy dose heterogeneity on estimates of α/β for prostate cancer. *Phys Med Biol* 2003;48:507–522.
96. Livsey JE, Cowan RA, Wylie JP, et al. Hypofractionated conformal radiotherapy in carcinoma of the prostate: five-year outcome analysis. *Int J Radiat Oncol Biol Phys* 2003;57:1254–1259.
97. Logue JP, Cowan RA, Hendry JH. Hypofractionation for prostate cancer. *Int J Radiat Oncol Biol Phys* 2001;49:1522–1523.
98. Lukka H, Hayter C, Julian JA, et al. Randomized trial comparing two fractionation schedules for patients with localized prostate cancer. *J Clin Oncol* 2005;23:6132–6138.
99. Maciejewski B, Taylor JMG, Withers HR. Alpha/beta value and the importance of

size of dose per fraction for late complications in the supraglottic larynx. *Radiother Oncol* 1986;7:323–326.

100. Maciejewski B, Withers H, Taylor J, et al. Dose fractionation and regeneration in radiotherapy for cancer of the oral cavity and oropharynx: tumor dose-response and repopulation. *Int J Radiat Oncol Biol Phys* 1989;16:831–843.

101. Mandell LR, Koadota R, Freeman C, et al. There is no role for hyperfractionated radiotherapy in the management of children with newly diagnosed diffuse intrinsic brainstem tumors: results of a Pediatric Oncology Group phase III trial comparing conventional vs. hyperfractionated radiotherapy. *Int J Radiat Oncol Biol Phys* 1999;43:959–964.

102. Marcial V, Pajak T, Chang C, et al. Hyperfractionated photon radiation therapy in the treatment of advanced squamous cell carcinoma of the oral cavity, pharynx, larynx, and sinuses, using radiation therapy as the only planned modality: (preliminary report) by the Radiation Therapy Oncology Group (RTOG). *Int J Radiat Oncol Biol Phys* 1987;13:41–47.

103. Merlano M, Benasso M, Corvo R, et al. Five-year update of a randomized trial of alternating radiotherapy and chemotherapy compared with radiotherapy alone in treatment of unresectable squamous cell carcinoma of the head and neck. *J Natl Cancer Inst* 1996;88:583–89.

104. Milas L, Mason K, Hunter N, et al. In vivo enhancement of tumor radio response by C225 antiepidermal growth factor receptor antibody. *Clin Cancer Res* 2000;6:701–708.

105. Mohan R, Qiuwen W, Manning M, et al. Radiobiological consideration in the design of fractionation strategies for intensity modulated radiation therapy of head and neck cancers. *Int J Radiat Oncol Biol Physics* 2000;46(3):619–630.

106. Munter MW, Thilmann C, Hof H, et al. Stereotactic intensity modulated radiation therapy and inverse treatment planning for tumors of the head and neck region: clinical implementation of the step and shoot approach and first clinical results. *Radiother Oncol* 2003;66(3):313–321.

107. Murray KJ, Scott C, Greenberg HM, et al. A randomized phase III study of accelerated hyperfractionation versus standard in patients with unresected brain metastases: a report of the Radiation Therapy Oncology Group (RTOG) 9104. *Int J Radiat Oncol Biol Phys* 1997;39(3):571–574.

108. Naslund I, Nilsson B, Littbrand B. Hyperfractionated radiotherapy of bladder cancer: a ten-year follow-up of a randomized clinical trial. *Acta Oncol* 1994;33:397–402.

109. Nguyen LN, Ang KK. Radiotherapy for cancer of the head and neck: altered fractionation regimens. *Lancet* 2002;3:693–701.

110. Notter G, Turesson I. Multiple small fractions per day versus conventional fractionation: comparison of normal tissue reactions and effect on breast carcinoma. *Radiother Oncol* 1984;1:299–308.

111. Olmi P, Crispino S, Fallai C, et al. Locoregionally advanced carcinoma of the oropharynx: conventional radiotherapy vs. accelerated hyperfractionated radiotherapy vs. concomitant radiotherapy and chemotherapy—a multicenter randomized trial. *Int J Radiat Oncol Biol Phys* 2003;55(1):78–92.

112. Overgaard J, Hansen HS, Grau C, et al. The DAHANCA 6 and 7 trial: a randomized multicenter study of 5 versus 6 fractions per week of conventional radiotherapy of squamous cell carcinoma (SCC) of the head and neck. *Radiother Oncol* 2000;56:S4.

113. Overgaard M. Spontaneous radiation-induced rib fractures in breast cancer patients treated with postmastectomy irradiation: a clinical radiobiological analysis of the influence of fraction size and dose-response relationships on late bond damage. *Acta Oncol* 1988;27:117–122.

114. Palcic B, Skarsgard L. Reduced oxygen enhancement ratio at low doses of ionizing radiation. *Radiat Res* 1984;100:328–339.

115. Paliament MB, Scrimger RA, Anderson SG, et al. Preservation of oral health-related quality of life and salivary flow rates after inverse-planned intensity-modulated radiotherapy (IMRT) for head-and-neck cancer. *Int J Radiat Oncol Biol Phys* 2004;58(3):663–673.

116. Peracchia G, Salti C. Radiotherapy with thrice-a-day fractionation in a short overall time: clinical experiences. *Int J Radiat Oncol Biol Phys* 1981;7:99–104.

117. Peters LJ. Accelerated fractionation using the concomitant boost: a contribution of radiobiology to radiotherapy. *Br J Radiol* 1992;24:200–203.

118. Peters LJ, Ang KK, Thames HD. Accelerated fractionation in the radiation treatment of head and neck cancer: a critical comparison of different strategies. *Acta Oncol* 1988;27:185–194.

119. Peters LJ, Brock WA, Travis EL. Radiation biology at clinically relevant fractions. In: DeVita V, Hellman S, Rosenberg SA, eds. *Important advances in oncology*. Philadelphia: J.B. Lippincott, 1991;65–83.

120. Peters LJ, Withers HR. Morbidity from large dose fractions in radiotherapy. *Br J Radiol* 1980;53:170–171.

121. Pignon JP, Bourhis J, Domenge C, et al. Chemotherapy added to locoregional treatment for head and neck squamous-cell carcinoma: three meta analyses of updated individual data. *Lancet* 2000;355:949–955.

122. Pinto L, Canary P, Araujo C, et al. Prospective randomized trial comparing hyperfractionated versus conventional radiotherapy in stages II and IV oropharyngeal carcinoma. *Int J Radiat Oncol Biol Phys* 1991;21:557–562.

123. Poulsen MG, Denham JW, Peters LJ, et al. A randomised trial of accelerated and conventional radiotherapy for stage III and IV squamous carcinoma of the head and neck: a Trans-Tasman Radiation Oncology Group Study. *Radiother Oncol* 2001;60:113–122.

124. Powell S, Cooke J, Parsons C. Radiation-induced brachial plexus injury: follow-up of two different fractionation schedules. *Radiother Oncol* 1990;18:213–220.

125. Prados MD, Wara WM, Sneed PK, et al. Phase III trial of accelerated hyperfractionation with or without difluoromethylornithine (DFMO) versus standard fractionated radiotherapy with or without DFMO for newly diagnosed patients with glioblastoma multiforme. *Int J Radiat Oncol Biol Phys* 2001;49:71–77.

126. Radiation Therapy Oncology Group. Available at: http://www.rtog.org/members/active.html#headneck.

127. Rezvani M, Alcock CJ, Fowler JF, et al. Normal tissue reactions in the British Institute of Radiology study of 3 fractions per week versus 5 fractions per week in the treatment of carcinoma of the laryngo-pharynx by radiotherapy. *Br J Radiol* 1991;64:1122–1133.

128. Rezvani M, Fowler JF, Hopewell JW, et al. Sensitivity of human squamous cell carcinoma of the larynx to fractionated radiotherapy. *Br J Radiol* 1993;66:245–255.

129. Rojas A, Joiner M, Ninis J. Rate of repair of radiation injury (kidney). *Gray Lab Ann Rep* 1986;42–43.

130. Sanchiz F, Milla A, Torner J, et al. Single fraction per day versus two fractions per day versus radiochemotherapy in the treatment of head and neck cancer. *Int J Radiat Oncol Biol Phys* 1990;19(6):1627–1628.

131. Sanguineti G, Richetti A, Bignardi M, et al. Accelerated versus conventional fractionated postoperative radiotherapy for advanced head and neck cancer: results of a multicenter phase III study. *Int J Radiat Oncol Biol Phys* 2006;61(3):762–771.

132. Saunders M, Dische S, Barrett A, et al. Continuous, hyperfractionated, accelerated radiotherapy (CHART) versus conventional radiotherapy in non-small cell lung cancer: mature data from the randomised multicentre trial. CHART Steering Committee. *Radiother Oncol* 1999;52:137–148.

133. Saunders M, Dische S, Fowler J. Radiotherapy with three fractions per day for twelve consecutive days for tumors of the thorax, head and neck. *Front Radiat Ther Oncol* 1988;22:99–104.

134. Saunders MI, Dische S, Fowler J. Radiotherapy employing three fractions on each of twelve consecutive days. *Acta Oncol* 1988;27:163–167.

135. Saunders MI, Dische S, Grosch EJ, et al. Experience with CHART. *Int J Radiat Oncol Biol Phys* 1991;21:871–878.

136. Sause W, Kolesar P, Taylor SIV, et al. Final results of phase III trial in regionally advanced unresectable non-small cell lung cancer: Radiation Therapy Oncology Group, Eastern Cooperative Oncology Group, and Southwest Oncology Group. *Chest* 2000;117:358–364.

137. Skladowski K, Maciejewski J, Golen M, et al. Randomized clinical trial on 7-day continuous accelerated irradiation (CAIR) of head and neck cancer: report on 3-year tumor control and normal tissue toxicity. *Radiother Oncol* 2000;55:93–102.

138. Staar S, Rudat V, Stuetzer H, et al. Intensified hyperfractionated accelerated radiotherapy limits the additional benefit of simultaneous chemotherapy—results of a multicentric randomized German trial in advanced head and neck cancer. *Int J Radiat Oncol Biol Physics* 2001;50:1161–71.

139. Stell PM, Morrison MD. Radiation necrosis of the larynx. *Arch Otolaryngol* 1973;98:111–113.

140. Strandqvist M. Studien über die kumulative Wirkung der Röntgenstrahlen bei Fraktionierung. *Acta Radiol* 1944;55[Suppl]:1.

141. Svoboda V. Accelerated fractionation: the Portsmouth experience 1971–1984. In: *Proceedings of Varian's fourth European Clinac users meeting*. 1984:70–75.

142. Tannehill SP, Mehta MP, Larson M, et al. Effect of amifostine on toxicities associated with sequential chemotherapy and radiation therapy for unresectable non–small-cell lung cancer: results of a phase II trial. *J Clin Oncol* 1997;15:2850–2857.

143. Taylor JMG, Mendenhall WM, Lavey RS. Dose, time, and fraction size issues for late effects in head and neck cancers. *Int J Radiat Oncol Biol Phys* 1992;22:3–11.

144. Terry NHA, Denekamp J. RBE values and repair characteristics for colorectal injury after cesium-137 gamma-ray and neutron irradiation: II. Fractionation up to ten doses. *Br J Radiol* 1984;57:617–629.

145. Thames HD, Bentzen SM. Factor for tonsillar carcinoma. *Int J Radiat Oncol Biol Phys* 1995;33:755–758.

146. Thames HD, Bentzen SM, Turesson I, et al. Time-dose factors in radiotherapy: a review of the human data. *Radiother Oncol* 1990;19:219–235.

147. Thames HD, Hendry JH. *Fractionation in radiotherapy*. London: Taylor Francis, 1987.

148. Thames HD, Peters LJ, Ang KK. Time-dose considerations for normal-tissue tolerance. *Front Radiat Ther Oncol* 1989;23:113–130.

149. Thames HD, Suit HD. Tumor radioresponsiveness versus fractionation sensitivity. *Int J Radiat Oncol Biol Phys* 1986;12:687–691.

150. Thames HD, Withers HR, Peters LJ. Tissue repair capacity and repair kinetics deduced from multi-fractionated or continuous irradiation regimens with incomplete repair. *Br J Cancer* 1984;49[Suppl VI]:263–269.

151. Thames HD, Withers HR, Peters LJ, et al. Changes in early and late radiation responses with altered dose fractionation: implications for dose-survival relationships. *Int J Radiat Oncol Biol Phys* 1982;8:219–226.

152. Travis E, Thames H, Watkins T. The kinetics of repair in mouse lung after fractionated irradiation. *Int J Radiat Biol* 1987;52:903–919.

153. Trott KR, Maciejewski B, Preuss-Bayer G. Dose-response curve and split-dose recovery in human skin cancer. *Radiother Oncol* 1984;2:123–130.

154. Turesson I, Thames HD. Repair capacity and kinetics of human skin during fractionated radiotherapy: erythema, desquamation, and telangiectasia after 3 and 5 year's follow-up. *Radiother Oncol* 1989;15:169–188.

155. van den Bogaert W, van der Schueren E, Horiot JC, et al. Early results of the EORTC randomized clinical trial on multiple fractions per day (MFD) and misonidazole in advanced head and neck cancer. *Int J Radiat Oncol Biol Phys* 1986;12:587–591.

156. van der Kogel AJ, Jarrett KA, Paciotti MA, et al. Radiation tolerance of the rat rectum to fractionated X-rays and pi-mesons. *Radiother Oncol* 1988;12:225–232.

157. van Dyk J, Mah K, Keane TJ. Radiation-induced lung damage: dose-time-fractionation considerations. *Radiother Oncol* 1990;18:184–187.

158. Vegesna V, Withers HR, Thames HD. Multifraction radiation response of mouse lung. *Int J Radiat Biol* 1985;47:413–422.

159. Wang CC. Local control of oropharyngeal carcinoma after two accelerated hyperfractionation radiation therapy schemes. *Int J Radiat Oncol Biol Phys* 1988;14:1143–1146.

160. Wang CJ, Leung SW, Chen HC, et al. The correlation of acute toxicity and late rectal injury in radiotherapy for cervical carcinoma: evidence suggestive of consequential late effect (CQLE). *Int J Radiat Oncol Biol Phys* 1998;40:85–91.

161. Wang RS, Liu WQ, Li J, et al. Acclerated fractionated radiotherapy with concurrent chemotherapy in advanced nasopharyngeal carcinoma. *Ai Zheng* 2003;22(9):982–984.

162. Watson ER, Halnan KE, Dische S. Hyperbaric oxygen and radiotherapy: a Medical Research Council trial in carcinoma of the cervix. *Br J Radiol* 1978;51:879–887.

163. Weber DP, Silverman LB, Catania L, et al. Outcomes of a randomized trial of hyperfractionated cranial radiation therapy for treatment of high-risk acute lymphoblastic leukemia: therapeutic efficacy and neurotoxicity. *J Clin Oncol* 2004;22(13):2701–2707.

164. Wendt TG, Grabenbauer GG, Rodel CM, et al. Simultaneous radiochemotherapy versus radiotherapy alone in advanced head and neck cancer: a randomized multicenter study. *J Clin Oncol* 1998;16:1318–1324.

165. Willers H, Liertz-Petersen C, Dubben HH, et al. Outcome of hyperfractionated radiation therapy in randomized clinical trials. *Int J Radiat Oncol Biol Phys* 1998;40:257–259.

166. Withers HR, Peters LJ, Taylor JM, et al. Local control of carcinoma of the tonsil by radiation therapy: an analysis of patterns of fractionation in nine institutions. *Int J Radiat Oncol Biol Phys* 1995;33:549–562.

167. Withers HR, Taylor JMG, Maciejewski B. The hazard of accelerated tumor clonogen repopulation during radiotherapy. *Acta Oncol* 1988;27:131–146.

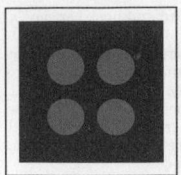

Chapter 12
Late Effects of Cancer Treatment on Normal Tissues

Louis S. Constine, Michael T. Milano, Debra Friedman, Monica Morris, Jacqueline P. Williams,
Philip Rubin, Paul Okunieff

The modern era of cancer therapy is predicated on the safe intensification of radiation, chemotherapy, and biologic adjuvants. This has resulted in a markedly increased survivorship, which now exceeds 64% overall, and is much higher for selected malignancies, such as 87% for breast cancer and 80% for all childhood cancers combined (287). Malignancies resistant to therapy have demanded an aggressive treatment approach that often resides on the edge of normal tissue tolerance, or even exceeds tolerance to some "acceptable" degree. Clearly, the potential to ameliorate or prevent such normal tissue damage, or to manage and rehabilitate affected patients, requires an understanding of tissue tolerance to therapy. Because "late effects" can manifest months or years after cessation of treatment, therapeutic decisions intended to obviate such effects can be based only on the probability, not the certainty, that such effects will develop. In making such decisions, the balance between efficacy and potential for toxicity should be considered and may be influenced by host, disease, and treatment-related risk factors.

Determining the frequency and pathogenesis of late effects is difficult for several reasons:

(a) Patients must survive long enough for damage to develop,
(b) The number of patients both affected and unaffected by therapy must be known, and
(c) The latent period to the manifestation of damage compromises discernment of the responsible component of multimodality therapy.

Further complicating our understanding of organ tolerance to therapy is that tumor and host factors interact with therapy in the causation of late effects. Tumor factors include direct tissue effects (e.g., extent of organ invasion), systemic effects of tumor-induced organ damage, and indirect mechanical effects (e.g., renal obstruction). Host factors include genetic (e.g., ataxia telangiectasia) and comedical (e.g., vascular disease, diabetes) predispositions, the developmental status when children are treated, and underlying structural abnormalities (e.g., horseshoe kidney). Therapeutic factors are the focus of this chapter. A recent report documents the high frequency of chronic health conditions in adult survivors of childhood cancer, many of which are severe or life-threatening. At 30 years, almost three-fourths of survivors had a chronic health condition, more than 40% had a serious health problem, and one-third had multiple conditions (256). These data underscore the importance of understanding the toxic effects of our therapy. The National Cancer Institute (NCI) and the major oncologic societies and cooperative groups have identified cancer survivorship as a target for education and research (142). The Children's Oncology Group committee on Late Effects has created risk-based guidelines for pediatric cancer survivors, many of which are applicable to adults (199).

Principles of Organ Tolerance to Therapy

From Classic to Contemporary/Molecular

The classic concepts of radiation pathophysiology are based on concepts of the normal anatomic–physiologic or functional unit of an organ. This traditional but still valuable view requires an appreciation of the relationship between the inherent structure of the organ at risk and the observed therapy-induced clinical and subclinical adverse effects (223,378). Of relevance are the target cells (e.g., parenchymal, vascular) in the organ, the distribution of function (homogeneous versus heterogeneous) in the organ, and the structural organization of the functional subunits (parallel or redundant versus in series or interdependent) (Fig. 12.1) (223). The traditional model also considers the proliferative dynamics of the target organ in order to understand both chemotherapy and radiation effects.

More recently, the traditional model for late effects has been brought into the modern era through the integration of molecular mechanisms that currently are under investigation. In brief, the classic concept of a single target cell explaining the dynamic sequence of events leading to organ damage has been supplanted by the interaction of multiple cellular systems through molecular signaling. Moreover, the perceived acute and late phases of adverse effects now are seen as manifestations of an ongoing sequence of events perpetuated through autocrine, paracrine, and endocrine messages that are initiated immediately after injury and persist until the clinical late effect events themselves. After irradiation, a variety of growth and inhibitory factors are released, cell receptors are altered, and the resulting dysregulation of the tissue environment is translated ultimately into postreceptor cytoplasmic, nuclear, and interstitial events (297) (Fig. 12.2). Thus, a combination of cell death, the production of reactive oxygen species, alterations in gene expression, and the expression of both proinflammatory and profibrotic cytokines are viewed as integral in the pathogenesis of late effects (250,299,350).

The importance of this new molecular concept is that it highlights the potential for interventions that can up-regulate or down-regulate cytokine responses, leading to modulation of the toxic reaction.

Modeling for Normal Tissue Damage

Rapid advances in radiation oncology, biology, and physics have led to an accumulation of information on the interactions of irradiation with other therapeutic modalities (e.g., chemotherapy, biologic response modifiers) and have had an impact on our understanding of normal tissue toxicities. Irradiation doses

		Function Distribution	
		Homogeneous	Heterogeneous
Organizational Structure	Parallel	Lung Liver Kidney	Diseased Lung Bone Brain
	Series	Esophagus Intestines	Optic Pathway Speech

FIGURE 12.1. The relationship between function distribution and tissue organization. (Redrawn from Marks LB. The impact of organ structure on radiation response. *Int J Radiat Oncol Biol Phys* 1996;34:1165–1171, with permission.)

customarily deemed "safe" may no longer be so when combined with another modality.

Although previously defined radiation tolerance doses (TD$_5$ and TD$_{50}$) remain as valuable guides, their applicability has changed (92). With the advent of three-dimensional planning, the volume of tissue receiving a given dose of radiation can be accurately quantified. As a result, more emphasis has been placed on the volume of the organ irradiated, and a construct relating global (whole-organ) and focal (partial-volume) injury as a function of the dose-volume histogram has been recognized. In addition to the structural and functional architecture of the organ, models for late effects now must consider the influence of volume irradiated, the threshold doses, and the clinical end points for assessment of late damage, including laboratory and imaging studies (312,380). In this regard, the nominal standard dose, the time-dose factor, the cumulative radiation effect, and the linear-quadratic equation become historical or contemporary participants in the normal tissue complication model, which seeks to describe causative relationships. Of course, these various models cannot supplant the understanding of normal tissue damage and the judgment regarding its

significance, which the clinician must possess. For example, as noted by Yorke (380), a 20% incidence of xerostomia is an acceptable risk, whereas that same likelihood of myelitis is unacceptable. In a similar sense, *severe* cardiac and *severe* mucosal injuries have entirely different connotations.

Scoring Late Effects

The ability to quantify and score late effects has been a concern of radiation oncologists. An abbreviated grading system was advocated by the Radiation Therapy Oncology Group (RTOG) and European Organization for Research and Treatment of Cancer, called *late effects morbidity scales*. The NCI consensus conferences have led to the introduction of SOMA classification for late toxicity: *s*ubjective, *o*bjective, *m*anagement criteria with *a*nalytic laboratory and imaging procedures. These scales, specific for each organ, form a scaffold for understanding the expression of later injury because their contents are the substance of late effects in normal tissue (LENT) expression (259,296). The NCI Common Terminology Criteria for Adverse Events (CTC v3.0) has recently been refined (354). These scales are generalized for combined modality therapy, and therefore not specific to radiation related effects. Although the CTC v3.0 does not clearly and consistently distinguish between early and late effects, it has been the first CTC scale to consider both early and long-term toxicity.

●● | Principles of Radiation Effects on Normal Tissues

Normal tissue responses to radiation can be divided into two categories: those that occur during the first days and weeks after treatment, often called *early effects,* and those that occur months, years, or even decades after irradiation, called *late effects.* "Consequential late effects" result from the host's reaction to severe acute toxicity. Certain organs are more prone to late toxicity (often termed *late responding tissues*) while others are more prone to acute toxicity (*early responding tissues*), although any organ can experience either acute and/or late effects. The type of effect expressed by an organ is generally a function of the tissue's renewal properties, but the clinical importance of the response typically depends on the critical biology of the organ. The most important modulators of radiation effects are the total radiation dose and fraction size, the duration of time during which the course of radiation is delivered, the interval between radiation fractions, the rate at which the radiation is given (dose rate), the specific organ being irradiated, and the volume. As previously stated, the organizational structure and the repair or compensatory capacities of the organ influence its tolerance to partial or whole-organ irradiation.

Dose Factors

Soon after the discovery of radiation, its effects on normal tissue became evident (130). Strandqvist (333) showed that a power law could be used to estimate the dose of radiation that would cause an equivalent level of toxicity to tumor or normal tissue if the total dose were delivered during different total times (130) (Fig. 12.3). Thus, if the log-dose is plotted against the log-time, a straight line is obtained. Strandqvist believed that the lines describing different levels of toxicity and tumor response were parallel, thus being a function of a constant exponential.

This simple observation was later modified by Ellis (90), who made two important improvements in our ability to predict radiation effects. First, the Ellis model dealt with the observation that different tissues clearly had different Strandqvist slopes, and that tumors had different slopes from many normal tissues.

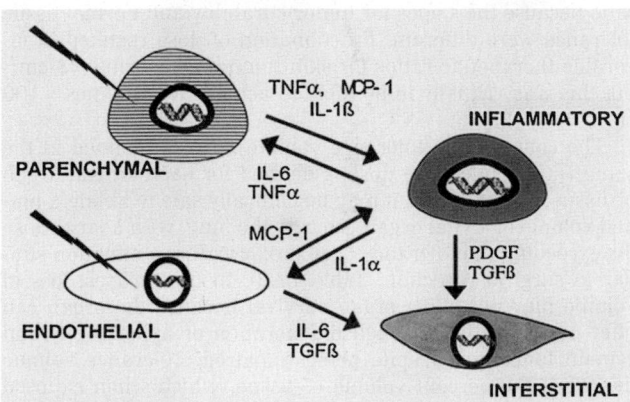

FIGURE 12.2. Pathway suggesting the chain of events beginning with the initial radiation injury and culminating in interstitial activity leading to fibrosis. TNFα, tumor necrosis factor-α; MCP-1, IL-6, interleukin 6; PDGF, TGFβ, tumor growth factor-β. (Modified from Rubin P, Finkelstein JN, Williams JP. Paradigm shifts in the radiation pathophysiology of late effects in normal tissues: molecular vs classic concepts. In: Tobias JS, Thomas PRM, eds. *Current radiation oncology.* London: Arnold; 1998:1–26, with permission.)

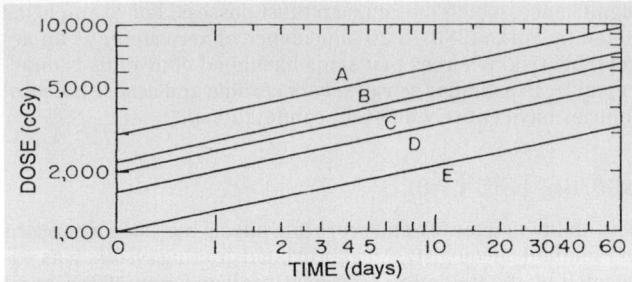

FIGURE 12.3. Strandqvist lines: The dose-time isoeffect line relates total dose delivered and total time independent of fractionation for different tissue end points: skin necrosis (**A**), cure of skin carcinoma (**B**), moist desquamation of skin (**C**), dry desquamation of skin (**D**), and skin erythema (**E**). (From Hall EJ. *Radiobiology for the radiologist*. Philadelphia: Lippincott Williams & Wilkins; 2000; redrawn from Strandqvist M. Studien uber die Kumulative Wirkung der Rontgenstrahlen bei Fraktion-ierung. *Acta Radiol* 1944;55[Suppl]:1–300, with permission.)

Table 12.1	PARAMETERS OF THERAPY: TOLERANCE DOSES ($TD_{5/5}$–$TD_{50/5}$)		
Single Dose (Gy)x		**Fractionated Dose (Gy)**	
Ovary	2–6	Testes	1–2
Bone marrow	2–10	Ovary	6–10
Testes	2–10	Eye (lens)	6–12
Eye (lens)	2–10	Kidney	20–30
Mucosa	5–20	Thyroid	20–40
Gastrointestinal	5–10	Lung	23–28
Lung	7–10	Skin	30–40
Colorectal	10–20	Liver	35–40
Kidney	10–20	Bone marrow	40–50
Vasculoconnective tissue	10–20	Heart	43–50
Liver	15–20	Gastrointestinal	50–55
Skin	15–20	Vasculoconnective tissue	50–60
Peripheral nerve	15–20	Spinal cord	50–60
Spinal cord	15–20	Brain	55–70
Brain	15–25	Peripheral nerve	65–77
Heart	18–20	Mucosa	65–77
Bone and cartilage	>30	Bone and cartilage	>70
Muscle	>70	Muscle	>70

From Rubin P. Law and order of radiation sensitivity: absolute versus relative. In: Vaeth JM, Meyer JL, eds. *Frontiers of radiation therapy and oncology*. Basel: Karger; 1989:7–40, with permission.

Second, he added a component related to the dose fraction; clinical experience and animal studies have demonstrated that fraction size alone is critical for late effects, whereas both fraction size and time are important for acute effects.

In the mid-1980s, the linear-quadratic model was used to model the shape of the experimentally observed radiation dose–response curve (340,377). This model proved simple to use because acute-reacting tissues and tumors demonstrated high alpha/beta (α/β) ratios (i.e., 7 to 10 Gy), whereas late-reacting tissues had low α/β ratios (i.e., <4 Gy). The mathematics associated with the quadratic formula made it simple to compare dose and fractionation schemes. Furthermore, the algorithms were found to be clinically reliable and acceptably safe.

The linear-quadratic formula, like the nominal standard dose formula, has undergone subsequent evolution. As with the power law formula, various modifiers have been created to account for dose rate, technical changes (e.g., brachytherapy), and proliferation during the course of radiation. However, all of these formulae are approximations, only because they are based on single-cell survival curves. Because it is unlikely that the underlying biology of radiation toxicity in normal tissues is simply a matter of survival of clonogenic cells, any use of the models must always be subject to clinical judgment. In general, the generated curves model early effects well, but are less effective for modeling late effects.

When using the terms TD_5 or TD_{50}, convention assumes the use of uniform irradiation of all or part of an organ, conventional fractionation schedules (1.8 to 2 Gy per fraction and five fractions per week), a relatively normal organ function as a baseline, no adjuvant drugs or surgical manipulations, and age ranges that exclude children and the elderly (Table 12.1). The following are tolerances with specific end points for single irradiation doses to whole organs:

- *1 to 10 Gy:* These organs are primarily composed of radiosensitive cells. Most affected are those of the lymphoid tissue (including lymphocytes), bone marrow hematopoietic stem cells, lens epithelium, ovaries (oocytes), testes (spermatogonia), lung type II cells, and gastrointestinal (GI) epithelium and villi. Most of these tissues include rapidly dividing stem cells and are affected directly without injury to the microvasculature or connective tissue stroma. Apoptotic death as opposed to mitotic death predominates in lymphoid tissue.
- *10 to 20 Gy:* Most other organ systems are in this category in terms of their sensitivity to irradiation, and include the upper aerodigestive mucosa, kidney, heart, liver, peripheral nerves, spinal cord, brain, and skin. The effects on these organs are related to radiation damage to microcirculation and connective tissue interstitium, as well as

parenchymal cells. When large single doses of radiation are used, it is difficult to differentiate the impact of indirect vascular injury from the direct effects on parenchymal cells, which are often slow-cycling.
- *More than 20 Gy:* At doses >20 Gy, a number of otherwise radioresistant structures may be affected, including bone and cartilage, muscle, endocrine organs such as the pituitary and adrenals, reproductive organs such as the uterus and prostate, and other organs such as the pancreas and biliary system.

Volume Factors

The volume of an organ or tissue exposed to radiation may be as important as fractionation in determining the induction of late effects (151). Paterson (264) first quantified the radiation response of normal skin, showing an inverse relationship between dose and volume using similar fractionation schemata. von Essen (366) demonstrated that an increase in the irradiated volume of tumor and normal skin led to an adverse therapeutic ratio because the slopes for tumor curability and normal tissue tolerance were different. Fractionation of dose resulted in favorable therapeutic ratios for skin tumors measuring <3 cm², but this was virtually impossible to achieve for volumes >100 cm³.

The concept of a tolerance volume must be defined in the same way as tolerance dose is defined for each critical organ or tissue. For example, it may be clinically safe to ablate a limited volume of a vital organ, such as the lung, with a large dose far exceeding the tolerance dose (i.e., creating a situation similar to surgical resection; Table 12.2). In these cases, loss of volume may not affect organ survival because the organ can offer compensation through regeneration or hypertrophy and remain functional despite being impaired. Tolerance volume describes the percent volume of tissue, which when exposed to radiation doses exceeding accepted tolerance can result in a life-threatening or lethal complication. For example, a tolerance volume 30% (TV_{30}) would result in severe toxicity with 30% of the volume of tissue irradiated to above threshold doses. The GI tract and the central nervous system (CNS) have low tolerance volumes (TV_{530}) as a small volume of suprathreshold radiation

Table 12.2 **NORMAL TISSUE TOLERANCE TO THERAPEUTIC IRRADIATION**

Organ	TD$_{5/5}$ Volume			TD$_{50/5}$ Volume			Selected End Point
	1/3	2/3	3/3	1/3	2/3	3/3	
Kidney	50	30	23	—	40	28	Clinical nephritis
Brain	60	50	45	75	65	60	Necrosis, infarction
Brainstem	60	53	50	—	—	65	Necrosis, infarction
Spinal cord	5 cm: 50	10 cm: 50	20 cm: 47	5 cm: 70	10 cm: 70	20 cm:—	Myelitis, necrosis
Lung	45	30	17.5	65	40	24.5	Pneumonitis
Heart	60	45	40	70	55	50	Pericarditis
Esophagus	60	58	55	72	70	68	Clinical stricture/perforation
Stomach	60	55	50	70	67	65	Ulceration, perforation
Small intestine	50	—	40	60	—	55	Obstruction, perforation/fistula
Colon	55	—	45	65	—	55	Obstruction, perforation/ulceration/fistula
Rectum	Volume: 100 cm^3		60	Volume: 100 cm^3		80	Severe proctitis/necrosis/fistula
Liver	50	35	30	55	45	40	Liver failure

TD, tolerance dose.
From Emami B, Lyman J, Brown A, et al. Tolerance of normal tissue to therapeutic irradiation. *Int J Radiat Oncol Biol Phys* 1991;21:109–122, with permission.

exposure in these organs would have disastrous outcomes. For most other organs that are considered dose-limiting, such as bone marrow, lung, kidney, and probably heart and liver, high doses to smaller volumes are tolerated; however, many organs decompensate when more than 40% to 60% of the total volume (as applied to paired organs) is exceeded.

Critical Organ Tolerance

Most organ systems are composed of multiple cell subpopulations, each performing an important activity. Organ tolerance is determined by the radiosensitivity of critical stem cell subpopulations that may not always be proliferating or dividing (130), and the most radiosensitive vital cell population determines the acute organ tolerance. Just as the degree of importance of an organ that has been irradiated determines the survival of an organism as a whole, the functional capacity of cells is often distinct from their regenerative capacity, permitting organ physiology to be preserved in the face of injury and allowing for recovery or repair from the insult.

The LENT Paradigm

Late effects syndromes at each organ site are not random events, but are specific entities that occur at certain times, are expressed in a recognizable fashion and, in many cases, can be ameliorated. A paradigm can be outlined that guides the clinical radiation oncologist to arrive at a correct diagnosis and management of specific complications. This 10-step diagnosis process will be designated as the *Late Effects of Normal Tissue (LENT)* paradigm and includes the following:

1. *Clinical detection:* Characteristic signs and symptoms that herald the onset of radiation-induced toxicities.
2. *Time course of events:* Recognition of the clinical pathologic time course, including the onset of subclinical and overt abnormalities.
3. *Dose/time/volume:* Identification of the relevant radiation parameters, with determination of whether these factors explain the sequelae under consideration.
4. *Chemical/biologic modifiers:* Identification of other relevant treatment components.

5. *Radiologic imaging:* Discernment of the abnormalities on imaging techniques.
6. *Laboratory tests:* Definition of the associated laboratory abnormalities.
7. *Differential diagnosis:* Distinction of therapy-associated sequelae from recurrence or metastatic cancer in the first 5 years, other degenerative or inflammatory diseases from 5 to 10 years, and second malignant tumors after 10 years.
8. *Pathologic diagnosis:* Consideration for tissue diagnosis of the adverse effect to confirm its presence versus disease recurrence or second malignant tumors.
9. *Management:* Use of restorative, ameliorative, or prophylactic treatment in the form of either medical or surgical intervention.
10. *Follow-up:* Consideration for nursing and medicolegal aspects.

Central Nervous System: Brain and Spinal Cord, and Special Senses (Eyes, Ears)

1. **Clinical Detection.** *Brain:* Headache, somnolence, intellectual deficits, functional neurologic losses, and memory alterations may occur during, shortly after, or, most often, as a delayed effect at 6 months. Objectively, depending on the site of the brain irradiation, neurologic deficit, loss of cognitive function, mood and personality changes, and focal to generalized seizures can occur. All gradations of effects are possible, depending on dose-volume factors. *Spinal cord:* Paresthesias (tingling sensation, shooting pain, and Lhermitte's syndrome), numbness, motor weakness, and loss of sphincter control have their counterparts in a neurologic examination to identify a specific cord level; these maladies progress through Brown-Séquard syndrome to total paraparesis and paraplegia.
2. **Time Course of Events.** *Brain:* Early during treatment, symptoms and signs reflect increased edema because of the tumor itself or secondary to the treatment of the brain lesion. Normally, brain necrosis and gliosis require 6 to 12 months to develop. *Spinal cord:* Lhermitte's syndrome occurs 2 to 4 months after irradiation and then persists or returns at 6 months. Paresis, numbness, altered sphincter control appearing at 6 to 12 months with progression comprise the classic onset of radiation-induced spinal cord transection.

3. **Dose/Time/Volume.** *Brain:* In general, doses of 50 Gy to whole brain in 1.8 to 2 Gy fractions are well tolerated, although in children the threshold dose is 30 to 35 Gy. The TD_5 in adults for necrosis is ~50 Gy (218); a threshold dose is 57.6 Gy (207) using 1.8 to 2 Gy fractions. With focal areas, the TD_{50} is between 70 and 80 Gy as evidenced by an RTOG study (373). With conformal radiotherapy, the risk of cerebral radiation necrosis increases approximately linearly in the dose range of 50 to 110 Gy, with corresponding risks of ~5% to 20% (293). Fraction size and the quotient of fraction size × total dose are also predictive of radiation necrosis (204,293). The extent to which therapeutic dose of radiation affects cognition and memory is somewhat controversial and not well characterized. Recent prospective studies have shown that, with partial brain irradiation with doses of 50 to 60 Gy, there is minimal-to-no discernable effect on memory and cognition (18,45,197,349,365). In children, dose-volume parameters of the whole brain, individual temporal lobes, supratentorial brain and infratentorial brain have been used to model changes in IQ as a function of time (232,233). *Spinal cord:* The most widely observed dose limit for spinal cord is 45 Gy in 22 to 25 fractions. Certainly a 5% risk of grade ≥2 spinal late spinal cord toxicity is unacceptable. Marcus and Million (217) found that 45 Gy conventionally fractionated is on the flat part of the dose–response curve and yields an incidence of myelopathy of <0.2%; the true TD_5 is 57 to 61 Gy. However, even a 5% likelihood of spinal cord necrosis is an unacceptable risk for most clinicians. The TD_{50} is 68 to 73 Gy (Fig. 12.4) (311). No volume effect is supported by current clinical data, nor is there evidence to suggest that one section of spinal cord is more sensitive than another. However, for the cervical spinal cord, doses of >50 Gy are generally considered safe (217,224). Shortening the treatment interval from 24 to 6 to 8 hours reduces spinal cord tolerance by 10% to 15%. In rhesus monkeys undergoing two courses of radiation (44 Gy followed by 57 to 66 Gy 1 to 3 years later), <10% of the monkeys developed paralysis (albeit with limited follow-up), suggesting repair of occult spinal cord injury in the intervening years between radiotherapy (10).

4. **Chemical/Biologic Modifiers.** *Brain:* Generally, concurrent nitrosoureas (i.e., BCNU) or temozolomide chemotherapy

is well tolerated, although there are data to suggest that alkylating chemotherapeutic agents can increase the risk of radionecrosis (293). The immediate subsequent use of methotrexate, intrathecally or intravenously, is of particular concern. Beta-interferon used concomitantly can lead to liquefaction necrosis of the tumor and surrounding brain tissue. Valproate use has been shown to be associated with a lower risk of radionecrosis (293). *Spinal cord:* Concomitant use of intrathecal and intravenous chemotherapeutic agents known to be associated with neurotoxicity include methotrexate, cisplatin, cytarabine, and others. However, the contribution of the intrathecal component is unclear.

5. **Radiologic Imaging.** *Brain:* Computed tomographic (CT) changes and magnetic resonance imaging (MRI) alterations are confined to high-dose volumes, showing changes in white matter and demyelination. Four stages have been described, from early whitening in the periventricular region to a diffuse coalescence of white and gray matter into an intense signal region and loss of structure. Interestingly, in one series, hyperintensity and white matter atrophy seen on serial T2-weighted MRIs did not correlate with whether or not patients underwent radiation, suggesting that late MRI changes are also attributable to surgical intervention (17). *Spinal cord:* CT scans are not worthwhile, but MRI may show cord swelling or atrophy, decreased intensity on T1-weighted images, or increased intensity on T2-weighted images, indicative of edema/necrosis/demyelination patterns (370).

6. **Laboratory Tests.** Myelin basic protein can be released into the cerebrospinal fluid in high concentrations when focal or diffuse demyelination is in progress, both in the transient and permanent phases.

7. **Differential Diagnosis.** *Brain:* Differentiation of late changes from tumor recurrence and progression may be difficult. Studies with positron emission tomography scans may be helpful and indicate hypometabolic zones for necrosis and hypermetabolic ones for tumor (57,129); single-photon emission CT scanning with ^{99m}Tc is less widely accepted. Diffusion-weighted MRI is an emerging approach to differentiating radiation changes from disease progression (23,139,328). *Spinal cord:* Epidural metastasis or compression secondary to vertebral metastases must be excluded for lymphoma and carcinoma. Exclusion diagnosis rules out degenerative spondylitis and hypertrophic arthritis in the intervertebral foramen.

8. **Pathologic Diagnosis.** Establishing diagnosis is hazardous and indicated only if tumor recurrence or progression is expected. Alterations in vasculature and loss of myelination due to oligodendrocytic death are well documented.

9. **Management.** *Brain:* This is often symptomatic with analgesics and antiseizure medications, such as phenytoin (Dilantin) and barbiturates, but as headaches and neurologic deficits increase, high-dose corticosteroids are used. Reoperation and evacuation may be required for accessible foci of necrosis, especially after interstitial implants. *Spinal cord:* Currently, corticosteroids are prescribed using an intensive intravenous schedule: 10 mg intravenously of dexamethasone (Decadron) for 1 day; the dose is then tapered to stabilize progress.

10. **Follow-up.** The patient is seen every day or week until relief is obtained and then at 1- to 3-month intervals. Intensive nursing and rehabilitative care are essential, and medicolegal implications should be carefully assessed.

Pathophysiology and Cellular Biology

In the first weeks after irradiation, early demyelinating changes are usually limited to scattered astrocytic or microglial reactions with occasional perivascular collections of mononuclear cells.

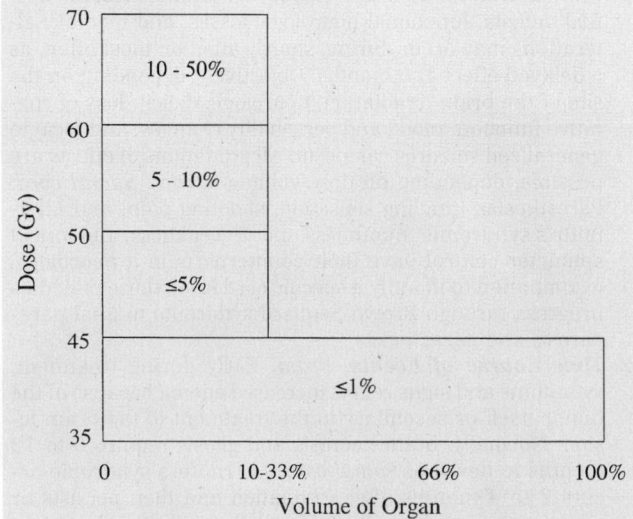

FIGURE 12.4. Schematic diagram depicting the dose-volume relationship to complication. Each box represents the percentage likelihood of developing damage according to the volume of the spinal cord irradiated (x-axis) and radiation dose administered (y-axis).

Table 12.3	TOLERANCE DOSES FOR THE CENTRAL NERVOUS SYSTEM
Site	**Dose/Reference**
Brain	52 Gy/5 wk at 2 Gy per fraction (318)
	50 Gy/25 F/35 days or 54 Gy/30 F/42 days (218)
Spinal cord	50 Gy/2 Gy fractions (371)
	50 Gy/25 F/35 days (1)
	ED_5 57–61 Gy (308)
	ED_{50} 68–73 Gy (308)
	ED_{50} 65 Gy (58–79 Gy) (285)

F, fractions; ED, estimated damage.
From Hopewell JW. Radiation injury to the central nervous system. *Med Pediatr Oncol Suppl* 1998;1:1–9, with permission.

Subsequently, neural tissue begins to break down, with the appearance of regions of myelin destruction, proliferative and degenerative changes in glial cells, and vascular changes such as endothelial cell loss, proliferation, capillary occlusion, degeneration, and hemorrhagic exudates. When a critical mass of capillary endothelial cells fails, vasogenic edema develops in response to the loss of essential support of dependent neurons, reflecting cerebral cortical atrophy. Intracerebral calcifications sometimes are present and presumably represent lesions of mineralizing microangiopathy. Recent data, in which endothelial cells in rat spinal cords were selectively irradiated, suggest that vascular endothelial damage is primarily responsible for white matter necrosis (63).

There is now a considerable body of work defining the tolerance doses for the CNS (Table 12.3). Data for single-dose irradiation are sparse, but when Hindo et al. (145) used single doses of 10 Gy in patients with brain metastases, 7% of patients died within 48 hours. After 10 Gy total body irradiation (TBI) in preparation for bone marrow transplantation (BMT), Thomas et al. (343) found a 7% incidence of leukoencephalopathy at 1 to 5 months in patients who were previously treated with 12 doses of 2 Gy for acute lymphocytic leukemia prophylaxis. In the spinal cord, a number of investigations have contributed to changing our concepts of tolerance. The most widely observed clinical dose limits are 45 Gy in 22 to 25 fractions of 1.8 to 2 Gy, and the tolerance dose (TD_5) of 50 Gy often is recommended as the maximum level when cord segments of <10 cm are irradiated.

In animal models, a large number of cytokines are being released immediately after CNS irradiation. When RNA protection techniques were used, increased expression of proinflammatory and profibrotic cytokines was shown in the CNS tissues within the first 24 hours after x-irradiation (150). Building on a late effect multicellular paradigm, the basis of demyelination can be seen as an interplay of growth factors expressed by endothelial cells, oligodendrocytes, astrocytes, and the microglia. Once disruption of the endothelium occurs, an infiltration of lymphocytes initiates the expression of immunologic mechanisms, which drives the pathogenesis of encephalopathy and myelopathy (59,196,258). Alternatively, other authors have suggested that the repair response initiated in the CNS after radiation injury leads to a secondary reactive process through the cytokine-signaling mechanisms, resulting in a persistent oxidative stress (348).

Combined Modalities

In contrast to radiation, it has been presumed that most drugs do not cause late effects because of their inability to cross the blood–brain barrier. However, it has been suggested that radiation alters and increases capillary permeability, facilitating the entry of systemically administered drugs into the brain (285). The best-recognized example of adverse combined radiation and drug effects involves methotrexate (37,38) (Fig. 12.5). Although large doses of methotrexate alone can lead to leukoencephalopathy, this complication is most often seen when

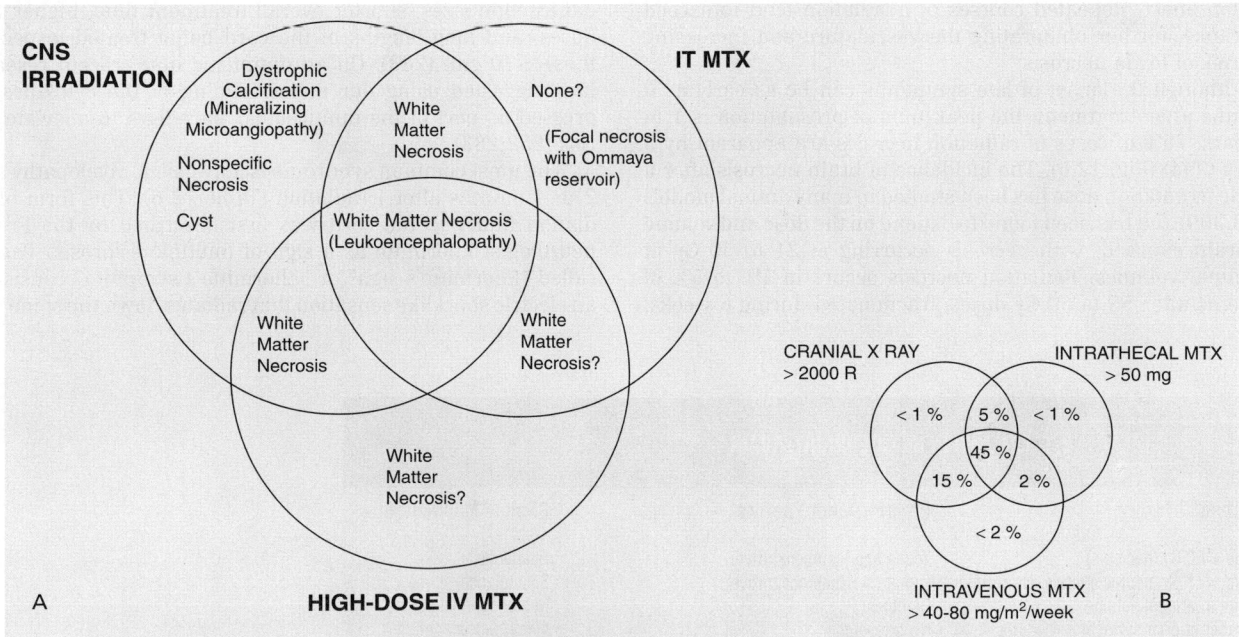

FIGURE 12.5. A: A Venn diagram illustrates the pathophysiology of late central nervous system (CNS) sequelae after radiation, intrathecal methotrexate (IT MTX), and high-dose intravenous methotrexate (IV MTX), administered either alone or in combination. (From Bleyer WA, Griffin TW. White matter necrosis, mineralizing microangiopathy and intellectual abilities in survivors of childhood leukemia: associations with central nervous system irradiation and methotrexate therapy. In: Gilbert HA, Kagan AR, eds. *Radiation damage to the nervous system.* New York: Raven Press; 1980:155–174, with permission.) **B:** The incidence is greatest when all modes are combined. (From Bleyer WA. Current status of intrathecal chemotherapy for human meningeal neoplasms. *Natl Cancer Inst Monogr* 1977;46:171–178, with permission.)

Techniques, Modalities, and Modifiers in Radiation Oncology

whole-brain irradiation is part of a regimen using methotrexate, particularly when high doses are given intravenously. Damage to the vascular choroid plexus may alter methotrexate clearance and decrease turnover, thereby leading to higher drug concentrations. The ependymal connective tissue layer also may be affected, allowing methotrexate to enter the ventricles and the CNS white matter. The incidence of injury is highest when all modalities are combined, and is not commonly seen when radiation or methotrexate are administered alone. Methotrexate can also be associated with neurocognitive deficits in children when doses above 1 g/m^2 are administered intravenously or when it is administered intrathecally in combination with cranial radiotherapy (36,84,288,367).

Increasing use of combined-modality therapy, particularly in the conditioning regimens for BMT and in the treatment of CNS tumors in young children, has led to a greater awareness of risk factors in children. The radiation oncologist must be alert to the signs of developmental difficulties and attempt to minimize the fields of irradiation in children at all times, particularly those younger than 3 years of age (169,326).

Clinical Syndromes

Brain

The initial response of the CNS to irradiation may be increased intracranial pressure due to radiation edema; however, clinicians should be aware that tumor-associated cerebral edema might exist before radiation treatment is undertaken. Headache and other expressions of increased intracranial pressure are frequently present (Table 12.4), in addition to focal deficits. It is not until the subacute period that the more severe manifestations of infarction and gliosis appear as brain necrosis. Children in the chronic clinical period show poor cerebration, and mental retardation may follow total-brain irradiation (e.g., as used for medulloblastoma) (281). However, pre-existing hydrocephalus resulting from posterior fossa tumors causes cerebral atrophy and poor mentation independent of, and augmenting, the radiation effect. Repeated courses of irradiation tend to exceed tolerance, further obliterating the vasculature and increasing the risk of brain necrosis.

Although the onset of late symptoms can be as early as 6 months after treatment, the peak time of presentation is 1 to 2 years; 75% of cases of radiation necrosis are apparent by 3 years (294) (Fig. 12.6). The incidence of brain necrosis after a single irradiation dose has been studied in many animal models (163,309) and has been found to depend on the dose and volume of brain exposed, with necrosis occurring at 21 to 50 Gy at maximal volumes. Radiation necrosis occurs in 1% to 5% of patients after 55 to 60 Gy doses, fractionated during 6 weeks;

in one of the few prospective studies, Marks et al. (218) reported a 5% incidence in patients treated with 54 Gy or more in 1.8 to 2 Gy fractions.

Radiation necrosis is visualized on MRI and CT as a mass lesion with surrounding edema. Radiation necrosis is often progressive and fatal, and surgical debulking is performed whenever possible; corticosteroids may offer transient relief. Reducing the volume of irradiation is presumed to decrease the risk for radiation necrosis, although this may not be true in children. Focal edema and necrosis after intensive irradiation (e.g., stereotactic radiosurgery [103]) can be seen earlier than 6 months (2 to 4 weeks) as MRI changes and persist for months to years into chronic necrosis.

The incidence and extent of cognitive and emotional dysfunction in patients treated with radiation are difficult to define. Variables include the underlying disease (brain tumor or leukemia), associated pathologic processes (hydrocephalus or increased intracranial pressure), and other therapies (surgery and chemotherapy); in children, age is an important variable (319). Recent studies using lower doses and more refined beams have demonstrated improved results (261,319,368). However, even conformal radiation therapy, particularly to central brain structures, impairs neurocognitive function such as attention and reaction time (179). Other adverse effects of CNS irradiation, such as stroke, are increasingly identified in survivors of malignancies (e.g., leukemia, brain tumors) treated with >30 Gy (41).

Spinal Cord

The spectrum of radiation injuries to the spinal cord includes both transient and irreversible syndromes (Table 12.5). A rapidly evolving permanent paralysis is seen rarely and is presumed to result from acute infarction of the cord. Chronic progressive radiation myelitis is rare. The initial symptoms are usually paresthesias and sensory changes that start 9 to 15 months after therapy and progress during the following year (308); longer intervals to initial symptoms have been seen. An increased risk of myelopathy is associated with higher individual fraction sizes, shorter overall treatment time, higher total doses, and long lengths of the cord being treated (especially those >10 cm) (283). On an optimistic note, recent research has suggested using our understanding of the cytokines expressed as part of the multicellular paradigm to alleviate this risk (252,283).

The most common syndrome is a transient myelopathy seen 2 to 4 months after irradiation (Table 12.6). This form of radiation injury to the cord was first described by the French neurologist Lhermitte as a sign of multiple sclerosis. The so-called "Lhermitte's sign" or "Lhermitte's symptom" consists of an electric shocklike sensation that radiates down the spine and,

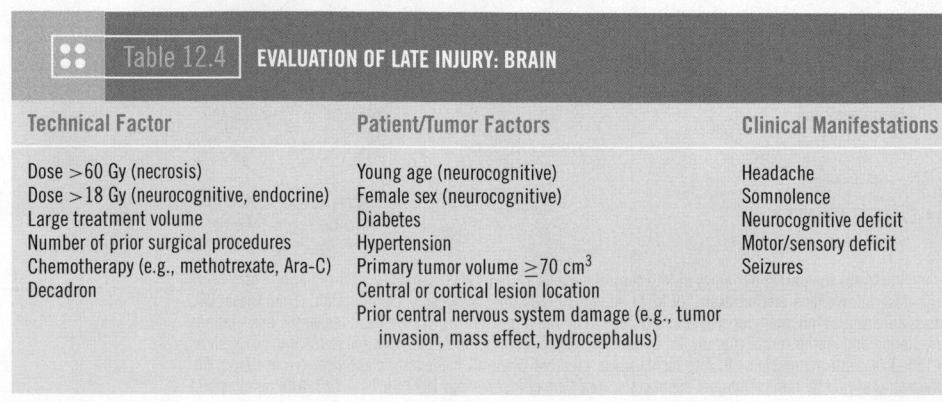

Table 12.4	EVALUATION OF LATE INJURY: BRAIN	
Technical Factor	**Patient/Tumor Factors**	**Clinical Manifestations**
Dose >60 Gy (necrosis)	Young age (neurocognitive)	Headache
Dose >18 Gy (neurocognitive, endocrine)	Female sex (neurocognitive)	Somnolence
Large treatment volume	Diabetes	Neurocognitive deficit
Number of prior surgical procedures	Hypertension	Motor/sensory deficit
Chemotherapy (e.g., methotrexate, Ara-C)	Primary tumor volume ≥ 70 cm^3	Seizures
Decadron	Central or cortical lesion location	
	Prior central nervous system damage (e.g., tumor invasion, mass effect, hydrocephalus)	

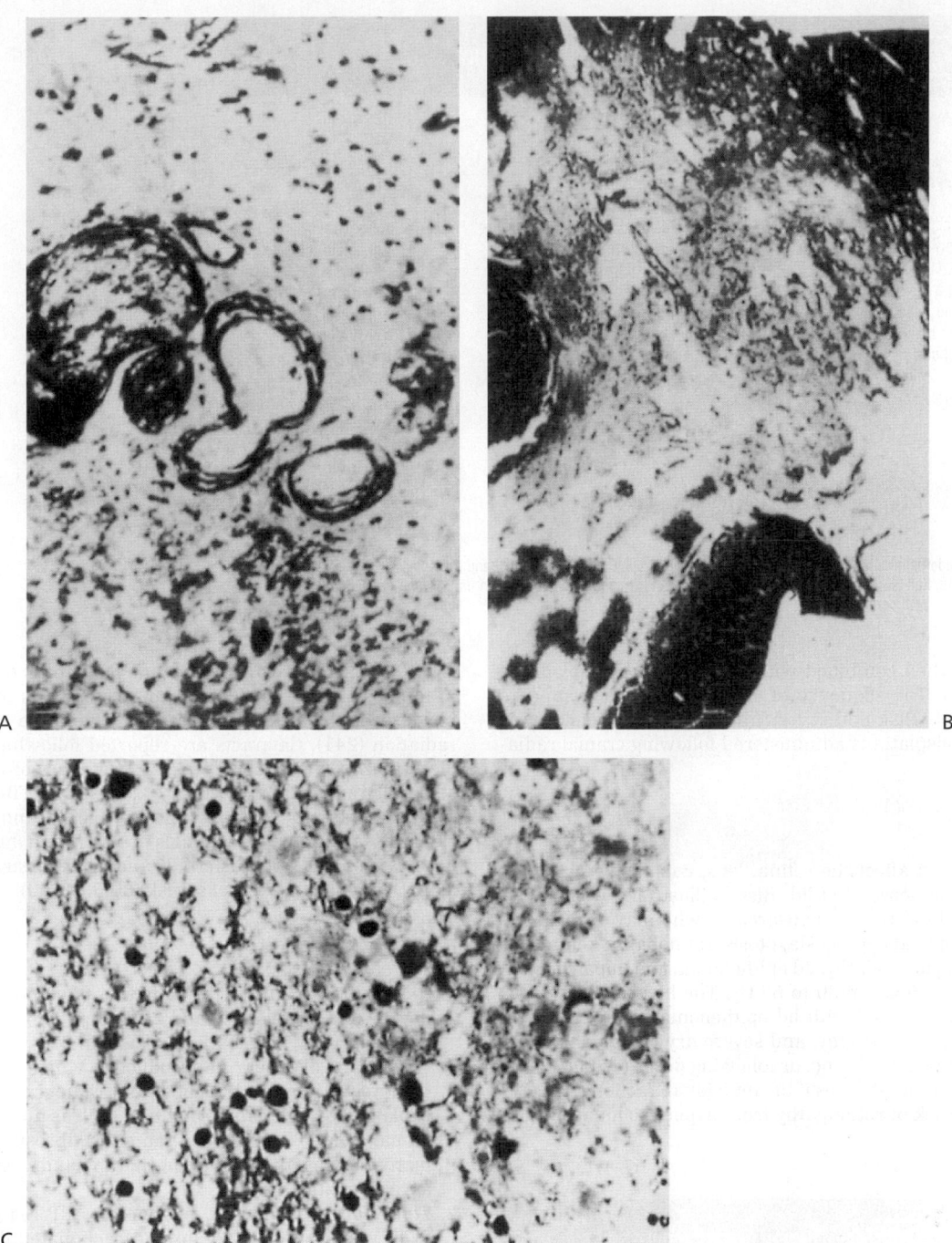

FIGURE 12.6. A, B: White matter necrosis is very common with methotrexate and is diffuse and unrelated to vascularization. (**A** and **B** from reference 37) **C:** In contrast, the radiation-induced lesions are oriented around vessels that are damaged, such as the dystrophic calcification of fine vessels referred to as *mineralizing microangiopathy.* (From Rubin P, Casarett GW. *Clinical radiation pathology.* Philadelphia: WB Saunders; 1968, with permission.)

frequently, into the limbs (173). The location of the sensation can change with time. The symptoms may be precipitated by flexion of the neck, walking on a hard surface, sitting on a hard surface, or other forms of physical exertion. The syndrome generally occurs a few months after spinal irradiation. The incidence after full-dose mantle irradiation for Hodgkin lymphoma may be on the order of 10% to 15%. The mechanism is thought to be transient demyelinization, although detailed human pathologic studies are lacking. There are no known CT or MRI correlations. Lhermitte's sign is also reported in association with cisplatin administration, where the results may be long-lasting (161).

Hearing

Radiotherapy can result in cochlear damage, with sensorineural hearing loss (SNHL) occurring in about 25% of patients treated with doses approaching 60 Gy, but SNHL has been considered infrequent at lower radiation therapy doses in the absence of cisplatin. Data suggest that cochlear doses of 30 to 50 Gy can cause intermediate frequency SNHL, and that cerebrospinal fluid shunting procedures increase the risk. Emerging data on adults treated for head and neck cancer also suggest that doses of >45 Gy impair hearing, particularly in the higher frequencies (262). Cisplatin, at doses as low as 270 mg/m^2, can result in

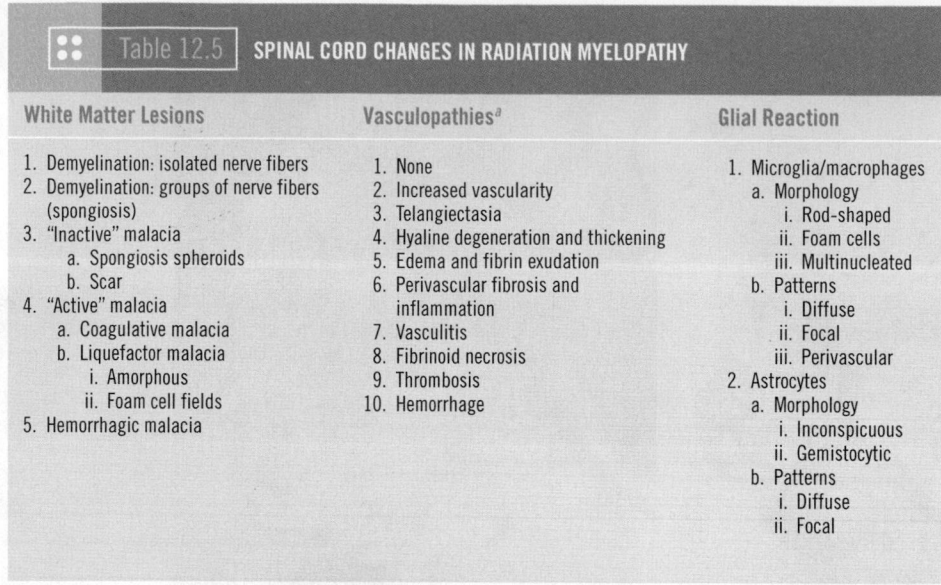

Table 12.5 SPINAL CORD CHANGES IN RADIATION MYELOPATHY

White Matter Lesions	Vasculopathies[a]	Glial Reaction

1. Demyelination: isolated nerve fibers
2. Demyelination: groups of nerve fibers (spongiosis)
3. "Inactive" malacia
  a. Spongiosis spheroids
  b. Scar
4. "Active" malacia
  a. Coagulative malacia
  b. Liquefactor malacia
    i. Amorphous
    ii. Foam cell fields
5. Hemorrhagic malacia
	1. None
	2. Increased vascularity
	3. Telangiectasia
	4. Hyaline degeneration and thickening
	5. Edema and fibrin exudation
	6. Perivascular fibrosis and inflammation
	7. Vasculitis
	8. Fibrinoid necrosis
	9. Thrombosis
	10. Hemorrhage
		1. Microglia/macrophages
		  a. Morphology
		    i. Rod-shaped
		    ii. Foam cells
		    iii. Multinucleated
		  b. Patterns
		    i. Diffuse
		    ii. Focal
		    iii. Perivascular
		2. Astrocytes
		  a. Morphology
		    i. Inconspicuous
		    ii. Gemistocytic
		  b. Patterns
		    i. Diffuse
		    ii. Focal

[a]With or without endothelial alterations of hyperchromasia, hypertrophy, anisokaryocytosis, and hyperplasia.
From Schultheiss TE, Kun LE, Ang KK, et al. Radiation response of the central nervous system. *Int J Radiat Oncol Biol Phys* 1995;31:1093–1112, with permission.

hearing loss, when combined with cranial radiotherapy doses of 40 to 50 Gy. The sequence of chemoradiotherapy appears to influence risk. Risk and severity of ototoxicity in children is greater when cisplatin is administered following cranial radiation (156,284).

Eye

Radiotherapy can affect the retina, lens, conjunctiva, lacrimal apparatus, optic nerve, and lid. Risk is illustrated well among survivors of orbital rhabdomyosarcoma who may develop dry eye, cataract, orbital hypoplasia, ptosis, retinopathy, keratoconjunctivitis, optic neuropathy, lid epithelioma, and impairment of vision, following doses of 30 to 65 Gy. The higher dose ranges (>50 Gy) are associated with lid epitheliomas, keratoconjunctivitis, lacrimal duct atrophy, and severe dry eye. Retinitis and optic neuropathy may also occur following doses of 50 to 65 Gy, and even at lower total doses if the individual fraction size is >2 Gy (182). The risk of retinopathy from hyperfractionated (dose

of 1.1 to 1.2 Gy twice daily) regimens appears to be negligible in to 50- to 60-Gy range, and appreciably less than comparable doses in the 60- to 70-Gy range delivered by standard daily radiation (241). Cataracts are reported following lower doses of 10 to 18 Gy (255,263,266,284). Survivors of hematopoietic stem cell transplantation who are treated with TBI are at known risk for cataracts. A shorter latency period and more severe cataracts are noted after single fraction and higher dose or dose-rate of TBI. Corticosteroids and graft-versus-host-disease (GVHD) may further increase risk (30,359,360).

Lung

1. ***Clinical Detection.*** Acute radiation pneumonitis (ARP) will develop in between 4% and 20% of patients receiving lung radiation (122,141,159,210). The clinical syndrome of ARP consists of dyspnea, nonproductive cough, pleuritic chest pain, fever, rales, and a consistent radiographic picture not explained by other abnormalities, such as pneumonia or pulmonary embolus. Delayed radiation fibrosis has an onset many months after radiation therapy and is often clinically asymptomatic.

2. ***Time Course of Events.*** In general, ARP reactions occur 8 to 16 weeks after single-dose or fractionated therapy. When chemotherapy has been used, as in TBI and BMT conditioning regimens, reactions can and do occur during treatment. ARP may precede its successor, radiation fibrosis, by many months.

3. ***Dose/Time/Volume.*** All three factors are important. With 30 to 50 Gy, radiographic changes are evident in 30% to 90% of patients. Where smaller lung volumes are irradiated in the setting of good functional reserve, as in irradiation for breast cancer, the reported rates of clinically evident pneumonitis are relatively low (<3%), and the pneumonitis is transient (210,211). Use of higher doses and treatment volumes in the setting of decreased anatomic and functional reserve, as in irradiation for lung cancer, is more likely to result in clinically evident pneumonitis with later delayed fibrosis (122,194).

The risk of late lung toxicity is a function of dose-volume histogram parameters (19,62,122,140,194,222,313,355, 381,382). These parameters include mean lung dose as well as the volume of lung receiving greater than a given

Table 12.6 EVALUATION OF LATE INJURY: SPINE

Technical Factors	Patient/Tumor Factors	Clinical Manifestations
Length (volume)	Primary spinal cord tumor (e.g., meningioma, astrocytoma)	Motor/sensory deficit
Chemotherapy (especially intrathecal, intraventricular, high dose methotrexate or Ara-C)	Diabetes, hypertension	Incontinence
Large dose or dose per fraction	Prior CNS damage (e.g., tumor invasion, mass effect)	Lhermitte's syndrome
Region treated (cervical spine vs. thoracolumbar spine)		

threshold dose (generally in 10 to 30 Gy range of threshold doses, expressed as V_X where X is the radiation dose). As a general rule, the risk of symptomatic radiation pneumonitis significantly increases with mean lung doses >10 to 20 Gy, V_{13} > 40%, V_{20} >25% to 30% and V_{30} >10% to 15%.

4. ***Chemical/Biologic Modifiers.*** Many chemotherapeutic agents alone produce pneumonopathies or can exaggerate responses to irradiation. These include actinomycin D, doxorubicin, bleomycin, busulfan, cyclophosphamide, BCNU, and the interferons (α, β, and ν).

5. ***Radiologic Imaging.*** Classically, a pneumonitic reaction appears to be limited to the irradiated field, with a geometric outline on chest radiograph and CT corresponding to the isodose distribution, although an abscopal effect, with pneumonitis extending outside the irradiated field, has been described (242). However, with increasingly complex dose distributions, the classic straight-edge sign on chest film becomes less reliable. Unlike late radiation fibrosis, ARP may be confused with malignancy.

6. ***Laboratory Tests.*** Late pulmonary toxicity, such as fibrosis and/or changes in lung perfusion, could impact pulmonary function tests. By 16 weeks, decreased lung volumes may be seen on pulmonary function testing; decreased lung perfusion is predictive of late fibrotic changes (221). Generally, radiation is associated with a decline in pulmonary function tests, although improvements in pulmonary function tests have also been noted in patients with thoracic tumors, perhaps as the result of reduction in tumor burden and or altering perfusion-ventilation ratios (219,220). Serum surfactant apoprotein, interleukin-6 (IL-6), IL-10, and transforming growth factor-β (TGF-β) plasma levels are undergoing testing as predictive markers (11,12,22,26,58,220,228).

7. ***Differential Diagnosis.*** Because combined-modality treatment regimens may lead to atypical timing of pneumonitis or fibrotic reactions, diagnosis can be misleading. Recurrence, persistent disease, metastatic spread, and infiltrates, such as lymphangitic spread patterns, must be considered. Opportunistic and secondary infection can mimic radiation reactions.

8. ***Pathologic Diagnosis.*** An invasive procedure is rarely indicated unless recurrent neoplasms are suspected and further treatment is possible, such as in Hodgkin lymphoma. Bronchoalveolar lavage fluids can be analyzed for cellular and cytokine responses. Typical hyaline membrane changes are characteristically described in ARP (94).

9. and 10. ***Management and Follow-up.*** Management most often entails the use of high-dose steroids, starting with prednisone (30 to 60 mg/day) or dexamethasone (16 to 20 mg/day) for pneumonitis. Symptoms clear rapidly within 24 to 48 hours. Steroids are very gradually tapered over months unless or until symptoms recur. The combination of pentoxifylline (Trental) and tocopherol (vitamin E) has been used with some success in the setting of fibrosis (80).

Pathophysiology and Cellular Biology

The first event seen after lung irradiation is the response to injury by the alveolar type II cells as an early release of surfactant (298). The initial events are readily detectable within minutes to hours, but have no evident clinical or radiographic manifestations. After these initial events, a latent period of 1 to 3 months occurs before detectable pathologic or clinical syndromes are seen as a result of the alveolar type II cell injury and subsequent loss. The next phase, proliferation of type II pneumocytes, occurs at 1 to 3 months, and there is a compensatory hypertrophy of lamellar bodies. The late fibrotic phase begins at 3 to 6 months and is recognized by sclerosis of the alveolar wall, extensive endothelial damage with loss, replacement of some capillaries, eventual replacement of alveolar spaces, and fibro-

sis with loss of function. Radiation therapy causes blistering of the capillary endothelial cells, which plays an independent role leading to both early and late pulmonary effects more readily detected by electron microscopy.

Investigators have demonstrated alterations in the expression of proinflammatory and profibrotic cytokines, chemokines, and growth factors in mouse models for lung radiation injury, including IL-1 and IL-6, tumor necrosis factor-α, TGF-β, and monocyte chemoattractant protein (100,170,171). Cytokines are released by macrophages, type II pneumocytes, and endothelial cells, stimulating the subsequent genetic expression of collagens I, III, and IV, as well as fibronectin. These cytokine cascades have been shown to persist, increase, or decrease, depending on the radiation dose and the mouse strain (172,267).

Supportive clinical data for these models are now beginning to accumulate. Elevated plasma TGF-β levels are an independent risk factor for symptomatic radiation-induced lung injury (11). Similar cytokine cascades occur with chemotherapeutic agents, biologic response modifiers, surgery, and infection, providing a molecular rationale for sensitization. A powerful association between native circulating IL-1 and IL-6 levels and radiation pneumonitis has been reported (58). There is a correlation of circulating levels of IL-10 and IL-6 with radiation pneumonitis (22).

Combined-Modality Therapy

The combination of both radiation and chemotherapy can produce an intensified response, and a "recall phenomenon" can appear when drugs are used after irradiation. Actinomycin D, used with radiation therapy for pulmonary metastases in Wilms' tumor, was shown to produce lethal radiation pneumonitis despite radiation doses within tolerance (336). However, an analysis among long-term Wilms' tumor survivors shows risk of late-occurring restrictive pulmonary disease to be related to the dose delivered to the lung, as well as use of cyclophosphamide (107). Administration of bleomycin and the nitrosoureas alone can produce severe pneumonopathies, and, when combined with radiation therapy, heighten radiation reactions and lead to increased mortality (71). Patients treated for Hodgkin lymphoma are at particularly increased risk for late-occurring pulmonary fibrosis with a decreased diffusion capacity. Bleomycin commonly used in chemotherapy regimens for Hodgkin lymphoma is also associated with pulmonary fibrosis and decreased diffusion capacity is most commonly seen following doses >200 to 400 U/m^2 (108,187).

Clinical Syndromes

Radiation therapy produces dramatic effects, both acute and late, in the lung (Table 12.7). Two distinct lung injuries occur after irradiation: the acute pneumonitic phase that occurs after 1 to 3 months and the delayed fibrotic phase that is seen after 2 to 4 months (94). Pulmonary function parameters include pulmonary ventilation tests, nuclear medicine techniques for aeration and blood flow, diffusion capacities, alveolar lavage for surfactant release and collagenase, and biopsy analyses for hydroxyproline content. Radiographic studies, including CT and MRI, differentiate normal from abnormal irradiated tissues in the intact organ, although work by Marks et al. (221) supports single photon emission CT perfusion as the most sensitive procedure at 85%. The disparity between clinical symptoms and radiographic findings is well illustrated; only 5% to 15% of patients will have clinically evident symptoms, and five times this number will have imaging abnormalities (Table 12.8). However, symptoms are usually minimal if fibrosis is limited to <50% of one lung.

The dose range for lethal radiation-induced pneumonitis for whole lung irradiation is 8.2 Gy for a 5%, 9.3 Gy for a 50%,

Table 12.7	EVALUATION OF LATE INJURY: LUNG	
Technical Factors	**Patient/Tumor Factors**	**Clinical Manifestations**
V_{13}, V_{20}, V_{30}, V_{eff}, mean lung dose	Preexisting cardiopulmonary disease	Cough Low-grade fever
Large dose per fraction	Smoking	Dyspnea
Dose rate	Age extremes	Chest pain
Chemotherapy (especially concomitant, e.g., bleomycin, doxorubicin, actinomycin)	Cytokine levels (e.g., interleukin-6, interleukin-10, transforming growth factor-β)	Pulmonary fibrosis
Region treated (base > mid > apex) ? Tamoxifen	? Lung levels of vitamin A	

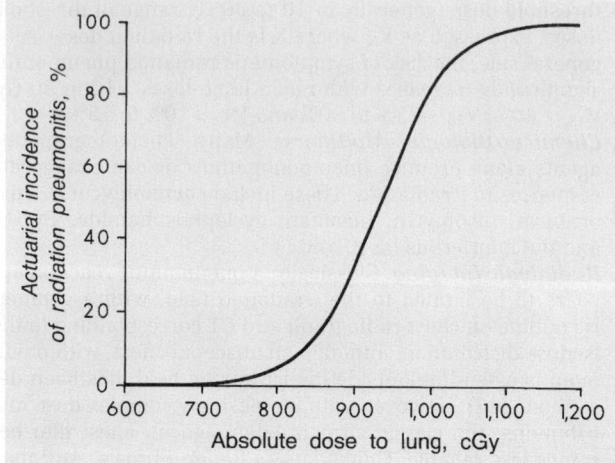

FIGURE 12.7. A best-fit curve based on a probit regression analysis of actuarial incidence of radiation pneumonitis versus absolute dose to lung for patients receiving upper hemibody irradiation. (From van Dyk J, Keane TJ, Kan S, et al. Radiation pneumonitis following large single dose irradiation: a re-evaluation based on absolute dose to lung. *Int J Radiat Oncol Biol Phys* 1981;7:461–467, with permission.)

and 11 Gy for an 80% incidence after a single high-dose-rate exposure (358) (Fig. 12.7). The dose-response relationship is shifted to the right for protracted low–dose-rate radiation as used in TBI for BMT. Fractionated irradiation dramatically improves tolerance, experimentally and clinically, although a high radiosensitivity of the lung has been noted in fractionated irradiation exposures as a component of TBI for BMT, with many patients suffering fatal interstitial pneumonitis (30,316). The clinical data for fractionated regimens have been carefully reconstructed, particularly for children with Wilms' tumor, and the dose modification factor for single versus fractionated doses has been shown to be 3.2, demonstrating a considerable increase in tolerance for the latter (229). This is consistent with the findings of a literature review by Bentzen et al. (31), concluding that the α/β ratio for normal lung tissue is low, possibly 2 to 3 Gy. Also important is the effect of dose rate because considerable protection is conferred by lowering the rate from 0.47 to 0.08 Gy/min; such a reduction in rate changes the $LD_{50/5}$ from 7.75 to 8.7 Gy, for a dose-modification ratio of 1.12.

Data on a specific range of injurious doses are beginning to accumulate with the increased use of three-dimensional conformal planning (Fig. 12.8). The findings are complicated in patients with lung cancer by the baseline pulmonary abnormalities resulting from changes produced by the cancer itself and, in many cases, by years of tobacco smoking that preceded the treatment. Other than smoking, which appears to confer a radioprotective effect on both tumor and normal tissue (34,168,342), patient factors have been difficult to correlate with symptomatic outcome, but seem to improve the pre-

dictive value of multivariate models (113,140). Demonstrated dosimetric predictors of radiation-induced pulmonary toxicity include mean lung dose, as well as the percentage of total lung volume treated to a minimum of 13, 20, or 30 Gy (V_{13}, V_{20}, and V_{30}, respectively) (109,122,140,220). For example, Graham et al. (122) demonstrated that a V_{20} of <22% correlated with an actuarial incidence of significant pneumonitis of 0%, whereas a V_{20} of >40% correlated with a 36% rate. Yorke et al. (381,382) have shown that mean lung dose as well as a V_X values in the range of V_{5-40} of total lung, V_{5-40} of ipsilateral lung, and V_{5-50} of lower lung were significant in predicting late pulmonary toxicity. With complication probability modeling, a mean lung dose of ~12 Gy or a V_{13} of >40% to ipsilateral lung results in a 5% risk of moderately severe, late complications. A V_{13} of 36% to the lower lung, 42% to the total lung, or 62% to the ipsilateral lung results in a 20% late complication risk. Patients with Hodgkin's disease who undergo mediastinal radiation appear to have a lower risk of radiation pneumonitis as compared with patients treated for lung cancer; data from Princess Margaret Hospital suggest a minimal risk of grade 2 radiation pneumonitis with a V_{20} <36% and mean lung dose <14 Gy (183).

With respect to the multifactorial paradigm for late effects, Fu et al. (109) found that patients with lung cancer with a low baseline plasma TGF-β1 level treated to V_{30} of <30% had a 7% rate of symptomatic pneumonitis, versus 43% in patients with both high V_{30} and elevated TGF-β1 level. In patients with one of these risk factors alone, pneumonitis developed at an intermediate rate of 23%.

Skin and Soft Tissue

1. **Clinical Detection.** Acute radiation skin reaction appears as erythema and hypersensitivity, edema, alopecia, and hyperpigmentation, with desquamation at higher doses. Prior to the advent of megavoltage radiation, acute skin toxicity was the most common dose-limiting factor. More delayed (late) effects can consist of telangiectasia, dense dermal fibrosis, sebaceous gland atrophy, loss of hair follicles, altered melanin deposition, and skin ulceration.

2. **Time Course of Events.** Erythema typically appears in the second or third week of a standard fractionated radiation therapy course as seen with modern megavoltage equipment. Epilation occurs in a dose-dependent fashion (with a threshold of 1 Gy) in the third week after conventional radiation, with regeneration of the hair follicles at 9 weeks

Table 12.8	RADIOLOGIC VERSUS SYMPTOMATIC CHANGES AFTER THORACIC IRRADIATION[a]	
Patient Group/Reference	**Frequency of of Radiographic Abnormalities (%)**	**Frequency of Clinical Pneumonitis (%)**
Breast cancer (118,275)	27–40	0–10
Lung cancer (126)	~65	5–15
Mediastinal lymphoma (317)	60–92	0
Miscellaneous (216,220)	67–87	0–18

[a]The data listed often represent approximate values, as precise information is not always reported. A variety of radiologic tests were used.
From McDonald S, Rubin P, Phillips TL, et al. Injury to the lung from cancer therapy: clinical syndromes, measurable endpoints, and potential scoring systems. *Int J Radiat Oncol Biol Phys* 1995;144:160–169, with permission.

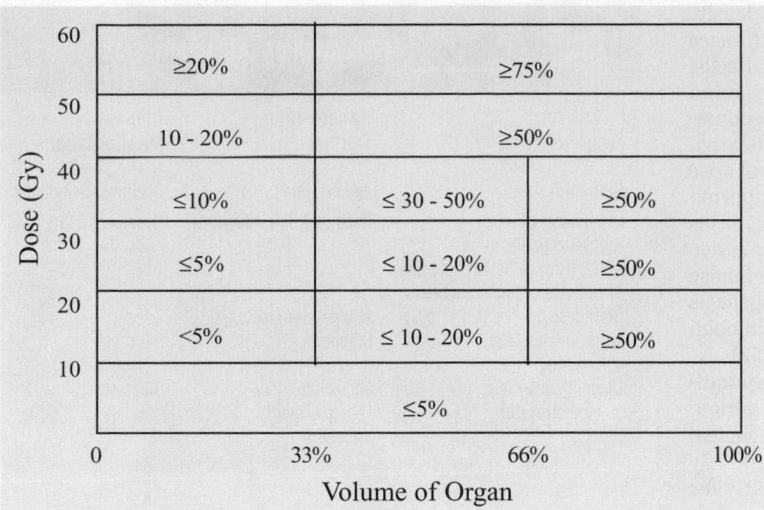

FIGURE 12.8. Schematic diagram depicting the dose-volume relationship to complication. Each box represents the percentage likelihood of developing damage according to the volume of the lung irradiated (x-axis) and radiation dose administered (y-axis).

(195). Late skin changes evolve during a period of months to years. The latency is 3 years for fibrosis, and 5 years for telangiectasia.

3. **Dose/Time/Volume.** Late skin toxicity is increased when therapy is delivered at doses of 2.5 Gy per fraction and above. The risk of telangiectasia and necrosis rises with increasing volume and increasing dose (92). Skin toxicity was seen more commonly before the modern era of high-energy linear accelerators because orthovoltage and cobalt machines offered little or no skin sparing. Recent data on the radiation therapy dose associated with permanent alopecia support a dose-response relationship with a hair follicle D_{50} of 43 Gy (200).

4. **Chemical/Biologic Modifiers.** Certain chemotherapy agents appear to increase the erythema response to radiation therapy, including methotrexate, actinomycin D, and doxorubicin.

5. **Radiologic Imaging.** Radiographic findings consist typically of thickening and increased density of skin and underlying soft tissue.

6. **Laboratory Tests.** There are no proven laboratory tests that have any predictive value, although at least one group has suggested that, similar to the lung, increases in systemic plasma levels of TGF-β may indicate a susceptibility to the development of radiation-induced fibrosis (257).

7. **Differential Diagnosis.** Erythema and fibrosis can be confused with recurrent inflammatory breast cancer, other malignancies involving the dermal lymphatics, and local inflammations due to infection, cellulitis, or allergy. Fat necrosis can be confused with a recurrent malignancy. Late ulcerations can be caused by radiation therapy, by recurrent cancer, or a new primary skin malignancy. Other medical illnesses may offer a similar appearance, including systemic sclerosis, lupus erythematosus, lichen sclerosus et atrophicus, and stasis dermatitis.

8. **Pathologic Diagnosis.** Acutely, radiation effects appear as a decrease in the number of basal epithelial cells and an increased mitotic index in the setting of edema, inflammation, and vascular dilatation. Later changes include destruction of the microvasculature, causing telangiectases, epidermal atrophy, dense dermal fibrosis, loss of pilosebaceous units, atrophic sweat glands, and progressive arterial and venous lesions (94).

9. **Management.** Although acute reactions can be painful, symptomatic treatment and careful skin care are sufficient because this is a self-limiting problem after standard dose, megavoltage radiation therapy. Careful wound care is re-

quired to promote reepithelialization from the field edges. Management of late reactions, such as fibrosis and necrosis, is aimed at symptom relief and prevention of infection. There are some data to suggest that a combination of tocopherol (vitamin E) and pentoxifylline (Trental) may be useful in the treatment of radiation fibrosis (80). Hyperbaric oxygen is an alternative strategy to promote healing of ulcerations. Surgical management with grafting of the irradiated area is a last resort in very severe cases.

10. **Follow-up.** Skin care guidance and close follow-up are warranted throughout the healing process.

Pathophysiology and Cellular Biology

The skin is essentially constructed of shells of varying thickness. These shells consist of the epidermis, the papillary dermis, the rete dermis, the dermal subcutaneous junction with the dermal plexus, and the subcutaneous layer. Much of the experimental data on skin irradiation come from work in swine, an important model because swine skin closely resembles that of humans. Archambeau et al. (16) defined the functional subunit (FSU) of skin as a single microvessel with associated epidermis and dermis, measuring approximately 30 μm in diameter by 350 μm in length. In swine skin, there are an estimated 30,000 FSU/cm^2.

In a study using 60 Gy in 30 fractions and repeated biopsies, Archambeau et al. (15) found that epidermal cell densities fell 50% before returning to normal 10 days after irradiation. In contrast, basal cell mitotic rate rose from 0.2% to 0.6% at the end of therapy and then returned to baseline; the number of basal cells did not fall until total doses of 20 to 25 Gy were administered. Microvascular changes were not seen. The group also demonstrated that early radiation injury of the basal epithelial cell correlated with visible erythema (15,16); later decreases in endothelial cells and vascular lumen densities correlated with moist desquamation or, after larger doses, skin necrosis. Telangiectases were formed when excessive loss of the microvascular endothelium occurred, causing capillary loops to contract and fuse into dilated channels beneath an atrophied overlying epidermis. In another experimental model using SCID (severe combined immunodeficiency) mice (195), it has been demonstrated that epilation results from the breaking of hairs when the hair width decreases to less than 20 μm. By 9 weeks, the follicle is in regeneration and hair growth activity is seen, although approximately one third of hairs did not regrow.

After a large single dose, there is loss of basal cells, reaching a nadir at approximately 21 days, followed by reepithelialization to baseline or above by 28 to 32 days. With standard fractionation, there is no observable change in basal cell density until total doses of 20 to 25 Gy are reached, after which there is a dose-dependent loss of basal cells. Surviving basal cells, scattered over a wide area, then repopulate the basal layer and preserve function. The survival of one cell per square centimeter is sufficient to permit epithelial regeneration in this area. Complete regeneration of the epidermis is produced at all dose fractions up to 45 Gy (16). After reepithelialization at approximately 30 days, the endothelial population density decreases abruptly, vessel diameter increases, and there is a progressive loss of lumen with an increase in microvessel diameter; these changes accompany clinically evident erythema. Angiogenesis and microvessel endothelial proliferation are not seen, although endothelial proliferation in larger vessels is reported (152).

Near-tolerance doses that are typically used in curative radiation therapy result in changes that occur during a long period. The α/β ratio for human skin has been estimated from clinical experience, with a value of 1.9 Gy for fibrosis, 2.8 to 3.9 Gy for telangiectasia, 7.5 to 8.8 Gy for erythema, and 12.2 Gy for desquamation (341,357).

Combined-Modality Therapy

An additive response between combined chemotherapy and radiation therapy is expected, but not well documented in the literature. For example, increased erythema is seen in patients receiving concurrent methotrexate for breast cancer and in children receiving actinomycin D. An erythematous "radiation recall" is reported in patients first irradiated, then subsequently given a course of doxorubicin, actinomycin D, paclitaxel, or other chemotherapy agents (40,110,154).

Clinical Syndromes

The first descriptions of radiation-induced injury were of the skin, appearing just 9 months after Roentgen's discovery of x-rays (237). The erythema dose, the treatment dose required to induce skin redness, was the first reported tolerance dose. In 1904, the first known death due to radiation was caused by a radiation-induced skin carcinoma in an early radiation worker, Clarence Dally (237).

Acute changes occur during the first 70 days after irradiation. The first manifestation of radiation dose is a reddening of the skin or erythema. The intensity of the erythema varies with the dose, although there is considerable interindividual variation. Skin erythema may be seen after a single low (3 Gy) dose of low-voltage radiation, but requires higher doses (20 to 40 Gy) with fractionated megavoltage radiation therapy. With increasing dose, hyperpigmentation, epilation, and desquamation appear. Epilation occurs at approximately 18 days after doses of $\geq$20 Gy; hyperpigmentation and dry desquamation occur after 45 Gy; moist desquamation may result if the dose is high enough (>45 Gy), and typically heals by 50 days after irradiation. At skin doses above 60 Gy, moist desquamation defies healing 50% of the time at 50 days.

A period of variable length follows the acute phase during which the skin appears normal. After periods as long as several years, late effect changes may appear, such as xerosis, atrophy, telangiectasia, subcutaneous fibrosis, and necrosis (Table 12.9). As early as 6 months after therapy, telangiectasia develops as an area of thinned epidermis with underlying multiple, prominent, thin-walled, and dilated vessels. The degree of telangiectasia continues to evolve and increase in severity during a period of up to 10 years (357). Fibrosis may develop, with progressive induration, edema, and thickening of the dermis and subcutaneous tissues. The onset and progression of fibrosis are dose-dependent and slowly progressive once underway.

If the doses delivered are significantly greater than the erythema dose, induration of the dermis is seen because of edema.

Table 12.9	EVALUATION OF LATE INJURY: SKIN	
Treatment Factors	**Patient/Tumor Factors**	**Clinical Manifestations**
High total dose	Age extremes	Scaliness/roughness
Low-energy photons High-energy electrons Obliquity of radiation field use of bolus or beam modifiers	Race (red hair, fair skin)	Hypersensitivity
High dose per fraction (2.5 Gy) Large volume (e.g., >60% to >40 Gy)	Ataxia-telangiectasia Diabetes	Edema Pain
Chemotherapy (e.g., methotrexate)	Microcirculatory impairment Infection	Ulceration

True radiodermatitis is a syndrome of pain, blister formation, erosions, and even ulcers. Healing of the less severe erythema results in dry, scaling, atrophic, and often pigmented skin, a condition termed *dry desquamation*. Healing of a true severe radiodermatitis may require months, with very severe cases requiring surgery and skin grafting. Permanent results of delayed radiation injury include skin atrophy, alopecia, dryness, and hypopigmentation, termed *poikiloderma*. This skin after delayed injury appears thin, inelastic, and excessively smooth and dry. It may be hyperpigmented or hypopigmented with higher doses (94).

Radiotherapy is also associated with increased risk of second malignancies of the skin, particularly nonmelanoma skin cancers, reported in survivors of childhood cancer as well as survivors of hematopoietic stem cell transplantation (208).

Heart

1. ***Clinical Detection.*** The spectrum of clinical manifestations of cardiac injury includes
   - (a) coronary artery disease (CAD)—silent, anginal pain, dyspnea, diaphoresis, sudden death;
   - (b) pericarditis—silent, chest pain, dyspnea, cyanosis, peripheral edema, muffled heart sounds, venous distension, pulsus paradoxus;
   - (c) cardiomyopathy—dyspnea on exertion, peripheral edema, tachypnea/rales, hepatomegaly, syncope, palpitations;
   - (d) valvular damage—weakness, cough, dyspnea, new murmur, pulsating liver; and
   - (e) arrhythmias—palpitations, dyspnea (2,4,39,118,300).
2. ***Time Course of Events.*** Pericardial disease usually appears within 6 months to 1 year, and may progress to a constrictive process. CAD appears 10 to 15 years after irradiation, but is affected by the usual cardiac risk factors of obesity, smoking, family history, and hypertension.
3. ***Dose/Time/Volume.*** The incidence of pericardial disease in patients treated for Hodgkin's disease decreases with subcarinal shields blocking the major ventricles at 20 to 30 Gy. In patients with breast cancer, left-sided cancers are associated with a higher cardiac exposure to radiation; left-sided breast cancers treated with radiation have been shown to increase the risk of coronary artery disease and myocardial infarction as compared with right-sided tumors; this was associated with a nonsignificantly increased risk of cardiac death (133,282). In patients treated for non-Hodgkin's lymphoma, doses >40 Gy to the mediastinum are associated with significantly increased risk of chronic

heart failure and myocardial infarction (244). Doses should be <40 Gy for <25% of cardiac volume and 30 Gy for larger volumes (111,332). Dose-volume tolerance is diminished by anthracycline administration.

4. ***Chemical/Biologic Modifiers.*** Anthracyclines are the best-recognized cardiotoxic agents, and dose modification to well below 500 mg/m² is currently recommended if radiation is part of the treatment protocol.

5. ***Radiologic Imaging.*** Chest films are used to identify increases in size of cardiac silhouette. Echocardiograms of specific structures (pericardium, valves, aorta, branch pulmonary arteries) are used to assess for pericardial effusion, cardiac function, ventricular thickness, and valvular function. Radionuclide studies, including stress perfusion scans, equilibrium radionuclide angiocardiography, and quantitative thallium scintigraphy (to assess myocardial function and blood flow), are helpful in establishing cardiac injury (119,120,206). Nonradiologic assessments includes include electrocardiograms, which can assess prior infarctions, rhythm abnormalities, and exercise stress testing, which can also be used to assess cardiac function (5,120).

6. ***Laboratory Tests.*** Heat-stable C-reactive protein may predict cardiovascular events and is a useful addition to lipid profiles (14,177).

7. ***Differential Diagnosis.*** Sensitive mediastinal tumors can trigger pericardial reactions in response to irradiation, occurring during or at the end of treatment, and are due to the tumor invading the pericardium. Primary Hodgkin and non-Hodgkin lymphoma, and recurrent cancers of lung and esophagus, can invade the pericardium. CAD is not unique or different in the irradiated patient.

8. ***Pathologic Diagnosis.*** When the differential diagnosis in constrictive pericarditis is secondary to irradiation or recurrent malignancy, open biopsy of the pericardium is advised.

9. ***Management.*** Most often, pericardial effusions are asymptomatic, but if tamponade develops, pericardiocentesis tapping is necessary. Preventive measures are desirable in reducing the incidence of CAD. Late cardiac toxicity is managed similarly to patients presenting with cardiac disease unrelated to prior cancer treatment.

10. ***Follow-up.*** Patients treated with mediastinal radiation as children or young adults should be screened for coronary artery disease. Screening stress echocardiography and radionuclide perfusion imaging can identify asymptomatic patients at high risk for myocardial infarction (138). The pediatric and young adult population, particularly girls <20 years of age, should be informed of the risks of late cardiac effects and encouraged to have a healthy lifestyle.

Pathophysiology and Cellular Biology

The severe cardiomyopathies encountered as a late effect of cancer treatment demonstrate the additive effects of both radiation and chemotherapy through their actions on two different populations of cells. Doxorubicin appears not to affect endothelial cells directly, whereas radiation's primary target is the endothelial cell, altering the fine vasculoconnective stroma of the myocardium (96). The histopathologic and ultrastructural changes of doxorubicin alone, irradiation alone, and irradiation and doxorubicin together dramatically show these independent and additive organ effects (95) (Fig. 12.9).

Radiation changes in the heart in humans are experimentally reproducible and similar in rabbits and other models (96,115). The hallmarks are seen as a pericardial effusion clinically and fibrosis pathologically, involving a thickened collagenous pericardium and an extensive fibrinous exudate. When the myocardium is involved, diffuse interstitial fibrosis occurs, which follows the pattern of septa in the myocardium. With therapeutic doses of radiation, direct damage to myocytes in humans

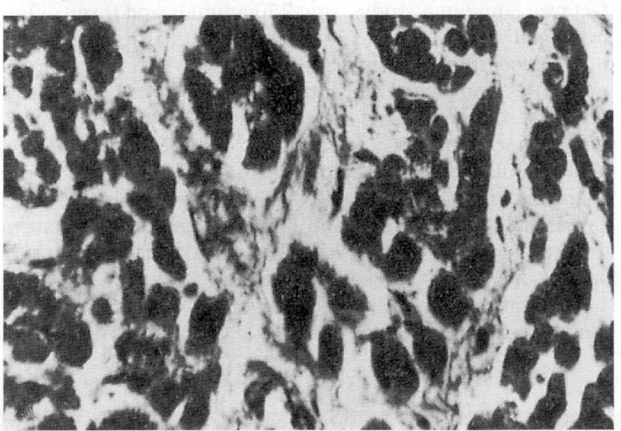

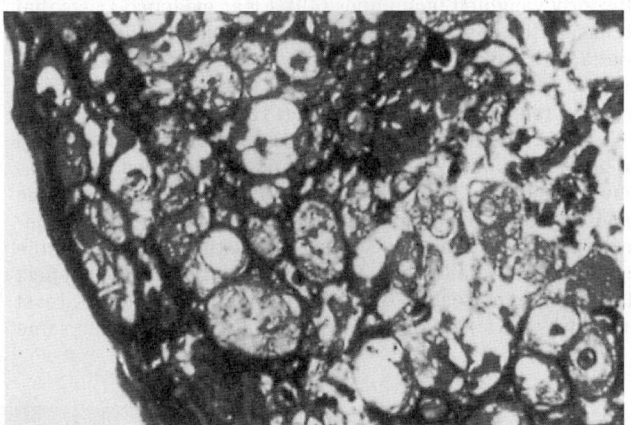

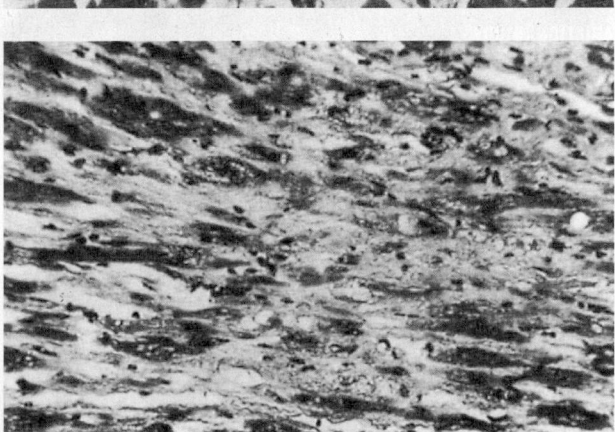

FIGURE 12.9. Pathologic late effects in the heart. **A:** Radiation therapy effects. The myocardium or cardiac myocytes are normal in appearance, with increased fibrosis in the interstitium and capillary and arterial narrowing. (From Fajardo LF, Stewart JR. Experimental radiation-induced heart disease: I. Light microscopic studies. *Am J Pathol* 1970;59:299–316, with permission.) **B:** Chemotherapy effects. The effect of doxorubicin is dramatic, with vacuolization localized to the cardiac myocytes. The interstitium is normal in appearance, showing vascular sparing despite dramatic cellular changes. **C:** Chemoradiation effects. Combined radiation and chemotherapy induce damage in both the vascular connective tissue stroma and the cardiac myocytes (**B** and **C** from Fajardo LF, Eltringham JR, Stewart JR. Combined cardiotoxicity of Adriamycin and x-radiation. *Lab Invest* 1976;34:86–96, with permission.)

and animals does not occur. The coronary arteries are large enough not to be the main focus of radiation lesions, and coronary thrombosis is a relatively infrequent occurrence, found in <5% of patients treated. Coronary thrombosis does not differ from spontaneous arteriosclerosis in unirradiated patients and is difficult to establish without a matched cohort of patients managed by other means.

After a variety of irradiation schedules, a serial sacrifice of rabbits yielded a predictable and identifiable sequence of lesions in the myocardial microvasculature (95). The hypothesis of Fajardo and Stewart (96) for the induction of coronary late effects is that the radiation insult results in latent damage to the capillary endothelial cells; severe alterations in myocardial capillaries, including irregularities of the endothelial cell membranes, cytoplasmic swelling, thrombosis, and rupture of the walls, have been reported. Quantitative studies also have shown that the ratio of capillaries to myocytes is reduced by approximately 50% over unirradiated controls at 120 to 540 days and, by pulse labeling with tritiated thymidine, a peak incorporation entirely within capillary endothelial cells was noted. A compensatory burst of endothelial cell proliferation occurs, and the cells die at mitosis. The resulting reduction in capillaries leads to ischemia and, in turn, myocardial fibrosis (96). A reduction in capillary size also occurs in experimental animals (115), with focal loss of endothelial cell alkaline phosphatase and 5'-nucleotidase in irradiated hearts. Enzyme activity is decreased and associated with foci of myocardial degeneration, supporting evidence that these changes are secondary to ischemic injury.

Studies in the rabbit model (96) found that single radiation doses of 18 to 20 Gy or fractionated doses of 54 Gy (4.5 Gy × 12) caused pericarditis in all animals, whereas <18 Gy (single dose) caused no damage. Pericarditis develops in <5% of patients treated for Hodgkin lymphoma when a radiation dose of <40 Gy is administered through equally weighted anterior and posterior portals, whereas a 30% incidence is seen with anteriorly weighted techniques (49). Clear evidence exists that increasing the dose per fraction increases the risk of CAD. Volume factors have been correlated with dose; the larger the irradiated cardiac volume, the smaller the dose that can cause cardiac damage, and vice versa (Fig. 12.10).

Table 12.10 denotes identifiable risk factors associated with the observed clinical incidence of radiation-induced complications of the heart (3), and Figure 12.11 shows the dose-volume response curves for the heart (111). The curves plotted for different partial volumes are similar, suggesting that the volume dependence is small (111). A comparison of cardiac late effect data on patients treated for Hodgkin lymphoma and for breast cancer was performed by Eriksson et al. (93). Using the same

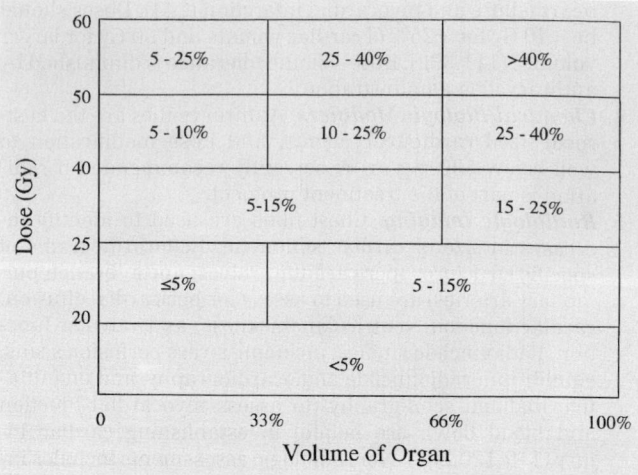

FIGURE 12.10. Schematic diagram depicting the dose-volume relationship to complication. Each box represents the percentage likelihood of developing damage according to the volume of the heart irradiated (x-axis) and radiation dose administered (y-axis).

volume parameters, significantly different TD_{50} values were obtained for treatment of the breast cancer versus Hodgkin lymphoma, suggesting that different portions of the heart were irradiated (93), although there may be other confounding variables not easily identified (e.g., patient age when irradiated and similar risk factors between breast cancer and cardiac disease).

Combined-Modality Therapy

The effect of combining radiation and chemotherapy has been studied intensively by Eltringham et al. (91), and an additive effect was found in a study using 350 animals and three different fractionation schedules. Histopathologic investigation showed both myocardial damage and interstitial fibrosis when both modalities were used, but no sensitization and enhancement occurred. On the basis of dose and interval of treatment used in these experiments, 1 Gy was considered equivalent to 10 mg/m^2 of doxorubicin; the threshold dose of 450 to 500 mg/m^2 for doxorubicin parallels the 45 to 50 Gy dose for radiation therapy. Recall of subthreshold radiation injury is time-independent, and doxorubicin administered 5 to 10 years after radiation therapy can produce cardiac decompensation.

Anthracycline-related cardiomyopathy is associated with female sex, cumulative doses >300 mg/m^2, younger age

Table 12.10	RISK FACTORS ASSOCIATED WITH CARDIAC LATE RADIATION INJURY					
Injury	Time Postradiation Therapy	Dose (Gy)/ Volume (%)	Tumor Location	Age	Chemotherapy	Other
Coronary artery disease	10–15 y	>40 Gy/>25%; >30 Gy/>50%; Increased dose per fraction	—	<20 y	Yes	Weighted portals (anterior > posterior); lack of subcarinal shields
Pericarditis	6 mo–1 y	>40 Gy/>25%	Proximity to pericardium	? <20 y	Yes	Lack of subcarinal shields
Cardiomyopathy	Any	>40 Gy/>25%	—	? <20 y	Yes	
Valvular damage	>10 y	>35 Gy	—	? <20 y	Yes	
Arrhythmias	>10 y	>40 Gy	—	? <20 y	Yes	QTC prolongation

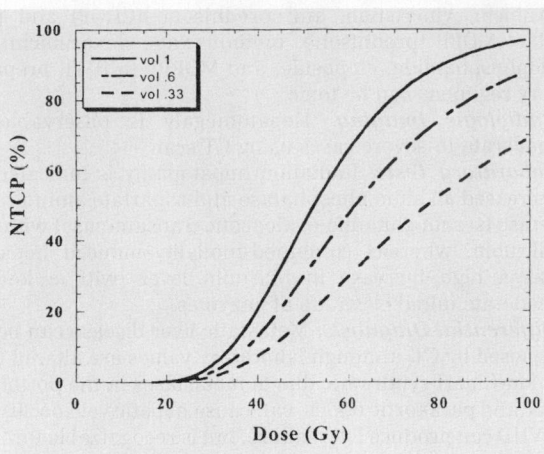

FIGURE 12.11. Dose-response curves for long-term cardiac mortality. The curves show 100%, 66%, and 33% of the heart volume. The clinical incidence data covered an interval from 0% to 8%. (From Gagliardi G, Lax I, Rutqvist LE. Partial irradiation of the heart. *Semin Radiat Oncol* 2001;11:224–233, with permission.)

Table 12.11	**EVALUATION OF LATE INJURY: HEART**	
Treatment Factors	**Patient Tumor Factors**	**Clinical Manifestations**
High total dose	Preexisting cardiopulmonary disease (e.g., pericarditis, myocardiopathy)	Angina pectoris
High dose per fraction	Age extremes	Pericardial pain
Large volume (e.g., >40 Gy to >60%)	Hypercholesterolemia	Dyspnea
Chemotherapy (e.g., doxorubicin)	Family history	Pedal edema
Left ventricle in treatment field	Diabetes	
Single vs. multiple fields treated per day	Hypertension Obesity	

at time of exposure, and increased time from exposure (188,189,212,269,331) A recent review on cardiotoxicity in childhood cancer revealed a dose response with ranges of subclinical cardiotoxicity of 15.5% to 27.8% and abnormal afterload of 19% to 52%, for those who received doses in excess of 300 mg/m² and abnormal left ventricular function of 0% to 15.2% in patients receiving lower doses (188). In one of the few studies to assess the combined effect of doxorubicin and radiation in patients, LaMonte et al. (198) reported on 20 adults treated with MOPP/ABVD (nitrogen mustard, vincristine, procarbazine, and prednisone/doxorubicin, bleomycin, vinblastine, and dacarbazine DTIC) and mantle irradiation, studied at a median of 39 months after treatment. Four patients had either a decreased left ventricular ejection fraction at rest or a decreased response to exercise, and one additional patient had congestive heart failure documented by radionuclide cardiac angiography. The mean cumulative dose of doxorubicin was 176 mg/m² and the irradiation dose was 20 Gy.

Clinical Syndromes

A classification system of radiation injuries modified from Fajardo and Stewart (96) includes acute pericarditis during irradiation (rare and associated with juxtapericardial cancer); delayed pericarditis that can present abruptly or as chronic pericardial effusion; pancarditis, which includes pericardial and myocardial fibrosis, with or without endocardial fibroelastosis (only after large doses); myopathy in the absence of significant pericardial disease; CAD, usually involving the left anterior descending artery (181) (Fig. 12.12); and functional valve injury and conduction defects (Table 12.11). Although CAD occurs, it is relatively uncommon and multifactorial. Several parameters must be considered in the evaluation of radiation injuries, including relative weighting of the irradiation portals and, thus, the amount of radiation delivered to different depths of the heart: presence of juxtapericardial tumor; volume and specific areas of the heart irradiated; total and fractionated irradiation dose; presence of other risk factors in each patient, such as age, weight, blood pressure, family history, lipoprotein levels, and habits such as smoking; and use of specific chemotherapeutic agents.

Delayed acute pericarditis can be symptomatically occult or can manifest suddenly with fever, dyspnea, pleuritic chest pain, friction rub, S and T wave changes, and decreased QRS voltage. Up to 30% of patients treated with radiation for Hodgkin lymphoma with a mean midplane heart dose of 46 Gy are affected; with equally weighted anterior and posterior fields and

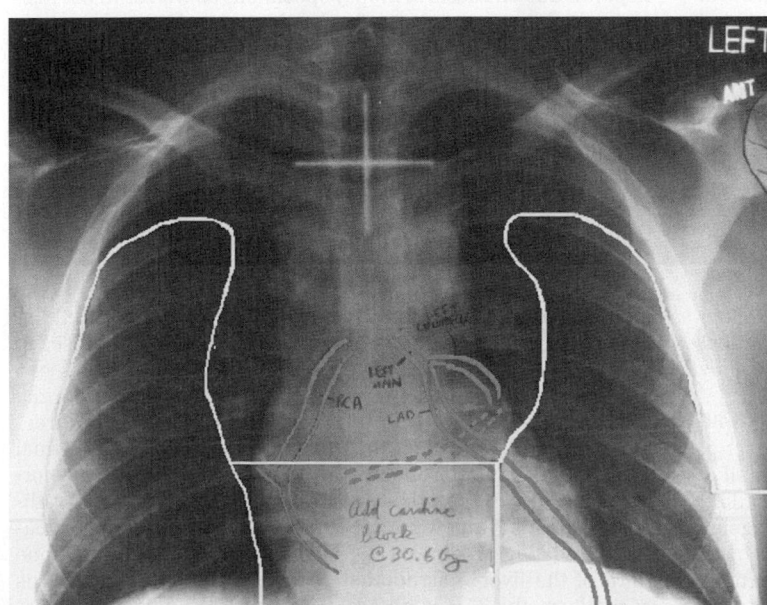

FIGURE 12.12. Location of the coronary vessels is indicated on a standard mantle field. (From King V, Constine LS, Clark D, et al. Symptomatic coronary artery disease after mantle irradiation for Hodgkin's disease. *Int J Radiat Oncol Biol Phys* 1996;36:881–889, with permission.)

the use of subcarinal blocking, the incidence decreases to 2.5%. The onset of delayed acute pericarditis averages 6 months, and 92% of effusions occur within 12 months; even though the effusion usually resolves within 1 to 10 months, it may persist for years. Up to 50% of patients have some degree of tamponade (paradoxic pulse, Kussmaul's sign), occasionally requiring pericardiocentesis. Chronic effusive-constrictive pericarditis develops in 10% to 15% of patients and may require pericardectomy. On the other hand, constriction may present 5 to 50 years after irradiation with no antecedent acute disease. Diuretics are sometimes necessary to control peripheral edema or ascites.

Pancarditis is both rare and severe and probably requires irradiation doses of at least 60 Gy; intractable congestive heart failure can result. Restrictive hemodynamics are demonstrated by catheterization. Myocardiopathy is highly potentiated by doxorubicin, but also occurs in its absence. Right ventricular end-diastolic function also may be reduced by up to 25% in asymptomatic patients, whereas ejection fractions may be decreased in up to 33%.

Fibrous valvular endocardial thickening is found in 80% of patients examined at autopsy who were treated with high irradiation doses. The mitral, aortic, and tricuspid valves are most frequently affected. High-degree atrioventricular conduction abnormalities are rarely seen and have been attributed to fibrosis of the atrioventricular node-conducting branches.

Concern has arisen over the increasing incidence of CAD in two patient populations as they become long-term survivors: early breast cancer survivors, particularly those with cancer of the left breast treated with tangential fields including the anterior portion of the heart, and Hodgkin lymphoma survivors. Among the latter group, several series demonstrate an increased relative risk for CAD of two to three times the normal control population (39,118,131,226). The real concern is among children, especially girls younger than 20 years of age, in whom the highest incidence of CAD is found and relative risk increases to 40% (181). With equilibrium radionuclide angiocardiography and quantitative thallium scintigraphy scans, asymptomatic patients with Hodgkin lymphoma treated at 30 Gy with cardiac shields showed minimal to no significant abnormalities at long-term follow-up (average 10 years) (67).

Eriksson et al. (93) and Rutqvist et al. (300) in Sweden noted an excess of CAD in breast cancer patients receiving postoperative irradiation versus surgery alone, with a relative risk of 3.2 in long-term follow-up of survivors. Of late, most drug–radiation protocols have dose-modified or eliminated doxorubicin, although three reports failed to show any relationship between myocardial infarction and chemotherapy, and one even suggested a decreased risk because the radiation dose to the mediastinum was lowered (39,119,131).

Liver

1. and 2. *Clinical Detection and Time Course of Events.* Radiation-induced liver disease presents as vague-to-intense right upper abdominal pain followed by abdominal swelling due to hepatomegaly and ascites, resulting in weight gain. It is characterized by the development of anicteric ascites 2 to 4 months after irradiation; chemoradiation-induced liver disease occurs more rapidly (e.g., 1 to 4 weeks in a BMT setting).
3. *Dose/Time/Volume.* The whole liver can receive 20 to 30 Gy, with an upper threshold of 33 to 35 Gy and onset of radiation hepatopathy at >35 Gy, whereas a third to half of the liver volume can receive >40 Gy without complication.
4. *Chemical/Biologic Modifiers.* A wide variety of agents have been reported to elevate liver enzymes: nitrosoureas (BCNU), methotrexate, and some combinations of chemotherapy agents such as cyclophosphamide, dox-

orubicin, vincristine, and prednisone (CHOP) and proMace-MOPP (prednisone, methotrexate, doxorubicin, cyclophosphamide, etoposide, and MOPP). In BMT, preparatory regimens can be toxic.
5. *Radiologic Imaging.* Hepatomegaly is observable in moderate-to-severe cases using CT scan.
6. *Laboratory Tests.* Radiation hepatopathy is indicated by increased alkaline phosphatase and aspartate aminotransferase (serum glutamic-oxaloacetic transaminase) with low bilirubin, whereas combined-modality–induced hepatitis has a high increase in bilirubin levels with a low-to-moderate initial elevation of enzymes.
7. *Differential Diagnosis.* Metastatic liver disease can be diagnosed by CT, although laboratory values are altered late. Budd-Chiari syndrome, due to metastases in the portohepatic and paraaortic nodes, can cause hepatic vein occlusion. GVHD can produce liver failure, but is recognizable through the associated features of anemia, leukopenia, skin rash, and adenopathy.
8. *Pathologic Diagnosis.* The characteristic lesion is central vein occlusive disease (VOD) characterized by occlusion and obliteration of the central veins of the hepatic lobules with retrograde congestion and secondary necrosis of hepatocytes. Liver biopsy can yield diagnosis and several characteristic patterns.
9. *Management.* There is no effective treatment to reverse the process; therefore, prophylaxis and prevention are best. Anticoagulants, paracentesis, and diuretics can be used. Liver transplantation is required for frank radiation hepatopathy.
10. *Follow-up.* Intensive medical and nursing care is required to ameliorate the disease, especially if part of the liver has been spared.

Pathophysiology and Cellular Biology

The basic lesion is central vein thrombosis at the lobular level, which results in retrograde congestion leading to hemorrhage and secondary alterations in surrounding hepatocytes (98) (Fig. 12.13). Severe acute hepatic changes often progress to fibrosis or cirrhosis and liver failure.

The pathogenesis of VOD is still obscure, in part because of the difficulty of inducing a radiation hepatopathy in animals. Recently, TGF-β has been implicated as having a role in fibrogenesis, and has been shown to be elevated in the setting of chronic hepatitis and cirrhosis in biopsy specimens as well as in BMT recipients who are at high risk for development of VOD after an intensive chemoradiation conditioning regimen (13,248). VOD is an uncommon, but severe, complication of high-dose chemoradiation administered in preparation for BMT, especially in children (104,136). Thomas et al. (345), studying changes in function in children >5 years of age, observed that fractionated radiation doses of <25 Gy caused abnormal liver function test results and radionuclide scans in approximately 50% of patients, whereas 25 to 35 Gy doses caused abnormalities in 63%, and doses of >35 Gy were highly toxic to 86% of patients.

An increasing number of investigators have emphasized the effect of volume in addition to dose (47,77,78,92,165,338) because although radiation hepatopathy can occur with doses of 35 to 40 Gy to the entire liver, significantly higher doses can be given with few clinical complications if sufficient normal tissue is spared (Fig. 12.14). Of great interest are the three-dimensional dose-volume histogram data in which a normal tissue complication probability model has shown excellent correlation between the calculated and observed incidence of radiation hepatitis (Table 12.12). Normal tissue complication probability modeling predict a TD_5 in excess of 80 Gy if less than one third of the liver is irradiated. With irradiation of two thirds of the liver, the TD_5 is about 50 Gy and TD_{50} is about 60 Gy.

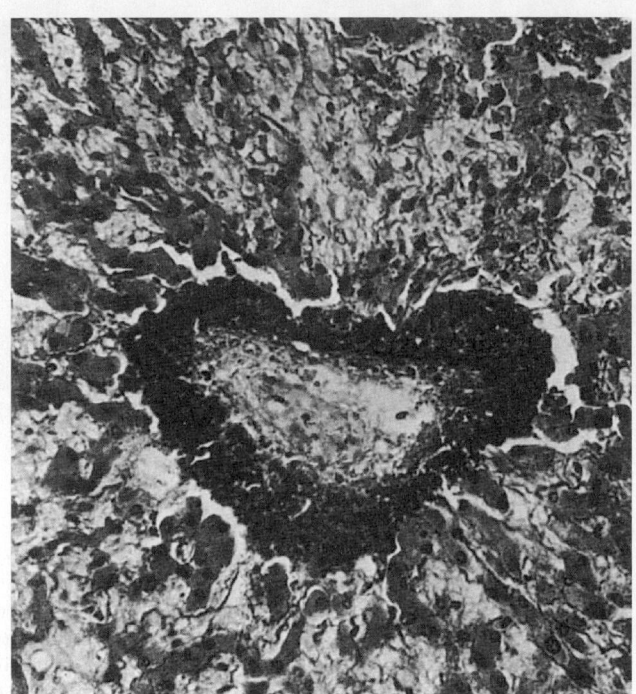 A

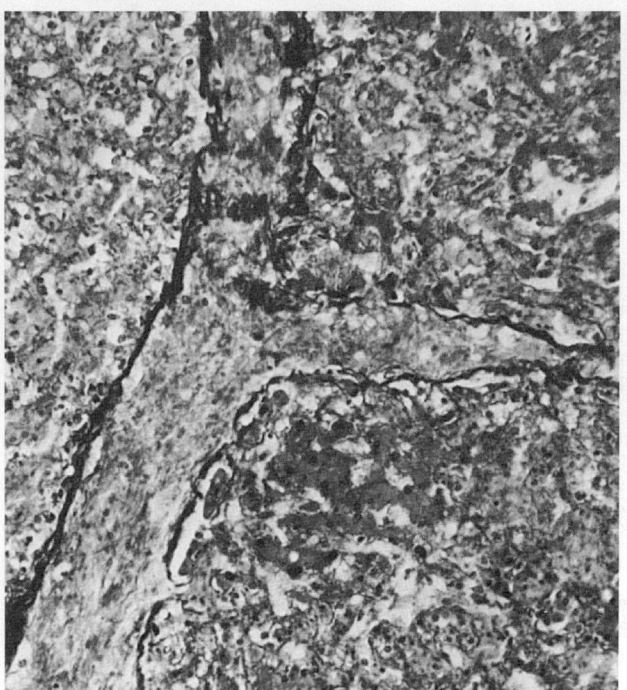 B

FIGURE 12.13. Veno-occlusive liver disease caused by radiation. **A:** Transverse section of a sublobular vein almost completely obstructed by proliferation of fine collagen fibers. The afferent sinusoids are markedly dilated and there is advanced atrophy of the liver cell plates (Gomori's trichrome stain, original magnification ×224). **B:** Longitudinal section of a central vein at the point of confluence with a large vein. The lumen of both veins is totally obliterated by a gray, granular material, which is composed of a mesh of fine reticulin fibers and trapped red cells. The surrounding liver plates are atrophic (Gomori's trichrome stain, original magnification ×160). (From King V, Constine LS, Clark D, et al. Symptomatic coronary artery disease after mantle irradiation for Hodgkin's disease. *Int J Radiat Oncol Biol Phys* 1996;36:881–889, with permission.)

Smaller volumes of liver can receive doses as high as >150 Gy using ^{90}Yttrium glass microspheres delivered via the hepatic artery (51,209,302). Dose = volume constraints have not been published using this approach.

Combined-Modality Therapy

VOD in the setting of BMT is a result of aggressive chemotherapy and TBI, the combination of which has proven additive for untoward effects in the liver, kidney, and lung. Veno-occlusive disease is characterized by occlusion and obliteration of the central veins of the hepatic lobules with retrograde congestion and sec-

ondary necrosis of hepatocytes. Although there may be a dose effect of radiotherapy, this complication is also reported following conditioning regimens with cyclophosphamide and busulfan alone. Pre-existing hepatic disease, including infection, and GVHD may increase the risk. Long-term complications of VOD depend on the severity, but can include hepatic insufficiency or failure and portal hypertension (28,52).

Most studies have supported the view that the dose of radiation in the conditioning regimen is an independent factor in producing VOD (52,273). However, it must be noted that a recent study suggested that the radiation component of the conditioning regimen may be less important than the drug because TBI alone was shown to have a better survival rate and induce less VOD than busulfan/cyclophosphamide (135).

TGF-β acts as a predictor of BMT recipients at risk for VOD (13); Anscher et al. (13) have demonstrated that patients with pretransplantation plasma values of TGF-β greater than two deviations above the mean established for normal control subjects had a 90% probability for development of VOD. The increase in plasma TGF-β after induction chemotherapy also correlated with a patient's risk.

Hepatopathy has been reported in children treated with radiotherapy to the liver for Wilms' tumor and neuroblastoma when radiosensitizing agents such as doxorubicin or dactinomycin are administered as part of the multimodality treatment regimen (345).

Clinical Syndromes

The acute clinical period tends to be silent in the liver; however, progressive damage in the fine vasculature of the liver eventually leads to clinically significant secondary degeneration late in the acute clinical period and beyond, depending on the dose and rate of progression of vascular damage. The sensitivity of

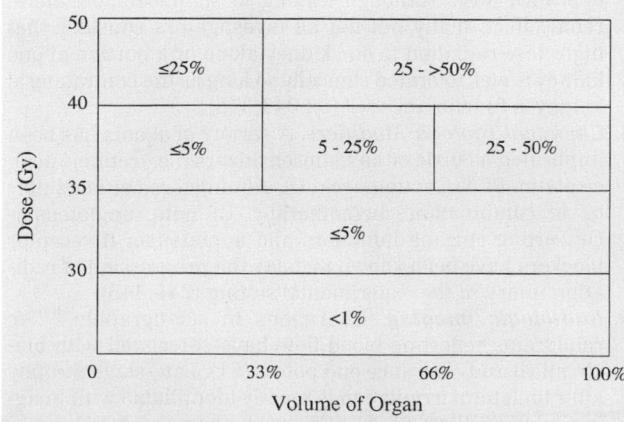

FIGURE 12.14. Schematic diagram depicting the dose-volume relationship to complication. Each box represents the percentage likelihood of developing damage according to the volume of the liver irradiated (x-axis) and radiation dose administered (y-axis).

Table 12.12 THE ESTIMATED 50% RISK OF RADIATION-INDUCED LIVER DISEASE FOR UNIFORM IRRADIATION OF ONE-THIRD, TWO-THIRDS, AND THE WHOLE LIVER[a]

| Year/Reference | No. of Patients | | NTCP Model | 50% Risk of RILD | | |
	With RILD	Total		One-Third Liver	Two-Thirds Liver	Whole Liver
1991 (92)	27[b]	407[b]	None	55 Gy[c]	45 Gy[c]	40 Gy[c]
1991 (47)	27[b]	407[b]	Lyman	57 Gy[c]	46 Gy[c]	40 Gy[c]
1992 (201)	9	79	Lyman	95 Gy	60 Gy	45 Gy
1995 (165)	9	93	D-I	No limit	75 Gy	41 Gy
2000 (338)	19	183	Lyman	>118 Gy	62 Gy	43 Gy
2000 (338)	19	183	D-I	No limit	61 Gy	42 Gy
2000 (338)	19	183	Mean dose	—	—	43 Gy
2002 (77)	19	203	Lyman	>118 Gy	60–70 Gy	40–46 Gy

RILD, radiation-induced liver disease; NTCP, normal tissue complication probability.
[a]In 1.5-Gy twice-daily equivalent dose.
[b]Estimates based on pooled data from multiple publications. Exact number of patients on which partial liver tolerance estimates were based is not available.
[c]2-Gy once-daily equivalent dose.
Adapted from Dawson LA, Ten Haken RK, Lawrence TS. Partial irradiation of the liver. *Semin Radiat Oncol* 2001;11:240–246, with permission.

the liver to radiation injury precludes eradication of infiltrating tumors from this organ by high doses to the total liver. After such doses, a series of pathologic changes occurs in the liver, such as hyperemia, increase in volume, dilatation, congestion of sinusoids, atrophy of hepatocytes, and veno-occlusive lesions appearing as early as 2.5 to 6 months after irradiation (294). Ascites develop, and there is an increase in hepatic size with an increase in alkaline phosphatase levels. When right upper quadrant pain occurs, liver congestion and necrosis can lead to jaundice or the gradual onset of jaundice-related events.

Hepatopathy induced by combined-modality therapy occurs with allogenic BMT, which includes aggressive conditioning regimens and TBI. In contrast to radiation hepatitis, which is expressed months after irradiation, the onset of symptoms typically occurs 1 to 2 weeks after TBI, with jaundice occurring in 98% of patients, in addition to weight gain, right upper quadrant pain, ascites, and hepatomegaly (Table 12.13). Encephalopathy can occur in approximately half of the patients. Combined-modality–induced liver disease differs from subacute radiation-induced liver disease with a significant elevation of bilirubin and subtly elevated alkaline phosphatase levels, whereas the reverse is seen in the latter (273). Other causes of hepatitis must be excluded, such as hepatic vein occlusion due to metastatic retroperitoneal nodes, metastatic liver disease, viral hepatitis, intra-abdominal sepsis, or interstitial infarction.

Kidney

1. ***Clinical Detection.*** Radiation nephropathy is an uncommonly reported toxicity, not because kidneys are radioresistant, but because clinicians carefully respect renal tolerance doses. Five distinct clinical syndromes may overlap in symptoms, signs, and time sequence: acute radiation

Table 12.13 EVALUATION OF LATE INJURY: LIVER

Treatment Factors	Patient/Tumor Factors	Clinical Manifestation
Large volume or dose:	Cirrhosis	Edema
Whole liver >25 Gy	Hepatitis	Weight gain
One-third liver >40 Gy	Tumor-related organ damage	Bleeding
Chemotherapy	Other decreased functional reserve	

nephropathy, chronic radiation nephropathy, benign or malignant hypertension, and hyperreninemic hypertension (Goldblatt's kidney). The signs and symptoms of radiation nephropathy are not distinguishable from other causes of renal damage, and these should be excluded.

2. ***Time Course of Events.*** There is a 6 to 12 month latency period before the expression of acute radiation nephropathy. Chronic radiation nephropathy and hypertension do not develop until after 12 to 18 months. Because renal damage may not manifest for years after treatment, long-term follow-up is important. In one long-term study, the latent period in nearly half of the patients was >10 years (346).

3. ***Dose/Time/Volume.*** With conventional fractionation and normal baseline renal function, the threshold of adult kidney damage is approximately 15 Gy, although there are reports of impaired renal function in children occurring with 12 to 14 Gy (272). Renal tolerance (TD$_{5/5}$, 5% incidence at 5 years) is 20 Gy when both kidneys are irradiated, and doses of more than 25 to 30 Gy to both kidneys are likely to eliminate clinically relevant function in the long term (26,102,162). A pooled analysis of studies in patients treated with TBI (with doses normalized using the linear quadratic model) has shown that a BED of >16 Gy is associated with an increased risk of >16 Gy (175). There is very little published on dose-volume parameters to predict late renal toxicity, in part because clinicians make an effort to minimize the volume of kidney exceeding the accepted tolerance dose. Although leading to significant unilateral renal effect, many but not all investigators consider that high-dose radiation to one kidney alone or a portion of one kidney is well tolerated clinically so long as the contralateral kidney is functioning well (82,243,375).

4. ***Chemical/Biologic Modifiers.*** A variety of agents has been implicated as toxic or as radiosensitizers (i.e., retinoic acid, cisplatin, BCNU, actinomycin D), administered either singly or in combination chemotherapy. Of note, angiotensin-converting enzyme inhibitors and angiotensin II receptor blockers have been shown to delay the progression of radiation injury in the experimental setting (245,246).

5. ***Radiologic Imaging.*** Alterations in scintigraphic ^{99m}Tc renograms reflecting blood flow have correlated with biochemical and clearance end points (81). Late-stage atrophy after unilateral irradiation is readily identifiable with imaging, such as ultrasound or CT.

6. ***Laboratory Tests.*** Alterations in blood urea nitrogen (BUN), creatinine, and creatinine clearance rarely occur in the first 6 months after treatment, but progressive

abnormalities show over time (243,375). Urinary findings consist of microscopic hematuria, proteinuria, and urinary casts. Blood alterations in β_2-microglobulin correlate linearly with both inulin and creatinine clearance, and with later elevations of BUN. Investigators have noted an initial 15% to 20% rise in glomerular filtration rate during a course of treatment to >20 Gy, followed in most cases by a decrease of 20% to 25% of baseline in the following months (24).

7. ***Differential Diagnosis.*** It is unlikely that recurrent cancers in the upper abdomen will mimic these syndromes. Radiation nephropathy should be differentiated from other, more common, causes of renal damage.

8. ***Pathologic Diagnosis.*** Glomerular tuft obliteration and tubular degeneration contribute to the diagnosis and are consistent with radiation nephropathy.

9. ***Management.*** A reduction in renal workload, bed rest, a low-protein diet, and fluid and salt restrictions are required. Correction of anemia using erythropoietin has been recommended. Dialysis and renal transplantation are possible correctional procedures in long-term survivors free of recurrent cancer. Decadron, aspirin, angiotensin-converting enzyme inhibitors, and hyperbaric oxygen all have been proposed to effect some improvement, or at least slow the progression of injury (225,245,364). Vascular surgical approaches or nephrectomy may be curative for hypertension in cases due to renal artery stenosis/fibrosis (289).

10. ***Follow-up.*** Once radiation-induced disease is detected, repeat examination of urinary and serum values and monitoring of blood pressure should be performed.

Pathophysiology and Cellular Biology

The initial injury is clinically silent, and the major focus of change is in the arteriolar-glomerular area rather than the tubular epithelium (97) (Fig. 12.15A). The cortical rather than the medullary tubules are involved, and this involvement usually follows, rather than precedes, vascular alterations. Microangiography dramatically indicates glomerulosclerosis as a function of increasing dose, so that complete obliteration of glomeruli occurs at single doses of 5 to 20 Gy (97) (Fig. 12.15B).

Radiation-induced lesions in the kidney are detected by light microscopy and occur as a progressive replacement of capillary walls and lumina leading to glomerular sclerosis, which precedes tubular atrophy (121). Larger arteries are not affected, whereas glomeruli are being lost. Blood flow was reduced significantly, although variably, 2 to 3 months after irradiation. The evidence suggests that a functional lesion is occurring in the glomerular capillaries and precedes tubular depletion.

After TBI, nephrosclerotic changes occur that are consistent with progressive arteriolonephrosclerosis due to degeneration of arterioles or capillaries. Experiments in mice show that single radiation doses of more than 19 Gy to both kidneys caused renal failure and death, whereas 11 Gy allowed a 90% survival rate (121). Months after single doses of up to 15 Gy to both kidneys in rats, the glomerular filtration rates and urine osmolality progressively deteriorated and the systolic blood pressure increased. However, recovery was observed after lower doses (174).

Renal tolerance ($TD_{5/5}$) is 20 Gy when both kidneys are irradiated (54). A dose-response curve (24,54,81,180,203,213,346) (Fig. 12.16) shows an approximate threshold dose of 15 Gy (conventional fractionation) and a plateau at 40 Gy. Pediatric radiation tolerance in the kidney is somewhat lower than it is in adults, but is surprisingly closer than in most other organs. Doses to infants of 12 to 14 Gy lead to chemical alterations (272,327). Growth arrest occurs in developing kidneys at 20 to 30 Gy after unilateral irradiation (301). There also are data to suggest that unilateral irradiation to doses of 14 to 20 Gy may reduce or eliminate the ability of the contralateral (untreated) kidney to undergo compensatory hypertrophy (53). Minimum periods of follow-up of 8 years have been possible in patients receiving unilateral irradiation of the stomach (for peptic ulcer to suppress acid formation) compared with bilaterally irradiated patients (346). A 17% incidence of symptomatic renal disease at 20 Gy was found, with the majority of patients dying of related renal disease; 46% had measurable abnormalities.

Combined-Modality Therapy

When combined-modality treatment is used, additive or enhanced effects can occur. Of concern are multidrug

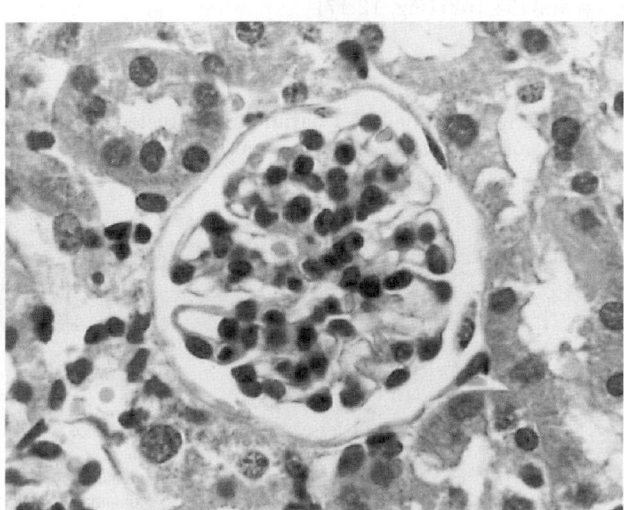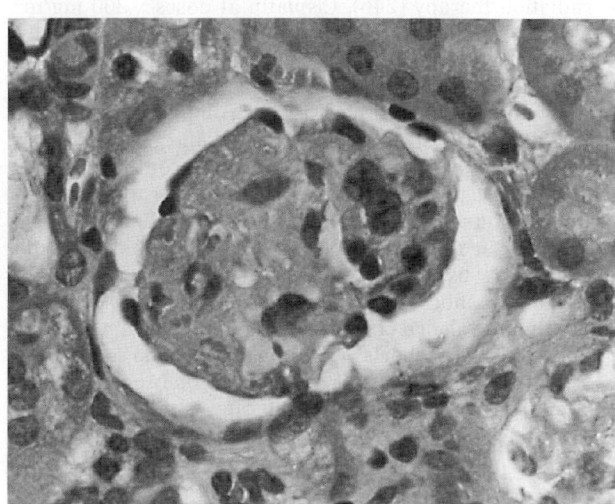

A   B

FIGURE 12.15. Radiation nephropathy. **A:** A section of normal murine kidney, with a glomerulus in the center, surrounded by tubules (mainly proximally convoluted). Notice the regular distribution of small, dense nuclei in the glomerular tuft and the multiple, well-defined capillary lumina. **B:** Section of a kidney 9 months after 4,500 cGy in 10 fractions given to the kidneys *in situ.* Notice the increase in the density of the glomerular tuft, which no longer has capillary lumina. Glomerular nuclei are irregularly distributed, and some are also enlarged. Some of the tubules (*upper left, lower right*) are atrophic. Radiation nephropathy in humans and other mammals affects primarily glomeruli and tubules and eventually results in atrophy with fibrosis. Arteries are compromised secondarily, probably as the result of hypertension (**A** and **B**, hematoxylin and eosin, original magnification ×650). (From Fajardo LF. Morphology of radiation effects on normal tissues. In: Perez CA, Brady LW, eds. *Principles and practice of radiation oncology,* 2nd ed. Philadelphia: JB Lippincott; 1992:114–123.)

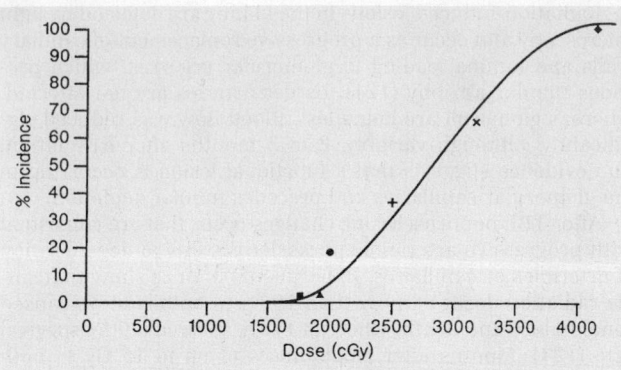

FIGURE 12.16. Dose-response curve for renal intolerance (TD$_{5/5}$) generated from data presented in several series in the literature (54). Thompson et al. (346); ν, Dewit et al. (81); σ, Avioli et al. (24); $+$, Luxton (213); υ, Lebesque (203); and X, Kim et al. (180).

combinations used in children requiring BMT. Hemolytic anemia and renal insufficiency using combinations, such as VM-26, cytarabine, and cyclophosphamide or VM-26, melphalan, and cisplatin, develop in almost one third of the patients receiving these agents with TBI of 12 to 14 Gy given in six to eight fractions (127). However, such concerns are not limited to children. A 14% incidence of renal dysfunction occurred in adults receiving transplants, primarily for leukemia and non-Hodgkin's lymphoma (202). In 79 patients treated with TBI to 10 to 13.5 Gy with conditioning consisting of high-dose cyclophosphamide, with or without other chemotherapy agents, 77% were free of renal dysfunction at 18 months. TBI dose and the presence of GVHD were significantly correlated with renal dysfunction so that patients receiving a high dose of radiation and GVHD had a 48% predicted rate of renal dysfunction (239).

Agents used in the treatment of Wilms' tumor, such as dactinomycin, vincristine, cyclophosphamide, and doxorubicin, lead to little injury when combined without irradiation; however, they lead to earlier appearance of lesions when administered with low, nontoxic irradiation doses. Changes usually seen at threshold doses of 20 Gy can occur at 10 Gy with multiagent chemotherapy. In a rat model, the most toxic sequence occurred when chemotherapy (cisplatin) was given before rather than after radiation therapy (246). Cisplatin at doses >200 mg/m^2 can result in glomerular or tubular injury and renal insufficiency. Other nephrotoxic agents such as aminoglycosides, amphotericin, and ifosfamide may further increase risk. Effects can be seen acutely and may progress after completion of therapy (33,160,230). Ifosfamide can also cause glomerular and tubular toxicity, with renal tubular acidosis and Fanconi's syndrome. Doses >60 to 100 g/m^2, age under 5 years at time of treatment, and combination with cisplatin and carboplatin increase risk. Abnormalities in glomerular filtration are less common, and when found are usually not clinically significant. More common are abnormalities with proximal > distal tubular function, although the prevalence of these findings is uncertain and further study of larger cohorts with longer follow-up is required (20,21,279,321). The effects of these chemotherapeutic agents may be more relevant when radiotherapy is delivered to the kidneys.

Renal Dysfunction after Irradiation

Rubin and Casarett (294) combined autopsy and clinical data to define different periods in the progression of renal dysfunction after irradiation:

- The acute period (up to 6 months) is rarely symptomatic, and a decreased glomerular filtration rate may be present.

- In the subacute period (6 to 12 months), the signs and symptoms include dyspnea on exertion, headaches, ankle edema, lassitude, anemia, hypertension, albuminuria, papilledema, elevated blood urea, and urinary abnormalities (granular and hyalin casts, red blood cells). Death may occur from chronic uremia or left ventricular failure, pulmonary edema, pleural effusion, and hepatic congestion.
- In the chronic period (usually after 18 months), either benign or malignant hypertension is seen, depending on the severity of the renal insult.
- Chronic radiation nephropathy in its mildest form is referred to as hyperreninemic hypertension secondary to a scarred encapsulated kidney (Goldblatt's kidney) and may not be diagnosed until 10 to 14 years after therapy (54,180). The only abnormalities may be proteinuria and azotemia with urinary casts, and mild or no hypertension. A contracted renal size (mild atrophy) is seen on intravenous pyelography. When chronic nephropathy is severe, death may result.

Clinical Syndromes

In a typical acute course with alterations in renal parameters there is an initial increase in glomerular filtration rate and renal plasma flow due to glomerular vasodilatation and permeability, which later decreases as tuft scarring occurs (Table 12.14). More conventional measurements (BUN, creatinine serum, and clearance) are not altered. Analytic scales note proteinuria at <3 g/L, 3 to 10 g/L, and >10 g/L for grades 1, 2, and 3, respectively, with nephrotic syndrome as grade 4.

In humans, dose-response data after high single-dose exposure to both kidneys are scarce. Fractionated doses of 10 to 20 Gy cause a decrease in the glomerular filtration rate, a 38% to 87% reduction in renal plasma flow, and suppression of tubular excretory capacity up to 12 months after therapy. However, the BUN and maximum urinary concentrating ability remain normal after these doses. If the entire single kidney is treated with fractionated doses of >26 Gy, a laboratory trend to increased creatinine clearance is seen that does not translate into a clinically relevant alteration in renal function (Table 12.15). Overall, kidney failure after fractionated irradiation was calculated to be 23 Gy for a TD$_{5/5}$ and 28 Gy for a TD$_{50/5}$ (50% incidence at 5 years) (54,102) (Fig. 12.17).

Gastrointestinal Tract and Dentition

The description of the LENT paradigm is directed at the longest sections of the GI tract and those most vulnerable to radiation injury: the small and large intestines.

	Table 12.14	**EVALUATION OF LATE INJURY: KIDNEY**	
Treatment Factors	**Patient/Tumor Factors**	**Clinical Manifestations**	
Large volume	Decreased functional reserve	High blood pressure	
High dose	Nephrectomy	Hematuria	
Chemotherapy (e.g., cisplatin, ifosfamide)	Chronic renal failure or insufficiency	Oliguria	
Region irradiated:	Tumor-related damage or obstruction	Edema	
Hilum vs. parenchymal	Infancy	Obtundation	
Bilateral vs. unilateral	Hypertension		

Table 12.15	DECREASE IN MEAN CREATININE CLEARANCE AFTER UNILATERAL RADIATION THERAPY TO >26 GY			
Time	N	Mean Creatinine	Mean Creatinine Clearance	% Change Mean Creatinine Clearance
Before radiation therapy	86	1.0	79	
Years 1–5	86	1.1	65	−15
Years 6–10	27	1.2	64	−22
Years >10	17	1.3	51	−37

N, number of observations.
From Morris MM, Willett CG. Late renal function after upper abdominal irradiation. *Int J Radiat Oncol Biol Phys* 1997;39[Suppl 2]:284(abstr); and Willett CG, Tepper JE, Orlow EL, et al. Renal complications secondary to radiation treatment of upper abdominal malignancies. *Int J Radiat Oncol Biol Phys* 1986;12:1601–1604, with permission.

1. **Clinical Detection.** Onset of symptoms in the acute phase is increased stool frequency, with a loss of form into diarrheal fluid. Late effects could persist in this fashion, but melena, obstruction, and weight loss may also be present. With increasing understanding and the use of conformal treatments, late obstructions and fistula formation are becoming rare as late complications. Bleeding is the most distressing symptom, and changes from melena to bright red blood if the injury is to the rectosigmoid or lower in the bowel.

2. **Time Course of Events.** Acute symptoms of diarrhea during therapy bear no relation to late effects of stricture and ulceration, which may present anywhere from 6 months to 3 years after therapy.

3. **Dose/Time/Volume.** Tolerance doses range between 45 and 70 Gy in the absence of other predisposing factors. In general, stomach and small bowel dose should be limited to 45 Gy and colon to 50 to 54 Gy, whereas esophagus and rectum can tolerate doses of 60 to 70 Gy. Volume and circumference exposure play a critical role.

4. **Chemical/Biologic Modifiers.** Most often, 5-fluorouracil (5-FU) infusions are well tolerated with irradiation, but prolonged maintenance on high doses of chemotherapy can lead to injury when the irradiation threshold is reached. Patients with pre-existing inflammatory bowel disease, prior pelvic surgery, pelvic inflammatory disease, or di-

abetes have demonstrated increased risk of GI toxicity (86,270,330,374). Future strategies to reduce bowel toxicity include the use of radiation protectors, cytokines, enterotrophic interventions, as well as modulators of intraluminal factors, endothelial dysfunction, and neuroimmune interactions (137).

5. **Radiologic Imaging.** Plain films of the abdomen can show obstruction patterns of dilated bowel loops. Barium meals can identify a loss of the feathery mucosal surface on the haustral markings after persistent stricture and narrowing or shallow ulceration with perforation. CT and MRI can show ulceration and fused bowel loops.

6. **Laboratory Tests.** The most frequent abnormal findings are malabsorption of bile salts and fat.

7. **Differential Diagnosis.** Recurrent abdominal malignancies can lead to obstruction and stricture and must be excluded. Hemorrhoids are a more common cause of rectal bleeding than postradiation therapy injury.

8. **Pathologic Diagnosis.** The classic lesion in resected specimens of intestine is infarction necrosis associated with arterial thromboses and sclerosis or gliosis and microvasculature obliteration in the bowel wall. Confluent regions of telangiectatic submucosal vessels correlate with rectal bleeding.

9. **Management.** Conservative measures are antiemetic and antidiarrheal agents in the acute phase. Low-grade rectal bleeding is transient and responsive to steroids. Higher-grade late rectal bleeding may require transfusion or coagulation procedures. Once serious bleeding occurs and the danger of ulceration and perforation exists, surgical resection of the affected loops can be lifesaving.

10. **Follow-up.** Once detected, the radiation injury needs careful scrutiny.

Pathophysiology and Cellular Biology

The mucosa is a rapid renewal system, with dramatic mucosal changes appearing within 7 to 14 days, with regenerating foci of epithelium occurring with zones of complete denudation. Indeed, complete epithelial regeneration of the esophagus can occur 3 months to 2 years after irradiation.

Progressive endarteritis is the critical radiation lesion for late effects in the alimentary tract (97) (Fig. 12.18). It results in either ulceration and infarction necrosis with more rapid obliteration of vessels or an increasing slow fibrosis and stricture of the bowel with gradual narrowing of the fine vasculature. Unlike the acute mucosal loss and gradual return of regenerative epithelial clonogenic clusters in bowel crypts after irradiation, late ulceration is spotty and focal. The long axis of the ulcer is transverse, similar to ulcers that occur in obliterative vasculitis of other origins. Gastric ulcers are typically antral and solitary and measure 0.5 to 2 cm in size (94). Fistulae and perforations are focal and transmural, representing geographic loss of a segment of mucosa and its smooth musculature. However, this cannot be explained in classic fashion by the simultaneous cellular hypoplasia of two different cell populations (i.e., the mucosa and the smooth muscle cells). Indeed, the association of obliterative endoarteritis with zones of necrosis and perforation indicates infarction necrosis of the supplying vessels as an essential mechanism. In addition, if mucosal surfaces are intact with endoarteritis as an underlying defect, it requires an event such as surgical handling or trauma to result in the clinical manifestation of late effects. Thus, surgical handling of bowel and freeing of adhesions months to years after irradiation may interfere with a tenuous blood supply and precipitate alterations in hemodynamics, leading to repeated operations for infarction necrosis.

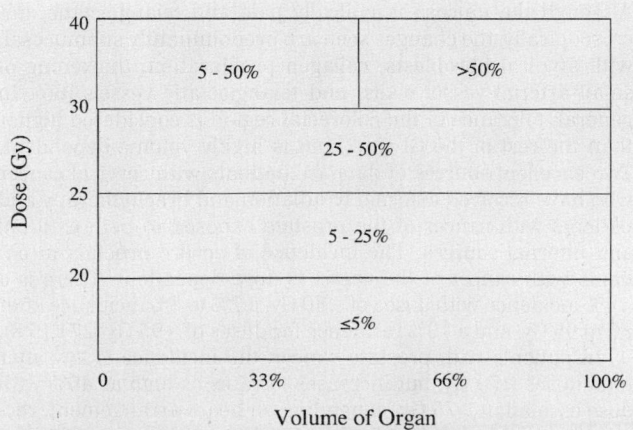

FIGURE 12.17. Schematic diagram depicting the dose-volume relationship to complication. Each box represents the percentage likelihood of developing damage according to the volume of the single kidney irradiated (x-axis) and radiation dose administered (y-axis).

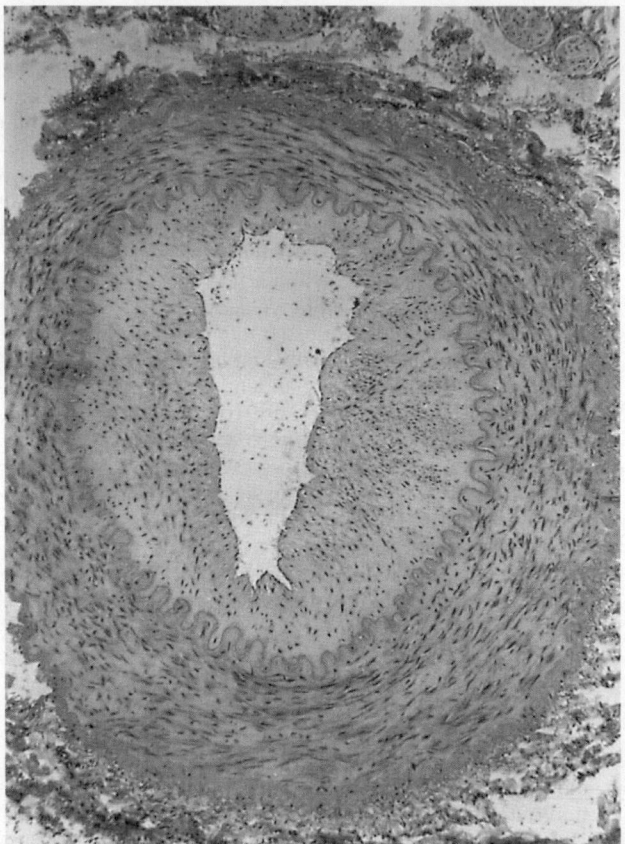

FIGURE 12.18. Gastric artery showing concentric myointimal proliferation years after therapy (unknown dose) for adjacent neoplasm. Most of the tissue between the wavy internal elastic membrane and the reduced lumen is an abnormal growth of myocytes, fibroblasts, and collagen. (From Fajardo LF. Morphology of radiation effects on normal tissues. In: Perez CA, Brady LW, eds. *Principles and practice of radiation oncology*, 2nd ed. Philadelphia: JB Lippincott; 1992:114–123.)

Esophagus

An RTOG study reported an incidence of pharyngeal/cervical esophageal late effects in 6% of patients treated after surgery with 60 Gy during 6 weeks versus 1% treated to 50 Gy for 5 weeks before surgery (186). Higher rates of delayed stricture, up to 20%, are reported when chemotherapy is added to 60 Gy irradiation (66). Emami and colleagues (92) calculated the tolerance doses ($TD_{5/5}$) for strictures or ulceration as 60 Gy for a third of the esophagus and 55 Gy when the whole esophagus was treated. Supplemental intraluminal brachytherapy as a boost after irradiation also confers an increased risk of ulceration and perforation: A 90% rate of ulceration occurred when a single fraction of 20 Gy given intraluminally supplemented a fractionated 60 Gy dose, according to Hishikawa et al. (146). Dosimetric parameters shown to significantly influence risk of late toxicity are maximal and mean esophageal dose, as well as the volume, surface and length of esophagus receiving >50 to 60 Gy (7,215,320). Duke University research has shown that with 32% of the volume or 32% of the surface receiving >50 Gy, the risk of late toxicity is predicted to be ~30% versus 7% in those with less volume or surface receiving >50 Gy (215).

After radiation treatment, abnormal peristalsis starts at the site of irradiation and progresses caudally. The cause of this esophageal dysmotility is thought to be the microscopic hyalinization of the muscularis propria layer, although manometry findings support neuronal damage as the culprit (98). Strictures are the end result of progressive, severe submucosal fibrosis.

Stomach

Considerable data have been gathered since the original Walter Reed Army Medical Center experience, when the treatment of testicular tumors with 40 to 60 Gy led to incidental gastric hemorrhage (44). The LENT review showed that at low doses of 40 to 50 Gy, ulcerations and perforations were uncommon (~5%); 50 to 60 Gy resulted in a 10% rate of ulcers within 5 months; doses of 55 to 64 Gy resulted in a 14% rate of ulceration associated with a 64% rate of gastric injury and a 34% rate of gastritis, whereas no ulcers occurred with doses below 45 Gy (66). Studies in patients with Hodgkin lymphoma have demonstrated the effect of prior surgery and dose fractionation as factors in gastric tolerance (112,178). Ulcerations were seen at a rate of 42% in patients undergoing staging laparotomy and a dose per fraction of 3.3 Gy, whereas the rate was 5% for those without laparotomy and a dose per fraction of 2.5 Gy.

Small Intestine

The threshold for minimal effect is 50 Gy, but there is a steep dose-response curve using daily conventional fractions of 1.8 to 2 Gy. The incidence of small bowel injury is 15% to 25% if paraaortic irradiation doses are 50 to 55 Gy (277), whereas 45 to 50 Gy is well tolerated (274). Perez and colleagues (271) found a 1% incidence of small bowel toxicity with a pelvic sidewall dose of ≤50 Gy and a 5% incidence at >70 Gy; fractionated doses induce a 15% increased incidence of severe late complications when more than 2 Gy per fraction is used (132). Eifel and associates (86), in a 20-year follow-up study of patients with cervical cancer, noted an increase in the complication rate over time. Again, dose per fraction is an important determinant of radiation-related duodenal ulcers.

The terminal ileum is most frequently symptomatically damaged; cell turnover rate is the principal factor in the temporal chain because cell replacement in the crypts and villi occurs every 3 to 6 days. Pathologic changes include a cessation of mitosis, crypt cell pyknosis, fragmentation, and swelling and vacuolation of the cells in the enteric mucosa. After 6 to 8 hours, mucosal cells demonstrate a transient proliferation with a burst of atypical mitoses and, over the next 48 hours, cell loss without renewal is progressive with shortening of the crypts and villi. Subsequently, the villi show progressive denudation resulting in a loss of protein and electrolytes. With lower doses, recovery with a chronic reaction may ensue; the submucosa is most severely affected. Collagen and bizarre fibroblasts replace fatty tissue, and vascular lesions occur. Delayed effects can take 10 years or more to develop.

Colorectum

Although the mucosa is typically pale and telangiectatic, microscopically, the changes seen are predominantly submucosal, with atypical fibroblasts, collagen proliferation, thickening of small arterial vessel walls, and telangiectatic vessels (66). In general, tolerance in the colorectal region is considered higher than the rest of the GI tract, but is highly volume-dependent. Two excellent sources of data are patients with cervical cancer who have received external irradiation and brachytherapy and patients with cancer of the prostate exposed to both external and internal sources. The incidence of severe proctitis in patients with cancer of the cervix is dose-dependent: There is a <4% incidence with doses of <80 Gy, a 7% to 8% incidence after 80 to 95 Gy, and a 13% incidence for doses of ≥95 Gy (271,278).

In patients with prostate cancer, the incidence is low after total doses <70 Gy, but increases to rates as high as 40% with dose escalation >75 Gy, depending on beam arrangement, rectal shielding, and dose (35,134,310). Volume is particularly important with dose escalation using three-dimensional dynamic conformal therapy with doses of ≤80 Gy to the prostate. Less than a third of the circumference exposure to high dose is

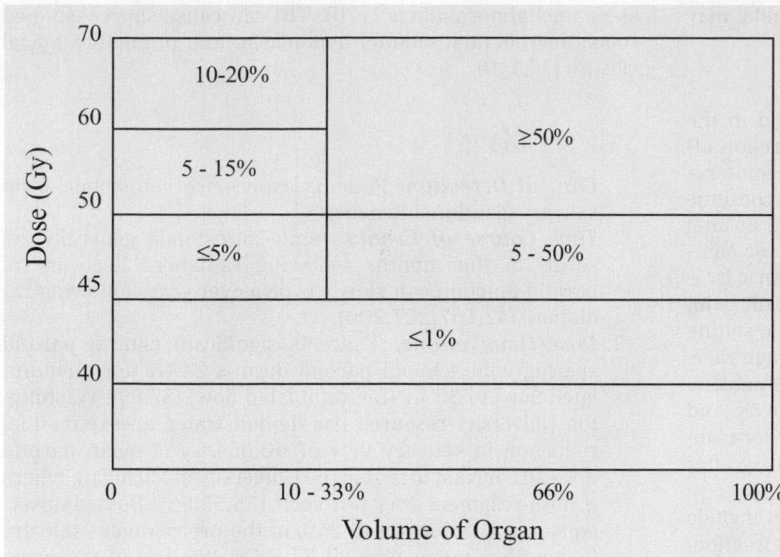

FIGURE 12.19. Schematic diagram depicting the dose-volume relationship to complication. Each box represents the percentage likelihood of developing damage according to the volume of the gastrointestinal tract irradiated (x-axis) and radiation dose administered (y-axis).

essential, but the smaller the circumference and the lower the volume irradiated, the better higher doses are tolerated (Fig. 12.19). Studies from Pollack et al. (276) and Huang et al. (157) have shown that the risk of late rectal complications is a continuous function of dose and volume; in one study the risk was 46% if ≥25% of the rectal volume received ≥70 Gy as opposed to 16% if <25% received ≥70 Gy. Several other groups have confirmed the importance of dose-volume histogram values in predicting late toxicity, with both the volume of rectum and volume of rectal wall being predictive (101,164,193,325,363,369). Preliminary results suggest a drastic reduction in GI toxicity for prostate therapy with intensity modulated radiation therapy owing to the increased ability to spare normal tissues (383).

Combined-Modality Therapy

Chemotherapy alone does not appear to produce significant late GI complications with any frequency, despite the well-documented acute toxicity caused by a long list of agents (240). Late effects such as GI bleeding and damage to the small and large bowel, with chronic malabsorption related to radiotherapy, may be worsened with administration of radiation sensitizing agents such as doxorubicin or dactinomycin.

Esophagus

Acute radiation effects in the esophagus are enhanced by cisplatin, 5-FU, actinomycin D, doxorubicin, bleomycin, taxanes, and methotrexate, with only a 1.6% incidence of severe esophagitis with doses <60 Gy. The simultaneous delivery of ≥60 Gy of radiation and systemic chemotherapy agents increases the incidence of esophagitis and late benign stricture to 11% (65), with doxorubicin being of special concern, with an increased incidence of 20% (123). Bougienage relieves benign stricture in 85% of patients, allowing for a return to a normal diet; when dilatation is used, the most effective median interval between dilatations is 5 months, with 2.5 dilatations as the median number required for success (254).

Stomach

There is no apparent increase in late gastric injury after doses of 45 to 50 Gy with concurrent 5-FU compared with similar doses without the drug. In pancreatic cancers, doxorubicin and mitomycin-C in combination with irradiation have been well tolerated (66).

Small Intestine

Most of the evidence suggests 5-FU infusion as a bolus with irradiation doses ranging from 45 to 50 Gy is well tolerated, with few reports of late toxicity. However, concurrent doxorubicin and actinomycin D enhance risk for intestinal complications (253).

Colorectum

The absence of predictive parameters for late intestinal events was demonstrated in the catastrophic complications that occurred in a carefully piloted Eastern Cooperative Oncology Group study using split-course irradiation (60 Gy in 10 weeks, 20 Gy per 2-week courses × 3 with 2-week rest intervals) and maintenance chemotherapy (5-FU and methyl CCNU [semustine]) for 1 year (75,76). Although no undue acute toxicity occurred with either radiation therapy or chemotherapy, fistulization and necrosis occurred in 29% of patients 6 months to 2 years after all therapy ceased. In general, 5-FU alone added to 45 to 50 Gy is well tolerated, but the addition of mitomycin-C raises the rate of grade 3 toxicity to 25% (72) and the addition of cisplatin in cervix cancer leads to an 18% large bowel complication rate (125).

Clinical Syndromes

Esophagus

Acutely, odynophagia and dysphagia are seen and may relate to either focal erosions or abnormal esophageal peristalsis. Dysmotility is seen, with an onset of 4 to 12 weeks after the start of radiation therapy and earlier with concurrent chemotherapy. In the long term, dysphagia is the most common symptom and reflects continued abnormal peristalsis. Severe submucosal fibrosis can lead to stricture in 1% to 5% of patients, with a typical onset at 3 to 18 months after treatment; risk may be further increased by coexisting inflammatory conditions (e.g., acquired immunodeficiency syndrome) (70). However, strictures can occur many years after therapy (98,158). Late ulceration, particularly at the gastroesophageal junction, is uncommon, but may occur with higher doses, particularly after intraluminal brachytherapy, after which pseudodiverticula, sinus tracts, and fistula formation are also possible.

Management of acute esophagitis can include analgesics, topical anesthetics, sucralfate, and nystatin. Antacids or histamine-2 blockers can be helpful in patients with a component of gastric reflux. Late stricture is managed by esophageal dilatation, and prokinetic drugs, such as metoclopramide, may lessen gastroesophageal reflux.

Stomach

The radiosensitivity of the gastric mucosa is reflected in the early depression of hydrochloric acid and pepsin secretion after modest radiation doses of 15 to 20 Gy. Although some recovery of cellular structure occurs, suppression can continue for 6 months to many years after irradiation. Usually, at total doses ≥50 Gy, cellular and functional recovery is never complete. Ulcers are the most common complication of gastric irradiation, and present clinically with dyspepsia, significant pain, and sometimes hemorrhage. An ulcer in this anatomic setting can lead to hemorrhage and perforation which, although rare, can be fatal. Ulcerations have been described as typically antral, perhaps because of placement of radiation therapy fields, and develop as early as 2 to 12 months after treatment. Pyloric obstruction may be a late development related to fibrosis after ulcer healing.

Management of acute nausea and vomiting should include antiemetics and consideration of a reduced dose per fraction. However, there are few data on the management of late toxicities from radiation therapy. Severe complications may require surgical management, such as a partial gastrectomy.

Small Intestine

The early onset of malabsorption of fat and hypermotility after modest doses of radiation illustrates the radiosensitivity of the small intestine. Usually, recovery at dose levels below 40 to 45 Gy occurs, although some persistence of small bowel dysfunction and mesenteric cramping may be noted. Surgical intervention and adhesions can precipitate a more serious course of events. Higher doses result in diarrhea, malabsorption of fat, and leakage of albumin into the bowel. If an obliterative arteritis develops, the risk of infarction and perforation remains despite recovery. The underlying lesion is one of ulceration and segmental enteritis that can lead to stenosis of the bowel lumen, with varying degrees of obstruction during the chronic period.

Management of mild late injury is best with a low-residue diet and stool softeners, and loperamide as needed. Cholestyramine can be useful for diarrhea caused by small bowel injury. Where required for small bowel obstruction, a conservative bypass surgical approach should be favored over aggressive lysis of adhesions and resection (66).

Colorectum

The manifestations of radiation injury in the colon and rectum are less marked than those in the small intestine after similar doses. The initial reaction of hypermotility at modest levels of 10 to 20 Gy rapidly disappears. However, if constipation is a later complication, roughage can traumatize the bowel surface mucosa. Tenesmus may be obscured by the simultaneous onset of diarrhea if a large segment of small bowel is treated in addition to the rectum. Higher doses can cause painless rectal bleeding that is rarely fatal, and can occur at a median of 12 months but up to 3 years or more after treatment (339). Segmental colitis and rectal strictures are major concerns (164,310).

Management of low-grade rectal bleeding with steroids is often successful. Unresponsive bleeding from ulcerated areas may be cauterized or controlled by endoscopic laser treatment. Rectal bleeding may require transfusion (166).

Dentition

In children, doses of 20 to 40 Gy can cause root shortening or abnormal curvature, dwarfism, and hypocalcification (214). Doses of >40 Gy may result in mandibular or maxillary hypoplasia, increased caries, hypodontia, microdontia, root stunting, and xerostomia (266). Chemotherapy for the treatment of leukemia can cause shortening and thinning of the premolar roots, as well

as enamel abnormalities (176). TBI can cause short V-shaped roots, microdontia, enamel hypoplasia, and premature apical closure (74,149).

Salivary Glands

1. *Clinical Detection.* Patients experience xerostomia from salivary gland insufficiency.
2. *Time Course of Events.* Acute xerostomia generally resolves in the months following radiation. Recovery of parotid function can slowly evolve over years following radiation. (42,167,227,290).
3. *Dose/Time/Volume.* There is significant clinical parotid sparing with a mean parotid dose < 24 Gy (for unstimulated flow) to 26 Gy (for stimulated flow) (87,89). Washington University research has demonstrated an exponential reduction in salivary flow of ~0.054/Gy of mean parotid dose, in contrast to that of the University of Michigan, where a dose-response was not seen (35,55,56). Both datasets equate to a reduction to 25% of the pretreatment salivary flow with a mean dose of 25.8 Gy. Because of the proximity of the parotid to the level II lymphatics, intensity-modulated radiation therapy is often used in the treatment of head and neck patients to reduce the parotid dose and prevent xerostomia. Other groups have corroborated the mean dose as a significant variable impacting salivary function (8,48,247,260,291). Animal data suggest the possibility of regional variation of parotid gland susceptibility to damage, which would imply that a mean dose model may not be ideal for predicting xerostomia (184).
4. *Chemical/Biologic Modifiers.* Chemotherapy alone can result in xerostomia, although the effect is often less severe and temporary. Concurrent chemotherapy and radiation may exacerbate the risk of late xerostomia. Amifostine has been shown to be effective in reducing the risk of late xerostomia (87,185,304).
5. *Radiologic Imaging.* Quantitative salivary gland scintigraphy can be used to study salivary gland function, although it is not routinely used (247).
6. *Laboratory Tests.* Stimulated and unstimulated salivary flow can be used to quantify the extent of salivary flow (88). Pretreatment baseline and posttreatment salivary flow can be assessed.
7. *Differential Diagnosis.* Many prescription medications can cause xerostomia; these should be eliminated in patients with presumed radiation-induced xerostomia. Nerve damage after surgery can also hamper saliva production. Other common causes include dehydration, both autoimmune (i.e., Sjogren's syndrome) and idiopathic (often in the elderly).
8. *Pathologic Diagnosis.* This is generally unnecessary.
9. *Management.* Most patients opt to carry a water bottle with them. Other therapeutic options include mechanical stimulation (i.e., sugarless gum), cholinergic drugs (side effects include sweating and flushing), and artificial saliva or other oral lubricants. Patients with teeth should undergo routine dental evaluation; prophylactic fluoride treatments may be warranted. Patients should avoid sugary foods and drinks, and cleanse their mouth regularly after eating.
10. *Follow-up.* Patients should be seen for routine follow-up to address symptoms of late toxicity.

Pathophysiology and Cellular Biology

Late histopathologic changes associated with salivary radiation are characterized by loss of serous acini, dilation of the ducts, and fibrosis. The mucinous epithelium and ducts are less sensitive to radiation, resulting in more mucinous saliva production.

Clinical Syndrome

Parotid glands generate ~60% of saliva, and the majority of serous saliva, with the remainder of saliva secreted by submandibular, sublingual, and minor salivary glands. Therefore, the parotid glands have been a major focus of investigation. After radiation damage, salivary flow is reduced, the saliva is more mucinous and more concentrated, and has a lower pH. Patients are at a higher risk of oral candidiasis. Impaired salivary function can lead to difficulty chewing, swallowing, or talking. The risk of dental caries is increased.

The Endocrine System: Neuroendocrine

1. *Clinical Detection.* Growth hormone (GH) production is the more sensitive to radiation than adrenalcorticotropic hormone (ACTH) or thyrotropin-releasing hormone (TRH). GH deficiency results in inadequate growth velocity and inadequate pubertal growth spurt. In adults, GH deficiency may be asymptomatic or result in decreased muscle mass relative to adipose tissue. ACTH deficiency can cause muscle weakness, skin hyperpigmentation, hypotension, dehydration, and anorexia. TRH deficiency can result in classic symptoms of hypothyroidism such as weight gain, cold intolerance, dry skin, brittle hair, cold intolerance, menstrual irregularities, hypotension, and bradycardia; poor linear growth can also occur. Gonadotropin deficiency causes diminished sex hormone production, resulting in delayed puberty. Other signs and symptoms of sex hormone deficiency are discussed in the Reproductive Endocrine section. Precocious puberty can also be a result of radiation. The cause of this effect is unclear, although it relates to hypothalamic deregulation, and it seems to effect girls more so than boys. Radiation can also cause hyperprolactinemia, resulting in infertility and diminished libido; females can also experience menstrual irregularities, galactorrhea, hot flashes, and osteopenia.

2. *Time Course of Events.* The time course of events is highly variable, depending on the radiation dose, patient age during radiation, and patient age at assessment for late effects.

3. *Dose/Time/Volume.* GH deficiency and precocious puberty can occur after doses >18 to 20 Gy to the hypothalamic-pituitary axis, and TRH deficiency, ACTH deficiency, and hyperprolactinemia can occur after doses >40 to 50 Gy (see previous discussion).

4. *Chemical/Biologic Modifiers.* Busulfan and cyclophosphamide increase risk of late side effects (329).

5. *Radiologic Imaging.* Clinical assessment is based on clinical and laboratory testing. Plain radiographs of several growth centers (e.g., wrist and elbow) can be used to assess bone age.

6. *Laboratory Tests.* GH can be assessed by an insulin stimulation test and analysis of pulsatile GH secretion. ACTH can be assessed by the insulin hypoglycemia and overnight metyrapone tests. TRH is most commonly indirectly assessed by Free T4, T3, thyroid-stimulating hormone (TSH).

7. *Differential Diagnosis.* Patients who have had pelvic radiotherapy and/or alkylating chemotherapy agents may develop late gonadal toxicity. Patients may have idiopathic hormonal deficiencies, such as congenital GH deficiency, Addison's disease, hypothyroidism, or other syndromes.

8. *Pathologic Diagnosis.* Pathologic confirmation is unnecessary.

9. *Management.* GH deficiency can be managed with GH replacement therapy; in prepubescent children, a gonadotropin releasing hormone (GnRH) agonist can be used to block puberty. A GnRH agonist can also be used in children with precocious puberty. For ACTH deficiency, hydrocortisone can be prescribed, and for TRH deficiency, thyroxine can be prescribed. Sex hormone replacement can be offered (as described in the next section). Dopamine agonists (such as bromocriptine) can be used to treat hyperprolactinemia.

10. *Follow-up.* Children should undergo at least a biannual growth assessment, with weight and height and Tanner staging. The NCI recommends that children with GH deficiency undergo bone age assessment at 9 years and annually until puberty. Laboratory assessment (discussed previously) should be performed every 3 to 5 years.

Clinical Syndromes

In pediatric patients, risk of GH deficiency is related to the dose and volume of the radiotherapy and the age at which it is delivered. The higher the radiation dose, the earlier the GH deficiency will occur after treatment. Therefore, this is most commonly reported among patients treated for brain tumors and acute lymphoblastic leukemia (61,231). Children who receive hematopoietic stem cell transplant (HSCT) with total body radiation (TBI) have a significant risk of growth hormone (GH) deficiency. Risk is increased with single-dose as opposed to fractionated radiation, pretransplant cranial irradiation, young age at transplant, and posttreatment complications such as GVHD (64,329,376).

Gonadotrophin deficiency can result from doses >50 Gy. Conversely, doses in the 18 to 47 Gy range can result in precocious puberty. In the pediatric population, girls who receive 24 Gy for leukemia appear to be at highest risk (315).

Adrenocorticotropin deficiencies and hyperprolactinemia may manifest with doses >50 Gy, such as that delivered for brain tumors and nasopharyngeal or paranasal sinus carcinoma (69,303).

Thyroid

1. *Clinical Detection.* Hypothyroidism or hyperthyroidism can develop after radiotherapy. Hyperthyroidism results from Grave's disease or thyroiditis, and the latter usually results in subsequent hypothyroidism. The manifestations of hypothyroidism are outlined in the preceding section. Hyperthyroidism is characterized by heat intolerance, weight loss, insomnia, increased appetite, diarrhea, moist skin, tachycardia, nervousness, tremors, exophthalmus, and goiter. Thyroid enlargement, and more frequently, thyroid nodularity, can also develop.

2. *Time Course of Events.* The time course of developing late thyroid effects is highly variable. The risk for both hypo- or hyperthyroidism reported in one study increased in the first 3 to 5 years since diagnosis, whereas the risk for nodules increased ≥10 years from diagnosis (322).

3. *Dose/Time/Volume.* Hypo- or hyperthyroidism results from fractionated radiation >20 Gy to the neck or cervical spine, or >7.5 Gy of TBI. Thyroid nodularity can occur after lower dose exposures (292). Recent data on patients with head and neck cancer support a radiation dose-response for hypothyroidism (337).

4. *Chemical/Biologic Modifiers.* In children treated for Hodgkin's disease, the addition of chemotherapy to radiation does not appear to increase the risk of hypothyroidism, although chemotherapy alone can result in hypothyroidism (322).

5. *Radiologic Imaging.* Thyroid nodules should be assessed by ultrasound, and an I-125 scan can be considered.

6. *Laboratory tests.* Free T4 and TSH should be used to monitor thyroid function.

7. *Differential Diagnosis.* Grave's disease, Hashimoto's thyroiditis, and idiopathic thyroid nodules can occur in the general population. Patients undergoing cranial irradiation

Techniques, Modalities, and Modifiers in Radiation Oncology

may have neuroendocrine deficiencies (namely TRH deficiency) as previously discussed.

8. *Pathologic Diagnosis.* Fine-needle aspiration of newly diagnosed thyroid nodules, particularly those that do not demonstrate I-125 uptake, is suggested. Suspicious nodules or biopsy-proven thyroid cancer should be resected. Interpretation of the fine-needle aspiration may be confounded by radiation-induced atypia.

9. *Management.* Thyroid shielding during therapeutic radiation should be considered if possible to lower the risk of late thyroid toxicity. Hypothyroidism can be managed with thyroxine replacement, and hyperthyroidism can be managed with propylthiouracil (PTU), propanol I-131, or thyroidectomy. Thyroid nodules should be managed as previously described.

10. *Follow-up.* Routine examination of the neck should be performed to assess for nodularity and/or growth. The NCI recommends annual laboratory assessment up to 10 years postradiation.

Clinical Syndromes

The frequency of central hypothyroidism following cranial irradiation relates to the dose to the hypothalamic pituitary axis with an increased likelihood after doses above 40 to 50 Gy. At the higher doses, as many as 65% of patients may have evidence of subclinical or clinical hypothyroidism, and at somewhat lower hypothalamic pituitary (HP) doses, the risk may be closer to 20% (68,128,307).

Survivors of Hodgkin lymphoma are at a uniquely increased risk of thyroid abnormalities as a result of cervical or mantle radiotherapy. The largest analysis of all thyroid abnormalities has been conducted among 1,791 childhood Hodgkin lymphoma survivors followed in the Childhood Cancer Survivor Study, in which 34% reported that they had been diagnosed with at least one thyroid abnormality (322). For hypothyroidism, there was a clear dose response with a 20-year risk of 20% for those who had received <35 Gy, 30% following 35 to 44.9 Gy and 50% following >45 Gy to the thyroid gland. Compared with the general age-matched population, the relative risk for hypothyroidism was 17.1; for hyperthyroidism, 8.0; and for thyroid nodules, 27.0. The risk for both hypo- or hyperthyroidism increased in the first 3 ti 5 years since diagnosis, whereas that for nodules increased ≥10 years from diagnosis (322). In patients with head and neck cancer, surgery involving the thyroid gland is documented to increase risk of hypothyroidism (337).

Reproductive Endocrine

1. *Clinical Detection.* Late effects from adult female ovarian radiation include infertility, oligomenorrhea/amenorrhea, hot flashes, atrophic vulvitis and vaginitis, changes in fat distribution, breast changes, bone demineralization, and diminished libido (124). In males, testicular germ cell damage can result in oligospermia/azospermia and testicular atrophy. Damage to the Leydig cells can cause testosterone deficiency, potentially resulting in diminished libido and impaired sexual performance. Delayed puberty can occur in male and female children.

2. *Time Course of Events.* Oligospermia can occur during the course of months, and can potentially recover after low-dose exposure. There is a lag between radiation exposure and effect of sperm production, which is a function of the time course of spermatozoa differentiation (the relatively radiosensitive spermatagonia differentiates to the relatively radioresistant spermatozoa during the course of ~70 days). There can also be recovery of ovarian function after low-dose exposures, following months to years of anovulation and amenorrhea.

3. *Dose/Time/Volume.* Radiotherapy delivered to the abdominopelvic fields with direct or scatter radiation to the gonads can result in gonadal failure. The germinal epithelium is exquisitely sensitive to radiation as opposed to the endocrine cells. Temporary oligospermia can occur after low radiation (<1 Gy) doses; permanent azoospermia results from doses of >3 to 4 Gy. The threshold doses of ovarian dysfunction are similar to those of testicular dysfunction.

4. *Chemical/Biologic Modifiers.* Alkylating chemotherapy agents can impair testicular and ovarian function, and thus the combination of chemotherapy and radiation is most significant. Data from Hodgkin lymphoma survivors illustrate this risk well.

5. *Radiologic Imaging.* Patients at risk for bone demineralization may benefit from bone densitometry.

6. *Laboratory Tests.* Serum follicle-stimulating hormone and luteinizing hormone (LH) as well as testosterone or estradiol should be followed. Semen analysis can quantify the extent of oligospermia.

7. *Differential Diagnosis.* Patients also undergoing cranial radiation may experience hypothalamic hypopituitarism. Treatment-related causes of female infertility also include uterine fibrosis; unrelated causes of fertility include polycystic ovarian disease, pelvic inflammatory disease, endometriosis, uterine fibroids, or retroverted uterus. Some unrelated causes of male infertility include chronic infection, chronic disease, retrograde ejaculation, and injury.

8. *Pathologic Diagnosis.* There is no role for pathologic diagnosis of reproductive impairment.

9. *Management.* Prevention of reproductive of failure, when possible, should be attempted in patients wishing to maintain their fertility (205). Testicular shielding can reduce exposure to radiation. Ovarian transposition and the use of extra shielding (10 half-value layers) can help shield the ovaries. Sperm banking and harvesting of oocytes should also be considered. In patients with diminished levels of sex hormone production, hormonal replacement therapy can be considered.

10. *Follow-up.* Children exposed to gonadal radiation should undergo routine Tanner staging. Testicular size should be assessed in males. The NCI recommends that girls should have serum follicle-stimulating hormone, LH, and estradiol levels drawn at age 12, followed by routine measurements for those who experience delayed puberty, and baseline levels should be drawn when they are fully mature. Boys should have serum LH and testosterone levels drawn at age 13, followed by routine measurements for those who experience delayed puberty, and baseline levels should be drawn when they are fully mature. Patients with delayed puberty should be followed by an endocrinologist. Patients with infertility should be referred to endocrine fertility specialists.

Male Gonadal Function

Spermatogenesis is highly sensitive to cyclophosphamide, procarbazine, and nitrogen mustard used to treat Hodgkin lymphoma. With therapies that contain these agents, even in the absence of radiotherapy, azoospermia rates of up to 86% occur (190,192,286,306). Review of the available studies suggests that males who receive <4 g/m^2 of cyclophosphamide, without testicular radiation or any other alkylating agent, are likely to retain their fertility. Cumulative doses above 9 g/m^2 are unlikely to result in any conservation of fertility (144,192,286,306).

The degree and permanency of radiotherapy-induced damage to the male reproductive system depend on dose, field, and schedule. The germinal epithelium is damaged by much lower doses (<1 Gy) of radiotherapy than are Leydig cells (20 to 30 Gy). Doses <30 Gy are unlikely to affect endocrine function and boys can progress through puberty normally. Although temporary oligospermia can occur after these very low radiation doses, permanent azoospermia results from doses of >3 to 4 Gy. The potential for a return of spermatogenesis in the intermediate dose range of 1 to 3 Gy is variable.

Female Gonadal Function

Risk of menstrual irregularity, ovarian failure, and infertility related to alkylating agent chemotherapy increases with age at treatment (27,144,347). Amenorrhea and premature ovarian failure occur more commonly in adult women treated with cyclophosphamide and other alkylating agents than in adolescents, and thus newer regimens have reduced such exposures (29,153). Two studies of childhood cancer survivors illustrate the risk of combined alkylating agent and radiation therapy. In a cohort treated between 1945 and 1975, the relative fertility of married survivors of childhood Hodgkin lymphoma was 0.77 (95% confidence interval: 0.64, 0.92), compared with sibling controls. The relative risk for premature ovarian failure between 21 and 30 years was 3.35 and between 31 and 40 years it was 1.27, compared with the sibling controls. Relative risk between the ages of 21 and 30 rose to 9.6 for those treated with radiotherapy below the diaphragm and alkylating agents (50). In another study of 719 survivors treated between 1964 and 1988, of whom 29% were lymphoma survivors, overall there was a 15.5% failure to conceive. Increasing doses of abdominopelvic radiotherapy and increasing doses of alkylating agents resulted in an increase in premature ovarian failure and a fertility deficit in the entire cohort (60).

Females exposed to pelvic radiation as children, who are able to conceive children as an adult, appear to have a greater risk of preterm offspring, although this was not associated with low–birth weight offspring (when corrected for preterm delivery). This is likely an effect of uterine radiation exposure (85).

Bone

1. *Clinical Detection.* Scoliosis, kyphosis, lordosis, and limb asymmetry can be assessed by clinical examination. Plain films can assess limb or spinal asymmetry, and impending epiphyseal slippage.
2. *Time Course of Events.* Late growth abnormalities occur as a result of impaired bone growth, and thus occur progressively until normal bone growth has ceased.
3. *Dose/Time/Volume.* Avoiding the growth plate can reduce the extent and risk of late growth defects. If the growth plate must be encompassed, it is best to avoid treating only a portion of the growth plate. With partial irradiation of the growth plate, a portion will likely grow more readily than the unirradiated portion, resulting in more severe growth abnormalities.
4. *Chemical/Biologic Modifiers.* Chemotherapy may potentiate the risk of late effects from radiation, but the data are not conclusive.
5. *Radiologic Imaging.* Plain films can assess bone length, femoral head angle, and epiphyseal width. Widened epiphyseal width may precede epiphyseal slippage. The extent of scoliosis, lordosis, and kyphosis can also be assessed. Skull films and panaramic x-ray films can be used to assess cephalometric measurements and tooth development.
6. *Laboratory Tests.* Endocrine testing is suggested in patients whose gonads or hypothalamic-pituitary axis were in the radiation field.
7. *Differential Diagnosis.* Growth hormone suppression can cause symmetric bony growth impairment.
8. *Pathologic Diagnosis.* Generally, late bone growth effects are based on clinical and radiographic assessment.
9. *Management.* For mild scoliosis, physical therapy and tailored exercise programs are suggested. Moderate scoliosis

may benefit from a brace. Severe scoliosis might require surgical intervention. Epiphyseal slippage is managed with surgical pinning, or in severe cases, osteotomy and osteoplasty. For leg-length discrepancy, shoe lifts may offer adequate correction.

10. *Follow-up.* Clinical assessment of weight, height, and limb length should be performed at every follow-up. Regular imaging to assess epiphyseal width is recommended for patients at risk for epiphyseal slippage. Periodic x-rays are also recommended to assess the limbs in spine included in the radiation field.

Clinical Syndromes

Clinically, radiation's effects on growing bone may be most simply characterized as shortening of long bones (i.e., femur, tibia, humerus) or hypoplasia of flat bones (i.e., ilium). For children treated with craniospinal radiotherapy for either acute lymphoblastic leukemia or CNS tumors, the cranial dose can result in decreased growth, as a result of growth hormone deficiency, and the spinal dose can result in stature loss due to the effect on the vertebral bodies (314,323,324). In children treated for Wilms' tumor, mathematical modeling has defined risk well. For those under 12 months of age at diagnosis who received >10 Gy, the estimated adult height deficit was 7.7 cm when contrasted with the nonradiation group. For those who received 10 Gy, the estimated trunk shortening was only 2.8 cm or less. For those who had height measurements in the teenage years available, patients who received 15 Gy or more of radiation therapy were 4 to 7 cm shorter on average than their nonirradiated counterparts, with a dose response evident (148).

Scoliosis and kyphosis can result from spinal or flank irradiation, causing asymmetric spinal growth. Prior to the recognition that an inhomogeneous dose across a growth plate may lead to curvature of bone growth, this was most frequently seen following irradiation for Wilms' tumor and neuroblastoma in children, where there has been flank surgery (e.g., nephrectomy) and radiation. However, with current doses and fields of radiotherapy employed in the treatment of Wilms' tumor, scoliosis and kyphosis are less common (265). If therapy is limited to half of the abdomen, it is advisable to bring the ports slightly beyond the midline so that the entire transverse diameter of the spine is included, receiving irradiation of fairly uniform intensity. If the entire abdomen requires treatment and it must be subdivided into quadrants, caution should be exercised in avoiding quadruple cross-firing of the spine producing a so-called hot spot in the region of the first or second lumbar vertebrae.

Avascular necrosis of the femoral or humeral heads can occur 2 to 3 years following irradiation following doses of 30 to 60 Gy (280). Corticosteroids also increase risk of avascular necrosis and are now implicated even in the absence or radiotherapy (114,147,334).

Bone Marrow

1. *Clinical Detection.* Bone marrow irradiation is incidental to the treatment of most malignancies, with clinical consequences dependent on the volume exposed, bone marrow reserve, and chemotherapy history. An exception is when TBI is used as a component of the conditioning regimen for BMT, when the bone marrow is specifically targeted for suppression. Neutropenia (granulocytes 500 to 1,000/mL) and lymphopenia increase the risk for infection; thrombocytopenia (platelets <20,000/mL) is associated with subclinical or overt bleeding; anemia has multiple consequences, including fatigue and hypoxemia.
2. *Time Course of Events.* For a single, large dose, the latent period is 1 to 2 weeks, after which a cascade of events occurs that can result in hemorrhage or infection.

Fractionation courses lower white blood cell and platelets counts over weeks to months, but there are rarely red blood cell effects with conventional schedules.

3. *Dose/Time/Volume.* For permanent suppression of a limited bone marrow volume by irradiation, doses >30 to 40 Gy are required.

4. *Chemical/Biologic Modifiers.* A large variety of antineoplastic agents are myelotoxic and have both short- and long-term effects.

5. *Radiologic Imaging.* Bone marrow imaging is best done with ^{99m}Tc-sulfur (^{99m}Tc-S) colloid, and patterns of bone marrow injury reflect suppression, followed by regeneration and extension into the femurs. MRI provides an alternative means of visualization and is excellent for limited volumes.

6. *Laboratory Tests.* Numerous bone marrow stem cell assays are available (colony-forming unit–granulocyte-macrophage [CFU-GM], burst-forming unit—erythroid [BFU-E], CFU-granulocyte-erythroid-macrophage-megakaryocyte [CFU-GEMM], CFU-fibroblast [CFU-F], high proliferative potential colony-forming cell [HPP-CFC], and long-term culture-initiating cell [LTC-IC]), as is a cell morphologic study of bone marrow aspirate. Hemograms show alterations in complete blood count weeks later, with leukopenia and thrombocytopenia.

7. *Differential Diagnosis.* Metastatic dissemination of cancer or lymphomas gradually eradicating bone marrow, coupled with the use of aggressive chemoradiation programs for treatment, can lead to severe bone marrow ablation. Radiation dose/time factors leading to bone marrow suppression must be distinguished from chemotherapy bone marrow suppression patterns.

8. *Pathologic Diagnosis.* Depending on the time after irradiation, there is immediate loss of lymphoid, myeloid, and erythroid blast progenitor cells, followed by a gradual loss of hematopoietic stem cells. Sinuses are gradually obliterated and replaced by a fatty and fibrous marrow that is acellular.

9. *Management.* A number of growth cytokines can be used to stimulate and radioprotect or chemoprotect bone marrow regeneration (i.e., IL-1, IL-4, IL-6, IL-11); these can be coupled with BMT.

10. *Follow-up.* Careful, detailed follow-up using bone marrow ^{99m}Tc-S colloid is best, correlated with peripheral blood counts.

Pathophysiology and Cellular Biology

The bone marrow compartment is defined by the cellular composition of its various cell lineages and the renewal ability of the stem cell population. Assay systems for progenitor cells, referred to as *bone marrow stem cells,* include CFU-GM, BFU-E, CFU-GEMM, and CFU-blast, the stromal cell assays (CFU-F), long-term bone marrow cultures, and primitive stem cell assays (HPP-CFC, CFU-Dexter, LTC-IC, somatic mutation analysis/DNA analyses). The regenerative activity of the bone marrow compartment depends more on volume than dose. This volume effect is best understood by reviewing the findings after subdividing clinical and experimental investigations into three arbitrary categories and examining the dose, time, and fractionation factors (305):

- When <10% to 15% of bone marrow volume is irradiated, permanent ablation of bone marrow occurs with fractionated doses beyond 30 Gy and single doses of 20 Gy. The ability of the protected bone marrow to compensate by accelerating its rate of hematopoiesis is sufficient.
- After the loss of activity in 10% to 25% of the bone marrow after irradiation, the unexposed bone marrow responds

by increasing its population of progenitor cells (295). In this situation, the bone marrow may fail to regenerate the ablated portion of marrow because the compensatory process is able to meet the demands for hematopoiesis.

- When 25% to 50% of bone marrow is exposed to radiation, permanent ablation occurs at similar dose levels as small fields. However, all of the unirradiated marrow becomes active and remains in this state of prolonged stimulus for the ablated segment. This is best demonstrated by the failure of bone marrow to regenerate in-field after mantle treatment in Hodgkin lymphoma with doses of 30 to 40 Gy (356).
- However, when a larger volume of bone marrow is irradiated ($\geq$50%), the paradoxic phenomenon of in-field regeneration is seen 2 to 5 years later, as well as extension of bone marrow into previously quiescent long bones within 1 to 2 years. This is well illustrated by the evaluation and mapping of bone marrow with nuclear scans using ^{99m}Tc-S colloid undertaken in Hodgkin lymphoma treated with different irradiation field arrangements (295).
- For subtotal bone marrow irradiation, in which 50% to 75% of the bone marrow is exposed, a complex series of events occurs to compensate for the large volume of bone marrow suppression (Table 12.16); the length of the process persists for years. Acutely, the nadir in the peripheral blood is manifested in 3 to 4 weeks, with a depression in white cells and platelets, followed by recovery in 1 to 2 months. Normal blood values persist for years after subtotal or total nodal irradiation in Hodgkin lymphoma, despite prolonged marrow cell suppression. Regeneration of the irradiated bone marrow is very gradual, as indicated, with recovery occurring at 1 to 5 years.

Different chemotherapeutic agents have been shown to act through similar cellular and molecular pathways. The combined use of these modalities in drug irradiation schedules sets up a competition for bone marrow compartments. Results of competitive repopulation assays show decreasing repopulation capacity of chemotherapeutically treated bone marrow cells (43).

Total-Body Irradiation and Bone Marrow Transplantation

TBI with conditioning chemotherapy programs and BMT, incidental exposure during space travel, and potential terrorist threats have stimulated an interest in the biologic effects of TBI. The lethal syndromes that follow high-intensity irradiation are related to the dose that the whole, specific, sensitive organ receives (98). Survival after TBI intentionally administered as preparation for BMT results from the infusion of viable bone marrow and intensive supportive care. Patients so treated demonstrate delayed adverse effects that depend on the tolerance of individual organs to irradiation.

After total-body doses of 1.5 to 7.5 Gy, there is a rapid depletion of vital stem cells within 1 week of exposure (356). Without hematopoietic stem cell rescue, death usually occurs as a result of granulocytopenia and thrombocytopenia, predisposing the patient to overwhelming infection and hemorrhage (9) (Fig. 12.20). Radiation doses of 3 to 5 Gy result in an $LD_{50/100}$, with death more frequently resulting from 7.5 to 10.5 Gy. With stem cell rescue, doses of 7.5 to 10.5 Gy are well tolerated, and the microvasculature of the marrow still allows for implantation and proliferation of transferred stem cells.

Fractionated radiation doses to the whole bone marrow organ are rarely used clinically except as TBI for treatment of leukemias, multiple myelomas, and lymphomas (46,117). However, TBI without stem cell rescue has been used occasionally and provides information on marrow tolerance. In chronic lymphocytic leukemia and non-Hodgkin lymphoma, daily doses of

Techniques, Modalities, and Modifiers in Radiation Oncology

| Table 12.16 | BONE MARROW REGENERATION PATTERNS AND COMPENSATORY MECHANISMS | | | | |

		Regeneration		Doses (Gy)	
Techniques of Irradiation	Exposed Bone Marrow	Unexposed Bone Marrow	Extension[a]	Daily	Total
Small field	N1	Locoregional ↑ BMR	N1	2	>30
Large field	N1	Generalized ↑↑ BMR	N1	2	>30
Segmental field (e.g., subtotal nodal)	Suppressed BMR which then recovers	Generalized ↑↑ BMR	↑↑	2	40
Total body	Active	—	N1	0.05–0.1	>1

N1, normal; ↑, increased activity; ↑↑, greatly increased activity; BMR, bone marrow regeneration.
[a]Extension: bone marrow activity in previously quiescent areas.
From Rubin P, Scarantino CW. The bone marrow organ: the critical structure in radiation–drug interaction. Sir Stanford Cade Memorial Lecture. *Int J Radiat Oncol Biol Phys* 1978;4:3–23, with permission.

0.05 to 0.15 Gy twice or three times per week have been used effectively to total doses of 0.5 to 1.5 Gy. Cycles of treatment are given monthly and can lead to total doses as high as 3 to 4.5 Gy; however, severe to life-threatening hematologic toxicity sometimes occurs. Titration of dose is essential because of thrombocytopenia, and treatment should be withheld if the platelet count decreases to less than 100,000/mL. Patients with multiple myeloma and chronic lymphocytic leukemia appear to exhibit more hematologic sensitivity to TBI than do those with normal bone marrow, and death has resulted after very modest irradiation doses.

Thomas (344) pioneered TBI using telecobalt units to deliver very low dose rates (0.05 Gy/min), but more recently the widespread use of TBI single-exposure techniques has been supplemented by safer fractionated schedules using both high and low dose rates. Total doses range from 5 to 10 Gy, fraction size varies from 1.2 to 4 Gy, and dose rates extend from 0.025 to 0.05 Gy/min (344,372). These fractionation schedules are designed to protect against lung toxicity when used in conjunction with lung shields, and are not designed to be of therapeutic advantage in bone marrow ablation.

Clinical Syndromes

Elements of the blood and bone marrow respond to irradiation by progressively decreasing in numbers because of the destruction of primitive radiosensitive precursor cells (9) (Fig. 12.20).

The neutropenia seen in the first week results from cessation of production and rapid turnover of these cells. This is followed in 2 to 3 weeks by thrombocytopenia and in 2 to 3 months by anemia. Recovery is related to the degree of initial response and usually begins with regeneration of the depleted stem cells. If large volumes of bone marrow have been irradiated, then a hypoplastic marrow can persist and occasionally become aplastic. The latter event also may result from an infiltration of the marrow and should be suspected if the depression in blood count does not occur at a predictable time or if only a limited volume of the bone marrow has been irradiated.

Second Malignant Neoplasms

Damage to normal tissues can manifest as organ dysfunction, as previously discussed, or as second malignant neoplasms, for which there are considerable data about the risks associated with both radiotherapy and chemotherapy.

Survivors of Hodgkin lymphoma appear to be at particularly increased risk. In an analysis of second malignant neoplasms in a multicenter study of all childhood cancer survivors, the highest reported standardized incidence ratio for secondary cancers (9.7) was found among survivors of Hodgkin lymphoma, where it was an independent risk factor even after adjusting for radiotherapy and chemotherapy exposures (249). The risk of leukemia is largely associated with exposure to alkylating agents and topoisomerase II inhibitors and appears to plateau at

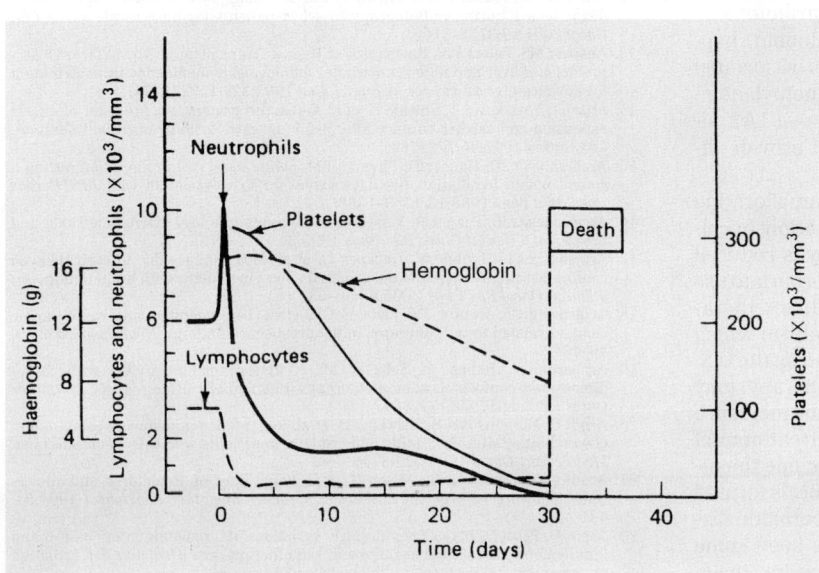

FIGURE 12.20. Expected hematologic response of a human after a single dose total-body exposure of 4.5 Gy. (From Andrews GA. Radiation accidents and their management. *Radiat Res Suppl* 1967;7:390–397, with permission.)

10 to 15 years after therapy, and the risk of second solid malignancies, associated with radiotherapy exposure, rises with ongoing follow-up and includes sarcoma, melanoma, breast, lung, thyroid, and gastrointestinal cancer (83,143,235,249,335,351–353,361,362,379).

Another group of survivors at particularly increased risk of second malignancies are hematopoietic transplant survivors, in whom excess risk has been reported for myelodysplasia, leukemia, lymphoma, liver, oral cavity, brain, bone, connective tissue, genitourinary, and skin cancer (6,25,32,73,79,99,105, 106,116,155,191,234,236,238,251,268). Although TBI is clearly a risk factor, particularly for the solid malignancies, other factors include GVHD, transplant type (autologous versus allogeneic), and chemotherapy used during the conditioning regimen (6,25,32,73,79,105,208). More recently, recapitulating what has been reported following treatment with conventional radiotherapy for Hodgkin lymphoma, HSCT survivors have been noted to be at increased risk for breast cancer, with TBI and ongoing follow-up time since transplant, significant risk factors (106,191).

Future Directions

The radiation oncologist must be familiar with the pathogenesis of normal tissue injury, the clinical experience with multimodality therapy in inducing such injury, and the management of established injury. Scientific directions to accomplish this are multiple and include:

- Identification of the incidence of key adverse effects
- Identification of associations of late events with specific components of therapy
- Dissection of the molecular pathogenesis of normal tissue injury
- Exploration of genetic predispositions (e.g., mutations or polymorphisms in candidate genes that predispose to damage)
- Exploration of gene–environment interactions that predispose to injury
- Using predictive models to identify patients at high risk of developing late toxicity.
- Developing and investigating agents that reduce the risk of late toxicity without compromising cancer control.

Cardiac toxicity after chemoradiation exemplifies these considerations. The incidence of anthracycline- and radiation-induced injury is becoming better defined, and several genes have been implicated in anthracycline-induced cardiotoxicity (e.g., the carbonyl reductase [S1] gene, metallothionein, hepcidin), together with the multiple polymorphisms associated with the risk of coronary artery disease (e.g., methylenetetrahydrofolate reductase, platelet glycoprotein IIIa—P1A2 allele). Further exploration of such associations will provide directions for amelioration and prevention.

However, at this moment the approach to ameliorating therapy-induced late effects accessible to all radiation oncologists is preventive. That is, the toxicity of therapy is reduced through safely minimizing field size through the appropriate use of conformal treatment-planning techniques. In addition, therapeutic approaches exist, such as identifying situations in which the radioprotector, amifostine (Ethyol, now approved by the U.S. Food and Drug Administration for use in radiation therapy) may be effective. This drug has been shown to decrease the incidence and severity of xerostomia in patients undergoing treatment of head and neck cancer. Other agents under study include the nitroxides, which, like aminothiols, scavenge free radicals formed by ionizing radiation. The antioxidant enzyme, superoxide dismutase, also works in this manner and there has been some work in the gene therapy field examining intratumoral injec-

tions of manganese superoxide dismutase–plasmid/liposome, with some success demonstrated in animal models.

Apart from these direct strategies, alternative methods that may have future application involve up-regulation or down-regulation of the many cytokines and growth factors that are expressed after radiation injury. Intentional dysregulation may be achieved through direct administration of either the cytokines themselves or blockers to the cytokines or their receptors through systemic application of antibodies or targeted gene therapy. Examples of cytokines of interest that are under investigation include TGF-β, a profibrogenic cytokine that has been shown to have multiple roles in both healing and downstream development of fibrosis, and keratinocyte growth factor, a potent mitogen for epithelial cells and a demonstrated potentiator of healing.

As our understanding of the cellular and molecular mechanisms that underlie the development of therapy-induced late effects increases, our potential for prevention and amelioration of normal tissue late effects will increase. This will lead to improved therapeutic ratios and quality of life after treatment, and may also permit enhanced tumor control as it increases our ability to deliver higher radiation doses with fewer normal tissue toxicities.

References

1. Abbatucci JS, Delozier T, Quint R, et al. Radiation myelopathy of the cervical spinal cord: time, dose and volume factors. *Int J Radiat Oncol Biol Phys* 1978;4:239–248.
2. Adams J, Hardenberg P, Constine L, et al. Radiation-associated heart disease. *Crit Rev Oncol Hematol* 2003;45:55–77.
3. Adams MJ, Constine LS, Lipshultz SE. Cardiac responses to environmental stress radiation. In: Crawford M, DiMarco J, eds. *Cardiology*. Philadelphia: Mosby, 2001; 1–8.
4. Adams MJ, Lipshultz SE, Schwartz C, et al. Radiation-associated cardiovascular disease: manifestations and management. *Semin Radiat Oncol* 2003;13: 346–356.
5. Adams MJ, Lipsitz SR, Colan SD, et al. Cardiovascular status in long-term survivors of Hodgkin's disease treated with chest radiotherapy. *J Clin Oncol* 2004;22:3139–3148.
6. Ades L, Guardiola P, Socie G. Second malignancies after allogeneic hematopoietic stem cell transplantation: new insight and current problems. *Blood Rev* 2002;16:135–146.
7. Ahn SJ, Kahn D, Zhou S, et al. Dosimetric and clinical predictors for radiation-induced esophageal injury. *Int J Radiat Oncol Biol Phys* 2005;61:335–347.
8. Amosson CM, Teh BS Van TJ, et al. Dosimetric predictors of xerostomia for head-and-neck cancer patients treated with the smart (simultaneous modulated accelerated radiation therapy) boost technique. *Int J Radiat Oncol Biol Phys* 2003;56:136–144.
9. Andrews GA. Radiation accidents and their management. *Radiat Res Suppl* 1967;7:390–397.
10. Ang KK, Jiang GL, Feng Y, et al. Extent and kinetics of recovery of occult spinal cord injury. *Int J Radiat Oncol Biol Phys* 2001;50:1013–1020.
11. Anscher MS, Kong FM, Andrews K, et al. Plasma transforming growth factor beta1 as a predictor of radiation pneumonitis. *Int J Radiat Oncol Biol Phys* 1998;41:1029–1035.
12. Anscher MS, Marks LB, Shafman TD, et al. Using plasma transforming growth factor beta-1 during radiotherapy to select patients for dose escalation. *J Clin Oncol* 2001;19:3758–3765.
13. Anscher MS, Peters WP, Reisenbichler H, et al. Transforming growth factor-β as a predictor of liver and lung fibrosis after autologous bone marrow transplantation for advanced breast cancer. *N Engl J Med* 1993;328:1592–1598.
14. Anzai T, Yoshikawa T, Shiraki H, et al. C-reactive protein as a predictor of infarct expansion and cardiac rupture after a first Q-wave acute myocardial infarction. *Circulation* 1997;96:778–784.
15. Archambeau JO, Hauser D, Shymko RM. Swine basal cell proliferation during a course of daily irradiation, five days a week for six weeks (6000 rad). *Int J Radiat Oncol Biol Phys* 1988;15:1383–1388.
16. Archambeau JO, Pezner R, Wasserman T. Pathophysiology of irradiated skin and breast. *Int J Radiat Oncol Biol Phys* 1995;31:1171–1185.
17. Armstrong CL, Hunter JV, Hackney D, et al. MRI changes due to early-delayed conformal radiotherapy and postsurgical effects in patients with brain tumors. *Int J Radiat Oncol Biol Phys* 2005;63:56–63.
18. Armstrong CL, Hunter JV, Ledakis GE, et al. Late cognitive and radiographic changes related to radiotherapy: initial prospective findings. *Neurology* 2002;59: 40–48.
19. Armstrong J, Raben A, Zelefsky M, et al. Promising survival with three-dimensional conformal radiation therapy for non-small cell lung cancer. *Radiother Oncol* 1997;44:17–22.
20. Arndt C, Morgenstern B, Hawkins D, et al. Renal function following combination chemotherapy with ifosfamide and cisplatin in patients with osteogenic sarcoma. *Med Pediatr Oncol* 1999;32:93–96.
21. Arndt C, Morgenstern B, Wilson D, et al. Renal function in children and adolescents following 72 g/m^2 of ifosfamide. *Cancer Chemother Pharmacol* 1994;34: 431–433.
22. Arpin D, Perol D, Blay JY, et al. Early variations of circulating interleukin-6 and interleukin-10 levels during thoracic radiotherapy are predictive for radiation pneumonitis. *J Clin Oncol* 2005;23:8748–8756.

23. Asao C, Korogi Y, Kitajima M, et al. Diffusion-weighted imaging of radiation-induced brain injury for differentiation from tumor recurrence. *Am J Neuroradiol* 2005;26:1455–1460.
24. Avioli LV, Lazor MZ, Cotlove E, et al. Early effects of radiation on renal function in man. *Am J Med* 1963;34:329–337.
25. Baker KS, DeFor TE, Burns LJ, et al. New malignancies after blood or marrow stem-cell transplantation in children and adults: incidence and risk factors. *J Clin Oncol* 2003;21:1352–1358.
26. Barthelemy-Brichant N, Bosquee L, Cataldo D, et al. Increased IL-6 and TGF-beta1 concentrations in bronchoalveolar lavage fluid associated with thoracic radiotherapy. *Int J Radiat Oncol Biol Phys* 2004;58:758–767.
27. Bath LE, Hamish W, Wallace B, et al. Late effects of the treatment of childhood cancer on the female reproductive system and the potential for fertility preservation. *Br J Obstet Gynaecol* 2002;109:107–114.
28. Bearman SI. The syndrome of hepatic veno-occlusive disease after marrow transplantation. *Blood Rev* 1995;85:3005–3020.
29. Behringer K, Breuer K, Reineke T, et al. Secondary amenorrhea after Hodgkin's lymphoma is influenced by age at treatment, stage of disease, chemotherapy regimen, and the use of oral contraceptives during therapy: a report from the German Hodgkin's Lymphoma Study Group. *J Clin Oncol* 2005;23:7555–7564.
30. Belkacemi Y, Labopin M, Vernant JP, et al. Cataracts after total body irradiation and bone marrow transplantation in patients with acute leukemia in complete remission: a study of the European Group for Blood and Marrow Transplantation. *Int J Radiat Oncol Biol Phys* 1998;41:659–668.
31. Bentzen SM, Skoczylas JZ, Bernier J. Quantitative clinical radiobiology of early and late lung reactions. *Int J Radiat Biol* 2000;76:453–462.
32. Bhatia S, Louie AD, Bhatia R, et al. Solid cancers after bone marrow transplantation. *J Clin Oncol* 2001;19:464–471.
33. Bianchetti MG, Kanaka C, Ridolfi-Luthy A, et al. Persisting renotubular sequelae after cisplatin in children and adolescents. *Am J Nephrol* 1991;11:127–30.
34. Bjermer L, Cai Y, Nilsson K, et al. Tobacco smoke exposure suppresses radiation-induced inflammation in the lung: a study of bronchoalveolar lavage and ultrastructural morphology in the rat. *Eur Respir J* 1993;6:1173–1180.
35. Blanco AI, Chao KS, El Naga I, et al. Dose-volume modeling of salivary function in patients with head-and-neck cancer receiving radiotherapy. *Int J Radiat Oncol Biol Phys* 2005;62:1055–1069.
36. Bleyer A, Robinson L, Fallovollita J, et al. Influence of age. sex and concurrent intrathecal methotrexate therapy on intellectual function after cranial irradiation during childhood. *Pediatr Hematol Oncol* 1990;7:329–338.
37. Bleyer WA, Griffin TW. In: Gilbert H, Kagan A, eds. *White matter necrosis, mineralizing microangiopathy and intellectual abilities in survivors of childhood leukemia: associations with central nervous system irradiation and methotrexate therapy radiation damage to the nervous system*. New York: Raven Press; 1980.
38. Bleyer WA. Current status of intrathecal chemotherapy for human meningeal neoplasms. *Natl Cancer Inst Monogr* 1977;46:171–178.
39. Boivin JF, Hutchison GB, Lubin JH, et al. Coronary artery disease mortality in patients treated for Hodgkin's disease. *Cancer* 1992;69:1241–1247.
40. Bokemeyer C, Lampe C, Heneka M, et al. Paclitaxel-induced radiation recall dermatitis. *Ann Oncol* 1996;7:755–756.
41. Bowers DC, Liu Y, Leisenring W, et al. Late-occurring stroke among long-term survivors of childhood leukemia and brain tumors: a report from the Childhood Cancer Survivor Study. *J Clin Oncol* 2006;24:5277–5282.
42. Braam PM, Roesink JM, Moerland MA, et al. Long-term parotid gland function after radiotherapy. *Int J Radiat Oncol Biol Phys* 2005;62:659–664.
43. Brecher G, Pallavicini MG, Cronkite EP. Competitive repopulation in leukemic and normal bone marrow. *Blood Cells* 1993;19:691–697.
44. Brick I. Effects of million volt irradiation on the gastrointestinal tract. *Arch Intern Med* 1955;96:26–31.
45. Brown PD, Buckner JC, O'Fallon JR, et al. Effects of radiotherapy on cognitive function in patients with low-grade glioma measured by the folstein mini-mental state examination. *J Clin Oncol* 2003;21:2519–2524.
46. Buchali A, Feyer P, Groll J, et al. Immediate toxicity during fractionated total body irradiation as conditioning for bone marrow transplantation. *Radiother Oncol* 2000;54:157–162.
47. Burman C, Kutcher GJ, Emami B, et al. Fitting of normal tissue tolerance data to an analytic function. *Int J Radiat Oncol Biol Phys* 1991;21:123–135.
48. Bussels B, Maes A, Flamen P, et al. Dose-response relationships within the parotid gland after radiotherapy for head and neck cancer. *Radiother Oncol* 2004;73:297–306.
49. Byhardt RW, Brace K, Ruckdeschel J, et al. Dose and treatment factors in radiation related pericardial effusion associated with the mantle technique for Hodgkin's disease. *Cancer* 1975;35:795–802.
50. Byrne J. Infertility and premature menopause in childhood cancer survivors. *Med Pediatr Oncol* 1999;33:24–28.
51. Carr BI. Hepatic arterial ^{90}Yttrium glass microspheres (Therasphere) for unresectable hepatocellular carcinoma: interim safety and survival data on 65 patients. *Liver Transpl* 2004;10[2 Suppl 1]:S107–110.
52. Carreras E, Bertz H, Arcese W, et al. Incidence and outcome of hepatic veno-occlusive disease after blood or marrow transplantation: a prospective cohort study of the European Group for Blood and Marrow Transplantation. European Group for Blood and Marrow Transplantation Chronic Leukemia Working Party. *Blood* 1998;92:3599–3604.
53. Cassady JR, Lebowitz RL, Jaffe N, et al. Effect of low dose irradiation on renal enlargement in children following nephrectomy for Wilms' tumor. *Acta Radiol Oncol* 1981;20:5–8.
54. Cassady JR. Clinical radiation nephropathy. *Int J Radiat Oncol Biol Phys* 1995;31:1249–1256.
55. Chao KS, Deasy JO, Markman J, et al. A prospective study of salivary function sparing in patients with head-and-neck cancers receiving intensity-modulated or three-dimensional radiation therapy: initial results. *Int J Radiat Oncol Biol Phys* 2001;49[4]:907–916.
56. Chao KS. Protection of salivary function by intensity-modulated radiation therapy in patients with head and neck cancer. *Semin Radiat Oncol* 2002;12[Suppl 1]:20–25.
57. Chao ST, Suh JH, Raja S, et al. The sensitivity and specificity of FDG PET in distinguishing recurrent brain tumor from radionecrosis in patients treated with stereotactic radiosurgery. *Int J Cancer* 2001;96:191–197.
58. Chen Y, Rubin P, Williams J, et al. Circulating IL-6 as a predictor of radiation pneumonitis. *Int J Radiat Oncol Biol Phys* 2001;49:641–648.
59. Chiang CS, Hong JH, Stalde A, et al. Delayed molecular responses to brain irradiation. *Int J Radiat Biol* 1997;72:45–53.
60. Chiarelli AM, Marrett LD, Darlington G. Early menopause and infertility in females after treatment for childhood cancer diagnosed in 1964–1988 in Ontario, Canada. *Am J Epidemiol* 1999;150:245–254.
61. Chow EJ, Friedman DL, Yasui Y, et al. Decreased adult height in survivors of childhood acute lymphoblastic leukemia: a report from the Childhood Cancer Survivor Study. *J Peds* 2007;150:370–375.
62. Claude L, Perol D, Ginestet C, et al. A prospective study on radiation pneumonitis following conformal radiation therapy in non-small-cell lung cancer: clinical and dosimetric factors analysis. *Radiother Oncol* 2004;71:175–181.
63. Coderre JA, Morris GM, Micca PL, et al. Late effects of radiation on the central nervous system: role of vascular endothelial damage and glial stem cell survival. *Radiat Res* 2006;166:495–503.
64. Cohen A, Rovelli A, Bakker B, et al. Final height of patients who underwent bone marrow transplantation for hematological disorders during childhood: a study by the Working Party for Late Effects-EBMT. *Blood* 1999;93:4109–4115.
65. Coia LR, Engstrom PF, Paul AR, et al. Long-term results of infusional 5-FU, mitomycin-C and radiation as primary management of esophageal carcinoma. *Int J Radiat Oncol Biol Phys* 1991;20:29–36.
66. Coia LR, Myerson RJ, Tepper JE. Late effects of radiation therapy on the gastrointestinal tract. *Int J Radiat Oncol Biol Phys* 1995;31:1213–1236.
67. Constine L, Schwartz R, Savage D, et al. Cardiac function, perfusion, and morbidity in irradiated long-term survivors of Hodgkin's disease. *Int J Radiat Oncol Biol Phys* 1997;39:897–906.
68. Constine LS, Donaldson SS, McDougall IR, et al. Thyroid dysfunction after radiotherapy in children with Hodgkin's disease. *Cancer* 1984;53:878–883.
69. Constine LS, Rubin P, Woolf PD, et al. Hyperprolactinemia and hypothyroidism following cytotoxic therapy for central nervous system malignancies. *J Clin Oncol* 1987;5:1841–1851.
70. Costleigh BJ, Miyamoto CT, Micaily B, et al. Heightened sensitivity of the esophagus to radiation in a patient with AIDS. *Am J Gastroenterol* 1995;90:812–814.
71. Crilley P, Topolsky D, Styler MJ, et al. Extramedullary toxicity of a conditioning regimen containing busulphan, cyclophosphamide and etoposide in 84 patients undergoing autologous and allogenic bone marrow transplantation. *Bone Marrow Transplant* 1995;15:361–365.
72. Cummings BJ, Keane TJ, O'Sullivan B, et al. Epidermoid anal cancer: treatment by radiation alone or by radiation and 5-fluorouracil with and without mitomycin C. *Int J Radiat Oncol Biol Phys* 1991;21:1115–1125.
73. Curtis RE, Rowlings PA, Deeg HJ, et al. Solid cancers after bone marrow transplantation. *N Engl J Med* 1997;336:897–904.
74. Dahllof G, Barr M, Balme P, et al. Disturbances in dental development after total body irradiation in bone marrow transplant recipients. *Oral Surg Oral Med Oral Pathol* 1988;65:41–44.
75. Danjoux CE, Catton GE. Delayed complications in colorectal carcinoma treated by combination radiotherapy and 5-fluorouracil: Eastern Cooperative Oncology Group (E.C.O.G.) pilot study. *Int J Radiat Oncol Biol Phys* 1979;5:311–315.
76. Danjoux CE. Delayed complications following combination of radiation and chemotherapy. *Int J Radiat Oncol Biol Phys* 1979;5:441–443.
77. Dawson LA, Normolle D, Balter JM, et al. Analysis of radiation-induced liver disease using the Lyman NTCP model. *Int J Radiat Oncol Biol Phys* 2002;53:810–821.
78. Dawson LA, Ten Haken RK, Lawrence TS. Partial irradiation of the liver. *Semin Radiat Oncol* 2001;11:240–246.
79. Deeg HJ, Socie G. Malignancies after hematopoietic stem cell transplantation: many questions, some answers. *Blood* 1998;91:1833–1844.
80. Delanian S, Balla-Mekias S, Lefaix JL. Striking regression of chronic radiotherapy damage in a clinical trial of combined pentoxifylline and tocopherol. *J Clin Oncol* 1999;17:3283–3290.
81. Dewit L, Anninga JK, Hoefnagel CA, et al. Radiation injury in the human kidney: a prospective analysis using specific scintigraphic and biochemical endpoints. *Int J Radiat Oncol Biol Phys* 1990;19:977–983.
82. Dewit L, Verheij M, Valdes Olmos RA, et al. Compensatory renal response after unilateral partial and whole volume high-dose irradiation of the human kidney. *Eur J Cancer* 1993;29A:2239–2243.
83. Dores GM, Metayer C, Curtis RE, et al. Second malignant neoplasms among long-term survivors of Hodgkin's disease: a population-based evaluation over 25 years. *J Clin Oncol* 2002;20:3484–3494.
84. Duffner PK, Cohen ME. The long-term effects of central nervous system therapy on children with brain tumors. *Neurol Clin* 1991;9:479–495.
85. Eifel P, Donaldson S, Thomas P. Response of growing bone to irradiation: a proposed late effects scoring system. *Int J Radiat Oncol Biol Phys* 1995;31:1301–1307.
86. Eifel PJ, Levenback C, Wharton JT, et al. Time course and incidence of late complications in patients treated with radiation therapy for FIGO stage IB carcinoma of the uterine cervix. *Int J Radiat Oncol Biol Phys* 1995;32:1289–1300.
87. Eisbruch A, Kim HM, Terrell JE, et al. Xerostomia and its predictors following parotid-sparing irradiation of head-and-neck cancer. *Int J Radiat Oncol Biol Phys* 2001;50:695–704.
88. Eisbruch A, Rhodus N, Rosenthal D, et al. How should we measure and report radiotherapy-induced xerostomia? *Semin Radiat Oncol* 2003;13:226–234.
89. Eisbruch A, Ten Haken RK, Kim HM, et al. Dose, volume, and function relationships in parotid salivary glands following conformal and intensity-modulated irradiation of head and neck cancer. *Int J Radiat Oncol Biol Phys* 1999;45:577–587.
90. Ellis F. Dose, time and fractionation: a clinical hypothesis. *Clin Radiol* 1969;20:1–7.
91. Eltringham JR, Fajardo LF, Stewart JR. Adriamycin cardiomyopathy: enhanced cardiac damage in rabbits with combined drug and cardiac irradiation. *Radiology* 1975;115:471–472.
92. Emami B, Lyman J, Brown A, et al. Tolerance of normal tissue to therapeutic irradiation. *International Journal of Radiation Oncology, Biology, Physics* 1991;21:109–122.
93. Eriksson F, Gagliardi G, Liedberg A, et al. Long-term cardiac mortality following radiation therapy for Hodgkin's disease: analysis with the relative seriality model. *Radiother Oncol* 2000;55:153–162.
94. Fajardo LF, Berthrong M, Anderson RE. *Radiation pathology*. New York: Oxford University Press; 2001.
95. Fajardo LF, Stewart JR. Experimental radiation-induced heart disease: I. Light microscopic studies. *Am J Pathol* 1970;59:299–316.

96. Fajardo LF, Stewart JR. Pathogenesis of radiation-induced myocardial fibrosis. *Lab Invest* 1973;29:244–257.

97. Fajardo LF. In: Perez C, Brady L, eds. *Morphology of radiation effects on normal tissues*, 2nd ed. Philadelphia: JB Lippincott; 1992, 114–123.

98. Fajardo LF. *Pathology of radiation injury. Principles and Practice of Radiation Oncology*, 2nd ed. New York: Masson Publishing 1982.

99. Fassas AB, Tricot G. Myelodysplastic syndromes complicating hematopoietic stem cell transplantation. *Cancer Treat Res* 2001;108:169–184.

100. Finkelstein JN, Johnston CJ, Baggs R, et al. Early alterations in extracellular matrix and transforming growth factor beta gene expression in mouse lung indicative of late radiation fibrosis. *Int J Radiat Oncol Biol Phys* 1994;28:621–631.

101. Fiorino C, Sanguineti G, Cozzarini C, et al. Rectal dose-volume constraints in high-dose radiotherapy of localized prostate cancer. *Int J Radiat Oncol Biol Phys* 2003;57:953–962.

102. Flentje M, Hensley F, Gademann G, et al. Renal tolerance to nonhomogenous irradiation: comparison of observed effects to predictions of normal tissue complication probability from different biophysical models. *Int J Radiat Oncol Biol Phys* 1993;27:25–30.

103. Flickinger JC, Lunsford LD, Kondziolka D, et al. Radiosurgery and brain tolerance: an analysis of neurodiagnostic imaging changes after gamma knife radiosurgery for arteriovenous malformations. *Int J Radiat Oncol Biol Phys* 1992;23:19–26.

104. Fried MW, Duncan A, Soroka S, et al. Serum hyaluronic acid in patients with veno-occlusive disease following bone marrow transplantation. *Bone Marrow Transplant* 2001;27:635–639.

105. Friedman DL, Leisenring W, Flowers MED, et al. Risk factors for second malignancies after transplantation differ between allogeneic and autologous recipients. Annual Meeting of the American Society of Hematology. Poster presentation, *Blood* 2005, 106: (abstract) 121 Atlanta, GA.

106. Friedman DL, Leisenring W, Schwartz J, et al. Is risk of secondary breast cancer increased following hematopoietic stem cell transplantation? Annual Meeting of the American Society of Hematology oral presentation *Blood* 2004;(abstract) 106:1121. Atlanta, GA.

107. Friedman DL, Qu A, Grigoriev YA, et al. Pulmonary complications in Wilms tumor survivors: a report from the National Wilms Tumor Study. 9th International Conference on Long-Term Complications of Treatment of Children and Adolescents for Cancer Niagara-On-The-Lake, Ontario, Canada, 2006.

108. Fryer C, Hutchinson RJ, Krailo M, et al. Efficacy and toxicity of 12 courses of ABVD chemotherapy followed by low-dose regional radiation in advanced Hodgkin's disease in children: a report from the Children's Cancer Study Group. *J Clin Oncol* 1990;8:1971–1980.

109. Fu XL, Huang H, Bentel G, et al. Predicting the risk of symptomatic radiation-induced lung injury using both the physical and biologic parameters V(30) and transforming growth factor beta. *Int J Radiat Oncol Biol Phys* 2001;50:899–908.

110. Gabel C, Eifel PJ, Tornos C, et al. Radiation recall reaction to idarubicin resulting in vaginal necrosis. *Gynecol Oncol* 1995;57:266–269.

111. Gagliardi G, Lax I, Rutqvist LE. Partial irradiation of the heart. *Semin Radiat Oncol* 2001;11:224–233.

112. Gallez-Marchal D, Fayolle M, Henry-Amar M, et al. Radiation injuries of the gastrointestinal tract in Hodgkin's disease: the role of exploratory laparotomy and fractionation. A study of 19 cases observed in a series of 134 patients treated at the Institut Gustave Roussy from 1972 to 1982. *Radiother Oncol* 1984;2:93–99.

113. Garipagaoglu M, Munley MT, Hollis D, et al. The effect of patient-specific factors on radiation-induced regional lung injury. *Int J Radiat Oncol Biol Phys* 1999;45:331–338.

114. Gaynon PS, Lustig RH. The use of glucocorticoids in acute lymphoblastic leukemia of childhood: molecular, cellular, and clinical considerations. *J Pediatr Hematol Oncol* 1995;17:1–12.

115. Gillette SM, Gillette EL, Shida T, et al. Late radiation response of canine mediastinal tissues. *Radiother Oncol* 1992;23:41–52.

116. Gilliland DG, Gribben JG. Evaluation of the risk of therapy-related MDS/AML after autologous stem cell transplantation. *Biol Blood Marrow Transplant* 2002;8:9–16.

117. Girinsky T, Benhamou E, Bourhis JH, et al. Prospective randomized comparison of single-dose versus hyperfractionated total-body irradiation in patients with hematologic malignancies. *J Clin Oncol* 2000;18:981–986.

118. Girinsky T, Cosset JM. Pulmonary and cardiac late effects of ionizing radiations alone or combined with chemotherapy. *Cancer Radiother* 1997;1:735–743.

119. Glanzmann C, Huguenin P, Lutolf UM, et al. Cardiac lesions after mediastinal radiation for Hodgkin's disease. *Radiother Oncol* 1994;30:43–54.

120. Glanzmann C, Kaufmann P, Jenni R, et al. Cardiac risk after mediastinal irradiation for Hodgkin's disease. *Radiother Oncol* 1998;46:51–62.

121. Glatstein E, Fajardo LF, Brown JM. Radiation injury in the mouse kidney: I. Sequential light microscopic study. *Int J Radiat Oncol Biol Phys* 1977;2:933–943.

122. Graham MV, Purdy JA, Emami B, et al. Clinical dose-volume histogram analysis for pneumonitis after 3D treatment for non-small cell lung cancer (NSCLC). *Int J Radiat Oncol Biol Phys* 1999;45:323–329.

123. Greco FA, Brereton HD, Kent H, et al. Adriamycin and enhanced radiation reaction in normal esophagus and skin. *Ann Intern Med* 1976;85:294–298.

124. Grigsby P, Russell A, Bruner D. Late injury of cancer therapy on the female reproductive tract. *Int J Radiat Oncol Biol Phys* 1995;31:1281–1299.

125. Grigsby PW, Perez CA. In: Rotman M, Rosenthal C, eds. *Efficacy of 5-fluorouracil by continuous infusion and other agents as radiopotentiators for gynecologic malignancies*. Medical Radiology: Concomitant continuous infusion chemotherapy and radiation Berlin: Springer-Verlag; 1991; 259–267.

126. Gross NJ. Pulmonary effects of radiation therapy. *Ann Intern Med* 1977;86:81–92.

127. Guinan EC, Tarbell NJ, Niemeyer CM, et al. Intravascular hemolysis and renal insufficiency after bone marrow transplantation. *Blood* 1988;72:451–455.

128. Gurney JG, Kadan-Lottick NS, Packer RJ. Endocrine and cardiovascular late effects among adult survivors of childhood brain tumors: Childhood Cancer Survivor Study. *Cancer* 2003;97:663–673.

129. Hagge RJ, Wong TZ, Coleman RE. Positron emission tomography: brain tumors and lung cancer. *Radiol Clin North Am* 2001;39:871–881.

130. Hall E. *Radiobiology for the radiologist*, 4th ed. Philadelphia: JB Lippincott; 1994.

131. Hancock S, Donaldson S, Hoppe R. Cardiac disease following treatment of Hodgkin's disease in children and adolescents. *J Clin Oncol* 1993;11:1208–1215.

132. Hanks GE, Kinzie JJ, White RL, et al. Patterns of care outcome studies: results of the national practice in Hodgkin's disease. *Cancer* 1983;51:560–573.

133. Harris EE, Correa C, Hwang WT, et al. Late cardiac mortality and morbidity in early-stage breast cancer patients after breast-conservation treatment. *J Clin Oncol* 2006;24:4100–4106.

134. Hartford AC, Niemierko A, Adams JA, et al. Conformal irradiation of the prostate: estimating long-term rectal bleeding risk using dose-volume histograms. *Int J Radiat Oncol Biol Phys* 1996;36:721–730.

135. Hartman AR, Williams SF, Dillon JJ. Survival, disease-free survival and adverse effects of conditioning for allogeneic bone marrow transplantation with busulfan/cyclophosphamide vs total body irradiation: a meta-analysis. *Bone Marrow Transplant* 1998;22:439–443.

136. Hasegawa S, Horibe K, Kawabe T, et al. Veno-occlusive disease of the liver after allogeneic bone marrow transplantation in children with hematologic malignancies: incidence, onset time and risk factors. *Bone Marrow Transplantation* 1998;22:1191–1197.

137. Hauer-Jensen M, Wang J, Denham JW. Bowel injury: current and evolving management strategies. *Semin Radiat Oncol* 2003;13:357–371.

138. Heidenreich PA, Schnittger I, Strauss HW, et al. Screening for coronary artery disease after mediastinal irradiation for Hodgkin's disease. *J Clin Oncol* 2007;25:43–49.

139. Hein PA, Eskey CJ, Dunn JF, et al. Diffusion-weighted imaging in the follow-up of treated high-grade gliomas: tumor recurrence versus radiation injury. *Am J Neuroradiol* 2004;25:201–209.

140. Hernando ML, Marks LB, Bentel GC, et al. Radiation-induced pulmonary toxicity: a dose-volume histogram analysis in 201 patients with lung cancer. *Int J Radiat Oncol Biol Phys* 2001;51:650–659.

141. Hernberg M, Virkkunen P, Maasilta P, et al. Pulmonary toxicity after radiotherapy in primary breast cancer patients: results from a randomized chemotherapy study. *Int J Radiat Oncol Biol Phys* 2002;52:128–136.

142. Hewitt M, Greenfield S, Stovall E, eds. *From cancer patient to cancer survivor: lost in transition*. Washington, DC: National Academy Press; 2006.

143. Hill DA, Gilbert E, Dores GM, et al. Breast cancer risk following radiotherapy for Hodgkin lymphoma: modification by other risk factors. *Blood* 2005;106:3358–3365.

144. Hill M, Milan S, Cunningham D, et al. Evaluation of the efficacy of the VEEP regimen in adult Hodgkin's disease with assessment of gonadal and cardiac toxicity. *J Clin Oncol* 1995;13:387–395.

145. Hindo WA, DeTrana FA, Lee MS, et al. Large dose increment irradiation in treatment of cerebral metastases. *Cancer* 1970;26:138–141.

146. Hishikawa Y, Izumi M, Kurisu K, et al. Esophageal ulceration following high-dose-rate intraluminal brachytherapy for esophageal cancer. *Radiother Oncol* 1993;28:252–254.

147. Hoelzer D, Gokbuget N, Ottmann O, et al. Acute lymphoblastic leukemia. *Hematology* 2002;162–192.

148. Hogeboom CJ, Grosser SC, Guthrie KA, et al. Stature loss following treatment for Wilms tumor. *Med Pediatr Oncol* 2001;36:295–304.

149. Holtta P, Alaluusua S, Saarinen-Pihkala UM, et al. Agenesis and microdontia of permanent teeth as late adverse effects after stem cell transplantation in young children. *Cancer* 2005;103:181–190.

150. Hong JH, Chiang CS, Campbell IL, et al. Induction of acute phase gene expression by brain irradiation. *Int J Radiat Oncol Biol Phys* 1995;33:619–626.

151. Hopewell JW, Trott KR. Volume effects in radiobiology as applied to radiotherapy. *Radiother Oncol* 2000;56:283–288.

152. Hopewell JW, van den Aardweg GJ. Studies of dose-fractionation on early and late responses in pig skin: a reappraisal of the importance of the overall treatment time and its effects on radiosensitization and incomplete repair. *Int J Radiat Oncol Biol Phys* 1991;21:1441–1450.

153. Horning SJ, Hoppe RT, Breslin S, et al. Stanford V and radiotherapy for locally extensive and advanced Hodgkin's disease: mature results of a prospective clinical trial. *J Clin Oncol* 2002;20:630–637.

154. Hortobagyi GN. Anthracyclines in the treatment of cancer: an overview. *Drugs* 1997;54[Suppl 4]:1–7.

155. Hosing C, Munsell M, Yazji S, et al. Risk of therapy-related myelodysplastic syndrome/acute leukemia following high-dose therapy and autologous bone marrow transplantation for non-Hodgkin's lymphoma. *Ann Oncol* 2002;13:450–459.

156. Huang E, The BS, Strother DR, et al. Intensity-modulated radiation therapy for pediatric medulloblastoma: early report on the reduction of ototoxicity. *Int J Radiat Oncol Biol Phys* 2002;52:599–605.

157. Huang EH, Pollack A, Levy L, et al. Late rectal toxicity: dose-volume effects of conformal radiotherapy for prostate cancer. *Int J Radiat Oncol Biol Phys* 2002;54:1314–1321.

158. Hui R, Bull CA, Gebski V, et al. Radiotherapy and concurrent chemotherapy for oesophageal carcinoma. *Australas Radiol* 1994;38:315–319.

159. Hurkmans CW, Borger JH, Bos LJ, et al. Cardiac and lung complication probabilities after breast cancer irradiation. *Radiother Oncol* 2000;55:145–151.

160. Hutchison FN, Perez EA, Gandara DR, et al. Renal salt wasting in patients treated with cisplatin. *Ann Intern Med* 1988;108:21–25.

161. Inbar M, Merimsky O, Wigler N, et al. Cisplatin-related Lhermitte's sign. *Anticancer Drugs* 1992;3:375–377.

162. Irwin C, Fyles A, Wong CS, et al. Late renal function following whole abdominal irradiation. *Radiother Oncol* 1996;38:257–261.

163. Ishikawa S, Otsuki T, Kaneki M, et al. Dose-related effects of single focal irradiation in the medial temporal lobe structures in rats: magnetic resonance imaging and histological study. *Neurol Med Chir* 1999;39:1–7.

164. Jackson A, Skwarchuk MW, Zelefsky MJ, et al. Late rectal bleeding after conformal radiotherapy of prostate cancer. II. Volume effects and dose-volume histograms. *Int J Radiat Oncol Biol Phys* 2001;49:685–698.

165. Jackson A, Ten Haken RK, Robertson JM, et al. Analysis of clinical complication data for radiation hepatitis using a parallel architecture model. *Int J Radiat Oncol Biol Phys* 1995;31:883–891.

166. Jackson A. Partial irradiation of the rectum. *Semin Radiat Oncol* 2001;11:215–223.

167. Jellema AP, Doornaert P, Slotman BJ, et al. Does radiation dose to the salivary glands and oral cavity predict patient-rated xerostomia and sticky saliva in head and neck cancer patients treated with curative radiotherapy? *Radiother Oncol* 2005;77:164–171.

168. Johansson S, Bjermer L, Franzen L. Effects of ongoing smoking on the development of radiation-induced pneumonitis in breast cancer and oesophagus cancer patients. *Radiother Oncol* 1998;49:41–47.

169. Johnson FL, Rubin CM. Allogeneic marrow transplantation in the treatment of infants with cancer. *Br J Cancer* 1992;18[Suppl]:S76–S79.
170. Johnston CJ, Piedboeuf B, Rubin P, et al. Early and persistent alterations in the expression of interleukin-1 alpha, interleukin-1 beta and tumor necrosis factor alpha mRNA levels in fibrosis-resistant and sensitive mice after thoracic irradiation. *Radiat Res* 1996;145:762–767.
171. Johnston CJ, Williams JP, Okunieff P, et al. Radiation-induced pulmonary fibrosis: examination of chemokine and chemokine receptor families. *Radiat Res* 2002;157:256–265.
172. Johnston CJ, Wright TW, Rubin P, et al. Alterations in the expression of chemokine mRNA levels in fibrosis-resistant and -sensitive mice after thoracic irradiation. *Exp Lung Res* 1998;24:321–337.
173. Jones AM. Transient radiation myelopathy (with reference to Lhermitte's sign of electrical paresthesia). *Br J Radiol* 1964;37:727–744.
174. Jongejan HT, van der Kogel AJ, Provoost AP, et al. Radiation nephropathy in young and adult rats. *Int J Radiat Oncol Biol Phys* 1987;13:225–232.
175. Kal HB, Loes Van Kempen-Harteveld L. Renal dysfunction after total body irradiation dose-effect relationship. *Int J Radiat Oncol Biol Phys* 2006;65:1228–1232.
176. Kaste S, Hopkins K, Crom D, et al. Dental abnormalities in children treated for acute lymphoblastic leukemia. *Leukemia* 1997;11:792–796.
177. Keane WF, Brenner BM, Mazzu A, et al. The CHORUS (Cerivastatin in Heart Outcomes in Renal Disease: Understanding Survival) protocol: a double-blind, placebo-controlled trial in patients with ESRD. *Am J Kidney Dis* 2001;37[Suppl]:S48–S53.
178. Kellum JM, Jaffe BM, Calhoun TR, et al. Gastric complications after radiotherapy for Hodgkin's disease and other lymphomas. *Am J Surg* 1977;134:314–317.
179. Kiehna EN, Mulhern RK, Li C, et al. Changes in attentional performance of children and young adults with localized primary brain tumors after conformal radiation therapy. *J Clin Oncol* 2006;24:5283–5290.
180. Kim T, Somerville P, Freeman C. Unilateral radiation nephropathy–the long-term significance. *Int J Radiat Oncol Biol Phys* 1984;10:2053–2059.
181. King V, Constine LS, Clark D, et al. Symptomatic coronary artery disease after mantle irradiation for Hodgkin's disease. *Int J Radiat Oncol Biol Phys* 1996;36:881–889.
182. Kline L, Kim J, Ceballos R. Radiation optic neuropathy. *Ophthalmology* 1985;92:1118–1126.
183. Koh ES, Sun A, Tran TH, et al. Clinical dose-volume histogram analysis in predicting radiation pneumonitis in Hodgkin's lymphoma. *Int J Radiat Oncol Biol Phys* 2006;66:223–228.
184. Konings AW, Cotteleer F, Faber H, et al. Volume effects and region-dependent radiosensitivity of the parotid gland. *Int J Radiat Oncol Biol Phys* 2005;62:1090–1095.
185. Koukourakis MI, Danielidis V. Preventing radiation induced xerostomia. *Cancer Treat Rev* 2005;31:546–554.
186. Kramer S, Gelber RD, Snow JB, et al. Combined radiation therapy and surgery in the management of advanced head and neck cancer: final report of study 73-03 of the Radiation Therapy Oncology Group. *Head Neck Surg* 1987;10:19–30.
187. Kreisman H, Wolkove N. Pulmonary toxicity of antineoplastic therapy. *Semin Oncol* 1992;19:508–520.
188. Kremer LC, Caron HN. Anthracycline cardiotoxicity in children. *N Engl J Med* 2004;351:120–121.
189. Kremer LC, van Dalen EC, Offringa M, et al. Anthracycline-induced clinical heart failure in a cohort of 607 children: long-term follow-up study. *J Clin Oncol* 2001;19:191–196.
190. Kreuser ED, Felsenberg D, Behles C. Long-term gonadal dysfunction and its impact on bone mineralization in patients following COPP/ABVD chemotherapy for Hodgkin's disease. *Ann Oncol* 1992;3[Suppl 4]:105–110.
191. Krishnan A, Bhatia S, Slovak M, et al. Predictors of therapy-related leukemia and myelodysplasia following autologous transplantation for lymphoma: an assessment of risk factors. *Blood* 2000;95:1588–1593.
192. Kulkarni S, Sastry P, Saikia T. et al. Gonadal function following ABVD therapy for Hodgkin's disease. *Am J Clin Oncol* 1997;20:354–357.
193. Kupelian PA, Reddy CA, Carlson TP, et al. Dose/volume relationship of late rectal bleeding after external beam radiotherapy for localized prostate cancer: absolute or relative rectal volume? *Cancer J* 2002;8:62–66.
194. Kwa SL, Lebesque JV, Theuws JC, et al. Radiation pneumonitis as a function of mean lung dose: an analysis of pooled data of 540 patients. *Int J Radiat Oncol Biol Phys* 1998;42:1–9.
195. Kyoizumi S, Suzuki T, Teraoka S, et al. Radiation sensitivity of human hair follicles in SCID-hu mice. *Radiat Res* 1998;149:11–18.
196. Kyrkanides S, Olschowka JA, Williams JP, et al. TNFα and IL-1β mediate ICAM-1 induction via microglia astrocyte interaction in CNS radiation injury. *J Neuroimmunol* 1999;95:95–106.
197. Laack NN, Brown PD, Ivnik RJ, et al. Cognitive function after radiotherapy for supratentorial low-grade glioma: a North Central Cancer Treatment Group prospective study. *Int J Radiat Oncol Biol Phys* 2005;63:1175–1183.
198. LaMonte CS, Yeh S, Straus D. Long-term follow-up of cardiac function in patients with Hodgkin's disease treated with mediastinal irradiation and combination chemotherapy including doxorubicin. *Cancer Treat Rep* 1986;70:439–444.
199. Landier W, Bhatia S, Eshelman DA. Development of risk-based guidelines for pediatric cancer survivors: the Children's Oncology Group Long-Term Follow-Up Guidelines from the Chidren's Oncology Group Late Effects Committee and Nursing Discipline. *J Clin Oncol* 2004;22:4979–4990.
200. Lawenda BD, Gagne HM, Gierga DP, et al. Permanent alopecia after cranial irradiation: dose-response relationship. *Int J Radiat Oncol Biol Phys* 2004;60:879–887.
201. Lawrence TS, Ten Haken RK, Kessler ML, et al. The use of 3-D dose volume analysis to predict radiation hepatitis. *Int J Radiat Oncol Biol Phys* 1992;23:781–788.
202. Lawton CA, Cohen EP, Barber-Derus SW, et al. Late renal dysfunction in adult survivors of bone marrow transplantation. *Cancer* 1991;67:2795–2800.
203. Lebesque JV, Stewart FA, Hart AA. Analysis of the rate of expression of radiation-induced renal damage and the effects of hyperfractionation. *Radiother Oncol* 1986;5:147–157.
204. Lee AW, Foo W, Chappell R, et al. Effect of time, dose, and fractionation on temporal lobe necrosis following radiotherapy for nasopharyngeal carcinoma. *Int J Radiat Oncol Biol Phys* 1998;40:35–42.
205. Lee SJ, Schover LR, Partridge AH, et al. American Society of Clinical Oncology recommendations on fertility preservation in cancer patients. *J Clin Oncol* 2006;24:2917–2931.
206. Lee TH, Boucher CA. Clinical practice: noninvasive tests in patients with stable coronary artery disease. *N Engl J Med* 2001;344:1840–1845.
207. Leibel SA, Sheline GE. In:Gutin P, Leibel S, Sheline G, eds. *Tolerance of the brain and spinal cord to conventional irradiation.* New York: Raven Press; 1991.
208. Leisenring W, Friedman DL, Flowers ME, et al. Nonmelanoma skin and mucosal cancers after hematopoietic cell transplantation. *J Clin Oncol* 2006;24:1119–1126.
209. Lewandowski RJ, Thurston KG, Goin JE, et al. ^{90}Y microsphere (TheraSphere) treatment for unresectable colorectal cancer metastases of the liver: response to treatment at targeted doses of 135-150 Gy as measured by [18F]fluorodeoxyglucose positron emission tomography and computed tomographic imaging. *J Vasc Interv Radiol* 2005;16:1641–1651.
210. Lind PARM, Marks LB, Hardenbergh PH, et al. Technical factors associated with radiation pneumonitis after local ± regional radiation therapy for breast cancer. *Int J Radiat Oncol Biol Phys* 2002;52:37–143.
211. Lingos TI, Recht A, Vicini F, et al. Radiation pneumonitis in breast cancer patients treated with conservative surgery and radiation therapy. *Int J Radiat Oncol Biol Phys* 1991;21:355–360.
212. Lipshultz S, Lipsitz S, Sallan S. Chronic progressive left ventricular systolic dysfunction and afterload excess years after doxorubicin therapy for childhood acute lymphoblastic leukemia. *Proceedings of American Society of Clinical Oncology,* 2000; 19: A-2281, 5800.
213. Luxton RW. Radiation nephritis: a long-term study of 54 patients. *Lancet* 1961;2:1221–1224.
214. Maguire A, Craft A, Evans R, et al. The long-term effects of treatment on the dental condition of children surviving malignant disease. *Cancer* 1987;60:2570–2575.
215. Maguire PD, Sibley GS, Zhou SM, et al. Clinical and dosimetric predictors of radiation-induced esophageal toxicity. *Int J Radiat Oncol Biol Phys* 1999;45:97–103.
216. Mah K, van Dyk J, Keane T, et al. Acute radiation-induced pulmonary damage: a clinical study on the response to fractionated radiation therapy. *Int J Radiat Oncol Biol Phys* 1987;13:179–188.
217. Marcus RB Jr, Million RR. The incidence of myelitis after irradiation of the cervical spinal cord. *Int J Radiat Oncol Biol Phys* 1990;19:3–8.
218. Marks JE, Baglan RJ, Prassad SC, et al. Cerebral radionecrosis: incidence and risk in relation to dose, time, fractionation and volume. *Int J Radiat Oncol Biol Phys* 1981;7:243–252.
219. Marks LB, Hollis D, Munley M, et al. The role of lung perfusion imaging in predicting the direction of radiation-induced changes in pulmonary function tests. *Cancer* 2000;88:2135–2141.
220. Marks LB, Munley MT, Bentel GC, et al. Physical and biological predictors of changes in whole-lung function following thoracic irradiation. *Int J Radiat Oncol Biol Phys* 1997;39:563–570.
221. Marks LB, Spencer DP, Bentel GC, et al. The utility of SPECT lung perfusion scans in minimizing and assessing the physiologic consequences of thoracic irradiation. *Int J Radiat Oncol Biol Phys* 1993;26:659–668.
222. Marks LB, Yu X, Vujaskovic Z, et al. Radiation-induced lung injury. *Semin Radiat Oncol* 2003;13:333–345.
223. Marks LB. The impact of organ structure on radiation response. *Int J Radiat Oncol Biol Phys* 1996;34:1165–1171.
224. Marucci L, Niemierko A, Liebsch NJ, et al. Spinal cord tolerance to high-dose fractionated 3D conformal proton-photon irradiation as evaluated by equivalent uniform dose and dose volume histogram analysis. *Int J Radiat Oncol Biol Phys* 2004;59:551–555.
225. Mathews R, Rajan N, Josefson L, et al. Hyperbaric oxygen therapy for radiation induced hemorrhagic cystitis. *J Urol* 1999;161:435–437.
226. Mauch P, Kalish LA, Marcus KC. Long-term survival in Hodgkin's disease: relative impact of mortality, second tumors, infection and cardiovascular disease. *Cancer J Sci Am* 1995;1:33–42.
227. McDonald S, Meyerowitz C, Smudzin T, et al. Preliminary results of a pilot study using WR-2721 before fractionated irradiation of the head and neck to reduce salivary gland dysfunction. *Int J Radiat Oncol Biol Phys* 1994;29:747–754.
228. McDonald S, Rubin P, Constine L, et al. Biochemical markers as predictors for pulmonary effects of radiation. *Radiat Oncol Invest* 1995;3:56–63.
229. McDonald S, Rubin P, Phillips T, et al. Injury to the lung from cancer therapy: clinical syndromes, measureable endpoints, and potential scoring systems. *Int J Radiat Oncol Biol Phys* 1995;31:1187–1203.
230. McKeage MJ. Comparative adverse effect profiles of platinum drugs. *Drug Safety* 1995;13:228–244.
231. Merchant TE, Goloubeva O, Pritchard DL, et al. Radiation dose-volume effects on growth hormone secretion. *Int J Radiat Oncol Biol Phys* 2002;52:1264–1270.
232. Merchant TE, Kiehna EN, Li C, et al. Modeling radiation dosimetry to predict cognitive outcomes in pediatric patients with CNS embryonal tumors including medulloblastoma. *Int J Radiat Oncol Biol Phys* 2006;65:210–221.
233. Merchant TE, Kiehna EN, Li C, et al. Radiation dosimetry predicts IQ after conformal radiation therapy in pediatric patients with localized ependymoma. *Int J Radiat Oncol Biol Phys* 2005;63:1546–1554.
234. Metayer C, Curtis RE, Vose J, et al. Myelodysplastic syndrome and acute myeloid leukemia after autotransplantation for lymphoma: a multicenter case-control study. *Blood* 2003;101:2015–2023.
235. Metayer C, Lynch CF, Clarke EA, et al. Second cancers amoung long-term survivors of Hodgkin's disease diagnosed in childhood and adolescence. *J Clin Oncol* 2000;18:2435–2443.
236. Micallef IN, Lillington DM, Apostolidis J, et al. Therapy-related myelodysplasia and secondary acute myelogenous leukemia after high-dose therapy with autologous hematopoietic progenitor-cell support for lymphoid malignancies. *J Clin Oncol* 2000;18:947–955.
237. Miller RW. Delayed effects of external radiation exposure: a brief history. *Radiat Res* 1995;144:160–169.
238. Milligan DW. Secondary leukaemia and myelodysplasia after autografting for lymphoma: is the transplant to blame? *Leuk Lymphoma* 2000;39:223–228.
239. Miralbell R, Bieri S, Mermillod B, et al. Renal toxicity after allogeneic bone marrow transplantation: the combined effects of total-body irradiation and graft-versus-host disease. *J Clin Oncol* 1996;14:579–585.
240. Mitchell EP. Gastrointestinal toxicity of chemotherapeutic agents. *Semin Oncol* 1992;19:566–579.

241. Monroe AT, Bhandare N, Morris CG, et al. Preventing radiation retinopathy with hyperfractionation. *Int J Radiat Oncol Biol Phys* 2005;61:856–864.
242. Monson JM, Stark P, Reilly JJ, et al. Clinical radiation pneumonitis and radiographic changes after thoracic radiation therapy for lung carcinoma. *Cancer* 1998;82:842–850.
243. Morris MM, Willett CG. Late renal function after upper abdominal irradiation. *Int J Radiat Oncol Biol Phys* 1997;39[Suppl 2]:284.
244. Moser EC, Noordijk EM, van Leeuwen FE, et al. Long-term risk of cardiovascular disease after treatment for aggressive non-Hodgkin lymphoma. *Blood* 2006;107:2912–2919.
245. Moulder JE, Fish BL, Regner KR, et al. Retinoic acid exacerbates experimental radiation nephropathy. *Radiat Res* 2002;157:199–203.
246. Moulder JE, Fish BL. Influence of nephrotoxic drugs on the late renal toxicity associated with bone marrow transplant conditioning regimens. *Int J Radiat Oncol Biol Phys* 1991;20:333–337.
247. Munter MW, Karger CP, Hoffner SG, et al. Evaluation of salivary gland function after treatment of head-and-neck tumors with intensity-modulated radiotherapy by quantitative pertechnetate scintigraphy. *Int J Radiat Oncol Biol Phys* 2004;58:175–184.
248. Murase T, Anscher MS, Petros WP, et al. Changes in plasma transforming growth factor beta in response to high-dose chemotherapy for stage II breast cancer: possible implications for the prevention of hepatic veno-occlusive disease and pulmonary drug toxicity. *Bone Marrow Transplant* 1995;15:173–178.
249. Neglia J, Friedman D, Yasui Y, et al. Second malignant neoplasms in five-year survivors of childhood cancer: Childhood Cancer Survivor Study. *J Nat Cancer Inst* 2001;93:618–629.
250. Neta R. Modulation with cytokines of radiation injury: suggested mechanisms of action. *Env Health Perspect* 1997;105[Suppl 6]:1463–1465.
251. Nichols G, de Castro K, Wei LX, et al. Therapy-related myelodysplastic syndrome after autologous stem cell transplantation for breast cancer. *Leukemia* 2002;16:1673–1679.
252. Nieder C, Ataman F, Price RE, et al. Radiation myelopathy: new perspective on an old problem. *Radiat Oncol Invest* 1999;7:193–203.
253. Novak JM, Collins JT, Donowitz M, et al. Effects of radiation on the human gastrointestinal tract. *J Clin Gastroenterol* 1979;1:9–39.
254. O'Rourke IC, Tiver K, Bull C, et al. Swallowing performance after radiation therapy for carcinoma of the esophagus. *Cancer* 1988;61:2022–2026.
255. Oberlin O, Rey A, Anderson J, et al. Treatment of orbital rhabdomyosarcoma: survival and late effects of treatment–results of an international workshop. *J Clin Oncol* 2001;19:197–204.
256. Oeffinger K, Mertens A, Sklar C, et al. Chronic health conditions in adult survivors of childhood cancer. *N Engl J Med* 2006;355:1572–1582.
257. Okunieff P, Rubin P, Williams JP, et al. TGF 1 involvement in the development of radiation-induced soft tissue fibrosis. *Radiat Res* In press.
258. Olschowka JA, Kyrkanides S, Harvey BK, et al. ICAM-1 induction in the mouse CNS following irradiation. *Brain Behav Immun* 1997;11:273–285.
259. Overgaard J, Bartelink H. Late effects consensus conference: RTOG/EORTC. *Radiother Oncol* 1995;35:1–82.
260. Pacholke HD, Amdur RJ, Morris CG, et al. Late xerostomia after intensity-modulated radiation therapy versus conventional radiotherapy. *Am J Clin Oncol* 2005;28:351–358.
261. Packer RJ, Goldwein J, Nicholson HS, et al. Treatment of children with medulloblastomas with reduced-dose craniospinal radiation therapy and adjuvant chemotherapy: a Children's Cancer Group Study. *J Clin Oncol* 1999;17:2127–2136.
262. Pan CC, Eisbruch A, Lee JS, et al. Prospective study of inner ear radiation dose and hearing loss in head-and-neck cancer patients. *Int J Radiat Oncol Biol Phys* 2005;61:1393–1402.
263. Parsons JT, Bova FJ, Mendenhall WM, et al. Response of the normal eye to high dose radiotherapy. *Oncology* 1996;10:837–847.
264. Paterson R. *The treatment of malignancy by radium and x-rays: being a practice of radiotherapy*. London: Edward Arnold; 1947.
265. Paulino AC, Wen BC, Brown CK, et al. Late effects in children treated with radiation therapy for Wilms' tumor. *Int J Radiat Oncol Biol Phys* 2000;46:1239–1246.
266. Paulino AC. Role of radiation therapy in parameningeal rhabdomyosarcoma. *Cancer Invest* 1999;17:223–230.
267. Pearlman SH, Rubin P, White HC, et al. Fetal hypothalamic transplants into brain irradiated rats: graft morphometry and host behavioral responses. *Int J Radiat Oncol Biol Phys* 1990;19:293–300.
268. Pederson-Bjergaard J, Andersen MK, Christianson DH. Therapy-related acute myeloid leukemia and myelodysplasia after high-dose chemotherapy and autologous stem cell transplantation. *Blood* 2000;95.
269. Pein F, Sakiroglu O, Dahan M, et al. Cardiac abnormalities 15 years and more after adriamycin therapy in 229 childhood survivors of a solid tumour at the Institut Gustave Roussy. *Br J Cancer* 2004;91:37–44.
270. Perez CA, Breaux S, Bedwinek JM, et al. Radiation therapy alone in the treatment of carcinoma of the uterine cervix: II. Analysis of complications. *Cancer* 1984;54:235–246.
271. Perez CA, Fox S, Lockett MA, et al. Impact of dose in outcome of irradiation alone in carcinoma of the uterine cervix: analysis of two different methods. *Int J Radiat Oncol Biol Phys* 1991;21:885–898.
272. Peschel R.E., Chen M., Seashore J. The treatment of massive hepatomegaly in stage IV-S neuroblastoma. *Int J Radiat Oncol Biol Phys* 1981;7:549–553.
273. Piedbois P, Ganem G, Cordonnier C, et al. Interstitial pneumonitis and venocclusive disease of the liver after bone marrow transplantation. *Radiother Oncol* 1990;18[Suppl 1]:125–127.
274. Pilepich MV, Krall JM, Sause WT, et al. Correlation of radiotherapeutic parameters and treatment related morbidity in carcinoma of the prostate: analysis of RTOG study 75–06. *Int J Radiat Oncol Biol Phys* 1987;13:351–357.
275. Polansky SM, Ravin CE, Prosnitz LR. Pulmonary changes after primary radiation for early breast carcinoma. *Am J Radiol* 1980;134:101–105.
276. Pollack A, Zagars GK, Starkschall G, et al. Prostate cancer radiation dose response: results of the MD Anderson phase III randomized trial. *Int J Radiat Oncol Biol Phys* 2002;53:1097–1105.
277. Potish RA, Jones TK Jr, Levitt SH. Factors predisposing to radiation-related small-bowel damage. *Radiology* 1979;132:479–482.
278. Pourquier H, Dubois JB, Delard R. Cancer of the uterine cervix: dosimetric guidelines for prevention of late rectal and rectosigmoid complications as a result of radiotherapeutic treatment. *Int J Radiat Oncol Biol Phys* 1982;8:1887–1895.
279. Prasad VK, Lewis IJ, Aparicio SR, et al. Progressive glomerular toxicity of ifosfamide in children. *Med Pediatr Oncol* 1996;27:149–155.
280. Prosnitz LR, Lawson JP, Friedlaender GE, et al. Avascular necrosis of bone in Hodgkin's disease patients with combined modality therapy. *Cancer* 1981;47:2793–2797.
281. Radcliffe J, Bunin GR, Sutton LN, et al. Cognitive deficits in long-term survivors of childhood medulloblastoma and other noncortical tumors: age-dependent effects of whole brain radiation. *Int J Dev Neurosci* 1994;12:327–334.
282. Ragaz J, Olivotto IA, Spinelli JJ, et al. Locoregional radiation therapy in patients with high-risk breast cancer receiving adjuvant chemotherapy: 20-year results of the British Columbia randomized trial. *J Natl Cancer Inst* 2005;97:116–126.
283. Rampling R, Symonds P. Radiation myelopathy. *Curr Opin Neurol* 1998;11:627–632.
284. Raney RB, Anderson JR, Kollath J. Late effects of therapy in 94 patients with localized rhabdomyosarcoma of the orbit: report from the Intergroup Rhabdomyosarcoma Study (IRS)-III, 1984–1991. *Med Pediatr Oncol* 2000;34:413–420.
285. Reinhold HS, Keyeux A, Dunjic A, et al. The influence of radiation on blood vessels and circulation: XII. Discussion and conclusions. *Curr Top Radiat Res Q* 1974;10:185–198.
286. Relander T, Cavallin-Stahl E, Garwicz S. Gonadal and sexual function in men treated for childhood cancer. *Med Pediatr Oncol* 2000;35:52–63.
287. Ries LA, Eisner MP, Kosary CL, *Cancer Statistics Review 1975–2003, SEE 2006*.
288. Riva D, Giorgi C, Nichelli F, et al. Intrathecal methotrexate affects cognitive function in children with medulloblastoma. *Neurology* 2002;59:48–53.
289. Robbins ME, Bonsib SM. Radiation nephropathy: a review. *Scanning Microsc* 1995;9:535–560.
290. Roesink JM, Moerland MA, Battermann JJ, et al. Quantitative dose-volume response analysis of changes in parotid gland function after radiotherapy in the head-and-neck region. *Int J Radiat Oncol Biol Phys* 2001;51:938–946.
291. Roesink JM, Schipper M, Busschers W, et al. A comparison of mean parotid gland dose with measures of parotid gland function after radiotherapy for head-and-neck cancer: implications for future trials. *Int J Radiat Oncol Biol Phys* 2005;63:1006–1009.
292. Ronckers C, Sigurdson A, Stovall M, et al. Thyroid cancer in childhood cancer survivors: a detailed evaluation of radiation dose response and its modifers. *Radiat Res* 2006;166:618–628.
293. Ruben JD, Dally M, Bailey M, et al. Cerebral radiation necrosis: incidence, outcomes, and risk factors with emphasis on radiation parameters and chemotherapy. *Int J Radiat Oncol Biol Phys* 2006;65:499–508.
294. Rubin P, Casarett GW. *Clinical radiation pathology,* vols I and II. Philadelphia: W.B.Saunders Co.; 1968.
295. Rubin P, Constine LS, Scarantino CW. The paradoxes in patterns and mechanism of bone marrow regeneration after irradiation: 2. Total body irradiation. *Radiother Oncol* 1984;2:227–233.
296. Rubin P, ed. Special issue: Late Effects of Normal Tissues (LENT) Consensus Conferene. *Int J Radiat Oncol Biol Phys* 1995;31:1037–1360.
297. Rubin P, Finkelstein JN, Williams JP. In: Tobias J, Thomas P, eds. *Paradigm shifts in the radiation pathophysiology of late effects in normal tissues: molecular vs. classic concepts.* London: Arnold; 1998.
298. Rubin P, Siemann DW, Shapiro DL, et al. Surfactant release as an early measure of radiation pneumonitis. *Int J Radiat Oncol Biol Phys* 1983;9:1669–1673.
299. Ruifrok AC, McBride WH. Growth factors: biological and clinical aspects. *Int J Radiat Oncol Biological Phys* 1999;43:877–881.
300. Rutqvist LE, Lax I, Fornander T, et al. Cardiovascular mortality in a randomized trial of adjuvant radiation therapy versus surgery alone in primary breast cancer. *Int J Radiat Oncol Biol Phys* 1992;22:887–896.
301. Sagerman RH, Berdon WE, Baker DH. Renal atrophy without hypertension following abdominal irradiation in infants and children. *Ann Radiol* 1969;12:278–284.
302. Salem R, Lewandowski RJ, Atassi B, et al. Treatment of unresectable hepatocellular carcinoma with use of ^{90}Y microspheres (TheraSphere): safe, tumor response, and survival. *J Vasc Interv Radiol* 2005;16:1627–1639.
303. Samaan NA, Vieto R, Schultz PN, et al. Hypothalmic pituitary and thyroid dysfunction after radiotherapy to the head and neck. *Int J Radiat Oncol Biol Phys* 1982;8:1857–1867.
304. Sasse AD, Clark LG, Sasse EC, et al. Amifostine reduces side effects and improves complete response rate during radiotherapy: results of a meta-analysis. *Int J Radiat Oncol Biol Phys* 2006;64:784–791.
305. Scarantino CW, Rubin P, Constine LS. The paradoxes in patterns and mechanism of bone marrow regeneration after irradiation: 1. Different volumes and doses. *Radiother Oncol* 1984;2:215–225.
306. Schellong G, Potter R, Bramswig J, et al. High cure rates and reduced long-term toxicity in pediatric Hodgkin's disease: the German-Austrian multicenter trial DAL-HD-90. The German-Austrian Pediatric Hodgkin's Disease Study Group. *J Clin Oncol* 1999;17:3736–3744.
307. Schmiegelow M, Feldt-Rasmussen U, Rasmussen AK, et al. A population-based study of thyroid function after radiotherapy and chemotherapy for a childhood brain tumor. *J Clin Endocrinol Metab* 2003;88:136–140.
308. Schultheiss TE, Higgins EM, El-Mahdi HM. The latent period in radiation myelopathy. *Int J Radiat Oncol Biol Phys* 1984;10:1109–1115.
309. Schultheiss TE, Kun LE, Ang KK, et al. Radiation response of the central nervous system. *Int J Radiat Oncol Biol Phys* 1995;31:1093–1112.
310. Schultheiss TE, Lee WR, Hunt MA, et al. Late GI and GU complications in the treatment of prostate cancer. *Int J Radiat Oncol Biol Phys* 1997;37:3–11.
311. Schultheiss TE. Spinal cord radiation tolerance. *Int J Radiat Oncol Biol Phys* 1994;30:735–736.
312. Schultheiss TE. The controversies and pitfalls in modeling normal tissue radiation injury/damage. *Semin Radiat Oncol* 2001;11:210–214.
313. Seppenwolde Y, Lebesque JV, de Jaeger K, et al. Comparing different NTCP models that predict the incidence of radiation pneumonitis: normal tissue complication probability. *Int J Radiat Oncol Biol Phys* 2003;55:724–735.
314. Shalet SM, Brennan BM. Growth and growth hormone status following treatment for childhood leukaemia. *Horm Res* 1998;50:1–10.
315. Shalet SM, Brennan BM. Puberty in children with cancer. *Horm Res* 2002;57[2 suppl]:39–42.
316. Shankar G, Cohen DA. Idiopathic pneumonia syndrome after bone marrow transplantation: the role of pre-transplant radiation conditioning and local cytokine dysregulation in promoting lung inflammation and fibrosis. *Int J Exp Pathol* 2001;82:101–113.

317. Shapiro SJ, Shapiro SD, Mill WB, et al. Prospective study of long-term manifestations of mantle irradiation. *Int J Radiat Oncol Biol Phys* 1990;19:707–714.
318. Sheline GE, Wara WM, Smith V. Therapeutic irradiation and brain injury. *Int J Radiat Oncol Biol Phys* 1980;6:1215–1228.
319. Silber JH, Radcliffe J, Peckham V, et al. Whole-brain irradiation and decline in intelligence: the influence of dose and age on IQ score. *J Clin Oncol* 1992;10:1390–1396.
320. Singh AK, Lockett MA, Bradley JD. Predictors of radiation-induced esophageal toxicity in patients with non-small-cell lung cancer treated with three-dimensional conformal radiotherapy. *Int J Radiat Oncol Biol Phys* 2003;55:337–341.
321. Skinner R, Pearson AD, English MW, et al. Risk factors for ifosfamide nephrotoxicity in children. *Lancet* 1996;348:578–580.
322. Sklar C, Whitton J, Mertens A, et al. Abnormalities of the thyroid in survivors of Hodgkin's disease: data from the Childhood Cancer Survivor Study. *J Clin Endocrinol Metab* 2000;85:3227–3232.
323. Sklar CA. Growth and neuroendocrine dysfunction following therapy for childhood cancer. *Pediatr Clin North Am* 1997;44:489–503.
324. Sklar CA. Growth following therapy for childhood cancer. *Cancer Invest* 1995;13:511–516.
325. Skwarchuk MW, Jackson A, Zelefsky MJ, et al. Late rectal toxicity after conformal radiotherapy of prostate cancer (I): multivariate analysis and dose-response. *Int J Radiat Oncol Biol Phys* 2000;47:103–113.
326. Smedler AC, Nilsson C, Bolme P. Total body irradiation: a neuropsychological risk factor in pediatric bone marrow transplant recipients. *Acta Paediatr* 1995;84:325–330.
327. Smith GR, Thomas PR, Ritchey M, et al. Long-term renal function in patients with irradiated bilateral Wilms tumor. National Wilms' Tumor Study Group. *Am J Clin Oncol* 1998;21:58–63.
328. Smith JS, Cha S, Mayo MC, et al. Serial diffusion-weighted magnetic resonance imaging in case of glioma: distinguishing tumor recurrence from postresection injury. *J Neurosurg* 2005;103:428–438.
329. Socié G, Salooja N, Cohen A, et al. Nonmalignant late effects after allogeneic stem cell transplantation. *Blood* 2003;101:3373–3385.
330. Song DY, Lawrie WT, Abrams RA, et al. Acute and late radiotherapy toxicity in patients with inflammatory bowel disease. *Int J Radiat Oncol Biol Phys* 2001;51:455–459.
331. Sorenson K, Levitt GA, Bull C, et al. Late anthracycline cardiotoxicity after childhood cancer: a prospective longitudinal study. *Cancer* 2003;97:1991–1998.
332. Stewart JR, Fajardo LF, Gillette SM, et al. Radiation injury to the heart. *Int J Radiat Oncol Biol Phys* 1995;31:1205–1211.
333. Strandqvist M. Studien uber die Kumulative Wirkung der Rontgenstrahlen bei Fraktion-ierung. *Acta Radiol* 1944;55[Suppl]:1–300.
334. Strauss AJ, Su JT, Dalton VM, et al. Bony morbidity in children treated for acute lymphoblastic leukemia. *J Clin Oncol* 2001;19:3066–3072.
335. Swerdlow AJ, Barber JA, Hudson GV, et al. Risk of second malignancy after Hodgkin's disease in a collaborative British cohort: the relation to age at treatment. *J Clin Oncol* 2000;18:498–509.
336. Tefft M. Radiation related toxicities in National Wilms' Tumor Study Number 1. *Int J Radiat Oncol Biol Phys* 1977;2:455–463.
337. Tell R, Lundell G, Nilsson B, et al. Long-term incidence of hypothyroidism after radiotherapy in patients with head-and-neck cancer. *Int J Radiat Oncol Biol Phys* 2004;60:395–400.
338. Ten Haken R, Dawson L, McGinn C, et al. Determination of model parameters for description of radiation induced liver disease. *Radiother Oncol* 2000;56[Suppl]:S115 (abstr).
339. Teshima T, Hanks GE, Hanlon AL, et al. Rectal bleeding after conformal 3D treatment of prostate cancer: time to occurrence, response to treatment and duration of morbidity. *Int J Radiat Oncol Biol Phys* 1997;39:77–83.
340. Thames HD Jr, Withers HR, Peters LJ. Changes in early and late radiation responses with altered dose fractionation: implications for dose-survival relationships. *Int J Radiat Oncol Biol Phys* 1982;8:219–226.
341. Thames HD, Bentzen SM, Turesson I, et al. Time-dose factors in radiotherapy: a review of the human data. *Radiother Oncol* 1990;19:219–235.
342. Theuws JC, Muller SH, Seppenwolde Y, et al. Effect of radiotherapy and chemotherapy on pulmonary function after treatment for breast cancer and lymphoma: a follow-up study. *J Clin Oncol* 1999;17:3091–3100.
343. Thomas ED, Sanders JE, Flournoy N, et al. Marrow transplantation for patients with acute lymphoblastic leukemia: a long-term follow-up. *Blood* 1983;62:1139–1141.
344. Thomas ED. Bone marrow transplantation: a review. *Semin Hematol* 1999;36[Suppl]:75–103.
345. Thomas PRM, Tefft M, D'Angio GJ, et al. Acute toxicities associated with radiation in the second National Wilms' Tumor Study. *J Clin Oncol* 1988;6:1694–1698.
346. Thompson PL, Mackay IR, Robson GSM, et al. Late radiation nephritis after gastric x-irradiation for peptic ulcer. *Q J Med* 1971;40:145–157.
347. Thomson AB, Critchley HO, Kelnar CJ, et al. Late reproductive sequelae following treatment of childhood cancer and options for fertility preservation. *Best Practice Res Clin Endocrinol Metab* 2002;16:311–334.
348. Tofilon PJ, Fike JR. The radioresponse of the central nervous system: a dynamic process. *Radiat Res* 2000;153:357–370.
349. Torres IJ, Mundt AJ, Sweeney PJ, et al. A longitudinal neuropsychological study of partial brain radiation in adults with brain tumors. *Neurology* 2003;60:1113–1118.
350. Travis EL. Organizational response of normal tissues to irradiation. *Semin Radiat Oncol* 2001;11:184–197.
351. Travis LB, Gospodarowicz M, Curtis RE, et al. Lung cancer following chemotherapy and radiotherapy for Hodgkin's disease. *J Natl Cancer Inst* 2002;94:182–192.
352. Travis LB, Hill D, Dores GM, et al. Cumulative absolute breast cancer risk for young women treated for Hodgkin lymphoma. *J Natl Cancer Inst* 2005;97:1428–1437.
353. Travis LB, Hill DA, Dores GM, et al. Breast cancer following radiotherapy and chemotherapy among young women with Hodgkin disease. *JAMA* 2003;290:465–475.
354. Trotti A, Colevas AD, Setser A, et al. CTCAE v3.0: development of a comprehensive grading system for the adverse effects of cancer treatment. *Semin Radiat Oncol* 2003;13:176–181.
355. Tsujino K, Hirota S, Endo M, et al. Predictive value of dose-volume histogram parameters for predicting radiation pneumonitis after concurrent chemoradiation for lung cancer. *Int J Radiat Oncol Biol Phys* 2003;55:110–115.
356. Tubiana M, Frindel E, Croizat H, et al. Effects of radiations on bone marrow. *Pathol Biol* 1979;27:326–334.
357. Turesson I, Thames HD. Repair capacity and kinetics of human skin during fractionated radiotherapy: erythema, desquamation, and telangiectasia after 3 and 5 year's follow-up. *Radiother Oncol* 1989;15:168–188.
358. van Dyk J, Keane TJ, Kan S, et al. Radiation pneumonitis following large single dose irradiation: a re-evaluation based on absolute dose to the lung. *Int J Radiat Oncol Biol Phys* 1981;7:461–467.
359. van Kempen-Harteveld ML, Struikmans H, Kal HB. Cataract after total body irradiation and bone marrow transplantation: degree of visual impairment. *Int J Radiat Oncol Biol Phys* 2002;52:1375–1380.
360. van Kempen-Harteveld ML, Struikmans H, Kal HB. Cataract-free interval and severity of cataract after total body irradiation and bone marrow transplantation: influence of treatment parameters. *Int J Radiat Oncol Biol Phys* 2000;48:807–815.
361. van Leeuwen FE, Klokman WJ, Stovall M, et al. Roles of radiation dose, chemotherapy, and hormonal factors in breast cancer following Hodgkin's disease. *J Natl Cancer Inst* 2003;95:971–980.
362. van Leeuwen FE, Klokman WJ, van't Veer MB, et al. Long-term risk of second malignancy in survivors of Hodgkin's disease treated during adolescence or young adulthood. *J Clin Oncol* 2000;18:487–497.
363. Vargas C, Martinez A, Kestin LL, et al. Dose-volume analysis of predictors for chronic rectal toxicity after treatment of prostate cancer with adaptive image-guided radiotherapy. *Int J Radiat Oncol Biol Phys* 2005;62:1297–1308.
364. Verheij M, Stewart FA, Oussoren Y, et al. Amelioration of radiation nephropathy by acetylsalicylic acid. *Int J Radiat Biol* 1995;67:587–596.
365. Vigliani MC, Sichez N, Poisson M, et al. A prospective study of cognitive functions following conventional radiotherapy for supratentorial gliomas in young adults: 4-year results. *Int J Radiat Oncol Biol Phys* 1996;35:527–533.
366. von Essen CF. Roentgentherapy of skin and lip carcinoma: factors influencing success and failure. *Am J Roentgenol* 1960;83:245–257.
367. Waber D, Tarbell N, Fairclough D, et al. Cognitive sequelae of treatment in childhood acute lymphoblastic leukemia: cranial radiation requires an accomplice. *J Clin Oncol* 1995;13;2490–2496.
368. Waber DP, Shapiro BL, Carpentieri SC, et al. Excellent therapeutic efficacy and minimal late neurotoxicity in children treated with 18 grays of cranial radiation therapy for high-risk acute lymphoblastic leukemia: a 7-year follow-up study of the Dana-Farber Cancer Institute Consortium Protocol 87-01. *Cancer* 2001;92:15–22.
369. Wachter S, Gerstner N, Goldner G, et al. Rectal sequelae after conformal radiotherapy of prostate cancer: dose-volume histograms as predictive factors. *Radiother Oncol* 2001;59:65–70.
370. Wang PY, Shen WC, Jan JS. Serial MRI changes in radiation myelopathy. *Neuroradiology* 1995;37:374–377.
371. Wara W, Phillips T, Sheline G, et al. Radiation tolerance of the spinal cord. *Cancer* 1975;35:1558–1562.
372. Weisdorf DJ, Woods WG, Nesbit Jr ME, et al. Allogeneic bone marrow transplantation for acute lymphoblastic leukaemia: risk factors and clinical outcome. *Br J Haematol* 1994;86:62–69.
373. Werner-Wasik M, Scott CB, Nelson DF. Final report of a phase I/II trial of hyperfractionated and accelerated hyperfractioned radiation therapy with carmustine for adults with supratentorial malignant gliomas: Radiation Therapy Oncology Group Study 83-02. *Cancer* 1996;77:1535–1543.
374. Willett CG, Ooi CJ, Zietman AL, et al. Acute and late toxicity of patients with inflammatory bowel disease undergoing irradiation for abdominal and pelvic neoplasms. *Int J Radiat Oncol Biol Phys* 2000;46:995–998.
375. Willett CG, Tepper JE, Orlow EL, et al. Renal complications secondary to radiation treatment of upper abdominal malignancies. *Int J Radiat Oncol Biol Phys* 1986;12:1601–1604.
376. Wingard JR, Plotnick LP, Freemer CS, et al. Growth in children after bone marrow transplantation: busulfan plus cyclophosphamide versus cyclophosphamide plus total body irradiation. *Blood* 1992;79:1068–1073.
377. Withers HR, Thames HD Jr, Peters LJ. Biological bases for high RBE values for late effects of neutron irradiation. *Int J Radiat Oncol Biol Phys* 1982;8:2071–2076.
378. Withers HR, Thames HD. Dose fractionation and volume effects in normal tissues and tumors. *Am J Clin Oncol* 1988;11:313–329.
379. Wolden S, Lamborn K, Cleary S, et al. Second cancers following pediatric Hodgkin's disease. *J Clin Oncol* 1998;16:536–544.
380. Yorke E. Modeling the effects of inhomogeneous dose distributions in normal tissues. *Semin Radiat Oncol* 2001;11:197–209.
381. Yorke ED, Jackson A, Rosenzweig KE, et al. Correlation of dosmetric factors and radiation pneumonitis for non-small-cell lung cancer patients in a recently completed dose escalation study. *Int J Radiat Oncol Biol Phys* 2005;63:672–682.
382. Yorke ED, Jackson A, Rosenzweig KE, et al. Dose-volume factors contributing to the incidence of radiation pneumonitis in non-small-cell lung cancer patients treated with three-dimensional conformal radiation therapy. *Int J Radiat Oncol Biol Phys* 2002;54:329–339.
383. Zelefsky MJ, Fuks Z, Happersett L, et al. Clinical experience with intensity modulated radiation therapy (IMRT) in prostate cancer. *Radiother Oncol* 2000;55:241–249.

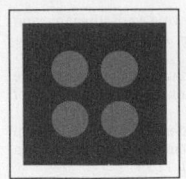

Chapter 13
Methodology of Clinical Trials

Shari B. Rudoler, Kathryn Winter, Walter J. Curran, Jr.

The accumulation of medical knowledge has undergone a significant change over the past 50 years, with de-emphasis on empiric or anecdotal observational learning to the now widespread acceptance of preplanned clinical trials as a means of establishing standards of care. Landmark controlled clinical trials in childhood acute leukemia in the 1950s set the stage for further prospective work in oncology. In the 1970s, many of today's cooperative multi-institutional groups were formed, including the Radiation Therapy Oncology Group (RTOG) in 1971.

"The purpose of a clinical trial is to provide valid and convincing evidence about the effects of medical therapy" (26). Many of the trial design principles we rely on today were developed for drug testing, but have been extrapolated and amended to evaluate all types of oncologic care, including radiation therapy, combined-modality therapy, and supportive therapies. To interpret these data effectively, the clinician must understand the key aspects of statistical analysis inherent in the design and analysis of clinical trials. Moreover, clinicians must be able to design trials properly, in conjunction with statisticians, so that the results are interpretable. "No amount of analysis can salvage a poorly designed study" (17).

Types of Study Design

The major categories of study design include retrospective studies, prospective studies, and meta-analyses. Each has strengths and weaknesses that must be taken into consideration when interpreting results.

Retrospective Studies

Retrospective studies review and make conclusions about the effectiveness of past treatment in patients who were not preselected for the treatment regimen in question. This type of analysis is best used as an important springboard to identify questions for future prospective study, rather than the sole evidence on which to base a change in clinical practice.

There are inherent problems in retrospective analysis. First, studies of past treatment try statistically to balance the patients to control for bias, but physician and patient preference in choosing the individual patient's treatment likely had an effect in shaping the characteristics each group. For example, Perez et al. (25) reported a radiation dose–response effect for the local control of stage III prostate cancer treated with definitive radiation therapy. The results showed increased local failure in patients who received <60 Gy. However, the policy for stage III patients at the Mallinckrodt Institute during the study period called for a minimum dose of 60 Gy to the prostate, with an additional 10-Gy boost based on prostate size. Therefore, patients who received less than the standard 60 Gy were probably discontinued early owing to poor toleration of treatment, poor overall performance status, or the development of disease progression during treatment. Thus, the claimed dose response may simply reflect differences in the patient populations.

Second, retrospective studies assume there have been no changes in the patient population over time. But we also know that patients are presenting earlier in the course of their disease than previously, especially in the case of sensitive screening tests, more widespread availability of screening, and heightened awareness in the lay public and among family physicians and internists. For example, patients presenting with prostate cancer before the routine use of prostate-specific antigen (PSA) screening in the 1990s may have had different disease biology than today's patients, who are diagnosed earlier. This phenomenon has been termed *lead time bias*. It refers to the idea that, within a given stage of disease, patients diagnosed earlier may initially appear to respond to treatment better than patients diagnosed later. But this effect may diminish or disappear as the natural history of the disease is followed over a longer period.

Third, retrospective studies cannot take into account the improvements in quality of care over time. Both advances in technology and in physician experience in delivering the treatment and managing the side effects contribute to improvement in patient outcome over time. Finally, individual retrospective studies may not be generalizable to the cancer population as a whole because of institutional differences and local patient population variability.

An example of effective use of retrospective data comes from investigation of fractionation issues in the treatment of squamous cell carcinoma of the head and neck. Three main altered fractionation regimens were established in the literature from three different institutions: University of Florida, Massachusetts General Hospital, and the M. D. Anderson Cancer Center. Each institution published retrospective data establishing the promising results of their altered fractionation schedules (14,24,35). This led to RTOG 90-03, a phase III randomized study comparing each of the three altered fractionation schedules with standard once-daily radiation (10). The results of the two best arms were sufficiently promising to warrant testing in new combined-modality regimens, thus taking the scientific process one step further (2).

Prospective Studies

"The major strength of prospective clinical trials is that the objectives are defined in advance. The patients can be selected, treated, and evaluated in accordance with standardized procedures, and the data can be recorded in a careful manner. When the treatments are randomly assigned, the resulting data are considered to be unbiased, which permits an immediate and straightforward interpretation of the study results" (23).

Important issues in trial design include proper framing of the scientific question, statistical control of error, ethical concerns for the patient, and the wise use of resources with collaborative groups. Ideally, prospective studies should be designed to answer one treatment question, or a limited number of questions. In this way, the required number of patients to statistically answer the question is achievable in a reasonable timeframe. In addition, the study should be designed so that the "result leads to a logical next question to be asked in a subsequent study" (17). Statistical parameters should be set in advance to control for both bias and variability. These include patient eligibility criteria, appropriate end points with expected differences to be detected, and preset descriptions of when interim analyses and follow-up analyses will be performed so as to avoid false-positive errors. Ethical considerations are addressed by the internal review board process, the use of informed consent, interim monitoring, and preselected early stopping rules should a given treatment prove significantly efficacious or unexpectedly toxic. Finally, because prospective trials require large numbers of patients and prolonged follow-up, most are carried out in a collaborative group setting. This type of arrangement allows for faster patient accrual, increased numbers of patients accrued, shorter trial duration, and broader clinical resources. Some of the disadvantages of the large group trial setting include difficulty with logistics, data management, financial cost, and quality control.

Meta-Analysis

A meta-analysis is a systematic overview of research in a particular area that is achieved by aggregating the results of many smaller studies in that area. The concept of meta-analysis originated in the 1970s, but became more widely accepted in the mid-1980s after the publication of the Oxford University group's overview of adjuvant therapy for breast cancer (3). This was the first major meta-analysis to influence standards of clinical care. Because most new interventions in cancer treatment are likely to produce a small or moderate effect on survival, the power of an individual trial to convincingly show a benefit is low. "As a consequence, trials demonstrating no apparent effect may merely lack sufficient numbers of patients for detection of the true underlying effect" (33).

The main benefit of a meta-analysis is that the combination of many individual trials can define a modest but real advantage associated with a new therapeutic approach. By comparison, a single study would require approximately 2,000 patients to detect a 5% difference between treatment arms, a nearly impossible task both logistically and financially. Small differences in survival not only are worthwhile to individual patients, but can have a significant impact on public health when the disease in question is common. For example, a 5% improvement in survival for patients with breast or lung cancer may translate into thousands of patient deaths prevented each year (4).

Another benefit of the meta-analysis is that the aggregation of data makes the result more generalizable to the overall population of patients with cancer and institutions (4). Finally, the combination of studies into a large data set allows more reliable analysis of well defined patient subsets (4).

A well designed meta-analysis should include only randomized clinical trials; should include all relevant randomized trials that have been initiated anywhere in the world, regardless of whether published; should not exclude any randomized patients from the aggregated analysis, even those patients excluded from the original analysis; and should assess therapeutic effectiveness based on the average results pooled across trials (31). These guidelines attempt to alleviate the main potential problems associated with meta-analyses, namely, publication bias, study selection, study comparability, and quality control.

Publication bias arises because journals are more likely to publish positive trials than negative trials. Therefore, if only published studies are included in a meta-analysis, the aggregated results may be biased toward a positive result. An exhaustive literature review on the topic at hand must be supplemented by detection of unpublished works, as well. However, when including unpublished trials, one must remember that they have not been peer reviewed, potentially making confidence in the data less compelling.

When selecting which studies collected should be included in the analysis, there should be consideration as to which are sufficiently similar in patient population, treatment intervention, and end points as to have meaningful results when combined. "The more varied are the studies contributing to an overview, the greater the concern that effective or ineffective therapies (or populations) will be lumped together and that the overall result will not provide a useful guide to practicing oncologists" (4). Finally, there should be an attempt to classify studies by their level of quality to determine if the lesser-quality studies inordinately affect the overall outcome of the meta-analysis.

In summary, meta-analysis can summarize the evidence about a treatment intervention and can reveal modest individual differences in outcome that may have a significant impact on public health. In some instances, such evidence may directly influence clinical practice, as in the case of the Early Breast Cancer Trialists' Collaborative Group (3). More often, the purpose of meta-analysis should not be to define a standard of care, but to formulate the direction of future research by summarizing current knowledge (4).

Types of Prospective Studies

Phase I

The main objective of the phase I trial is to determine the maximum safe, tolerable dose for later testing of efficacy. Although initially developed in the setting of drug testing, this concept has been adapted to test radiation alone and combined-modality regimens. The basic design is that of dose escalation in small patient cohorts until treatment toxicity reaches a predetermined level, or unexpected toxicity is seen (17). Thus, stepwise testing in phase I trials determines the maximum tolerated dose (MTD).

The key parameters that should be defined at the outset of a phase I trial include patient eligibility criteria, starting dose and the schedule of dose escalation, sample size at each dose level, and the expected or estimated MTD (26). It should be appreciated that the MTD is a relative concept that can change over time. For example, hematologic toxicity may be less dose limiting than it had been before the development of bone marrow stimulators such as erythropoietin and filgrastim.

Unlike chemotherapy trials, which usually evaluate acute or subacute toxicity, radiation therapy trials may evaluate early or late toxicity. Late toxicity may occur many years after the completion of radiation therapy. Consequently, the sample size requirements are much larger than for trials with an early end point because not all patients will survive beyond the latent period for late toxicity to be manifest. The follow-up period for such a trial also is significantly longer than for most chemotherapy trials (23).

Phase II

The main purpose of the phase II trial is to determine the response rate of certain tumor types to a given chemotherapy agent, radiation treatment regimen, or combination. Phase II trials can be conducted in either a single or cooperative setting. Early and late end points of the phase II trial can include tumor response, duration of response, overall locoregional control at a given time point, and toxicity. Survival is usually a secondary end point because phase II trials usually are not designed to allow convincing and unbiased detection of survival differences. Patient selection can influence the results (31), and overall response rates in single-institution phase II trials can be significantly higher than in phase III controlled trials (17). To avoid these causes of bias, phase II trials can be performed in a randomized fashion. This approach improves patient homogeneity and reduces bias between patient groups (26). The best treatment arm can then be tested in a phase III trial.

Phase III

Phase III trials are randomized comparisons between a new treatment regimen and the current best standard of care (i.e., the control). Typically, the experimental arm has already shown promise in phase I/II studies before randomized testing. Randomized trials offer three major advantages in terms of bias reduction over nonrandomized studies. First, randomization guarantees that treatments are assigned to patients independently of their known prognostic factors. Second, randomization homogenizes and balances the patients within each treatment arm, thereby minimizing or eliminating the unidentified nontreatment factors that may prejudice the results. Third, randomization can facilitate blinding techniques that also help eliminate bias (26). Finally, randomization in a cooperative group can balance any systematic bias of the treating physicians or institutions.

Phase III trials can address many types of questions. For example, a study can be designed to determine if standard treatment is better than best supportive care. An example is the Brain Tumor Study Group trial in which radiation therapy for gliomas was found to be superior to best supportive care (34). More often, phase III studies are designed to compare a new treatment with the current standard treatment. One example is the comparison of total mastectomy with breast-conserving surgery and radiation for patients with ductal carcinoma *in situ* (7). The result, showing equivalence of the two treatments, allowed for a new standard of care that included breast conservation in eligible women. Phase III studies can also compare two or three different regimens with each other, as well as with standard treatment. An example is RTOG trial 91-11 (9), which compared standard radiation for laryngeal carcinoma against induction chemotherapy followed by radiation or concurrent chemotherapy and radiation. This study found a significant improvement in organ preservation for the concurrent arm, again setting a new standard of care.

The major end point of a phase III trial is usually survival or disease-free survival. Important secondary end points can include locoregional control, tumor response, toxicity, or quality of life. Consequently, the maturation and follow-up period required for the phase III trial is much longer than with either phase I or phase II. Usually, the number of patients required to show the expected difference between arms is also larger for the Phase III trial.

Design of Phase III Clinical Trials

Eligibility Criteria and Patient Selection

Defining the eligibility criteria for a clinical study is very important. The patient population should be chosen in a way that is neither too exclusive nor too inclusive. If the primary end point is something other than a survival end point, such as late toxicity or 3-month complete response rate, the population should be chosen such that the patients have a high probability of surviving long enough to be evaluated for that end point. In addition, the eligible population should be large enough so that accrual to the study can be completed in a reasonable amount of time. For studies that are planned to accrue over a long period, usually phase III studies, the researcher must be aware of changes in eligibility variables over time. For example, if staging definitions change during the accrual period of a study, patients must continue to be staged with the original definitions, and be eligible based on the original staging criteria, not the more recent definitions.

Selection of End Points

The term *end point* refers to the outcome or event that is used to measure the efficacy or morbidity associated with the treatment. Clinical trials have a primary end point, on which the sample sized is based, and usually one or more secondary end points. The most common end point in phase III clinical trials is absolute survival, in which failure is defined as death due to any cause. In certain situations, using this end point can be somewhat misleading. For example, when the population in question has early disease, is elderly, and may very likely die from other causes not related to the disease, as in the case of men with low- to intermediate-stage prostate cancer, a more appropriate end point would be cause-specific survival, in which failure is defined as death due to the treated cancer. This allows the investigator to evaluate the effect of the treatment on the disease while adjusting for patients who die from non–cancer-related causes. A disadvantage of using cause-specific survival is the subjectivity involved in deciding the cause of death. This potential source of bias is avoided when using overall survival as the end point. If an investigator chooses to report cause-specific survival, absolute survival should also be reported along with a table showing the causes of death to allow the reader to decide if there are any biases in the data. For example, Laramore and associates used both end points and showed that fast neutron irradiation was superior to photon radiation therapy in patients with carcinoma of the prostate (16). On the other hand, McGowan reported only cause-specific survival while assessing the influence of prior transurethral resection on the prognosis of men with prostate cancer treated with irradiation (19). In the latter case, the reader was unable to judge if there were any biases introduced because no information was given about the total number of deaths and their causes.

Disease-free survival, also referred to as *relapse-free survival* or *no evidence of disease survival*, is another survival end point that is often reported. The definition of failure for this end point varies, and should be explicitly stated when the data are reported. Some consider a patient a failure at the time death due to any cause, as well as at the time of first local or distant recurrence. The National Surgical Adjuvant Breast Project (NSABP) also considers patients who are alive without local or distant recurrence failures if they have developed a secondary primary. Another issue is how to deal with patients whose original tumor never clears. There is no doubt that these patients are failures, but at what time point should they be considered such? RTOG defines patients with persistent disease as failures on day 1 for this end point (27). Disease-free survival is a commonly used end point when comparing two treatments used after treatment.

Response to the treatment being studied is another common end point. The most frequently used measures are complete and partial response. Complete response is defined as no evidence of the pretreatment tumor and symptoms and no recurrence within 1 month. A partial response is usually defined as a decrease in the size of the pretreatment measurable tumor of at least 50%. Frequency of tumor response evaluation, as well as the experience of the evaluator responsible for measuring the tumor, affect both of these responses. Partial response is particularly observer dependent. Evaluating the patients at the time points preselected in the protocol is also crucial to avoid bias.

Determining Sample Size

When a phase III clinical trial is designed, the sample size is based on the primary end point being evaluated by the study and is generated from the following parameters, which are specified by the investigator:

1. Type I error (α)
2. Type II error (β)
3. One-sided or two-sided test of significance
4. The expected failure rate on the standard arm
5. The minimum expected detectable difference in the primary end point between the two treatments

Type I error is the error of concluding that there is a significant difference based on the sample data when one really does not exist. It is expressed as the probability of the difference being due to chance alone versus being due to the treatment and is denoted by the Greek letter α. This can be thought of as a false-positive rate for the clinical trial. A standard value of α in medical research is 0.05.

Type II error is the error of concluding that there is not a significant difference based on the sample data when one really does exist. It is expressed as the probability of not detecting a difference due to the treatments when that difference really exists and is denoted by the Greek letter β. This can be thought of as a false-negative rate for the clinical trial. In clinical trials, it is common to set the type II error at 0.20, although possible definitive studies that will most likely not be repeated should have a lower type II error, for instance 0.10. This was done in an early Intergroup phase III study in head and neck cancer, testing the effectiveness of chemotherapy given between surgery and radiation therapy (29). To increase the sensitivity of the study, which had a limited number of available eligible patients and therefore a very small likelihood of being repeated, the study was designed using a type II error of 0.10 (29).

The type II error rate is often reported in terms of power. The power of a study is the probability of detecting a significant difference when one really does exist and is equal to $1 - \beta$. For a given sample size, type I and type II errors are inversely proportional. Therefore, as the type I error rate decreases, the type II error rate increases. Both rates can be set at a chosen level with the correct sample size.

If the investigator is comparing two accepted treatments and wants to detect a statistically significant difference between them, then a two-sided test is appropriate. Given treatments A and B, this allows for three possible conclusions:

1. Treatment A is significantly better than treatment B.
2. Treatment B is significantly better than treatment A.
3. Treatments A and B are not significantly different.

Note that the third conclusion is that the treatments are "not significantly different," which is not the same as saying that the treatments are equal. It only means that there was not sufficient evidence from the data to show them to be significantly different.

On the other hand, when an investigator is comparing an experimental treatment with a standard treatment, a one-sided test is appropriate. In this situation, the investigator assumes that it is not possible for the experimental treatment to be significantly worse than the standard treatment, otherwise it would not warrant testing. Therefore, there are only two possible outcomes:

1. The experimental treatment is significantly better than the standard and is therefore the treatment of choice.
2. The experimental treatment is not significantly better than the standard, in which case the standard remains the treatment of choice.

Many statisticians believe that one-sided tests should be used only if it is not possible for the difference to occur in two directions, because one-sided tests at the same significance level have a higher false-positive rate (5). If it is possible that an experimental treatment could be significantly worse than the standard treatment, some statisticians would argue that the one-sided test is not appropriate.

In a two-sided test, the type I error comprises two equal parts ($\alpha/2$). This means that the study may have the same chance of falsely detecting a benefit to treatment A as it may have of falsely detecting a benefit to treatment B. In a one-sided test, the entire type I error is given to concluding that the experimental treatment is significantly better than the standard treatment, when it is not. A compromise would be to do a one-sided test with a significance level of $\alpha/2$.

The primary failure rate on the standard arm usually comes from the literature or prior studies. The minimum amount of difference the investigators expect to be able to detect is often based on pilot data and should describe a clinically meaningful difference. The smaller the difference between the treatment arms, the more patients would be needed to detect it. Setting the difference too high in order to have a smaller sample size may be clinically unrealistic and a disservice to all the study participants. In an ideal trial design, the sample size should be large enough to demonstrate a statistically significant and clinically meaningful difference, yet represent a study population that can be realistically accrued in a timely fashion.

Table 13.1 shows the total required sample size when testing for an improvement in response rate with $\alpha = 0.05$ and $\beta = 0.10$ or 0.20. For example, if the response rate for standard arm is 0.45 and a study is being designed to detect a minimum improvement of 0.20 with $\alpha = 0.05$ and $\beta = 0.20$, the total required sample size is 212. The sample size is reduced by 36% (136 patients) when the minimum improvement is increased to 0.25. On the other hand, if the minimum improvement is decreased to 0.15, the required sample size is increased by 75% (372 patients).

Randomization and Stratification

When a clinical trial has two or more treatment arms, randomization is a key component. Patients entered onto a randomized study must be able to complete all possible courses of treatment because it is unknown to which treatment arm they will be assigned. Randomization helps to balance out both known and unknown prognostic factors as well as eliminating possible biases that could occur if the physician were subjectively to choose the treatment. Randomization allows the results of the study to be applicable over time as well as making them more reliable. The most basic way of randomizing patients to two treatment arms is the statistical equivalent of flipping a coin to determine their treatment. Although statistical theory guarantees that as the total number of patients increases, the number of patients on each arm will converge to an equal number, it does not guarantee that at a given time point, the accrual to the arms or the balance of prognostic factors will be equal (15).

A method to help balance the treatment arms at a given time point is the use of stratification variables. Important prognostic factors may be defined as stratification variables, and the combinations of the levels of these variables create a prognostic profile called a *stratum*. The treatment arms are assigned so that they are balanced after a specified number of patients is entered in each stratum, usually a multiple of the number of treatment arms. This group of patients is defined as a block. For a study with two treatment arms, blocks of size four or six are common. For example, RTOG 94-08, a study of prostate cancer, had two treatment arms: let X = radiation therapy + neoadjuvant total androgen suppression 2 months before and during radiation therapy; and Y = radiation therapy alone. Patients were stratified using the following important prognostic variables: PSA (<4 versus 4 to 20), differentiation (well versus moderately versus poorly), and nodal status (N0 versus NX). The combinations of the levels of these variables creates 12 strata: <4,

| Table 13.1 | TOTAL NUMBER OF PATIENTS REQUIRED TO DETECT AN IMPROVEMENT IN RESPONSE RATE (P_2) OVER THE SMALLER RESPONSE RATE (P_1) |

P_1 ⇩	\multicolumn{10}{c}{Improvement in Response Rate $P_2 - P_1$}
	0.05	0.10	0.15	0.20	0.25	0.30	0.35	0.40	0.45	0.50
0.05	1,240[a]	412	226	148	108	84	66	54	46	38
	946[b]	318	176	116	86	66	54	44	36	32
0.10	1,912	570	292	184	128	96	76	60	50	42
	1,448	436	224	142	100	76	60	48	40	34
0.15	2,500	708	348	212	146	106	82	66	52	44
	1,888	538	266	164	114	84	64	52	42	36
0.20	3,004	822	394	238	158	114	88	68	54	44
	2,264	626	302	182	124	90	68	54	44	36
0.25	3,424	918	432	254	168	120	90	70	56	46
	2,578	696	330	196	130	94	72	56	44	36
0.30	3,760	990	460	268	176	124	92	72	56	44
	2,828	750	350	206	136	96	72	56	44	36
0.35	4,012	1,044	478	276	178	126	92	70	54	44
	3,018	790	364	212	138	98	72	56	44	36
0.40	4,180	1,074	488	278	178	124	90	68	52	42
	3,142	814	372	214	138	96	72	54	42	34
0.45	4,264	1,086	488	276	176	120	88	66	50	38
	3,206	822	372	212	136	94	68	52	40	32
0.50	4,264	1,074	478	268	168	114	82	60	46	34
	3,206	814	364	206	130	90	64	48	36	28

[a]First row: $\alpha = 0.05$ and $\beta = 0.10$.
[b]Second row: $\alpha = 0.05$ and $\beta = 0.20$.

well, N0; <4, well, NX; <4, moderately, N0; <4, moderately, NX; <4, poorly, N0; <4, poorly, NX; 4 to 20, well, N0; 4 to 20, well, NX; 4 to 20, moderately, N0; 4 to 20, moderately, NX; 4 to 20, poorly, N0; 4 to 20, poorly, NX. Deciding at what point the treatment assignments should be balanced determines the size of the block. If a block of four is chosen, then the six possible combinations are XXYY, XYXY, XYYX, YYXX, YXYX, and YXXY. It is important that the investigators do not know the order of treatment assignments to avoid decisions that could compromise the integrity of the randomization procedure and hence the study.

Data Collection and Analyses

Data Collection

To evaluate the end points of a study, data should be collected in a timely and efficient manner. At the time of study design, it should be prospectively determined which data are to be collected and at what specific time points. Although it is possible to collect some data retrospectively, it is not always easy and in some cases may not be possible. One way to collect the data is to have questionnaires for the study that are filled out prospectively. The time interval between evaluations should be equivalent from patient to patient and is especially important in studies with more than one treatment arm. If patients on one treatment arm are seen less frequently than patients on another arm in the same study, it may introduce a bias in the treatment comparisons.

Interim Analyses

Studies should be monitored for accrual, safety, and efficacy. The plan for doing these analyses should be included in the initial protocol design. Analyses done after the accrual has been met and the patients have been followed for at least the spec-

ified amount of time usually are referred to as *final* analyses, whereas all analyses done before this time are referred to as *interim* analyses.

In all studies, the accrual should be monitored regularly. In the RTOG, accrual, pretreatment characteristics, and toxicity are routinely reported to the membership. Although it does not occur very often, when a study accrues too quickly, specifically for phase III studies whose designs depend on the accrual and the follow-up time, the follow-up may need to be lengthened to get efficacy estimates at the desired time points. When a study accrues too slowly, there is the possibility that it may not be able to reach its accrual goal. This could be due to a variety of reasons. For example, the eligibility criteria may be too restrictive or the patients may not be referred to the departments that are participating in the trial. Possible reasons should be investigated and appropriate changes made in the hopes of increasing accrual. Alternatively, a decision may be made to end the trial. Outcome and response data are reported only at times specified in the protocol, as described later, and then only to a selected committee, because results that are not significantly different may still introduce a bias with respect to investigators continuing to participate.

The main emphasis in phase III studies is on the difference in efficacy between the treatments being tested. Toxicity is also monitored as a secondary end point because these treatments have already been proven to be safe in phase I and II studies. Interim analyses for the efficacy end point are built into the study design to allow early stopping if the treatments are statistically significantly different from each other. The number and timing of these interim analyses affect the sample size. Too many analyses also increase the significance level (α), also called the *false-positive rate*, concluding that there is a difference between the treatments when one does not exist (20). For this reason, the interim analyses should be performed at prespecified time points. In addition, when the study is designed, the significance level of each planned interim analysis must be accounted for in the final overall significance level, so that there is no danger of increasing the chance of a false-positive result. That is, the sum of the significance levels for the planned interim analyses and the final analysis must equal α.

RTOG usually does the first interim analysis on phase III trials after at least 50% of the patients are accrued. The exact time point, based either on accrual or number of failures, is specified in the protocol. The blinded efficacy results of this interim analysis are reported to a data monitoring committee (DMC). If the treatment arms are significantly different at the significance level determined for that interim analysis, accrual to the study is stopped and an analysis done to investigate whether the difference is due to the treatment or some other factor. If the treatments are not significantly different at this analysis, then accrual continues until the total number of patients is accrued. The second interim analysis takes place sometime after the total accrual is met, also prespecified in the protocol. The blinded efficacy results are again presented to the DMC, and if the treatment arms are significantly different at this analysis, a full analysis is done to publish the results. If the treatment arms are not significantly different at this analysis, then the study continues in follow-up until the final analysis is due. RTOG 90-01 is an example of a study that had early reporting (22). This was a phase III study comparing pelvic radiation with concurrent chemotherapy to pelvic and paraaortic radiation alone for high-risk cervical cancer. The interim analysis conducted after the accrual was met showed a highly statistically significant difference in overall survival, the primary end point of the study. These blinded results were reported to the DMC, which recommended early reporting. For this particular study, the experimental arm was significantly better than the standard arm, but had it been in the other direction the results still would have been reported early.

Final Analyses

Before the final analysis, all outstanding data should be collected, and each patient's treatment should be reviewed for quality control. The following items are usually included in the final analysis:

1. The status of all of the cases entered with respect to their eligibility and whether they are included in the analysis, along with reasons for exclusion
2. A distribution of the important prognostic pretreatment characteristics for each treatment arm
3. The frequency and severity of the reported toxicities for each treatment arm
4. The rates for appropriate outcomes (e.g., survival, local control) for each treatment arm
5. Compliance rates for the treatment delivery relative to the prescribed protocol treatment

6. Comparisons for appropriate outcomes (e.g., survival, local control) between the treatment arms

To compare the important prognostic factors, the Pearson χ^2 test is usually used for categorical variables (e.g., sex, T-stage), whereas continuous variables (e.g., age) are usually compared with the t-test, assuming a normal distribution, or by nonparametric methods such as the Wilcoxon test.

Reporting the statistical methods used in the study design is critical to understanding the study's results. For example, the significance level used for testing (type I error) is often reported in the literature, yet the type II error is rarely defined. This is especially important in evaluating the results of a negative study. When a report concludes that there is no significant difference between treatments, the following question arises: "What was the probability of not detecting a treatment difference when one really existed?" This is the type II error. Suppose a study is designed to detect a 20% difference with 25 patients per treatment arm. The type II error rate is 0.80, meaning that if a difference exists, it will be missed 80 times out of 100. If this error rate is reported, the reader should not be surprised if the results indicate no treatment difference. If this same study is done with 50, 100, or 150 patients per treatment, the type II error rate is 0.56, 0.23, and 0.08, respectively. In the case of 150 patients per treatment, with a 20% treatment difference, a negative result is much more persuasive because if the difference really exists it will be missed only 8 times out of 100. Table 13.2 shows the Type II errors for various response rates and sample sizes.

Survival Analyses

When analyzing survival data, the most common approach is to use the Kaplan-Meier method (13) for estimating the survival rates and the log-rank test (18) to compare treatments. These analyses are appropriate for any end point where every patient will eventually fail, such as overall survival and disease-free survival. In fact, any end point that includes death from any cause as a failure falls into this category. However, certain end points, such as cause-specific survival, require different methods of calculation owing to the presence of competing risks for that end point. In this case, it is possible that the patient may die of non–cancer-related causes and hence is no longer at risk to die of cancer. The competing risk in this situation is death due to any cause other than cancer. The survival end point in this situation is best estimated using the cumulative incidence method and treatment differences tested with Gray's test (12) to adjust for the competing risk. In patients with prostate cancer, for example, there may be important differences between the overall survival rate and the cause-specific survival rate. Especially in the case of early-stage, low-risk prostate cancer,

| Table 13.2 | TYPE II ERRORS FOR VARIOUS RESPONSE RATES AND SAMPLE SIZES |

No. Patients per Arm	Observed Two Response Rates[a]			
	50% − 40% = 10%	55% − 40% = 15%	60% − 40% = 20%	65% − 40% = 25%
25	94/100[b]	88/100	80/100	69/100
50	88/100	75/100	56/100	36/100
100	63/100	49/100	23/100	7/100
150	37/100	30/100	8/100	1/100

[a]Type II errors (missing a treatment difference) were based on a binomial distribution with $\alpha = 0.05$ and the parameters specified in the table.
[b]A treatment difference of 10% will fail to be detected 94 out of 100 times with 25 patients per treatment arm.

patients are usually elderly and it is not uncommon for the patients to die from causes unrelated to cancer. In all situations, the survival time is measured from the date of randomization to the date of failure, or last follow-up if the patient did not fail.

Subset Analyses

If the overall results of a study show no statistically significant difference in the treatments, subset analyses often are performed to see if there is a difference in the treatments for a particular group of the patients. Even when there is a statistically significant difference in the treatments, subset analyses may be performed on groups of interest. Several problems may arise with subset analyses (8,30). Unless the study was designed to do subset analyses, there may not be sufficient patient numbers in each subset to have the statistical power to detect a difference. As previously discussed, as the sample size decreases, the difference that can be detected must increase. Another problem with subset analyses is that the balance of prognostic factors is no longer guaranteed between the treatments for the subset. Any subset analyses should include the distribution of the prognostic factors because differences in subsets may be due to an imbalance of prognostic factors. Finally, multiple testing may lead to an increased false-positive rate. As with interim analyses, the type I error rate (α) for the subset should be adjusted.

Because of these problems, results of unplanned subset analyses should not be considered definitive, but should be hypothesis-generating for future confirmation in phase III studies (11). For ethical reasons, this is possible only when the subset analysis results suggest a benefit for the patients. Two examples follow.

In a phase III trial for patients with rectal cancer at Princess Margaret Hospital (28), no overall survival difference was found between the treatments of 500 cGy of preoperative radiation versus none. Subsequent subset analysis with 22 patients from the radiation therapy arm and 16 patients from the surgery-only arm suggested a significant treatment difference in favor of the radiation for patients with Dukes stage C rectal cancer. However, a phase III trial performed by the Medical Research Council in the United Kingdom failed to confirm a difference in overall survival between these two treatments for patients with Dukes stage C rectal cancer (21).

The NSABP conducted a phase III study of the effects of postoperative adjuvant combination chemotherapy with semustine, vincristine, and 5-fluorouracil (MOF regimen) for rectal cancer (6). The results showed a statistically significant improvement in overall survival for the MOF regimen ($p = .01$). In a subset analysis looking at sex, the results were conflicting. The 5-year survival rate for the 119 male patients was 60% for those treated with the MOF and 37% for those not. In the 65 female patients, the 5-year survival rate was only 37% for those treated with the MOF and 60% for those not. A follow-up phase III study to investigate this result in the female patients would be unethical.

Conclusion/Future Directions

In summary, clinical trials over the past 30 years have helped shape oncologic practice. Unfortunately, only 2.5% of patients with cancer are enrolled on National Cancer Institute network–sponsored studies nationally (32). Although not all patients are candidates for protocol treatment, many patients who are eligible do not participate. Both physician and patient preferences are at fault for the low rate of trial participation, but clearly much more information could be gleaned in a timelier fashion if more patients participated in research. Therefore, one of the most important goals should be broadening access to and participation in clinical trials.

A special challenge in this regard relates to minority patients, who were historically underrepresented in national trials. Since 1993, the National Institutes of Health has published guidelines and special initiatives to encourage inclusion of minority and other underserved populations in research studies (1). These efforts have been shown to be successful in a few reports (32,1). In the RTOG, African Americans are appropriately represented in RTOG studies, compared with U.S. Census and Surveillance Epidemiology and End Results data (1). However, the same analysis in the RTOG has not yet been done for Hispanics and other minorities. Reaching out to these special populations is another challenge.

References

1. Chamberlain RM, Winter KA, Vijaykumar S, et al. Sociodemographic analysis of patients in Radiation Therapy Oncology Group clinical trials. *Int J Radiat Oncol Biol Phys* 1998;40:9–15.
2. Curran WJ. Medical research objectives. *Int J Radiat Oncol Biol Phys* 2001; 51[Suppl 2]:1–5.
3. Early Breast Cancer Trialists' Collaborative Group. Effects of adjuvant tamoxifen and of cytotoxic therapy on mortality in early breast cancer: an overview of 61 randomized trials among 28,896 women. *N Engl J Med* 1988;319:1681–1692.
4. Ellenberg SS. Meta-analysis: the quantitative approach to research review. *Semin Oncol* 1988;15:472–481.
5. Ellenberg S. Biostatistics in clinical trials: Part 2. Determining sample sizes for clinical trials. *Oncology* 1989;3:39–46.
6. Fisher B, Wolmark N, Rockette H, et al. Postoperative adjuvant chemotherapy or radiation therapy for rectal cancer: results from NSABP Protocol R-01. *J Natl Cancer Inst* 1988;80:21–29.
7. Fisher B, Dignam J, Wolmark N, et al. Lumpectomy and radiation therapy for the treatment of intraductal breast cancer: findings from National Surgical Adjuvant Breast and Bowel Project B-17. *J Clin Oncol* 1998;16:441–452.
8. Fleming TR, Watelet LF. Approaches to monitoring clinical trials. *J Natl Cancer Inst* 1989;81:188–193.
9. Forastiere AA, Berkey B, Maor M, et al. Phase III trial to preserve the larynx: induction chemotherapy and radiotherapy versus concomitant chemoradiotherapy versus radiotherapy alone. Intergroup trial R91-11. *Proc Am Soc Clin Oncol* 2001;20:4.
10. Fu K, Pajak T, Trotti A, et al. A Radiation Therapy Oncology Group (RTOG) phase III randomized study to compare hyperfractionation and two variants of accelerated fractionation to standard fractionation radiotherapy for head and neck squamous cell carcinomas: first report of RTOG 90-03. *Int J Radiat Oncol Biol Phys* 2000;48:7–16.
11. Gail M, Simon R. Testing for qualitative interactions between treatment effects and patient subsets. *Biometrics* 1985;41:361–372.
12. Gray RJ. A class of K-sample tests for comparing the cumulative incidence of a competing risk. *Ann Stat* 1988;16:1141–1154.
13. Kaplan EL, Meier P. Nonparametric estimation from incomplete observations. *J Am Stat Assoc* 1958;53:457–481.
14. Knee R, Shields RS, Peters LJ. Concomitant boost radiotherapy for advanced squamous cell carcinoma of the head and neck. *Radiother Oncol* 1985;4:1–7.
15. Lachin JM. Statistical properties of randomization in clinical trials. *Control Clin Trials* 1988;9:289–311.
16. Laramore GE, Krall J, Thomas FJ, et al. Fast neutron radiotherapy for locally advanced prostate cancer: results of an RTOG randomized study. *Int J Radiat Oncol Biol Phys* 1985;11:1621–1627.
17. Leventhal BG. An overview of clinical trials in oncology. *Semin Oncol* 1988;15:414–422.
18. Mantel N. Evaluation of survival data and two new rank order statistics arising in its consideration. *Cancer Chemother Rep* 1966;50:163–170.
19. McGowan DG. The adverse influence of prior transurethral resection on prognosis is carcinoma of prostate treated by radiation therapy. *Int J Radiat Oncol Biol Phys* 1980;6:1121–1126.
20. McPherson K. Interim analysis and stopping rules. In: Buyse ME, Staquet MJ, Sylvester RJ, eds. *Cancer clinical trials: method and practice*. Oxford: Oxford University Press, 1984;405–422.
21. Medical Research Council Working Party. The evaluation of low-dose preoperative x-ray therapy in the management of operable rectal cancer: results of a randomly controlled trial. *Br J Surg* 1984;71:21–25.
22. Morris M, Eifel P, Lu JD, et al. Pelvic radiation with concurrent chemotherapy versus pelvic and para-aortic radiation for high-risk cervical cancer: a randomized RTOG clinical trial. *N Engl J Med* 1999;340:1137–1143.
23. Pajak TF. Methodology of clinical trials. In: Perez CA, Brady LW, eds. *Principles and practice of radiation oncology*, 3rd ed. Philadelphia: Lippincott Williams & Wilkins,1998;231–242.
24. Parsons JT, Mendenhall WM, Cassisi NJ, et al. Hyperfractionation for head and neck cancer. *Int J Radiat Biol Phys* 1988;14:649–658.
25. Perez CA, Walz BJ, Zivnuska FR, et al. Irradiation of carcinoma of the prostate localized to the pelvis: analysis of tumor response and prognosis. *Int J Radiat Oncol Biol Phys* 1980;6:555–563.
26. Piantadosi S. Principles of clinical trial design. *Semin Oncol* 1988;15:423–433.
27. Pilepich MV, Krall JM, Johnson RJ, et al. Extended field (periaortic) irradiation in carcinoma of the prostate: analysis of RTOG 75-06. *Int J Radiat Oncol Biol Phys* 1986;12:345–351.
28. Rider WD, Palmer JA, Mahoney LJ, et al. Preoperative irradiation in operable

cancer of the rectum: report of the Toronto Trial. *Can J Surg* 1977;20:335–338.

29. Schuller DE, Laramore GE, Al-Sarraf M, et al. Combined therapy for resectable head and neck cancer: a phase 3 intergroup study. *Arch Otolaryngol Head Neck Surg* 1989;115:364–368.
30. Simon R. Patient subsets and variation in therapeutic efficacy. *Br J Clin Pharmacol* 1982;14:473–482.
31. Simon R. Design and conduct of clinical trials In: DeVita VT, Hellman S, Rosenberg SA, eds. *Cancer: principles and practice of oncology* 4th ed. PhiladelphiaJB Lippincott, 1993;418–440.

32. Tejeda HA, Green SB, Trimble EL, et al. Representation of African-Americans, Hispanics, and whites in National Cancer Institute cancer treatment trials. *J Natl Cancer Inst* 1996;88:812–816.
33. Tierney J. Meta-analysis in the research and treatment of cancer. *PPO Updates* 1999;13:1–12.
34. Walker MD, Alexander E Jr, Hunt WE, et al. Evaluation of BCNU and/or radiotherapy in the treatment of anaplastic gliomas: a cooperative clinical trial. *J Neurosurg* 1978;49:333–343.
35. Wang CC. Improved local control for advanced oropharyngeal carcinoma following twice daily radiation therapy. *Am J Clin Oncol* 1985;8:512–516.

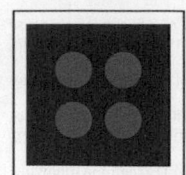

Chapter 14
Total-Body and Hemibody Irradiation

Kenneth B. Roberts, Zhe Chen, Stuart Seropian

Historically, total-body irradiation (TBI) has been used without stem cell support for palliation of radiation sensitive disease such as CLL or follicular lymphomas. Currently, TBI is mainly performed in the context of hematopoietic transplantation for its cytotoxic and immunologic effects. Normal bone marrow tolerance for radiation is exceeded, and the patient's hematopoietic system is reconstituted by the stem cell transplantation procedure. Hemibody irradiation (HBI) has a different therapeutic goal, which is generally for palliation of diffuse metastatic disease. Stem cell support is not required.

Total Body Irradiation

Historical Use of Total-Body Irradiation without Stem Cell Rescue

TBI has been used as a form of systemic therapy for various malignant diseases since the beginning of the 20th century (84). However, the usefulness of TBI without hematopoietic stem cell rescue is limited because the median lethal dose of whole-body radiation exposure given as a single fraction is approximately 4 Gy in humans. Given the radiosensitivity of chronic lymphocytic leukemia or low grade, advanced stage non-Hodgkin's lymphoma, TBI was an effective palliative modality using doses as low as 0.025 to 0.15 Gy several times a week, titrating total dose to clinical response (17,117). Because of myelosuppression—especially thrombocytopenia—the standard recommendation was to allow a 4- to 8-week treatment break be given after each cumulative 0.5 Gy of TBI (35,63). Johnson (63) reported in the 1970s that one third of patients with chronic lymphocytic leukemia attained complete remission with low-dose TBI alone, and slightly more when alkylating chemotherapy was added. These results were not supported by an Eastern Cooperative Oncology Group (ECOG) phase III trial, however (112), and the role for TBI without stem cell rescue has diminished further with the advances in cytotoxic chemotherapy since the 1960s as well as the recent availability of anti-CD20 antibody therapies, including radioimmunoconjugates.

Total-Body Irradiation in Stem Cell Transplantation

The conditioning regimen for hematopoietic stem cell transplantion has several functions. One is cytotoxicity: to contribute to the eradication of any residual cancer. Another important function of the conditioning regimen is immunosuppression so that the host does not reject the donor stem cells. TBI in the broad range of 2 to 15 Gy in conjunction with chemotherapy serves these functions well.

Radiobiologic Effects on Normal Hematopoietic System

Successful hematopoietic stem cell engraftment requires:

1. Eradication of the recipient bone marrow;

2. Immunosuppression to prevent rejection of donor marrow in the case of an allotransplant; and

3. Relative sparing of the recipient's bone marrow stromal cells.

The reported D_0 values of bone marrow stem cells usually range from 0.5 to 1.4 Gy, indicating intrinsic radiosensitivity (58,158). Although conventional wisdom assumes that recipient marrow cells must be removed to leave space for donor cells in stem cell microenvironmental conditions to favor the donor cells in a competitive repopulation, this concept has been challenged. In fact, mixed bone marrow chimerism resulting from a less cytotoxic nonmyeloablative transplantion may be acceptable or even desirable.

Immunosuppression in the setting of allogeneic bone marrow transplantation is necessary to avoid rejection of donor marrow, and TBI is a very efficient immunosuppressant. In animal work by Storb et al. (142,143), equivalent doses of fractionated TBI were significantly less effective than single dose TBI to condition DNA-identical littermate dogs before bone marrow transplantation. Their conclusion was that there was significant repair of DNA damage by lymphoid cells during interfraction intervals. In a murine model, Salomon et al. (122) looked at three TBI schemas from schedules that had been proposed for human TBI (8.5 Gy single-dose TBI, 2 Gy times six fractions of TBI, and 1.2 Gy times 12 fractions of hyperfractionated TBI). In terms of the immunosuppressive effects, the results favored single-dose TBI. A marked initial shoulder on the dose survival curve has been reported for T-lymphocyte precursors (156) and for a human lymphoblastoid cell line (108). There is a marked fractionation sensitivity of the immunosuppressive effect of TBI leading one to conclude that fractionated TBI would lead to more graft rejections than the same dose delivered in a single fraction. Clinical data confirm these findings in that fractionated TBI programs using total doses of 13 to 15 Gy are roughly equivalent to the efficacy of 10 Gy single-dose TBI.

If bone marrow stromal cells and their progenitors (colony forming units-fibroblast, or CFU-F) are damaged, delayed engraftment or even graft failure may follow (49). Progenitors of human bone marrow stromal cells have been found to have a D_0 of 1.46 Gy (47). They are also sensitive to dose-rate effects and fractionation; thus, fractionated TBI spares bone marrow stromal cells and their progenitors better than single-dose TBI (23).

Radiobiologic Effects on Leukemia

In the setting of stem cell transplantation procedures, TBI achieves significant leukemia cell killing, and in conjunction with chemotherapy and graft versus leukemia (GVL) effect, it leads to eradication of malignant clones in a significant portion of cases. The use of the D_0 value gives a rough indication of the radiosensitivity of various cell populations; most D_0 values for both animal and human leukemias cell lines range from 0.8 to 1.5 Gy (24,92,138,167), although extreme values range from 0.3 to >5 Gy. Leukemic cell lines frequently show a minimal initial shoulder in radiation cell survival curves, leading to the hypothesis that fractionation (or reduced dose rate exposure) should have only a minor effect on cell survival. Split dose radiation experiments lend further support to this hypothesis. Greater repair capacity is seen with more differentiated leukemias or lymphocytes (e.g., B- or T-cell phenotypes).

Graft versus Leukemia/Tumor Effects

Allogeneic stem cell transplantation is largely an immunologic therapy. Allogeneic hematopoietic cells must be matched with the recipient for the majority of the major histocompatability antigens to avoid rejection and minimize graft versus host disease, but minor HLA differences facilitate a GVL effect that enhances transplantation efficacy. Early studies demonstrated improved leukemia control with allogeneic bone marrow cells as compared to syngeneic (identical twin) donor cells. Further evidence for GVL effect derives from the efficacy of donor lymphocyte infusions after relapse of leukemia following allotransplant. In general with allogeneic transplantation, it is necessary to modulate the immune reconstitution during engraftment (for example, using cyclosporine) to produce a GVL effect while minimizing graft versus host disease.

Total-Body Irradiation Dose-Limiting Toxicity: Pneumonitis and Other Late Effects

Early in the history of TBI, grade 4 or 5 solid organ toxicities were found to be a major limitation, prompting a movement away from low-dose–rate single-fraction TBI to fractionated regimens and non-TBI regimens. Studies in mice and humans show that the toxicities of TBI can be improved further by fractionating the radiation as well as delivering radiation at a low dose rate. There is a high interfactional repair capacity of normal lung tissue. Thames and Hendry (148) reported a low alpha/beta value (3 to 6 Gy) for lung. This has been confirmed with both animal and human data (40,80,165). The lung sparing effect for fractionation has been shown to be important down to roughly 1 Gy (97). This dose roughly corresponds to the lowest fraction size in some hyperfractionated TBI schedules (129). The marked lung sparing effect of fractionation, or of a decrease in dose rate, has been confirmed by the work of Penney et al. (98), who showed a progressive sparing of the lung with increased fractionation for both early pneumonitis and late fibrosis. The rate of lung repair between fractions was reviewed by Travis (154), indicating the presence of two significantly different repair rates corresponding to a fast repair half time of 0.40 hours and a slow half time of 4.01 hours. The slow repair component needs to be kept in mind when designing TBI schedules that include two or three fractions per day (165).

The reduction of the risk of pneumonitis by fractionation is supported by a randomized clinical trial comparing low-dose–rate single-fraction TBI (9.2 or 10 Gy) with low-dose–rate fractionated TBI (12 Gy in six fractions over 3 days) for patients with acute myelogenous leukemia in first remission, which showed a significant improvement in event-free survival with fractionation, mainly because of a reduction in early mortality. Interstitial pneumonitis in these patients was decreased from 26% to 15% with fractionation (31). Other studies have confirmed that fractionated TBI regimens have markedly reduced the incidence of idiopathic interstitial pneumonitis (101,133,150) to <20% without increasing the rate of tumor recurrence. Within a range of conventional fraction sizes of 1.5 to 2 Gy given once or twice daily, no significant increase in the incidence of interstitial pneumonitis is noted up to total doses as high as 15 Gy (18,19,101).

Another radiobiologic approach to reduce the incidence of interstitial pneumonitis has been to lower the radiation dose rate, in essence a kind of continuous fractionation. Empirically

this was found to be efficacious (3,149), but treatment times of 2 to 3 hours or more are impractical for most radiotherapy departments. Moreover, patients find it difficult to tolerate such long treatment times. Fractionated TBI appears to be a better way of exploiting the potential advantages inherent in the different radiobiologic properties of tumor cells and the lung. Within the context of fractionated TBI schemes, instantaneous dose rates of 0.05 to 0.18 Gy have been generally employed, often determined by the available output of linear accelerators at extended treatment distances. It is unclear whether or not higher instantaneous dose rates are detrimental, despite theoretical concerns in this regard.

Clinical Myeloablative Stem Cell Transplantation

Bone marrow or stem cell transplantation was conceived as a method of rescuing patients from the lethal effects of dose-intensive chemoradiotherapy. TBI has been a central part of allogeneic transplantation for leukemias since the pioneering work of Thomas et al. beginning in the late 1950s (44a). A single dose of 9.2 Gy at a low-dose rate of 0.07 Gy per minute was required to obtain a consistent and sustained engraftment of allogeneic marrow in experimental animals. Consequently, a dose of 10 Gy at a dose rate of 0.07 to 0.10 Gy per minute using Cobalt teletherapy was used in humans.

The premise that TBI had to be given as a single fraction was challenged in the late 1970s when Peters (99) and Thomas et al. (149) demonstrated the marked sensitivity of most normal tissues to altered fractionation and dose rate with minimal effects on bone marrow progenitors and leukemic cells. It was concluded that with the same total dose an improved therapeutic ratio would be expected from a reduction in the dose rate of single fraction TBI or by TBI fractionation. Calculations of various fractionation schemes and dose rates have been published based on the linear quadratic model (2,28,93). O'Donoghue (93) calculated that for very low-dose–rate TBI to be equivalent radiobiologically to the more common fractionated TBI schedules, an unreasonable radiation time of 20 to 24 hours would be necessary. With concepts of both radiobiology and practicality in mind, a large variety of fractionated TBI schedules have been used. After a generation of clinical investigation, no one regimen is clearly superior to another; so many confounding variables exist (including TBI technique, disease and patient heterogeneity, chemotherapy, supportive care, and immunosuppression) that it is impossible to clearly demonstrate the superiority of a particular regimen. Currently, most myeloablative TBI programs use a twice or three times a day fractionation scheme over 3 to 4 days to deliver a total dose of 12 to 15 Gy.

Chemotherapy Used with Total-Body Irradiation

Chemotherapy agents used in conjunction with TBI include cyclophosphamide, etoposide, and Ara-C, with cyclophosphamide at 120 mg/kg over 2 days being the most common based on early work from the Seattle group. Programs adding in other agents have been used primarily in high-risk transplant settings, but cyclophosphamide remains a backbone given its effectiveness in immunosuppression and cytotoxicity. Reduced intensity or nonmyeloablative transplant regimens using low-dose TBI that have been developed in recent years have sometimes used fludarabine or pentostatin in place of cyclophosphamide (86). Chemotherapy and TBI are given sequentially rather than concurrently to avoid any potential increase in normal tissue toxicity. Whether chemotherapy should be given before or after TBI is unclear, and in the absence of clinical data showing which is best, logistic issues are the main consideration. Typically, TBI over 3 to 4 days is best delivered during the regular work week, when the full technical support staff is available. TBI may be better tolerated if given first when the patient is less fatigued and not sick from the effects of chemotherapy. The risk of nosocomial infections may be marginally lower when the patient travels to the radiotherapy department before becoming neutropenic later in the conditioning course. Alternatively, TBI at the end of the preparative regimen allows the stem cell transplant to proceed immediately thereafter; unlike chemotherapy, there is no washout period for elimination of the cytotoxic agent that would otherwise be harmful to the stem cells, thus saving a day or so of expected neutropenia while awaiting engraftment.

Non-Total-Body Irradiation Conditioning Regimens

Although the evolution of TBI has lead to significant reduction in toxicities, the initial concern about risk for fatal radiation pneumonitis lead to the development of non-TBI regimens. For example, Santos (125) at Johns Hopkins and other groups administered busulfan in place of radiotherapy (21,131,157). A French randomized clinical trial compared busulfan and cyclophosphamide (BuCy) to cyclophosphamide TBI before allogeneic bone marrow transplantation for adult acute myeloblastic leukemia (AML) in first remission (9). The results showed that cyclophosphamide-TBI was superior for disease-free survival, relapse, and transplant mortality. This result was confirmed in another French (nonrandomized) study of allogeneic bone marrow transplantation in childhood AML (85). In a small trial of 35 AML patients, Dusenbery et al. (41) concluded that cyclophosphamide TBI provided an equivalent or better outcome than BuCy. Although retrospective data from the International Bone Marrow Tumor Registry suggested similar results from TBI and non-TBI regimes for acute leukemias (21), a Japanese bone marrow transplant (BMT) registry showed an advantage for TBI in terms of overall survival and leukemia relapse rates (60). A meta-analysis comparing BuCy and cyclophosphamide TBI shows trends not reaching statistical significance in favor of TBI for both overall survival and disease-free survival (55).

In contrast, in chronic phase myeloid leukemia (CML), the Seattle group demonstrated that BuCy was better tolerated and associated with a survival and relapse probability that was comparable to cyclophosphamide TBI (20). Studies on either side of the question have held very few variables constant, making the data almost impossible to interpret. The choice of conditioning regimen prior to transplantation depends on a variety of factors that include the type of transplantation (allogeneic or autologous), the disease type (BuCy might be better in CML and cyclophosphamide TBI might be better for AML) (9), and the status of disease (cyclophosphamide TBI for patients with more advanced disease) (109).

Relative Advantage of Total-Body Irradiation—Based Regimens and Dose Tailoring

Toxicity concerns now tend to favor TBI containing regimens. As TBI techniques have evolved, the risk of pneumonitis is similar between TBI and non-TBI regimens. Prior thoracic radiotherapy is a risk factor for fatal pneumonitis (32% risk after TBI in patients with prior chest radiation doses above 20 Gy in one study) and would be a reason to avoid TBI (159). On the other hand, there is also a significantly higher risk of hepatic veno-occlusive disease and hemorrhagic cystitis with BuCy, compared with TBI-based regimens (55,89). The Nordic Bone Marrow Transplantation Group published a randomized trial comparing BuCy and cyclophosphamide TBI (109). The BuCy-treated patients had a veno-occlusive disease (VOD) incidence of 12% compared to 1% for the TBI-treated patients ($p = 0.009$). Hemorrhagic cystitis risk was 24% for busulfan-based therapy

versus 8% for TBI ($p = 0.002$). BuCy conditioning regimens also have an appreciable risk for seizures (30).

A relative advantage in using TBI for stem cell transplantation is that the dose delivery throughout the body is highly controllable. In contrast to chemotherapy, dose distribution is independent of such factors as blood supply, and there are no concerns about agent activation, metabolism, excretion, or dose modifications based on liver or kidney function. TBI may also reach chemotherapy sanctuary sites, which is of particular concern, for example, in patients at risk for or with central nervous system (CNS) involvement.

Historically, radiation oncologists have aimed to deliver a relatively homogenous dose of TBI throughout the whole body given the concern that leukemias are systemically distributed. Whether this is always an important goal is unclear, since microscopic disease burden during remission may not be uniform throughout the body. Some TBI programs use photon energies above 20 MV, which may theoretically deliver higher marrow doses due to increased pair production and higher bone absorption (12). Many correct for skin sparing effects of megavoltage irradiation, for instance with use of beam spoilers, although this is probably not necessary for low energy photons in the absence of leukemia cutis or a trophism for skin involvement such as in monocytic leukemias. Where there is concern for a higher burden of disease, boost radiation fields may be added to TBI. Augmented doses of radiation may be delivered to the head in the setting of CNS relapse or prophylaxis or to the testes in males with acute lymphoblastic leukemia (ALL), as examples.

Clinical Data Regarding Total-Body Irradiation Dose and Fractionation Schedule

A randomized study from Seattle in the setting of AML compared single-dose TBI (10 Gy) to a fractionated schedule (2 Gy for six fractions). The last update of this trial showed significant superiority of the fractionated scheme in terms of event-free survival (151). Investigators from France (95) and from Italy (126) reported that dose rate did not influence the relapse rate. Another Seattle randomized trial of AML in first remission compared fractionated TBI doses of 12 Gy with 15.75 Gy, showing a decreased relapse rate from 35% to 12%, but at the expense of a significant increase in therapy-related mortality, resulting in no survival advantage to a higher radiation dose (18). In short, in the setting of AML:

1. Fractionated TBI appears superior to 10 Gy single dose TBI in terms of leukemia-free survival; and
2. Dose rate has little impact on leukemia-free survival.

In contrast, a significant dose–rate effect has been found for CML in chronic phase treated with allotransplant. A higher dose rate correlated with a decreased relapse rate (65,126). As well, a multi-institutional nonrandomized French study of 180 patients with CML showed that TBI fractionation was associated with an increase in relapse rate (137). In a French trial comparing BuCy and cyclophosphamide TBI, the actuarial risk of relapse was 11.1% after single dose TBI (10 Gy) and 31% after fractionated TBI (37). The same trend is seen for patients receiving T-cell depleted marrow. In summary, a decrease in dose rate for single fraction schemes or TBI fractionation in CML in chronic phase may lead to reduced leukemic cell killing (23).

For ALL there is a paucity of clinical data regarding the optimal dose fractionation schedule for TBI. In a series from the City of Hope Medical Center, there was no significant difference in relapse rate between single dose (10 Gy) and hyperfractionated TBI (1.2 Gy times 11 fractions over 4 days) (10). A multicenter French study, however, showed a high likelihood of relapse for patients who received fractionated TBI, with graft versus host disease (GVHD) prophylaxis mainly via T-cell depletion (166).

Together with elimination of GVHD, T-cell depletion also results in the loss of the GVL effect, which may unmask the known differences in antileukemic efficacy of TBI schedules that otherwise might be obscured by the combined efficacy of the conventional chemotherapy–irradiation–GVL association (79). In fact, there is evidence of both a dose-rate effect (less relapse with dose rates higher than 14 cGy per minute) and fractionation effect (more relapse with fractionation), suggesting a repair capacity of some leukemic cells (23).

Nonmyeloablative or Reduced Intensity Stem Cell Transplantation

In the past decade, growing recognition of the immunotherapeutic potential of allografts has led to a reconsideration of the need for the high-dose myeloablative conditioning regimens traditionally administered prior to transplantation. Pioneering work of Storb et al. (143,144) in canine models established that highly immunosuppressive but nonmyeloablative regimens could establish stable mixed hematopoietic chimerism in major histocompatability complex matched littermates using one sixth of the usual ablative dose of TBI in combination with postgrafting immunosuppressive drugs. Subsequently, numerous clinical trials have established that a spectrum of subablative conditioning regimens of varying intensity may allow engraftment of donor cells with reduction in regimen-related toxicity, permitting transplantation of patients traditionally excluded from allografting because of age or medical condition (67,78,83,136,139,140). In essence, allogeneic-reduced intensity transplantation is a form of immunotherapy. The primary purpose of the nonmyeloablative preparatory regimen is to suppress the patient's immune system sufficiently to allow the engraftment of donor cells with minimum host toxicity. The GVT effect leads to eradication of tumor cells.

Common to these regimens is sufficient immunosuppression to overcome host resistant to engraftment using either antimetabolites such as fludarabine, TBI, or both, in combination with other agents. Other factors, such as patient age, HLA disparity with the donor, tumor burden, and prior therapy may also affect the degree of engraftment. A series of clinical studies by the Seattle transplant group, for example, demonstrated that a single 2 Gy fraction of TBI, in combination with postgrafting cyclosporine and mycophenolate, is sufficient to achieve a high rate of donor engraftment in patients with a prior history of autologous stem cell transplantation, but additional immunosuppression in the form of fludarabine is necessary to ensure engraftment in less heavily pretreated patients or patients receiving unrelated donor grafts.

Reduced-intensity transplants now account for roughly 25% of all allotransplants being performed. Efficacy is difficult to evaluate in the absence of randomized trials, but reduced intensity conditioning regimens have allowed for an expanded use of transplants in high-risk populations. As an example, elderly patients with acute leukemias in first remission have long-term survival rates over 40% with nonmyeloablative transplants, which would be considered a remarkable achievement compared to historical experience in which very few patients would be expected to survive (90). Toxicity is significantly lower than the traditional myeloablative transplants. The Seattle group has reported a 1-year nonrelapse-related mortality of allotransplants of 30% for ablative regimens compared to 16% for reduced intensity conditioning regimens ($p = 0.04$) (38). Certainly based on first principles, the toxicity of a single dose of 2 Gy of TBI should be minimal. Most transplant centers delivering this dose of TBI would dispense with the complexities of lung blocks as well as compensating filters to optimize dose homogeneity.

Total-Body Irradiation Technique

Basic Requirements

Technically, the goal of TBI is to deliver as uniform and accurate a dose as possible to the entire body while not exceeding the radiation tolerance of any organs. Because of the large variation in geometry and tissue density throughout the patient's body, dose delivery within $\pm 10\%$ of the prescription dose is standard, while higher dose deviations confined to smaller volumes particularly in the extremities are acceptable. Therefore, any TBI technique must undergo a rigorous dosimetry commissioning, and a quality assurance program must be in place when establishing a TBI program in a radiotherapy department. Because of the strict time constraints imposed by the bone marrow transplantation protocols, once a patient begins a course of TBI the timing of successive fractions becomes critical to the outcome of the procedure. Therefore, another important consideration when embarking on a TBI program is to establish a backup TBI system. If the primary system is down, a fully commissioned backup TBI system must be available to complete the remaining treatment.

Current Total-Body Irradiation Techniques

Many different techniques have been described for effective irradiation of the whole body and, indeed, improvements in both the irradiation technique and physical dosimetry are still being reported (39,44,59,72). Much of the early clinical experience with TBI and HBI procedures was gained at centers with facilities specifically designed for large field irradiation (160). Although a few dedicated systems still exist, most of the current TBI procedures are based on techniques established on linear accelerators that are used for conventional radiotherapy. Common to most of the TBI techniques is the use of radiation fields that are larger than the maximum field size ($\sim$40 by 40 cm^2) available at standard source-to-surface distance (SSD) treatment distance ($\sim$100 cm) in conventional radiotherapy. The large photon fields are generally achieved by treating the patient at extended SSD ($\sim$200 to 600 cm) with standard linear accelerators or with special dedicated machines with the conventional collimator removed (100). On a standard linear accelerator a SSD of 5 m or more is needed to produce a field size large enough to completely encompass most of the patient along the diagonal of a square radiation field. Although such a large SSD can be accommodated when new treatment rooms are being designed, existing radiotherapy facilities often have treatment rooms with SSD less than ideal. The variable SSD available at current radiotherapy facilities is partially responsible for the variation in TBI techniques and procedures.

Current TBI techniques can be classified into two main groups based on the radiation field size: those that utilize a large field size that encompasses the entire patient body and those that use less-than-whole-body field sizes, as shown in Figure 14.1. Patients are irradiated with a parallel-opposed beam configuration. These stationary TBI configurations include single or dual fixed beam dedicated units with patient in supine position and horizontal beams from conventional linear accelerators (LINACs) with patients in supine, upright, or lateral decubitus positions (73,76). When treatment room constraints necessitate less-than-whole-body fields (Fig. 14.2), irradiation of the whole body can be achieved by translating the radiation field (25) or the patient (106) or by sweeping the radiation field over a stationary patient (103).

The extended SSD technique using a single large field encompassing the entire patient is by far the simplest and the most prevalent TBI technique used today. It eliminates the dosimetry complications in regions of field junctions introduced by

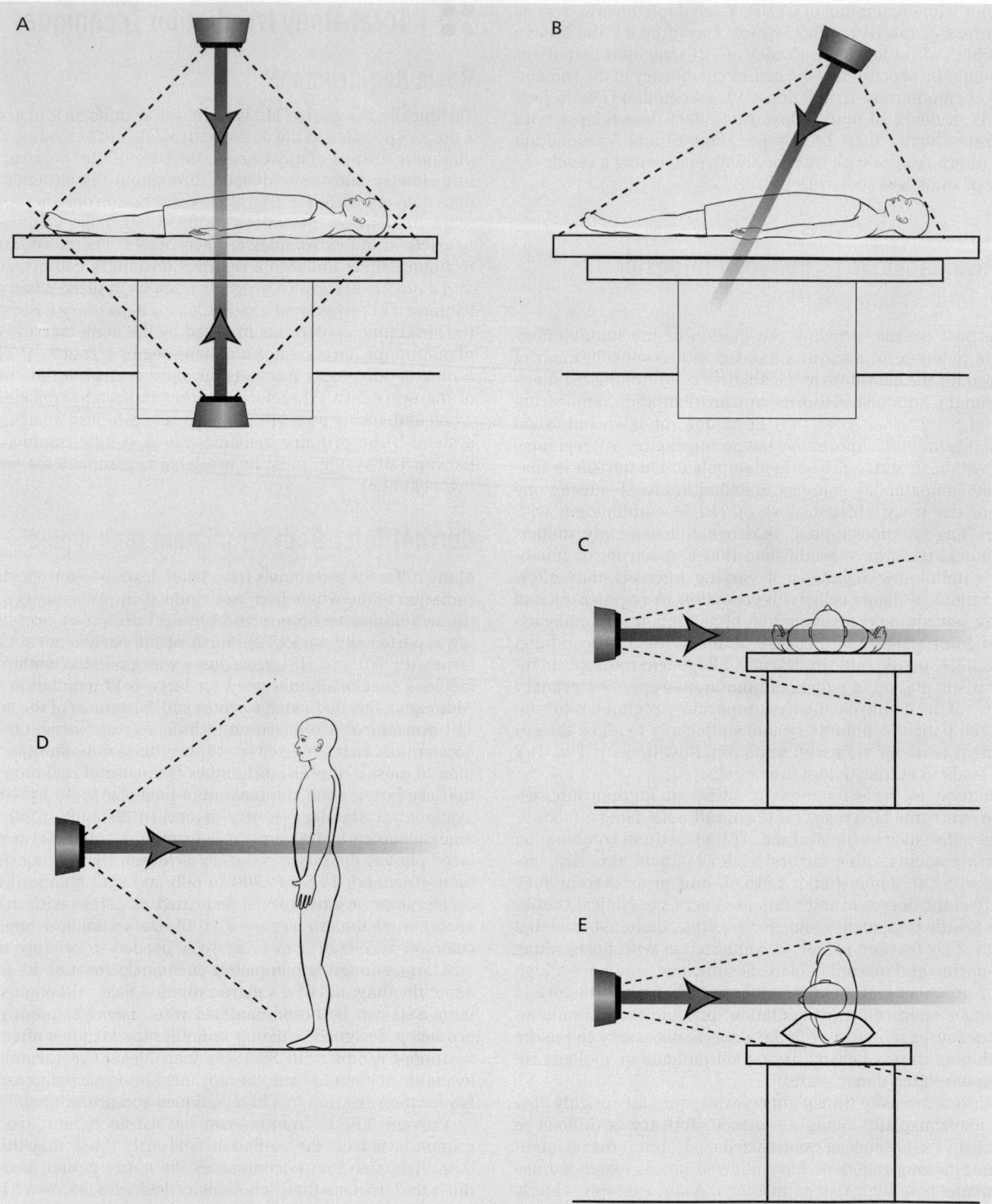

FIGURE 14.1. Illustration of some of the current large-field total-body irradiation techniques in which patient and beams are stationary. **A:** Two vertical beams. **B:** One vertical beam. **C:** One horizontal beam, patient in supine position. **D:** One horizontal beam, patient standing or sitting. **E:** One horizontal beam; patient in lateral decubitus position.

using multiple small fields and the concern that cells circulating through the body could potentially receive a reduced dose. These techniques use standard radiotherapy LINACs and rely on a maximum collimator setting, a large SSD, and beam divergence to produce the large irradiation field required for TBI. Treatment is typically delivered with a horizontal beam directed toward the primary shielding wall. At SSDs of 500 cm or more, the patient placed along the diagonal of the square field will be completely covered by the radiation.

Total-Body Irradiation Dosimetry

The dosimetry of TBI has been reviewed in several reports (15,160,162). In particular, the American Association of Physicists in Medicine (AAPM) task group 29 (TG-29) report on the physical aspects of total and half-body photon irradiation has discussed many dosimetry issues and techniques specific to large field TBI (160). Since the publication of TG-29, the basic reference dosimetry protocol for external beams, known as the

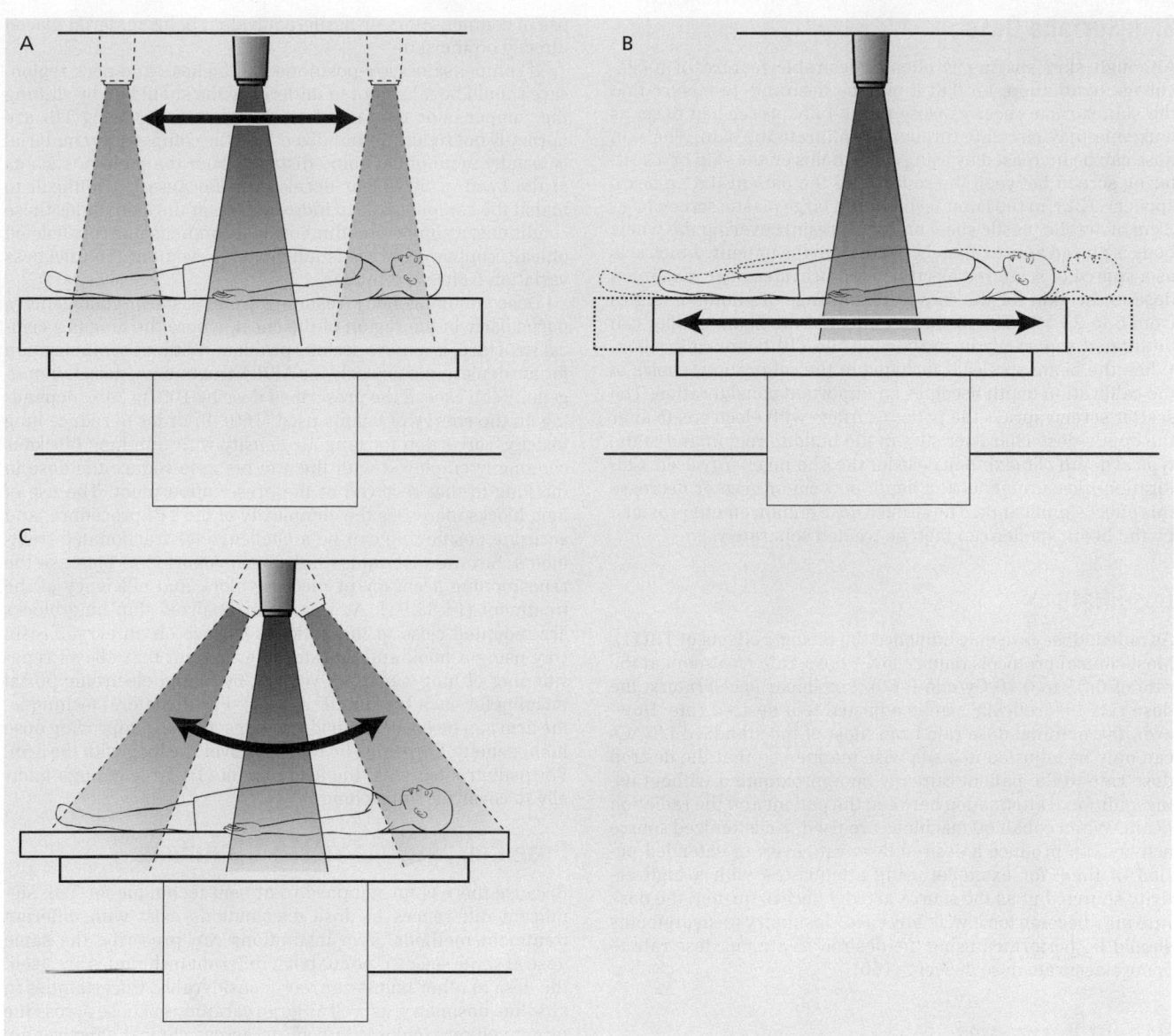

FIGURE 14.2. Illustration of some of the small-field total-body irradiation techniques in which patient or beam moves. **A:** Source scans horizontally. **B:** Patient moves horizontally. **C:** Sweeping beam.

TG-21 protocol, has been updated, and a new calibration protocol (TG-51) is being adopted by most radiotherapy departments. For photon beams, the TG-51 protocol produces similar results as the TG-21 protocol. Many of the discussions contained in the TG-29 report are still relevant when considering the dosimetric effects of large fields. The general approach recommended by TG-29 in determining the dose delivered to a patient involves three steps:

1. Absolute dose calibration of the large-field TBI beam at the TBI treatment distance using water or water-equivalent phantoms of a minimum size of 30 by 30 by 30 cm^3;
2. Dose corrections obtained for a standard phantom that covers entire the beam in full scattering conditions; and
3. Dose corrections for individual size variation in the area of the patient intersecting the beam as well as for patient thickness.

With this general approach, the effect of room scatter is taken into account because the same conditions are used for calibration and treatment, and the difference in patient scatter is also corrected in the final step. Calibration should be performed under treatment conditions (compensating filters that may be at the linear accelerator head or close to the patient, beam spoiler

to increase skin dose, etc.) to ensure accurate dose delivery. An alternative approach has been proposed by Curran et al. (26) to calibrate TBI photon beams using the standard AAPM TG-21 protocol geometry (now the TG-51 geometry) followed by application of various correction factors to account for the TBI geometry and scattering conditions. In this approach, directly measured correction factors should be used. For example, the reduction of the dose rate with distance from a treatment machine follows the inverse square rule only approximately and can differ by as much as 5% at a treatment distance of 300 cm. The conventional percentage depth dose (PDD) or tissue maximum ratio (TMR) tables may not be appropriate for TBI configuration (51). PDD or TMR should be measured under treatment conditions in a phantom with a size similar to that of the typical patient. In-phantom beam profiles at treatment distance, especially along the diagonal near the corners of the field, also should be measured to evaluate the dose variation across the radiation beam. Regardless of which approach is adopted, dose verification also should be performed on an anthropomorphic phantom (69,127,145,146). Thermoluminescent dosimeter measurements can be used to verify point doses, and film may be used to assess dose distributions (123).

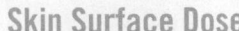

Skin Surface Dose

Although skin sparing is often a desirable feature of megavoltage irradiation, for TBI it may be desirable to ensure that the skin surface receives close to the fully prescribed dose, as leukemia may circulate through or infiltrate the skin. The skin dose can be increased by using either bolus on the skin or a scattering screen between the source and the patient (i.e., a beam spoiler) (132). In the latter technique, a large plastic screen (e.g., 2 cm of acrylic plastic sheet or acrylic resin) covering the whole body is placed approximately 10 cm from the patient, which acts as a source of scattered electrons and provides near maximum dose to the skin for the conventional range of photon energies from 6 to 25 MV. The dosimetry effect of the beam spoiler can be treated separately or included in the TBI beam calibration. When the beam spoiler is included in the calibration, choice of the calibration depth becomes an important consideration. The scatter screen sprays the patient surface with electrons to alter the depth–dose characteristics in the buildup region and at the typical depth of maximum dose for the photon energy used. Calibration measurements at a depth of 5 cm or greater decrease this effect significantly. The surface dose enhancement provided by the beam spoiler can then be treated separately.

Dose Rate

As noted, dose rate may influence the biologic effects of TBI (1). Most clinical protocols require low—dose–rate treatment at the rate of 0.05 to 0.10 Gy/min (160). For linear accelerators, the dose rate theoretically can be adjusted to a desired rate. However, the nominal dose rate from most of the standard LINACs can only be adjusted in a stepwise manner, so that the desired dose rate to the patient can only be approximated without using additional attenuation between the patient and the radiation beam. When cobalt 60 machines are used, a customized source activity can produce a desired dose rate over an extended period of time, for example, using attenuators with a high activity source, but as the source activity decays further, the dose rate may become too low. In any case, dosimetry measurements should be performed using the desired treatment dose rate to ensure accurate dose delivery (160).

Patient Positioning

As treatment times may last up to 30 or 40 minutes for each fraction of TBI (or longer for single fraction techniques), patients must be in comfortable and reproducible positions. Although it may be ideal to deliver TBI with the patient in the supine position, anterior-posterior/posterior-anterior (AP/PA) techniques tend to have more desirable dosimetry and are frequently achievable with horizontal beams due to room and LINAC geometry. With that setup, patients need to be in lateral decubitus, sitting, or even standing position. Since clinical problems with patient fatigue and orthostatic hypotension are not uncommon, some centers have special patient stands to facilitate an upright patient positioning.

Dose Homogeneity

Variation in patient thickness is the major factor contributing to dose inhomogeneity. As a result, an AP/PA technique is best as the dose variation will generally be on the order of ± 7% to 10% owing to a smaller variation in patient thickness in the anterior-posterior direction (160). For adults, lateral fields can have dose variations up to 50% in the head and neck region and 10% in other parts of the body. This dose variation decreases with increasing beam energy and with the use of larger treatment distances (160). Dose variation can be decreased with the use of compensators or tissue-equivalent bolus material placed directly on the skin.

If compensators are positioned in the head and neck region, care should be taken not to underdose the shoulders by shifting the compensator too far inferiorly. Patients receiving TBI are normally not rigidly immobilized, and the compensator material is usually mounted at some distance from the patient, such as at the head of the linear accelerator. Because it is difficult to match the compensator to index marks on the skin under these conditions, a simple one-dimensional compensator constructed of lead, copper, or brass is adequate to even out the thickness variation from head to toe.

Dose inhomogeneity resulting from tissue inhomogeneity, particularly in the region of the chest, where the lung is a critical structure, is a more serious problem. Without compensation for air density, particularly for AP/PA treatments, dose inhomogeneity can exceed the prescribed dose by 10% to 24%, depending on the energy of beams used (160). In order to reduce lung toxicity, correction for lung air density with thin lung blocks is commonly employed with the aim being to reduce the dose in the lung to that received at the prescription point. The use of lung blocks increases the complexity of the TBI procedure, and accurate positioning can be a challenge for fractionated treatments. Several techniques have been reported to increase the repositioning accuracy of the lung block and efficiency of the treatment (14,88,91). At Yale, individualized thin lung blocks are mounted close to the patient's surface on an acrylic resin tray using a hook and loop fastener system that allows repositioning of lung blocks as verified by online electronic portal imaging for each fraction (Fig. 14.3). For the lateral technique, the arm can be used to shield the lungs, thereby improving dose homogeneity. Care must be taken to cover the lung with the arm. For pediatric patients, the arm may not be large enough laterally to cover the entire lung.

Dose Comparisons among Institutions

Because there is no standard treatment technique for TBI, significant differences in dose distributions exist with different treatment methods. Two institutions can prescribe the same dose at some selected point, but if different techniques are used, the dose to other points can vary considerably. Uncertainties in absolute dosimetry, as well as large variations of dose across the target volume, make it difficult to assess clinical effectiveness when results from different treatment centers are compared.

To facilitate comparisons among institutions, various methods for describing the dose from large-field treatments have been reported (50,68). One approach uses a single-point prescription and specifies limits for the highest and lowest dose levels acceptable for any point in the body. Dose limits are also set for certain specific tissues such as the lungs. A good example of a TBI prescription is given in AAPM TG-29, using the midpoint at the level of the umbilicus as a convenient prescription point. A typical prescription might read the dose to the midpoint at the level of the umbilicus as 12 Gy in six to eight fractions. All points in the body should fall within the limits of 12.6 and 10.8 Gy, or +5% and –10%. The dose to more than half the lung volume should not exceed 12 Gy.

Quality Assurance

To improve the dosimetry accuracy and consistency, *in vivo* verification should be required when setting up any new TBI technique (160). In addition, *in vivo* dosimetry is a good practice to perform on the first treatment fraction for all TBI patients. Changes in patient position can alter dose distributions dramatically. Thermoluminescent dosimeters and diodes are typical choices for monitoring the dose to the patient (123,145). They may be used at entrance and exit, but scatter from the

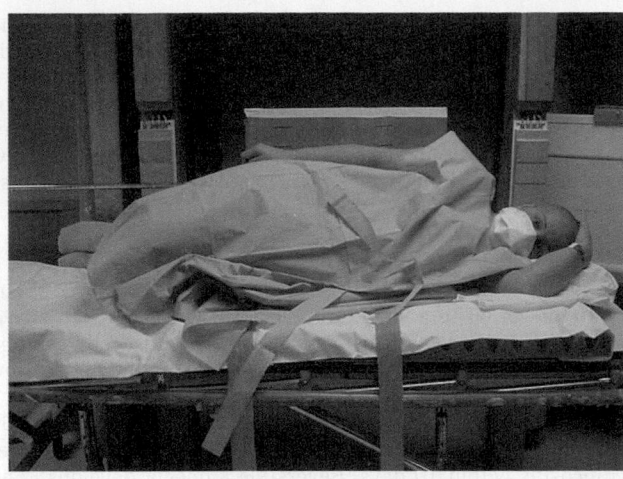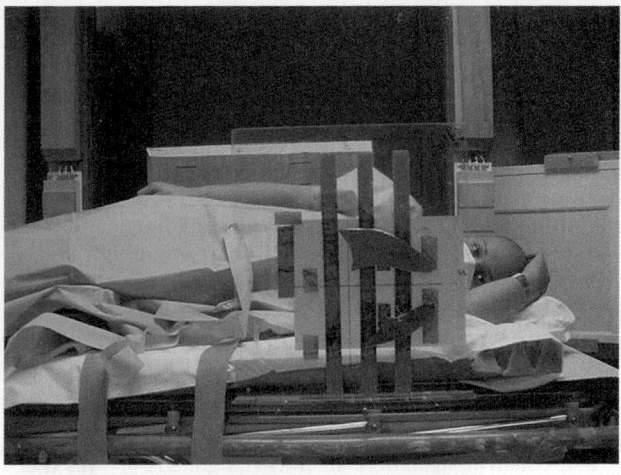

A   B

FIGURE 14.3. A: Patient in decubitus position for total-body irradiation, anterior beam. **B:** Thin lung blocks placed close to thorax using hook and loop fasteners/transparent resinous board system to reposition blocks with each fraction.

room must be carefully considered. Multiple-diode systems are convenient for these types of measurements because they allow simultaneous dose estimation at more than one anatomic site. At Yale, dose verification using a multidiode system is performed for each patient on the first treatment fraction. Significant dose deviations can be adjusted by changing the compensation filters or monitor units (output).

Lung (and Other Organ) Dose Attenuation

Many transplant centers use lung blocks during TBI in order to correct for the dosimetric effects of lung density or to specifically reduce the dose to a majority of lung tissue, thereby reducing the risk for pneumonitis. Overcompensation, however, risks an increase in leukemia recurrence (52). Specifically, a study from the Institut Gustave-Roussy delivering 10 Gy as a single fraction of TBI over 4 hours showed a higher incidence of relapse in patients whose lung dose is limited by lung blocks to 6 Gy instead of 8 Gy (52). The technique at Yale utilizes one-eighth–inch lead filters that attenuate the dose by 10% to 15%, in essence a slight overcorrection for the dosimetric effects of pulmonary air density (43) (Fig. 14.4). The Memorial Sloan Kettering Cancer Center (MSKCC) group utilizes one half-value layer (HVL) shielding (133) with the use of electron boosts of the chest wall under

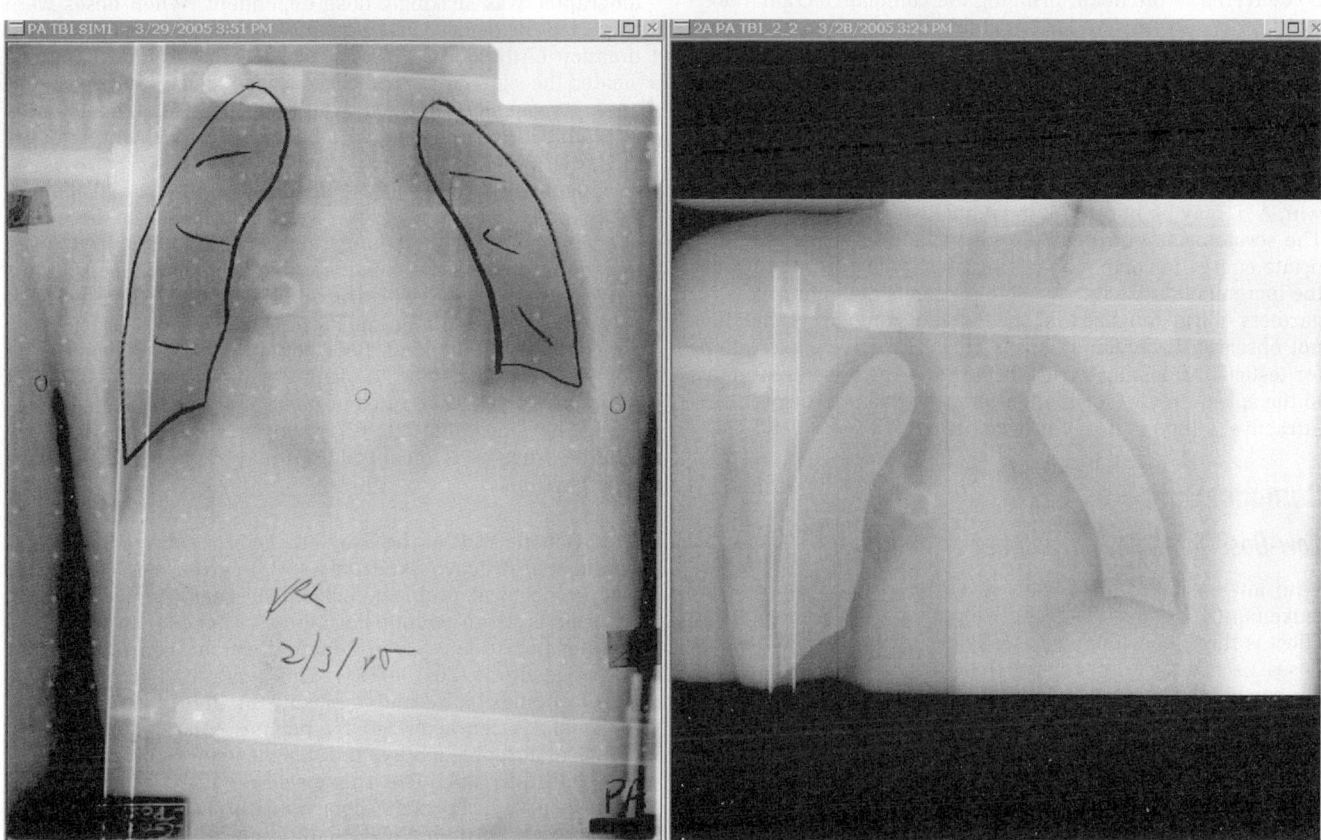

FIGURE 14.4. Thin lung blocks (eighth-inch lead) used at Yale to attenuate dose under block by 10% to 15%, primarily to compensate for air density inhomogeneity in total-body irradiation dosimetry. Left panel is megavoltage simulation film taken in decubitus position. Right panel is treatment portal imaging.

the lung blocks. There are considerable dosimetric problems with this technique: electrons treatments are planned in supine position, yet delivered standing; overlap issues of photon and electron fields; surface contour variability especially from breast tissue in women, while still delivering unwanted radiation dose to some limited volume of lungs. The Institut Gustave-Roussy has reported no clinical benefit to electron boosts to chest wall under such lung blocks (22). The Johns Hopkins group has reported using thick (7 HVL) blocks for just one fraction of their TBI course over several days (102). The Seattle group uses 1 HVL block for roughly half of the TBI fractions without a chest wall boost. Other transplant groups such as at the University of Minnesota have reported using partial transmission blocks to the liver and kidneys to reduce the risk of hepatic veno-occlusive disease or nephropathy (70,71). When TBI is used for nonneoplastic diseases (e.g., aplastic anemia), where the main objective is immunosuppression, one may also consider shielding radiosensitive structures such as the gonads or eyes (i.e., the lens) (130).

Boosting of Selected Organs with Total-Body Irradiation

A relative advantage of TBI is the treatment of chemotherapy sanctuary sites, of particular concern in patients at high risk for CNS relapse. Theoretically, regions of the body where there is a higher burden of disease at the time of transplant may be boosted with additional radiation fields to supplement TBI. In selected patients with lymphoblastic leukemia, CNS preventative therapy includes cranial radiation. When such patients are determined at diagnosis to be best managed with an allogeneic transplant, it is reasonable to defer prophylactic cranial radiation until the time of TBI. Augmented doses of radiation may be delivered to the head, bringing the cumulative cranial dose to 18 Gy (a current standard in children and many adults with ALL). Higher total doses to the head and perhaps the spine can be contemplated in patients being managed for CNS leukemia. Boost doses to the head using lateral fields may be given in 1.8 to 2.0 Gy fractions. Caution is necessary for additional CNS boost treatments when patients have received prior cranial irradiation due to toxicity concerns. Similarly, the testes in males with ALL may be boosted to a cumulative dose of 16 to 18 Gy. The scrotum may be treated with en face electrons of appropriate energy (or orthovoltage x-rays in young boys). Because the incremental toxicity of such testicular irradiation is low regardless of fraction size and the fact that some programs have not observed testicular relapses after TBI, dose prescriptions for testicular boosting varies from 0 to 4 Gy. Boost treatments to the spleen in CML or to chloromas in AML are theoretically attractive, although not of proven benefit (42,53).

Complications

Low-Dose Total-Body Irradiation

With low-dose TBI historically given for chronic lymphocytic leukemia (CLL) and low-grade lymphomas, the principal side effect is thrombocytopenia, usually occurring after cumulative doses exceeding 1 to 1.5 Gy (62,84). Nausea and vomiting are sometimes observed, controllable by standard antiemetics. When used with alkylating agent chemotherapy, a significant risk of acute leukemia or myelodysplasia has been observed, on the order of 8% to 9% at 15 years of follow-up (155).

High-Dose Total-Body Irradiation

Side effects from TBI used with stem cell transplantation have complex interactions with cytotoxic drugs and other support-

ive care or immunosuppressive agents. In addition, GVHD has its own set of toxicities, which have complex interactions with the conditioning regimen. Infectious complications also have a significant role in transplant-related toxicities. Isolating what toxicities are strictly related to TBI is not straightforward; nevertheless, the randomized trials from Seattle comparing 12 Gy versus 15 Gy, showed that nontransplant mortality increases with higher radiation doses (18,19).

Acute Toxicity

Nausea, vomiting, and diarrhea are the most common early side effects when a single fraction of 8 to 10 Gy TBI is given (7,16,149). These side effects also can be caused by cytotoxic drugs if given prior to TBI. The use of fractionated or low-dose–rate TBI reduces the incidence as well as the severity of these and other side effects (16,150). Patients also develop dry mouth, a reduction in tear formation, and oral and esophageal mucositis within 10 days. Reversible alopecia develops at approximately 2 weeks in all patients (149). One side effect that is unique to TBI is parotitis, which usually occurs after the first day of irradiation and subsides within 24 to 48 hours (33).

Delayed Toxicity

Lung. Interstitial pneumonitis is the major dose-limiting toxicity for TBI and upper HBI. The radiobiology of lung tolerance has been extensively studied (161,165). Published experience from the Princess Margaret Hospital in Toronto provides some of the best data regarding lung tolerance. A cohort of 245 patients with metastatic solid tumors received a variety of single fraction upper HBI doses up to 10 Gy at dose rates of 0.3 to 0.8 Gy/min. The actuarial incidence of acute radiation pneumonitis, defined as the sudden onset roughly 16 weeks after irradiation of cough, dyspnea, and opacities visible on chest radiographs, was strikingly dose dependent. When doses were corrected for density heterogeneity, producing an upward estimation of the doses actually received by the lungs, analysis yielded the sigmoid-shaped curve as shown in Figure 14.5. Using heterogeneity-corrected data, the incidence of pneumonitis is estimated to be negligible for single doses less than about 7.5 Gy (163).

Pneumonitis in the BMT setting has a multifactorial etiology, reflecting not only the effects of radiation, but also the effects of chemotherapy, GVHD, lung injury from tumor, opportunistic infections, and other risk factors. Cyclophosphamide is almost universally given with TBI. The addition of other drugs is based on institutional treatment policies. Many anticancer drugs are known to injure the lung. BMT conditioning regimens that do not use TBI (which tend to use high-dose busulfan in place of radiation) in fact have rates of interstitial pneumonitis similar to regimens including TBI. GVH may cause lung injury directly and the drugs used to control GVH may also cause pulmonary toxicity (168).

Liver. Hepatic VOD of the liver has been recently renamed sinusoidal obstructive syndrome (SOS), given the recognition that this clinical problem, principally seen in myeloablative transplants, is an endothelial injury to hepatic sinusoids and that hepatocyte injury and hepatic thrombosis are secondary late stage effects (36,134,171). This syndrome, accounting for significant morbidity and mortality in high dose transplant regimens, is characterized by hepatic enlargement, ascites, jaundice, encephalopathy, and weight gain in 10% to 40% of patients (16,81,111,171). This disease, which needs to be distinguished from cholestatic drug injury and acute GVHD, is best diagnosed by transvenous hepatic biopsy where an elevated hepatic venous pressure gradient is documented along with characteristic histology, showing hepatic sinusoidal and central vein fibrosis and accompanying hepatocyte necrosis. The

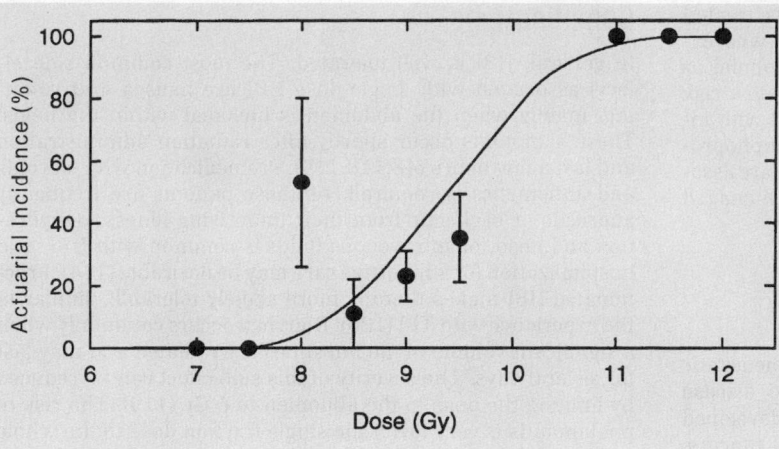

FIGURE 14.5. Incidence of radiation pneumonitis in patients receiving single-dose, whole-lung irradiation at dose rates of 0.3 to 0.8 cGy/min. Doses are corrected for tissue–air heterogeneity. (Figure reproduced from: Rockwell S, Roberts KB. "Radiation Pneumonitis, In: *Fishman's Pulmonary Diseases and Disorders*, 3rd ed. Fishman AP, Elias JA, et al., eds., Mcgraw-Hill, Inc., Philadelphia, PA, 1998.) (Data are redrawn from Van Dyk J, Keane TJ, Kan S, et al. Radiation pneumonitis following large single dose irradiation: a re-evaluation based on absolute dose to lung. *Int J Radiat Oncol Biol Phys* 1981;7[4]:461–467.)

etiology of SOS/VOD is thought to be related to acrolein, a cyclophosphamide metabolite also implicated in causing hemorrhagic cystitis, which acts as an endothelial toxin. Other toxic agents give rise to this disease, but in the transplant setting TBI, busulfan, cytosine arabinoside, and pre-existing or concomitant liver disease are cofactors possibly due to depletion of intracellular glutathione levels or matrix metalloproteinase activity. Radiobiologically, hepatocytes respond to dose fractionation (or dose rate) in a manner similar to late responding tissue with large variations of the isoeffect dose when fraction size (or dose rate) is modified (45,148). An alpha/beta ratio of 1 to 2 Gy has been estimated (46).

Clinically, in the transplant setting, the incidence of SOS/VOD has been minimized by fractionating TBI and keeping total doses below 13.2 Gy. The Seattle group has reported considerably more SOS/VOD after 10 Gy single-fraction TBI than after 12-Gy fractionated TBI in a randomized trial (31). A nonrandomized retrospective study found that fractionated TBI resulted in less SOS/VOD disease but with borderline significance (6). Barrett (4) showed a decrease in the incidence of SOS/VOD with a lower dose rate. Others have shown that modifications of chemotherapy dosing and scheduling based on individual pharmacodynamics may also lower the risk (109,171). Other prevention strategies for SOS/VOD include the administration of low molecular weight heparin and ursodiol as part of the pretransplant supportive care regimen (171). In one well-designed clinical trial, ursodiol prevented cholestatic liver injury and GVHD, but had no effect on SOS/VOD (115). Treatment is mainly supportive care, but there is some limited evidence that defibrotide, a single-stranded polydeoxyribonucleotide drug with antithrombotic and anti-ischemic properties may be helpful (107).

Lens. There is a high intrinsic radiation sensitivity of the lens. Schenken and Hagemann (128) derived an alpha/beta ratio of 1.2 Gy (0.6 to 2.1), suggesting a high fractionation or dose-rate sensitivity for cataract induction. In the first Seattle experience, >75% of patients developed cataracts 5 years after single dose TBI (33). The introduction of fractionated TBI in the 1980s has significantly reduced this risk. Ozsahin et al. (94) calculated a difference in the 5-year estimated cataract incidence between single dose TBI (39%) and in fractionated TBI (13%) while also showing a beneficial effect of lower dose rate. Bray et al. (13) reported a 63% cataract induction rate from TBI, but that risk was lower with fractionation TBI. Tichelli et al. (152) reported that the probability of requiring cataract surgery was 85% after single-dose TBI and 20% after fractionated TBI. This has been confirmed in the Seattle long-term analysis showing that fractionated TBI was much less toxic to the lens than a single-

dose regimen (8). Steroid therapy is an independent risk factor for cataract formation after bone marrow transplantation, even in the absence of TBI. Lens shielding during TBI is not recommended because of the risk of retro-ocular relapse of leukemia, but is a consideration in aplastic anemia and other nonneoplastic disease managed with stem cell transplantation.

Kidney. Renal toxicity has been underreported as a major late complication of bone marrow transplantation. A report by Tarbell et al. (147) in 1988 showed a 35% rate of renal dysfunction in ALL patients receiving transplants. Alpha/beta ratio calculations for kidney in a variety of animal and human systems consistently show relatively low values indicative of fractionation and dose rate radiosensitivity (61,64,170). A protracted value of the half-time for repair (T $^1/_2$) for late damage of 2.10 hours (1.90 to 2.34) was found by von Rongen et al. (164). Because transplant patients have often also received various nephrotoxic drugs (etoposide, teniposide, amphotericin B, aminoglycoside antibiotics) before, during and after intensive cytoreductive therapy, the contribution of TBI to renal dysfunction is not clearly established (54). GVHD also has complex interactions with radiation dose in determining the risk of transplant related nephritis (87). Helenglass et al. (57) reported a trial comparing cyclophosphamide TBI with melphalan TBI. The benefit obtained by melphalan in reducing the relapse rate was offset by its nephrotoxic effect. Some transplant programs have used partial transmission blocks over the kidneys, suggesting that kidney doses over 12 Gy are associated with increased risks of nephropathy (71). There is no standard recommendation in this regard, however.

Growth, Gonadal, and Endocrine Effects

Almost all children who undergo bone marrow transplantation with TBI experience decreased growth velocity, which is less with fractionated than single dose TBI (66,124). High-dose TBI produces primary gonadal failure in almost all patients, but recovery may occur (124). In children, puberty is usually delayed but can be induced by appropriate hormone replacement (5,34). Thyroid dysfunction is reported in as many as 43% of patients after TBI (66,135). Subclinical hypothyroidism is the most common picture, with raised thyroid-stimulating hormone and normal thyroxine levels. The incidence of thyroid dysfunction is lower when hyperfractionated TBI is used (11).

Secondary Cancers

The risk for development of a second tumor 10 to 15 years after intensive chemoirradiation and stem cell transplantation is estimated to be approximately 20% (5,27,29,32,34,75,141,172). Myelodysplastic syndrome and acute myelogenous leukemia are the most common secondary tumors in patients treated for lymphoid malignancies. Patients who are older, who experienced acute GVHD treated with antithymocyte globulin or anti-CD3 antibodies, or who receive TBI are at greatest risk (5,32,75,141,172). Higher TBI doses were associated with increased risk of solid cancers in one study (27). Some lymphoproliferative disorders that occur after allotransplantation are associated with Epstein Barr virus and may be successfully managed with donor lymphocyte transfusions (96).

Hemibody Irradiation

HBI has been used for many years to palliate widely metastatic solid tumors, often very late in the course of the disease (48,116,153). As the field of medical oncology has developed a larger array of systemic therapies for disseminated cancers, this form of radiotherapy has been less frequently employed.

Applications

Patients with osseous metastases tend to have multiple sites of disease, with multiple areas of pain developing over the course of their illness in up to 75% of patients (104). The pain relief produced by single fraction HBI for skeletal metastases involving several sites is fast, with nearly 50% of all responding patients doing so within 48 hours and 80% within 1 week after treatment (118,119). More than 70% of treated patients experience pain relief as documented in a number of studies including various Radiation Therapy Oncology Group (RTOG) trials from the 1980s (104,105,110,119,169). The duration of pain relief persists for at least 50% of the patient's remaining life (48,119). The most effective HBI doses found by the RTOG study are 6 Gy for upper HBI and 8 Gy for lower and middle HBI. Doses beyond these levels do not appear to increase pain relief or its duration or give a faster response (119).

When treatment of the other half of the body is indicated, it is advisable to wait 6 to 8 weeks to allow a sufficient recovery of blood cells and irradiated marrow to take place (48). Planned sequential upper and lower HBI 6 to 8 weeks apart has been used to treat multiple myeloma, malignant lymphoma, and other widely disseminated tumors (48,74,77,82,113,121). HBI appears to be capable of delaying the progression of existing asymptomatic metastasis and the clinical development of new metastases (56,74,77,104), which eliminates or reduces the need for patients to spend a substantial portion of their remaining lives commuting to treatment centers. At least for multiple myeloma, however, a randomized trial did not support routine use of hemibody radiotherapy (121).

Technique

The physical considerations for HBI are similar to those for TBI, as already discussed; however, as field size required for HBI is much smaller than that for TBI, and HBI can often be delivered on a conventional linear accelerator, albeit using extended distances. By convention, subtotal-body irradiation is usually divided into upper HBI, lower HBI, and middle HBI (114,119). An arbitrary line at the bottom of L4 is commonly used to separate upper and lower HBI (114), although this may be modified based on individual circumstances. Treatment is delivered using anteroposterior parallel-opposed fields. The patient is positioned with a vertical beam allowing coverage of the hemibody, and the treatment table is lowered to the appropriate level or to the floor. Shielding of previously irradiated areas or other body regions to reduce toxicity, such as the salivary glands and the lungs, may be employed. The dose is prescribed to the midplane of the patient at the central axis of the beam.

Complications

In general, HBI is well tolerated. The most common side effects associated with single-dose HBI are nausea and vomiting, mainly when the abdomen is included within the fields. These symptoms occur shortly after radiation administration and last a few hours (48,118,119). Premedication with steroids and antiemetics is required. As these patients are frequently anorectic or cachectic from their underlying illness, dehydration and need for intravenous fluids is common with HBI, and hospitalization for supportive care may be desirable (114). Fractionated HBI makes therapy more acutely tolerable, similar to the experience with TBI (120). Diarrhea occurs commonly when a significant volume of the intestines is irradiated and may last for several days. The severity of this side effect can be reduced by limiting the dose to the abdomen to 6 Gy (119). The risk of pneumonitis is very low if the single fraction dose to the whole lungs is limited to 7 Gy (uncorrected for air density). If 8 Gy is delivered to the upper body, partial transmission lung blocks to limit the lung dose at 6 to 7 Gy is recommended. Hematologic recovery usually occurs in 4 to 6 weeks.

References

1. Appelbaum FR. The influence of total dose, fractionation, dose rate, and distribution of total body irradiation on bone marrow transplantation. *Semin Oncol* 1993;20[4 Suppl 4]:3–10; quiz 1.
2. Barendsen GW. Dose fractionation, dose rate and iso-effect relationships for normal tissue responses. *Int J Radiat Oncol Biol Phys* 1982;8(11):1981–1997.
3. Barrett A, Depledge MH, Powles RL. Interstitial pneumonitis following bone marrow transplantation after low dose rate total body irradiation. *Int J Radiat Oncol Biol Phys* 1983;9(7):1029–1033.
4. Barrett A. Total body irradiation (TBI) before bone marrow transplantation in leukaemia: a co-operative study from the European Group for Bone Marrow Transplantation. *Br J Radiol* 1982;55(656):562–567.
5. Barrett AJ. Bone marrow transplantation. *Cancer Treat Rev* 1987;14(3–4):203–213.
6. Baume D, Cosset JM, Pico JL, et al. [Veno-occlusive disease of the liver after bone marrow graft. Possible value of fractionation of whole body irradiation]. *Presse Med* 1987;16(35):1759.
7. Bearman SI, Appelbaum FR, Back A, et al. Regimen-related toxicity and early post-transplant survival in patients undergoing marrow transplantation for lymphoma. *J Clin Oncol* 1989;7(9):1288–1294.
8. Benyunes MC, Sullivan KM, Deeg HJ, et al. Cataracts after bone marrow transplantation: long-term follow-up of adults treated with fractionated total body irradiation. *Int J Radiat Oncol Biol Phys* 1995;32(3):661–670.
9. Blaise D, Maraninchi D, Archimbaud E, et al. Allogeneic bone marrow transplantation for acute myeloid leukemia in first remission: a randomized trial of a busulfan-cytoxan versus cytoxan-total body irradiation as preparative regimen: a report from the Group d'Etudes de la Greffe de Moelle Osseuse. *Blood* 1992;79(10):2578–2582.
10. Blume KG, Forman SJ, Snyder DS, et al. Allogeneic bone marrow transplantation for acute lymphoblastic leukemia during first complete remission. *Transplantation* 1987;43(3):389–392.
11. Boulad F, Bromley M, Black P, et al. Thyroid dysfunction following bone marrow transplantation using hyperfractionated radiation. *Bone Marrow Transplant* 1995;15(1):71–76.
12. Bradley J, Reft C, Goldman S, et al. High-energy total body irradiation as preparation for bone marrow transplantation in leukemia patients: treatment technique and related complications. *Int J Radiat Oncol Biol Phys* 1998;40(2):391–396.
13. Bray LC, Carey PJ, Proctor SJ, et al. Ocular complications of bone marrow transplantation. *Br J Ophthalmol* 1991;75(10):611–614.
14. Breneman JC, Elson HR, Little R, et al. A technique for delivery of total body irradiation for bone marrow transplantation in adults and adolescents. *Int J Radiat Oncol Biol Phys* 1990;18(5):1233–1236.
15. Briot E, Dutreix A, Bridier A. Dosimetry for total body irradiation. *Radiother Oncol* 1990;18[Suppl 1]:16–29.
16. Buchali A, Feyer P, Groll J, et al. Immediate toxicity during fractionated total body irradiation as conditioning for bone marrow transplantation. *Radiother Oncol* 2000;54(2):157–162.
17. Chaffey JT, Rosenthal DS, Moloney WC, et al. Total body irradiation as treatment for lymphosarcoma. *Int J Radiat Oncol Biol Phys* 1976;1(5–6):399–405.
18. Clift RA, Buckner CD, Appelbaum FR, et al. Allogeneic marrow transplantation in patients with acute myeloid leukemia in first remission: a randomized trial of two irradiation regimens. *Blood* 1990;76(9):1867–1871.
19. Clift RA, Buckner CD, Appelbaum FR, et al. Allogeneic marrow transplantation in patients with chronic myeloid leukemia in the chronic phase: a randomized trial of two irradiation regimens. *Blood* 1991;77(8):1660–1665.
20. Clift RA, Buckner CD, Thomas ED, et al. Marrow transplantation for chronic myeloid leukemia: a randomized study comparing cyclophosphamide and total body irradiation with busulfan and cyclophosphamide. *Blood* 1994;84(6):2036–2043.
21. Copelan EA, Deeg HJ. Conditioning for allogeneic marrow transplantation in patients with lymphohematopoietic malignancies without the use of total body irradiation. *Blood* 1992;80(7):1648–1658.
22. Cosset JM, Baume D, Pico JL, et al. Single dose versus hyperfractionated total body irradiation before allogeneic bone marrow transplantation: a non-randomized

comparative study of 54 patients at the Institut Gustave-Roussy. *Radiother Oncol* 1989;15(2):151–160.
23. Cosset JM, Socie G, Dubray B, et al. Single dose versus fractionated total body irradiation before bone marrow transplantation: radiobiological and clinical considerations. *Int J Radiat Oncol Biol Phys* 1994;30(2):477–492.
24. Cosset JM, Socie G, Girinsky T, et al. Radiobiological and clinical bases for total body irradiation in the leukemias and lymphomas. *Semin Radiat Oncol* 1995;5(4):301–315.
25. Cunningham JR, Wright DJ. A simple facility for wholebody irradiation. *Radiology* 1962;78:941–949.
26. Curran WJ Jr, Galvin JM, D'Angio GJ. A simple dose calculation method for total body photon irradiation. *Int J Radiat Oncol Biol Phys* 1989;17(1):219–224.
27. Curtis RE, Rowlings PA, Deeg HJ, et al. Solid cancers after bone marrow transplantation. *N Engl J Med* 1997;336(13):897–904.
28. Dale RG. The application of the linear-quadratic model to fractionated radiotherapy when there is incomplete normal tissue recovery between fractions, and possible implications for treatments involving multiple fractions per day. *Br J Radiol* 1986;59(705):919–927.
29. Darrington DL, Vose JM, Anderson JR, et al. Incidence and characterization of secondary myelodysplastic syndrome and acute myelogenous leukemia following high-dose chemoradiotherapy and autologous stem-cell transplantation for lymphoid malignancies. *J Clin Oncol* 1994;12(12):2527–2534.
30. De La Camara R, Tomas JF, Figuera A, et al. High dose busulfan and seizures. *Bone Marrow Transplant* 1991;7(5):363–364.
31. Deeg HJ, Sullivan KM, Buckner CD, et al. Marrow transplantation for acute nonlymphoblastic leukemia in first remission: toxicity and long-term follow-up of patients conditioned with single dose or fractionated total body irradiation. *Bone Marrow Transplant* 1986;1(2):151–157.
32. Deeg HJ, Witherspoon RP. Risk factors for the development of secondary malignancies after marrow transplantation. *Hematol Oncol Clin North Am* 1993;7(2):417–429.
33. Deeg HJ. Acute and delayed toxicities of total body irradiation. Seattle Marrow Transplant Team. *Int J Radiat Oncol Biol Phys* 1983;9(12):1933–1939.
34. Deeg HJ. Delayed complications and long-term effects after bone marrow transplantation. *Hematol Oncol Clin North Am* 1990;4(3):641–657.
35. Del Regato JA. Proceedings: total body irradiation in the treatment of chronic lymphogenous leukemia. *Am J Roentgenol Radium Ther Nucl Med* 1974;120(3):504–520.
36. DeLeve LD, Shulman HM, McDonald GB. Toxic injury to hepatic sinusoids: sinusoidal obstruction syndrome (veno-occlusive disease). *Semin Liver Dis* 2002;22(1):27–42.
37. Devergie A, Blaise D, Attal M, et al. Allogeneic bone marrow transplantation for chronic myeloid leukemia in first chronic phase: a randomized trial of busulfan-cytoxan versus cytoxan-total body irradiation as preparative regimen: a report from the French Society of Bone Marrow Graft (SFGM). *Blood* 1995;85(8):2263–2268.
38. Diaconescu R, Flowers CR, Storer B, et al. Morbidity and mortality with nonmyeloablative compared with myeloablative conditioning before hematopoietic cell transplantation from HLA-matched related donors. *Blood* 2004;104(5):1550–1558.
39. Dominique C, Schwartz LH, Lescrainier J, et al. A modified 60C teletherapy unit for total body irradiation. *Int J Radiat Oncol Biol Phys* 1995;33(4):951–957.
40. Dubray B, Henry-Amar M, Meerwaldt JH, et al. Mediastinitis after irradiation for Hodgkin's disease: the role of fractionation. *Eur J Cancer* 1991;2[Suppl 2]:270.
41. Dusenbery KE, Daniels KA, McClure JS, et al. Randomized comparison of cyclophosphamide-total body irradiation versus busulfan-cyclophosphamide conditioning in autologous bone marrow transplantation for acute myeloid leukemia. *Int J Radiat Oncol Biol Phys* 1995;31(1):119–128.
42. Dusenbery KE, Howells WB, Arthur DC, et al. Extramedullary leukemia in children with newly diagnosed acute myeloid leukemia: a report from the Children's Cancer Group. *J Pediatr Hematol Oncol* 2003;25(10):760–768.
43. Dutreix J, Janoray P, Bridier A, et al. Biologic and anatomic problems of lung shielding in whole-body irradiation. *J Natl Cancer Inst* 1986;76(6):1333–1335.
44. Engler MJ, Feldman MI, Spira J. Arc technique for total-body irradiation by a 42-MV betatron. *Med Phys* 1977;4(6):524–525.
44a. Ferrebee JW, Thomas ED. Factors affecting the survival of transplanted tissues. *Am Journal of Med Sci* 235:369–386.
45. Fisher DR, Hendry JH, Scott D. Long-term repair in vivo of colony-forming ability and chromosomal injury in x-irradiated mouse hepatocytes. *Radiat Res* 1988;113(1):40–50.
46. Fisher DR, Hendry JH. Dose fractionation and hepatocyte clonogens: alpha/beta congruent to 1-2 Gy, and beta decreases with increasing delay before assay. *Radiat Res* 1988;113(1):51–57.
47. FitzGerald TJ, Santucci MA, Harigaya K, et al. Radiosensitivity of permanent human bone marrow stromal cell lines: effect of dose rate. *Int J Radiat Oncol Biol Phys* 1988;15(5):1153–1159.
48. Fitzpatrick PJ, Rider WD. Half body radiotherapy. *Int J Radiat Oncol Biol Phys* 1976;1(3–4):197–207.
49. Gallini R, Hendry JH, Molineux G, et al. The effect of low dose rate on recovery of hemopoietic and stromal progenitor cells in gamma-irradiated mouse bone marrow. *Radiat Res* 1988;115(3):481–487.
50. Galvin JM. Calculation and prescription of dose for total body irradiation. *Int J Radiat Oncol Biol Phys* 1983;9(12):1919–1924.
51. Gerig LH, Szanto J, Bichay T, et al. A translating-bed technique for total-body irradiation. *Phys Med Biol* 1994;39(1):19–35.
52. Girinsky T, Socie G, Ammarguellat H, et al. Consequences of two different doses to the lungs during a single dose of total body irradiation: results of a randomized study on 85 patients. *Int J Radiat Oncol Biol Phys* 1994;30(4):821–824.
53. Gratwohl A, Hermans J, von Biezen A, et al. No advantage for patients who receive splenic irradiation before bone marrow transplantation for chronic myeloid leukaemia: results of a prospective randomized study. *Bone Marrow Transplant* 1992;10(2):147–152.
54. Guinan EC, Tarbell NJ, Niemeyer CM, et al. Intravascular hemolysis and renal insufficiency after bone marrow transplantation. *Blood* 1988;72(2):451–455.
55. Hartman AR, Williams SF, Dillon JJ. Survival, disease-free survival and adverse effects of conditioning for allogeneic bone marrow transplantation with busulfan/cyclophosphamide vs total body irradiation: a meta-analysis. *Bone Marrow Transplant* 1998;22(5):439–443.
56. Hazra TA, Giri S. Prophylactic pelvic girdle irradiation in the treatment of prostatic carcinoma. *Int J Radiat Oncol Biol Phys* 1981;7(6):817–819.
57. Helenglass G, Powles RL, McElwain TJ, et al. Melphalan and total body irradiation (TBI) versus cyclophosphamide and TBI as conditioning for allogeneic matched sibling bone marrow transplants for acute myeloblastic leukaemia in first remission. *Bone Marrow Transplant* 1988;3(1):21–29.
58. Hendry JH. The cellular basis of long-term marrow injury after irradiation. *Radiother Oncol* 1985;3(4):331–338.
59. Hussein S, el-Khatib E. Total body irradiation with a sweeping 60Cobalt beam. *Int J Radiat Oncol Biol Phys* 1995;33(2):493–497.
60. Inoue T, Ikeda H, Yamazaki H, et al. Role of total body irradiation as based on the comparison of preparation regimens for allogeneic bone marrow transplantation for acute leukemia in first complete remission. *Strahlenther Onkol* 1993;169(4):250–255.
61. Jen YM, Hendry JH. Dose-fractionation sensitivity of mouse kidney clonogens measured using different interfraction intervals and postirradiation assay times. *Radiother Oncol* 1993;26(2):117–124.
62. Johnson RE, Ruhl U. Treatment of chronic lymphocytic leukemia with emphasis on total body irradiation. *Int J Radiat Oncol Biol Phys* 1976;1(5–6):387–397.
63. Johnson RE. Treatment of chronic lymphocytic leukemia by total body irradiation alone and combined with chemotherapy. *Int J Radiat Oncol Biol Phys* 1979;5(2):159–164.
64. Jordan SW, Anderson RE, Lane RG, et al. Fraction size, dose and time dependence of x-ray induced late renal injury. *Int J Radiat Oncol Biol Phys* 1985;11(6):1095–1101.
65. Keane TJ, Van Dyk J. TBI schedules prior to bone marrow transplantation: requirements for comparison. *Radiother Oncol* 1989;15(2):207–212.
66. Keilholz U, Korbling M, Fehrentz D, et al. Long-term endocrine toxicity of myeloablative treatment followed by autologous bone marrow/blood derived stem cell transplantation in patients with malignant lymphohematopoietic disorders. *Cancer* 1989;64(3):641–645.
67. Khoury H, Adkins D, Brown R, et al. Low incidence of transplantation-related acute complications in patients with chronic myeloid leukemia undergoing allogeneic stem cell transplantation with a low-dose (550 cGy) total body irradiation conditioning regimen. *Biol Blood Marrow Transplant* 2001;7(6):352–358.
68. Kim TH, Khan FM, Galvin JM. Total Body Irradiation Conference: a report of the work party: comparison of total body irradiation techniques for bone marrow transplantation. *Int J Radiat Oncol Biol Phys* 1980;6(6):779–784.
69. Kirby TH, Hanson WF, Cates DA. Verification of total body photon irradiation dosimetry techniques. *Med Phys* 1988;15(3):364–369.
70. Lawton CA, Barber-Derus S, Murray KJ, et al. Technical modifications in hyperfractionated total body irradiation for T-lymphocyte depleted bone marrow transplant. *Int J Radiat Oncol Biol Phys* 1989;17(2):319–322.
71. Lawton CA, Cohen EP, Murray KJ, et al. Long-term results of selective renal shielding in patients undergoing total body irradiation in preparation for bone marrow transplantation. *Bone Marrow Transplant* 1997;20(12):1069–1074.
72. Leer JW, Broerse JJ, De Vroome H, et al. Techniques applied for total body irradiation. *Radiother Oncol* 1990;18[Suppl 1]:10–15.
73. Leung PM, Rider WD, Webb HP, et al. Cobalt-60 therapy unit for large field irradiation. *Int J Radiat Oncol Biol Phys* 1981;7(6):705–712.
74. Lombardi F, Rottoli L, Gianni C, et al. Advanced neuroblastoma: results of two treatment programs including sequential hemibody irradiation. *Int J Radiat Oncol Biol Phys* 1989;17(3):485–491.
75. Lowsky R, Lipton J, Fyles G, et al. Secondary malignancies after bone marrow transplantation in adults. *J Clin Oncol* 1994;12(10):2187–2192.
76. Lutz WR, Dougan PW, Bjarngard BE. Design and characteristics of a facility for total-body and large-field irradiation. *Int J Radiat Oncol Biol Phys* 1988;15(4):1035–1040.
77. MacLennan I, Selim HM, Rubin P. Sequential hemibody radiotherapy in poor prognosis localized adenocarcinoma of the prostate gland: a preliminary study of the RTOG. *Int J Radiat Oncol Biol Phys* 1989;16(1):215–218.
78. Maris MB, Sandmaier BM, Storer BE, et al. Allogeneic hematopoietic cell transplantation after fludarabine and 2 Gy total body irradiation for relapsed and refractory mantle cell lymphoma. *Blood* 2004;104(12):3535–3542.
79. Marmont AM, Horowitz MM, Gale RP, et al. T-cell depletion of HLA-identical transplants in leukemia. *Blood* 1991;78(8):2120–2130.
80. McChesney SL, Gillette EL, Powers BE. Response of the canine lung to fractionated irradiation: pathologic changes and isoeffect curves. *Int J Radiat Oncol Biol Phys* 1989;16(1):125–132.
81. McDonald GB, Sharma P, Matthews DE, et al. The clinical course of 53 patients with venocclusive disease of the liver after marrow transplantation. *Transplantation* 1985;39(6):603–608.
82. McSweeney EN, Tobias JS, Blackman G, et al. Double hemibody irradiation (DHBI) in the management of relapsed and primary chemoresistant multiple myeloma. *Clin Oncol (R Coll Radiol)* 1993;5(6):378–383.
83. McSweeney PA, Niederwieser D, Shizuru JA, et al. Hematopoietic cell transplantation in older patients with hematologic malignancies: replacing high-dose cytotoxic therapy with graft-versus-tumor effects. *Blood* 2001;97(11):3390–3400.
84. Mendenhall NP, Noyes WD, Million RR. Total body irradiation for stage II-IV non-Hodgkin's lymphoma: ten-year follow-up. *J Clin Oncol* 1989;7(1):67–74.
85. Michel G, Gluckman E, Esperou-Bourdeau H, et al. Allogeneic bone marrow transplantation for children with acute myeloblastic leukemia in first complete remission: impact of conditioning regimen without total-body irradiation—a report from the Societe Francaise de Greffe de Moelle. *J Clin Oncol* 1994;12(6):1217–1222.
86. Miller KB, Roberts TF, Chan G, et al. A novel reduced intensity regimen for allogeneic hematopoietic stem cell transplantation associated with a reduced incidence of graft-versus-host disease. *Bone Marrow Transplant* 2004;33(9):881–889.
87. Miralbell R, Bieri S, Mermillod B, et al. Renal toxicity after allogeneic bone marrow transplantation: the combined effects of total-body irradiation and graft-versus-host disease. *J Clin Oncol* 1996;14(2):579–585.
88. Miralbell R, Rouzaud M, Grob E, et al. Can a total body irradiation technique be fast and reproducible? *Int J Radiat Oncol Biol Phys* 1994;29(5):1167–1173.
89. Nevill TJ, Barnett MJ, Klingemann HG, et al. Regimen-related toxicity of a busulfan-cyclophosphamide conditioning regimen in 70 patients undergoing allogeneic bone marrow transplantation. *J Clin Oncol* 1991;9(7):1224–1232.
90. Niederwieser D, Gentilini C, Hegenbart U, et al. Allogeneic hematopoietic cell transplantation (HCT) following reduced-intensity conditioning in patients with acute leukemias. *Crit Rev Oncol Hematol* 2005;56(2):275–281.

91. Niroomand-Rad A. Physical aspects of total body irradiation of bone marrow transplant patients using 18 MV x rays. *Int J Radiat Oncol Biol Phys* 1991;20(3):605–611.

92. O'Donoghue JA, Wheldon TE, Gregor A. The implications of in-vitro radiation-survival curves for the optimal scheduling of total-body irradiation with bone marrow rescue in the treatment of leukaemia. *Br J Radiol* 1987;60(711):279–283.

93. O'Donoghue JA. Fractionated versus low dose-rate total body irradiation. Radiobiological considerations in the selection of regimes. *Radiother Oncol* 1986;7(3):241–247.

94. Ozsahin M, Belkacemi Y, Pene F, et al. Total-body irradiation and cataract incidence: a randomized comparison of two instantaneous dose rates. *Int J Radiat Oncol Biol Phys* 1994;28(2):343–347.

95. Ozsahin M, Pene F, Touboul E, et al. Total-body irradiation before bone marrow transplantation. Results of two randomized instantaneous dose rates in 157 patients. *Cancer* 1992;69(11):2853–2865.

96. Papadopoulos EB, Ladanyi M, Emanuel D, et al. Infusions of donor leukocytes to treat Epstein-Barr virus-associated lymphoproliferative disorders after allogeneic bone marrow transplantation. *N Engl J Med* 1994;330(17):1185–1191.

97. Parkins CS, Fowler JF, Maughan RL, et al. Repair in mouse lung for up to 20 fractions of x rays or neutrons. *Br J Radiol* 1985;58(687):225–241.

98. Penney DP, Siemann DW, Rubin P, et al. Morphological correlates of fractionated radiation of the mouse lung: early and late effects. *Int J Radiat Oncol Biol Phys* 1994;29(4):789–804.

99. Peters L. Total Body Irradiation Conference: discussion: the radiobiological bases of TBI. *Int J Radiat Oncol Biol Phys* 1980;6(6):785–787.

100. Peters VG, Herer AS. Modification of a standard cobalt-60 unit for total body irradiation at 150 cm SSD. *Int J Radiat Oncol Biol Phys* 1984;10(6):927–932.

101. Phillips GL, Herzig RH, Lazarus HM, et al. Treatment of resistant malignant lymphoma with cyclophosphamide, total body irradiation, and transplantation of cryopreserved autologous marrow. *N Engl J Med* 1984;310(24):1557–1561.

102. Pinoy Torres JL, Bross DS, Lam WC, et al. Risk factors in interstitial pneumonitis following allogenic bone marrow transplantation. *Int J Radiat Oncol Biol Phys* 1982;8(8):1301–1307.

103. Pla M, Chenery SG, Podgorsak EB. Total body irradiation with a sweeping beam. *Int J Radiat Oncol Biol Phys* 1983;9(1):83–89.

104. Poulter CA, Cosmatos D, Rubin P, et al. A report of RTOG 8206: a phase III study of whether the addition of single dose hemibody irradiation to standard fractionated local field irradiation is more effective than local field irradiation alone in the treatment of symptomatic osseous metastases. *Int J Radiat Oncol Biol Phys* 1992;23(1):207–214.

105. Qasim MM. Half body irradiation (HBI) in metastatic carcinomas. *Clin Radiol* 1981;32(2):215–219.

106. Quast U. Physical treatment planning of total-body irradiation: patient translation and beam-zone method. *Med Phys* 1985;12(5):567–574.

107. Richardson PG, Murakami C, Jin Z, et al. Multi-institutional use of defibrotide in 88 patients after stem cell transplantation with severe veno-occlusive disease and multisystem organ failure: response without significant toxicity in a high-risk population and factors predictive of outcome. *Blood* 2002;100(13):4337–4343.

108. Rigaud O, Papadopoulo D, Moustacchi E. Decreased deletion mutation in radioadapted human lymphoblasts. *Radiat Res* 1993;133(1):94–101.

109. Ringden O, Ruutu T, Remberger M, et al. A randomized trial comparing busulfan with total body irradiation as conditioning in allogeneic marrow transplant recipients with leukemia: a report from the Nordic Bone Marrow Transplantation Group. *Blood* 1994;83(9):2723–2730.

110. Rowland CG, Bullimore JA, Smith PJ, et al. Half-body irradiation in the treatment of metastatic prostatic carcinoma. *Br J Urol* 1981;53(6):628–629.

111. Rozman C, Carreras E, Qian C, et al. Risk factors for hepatic veno-occlusive disease following HLA-identical sibling bone marrow transplants for leukemia. *Bone Marrow Transplant* 1996;17(1):75–80.

112. Rubin P, Bennett JM, Begg C, et al. The comparison of total body irradiation vs chlorambucil and prednisone for remission induction of active chronic lymphocytic leukemia: an ECOG study. Part I: total body irradiation-response and toxicity. *Int J Radiat Oncol Biol Phys* 1981;7(12):1623–1632.

113. Rubin P, Heilmann HP. International clinical trials in radiation oncology. Large field trials. *Int J Radiat Oncol Biol Phys* 1988;14[Suppl 1]:S65–S76.

114. Rubin P, Salazar O, Zagars G, et al. Systemic hemibody irradiation for overt and occult metastases. *Cancer* 1985;55[9 Suppl]:2210–2221.

115. Ruutu T, Eriksson B, Remes K, et al. Ursodeoxycholic acid for the prevention of hepatic complications in allogeneic stem cell transplantation. *Blood* 2002;100(6):1977–1983.

116. Saenger EL, Silberstein EB, Aron B, et al. Whole body and partial body radiotherapy of advanced cancer. *Am J Roentgenol Radium Ther Nucl Med* 1973;117(3):670–685.

117. Safwat A. The role of low-dose total body irradiation in treatment of non-Hodgkin's lymphoma: a new look at an old method. *Radiother Oncol* 2000;56(1):1–8.

118. Salazar OM, DaMotta NW, Bridgman SM, et al. Fractionated half-body irradiation for pain palliation in widely metastatic cancers: comparison with single dose. *Int J Radiat Oncol Biol Phys* 1996;36(1):49–60.

119. Salazar OM, Rubin P, Hendrickson FR, et al. Single-dose half-body irradiation for palliation of multiple bone metastases from solid tumors. Final Radiation Therapy Oncology Group report. *Cancer* 1986;58(1):29–36.

120. Salazar OM, Rubin P, Keller B, et al. Systemic (half-body) radiation therapy: response and toxicity. *Int J Radiat Oncol Biol Phys* 1978;4(11–12):937–950.

121. Salmon SE, Tesh D, Crowley J, et al. Chemotherapy is superior to sequential hemibody irradiation for remission consolidation in multiple myeloma: a Southwest Oncology Group study. *J Clin Oncol* 1990;8(9):1575–1584.

122. Salomon O, Lapidot T, Terenzi A, et al. Induction of donor-type chimerism in murine recipients of bone marrow allografts by different radiation regimens currently used in treatment of leukemia patients. *Blood* 1990;76(9):1872–1878.

123. Sanchez-Doblado F, Terron JA, Sanchez-Nieto B, et al. Verification of an on line in vivo semiconductor dosimetry system for TBI with two TLD procedures. *Radiother Oncol* 1995;34(1):73–77.

124. Sanders JE, Buckner CD, Leonard JM, et al. Late effects on gonadal function of cyclophosphamide, total-body irradiation, and marrow transplantation. *Transplantation* 1983;36(3):252–255.

125. Santos GW. The development of busulfan/cyclophosphamide preparative regimens. *Semin Oncol* 1993;20[4 Suppl 4]:12–16; quiz 7.

126. Scarpati D, Frassoni F, Vitale V, et al. Total body irradiation in acute myeloid leukemia and chronic myelogenous leukemia: influence of dose and dose-rate on leukemia relapse. *Int J Radiat Oncol Biol Phys* 1989;17(3):547–552.

127. Scarpati D, Mancini G, Corvo R, et al. Tissue air ratio in total body irradiation. An in vivo evaluation. *Acta Oncol* 1989;28(2):283–285.

128. Schenken LL, Hagemann RF. Time/dose relationships in experimental radiation cataractogenesis. *Radiology* 1975;117(1):193–198.

129. Shank B, Brochstein JA, Castro-Malaspina H, et al. Immunosuppression prior to marrow transplantation for sensitized aplastic anemia patients: comparison of TLI with TBI. *Int J Radiat Oncol Biol Phys* 1988;14(6):1133–1141.

130. Shank B, Chu FC, Dinsmore R, et al. Hyperfractionated total body irradiation for bone marrow transplantation. Results in seventy leukemia patients with allogeneic transplants. *Int J Radiat Oncol Biol Phys* 1983;9(11):1607–1611.

131. Shank B, Hopfan S, Kim JH, et al. Hyperfractionated total body irradiation for bone marrow transplantation: I. Early results in leukemia patients. *Int J Radiat Oncol Biol Phys* 1981;7(8):1109–1115.

132. Shank B. Can total body irradiation be supplanted by busulfan in cytoreductive regimens for bone marrow transplantation? *Int J Radiat Oncol Biol Phys* 1995;31(1):195–196; discussion 202–203.

133. Shank B. Techniques of magna-field irradiation. *Int J Radiat Oncol Biol Phys* 1983;9(12):1925–1931.

134. Shulman HM, Fisher LB, Schoch HG, et al. Veno-occlusive disease of the liver after marrow transplantation: histological correlates of clinical signs and symptoms. *Hepatology* 1994;19(5):1171–1181.

135. Sklar CA, Kim TH, Ramsay NK. Thyroid dysfunction among long-term survivors of bone marrow transplantation. *Am J Med* 1982;73(5):688–694.

136. Slavin S, Nagler A, Naparstek E, et al. Nonmyeloablative stem cell transplantation and cell therapy as an alternative to conventional bone marrow transplantation with lethal cytoreduction for the treatment of malignant and nonmalignant hematologic diseases. *Blood* 1998;91(3):756–763.

137. Socie G, Devergie A, Girinsky T, et al. Influence of the fractionation of total body irradiation on complications and relapse rate for chronic myelogenous leukemia. The Groupe d'Etude des greffes de moelle osseuse (GEGMO). *Int J Radiat Oncol Biol Phys* 1991;20(3):397–404.

138. Song CW, Kim TH, Khan FM, et al. Radiobiological basis of total body irradiation with different dose rate and fractionation: repair capacity of hemopoietic cells. *Int J Radiat Oncol Biol Phys* 1981;7(12):1695–1701.

139. Sorror ML, Maris MB, Sandmaier BM, et al. Hematopoietic cell transplantation after nonmyeloablative conditioning for advanced chronic lymphocytic leukemia. *J Clin Oncol* 2005;23(16):3819–3829.

140. Spitzer TR, McAfee S, Sackstein R, et al. Intentional induction of mixed chimerism and achievement of antitumor responses after nonmyeloablative conditioning therapy and HLA-matched donor bone marrow transplantation for refractory hematologic malignancies. *Biol Blood Marrow Transplant* 2000;6(3A):309–320.

141. Stone RM, Neuberg D, Soiffer R, et al. Myelodysplastic syndrome as a late complication following autologous bone marrow transplantation for non-Hodgkin's lymphoma. *J Clin Oncol* 1994;12(12):2535–2542.

142. Storb R, Raff RF, Appelbaum FR, et al. Comparison of fractionated to single-dose total body irradiation in conditioning canine littermates for DLA-identical marrow grafts. *Blood* 1989;74(3):1139–1143.

143. Storb R, Raff RF, Appelbaum FR, et al. Fractionated versus single-dose total body irradiation at low and high dose rates to condition canine littermates for DLA-identical marrow grafts. *Blood* 1994;83(11):3384–3389.

144. Storb R, Yu C, Wagner JL, et al. Stable mixed hematopoietic chimerism in DLA-identical littermate dogs given sublethal total body irradiation before and pharmacological immunosuppression after marrow transplantation. *Blood* 1997;89(8):3048–3054.

145. Svahn-Tapper G, Nilsson P, Jonsson C, et al. Calculation and measurements of absorbed dose in total body irradiation. *Acta Oncol* 1990;29(5):627–633.

146. Syh HW, Chu WK, Kumar PP, et al. Estimation of the mean effective organ doses for total body irradiation from random phantom measurements. *Med Dosim* 1992;17(2):103–106.

147. Tarbell NJ, Guinan EC, Niemeyer C, et al. Late onset of renal dysfunction in survivors of bone marrow transplantation. *Int J Radiat Oncol Biol Phys* 1988;15(1):99–104.

148. Thames HD Jr, Hendry JH. *Fractionation in radiotherapy*. London: Taylor and Francis, 1987.

149. Thomas E, Storb R, Clift RA, et al. Bone-marrow transplantation (first of two parts). *N Engl J Med* 1975;292(16):832–843.

150. Thomas ED, Clift RA, Hersman J, et al. Marrow transplantation for acute nonlymphoblastic leukemic in first remission using fractionated or single-dose irradiation. *Int J Radiat Oncol Biol Phys* 1982;8(5):817–821.

151. Thomas ED. Total body irradiation regimens for marrow grafting. *Int J Radiat Oncol Biol Phys* 1990;19(5):1285–1288.

152. Tichelli A, Gratwohl A, Egger T, et al. Cataract formation after bone marrow transplantation. *Ann Intern Med* 1993;119(12):1175–1180.

153. Tobias JS, Richards JD, Blackman GM, et al. Hemibody irradiation in multiple myeloma. *Radiother Oncol* 1985;3(1):11–16.

154. Travis EL. The sequence of histological changes in mouse lungs after single doses of x-rays. *Int J Radiat Oncol Biol Phys* 1980;6(3):345–347.

155. Travis LB, Weeks J, Curtis RE, et al. Leukemia following low-dose total body irradiation and chemotherapy for non-Hodgkin's lymphoma. *J Clin Oncol* 1996;14(2):565–571.

156. Triebel F, Gluckman JC, Chapuis F, et al. T-lymphocyte progenitors in man: phenotypic characterization of blood and bone marrow T-colony forming cells. *Immunology* 1985;54(2):241–247.

157. Tutschka PJ, Copelan EA, Kapoor N. Replacing total body irradiation with busulfan as conditioning of patients with leukemia for allogeneic marrow transplantation. *Transplant Proc* 1989;21(1 Pt 3):2952–2954.

158. Uckun FM, Song CW. Radiobiological features of human pluripotent bone marrow progenitor cells (CFU-GEMM). *Int J Radiat Oncol Biol Phys* 1989;17(5):1021–1025.

159. Van Der Jagt RH, Appelbaum FR, Petersen FB, et al. Busulfan and cyclophosphamide as a preparative regimen for bone marrow transplantation in patients with prior chest radiotherapy. *Bone Marrow Transplant* 1991;8(3):211–215.

160. Van Dyk J, Glavin JM, Glasgow GP. *The physical aspects of total and half body photon irradiation: a report of Task Group 29 Radiation Therapy Committee*. American Association of Physicists in Medicine, 1986.

161. Van Dyk J, Keane TJ, Kan S, et al. Radiation pneumonitis following large single dose irradiation: a re-evaluation based on absolute dose to lung. *Int J Radiat Oncol Biol Phys* 1981;7(4):461–467.

162. Van Dyk J, Keane TJ. Determination of parameters for the linear-quadratic model for radiation-induced lung damage. *Int J Radiat Oncol Biol Phys* 1989;17(3):695.

163. Van Dyk J. Dosimetry for total body irradiation. *Radiother Oncol* 1987;9(2):107–118.

164. van Rongen E, Kuijpers WC, Madhuizen HT. Fractionation effects and repair kinetics in rat kidney. *Int J Radiat Oncol Biol Phys* 1990;18(5):1093–1106.

165. Vegesna V, Withers HR, Thames HD Jr, et al. Multifraction radiation response of mouse lung. *Int J Radiat Biol Relat Stud Phys Chem Med* 1985;47(4):413–422.

166. Vernant JP, Sutton L, Kuentz M. Allogeneic bone marrow transplantation in 184 adults with acute lymphoid leukemia in first complete remission. *Proc Am Soc Clin Oncol* 1990;9:12.

167. Weichselbaum RR, Greenberger JS, Schmidt A, et al. In vitro radiosensivity of human leukemia cell lines. *Radiology* 1981;139(2):485–487.

168. Weiner RS, Bortin MM, Gale RP, et al. Interstitial pneumonitis after bone marrow transplantation. Assessment of risk factors. *Ann Intern Med* 1986;104(2):168–175.

169. Wilkins MF, Keen CW. Hemi-body radiotherapy in the management of metastatic carcinoma. *Clin Radiol* 1987;38(3):267–268.

170. Williams MV, Denekamp J. Radiation induced renal damage in mice: influence of fraction size. *Int J Radiat Oncol Biol Phys* 1984;10(6):885–893.

171. Wingard JR, Nichols WG, McDonald GB. Supportive care. *Hematology (Am Soc Hematol Educ Program)* 2004:372–389.

172. Witherspoon RP, Fisher LD, Schoch G, et al. Secondary cancers after bone marrow transplantation for leukemia or aplastic anemia. *N Engl J Med* 1989;321(12):784–789.

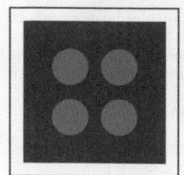

Chapter 15
Stereotactic Radiosurgery and Radiotherapy

John C. Flickinger, Ajay Niranjan

Stereotactic radiosurgery and radiotherapy are techniques to administer precisely directed, high-dose irradiation that tightly conforms to an intracranial target to create a desired radiobiologic response while minimizing radiation dose to surrounding normal tissue. These techniques exploit the fact that the radiation tolerance of normal tissue is volume-dependent. With these techniques the complication risks for any radiation dose delivered are reduced by minimizing or eliminating the margin of normal tissue otherwise included in the radiation treatment volume with conventional radiotherapy techniques. In the case of radiosurgery, all of the irradiation is done in a single session or fraction, while in stereotactic radiotherapy (SRT), more than one fraction of irradiation is administered. Table 15.1 lists the key requirements for successful stereotactic irradiation. Advances in imaging, computers, and treatment planning in the last 2 decades have led to the development of a variety of different stereotactic radiosurgery/radiotherapy techniques and their wider applications. Successful clinical experience with intracranial radiosurgery for a variety of applications has led to a re-examination of radiobiology and exploration of both fractionated approaches and extracranial applications. Margin reduction with radiosurgery and fractionated stereotactic irradiation techniques makes target definition accuracy more critical. Drawing contours from different imaging techniques or by different physicians are approaches to reduce target definition error (Fig. 15.1).

Terminology

Stereotactic refers to using a precise three-dimensional mapping technique to guide a procedure. The terminology used in stereotactic irradiation can be confusing. The term *radiosurgery* or *stereotactic radiosurgery* (SRS) is used for stereotactically guided conformal irradiation of a defined target volume in a single session. Radiosurgery or SRS can be delivered with Gamma Knife (Elekta Inc., Norcross, GA) modified LINAC radiosurgery systems (including Cyberknife (Accuray Inc., Sunnyvale, CA) and image-guided radiotherapy systems), tomotherapy, or proton beam systems. The term *stereotactic radiation therapy* (SRT) refers to stereotactically guided delivery of highly conformal radiation to a defined target volume in multiple fractions, typically using noninvasive positioning techniques. The term *fractionated stereotactic radiosurgery* (FSR) is limited to stereotactically guided high-dose conformal radiation administered to a precisely defined target volume in two to five sessions. Although it would have been less confusing to refer to this as *hypofractionated* SRT and reserve the term *radiosurgery* for single-fraction irradiation, the terminology is already in use. Adding intensity-modulated radiation therapy (IMRT) to the nomenclature can further complicate or confuse the terminology. Any radiation treatment plan that uses individual treatment beams that irradiate only part of the target at a time is IMRT. Strictly speaking, multiple isocenter radiosurgery (of a single target volume) meets the criteria for IMRT or stereotactic IMRT (SIMRT), but the term *SIMRT* is usually only used when multileaf collimators are employed. The terminology is useful to distinguish when the same linear accelerator is equipped to treat with either fixed circular collimators for radiosurgery (SRS or SRT mode), or to deliver IMRT using multileaf collimators (SIMRT mode).

Radiobiologic Considerations

Prior to the introduction of radiosurgery, essentially all clinical irradiation was administered with radiation dose fractions between 1.2 and 3 Gy for intracranial targets. Extracranial targets were usually treated with 1.2- to 4-Gy fractions with 6- to 8-Gy fractions used occasionally for treatment of bone metastases or malignant melanoma. Before the rapid adaption of radiosurgery into the clinic in the late 1980s, most radiation oncologists and radiation biologists believed that fractionating radiation treatment lessens the relative risk of injury to normal tissue compared with tumor in essentially all circumstances. Radiobiologic analysis of a limited number of malignant tumors in cell culture and clinical experience with conventionally fractionated radiotherapy of fast-growing malignant tumors established this radiobiologic dogma. Increasing the fractionation of radiotherapy for slow-growing benign tumors may not necessarily improve the balance between tumor control and radiation complication. Slow-growing benign tumors are difficult to study in either cell culture or animal models, so the effect of fractionation has not been well delineated. Stereotactic radiosurgery allowed clinicians to administer high single doses of radiation to intracranial targets with relative safety, thereby leading to a new appreciation of the underlying radiobiology. Laboratory studies that suggest that the radiation response for the high-dose single fractions used in radiosurgery is predominantly related to the supporting endothelial cells (25). Pathology studies of benign and malignant tumors treated by radiosurgery also support a vascular response (109).

Analysis of clinical data from radiosurgery to delineate dose-response relationships and define radiobiologic parameters is fraught with difficulties. Typical radiosurgery treatment plans use inhomogeneous dose distributions with the prescription isodose covering anywhere from 90% to 100% of the target volume. The absolute minimum dose to the target typically is 5% to 30% lower than the prescription dose. Contours of the same tumor/target volume or critical structures may vary slightly from one clinician to another. Using the linear-quadratic formula to extrapolate from experience with conventional radiotherapy experience with low-dose fractions to high-dose single fractions for radiosurgery appears problematic. Using single-fraction radiosurgery dose-response curves for arteriovenous malformation (AVM) obliteration, radiation injury to brain parenchyma and cranial nerves to calculate α/β ratios yields values of negative 30 to negative 60 rather than 2 to 3 as expected from conventional fractionated radiotherapy data (19,21). Comparing dose responses for fractionated SRT to radiosurgery is hampered by limited data with dose-response curves that have insufficient slopes for accurate comparison.

Table 15.1	**KEY REQUIREMENTS FOR OPTIMAL STEREOTACTIC IRRADIATION**

Requirement	Rationale
Small target/treatment volume	Reducing the volume of normal and target tissue irradiated to high doses improves tolerance
Sharply defined target	Can be treated with little or no extra margin of surrounding normal tissue and/or without unintentional under-dosage of the target (marginal miss)
Accurate radiation delivery	No margin of normal tissue needed for setup error and/or reduced chance of underdosing target
High conformality	Reduces the treatment volume to match the target volume
Sensitive structures excluded from target	Dose-limiting structures (such as optic chiasm, spinal cord) should be able to be defined and excluded from the target volume to limit the risk of radiation injury

Radiosurgical Techniques

Radiosurgery was originally envisioned to treat intracranial lesions by delivering a high dose of ionizing radiation in a single-treatment session using multiple beams precisely collimated to the target inside the cranium. Advances in both imaging and computer technologies resulted in wider applications of radiosurgery. There are now a variety of different radiosurgery and SRT techniques available for intracranial and extracranial use.

Gamma Knife Radiosurgery

After prior experience with stereotactic treatment using orthovoltage radiotherapy and proton beam irradiation, Leksell and Larson created the first prototype of the gamma knife in 1967. The gamma knife uses a relatively hemispherical array of multiple fixed cobalt-60 beams (201 in most models) that are sharply collimated to create small, relatively spherical treatment volumes of varied diameter with sharp dose falloff. The earlier model originally was referred to as the *U-style* and contained cobalt sources arranged in hemispherical array,

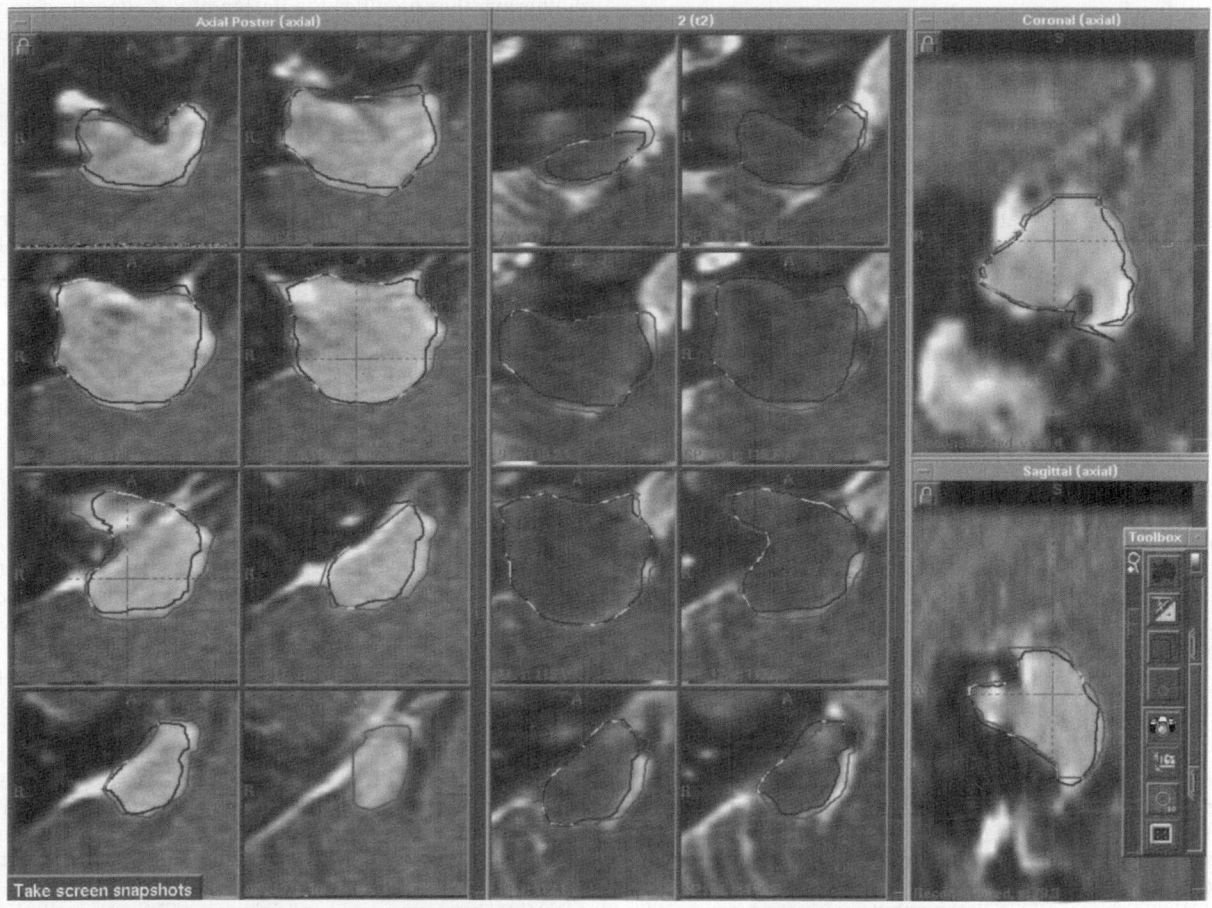

FIGURE 15.1. Comparisons of acoustic schwannoma contours drawn from T1-contrast magnetic resonance (MR) images (eight axial images on the left side, with coronal and sagittal images on the right side) with contours drawn from T2 MR images (the darker eight axial images in the center). T1 contours can sometimes slightly overestimate extension into the internal auditory canal and unnecessarily include adjacent blood vessels.

including sources at the pole of the hemisphere. These units present challenging loading and reloading issues with the cobalt-60 sources, particularly with radiation protection. To eliminate this problem, the B-unit (Elekta, Inc., Norcross, GA) (after Bergen, Norway, the first site) was redesigned so that sources were arranged in an annular section of a hemisphere, similar to the Northern Hemisphere with the Arctic Circle excluded. In 1999, the model C version of the gamma knife was introduced with the option to use robotic positioning to set treatment coordinates. This expedites execution of multiple-isocenter treatment plans. Manual positioning is still needed for some targets far from the center of the head. The model 4-C, introduced in 2005, was equipped with enhancements designed to improve workflow, increase accuracy, and provide integrated imaging capabilities. The Perfexion model introduced in 2006 uses a larger patient aperture and internally mounted secondary collimators. Because of the larger patient aperture, it is able to treat all intracranial and even cervical spine targets quickly and efficiently with robotic positioning.

Rotating Gamma System

A radiosurgery device called the *rotating gamma system* (RGS) was developed in China. The rotating gamma system (OUR International Inc., Shenzen, China) employs 30 cobalt-60 radiation sources in a revolving hemispherical shell. The secondary collimator is a coaxial hemispheric shell with six groups of five different collimators to produce spherical treatment volumes of different diameter. The experience with this system is somewhat limited.

Proton Radiosurgery

The chief advantage of charged proton radiosurgery is that the beams stop at a depth related to the beam's energy. Electron beams also use charged particles but lack the sharp beam edge of the proton beam. The lack of an exit dose and the sharp beam profile of protons allow target irradiation with lower integral doses than are delivered with photon (Linac x-ray or cobalt-60 gamma) irradiation. An unmodified proton beam irradiation deposits increased energy in the last couple of millimeters of the path length. This area of increased ionization, where cell killing is even higher because of an increased radiobiologic effect, is termed the *Bragg peak* or *Bragg-Gray peak*. To allow homogeneous irradiation of targets greater than a millimeter or two, the Bragg peak is normally modulated or spread out throughout the target, essentially eliminating its effect. The first treatment of a malignant tumor by irradiation with a proton beam Bragg peak was carried out in 1957 and followed by functional neurosurgery for advanced Parkinson's disease in 1958. Presently, proton beam irradiation is available at a limited number of centers because of the high cost of equipment and maintenance. If technical improvements and increased competition lead to continued cost reductions, proton beam irradiation will become increasingly used because of its dosimetric advantages

LINAC Radiosurgery

The pioneering work of many researchers in 1980s led to the gradual modifications of linear accelerators (LINACs) designed for conventional radiotherapy to be used for radiosurgery. LINAC technologies were modified by incorporating improved guiding (stereotactic) devices and methods to measure and improve accuracy of various components. Unmodified LINACs for conventional radiotherapy tend to deviate from alignment with the isocenter at different gantry angles. Most early LINAC-based radiosurgery techniques used multiple radiation arcs with circular secondary collimators to create spherical dose distributions for stereotactically defined three-dimensional targets. Improved hardware and advanced dose-planning software have been developed to enhance conformity. These include beam shaping with micromultileaf collimators, intensity modulation with inverse treatment-planning algorithms. Many LINAC-based systems such as Xknife (Radionics Inc., Burlington, MA), Novalis (BrainLAB, Heimstetten, Germany), the Peacock System (NOMOS Corp., Sewickley, PA), and Cyberknife (Accuray Inc., Sunnyvale, CA) are commercially available. The Peacock system uses inverse planning and multileaf wedge-generated intensity-modulated beams to obtain target conformity. The Cyberknife combines a miniaturized LINAC mounted on an industrial robot with a system for target tracking and beam realignment. This system uses a 6-MeV LINAC with different-sized circular collimators attached to a six-axis robotic manipulator. Stereotactic frames are not normally used for targeting. Cyberknife plans use multiple fixed-beam positions and multiple isocenters. Before the radiation is delivered from any beam position, the target position is tracked using an integrated x-ray image processing system, consisting of two orthogonal diagnostic x-ray cameras and an optical tracking system. During treatment, the image processing system acquires x-ray images of the patient's body multiple times throughout the treatment, while stealth tracking software compares the actual images with the target images to correct alignment of the beam.

Tomotherapy

Tomotherapy, literally "slice" therapy, is a new form of radiotherapy that modifies the design of a diagnostic computerized tomography (CT) scan into a treatment-delivery machine, thereby combining the precision of CT imaging with the radiation treatment. This is done by adding a LINAC megavoltage treatment beam to the rotating x-ray source and moving table design of diagnostic CT unit, which normally uses only a kilovoltage diagnostic x-ray beam. Unlike traditional radiation therapy systems with a slow-moving external gantry designed for positioning individual beams onto the tumor from a few different directions, tomotherapy rapidly rotates the beam around the patient (and inside the housing of the unit), thus allowing the beam to enter the patient from many different angles in succession. Beam intensity modulation (IMRT) is possible through the use of a multileaf collimator system. The inclusion of CT imaging technology within the tomotherapy unit allows precise localization of the target before and during treatment.

LINAC Image-Guided Radiotherapy

The combination of diagnostic three-dimensional imaging with highly conformal treatment delivery in a single unit to maintain accuracy is the basis of various treatment techniques and processes collectively known as *image-guided radiation therapy* (IGRT). Although tomotherapy (which is also a type of IGRT) accomplishes this by modifying a CT unit into a megavoltage radiotherapy machine, most other IGRT techniques add CT imaging capability to a LINAC radiotherapy unit equipped for stereotactic and IMRT use. Because any patient movement between image acquisition and treatment delivery (or during treatment delivery) can introduce error, these IGRT systems use noninvasive immobilization devices and patient position tracking systems. Several manufacturers currently offer IGRT using LINAC technology capable of delivering SRS and radiotherapy, including the Trilogy (Varian Medical Systems, Inc.) and the SynergyS (Elekta, Inc.) equipped with cone-beam CT imaging capability.

Techniques, Modalities, and Modifiers in Radiation Oncology

Normal Tissue Tolerance in SRS and SRT

Radiosensitivity

Estimating the risks of a proposed treatment plan with various doses is an essential part of treatment planning and dose prescription for SRS and SRT. The ability of normal tissue to tolerate radiation without injury depends on the radiation dose administered, the volume of tissue irradiated, the sensitivity of the tissue affected, history of any prior radiation treatment to the region, as well as any individual variation in radiation sensitivity between different people. At present, with the exception of patients with known increased radiation sensitivity, such as those with ataxia telangiectasia, there is usually no information available to modify treatment plans for individual differences in radiosensitivity. Prior fractionated radiotherapy appears to have limited effects on the risks of developing postradiosurgery parenchymal edema and neurologic sequelae after radiosurgery, but has been observed to effect optic nerve tolerance.

Location Effects

Analysis of postradiosurgery injury reactions in AVM patients revealed no difference in the likelihood of postradiosurgery injury imaging changes (increased signal developing in surrounding brain on long relaxation time or T2-weighted images) in different regions of the brain (15,19). Dramatic differences were seen in the rates of developing neurologic sequelae between different regions of the brain (as shown in Fig. 15.2).

Radiation Therapy Oncology Group (RTOG) Dose-Escalation Studies

The RTOG Radiosurgery Dose-Escalation Study established tolerance doses for radiosurgery of recurrent brain metastases and high-grade gliomas not involving the brainstem (103). They administered radiosurgery to 156 patients with brain metastases or primary brain tumors that recurred or progressed after conventional radiotherapy following a dose-escalation protocol. Starting with initial doses of 18, 15, and 12 Gy for diameters <20, 21 to 30, and 31 to 40 mm, respectively, they escalated prescription doses in 3-Gy intervals until irreversible toxicity was

seen in >20% of patients within 3 months. The exception was with tumors <20 mm in diameter where dose-limiting toxicity was not reached and investigators were reluctant to escalate above 24 Gy to 27 Gy. The recommended tolerance doses from that protocol were 24, 18, and 15 Gy for diameters of <20 mm, 21 to 30, and 31 to 40 mm, respectively. The data with longer follow-up beyond 3 months to assess late toxicity were fitted to individual logistic dose-response curves shown in Figure 15.3. These tolerance doses have been widely used as dose guidelines for radiosurgery of malignant tumors, often with interpolation for tumors close to 20 and 30 mm in diameter (e.g., 20 Gy for 18- to 22-mm diameter and 16.5 Gy for 28- to 32-mm diameter treatment volumes).

Optic Nerve Tolerance for Radiosurgery

The first analysis of optic nerve tolerance to radiosurgery—a combined Harvard and University of Pittsburgh study of patients with cavernous sinus meningiomas, craniopharyngioma, and pituitary adenomas—recommended 8 Gy as a safe maximum dose limit for the optic nerves/chiasm (110). The lowest optic chiasm dose at which optic neuropathy developed in that study was reported as being 9.7 Gy. Optic nerve/chiasm doses were estimated from isodose distributions overlaid on CT images, unlike the present day when the entire optic system is usually outlined on detailed magnetic resonance (MR) images and maximum doses are assessed from dose-volume histograms. It is highly likely that the true maximum doses to the optic system were higher and lay in portions of the nerve that were poorly visualized.

Stafford et al. (108) reported a later analysis of four cases of optic neuropathy occurring out of 215 Mayo Clinic radiosurgery patients with a median dose of 10 Gy to the optic chiasm. One case developed after an optic nerve/chiasm dose of 12.8 Gy with radiosurgery alone, at which the risk level appeared to be approximately 3%. The other cases developed in patients with prior fractionated radiotherapy (7 Gy after 58.8 Gy, 9 Gy after 45 Gy, and two procedures delivering 9 and later 12 Gy to the optic system after 50.4 Gy).

Leber et al. (56)' analyzed optic nerve injury risks in 50 patients with 24- to 60-month follow-up (median, 40 months) who underwent gamma knife radiosurgery for benign skull base tumors. Their risks of optic neuropathy were 0% with <10 Gy, 27% with 10 to 15 Gy, and 78% with >15 Gy. They found no cavernous sinus nerve injury with doses of 5 to 30 Gy.

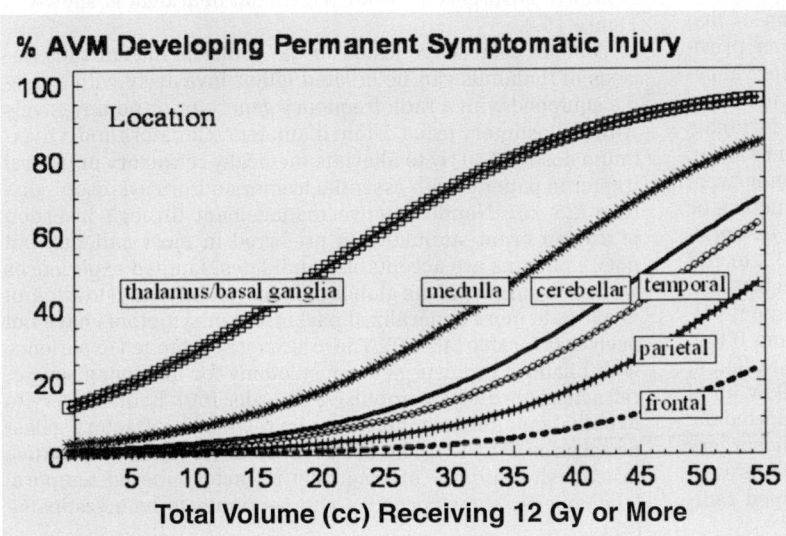

FIGURE 15.2. Effect of location on the risk of developing permanent symptomatic neurologic injury following arteriovenous malformation (AVM) radiosurgery.

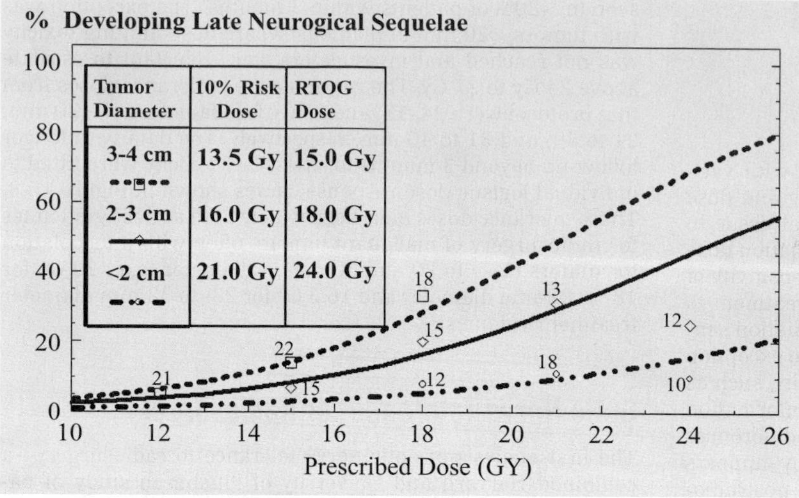

FIGURE 15.3. Phase 1 Radiation Therapy Oncology Group (RTOG) dose-escalation data for radiosurgery of recurrent brain metastases and glioblastoma fit to logistic dose-response curves. The numbers at each data point indicate the number of patients in each dose/diameter group (103).

Considering these data and published risks of optic neuropathy for conventional fractionated radiotherapy, α/β ratios in the range of 0 to 1 seem reasonable for estimating fractionated radiotherapy dose-equivalents for radiosurgery doses for the optic nerve and probably other cranial nerves

Tolerance of Other Cranial Nerves

From clinical experience with fractionated conventional radiosurgery and radiosurgery, it appears that special sensory nerves (optic and auditory) are the most radiosensitive, followed by somatic sensory nerves (trigeminal) and finally the motor nerves (cranial nerves 2, 4, 6, 7, and 9 through 12). After acoustic schwannoma radiosurgery to doses of 12 to 13 Gy, FSR to 18 Gy in three fractions or SRT to 45 to 50 Gy in 25 to 28 fractions, decreased hearing develops in 30% to 50% of patients, facial numbness in 2% to 3%, and facial weakness in ≤0.5%. Radiosurgery with present techniques for meningiomas involving the cavernous sinus is associated with a risk of trigeminal neuropathy of approximately 3% of patients, with radiation injuries to cranial nerves III, IV, or VI more uncommon (11–15)

Spinal Cord Tolerance

The tolerance of the spinal cord to SRS or SRT depends on the volume of spinal cord irradiated, the distribution of that radiation (e.g., maximum dose), the dose of radiation previously administered to the spinal cord, and the time interval between initial radiation and retreatment. Spinal cord tolerance to SRS or SRT has not been well defined because of a fortunate paucity of radiation injury reactions in clinical experience so far. Gerszten et al. (28) reported on 125 patients who underwent Cyberknife spine radiosurgery (17 benign and 108 metastatic cases). Seventy-eight lesions had previously received external-beam radiotherapy. Treatment volumes varied from 0.3 to 232 mL, with a mean of 27.8 mL. Prescription doses varied between 12 and 20 Gy (mean, 14 Gy) to an 80% isodose treatment volume. Spinal cord volumes receiving >8 Gy varied from 0.0 to 1.7 mL, with a mean, 0.2 mL. They identified no acute radiation toxicity or new neurologic deficits after a median follow-up of 18 months (range, 9 to 30 months). Benzil et al. (6) reported the New York Medical College experience with spine radiosurgery in 31 patients using a Novalis LINAC unit. Two patients who received biologic equivalent doses of >60 Gy developed radiculitis.

Clinical Uses of SRS and SRT

Table 15.2 lists the most commonly used indications for radiosurgery, with representative references. Except for functional radiosurgery, there are varied levels of experience with SRT for each of these indications.

Functional Radiosurgery

The most widely used functional application for radiosurgery is in the management of typical trigeminal neuralgia refractory to medical therapy (18–22). Atypical or constant pain does not respond. Other alternatives for managing typical trigeminal neuralgia are medication, open surgery with microvascular decompression, and rhizotomy procedures using glycerol injection, balloon compression, or radiofrequency injury to the nerve. Typically, 4-mm collimators are used for radiosurgery to a maximum dose of 80 Gy. Response rates reach approximately 85%, typically 1 week to 4 months after the procedure, but can develop as late as 6 months later. Approximately 50% of typical trigeminal neuralgia patients remain pain-free and off medication 5 years following radiosurgery. A typical radiosurgery plan for trigeminal neuralgia is shown in Figure 15.4.

A small destructive lesion in the ventralis intermedius nucleus of thalamus can be created either invasively with a needle equipped with a radiofrequency generator or noninvasively with radiosurgery using 4-mm diameter collimators and a maximum dose of 130 Gy to alleviate medically refractory unilateral tremor in patients with essential tremor and/or Parkinson's disease (23–26). Nondestructive management through insertion of a deep brain stimulator is preferred in most patients, but not all patients are acceptable candidates. Limited experiences with radiosurgery of the globus pallidus (pallidotomy) to attempt to alleviate more generalized parkinsonian symptoms have not been as favorable (48–50). There is favorable limited experience with bilateral radiosurgical capsulotomy for managing severe, refractory obsessive-compulsive disorder (60). Radiosurgery to hypothalamic hamartomas may help control refractory gelastic seizures (94,112). The use of radiosurgery as an alternative to extensive surgery in medically refractory mesial temporal lobe epilepsy shows promise and continues to be investigated (97).

	Table 15.2	COMMON INDICATIONS FOR RADIOSURGERY OR HYPOFRACTIONATED STEREOTACTIC RADIOTHERAPY		
Indication	**Experience**	**Value**	**References**
Functional a. Trigeminal neuralgia b. Unilateral tremor	a. Extensive b. Moderate	1. Less numbness than rhizotomy 2. In poor candidates for deep brain stimulation	a. 1822 b. 23–26
Vascular a. AVM b. Cavernous	a. Extensive b. Moderate	a. High b. Controversial	a. 4, 27–29 b. 30–32
Benign tumors: schwannoma, pituitary adenoma, meningioma, and others	Extensive	High tumor control, acceptable morbidity for selected small tumors	11–13, 33–36, 71–98
Brain metastases	Extensive	Control rates equal to or higher than those for surgery for small mets	37–38
Primary malignant brain tumors	Extensive for GBM; limited with other uses	Initial SRS appears ineffective for GBM; helpful for recurrent tumors, possibly initial pilocytic, neurocytoma	39–47
Spinal metastases	Moderate	High for recurrent tumors; no phase 3 comparison with conventional XRT for initial treatment	16–17

AVM, arteriovenous malformation; GBM, glioblastoma multiforme; SRS, stereotactic radiosurgery; XRT, radiotherapy.

Vascular Malformations

Untreated intracranial AVMs have a bleeding risk of approximately 3% per year, or higher if prior bleeds have occurred (83,86). This results in an average of 1% of untreated AVM patients dying each year from hemorrhage. Management options include observation, surgical resection, embolization, and radiosurgery. Radiosurgery can dramatically reduce the risk of hemorrhage. Radiosurgery obliterates the AVM nidus in approximately 75% of patients within 3 years of the procedure

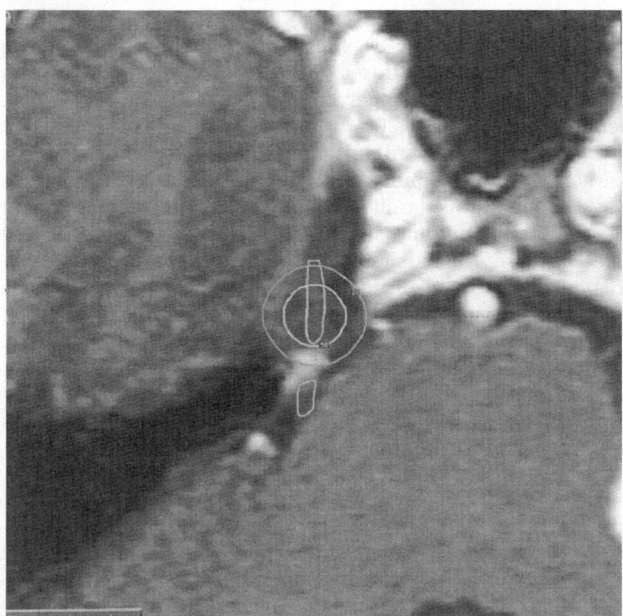

FIGURE 15.4. Typical radiosurgery plan for right trigeminal neuralgia. The right trigeminal nerve is outlined in white. The 30% and 50% isodose volumes from treating a single isocenter with 4-mm diameter collimators with a gamma unit are shown. A maximum dose of 80 Gy will deliver 40 Gy to the 50% isodose volume and 16 Gy to the 20% volume.

(21,39,69). Individual obliteration rates vary from 50% to 88% depending on marginal dose administered, as shown in the dose-response curve illustrated in Figure 15.5. Although AVM obliteration rates appear to be optimized with marginal doses of approximately 23 Gy, lower doses are selected for most patients to minimize complications. The risk of neurologic sequelae from radiosurgery averages approximately 3% but varies with treatment volume, dose, and location (Fig. 15.2). The risk of hemorrhage while waiting for complete obliteration to develop seems unaltered (86). All of these risks and benefits of radiosurgery need to be considered together to optimize management of individual AVM patients.

When an AVM nidus fails to completely obliterate by 3 years after radiosurgery, irradiation can be repeated with acceptable morbidity (87). Although some residual radiation injury effect would be expected within the previously irradiated, unobliterated AVM nidus vasculature, retreatment appears to require similar, if not higher, doses to achieve similar rates of complete obliteration as initial radiosurgery (87).

Management of large AVMs is presently difficult because radiosurgery may be associated with high complication risks and low obliteration rates. Recent improvements in embolization with liquid glue or (ev3, Inc., Plymouth, MN) polymer can sometimes help reduce the target volume, but adds to the total risks of the overall management (65). Another promising approach is staged radiosurgery, in which large AVMs are treated in two or three sections separated by 4- to 6-month intervals to reduce acute toxicity. Whether there is any benefit to fractionating stereotactic irradiation of AVMs is presently unclear (106).

Cavernous malformations do not show detectable flow on angiography but nevertheless are vascular lesions with annual hemorrhage risks of 0.5% per year with no prior bleed, 4.5% with one prior hemorrhage, and approximately 32% per year after a history of two or more hemorrhages (61–65). Lower pressures in these lesions lead to smaller bleeds than are typically seen with AVM. Repeated bleeds from brainstem cavernous malformations can cause considerable neurologic morbidity. Symptomatic, surgically accessible lesions should be resected. Radiosurgery of brainstem cavernous malformations with a history of two or more prior hemorrhages appears to reduce the

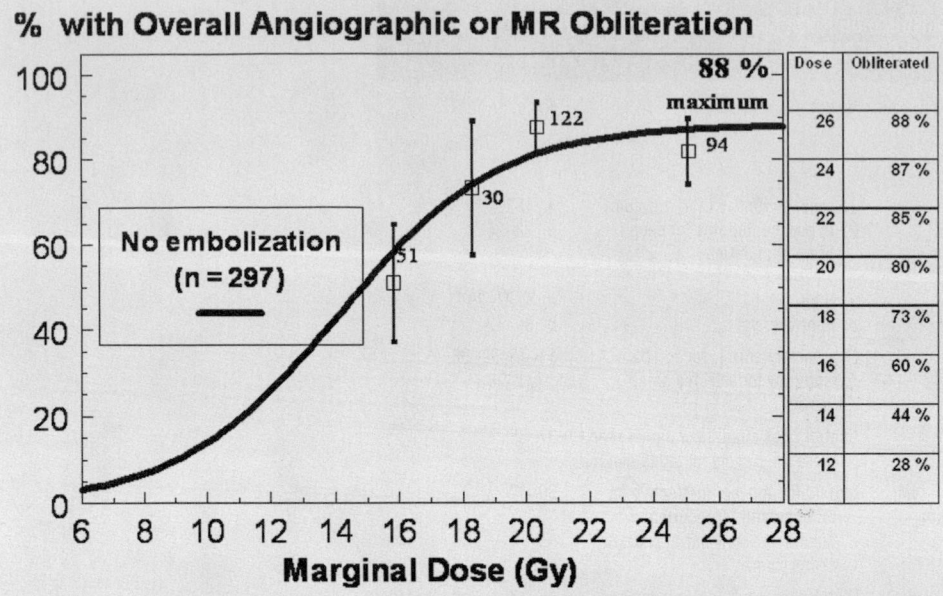

FIGURE 15.5. Dose response for obliteration of arteriovenous malformation after radiosurgery from 297 patients treated at University of Pittsburgh without embolization (21). MR, magnetic resonance.

risk of subsequent bleeds to approximately 1% per year with acceptable morbidity (63,66–69).

Benign Tumors

Most small benign intracranial tumors are well managed with radiosurgery, FSR, or SRT. Radiosurgery control rates are high with radiosurgery, with prescription doses on the order of 12–14 Gy (11–13,33–37). Kondziolka et al. (51) evaluated long-term tumor control in 285 consecutive patients who underwent radiosurgery for benign intracranial tumors between 1987 and 1992, with a median follow-up period of 10 years. This included 157 patients with vestibular schwannomas, 10 with other cranial nerve schwannomas, 85 with meningiomas, 28 with pituitary adenomas, and 5 with craniopharyngiomas. Forty-four percent of the patients had prior surgical resection and 5% had prior fractionated radiotherapy. They found that 95% of the 285 patients had imaging-defined local tumor control (63% had tumor regression and 32% had no further tumor growth). The crude tumor control was 95% (271/285 patients) with a 15-year actuarial tumor control rate of 93.7%. In 5% of the patients, delayed tumor growth was identified. Resection was performed after radiosurgery in 13 patients (5%) for tumor growth.

Vestibular Schwannomas

Vestibular schwannomas, also known as *acoustic neuromas*, are benign tumors arising from Schwann cells. They are associated with loss of genetic information on chromosome 22 (78). Vestibular schwannomas either occur on one side as spontaneous mutations or bilaterally as the hallmark of type 2 neurofibromatosis (NF-2). Vestibular schwannomas usually arise within the internal auditory canal and later extend intracranially into the cerebellar pontine angle. Because these tumors lack the ability to invade bone, the portion of tumor outside the canal in the cerebellar pontine angle eventually grows into a globular extension that is larger than the intracanalicular portion (Fig. 15.1). The differential diagnosis of a cerebellar-pontine angle tumor includes vestibular schwannoma (90%), meningioma (close to 10%), cholesteatomas, facial or trigeminal schwannoma, and rare primary or metastatic malignant tumors. Cerebellar pontine angle meningiomas (which can be managed similarly to vestibular schwannomas) also may in-

volve the internal auditory canal, but are usually distinguished by a broad, flat, dural attachment that is lacking in vestibular schwannomas.

Observation or surgical resection were essentially the only management strategies offered to acoustic schwannoma patients until favorable experiences with gamma knife radiosurgery were reported in the 1980s. Observation may be appropriate in selected NF-2 patients and some elderly patients with small, minimally symptomatic vestibular schwannomas, but early intervention appears to be the best strategy for long-term hearing preservation for most patients (99,105). Surgery appears to be the best initial strategy in patients with vestibular schwannomas large enough to cause symptomatic brainstem compression with obstructive hydrocephalus. For small-to-medium vestibular schwannomas, tumor control rates with radiosurgery or SRT are comparable to those of surgical resection (71–94).

Early radiosurgery series including patients treated during the 1980s with higher doses (14 to 18 Gy) and less conformal treatment plans had higher rates of postradiosurgery cranial neuropathies (15% to 20% trigeminal and/or facial and 67% with a drop in their Gardner-Robertson hearing level) (49). This led some groups to pursue SRT for vestibular schwannomas, while others pursued radiosurgery with refined techniques and lower doses. Both approaches led to improved results (71–94). The University of Pittsburgh reported on 313 previously untreated unilateral acoustic schwannoma patients who underwent gamma knife radiosurgery doses of 12 to 13 Gy between February 1991 and February 2001 (18). Median follow-up was 24 months, maximum follow-up was 115 months, and 36 patients had >60 months of follow-up. The actuarial clinical tumor control rate, free of surgical intervention, was 98.6% at 7 years. One patient's growing tumor was subsequently completely resected. The only other failure required a partial resection because of an enlarging adjacent subarachnoid cyst, despite control of the irradiated tumor. The 7-year actuarial rates for unchanged facial strength, unchanged facial sensation, unchanged hearing level, and useful hearing preservation were 100%, 95.6%, 70.3%, and 78.6%, respectively. Eight patients developed new trigeminal neuropathy, six of whom developed numbness (7-year actuarial rate = 2.5%), and the other two developed new typical trigeminal neuralgia (7-year actuarial rate = 1.9%). The risk of developing postradiosurgery trigeminal neuropathy was associated with increasing tumor volume ($p = .038$). Similar results with low-dose radiosurgery of vestibular schwannomas were reported by Iwai et al. (38), Paek et al. (84), Muacevic et al. (77), and Rowe et al. (98).

Various fractionation schemes (18 Gy/3, 20 Gy/4 to 5, 25 Gy/5, 45 to 50 Gy/25, and 54 Gy/30) have been used with vestibular schwannoma with minor differences in results. After accounting for length and quality of follow-up, treatment results seem similar to those of radiosurgery with 12 to 13 Gy, but an advantage for fractionation cannot be excluded entirely (14). Combs et al. (12) from Heidelberg reported seemingly better useful hearing preservation (94%) in 106 acoustic schwannoma patients managed with FSRT to a median dose of 57.6 Gy with 1.8 Gy fractions. They reported 98% actuarial hearing preservation for non-NF2 patients compared to 68% for NF-2 patients. These numbers were based on telephone questioning rather than audiograms, making comparison to radiosurgery series difficult. Their 5-year actuarial tumor control rate was 93%, and postradiation trigeminal and facial neuropathy rates were 3.4% and 2.3%, respectively. The University of California, Los Angeles, also reported unusually good hearing preservation (93%) for their experience with 50 unilateral acoustic schwannoma patients irradiated to 54 Gy in 30 fractions to a 90% isodose treatment volume including a 1- to 3-mm margin around gross tumor (59). All tumors were controlled with a median follow-up of 36 months (range, 6 to 74 months). They defined useful hearing preservation as the ability to talk on the telephone and listen with the affected ear. New facial numbness developed in one patient (2%) and facial weakness also developed in one patient (2%) after radiotherapy.

Andrews et al. (3) analyzed the Jefferson vestibular schwannoma experience, comparing 69 radiosurgery patients with 50 SRT patients who received 50 Gy in 25 fractions. Their first 25 vestibular schwannoma patients were treated using a linear accelerator, and later radiosurgery patients were treated with gamma knife radiosurgery. They authors had similar facial and trigeminal neuropathy rates for the radiosurgery and fractionated radiotherapy groups but the rate of hearing loss was significantly higher in their radiosurgery group. There were only a small number of patients with serviceable (useful) hearing in each group prior to irradiation (12 in the radiosurgery and 21 in the FSRT groups) and follow-up was limited. Meijer et al. (73), from Amsterdam, also reported a single-institution comparison of radiosurgery (LINAC to 10 or 12.5 Gy) and SRT (20 Gy/4 to 5 fractions) for vestibular schwannoma. They selected 49 edentulous patients (mean age, 63 years) for radiosurgery and 80 patients (mean age, 43 years) with intact dentition for SRT. They found a higher rate of trigeminal neuropathy following radiosurgery (8%) than SRT (2%) at 5 years ($p = .048$), but similar hearing loss with radiosurgery (25%) than SRT (39% FSRT; $p > .05$), similar, but higher than usual rates of new facial neuropathy (7% radiosurgery vs. 3% FSRT; $p > .05$), and similar 5-year actuarial tumor control rates (100% with radiosurgery vs. 94% with SRT).

Nonacoustic Schwannomas

Schwannomas may occasionally involve other cranial nerves, particularly V, VII, and XI through XII in the jugular foramen. Tumor control rates are similar, but postradiosurgery neuropathies seem less common as somatic sensory and particularly motor nerves seem less sensitive to radiation injury than special sensory nerves like VIII (95–98).

Meningiomas

Radiosurgery and SRS are both excellent management options for most small benign meningiomas, with in-field tumor control rates well above 90%, as has been seen with most other benign tumors (17,51). Marginal recurrences rates as high as 25% may develop because of the tight margins used for radiosurgery or SRT treatment volumes limited to small recurrences or residual tumor after resection of large parasagittal meningiomas (11,33,99–101). Marginal recurrences are far less of a problem with unresected (and usually unbiopsied) meningiomas. A University of Pittsburgh study (17) analyzed 219 imaging-diagnosed meningiomas (unbiopised) managed with gamma knife radiosurgery to a prescription dose of 8.9 to 20 Gy (median, 14 Gy), treatment volumes of 0.47 to 56.5 mL (median, 5.0 mL) with 2 to 164 months of follow-up (median, 29 months). Tumors progressed in seven patients; two of the tumors proved to be different ones (metastatic nasopharyngeal adenoid cystic carcinoma and chondrosarcoma). Another patient with local control of the lesion developed a subsequent brain metastasis, changing the diagnosis of the first lesion to the same. The actuarial tumor control rate was 93.2% at both 5 and 10 years. The actuarial rate of identifying a diagnosis other than meningioma was at both 5 and 10 years. No pretreatment variables, including dose, correlated with tumor control in univariate or multivariate analysis. The actuarial rate for developing any postradiosurgical injury reaction was 8.8% at 5 and 10 years. The risk of postradiosurgery sequelae was lower (5.3%) after 1991 (with stereotactic MR imaging and lower doses; $p = .0104$).

Atypical and malignant (anaplastic) meningiomas have higher rates of local and marginal recurrence after therapeutic intervention. Complete surgical resection is advocated whenever possible, followed by a full course of conventional radiotherapy with at least 1-cm margins around the tumor volume. Radiosurgery has been recommended to improve local control of unresectable tumor (101–104). Malik et al. (67) reported 5-year actuarial control rates of 87% for typical meningiomas, 49% for atypical, and 0% for malignant meningioma in the Sheffield gamma knife experience. Harris et al. (30) reported on the Pittsburgh gamma knife experience in 12 malignant and 18 atypical meningiomas. Their 5-year local tumor control was 72% for malignant and 83% for atypical meningiomas; however, 10-year actuarial survival rates were only 59% and 0%, respectively. Katz et al. (40) could not substantiate that either accelerated fractionated radiotherapy or a radiosurgery boost improved tumor control or survival in their analysis of 27 atypical and 9 malignant meningioma patients managed at the University of Florida.

Pituitary Adenoma

Management of pituitary adenomas requires a multidisciplinary approach to properly select which patients are suitable for different approaches with medical therapy, surgery, fractionated radiotherapy, and radiosurgery, or combinations of these. Most patient with visual compromise, particularly with a hemianopsia or greater, will do better with initial surgical decompression. Prolactinomas are usually initially managed with medical therapy (92). Most other small pituitary adenomas, where the target volume can be separated from the optic nerves, are reasonable candidates for radiosurgery (11,34–36).

Sheehan et al. (104) performed a review of 35 peer-reviewed reports of radiosurgery for pituitary adenoma that included 1,621 patients. Most studies reported >90% control of tumor size (range, 68% to 100%). The weighted average tumor control rate for all published series (encompassing 1,283 patients) was 96%. In eight published series with mean or median patient follow-up periods of ≥ 4 years, tumor growth control rates varied from 83% to 100%.

Twenty-two series have published radiosurgery results for 314 Cushing's disease patients. The mean radiosurgical prescription (margin) doses for these series varied from 15 to 32 Gy. In those series with at least 10 patients and a median follow-up of 2 years, endocrinologic remission rates range from 17% to 83%. Many of the patients in older series were treated in the pre-CT and MR imaging era of radiosurgery, sometimes as often as many as four times before their Cushing's disease went into remission.

Malignant Tumors

Brain Metastases

Brain metastases are the most common and best studied of the indications for radiosurgery (71). Early clinical investigations found impressive tumor control with radiosurgery for brain metastases that progressed after prior whole-brain radiotherapy (WBXRT). The RTOG phase I dose-escalation trial in recurrent brain tumors to some degree standardized dose prescription for brain metastasis radiosurgery (21). Because of the success of radiosurgery in controlling brain metastases after whole-brain radiotherapy and the high rate of eventual local tumor progression in brain metastases after conventional WBXRT, radiosurgery has been increasingly used in initial management of brain metastases (21). The subsequent phase III randomized trial, RTOG 95-08, established that radiosurgery immediately following standard WBXRT (37.5 Gy in 15 fractions) improves local control and quality of life for patients with one to three brain metastases while also improving overall survival for patients with solitary metastasis, all compared with patients initially managed with WBXRT only (2).

Although RTOG 95-08 established the role of radiosurgery after WBXRT in managing one to three brain metastases, questions remained about managing brain metastases with radiosurgery alone, preserving full-dose WBXRT as an option for later managing cases with subsequent progression. Aoyama et al. (4) recently published the outcome of a prospective randomized controlled trial to evaluate whether initial WBXRT provides better outcomes when added to SRS compared to using SRS alone. The 11-hospital study done by Aoyama et al. (4) randomized 132 patients with one to four brain metastases <3 cm in diameter to radiosurgery either with or without initial WBXRT. They found that the median survival time and the 1-year actuarial survival rates were not significantly different with or without WBXRT. The 1-year brain tumor "recurrence rate" (corresponding to the development of additional brain metastases) was higher in the SRS-alone group compared with the patient group that received both WBRT and SRS. Earlier retrospective studies had similar observations. The most common primary site in these studies was lung. Separate analyses of radiosurgery of brain metastases of different histologies with and without WBXRT found that WBXRT reduced subsequent development of brain metastases in lung cancer patients but not patients with melanoma or renal cell carcinoma. Administering initial WBXRT and waiting a month before radiosurgery for subsequent tumor shrinkage is a reasonable strategy for limiting radiation injury reactions and/or to improve tumor control for brain metastases >3 cm in diameter and for brainstem metastases >2 cm in diameter.

There is no clear limit as to how many metastases and what total volume of metastases can or should be treated by radiosurgery. RTOG 9508 was limited to one to three metastases, while the trial of Aoyama et al. (4) and a smaller University of Pittsburgh trial included patients with up to four brain metastases (52). Bhatnagar et al. (7) analyzed 205 patients who underwent radiosurgery for 4 to 18 brain metastases (median, 5). They reported a median survival of 8 months after radiosurgery and found that survival correlated with the total volume of metastases, age, and RTOG-RPA class, but not the total number of brain metastases. Presently, many centers use WBXRT alone to initially manage patients with five or more metastases, and subsequently consider radiosurgery for patients who are unable to be withdrawn from steroid medication and for patients whose brain metastases progress after WBXRT.

Glioblastomas

During the late 1980s and 1990s, many centers that had been using brachytherapy for recurrent high-grade gliomas and as boosts after conventional radiotherapy switched to radiosurgery (72,107). Although retrospective series appeared to show that initial brachytherapy or radiosurgery boosts after conventional radiotherapy improved survival of glioblastoma patients, prospective randomized trials of both modalities used prior to conventional radiotherapy of glioblastoma patients were negative (72,107). Radiosurgery appears to be a reasonable option for small, well-circumscribed, high-grade gliomas that recur after prior conventional large-field radiotherapy and chemotherapy.

Radiosurgery of Spinal Metastases

Radiosurgery has been used to treat spinal tumors, mostly metastases, either as initial treatment or for recurrence after prior fractionated radiotherapy (6,26-28). By limiting spinal cord radiation dose with radiosurgery techniques, higher doses can be safely given to the tumor target volume with the hope of achieving greater local tumor control and higher response rates. Spinal cord tolerance in the experience of Gerzsten et al. (28) with 125 Cyberknife spine radiosurgery procedures in 17 benign and 108 metastatic cases was previously discussed in this chapter. Gerzsten et al. (26) separately reported results for single-fraction Cyberknife radiosurgery of 68 breast carcinoma metastases to the spine in 50 patients after 6 to 48 months of follow-up (median, 16 months). Pain was the most common indication for radiosurgery (in 57 lesions). Radiosurgery was delivered for radiographic tumor progression, as a postsurgical boost and for a progressive neurologic deficit in one case each. Radiosurgery was used as primary management in eight patients. Target volumes varied from 0.8 to 197 mL (mean, 27.7 mL). Maximum tumor doses were 15 to 22.5 Gy (mean, 19 Gy). No radiation-induced toxicity occurred during the follow-up period (6 to 48 months). Cyberknife radiosurgery achieved long-term pain improvement in 55 of the 57 patients (96%) who were treated primarily for pain. Long-term radiographic tumor control was seen in all patients who underwent primary radiosurgery as well as those treated for radiographic tumor progression after radiotherapy or as a postsurgical treatment. Similar results were seen in separate reports for spine radiosurgery of melanoma metastases (27). Randomized trials are needed to prove that SRS or hypofractionated SRT improve results compared with conventionally fractionated radiotherapy or IMRT with conventional immobilization (8).

Stereotactic Irradiation of Lung Tumors

Hypofractionated SRT has been used for treatment of small, medically inoperable non–small lung cancer primary tumors and to manage lung metastases in patients with limited metastatic disease (112–114). Beitler et al. (5) reported the Staten Island experience with SRT using five fractions of 8 Gy each in 75 patients (67 SRS alone and 8 with SRS boost after conventional radiotherapy) with 1 to 92 months of follow-up (median, 17 months). Treatment volumes varied from 0.26 to 1197 mL, with a median of 26.8 mL. Complete responses developed in 7 patients, tumor shrinkage in 25, stable disease in 22, and tumor progression in 9; 12 lacked follow-up. Radiation pneumonitis was reported in two patients. Patients with tumors <65 mL had a median survival of 26 months compared with 10 months for those with tumors >65 mL.

Ernst-Stecken et al. (13) reported results with hypofractionated stereotactic irradiation of 39 primary or secondary lung tumors in 21 patients. They delivered five fractions of either 7 Gy (n = 21) or 8 Gy (n = 18) to median tumor volumes of 2.9 mL (0.15 to 67.9 mL) using planning target volumes of 7.2 to 124.0 mL (median, 25.8 mL). They reported completed remission in 51%, partial in 33%, no change in 3%, and progressive disease in 13%. Most patients experienced grade 1 toxicity; none developed grade 2 or 4, but one patient developed grade 3 dyspnea 6 months after SRT.

Schefter et al. (100) reported a phase 1-2 dose escalation study of stereotactic body radiotherapy for lung metastases in 25 patients. Using 5-mm radial and 10-mm cranial-caudal margins, they administered three fractions of 16, 18, or 20 Gy while restricting the percentage of normal lung receiving >15 Gy to under 35%. Fourteen patients were in the phase 1 part of the study: six at 48 Gy, four at 54 Gy, and four at 60 Gy. Afterward, 14 patients were enrolled in the phase 2 part and received 60 Gy in three fractions, but follow-up was insufficient to report toxicity. Dose-limiting toxicity, defined as grade >3 lung, esophageal, or spinal toxicity occurring in any single patient, never developed in this study. Grade 1-2 esophagitis developed in three-fourths of the patients in the lowest dose group only. Grade 1 dermatitis developed in one fourth of the patients receiving 18 Gy × 3 and in one fourth of the patients with 20 Gy × 3. Grade 1 pain developed in one fourth of the patients within each dose level.

Miscellaneous Uses

Radiosurgery and hypofractionated SRT have been used as a substitute for brachytherapy in the management of recurrent head and neck tumors (50,113). Liver metastases can also be irradiated with these techniques (101). Hypofractionated prostate SRT is also being explored (43,64).

References

1. Aiba T, Tanaka R, Koike T, et al. Natural history of intracranial cavernous malformations. *J Neurosurg* 1995;83:56–59.
2. Andrews DW, Scott CB, Sperduto PW, et al. Whole brain radiation therapy with or without stereotactic radiosurgery boost for patients with one to three brain metastases: phase III results of the RTOG 9508 randomized trial. *Lancet* 2004;363:1665–1672.
3. Andrews DW, Suarez O, Goldman HW, et al. Stereotactic radiosurgery and fractionated stereotactic radiotherapy for the treatment of acoustic schwannomas: comparative observations of 125 patients treated at one institution. *Int J Radiat Oncol Biol Phys* 2001;50:1265–1278.
4. Aoyama H, Shirato H, Tago M, et al. Stereotactic radiosurgery plus whole-brain radiation therapy vs stereotactic radiosurgery alone for treatment of brain metastases: a randomized controlled trial. *JAMA* 2006;295:2483–2491.
5. Beitler JJ, Badine EA, El-Sayah D, et al. Stereotactic body radiation therapy for nonmetastatic lung cancer: an analysis of 75 patients treated over 5 years. *Int J Radiat Oncol Biol Phys* 2006;65:100–106.
6. Benzil DL, Saboori M, Mogilner AY, et al. Safety and efficacy of stereotactic radiosurgery for tumors of the spine. *J Neurosurg* 2004;101[Suppl 3]:413–418.
7. Bhatnagar AK, Flickinger JC, Kondziolka D, et al. Stereotactic radiosurgery for four or more intracranial metastases. *Int J Radiat Oncol Biol Phys* 2006;64(3):898–903.
8. Bilsky MH, Yamada Y, Yenice KM, et al. Intensity-modulated stereotactic radiotherapy of paraspinal tumors: a preliminary report. *Neurosurgery* 2004;54:823–831.
9. Bush DA, McAllister CJ, Loredo LN, et al. Fractionated proton beam radiotherapy for acoustic neuroma. *Neurosurgery* 2002;50:270–273.
10. Chang SD, Gibbs IC, Sakamoto GT, et al. Staged stereotactic irradiation for acoustic neuroma. *Neurosurgery* 2005;56:1254–1263.
11. Combs SE, Thilmann C, Edler L, et al. Efficacy of fractionated stereotactic reirradiation in recurrent gliomas: long-term results in 172 patients treated in a single institution. *J Clin Oncol* 2005;23:8863–8869.
12. Combs SE, Volk S, Schulz-Ertner D, et al. Management of acoustic neuromas with fractionated stereotactic radiotherapy (FSRT): long-term results in 106 patients treated in a single institution. *Int J Radiat Oncol Biol Phys* 2005;63:75–81.
13. Ernst-Stecken A, Lambrecht U, Mueller R, et al. Hypofractionated stereotactic radiotherapy for primary and secondary intrapulmonary tumors: first results of a phase i/ii study. *Strahlenther Onkol* 2006;182:696–702.
14. Flickinger JC, Kondziolka D, Lunsford L. Fractionation of radiation treatment in acoustics. Rationale and evidence in comparison to radiosurgery. *Neurochirurgie* 2004;50:421–426.
15. Flickinger JC, Kondziolka D, Lunsford LD, et al. Development of a model to predict permanent symptomatic postradiosurgery injury for arteriovenous malformation patients. Arteriovenous Malformation Radiosurgery Study Group. *Int J Radiat Oncol Biol Phys* 2000;15;46:1143–1148.
16. Flickinger JC, Kondziolka D, Lunsford LD. Radiobiological analysis of tissue responses following radiosurgery. *Technol Cancer Res Treat* 2003;2:87–92.
17. Flickinger JC, Kondziolka D, Maitz AH, et al. Gamma knife radiosurgery of imaging-diagnosed intracranial meningioma. *Int J Radiat Oncol Biol Phys* 2003;56:801–806.
18. Flickinger JC, Kondziolka D, Niranjan A, et al. Acoustic neuroma radiosurgery with marginal tumor doses of 12 to 13 Gy. *Int J Radiat Oncol Biol Phys* 2004;60:225–230.
19. Flickinger JC, Kondziolka D, Pollock BE, et al. Complications from arteriovenous malformation radiosurgery: multivariate analysis and risk modeling. *Int J Radiat Oncol Biol Phys* 1997;38:485–490.
20. Flickinger JC, Pollock BE, Kondziolka D, et al. Does increased nerve length within the treatment volume improve trigeminal neuralgia radiosurgery? A prospective double-blind, randomized study. *Int J Radiat Oncol Biol Phys* 2001;51:449–454.
21. Flickinger JF, Kondziolka D, Maitz AH, et al. An analysis of the dose-response for arteriovenous malformation radiosurgery and other factors affecting obliteration. *Radiother Oncol* 2002;63:347–354.
22. Florio F, Lauriola W, Nardella M, et al. Endovascular treatment of intracranial arterio-venous malformations with Onyx embolization: preliminary experience. *Radiol Med (Torino)* 2003;106:512–520.
23. Foote KD, Friedman WA, Buatti JM, et al. Analysis of risk factors associated with radiosurgery for vestibular schwannoma. *J Neurosurg* 2001;95:440–449.
24. Friedman DP, Goldman HW, Flanders AE, et al. Stereotactic radiosurgical pallidotomy and thalamotomy with the gamma knife: MR imaging findings with clinical correlation—preliminary experience. *Radiology* 1999;212:143–150.
25. Garcia-Barros M, Paris F, Cordon-Cardo C, et al. Tumor response to radiotherapy regulated by endothelial cell apoptosis. *Science* 2003;300:1155–1159.
26. Gerszten PC, Burton SA, Ozhasoglu C, et al. Stereotactic radiosurgery for spinal metastases from renal cell carcinoma. *J Neurosurg Spine* 2005;3:288–295.
27. Gerszten PC, Burton SA, Quinn AE, et al. Radiosurgery for the treatment of spinal melanoma metastases. *Stereotact Funct Neurosurg* 2005;83:213–221.
28. Gerszten PC, Ozhasoglu C, Burton SA, et al. CyberKnife frameless stereotactic radiosurgery for spinal lesions: clinical experience in 125 cases. *Neurosurgery* 2004;55:89–98.
29. Hadjipanayis CG, Kondziolka D, Flickinger JC, et al. The role of stereotactic radiosurgery for low-grade astrocytomas. *Neurosurg Focus* 2003;14:1–7.
30. Harris AE, Lee JY, Omalu B, et al. The effect of radiosurgery during management of aggressive meningiomas. *Surg Neurol* 2003;60:298–305.
31. Hasegawa T, Kondziolka D, Spiro R, et al. Repeat radiosurgery for refractory trigeminal neuralgia. *Neurosurgery* 2002;50:494–502.
32. Hasegawa T, McInerney J, Kondziolka D, et al. Long-term results after stereotactic radiosurgery for patients with cavernous malformations. *Neurosurgery* 2002;50:1190–1198.
33. Hasegawa T, McInerney J, Kondziolka D, et al. Long-term results after stereotactic radiosurgery for patients with cavernous malformations. *Neurosurgery* 2002;50:1190–1197.
34. Henson CF, Goldman HW, Rosenwasser RH, et al. Glycerol rhizotomy versus gamma knife radiosurgery for the treatment of trigeminal neuralgia: an analysis of patients treated at one institution. *Int J Radiat Oncol Biol Phys* 2005;63:82–90.
35. Hsieh PC, Chandler JP, Bhangoo S, et al. Adjuvant gamma knife stereotactic surgery at the time of tumor progression potentially improves survival for patients with glioblastoma multiforme. *Neurosurgery* 2005;57:684–692.
36. Huang YC, Tseng CK, Chang CN, et al. LINAC radiosurgery for intracranial cavernous malformation: 10-year experience. *Clin Neurol Neurosurg* 2006;108:750–756.
37. Inoue HK. Low-dose radiosurgery for large vestibular schwannomas: long-term results of functional preservation. *J Neurosurg* 2005;102[Suppl]:111–113.
38. Iwai Y, Yamanaka K, Shiotani M, et al. Radiosurgery for acoustic neuromas: results of low-dose treatment. *Neurosurgery* 2003;53:282–288.
39. Karlsson B, Lindquist C, Steiner L. Prediction of obliteration after gamma knife surgery for cerebral arteriovenous malformations. *Neurosurgery* 1997;40:425–430.
40. Katz TS, Amdur RJ, Yachnis AT, et al. Pushing the limits of radiotherapy for atypical and malignant meningioma. *Am J Clin Oncol* 2005;28:70–74.
41. Kim DS, Park YG, Choi JU, et al. An analysis of the natural history of cavernous malformations. *Surg Neurol* 1997;48:9–17.
42. Kim MS, Pyo SY, Jeong YG, et al. Gamma knife surgery for intracranial cavernous hemangioma. *J Neurosurg* 2005;102[Suppl]:102–106.
43. King CR, Lehmann J, Adler JR, et al. CyberKnife radiotherapy for localized prostate cancer: rationale and technical feasibility. *Technol Cancer Res Treat* 2003;2:25–30.
44. Kondziolka D, Flickinger JC, Perez B. Judicious resection and/or radiosurgery for parasagittal meningiomas: outcomes from a multicenter review. Gamma Knife Meningioma Study Group. *Neurosurgery* 1998;43:405–413.
45. Kondziolka D, Levy EI, Niranjan A, et al. Long term outcomes after meningioma radiosurgery: physician and patient perspectives. *J Neurosurg* 1999;91:44–50.
46. Kondziolka D, Lunsford LD, Flickinger JC, et al. Reduction of hemorrhage risk after stereotactic radiosurgery for cavernous malformations. *J Neurosurg* 1995;83:825–831.
47. Kondziolka D, Lunsford LD, Flickinger JC. Stereotactic radiosurgery for the treatment of trigeminal neuralgia. *Clin J Pain* 2002;18:42–47.
48. Kondziolka D, Lunsford LD, Kestle JR. The natural history of cerebral cavernous malformations. *J Neurosurg* 1995;83:820–824.
49. Kondziolka D, Lunsford LD, McLaughlin MR, et al. Long-term outcomes after radiosurgery for acoustic neuromas. *N Engl J Med* 1998;339:1426–1433.
50. Kondziolka D, Lunsford LD. Stereotactic radiosurgery for squamous cell carcinoma of the nasopharynx. *Laryngoscope* 1991;101:519–522.
51. Kondziolka D, Nathoo N, Flickinger JC, et al. Long-term results after radiosurgery for benign intracranial tumors. *Neurosurgery* 2003;53:815–822.
52. Kondziolka D, Patel A, Lunsford LD, et al. Stereotactic radiosurgery plus whole brain radiotherapy versus radiotherapy alone for patients with multiple brain metastases. *Int J Radiat Oncol Biol Phys* 1999;45:427–434.
53. Niranjan A. Gamma knife thalamotomy for disabling tremor. *Arch Neurol* 2002;59:1660.
54. Kupersmith MJ, Kalish H, Epstein F, et al. Natural history of brainstem cavernous malformations. *Neurosurgery* 2001;48:47–53.
55. Lax I, Karlsson B. Prediction of complications in gamma knife radiosurgery of arteriovenous malformation. *Acta Oncol* 1996;35:49–55.

Techniques, Modalities, and Modifiers in Radiation Oncology

56. Leber KA, Bergloff J, Pendl G. Dose-response tolerance of the visual pathways and cranial nerves of the cavernous sinus to stereotactic radiosurgery. *J Neurosurg* 1998;88:43–50.

57. Lederman G, Lowry J, Wertheim S, et al. Acoustic neuroma: potential benefits of fractionated stereotactic radiosurgery. *Stereot Funct Neurosurg* 1997;69(1–4 Pt 2):175–82.

58. Lee JY, Niranjan A, McInerney J, et al. Stereotactic radiosurgery providing long-term tumor control of cavernous sinus meningiomas. *J Neurosurg* 2002;97(1):65–72.

59. Lin VY, Stewart C, Grebenyuk J, et al. Unilateral acoustic neuromas: long-term hearing results in patients managed with fractionated stereotactic radiotherapy, hearing preservation surgery, and expectantly. *Laryngoscope* 2005;115:292–296.

60. Lippitz BE, Mindus P, Meyerson BA, et al. Lesion topography and outcome after thermocapsulotomy or gamma knife capsulotomy for obsessive-compulsive disorder: relevance of the right hemisphere. *Neurosurgery* 1999;44:452–460.

61. Liscak R, Vladyka V, Simonova G, et al. Gamma knife surgery of brain cavernous hemangiomas. *J Neurosurg* 2005;102[Suppl]:207–213.

62. Liu KD, Chung WY, Wu HM, et al. Gamma knife surgery for cavernous hemangiomas: an analysis of 125 patients. *J Neurosurg* 2005;102[Suppl]:81–86.

63. Mabanta SR, Buatti JM, Friedman WA, et al. Linear accelerator radiosurgery for nonacoustic schwannomas. *Int J Radiat Oncol Biol Phys* 1999;43:545–548.

64. Madsen BL, Hsi RA, Pham HT, et al. Intrafractional stability of the prostate using a stereotactic radiotherapy technique. *Int J Radiat Oncol Biol Phys* 2003;57:1285–1291.

65. Maesawa S, Flickinger JC, Kondziolka D, et al. Repeated radiosurgery for incompletely obliterated arteriovenous malformations. *J Neurosurg* 2000;92:961–970.

66. Mahajan A, McCutcheon IE, Suki D, et al. Case-control study of stereotactic radiosurgery for recurrent glioblastoma multiforme. *J Neurosurg* 2005;103:210–217.

67. Malik I, Rowe JG, Walton L, et al. The use of stereotactic radiosurgery in the management of meningiomas. *Br J Neurosurg* 2005;19:13–20.

68. Martin JM, Katati M, Lopez E, et al. Linear accelerator radiosurgery in treatment of central neurocytomas. *Acta Neurochir (Wien)* 2003;145:749–754.

69. Maruyama K, Kawahara N, Shin M, et al. The risk of hemorrhage after radiosurgery for cerebral arteriovenous malformations. *N Engl J Med* 2005;352:146–153.

70. McDermott MW, Berger MS, Kunwar S, et al. Stereotactic radiosurgery and interstitial brachytherapy for glial neoplasms. *J Neurooncol* 2004;69:83–100.

71. Mehta MP, Tsao MN, Whelan TJ, et al. The American Society for Therapeutic Radiology and Oncology (ASTRO) evidence–based review of the role of radiosurgery for brain metastases. *Int J Radiat Oncol Biol Phys* 2005;63:37–46.

72. Mehta MP, Tsao MN, Whelan TJ, et al. The American Society for Therapeutic Radiology and Oncology (ASTRO) evidence-based review of the role of radiosurgery for brain metastases. *Int J Radiat Oncol Biol Phys* 2005;63:37–46.

73. Meijer OW, Vandertop WP, Baayen JC, et al. Single-fraction vs. fractionated linac-based stereotactic radiosurgery for vestibular schwannoma: a single-institution study. *Int J Radiat Oncol Biol Phys* 2003;56:1390–1396.

74. Mingione V, Yen CP, Vance ML, et al. Gamma surgery in the treatment of nonsecretory pituitary macroadenoma. *J Neurosurg* 2006;104:876–883.

75. Modha A, Gutin PH. Diagnosis and treatment of atypical and anaplastic meningiomas: a review. *Neurosurgery* 2005;57:538–550.

76. Morita A, Coffey RJ, Foote RL, et al. Risk of injury to cranial nerves after gamma knife radiosurgery for skull base meningiomas: experience in 88 patients. *J Neurosurg* 1999;90:42–49.

77. Muacevic A, Jess-Hempen A, Tonn JC, et al. Results of outpatient gamma knife radiosurgery for primary therapy of acoustic neuromas. *Acta Neurochir Suppl* 2004;91:75–78.

78. Narod SA, Parry DM, Parboosingh J, et al. Neurofibromatosis type 2 appears to be a genetically homogeneous disease. *Am J Hum Genet* 1992;51:486–496.

79. Nicolato A, Foroni R, Alessandrini F, et al. The role of Gamma Knife radiosurgery in the management of cavernous sinus meningiomas. *Int J Radiat Oncol Biol Phys* 2002;53:992–1000.

80. Niranjan A, Jawahar A, Kondziolka D, et al. A comparison of surgical approaches for the management of tremor: radiofrequency thalamotomy, gamma knife thalamotomy and thalamic stimulation. *Stereotact Funct Neurosurg* 1999;72:178–184.

81. Ohye C, Shibazaki T, Sato S. Gamma knife thalamotomy for movement disorders: evaluation of the thalamic lesion and clinical results. *J Neurosurg* 2005;102[Suppl]:234–240.

82. Okun MS, Stover NP, Subramanian T, et al. Complications of gamma knife surgery for Parkinson disease. *Arch Neurol* 2001;58:1995–2002.

83. Ondra SL, Troupp H, George ED, et al. The natural history of symptomatic arteriovenous malformations of the brain: a 24-year follow-up assessment. *J Neurosurg* 1990;73:387–391.

84. Paek SH, Chung HT, Jeong SS, et al. Hearing preservation after gamma knife stereotactic radiosurgery of vestibular schwannoma. *Cancer* 2005;104:580–590.

85. Pan L, Wang EM, Zhang N, et al. Long-term results of Leksell gamma knife surgery for trigeminal schwannomas. *J Neurosurg* 2005;102[Suppl]:220–224.

86. Pollock BE, Flickinger JC, Lunsford LD, et al. Factors that affect the hemorrhage risk of arteriovenous malformations. *Stroke* 1996;27:1–6.

87. Pollock BE, Flickinger JC, Lunsford LD, et al. Hemorrhage risk after radiosurgery for arteriovenous malformations. *Neurosurgery* 1996;38:.

88. Pollock BE, Garces YI, Stafford SL, et al. Stereotactic radiosurgery for cavernous malformations. *J Neurosurg* 2000;93:987–991.

89. Pollock BE, Kondziolka D, Flickinger JC, et al. Preservation of cranial nerve function after radiosurgery for nonacoustic schwannomas. *Neurosurgery* 1993;33:597–601.

90. Pollock BE, Lunsford LD, Kondziolka D, et al. Outcome analysis of acoustic neuroma management: a comparison of microsurgery and stereotactic radiosurgery. *Neurosurgery* 1995;36:215–225.

91. Pollock BE, Stafford SL. Results of stereotactic radiosurgery for patients with imaging defined cavernous sinus meningiomas. *Int J Radiat Oncol Biol Phys* 2005;62:1427–1431.

92. Pouratian N, Sheehan J, Jagannathan J, et al. Gamma knife radiosurgery for medically and surgically refractory prolactinomas. *Neurosurgery* 2006;59:255–266.

93. Rades D, Schild SE. Value of postoperative stereotactic radiosurgery and conventional radiotherapy for incompletely resected typical neurocytomas. *Cancer* 2006;106:1140–1143.

94. Regis J, Hayashi M, Eupierre LP, et al. Gamma knife surgery for epilepsy related to hypothalamic hamartomas. *Acta Neurochir Suppl* 2004;91:33–50.

95. Regis J, Metellus P, Hayashi M, et al. Prospective controlled trial of gamma knife surgery for essential trigeminal neuralgia. *J Neurosurg* 2006;104:913–924.

96. Regis J, Pellet W, Delsanti C, et al. Functional outcome after gamma knife surgery or microsurgery for vestibular schwannomas. *J Neurosurg* 2002;97:1091–1100.

97. Regis J, Rey M, Bartolomei F, et al. Gamma knife surgery in mesial temporal lobe epilepsy: a prospective multicenter study. *Epilepsia* 2004;45:504–515.

98. Rowe JG, Radatz MW, Walton L, et al. Gamma knife stereotactic radiosurgery for unilateral acoustic neuromas. *J Neurol Neurosurg Psychiatr* 2003;74:1536–1542.

99. Sakamoto T, Shirato H, Takeichi N, et al. Annual rate of hearing loss falls after fractionated stereotactic irradiation for vestibular schwannoma. *Radiother Oncol* 2001;60:45–48.

100. Schefter TE, Kavanagh BD, Raben D, et al. A phase I/II trial of stereotactic body radiation therapy (SBRT) for lung metastases: Initial report of dose escalation and early toxicity. *Int J Radiat Oncol Biol Phys* 2006;66(4 Suppl):S120.

101. Schefter TE, Kavanagh BD, Raben D, et al. A phase I/II trial of stereotactic body radiation therapy (SBRT) for lung metastases: Initial report of dose escalation and early toxicity. *Int J Radiat Oncol Biol Phys* 2006;66(4 Suppl):S120.

102. Selch MT, Pedroso A, Lee SP, et al. Stereotactic radiotherapy for the treatment of acoustic neuromas. *J Neurosurg* 2004;101[Suppl 3]:362–372.

103. Shaw E, Scott C, Souhami L, et al. Single dose radiosurgical treatment of recurrent previously irradiated primary brain tumors and brain metastases: final report of RTOG protocol 90–05. *Int J Radiat Oncol Biol Phys* 2000;47:291–298.

104. Sheehan JP, Niranjan A, Sheehan JM, et al. Stereotactic radiosurgery for pituitary adenomas: an intermediate review of its safety, efficacy, and role in the neurosurgical treatment armamentarium. *J Neurosurg* 2005;102:678–691.

105. Shirato H, Sakamoto T, Sawamura Y, et al. Comparison between observation policy and fractionated stereotactic radiotherapy (SRT) as an initial management for vestibular schwannoma. *Int J Radiat Oncol Biol Phys* 1999;44:545–550.

106. Sirin S, Kondziolka D, Niranjan A, et al. Prospective staged volume radiosurgery for large arteriovenous malformations: indications and outcomes in otherwise untreatable patients. *Neurosurgery* 2006;58:17–27.

107. Souhami L, Seiferheld W, Brachman D, et al. Randomized comparison of stereotactic radiosurgery followed by conventional radiotherapy with carmustine to conventional radiotherapy with carmustine for patients with glioblastoma multiforme: report of Radiation Therapy Oncology Group 93-05 protocol. *Int J Radiat Oncol Biol Phys* 2004;60:853–860.

108. Stafford SL, Pollock BE, Leavitt JA, et al. A study on the radiation tolerance of the optic nerves and chiasm after stereotactic radiosurgery. *Int J Radiat Oncol Biol Phys* 2003;55:1177–1181.

109. Szeifert GT, Massager N, DeVriendt D, et al. Observations of intracranial neoplasms treated with gamma knife radiosurgery. *J Neurosurg* 2002;97:623–626.

110. Tishler RB, Loeffler JS, Lunsford LD, et al. Tolerance of cranial nerves of the cavernous sinus to radiosurgery. *Int J Radiat Oncol Biol Phys* 1993;27:215–221.

111. Tyler-Kabara E, Kondziolka D, Flickinger JC, et al. Stereotactic radiosurgery for residual neurocytoma. Report of four cases. *J Neurosurg* 2001;95:879–882.

112. Unger F, Schrottner O, Feichtinger M, et al. Stereotactic radiosurgery for hypothalamic hamartomas. *Acta Neurochir Suppl* 2002;84:57–63.

113. Voynov G, Heron DE, Burton S, et al. Frameless stereotactic radiosurgery for recurrent head and neck carcinoma. *Technol Cancer Res Treat* 2006;5:529–535.

114. Weber DC, Chan AW, Bussiere MR, et al. Proton beam radiosurgery for vestibular schwannoma: tumor control and cranial nerve toxicity. *Neurosurgery* 2003;53:577–586.

115. Williams JA. Fractionated stereotactic radiotherapy for acoustic neuromas. *Int J Radiat Oncol Biol Phys* 2002;54:500–504.

116. Wowra B, Muacevic A, Jess-Hempen A, et al. Outpatient gamma knife surgery for vestibular schwannoma: definition of the therapeutic profile based on a 10-year experience. *J Neurosurg* 2005;102[Suppl]:114–118.

117. Young RF, Jacques S, Mark R, et al. Gamma knife thalamotomy for treatment of tremor: long-term results. *J Neurosurg* 2000;93[Suppl 3]:128–135.

118. Young RF, Vermeulen S, Posewitz A, et al. Pallidotomy with the gamma knife: a positive experience. *Stereotact Funct Neurosurg* 1998;70[Suppl 1]:218–228.

119. Zabel A, Debus J, Thilmann C, et al. Management of benign cranial nonacoustic schwannomas by fractionated stereotactic radiotherapy. *Int J Cancer* 2001;96:356–362.

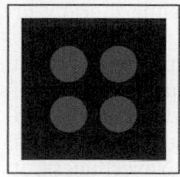

Chapter 16
Stereotactic Irradiation of Tumors Outside the Central Nervous System

Brian D. Kavanagh, Jeffrey D. Bradley, Robert D. Timmerman

Departing from the established traditions of conventionally fractionated external beam radiotherapy, in the late 1980s and early 1990s groups of investigators in Sweden and Japan began to explore the use of alternative hypofractionated radiation treatment regimens for lung, liver, and selected other malignant extracranial tumors. In essence these clinical researchers were modifying techniques proven clinically valuable in the context of cranial and spine stereotactic radiosurgery in an effort to exploit the efficiency and biological potency of high–dose-per-fraction irradiation (23). This idea was soon also appreciated for its clinical promise by researchers in Germany and the United States, and interest has now spread to numerous centers worldwide.

Pioneers in this field initially used customized ancillary equipment constructed in their own institutions to immobilize patients and to adapt ordinary linear accelerators for the task of precise internal tumor targeting. Now, however, the administration of high-dose, tightly focused external radiation treatment is greatly facilitated by a wide assortment of commercially available systems that immobilize patients, address the problem of respiratory motion during treatment, and ensure accurate treatment with the use of image guidance. The newest generation of linear accelerators from several manufacturers are either exclusively dedicated to cranial or extracranial stereotactic radiotherapy or are equipped with a built-in package of features that provide an easy means of administering this type of treatment.

Stereotactic body radiation therapy (SBRT) is the term applied in the United States by the American Society of Therapeutic Radiology and Oncology (ASTRO) for the management and delivery of image-guided high-dose radiation therapy with tumor-ablative intent within a course of treatment that does not exceed 5 fractions (29). Other terms have been variously applied in the past to describe what is now called SBRT (for example, extracranial radiosurgery and extracranial stereotactic radioablation), and for simplicity we will apply the term SBRT throughout in the description of techniques that might have been described otherwise in the past but now fall under the current definition of SBRT.

Biological and Oncological Rationale for Stereotactic Body Radiation Therapy

The appeal of SBRT is based upon the nonlinear relationship between radiation dose and cytotoxic effect, whereby one or a few large individual doses of radiation therapy have substantially more cell-killing effect than the same dose of radiation given in smaller individual doses. This concept has been extensively reviewed (9) and is largely predicated upon the linear-quadratic (LQ) model of radiation dose response that has become widely accepted for the purpose of comparing the biological potency of different schedules of conventionally fractionated radiation therapy.

Although preclinical and clinical data support the concept that treatments using large dose per fraction are more tumorici-dal than the same total dose given with conventionally fractionated regimens, mathematically modeling the complex biological interactions with radiation is inherently difficult. Furthermore, some have questioned whether the LQ model is accurate in the range of the high doses applied with SBRT, especially given that only limited data are available to characterize clinical outcomes following multiple radiation doses in the range of 10 to 20 Gy, as are commonly applied with SBRT. Guerrero and Li (13), for example, have argued that it would be appropriate to modify the LQ model to incorporate features of the lethal–potentially lethal (LPL) model, also called the Curtis model (5). One key difference between the Curtis LPL model and the LQ model is that the former more thoroughly accounts for ongoing radiation repair processes that occur *during* the individual radiation treatment. The net result is a substantial difference in the predicted tumor cell kill at SBRT-level doses: for a dose of approximately 20 Gy, for example, the LQ model predicts several orders of magnitude greater cell kill than the Curtis model (13).

An experimental model of the effect of intrafraction radiation repair during cranial stereotactic radiosurgery supports the notion that significant repair can occur within the clinically realistic variations of time of an individual high-dose treatment. In this context Benedict et al. (1) demonstrated that for a dose of 18 Gy, increasing the length of treatment from approximately 30 minutes to 2 hours corresponded to an order of magnitude decrement in cytotoxicity. It is plausible that a similar degree of intrafractional repair could occur during SBRT, where the total length of time for an individual treatment can vary widely depending on the complexity of the beam arrangement and particular technique employed. Other theoretical analyses are concordant with this concern (10).

The rationale for evaluating SBRT for prostate cancer is based on a fundamentally different consideration. Here, applying the LQ model-based assumptions and interpretation, Fowler et al. (8) have contended that since prostate cancer is believed to have a relatively low α/β ratio, likely in the range of 1 to 2 Gy, a hypofractionated course of therapy should be advantageous. If this estimate of α/β for prostate cancer is correct, then high doses per fraction, for example in the range of 6 to 9 Gy per fraction, should provide a more favorable therapeutic ratio than a conventionally fractionated regimen.

This proposition is at first counterintuitive to traditional dogma concerning the normal tissue late effects risks associated with high–dose-per-fraction treatment. However, it should be appreciated that this concern applies only for the situation in which the α/β ratio of adjacent normal tissue is markedly lower than the tumor α/β ratio, in which case a large dose per fraction would have a disproportionately greater impact upon the normal tissues.

SBRT has also been used as a noninvasive and efficient means of eradicating discrete metastatic tumors, and the case for this application can be constructed in accordance with any of numerous overlapping lines of evidence or conceptual theories of cancer growth and dissemination, listed here in order of increasing complexity: (a) the phenomenological, (b) the patterns of failure concept, (c) the theory of oligometastases, or (d) the Norton-Simon hypothesis.

The most straightforward argument for SBRT in the setting of isolated sites of metastatic disease is what might be termed the phenomenological. There have been numerous reports of patients enjoying a high rate of 3- to 5-year survival following other forms of aggressive local treatment (surgical resection, radiofrequency ablation, cryotherapy, and so forth) for limited metastases in the liver or lung from an assortment of solid tumor types. On one level, then, SBRT can be considered a noninvasive substitute for other local modalities if it can be demonstrated to provide similar efficacy and the same or less toxicity.

The use of SBRT in the setting of metastatic disease might be alternatively couched in terms of a patterns-of-failure model. An example of one application of this concept already commonplace in radiation oncology would be the practice patterns that have been employed for many years in the combined modality treatment of lymphomas. Here, systemic treatment with chemotherapy is combined with involved field radiotherapy on the supposition that the sites of disease that were grossly evident at the time of diagnosis contain the highest number of clonogenic cells and are thus least likely to be completely eliminated by the chemotherapy. Involved field radiotherapy is then given in an effort to eradicate tumor cells in the sites most likely to harbor residual disease. SBRT given to sites of residual disease following some form of systemic therapy might be given with this goal in mind.

Yet another argument that has been advanced in support SBRT in this setting can be called the theory of oligometastases. As articulated by Hellman and Weichselbaum (16), this viewpoint considers that there could be a subgroup of patients with metastatic disease that is intermediate between completely absent and widely metastatic. For such patients the entire systemic disease burden is then entirely contained within the finite number of individual sites of gross disease recognized by the pertinent imaging studies. This condition would reflect an intermediate point in the natural history of that individual's cancer; therefore, these patients might be cured if their limited numbers of metastatic sites are eradicated.

A fourth, perhaps more nuanced oncology theory offered in support of SBRT in this setting is a modification of the Norton-Simon hypothesis. This conjecture is based on the experimental observation that in animal models, the total burden of cancer cells increases in a manner described by Gompertzian kinetics from beneath the threshold of detectability through a phase of rapid growth and onward toward a plateau level that is lethal to the host (28). This observation was translated into clinical trials by postulating that traditional DNA-targeted chemotherapy is expected to render the greatest degree of cytotoxicity to cancer cells in the rapid phase of growth, when there is higher mitotic activity that renders DNA more vulnerable. Trials testing "dose-dense" chemotherapy were designed to exploit the enhanced chemosensitivity of rapidly growing cancer cells with the use of frequent dosing schedules that capture tumors repeatedly at relatively smaller volume, without allowing as much time for regrowth into relatively less sensitive, near-plateau tumor volumes (7).

Bolstered by the success of dose-dense chemotherapy in the treatment of breast cancer, SBRT given according to the tenets of the Norton-Simon hypothesis would have two goals:

1. to reduce the patient's total burden of disease in such a way that the remaining cancer within the patient's body enters into a state of relatively higher growth fraction and is thus more susceptible to cytotoxic systemic agents; and, more importantly,
2. to prevent or delay as long as possible the condition of lethal tumor burden that is fatal to the patient (21).

SBRT could be construed in this sense as a local therapy used for the purpose of systemic disease-burden cytoreduction, possibly as a complement to traditional cytotoxic systemic therapy or novel molecularly targeted agents.

There is overlap among all of these perspectives, and it would be nearly impossible to prove the exclusive validity of any one above another. For example, improved disease-free and overall survival following the use of SBRT to metastatic sites of disease would support any of these theories. Nevertheless, it is very important to consider the larger context of cancer treatment in which SBRT is applied for metastatic disease, and these theories can serve to frame the stated primary objectives of clinical trials in which SBRT is studied as a treatment for metastatic disease, either alone or in combination with a systemic agent.

●● Practical Stereotactic Body Radiation Therapy Physics and Dosimetry

In 2003 the American Association of Physicist in Medicine (AAPM) formed a task group (TG101; S. Benedict, Chair) that was charged with cataloging and synthesizing the published literature of SBRT, with aims that included determining the appropriate criteria for establishing an SBRT program, the necessary components of proper quality assurance for SBRT, and standards for adequate documentation of SBRT. The AAPM TG101 report will serve to expand and augment the ASTRO guidelines, which include the recommendations that the following components must be in place for an institution initiating an SBRT program (23):

1. Qualified personnel:
   a. Board-certified radiation oncologist
   b. Qualified medical physicist
   c. Licensed radiation therapist
   d. Other support staff as indicated (dosimetrists, oncology nurses, and so forth);
2. Ongoing machine quality assurance program;
3. Documentation in accordance with the *ACR Practice Guideline for Communication: Radiation Oncology*;
4. Quality control of treatment accessories;
5. Quality control of planning and treatment images;
6. Quality control of treatment planning system;
7. Simulation and treatment systems that account for systematic and random errors associated with setup and target motion in a manner that is based on actual measurement of organ motion and setup uncertainty.

Proper patient repositioning, target localization, and management of breathing-related motion are essential for SBRT. A variety of patient immobilization devices are available, including several types of body frames with external fiducial markers. So-called frameless systems incorporate ultrasound, kilovolt, or near real-time computed tomography (CT) scanning to verify the location of internal targets relative to the beams to be used. It should be appreciated that since SBRT treatment sessions are lengthier than conventional external beam treatments, patient comfort is an important issue.

Breathing-related motion control devices and systems fall into three general categories: (a) dampening, (b) gating, and (c) tracking or "chasing." Respiratory dampening techniques include systems of abdominal compression intended to diminish one of the largest contributors to breathing-related motion, namely diaphragmatic excursion, by obliging the inspiratory–expiratory lung motion pattern to involve more intracostal expansion and shallower breathing overall. Also included in this category are the systems employing breath-holding maneuvers to stabilize the tumor in a reproducible stage of the respiratory cycle (e.g., deep inspiration). Gating systems for SBRT, as for any radiotherapy application, follow the respiratory cycle using a surrogate indicator for respiratory motion, for example, chest wall motion, and employ an electronic beam activation trigger allowing irradiation to occur only during a specified range of expected tumor locations. Tracking or "chasing" systems move the radiation beam or patient to follow the movement of the tumor.

Regardless of the system employed, the procedure of treatment planning must include the same consideration for respiratory motion management to be used during treatment. Despite available motion control equipment, some positional uncertainty will remain. The planning target volume (PTV) margins used to account for this residual motion of the gross tumor volume (GTV) will typically range from 5 to 10 mm.

The word "stereotactic" has heretofore usually implied that some sort of external reference markers indexed to internal structures facilitate internal target relocalization, although the definition has loosened to include systems of image-guided radiation therapy (IGRT). Indeed, implicit in the current definition of SBRT is the assumption that some form of IGRT will be used for treatment delivery.

Most reports describing SBRT published to date have employed high-energy photons (x-rays) as the source of therapeutic radiation, although other particles could also be used. There is no absolute standard for the combination of beam or arc angles ideal for any given clinical situation, and each case can present unique challenges. In general to achieve a tightly focused high-dose distribution within the PTV and rapid dose falloff outside the PTV, a combination of multiple (often seven to 10) noncoplanar beams or multiple arcs are required. Intensity modulation across the individual beams or arc segments can be incorporated within SBRT.

Clinical Experience with Stereotactic Body Radiation Therapy in Selected Sites

Liver

The two major reasons for considering SBRT for hepatocellular cancer (HCC) is that underlying severe liver disease often renders patients medically inoperable and that other nonsurgical therapies have generally achieved at best rather modest success in that setting. Blomgren et al. (14) reported the outcomes following SBRT of nine patients with HCCs and two with other primary intrahepatic cancers. Twenty discrete tumors were treated in these patients, and a widely variable dose schedule was employed (minimum total doses, 14 to 45 Gy in 1 to 3 fractions). Partial or complete response was observed in 70% of the lesions. Currently, there is an ongoing trial of SBRT for HCC at the Princess Margaret Hospital.

There have been three studies of SBRT for liver tumors in which local control is reported as an actuarial estimate more than 1 year after SBRT. In 2001 Wulf et al. (39) from Würzburg reported outcomes for the treatment of 24 liver tumors—23 metastases and one cholangiocarcinoma. Tumor volumes were not reported. A clinical target volume (CTV) was defined as the GTV plus 2- to 3-mm margin in all directions. The median CTV was 50 cm^3 (range, 9 to 516 cm^3). The PTV was then created by adding 5 mm radially and 10 mm superiorly and inferiorly to the CTV. The PTV received a dose of 30 Gy in three fractions, generally prescribed to the 65% isodose line. The 18-month actuarial control rate was 61%.

In 2005 Herfarth and Debus (17) reported an experience that included patients enrolled within a prospective phase II trial of liver SBRT plus others treated in the same manner following completion of enrollment in the trial. The 70 patients were treated with a single fraction of liver SBRT, sometimes termed liver radiosurgery. Details of tumor volume were not reported. After a median dose of 22 Gy, the 18-month actuarial control rate was 66%. Patients with metastases from colorectal primaries experienced lower tumor control rates than others.

In 2006 investigators from the University of Colorado and collaborating institutions reported an interim analysis of a phase I or II trial of liver SBRT (22). The trial was a continuation of a previously reported phase I study in which it had been demonstrated that dose escalation to a level of 60 Gy in three fractions of liver SBRT was safe and feasible (33). Patients with liver metastases were eligible if they met the following criteria: (a) maximum tumor diameter <6 cm; (b) ≤3 discrete lesions; (c) treatment planning confirmed ≥700 cm^3 of normal liver receives ≤15 Gy over the entire course of SBRT. The GTV was expanded 5 to 10 mm to yield the planning target volume, which received 60 Gy in three fractions of SBRT over 3 to 14 days in the phase II component of the study. For 28 discrete lesions evaluable for analysis (median GTV 14 cm^3, range 1 to 98), the 18-month actuarial local control estimate was 93%. Toxicity was generally mild, with only one instance of grade 3 toxicity in subcutaneous tissue that resulted from an unintentional dose hot spot. In retrospect, the authors concluded that this specific instance of toxicity could likely have been easily avoided with the use of extra beams that avoided overlapping entrance and exit doses so that the dose falloff would be more isotropic within the normal tissues superficial to the tumor.

The normal liver tissue dose constraint applied in the University of Colorado SBRT trials is noteworthy insofar as it differed from what has been applied in trials of conventionally fractionated radiotherapy to liver tumors. Rather than an application of the normal tissue complication probability (NTCP) formalism, the approach taken was an application of the critical volume model, initially conceived by Yaes and Kalend (42). Applicable for organs of parallel structure, the crux of this application is to work backward, in a sense, from an estimate of how much volume of the organ is essential and must be protected from functional ablation. The estimate for liver that at least 700 cm^3 should receive <15 Gy during a three-fraction SBRT course was derived from a combination of prior reports of outcomes after partial hepatectomy documenting approximate minimum volumes required and estimates of the effects of that dose of radiation extrapolated from prior reports of conventionally fractionated treatment (33).

One feature of the normal tissue effect of liver SBRT consistently observed within the first few months after SBRT is a zone of hypodensity observed on follow-up CT scans corresponding to the volume that received approximately 30 Gy (33). This phenomenon, first described by Herfarth et al. (18) following single dose liver SBRT, is of uncertain etiology. There is no known clinical consequence associated with the finding, but it can cloud the assessment of tumor response within the first few months after liver SBRT. Herfarth labeled this initial appearance a type I reaction, characterized by hypodensity in the portal-venous phase and isodensity in the late phase of a contrast-enhanced scan. A type 2 reaction, typically occurring later, involves hypodensity in the portal-venous phase followed by hyperdensity in late phase, and a type 3 reaction includes isodensity or hyperdensity in the portal-venous phase and hyperdensity in the late phase.

Case Study

Liver Stereotactic Body Radiation Therapy

A 45-year-old female had been diagnosed with stage IV breast cancer 2 years previously. Biopsy-proven liver metastases were present at the time of diagnosis. Numerous systemic agents had been given, most recently gemcitabine and trastuzumab. Although all other measurable or assessable sites of disease were stable or regressing, a mass in the liver had progressed from 2.5 by 2.9 cm to 6.0 by 4.2 cm within the past 3 months. Because the patient was tolerating the regimen well and apparently having a response in most sites, she was offered SBRT in an effort to eradicate tumor in the liver.

The lesion diameter (>6 cm) rendered the patient ineligible for the ongoing University of Colorado phase II trial of SBRT for liver metastases, and the dose given was lower than the protocol doses (Fig. 16.1). The 53 cm^3 GTV was expanded by 5 mm radially and 10 mm in the superior-inferior direction to generate the PTV. The dose distribution shown was administered in three fractions within 1 week using multiple dynamic conformal arcs and a controlled breath-holding device. The nominal prescription dose was 45 Gy. The maximum point dose was 59 Gy, and the equivalent uniform dose was 54 Gy. The volume of normal liver receiving <15 Gy was 273 cm^3. The portion of the right kidney receiving above 15 Gy was 13%.

Follow-up scans at 6 months and 10 months show a Herfarth type 2 reaction with hyperdensity in the treated normal liver (18). There is also the development of atrophy in the ablated normal liver parenchyma surrounding the lesion, a phenomenon that has also been reported (22).

Lung

Among the early exploratory studies of lung SBRT for stage I non–small-cell lung cancer were the experiences from Karolinska Hospital in Stockholm (3) and from the National Medical Defense Hospital in Saitama (37), which prompted others to initiate prospective clinical trials. Numerous formal prospective studies of SBRT for medically inoperable non–small-cell lung cancer have been now been reported (23–29), and they are summarized in Table 16.1.

One important observation from the Indiana University studies was that although the treatment was generally well tolerated, tumor location near large airways in the vicinity of the pulmonary hilum (called the zone of the proximal bronchial tree) was associated with a markedly higher risk of toxicity. For this reason, in the RTOG 0236 study (R. Timmerman, PI) of SBRT for medically inoperable NSCLC, patients with tumors located in the zone of the proximal bronchial tree were excluded. Accrual to RTOG 0236 was completed in late 2006. The primary end point was local control, and the secondary end points included disease-free survival and overall survival. The SBRT dose used was 20 Gy in three fractions (60 Gy total). The maximum tumor diameter was 5 cm.

A Japanese Cooperative Oncology Group study of lung SBRT for stage I lung cancer modeled after the Kyoto University trial is now ongoing, and three more RTOG studies are in development. First, as a follow-up to RTOG 0236, RTOG 0624 (B. Kavanagh, PI) is planned to have the same fundamental study design and SBRT specifications but will involve the addition of systemic agents to the SBRT. Another, RTOG 0618 (R. Timmerman, PI) will be very similar to RTOG 0236 except that medically operable patients will be eligible. There will be close surveillance following SBRT, and surgical salvage will be offered for patients with suspected local failure. Finally, RTOG 0633 (A. Bezjak, J. Bradley, L. Gaspar, co-PIs) will be a phase I dose escalation study for patients with tumors located within the zone of the proximal bronchial tree.

In the realm of SBRT for lung metastases, fewer prospective studies have been reported. In the University of Colorado phase I SBRT trial for lung metastases (34), eligible patients had one to three pulmonary metastases from a solid tumor, cumulative tumor diameter <7 cm, and adequate pulmonary function (FEV1 >1.0 L). The PTV was typically constructed from the GTV by adding a 5 mm radial and 10 mm cranio-caudal margin. The first cohort received 48 Gy to the PTV in three fractions. The SBRT dose was escalated in subsequent cohorts up to a preselected maximum of 60 Gy in three fractions. The percentage of normal lung receiving more than 15 Gy (V15) was restricted to <35%. Dose-limiting toxicity (DLT) included acute grade 3 lung or esophageal toxicity or any acute grade 4 toxicity. No patient experienced a DLT, and the SBRT dose was escalated to 60 Gy in three fractions without reaching a maximum tolerated dose. No consistent significant effects upon pulmonary functions tests were noted. The trial continues on now as a phase II study, with local control as a primary end point. The RTOG will also be launching a phase I to II trial of SBRT for lung metastases (V. Stieber, PI).

Characteristic normal tissue changes in surrounding parenchyma have been observed in this trial. Typically, a brisk fibrotic response will develop in the vicinity of the treated lesion. The tumor itself becomes less well defined. Ultimately, residual fibrosis in a configuration that recapitulates the region of lung that received approximately 20 Gy or more can develop, and faint residual metabolic activity can sometimes be observed in this volume for many months on positron emission tomography scan. Traditional CT scan-based tumor response criteria are not easily applied.

Case Study

Lung Stereotactic Body Radiation Therapy

A 74-year-old female had undergone wedge resection for a pT1N0M0 non–small-cell cancer of the right lung 7 years previously. She had a right pneumonectomy 3 years later as salvage treatment for a locoregional recurrence. She was later observed to have developed a left lung nodule on a surveillance chest x-ray, and needle biopsy proved it to be a non–small-cell lung cancer, presumed to be a second primary. Staging studies revealed no other sites of disease. She was given systemic therapy and enjoyed a transient minor response and then regrowth of the lesion (Fig. 16-2).

The patient used supplemental oxygen, 2 L per minute at bedtime and occasionally during the day. She was offered SBRT as potentially curative therapy for a new T1N0M0 lung cancer. The 4 cm^3 GTV was expanded by 5 mm radially and 10 mm in the superior-inferior direction to generate the 29 cm^3 PTV. The dose distribution shown was administered in three fractions within 1 week using multiple dynamic conformal arcs. The patient did not comfortably tolerate a breath-holding technique because of her supplemental oxygen requirements; therefore, an abdominal compression technique was used during simulation and treatment. The nominal prescription dose was 60 Gy. The maximum point dose was 79 Gy, and the equivalent uniform dose was 72 Gy. The portion of normal lung receiving <15 Gy was 12.7%.

Spine

Spinal SBRT has also been labeled spinal radiosurgery when treatment is given in a single fraction. The earliest investigation into this area was that of Hamilton et al. (14,15), who used a rigid immobilization with a device surgically attached to the spinal column. Conservative doses in the range of 8 to 10 Gy were given in one fraction to nine patients with recurrent lesions in the spine following prior conventional radiotherapy. Spinal cord doses were very low using this technique (0.5 to 3.2 Gy). Limited follow-up suggested a favorable clinical effect in some patients, and no complications were observed. More recently, less invasive techniques have been investigated.

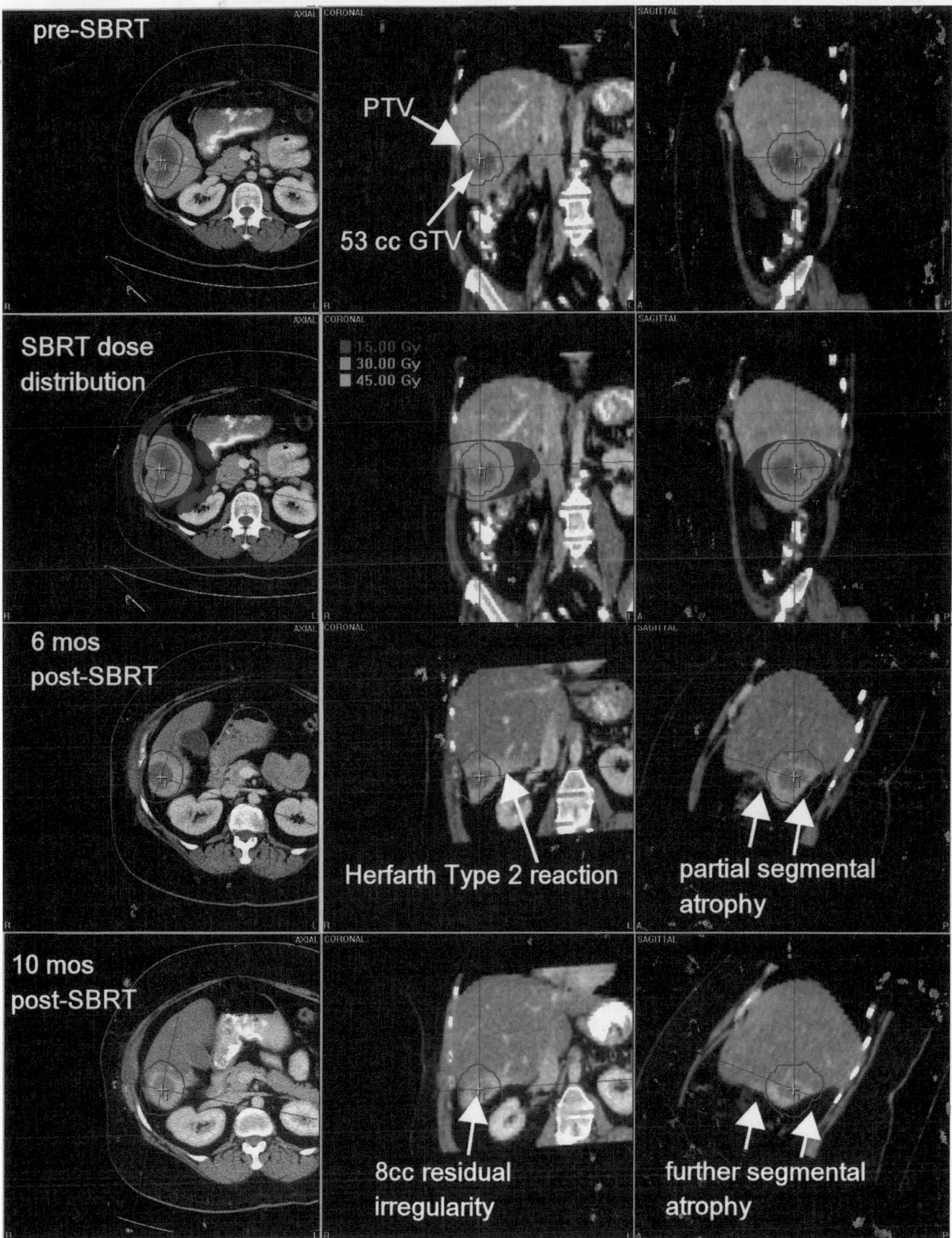

FIGURE 16.1. Example of liver stereotactic body radiation therapy (SBRT). Top panel, pre-SBRT planning CT images with thin arrow pointing to the gross tumor volume (GTV) and wide arrow showing the planning target volume (PTV), which is outlined. Second panel, SBRT composite dose distribution. Third panel, images obtained 6 months (mos) post-SBRT illustrating a Herfarth type 2 reaction in adjacent parenchyma and partial segmental atrophy. The bottom panel shows images 10 months post-SBRT, indicating continued tumor regression as the ablated liver volume continues to recede.

Table 16.1	PROSPECTIVE STUDIES OF STEREOTACTIC BODY RADIATION THERAPY FOR PRIMARY LUNG CANCER			
Institution (Reference)		N	SBRT Dose and Fractionation	Results
Indiana University (26,36)		47	24–66 Gy/3 fractions	Phase I study; MTD not reached for T1 lesions; MTD 66 Gy for T2 lesions
Indiana University (35)		70	60–66 Gy/3 fractions	1-y local control 98%
Aarhus University (19)		40	45 Gy/3 fractions	2-y local control 85%
Kyoto University (27)		45	48 Gy/4 fractions	2-y local control 95%
Air Force General Hospital, Beijing (40)		43	50 Gy/10 fractions	1-y local control 95%
University of Marburg (11)		33	30 Gy/1 fraction	1-y local control 94%

MTD, maximum tolerated dose; *N*, number of patients enrolled; SBRT, stereotactic body radiation therapy

Ryu et al. (30) at the Henry Ford Hospital initially studied the treatment of spine metastases with initial fractionated radiotherapy followed by a spinal radiosurgery boost (6 to 8 Gy), observing prompt relief of pain in nearly all 10 treated patients. In a subsequent study of single fraction spinal radiosurgery alone (10 to 16 Gy), this group observed complete or partial pain relief in 85% of the 49 patients treated (31). Perhaps even more importantly, pain relief was rapid after SBRT, sometimes within hours of treatment.

Chang et al. (4) at the M.D. Anderson Cancer Center performed a prospective phase I dose escalation study in treating spinal metastases. The equipment used included a "CT on rails" that allowed for imaging immediately to guide patient repositioning. Thirteen patients received 30 Gy total dose (6 Gy per fraction). Two patients received 20 Gy in order to limit the maximum dose to the spinal cord to 10 Gy. The maximum spinal cord point dose was limited to 2 Gy per fraction. Five patients had received prior external beam radiation therapy. No neurological toxicity was detected with median follow-up of 9 months.

At other centers similar stereotactic treatments have been given to paraspinal tumors. The group from Memorial Sloan-Kettering Cancer Center reported an experience that included 35 patients with either primary or metastatic tumors of the paraspinal region who received a hypofractionated SBRT-like regimen or a more protracted conventionally fractionated treatment regimen (41). Patients were immobilized in a customized frame developed at the institution. The PTV was constructed by adding by 1.0 cm in all directions to the GTV without overlapping any portion of the spinal cord. Many of the patients had undergone previous radiotherapy. Spinal cord doses could be kept low with attention to technique. Likewise, at the University of Pittsburgh, Gerszten et al. (12) have published results of a series of over 100 patients with either primary or metastatic tumors of the spine. Single fraction spine radiosurgery doses of 12 to 20 Gy were administered while maintaining the volume of tissue inside the spinal canal getting 8 Gy or more as low as possible. Each of these reports mentioned generally favorable clinical effects, though follow-up is limited.

Clear dosimetric predictors of toxicity after spinal SBRT have not yet been identified given that few instances of significant toxicity have been observed. However, the experience reported by Dodd et al. (6) from Stanford is noteworthy in this regard. Among 51 patients treated with spinal radiosurgery for benign spinal tumors (30 schwannomas, nine neurofibromas, 16 meningiomas), there was one case of radiation myelopathy observed. The patient had a recurrent C7-T1 spinal meningioma and developed new onset posterior column dysfunction 8 months after receiving a peripheral tumor dose of 24 Gy in three fractions to a 7.6 cm³ lesion. The dose volume histogram revealed that approximately 1.7 cm³ of the spinal cord received >8 Gy per fraction.

Other Sites

SBRT has also been investigated for prostate cancer, renal cell carcinoma (RCC), and pancreatic cancer, among other sites. Reports of SBRT for prostate cancer are largely limited to descriptions of technical aspects of treatment to document feasibility (25,38). Because prostate cancer tumor control outcomes are slow to mature, extended follow-up will be needed to evaluate the clinical efficacy. The largest single institutional experience of SBRT applied for RCC has been achieved at the Karolinska Institute, where 50 patients with metastatic and eight patients with inoperable primary tumor were treated with SBRT between 1997 and 2003 (38). A variety of dose regimens were used, typically amounting to a total dose of 32 to 45 Gy in three or four fractions. A very high rate of in-field control was observed.

Koong et al. (24) have reported a phase II study of single fraction SBRT in patients with locally advanced pancreatic to determine the efficacy of concurrent 5-fluorouracil (5-FU) and intensity-modulated radiotherapy (IMRT) followed by single fraction SBRT. Nineteen patients received 45 Gy of conventionally fractionated IMRT with concurrent 5-FU followed by a 25 Gy SBRT boost to the primary tumor. Based on comparisons with other patients treated at the institution with SBRT alone, the investigators concluded that it was unclear whether the IMRT and 5-FU added meaningful benefit beyond the SBRT alone. The Aarhus University group has also investigated the use of SBRT for pancreatic carcinoma (20). Twenty-two patients with locally advanced primary pancreatic carcinoma were treated to a dose of 45 Gy in three fractions. The investigators observed substantial acute toxicity and no convincing evidence of important clinical benefits with SBRT given in that schedule.

Conclusions

SBRT is an emerging technology with the potential to benefit cancer patients in many ways. As SBRT is implemented more widely throughout the field, radiation oncologists are encouraged to participate in formal clinical trials whenever possible so that the knowledge base concerning the strengths and limitations of SBRT can continue to broaden. Outside of formal clinical trials, the same level of discipline and quality assurance measures should be applied so that patients may receive this novel, technically complex treatment as safely and effectively as possible.

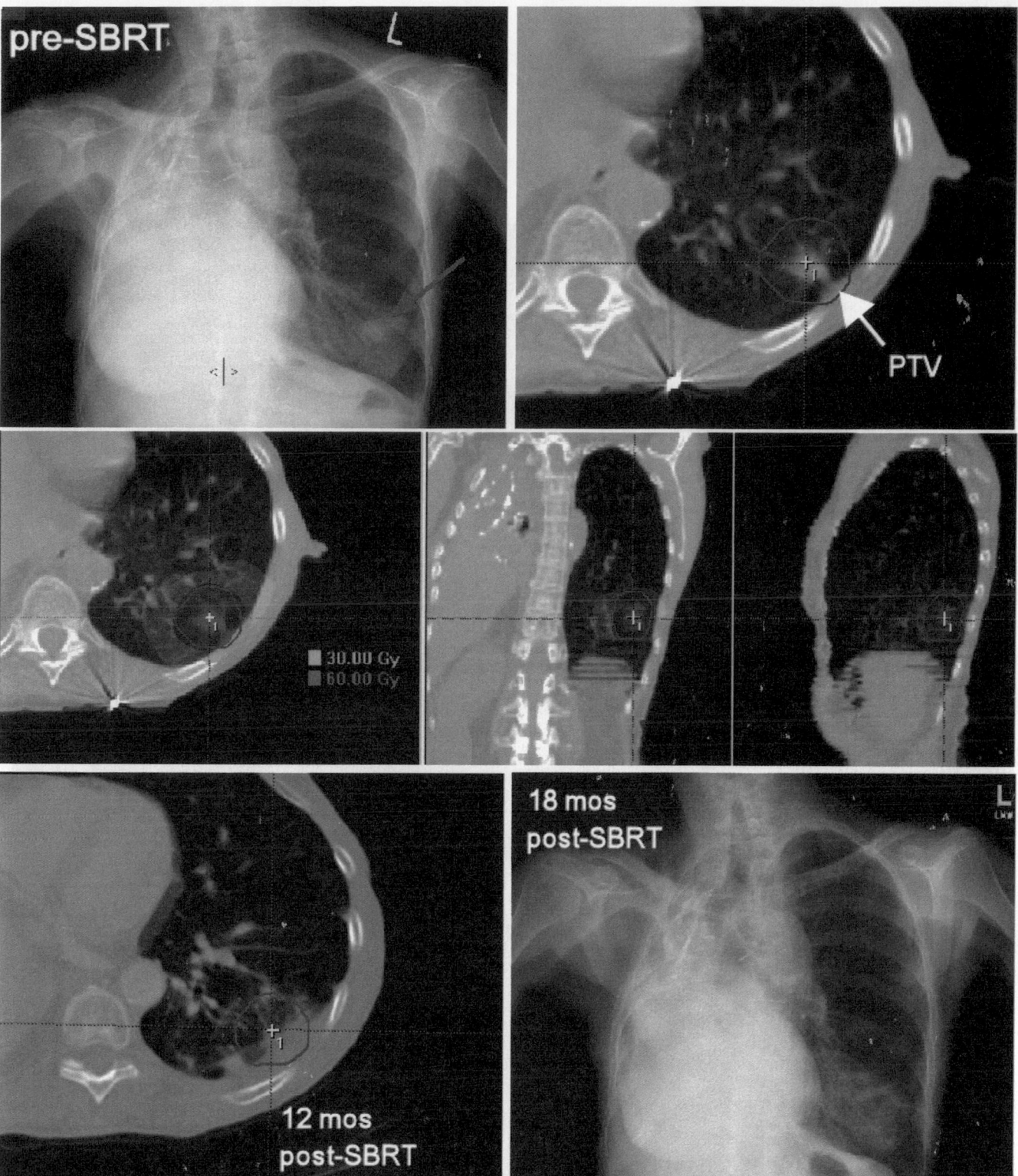

FIGURE 16.2. Example of lung stereotactic body radiation therapy (SBRT). Top panel, pre-SBRT chest x-ray showing the left lung nodule (*red arrow*) and axial planning computed tomography (CT) image with white arrow pointing to the planning target volume (PTV), which is outlined. Middle panel, SBRT composite dose distribution shown in axial, coronal, and sagittal perspectives. Bottom panel, follow-up CT scan axial image obtained 12 months (mos) post-SBRT illustrating stable patchy fibrosis in the high dose region (*left*) and chest x-ray obtained 12 months post-SBRT, indicating minimal residual haziness in the region treated.

References

1. Benedict SH, Lin PS, Zwicker RD, et al. The biological effectiveness of intermittent irradiation as a function of overall treatment time: development of correction factors for LINAC-based stereotactic radiotherapy. *Int J Radiat Oncol Biol Phys* 1997;37:765–769.
2. Blomgren H, Lax I, Naslund I, et al. Stereotactic high dose fraction radiation therapy of extracranial tumors using an accelerator: clinical experience of the first thirty-one patients. *Acta Oncol* 1995;34:861–870.
3. Blomgren, H, Lax, I, Goranson, H, et al. Radiosurgery for tumors in the body: clinical experience using a new method. *J Radiosurg* 1998;1:63–74.
4. Chang EL, Shiu AS, Lii MF, et al. Phase I clinical evaluation of near-simultaneous computed tomographic image-guided stereotactic body radiotherapy for spinal metastases. *Int J Radiat Oncol Biol Phys* 2004;59:1288–1294.
5. Curtis SB. Lethal and potentially lethal lesions induced by radiation—a unified repair model. *Radiat Res* 1986;106:252–270.
6. Dodd RL, Ryu MR, Kamnerdsupaphon P, et al. CyberKnife radiosurgery for benign intradural extramedullary spinal tumors. *Neurosurgery* 2006;58:674–685.
7. Fornier M, Norton L. Dose-dense adjuvant chemotherapy for primary breast cancer. *Breast Cancer Res* 2005;7(2):64–69.
8. Fowler JF, Ritter MA, Chappell RJ, et al. What hypofractionated protocols should be tested for prostate cancer? *Int J Radiat Oncol Biol Phys* 2003;56(4):1093–1104.
9. Fowler JF, Tome WA, Welsh JS. Estimation of required doses in stereotactic body radiation therapy. In: Kavanagh BD, Timmerman RD, eds. *Stereotactic body radiation therapy.* New York: Lippincott Williams & Wilkins, 2005; .
10. Fowler JF, Welsh JS, Howard SP. Loss of biological effect in prolonged fraction delivery. *Int J Radiat Oncol Biol Phys* 2004;59:242–249.
11. Fritz P, Kraus HJ, Muhlnickel W, et al. Stereotactic, single-dose irradiation of stage I non-small cell lung cancer and lung metastases. *Radiat Oncol* 2006;1:30.
12. Gerszten PC, Ozhasoglu C, Burton SA, et al. CyberKnife frameless stereotactic radiosurgery for spinal lesions: clinical experience in 125 cases. *Neurosurgery* 2004;55(1):89–98.
13. Guerrero M, Li X. Extending the linear–quadratic model for large fraction doses pertinent to stereotactic radiotherapy. *Phys Med Biol* 2004;49:4825–4835.
14. Hamilton AJ, Lulu BA, Fosmire H, et al. LINAC-based spinal stereotactic radiosurgery. *Stereotact Funct Neurosurg* 1996;66:1–9.
15. Hamilton AJ, Lulu BA, Fosmire H, et al. Preliminary clinical experience with linear accelerator-based spinal stereotactic radiosurgery. *Neurosurgery* 1995;36(2):311–319.
16. Hellman S, Weichselbaum RR. Oligometastases. *J Clin Oncol* 1995;13(1):8–10.
17. Herfarth KK, Debus J. [Stereotactic radiation therapy for liver metastases]. *Chirurg* 2005;76(6):564.
18. Herfarth KK, Hof H, Bahner ML, et al. Assessment of focal liver reaction by multiphasic CT after stereotactic single-dose radiotherapy of liver tumors. *Int J Radiat Oncol Biol Phys* 2003;57:444–451.
19. Hoyer M, Roed H, Hansen AT, et al. Prospective study on stereotactic radiotherapy of limited stage non-small cell lung cancer. *Int J Radiat Oncol Biol Phys* 2005;63: S396.
20. Hoyer M, Roed H, Sengelov L, et al. Phase-II study on stereotactic radiotherapy of locally advanced pancreatic carcinoma. *Radiother Oncol* 2005;76:48–53.
21. Kavanagh BD, Kelly KA, Kane M. The promise of stereotactic body radiation therapy in a new era of oncology. In: Meyer JL, ed. *Frontiers of radiation therapy and oncology*, Vol. 40: *Proceedings of the 38th San Francisco Radiation Oncology Conference.* Berlin: Karger, 2007; .
22. Kavanagh BD, Schefter TE, Cardenes HR, et al. Interim analysis of a prospective phase I/II trial of SBRT for liver metastases. *Acta Oncol* 2006;45:848–855.
23. Kavanagh BD, Timmerman RD. Stereotactic radiosurgery and stereotactic body radiation therapy: an overview of technical considerations and clinical applications. *Hematol Oncol Clin North Am* 2006;20(1):87–95.
24. Koong AC, Christofferson E, Le QT, et al. Phase II study to assess the efficacy of conventionally fractionated radiotherapy followed by a stereotactic radiosurgery boost in patients with locally advanced pancreatic cancer. *Int J Radiat Oncol Biol Phys* 2005;63:320–323.
25. Madsen BL, Hsi RA, Pham HT, et al. Intrafractional stability of the prostate using a stereotactic radiotherapy technique. *Int J Radiat Oncol Biol Phys* 2003;57:1285–1291.
26. McGarry R McGarry RC, Papiez L, et al. Stereotactic body radiation therapy of early-stage non-small-cell lung carcinoma: phase I study. *Int J Radiat Oncol Biol Phys* 2005;63(4):1010–1015.
27. Nagata Y, Takayama K, Matsuo Y, et al. Clinical outcomes of a phase I/II study of 48 Gy of stereotactic body radiotherapy in 4 fractions for primary lung cancer using a stereotactic bodyframe. *Int J Radiat Oncol Biol Phys* 2005;63:1427–1431.
28. Norton L, Simon R, Brereton HD, et al. Predicting the course of Gompertzian growth. *Nature* 1976;264(5586):542–545.
29. Potters L, Steinberg M, Rose C, et al. American Society the Therapeutic Radiology and Oncology and American College of Radiology practice guidelines for the performance of stereotactic body radiation therapy. *Int J Radiat Oncol Biol Phys* 2004;60:1026–1032.
30. Ryu S, Fang Yin F, Rock J, et al. Image-guided and intensity-modulated radiosurgery for patients with spinal metastasis. *Cancer* 2003;97(8):2013–2018.
31. Ryu S, Rock J, Rosenblum M, et al. Patterns of failure after single-dose radiosurgery for spinal metastasis. *J Neurosurg* 2004;101[Suppl 3]:402–405.
32. Schefter TE, Cardenes HR, Kavanagh BD. Stereotactic body radiation therapy for primary and metastatic liver tumors. In: Kavanagh BD, Timmerman RD, eds. *Stereotactic body radiation therapy.* New York: Lippincott Williams & Wilkins, 2005;6(45):5120–5127.
33. Schefter TE, Kavanagh BD, Timmerman RD, et al. A phase I trial of stereotactic body radiation therapy (SBRT) for liver metastases. *Int J Radiat Oncol Biol Phys* 2005;62:1371–1378.
34. Schefter TE, Kavanagh BD. A phase I/II trial of stereotactic body radiation therapy (SBRT) for lung metastases: initial report of dose escalation and early toxicity. *Int J Radiat Oncol Biol Phys* 2006; .
35. Timmerman R, McGarry R, Papiez L, et al. Initial report of a prospective phase II trial of stereotactic body radiation therapy for patients with medically inoperable stage I non-small cell lung cancer. *Int J Radiat Oncol Biol Phys* 2005;63:S99.
36. Timmerman R, Papiez L, McGarry R, et al. Extracranial stereotactic radioablation: Results of a phase I study in medically inoperable stage I non-small cell lung cancer patients. *Chest* 2003;124:1946–1955.
37. Uematsu M, Shioda A, Tahara K, et al. Focal, high dose, and fractionated modified stereotactic radiation therapy for lung carcinoma patients: a preliminary experience. *Cancer* 1998;82:1062–1070.
38. Wersall PJ, Blomgren H, Lax I, et al. Extracranial stereotactic radiotherapy for primary and metastatic renal cell carcinoma. *Radiother Oncol* 2005;77(1):88–95.
39. Wulf J, Hadinger U, Oppitz U, et al. Stereotactic radiotherapy of targets in the lung and liver. *Strahlenther Onkol* 2001;177:645–655.
40. Xia T, Li H, Sun Q, et al. Promising clinical outcome of stereotactic body radiation therapy for patients with inoperable Stage I/II non-small-cell lung cancer. *Int J Radiat Oncol Biol Phys* 2006;66:117–125.
41. Yamada Y, Lovelock DM, Yenice KM, et al. Multifractionated image-guided and stereotactic intensity-modulated radiotherapy of paraspinal tumors: a preliminary report. *Int J Radiat Oncol Biol Phys* 2005;62:53–61.
42. Yeas RJ, Kalend A. Local stem cell depletion model for radiation myelitis. *Int J Radiat Oncol Biol Phys* 1988;14:1247–1259.

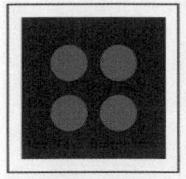

Chapter 17
Intraoperative Radiotherapy

Felipe A. Calvo, Rosa M. Meirino, M. Dolores de la Mata, F. Javier Serrano, Mirian Gálvez

In the last 2 decades, advances in the radiation component of cancer treatment have been the result of improvements in dose distribution between tumor and dose-limiting normal tissues. In many clinical situations, however, the dose that can be delivered safely to the tumor volume is limited by dose-limiting normal tissues in close proximity to the tumor volume. Intraoperative irradiation (IORT) in its broadest sense refers to the delivery of radiation at the time of an operation. In this chapter, we discuss the rationale for and use of intraoperative electron irradiation (IOERT) in conjunction with surgical exploration with or without external-beam irradiation (EBRT) and chemotherapy

Modern ERA: IOERT or Orthovoltage

The modern approach to IORT began with studies made by Abe and Takahashi (1) at the University of Kyoto in the early 1960s. The first human IOERT treatment was given at Howard University in November 1976, and by December 1982, 114 patients had been treated with variable electron energies (38). The National Cancer Institute (NCI) began using IOERT in September 1979 (109). In the early 1980s, IORT programs also became active at the Mayo Clinic (April 1981) and the New England Deaconess Hospital division of the Joint Center for Radiation Therapy (86) (January 1982). At Mayo Clinic, IOERT was incorporated as a component of treatment with the same general approach and philosophy as at the Massachusetts General Hospital (MGH).

In the early 1980s, several European institutions implemented IORT programs using either high-energy electron beam or orthovoltage. What follows is a chronology of the historical origins of European IOERT: Caen (France), 1983; Pamplona (Spain), 1984; Innsbruck (Austria), 1984; Lyon (France), 1985; Milan (Italy), 1985; Muchen (Germany), 1986; Brussels (Belgium), 1987; Groningen (Holland), 1988; Oslo (Norway), 1990; and Stockholm (Sweden), 1990. A modern orthovoltage IORT program was instituted in Montpelier (France) in 1984 with transition to a dedicated IOERT facility in 1996 (Fig. 17.1).

Rationale for IORT

The combination of IOERT with EBRT has the potential to improve the therapeutic ratio of local control versus complications by: (a) decreasing the volume of the irradiation boost field, (b) excluding all or part of dose-limiting sensitive structures, and (c) increasing the effective dose by virtue of factors 1 and 2 (Fig. 17.2).

Impact of Local Tumor Control

Improved local control (LC) of cancer often improves survival (29,30,107,110). If microscopic residual exists after gross total resection, EBRT doses necessary to achieve LC are ≥60 Gy in 1.8- to 2-Gy fractions. Although an aggressive EBRT philosophy may allow better local tumor control, it may also cause severe treatment-related complications. A preferred treatment alternative for patients with locally advanced malignancies is to give tolerable EBRT doses of 45 to 50 Gy preoperatively (1.8-

Gy fractions) and deliver IORT. This unique approach allows an increase in LC with a lower risk of complications than with an EBRT-only approach.

Patient Selection Criteria

Appropriateness for IORT should be determined by the surgeon and radiation oncologist in the setting of a joint preoperative consultation. Several general criteria guide the selection of appropriate patients for IORT:

- Surgery alone will not achieve acceptable LC.
- EBRT doses needed for adequate LC after subtotal resection or no resection would exceed normal tissue tolerance.
- IORT will be performed at the time of a planned operative procedure.
- There is no evidence of distant metastases or peritoneal seeding.
- An informed consent can be obtained.

Patient Evaluation

The pretreatment patient work-up should include a detailed evaluation of the extent of the locally advanced primary or recurrent lesion combined with studies to rule out hematogenous or peritoneal spread of disease. Computed tomography can confirm lack of free space between the malignancy and a structure that may be surgically unresectable for cure (e.g., presacrum, pelvic side wall). In such patients, preoperative EBRT with or without chemotherapy should be given before an attempt at resection

Radiation Doses and Techniques

The method of EBRT has been fairly consistent in most U.S. and European IORT studies. In patients who have had no prior irradiation, doses of 40 to 54 Gy are delivered in 1.8-Gy fractions 5 days per week during 5 to 6 weeks.

For previously irradiated patients, an attempt is made to reirradiate with low-dose preoperative EBRT doses of 20 to 30 Gy in 1.8- to 2.0-Gy fractions (with chemotherapy).

The biologic effectiveness of a single dose of IORT is estimated to be equivalent to 1.5 to 2.5 times the same total dose of fractionated EBRT (45,73,79). The effective dose in the IORT boost field, when added to the 45 to 50 Gy given EBRT, is 70 to 80 Gy with 10 Gy IORT, 75 to 87.5 Gy with 15 Gy, and 85 to 100 Gy with 20 Gy.

IORT Tolerance and Dose-Limiting Structures, Late Effects, Risk of Tumor Recurrence, and Second Malignancies

In patients with locally advanced malignancies, the issue of morbidity after aggressive treatment is placed into clearer perspective by a comparison with tumor-related morbidity and mortality.

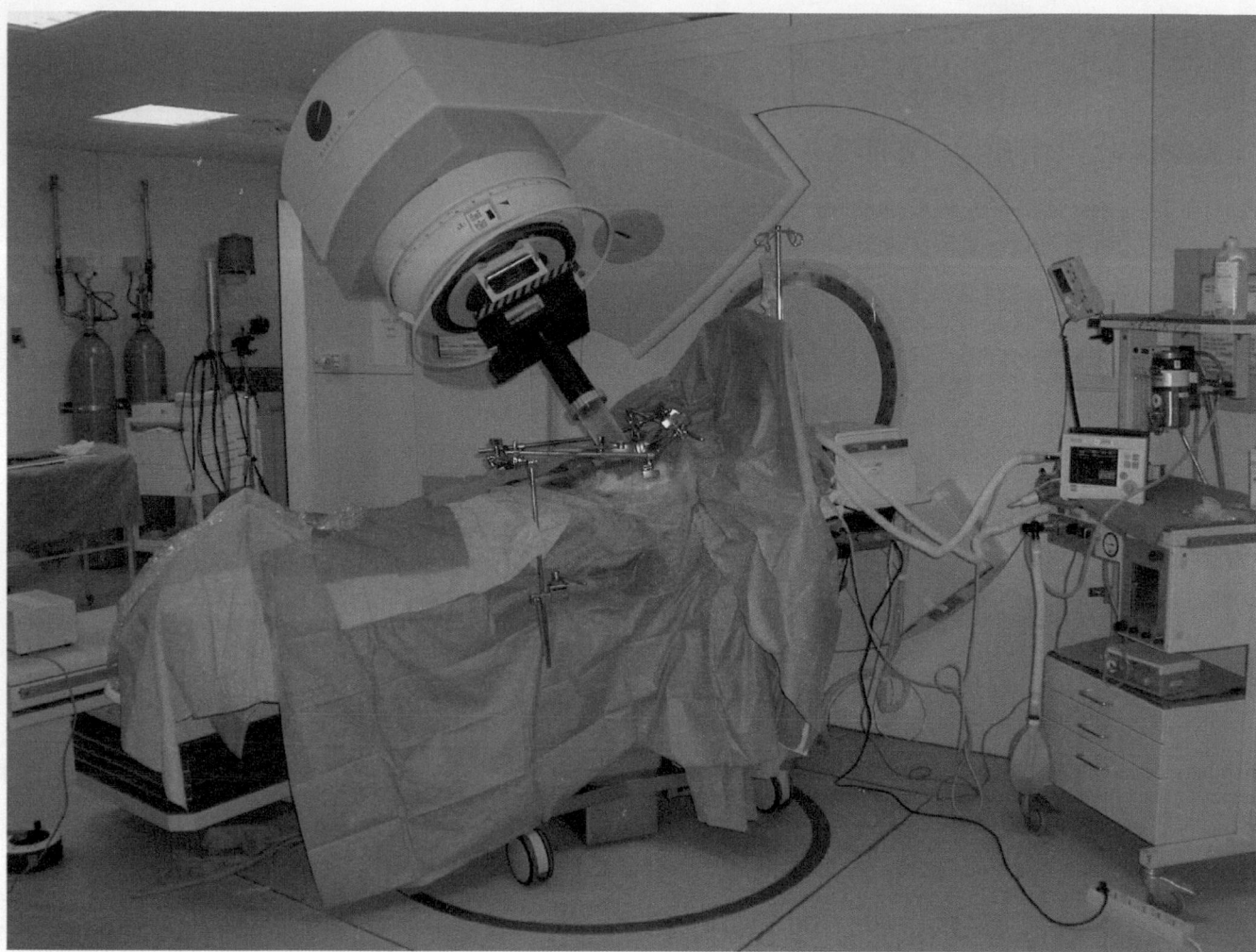

FIGURE 17.1. Overview of an intraoperative electron irradiation (IOERT) procedure generated in a nondedicated linear accelerator. The treatment room is temporarily transformed into a surgical room with full anesthesia support and visual control of the patient/IOERT field.

IOERT tolerance for intact or surgically manipulated organs or structures in animals is seen in Table 17.3. This information has largely been derived from studies at the NCI (20,56,57,98) and Colorado State University (34). Dose-sensitive structures identified in previous IOERT analyses include ureter and bile duct. Neither structure is dose-limiting because stents can be inserted to overcome obstruction and preserve renal or liver function. In a published Mayo Clinic analysis (94), 44% of previously unobstructed ureters became partially or totally obstructed when included in the IOERT field.

Peripheral nerve is the principal dose-limiting normal tissue for IOERT in the pelvis, retroperitoneum, and extremities. The anatomic location of the peripheral nerve often places it adjacent to or involved by a sarcoma, and usually it has to be irradiated because the sarcoma is marginally resected near neurovascular structures. On the basis of both human and animal data, when a full dose of EBRT option exists (i.e., 45 to 55 Gy fractionated EBRT), an IORT boost dose of 10 to 20 Gy should be used depending on the amount of tumor remaining after maximal resection (≤15 Gy with IORT/intraoperative hyperthermia [IOHT] combined). IORT doses ranging from 21 Gy to 25 Gy are used only when EBRT doses must be limited because of prior treatment.

Early reports on *late normal tissue complications* potentially related to IOERT were focused on the description of unexpected findings derived from the radiobiology of high single-dose electron irradiation. Early and late effects of IOERT have been extensively investigated in animals including ureteral changes

(71), peripheral nerve (35,54,70,115), and damage to other anatomic structures (24,83). Experiments in large and smaller animals tested the tolerance to IOERT with or without external irradiation in surgically manipulated organs and tissues (58,93). The late effects observed in animals suggest that 10 to 20 Gy of IOERT plus external fractionated irradiation (45 to 50 Gy) do not compromise the outcome of healthy young adult dogs. On the other hand, the *volume* of tissue treated with IOERT is critical, in particular the length of tubular structures irradiated (such as large vessels and ureters). The tissues at risk from IOERT were late-responding. Damage to the intrinsic vasculature and connective tissue of organs observed in the examined specimens seems to be responsible for the damage to the organ with an increasing degree of severity depending IOERT dose escalation.

The analysis by Azinovic et al. (9) revealed that long-term normal tissue tolerance in patients treated with multimodality therapy should be interpreted as secondary to multifactorial molecular, cellular, and tissue-damage mechanisms and its implications in late-repair capacity. Their experience correlated the estimation of risk of normal tissue damage (calculated by the additive effect from treatment modalities) with the relative incidence of grade 3–4 toxicities.

Neuropathy is the dominant IOERT-related late normal tissue complication observed in patients surviving >5 years. This event appeared most frequently at locations in which a peripheral nerve is commonly found in the surgical bed. Because most patients (65%) received doses on a 15 Gy, the length

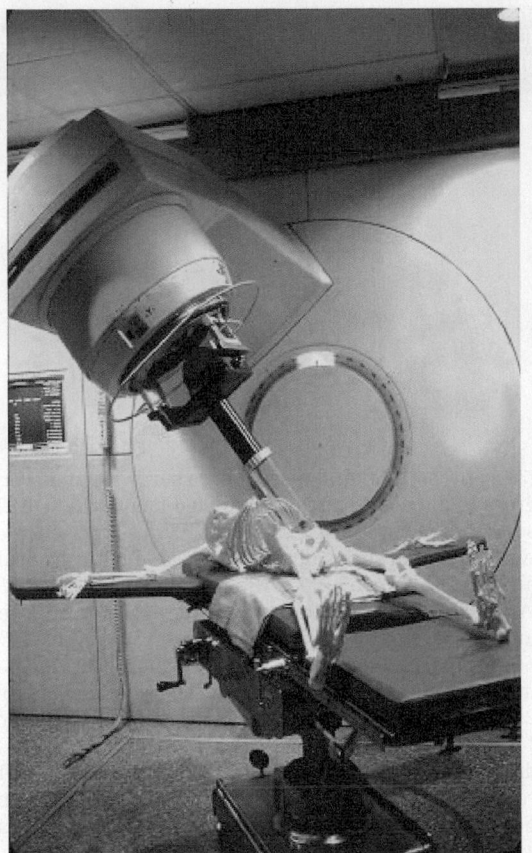

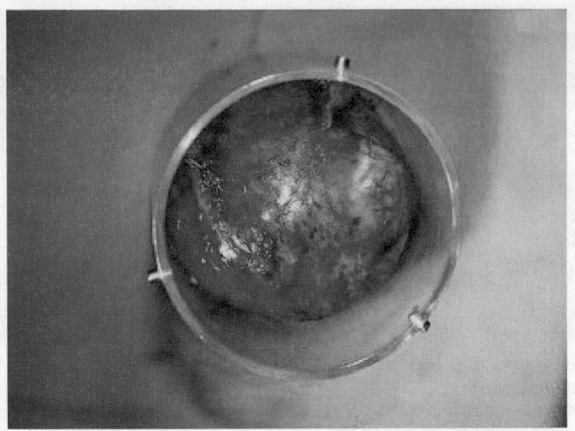

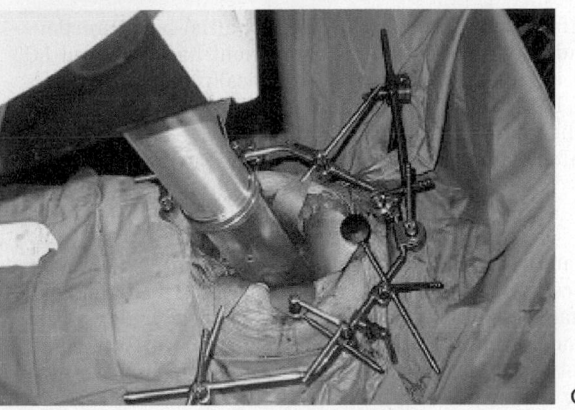

FIGURE 17.2. Basic method description of intraoperative irradiation with high-energy electrons: **(A)** the bone structure is the limiting factor for positioning applicators; **(B)** the tumor bed size can be estimated after tumor resection (surgical specimen); and **(C)** the use of surgical retractors helps the displacement and protection of uninvolved tissue.

of the irradiated nerve may be of critical importance. There may be an additive effect when IOHT is combined with IOERT (34,35,115). An area for future research is the potential contribution of intra-arterial cisplatinum preoperatively, the role of other neurotoxic agents, and/or the influence of extensive surgical manipulation (70).

Second malignancies were described early in animal experiments using IOERT. This was of concern, particularly because of the development of undifferentiated (occasionally sarcoma-like) tumors inside the IOERT field (36,55). Similar events have never been reported in clinical IOERT. The University of Navarra (9) analysis identified eight patients with second tumors after IOERT, three were marginal to the EBRT volume (two bladder cancers after IOERT prostate cancer and one right renal cancer after IOERT for bile duct carcinoma). All were outside the IOERT-boosted region. Although the median follow-up for this series is 94 months, further time might be required to better address the risk of second malignancies.

Finally, *late recurrences* of the originally IOERT-treated tumor may be seen in long-term surviving patients. Long-term analysis is needed to evaluate precisely the patterns of failure. This may help to delineate new treatment strategies.

:: | RESULTS

Pancreas

The combination of EBRT plus IOERT has resulted in improved LC in cancer of the pancreas in series from the MGH (46) and Mayo Clinic (42,87). This has not translated into an improve-

ment in either median or 5-year survival because of a high incidence of liver and peritoneal cavity relapse (21,72).

Results are influenced by the extent of tumor resection (111). In patients treated with advanced unresectable pancreatic cancer (IORT doses 10 to 40 Gy + EBRT +/− chemotherapy), the median survival time ranged from 8 to 16 months and abdominal pain relief was achieved in 57% to 89%. In resectable pancreatic cancer, median survival time ranged from 9 to 39 months.

The M.D. Anderson Cancer Center experience was updated by Pisler et al. using rapid-fractionation with chemotherapy (30 Gy/10 fraction + daily infusion of 5-fluorouracil [5-FU]) and surgery together with IORT boost (10 to 15 Gy). The median survival time for resected group was 24 months, 3-year actuarial survival rate was 23%, and the local relapse rate was 10%.

The MGH reviewed 150 patients with unresectable pancreatic cancer between 1978 and 2001 who were treated with combined therapy (5-FU + EBRT + IORT) achieving a median survival of 17 months. There was a significantly better prognosis when a smaller applicator was used (probably a surrogate for tumor size applicator size <8 cm) (118).

For pancreatic cancer patients, IORT contributes to modestly prolonged survival in unresectable patients and aids abdominal pain control in a high proportion of cases, with durable effect (21,72).

Stomach

IORT is a feasible technique to be incorporated in gastric cancer surgery and seems to promote LC (20). Severe vascular toxicity has been reported in IORT gastric trial with an incidence of 3% to 12% (14). High-risk gastric cancer requires multimodality

| Table 17.1 | EUROPEAN EXPERIENCES WITH PREOPERATIVE RADIOTHERAPY OR CHEMORADIATION + RESECTION + INTRAOPERATIVE IRRADIATION (IORT) BOOST IN PRIMARY ADVANCED DISEASE | | | | | |

Study	N	Dose IORT (Gy)	Dose EBRT (Gy)	In-Field Relapse (%)	Pelvic Relapse (%)	Survival at 5 Yr (%)
Mannaerts et al. (63)	38	10–17	50.4	7	13	72***
Valentini et al. (113)	69	10	38	—	6.6	81.4*
Eble et al. (27)	45	10–15	41	—	4	82***
Huber et al. (53)	19	15	50	0	10	60
Calvo et al. (16)	62	10–15	45–50	1	4	76.5
Canon et al. (19)	66	10–15	45–54	—	5	76

EBRT, external-beam radiation therapy.
*Disease-specific survival.
**High-dose-rate IORT (flab technique).
***3 years.

therapy, including chemotherapy and external-beam fractionated irradiation (62). The IORT component has improved LC rates in recurrent tumors (51) and locally advanced cases (37,104). IORT boosts have been piloted in the context of neoadjuvant chemotherapy, surgical resection, and external-beam fractionated irradiation with acceptable tolerance (117).

Lung

The intrathoracic high-risk regions for residual disease after lung cancer surgery can be treated by an IOERT electron field. Unresectable tumors, postresected right and left hilar region and/or mediastinum, and posterior or apex chest wall zones are target areas for an IORT boost (112). European investigators have used IORT as a radiation-boosting technique, complemented with external irradiation alone or in the context of induction systemic chemotherapy (8). Pancoast tumors seem particularly appropriate for IORT boost, with actuarial LC rates of 91% and overall survival of 56% (66). Moderate results for pleural mesothelioma have been achieved with high-dose-rate (HDR) IORT (88).

Esophagus

A large experience in the IORT boosting of the upper mediastinum during esophagectomy and lymphadenectomy with a nerve-sparing approach in esophageal cancer has been reported recently (7,52) with successful LC results (94% to 100%). The main complication was tracheal damage with an IOERT dose >20 Gy.

Colon and Rectum

Primary Locally Advanced Cancers

In MGH IOERT analysis of 64 patients with locally advanced primary lesions, 5-year actuarial disease-free survival was 43%

(39), and both LC and disease-free survival rates were higher if gross total resection was completed before the IOERT. Gunderson et al. (42) reported the Mayo Clinic experience comparing two sequential series of patients treated with surgical resection and EBRT alone (n = 17) or in conjunction with IOERT (n = 56). With IOERT, the 3-year actuarial survival was 55% versus 24%, and the 3-year actuarial LC rate was 85% versus 24%.

European institutions have explored strategies including preoperative radiotherapy or chemoradiation (16,19,25,27,53,63,64,81) followed by resection and IORT boost (Table 17.1). Calvo et al. (16) and Diaz-Gonzalez et al. (25) have addressed the question of IORT boost target volume after radical resection in primary rectal cancer. Using an adjuvant electron boost on the presacral space, only one in-field relapse was observed in 62 patients treated, with a median follow-up time of 46 months. The Catholic University School of Medicine (Italy) (81) has recently reported the results in 113 patients treated with (n = 69) or without (n = 44) preoperative EBRT plus IOERT (10 Gy) and total mesorectal resection. The 5-year disease-specific survival and LC rates were 81% versus 58% and 93% versus 77% in the IOERT group and resection alone arm, respectively.

Locally Recurrent Cancers

There is a 5-year survival improvement of 20% with the addition of IOERT to standard treatment (2,41,44,116,120). Data supporting the use of IOERT for locally recurrent disease are also found in Mayo Clinic analysis of 106 patients treated with palliative resection alone (n = 64) or including a 15 to 20 Gy of IOERT boost (n = 42). Significant factors that impact 5-year survival included the amount of residual tumor (microscopic vs. gross; 33% vs. 9%: $p = .032$) and IOERT versus none (19% vs. 7%; $p = 0.0006$) (119). Analyses of preoperative radiotherapy, chemoradiation, extended surgery, HDR-IORT or ^{125}Iodine low-dose-rate brachytherapy (48,50,61,64,68,69,97,108,113). Generally, validate the hypothesis that postresection residual

| Table 17.2 | SIDE EFFECTS FROM INTRAOPERATIVE RADIOTHERAPY WITH ELECTRONS DURING BREAST-CONSERVING SURGERY IN THE MILAN EXPERIENCE | |

Side Effect (590 Patients)	N	%
Severe fibrosis	1	0.2
Mild fibrosis	18	3.0
Liponecrosis	15	2.5
Hematoma	2	0.3
Skin retraction	2	0.3
Total	38	6.3

Table 17.3	NORMAL TISSUE TOLERANCE TO INTRAOPERATIVE ELECTRON IRRADIATION IN ANIMALS (MOST COMMONLY IN DOGS)			
Tissue	Maximun Tolerated Dose (Gy)	Tissue Effect	Dose (Gy)
Intact structure			≥ 30
Aorta, vena cava	50	Fibrosis of wall	≥ 20
Peripheral nerve	15	Neuropathy, sensory motor	≥ 25
Bladder	30	Contraction and ureterovesical narrowing	≥ 30
Ureter	30	Fibrosis and stenosis	≥ 20
Kidney	≤ 15	Atrophy and fibrosis	≥ 30
Bile duct	20	Fibrosis and stenosis	≥ 20
Small intestine	≤ 20	Ulceration, fibrosis, and stenosis	≥ 17.5
Large bowel	15	Ulceration, fibrosis, and stenosis	50
Esophagus			
Full thickness	≤ 20	Ulceration, stricture	≥ 30
Partial thickness	10	No sequelae at this dose	≥ 40
Muscle (psoas)	23	50% decrement muscle fibers	38
Heart	20	Fibrosis	≥ 30
Lung	20	Fibrosis	≥ 20
Trachea	30	Submucosal fibrosis	≥ 30
Surgically manipulated			
Aorta anastomosis	20	Fibrosis and stenosis	≥ 20
			≤ 45
Aortic prosthetic graft	25	No anastomosis	25
Portal vein anastomosis	40	Graft occlusion	> 40
Biliary-enteric anastomosis	≤ 20	Stenosis	≥ 20
		Anastomotic breakdown	
Small intestine defuntionalized	45	Fibrosis and stenosis	≤ 20
		No suture line breakdown	≤ 45
Bladder	30	Healing but contraction	≥ 30
Bronchial stump	40	Absence of air leak	40

Data from Gillette EL, Gillette SM, Powers BE. Studies at Colorado State University of normal tissue tolerance of beagles to IOERT, EBRT or a combination. In Gunderson LL, Willet CG, Harrison LB, et al. eds. *Intraoperative irradiation. Techniques and results.* Totowa, NJ: Humana Press; 1999:147–164.

disease is a determinant for survival and LC (ranging from 43% to 80% in R0, 26% to 55% in R1, and 0% to 20% in R2). It is important to emphasize that some long-term survivors are consistently reported if an IORT component is added.

Recurrent disease in previously irradiated patients is a challenging situation in which the treatment should be individualized (Fig. 17.3). Researchers of the Mayo Clinic have reported long-term LC in 60% of patients, and there was a trend to improved LC with moderate doses of external reirradiation (>30 Gy, 81% vs. 54%). The incidence of neuropathy was 32% (48).

HDR-IORT (flab method) is a well-adapted boosting technique in the pelvic region for rectal cancer patients (53), but the relatively frequent gross residual disease postresection bias the modality selection to IOERT to assure enough beam depth penetration.

Retroperitoneal and Pelvic Soft Tissue Sarcomas

The NCI conducted a randomized trial in 35 patients with primary retroperitoneal sarcomas (all had gross total resection) using EBRT (35 to 40 Gy) followed by IOERT boost (20 Gy) or reduced-field external radiation (15 Gy) (99), showing a locoregional relapse rate within the irradiation fields of 20% versus 80% in IOERT and non-IOERT groups, respectively (*p* <.001).

Resection plus IOERT has been given to 87 Mayo Clinic patients with primary (n = 43) or locally recurrent (n = 44) retroperitoneal/pelvic sarcoma (82). Local relapse occurred in only 3 of 43 patients (7%) with primary lesions versus 17 of 44 (39%) with recurrent disease. Initial lesion size ≤ 10 cm and the surgeon's ability to achieve a gross total resection have a favor-

able impact on 5-year survival (60% vs. 28% and 52% vs. 37%, respectively). In the MGH experience in 37 patients treated with curative intent (33), 5-year actuarial survival was 50% and LC was 38%. Better outcome was observed in the subgroup undergoing gross total resection, with LC of 83% and survival of 74%.

The use of adjuvant EBRT alone in retroperitoneal/pelvic sarcomas after marginal resection could be questioned because of the high rate of tumor bed relapse (80%) (99). IORT combined with resection and EBRT offers a more effective approach to improve LC, as seen in randomized trials and single-institution studies (4,11,15,26,43,74,121).

Extremity Sarcomas

The management of soft tissue sarcomas of the extremities requires postresection radiotherapy for extremity preservation. A component of the total radiation dose can be delivered as an intraoperative boost, IOERT, or IOHDR (59,84). At the Technical University Munich (59), an IORT electron boost was used in 28 patients and the overall actuarial recurrence rate after 5 years was 16%. At the University of Innsbruck, 39 adult patients were treated in an 8-year period and no local recurrence was detected using IOHDR boost. No vascular, nerve, or soft tissue radiation-induced damage was reported. Functional status of the extremity was excellent (84). At the University of Navarra, results observed with IOERT electron boost in 45 patients (median follow-up, 93 months) with primary and recurrent sarcoma showed 20% local recurrence rate and 11% peripheral neuropathy (7-year actuarial survival rate of 75%) (10).

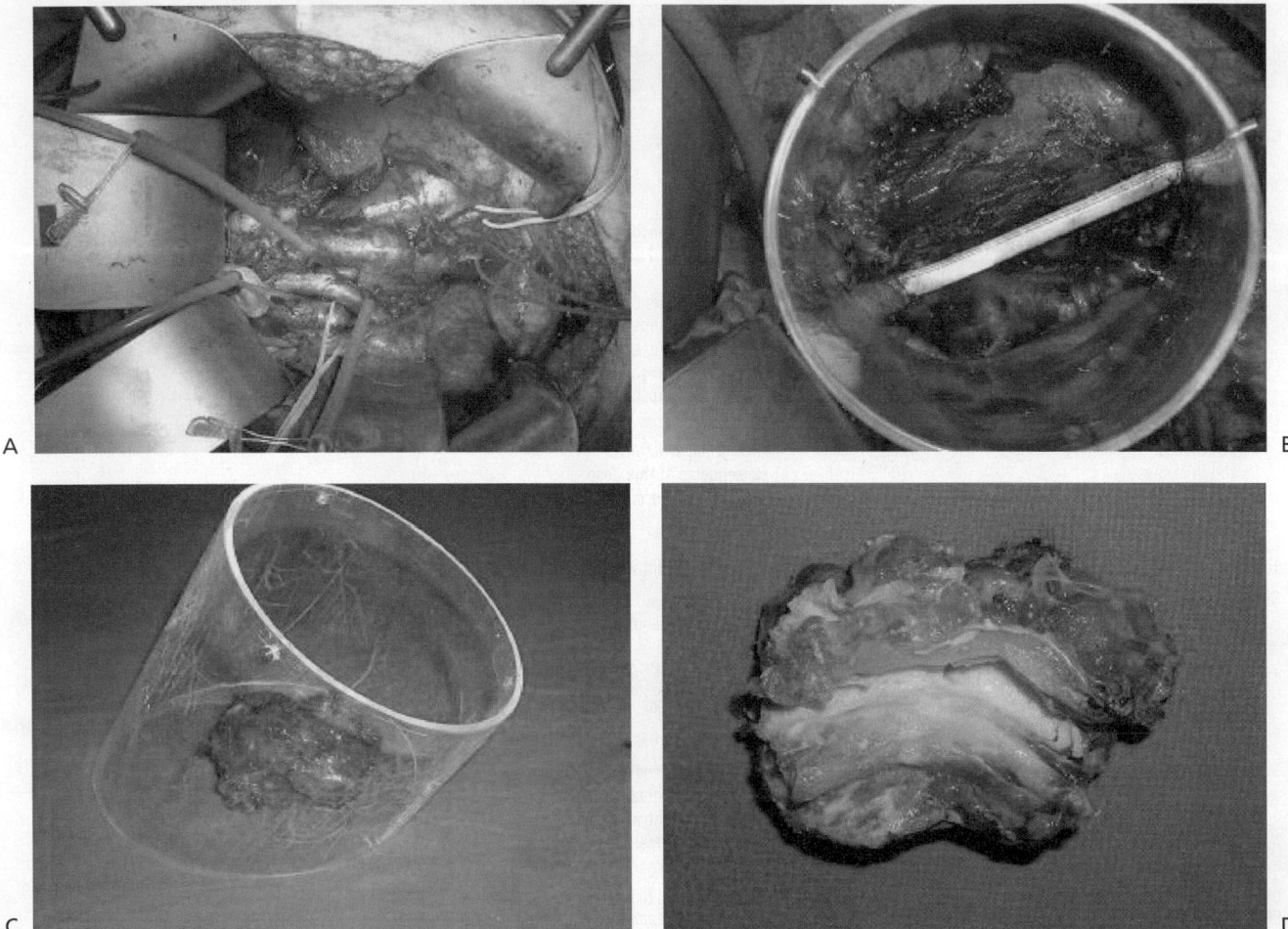

FIGURE 17.3. A: Surgical field view of a recurrent rectal cancer with unilateral involvement of the pelvic vascular structures. **B:** Macroscopic tumor resection requiring vascular graft reconstruction. **C:** The tumor bed was treated with an intraoperative irradiation boost (15 Gy, 10-cm diameter applicator, 30 degree beveled, 12-MeV electron beam). Except for the lateral pelvic wall soft tissues and bone, the remaining normal uninvolved intrapelvic tissues and organs are protected from the electron beam. **D:** Surgical specimen showing vascular segment surrounded by recurrent cancer.

Pediatric Tumors

IORT in pediatric patients represents a means of improving precision in dose deposition, protection of normal uninvolved tissues and, moreover, radiation treatment design in which the EBRT can be either omitted or decreased in total dose. HDR brachytherapy or IOERT are selected for pediatric patients depending on tumor location and surgical accessibility (74,75,77). Neuroblastoma (high-risk category) is a disease approached with an IOERT component (7 to 16 Gy) (3,47), addressing a total local failure rate (100%) in gross residual tumor postresection patients. In bone sarcomas (both Ewing and osteosarcoma), IOERT-augmented extremity preservation surgical management was able to promote high LC rates (95% Ewing and 95% osteosarcoma) (17).

Bladder and Kidney

Rostom et al. (89) have reported the potential role of IOERT in the radical treatment of infiltrating bladder cancer using chemoradiation and conservative surgery (TUR plus cystostomy for tumor exposure) showing 5-year overall and cystectomy-free survivals of 53% and 48%, respectively (89). In locally advanced or recurrent renal cell cancer, LC can be achieved using IOERT (15 to 20 Gy) after incomplete tumor resection, with minimal therapy-related side effects (28).

Breast

Several randomized trials with very long follow-up have established the equivalence of breast-conserving therapy to mastectomy in terms of overall survival. Breast-conserving therapy computed tomography followed by a course of postoperative radiotherapy is now considered standard of care for patients with early operable breast cancer.

Several trials (6) have demonstrated that the addition of a localized dose to the tumor bed reduces local recurrences. Typical radiation therapy after breast-conserving surgery includes the whole remaining breast to a total of 50 Gy in a 2-Gy daily fraction and a boost to the tumor bed using electrons. This is obvious, considering the application of a total dose of 60 Gy or more to the tumor bed for a high local tumor control, maintaining a good cosmetic outcome.

Clinical delineation of the tumor bed not only carries a significant risk of missing the target, but also unnecessarily treats breast tissue that may be spared. In this regard, IORT, given as a boost, has demonstrated a high ability to prevent local recurrence in early breast cancer with good cosmetic results (60,12,85).

In Montpelier (France) in 50 patients with early breast cancer, the treatments were delivered using 6 to 13 MeV electron beam at doses of 9 to 20 Gy to the 90% reference isodose. All patients received postoperative EBRT (50 Gy in 2-Gy fractions);

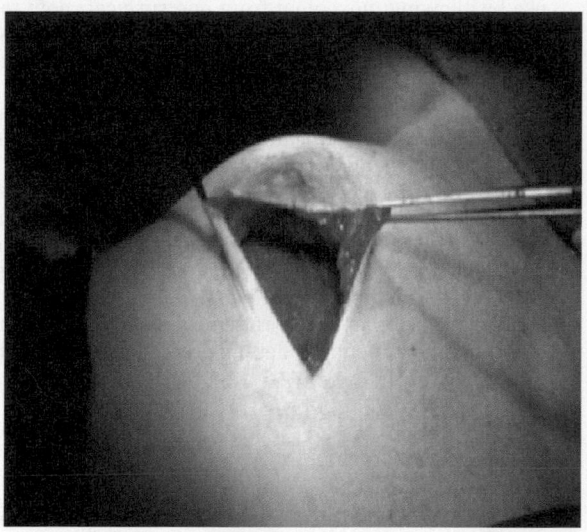 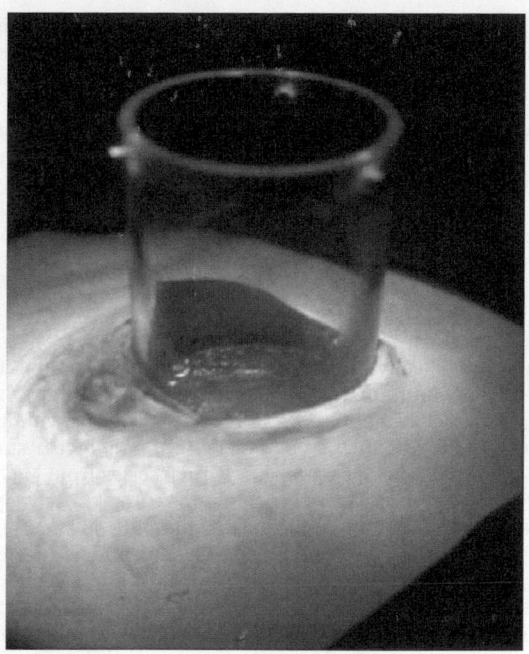

FIGURE 17.4. Simulation of an intraoperative irradiation procedure in early breast cancer after tumorectomy. **A:** Surgical incision in tumor bed area. **B:** Applicator encompassing the tumorectomy postsurgical bed.

after a median follow-up of 9.1 years, two local recurrences were observed within the primary tumor bed. Cosmesis was good-to-excellent in the evaluated patients. Six patients had grade 2 late subcutaneous fibrosis on the boost area. In Salzburg, 156 women were treated with IORT for stage I and II breast cancer; a single dose of 9 Gy was applied to the 90% reference isodose with energies ranging from 4 to 15 MeV. The applicator tubes were placed so that the whole tumor and surrounding tissue of approximately 2 to 4 cm were in the radiation target volume. After a mean follow-up 18 moths, no local recurrences were observed. Cosmesis of the breast was very good and comparable to that of patients without IORT. The late complications were two rib necroses.

There is an important controversy surrounding the optimal minimum treatment required for adequate LC without compromising therapeutic effect (Fig. 17.4). Long-term results of the Milan III trial showed that about 86% of recurrences in the ipsilateral breast occur in the previously involved quadrant. This is the rationale for partial breast irradiation: a more limited radi-

ation treatment aimed at the elimination of potentially residual cancer cells in the vicinity of the primary tumor, while avoiding irradiation of the whole breast.

IOERT in the Milan experience (12,13,114) has demonstrated its capacity for safely delivering relatively high single doses of irradiation directly to the tumor bed at the time of an operation while sparing adjacent normal surrounding tissues. From 1999 to 2003, 590 breast cancer patients (mean age, 59 years) received IOERT after breast-conserving surgery as sole radiation treatment modality (574 patients) or as an anticipated boost followed by external radiotherapy (16 patients). All patients had unicentric primary carcinoma, ≤2.5 cm in largest diameter. The dose delivered was 21 Gy in 559 patients, 19 Gy in 6 patients, and 17 Gy in 9 patients prescribed at the 90% using 3 to 10 MeV electron beams. With a mean of follow-up of 24 months (range, 4 to 57 months), there were 3 local recurrences (0.5%); 3 (0.5%) patients presented with ipsilateral second breast carcinoma and (0.8%) with contralateral carcinoma; 1 patient developed axillary lymph node metastases

Table 17.4	INTRAOPERATIVE IRRADIATION (IORT) FOLLOWING PANCREATIC CANCER RESECTION				
Author	N	Dose IORT (Gy)	N Receiving EBRT	Local Recurrence % (2y.)	Median Survival (months)
Zerbi[121a]	43	12.5–20	0	27	19
	47	Control		56	12
	30	10–25	10	27	24
	19		2	60	14
Valentini[110a]	17	10	0	18	18
Calvo[16]	15	10–15	0	47	17
Coquard[22]	25	12–25	20	36	15
Sindelar[97]	12	20	0	33	18
	12	Control	12	100	12

N = Number

and 13 (2.2%) distant metastases. The side effects included fibrosis and liponecrosis (Table 17.2). These complications resolved with conservative care; one case required surgical curettage.

Finally, the Milan clinical experience (12) contains an interesting nipple-sparing mastectomy study testing a new technique to preserve the nipple and areola complex during mastectomy, which included delivery of a 16-Gy single dose to this anatomic area. Results are promising, but the follow-up period was too short to reach definitive conclusions.

Gynecologic Sites

In patients with locally recurrent gynecologic cancer in the pelvic side walls, para-aortic nodes, or pelvic lymph nodes, the use of aggressive salvage surgery and IOERT with or without EBRT or chemotherapy may be beneficial (23). The 5-year survival is 27% and 32% in separate U.S. IOERT series from Mayo Clinic (32) and the University of Washington (106), respectively. The University of Navarre (Pamplona) is evaluating the incorporation of preoperative EBRT with cisplatin plus infusion 5-FU, resection, and IOERT in the treatment of locally advanced primary cervical cancers (67). An update of this experience reports 10-year in-field control rates of 92% and 46% for primary and recurrent disease, respectively.

Researchers at Stanford University have published a study in patients with recurrent ovarian cancer treated with cytoreductive surgery and IORT with orthovoltage x-rays. IORT doses ranged from 9 to 14 Gy. At a median follow-up of 24 months, 5 patients remained free of disease and 17 patients had recurrences, of whom 4 are alive with disease.

Miscellaneous Indications

Brain tumors have been approached with IORT in some European and Japanese institutions (90,91). Metastatic spinal tumors have been treated with IORT (20 Gy) during surgical resection (78). In head and neck cancer patients, most investigators have use IORT in the context of the salvage treatment of recurrent disease (76).

Summary

In the past 25 years, the understanding of the potential contribution of IORT has improved and the rational basis for its use has aided the general progress of oncology, in particular the concept of multimodal treatment. In IORT, institutional programs with a dedicated portable linear accelerator, HDR brachytherapy device, or fixed conventional linear accelerator in a surgical area, or all of these devices, is a real test of teamwork (80).

IORT is now accepted as a locoregional treatment modality that produces local effects and contributes to treatment success by increasing LC without major treatment morbidity (18). In the future, the effectiveness of radiation treatment may be further increased by the application of IOHT during IORT or the selective use of radiation protectors or radiation sensitizers.

To demonstrate the IORT therapeutic benefit, meticulous methods are needed and randomized controlled clinical trials are required to accelerate the introduction of IORT into the clinical practice. Randomized trials were initiated in the mid-1980s at the NCI (Bethesda, MD) in resectable and unresectable pancreatic cancer, postresected gastric cancer, and resectable retroperitoneal sarcomas (99,100,101). The results showed method limitations with a small number of patients, heterogeneous stage, and treatment factors, but also a trend toward improved LC without differences in treatment-related complications.

IOERT was handicapped by the need for patient transportation at the time of surgical operation. There are mobile linear accelerators able to produce high-energy electron beams of up to 9 to 12 MeV that overcome this limitation, increase its potential use by allowing movement from one surgical room to another, and make IORT significantly less time-consuming, less costly, and less risky to administer. Portable HDR brachytherapy devices using molds and flaps are extremely accurate in adapting the dosimetrically useful volume to target regions that are not accessible to electron beams because of anatomic restrictions or unacceptable dosimetric inhomogeneities (49).

Specific IORT dosimetric treatment-planning systems, preplanning IORT virtual simulation, two-dimensional and three-dimensional real-time isodose distribution, documentation of final dosimetric treatment characteristics, and integration of IORT boost into the external-beam component of treatment are valuable developments in radiation physics, emerging as research projects pending definitive validation and commercial availability (5,95).

References

1. Abe M, Takahashi M, eds. Intraoperative radiation therapy. *Proceedings of the Third International Symposium on Intraoperative Radiation Therapy.* Philadelphia: Pergamon Press; 1991.
2. Abuchaibe O, Calvo FA, Tangeo E, et al. Intraoperative irradiation in locally advanced recurrent colorectal cancer. *Int J Radiat Oncol Biol Phys* 1993;26:859–867.
3. Aitken DR, Hopkins GA, Archambeau JO, et al. Intraoperative radiotherapy in the treatment of neuroblastoma: report of a pilot study. *Ann Surg Oncol.* 1995;2:343–350.
4. Alektiar KM, Hu K, Anderson L, et al. High-dose-rate intraoperative radiation therapy (HDR-IORT) for retroperitoneal sarcomas. *Int J Radiat Oncol Biol Phys* 2000;47:157–163.
5. Anderson LL, Harrington PJ, St Germain J. Physics of intraoperative high-dose-rate brachytherapy. In: Gunderson LL, Willet CG, Harrison LB, Calvo FA (eds). *Intraoperative irradiation. Techniques and results.* Totowa, NJ: Humana Press; 2000;87–104.
6. Antonini N, Horiot JC, Poortmans P, et al. Local control and age after breast conserving treatment with complete resection; EORTC Trial 22881. *Radiother Oncol* 2004;73:281(abstr).
7. Arimoto T, Takamura A, Tomita M, et al. Intraoperative radiotherapy for esophageal carcinoma–significance of IORT dose for the incidence of fatal tracheal complication. *Int J Radiat Oncol Biol Phys* 1993;27:1063–1067.
8. Aristu J, Rebollo J, Martinez-Monge R, et al. Cisplatin, mitomycin, and vindesine followed by intraoperative and postoperative radiotherapy for stage III non-small cell lung cancer: final results of a phase II study. *Am J Clin Oncol* 1997;20:276–281.
9. Azinovic I, Calvo FA, Puebla F, et al. Long-term normal tissue effects of intraoperative electron radiation therapy (IOERT): late sequelae, tumor recurrence, and second malignancies. *Int J Radiat Oncol Biol Phys* 2001;49:597–604.
10. Azinovic I, Martinez Monge R, Javier Aristu J, et al. Intraoperative radiotherapy electron boost followed by moderate doses of external beam radiotherapy in resected soft-tissue sarcoma of the extremities. *Radiother Oncol* 2003;67:331–337.
11. Bobin JY, Al-Lawati T, Granero LE, et al. Surgical management of retroperitoneal sarcomas associated with external and intraoperative electron beam radiotherapy. *Eur J Surg Oncol* 2003;29:676–681.
12. BR2; Orecchia R, Ciocca M, Lazzari R, et al. Intraoperative radiation therapy with electrons (ELIOT) in early-stage breast cancer. *Breast* 2003;12:483–490.
13. BR5; Orecchia R, Ciocca M, Tosi G, et al. Intraoperative electron beam radiotherapy (ELIOT) to the breast: a need for a quality assurance programme. *Breast* 2005;14:541–546.
14. Calvo FA, Aristu JJ, Azinovic I, et al. Intraoperative and external radiotherapy in resected gastric cancer: updated report of a phase II trial. *Int J Radiat Oncol Biol Phys* 1992;24:729–736.
15. Calvo FA, Azinovic I, Martinez R, et al. Intraoperative radiotherapy for the treatment of soft tissue sarcomas of central anatomical sites. *Radiat Oncol Invest* 1995;3:90–96.
16. Calvo FA, Gomez-Espi M, Diaz-Gonzalez JA, et al. Intraoperative presacral electron boost followed by preoperative chemoradiation in T3–4Nx rectal cancer: initial local effects and clinical outcome analysis. *Radiother Oncol* 2002;62:201–206.
17. Calvo FA, Ortiz de Urbina D, Sierrasesumaga L, et al. Intraoperative radiotherapy in the multidisciplinary treatment of bone sarcomas in children and adolescents. *Med Pediatr Oncol* 1991;19:478–485.
18. Calvo FA, Santos M, Brady LW, eds. *Intraoperative radiotherapy: clinical experiences and results.* Heidelberg, Germany: Springer-Verlag; 1992.
19. Canon R, Azinovic I, Aristu JJ, et al. Long-term results after preoperative chemorradiation with or without intraoperative chemoradiation (IORT) in locally advanced rectal carcinoma. In: *Proceedings of the International Society of Intraoperative Radiation Therapy.* Boston: 2000:68.
20. Carter YM, Jablons DM, DuBois JB et al. intraoperative radiation therapy in the multimodality approach to upper aerodigestive tract cancer. *Surg Oncol Clin North Am* 2003;12:1043–1063.
21. Cienfuegos JA, Manuel FA, et al. Analysis of intraoperative radiotherapy for pancreatic carcinoma. *Eur J Surg Oncol* 2000;26[Suppl A]:S13–15.

22. Coquard R, Ayzac L, Gilly FN, et al. Intraoperative Radiotherapy in Resected Pancreatic Cancer: feasibility and results. *Radiother Oncol* 1997;44:271–275.
23. del Carmen MG, Eisner B, Willet CG, et al. Intraoperative radiation therapy in the management of gynecologic and genitourinary malignancies. *Surg Oncol Clin North Am.* 2003;12:1031–1042.
24. DeLuca AM, Johnstone PA, Ollayos CW, et al. Tolerance of the bladder to intraoperative radiation in a canine model: a five-year follow-up. *Int J Radiat Oncol Biol Phys* 1994;30:339–345.
25. Diaz-Gonzalez JA, Calvo FA, Cortes J, et al. Preoperative chemoradiation with oral tegafur within a multidisciplinary therapeutic approach in patients with T3–4 rectal cancer. *Int J Radiat Oncol Biol Phys* 2005;61:1378–1384.
26. Dubois JB, Hay MH, Gely S, et al. The intraoperative radiation therapy (IORT) in soft tissue sarcomas. IORT 94th-5th International Symposium Abstracts. *Hepatogastroenterology* 1994;41:3.
27. Eble MJ, Lehnert T, Herfarth C, et al. IORT as adjuvant treatment in primary rectal carcinomas: multi-modality treatment. *Front Radiat Ther Oncol* 1997;31:200–203.
28. Eble MJ, Staehler G, Wannenmacher M. The intraoperative radiotherapy (IORT) of locally spread and recurrent renal-cell carcinomas. *Strahlenther Onkol* 1998;174:30–36.
29. Fletcher GH, Shukovsky LJ. The interplay of radiocurability and tolerance in the irradiation of human cancers. *J Radiol Electrol* 1975;56:383–400.
30. Fletcher GH. Clinical dose response curves of human malignant epithelial tumors. *Br J Radiol* 1973;46:1–12.
31. Garton GR, Gunderson LL, Nagorney DM, et al. High-dose preoperative external beam and intraoperative irradiation for locally advanced pancreatic cancer. *Int J Radiat Oncol Biol Phys* 1993;27:1153–1157.
32. Garton GR, Gunderson LL, Webb MJ, et al. lntraoperative irradiation in Gynecologic cancer: The Mayo Clinic experience. *Gynecol Oncol* 1993;48:328–332.
33. Gieschen HL, Spiro IJ, Suit HD, et al. Long-term results of intraoperative electron beam radiotherapy for primary and recurrent retroperitoneal soft tissue sarcoma. *Int J Radiat Oncol Biol Phys* 2001;50:127–131.
34. Gillette EL, Gillette SM, Powers BE. Studies at Colorado State University of normal tissue tolerance of beagles to IOERT, EBRT or a combination. In: Gunderson LL, Willet CG, Harrison LB, Calvo FA, eds. *Intraoperative irradiation. Techniques and results.* Totowa, NJ: Humana Press; 1999:147–164.
35. Gillette EL, Powers BE, Gillette SM, et al. Peripheral nerve tolerance: experimental and clinical. In: Gunderson LL, Willet CG, Harrison LB, Calvo FA, eds. *Intraoperative irradiation. Techniques and results.* Totowa, NJ: Humana Press; 2000:165–174.
36. Gillette SM, Gillette EL, Powers BE, et al. Radiation-induced osteosarcoma in dogs after external beam or intraoperative radiation therapy. *Cancer Res* 1990;50:54–57.
37. Glehen O, Beaujard AC, Romestaing P, et al. Patterns of failures in gastric cancer patients with lymph node involvement treated by surgery, intraoperative and external beam radiotherapy. *Radiat Oncol* 2003;67:171–175.
38. Goldson AL. Preliminary clinical experience with intraoperative radiotherapy. *J Natl Med Assoc* 1978;70:493–495.
39. Goldson AL. Update on 5 years of pioneering experience with intraoperative electron irradiation. In: *Session II. Intraoperative electron therapy. Varian Users Proceedings.* 1982:21–27.
40. Gunderson LL, Haddock MG, Burch P, et al. Future role of radiotherapy as a component or treatment in biliopancreatic cancers. *Ann Oncol* 1990;10[Suppl 4]: 291–5.
41. Gunderson LL, Haddock MG, Nelson H, et al. cally recurrent colorectal cancer: IOERT and EBRT +/-5-FU and maximal resection. *Front Radiat Ther Oncol* 1997;31:224–228.
42. Gunderson LL, Nagorney DM, Martenson JA, et al. External beam plus intraoperative irradiation for gastrointestinal cancers. *World J Surg* 1995;19:191–197.
43. Gunderson LL, Nagorney DM, McIlrath DC, et al. External beam and intraoperative electron irradiation for locally advanced soft tissue sarcomas. *Int J Radiat Oncol Biol Phys* 1993;25:647–656.
44. Gunderson LL, Nelson H, Martenson JA, et al. Intraoperative electron and external beam irradiation with or without 5-fluorouracil and maximum surgical resection for previously unirradiated, locally recurrent colorectal Cancer. *Dis Colon Rectum* 1996;39:1379–1395.
45. Gunderson LL, Shipley WU, Suit HD, et al. Intraoperative irradiation: a pilot study combining external beam photons with 'boost" dose intraoperative electrons. *Cancer* 1982;49:2259–2266.
46. Gunderson LL, Willet C. Pancreas and hepatobiliary tract cancer. In: Perez CA, Brady LW, eds. *Principles and practice of radiation oncology*, 3rd ed. Philadelphia: JB Lippincott; 1997:1467–1488.
47. Haas-Kogan DA, Fisch BM, Wara WM, et al. Intraoperative radiation therapy for high-risk pediatric neuroblastoma. *Int J Radiat Oncol Biol Phys* 2000 1;47:985–992.
48. Haddock MG, Gunderson LL, Nelson H, et al. Intraoperative irradiation for locally recurrent colorectal cancer in previously irradiated patients. *Int J Radiat Oncol Biol Phys* 2001;49:1267–1274.
49. Harrison LB, Cohen AM, Enker WA. High-dose-rate intraoperative irradiation (HDR'IORT): technical factors. In: Gunderson LL, Willet CG, Harrison LB, Calvo FA, eds. *Intraoperative irradiation. Techniques and results.* Totowa, NJ: Humana Press; 2000;105–110.
50. Hashiguchi Y, Sekine T, Sakamoto H, et al. Intraoperative irradiation after surgery for locally recurrent rectal cancer. *Dis Colon Rectum* 1999;42:886–893.
51. Henning GT, Schild SE, Gunderson LL et al. Results of irradiation or chemoirradiation for primary unresectable, locally recurrent or grossly incomplete resection of gastric adenocarcinoma. *Int J Radiat Oncol Biol Phys* 2000;46:109–118.
52. Hosokawa M, Shirato H, Ohara M, et al. Intraoperative radiation therapy to the upper mediastinum and nerve-sparing three-field lymphadenectomy followed by external beam radiotherapy for patients with thoracic esophageal carcinoma. *Cancer* 19991;86:6–13.
53. Huber FT, Stepan R, Zimmerman F, et al. Locally advanced rectal cancer: resection and intraoperative radiotherapy using the flab method combined with preoperative or postoperative radiochemotherapy. *Dis Colon Rectum* 1996;39:774–779.
54. Johnstone PA, DeLuca AM, Bacher JD, et al. Clinical toxicity of peripheral nerve to intraoperative radiotherapy in a canine model. *Int J Radiat Oncol Biol Phys* 1995;32:1031–1034.
55. Johnstone PA, Laskin WB, DeLuca AM, et al. Tumors in dogs exposed to experimental intraoperative radiotherapy. *Int J Radiat Oncol Biol Phys* 1996;34:853–857.
56. Johnstone PA, Rohde DC, Saunders EL, et al. Combining intraoperative and conventional external radiotherapy doses: a biology-based approach. *Front Radiat Ther Oncol* 1997;31:18–21.
57. Johnstone PA, Sindelar WF, Kinsella TJ. Experimental and clinical studies of intraoperative radiation therapy. *Curr Probl Cancer* 1994;18:249–292.
58. Johnstone PA, Sprague M, DeLuca AM, et al. Effects of intraoperative radiotherapy on vascular grafts in a canine model. *Int J Radiat Oncol Biol Phys* 1994;29:1015–1025.
59. Kretzler A, Molls M, Gradinger R, et al. Intraoperative radiotherapy of soft tissue sarcoma of the extremity. *Strahlenther Onkol* 2004;180:365–370.
60. Lemanski C, Azria D, Thezenas S, et al. Intraoperative radiotherapy given as a boost for early breast cancer: long-term clinical and cosmetic results. *Int J Radiat Oncol Biol Phys* 20061;64:1410–1415.
61. Lindel K, Willett CG, Shellito PC, et al. Intraoperative radiation therapy for locally advanced recurrent rectal or rectosigmoid cancer. *Radiother Oncol* 2001;58:83–87.
62. Macdonald JS, Smalley SR, Benedetti J, et al. Chemoradiotherapy after surgery compared with surgery alone for adenocarcinoma of the stomach or gastroesophageal junction. *N Engl J Med* 2001;345:725–730.
63. Mannaerts GH, Martijn H, Crommelin MA, et al. Feasibility and first results of multimodality treatment, combining EBRT, extensive surgery, and IOERT in locally advanced primary rectal cancer. *Int J Radiat Oncol Biol Phys* 2000;47:425–433.
64. Mannaerts GH, Rutten HJ, Martijn H, et al. Comparison of intraoperative radiation therapy-containing multimodality treatment with historical treatment modalities for locally recurrent rectal cancer. *Dis Colon Rectum* 2001;44:1749–1758.
65. Martinez-Monge R, Calvo FA, Azinovic I, et al. Patterns of failure and long-term results in high-risk resected gastric cancer treated with postoperative radiotherapy with or without intraoperative electron boost. *J Surg Oncol* 1997;66:24–29.
66. Martinez-Monge R, Herreros J, Aristu JJ, et al. Combined treatment in superior sulcus tumors. *Am J Clin Oncol* 1994;17:317–322.
67. Martinez-Monge R, Jurado M, Aristu JJ, et al. Intraoperative electron beam radiotherapy during radical surgery for locally advanced and recurrent cervical cancer. *Gynecol Oncol* 2001;82:538–543.
68. Martinez-Monge R, Nag S, Martin EW. 125Iodine brachytherapy for colorectal adenocarcinoma recurrent in the pelvis and paraortics. *Int J Radiat Oncol Biol Phys* 1998;42:545–550.
69. Martinez-Monge R, Nag S, Martin EW. Three different intraoperative radiation modalities (electron beam, high-dose-rate brachytherapy, and iodine-125 brachytherapy) in the adjuvant treatment of patients with recurrent colorectal adenocarcinoma. *Cancer* 1999;86:236–247.
70. McMahon SB, Priestley JV. Peripheral neuropathies and neurotrophic factors: animal models and clinical perspectives. *Curr Opin Neurobiol* 1995;5:616–624.
71. Miller RC, Haddock MG, Gunderson LL et al. Intraoperative electron-beam radiotherapy and ureteral obstruction. *Int J Radiat Oncol Biol Phys* 2006;64:792–8.
72. Mulcahy MF, Wahl AO, Small W Jr. The current status of combined radiotherapy and chemotherapy for locally advanced or resected pancreas cancer. *J Natl Compr Cancer Netw* 2005;3:637–642.
73. Nag S, Gunderson LL, Willett CG, et al. Intraoperative irradiation with electron beam or high dose rate brachytherapy: methodological comparisons. In: Gunderson LL, Willet CG, Harrison LB, Calvo FA, eds. *Intraoperative irradiation. Techniques and results.* Totowa, NJ: Humana Press; 1999:111–130.
74. Nag S, Orton C. Development of Intraoperative high dose rate brachy-therapy for treatment of resected tumor beds in anesthetized patients. *Endcurieth Hyperth Oncol* 1993;9:187–193.
75. Nag S, Retter E, Martinez-Monge R, et al. Feasibility of intraoperative electron beam radiation therapy in the treatment of locally advanced pediatric malignancies. *Med Pediatr Oncol* 1999;32:382–384.
76. Nag S, Schuller DE, Rodriguez-Villalba S, et al. Intraoperative high dose rate brachytherapy can be used to salvage patients with previously irradiated head and neck recurrences. *Rev Med Univ Navarra* 1999;43:56–61.
77. Nag S, Tippin D, Smith S, et al. Intraoperative electron beam treatment for pediatric malignancies: the Ohio State University experience. *Med Pediatr Oncol* 2003;40:360–366.
78. Nemoto K, Ogawa Y, Matsushita H, et al. Intraoperative radiation therapy (IORT) for previously untreated malignant gliomas. *BMC Cancer.* 2002;2:1.
79. Okunieff P, Sundararaman S, Chen Y. Biology of large dose per fraction radiation therapy. In: Gunderson LL, Willet CG, Harrison LB, Calvo FA, eds. *Intraoperative irradiation. Techniques and results.* Totowa, NJ: Humana Press; 1999:25–46.
80. Ortiz de Urbina D, Tangco E, Arroyo JL, et al. Anesthesia and hospital coordination. In: Calvo FA, Santos M, Brady LW, eds. *Intraoperative radiotherapy.* Heidelberg: Springer Verlag; 1992;25–30.
81. Pacelli F, Di Giorgio A, Papa V, et al. Preoperative radiotherapy combined with intraoperative radiotherapy improve results of total mesorectal excision in patients with T3 rectal cancer. *Dis Colon Rectum* 2004;47:170–179.
82. Petersen IA, Haddok MG, Denohne JH, et al. Use of intraoperative electron beam radiotherapy in the management of retroperitoneal soft tissue sarcomas. *Int J Radiat Oncol Biol Phys* 2002;52:469–475.
83. Powers BE, Gillette EL, Gillette SL, et al. Muscle injury following experimental intraoperative irradiation. *Int J Radiat Oncol Biol Phys* 1991;20:463–471.
84. Rachbauer F, Sztankay A, Kreczy A, et al. High-dose-rate intraoperative brachytherapy (IOHDR) using flab technique in the treatment of soft tissue sarcomas. *Strahlenther Onkol* 2003;179:480–485.
85. Reitsamer R, Peintinger F, Sedlmayer F, et al. Intraoperative radiotherapy given as a boost after breast-conserving surgery in breast cancer patients. *Eur J Cancer* 2002;38:1607–1610.
86. Rich TA, Cady D, McDermott W, et al. Orthovoltage intraoperative radiotherapy: a new look at an old idea. *Int J Radiat Oncol Biol Phys* 1984;10:1951–1965.
87. Roldan GE, Gunderson LL, Nagorney DM,et al: External beam vs intraoperative and external beam irradiation for locally advanced pancreatic cancer. *Cancer* 1988;16:1110–1116.
88. Rosenweig KE, Fox JL, Zelefsky MJ, et al. A pilot trial of high-dose-rate intraoperative radiation therapy for malignant pleural mesothelioma. *Brachytherapy* 2005;4:30–33.

89. Rostom YA, Chapet O, Russo SM, et al. Intra-operative electron radiotherapy as a conservative treatment for infiltrating bladder cancer. *Eur J Cancer* 2000;36:1781–1787.

90. Saito T, Kondo T, Hozumi T, Karasawa K, et al. Results of posterior surgery with intraoperative radiotherapy for spinal metastases. *Eur Spine J* 2006;15: 216–222.

91. Schueller P, Micke O, Palkovic S, et al. 12 years' experience with intraoperative radiotherapy (IORT) of malignant gliomas. *Strahlenther Onkol* 2005;181:500–506.

92. Schwarz RE, Smith DD, Keny H, et al. impact of intraoperative radiation on postoperative and disease-specific outcome after pancreatoduidenectomy for adenocarcinoma: a propensity score analysis. *Am J Clin Oncol* 2003;26:16–21.

93. Seifert WF, Biert J, Wobbes T, et al. Late effects of intraoperative radiation therapy in anastomotic rat colon. *Int J Radiat Oncol Biol Phys* 1998;42:623–629.

94. Shaw EG, Gunderson LL, martin JK, et al. Peripheral nerve and ureteral tolerance of intraoperative radiation therapy: clinical and dose response analysis. *Radiother Oncol* 1990;18:247–255.

95. Shibata D, Guillem JG, Lanouette N, et al. Functional and quality-of-life outcomes in patients with rectal cancer after combined modality therapy, intraoperative radiation therapy, and sphincter preservation. *Dis Colon Rectum* 2000;43:752–758.

96. Shoup M, Guillem JG, Alektiar KM, et al. Predictors of survival in recurrent rectal cancer after resection and intraoperative radiotherapy. *Dis Colon Rectum* 2002;45:585–592.

97. Sindelar WF, Johnstone PA, Hoekstra H, et al. Normal tissue tolerance to IORT: The NCI experimental studies. In: Gunderson LL, Willett CG. Harrison LB, Calvo FA, eds. *Intraoperative irradiation. Techniques and results.* Totowa, NJ: Humana Press; 1999:131–146.

98. Sindelar WF, Kinsella TJ, Chen PW, et al. Intraoperative radiotherapy in retroperitoneal sarcomas: final results of a prospective, randomized trial. *Arch Surg* 1993;128:402–410.

99. Sindelar WF, Kinsella TJ, Tepper JE, et al. National Cancer Institute randomized trial of intraoperative radiotherapy in resectable cancer. *Hepato-Gastroenterol* 1994;41:2.

100. Sindelar WF, Kinsella TJ, Tepper JE, et al. Randomized trial of intraoperative radiotherapy in carcinoma of the stomach. *Am J Surg* 1993;165:178–187.

101. Skoropad VY, Berdov BA, Mardynski YS, et al. A prospective, randomized trial of pre-operative and intraoperative radiotherapy versus surgery alone in resectable gastric cancer. *Eur J Surg Oncol* 2000;26:773–779.

102. Staley CA, Lee JE, Clark KR, et al. Preoperative chemoradiation, pancreaticoduodenectomy and intraoperative radiation therapy for adenocarcinoma of pancreatic head. *Ann J Surg* 1996;171:118–125.

103. Stelzer K, Koh W, Greer B, et al. Intraoperative electron beam therapy (IOEBT) as an adjunct to radical surgery for recurrent cancer of the cervix. In: Schildberg FW, Willich N, Kramling H, eds. *Intraoperative radiation therapy.* Essen, Germany: Verlag Die Blaue Hule; 1993:411–414.

104. Suit HD. Potential for improving survival rates for the cancer patient by increasing the efficacy of treatment of the primary lesion. *Cancer* 1982;50:1227–1234.

105. Taylor WE, Donohue JH, Gunderson LL, et al. The Mayo Clinic experience with multimodality treatment of locally advanced or recurrent colon cancer. *Ann Surg Oncol* 2002;9:177–185.

106. Tepper JE, Sindelar W. A summary on intraoperative radiation therapy. *Cancer Treat Rep* 1981;65:911–918.

107. Tepper JE. Clonogenic potential of human tumors: a hypothesis. *Acta Radiol Oncol* 1981;20:283–288.

108. Termehler PM, Evans DB, Willet CG. IORT in pancreatic cancer. In: Gunderson LL, Willet CG, Harrison LB, Calvo FA, eds. *Intraoperative irradiation. Techniques and results.* Totowa, NJ: Humana Press; 1999:201–202.

109. Tochner ZA, Pass HI, Sindelar WF, et al. Long term tolerance of thoracic organs to intraoperative radiotherapy. *Int J Radiat Oncol Biol Phys* 1992;22:65–69.

110. Valentini V, Morganti AG, De Franco A, et al. Chemoradiation with or without intraoperative radiation therapy in patients with locally recurrent rectal carcinoma: prognostic factors and long-term outcome. *Cancer* 1999;86:2612–2624.

110a. Valentini V, Balducci M, Tortoreto F, Morganti AG, De Giorgi U, Fiorentini G. Intraoperative radiotherapy: current thinking. *Eur J Surg Oncol.* 2002 Mar;28(2): 180–185.

111. Veronesi U, Orecchia R, Luini A, et al. Full-dose intraoperative radiotherapy with electrons during breast-conserving surgery: experience with 590 cases. *Ann Surg* 2005;242:101–106.

112. Vujaskovic Z, Powers BE, Paardekoper G, et al. Effects of intraoperative irradiation (IORT) and intraoperative hyperthermia (IOHT) on canine sciatic nerve: histopathological and morphometric studies. *Int J Radiat Oncol Biol Phys* 1999;43:1103–1109.

113. Wallace HJ, Willett CG, Shellito PC, et al. Intraoperative radiation therapy for locally advanced recurrent rectal or rectosigmoid cancer. *J Surg Oncol* 1995;60:122–127.

114. Weese JL, Harbison SP, Stiller GD, et al. Neoadjuvant chemotherapy, radical resection with intraoperative radiation therapy (IORT): improved treatment for gastric adenocarcinoma. *Surgery* 2000;128:564–571.

115. Willet CG, Del Castillo CF, Shis HA et al. Long-term results of intraoperative electrón beam irradiation (IOERT) for patients with unresectable pancreatic cancer. *Ann Surg* 2005;241:295–299.

116. Willett CG, Shellito PC, Gunderson LL. Primary colorectal EBRT and IOERT. In: Gunderson LL, Willet CG, Harrison LB, Calvo FA, eds. *Intraoperative irradiation. Techniques and results.* Totowa, NJ: Humana Press; 1999:249–272.

117. Willett CG, Shellito PC, Tepper JE, et al. Intraoperative electron beam radiation therapy for primary locally advanced rectal and rectosigmoid carcinoma. *J Clin Oncol* 1991;9:843–849.

118. Willett CG, Suit HD, Tepper JE, et al. Intraoperative electron beam radiation therapy for retroperitoneal soft tissue sarcoma. *Cancer* 1991;68:278–283.

119. Willett CG, Warshaw A. Intraoperative radiation therapy of pancreatic cancer. In: Begen HG, Warshaw Al, Carr-Locke DL, et al, eds. *The pancreas: a clinical textbook.* Cambridge, MA: Blackwell Scientific; in press.

120. Yap OW, Kapp DS, Teng NN, et al. Intraoperative radiation therapy in recurrent ovarian cancer. *Int J Radiat Oncol Biol Phys* 200515;63:1114–1121.

121. Zelefsky MJ, LaQuaglia MP, Ghavimi F, et al. Preliminary results of phase I/II study of high-dose-rate intraoperative radiation therapy for pediatric tumors. *J Surg Oncol* 1996;62:267–272.

121a. Zerbi A, Fossati V, Parolini D, Carlucci M, Balzano G, Bordogna G, Staudacher C, Di Carlo V. Intraoperative radiation therapy adjuvant to resection in the treatment of pancreatic cancer. *Cancer* 1994 Jun 15;73(12):2930–2935.

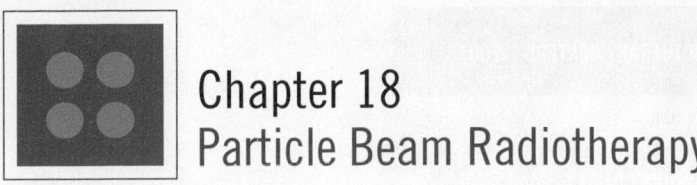

Chapter 18
Particle Beam Radiotherapy

George E. Laramore, Mark H. Phillips, Thomas F. DeLaney

This chapter concerns the clinical use of the more exotic "heavier" nuclear particles in radiation oncology. Although the electron is certainly a "particle," it is used routinely in clinical practice, has no extraordinary radiobiologic properties, and will not be considered here. Particles currently used in radiation oncology are neutrons, which are uncharged and have high linear energy transfer (LET) characteristics; protons and α-particles, which are "charged" but have the same low LET radiobiologic properties as x-rays; and heavy charged particles such as carbon and neon ions, which have high LET properties. For historical interest we also briefly will describe the clinical work using π-mesons, which are a "hybrid" form of high and low LET radiation no longer used in clinical practice and some of the early work with neon ions. Due to space limitations we will not discuss the very specialized area of neutron capture therapy or its application to locally enhancing the dose delivered by a fast neutron therapy beam (3,76).

The initial clinical studies on particle radiation used laboratory-based accelerators or cyclotrons located in physics research laboratories, but now this work has shifted to the setting of major medical centers. Two main factors have motivated this research. One is the better depth-dose distribution and reduced penumbra that is achieved with charged particles of proton mass or greater. In principle, this allows for the ultimate expression of intensity modulated, conformal radiotherapy. The other factor relates to the more favorable radiobiologic properties of high LET radiation. This provided the impetus for the clinical studies using fast neutron beams, which, at best, have dose localization properties approximating those of megavoltage photon beams.

Basic Radiobiology Relating to Particle Radiotherapy

The rate of energy transferred by ionizing radiation along its path is referred to as *linear energy transfer*. Conventional photon and electron beams used in therapy typically have LETs in the range of 0.2 to 2 keV/μ, whereas a high LET form of radiation such as a fast neutron typically has an LET in the range of 20 to 100 keV/μ. Heavy, stripped ions have LETs in the range of 100 to 1,000 keV/μ. The biologic effect of radiation is highly dependent on its LET. This is characterized by the relative biologic effectiveness (RBE) factor, which is the ratio of the dose of ^{60}Co radiation to the dose of particle radiation producing the same biologic end point. The RBE versus LET curve for most systems peaks at about 160 keV/μ (52). The RBE of a given type of radiation is, of course, dependent upon many factors such as the tissue type, chosen end point, dose fractionation schema, and so forth. However, for practical clinical work using common fractionation schedules, one can use a set of simple numbers in comparing the effective doses of the various types of particle radiotherapy beams. Compared to standard forms of radiotherapy taken to have an RBE of 1, protons and α-particles also are considered to be low LET particles with an RBE of 1.1 to 1.2. Fast neutrons are high LET particles with an RBE in the range

of 3 to 3.5 in terms of most normal tissue late effects, an RBE in the range of 4 to 4.5 in terms of damage to the central nervous system (CNS), and an RBE in the range of 8 for salivary gland malignancies (4,52,77). Heavy charged particles are also high LET particles with RBEs in the range of 2 to 4 for most normal tissues (52,90,105,118). Therefore, the radiobiology of protons and α-particles is considered to be essentially the same as that of standard radiotherapy except at the very end of the Bragg peak, where the LET increases. The high LET forms of radiation offer potential therapeutic advantages in several clinical situations.

Low LET radiation primarily kills cells via an indirect, free radical mediated mechanism. These free radicals are produced predominantly in the cell cytoplasm and then have to diffuse to the nuclear DNA (or other critical target) to damage it (52). For this to be effective, a long free radical lifetime is desirable. Oxygen acts as an electron scavenger; hence, free radical lifetimes are longer in cells that are well oxygenated. Oxygen also acts to stabilize the free radical damage. In hypoxic cells, the free radical lifetimes are shorter; hence, these cells are "protected" from much of the damage. Thus it takes a higher radiation dose in hypoxic cells to achieve the same biologic end point compared to the required dose in well-oxygenated cells. High LET radiation causes a higher proportion of direct damage to the critical cellular targets and therefore is not as dependent on the free radical intermediary. The oxygen enhancement ratio (OER) is the ratio of the radiation dose required to produce a specific biologic effect under anoxic conditions to the dose required to produce the same effect under well-oxygenated conditions. For most mammalian cells, the OER for conventional low LET radiation is in the range of 2.5 to 3, whereas for clinically used high LET radiation, the OER is in the range of 1.4 to 1.7 (2,8,52). Although the lower OER was one of the primary motivating factors in using high LET radiation, its actual importance in most clinical settings may not be that great because of reoxygenation during a course of fractionated radiotherapy.

Another potential advantage to high LET radiation relates to the reduced ability of cells to repair the radiation damage it produces. The dense chain of ionization events produced by high LET radiation causes simultaneous damage to both strands of the cellular DNA. Cell survival curves for low LET radiation characteristically exhibit a shoulder at low radiation doses, indicating the ability of the cells to repair this "sublethal" damage. High LET radiation, however, exhibits a very reduced shoulder, resulting in a cell survival curve that is almost log-linear in shape over the range of radiation doses of clinical relevance (45,52). One therefore would expect tumors having a large capacity for radiation damage repair to be among those best treated with high LET radiation (4). Although the cell survival curves for experimental tumor types can vary considerably, it does appear that tumors where there is a clinically proven advantage for high LET radiation fall into this category. Another type of radiation damage is "potentially lethal" damage, which occurs in cells that are in a noncycling, plateau phase (45,52,53). This has been demonstrated in the laboratory and may be important in tumors having a large fraction of cells in the G0 phase of the cell cycle. This type of repair is less pronounced for high LET radiation than for low LET radiation.

Table 18.1	LOCATION OF OPERATING FAST NEUTRON RADIOTHERAPY CENTERS—2007	
Location	**Beam Reaction**	**Comments**
United States		
University of Washington Medical Center—Seattle	50 MeV p→Be	Isocentric gantry and multileaf collimator
Harper-Grace Hospital—Detroit, MI	48 MeV d→Be	Isocentric gantry and multileaf collimator. Converted from multirod collimator in 2005
Fermi Laboratories—Batavia, IL	66 MeV p→Be	Horizontal beam, fixed collimators with blocking inserts
Europe		
Centre Hospitalier Regional—Orleans, France	34 MeV p→Be	Vertical beam, fixed collimators with blocking inserts
University of Essen—Essen, Germany	14 MeV d→Be	Isocentric gantry with collimator inserts and wedge capability
Africa		
National Accelerator Centre—Faure, South Africa	66 MeV p→Be	Isocentric gantry and jaw collimator

A final point relates to the variation of radiosensitivity across the cell cycle. Mammalian cells are more radiosensitive in M and late G1/early S phases than in early G1 and G2. If radiation is given to an asynchronously dividing cell population, then cells in the sensitive portions of the cycle are killed preferentially. Over a course of fractionated radiotherapy, cells continue through the cycle, and when other fractions of radiation are delivered, many of the formerly resistant cells are in the more sensitive phases of the cycle. The variation in radiosensitivity across the cell cycle is about a factor of 4 less with high LET radiation (46,52). Hence, tumors with long cell-cycle times theoretically would be better treated with high LET radiation.

With this as background, we now will discuss the clinical results for the various types of particle radiation. Because of space limitations, we will focus on the more promising areas or those of special importance from a historical perspective.

Fast Neutron Radiotherapy

Between 1938 and 1943 Robert Stone (117) treated 240 patients with fast neutron radiotherapy at the Crocker Radiation Laboratory, which was the forerunner of the Lawrence Berkeley Laboratory (LBL). The beams he used had depth-dose properties similar to those of orthovoltage x-rays, and many of his patients had received prior radiotherapy. There were few long-term survivors, and the patients who did survive experienced severe radiation sequelae. Further clinical work was suspended for almost 20 years when a review of Stone's work by Brennan and Phillips (6) showed that an inappropriate value for the RBE had been used and therefore Stone's patients inadvertently had been overdosed. Based on this new knowledge, in the 1960s Catterall et al. (16–18) resumed neutron clinical trials at Hammersmith Hospital in London, England. After treating several hundred patients, the authors concluded that with appropriate fractionation schemas, neutron radiation was well tolerated and many advanced tumors responded extremely well. Following their initial reports, clinical trials were instituted at many other facilities throughout the world. At one time or another, 39 different centers in North America, Europe, Asia, and Africa treated patients with fast neutrons. To date approximately 30,000 patients have received neutron radiotherapy as all or part of their cancer therapy. Although neutron radiotherapy has demonstrated clinical utility in the treatment of certain tumors, it has not proven to be as effective a panacea as was originally hoped. There are currently five operating neutron radiotherapy facilities, which

are listed in Table 18.1 along with some of their more important characteristics. The more important conclusions from the neutron clinical trials are discussed later in this chapter. Because space does not permit us to be all-inclusive, we will emphasize the areas where neutrons show therapeutic benefit compared to conventional radiotherapy.

Salivary Gland Tumors

Although fast neutron radiotherapy has been used in the treatment of many different types of tumors, their major therapeutic advantage has been demonstrated for salivary gland tumors. In retrospect, this could have been predicted from the early radiobiologic work of Battermann, et al. (4), in which the RBE for fractionated radiotherapy was found to be approximately eight, compared to values in the range of 3 to 3.5 expected for late damage in most normal tissues. With appropriate field shaping, one can deliver neutron radiation doses of approximately 20 $Gy_{n\gamma}$ (by convention the γ-rays produced by the neutron interactions are included in the physical dose measurement) to the head and neck region with blocking to reduce the dose to the spinal cord (54). This roughly corresponds to an equivalent photon dose of 60 to 70 Gy-equivalent (Gy-equivalent equals the physical dose multiplied by RBE) as far as normal tissues are concerned but approximately 160 Gy-equivalent as far as the tumor is concerned. The therapeutic gain factor for salivary gland tumors thus is in the range of 2.3 to 2.6.

Early single-institution series seemed to confirm this therapeutic advantage, and the Radiation Therapy Oncology Group (RTOG) and the Medical Research Council of Great Britain conducted a prospective randomized trial for this disease site. A final report on this study showed improved local regional control at 10 years (56% vs. 17%; $p = 0.009$) but no improvement in long-term survival due to distant metastases (81). This study was stopped early for ethical reasons when 2-year survival data showed a strong trend in favor of the neutron patients. At the 10-year end point there was a slight (but not statistically significant) benefit to median patient survival on the neutron arm of about 8 months but, with the patients living longer as a result of controlled local/regional disease, the subsequent development of distant metastases became the dominant cause of death. The final local-regional control curve from this study is shown in Fig. 18.1.

More recent single-institution data continue to support the efficacy of fast neutron radiotherapy in the treatment of salivary gland tumors. Douglas et al. (26) have analyzed their results for

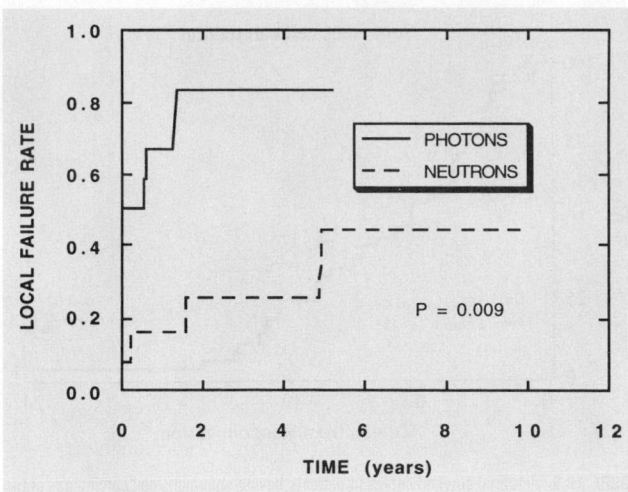

FIGURE 18.1. Actuarial local/regional control rates for patients with unresectable salivary gland tumors who were treated on the RTOG/MRC randomized trial (80-01). The neutron curve is shown as the dashed line and the photon curve is shown as the solid line. The difference between the two curves is statistically significant at the $p = 0.009$ level. (Reprinted from Laramore GE, Krall JM, Griffin TW, et al. Neutron versus photon irradiation for unresectable salivary gland tumor: Final report of an RTOG-MRC randomized clinical trial. *Int J Radiat Oncol Biol Phys* 1993;27:235–240, with permission.)

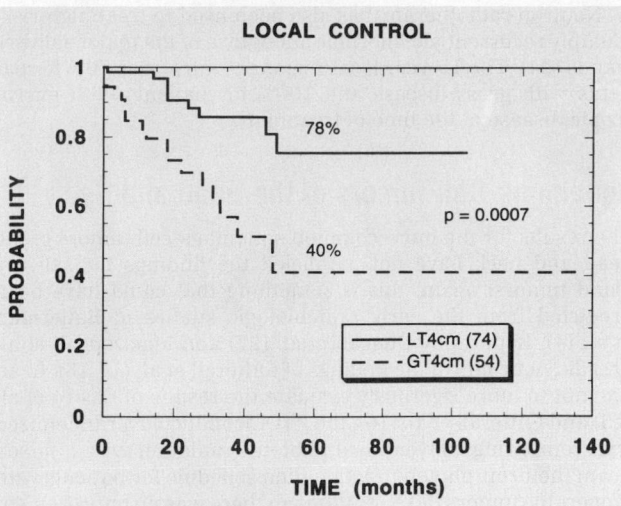

FIGURE 18.2. Actuarial local/regional control rates for patients with major salivary gland tumors who were treated at the University of Washington Fast Neutron Radiotherapy facility. On both univariate and multivariate analysis, tumor size was a predictive factor for local/regional control. The solid curve depicts the results for patients with tumors <4 cm in extent, whereas the dashed curve depicts the results for tumors >4 cm in extent. (Reprinted from Douglas JD, Lee S, Laramore GE, et al. Neutron radiotherapy for the treatment of locally advanced major salivary gland tumors. *Head Neck* 1999;21:255–263, with permission.)

tumors of the major salivary gland (all histologies) and found that if the overall tumor size was <4 cm, the local control rate at 9 years was 78%. The control rate was about 40% for the larger tumors. Figure 18.2 shows actuarial local control probabilities as a function of tumor size as taken from this analysis. Tumor size and location (parotid versus submandibular and sublingual) were factors affecting local regional control and survival. Another analysis of Douglas et al. (25) focused specifically on patients with adenoid cystic carcinoma. Control rates and cause-specific survival as a function of tumor location are given in Table 18.2. The lower local/regional control rates for tumors arising in the paranasal sinuses or nasopharynx are attributable to tumors invading the cavernous sinus or skull base where the proximity of critical CNS structures limited the neutron dose that could be given relative to tumors in other sites. On multivariate analysis, the presence of base-of-skull involvement was found to be a statistically significant adverse factor for local/regional control at the $p \leq 0.01$ level. A gamma knife boost is currently being used to boost areas of skull base disease but follow-up is too short to know whether or not this has solved the problem. The risk of developing distant metastases was approximately 50% at 2 years for node positive patients,

and for node negative patients the risk also reached approximately 50% but took 10 years to do so. Clearly better systemic therapy is needed for this tumor.

To reduce the side effects associated with the poorly penetrating properties of the early beams, early neutron work often involved treating patients with a combination of neutrons and photons (known as a *mixed beam regimen*) rather than with neutrons alone. There is a concern that this approach also might reduce the tumor-control probability in the case of adenoid cystic carcinomas where there is a high therapeutic gain factor. Huber et al. (59) reported on a series of patients with adenoid cystic carcinomas treated at the Heidelberg neutron facility and found a 5-year local control rate of 75% for patients treated with neutrons alone compared to 32% for groups of patients treated with a mixed beam regimen or with photons alone. In settings where treatment morbidity is not a major problem, it appears advantageous to use the more effective modality (e.g., neutrons, for the entire treatment). Like other investigators, they also found that a high rate of distant metastases prevented improved local/regional control from being translated into improved survival.

Table 18.2	FIVE-YEAR ACTUARIAL LOCAL/REGIONAL CONTROL RATES AND CAUSE SPECIFIC SURVIVAL AS A FUNCTION OF PRIMARY SITE FOR PATIENTS WITH ADENOID CYSTIC CARCINOMAS TREATED WITH FAST NEUTRONS		
Site	Patient Number	Local/Regional Control (%)	Cause-Specific Survival (%)
Paranasal sinus	32	43	67
Parotid	27	67	82
Oral cavity	26	68	87
Oropharynx	19	75	92
Submandibular/sublingual	15	59	83
Nasopharynx	15	21	35
Lacrimal gland	7	80	100
Trachea	4	25	75
Other	6	100	100

From Douglas JD, Laramore GE, Austin-Seymour M, et al. Treatment of locally advanced adenoid cystic carcinoma of the head and neck with neutron radiotherapy. *Int J Radiat Oncol Biol Phys* 2000;46:551–557, with permission.

Neutron radiotherapy has also been used to treat high-risk, multiply recurrent pleomorphic adenomas of the major salivary glands (24). The 15-year local/regional control was 76% for patients with gross disease and 100% for patients with microscopic disease at the time of treatment.

Squamous-Cell Tumors of the Head and Neck

The results for the more common squamous-cell tumors of the head and neck have not paralleled the findings for salivary gland tumors; again, this is something that could have been predicted from the early radiobiologic studies of Batterman et al. (4). Reports by Duncan et al. (27) and MacDougall et al. (91) did not confirm the findings of Catterall et al. (17,18). In an attempt to more rigorously evaluate the results of Castro et al. (15) and Catterall et al. (16), the RTOG conducted a randomized trial comparing conventional photon irradiation with a mixed beam (neutron/photon) fractionation schedule for patients with inoperable tumors (50,51). Although there was no improvement in terms of local control of the primary tumor or in survival, there was an apparent benefit in terms of improved regional control in the neck for patients presenting with clinically positive adenopathy. In contrast to the results of Catterall et al. (17,18), many patients who had an initial apparent complete local/regional response with fast neutrons developed failures within the radiation fields with passage of time—just as occurred for those patients on the photon control arm. The results of this trial were criticized because its neutron arm did not correspond to the particular regimen used at Hammersmith Hospital. Instead it was "diluted" with photon irradiation and also had a substantially longer overall treatment time of 7 weeks compared to the 4-week fractionation schema used at Hammersmith. The Neutron Therapy Cooperative Working Group (NTCWG) therefore repeated this study using the second generation, hospital-based facilities located in the United States and Great Britain with the experimental neutron arm being identical to that used by Catterall et al. The results of this second randomized trial also showed no benefit in either local/regional control or survival for the neutron-treated patients (92). There was a suggestion of improved regional control of clinically positive nodes with fast neutrons, but it did not achieve clinical significance. Late complications graded "severe or greater" according to the joint RTOG/EORTC (European Organization of Radiation Treatment Centers) scoring schema were 40% on the neutron arm compared to 17% on the photon arm ($p = 0.008$). Hence, it currently is felt that neutron radiotherapy is of limited utility in the treatment of head and neck squamous-cell tumors with the possible exception of patients with massive cervical adenopathy.

Non–Small-Cell Lung Cancer

The first reported experience using fast neutron radiotherapy for non–small-cell lung cancer was from Eichhorn (30), who used a very low energy neutron beam. Autopsy rates showed higher rates of tumor sterilization as the percentage of the dose given with neutrons increased: Photons alone produced a 33% sterilization rate in 149 patients, mixed beam (20% neutrons and 80% photons) produced a sterilization rate of 48% in 75 patients, and mixed beam (37% neutrons and 63% photons) produced a sterilization rate of 57% in 49 patients. There have been two reported series that showed exceptionally high local control rates for Pancoast's or superior sulcus tumors: Komaki et al. (75) found a 91% local control rate, which translated into improved survival relative to a group of photon treated patients, and Sawada et al. (108) found a mean survival of 11.5 months for 18 patients treated with neutrons compared to four months for five patients treated with conventional photon irradiation.

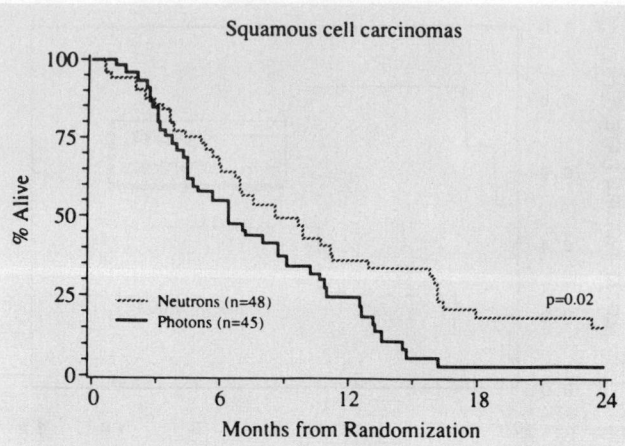

FIGURE 18.3. Actuarial survival curves in patients having squamous cell carcinomas of the lung treated on an NTCWG study (85-24). The neutron-treated group is shown as the dotted curve, and the photon-treated group is shown as the solid curve. The difference between the two curves is statistically significant at the $p = 0.02$ level. (Reprinted from Koh WJ, Krall JM, Peters LJ, et al. Neutron versus photon radiation therapy for inoperable regional non–small cell lung cancer: Results of a multicenter randomized trial. *Int J Radiat Oncol Biol Phys* 1993;27:499–505, with permission.)

There have been two randomized clinical trials for inoperable, non–small-cell lung cancer. The first was a three-armed study comparing conventional photon radiation versus mixed (neutron/photon) radiation versus neutron radiation alone (78). The complication rate was higher on the neutron-only arm (perhaps due in part to the relatively low-energy neutron beams in use at that time), and there was no difference in overall survival. A second randomized trial was conducted using the modern hospital-based facilities, which compared a neutron-only regimen with conventional photon irradiation (74). For the entire cohort of patients there was no difference in overall survival. However, there was a statistically significant survival advantage for the subset of patients having squamous-cell histology. The survival curves for this subset of patients is shown in Fig. 18.3. There was also a nonsignificant trend toward increased survival ($p = 0.15$) for patients of all histologies with favorable prognostic factors (no pleural effusion, not T4 or N3 in stage, weight loss <5% of normal body weight). Except for skin and subcutaneous changes, which were more severe on the neutron arm, acute and late toxicity were comparable.

The overall results are consistent with the conclusions of conventional photon therapy—namely, that a more aggressive form of radiation treatment delivering higher doses resulting in improved local control will only affect survival in a favorable subgroup of patients that is not prone to early distant metastases. There have been no reported studies in which chemotherapy was used along with neutron irradiation.

Prostate Cancer

There have been two important randomized clinical trials comparing neutron radiotherapy versus conventional photon radiotherapy for patients with locally advanced prostate cancer. In the late 1970s and early 1980s, the RTOG conducted a study (77-04) comparing mixed (neutron/photon) beam radiation with standard external beam radiotherapy for patients with stages C and D1 tumors (80). At the 10-year end point there was both improved local/regional control (70% vs. 58%; $p = 0.03$) and survival (46% vs. 29%; $p = 0.04$) in favor of the mixed beam arm. The survival curves from this study are reproduced in Fig. 18.4. There was no difference in the rate of significant complications between the two arms. This is one of the few published studies showing improved survival with an experimental form of

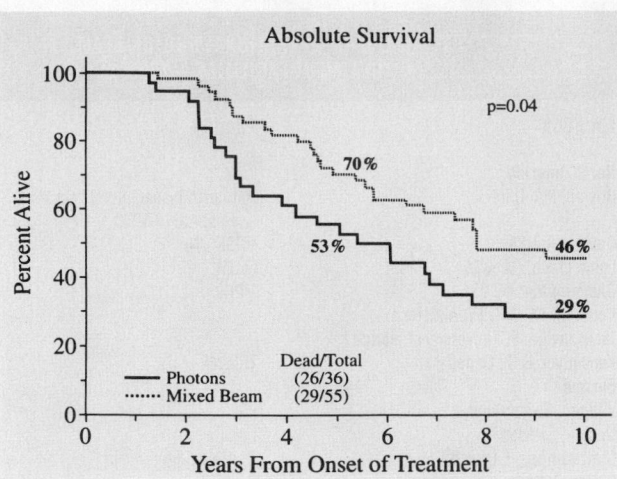

FIGURE 18.4. Actuarial survival curves for patients with locally advanced prostate cancer treated on an RTOG protocol (77-04). The curve for the mixed beam (neutron/photon) group is shown as the dashed line, and the curve for the photon group is shown as the solid line. The difference between the two curves is statistically significant at the $p = 0.04$ level. (Reprinted from Laramore GE, Krall JM, Griffin TW, et al. Fast neutron radiotherapy for locally-advanced prostate cancer. *Am J Clin Oncol (CCT)* 1993;16:164–167, with permission.)

treatment for prostate cancer. This study was criticized because of its relatively small size (91 evaluable patients), its unbalanced randomization (3:2 in favor of the experimental arm), and the fact that the photon control group appeared to do somewhat worse than would have been expected for supposedly comparable patients based on historical results. Hence, while this study was maturing, a second randomized trial comparing fast neutron radiotherapy alone versus conventional photon radiotherapy was initiated by the NTCWG for patients with high grade T2 or any grade T3 to T4, N0 to N1, or M0 tumors. One hundred seventy-two evaluable patients were entered into the study, and 5-year data have been reported (107). A routine, posttreatment biopsy was designed into the study to assay for local control in the pre-PSA (prostate-specific antigen) era. Unfortunately, all patients at risk for failure at the 2-year end point did not undergo this biopsy. The clinical local failure rate in the neutron arm of this study was 11%, compared to 32% for the photon control arm (p <0.01). Thus, the control arm of this study had a comparable rate of local tumor control to that of other published literature. However, there was no statistical difference in either actual survival or cause-specific survival between the two arms of NTCWG protocol 85-23. Posttreatment PSA levels in those patients at risk at 5-plus years were elevated in 17% of patients on the neutron arm, compared to 45% of patients on the photon arm (p <0.001). Although there was increased treatment morbidity on the neutron arm, it appeared to be confined to those neutron facilities not having a multileaf collimator to shape precisely the radiation fields (1,107). Given the steepness of the neutron dose-response curves for both tumor control and normal tissue damage, precise field shaping is a prerequisite for safe treatment delivery.

Considerable work has been done by the Wayne State University group using a combination of neutrons and photons (mixed beam) to treat prostate cancer (21,39–41,56,94). This work was done using a multirod collimator for field shaping and achieved an acceptable level of morbidity with over 1,500 patients having been treated at the present time. Forman (38) has summarized this work and discussed the sequence of studies that have lead to their current treatment regime. Following dose escalation studies to determine the maximum safe radiation doses, the Wayne State group compared two different treatment schemas: (a) giving the neutron portion of the treatment before the photon portion and (b) giving the photon por-

tion prior to the neutron portion. Interestingly, they found a higher therapeutic advantage when the neutron radiotherapy was given prior to the photon radiotherapy with disease-free survival being 93% if the neutron radiation was given initially versus 73% if the photon radiation was given initially. Furthermore, they found that the overall complication rate was about the same as that expected using conventional photon irradiation delivered via a three-dimensional conformal schema. The Wayne State group now uses 10 $Gy_{n\gamma}$ followed by 40 Gy photon as its "standard" mixed beam treatment for prostate cancer.

There also have been several reported single institution studies from Europe (35,103,109,113), and Asia (42,120,121) that show high local control rates with fast neutrons and support the results of the two randomized trials. Among these was a major review of prostate cancer patients using the cyclotron at the Universite Catholique de Louvain (109). Five hundred thirty-three patients were treated between 1978 and 1998 with a mixed-beam combination of neutrons and photons with three neutron treatments of 0.7 $Gy_{n\gamma}$ and two photon treatments of 2 Gy given per week on a daily basis. The total dose was felt to be equivalent to 66 Gy-photon based upon RBE estimates for their neutron beam. Prior to 1992 only simple field blocking was available; after 1992 a multileaf collimator was used for more precise field shaping. The review consisted of 308 consecutive patients treated from 1990 to 1996 with either the mixed beam regimen or with photon radiotherapy alone. Of these, 262 were presumed alive and quality of life (QOL) questionnaires were mailed to them. There were 230 responses: 20 in the photon group and 210 in the mixed beam group. Bowel problems, nocturia and urinary incontinence, and loss of sexual potency were present in each group. There were more patient reported side effects in the mixed-beam group with the difference in bowel problems felt to be significant ($p = 0.003$). The authors acknowledge that this was likely due to unsophisticated rectal blocking utilized for the lateral fields.

Although there is certainly increased risk of rectal complications with the use of high LET neutron radiotherapy, the aggregate data also show improved local regional control. This is consistent with more recent radiobiological models showing a low α/β ratio in the range of 1.5 to 3 for prostate cancer based upon fits to clinical data (7,122). High values of β indicate a tumor's ability to repair sublethal damage from conventional photon irradiation, and it is exactly this situation where high LET radiotherapy would be of benefit. It should also be noted that the neutron studies were generally done in the absence of antiandrogen therapy, which has been shown to be advantageous in improving survival in photon-treated patients. This may be an avenue for future investigation.

Sarcomas

Sarcomas generally are thought to be "radioresistant" and have many of the characteristics noted by Battermann et al. (4) as being favorable for high RBEs for neutron radiotherapy. A review of this historical data for neutron radiotherapy seems to show a probable benefit for high LET radiotherapy with comparative local control rates (neutrons versus photons) for patients treated for inoperable gross disease being 53% versus 38% for soft-tissue sarcomas, 55% versus 21% for osteogenic sarcomas, and 49% versus 33% for chondrosarcomas (79). In 1996 Schwarz et al. (112) summarized the results of 1,171 patients treated between 1972 and 1990 at 11 European neutron radiotherapy centers. For patients treated following primary resection with either clear or microscopically positive margins (categories R0 to R1), the local control rate was about 90%—about the same as would be expected for conventional postoperative photon irradiation. For patients with unresectable tumors (category R2) the approximate control rate was 47%. Complication rates ranged between 7% and 29% and were correlated with field size and the limited degree of technical sophistication available at some of the treatment centers. Clearly the results are inferior to those expected using a "clean" resection followed by conventional postoperative radiotherapy, but neutron radiotherapy appears to be more effective than photon radiation alone for those tumors where a surgical resection is not an option.

Charged Particle Radiotherapy

When charged particles pass through tissue, they deposit most of their energy at the end of their path, producing a so-called *Bragg peak*. The particular depth at which this occurs depends on the energy, mass, and charge of the particle. The main advantage of charged particle radiotherapy lies in the sharp falloff of dose beyond this Bragg peak and the smaller amount of energy deposited in intervening tissue. The lateral edges of the fields can also be sharper up to certain depths in tissue because of less large-angle scattering. The size of the Bragg peak along the axis of the beam is only a few millimeters, as is the cross section of the beam as it exits the accelerator. Applying such beams to cancer therapy requires specialized technology in order to match the dose distribution to the size, location, and shape of the tumor.

Historically, the particle beam was shaped to the tumor size by passive scattering and collimation methods, and this is the method currently used in the majority of charged particle facilities. Improvements in magnets, computers and control systems have recently made it practical to actively scan the small Bragg peak throughout the tumor volume. The Paul Scherrer Institute (PSI) in Villigen, Switzerland, and the Gesellschaft für Schwerionenforschung (GSI) in Darmstadt, Germany, have implemented some aspects of these advanced methods. Active scanning allows the high-dose Bragg peak region to be more tightly confined to the tumor volume and scatter to be reduced. There is also the potential for intensity modulated proton therapy (IMPT). The disadvantages are the increased technology and the fact that the dose is delivered at different times to different parts of the tumor, which can be problematic if there is tissue movement. These are the same problems faced in using intensity modulated photon therapy (IMRT).

IMRT offers some of the dose localization advantages of charged particles, particularly when passive scattering and collimation methods are utilized. However, charged particles still appear superior in terms of reducing the integral dose, reducing the time needed to treat (since fewer beams are needed), and using the Bragg peak to provide near total sparing of selected normal tissues. These advantages suggest applications to the treatment and retreatment of tumors adjacent to critical structures already at tolerance doses, of pediatric tumors, and of lung tumors where normal tissue integral dose constraints are important. IMPT theoretically will increase these advantages.

In the 1950s clinical trials using charged particles began at LBL first with protons and then with α-particles. Both high-energy protons and α-particles are considered to be low LET particles with clinical RBEs in the range of 1.1 to 1.2; therefore, their advantage over conventional photon radiotherapy lies entirely in their better dose-localization properties. Although there are no facilities currently using α-particles for therapy, there is burgeoning interest in the use of proton beams. As of July 2005 there were 19 treatment centers using proton radiotherapy throughout the world (Table 18.3). In addition, approximately 20 facilities are in various stages of the planning or construction process. Many of the older centers use fixed, horizontal beams, with eye tumors and arteriovenous malformations (AVMs) of the CNS being the most common entities treated. The newer, more modern centers have higher energy beams coupled with isocentric gantries, making it possible to treat tumors located anywhere in the body.

Table 18.3	LIST OF OPERATIONAL PROTON BEAM TREATMENT FACILITIES—2005	
Location	**Facility**
North America	
Boston, MA, USA	Harvard/Massachusetts General Hospital—NPTC
Davis, CA, USA	UCSF-CNL
Loma Linda, CA, USA	LLUML
Bloomington, IN, USA	MPRI
Houston, TX, USA/MD Anderson	
Jacksonville, FL/University of Florida	
Vancouver, B.C., Canada	TRIUMF
Europe	
Villigen, Switzerland	PSI
Upsala, Sweden	Upsala
Clatterbridge, England	Clatterbridge
Berlin, Germany	Berlin
Nice, France	Nice
Orsay, France	Orsay
St. Petersburg, Russia	St. Petersburg
Moscow, Russia	ITEP
Dubna, Russia	Dubna
Orsay, France	Proton therapie—Institute Curie
Goyang, Korea/National Cancer Center	
Asia	
Chiba, Japan	NIRS
Hyogo, Japan	HARIMAC
Kashiwa, Japan	NCC
Tsukuba, Japan	PMRC
Wakasa Bay, Tsurga, Japan	WERC
Shizuoka, Japan	SCC
Wanjie, China	WPTC
Africa	
Faure, South Africa	NAC

"Heavy" ions such as carbon, nitrogen, argon, neon, and silicon nuclei stripped of their electrons are high LET particles and combine the depth-dose localization properties of protons and α-particles with the RBE advantage of fast neutrons. Clinical trials using heavy, charged particles began at LBL in 1975 with a total of 433 patients being treated before the project was discontinued. Currently there are three active centers treating with heavy particles: HIMAC in Chiba, Japan; HARIMAC in Hyogo, Japan; and GSI in Darmstadt, Germany. Most of the ongoing clinical work utilizes carbon nuclei. A new combined proton-heavy ion radiotherapy center is being planned in Heidelberg, Germany.

π-mesons are a third category of particle radiation that has been used clinically. π-mesons mediate the binding force between nuclear particles and can be produced in significant quantities when a high-energy proton beam impacts a suitable target. Although there are three charge states for the π-meson, only the π^--meson has been used clinically. It is attractive for radiotherapeutic purposes because when it "slows down" it is captured by a nucleus, causing it to "explode" in a shower of charged particles and neutrons. It provides a mixture of high and low LET components as a result of its high energy and low mass compared to the proton. It deposits low LET events along its entry path, with the high LET events being confined to the "peak" region at the end of its path. Clinical trials using π-mesons began at Los Alamos, New Mexico, in 1974, with 272 patients being treated before 1982 when the project was closed because of lack of accrual. Other π-meson projects were carried out at the TRIUMF facility in Vancouver, British Columbia, and at the Swiss Institute for Nuclear Physics Research (SIN) facility in Villigen, Switzerland. There are no clinical centers currently treating with π-mesons.

According to unpublished data compiled by the Proton Therapy Co-Operative Group (PTCOG), as of July 2005 a total of 48,386 patients had received some form of particle radiotherapy: 1,100 with π-mesons, 4,520 with heavy ions or α-particles, and 42,766 with protons. In the following sections we will review the clinical results for each of these modalities. Because of their similar properties, we will discuss protons and α-particles together.

Proton and α-Particle Radiotherapy

Although there is a slight difference in the clinically employed RBEs of protons and α-particles, 1.1 and 1.3 respectively, both are considered "low LET" forms of radiation. Doses are typically specified in terms of "cobalt gray equivalent" (CGE) where CGE equals the physical dose multiplied by RBE. The first clinical trials in the United States using these particles began in the 1970s with α-particles at LBL and with protons at the Massachusetts General Hospital–Harvard Cyclotron Laboratory (MGH–HCL). The majority of treated patients had tumors adjacent to critical structures and so in most cases it was not felt possible to conduct randomized trials with photon radiotherapy. With the advent of photon IMRT, it now may be possible to conduct certain trials and directly compare the two modalities. However, it is important to recognize that the better target volume dose of photon IMRT comes at the price of increased doses to normal tissue at low to moderate levels. This increased "integral dose" associated with IMRT may put patients at increased risk for secondary radiation-induced malignancies (54). This is particularly important in the treatment of pediatric patients, where other consequences of radiation dose to normal tissue such as growth retardation or arrest, gonadal injury, pneumonitis, or late cardiac injury might be eliminated or reduced with protons.

Uveal Melanoma

Uveal melanoma is the most common primary ocular tumor. For many years the standard therapy has been surgical enucleation, with distant metastases being the most common form of failure. Given the close proximity of critical structures of the eye (cornea, lens, retina, fovea, and optic nerve) to the tumor, it was felt that standard external beam radiotherapy would not be able to preserve useful vision. Radioactive plaque brachytherapy has been used successfully, but presently its applicability is limited to lesions <8 mm in thickness. The superficial location of these tumors makes it feasible to treat them with relatively low-energy particle beams, and the relative ease of immobilization of the head compared to other parts of the body made these tumors attractive for proton and α-particle therapy.

Between 1978 and 1988, 307 patients with uveal melanoma were treated with α-particles at LBL (87). At 10 years on an actuarial basis, local tumor control was 97%, the eye retention rate was 83%, and the determinant survival rate was 81%. Of patients with a minimum follow-up of 5 years, 47% retained a visual acuity of 20/200 or better. Neovascular glaucoma occurred in 84 patients, with 35 of these subsequently requiring an enucleation.

Massachusetts General Hospital in collaboration with Massachusetts Eye and Ear Infirmary reported the results on an analysis of 2,069 patients treated with proton therapy between 1975 and 1997; at a median follow-up of 9.4 years 95% of tumors were locally controlled (48). The probability of eye retention at 5 years was estimated to be 90% for the entire group and 97%, 93%, and 78% for patients with small (height $\leq$3 mm and diameter $\leq$10 mm), intermediate, and large (height $\geq$8 mm and diameter $\geq$30 mm tumors, respectively (28). Independent risk factors for enucleation identified by multivariate analysis were involvement of the ciliary body, tumor height >8 mm, and

tumor proximal to the fovea. Seventy CGE in five fractions was used to treat the majority of patients. A randomized dose de-escalation trial was conducted between 1989 and 1994 to determine if visual morbidity could be decreased while maintaining local control (47). One hundred and eighty-eight patients with small and intermediate-sized lesions located near the optic disc or macula (within 4 disc diameters of either structure) were treated to a dose of 50 CGE. Interim analysis at a median follow-up of 60 months suggests that local control and survival were not compromised by this decrease in dose. No significant improvement in visual acuity was seen. However, visual field analysis did show a smaller mean defect in the patients randomized to 50 CGE.

The Nice group has reported on 538 patients treated between 1991 and 1996 (23). At 78 months they found a local control rate of 89%, a cause-specific survival rate of 77%, and a rate of distant metastases of 8%.

Between 1984 and 1998, 2,435 patients with uveal melanoma were treated with protons at PSI (29). At 10 years actuarial data show a local tumor-control rate of 94.8%, an eye retention rate of 94%, and a cause-specific survival rate of 73% for patients with controlled tumors compared to 48% for patients with uncontrolled tumors. There was evidence of a "learning curve" with the local control rate at 5 years being 99% for patients treated after 1994. PSI currently treats approximately 600 uveal melanoma patients per year.

An example of the radiation dose distribution that can be achieved with a proton beam is shown in Fig. 18.5 (see color Fig. 18.5). Note the ability to treat the tumor with a minimal dose to the lens and anterior chamber structures.

Optic Pathway Gliomas

At Loma Linda University (LLU), seven children with optic pathway gliomas were treated with proton radiation therapy (43). At a median follow-up of 37 months, all patients were locally controlled. A reduction in tumor volume was seen in three patients and was stable in the other four. Visual acuity was stable in those that presented with useful vision. Proton plans were compared to photon plans for individual patients. With proton therapy radiation, there was a 47% reduction in the dose to the contralateral optic nerve. There was an 11% reduction to the chiasm and a 13% reduction in dose to the pituitary gland. There was also a reduction in the dose to the temporal lobes and frontal lobes.

Skull-Base Tumors

Base-of-skull tumors, although often "benign" histologically, present a complex problem in clinical management. These tumors generally cannot be resected with adequate margins, and the location of these tumors limits the dose of conventional photon radiation that can be delivered adjuvantly. The results of conventional photon irradiation are generally suboptimal, and as for uveal melanomas, the ease of patient immobilization and the relatively shallow tumor depths made this set of tumors amenable to treatment with the early charged-particle beams.

LBL, MGH–HCL, and Loma Linda have reported excellent local control rates, as shown in Table 18.4. Total doses in the range of 60 to 80 CGE were given with patients being treated 5 days per week. Local control rates for clival chordomas and chondrosarcomas have been estimated to be in the range of 35% with standard radiotherapy (98), which would make it difficult to undertake a randomized trial. For chordomas of the clivus, female gender was found to be a significant adverse prognostic factor in the MGH–HCL series and a nonsignificant trend was noted in the LBL series (55,98). A report from Loma Linda indicates that all "small and medium size" tumors without brainstem involvement were controlled and there was only a 7% incidence of significant late toxicity (63). Figure 18.6 shows an

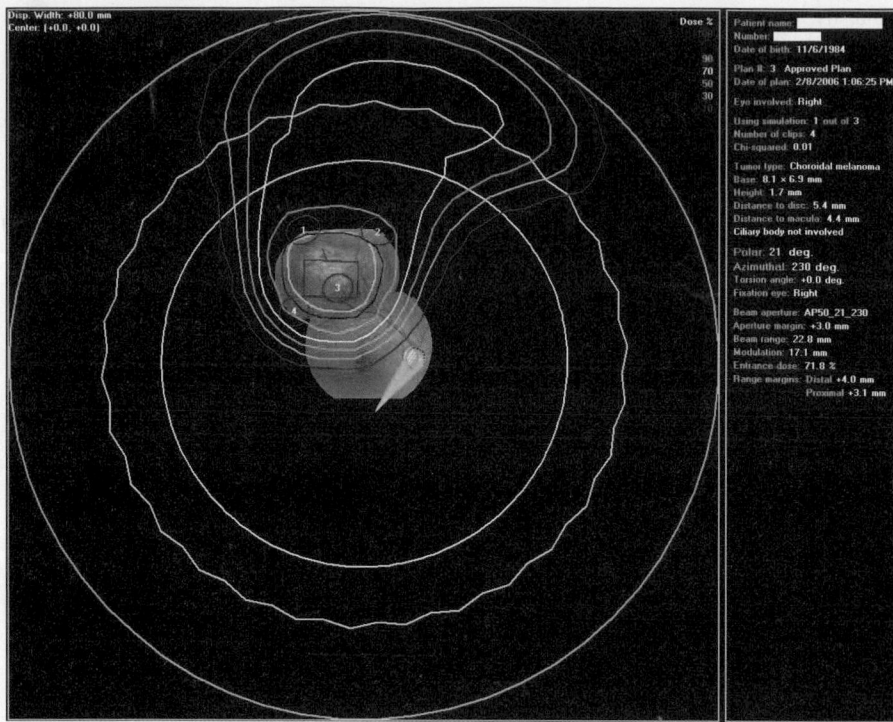

FIGURE 18.5. Proton treatment plan for a patient with an 8.1 × 6.9 mm uveal melanoma of 1.7 mm thickness which is 5.4 mm from the disc, outlined by four tantalum clips (1–4) and green contour. The lesion is encompassed by the 97% isodose line. Note the sparing of the optic disc. The dose to the fovea is in the range of 20%. (Courtesy of J. Michael Collier, Ph.D.)

example of a proton beam distribution for a patient with a chordoma of the clivus.

Benign and malignant meningiomas of the skull base are also of interest for proton beam radiotherapy. Benign meningiomas constitute approximately 20% of all intracranial neoplasms. Although histologically benign, they may cause significant morbidity as a result of their frequent proximity to the optic structures. Although postoperative radiotherapy has been demonstrated to improve local control rates at 5 and 10 years (44,123), with a "safe" dose of 55.8 Gy, the 10-year local control rate is still only about 50%. At the MGH–HCL a series of 46 patients with recurrent and/or partially resected/biopsied tumors was treated with a combination of protons and photons to a median dose of 59.8 CGE with a recurrence-free survival at 10 years of 88% (126). However, in this patient group there were eight patients who developed a significant long-term morbidity as a result of the treatment and one patient died of a brainstem necrosis. Investigators from PSI recently reported on the treatment with proton spot scanning of 16 patients with recurrent, residual, or untreated intracranial meningiomas (124). The median prescribed dose was 56 CGE (52 to 64) at 1.8 to 2 CGE per fraction. Cumulative 3-year local control, progression-free survival, and overall survival were 91%, 91%, and 92%, respectively. No patient died of recurrent meningioma. Radiographic follow-up (34-month median) revealed an objective response in three patients and stable disease in 12 patients. Cumulative

3-year toxicity-free survival was 76%. No radiation-induced hypothalamic/pituitary dysfunction was observed.

At the National Accelerator Centre (NAC, South Africa) patients with skull base meningiomas were treated with protons using either a stereotactic radiosurgical approach (20 CGE/3 fractions) or via a more conventional fractionation approach (61.6 CGE/16 fractions). In the prolonged fractionation group the radiologic control rate was 88% (16 of 18 patients), whereas the radiologic control rate was 100% (five patients) in the radiosurgically treated group. Three patients suffered permanent neurologic deficits. In the case of atypical and malignant meningiomas, the 5-year local control rate with comparable radiation doses is only about 25% (61).

Pituitary Tumors

Whereas for nonsecreting pituitary tumors "standard treatment" consisting of a transsphenoidal resection followed by postoperative radiotherapy gives excellent results, for secretory tumors the results are less optimal. Large series of patients with these histologies have been treated at MGH–HCL and LBL. Five hundred ten patients with growth hormone-secreting tumors were treated over a 20-year period with proton radiosurgery being used as the primary treatment modality in 67% of patients. The overall follow-up rate was 85%, and the mean human growth hormone (HGH) levels decreased by 80% at 2 years,

Table 18.4	**LOCAL CONTROL RATES FOR BASE-OF-SKULL TUMORS ACHIEVED WITH ALPHA-PARTICLES (13) OR PROTONS (32, 63, 98, 126)**		
Tumor Histology	Lawrence Berkeley National Laboratory (%)	Harvard/Massachusetts General Hospital (%)	Loma Linda (%)
Meningioma	85	88	—
Chordoma	63	59	76
Chondrosarcoma	78	99	92
Sarcoma (other)	58	—	—

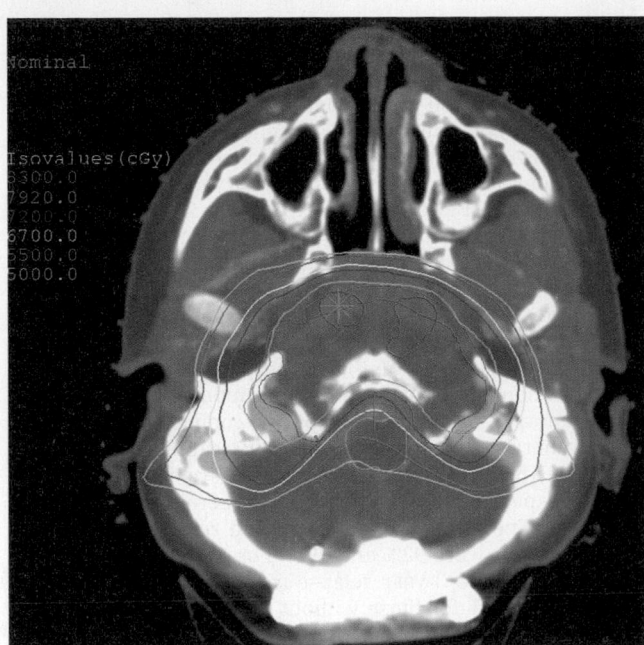

FIGURE 18.6. Proton treatment plan for an 8-year-old with a clivus chordoma. Prescription dose is 79.2 CGE at 1.8 CGE per fraction. Dose constraint was set at 67 CGE to the brainstem surface and 55 CGE to the brainstem center. (Courtesy of Norbert Liebsch M.D., Ph.D. and Judith Adams, C.M.D.)

reaching an average decrement of 98% by 20 years. The decline in HGH was slow, with values <5 ng/mL being found in 27.5% at 2 years, 75% at 10 years, and 92.5% at 20 years (73). The LBL experience is similar; by 4 years after treatment, the median HGH level had fallen below 5 ng/mL in their cohort of 220 acromegalic patients (83).

In the case of patients with Cushing's disease, the MGH–HCL experience is based on the treatment of 145 patients over 20 years. Stereotactic proton radiosurgery was used, giving 120 to 140 CGE in a single fraction. Taking a fasting serum cortisol of <10 ng/dL as indicating tumor remission, Kjellberg (72) reported remission rates of 55% at 2 years and 80% at 5 years. At LBL, 64 patients with Cushing's disease were treated with helium ions to a dose of 50 to 150 CGE in three or four daily fractions. Reported remission occurred in 55 of 64, although criteria for remission were not stated explicitly (82,86). Failures predominantly occurred in the early treatment group, where six treatment fractions were used.

More recently, fractionated proton beam radiotherapy has been used for treatment of pituitary adenomas. Loma Linda reported treatment of 47 patients with pituitary adenomas, 42 prior to surgical resection and five with primary radiation (106). Approximately half the tumors were functional and the median dose was 54 CGE. Tumor stabilization occurred in all 41 patients for whom there was follow-up imaging; 10 patients had no residual tumor, and three had >50% reduction in tumor size. Seventeen patients with functional adenomas had normalized or decreased hormone levels; progression occurred in three patients. Six patients died; two deaths were attributed to functional progression. Complications included temporal lobe necrosis in one patient, new significant visual deficits in three patients, and incident hypopituitarism in 11 patients. Postradiation hypopituitarism, attributed in part to concomitant risk factors for hypopituitarism in the patient population, was the most common side effect.

Pituitary adenomas recurrent after standard radiotherapy represent another treatment challenge. Two series suggest that repeat irradiation may have a useful role in patients who achieved long-term (>3 years) control of their disease with their initial treatment, but the risk of temporal lobe injury is significant (36,110). Proton reirradiation offers the possibility of re-treating a proportion of these patients with minimal dose to the chiasm. Furthermore, by using off-axial, noncoplanar beams, previously irradiated brain parenchyma may be avoided to a significant degree. A protocol to re-treat recurrent pituitary adenomas currently is under way at Massachusetts General Hospital—Francis H. Bitler Proton Therapy Center (MGH–FHBPTC) for patients for whom there is a separation of 5 mm or more between the optic system and the tumor (57).

Acoustic Neuromas

For acoustic neuromas that are especially large and have an irregular shape, the highly conformal properties of the proton beam may offer some advantages over stereotactic radiosurgery using a linear accelerator or a gamma knife. The ability to control the depth of the proton beam significantly restricts the unintended irradiation to adjacent fifth and seventh cranial nerves and adjacent structures. Loma Linda has reported treatment results with fractionated proton radiotherapy and MGH has reported results with stereotactic proton radiosurgery. Loma Linda University reported their experience with fractionated proton radiation for vestibular schwannomas. Thirty patients received treatment between 1991 and 1999. The mean tumor volume in this study was 4.3 cm^3. Patients with useful hearing were treated with standard fractionation to a dose of 54 CGE, and those without functional hearing received a dose of 60 CGE. At a mean follow-up of 34 months, no patients demonstrated tumor progression and 11 tumors were found by imaging studies to have decreased in size. Of the 13 patients with functional hearing, 31% maintained functional hearing. No transient or permanent facial or trigeminal nerve dysfunction was observed (58).

Between 1992 and 2000, 88 patients with vestibular schwannomas were treated at MGH–HCL using proton beam stereotactic radiosurgery. The median tumor volume was 1.4 cm^3 and median transverse diameter was 16 mm. A median dose of 12 CGE was prescribed to the 70% isodose line. At 38.7 months follow-up, 94.3% of tumors were locally controlled. Five patients required some form of salvage therapy and no radiation-induced malignancies have been observed. The actuarial 2- and 5-year tumor control rates were 95.3% and 93.6%, respectively. Twenty-one patients had functional hearing at the time of treatment with 33.3% retaining functional hearing at a follow-up of 31.8 months (58).

Astrocytomas

At MGH–HCL, a phase II study was undertaken to assess whether dose escalation to 90 CGE with conformal protons and photons in accelerated fractionation (twice a day) would improve local tumor control and survival (33). A total of 23 patients were enrolled, ages 18 to 70 years. Actuarial survival rates at 2 and 3 years were 34% and 18%, respectively. The median survival time was 20 months, with four patients alive 22 to 60 months postdiagnosis. All patients developed new areas of gadolinium enhancement during the follow-up period. Histological examination of tissues obtained at biopsy, resection, or autopsy was conducted in 15 patients. Radiation necrosis without recurrent tumor was demonstrated in seven patients, and their survival was significantly longer than patients with recurrent tumors. Tumor regrowth occurred most commonly in areas that received doses of 60 to 70 CGE or less; recurrent tumor was found in only one case in the 90 CGE volume. The authors concluded that attempts to extend local control by enlarging the volume would likely be complicated by a high incidence of radionecrosis.

Paranasal Sinus and Nasopharyngeal Tumors

Tumors of the paranasal sinuses have a relatively sparse lymphatic drainage pattern and may well represent a category of head and neck tumors for which increased local control translates into increased survival. There is currently a hyperfractionated/accelerated fractionation trial combining photons and protons under way at MGH–HCL for patients with advanced malignancies of the paranasal sinuses. Using a three-dimensional treatment planning approach, it appears feasible to deliver approximately 76 CGE to the primary target volume instead of the 65 Gy that usually is given with conventional radiotherapy. Model calculations indicated that this may improve the local control rate by about 35% (104). Between 1988 and 2002, 91 patients with newly diagnosed nonmetastatic (AJCC) stage III to IV paranasal sinus cancer received combined conformal proton and photon radiotherapy at MGH (19). The histology was squamous cell carcinoma in 28, carcinoma with neuroendocrine differentiation in 34, adenoid cystic carcinoma in 20, and sarcoma in nine patients. Sixty-seven percent of patients underwent surgical resection before radiation. The median total prescribed dose to the primary target volume was 73.6 CGE (range 59.40 to 77.80). The median proportion of proton dose was 49% (range 23 to 84). Eighty-seven percent of patients received continuous accelerated hyperfractionated radiotherapy and 32 patients received chemotherapy. With a mean follow-up of 45 months, 11, six, and 19 patients had developed local recurrence, neck recurrence, and distant metastasis, respectively, as their first site of failure. Distant metastasis was the predominant pattern of relapse for squamous cell carcinoma, carcinoma with neuroendocrine differentiation, and adenoid cystic carcinoma. At 3 and 5 years, overall survival rates were 65% and 58%, respectively. The disease-free survival rates at 3 and 5 years were 59% and 52%, respectively. The overall freedom from distant metastatic rates at 3 and 5 years were 79% and 75%, respectively. The 3- and 5-year actuarial local control rates were 87% and 82%, respectively. The local control rate at 3 years was 83% for squamous cell carcinoma, 91% for carcinoma with neuroendocrine differentiation, 86% for adenoid cystic carcinoma, and 88% for sarcoma. The ultimate local control rate after salvage treatment was 89% and 86% at 3 and 5 years respectively. The neck control rate was 91% and 89% at 3 and 5 years, respectively. Visual complications appear to be modest (34).

Nasopharyngeal tumors recurrent after initial radiotherapy and/or chemoradiation present a difficult problem in medical management. At Loma Linda a small group of 16 patients with recurrent nasopharyngeal tumors were re-treated with protons to additional doses of 59.4 to 70.2 CGE (85). At 2 years the actuarial survival and progression-free survival rates were 50% and no central nervous system side effects were reported.

Chan et al. (20) reviewed the experience of patients treated with protons for treatment of nasopharyngeal cancer at the HCL and the FHBPTC between 1990 and 2002 (20). During that period, 17 patients with newly diagnosed T4 N0 to N3 nasopharyngeal carcinoma received combined conformal proton and photon radiotherapy. Seventy-one percent of the patients had World Health Organization (WHO) type 2 or 3 histology. The median prescribed dose to the gross target volume was 73.6 CGE (range 69 to 76.8). Eleven patients received twice-daily radiation and 10 patients received induction or concurrent chemotherapy. All patients except one completed the planned concurrent radiation and chemotherapy treatments. With a median follow-up of 43 months, one patient developed local failure and two experienced systemic failures. There were no neck recurrences. The locoregional control and relapse-free survival rates at 3 years were 92% and 79%. For patients who received chemotherapy, the 3-year relapse-free survival rate was 91% compared to 50% for those without chemotherapy ($p = 0.09$). The 3-year overall survival rate was 74%. For patients who received chemotherapy, the 3-year overall survival rate was 91% compared to 40% for those without chemotherapy ($p = 0.01$). Late toxicities included five patients with radiographic changes of the temporal lobes and one osteoradionecrosis of the mandible.

Juxtaspinal Cord Tumors

A complete surgical resection of juxtaspinal cord tumors is generally impossible because of tumor invasion or adherence to the vertebrae, spinal cord, or peripheral nerve roots. The spinal cord serves as the main dose-limiting organ for conventional photon radiotherapy, with doses in the range of 50 to 55 Gy generally being the maximum that can be given safely. This is too low to sterilize gross residual disease for most tumor histologies, so treatment results are generally unsatisfactory. With the use of charged particle radiotherapy, one literally can "wrap" the isodose distribution around the spinal cord, keeping it within tolerance levels and at the same time taking the tumor mass to a considerably higher dose. Figure 18.7 compares photon

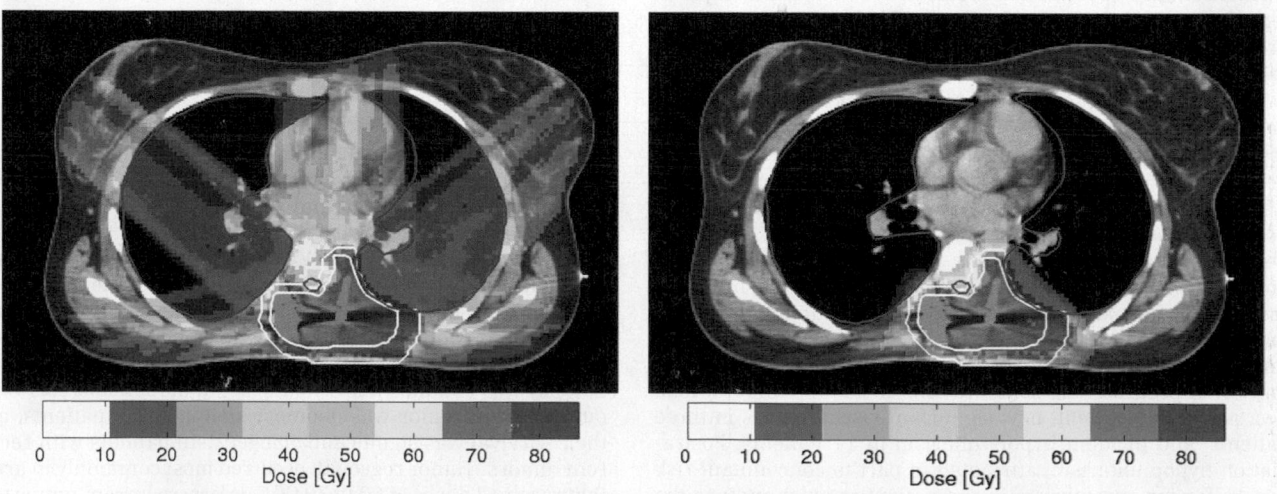

FIGURE 18.7. Color wash dose distributions comparing intensity modulated radiotherapy (IMRT) with photons **(A)** and intensity modulated proton therapy (IMPT) **(B)** for the planning target volumes (PTV) for a patient with a supradiaphragmatic epithelioid sarcoma, with dose to the areas of gross tumor prescribed to 77.4 CGE. Note the dramatic reduction in integral dose with the proton plan. (Reprinted from Weber DC, Trofimov AV, DeLaney TF, et al. A treatment planning comparison of intensity modulated photon and proton therapy for paraspinal sarcomas. *Int J Radiat Oncol Biol Phys* 2004;58:1596–1606, with permission.)

IMRT and proton IMPT isodose distributions for a paraspinal sarcoma. The need for accurate and reproducible patient immobilization makes it easier to apply this technique in the cervical region compared to the thoracic and lumbar regions.

Between 1976 and 1987, 52 patients with juxtaspinal cord tumors were treated with α particles at LBL (99). A mix of tumors was involved consisting of chordomas, chondrosarcomas, and other types of sarcomas, and there were patients with metastatic lesions. The tumors were distributed along the cord, with 16 occurring in the cervical spine, 23 in the thoracic spine, 11 in the lumbar spine, and two in both the thoracic and lumbar spine. The median tumor dose was 70 CGE. An overall local control rate of 52% was achieved. Only one patient developed a radiation myelitis. Fifty-one patients with chordomas of the cervical spine were treated at MGH–HCL between 1975 and 1993. A local control rate of 65% was achieved (32). Hug et al. (62) presented results on combined photon/proton treatment of 47 patients with osteo- and chondrogenic tumors of the axial skeleton. Actuarial local control (5-year) and survival for patients with chondrosarcoma were 100% and 100%, and with chordoma were 53% and 50%. Actuarial 5-year local control for patients with osteosarcoma was 59%.

Weber et al. (125) carried out a treatment planning comparison of IMRT and IMPT for paraspinal sarcomas. Plans for five patients were computed for IM photons (seven coplanar fields) and protons (three coplanar beams). Prescribed dose was 77.4 CGE for protons to the gross tumor volume. Surface and center spinal cord dose constraint for all techniques was 64 and 53 CGE, respectively. Gross tumor volume coverage was optimal and equally homogeneous with both IM photon and IM proton plans. Median heart, lung, kidney, stomach, and liver mean dose and dose at the 50% volume level were consistently reduced by a factor of 1.3 to 25. Tumor dose homogeneity in IMPT plans was always better than IMRT plans. IMPT dose escalation (to 92.9 CGE to the GTV) was possible in all patients without exceeding the normal-tissue dose limits.

Prostate Cancer

Prostate cancer continues to be the subject of numerous clinical investigations. It is the only tumor system to date where there has been a randomized trial testing the effect of dose escalation with a proton beam relative to a conventional, radiotherapeutic treatment (5,114). The experimental arm was not a pure proton treatment in that patients were first given 50.4 Gy photon dose to the pelvis and then were randomized to receive either a 25.2 CGE proton boost or a 16.8 Gy photon boost. Ninety-four evaluable patients were randomized to the photon arm, and 103 were randomized to the proton arm. There was no difference between the two groups in terms of local control, survival, or disease-specific survival. On subset analysis, it turned out that patients with poorly differentiated tumors had better local control with proton treatment, but only 57 patients fell into this category. Unfortunately, the complication rate was higher on the proton arm, with a 32% incidence of rectal bleeding on the proton arm compared to a 12% incidence on the photon arm ($p = 0.002$). There was also an increased incidence of urethral stricture on the proton arm (19% versus 8%), but this did not achieve statistical significance ($p = 0.07$). Parameters relating to the posttreatment incidence of rectal bleeding were analyzed, and a dose-volume histogram for the anterior rectal wall was the most significant variable.

Studies utilizing more modern proton facilities have now been reported. At Loma Linda 319 patients with early-stage tumors (T1 to T2b, PSA <15 ng/mL) were treated with conformal photon or proton fields to doses of 74 to 75 CGE (115). At 5 years the overall survival was 97% and the biochemical disease-free survival was 88%, which are comparable to rates achieved with radical prostatectomy and seed brachytherapy. No se-

vere treatment-related morbidity was noted. In the randomized, phase III, Proton Radiation Oncology Group (PROG, 95-09 study), 393 patients with stage T1b through T2b prostate cancer and PSA levels <15 ng/mL were randomized to receive external beam radiation to a total dose of either 70.2 or 79.2 CGE at 1.8 CGE per day, with 50.4 Gy given with conformal photons and a boost of either 19.8 CGE or 28.8 CGE delivered with protons (127). The proportions free from biochemical failure at 5 years were 61.4% for conventional-dose and 80.4% for high-dose therapy ($p <0.001$). The advantage to high-dose therapy was observed in both the low-risk and the higher-risk subgroups. To date, there has been no significant difference in overall survival rates between the treatment groups. Only 1% of patients receiving conventional dose and 2% receiving high-dose radiation experienced acute urinary or rectal morbidity of grade 3 or greater using the Radiation Therapy Oncology Group (RTOG) criteria. So far, only 2% and 1%, respectively, have experienced late morbidity of RTOG grade 3 or greater, indicating the safety of the dose escalation. MGH and Loma Linda have recently completed accrual to a phase II study of proton beam for patients with T1C to T2A prostate cancer and PSA values ≤15 ng/mL, treating the prostate and seminal vesicles to 50 CGE and then boosting the prostate with another 32 Gy at 2 CGE per fraction. Results on this study have not yet been reported.

Arteriovenous Malformations of the Brain

Surgery has been the most widely used method for treating AVMs, with its primary advantage being its ability to reduce the risk of immediate hemorrhage. Surgery, however, is associated with varying degrees of morbidity, dependent largely on location and size of the AVM. Radiation therapy in the form of stereotactic radiotherapy also has been used in the treatment of AVMs, especially in deeply seated lesions ill suited for surgical resection. Both charged particles and photons from either a gamma knife or a specially modified linear accelerator have been used in this manner.

Success rates with radiosurgery are highly dependent on the volume of the AVM treated. Using gamma knife technology, researchers at the University of Pittsburgh have demonstrated 2-year obliteration rates of 100% for lesions smaller than 1 cm in diameter, 85% for those 1 to 4 cm, and 58% for those larger than 4 cm (89). Stereotactic radiosurgery using modified linear accelerators yields similar 2-year complete obliteration rates in the range of 29.4% to 84%. In particular, Colombo et al. (22) report complete obliteration rates of 96% for lesions <1.5 cm diameter, 74% for those 1.5 to 2.5 cm, and 33% for those larger than 2.5 cm. Protons and other charged particles have been used in the treatment of AVMs since 1965. Kjellberg et al. (70,71) have treated more than 1,000 patients with AVMs using protons generated from the 160 MeV Harvard Cyclotron, reporting a 20% complete angiographic obliteration rate, with 56% of AVMs showing a reduction in volume of more than 50%. Charged-particle therapy at LBL has been used to treat more than 400 patients. Published results demonstrate complete, angiographically determined obliteration rates at 3 years of 100% for lesions smaller than 4 cc volume, 95% for those 4 to 25 cm^3, and 70% for lesions larger than 25 cm^3 (31). Smaller lesion size and higher radiation doses correlated with a more rapid response. The complication rate correlated directly with AVM size and dose received. Large AVMs (diameters >3 cm) may be better treated with charged particles due to their dose-localization properties.

Lung Cancer

Bush et al. (11) performed a prospective study to assess the efficacy and toxicity of proton beam therapy for patients with inoperable stage I to IIIA non–small-cell lung cancer (27 stage

I, 2 stage II, 8 stage IIIA). Thirty-seven patients were treated with either 45 Gy photon therapy to the primary tumor and mediastinum followed by 28.8 CGE boost to the primary with protons, or in cases of limited cardiopulmonary reserve, 51 CGE proton therapy in 10 fractions only to the primary site. At a median follow up of 14 months, actuarial disease-free survival was 63% for the entire group and 86% for patients with stage I disease. Two cases of radiation pneumonitis were diagnosed with both responding to a short course of steroids. The authors concluded that high dose proton radiation could be delivered safely to patients with poor pulmonary function.

Gastrointestinal Cancer

Surgery provides the best outcome for patients with hepatocellular carcinoma; however, many patients are not considered surgical candidates due to underlying cirrhosis (102). Radiation therapy doses are limited due to the risk of hepatic toxicity in the usual setting of underlying hepatic dysfunction secondary to hepatitis. Investigators at Tsukuba University in Japan have reported impressive long-term control and survival results in 122 patients with primary hepatocellular carcinoma treated with proton radiotherapy (93). Seventy-two CGE was delivered at 4 CGE per fraction. The 7-year local control and survival were 94% and 27%, respectively. Proton irradiation did not cause clinically symptomatic changes in liver function with only a transient increase in liver transaminases being observed. LLU has also examined the efficacy and toxicity of proton beam therapy in 34 patients with localized hepatocellular carcinoma (9). Patients with distant metastases, positive lymph nodes, and a Child-Pugh score exceeding 10 were excluded. Computed tomography (CT) scans were obtained prior to enrollment; patients with more than 30% of the liver within the 50% isodose line were excluded. Treatment was prescribed to the gross tumor volume plus a 1- to 2-cm margin to a total dose of 63 CGE in 15 fractions at 4.2 CGE per fraction. The average tumor volume was 5.6 cm^3 (range 1 to 10 cm^3) and median follow-up was 20 months. Two-year actuarial data showed a 75% local control rate and an overall survival of 55%. Six patients subsequently underwent liver transplantation. Two of these patients had no evidence of tumor, one showed only microscopic residual tumor, and the others showed gross residual tumor.

Pediatric Malignancies

Investigators at PSI looked at the potential influence of improved dose distribution with proton beams compared to conventional or IMRT x-ray beams on the incidence of treatment-induced secondary cancers in children (95). Two children, one with parameningeal rhabdomyosarcoma (RMS) and another with medulloblastoma, were used as models for this study. After defining the target and critical structures, treatment plans were calculated and optimized, four for the RMS case (conventional x-ray, IMRT, protons, and IMPT) and three for the irradiation of the spinal axis in medulloblastoma (conventional x-ray, IMRT, protons). The secondary cancer incidence was estimated using a model by the International Commission on Radiologic Protection. This model allowed estimation of absolute risks of secondary cancer for each treatment plan based on dose-volume distributions for nontarget organs. Proton beams reduced the expected incidence of radiation-induced secondary cancers for the RMS patient by a factor equal or >2, and for the medulloblastoma cases, a factor of 8 to 15 when compared with either IM or conventional x-ray plans. This study underscores the concern with using radiation therapy in the treatment of pediatric malignancies. It is the goal of clinicians not only to eradicate the primary tumor but also to minimize the risk of radiation-induced malignancies over the lifetime of these patients.

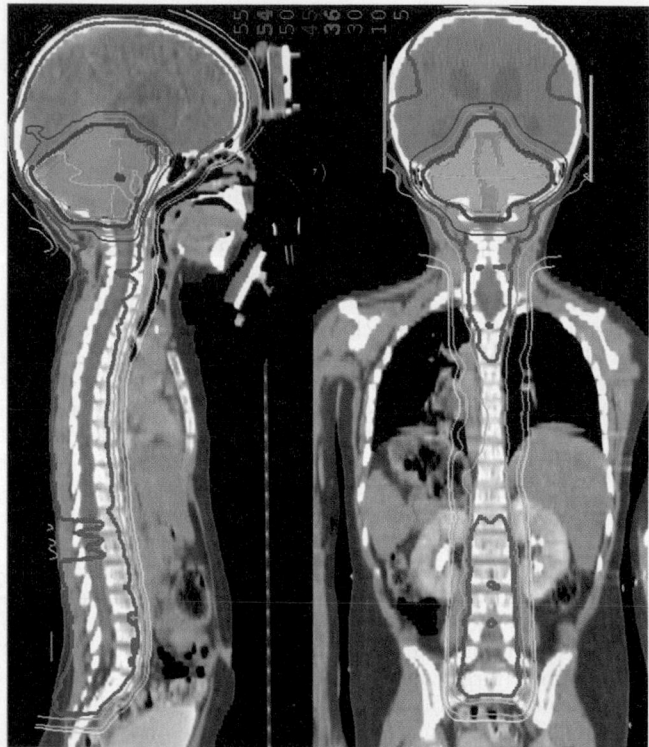

FIGURE 18.8. Sagittal and coronal composite dose displays for a child with high-risk medulloblastoma undergoing craniospinal irradiation with protons. Prescription dose to the craniospinal axis for this child with high-risk disease is 36 CGE and the dose to the posterior fossa is 54 CGE. Note the absence of significant exit dose beyond the anterior border of the vertebral bodies, thus sparing the bowel, heart, and mediastinum from potential acute and late side effects of radiotherapy. (Reprinted from Levin WP, Kooy H, Loeffler JS, et al. Proton beam therapy. *Br J Cancer* 2005;93:849–54, with permission.)

In a study done at MGH, treatment plans were compared using standard photon therapy, IMRT, and protons for craniospinal axis irradiation and posterior fossa boost in a patient with medulloblastoma (116). Substantial normal tissue sparing was realized with IMRT and proton irradiation of the posterior fossa and spinal axis as shown in Fig. 18.8. The dose to 90% of the cochlea was reduced from 101% of the prescribed posterior fossa boost dose from conventional x-rays to 33% and 2% from IMRT and protons, respectively. Dose to 50% of the heart volume was reduced from 72% for photons to 30% for IMRT and 0.5% for protons.

The LLU group also compared photon and proton plans for pediatric patients receiving posterior fossa irradiation (84). Using the original planning CT scans, the posterior fossa, inner and middle ear, and temporal lobes were delineated. The 95% isodose encompassed the posterior fossa in all plans. Normal structures received markedly less radiation from proton plans than from photon plans. The cochlea received an average mean of 25% of the prescribed dose from the proton plan and 75% from the photons. Forty percent of temporal lobe volume was completely excluded using protons; with photons, 90% of the temporal lobe received 31% of the dose.

LLU investigators evaluated the safety and efficacy of proton beam irradiation in the treatment of pediatric patients with intracranial low-grade astrocytoma (65). Between 1991 and 1997, 27 patients between 2 and 18 years old underwent fractionated proton radiation therapy for progression of recurrent low-grade astrocytoma. Twenty-five of the 27 patients (92%) were treated for progressive, unresectable, or residual disease following subtotal resection. Mean target dose was 55.2 CGE (50.4 to 63) and fraction size was 1.8 CGE. At a mean follow-up period of 3.3 years (0 to 6.8 years), six of the patients experienced local failure within the irradiated field and four had died. Local control and survival was 87% and 93%, respectively, for centrally located tumors, 71% and 86% for hemispheric tumors, and 60% and 60% for tumors of the brainstem. All children with local control maintained their performance status, except one, who developed Moyamoya disease. All six patients with optic pathway tumors and useful vision maintained or improved their visual status.

Work has also been done in evaluating proton radiotherapy for pediatric patients with skull base tumors, retroperitoneal neuroblastomas, and orbital rhabdomyosarcomas (60,64,66). In all cases there was significant sparing of critical normal structures compared to plans utilizing photon radiotherapy.

Breast Cancer

Some patients with breast cancer have anatomic configurations that make it difficult to adequately treat the breast while sparing the underlying lung and heart. A treatment planning exercise was undertaken comparing standard photon therapy to IMRT and proton therapy in the treatment of breast cancer (37). Using CT data from a breast cancer patient, treatment plans were computed for the different treatment techniques. A dose of 50 Gy was prescribed to the target volume consisting of the involved breast, internal mammary, supraclavicular, and axillary nodes. Lung dose volume histograms (DVH) for the photon and IMRT plans were comparable, while the proton plan showed the best sparing overall dose levels. Mean doses to the ipsilateral lung for the three plans were 17 Gy, 15 Gy, and 13 Gy, for the photon, IMRT, and proton plans, respectively. For the heart, the IMRT plan delivered the highest mean dose (16 Gy), reflecting the extra dose delivered through this organ to spare the lungs. This was reduced somewhat by the standard plan (15 Gy), with the best sparing being provided by the proton plan (6 Gy). When the IMRT plan was reoptimized with an increased precedence to the normal tissues, the mean doses to all neighboring organs at risk could be reduced, but only at the cost of substantial target dose heterogeneity. Only the two-field, energy-modulated proton plan had the potential to preserve target dose homogeneity while simultaneously minimizing the dose delivered to lungs, heart, and the contralateral breast.

:: | Heavy Ion Radiotherapy

The first published clinical results using heavy ion radiotherapy were from the Bevalac facility at LBL (14,15,88). Stripped carbon and neon nuclei were used clinically, but as a result of beam time constraints, most of the patients had a component of low LET α-particle or photon radiation as well. Hence, it is difficult to assign any benefit or adverse effect to the heavy ions themselves in the LBL work.

Thirty-nine patients with high-grade gliomas of the brain were treated wholly or in part with charged-particle radiation (14). Six patients had recurrent tumor after prior photon irradiation, and 33 patients were treated de novo. The treatment techniques were quite varied, with three patients being treated with only α-particles, 10 receiving an α-particle boost after photon irradiation, 12 receiving both photon irradiation and either carbon or neon ions as a boost, and only 14 patients receiving a "pure" heavy ion treatment with neon ions alone. Relative to megavoltage photons, the RBE of the α-particles was taken to be 1.2 and that of the heavier carbon and neon ions was taken to be 3. Of the 33 previously untreated patients, 17 patients had glioblastoma multiforme, 15 died, and 13 had evidence of tumor progression at the time of analysis. The overall median survival for the glioblastoma multiforme patients was 13.9 months. Eleven patients had anaplastic astrocytomas and of these, nine

| Table 18.5 | OUTCOME FOR SELECTED PATIENT GROUPS TREATED WITH NEON IONS AT THE BEVALAC |

Tumor Type	Patient Number	5-Year Local Control (%)
Salivary gland	18	61
Paranasal sinus	12	69
Soft-tissue sarcoma	12	56
Bone sarcoma	19	59
Prostate cancer (locally advanced)	12	75
Biliary tract	8	44

From Linstadt DE, Castro JR, Phillips TL. Neon ion radiotherapy: Results of the phase I/II clinical trial. *Int J Radiat Oncol Biol Phys* 1991;20:761–769, with permission.

died with local failure. The overall median survival for this subgroup of patients was only 7.6 months. Five other patients in the previously untreated group had low-grade tumors with local failures occurring in two of these. Although radionecrosis of the brain was minimal in this patient series, there was no evidence for any improvement in therapeutic outcome.

The outcome of the Bevalac studies for other tumor types has been reported by Linstadt et al. (88). As was the case for the patients with brain tumors, it is difficult to interpret these results because the majority of patients also received photon or α-particle radiation. A total of 239 patients had received a minimum of 10 Gy neon dose; evaluating the outcome for these patients, the authors concluded that there was improved outcome, relative to historically expected results, for advanced salivary gland tumors, paranasal sinus tumors, soft-tissue sarcomas, bone sarcomas, locally advanced prostate cancer, and biliary tract carcinomas. The 5-year local control rates for these tumors as well as the number of patients treated for each tumor type are summarized in Table 18.5. Although the number of patients in each category is small, it is interesting to note that in general, these tumors are the same types as are felt to be advantageously treated with fast neutrons, another form of high LET radiotherapy. Results also were reported for malignant gliomas, pancreatic carcinoma, esophageal cancer, lung cancer, and squamous-cell tumors of the head and neck, but these were felt to be no better than would be expected using conventional photon radiation therapy. Bevalac is no longer treating patients, and there are no heavy ion facilities operating in the United States.

The Heavy Ion Medical Accelerator in Chiba (HIMAC) facility at the National Institute of Radiological Sciences in Chiba, Japan, can treat patients with α-particles and the nuclei of carbon, neon, silicon, and argon. Currently, fully ionized ^{12}C is the "ion of choice" for clinical work. Considerable laboratory work has been done on the radiobiology of such beams, but space does not permit our delving into this here other than to note that a ^{12}C beam of 80 keV/μ in the spread Bragg peak has approximately equivalent RBE as the 30 MeV d$\rightarrow$Be neutron beam produced at the National Institute for Radiological Sciences neutron facility (68,118). Clinically, an approximate RBE equal to 3 is used for setting doses. No randomized clinical trials have been carried out, but several phase I/II trial reports have been published. As of 2005, approximately 2,300 patients had been treated (119). There is a preliminary indication that nonsquamous tumors responded better than squamous-cell carcinomas. Kamada et al. (67) have reported on a phase I/II study using ^{12}C beams to treat patients with inoperable sarcomas. Sixty-four lesions were treated in 57 patients using spread Bragg peaks. The applied dose was escalated from 17.6 Gy to 24.5 Gy in 16 fractions over 4 weeks. Grade 3 skin reactions at the highest dose level prevented the investigators from further increasing the dose. The median tumor size was 559 cm^3 (range 20 to

2,290 cm^3) and the minimum follow-up time for the surviving patients was 18 months. The local control rate at 3 years was 73%, with the overall survival rate being 46%. Mizoe et al. (97) reported on a phase I/II dose escalation study for patients with locally advanced head and neck cancers. Two different dose escalation protocols were utilized: 18 fractions over 6 weeks or 16 fractions over 4 weeks. A spectrum of different tumor histologies were treated with the overall 5-year local control rate being 75% for the 34 patients who were analyzed. The authors concluded that toxicity was acceptable and that there was improved local control for nonsquamous cell tumors such as melanomas and salivary gland tumors compared to that expected with standard photon radiotherapy. Eighty-one patients with non–small-cell lung cancer were also treated with doses ranging between 19.8 Gy to 31.8 Gy to the primary target volume using either 18 fractions over 6 weeks or 9 fractions over 3 weeks (96). Treatment-related reactions were quite modest with grade 2 pneumonitis being only 10% overall and grade 3 pneumonitis being only 4% overall. The tolerance dose was felt to be 26.4 Gy for the shorter fractionation schema and 31.8 Gy for the longer treatment course. Pulmonary function testing indicated that little change from baseline was measured at 6 and 12 months, and, furthermore, that the use of respiratory gating was associated with reduced side effects.

The GSI group has reported on 37 patients with skull base tumors treated with ^{12}C ions between 1998 to 2000 (111). There were 24 patients with chordomas and 13 patients with chondrosarcomas. The clinical target volume received 15 Gy followed by a 5 Gy boost to areas of gross disease (total dose 60 Gy-equivalent). Patient positioning was verified using orthogonal x-rays with digitally reconstructed images and the beam was delivered using a scanning mode. With a mean follow-up time of 13 months, the progression-free survivals at 2 years were 100% for the chondrosarcoma patients and 83% for the chordoma patients. Treatment toxicity was characterized as "mild." Clearly more follow-up time is required to determine whether there is any advantage compared to proton beam radiotherapy, but the absence of toxicity means that further dose escalation is possible.

π-Meson Radiotherapy

Although various types of tumors have been treated, the majority of the published or presented clinical results from the π-meson program are for the treatment of high-grade gliomas of the brain. Bush et al. (12) reported on 42 patients treated at LAMPF. Tumors were graded according to the Kernohan schema (69), with 27 patients having grade IV tumors and 15 patients having grade III lesions. Seventeen patients had a whole-brain, photon component to their treatment. At the time of publication the median survival of the patients with grade IV tumors was 14 months, and the survival of the patients with grade III tumors was about 56% at 28 months. There was one reported case of radiation necrosis in a woman who had received 37 Gy-pion (no photon irradiation), but local tumor recurrence also was present.

Greiner et al. (49) reported on 56 patients with malignant gliomas of the brain treated with π-mesons at SIN. Forty patients received doses of 27.2 to 34.2 Gy-pion dose delivered for 4 to 5 weeks, and 12 patients were treated with an accelerated fractionation scheme of 32.8 Gy-pion dose in 2 to 3 weeks. Acute effects were well tolerated. Three patients were excluded from analysis because they had extremely large tumors involving the central regions of the brain with extremely short survival times. There was no statistically significant difference in outcome between the two patient groups, with the overall median survival being approximately 12 months. At the time of analysis six of 32 patients with glioblastoma multiforme were alive but all had

evidence of active tumor. Three of the 17 patients with anaplastic astrocytoma appeared to have local control of tumor. Seventeen patients had posttreatment histologic investigation, with 10 having no gross evidence of tumor. In the other seven cases, active tumor was identified within the 90% isodose line. Unlike the early neutron studies, there was no evidence of either radiation necrosis or demyelination extending far from the original tumor volume.

Pickles et al. (101) have reported on the final outcome of a randomized trial conducted at TRIUMF. Eighty-one evaluable patients with high-grade gliomas were randomized to either 33 to 34.5 Gy-pion dose given over 3 weeks or 60 Gy photon dose given over 6 weeks. Median survival was 10 months on each arm, and there was no difference in terms of time to progression, radiation toxicity, serial Karnofsky performance scores, or serial quality-of-life assessments. Although the pion radiation schema appeared safe, there was no demonstrable benefit to its use.

In 1999 the TRIUMF group reported on the outcome of a phase III clinical trial for patients with locally advanced prostate cancer (100). Patients were randomized to receive either 66 Gy in 33 fractions conventional photon irradiation versus 37.5 Gy-pion dose in 15 fractions with appropriate field reductions taking place during therapy. There were 213 analyzable patients entered into the study. With a median follow-up time of 3.75 years, there was more acute grade 3 or 4 bladder toxicity on the pion arm (12% vs. 6%, $p = 0.002$), no difference in significant late toxicities (RTOG/EORTC grades 3+), and no difference in local control or survival. Clinical local failure was about 50% at 5 years for both arms, indicating perhaps the advanced nature of the tumors being treated.

Summary and Future Directions

In this chapter we have discussed the basic physical and radiobiologic properties of particle beams and related these to the clinical interest in using them for radiotherapeutic purposes. Neutrons were the first of these particles to enter widespread clinical trials. These are a high LET form of radiation with different radiobiologic properties compared to more conventional radiotherapeutic modalities. Despite initial promise, neutrons have not been shown to have widespread applicability. However, they have an established role in the treatment of some so-called radioresistant tumors such as salivary gland malignancies; sarcomas of bone and soft tissue; nonhormonally responsive, locally advanced prostate cancers; and perhaps certain other tumors such as renal cell cancer, melanomas, and thyroid cancers. There are no ongoing multi-institutional clinical trials taking place using neutrons, but there are continuing studies taking place at those institutions where neutrons are used clinically in order to refine their use.

Charged-particle radiotherapy is an exciting contemporary area of radiotherapy clinical research. The majority of this work is being done with proton beams having essentially the same radiobiologic properties as conventional photon/electron radiation but allowing a much more precise control of the radiation dose distribution. These beams are ideal for the treatment of well-defined lesions in critical locations. Such tumors do not lend themselves well to randomized phase III trials, but with IMRT photon beams, this may change. There are also a small number of centers using heavy ion beams to treat cancers. In principle, such beams offer the best of both worlds—the radiobiologic advantage of high LET radiotherapy and the precise dose delivery of proton beams. Given the small number of such centers, it will be especially important that they conduct well-designed and well-executed clinical studies to determine whether the cost of additional facilities is clinically justified.

References

1. Austin-Seymour M, Caplan R, Russell K, et al. Impact of a multileaf collimator on treatment morbidity in localized carcinoma of the prostate. *Int J Radiat Oncol Biol Phys* 1994;30:1065–1071.
2. Barendsen GW, Koot CJ, Van Kersen GR, et al. The effect of oxygen on impairment of the proliferative capacity of human cells in culture by ionizing radiations of different LET. *Int J Radiat Biol* 1966;10:317–327.
3. Barth RF, Codere JA, Vicente MG, et al. Boron neutron capture therapy of cancer: current status and future prospects. *Clin Cancer Res* 2005;11:3987–4002.
4. Battermann JJ, Breur K, Hare GAM, et al. Observations on pulmonary metastases in patients after single doses and multiple fractions of fast neutrons and cobalt-60 gamma rays. *Eur J Cancer* 1981;17:539–548.
5. Benk VA, Adams JA, Shipley WU, et al. Late rectal bleeding following combined x-ray and proton high dose irradiation for patients with stages T3-T4 prostate cancer. *Int J Radiat Oncol Biol Phys* 1993;26:551–557.
6. Brennan JT, Phillips TL. Evaluation of past experience with fast neutron teletherapy and its implications for future applications. *Eur J Cancer Clin Oncol* 1971;7:219–225.
7. Brenner DJ, Hall EJ. Fractionation and protraction for radiotherapy of prostate carcinoma. *Int J Radiat Oncol Biol Phys* 1999;43:1095–1101.
8. Broerse JJ, Barendsen GN, van Kersen GR. Survival of cultured human cells after irradiation with fast neutrons of different energies in hypoxic and oxygenated conditions. *Int J Radiat Biol* 1967;13:559–572.
9. Bush DA, Hillebrand DJ, Slater JM, et al. High-dose proton beam radiotherapy of hepatocellular carcinoma: preliminary results of a phase II trial. *Gastroenterology* 2004;127:S189–S193.
10. Bush DA, McAllister CJ, Loredo LN, et al. Fractionated proton beam radiotherapy for acoustic neuroma. *Neurosurgery* 2002;50:270–273.
11. Bush, DA, Slater, JD, Bonnet, R, et al. Proton-beam radiotherapy for early-stage lung cancer. *Chest* 1999;116:1313–1319.
12. Bush SE, Smith AR, Zink S. Pion radiotherapy at LAMPF. *Int J Radiat Oncol Biol Phys* 1982;8:2181–2186.
13. Castro JR, Linstadt DE, Bahary JP, et al. Experience in charged particle irradiation of tumors of the skull base: 1977–1992. *Int J Radiat Oncol Biol Phys* 1994;29:647–655.
14. Castro JR, Saunders WM, Austin-Seymour MM, et al. A phase I-II trial of heavy charged particle irradiation of malignant glioma of the brain: A Northern California Oncology Group study. *Int J Radiat Oncol Biol Phys* 1985;11:1795–1800.
15. Castro JR, Saunders WM, Tobias CA, et al. Treatment of cancer with heavy charged particles. *Int J Radiat Oncol Biol Phys* 1982;8:2191–2198.
16. Catterall M. The treatment of advanced cancer by fast neutrons from the Medical Research Council's cyclotron at Hammersmith Hospital, London. *Eur J Cancer Clin Oncol* 1974;10:343–347.
17. Catterall M, Bewley DK, Sutherland I. Second report on results of a randomized clinical trial of fast neutrons compared with x or gamma rays in treatment of advanced tumor of head and neck. *BMJ* 1977;1:1642.
18. Catterall M, Sutherland I, Bewley DK. First results of a randomized clinical trial of fast neutrons compared with x or gamma rays in treatment of advanced tumors of the head and neck. *BMJ* 1975;2:653–656.
19. Chan A, Pommier P, Deschler DG, et al. Change in patterns of relapse after combined proton and photon irradiation for locally advanced paranasal sinus cancer. *Int J Radiat Oncol Biol Phys* 2004;60:S320.
20. Chan AW, Lidbsch NJ, Deschler DG, et al. Proton radiotherapy for T4 nasopharyngeal carcinomas. *Proc ASCO* 2004;23:504 (abstr 5574).
21. Chuba PJ, Maughan R, Forman JD. Three dimensional conformal neutron radiotherapy for prostate cancer. *Strahlenther Onkol* 1999;175:79–81.
22. Colombo F, Pozza F, Chierego G, et al. Linear accelerator radiosurgery of cerebral arteriovenous malformations: An update. *Neurosurgery* 1994;34:14–20.
23. Courdi A, Caujolle JP, Grange JD, et al. Results of proton therapy of uveal melanomas treated in Nice. *Int J Radiat Oncol Biol Phys* 1999;45:5–11.
24. Douglas JG, Einck J, Austin-Seymour M, et al. Neutron radiotherapy for recurrent pleomorphic adenomas of major salivary glands. *Head Neck* 2001;23:1037–1042.
25. Douglas JD, Laramore GE, Austin-Seymour M, et al. Treatment of locally advanced adenoid cystic carcinoma of the head and neck with neutron radiotherapy. *Int J Radiat Oncol Biol Phys* 2000;46:551–557.
26. Douglas JD, Lee S, Laramore GE, et al. Neutron radiotherapy for the treatment of locally advanced major salivary gland tumors. *Head Neck* 1999;21:255–263.
27. Duncan W, Arnott SJ, Batterman JJ, et al. Fast neutrons in the treatment of head and neck cancers: The results of a multi-centre randomly controlled trial. *Radiother Oncol* 1984;2:293–300.
28. Egan, KM, Gragoudis ES, Seddon JM, et al. The risk of enucleation after proton beam irradiation of uveal melanoma. *Ophthalmology.* 1989;96:1377–1382.
29. Egger E, Schalenbourg A, Zografos L, et al. Maximizing local tumor control and survival after proton beam radiotherapy of uveal melanoma. *Int J Radiat Oncol Biol Phys* 2001;51:138–147.
30. Eichhorn HJ. Results of a pilot study on neutron radiotherapy with 600 patients. *Int J Radiat Oncol Biol Phys* 1981;8:1561–1565.
31. Fabrikant JI, Levy RP, Steinberg GK, et al. Charged-particle radiosurgery for intracranial vascular malformations. *Neurosurg Clin North Am* 1992;3:99–139.
32. Fagundes MA, Hug EB, Liebsch NJ, et al. Radiation therapy for chordomas of the base of skull and cervical spine: Patterns of failure and outcome after relapse. *Int J Radiat Oncol Biol Phys* 1995;33:579–584.
33. Fitzek MM, Thornton AF, Rabinov JD, et al. Accelerated fractionated proton/photon irradiation to 90 cobalt gray equivalent for glioblastoma multiforme: results of a phase II prospective trial. *J Neurosurg* 1999;91:251–260.
34. Fitzek, MM, Thornton AF, Varvares M, et al. Neuroendocrine tumors of the sinonasal tract. Results of a prospective study incorporating chemotherapy, surgery, and combined proton-photon radiotherapy. *Cancer* 2002;94:2623–2634.
35. Fleurette F, Charvet-Protat S. Proton and neutron radiation in cancer treatment: Clinical and economic outcomes. *Bull Cancer Radiother* 1996;83S:223–227.
36. Flickinger JC, Deutsch M, Lundsford LD. Repeat megavoltage irradiation of pituitary and suprasellar tumors. *Int J Rad Oncol Biol Phys* 1989;17:171–175.
37. Fogliata A, Bolsi A, Cozzi L. Critical appraisal of treatment techniques based on conventional photon beams, intensity modulated photon beams and proton beams for therapy of intact breast. *Radiother Oncol* 2002;62:137–145.
38. Forman JD. Neutron radiotherapy for prostate cancer. *Pros J* 1999;1:8–14.
39. Forman JD, Duclos M, Sharma R, et al. Conformal mixed neutron and photon irradiation in localized and locally advanced prostate cancer: Preliminary estimates of the therapeutic ratio. *Int J Radiat Oncol Biol Phys* 1996;35:259–266.
40. Forman JD, Porter AT. The experience with neutron irradiation in locally advanced adenocarcinoma of the prostate. *Semin Urol Oncol* 1997;15:239–243.
41. Forman JD, Yudelev M, Bolton S, et al. Fast neutron irradiation for prostate cancer. *Cancer Metastasis Rev* 2002;21:131–135.
42. Fuse H, Katayama T, Akimoto S, et al. Radiotherapy of prostatic carcinoma [in Japanese]. *Hinyokika Kiyo* 1991;37:801–808.
43. Fuss M, Hug EB, Schaefer RA, et al. Proton radiation therapy (PRT) for pediatric optic pathway gliomas: comparison with 3D planned conventional photons and a standard photon technique. *Int J Radiat Oncol Biol Phys* 1999;45:1117–1126.
44. Goldsmith BJ, Wara WM, Wilson CB, et al. Post-operative irradiation for subtotally resected meningiomas. A retrospective analysis of 140 patients treated from 1967 to 1990. *J Neurosurg* 1994;80:195–201.
45. Gragg RL, Humphrey RM, Meyn RE. The response of Chinese hamster ovary cells to fast neutron radiotherapy beams. II. Sublethal and potentially lethal damage recovery capabilities. *Radiat Res* 1977;71:461–470.
46. Gragg RL, Humphrey RM, Meyn RE. The response of Chinese hamster ovary cells to fast neutron radiotherapy beams. III. Variations in relative biological effectiveness with position in the cell cycle. *Radiat Res* 1978;76:283–291.
47. Gragoudas ES, Lane AM, Regan S, et al. A randomized controlled trial of varying radiation doses in the treatment of choroidal melanoma. *Arch Opthalmol* 2000;118:773–778.
48. Gragoudas ES, Li W, Goitein M, et al. Evidence-based estimates of outcome in patients irradiated for intraocular melanoma. *Arch Opthalmol* 2002;120:1665–1671.
49. Greiner R, Blattman H, Thum P, et al. Anaplastic astrocytoma and glioblastoma: Pion irradiation with the dynamic conformation technique at the Swiss Institute for Nuclear Physics Research (SIN). *Radiother Oncol* 1990;17:37–46.
50. Griffin TW, Davis R, Laramore GE, et al. Fast neutron radiotherapy of metastatic cervical adenopathy: The results of a randomized RTOG study. *Int J Radiat Oncol Biol Phys* 1983;9:1267–1270.
51. Griffin TW, Pajak TF, Maor MH, et al. Mixed neutron/photon irradiation of unresectable squamous cell carcinomas of the head and neck. The final report of a randomized cooperative trial. *Int J Radiat Oncol Biol Phys* 1989;17:959–965.
52. Hall EJ. *Radiobiology for the Radiologist*. 4th ed. Philadelphia: Lippincott, 1992. (See in particular Chaps. 9 and 14.)
53. Hall EJ, Kraljevic J. Repair of potentially lethal radiation damage: Comparison of neutron and x-ray RBE and implications for radiation therapy. *Radiology* 1976;121:731–735.
54. Hall EJ, Wuu C-S. Radiation-induced second cancers: The impact of 3D-CRT and IMRT. *Int J Radiat Oncol Biol Phys* 2003;56:83–88.
55. Halperin EC. Why is female sex an independent predictor of shortened overall survival after proton/photon radiation therapy for skull base chordomas? *Int J Radiat Oncol Biol Phys* 1997;38:225–230.
56. Haraf DJ, Rubin SJ, Sweeney P, et al. Photon neutron mixed-beam radiotherapy of locally advanced prostate cancer. *Int J Radiat Oncol Biol Phys* 1995;33:3–14.
57. Harsh G, Loeffler JS, Thornton A, et al. Stereotactic proton radiosurgery. *Neurosurg Clin North Am* 1999;10:243–256.
58. Harsh GR, Thornton AF, Chapman PH, et al. Proton beam stereotactic radiosurgery of vestibular schwannomas. *Int J Radiat Oncol Biol Phys* 2002;54:35–44.
59. Huber PE, Debus J, Latz D, et al. Radiotherapy for advanced adenoid cystic carcinoma: Neutrons, photons, or mixed beam? *Radiother Oncol* 2001;59:161–167.
60. Hug EB, Adams J, Fitzek M, et al. Fractionated, three-dimensional, planning-assisted proton-radiation therapy for orbital rhabdomyosarcoma: a novel technique. *Int J Radiat Oncol Biol Phys* 2000;47:979–984.
61. Hug EB, deVries A, Thornton AF, et al. Management of atypical and malignant meningioma: Role of high dose, 3D-conformal radiation therapy. *J Neurooncol* 2000;48:151–160.
62. Hug EB, Fitzek MM, Liebsch NJ. Locally challenging osteo- and chondrogenic tumors of the axial skeleton: Results of combined proton and photon radiation therapy using three-dimensional treatment planning. *Int J Radiat Oncol Biol Phys* 1995;31:467–476.
63. Hug EB, Loredo LN, Slater JD, et al. Proton radiation therapy for chordomas and chondrosarcomas of the skull base. *J Neurosurg* 1999;91:432–439.
64. Hug EB, Muenter MW, Adams JA, et al. 3-D-conformal radiation therapy for pediatric giant cell tumors of the skull base. *Strahlenther Onkol* 2002;178:239–244.
65. Hug EB, Muenter MW, Archambeau JO, et al. Conformal proton radiation therapy for pediatric low-grade astrocytomas. *Strahlenther Onkol* 2002;178:10–17.
66. Hug EB, Nevinny-Stickel M, Fuss M, et al. Conformal proton radiation treatment for retroperitoneal neuroblastoma: introduction of a novel technique. *Med Pediatr Oncol* 2001;37:36–41.
67. Kamada T, Tsujii H, Tsuji H, et al. Efficacy and safety of carbon ion radiotherapy in bone and soft tissue sarcomas. *J Clin Oncol* 2002;20:4466–4471.
68. Kanai T, Endo M, Minohara S, et al. Biophysical characteristics of HIMAC clinical irradiation system for heavy ion radiation therapy. *Int J Radiat Oncol Biol Phys* 1999;44:201–210.
69. Kernohan JW, Sayre GP. Tumors of the central nervous system. In: *Atlas of Tumor Pathology, Fasc. 35 & 37*. Washington, DC: Armed Forces Institute of Pathology, 1952: 17–42.
70. Kjellberg RN. Stereotactic Bragg peak proton beam radiosurgery for cerebral arteriovenous malformations. *Ann Clin Res* 1986;18:17–19.
71. Kjellberg RN, Hanamura T, Davis KR, et al. Bragg-peak proton-beam therapy for arteriovenous malformations of the brain. *N Engl J Med* 1983;309:269–274.
72. Kjellberg RN, Kliman B, Swisher B, et al. Proton beam therapy of Cushing's disease and Nelson's syndrome. In: Black P McL, ed. *Secretory Tumors of the Pituitary Gland*. New York, Raven Press, 1984:295–307.
73. Kliman B, Kjellberg RN, Swisher B, et al. Proton beam therapy of acromegaly: A 20-year experience. In: Black P McL, ed. *Secretory Tumors of the Pituitary Gland*. New York: Raven Press, 1984: 191–211.
74. Koh W-J, Krall JM, Peters LJ, et al. Neutron vs photon radiation therapy for inoperable regional non-small cell lung cancer: Results of a multicenter randomized trial. *Int J Radiat Oncol Biol Phys* 1993;27:499–505.
75. Komaki R, Mountain C, Holbert J, et al. Superior sulcus tumors: Treatment selection and results for 85 patients without metastases (M_0) at presentation. *Int J Radiat Oncol Biol Phys* 1990;19:31–36.

76. Laramore GE. The use of neutrons in cancer therapy: A historical perspective through the modern era. *Semin Oncol* 1997;24:672–685.

77. Laramore GE, Austin-Seymour MM. Fast neutron radiotherapy in relation to the radiation sensitivity of human organ systems. *Adv Radiat Biol* 1992;15:153–193.

78. Laramore GE, Bauer M, Griffin TW, et al. Fast neutron and mixed beam radiotherapy for inoperable non-small cell carcinoma of the lung. *Am J Clin Oncol (CCT)* 1986;9:233–243.

79. Laramore GE, Griffith JT, Boesplflug M, et al. Fast neutron radiotherapy for sarcomas of soft tissue, bone, and cartilage. *Am J Clin Oncol (CCT)* 1989;12:320–326.

80. Laramore GE, Krall JM, Griffin TW, et al. Fast neutron radiotherapy for locally-advanced prostate cancer. *Am J Clin Oncol (CCT)* 1993;16:164–167.

81. Laramore GE, Krall JM, Griffin TW, et al. Fast neutron irradiation for unresectable salivary gland tumors: Final report of an RTOG-MRC randomized clinical trial. *Int J Radiat Oncol Biol Phys* 1993;27:235–240.

82. Lawrence JH, Linfoot JA. Treatment of acromegaly, Cushing's disease and Nelson syndrome. *West J Med* 1980;133:197–202.

83. Levy RP, Fabrikant JI, Frankel KA. Particle-beam irradiation of the pituitary gland. In: Alexander E III, Loeffler JS, Lunsford LD, eds. *Stereotactic Radiosurgery.* New York: McGraw-Hill, 1993:157–165.

84. Lin R, Hug EB, Schaefer RA, et al. Conformal proton radiation therapy of the posterior fossa: a study comparing protons with three-dimensional planned photons in limiting dose to auditory structures. *Int J Radiat Oncol Biol Phys* 2000;48:1219–1226.

85. Lin R, Slater JD, Yonemoto LT, et al. Nasopharyngeal carcinoma: Repeat treatment with conformal proton therapy—dose-volume histogram analysis. *Radiology* 1999;213:489–494.

86. Linfoot JA, Lawrence JH, Born JL, et al. The alpha particle or proton beam in radiosurgery of the pituitary gland for Cushing's disease. *N Engl J Med* 1963;269:597–601.

87. Linstadt D, Castro J, Char D, et al. Long-term results of helium ion irradiation of uveal melanoma. *Int J Radiat Oncol Biol Phys* 1990;19:613–618.

88. Linstadt DE, Castro JR, Phillips TL. Neon ion radiotherapy: Results of the phase I/II clinical trial. *Int J Radiat Oncol Biol Phys* 1991;20:761–769.

89. Lunsford LD, Kondziolka D, Flickinger JC, et al. Stereotactic radiosurgery for arteriovenous malformations of the brain. *J Neurosurg* 1991;75:512–524.

90. Lyman JT. Computer modeling of heavy charged particle beams. In: Skarsgard LD, ed. *Pion and Heavy Ion Radiotherapy: Preclinical and Clinical Studies.* New York: Elsevier Science Publishing, 1983:139–147.

91. MacDougall RH, Orr JA, Kerr GR, et al. Fast neutron treatment for squamous cell carcinoma of the head and neck: Final report of the Edinburgh randomized trial. *BMJ* 1990;301:1241–1242.

92. Maor MH, Errington RD, Caplan RJ, et al. Fast-neutron therapy in advanced head and neck cancer: A collaborative international randomized trial. *Int J Radiat Oncol Biol Phys* 1995;32:599–604.

93. Matsuzaki Y, Osuga T, Chiba T, et al. New, effective treatment using proton irradiation for unresectable hepatocellular carcinoma. *Intern Med* 1995;34:302–307.

94. Maughan RL, Brambs B, Porter AT, et al. The cost-effectiveness of mixed beam neutron-photon radiation therapy in the treatment of adenocarcinoma of the prostate. *Strahlenther Onkol* 1999;175:104–107.

95. Miralbell R, Lomax A, Cella L, et al. Potential reduction of the incidence of radiation-induced second cancers by using proton beams in the treatment of pediatric tumors. *Int J Radiat Oncol Biol Phys* 2002;54:824–829.

96. Miyamoto T, Yamamoto N, Nishimura H, et al. Carbon ion radiotherapy for stage I non-small cell lung cancer. *Radiother Oncol* 2003;66:127–140.

97. Mizoe J, Tsujii H, Kamada T, et al. Dose escalation study of carbon ion radiotherapy for locally advanced head and neck cancer. *Int J Radiat Oncol Biol Phys* 2004;60:358–364.

98. Munzenrider JE, Liebsch NJ. Proton therapy for tumors of the skull base. *Strahlenther Onkol* 1999;175:57–63.

99. Nowakowski VA, Castro JR, Petti PL, et al. Charged particle radiotherapy of paraspinal tumors. *Int J Radiat Oncol Biol Phys* 1991;22:295–303.

100. Pickles T, Goodman GB, Fryer CJ, et al. Pion radiation for locally advanced prostate cancer: Results of a randomized trial. *Int J Radiat Oncol Biol Phys* 1999;43:47–55.

101. Pickles T, Goodman GB, Rheaume DE, et al. Pion radiation for high grade astrocytoma: Results of a randomized trial. *Int J Radiat Oncol Biol Phys* 1997;37:491–497.

102. Poon RT, Fan ST, Tsang FH, et al. Locoregional therapies for hepatocellular carcinoma: a critical review from the surgeon's perspective. *Ann Surg* 2002;235:466–486.

103. Richard F, Renard L, Wambersie A. Current results of neutron therapy at the UCL, for soft tissue sarcomas and prostatic adenocarcinomas. *Bull Cancer (Paris)* 1986;73:562–568.

104. Roa WH, Hazuka MB, Sandler HM, et al. Results of primary and adjuvant CT-based 3-dimensional radiotherapy for malignant tumors of the paranasal sinuses. *Int J Rad Oncol Biol Phys* 1994;28:857–865.

105. Rodriguez A, Alpen EL, Powers-Risius P. The RBE-LET relationship for rodent intestinal crypt cell survival, testes weight loss, and multicellular spheroid cell survival after heavy-ion irradiation. *Radiat Res* 1992;132:184–192.

106. Ronson BB, Schulte RW, Han KP, et al. Fractionated proton beam irradiation of pituitary adenomas. *Int J Radiat Oncol Biol Phys* 2006;64:425–434.

107. Russell KJ, Caplan RJ, Laramore GE, et al. Photon versus fast neutron external beam radiotherapy in the treatment of locally advanced prostate cancer: Results of a randomized prospective trial. *Int J Radiat Oncol Biol Phys* 1993;28:47–54.

108. Sawada K, Fukuma S, Seki Y, et al. Clinical experience with Pancoast tumor treated by fast neutron radiotherapy. *Gan No Rinsho* 1983;A7:111–114(abstr).

109. Scalliet PG, Remouchamps V, Lhoas F, et al. A retrospective analysis of the results of p(65) + Be neutron therapy for the treatment of prostate adenocarcinoma at the cyclotron of Louvain-la-Neuve. Part I: Survival and progression-free survival. *Cancer Radiother* 2001;5:262–272.

110. Schoenthaler R, Albright NW, Wara WM, et al. Reirradiation of pituitary adenoma. *Int J Rad Oncol Biol Phys* 1992;24:307–314.

111. Schulz-Ertner D, Haberer T, Jalel O, et al. Radiotherapy for chordomas and low-grade chondrosarcomas of the skull base with carbon ions. *Int J Radiat Oncol Biol Phys* 2002;53:36–42.

112. Schwarz R, Krull A, Heyer D, et al. Neutron therapy in soft tissue sarcomas: a review of European results. *Bull Cancer/Radiother* 1996;83[Suppl]:110–114.

113. Schwarz R, Krull A, Heyer D, et al. Present results of neutron therapy. The German experience. *Acta Oncol* 1994;33:281–287.

114. Shipley WU, Verhey LJ, Munzenrider JE, et al. Advanced prostate cancer: The results of a randomized comparative trial of high dose irradiation boosting with conformal protons compared with conventional dose irradiation using photons alone. *Int J Radiat Oncol Biol Phys* 1995;32:3–12.

115. Slater JD, Rossi CJ, Yonemoto LT, et al. Conformal proton therapy for early-stage prostate cancer. *Urology* 1999;53:978–98.

116. St Clair WH, Adams JA, Bues M, et al. Advantage of protons compared to conventional x-ray or IMRT in the treatment of a pediatric patient with medulloblastoma. *Int J Radiat Oncol Biol Phys* 2004;58:727–734.

117. Stone RS. Neutron therapy and specific ionization. *Am J Roentgenol* 1948;59:771–785.

118. Suzuki M, Kase Y, Yamaguchi H, et al. Relative biological effectiveness for cell-killing effect on various human cell lines irradiated with heavy-ion medical accelerator in Chiba (HIMAC) carbon-ion beams. *Int J Radiat Oncol Biol Phys* 2000;48:241–250.

119. Tsujii H. PTOCG 43, Munich, Germany, December 10–14, 2005, Abstract VIII/5.

120. Tsunemoto H, Morita S, Shimazaki J. Fast neutron therapy for carcinoma of the prostate. In: Karr JP, Yamanaka H, eds. *Prostate Cancer: The Second Tokyo Symposium.* New York: Elsevier Science Publishing, 1989:383–391.

121. Tsunemoto H, Yoo SY. Present status of fast neutron therapy in Asian countries. *Bull Cancer Radiother* 1996;83S:93–100.

122. Wang JZ, Guerrero M, Li XA. How low is the α/β ratio for prostate cancer? *Int J Radiat Oncol Biol Phys* 2003;55:194–203.

123. Wara WM, Sheline GE, Newman HJ, et al. Radiation therapy of meningiomas. *Am J Roentgenol Rad Ther Nucl Med* 1975;123:453–458.

124. Weber DC, Lomax AJ, Rutz HP. Spot-scanning proton radiation therapy for recurrent, residual or untreated intracranial meningiomas. *Radiother Oncol* 2004;71:251–258.

125. Weber DC, Trofimov AV, Delaney TF, et al. A treatment planning comparison of intensity modulated photon and proton therapy for paraspinal sarcomas. *Int J Radiat Oncol Biol Phys* 2004;58:1596–1606.

126. Wenkel E, Thornton AF, Finkelstein D, et al. Benign meningioma: Partially resected, biopsied, and recurrent intracranial tumors treated with combined proton and photon radiotherapy. *Int J Radiat Oncol Biol Phys* 2000;48:1363–1370.

127. Zeitman AL, DeSilvo ML, Slater JD, et al. Comparison of conventional-dose vs high-dose conformal radiation therapy in clinically localized adenocarcinoma of the prostate: A randomized controlled trial. *JAMA* 2005;294:1233–1239.

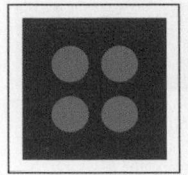

Chapter 19
Physics and Biology of Brachytherapy

Jeffrey F. Williamson, David J. Brenner

Brachytherapy (*brachy* is from the Greek for short distance) consists of placing sealed radioactive sources very close to or in contact with the target tissue. Because the absorbed dose falls off rapidly with increasing distance from the sources, high doses may be delivered safely to a localized target region over a short time. This chapter reviews the properties and applications of commonly used sealed radionuclides and sources, the basic biologic principles governing clinical response to brachytherapy, methods of dose calculation and source-strength specification, and implant design and dose specification for interstitial and intracavitary brachytherapy.

Basic Terminology

Implantation techniques may be classified in terms of surgical approach to the target volume (interstitial, intracavitary, transluminal, or mold techniques); The means of controlling the dose delivered (temporary or permanent implants); The source loading technology (preloaded, manually afterloaded, or remotely afterloaded); And the dose rate (low, medium, or high).

Intracavitary insertion consists of positioning applicators (bearing the radioactive sources) into a body cavity in close proximity to the target tissue. Intracavitary brachytherapy is used most widely for treatment of localized gynecologic malignancies. All intracavitary implants are *temporary implants*; They are left in the patient for a specified time needed to deliver the prescribed dose. With a few exceptions, during temporary implantation, the patient must be confined to a controlled, if not shielded, area in the hospital to manage the radiation safety hazard posed by the large ambient exposure rates around the implant.

Interstitial brachytherapy consists of surgically implanting small radioactive sources directly into the target tissues. A *permanent* interstitial implant remains in place indefinitely and is not removable; The initial source strength is chosen so that the prescribed dose is fully delivered only when the implanted radioactivity has decayed to a negligible level.

Surface-dose applications (sometimes called plesiocurie therapy or mold therapy) consist of an applicator containing an array of radioactive sources usually designed to deliver a uniform dose distribution to a skin or mucosal surface. *Transluminal* brachytherapy consists of inserting a single line source into a body lumen to treat its surface and adjacent tissues.

Until the early 1960s, radioactive sources (needles for interstitial therapy or preloaded applicators for intracavitary therapy) were implanted directly into the patient. Radiation exposure to the brachytherapist and operating room staff was reduced significantly with the advent of *afterloading* technology (111,264). *Manual afterloading* consists of implanting nonradioactive tubes or intracavitary applicators into the patient. Following transport of the patient to his or her room, sources are manipulated into the applicators by means of forceps and other hand-held tools. Exposure to staff responsible for source loading and the care of brachytherapy patients can be greatly reduced or eliminated by use of a *remote afterloading system*, which consists of a pneumatically driven or motor-driven source

transport system for robotically transferring radioactive material between a shielded safe and each treatment applicator (see Chapters 20 and 21).

According to Report No. 38 of the International Commission on Radiation Units and Measurements (ICRU) (122), *low–dose-rate* (LDR) implants deliver doses at the rate of 40 to 200 cGy/h (0.4 to 2 Gy/h), requiring treatment times of 24 to 144 hours, during which the patient is confined to an inpatient treatment room. At the other extreme, *high–dose-rate* (HDR) brachytherapy uses dose rates in excess of 0.2 Gy/min (12 Gy/h). In fact, modern HDR remote afterloaders deliver instantaneous dose rates as high as 0.12 Gy/sec (430 Gy/h) at a distance of 1 cm, resulting in treatment times of a few minutes. Such treatments must be delivered in heavily shielded vaults using remote afterloading devices, but that allow fractionated brachytherapy to be delivered on an outpatient basis. Medium–dose-rate delivery, defined as the 2 to 12 Gy/h range, rarely is used. Although not recognized by ICRU Report No. 38, the ultralow–dose-rate (ULDR) range (0.01 to 0.3 Gy/h) is of great importance; It is the dose-rate domain used in permanent implants with ^{125}I and ^{103}Pd seeds.

Properties of Brachytherapy Sources and Radionuclides

The clinical utility of any radionuclide depends on physical properties such as half-life, radiation output per unit activity, specific activity (Ci/g), and photon energy. In addition, the methods of producing the radionuclide and its physical or chemical form strongly influence cost effectiveness, safety, and toxicity. Detailed properties of brachytherapy radionuclides are listed in Table 19.1.

Photon Spectrum and Dosimetric Characteristics of Brachytherapy Sources

The dose delivered with a brachytherapy procedure depends on the individual source strengths, source arrangement, and implant duration as well as the dosimetric characteristics of the implanted sources. These dosimetric characteristics are described by specifying the distribution of dose rates per unit strength about the source, often in terms of an "away-and-along" table (294) in Cartesian coordinates or in terms of the Task Group 43 protocol (245) described later in this chapter. The single-source dose distribution is of central importance to treatment planning because commercial computer planning systems estimate dose distribution from the spatial coordinates of the implanted sources using the principle of superposition. The source superposition algorithm estimates the contribution of each source, given its tip-and-end coordinates and the single-source dose-rate array, to each point of interest. These contribution estimates are summed to estimate the total dose rate at each point. Often, total dose rates are calculated over a two-dimensional (2D) grid of points and are represented as isodose-rate curves.

Table 19.1   PHYSICAL PROPERTIES AND USES OF BRACHYTHERAPY RADIONUCLIDES

Element	Isotope	Energy (MeV)	Half-Life	HVL-Lead (mm)	Exposure Rate Constant[a] Γ_δ	Source Form	Clinical Application
Obsolete Sealed Sources of Historical Significance							
Radium	^{226}Ra	0.83 (average)	1,626 y	16	8.25[b]	Tubes and needles	LDR intracavitary and interstitial
Radon	^{222}Rn	0.83 (average)	3.83 d	16	8.25[b]	Gas encapsulated in gold tubing	Permanent interstitial Temporary molds
Currently Used Sealed Sources							
Cesium	^{137}Cs	0.662	30 y	3.28		Tubes and needles	LDR intracavitary and interstitial
Cesium	^{131}Cs	0.030	9.69 d	0.030	0.64	Seeds	LDR permanent implants
Iridium	^{192}Ir	0.397 (average)	73.8 d	6	4.69	Seeds in nylon ribbon; Metal wires	LDR temporary interstitial Intravascular brachytherapy; Cardiac
						Encapsulated source on cable	HDR interstitial and intracavitary Intravascular brachytherapy: peripheral
Cobalt	^{60}Co	1.25	5.26 y	11	13.07	Encapsulated spheres	HDR intracavitary
Iodine	^{125}I	0.028	59.6 d	0.025	1.45	Seeds	Permanent interstitial
Palladium	^{103}Pd	0.020	17 d	0.013	1.48	Seeds	Permanent interstitial
Gold	^{198}Au	0.412	2.7 d	6	2.35	Seeds	Permanent interstitial
Strontium/Yttrium	^{90}Sr–^{90}Y	2.24 β_{max}	28.9 y	—		Plaque	Treatment of superficial ocular lesions
						Seeds	Intravascular brachytherapy
Developmental Sealed Sources							
Americium	^{241}Am	0.060	432 y	0.12	0.12	Tubes	LDR intracavitary
Ytterbium	^{169}Yb	0.093	32 d	0.48	1.80	Seeds	HDR interstitial
Californium	^{252}Cf	2.4 (average) neutron	2.65 y	—	—	Tubes	High-LET LDR intracavitary
Samarium	^{145}Sm	0.043	340 d	0.060	0.885	Seeds	LDR temporary interstitial

HDR, high dose rate; HVL, half-value layer; LDR, low dose rate; LET, linear energy transfer.
[a]No filtration in units of R · cm^2 · mCi^{-1} · h^{-1}.
[b]0.5 mm platinum filtration; Units of R · cm^2 · mg^{-1} · h^{-1}.

For conventional brachytherapy, for which the therapeutically relevant distance range is 3 to 20 mm, only photons (γ-rays or characteristic x-rays) with energies in excess of 15 keV (kiloelectron volts) contribute to the therapeutic effect. In general, four factors influence the single-source dose distribution for photon-emitting sources:

1. Distance (inverse-square law);
2. Absorption and scattering in the source core and encapsulation;
3. Photon attenuation; And
4. Scattering in the surrounding medium (Fig. 19.1).

Encapsulation prevents radioactive material from leaking out of the source and absorbs nonpenetrating radiation (β-rays, α-rays, and low-energy photons), which would otherwise give rise to high-surface doses while contributing nothing to the therapeutic effect.

Each voxel of radioactive core material shown in Figure 19.1 can be assumed to be an isotropic point source (Fig. 19.2). Because of the straight-line emission of photons in all directions, photon intensity or fluence, $\Phi(r)$, at any point is proportional to the inverse square of its distance, r:

$$\Phi(r) = \frac{\text{no. incident photons}}{\text{unit area irradiated}} = \frac{\text{no. photons emitted}}{4\pi r^2} \qquad (1)$$
$$\propto \text{dose}(r) \propto \text{exposure}(r)$$

assuming that attenuation and scattering can be neglected.

As a result of this purely geometric effect, the absorbed doses $D(r_1)$ and $D(r_2)$ at the two distances r_1 and r_2 (Fig. 19.2) are

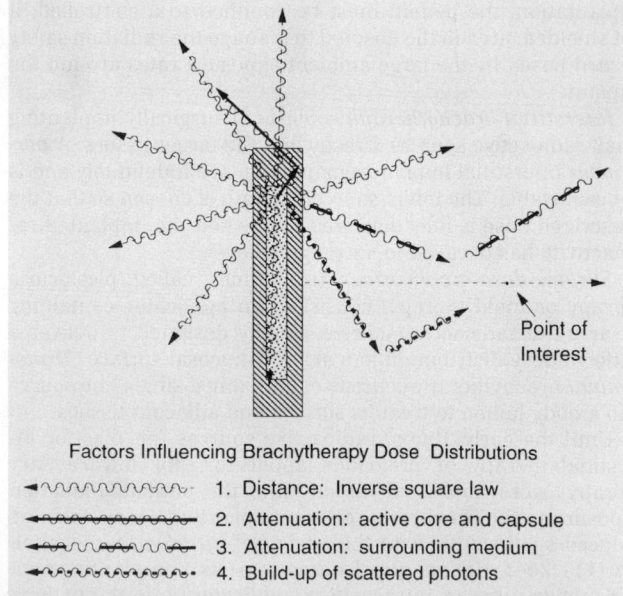

Factors Influencing Brachytherapy Dose Distributions

1. Distance: Inverse square law
2. Attenuation: active core and capsule
3. Attenuation: surrounding medium
4. Build-up of scattered photons

FIGURE 19.1. Typical cylindrical brachytherapy source, consisting of an active core (inner cylinder within which radioactivity is uniformly distributed) and the surrounding encapsulation (usually stainless steel or titanium for modern sources). The four principal factors influencing the dose distribution are: (1) distance, (2) attenuation and scattering of photons by the source structure and (3) two competing effects of the surrounding medium: attenuation of primary photons and (4) accumulation of scattered photons originating throughout the medium.

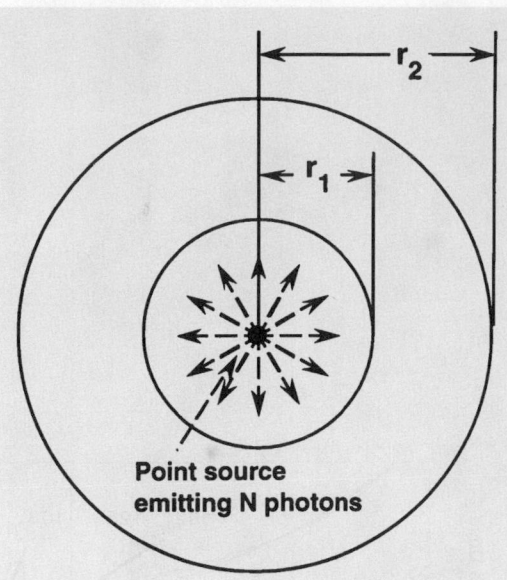

FIGURE 19.2. An isotropic point source of activity. To illustrate the derivation of inverse-square law, the source is surrounded by a vacuum and placed at the center of two concentric spherical surfaces of radii r_1 and r_2. By definition, an isotropic point source has no extension and radiates photons with equal likelihood in all directions in straight-line paths.

related by:

$$\frac{D(r_1)}{D(r_2)} = \frac{\Phi(r_1)}{\Phi(r_2)} = \left(\frac{r_2}{r_1}\right)^2 \quad (2)$$

This fundamental law applies exactly to each point of the radioactive core of the source shown in Figure 19.1, assuming that there is no attenuation and scattering of photons by the surrounding medium. However, equation 2 will not accurately describe the "collective" dose fall-off arising from the combined action of the point sources distributed throughout the core, unless both r_1 and r_2 are large relative to the active source dimensions. Of the four factors influencing the dose distribution (Fig. 19.1), inverse-square law is by far the most important. For a pure isotropic point source, the dose will decrease by a factor of 100 between the distances of 0.5 and 5 cm. The influence of the remaining factors over the same distance range rarely exceeds a factor of 2 or 3. Consequently, most of the clinical characteristics of implants (e.g., the heterogeneous dose distribution within the target tissue and rapid fall-off of dose outside the implanted volume) can be accounted for by applying inverse-square law to each pointlike element of radioactivity within the implant. Control of intersource spacing and positioning relative to the target and dose-limiting tissues is the most challenging issue in delivering brachytherapy.

Although inverse-square law dominates the dose distribution, the surrounding medium and the source structure both significantly affect the dose distribution (Fig. 19.1). The source core and surrounding capsule reduce the dose at the point of interest through absorption and scattering of primary photons. Primary photons contributing dose to points located near the longitudinal source axis (cylindrical axis of the source or axis of rotation) must traverse longer path lengths of capsule and core material and therefore experience more attenuation than photons contributing dose to equidistant points on the transverse source axis (plane perpendicular to the longitudinal source axis that bisects its active core). At a fixed distance from the source center, the dose near the longitudinal axis is usually smaller than on the transverse axis. This phenomenon is known as *oblique filtration* and is the main cause of dose *anisotropy* (variation of

dose as a function of polar angle at each fixed distance relative to the source center) characteristic of extended brachytherapy sources. Because brachytherapy sources are cylindrically symmetric, the dose distribution will be equatorially isotropic (constancy of dose as a function of azimuthal angle for each fixed polar angle and distance).

The tissue-equivalent medium surrounding the source affects the dose distribution in two important and competing ways (factors 3 and 4 of Fig. 19.1). At each point of interest, the intervening medium reduces the dose distribution by attenuating primary photons (deflecting them from their straight-line trajectories). At the same time, photons are being emitted in all directions from the source and are interacting with the medium by means of Compton scattering and photoelectric absorption. Thus, each volume element of tissue is effectively radiating scattered photons in all directions, many of which contribute to the dose at the point of interest. This mechanism, known as scattered-photon buildup, enhances the dose. The overall influence of the surrounding medium is the combined effect of these two competing processes: photon attenuation and scattered-photon buildup. In contrast to external-beam therapy, in which the scattering volume is limited to a narrow cone, scattered photons dominate brachytherapy dose distributions at distances >2 cm. Photon scattering is the main source of complexity in brachytherapy dose measurement and algorithm development.

Figure 19.3 demonstrates that the relative dose versus distance from the source is nearly independent of its photon energy so long as the average photon energy is >200 keV. In this energy range, dose deviates from inverse-square law by <5% over the 1- to 5-cm distance range. All of the "radium substitute" isotopes, including ^{137}Cs, ^{192}Ir, and ^{198}Au, fall into this energy range. This behavior, which greatly simplifies brachytherapy dosimetry, is the result of equilibrium between primary photon attenuation and buildup of scattered photons. Only for low-energy sources (e.g., ^{103}Pd and ^{125}I) does the depth-dose curve significantly deviate from inverse-square law. Because photon absorption rather than Compton scattering dominates energy deposition below 40 keV, scatter buildup is unable to compensate for loss of dose resulting from attenuation.

For radium-substitute radionuclides Figure 19.4A and B show that the absolute dose rate (cGy/h to fat or water tissue per mg Ra Eq or unit air-kerma strength [S_K]), as well as the relative dose distribution, is nearly independent of both energy and composition of the surrounding medium. Compton scattering, which dominates photon absorption and scattering above 100 keV, depends mainly on electron density (electrons/g) of the medium, which is nearly constant for all biologic materials. Below the radium-substitute energy range, absolute and relative dose distributions become highly dependent on both energy and composition (atomic number) of the surrounding medium. Implanting an ^{125}I seed in fat medium ($Z_{eff} = 6$) will deliver about half the absorbed dose at 1 cm, which is expected on the basis of dose measurements or calculations in water ($Z_{eff} = 7.5$). This is because energy absorption per unit mass from photoeffect interactions is proportional to the cube of the atomic number (Z_{eff}^3) of the medium. Figure 19.4B demonstrates that the inverse-square law actually underestimates relative dose at 5 cm by as much as a factor of 2 in the 60-keV to 100-keV energy range. In this narrow energy range, called the *intermediate low-energy range*, photoelectric effect is negligible, whereas Compton scattering transfers most of the colliding primary photon energy to the scattered photon rather than to the Compton electron. As a result of this imbalance between energy absorption and photon scattering, buildup of scattered photons overcompensates for loss of dose as a result of primary photon attenuation out to distances of 4 to 6 cm.

Above the 100-keV threshold, the photon-energy spectrum is much less important to optimizing brachytherapy dose-rate distributions than in external-beam therapy. Because artificial

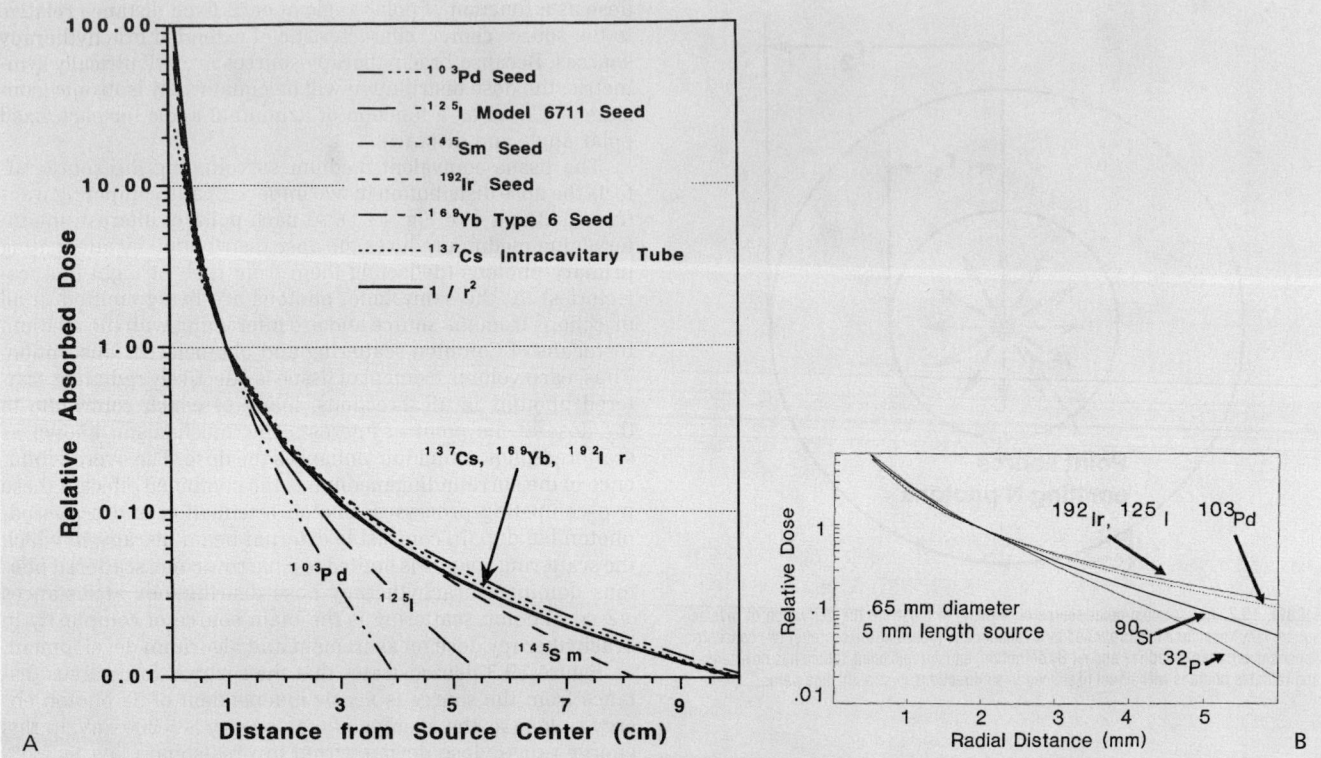

FIGURE 19.3. A: Variation of dose as a function of distance for point sources of ^{60}Co, ^{226}Ra, ^{137}Cs, ^{198}Au, ^{192}Ir, and ^{125}I. The results are normalized to 100% at 1-cm distance. The function (1/r^2) is plotted for comparison. **B:** Relative dose (normalized to 1.0 at 1 mm) versus distance for various cylindric sources (0.65 mm diameter and 5 mm long) over the 1 to 5 mm distance range. (From Amols HI, Zaider M, Weinberger J, et al. Dosimetric considerations for catheter-based beta and gamma emitters in the therapy of neointimal hyperplasia in human coronary arteries. *Int J Radiat Oncol Biol Phys* 1996;36:913–921, with permission.)

brachytherapy radionuclides in this energy range (^{60}Co, ^{137}Cs, ^{192}Ir, ^{198}Au) have dose-rate distributions nearly identical to those of ^{226}Ra in the 1- to 5-cm distance range, they are referred to as *radium substitutes*.

Figure 19.4C demonstrates that although photon energy is a relatively unimportant determinant of tissue dosimetry, it significantly influences the cost, weight, and thickness of shielding required to protect both critical anatomic structures in the patient and personnel involved in patient care. The half-value layer (HVL) in lead varies from 0.5 mm for a 100-keV source to 12 mm for ^{60}Co brachytherapy sources. Thus, for classical radium-equivalent brachytherapy, a radionuclide with a mean energy of about 100 to 200 keV is optimal. The major benefit of ^{125}I and ^{103}Pd as a brachytherapy source is the ability to provide complete protection by thin lead foils (0.1 to 0.2 mm), greatly reducing exposure to physicians during the implant procedure and allowing permanent-implant patients to be released from medical confinement without posing a radiation safety hazard to the general public. Recently, interest has been expressed in using radionuclides in the intermediate low-energy range (60 to 120 keV) (183,202,223). Tissue dose distributions are still approximately radium equivalent in this energy range, and thin layers of lead provide significant sparing of dose-limiting normal tissues near the implanted volume.

Sources for Low–Dose-Rate Intracavitary Brachytherapy

Since the 1930s, sources for classical LDR intracavitary brachytherapy have taken the form of "tubes" having a physical length of 2 to 2.5 cm and an external diameter of about 3 mm. For treatment systems influenced by the Manchester

(271) and Anderson (84) treatment techniques, active lengths of 1.3 to 1.5 cm are typical. Radionuclides for intracavitary applications should have a half-life long enough to support a 5- to 10-year working life without large variations in prescription dose rate so that the high cost of these reusable sources can be amortized over a large number of patient treatments. The average photon energy should be at least 60 to 100 keV, as the dose fall-off for lower energy sources (e.g., ^{125}I) is too rapid to adequately treat the target volume periphery (2 to 5 cm from the applicator center) without overtreating the mucosal tissues in contact with the applicator system.

Radium 226 Sources

Radium 226, a naturally occurring radionuclide, was the first radionuclide isolated, intensively investigated, and used in clinical brachytherapy. The unit of activity, the curie (Ci), originally was defined as the rate of disintegration within 1 g of ^{226}Ra. Radium 226 has a complex decay scheme, consisting of a cascade of transformations from one daughter product to another, ending with a stable isotope of lead, $^{206}_{82}$Pb. Radium decays to gaseous ^{222}Rn by means of α decay with a half-life of 1,626 years. Approximately 75 γ-rays are emitted by radium and its decay products, ranging in energy from about 0.05 to 2.4 MeV, give an average energy of about 0.8 MeV. The maximum β-ray energy is about 3.26 MeV. The exposure-weighted average energy of ^{226}Ra is 1.25 MeV when its photon spectrum is filtered by 0.5 mm of platinum. Nearly all ^{226}Ra brachytherapy sources are filtered by at least 0.5 mm Pt, which reduces the surface dose contributed by β-particles to a negligible level.

Radium 226 sources consist of discrete cells of radium salt (radium sulfate plus filler) that are placed in needles or tubes with platinum walls of thickness of 0.5 and 1.0 mm, respectively.

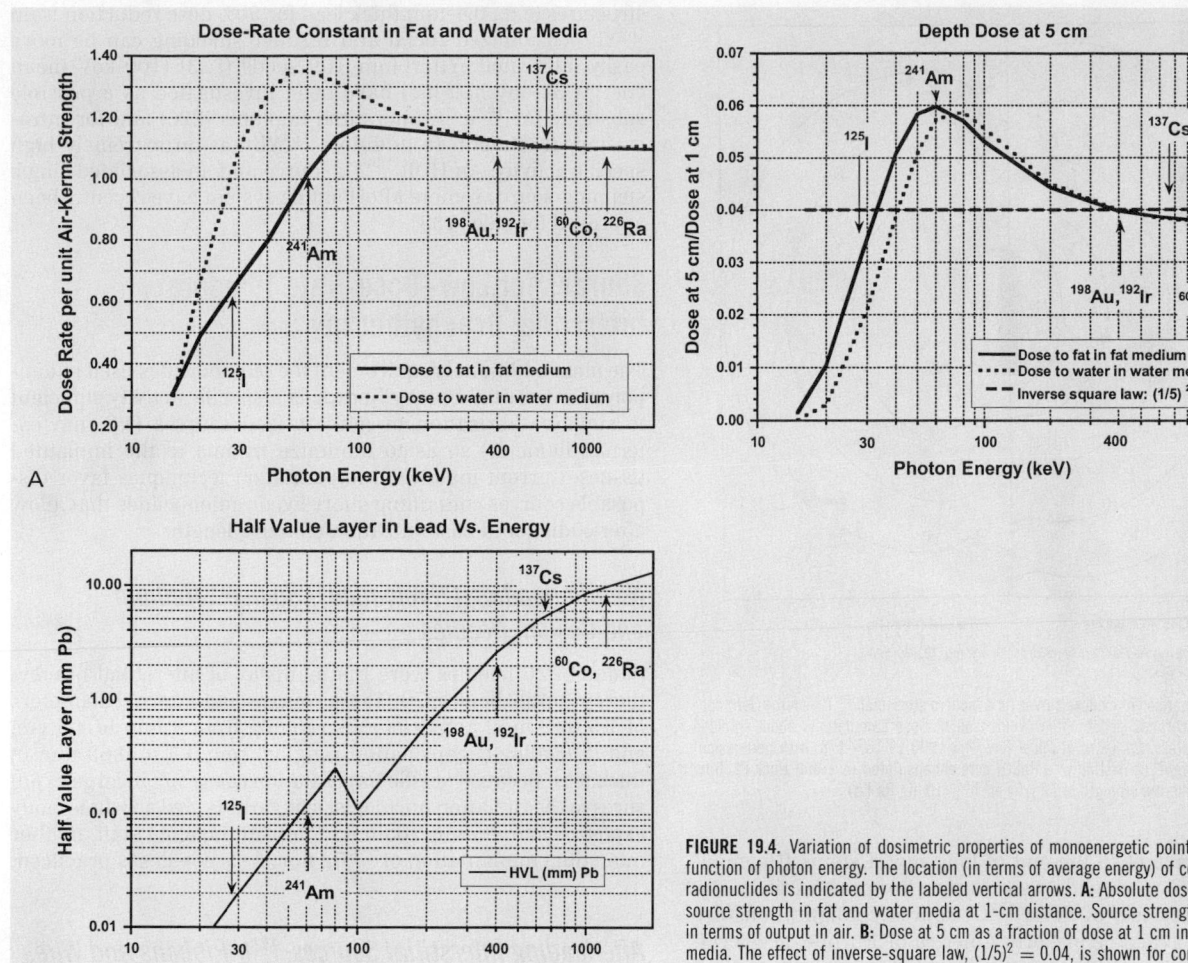

FIGURE 19.4. Variation of dosimetric properties of monoenergetic point sources as a function of photon energy. The location (in terms of average energy) of commonly used radionuclides is indicated by the labeled vertical arrows. **A:** Absolute dose rate per unit source strength in fat and water media at 1-cm distance. Source strength is specified in terms of output in air. **B:** Dose at 5 cm as a fraction of dose at 1 cm in fat and water media. The effect of inverse-square law, $(1/5)^2 = 0.04$, is shown for comparison as a broken line. **C:** Half-value layer in lead, the thickness (mm) in lead required to reduce primary dose by a factor of 2.

Intracavitary radium tubes were usually 22 mm long, contain 5 to 30 mg of radium (S_K = 30 to 200 μGy m$^2 \cdot$h^{-1}), and have active lengths of 15 mm. For interstitial brachytherapy, the full-, half-, and quarter-intensity needles popularized by the Manchester LDR implant system typically contain 0.66 mg, 0.33 mg, or 0.165 mg of radium per centimeter of active length, respectively.

The clinical use of radium has almost disappeared and is now only of historic interest. The potential of damaged sources to leak radioactive salts or emit radon gas (^{222}Rn) is the major reason for its decline, and the exposure hazard to interstitial brachytherapy practitioners (298). Another factor is the high cost of extracting radium from pitchblende ore in comparison with the cost of radium-substitute sources. Finally, the safe disposal of spent ^{226}Ra sources is a significant financial liability. However, because of its many years of therapeutic use, several widely used quantities for source strength specification and prescription of intracavitary treatment are derived from the early experience with ^{226}Ra.

Cesium 137 Sources

Cesium 137, a fission by-product, is a popular radium substitute because of its 30-year half-life. Its single γ-ray (0.66 MeV) is less penetrating (HVL$_{Pb}$ = 0.65 cm) than the γ-rays from radium (HVL$_{Pb}$ = 1.4 cm) or ^{60}Co (HVL$_{Pb}$ = 1.1 cm). Because ^{137}Cs decays to solid barium 137, ^{137}Cs sources have virtually replaced ^{226}Ra intracavitary tubes in LDR gynecological applications.

Cesium 137 brachytherapy sources were introduced in the early 1960s (119,120). Recently marketed sources (e.g., the Amersham model CDCS-J tube and 3M model 6500 intracavitary tube) consist of radioactive cesium distributed within an insoluble glass or ceramic matrix (294), which produces far less radiochemical hazard from ruptured sources than does the radon gas or cesium salts. These sources are encapsulated in stainless-steel sheaths with wall thicknesses of 0.5 to 1.0 mm, active lengths of 13.5 to 15 mm, diameters of 2.6 to 3.1 mm, and total lengths of about 20 mm. Figure 19.5 shows that cesium and radium sources produce nearly identical transverse-axis dose-rate distributions when their active lengths and source strengths are the same. However, the ^{226}Ra tube isodose curves exhibit significant retraction along the longitudinal source axis as a result of oblique filtration of ^{226}Ra γ-rays through the dense ($\rho = 21$ g $\cdot$ cm^{-3}) 1-mm thick platinum capsule. In contrast, lightly filtered ^{137}Cs tubes produce nearly elliptical isodose curves. Consequently, vaginal applicator systems containing modern ^{137}Cs sources with their axes positioned perpendicular to the coronal patient plane (e.g., the Fletcher colpostat) always will give rise to higher bladder and rectal doses than when loaded with ^{226}Ra tubes (291).

Many other ^{137}Cs source designs have been used over the past 20 years including spherical steel-encapsulated ^{137}Cs pellets for the Selectron-composable source-train remote afterloader (97). For preoperative treatment of endometrial cancer (259) or definitive treatment of medically inoperable endometrial cancer, afterloading sources with nominal strengths of 72 μGy m^2 h^{-1}, external diameters of about 1.2 mm, and lengths

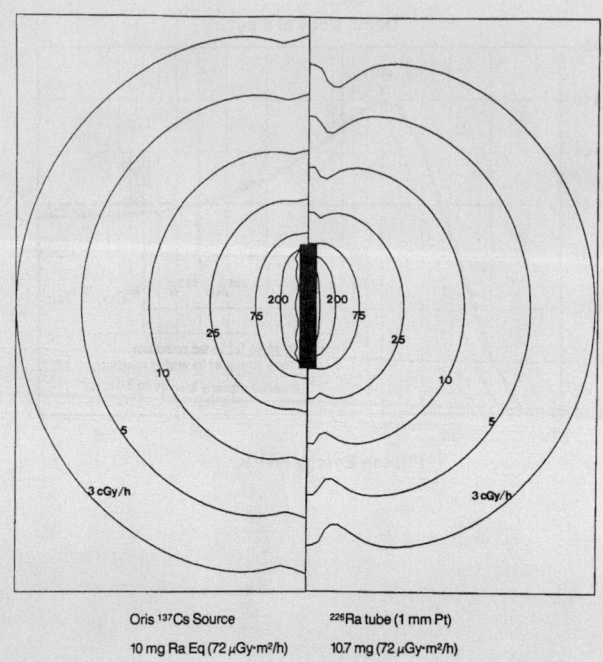

Oris ^{137}Cs Source ^{226}Ra tube (1 mm Pt)

10 mg Ra Eq (72 μGy·m^2/h)   10.7 mg (72 μGy·m^2/h)

FIGURE 19.5. Comparison of isodose curves for a modern steel-clad ^{137}Cs source (*left*) containing radioactive ceramic pellets (from Williamson JF. Dose calculations about shielded gynecological colpostats. *Int J Radiat Oncol Biol Phys* 1990;19:167–178, with permission) and a ^{226}Ra tube (*right*) consisting of a RaSO$_4$ core encapsulated in 1-mm thick Pt. Both sources have an air-kerma strength of 72 μGy m^2 h^{-1} (10 mg Ra Eq).

of 12 mm attached to the end of long metal stems (Heyman-Simon sources) were widely used up to the present time. Unfortunately, very few of these ^{137}Cs source configurations are commercially available in North America or Europe, accelerating the conversion of LDR intracavitary brachytherapy to HDR techniques. As of this writing, only 3M-like intracavitary tubes are being manufactured (70a).

Experimental Intracavitary Brachytherapy Radionuclides

Californium 252 is a unique radionuclide that decays by α-emission with a half-life of 2.65 years and emits neutrons by spontaneous fission with average energies of 2.1 to 2.3 MeV. Depending on the distance from the source, one half to two thirds of the total dose is the result of the neutron component. However, assuming a relative biologic effectiveness (RBE) of six for the neutron component, approximately 90% of the biologically effective dose derives from the neutron component. The radiobiologic rationale for using ^{252}Cf, especially in treating bulky gynecologic malignancies, is that the high linear energy transfer (LET) neutron component more effectively depopulates the tumor's radioresistant hypoxic core, thereby improving local control, while the rapid dose fall-off maintains an acceptable level of late complications (182). Californium 252 sources require more complex radiation protection and source handling procedures to reduce radiation exposure hazards to an acceptable level, due to the high neutron quality factor of 10 to 20 that is assumed by radiation protection standards (286). As of this writing, one group has designed a practical HDR ^{252}Cf source (244).

Ytterbium 169 (223) and Americium 241 (202) are examples of so-called intermediate low-energy photon emitters, giving rise to 60-keV and 100-keV photons, respectively. The emitted photon energy is low enough that relatively thin lead foils can be used to shield personnel and dose-limiting tissues in the patient, but high enough that the resultant dose distributions in tissue remain approximately radium equivalent (297). Since relatively thin lead sheets can be used to shield critical

structures (e.g., 0.4-mm thick lead for 50% dose reduction from ^{169}Yb), customized rectal and bladder shielding can be more easily fabricated. Ytterbium 169 seeds (223) (100-keV mean energy, 32-day half-life) have been investigated as a possible substitute for ^{192}Ir in interstitial implants (226) and for intracavitary treatment. In addition, ^{169}Yb has an extremely high specific activity. An HDR ^{169}Yb source and an associated single stepping-source remote afterloading system have recently been approved for sale (183).

Sources for Low–Dose-Rate Temporary Interstitial Brachytherapy

The main additional requirement for radionuclides used in temporary interstitial brachytherapy is a specific activity sufficient to support fabrication of miniaturized sources (<2 mm external diameter) so as to minimize trauma to the implanted tissues. Current interstitial implantation techniques favor disposable sources containing short-lived radionuclides that allow afterloading and customization of active length.

Nonafterloading ("Preloaded") Sources: Radium and Cesium Needles

Radium 226 needles were the mainstay of interstitial brachytherapy until about 1970. These sources had external diameters of 1.5 to 2 mm, active lengths ranging from 3 mm to 4.5 cm, and Pt-Ir alloy encapsulation ranging from 0.5 to 0.65 mm in thickness. Because needle implantation can result in large exposures to the radiation oncologist's fingers, as well as whole-body exposure to operating room and implant imaging staff, neither interstitial implantation of ^{226}Ra nor ^{137}Cs needles is practiced.

Afterloading Interstitial Sources: ^{192}Ir Ribbons and Wires

Temporary interstitial brachytherapy experienced a renaissance in the 1960s because of the introduction of ^{192}Ir (298). This useful radionuclide is produced by bombarding nonradioactive ^{191}Ir with thermal neutrons in a nuclear reactor, which is available in relatively pure form, has an extremely large neutron-capture cross-section, and produces no significant contaminant radioisotopes. Because of these properties, very high-specific activities can be achieved. Miniaturized interstitial sources can be fabricated relatively cheaply. The use of ^{192}Ir in brachytherapy was pioneered by Ulrich Henschke et al. (112), who developed a family of widely used afterloading techniques, and to Pierquin and Dutreix (228), who developed the ^{192}Ir-based Paris interstitial system in the early 1960s.

Iridium 192 has a 73.8-day half-life and a complex decay scheme, dominated by β decay to ^{192}Pt, but also including some electron capture and $\beta+$ decay. Its photon spectrum includes characteristic x-rays and γ-rays ranging from 63 keV to 1.4 MeV and has an exposure-weighted average energy of 397 keV. Compared with higher energy ^{137}Cs, the thicknesses of lead and concrete shielding can be reduced by 33% and 20%, respectively (208). More important advantages of ^{192}Ir sources are compatibility with afterloading techniques, technical flexibility, and patient comfort.

In the United States, ^{192}Ir is available in the form of seeds, 0.5 mm in diameter and 3 mm long, for LDR brachytherapy (Fig. 19.6). Iridium seeds, encapsulated in a 0.8-mm diameter nylon ribbon and spaced at 1- or 0.5-cm center-to-center intervals, are available in strengths of 1 to 150 μGy · m^2·h^{-1} (0.1 to 20 mg Ra Eq). In Europe ^{192}Ir is used in the form of a wire (0.3-mm or 0.6-mm outer diameter) consisting of an iridium-platinum radioactive core encased in a 0.1-mm sheath of platinum. In addition to eliminating radiation exposure hazards in the operating room, ^{192}Ir ribbons and wires can be trimmed to the

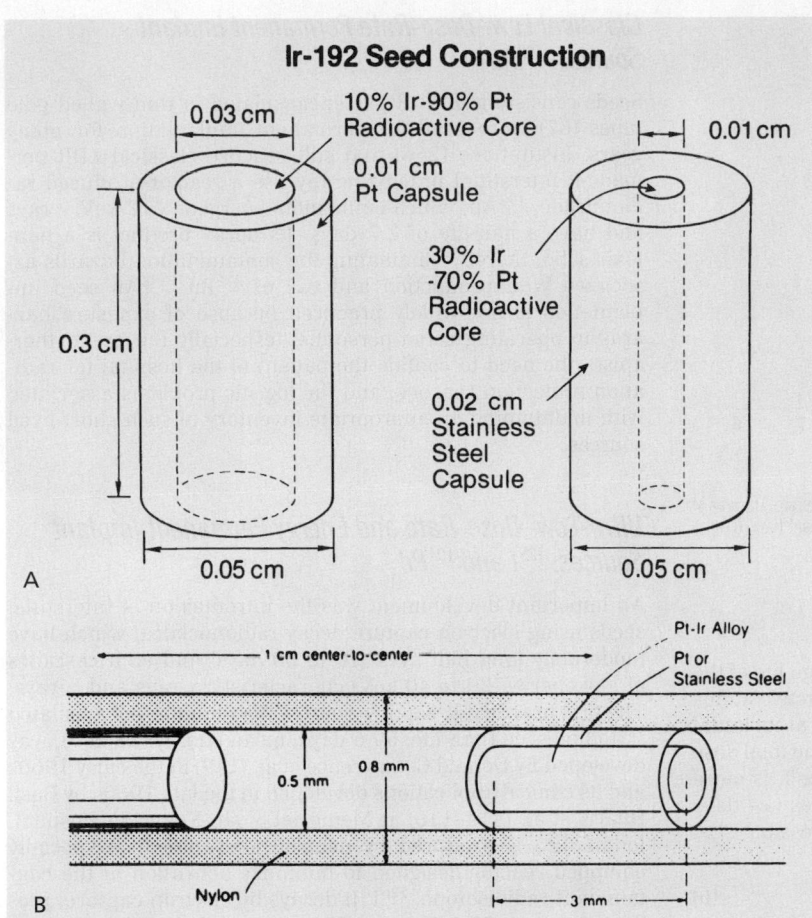

FIGURE 19.6. A: Construction and dimensions (in mm) of the two types of commercially available ^{192}Ir seeds. (From Williamson JF. The accuracy of the line and point dose approximation in Ir-192 dosimetry. *Int J Radiat Oncol Biol Phys* 1986;12:409, with permission.) **B:** The 0.8-mm external diameter nylon carrier or ribbon in which the seeds are "encapsulated." (From Anderson LL, Nath R, Weaver KA, et al. *Interstitial brachytherapy: Physical, biological and clinical considerations.* New York: Raven, 1990, with permission.)

appropriate active length for each catheter. Generally, ^{192}Ir ribbons or wires are used only for one to three patient procedures and then returned to the vendor for disposal.

Low-Energy Sources for Temporary Interstitial Brachytherapy

High-intensity ^{125}I sources (166) have been proposed for temporary interstitial implantation at classical dose rates. High-intensity model 6711 (GE Healthcare Fairfield, CT) or 3631 (North American Scientific, Chatsworth, CA) A/M ^{125}I seeds now are used routinely as temporary interstitial sources for episcleral plaque treatment of intraocular choroidal melanoma (41). By placing a 0.5-mm thick gold shield over the episcleral plaque, tissues posterior to the eye are shielded, and radiation directed toward the tumor is partially collimated (136). A disadvantage of high-intensity ^{125}I seed therapy is its high cost relative to ^{192}Ir seeds.

Sources for Permanent Interstitial Brachytherapy

There are two basic approaches to permanent implantation. Classical LDR permanent brachytherapy originally used [222]Rn seeds, and more recently [198]Au seeds, both of which have half-lives of a few days. To manage the radiation hazard as a result of the high-energy γ-rays emitted by these sources, the patient must be confined to the hospital until the source strength decays to a safe level (two to three half-lives or about 10 days). The contemporary approach to permanent implantation, ULDR brachytherapy, uses longer-lived but low-energy photon emitters (e.g., [103]Pd and ^{125}I). The patient's tissues or a thin lead foil

are sufficient to limit ambient exposure rates to negligible levels, eliminating the need to hospitalize patients solely for radiation protection. During the implant procedure, low-energy photon sources markedly reduce radiation exposure to operating room personnel and to the radiation oncologist's hands.

Mathematics of Radioactive Decay

The phenomenon of exponential decay results in a reciprocal relationship between dose rate achieved and radionuclide half-life. The total activity, A(t), present in the implant after an interval of time (T) has elapsed after source insertion, is given by Figure 19.7:

$$A(t) = A(0) \cdot e^{-\ln 2 \cdot t / T_{1/2}} \tag{3}$$

where A(0) is the activity at the time of insertion, ln2 is the natural logarithm of 2 (equal to 0.693), and $T_{1/2}$ is the half-life of the radionuclide. The quantity $\ln 2 / T_{1/2}$, represented by the symbol λ, is called the decay constant. Equation 3 is applicable to any measure of source strength (S_K, equivalent mass of radium, etc.). Because dose rate, $\dot{D}(t)$ at time t is proportional to activity, that is, $\dot{D}(t) \propto A(t)$, we can write:

$$\dot{D}(t) = \dot{D}(0) \cdot e^{-t \cdot \ln 2 / T_{1/2}} \tag{4}$$

where $\dot{D}(0)$ is the dose rate at the time of source insertion. The total dose, D(T), accumulated over time interval T after source insertion, is the shaded area under the curve of Fig. 19.7 and can be obtained by integrating equation 4:

$$
\begin{aligned}
D(T) &= \dot{D}(0) \cdot \int_0^T e^{-t \cdot \ln 2 / T_{1/2}} \cdot dt \\
&= \dot{D}(0) \cdot T_{1/2} \cdot 1.443 \cdot [1 - e^{-T \cdot 0.693 / T_{1/2}}]
\end{aligned}
\tag{5}
$$

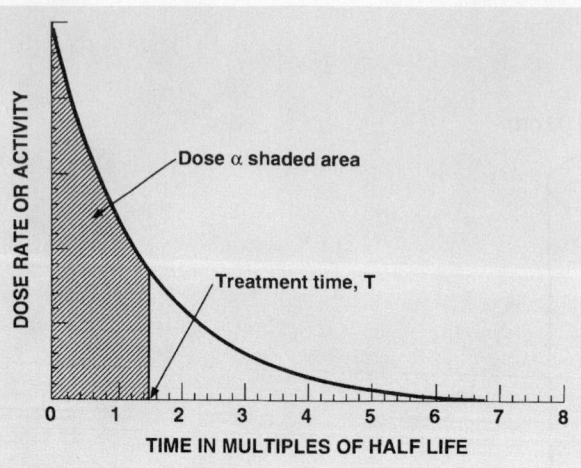

FIGURE 19.7. Illustration of exponential decay of source strength and dose rate. The area of the shaded region is the total dose administered to the patient over treatment time, T.

The product $T_a = 1.443 T_{1/2} \cdot$ is called the average life of the radionuclide and is the time required for all radioactive atoms to decay assuming the rate of decay remains fixed at its initial value, A(0). Equation 5 should be used to calculate the total dose delivered by any implant when the treatment time, T, is more than 5% of the half-life. For shorter treatment times (<4 days for ^{192}Ir or <3 days for ^{125}I), the approximate expression

$$D(T) = \dot{D}(0) \cdot T \qquad (6)$$

is accurate within 2% and may be used.

For permanent implants, the total dose administered to the patient, D_{tot}, resulting from complete decay of the implant can be derived from equation 5:

$$D_{tot} = \lim_{T \to \infty} D(T) = 1.443 \cdot T_{1/2} \cdot \dot{D}(0) = T_a \cdot \dot{D}(0) \qquad (7)$$

This equation demonstrates that initial dose rate and radionuclide half-life are in reciprocal relationship with one another: the longer the half-life, the lower the dose rate will be. Typical total dose rates and total doses are given in Table 19.2 for commonly used permanent implant sources. These sources fall into two categories: short-lived radium-substitute sources with initial dose rates within the classical LDR range and longer lived low-energy sources with dose rates below the classical range (ULDR).

Classical Low–Dose-Rate Permanent Implant Sources: ^{198}Au

Seeds consisting of ^{222}R gas encapsulated in thin-walled gold tubes (67) were used for permanent implantation for many years. Institutions (266) that still practice classical LDR permanent interstitial brachytherapy use a reactor-produced radionuclide, ^{198}Au, which emits monoenergetic 412-keV γ-rays and have a half-life of 2.7 days. Its decay product is a nontoxic solid, thereby eliminating the contamination hazards associated with production and use of ^{222}Rn. ^{198}Au seed implantation is not widely practiced because of exposure hazards to operating room personnel (especially the brachytherapist), the need to confine the patient to the hospital for radiation protection reasons, and the logistic problems associated with maintaining an appropriate inventory of such short-lived sources.

Ultra-Low–Dose-Rate and Energy Permanent Implant Sources: ^{125}I and ^{103}Pd

An important development was the introduction of interstitial seeds using electron-capture decay radionuclides, which have moderately long half lives (10 to 60 days) and emit cascades of low energy (20 to 40 keV) characteristic x-rays and γ-rays. The first practical K-capture source, the titanium-encapsulated ^{125}Iodine seed (half life: 59.6 days, mean energy: 28 keV), was developed by Donald C. Lawrence et al. (149) in the early 1960s and its clinical applications developed in the late 1960s by Basil Hilaris et al. (114–116) at Memorial Sloan-Kettering Hospital. Iodine 125 is produced by neutron activation in a specially equipped reactor designed to minimize activation of the contaminant radioisotope, ^{126}I. It decays by electron capture, producing a single 35-keV γ-ray. The captured K-shell electron produces a cascade of 27-keV to 32-keV characteristic x-rays. In addition, 93% of the γ-rays are internally converted, producing a second characteristic x-ray cascade. Thus, ^{125}I is an "x-ray emitter" because 95% of the useful primary photons are characteristic x-rays of atomic rather than nuclear origin.

Other important radionuclides are ^{103}Pd (^{103}Palladium, 17.0 day half-life and 22 keV mean energy), commercially realized in 1987, and ^{131}Cs (^{131}Cesium, 9.7 day half-life and 29 keV mean energy), which was initially proposed by Henschke and Lawrence (113) but has only recently become available commercially (196). The low-energy photons emitted by these sources (including ^{125}I) dramatically reduce external exposure hazards: an 8-cm thickness of tissue reduces exposure 10-fold. Thin (0.2 mm) lead foils also produce almost complete shielding. Thus, there is usually no need to confine patients to the hospital solely for radiation safety reasons. As a result of the rapidly increasing popularity of transperineal ultrasound (TRUS)-guided permanent implant (19,117) for definitive treatment of low- and intermediate-risk prostate cancer (99,265), approximately 25 different models of ^{125}I and ^{103}Pd sources have been introduced to the market since 1999. (See the American Association of Physicists in Medicine [AAPM] revised TG-43 Report [245] and the Joint AAPM/Radiological Physics Center (RPC) Source Registry (2) for a review of many of the available sources.) Most of these interstitial seeds are encapsulated in thin (0.05-mm to 0.10-mm thick) titanium tubing (see Wang et al. [282] for an exception) with external dimensions of approximately 0.8 by 4.5 mm (Fig. 19.8). The widely used model 6711 seed (167), the only ^{125}I source available from 1983 to 1998, contains a 3-mm-long silver rod on which radioactive iodine is absorbed and is available in strengths of 0.5 to 7 μGy m^2 h^{-1} (0.5 to 5 mCi) (Fig. 19.8A, top). The silver rod is radio opaque, so that the seeds can be visualized on orthogonal or stereoshift radiographs. Figure 19.8A (center) illustrates the more recent I-Seed ^{125}I source (109) product, which consists of radioactive iodine

	Mean Photon Energy	$T_{1/2}$	Typical Prescribed Dose	Initial Dose Rate
Table 19.2	**TOTAL DOSE AND INITIAL DOSE RATES FOR PERMANENTLY IMPLANTED RADIONUCLIDES**			
Radionuclide				
^{222}Rn	1.2 MeV	3.83 days	100 Gy	75 cGy $\cdot$ h^{-1}
^{198}Au	412 keV	2.70 days	100 Gy	107 cGy $\cdot$ h^{-1}
^{131}Cs	29 keV	9.7 days	115 Gy	34.2 cGy $\cdot$ h^{-1}
^{125}I	28 keV	59.6 days	145 Gy	7.0 cGy $\cdot$ h^{-1}
^{103}Pd	22 keV	17 days	125 Gy	21.2 cGy $\cdot$ h^{-1}

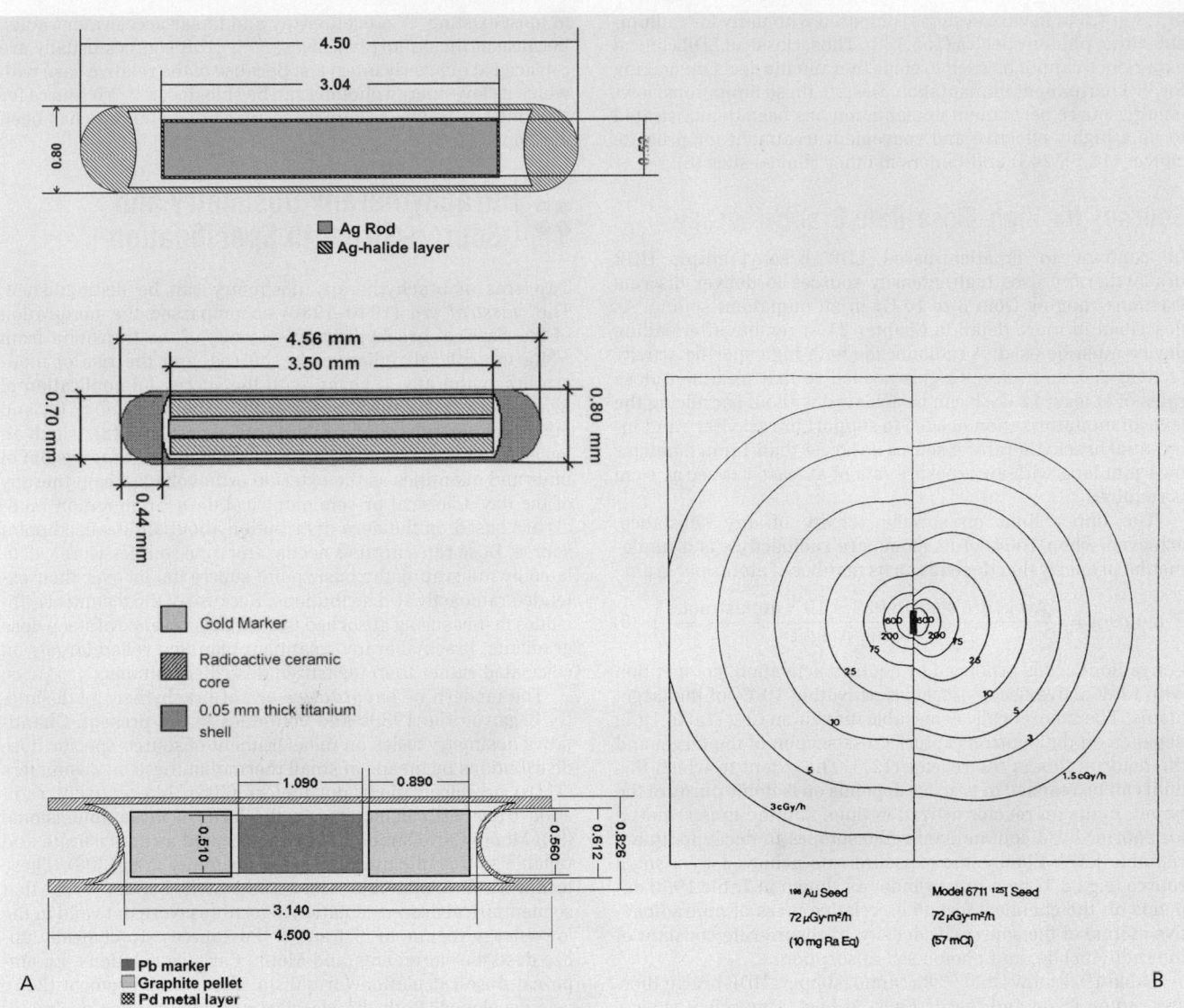

FIGURE 19.8. A: Design characteristics of the GE Healthcare (Fairfield, CT) (formerly [Amersham Health, Princeton, NJ] and 3M [Amersham Health, St. Paul, MN]) Model 6711 ^{125}I seed (*top*), the Theragenics (Theragencies Corporation Buford, GA)(formerly Bebig) I-Seed (formerly Symmetra) Model I25.S06 ^{125}I seed (*center*), and the Theragenics Model 200 [103]Pd seed (*bottom*). (Figures reproduced from Williamson JF, Rivard MJ. Quantitative dosimetry methods for brachytherapy. In: Thomadsen BR, Rivard MJ, Butler WM, eds. *Brachytherapy physics.* 2nd ed. Madison, WI: Medical Physics Publishing, 2005:233–294; Hedtjärn H, Carlsson GA, Williamson JF. Monte Carlo-aided dosimetry of the UroMed/Bebig Symmetra I-125, Model I25.S06 interstitial brachytherapy seed. *Med Phys* 2000;27:1076–1085; Monroe JI, Williamson JF. Monte Carlo-aided dosimetry of the Theragenics TheraSeed® Model 200 [103]Pd interstitial brachytherapy seed. *Med Phys* 2002;29:609–621, with permission.) **B:** Isodose curves for a [198]Au seed (*left half*) and Model 6711 ^{125}I seed (*right half*) both with air-kerma strengths of 72 μGy $\times$ m^2 $\times$ h^{-1} (equivalent to 35 mCi of [198] and 57 mCi of ^{125}I).

distributed in a low density cylindrical annulus that fits over a gold rod used for radiographic localization.

[103]Pd decays by K-electron capture and emits characteristic x-rays of 21 keV. It has all of the radiation protection advantages of ^{125}I along with a significantly shorter half-life of 17 days. With this source, an implant can deliver 112 Gy (90% of prescribed dose) in approximately 8 weeks at an initial peripheral dose rate of 21 cGy/h. The Model 200 seed (Fig. 19.8A) was the only commercially available [103]Pd seed from 1988 to 1999. The radioactive palladium is distributed within a thin Pd metal coating of the two graphite pellets, which are encapsulated in Ti tubing of the same dimensions as ^{125}I seeds. As of July 2006, there are approximately seven different [103]Pd seed models commercially available. The biological rationale for using shorter-lived [103]Pd and [131]Cs interstitial sources is discussed below in the Biology section of this chapter.

Low-energy seed implantation poses a number of challenges. There dose distributions are not radium equivalent (Fig. 19.8B),

falling off more rapidly with distance. Dose estimation is inherently more complex, depending significantly on photon energy and composition of the surrounding medium (Fig. 19.4) (48,55) and are more sensitive to the internal seed geometry (193,308). Because of shifts in calibration standards, large uncertainties in dose measurement, and questionable applicability of classical dose-calculation model, ^{125}I and [103]Pd dosimetry has been uncertain and variable over most of the clinical life of these products (292). Between 1975 and 1999, the ^{125}I dose-rate constant was revised downward, in several steps, by nearly 50% (298). Only with development and validation of more sophisticated experimental and computation dosimetry techniques in the past 10 to 15 years can we claim to know low energy seed dose-rate distributions with an uncertainty of 3% to 7% (245). Because of the low dose rates used, low energy seed implantation is effectively a different therapeutic modality than classical LDR brachytherapy. In addition, 20- to 30-keV photons have a significantly higher LET spectrum, which results in an RBE for ^{125}I of 1.3 to 1.5 in in vitro systems compared with unity for radium-substitute photon spectra (165,178). Thus, classical LDR clinical experience cannot be used to guide therapeutic decision making for ^{125}I permanent implantation. Despite these limitations, low-energy source permanent implantation has been demonstrated to be a highly effective and convenient treatment for prostate cancer (18,98,243) and tumors in other clinical sites (8).

Sources for High–Dose-Rate Brachytherapy

In contrast to inpatient-based LDR brachytherapy, HDR brachytherapy uses high-intensity sources to deliver discrete fractions ranging from 3 to 10 Gy in an outpatient setting. As described in more detail in Chapter 21, a remote afterloading device must be used. A radionuclide with high specific activity (activity per unit mass; Ci/g) is needed so that treatment dose rates of at least 12 Gy/h can be achieved without sacrificing the level of miniaturization needed to support intracavitary and interstitial brachytherapy. A source no larger than 1 mm diameter by 4 mm long with an exposure rate of at least 1 R/sec at 1 cm is required.

The upper limit on specific activity of any substance, achieved when 100% of its atoms are radioactive, is a fundamental property that depends on its number of atoms per gram:

$$\text{atoms/g} = \left(\frac{\text{Avogadro's no. } (6.023 \times 10^{23} \text{ atoms/mole})}{\text{Atomic Weight}} \right) \quad (8)$$

For radionuclides produced by neutron activation, competition with radioactive decay precludes activating 100% of the target atoms. The theoretically achievable maximum Ci/g (Table 19.3) depends on the neutron capture cross-section of the target and the neutron flux in the reactor (127). The extent to which this limit can be reached in practice depends on isotopic purity of the target, limits on reactor activation time, and the time required for shorter-lived contaminant radioisotopes to decay to an acceptable level. Finally, the exposure rate achieved by a small source (e.g., a 1- by 4-mm cylinder as shown in Table 19.3) depends on the chemical form (i.e., relative mass of nonradioactive atoms) of the source, its density, exposure-rate constant of the radionuclide, and photon self-absorption.

Table 19.3 shows that ^{226}Ra cannot support HDR brachytherapy radionuclide and that ^{137}Cs is, at best, a marginal choice. Cobalt 60 (5.26-year half-life and γ-rays of 1.17 and 1.33 MeV) has been widely used as an intracavitary HDR source in the form of small spherical pellets. Based solely on specific activity considerations, ^{192}Ir is the optimal choice for HDR brachytherapy and is the most widely used radionuclide for this application. Sources with external diameters as small as 0.6 mm are now available for use in single-stepping source remote afterloading devices. In contrast to ^{60}Co, the lower energy ^{192}Ir photons are shielded effectively by the scatter and leakage barriers present

in most existing ^{60}Co teletherapy and linear accelerator vaults. Because of their short half-lives, ^{192}Ir HDR sources usually are replaced at quarterly intervals. Because of the relative ease with which its low-energy photons can be shielded, a ^{169}Yb source for HDR intraoperative and intravascular brachytherapy has been developed (183).

Brachytherapy Dosimetry and Source-Strength Specification

Two eras of brachytherapy dosimetry can be distinguished. The *classical era* (1940–1980) encompassed the maturation of the classical brachytherapy systems, of the transition from ^{226}Ra to artificial radionuclide sources, and the rise of modern brachytherapy. It began with the successful application of Bragg-Gray cavity theory (95) to the calibration of ^{226}Ra and other high-energy sources in terms of exposure (148), which allowed brachytherapy to be quantified using the same system of units and quantities as the external orthovoltage-beam therapy of the day. Classical or semiempirical dose-computation models are based on the dose distribution about an idealized point source. Dose rates around needle and tube sources were calculated by integrating the basic point source model over their extended radioactivity distributions. Because of the technical difficulties in measuring absorbed dose in the presence of steep dose gradients, brachytherapy treatment planning relied largely on calculated rather than measured dose distributions.

The modern or *quantitative* era of brachytherapy dosimetry began in the 1980s and continues to the present. Quantitative dosimetry relies on measurement of source-specific dose distributions by means of small thermoluminescent dosimeters (TLDs) or silicon diode dosimeters (308). Alternatively, radiation transport calculations in the form of three-dimensional (3D) Monte Carlo simulations are accepted as an accurate and reliable source of clinically useful dosimetry data (308). These technical developments were motivated by concerns that semiempirical dose-calculation algorithms were not valid in the low-energy regime of ^{125}I and ^{103}Pd sources. To clinically utilize dose measurements and Monte Carlo calculations, an empirical dose-calculation formalism, the TG-43 protocol (245), was developed. Both the classical and quantitative dosimetry methods are based on the principle that brachytherapy source strength should be specified in terms of radiation output in free air.

Source-Strength Specification Quantities and Units

Brachytherapy calibration is an unnecessarily confusing topic because of the many quantities that have been used to specify source strength throughout the history of brachytherapy. Many of the historically obsolete (but still widely used) quantities were defined in terms of ^{226}Ra properties, the only brachytherapy radionuclide intensively studied until about 1940. Obsolete quantities (e.g., apparent activity and equivalent mass of radium [mg Ra Eq]) often obscure the experimental origin of calibration measurements by describing output measurements in activity units. Finally, the brachytherapy literature has added to the lack of conceptual clarity by obscuring the important distinction between quantities and units. A *quantity* is a property of nature that is directly or indirectly measurable (e.g., kerma, equivalent mass of radium, length, time), whereas a *unit* is a selected sample of a quantity to which the magnitude unity (1.0) is assigned (e.g., gray, mg Ra Eq, meter, second). A quantity such as absorbed dose can have many units (e.g., rad, cGy, Gy, J/kg).

Regardless of the units and quantities used to describe calibrations, all photon-emitting sealed brachytherapy sources are

Table 19.3	SPECIFIC ACTIVITIES AND MAXIMUM EXPOSURE RATES ACHIEVABLE FOR DIFFERENT RADIONUCLIDES		
Radionuclide	**Maximum Ci/g Possible**	**Fraction Practicably Achievable (%)**	**Exposure Rate[a] (R/s) at 1 cm From 1 mm × 4 mm Seed**
^{226}Ra	0.98	100	0.04 R · cm^2 · s^{-1}
^{137}Cs	87	23	0.22 R · cm^2 · s^{-1}
^{60}Co	1,020[b]	49	50 R · cm^2 · s^{-1}
^{192}Ir	7,760[b]	35	248 R · cm^2 · s^{-1}
^{169}Yb	33,700[b]	14	51 R · cm^2 · s^{-1}

[a]Neglecting self absorption.
[b]Reactor-produced by neutron activation: a flux $\phi = 10^{14}$ n · cm^{-2} · s^{-1} and 100% target purity are assumed.

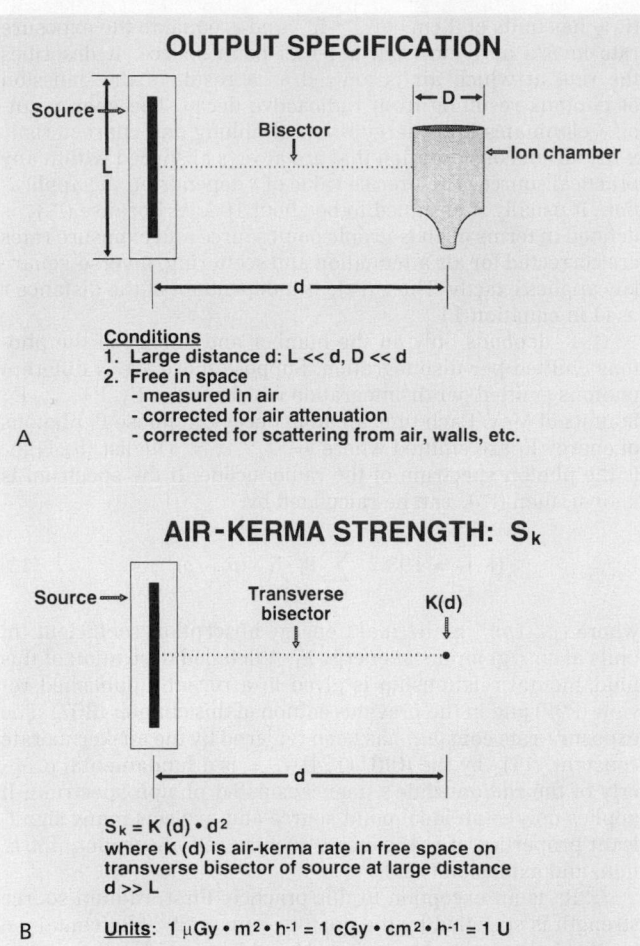

OUTPUT SPECIFICATION

Source

L

Bisector

D

Ion chamber

d

Conditions
1. Large distance d: L << d, D << d
2. Free in space
   - measured in air
   - corrected for air attenuation
   - corrected for scattering from air, walls, etc.

A

AIR-KERMA STRENGTH: S_k

Source →

Transverse bisector

K(d)

d

$S_k = K(d) \cdot d^2$

where K (d) is air-kerma rate in free space on transverse bisector of source at large distance d >> L

B

Units: $1\ \mu Gy \cdot m^2 \cdot h^{-1} = 1\ cGy \cdot cm^2 \cdot h^{-1} = 1\ U$

FIGURE 19.9. A: Illustration of a free-air geometry for measuring brachytherapy source strength in terms of a radiation output quantity such as air-kerma. In practice, the source and cavity chamber are suspended in air in a large room and separated by 20-cm to 100-cm distance (which must be large in relation to the detector and source dimensions). The measured air kerma must be corrected for photon scattering from walls, floor, and ceiling and for photon scattering and attenuation by the intervening air. **B:** Definition of air-kerma strength. For an actual source, the air-kerma rate must be measured at a distance, d, which is large in relation to the source dimensions.

calibrated in terms of output (kerma rate, dose rate, or exposure rate) in air at a specific reference point on the transverse bisector of the source. Much like superficial x-ray beam calibration, a calibrated ion chamber (Fig. 19.9) is used to measure the brachytherapy source output in a free-air geometry in which the source and chamber are suspended in air in a large room.

Air-Kerma Strength

In North America, photon-emitting source strength is specified in terms of air-kerma strength, denoted by S_K, a practice that was introduced by the AAPM in 1987 (199). The AAPM (245) currently defines S_K as the air-kerma rate, $\dot{K}_{\delta,air}$ (d) at distance d, *in vacuo* and due to photons of energy greater than δ, multiplied by the square of this distance, d^2.

$$S_K = \dot{K}_{\delta,air}(d) \cdot d^2 \qquad (9)$$

The distance d is the distance from the source center to the point of air-kerma rate specification (usually but not necessarily the point of measurement), which must be in the transverse plane of the source (the plane normal to the long axis of the source that bisects its radioactivity distribution) where d can be any distance that is large relative to the maximum linear dimen-

sion of the radioactivity distribution so that S_K is independent of its value. $\dot{K}_{\delta,air}$ (d) is usually inferred from transverse-plane air-kerma rate measurements performed in a free-air geometry (see Fig. 19.9) at distances large in relation to the maximum linear dimensions of the detector and source, typically of the order of 1 m. The "in vacuo" qualifier (equivalent in meaning to "in free space") means that $\dot{K}_{\delta,air}$ (d) must be specified as if the source and small mass of air, producing ionization at distance d, were immersed in a vacuum. Air-kerma rate measurements must be corrected for photon attenuation and scattering by the surrounding air as well as for scattering from nearby objects. The energy cutoff, δ, is intended to exclude low-energy or contaminant photons (e.g., characteristic x-rays originating in the outer layers of steel or titanium source cladding (290) that increase $\dot{K}_{\delta,air}$ (d) without contributing significantly to the dose at distances >0.1 cm in tissue. The value of δ is typically 5 keV for low-energy photon-emitting brachytherapy source, and is dependent on the application. The unit of air-kerma strength is $\mu Gy \cdot m^2 \cdot h^{-1}$ and is often denoted in the literature by the symbol "U": where $1\ U = 1\ cGy \cdot cm^2 \cdot h^{-1} = 1\ \mu Gy \cdot m^2 \cdot h^{-1} = 1\ U$.

Air-kerma strength is numerically (but not dimensionally) equal to the quantity reference air-kerma rate, $\dot{K}_{ref}$, a very similar quantity defined by the ICRU (122) and used outside North America. $\dot{K}_{ref}$ is defined as the air-kerma rate in free space at a reference distance, l (taken to be 1 m), on the transverse axis; It has units of $\mu Gy\ h^{-1}$ at 1 m. Thus, $\dot{K}_{ref} = S_K/\ell^2$. The procedures for standardizing and measuring $\dot{K}_{ref}$ and S_K are identical.

The U.S. National Institute of Standards and Technology (NIST) maintains primary S_K standards for commercially available ^{137}Cs sources (171), LDR ^{192}Ir seeds (172), and all ^{103}Pd, ^{131}Cs, and ^{125}I seeds (254). A *primary standard* is an instrument against which all other S_K measurement devices, called secondary or tertiary standards, must be intercompared. Such instruments are designed to permit inference of air-kerma values from the measured charge and instrument design using first principles. For ^{137}Cs and ^{192}Ir sources, the S_K standard is based on transverse-axis air-kerma measurements using spherical ion chambers with carbon walls—the same instruments used to maintain the ^{60}Co teletherapy air-kerma standard. For low energy interstitial seeds, a special free-air chamber (254), called the wide-angle free-air chamber (WAFAC), is used. Brachytherapy sources calibrated directly by the NIST standard or one of the AAPM-Accredited Dosimetry and Calibration Laboratories (ADCL), are said to have *directly NIST-traceable calibrations*. Sources that are calibrated against sources or ion chambers, which themselves have directly traceable NIST calibrations, are said to have *indirectly NIST-traceable* calibrations. A recent review by DeWerd (62) is a more detailed description of air-kerma–based standards, measurement techniques, and traceability requirements. The AAPM recommends (201) that individual clinics using brachytherapy sources maintain instrumentation that is able to make indirectly traceable calibration measurements for verification of vendor-supplied calibrations.

Kerma (kinetic energy released in the medium), K_x, is the ratio $\Delta E_{tr}/\Delta m$, where ΔE_{tr} is the total kinetic energy transferred to charged particles by photon interactions with atoms in small mass, Δm, of medium x (124). For photons, ΔE_{tr} includes the initial kinetic energies of any secondary charged particles (e.g., Compton electrons, photoelectrons, and positrons) liberated by Compton, photoelectric, and pair production interactions. Kerma is defined only for indirectly ionizing radiations (e.g., photons and neutrons) and quantifies the transfer of energy from these radiation fields to matter. It takes the same units (cGy and Gy) as the related quantity absorbed dose. Although kerma can be specified in any medium x, usually air medium (x = air) is assumed for radiation metrology. K_{air} replaces the obsolete quantity exposure and is closely related to absorbed dose, D: the ratio, $\Delta E_{ab}/\Delta m$, where ΔE_{ab} is the energy imparted to Δm by the radiation field. Because the secondary electrons released by photon collisions may travel a significant distance before depositing their energy and may convert some of their kinetic energy to Bremsstrahlung radiation, D_{air} and K_{air} are not necessarily equal. When kerma remains relatively constant over the range of the secondary electrons, a special condition, secondary charged particle equilibrium (CPE), exists (11,127). When the CPE obtains, the rates of energy absorption and energy transfer are approximately equal, so that kerma closely approximates absorbed dose:

$$D_{air} = X \cdot \left(\frac{W}{e}\right) = K_{air} \cdot (1 - g) \qquad (10)$$

where X represents the quantity exposure. The quantity (W/e) is the average energy imparted to air per ion pair created and is a constant, independent of photon energy: $(W/e) = 33.97$ eV/ion pair $= 33.97$ J/C $= 0.876$ cGy/R (20). The factor g is the fraction of kinetic energy transferred to the medium converted back to radiant energy (photons) by the Bremsstrahlung process; g is less than 0.001 at brachytherapy energies and usually is ignored, further simplifying equation 10. Virtually all brachytherapy dose-calculation algorithms and dosimetric analyses assume that CPE obtains and that dose, D, can be well approximated by kerma, K, everywhere. Although generally valid, CPE can be expected to break down in the presence of steep dose gradients near sources (246); Near metal-tissue interfaces (206); And within the active elements of thin, bounded detectors (35).

Activity

To define the obsolete quantities for describing source output, the quantity activity, A, must be introduced. It is defined as the rate of nuclear disintegration or transformation within a radioactive source. The contemporary unit of activity is the becquerel (1 Bq = 1 disintegration/sec). We will freely use the more traditional but obsolete unit, the curie (1 Ci = 3.7×10^{10} disintegrations/s = 3.7×10^{10} Bq). A more convenient multiple of the curie, the millicurie, is defined as 1 mCi = 10^{-3} Ci = 3.7×10^{7} disintegrations/s. Each disintegration represents the spontaneous transformation of an atom from one nuclear state to another. For most brachytherapy radioisotopes, such transformations of nuclear state give rise to photons in the form of unconverted γ-rays, annihilation photons, characteristic x-rays, and Bremsstrahlung photons. Activity is measured by counting the number of photons, β-particles, and so on emitted by an unencapsulated point source of the radionuclide by means of scintillation or proportional counters, from which its activity is inferred (209). For sealed brachytherapy sources, A refers to activity contained inside the sealed source.

Activity, as defined in this strict sense, is no longer used in brachytherapy dosimetry. However, activity continues to serve as the basis for treatment specification and dosimetry of unsealed radiopharmaceuticals used for diagnosis and therapy and may play a future role in dosimetry of sealed β-emitting sources for intravascular brachytherapy and other clinical applications. NIST maintains contained activity standards for a wide variety of radionuclides in aqueous solution (45).

Relationship Between Activity and Exposure Rate

The activity, A, of a radioactive nuclide emitting photons and the exposure rate in free space, $\dot{X}_\delta(r)$, (in R/h) at distance r (in centimeters) due to photons of energy greater than δ are related by a fundamental quantity, the exposure rate constant, $(\Gamma_\delta)_X$, defined as follows (124):

$$(\Gamma_\delta)_X = \frac{\dot{X}_\delta(r) \cdot r^2}{A} \qquad (11)$$

$(\Gamma_\delta)_X$ has units of R cm² mCi⁻¹ h⁻¹ and is equal to the exposure rate in R/h at 1 cm from a 1-mCi point source. It describes the rate at which air is ionized as a result of the emission of photons resulting from radioactive decay. The energy cutoff δ eliminates low-energy Bremsstrahlung and characteristic x-rays from consideration that are always absorbed within any practical source. The precise value of δ depends on the application; It usually is assumed to be about 10 keV. Because $(\Gamma_\delta)_X$ is defined in terms of an isotropic point source and exposure rates are corrected for air attenuation and scattering, inverse-square law applies exactly. Thus, $(\Gamma_\delta)_X$ is independent of the distance r used in equation 11.

$(\Gamma_\delta)_X$ depends only on the number and energy of the photons emitted per disintegration. Suppose there are N different photons emitted per disintegration with energies $E_1, E_2, \ldots, E_N$ in units of MeV. Each time an atom decays, suppose P_i photons of energy E_i are emitted where i = 1, ..., N. The list $\{E_i, P_i\}_{i=1}^{N}$ is the photon spectrum of the radionuclide. If the spectrum is known, then $(\Gamma_\delta)_X$ can be calculated by:

$$(\Gamma_\delta)_X = 193.7 \cdot \sum_{i=1}^{N} P_i \cdot E_i \cdot (\mu_{en}/\rho)_i^{air} \qquad (12)$$

where $(\mu_{en}/\rho)_i^{air}$ is the mass energy absorption coefficient (in units of cm²/g) for air at energy E_i. A detailed derivation of this fundamental relationship is given in a recently published review (297) and in the previous edition of this chapter (307). The exposure-rate constant has been replaced by the air-kerma rate constant, $(\Gamma_\delta)_K$ by the ICRU (124). $(\Gamma_\delta)_X$ is a fundamental property of the radionuclide's unencapsulated photon spectrum; It applies only to an ideal point source and neglects many significant properties of real sources such as self-absorption, filtration, and extension (124).

^{226}Ra is an exception to this practice. First, radium source strength is specified by the quantity—mass of ^{226}Ra contained inside the source—denoted by M_{Ra}. M_{Ra} excludes the nonradioactive core components as well as radioactive decay products. Historically, M_{Ra} was introduced and widely used before the more general activity standards were available. Indeed, the unit curie originally was defined as the number of disintegrations produced by 1 g of ^{226}Ra. M_{Ra} standards were prepared by carefully weighing pure ^{226}Ra samples in an analytical balance. The first M_{Ra} standard was prepared by Marie Curie in 1913 and the currently used NIST standard was prepared by Hönigschmidt in 1934. To calibrate a user's source in M_{Ra}, its radiation output is compared with that of the NIST radium standard by means of an ion chamber. NIST no longer offers an M_{Ra} calibration service. In contrast to the other radionuclides, exposure-rate constant of ^{226}Ra—denoted by the special symbol $(\Gamma_\delta)_{Ra,t}$ in this chapter—is tabulated as a function of its effective capsule thickness, t, in millimeters of platinum. $(\Gamma_\delta)_{Ra,t}$ is normalized to the mass of radium contained in the source and has units of R cm² mg⁻¹ h⁻¹.

Obsolete Quantities for Specifying Source Output

Because of the close association of early brachytherapy with ^{226}Ra, it is not surprising that the measured output of brachytherapy sources continues to be expressed as multiples of the output of a 1-mg radium needle. This quantity, equivalent mass of radium (M_{eq}), was introduced when artificial radioisotopes, such as ^{60}Co and ^{137}Cs, were developed as radium replacements. It allowed old implant and radium needle dosimetry tables, which gave dose per milligram-hour (mg-h) of ^{226}Ra, to be used without modification for these new sources. M_{eq} is that mass of ^{226}Ra filtered by 0.5 mm Pt that has the same S_K as that of the given source. Because M_{eq} is simply a statement of S_K relative to that of a hypothetic radium needle, the given source being quantified need not contain ^{226}Ra, be encapsulated in Pt, nor have a wall thickness of 0.5 mm. Because $K_{air} = X \cdot (W/e)$ and $(\Gamma_\delta)_{Ra,0.5} = 8.25 \, R \cdot cm^2 \cdot mg^{-1} \cdot h^{-1}$ for ^{226}Ra filtered by 0.5 mm Pt[12], S_K and M_{eq} are related by:

$$S_K = M_{eq} \cdot (\Gamma_\delta)_{Ra,0.5} \cdot (W/e) = M_{eq} \cdot 7.223$$

$$M_{eq} = \frac{S_K}{(\Gamma_\delta)_{Ra,0.5} \cdot (W/e)} = \frac{S_K}{7.223} \quad (13)$$

where $(W/e) = 33.97$ eV/ion pair. M_{eq} continues to be widely used to specify strength of intracavitary and interstitial brachytherapy radium-substitute sources such as ^{137}Cs and ^{192}Ir.

Similar to the philosophy of M_{eq}, apparent activity, A_{app}, is a statement of source output relative to that of a hypothetic unfiltered point source. A_{app} is the activity of a hypothetic unfiltered point source that has the same S_K as that of the given source.

$$A_{app} = \frac{S_K}{(\Gamma_\delta)_X \cdot (W/e)} \quad (14)$$

Apparent activity in units of mCi continues to be widely used for specifying strength for permanent interstitial implants (e.g., ^{125}I and ^{103}Pd sources). In contrast to M_{eq}, which is based on the universally accepted $(\Gamma_\delta)_{Ra,0.5}$ value of $8.25 \, R \cdot cm^2 \cdot mCi^{-1} \cdot h^{-1}$ (12), no consensus as to $(\Gamma_\delta)_X$ values for the other radionuclides exists. Often different vendors will assume different $(\Gamma_\delta)_X$ values for the same radionuclide. Thus, A_{app} is an inherently ambiguous means of describing source strength. In an effort to reduce low-energy dose-calculation errors associated with this ambiguity, the AAPM recently recommended (303) that the $(\Gamma_\delta)_X$ values of 1.476 and 1.45 $R \cdot cm^2 \cdot mCi^{-1} \cdot h^{-1}$ for ^{103}Pd and ^{125}I sources, respectively, be used universally for specification of A_{app}. Nearly all scientific societies involved in brachytherapy (34,201,299) including the ICRU (122) recommend that M_{eq} and A_{app} be abandoned in favor of S_K for source ordering, dose calculation, and implant prescription.

Milligram-Hours and Integrated Reference Air-Kerma

In gynecologic intracavitary therapy, the quantities M_{Ra} and M_{eq} are used both to describe source loadings and to prescribe individual treatments. For prescribing therapy, these quantities, in units of milligrams of ^{226}Ra (or mg Ra Eq) are integrated over treatment time yielding the so-called quantities mg-h and mg Ra Eq-h. As the product of total source strength and treatment time, mg-h and mg Ra Eq-h represent the total exposure or air-kerma accumulated at a distance of 1 m from the implant, under the assumptions that the implant is a point source and that tissue attenuation is negligible. Both the ICRU (122) and the American Endocurietherapy Society (AES, now known as American Brady Therapy Society; 299) recommend that mg-h be abandoned as a prescription or reporting quantity in favor of quantities defined in terms of air-kerma. The AES has proposed the quantity integrated reference air-kerma (IRAK), K_{ref}:

$$K_{ref} = \sum_{i=1}^{N} S_{K,i} \cdot t_i \quad (15)$$

where $S_{K,i}$ and t_i are the air-kerma strength and treatment time in hours, respectively, of the i-th source. Thus, 1 unit of IRAK = $1 \, cGy \, cm^2 = 1 \, \mu Gy \, m^2 = 1$ U-h. A numerically identical quantity, total reference air-kerma (TRAK), with units of μGy at 1 m, has been recommended by the ICRU (122). IRAK and TRAK are related to mg-h and mg Ra Eq-h:

$$K_{ref} = \begin{cases} mg\text{-}h \cdot 6.754 & \text{for filtration } t = 1 \, mm \, Pt \\ mgRaEq\text{-}h \cdot 7.227 & \text{for filtration } t = 0.5 \, mm \, Pt \end{cases} \quad (16)$$

Intracavitary treatment systems (84) historically based on ^{226}Ra tubes (1 mm Pt encapsulation) typically use mg-h, whereas systems based on ^{137}Cs or other radium substitutes prescribe therapy in units of mg Ra Eq-h. Because of the difference in platinum filtration assumed by these two milligram-based quantities, numerically identical prescriptions can deliver quantities of IRAK that differ by 7%. Use of IRAK as an integrated output reporting quantity eliminates this 7% ambiguity that has confused comparison of different implant systems since the appearance of radium-substitute sources for brachytherapy.

Classical Dose-Calculation Formalism: Isotropic Point Source

Consider an unencapsulated point source with an air-kerma strength of S_K, illustrated in Fig. 19.10. Because this source has no extension, there is no attenuation of the emitted radiation by the source itself. Isotropy (Fig. 19.2) implies that photons are emitted with equal likelihood in all directions and travel in straight lines. In contrast, actual brachytherapy sources are encapsulated, have finite dimensions, and usually are cylindrically rather than spherically symmetric. The dose rate, $\dot{D}(r) \, (cGy/h)$, at distance r (cm) in the water-equivalent medium surrounding the source is given by:

$$\dot{D}_{med}(r) = S_K \cdot \frac{\overline{\left(\mu_{en}/\rho\right)_{air}^{med}}}{r^2} \cdot T(r) \quad (17)$$

The inverse-square law term corrects for the difference in dose-specification distance, r, and the 1-cm reference point assumed by the units of air-kerma strength. The quantity $\overline{\left(\mu_{en}/\rho\right)_{air}^{med}}$ is the ratio of mass-energy absorption coefficients in medium compared to that in air averaged over the photon spectrum in free space. This correction, equal to $\dot{K}_{med}/\dot{K}_{air}$ in free space, is a consequence of the fundamental relationship between particle fluence and dose (297,307). It corrects for the efficiency with which the medium extracts energy from the emitted photons compared with air. For all radionuclides emitting photons with energies >200 keV, including all radium substitutes, $\overline{\left(\mu_{en}/\rho\right)_{air}^{med}}$ has the value 1.11 in water medium.

The last term of equation 17—the kerma-to-dose conversion factor, T(r)—describes the net influence of primary photon

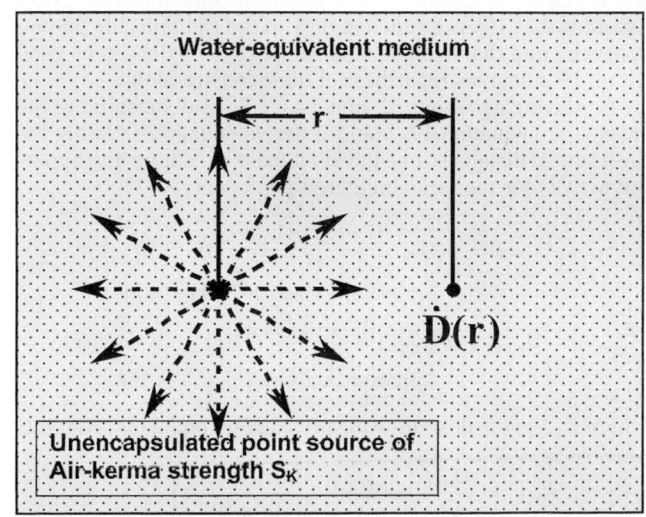

FIGURE 19.10. Unencapsulated point source of strength S_K immersed in an unbounded water-equivalent medium.

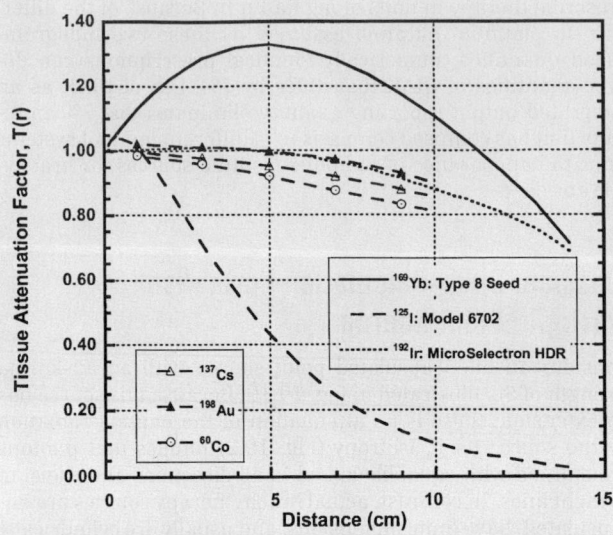

FIGURE 19.11. Photon attenuation and scatter factors, T(r), for a number of brachytherapy radionuclides. The left panel shows T(r) for a number of radium-equivalent radionuclides, as presented in the classic paper of Meisberger et al. The right panel shows T(r) for several low-energy radionuclides. Meisberger et al. fit their data to a third-degree polynomial $T(r) = A + B \cdot r + C \cdot r^2 + D \cdot r^3$, which is widely used to represent T(r) in modern treatment planning systems. (From Meisberger LL, Keller RJ, Shalek RJ. The effective attenuation in water of the δ-rays of gold-198, iridium-192, cesium-137, radium-226, and cobalt-60. *Radiology* 1968;90:953, with permission.)

attenuation and buildup of scattered photons in the surrounding medium. Sometimes this factor is termed the effective attenuation factor or the scatter-buildup factor.

$$
\begin{aligned}
T(r) &= \frac{\text{Dose in medium}}{\text{Medium} - \text{kerma in free space}} \\
&= \left.\frac{\text{Exposure in medium}}{\text{Exposure in air}}\right\} \begin{array}{l}\text{at distance r} \\ \text{from a point source}\end{array}
\end{aligned}
\tag{18}
$$

Figure 19.11 shows T(r) for several radium-substitute radionuclides as well as for a few low-energy radionuclides. For ^{226}Ra-equivalent radionuclides, T(r) deviates <5% from unity (1.00) out to distances, r, of 5 cm. Numerous tabulations of T(r) are available in the literature; Those of Meisberger et al. (186), Berger (15), and Van Kleffens and Star (275) are among the best known. Most of these data are derived from theoretic photon transport calculations. The classical semiempirical model assumes that T(r) is a function only of the radionuclide photon spectrum and that a single data set (e.g., for ^{192}Ir) can be used for all ^{192}Ir sources regardless of their construction.

By solving equations 13 and 14 for S_K and substituting the results into equation 17, one can derive equations relating the dose rate at distance r to equivalent mass of radium and apparent activity for the same unfiltered point source:

$$
\begin{aligned}
\dot{D}_{med}(r) &= M_{eq} \cdot \frac{(\Gamma_\delta)_{Ra,0.5} \cdot f_{med}}{r^2} \cdot T(r) \\
&\qquad \text{Equivalent Mass of } ^{226}\text{Ra} \qquad \text{(a)}
\end{aligned}
\tag{19}
$$

$$
\begin{aligned}
\dot{D}_{med}(r) &= A_{app} \cdot \frac{(\Gamma_\delta)_X \cdot f_{med}}{r^2} \cdot T(r) \\
&\qquad \text{Apparent Activity} \qquad \text{(b)}
\end{aligned}
$$

where f_{med} is the dose-to-exposure conversion factor given by:

$$
\begin{aligned}
f_{med} &= \frac{D_{med}}{X} = (W/e) \cdot \overline{\left[\frac{(\mu_{en}/\rho)^{med}}{(\mu_{en}/\rho)^{air}}\right]} \\
&= 0.876 \frac{cGy}{R} \cdot \overline{(\mu_{en}/\rho)^{med}_{air}} \Big\} \text{ in free space}
\end{aligned}
\tag{20}
$$

For all ^{226}Ra substitutes (radionuclides with photon energies of more than 200 keV), f_{med} has the value 0.974 cGy R^{-1} for water and 0.966 cGy $\cdot$ R^{-1} for muscle medium (127).

Equations 17 and 19 give the dose rate, $\dot{D}_{med}(r)$, for a point source surrounded by an arbitrary medium that has been specified in terms of equivalent mass of radium, apparent activity, and S_K. Assuming that the same exposure rate constants, $(\Gamma_\delta)_{Ra,0.5}$ and $(\Gamma_\delta)_X$, were used to evaluate absorbed dose as were used to convert the measured air-kerma strength to M_{eq} and A_{app} via equations 13 and 14, all three equations should give numerically identical dose rates. This demonstrates that Γ_δ is, in fact, a "dummy" constant that plays no physical role in the dosimetry of output-calibrated sealed sources because any arbitrary, but consistently used, value will yield identical dose-rate distributions. These unit conversions may not be performed by the same individual. For example, the vendor calibrates ^{125}I sources by intercomparing them with the NIST S_K standards. The vendor calculates A_{app} from the measured S_K by equation 14 using an assumed $(\Gamma_\delta)_X$ value and records the result on the source's calibration certificate. The hospital physicist, in calculating dose rates by equation 19, also must use an assumed $(\Gamma_\delta)_X$ value. If the physicist fails to use the same value as the vendor, significant dose-calculation errors may result. Use of S_K for clinical source-strength specification eliminates these dummy constants, thereby eliminating errors resulting from inconsistent conventional choices.

Modeling of Source Anisotropy: The Anisotropy Factor

Despite its simplicity, the classical isotropic point-source model, equation 17, accurately predicts the transverse-axis dose-rate distributions of most actual radium-substitute sources. Simply by using an output quantity to calibrate the source, rather than contained activity, A, the influence of its internal structure (filtration and self-absorption) has been implicitly accounted for. Had true activity, A, instead of A_{app} been used in equation 19 (b), then the expression for $(\Gamma_\delta)_X$ (Eq. 12) would require correction for attenuation and scattering in the radioactive core and surrounding encapsulation. Any uncertainties in $\{E_i, P_i\}_{i=1}^N$ (which are large for many radionuclides) and filtration corrections would directly degrade dose-calculation accuracy. In addition, fundamental activity measurements are technically difficult for the high-intensity sources used in brachytherapy. For this reason, contained activity does not play a role in photon brachytherapy dosimetry. In contrast, equation 17 infers dose rate from a quantity measured outside the source, which is not influenced significantly by knowledge of the unfiltered photon spectrum. The required quantities, $\overline{(\mu_{en}/\rho)}^{med}_{air}$ and T(r), are ratios and are therefore insensitive to errors in the assumed spectrum.

Practically all brachytherapy sources are cylindrical, giving rise to anisotropic dose distributions. In addition, some sources, especially those used in intracavitary brachytherapy, have active lengths that are comparable to typical calculation distances. Thus the dose rate, $\dot{D}(r,\theta)$, around a brachytherapy source depends both on distance r, and polar angle, θ (Fig. 19.8B). $\dot{D}(r,\theta)$ may deviate significantly from the transverse-axis dose rate, $\dot{D}(r,\pi/2)$, predicted by equation 17, especially near the long axis of the seed.

In the case of implants consisting of many randomly oriented seeds with active lengths less than the minimum distance of interest, equation 17 will accurately represent the multiple-seed dose distribution if an average correction for single-seed dose anisotropy is applied (288). This correction factor, called the anisotropy factor, $\phi_{an}(r)$, is defined by averaging the dose at each fixed distance r with respect to solid angle, Ω:

$$\phi_{an}(r) = \frac{\text{Average dose at r}}{\text{Transverse–axis dose at r}}$$

$$= \frac{\int_{4\pi} \dot{D}(r,\theta) \cdot d\Omega}{4\pi \dot{D}(r,\pi/2)} \qquad (21)$$

$$= \frac{\int_0^\pi \dot{D}(r,\theta) \cdot \sin\theta \cdot d\theta}{2 \cdot \dot{D}(r,\pi/2)}$$

Often a distance-independent average value of $\phi_{an}(r)$, called the anisotropy constant, $\overline{\phi}_{an}$, is used. Incorporating this average correction into equation 17, leads to:

$$\dot{D}_{med}(r) = \frac{S_K \cdot \overline{(\mu_{en}/\rho)}_{air}^{med}}{r^2} \cdot T(r) \cdot \overline{\phi}_{an} \qquad (22)$$

For radium-substitute sources, $\overline{\phi}_{an}$ was often evaluated by measuring relative photon fluence in air at relatively large distances (30 to 100 cm) using a NaI or GeLi scintillation detector (163,167).

Equation 22 implies that source strength should be increased by a constant fraction ranging from 2% (^{192}Ir seeds) to 10% ([103]Pd seeds) to correct for polar anisotropy effects. Lindsay et al. (162) compared prostate implant 3D dose distributions derived from the isotropic point-source model, $\dot{D}(r)$, to those derived from the full 2D single-source dose-calculation model, $\dot{D}(r,\theta)$. Based on voxel-by-voxel comparisons, they found that the isotropic point-source model introduced errors exceeding 10% of the D_{90} (see section on dose specification) in 8% and 33% of the target volume for the model 6711 ^{125}I and model 200 [103]Pd sources. Corbett et al. (44) found that despite local large local dose-distribution differences, including 2D anisotropy effects did not alter the dose-volume histogram (DVH): neither the V_{100} nor the margin between D_{100} and prostate boundary was altered significantly. For volume implants consisting of parallel arrays of ^{192}Ir seeds, a similar finding has been reported (288).

Dose Calculation for Extended Sources: The Sievert Integral Model

Dose distributions around larger sources, such as intracavitary tubes and interstitial needles, are calculated by partitioning the extended source into a set of point sources to which corrections for distance, oblique filtration, attenuation, and scattering are applied separately. By summing these point-source contributions, the dose at point P can be estimated. This class of algorithms, first described by Rolf Sievert in 1921 (258), is known as the Sievert integral algorithm, or more generally, the 1-D pathlength model (293,297).

Assume that the source illustrated in Figure 19.12 has an air-kerma strength, S_K, and contained activity, A. The classical Sievert model approximates the cylindrical active core by a line of radioactivity positioned along its axis. The axial length of the core is called the active length, L. Oblique filtration is modeled by assuming that the capsule reduces dose by exponential attenuation using an effective filtration coefficient, μ'. The dose rate $\Delta\dot{D}(x, y)$ at point (x, y) from the incremental source ΔL located at angle θ is

$$\Delta\dot{D}(x,y) = A \cdot \frac{\Delta L}{L} \cdot \frac{(\Gamma_\delta)_X \cdot f_{med}}{(x/\cos\theta)^2} \cdot T(x/\cos\theta) \cdot e^{-\mu' \cdot t/\cos\theta} \qquad (23)$$

where $(\Gamma_\delta)_X$ is the exposure rate constant of the unfiltered source material. Because $S_K = A \cdot (W/e) \cdot (\Gamma_\delta)_X \cdot e^{-\mu' t}$, equation 23 becomes:

$$\Delta\dot{D}(x,y) = S_K \cdot \frac{\Delta L}{L} \cdot e^{\mu' \cdot t} \cdot \frac{\overline{(\mu_{en}/\rho)}_{air}^{med}}{(x/\cos\theta)^2} \cdot T(x/\cos\theta) \cdot e^{-\mu' \cdot t/\cos\theta} \qquad (24)$$

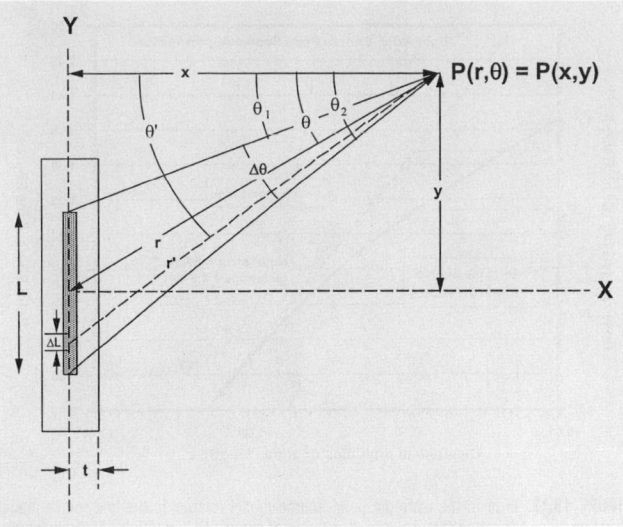

FIGURE 19.12. A typical encapsulated line source, illustrating calculation of dose rate at point P at (x,y) relative to the source center by the Sievert integral method. The active length and radial encapsulation thickness are denoted by L and t, respectively. The distances x and y are referred to as "distance away" and "distance along," respectively, in the literature.

By summing over all these incremental sources (i.e., integrating with respect to θ') and transforming to polar coordinates, we obtain the Sievert integral:

$$\dot{D}(r,\theta) = \frac{S_K \cdot \overline{(\mu_{en}/\rho)}_{air}^{med} \cdot e^{\mu' \cdot t}}{L \cdot r \cdot \cos\theta} \cdot \int_{\theta_1}^{\theta_2} e^{-\mu' t \cdot \sec\theta} \cdot T(x \cdot \sec\theta) \cdot d\theta \qquad (25)$$

The extra $e^{\mu' t}$ term outside the integral is needed to avoid global "double correction" for filtration.

Variants of equation 25 applicable to the regions near the source capsule ends are available. Numerous improvements to the basic model have been introduced over the years (94,255), including modeling of photon absorption by the source core, extension to noncylindrical sources, generalization to radioactivity distributed over a volume (294), extension to low energy sources (293), and treatment of applicator shielding and attenuation (274,284).

The Sievert algorithm is widely used to model 2D dose distributions around ^{137}Cs tubes and needles for clinical treatment planning. Both experimental (65,135) and Monte Carlo studies (289,294) have demonstrated that the Sievert model accurately predicts dose-rate distributions in this energy range. When the filtration coefficient μ' is approximated (17) by the linear energy absorption coefficient, μ_{en} (0.023 mm^{-1} for steel-clad ^{137}Cs sources), maximum errors are no larger than 5% to 8% and are much smaller (<3%) near the transverse axis. Published dose-rate distributions derived from the Sievert model, tabulated in terms of distances away and along, are available for several types of ^{137}Cs sources (289,294) and [226]Ra sources (262). Williamson (293) showed that the classical Sievert integral gives rise to large errors (20% to 37% maximum error, 7% to 16% average error) when applied to lower energy sources of ^{192}Ir, [169]Yb, and [125]I. Although accuracy can be improved by modifying the basic model (293), classical semiempirical models should be used cautiously at photon energies below [137]Cs. Tabulated dose-rate distributions derived from direct measurement or Monte Carlo simulation are preferable for these sources.

If the encapsulation thickness is set to zero (t = 0) in equation 25, the Sievert integral reduces to a simple closed-form analytic expression:

$$\dot{D}(x,y) = S_K \cdot \overline{(\mu_{en}/\rho)}_{air}^{med} \cdot \frac{\Delta\theta}{L \cdot x} \qquad (26)$$

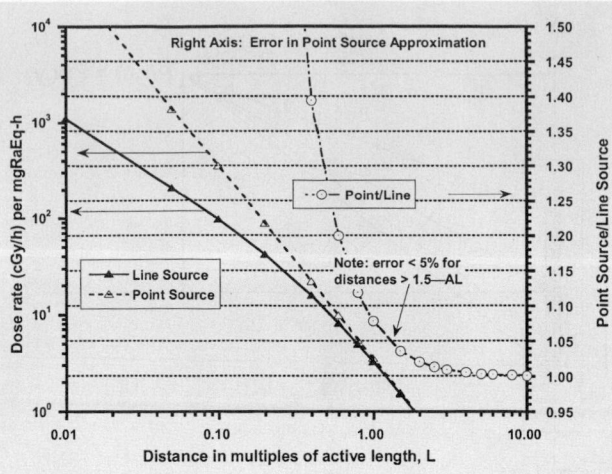

FIGURE 19.13. Error in the isotropic point source-model relative to the line source model equation 26 as a function of transverse-axis distance expressed in multiples of active length.

where $\Delta\theta$ is the angle, in radians, subtended by the active length, L, with respect to the point of interest (Fig. 19.12). When the interest point lies on the transverse axis (y = 0), then $\Delta\theta = 2 \cdot \tan^{-1}(L/2x)$, where $\tan^{-1}$ denotes the inverse tangent or arctan function. Angles must be specified in units of radians rather than degrees (180 degrees = π radians). This approximation is extremely useful as a manual calculation aid and is highly accurate near the transverse axis of lightly encapsulated ^{137}Cs sources.

Figure 19.13 shows that as the distance $r = \sqrt{(x^2 + y^2)}$ becomes large in relation to active length, L, equation 26 reduces to the point-source formula. For distances less than L (1.5 cm for intracavitary tubes), use of equation 17 will yield errors of at least 10%. For distances >1.5 L (2 to 2.5 cm for gynecologic tubes), the point-source approximation is accurate within 5%.

Modern Quantitative Dosimetry

In contrast to classical dose-calculation models, which assume that the parameters T(r) and $\overline{(\mu_{en}/\rho)}_{air}^{wat}$ depend only on the radionuclide used, quantitative dosimetry methods assume that dosimetry parameters are source-geometry specific and should be measured or calculated specifically for each type of source. Classical approaches to brachytherapy dosimetry began to break down with the introduction of ^{125}I interstitial seeds in the early 1970s, as this 30 keV x-ray emitter clearly fell outside the scope of validated analytic models (298). Although ^{125}I dose distributions derived from semiempirical models were published (138) and widely used, it was recognized (167) that internal seed structure could modulate the emitted photon spectrum and significantly alter the absorbed dose distribution. The growing use of ^{125}I and the introduction of a primary exposure standard in 1985 (173) motivated investigation of more quantitative dosimetry methods. Appendix C of the original TG-43 report gives a more detailed discussion of early ^{125}I dosimetry (200). Currently, both experimental methods and sophisticated computational dosimetry approaches are routinely used to derive such source-specific parameters. Both the classical and quantitative dosimetry approaches are based on the NIST air-kerma strength standards.

Experimental Brachytherapy Dosimetry

Clinical acceptance of measured dose rates in brachytherapy is a relatively recent phenomenon, beginning in the mid-1980s.

Historically, this is due not only to the difficulties and labor-intensity attending such measurements, but to a consensus that dose measurement was so difficult and intrinsically inaccurate that even simplistic theoretic models were more reliable. Brachytherapy dose measurement does indeed place severe demands on detectors because the dose distributions are characterized by large dose gradients, a large range of dose rates, and relatively low photon energies. The most severe measurement artifact is the exquisite sensitivity of detector response to positioning errors; Measurement of dose near a point source with 2% accuracy requires that the source-to-detector distance be specified with accuracy of 20, 50, 100, and 200 μm, respectively, at distances of 2, 5, 10, and 20 mm.

Commonly used dose detectors include thermolumiscent detectors (TLD), small ion chambers, diode detectors, and silver-halide radiographic film. Radiochromic film (61,192,213) and plastic scintillator detectors (14,224) show promise as planar dose measurement systems. Three-dimensional dose measurement technologies under investigation include liquid scintillation cocktails (133) with dose distributions reconstructed by optical emission tomography and polymer gel dosimetry (57,79) using magnetic resonance imaging (MRI) to quantify the detector signal. One consideration in selecting a detector for brachytherapy dosimetry is minimizing energy-response artifacts, which arise from compositional differences between water and the detector and can result in variation of detector reading/unit dose in medium as the photon spectrum changes with position. Silicon diodes are useful detectors for measuring relative dose distributions around ultralow-energy sources (e.g., ^{103}Pd and ^{125}I) because diode sensitivity is nearly independent of measurement point location (42,160) but are not recommended for higher energy brachytherapy sources, as variations in sensitivity with position in the phantom as large as 15% for ^{137}Cs and 75% for ^{192}Ir have been reported (306).

Among the established dosimetric techniques, LiF TLD dosimetry is considered to offer the best compromise between sensitivity, small size, and freedom from energy-response artifacts (8,308) and is currently considered to be standard of practice (245). The acceptance of TLD dosimetry owes much to a 3-year (1987–1989) multi-institutional contract to perform a definitive review of low-energy seed dosimetry that was funded by the National Cancer Institute. The three institutions, collectively called the Interstitial Collaborative Working Group (ICWG), consisted of Memorial Sloan-Kettering, Yale, and UCSF led by principal investigators Lowell Anderson, Ravinder Nath, and Keith Weaver, respectively (8). Using TLD-100 thermoluminescent chips and powder capsules, embedded in machined solid-water phantoms, the ICWG developed procedures, including TLD dose calibration and energy-response correction, for making quantitative estimates of absolute dose rates in water. Each of the three ICWG investigator groups independently measured transverse-axis dose distributions for the ^{125}I and ^{192}Ir then available to validate their TLD measurement methodology (8). This was followed by more complete 2D dose distributions about ^{125}I, ^{192}Ir, and ^{103}Pd brachytherapy sources then available (40,42,204). The results showed good agreement among the different measurements and overall substantial differences between measured and classically computed dose rates for ^{125}I seeds [when normalized to the air-kerma strength standard (173), $S_{K,N85}$, then available], but good agreement between the classical and experimental approaches for ^{192}Ir. With careful correction for TLD linearity, perturbation of the photon field by the detectors, and relative energy response, absolute dose rate (cGy/h in tissue per unit S_K) can be measured with a total uncertainty of 7% to 9% in the 1 to 5 cm distance range (245,308).

Measured dose-rate distributions using TLD detectors are available for many common brachytherapy sources, including nearly all commercially available ^{125}I and ^{103}Pd sources (see the revised TG-43 Report [245] and a recent review article [308] for more comprehensive discussions); Many LDR ^{192}Ir sources for LDR, HDR, and pulsed–dose-rate (PDR) sources; As well as for many investigational sources (308). For radium-substitute sources, the measurements are in close agreement with the classical semiempirical models: isotropic point source and Sievert integral models (293,294,297). For ^{125}I sources normalized to the 1984 Loftus (173) S_K standard, measured dose rates were found to be 10% to 20% lower than those predicted by equation 17 (245,292). Better agreement (300) is observed between classical models and measurements when calibrations are traceable to the 1999 WAFAC standard ($S_{K,N99}$) (254). However, classical models such as the Sievert integral are not recommended for the low energy source regime as they poorly predict low-energy anisotropy (293) and do not take into account modulation of the dose distribution by internal source geometry.

Computational Dosimetry Methods: Monte Carlo Photon Transport Simulation

Concurrently with the development of TLD dosimetry in the 1990s, other investigators used Monte Carlo photon-transport techniques as tools for quantitative evaluation of single-source dose distributions. Based on an accurate and detailed mathematical model of the internal structure of the source, photon histories can be generated and then evaluated to assess absorbed dose. Monte Carlo techniques are now accepted as a reliable and probably the most accurate source of brachytherapy dosimetry data (245,308). As illustrated in Figure 19.14, this theoretical method uses a digital computer to randomly select a small number (10^5 to 10^7) of photon trajectories or

"histories." A geometric model indicating the location of all media boundaries and photon sources must be available. By using probability distributions derived from total and differential cross-sections, a photon is randomly constructed by following each photon from birth history through successive scattering events and, eventually, to absorption or escape from the system. At each decision point, random sampling is used to decide the fate of the photon. The process of randomly constructing photon trajectories is equivalent to selecting photon histories from the set of all those possible. To statistically estimate the dose rate at a specified point, the dose contributed by each simulated collision is estimated and then averaged over all collisions. Monte Carlo simulation techniques are reviewed in more detail elsewhere (276,308). Because particle histories can be accurately and efficiently constructed even in the presence of complex 3D geometries, approximation-free but statistically inexact solutions, derived from first principles, are possible for a wide range of geometrically complex but clinically relevant brachytherapy problems.

The dosimetric accuracy of Monte Carlo simulation has been confirmed across the entire energy spectrum from ^{125}I to [137]Cs. Agreement between Monte Carlo and TLD measurement ranges from 2% to 6%, both in homogeneous medium and in the presence of tissue and applicator heterogeneities (55,134,184,223,292,306). In contrast to experimental methods, Monte Carlo accuracy is not limited by dosimeter artifacts such as energy response and volume averaging. Because the geometric model can be specified exactly, detector positioning error is not an issue in Monte Carlo. Recent analyses (245,308) have shown that the uncertainty (including all known systematic

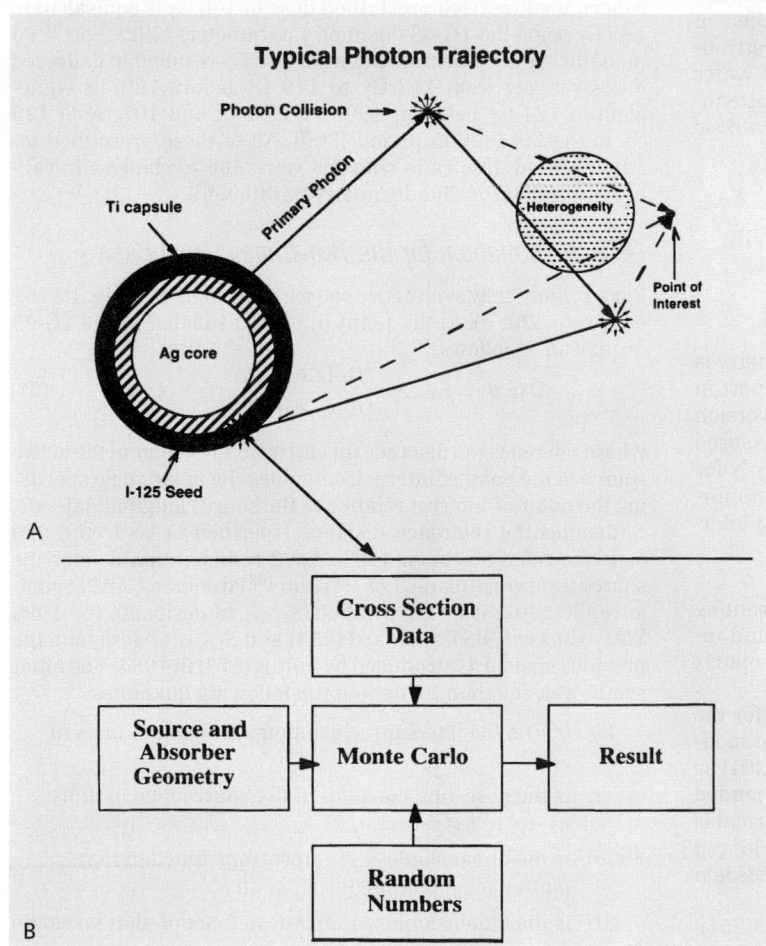

Typical Photon Trajectory

FIGURE 19.14. **A:** Two-dimensional representation of a typical photon history. The heavy solid lines illustrate the origin of the primary photon (randomly selected from the assumed distribution of radioactivity), and each successive collision, which is randomly selected from the competing collision mechanisms (photo-effect, Compton scattering, and coherent scattering), is based on their relative probabilities. The dashed lines illustrate the problem of estimation (i.e., calculating the probable contribution of each simulated collision to the point of interest). **B:** Functional diagram of a Monte Carlo code illustrating the required input data. Cross-section data include total attenuation coefficients, total cross sections for each collision process, and differential cross sections, which are used to randomly sample the distance between successive collisions, the interaction mechanism at each collision, and the angle and energy of the scattered photon leaving each collision, respectively. Sequences of random numbers are obtained from a "random number generator," a computer program designed to generate a pseudorandom sequence of numbers uniformly distributed between 0 and 1.

and random error sources) of Monte Carlo absolute dose-rate estimates on the transverse axis of ^{125}I seeds is 2.5% to 5% over the 1 to 5 cm distance range. Unlike dose measurements, Monte Carlo dose calculations cannot account for unsuspected deviations from the design specifications of the problem (e.g., a contaminant radionuclide in the source or an error in measuring its source strength).

Currently, the most important role of Monte Carlo simulation is calculation of reference-quality transverse-axis dose-rate distributions and anisotropy functions for low and medium-energy brachytherapy sources (293). For low-energy interstitial seeds for routine clinical use, both experimental and Monte Carlo–based published dosimetry studies in peer-reviewed journals are required for developing AAPM-approved consensus data sets or posting the interstitial seed product on the Joint AAPM/RPC Source Registry (245,301). Monte Carlo simulation is a useful alternative to dose measurement in many other applications such as characterizing the effects of applicator shielding materials (223,306) and tissue heterogeneities (55) on brachytherapy dose distributions; validating heuristic dose-calculation algorithms (37); and optimizing new source and applicator designs (185).

Because statistical precision increases with the square root of computing time, long computing times on the order of several hours, even days, may be needed to obtain sufficiently accurate dose distributions, limiting Monte Carlo–based treatment planning (60) to the experimental setting. However, several groups are investigating variance reduction techniques (108) and deterministic transport solutions (56) for more efficient but quantitatively accurate dose calculation for clinical treatments. At least one group has reported single-processor calculation times of the order of a minute for clinical prostate seed implants (39). Unlike current TG-43 clinical dose computations, Monte Carlo or deterministic transport solutions account for the perturbing effect of multiple implanted sources on the single-source dose distributions, deviations in tissue composition from the assumed water medium, and the influence of applicator shielding and attenuation. These phenomena have been shown to introduce dose estimation as large as a factor of 2.

American Association of Physicists in Medicine Task Group 43 Report: A Table-Based Dose-Calculation Formalism

An important milestone in modern brachytherapy dosimetry is the publication of the original AAPM Task Group 43 Report in 1995 (200) and a substantially revised and expanded version in 2004 (245). The TG-43 approach consists of using measured and Monte Carlo–generated dose-rate distributions directly for clinical dose calculation aided by a standard table-lookup formalism. The revised TG-43 report includes the following information:

1. A recommended dose-calculation formalism for representing 2D and one-diminsional (1D) dose distributions around interstitial sources specifically designed to use a sparse matrix of Monte Carlo or measured dose rates as its input.
2. A critically reviewed set of 2D dose-distribution data for the source models (6 ^{125}I seed models and two ^{103}Pd seed models) that satisfied the AAPM dosimetric prerequisites (301) as of July 2003. For each of these source types, a recommended or consensus dose-distribution in TG-43 formalism format is presented based on "merging" published Monte Carlo and experimental dosimetry data sets that met the standards laid out in Section V of the report.
3. A history of air-kerma strength primary standards (173,254), which summarizes previous AAPM guidance (302,304),

including the impact of calibration shifts on the delivered-to-prescribed dose ratio.
4. Methodological recommendations for obtaining TG-43 dosimetry parameters from TLD measurements or Monte Carlo simulations, including uncertainty analyses.
5. Guidance on clinical implementation of TG-43 report recommendations.

The TG-43 report recommends that treatment-planning software vendors accept the TG-43 formalism as the basis of dose calculation or at least for data entry, allowing users to easily input the new data into their systems. With the introduction of the new WAFAC-based air-kerma strength standard by NIST and the growing number of low-energy interstitial brachytherapy sources commercially available, the radiotherapy community has embraced the TG-43 dose-calculation formalism, described below. Important AAPM recommendations address:

a. Clinical implementation of TG-43 dose calculations and revised S_K standard for ^{125}I brachytherapy (302);
b. Implementation of NIST-traceable standards for ^{103}Pd brachytherapy (300); And
c. Dosimetric prerequisites for routine clinical use of low-energy sources (301).

For routine non-IRB approved brachytherapy sources, the AAPM recommends using only sources with NIST-traceable S_K calibrations (including periodic source-strength intercomparisons among NIST, the ADCLs, and the vendor [63]) and the two independent Monte Carlo and experimental dosimetry studies mentioned previously. It is important for physicians to realize that acceptance of new dosimetry systems and source-strength standards can have important implications for selection of prescribed dose. For example, in ^{125}I monotherapy for prostate cancer, the Pre-TG43 prescribed dose of 160 Gy is equivalent to 145 Gy using the TG-43 dosimetry parameters (302). For ^{103}Pd monotherapy, a prescribed dose of 115 Gy resulted in delivered doses ranging from 113 Gy to 119 Gy before 1997 is equivalent to 124 Gy between 1997 and 2000, and 107 Gy to 125 Gy in the 2001–2005 period (300). All of these prescribed-to-administered dose ratio changes were due to changes in calibration standards and dosimetry parameters.

General Formalism for the Two-Dimensional Case

For a cylindrically symmetric source of strength S_K, (Fig. 19.15), dose rate, $\dot{D}(r, \theta)$, at the point (r, θ) is calculated in the TG-43 formalism as follows:

$$\dot{D}(r, \theta) = S_K \cdot \Lambda \cdot \frac{G_L(r, \theta)}{G_L(r_0, \theta_0)} \cdot g_L(r) \cdot F(r, \theta) \qquad (27)$$

where r denotes the distance (in cm) from the center of the active source to the point of interest, θ denotes the polar angle specifying the point-of-interest relative to the source longitudinal-axis, r_0 denotes the reference distance (specified to be 1 cm), and θ_0 is the reference angle (90° or $\pi/2$ radians) that defines the source transverse plane. For ^{125}I and ^{103}Pd sources, AAPM guidance (300,302) uses the symbols $S_{K,N99}$ to designate the 1999 WAFAC-based NIST standard (254) and $S_{K,N85}$ to designate the previous standard introduced by Loftus (173) in 1984. The other symbols in equation 27 denote the following quantities:

G_L (r, θ) is the line-source geometry function in units of cm^{-2}

Λ is the dose-rate constant of the source type in units of cGy h^{-1} U^{-1}

$F(r, \theta)$ is the dimensionless 2D anisotropy function that takes the value unity for θ_0 at all r

$g(r)$ is the dimensionless radial dose function that takes the value unity at r = r_0

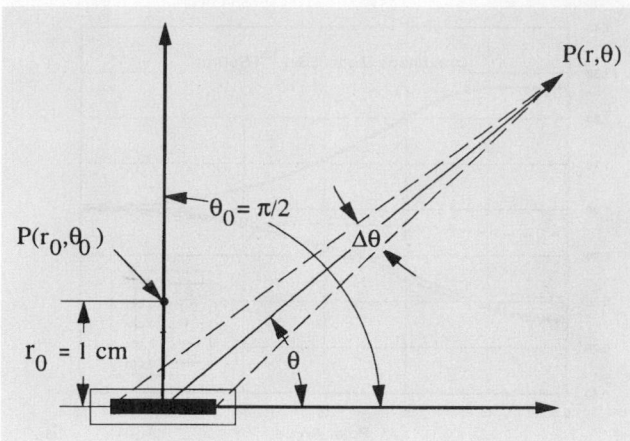

FIGURE 19.15. Illustration of TG-43 formalism for calculation of absorbed dose rate, $\dot{D}(r, \theta)$, at (r, θ), in a polar coordinate system centered about the source active core.

The dose-rate constant is defined by:

$$\Lambda = \frac{\dot{D}(r_0, \theta_0)}{S_K} = \frac{\dot{D}(1 \text{cm}, 90°)}{S_K} \qquad (28)$$

where $\dot{D}(r_0, \theta_0)$ is the measured dose rate at the reference point. Λ depends on the medium surrounding the source and includes the effects of source geometry, spatial distribution of radioactivity, encapsulation, self-filtration in the source, and attenuation and scattering of photons in the surrounding medium. It also depends on the standardization measurements to which the S_K calibration of the source is traceable. TG-43 recommends that liquid water be used as the medium for specification of absorbed dose in clinical brachytherapy. For radium-substitute point sources, $\Lambda = \overline{(\mu_{en}/\rho)}_{air}^{med} \cdot T(r)$. Table 19.4 shows that during the era (1984–1999) of the $S_{K,N85}$ standard, the classical point-source model overestimated absolute doses, relative to

TLD measurements and Monte Carlo calculations, by as much as 15% for ^{125}I sources. In 1999, the $S_{K,N85}$ standard was replaced by the WAFAC ($S_{K,N99}$), which required an upward adjustment of these values, bringing the classical and quantitative values closer together. The old and new dose calculations are in close agreement for ^{192}Ir and other radium substitutes. This table shows that for both ^{103}Pd and ^{125}I sources, that average agreement between TLD and Monte Carlo is about 5%, well within the total uncertainty of these comparisons (308).

The purpose of the geometry function $G_X(r, \theta)$ (where the subscript X denotes point or line source) is to improve the accuracy with which dose rates can be estimated by interpolation from data tabulated at discrete points. Physically, $G_X(r, \theta)$ neglects scattering and attenuation and provides an effective inverse square-law correction based on an *approximate model* of the spatial radioactivity distribution within the source. Because the geometry function is used only to interpolate between tabulated dose-rate values at defined points, highly simplistic approximations yield sufficient accuracy for treatment planning (245). Because the line source greatly improves the accuracy of linear interpolation near the source, the AAPM protocol requires use of (r, θ) for 2D calculations and prefers $G_L(r, \theta)$ over $G_P(r, \theta)$ for 1D calculations. For small cylindrical seeds, $G_X(r, \theta)$ is approximated by a line source.

$$G_P(r, \theta) = r^{-2} \qquad \text{point-source approximation}$$

$$G_L(r, \theta) = \begin{cases} \dfrac{\Delta\beta}{Lr\sin\theta} & \text{if } \theta \neq 0° \\ (r^2 - L^2/4)^{-1} & \text{if } \theta = 0° \end{cases} \quad \text{line-source approximation}$$

$$(29)$$

where $\Delta\beta = \theta_2 - \theta_1$ is the angle subtended by the active source with respect to the point (r, θ). For sources where the radioactivity is distributed over or within a right-cylindrical volume or annulus, L can be taken as the length of this cylinder. For sources containing uniformly spaced multiple radioactive components, L should be taken as the effective length, L_{eff}, given by, $L_{eff} = \Delta S \times (N)$, where N represents the number of discrete pellets contained in the source with a nominal pellet center-to-center

	Table 19.4	DOSE-RATE CONSTANTS FOR SELECTED INTERSTITIAL SEEDS		
		Λ (cGy h^{-1} U^{-1})[a]		
Source	2004 TG-43	Classical Model (Ref.)	Quantitative	Author/Method
Best Medical (Springfield, VA) ^{192}Ir (Fe Clad)	—	1.12 (186)	1.11 1.11	TLD: ICWG (8) MC: Williamson (292)
Amersham Health ^{125}I (Model 6711)	0.965	1.04 (167)	0.877 ($S_{K,N85}$)[b] 0.935[b] ($S_{K,N99}$)[c] 0.879 ($S_{K,N85}$)[b] 0.980 ($S_{K,N99}$)[c]	MC: DLC-99 (292) MC: DLC-146 (295) TLD: ICWG (8) TLD: ICWG (8)
Theragenics I-Seed ^{125}I (Model I25.S06)	1.012	1.029 (296)	1.033[c] 0.991[c]	TLD (217) MC: DLC-146 (109)
Theragenics ^{103}Pd (Model 200)	0.686	0.683 (193)	0.74 ($S_{K,T88}$)[d] 0.68[c] 0.691[c]	TLD: 1995 TG-43 (200) TLD (207) MC: DLC-146 (193)
North American Scientific (Chatsworth, CA) ^{103}Pd (MED 3633)	0.688	0.683 (193)	0.68[c] 0.677[c]	TLD (278) MC: DLC-99 (159)

DLC, Data Code Library indicating vintage of cross-section library; MC, Monte Carlo; TLD, Measured by Thermoluminescent Dosimetry
[a]All measured Λ include solid-to-liquid water conversion factors.
[b]Denotes National Institute of Standards and Technology (NIST) 1985 standard, $S_{K,N85}$.
[c]Normalized to NIST 1999 standard, $S_{K,N99}$
[d]Denotes original vendor-maintained standard implemented in 1988.

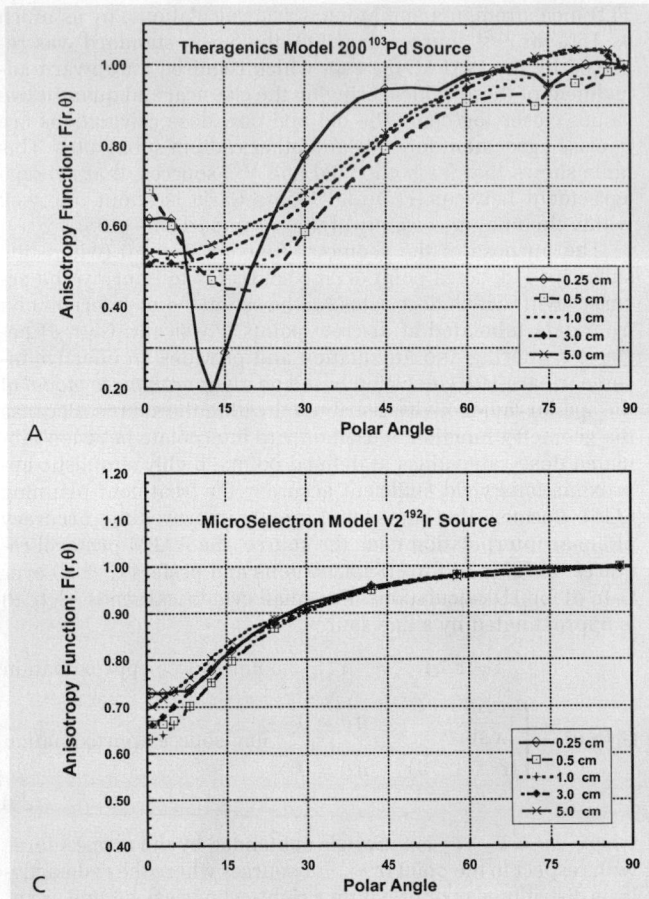

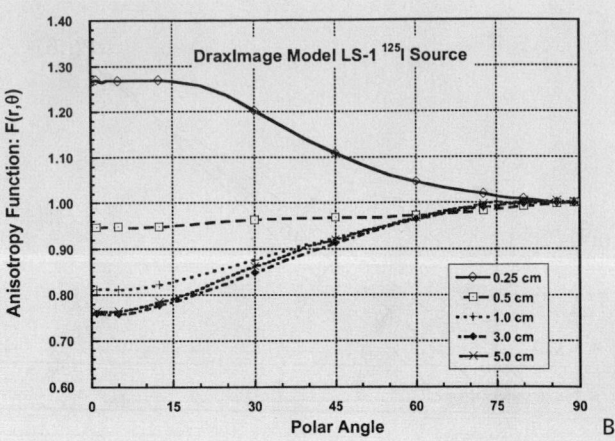

FIGURE 19.16. Examples of anisotropy functions evaluated for three different interstitial sources by the author's group. **A:** Theragenics Model 200 "light seed" ^{103}Pd source. (From Monroe JI, Williamson JF. Monte Carlo-Aided dosimetry of the Theragenics TheraSeed® Model 200 ^{103}Pd interstitial brachytherapy seed. *Med Phys* 2002;29:609–621, with permission.) **B:** DRAXIMAGE Model LS-1 ^{125}I seed. (From Williamson JF. Dosimetric characteristics of the DraxImage Model LS-1 I-125 interstitial brachytherapy source design: A Monte Carlo investigation. *Med Phys* 2002;29:509–521, with permission.) **C:** Nucletron MicroSelectron Model V2 high dose-rate ^{192}Ir source. (From Daskalov GM, Loffler E, Williamson JF. Monte Carlo-aided dosimetry of a new high dose-rate brachytherapy source. *Med Phys* 1998;25:2200–2208, with permission.)

spacing, ΔS. If L_{eff} is greater than the physical length of the source capsule (usually ~ 4.5 mm), the maximum distance between proximal and distal aspects of the activity distribution should be used as the active length, L.

The 2D anisotropy function $F(r, \theta)$ gives the angular variation of dose about the source at each distance as a result of self-filtration, oblique filtration of primary photons through the encapsulating material, and photon attenuation and scattering in the surrounding medium.

$$F(r, \theta) = \frac{\dot{D}(r, \theta)}{\dot{D}(r, \theta_0)} \frac{G_L(r, \theta_0)}{G_L(r, \theta)} \quad (30)$$

where the dose rates, $\dot{D}(r, \theta)$, are obtained by measurement or Monte Carlo simulation. The line-source geometry function is used to suppress the influence of inverse-square law on the angular dose distribution at short distances. Thus, $F(r, \theta)$ need be tabulated only at a few distances, r, to facilitate accurate interpolation at all distances. Examples of anisotropy functions for various interstitial sources are illustrated in Figure 19.16 and in Table 19.5.

The radial dose function, $g_X(r)$, accounts for the fall off of dose along the transverse axis as a result of attenuation and scattering in the medium, capsule filtration, and self-absorption.

$$g_X(r) = \frac{\dot{D}(r, \theta_0)}{\dot{D}(r_0, \theta_0)} \frac{G_X(r_0 \, \theta_0)}{G_X(r, \theta_0)} \quad (31)$$

$g_X(r)$ is normalized to unity at 1 cm distance and is illustrated by Table 19.6. For 2D dose calculations, TG-43 recommends that $X = L$.

One-Dimensional Isotropic Source Approximation

Most commercial treatment planning systems used for permanent implant dose computation support only 1D isotropic point-source calculations. Thus, the TG-43 formalism includes a 1D equation analogous to the classical isotropic point-source model, as shown in equation 22. Two forms of the 1D model are recognized by the TG-43 protocol:

$$\dot{D}(r) = S_K \cdot \Lambda \cdot \left(\frac{r_0}{r}\right)^2 \cdot g_P(r) \cdot \phi_{an}(r)$$

$$\dot{D}(r) = S_K \cdot \Lambda \cdot \frac{G_L(r, \theta_0)}{G_L(r_0, \theta_0)} \cdot g_L(r) \cdot \phi_{an}(r) \quad (32)$$

where $\phi_{an}(r)$ is the 1D anisotropy function defined by equation 21 and illustrated by Table 19.6. The AAPM protocol prefers the line-source version of equation 32 but allows use of the simpler point-source formalism.

:: | Interstitial Implantation

The traditional implant systems (Manchester, Quimby, and Paris), which arose early in the 20th century, were used to guide the radiation oncologist in arranging and positioning radium needles within the surgically identified target volume. In contrast, the most frequently practiced implant procedure today, transperineal permanent implants of the prostate, uses image guidance to position the sources. In place of nomograms and classical system lookup tables, 3D computerized planning is used to prescribe the dose and to optimize the implant geometry. However, the most sophisticated optimization software that is widely available, dwell-weight optimization used with

Table 19.5	EXAMPLE OF A TABULATED 2D ANISOTROPY FUNCTION, $F(r, \theta)$ TABLE, ALONG WITH ITS ASSOCIATED 1D ANISOTROPY FUNCTION, $\phi_{an}(r)$, VALUES FOR A THERAGENICS I-SEED (MODEL I25.S06) ^{125}I SOURCE

Polar Angle θ (degrees)	r [cm]							
	0.25	*0.5*	*1*	*2*	*3*	*4*	*5*	*7*
0	*0.302*	*0.429*	0.512	0.579	0.610	0.631	*0.649*	*0.684*
5	*0.352*	*0.436*	0.509	0.576	0.610	0.635	*0.651*	*0.689*
10	*0.440*	*0.476*	0.557	0.622	0.651	0.672	*0.689*	*0.721*
20	*0.746*	*0.686*	0.721	0.757	0.771	0.785	*0.790*	*0.807*
30	*0.886*	*0.820*	0.828	0.846	0.857	0.862	*0.867*	*0.874*
40	*0.943*	*0.897*	0.898	0.907	0.908	0.913	*0.918*	*0.912*
50	*0.969*	*0.946*	0.942	0.947	0.944	0.947	*0.949*	*0.946*
60	*0.984*	*0.974*	0.970	0.974	0.967	0.966	*0.967*	*0.976*
70	*0.994*	*0.989*	0.988	0.990	0.984	0.985	*0.987*	*0.994*
80	*0.998*	*0.998*	0.998	1.000	0.994	1.000	*0.993*	*0.999*
$\phi_{an}(r)$	*1.122*	*0.968*	0.939	0.939	0.938	0.940	*0.941*	*0.949*

Reproduced from Rivard MJ, Coursey BM, DeWerd LA, et al. Update of AAPM Task Group No. 43 Report: A revised AAPM protocol for brachytherapy dose calculations. *Med Phys* 2004;31(3):633–674, with permission.

single-stepping source remote afterloaders (See Chapters 20 and 21), still relies on the operator to specify the source and needle locations. To guide source positioning, we continue to rely on the classical systems of brachytherapy and their later variants.

Classical Systems for Interstitial Brachytherapy with Radium-Substitute Sources

The Manchester and Quimby systems were developed before the advent of computer-aided dosimetry in implant therapy, whereas the Paris system relies on multiplanar isodose distributions. All interstitial implant systems consist of the following components:

1. *Distribution rules:* Given a target volume, the distribution rules determine how to distribute the radioactive sources and applicators in and around the target volume.
2. *Dose-specification and implant-optimization criteria:* At the heart of each system is a dose-specification criterion (i.e., a definition of prescribed dose). In the Manchester or Paterson-Parker system, for example, the prescribed dose is the modal dose in the volume bounded by the peripheral sources. The distribution rules and dose-specification criterion together often reflect a compromise between mutually exclusive goals such as dose homogeneity, normal tissue sparing, number of catheters implanted, dosimetric margins around the target, and presence of high-dose regions outside the target.
3. *Dose calculation aids:* These devices are used to estimate the source strengths required to achieve the prescribed dose

Table 19.6	LINE-SOURCE RADIAL DOSE FUNCTIONS FOR VARIOUS ^{125}I SEED SOURCES

	Line Source Approximation					
r [cm]	Amorsharn 6702 $L = 3.0$ mm	Amersharn 6711 $L = 3.0$ mm	Best 2301 $L = 3.0$ mm	NASI MED3631-A/M $L = 4.2$ mm	Theragenics 125.S06 $L = 3.5$ mm	Imagyn 1S12501 $L = 3.4$ mm
0.10	1.020	1.055	1.033		*1.010*	*1.022*
0.15	1.022	1.078	1.029		**1.018**	*1.058*
0.25	**1.024**	1.082	1.027	*0.998*	*1.030*	*1.093*
0.50	1.030	1.071	1.028	*1.025*	*1.030*	1.080
0.75	1.020	**1.042**	1.030	*1.019*	**1.020**	**1.048**
1.00	1.000	1.000	1.000	1.000	1.000	1.000
1.50	0.935	0.908	0.938	**0.954**	0.937	0.907
2.00	0.861	0.814	0.866	0.836	0.857	0.808
3.00	0.697	0.632	0.707	0.676	0.689	0.618
4.00	0.553	0.496	0.555	0.523	0.538	0.463
5.00	0.425	0.364	0.427	0.395	0.409	0.348
6.00	0.322	0.270	0.320	0.293	0.313	0.253
7.00	0.241	0.199	0.248	0.211	0.232	0.193
8.00	0.179	0.148	0.187		0.176	0.149
9.00	0.134	0.109	0.142		0.134	0.100
10.00	0.0979	0.0803	0.103		0.0957	0.075

Bolded entries indicate interpolated values while italicized entries indicate extrapolated values.
Reproduced from Rivard MJ, Coursey BM, DeWerd LA et al. Update of AAPM Task Group No. 43 Report: A revised AAPM protocol for brachytherapy dose calculations. *Med Phys* 2004;31(3):633–674, with permission.

rate as defined by the system for source arrangements satisfying its distribution rules. Older systems (Manchester and Quimby) use tables that give dose delivered per mg Ra Eq-h as a function of treatment volume or area. The more recent Paris system makes extensive use of computerized treatment planning to relate absorbed dose to source strength and treatment time.

The Manchester System

The Manchester system was developed by Ralston Paterson (radiation oncologist) and Herbert Parker (physicist) in the 1930s (216,218–220) and often is called the Paterson-Parker (P-P) system. The P-P system remains relevant to today's practice patterns: Its distribution rules, anticipating the "peripheral loading technique," were designed to maximize dose homogeneity inside the implanted volume for volume implants and in the treatment plane (plane parallel to the needles at the treatment distance) for mold or planar implants (Fig. 19.17). Its volume and area lookup tables remain useful as quality assurance tools for optimized HDR volume implants.

The P-P system rules preferentially concentrate radioactivity in the rind or periphery of the implant, compensating for the dose fall-off characteristic of a uniform density implant, thereby improving dose uniformity. After deriving the optimal fraction of radioactivity to be implanted in the rind and core (4:2 ratio), Parker coalesced the continuous radioactivity distribution into several concentric cylindrical surfaces and then further discretized these surfaces into individual needles. The derivation of the volume and planar rules and tables was reviewed by Anderson and Presser (9). Table 19.7 lists the rules of the Manchester system, and Table 19.8 lists the stated dose per mg Ra Eq-h and unit IRAK as a function-treated area or volume.

The P-P rules are designed to yield target area or volume dose distribution that deviates by no more than ±10% of the stated dose, excluding cold spots in the corners and local hotspots at distances <5 mm from the source centers. For pla-nar implants, the target or treatment surface (Fig. 19.17) is that area bounded by the peripheral needles, which is parallel to and 5 mm from the needle plane. For volume implants, the target volume is that region bounded by the peripheral sources. The distribution rules assume that both planar and volume implants will be crossed at both ends by needles placed orthogonal to the predominant direction of insertion and at the level of the belt needle active tips. Fixed 1-cm needle spacing is recommended, with full-intensity sources placed on the periphery of planar implants and partial-strength needles used as central needles. For volume implants, these two groups of sources are called *belt* and *core* sources, respectively. The stated or prescribed dose is the modal dose in the target region and is approximately 10% higher than the minimum peripheral dose (minimum dose to the implanted volume or area) and 10% below the effective maximum dose.

In effect, single-plane interstitial implants with crossed ends treat a 1-cm thick target volume with an area equal to that bounded by the peripheral sources. Thicker target volumes (>1 cm) must be treated by using two parallel planes of needles placed on the target volume boundaries (double-plane implant), with source strength arranged according to the single-plane rules. The mg Ra Eq-h is calculated from the 0.5-cm single-plane table, multiplied by the appropriate two-plane separation factor, and divided between the two planes. The dose actually is delivered to the inner plane 0.5 cm from each needle plane, resulting in mid-plane cold spots ranging from 10% to 30% for separations of 1.5 to 2.5 cm. Target volumes thicker than 2.5 cm must be treated by the volume implant system.

Volume implants can treat cylindrical, spherical, or cubic target volumes in which needles or seeds are arranged on concentric cylinders, concentric spheres, or parallel planes, using a 1-cm needle-to-needle spacing when possible. The target region is the volume encompassed by the peripheral sources. Regardless of implant size, 75% of the source strength should be placed in the rind and 25% in the core, with more specific rules for cylinder implants.

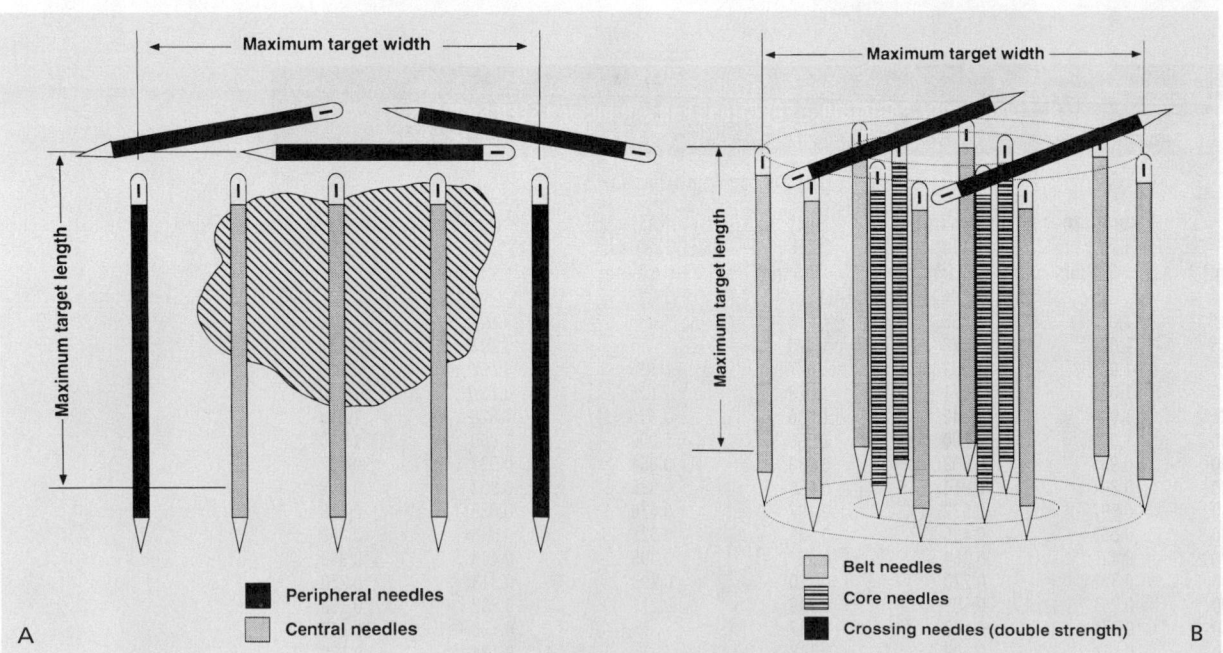

FIGURE 19.17. A: Relationship between target volume or area and peripheral needles (*solid color active regions*) and central needles (*hatched active regions*). Notice that peripheral needles always are placed on the boundary of the target region. **B:** For a cylindric volume implant, the peripheral needles distributed on the cylindric surface of the target are called *belt* needles, whereas those at right angles are called *end* or *crossing* needles. Because the inferior end of the implant is uncrossed, the target volume effectively treated is 7.5% shorter than the active length of the belt needles.

Table 19.7	MANCHESTER SYSTEM RULES

Feature	Paterson and Parker (Manchester System) Rules
Dose and dose rate	6,000 R to 8,000 R in 6–8 days (1,000 R/day; 40 R/h)
Dose specification criterion	Effective minimum dose is 10% above the absolute minimum dose in treatment plane or volume.
Dose gradient	Dose in treatment volume or plane varies by no more than ± 10% from stated dose except for localized hot spots.
	For double-plane implants with a separation >1 cm, dose is specified on interior plane 0.5 cm from implanted plane resulting in 10% to 30% midplane cold spot. Single plane mg Ra Eq-h are multiplied by a separation factor to obtain total double-plane mg Ra Eq-h.
Linear activity	Variable: 0.66 and 0.33 mg Ra Eq/cm
Source strength distribution: planar	Area <25 cm^2: 2/3 periphery; 1/3 center 25 <Area <100 cm^2: 1/2 periphery; 1/2 center Area >100 cm^2: 1/3 periphery; 2/3 center
Source strength distribution: volume	Cylinder: belt: core: end: end = 4:2:1:1 Sphere: belt: core = 6:2 Cube: 1/8 of the activity in each face 2/8 of the activity in the core
Source implant pattern and spacing between sources	Constant uniform spacing: 1-cm separation between sources recommended. Smaller spacings must be used to satisfy distribution rules for small implants.
Crossing needles	Perpendicular to and at the active ends of the parallel needles; If placed beyond the active ends of the needles, should be double strength. Crossing needles used when possible. Planar implant: Target area effectively treated is reduced in length by 10% per uncrossed end. Volume Implant: Target volume effectively treated is reduced by 7.5% per uncrossed end. 1 uncrossed end: belt: core = 4:2:1 2 uncrossed end: belt: core = 4:2
Elongation corrections	Long: short dimension: 1.5:1 2:1 2.5:1 3:1 4:1 Correction factors (applied to mg Ra Eq-h, not area or volume) Planar 1.025 1.05 1.07 1.09 1.12 Volume 1.03 1.06 1.10 1.15 1.23
Relation between implanted volume/area and treated (target) volume/area	Peripheral and crossing needles placed on the target volume boundaries. Active length determines target length.

To apply the P-P system, the relationship between target volume, implanted volume (region enclosed by peripheral sources), and treated volume (region receiving 90% of the stated dose) must be appreciated for crossed and uncrossed end cases. The treated volume may be larger than the target volume but always should contain the latter. When both ends are crossed, the active length (AL) required and target length (TL) are identical. For volume implants, AL should be at least 7.5% longer than TL for each uncrossed end. For planar implants, the Al

Two crossed ends AL = TL planar and volume

One crossed end   AL = $\begin{cases} \text{TL}/0.90 & \text{planar} \\ \text{TL}/0.925 & \text{volume} \end{cases}$ (33)

No crossed ends   AL = $\begin{cases} \text{TL}/0.81 & \text{planar} \\ \text{TL}/0.85 & \text{volume} \end{cases}$

Conversely, given AL, the length of the treated volume always can be calculated by solving the appropriate equation 33 for TL. The area and volume used for looking up dose per mg Ra Eq-h from Table 19.8 should be calculated using the treated length. For example, for a single-plane implant with two uncrossed ends, width, W, and needles of active length AL, the area, A, used for table lookup is given by A = W × AL × 0.81.

To apply P-P tables to modern implants using ^{192}Ir wires or ribbons, several corrections must be applied. The 1938 P-P tables assumed a Γ value of 8.4, ignored attenuation and scattering, neglected oblique filtration, and specified treatment in

terms of exposure rather than absorbed dose. For ^{226}Ra needles, an average correction of 0.90 (262) applied to the original P-P tables to estimate absorbed dose. Modifying these corrections for ^{137}Cs needles and ^{192}Ir seeds and adding an additional factor of 10% to convert from stated (modal target dose) to minimum target volume dose, we obtain the following equivalencies:

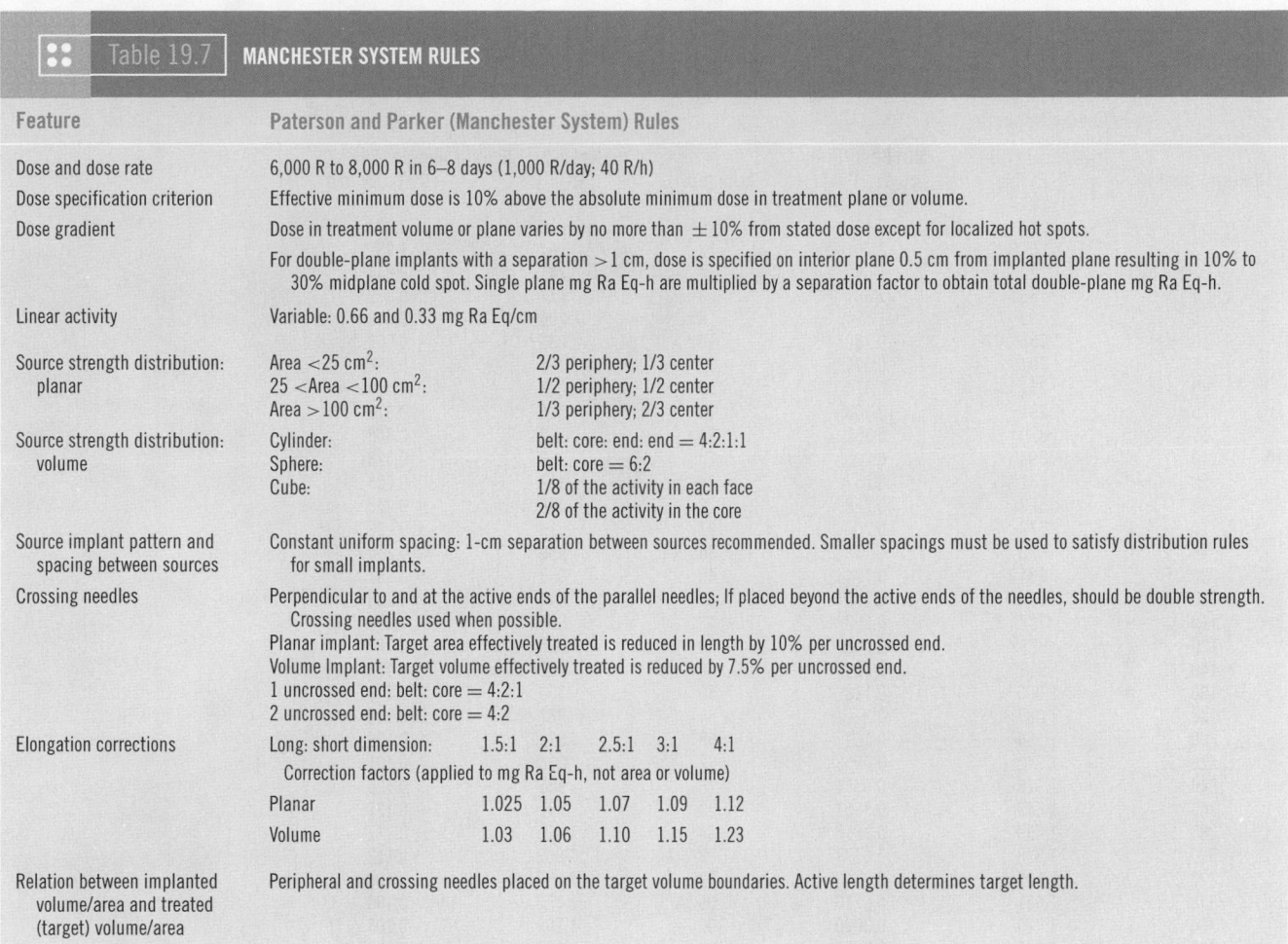

$$1'P - P'R = \begin{cases} 0.97 \cdot \frac{8.25}{8.4} & 0.98 & 0.98 & 0.90 \\ 0.97 \cdot \frac{8.25}{8.4} & 1.00 & 0.98 & 0.90 \\ 0.97 \cdot \frac{8.25}{8.4} & 1.00 & 1.00 & 0.90 \\ \text{(cGy/R)} \cdot \left(\frac{\Gamma_{new}}{\Gamma_{old}}\right) & \text{(filtration)} & \text{(attenuation/buildup)} & \left(\frac{min}{stated}\text{dose}\right) \end{cases}$$

$$= \begin{cases} 0.82 \text{ cGy radium needles} \\ 0.84 \text{ cGy cesium needles} \\ 0.86 \text{ cGy iridium ribbons} \\ \left(\frac{\text{Modern cGy}}{'P - P'R}\right) \end{cases} \quad (34)$$

Using the 0.90 cGy/P-P R conversion factor, Stovall and Shalek (262) found excellent agreement between computer calculations and the P-P tables for a variety of planar and cylindrical implants following the Manchester distribution rules. For single-plane implants, 90% of the stated dose in cGy covers 94% to 99% of the target area. For cubic arrays of seeds using fixed 1-cm spacing, agreement between the tables and computer

	Volume Implants			**Planar Implants**	
Volume (cm³)	**mgRaEq-h/1,000 'P-P' R[a]**	**Min Dose/IRAK[b] cGy/(μGy m²)**	**Area (cm²)**	**mgRaEq-h/1,000 'P-P' R[a]**	**Min Dose/IRAK[b] cGy/(μGy m²)**
1	34	3.49	0	30	3.97
2	54	2.20	2	97	1.23
3	70	1.68	4	141	0.844
4	85	1.38	6	177	0.672
5	99	1.194	8	206	0.578
10	158	0.752	10	235	0.506
15	207	0.574	12	261	0.456
20	251	0.474	14	288	0.413
25	291	0.408	16	315	0.378
30	329	0.361	18	342	0.348
40	398	0.298	20	368	0.323
50	462	0.257	24	417	0.285
60	522	0.228	28	466	0.255
70	579	0.206	32	513	0.232
80	633	0.188	36	558	0.213
90	684	0.174	40	603	0.197
100	734	0.162	44	644	0.185
110	782	0.152	48	685	0.174
120	829	0.143	52	725	0.164
140	919	0.129	56	762	0.156
160	1,005	0.118	60	800	0.149
180	1,087	0.110	64	837	0.142
200	1,166	0.102	68	873	0.136
220	1,242	0.0958	72	908	0.131
240	1,316	0.0904	76	945	0.126
260	1,389	0.0857	80	981	0.121
280	1,459	0.0815	84	1,016	0.117
300	1,528	0.0779	88	1,052	0.113
320	1,595	0.0746	92	1,087	0.109
340	1,661	0.0716	96	1,122	0.106
360	1,725	0.0690	100	1,155	0.103
380	1,788	0.0665	120	1,307	0.0910
400	1,851	0.0643	140	1,463	0.0813
—	—	—	160	1,608	0.0740
—	—	—	180	1,746	0.0682
—	—	—	200	1,880	0.0633
—	—	—	220	2,008	0.0593
—	—	—	240	2,132	0.0558
—	—	—	260	2,256	0.0527
—	—	—	280	2,372	0.0502
—	—	—	300	2,495	0.0477

Table 19.8 **MANCHESTER IMPLANT TABLES**

[a]Original Manchester Values from Paterson R, Parker HM. A dosage system for interstitial radium therapy. *Br J Radiol* 1938;11:313–339.
[b]Modified from original values for ^{192}Ir assuming 860 cGy minimum peripheral dose per 1,000 'P-P' R and 7.227 μGy m²/mg Ra Eq-h.

calculations is excellent for treatment volumes of more than 100 cm³ (147,256), but results in errors ranging from 10% to 40% for smaller arrays. These discrepancies probably result from deviations from the 4:2 activity ratio and use of a dose-specification criterion incompatible with the Manchester system.

The classical implant systems are based on ^{192}Ir wires or interstitial needles, consisting of continuous distributions of radioactivity (i.e., line sources) with well-defined active lengths. To apply the classical systems to modern interstitial sources consisting of discrete seeds, the dosimetric equivalence between ribbons of discrete seed sources and line sources must be appreciated (Fig. 19.18). A ribbon consisting of N seeds with center-to-center separations, S, has a dose distribution that closely approximates that of a continuous line source of length, AL and strength $(S_k)_{line}$ (179,288):

$$\left. \begin{array}{l} AL = N \cdot S \\ (S_K)_{line} = N \cdot (S_K)_{seed} \end{array} \right\} \quad (35)$$

This equivalence tends to break down at distances less than S/2: the cylindrical isodose curves break up into ellipsoidal shapes centered about each seed. In addition, the ribbon isodose curves undulate significantly at distances comparable with or less than

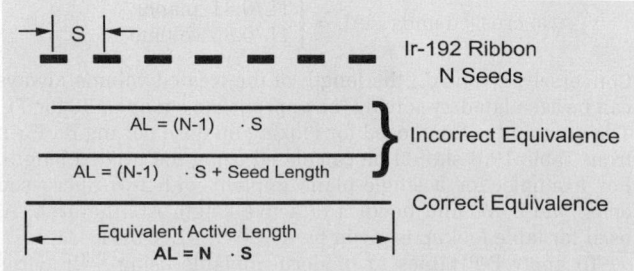

FIGURE 19.18. Relationship between a linear array of equally spaced discrete seeds and its dosimetrically equivalent line source. Both sources are assumed to have the same total strength. Common errors in defining this equivalence are illustrated.

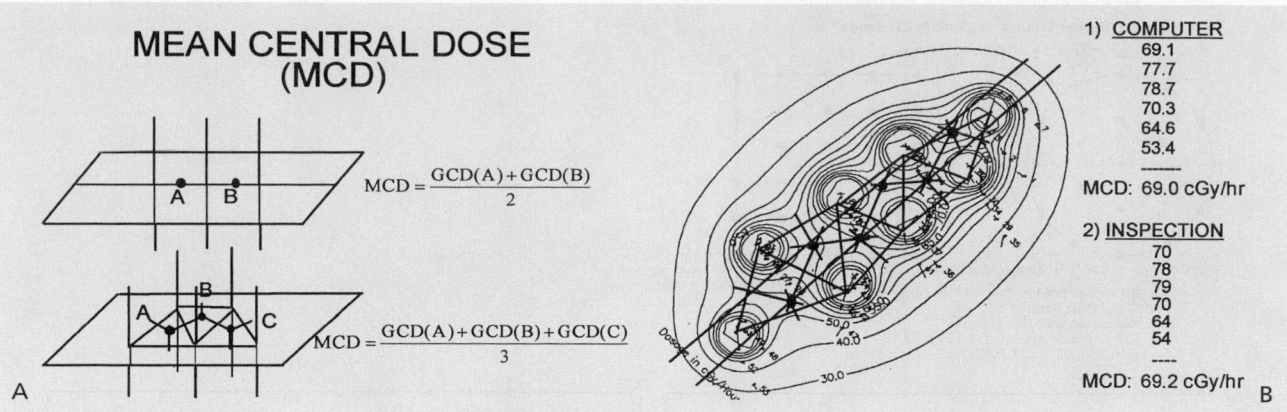

FIGURE 19.19. A: Calculation of mean central dose (MCD) as the arithmetic mean of the doses at mid-distance between each pair of adjacent sources for single-plane implants and the mean of the local minimum doses between each group of three adjacent sources in a multiple-plane implant. All local minimum doses are specified in the "central transverse" plane, which is normal to and bisects the source axes. Practical specification of MCD for a computer plan is illustrated in (**B**).

the gap, S, between adjacent seeds, although on average the equivalence remains accurate. For this reason, use of standard ^{192}Ir ribbons (S = 1.0 cm, seed length = 0.3 cm) is thought to lead to an unacceptably inhomogeneous dose distribution for Paris system implants (179).

Because the P-P system uses 1-cm interneedle spacing, the fraction of sources in the core (vs. periphery) increases as volume increases. Thus, using uniform-strength ^{192}Ir ribbons and fixed spacing results in underloading the core for very small implants and overloading the core for very large implants, relative to the P-P distribution rules. In the latter case, the gap between minimum peripheral dose and central maximum dose widens. An alternative to the differential loading method is to vary the ribbon spacing with implant size, using smaller (<1 cm) spacing for very small implants and larger spacing (up to a limit of 1.5 cm) for larger implants, so that the relative number of central ribbons complies approximately with the P-P rules, allowing uniform seed strengths to be used. Two examples of this strategy are given in the next section.

To use the Manchester tables for verification of computerized dose calculations requires a method for objectively identifying the computer-generated isodose surface that corresponds to the minimum peripheral dose rate predicted by the Manchester system. For volume implants, mean central dose (MCD), a quantity proposed by the ICRU report on dose specification in interstitial brachytherapy, is useful (123) (Fig. 19.19). In our experience, the maximum dose (110% of stated dose) of the Manchester system is closely approximated by MCD. Minimum peripheral dose and stated dose are given by 80% and 89%, respectively, of MCD. For planar implants, the minimum dose/MCD ratio varies from 55% to 70%, depending on catheter spacing and is of limited value.

Manchester Volume Implant Example

A 5-cm high by 5-cm diameter cylindrical target volume is to be treated using ^{192}Ir ribbons with seed-to-seed and intercatheter spacings of 1 cm and 1.3 cm, respectively (Fig. 19.20). Calculate the (a) minimum ribbon length needed, (b) the required ribbon arrangement, and (c) the strength/seed needed to deliver 45 cGy/h to the P-P minimum dose specification volume.

a. There are two approaches: treating the ribbons as needles with uncrossed ends or treating the proximal and distal seeds of each ribbon as crossing sources. In the uncrossed

end approach, equation 33 implies that

$$AL = \text{target length}/0.925^2 = 5\,\text{cm}/0.85 = 5.9\,\text{cm}$$

Equation 35 implies that N = 6 seeds/ribbon are required. In the crossed-end approach, the first and last seeds must be placed at the target volume surfaces, again requiring six seeds/ribbon.

b. To satisfy the 1.3-cm ribbon-spacing requirement, 12 ribbons must be placed on the cylindrical target boundary, six ribbons must be placed on an inner cylindrical surface, and there should be one central ribbon. Treating the ends as uncrossed and assuming that the ribbons have uniform strengths, the belt-to-core ratio is 0.63:0.37, which is close to the P-P 4:2 ratio. Again assuming all seeds have the same strength, Figure 19.20 shows that the required crossed-end ratios are also closely approximated. This illustrates that ribbon spacing can be manipulated to adhere to the P-P distribution rules with uniform strength sources.

c. Assuming the uncrossed end point of view:

$$TL = AL \times 0.85 = (1\,\text{cm}) \times 0.85 = 5.1\,\text{cm}$$

Treated (lookup) Volume $= \pi \times (2.5)^2 \times 5.1 = 100.1\,\text{cm}^3$

Hence:

$$\frac{734\,\text{mg}-\text{h}}{1000'P-P'R} = \frac{734\,\text{mg}-\text{h}}{860\,\text{cGy minimum dose}} = \frac{1\,\mu\text{Gy}\cdot\text{m}^2}{0.162\,\text{cGy}}$$

Differential loading:

$$S_K/\text{seed} = \frac{45\,\text{cGy/h}}{0.162\,\text{cGy}}\cdot\times$$

$$\begin{cases} \frac{2}{3}\cdot\frac{1\,\mu\text{Gy}\cdot\text{m}^2}{12\,\text{ribbons}\times6\,\text{seeds/ribbon}} = 2.6\,\mu\text{Gy}\cdot\text{m}^2\cdot\text{h}^{-1}\ \text{periphery} \\ \frac{1}{3}\cdot\frac{1\,\mu\text{Gy}\cdot\text{m}^2}{7\,\text{ribbons}\times6\,\text{seeds/ribbon}} = 2.2\,\mu\text{Gy}\cdot\text{m}^2\cdot\text{h}^{-1}\ \text{core} \end{cases}$$

Uniform loading:

$$S_K/\text{seed} = \frac{45\,\text{cGy/h}}{0.162\,\text{cGy/h}}\cdot\frac{1\,\mu\text{Gy}\cdot\text{m}^2}{19\,\text{ribbons}\times6\,\text{seeds/ribbon}}$$
$$= 2.4\,\mu\text{Gy}\cdot\text{m}^2\cdot\text{h}^{-1}$$

The Quimby System

The Quimby system was developed by Edith Quimby et al. (240–242) at New York Memorial Hospital from 1920 to 1940. Unlike the Manchester system, equal linear intensity (mg Ra Eq/cm)

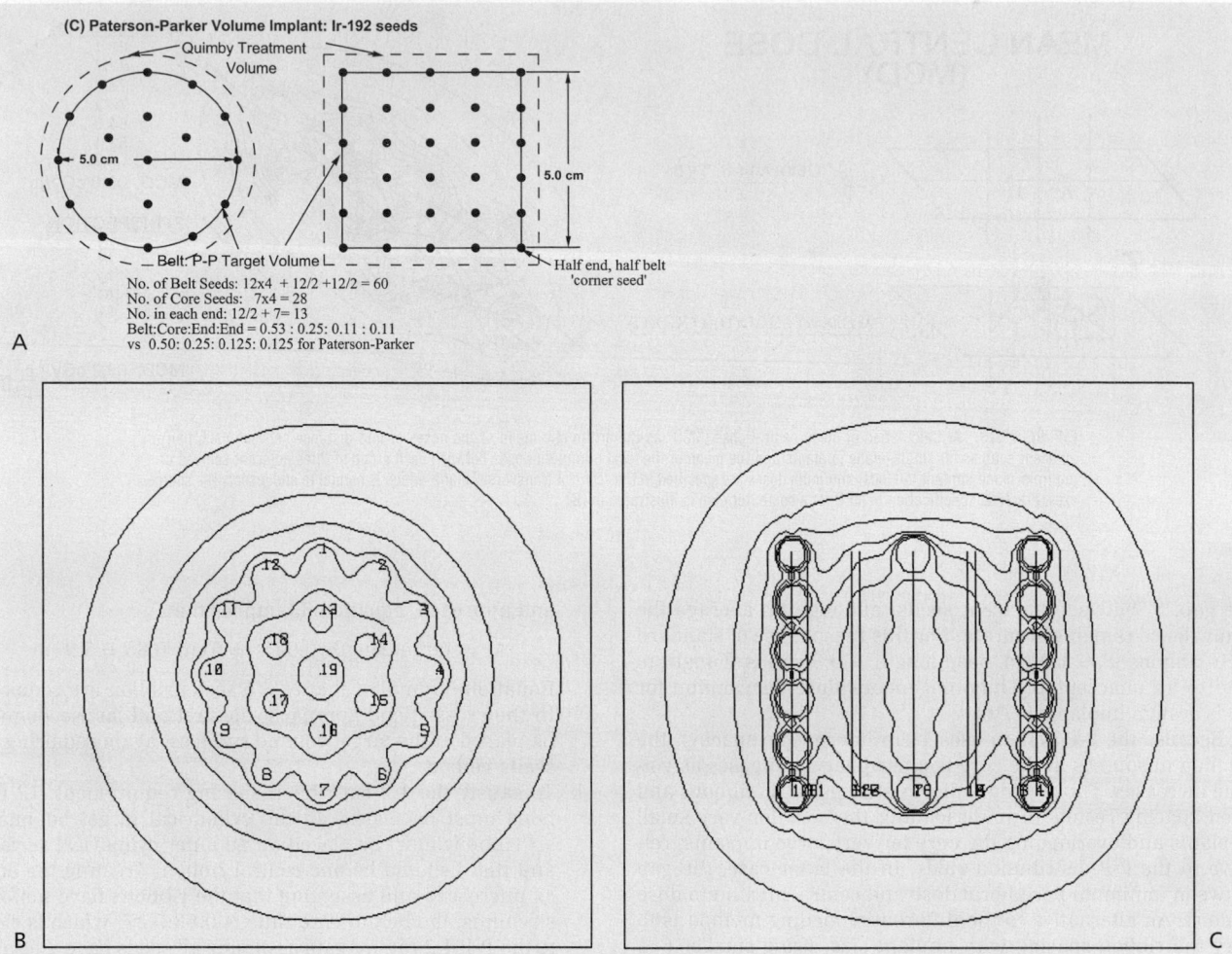

FIGURE 19.20. **A:** Cylindric volume implant, example **(C)**, using uniform strength ^{192}Ir ribbons spaced at 1.3-cm intervals. Central transverse **(B)** and Coronal **(C)** isodose curves are plotted normalized to the mean central dose (MCD) = 58.9 cGy/h = 100%: 115% (68 cGy/h), 100% (59 cGy/h), 90% (53 cGy/h), 80% (47 cGy/h), 60% (35 cGy/h), 40% (24 cGy/h), 20% (12 cGy/h). Note that 80% of MCD, 47 cGy/h, agrees closely with the minimum peripheral dose rate of 45 cGy/h predicted by the Paterson-Parker tables.

needles are distributed uniformly (fixed spacing) in each implant. Like the Manchester system, the associated Quimby tables give the mg Ra Eq-h needed to deliver a stated exposure of 1,000 R as a function of target volume or area.

The so-called planar implant tables were intended for surface molds; None of the early Memorial publications suggest that it was used for single-plane interstitial implants. In part because Quimby's stated dose is the maximum dose in the treatment plane, Quimby planar implants deliver 30% to 40% less radiation (IRAK) per unit stated dose than an equivalent Manchester implant delivers. Rules for distributing radium needles (relationship to target-area boundaries, crossed ends, spacing, and so forth) are not clearly described. Volume implant needle arrangements are similar to their Manchester counterparts; Both systems recommend crossed ends and placing peripheral needles on or beyond the target volume boundaries. However, Quimby allows the needle spacing to vary with implant size and specifies dose as the absolute minimum to the target volume. The physical and mathematical origins of the widely cited Quimby volume implant table are obscure; The tables published in the 1952 edition of *Physical Foundations of Radiology* (241) deliver 25% to 90% more mg Ra Eq-h per unit dose than P-P volume implants of similar size. Because they are evenly spaced, uniform-strength sources approximate the Manchester distribution rules for medium-size volumes, and

these differences are likely a result of differences in the definition of "minimum dose" used by the two systems. Although vague on the subject, Quimby appears to specify minimum dose at a point located 3 to 5 mm from the peripheral needles (and therefore outside the target volume) near their active tips (242). This corresponds to a treatment volume (volume encompassed by prescription isodose surface) that is 6 to 10 mm larger than the implanted volume (used for table lookup) in each linear dimension. The Quimby planar and volume dose specification criteria are clearly inconsistent, and a detailed-derivation of the associated tables is lacking. For these reasons, we do not recommend Quimby tables for clinical use. Zwicker (321) has recently reviewed implant systems based on the widely used Quimby-like source arrangements.

The Paris System

The Paris system, developed in the early 1960s by Pierquin et al. (229) and Dutreix and Marinello (70), was motivated by the ^{192}Ir afterloading techniques developed by Henschke (112). Outside the United States, the Paris system is used widely for definitive brachytherapy of localized lesions in the head and neck, breast, and many other sites. An up-to-date summary of the system has been published by Gillin and Mourtada (92).

Table 19.9	PARIS SYSTEM CHARACTERISTICS

Feature	Paris System Rules
Dose and dose rate	6,000 cGy to 7,000 cGy in 3–11 days (25 cGy/h to 90 cGy/h).
Dose specification criterion	Reference dose (prescribed dose) is 85% of the basal dose and encompasses the target volume when distribution rules are followed. Basal dose is the average of the minimum doses between pairs or groups of adjacent sources in the central transverse plane.
Dose gradient	Fixed 15% gradient between reference dose and basal dose. The "hyperdose sleeve" (region receiving at least twice the reference dose) diameter should be <8–10 mm.
Linear activity	Constant (4–14 μGy m^2 h^{-1}/cm) linear density Ir-192 wires used.

Source arrangement geometry for target volume of thickness, width, and length of T × W × L	Only single and double plane implants allowed. Spacing, S, and lateral margin (called "safety margin" for double-plane case), M, are fixed fractions of T and constant within a given implant. Active length, AL, is a fixed fraction of L, which varies with S.
	Single plane: T = 12 mm
	S = 2 × T (2 sources)
	S = 1.67 × T (3 sources)
	M = 0.37 × T
	AL = (1.3 – 1.49) × T
	Double plane: (square pattern) (triangle pattern)
	    S = 0.62 × T S = 0.77 × T
	    M = 0.27 × T M = 0.15 × T
	    AL = (1.37 – 1.62) × L AL = (1.33 – 1.49) × L

Source spacing, S, limits	Short sources (1–4 cm): 8 mm $\leq$ S $\leq$ 15 mm Long sources ($\leq$10 cm): 15 mm $\leq$ S $\leq$ 22 mm
Crossing needles	Generally not used; AL $\sim$ 1.45 × L to compensate for uncrossed ends. For oral cavity implants, hairpins are common, which approximate crossed ends.
Relation between target volume and implanted volume	W = distance between outermost sources + 2 × M L = (1.3 – 1.62) × L $$T = \begin{cases} S/1.67 & \text{Single plane} \\ S + 2 \times M & \text{Double plane: squares} \\ S \times \cos 30^\circ + 2 \times M & \text{Double plane: triangles} \end{cases}$$

The starting point of the Paris system is the definition of the target volume, which is described in terms of thickness, T, length, L, and width, W. The system provides rules for constructing implants, which, if followed, guarantee that the target volume is completely covered by the prescription isodose surface (Table 19.9). The prescription dose level, called the *reference dose*, is a fixed percentage (85%) of the basal dose (Fig. 19.21, which closely resembles the more general concept of mean central dose in Fig. 19.19). ^{192}Ir wire sources are arranged in parallel rectilinear arrays with their centers located in the central plane, which is perpendicular to the sources. Adjacent sources must be equidistant from one another, resulting in single-plane implants with equal spacing and double-plane implants with groups of adjacent sources arranged in equilateral triangles or squares in the central plane. The linear density (μGy · m^2 · h^{-1}/cm) must be uniform and the same for all sources. Interneedle spacing scales with the thickness, T, of the target volume. The number of sources is determined largely by the relative shape of the target volume cross-sectional area, W × T. In contrast, the Manchester system uses fixed spacing and increases the number of sources as the cross-sectional area of the target volume increases.

Table 19.9 shows that the location of the peripheral sources relative to the treated volume (region encompassed by the reference isodose-rate surface, as shown in Fig. 19.22) differs from the Manchester system, which implants to the boundary of the treated tissue. In the transverse plane, the peripheral sources lie 2 to 4 mm (the lateral margin distance, M) inside the treatment surface, whereas longitudinally the AL extends 15% to 20% beyond the distal and proximal margins of the target volume. In practice, the margin, M, is treated as a safety margin,

and the peripheral needles are implanted along the margins of the clinical target volume (CTV). The maximum thickness, T, of a target volume treatable in the Paris system is about 2.5 cm. An example of a double-plane implant arranged in squares is shown in Figure 19.23.

To apply the Paris system, the target thickness, T, must be known, which defines the spacing and determines whether single-plane or double-plane geometry is required. The number of sources and selection of a square or triangular arrangement are defined by the relative cross-sectional shape of the target volume in the central plane perpendicular to the sources. Finally, the active length is calculated. The source tip and end coordinates are reconstructed from orthogonal radiographs and the dose distribution and basal dose are calculated by computer for the actual implant geometry realized in the patient, not the idealized implant of clinical intention. This approach differs from the classical Manchester method, which bases dose prescription on the P-P table and, in general, ignores deviations of the actual implant geometry from the ideal. The Paris system addresses only single- and double-plane implants; Large volume implants for treating pelvic masses and brain tumors were not part of the original system. Extensions of Paris system principles to large-volume implants are discussed by Leung (157) and Gillin et al. (91).

Dose Specification in Interstitial Brachytherapy

Many of the differences between the Manchester, Paris, and Quimby systems can be attributed to fundamental differences in dose specification. Because of the high-dose gradients near the peripheral sources or the target volume boundary,

Table 19.10 SIMPLIFIED FLETCHER SYSTEM PRESCRIPTIONS

Treatment Scheme	Indications	External Beam		Intracavitary Maximum		Range: Smallest to Largest Insertion		
		Whole Pelvis (Gy)s	Split Field (Gy)	mg-h[a]	Time (h)	Point A (Gy)	Point B (Gy)[b]	mg-h[a]
A	<1 cm tumor	0	0	6,000 / 4,000	72 / 48	59–63	17–22	6,600–10,000
B	IB/IIB 1–3 cm tumor	0	<40	5,400 / 3,600	72 / 48	56–59	57–60	6,600–9,000
C	IB/IIB 1–3 cm tumor	20	<20	3,600 / 3,900	48 / 52	67–69	54–56	5,500–7,500
D	Endocervical tumor; IB/IIB moderate bulk (3–6 cm) disease; IIB/IIIB bulky (>6 cm) tumor with good regression	40	<10[c]	3,250 / 3,250	48 / 48	81–90	63–64	5,280–6,500
E	Bulky disease with poor regression	50	0	2,500 / 2,500 or 5,000	48 / 48 or 72	81–94	62	5,000

[a]Radium tubes with 1 mm platinum filtration.
[b]With maximum split field dose.
Adapted from Potish RA, Gerbi BJ. Cervical cancer intracavitary dose specification and prescription. *Radiology* 1987;165:555–560, with permission.

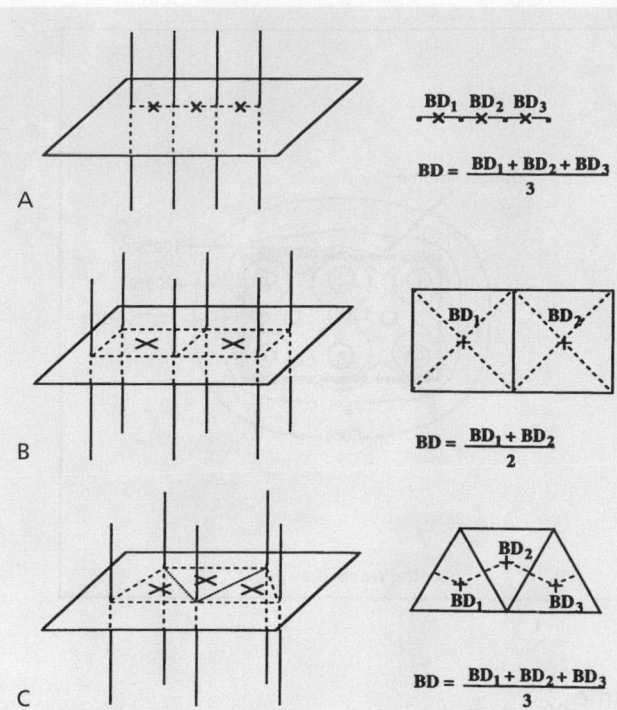

FIGURE 19.21. The three central plane configurations allowed by the Paris system: **(A)** single-plane implant, **(B)** double-plane implant using the pattern of squares; And **(C)** double-plane implant using the pattern of equilateral triangles. The calculation of basal dose rate at a point equidistant from each group of adjacent sources is illustrated for each configuration. (From Gillin MT, Albano KS, Erickson B. Classical systems II for planar and volume temporary interstitial implants: The Paris and other systems. In: Williamson JF, Thomadsen BR, Nath R, eds. *Brachytherapy physics.* Madison, WI: Medical Physics Publishing, 1995;232–343, with permission.)

the quantity of radiation actually delivered to the patient, or for reporting. The *specified dose* sometimes is called the *reference dose*. The dose that an implant actually delivers to the patient, based on postinsertion treatment planning, may differ significantly from the dose prescribed for a variety of reasons. For example, anatomic or technical constraints may preclude accurate positioning of sources at their intended locations, resulting in a partial geometric miss or underdose of the specified volume. Dose specification for reporting purposes usually refers to efforts to develop reproducible and system-independent specification schemes to promote comparison of different implantation systems so as to minimize patient-to-patient and operator-to-operator variability in level of treatment delivered. The ability to objectively compare different interstitial implant plans as to target volume coverage, normal tissue sparing, and dose homogeneity depends on dose specification. Several divergent and rather abstract approaches to dose specification have been developed and promoted by various national and international advisory groups; No single approach to dose specification has been widely accepted within the brachytherapy community.

Minimum Dose to an Anatomically Defined Target Volume

The minimum dose to the anatomically defined target volume harboring malignant cells is conceptually attractive because it is based on the intuitively satisfying premise that local tumor control will be determined by the minimum dose received by tumor cells. The American Brachytherapy Society (ABS) recommends that the minimum dose should be identified as accurately as possible by the best means available and should be used for dose prescription, evaluation, and reporting (7). In practice, minimum target dose specification is difficult to implement clinically for many implants. In the prostate brachytherapy literature (317), minimum target dose usually is called *minimum peripheral dose*, or mPD, when used for prescription and D_{100} (see discussion on dose-volume histograms) when used for postimplant dose evaluation. Except for image-guided prostate implants, imaging data showing the target volume in relation to the sources is frequently not available. In such cases, ABS recommends approximate target localization by means of intraoperatively placed surgical clips, orthogonal planar imaging, or measurements relative to peripheral sources. A clear disadvantage of minimum dose specification is that the target volume surface lies within the zone of largest dose gradient. This can

reproducible specification of dose and evaluation of implant quality is difficult. Conversely, small differences in dose-specification criteria can lead to large differences in treatment time or in the geometric relationship between implanted and treated volume. The term *dose specification* means objective identification of a spatial volume or location for evaluating absorbed dose for the purposes of prescription (defining the dose that the radiation oncologist intends to deliver), for describing

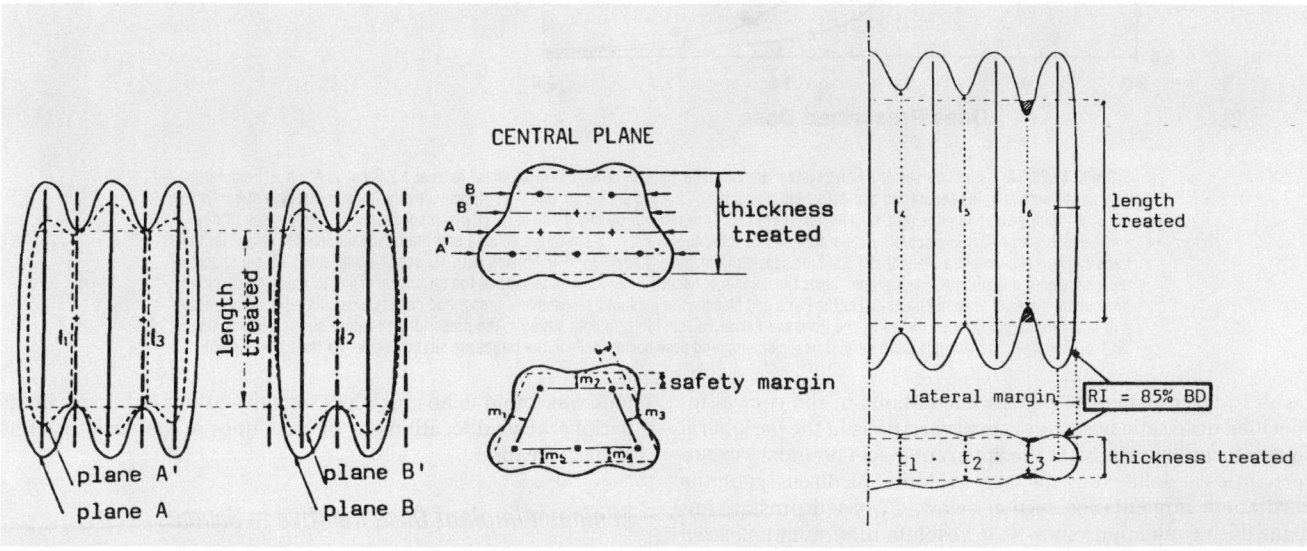

FIGURE 19.22. Relationship of the reference isodose, source locations, and target volume dimensions for each of the basic implant configurations allowed by the Paris system. The concept of safety margin (lateral margin, M) is illustrated. (From Pierquin B, Wilson JF, Chassange D. *Modern brachytherapy.* New York: Masson, 1987, with permission.)

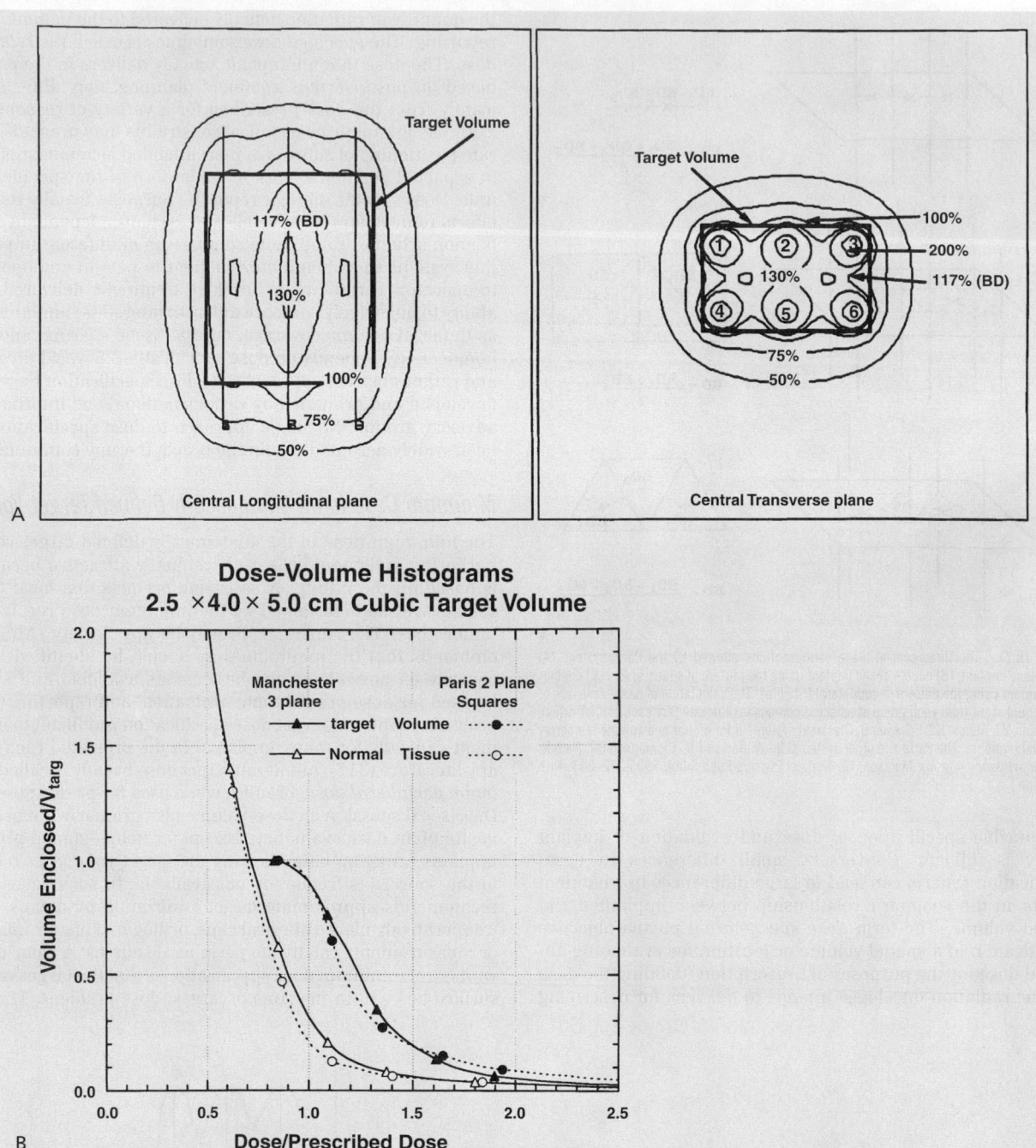

FIGURE 19.23. A: Isodose curves of a Paris system double-plane implant arranged "in squares" to treat a 2.5-cm × 4-cm × 5-cm target volume (*heavy lines*). The separation and active lengths of the ^{192}Ir wires are 1.6 cm and 7.3 cm, respectively. A linear strength of 6 μGy × m² × h⁻¹/cm gives reference (100%) and basal (117%) dose rates of 60 cGy/h and 70.6 cGy/h, respectively. **B:** Comparison of dose-volume histograms (DVHs) calculated separately for the 2.5-cm × 4-cm × 5-cm target volume and the tissue outside the target for the Paris implant shown and a Manchester implant consisting of three planes, 15 ^{192}Ir ribbons with six seeds each, and 1.25-cm spacing between planes and ribbons. Each graph shows the volume of tissue (in multiples of volume of the target) receiving at least the specified dose (in multiples of prescribed dose). For the Paris and Manchester implants, respectively, prescribed dose is a calculated reference dose and minimum target dose predicted by the Paterson-Parker volume table. In both systems, the prescription isodose surface covers about 90% of the target. Surprisingly, both normal tissue sparing and dose homogeneity in the target are slightly better for the Paris implant.

result in large patient-to-patient fluctuations in the central-to-specified dose ratio because of small variations in the peripheral source locations relative to the apparent target boundary or uncertainties in delineating the target volume. As discussed in the Permanent Implantation section below, CT-based prostate implant dose evaluations show that absolute minimum delivered doses (D_{100}) relative to the prescribed dose show large patient-to-patient variabilities and average 30% to 60% (188,249). The minimum dose covering at least 99% (or 95%) of the target volume was found to be much less sensitive to small changes in the peripheral seed locations or uncertainties in the target volume surface location.

Minimum Implant Dose Relative to Sources

Traditional treatment planning uses planar radiographs for 3D reconstruction of radioactive source positions, yielding accurate dose estimates relative to the sources but not relative to an anatomic target volume (161). Thus, it is natural to prescribe treatment to a point or surface that has a fixed relationship to the peripheral sources. The minimum implant dose (MID) is the minimum dose received by the "target" volume defined relative to the implanted volume, the smallest regular geometric shape circumscribing the peripheral sources. Often this specification volume is taken to be that volume that is 2 to 5 mm larger in each linear dimension relative to the implanted volume, as in the Paris and Quimby systems. With the exception of image-guided prostate implants, MID is perhaps the most widely used specification approach and is the basis of the classical systems and the U.S. practice of selecting prescription isodose surfaces from 2D isodose curve plots. However, MID yields information about tumor coverage only to the extent that the radiation oncologist has implanted peripheral sources at known distances from the anatomic target volume boundaries. In addition, MID lies in the zone of maximum dose gradient and can be difficult to evaluate objectively for an implant of irregular shape, again leading to large patient-to-patient variations and variations in the central-to-prescribed dose ratio. The Paris and Manchester systems eliminate the possibility of subjective isodose selection by rigidly specifying dose rate by means of basal dose rate and implant tables, respectively.

Mean Central Dose

The ICRU report on dose specification in interstitial brachytherapy (123) emphasizes reporting mean central dose (MCD; See Fig. 19.19), although it recommends reporting the prescribed dose, the peripheral dose (minimum target dose), and a description of dose uniformity as well. MCD specifies dose in the low-gradient regions located between adjacent source locations in the central plane of the implant. Thus, MCD is relatively free of the variability inherent in minimum peripheral or target dose specification. It is a generalization of the Paris system basal dose. As a reporting parameter, MCD can be reproducibly estimated from 2D central transverse-plane isodoses and should be very useful for comparing implants performed using different clinical systems. However, for systems other than the Paris and Manchester systems (which rigidly specify how sources are to be arranged relative to the target volume), MCD does not have a known relationship to minimum peripheral or target dose. Thus, its value as a prescription parameter is limited.

Three-Dimensional Dose-Volume Histogram Representations

DVHs are 1D plots that describe the distribution of tissue volumes, V, irradiated by the implant with respect to dose, D. DVHs can be presented in either differential, $\Delta V(D)/\Delta D$, or cumulative, V(D), forms. DVH computation involves calculating dose over a fine 3D grid extending at least 2 cm beyond the peripheral seeds, dividing the dose axis into small bins of width ΔD, and then counting the number of voxels falling into each dose interval. The cumulative DVH gives the volume of tissue, V(D), receiving a dose of at least D.

DVHs can be evaluated for specific anatomic regions (e.g., target and normal tissue as illustrated by Fig. 19.23) or can be evaluated for tissue irradiated by the implant without regard to anatomic boundaries. For bounded volumes, V(D) is flat below the minimum dose received by the structure. When evaluated over unbounded space, V(D) steeply increases with decreasing dose and asymptotically approaches the central point-source DVH, $V_{point}(\dot{D}) = (4\pi/3) \cdot [S_K \cdot \Lambda/\dot{D}]^{3/2}$. The use of DVHs has enriched discussions of dose specification by focusing attention on describing the 3D dose distribution rather than on single parameters. However, in the absence of target volume and nor-

mal tissue geometry, DVHs in themselves do not solve the dose-specification problem.

Because a quantitative description of the patient's anatomy is often lacking, several investigators have proposed figures of merit (FOMs) derived from DVHs that can be calculated without an anatomically defined target volume. Such FOMs may be useful for ranking the quality of competing implant geometries in terms of uniformity and normal-tissue sparing or for optimally selecting a specification dose rate for a given implant geometry. An important contribution is the "natural" DVH introduced by Anderson et al. (4,5). The natural DVH is a plot $\Delta V(u)/\Delta u$ where $u = D^{-3/2}$. The natural DVH plots as a horizontal line for a central point source. It suppresses r^{-2} effects, which dominate the conventional V(D) plot, making its detailed implant geometry–specific structure more evident. Low and Williamson (175) introduced an alternative modified DVH, $R_p(D) = V_{impl}(D)/V_{point}(D)$. Both of these modified DVHs show a sharply defined peak centered about MCD, the width and height of which quantify the volume of tissue receiving an approximately uniform dose. Other useful quality measures include the uniformity index (221) and the dose nonuniformity ratio (DNR) (252). The DNR, usually plotted as a function of reference dose, D_r, is defined as the ratio of volume receiving a specified multiple of D_r (usually 1.25 or 1.5) to that receiving at least D_r.

Target-volume–dependent DVH quality indices were introduced by Saw and Suntharalingam (251). For single- and double-plane implants designed to cover specified cubic target volumes, respectively, they defined three indices as a function of reference dose D_r. The coverage index, $CI(D_r)$, is that fraction of the target tissue receiving a dose $\geq D_r$. The homogeneity index, $HI(D_r)$, is the fraction of target volume receiving doses between D_r and 1.5 D_r. The external volume index, $EI(D_r)$, is the volume of tissue outside the target volume, expressed in multiples of the target volume, receiving dose rates $\geq D_r$. When these indices are plotted (Fig. 19.24), the tradeoffs among these clinical end points are evident. If a prescription dose rate is selected to maximize dose homogeneity (i.e., maximize HI), then 85% to 95% coverage of the target must be accepted. To minimize irradiation of tissue outside the target, both target coverage and dose homogeneity must be compromised. Low and Williamson (175) suggested ranking competing implant geometries by specifying the HI achieved for the maximum reference dose level that yields a CI of unity. Zwicker and Schmidt-Ullrich (322) have applied this general approach to the problem of identifying optimal interplane separations in double-plane implants.

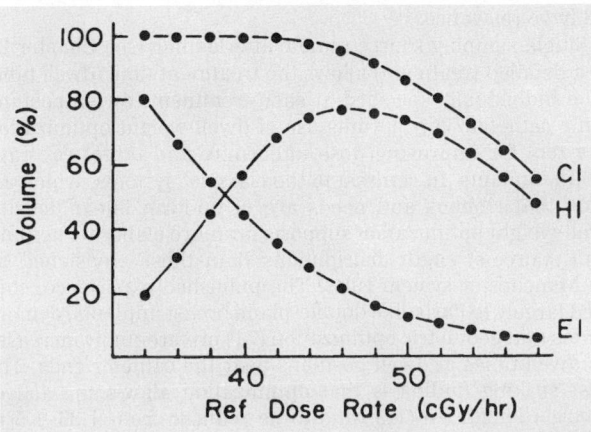

FIGURE 19.24. Plot of coverage index (CI), external index (EI), and homogeneity index (HI) as a function of reference dose rate for double-plane implant consisting of five ^{192}Ir ribbons with seven 1-mCi seeds in each plane and a 6-cm × 6-cm × 2.5-cm target volume. Ribbon and plane spacings of 1.5 cm were used. (From Saw CB, Suntharalingam N. Reference dose rates for single and double plane ^{192}Ir implants. *Med Phys* 1988;15:391, with permission.)

For TRUS-guided prostate implantation, DVH metrics such as D_{100}, D_{99}, and D_{90}, denoting the minimum doses administered to the highest dose volumes covering 100%, 99%, and 90% of the contoured CTV or PTV (planned target volume), respectively, have become widely accepted as reporting parameters (197). Volumetric indices, such as the V_{150}, V_{100}, and V_{90}, which denote the fraction of the CTV or PTV receiving at least 150%, 100%, and 90%, respectively, of the prescribed dose, are recommended to assess dose homogeneity and to assess adequacy with which the prescription has been fulfilled.

Modern Developments in Temporary Interstitial Brachytherapy

Three modern developments in brachytherapy planning and delivery technology have significantly influenced implant design and utilization of classical system rules. They include computer isodose calculations, dwell-weight optimization of single-stepping source remotely afterloaded implants, and utilization of 3D imaging to define target volumes and to guide applicator insertion.

Computer isodose calculations for interstitial implants were introduced in the early 1960s (298) and, along with software for reconstructing implant geometry from radiographs, have been routinely available for about 25 years. In contrast to the older classical systems, which are based on idealized geometries, computer-assisted planning capability permits evaluation of the dose distribution for the implant geometry actually realized in the patient. Thus the brachytherapist can compensate for deviations between the actual and intended implant geometries through selection of the prescription isodose or by modifying the catheter loadings or locations. In principle, dose calculation capability permits preprocedure customization of catheter spacings, loadings, and locations relative to the target boundary as an alternative to classical system distribution rules. Because manual forward planning is so time intensive, only a small number of alternative plans can be compared in practice. However, use of computer dose calculation to design implants and to specify dose has displaced the tables and implant rules of the classical systems in many U.S. centers. Khan (130) calls this approach the "computer system" and points outs that, in fact, it does assume simple guidelines for distributing the sources. These include 1-cm intercatheter spacing, uniform loading, and implanting to the margin of the tumor. Dose specification usually is based on the concept of MID, described earlier. Thus, even in the era of computerized dose calculation, distribution rules derived from one of the historical implant systems still have relevance.

Single-stepping source remote afterloading (see Chapter 21 for a detailed treatment) allows the treatment time (dwell time) to be individually specified at each treatment (dwell) position in the catheter. This permits use of dwell-weight optimization as a tool for improving dose uniformity and target coverage within implants. In contrast to the classical systems, which assume that ribbons and needs are of uniform linear density, dwell-weight optimization supports far more elaborate nonuniform source-strength distributions than those envisioned by the Manchester system rules. The published experience, confined largely to Paris-like double-plane breast implants, demonstrates that geometric optimization (71) preferentially increases the dwell times at dwell positions near the catheter ends. The most striking finding is that optimization allows the active-to-target length (AL/TL) ratio to be reduced from 1.33–1.5 to 1.1–1.25 (2,137,230). In the transverse plane, target coverage remains unchanged, whereas dose homogeneity is improved modestly, depending on the figure of merit used to quantify this effect. When dose-point optimization (specifying dose constraints at dose calculation points throughout the treatment

volume) is used, acceptable dose homogeneity results with even smaller AL/TL ratios, even when all peripheral dwell positions are placed inside the target volume (AL/TL = 1.0) (76,175) for idealized volume implants and clinical volume implants (137). These early efforts did not address the practical problem of how to distribute dose-constraint points in clinical volume implants with irregular catheter spacings and how to select dwell positions to be activated in each catheter. Although dwell-weight optimization techniques have the potential to reduce AL/TL ratios to near unity with good CI and HI, the direction and location of the catheters relative to the target, they thus require distribution rules drawn from the classical systems or one's own clinical experience.

The use of 3D imaging to preplan implants or intraoperatively guide catheter or seed insertion is growing rapidly. The most widely practiced form of image-guided brachytherapy is use of intraoperative TRUS to guide transperineal insertion of needles used to implant the prostate gland with low-energy seeds (19,117). However, image-guided implant methodologies have been developed for HDR interstitial implantation of breast (277) and prostate cancers (72). All of these approaches require delineation of the target volume and critical structure surfaces from 3D imaging studies. Then catheter or needle trajectories and, ultimately, seed or dwell position locations can be selected to improve target volume coverage while minimizing unnecessary dose to critical structures.

As practiced by most brachytherapists, image-guided, intraoperatively planned implants continue to rely on the planner's judgment for selecting source locations. These decisions are guided by a "loading approach," or set of guidelines that specify margins, seed locations relative to the target boundary, spacings, and approximate periphery-to-core loading ratios (36,72). Dose calculations and DVH quality indices often are used to guide manual source position adjustments to improve target volume coverage, improve dose homogeneity, and select source strengths (or dwell times) and the prescription isodose.

An important advance is anatomy-based optimization in which constraints and treatment goals are defined in terms of doses to the CTV or normal tissues. For example, in the simulated annealing HDR dwell-time optimization technique developed by Lessard and Pouliot (155), the objective function to be minimized consists of penalty factors summed over dose calculation points in the CTV, urethra, rectum, and other organs. The penalty factors are functions that increase linearly for doses that fall outside the dose range specified by the physician. Other authors have investigated anatomy-based multiobjective gradient-descent optimization algorithms (146,189) for HDR brachytherapy while others have applied simulated annealing (238), genetic algorithms (319), and mixed-integer programming (153) to the problem of selecting optimal source locations in permanent seed brachytherapy (see Ezzell's review [77] for a highly readable introduction to optimization techniques). The inverse planning technique for HDR brachytherapy developed by Lessard and Pouliot (155) shows significantly reduced CTV dose heterogeneity (V150 of 29% vs. 50%) and urethral doses in clinical prostate implants compared to geometric optimization (145). Anatomy-based optimization also solves the problem of selecting active dwell positions and locations for dose-constraint points faced by the older dose-point optimization algorithms. Although anatomy-based inverse planning does not optimize catheter trajectories, its proponents argue that it reduces the dependence of implant quality on distribution used and deviations of actual from intended catheter positions (237). In support of this hypothesis, they present data showing that the favorable dose homogeneity, prostate coverage, and normal tissue avoidance achieved in inverse-planned prostate implants are independent of the number of catheters implanted in the 9 to 21 range. If this hypothesis is validated, inverse planning could reduce the importance of system-based implant guidelines and distribution rules.

In summary, computerized dose calculation, dwell-weight optimization, and image-guided brachytherapy have made anatomy-based dose specification and meaningful implant optimization a reality in some clinical settings. However, as currently available, these innovations still require users to conceptually plan implants in terms of specified source- and needle-distribution patterns, implant-target volume margins, and loading ratios. Specific rules borrowed from the classical systems (e.g., AL/TL ratios) may require significant modification when adapted to these modern technologies.

Permanent Implantation

In contrast to temporary implantation, in which treatment time is varied to control the total dose delivered, the dose delivered by a permanent implant is determined by the initial geometric arrangement of sources and S_K per source: once the patient is implanted, neither the total dose delivered nor the relative distribution can be modified easily. Up through the mid-1980s, manual planning and dose-calculation tools were used widely to estimate the number and density of sources needed to deliver the prescribed dose or to intraoperatively correct for deviations between the planned actual source locations. For radium-substitute sources (e.g., ^{198}Au), the Manchester Laughlin et al. (147) or Shalek et al. (256) tables and associated distribution rules have been used.

Manual planning aids for radium-equivalent sources cannot be applied to low-energy seed (^{125}I and ^{103}Pd) implants because of the importance of tissue attenuation in this energy range. The influence of photon energy on the relationship between dose rate, $\dot{D}$, and implanted volume, V, is illustrated by Figure 19.25. Parker (216) recognized that this relationship can be described accurately by a power-law formula, of the form

$$\dot{D} = \alpha \cdot S_K \cdot V^{-\beta} \qquad (36)$$

In fact, the original Manchester table (Table 19.8), converted to modern units and quantities, can be derived from equation 36 by setting $\alpha = 3.49$ and $\beta = 2/3$. As the data from Anderson et al. (6) and Yu et al. (318) illustrate, ^{103}Pd and ^{125}I volume implants also can be described in terms of a power-law formula. Low-energy seed implants have somewhat larger exponents, β, demonstrating that dose rate falls off faster with increasing volume than for radium-substitute sources. The proportionality constants, α, are substantially lower, indicating that low-energy seed implants require higher source strengths to achieve a stated dose rate. The author-to-author variations in α values for the same radionuclide are due, in part, to differences in dose specification and implant construction. The data from Anderson et al., based on the pre-TRUS era Memorial nomogram, assume that dose is specified in terms of matched peripheral dose (MPD) and that all seeds are implanted 2 to 5 mm inside the target (prostate) boundary, whereas the analysis of Yu et al. assumes that peripheral seeds are implanted on or outside the boundary and that minimum target dose is specified. Such manual planning tools (139,203,312,318) are available for various types of prostate implants. These planning tools assume a variety of underlying single-source dose-rate distributions, seed arrangements, dose-specification criteria, and absolute prescribed doses, yielding estimated seed strengths that differ significantly from one another. Before using one of these methods for quality assurance checks or preplanning, it is important to assess carefully its consistency with dose calculation and the planning methods used in specific clinical practices.

The best-known manual planning tool for permanent ^{125}I implantation is the Memorial dimension averaging method (3,6). The associated nomogram was used for manual intraoperative planning of implants delivered by directly implanting seeds into

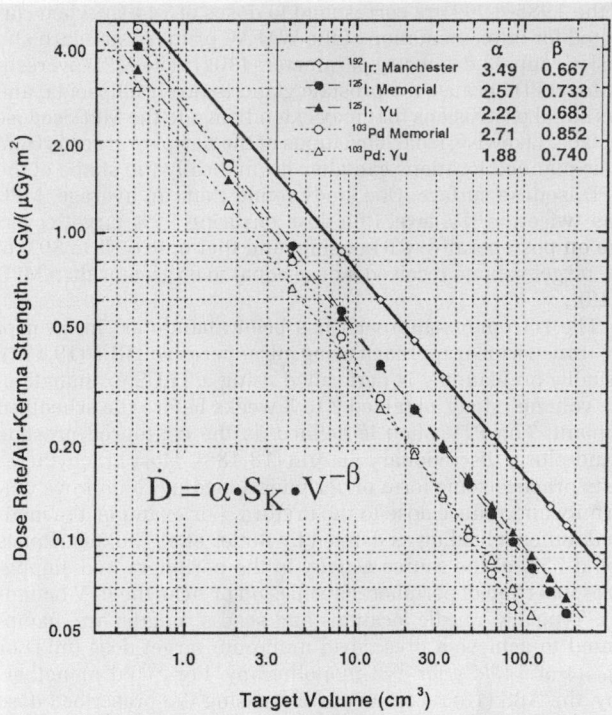

FIGURE 19.25. Comparison of reference dose rate per unit air-kerma strength versus volume of the target volume for Manchester volume implants and ^{103}Pd and ^{125}I permanent prostate implants. The inset gives the exponents and proportionality constants needed to describe these relationships in terms of a simple power-law equation 36. (The data in the figure are from Yu Y, Waterman FM, Suntharalingham N, et al. Limitations of the minimum peripheral dose as a parameter for dose specification in permanent ^{125}I prostate implants. *Int J Radiat Oncol Biol Phys* 1996;34:717–725; Anderson LL, Moni JV, Harrison LB. A nomograph for permanent implants of Palladium-103 seeds. *Int J Radiat Oncol Biol Phys* 1993;27:129–135; and Parker HM. A dosage system for interstitial radium therapy. II. Physical aspects. *Br J Radiol* 1938;11:252–266.)

the surgically exposed prostate, known as the retropubic approach. After surgical exposure of the target volume (prostate), the three orthogonal dimensions of target volume are measured, and the arithmetic mean of these measurements, or average diameter, d_a, in units of centimeter, is calculated. Next, the total apparent activity, A_{app} (in mCi units), to be implanted is calculated as follows:

$$A_{app} = \begin{cases} 5 \cdot d_a & d_a < 3\,\text{cm} \\ 1.34 \cdot d_a^{2.2} & d_a \geq 3\,\text{cm} \end{cases} \qquad (37)$$

Then, using a nomogram, consisting of several juxtaposed logarithmic scales, the total number of seeds needed is estimated graphically given the strength per seed. Other nomogram scales were used to estimate the spacing between needles given the seed spacing along each needle track. The seeds are to be implanted inside the target volume boundary, such that peripheral needle-to-target boundary distance is <50% of the interneedle spacing. Anderson et al. (6) have extended the dimension-averaging nomogram to ^{103}Pd and reviewed the underlying assumptions of this method.

Equation 37 is designed to deliver an MPD of 160 Gy over the life of the implant when d_a is more than 3 cm (6). MPD is defined as the dose level whose corresponding 3D isodose surface encompasses a volume, V_E, equal to that of an ellipsoid having the same orthogonal dimensions as the originally measured target volume ($V_E = \pi d_x d_y d_z /6$). For a given implant, MPD is derived from the corresponding cumulative DVH, V(D), according to $V_E = V(MPD)$. By design, the Memorial nomogram delivers significantly higher MPDs to target volumes with average dimensions <3 cm. Prescribed doses of 160 Gy delivered in the 1985–1999 era correspond to doses of 144 Gy when corrected for implementation of the WAFAC primary standard and Task Group 43 dosimetry parameters (302). The MPD overestimates mPD because the prostate gland is rarely ellipsoidal and has small protrusions that may extend outside the MPD isodose surface. Likewise, small deviations of the peripheral seeds from their planned locations can alter dramatically the shape of the MPD isodose surface. One study found that, on average, MPD was twice the D_{99} level (the dose ensuring 99% target coverage on postoperative CT imaging) and that only 69% to 89% of the target volume received a dose equal to or greater than MPD (249).

The retropubic approach has been abandoned in favor of the transperineal approach using intraoperative TRUS (19,117). Usually, preplanning is performed using a TRUS examination, or "volume" study, obtained 2 to 3 weeks before the scheduled implant. The PTV often is defined as the contoured prostate gland plus a discretionary margin (18,188). Most brachytherapists practice some form of peripheral loading to improve uniformity and reduce dose to the urethra. For example, the modified uniform loading as defined by Butler et al. (36) distributes about 75% of the source activity in the periphery and emphasizes insertion of peripheral needles on or near the PTV boundary. Typically, needle locations and seed strengths are manipulated to achieve a prescribed minimum target dose (mPD or $D_{100\%}$) of 145 Gy for ^{125}I monotherapy. For ^{103}Pd monotherapy, the ABS (16) recommends increasing the prescribed dose from historically used 115 Gy to 125 Gy following implementation of the NIST $S_{K,N99}$ standard and recently revised TG-43 parameters, based on the AAPM's analysis (304) of the impact of historical changes in calibration standards and dosimetry practice. AAPM's most recent historical analysis of ^{103}Pd prescribed-to-administered doses (300) indicates that a 120 Gy prescribed dose may better reproduce the published clinical experience.

Dose specification, for recording and reporting doses actually administered by a permanent implant, is based on postimplant dose evaluation (317). Following the implant procedure, a CT scan is obtained; The prostate gland, rectum, and bladder are contoured; And the seed locations are identified from the transverse images. The choice of dose-specification parameter for this purpose has been the subject of intense investigation. Based on analysis of both idealized and actual implants, Yu et al. (318) found that the postinsertion D_{100} was very sensitive to small random displacements of the seeds from their intended positions, which resulted in underdoses of 15% or more to small volumes in the target periphery. However, they found that the mPD of the idealized implant (no seed displacement) covered at least 90% of the target (i.e., $D_{90} \geq$ mPD and $V_{100} \geq$ 90%), even in the face of 6-mm seed displacements. In a study of 60 consecutive implant patients, Merrick et al. (188) found mean V_{100} and D_{90} values of 94% of the CT prostate volume and 108% of the prescribed dose (mPD of preplanned implant), respectively. Of the patients, 82% had a D_{90} exceeding the preplanned mPD and no patient had a D_{90} smaller than 90% of mPD. In contrast, D_{100} was only 68% of the prescribed mPD, on average. Two groups (236,261) have found a correlation between prostate-specific antigen (PSA) relapse-free survival at 4 years and D_{90}. In particular, Potters et al. (236) found a D_{90} dose-response cutoff of 90% of the prescribed dose but could find no statistically significant cutoffs for D_{100} and V_{100}. The clinical significance of such limited-volume underdosages is not clear. Based on LQ theory, Ling et al. (164) argued that larger tumor kills in central voxels irradiated to doses 20% to 30% above D_{100} can partially offset the loss of tumor-control probability as a result of large but focal underdosages near the tumor periphery. For postimplant CT-based dose evaluation, the ABS recommends that D_{100}, D_{90}, and D_{80} be reported along with V_{80}, V_{90}, V_{100}, V_{150}, and V_{200} (197).

Intracavitary Brachytherapy

In contrast to the comparatively uniform dose distributions of interstitial brachytherapy, the unidirectional source arrangements used in gynecologic intracavitary brachytherapy give rise to dose distributions that fall off rapidly with distance from the applicator surface, producing large dose gradients across the target volume. Such large dose gradients make target volume-based dose specification difficult and give this treatment modality a highly empirical character. Numerous parameters have been used to prescribe, constrain, or report intracavitary therapy applications, including mg-h, mg Ra Eq-h, reference point doses (points A and B), bladder and rectal reference point doses, vaginal surface dose, treatment time, and the ICRU Report No. 38 (122) 60-Gy reference volume. This section will emphasize the physical relationships among these parameters and their dependence on applicator characteristics. Systems for treating carcinoma of the cervix, the most intensively studied form of intracavitary therapy, will be reviewed. Our focus will be further restricted to applicator geometries and treatment systems (e.g., Fletcher and Washington University/Mallinckrodt systems) derived from the Manchester system. This limited focus is justified by the fact that Manchester- or Fletcher-style applicators continue to be the dominant choice across the world for both HDR and LDR treatments.

The Manchester Family of Intracavitary Therapy Systems

The Manchester system, developed in 1938 by Tod and Meredith (271), has heavily influenced intracavitary treatment practice patterns throughout the world, especially in North America. The widely used Fletcher-Suit applicator system, the Fletcher loadings, and the point A and B reference points are all derived from the Manchester system. This system was the first to use applicators and loadings designed to satisfy specific dosimetric constraints (271,272). It was the first system to use a radiation field quantity, exposure at point A, rather than mg-h, to specify treatment.

The Classical Manchester System

The original Manchester applicator system consisted of a rubber intrauterine tandem and two vaginal "ovoids," whose ellipsoidal shape was designed to conform to the isodose curves arising from ^{226}Ra tubes placed along their long axes. The applicators were designed for use with ^{226}Ra tubes 2.2-cm long with 1-mm platinum filtration and an active length between 1 and 1.5 cm. The small, medium, and large ovoid minimum diameters were 2, 2.5, and 3 cm, respectively, and are the same as Fletcher's small, medium, and large colpostats (83). The preloaded ovoids contained no shielding and relied on extensive anterior and posterior packing to spare bladder and rectal tissue.

The reference point A (Fig. 19.26) originally was defined as the point "2 cm lateral to the center of the uterine canal and 2 cm from the mucous membrane of the lateral fornix in the plane of the uterus" (271). This seemingly arbitrary definition reflected the system developers' view that "radiation necrosis is not the result of direct effects of radiation on the bladder and rectum, but high dose effects in the area in medial edge of the broad ligament where the uterine vessels cross the ureter" (187). They believed the radiation tolerance of this area, termed "the paracervical triangle," to be the limiting factor in the treatment of cervical cancer and used point A exposure to represent its average dose. In current practice, point A dose is used to approximate the average or minimum dose to the tumor. Point B, defined to be 5 cm from the patient's midline at the same

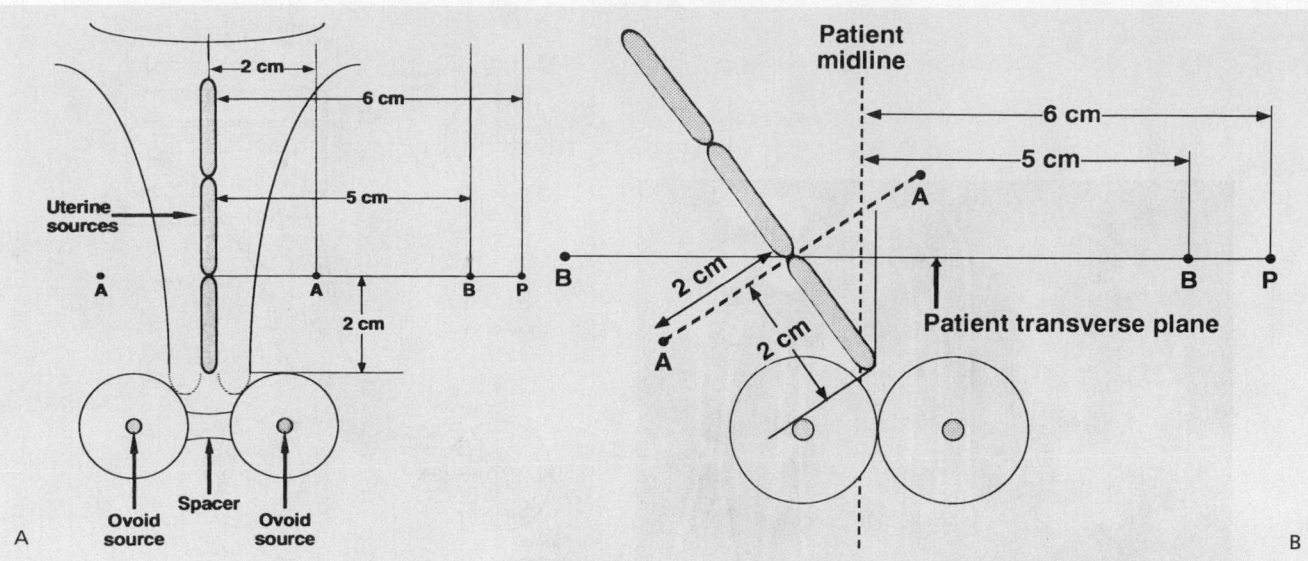

FIGURE 19.26. Definition of points A and B in an ideal application **(A)** and a distorted application **(B)**, which is displaced to the left of the patient's midline, and a uterus, which is tilted toward the right. Note that point A is carried with the uterus, whereas points B and P are defined to be 5 and 6 cm, respectively, to the right and left of patient midline. Point P is used by the Mallinckrodt Institute of Radiology System to specify minimum dose to the pelvic lymph nodes. (Adapted from Meredith WJ. Dosage for cancer of cervix uteri. In: Meredith WJ, eds. *Radium Dosage: The Manchester System,* 2nd ed. Edinburgh: E. & S. Livingston, Ltd, 1967;42–50, with permission.)

level as point A, was intended to quantify the dose delivered to the obturator lymph nodes.

The Manchester ovoid dimensions and applicator loadings were designed to ensure that the point A dose rate, about 0.52 Gy/h in modern units, remained constant for all allowed applicator loadings and combinations. The design also ensured that the vaginal contribution to point A was limited to 40% of the total dose. Small, medium, and large ovoids were loaded with 17.5, 20, and 22.5 mg of radium, respectively, to compensate for the greater source-to-point A treatment distances with the larger ovoids. Medium (4-cm long) and long (6 cm) tandems were loaded, os to fundus, with source trains consisting of 10 and 15 mg sources and 10, 10, and 15 mg sources, respectively, whereas the short tandem (used for cervical stump cancer) was loaded with a single 20-mg radium tube. With the exception of the short tandem, these loadings satisfied the dosimetric constraints within 2%. The point B dose, determined largely by inverse-square law, was calculated by the formula 9 Gy to point B for every 4,000 mg-h administered.

Without external-beam treatment to the whole pelvis, a total point A exposure of 8,000 R (72.8 Gy) in 140 hours split between two applications traditionally was prescribed (272). Because the point A dose rate is constant whether the application contains 60 mg of ^{226}Ra (small ovoids, medium tandem) or 80 mg (large ovoids, long tandem), delivery of a fixed point A dose amounts to using time, not mg-h, as the factor that terminates the treatment. In contrast to the Paris and Stockholm systems, which prescribed a fixed number of mg-h, equivalent Manchester treatment regimens could deliver from 8,400 to 11,200 mg-h—a variation of 33%.

As the size of an intracavitary application (i.e., colpostat diameter and tandem length) increases, the penetration or "lateral throw-off" of the dose distribution increases. As colpostat diameter increases from 2 to 3 cm, the vaginal surface dose decreases by 35% relative to the dose 2 cm from the applicator surface; This is simply a consequence of increasing the source-to-surface distance. Similarly, increasing the tandem length increases the point B contribution relative to the uterine cavity surface dose; The radioactivity near the ends of the long tandem contributes little to the surface dose (because of inverse-square

law), whereas each tandem segment makes roughly equal contributions to points remote from the applicator. These physical principles underlie the practice of using the largest colpostats and longest tandem that the patient's anatomy can accommodate (84,272).

Modern Fletcher-Suit Applicator Systems

The Fletcher applicator system (Fig. 19.27A) adhered to the basic Manchester design while incorporating many improvements including internal shielding. These shields are located on the medial aspects of the anterior and posterior colpostat faces (Fig. 19.27B) and consist of 180-degree and 150-degree disc-shaped 3- to 5-mm thick tungsten sectors to shield the rectum and bladder respectively (83). The cylindrical colpostat body has a diameter of 2 cm that can be increased to 2.5 and 3 cm by use of small and large slip-on plastic caps, thereby retaining the Manchester ovoid dimensions. Afterloading capability was added to the Fletcher applicator by Suit et al. (264). The Fletcher loadings—15, 20, and 25 mg for small, medium, and large colpostats, respectively—are similar to those of the Manchester system, whereas tandem loadings are identical to their Manchester counterparts. Because of the similarity of Fletcher loadings (55 to 85 mg) to the Manchester loadings, point A dose rates are nearly independent of applicator dimensions.

The shielded Fletcher colpostat was designed to reduce the dose to the bladder trigone and the anterior rectal wall without decreasing irradiation to the uterosacral and broad ligaments, thereby reducing the need for extensive vaginal packing characteristic of Manchester insertions (83). For a single colpostat (Fig. 19.27B–D), the maximum dose reduction varies from 40% to 50% (58,100,291). When the effects of the intrauterine tandem and the contralateral colpostat are included, applicator shielding reduces midline rectal and bladder doses by 21% to 34% relative to conventional treatment planning calculations, which ignore shielding and include only the effects of source encapsulation (180). CT-based dose evaluation studies reveal that colpostat shielding modestly reduces rectal doses, reducing the rectal $D_{2\%}$ by 2% to 11% (260) and D_{2cc} by 10% (90). Modern versions of the shielded Fletcher colpostat for LDR brachytherapy

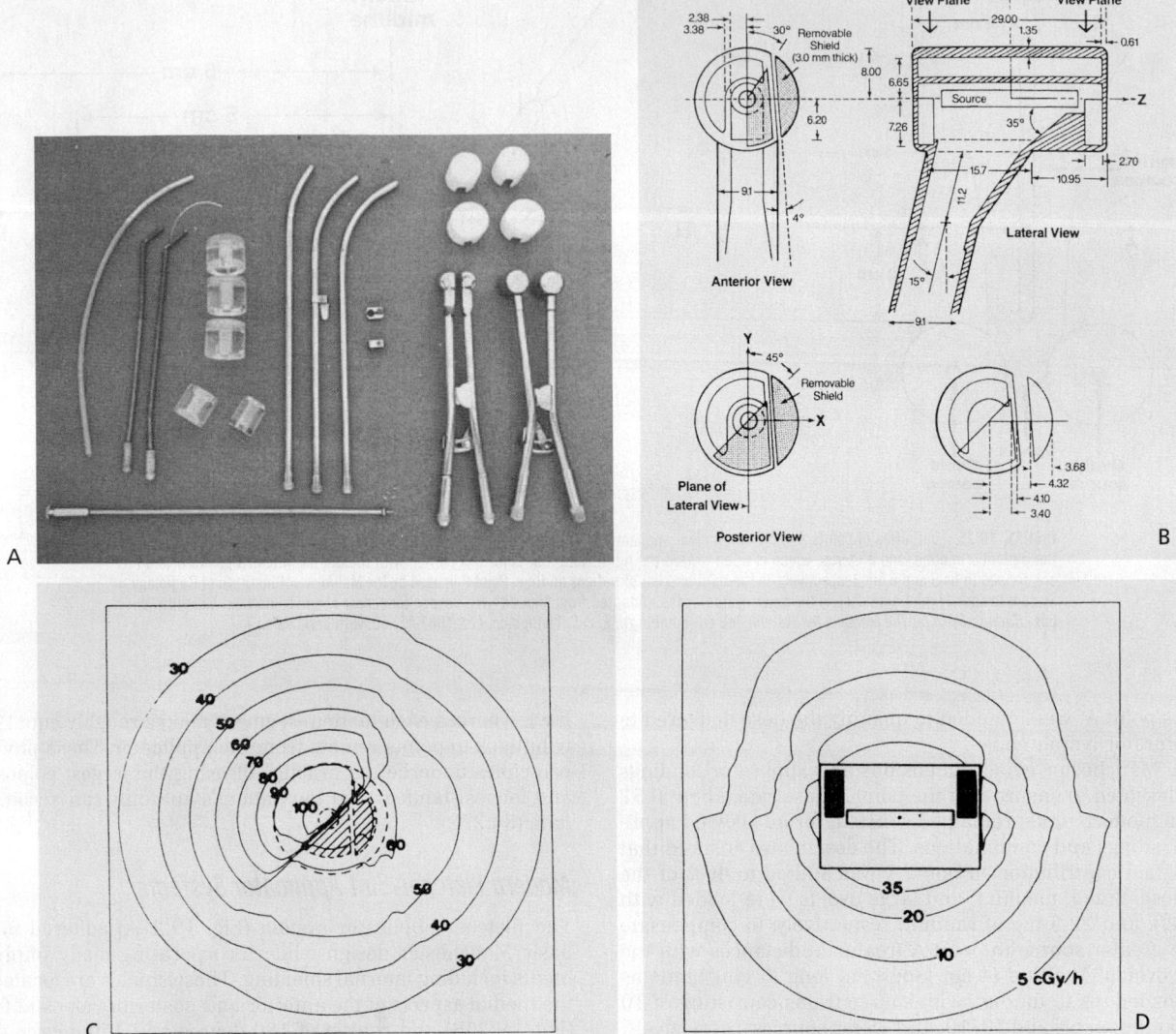

FIGURE 19.27. A: Fletcher-Suit applicator system. From left to right are tandem insert loaded with dummy sources, colpostat source holders, vaginal cylinder sleeves, three curvatures of intrauterine tandems, cervical collars, Delclos mini-colpostats, and round-handled Fletcher-Suit colpostats with small and medium caps. The tubelike instrument in the left foreground is a cervical localization seed implanter. (From Fletcher GH, Hamberger AD. Squamous cell carcinoma of the uterine cervix: Treatment techniques according to size of the cervical lesion and extension. In: Fletcher GD, eds. *Textbook of radiotherapy.* 3rd ed. Philadelphia: Lea & Febiger, 1980;732–772, with permission). **B:** Three orthogonal views of the 3M Fletcher-Suit Delclos colpostat, consisting of a stainless steel body. The removable parts of the tungsten alloy shield, which allow conversion of the applicator to a shielded Delclos mini-colpostat, are inset into a nylon cap (not shown) with an outer diameter of 2 cm. Shown are isodose curves **(C)** in the coronal plane 10 mm from the posterior face of the applicator and **(D)** in the transverse plane of the colpostat for a 72 μGy $\times$ m^2 $\times$ h^{-1} ^{137}Cs tube. (Figures B–D reproduced from Williamson JF. Dose calculations about shielded gynecological colpostats. *Int J Radiat Oncol Biol Phys* 1990;19:167–178, with permission.)

include the LDR 3M (3M Corporation, St. Paul, MN) Fletcher-Suit-Delclos (FSD) (291) and reproductions of the round-handled Fletcher-Suit (58) colpostats. For HDR brachytherapy, the Fletcher-Williamson applicator duplicates the original Fletcher shielding configuration (239). Weeks and Montana (285) have designed a CT-compatible version with afterloadable shields and an aluminum body having the same dimensions as the FSD applicator.

Dose Specification in Intracavitary Brachytherapy

Point A Dose and Milligram-Hours

Two quantities are used widely to prescribe intracavitary brachytherapy: mg-h (or its modern equivalent, IRAK) is used in

practices influenced by the M.D. Anderson Cancer Center system (84,118,225) and Table 19.10, whereas some form of the Manchester point A dose specification is used by most other practitioners. Efforts to unify these two prescription practices by identifying a linear relationship between these quantities are misguided from the perspective of the Manchester system (232). The Manchester-like loadings specified by the Washington University/Mallinckrodt Institute of Radiology (WU) clearly show (Fig. 19.28) that despite a twofold variation in source strength loaded into the smallest versus the largest applicator system, the point A dose rate varies by only 15%. To deliver a fixed point A dose of 65 Gy with WU loadings, a constant total treatment time of approximately 100 hours is needed, resulting in delivery of mg Ra Eq-h ranging from 5,200 to 10,000 in any sample of patients characterized by a range of applicator sizes. Conversely, for fixed mg Ra Eq-h, prescription would result in

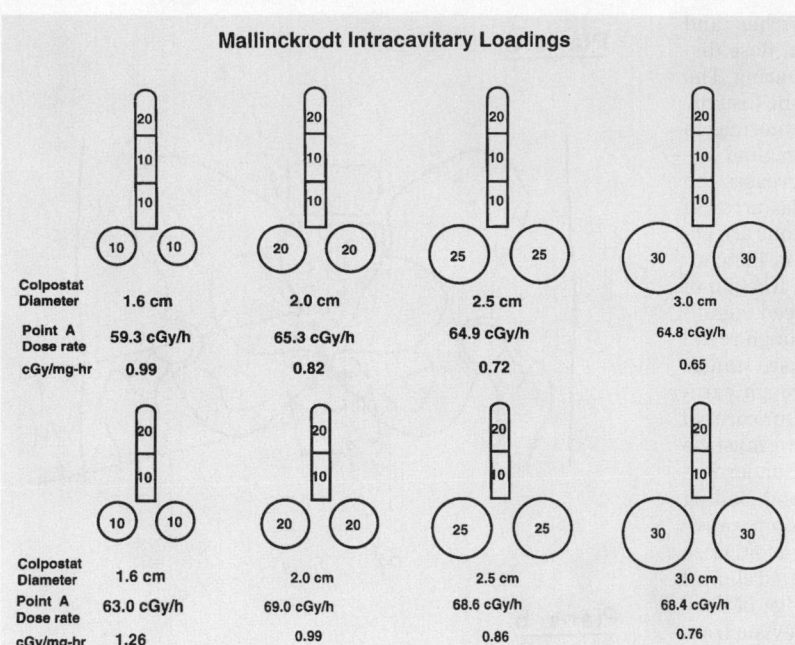

FIGURE 19.28. Mallinckrodt Institute of Radiology/Washington University (WU) applicator loadings used with Fletcher-Suit applicators for treatment of cervix carcinoma. Because the WU system uses Model 6500 3M ^{137}Cs tubes, equivalent mass of radium is used to specify loadings and mg Ra Eq-h, rather than mg-h, to prescribe intracavitary therapy. The point A dose rates assume the classical Manchester definition and average colpostat separations and tandem-colpostat alignments.

a nearly twofold variation in total treatment time and point A dose.

The proportionality of point A dose and treatment time applies only to the classical (Manchester) definition of point A. Many radiation oncologists use a revised definition of point A (Fig. 19.29) that references its location to the cervical os (tandem collar, proximal aspect of the most caudal tandem source, or a gold seed implanted in the cervix) rather than to the lateral fornix. This practice obscures the relationship between point A and mg-h prescription philosophies. Potish and Gerbi's (232) study of 90 Fletcher applications demonstrates that the revised point A dose rates vary widely from patient to patient and are, on average, significantly higher than the classical Manchester value. Because point A is fixed to the tandem and the vertical tandem-to-colpostat displacement varies with each patient, the vaginal contribution to point A is highly variable. In contrast, classically defined point A dose rates are tightly grouped, are independent of the loading, and are in close agreement with the Tod-Meredith value. The vaginal contribution to classical point A is fixed by definition, whereas the intrauterine contribution is insensitive to colpostat-to-tandem displacement because of the parallel tandem isodose curves. Thus, the revised point A definition does not have the physical significance of the classical quantity. Use of revised point A dose to prescribe therapy for "free-floating" tandem and colpostat insertions may introduce large patient-to-patient fluctuations in treatment times because of small, clinically insignificant variations in implant geometry.

The previous discussion is applicable only to the Fletcher applicator system with relative loadings approximating those of the Manchester system. As the intrauterine-to-vaginal loading ratio (1:1 for the Manchester system) increases, and the maximum width of the pear-shaped reference isodoses falls and the rectal dose increases (38). Appreciation of how loading influences isodose shape and normal-tissue doses is especially important in HDR brachytherapy because availability of dwell-weight optimization invites deviation from classical loading rules. Using judiciously placed dose points to control the relative dimensions of the point A isodose surface, Mai et al. (177) were able to increase tapering near the cephalad aspect of the tandem to reduce the vaginal surface dose and to modestly reduce the rectal dose with only slight loss of the maximum width of the pear-shaped isodose. These considerations suggest that dose-point driven optimization of the dwell-weight distribution should be accompanied by a geometric analysis of the point A isodose surface (see ICRU Report 38 discussion later in this chapter) so that changes to target coverage can be assessed at least approximately.

Other applicators in current use include the HDR tandem and ring applicator (121) and the LDR Henschke applicator (111). The latter consists of hemispheric colpostats rigidly attached to the tandem with the vaginal source axes parallel to the intrauterine sources rather than transverse as in the Fletcher system. Henschke colpostats with internal shielding (191) are

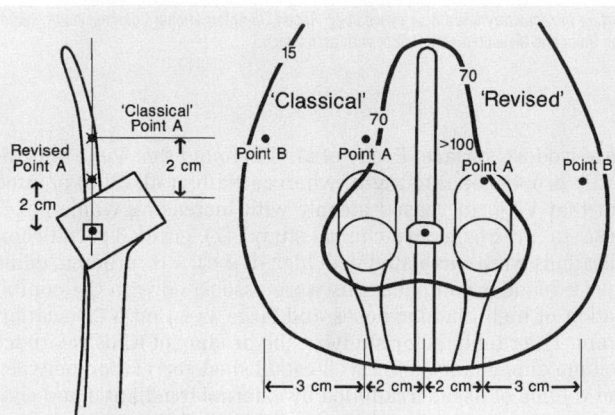

FIGURE 19.29. Radiographic definition of classical point A (2 cm above the cephalic-most aspect of the colpostat in the tilted coronal plane) and the revised point A (2 cm above the cervical collar top or center). Because the distance from caudal-most intrauterine source tip to colpostat center (tandem-to-colpostat displacement) varies from patient to patient, the vaginal contribution to revised point A is highly variable. (From Potish RA, Gerbi BJ. Role of point A in the era of computerized dosimetry. *Radiology* 1986;158:827–831, with permission.) The revised definition was suggested in Tod M, Meredith WJ. Treatment of cancer of the cervix uteri: A revised Manchester method. *Br J Radiol* 1953;26:252–257.

available. Delclos et al. (58) note that the Fletcher and Henschke applicators system do not yield equivalent dose distributions, especially with respect to normal tissue sparing. The vaginal ring applicator consists of a circular guide tube (usually 34-mm outer diameter) with its plane fixed rigidly normal to the tandem. It is placed up against the cervix and vaginal fornices with a donut-shaped cap attached, which increases the distance between the vaginal mucosa and the circular array of dwell positions (of which only the lateral dwell positions are activated) to 7 mm (compared to 10 to 15 mm for the Fletcher colpostat). Analyses demonstrate (177,214) that the fraction of source strength loaded into the ring must be reduced significantly to avoid overdosing the vaginal mucosa. Although rectal and vaginal vault doses, relative to the point A dose, similar to that of the Fletcher system can be achieved through careful optimization, the lateral coverage, (i.e., maximum coronal width of the point A isodose) is reduced (177). Care must be taken in positioning the applicator system to avoid underdosing the gross tumor volume. Applicator geometry and loading practices should be changed only after extensive comparative evaluation of the old and new dose distributions to avoid dose distribution changes that would invalidate the evaluated clinical experience on which the brachytherapist's knowledge of dose response rests. Finally, for applicator systems that deviate from the classical Manchester geometry or relative loading rules, one cannot assume that point A dose is proportional to treatment time over all allowed variations of applicator sizes and loadings.

Volumetric Specification of Intracavitary Treatment: ICRU Report No. 38 Recommendations

The ICRU (122) introduced the concept of reference volume enclosed by the reference isodose surface for reporting and comparing intracavitary treatments performed in different centers regardless of the applicator system, insertion technique, and method of treatment prescription used. Specifically, ICRU Report No. 38 recommended that the reference volume be taken as the 60-Gy isodose surface, resulting from the addition of dose contributions from any external-beam whole-pelvis irradiation and all intracavitary insertions. The ICRU proposed that this pear-shaped reference volume (Fig. 19.30) be described in terms of its three orthogonal maximal dimensions: height (d_h), width (d_w), and thickness (d_t), measured in the oblique coronal and sagittal planes containing the intrauterine sources. Figure 19.31 illustrates the bladder and rectal reference points recommended by the ICRU.

In contrast to point A dose and mg Ra Eq-h, the ICRU proposal is only a means of describing or reporting treatment. No guidance is given as to how to prescribe treatment, use these measurements to evaluate implant quality, or correlate reference volume dimensions with clinical outcome. The 60 Gy dose-level choice appears to have been motivated by the preoperative radiotherapy regimen popular within the French school of radiotherapy (227). Descriptions of institution-specific treatment techniques for early-stage cervical cancer patients include rules for evaluating the 60-Gy reference volume dimensions and offsets relative to the applicator system for the allowed combinations of applicator dimensions and loadings (227). Subsequent investigation has followed two pathways. Potish et al. (231,233), and later Eisbruch et al. (73), investigated the relationship between the individual ICRU reference volume dimensions and the geometric characteristics of Fletcher implants (such as colpostat separation and vertical and horizontal displacement of the tandem from the colpostat centers) and found them to be moderately well correlated. Other investigators (47,75,205) have proposed using the product of ICRU dimensions, $V_{ICRU} = d_t \times d_w \times d_h$, to estimate the relative volume contained within the refer-

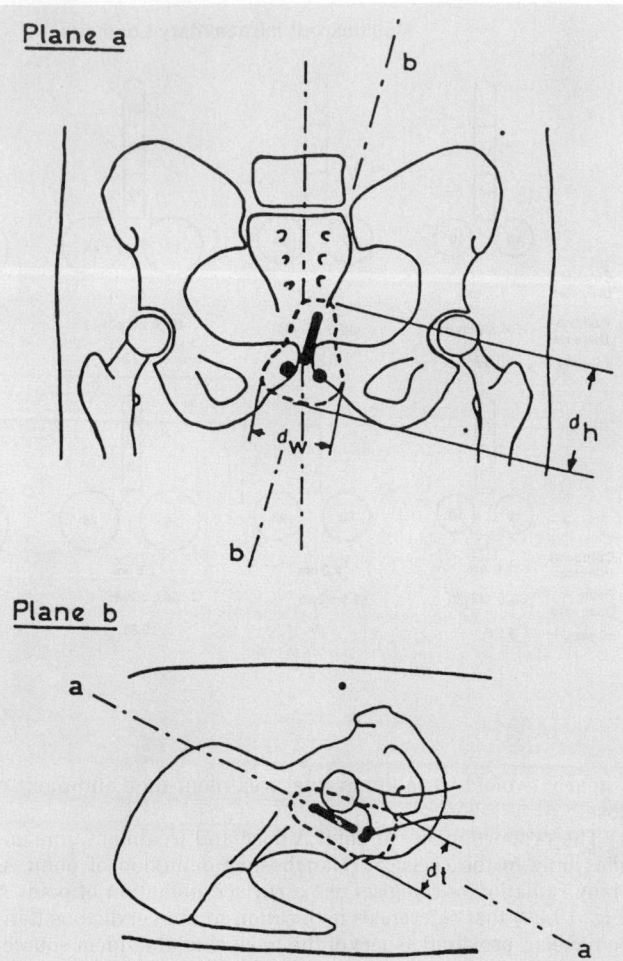

FIGURE 19.30. Geometry for measuring the three orthogonal dimensions of the pear-shaped ICRU (International Commission on Radiation Units and Measurements) reference isodose surface (*broken line*) in a typical treatment of cervix carcinoma using one rod-shaped uterine applicator and two vaginal applicators. Plane a (*top*) is the "oblique" frontal plane that contains the intrauterine device. The oblique frontal plane is obtained by rotation of the frontal plane around a transverse axis. Plane b (*bottom*) is the "oblique" sagittal plane that contains the intrauterine device. The oblique sagittal plane is obtained by rotation of the sagittal plane around the AP axis. The height (d_h) and the width (d_w) of the reference volume are measured in plane a as the maximal sizes parallel and perpendicular to the uterine applicator, respectively. The thickness (d_t) of the reference volume is measured in plane b as the maximal size perpendicular to the uterine applicator. (From ICRU. *Dose and volume specification for reporting intracavitary therapy in gynecology: Report 38.* International Commission of Radiation Units and Measurements, 1985, with permission.)

ence isodose surface. Esche et al. (75) found that V_{ICRU} was directly proportional to mg-h, whereas Nath et al. (205) pointed out that V_{ICRU} increased steeply with increasing whole-pelvis dose. In a retrospective clinical study (47), grade 3 rectal complications were correlated with high $d_t \times d_w \times d_h$ product, while severe bladder complications were associated with the combination of high bladder doses and large V_{ICRU} on a 2D scattergram. The rationale for studying the product of ICRU reference volume dimensions is the well-established correlation between the volume of tissue irradiated by external irradiation and clinical outcome (156). In contrast to ICRU 38 (122), which defines reference isodose surface dimensions for a single fixed dose level, these studies treat ICRU reference volume dimensions as functions of total dose or intracavitary dose.

The ICRU reference volume concept appropriately emphasizes that volume of tissue irradiated, as well as dose, is an important predictor of clinical response to intracavitary irradiation. Wilkinson and Ramachandran (287) and Eisbruch et al.

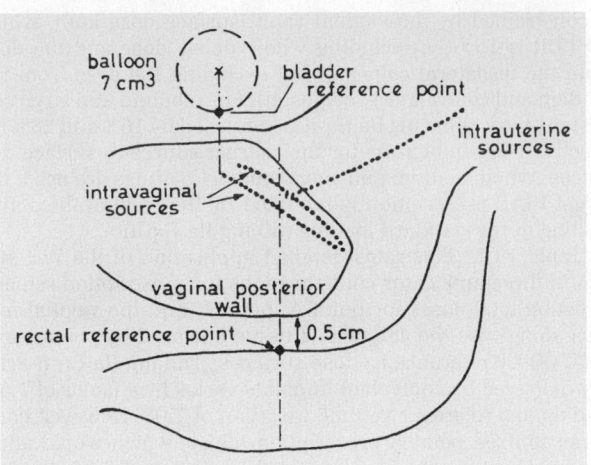

FIGURE 19.31. Reference points for bladder and rectal brachytherapy doses proposed by International Commission on Radiation Units and Measurements Report 38. (From ICRU. *Dose and volume specification for reporting intracavitary therapy in gynecology: Report 38.* International Commission of Radiation Units and Measurements, 1985, with permission.)

(73) used DVHs to study the correlation between volume enclosed by intracavitary isodose surfaces and other prescription parameters. The latter analyzed the volumetric characteristics of 204 intracavitary insertions in 128 patients with carcinoma of the cervix and demonstrated that intracavitary implants delivering the same mg Ra Eq-h have nearly identical DVHs over the dose range of clinical interest despite significant differences in geometry and loadings (Fig. 19.32). They also showed that the volume, V(D,M), enclosed by isodose surfaces can be estimated accurately from a modified power-law model requiring knowledge of only the intracavitary dose in cGy (D) and mg Ra

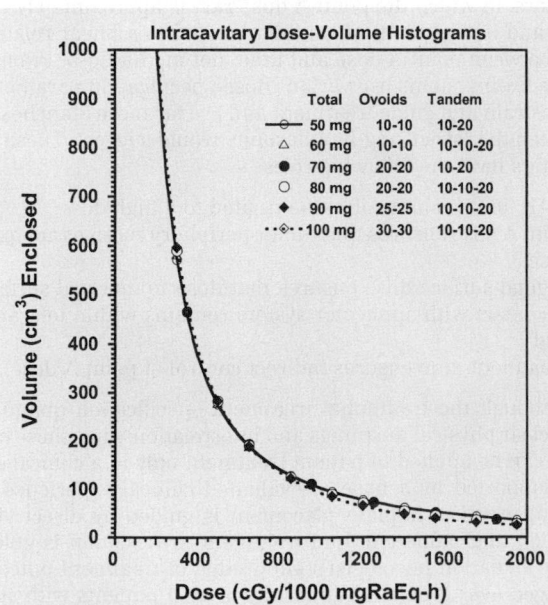

FIGURE 19.32. Dose-volume histograms for seven Mallinckrodt Institute of Radiology/Washington University (WU) intracavitary insertions using 1.4 cm active length ^{137}Cs sources. The strength of each source was determined by the loading rules for WU schema C (20 Gy, whole pelvis plus 8,000 mg Ra Eq-h) and then was scaled down to 1,000 mg Ra Eq-h. Note that as the size of the insertion increases, the volume of tissue encompassed by the high-dose isosurfaces decreases. Point A doses ranged from 8.28 to 11.35 Gy.

Eq-h (M):

$$V(D, M) = \left[104.8 - 8.103 \left(\frac{M}{D} \right) + 0.437 \left(\frac{M}{D} \right)^2 \right] \cdot \left(\frac{M}{D} \right)^{1.635}$$

(38)

The volume predicted by this simple model is accurate within ±10% in 95% of the implants when M/D is more than 0.8, which corresponds to an intracavitary dose of 100 Gy for 8,000 mg Ra Eq-h of intracavitary therapy. In addition, the practice of using the product of ICRU orthogonal dimensions to estimate the volume receiving a given intracavitary dose was found to be without physical foundation. The ratio of ICRU dimension product to the true volume given by DVH analysis, $d_t \times d_w \times d_h / V(D,M)$, varied widely from patient to patient and differed systematically from one implant type to another.

The consequences of equation 38 can be summarized as follows:

1. Volumetrically, an intracavitary implant behaves like a central point source:

$$V(D, M) \propto (M/D)^{3/2}$$

2. Describing an implant in terms of volume contained within its isodose curves carries no more information content than a statement of mg Ra Eq-h or total reference air-kerma.
3. The volume of tissue irradiated to a specified dose is closely related to total exposure given by the implant in terms of mg Ra Eq-h, TRAK, or IRAK.

The second consequence suggests that the correlation between clinical outcome, in terms of tumor control and complications, and isodose surface volume should be no better or worse than the correlation between clinical outcome and mg Ra Eq-h for a fixed external pelvis dose. Consequence three suggests a new and fundamental physical interpretation of mg Ra Eq-h or its derivative, total reference air-kerma. Prescribing intracavitary brachytherapy by mg Ra Eq-h is equivalent to treating until each specified isodose surface achieves a fixed volume independent of the underlying implant geometry. Use of mg Ra Eq-h to constrain intracavitary treatment therefore limits the volume of tissue irradiated to high doses. This observation may help explain the clinical utility of mg Ra Eq-h as a dose-specification parameter. Finally, the individual reference isodose dimensions, which are more strongly influenced by implant geometry than their product, clearly convey additional information about the spatial extension of the reference isodose surface in their respective planes, cannot be reduced to a statement of total exposure from the implant, and may have additional prognostic significance.

Practical Systems for Intracavitary Prescription and Reporting

For Manchester-like loadings and applicators, if treatment were to be prescribed as a fixed number of mg Ra Eq-h or IRAK without regard to the diameter and length of the applicators, the treatment times and total point A doses would differ by the ratio of total source strengths in the applications. Small applications would have unacceptably high point A and vaginal vault surface doses and excessively long treatment times. In contrast, large applications treated to a fixed mg Ra Eq-h prescription would underdose these reference points. In contrast, the ICRU reference volume for fixed levels of whole pelvic irradiation and mg Ra Eq-h would be independent of the loading because the mg Ra Eq-h is constant. Conversely, when the point A dose is held constant, the mg Ra Eq-h needed to deliver these doses will vary significantly, introducing corresponding variations in the volume of the ICRU reference isodose.

Clearly, no IRAK-based system would endorse such a naive approach. Actual mg Ra Eq-h–based systems use a combination of parameters. Physically, mg Ra Eq-h or IRAK controls the volume of tissue treated to high doses, and parameters such as time, colpostat surface dose, and point A are used to control doses at points near the applicator to ensure that surface tolerance is not exceeded and that the tumor is not undertreated. For each applicator combination and choice of external-beam dose, a compromise between volume of tissue treated and dose delivered near the applicator must be reached. For example, the Fletcher system (84,233) specifies both a maximum treatment time and maximum mg-h constraint for each combination of external-beam and intracavitary therapy (Table 19.10). Whichever constraint is reached first terminates the application. Small applications tend to be terminated by the maximum time constraint, which limits the mg-h and prevents tissues near the applicator from exceeding tolerance doses, whereas larger applications are terminated by the mg-h constraint, ensuring adequate dose to the tumor. Although the historical Fletcher system does not use point A dose either for prescription or reporting, the total point A dose is constant within 12% for allowed tandem and colpostat loadings within each treatment scheme (A–E) of Table 19.10. The reader should note that the Fletcher system is a complex, highly individualized treatment system that resists formulation in terms of a few rules. Table 19.10 is a highly condensed and simplified summary derived from the literature, not from observation of current M.D. Anderson Cancer Center practice patterns.

The WU system for prescribing intracavitary therapy illustrates another empirical approach for ensuring adequate dose delivery to the tumor while limiting the volume of tissue treated to high doses. Like the Fletcher system, intracavitary brachytherapy prescriptions are stated in mg Ra Eq-h. Historically, the WU system used Manchester-like applicators and loadings preloaded with ^{226}Ra or ^{60}Co tubes, until the late 1950s when the Ter-Pogossian applicator was introduced. The system changed with the introduction of high-energy x-ray external-beam therapy in 1958, the adoption of the Fletcher-Suit applicator in 1965, and the acquisition of ^{137}Cs tubes in 1971 (225). Because of the long association of the WU system with artificial radionuclides, equivalent mass of radium rather than mass of radium is used to specify source strength; Hence, 1 mg Ra Eq-h in the WU system is equivalent to 1.07 mg-h in the Fletcher system, which, in turn, is equivalent to an IRAK of 0.00723 mGy m^2.

Manchester-like applicator loadings (Fig. 19.28) currently are used for LDR applications, yielding an approximately constant point A dose rate of 65 cGy/h. For HDR applications, the dwell weights are selected to duplicate the relative Manchester loadings and the IRAK per insertion is reduced to reflect the increased radiobiologic effectiveness of the HDR fractionation schedule relative to the LDR regimen. Classically defined point A doses are calculated for reporting purposes for all patients, although this quantity plays no role in prescribing therapy. Dose to the pelvic lymph nodes is calculated at point P, located 2 cm superior to the lateral fornix and 6 cm lateral to the patient's midline. Bladder and rectal reference points (Fig. 19.31) are defined according to ICRU Report No. 38 (122). The prescribed doses for the external-beam and intracavitary (delivered in two LDR insertions) components of treatment are listed in Table 19.11 as a function of extent and stage of disease. The mg Ra Eq-h prescription is divided equally between the vaginal and uterine components and is delivered exactly as prescribed only in the case of the standard 80 mg Ra Eq-h application (2-cm diameter colpostats and long tandem, loaded 20-10-10). For nonstandard loadings using minicolpostats, the vaginal and intrauterine IRAK prescriptions are modified independently. When Delclos minicolpostats are used, vaginal IRAK is constrained by the vaginal vault, surface dose limit, which for LDR is 150 Gy (including whole pelvic dose and the dose from the ipsilateral colpostat but excluding the dose from the tandem and contralateral colpostat). For medium and large colpostats, the vaginal mg Ra Eq-h is increased by 16% and 28% respectively to compensate for their larger source-to-surface distances. When medium and short tandem loadings are used, the target IRAK prescription is modified by the ratio of the actual loading to the standard loading (80 mg Ra Eq-h).

Table 19.12 illustrates detailed application of the WU system to three applicator configurations for prescription schema C, listing total doses for point A, point P, and the vaginal mucosa along with the volumes of tissue enclosed by point A and ICRU 60-Gy reference isodose surfaces. The mg Ra Eq-h actually delivered by equivalent implants varies by a factor of 1.62, leading to a reference volume variation of 2.08. However, compared to fixed point A prescription 65 Gy, which would allow administered mg Ra Eq-h to vary by a factor of 2.31, the WU rules limit the variation of irradiated volume. These rules represent an empirically developed compromise between limiting volume of tissue treated and maintaining a tumoricidal dose contribution to the colpostat surface and to point A.

Table 19.11 shows that as tumor size increases and therapeutic emphasis shifts from intracavitary insertions to external-beam therapy, the point A dose increases, from 58 Gy for small IB lesions (schema A) to 94 Gy for stage IV lesions (schema E). The mg Ra Eq-h actually administered within a given treatment group may deviate from the target mg Ra Eq-h prescriptions by as much as –30% to +40% for very small and large insertions, respectively. Despite reliance on the mg Ra Eq-h prescription philosophy, treatment times are approximately constant and total point A doses are nearly independent of applicator size, the defining features of the Manchester system.

Summary Principles: Intracavitary Brachytherapy Dose Specification

The most widely used intracavitary brachytherapy systems in North America are based on Manchester-type loadings and applicators, in which the point A dose rate is approximately constant and independent of loading, leading to a linear relationship between point A dose and time, not mg Ra Eq-h. Practical mg Ra Eq-h systems use various dose-specification parameters to constrain and guide treatment and are far more Manchester-like than the "strict" mg-h philosophy would suggest. These parameters have the following roles:

a. IRAK limits volume of tissue treated to a high dose;
b. Point A dose ensures that tumor periphery receives adequate dose;
c. Vaginal surface dose ensures that dose to mucosal surfaces in contact with applicator system remains within tolerance; And
d. Treatment time ensures indirect control of point A dose.

Although the traditional treatment specification quantities have clear physical meanings and interrelationships, these concepts can be applied to patient treatment only in a clinical system supported by a base of evaluated clinical experience. In current practice, implant placement is guided by direct visualization and palpation, and treatment prescription is guided by the radiation oncologist's knowledge of treatment outcome averaged over groups of uniformly treated patients with similar tumor size and location and medical condition. This implies that the implant system must be applied as a whole: Mixing dose specification methods, insertion techniques, and normal-tissue dose-response relationships from different clinical systems is a dangerous practice that can lead to suboptimal or

Table 19.11 WASHINGTON UNIVERSITY PRESCRIPTIONS FOR CARCINOMA OF THE CERVIX: LOW DOSE-RATE APPLICATIONS

Treatment Scheme	Indication	External Beam Treatment		Intracavitary Treatment		Range: Smallest to Largest Insertion		
		Whole Pelvis (Gy)	Split Field (Gy)	Target mg Ra Eq-h	Maximum Vaginal Vault Dose (Gy)	Point A Dose (Gy)	Point P Dose (Gy)	mg Ra Eq-h
A	IB ≤2 cm	0	45	7,000	150	58–60	56–60	5,580–7,980
B	IB 2–4 cm	10	40	7,500	150	71–72	61–66	5,580–8,550
C	IB/IIA/IIB/IIIA bulky (>4 cm) limited parametrial extension	20	30	8,000	150	84–86	61–67	5,600–9,100
D	IIB/IIB bulky extensive parametrial extension	20	40	8,000	150	84–86	71–77	5,600–9,100
E	IIB, IIIB, IV poor anatomy, poor regression	40	20	6,500	150	92–94	69–74	4,610–7,410

Table 19.12 WASHINGTON UNIVERSITY SCHEMA C: 8,000 mg-h, 20 Gy WHOLE PELVIS, AND 30 Gy SPLIT PELVIS

Applicator	Loading	Time	mg Ra Eq-h	Vaginal[a] Surface Dose (Gy)	Total Point A Dose (Volume)	Total Point P Dose (Gy)	ICRU[b] Volume (40 Gy)
Small tandem	20 } 10	× 100 h =	3,000	152.3	83.5 Gy (85 cm³)	61.0	165 cm³
Miniovoids	10 10	× 130 h =	2,600				
			5,600				
Standard tandem	20 } 10 } 10	× 100 =	4,000	150.1	86.3 Gy (131 cm³)	65.2	281 cm³
2-cm colpostats	20 20	× 100 h =	4,000				
			8,000				
Standard tandem	20 } 10 } 10	× 100 h =	4,000	98.6	85.6 Gy (160 cm³)	66.9	343 cm³
3-cm colpostats	30 30	× 85 h =	5,100				
			9,100				

[a]On surface of single colpostat, neglecting other sources.
[b]ICRU, International Commission on Radiation Units and Measurements.

indeterminate clinical outcomes. For example, use of the WU maximum rectal tolerance dose (75 to 80 Gy) to guide prescription in a system using higher whole-pelvis doses or less packing will not guarantee an acceptable level of complications. Second, because classical dose-specification quantities fail to completely describe the dose distribution, a radiation oncologist must be trained in all details of an intracavitary system to duplicate the results of its developers. Finally, for the clinical physicist, consistency of current dosimetric practice with past clinical experience is often more important than absolute accuracy of the computed dose distributions or consistency with some practice standard or definition external to the treatment system.

Image-Guided Intracavitary Brachytherapy

Classical brachytherapy prescription techniques rely on empirically based rules, prescription practices, operator experience, and feedback derived from patient follow-up to shape and position intracavitary dose distributions so as to produce acceptable clinical outcomes. In contrast to external beam therapy, 3D imaging rarely is used for planning or evaluating dose distributions. The combination of potential radiocurability of locally advanced lesions, high local failure rates, high rates of complications, and poor correlation between dose specification indices and 3D anatomy has led a number of investigators (80,89,190,253) to investigate anatomy-based dose specification using 3D x-ray CT or MRI studies acquired with the applicator system in place. These studies, based on small numbers of single-insertion image sets, consistently show that conventional orthogonal film-based reference points overestimate minimum doses to the cervix and underestimate maximum doses to critical structures by factors of 1.5 to 2.3 with large patient-to-patient variations. Because MRI has been shown to be far superior to CT for distinguishing tumor from normal cervical stroma (96), advisory groups (101,198) recommend using T2-weighted MRI studies acquired prior to imitating treatment and after each intracavitary insertion for reconstructing the doses delivered to both the pretreatment CTV and to the regressing CTVs derived from MRI and clinical findings acquired at the time of each insertion. One such group, the gynecological GEC-ESTRO Working Group, has proposed target volume nomenclature (high risk, intermediate risk, and low risk CTVs) (101) and specific dose-volume histogram parameters (234) for assessing

the correlation between clinical outcome and the delivered dose distribution.

Many problems remain to be solved in carrying forward the program of MRI-guided or -evaluated definitive radiotherapy. First, routine MRI for intracavitary brachytherapy is not available in most centers due to its expense and logistical challenges. Second, applicator insertion and removal, tumor regression, and bladder and rectal filling variations produce substantial soft-tissue deformation in the pelvis, making it difficult to meaningfully evaluate cumulative dose distributions. An important area of research is application of deformable image registration to account explicitly for the temporal sequence of deforming 3D anatomies needed to accurately characterize a multiple insertion course of intracavitary and external beam therapy (43). As intensity-modulated radiation therapy (IMRT) is use to create more conformal external-beam dose distributions (194), the need to account for local tissue deformation will become more acute. Finally, metal intracavitary applicators, especially shielded applicators, produce severe streaking artifacts on conventionally reconstructed CT images and distortions on MRIs as well. Despite these challenges, integration of 3D imaging into intracavitary brachytherapy treatment planning remains an active and promising area of research.

The Radiobiology of Brachytherapy

The development of high-intensity remote-afterloading stepping sources and low-energy permanently implantable sources has resulted in clinical utilization of dose rates and dose-time-fractionation patterns that can differ radically from conventional LDR brachytherapy protocols. A clear understanding of the principles governing selection of dose-time-fractionation protocols in brachytherapy has become an essential clinical tool.

Brachy means short, and with regard to key radiobiological advantages, refers both to short treatment times and short treatment distances. Short overall treatment times, compared to external-beam radiation therapy (EBRT), minimizes tumor repopulation in rapidly growing tumors. In addition, the excellent dose distributions characteristic of low-energy short-ranged brachytherapy sources significantly reduce the exposed volume, and often the maximum dose, in adjacent normal tissues, compared to EBRT. As well as diminishing late-responding normal-tissue complications, such dose sparing keeps early-responding normal tissue sequelae to acceptable levels, making the short treatment times used in brachytherapy tolerable. This is in contrast to EBRT, where the risk of early responding tissue sequelae requires treatment times to be prolonged for a minimum of about 6 weeks, with the corresponding potential lost of tumor control through repopulation. The short overall treatment times used in brachytherapy are likely to contribute significantly to clinical efficacy for those tumor sites (e.g., cervix, head and neck, and lung) where long overall treatment time is associated with reduced local control.

Biophysical Modeling of Brachytherapy

In parallel with the emergence of a clear radiobiologic rationale for brachytherapy, biophysical models for predicting responses to alternative protraction schemes have been developed. In the 1970s, before the differential response of early- and late-responding tissues was understood, the most widespread approach for designing alternative fractionation schemes was the nominal standard dose (NSD) equation, developed by Ellis (74). This empirical equation was based on data from early responding tissues, and it does not account for the differential response to fraction size/dose rate of early versus late effects.

By contrast, the currently used linear quadratic (LQ) model unequivocally distinguishes between early and late responses and is based on mechanistic notions about how cells are killed by radiation. After several decades of investigation and use, the basic ideas and parameters in the LQ model have been well supported by clinical experience and outcome data.

The Linear-Quadratic Model and Its Mechanistic Basis

Central to the LQ approach is a biologic model of radiation action, which was spelled out in detail more than 50 years ago by Lea and Catcheside (150,151), based on a mechanistic analysis of radiation-induced chromosome aberration induction. The application of the LQ formalism to radiation therapy has been reviewed by Thames and Hendry (267), Dale (51), Fowler (86), and many others.

In this approach, radiotherapeutic response is primarily related to cell survival (or survival of groups of cells). Although not the sole determinant of biologic response, there is now a wealth of evidence that cell killing (i.e., loss of reproductive integrity) is the dominant determinant of radiotherapeutic response, both for early- and late-responding end points (267).

In the most basic LQ approach, cellular survival, S, at a dose D is written as

$$S(D) = \exp(-\alpha D - \beta D^2) \quad (39)$$

The mechanistic interpretation of equation 39 is that cell killing results from the interaction of two elementary damaged species, most often DNA double-strand breaks (DSBs), to produce species that cause cell lethality, such as dicentric chromosomal aberrations. The two terms in equation 39 indicate that the two DSB may be produced by the passage of the same photon (linear term in dose) or by two independent photons (quadratic term).

Equation 39 is applicable to a single acute radiation exposure. If the two DSBs are formed at different times, there exists the possibility of the first being repaired before it has a chance to interacting with the second. This will not effect the first term in equation 39, because the two DSBs are formed simultaneously from a single photon, but DSB repair during a prolonged exposure will result in a reduction of the second, quadratic term in equation 39 by a factor denoted "G" by Lea and Catcheside (150,151):

$$S(D) = \exp(-\alpha D - G \cdot \beta D^2), \quad (40)$$

where, for acute exposures, $G \rightarrow 1$, and for very long exposures, $G \rightarrow 0$. In this context, "acute" and "long" are defined relative to the half-time ($T_{1/2}$) for DSB repair of sublethal damage. In general, the G factor in equation 40 will depend on the details of the temporal distribution of the dose, as well as on $T_{1/2}$. For many simple cases, G can be calculated analytically. For example, for a permanent exponentially decaying implant, G is simply $\lambda/(\mu + \lambda)$ where λ is the radioactive decay constant of the particular nuclide used, and $\mu = 0.693/T_{1/2}$. Formulae for G for many other standard schemes also have been derived (49,151), as has a general formalism for any possible protraction scheme (25).

It is important to note that equation 40 is not simply a convenient formula for fitting cellular survival curves; But can be derived from a variety of underlying mechanistic models. The theory of dual radiation action (129), for example, represents only one of several different approaches to describing radiobiologic damage mechanistically. The approach devised by Lea and Catcheside (150,151) deals instead with the kinetics of damage development. Typical kinetic models track the temporal evolution of lesions as a cell gradually repairs or misrepairs initial damage (82,250,270). Many different molecular mechanisms have been studied kinetically, such as pairwise misrepair of DNA DSBs, direct one-hit induction of lethal lesions, and saturable repair pathways in which the repair enzyme system can be overloaded.

It is now well established that a surprisingly broad spectrum of such kinetic models lead to the LQ formalism, reducing to equations 39 and 40 via first-order time-dependent perturbation theory when the dose or dose rate are not too high, a constraint that includes most clinically and experimentally relevant doses and dose rates (28).

Practical Applications of the Linear Quadratic Model

Equation 40 can be used in two different ways: We either can design "equivalent" dose protraction protocols (i.e., design a regimen with the same tumor response, or the same late complications, as a "tried and tested" regimen), or we can try to predict absolute radiotherapeutic responses. We will discuss both approaches here, although we will argue that designing equivalent protraction schemes is a considerably more robust procedure.

In order to design a new dose protraction protocol (labeled "2"), which will have the same effect as a current protocol (labeled "1"), based on equation 40, we need to ensure the quantity $(\alpha D + G\beta D^2)$ is equal for the two protocols, that is:

$$D_1\left(1 + G_1 D_1/(\alpha/\beta)\right) = D_2\left(1 + G_2 D_2/(\alpha/\beta)\right) \quad (41)$$

The quantity on either side of equation 41 is often called the biologically effective dose (BED) (86), so generating a new "equivalent" regime amounts to matching BEDs for the old and new regimes.

By contrast, to use the LQ model to calculate absolute tumor-control probabilities (TCP) or normal-tissue complication probabilities (NTCP), we need additional models relating cellular survival (S) with TCP or with NTCP. The simplest approach, originating with Munro and Gilbert (195), equates TCP with the probability that, after radiation treatment, there are no remaining tumor stem cells capable of initiating tumor regrowth. Let us suppose that a dose, D, delivered in a given protraction pattern, produces a stem-cell survival probability, S. Let K be the initial number of potential stem cells in the tumor. Then the probability that any given stem cell will be unable to initiate tumor regrowth is $(1 - S)$. Thus the TCP for the irradiated tumor is simply $(1 - S)^k$ which, for small values of S can be approximated as:

$$TCP = \exp(-S \cdot K) \qquad (42)$$

Thus, if cell survival, S, is described by equation 40, then

$$TCP(D) = \exp\left(-K \cdot \exp\left[-\alpha D - G - \beta D^2\right]\right)$$
$$= \exp\left(-\exp\left[\ln K - \alpha D - G \cdot \beta D^2\right]\right) \qquad (43)$$

Equation 43 may also be used to calculate NTCP, except that now the parameter K does not refer to the number of tumor cells that need to be sterilized, but rather to the number of groups of cells in the normal tissue ("tissue-rescuing units") (110), whose destruction would result in the late complication.

The difficulty with using equation 43, or similar approaches, to estimate, de novo, absolute values of TCP or NTCP is that the results are exquisitely sensitive to the parameter values, particularly the K parameter; This severely limits the utility of such equations for absolute TCP or NTCP estimation. Rather, the most robust applications of the LQ model are for comparisons between protraction regimens (equation and its extensions described below), which are much less sensitive to the LQ parameter values (68).

Use of the Linear-Quadratic Model in Brachytherapy

Quantifying the Rationale for Low–Dose-Rate Brachytherapy

It has long been known that lowering the dose rate generally reduces radiobiologic damage (102). The explanation of this effect, relating to sublethal damage repair, also has been long understood (150,151). It also has been clear since the pioneering work of Coutard (46) that fractionating or protracting a radiotherapeutic exposure can give a therapeutic advantage between tumor control and normal tissue sequelae. However, the exact link between these observations was not clearly made until the 1980s by Withers et al. (268,309).

To understand their insight, consider the isoeffect curves in Figure 19.33, representing "equivalent" schemes for either early- or late-responding end points, as a function of treatment time. For higher dose rates, the dose reduction needed to match the late effects is larger than the dose reduction needed to match tumor control. For any selected dose, increasing the dose rate will increase late effects much more than it will increase tumor control. Conversely, decreasing the dose rate will decrease late effects much more than it will decrease tumor control. Thus the *therapeutic ratio* (ratio of tumor control to complications) increases as the dose rate decreases.

These observations can be interpreted in terms of the α/β ratio (268) in the linear-quadratic equation 40. In terms of survival curves (Fig. 19.34), the α/β ratio essentially describes the degree of "curviness" of the acute survival curve. A small value of α/β means that the β (dose squared) term is dominating at radiotherapeutic doses, resulting in a curvy survival curve (Fig. 19.34). A large value of α/β means the α (linear in dose) term is dominating, resulting in a straighter semilog survival curve. Now, as a first approximation, the dose-response relation for a fractionated (or LDR) regimen can be thought of as simply the result of multiple repeats of the initial part of the survival curve. It is clear that repeating the early part of a curvy survival curve many times will result in far more sparing than repeating the early part of a straighter survival curve.

Thus, late effects, which are very sensitive to changes in fractionation, are characterized by small values of α/β (a typical value is 3 Gy), and early effects (tumor control or early responding normal sequelae) are characterized by large values of α/β, a

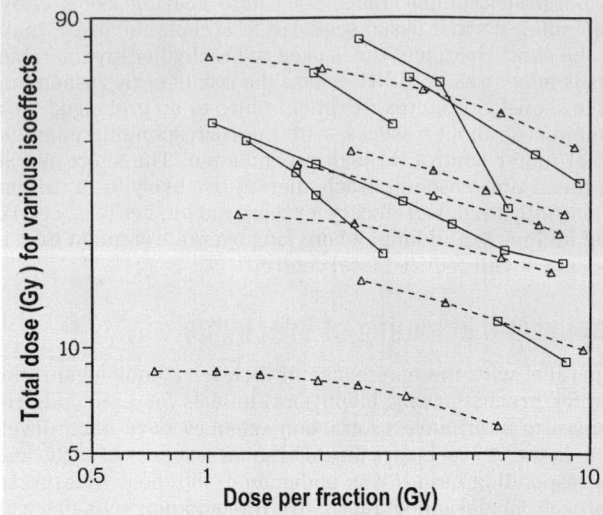

FIGURE 19.33. Isoeffect curves (adapted from Withers HR, Taylor JMG, Maciejewski B. The hazard of accelerated tumor clonogen repopulation during radiotherapy. *Acta Radiol* 1988;27:131–146, with permission) showing the total dose to produce a given end point, plotted against dose per fraction, a surrogate, in this context, for dose rate. The triangles, joined by dashed lines, refer to a variety of different early responding end points (of which tumor control is an example), whereas the squares, joined by solid lines, refer to a variety of different late-responding sequelae. Note the generally steeper slopes of the solid lines, suggesting that late-responding tissues are more sensitive than early responding tissues to changes in the protraction of a given radiation dose.

typical value for most tumors being about 10 Gy. As clinical data from which α/β ratios can be derived have accumulated, the dichotomy between α/β ratios for early and late effects has held up remarkably well. Consequently, when using the LQ model, it is essential to be clear about whether the calculation is designed to refer to early- or late-responding tissue, and to then use the appropriate α/β value. From equation 41, it is clear that use of different values of α/β will result in different predictions for the isoeffect dose.

Modeling the Effect of Treatment Time

For temporary implants or HDR, the effect of tumor repopulation is generally small, but this is not necessarily the case with longer permanent implants. Equation 40 can be simply modified to take into account the effects of tumor repopulation (i.e., the effects of overall time). Following the original formulation by Travis and Tucker (273), repopulation is taken into account by increasing the surviving fraction by a factor $\exp(\gamma T)$, where T is the overall treatment time. One can also take into account delay in the onset of accelerated repopulation, by replacing T with $(T - T_D)$, where T_D is the delay after the beginning of the treatment before tumor-cell proliferation begins (86). Then the surviving fraction is given by:

$$S = \exp\left(-\alpha D - G \cdot \beta D^2 + \gamma\left[T - T_p\right]\right) \qquad (44)$$

The parameter γ determines the speed of repopulation, and is given by $\gamma = 0.693/T_P$, where T_P is the effective doubling time of cells in the tumor. If we can ignore cell loss, T_P is the same as T_{POT}, which is the measurable (107) *in vitro* doubling time of the tumor cells.

If tumor repopulation is relevant, then, in order to designed a new equivalent regimen, rather than match the quantity $(\alpha D + G \cdot \beta D^2)$, we need to match the quantity $(\alpha D + G \cdot \beta D^2 - \gamma[T - T_P])$, and equations 41 or 43 can be modified correspondingly.

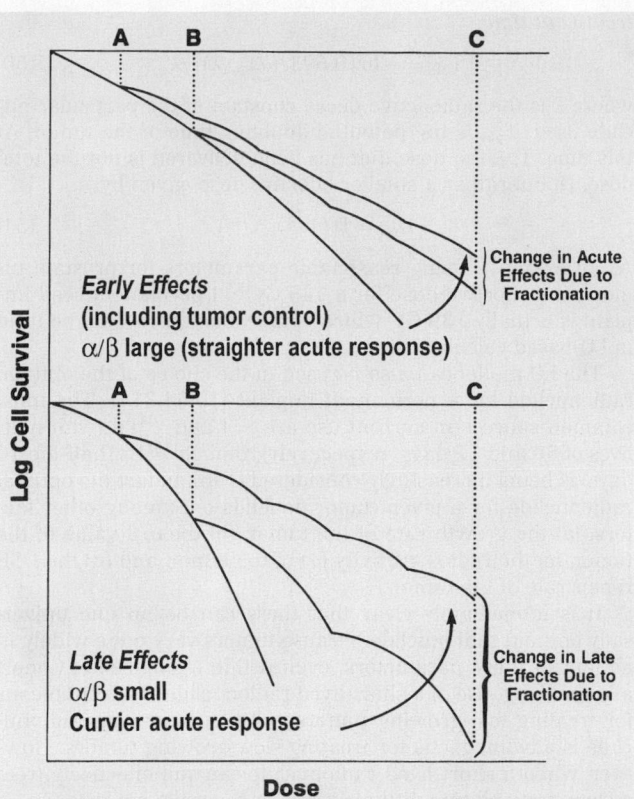

FIGURE 19.34. Illustrating the differing effects of protraction on early and late responding tissues, as elucidated by Thames et al. (From Thames HD, Withers HR, Peters LJ, et al. Changes in early and late radiation responses with altered dose fractionation: Implications for dose-survival relationships. *Int J Radiat Oncol Biol Phys* 1982;8(2):219–226, with permission.)

Redistribution and Reoxygenation

Radiobiological response is dominated by the four Rs: repair, repopulation, redistribution, and reoxygenation (310). Equation 40 describes repair, which is extended using equation 44 to include repopulation. Further extensions to include the remaining two Rs, cell-cycle redistribution and reoxygenation, are also possible (27). This approach treats both redistribution (as a result of progression through the cell cycle) and reoxygenation as aspects of a single phenomenon, termed resensitization, which occurs when a radiation exposure preferentially kills the more radiosensitive cells in a diverse population, leaving a cell population with decreased average radiosensitivity. Subsequent biologically driven changes then tend to gradually restore the original population average radiosensitivity.

In contrast to some multiparametric approaches, the LQR approach uses only two additional adjustable parameters—an overall resensitization time and overall resensitization amplitude. The LQR model replaces the LQ equation 40 with:

$$S(D) = \exp(-\alpha D - G\beta D^2 + \tfrac{1}{2}\sigma^2 \hat{G} D^2). \quad (45)$$

The new term, $\tfrac{1}{2}\sigma^2 \hat{G} D^2$, contains the resensitization magnitude, $\tfrac{1}{2}\sigma^2$, which is positive. This resensitization magnitude represents the average of the dominant resensitization effects present in a heterogeneous tumor. The factor $\hat{G}$ models the influence of fractionation on resensitization and depends on a characteristic resensitization time, τ_S. In fact, $\hat{G}$ has exactly the same form as the G function used to account for sublethal damage repair (Eq. 40), except that the characteristic repair time is replaced with the characteristic resensitization time, τ_S. However, in contrast to repair, resensitization tends to increase radiosensitivity as the overall time increases. For example, tumor

cells, which were in a resistant part of the cell cycle at the beginning of the treatment and were thus preferentially spared, may move to a more sensitive part of the cell cycle as the treatment progresses. Although mechanistically driven, LQR is sufficiently simple that it can be used for isoeffect calculations in radiation therapy. Its idealized treatment parallels that of the standard LQ model of repair. The model gives reasonable fits to relevant experimental data in the literature (27).

If reoxygenation or repopulation are relevant, then, in order to designed a new equivalent regimen, rather than match the quantity $(\alpha D + G\beta D^2)$, we need to match the quantity $(\alpha D + G\beta D^2)^2 - (\alpha D + G\beta D^2 - \tfrac{1}{2}\sigma^2 \hat{G} D^2)$, and equations 41 or 43 can be modified correspondingly.

The Effects of Tumor Shrinkage

If the reference surface, to which dose is prescribed, diminishes in size during the treatment as a result of tumor shrinkage, then an increase in physical dose rate results because cells near the dose-specification point will move closer to the sources and will receive a higher dose. The radiobiologic consequences of this phenomenon have been modeled in detail by Dale et al. (52,54) using the LQ formalism. For permanent implants in tumors with long doubling times, tumor shrinkage may significantly enhancing the clinical potential of long-lived nuclides such as ^{125}I, but tumor shrinkage would be expected to have much less effect for short-lived nuclide such as ^{103}Pd or ^{131}Cs, or for rapidly growing tumors. In fact, this is one argument against the use of long-lived nuclides for permanent-implant brachytherapy, in that the outcome may depend on shrinkage parameters that we are not able to predict.

Nonuniform Dose Distributions

Thus far, our radiobiologic models have assumed that an implant can be characterized by a single prescribed dose, an assumption that ignores the highly nonuniform dose distributions produced by brachytherapy. As discussed earlier, radiobiologic modeling can be used either to compare (and potentially equate) different protraction schemes or to make absolute predictions of TCP or NTCP. As discussed earlier, the latter application is far less robust.

When the goal is to match tumor control for two different protraction schemes, each of which have similar relative dose distributions across the tumor, the use of mean dose or minimum dose (21) or equivalent uniform dose (211) (EUD; the uniform dose that produces the same cell survival in the tumor as the given inhomogeneous dose distribution), is likely to give reasonable results in any dose measurement. Equation 41 implies that, when matching protraction schemes, the lower the dose rate, the less important will be the effects of dose inhomogeneity.

Absolute TCP and NCTP models can be extended to inhomogeneous dose distributions by dividing the tumor into many voxels, each with its own dose, D_i, and each containing K_i target cells (21,212,283). It then is assumed that each tumor voxel must be controlled independently if tumor control is to be achieved. Then the overall tumor control can be written:

$$TCP = \exp\left[-\sum_i K_i \cdot \exp\left(-\alpha \cdot D_i - \beta \cdot D_i^2\right)\right] \quad (46)$$

where the summation is over the total number of voxels. Typically the D_i are derived from dose-volume histogram data. Several authors (212,283) have extended this approach also to include the possibility of an inhomogeneous distribution of target cells within the tumor.

The approach to extending TCP to inhomogeneous dose distributions, embodied in equation 46, can also be applied to

NTCP models (315) based on the survival of functional subunits (FSU). Many organs are best modeled by FSUs organized with a parallel architecture such that a complication results only if when sufficiently large number of FSUs are inactivated (125), although serial architectures, such as the spine, can also be modeled (212).

The Relative Effectiveness of Different Radioisotopes Used in Brachytherapy

As discussed earlier in this chapter, a wide variety of radionuclides are used in brachytherapy, with mean photon energies ranging from 398 keV (^{192}Ir) down to 21 keV (^{103}Pd). It is well established that biological effectiveness varies with photon energy, as a result of different patterns of energy deposition produced by the different photon spectra (30,313). It is possible, however, to estimate the RBE of these different isotopes directly from the energy deposition patterns—the subject matter of microdosimetry (247). In this approach, the response per unit dose at low dose rates (or low doses), R_i, to a particular radiation, i, can be written as (33):

$$R_i = \int w(y) \cdot d_i(y) \cdot dy \qquad (47)$$

where y is the stochastic quantity, lineal energy (247), defined as the energy deposited by a single photon track, divided by the average path length in the cellular target, and $d_i(y)$ is the dose-weighted probability that a photon will deposit lineal energy y in the target volume of interest. The quantity $d_i(y)$ often is referred to as the microdosimetric single-event spectrum. It can be measured using a low-pressure proportional counter or calculated (247). The quantity w(y) describes the response of an individual cellular target to a lineal energy deposition, y. For photons (although not for densely ionizing radiations such as neutrons), it is reasonable to assume that w(y) is proportional to y (247). Thus, at low doses rates:

$$RBE_i \propto \int y \cdot d_i(y) \cdot dy \qquad (48)$$

where $d_i(y)$ is the dose-averaged lineal energy. Based on this approach, RBE values have been estimated from measured or calculated microdosimetric data (313,320). For example, Wuu et al. (313) report low dose rate RBE values relative to ^{60}Co of 1.3, 2.1, 2.1, and 2.3 for ^{192}Ir, ^{241}Am, ^{125}I, and ^{103}Pd, respectively. These values are comparable to those obtained experimentally. The approach outlined above is applicable only to LDR brachytherapy, but it can be generalized to HDR regimens (33).

Incorporating the low-dose-rate RBE into the LQ equations is surprisingly easy (Dale and Jones 1988), requiring a simple modification of the BED (biological effective dose) equation embodied in equation 41. Specifically, the BED now becomes:

$$BED = D\left[RBE + G \cdot D/(\alpha/\beta)\right] \qquad (49)$$

The LQ Model for Permanent Implants

As seen in equation 41 and 44, to generate a new protocol that has equivalent effects to a current one, we need to match the quantity ($\alpha D + G\beta D^2 - \gamma[T - T_D]$), where T is the treatment time. When comparing permanent implant, it is important to note that the effective treatment time for a permanent implant is not infinite (50), because when the dose rate becomes sufficiently low that more tumor cells are being born by repopulation than are being killed, the treatment is effectively over, and any dose given after that time is probably irrelevant to tumor cure. The time, postimplant, when this occurs is called the *effective*

treatment time:

$$T_{eff} = -\ln\left[0.693/(\alpha T_{pot}\lambda)\right]/\lambda \qquad (50)$$

where λ is the radioactive decay constant of the particular nuclide used, T_{pot} is the potential doubling time of the tumor. At this time, T_{eff}, the dose that has been delivered is not the total dose, D, but rather a smaller effective dose, given by:

$$D_{eff} = D\left(1 - e^{-\lambda T_{eff}}\right) \qquad (51)$$

As an example, using reasonable parameters for prostate tumors, the effective dose for a 145 Gy ^{125}I permanent seed implant is actually 139 Gy, which is the value that would be used in LQ-based calculations.

The LQ model can also be used in the choice of the optimal radionuclide for a permanent implant (10,64,314). The most common sources in current use are ^{125}I and ^{103}Pd (with half-lives of 59 and 17 days, respectively), though ^{131}Cs (half-life 10 days) is being increasingly considered (196). In fact the optimal radionuclide for a given tumor depends on, among other factors: (a) the growth rate of the tumor, (b) the α/β value of the tumor, (c) the radiosensitivity (α) of the tumor, and (d) the DSB repair rate of the tumor.

It is immediately clear that there can be no one universally optimal radionuclide because tumors vary quite widely in all four of these parameters, even within a single site. Generally speaking, use of a short-lived radionuclide is advantageous for treating fast-growing tumors, while a long-lived radionuclide is advantageous for treating slow-growing tumors. However, while a short-lived radionuclide can still effectively treat a slow-growing tumor, the reverse is generally not true (i.e., a long-lived radionuclide is not well suited to treat a fast-growing tumor) (10,64). In addition, the outcomes of treatments using short-lived radionuclides are generally much less sensitive to the tumor properties than is the case for long-lived radionuclides. These considerations suggest that short-lived radionuclides such as ^{103}Pd and ^{131}Cs are better suited, radiobiologically, for treating a broad spectrum of tumor types through permanent implants.

High–Dose-Rate Intracavitary Brachytherapy for Cervical Cancer

There has been a trend in the past few years toward increased use of HDR brachytherapy in some tumor sites, driven largely by the economic and logistical benefits of outpatient-based fractionated HDR brachytherapy. Although sometimes delivered in a single fraction, more often 3 to 12 HDR fractions are used.

In some situations, such as palliative or intraoperative brachytherapy, the therapeutic ratio between tumor control and late sequelae is not a prime consideration; But in general, when the treatment is designed to be curative, as we have discussed earlier, increasing the dose rate is likely to *decrease* the therapeutic advantage between tumor control and late sequelae. However, there are two curative applications (intracavitary implants for cancer of the uterine cervix and implant therapy for prostate cancer) where, for differing reasons, HDR brachytherapy is as effective, or potentially even more effective, compared to LDR brachytherapy.

The radiobiological principles involved in moving from LDR to HDR are illustrated schematically in Figure 19.35, which shows typical dose-response relationships for early and late-responding tissues. As we have discussed, the dose-response relations for late effects are significantly "curvier" (smaller α/β ratio) than for early-responding tissues such as tumors, which have a larger α/β ratio. Let us assume we have used an LDR treatment dose, D, and that we want to produce the same tumor control with HDR: As illustrated in the left panel of Fig. 19.35, we need to reduce the dose by reduction factor DRF (see

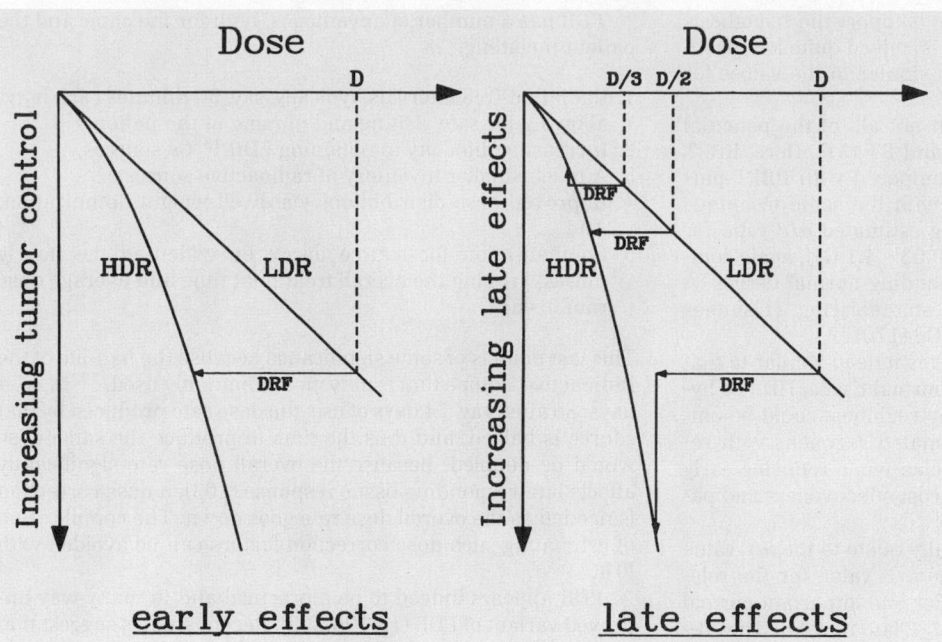

FIGURE 19.35. Illustration of the interplay between early and late effects for low–dose-rate (LDR) and high–dose-rate (HDR) brachytherapy for cervical cancer. DRF is the dose reduction factor that produces the same early effects (tumor control) for HDR as LDR. If D is the LDR giving rise to late effects, then reducing D by DRF for HDR will result in more late effects than at LDR. As the HDR dose to late-responding tissue is reduced by treatment planning, then reducing that dose by the factor DRF no longer produces worse late effects than at LDR.

left panel). From the right panel of Fig. 19.35, however, it can be seen that this same reduction in dose from dose D will result in increased late effects compared to LDR. Thus there is an expected increase in late effects when moving from LDR to HDR. But now let us suppose that the LDR dose causing the late effects is not the treatment dose D but some lower dose. This is the case for cervical brachytherapy because the bladder and rectum are generally some significant distance from the cervical implant. To be specific, let us suppose that the dose responsible for late effects is half the treatment dose (i.e., D/2). From the right-hand panel in Fig. 19.35, we see that if we move to HDR and reduce this reduced rectal dose (D/2) by the factor DRF needed to match tumor control, because we are further up the survival curve, we will *not* get more late effects for HDR compared to LDR, but actually a similar late-effect probability. Indeed, if the rectal dose were an even smaller fraction of the treatment dose (say D/3, in Fig. 19.35), we could even be in a situation where we have *less* late effects at HDR than at LDR—all for the same level of tumor control.

In fact, if the cervical brachytherapy results in a dose to the bladder/rectum that is less than about three fourths of the treatment dose, then if the HDR dose is reduced to give equal tumor control compared with LDR, the HDR late effects should not be worse than the LDR late effects (25,29).

Of course there is another related factor to consider, which is that the short treatment time characteristic of HDR allows packing and retraction of the sensitive organs, which typically results in a 20% further decrease in the rectal/bladder dose compared to that achievable with LDR (215). This gives an extra physically based advantage to HDR, in addition to the biological factors discussed here.

In summary, these radiobiological considerations lead to explicit recommendations about the appropriate usage of HDR versus LDR for cervical cancer brachytherapy: When the dose to the dose-limiting critical normal tissues (bladder/rectum) is less than about three fourths of the prescribed dose, HDR (with at least about five fractions to ensure adequate tumor reoxygenation) results in comparable (or less) late effects than LDR for the same level of tumor control. For less advantageous geometries (i.e., for those patients where the dose to the bladder/rectum is comparable to the prescribed dose), HDR would be expected to give a worse therapeutic advantage compared with LDR.

These considerations are supported by a number of clinical studies (59,78,81,104,141,152,235). These reports generally show that HDR and LDR for cervical brachytherapy produce similar local control and late complications.

Optimized Dose Protraction for Prostate Cancer Brachytherapy

As discussed above, one of the main reasons for protracting any radiotherapeutic exposure is that late sequelae are generally more sensitive than early effects (such as tumor control) to changes in protraction. So lowering the dose rate generally spares late-responding tissues more than the tumor. The reason for this difference in response to changes in protraction is generally assumed to be related to the larger proportion of cycling cells in tumors compared with normal tissues. Because prostate tumors contain unusually small fractions of cycling cells (107), it was suggested that prostate tumors might respond to changes in protraction more like late-responding normal tissues rather than typical tumors (26,69). In terms of the LQ model, the suggestion was that the α/β ratio for prostate cancer might be low, comparable to that for late sequelae. If so, much of the rationale for using low dose rate, or using many fractions, would disappear for prostate radiotherapy.

A first estimate of α/β ratio for prostate cancer was made in 1999 (26), by comparing results from external beam RT (EBRT) with those from permanent seed ^{125}I brachytherapy (BT). Consistent with the theoretical hypotheses (see above), the estimated value of α/β ratio was 1.5 Gy (95% confidence interval (CI): 0.8 – 2.2 Gy), indeed comparable to α/β values for late-responding normal tissues, and much smaller than those for most tumors.

The problem with this α/β estimate, and almost all subsequent ones (85,128,132,154,174,280,281), is that they involved comparing or equating EBRT results with permanent implantation results. There are many pertinent differences between EBRT and BT (different dose distributions, different RBEs, different overall times, different institutions, different PSA distributions, hypoxia), any or all of which could bias the α/β estimate. Much debate has centered around the significance of these biases, and how to take them into account. Despite these problems, most of the analyses above support the hypothesis that the α/β value for prostate cancer is indeed quite low, probably in the 1 to 4 Gy range, which is similar to the values for most late-responding tissues.

One analysis avoids many, though not all, of the potential biases involved in comparing EBRT and BT (31). Here, EBRT plus two HDR boost fractions was compared with EBRT plus three HDR boost fractions, all done with the same technique at the same institution. The resulting estimated α/β ratio for prostate cancer was 1.2 Gy (95% CI : 0.03 – 4.1 Gy], again comparable with α/β values for late-responding normal tissues. A recent meta-analysis of four reports summarizing 21 studies yielded an estimated α/β ratio of 1.3 Gy (170).

If the α/β value for prostate cancer is indeed similar to that for the surrounding late-responding normal tissue, HDR or hypofractionated external beam therapy regimens could be employed to match conventional fractionated regimens with respect to tumor control and late sequelae while reducing early urinary sequelae (22) and improving cost effectiveness and patient convenience.

The arguments presented here really relate to the α/β value for prostate cancer in relation to the α/β value for the relevant late-responding normal tissue. For one important normal tissue complications end point, grade ≥ 2 late rectal toxicity, recent analyses of clinical data suggest that the α/β ratio is in fact higher than for most late-responding tissue, and indeed higher than recent estimates of prostate tumor α/β ratio. Specifically, the estimated value of α/β value for RTOG grade ≥ 2 late rectal toxicity was 5.4 $\pm$ 1.5 Gy (23), which is intermediate between typical values for early and late responding tissues, giving credence to the notion that at least some late rectal damage is a direct consequence of early responding damage (66,126,279). This suggests that HDR prostate brachytherapy, as well as being logistically convenient, might actually improve the therapeutic outcome of prostate cancer brachytherapy.

HDR (or hypofractionation) in a curative setting, even when the dose is appropriately lowered, is a prima facie unsettling idea. However, there is now a significant body of clinical evidence suggesting that these approaches do not lead to increased early or late sequelae after prostate radiotherapy, either for external beam RT or for brachytherapy, providing further evidence to support the underlying radiobiological rationale. For external beam radiotherapy, in those hypofractionation studies that have reported on potential late sequelae, there is to date little indication of any unexpected late sequelae after median follow-up periods of 21 months (142), 31 months (1), 48 months (168), 59 months (176), 66 months (143), and 97 months (169). HDR has been used in prostate brachytherapy both as a monotherapy (181,316) and, more commonly, as a boost to external beam radiotherapy (88,210,222,257). In both cases the results are promising, with no evidence for excessive normal tissue sequelae.

Pulsed Brachytherapy

The motivation for PDR is to combine the radiobiological benefits of LDR with the practical advantages of computer-controlled remote afterloader technology. PDR works by replacing a continuous LDR treatment lasting several days with a series of short HDR irradiations, often using the same overall time. LQ analyses using equation 40 suggest that this can be done without significant loss of therapeutic advantage by delivering a series of 5- to 10-minute pulses, delivered every hour (24).

Thus a PDR irradiator consists of a single high-activity radioactive source that, typically once each hour, steps, under computer control, through the catheters of an implant, with dwell times in each position adjusted to obtain the required dose distribution. When the source is not stepping through the implant (typically most of the time), it is retracted into its safe.

PDR has a number of advantages, both for the clinic and the patient including:

1. Radiation-free intervals, typically, say, 50 minutes each hour, allowing for safe visiting and nursing of the patient;
2. Increasing difficulty in obtaining LDR ^{137}Cs sources;
3. A much smaller inventory of radioactive sources;
4. Improved dose distributions via dwell weight optimization; And
5. Compensation for source decay by widening the hourly pulses, keeping the overall treatment time and average dose rate fixed.

This last point is of some significance because the half-life of the radioactive isotope that is now most commonly used, ^{192}Ir, is 74 days. So after, say, 74 days of use, the dose rate produced by that source is halved, and thus the time to produce the same dose would be doubled. Because the overall dose rate significantly affects late-responding tissue response (103), a dose correction is needed as the overall dose rate goes down. The complication of estimating such dose correction factors can be avoided with PDR.

PDR appears indeed to be a practical and in many way improved variant of LDR (13,106,263). Recent studies suggest that it may well be possible to use PDR only during "office hours," rather than on a day-and-night basis, by incorporating minor adjustments to the overall dose and time (32,105,158). If such suggestions turn out to be practical, PDR may well have the potential to replace LDR in many situations, which is of some practical importance as ^{137}Cs LDR sources are becoming increasing difficult to obtain.

:: | Conclusions

This chapter has focused on several basic topics, including the interplay between physical properties, single-source dosimetry, source-strength specification, classical interstitial and intracavitary brachytherapy systems and dose specification, and biologic effects and clinical utility of brachytherapy sources. Many topics usually covered in an introductory survey have been omitted. For a review of radiographic imaging and localization of brachytherapy sources, the reader is referred to more specialized recent reviews (161,248). For discussions on quality assurance of manually and remotely afterloading brachytherapy and treatment planning, the reader is referred to Chapters 20, 21, and 22 of this text as well as a number of excellent reviews (87,140,144,201,305) including appropriate chapters from *Brachytherapy Physics* second edition (269). For useful reviews of the radiobiology of brachytherapy, the reader is referred to excellent reviews by Dale (53) and by King (131). For a discussion of brachytherapy licensing and regulatory issues, the review by Glasgow (93) is suggested.

References

1. Akimoto T, Muramatsu H, Takahashi M, et al. Rectal bleeding after hypofractionated radiotherapy for prostate cancer: correlation between clinical and dosimetric parameters and the incidence of grade 2 or worse rectal bleeding. *Int J Radiat Oncol Biol Phys* 2004;60(4):1033–1039.
2. Anacak Y, Esassolak M, Aydin A, et al. Effect of geometrical optimization on the treatment volumes and the dose homogeneity of biplane interstitial brachytherapy implants. *Radiother Oncol* 1997;45:71–76.
3. Anderson LL. Spacing nomograph for interstitial implants of I-125 seeds. *Med Phys* 1976;3:48.
4. Anderson LL. A natural volume-dose histogram for brachytherapy. *Med Phys* 1986;13:898–903.
5. Anderson LL. Dose specification and quantification of implant quality. In: Williamson JF, Thomadsen BR, Nath R, eds. *Brachytherapy physics*. Madison, WI: Medical Physics Publishing Company, 1995;343–361.
6. Anderson LL, Moni JV, Harrison LB. A nomograph for permanent implants of Palladium-103 seeds. *Int J Radiat Oncol Biol Phys* 1993;27:129–135.

7. Anderson LL, Nath R, Olch AJ, et al. American Endocurietherapy Society recommendations for dose specification in brachytherapy. *Endocurietherapy Hyperther Oncol* 1991;7:1–12.
8. Anderson LL, Nath R, Weaver KA, et al. *Interstitial brachytherapy: physical, biological and clinical considerations*. New York: Raven, 1990.
9. Anderson LL, Presser JE. Classical systems I for temporary interstitial implants: Manchester and Quimby systems. In: Williamson JF, Thomadsen BR, Nath R, eds. *Brachytherapy physics*. Madison, WI: Medical Physics Publishing Company, 1995;301–323.
10. Armpilia CI, Dale RG, Coles IP, et al. The determination of radiobiologically optimized half-lives for radionuclides used in permanent brachytherapy implants. *Int J Radiat Oncol Biol Phys* 2003;55(2):378–385.
11. Attix FH. *Introduction to radiological physics and radiation physics*. New York: Wiley, 1986.
12. Attix FH, Ritz VH. A determination of the gamma-ray emission of radium. *J Res Natl Bureau Stand* 1957;59:293–305.
13. Bachtiary B, Dewitt A, Pintilie, M, et al. Comparison of late toxicity between continuous low-dose-rate and pulsed-dose-rate brachytherapy in cervical cancer patients. *Int J Radiat Oncol Biol Phys* 2005;63(4):1077–1082.
14. Bambynek M, Fluhs D, Quast U, et al. A high-precision, high-resolution and fast dosimetry system for beta sources applied in cardiovascular brachytherapy. *Med Phys* 2000;27(4):662–667.
15. Berger MJ. Energy deposition in water by photons from point isotropic sources. *J Nucl Med* 1968;[Suppl 1]:17–25.
16. Beyer D, Nath R, Butler W, et al. American Brachytherapy Society recommendations for clinical implementation of NIST-1999 standards for ^{103}palladium brachytherapy. The clinical research committee of the American Brachytherapy Society. *Int J Radiat Oncol Biol Phys* 2000;47(2):273–275.
17. BIR/IPSM. *Recommendations for brachytherapy dosimetry: report of a joint working party*. London: British Institute of Radiology and Institute of Physical Sciences in Medicine, 1993.
18. Blasko JC, Grimm PD, Sylvester JE, et al. Palladium-103 brachytherapy for prostate carcinoma. *Int J Radiat Oncol Biol Phys* 2000;46(4):839–850.
19. Blasko JC, Radge H, Schumacker D. Transperineal percutaneous Iodine-125 implantation for prostatic carcinoma using transrectal ultrasound and template guidance. *Endocurietherapy Hyperther Oncol* 1987;3:131–139.
20. Boutillon M, Perroche-Roux AM. Re-evaluation of the W value for electrons in dry air. *Phys Med Biol* 1987;32:213–219.
21. Brahme A. Dosimetric precision requirements in radiation therapy. *Acta Radiol Oncol* 1984;23(5):379–391.
22. Brenner DJ. Toward optimal external-beam fractionation for prostate cancer. *Int J Radiat Oncol Biol Phys* 2000,48(2):315–316.
23. Brenner DJ. Fractionation and late rectal toxicity. *Int J Radiat Oncol Biol Phys* 2004;60(4):1013–1015.
24. Brenner DJ, Hall EJ. Conditions for the equivalence of continuous to pulsed low dose rate brachytherapy. *Int J Radiat Oncol Biol Phys* 1991;20(1):181–190.
25. Brenner DJ, Hall EJ. Fractionated high dose-rate versus low dose-rate brachytherapy of the cervix. I. General considerations based on radiobiology. *Br J Radiol* 1991;64:133.
26. Brenner DJ, Hall EJ. Fractionation and protraction for radiotherapy of prostate carcinoma. *Int J Radiat Oncol Biol Phys* 1999;43(5):1095–1101.
27. Brenner DJ, Hlatky LR, Hahnfeldt JP, et al. A convenient extension of the linear-quadratic model to include redistribution and reoxygenation. *Int J Radiat Oncol Biol Phys* 1995;32:379–390.
28. Brenner DJ, Hlatky LR, Hahnfeldt PJ, et al. The linear-quadratic and most other common radiobiological models predict similar time-dose relationships. *Radiat Res* 1998;150:83–88.
29. Brenner DJ, Huang Y-P, Hall EJ. Fractionated high dose-rate versus low dose-rate regimens for intracavitary brachytherapy of the cervix: equivalent regimens for combined brachytherapy and external irradiation. *Int J Radiat Oncol Biol Phys* 1991;21:1415–1423.
30. Brenner DJ, Leu CS, Beatty JF, et al. Clinical relative biological effectiveness of low-energy x-rays emitted by miniature x-ray devices. *Phys Med Biol* 1999;44(2):323–333.
31. Brenner DJ, Martinez AA, Edmundson GK, et al. Direct evidence that prostate tumors show high sensitivity to fractionation (low alpha/beta ratio), similar to late-responding normal tissue. *Int J Radiat Oncol Biol Phys* 2002;52(1):6–13.
32. Brenner DJ, Schiff PB, Huang Y, et al. Pulsed-dose-rate brachytherapy: design of convenient (daytime-only) schedules. *Int J Radiat Oncol Biol Phys* 1997;39(4):809–815.
33. Brenner DJ, Zaider M. Estimating RBEs at clinical doses from microdosimetric spectra. *Med Phys* 1998;25(6):1055–1057.
34. British Committee on Radiation Units and Measurements. Specification of brachytherapy sources. *Br J Radiol* 1984;57:941.
35. Burlin TE. A general theory of cavity ionization. *Br J Radiol* 1966;39:361.
36. Butler WM, Merrick GS, Lief JH. Comparison of seed loading approaches in prostate brachytherapy. *Med Phys* 2000;27:381–392.
37. Carlsson AK, Ahnesjo A. The collapsed cone superposition algorithm applied to scatter dose calculations in brachytherapy. *Med Phys* 2000;27(10):2320–2332.
38. Cetingoz R, Ataman OU, Tuncel N, et al. Optimization in high dose rate brachytherapy for utero-vaginal applications. *Radiother Oncol* 2001;58(1):31–36.
39. Chibani O, Williamson JF. MCPI: a sub-minute Monte Carlo dose calculation engine for prostate implants. *Med Phys* 2005;32(12):3688–3698.
40. Chiu-Tsao S-T. Thermoluminescent dosimetry for Pd-103 seeds (model 200) in solid water phantom. *Med Phys* 1991;18:449–452.
41. Chiu-Tsao S-T. Episcleral eye plaques for treatment of intra-ocular malignancies and benign diseases. In: Thomadsen BR, Rivard MJ, Butler WM eds. *Brachytherapy physics*. 2nd ed. Madison, WI: Medical Physics Publishing, 2005;673–706.
42. Chiu-Tsao S-T, Anderson LL, O'Brien K, et al. Dose rate determination for I-125 seeds. *Med Phys* 1990;17:815–825.
43. Christensen GE, Carlson B, Chao KS, et al. Image-based dose planning of intracavitary brachytherapy: registration of serial-imaging studies using deformable anatomic templates. *Int J Radiat Oncol Biol Phys* 2001;51(1):227–243.
44. Corbett JF, Jezioranski JJ, Crook J, et al. The effect of seed orientation deviations on the quality of ^{125}I prostate implants. *Phys Med Biol* 2001;46(11):2785–2800.
45. Coursey BM. Needs for radioactivity standards and measurements in the life sciences. *Appl Radiat Isot* 2000;52(3):609–614.
46. Coutard H. Roentgentherapy of epitheliomas of the tonsillar region, hypopharynx and larynx, from 1920–1926. *Am J Roentgenol* 1932;28:313–331, 343–348.
47. Crook JM, Esche BA, Chaplain G, et al. Dose-volume analysis and the prevention of radiation sequelae in cervical cancer. *Radiother Oncol* 1987;8:321–332.
48. Dale RG. Some theoretical deviations relating to the tissue dosimetry of brachytherapy nuclides, with particular reference to Iodine-125. *Med Phys* 1983; 10:176.
49. Dale RG. The application of the linear-quadratic dose-effect equation to fractionated and protracted radiotherapy. *Br J Radiol* 1985;58:515–528.
50. Dale RG. Radiobiological assessment of permanent implants using tumour repopulation factors in the linear-quadratic model. *Br J Radiol* 1989;62(735):241–244.
51. Dale RG. The use of small fraction numbers in high dose-rate gynecological afterloading: some radiobiological considerations. *Br J Radiol* 1990;63:290.
51a. Dale RG, Jones B. The assessment of RBE effects using concept of biologically effective dose. IJROBP 1999;43:639–645.
52. Dale RG, Jones B. The effect of tumour shrinkage on biologically effective dose, and possible implications for fractionated high dose rate brachytherapy. *Radiother Oncol* 1994;33:125–132.
53. Dale RG, Jones B. The clinical radiobiology of brachytherapy. *Br J Radiol* 1998;71(845):465–483.
54. Dale RG, Jones B, Coles IP. The effect of tumour shrinkage on biologically effectiveness of permanent brachytherapy implants. *Br J Radiol* 1994;67:639–647.
55. Das RK, Keleti D, Zhu Y, et al. Validation of Monte Carlo dose calculations near I-125 brachytherapy sources in the presence of bounded tissue heterogeneities. *Int J Radiat Oncol Biol Phys* 1997;38:843–853.
56. Daskalov GM, Baker RS, Rogers DW, et al. Multigroup discrete ordinates modeling of ^{125}I 6702 seed dose distributions using a broad energy-group cross section representation. *Med Phys* 2002;29:113–124.
57. De Deene Y, Reynaert N, De Wagter C. On the accuracy of monomer/polymer gel dosimetry in the proximity of a high-dose-rate ^{192}Ir source. *Phys Med Biol* 2001;46(11):2801–2825.
58. Delclos L, Fletcher GH, Sampiere V. Can the Fletcher gamma ray colpostat system be extrapolated to other systems? *Cancer* 1978;41:970.
59. Demanes DJ, Rodriguez RR, Bendre DD, et al. High dose rate transperineal interstitial brachytherapy for cervical cancer: high pelvic control and low complication rates. *Int J Radiat Oncol Biol Phys* 1999;45(1):105–112.
60. DeMarco JJ, Smathers JB, Burnison CM, et al. CT-based dosimetry calculations for ^{125}I prostate implants. *Int J Radiat Oncol Biol Phys* 1999;45(5):1347–1353.
61. Dempsey JF, Low DA, Mutic S, et al. Validation of a precision radiochromic film dosimetry system for quantitative two-dimensional imaging of acute exposure dose distributions. *Med Phys* 2000;27(10):2462–2475.
62. DeWerd LA. Calibration of brachytherapy sources. In: Thomadsen BR, Rivard MJ, Butler WM, eds. *Brachytherapy physics*. 2nd ed. Madison, WI: Medical Physics Publishing, 2005;153–172.
63. DeWerd LA, Huq MS, Das IJ, et al. Procedures for establishing and maintaining consistent air-kerma strength standards for low-energy, photon-emitting brachytherapy sources: recommendations of the Calibration Laboratory Accreditation Subcommittee of the American Association of Physicists in Medicine. *Med Phys* 2004;31(3):675–681.
64. Dicker AP, Lin CC, Leeper DB, et al. Isotope selection for permanent prostate implants? An evaluation of ^{103}Pd versus ^{125}I based on radiobiological effectiveness and dosimetry. *Semin Urol Oncol* 2000;18(2):152–159.
65. Diffey BL, Levenhagen SC. An experimental and calculated dose distribution in water around CDC-K type cesium-137 sources. *Med Phys* 1975;20:446.
66. Dorr W, Hendry JH. Consequential late effects in normal tissues. *Radiother Oncol* 2001;61(3):223–231.
67. Duane W. Methods of preparing and using radioactive substances in the treatment of malignant disease and estimating suitable doses. *Boston Med Surg J* 1917;177:787–799.
68. Dubray BM, Thames HD. The clinical significance of ratios of radiobiological parameters. *Int J Radiat Oncol Biol Phys* 1996;35(5):1099–1111.
69. Duchesne GM, Peters LJ. What is the alpha/beta ratio for prostate cancer? Rationale for hypofractionated high-dose-rate brachytherapy. *Int J Radiat Oncol Biol Phys* 1999;44(4):747–748.
70. Dutriex A, Marinello G. The Paris system. In: Pierquin, Wilson JF, Chassagne D, eds. *Modern brachytherapy* New York: Masson, 1987;25–42.
70a. Eckert & Ziegler Isotope Products website. Available at: http://www.ipl.isotopeproducts.com/new_ipl_site/html/products_medical.asp
71. Edmundson GK. Geometry-based optimization for stepping source implants. In: Martinez AA, Orton CG, Mould RF eds. *Brachytherapy: HDR and LDR*. Columbia, MD: Nucletron Corporation, 1992:184–192.
72. Edmundson GK, Yan D, Martinez A. Intraoperative optimization of needle placement and dwell times for conformal prostate brachytherapy. *Int J Radiat Oncol Biol Phys* 1995;33:1257–1263.
73. Eisbruch A, Williamson JF, Dickson R, et al. Estimation of tissue volume irradiated by intracavitary implants. *Int J Radiat Oncol Biol Phys* 1993;25:733–744.
74. Ellis F. Dose, time and fractionation in radiotherapy. In: Ebert M, Howard A, eds. *Current topics in radiation research*. Amsterdam: North Holland Publishing Company, 1968;359–397.
75. Esche BA, Crook JM, Isturiz J, et al. Reference volume, milligram-hours and external irradiation for the Fletcher applicator. *Radiother Oncol* 1987;9:255–261.
76. Ezzell GA. Clinical implementation of dwell-time optimization techniques. In: Williamson JF, Thomadsen BR, Nath R, eds. *Brachytherapy physics: American Association of Physicists in Medicine, 1994 summer school*. Madison, WI: Medical Physics Publishing Corporation, 1995;617–639.
77. Ezzell GA. Optimization in Brachytherapy. In: Thomadsen BR, Rivard MJ, Butler WM, eds. *Brachytherapy physics*. 2nd ed. Madison, WI: Medical Physics Publishing, 2005;415–434.
78. Falkenberg E, Kim RY, Meleth S, et al. Low-dose-rate vs. high-dose-rate intracavitary brachytherapy for carcinoma of the cervix: the University of Alabama at Birmingham (UAB) experience. *Brachytherapy* 2006;5(1):49–55.
79. Farajollahi AR, Bonnett DE, Ratcliffe AJ, et al. An investigation into the use of polymer gel dosimetry in low dose rate brachytherapy. *Br J Radiol* 1999;72(863):1085–1092.
80. Fellner C, Potter R, Knocke TH, et al. Comparison of radiography- and computed tomography-based treatment planning in cervix cancer in brachytherapy with specific attention to some quality assurance aspects. *Radiother Oncol* 2001;58(1);53–62.

81. Ferrigno R, Nishimoto IN, Novaes PE, et al. Comparison of low and high dose rate brachytherapy in the treatment of uterine cervix cancer. Retrospective analysis of two sequential series. *Int J Radiat Oncol Biol Phys* 2005;62(4);1108–1116.

82. Fertil B, Reydellet I, Deschavanne PJ. A benchmark of cell survival models using survival curves for human cells after completion of repair of potentially lethal damage. *Radiat Res* 1994;138:61–69.

83. Fletcher GH. Cervical radium applicators with screening in the direction of bladder and rectum. *Radiology* 1953;60:77.

84. Fletcher GH, Hamberger AD. Squamous cell carcinoma of the uterine cervix: treatment techniques according to size of the cervical lesion and extension. In: Fletcher GD, ed. *Textbook of radiotherapy*. 3rd ed. Philadelphia: Lea & Febiger, 1980;732–772.

85. Fowler J, Chappell R, Ritter M. Is alpha/beta for prostate tumors really low? *Int J Radiat Oncol Biol Phys* 2001;50(4):1021–1031.

86. Fowler JF. The linear-quadratic formula and progress in fractionated radiotherapy. *Br J Radiol* 1989;62:679–694.

87. Fraass B, Doppke K, Hunt M, et al. American Association of Physicists in Medicine Radiation Therapy Committee Task Group 53: quality assurance for clinical radiotherapy treatment planning. *Med Phys* 1998;25(10):1773–1829.

88. Galalae RM, Martinez A, Nuernberg N, et al. Hypofractionated conformal HDR brachytherapy in hormone naive men with localized prostate cancer. Is escalation to very high biologically equivalent dose beneficial in all prognostic risk groups? *Strahlenther Onkol* 2006;182(3):135–141.

89. Gebara WJ, Weeks KJ, Hahn CA, et al. Computed axial tomography tandem and ovoids (CATTO) dosimetry: three-dimensional assessment of bladder and rectal doses. *Radiat Oncol Invest* 1998;6(6):268–275.

90. Gifford KA, Horton JL Jr, Pelloski CE, et al. A three-dimensional computed tomography-assisted Monte Carlo evaluation of ovoid shielding on the dose to the bladder and rectum in intracavitary radiotherapy for cervical cancer. *Int J Radiat Oncol Biol Phys* 2005;63(2),615–621.

91. Gillin MT, Albano KS, Erickson B. Classical systems II for planar and volume temporary interstitial implants: the Paris and other systems. In: Williamson JF, Thomadsen BR, Nath R., eds. *Brachytherapy physics*. Madison, WI: Medical Physics Publishing, 1995;232–343.

92. Gillin MT, Mourtada F. Manchester planar and volume implants and the Paris system. In: Thomadsen BR, Rivard MJ, Butler WM, eds. *Brachytherapy physics*. 2nd ed. Madison, WI: Medical Physics Publishing, 2005;351–372.

93. Glasgow GP. An apercu of codes, directives, guidances, notices, and regulations in brachytherapy. In: Thomadsen BR, Rivard MJ, Butler WM, eds. *Brachytherapy physics*. 2nd ed. Madison, WI: Medical Physics Publishing, 2005;173–186.

94. Gooden TJ. *Physical aspects of brachytherapy* (Medical Physics Handbook 19). Bristol: Adam Hilger, 1988.

95. Gray LH. An ionization method for the absolute measurement of gamma-ray energy. *Proc R Soc* 1936;A156:578.

96. Greco A, Mason P, Leung AWL, et al. Staging of carcinoma of the uterine cervix: MRI-surgical correlation. *Clin Radiol* 1989;40:401–405.

97. Grigsby PW, Williamson JF, Perez CA. Source configuration and dose rates for the Selectron afterloading equipment for gynecologic applicators. *Int J Radiat Oncol Biol Phys* 1992;24(2):321–327.

98. Grimm P, Sylvester J. Advances in brachytherapy. *Rev Urol* (Cryosurgery and Brachytherapy) 2004;6:37–48.

99. Grimm PD, Blasko JC, Sylvester JE, et al. 10-year biochemical (prostate-specific antigen) control of prostate cancer with (125)I brachytherapy. *Int J Radiat Oncol Biol Phys* 2001;51(1):31–40.

100. Haas JS, Dean RD, Mansfield CM. Dosimetry comparison of the Fletcher family of gynecologic colpostats 1950–1980. *Int J Radiat Oncol Biol Phys* 1985;11:1317–1321.

101. Haie-Meder C, Potter R, Van Limbergen E, et al. Recommendations from Gynaecological (GYN) GEC-ESTRO Working Group (I): concepts and terms in 3D image based 3D treatment planning in cervix cancer brachytherapy with emphasis on MRI assessment of GTV and CTV. *Radiother Oncol* 2005;74(3):235–245.

102. Hall EJ, Bedford JS. Dose-rate: its effect on the survival of HeLa cells irradiated with gamma-rays. *Radiat Res* 1964;22:305–315.

103. Hall EJ, Brenner JD. The dose-rate effect in interstitial brachytherapy: a controversy resolved. *Br J Radiol* 1992;65(771):242–247.

104. Hareyama M, Sakata K, Oouchi A, et al. High-dose rate versus low-dose-rate intracavitary therapy for carcinoma of the uterine cervix: randomized trial. *Cancer* 2002;94(1):117–124.

105. Harms W, Krempien R, Grehn C, et al. Daytime pulsed dose rate brachytherapy as a new treatment option for previously irradiated patients with recurrent oesophageal cancer. *Br J Radiol* 2005;78(927):236–241.

106. Harms W, Krempien R, Hensley FW, et al. 5-year results of pulsed dose rate brachytherapy applied as a boost after breast-conserving therapy in patients at high risk for local recurrence from breast cancer. *Strahlenther Onkol* 2002;178(11):607–614.

107. Haustermans KM, Hofland I, Van Poppel H, et al. Cell kinetic measurements in prostate cancer. *Int J Radiat Oncol Biol Phys* 1997;37(5):1067–1070.

108. Hedtjärn H, Carlsson GA, Williamson JF. Accelerated Monte Carlo-based dose calculations for brachytherapy planning using correlated sampling. *Phys Med Biol* 2002;47:351–376.

109. Hedtjärn H, Carlsson GA, Williamson JF. Monte Carlo-aided dosimetry of the UroMed/Bebig Symmetra I-125, Model I25.S06 interstitial brachytherapy seed. *Med Phys* 2000;27:1076–1085.

110. Hendry JH, Thames HD. The tissue rescuing unit. *Br J Radiol* 1986;59:628–630.

111. Henschke UK. "Afterloading" applicator for radiation therapy of carcinoma of the uterus. *Radiology* 1960;74:834.

112. Henschke UK, Hilaris BS, Mahan GD. Afterloading in interstitial and intracavitary radiation therapy. *Am J Roentgenol* 1963;90:386–395.

113. Henschke UK, Lawrence DC. Cesium-131 seeds for permanent implants. *Radiology* 1965;85,1117–1119 (1965).

114. Hilaris BS, Henschke UK, Holt JG. Clinical experience with long half-life and low-energy encapsulated radioactive sources in cancer radiation therapy. *Radiology* 1968;91,1163–1167.

115. Hilaris BS, Holt GJ, St. Germain J. *The use of Iodine-125 for interstitial implants*. Rockville, MD: Department of Health, Education and Welfare, Publication (FDA) 76-8022, 1975.

116. Hilaris BS, Nori D, Anderson LL. *Atlas of brachytherapy*. New York: Macmillan Publishing Co., 1988.

117. Holm HH, Juul N, Pederson JF, et al. Transperineal Iodine-125 seed implantation in prostatic cancer guided by transrectal ultrasonography. *J Urol* 1983;130:283–286.

118. Horiot JC, Pigneux J, Pourquier H, et al. Radiotherapy alone in carcinoma of the intact uterine cervix according to G. H. Fletcher guidelines: a French cooperative study of 1383 cases. *Int J Radiat Oncol Biol Phys* 1988;14(4):605–611.

119. Horsler AFC, Jones JC, Stacey AJ. Cesium-137 sources for use in intracavitary and interstitial radiotherapy. *Br J Radiol* 1964;37:385.

120. Horwitz H, Kereiakes JG, Bahr GK, et al. An after-loading system utilizing Cesium 137 for the treatment of carcinoma of the cervix. *Am J Roentgenol Radium Ther Nucl Med* 1964;91:176–191.

121. Houdek PV, Schwade JG, Abitbol AA, et al. Optimization of high dose-rate cervix brachytherapy; Part I: dose distribution. *Int J Radiat Oncol Biol Phys* 1991;21(6):1621–1625.

122. ICRU. *Dose and volume specification for reporting intracavitary therapy in gynecology: Report 38*. Bethesda, MD: International Commission of Radiation Units and Measurements, 1985.

123. ICRU. *Dose and volume specification for reporting interstitial therapy, Report 58*. Bethesda, MD: International Commission on Radiation Units and Measurements, 1997.

124. ICRU. *Fundamental quantities and units for ionizing radiation, Report 58*. Bethesda, MD: International Commission on Radiation Units and Measurements, 1998.

125. Jackson A, Kutcher GJ, Yorke ED. Probability of radiation-induced complications for normal tissues with parallel architecture subject to non-uniform irradiation. *Med Phys* 1993;20(3):613–625.

126. Jereczek-Fossa BA, Jassem J, Badzio A. Relationship between acute and late normal tissue injury after postoperative radiotherapy in endometrial cancer. *Int J Radiat Oncol Biol Phys* 2002;52(2):476–482.

127. Johns HE, Cunningham JR. *The physics of radiology*. Springfield, IL: Charles C. Thomas, 1983.

128. Kal HB, Van Gellekom MP. How low is the alpha/beta ratio for prostate cancer? *Int J Radiat Oncol Biol Phys* 2003;57(4):1116–1121.

129. Kellerer AM, Rossi HH. The theory of dual radiation action. *Curr Top Radiat Res* 1972;8:85–158.

130. Khan FM. *The physics of radiation therapy*. 2nd ed. Baltimore: Wilkens & Wilkens, 1994.

131. King CR. LDR vs. HDR brachytherapy for localized prostate cancer: the view from radiobiological models. *Brachytherapy* 2002;1(4):219–226.

132. King CR, Fowler JF. A simple analytic derivation suggests that prostate cancer alpha/beta ratio is low. *Int J Radiat Oncol Biol Phys* 2001;51(1):213–214.

133. Kirov AS, Shrinivas S, Hurlbut C, et al. New water equivalent liquid scintillation solutions for 3D dosimetry. *Med Phys* 2000;27(5):1156–1164.

134. Kirov AS, Williamson JF, Meigooni AS. Measurement and calculation of heterogeneity correction factors for an Ir-192 high dose-rate brachytherapy source behind tungsten alloy and steel shields. *Med Phys* 1996;23:911–916.

135. Klevenhagen SL. An experimental study of dose distribution in water around ^{137}Cs tubes used in brachytherapy. *Br J Radiol* 1973;46:1073.

136. Kline RW, Yeakel PD. Ocular melanoma I-125 plaques. *Med Phys* 1987;14:475.

137. Kolkman-Deurloo IKK, Visser AG, Niel CGJH, et al. Optimization of interstitial volume implants. *Radiother Oncol* 1994;31:229–239.

138. Krishnaswamy V. Dose distribution around an I-125 seed source in tissue. *Radiology* 1978;126:489.

139. Krishnaswamy V. Dose tables for ^{125}I seed implants. *Radiology* 1979;132:727–730.

140. Kubo HD, Glasgow GP, Pethel TD, et al. High dose-rate brachytherapy treatment delivery: report of the AAPM Radiation Therapy Committee Task Group No. 59. *Med Phys* 1998;25(4):375–403.

141. Kucera H, Potter R, Knocke TH, et al. High-dose versus low-dose rate brachytherapy in definitive radiotherapy of cervical cancer. *Wien Klin Wochenschr* 2001;113(1–2):58–62.

142. Kupelian PA, Reddy CA, Carlson TP, et al. Preliminary observations on biochemical relapse-free survival rates after short-course intensity-modulated radiotherapy (70 Gy at 2.5 Gy/fraction) for localized prostate cancer. *Int J Radiat Oncol Biol Phys* 2002;53(4):904–912.

143. Kupelian PA, Thakkar VV, Khuntia D, et al. Hypofractionated intensity-modulated radiotherapy (70 Gy at 2.5 Gy per fraction) for localized prostate cancer: long-term outcomes. *Int J Radiat Oncol Biol Phys* 2005;63(5):1463–1468.

144. Kutcher GJ, Coia L, Gillin M, et al. Comprehensive QA for radiation oncology: report of AAPM Radiation Therapy Committee Task Group 40. *Med Phys* 1994;21(4):581–618.

145. Lachance B, Beliveau-Nadeau D, Lessard E, et al. Early clinical experience with anatomy-based inverse planning dose optimization for high-dose-rate boost of the prostate. *Int J Radiat Oncol Biol Phys* 2002;54(1):86–100.

146. Lahanas M, Baltas D, Giannouli S. Global convergence analysis of fast multiobjective gradient-based dose optimization algorithms for high-dose-rate brachytherapy. *Phys Med Biol* 2003;48(5):599–617.

147. Laughlin JS, Siler WM, Holodny EI. A dose description system for interstitial radiation therapy: seed implants. *Am J Roentgenol Radiat Ther Nucl Med* 1963;89:470.

148. Laurence GC. Measurement of extra hard x-rays and gamma rays in roentgens. *Can J Res* 1937;A15:67–78.

149. Lawrence DC, Sondhaus CA, Feder B, et al. Soft x-ray "seeds" for cancer therapy. *Radiology* 1966;86:143.

150. Lea DE. *Actions of radiations on living cells*. London: Cambridge University Press, 1946.

151. Lea DE, Catcheside DG. The mechanism of the induction by radiation of chromosome aberrations in *Tradescantia*. *J Genet* 1942;44:216–245.

152. Leborgne F, Leborgne JH, Zubizarreta E, et al. High-dose-rate brachytherapy at 14 Gy per hour to point A: preliminary results of a prospectively designed schedule for cancer of the cervix based on the linear-quadratic model. *Int J Gynecol Cancer* 2001;11(6):445–453.

153. Lee EK, Gallagher RJ, Silvern D, et al. Treatment planning for brachytherapy: an integer programming model, two computational approaches and experiments with permanent prostate implant planning. *Phys Med Biol* 1999;44(1):145–165.

154. Lee WR. In regard to Brenner et al. Direct evidence that prostate tumors show high sensitivity to fractionation (low alpha/beta ratio) similar to late-responding normal tissue. *Int J Radiat Oncol Biol Phys* 2002;53(5):1392; Author reply 1393.

155. Lessard E, Pouliot J. Inverse planning anatomy-based dose optimization for HDR-brachytherapy of the prostate using fast simulated annealing algorithm and dedicated objective function. *Med Phys* 2001;28:773–779.
156. Letschet JGJ, Lebesque JV, de Boer RW, et al. Dose-volume correlation in radiation-related late small-bowel complications: a clinical study. *Radiother Oncol* 1990;18:307–320.
157. Leung S. Perineal template techniques for interstitial implantation of gynecological cancers using the Paris system of dosimetry. *Int J Radiat Oncol Biol Phys* 1990;19:769–774.
158. Levendag PC, Schmitz PI, Jansen PP, et al. Fractionated high-dose-rate and pulsed-dose-rate brachytherapy: first clinical experience in squamous cell carcinoma of the tonsillar fossa and soft palate. *Int J Radiat Oncol Biol Phys* 1997;38(3):497–506.
159. Li Z, Palta JR, Fan JJ. Monte Carlo calculations and experimental measurements of dosimetry parameters of a new 103Pd source. *Med Phys* 2000;27(5):1108–1112.
160. Li Z, Williamson JF, Perera H. Monte Carlo calculation of kerma to a point in the vicinity of media interfaces. *Phys Med Biol* 1993;38:1825–1840.
161. Lief EP. Localization I: radiographic methods and accuracy. In: Thomadsen BR, Rivard MJ, Butler WM, eds. *Brachytherapy physics*. 2nd ed. Madison, WI: Medical Physics Publishing, 2005;173–186.
162. Lindsay P, Battista J, Van Dyk J. The effect of seed anisotropy on brachytherapy dose distributions using ^{125}I and ^{103}Pd. *Med Phys* 2001;28(3):336–345.
163. Ling CC, Anderson LL, Shipley WU. Dose inhomogeneity in interstitial implants using ^{125}I seeds. *Int J Radiat Oncol Biol Phys* 1979;5:419–425.
164. Ling CC, Roy J, Sahoo N, et al. Quantifying the effect of dose inhomogeneity in brachytherapy: application to permanent prostatic implant with ^{125}I seeds. *Int J Radiat Oncol Biol Phys* 1994;28:971–977.
165. Ling CC, Roy JN. Radiobiophysical aspects of brachytherapy. In: Williamson J, Thomadsen BR, Nath R, eds. *Brachytherapy physics: American Association of Physicists in Medicine, 1994 summer school*. Madison, WI: Medical Physics Publishing, 1995;39–71.
166. Ling CC, Yorke ED, Schell MC, et al. Physical advantages of using Iodine-125 in temporary implants of the breast. *Endocurie Hypertherm Oncol* 1986;2:216–217.
167. Ling CC, Yorke Ed, Spiro IJ. Physical dosimetry of I-125 seeds of a new design for interstitial implant. *Int J Radiat Oncol Biol Phys* 1983;9:1747.
168. Livsey JE, Cowan RA, Wylie JP, et al. Hypofractionated conformal radiotherapy in carcinoma of the prostate: five-year outcome analysis. *Int J Radiat Oncol Biol Phys* 2003;57(5):1254–1259.
169. Lloyd-Davies RW, Collins CD, Swan AV. Carcinoma of prostate treated by radical external beam radiotherapy using hypofractionation. Twenty-two years' experience (1962–1984). *Urology* 1990;36(2):107–111.
170. Loblaw DA, Cheung P. External beam irradiation for localized prostate cancer—the promise of hypofractionation. *Can J Urol* 2006;13[Suppl 1]:62–66.
171. Loftus TP. Standardization of Cesium-137 gamma-ray sources in terms of exposure units (roentens). *J Res Natl Bureau Stand* 1970;74:1–6.
172. Loftus TP. Standardization of Iridium-192 gamma-ray sources in terms of exposure. *J Res Natl Bureau Stand* 1980;85:19–25.
173. Loftus TP. Exposure standardization of Iodine-125 seeds used for brachytherapy. *J Res Natl Bureau Stand* 1984;89:295–303.
174. Logue JP, Cowan RA, Hendry JH. Hypofractionation for prostate cancer. *Int J Radiat Oncol Biol Phys* 2001;49(5):1522–1523.
175. Low DA, Williamson JF. Objective evaluation of optimized planar implants. *Med Phys* 1995;22:1477–1485.
176. Lukka H, Hayter C, Julian JA, et al. Randomized trial comparing two fractionation schedules for patients with localized prostate cancer. *J Clin Oncol* 2005;23(25):6132–6138.
177. Mai J, Erickson B, Rownd J, et al. Comparison of four different dose specification methods for high-dose–rate intracavitary radiation for treatment of cervical cancer. *Int J Radiat Oncol Biol Phys* 2001;51(4):1131–1141.
178. Marchese MJ, Goldhagen PE, Zaider M, et al. The relative biological effectiveness of photon radiation from encapsulated Iodine-125, assessed in cells of human origin. I. Normal diploid fibroblasts. *Int J Radiat Oncol Biol Phys* 1990;18:1407–1413.
179. Marinello G, Valero M, Levng S, et al. Comparative dosimetry between iridium wire and seed ribbons. *Int J Radial Oncol Biol Phys* 1985;11:1733.
180. Markman J, Williamson JF, Dempsey JF, et al. On the validity of the superposition principle in dose calculations for intracavitary implants with shielded vaginal colpostats. *Med Phys* 2001;28(2):147–155.
181. Martin T, Baltas D, Kurek R, et al. 3-D conformal HDR brachytherapy as monotherapy for localized prostate cancer. A pilot study. *Strahlenther Onkol* 2004;180(4):225–232.
182. Maruyama Y, Vtyurin BM, Kaneta K, et al. Californium-252 brachytherapy. In: Nag S, ed. *Principles and practice of brachytherapy*. Armonk, NY: Futura, 1997;649–687.
183. Medich DC, Tries MA, Munro JJ 2nd. Monte Carlo characterization of an ytterbium-169 high dose rate brachytherapy source with analysis of statistical uncertainty. *Med Phys* 2006;33(1):163–172.
184. Meigooni AS, Bharucha Z, Yoe-Sein M, et al. Dosimetric characteristics of the bests double-wall 103Pd brachytherapy source. *Med Phys* 2001;28(12):2568–2575.
185. Meigooni AS, Zhu Y, Myerson RJ, et al. Design, construction and dosimetry of a rectal applicator for a high dose-rate remote afterloading system. *Int J Radiat Oncol Biol Phys* 1996;34:1153–1164.
186. Meisberger LL, Keller RJ, Shalek RJ. The effective attenuation in water of the g-rays of gold-198, iridium-192, cesium-137, radium-226, and cobalt-60. *Radiology* 1968;90:953.
187. Meredith WJ. Dosage for cancer of cervix uteri. In: Meredith WJ, ed. *Radium dosage: the Manchester system*. 2nd ed. Edinburgh: E & S Livingston, Ltd, 1967;42–50.
188. Merrick GS, Butler WM, Dorsey AT, et al. Potential role of various dosimetric quality indicators in prostate brachytherapy. *Int J Radiat Oncol Biol Phys* 1999;44(3):717–724.
189. Milickovic N, Lahanas M, Papagiannopoulo M, et al. Multiobjective anatomy-based dose optimization for HDR-brachytherapy with constraint free deterministic algorithms. *Phys Med Biol* 2002;47(13):2263–2280.
190. Mizoe J. Analysis of the dose-volume histogram in uterine cervical cancer by diagnostic CT. *Strahlenther Onkol* 1990;166:279–284.
191. Mohan R, Ding, IY, Martel MK. Measurement of radiation dose distribution of shielded cervical applicators. *Int J Radial Oncol Biol Phys* 1985;11:861.
192. Monroe JI, Dempsey JF, Dorton JA, et al. Experimental validation of dose calculation algorithms for the GliaSite RTS, a novel 125I liquid-filled balloon brachytherapy applicator. *Med Phys* 2001;28(1):73–85.
193. Monroe JI, Williamson JF. Monte Carlo-aided dosimetry of the Theragenics TheraSeed ®Model 200 ^{103}Pd Interstitial Brachytherapy Seed. *Med Phys* 2002;29:609–621.
194. Mundt AJ, Mell LK, Roeske JC. Preliminary analysis of chronic gastrointestinal toxicity in gynecology patients treated with intensity-modulated whole pelvic radiation therapy. *Int J Radiat Oncol Biol Phys* 2003;56(5):1354–1360.
195. Munro TR, Gilbert CW. The relation between tumour lethal doses and the radiosensitivity of tumour cells. *Br J Radiol* 1961;34:246–251.
196. Murphy MK, Piper RK, Greenwood LR, et al. Evaluation of the new cesium-131 seed for use in low-energy x-ray brachytherapy. *Med Phys* 2004;31(6):1529–1538.
197. Nag S, Bice W, DeWyngaert K, et al. The American Brachytherapy Society recommendations for permanent prostate brachytherapy postimplant dosimetric analysis. *Int J Radiat Oncol Biol Phys* 2000;46(1):221–230.
198. Nag S, Cardenes H, Chang S, et al. Proposed guidelines for image-based intracavitary brachytherapy for cervical carcinoma: report from Image-Guided Brachytherapy Working Group. *Int J Radiat Oncol Biol Phys* 2004;60(4):1160–1172.
199. Nath R, Anderson L, Jones D, et al. *Specification of brachytherapy source strength: a report by Task Group 32 of the American Association of Physicists in Medicine. Report No. 21*. New York: American Institute of Physics, 1987.
200. Nath R, Anderson LL, Luxton G, et al. Dosimetry of interstitial brachytherapy sources: recommendations of the AAPM Radiation Therapy Committee Task Group No. 43. *Med Phys* 1995;22(2):209–234.
201. Nath R, Anderson LL, Meli JA, et al. Code of practice for brachytherapy physics: report of the AAPM Radiation Therapy Committee Task Group No. 56. American Association of Physicists in Medicine. *Med Phys* 1997;24(10):1557–1598.
202. Nath R, Gray L. Dosimetric studies on a prototype 241Am source for brachytherapy. *Int J Radial Oncol Biol Phys* 1987;13:897.
203. Nath R, Meigooni AS, Melillo A. Some treatment planning considerations for ^{103}Pd and ^{125}I permanent interstitial implants. *Int J Radiat Oncol Biol Phys* 1992;22:1131–1138.
204. Nath R, Meigooni AS, Muench P, et al. Anisotropy functions for ^{103}Pd, ^{125}I, and ^{193}Ir interstitial brachytherapy sources. *Med Phys* 1993;20:1465–1473.
205. Nath R, Urdaneta N, Bolanis N, et al. A dosimetric analysis of Morris, Fletcher and Henschke systems for treatment of uterine cervix carcinoma. *Int J Radiat Oncol Biol Phys* 1991;21:995–1003.
206. Nath R, Yue N, Liu L. On the depth of penetration of photons and electrons for intravascular brachytherapy. *Cardiovasc Radiat Med* 1999;1:72–79.
207. Nath R, Yue N, Shahnazi K, et al. Measurement of dose-rate constant for Pd^{103} seeds with air kerma strength calibration based upon a primary national standard. *Med Phys* 2000;27(4):655–658.
208. NCRP. *Structural shielding design and evaluation for medical use of x-rays and gamma rays up to 10 MeV. Report No. 49*. Bethesda, MD: National Council on Radiation Protection and Measurements, 1976.
209. NCRP. *A handbook of radioactivity measurements procedures. Report No. 5*. Bethesda, MD: National Council on Radiation Protection and Measurements, 1985.
210. Nickers P, Thissen B, Jansen N, et al. 192Ir or 125I prostate brachytherapy as a boost to external beam radiotherapy in locally advanced prostatic cancer: a dosimetric point of view. *Radiother Oncol* 2006;78(1):47–52.
211. Niemierko A. Reporting and analyzing dose distributions: a concept of equivalent uniform dose. *Med Phys* 1997;24(1):103–110.
212. Niemierko A, Goitein M. Implementation of a model for estimating tumor control probability for an inhomogeneously irradiated tumor. *Radiother Oncol* 1993;29(2):140–147.
213. Niroomand-Rad A, Blackwell CR, Coursey BM, et al. Radiochromic film dosimetry: recommendations of AAPM Radiation Therapy Committee Task Group 55. American Association of Physicists in Medicine. *Med Phys* 1998;25(11):2093–2115.
214. Noyes WR, Peters NE, Thomadsen BR, et al. Impact of "optimized" treatment planning for tandem and ring, and tandem and ovoids, using high dose rate brachytherapy for cervical cancer. *Int J Radiat Oncol Biol Phys* 1995;31(1):79–86.
215. Orton C. High and low dose-rate brachytherapy for cervical carcinoma. *Acta Radiol* 1998;37(2):117–125.
216. Parker HM. A dosage system for interstitial radium therapy. II. Physical aspects. *Br J Radiol* 1938;11:252–266.
217. Patel NS, Chiu-Tsao ST, Williamson JF, et al. Thermoluminescent dosimetry of the Symmetra ^{125}I model I25.S06 interstitial brachytherapy seed. *Med Phys* 2001;28(8):1761–1769.
218. Paterson R. *The treatment of malignant disease by radiotherapy*. 2nd ed. London: Edward Arnold, 1963.
219. Paterson R, Parker HM. A dosage system for g-ray therapy. *Br J Radiol* 1934;7:592.
220. Paterson R, Parker HM. A dosage system for interstitial radium therapy. *Br J Radiol* 1938;11:313–339.
221. Paul JM, Koch RF, Philips PC, et al. Uniformity of dose distribution in interstitial implants. *Endocurie Hyper Oncol* 1986;2:107.
222. Pellizzon AC, Salvajoli JV, Maia MA, et al. Late urinary morbidity with high dose prostate brachytherapy as a boost to conventional external beam radiation therapy for local and locally advanced prostate cancer. *J Urol* 2004;171(3):1105–1108.
223. Perera H, Williamson JF, Li Z, et al. Dosimetric characteristics, air-kerma strength calibration and verification of Monte Carlo simulation for a new Ytterbium-169 brachytherapy source. *Int J Radiat Oncol Biol Phys* 1994;28:953–971.
224. Perera H, Williamson JF, Monthofer SP, et al. Rapid two-dimensional dose measurement in brachytherapy using plastic scintillator sheet: linearity, signal-to-noise ratio and energy response characteristics. *Int J Radiat Oncol Biol Phys* 1992;23:1059–1069.
225. Perez CA, Camel HM, Kuske RR, et al. Radiation therapy alone in treatment of the uterine cervix: a 20 year experience. *Gynecol Oncol* 1986;23:127.
226. Piermattei A, Azario L, Montemaggi P. Implantation guidelines for Yb-169 seed interstitial treatments. *Phys. Med. Biol.*40,1331–1338 (1995).
227. Pierquin B. Cervix. In: Pierquin B, Marinello G, eds. *A practical manual of brachytherapy*. Madison, WI: Medical Physics Publishing, 1997;165–196.
228. Pierquin B, Dutreix A. Towards a new system in curietherapy endocurietherapy and plesiotherapy with non-radioactive preparation. *Br J Radiol* 1967;40:184.
229. Pierquin B, Wilson JF, Chassange D. *Modern brachytherapy*. New York: Masson, 1987.

230. Pieters BR, Saarnak AE, Steggerda MJ, et al. A method to improve the dose distribution of interstitial breast implants using geometrically optimized stepping source techniques and dose normalization. *Radiother Oncol* 2001;58:63–70.
231. Potish RA. The effect of applicator geometry on dose specification in cervical cancer. *Int J Radiat Oncol Biol Phys* 1990;18:1513–1520.
232. Potish RA, Gerbi BJ. Role of point A in the era of computerized dosimetry. *Radiology* 1986;158:827–831.
233. Potish RA, Gerbi BJ. Cervical cancer intracavitary dose specification and prescription. *Radiology* 1987;165:555–560.
234. Potter R, Haie-Meder C, Van Limbergen E, et al. Recommendations from gynaecological (GYN) GEC ESTRO working group (II): concepts and terms in 3D image-based treatment planning in cervix cancer brachytherapy-3D dose volume parameters and aspects of 3D image-based anatomy, radiation physics, radiobiology. *Radiother Oncol* 2006;78(1):67–77.
235. Potter R, Knocke TH, Fellner C, et al. Definitive radiotherapy based on HDR brachytherapy with iridium 192 in uterine cervix carcinoma: report on the Vienna University Hospital findings (1993–1997) compared to the preceding period in the context of ICRU 38 recommendations. *Cancer Radiother* 2000;4(2):159–172.
236. Potters L, Cao Y, Calugaru E, et al. A comprehensive review of CT-based dosimetry parameters and biochemical control in patients treated with permanent prostate brachytherapy. *Int J Radiat Oncol Biol Phys* 2001;50:605–614.
237. Pouliot J, Lessard E, Hsu IC. Advanced 3D planning. In: Thomadsen BR, Rivard MJ, Butler WM, eds. *Brachytherapy physics*. 2nd ed. Madison, WI: Medical Physics Publishing, 2005;233–294.
238. Pouliot J, Tremblay D, Roy J, et al. Optimization of permanent ^{125}I prostate implants using fast simulated annealing. *Int J Radiat Oncol Biol Phys* 1996;36:711–720.
239. Price MJ, Horton JL, Gifford KA, et al. Dosimetric evaluation of the Fletcher-Williamson ovoid for pulsed-dose-rate brachytherapy: a Monte Carlo study. *Phys Med Biol* 2005;50(21):5075–5087.
240. Quimby EH. Physical factors in interstitial radium therapy. *Am J Roentgenol Radium Ther* 1935;33:306–316.
241. Quimby EH. Dosage calculations in radium therapy. In: Glasser O, Quimby EH, Taylor LS, et al. eds. *Physical foundations of radiology*. New York: Paul B. Hoeker, 1952;339–372.
242. Quimby EH, Castro V. The calculation of dosage in interstitial radium therapy. *Am J Roentgenol* 1953;70:739–749.
243. Ragde H, Korb LJ, Elgamal AA, et al. Modern prostate brachytherapy. Prostate specific antigen results in 219 patients with up to 12 years of observed follow-up. *Cancer* 2000;89(1):135–141.
244. Rivard MJ. Burst calculations for 252Cf brachytherapy sources. *Med Phys* 2000;27(12):2816–2820.
245. Rivard MJ, Coursey BM, DeWerd LA, et al. Update of AAPM Task Group No. 43 Report: a revised AAPM protocol for brachytherapy dose calculations. *Med Phys* 2004;31(3):33–74.
246. Roesch WC. Dose for nonelectronic equilibrium conditions. *Radit Res* 1958;9:399–410.
247. Rossi HH, Zaider M. *Microdosimetry and its applications*. Berlin: Springer-Verlag, 1996.
248. Rownd J. Localization II: volume imaging techniques. In: Thomadsen BR, Rivard MJ, Butler WM, eds. *Brachytherapy physics*. 2nd ed. Madison, WI: Medical Physics Publishing, 2005:187–200.
249. Roy JN, Wallner KE, Harrington PJ, et al. A CT-based evaluation method for permanent implants: application to prostate. *Int J Radiat Oncol Biol Phys* 1993;26:163–169.
250. Sachs RK, Hahnfeldt PJ, Brenner JD. Review: the link between low-LET dose-response relations and the underlying kinetics of damage production/repair/misrepair. *Int J Radiat Oncol Biol Phys* 1997;72:351–374.
251. Saw CB; Suntharalingam N. Reference dose rates for single and double plane ^{192}Ir implants. *Med Phys* 1988;15:391.
252. Saw CB, Suntharalingam N. Quantitative assessment of interstitial implants. *Int J Radiat Oncol Biol Phys* 1991;20:135–139.
253. Schoeppel SL, La Vigne ML, Martel MK, et al. 3-D treatment planning of intracavitary gynecologic implants: analysis of ten cases and implications for dose specification. *Int J Radiat Oncol Biol Phys* 1993;28:277–283.
254. Seltzer SM, Lamperti PJ, Loevinger R, et al. New national air-kerma-strength standards for ^{125}I and ^{103}Pd brachytherapy seeds. *J Res Natl Inst Stand Technol* 2003;108:337–358.
255. Shalek RJ, Stovall M. The MD Anderson method for the computation of isodose curves around interstitial and intracavitary radiation sources. I. Dose from linear sources. *Am J Roentgenol Radium Ther* 1968;102:662–672.
256. Shalek RJ, Stovall MA, Sampiere VA. The radiation distribution and dose specification in volume implants of radioactive seeds. *Am J Roentgenol Radium Ther* 1957;77:863–868.
257. Shigehara K, Mizokami A, Komatsu K, et al. Four year clinical statistics of iridium-192 high dose rate brachytherapy. *Int J Urol* 2006;13(2):116–121.
258. Sievert RM. Die Intensitatsverteilung der primaren: strahlung in der Nahe medizinischer Radiumpraparate. *Acta Radiol* 1921;1:89–128.
259. Simon N, Silverstone SM. Intracavitary therapy of endometrial cancer by afterloading. *J Gynecol* 1972;1:13.
260. Steggerda MJ, Moonen LM, Damen EM, et al. An analysis of the effect of ovoid shields in a selectron-LDR cervical applicator on dose distributions in rectum and bladder. *Int J Radiat Oncol Biol Phys* 1997;39(1):237–245.
261. Stock EG, Stone NN, Tabert A, et al. A dose-response study for I-125 prostate implants. *Int J Radiat Oncol Biol Phys* 1998;41:101–108.
262. Stovall M, Shalek RJ. The MD Anderson method for the computation of isodose curves around interstitial and intracavitary radiation sources. III. Roentgenograms for input data and the relation of isodose calculations to the Paterson-Parker system. *Am J Roentgenol Radium Ther* 1968;102:677–687.
263. Strand V, Melzner W, Geiger M, et al. Role of interstitial PDR brachytherapy in the treatment of oral and oropharyngeal cancer. A single-institute experience of 236 patients. *Strahlenther Onkol* 2005;181(12):762–767.
264. Suit HD, Moore EB, Fletcher GH, et al. Modification of the Fletcher ovoid system for afterloading, using standard sized radium tubes. *Radiology* 1963;81:126–131.
265. Sylvester JE, Blasko JC, Grimm PD, et al. Ten-year biochemical relapse-free survival after external beam radiation and brachytherapy for localized prostate cancer: the Seattle experience. *Int J Radiat Oncol Biol Phys* 2003;57(4):944–952.
266. Teh BS, Berner BM, Carpenter LS, et al. Permanent gold-198 implant for locally recurrent adenocarcinoma of the prostate after failing initial radiotherapy. *J Brachytherapy Int* 1998;14:233–240.
267. Thames HD, Hendry JH. *Fractionation in radiotherapy*. London: Taylor and Francis, 1987.
268. Thames HD, Withers HR, Peters LJ, et al. Changes in early and late radiation responses with altered dose fractionation: implications for dose-survival relationships. *Int J Radiat Oncol Biol Phys* 1982;8(2):219–226.
269. Thomadsen BR, Rivard MJ, Butler WM. Localization II: volume imaging techniques. In: Thomadsen BR, Rivard MJ, Butler WM, eds. *Brachytherapy physics*. 2nd ed. Madison, WI: Medical Physics Publishing, 2005;965.
270. Tobias CA. The repair-misrepair model in radiobiology: comparison to other models. *Radiat Res* 1985;8:S77–S95.
271. Tod MC, Meredith WJ. A dosage system for use in the treatment of cancer of the uterine cervix. *Br J Radiol* 1938;11:809.
272. Tod M, Meredith WJ. Treatment of cancer of the cervix uteri: a revised Manchester method. *Br J Radiol* 1953;26:252–257.
273. Travis EL, Tucker SL. Isoeffect models and fractionated radiation therapy. *Int J Radiat Oncol Biol Phys* 1987;13(2):283–287.
274. Van der Laars R, Meertens H. An algorithm for ovoid shielding of a cervix applicator. In: Cunningham JR, Ragan D, Van Dyke D, eds. *The Proceedings of 8th International Conference on the Use of Computers in Radiation Therapy*. IEEE Computer Society, Toronto, Canada, Los Angeles, 1984;365–369.
275. Van Kleffens HJ, Star WM. Application of stereo x-ray photogrammetry (SRM) in the determination of absorbed dose values during intracavitary radiation therapy. *Int J Radiat Oncol Biol Phys* 1979;5:557.
276. Verhaegen F, Seuntjens J. Monte Carlo modelling of external radiotherapy photon beams. *Phys Med Biol* 2003;48(21):R107–164.
277. Vicini FA, Jaffray DA, Horwitz EM. Implementation of 3D-virtual brachytherapy in the management of breast cancer: a description of a new method of interstitial brachytherapy. *Int J Radiat Oncol Biol Phys* 1998;40:629–635.
278. Wallace RE, Fan JJ. Dosimetric characterization of a new design palladium-103 brachytherapy source. *Med Phys* 1999;26(11):2465–2470.
279. Wang CJ, Leung SW, Chen HC, et al. The correlation of acute toxicity and late rectal injury in radiotherapy for cervical carcinoma: evidence suggestive of consequential late effect (CQLE). *Int J Radiat Oncol Biol Phys* 1998;40(1):85–91.
280. Wang JZ, Guerrero M, Li XA. How low is the alpha/beta ratio for prostate cancer? *Int J Radiat Oncol Biol Phys* 2003;55(1):194–203.
281. Wang JZ, Li XA, Yu CX, et al. The low alpha/beta ratio for prostate cancer: what does the clinical outcome of HDR brachytherapy tell us? *Int J Radiat Oncol Biol Phys* 2003;57(4):1101–1108.
282. Wang Z, Hertel NE. Determination of dosimetric characteristics of OptiSeed^{TM} a plastic brachytherapy ^{103}Pd source. *Appl Radiat Isot* 2005;63(3):311–321.
283. Webb S, Nahum AE. A model for calculating tumour control probability in radiotherapy including the effects of inhomogeneous distributions of dose and clonogenic cell density. *Phys Med Biol* 1993;38(6):653–666.
284. Weeks KJ, Dennett JC. Dose calculation and measurements for a CT-compatible version of the Fletcher applicator. *Int J Radiat Oncol Biol Phys* 1990;18:1191–1198.
285. Weeks KJ, Montana GS. Three-dimensional applicator system for carcinoma of the uterine cervix. *Int J Radiat Oncol Biol Phys* 1997;37(2):455–463.
286. Wierzbicki J, Maruyama Y, Feola JM, et al. Facility and clinical handling of Californium-252 sources for brachytherapy. *Endocuriether Hypertherm Oncol* 1992;8:131–135.
287. Wilkinson JM, Ramachandran TP. The ICRU recommendations for reporting intracavitary therapy in gynaecology and the Manchester method of treating cancer of the cervix uteri. *Br J Radiol* 1989;62:362–365.
288. Williamson JF. The accuracy of the line and point dose approximation in Ir-192 dosimetry. *Int J Radiat Oncol Biol Phys* 1986;12:409.
289. Williamson JF. Monte Carlo and analytic calculation of absorbed dose near ^{137}Cs intracavitary sources. *Int J Radiat Oncol Biol Phys* 1988;15:227–237.
290. Williamson JF. Monte Carlo evaluation of specific dose constants in water for ^{125}I seeds. *Med Phys* 1988;15:686.
291. Williamson JF. Dose calculations about shielded gynecological colpostats. *Int J Radiat Oncol Biol Phys* 1990;19:167–178.
292. Williamson JF. Comparison of measured and calculated dose rates in water near I-125 and Ir-192 seeds. *Med Phys* 1991;28:776–786.
293. Williamson JF. The Sievert integral revised: evaluation and extension to low energy brachytherapy sources. *Int J Radiat Oncol Biol Phys* 1996;36:1239–1250.
294. Williamson JF. Monte Carlo-based dose-rate tables for the Amersham CDCS. J and 3M model 6500 137Cs tubes. *Int J Radiat Oncol Biol Phys* 1998;41(4):959–970.
295. Williamson JF. Monte Carlo modeling of the transverse-axis dose distribution of the Model 200 ^{103}Pd interstitial brachytherapy source. *Med Phys* 2000;27:643–654.
296. Williamson JF. Dosimetric characteristics of the DraxImage Model LS-1 I-125 interstitial brachytherapy source design: a Monte Carlo investigation. *Med Phys* 2002;29:509–521.
297. Williamson JF. Semi-empirical dose-calculation models in brachytherapy. In: Thomadsen BR, Rivard MJ, Butler WM, eds. *Brachytherapy physics*. 2nd ed. Madison, WI: Medical Physics Publishing, 2005;201–232.
298. Williamson JF. Brachytherapy technology and physics practice since 1950: a half-century of progress. *Phys Med Biol* 2006;51:R1–R23.
299. Williamson JF, Anderson LL, Grigsby PW, et al. American Endocurietherapy Society recommendations for specification of brachytherapy source strength. *Endocuriether Hypertherm Oncol* 1993;9:1–7.
300. Williamson JF, Butler W, Dewerd LA, et al. Recommendations of the American Association of Physicists in Medicine regarding the impact of implementing the 2004 task group 43 report on dose specification for ^{103}Pd and ^{125}I interstitial brachytherapy. *Med Phys* 2005;32(5):1424–1439.
301. Williamson JF, Coursey BM, DeWerd LA, et al. Dosimetric prerequisites for routine clinical use of new low energy photon interstitial brachytherapy sources. *Med Phys* 1998;25(12):2269–2270.
302. Williamson JF, Coursey BM, DeWerd LA, et al. Guidance to users of Nycomed Amersham and North American Scientific, Inc. I-125 interstitial sources: dosimetry and calibration changes: recommendation of the American Association of Physicists in Medicine Radiation Therapy Committee Ad Hoc Subcommittee on Low-Energy Seed Dosimetry. *Med Phys* 1999;26:570–573.
303. Williamson JF, Coursey BM, DeWerd LA, et al. On the use of apparent

activity (A_{app}) for treatment planning of 125I and 103Pd interstitial brachytherapy sources: recommendations of the American Association of Physicists in Medicine radiation therapy committee subcommittee on low-energy brachytherapy source dosimetry. *Med Phys* 1999;26(12):2529–2530.

304. Williamson JF, Coursey BM, DeWerd LA, et al. Recommendations of the American Association of Physicists in Medicine on [103]Pd Interstitial Source Calibration and Dosimetry: implications for dose specification and prescription. *Med Phys* 2000;27:634–642.

305. Williamson JF, Ezzell GA, Olch A, et al. Quality assurance for high dose-rate brachytherapy. In: Nag S, ed. *Textbook on high dose rate brachytherapy*. Armonk, NY: Futura, 1994;147–212.

306. Williamson JF, Perera H, Li Z, et al. Comparison of calculated and measured heterogeneity correction factors for ^{125}I, ^{137}Cs and ^{192}Ir brachytherapy sources near localized heterogeneities. *Med Phys* 1993;20:209–222.

307. Williamson JF, Brenner, DJ. Physics and biology of brachytherapy. In: Perez CA, Brady LW, Halperin E, et al., eds. *Principles and practice of radiation oncology*. 4th ed. Philadelphia: J.B. Lippincott Company, 2003;472–537.

308. Williamson JF, Rivard MJ. Quantitative dosimetry methods for brachytherapy. In: Thomadsen BR, Rivard MJ, Butler WM, eds. *Brachytherapy physics*. 2nd ed. Madison, WI: Medical Physics Publishing, 2005;233–294.

309. Withers HR. Biologic basis for altered fractionation schemes. *Cancer* 1985;55: 2086–2095.

310. Withers HR. Biological basis of radiation therapy for cancer. *Lancet* 1992; 339(8786):156–159.

311. Withers HR, Taylor JMG, Maciejewski B. The hazard of accelerated tumor clonogen repopulation during radiotherapy. *Acta Radiol* 1988;27:131–146.

312. Wu A, Zwicker RD, Sternick ES. Tumor dose specification of I-125 seed implants. *Med Phys* 1985;12:27.

313. Wuu CS, Kliauga P, Zaider, M, et al. Microdosimetric evaluation of relative biological effectiveness for 103Pd, 125I, 241Am, and 192Ir brachytherapy sources. *Int J Radiat Oncol Biol Phys* 1996;36(3):689–697.

314. Yaes RJ. Late normal tissue injury from permanent interstitial implants. *Int J Radiat Oncol Biol Phys* 2001;49(4):1163–1169.

315. Yorke ED. Modeling the effects of inhomogeneous dose distributions in normal tissues. *Semin Radiat Oncol* 2001;11(3):197–209.

316. Yoshioka Y, Nose T, Yoshida K, et al. High-dose-rate interstitial brachytherapy as a monotherapy for localized prostate cancer: treatment description and preliminary results of a phase I/II clinical trial. *Int J Radiat Oncol Biol Phys* 2000;48(3):675–681.

317. Yu Y, Anderson LL, Li Z, et al. Prostate seed implant brachytherapy: report of the American Association of Physicists in Medicine Task Group No. 64. Med Phys 1999;26:2054–2076.

318. Yu Y, Waterman FM, Suntharalingham N, et al. Limitations of the minimum peripheral dose as a parameter for dose specification in permanent ^{125}I prostate implants. *Int J Radiat Oncol Biol Phys* 1996;34:717–725.

319. Yu Y, Zhang JBY, Brasacchio RA. Automated treatment planning engine for prostate seed implant brachytherapy. *Int J Radiat Oncol Biol Phys* 1999;43:647–652.

320. Zellmer DO, Gillin MT, Wilson JF. Microdosimetric single event spectra of Ytterbium-169 compared with commonly used brachytherapy sources and teletherapy beams. *Int J Radiat Oncol Biol Phys* 1992;23(3):627–632.

321. Zwicker RD. Quimby-based brachytherapy systems. In: Thomadsen BR, Rivard MJ, Butler WM, eds. *Brachytherapy physics*. 2nd ed. Madison, WI: Medical Physics Publishing, 2005;373–388.

322. Zwicker RD, Schmidt-Ullrich R. Dose uniformity in a planar interstitial implant system. *Int J Radiat Oncol Biol Phys* 1995;31(1):149–155.

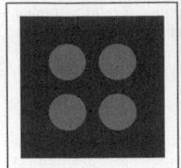

Chapter 20
Clinical Applications of Brachytherapy: Low–Dose-Rate and Pulse–Dose-Rate

Paolo Montemaggi, Patrizia Guerrieri, Mario Federico, Gianluca Mortellaro

Brachytherapy was used increasingly in the treatment of malignant tumors shortly after the discovery of radium by Marie Curie and Henri Becquerel. The first report on the use of radiation in the treatment of carcinoma of the uterine cervix was presented in La Halle in 1913 (43). In 1960, Henschke (139) published the first paper on afterloading brachytherapy in gynecologic malignancies and later in other tumors, followed shortly by a publication describing the Fletcher-Suit afterloading applicators (70,322). The widespread use of brachytherapy in the United States declined, as noted by Nag et al. (244), but it is undergoing a remarkable revival.

Reactor-produced isotopes became available for brachytherapy, including gold-198 (^{198}Au), cobalt-60 (^{60}Co), cesium-137 (^{137}Cs), and iridium-192 (^{192}Ir). A few years later, iodine-125 (^{125}I) and californium-252 (^{252}Cf) became available, and more recently americium-241 (^{241}Am), palladium-103 (^{103}Pd), ytterbium-169 (^{169}Yb), selenium-75 (^{75}Se), and samarium-145 (^{145}Sm) (158) became available. The combined administration of superficial and interstitial thermoirradiation in a variety of lesions has gained popularity (82).

Computers have enhanced the ability to more efficiently generate precise dosimetric calculations. Hall (130) and Hall and Brenner (132) published excellent reviews on the biologic basis of brachytherapy and clinical implications of dose rate, including pulse dose rate (PDR).

The widespread use of remote afterloading devices has enhanced the clinical applications of brachytherapy and practically has eliminated radiation exposure to the operators. Furthermore, in many parts of the world high–dose-rate (HDR) brachytherapy has supplanted low–dose-rate (LDR) brachytherapy with equivalent clinical results.

According to International Commission on Radiation Units (ICRU) Report No. 38 (157), dose rates of 0.4 to 2 Gy per hour are referred to as LDR, those in the range of 2 to 12 Gy per hour as medium dose rate (MDR), and those >12 Gy per hour are HDR. PDR will be defined later in the chapter.

The distribution of dose around radioactive sources depends on the physical properties of the isotopes, including the encapsulation and activity of the sources, and the inverse-square law. At distances greater than three times the physical length of a source, the inverse-square law applies within practical approximation; at closer distances the dosimetry is more complex.

Giap and Massulo (116) used the linear-quadratic model based on Dale's formalism to derive the brachytherapy dose rate at which biologic effectiveness is equivalent to that of external beam radiation therapy (EBRT). The functional dependencies of brachytherapy, relative effectiveness on dose rate, α/β ratio, and implant duration were investigated. The isoeffect dose rate depends only on the dose per fraction, the sublethal damage repair constant, and the implant duration, but it does not depend on α/β ratio. For sufficiently long implant duration of more than 10 to 15 hours, the value for isoeffect dose rate approaches a constant value around 40 to 50 cGy per hour. However, Dale and Jones (63) caution that such studies should be based on averaged biologically effective dose (BED) representative of the entire treated volume rather than the lower prescribed dose at the surface.

Selection of Radioactive Material

To meet all clinical situations, a variety of radioisotopes must be available. The Amersham (Amersham, U.K.) ^{137}Cs stainless steel encapsulated sources have been widely used in LDR brachytherapy with manual or remote afterloading. Casal et al. (37) presented Monte Carlo calculations of absolute dose rate in water around this source using a Monte Carlo code in the form of along-away tables and in the TG43 formalism, which can be used as benchmark data to verify treatment planning system calculations or directly as input data for treatment planning.

Afterloaded ^{192}Ir wires or seeds (in nylon strands) have been used in many sites (Fig. 20.1). Because iridium has a relatively short half-life, the wires must be calibrated often, which involves a fairly elaborate bookkeeping system. ^{125}I seeds are used widely for permanent implants in less accessible areas and for tumors that require surgical exposure at laparotomy or thoracotomy, such as the pancreas or lung. Other isotopes such as ^{103}Pd, ^{241}Am, and ^{152}Cf were introduced in clinical practice.

Anderson et al. (9) developed a nomographic planning guide to be used for planar implants of ^{192}Ir seeds in ribbons. Planar interstitial dosimetry systems also have been described by Zwicker et al. (365,366) and Kwan et al. (182). A simplified dosimetry system for ^{192}Ir volume implants was designed by Olch et al. (254). Dose parameters of ^{192}Ir and ^{125}I seeds have been reported by Weaver et al. (352).

Karaiskos et al. (168) evaluated the American Association of Physicists in Medicine (AAPM) Task Group 43 dosimetric formalism for ^{192}Ir wires used as interstitial sources in LDR brachytherapy applications. Results were presented in look-up tables that allow interpolation for dose-rate calculations around all practically used wire lengths, with accuracy acceptable for clinical applications.

As longer iridium wires have become available, the necessity for crossing one or both ends of the implant almost has disappeared. Sources of 0.4 to 0.5 mCi Ra Eq/cm are used for single-plane arrangements, and sources of 0.25 to 0.35 mCi Ra Eq/cm linear intensity are used for multiple-plane or volume implants. The two intensities are combined for complex implants (72).

Afterloading Interstitial Brachytherapy

The flexible carrier method was first used with radon seeds by Hames (134) in 1937. Afterloading was systematized by Henschke et al. (141) and Suit et al. (322). In the early 1960s, Pierquin et al. (271) popularized the Henschke techniques with modifications and contributed the use of "hairpins" for afterloading with thicker iridium wires (0.5 mm diameter), mainly for lesions of the oral cavity and oropharynx.

Kolotas and Zamboglou (172) recently reviewed the current status of interstitial brachytherapy. Modern techniques involve the use of ^{192}Ir in computer-controlled remote afterloading machines, which can deliver HDR, PDR, or LDR brachytherapy. Treatment planning is undertaken with computers and anatomic cross-section images using computed tomography

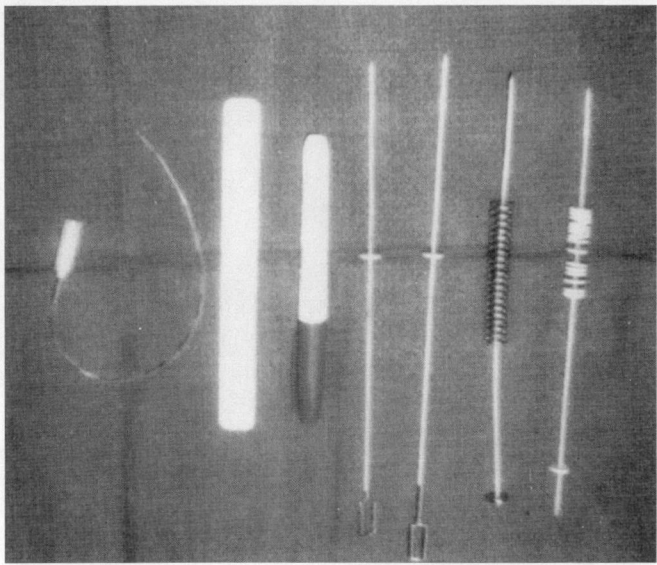

FIGURE 20.1. Operating room tray showing items used for manual interstitial implants (*left to right*): nylon tubing with dummy sources, metallic ruler, marking pencil, several plastic catheters with metallic guides, and plastic buttons.

(CT), ultrasound, and magnetic resonance imaging (MRI). Several reports in the literature describe techniques and instrumentation for the use of afterloading interstitial therapy with other isotopes such as tantalum wires (215), ^{125}I seeds, and ^{103}Pd (3,140,229).

Afterloading Iridium-192 Wires or Ribbons

Removable implants are performed with either stainless steel needles or semiflexible Teflon or nylon catheters with metallic guides (Fig. 20.2).

Stainless Steel Guides

Stainless steel or Teflon 16-gauge tubing (1.6 mm in outer diameter) is cut into the desired length. The distal end of the tubing is beveled at a 30- or 45-degree angle and is crimped but not closed to hold the afterloaded iridium insert in place, still allowing repositioning should it be required. A nylon or Teflon ball or a metallic button is fitted snugly at the proximal end (Fig. 20.3) (71). In this Teflon ball—a further development of the glass ball used by Hames (134)—or metallic button, a hole is inserted to thread the suture, and a lead bead is added for x-ray localization. Figure 20.4 shows the procedures followed for insertion and afterloading of the rigid guides in tumors approachable from one side only (e.g., tumors of the columella and nasal septum, base of the tongue, female urethra, and anal margin). This technique also can be used to treat the parotid gland or involved lymph nodes in the neck or for primary breast cancer.

Through-and-Through Plastic Tubing Technique

The through-and-through plastic tubing technique is used when a tumor can be transfixed from both sides (e.g., lower and upper lip, buccal mucosa, breast, or neck masses). In locations in which the guide can be placed through the tumor or normal tissues, the 16-gauge metallic guides are inserted at the appropriate distances to achieve the desired distribution (Fig. 20.5). After this, the lead of the nylon tube that will contain the ^{192}Ir nylon thread is inserted through the metallic guide and is progressively pushed all the way through along with the nylon tube. When the nylon tube is in place, a metallic button is crimped or a Teflon ball is placed at the distal end to secure it. When all of the nylon tubing has been implanted, the desired length of the active wire is measured by using a "dummy" wire (to 0.5 cm below the skin at the opposite end) and cut a few centimeters longer so that it will protrude beyond the skin and will be easier to manipulate. After localization, x-ray films are taken with inactive wires (or seeds) used to determine the length and

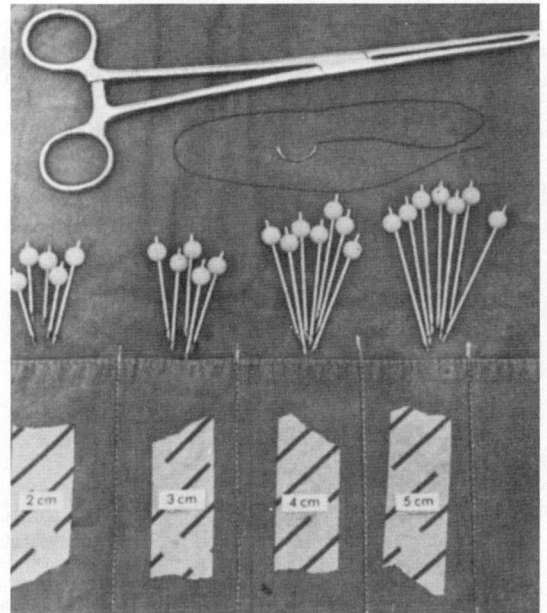

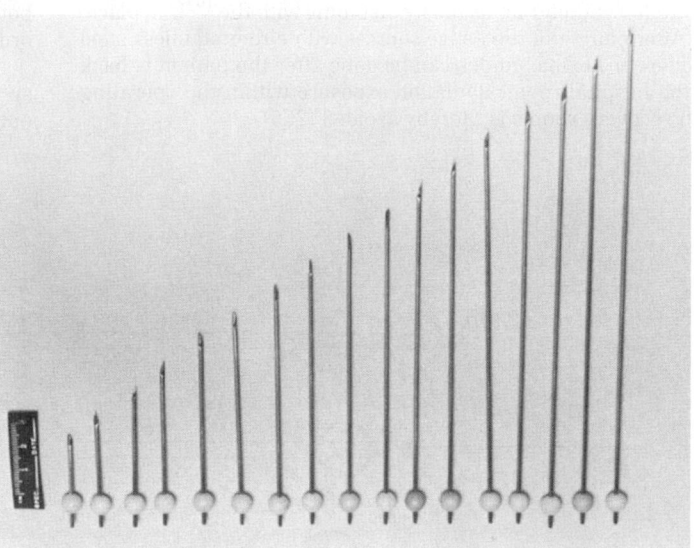

FIGURE 20.2. **A:** Stainless steel needles are manufactured to any desired length; a Teflon or nylon button with a hole for suturing and a lead pellet for radiographic identification are incorporated at the ball. The distal end is crimped to position the ^{192}Ir insert and to prevent it from dropping out. The needles are inserted with a standard needle-inserting forceps (Radium Chemical Co., NY) and sutured into place with a C-0 suture. The Teflon ball, which causes less trauma, substitutes for the metal flange used earlier. (From Delclos L. Afterloading method for interstitial gamma-ray therapy. In: Fletcher GH, ed. *Textbook of radiotherapy*, 3rd ed. Philadelphia: Lea & Febiger, 1980; with permission.) **B:** Stainless steel needle guides of various lengths with Teflon ball used for breast implant at M.D. Anderson Hospital. (Courtesy of Luis Delclos, M.D.)

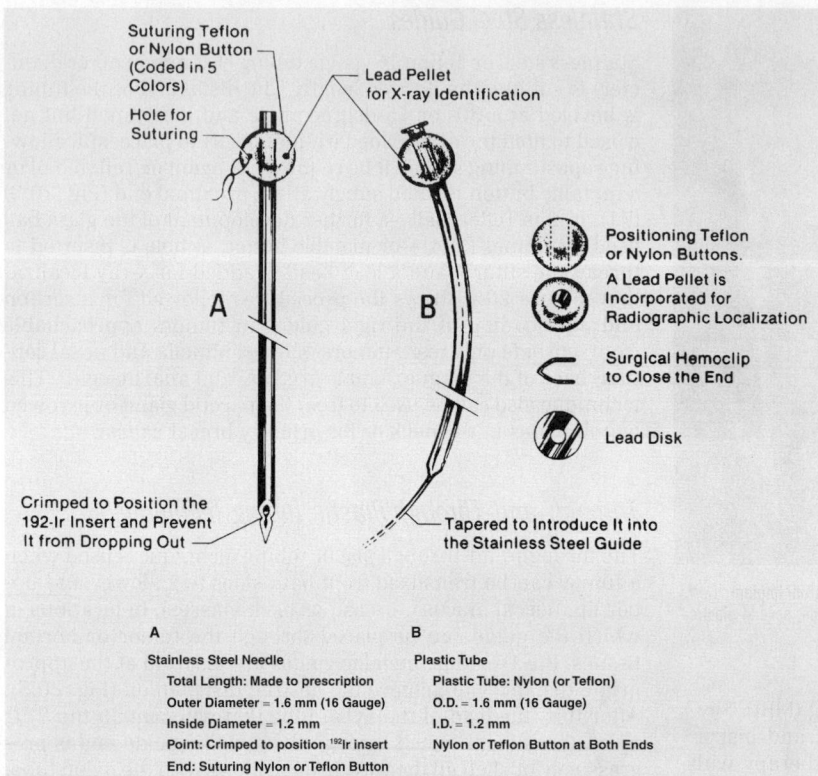

FIGURE 20.3. A: Stainless steel afterloadable needle with plastic, Teflon, or nylon buttons. The needles are made to any desired length. **B:** Teflon or nylon tube, closed-end variety, used for the through-and-through technique. A stainless steel guide of the same outside diameter is inserted first. (From Delclos L. Interstitial irradiation of the penis. In: Johnson DE, Boileau A, eds. *Genitourinary tumors: fundamental principles and surgical techniques.* New York: Grune & Stratton, 1982; with permission.)

position of the tubes, the ^{192}Ir active sources are prepared and inserted, and the proximal end of the tubing is crimped with a metallic button. Each dummy and corresponding active source or wire is marked with different color threads and buttons and specific radiopaque patterns to identify each tube or loading on the patient or the implant radiographs.

If thermoirradiation is planned, the technique is modified. Teflon catheters with a B-D lock and a special plastic insert to secure the catheter to the skin are used. An adapter that locks in the Teflon catheter holds the nylon tubing with the ^{192}Ir in place.

Afterloading of the active sources with either stainless steel needles or flexible guides can be done after the patient is back in the hospital room. Radiation exposure within the operating and recovery rooms is thereby avoided (265).

Suturing of Needles or Guides or Plastic Buttons

Needles or guides are sutured to the implanted tissues in various ways (97). Separate 2-0 silk or cotton sutures permanently attached to a half-circle taperpoint needle, which is threaded through the loop of the color-coded silk before insertion, are preferred.

Color-coded silk threads are used to identify the different lengths and strengths of the radioactive sources. This facilitates both the selection of sources at the time of the implant and the orderly removal of the implant.

Needles or buttons holding the catheters should be sutured systematically. For a double-plane implant, all suturing is done outside the needle rows to simplify removal.

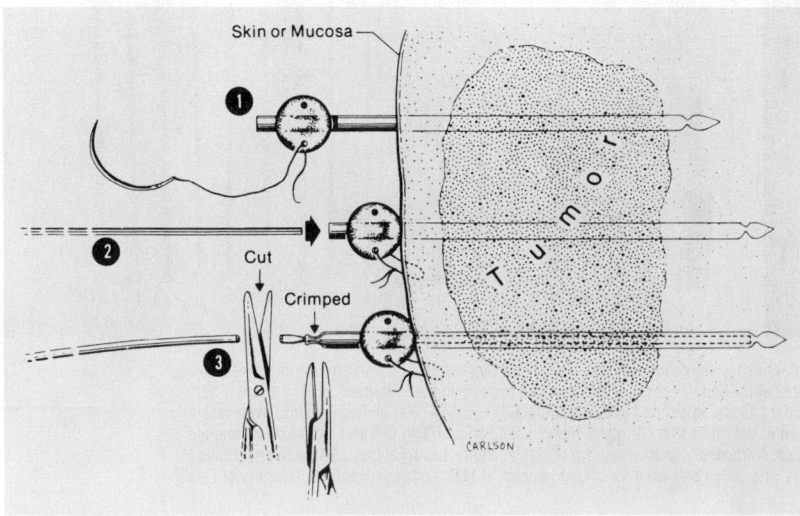

FIGURE 20.4. One-end implant technique for tumors approached from one side. **1:** Insertion of empty stainless steel needle with nylon button. The needle is sutured to the skin or mucosa through a hole in the nylon button. **2:** The iridium wire mounted in plastic tube carrier is introduced into the stainless steel needle. **3:** The open end is crimped to close it. The plastic tube carrier is cut, leaving about 0.5 cm protruding to facilitate removal of the iridium wire when indicated. To remove it, one can either cut the suture and remove the needle with the iridium inside, then deposit it in the lead carrier for transportation and further manipulation in the laboratory, or uncrimp the end of the stainless steel needle with a specially designed uncrimper and pull out the plastic tube carrier with the iridium insert inside. (From Delclos L. Afterloading method for interstitial gamma-ray therapy. In: Fletcher GH, ed. *Textbook of radiotherapy,* 3rd ed. Philadelphia: Lea & Febiger, 1980; with permission.)

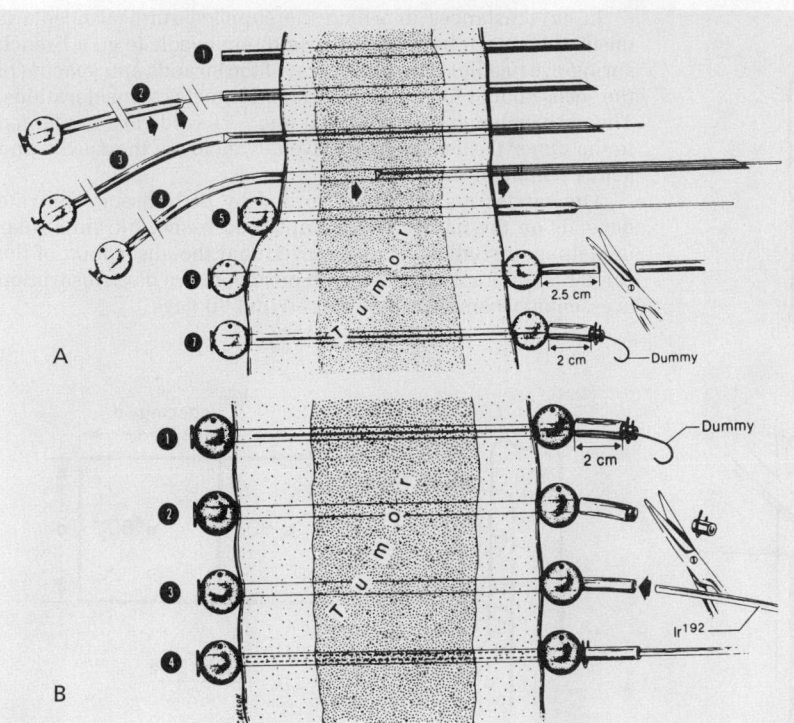

FIGURE 20.5. Through-and-through implant technique for tumors approachable from two sides. **A:** To insert (*1*) the stainless steel guide is introduced; (*2*) the leader (tapered end) of the nylon implant tube is introduced and (*3*) passed down the guide until the plastic tube is in contact with the end of the stainless steel guide; (*4*) both the stainless steel guide and the tapered end (leader) of the nylon implant tube are pulled through the other end; (*5*) when the stainless steel guide is out, the nylon tube is pulled until the closed-end nylon implant tube with the nylon button is in contact with the surface; (*6*) another nylon button is inserted at the opposite end of the nylon implant tube (the nylon tube is cut at about 2.5 cm from the nylon button surface); (*7*) a larger nylon tube 2 cm in length is placed on top of the protruding end of the nylon tube. A dummy wire is placed inside, protruding 1 cm, for localization. A hemoclip is placed at the end to prevent the nylon tube from slipping out during manipulation. **B:** To load: (*1*) the dummy wire is removed; (*2*) the nylon end of the implant tube is cut with the hemoclip; (*3*) the ¹⁹²Ir wire in plastic tube carrier (*insert*) is inserted into the nylon implant tube; (*4*) a hemoclip is placed near the nylon button, to close the nylon tube. (From Delclos L. Afterloading method for interstitial gamma-ray therapy. In: Fletcher GH, ed. *Textbook of radiotherapy*, 3rd ed. Philadelphia: Lea & Febiger, 1980; with permission.)

Removable Iridium-192 Hairpin Technique

The physical characteristics of the Paris technique have been described elsewhere (see Chapter 16). Metallic gutter guides have been constructed to facilitate insertion of the iridium wires (Fig. 20.6) (273). The usual separation of the legs is 1.2 cm, although 0.9 or 1.5 cm separation can be used. The standard gutter length is 2.5, 3, 4, or 5 cm. Iridium wire ends are inserted along the gutters and held in place with a fine-tip clamp while the gutter guide is removed (Fig. 20.7). Gutter guides should allow for a predictable insertion of the hairpin, which will result in an acceptable geometry and homogeneous dose distribution of the implant (Fig. 20.8). The gutter guide technique is used primarily in smaller tumors of the oral cavity and in the anal region.

Removable Iodine-125 Plastic Tube Implants

Clarke et al. (49) described a temporary removable ¹²⁵I plastic tube implant technique. ¹²⁵I seeds were 4.5 mm in length, and the interseed spacing within the ribbons (from seed center to seed center) ranged from 4.5 (seeds back to back) to 12.5 mm (8-mm spacers). The operative technique using hollow stainless steel 18-gauge trocars is identical to the ¹⁹²Ir implant procedure. ¹²⁵I dosimetry is somewhat more complex because iodine seed dose distributions are more anisotropic, fall off more rapidly with distance, and are more sensitive to tissue heterogeneities than ¹⁹²Ir sources. However, the ¹²⁵I tubes must have a greater diameter to house the ¹²⁵I seed ribbons, which are larger than the ¹⁹²Ir ribbons. The seed ribbons are prepared by loading loose seeds into the hollow ribbons; the seeds are

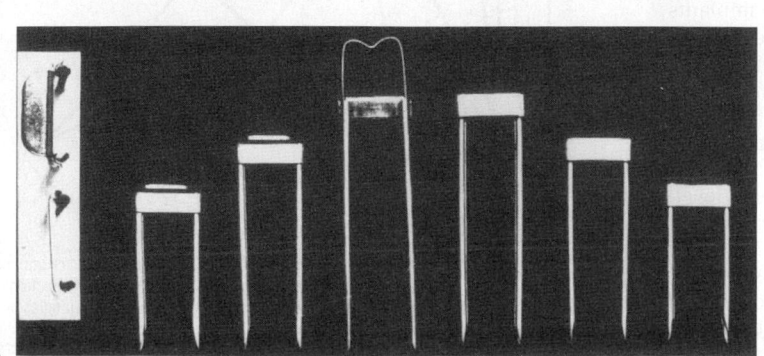

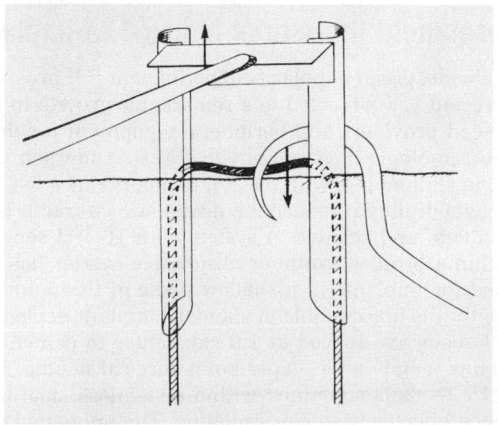

FIGURE 20.6. A: Hairpins of different sizes and iridium wire (*center*). **B:** Diagram of gutter guide used by Pierquin and small hook to hold the iridium wire in place while the guide is being removed with a clamp. (From Pierquin B, Wilson JF, Chassagne D. *Modern brachytherapy.* New York: Masson, 1987; with permission.)

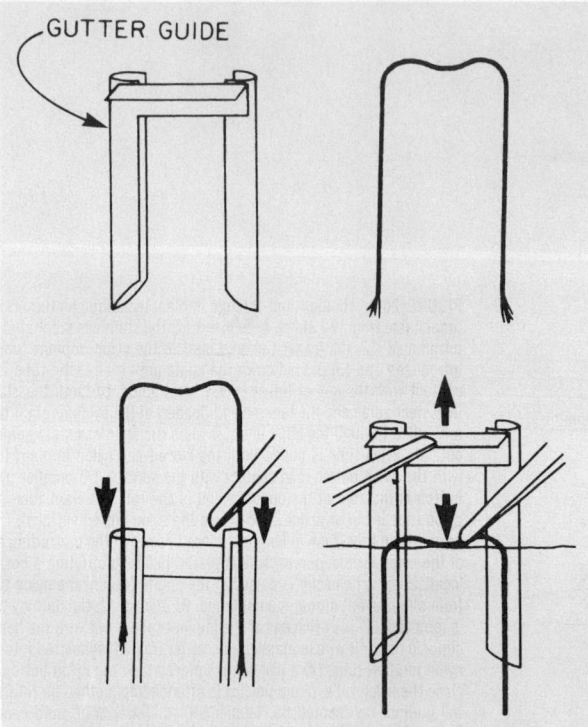

FIGURE 20.7. Diagram showing basic design of gutter guide and technique for insertion of the iridium wire and subsequent removal of the guide while holding the wire with a clamp.

separated by spacers and held in position by a "pusher." The open end of the seed ribbon is heated for sealing. The seed separation varies depending on the activity, the geometry of the implant, and the desired dose rate, which is individualized for each patient and determined after the procedure in the operating room is completed. The most common clinical applications of temporary ^{125}I seeds are episcleral plaque therapy for ocular melanoma and volume implants in the brain.

Compared with the ^{192}Ir implants, use of the ^{125}I seed ribbons requires additional physicist or dosimetrist time to assemble and disassemble the ribbons. However, this is offset by a compensatory decrease in other tasks that are required for the preparation of the ^{192}Ir seeds or wires. Because of the lower energy of ^{125}I, shielding is accomplished easily, which increases safety during the operation and for the nurses caring for the patient.

Permanent Interstitial Iodine-125 Implants

The widespread popularity of permanent ^{125}I prostate implants in recent years has led to a remarkable growth in the number of seed providers and peripheral equipment for this modality. The radiologic Physics Center at M.D. Anderson Cancer Center, in conjunction with the AAPM, maintains a list of ^{125}I seeds for which they consider the dosimetric characterization to be complete and reliable. A system with 10 ^{125}I seeds contained within a braided synthetic absorbable carrier has been developed for implants in a shallow plane of tissue or for a tumor site that is inaccessible to standard implant devices (137). The ^{125}I seeds are spaced at 1.0 cm, center to center. The carrier retains a half-circle, taper-point surgical needle. Each strand of 10 seeds is contained within a stainless steel tubular ring, which effectively shields radiation. The unopened package has a surface dose rate of <0.2 mR per hour for a loading of 10 0.5-mCi seeds. Consequently, it can be handled and stored without additional shielding.

In circumstances in which the supplied surgical needle is unsuitable, it can be replaced by a tie-on needle (e.g., a French spring-eye needle). The placement of the strands and spacing of the seeds should follow appropriate dosimetric considerations. The absorbable carrier material and ^{125}I seeds are implanted in the tumor tissues by successive advancing of the needle and gentle pulling of the carrier.

The carrier material is absorbed by body tissue; the rate depends on the nature of the implanted tissue. Intramuscular implantation studies in rats showed that the absorption of the carrier is minimal until the 40th postoperative day. Absorption is essentially complete between 60 and 90 days.

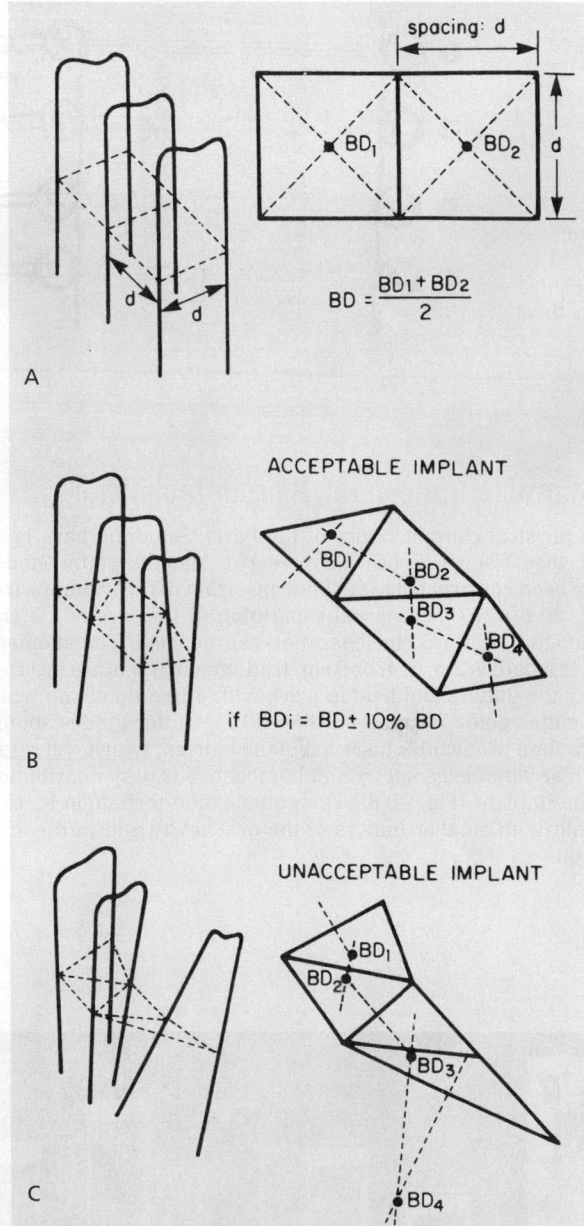

FIGURE 20.8. Diagrams illustrating dosimetry principles of Paris system. **A:** For implants containing more than one plane, equidistant radioactive lines imply that the intersections of the lines with the central plane will be arranged as the apices of equilateral triangles or as the corners of squares. Calculation of basal dose (BD) rate is made at various points. Dose is specified along an isodose surface defined as a given proportion of the basal dose rate calculated inside the implant volume (reference isodose, which should encompass target volume as closely as possible). In practice, the value of the reference isodose is fixed at 85% of the basal dose rate. **B:** Geometry of acceptable implant. **C:** Geometry of unacceptable implant.

Goffinet et al. (118) reported on 64 intraoperative ^{125}I implants with absorbable Vicryl suture carriers performed in 53 patients with head and neck cancers, many of them recurrent after initial definitive radiation therapy. A variation of this technique was described by Greenblatt et al. (120), who sewed the ^{125}I suture material through Gelfoam, which in turn was secured to the tumor bed with special clips.

Templates

A variety of templates have been designed in an attempt to more easily place interstitial sources and to obtain more homogeneous doses with implants.

Syed-Neblett Templates

Several Syed-Neblett templates are commercially available. A template primarily used for gynecologic tumors consists of two Lucite plates joined by six screws that tighten to grasp as many as 38 afterloading, hollow, stainless steel needles. An additional six needles fit into grooves of a 2-cm diameter plastic vaginal cylinder that is placed inside an opening in the middle of the template. These needles are arranged in concentric circles or arcs with a spacing of 1 cm between adjacent needles (Fig. 20.9) (11). A 4- by 10-cm area can be implanted in a butterfly distribution. The 18-gauge needles supplied with the templates are 20 cm long, but they can be shortened to treat more shallow areas. The vaginal cylinder has a central opening for placement of a tandem if desired.

A rectal template is similar to the one just described, but the two plates contain three concentric circular rings with a total of 36 needles with 1-cm spacing. Cylindrical volumes with diameters of 2, 4, or 6 cm can be implanted. A rectal tube can be placed in the central hole if necessary, but this hole can be left open if the template is placed in an area not covering the anus, such as the vulva.

Syed et al. (325) described a prostate template used to guide the insertion of metallic source guides transperineally. The template consists of two concentric rings with radii of 1 cm and 2 cm, containing 6 and 12 guide holes, respectively (Fig. 20.10) (289,325). Up to 18 metallic source guides (18-gauge, 20-cm long needles) are inserted transperineally through the prostate and seminal vesicles as indicated. The tips of the guides are usually 1 cm above the level of the bladder neck. The template is fixed to the perineum by "00" silk sutures, and the space between the perineum and the template is filled with gauze soaked in antibiotic cream.

The urethral template has two concentric rings with a total of 18 needles with the same 1-cm spacing as the rectal template. A cylindrical volume with either a 2- or 4-cm diameter is implanted with this template. This is a single plate with no machine screws to other plates. A Foley urethral catheter is inserted through the central opening to drain the urinary bladder.

Höckel and Muller (151) described a modified Syed-Neblett type perineal template for HDR interstitial brachytherapy of gynecologic malignancies. The template can be disassembled easily after insertion of the central needles into the pelvis, allowing cystoscopic and rectoscopic control of the needle positions. Needles penetrating the bladder or the rectum can be repositioned before reassembling the template, eliminating a high-irradiation zone in tumor-free bladder and rectum walls.

Martinez Universal Perineal Interstitial Template

The Martinez Universal Perineal Interstitial Template (MUPIT) was designed to treat locally advanced or recurrent tumors in the prostatic, anorectal, perineal, or gynecologic areas. The device consists of two acrylic cylinders (one that can be placed in the vagina and the other in the rectum), an acrylic template with an array of holes that allow placement of the metallic guides in the tissues to be implanted, and a cover plate (Fig. 20.11) (205). The cylinders are placed in the vagina, rectum, or both and fastened to the template so that a fixed geometric relationship among the tumor volume, normal structures, and source placement is preserved throughout the course of the implantation. When the MUPIT interstitial template is used, no central intracavitary sources are inserted, except in some patients requiring an intrauterine tandem (beyond the volume treated with the interstitial sources).

Gaddis et al. (111) reported on their experience with perineal interstitial implants in 75 women with squamous cell carcinoma of the cervix. Follow-up ranged from 3 to 60 months with a median of 18 months. The recurrence rate in the pelvis was 46.2% (12/26) for patients with stage IIIB and 20% (5/25) for patients with stage IIB tumors. The non–tumor-associated fistula rate was 13.3%. Severe (grade 3) nonfistula complications occurred in six additional patients; thus, 16/75 (21.3%) patients had severe morbidity.

Molds

Molds have been used for the treatment of patients with skin cancer of the face or hands or other anatomic locations and for lesions of the lip and oral cavity (260). The mold can be constructed from plastic or acrylic, after initially obtaining the configuration of the anatomic area to be molded with a liquid plaster cast to form a negative plaster mold. Computations for the dose desired are carried out, and optimal placement of the sources is determined. Small holes are drilled in the mold to contain the nylon ribbons or catheters with the radioactive sources or the rigid radium (or cesium) needles. These techniques have been extensively used by Patterson (260) and Fletcher (99).

Marchese et al. (199) described a technique using ^{125}I sources embedded in Gelfoam to permanently implant small residual tumors or tumor margins in anatomic locations where standard implant techniques may not be feasible—for instance, at sites involving tissues adjacent to major blood vessels, the vertebral column, or the brain. The technique consists of preparing an adequate size and thickness of Gelfoam and fixing it to the implant site. Catheters with ^{125}I seeds inserted into the Gelfoam are placed at 1-cm intervals. The absorbable Gelfoam mesh is

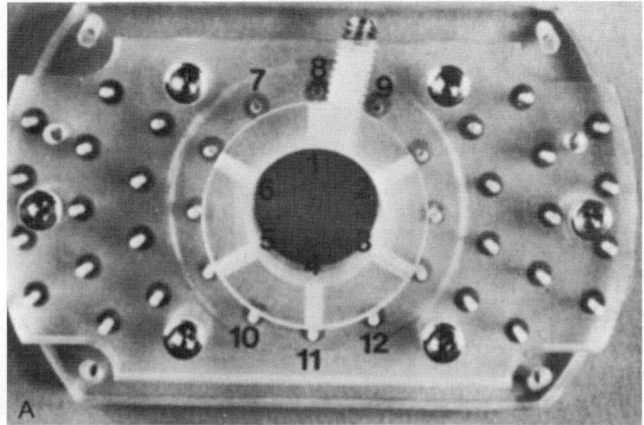

FIGURE 20.9. Syed-type perineal template used for interstitial parametrial irradiation. (From Aristizabal SA, Valencia A, Ocampo G, et al. Interstitial parametrial irradiation in cancer of the cervix IIB-IIIB. *Endocurie Hypertherm Oncol* 1985;1:41, with permission.)

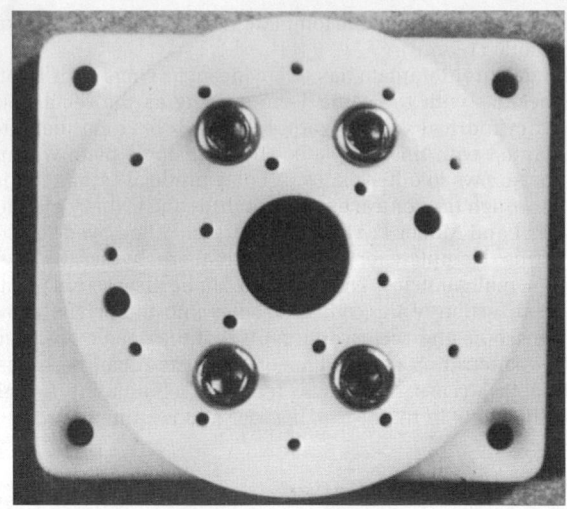

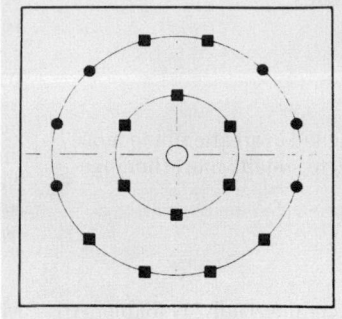

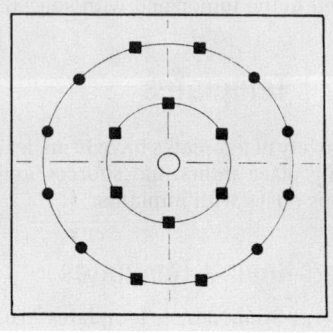

FIGURE 20.10. A: Syed/Neblett prostate template. (From Syed AMN, Puthawala AA, Tansey LA, et al. Temporary iridium-192 implantation in the management of carcinoma of the prostate. In: Hilaris BS, Batata MA, eds. *Brachytherapy oncology—1983*. New York: Memorial Sloan-Kettering Cancer Center, 1983;83, with permission.) **B:** Example of different intensity sources used with Syed template to decrease doses to urethra, bladder, and rectum. (From Puthawala AA, Syed AM, Tansey LA, et al. Temporary iridium-192 implant in the management of carcinoma of the prostate. *Endocurie Hypertherm Oncol* 1985;1:25, with permission.)

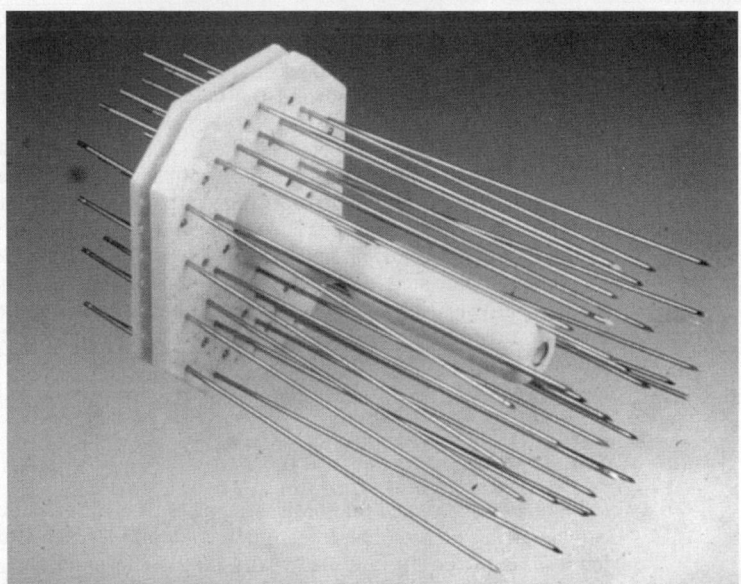

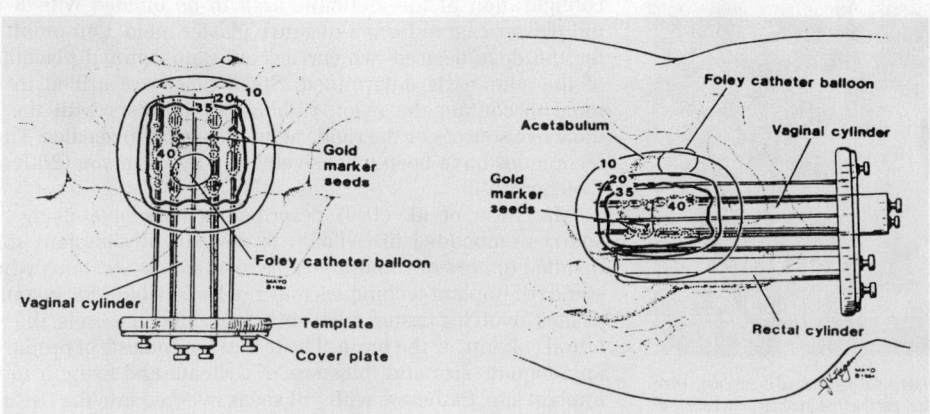

FIGURE 20.11. A: Martinez Universal Perineal Interstitial Template (MUPIT). (Courtesy of Dr. Alvaro Martinez, William Beaumont Hospital, Detroit, MI.) **B:** Diagrammatic representation in coronal and sagittal planes of same template. (From Martinez A, Edmundson GK, Cox RS, et al. Combination of external beam irradiation and multiple-site applicator (MUPIT) for treatment of locally advanced or recurrent prostatic, anorectal, and gynecologic malignancies. *Int J Radiat Oncol Biol Phys* 985;11:391–398, with permission.)

sutured with catgut absorbable material, and both are absorbed for 6 weeks.

Acrylic molds have been used for the treatment of vaginal or uterine cervix lesions. Lichter et al. (188) described the use of thermoplastic vaginal molds for this purpose. The locations of the channels for insertion of the sources and for the central tandem (if desired) are determined by the topography of the tumor. The central tandem can be placed in the uterus or the vagina, through the vaginal mold, and locked into position.

Remote-Control Afterloading

Remote-control afterloading brachytherapy for interstitial and intracavitary applications is used with increasing frequency for both LDR and HDR implants. Glasgow (117) reviewed the developmental aspects of remote afterloading and described the characteristics of several commercially available systems. The special features of three LDR systems are detailed in Table 20.1.

LDR units use ^{137}Cs or ^{192}Ir, whereas HDR systems are built for either ^{60}Co or ^{192}Ir sources. Shielded rooms equivalent to ^{60}Co are necessary for HDR procedures.

The advantages of LDR remote control afterloading include:

1. Radiation exposure to hospital personnel virtually eliminated,
2. Improved control of isodose distributions,
3. Low probability of misplacing or losing sources,
4. Less source preparation work for the source curator,
5. Medical and nursing staff not rushed; no fear of exposure while caring for the patient, and
6. Source loading, unloading, and recording performed automatically.

After the unloaded applicators are placed in the patient, the sources are loaded under pneumatic or mechanical control through hollow tubes connected to the applicators by a remotely activated system. A sorting and selection device and transport train for the sources are available. Safety mechanisms for checking correct connection of the applicator and the position of the sources are integral components of the system (357,358). Most units produce a hardcopy of the treatment at completion of the procedure. Equipment for remote-control afterloading brachytherapy is available for multiple anatomic sites and applications (Fig. 20.12).

A special problem with remote afterloading equipment for gynecologic use is reproduction of the isodose distributions obtained with standard 2-cm cesium tubes and the Fletcher-Suit-Delclos tandem, ovoids, and vaginal cylinders. A fixed source train decreases flexibility unless several source trains are in inventory. A system of active and inactive pellets (Selectron, Veenendaal, The Netherlands) requires the compilation of a dose-distribution atlas to duplicate the standard 2-cm cesium tube dose distribution of the Fletcher-Suit applicators (124).

Wilkinson et al. (356) and Jones et al. (165) described the use of Selectron afterloading equipment to simulate the Manchester system for intracavitary therapy. Dean et al. (65) adapted its use with the Newcastle system.

Few studies compare results of therapy with LDR remote afterloading implants with those for manual afterloading systems because there are no significant changes in isotopes or dose rates. Battermann and Szabol (22) reported their experience with the Selectron afterloading machine for patients with cancer of the cervix using the same treatment policy as previously used for manual afterloading. Local tumor control and complications were the same for both groups.

Scalliet et al. (301), Fu and Phillips (109), and Petereit et al. (269) compared HDR and LDR in gynecologic brachytherapy, especially regarding the conversion of LDR total dose into equivalent HDR dose per fraction and total dose. The reported clinical experience with HDR is equivalent to that of classic LDR. Treatment with LDR has proven to be quite tolerant to a lack of absolute precision, something that would be disastrous with HDR techniques.

Pulsed–Dose-Rate

PDR was proposed (34) to exploit the advantages of HDR computer-controlled remote afterloading technology. It was noted that by varying the dwell times of the stepping source, dose optimization could be achieved, which maintained the potential benefits of LDR, including improved radiation protection. The inactive source times, when the sources are in the safe between pulses, should allow for better nursing care and visiting of the patients. A stepping source of 1 Ci carries a sphere of "HDR" of radius 20 mm within its track through tissue. The pulse initially delivers about 0.6 Gy per 10-minute exposure every hour. As the dose rate gradually decreases because of radioactive decay of the source, somewhat longer periods of pulsed times are required (Fig. 20.13) (132).

High ratios of PDR/LDR effect can be avoided by keeping dose per pulse below 1 Gy. About 75% of the total dose is delivered at HDR in a PDR implant of moderate volume, reducing to 40% as a source decays from 1 to 0.3 Ci. Even so, restricting the dose per pulse to 0.5 or 0.6 Gy should avoid ratios of increased effect larger than about 10%. It appears that PDR delivered by stepping source might behave more like HDR than LDR, especially for tissues with a substantial component of repair of very short T1-2.

Based on linear quadratic formalism, the late normal tissue damage and tumor control were assumed by Brenner et al. (33) to be determined primarily by the level of cellular survival. PDR schedules were designed in which pulses are delivered during "extended office hours" (8 AM to 8 PM) with no irradiation overnight. Generally, the proposed PDR regimens last the same number of treatment days as the corresponding LDR (CLDR) regimen, but the PDR treatment lasts longer on the final day. The protocols could allow the patient to go home overnight, or to stay overnight in an adjacent medical inn or hospital-associated hotel, rather than in a hospital bed, which has major economic benefits. In such an economic situation, an extra treatment day for the daytime PDR could well be considered, which would virtually guarantee an improved clinical advantage relative to LDR.

Using the linear-quadratic formula, Brenner and Hall (32) determined the pulse lengths and frequencies based on radiobiologic data that were equivalent to conventional continuous LDR irradiation. They noted that for a regimen of 30 Gy in 60 hours, a 1-hour period between 10-minute pulses might produce up to a 2% increase in late effects probability.

Visser et al. (341) described a radiobiologic model and equations to determine the HDR or PDR schedules equivalent to certain LDR schedules, similar to that proposed by Brenner and Hall (32), by applying probable ranges for the values for α/β ratio and repair time. They concluded that eight fractions of 1 to 1.5 Gy per 24 hours, up to 3 hours apart, would be equivalent to commonly used LDR treatment schedules.

Erickson and Shadley (83), using *in vitro* irradiation experiments on rodent tumor cell lines, showed that there was a slight increase in cell killing with PDR relative to continuous LDR irradiation of hourly 5-, 10-, or 20-minute pulses, or a 20-minute pulse every 2 hours. In no case were the increases statistically significant, and they did appear to be clinically indistinguishable as determined by the Brenner and Hall criteria.

Narayana and Orton (247) developed a generalized extrapolated response dose (ERD) equation based on the linear quadratic model to account for the variation in the dose rate to maximize the therapeutic advantage (TA). They noted that with

▣▣ Table 20.1 | SPECIAL FEATURES OF LOW–DOSE–RATE REMOTE AFTERLOADING DEVICES

Characteristics	MINIRAD Isotopen-Technik Dr. Sauerwein GmbH Germany	Manufacturer or Vendor Selectron (LDR) Nucletron Engineering BV Netherlands	MicroSelectron (LDR) Nucletron Engineering BV Netherlands
Number of sources and container maximum storage activity	16 sources in unit; 16 in each storage container	48 ^{137}Cs pellets in unit 2.2 Ci	15 sources in unit; ^{137}Cs: 1 Ci ^{192}Ir: 5 Ci 45 sources in mobile safe ^{137}Cs: 3 Ci ^{192}Ir: 15 Ci
Physical size of sources	0.9 mm OD × 120 or 200 mm L; uses ^{192}Ir or ^{137}Cs wires	Spherical pellets 2.5 mm OD	^{137}Cs: Mini seeds up to 140 mm L × 0.8 mm OD in 1.3 mm OD train ^{192}Ir: Ribbons (wire, seed) up to 140 mm L × 1.1 mm OD
Smallest outside diameter of applicator	1.6 mm	6.0 mm	^{192}Ir: 1.5 mm ^{137}Cs: 1.9 mm
Method of source attachment or control	Sources magnetically connect to cables	Sources trains with 48 pellets/120 mm; any pellet may be programmed to be active/inactive	Sources autoconnect to drive cable; monitored by microprocessor
Number of applicator channels	16	3 (one patient) or 6 (two patients)	15
Method of source movement	Stationary linear sources, or seed arrays motor driven to single treatment position	Pneumatically transported to single treatment position	Stationary linear sources, or seed arrays motor drive to single treatment position
Method of source retraction in the event of failure	Not stated	Emergency battery to operate air reservoir for pneumatic return	Backup battery
Control unit and isodose planner system	LOWDOT, uses MS-DOS operating system with IBM-compatible computer	PLATO-BPS	PLATO-BPS
Dose optimization	Yes; optimization of individual catheter treatment times	Menu choice of multiple optimization routines	Menu choice of multiple optimization routines
Special features	Allows several patients to be sequentially loaded or continuous treatment of single patient including elective interruptions and automatic source retraction at end of treatment	Pneumatic checks of source positions. Closed system: sources not accessible to user. Independently programmed times for each applicator.	Open system: Standard LDR ^{192}Ir ribbons/wires with special adapters inserted into storage container by user All applicators have same treatment time.

Ci, curie; Cs, cesium; Ir, iridium; LDR, low dose rate; mm L, millimeters in length; mm OD, millimeters in outer diameter.

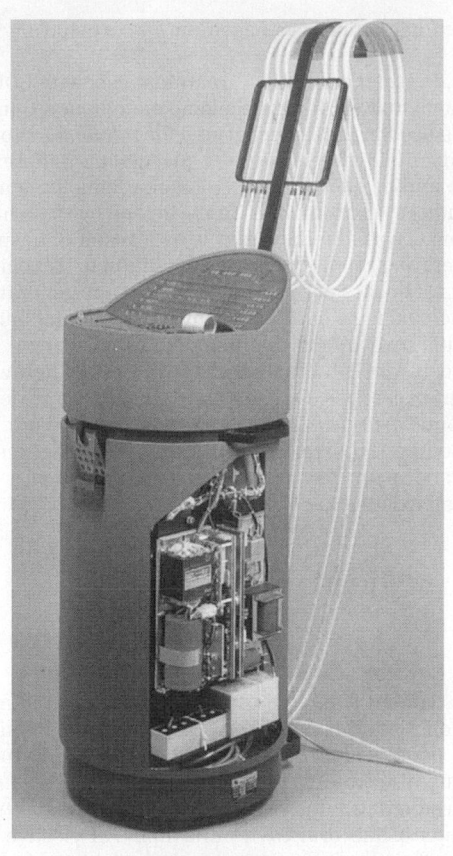
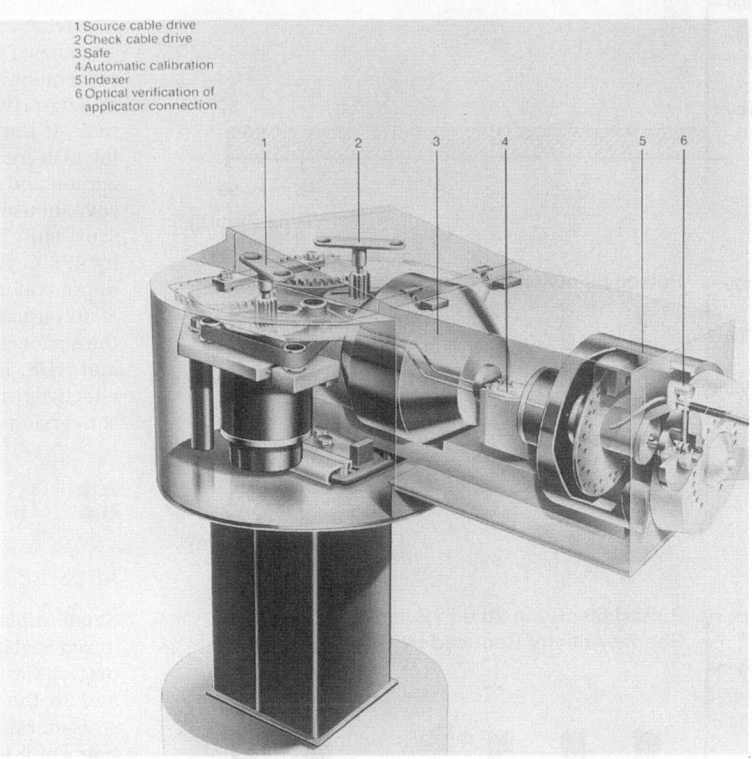

1 Source cable drive
2 Check cable drive
3 Safe
4 Automatic calibration
5 Indexer
6 Optical verification of applicator connection

A   B

FIGURE 20.12. **A:** Remote afterloader used for intracavitary low–dose-rate brachytherapy. **B:** System layout for a high–dose-rate remote afterloader for interstitial and intracavitary brachytherapy using a single high-activity (10 Ci) ^{192}Ir source. (Courtesy of Nucletron Engineering BV, The Netherlands.)

a careful choice of pulse length and frequency and using the ERD bioeffect dose model, TA values >1 might be possible, depending on the repair rate constants assumed for the tissues involved. Furthermore, for PDR treatments the dose rate at a point of interest during each pulse is not uniform because the treatment involves a single stepping source. Narayana and Orton's calculations indicated that PDR performed with 40 pulses in 120 hours with an irradiation time of 30 minutes per pulse with a delay time of 2.5 hours is the best replacement for a LDR treatment that delivers 60 Gy in 120 hours.

Fowler and Van Limbergen (105) explored the possible increase of radiation effect in tissues irradiated by PDR brachytherapy for local tissue dose rates between those "averaged over the whole pulse" and the instantaneous high-dose rates close to the dwell position. Increased effect is more likely for tissues with a short half-life of repair of the order of a few minutes, similar to pulse durations. Calculations were done assuming the linear quadratic formula for radiation damage, in which only the dose-squared term is subject to exponential repair. A constant overall time of 140 hours and a constant total dose of 70 Gy were assumed throughout, with the continuous LDR of 0.5 Gy per hour, providing the unitary standard effects for each PDR condition. Effects of dose rates ranging from 4 Gy per hour to 120 Gy per hour (HDR at 1 Gy per minute) were studied, covering the gap in an earlier publication. Four schedules were examined: doses per pulse of 0.5, 1, 1.5, and 2 Gy given at repetition frequencies of 1, 2, 3, and 4 hours, respectively, each with a range of an assumed half-life of repair of 4 minutes to 1.5 hours. Ratios as high as 1.5 can be found for large doses per pulse (2 Gy) if the half-life of repair in tissues is as short as a few minutes. The major influences on biologic effect are doses per pulse, half-life of repair in tissues, and—when

T1-2 is short—the instantaneous dose rate. Maximum ratios of PDR/LDR occur when the dose rate is such that pulse duration is approximately equal to T1-2. As dose rate in the pulse is increased, a plateau of effect is reached for most T1-2s, above 10 to 20 Gy per hour, which is radiobiologically equivalent to the highest HDR.

In an editorial, Hall and Brenner (131) noted that although the linear-quadratic model has been widely used and accepted, it has not been tested in extreme cases, and the biologic data needed for the modal calculations are not very well known. They also pointed out that Visser et al. (341) showed that the more different the proposed regimen is from continuous LDR, the longer the overall treatment time needs to be extended to preserve the therapeutic ratio.

Although PDR has prospered in Europe and Asia, unfortunately in the United States it has floundered because the Nuclear Regulatory Commission (NRC) requires that a physicist and/or radiation oncologist (or other suitably qualified person) be present throughout the treatment, which is almost impossible to accomplish in a long treatment schedule in a hospital setting (313). Williamson et al. (359) described the procedures and quality assurance regulations for PDR brachytherapy.

Swift et al. (323) at the University of California, San Francisco, described results in 65 patients who underwent 77 PDR brachytherapy procedures as part of their treatment for pelvic malignancies. PDR brachytherapy showed no significant increased toxicity above that seen with the standard continuous LDR approach. Further trials will need to be carried out to determine if larger doses per pulse and shorter total treatment times have comparable therapeutic ratios.

Peiffert et al. (262) prospectively evaluated PDR brachytherapy in 30 patients and concluded that PDR is feasible in

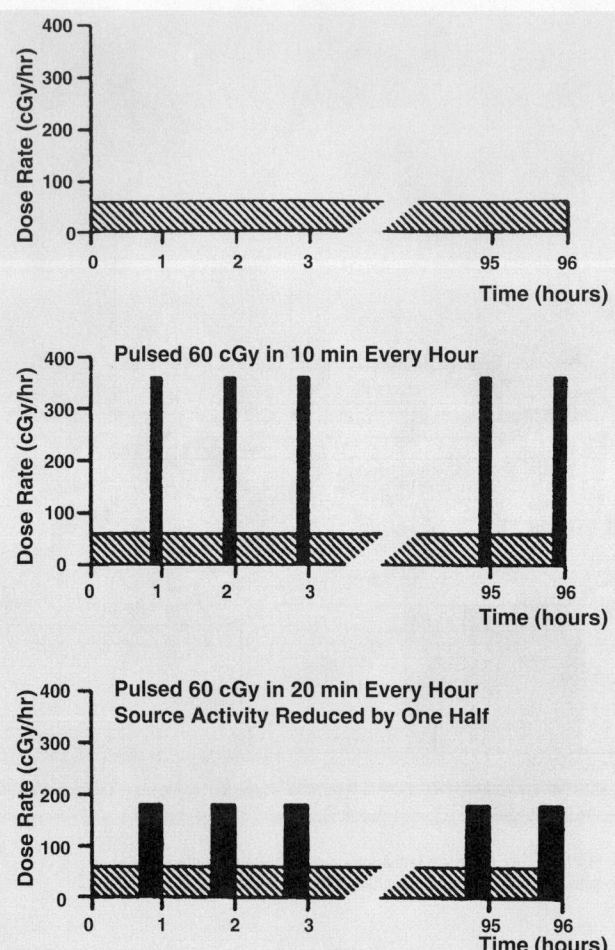

FIGURE 20.13. Principles of pulsed brachytherapy. A continuous low dose rate of 0.6 Gy per hour, for example, is replaced by a pulse of 0.6 Gy delivered in 10 minutes. As the single ^{192}Ir source decays with a half-life of 74 days, the pulse length is adjusted to maintain the dose per pulse to precisely 0.6 Gy. Thus, the average dose rate is maintained, and the overall treatment time for a given total dose remains fixed. (From Hall EJ, Brenner DJ. The dose-rate effect in interstitial brachytherapy: a controversy resolved. *Br J Radiol* 1992;65:242–247, with permission.)

patients with head and neck tumors but necessitates improvement of the quality of the plastic tubes. De Pree et al. (64) reported on 43 patients treated with PDR interstitial brachytherapy (24 with pelvic cancer, 17 with head and neck cancer, and two with breast cancer). Of 14,499 source and 14,399 dummy source transfer procedures, three technical machine failure events were observed (0.02%). Grade 3 or 4 late complications were observed in 4/41 (9.8%) patients.

Financial Considerations

Grigsby and Perez (123) published a financial analysis of LDR remote afterloading brachytherapy devices. Jones et al. (164) and Abrath et al. (1) compared the costs of HDR and LDR treatment (capital, maintenance, source, and operating costs) for Nucletron intracavitary equipment under alternative assumptions (three HDR fractions compared with one LDR fraction). The LDR-3 (Nucletron, Veenendaal, The Netherlands) is the most cost-effective, practical machine for up to 40 patients per year. Although LDR-3 is more cost effective for a greater number of patients, HDR would be recommended for more than 40 patients a year for practical reasons. Similarly, for five HDR compared with two LDR fractionations, LDR-3 was recommended for up to 20 patients per year, and HDR for a greater number of

patients. Recommendation was based on no cost sharing with other sites.

Bastin et al. (18) compared HDR treatment cost with LDR intracavitary brachytherapy for gynecologic malignancy. General anesthesia was used in 95% of programs for tandem and ovoid placement and in 31% for ovoid-only placement. Differences among private and academic practice respondents were minimal. At the authors' institution, a 244% higher overall charge for LDR treatment was noted, primarily as a result of hospitalization and operating room expenses. In addition to its ability to save thousands of dollars per patient, HDR therapy generated a "cost-shift," increasing radiation therapy departmental billings by 438%. Capital investment, maintenance requirements, and depreciation costs for HDR brachytherapy are lower because it is an outpatient procedure. Grigsby and Baker (121) reviewed the socioeconomic aspects of remote afterloading for both LDR and HDR, including required resources, reimbursement, cost-effectiveness, and a *pro forma* analysis of a new facility and conversion of an existing facility.

Implantation Techniques

Anesthesia

Small implants can be done under local anesthesia (and monitored sedation). General anesthesia, however, is sometimes preferable for good visualization and palpation of the tumor and for the patient's comfort.

General anesthetic is administered by nasotracheal intubation for implants of the oral cavity and lips. An elective tracheostomy initially is performed in patients with extensive oral cavity lesions requiring large implants and for all tumors of the glossopalatine sulcus, base of the tongue, or vallecula because the associated edema may cause serious breathing difficulties (72).

Breast implants can be done with local or general anesthesia. For brachytherapy procedures in the pelvis, general or spinal anesthesia is administered. Occasionally, a pudendal nerve block may be used.

Preoperative and Postoperative Orders

The radiation oncologist must assess the condition of the patient before the brachytherapy procedure is performed and log in the chart detailed instructions for nursing personnel, including tests results to be obtained, medications to be administered, preparation procedures for the operating room, and radiation safety measures. After the procedure is completed, a description of it should be recorded in the chart, including a diagram illustrating the exact location and pattern of placement as well as characteristics of the sources (length, strength, etc.). Clear postoperative orders are necessary, including time of removal of radioactive sources, appropriate medications, and special precautions.

Radiation Safety in the Operating Room

If high-energy radioactive sources such as ^{192}Ir or ^{137}Cs are prepared in the operating room (rarely done in the United States today), a workbench with shielding should be placed in one corner of the room so no one except the brachytherapy technician preparing them is exposed to radiation. The workbench is designed with a frontal working area with an L-shaped lead screen to protect the trunk, lower extremities, and medial aspect of the arms. In addition, a leaded-glass screen reduces exposure to the eyes.

Behind the barrier, there should be a lead well to store the remaining radioactive material while the individual needles, wire, grains, or seeds are being prepared for insertion into the patient. The bench should be covered with sterile drapes.

Sterilization of the radioactive sources is done by soaking the cesium needles in a germicidal solution such as CyDex. Gold-grain magazines and iridium wires are sterilized by gas.

When using radioactive sources, the operating physician, assistants, and anesthesiologist should work behind individual lead barriers. Exposure to the eyes and hands can be reduced only by distance and by dexterity gained through experience. All radioactive sources should be handled with long instruments. Because most procedures are performed with afterloading techniques, exposure to the fingers during manipulation is minimal. After insertion of the sources and removal of the patient, the remaining sources should be inventoried carefully and the operating room should be surveyed using a Geiger-Müller detector.

The details of protective procedures used during the preparation and transportation of radioactive materials and the regulations governing them were described in detail by Pierquin et al. (274) and Van Roosenbeek and Delclos (334). Compliance with NRC procedures and regulations is mandatory in the United States.

Removal of Implants

Interstitial needle sources generally can be removed in the treatment room and should not be removed in the patient's room. For patients with standard needles directly implanted in the posterior tongue and for less-than-cooperative patients, it is preferable, and sometimes essential, to remove the implant in the operating room, at times with the patient under general anesthesia; thus, adequate lighting, suction, and assistants are available. Bleeding at the time of needle removal is infrequent, but when it occurs, it may cause the patient or the assisting staff to panic. Firm and steady pressure with a finger on a compress over the bleeding point for several minutes usually is adequate treatment; occasionally, suturing of the blood vessel area with absorbable catgut may be necessary. It is not uncommon for the needle thread to be accidentally cut instead of the suture, and finding the needle requires an optimal surgical environment because the task is complex and time-consuming. Radiographic localization of the needle may be required before the needle base can be surgically exposed.

The afterloading nylon tubing is removed more easily. For the sake of radiation protection, it is advisable initially to un-crimp the metallic buttons and carefully remove the radioactive sources, which are accounted for and immediately placed in a portable safe or shielded cart. After this is done, each individual tube is removed by freeing one end. For oral cavity or oropharynx implants, it is preferable to cut the two ends of the tubing at the skin and pull it out through the oral cavity. A previously tied silk thread inside the cavity on the nylon tube loop is helpful in this maneuver.

After all needles or tubes are removed, the implanted site may be palpated gently to verify that all implant materials have been removed. The patient and, after the radioactive sources are taken out of the room, the room should be surveyed with a Geiger-Müller counter or some other radiation detector to make sure that there is no residual radioactivity. Appropriate notes in the patient's chart, an isotope form, and a radiation survey form should be completed to record all procedures performed.

Feeding the Patient with a Head and Neck Implant

Although some patients undergoing head and neck implants can be allowed to sip a liquid formula through a straw, most are fed through a nasogastric tube. This is a strict necessity when the lips have been sutured together for implants involving the buccal commissure.

Low–Dose-Rate Brachytherapy Techniques for Specific Sites

Interstitial Brain Implants

Radiation therapy is the only treatment option that has shown to have, even as single modality, an impact on survival of patients with malignant gliomas (344). This in addition to the observation that 80% of malignant gliomas recurrences occur within 2 cm from the original site led to the introduction of stereotactic techniques to focus higher radiation doses on the tumor bed while sparing surrounding brain in the attempt to improve local control and survival. Brachytherapy is one of these techniques and has a long history in the treatment of CNS tumors with the first treatment being carried out by Hirsch in 1912 (27). Although this first treatment by Hirsch was for a pituitary tumor, the first glioma treated with a radioactive source directly implanted into the tumor cavity was carried out by Frazier in 1914 (106). The era between the 1960s and the end of the 1980s saw the development of new and more sophisticated stereotactic implantation techniques as well as the development of new radioisotopes, which brought a renewed interest in brachytherapy for the treatment of brain tumors. Brachytherapy seemed to offer the chance to treat patients with higher doses while exploiting the advantages that altered fractionations allows. Interstitial irradiation, in fact, has two advantages over external radiotherapy: first, from a dosimetric point of view the implantation of low energy sources into the tumor allows irradiation tumor volume at the desired dose level with a steep dose falloff at the tumor edge that is much more pronounced than what is obtained with external stereotactic radiosurgery. Second, brachytherapy has related to the favorable radiation biology of the LDR irradiation, which tends to increase the damage to proliferating tumor cells while allowing normal tissue the chance for repair of sublethal damage. Actually, it has been demonstrated that altered fractionations in adult patients with supratentorial high-grade gliomas does not allow any significant survival improvement (252) as well as doses higher than 60 Gy (38). Beside the technical improvement, the initial reports from retrospective single institution experiences (126,197,231,304,326), showing improvement in survival, created a great interest in brain brachytherapy and led several authors to explore this new approach in high-grade and low-grade gliomas as well as in metastatic tumors. Several implantation techniques and radiobiologic strategy have been explored. First, a distinction can be made between temporary and permanent implants; while in a temporary ^{192}Ir implant the dose–rate range between 40 to 90 cGy per hour in a permanent ^{125}I implant the dose rate is around 2.5 to 3 cGy per hour. Even if *in vitro* studies demonstrate a sure dose–rate effect on glioma cells' radiosensitivity (25), such a dose–rate effect has not been shown in clinical trials comparing permanent and temporary implants brachytherapy implants (173).

Second, the radiation sources' implantation techniques can be divided into two categories: open techniques, in which individual seeds or imbedded in Vicryl suture seeds are placed via craniotomy (91,133,259), and stereotactic techniques (Fig. 20.14A,B,C,D; Fig. 20.15A,B,C,D) (171,197,303). A new technique, based on a new inflatable silicone balloon reservoir (GliaSite RTS, Cytye, Marlborough, MA) attached to a positionable catheter that is intraoperatively implanted into the resection cavity and postoperatively filled with a liquid radionuclide solution (liquid ^{125}I), has been developed. The dosimetric strengths

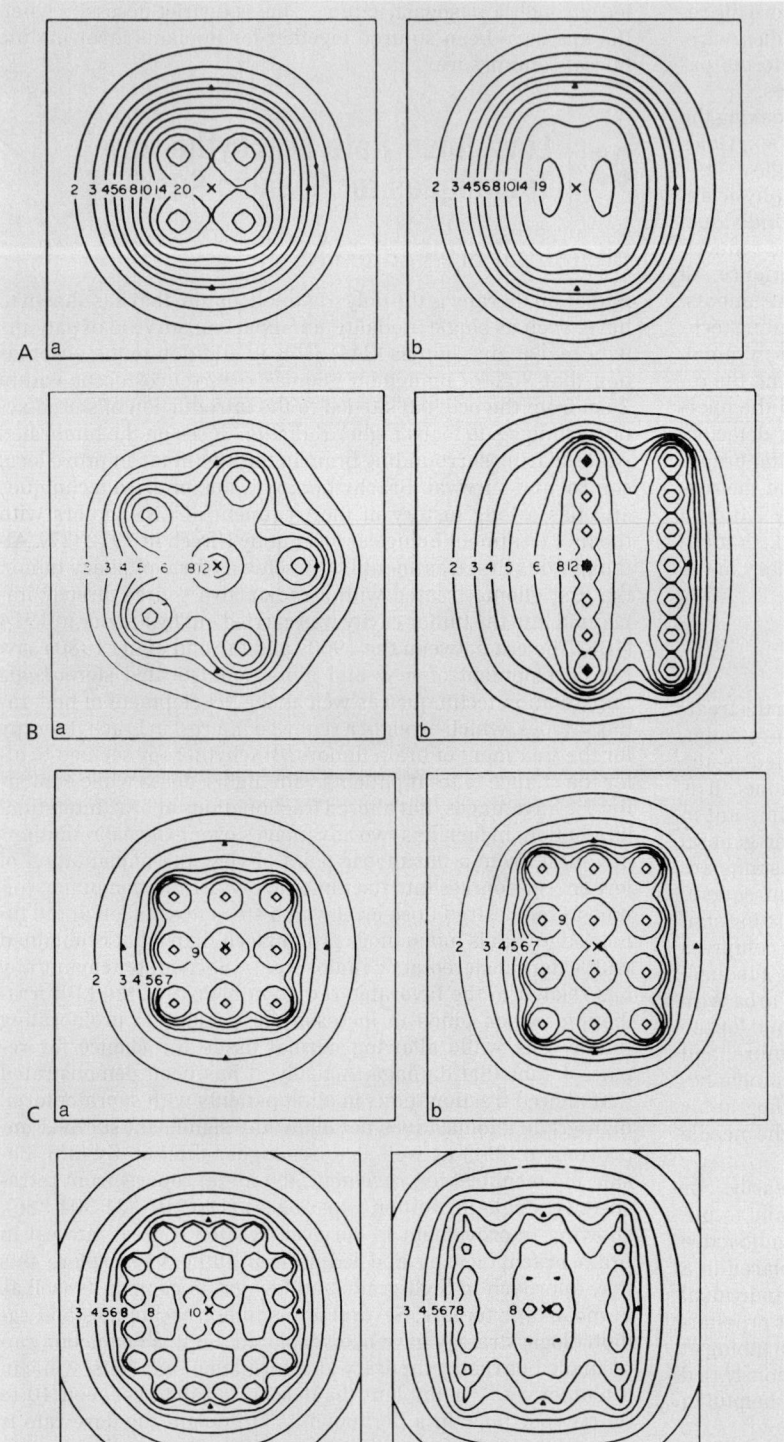

FIGURE 20.14. A: Dose distributions of brain implant at Institution A in two orthogonal planes: (a) the transverse plane and (b) the longitudinal plane, both bisecting the implant. Isodose rates in 0.1 Gy per hour are labeled. **B:** Dose distributions of the implant at Institution B in two orthogonal planes: (a) the transverse plane, taken 0.5 cm above the central plane, and (b) the longitudinal plane. Isodose rates in 0.1 Gy per hour are labeled. **C:** Dose distribution of the implant at Institution C in two orthogonal planes: (a) the transverse plane, bisecting the implant, and (b) the longitudinal plane. Isodose rates in 0.1 Gy per hour are labeled. **D:** Dose distributions of the implant at Institution D in two orthogonal planes: (a) the transverse plane and (b) the longitudinal plane, both bisecting the implant. Isodose rates in 0.1 Gy per hour are labeled. (From Saw CB, Suntharalingam N, Ayyangar KM, et al. Dosimetric considerations of stereotactic brain implants. *Int J Radiat Oncol Biol Phys* 1989;18:887–891, with permission.)

of this new applicator in comparison to traditional ^{125}I interstitial seed implants seems to be a more conformal therapy with no target-volume underdosing with an improved target-volume dose homogeneity with no healthy tissue "hot spots." On the contrary, the main weakness of the GliaSite applicator versus a traditional implant is the increased volume of healthy tissue receiving doses between 50% and 100% of the prescribed dose (73). Actually, the interest on central CNS brachytherapy is generally decreased mainly because randomized studies (183,309) failed to show a significant survival benefit and because of the

steep increase of stereotactic external beam irradiation techniques. On the other hand, brain brachytherapy has dosimetric and radiobiologic features that still make it an interesting field of study and research. Typically, candidates for brachytherapy should have a solitary lesion that is <6 cm in maximum diameter and noninvolvement of the corpus callosum as well as leptomeningeal or ependymal spreading (28,303,315). The treatment of lesions in the deep gray matter nuclei and infratentorial structures such as the brainstem vary from center to center but are generally excluded from prospective studies (342); however,

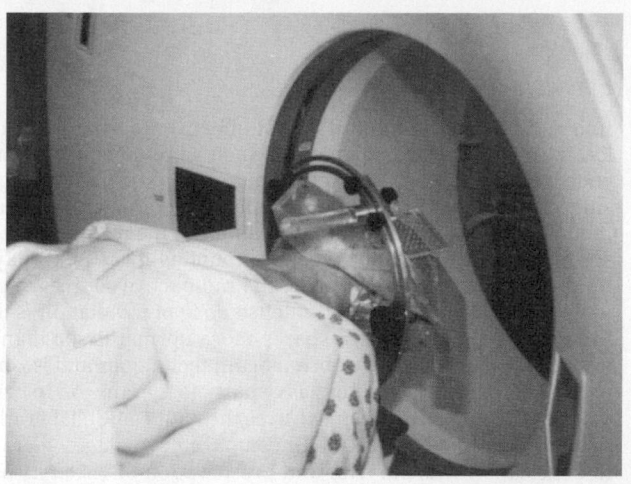
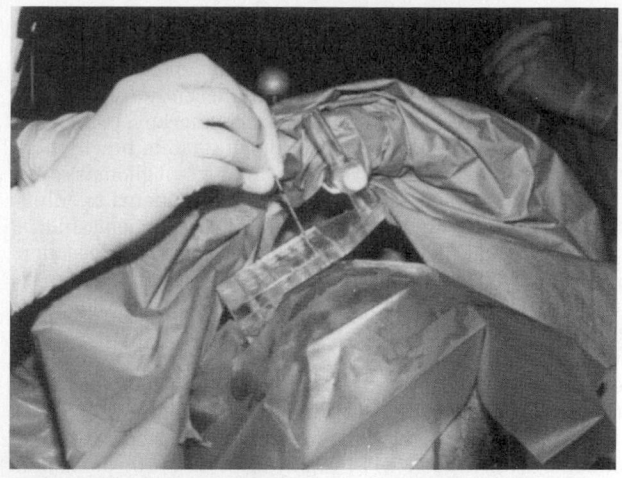
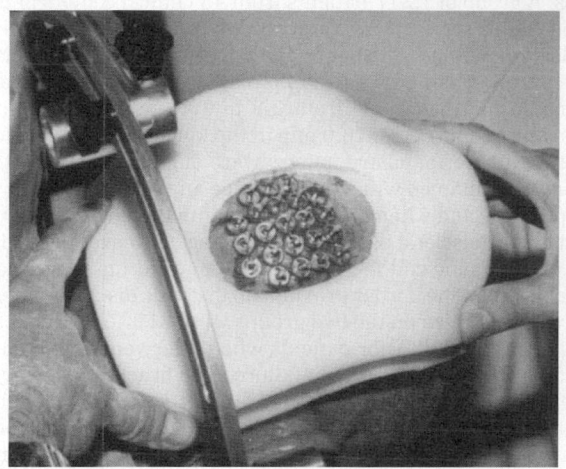
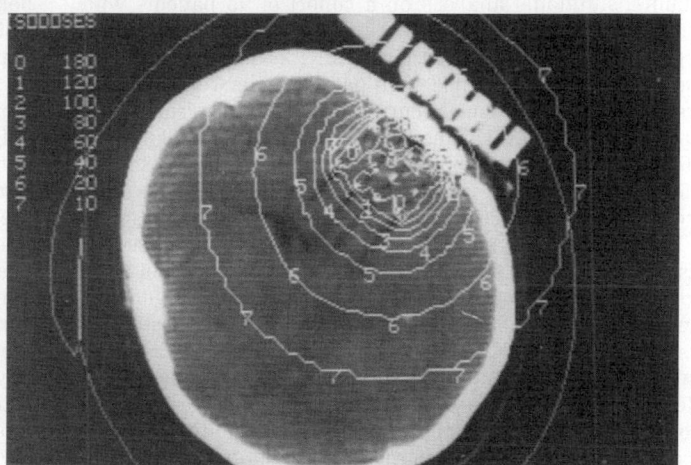

FIGURE 20.15. A: Patient on computed tomography (CT) scanner in position for ^{192}Ir brain implant. Stereotactic ring and plastic template to direct placement of catheters are shown. **B:** Insertion of afterloading plastic catheter with metallic guide into the brain through small burr holes in the skull. A plastic template is used to determine exact positioning of catheters **C:** Patient after implant is finished, demonstrating metallic buttons sewn to scalp to secure catheters in place. **D:** CT scan of skull with ^{192}Ir sources in place and isodose curve.

several authors have treated these lesions with extremely low–dose-rate permanent implants in an attempt to control growth of the lesion without causing necrosis (133,259).

The first published data on brachytherapy treatments of primary high-grade gliomas comes from UCSF. In 1991, Gutin et al. (127) published the results of 63 patients with newly diagnosed glioblastoma multiforme (GBM) or anaplastic astrocytomas (AA), treated with temporary ^{125}I implantation. Patients were treated with surgery followed by EBRT (60 Gy) with concomitant hydroxyurea followed by brachytherapy (BRT) (60 Gy) and then chemotherapy with CCNU (lomustine) and PVC. No major surgical complications were reported, and survival for patients undergoing implantation was 22 months for GBM and 39.3 for AA. Forty-eight percent required reoperation, and this was found to be associated with improved survival only for GBM patients. Scharfen et al. (303) retrospectively reviewed the outcomes of 307 patients (GBM: 106 primary, 66 recurrent; AA: 52 primary, 45 recurrent; moderately AA: 16 primary, 22 recurrent) treated with temporary ^{125}I implants. Survival rates were similar to Gutin's results. The authors concluded that compared with several historical studies, their survival for primary and recurrent GBM was superior to other treatment modalities, while the results for primary or recurrent AA were not superior to standard treatments. Wen et al. (353) treated 56 patients with newly diagnosed GBM were treated with surgery, limited field

EBRT (60 Gy), and stereotactic brachytherapy with temporary high activity ^{125}I sources giving an additional 50 Gy to the tumor bed. Median survival for patients undergoing BRT was 18 months compared with 11 months for a matched control group with similar clinical and radiologic features. Survival rates at 1, 2, and 3 years after diagnosis as high as 83%, 34%, and 27%, respectively, for patients receiving brachytherapy were significantly increased compared with survival rates of 40%, 12.5%, and 9%, respectively, for control subjects. Thirty-six patients (64%) underwent reoperation for symptomatic radiation necrosis from 3 to 42 months (median 11 months) after brachytherapy. The median survival of patients undergoing reoperation was 22 months, compared with 13 months for those who did not have further surgery. Such encouraging single institution retrospective results were not confirmed by two randomized trials. In the first one, from the University of Toronto (183), patients with primary malignant gliomas were randomized to receive EBRT (50 Gy) alone or EBRT (50 Gy) followed by BRT (60 Gy) with temporary ^{125}I and analyzed on the intent-to-treat. The median survivals of the two arms were 13.8 and 13.2 months. If only those patients who were actually implanted were considered, then the survival of the implant group is increased to 15.7 months. The second randomized trial was a multicentric study by the Brain Tumor Cooperative Group (309) evaluating surgery plus EBRT (60 Gy) plus BCNU (methotrexate, cytarabine, thioguanine, asparaginase, carmustine) with and without temporary ^{125}I brachytherapy (60 Gy) to treat newly diagnosed malignant gliomas. Also this trial demonstrated no survival advantages for interstitial BRT arm. Recently, GliaSite has given a new impulse to brain tumors brachytherapy; in the past few years several studies on the results of GliaSite brachytherapy approach to treatment of recurrent malignant gliomas came out in literature. Chan et al. (39) treated 24 patients at Johns Hopkins Hospital with recurrent GBM. Those patients had a prior surgery and EBRT (60 Gy) and, after relapse, a reresection and GliaSite BRT to a mean dose of 53.1 Gy. Median diagnosis for all patients was 23.3 months and median survival after GliaSite BRT was 9.1 months. Patients with a KPS ≥70 had a median survival of 9.3 months, whereas patients with KPS <70 had a median survival of 3.1 months. The authors conclude that GliaSite confers a prolongation of survival in patients with recurrent GBM compared to historical controls with recurrent GBM in patients with a good KPS. Gabayan et al. (110) published a multi-institutional analysis on a cohort of 95 patients with recurrent grade 3 or 4 gliomas. All patients had previously undergone resection and had received EBRT as part of their initial treatment. After recurrence each patient underwent maximal surgical debulking of their recurrent lesion and placement of a GliaSite catheter in the tumor cavity to deliver a median dose of 60 Gy to an average depth of 1 cm with a median dose rate of 53 Gy per hour. The median survival for all patients, measured from the date of GliaSite placement, was 36.3 weeks with an estimated 1 year survival of 31.1%. The median survival was 35.9 weeks for patients with an initial diagnosis of GBM and 43.6 weeks for those with non-GBM malignant gliomas. Analysis of the influence of various individual prognostic factors on patients survival demonstrated that only KPS significantly predicted for improved survival. A large number of articles in literature also deal with low-grade gliomas, reporting interesting data for brachytherapy as single modality treatment, an option that has been explored by several groups. Scerrati et al. (302) historically reviewed a group of 36 patients affected by low-grade gliomas (two pilocytic astrocytomas, 23 astrocytomas, and 11 oligodendrogliomas) with a location that made surgical removal not advisable, at least as first choice treatment. Permanent implants were performed in 22 patients and temporary implants in the remaining 14 patients. The mean peripheral dose was 89.71 Gy for the permanent implants and 42.8 Gy (32.05 cGy per hour) for the temporary implants. External beam irradiation was added in 15 cases in which primary tumor volume was >35 cc; the PTV expansion included 2 cm surrounding the gross tumor volume (GTV). Survival rates at 66, 84, and 100 months were 91.67%, 76.39%, and 50.93%, respectively. Encouraging data came from other authors, but the optimal treatment strategy for low-grade gliomas still remains controversial. Table 20.2 lists isotopes available and used for brain brachytherapy.

Eye

Episcleral Plaque

Episcleral plaque therapy is a cost-effective approach to treat localized intraocular malignancies such as retinoblastoma and choroidal melanoma. The technique consists of fabricating a small, spherically curved plaque containing radioactive sources, immobilizing the patient's eye, and suturing the plaque onto the sclera opposite the tumor where it remains for 3 to 10 days. Because of the close proximity of the radioactive sources to the tumor, a highly localized and intense dose of irradiation is delivered to the tumor, which spares more normal tissue than is possible by conventional external beam techniques and is competitive with the precision of heavy particle therapy. An interinstitutional randomized clinical trial through the Collaborative Ocular Melanoma Study (COMS) compared eye plaque therapy to enucleation with survival and preservation of vision as end points. A group of 1,317 patients from 43 clinical centers in the United States an Canada were randomly assigned to receive enucleation (660 patients) or ^{125}I brachytherapy (657 patients). To be enrolled, patients had to be diagnosed with a choroidal melanoma that had to be from 2.5 to 10.0 mm in the apical height and no more than 16.0 mm in the longest basal diameter. Patients with peripapillary tumors were eligible only when the tumor was contained within a 90-degree angle, with the apex at the optic disc, and when the enrolling ophthalmologist was confident that a episcleral plaque could be placed to cover the entire base of the tumor and a 2-mm margin beyond the tumor borders apart from the border proximal to the optic disc. The 5-year survival rates between the two groups were 81% for the enucleated patients and 82% for patients who underwent brachytherapy (52). The risk of treatment failure after brachytherapy was estimated to be 10.3%. Treatment failure was the most common reason for enucleation within 3 years of treatment; beyond 3 years ocular relapses resulted the most common cause for a enucleation procedure. Risk factors for treatment failure were older age, greater tumor thickness, and proximity of the tumor to the foveal avascular zone. Local treatment failure was associated weakly with reduced survival (53). Almost all surviving patients retained good visual acuity in the fellow eyes throughout 5 years of follow-up after treatment for choroidal melanoma. These findings persisted through 10 years of follow-up (51), in fact there was no evidence that fellow eyes of patients whose effected eye was treated with ^{125}I brachytherapy were at great risk of loss of visual acuity or new ophthalmic diagnoses than eyes of patients treated with enucleation alone (175). Historically, plaque therapy has been delivered using the ^{60}Co plaque system originally developed by Stallard (316) for treatment of retinoblastoma. These plaques (Fig. 20.16) are available in a limited range of sizes (8 to 12 mm diameter). Both circular and semicircular notched plaques are available for treatment

	Table 20.2	CHARACTERISTICS OF ISOTOPES COMMONLY USED IN BRAIN BRACHYTHERAPY			
Element		Isotope	Energy	Half-Life	Half-Value in Tissue (mm)
Interstitial brachytherapy					
Iodine		Iodine-125	0.028 MeV	59.6 days	20.0 mm
Iridium		Iridium-192	0.380 MeV	73.8 days	70.0 mm
Intracavitary brachytherapy					
Yttrium		Yttrium-90	0.93 MeV β-mean	64.0 hours	
Phosphorus		Phosphorus-32	0.69 MeV β-mean	14.3 days	0.8 mm
Iodine		Iodine-125	0.028 MeV	59.6 days	20.0 mm

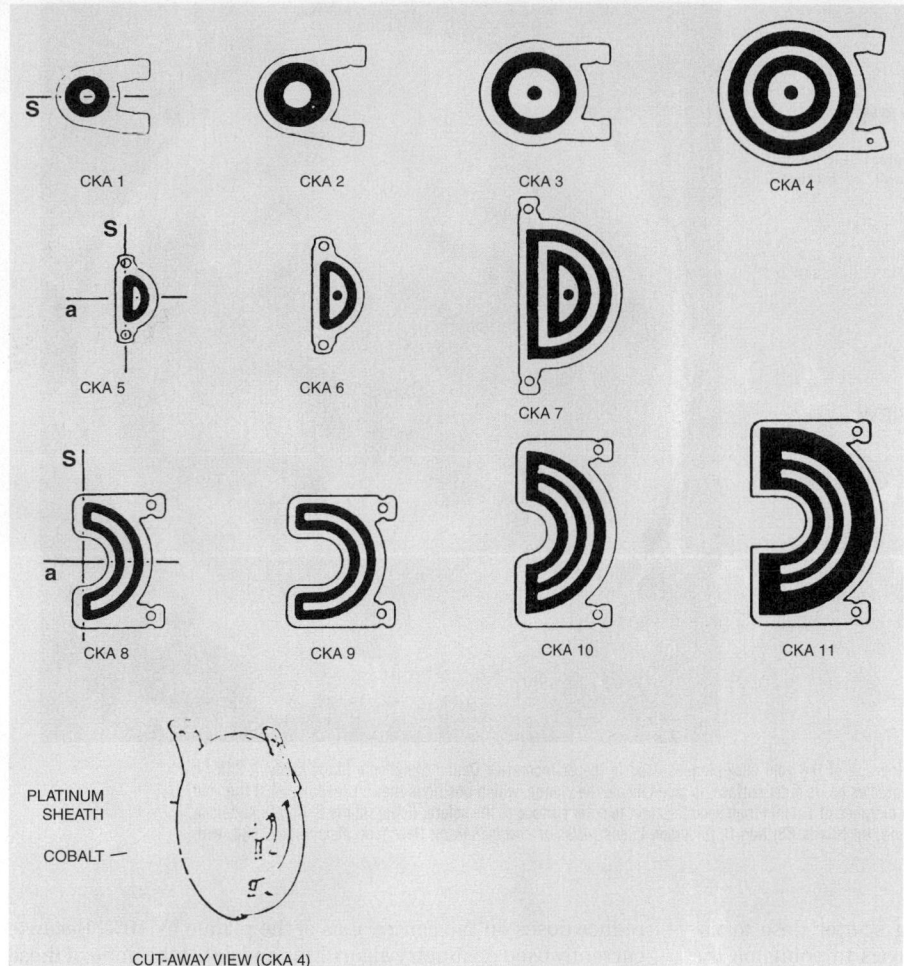

CKA 1   CKA 2   CKA 3   CKA 4

CKA 5   CKA 6

CKA 7

CKA 8   CKA 9   CKA 10   CKA 11

PLATINUM
SHEATH

COBALT

CUT-AWAY VIEW (CKA 4)

FIGURE 20.16. Axial views of the standard Stallard plaques used for treatment of intraocular malignancies. The ^{60}Co, distributed evenly over the blackened rings, is encapsulated in a platinum sheath. (From Stallard HB. Malignant melanoma of the choroid treated with radioactive applicators. *Ann R Coll Surg Engl* 1961;29:180, with permission.)

of posterior lesions abutting the optic nerve. Although easy to prepare and use, ^{60}Co plaques do not allow customization of the dose distribution, shielding of critical structures, or treatment of eye tumors on an outpatient basis. Packer et al. (255) used ^{125}I seeds as a substitute for ^{60}Co plaques in the treatment of ocular melanoma. In the COMS clinical trial, ^{125}I seeds are being used in conjunction with standardized gold-alloy plaques ranging from 12 to 20 mm in diameter (46). Each plaque is accompanied by a silastic insert with precut channels for reproducibly positioning the seeds in concentric circles (Fig. 20.17) (147). After the seeds are positioned in the insert, they are securely glued to the plaque so that the seeds are "sandwiched" between a 1-mm thick layer of plastic and the gold backing of the plaque. A COMS plaque can be assembled within 30 minutes, almost entirely eliminates the possibility of seed loss during treatment, fixes the seeds in a rigid geometry, and retains a high degree of individualization. Notched or noncircular plaques can be fabricated using dental casting techniques. Before plaque fabrication, all relevant imaging studies should be examined to define the basal dimensions and location of the tumor. A-mode ultrasound studies are used to define the maximum height of the tumor. Fluorescein angiograms often are helpful in determining the posterior boundary of the tumor. The fundus-view diagram, used by the ophthalmologist to record clinical impressions, represents a polar plot of the surface anatomy of the retina with its origin at the macula. When the anterior margin of the tumor is anterior to the equator, every attempt should be made to localize this margin relative to the ora serrata using transillumination. After the basal diameters, height, and location of the tumor are defined, a plaque is fabricated such that its diameter

is 4 to 8 mm larger than the assumed diameter of the tumor. A dummy plaque of identical size is used to define the plaque position in the operating room using transillumination as the definitive guide to tumor localization and size. A small caliper should be available for measuring the orthogonal dimensions and location of the tumor relative to the ora serrata. These data should be used as the basis for the final treatment plan. Both fundus-view isodose curves, which give the dose distribution on the retinal surface, and conventional transverse view are useful. Luxton et al. (194) and Chiu-Tsao et al. (44) demonstrated that ^{125}I plaques give dose distributions very similar to those of ^{60}Co plaques. [125]I plaque therapy delivers retinal surface doses of 270 to 400 Gy for a prescribed dose of 100 Gy to the tumor apex (Fig. 20.18) (194). [125]I plaques offer several dosimetric advantages over ^{60}Co plaques. The 0.5-mm thick gold plaque almost completely attenuates ^{125}I primary x-rays, providing a high degree of protection (95%) to tissue posterior to the eye. The 2.5-to 3.3-mm high lip of the COMS plaque produces limited collimation of the [125]I x-rays, which reduces the area of the retina treated to a high dose. Moreover, a thin lead foil (0.2 mm thick) placed over the patient's eye affords substantial radiation protection, making it possible to treat with plaques on an outpatient basis. When using ^{125}I plaques, physicists and clinicians should be aware that Williamson (357), Weaver et al. (352), and Nath et al. (248) showed that conventional ^{125}I data overestimate the dose rate in water at 1 cm from a model 6711 seed by 13% to 20%. As discussed in Chapter 16, the AAPM (5) has incorporated these differences into a new interstitial brachytherapy dosimetry protocol applicable to all tumor sites. Weaver (351) demonstrated that the gold backing of the plaque, which significantly

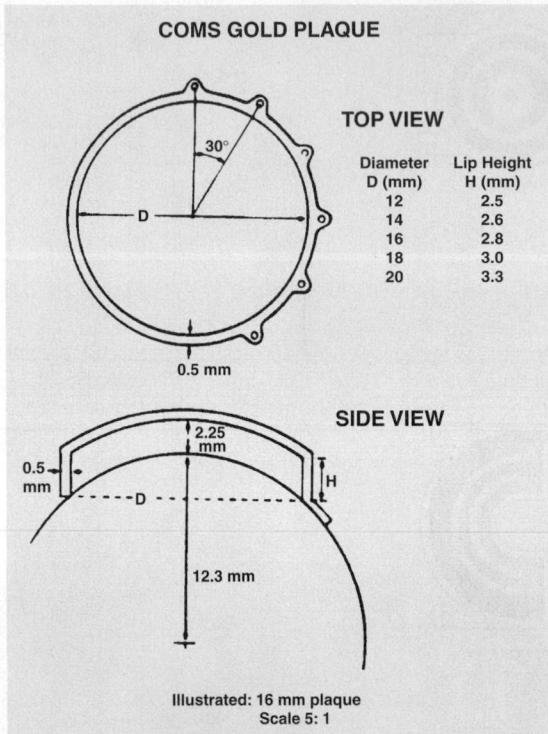

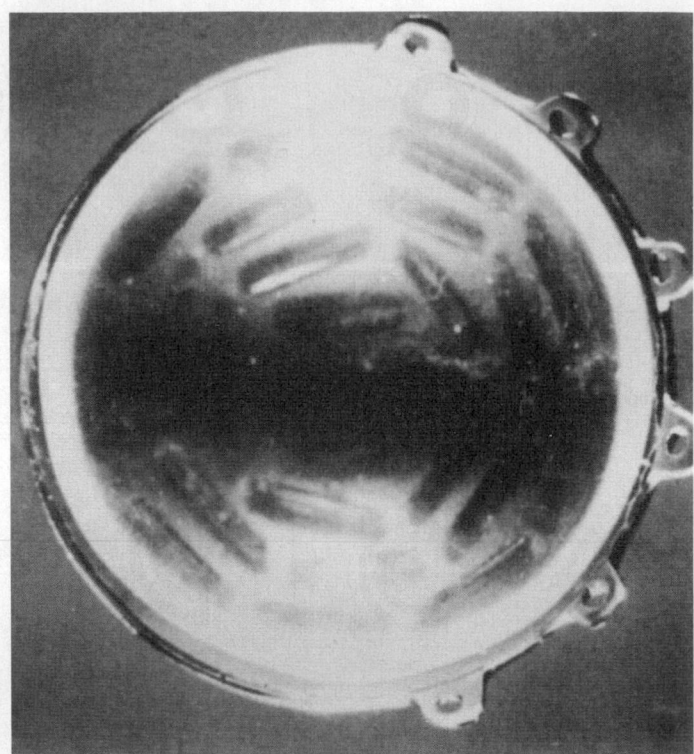

FIGURE 20.17. Drawings and photograph of the gold alloy plaques used in the Collaborative Ocular Melanoma Study study. A Silastic plastic insert, containing seed receptacles on its outer surface, is glued inside the plaque, which positions the ^{125}I seeds against the gold backing and maintains a treatment distance of 1.4 mm from seed to center to outer surface of the sclera. (From Hilaris B, Nori D, Anderson L. Brachytherapy of ocular melanoma. In: Hilaris BS, Nori D, Anderson L, eds. *Atlas of brachytherapy.* New York: Macmillan, 1988; with permission.)

reduces the volume of tissue contributing scatter dose to tissue anterior to the plaque, may reduce doses to points on the plaque axis by an additional 5% to 8%. Chiu-Tsao et al. (45) have shown that the 1-mm thick silastic insert, which has an effective atomic number (11.2) higher than that of tissue, may reduce doses on the central axis of the plaque by 10%. Because currently used dosimetry algorithms and data take none of these effects into account, minimum tumor doses delivered by COMS plaques are probably no >75% of the normally prescribed values (46). Krintz et al. (175) recalculated the dosimetric data of

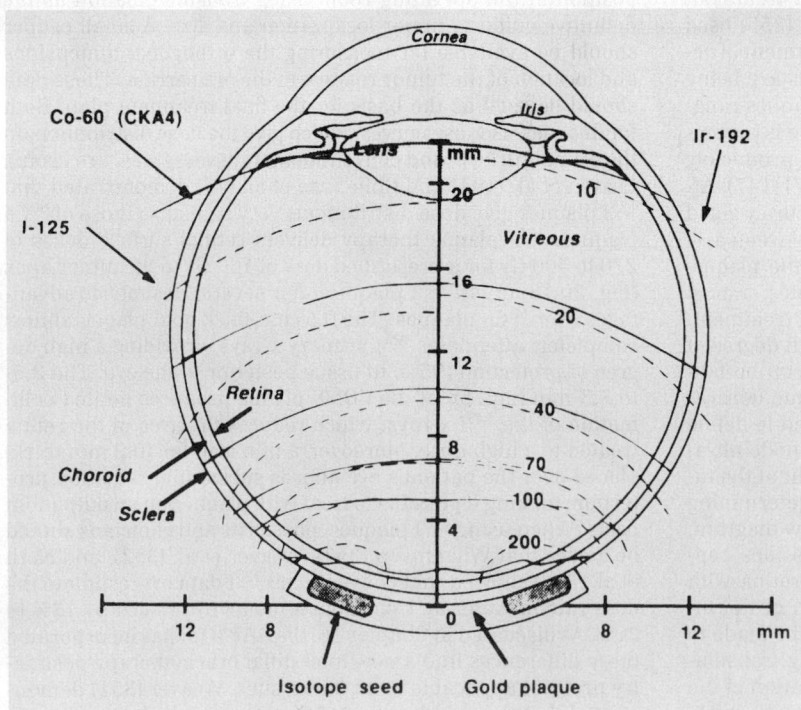

FIGURE 20.18. Isodose curves in the transverse plane of the eye for a 12-mm diameter plaque. The solid lines indicate isodoses arising from the CKA-4 ^{60}Co plaque, whereas the dashed lines on the right and left denote isodose curves arising from ^{192}Ir and ^{125}I seeds, respectively. All isodoses are normalized to 100% on the central axis 5 mm from the plaque surface. (From Luxton G, Astrahan MA, Liggett PE, et al. Dosimetric calculations and measurements of gold plaque ophthalmic irradiators using ^{192}Ir and ^{125}I seeds. *Int J Radiat Oncol Biol Phys* 1988;15:167, with permission.)

the brachytherapy arm for patients enrolled in the Collaborative Ocular Melanoma Study Medium Tumor Trial. By using an eye plaque radiotherapy planning system (plaque simulator) that incorporates all the dosimetric corrections including line source approximations, anisotropy, silastic attenuation, and gold shield attenuation, they found that the dose delivered to the structures of interest within the eye was significantly lower (7% to 21%) than the prescribed dose (175). Astrahan (14), by using an ophthalmic plaque planning system modified to incorporate additional scatter and attenuation correction factors that take into account the path length of primary radiation in the silastic seed carrier and the distance between the dose calculation point and the eye–air interface, found that the dose to critical ocular structures ranged from 16% to 50% less than would have been calculated using the standard COMS dose calculation protocol. A further element that has been investigated is the optimal dose–rate value of a ^{125}I brachytherapy treatment. Ocular melanoma patients may safely choose to retain the affected eye, but the benefits of organ preservation are dramatically reduced by lost visual function and symptomatic radiation toxicities. The COMS, in fact, reported that 43% of treated eyes had a visual acuity of 20/200 or worse by 3 years posttreatments. Jensen et al. (161) found in a cohort of 156 patients who underwent ^{125}I episcleral plaques for ocular melanoma that vision losses were associated with dose and dose rate to the lens as well as proximity and, hence, dose to the macula, optic disc, and fovea. Similarly, the development of distant metastasis as well as the melanoma-related mortality was associated with low-dose rates to the tumor apex (161). Current data suggest that low dose rates (<75-90 cGy per hour) to the tumor apex reduce systemic control; on the contrary, higher radiation dose rates are associated with worse results regarding residual ocular function. The ideal dose and dose rate for achieving local and systemic control without incurring a high risk of decreased visual acuity remains undefined. Although in North America the ^{125}I episcleral applicator has become the primary choice for brachytherapy, many institutions in Europe have gained a large experience using ruthenium-106 ([106]Ru) since it was introduced in the 1960s by Lommatzsch (192), for treating small to medium melanomas. Bergman et al. (26) from Karolinska Hospital recently published their 20-year experience on 579 patients, demonstrating similar results in terms of local control but better results in terms of visual acuity retain.

Pterygium

After surgical resection of the pterygium, because of the high recurrence rate (20% to 69%), it was for many years common practice to administer radiation therapy (55,331,364). In most institutions, a strontium-90 (^{90}Sr) β-ray applicator is used for treatment of these patients. The overall diameter of the applicator is 12.7 mm; the center is a circular radioactive disk 5 mm in diameter containing the isotope. The dose rate is generally about 5 Gy per minute. In some models, a Lucite disk on the shaft of the applicator shields the operator's hands (Fig. 20.19A) (273). Irradiation is begun within 24 hours after resection because failure increases with greater time delays (331). The patient is placed in a comfortable supine position with the head slightly tilted for optimal positioning of the medial portion of the eye. A lid retractor is inserted to hold the eye open. The cornea and conjunctiva are anesthetized with a few drops of 0.5% to 1% lidocaine. After 30 seconds to 1 minute, to allow for the anesthetic to take effect, the applicator is applied carefully on the surface of the resected sclera (Fig. 20.19B). Doses of about 10 Gy are delivered. The application is repeated in three consecutive weekly fractions for a total of 30 Gy. If a larger area of resection is to be irradiated, it may require application to two contiguous areas, each receiving the same dose. The lens, which is located at the depth of 3.5 to 5 mm from the surface, receives <5% of the dose (119). Monteiro-Grillo et al. (223) reported on 94 patients (100 eyes) treated with [90]Sr β-radiation— 37 eyes for primary and 63 for recurrent pterygium. Radiation doses were 30 Gy for three fractions per 5 days in 17 patients, 60 Gy for six fractions per 6 weeks in 80 patients, and 20 Gy for one fraction in three patients. Of the 100 eyes treated, 14% developed a recurrence of the pterygium. The 5-year local control rates were 94% for patients with primary pterygium and 76.9% for patients with recurrence. No late sequelae have been observed.

Head and Neck

The role of brachytherapy and philosophy of management for primary tumors in various anatomic locations and for different stages are analyzed in detail throughout this book and will not be discussed in this chapter. A complete review of the management principles, brachytherapy techniques, and treatment

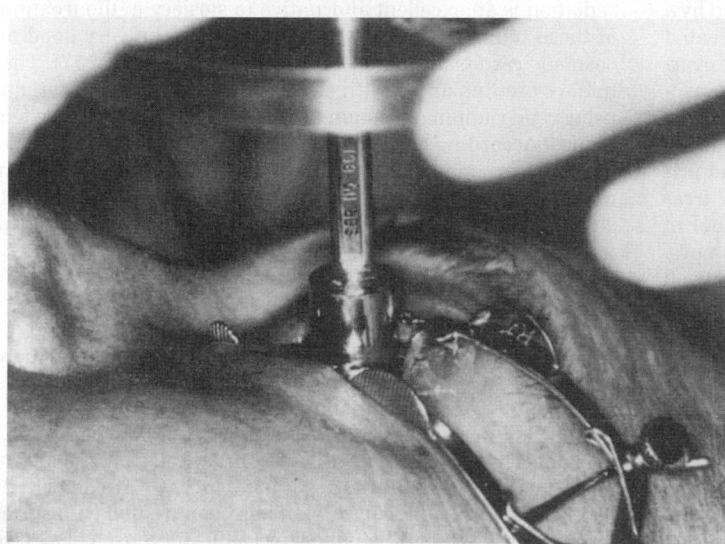
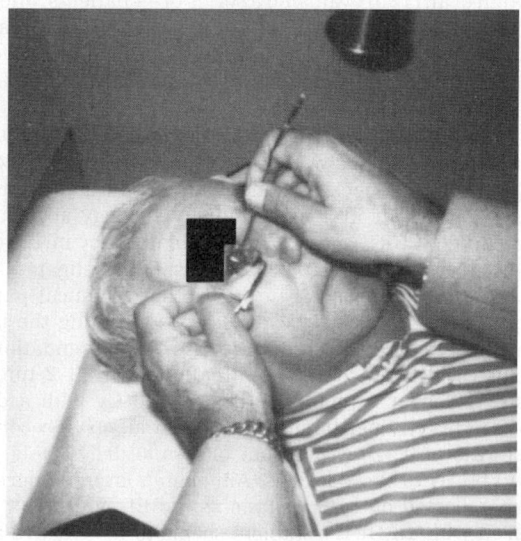

FIGURE 20.19. A: Patient undergoing ^{90}Sr application with eyelids retracted. Applicator has plastic shielding to protect operator's hands. (From Pierquin B, Wilson JF, Chassagne D. *Modern brachytherapy.* New York: Masson, 1987; with permission.) **B:** Similar ^{90}Sr application without shielding on applicator.

results for various tumors of the head and neck is available (207). It is enough to say that radiotherapy and surgery allows 80% of local control rate in T1-2 tumors with limited neck node involvement (225), and that brachytherapy represent a valid option as exclusive modality treatment for early stage head and neck tumors. Exclusive brachytherapy, in fact, offers comparable results to surgery in terms of local control and survival in small tumors without the side effects (both cosmetic and functional) that surgery usually carries. In 1987, the GEC-ESTRO (Groupe Europeen de Curietherapie), reviewing more than 2,000 cases from all over Europe, demonstrated that exclusive brachytherapy offers better local control rates than the integration of brachytherapy plus EBRT (209,224) for T1-2 lesions of mobile tongue probably due to the shortening of the total treatment time that, usually, exclusive brachytherapy allows, and to the minor probability of " geographical missing" in the treatment planning that an up-front technique carries. Such data have been confirmed recently by several authors from leading institutions. Marsiglia et al. (202) from Gustave-Roussy Institute published a retrospective analysis on 160 patients who underwent radical LDR brachytherapy for a T1-2 floor of the mouth cancer. They found that 89% of the patients were disease-free 5 years after treatment. The rates of local tumor failure were 10% for all patients, 7% of T1 tumors, and 12% of T2. The 5-year actuarial survival rate for all patients was 76%, 88% for T1, and 74% for T2. Pernot et al. (268) analyzed a cohort of 207 patients affected by a squamous tumor floor of the mouth treated with exclusive irradiation. The treatment consisted of a combination of external beam irradiation to the tumor bed and the node areas and complementary LDR brachytherapy to the primary tumor in 105 cases and of exclusive LDR brachytherapy to the tumor with or without neck dissection of the node areas in the remaining 102 cases. The brachytherapy was performed initially according to the hairpin technique and later with the plastic tubes following the Paris system rules. The local control rates at 5 years were 97% and 72%, respectively, for T1-2 tumors, while the 5-year specific survival rates were 88% and 47%, respectively. It was also found that the patients treated by exclusive brachytherapy for T1-2 N0 tumors had better 5-year results (92% local control; 76% specific survival) than those treated by combined therapy (63% local control; 35% specific survival). Similar rates of local control and survival were obtained by Wadsley et al. (343). Exclusive brachytherapy has been demonstrated to be effective and safe also in locations in which a treatment is technically more difficult to be arranged. Le Scodan et al. (185) evaluated a series of 44 patients, affected by a T1 or T2 squamous carcinoma of the velotonsillar area, treated with exclusive interstitial brachytherapy and found 5-year overall and progression-free survival rates of 76% and 68%, respectively.

Brachytherapy may also provide a useful method for the retreatment of patients with recurrent, persistent, or second primary head and neck malignant tumors in a previously irradiated region, or in a multimodality strategy a useful tool in addiction to EBRT, surgery, and chemotherapy in T3-4 tumors. Another aspect that has been intensely investigated has been the optimal dose, dose rate, and other technical parameters to maximize the tumor response without rising the incidence of treatments complication. The GEC recommendations for an exclusive LDR brachytherapy treatment for T1-2 tumors suggests to deliver a total dose of not <70 Gy with a dose rate of 45 to 60 cGy per hour. Fontanesi et al. (103) recommend a dose rate of 0.42 Gy per hour or less to deliver total doses of 50 to 60 Gy to these lesions. Although a larger experience has been collected on LDR treatments, a BED-equivalent dose delivered with an HDR treatment seems to be effective and safe. Inoue et al. (155,156) from Osaka University compared LDR and HDR exclusive brachytherapy for mobile tongue T1-2 tumors. In a group of 59 patients, they found that the 5-year local

control rate was not different between the two groups (77% vs. 76%, respectively) and, although the incidence of acute adverse effects was higher in the HDR group, no difference was evidenced in terms of late toxicities. Interesting results regarding PDR brachytherapy have been reported by Strnad et al. (318) from Erlangen-Nurnberg University. Analyzing retrospectively a group of 47 patients with head and neck cancers treated with BRT alone (24 patients) or BRT plus EBRT (23 patients) delivered with an effective dose rate of 0.5 to 0.7 Gy per hour they found toxicity rates comparable with LDR regimens.

Maxillary Sinus

Rosenblatt et al. (293) described the use of a surgical obturator made of vinyl polysiloxane as a carrier for afterloading ^{192}Ir seed ribbons to treat patients with maxillary antrum tumors after partial or total maxillectomy. Two weeks after the surgical procedure, an impression was made of the maxillary cavity and the obturator mold was built. Multiple nylon catheters were inserted, depending on the geometry and dosimetry of the implant. The inner aspect of the impression was coated with a sheet of visible light cure denture material, the obturator was placed in an oven for 5 minutes, and the device was trimmed and polished. After the obturator was inserted into the patient, isodose distributions were obtained. Prescribed doses were 45 to 70 Gy (modal dose of 60 Gy) at 0.5 cm from the outermost source plane. Iridium seed activity was 0.7 to 1 mg Ra Eq per seed. The obturator mold previously loaded with ^{192}Ir was coated with acrylmethacrylate resin to secure it in place and prevent disturbance of the dosimetry once inserted in the surgical cavity. The approximate dose rate per day was 10 to 15 Gy. Intracavitary therapy was combined with external irradiation in five patients (mean dose, 53 Gy in 2-Gy fractions). After a median follow-up of 35 months, 9/11 patients were alive without evidence of disease; one patient developed a local recurrence, and another patient developed a new lesion in the lower buccal mucosa. One patient required orbital exenteration. One patient developed bilateral cataracts, and another developed blurred vision in the homolateral eye after an estimated dose of 7 Gy.

Nasal Vestibule

Small lesions of the nasal vestibule can be treated adequately with either external or interstitial irradiation, whereas more advanced lesions require a combination of both modalities. Irradiation is an excellent alternative to surgery in the treatment of these tumors because tumor control can be very good and cosmetic results are better than with surgery (216,217). These tumors are implanted with single- or double-plane techniques using rigid radium or cesium needles or ^{192}Ir nylon tubing techniques. According to Mendenhall et al. (216), the distal vertical needles (perpendicular to the dorsum of the nose) in each plane may be mounted in a nylon bar to stabilize the distal needles and adequately cover the tumor involving the opening of the nasal vestibule (258).

Skin and Lip

Brachytherapy for treatment of skin and lip tumors was popular before the advent of external irradiation techniques. Interstitial single- or double-plane implants could be performed to encompass the tumor with a safe margin, following the basic principles of brachytherapy (Paterson-Parker, Quimby, or Paris technique) (Fig. 20.20A,B). Doses of 50 to 70 Gy are delivered in 5 to 7 days. Carcinoma of the skin has been treated with surface molds or interstitial brachytherapy (199). Jorgensen et al. (166) reported on 869 patients with squamous cell carcinoma of the lip for whom irradiation was the initial form of treatment in all but 25. Radium implants were used in 766 patients with local

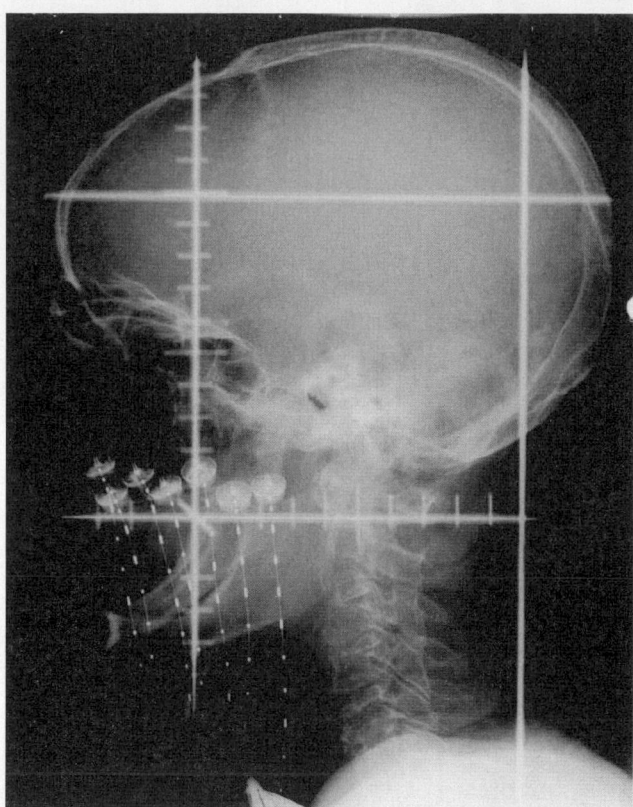

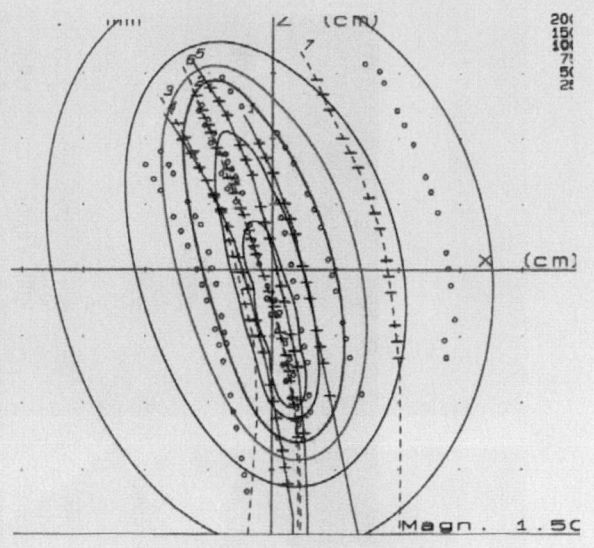

FIGURE 20.20. A: Sagittal view of in interstitial implant of a tick lesion of the left cheek. Tumor was staged as a T3 lesion and treated with a combination of external and interstitial radiotherapy. **B:** Sagittal isodose distribution of the implant shown in (A).

tumor-control rates of 93% in T1, 87% in T2, and 75% in T3 tumors. Similar results were described by Pigneux et al. (275). Tombolini et al. (329) described the technique and results in 57 patients with squamous cell carcinoma of the lower lip treated with LDR interstitial brachytherapy. The median tumor dose was 62 Gy (range, 44–96): 10 patients (18%) received a total dose <50 Gy, 28 (59%) between 50 and 70 Gy, and 19 (33%) more than 70 Gy. The clinical N+ cases were irradiated to total doses of 65 to 70 Gy on the involved station. Actuarial disease-free survival at 5 and 10 years was 81% and 81%, respectively. Actuarial local tumor control was 90% at 3 and 5 years, rising to 94% with salvage surgery.

Nasopharynx

Erickson and Wilson (84) summarized the techniques for management of patients with carcinoma of the nasopharynx (Table 20.3). Some authors have used interstitial techniques, which are more laborious to carry out because of difficulty in positioning the applicator in the tumor area, dosimetric problems related to the irregular mucosal surface of the nasopharynx, and limitation of effective depth dose versus surface dose (85). Palatal fenestration may be required in patients with lesions in the superior and high posterior nasopharyngeal walls, which are more difficult to reach through the nasal or oral cavities (85,138). Scott (307) described temporary interstitial techniques transversing the lesion with sutures containing iridium seeds accessed through the oropharynx and subsequently removed. The use of ^{103}Pd seeds for permanent implant of nasopharyngeal tumors has been described by Porrazzo et al. (281). Wang (347) described use of intracavitary brachytherapy alone or combined with external irradiation to boost the dose to the nasopharynx, in conjunction with external beam irradiation. Two pediatric endotracheal tubes with inner and outer diameters of 5 mm and 6.9 mm, respectively, and loaded

with two 20 mg Ra Eq ^{137}Cs sources are used. Local anesthesia of the nasal cavity is achieved with cocaine. The endotracheal tubes are introduced through the nares into the nasopharynx with the head hyperextended. Under fluoroscopic control on the simulator, the tips of the cesium sources are placed at the free edge of the soft palate posteriorly and behind the posterior wall of the maxillary sinus anteriorly. A 5-cc balloon attached to the distal end of the endotracheal tube is inflated for anchoring purposes and to improve the dose to the nasopharynx (by increasing the distance from the source). The dose reference point is 0.5 cm below the mucosa of the nasopharyngeal vault; the dose rate is approximately 1.2 Gy per hour. Denham et al. (74) described a technique for intracavitary irradiation of the nasopharynx with afterloading catheters of different curvatures that are introduced into the nasopharynx via the nasal cavity, with appropriate anesthesia. The major difficulty with this technique is the successful rigid anchoring of the catheters to prevent movements that could be potentially injurious to the nasal cavity or nasopharynx. For this purpose, a special plastic face mask was constructed with adjustable universal joint fittings for rigid attachment of the catheters with minimal discomfort to the patient. Because of asymmetry of the nasopharynx, different angle catheters can be used (22.5, 40, or 50 degrees). Levendag et al. (187) designed an inexpensive, reusable, and flexible silicone applicator, tailored to the shape of the soft tissues of the nasopharynx, which can be used with either LDR brachytherapy or high (pulsed) dose rate remote-controlled afterloaders. The applicator proved to be easy to introduce and patient friendly, and it can remain *in situ* for the duration of the treatment (2 to 6 days).

Oral Cavity

The oral cavity should be kept dry with adequate preanesthesia medication, including scopolamine, and suction. It is desirable to outline the tumor with gentian violet, Castellani's paint, or a

Table 20.3 INTRACAVITARY LOW–DOSE-RATE/MEDIUM–DOSE-RATE TECHNIQUES IN CARCINOMA OF NASOPHARYNX

Author (Reference)	Technique	Dose/Prescription Point	Timing	External Beam Dose	D/E/R
Wang and Schultz (349)	^{226}Ra pack	20–40 Gy	—	± 22–58 Gy	R
Patterson (261)	^{226}Ra in cork (15 mg)	80 Gy/7 days at 0.5 cm	—	±	D, P
Martin & MacComb (203)	^{226}Ra needles (10 mg) or ^{226}Ra seeds in lead capsule ball	2,500–3,000 mgh (with external), 3,500 mgh (definitive) over 20 days with 48-h break every 5 days	Before external	± 30 Gy	D, E, R
Henschke et al. (141)	Plastic sphere (^{192}Ir, ^{60}Co)	1,000 mgh/2 applications		±	E, R
Pryzant et al. (288)	Teflon balls (^{137}Cs)	20–50 Gy/2–5 days at applicator surface	After external	+	R
Suit et al. (321)	Acrylic resin mold (^{226}Ra tubes)	30 Gy/2 Fx every 10 days; at 1 cm	After external	50 Gy	P
Yan et al. (361); Qin et al. (291)	Mold (^{226}Ra needles)	40 Gy/2 Fx at surface, 7–10 days apart	After external	±(R); 70 Gy (P)	E, P, R
McNeese Fletcher (214)	Mold (^{226}Ra)	30–35 Gy at surface	After external	40 Gy	R
Chassagne et al. (42); Pierquin et al. (270); Gerbaulet et al. (114)	Mold (^{192}Ir)	30 Gy (E); 40–98.5 Gy (P, R)	After external	45 Gy (E); ±(P, R)	E, P, R
Deutsch et al. (77)	Mold (^{60}Co), palatal fenestration	60 Gy at 1.5 cm at 0.5 Gy/h/14 h/day × 8 days	—	—	R
Ashayeri et al. (13)	Foley catheter (^{192}Ir)	21 Gy	—	—	E, R
Wang (348)	Endotracheal tube (^{137}Cs)	20 Gy at 0.5 cm at 1.2 Gy/h, 1–2 Fx 1 week apart	10–14 days after external	40 Gy	R
Wang (348)	Endotracheal tube (^{137}Cs)	7 Gy at 0.5 cm in 5 hours	2–3 weeks after external	65 Gy	E
Flores (102)	Endotracheal tube (^{226}Ra, ^{137}Cs)	60 Gy/58 h at 1.5 cm		40 Gy	R
Flores (102)	Endotracheal tube (^{137}Cs)	26 Gy/1.77 h at 1.5 cm		± 40 Gy	R
Shankar et al. (311)	Endotracheal tube + mold (^{137}Cs + ^{192}Ir)	21 Gy/30 h at surface		—	P
Harrison et al. (136)	Endotracheal tube (^{192}Ir); plastic tube (^{192}Ir)	15–20 Gy		45 Gy	R
Sham et al. (310)	Latex tube (^{137}Cs)	20–30 Gy/2–3 Fx/every week 4–5 h/Fx	During external (after 2 weeks)	–(P); 40–50 Gy (R)	P, R
Yamashita et al. (360)	Double lumen-plastic tube (^{60}Co)	8 Gy/2 Fx at 0.5 cm 1 week apart		66–70 Gy	E
Denham et al. (74)	2 uterine tandems (^{192}Ir)	7.2 Gy/16 h		64.5 Gy	E
Haghbin et al. (129)	Intracavitary (^{226}Ra, ^{137}Cs)	40–60 Gy		—	R

Co, cobalt; Cs, cesium; D, definitive; E, elective boost; Fx, fraction; Ir, iridium; P, persistent; R, recurrent; Ra, radium.
Modified from Erickson BA, Wilson JP. Nasopharyngeal brachytherapy. *Am J Clin Oncol* 1993;16:424–443.

surgical marker before starting the implantation of sources. A metric ruler always should be on the implant tray. When rigid needles are being implanted in the oral cavity, one assistant retracts the patient's lips and another either pulls or depresses the tongue while the operating radiation oncologist performs the implant. The anterolateral needles of an implant of the oral cavity should be kept away from the thin mucous membrane that covers the bone in the upper and lower gum, as well as from the periosteum, teeth, and bone. To increase and maintain the distance, a regular fluoride carrier is thickened on the inside by one to four layers (one layer = 2 mm) to increase the distance so that the unavoidable "hot spot" around each needle is kept away from the adjacent normal mucosa. Miura et al. (221) reported on 103 patients with T1 or T2 tongue carcinoma treated by a single-plane implantation of ^{192}Ir pins (60 treated by BRT alone, and the rest were combined with external irradiation and/or chemotherapy); 48 and 55 patients were given BRT with and without a spacer, respectively. Spacers were individually made of acrylic resin according to a prosthetic technique to obtain the thickness of 7 to 10 mm at the lingual part of the implanted side. The spacer reduced about 50% of the absorbed dose at the lingual side surface of the lower gingival to that in the absence of a spacer. Absolute incidence of mandibular osteonecrosis was 2.1% (1/48) and 40.0% (22/55), with and without a spacer, respectively ($p = .0004$).

Tongue and Floor of Mouth

Lesions beneath the tongue, or in the floor of the mouth, usually are implanted through the dorsum of the tongue if standard needles (or substitutes) are used. The anterolateral needles emerge from the undersurface of the tongue and are reinserted into the floor of the mouth. The implants should extend beyond the visible or palpable tumor by at least 1 cm in all directions. A popular technique of interstitial implants with nylon tubing and ^{192}Ir sources for lesions of the oral tongue or floor of the mouth uses a submental or submaxillary approach for the insertion of metallic guides into the oral cavity with one hand. The exit points of the guides in the oral cavity are carefully verified with the index finger of the other hand (through-and-through technique).

The major nylon tubing is threaded through the metallic guides and looped around the dorsum of the tongue and then exits through a parallel metallic guide. The metallic guides are pulled out externally, and the nylon thread is secured by crimping with a metallic button at one end. The procedure continues as described previously leaving the other end open momentarily for insertion of the radioactive sources. Tying a silk thread on the loop of each nylon tube inside the oral cavity facilitates removal.

After position of the sources is verified on x-ray films using radiopaque inactive dummy sources, the appropriate ^{192}Ir wires (or seeds in nylon tubing) are inserted, and the other end of the larger nylon tube is crimped. The sequence of needle implantation for lesions involving the oral tongue and the anterior floor of the mouth is illustrated in Figure 20.21.

Mendenhall et al. (216) described a template for floor-of-the-mouth implants made of aluminum, stainless steel, or nylon that is individually customized to fit the lesion of each patient (Fig. 20.22) (200). The device is inserted into the floor of the mouth under general anesthesia and is secured by one suture through the submental area, which is tied to a cotton roll. The active ends of the radium needles may be positioned above the level of the mucosa to ensure an adequate surface dose. Crossing is accomplished by placing a needle parallel to the mucosal surface on the implant device. The system is not afterloaded, but the procedure can be performed rapidly with predictable geometry so irradiation exposure to the operating staff is lower than with the hairpin technique. According to the authors, the advantage of this technique over use of iridium hairpins is that

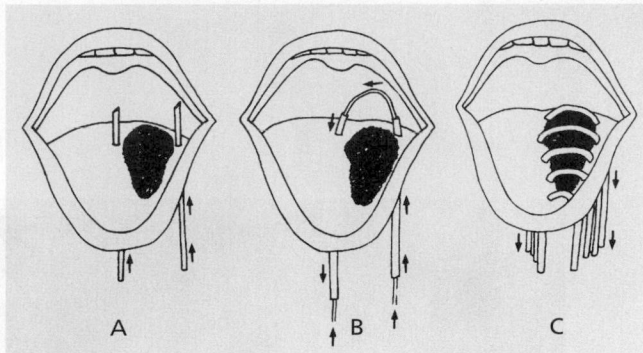

FIGURE 20.21. Diagram illustrating submental or submaxillary approach for insertion of Teflon catheters with metallic guides (for ^{192}Ir) into oral cavity for lesions for the floor of the mouth or lateral border of the tongue. **A:** Metallic guides are introduced, with one hand guiding the position of the guide inside the oral cavity. **B:** Introduction of nylon strand for placement of the ^{192}Ir wire or seeds, looped over dorsum of the tongue. **C:** Various nylon tubes in position on dorsum of the tongue. At this point, the metallic guides have been withdrawn from the submaxillary region. After position of the radioactive sources is radiographically determined using dummy sources, active sources are inserted, and the ends of the plastic tubes are crimped with metallic buttons.

all needles with the template are rigidly fixed in relationship to one another, and the isodose distributions can be calculated before the procedure or can be modified if necessary by adjusting the arrangement of the needles.

Implantation with rigid needles of the posterolateral border of the tongue via the oral cavity requires pulling the tongue forward to start the implant at the base of the tongue. The first needle is inserted pointing posteriorly and inferiorly at about 45 degrees; a lesser angle is used for successive needles. At the end of the implant, when the tongue returns to its normal position, the implant needles adopt a vertical position.

At the University of Florida a technique has been used with radium or cesium needles mounted on rigid bars made of stainless steel or nylon; the number of needles depends on the diameter of the lesion (216). A crossing needle usually is added to one or both bars to ensure adequate irradiation dose to the dorsal mucosal surface of the tongue. Another technique described by Baillet et al. (17) uses the ^{192}Ir hairpin technique. Inactive gutter guides are placed into the tongue, and under fluoroscopic control it is verified that the gutter guides are parallel. The iridium hairpins are afterloaded into the guides, which are removed at that time. A suture is used to secure each hairpin to the tongue. A cotton roll sutured between the tongue and the mandible with either technique displaces the tongue medially and decreases the irradiation given to the mandible. The advantage of the iridium hairpin technique over the radium or cesium rigid needles is that the overall source length is shorter for the same active length because of the 6-mm inactive tips at either end of the rigid needles. Furthermore, there are only two vertical sources per hairpin as opposed to three or four radium or cesium needles on each bar so that it is easier to position the hairpins in the tongue (Fig. 20.23) (257). This is particularly helpful in patients with small mouths, trismus, or full dentition, where it is very difficult to adequately position the rigid needles. An effort should be made to reduce treatment morbidity. Lozza et al. (193) noted mandibular necrosis in 10/100 patients with oral cancer treated with LDR brachytherapy; median follow-up was 38 months. No significant incidence of this complication was observed when tumor site (mobile tongue vs. floor of mouth), dental status, or total physical dose was considered. A significant correlation between the incidence of bone necrosis and two main parameters was found (i.e., dose rate is $p < .02$ and reference volume is $p < .05$). A threshold value may be suggested both for dose rate (50 cGy per hour) and reference volume (25,000 mm^3).

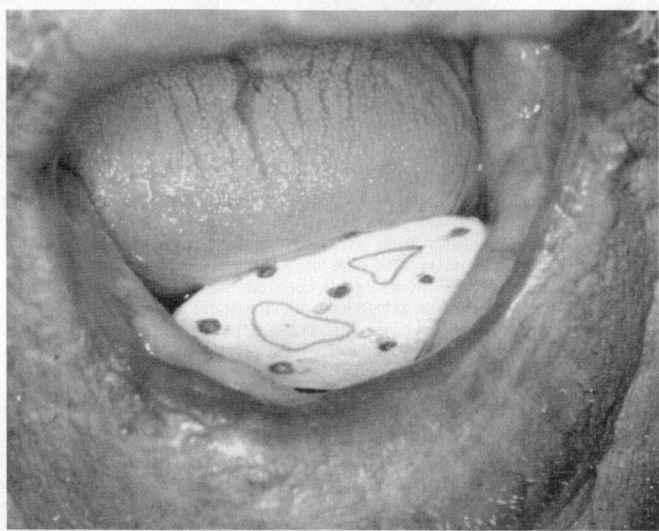

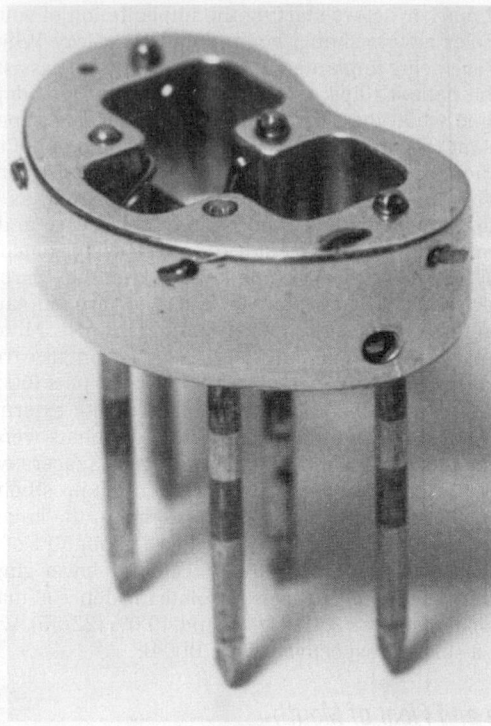

FIGURE 20.22. A: Cardboard template is cut to fit the lesion in floor of mouth. **B:** Customized floor-of-mouth implant device. Needles are secured to the implant device with stainless steel wire passed through the needle eyes. A crossing needle can be mounted through the device if desired. (From Marcus RB Jr., Million RR, Mitchell TP. A preloaded, custom-designed implantation device for stage T1-T2 carcinoma of the floor of mouth. *Int J Radiat Oncol Biol Phys* 1980;6:111–113, with permission.)

Base of Tongue

Because of the possibility of airway obstruction, it is imperative to perform an elective temporary tracheostomy before the implant procedure is initiated. Implantation of the base of the tongue (and sometimes the posterolateral border of the oral tongue) is best accomplished by using long metallic or Teflon catheters with guides inserted through the submaxillary/subdigastric region, with the index finger of the other hand in the oropharynx to verify the position of the guide at the exit point, the base of the tongue. As described earlier, the nylon thread is inserted through the tubing into the oropharynx, looped around, and brought out through the opposite guide, thus providing the equivalent of a "crossing needle" in the cephalad end of the implant (Fig. 20.24A). The metallic guides are withdrawn from the submental region (Fig. 20.24B–D), and

the nylon tubes are secured externally with metallic buttons as described earlier. Occasionally, it is not possible to open the oral cavity adequately, and the only recourse is to perform a submandibular implant with metallic guides and afterloading ^{192}Ir (Fig. 20.25). Double-plane or volume implants can be performed easily. After implant localization x-ray films with dummy sources are taken, afterloading ^{192}Ir wire or seeds in nylon threads are inserted into the nylon tubing or metallic guides, and isodose distributions are obtained (Fig. 20.26A,B).

Tonsillar Region Including Faucial Arch

Fletcher and MacComb (97) described a double-plane pterygomaxillary implant with radium needles to boost the dose in patients with carcinoma of the faucial arch or tonsillar region

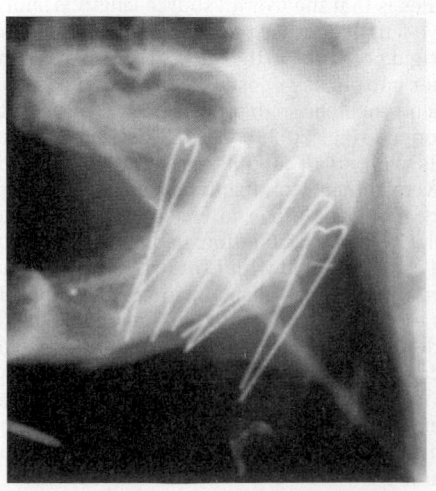

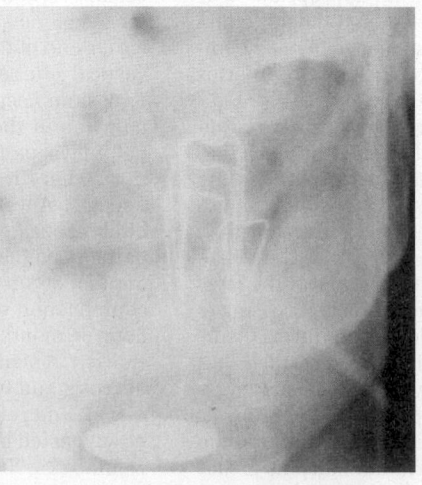

FIGURE 20.23. Roentgenograms of ^{192}Ir hairpin implant for carcinoma of the left side of the oral tongue, stage T2 N0, measuring 3.5 by 2.0 by 2.0 cm, with submucosal extension to within 0.5 cm of the midline of the tongue. Treatment consisted of 30 Gy in 10 fractions, followed by an ^{192}Ir implant using the gutter-guide technique with the patient in a sitting position. A gauze pack was secured onto the lateral floor of the mouth to displace the tongue medially away from the mandible. The implant delivered 40 Gy tumor dose to the area of gross disease (0.55 Gy per hour). The patient remained free of disease at 36 months. (From Parsons JT, Mendenhall WM, Bova FJ, et al. Irradiation techniques for head and neck cancer. In: Levitt SL, Khan FM, Potish RA, eds. *Technological basis of radiation therapy: practical clinical applications*, 2nd ed. Philadelphia: Lea & Febiger, 1992; with permission.)

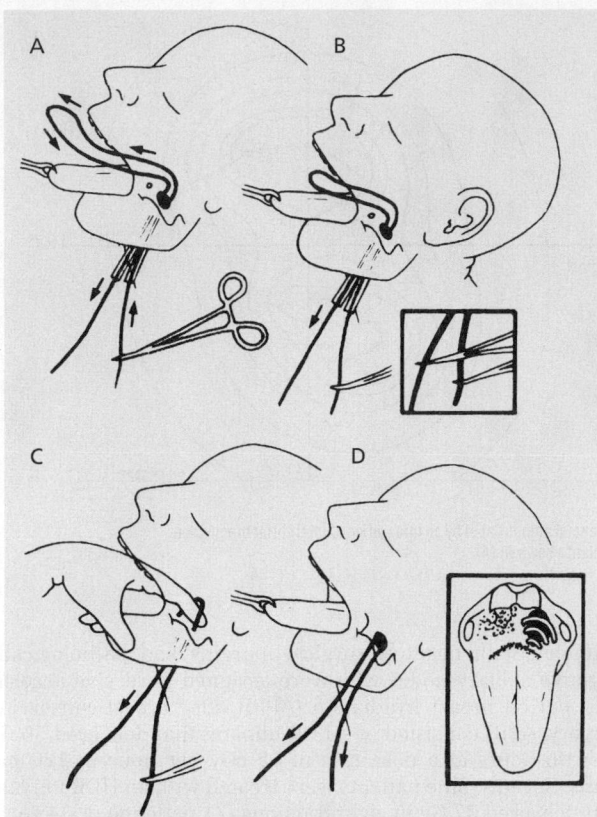

FIGURE 20.24. Diagram illustrating the use of stainless steel guides inserted through the submaxillary region for patients with carcinoma of the left base of the tongue. **A,B:** As described in Fig. 20.21, the nylon tubing is looped around the dorsum of the tongue (**C**), the stainless steel guides are removed, and dummy and later radioactive sources are inserted and secured with metallic buttons (**D**).

with extension into the tongue. ^{192}Ir hairpin or plastic tube techniques have been used by Pierquin et al. (272) and Mazeron et al. (212). The nylon tube technique also may be used to implant the soft palate (86). The iridium hairpin technique is used with one gutter guide placed in the soft palate in the transverse plane and additional gutter guides placed vertically into the anterior tonsillar pillars, depending on the extent of the lesion. Iridium hairpins are afterloaded into the gutter guides, which are removed as described earlier. If the uvula is involved by tumor, it should be amputated before implantation (87). Mendenhall et al. (216) reviewed the techniques for implantation of the anterior tonsillar pillars, soft palate, or tonsillar

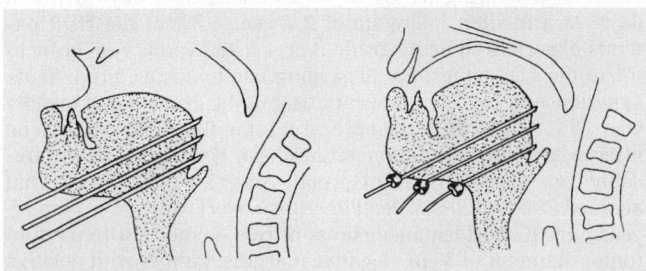

FIGURE 20.25. Submandibular implant with metallic guides in which it was not possible to "loop around" nylon strands over the base of the tongue (one-end technique). The nylon tubing is cut to fit desired tumor volume to be implanted, and metallic buttons are used to secure nylon tubes and guides in position. The buttons are sutured to the skin to ensure the placement of the stainless steel guides.

region using two nylon bars, each containing three full-intensity, 2- to 3-cm active-length radium or cesium needles implanted into the anterior tonsillar pillar and the other 1 cm medial to the tonsillar pillar bar, in the base of the tongue. A crossing needle sometimes is included in the anterior pillar bar to ensure adequate mucosal dose.

Breast

Since 1977, breast conserving surgery plus radiotherapy can be considered as the standard of care for the treatment of early stage breast cancer (93,94,335,336). The standard radiation schedule consist of 45 to 50 Gy delivered after conservative surgery to the whole residual breast parenchyma, with or without the addition of a tumor bed boost. Interstitial brachytherapy has long been in use as boost therapy after whole breast external beam radiotherapy, and, more recently, has been investigated as a possible technique to deliver single modality radiation therapy after lumpectomy (partial breast irradiation) in selected patients.

Partial Breast Brachytherapy Irradiation

The rationale for giving adjuvant whole breast radiotherapy (WBRT) after breast conserving surgery is the attempt to sterilize areas of residual microscopic disease after tumor excision, for frequent multifocality and/or multicentricity of breast cancer. It is well known, in fact, from single institution trials (190,337) as well as from large meta-analysis (81) that postoperative radiation therapy reduce the incidence of local recurrence from 20% to 30% to <10%. In contrast to what has been suggested several times in the past, it has been recently demonstrated that local recurrence has a negative impact on survival (50). If radiotherapy can be considered unavoidable after conservative breast surgery, some questions are raised on the volume of breast parenchyma that has to be treated. The compelling evidence that the vast majority of local recurrences occur in close proximity of the tumor bed (48,95,96,104,178,189,190,305,314,330,338) suggested the possibility to achieve a good local control by irradiating just the tumor bed and the surrounding tissues in the close proximity. On the other hand, in the quadrantectomy arm of the Milan III trial by Veronesi et al. (337), the local recurrence rate outside the tumor bed was only 15%, and this value was no different from the incidence of a contralateral breast cancer. Basically, a certain uniformity emerge in considering the tumors developed in a different quadrant than the primary tumor as second tumors rather than true recurrences (314). WBRT, on the other hand, was demonstrated to have a protective effect on the incidence of ipsilateral recurrence away from the primary site (7%) in comparison to the rate of a new breast cancer in the contralateral breast (14%) (107), but this gain seems to be reduced when we consider the long-term overall survival that seems to be reduced by the insurgence of long-term vascular toxicity that affects women who undergo a total breast irradiation as demonstrated by the Early Breast Cancer Trialists Collaborative Group (81). A brachytherapy partial breast irradiation could offer the chance of reducing the incidence of such long-term vascular side effects by reducing the irradiated volume of chest wall and lung. Besides that, a BRT partial breast approach, if effective, could reduce significantly the overall treatment time from the usual 5 to 6 weeks to <10 days with a consistent reduction of the delay for the other planned adjuvant treatments (chemotherapy). It has also been suggested that partial breast irradiation could reduce the treatment costs, but it seems to be true just for three-dimensional conformal radiation therapy partial breast irradiation and not for the BRT approach (320). Historically, several pioneeristic works were carried out at the beginning of the 1990s: Cionini et al. (47) from the University

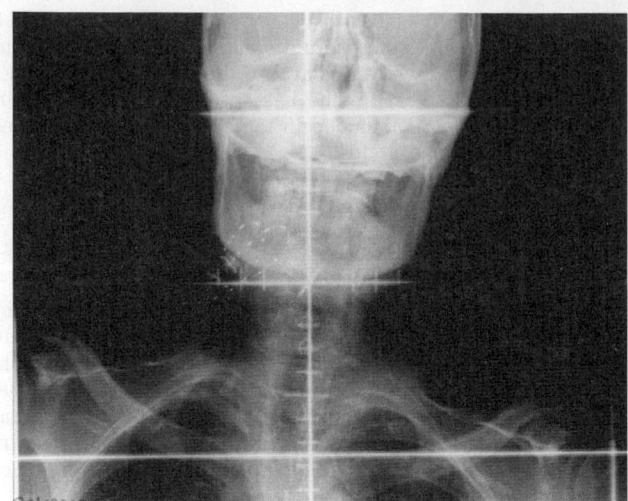
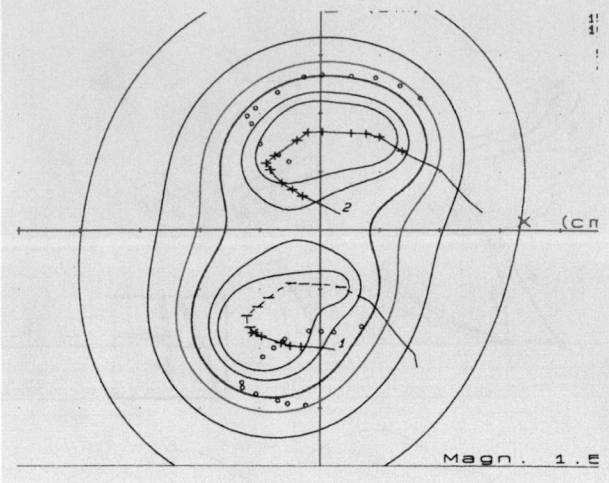

FIGURE 20.26. A: Coronal view of an interstitial implant of a T1 lesion of the faucial arch, treated by an integration of interstitial brachytherapy and external beam. **B:** Coronal view of the isodose distribution of the implant shown in (**A**).

of Pisa treated 115 patients T1-2 N0-1 tumors with quadrantectomy, axillary dissection, and LDR of the involved quadrant, delivering a total dose of 50 to 60 Gy. The study accrued patients independently from their menopausal status. Patients with axillary node involvement received chemotherapy or tamoxifen. Fifteen percent of patients had positive or unknown margins after surgery and 20% had invasive lobular carcinoma. The reported 5-year local recurrence, disease-free survival and overall survival were 6%, 83%, and 96%, respectively. Kuske et al. (179) and King et al. (170) treated 50 patients who had received breast-conserving surgery with brachytherapy alone. Patients were assigned to receive a LDR implant (45 Gy over 3.5 to 6 days) or HDR implant (32 Gy in 8 fractions twice a day). The treated volume included 2 cm of breast parenchyma surrounding the surgical cavity. All patients had tumors smaller than 4 cm with negative margins, one to three axillary node positive patients were admitted as well as ductal carcinoma *in situ* patients. At a median follow-up of 75 months one breast recurrence (2%) and three nodal recurrences (6%) were reported. The most recent update of their experience has been published recently (177), including 150 patients with a mean follow-up of 46 months. They reports 1% of breast failure and 3% of regional node failure. Cosmetic outcomes were good or excellent in 75% of patients. Fentiman et al. (90), from the Guy's Hospital of London, performed two consecutive pilot trials. In the first one (conducted from May 1987 to November 1988), 27 patients were treated with two or three plane LDR implants including a 2-cm margin surrounding the tumor bed. All the implants delivered 55 Gy over 5 to 6 days according the dosimetric rules of the Paris system. With a median follow-up of 6 years, 10/27 (37%) patients experienced a local recurrence (89). In the second study, due to the unacceptable incidence of local failures, adjuvant chemotherapy was administered to the 92% of the 50 enrolled patients. Patients' selection criteria and surgical and implant techniques were similar to the previous study, but in this second study a MDR remote-controlled afterloading system employing ^{137}Cs was used to deliver a total dose of 45 Gy in four fractions over 4 days. At a median follow-up of 6.3 years, 18% of the eligible patients developed a breast relapse. Only one local recurrence (4%) occurred among patients with tumors smaller than 2 cm, whereas the rate of incidence grew to 35% among patients with tumors of 2 cm or larger (88). One of the largest single institution experiences has been recently published by Vicini et al. (339,340). The group was comprised of 199 patients older than 40 years, with infiltrating ductal carcinomas <3 cm in

diameter, with negative surgical margins and pathologically negative axillary nodes who were assigned to receive accelerated partial breast irradiation (APBI) after breast-conserving surgery. APBI consisted of a LDR implant that delivered 50 Gy over 96 hours at a dose rate of 52 cGy per hour in 120 patients. Seventy-nine patients were treated with an HDR implant that delivered 32 Gy in eight fractions (71 patients) or 34 Gy in 10 fractions (eight patients). The treated volume encompassed the surgical margin plus a 2 cm surrounding margin. Seventy percent of the patients received adjuvant chemo- or hormonal therapy. The reported 5-year actuarial ipsilateral recurrence rate was 1%, cosmetic results in those patients who had been followed for 5 years or more were considered to be good or excellent in 99% of cases. These results were compared with those in a matched cohort of 199 patients treated with conventional whole breast RT at the same institution; there were no statistical differences between the two groups in terms of local failure, regional local failure, distant metastases, disease-free survival, overall survival, and cause-specific rates. After these and many other encouraging single institutional experiences, several large multi-institutional trials have been designed.

The Radiation Therapy Oncology Group (RTOG) promoted the first prospective phase I and II trial (RTOG 95-17) of APBI alone after lumpectomy (181). The inclusion criteria included invasive nonlobular tumors ≤3 cm after lumpectomy with negative surgical margins and axillary dissection with zero to three positive axillary nodes without extra capsular extension. One hundred patients were enrolled and received LDR (33 patients) implant delivering 45 Gy in 3.5 to 5 days or HDR implants (66 patients) delivering 34 Gy in 10 fractions in 5 days (twice a day). At a median follow-up of 2.7 years, 3% of the HDR patients experienced acute grade 3 or 4 toxicity, this rate grew to 9% in the LDR subgroup. Regarding late toxicities, no patients experienced grade 4 complications, but the grade 3 late toxicity was 18% for the LDR group and 4% for the HDR group. The interim analysis of another large phase II trial has been published recently (318). The German Austrian multicentric trial accrued 206 patients, selection criteria were: age older than 35 years, ECOG performance status of two or more, a maximum tumor diameter of 3 cm, negative margins, tumors with positive hormones receptors, negative axillary nodes or presence of a single micrometastasis with at least nine nodes having been removed. Irradiation was performed using a PDR technique (0.60 median dose per pulse each hour until a prescribed median total dose of 49.8 Gy) or HDR afterloading device (32 Gy in eight twice-daily fractions). At a median follow-up of 12 months, no patients developed ipsilateral recurrence. One hundred patients were valuable for complications and cosmetic results. Acute toxicity was low: 5% experienced mild radiodermatitis and 1% experienced moderate radiodermatitis. Late toxicity rates were comparably low: 7% of patients experienced mild pain in the irradiated area and 1% developed intermittent but tolerable pain. Mild or moderate fibrosis was palpable in 18% of cases, mild to moderate telangiectasia were found in 8% of patients. On the whole, the cosmetic result was judged good or excellent in 93% of patients. The National Institute of Oncology in Budapest promoted the first phase III trial (279). From 1998 and 2004, 255 patients with unifocal tumors, tumor size of 20 mm or smaller, negative margins, negative axillary nodes (but admitting axillary micrometastases), and histological grade of 1 or 2, were randomized to receive either 50 Gy whole breast radiotherapy or partial breast irradiation. The majority of patients in both arms (70%) received adjuvant hormone therapy. The first interim analysis has not yet been published. Other phase III trials are currently under way: based on the success of the German-Austrian study (318), the Breast Cancer Working Group of the Groupe European de Curietherapie-European Society for Ther-

apeutic Radiology and Oncology is promoting a phase III trial in which patients will be randomized to receive APBI (HDR/PDR implant) or whole breast irradiation (50 to 50.4 Gy plus 10 Gy electron boost). The planned accrual is 1,170 patients. The first patients were randomized in May 2004.

Technically, the major concern in manufacturing a partial breast implant is the adequate coverage of the tumor bed, and it depends basically on a good outline of the surgical cavity. Preplanning of the implant can provide important information on the target geometry and required placement of the source guides. This information may be critical in achieving acceptable target coverage, critical structure avoidance, and dose uniformity throughout the irradiated volume (Fig 20.27A,B,C,D). DeBiose et al. (66) reviewed 60 patients with early stage breast cancer, a portion of whom underwent ultrasonography-assisted placement of interstitial brachytherapy needles. The lumpectomy cavity was outlined in all dimensions, and corresponding skin marks were placed for reference at time of implantation. These dimensions were compared to the physician's clinical estimate of the location of the lumpectomy cavity, the patient's presurgical mammograms, and the position of the scar. In the intraoperative setting, the dimensions of the lumpectomy cavity

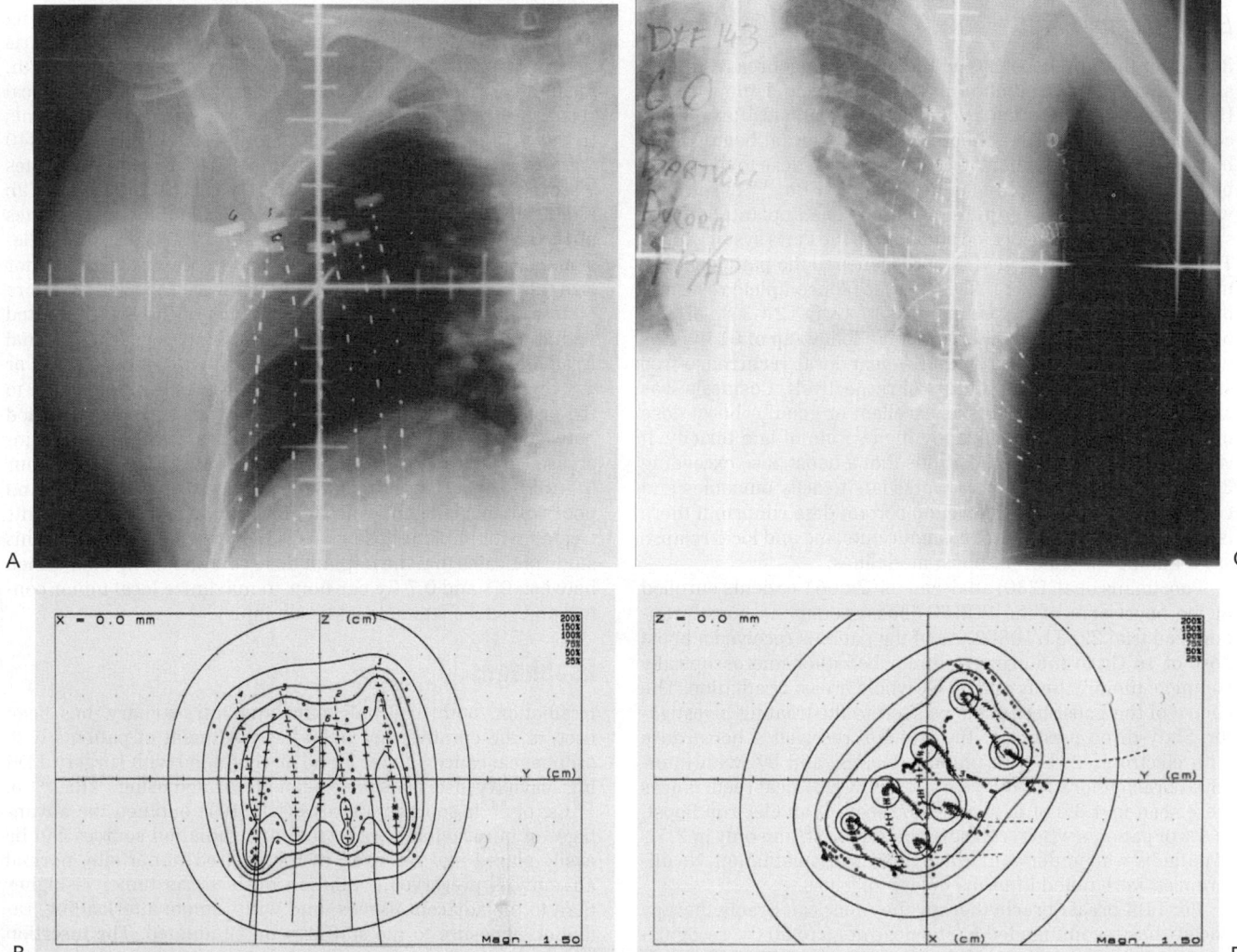

FIGURE 20.27. A: Coronal view of an interstitial implant of breast carcinoma as a boost after external tangential fields. **B:** Coronal isodose distribution of the implant shown in (**A**). **C:** Coronal view of a perioperative implant of breast cancer. The implant was done at the time of surgery and used as a reverse boost, followed by tangential fields external beam radiotherapy. **D:** Isodose distribution on the axial plane for the implant shown in (**C**).

were obtained, and the placement of the deep plane of interstitial needle was verified by ultrasound (350). The full extent of the lumpectomy cavity was underestimated by clinical examination (physical examination, operative report, mammographic information, and location of the scar) in 33/38 patients (87%). The depth of the chest wall also was estimated incorrectly in 34 patients (90%) when compared to ultrasound examination. Intraoperatively, ultrasound was performed on nine patients and was useful in verifying the accurate placement of the deepest plane of interstitial brachytherapy needles. In seven of nine patients, the posterior extent of the lumpectomy cavity was visualized by the intraoperative ultrasound. A variety of modalities have been used for identification of the target volume in preparation for the implant. These include the use of surgical clips, ultrasound, CT, MRI, and intraoperative visualization of the lumpectomy cavity. RTOG 95-17 required that at least six radiopaque clips be left in the cavity at the time of surgery to define the maximal extent of the cavity in three dimensions. Visualization of the clips under fluoroscopy allows the determination of an advantageous direction of approach for the source guides, which may achieve the most conformal coverage of the target volume with the minimum number of source ribbons or wires. Skin marks then are placed to guide the needle insertions. CT, MRI, or ultrasound can be used for the same purpose, with even better visualization of the excision cavity geometry.

Brachytherapy Boost

Radiation therapy boost to the tumor bed after breast surgery and whole breast irradiation have been largely demonstrated. Harms et al. (135) treated a cohort of 113 patients after breast-conserving surgery. All patients received external beam whole breast irradiation (median 50 Gy) plus a boost dose to the tumor bed delivered by PDR brachytherapy (37 G/Bq, ^{192}Ir sources) with a dose rate of 1 Gy/pulse per hour. The implantation and specification were performed similarly to the Paris system rules. The boost dose was graded in accordance to the pathologic tumor characteristics: 20 to 25 Gy in case of incomplete resection or vascular invasion or close margins, 15 Gy in T2-G3 stage. The overall local failure rate after a median follow-up of 61 months was 4.4%. The actuarial 5- and 8-year local recurrence-free survival rates were 95% and 93%, respectively. Cosmesis was rated in 90% of the patients as excellent or good. A boost dose of 25 Gy resulted in significantly higher rate of late toxicity. It was demonstrated since the 1980s that a boost dose exceeding 20 to 25 Gy correlates with a worse late toxicity outcomes and cosmetic results. Furthermore, no certain data confirm if there is any difference in terms of cosmetic outcome and local relapse rates among the different boost modalities.

Poortmans et al. (280) analyzed the 2m661 patients enrolled in the boost arm of the EORTC "boost versus no boost" randomized trial 22881/10882. All of the patients received a boost dose of 16 Gy to the primary tumor bed after microscopically complete tumorectomy and 50 Gy whole breast irradiation. The choice of the boost technique was left to the treating investigator. Sixty-three percent of the patients received a boost dose with electrons, 28% with photons beams, and 9% with interstitial brachytherapy. At 5 years of follow-up, local recurrences were seen in 4.8% of patients who received an electron boost, in 4% of patients who received a photon boost, and only in 2.5% of patients who underwent brachytherapy implantation. No differences were noted in terms of late toxicities.

For LDR breast brachytherapy the American Brachytherapy Society has recommended a total dose of 45 to 50 Gy, recognizing that the dose traditionally has been given at about 10 Gy per day, with a range of about 30 to 70 cGy per hour. Source positioning should be such that the maximum skin dose is no higher than the prescription dose. For brachytherapy used as a boost following 45 to 50 Gy of external beam radiation, a total dose

of 10 to 20 Gy is recommended, also at a rate of 30 to 70 cGy per hour. Typical maximum skin doses for boost implants are about 50% of the prescription dose. A number of variants of the breast implant technique have been described in the literature. In some centers, templates are used to control the spacing of the guide needles. Delclos (72) used only one point of entrance for the guide needles to improve the cosmetic results. Mansfield et al. (198) described an intraoperative technique placing four or five plastic tubes, 2 cm apart, in each of two planes separated by 2 cm at the time of the breast tumor excision. ^{192}Ir seeds, spaced 0.5 cm and with activity of 0.5 mCi per seed per 1 cm, were inserted after the wound was closed, and the position of the dummy sources was determined on localization radiographs. The plastic tubes were loaded with the active sources within 6 hours of surgery. The dose rate was 0.3 to 0.5 Gy per hour; usual dose was 20 Gy delivered in 50 to 60 hours. Ten days later, breast irradiation was begun with tangential fields, 6-MV photons, to deliver 45 Gy at 1.8 Gy per day. The 10-year local tumor-control rates for stage T1 and T2 were 93% and 87%, respectively, and the 10-year disease-free survival rates were 82% and 75%, respectively. Mazeron et al. (213) used a technique for interstitial brachytherapy of the breast with rigid metallic needles inserted through a template in single or double planes. After breast irradiation (45 Gy in 25 fractions), a boost to the primary tumor was prescribed at the 85% basal dose rate (Paris system). Intersource spacing varied from 1.5 to 2 cm. Implanted volume was adapted to tumor extent by varying the number of sources and active length according to the Paris system rules. Linear activity ranged from 1.3 to 1.8 mCi/cm. Mean dose rates were 0.53 Gy per hour for patients with local recurrence and 0.56 Gy per hour for recurrence-free patients ($p <.01$). Of patients, 58 were treated with single-plane and 340 were treated with two-plane implants. Local recurrence rates were 10% for T1 (2/20), 15% for T2a (21/138), 23% for T2b (30/129), and 25% for T3 (13/53). The local tumor-control rates at 15 years were 76% for T1 and T2a and 70% for T2b and T3 lesions. Local tumor control correlated with dose rate and tumor size (Fig. 20.28). Similar observations were reported by Deore et al. (76) in 118 T1 and 171 T2 lesions of the breast treated with radiation therapy after conservative surgery. The external irradiation dose of 43 Gy was delivered with either 2.5 Gy or 1.8 Gy per fraction. A boost dose of 15 to 30 Gy was given to the primary tumor, using interstitial implants; dose rate varied between 0.2 and 1.6 Gy per hour. The local failure rate was increased significantly with implant dose rates <0.3 Gy per hour ($p <.05$). The incidence of late normal tissue complications and poor cosmetic outcome was significantly higher in the patients treated with implant dose rates >1 Gy per hour ($p <.05$). This study indicates that the implant dose rate should be maintained between 0.3 and 0.7 Gy per hour to maximize local tumor control and reduce late normal tissue injury.

Esophagus

Irradiation, both external beam and intracavitary, has been used in the curative and palliative treatment of patients with esophageal cancer, either alone or combined with surgery. LDR intracavitary insertions have been performed using ^{226}Ra, ^{60}Co, ^{137}Cs, or ^{192}Ir sources. Flores et al. (101) outlined the advantages of intracavitary brachytherapy: radiation sources can be easily placed and removed at the desired tumor site; normal anatomy is preserved; radiation dose to the tumor is higher than to the adjacent tissues; and with remote afterloading, radiation exposure to the staff can be eliminated. The insertion technique can be performed as an outpatient procedure under local anesthesia, usually xylocaine spray (1% to 2%), or mild sedation. A soft rubber bougie or French catheter (no. 24 to 26) is inserted, preferably through the nose. The rubber tube is removed, and a 260-cm Teflon-coated guidewire in a 60-cm

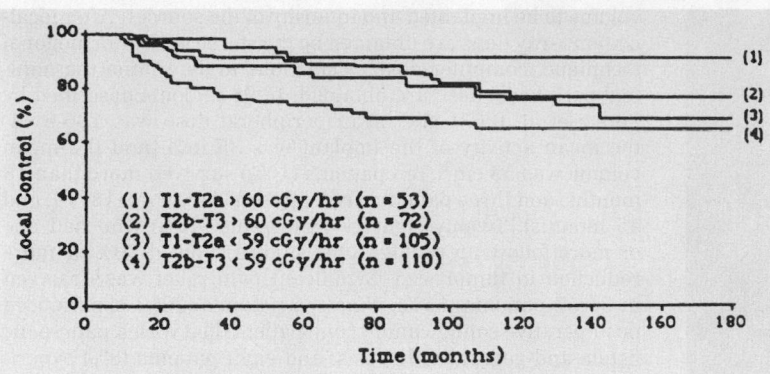

FIGURE 20.28. Local tumor control in patients with breast cancer correlated with dose rate and tumor size (adjusted log rank test). For tumors ≤3.5 cm, local control was 91% for dose rates >0.6 Gy per hour and 69% for dose rates <0.6 Gy per hour. For tumors >3.5 cm local control was 77% and 65%, respectively. The difference is statistically significant at 15 years (p <.05). (From Mazeron JJ, Simon JM, Crook J, et al. Influence of dose rate on local control of breast carcinoma treated by external beam irradiation plus iridium 192 implant. *Int J Radiat Oncol Biol Phys* 1991;21:1183–1187, with permission.)

FA-f10 cut-end feeding tube is inserted to the stomach. The cut-end feeding tube is removed, and the esophageal stricture is dilated to f32 by a balloon dilator (2 minutes required). The balloon dilator is removed, and the esophageal bougie containing dummy markers for intracavitary treatment is placed and secured in the desired position using fluoroscopy. After the position of the dummy sources is verified on radiograph, the patient is taken to the treatment room, where the remote-controlled afterloading device is connected for treatment. If LDR sources are used, the usual dose rate is 0.4 Gy per hour at 0.5 to 1 cm. Depending on the external beam dose given, the total intracavitary dose is prescribed to complete 65 to 70 Gy to the tumor volume. With higher dose rates, corresponding lower treatment times and total doses are used. Isoeffect curves are illustrated in Figure 20.29.

Syed et al. (324) described a comparable technique used in 47 patients with carcinoma of the esophagus (37 with primary and 10 with recurrent lesions). After completion of external irradiation, patients received intraluminal brachytherapy to deliver 30 to 40 Gy at 0.5 cm from the surface of the applicator in two applications, 2 weeks apart. In patients with minimum residual tumor, only one application was used to deliver 20 to 25 Gy minimal tumor dose. Most patients also received concomitant 5-fluorouracil infusion. Intraluminal application was performed with a Syed-Puthawala-Hedger esophageal applicator (Fig. 20.30) consisting of a special tube made of silicone rubber (outer diameter 1 cm) with a conical smooth tip for easy insertion. The central nasogastric tube has six longitudinally placed afterloading catheters to accommodate various radionuclide sources. The total length of the applicator is 65 cm. Marked

rings are present at 10-cm intervals from the tip of the applicator for identification on localization films. The central nasogastric tube can be used for both feeding and suction. The procedure is performed under either general anesthesia or deep sedation and local anesthesia. Determination is made of the proximal and distal end of the tumor from the level of the incisor teeth, on endoscopy, and on review of the initial barium swallow x-ray films. A Robinson catheter (no. 14 or 16) is inserted through one of the nostrils, and its tip is brought out through the mouth. The tip of the esophageal applicator is sutured to the proximal end of the Robinson catheter using "00" silk sutures (Fig. 20.31A). The Robinson catheter is pulled through the mouth until the tip of the esophageal applicator enters the oral cavity. The suture is cut, and the Robinson catheter is discarded while the tip of the esophageal applicator is inserted into the oropharynx and guided along the hypopharynx and esophagus into the stomach (Fig. 20.31B). The esophageal applicator is secured in position by "00" silk sutures through the nasal septum and around the applicator or adhered by adhesive tape. Orthogonal anteroposterior and lateral x-ray films of the chest are obtained after inactive dummy sources have been inserted into the afterloading catheters in the applicator. The location of the tumor is marked on the x-ray films, and appropriate margins are determined to carry out the dose calculations. Radioactive sources are spaced 0.5 to 1 cm, and margins of 3 cm above and below the tumor are allowed. When the dose calculations are completed, the treatment with the active sources is initiated (Fig. 20.31C). A total of 74 procedures were performed. Average survival was 13 months in patients with primary tumors. There were two esophageal strictures, and one patient died of

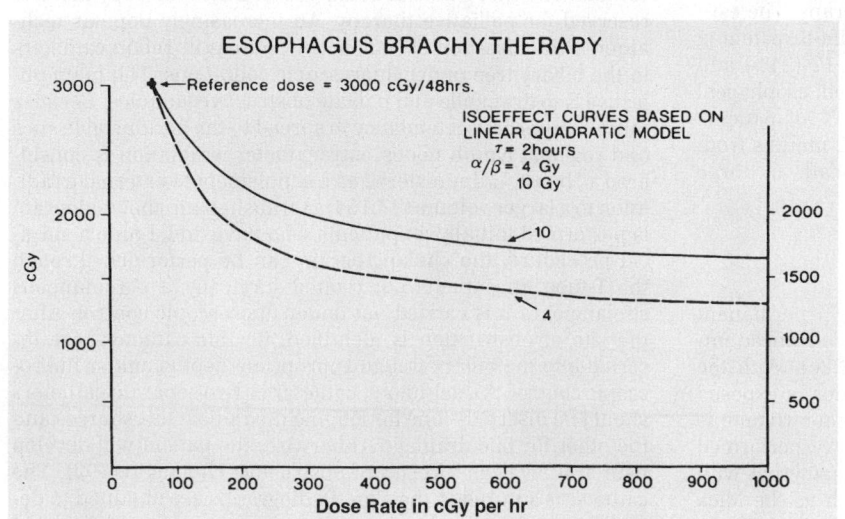

FIGURE 20.29. Isoeffect curves correlated with dose rates. (From Flores AD, Nelems B, Evans K, et al. Impact of new radiotherapy modalities on the surgical management of cancer of the esophagus and cardia. *Int J Radiat Oncol Biol Phys* 1989;18:937–944, with permission.)

Techniques, Modalities, and Modifiers in Radiation Oncology

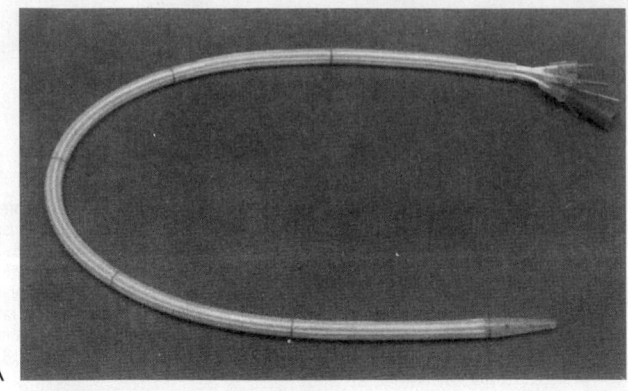

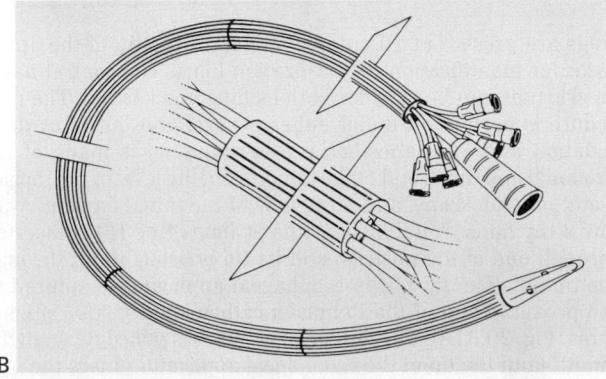

FIGURE 20.30. Syed-Puthawala-Hedger esophageal applicator. (From Syed AMN, Puthawala AA, Severance SR, et al. Intraluminal irradiation in the treatment of esophageal cancer. *Endocurie Hypertherm Oncol* 1987;3:105–113, with permission.)

tracheoesophageal fistula (tumor invaded trachea before treatment).

Gaspar et al. (112) reported on an RTOG study delivering 50-Gy external beam radiation (25 fractions in 5 weeks) followed 2 weeks later by esophageal brachytherapy, either HDR 6 Gy during weeks 8, 9, and 10, for a total of 15 Gy, or LDR 20 Gy during week 8, in patients with esophageal cancer; 45 (92%) had squamous histology and four (6%) had adenocarcinoma. Chemotherapy was given during weeks 1, 5, 8, and 11, with cisplatin 75 mg/m^2 and 5-fluorouracil 1,000 mg/m^2/ 24 hours in a 96-hour infusion; 47 patients (96%) completed external beam radiation plus at least two courses of chemotherapy, whereas 34 patients (69%) were able to complete external beam radiation, and at least two courses of chemotherapy. The estimated survival rate at 12 months was 49%. Life-threatening toxicity or treatment-related death occurred in 12 (24%) and five (10%) cases, respectively. Treatment-related esophageal fistulas occurred in six cases (12% overall, 14% of patients starting esophageal brachytherapy) at 0.5 to 6.2 months from the first day of brachytherapy, leading to death in three cases.

Pancreas

Interstitial irradiation, most frequently using ^{125}I permanent implants, has been used in patients with locally advanced unresectable carcinoma of the pancreas (78,148,226). With the patient under general anesthesia, after the tumor is exposed by the surgeon and biopsies are performed, tumor volume is evaluated and biliary and/or gastric bypasses are performed as required. Multiple seeds are implanted in the pancreas with ^{125}I implantation techniques (with a device such as the Mick applicator), usually at 0.5- or 1-cm intervals, depending on the

volume to be implanted and intensity of the sources. After localization x-ray films are obtained by the stereo shift or orthogonal technique, computer dose calculations to determine the minimal peripheral dose are obtained. In 98 patients described by Peretz et al. (263), the mean peripheral dose was 136.6 Gy, the mean activity of the implant was 35 mCi, and the mean volume was 53 cm^3. Ten patients (10%) survived more than 18 months, and three patients are long-term survivors (18, 19, and 45 months). Twenty-eight of 68 patients (45%) who had one or more follow-up radiographic studies showed 30% or more reduction in tumor size. Significant pain relief was observed in 37/57 patients (65%). Nineteen patients (20%) experienced postoperative complications: one patient died with a pancreatic fistula and generalized sepsis, and eight patients (8%) experienced major complications that included fistula formation, gastrointestinal bleeding, gastrointestinal obstruction, and intra-abdominal abscess. Similar survival results in groups of 12 to 18 patients have been reported by Mohiuddin et al. (222) and Montemaggi et al. (226). Because of putative potential biologic disadvantages of ^{125}I (long half-life and low dose rate), Peretz et al. (263) introduced ^{103}Pd (half-life of 18 days and 20 to 23 keV) as a new isotope for pancreatic implants. Nickers et al. (253) treated 15 patients with biopsy-proven unresectable adenocarcinoma of the pancreas with interstitial ^{103}Pd implants during laparotomy. In 13 patients, the lesion was located in the head of the pancreas, in one patient in the uncinate process, and in one patient in the body of the pancreas. The stage distribution was for T1, two patients; for T2, six patients; and for T3, seven patients. In addition, all patients underwent biliary and gastric bypass. The mean number of ^{103}Pd pellets was 45; the mean total activity to obtain a matched peripheral dose (MPD) of 11,000 cGy was 68.9 mCi. The mean tumor volume encompassing the MPD was 16.5 cc. All patients received postoperative external beam radiation (4,500 cGy over 4.5 weeks) and chemotherapy (5-fluorouracil and mitomycin C). This combined treatment was well tolerated in all patients. Pain relief was obtained within 3 to 6 weeks in 10/12 patients presenting with pain. Survival ranged from 6 to 24 months (median 10 months). Symptom relief appeared to occur faster and complications are significantly less compared to ^{125}I.

Biliary Tree

Erickson and Nag (82) reviewed the use of intraluminal brachytherapy as definitive treatment for unresectable bile duct tumors or as adjuvant therapy after resection. External beam irradiation (45 to 50 Gy) generally is given. Brachytherapy can be given using LDR or HDR via an indwelling biliary drainage catheter to boost external beam doses. Brachytherapy alone is reserved for palliative therapy. An increasingly popular technique is the insertion of radioactive sources in Teflon catheters in the biliary tree under fluoroscopic conditions. The main objective is to drain bile and palliate obstructive jaundice. Because these tumors have a tendency to spread to the periductal tissues and regional lymph nodes, intracatheter irradiation is considered a "boost," administered as a supplement to external irradiation to a larger volume (92,154). A transhepatic cholangiogram is performed initially; in patients who have undergone a surgical procedure, the cholangiogram can be performed through the T-tube. In patients not treated surgically, a percutaneous cholangiogram is carried out under fluoroscopic control. After the site of obstruction is identified, flexible catheters are inserted into the biliary tree to appropriate depths, under fluoroscopic control. A dual-lumen catheter or two separate catheters should be inserted—one for lodging the radioactive sources and the other for bile drainage. Otherwise, the patient will develop pain and fever as a result of obstructive cholangitis (92). The catheter is sutured to the skin. Radiographs are obtained to determine the length of active radioactive sources to be inserted

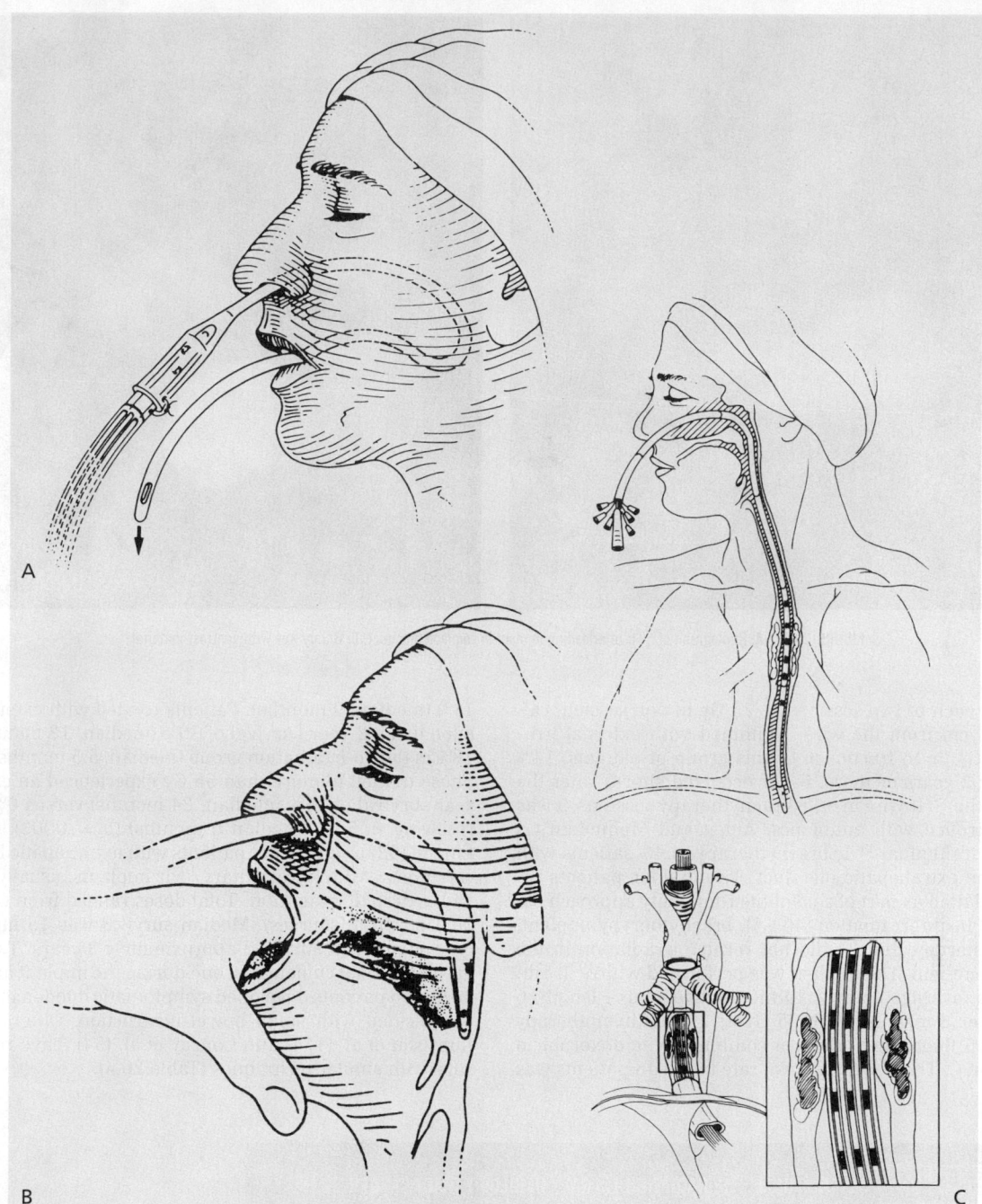

FIGURE 20.31. A: The tip of the applicator is sutured to the Robinson catheter. **B:** Esophageal applicator is being guided into the hypopharynx and the esophagus. **C:** Radioactive sources shown against the tumor. (Syed AMN, Puthawala AA, Severance SR, et al. Intraluminal irradiation in the treatment of esophageal cancer. *Endocurie Hypertherm Oncol* 1987;3:105–113, with permission.)

and the exact position of the catheter for dosimetric purposes (Fig. 20.32). Doses of 20 to 30 Gy are delivered at 1 cm from the catheter. This is combined with external irradiation (45 to 50 Gy) to encompass the periductal tissues and regional lymph nodes. If intracavitary irradiation alone is used, the doses with this modality are 60 to 65 Gy at 1 cm. Montemaggi et al. (227) evaluated 31 patients with unresectable extrahepatic bile duct or pancreatic cancer treated with intraluminal brachytherapy (ILBT) exclusively or as part of a definitive treatment regimen. ILBT was performed with transhepatic percutaneous drainage in four patients and with endoscopic retrograde cholangiopancreatography in 27. Fourteen patients with no metastases, an Eastern Cooperative Oncology Group performance score of ≤2,

and good hematologic parameters received combined modality treatment: 30-Gy ILBT and 45-Gy external beam radiation therapy with continuous infusion of 5-fluorouracil. Seventeen patients underwent 50-Gy ILBT alone for palliation. No direct treatment-related acute toxic reactions were seen. Three patients had cholangitis early in the study. Three patients had late gastrointestinal bleeding. Jaundice was palliated in all patients; pain in 11/13 patients. The survival rate in patients with extrahepatic bile duct cancer was 62% at 2 years for combined modality treatment. No patient with pancreatic cancer lived for longer than 2 years. Meerwaldt et al. (215) reported on 42 patients with bile duct tumors treated with one or two brachytherapy sessions and external irradiation. A dose of 15 Gy was

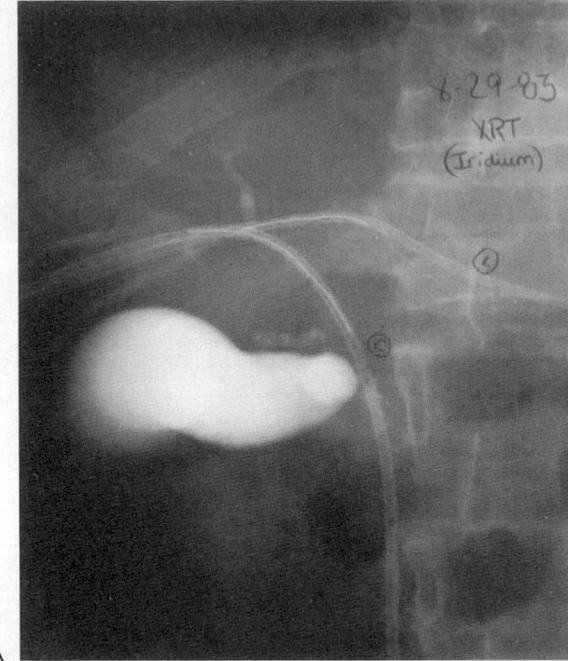 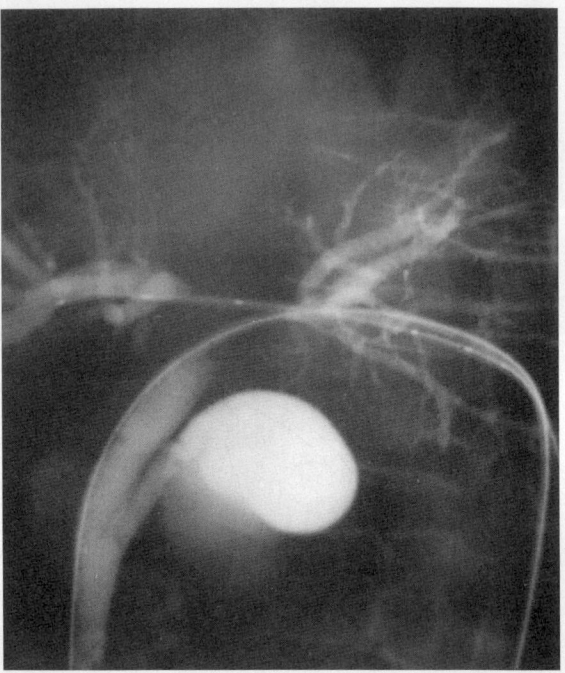

FIGURE 20.32. A: Radiograph of ^{192}Ir afterloading implant in common bile duct. **B:** Biliary tree with contrast material.

delivered at each of two sessions or 25 Gy in one session, calculated at 1 cm from the wire, combined with external irradiation (40 Gy in 16 fractions). Of this group of patients, 14% survived for 2 years or more. Fever occurred shortly after the insertion of the ^{192}Ir wire in 6/38 brachytherapy sessions; it was usually controlled with antibiotics. Alden and Mohiuddin (2) evaluated intraluminal ^{192}Ir brachytherapy in 48 patients with cancer of the extrahepatic bile duct. Twenty-four patients received irradiation as part of a combined-modality approach using external beam irradiation (46 Gy), brachytherapy implant, and chemotherapy, and 24 did not receive irradiation in the course of treatment. The implant was performed with ^{192}Ir ribbon sources (average activity, 29 mCi; active source length, 6 cm) to deliver a mean dose of 25 Gy at 1 cm. Chemotherapy consisted of 5-fluorouracil alone or combined with doxorubicin or mitomycin C. The 2-year survival rate for all 48 patients was

18% (median, 9 months). Patients treated with external irradiation had a 2-year survival of 30% (median, 12 months) versus 18% in the no-irradiation group (median, 5.5 months) ($p = .01$). Those treated to more than 55 Gy experienced an extended 2-year survival of 48% (median, 24 months) versus 0% for those receiving <55 Gy (median 6 months) ($p = .0003$). Fields and Emami (92) treated eight patients with extrahepatic biliary duct carcinomas with intracavitary ^{192}Ir implants, usually combined with external irradiation. Total doses ranged from 60 to 76 Gy (at 1 cm from sources). Median survival was 15 months, and only one patient survived approximately 3 years. Two patients developed fatal cholangitis, one during the implant and another later; two patients developed symptomatic duodenal ulcers, one complicated with small bowel obstruction. Others, including Kopelson et al. (174) and Conroy et al. (54), have reported results with similar techniques (Table 20.4).

Table 20.4	**INTRALUMINAL [192]IR RADIATION THERAPY IN BILIARY TRACT CANCER**				

Author (Reference)	No. of Patients	Radiation Dose (Gy)	Patients with External Beam Also	Local Failures	Alive ≥2 Years
Fletcher (100)	8	40 to 48	0/8	3	0[a]
Herskovic et al. (142)[b]	15	50 + 10 to 16	11/15	3	0[c]
Alden & Mohiuddin (2)	48	46	24/48	—	18%
Fritz et al. (108)	30	45 + 20	21/30	—	18%
Meerwaldt et al. (215)	35	40 + 25	35/35	—	14%
Fields & Emami (92)	8	60 to 75	8/8	6	1 patient
Druy et al. (79)[d]	7	19.5 to 46.69	6/7	5[e]	0

[a]Two alive at 22+ and 23+ months.
[b]Data from Duke University include only primary bile duct cases.
[c]One alive at 18+ months.
[d]The data of Druy et al. include five extrahepatic biliary duct primary tumors and two local recurrences of adenocarcinoma of the ampulla of Vater.
[e]Including local persistence and local recurrence.
Modified from Kopelson G, Gunderson LL. Primary and adjuvant radiation therapy in gallbladder and extrahepatic biliary tract carcinoma. *J Clin Gastroenterol* 1983;5:43–50.

Soft-Tissue Sarcomas

External radiation therapy in soft-tissue sarcomas combined with limb-preservative surgery has been successful in achieving the same results as those obtained with radical surgical resection. Interstitial brachytherapy can successfully eradicate microscopic or minimal macroscopic residual sarcomas. The theoretic advantages of such a combination include:

(a) Less extensive surgery;

(b) Synchronous brachytherapy, which allows aggressive treatment of residual malignant cells at a time when these cells still are oxygenated and before they are embedded in scar tissue;

(c) Placing of the implant plane(s) on the residual tumor (bed), which ensures that this site will receive the highest irradiation dose;

(d) Short treatment (4 to 5 days) completed before the discharge of the patient from the hospital, which presents a considerable medical, psychologic, and economic advantage; and

(e) Feasibility even when surgery and external beam irradiation have previously failed (246).

The American Brachytherapy Society (ABS) guidelines recommend brachytherapy as the sole radiation therapy only for patients with completely resected intermediate or high-grade sarcomas of the extremity or superficial trunk, with negative margins (246). Contraindications for sole therapy include the inability to cover the entire target volume, normal tissue tolerance concerns, positive margins, or skin ulceration indicating extensive cutaneous spread via lymphatics. Brachytherapy as a boost to wide-field external beam therapy is recommended for patients with intermediate or high-grade sarcoma with either negative or positive margins, and it can be considered for patients with low-grade sarcoma and postoperatively for patients with small lesions having positive or uncertain margins, possible surgical field contamination, or deep lesions. [192]Ir seeds or wire usually are used for soft-tissue sarcoma implants, but ^{125}I also has been used and may be advantageous. After surgical removal of the tumor, the overlying skin and soft tissues collapse onto the underlying structures. This composite slab of tissues forms the clinical target volume (CTV). Radiopaque markers such as surgical clips should be placed at the time of surgery to identify the extent of the CTV radiographically. The

guide needles are inserted through the normal skin (at least 1 cm from the incision) after surgical resection but before completion of any reconstruction and wound closure. The parallel needles are spaced uniformly at 1.0 to 1.5 cm apart and embedded in the depth of the operative field. If preordered seeds or wires of known activity are to be used, the needle spacing required to deliver a dose of about 10 Gy per day to the CTV can be estimated using the Anderson planar implant nomogram or comparable dosimetry system (327). The ABS recommends that catheter placement should extend at least 1 to 2 cm outside the CTV in the direction lateral to the catheters and 2 to 5 cm along the catheter length (246). After placement of the guide needles, the closed end of each afterloading catheter is threaded through the needle until it emerges from the opposite end of the needle. The needle is withdrawn while holding the catheter in place until the needle is out of the skin. Radiopaque clips are placed near the blind end of each afterloading catheter for later identification of this end on localization radiographs. The catheters are individually secured to the skin by means of a stainless steel button that is threaded over the catheter, fixed to it by crimping, and anchored to the underlying skin by silk sutures. Because of the anticipated effects of the radiation, wound closure requires extra planning and care to avoid undue tension predisposing to wound breakdown. To further diminish wound complications, the ABS recommends that the loading of the radioactive sources should be delayed at least 5 days after surgery for implants used as sole radiotherapy but that loading may take place within 2 to 3 days of surgery if a brachytherapy dose <20 Gy is to be given as a supplement to EBRT. After the surgical procedure is completed, orthogonal radiographs of the CTV with dummy seeds inserted in the catheters are obtained for treatment planning purposes (Fig. 20.33A,B). If available, CT or MRI images can provide more detailed information for treatment planning. Isodose curves should be generated in planes approximately perpendicular to the source ribbons at intervals of 1.0 cm or less. The CTV should be drawn on the isodose planes, and the isodose line giving satisfactory coverage of the CTV on all planes should be selected as the prescription. Sources can be especially ordered with activities selected to scale the prescription dose rate to deliver 10 Gy per day (or any other desired dose rate), or if preordered sources are used, the calculated prescription dose rate must be used to determine the required treatment time. For LDR brachytherapy as sole

Techniques, Modalities, and Modifiers in Radiation Oncology

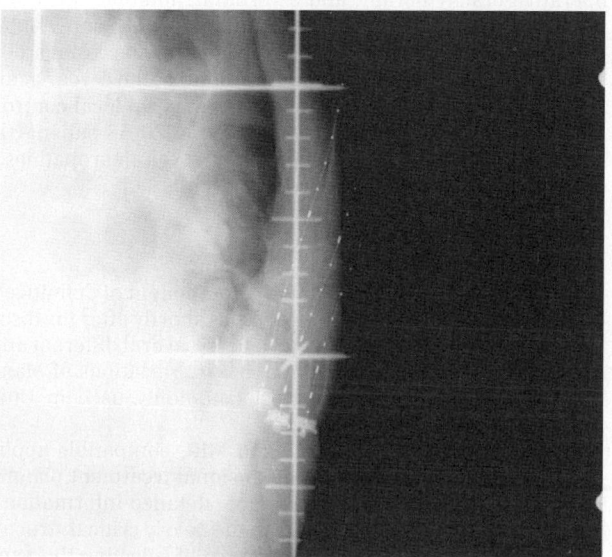
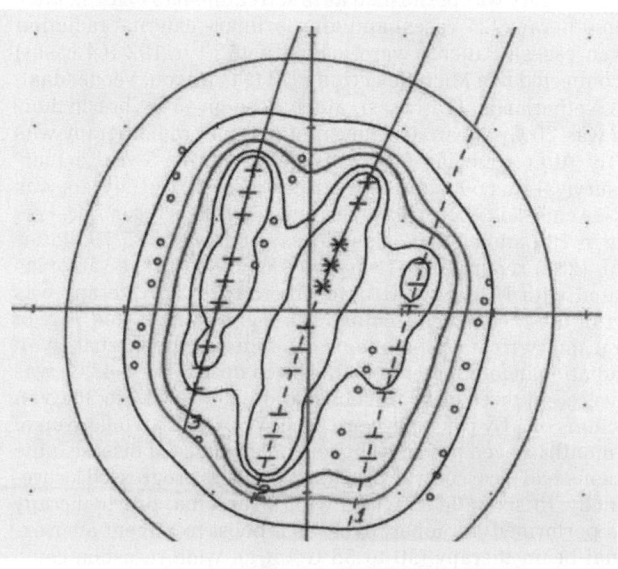

FIGURE 20.33. A: Anterior posterior oblique of a perioperative interstitial implant of a high-grade, small-dimension, soft-tissue sarcoma of the right arm. **B:** Isodose distribution on a coronal plane of the implant shown in **(A)**.

adjuvant radiotherapy, the ABS recommends a dose of 45 to 50 Gy delivered over 4 to 6 days. For implants providing a boost to an external beam dose of 45 to 50 Gy at 1.8 to 2.0 Gy per day, a boost dose of 15 to 25 Gy should be delivered in 2 to 3 days. For correlation of implant quality with clinical outcome, the ABS encourages the calculation of dose–volume histograms for the CTV and suggests that the dose covering 90% and 100% of the CTV should be recorded along with the percentage of the CTV receiving 100%, 150%, and 200% of the prescribed dose (246). For additional technical details the reader is referred to Hilaris et al. (146). Pisters et al. (276) reported on 164 patients with soft-tissue sarcomas randomized to receive or not receive brachytherapy after complete wide local tumor resection (78 and 86 patients in either group, respectively). A target region in the tumor bed was identified by adding 2 cm to the superior and inferior dimensions and 1.5 to 2 cm in the medial and lateral directions. Afterloading catheters were placed approximately 1 cm apart. Implant dose was 42 to 45 Gy for 4 to 6 days using ^{192}Ir. Sources were loaded on the fifth or sixth postoperative day to decrease interference with wound healing. There were 13/78 local recurrences in patients (16%) receiving brachytherapy and 25/86 in patients (29%) treated with surgery only. Actuarial estimates of local recurrence at 60 months were 18% in the brachytherapy and 31% in the no-irradiation group. It is likely that the prescribed dose of irradiation was not adequate to eliminate microscopic disease, and higher doses (55 to 60 Gy) would have been more effective.

Kaled et al. (167) evaluated 202 adult patients with primary high-grade soft-tissue sarcoma of the extremities treated with limb-sparing surgery and adjuvant brachytherapy. All patients underwent complete gross resection, but the margin of resection was microscopically positive in 18% of patients. The median dose of brachytherapy was 45 Gy delivered over 5 days. Tumors located in the shoulder or groin were defined as central location. With a median follow-up of 61 months, the 5-year local control, distant relapse–free survival, and overall survival rates were 84%, 63%, and 70%, respectively. The 5-year actuarial rates of wound complications requiring reoperation, bone fracture, and grade ≥3 nerve damage were 12%, 3%, and 5%, respectively. Llacer et al. (191) evaluated intraoperative brachytherapy in the management of soft-tissue sarcomas involving neurovascular structures. Ninety-eight patients received an intraoperative implant in conjunction with conservative surgery. Brachytherapy was part of the initial treatment (79 cases) or performed in recurrent disease (19 cases). Conservative surgery was performed as first treatment (51 cases), after chemotherapy (21 cases) and after primary external radiation (seven cases). Patients were loaded with ^{192}Ir 192 (64 cases) or connected to a MicroSelectron PDR (NucleTron, Veenendaal, The Netherlands) (15 cases). Mean dose given by brachytherapy was 20 Gy. Mean dose given of external radiotherapy was 46 Gy. After a median follow-up of 58 months, 5-year actuarial survival was 69% and local disease-free rate at 5 years was 90%. Acute side effects occurred in 22/79 requiring surgical repair in 10 patients. Late side effects occurred in 35/79. Potter et al. (283) reported on 12 patients with soft-tissue sarcomas treated with HDR or PDR brachytherapy. Brachytherapy was part of the recurrence treatment in eight patients and part of the primary treatment alone or combined with external beam irradiation in four patients. With HDR a dose of 15 to 43 Gy was delivered in three to 16 fractions, and with PDR 13 to 36 Gy in fractions of 1 Gy per hour were used. With median follow-up of 14 months, seven patients showed no evidence of disease, nine patients had local control, and three patients progressed locoregionally. In six patients with Ewing's sarcoma, brachytherapy was performed intraoperatively as a boost treatment after external beam therapy (50 to 55 Gy) if no wide resection could be achieved. A dose of 10 to 12 Gy was applied in one fraction to a limited volume (20 to 50 cm^3) at the time of surgery with

median follow-up of 21 months. All patients were disease free, and perioperative and subacute morbidity were not increased. Lazzaro (184) evaluated 42 patients treated with a combination of surgery and BRT alone (18 patients) or BRT/external beam radiotherapy (24 patients) for the treatment of primary ($n = 32$) and recurrent ($n = 10$) soft-tissue sarcomas located in the proximal extremity ($n = 17$), distal extremity ($n = 17$), and trunk ($n = 8$). The median BRT dose delivered was 15 Gy, and the median external beam irradiation dose was 50 Gy. With a median follow-up of 34 months, the 36-month survival was 83.9%, and the local control was 89%. Brachytherapy (15 to 20 Gy with LDR) was combined with external irradiation (45 to 50 Gy) either preoperatively or postoperatively by Schray et al. (306). Margins beyond the tumor were 5 to 10 cm axially or along tissue planes and 2 to 4 cm radially or perpendicular to tissue planes. Brachytherapy was performed with standard nylon afterloading tubes positioned to encompass the boost volume with a 2- to 4-cm margin. The boost volume was considered to be the tumor bed after preoperative irradiation and the surgical bed and incision if no previous irradiation had been given. With rare exceptions (distal extremities, groin), needles were placed transversely to the incision (and axis of the extremity) under direct visualization of the tumor bed and with entry and exit points outside the tumor and surgical bed. Needles commonly were placed in contact with bone and neurovascular structures and were maintained in place by skin fascia and muscle; sutures rarely were used. After the implant was in place, skin was closed with sutures. Implants were loaded postoperatively with ^{192}Ir 72 to 96 hours later; the sources were placed 1 cm deep to the skin surface along the tube axis. Average implant activity was 107 mCi, and a portion of the implants used two or more planes. The average dose rate was 48.6 cGy per hour, average time was 44.2 hours, and dose was 20.52 Gy. In 63 patients, 65 brachytherapy procedures were performed. With median follow-up of 20 months, there were two local failures in 56 patients (4%) initially treated and in three of nine patients treated for recurrent tumors. Two of 40 implants (5%) performed at initial resection followed by postoperative irradiation led to wound complications, in contrast to 4/16 implants (25%) performed at resection after preoperative external irradiation. LDR intraoperative brachytherapy has been used as a boost in primary tumors. The mean brachytherapy dose was 20 Gy and external beam irradiation dose was 45 Gy. Delannes et al. (67) reported on a group of 58 patients with primary sarcomas treated by a combination of conservative surgery, intraoperative brachytherapy, and external irradiation. Most of the tumors were located in the lower limbs (46/58, or 79%). Median size of the tumor was 10 cm, most of the lesions being T2-3. With a median follow-up of 54 months, the 5-year actuarial survival was 64.9%, with a 5-year actuarial local control of 89%. Wound healing problems occurred in 20/58 patients, late side effects occurred in 16/58 patients (seven neuropathies G2 to G4). No amputations were required.

Uterine Cervix

Brachytherapy has been a standard component of definitive radiation therapy for cervical cancer since shortly after the discovery of radium. Although there have been several different applicator systems and prescription methods, variations of Manchester system have been the most commonly used in United States.

With the development of CT and MRI, compatible applicators, and computerized three-dimensional treatment planning, it is now possible to obtain much mote detailed information regarding tumor coverage and dose to the nearly critical structure. Fletcher (98) illustrated the importance of selecting the appropriate diameter for cylinders or colpostats and the length for intrauterine tandems. Use of a colpostat or vaginal cylinder with the largest clinically indicated diameter will yield the highest tumor dose at the depth for a given mucosal dose. It is extremely important to keep in mind the surface dose because excessive irradiation to the vaginal mucosa (maximum 150 Gy total dose to the proximal and 90 Gy total dose to the distal vagina) may result in severe mucosal atrophy, fibrosis, and vaginal stenosis or necrosis (150). Similarly, longer tandems will result in improved doses delivered to the lateral parametrium and pelvic lymph nodes. The internal radiation treatments are delivered in a dedicated surgical suite in the department of radiation oncology. Intracavitary insertions in carcinoma of the cervix are performed under general, spinal, or local (block) anesthesia. The patient is placed in the lithotomy position, and a complete bimanual pelvic and rectal examination is performed. After adequate preparation, sterile fields are draped, the cervix is grasped with a tenaculum, and the uterus is sounded carefully to prevent a perforation. Bimanual pelvic examination is extremely helpful in determining the position of the uterus and the probe or sound. In most patients, dilatation and curettage is performed at the time of the first intracavitary insertion (if not performed at initial workup). Mayr et al. (208) described the use of osmotic dilators (laminaria) for gradual nontraumatic dilation of the cervical canal for brachytherapy in gynecologic cancer patients without the use of general/regional anesthesia. Discomfort is minimal in all cases. Radiopaque markers (lead shots or metallic clips) are placed in the anterior and posterior lips of the cervix. The tandem is inserted into the uterus to the appropriate depth (as determined by a stopper), and subsequently each ovoid is inserted gently to prevent injury to the vaginal mucosa. If ideally inserted in the patient, the tandem should be in the midline or as nearly as possible equidistant from the lateral pelvic wall, and the vaginal colpostats should be symmetrically positioned against the cervix in relation to the tandem (Fig. 20.34A,B). The tandem should be kept along the sagittal axis of the pelvis, equidistant from the pubis, sacral promontory, and lateral pelvic wall as allowed by the geometry of the patient and the tumor to avoid overdosage to the bladder, rectosigmoid, or either ureter. After the tandem and colpostat positions are judged to be correct, careful packing of the vagina with iodoform gauze should be performed. A small amount of packing in front of and behind the colpostats (mak-

ing sure overpacking will not separate the cervix from the colpostats) will decrease the dose to the bladder base and the anterior rectal wall. An indwelling Foley catheter should be inserted into the bladder; 7 mL of radiopaque contrast material in the Foley balloon will aid in determining a point dose to the bladder neck (157). After the patient recovers from anesthesia, anteroposterior and lateral x-ray films of the pelvis are obtained to document the position of the applicator, and isodose curves are generated. Doses are prescribed as indicated (see Chapters 6 and 61). Corn et al. (57), in a prospective study of 15 patients with cervical cancer treated with external irradiation and brachytherapy on whom pelvic radiographs were obtained before afterloading and after removal of the ^{137}Cs sources (median duration of insertion, 56.5 hours), documented an average 3-mm shift of the applicator. The changes in median dose resulting from source movement were 1.4% to point A, 1.7% to point B, 0.9% to pelvic lymph nodes, 1.9% to the bladder, and 2.6% to the rectum. Thus, applicator movement during LDR brachytherapy does not result in significant dose changes that could have an impact on tumor control or complication rate. Corn et al. (58,59) used a database from two Philadelphia institutions to assess the acute morbidity associated with the implantation of tandems and colpostats in women with carcinoma of the cervix; to determine factors that predispose to the development of such complications; and to assess whether the use of ultrasound allowed the apparatus to be safely implanted in women at relatively high risk for perforation of hollow viscous organs among 143 tandems/colpostats inserted into 100 women. Twenty patients had insertion under ultrasound guidance because of stenotic cervical os, fibrosis from external beam irradiation, indeterminate orientation of endometrial cavity axis, or previous perforation. Intraoperative complications occurred in 7/143 placements (5%). These included uterine perforations, vaginal lacerations, and one instance of bladder perforation. Only older age, whether entered as a continuous or a dichotomous variable, was associated statistically with these complications. Perioperative complications (e.g., fever, bowel obstruction, exacerbation of chronic obstructive pulmonary disease, cardiac complication) occurred in 54/143 implanted women. In univariate analysis, older age and underlying chronic obstructive pulmonary disease appeared to be associated with

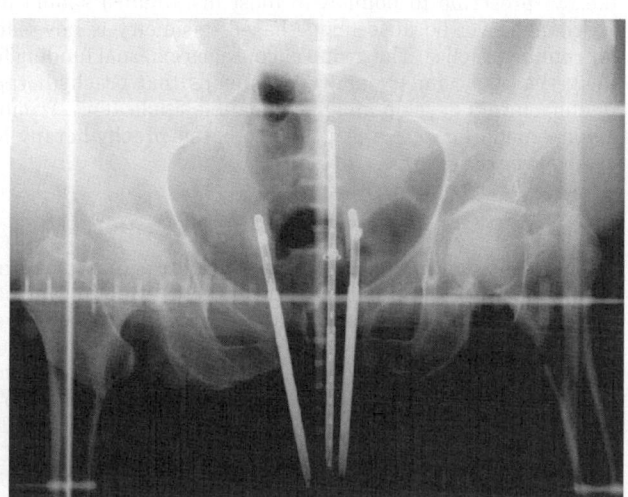

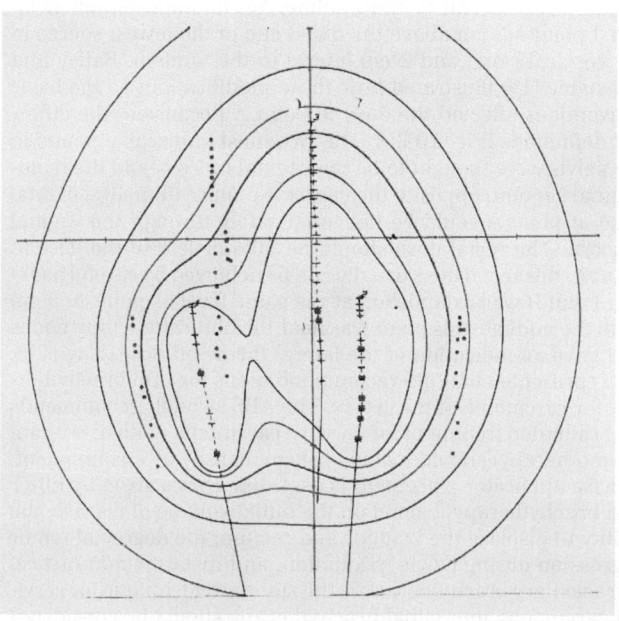

A   B

FIGURE 20.34. A: Anteroposterior view of intracavitary insertion for carcinoma of the uterine cervix. **B:** Coronal isodose distribution of the implant shown in **(A)**.

perioperative complications. A multivariate analysis showed that underlying chronic obstructive pulmonary disease predisposed to perioperative complications during the first implant, and that age over 60 years independently predicted for complications during any implant. Intraoperative complications are relatively rare events. Ultrasonography seems to allow safe intrauterine insertion of the tandem despite the selection of difficult cases for this adjunctive imaging tool. Patient age over 60 years independently predicts for perioperative complications. Chronic obstructive pulmonary disease predicts for perioperative complications during the first but not the second implant, implying that physicians are able to optimize the medical management of pulmonary disease to allow a second implant to be performed more safely (59).

Brachytherapy Systems for Carcinoma of the Cervix

Initially, three systems for brachytherapy in carcinoma of uterine cervix were developed: the Paris, the Swedish, and the Manchester systems (Fig. 20.35) (218,230). The systems differ in the type of applicator used, strength of the source, and time of administration (230). In the United States, most systems used are derivations of the Manchester technique. Dosimetric systems are set of rules, specific to a radioisotope and its spatial distribution in the applicator to deliver a defined dose to a designated region. The Manchester intracavitary system, introduced by Tod and Meredith (328) in 1938, define treatments in terms of dose to a point representative of the target using a dosimetric field quantity, total exposure at point A, to prescribe treatment rather than milligram hours. To define the actual dose delivered in "fixed mg-hour systems" in a more meaningful way, Tod and Meredith began to calculate the dose (in roentgens) to various sites in the pelvis by defining a series of points anatomically comparable from patient to patient. Limiting dose factor was not the dose to the critical structures, such as the rectum or bladder, but to the area, paracervical triangle, in the medial edge of the broad ligament where uterine vessels cross the ureter. Point A was defined as being 2 cm above the mucous membrane of the lateral vaginal fornix and 2 cm lateral to the center of the uterine canal. It was considered that the tolerance of this paracervical triangle is the main limiting factor in the irradiation of uterine cervix. A subsequent arbitrary convention defined point A as being 2 cm above the external cervical os and 2 cm lateral to the midline. Yet another definition located point A 2 cm above the distal end of the lowest source in the cervical canal and 2 cm lateral to the tandem. Batley and Constable (19) illustrated how these modifications to the basic conventions affected the dose to point A because of the different definitions (Fig. 20.36). The two most vulnerable points in the pelvis were thought to be the vaginal mucosa and the rectovaginal septum, opposite the cervix. No more than 40% of total dose at point A could be delivered safely through the vaginal mucosa. The rectal dose should be 80% or less of the dose at point A; this rectal dose usually can be achieved by careful packing. Point B was established at the same level as point A, 5 cm from the midline; this point was near the obturator lymph nodes and gave an indication of the lateral throw-off dose. Nag et al. (237) presented the ABS recommendations for LDR brachytherapy for carcinoma of the cervix. The ABS strongly recommends that radiation treatment for cervical carcinoma (with or without chemotherapy) should include brachytherapy as a component. Precise applicator placement is essential. Doses given by EBRT and brachytherapy depend on the initial volume of disease, the ability to displace the bladder and rectum, the degree of tumor regression during pelvic irradiation, and institutional practice. Intracavitary brachytherapy is the standard technique for cervical carcinoma; interstitial brachytherapy should be considered for patients with disease that cannot be optimally encompassed by intracavitary brachytherapy. The ABS recommends completion of treatment within 8 weeks because prolonging total treatment duration can adversely affect local tumor control and survival. Suggested dose and fractionation schemes for combining the EBRT with LDR brachytherapy for each stage of disease are presented. Dose rates of 0.50 to 0.65 Gy per hour are suggested for intracavitary brachytherapy. Dose rates of 0.50 of 0.70 Gy per hour to the periphery of the implant are suggested for interstitial implant. Use of differential source activity minimizes excessive central dose rates. The dose prescription point (point A) is defined for intracavitary insertions. The ABS recommends reporting the following parameters:

1. For intracavitary insertions: the prescription, including the prescribed dose to point A, dose rate, implant duration, radionuclide used, sources' strengths, and loading pattern; the type of applicator used; doses to vaginal dose points (vaginal surface and depth); doses to rectal and bladder points; and dose to the pelvic wall, point PW.
2. For interstitial implants: the prescription, including the prescribed dose, dose rate, implant duration, radionuclide used, sources' strengths, and loading patterns; the type of applicator used; the volume encompassed by the prescribed isodose surface; the maximum significant dose; and the rectal and bladder doses if assessed.

Considerations for future image-based dosimetry also are noted. Nag et al. (236) recommended T_2-weighted MRI using a pelvic surface coil with MRI-compatible brachytherapy applicators in place for image-based intracavitary brachytherapy for cervical cancer. Imaging must be performed with the patient in the treatment position. Future use of PET or PET/CT may obviate the need for special applicators. The GTV((I)) is defined as the gross tumor volume assessed through imaging, GTV is defined as the GTV((I)) plus any clinically visualized or palpable tumor extensions, and GTV + cx is defined as the GTV plus the entire cervix. The dose-volume histograms (DVH) of the GTV, GTV((I)), GTV + cx should be performed, and the dose to 100%, 95%, or 90% of the GTV (D(100), D(95), and D(90), respectively) and the percentage of the GTV covered by point A dose (V(100)) should be reported. Similarly, the DVH of the bladder and rectum wall should be performed, and the maximal dose at any point within the bladder and rectal wall should be reported, along with the maximal dose to a contiguous 1, 2, and 5 cm (3) volume of the bladder and rectum, respectively. In addition, the dose at the International Commission on Radiation Units and Measurements reference point for the bladder and rectum should be reported. This group thought that the current dose prescription method in use for cervical cancer brachytherapy (i.e., to prescribe to point A in most institutions) should not be changed yet because image-based dosimetry is not ready for routine practice. The group encourages external funding for image-based dosimetry and recommends that brachytherapy manufacturers develop image-compatible applicators. Proposals are made for research in image-based brachytherapy for cervical cancer (236).

Applicators for Carcinoma of the Cervix

Applicators used to insert intracavitary sources into the uterus and vagina included rubber catheters and ovoids developed by French researchers, metallic tandems and plaques designed in Sweden, and plastic tandems and ovoids of the Manchester system. Fletcher (98) designed a preloadable colpostat, which Suit et al. (322) modified and adapted to afterloading. Intracavitary vaginal colpostats typically incorporate internal shielding to reduce dose to the bladder and rectum. Markman et al. (201) evaluated the dosimetric effects of inhomogeneities in brachytherapy using Monte Carlo calculations to model dose distributions about both a Fletcher-Suit-Delclos (FSD) LDR system and the MicroSelectron HDR remote afterloading system.

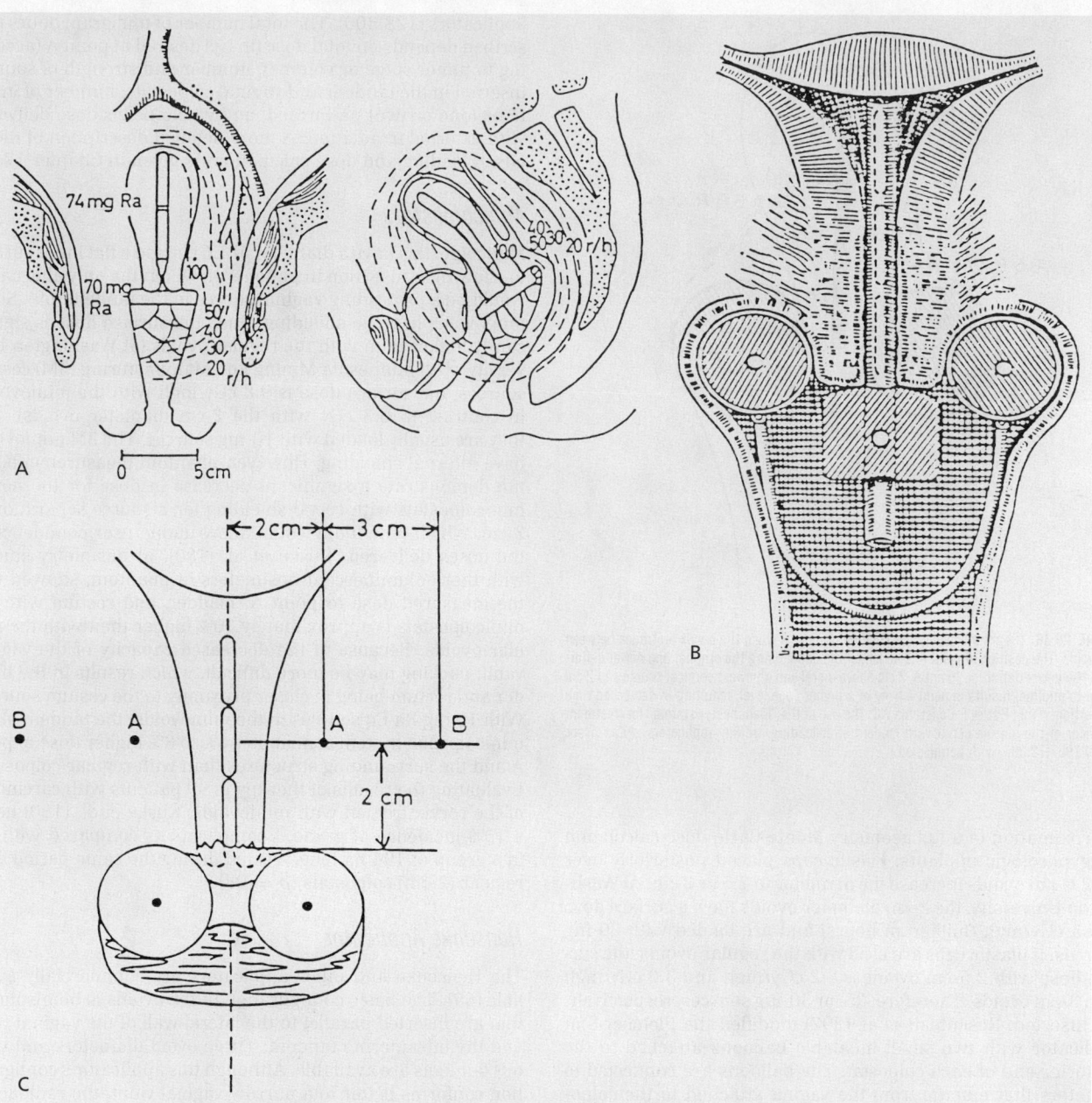

FIGURE 20.35. A: The Stockholm system. The intrauterine rod-shaped applicator is loaded with 53 to 88 mg of radium (74 mg in the example shown). The vaginal applicator usually consists of a flat box containing 60 to 80 mg of radium (70 mg in the example shown), but in special cases other forms of vaginal applicators may be used. Classically, the two applicators are not fixed to each other, but fixed or semifixed combinations have been developed. The vaginal applicator is held against the cervix and lateral fornices by careful and systematic gauze packing. Typically, two or three applications are given with 3-week intervals, each application lasting for 27 to 30 hours. (From Walstam R. The dosage distribution in the pelvis in radium treatment of carcinoma of the cervix. *Acta Radiol* 1954;42:237, with permission.) **B:** The Paris system. Typical radium application for a treatment of cervix carcinoma consisting of three individualized vaginal sources (one in each lateral fornix and one central in front of the cervical os) and one intrauterine source made of three radium tubes (in so-called tandem position). The active length of the sources is usually 16 mm, their linear activity is between 6 and 10 mg/cm, and their strength is 10 to 15 mg of radium. The total activity is one of the lowest in use for such treatments and implies a typical duration of the application of 6 to 8 days. Typically, the ratio of the total activity of the vaginal sources to the total activity of the uterine sources should be 1 (with variations between 0.66 and 1.5). (From Pierquin B. *Precis de curietherapie, endocurietherapie et plesiocurietherapie.* Paris: Masson, 1964, with permission.) **C:** The Manchester system. Definitions of points A and B in the classic Manchester system are found in the text. In a typical application, the loading of intrauterine applicators varies between 20 and 35 mg of radium and between 15 and 25 mg of radium for each vaginal ovoid. The resultant treatment time to get 8,000 R at point A is 140 hours. (From Meredith WJ. *Radium dosage: the Manchester system.* Edinburgh: Livingston, 1967, with permission.)

Errors were largely dominated by the primary photon attenuation and were largest behind the shields and tandem. For the FSD applicators, applicator superposition showed differences ranging from a mean of 2.6% at high doses (greater than Manchester point A dose) to 4.3% at low doses (less than Manchester point A dose) compared to the full geometry simulation. Source-only superposition yielded errors higher than 10% throughout the dose range. For the HDR applicator system, applicator superposition-induced errors ranged from 3.6% to 6.3% at high and low doses, respectively. Source superposition caused errors of 5% to 11%. These results indicated that precalculated applicator-based dose distributions can provide an excellent

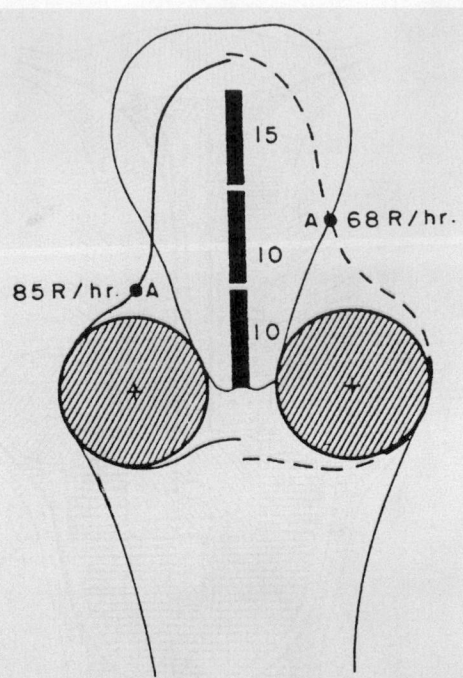

FIGURE 20.36. Diagram showing the position of point A when the cervix protrudes between the ovoids. The position of point A is no longer the same using the original and newer definitions. The newer definition (point A, 2 cm above distal end of lowest cervical source and 2 cm lateral to midline) results in point A lying at a higher dose level, resulting in decreased time of insertion. (From Batley F, Constable WC. The use of the "Manchester system" for treatment of cancer of the uterine cervix with modern after-loading radium applicators. *J Can Assoc Radiol* 1967;18:396, with permission.)

approximation of a full geometry Monte Carlo dose calculation for gynecologic implants. Plastic caps placed posteriorly over the 2.0-cm ovoids increase the diameter to 2.5 or 3 cm. At Washington University, the 2-cm diameter ovoids have a surface dose of 6.3 cGy/mgh (milligram hours) and are loaded with 20 mg sources. If plastic caps are used with the regular ovoids, the surface dose with 2.5-cm ovoids is 4.2 cGy/mgh and 3.0 cGy/mgh with 3-cm ovoids. Therefore, 25- or 30-mg sources, respectively, are inserted. Rosenblatt et al. (292) modified the Fletcher-Suit applicator with two small inflatable balloons attached to the posterior end of each colpostat. The balloons are connected to catheters that emerge from the vagina attached to the colpostat's handles. The balloons were affixed to the colpostats with a plastic adaptor and are inserted empty. The balloons are filled with radiologic contrast material, and lateral film usually shows a significant posterior displacement of the anterior rectal wall away from the vaginal sources. In 90 brachytherapy applications using this device for cervical cancer and vaginal applications for endometrial carcinoma following total abdominal hysterectomy, on average, the ICRU rectal point was displaced 14 mm posterior from the colpostats, reducing the dose rate by 60% and resulting in an average dose sparing of about 10 Gy to the anterior rectal wall. The Fletcher tandems, about 6 mm in diameter, are available in three curvatures. A flange or stopper is used to keep the uterine tandem in the selected position; a keeled flange can be used to avoid rotation of the tandem. A special yoke was designed to maintain the position between the intrauterine tandem and the colpostats (72). In general, the loading in the tandem is with 20-10-10 mg Ra Eq ^{137}Cs sources. It is extremely important when applicators are purchased to examine the design, to obtain radiographs to identify the position of the shielding (69), and to take dosimetric measurements after determining the diameter and thickness of the walls of the applicator to determine exactly the dose distribution around the

applicators (128,300). The total number of milligram hours prescribed depends on total dose (in Gy) desired at point A (according to tumor stage or volume), number and strength of sources inserted in the tandem and vaginal colpostats, number of insertions (one or two) performed, and whole-pelvis dose delivered with external irradiation. A more detailed description of methods of loading and dose calculations is given in Chapter 17.

Minicolpostats

Minicolpostats have a diameter of 1.6 cm and a flat inner surface to allow their insertion in patients on whom the only alternative would be a protruding vaginal source in the tandem (69). Some miniovoids have no shielding; thus, the surface dose is significantly higher than with the regular ovoids (at Washington University, with Minnesota Mining and Manufacturing (3M) cesium sources, the surface dose is 9.8 cGy/mgh with the miniovoids, in contrast to 6.3 cGy with the 2-cm diameter ovoids), and they are usually loaded with 10-mg sources. The 3M miniovoids have internal shielding. However, phantom measurements did not demonstrate a significant decrease in dose for the newer minicolpostats with rectal shielding for a source separation of 3 cm, which potentially could allow undue user confidence in the doses delivered. Kuske et al. (180), in dosimetry studies with thermoluminescent dosimeters in phantom, showed that the measured dose to point A, bladder, and rectum with the minicolpostats is approximately 10% higher than with the regular ovoids. Because of the decreased capacity of the vaginal vault, packing may be more difficult, which results in the bladder and rectum being in closer proximity to the cesium sources. With 10 mg Ra Eq sources in the miniovoids, the tandem in the minicolpostat system contributes 6% to 8% higher dose to point A and the surrounding structures than with regular colpostats. Evaluating the results of therapy in 99 patients with carcinoma of the cervix treated with miniovoids, Kuske et al. (180) noted a 15% incidence of grade 3 complications compared with 8% in a group of 194 patients treated during the same period with regular (2-cm) colpostats (*p* = .08).

Henschke Applicator

The Henschke and other applicators are commercially available (69). The basic configuration of the ovoids is hemispheres that are inserted parallel to the lateral wall of the vaginal vault and the intrauterine tandem. Three ovoid diameters and various tandems are available. Although this applicator's configuration conforms better to a narrow vaginal vault, the radioactive sources are placed parallel to the long axis of the bladder and the rectum and do not have any shielding, thus potentially delivering a higher dose to these organs. Users should familiarize themselves with the dosimetric aspects of these devices. Delclos et al. (69) emphasized that the dosimetry with the Fletcher colpostats is unique and that treatment techniques and tables derived for this applicator should not be used with other applicators because this might result in significantly higher doses to the vagina, bladder, or rectum. Figure 20.37 illustrates the differences in dose delivered to the bladder or rectum with the Fletcher or the Henschke applicator for a normalized dose of 70 Gy to point A. Appropriate source loading and dose prescription will produce satisfactory clinical results.

Interstitial Implants for Cervical Carcinoma

Metallic needles containing ^{137}Cs or more recently afterloading metallic guides or Teflon catheters for insertion of ^{192}Ir wires or seeds have been implanted in the parametrium or cervix, using a transvaginal or transperineal approach (sometimes in lieu of intracavitary insertions when the cervical canal cannot be identified) frequently with the aid of templates (285). The

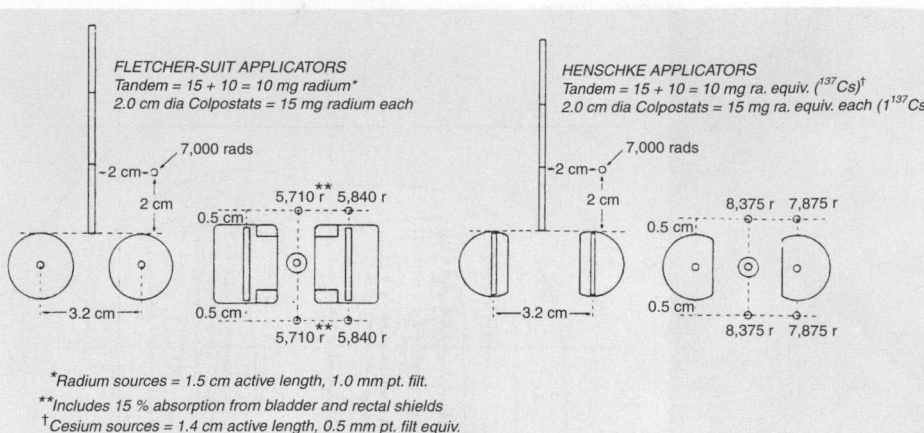

FIGURE 20.37. Comparison of doses delivered by Fletcher or Henschke colpostats to a plane 0.5 cm anterior and 0.5 cm posterior to the poles of the colpostats with the dose normalized at 70 Gy to point A. It is obvious that the number of milligram hours (mgh) must be reduced in the Henschke system to bring the dose to the bladder and rectum more in line with that obtained with the Fletcher applicator. (From Delclos L, Fletcher GH, Sampiere V, et al. Can the Fletcher gamma ray colpostat system be extrapolated to other systems? *Cancer* 1978;41:970, with permission.)

procedure is similar to that followed for intracavitary insertions. The operator should keep in mind the expected anatomic location of the major pelvic vessels, especially veins (because arteries are more difficult to pierce). For implants in the cervix itself, the needles or nylon catheters with metallic guides (5 to 6 cm long) are inserted straight, about 1.2 cm apart, following the position of the uterus (which can be verified with a finger in the rectum) in a single- or double-circle arrangement. If a single circle is used, full-intensity sources are required. If a double circle is implanted, the central one should have half-intensity sources (usually four) and the periphery should have full-intensity sources. At Washington University, the parametrial Teflon catheters (with metallic guides), usually 12 to 15 cm long, are inserted through the vaginal fornices. A double-plane or volume implant usually can be placed in each parametrium.

The catheters are implanted starting at 1 o'clock on the patient's left side and at 11 o'clock on the right, directed parallel to the coronal plane of the patient and 5 to 10 degrees lateral toward the pelvic wall. The peripheral planes should be placed 1.2 to 1.5 cm lateral to the more medial planes, and the catheters should be inserted in the same fashion, about 10 degrees divergent in the cephalad direction from the midline. Insertion of the needles into the bladder should be avoided, unless it is necessary to cover the tumor volume. When the uterosacral ligament area is to be implanted, the catheters are directed 5 to 10 degrees posteriorly. In general, 6 to 10 catheters can be implanted easily in each parametrium. We prefer to implant the interstitial catheters alone, without vaginal colpostats or cylinders, to prevent displacement or enhanced penetration of the needles (Fig. 20.38). Gentle packing with iodoform gauze will keep the

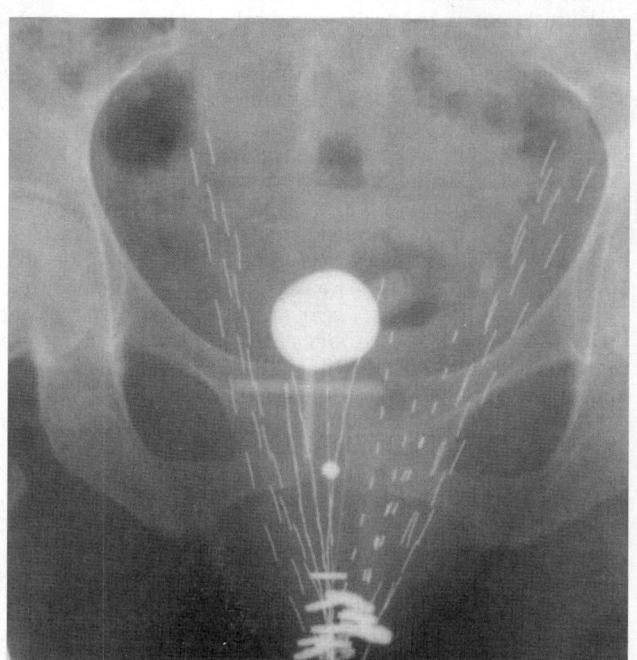

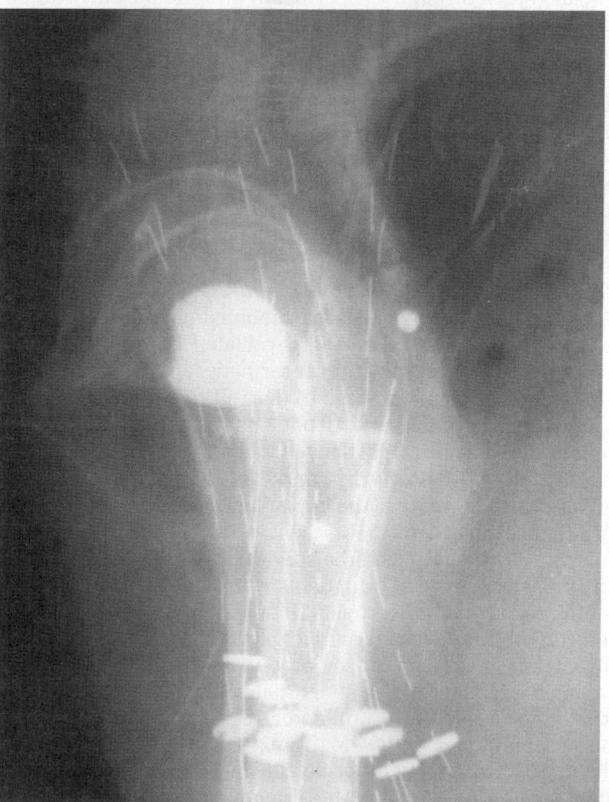

FIGURE 20.38. Anteroposterior (**A**) and lateral (**B**) radiographs of the pelvis illustrating bilateral parametrial implant (with sources extending into vaginal walls) for extensive carcinoma of the uterine cervix. The upper radiopaque marker indicates the position of the cervix. The lower radiopaque marker denotes the distal margin of vaginal tumor extension.

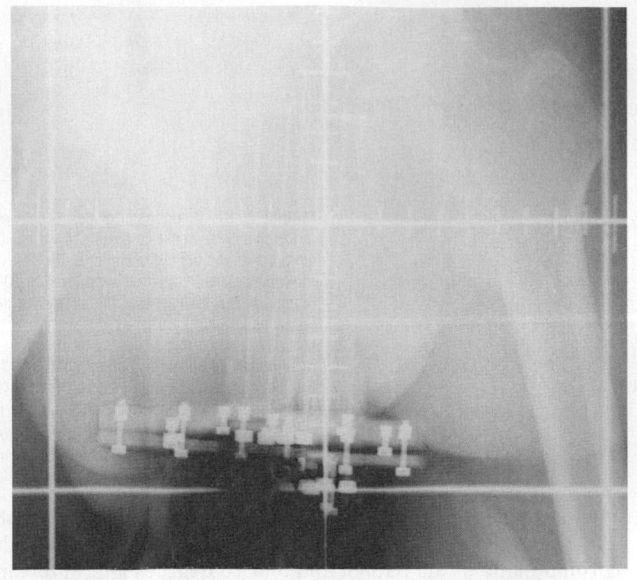
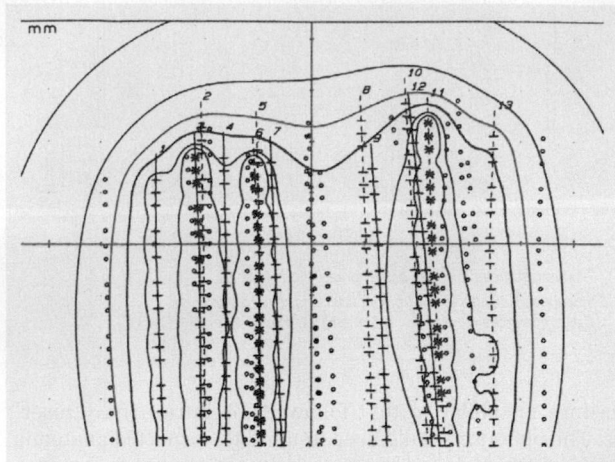

FIGURE 20.39. A: Left anterior posterior oblique view of an interstitial implant using Martinez Universal Perineal Interstitial Template. **B:** Coronal isodose distribution of the implant shown in **(A)**.

needles in place. Cystoscopy and a careful rectal examination at the completion of the procedure will help identify any misplaced needles, which should be withdrawn or replaced immediately. A digital rectal examination is performed (with a second glove, to be discarded) to ensure that there are no catheters where radioactive sources would be placed in the rectum. Aristizabal et al. (11), Martinez et al. (205), and Syed et al. (325) have popularized the use of interstitial implants, using perineal templates for guidance of spacing and alignment, with introduction of long metallic guides through the perineum into the parametrial tissues (Fig. 20.39). [192]Ir seeds or ^{137}Cs microspheres in nylon tubes are inserted in an afterloading fashion after x-ray films are obtained with dummy sources for dosimetry computations. Aristizabal et al. (11) modified their technique by deleting three anteriorly and three posteriorly placed needles in the central row; the central tandem also was omitted in an effort to decrease an initial high incidence of vesicovaginal or rectovaginal fistula. The authors reported about 75% pelvic tumor control in 118 patients with stage IIB and III carcinoma of the uterine cervix. The major complication rate was 6% with <4,500 mgh, 16% with 4,500 to 4,999 mgh, 28% with 5,500 mgh, and 87% with higher intracavitary doses (combined with 45 to 50 Gy to the whole pelvis). Syed et al. (324) evaluated 185 previously untreated patients with cervical cancer between 1977 and 1997. Twenty-one patients had stage IB (barrel), 77 stage II, 77 stage III, and 10 stage IV disease. All patients were treated by a combination of external megavoltage irradiation to the pelvis to a dose of 5,040 cGy followed by interstitial-intracavitary implants to a dose of 40 to 50 Gy to the implanted volume in two applications. Clinical local control was achieved in 152 (82%) of the 185 patients. A 5-year disease-free survival rate of 65%, 67%, 49%, and 17% was achieved for patients with stage IB, II, III, and IV disease, respectively. Eighteen (10%) of the 185 patients developed RTOG grade 3 or 4 late complications. Patients with locally advanced cervical cancer, or with distorted anatomy, may be treated adequately with interstitial brachytherapy to achieve excellent locoregional control and a reasonable chance of cure with acceptable morbidity. Martinez et al. (205) described results in 104 patients with locally advanced or recurrent pelvic tumor using a universal perineal template combined with external irradiation (36 Gy to the whole pelvis and 14 Gy to the pelvic sidewall with midline block using four-field techniques, 4- or 10-MV photons). Local tumor control was obtained in 82%

of 63 patients with gynecologic lesions. The major complication rate was 3.2%. Jensen et al. (162), between June 1993 and August 1996, treated 34 patients with gynecologic malignancies (22 pelvic recurrences, 12 primary locally advanced) with external irradiation, four-field box technique, to 46 Gy in 23 fractions, 5 fractions per week and ^{192}Ir interstitial PDR brachytherapy in pulses of 0.6 Gy, one pulse per hour to a total of 30 Gy. The MUPIT applicator was used for all implantations. The overall complete response rate was 74%. At median 14 months follow-up (range 3 to –40 months), 15 patients were alive with no evidence of disease. Seven of 14 patients with a second recurrence or progressive disease were still alive. The overall 1- and 2-year survival was 71% and 63%, respectively. There was no difference in survival probability when stratifying the patients by primary diagnosis (recurrent vs. primary advanced), relapse locations (central vs. central + pelvic wall mass), or treatment volume. Seventeen chronic grade III complications were observed in 10 patients. Large treatment volumes significantly correlated to severe gastrointestinal complications. Fifteen of 17 chronic grade III complications were observed in patients treated for recurrent disease. Hughes-Davies et al. (153) reported on 139 patients treated with transperineal template interstitial brachytherapy for locally advanced or recurrent pelvic cancer. Most patients received external pelvic irradiation (median dose, 42 Gy) followed by an implant (median dose, 30 Gy, 48 hours). The dose rate was 0.4 to 1 Gy per hour. Implant geometry was based on CT scan or MRI studies. An acrylic template was sutured in place, and a bladder catheter was inserted. Blind-ended hollow plastic afterloading catheters were inserted in the pelvic tissues. With median follow-up of 57 months in the survivors, the 5-year local tumor-control rate was 25% and the disease-free survival rate was 22%. Eighteen patients (13%) developed fistula. Late bladder complications were observed in 18 patients (12%), and bowel complications were seen in 28 patients (20%). Two patients developed pathologic fracture of the pubic ramus. Bachitiary et al. (15) reported on 166 patients with cervical cancer who underwent primary radiotherapy with or without concurrent cisplatin. In the group, 109 (65.7%) received LDR brachytherapy and 57 (34.3%) received PDR brachytherapy. The 3-year overall survival and disease-free survival rates were 70% and 57% for the LDR group and 82% and 70% for the PDR group, respectively. The 3-year probability rate for late grade 3 or worse toxicity was 7.4% for LDR brachytherapy

	RESULTS WITH EXTERNAL BEAM IRRADIATION AND TEMPLATE FOR LOCALLY ADVANCED (IIB AND IIIB) CERVICAL CANCER		
Table 20.5			
Author (Reference)	No. of Patients	Local Recurrence	Complications
Aristizabal et al. (11)	118	30 (25%)	25 (21%)
Martinez et al. (205)	37	6 (16%)	2 (5.4%)
Gaddis et al. (111)	51	18 (33%)	8 (16%)
Ampuero et al. (7)	24	9 (38%)	7 (29%)
Total	265	76 (29%)	45 (18%)

patients and 7.6% for PDR brachytherapy patients, respectively, and 6.9% and 7.6%, respectively, for concurrent chemotherapy versus none. No difference was found in severe late toxicity, overall survival, or disease-free survival between the LDR and PDR groups. Nag et al. (243) used fluoroscopy to guide the needles for interstitial brachytherapy with ^{192}Ir using a Syed template to treat various gynecologic malignancies. The brachytherapy dose (prescribed to the periphery of the implant) was 40 to 55 Gy when used alone (15 patients) and 22 to 40 Gy when used as a boost to 34.2 to 59.4 Gy of pelvic EBRT (56 patients). Nag et al. (243) also reported on 31 patients with carcinoma of the cervix and eight patients with vaginal carcinoma treated with EBRT and fluoroscopic-guided interstitial brachytherapy. Clinical indications for interstitial brachytherapy were extensive parametrial involvement in 22 patients, extensive vaginal involvement in 10 patients, and poor vaginal anatomy in seven patients. With a median follow-up of 36 months, 16 patients (51%) with cervical carcinomas and five patients (62.5%) with vaginal carcinomas had local tumor control. Only one patient experienced grade 3 complications (2.5%). Results reported by several authors using templates in locally advanced uterine carcinoma are shown in Table 20.5.

Other Brachytherapy Techniques in Carcinoma of the Cervix

A report by Sherrah-Davies (312) illustrates the importance of recognizing variations in techniques when new devices are introduced into clinical use. At the Christie Hospital, it was customary to deliver 75 Gy to point A using ^{226}Ra sources in two insertions of 70 hours each, with a week interval between insertions, without supplemental external irradiation in patients with stage I and IIA disease. In 1979, the sources were changed to ^{137}Cs, and patients were given one brachytherapy fraction of 37.5 Gy to point A with ^{226}Ra and a second insertion of 35 Gy with ^{137}Cs (to account for 10% higher dose rate for cesium sources). Subsequently, 12 patients were treated with two ^{137}Cs insertions for a dose of 70 Gy to point A. After the short pilot study, patients were randomly allocated to be treated with 75 Gy with ^{226}Ra or 75 Gy to point A with ^{137}Cs sources. At the same time, patients received external irradiation using two techniques, one with wedges and the other with four hexagonal fields, with different doses of irradiation. The incidence of bowel damage in patients treated with ^{137}Cs alone was 27% (7/26 patients) compared with 3% (1/33) with ^{226}Ra alone or in the group combined with ^{137}Cs intracavitary insertion. It was concluded that dose rate may have contributed to the increased morbidity with the cesium sources but to a smaller extent than radiobiology predicted. The author ascertained that bowel damage seemed to be associated with use of long (6-cm) intrauterine tubes in 98% of patients treated with ^{137}Cs to 75 Gy to point A. With new 40-degree angle tubes, less use of the long tubes, and a decreased dose to 65 to 70 Gy to point A, the incidence of bowel damage was reduced to 0.5%. Leborgne et al. (186) reported their experience with dose fractionation schedules using MDR brachytherapy (1 to 12 Gy per hour) in 42 patients with stage IB, IIA, and IIB carcinoma of the cervix. External irradiation with a central block was given to the pelvis (40 Gy at 2 Gy per fraction), and patients with stage IIB disease received an additional 20 Gy to the whole pelvis without central shielding. The MDR group was treated at 1.6 to 1.7 Gy per hour to point A; treatment factors are summarized in Table 20.6. A control group of 102 patients was treated with LDR brachytherapy (average dose rate was 0.44 Gy per hour, two 32.5 Gy fractions to point A in 74 hours each, 2 weeks apart). Grades 2 and 3 sequelae at 2 years were noted in 1% of patients treated with LDR brachytherapy and in 2.4% treated with MDR. The average nominal BED for the various groups ranged from 78 to 124 Gy. The incidence of late rectal complications was zero for patients receiving rectal BED of <50 Gy, 24% to 36% (53/184) for 50 to 199 Gy, and 67% (four of six) for doses of 200 Gy BED or greater. The authors concluded that the safest schedule was to deliver 18 Gy to the whole pelvis with external irradiation and brachytherapy, delivering a dose rate to point A of 1.6 Gy per hour, in six fractions of 8 Gy, two in each treatment day, 10 days apart. Two fractions are given on a single day, 6 hours apart, to reduce the number of insertions to three. This study emphasizes the importance of conducting prospective dose fractionation studies based on sound biologic data.

	TREATMENT FACTORS IN LOW–DOSE-RATE OR MEDIUM–DOSE-RATE BRACHYTHERAPY				
Table 20.6					
	Low Dose Rate	Medium Dose Rate 1	Medium Dose Rate 2	Medium Dose Rate 3	Medium Dose Rate 4
Dose rate (median Gy/hour)	0.44	1.68	1.65	1.64	1.61
Brachytherapy fractions	2	2	2	3	6
Mean dose/fraction	32.6	31.3	24.1	15.3	7.7
Brachytherapy total dose	65.1	62.5	48.2	46.0	46.2
External dose to point A (two fractions)	15.2	18.9	10.0	12.4	9.3
Total dose to point A	80.3	80.4	58.2	58.4	55.5
Coefficient of variation (= SD/mean)	13%	10%	18%	22%	21%

SD, standard deviation.
From Leborgne F, Fowler JF, Leborgne JH, et al. Fractionation in medium-dose rate brachytherapy of cancer of the cervix. *Int J Radiat Oncol Biol Phys* 1996;35:907–914, with permission.

Techniques, Modalities, and Modifiers in Radiation Oncology

Endometrium

Carcinoma of the endometrium may grow irregularly into the uterine cavity and produce deformity of the lumen from exophytic tumor, thickening of the uterine wall caused by myometrial infiltration, or uterine enlargement. It is important to determine the size and shape of the uterus; this can be accomplished by rotating the uterine sound and measuring the width and depth of the uterine cavity as well as by bimanual palpation or hysterogram. Special care should be taken to avoid a perforation because, if this occurs, packing with Heyman capsules should not be performed at that time. However, a carefully inserted tandem may be used, avoiding the site of perforation. Ultrasound may help in ascertaining the exact position of the tandem. Rutledge and Delclos (298) also cautioned against rupture (splitting) of the cervix, which may be caused by excessive careless dilatation. Uterine packing with capsules was described by Heyman et al. (144) in 1934. The practice of introducing as many capsules as possible to stretch the wall of the uterus has several advantages, as outlined by Rutledge and Delclos (298): a bulky tumor can be flattened out, allowing the base of the lesion to be more effectively irradiated; stretching of the uterine wall to make it thinner permits higher doses to be delivered to the serosa of the organ; and a more uniform distribution of the radiation is delivered to the entire myometrium. Afterloading Heyman-Simon capsules are available in 6, 8, and 10 mm diameters and 2 to 3 cm length. Inactive metallic guides and later ^{137}Cs sources are inserted. When capsules are used, it is convenient to insert an afterloading tandem to cover the lower uterine segment because this permits more flexibility in the loading to obtain improved coverage of this portion of the uterus and the cervical canal. Afterloading colpostats should be used routinely to irradiate the vaginal cuff (Fig. 20.40). A technical problem with the afterloading Heyman-Simon capsules is the relatively large thickness of the stems, which requires continued dilatation of the cervical canal (Hegar dilators) after a few capsules have been inserted. It is critical to record the order of insertion of the capsules (by numbers that are printed on each capsule) so that removal is done in the reverse order of insertion. Otherwise, the capsules may become jammed, making removal more difficult. Ideally, a minimum of four capsules should be inserted. If fewer are allowed by the size of the endometrial cavity, it may be better to insert an afterloading tandem. The dose of irradiation delivered with this system is somewhat empirically derived. In general, in preoperative insertions (currently rarely used) we use 3,500 mgh in the uterine cavity; however, cavities larger than 8 cm receive doses of approximately 4,000 mgh. Doses of about 65 Gy to the mucosal surface of the vagina are delivered (1,900 to 2,000 mgh) with 2-cm diameter vaginal ovoids. Grigsby et al. (122) reported higher survival and fewer pelvic recurrences and distant metastases in patients with stage I poorly differentiated endometrial carcinoma when doses higher than 3,500 mgh were delivered in the uterus. A lesser beneficial impact was noted in moderately differentiated tumors. In patients treated with radiation therapy alone (because of medical condition), higher intracavitary doses (in the range of 8,000 mgh) are given in two or three insertions. This is combined with external irradiation (20 Gy whole pelvis and an additional 30 Gy to the parametria with midline shielding). For postoperative irradiation in endometrial carcinoma, if no preoperative irradiation was delivered, we use afterloading colpostats to deliver 60 to 70 Gy to the vaginal mucosa (1,900 to 2,000 mgh) with LDR brachytherapy in patients with poorly differentiated tumors even in the absence of deep myometrial invasion. When there is deep myometrial invasion (>50%), regardless of the histologic features, the intracavitary therapy is combined with external irradiation (20 Gy whole pelvis and an additional 30 Gy to parametria with midline shielding). If a preoperative implant was performed, only external irradiation is administered postoperatively, as outlined. Nag et al. (241,242) treated 15 patients with locally recurrent endometrial adenocarcinoma with perineal template interstitial irradiation with LDR brachytherapy (^{192}Ir/^{137}Cs). Five of the seven previously unirradiated patients received pelvic EBRT of 45 to 50 Gy, with

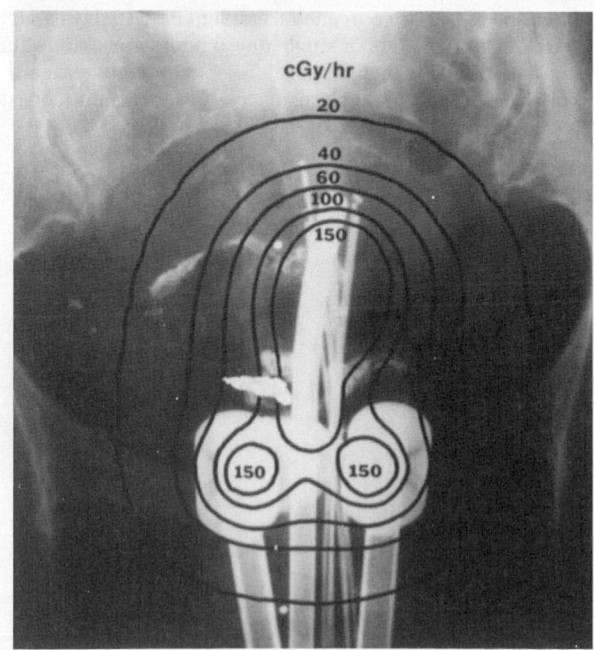

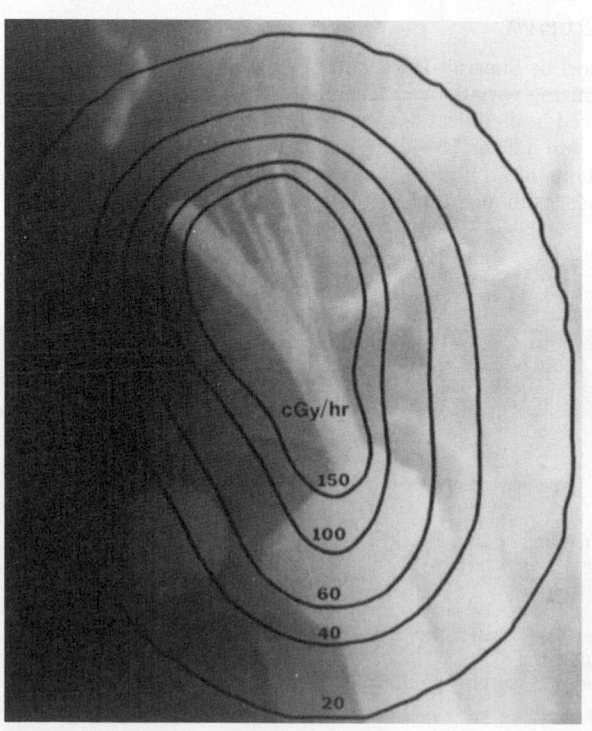

FIGURE 20.40. Anteroposterior (**A**) and lateral (**B**) views of implant for treatment of carcinoma of the endometrium using Heyman-Simon capsules, afterloading tandem, and vaginal colpostats. Isodose curves (cGy/h) are superimposed.

standard fractionation followed by an interstitial brachytherapy boost dose of 30 Gy (range 25 to 35 Gy). The other two patients received only brachytherapy of 40 Gy (palliative) and 50 Gy. Eight previously irradiated patients received only brachytherapy of 50 to 55 Gy. After a median follow-up of 47 months (range 14 to 81), the actuarial local tumor-control rate was 66.6% (for patients treated with interstitial irradiation only, it was 64.3% and for patients treated with interstitial irradiation plus EBRT, it was 100%). Actuarial overall and disease-specific 5-year survival rates were 42.3 and 67.5%, respectively. Toxicity has been minimal, with six patients complaining of vaginal/rectal (RTOG) grade 1 to 3 complications (five patients grade 1 to 2, one patient grade 3). Nag et al. (239), with members of ABS, performed a literature review, supplemented their clinical experience, and formulated recommendations for endometrial HDR brachytherapy. The ABS made specific recommendations for HDR applicator selection, insertion techniques, target volume definition, dose fractionation, and specifications for postoperative adjuvant vaginal cuff therapy, for vaginal recurrences, and for medically inoperable primary endometrial cancer patients. The ABS recommends that applicator selection should be based on patient and target volume geometry. The dose prescription point should be clearly specified. The treatment plan should be optimized to conform to the target volume whenever possible, while recognizing the limitations of computer optimization. Suggested doses were tabulated for treatment with HDR alone, and in combination with EBRT, when applicable. For intravaginal brachytherapy, the largest diameter applicator should be selected to ensure close mucosal apposition. Doses should be reported both at the vaginal surface and at 0.5-cm depth irrespective of the dose prescription point. For vaginal recurrences, intracavitary brachytherapy should be restricted to patients with nonbulky (<0.5-cm thick) disease. Patients with bulky (>0.5-cm thick) recurrences should be treated with interstitial techniques. For medically inoperable patients, an appropriate applicator that will allow adequate irradiation of the entire uterus should be selected (239).

Iridium-192 Interstitial Brachytherapy for Locally Advanced or Recurrent Gynecologic Malignancies

Gupta et al. (125) assessed treatment outcome in 69 patients with either locally advanced or recurrent malignancies of the cervix, endometrium, vagina, or urethra treated using the MUPIT with (24 patients) or without (45 patients) interstitial hyperthermia. Fifty-four patients had no prior treatment with radiation and received a combination of EBRT and an interstitial implant. The combined median dose was 71 Gy (range 5 to 99 Gy), median EBRT dose was 39 Gy (range 30 to 74 Gy), and the median implant dose was 32 Gy (range 18 to 40 Gy). Fifteen patients with prior radiation treatment received an implant alone. The total median dose including previous EBRT was 91 Gy (range 70 to 130 Gy) and the median implant dose was 35 Gy (range 25 to 55 Gy). With a median follow-up of 4.7 years in survivors, the 3-year actuarial local control, disease-specific survival, and overall survival for all patients were 60%, 55%, and 41%, respectively. The clinical complete response rate was 78%, and in these patients the 3-year actuarial local control, disease-specific survival, and overall survival rates were 78%, 79%, and 63%, respectively. On univariate analysis for local tumor control, tumor volume and hemoglobin levels were found to be statistically significant. On multivariate analysis, however, only tumor volume remained significant ($p = .011$). The grade 4 complication rate (small bowel obstruction requiring surgery, fistulas, soft-tissue necrosis) for all patients was 14%. With a dose rate <70 cGy per hour, the grade 4

complication rate was 3% versus 24% with dose rate of 70 cGy per hour or more ($p = .013$).

Acute Morbidity of Brachytherapy

Chao et al. (40) described the medical complications associated with 150 intracavitary implants performed in 96 patients treated with irradiation alone for inoperable carcinoma of the endometrium. General anesthesia was used in 98 implants, spinal anesthesia was used in 26, local anesthesia was used in 25, and epidural anesthesia was used in one. Preventive measures included low-dose cutaneous heparin (5,000 units every 8 to 12 hours) in 55 patients and intermittent pneumatic compression boots in 29. Four patients (4.2%) developed life-threatening complications (myocardial infarction in two, congestive heart failure in one, and pulmonary embolism in one patient). Two patients died (myocardial infarction and pulmonary embolism). Dusenbery et al. (80) also reported complications of gynecologic brachytherapy. Cardiovascular complications accounted for 16/21 patients with life-threatening brachytherapy sequelae; cardiac disease history was present in nine patients. Rotte (294) reported an incidence of 7.5% thromboembolic complications in 106 patients with carcinoma of the endometrium undergoing LDR implants. In contrast, none of the patients treated at the institution with HDR devices had thromboembolic phenomena. It is important to identify high-risk patients for thromboembolic complications, such as those with trauma to the lower extremities or pelvis, obesity, advanced age, history of prior thromboembolism, and need for prolonged bed rest. Adequate preventive measures should lower the already low incidence of this complication. Jhingran and Eifel (163) evaluated perioperative and postoperative complications of LDR intracavitary radiation therapy in 4,043 patients with International Federation of Gynecology and Obstetrics (FIGO) stage I to stage III carcinoma of the uterine cervix who had undergone 7,662 intracavitary procedures; 11 (0.3%) patients had documented or suspected cases of thromboembolism resulting in four deaths; of the 11, eight had clinical or radiographic evidence of tumor involving pelvic nodes or fixed pelvic wall. The risk of postoperative thromboembolism did not decrease significantly with the routine use of minidose heparin prophylaxis ($p = .3$). Other life-threatening perioperative complications included myocardial infarction (one death in five patients), cerebrovascular accident (two patients), congestive heart failure or atrial fibrillation (three patients), and halothane liver toxicity (two patients). Intraoperative complications included uterine perforation (2.8%) and vaginal laceration (0.3%), which occurred more frequently in patients 60 years old or older ($p < .01$). Of patients, 14% had a temperature of 100°F or higher during at least one hospital stay. The only correlation between minor intraoperative complications and disease-specific survival was found in patients who had stage III disease and uterine perforation; survival was significantly ($p = .01$) decreased in these patients. Deep venous thrombosis and pulmonary embolism did not occur in otherwise healthy patients with early disease and were rare even when disease was more advanced. Minor perioperative complications were not correlated with serious late complications or with death from disease.

Vagina, Vulva, and Female Urethra

Indications for and techniques of interstitial therapy for carcinoma of the vagina, vulva, and urethra have been described (264,266). Use of interstitial implants ideally should be limited to a volume encompassing 75% or less of the circumference of the vagina, particularly when the lesion involves the posterior wall and rectovaginal septum. The remaining normal tissues should be kept away from the implanted area as much as possible, with the judicious use of gauze packing, cylinders,

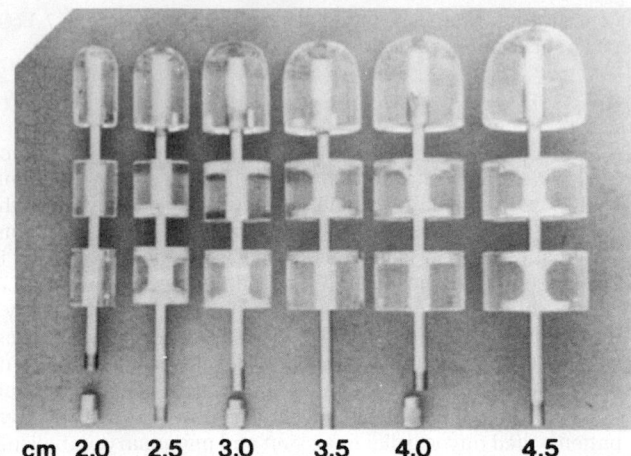
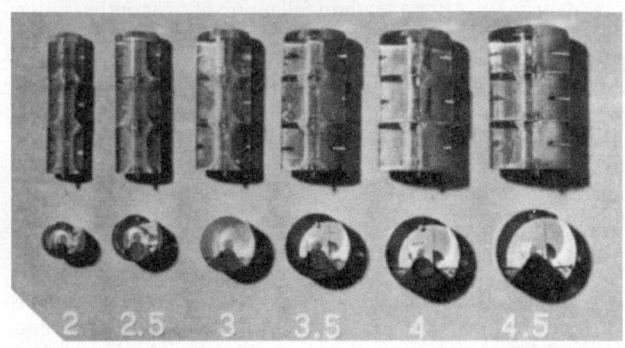

A cm 2.0 2.5 3.0 3.5 4.0 4.5 **B**

FIGURE 20.41. A: Dome colpostats to treat vaginal cuff alone or vaginal cuff and any selected vaginal length in a patient who had a hysterectomy. The curvature of each dome cylinder follows an isodose of a ^{137}Cs minisource placed at an adequate distance from the dome in the afterloading stem. Vaginal cylinders can be added to the dome cylinders, as shown. Any length of vaginal surface can be treated by combining a ^{137}Cs minisource with radium tubes or cesium sources. (From Delclos L, Wharton JT, Rutledge FN. Tumors of the vagina and female urethra. In: Fletcher GH, ed. *Textbook of radiotherapy,* 3rd ed. Philadelphia: Lea & Febiger, 1980;, with permission.) **B:** Cylinders with a segment of lead incorporated to shield part of the vaginal wall, rectum, or urinary bladder and urethra. (From Delclos L, Fletcher GH, Moore EB, et al. Minicolpostats, dome cylinders, other additions and improvements of the Fletcher-Suit after loadable system: indications and limitations of their use. *Int J Radiat Oncol Biol Phys* 1980;6:1195–1206, with permission.)

or templates. Two rolls of gauze are placed on top of and between the thighs, so that when the legs are brought down from the lithotomy position (in which the implant is done), the inside surfaces of the thighs are separated as much as possible from the radioactive sources.

Vaginal Cylinders

Carcinomas of the vagina are uncommon tumors comprising 1% to 2% of gynecologic malignancies. They can be effectively treated, and when found in early stages are often curable. Therapeutic alternatives depend on stage; surgery or radiation therapy is highly effective in early stages, while radiation therapy is the primary treatment of more advanced stages (264,299).

Afterloading vaginal cylinders have a central, hollow metallic cylinder, in which the sources are placed, and plastic rings 2.5 cm in length and of varying diameters are inserted over the cylinder. Domed cylinders are used to irradiate the vaginal cuff homogeneously, when indicated (Fig. 20.41A). Delclos et al. (68) recommend that a short cesium source be used at the top to obtain a uniform dose around the dome because a lower dose is noted at the end of the linear cesium sources. In some instances the cylinders have lead shielding to protect selected portions of the vagina (Fig. 20.41B). A flange with a keel is placed over the tandem after the last plastic cylinder has been inserted to secure the system in place and avoid rotation. The Bloedorn applicator consisted of a device incorporating the configuration of vaginal colpostats or a single midline ovoid and vaginal cylinders. Although extensively used, it was never described in detail; the Bloedorn applicator was later adapted for afterloading (68).

Perez et al. (267) designed a vaginal applicator that incorporated two ovoid sources and a central tandem that can be used to treat the entire vagina (alone or in combination with the uterine cervix). The applicator has vaginal apex caps and additional cylinder sleeves that allow for increased dimensions (Fig. 20.42). The dosimetry and dose specifications for this applicator have been published (227), showing that the applicator delivers 1.1 to 1.2 Gy per hour to the vaginal apex and 0.95 to 1 Gy per hour to the distal vaginal surface when loaded with 20 mg Ra Eq ^{137}Cs tubes in each ovoid and 10, 10, and 20 mg Ra Eq tubes in the vaginal cylinder (Fig. 20.43). The tandem

in the uterus can be used when clinically indicated with standard loadings, depending on the depth of the uterus (20-10-10 or 20-10 mg Ra Eq). When the tandem and vaginal cylinder are used, the strength of the sources in the ovoids should always be 15 mg Ra Eq. The vaginal cylinder or uterine tandem *never* carries an active source at the level of the ovoids. Armadur et al. (12) described a simple, inexpensive custom-made applicator for irradiation of localized areas of the vagina with intracavitary brachytherapy that allowed the higher dose to be limited to the portion of the vagina at risk for residual disease. The applicator was fabricated from a clear case acrylic (Lucite) rod, 3.5 cm diameter by 5 cm long. The applicator contained 11 parallel grooves, each 1.8 mm deep by 2.2 mm wide, machined along the surface of the cylinder parallel to its long axis at 1.0-cm increments. Plastic needles (15-gauge) were inserted into the grooves along the surface of the acrylic cylinder and held in place with heat shrink tubing. The applicator was inserted easily and positioned without anesthesia. Standard LDR ^{192}Ir ribbons were inserted into the plastic needles after

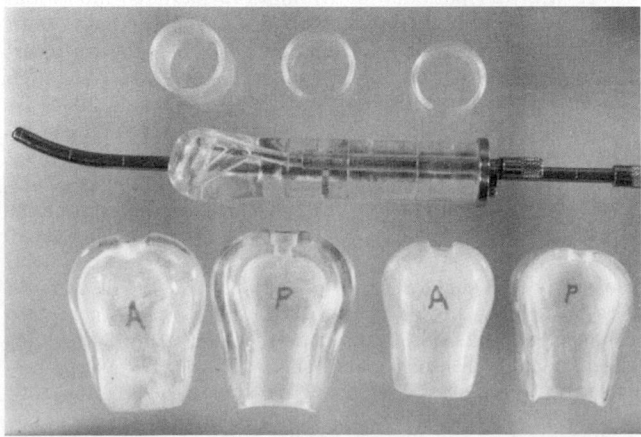

FIGURE 20.42. MIRALVA applicator with plastic sleeves to increase diameter of vaginal cylinder, afterloading tandem, and plastic caps (A–P) of different sizes to increase diameter of vaginal cuff portion of applicator. (From Perez CA, Slessinger E, Grigsby PW. Design of an afterloading vaginal applicator (MIRALVA). *Int J Radiat Oncol Biol Phys* 1990;18:1503–1508, with permission.)

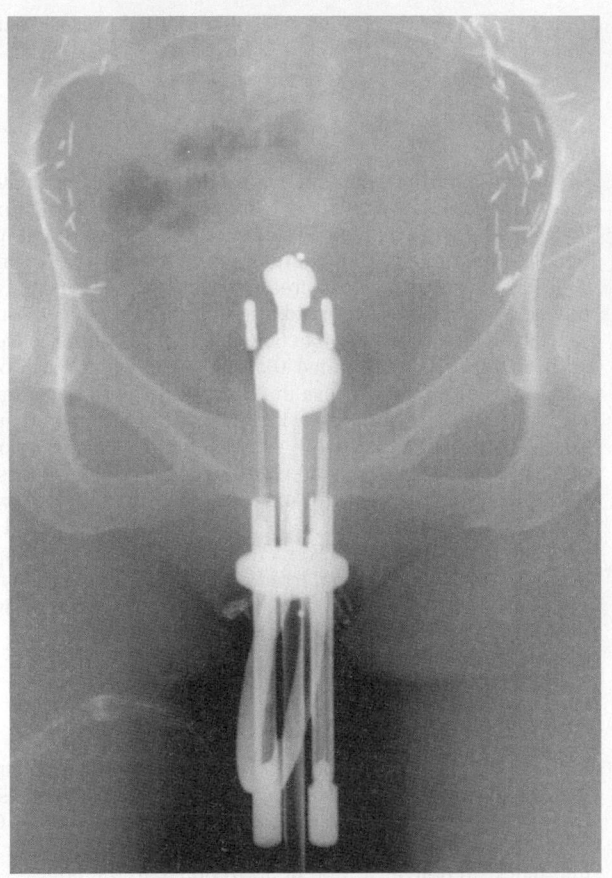

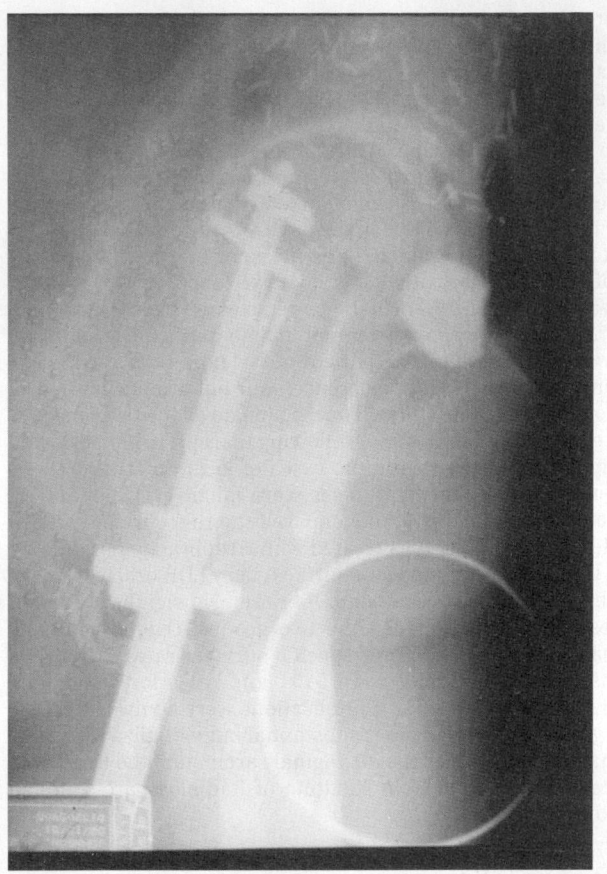

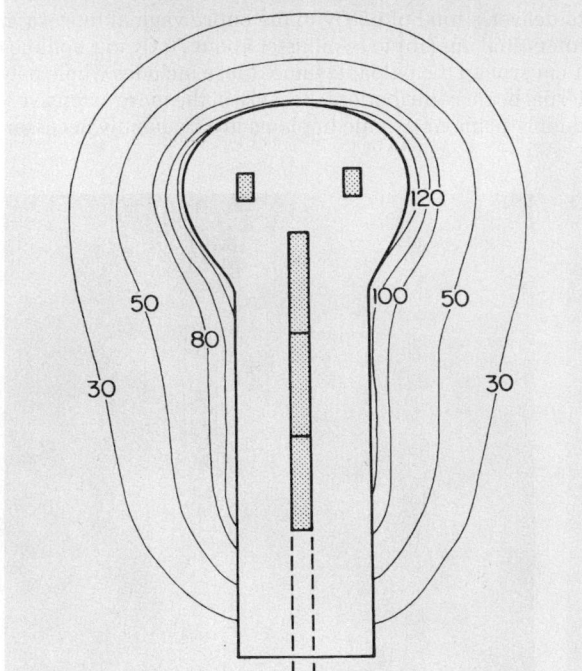

FIGURE 20.43. Anteroposterior **(A)** and lateral **(B)** radiographs depicting position of MIRALVA applicator for treatment of patient with vaginal recurrence of carcinoma of uterine cervix previously treated with a radical hysterectomy. **C:** Isodose curves of the MIRALVA applicator. (Perez CA, Slessinger E, Grigsby PW. Design of an afterloading vaginal applicator (MIRALVA). *Int J Radiat Oncol Biol Phys* 1990;18:1503–1508, with permission.)

positioning the applicator in the vagina. Fabrication of this applicator requires a few weeks' notice and is a routine task for a workshop with a milling machine; the cost is approximately $150. Seeger et al. (308) treated 22 patients with vulvar (nine) and vaginal (13) malignancies using interstitial pulsed dose rate brachytherapy. Twelve out of 22 patients were additionally treated using external beam therapy to the pelvis and regional lymph nodes. The median total dose of pulsed dose rate brachytherapy was 55 Gy for vulvar carcinoma and 20.25 Gy for PDR treatment of vaginal malignancies. After a median follow-up of 19 months for patients with vulvar cancer and 27 months for vaginal cancer, 77.8% of the patients with vulvar cancer and 100% of the patients with vaginal malignancies achieved complete local remission. One patient out of nine with vulvar carcinoma developed local recurrence, four out of nine developed regional recurrence, and two out of nine developed regional recurrence and had local tumor following therapy. In patients with malignancies of the vagina, no cases of local recurrence were observed, but distant metastases were found in five out of 13 patients. Kucera et al. (176) compared the role of remote afterloaded HDR in 80 patients treated with HDR brachytherapy and 110 LDR patients treated with intracavitary LDR brachytherapy (with or without external beam therapy). No significant differences were found between the two groups. Overall actuarial 3-year survival and disease-specific survival rates for all patients in the HDR series were 51%, and rates for patients in the LDR series were 66%. Complications were equivalent in the two groups. Because there is substantial individualization in the management of patients with vaginal carcinoma, the treatment guidelines at Mallinckrodt Institute of Radiology are summarized for each stage.

Carcinoma In Situ

An intracavitary application with a vaginal cylinder or similar applicator (i.e., Bloedorn, Burnett, Delclos, MIRALVA) delivering about 70 to 80 Gy to the mucosa is adequate to control carcinoma *in situ*. Higher doses of irradiation may result in significant vaginal fibrosis and stenosis. Because of the multi-centric nature of this tumor, the entire vaginal mucosa must be treated.

Stage I

The most superficial tumors are treated with an intracavitary insertion alone, usually with a cylinder 2.5 to 3 cm in diameter covering the entire vagina. If the lesion is thicker, a single-plane needle implant is used in addition to the intracavitary cylinder. This has the advantage of increasing the tumor depth dose without delivering excessive irradiation to the uninvolved vaginal mucosa, which receives 60 to 65 Gy. The gross tumor is treated with 65 to 70 Gy calculated 0.5 cm beyond the plane of the implant; the vaginal mucosa in this area receives an estimated 80 to 120 Gy, depending on the size of the lesion and tumor dose prescribed (Fig. 20.44). At Washington University, more extensive tumors are treated with intracavitary and interstitial therapy supplemented with external beam irradiation (whole pelvis dose of 10 or 20 Gy, with an additional parametrial dose with a midline block, to deliver a total of 45 to 50 Gy to the lateral pelvic wall). When external irradiation is used, the brachytherapy dose is adjusted downward, adding it to the whole pelvis to achieve the prescribed total vaginal tumor dose.

Stage II

Patients with more advanced paravaginal tumors without extensive parametrial infiltration (stage II lesions) always are treated with a greater external irradiation dose (20 to 40 Gy to the whole pelvis) and an additional parametrial dose with midline block, to deliver a total of 50 to 60 Gy to the lateral pelvic wall. In these patients, intracavitary therapy also should be used to deliver a total of 65 Gy to the entire vaginal mucosa and an interstitial implant to administer about 70 Gy to a volume 0.5 to 1 cm around the palpable tumor (dose includes whole pelvis external beam contribution). Because of the more extensive tumor, double-plane or volume implants are frequently necessary.

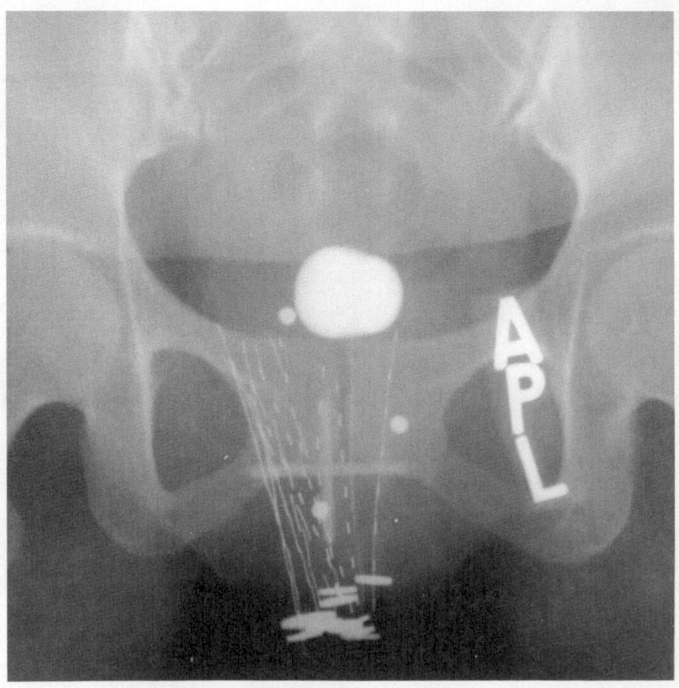
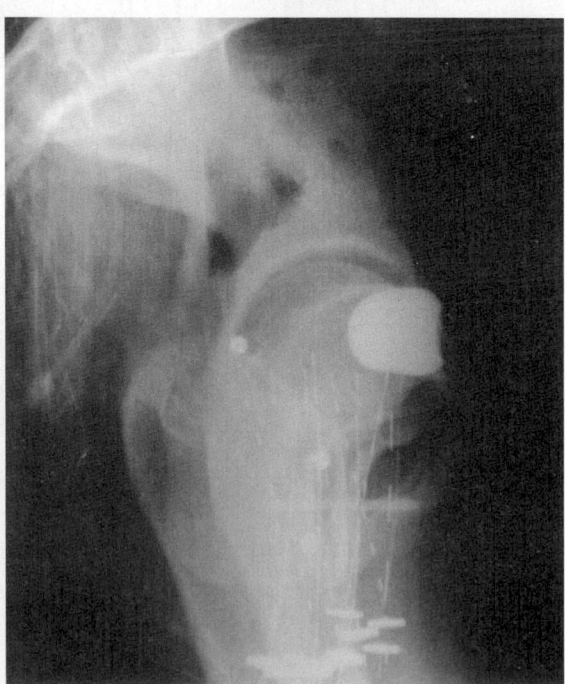

FIGURE 20.44. A: Anteroposterior and **(B)** lateral radiographs of the pelvis illustrate interstitial implant performed in a patient with carcinoma of right vaginal wall (intracavitary cylinder omitted).

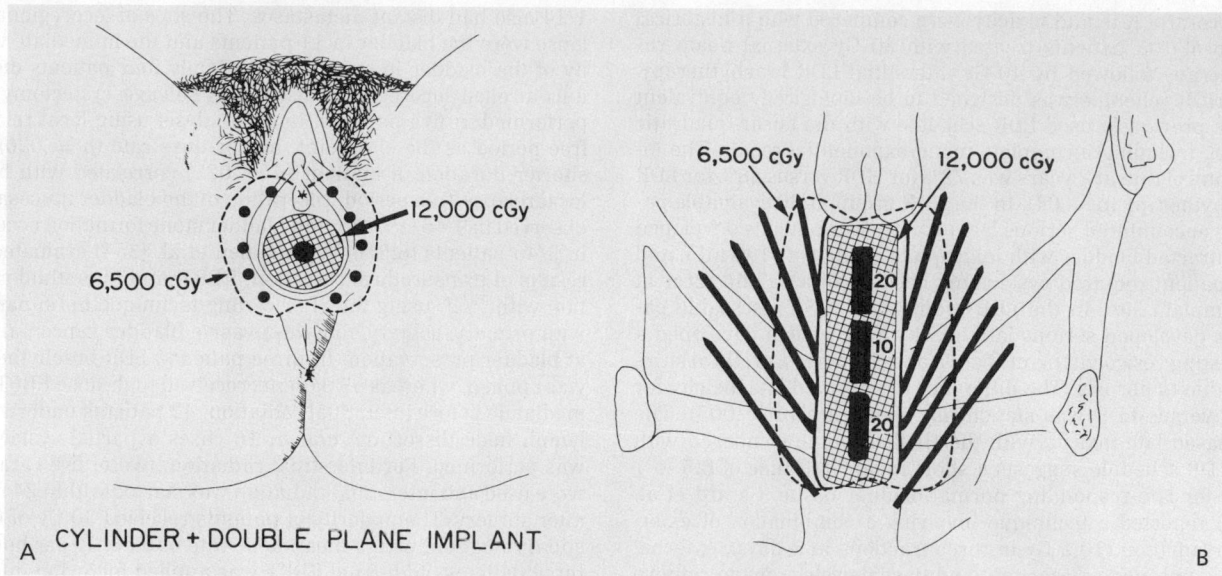

FIGURE 20.45. A: Cross-section (perineal) view of source arrangement for interstitial and intracavitary implant in a patient with involvement of the right and left lateral vaginal walls and paravaginal tissues. **B:** Coronal illustration of interstitial and intracavitary implant for same patient.

Stages III and IV

For stage III and IV tumors, 40 Gy to the whole pelvis and a total of 55 to 60 Gy parametrial dose with a midline block are administered. As in stage IIA tumors, a vaginal cylinder and an interstitial implant are used to complete total doses of 75 to 80 Gy to the tumor volume and 65 to 70 Gy to the uninvolved vaginal mucosa. If the tumor is located in the middle or lower third of the vagina, it is possible to combine in one procedure the insertion of a cylinder with the ^{192}Ir implant along the vaginal walls. However, if the tumor is in the upper third or involves the parametrium, it is preferable to perform two procedures because of concern that the cylinder will displace the interstitial catheters and distort the geometry of the implant. In patients with parametrial infiltration, in addition to the above doses, it is advisable to deliver an additional 15 to 20 Gy with an interstitial implant (Fig. 20.45).

Tumors of the Rectovaginal Septum

When the catheters and needles are inserted in the thin rectovaginal septum, one finger (covered with a second glove) should be inserted into the rectum to ensure that the catheters do not protrude beyond the rectal mucosa. If this occurs, the catheters should be withdrawn and reinserted in a satisfactory position. When needles or stainless steel guides are implanted for tumors of the posterior vaginal wall, the rectal ampulla is kept distended for the duration of the implant with a 30-mL Foley double-lumen catheter to minimize irradiation to the lateral and posterior rectal walls.

Lesions of the Bladder or Proximal Female Urethra

An open-bladder implant may be necessary for lesions of the bladder or proximal portion of the female urethra that extend into the bladder neck. This procedure also allows direct visualization of tumor extension into the bladder (70). If the tumor has extended beyond the vesical wall, the implant procedure is stopped and external irradiation is used. In a series of 160 patients, the mean hospitalization was 36 days after the operation. In 10% of the patients, the abdomen had to be reopened to remove one or more needles (20,22). Van der Werf-Messing

et al. (332) used radium implants in 328 patients with T2 and 63 patients with T3 bladder tumors after preoperative irradiation (3.5 Gy for three fractions). The recurrence rates were 16% for the T2 and 28% for the T3 tumors. Disease-free survival rates were 75% and 62%, respectively. Battermann and Tierie (23), using a similar technique, obtained local tumor control in 69/85 patients (81%) with T2 tumors and a 10-year disease-free survival rate of 56%. Subsequently, van der Werf-Messing and van Putten (333) used 40 Gy external irradiation followed by ^{137}Cs implants in 48 patients with T2 and 42 patients with T3 bladder cancer. The 5-year disease-free survival rate was 70%. A different method using iridium wires was designed in France and modified by Battermann and Boon (21) to overcome most of the disadvantages of the rigid needle technique. After a lower abdominal incision, the bladder is opened to visualize the tumor area. Plastic carriers consisting of a hollow part and a thinner leading end are inserted 1.5 cm apart. The tubes penetrate the abdominal wall, are tunneled in the bladder muscle through the tumor and out of the bladder, and penetrate the abdominal wall again. The catheters should be placed in such a way that removal is feasible without a second laparotomy, although in more complex cases this may be necessary. Dummy sources are introduced in the carriers to visualize the length of the source to be used while the bladder is still open. After the position of the sources is checked, the bladder is closed, and subsequently the abdomen is closed. A Foley catheter is placed for drainage. After film localization, the dose distribution is determined. The carriers are connected to the MicroSelectron, and the radioactive phase of the procedure is started. The tubes are well tolerated and, after completion of irradiation, can be removed easily. All patients receive preoperative external irradiation to prevent tumor seeding during operation (30 Gy). A dose of 40 Gy is given by brachytherapy at a dose rate of 0.3 to 0.5 Gy per hour. Pos et al. (282) determined the efficacy and safety of an HDR brachytherapy schedule in the treatment of bladder cancer and investigated the impact of different values of repair half-times and α/β ratios on the design of the HDR schedule. Between 2000 and 2002, 40 patients with T1 G3 and T2 bladder carcinoma were treated with 30 Gy external beam radiotherapy followed by interstitial HDR brachytherapy to a total dose of 32 Gy in 10 sessions of 3.2-Gy fractions in two fractions daily with a 6-hour interfraction interval. The local control rate and toxicity were compared with a historical group of 108 patients treated with 30 Gy external beam radiotherapy followed by 40-Gy interstitial LDR brachytherapy. The HDR schedule was designed to be biologically equivalent to the previously used LDR schedule with the linear-quadratic model, including incomplete mono-exponential repair. The local control rate at 2 years was 72% for HDR versus 88% for LDR brachytherapy ($p = .04$). In the HDR group, 5/30 evaluable patients encountered serious late toxicity: four patients developed a contracted bladder with inadequate capacity (<100 mL), and one patient required cystectomy because of a painful ulcer at the implant site. In the LDR group, only 2/84 assessable patients developed serious late toxicity. One patient developed a persisting vesicocutaneous fistula and the other a urethral stricture due to fibrosis. The difference in observed late toxicity for HDR versus LDR was statistically significant ($p = .005$). The increased late toxicity with the HDR schedule compared with the LDR schedule suggests a short repair half-time of 0.5 to 1 hour for late-responding normal bladder tissue. Gerard et al. (113) reported a technique involving a combination of external irradiation (10.5 Gy in three fractions in 3 days), external iliac lymph node dissection, and partial cystectomy to remove the tumor, in addition to a ^{192}Ir implant using a nylon thread technique or a specially designed curved needle to implant the nylon thread. Radiopaque markers help to accurately position the ^{192}Ir wires, which are 5 to 9 cm in length, with a linear activity of 1.2 to 2 mCi/cm. The thickness of the treated volume depends on the spacing of the wires (6 to 10 mm). The dose is calculated using the Paris system (40 to 50 Gy specified on the 85% isodose of the basal dose). The brachytherapy application lasts 2 to 5 days depending on the dose desired, and removal is accomplished simply by pulling the plastic tubes. Somewhat comparable brachytherapy techniques for treatment of carcinoma of the bladder have been described by Moonen (228), Maat and Venselaar (196), and Wijnmaalen et al. (355).

Rozan et al. (297) report the data on 205 patients (177 men and 28 women) treated in eight French centers. The patients had received the following treatment: a short course of preoperative pelvic irradiation, followed by surgery consisting of partial cystectomy or tumor resection, and implantation of plastic tubes filled with inactive lead wires, which were replaced by ^{192}Ir wires. The tumor characteristics were transitional cell carcinoma, 88.8%; mean size of the tumor, 29 mm; pathological stages: pTis, 1; pT1, 98; pT2, 66; pT3a, 26; pT3b, 9; pT4, 1; unknown, four, respectively; surgical lymph node status: N+, 3; N−, 118; no node dissection, 84. The mean follow-up was 51 months. Intravesical failures were seen in 35 patients (17.0%), 25 (71.4%) of them without metastases or regional recurrences. Twenty-one patients (10.2%) presented distant metastases, two-thirds of them suffered no bladder relapse. The 5-year survival rate was 77.4% for the T1, 62.9% for the T2, and 46.8% for the T3. Fifty-three patients had immediate side effects and three died from surgical complications. Twenty-nine patients had delayed bladder side effects (hematuria, fistula, chronic cystitis). Six patients presented with ureteral stenosis. Of the disease-free survivors, 96.1% retained their bladder function. Three factors were significantly predictive of delayed side effects: partial cystectomy, preoperative radiotherapy total dose, and linear activity of the wires ($p < .01$). Straus et al. (317) also used preoperative external irradiation (10 to 15 Gy for tumors <3 cm or 36 to 50 Gy for tumors 3 to 5 cm) and ^{192}Ir afterloading implants. The 2-year survival rate in 11 patients with T2 and T3a tumors was 72%. Forty-six patients with stage T1 or T2 cancer of the urinary bladder and one with stage T3 were treated with an interstitial implant (195). Before implantation, one patient received no external radiation therapy; the other 46 patients were treated with either a low dose (40 patients, 12 Gy median) or an intermediate dose (six patients, 38 to 40 Gy) of external irradiation. Locoregional relapse was observed in 14/47 patients (30%), and

1/14 also had distant metastases. The sites of locoregional relapse were the bladder in 11 patients and the immediate vicinity of the bladder in three patients. Only four patients died of uncontrolled locoregional disease. A salvage cystectomy was performed in five patients. In an analysis using local relapse-free period as the end point, higher dose rate ($p = .026$) and shorter duration of implant ($p = .021$) correlated with better local relapse-free period. Ulceration of the bladder mucosa was observed in 9/46 (19.6%), and bladder stone formation occurred in 3/46 patients (6.5%). Wijnmaalen et al. (354) evaluated the results of transurethral resection, EBRT, and interstitial radiation with ^{192}Ir, using the afterloading technique in 66 patients with primary, solitary, muscle-invasive bladder cancer, aiming at bladder preservation. In three patients, LDR brachytherapy was applied, whereas 63 patients received high-dose EBRT. Immediately before interstitial radiation, 42 patients underwent a lymph node dissection, and in 16 cases a partial cystectomy was performed. For interstitial radiation, two of five catheters were used and interstitial radiation was started within 24 hours after surgery. The majority of patients received 30 Gy of interstitial radiation, with a mean dose rate of 0.58 Gy per hour. In three patients, additional EBRT was applied following interstitial radiation. Follow-up consisted of cystoscopies, mostly done during joint clinics of urologists and radiation oncologists, with urine cytology routinely performed. With a median follow-up of 26 months, in seven patients a bladder relapse developed. The probability of remaining bladder relapse free at 5 years was 88%, and the bladder was preserved in 98% of the surviving patients. Metastases developed in 16 patients, and the probability of remaining metastasis-free at 5 years was 66%. The cumulative 5-year overall and bladder and distant relapse-free survival were 48% and 69%, respectively. Surgical correction of a persisting vesicocutaneous fistula was necessary in two patients, and a wound toilet had to be performed in another patient. Serious late toxicity (bladder, RTOG grade 3) was experienced by only one patient.

Tumors of the Vulva or Distal Urethra

Vulvar or distal urethral tumors can be treated with similar brachytherapy techniques. Erickson (85) has published a historical review of interstitial implants for vulvar carcinoma. The patient is placed in a lithotomy position, and single, double-plane, or volume implants can be designed around the urethra or in the vulvar labia. It is preferable to carefully place a no. 8 or no. 10 Hegar dilator in the urethra during the procedure for orientation of the planes of the implant. If the proximal urethra is involved, the radioactive sources must be inserted reaching the bladder. When the procedure is completed, the Hegar dilator is withdrawn; cystoscopy is performed to ascertain the position of the catheters in the bladder, and an indwelling three-way catheter is inserted. If there is intravesical bleeding, periodic irrigation of the bladder is necessary while the implant is in place, and it is preferable to leave a three-way catheter in place for a few days (up to 1 week) to facilitate bladder irrigation and avoid clot formation with bladder neck obstruction. When the vulva is involved, the sources must protrude into the perineum. If the tumor extends into the vagina, an intravaginal cylinder with some sources may be necessary to increase the dose to the vaginal mucosa (Fig. 20.46). The design of the implant, placement of the radioactive sources, and tumor doses are similar to those for comparable lesions in the vagina.

Pohar et al. (277) treated 34 patients with ^{192}Ir brachytherapy for vulvar cancer between 1975 and 1993 at Centre Alexis Vautrin. Twenty-one patients were treated at first presentation when surgery was contraindicated or declined. Of these patients, 12 had stage III or IV disease, eight were stage II, one was stage I, and one was stage 0. Thirteen patients were treated for recurrent disease. Paris system rules for implantation and

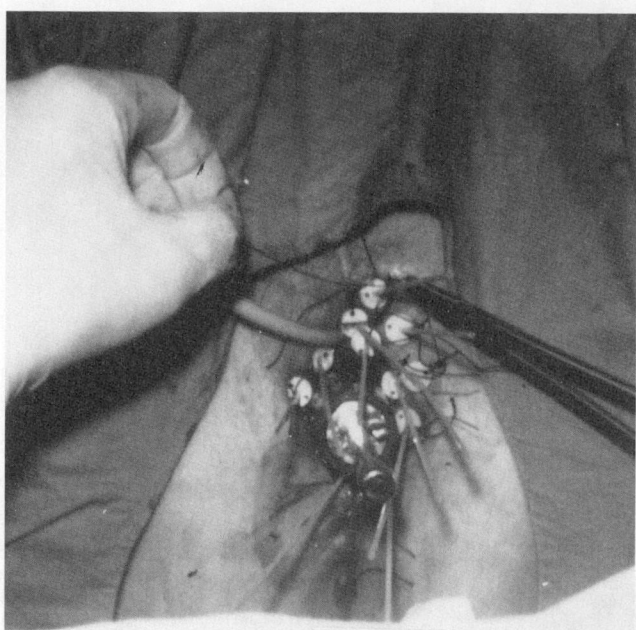

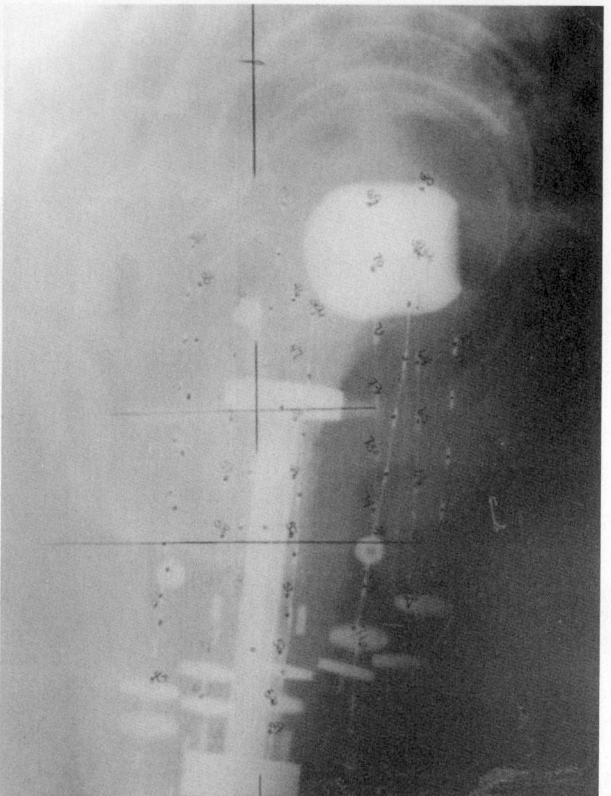

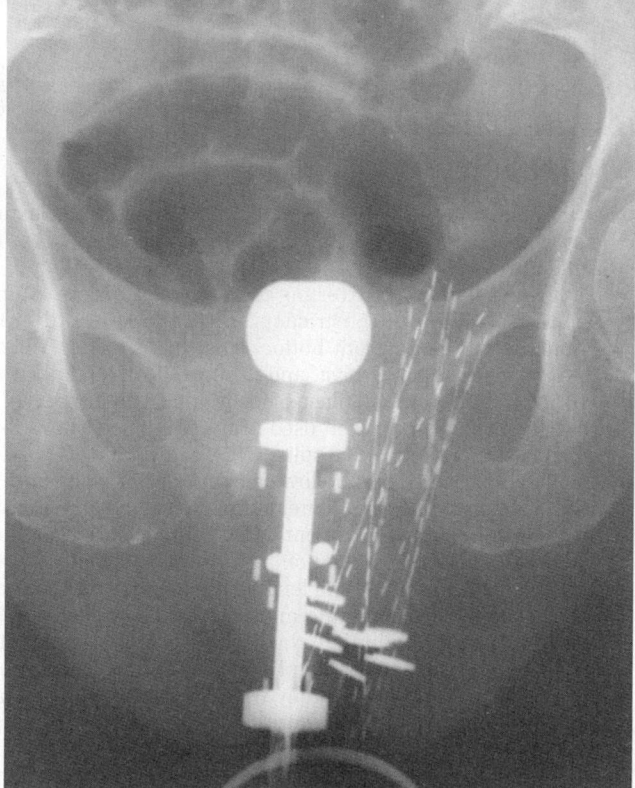

FIGURE 20.46. A: Patient at completion of interstitial implant and intracavitary insertion with stainless steel guides for ^{192}Ir tubing and Delclos vaginal cylinder. A bladder catheter is in place. The metallic buttons on the plastic catheters are being sutured to the skin to secure the position of the implant. Anteroposterior (**B**) and lateral (**C**) radiographs of implant for urethral tumor with left paraurethral extension.

dose prescription were followed. The median reference dose was 60 Gy (range 53 to 88 Gy). At the time of analysis, 10/34 patients were alive. Median follow-up in these 10 patients was 31 months (range 21 to 107 months). Fourteen of the 24 deaths were from causes other than vulvar cancer. Kaplan-Meier actuarial 5-year local control was 47% (95% confidence interval [CI], 23% to 73%) and 5-year actuarial locoregional control was 45% (95% CI, 21% to 70%). Kaplan-Meier actuarial 5-year disease-

specific survival was 56% (95% CI, 33% to 76%) and actuarial 5-year survival was 29% (95% CI, 15% to 49%). Median time to death was 14 months. Subset analysis revealed a higher actuarial 5-year local control in patients treated at first presentation than those treated for recurrence (80 vs. 19%, log rank; $p = .04$). Similarly, actuarial 5-year locoregional control was higher in patients treated at first presentation (80 vs. 16%, log rank; $p = .01$). The two groups did not differ significantly in

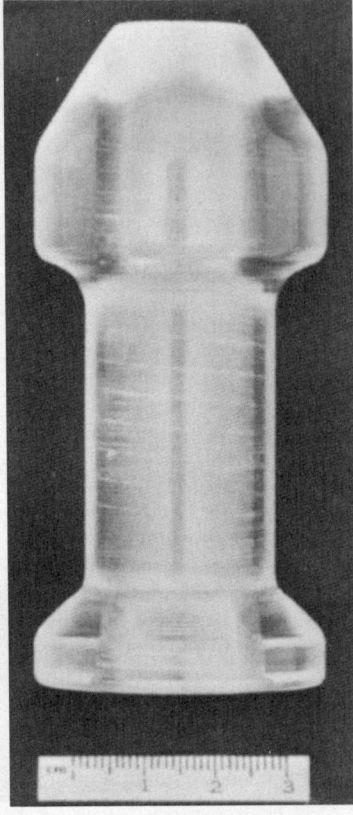

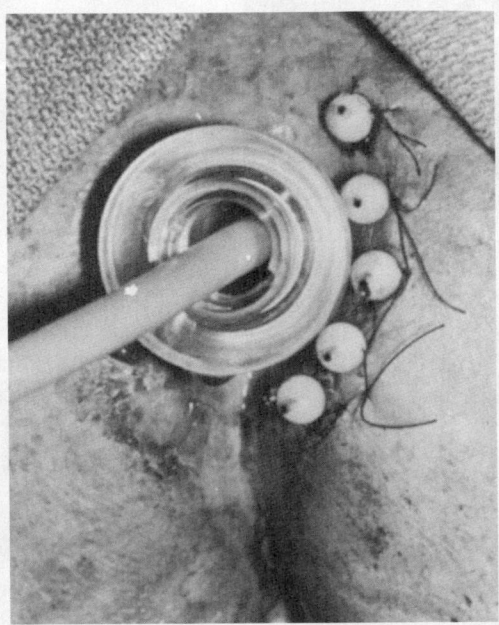

FIGURE 20.47. A: For implants of the anal canal, a hollow rectal plug that reduces the dose to the opposite side of the implant can be used. Several sizes are available. **B:** A single-plane implant of the anal canal, using stainless steel needles with Teflon balls. Note the rectal plug in place. In addition, the patient has a Foley catheter inserted into the rectum to keep the rectum distended. The catheter retractor is recommended only for implants performed with long guides. (From Delclos L. A second look at interstitial irradiation. In: Deeley TJ, ed. *Topical reviews in radiotherapy and oncology—2*. London: John Wright & Sons, 1982; with permission.)

disease-specific or overall survival. The actuarial 5-year disease specific survival of 56% is somewhat less than the expected 5-year disease-specific survival after surgery in a group having a similar proportion of early stage, advanced stage, and recurrent vulvar cancer. Micaily et al. (220) evaluated uncommon carcinoma of the female urethra. The review of literature and their experience indicate that early distal urethral cancers (squamous and adenocarcinoma) can be treated either with surgery (70% to 80% 5-year survival) or with radiotherapy (brachytherapy) with excellent results (75% 5-year survival). Early proximal or entire urethral cancers (squamous and adenocarcinoma), if treated surgically, will require exenterative procedures. Alternatively, these cancers can be treated with a combination of external beam and brachytherapy with or without chemotherapy with good results and preservation of organs. Surgery can be used for failures or persistent tumors. Advanced cancers require a multimodality approach, and a combination of radiation and chemotherapy appears to be the optimal way to treat these patients, with surgery to be used for biopsy-proven persistent tumors or recurrences.

Anal Canal and Rectum

Interstitial and intracavitary techniques have been used for many years for the treatment of anorectal carcinoma. Ideally, implants should be restricted to lesions that require implantation of no more than half the circumference of the anal canal for preservation of sphincter function (160). Single, double-plane, or volume implants may be necessary, depending on the extent of the tumor. The catheters are inserted through the perianal area in the central plane 0.5 cm away from the anal or rectal mucosa with one finger (double gloved) in the rectum to verify appropriate placement. Peripheral planes are placed at 1- to 1.5-cm spacing. The anal canal is kept distended with a custom-designed rectal plug, which reduces the dose to the opposite side of the canal to <15% of the minimum tumor dose

at the implanted area (Fig. 20.47) (70). Although a colostomy may be avoided with diligent care of the implanted area, this is not always practical. It may be necessary to precede the implant with a temporary diverting colostomy, regardless of tumor size or lack of bowel constriction. It is important to decrease irradiation of the adjacent buttock and thighs as described in the section on vagina, vulva, and urethra. IVALON (Fabco, Old Mystic, CT) or gauze is placed in the intergluteal space. The MUPIT applicator has been used in the treatment of anorectal tumors with satisfactory results (217). Kin et al. (169) used a template for insertion of hollow steel needles to place the ^{192}Ir and a rubber drain for treatment of patients with carcinoma of the anal canal; in some patients, this approach was combined with external beam irradiation. A ring-shaped template with the appropriate number and lengths of radioactive hollow steel needles was placed over the anus, and the needles were implanted successfully through the corresponding holes (about 1 cm apart) into the anal or rectal wall. The template and rubber drain were withdrawn carefully while the needles were maintained in place. The needles were secured, and the whole applicator was held in place by suturing the drain and the template to the perianal skin. Later orthogonal x-ray films were obtained, and dose calculations were performed. The total tumor dose from the external beam and interstitial irradiation ranged from 54 to 80 Gy (mean 64.2 Gy). Of 32 patients treated, 24 (74%) had local tumor control. Four patients had severe complications (two radionecrosis, one atony of the sphincter, and one severe rectitis); one patient required colostomy and another an abdominoperineal resection. Fourteen other patients had less severe complications. The probability of preserving good or acceptable anal function was 69% (22/32). Papillon et al. (256) reported on 221 patients with epidermoid carcinoma of the anal canal treated with a combination of external irradiation (35 Gy) and 5-fluorouracil and mitomycin-C, followed by an ^{192}Ir implant 2 months later. The implants were performed with either a plastic template or a steel fork, using four to eight wires, 5 to 7 cm long, adapted to the tumor extent and covering the quadrants of the anal circumference involved by the tumor. A minimum dose of 15 to 20 Gy was delivered in 15 to 28 hours. Of 189 patients followed for 5 years, 118 (65.9%) were alive and well, and 110 (61.4%) had anal preservation. Thirty-three patients (20.4%) died of cancer. In patients with tumors <4 cm, 50/66 (75.7%) were alive with anal preservation at the time of the report, and only five (7.5%) died of cancer. Papillon et al. (256) also reported on 90 patients with T1 or T2 rectal carcinoma treated with contact x-ray endocavitary therapy followed by ^{192}Ir implant with an iridium fork. Doses were similar to those administered to the patients with anal carcinoma. The 5-year survival rate was 77.8%; 67 (74%) were alive with anal preservation, and only 10 (11.1%) died of cancer. They also reported on a third group of patients with more advanced, moderately infiltrating low-lying T2 or T3 tumors, who would have been treated by abdominoperineal resection but because of age or poor operative risk were treated with radiation therapy including interstitial implants. At 4 years, 37/62 patients (59.6%) were alive, and 36 (58%) had anal preservation. Only nine patients (14.5%) died of cancer; three had unresectable lesions, and one died after major surgery. Bruna et al. (35) reported on 71 patients (14 T1, 41 T2, 15 T3, and one T4, 52 N0, 13 N1, three N2, and three N3. All the patients were M0 with squamous cell anal canal carcinoma treated with external irradiation to the posterior pelvis (mean dose 45.5 Gy). After an interval of 2 to 6 weeks, PDR interstitial brachytherapy was performed with a mean dose of 17.8 Gy to the 85% reference isodose of the Paris system. Forty-seven patients received chemotherapy (neoadjuvant/concomitant or both). With a median follow-up of 28.5 months, 2-year actuarial overall survival was 90% with 14 relapses, 10 patients with a grade III complication, and two with a grade IV complication. Price et al. (287) described 44 patients with inoperable anorectal carcinoma treated with interstitial implants using ^{226}Ra or ^{137}Cs needles to doses of 50 to 60 Gy (in five patients preceded by external irradiation). They recommended a dose of 60 Gy at 0.5 cm when external irradiation is not used. Local tumor control was achieved in 16/31 patients (52%) assessed for response. Late morbidity was observed in 12 patients: five had occasional bleeding or diarrhea; one had mucoid discharge; three developed stricture requiring surgery, and three had necrosis requiring surgery. Most patients who developed complications received total tumor doses above 80 Gy. Puthawala et al. (290) reported on 40 patients with anorectal cancer treated with external irradiation (40 to 50 Gy in 25 to 30 fractions) followed by two ^{192}Ir implants using the Syed template to deliver a total tumor dose of 65 to 75 Gy. Local tumor control was achieved in 70% of tumors with 20% major morbidity. Deniaud-Alexandre et al. (75), between June 1972 and January 1997, treated 305 patients with curative-intent radiation therapy. The T-stages were 26 T1, 141 T2, 104 T3, and 34 T4. There were 49 patients with nodal involvement at presentation. Pretreatment anal function scoring according to their in-house system was: 22 scored 0, 182 scored 1, 74 scored 2, seven scored 3, 11 scored 4, and nine not available. The treatment started with external beam radiation therapy in 303 patients (median dose 45 Gy). After a rest period of 4 to 6 weeks, a boost of 20 Gy was delivered by EBRT in 279 patients and by interstitial ^{192}Ir brachytherapy in 17 patients. Seven patients received only one course of EBRT (mean dose 49.5 Gy) and two patients were treated with interstitial ^{192}Ir brachytherapy alone (55 and 60 Gy, respectively). Concomitant chemotherapy (5-fluorouracil and either mitomycin C or cisplatin) was delivered to 19 patients. Mean follow-up was 103 months. At the end of radiation therapy, local tumor clinical complete response rate was 80%. Out of 61 nonresponders or local progressive tumors, 27 (44%) were salvaged with abdominoperineal resection. The rate of local tumor relapse was 12%. Out of 37 local tumor relapse, 20 (54%) were salvaged with abdominoperineal resection

and one with interstitial ^{192}Ir brachytherapy. The overall local tumor control rate with or without salvage local treatment was 84%. Local control rate with a good anal function scoring (score 0 and 1) was 56.5%. Among 181/186 available patients who preserved their anuses, 94% had a good anal function. For a subgroup of 15 patients with length tumor <2 cm N0, the local control rate after the end of radiation therapy was 100%, the local control rate with or without local salvage treatment was 100%, and among 13 available patients who preserved their anuses, the anal function scoring was good in 12 patients (92%). The 10-year disease-free survival was 74%. After multivariate analysis, three independent factors significantly influenced the disease-free survival: gap duration between two courses of radiation therapy (>38 days vs. ≤38 days; $p = .0025$), pretreatment anal function scoring (0 vs. 1 vs. 2 vs. 3 vs. 4; $p = 4.4$ 10^{-6}), and clinical complete response after the end of radiation therapy (no complete response vs. complete response; $p = 2.5$ 10^{-14}). Interstitial implants with 10- to 15-cm nylon catheters for ^{192}Ir ribbons are used to treat patients with recurrent carcinoma of the rectum in the perineal and presacral fossa after abdominoperineal resection. Care should be exercised to direct the metallic guides initially inserted or catheters with a posterior orientation (5 to 10 degrees from the horizontal plane). In many instances, the needles find resistance from the sacrum; occasionally, the sources are inadvertently placed in the bladder. Occasionally, intraoperative implants have been performed at the time of resection of the recurrent tumor, which allows for better identification of the volume to be treated and placement of the catheters (Fig. 20.48).

A technique was described using intraoperative permanent ^{125}I brachytherapy in colorectal cancers recurrent in the pelvis and para-aortic nodes in 29 patients (206). All patients had undergone prior surgery; 72% had prior EBRT. The implanted residual tumor volume was microscopic in 38% and gross in 62%. The implanted area (median 25 cc) received a median minimal peripheral dose of 140 Gy. An omental pedicle was used to minimize irradiation of the bowel. Five patients received additional postimplant EBRT (20 to 50 Gy; median 30 Gy). The 4-year actuarial locoregional control rate was 18%, with a median time to local failure of 11 months (95% CI, 10 to 12 months). The first manifestation of disease progression in 52% of the patients was locoregional. In addition, 22 patients (75%) developed distant metastases. Overall survival was better for patients with smaller volume implants ($p = .007$), with a lower total activity implanted ($p = .0003$), with a smaller number of implanted sites ($p = .004$), and with microscopic residual disease ($p = .01$). Patients receiving additional EBRT also had a better prognosis ($p = .005$). Of the patients, 13 (45%) experienced 15 toxic events, including three patients (10%) with enteric fistula.

Penis and Male Urethra

Carcinoma of the penis is rare in the United States; therefore, experience in its treatment is scarce. Interstitial therapy with single- or double-plane implants has been used for small lesions of the glans or distal penis (Fig. 20.49). Doses of 60 to 70 Gy are delivered in 6 to 7 days with a dose rate of about 0.45 to 0.5 Gy per hour. Molds have been used, particularly in earlier years in Europe, but tumor control and functional results were not as satisfactory as with other irradiation techniques (159). Crook et al. (60) report results for 49 men with squamous cell carcinoma of the penis treated with primary penile interstitial brachytherapy. Fifty-one percent of tumors were T1, 33% T2, and 8% T3; 4% were *in situ* and 4% Tx. Grade was well differentiated in 31%, moderate in 45%, and poor in 2%; grade was unspecified for 20%. One tumor was verrucous. Four patients had a single plane implant with a plastic tube technique, and all others had a volume implant with predrilled acrylic templates and two or three parallel planes of needles. Dose rates

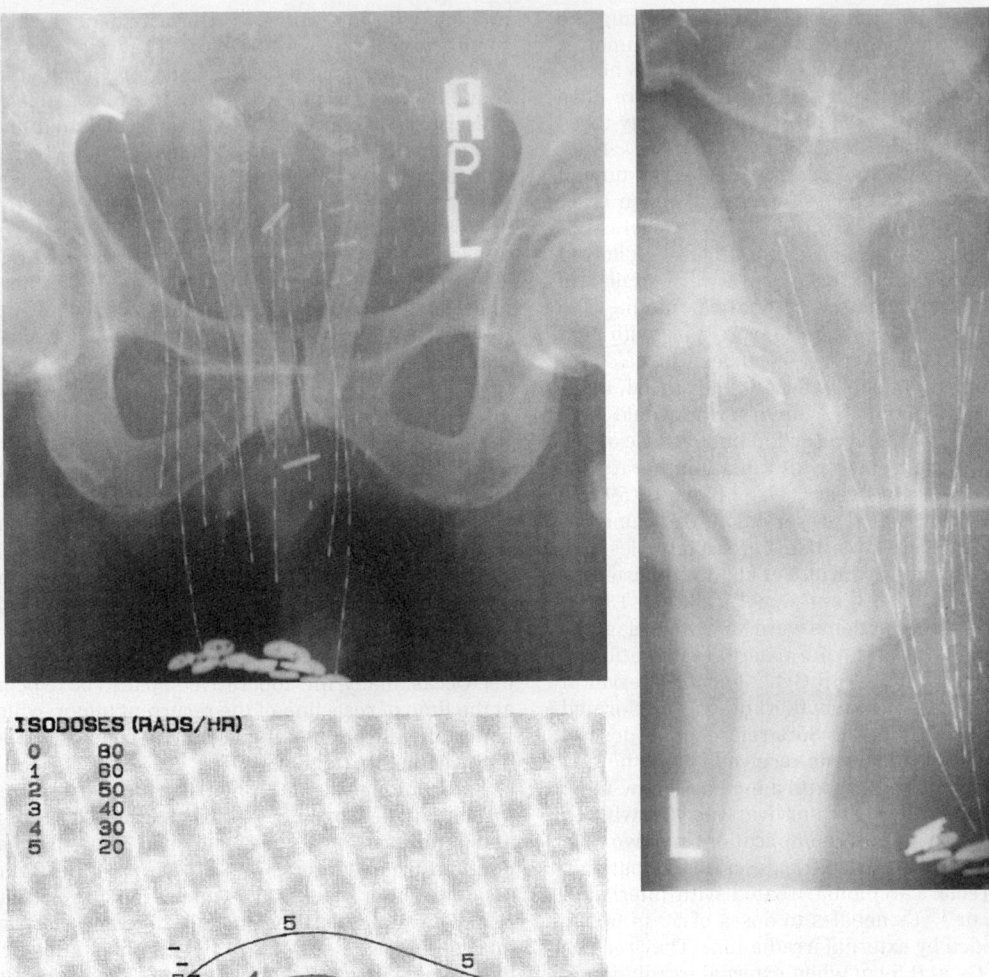

ISODOSES (RADS/HR)

0	80
1	60
2	50
3	40
4	30
5	20

FIGURE 20.48. Anteroposterior (**A**) and lateral (**B**) radiographs of interstitial implant performed intraoperatively with plastic catheters and ^{192}Ir in patient with recurrent carcinoma of the rectum in the posterior pelvis. The patient had received 45 Gy preoperatively a year earlier. **C:** Cross-section isodose curves of implant showing dose rate of approximately 40 cGy per hour. Additional 50 Gy was administered with the interstitial implant.

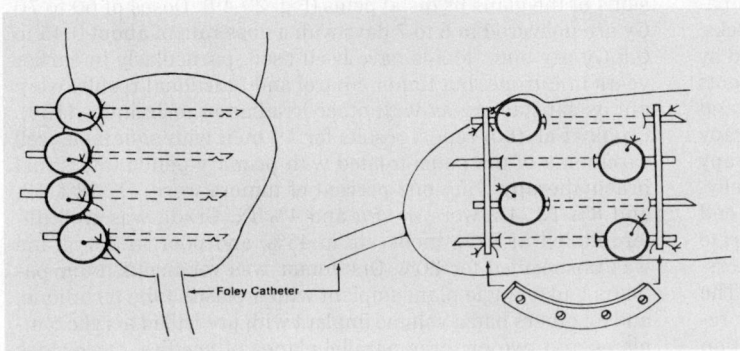

FIGURE 20.49. Diagram illustrating a one-end interstitial implant (*left*) or through-and-through interstitial implant with crossing needles and plate to secure the position of implant in carcinoma of the penis.

for PDR brachytherapy were 50 to 61.2 cGy per hour, with no correction in total dose, which was 60 Gy in all cases. After a median follow-up of 33.4 months, 5-year actuarial overall survival was 78.3% and cause-specific survival 90.0%. Four men died of penile cancer, and six died of other causes with no evidence of recurrence. The cumulative incidence rate for never having experienced any type of failure at 5 years was 64.4% and for local failure was 85.3%. All five patients with local failure were successfully salvaged by surgery; two other men required penectomy for necrosis. Of 49 men, 42 had an intact and tumor-free penis at last follow-up or death. The actuarial penile preservation rate at 5 years was 86.5%. Brachytherapy plays a significant role, often associated with external beam irradiation and surgery, in the conservative management of the male urethra cancer. Gerbaulet et al. (115) use a catheter or a vaginal mold applicator for intraluminal/intracavity brachytherapy, and hypodermic needles or guide gutters for the interstitial portion. The radioactive source usually employed is ^{192}Ir. The total dose administered is usually between 60 and 70 Gy. Disease-free survival is 50%, local control 70%, and the complication rate is 20%.

Prostate

The older retropubic techniques have been replaced by ultrasound or CT-guided transperineal techniques. Prostate brachytherapy may be temporary or permanent, and the planning techniques for either approach are similar. Nori and Moni (253) briefly discussed the advantages and limitations of each. Temporary techniques may be used with LDR or HDR applications. The basic steps include assessing prostate volume by any diagnostic modality (CT or ultrasonography), determining total activity needed to encompass the gland and deliver the appropriate minimum peripheral dose, and determining the pattern of placement of seeds within the gland. Preplanning may be done either by ultrasound or by CT. The operative technique requires the visualization of the prostate in three dimensions and usually is performed using a combination of ultrasound and fluoroscopy. Special circumstances that necessitate neoadjuvant hormonal therapy include interference from the pubic arch and large volume glands. Potency is preserved in >80% of patients. Patient selection criteria include the pretreatment prostate-specific antigen (PSA) level, tumor grade (Gleason), stage of disease, and presence or absence of bilateral positive biopsies and/or perineural invasion. We have divided patients with prostate cancer into good, intermediate, and poor risk groups. We recommend brachytherapy as the sole procedure for good risk patients and a combination of EBRT and brachytherapy for the intermediate risk group. Selection criteria for permanent implants are summarized in Table 20.7 (234). Currently, ^{125}I or ^{103}Pd are used for permanent implants (Table 20.8). Holm et al. (152) developed the transperineal implant technique for prostate cancer. Blasko et al. (29) popularized the technique in the United States. Nag et al. (233) and Potters (284) have reviewed the current status of permanent prostate brachytherapy.

Permanent Iodine-125 Implants: Retropubic Technique

Hilaris et al. (149) popularized the use of ^{125}I seeds for treatment of stage A (T1), B (T2), or occasionally C (T3) prostate carcinoma when the tumor size did not exceed 5 to 6 cm in average dimension. In patients with stage C tumors, implants with ^{125}I seeds are discouraged because of the difficulty of adequately irradiating the periprostatic extent of the tumor. The ^{125}I seeds were implanted permanently in the prostate through open retropubic laparotomy incision with the patient in a modified lithotomy position. An extraperitoneal bilateral pelvic lymphadenectomy was performed. Hilaris and Batata (145) described the implant

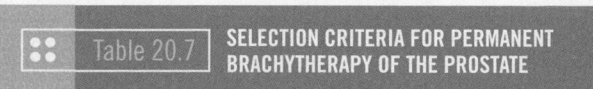

Table 20.7	SELECTION CRITERIA FOR PERMANENT BRACHYTHERAPY OF THE PROSTATE

Brachytherapy as monotherapy:
Stage: T1 to T2a and
Grade: Gleason sum 2–6 and
PSA ≤10 ng/mL

Brachytherapy as a boost to EBRT:
Stage: Clinical T2b, T2c *or*
Grade: Gleason sum 7–10 *or*
PSA >10 ng/mL

Brachytherapy (including boosting EBRT) in conjunction with androgen deprivation:
Patients with initially large prostate (>60 cc) that have downsized sufficiently
Clinical exclusion criteria:
Life expectancy <5 years
Large or poorly healed TURP defect
Unacceptable operative risks
Distant metastases

Relative contraindications for brachytherapy:
Patients not ideal candidates for brachytherapy, but nevertheless have been successfully implanted. Beginners should not implant these patients at increased risk of developing complications:
Large median lobes
High AUA score
History of multiple pelvic surgeries
Severe diabetes with healing problems

Technical difficulties that may result in inadequate dose coverage:
Gland size >60 cc at time of implantation
Positive seminal vesicles

AUA, American Urological Association; EBRT, external beam radiation therapy; PSA, prostate-specific antigen; TURP, transurethral resection of prostate.
Modified from Nag S, Beyer D, Friedland J, et al. American Brachytherapy Society (ABS) recommendations for transperineal permanent brachytherapy of prostate cancer. *Int J Radiat Oncol Biol Phys* 1999;44:789–799.

technique in detail. The methods for dose calculation and specification for ^{125}I implants were specified by Anderson (10) and Anderson and Aubrey (8). The MPD, defined as the dose enclosing a volume equal to the target volume, was recorded along with the integral dose within the MPD isodose surface. The prescribed dose for prostate treatment by implant only was 160 Gy in pre-TG-43 dose units (now more accurately identified as 145 Gy). Lower doses were prescribed for implants used as a boost to external beam therapy. The retropubic technique now has been replaced by the ultrasound-guided transperineal approach.

Transperineal Iodine-125 Implants

Several authors, including Blasko et al. (31), Holm et al. (152), and Wallner et al. (345), described the technique for ^{125}I or ^{103}Pd implants of the prostate using a transperineal approach under transrectal ultrasonography guidance. Implants are recommended for patients with a prostate volume <60 cm^3, no severe pubic arch interference, no severe urinary obstructive symptoms, and clinically intracapsular disease. Prior transurethral resection of the prostate is discouraged. The ABS has issued a detailed set of guidelines for transperineal prostate implants (233,234). The standard technique for transrectal ultrasonography–guided prostate implants involves a two-step approach. The initial step is a volume study of the prostate obtained for treatment planning purposes. The patient is placed in the lithotomy position, and a rectal ultrasound probe is inserted. The probe is part of a larger positioning system that includes a special needle-guidance template, which will be locked into a fixed position relative to the probe during the implant procedure (Fig. 20.50). The projected position of the template relative to the prostate images is shown on the ultrasound screen. After a near-central transverse image of the prostate is obtained, the probe can be repositioned with the aim of centralizing the

Table 20.8	RADIOISOTOPES USED FOR PROSTATE BRACHYTHERAPY					
	Energy (keV)	Half-Life (Days)	Initial Dose Rate (cGy/h)	Mean Activity Per Seed (mCi)	Monotherapy Dose (Gy)	Dose (Gy) Combined with EBRT[a]
Permanent						
Iodine-125	27	60.0	8	0.42	145	110
Palladium-103	21	17.0	20	1.30	125	100
Gold-198	412	2.7	64	—	60	—
Temporary						
Iridium-192	340	70.0	Highly variable	—	Variable (about 60)	20–25

EBRT, external beam radiation therapy.
[a]EBRT—Pelvis external irradiation, 40–45 Gy in 20–25 fractions.
Modified from Porter AT, Blasko JC, Grimm PD, et al. Brachytherapy for prostate cancer. *Ca Cancer J Clin* 1995;45:165–178.

prostate in the image and minimizing distortion by the probe. Further images can be obtained and repositioning can be carried out to ensure that through the course of images the urethra position does not move significantly relative to the template guide holes, which could obstruct the placement of needles in critical locations. After positioning is completed, a set of transverse images is recorded at 5-mm increments from the base to the apex (Fig. 20.51A). The patient then is released, and treatment planning is carried out. Using the projected guide hole locations as constraints, a seed distribution is generated, which is optimized in terms of prostate coverage while limiting the doses to the urethra and rectum. This generally will require that a large percentage of the seeds be placed at the periphery of the prostate capsule. Recommended prescribed doses for ^{125}I prostate implants are 145 Gy for implants used as the sole radiotherapy and 100 to 110 Gy for implants used as a boost to 40 to 50 Gy of external beam radiation. Seeds of the required number and activity to deliver the prescribed dose are ordered and, on receipt, calibrated and loaded in sterile needles (typically 18 gauge) along with absorbable spacers, according to the treatment plan. Sterile bone wax or other biodegradable material is used to stopper the ends of the needles. At the time of the implant, the patient again is placed in the lithotomy position, usually under spinal epidural anesthesia, and after appropriate sterilization of the skin and sterile draping, the rectal ultrasound probe is inserted and moved as nearly as possible to the same position used for the volume study. The template is locked into position against the perineum, and special fixation

needles are inserted (through guide holes not planned for use in the implant) to hold the prostate in position during the implant. With the ultrasound probe imaging the cephalad portion of the target volume first, loaded needles that have been planned to reach that depth are inserted one at a time, their position verified under ultrasound, and then withdrawn while holding the stylet in place to leave the seeds and spacers behind in the prostate. The probe then is withdrawn to the next image plane (usually 5 mm), and needles reaching that depth are inserted. The procedure is repeated until the entire prostate is filled with seeds according to the treatment plan. C-arm fluoroscopy often is used to check seed positions during and on completion of the planned implant. Extra seeds sometimes are inserted at this point to avoid underdosing in regions that appear to be deficient in seeds, possibly as a result of needle bending or unintended movement of the prostate during the implant. A few seeds may be placed in the urethra, and they usually are expelled within 24 hours, necessitating urine collection and monitoring after implantation. Merrick et al. (219) reported that about 10% of seeds lost from the pelvis were found to embolize to the lungs. The use of seeds in suture was found to minimize seed loss. A cystoscopy sometimes is carried out after the implant is completed to remove misplaced seeds and detect other possible problems. Many variants of the transperineal implant technique have been introduced, including the use of the Mick applicator for seed insertion instead of preloaded needles. Wallner et al. (345) described a CT method for transperineal implants that is integrated with transrectal ultrasonography for verification of correct needle placement at implantation. A more recent development features an intraoperative approach in which the volume study, treatment planning, applicator preparation, and implantation are carried out in a single operating room procedure. This technique offers a number of advantages over the two-step procedure. In addition to sparing the patient a second ultrasound probe insertion, it also eliminates the requirement for accurate repositioning of the patient and probe in the planned position before the implant. It further allows for possible modification of the treatment plan in response to needle divergence and other problems arising during the implant procedure. Zelefsky et al. (363) have reported significant improvement in target coverage using this technique. An ABS report on intraoperative planning and dosimetry for prostate implants has been published by Nag et al. (237). An intraoperative technique carried out under MRI has been described (56,62). MRI offers the advantages of excellent soft-tissue resolution with arbitrary imaging planes, although seed imaging with MRI is generally inferior to CT. A technique using magnetic resonance spectroscopy imaging also has been proposed for prostate implants (362). This technique introduces the possibility of identifying and applying elevated doses to small localized high-risk areas within the prostate capsule. Postimplant image-based dosimetry

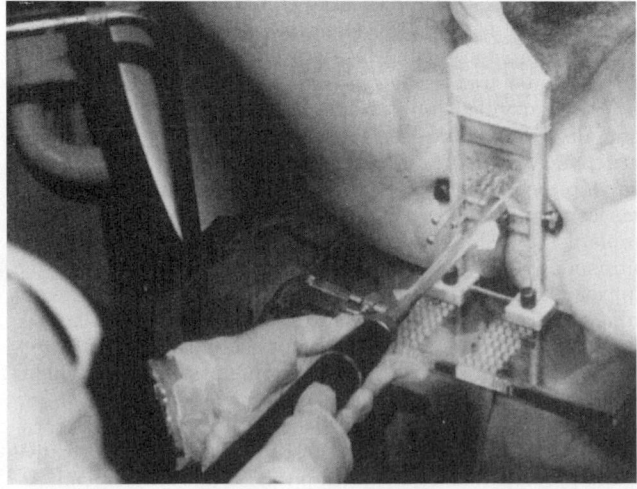

FIGURE 20.50. Prostate implant system including ultrasound unit with rectal probe, stepper unit controlling probe movement, and perineal template.

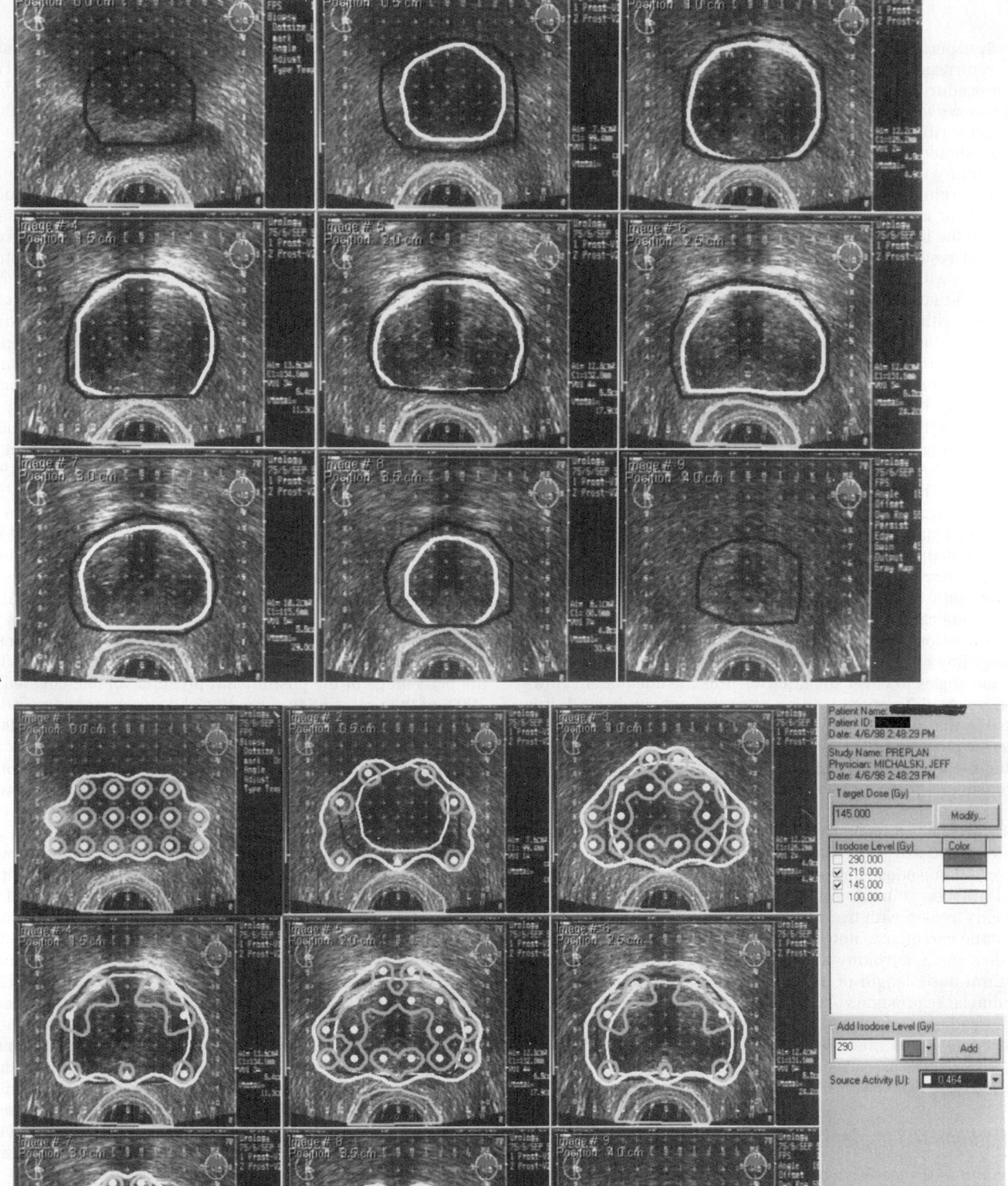

FIGURE 20.51. **A:** Ultrasound volume study for preimplant dosimetry. The prostate is contoured in white, and the planning target volume margin is in black. The margin is larger at the prostate base and apex to account for three-dimensional changes in the gland contours. Posteriorly, there is no margin because the ultrasound probe contacts the rectal wall and prostate directly. **B:** A preplant treatment plan using the modified uniform loading technique described by Merrick et al. (Merrick GS, Butler WM, Dorsey AT, et al. Prostatic conformal brachytherapy: [125]I [103]Pd postoperative dosimetric analysis. *Radiat Oncol Invest* 1994;5:305–313). Isodose curves displayed are 150% and 100%. Source positions are represented by the points on the grid. Alternate slices are loaded heavily or peripherally. The periurethral sources have been removed to decrease the dose to that organ. (From Perez CA, Michalski JM, Martinez AA. Prostate. In: Levitt SH, Kahn FM, Potish RA, et al., eds. *Levitt & Tapley's technological basis of radiation therapy clinical applications*, 3rd ed. Philadelphia: Lippincott Williams & Wilkins, 1999;435–465, with permission.)

usually is performed on every patient. For this purpose, the patient returns a few days or weeks after the implant for an imaging procedure, usually CT and/or orthogonal films. The films may be used for planning but are more useful for seed count and position verification when CT or MRI planning is used. The CT images should include all relevant critical structures and seeds in proximity to the prostate. ABS guidelines (233) recommend that a margin of at least 2 cm should be added to the superior and inferior aspects of the prostate. The optimal time interval between the implant procedure and postimplant dosimetry has not been resolved at this time. Postoperative edema appears to resolve with a half-life of about 10 days (235). It has been suggested that the most reproducible dosimetric results can be obtained with a postoperative interval of 1 month. After the seeds have been identified on the cross-sectional images, isodose curves are generated on all slices imaging the prostate (Fig. 20.51B). The original ABS guidelines for transperineal prostate implants (234) recommended that the items to be recorded and correlated with outcome were the prescribed dose, the MPD, the dose covering 90% of the prostate volume (D90), and the percentage of the prostate volume receiving the prescription dose or greater (V100). The later ABS report on postimplant dosimetry (235) suggested a much more elaborate reporting scheme based on detailed information from dose–volume histograms and included urethral and rectal doses. Several technical details may have an impact on tumor control of prostate cancer treated with brachytherapy. Because of patient anatomy, the pubic bone can interfere with the direct placement of sources in the interior prostate, and this potentially can cause underdosing. Roy et al. (295) recommend that needles be placed at oblique angles to cover the anterior prostate adequately. However, unless differential loading of source activity is used, it is possible that high doses may be delivered to the central and anterior portions of the gland (61). However, rapid dose falloff in the most peripheral portion of the gland may result in underdosing of posterior, peripheral prostate cancer or overdosing of the anterior rectal wall. Roy et al. (296), in an analysis of 10 prostate implants with CT-planned and fluoroscopically guided radioactive ^{125}I seed placement, found that the 150 Gy prescription isodose line encompassed only 78% to 96% of the total prostate volume. Wallner et al. (346), in a review of 65 patients treated with transperineal ^{125}I implants for T1 and T2 prostatic carcinoma, noted that a greater incidence of urinary grade 2 and 3 morbidity was associated with maximum central urethral dose, length of urethra that received more than 400 Gy, and large prostate volume. Rectal ulceration was associated with irradiation of the rectal wall to doses of more than 100 Gy. Efforts should be made to keep the central urethral dose below 150% of the prescribed minimal peripheral dose and rectal surface dose below 80% to decrease toxicity.

Palladium-103 Implants

Palladium-103 seeds have been in use for permanent implants for a number of years. The ^{103}Pd seeds are physically similar to ^{125}I seeds, so the equipment and implant techniques used with ^{125}I seeds also can be used with ^{103}Pd. The main differences in the seeds are the cost (^{103}Pd is more expensive) and the fact that the ^{103}Pd seed has a slightly lower photon energy (21 keV vs. 28 keV for ^{125}I seeds) and a significantly shorter half-life at 18 days (compared with 60 days for ^{125}I seeds). These differences in energy and half-life require corresponding changes in dose prescription and planning techniques. Because tissue tolerance is a function of dose rate as well as total dose, an adjustment of the prescription dose must be made when using ^{103}Pd rather than ^{125}I for an implant. Radiobiologic modeling suggests that a prescription dose of 125 Gy with ^{103}Pd should be equivalent to the 145 Gy prescribed with ^{125}I for implants alone. For implants used as a boost to 40 to 50 Gy of external beam ther-

apy, a ^{103}Pd prescription dose of 90 to 100 Gy is recommended (30,234,250). Because of its shorter half-life, a higher initial activity of ^{103}Pd must be used, resulting in a typical initial dose rate of about 18 to 20 cGy per hour for ^{103}Pd used as sole therapy, compared with about 7 cGy per hour for ^{125}I. At 5 weeks after implantation, the ^{103}Pd will have delivered approximately 76% of the total dose, whereas an ^{125}I implant will have delivered only 33% of its intended total dose. Because of the more rapid dose delivery with ^{103}Pd, this isotope is more commonly used for higher grade malignancy (Gleason score >6), whereas ^{125}I is preferred for lower grades (286). Although some studies have tended to confirm the greater effectiveness of ^{103}Pd in poorly differentiated tumors (245), further work is needed to demonstrate this advantage conclusively. The lower photon energy of ^{103}Pd results in a greater degree of attenuation of the dose relative to ^{125}I. This difference in dose falloff becomes more pronounced as the distance from the seed increases, and it must be taken into consideration in treatment planning for ^{103}Pd implants (30,249,250). ABS guidelines recommend a seed spacing no >1.7 cm when ^{103}Pd is used (234). Herstein et al. (143) evaluated 352 of a planned total of 600 patients with 1997 American Joint Committee on Cancer (AJCC) clinical stage T1c or T2a prostatic carcinoma (Gleason grade 2 to 6, PSA 4 to 10 ng/mL) had been randomized to implantation with ^{125}I (144 Gy, TG-43) or ^{103}Pd (125 Gy, NIST-99). Treatment-related morbidity was monitored by questionnaires based on standard American Urologic Association (AUA) and RTOG criteria that were mailed at 1, 3, 6, 12, 18, and 24 months after implant. All patients reported here had a minimum follow-up of 2 years. Dosimetric parameters analyzed included the V100, which was defined as the percentage of the postimplant prostate volume covered by 100% of the prescription dose. Rectal doses were expressed as the R100, defined as the rectal volume (cc) that received at least 100% of the prescription dose. The AUA scores peaked at the 1-month postimplant time point for both isotopes and gradually declined. The difference in AUA scores between patients who received ^{125}I versus those who received ^{103}Pd was greatest at 1 and 6 months following implantation. At 1 month, ^{125}I patients had a mean AUA score of 14.8 (+/– 9.5) compared with 20.6 (+/– 9.8) for the ^{103}Pd patients ($p = .0009$). By 6 months, mean AUA scores for the ^{125}I patients had decreased to 12.0 (+/– 9.1) compared with 9.9 (+/– 8.7) for the ^{103}Pd patients ($p = .04$). Radiation proctitis (persistent bleeding) occurred in 29/314 patients (9%). There was an overall trend toward more proctitis in ^{125}I patients ($p = .21$). However, 4/163 patients (2%) with an R100 below the recommended 1.0 cc developed bleeding, which did not differ between isotopes ($p = .49$). Patients treated with ^{103}Pd had more intense radiation prostatitis in the first month after implantation, but they recovered from their radiation-related symptoms sooner than ^{125}I patients, consistent with palladium's shorter half-life. The trend toward more proctitis in the ^{125}I patient group likely reflects their higher R100 values due to less rapid dose falloff that can be overcome with judicious treatment planning and implant execution.

Gold Grain Permanent Implants

Carlton et al. (36) described a technique to implant a smaller number of radioactive colloidal gold grains in the prostate gland to deliver approximately 35 Gy. This was combined with 40 Gy of external irradiation.

Removable Interstitial Implants with Iridium-192

Charyulu (41) and Syed et al. (325) developed an interstitial implant technique using removable ^{192}Ir sources with a transperineal template for the treatment of carcinoma of the prostate. In the technique of Syed et al., a bilateral pelvic lymphadenectomy is carried out without mobilization of the prostate. With

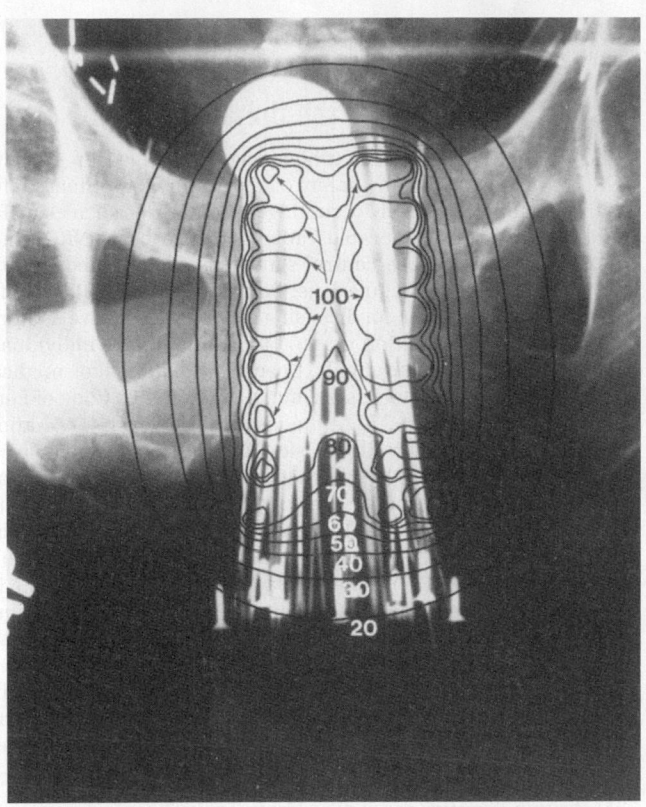
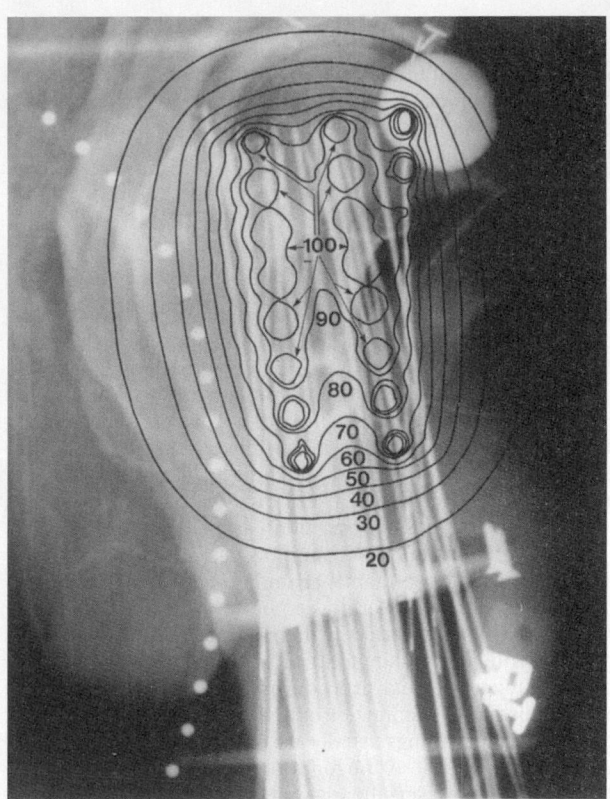

FIGURE 20.52. Postimplant isodose curves for ultrasound-guided ^{192}Ir transperineal prostate implant.

the patient in a semilithotomy position, a bladder catheter with a Foley bag containing 10 mL of Hypaque solution is inserted. The prostate template is placed in the perineum, and metallic guides are inserted transperianally through the prostate and seminal vesicles (if indicated). The tip of the source guides is usually 1 cm above the level of the bladder neck. The template is fixed to the perineum by 2-0 silk sutures. The hollow guides are loaded with inactive dummy sources for x-ray localization films, which are taken in anteroposterior and lateral orthogonal projections. Usually seven seeds of radioactive ^{192}Ir, spaced 1 cm apart in either ribbon, are loaded into each of 18 guides placed through the template (Fig. 20.52). Activity of the iridium sources in the central guides is about 0.25 to 0.3 mg Ra Eq and in the outer 12 guides, 0.4 to 0.5 mg Ra Eq per seed. Dose rate per hour is 0.7 to 0.9 Gy, with the bladder neck and rectum receiving only 0.3 to 0.4 Gy per hour. The implant is removed after 30 to 35 Gy are delivered (40 to 45 hours). After the interstitial irradiation is completed, the radioactive sources are withdrawn with long forceps, and the template is removed with all guides in place, after the perineal sutures are transected. The Foley catheter is removed 1 day later. This interstitial therapy is combined with 40 Gy of external irradiation to the pelvis. Their results and some modification of technique have been updated by Puthawala et al. (289). Martinez et al. (204) and Brindle et al. (34), in an update of the initial publication, described implantation of the prostate with a perineal template (MUPIT). A bilateral staging pelvic lymphadenectomy is performed; the length of metallic guides is determined by palpation, and palpable tumor margins are identified with inactive gold seeds. In a modification of the technique, the first needle is placed with the guidance of a finger in the rectum to prevent piercing of that organ. A rectal tube is inserted to help position the template to allow for proper spacing of the rest of the needles. The template is aligned parallel to the floor of the pelvis, not conforming to the perineal slope, to avoid posterior angling of the

needles. The needles are differentially loaded with ^{192}Ir seeds on nylon ribbons on which activity, number of seeds, and the use of ribbon spacers all vary. The posterior needles, in particular, which are primarily directed to the seminal vesicles, are loaded only in the superior half. The implant dose is 33 Gy, which is combined with external irradiation (5 Gy in one dose before the implant and 30 Gy in 18 fractions after the implant). Nickers et al. (251) evaluated the feasibility of combining EBRT and LDR brachytherapy in 71 patients with prostate cancer in a dose escalation trial from 74 to 85 Gy performed in four groups. Shifting from intraoperative placement of source vectors (group I) to positioning under ultrasound controls (groups II to IV), improving the implantation shape, and optimizing radiation delivery to the urethral bed reduced the total dose to the rectal wall to <65 Gy and to the urethra to <100 Gy. Rectal/prostate dose ratio was lowered from 0.7 (groups I to II) to 0.58 (groups III to IV) while avoiding problems resulting from pelvic bone arch interference, prostate volume, or location of seminal vesicles. The mean and median follow-up periods are 28 and 18 months. In groups III and IV, 85% of patients without hormone therapy treated with 80 to 85 Gy experienced a normalized PSA under 1 ng/mL within 6 months. No severe late effect had been noted for patients implanted under echographic control. Longer follow-up is needed, but the dose delivered up to 85 Gy was not expected to induce prohibitive side effects.

Interstitial Irradiation and Hyperthermia

Bagshaw et al. (16) reported a combination of ^{192}Ir and hyperthermia in 13/32 patients treated with brachytherapy. The technique is similar to that described by other authors, except for the introduction of the hyperthermia trocars, which are energized with 0.5 MHz microwave radio frequency for 45 minutes to achieve 42°C to 44.5°C throughout the prostate.

Endovascular Brachytherapy

A new application of brachytherapy is to prevent restenosis after coronary angioplasty, stenting, peripheral vascular bypass surgery, or access procedures for renal dialysis. This topic is discussed in detail in Chapter 86.

Quality Assurance and Radiation Safety in Brachytherapy

It is extremely important in the use of brachytherapy to formulate and strictly observe radiation safety procedures at each institution in compliance with U.S. NRC regulations. The safety of personnel, patients, and visitors is based on three factors: keeping time of radiation exposure as short as possible, making distance as great as practically allowed between the radioactive sources and the operator, and shielding to diminish radiation exposure to all concerned. Careful quality control procedures should be followed in the prescription and calculation of doses; preparation, calibration, and handling of radioactive sources; and verification of treatment parameters. If promptly discovered, an error in brachytherapy can be corrected, but it is more difficult to do than in external beam irradiation. At the Radiation Oncology Center of Washington University's Mallinckrodt Institute of Radiology, formal procedures for brachytherapy have been established to minimize treatment errors. For temporary implants, source loadings usually are prescribed after the physician has reviewed the orthogonal dummy source-localization radiographs. The prescription is written on a form that is given to the brachytherapy source curator specifying the configuration of source strengths for intracavitary treatment or the array of active lengths and linear activity if iridium wires or seed ribbons are used for interstitial techniques (Fig. 20.53). Treatment duration generally is determined after reviewing the computer planar isodose rate distributions and is double-checked with "hand calculations." The source curator documents the preparation of sources in a treatment logbook, on a source inventory sheet that is to be posted on the patient's door, and also on a magnetic source inventory board in the radioactive source room. If iridium is used, the vendor's lot identification code also is documented. A well-type re-entrant ion chamber is used to verify the source activity in accord with the recent AAPM recommendations (4,358). When manual intracavitary afterloading is used, for the sake of prompt patient loading, the various cesium tubes are color coded. The attending physician or resident (after verifying the source loading) and the source curator load the applicator into the patient. The loading time is documented by the physician, and the curator or physicist measures the radiation exposure levels around the patient and arranges lead shields appropriately. The nursing division is also actively involved in checking every 3 to 4 hours that applicators or sources do not become dislodged over the course of treatment. For further discussion of LDR brachytherapy quality assurance techniques and programs, the reader is referred to a review by Williamson et al. (359) and published AAPM recommendations (4–6). The physician's orders sheet contains the home telephone number and the pager number of at least two physicians who can be contacted in an emergency if source removal is required. The attending physician or resident is responsible for the unloading of the implant. The physician counts the sources as they are removed and places them in a lead carrier. After removal of the sources, the patient is surveyed to ensure that no sources remain in the patient or in the patient's room. The time of unloading is documented, and all radiation warning signs are removed from the patient's door. The source curator checks that all sources have been recovered and returns the sources to their designated storage area. The magnetic inventory board is revised to show that the sources have been returned to their storage area. Additionally, source recovery is documented in the source logbook.

Safety Regulations in the United States

The U.S. NRC and states that have negotiated agreements with NRC regulate the use and safety of all reactor by-product materials (excluding naturally occurring radionuclides such as ^{226}Ra and electronically generated radiation). The basic NRC functions such as exposure control standards are outlined in Title 10 Code of Federal Regulations, Part 20 (10 CFR 20). Specific regulations also exist for licensing use of radioactive materials through authorization granted to institutions or individuals meeting specific requirements. Specific regulations for medical use of by-product materials are outlined in Title 10 Code of Federal Regulations, Part 35. At the institutional level, a radiation safety committee and radiation safety officer are responsible for supervising the use of by-product materials and seeing that all NRC license requirements are in compliance. The NRC mandates an institutional Quality Management Program philosophy aimed to zero incidence of misadministrations or recordable events (see Table 20.7). When misadministration occurs, the licensee is required to report to NRC by phone within 24 hours and in writing within 15 days; the patient and referring physician should be informed verbally within 24 hours and by written report within 15 days, or if informing the patient is medically harmful, a relative or friend of the patient must be selected to receive this information. The Quality Management Program must include procedures to meet the following goals:

(a) Written directive is prepared before initiating each radionuclide treatment (sealed or unsealed sources);

(b) Patient is identified before treatment by at least two different methods;

(c) Plan of treatment and calculations agree with the written directive;

(d) Each administration is in accord with the written directive; and

(e) All unintended deviations from the written directive are identified.

A Quality Management Program review must be conducted at least annually to determine compliance and whether modifications are required. Review should include all recordable events and misadministrations and an audit of representative sample cases treated. For HDR or PDR procedures, the NRC requires the presence of an authorized radiation oncologist and physicist at all times when a procedure is being performed. Imaging or techniques must be in place to verify source position and accuracy before performing a procedure. A physicist must verify the accuracy of plan input data, dose calculation, and information transfer. Before treatment, the technologist verifies treatment site, isotope, total dose, dose per fraction and treatment modality, program sequence of source positions, and dwell times (which must agree with the treatment plan calculation); the technologist also must verify that HDR treatment channels are correctly connected to corresponding applicators. After treatment, the attending physician must review the record and sign forms as required. A more detailed review of NRC regulations on medical use of by-product materials is given by Benedetto (24). For other (non-HDR) brachytherapy procedures, there are similar requirements. In addition, for manual afterloading intracavitary sources color coding or serial number must identify the sources; ideally, a second person should verify the correct loading of the applicator. For ^{192}Ir, ^{103}Pd, ^{125}I, or other radionuclides, verification of batch number and a pot calibration check must be performed. Misadministrations with remote afterloading devices occur, although fortunately they are rare. These devices and their operation are complex, and a mishap may have severe or fatal complications.

A

Barnes Radiation Oncology Center
Mallinckrodt Institute of Radiology

CAUTION

Intracavitary LDR Brachytherapy Prescription

Name: ________ Birthdate: ___/___/___ SS#: ___/___/___
Rad. Onc. No.: ________ Ref. Physician: ________ Implant No: ________
Primary Site: ________ ☐ Manual Afterloading ☐ Remote Afterloader
Applicators: ________ ☐ LDR-6 (SN 0264) ☐ LDR-3 (SN 0296)

Sounding ____ cm Nominal Source Configuration		Order of Heyman Capsule Insertion	Channel No.	Selectron Remote Afterloading Source Configuration (Indicate Radioactive Pellets •) Channel ___	Channel ___	Channel ___
Preplanned	Actual					
		1				
		2				
		3				
		4				
		5				
		6				
		7				
		8				
		9				
		10				
		11				
		12				
		13				
		14				
		15				
		16				
		17				
		18				
		19				
		20				

Isotope ____ No. Sources: ________
Total Source Strength ________ mgRaEq
Prescription approved: ________ ,MD ____ Date
Modifications: ________
________ , MD ____ Date
Implant removed Time ____ Date ____ by ____
Actual treatment. hrs ____
mR/h over Bkgd on surface, post-treatment: ________
Treatment delivered as prescribed:
________ , MD ____ Date

Applicator				
Trmnt. Time (hrs)				
RSD (cGy)		XXX		
mgRaEq-h				
Total mgRaEq-h				
I	Time			
N	Day			
	Date			
O	Time			
U	Day			
T	Date			

Physicist Review: ________ Date ________

2751-36 rev. 7/94

B

Barnes Radiation Oncology Center
Mallinckrodt Institute of Radiology

CAUTION

Interstitial Brachytherapy Prescription

Name: ________ Birthdate: ___/___/___ SS#: ___/___/___
Rad. Onc. No.: ________ Ref. Physician: ________ Implant No: ________
Primary Site: ________ Applicators: ________
☐ Temporary ☐ Permanent Seed Spacing in Ribbon ________

Implant Geometry	Catheter Number	Model No.	Batch No.	☐mCi ☐ mgRaEq per seed at loading	Number of Seeds	Spacer Length
Preplanned	1					
	2					
	3					
	4					
	5					
	6					
	7					
	8					
	9					
Actual	10					
	11					
	12					
	13					
	14					
	15					
	16					
	17					
	18					
	19					
	20					

Isotope ________ Total No. Seeds ________
Treatment Time ☐ ____ hours (Temporary) ☐ Forever (Permanent)
Total ☐ mCi ☐ mgRaEq at Loading: ________
Prescribed dose for temporary implant: ____ cGy
☐ to ____ cGy/h isodose or ☐ to ________

	IN	OUT
TIME		
DAY		
DATE		

Prescription approved: ________ , MD Date ____ Physicist Review ____ Date ____
Prescription Modifications: ________
________ MD Date ____

Implant Removal (Temporary only)
Sources removed at: Date ____ Time: ____ Actual Treatment Time: ____ hours
Patient Survey: mR/h above background at surface: ____ Signed: ________

Treatment Delivered As Prescribed: ________ ,MD ____ Date

2751-35 rev. 7/94

C

Barnes Radiation Oncology Center
Mallinckrodt Institute of Radiology

RADIOPHARMACEUTICAL THERAPY CAUTION
Prescription and Treatment Record

Name: ________ Birthdate: ___/___/___ SS#: ___/___/___
Rad. Onc. No.: ________ Ref. Physician: ________ Fraction No: ____ of ____
Primary Site: ________

PRESCRIPTION

Agent		Form		Route of Administration	
Sodium Iodide (I-131)	☐	Solution	☐	Oral	☐
Chromic Phosphate (P-32)	☐	Colloid	☐	Instillation	☐
Sodium Phosphate (P-32)	☐	Solution	☐	Intravenous	☐
Strontium Chloride (Sr-89) (Metastron)	☐	Solution	☐	Intravenous	☐
Other: ________	☐	____	☐	____	☐

Prescribed Activity ____ mCi

Physician Signature ________ Date ________

Measured Activity ____ mCi on treatment date ____ for proposed administered volume of ____ ml
Physicist Signature ________ Date ________

ADMINISTRATION

Agent Administered		Form used		Route of Administration	
Sodium Iodide (I-131)	☐	Solution	☐	Oral	☐
Chromic Phosphate (P-32)	☐	Colloid	☐	Instillation	☐
Sodium Phosphate (P-32)	☐	Solution	☐	Intravenous	☐
Strontium Chloride (Sr-89) (Metastron)	☐	Solution	☐	Intravenous	☐
Other: ________	☐	____	☐	____	☐

Quantity Administered
Activity Administered ____ mCi
Volume Administered ____ ml
Administered by ________
Date ____ Time ____
Initial mR/h @1 m (^{131}I only) ____

POST TREATMENT REVIEW

Exposure Rate (mR/h @ 1 m) at discharge (^{131}I only) ____ Date ____ Time ____
☐ Treatment delivered as prescribed ________ , MD Date ________

2751-32 rev. 7/94

D

BARNES RADIATION ONCOLOGY CENTER
MALLINCKRODT INSTITUTE OF RADIOLOGY
RADIOPHARMACEUTICAL THERAPY
QUALITY ASSURANCE CHECK-OFF LIST

Name: ________ Radiation Oncology No.: ________
Date of Procedure: ________ Isotope: ________ Form: ________

Pre-Treatment Checklist: ^{131}I ONLY
☐ TSH Date ____ Value ____ | ☐ Thyroglobulin Value ____ | ☐ On Synthroid? ☐ Yes ☐ No | ☐ Diagnostic Scan ☐ Done ☐ NA

Pre-Treatment Checklist: All Radiopharmaceuticals
☐ Pregnancy Test ☐ Negative ☐ Positive | ☐ Breast Feeding ☐ Yes ☐ No | ☐ Lactating ☐ Yes ☐ No | ☐ Diagnosis of Malignancy Verfied Path Report No. ________ Hospital ________

PREPARATION

☐ Procedure Scheduled ☐ Isotope Ordered (Date: ____ / ____ mCi) ☐ Room Assigned ☐ Isotope Calibrated

EXECUTION OF TREATMENT
☐ Informed consent signed
☐ Prescription signed and dated by authorized physician
☐ Prescribed and labeled activity compared by physician (outside patient's room)
☐ For γemitters: measured and prescribed activity agree within 10%
☐ For βemitters: vendor and prescribed activity agree within 10%
☐ Patient identified by two methods (check two) (☐ name, ☐ SS#, ☐ DOB ☐ photo, ☐ other ____)

TREATMENT EXECUTION
☐ Nursing orders written
☐ Source Preparation Area Surveyed
☐ Room posted
☐ Radiation survey completed (^{131}I only)

DISCHARGE INFORMATION (^{131}I only)
☐ Patient survey completed
☐ Initial survey
☐ 2nd day survey
☐ Discharge survey
☐ Physician aware of final survey exposure rate
☐ <5 mR/h at 1 m
☐ <30 mCi
☐ Room posted for radiation safety; survey forms completed and filed
☐ Scan scheduled prior to discharge ☐ Yes ☐ No

POST TREATMENT DOCUMENTATION AND AUDIT
☐ Procedure billed
☐ Administration documented on treatment record
☐ Signatures completed including post treatment signatures
☐ Filed in therapy chart

COMMENTS: ________

2751-51 Rev 7/94

FIGURE 20.53. Brachytherapy prescription sheet used at Mallinckrodt Institute of Radiology. The configuration of the source loading in the various channels of remote-control afterloading applications can be indicated in the appropriate section. **A:** Low–dose-rate intracavitary brachytherapy. **B:** Interstitial brachytherapy. **C:** Radiopharmaceutical therapy. **D:** Quality assurance checklist.

To prevent such occurrences, strictly followed safety and quality assurance procedures are mandatory. For a concise review, the reader is referred to a publication by Glasgow (117).

References

1. Abrath FG, Henderson SD, Simpson JR, et al. Dosimetry of CT-guided volumetric Ir-192 brain implant. *Int J Radiat Oncol Biol Phys* 1986;12:539.
2. Alden ME, Mohiuddin M. The impact of radiation dose in combined external beam and intraluminal Ir-192 brachytherapy for bile duct cancer. *Int J Radiat Oncol Biol Phys* 1994;28:945–951.
3. Allt WEC, Hunt JW. Experience with radioactive tantalum wire as a source for interstitial therapy. *Radiology* 1963;80:581.
4. American Association of Physicists in Medicine. *Comprehensive QA for radiation oncology.* Report of the AAPM Radiation Therapy Committee Task Group 40 (J Kutcher, Chairman). *Med Phys* 1994;21:581–618.
5. American Association of Physicists in Medicine. Dosimetry of interstitial brachytherapy sources. Recommendations of the AAPM Radiation Therapy Committee Task Group No. 43. (R. Nath, Chairman). *Med Phys* 1995;22:209–234.
6. American Association of Physicists in Medicine. Remote afterloading technology. Report of the Radiation Therapy Task Group No. 41 (G. Glasgow, Chairman). New York: American Institute of Physics, 1993.
7. Ampuero F, Doss LL, Khan LM, et al. The Syed-Neblett interstitial template in locally advanced gynecological malignancies. *Int J Radiat Oncol Biol Phys* 1983;9:1897–1903.
8. Anderson LL, Aubrey RF. Computerized dosimetry for ^{125}I prostate implants. In: Hilaris BS, Batata MA, eds. *Brachytherapy oncology—1983.* New York: Memorial Sloan-Kettering Cancer Center, 1983;57–63.
9. Anderson LL, Hilaris BS, Wagner LK. A nomograph for planar implant planning. *Endocurie Hypertherm Oncol* 1985;1:9–15.
10. Anderson LL. A spacing nomograph for interstitial implants of I-125 seeds. *Med Phys* 1976;3:48–51.
11. Aristizabal SA, Valencia A, Ocampo G, et al. Interstitial parametrial irradiation in cancer of the cervix stage IIB–IIIB. *Endocurie Hypertherm Oncol* 1985;1:41.
12. Armadur RJ, Piontek R, Hadley VE, et al. A simple, inexpensive applicator for irradiation of localized areas of the vagina with intracavitary brachytherapy. *Int J Radiat Oncol Biol Phys* 1997;37:965–969.
13. Ashayeri E, Collier-Manning J, Nibhanupudy JR, et al. Localization technique and afterloading intracavitary irradiation in the treatment of nasopharyngeal carcinoma. *Endocurie Hypertherm Oncol* 1987;3:115–119.
14. Astrahan MA. Improved treatment planning for COMS eye plaques. *Int J Radiat Oncol Biol Phys* 2005;61(4):1227–1242.
15. Bachtiary B, Dewitt A, Pintilie M, et al. Comparison of late toxicity between continuous low-dose-rate and pulsed-dose-rate brachytherapy in cervical cancer patients. *Int J Radiat Oncol Biol Phys* 2005;63(4):1077–1082.
16. Bagshaw MA, Kaplan ID, Cox RC. Radiation therapy for localized disease. *Cancer* 1993;71:939–952.
17. Baillet F, Decroix Y, Mazeron JJ. Oral tongue. In: Pierquin B, Wilson J-F, Chassagne D, eds. *Modern brachytherapy.* New York: Masson, 1987;107–118.
18. Bastin K, Buchler D, Stitt J, et al. Resource utilization: high dose rate versus low dose rate brachytherapy for gynecologic cancer. *Am J Clin Oncol* 1993;16:256–263.
19. Batley F, Constable WC. The use of the "Manchester system" for treatment of cancer of the uterine cervix with modern after-loading radium applicators. *J Can Assoc Radiol* 1967;18:396.
20. Battermann JJ, Boon TA. Interstitial therapy in the management of T2 bladder tumors. *Endocurie Hypertherm Oncol* 1988;4:1–6.
21. Battermann JJ, Boon TA. Treatment of T2 bladder tumours with interstitial therapy: the role of lymph node dissection. In: Mould RF, ed. *Brachytherapy 2.* Leersum, The Netherlands: Nucletron International BV, 1989;187–191.
22. Battermann JJ, Szabol B. Preliminary results of radiation therapy for carcinoma of the uterine cervix, using the Selectron afterloading machine. In: Mould RF, ed. *Brachytherapy 2.* Leersum, The Netherlands: Nucletron International BV, 1989;229–234.
23. Battermann JJ, Tierie AH. Results of implantation for T1 and T2 bladder tumours. *Radiother Oncol* 1986;5:85–90.
24. Benedetto A. The brachytherapy regulatory environment: organization of radiation safety program. In: Williamson JF, Thomadsen BR, Nath R, eds. *Brachytherapy physics.* American Association of Physicists in Medicine, 1994 Summer School. Madison, WI: Medical Physics Publishing, 1995;163–184.
25. Benedict SH, Lin PS, Zwicker RD, et al. The biological effectiveness of intermittent irradiation as a function of overall treatment time: development of correction factors for linac based stereotactic radiotherapy. *Int J Radiat Oncol Biol Phys* 1997;37(4):765–769.
26. Bergman L, Nilsson B, Lundell G. Ruthenium brachytherapy for uveal melanoma 1979–2003. Survival and functional outcomes in the Swedish population. *Ophthalmology* 2005;112:5;834–840.
27. Bernstein M, Gutin PH. Interstitial irradiation of brain tumors: a review. *Neurosurgery* 1981;9:741–750.
28. Bernstein M, Laperriere N. Indications for brachytherapy for brain tumors. *Acta Neurochir* 1995;63:25–28.
29. Blasko J, Ragde H, Grimm PD. Transperineal ultrasound-guided implantation of the prostate: morbidity and complications. *Scand J Urol Nephrol* 1991;137[Suppl]:113–118.
30. Blasko JC, Grimm PD, Sylvester JE, et al. Palladium-103 brachytherapy for prostate carcinoma. *Int J Radiat Oncol Biol Phys* 2000;46:839–850.
31. Blasko JC, Radge H, Schumacher D. Transperineal percutaneous iodine-125 implantation for prostatic carcinoma using transrectal ultrasound and template guidance. *Endocurie Hypertherm Oncol* 1987;3:131–139.
32. Brenner DJ, Hall EJ. Conditions for the equivalence of continuous to pulsed low dose rate brachytherapy. *Int J Radiat Oncol Biol Phys* 1991;20:181–190.
33. Brenner DJ, Schiff PB, Huant Y, et al. Pulsed-dose-rate brachytherapy: design of convenient (daytime-only) schedules. *Int J Radiat Oncol Biol Phys* 1997;39:809–815.
34. Brindle JS, Martinez A, Schray M, et al. Pelvic lymphadenectomy and transperineal interstitial implantation of ^{192}Ir combined with external beam radiotherapy for bulky stage C prostatic carcinoma. *Int J Radiat Oncol Biol Phys* 1989;18:1063–1066.
35. Bruna A, Gastelblum P, Thomas L, et al. Treatment of squamous cell anal canal carcinoma (SCACC) with pulsed dose rate brachytherapy: a retrospective study. *Radiother Oncol* 2006;79(1):75–79.
36. Carlton CE Jr., Dawoud F, Hudgins PT, et al. Irradiation treatment of carcinoma of the prostate: a preliminary report based on 8 years of experience. *J Urol* 1972;108:924.
37. Casal L, Ballester F, Lluch JL, et al. Monte Carlo calculations of dose rate distributions around the Amersham CDCS-M-type ^{137}Cs source. *Med Phys* 2000;27:132–140.
38. Chan JL, Lee SW, Fraass BA, et al. Survival and failure patterns of high grade gliomas after three-dimensional conformal radiotherapy. *J Clin Oncol* 2002;20:1635–1642.
39. Chan TA, Weingart JD, Parisi M, et al. Treatment of recurrent glioblastoma multiforme with Gliasite Brachytherapy. *Int J Radiat Oncol Biol Phys* 2005;62(4):1133–1139.
40. Chao CKS, Grigsby PW, Perez CA, et al. Brachytherapy-related complications for medically inoperable stage I endometrial carcinoma. *Int J Radiat Oncol Biol Phys* 1995;31:37–42.
41. Charyulu KKN. Transperineal interstitial implantation of prostate cancer: a new method. *Int J Radiat Oncol Biol Phys* 1980;6:1261.
42. Chassagne D, Janvier L, Pierquin B, et al. La plesiotherapie des cancers du cavum avec support-moule et iridium 192. *Ann Radiol* 1963;6:719–726.
43. Cheron H, Rubens-Duval H. Apercu sur les resultants de la radiumtherapie des cancers d l'uerus et du vagin. *Bull Soc de'Obst et de Gynec de Par* 1913;2:418–429.
44. Chiu-Tsao S-T, Anderson LL, Stabile L. TLD dosimetry for ^{125}I eye plaque. *Phys Med Biol* 1988;33:28.
45. Chiu-Tsao S-T, Tsao HS, Vialotti C, et al. Monte Carlo dosimetry for ^{125}I and ^{60}Co in eye plaque therapy. *Med Phys* 1986;13:678.
46. Chiu-Tsao S-T. ^{125}I episcleral eye plaques for treatment of intra-ocular malignancies. In: Williamson JF, Thomadsen BR, Nath R, eds. *Brachytherapy physics.* Madison, WI: Medical Physics Publishing Company, 1995;451–485.
47. Cionini L, Marzano S, Pacini P, et al. Iridium implant of the surgical bed as the sole radiotherapeutic treatment after conservative surgery for breast cancer. *Radiother Oncol* 1995;35:S1.
48. Clark RM, McCulloch PB, Levine M. Randomized clinical trial to assess the effectiveness of breast irradiation following lumpectomy and axillary dissection for node negative breast cancer. *J Natl Cancer Inst* 1992;84:683–689.
49. Clarke DH, Edmundson GK, Martinez A, et al. The clinical advantages of I-125 seeds as a substitute for Ir-192 seeds in temporary plastic tube implants. *Int J Radiat Oncol Biol Phys* 1989;18:859–863.
50. Clarke M, Collins R, Darby S, et al. EBCTCG. Effects of radiotherapy and of differences in the extent of surgery for early breast cancer on local recurrence and 15-year survival: an overview of the randomised trials. *Lancet* 2005;366:2087–2106.
51. Collaborative Ocular Melanoma Study Group. Ten-year follow-up of fellow eyes of patients enrolled in Collaborative Ocular Melanoma Study randomized trials. COMS report no. 22. *Ophthalmology* 2004;111(5):966–976.
52. Collaborative Ocular Melanoma Study Group. COMS randomized trial of iodine 125 brachytherapy for choroidal melanoma, III: initial mortality findings. COMS report no. 18. *Arch Ophthalmol* 2001;119:969–982.
53. Collaborative Ocular Melanoma Study Group. COMS randomized trial of iodine 125 brachytherapy for choroidal melanoma, IV: local treatment failure and enucleation in the first 5 years after brachytherapy. COMS report no. 19. *Ophthalmology* 2002;109(12):2197–2206.
54. Conroy RM, Shahbazian AA, Edwards KC, et al. A new method for treating carcinomatous biliary obstruction with intracatheter radium. *Cancer* 1982;49:1321.
55. Cooper FS. Postoperative irradiation of pterygia: ten more years of experience. *Radiology* 1978;128:753–756.
56. Cormack RA, Kooy H, Tempany CM, et al. A clinical method for real-time dosimetric guidance of transperineal I-125 prostate implants using interventional magnetic resonance imaging. *Int J Radiat Oncol Biol Phys* 2000;46:207–214.
57. Corn BW, Galvin JM, Soffen EM, et al. Positional stability of sources during low-dose-rate brachytherapy for cervical carcinoma. *Int J Radiat Oncol Biol Phys* 1993;26:513–518.
58. Corn BW, Hanlon AL, Pajak TF, et al. Technically accurate intracavitary insertions improve pelvic control and survival among patients with locally advanced carcinoma of the uterine cervix. *Gynecol Oncol* 1994;53:294–300.
59. Corn BW, Shaktman BD, Lanciano RM, et al. Intra- and perioperative complications associated with tandem and colpostat application for cervix cancer. *Gynecol Oncol* 1997;64(2):224–229.
60. Crook JM, Jezioranski J, Grimard L, et al. Penile brachytherapy: results for 49 patients. *Int J Radiat Oncol Biol Phys* 2005;62(2):460–467.
61. D'Amico AV, Coleman CN. Role of interstitial radiotherapy in the management of clinically organ-confined prostate cancer: the jury is still out. *J Clin Oncol* 1996;14:304–315.
62. D'Amico AV, Cormack RA, Tempany CM, et al. The use of real time MR guided interstitial brachytherapy in select patients with localized prostate cancer. *Int J Radiat Oncol Biol Phys* 1998;42:507–515.
63. Dale RG, Jones B. Regarding Giap and Massullo. *Int J Radiat Oncol Biol Phys* 2000;48:304–305.
64. de Pree C, Popowski Y, Weber D, et al. Feasibility and tolerance of pulsed dose rate interstitial brachytherapy. *Int J Radiat Oncol Biol Phys* 1999;43:971–976.
65. Dean E, Lambert G, Dawes P. Gynaecological treatments using the Selectron remote afterloading system. *Br J Radiol* 1988;61:1053–1057.
66. DeBiose DA, Horwitz EM, Martinez AA, et al. The use of ultrasonography in the localization of the lumpectomy cavity for interstitial brachytherapy of the breast. *Int J Radiat Oncol Biol Phys* 1997;38:755–759.
67. Delannes M, Thomas L, Martel P, et al. Low-dose-rate intraoperative brachytherapy combined with external beam irradiation in the conservative treatment of soft tissue sarcoma. *Int J Radiat Oncol Biol Phys* 2000;47:165–169.
68. Delclos L, Fletcher GH, Moore EB, et al. Minicolpostats, dome cylinders, other

additions and improvements of the Fletcher-Suit after loadable system: indications and limitations of their use. *Int J Radiat Oncol Biol Phys* 1980;6:1195–1206.
69. Delclos L, Fletcher GH, Sampiere V, et al. Can the Fletcher gamma ray colpostat system be extrapolated to other systems? *Cancer* 1978;41:970–979.
70. Delclos L. A second look at interstitial irradiation. In: Deeley TJ, ed. *Topical reviews in radiotherapy and oncology—2*. London: John Wright & Sons, 1982;.
71. Delclos L. Interstitial irradiation of the penis. In: Johnson DE, Boileau MA, eds. *Genitourinary tumors: fundamental principles and surgical techniques*. New York: Grune & Stratton, 1982;219–226.
72. Delclos L. Interstitial irradiation techniques. In: Levitt SH, Tapley N duV, eds. *Technological basis of radiation therapy: practical clinical applications*. Philadelphia: Lea & Febiger, 1984;55–84.
73. Dempsey JF, Williams JA, Stubbs JB, et al. Dosimetric properties of a novel brachytherapy ballon applicator for the treatment of malignant brain-tumor resection cavity margins. *Int J Radiat Oncol Biol Phys* 1998;42(2):421–429.
74. Denham JW, Baldacchino AC, Gutte J, et al. Remote afterloading techniques for the treatment of nasopharyngeal and endometrial cancer. *Int J Radiat Oncol Biol Phys* 1988;14:191–195.
75. Deniaud-Alexandre E, Touboul E, Tiret E, et al. Epidermoid carcinomas of the anal canal treated with definitive radiation therapy in a series of 305 patients. *Cancer Radiother* 2003;7(4):237–253(in French).
76. Deore SM, Sarin R, Dinshaw KA, et al. Influence of dose-rate and dose per fraction on clinical outcome of breast cancer treated by external beam irradiation plus iridium-192 implants: analysis of 289 cases. *Int J Radiat Oncol Biol Phys* 1993;26:601–606.
77. Deutsch M, Segall BW, Leen R, et al. Retreatment of recurrent nasopharyngeal malignancy using a radium mold. *J Prosthet Dent* 1973;30:315–320.
78. Dobelbower RR, Merrick HW, Ahuja RK, et al. I-125 interstitial implant, precision high-dose external beam therapy, and 5-FU for unresectable adenocarcinoma of pancreas and extrahepatic biliary tree. *Cancer* 1986;58:2185–2195.
79. Druy EM, Carabell SC, Ling CC. Treatment of bile duct tumors with ^{192}Ir. Presented at the 67th Annual Meeting of the Radiological Society of North America. Chicago; November 19, 1981.
80. Dusenbery K, Carson L, Potish R. Perioperative morbidity and mortality of gynecologic brachytherapy. *Cancer* 1991;67:2786–2790.
81. Emami B, Perez CA. Interstitial thermoradiotherapy in the treatment of malignant tumors. In: Sauer R, ed. *Interventional radiation therapy techniques: brachytherapy*. Berlin: Springer-Verlag, 1991;159–169.
82. Erickson BA, Nag S. Biliary tree malignancies. *J Surg Oncol* 1998;67:203–210.
83. Erickson BA, Shadley JD. *In vitro* test of the cytotoxic equivalence between pulsed dose rate and continuous low dose rate. *Radiat Oncol Invest* 1996;3:218–224.
84. Erickson BA, Wilson JF. Nasopharyngeal brachytherapy. *Am J Clin Oncol* 1993;16:424–443.
85. Erickson BA. Interstitial implantation of vulvar malignancies: an historical perspective. *Endocurie Hypertherm Oncol* 1996;12:101–112.
86. Esche BA, Haie CM, Gerbaulet AP, et al. Interstitial and external radiotherapy in carcinoma of the soft palate and uvula. *Int J Radiat Oncol Biol Phys* 1988;15:619–625.
87. Early Breast Cancer Trialists Collaborative Group. Favourable and unfavourable effects on long-term survival of radiotherapy for early breast cancer: an overview of the randomised trials. *Lancet* 2000;355:1757–1770.
88. Fentiman IS, Deshmane V, Tong D, et al. 137-caesium implant as sole radiation therapy for operable breast cancer: a phase II trial. *Radiother Oncol* 2004;71:281–285.
89. Fentiman IS, Poole C, Tong D, et al. Inadequacy of Iridium implant as a sole radiation treatment for operable breast cancer. *Eur J Cancer* 1996;32A:608–611.
90. Fentiman IS, Poole C, Tong PJ, et al. Iridium implant treatment without external radiotherapy for operable breast cancer: a pilot study. *Eur J Cancer* 1991;27:447–450.
91. Fernandez PM, Zamorano L, Yakar D, et al. Permanent iodine-125 implants in the up-front treatment of malignant gliomas. *Neurosurgery* 1995;36:467–473.
92. Fields JN, Emami B. Carcinoma of the extrahepatic biliary system: results of primary and adjuvant radiotherapy. *Int J Radiat Oncol Biol Phys* 1987;13:331–338.
93. Fisher B, Anderson S, Bryant J, et al. Twenty year follow up of a randomized trial comparing total mastectomy, lumpectomy plus irradiation for the treatment of invasive breast cancer. *N Engl J Med* 2002;347:1233–1241.
94. Fisher B, Montagne E, Redmond C, et al. Comparison of radical mastectomy with alternative treatments for primary breast cancer. A first report of results from a prospective randomized clinical trial. *Cancer* 1977;39:2827–2839.
95. Fisher ER, Anderson S, Redmond C, et al. Ipsilateral breast tumor recurrence and survival following lumpectomy and irradiation: pathological findings from NSABP protocol B-06. *Semin Surg Oncol* 1992;8:161–166.
96. Fisher ER, Sass R, Fisher B, et al. Pathologic findings from the National Surgical Adjuvant Breast Project (protocol 6). Relation of local breast recurrence to multicentricity. *Cancer* 1986;57:1717–1724.
97. Fletcher GH, MacComb WS. *Radiation therapy in the management of cancers of the oral cavity and oropharynx*. Springfield, IL: Charles C Thomas, 1962.
98. Fletcher GH. Cervical radium applicators with screening in the direction of bladder and rectum. *Radiology* 1953;60:77–84.
99. Fletcher GH. Oral cavity and oropharynx. In: Fletcher GH, ed. *Textbook of radiotherapy,* 3rd ed. Philadelphia: Lea & Febiger, 1980;286–329.
100. Fletcher MS. Treatment of high bile duct carcinoma by internal radiotherapy with ^{192}Ir wire. *Lancet* 1981;2:182.
101. Flores AD, Nelems B, Evans K, et al. Impact of new radiotherapy modalities on the surgical management of cancer of the esophagus and cardia. *Int J Radiat Oncol Biol Phys* 1989;18:937–944.
102. Flores AD. Remote afterloading intracavitary irradiation for carcinoma of the nasopharynx. In: Mould RF, ed. *Brachytherapy 2*. Leersum, The Netherlands: Nucletron, 1988;49–66.
103. Fontanesi J, Hetzler D, Ross J. Effect of dose rate on local control and complications in the reirradiation of head and neck tumors with interstitial iridium-192. *Int J Radiat Oncol Biol Phys* 1989;18:365–369.
104. Fowble B, Solin LJ, Schultz DJ, et al. Breast recurrence following conservative surgery and radiation: patterns of failure, prognosis, and pathologic findings from mastectomy specimens with implications for treatment. *Int J Radiat Oncol Biol Phys* 1990;19:833–842.
105. Fowler JF, Van Limbergen EF. Biological effect of pulsed dose rate brachytherapy with stepping sources if short half-times of repair are present in tissues. *Int J Radiat Oncol Biol Phys* 1997;37:877–883.
106. Frazier C. The effects of radium emanations upon brain tumors. *Surg Gynecol Obstet* 1920;31:236–239.
107. Friedman GM, Hanlon AL, Anderson PR. Pattern of local recurrence after conservative surgery and whole breast radiation: implications for partial breast irradiation. *Int J Radiat Oncol Biol Phys* 2003;57[Suppl 2]:S171.
108. Fritz P, Brambs HJ, Schraube P, et al. Combined external beam radiotherapy and intraluminal high dose rate brachytherapy on bile duct carcinomas. *Int J Radiat Oncol Biol Phys* 1994;29:855–861.
109. Fu KK, Phillips TL. High-dose rate versus low-dose rate intracavitary brachytherapy for carcinoma of the cervix. *Int J Radiat Oncol Biol Phys* 1990;19:791–796.
110. Gabayan AJ, Green SB, Sanan A, et al. GliaSite brachytherapy for treatment of recurrent malignant gliomas: a retrospective multi-institutional analysis. *Neurosurgery* 2006;58(4):701.
111. Gaddis O Jr., Morrow CP, Klement V, et al. Treatment of cervical carcinoma employing a template for transperineal interstitial ^{192}Ir brachytherapy. *Int J Radiat Oncol Biol Phys* 1983;9:819–827.
112. Gaspar LF, Winter K, Kocha WI, et al. A phase I/II study of external beam radiation, brachytherapy, and concurrent chemotherapy for patients with localized carcinoma of the esophagus. *Cancer* 2000;88:988–995.
113. Gerard JP, Rozan R, Mazeron JJ, et al. Iridium-192 brachytherapy in urinary bladder cancer: the French experience. In: Mould RF, ed. *Brachytherapy 2*. Leerum, The Netherlands: Nucletron International BV, 1989;189–192.
114. Gerbaulet A, Haie-Meder C, Marsiglia H, et al. The role of brachytherapy in treatment of head and neck cancer: Institut Gustave Roussy experience with 1140 patients. In: Mould RF, ed. *International brachytherapy*. Leerum, The Netherlands: Nucletron, 1992;49–66.
115. Gerbaulet A, Haie-Meder C, Marsiglia H, et al. Brachytherapy in cancer of the urethra *Ann Urol (Paris)* 1994;28(6–7):312–317(review in French).
116. Giap HB, Massulo V. Derivation of isoeffect dose rate for low–dose-rate brachytherapy and external beam irradiation. *Int J Radiat Oncol Biol Phys* 1999;45:1355–1358.
117. Glasgow GP. Radiation control, personnel training, and emergency procedures for remote afterloading units. *Endocurie Hypertherm Oncol* 1996;12:67–79.
118. Goffinet DR, Martinez A, Fee WE Jr. 125I Vicryl suture implants as a surgical adjuvant in cancer of the head and neck. *Int J Radiat Oncol Biol Phys* 1985;11:399.
119. Greenberg M. Eye: choroidal melanomas and pterygium. In: Pierquin B, Wilson J-F,Chassagne D, eds. *Modern brachytherapy*. New York: Masson, 1987;301–314.
120. Greenblatt DR, Nori D, Tankenbaum A, et al. New brachytherapy techniques using iodine-125 seeds for tumor bed implants. *Endocurie Hypertherm Oncol* 1987;3:73–80.
121. Grigsby PW, Baker S. Socioeconomic aspects of remote afterloading. In: Williamson JF, Thomadsen BR, Nath R, eds. *Brachytherapy physics*. Madison, WI: Medical Physics Publishing Company, 1995;699–708.
122. Grigsby PW, Perez CA, Kuten A, et al. Clinical stage I endometrial cancer: results of adjuvant irradiation and patterns of failure. *Int J Radiat Oncol Biol Phys* 1991;21:379–385.
123. Grigsby PW, Perez CA. The costs of low dose rate remote afterloading compared to manual afterloading brachytherapy. *Admin Radiol* 1990;9:61–67.
124. Grigsby PW, Williamson JF, Perez CA. Source configuration and dose rates for the Selectron afterloading equipment for gynecologic applicators. *Int J Radiat Oncol Biol Phys* 1992;24:423–430.
125. Gupta AK, Vicini FA, Frazier AJ, et al. Iridium-192 transperineal interstitial brachytherapy for locally advanced or recurrent gynecological malignancies. *Int J Radiat Oncol Biol Phys* 1999;43:1055–1060.
126. Gutin PH, Phillips TL, Wara WM, et al. Brachytherapy of recurrent malignant brain tumors with removable high activity iodine 125 sources. *J Neurosurg* 1984;60:61–68.
127. Gutin PH, Prados MD, Phillips TL, et al. External irradiation followed by interstitial high activity iodine-125 implant "boost"in the initial treatment of malignant gliomas: NCOG study 6G-82-2. *Int J Radiat Oncol Biol Phys* 1991;21:601–606.
128. Haas JS, Dean RD, Mansfield CM. Dosimetric comparison of the Fletcher family of gynecologic colpostats, 1950–1980. *Int J Radiat Oncol Biol Phys* 1985;11:1318–1321.
129. Haghbin M, Kramer S, Patchefsky AS, et al. Carcinoma of the nasopharynx: a 25-year study. *Am J Clin Oncol* 1985;8:384–392.
130. Hall E. The biological basis of endocurie therapy. *Endocurie Hypertherm Oncol* 1985;1:141.
131. Hall EJ, Brenner DJ. Pulsed dose rate brachytherapy: can we take advantage of new technology? *Int J Radiat Oncol Biol Phys* 1996;34:511–512.
132. Hall EJ, Brenner DJ. The dose-rate effect in interstitial brachytherapy: a controversy resolved. *Br J Radiol* 1992;65:242–247.
133. Halligan JB, Stelzer KJ, Rostomily RC, et al. Operation and permanent low activity ^{125}I brachytherapy for recurrent high grade astrocytomas. *Int J Radiat Oncol Biol Phys* 1996;35:541–547.
134. Hames F. A new method in the use of radon gold seeds. *Am J Surg* 1937;38:235.
135. Harms W, Krempien R, Hensley FW, et al. 5-year results of pulsed dose rate brachytherapy applied as boost after breast conserving therapy in patients at high risk for local recurrence from breast cancer. *Stralenther Onkol* 2002;11:607–614.
136. Harrison LB, Nori D, Hilaris BS, et al. Nasopharynx. In: Interstitial Collaborative Working Group, eds. *Interstitial brachytherapy*. New York: Raven Press, 1990;95–109.
137. Harrison LB, Weissberg JB. A technique for interstitial nasopharyngeal brachytherapy. *Int J Radiat Oncol Biol Phys* 1987;13:451–453.
138. Harter DJ, Delclos L. Sealed sources in synthetic absorbable suture. *Radiology* 1975;116:727.
139. Henschke UK. Afterloading applicator for radiation therapy of carcinoma of the uterus. *Radiology* 1960;74:834.
140. Henschke UK. *Artificial radioisotopes in nylon ribbons for implantation in neoplasms*. International Conferences on the Peaceful Uses of Atomic Energy. New York: United Nations, 1956.

141. Henschke UK, Hilaris BS, Mahan GD. Afterloading in interstitial and intracavitary radiation therapy. *Am J Roentgenol* 1963;90:386–395.

142. Herskovic A, Heaston D, Engler MJ, et al. Irradiation of biliary carcinoma. *Radiology* 1981;139:219.

143. Herstein A, Wallner K, Merrik G, et al. I-125 versus Pd-103 for low-risk prostate cancer: long-term morbidity outcomes from a prospective randomized multicenter controlled trial. *Cancer J* 2005;11(5):385–389.

144. Heyman J, Reuterwall O, Benner S. The Radiumhemmet experience with radiotherapy in cancer of the corpus of the uterus: classification, method of treatment and results. *Acta Radiol* 1941;11:11.

145. Hilaris BS, Batata MA. Brachytherapy techniques. In: Hilaris BS, Batata MA, eds. *Brachytherapy oncology—1983*. New York: Memorial Sloan-Kettering Cancer Center, 1983;41–56.

146. Hilaris BS, Nori D, Anderson LL. Brachytherapy for soft tissue sarcomas. In: Hilaris BS, Nori D, Anderson LL, eds. *Atlas of brachytherapy*. New York: Macmillan, 1988;180–182.

147. Hilaris BS, Nori D, Anderson LL. Brachytherapy of ocular melanoma. In: Hilaris BS, Nori D, Anderson LL, eds. *Atlas of brachytherapy*. New York: Macmillan, 1988;304–310.

148. Hilaris BS, Roussi K. Cancer of the pancreas. In: Hilaris BS, ed. *Handbook of interstitial brachytherapy*. Acton, MA: Acton Publishing Science Group, 1975;251–262.

149. Hilaris BS, Whitmore WF, Batata MA, et al. Behavioral patterns of prostate adenocarcinoma following an I-125 implant and pelvic node dissection. *Int J Radiat Oncol Biol Phys* 1977;2:631.

150. Hintz BL, Kagan AR, Chan P, et al. Radiation tolerance of the vaginal mucosa. *Int J Radiat Oncol Biol Phys* 1980;6:711–716.

151. Höckel M, Muller T. A new perineal template assembly for high–dose-rate interstitial brachytherapy of gynecologic malignancies. *Radiother Oncol* 1994;31:262–264.

152. Holm HH, Juul N, Pedersen JF, et al. Transperineal 125 iodine seed implantation in prostatic cancer guided by transrectal ultrasonography. *J Urol* 1983;130:283–286.

153. Hughes-Davies L, Silver B, Kapp KS. Parametrial interstitial brachytherapy for advanced or recurrent pelvic malignancy: the Harvard/Stanford experience. *Gynecol Oncol* 1995;58:24–27.

154. Ikeda H. Intraluminal irradiation with ^{192}Ir wires for extrahepatic bile duct carcinoma. *Nippon Igaku Hoshasen Gakkai Zasshi* 1979;39:1356.

155. Inoue T, Yoshiaka Y, et al. High dose rate interstitial brachytherapy for mobile tongue cancer: part three. Comparative study of early mucosal reaction and late tongue trophy between LDR and HDR Ir 192 interstitial brachytherapy for patients with carcinoma. *Gan To Kagaku Ryoho* 2000;27[Suppl 2]:296–300.

156. Inoue T, Teshima T, et al. Phase III trial of high versus low dose rate interstitial radiotherapy for early mobile tongue cancer. *Int J Radiat Oncol Biol Phys* 2001;51(1):171–175.

157. International Commission on Radiation Units. ICRU Report No. 38: *Dose and volume specification for reporting intracavitary therapy in gynecology*. Bethesda, MD: ICRU, 1985;1–16.

158. Iyer PS, Shanta A. Update of radionuclides used in endocurietherapy. *Endocurie Hypertherm Oncol* 1994;10:161–165.

159. Jackson SM. The treatment of carcinoma of the penis. *Br J Surg* 1966;53:33–35.

160. James RD, Pointon RS, Martin S. Local radiotherapy in the management of squamous carcinoma of the anus. *Br J Surg* 1985;72:282–285.

161. Jensen AW, Petersen IA, Kline RW, et al. Radiation complications and tumor control after 125-I plaque brachytherapy for ocular melanoma. *Int J Radiat Oncol Biol Phys* 2005;63:1:101–108.

162. Jensen PT, Roed H, Engelholm SA, et al. Pulsed dose rate (PDR) brachytherapy as salvage treatment of locally advanced or recurrent gynecologic cancer. *Int J Radiat Oncol Biol Phys* 1998;42(5):1041–1047.

163. Jhingram A, Eifel PJ. Perioperative and postoperative complications of intracavitary radiation for FIGO stage I-III carcinoma of the cervix. *Int J Radiat Oncol Biol Phys* 2000;46:1177–1183.

164. Jones C, Lukke H, O'Brien B. High dose rate versus low dose rate brachytherapy for squamous cell carcinoma of the cervix: an economic analysis. *Br J Radiol* 1994;67:1113–1120.

165. Jones D, Notley H, Hunter R. Geometry adopted by Manchester radium applicators and Selectron afterloading applicators in intracavitary treatment for carcinoma cervix uteri. *Br J Radiol* 1987;60:481–485.

166. Jorgensen K, Elbrond O, Andersen AP. Carcinoma of the lip: a series of 869 cases. *Acta Radiol Ther Phys Biol* 1973;12:187–190.

167. Kaled M, Alektiar MD, Leung D, Zelefsky MJ, et al. Adjuvant brachytherapy for primary high-grade soft tissue sarcoma of the extremity. *Ann Surg Oncol* 2002;9:48–56.

168. Karaiskos P, Papagiannis P, Angelopoulas A, et al. Dosimetry of ^{192}Ir wires for LDR interstitial brachytherapy following the AAPM TG-43 dosimetric formalism. *Med Phys* 2001;28:156–166.

169. Kin NYK, Pigneux J, Auvray H, et al. Our experience of conservative treatment of anal canal carcinoma combining external irradiation and interstitial implant: 32 cases treated between 1973 and 1982. *Int J Radiat Oncol Biol Phys* 1988;14:253–259.

170. King TA, Bolton JS, Kuske RR, et al. Long term results of wide field brachytherapy as the sole method of radiation therapy after segmental mastectomy for Tis, 1,2, breast cancer. *Am J Surg* 2000;180:299–304.

171. Koken PW, de Vos RJ. A straightforward implantation method of radioactive sources by means of the Leksell frame. *Stereotact Funct Neurosurg* 1995;64:202–213.

172. Kolotas C, Zamboglou N. Role of interstitial brachytherapy in the treatment of malignant disease. *Onkologie* 2001;24:222–228.

173. Koot RW, Maarouf M, Hulshof MCCM, et al. Brachytherapy: results of two different therapy strategies for patients with primary glioblastoma multiforme. *Cancer* 2000;88(12):2796–2802.

174. Kopelson G, Harisiadis L, Tretter P, et al. The role of radiation therapy in cancer of the extrahepatic biliary system: an analysis of 13 patients and a review of the literature of the effectiveness of surgery, chemotherapy and radiotherapy. *Int J Radiat Oncol Biol Phys* 1977;2:883–894.

175. Krintz AL, Hanson WF, Ibbot GS, et al. A reanalysis of the collaborative ocular melanoma study medium tumor trial eye plaque dosimetry. *Int J Radiat Oncol Biol Phys* 2003;56(3):889–898.

176. Kucera H, Mock C, Knocke TH, et al. Radiotherapy alone for invasive vaginal cancer: outcome with intracavitary high dose rate brachytherapy versus conventional low dose rate brachytherapy. *Acta Obstet Gynecol Scand* 2001;80:355–360.

177. Kuske RR, Bolton JS, Fuhrman G, et al. Wide volume brachytherapy alone for selected breast cancers: the 10 year experience of the Ochsner Clinic. *Int J Radiat Oncol Biol Phys* 2000;48[Suppl 3]:296.

178. Kuske RR, Bolton JS, Hanson W. *RTOG 95-8: a phase I/II trial to evaluate brachytherapy as the sole method of radiation therapy for stage I and II breast carcinoma*. Philadelphia: Radiation Therapy Oncology Group, 1998;1–34.

179. Kuske RR, Bolton JS, Wilenzick RM, et al. Brachytherapy as the sole method of breast irradiation in T1S, T1, T2, N0-1 breast cancer. *Int J Radiat Oncol Biol Phys* 1994;30[Suppl 1]:245.

180. Kuske RR, Perez CA, Jacobs AJ, et al. Mini-colpostats in the treatment of the uterine cervix. *Int J Radiat Oncol Biol Phys* 1988;14:899–906.

181. Kuske RR, Winter K, Arthur DW, et al. Phase II trial of brachytherapy alone after lumpectomy for selected breast cancer: toxicity analysis or RTOG 95-17. *Int J Radiat Oncol Biol Phys* 2006;65(1):45–51.

182. Kwan DK, Kagan AR, Olch AJ, et al. Single and double plan iridium-192 interstitial implants: implantation guidelines and dosimetry. *Med Phys* 1983;10:456–461.

183. Laperriere N, Leung P, McKenzie S, et al. Randomized study of brachytherapy in the initial management of patients with malignant astrocytoma. *Int J Radiat Oncol Biol Phys* 1998;41:1005–1011.

184. Lazzaro G. Pulsed dose-rate perioperative interstitial brachytherapy for soft tissue sarcomas of the extremities and skeletal muscles of the trunk. *Ann Surg Oncol* 2005;12(11):935–942.

185. Le Scodan R, Pommier P, Ardiet JM, et al. Exclusive brachytherapy for T1 and T2 squamous cell carcinomas of the velotonsillar area: results in 44 patients. *Int J Radiat Oncol Biol Phys* 2005;63(2):441–448.

186. Leborgne F, Fowler JF, Leborgne JH, et al. Medium-dose-rate brachytherapy of cancer of the cervix: preliminary results of a prospectively designed schedule based on the linear-quadratic model. *Int J Radiat Oncol Biol Phys* 1999;43:1061–1064.

187. Levendag FC, Peters R, Meelwis CA, et al. A new applicator design for endocavitary brachytherapy of cancer in the nasopharynx. *Radiother Oncol* 1997;45:95–98.

188. Lichter AS, Dillon MB, Rosenshein NB, et al. The use of custom molds for intracavitary treatment of carcinoma of the cervix. *Int J Radiat Oncol Biol Phys* 1978;4(9–10):876.

189. Liljegren G, Holmberg L, Adami HO, et al. Sector resection with or without II postoperative radiotherapy for stage I breast cancer: five years results of a randomized trial. Uppsla-Orebro Breast Cancer Study Group. *J Natl Cancer Inst* 1994;86:717–722.

190. Liljegren G, Holmberg L, Bergh J, et al. 10 years results after sector resection with or without postoperative radiotherapy for stage I breast cancer: a randomized trial. *J Clin Oncol* 1999;17:2326–2333.

191. Llacer C, Delannes M, Minsat M, et al. Low-dose intraoperative brachytherapy in soft tissue sarcomas involving neurovascular structure. *Radiother Oncol* 2006;78(1):10–16.

192. Lommatzsch PK. Results after beta-irradiation (^{106}Ru/^{106}Rh) of choroidal melanomas: 20 years experience. *Br J Ophthalmol* 1986;70:844–851.

193. Lozza L, Cerrota A, Gardani G, et al. Analysis of risk factors for mandibular bone radionecrosis after exclusive low dose-rate brachytherapy for oral cancer. *Radiother Oncol* 1997;44:143–147.

194. Luxton G, Astrahan MA, Liggett PE, et al. Dosimetric calculations and measurements of gold plaque ophthalmic irradiators using ^{192}Ir and ^{125}I seeds. *Int J Radiat Oncol Biol Phys* 1988;15:167.

195. Lybeert ML, Ribot JG, de Neve W, et al. Carcinoma of the urinary bladder: long-term results of interstitial radiotherapy. *Bull Cancer Radiother* 1994;81:33–40.

196. Maat B, Venselaar JLM. Improved afterloading technique for interstitial brachytherapy of bladder cancer. In: Mould RF, ed. *Brachytherapy 2*. Leerum, The Netherlands: Nucletron International BV, 1989;183–186.

197. Malkin MG. Interstitial brachytherapy of malignant gliomas: the Memorial Sloan-Kettering Cancer Center experience. *Recent Results Cancer Res* 1994;135:117–125.

198. Mansfield CM, Komarnicky LT, Schwartz GF, et al. Perioperative implantation of iridium-192 as the boost technique for stage I and II breast cancer: results of a 10-year study of 655 patients. *Radiology* 1994;192:33–36.

199. Marchese MJ, Nori D, Anderson LL, et al. A versatile permanent planar implant technique utilizing iodine-125 seeds imbedded in Gelfoam. *Int J Radiat Oncol Biol Phys* 1984;10(5):747.

200. Marcus RB Jr, Million RR, Mitchell TP. A preloaded, custom-designed implantation device for stage T1-T2 carcinoma of the floor of mouth. *Int J Radiat Oncol Biol Phys* 1980;6:111–113.

201. Markman J, Williamson JF, Dempsey JF, et al. On the validity of the superposition principle in dose calculations for intracavitary implants with shielded vaginal colpostats. *Med Phys* 2001;28:147–155.

202. Marsiglia H, Haie-Meder C, Sasso G, et al. Brachytherapy for T1-T2 floor of the mouth cancers: the Gustave Roussy Institute Experience. *Int J Radiat Oncol Biol Phys* 2002;52(5):1257–1263.

203. Martin HE, MacComb WS. Protracted irradiation by radium. *Am J Roentgenol Radium Ther* 1937;37:224–233.

204. Martinez A, Benson RC, Edmundson GK, et al. Pelvic lymphadenectomy combined with transperineal interstitial implantation of iridium-192 and external beam radiation for locally advanced prostatic carcinoma: technical description. *Int J Radiat Oncol Biol Phys* 1985;11:841–847.

205. Martinez A, Edmundson GK, Cox RS, et al. Combination of external beam irradiation and multiple-site perineal applicator (MUPIT) for treatment of locally advanced or recurrent prostatic, anorectal, and gynecologic malignancies. *Int J Radiat Oncol Biol Phys* 1985;11:391–398.

206. Martinez-Monge R, Nag S, Martin EW. ^{125}Iodine brachytherapy for colorectal adenocarcinoma recurrent in the pelvis and para-aortics. *Int J Radiat Oncol Biol Phys* 1998;42:545–550.

207. Martini N. Clinical application of interstitial implantation in carcinoma of the lung. In: Hilaris B, Nori D, eds. *Brachytherapy—1984*. New York: Memorial Sloan-Kettering Cancer Center, 1984;23–27.

208. Mayr NA, Sorosky JI, Zhen W, et al. The use of laminarias for osmotic dilation of

the cervix in gynecological brachytherapy applications. *Int J Radiat Oncol Biol Phys* 1998;42:1049–1053.

209. Mazeron JJ. Exclusive brachytherapy in oral tongue cancer: analysis of the GEC questionnaire for the 1988 annual meeting. Proceedings of the XXV GEC Annual Meeting. Stiges, 1988.

210. Mazeron JJ. Nasopharynx. In: Pierquin B, Wilson JF, Chassagne D, eds. *Modern brachytherapy.* New York: Masson, 1987;155–162.

211. Mazeron JJ, Crook J, Chopin D, et al. Conservative treatment of bladder carcinoma by partial cystectomy and interstitial iridium 192. *Int J Radiat Oncol Biol Phys* 1988;15:1323–1330.

212. Mazeron JJ, Lusichini A, Marinello G, et al. Interstitial radiation therapy for squamous cell carcinoma of the tonsillar region: the Creteil experience (1971–1981). *Int J Radiat Oncol Biol Phys* 1986;12:895–900.

213. Mazeron JJ, Simon J-M, Crook J, et al. Influence of dose rate on local control of breast carcinoma treated by external beam irradiation plus iridium 192 implant. *Int J Radiat Oncol Biol Phys* 1991;21:1183–1187.

214. McNeese MD, Fletcher GH. Retreatment of recurrent nasopharyngeal carcinoma. *Radiology* 1981;138:191–193.

215. Meerwaldt JH, Veeze-Kuijpers B, Visser AG, et al. Combined modality radiotherapy in the treatment of bile duct carcinoma. In: Mould RF, ed. *Brachytherapy 2.* Leersum, The Netherlands: Nucletron International BV, 1989;577–583.

216. Mendenhall NP, Parsons JT, Cassisi NJ, et al. Carcinoma of the nasal vestibule. *Int J Radiat Oncol Biol Phys* 1984;10:627–637.

217. Mendenhall NP, Parsons JT, Cassisi NJ, et al. Carcinoma of the nasal vestibule treated with radiation therapy. *Laryngoscope* 1987;97:626–632.

218. Meredith WJ. *Radium dosage: the Manchester system.* Edinburgh: Livingstone, 1967.

219. Merrick GS, Butler WM, Dorsey AT, et al. Seed fixity in the prostate/periprostatic region following brachytherapy. *Int J Radiat Oncol Biol Phys* 2000;462:215–220.

220. Micaily B, Dzeda MF, Miyamoto CT, et al. Brachytherapy for cancer of the female urethra. *Semin Surg Oncol* 1997;13(3):208–214(review).

221. Miura M, Takeda M, Sasaki T, et al. Factors affecting mandibular complications in low dose rate brachytherapy for oral tongue carcinoma with special reference to spacer. *Int J Radiat Oncol Biol Phys* 1998;41:763–770.

222. Mohiuddin M, Canton RJ, Bierman W, et al. Combined modality treatment of localized unresectable adenocarcinoma of the pancreas. *Int J Radiat Oncol Biol Phys* 1988;14:79–84.

223. Monteiro-Grillo I, Gaspar L, Monteiro-Grillo M, et al. Postoperative irradiation of primary or recurrent pterygium: Results and sequelae. *Int J Radiat Oncol Biol Phys* 2000;48:865–869.

224. Montemaggi P, Thorud E. Integrated external beam and brachytherapy in oral tongue cancer: analysis of the GEC questionnaire for the 1988 annual meeting. Proceedings of the XXV GEC Annual Meeting. Stiges, 1988.

225. Montemaggi P, Smaniotto D, Luzi S, et al. Long term analysis of surgery plus radiotherapy versus radiotherapy alone in oral cavity and oropharyngeal cancer. Proceedings ICRO Meeting 1993, Kyoto.

226. Montemaggi P, Dobelbower R, Crucitti F, et al. Interstitial brachytherapy for pancreatic cancer: report of seven cases treated with ^{125}I and a review of the literature. *Int J Radiat Oncol Biol Phys* 1991;21(2):451–457(review).

227. Montemaggi P, Morganti AG, Dobelbower RR Jr, et al. Role of intraluminal brachytherapy in extrahepatic bile duct and pancreatic cancers: is it just for palliation? *Radiology* 1996;199(3):861–866.

228. Moonen L. Brachytherapy in the management of bladder cancer. In: Mould RF, ed. *Brachytherapy 2.* Leersum, Netherlands: Nucletron International BV, 1989;184–188.

229. Morphis OL. Teflon tube method of radium implantation. *Am J Roentgenol* 1960;83:455.

230. Moss WT, Brand WN, Battifora H, eds. *Radiation oncology: rationale, technique, results,* 5th ed. St. Louis, MO: CV Mosby, 1979.

231. Mundinger F, Braus DF, Kraus JK, et al. long term outcome of 89 low grade brainstem gliomas after interstitial radiation therapy. *J Neurosurg* 1991;75:740–746.

232. Nag S. Brachytherapy for prostate cancer: summary of American Brachytherapy Society recommendations. *Semin Urol Oncol* 2000;18:133–136.

233. Nag S, Baird M, Blasko J, et al. American Brachytherapy Society (ABS) survey of current clinical practice for permanent brachytherapy of prostate cancer. *J Brachy Int* 1997;13:243–251.

234. Nag S, Beyer D, Friedland J, et al. American Brachytherapy Society (ABS) recommendations for transperineal permanent brachytherapy of prostate cancer. *Int J Radiat Oncol Biol Phys* 1999;44:789–799.

235. Nag S, Bice W, DeWyngaert K, et al. American Brachytherapy Society recommendations for permanent prostate brachytherapy post-implant dosimetric analysis. *Int J Radiat Oncol Biol Phys* 2000;46:221–223.

236. Nag S, Cardenes H, Chang S, et al. Image-Guided Brachytherapy Working Group. Proposed guidelines for image-based intracavitary brachytherapy for cervical carcinoma: report from Image-Guided Brachytherapy Working Group. *Int J Radiat Oncol Biol Phys* 2004;60(4):1160–1172.

237. Nag S, Chao C, Erickson B, Fowler J, et al. The American Brachytherapy Society recommendations for low dose rate brachytherapy for carcinoma of the cervix. Clinical Research Committee. *Int J Radiat Oncol Biol Phys* 2002;52(1): 33–48.

238. Nag S, Ciezki JP, Cormack R, et al. Intraoperative planning and evaluation of permanent prostate brachytherapy: report of the American Brachytherapy Society. *Int J Radiat Oncol Biol Phys* 2001;51:1422–1430.

239. Nag S, Erickson B, Parikh S, et al. The American Brachytherapy Society recommendations for high-dose-rate brachytherapy for carcinoma of the endometrium. *Int J Radiat Oncol Biol Phys* 2000;48(3):779–790.

240. Nag S, Kuske RR, Vicini FA, et al. Brachytherapy in the treatment of breast cancer: recommendations from the American Brachytherapy Society. *Oncology* 2001;15:195–205.

241. Nag S, Martinez-Monge R, Copeland LJ, et al. Perineal template interstitial brachytherapy salvage for recurrent endometrial adenocarcinoma metastatic to the vagina. *Gynecol Oncol* 1997;66:16–19.

242. Nag S, Martinez-Monge R, Ellis R, et al. The use of fluoroscopy to guide needle placement in interstitial gynecological brachytherapy. *Int J Radiat Oncol Biol Phys* 1998;40:415–420.

243. Nag S, Martinez-Monge R, Selman AE, et al. Interstitial brachytherapy in the management of primary carcinoma of the cervix and vagina. *Gynecol Oncol* 1998;70:27–32.

244. Nag S, Owen JB, Farnan N, et al. Survey of brachytherapy practice in the United States: a report of the Clinical Research Committee of the American Endocurietherapy Society. *Int J Radiat Oncol Biol Phys* 1995;31:103–107.

245. Nag S, Ribovich M, Cai JZ, et al. Palladium-103 vs iodine-125 brachytherapy in the Dunning-PAP rat prostate tumor. *Endocurie Hypertherm Oncol* 1996;12:119–124.

246. Nag S, Shasha D, Janjan N, et al. The American Brachytherapy Society recommendations for brachytherapy of soft tissue sarcomas. *Int J Radiat Oncol Biol Phys* 2001;49:1033–1043.

247. Narayana Y, Orton CG. Pulsed brachytherapy: a formalism to account for the variation in dose rate of the stepping source. *Med Phys* 1999;26:161–165.

248. Nath R, Meigooni AS, Meli JA. Dosimetry on the transverse axes of ^{125}I and ^{192}Ir interstitial brachytherapy sources. *Med Phys* 1990;18:1032–1040.

249. Nath R, Meigooni AS. Some treatment planning considerations for palladium-103 and iodine-125 permanent interstitial implants. *Endocurie Hypertherm Oncol* 1989;5:244(abstr).

250. Nath R, Meigooni AS, Melillo A. Some treatment planning considerations for Pd-103 and I-125 permanent interstitial implants. *Int J Radiat Oncol Biol Phys* 1992;22:1131–1138.

251. Nickers P, Coppers L, Beauduin M, et al. Feasibility study combining low dose rate ^{192}Ir brachytherapy and external beam radiotherapy aiming at delivering 80–85 Gy to prostatic adenocarcinoma. *Radiother Oncol* 2000;55:41–47.

252. Nieder C, Andratschke N, Wiedenmann N, et al. Radiotherapy for high-grade gliomas: does altered fractionation improve the outcome? *Strahlenther Onkol* 2004;180:401–407.

253. Nori D, Moni J. Current issues in techniques of prostate brachytherapy. *Semin Surg Oncol* 1997;13:444–453.

254. Olch AJ, Kagan AR, Wollin M, et al. A simple volume iridium implant dosimetry system. *Endocurie Hypertherm Oncol* 1987;3:183–191.

255. Packer S, Rotman M, Salanitro P. Iodine-125 irradiation of choroidal melanoma: clinical experience. *Ophthalmology* 1984;91:1800.

256. Papillon J, Montbarbon JR, Gerard JP, et al. Interstitial curietherapy in the conservative treatment of anal and rectal cancers. *Int J Radiat Oncol Biol Phys* 1989;18:1161–1169.

257. Parsons JT, Mendenhall WM, Bova FJ, et al. Head and neck cancer. In: Levitt SL, Khan FM, Potish RA, eds. *Levitt and Tapley's technological basis of radiation therapy: practical clinical applications,* 2md ed. Philadelphia: Lea & Febiger, 1992;203–231.

258. Parsons JT, Stringer SP, Mancuso AA, et al. Nasal vestibule, nasal cavity and paranasal sinuses. In: Million RR, Cassisi NJ, eds. *Management of head and neck cancer: a multidisciplinary approach,* 2nd ed. Philadelphia: J.B. Lippincott, 1994;551–598.

259. Patel S, Breneman JC, Warnick RE, et al. Permanent iodine 125 interstitial implants for the treatment of recurrent glioblastoma multiforme. *Neurosurgery* 2000;46:1123–1128.

260. Patterson R. *The treatment of malignant disease by radiotherapy,* 2nd ed. Baltimore: Williams & Wilkins, 1963.

261. Patterson R. *The treatment of malignant disease by radium and x-rays being a practice of radiotherapy.* Baltimore: Williams & Wilkins, 1948;254–255.

262. Peiffert D, Castelain B, Thomas L, et al. Pulsed dose rate brachytherapy in head and neck cancers. Feasibility study of a French cooperative group. *Radiother Oncol* 2001;58:71–75.

263. Peretz T, Nori D, Hilaris B, et al. Treatment of primary unresectable carcinoma of the pancreas with I-125 implantation. *Int J Radiat Oncol Biol Phys* 1989;18:931–935.

264. Perez CA, Camel HM, Galakatos AE, et al. Definitive irradiation in carcinoma of the vagina: long-term evaluation of results. *Int J Radiat Oncol Biol Phys* 1988;15:1283–1290.

265. Perez CA, Grigsby PW, Williamson JF. Clinical applications of brachytherapy I. Low dose rate. In: Perez CA, Brady LW, eds. *Principles and practice of radiation oncology,* 3rd ed. Philadelphia: J.B. Lippincott, 1998;487–559.

266. Perez CA, Kuske R, Glasgow GP. Review of brachytherapy for gynecologic tumors. *Endocurie Hypertherm Oncol* 1985;1:153.

267. Perez CA, Slessinger E, Grigsby PW. Design of an afterloading vaginal applicator (MIRALVA). *Int J Radiat Oncol Biol Phys* 1990;18:1503–1508.

268. Pernot M, Hoffstetter S, Peiffert D, et al. Epidermoid carcinomas of the floor of the mouth treated by exclusive irradiation: statistical study of a series of 207 cases. *Radiother Oncol* 1995;35:177–185.

269. Petereit DG, Sarkaria JN, Potter DM, et al. High–dose-rate versus low–dose-rate brachytherapy in the treatment of cervical cancer: analysis of tumor recurrence—the University of Wisconsin experience. *Int J Radiat Oncol Biol Phys* 1999;45:1267–1274.

270. Pierquin B, Cachin Y, Chassagne D, et al. Etude de 49 cas de carcinomes epidermides du cavum traites a l'institut Gustav-Roussy de 1960 a 1965. *Presse Med* 1968;76:1565–1566.

271. Pierquin B, Chassagne D, Baillet F, et al. The place of implantation in tongue and floor of mouth cancer. *JAMA* 1971;215:961.

272. Pierquin B, Pernot M, Baillet F. Tonsillar region. In: Pierquin B, Wilson J-F, Chassagne D, eds. *Modern brachytherapy.* New York: Masson, 1987;141–145.

273. Pierquin B, Wilson J-F, Chassagne D, eds. *Modern brachytherapy.* New York: Masson, 1987.

274. Pierquin B, Wilson J-F, Chassagne D. Radiation protection and the organizational plan of a brachytherapy department. In: Pierquin B, Wilson J-F, Chassagne D, eds. *Modern brachytherapy.* New York: Masson, 1987;43–59.

275. Pigneux J, Richaud PM, Largade C. The place of interstitial therapy using ^{192}Ir in the management of carcinoma of the lip. *Cancer* 1979;43:1073–1077.

276. Pisters PWT, Harrison LB, Leung DHY, et al. Long-term results of a prospective randomized trial of adjuvant brachytherapy in soft tissue sarcoma. *J Clin Oncol* 1995;14:859–868.

277. Pohar S, Hoffstetter S, Peiffert D, et al. Effectiveness of brachytherapy in treating carcinoma of the vulva. *Int J Radiat Oncol Biol Phys* 1995;32(5):1455–1460.

278. Polgar C, Fodor J, Orosz Z, et al. Electron and high dose rate brachytherapy boost in the conservative treatment of stage I-II breast cancer. *Stralenther Onkol* 2002;11:615–623.

279. Polgar C, Major T, Fedor J, et al. HDR brachytherapy alone versus whole breast radiotherapy with or without tumor bed boost after breast conserving surgery: seven years results of a comparative study. *Int J Radiat Oncol Biol Phys* 2003;56:681–689.

280. Poortmans P, Bartelink H, Horiot JC, et al. The influence of the boost technique on local control in breast conserving treatment in the EORTC "boost vs non boost" randomised trial. *Radiother Oncol* 2004;72:25–33.
281. Porrazzo MS, Hilaris BS, Moorthy CR, et al. Permanent interstitial implantation using palladium-103: the New York Medical College preliminary experience. *Int J Radiat Oncol Biol Phys* 1992;23:1033–1036.
282. Pos FJ, Horenblas S, Lebesque J, et al. Low-dose-rate brachytherapy is superior to high-dose-rate brachytherapy for bladder cancer. *Int J Radiat Oncol Biol Phys* 2004;59(3):696–705.
283. Potter R, Knocke TH, Kovacs G, et al. Brachytherapy in the combined modality treatment of pediatric malignancies: principles and preliminary experience with treatment of soft tissue sarcoma (recurrence) and Ewing's sarcoma. *Klin Padiatr* 1995;207:164–183.
284. Potters L. Permanent prostate brachytherapy: lessons learned, lessons to learn. *Oncology* 2000;14:981–991.
285. Prempree T. Parametrial implant in stage IIIB cancer of the cervix. III. A five-year study. *Cancer* 1983;52:748.
286. Prestidge BR, Prete JJ, Buchholz TA. A survey of current clinical practice of permanent prostate brachytherapy in the United States. *Int J Radiat Oncol Biol Phys* 1998;40:461–465.
287. Price A, Kerr GR, Arnott SJ. Radioactive needle implants in the treatment of anorectal cancer. *Clin Radiol* 1988;39:186–189.
288. Pryzant RM, Wendt CD, Delclos L, et al. Re-treatment of nasopharyngeal carcinoma in 53 patients. *Int J Radiat Oncol Biol Phys* 1992;22:941–947.
289. Puthawala AA, Syed AM, Tansey LA, et al. Temporary iridium-192 implant in the management of carcinoma of the prostate. *Endocurie Hypertherm Oncol* 1985;1:25.
290. Puthawala AA, Syed AMN, Gates TC, et al. Definitive treatment of extensive anorectal cancer by external and interstitial irradiation. *Cancer* 1982;50:1846–1850.
291. Qin D, Hu Y, Yan J, et al. Analysis of 1,379 patients with nasopharyngeal carcinoma treated by radiation. *Cancer* 1988;61:1118–1124.
292. Rosenblatt E, Cederbaum M, Yereslav N, et al. Reduction of the rectal dose in gynecological brachytherapy: modification of the Fletcher-Suit applicator. *Med Dosim* 1996;21:139–143.
293. Rosenblatt E, Rachmiel A, Blumenfeld I, et al. Intracavitary mould brachytherapy in malignant tumors of the maxilla. *Endocurie Hypertherm Oncol* 1996;12:25–34.
294. Rotte K. Technique and results of HDR afterloading in cancer of the endometrium. In: Martinez AA, Orton CG, Mould RF, eds. *Brachytherapy: HDR and LDR*. Columbia, MD: Nucletron Corporation, 1990;68–79.
295. Roy JN, Wallner KE, Chiu-Tsao S, et al. CT-based optimized planning for transperineal prostate implant with customized template. *Int J Radiat Oncol Biol Phys* 1991;21:483–489.
296. Roy JN, Wallner KE, Harrington PJ, et al. A CT-based evaluation method for permanent implants: application to prostate. *Int J Radiat Oncol Biol Phys* 1993;26:163–169.
297. Rozan R, Albuisson E, Donnarieix D, et al. Interstitial iridium-192 for bladder cancer (a multicentric survey: 205 patients). *Int J Radiat Oncol Biol Phys* 1992;24(3):469–477.
298. Rutledge FN, Delclos L. Adenocarcinoma of the uterus. In: Fletcher GH, ed. *Textbook of radiotherapy*, 3rd ed. Philadelphia: Lea & Febiger, 1980;798–808.
299. Ryan TP, Taylor JH, Coughlin CT. Interstitial microwave hyperthermia and brachytherapy for malignancies of the vulva and vagina. I. Design and testing of a modified intracavitary obturator. *Int J Radiat Oncol Biol Phys* 1992;23:189–199.
300. Saylor WL, Dillard M. Dosimetry of ^{137}Cs sources with Fletcher-Suit gynecological applicator. *Med Phys* 1976;3:118–119.
301. Scalliet P, Gerbaulet A, Dubray B. HDR versus LDR in gynecological brachytherapy revisited. *Radiother Oncol* 1993;28:118–126.
302. Scerrati M, Montemaggi P, Roselli R. Long-term results of interstitial brachytherapy for well differentiated cerebral tumors. *Acta Neurochirurgica* 1992; 117:1.
303. Scharfen CO, Sneed PK, Wara WM, et al. High activity iodine 125 interstitial implants for gliomas. *Int J Radiat Oncol Biol Phys* 1992;24:583–591.
304. Schatz CR, Kreth FW, Faist M, et al. Interstitial 125-iodine radiosurgery of low grade gliomas of the insula of Reil. *Acta Neurochir* 1984;130:80–89.
305. Schnitt SJ, Hayman J, Gelman R, et al. A prospective study of conservative surgery alone in the treatment of selected patients with stage I breast cancer. *Cancer* 1996;77:1094–1100.
306. Schray MF, Gunderson LL, Sim FH, et al. Soft tissue sarcoma: integration of brachytherapy, resection, and external irradiation. *Cancer* 1990;66:451–456.
307. Scott WP. Interstitial therapy using non-absorbable (Ir 192 nylon ribbon) and absorbable (I125 "Vicryl") suturing techniques. *Am J Roentgenol* 1975;124:560–564.
308. Seeger AR, Windschall A, Lotter M, et al. The role of interstitial brachytherapy in the treatment of vaginal and vulvar malignancies. *Strahlenther Onkol* 2006;182(3):142–148.
309. Selker RG, Shapiro WR, Burger PC, et al. The Brain Cooperative Group NIH trial 87-01: a randomized comparison of surgery, external radiotherapy and carmustine versus surgery, interstitial radiotherapy boost, external radiotherapy and carmustine. *Neurosurgery* 2002;51:343–355.
310. Sham JST, Wei WI, Choy D, et al. Treatment of persistent and recurrent nasopharyngeal carcinoma by brachytherapy. *Br J Radiol* 1989;62:355–361.
311. Shankar PG, Wolf D, Cytacki EP. Brachytherapy as boost for advanced tumors involving the oropharynx. *Endocurie Hypertherm Oncol* 1991;7:53–56.
312. Sherrah-Davies E. Morbidity following low-dose rate Selectron therapy for cervical cancer. *Clin Radiol* 1985;36:131–139.
313. Sminia P, Schneider CJ, van Tienhoven G, et al. Office hours pulsed brachytherapy boost in breast cancer. *Radiother Oncol* 2001;59:273–280.
314. Smith TE, Lee D, Turner BC, et al. True recurrence vs. new primary ipsilateral breast tumor relapse: an analysis of clinical and pathologic differences and their implications in natural history, prognosis, and therapeutic management. *Int J Radiat Oncol Biol Phys* 2000;48:1281–1289.
315. Sneed PK, Russo C, Scharfen CO, et al. Long-term follow-up after high activity ^{125}I brachytherapy for pediatric brain tumors. *Ped Neurosurg* 1996;24:314–322.
316. Stallard HB. Malignant melanoma of the choroid treated with radioactive applicators. *Ann R Coll Surg Engl* 1961;29:180.
317. Straus KL, Littman P, Wein AJ, et al. Treatment of bladder cancer with interstitial iridium-192 implantation and external beam irradiation. *Int J Radiat Oncol Biol Phys* 1988;14:265.
318. Strnad V, Lotter M, Grabenbauer G, et al. Early results of pulsed dose rate interstitial brachytherapy for head and neck malignancies after limited surgery. *Int J Radiat Oncol Biol Phys* 2000;46(1):27–30.
319. Strnard V, Ott O, Potter R, et al. Interstitial brachytherapy alone after breast conserving surgery: interim results of 2 German Austrian multicenter phase II trial. *Brachytherapy* 2004;3:115–119.
320. Suh WW, Pierce LJ, Vicini FA, et al. A cost comparison analysis of partial versus whole breast after breast conserving surgery for early stage breast cancer. *Int J Radiat Oncol Biol Phys* 2005;62(3):790–796.
321. Suit HD, Lloyd RS, Andrews JR, et al. Technique for intracavitary irradiation of the nasopharynx. *Am J Roentgenol* 1960;84:629–631.
322. Suit HD, Moore EB, Fletcher GH, et al. Modifications of Fletcher ovoid system for afterloading using standard sized radium tubes (milligram and microgram). *Radiology* 1963;81:126.
323. Swift, PS, Purser P, Roberts LW, et al. Pulsed low dose rate brachytherapy for pelvic malignancies. *J Radiat Oncol Biol Phys* 1997;37:811–818.
324. Syed AM, Puthawala AA, Abdelaziz NN, et al. Long-term results of low-dose-rate interstitial-intracavitary brachytherapy in the treatment of carcinoma of the cervix. *Int J Radiat Oncol Biol Phys* 2002;54(1):67–78.
324a. Syed AM, Puthawala AA, Severance SR, et al. Intraluminal irradiation in the treatment of esophageal cancer. *Endocurie Hyperterm Oncol* 1997;3:105–113.
325. Syed AMN, Puthawala AA, Tansey LA, et al. Temporary iridium-192 implantation in the management of carcinoma of the prostate. In: Hilaris BS, Batata MA, eds. *Brachytherapy oncology—1983*. New York: Memorial Sloan-Kettering Cancer Center, 1983;83–91.
326. Szikla G, Schlienger M, Blond S, et al. interstitial and combined interstitial and external irradiation of supratentorial gliomas. Results of 61 cases treated 1973–1981. *Acta Neurochirurg Suppl* 1984;33:355–362.
327. Thomadsen B, Ayyangar K, Anderson L, et al. Brachytherapy treatment planning. In: Nag S, ed. *Principles and practice of brachytherapy*. Armonk NY: Futura Publishing, 1997;127–199.
328. Tod MC, Meredith WJ. A dosage system for use in the treatment of cancer of the uterine cervix. *Br J Radiol* 1938;11:809.
329. Tombolini V, Bonanni A, Valeriani M, et al. Brachytherapy for squamous cell carcinoma of the lip. The experience of the Institute of Radiology of the University of Rome "La Sapienza." *Tumori* 1998;84:478–482.
330. Vaidya JS, Vyas JJ, Chinoy RF, et al. Multicentricity of breast cancer: whole organ analysis and clinical implications. *Br J Cancer* 1996;74:820–824.
331. van den Brenk HAS. Results of prophylactic postoperative irradiation in 1,300 cases of pterygium. *Am J Roentgenol* 1968;103:723–733.
332. van der Werf-Messing B, Menon RS, Ho WCJ. Cancer of the urinary bladder category T2, T3, (NxM0) treated by interstitial radium implant: second report. *Int J Radiat Oncol Biol Phys* 1983;9:481.
333. van der Werf-Messing B,van Putten WLJ. Carcinoma of the urinary bladder category T2,3Nx M0 treated by 40 Gy external irradiation followed by cesium 137 implant at reduced dose (50%). *Int J Radiat Oncol Biol Phys* 1989;16: 369.
334. Van Roosenbeek E, Delclos L. *The radioactive patient: care, precautions, and procedures in diagnosis and therapy*. Flushing, NY: Medical Examination Publishing, 1975.
335. Veronesi U, Banfi A, Saccozzi R, et al. Conservative treatment of breast cancer. A trial in progress at the Cancer Institute of Milan. *Cancer* 1977;39:2822–2826.
336. Veronesi U, Cascinelli N, Mariani L, et al. Twenty year follow up of a randomized study comparing breast conserving surgery with radical mastectomy for early breast cancer. *N Engl J Med* 2002;347:1227–1232.
337. Veronesi U, Marubini E, Mariani L, et al. Radiotherapy after breast conserving surgery in small breast carcinoma: long-term results of a randomized trial. *Ann Oncol* 2001;12:997–1003.
338. Veronesi U, Salvadori, Luini A, et al. Conservative treatment of early breast cancer. Long term results of 1,232 cases treated with quadrantectomy, axillary dissection and radiotherapy. *Ann Surg* 1990;211:250–259.
339. Vicini FA, Chen PY, Fraile M, et al. Low dose rate brachytherapy as the sole radiation modality in the management of patients with early stage breast cancer treated with breast conserving therapy: preliminary results of a pilot trial. *Int J Radiat Oncol Biol Phys* 1997;38:301–310.
340. Vicini FA, Kestin L, Chen P, et al. Limited field radiation therapy in the management of early stage breast cancer. *J Natl Cancer Inst* 2003;95:1205–1210.
341. Visser AG, van den Aardweg GJMJ, Levendag PC. Pulsed dose rate and fractionated high dose rate brachytherapy: choice of brachytherapy schedules to replace low dose rate treatments. *Int J Radiat Oncol Biol Phys* 1996;34:497–505.
342. Vitaz TW, Warnke PC, Tabar V, et al. Brachytherapy for brain tumors. *J Neuro-Oncol* 2005;73:71–86.
343. Wadsley JC, Patel M, Tomlins CDC, et al. Iridium-192 implantation for T1 and T2 carcinomas of the tongue an floor of the mouth. Retrospective study of the results of treatment at the Royal Berkshire Hospital. *Br J Radiol* 2003;76:414–417.
344. Walker M, Alexander E, Hunt WE, et al. Evaluation of BCNU and/or radiotherapy in the treatment of anaplastic gliomas. *J Neurosurg* 1978;49:333–343.
345. Wallner K, Chiu-Tsao S-T, Roy J, et al. An improved method for computerized tomography-planned transperineal 125-iodine prostate implants. *J Urol* 1991;146:90–95.
346. Wallner K, Roy J, Harrison L. Dosimetry guidelines to minimize urethral and rectal morbidity following transperineal I-125 prostate brachytherapy. *Int J Radiat Oncol Biol Phys* 1995;32:465–471.
347. Wang CC. Re-irradiation of recurrent nasopharyngeal carcinoma: treatment techniques and results. *Int J Radiat Oncol Biol Phys* 1987;13:953–956.
348. Wang CC. Treatment of malignant tumors of the nasopharynx. *Otolaryngol Clin North Am* 1980;13:477–481.
349. Wang CC, Schultz MD. Management of locally recurrent carcinoma of the nasopharynx. *Radiology* 1966;86:900–903.
350. Waterman FM, Mansfield CM, Komarnicky L, et al. A dosimetry system for Ir-192

interstitial breast implants performed at the time of lumpectomy. *Int J Radiat Oncol Biol Phys* 1997;37:229–235.

351. Weaver K. The dosimetry of ^{125}I seed eye plaques. *Med Phys* 1986;13:78.
352. Weaver K, Smith V, Huang D, et al. Dose parameters of ^{125}I and ^{192}Ir seed sources. *Med Phys* 1989;16:636.
353. Wen PY, Alexander E, Black PM, et al. Long term results of stereotactic brachytherapy used in the initial treatment of patients with glioblastomas. *Cancer* 1994;73(12):3029–3036.
354. Wijnmaalen A, Helle PA, Koper PC, et al. Muscle invasive bladder cancer treated by transurethral resection, followed by external beam radiation and interstitial iridium-192. *Int J Radiat Oncol Biol Phys* 1997;39:1043–1052.
355. Wijnmaalen AJ, Helle PA, Koper PCM, et al. Combined external beam and interstitial radiation for bladder cancer. In: Mould RF, ed. *Brachytherapy 2*. Leerum, The Netherlands: Nucletron International BV, 1989;192–195.
356. Wilkinson J, Moore C, Notley H, et al. The use of Selectron afterloading equipment to simulate and extend the Manchester system for intracavitary therapy of the cervix uteri. *Br J Radiol* 1983;56:409–414.
357. Williamson JF. Monte Carlo evaluation of specific dose constants in water for ^{125}I seeds. *Med Phys* 1988;15:686.
358. Williamson JF. Practical quality assurance in low-dose rate brachytherapy. In: *Proceedings of American College of Medical Physics—sponsored symposium on quality assurance in radiotherapy physics*. Madison, WI: Medical Physics Publishing Company, 1991;139–182.

359. Williamson JF, Grigsby PW, Meigooni AS, et al. Clinical physics of pulsed dose-rate remotely-afterloaded brachytherapy. In: Williamson JF, Thomadsen BT, Nath R, eds. *Brachytherapy physics*. Madison, WI: Medical Physics Publishing Company, 1995;577–616.
360. Yamashita S, Kondo M, Inuyama Y, et al. Improved survival of patients with nasopharyngeal squamous cell carcinoma. *Int J Radiat Oncol Biol Phys* 1986;12:307–312.
361. Yan JH, Hu YH, Gu XZ. Radiation therapy of recurrent nasopharyngeal carcinoma: report on 219 patients. *Acta Radiol Oncol* 1983;22:23–28.
362. Zaider M, Zelefsky MJ, Lee EK, et al. Treatment planning for prostate implants using magnetic resonance spectroscopy imaging. *Int J Radiat Oncol Biol Phys* 2000;47:1085–1096.
363. Zelefsky JM, Yamada Y, Cohen, et al. Postimplantation dosimetric analysis of permanent transperineal prostate implantation: improved dose distributions with an intraoperative computer-optimized conformal planning technique. *Int J Radiat Oncol Biol Phys* 2000;48:602–608.
364. Zolli CI. Experience with the avulsion technique in pterygium surgery. *Ann Ophthalmol* 1979;11:1569–1576.
365. Zwicker RD, Schmidt-Ullrich R. Dose uniformity in a planar interstitial implant system. *Int J Radiat Oncol Biol Phys* 1994;31:149–155.
366. Zwicker RD, Schmidt-Ullrich R, Schiller B. Planning of Ir-192 seed implants for boost irradiation to the breast. *Int J Radiat Oncol Biol Phys* 1985;11:2163–2180.

Techniques, Modalities, and Modifiers in Radiation Oncology

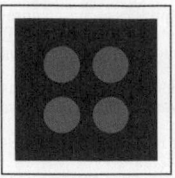

Chapter 21
The Physics and Dosimetry of High–Dose-Rate Brachytherapy

Bruce Thomadsen, Rupak Das

Introduction

Nature of High–Dose-Rate Brachytherapy

Conventional brachytherapy was developed very shortly after the discovery of radium. The limited amount of radium that could be packed into the needles and tubes dictated the use of many sources to deliver a treatment dose through a target volume, and even with many sources, the delivery of the dose required durations from a day to a week. For the most part, when new radionuclides became available, they matched the strength of the radium sources to facilitate application of the clinical experience gained through the decades of radium treatments. This conventional treatment format describes low–dose-rate (LDR) brachytherapy.

Beginning around 1962, a new approach to brachytherapy developed. Using very intense, small sources (usually of ^{60}Co in the early machines and often three in number) on the ends of cables, a treatment unit would move the source through the volume to be treated, delivering the radiation in a relatively short time (less than an hour). The rapid treatment delivery gave these treatments the name high–dose-rate (HDR) brachytherapy. The original units mostly oscillated the source through a catheter's treatment length, a method in common use until the modern generation of units developed in the early 1980s, described below. The treatments took so little time that the therapy proceeded on an outpatient basis. However, for reasons discussed later in this section, the treatment regimen usually entailed several fractions delivered over days or weeks.

The modern HDR units move a single source through the treatment volume in a stepwise fashion, moving at intervals determined by the machine construction and the operator to positions where the source pauses (dwell positions) for durations (dwell times) determined through optimization procedures.

High–Dose-Rate Devices

Remote Afterloaders

A remote afterloader (RAL) is a computer-driven system that transports the radioactive source from a shielded safe into the applicator placed in the patient. Upon termination or interruption of the treatment, the source is driven back to its safe. The device may move the source by one of several methods, most commonly pneumatic air pressure or cable drives. A stepping-source RAL is a particular design of the treatment unit that consists of a single source at the end of a cable that moves the source through applicators placed in the treated volume. The treatment unit can treat implants consisting of many needles or catheters in the patient. Multiple catheters are often required to cover the target with uniform radiation doses. Each catheter or part of an applicator is connected to the RAL through a channel. The computer drives the cable so that the source moves from the safe through a given channel to the programmed dwell position for a specific dwell time. In any applicator, there may be many dwell positions. After treating all the positions in a given catheter (channel) the source is retracted to its safe and then driven to the next channel. The dwell positions and the dwell time in each channel are programmable independently, thereby giving a high level of flexibility of dose delivery. All currently available HDR RALs use the stepping-source design. Currently there are three models of HDR RALs available in the market: MicroSelectron (Nucletron, Veenendaal, Netherlands), Gamma-Med and VariSource (both Varian Associates, Palo Alto, CA). Figure 21.1 shows two of the units. Even though they may vary in details, all available HDR RALs consist of the same general components (Fig. 21.2): (a) shielded safe, (b) radioactive source, (c) source drive mechanism, (d) indexer, (e) transfer tube, (f) treatment control station, and (g) treatment control panel.

Sources

While delivering the HDR brachytherapy requires an intense source, passing the source through needles placed through a tumor requires one of a small size. The radioactive source in an HDR RAL is usually 3 to 10 mm in length and <1 mm in diameter, fixed at the end of a steel cable. The Nucletron source is placed in a stainless steel capsule and welded to the cable, while the Varian source is placed in a hole drilled into the cable and closed by welding. Figure 21.3 shows diagrams of the sources. ^{192}Ir is now used for almost all HDR RALs, although early versions of HDR RAL used ^{60}Co. ^{192}Ir emits many photon energies, mostly between 110 and 704 keV, with an effective energy around 380 keV. A new source has an activity near 0.37 TBq (10 curies, approximately 44 mGy m^2 h^{-1}). Since ^{192}Ir has a half-life of 74 days, the source should be replaced every 3 months to keep the treatment in the HDR radiobiological regime (see below). A trained medical physicist calibrates the source after each installation using a reentrant, well-type ionization chamber, as discussed below. The resulting source calibration is verified against the manufacturer's source calibration.

Recently, an afterloader came to market using a ^{169}Yb source. The advantage of this source comes from the lower energy of its emissions, dominated by 63 keV (44% of the time) and 198 keV (36% of the time). The lower energy implies that shielding in any applicator reduces the intensity of the radiation more than for ^{192}Ir and also opens the possibility of including shielding in smaller structures, such as an intrauterine tandem.

Applicators

An array of applicators for different treatment sites are marketed by each vendor. Each vendor designs their own applicators that can only be used with their transfer tubes and their HDR RALs. Before an applicator is used clinically, tests should be performed to verify the functionality of the applicator. It should also be radiographed with dummy sources (ribbons) to verify agreement with the vendor's specifications. The length of each applicator, location of the dwell positions with respect to the applicator, and integrity of the applicators should be a part of the routine quality assurance (QA) program to ensure

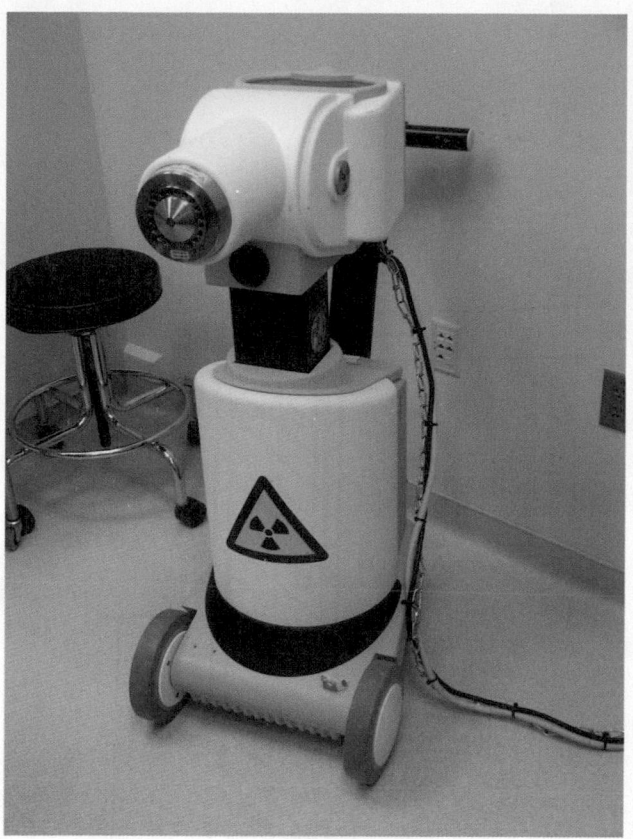
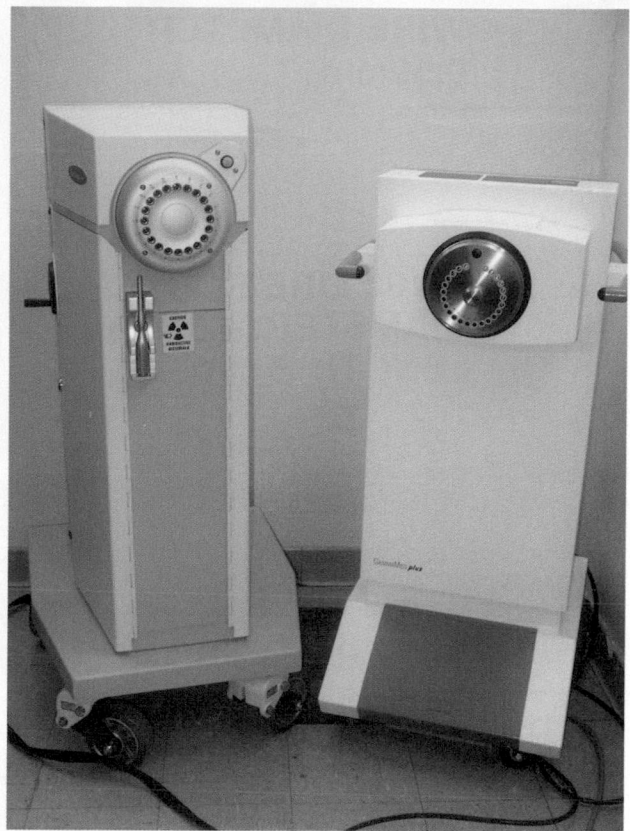

A   B

FIGURE 21.1. A: The Nucletron MicroSelectron. **B:** The Varian VariSource and the GammaMed.

safe and precise delivery of the radiation treatment plan. Figure 21.4 shows a comparison between an HDR and a LDR intrauterine cervical tandem. The smaller diameter of the HDR applicator leads to greater patient comfort during the procedure. Since high–dose-rate iridium source is much smaller than the low–dose-rate cesium tubes, high–dose-rate applicators have a smaller radius.

Advantages and Disadvantages

Advantages of HDR brachytherapy over LDR include:

1. *Optimization.* The stepping-source design permits very fine control of the source position through the target volume. In most treatments, the determination of the dwell times comes from inverse planning, that is, specifying the doses desired at various locations and using some algorithm to calculate the dwell times that best fit the dose specifications. The map of how long the source dwells at each possible dwell position can be finely tailored to the geometry and needs of the particular patient because of the wide range of dwell times available. This process constitutes *optimization.* Although optimization is possible and frequently used with LDR applications, it forms a more natural part of the planning process with HDR brachytherapy.

2. *Immobilization and stability.* The relatively short duration of the HDR treatments allows better stability of many intracavitary treatment applicators during the treatment, and thus, higher precision in conforming the dose to the target. In addition to simply not giving much time for applicator motion,

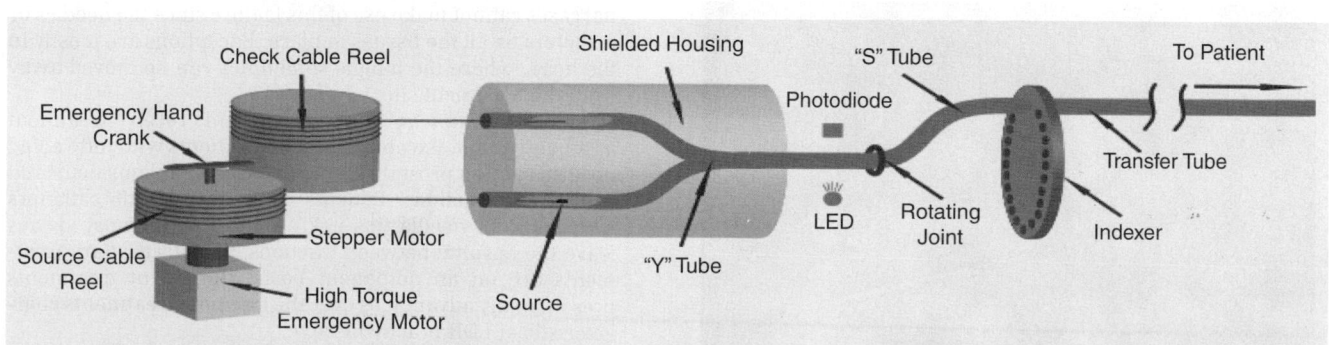

FIGURE 21.2. Components of a high dose-rate brachytherapy remote afterloader. (Figure by Adam Uselmann after the draft by Liyong Lin).

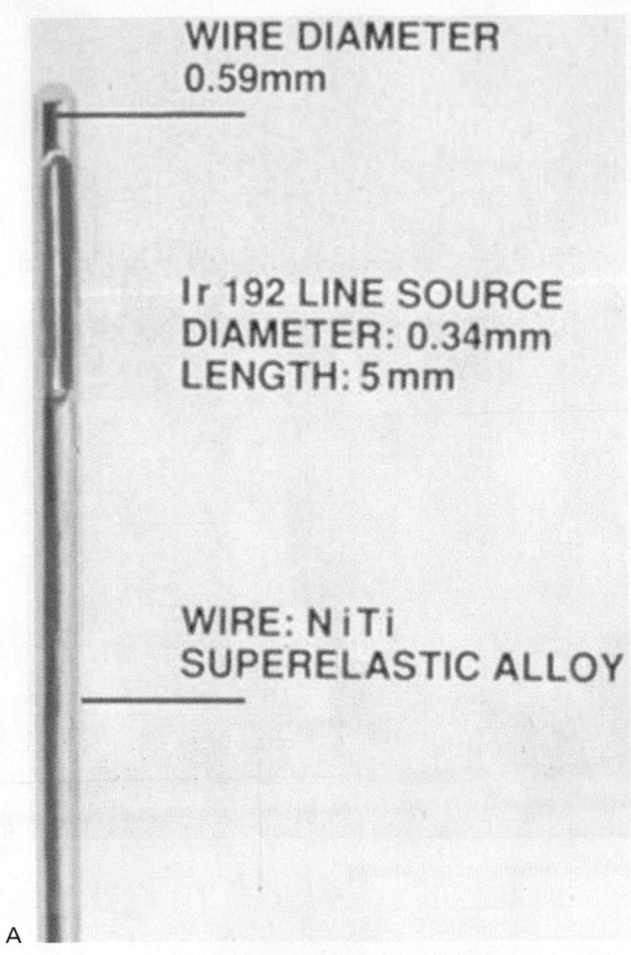

WIRE DIAMETER
0.59mm

Ir 192 LINE SOURCE
DIAMETER: 0.34mm
LENGTH: 5mm

WIRE: NiTi
SUPERELASTIC ALLOY

A

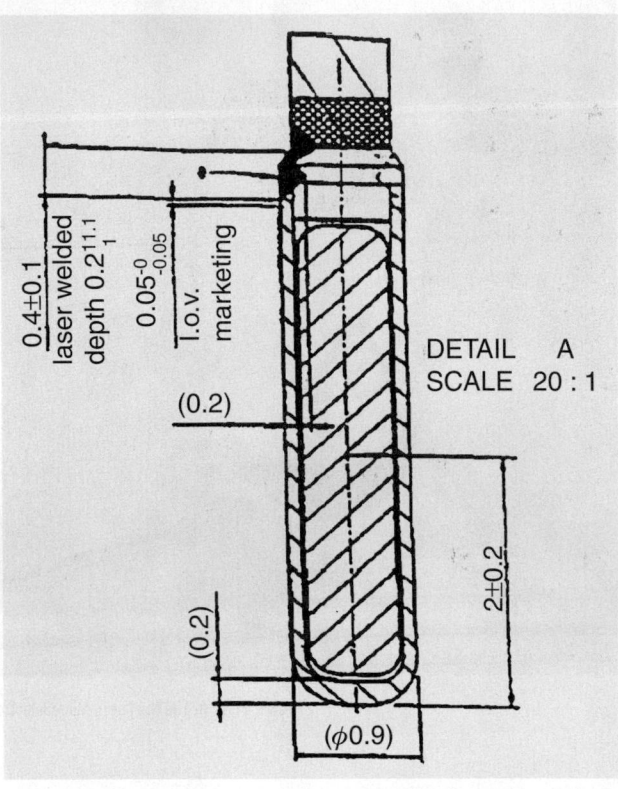

DETAIL   A
SCALE   20 : 1

B

FIGURE 21.3. Diagrams of two HDR brachytherapy sources: **(A)** for the VariSource (figure provided courtesy of Varian Associates, Palo Alto, CA); **(B)** for the MicroSelectron (figure provided courtesy of Nucletron, Veendendaal, The Netherlands).

the applicator and the patient can both be immobilized with respect to the treatment table over the duration of the treatment. Such fixation is not possible with LDR brachytherapy because the patient would not tolerate the immobility for long periods. Interstitial cases may or may not exhibit better stability. The needles often tend to slide outward over the time that prostate implants remain in the patient, even with a template that fixes the needles sutured to the patient. In such a patient, the needles' positions require adjustment before each fraction but move very little during the treatment deliv-

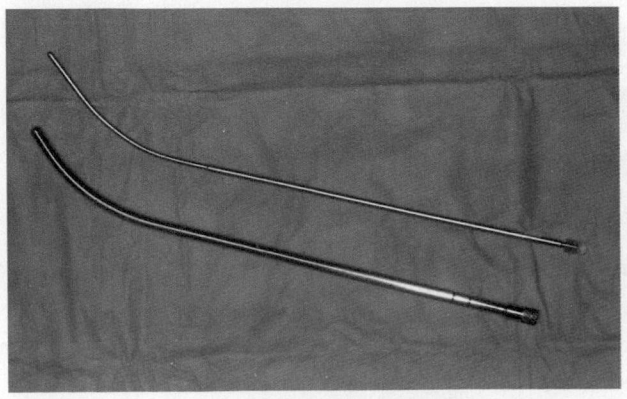

FIGURE 21.4. HDR (*top*) and LDR (*bottom*) intrauterine tandems.

ery. Performing the same treatment using LDR brachytherapy would cause needle movement during the long, slow delivery. On the other hand, head and neck implants with buttons anchoring the catheters at both ends may allow very little movement from the time of insertion through removal. Such cases would not find improvement in stability with HDR brachytherapy.

3. *Dose reduction to normal tissue.* Again, the short duration of HDR intracavitary treatments often allows displacement of normal tissue structure to a greater extent than with LDR treatments. This holds true for gynecological and oral intracavitary cases, but not for intraluminal applications, such as endoesophageal or endobronchial treatments. Most interstitial cases cannot make use of this feature since the needles or catheters fix all the tissues in place. Exceptions are mostly in the head, where the tongue sometimes can be moved away from the treatment site.

4. *Outpatient treatment.* Most HDR patients receive treatment as an outpatient. Exceptions include patients with indwelling needles such as prostate or gynecological implants delivered in multiple fractions. Patients containing plastic catheters (i.e., not with needle tips poking into flesh) almost always leave the hospital between fractions. All intracavitary treatments are on an outpatient basis. Outpatient treatments present many advantages over the inpatient treatments characteristic of LDR brachytherapy:

   • *Patient comfort.* Patients confined to a room during LDR treatments often feel closed in. Compounding the claustrophobic effects, radiation safety considerations limit the time nursing staff can spend with the patient (sometime very severely), leading patients to feel like a pariah.

- *Patient health*. Many LDR brachytherapy applications require the patients to stay in bed, increasing the probability of thrombosis or bed soars. Although pneumatic socks greatly reduce the likelihood of thrombosis, aching muscles from immobility still create discomfort. In many cases, patients who could not tolerate protracted LDR treatments will be able to receive their treatments using HDR techniques.

- *Economics*. The cost of staying in the hospital greatly exceeds outpatient treatment. Counterbalancing the cost of hospitalization, the costs of the HDR remote afterloading equipment far exceeds that for LDR applications. However, the HDR equipment costs quickly become amortized with a modest patient load, while the hospitalization costs remain constant for each patient.

5. *Less discomfort due to small size*. Because the encapsulated HDR source is only 1 mm or less in diameter, the gynecological intrauterine tandem need only be 3 mm in diameter compared with 7 mm for the standard LDR tandem. Another way of looking at this comparison is to recognize that the diameter of the HDR tandem equals the smallest-size dilator used to stretch the cervical os to accept the LDR tandem. Much of the pain and discomfort from a cervical cancer treatment comes during the dilation. Eliminating that step eliminates much of that pain. As a result, some facilities use only light sedation for the HDR tandem insertion rather than a general anesthetic, as is common with LDR procedures.

6. *Elimination of delays*. When applications fail to follow a plan or when plans have to change, HDR treatments can still proceed following localization with little, if any, delay. LDR treatments likely would require ordering new sources to match the new situation, and a delay in treatment to await delivery. The HDR model eliminates extra charges accruing from multiple-source orders.

7. *Intraoperative procedures*. HDR brachytherapy allows treatment intraoperatively, with suitable shielding in the operating room. With the short duration for dose delivery, a surgeon can add placement of the applicator and treatment of the patient to surgery with little additional time.

8. *Radiation safety*. HDR brachytherapy eliminates radiation exposure to personnel.

Unfortunately, HDR brachytherapy carries with it the following disadvantages:

1. *Radiobiology*. Compared with low–dose-rate brachytherapy, HDR treatments have worse therapeutic ratios, that is the amount of damage to tumor cells compared with damage to normal tissue cells for the same dose. The damage to both types of cells per unit dose increases with dose rate, but the increase is greater for normal cells. Just as with external-beam radiotherapy, which also is high–dose-rate delivery, an approach to mitigating this effect is to fractionate the treatment. Although LDR therapy usually entails a single session, or possibly two, most curative HDR regimens use five fractions.

2. *Error hazard*. The increased complexity of the procedures and the compressed time frame of delivery increase the probability of errors in the treatment compared with LDR therapy.

3. *Potential for very high radiation doses to patients and unit operators following failure of the source to retract*. The HDR source can deliver 7.4 Gy/min at 1 cm in the patient. If the source stops moving or separates from the drive cable, serious injury occurs in a short time.

4. *Resources*. HDR treatments demand more resources that LDR treatments:
   - *Personnel*. Because many HDR treatments proceed quickly from placement of the treatment appliance to delivery of

the treatment, all the persons involved with the treatment must be available at the same time or in relatively quick secession. That means that the facility must have sufficient staffing to release these persons on demand of the HDR brachytherapy cases.

- *Economics*. The HDR afterloading equipment comes with a large initial investment (at the time of writing approximately $300,000 to $500,000), not including the significant costs of shielding the treatment room and the increased cost for all the treatment applicators and supplies.

Radiobiological Dosimetry

Because of the radiobiological disadvantage of HDR treatments, considerable care must be taken in planning the time course of the therapy regimen. One of the important tools for such planning is the linear-quadratic model for biological response.

The Linear-Quadratic Model

The basis for the model for biological response to radiation stems from an approximation to the cell survival curves as shown in Fig. 21.5.

Several models have been used over the years to describe the shape of the curve, each giving different insights into the interaction of the radiation and the organism irradiated. One of the more useful when investigating radiotherapy regimen has been the linear-quadratic (LQ) model. This model approximates the cell survival, S, as

$$S = e^{-\alpha D - \beta D^2} \tag{1}$$

Like any model, this equation fits the curves well over a particular range, which makes it useful. It can also shed some light on biological underpinnings. However, the model should not be seen as a true and complete description and explanation of a complex biological phenomenon.

The curves shown apply to a single exposure of the cells over a short period of time at given dose rate. As can be seen, the effect of dose rate markedly changes the survival of the cells. This discussion need only consider the two components of the exponent in equation 1. Conceptually, the first term, αD, corresponds to damage to the cells when a single charged-particle track breaks both sides of a DNA molecule rung (for example, both a guanine and a cytosine), referred to as a double-strand break. Killing the cells requires a double-strand break. The surviving fraction depends only on the dose, and the effect does not depend on the dose rate. The second term, βD^2 represents damage done when one charged-particle path breaks one side of the DNA rung, say the guanine, and a different track breaks the other side (the cytosine). Following the first side break, called a single-strand break, the DNA attempts repair. Because of the remaining cytosine on the opposite side, only a guanine will fit into the hole left on the damaged side. The nucleus contains many free guanine molecules and one will be attracted to the opening and heal the wound. The repair takes place with a half time of T_{bio}, which corresponds to a repair rate of:

$$\mu = 0.693/T_{bio}. \tag{2}$$

Since the repair takes some time, there is a window in which the second break must take place for the entire rung to be removed. If the second hit takes place after repair of the first, the damage still only forms a single-strand break, and the opposite side must be hit again to form a double-side break. Because forming a double-strand break this way requires two independent hits, the probability follows D^2. Because the second hit must occur before the repair of the first, the incidence of double-strand breaks depends on the dose rate. Frequently, a value for T_{bio} of 1.5 hours is used in calculations, although most tissues probably

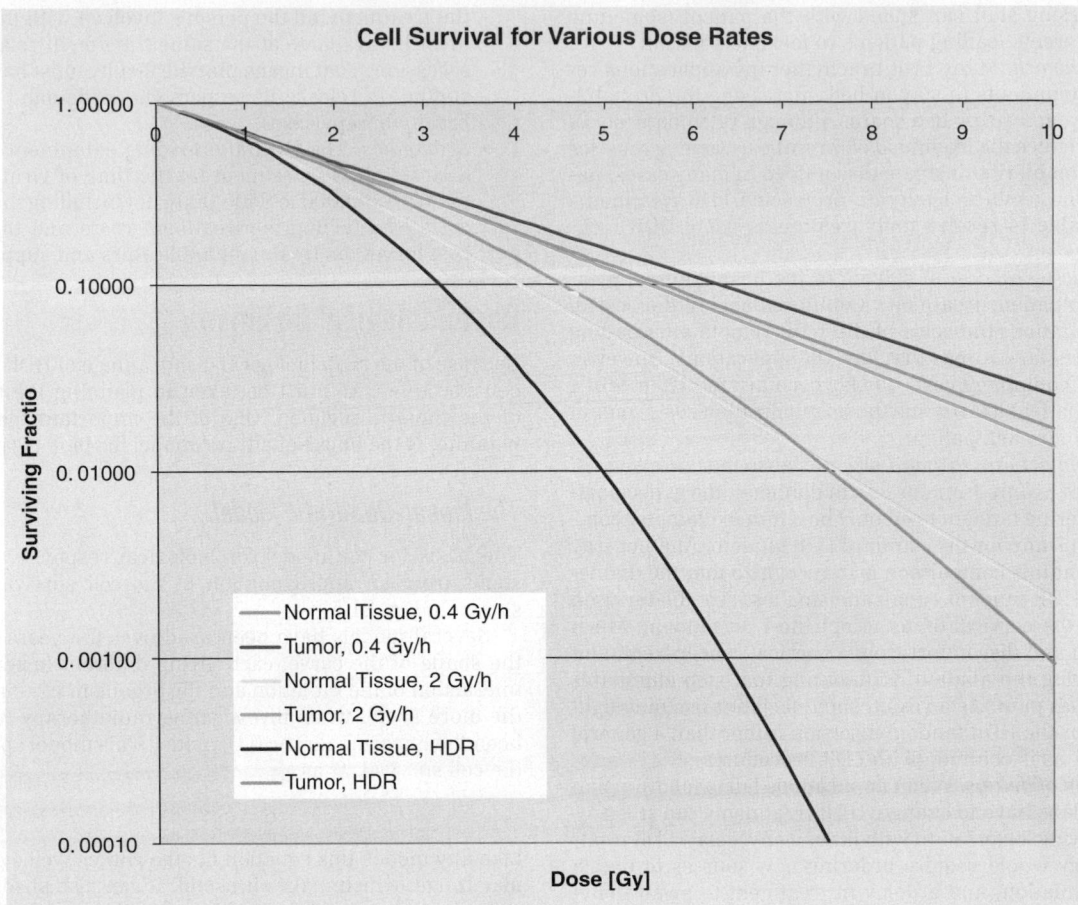

FIGURE 21.5. Typical cell survival curves with dose on the abscissa and surviving fraction on the ordinate, for three dose rates. The curves in the figure used α/β values of 3 Gy for normal tissue, 10 Gy for the tumor, and an α of 0.35 Gy^{-1} and μ of 1.5 h^{-1} for both types of tissue.

have a more complicated repair pattern, with a fast component of about 20 minutes, and a longer one of about 2.2 hours.

The surviving fraction also depends on the values of α and β. These parameters are characteristic of the tissue being irradiated and the type of tissue injury being caused. The actual values are often not well known, and large variations in most tissues have been reported. However, in general, the values of α tend to be very similar for most tissues (within the uncertainties), with most of the variations being in the β term. Although the variations in the values determined for the two parameters tend to be large, smaller variation characterizes the ratio of α/β, the quantity most often given in the literature. For the most part, this ratio tends to be on the order of 2 to 3 for late effects in normal tissues, and 5 to 20 for early effects. In general, tissues exhibiting less mitotic activity show lower values. Most tumors behave similarly to normal tissue early effects, but with a much wider range of values. Prostate cancer forms a notable exception, with an α/β between 1.5 and 2.

Figure 21.5 shows that as the dose rate increases, the fraction survival decreases for a given dose, and this effect is more marked for tissues with a low value for α/β. Thus, as stated above, compared with low–dose-rate brachytherapy, normal tissue has a comparative disadvantage for high–dose-rate brachytherapy. The usual approach to overcome the disadvantage fractionates the dose delivery. Figure 21.6 shows a survival curve with the dose delivered in several fractions. The pauses in the delivery allows repair of those single-strand breaks not converted into double-strand breaks by a second hit. Thus, at the beginning of each fraction the curve exhibits a new shoulder as the first single-strand breaks begin accumulating. The

fractionation has no affect on the α term. Fractionation has a long history in external-beam radiotherapy, which also is high–dose-rate delivery. Understanding the repair mechanism allows for a definition of what dose rates qualify as "high": when the delivery duration remains much less than T$_{bio}$, or about 30 minutes.

Surviving fraction does not depend directly on dose; rather the whole exponent forms the independent variable. Because the α tends to be constant, it is often pulled out, leaving what is called the biologically effective dose (BED) or equivalently the effective radiation dose (ERD) as:

$$BED = D + \frac{D^2}{\left(\frac{\alpha}{\beta}\right)} = D \left[1 + \frac{D}{\left(\frac{\alpha}{\beta}\right)} \right] \tag{3}$$

For the fractionated, high–dose-rate irradiations, each new fraction starts the curve over but at the surviving fraction level where it left off at the end of the previous fraction (in the absence of proliferation), and the equation becomes:

$$BED_{HDR} = n \left[d \left(1 + \frac{d}{\left(\frac{\alpha}{\beta}\right)} \right) \right] = nd \left(1 + \frac{d}{\left(\frac{\alpha}{\beta}\right)} \right) \tag{4}$$

where n equals the number of fractions and d equals the dose per fraction.

The LDR situation becomes more complicated because repair takes place during the irradiation, reducing the effectiveness.

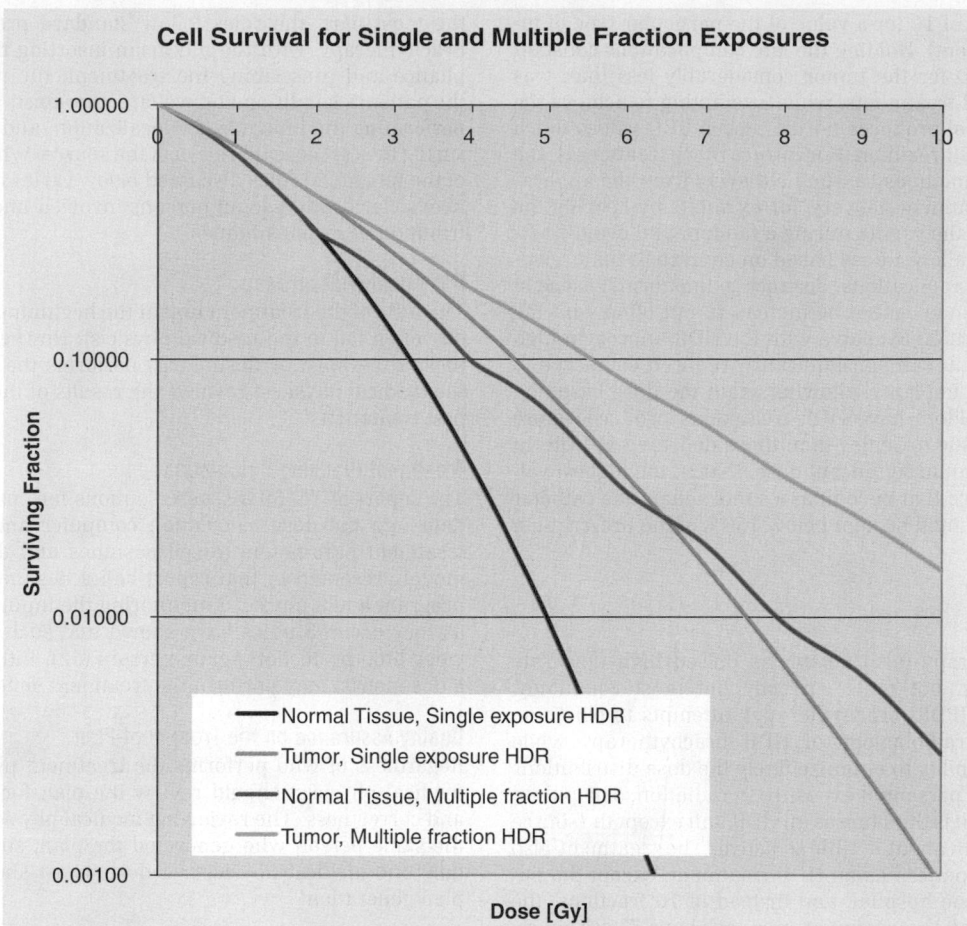

Cell Survival for Single and Multiple Fraction Exposures

FIGURE 21.6. Survival curves illustrating the effects of fractionation. The cell parameters are the same as in Figure 21.5.

In this case, BED becomes:

$$BED_{LDR} = D \left\{ 1 + \left[\frac{2R}{\left(\frac{\alpha}{\beta}\right)\mu} \right] \bullet \left[\frac{1 - e^{-\mu T}}{\mu T} \right] \right\} \quad (5)$$

where T equals the duration of the treatment and R equals the dose rate. Because the BED depends on the α/β used, the convention when giving a BED specifies the value in units of gray with a subscript of the α/β, for example, the BED for late responding tissue with an α/β of 3 might be stated as BED = 10 Gy_3.

In fact, the equations for both modalities also contain a term, not shown in the equations:

$$- \frac{0.693T}{\alpha T_{pot}} \quad (6)$$

to account for cell repopulation over the total treatment duration. T_{pot} represents the potential cell doubling time. Most applications ignore this term because of the large uncertainties in the values for α and T_{pot}. In situations comparing the BED of low– and high–dose-rate application where the total duration of the therapy would be approximately the same, this omission probably causes no significant loss of information.

Conversion from Low– to High–Dose-Rate Brachytherapy

Often, when beginning an HDR brachytherapy program, the question as to the type of treatment becomes how many fractions to use and what dose per fraction. The larger the number of fractions, the better the therapeutic effect, that is the ratio

of the damage to tumor cells to the damage to normal tissue cells. This ratio improves with each additional fraction, but the incremental increase decreases with each added fraction. For example, going from four to five fractions improves the therapeutic ratio by 4%. Adding a sixth fraction imposes the therapeutic ratio, but only by another 3.5%. Each additional fraction carries with it costs in departmental resources (particularly the time of those persons involved) and inconvenience (and possibly discomfort) to the patient. Thus, selecting the number of fractions becomes a compromise. Most curative regimens use five or six fractions if applicator insertion procedures are involved, or eight to 12 fractions if the applicator can be left in place and the patient simply treated. Small volume applications, such as vaginal cuff or most endobronchial treatments, may require only three of four fractions. After establishing the number of fractions, determining the dose per fraction comes next. One method that utilizes the LDR experience sets the BED equal for the two modalities and then solves for the dose per fraction:

$$BED_{HDR} = BED_{LDR} \quad (7a)$$

$$nd\left[1 + \frac{d}{\frac{\alpha}{\beta}}\right] = D \left\{ 1 + \left[\frac{2R}{\frac{\alpha}{\beta}\mu} \right] \bullet \left[\frac{1 - e^{-\mu T}}{\mu T} \right] \right\} \quad (7b)$$

$$d = \frac{-\frac{\alpha}{\beta} + \sqrt{\left(\frac{\alpha}{\beta}\right)^2 + \left(\frac{4D}{n}\right)\left(\frac{\alpha}{\beta}\right)\left\{1 + \left(\frac{2R}{\mu}\right)\left(\frac{\beta}{\alpha}\right)\left[1 - \frac{1 - e^{-\mu T}}{\mu T}\right]\right\}}}{2} \quad (7c)$$

The absolute value for the dose per fraction depends on the α/β, thus requiring another decision. Projecting d from the LDR experience, the normal tissue toxicities could be held constant and an α/β of three used, or tumor cure could be the end point, suggesting an α/β of 10 (or a value of the particular type of tumor under treatment). Holding the late complications constant will lead to a BED for the tumor considerably less than was used with the LDR treatments, while attempting to achieve the same tumor control produces normal tissue BED values much higher than the LDR regimen. For intracavitary treatments, the normal tissues sometimes can be held away from the applicator during the treatment delivery, for example, by keeping the rectal retractor in the vagina during a tandem and ovoid treatment. This would allow a dose based on equivalent tumor control. In interstitial applications, distance to the normal tissue in the implanted volume cannot be increased, but often with the improved optimization available with the HDR approach, high doses in the implant can be significantly reduced compared to conventional LDR implants, allowing again the dose based on tumor control. Seldom have HDR treatments produced more severe normal tissue toxicities than those delivered at LDR. In general, the maximum significant dose, that is, the highest valued isodose surface that encompasses more than one catheter or needle track, should be kept below 150% of the prescription dose.

Pulsed Brachytherapy

Pulsed brachytherapy (also known as pulsed high–dose-rate brachytherapy, or, not quite correctly but most commonly, pulsed–dose-rate [PDR] brachytherapy), attempts to eliminate the unfavorable radiobiology of HDR brachytherapy while maintaining the ability to optimize finely the dose distributions and eliminate the personnel exposure to radiation. The pulsed brachytherapy unit is the same as an HDR unit except the source is shorter and only about a 10th as active. The treatment also follows the same pattern as an HDR treatment, except the patient remains in the hospital, and instead of 10 fractions, the source runs through the treatment once each hour. These hourly treatment pulses last only a few minutes, but the overall duration usually covers 1 or 2 days. Thus, biologically, since each fraction comes before complete repair of sublethal cellular damage, the tissues experience the radiation as almost continuous, mimicking LDR brachytherapy.

Although this approach incorporates the biological advantages of LDR treatments and the optimization advantage of HDR brachytherapy, it also has many of the disadvantages of both modalities, including: (a) inpatient treatments, (b) lack of applicator stabilization, and (c) possibility of mechanical failures. Because the source treats the patient 24 times per day, and each treatment includes three or more catheters, the number of source transits becomes quite large and many times more than for a normal HDR regimen. Such frequent source use increases the likelihood of source failure during a treatment. Should a source become caught during transit, the dose to the patient could become quite large. Unlike HDR procedures, the operator does not sit at the control panel always ready to retrieve a stuck source. Limiting the activity of the source to a 10th of the normal HDR source allows 10 times the response time for a stuck source before significant injury to the patient. The other reason for the low activity is that, with the treatment divided into so many small fractions, the dwell times become too short for the treatment unit to control with a very active source. In summary, pulsed brachytherapy presents opportunities to potentially improve brachytherapy, but it also comes with detriments.

Operation

Personnel Roles

The report of Task Group 59 of the American Association of Physicists in Medicine discusses the roles of the members of the treatment team for high dose-rate brachytherapy (23). For the most part, the roles follow standard procedures for any brachytherapy, with the physician inserting the treatment appliance and prescribing the treatment; the nurse monitoring the patient's condition and welfare; therapists or radiographers performing the imagines for localization; and the physicist assuring the correct calibration of the source. Who performs some of the functional roles discussed below varies by institution, but needs clarification so all persons involved understand the distribution of responsibilities.

Daily Quality Assurance

The tests of the treatment unit at the beginning of the treatment day often fall to the medical physicist. However, in some facilities, a therapist or dosimetrist performs the actual tests, and the medical physicist reviews the results of the tests before the first treatment.

Treatment Planning Calculation

The report of TG-59 discusses options for entering the patient data into the dose calculation computer and generating the treatment parameters (dwell positions and dwell times). One model presented in that report had a dosimetrist running the program and a physicist monitoring the input to correct errors as they occur. Studies have shown that such supervision provides little protection against errors (52). Either a physicist or a dosimetrist may perform the treatment generation.

Quality Assurance on the Treatment Plan

Regardless of who performs the treatment plan generation, a medical physicist should review the plan for appropriateness and correctness. The reviewing medical physicist should *not* be the same person who generated the plan, so in facilities with only one medical physicist, a dosimetrist should perform the plan generation.

Delivery of the Treatment

Several factors enter into considerations of who should staff the control panel during the treatment. In some states, regulations dictate that only therapists may deliver treatments and control treatment units. The regulations in most states, and from the U.S. Nuclear Regulatory Commission, are silent on the issue. At the time of writing, regulations almost uniformly require the attendance of a medical physicist at the treatment (or within unamplified voice communication of the unit operator). As a result, many facilities have the medical physicist operate in the unit during treatments. One important consideration is that at least one person in the control area during treatments must be ready and willing to enter the room and take appropriate actions in case the source becomes stuck in the patient.

Normal Procedures

When the afterloader receives a command from the treatment control panel to initiate a treatment, the source cable advances from the shielded safe through the S tube to the first channel in the indexer, and then along a path constrained by transfer tubes to the first treated dwell position in the applicator. The source dwells at that position for a predetermined duration. After completing that dwell it goes on to the subsequent dwell positions. Some units step as the source drives out (MicroSelectron and Gamma-Med), stopping first at the dwell position most proximal to the afterloader, while in the other (VariSource) the source travels first to the most distal dwell (toward the tip of the applicator), and a bit farther, and then steps as the source returns toward the safe. Stepping on the outward drive obviates any concern about the effect of slack in the drive mechanism affecting the accuracy of the source position. The unit that steps on the way back into the unit includes correction for slack in the calibration of the source location. Upon completion of the treatment for the first channel, the source is retracted into the safe and redirected to travel to the second channel. The process is repeated for all the subsequent treatment channels. The programmed movement of the source is verified by means of an optical encoder or other devices that compare the angular rotation of a stepper motor or cable length ejected or retracted with the number of pulses sent to the drive motor. This system is capable of detecting catheter obstruction or constriction as increased friction in the cable movement. Under certain fault conditions, such as if the stepper motor fails to retract the source, a high-torque direct current emergency motor will retract the source.

The confirmation of the source exit from and return to the safe is carried out by an opto-pair, consisting of a pair of light-sensitive detector and infrared light source, which detect the cable when its tip obstructs the light path. All the currently marketed afterloaders are also equipped with check cables, or "dummy sources." The check cable is an exact duplicate of the radioactive source along with its cable, except it is not radioactive. Before the ejection of the radioactive source, the check cable is first ejected to check the integrity of the catheter system. After a noneventful check by this dry run with the dummy source, the radioactive source is then sent for treatment.

Emergency Procedures

Since HDR RALs are complicated devices containing very high activity radioactive sources, serious accidents can happen very quickly, thereby demanding many safety features and operational interlocks to prevent erroneous source movement or facilitate rapid operator response in the event of a system failure.

Door Interlock

Interlock switches prevent initiation of a treatment with the door open. Opening the door interrupts the treatment's progress. This safety feature protects the medical personnel from radiation exposure, in the event somebody enters the treatment room without the knowledge of the operator. If a door is opened inadvertently during the treatment, the treatment is interrupted and the source returns to the safe. The treatment can be resumed at the same point where it was interrupted by closing the door and pressing the start or the resume button at the control panel.

Emergency Switches

Numerous emergency off switches are located at convenient places and are easily accessible in case a situation arises. One is located on the control panel for the HDR operator. Another is located on the top of the remote afterloader treatment head. Vendors also install two or more switches in the walls of the treatment room. In the event a treatment is initiated with someone other than the patient in the treatment room, that person can stop the treatment and retract the source by pressing the emergency off button.

Emergency Crank

In the event of the failure of a source to retract normally as well as the failure of the emergency motor, all HDR RALs have emergency cranks to retract the source cable. Using the crank requires the operator to enter the room with the source unshielded.

Emergency Service Instruments

If the radioactive source fails to retract after termination or interruption, pushing the emergency switch or cranking the stepper motor manually, the immediate priority is to remove the source from the patient. Since the source is in contact with the patient, it can cause severe injury in a very short time. But working at a greater distance, it is unlikely that the operator will receive a dose exceeding regulatory limits for a year, let alone one that would cause health problems. Once the source is removed from the patient and moved to the distance of even a meter, the exposure rate drops drastically and actions can then be taken to remove the patient from the room safely.

The safest approach to a source that will not retract by any of the methods is to remove the applicator from the patient as quickly as possible and place the applicator containing the source in a shielded container. If it is clear that the cable is caught in the transfer tube and not in the applicator itself, the applicator may be disconnected from the transfer tube and the patient removed from the treatment room. In some cases, this will be faster than removing the applicator. The reason to avoid disconnecting the applicator from the transfer tube is that a source may stay in the applicator if the source capsule shatters. In that case, removing the applicator attached to the transfer tube keeps the system closed, while disconnecting the two opens a path for parts of a broken source to fall from the applicator into body cavities or crevices, or roll onto the floor.

A situation may arise when the source needs to be detached manually from the treatment unit. Such a rare situation might be if the unit with an unretractable source fell on a person and could not be moved by hand (perhaps by something else falling on the unit). The source could be close to the person, but not inside. In this situation, the source cable should be cut from the unit and the source placed in the shielded container always present in the room. In cutting the source cable, it must be clear that the cut is *not* through the source capsule. For units with the capsule welded on the cable, the cut must be through the braided cable as opposed to the smooth steel capsule. For sources imbedded in the cable, a sufficient length of the cable must be seen to ensure the cut occurs behind the source. Thus, emergency tools that must be present in the treatment room and always readily accessible include a wire cutter, a pair of forceps, and a shielded service container. The source should *never* be cut from the cable while the source is still in an applicator in the patient!

Facility Design

The radioactive source in the high dose rate machine starts about at 10 Ci with an in-airdose equivalent rate at a distance of 1 m from the source of about 44 mSv/h. According to the rules and regulations of the Nuclear Regulatory Commission (NRC), the annual limit for radiation exposure to the public is 1 mSv and the annual occupational limit is 5 mSv. (The actual limit for occupationally exposure persons is 50 mSv/y, but following the principle of maintaining exposures as low as reasonable achievable, the NRC usually holds licensees to exposure 0.1 of the actual limit.) In addition to the annual limit, NRC requires that in an unrestricted area the dose equivalent rate should not be more than 0.02 mSv in any hour. Thus, the high dose-rate machine needs to be housed in an adequately shielded room. To meet these requirements in an HDR suite, where the walls and the ceiling are at least 5 feet from the machine head, concrete walls of about 43 to 50 cm (or 4 to 5 cm of lead) are needed. For larger rooms the concrete wall thickness will be lower since the exposure rate is inversely proportional to the square of the distance from the radioactive source. The 10th value layer thicknesses for ^{192}Ir are 1.6 cm and 15 cm of lead and concrete respectively. For details on the procedures for calculating the thickness of barriers for a particular facility, see health physics texts such as Cember (2) or McGinley (28).

Imaging plays an important part in most brachytherapy nowadays, so consideration of required imaging modalities should enter into the room design. If the facility will perform a significant amount of gynecological intracavitary insertions, fluoroscopic and radiographic equipment in the room saves a considerable amount of time and eliminates the motion inherent in moving the patient between rooms for imaging and treatment. Space and access for anesthesia in the room facilitates HDR brachytherapy for prostate cases.

All HDR brachytherapy rooms must have video and audio communication for monitoring the patient. Radiation detectors for monitoring the radiation levels in the room and indicating when the source is out of its shielding also are required.

Quality Control of the Remote Afterloading Device

Several of the disadvantages of HDR brachytherapy concerned the probability of failure, either human or mechanical. Both aspects of the treatments require effective quality management. This section deals with quality assurance for the treatment unit. One report from the American Association of Physicists in medicine discusses this topic (23), as well as fundamental publications by Ezzell (13,15), Chenery et al. (4), Flynn (16), Grigsby (17), Jones (20), and Meigooni et al. (31). Williamson et al. (58) assembled much of the important material into a chapter. For a fairly comprehensive discussion, the reader is directed to Thomadsen (50).

As with any piece of radiotherapy equipment, the QA begins with acceptance testing and commissioning. Periodic QA includes tests performed with each new source (approximately quarterly for most units) and those at the beginning of each treatment day. Of all of these, the daily morning checks form the basic set of essential tests.

Morning Checks

Although the list of safety checks seems long, the evaluation need not consume a great deal of time. At our facility, the entire morning routine takes about 10 to 15 minutes. Most of the items could be tested in numerous manners, but only one set of techniques will be discussed here. Individual units may differ in the exact methods. The procedure in the list often assumes the successful completion of all of the items going before. Failure of *any* item requires evaluation by the physicist of the appropriateness of continuing with patient treatments in light of the particular failure. The morning checks focus on ensuring that the unit is operating safely and correctly.

Safety Checks

The following items should be considered in a safety check:

Communication equipment. See that the television and intercom systems function.

Catheter attachment lock. Attach a transfer tube to one of the channels of the unit, but do not lock the transfer tube in place (often accomplished by the locking ring). Program the unit to send the source to a dwell position that would be in an applicator were one attached, and initiate a source run. A program time for a single dwell of about 20 s would allow execution of the tests to follow. The unit should detect that the transfer tube has not been locked in place and prevent the source run. Were a treatment to take place in this condition, the source cable could push the transfer tube out of the unit and never enter the applicator.

Applicator attachment. Keeping the same program, lock the transfer tube in place but still do *not* attach an applicator to the transfer tube. Again attempt to initiate a source run. The check cable run should detect the absence of an applicator and prevent sending out the source. Failure of the unit to detect this situation could lead to the source indicating that it treated a catheter when in reality the catheter was never attached. This test also checks that the unit will not send out a source if the pathway is blocked, since for most

transfer tubes, the applicators push aside a blockage of the tube when they lock in place.

Door interlock. Lock an applicator into the transfer tube. For future tests it is convenient to use a needle in a well-type ionization chamber. Keeping the same program as in the previous tests and with the door to the room open, try to initiate a run. The unit should refuse to initiate the treatment and indicate that the door is open.

Source-out indicators. Close the door, and initiate the source run. Observe that the indication lamps operate. Most rooms have three beam-on indicator lamps: one connected to a treatment-unit microswitch that triggers when the source leaves its shielded housing, one that lights when the signal on the radiation detector in the room exceeds its trip level, and one from the on-board Geiger counter. Let the exposure continue for the next test.

Room monitor audio operation. Listen through the intercom for the sound of the room radiation monitor. It should make a mild, but clearly audible sound. It should not be too loud, for that would disturb the patient. There is no regulation in most states or with the NRC that the in-room monitor provide any audible signal. The presence of such a signal would alert anyone in the room unintentionally when the source is out. Some practitioners feel that any such signal causes concern on the part of the patient. We have tried both situations and have not found that patients mind the signal if they have been informed that it would occur. Continue the exposure.

Room monitor visual operation. Open the door to the room and observe the visual indicators on the room monitor. The room design should provide protection to a person in the doorway until the source retracts. At the same time as this test is performed, so is the next.

Hand-held monitor. Immediately on opening the door during the previous test, hold the hand-held monitor in the doorway and see if it indicates the presence of radiation. The hand-held detector is to be carried upon entry to the treatment room any time after a source run. Alternatively, the detector could be tested with a dedicated check source at the beginning of each day. Performing the test along with the room monitor makes the treatment unit the dedicated check source.

Door interrupt. During the previous two tests, the unit should have been retracting the source, beginning from the opening of the door. The retraction should take no longer than 4 to 6 seconds to return the source to its shielded location.

Emergency stop. Close the door and reinitiate the exposure. Once the source reaches the dwell position, press the emergency off button. The unit must immediately retract the source and likely require a reset.

Treatment interrupt. Reinitiate the exposure and once the source again reaches the dwell position, press the treatment interrupt button. Again, the unit must immediately retract the source.

Timer termination. Reinitiate the exposure and let it continue until the elapsed duration equals the time set on the timer. At that time, the unit stops the exposure and retracts the source.

Dosimetry Checks

The thrust of the dosimetry checks focuses on the delivery of the correct dose to the proper location.

Source Positioning Accuracy

Proper treatment requires that the source occupy the position along the catheter corresponding to that used in the treatment plan. The uncertainty of the determination of the dwell positions on the treatment plan is discussed elsewhere in this chapter. Here, the issue becomes duplicating the dwell locations on the treatment plan during execution. A usual criterion for coincidence with the planned treatment dwells is 2 mm, although the HDR units are able to place the source in a given location within 1 mm. Reproducibility below 0.5 mm begins to be less ensured. To direct the source to correct locations corresponding to each dwell position, the source controller requires the distance along the catheter corresponding to the first dwell position. The distance may refer to the length from some part of the unit (such as the front face, the point of catheter insertion, or a microswitch that tells the unit when the source enters the catheter), or it may be from some fictitious point (similar in concept to the effective source for electron beams). Verifying that the source can place the center at a specified distance becomes an important part of the morning QA.

Three methods for verifying the source placement accuracy will be discussed here, although many others exist. The first method makes an autoradiograph of the source. After taping a clear catheter to a piece of paper-jacketed film (e.g., XV-2 "ready pac," Kodak, Rochester, NY) and inserting the x-ray marker wire, mark the position of the first dwell marker on the film. (This method assumes the x-ray marker to be correct. Verification of that is discussed with tests following a source replacement.) This can be done by pinpricks or pressing hard with a ballpoint pen. If using a pinprick, the lights in the room should be dimmed and the film processed immediately after exposure. A pinprick at a farther distance from the source track gives an indication of the amount of signal due to light exposures. If using a pen, lines about 1-cm long with an end at the center of the marker help to see the actual position. Pen marks must be strong enough to etch the film through the jacket but not so strong as to tear the jacket. With either technique, marking both sides of the catheter makes determining the center of the marker on the film easier. Establishing that the unit not only places the source at the correct location for the first dwell position but also keeps track of relative positions is a good idea. To do this, also mark some additional dwell positions, such as dwell positions 5 cm and 10 cm from the first. Program the source to stop at the marked positions for about 2 seconds each for a source with a strength of 0.04 Gy m²/h. The times for other source strengths vary in inverse proportion. Deliver the exposure and process the film. The resultant image looks like a dark blot, where the centroid indicates the effective center of the source. This centroid should fall between the marks, plus or minus the allowed tolerance. The distance to the centroid of other marked dwell positions should be much better than the absolute tolerance for hitting the first dwell position. Many factors influence the results of this method and interpretation of the results. One is the effect of light exposing the film when using pinpricks. To assess the size of the exposure due to light, poke a hole in the film well away from the catheter path. After processing, the dark blot by this hole should remain less than half the diameter of the holes marking dwell positions. If the light-leak hole shows a blot about the same size as the actual test holes, then the test holes mostly just indicate room light and provide no information about source positioning. Figure 21.7 shows a typical test film.

Another method uses the ruler provided with the unit. Such a ruler provides a channel for the source to follow alongside a scale marked in the distance. Using any ruler requires a good television system able both to distinguish the source capsule clearly and to resolve the markers on the ruler. The lighting of the ruler becomes an important variable. For one unit, a televised check of the source positions on a ruler forms a routine part of any treatment. For another, the ruler is just part of the unit QA equipment and requires a separate television system, such as that used to monitor the patient. To perform the check, attach the ruler as appropriate for the unit and program the

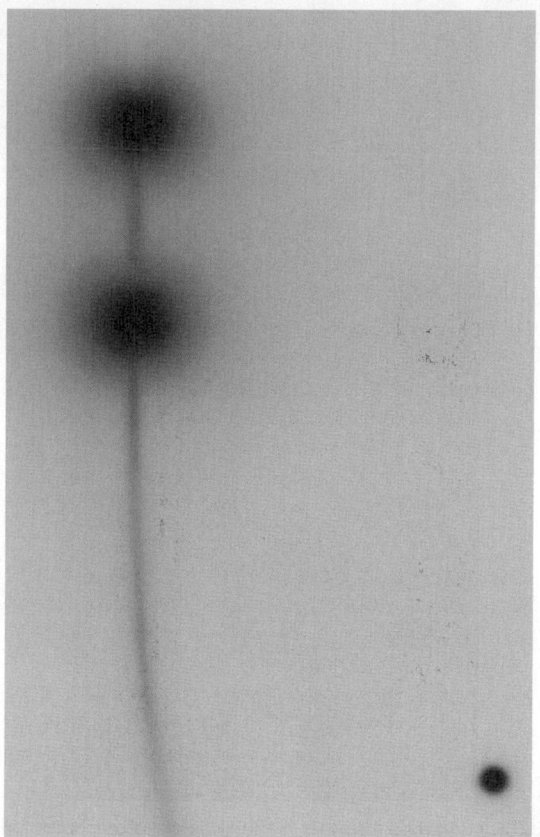

FIGURE 21.7. A typical image made to test the accuracy of the high–dose-rate unit source positioning.

source to a distance that shows on the rule. Watch on the video screen as the source moves into position. The tip of the source will be seen at some distance that should be farther than that distance programmed. From the distance of the tip, subtract the distance from the tip to the center of the source as shown in Figure 21.3.

A simpler and more precise method of verifying the positioning of the source follows the technique determined by DeWerd et al. (11). This procedure uses a well-type ionization chamber with a special insert that includes lead attenuators and plastic transmission disks, and shown in Figure 21.8. The lead attenuators reduce the signal from the source to approximately one-third its unshielded value, while the plastic discs have little affect. As the source passes through the needle centered in this insert, the measured signal appears as in Figure 21.9. The peaks occur when the source is centered on the plastic discs, and the greatest gradient when half the source is shielded and half is on the plastic. At these points, the signal depends critically on the precise position of the source, with the signal changing approximately 3.5%/mm. The signal at the plateau changes little over 2 mm. Dividing the current signal at the high-gradient point by that at the plateau removes any variations in the reading due to source decay, timer miscalibration, or atmospheric density. The ratio of signals, thus, gives a sensitive indication of whether the unit accurately places the source to the correct location. Making measurements at two high-gradient points and the peak not only assesses the correct placement of the source at the one point but also the correct interval between. Use of this method requires measurement of the signal profile as a function of distance along the axis of the well chamber after initial verification of the source position using one of the other methods. Once put in place, this approach takes less than a minute. If the insert is left in the well chamber, the needle can be used for the

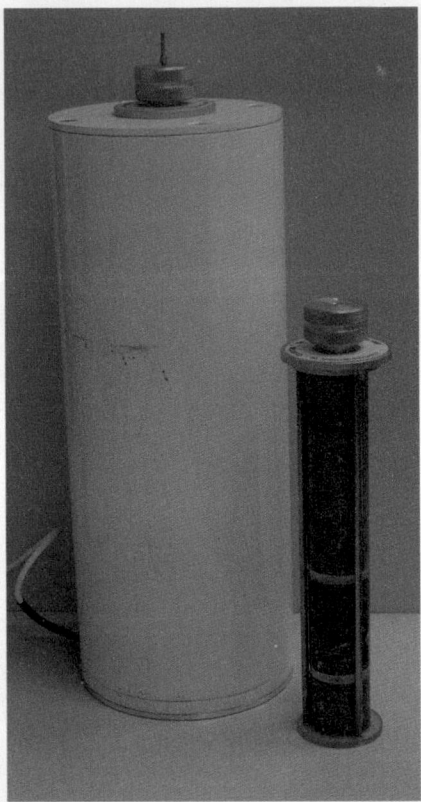

FIGURE 21.8. A special insert designed to assist in the evaluation of source positioning accuracy, with large lead cylinders separated by a plastic disc.

safety checks and this test can follow the safety checks without reentering the room.

Dose Consistency

Correct dose delivery hinges on the proper operation of the timer controlling the exposure. The proper operation does *not* depend on the timer accurately keeping true clock time. The only important features of the timer are that it operates linearly and that its operation remains consistent over time. The daily QA generally need only check two times to evaluate timer consistency and linearity, compared with the tests performed during the source exchange. The uncertainty in the measurement should be on the order of a few 10th of a second in order to check the shorter times.

One technique for checking the timer observes the reading produced in a radiation detector as a function of the timer settings. To evaluate the timer, the measurement system must respond linearly to radiation dose and the setup provide a stable and reproducible geometry. A well chamber, such as that used for calibration, performs this function well. Such measurements in a well chamber include the effects of source decay and the source transit time. For the most part, source decay seldom deviates from the expected but should be checked because there have been sources with contaminant radionuclides that produce an anomalous decay. Because the reading varies directly with the set exposure time, these readings can form a check of the timer. The chamber reading needs a baseline, for example, a reading taken immediately after the initial calibration of the source. The expected reading can be tabulated as a function of day by correcting the initial reading by the decay factor, $e^{-0.693t/73.8 \text{ days}}$, where t equals the time in days since the initial reading. The reading should remain within $\pm 2\%$ of the projected reading, values that also could be in the table. Deviations from the projected values indicate changes in the timer operation (linearity or consistency), changes in the unit's transit time, or anomalous decay. Further tests would be required to sort out the actual problem.

Source Strength Value

The value for the source strength at any time should be the same in the treatment-planning computer as in the treatment unit computer to within 0.5%. The date and time in the treatment unit must be correct for the unit to calculate the source decay correctly. The format of the date, American or European, must be the same as that expected by the computer.

Initial Checks

Each source change requires a number of procedures in addition to the daily checks.

Safety Checks

The initial safety checks include:

Treatment unit backup batteries. In case of loss of power to the treatment unit, the machine has backup batteries to retract the source and save the record of the treatment up to the time of retraction. Checking the batteries entails initiating a source run, pulling the circuit breaker for power to the unit, and verifying that the source retracts; the history is then saved, and the unit resumes the program where it left off when restarted after restoring the power.

In-room radiation monitors backup batteries. The in-room radiation monitor also has backup batteries allowing it to continue functioning in case of a power loss. Continued operation at such times becomes extremely important in case the source fails to retract. Verifying operation of these batteries simply requires unplugging the unit from the wall socket and performing the usual check for the monitor.

Dosimetry Checks

The following are the initial dosimetry checks:

Calibration. The accepted method for calibration of an HDR source uses a well-type ionization chamber that has itself been calibrated in terms of HDR source strength per unit current. The calibration factor for the same chamber will differ for low–dose-rate and high–dose-rate ^{192}Ir sources because of differences in source construction. The uncertainty in source strength calibrations using such chambers usually runs around 1% from national standards plus an additional 5% in the national standard with respect to absolute measures of energy absorbed per unit mass. The source strength is in terms of air-kerma strength, S_K, with units of μGy m^2 h^{-1} (34), often called a U for convenience. This unit gives numbers that become very large, so sometimes units of mGy m^2 h^{-1} (called U$_h$) are used. Most treatment planning computers accommodate at least one of these units; However, many practitioners still relate better to source strength converted into Ci, derived simply by multiplying S_K by a constant that must be the same as that used by the manufacture in the treatment planning program.

Timer linearity. The verification for timer linearity uses several readings, R_i, for various, increasing times, t_i taken in the well chamber. The free-running reading rate can be defined as:

$$\dot{R}_i = \frac{(R_{i+1} - R_i)}{(t_{i+1} - t_i)} \qquad (8)$$

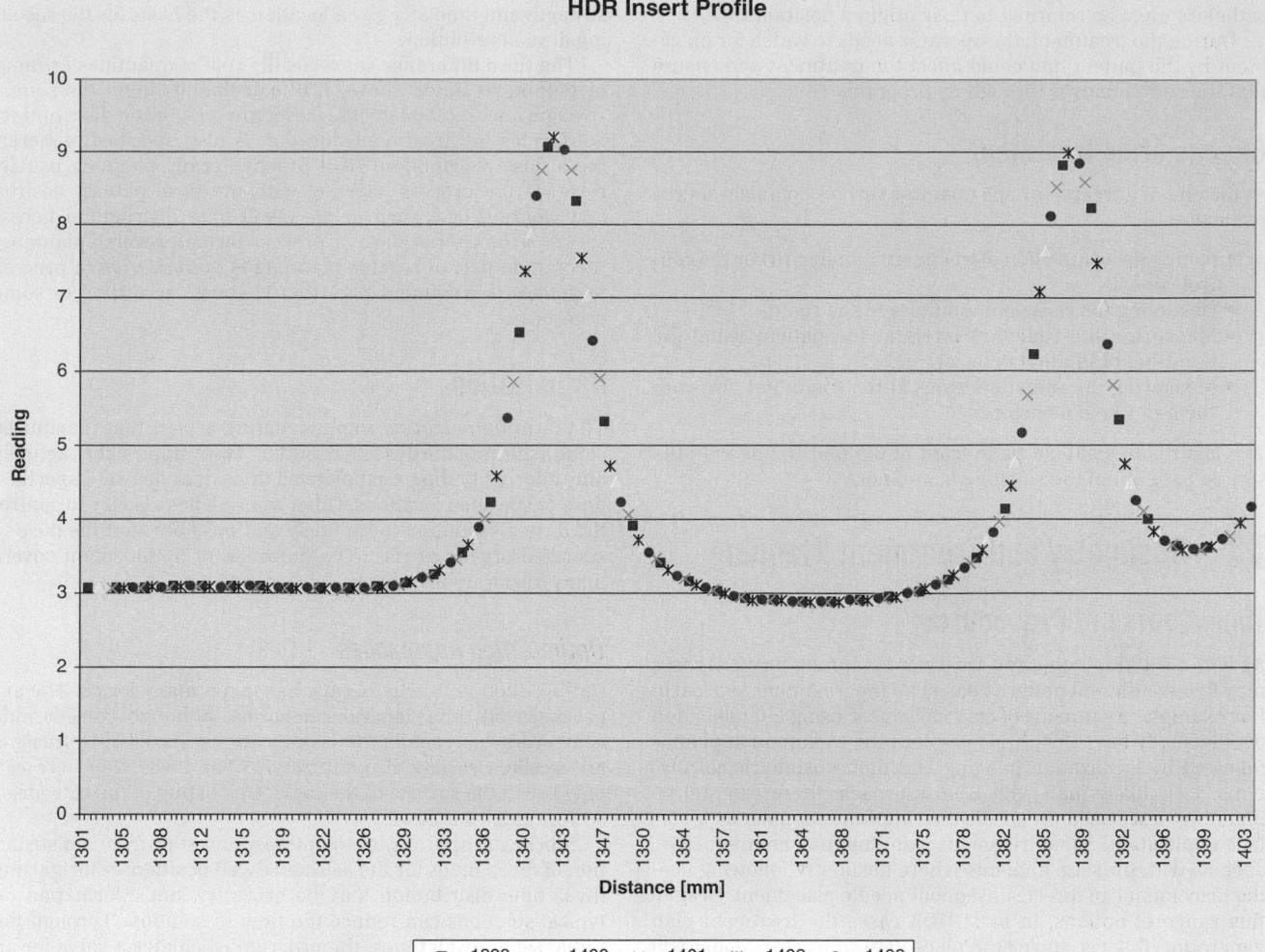

FIGURE 21.9. The signal produced as the source passes through the insert shown in Figure 21.7. Notice the high signal gradient that corresponds to the source centered on the plastic-lead interface.

which contains no effect from the source transit time and cancels during the subtractions. Taking approximately five readings covering the range of dwell times common in treatments gives four values for the free-running reading rate using adjacent times. These values should differ by <0.5%.

The transit time from the unit to the dwell position is hard to measure and is not important directly. What is important is that the transit time remains constant. An effective transit time can be defined as the time it would take to deliver the extra reading in the chamber due to the irradiation during the time the source moves into, and then leaves, the measurement dwell position, *if* the extra reading were delivered at the free-running reading rate. One expression for the effective transit time, t_ε, becomes:

$$t_\varepsilon = \frac{R_i}{\dot{R}} - t_i \qquad (9)$$

An alternative expression for evaluating the timer linearity calculates ζ, defined as:

$$\zeta = \frac{(R_i/R_{i+1})}{((t_i - t_\varepsilon)/(t_{i+1} - t_\varepsilon))} \qquad (10)$$

In general, ζ should remain between 0.99 and 1.01.

Entry of data into computers. The new source strength must be entered into the treatment planning computer and the treatment unit computer. Special attention needs to be paid to selecting the units for the source strength, particularly if the system automatically defaults to given units.

Checks Just Before and During Treatment

Other than the check performed on the treatment plan just before treatment, connecting the patient also requires care and verification. For gynecological applicators the three parts of a tandem and ovoid set have coded connectors that only allow the correct transfer tubes to attach, and the transfer tubes also can only connect to the correct holes in the indexer. However, for implants with needles or catheters, no interlocking prevents mismatches between channels and catheter or needle tracks. For large implants, the treatments often require first connecting the number of catheters equal to the number of channels and delivering the part of treatment that uses those channels. Those channels are then disconnected and the next set of catheters is then connected to the indexers starting again with channel number 1. One of the most likely errors would be connecting a channel during the second set to a catheter from the first, or vice versa.

Also in interstitial implants, between fractions the catheters often move from the position they occupied during the imaging used for treatment planning. Immediately before treatment, the catheters must be returned to their original position.

During the treatment, the operator needs to watch for movement by the patient that could affect the treatment and ensure that the source moves through its program.

Checks After Treatment

At the end of a treatment, the operator verifies complete source retraction by:

- Noting the completion of treatment as indicated by the control console,
- Observing the radiation monitors in the room,
- Measuring the radiation levels at the patient using the hand-held radiation detector, and
- Measuring the radiation levels at the treatment unit with the hand-held detector.

The last reading should be in front of the unit in line with the source path out of the shielding container.

:: | Dosimetry and Treatment Planning

Time-Course of Procedures

As with LDR brachytherapy, treatment planning for HDR cases may follow different patterns based on the treatment approach. For example, treatments of cervical cancer using a tandem and ovoid usually have the physician place the treatment appliance followed by localization imaging and then dosimetric calculations. Less likely than with LDR approach, there can still be planning first based on an idealize application, such as a surface application. Some treatment planning may be interactive, such as with prostate implants where dosimetry following needle placement can direct subsequent needle placement. Despite this range of options, in most HDR cases the treatment plan generation follows applicator placement, and that model will be assumed in this discussion.

Differences Between Low– and High–Dose-Rate Brachytherapy Treatment Planning

HDR brachytherapy treatment planning differs from LDR brachytherapy in three ways. The first difference results from the time course of the treatments. In treatments of several sites, particularly most gynecological applications and some methods for treatment of prostates, the patient waits in the treatment position during the treatment plan generation. Most interstitial and intraluminal treatments differ little from the LDR varieties, with treatment plan generation performed with the patient elsewhere. For those cases with the patient waiting in the treatment position, time becomes an important factor. If the plan generation takes too long, the patient will begin moving with respect to the applicator even though both may be "immobilized." Additional problems with excessively long dosimetry sessions include patient discomfort (other than leading to movement) or, alternatively, cost of support staff such as anesthesiologists.

A second difference entails the quantities involved with the dose calculation. LDR applications often use input source strength, for example, cesium sources used in a tandem and ovoid, and calculate resulting dose rates based on the source configuration. The problem in many cases, particularly in interstitial implants, becomes selecting the dose rate isodose surface on which to base the treatment duration. The case may have many sources, possibly of various strengths, but only a single duration for all sources. High–dose-rate brachytherapy has one source strength and many different dwell times. In both cases,

the dose calculation algorithm uses the product of the source strength and time at a given location as the basis for the resulting dose distribution.

The third difference concerns the role of quantities as input or output. As noted above, LDR calculations input the source strengths and calculate the resultant dose-rate distribution. Sometimes the treatment duration is also specified, generating a dose distribution. HDR brachytherapy planning usually reverses the process, starting with the dose pattern desired and working backward to the dwell time distribution necessary to achieve that dose, a process termed reverse planning. A common part of reverse planning is *optimization*, a process to achieve a treatment plan that is "best" according to some criteria.

Optimization

The term *optimization* implies finding a plan that maximizes some aspects of the dose distribution. Many approaches actually only address finding a set of dwell times that deliver a specified dose to specified locations. Other approaches also try to control the dose distribution more finely and possibly limit the dose to specified organs at risk. The umbrella of optimization covers many disparate processes.

Optimization Approaches

Optimization in brachytherapy has taken many forms. The approaches fall into general categories, although considerable controversy surrounds the classifications. Ezzell (14) presents an excellent review of optimization. The discussion here can only brush the surface of the topic. One listing of the categories with examples follows.

Stochastic approaches to optimization start from a distribution of dwell times for the selected dwell positions. The starting dwell-time distribution may be arbitrary, but information on typical solutions can reduce the time to solution. Through the initial set of dwell times, the program calculates a value for an *objective function*. An objective function assigns a numerical value to the solution set that allows ranking the set according to quality. The objective function may be as simple as the difference between the value of dose calculated at a set of point and the dose desired. Objective functions often become more complicated, as in equation 11.

$$OF = w_t(0.95D_{pre} - D_{t,m})_{D_{t,m} < 0.95D_{pre}} \qquad (11)$$
$$+ \sum_i w_{OAR,i}(\overline{D}_{OAR,i,calc} - D_{OAR,i,limit})^2_{\overline{D}_{OAR,i,calc} > D_{OAR,i,limit}}$$

In equation 11, D_{pre} represents the prescription dose and $D_{t,m}$ stand for the minimum dose in the planning target volume. In this example, the person running the optimization wants to evaluate whether the dwell time set results in part of the target receiving <95% of the prescribed dose, and if so, to keep track of how much less. The second term considers the average doses ($\overline{D}$) to each of the organs at risk (OAR), and determines for each the amount over some limiting dose assigned for that organ. The objective function, OF, in this case is a penalty paid for the dwell-time distribution. The first term would be omitted as long as the minimum target dose equaled or exceeded 95% of the prescription dose, and the term for any of the organs at risk would be zero as long as the dose remained below the limiting value. The power of 2 in the exponent indicates tolerance of a little excess dose, but imposes serious penalties for larger values. The weighting factors, w, allow a differentiation between the importance given to achieving the desired dose distribution and limiting the dose to a given organ at risk. In addition to the objective function, the dwell-time set might also be subject to *hard constraints* that would reject the set outright if the target dose fell below 90% of the prescribed dose or an organ at risk exceeded a different, maximum limit. Because the value increases as the dose distribution gets worse, the program tries to minimize this function. Please keep in mind that this equation only illustrates the concepts and is not intended to serve as a model of a good objective function.

The methodology for finding the best set of dwell times differs among the stochastic approaches. In *simulated annealing* (40,41,47,48), random changes, often sizable, will be made from the initial solution of the program in the dwell times of some or all of the dwell positions. Following the changes and recalculation of the objective function, the program will hold on to the better of the two dwell-time sets. New random changes will be made from the better set, and again the sets with be compared using the objective function. As this process continues, the allowed changes become smaller and the objective function should be improving as the process moves toward the solution—the set with the best objective function. The process as described can fall into a local minimum for the objective function, where any changes make the function worse, while somewhere distant to this local minimum, lower values obtain. To avoid such traps, the program periodically allows big jumps in the dwell times to investigate completely different regions of dwell times. If the new region does not seem promising because the objective functions are worse, the program goes back to the better region.

Often, the value of the objective function changes little with fairly large changes in individual dwell times in the neighborhood of the optimal solution. Going from a close dwell-time set to the true optimum can require a considerable amount of computer time, and often more than getting close in the first place. Most programs contain a criterion for stopping the process once the objective function finds an adequate solution, instead of continuing to the true optimum.

Other stochastic approaches, such as the *genetic algorithm* (25), use different search mechanisms, but the overall procedures tend to be similar.

Instead of solving in terms of dose, geometric optimization (12) solves for dwell times that would give the same doses to the vicinities around each of the dwell positions, based on several simplifying assumptions. This approach recognizes that the dose near any dwell position results not only from the nearby dwell but also from the sum of the contributions from all the other sources. To produce a uniform dose through the implanted volume, this method posits, first calculate how much dose comes to a dwell position from all the other dwell positions, and then weight the dwell time at the dwell position under consideration by the inverse of this dose. Thus, each dwell position needs only make up for the difference between the dose it already receives from the other positions and the dose desired.

The first step sets the dwell weight, τ, (the relative dwell time, normalized as described below) for dwell position i, with the geometric contributions of the other positions, in the formalism of AAPM Task Group 43 (35), as:

$$\tau_i = \left[\sum_{j \neq i} \frac{g(r_{i \leftarrow j}) \cdot \phi(r_{i \leftarrow j})}{r_{i \leftarrow j}^2} \right]^{-1} \quad (12)$$

where $r_{i \leftarrow j}$ equals the distance between dwell positions i and j, $g(r_{i \leftarrow j})$ equals the radial dose function, and $\phi(r_{i \leftarrow j})$ equals the anisotropy factor. This equation assumes that the dose rate follows the inverse square law (i.e., approximates the source as a point). Commercial versions of this algorithm usually ignore the radial-dose function, which remains within 2% of unity out to a distance of 5 cm, and the anisotropy factor, which fall within 3.5% of 0.98 over that same range. The errors from these omissions and the point source approximation (inherent in the inverse square relationship) remain smaller than errors that creep in later.

Determining the absolute dwell times then requires specifying the dose desired to a point, or the average of several points. For the average dose to several points (indicated by k), the equation for the average dose to the points is:

$$\overline{D}_{initial\ pass} = \frac{S_K \cdot \Lambda}{n} \sum_{k=n}^{1} \sum_{j=m}^{1} \frac{\tau_j \cdot g(r_{k \leftarrow j}) \cdot \phi(r_{k \leftarrow j})}{r_{k \leftarrow i}^2} \quad (13)$$

where S_K equals the source strength in mGy m^2 h^{-1}, Λ equals the dose rate constant in Gy cm^2/unit source strength, n equals the number of dose points in the average, m equals the number of dwell positions, and serves as the dwell weights dwell times.

Adjusting $\overline{D}_{initial\ pass}$ to become $D_{prescribed}$ requires scaling the dwell times. Letting each of the t_j be the time to deliver $D_{prescribed}$, and c the scaling factor such that $t_j = c\,\tau_j$, then:

$$c = \frac{\overline{D}_{initial\ pass}}{D_{prescribed}} \quad (14)$$

This process assumed the equality of all the dwell times at the first step when calculating the dwell weights. Yet, when using the dwell weights in equation 13, and then scaling them by a constant, each dwell time in the equation had individual values. Thus, the situation for which equation 12 applies never obtains, compromising the uniformity of dose through the volume. The uniformity could improve by iterating the process, at the sacrifice of its very high speed. The process also assumes that the implant, and particularly the dwell positions, matches the target volume.

Adjacent dwell positions along the same catheter track can produce the greatest affect on the dwell weights, resulting in isodose surfaces that tend to follow the catheters rather than conform to the shape of the implanted volume as a whole. This is especially the case if the separation between dwell positions along a catheter is much less than the separation between catheters. To reduce this effect, a version of the algorithm neglects all other dwell positions along the same catheter track when calculating the dwell weights in a given catheter. This variation is called *volume optimization* because it tends to spread the doses throughout the implanted volume. The original version, which includes the contributions of all other dwell positions for the calculation of any dwell weight, is called *distance optimization* because the isodose surfaces tend to follow a catheter at a constant distance.

The analytic approach, also known as *point optimization* or *point-dose optimization*, attempts to solve algebraically for the set of dwell times that produce the desired dose distribution, as represented by a set of points, called *optimization points*, each with their own specified desired dose. In the most basic form (55,56), the specified doses and the dwell times establish a set of simultaneous equations of the form:

$$D_i = \sum_{j=1}^{m} C_{i,j} \cdot t_j \quad (15)$$

where D_i equals the dose specified to point i, m equals the number of dwell positions, t_j equals the dwell time at position j, and C_{ij} equals the factors that give the dose contribution at i due to the source at position j, with the sum over all sources. The source strength at each source position forms a variable (unknown), and each dose-specification point yields an equation. Equal numbers of dwell times and dose points form a *determined* system with an exact solution. In more complex cases, there may be more optimization points than source positions, resulting in an *overdetermined* system (more equations than variables). This would be the situation where optimization points were spread around the contour of a region of interest and scattered through the volume. Faced with this situation, the source strengths can be varied to minimize the square of the differences between the desired and calculated doses at the optimization points. At the other extreme, a case may have more source positions than optimization points (more variables than equations), resulting in an *underdetermined* system. This situation most often happens with large implants and a minimum of optimization points or complicated gynecological applicators with only a few dose-control points. With this situation the source strengths have no well-defined values; many solutions would possibly exist with the same value for the square of the difference between the doses desired and those calculated. Distinguishing between the solutions requires some other criteria. One often is a minimization of the total dwell time, under the assumption that such would also minimize the integral dose to the patient.

Determined and overdetermined systems can (and often do) generate solutions with negative dwell times. Simply truncating the negative dwell times often results in a very unsatisfactory dose distribution. Avoiding this nonphysical situation also requires an additional criterion. One possible criterion minimizes the differences between adjacent source strengths. For *m* dwell positions, this term becomes:

$$\delta = \sum_{j=1}^{m-1} (t_j - t_{j+1})^2. \tag{16}$$

Including this term in the optimization limits the fluctuations between adjacent sources. In order to deliver a dose to the target volume requires a net positive total dwell time, so limiting the amount of differences between the dwell times eventually results in all positive times. An additional condition for underdetermined systems selects solutions that minimize the total radiation to the patient as a whole, which depends directly on the total source strength. The final optimization becomes minimizing the chi squared value in:

$$X^2 = \sum_{i=1}^{m} w_i \left(D_i - C_{ij} \sum_{j=1}^{n} t_j \right)^2 + v \sum_{j=1}^{n-1} \left(t_j - t_{j+1} \right)^2$$
$$+ u \sum_{j=1}^{n} t_j \tag{17}$$

where, in addition to those quantities defined above, *n* equals the number of dose points specified, w_i equals the weighting

given to the dose specification at point *i* (how much the operator wants the correct dose there), *v* equals the importance in minimizing the fluctuations between adjacent sources, and *u* equals the importance of minimizing the integral dose to the patient.

With a large number of optimization points or source positions, or both, the running of the program solving the equations becomes long, and approximations cut the calculational time greatly, without significantly compromising the accuracy of the final dose distribution. By setting the dwell time:

$$t_i = \sum_{k=1}^{p} a_k \cdot F_k(j-1), \tag{18}$$

where *F* is a fitting function, such as a Fourier series of order p, and a_k is the coefficient for the kth element, and substituting that into the X^2 equation 17, the optimization now need only solve for the fitting coefficients, assumedly a much smaller set of values. An alternative approach to solving the equation follows Newton's method (19,26).

Obviously, the selection of the optimization points becomes very important. The number of points must adequately describe the shape of the dose distribution desired. The dose distributions may satisfy the specifications established for the optimization points, but leave portions of the target without dose specification points untreated. However, the points should avoid regions of large dose gradients, since specification there can produce unexpected and inappropriate results.

In general, lower values for *v* allow better conformality of the dose distribution, and the optimum value often is that just sufficient to prevent negative strengths. However, simply solving for the dose to specified points can produce unwanted dose distribution, even when the points seem to follow normal guidelines. van der Laarse (55) gives the example similar to that in Figure 21.10. Here, the dose points mirror the basal doses equidistant from the surrounding catheters. With a low value for *v* in the optimization equation, the simple solution places all of the source material in the center, bottom needle—not at all what was really desired. The situation could be avoided by limiting the dwell-time variations, or using more dose points, particularly

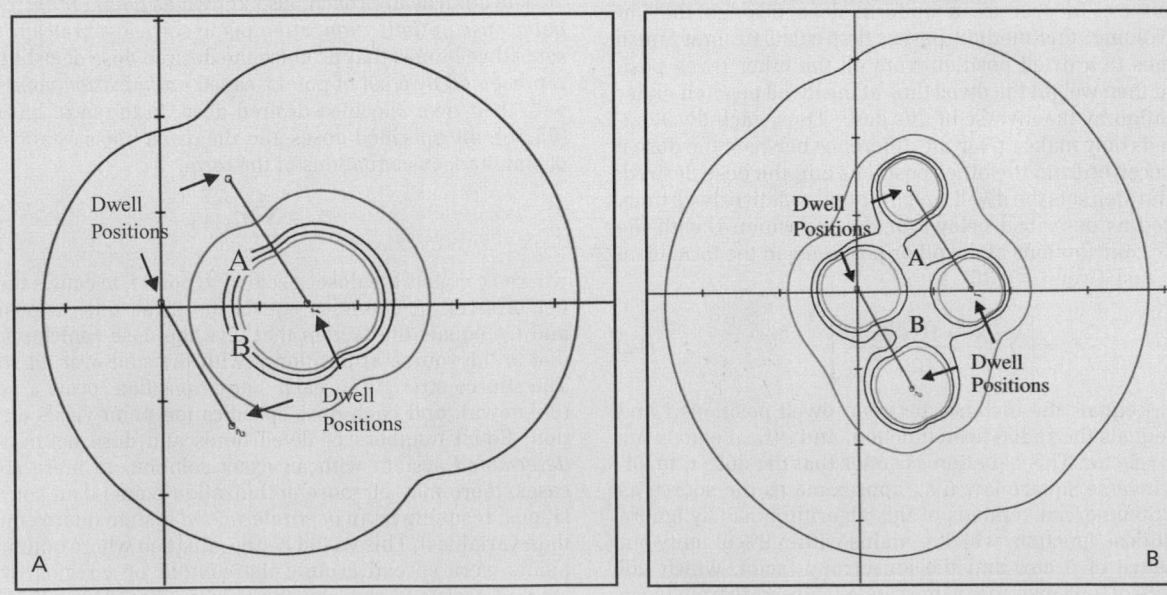

FIGURE 21.10. An example of potential optimization problem. The criterion used for **(A)** was that the two optimization points (*marked a and b*) receive the same dose, which was satisfied by a single active dwell position. **B:** Adding constrains on the dwell time variation solved the problem. (Example inspired by van der Laage [55].)

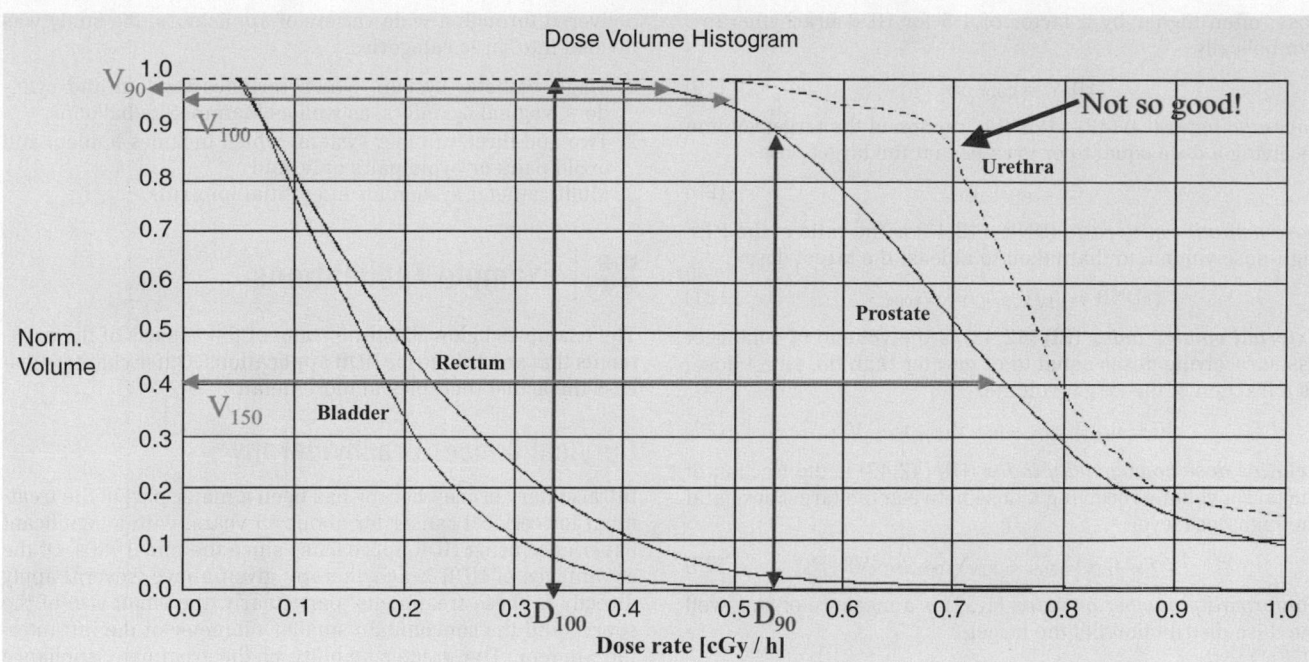

FIGURE 21.11. A volume-dose histogram for an HDR implant of the prostate.

on the outside of the implant. Alternatively, performing a geometric optimization first to obtain an approximate source distribution, followed by optimization on the points, also alleviates the problem.

The output of any optimization approach may leave the operator wishing to make modifications. One method commercially available works on the computer-screen display of the dose distribution and allows the operator to "grab" a dose line on the display with the cursor and move the line to a desired location. These fine adjustments make changes that would be difficult to describe in the optimization routine's specifications. Most of the programs allow adjusting the impact of any change between changing all of the dwell times (scaling the distribution, making the whole larger or smaller) and changing a single dwell time (affecting very local changes). Even local changes, however, result in changes in image planes other than the one which the change has made because the radiation carries the dose beyond the immediate locale.

Changes in the dose distribution to produce desired modifications can also produce unintended changes. Of particular concern would be expending the prescription isodose surface and inadvertently also expending the higher dose surfaces, possibly into a significant volume. During any manipulation of the isodose surfaces, the display should also show the higher doses. Assuming that most of the manipulation occurs with the 100% surface, the 150% should also be on display.

Evaluation of Dose Distributions

Optimization calculations compute relative dose distributions and require only spatial dose information. After establishing the shape of the dose distribution, the entire distribution must be raised or lowered to give the correct absolute dose or dose rate to a specified point, or the average at a number of specified points. This process requires some evaluation of the dose distribution.

Other than visually examining the isodose distribution resulting from the optimization routine, there are some tools that provide quantitative assessments of various aspects. Much of

the analysis remains the same as for the low dose-rate situation, so it will not be considered here. Thomadsen (50) provides a fuller discussion. Intracavitary evaluation mostly relies on visual interpretation, so the discussion below focuses on evaluation of the dose distribution for interstitial implants.

The *maximum significant dose* (MSD) refers to the highest-level isodose surface that encompasses more than one needle track. The dose very close to the needle track becomes very high, but the body seems to tolerate these small local volumes. The MSD provides a convenient criterion for when the high-dose volumes become "significant" and likely to produce biological consequences. For most implants, the MSD should remain below 150% of the prescription dose, assuming that the prescription dose encompasses the target volume. For vary large volumes, the limiting value should decrease to about 125%.

Figure 21.11 shows a typical volume-dose histogram for a prostate implant. The histogram proved the basis for many of the analytical quantities. Ideally, the target structure curve should follow the 100% (or 1.00) level (top of the graph) from the low doses on the left through the target dose, indicating that the entire target receives at least the target dose. In practice, such coverage often becomes challenging. The volume of the target receiving at least a dose "x" is indicated by the symbol V_x, where the x can be either a percentage of the prescription dose or an absolute dose. Alternatively, sometime the quantity of interest is the dose received by a volume "y," indicated as D_y, where y can be either the fraction of the region of interest or an absolute volume. In this chapter (although not a very common practice) a preceding subscript indicates delimitations, such as confining the value to the planned target volume (PTV) or looking at the value through the entire universe ("total").

Competing treatment plans may have quite different features. Some quantities that can help condense some characteristics into values include the following. It should be noted that some of the quantities originally applied to the dose distribution in the absence of any regions of interest, but have been adapted to the modern situation where volume images provide a context for assessment and evaluation.

High dose volume (HDV) (38,39,43) is the volume of a region of interest raised to a dose significantly higher than the target dose, often higher by a factor of 1.5 for HDR brachytherapy. Symbolically:

$$HDV = {}_{ROI}V_{150\%}. \qquad (19)$$

Coverage index (CI) (42–44) is the fraction of the target volume receiving a dose equal to or greater that the target dose:

$$CI = {}_{PTV}V_{100\%}. \qquad (20)$$

Dose nonuniformity ratio (DNR) (42,43) is the ratio of the PTV high-dose volume to that taken to at least the target dose:

$$DNR = {}_{PTV}V_{150\%}/{}_{PTV}V_{100\%} \qquad (21)$$

External volume index (EI) (42,43) is the volume of nontarget tissue receiving doses equal to or greater than the target dose, as a fraction of the target volume.

$$EI = ({}_{total}V_{100\%} - {}_{PTV}V_{100\%})/{}_{PTV}V \qquad (22)$$

Relative dose homogeneity index (HI) (42,43) is the fraction of the target volume receiving a dose between the target dose and the high dose level:

$$HI = ({}_{PTV}V_{150\%} - {}_{PTV}V_{100\%}/{}_{PTV}V) \qquad (23)$$

Conformality number or index (1,57) is a measure of how well the dose distribution fits the target:

$$CN = \frac{{}_{PTV}V_{100\%}}{{}_{total}V_{100\%}} \cdot \frac{{}_{PTV}V_{100\%}}{{}_{PTV}V} \qquad (24)$$

Each of these quantities tells a small part of the dose distribution's entire story. Each can help in the evaluation of a dose distribution, and all together give a better picture. However, none of the indices—even together—capture the complexity and nuances of the total dose distribution. Inspection of the results of the optimization remains a necessity.

Quality Control of Treatment Plan

The use of HDR brachytherapy in the definitive management of gynecological cancer (49), early stage breast cancer (5,24) and prostate cancer (27), has made the HDR RAL a very common treatment modality in most radiotherapy clinics. Treatment planning systems for HDR RALs are now interfaced with multimodality images (computed tomography [CT], magnetic resonance imaging [MRI], and ultrasound) and sophisticated dose optimization software like inverse planning or interactive graphical optimizers, which enable the planner to maximize the dose uniformity, while minimizing the implant volume needed to adequately cover the target volume and at the same time reduce the dose to the organs at risk. Such flexibility creates a challenge for the verification of the optimized calculations with practical manual calculation techniques. With the time constraint between HDR planning and the delivery of treatment while the patient is in the operating room, an efficient, precise, and easy method for checking the complex computer calculation is necessary for quality control of the treatment plan. Every institution should have an established quality control program that takes only a few minutes but at the same time gives a high probability of detecting significant errors since the NRC considers a difference between the administered dose and calculated dose of 20% a reportable medical event (54).

Simplistic models to verify computer calculations quickly have drawbacks since applicators or interstitial implants used in HDR treatments are complex in design, and simple point dose or linear source calculations tends to fall apart in most circumstances (22,53,58). Today, since all treatment planning systems have the capability of generating dose volume histogram, it is logical that volume-based QA should be the choice. Recently, Das et al. (10) has addressed this possibility, and provided an easy and quick calculation check for most HDR interstitial and intracavitary implants. Since HDR treatments are delivered through a wide variety of applicators, the study was divided into three categories:

1. Single catheter system, which includes tandem and cylinders, vaginal cylinders, as well as MammoSite balloons,
2. Two and three catheter system, which includes tandem and ovoid pairs or ovoid pairs only, and
3. Multi-catheter system for interstitial implants.

Example Applications

The examples below illustrate some of the aspects of the treatments that are unique for HDR applications. Other chapters discuss the actual therapies in more detail.

Cervical Cancer Brachytherapy

Intracavitary brachytherapy has been a major part of the treatment for cervical cancer for about 85 years, with a significant experience using HDR approaches since the mid-1980s. Of the advantages of HDR brachytherapy given above, several apply directly to these treatments, particularly, the small size of the source and the concomitant smaller diameter of the intrauterine tandem; The greater stability of the treatment appliance and higher accuracy and relevance of the calculated dose distribution; And the ability to hold organs at risk away from the applicator and source track. Imaging plays a major role in these treatments with the future seeing an increase in that role. Ultrasound often provides guidance during the placement of the intrauterine tandem, particularly when the tumor obliterates the external cervical os. Fluoroscopy provides guidance during placement of the appliance, assisting the assessment of applicator geometry (e.g., evaluating the centering of the tandem with the ovoids in both the anteroposterior and the lateral projections) and the positions of the rectum and bladder. Most commonly, images after fluoroscopy indicate a satisfactory placement, and radiographic images are made for dosimetric localization and reconstruction.

Imaging for gynecological brachytherapy is evolving very rapidly at the present (51), particularly for HDR approaches. Both the brachytherapy arm of the European Society for Therapeutic Radiology and Oncology (Groupe Européen de Curiethérapie, or GEC-ESTRO) (18) and a group sponsored by several U.S. organizations, principally the Gynecological Oncology Group (31), both have recommended moving toward image-based target prescriptions. Identifying the target, that is tumor tissue in the uterus, requires MRI, the only form of imaging that also reliably differentiates the uterus from other pelvic tissues. The U.S. group felt that it was premature to prescribe the dose to the target identified on MRI because there was no information on what doses tumors had been receiving historically, and they believed that protocols should gather data on tumor doses based on conventional treatment approaches. GEC-ESTRO, on the other hand, proposed using the doses conventionally delivered to Manchester points A, approximately 85 Gy, including the external beam contribution, as the dose to the identified clinical target volume.

Although only MRI identifies the target and the uterus, CT images the rectum and the bladder well. Using CT localization does not permit target-based prescription, but does facilitate determining the doses to the organs at risk, when using conventional treatment prescriptions (45,46). Dose calculations based on either CT or MRI often indicate the maximum dose to the bladder falls 2 to 4 cm superior to the conventional point indicated following Report 38 of the International Commission on Radiation Units and Measurement (ICRU) (3), and may be 2 to 4 times the dose to the conventional point. The ICRU indicated rectal point differs less than the bladder point, with the true

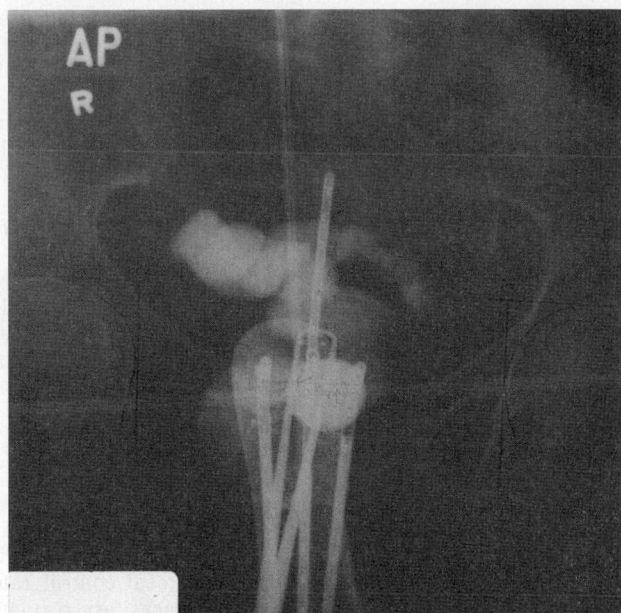
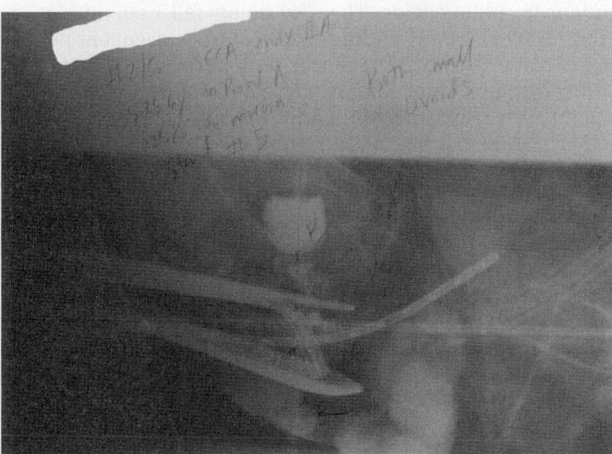

FIGURE 21.12. Radiographs of an HDR application using a tandem and ovoids for the treatment of cervical cancer, with a anteroposterior on the left and lateral on the right.

maximum falling between 1 and 3 cm superiorly and the true maximum dose being 1 to 3 times the conventional point.

The accuracy and precision of determining the dose matters much more in HDR intracavitary brachytherapy for the cervix than for LDR treatments for two reasons. The first concerns the precision of dose delivery. King et al. (21) demonstrated that the typical LDR tandem and ovoids move an average of 2 cm over the course of treatment. HDR tandems and ovoids move a maximum of 3 mm when not moving the patient (53). Thus, the added precision of volume-imaged–based dose calculations would be lost in the general positional uncertainty of LDR intracavitary brachytherapy. In the second place, HDR applications not only can utilize the dosimetric accuracy, but may require it. Because of the radiobiological disadvantage of HDR brachytherapy, knowing the dose distribution with a high certainty is necessary to avoid complications.

Avoiding complications leads to several differences between the cervical applications with HDR compared to LDR brachytherapy. To prevent rectal complications, the dose to the rectum should remain <70% of the dose to the Manchester point A (49). Treating with the rectal retractor in place usually accomplishes this goal. As noted under the advantages of HDR brachytherapy, patients would not tolerate such a practice over the long durations with LDR applications. Adding distance to the bladder generally uses copious packing anterior to the ovoids, taking care not to let the packing slip between the ovoid surface and the superior or lateral fornices. An unpublished 1988 review of LDR cervical cases at the University of Wisconsin found the beginning of late complications in the superior bowel (fistulae) at about 13 years after treatment, and that the prevalence increased continually with time out. That problem with LDR treatments generated concern that the situation might be worse with HDR treatments due to the unfavorable radiobiology. Thus, in the early approach, the dose to the superior bowel was reduced by pulling the uterus low into the vagina during treatment (49) and making the dose distribution more square than the LDR applications, so less unnecessary dose extended into the upper uterus and into the superior bowel. The current practice at the University of Wisconsin is to leave the uterus in a neutral position and simply not use the first few dwell positions. Most commonly, the first dwell position used is 1 cm from dwell

position number 1, but that varies with the extent of the disease and the patient's anatomy. Figure 21.12 shows radiographs of a typical case. Figure 21.13 compares a conventional LDR application with a HDR treatment, both normalized to point A, defined as per the American Brachytherapy Society (32,33).

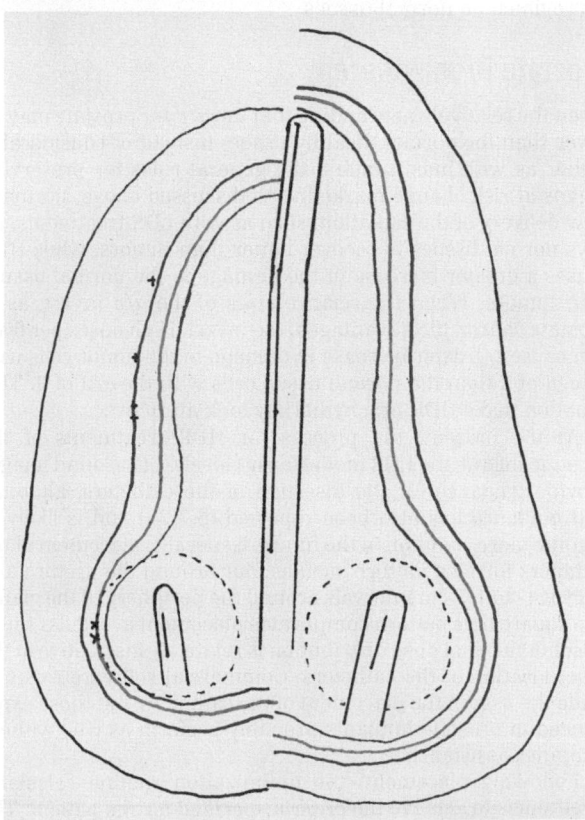

FIGURE 21.13. Comparison of an LDR (*left*) and an HDR (*right*) dose distribution for a tandem and ovoid application for cervical cancer. The HDR dose distribution also shows the locations of the optimization points.

At Wisconsin, these cases use point-dose optimization. For a tandem and ovoid, the optimization starts 1 cm below the first dwell position used (which normally is 2 cm below the dwell position number 1) with optimization points 18 cm lateral to the tandem on both sides. Placing the points on both sides gives an average correcting for any twist of the tandem or varying contributions from the ovoids. The next points fall 1 cm inferior to the first at 2 cm lateral to the tandem, with subsequent points also 2 cm lateral and 1 cm inferior to the previous points until reaching the position of point A. Regardless of where the previous points were, optimization points are placed at point A and also 2 cm lateral to the next dwell position. Placing any more points along the tandem tends to interfere with the dose distribution around the ovoids. For the ovoids, optimization points are placed on the lateral ovoid surface a quarter of a centimeter posterior and anterior of the center.

The optimization process assumes that the anatomy follows the applicator since the dose distribution conforms to the treatment appliance. When MRI targeting becomes more widely available, the optimization process would be customized to the patient's disease and limited by the normal anatomy. At the time of writing, the expense and design of MRI and CTI compatible applicators prevents wide use, as does the limitations on access to, and the price of, MR imaging. All of these impediments should resolve in the very near future.

The absolute dose used may depend on the stage of disease, the number of fractions used, and concomitant other therapy, including external beam and chemotherapy. The dose also tends to change with long-term follow-up and observation. Currently at Wisconsin, 26.25 Gy over five 5.25 Gy fractions serves for most patients, differences based on stage occurs with the external-beam portion of the treatments. Orton et al. (36) cautioned not to exceed 7 Gy per fraction based on a survey of users, but it was unclear if the users who had problems with the higher doses per fraction had calculated the biological equivalency of the regimen on normal tissues.

Prostate Brachytherapy

Given the relatively new finding that the α/β for prostate may be lower than for normal, healthy tissue, instead of considerably higher as with most tumors, the general rules for preserving organs at risk change markedly. As discussed above, normally slow delivery of the radiation, such as with LDR treatments, allows normal tissues to recover better than tumors, while HDR causes a greater increase in the damage to the normal tissues than tumors. When the relative sizes of the α/β invert, as in prostate cancer, the advantages also invert. High doses per fraction cause a greater increase in damage to the tumor cells with an α/β of 2 than the normal tissue cells with the α/β of 3. This situation make HDR brachytherapy look attractive.

At the present, the process for HDR treatments of the prostate follows the LDR model fairly closely. Ultrasound images provide guidance for the insertion of the catheters, although MRI guidance has also been reported (6,7,30) and is likely to become more common in the future. Generally, placement of the catheters follow a pattern such as four around the urethra and then at 1- to 1.5-cm intervals around the periphery of the gland. The square hole pattern complicates placement at regular intervals, but the final dose distribution is relatively insensitive to the exact location of the catheters. Commercial software exists to guide the user in the placement of the catheters, but those experienced in prostate implants probably perform as well without computer assistance.

Following placement, the optimization routine calculates dwell times to achieve the criteria specified for the patient. The resultant dose distribution may still require adjustment through graphical optimization. Upon approval of the plan, the operator connects the needles to the treatment unit using the transfer tubes. Because the needles have no inherent numbering, great care must be taken during this process to ensure correct correlation between the needles in the patient and those in the treatment plan.

The location of the first dwell position in the needles would have been determined previously. Radiographing the needles with the x-ray markers in place forms one of the simplest methods. If the treatment unit does not seek the end of the needle to establish the first dwell position, all needles must be tested for uniformity of length.

Treating multiple fractions with the same insertion requires verification of the needle depth. Between fractions the needles tend to work toward the surface and may need repositioning under ultrasound or fluoroscopic guidance. Marks on the needles where they enter a template also can serve as indicators of the needle for repositioning.

Breast Brachytherapy

Accelerated partial breast irradiation (APBI) for breast cancer patients with HDR brachytherapy as monotherapy, following lumpectomy, has produced excellent local control rates and cosmesis (10,37). Interstitial and intracavitary (catheter balloon) implants are commonly being used for this treatment modality. Usually within 8 weeks of lumpectomy and axillary nodal evaluation, the patient undergoes an interstitial implant with one of two methods: a prone, stereotactic, template method with digital mammographic guidance or a supine, ultrasound-guided technique, both under local anesthesia. Due to the perceived technical challenge of multicatheter interstitial implants, an alternative method for APBI has been developed using an intracavitary balloon catheter treatment device known as MammoSite (CYTYC, Alpharetta, GA). The system is comprised of a single catheter located centrally within a balloon that is placed and inflated within the lumpectomy cavity and is placed postoperatively with the cavity often closed, under ultrasound guidance. CT-based treatment planning with interactive graphical optimization to cover the PTV and at the same time avoid critical structures like lung, heart, and skin is becoming increasingly popular in radiotherapy clinics. Greater emphasis should be given to the quality control of the treatment plan since the dose per fraction is very large for this accelerated fractionation scheme. Das et al. (8) has published a recipe to derive an estimated irradiation time based on the prescription isodose volume, which can easily be achieved by the dose volume histogram of the implant. This provides an important tool for the quality control of the treatment plan. Similarly, percentage of PTV coverage, dose homogeneity index, congruency of the PTV, and 100% isodose volume should also be considered for comprehensive quality control (11).

Acknowledgement

The authors thank Adam Uselmann and Liyong Lin for the artwork they contributed to this chapter.

References

1. Baltas D, Kolotas C, Geramani K, et al. A conformal index (COIN) to evaluate implant quality and dose specification in brachytherapy. *Int J Radiat Oncol Biol Phys* 1998;40:515–524.
2. Cember H. *Introduction to health physics*. 3rd ed. New York: McGraw-Hill, 1996.
3. Chassagne D, Dutreix A, Almond P, et al. International Commission of Radiation Units and Measurements: Report 38. *Dose and volume specification for reporting intracavitary therapy in gynecology*. Bethesda, MD: International Commission of Radiation Units and Measurements, 1985.
4. Chenery S, Pla M, Podgorsak E. Physical characteristics of the Selectron high dose rate intracavitary afterloader. *Br J Radiol* 1985;58:735–740.

5. Clarke DH, Vicini FA, Jacobs H, et al. High dose rate brachytherapy for breast cancer. In: Nag S, ed. *High dose rate brachytherapy: a textbook.* Armonk, NY: Futura Publishing Co, 1994;321–329.

6. Cormack R, Kooy H, Tempany C, et al. A clinical method for real-time dosimetric guidance of transperineal ^{125}I prostate implants using interventional magnetic resonance imaging. *Int J Radiat Oncol Biol Phys* 2000;46:207–214.

7. D'Amico A, Cormack R, Kumar S, et al. Real-time magnetic resonance imaging-guided brachytherapy in the treatment of selected patients with clinically localized prostate cancer. *J Endourol* 2000;14:367–370.

8. Das RK, Bradley KA, Nelson IA, et al. Quality assurance of treatment plans for interstitial and intracavitary high–dose-rate brachytherapy. *Brachytherapy* 2006;5:56–60.

9. Das RK, Patel R. Breast interstitial implant and treatment planning. In: Thomadsen B, Rivard M, Butler W, eds. *Brachytherapy physics.* 2nd ed. Madison, WI: Medical Physics Publishing Co, 2005;755–766.

10. Das RK, Patel R, Shah H, et al. 3D CT-based high–dose-rate breast brachytherapy implants: treatment planning and quality assurance. *Int J Radiat Oncol Biol Phys* 2004;59:1224–1228.

11. DeWerd L, Jursinic P, Kitchen R, et al. Quality assurance tool for high dose rate brachytherapy. *Med Phys* 1995;22:435–440.

12. Edmundson GK. Geometry based optimization for stepping source implants. In: Martinez A, Orton C, Mould R, eds. *Brachytherapy HDR and LDR.* Columbia, MD: Nucletron, 1990;184–192.

13. Ezzell G. Acceptance testing and quality assurance for high dose-rate remote afterloading systems. In: Martinez A, Orton C, Mould R, eds. *Brachytherapy HDR and LDR.* Columbia, MD: Nucletron, 1990;138–159.

14. Ezzell G. Optimization in brachytherapy. In: Thomadsen B, Rivard M, Butler W, eds. *Brachytherapy physics.* 2nd ed. Madison, WI: Medical Physics Publishing Co, 2005;415–434.

15. Ezzell G. Quality assurance in HDR brachytherapy: physical and technical aspects. *Act—Selectron Brachytherapy J* 1991;5:59–62.

16. Flynn A. Quality assurance checks on a microSelectron-HDR. *Act—Selectron Brachytherapy J* 1990;4:112–115.

17. Grigsby P. Quality assurance of remote afterloading equipment at the Mallinckrodt Institute of Radiology. *Act—Selectron User's Newsl* 1989;1:15.

18. Haie-Meder C, Pötter R, Van Limbergen E, et al. Recommendations from Gynaecological (GYN) GEC-ESTRO Working Group (I): concepts and terms in 3D image based 3D treatment planning in cervix cancer brachytherapy with emphasis on MRI assessment of GTV and CTV. *Radiat Oncol* 2005;74:235–245.

19. Holms TW, Mackie TR. A comparison of three inverse treatment planning algorithms. *Phys Med Biol* 1994;39:91–106.

20. Jones C. Quality assurance in brachytherapy using the Selectron LDR/MDR and microSelectron-HDR. *Selectron Brachytherapy J* 1990;4:48–52.

21. King C, Stockstill T, Bloomer W, et al. Point dose variations with time in brachytherapy for cervical carcinoma. *Med Phys* 1992;19:777(abstr).

22. Kubo H, Chin RB. Simple mathematical formulas for quick-checking of single catheter high dose rate brachytherapy plans. *Endocuriether/Hyperthermia Oncol* 1992;8:165–169.

23. Kubo H, Glasgow G, Pethel T, et al. American Association of Physicists in Medicine: Report 61 (Task Group 59): high dose-rate brachytherapy delivery. *Med Phys* 1998;25:375–403.

24. Kuske R, Bolton J, Wilenzick R, et al. Brachytherapy as the sole method of breast irradiation in Tis, T_1, T_2, $N_{0,1}$ breast cancer. *Int J Radiat Oncol Biol Phys* 1994;30[Suppl 1]:245 (abstr).

25. Lahanas M, Baltas D, Zamboglou N. Anatomy-based three dimensional dose optimization in brachytherapy using multiobjective genetic algorithms. *Med Phys* 1999;26:1904–1918.

26. Luenberger DG. In: *Linear and nonlinear programming.* 2nd ed. Reading, MA: Addison and Wesley, 1989;261–288.

27. Martinez AA, Pataki I, Edmunson G, et al. Interim report of image-guided conformal high–dose-rate brachytherapy as monotherapy for the treatment of favorable stage prostate cancer: a feasibility report. *Int J Radiat Oncol Biol Phys* 2001;49:61–69.

28. McGinley P. *Shielding techniques for radiation oncology facilities.* 2nd ed. Madison, WI: Medical Physics Publishing, 2002.

29. Meigooni A, Williamson J, Slessinger E. Practical quality assurance tests for positional and temporal accuracy of HDR remote afterloaders. *Endocuriether/Hyperthermia Oncol;*9:46–(abstr).

30. Menard C, Susil R, Choyke P, et al. MRI-guided HDR prostate brachytherapy in standard 1.5T scanner. *Int J Radiat Oncol Biol Phys* 2004;59:1414–1423.

31. Nag S, Cardenes H, Chang S, et al. Proposed guidelines for image-based intracavitary brachytherapy for cervical carcinoma: report from Image-Guided Brachytherapy Working Group. *Int J Radiat Oncol Biol Phys* 2004;60:1160–1117.

32. Nag S, Chao C, Erickson B, et al. The American Brachytherapy Society recommendations for low dose rate brachytherapy for carcinoma of the cervix. *Int J Radiat Oncol Biol Phys* 2002;52:33–48.

33. Nag S, Erickson B, Thomadsen B, et al. The American Brachytherapy Society recommendations for high-dose-rate brachytherapy for carcinoma of the cervix. *Int J Radiat Oncol Biol Phys* 2000;48:201–211.

34. Nath R, Anderson L, Jones D, et al. American Association of Physicists in Medicine: Report 21: Task Group 32. *Specification of brachytherapy source strength.* College Park, MD: American Institute of Physics, 1987.

35. Nath R, Lowell L, Anderson L, Luxton G, et al. American Association of Physicists in Medicine: Report 61 (Task Group 43): dosimetry of interstitial brachytherapy sources. *Med Phys* 1995;22:209–234.

36. Orton C, Seyedsadr M, Somnay A. Comparison of high and low dose rate remote afterloading for cervix cancer and the importance of fractionation. *Int J Radiat Oncol Biol Phys* 1991;21:1425–1434.

37. Patel R, Das RK. Image-guided breast brachytherapy: an alternative to whole breast radiotherapy. *Lancet Oncol* 2006;7:407–415.

38. Pierquin B, Chassagne D, Chahbazian C, et al. *Brachytherapy.* St. Louis: Warran H. Green, 1978.

39. Pierguin B, Dutreix A, Paine C, et al. The Paris system in interstitial radiation therapy. *Acta Radiol Oncol* 1978;17:33–48.

40. Pouliot J, Kim Y, Lessard E, et al. Inverse planning for HDR prostate brachytherapy use to boost dominant intra-prostatic lesion defined by magnetic resonance spectroscopy imaging. *Int J Radiat Oncol Biol Phys* 2004;54:1196–1207.

41. Pouliot J, Lessard E, Hsu I-C. Number of catheters in prostate high dose rate brachytherapy: the role of inverse planning. Joint Brachytherapy Meeting GEC/ESTRO-ABS-GLAC, Barcelona, Spain, May 2004.

42. Saw C, Suntharalingam N. Qualitative assessment of interstitial implants. *Int J Radiat Oncol Biol Phys* 1991;20:135–139.

43. Saw C, Suntharalingam N. Reference dose rates for single- and double-plane ^{192}Ir implants. *Med Phys* 1988;15:391–396.

44. Saw C, Waterman F, Ayyangar K, et al. Qualitative evaluation of planar ^{192}Ir implants. *Med Phys* 1986;3:580(abstr).

45. Schoeppel S, Frasss B, Hopkins M, et al. A CT-compatible version of the Fletcher system intracavitary applicator: clinical application and 3-dimensional treatment planning. *Int J Radiat Oncol Biol Phys* 1989;17:1103–1109.

46. Schoeppel S, LaVigne M, Martel M, et al. Three-dimensional treatment planning of intracavitary gynecologic implants: analysis of ten cases and implications for dose specification. *Int J Radiat Oncol Biol Phys* 1994;28:277–283.

47. Sloboda RS. Optimization of brachytherapy dose distributions by simulated annealing. *Med Phys* 1992;19:955–964.

48. Sloboda RS, Pearcey RG, Gillan SJ. Optimized low dose rate pellet configuration for intravaginal brachytherapy. *Int J Radiat Oncol Biol Phys* 1993;26:499–511.

49. Stitt J, Fowler J, Thomadsen B, et al. High dose rate intracavitary brachytherapy for carcinoma of the cervix: the Madison system: I. clinical and radiobiological considerations. *Int J Radiat Oncol Biol Phys* 1992;24:335–348.

50. Thomadsen B. Quality management for high-dose-rate units. In: *Achieving quality on brachytherapy.* Bristol: Institute of Physics Press, 1999;97–125.

51. Thomadsen B. Volume imaging in gynecological brachytherapy. In: Thomadsen B, Rivard M, Butler W, eds. *Brachytherapy physics.* 2nd ed. Madison, WI: Medical Physics Publishing Co, 2005;785–796.

52. Thomadsen B, Lin S-W, Laemmrich P, et al. Analysis of treatment delivery errors in brachytherapy using formal risk analysis techniques. *Int J Radiat Oncol Biol Phys* 2003;57:1492–1508.

53. Thomadsen B, Shahabi S, Stitt J, et al. High dose rate intracavitary brachytherapy for carcinoma of the cervix: the Madison system. II. Procedural and physical considerations. *Int J Radiat Oncol Biol Phys* 1992;24:349–351.

54. U.S. Nuclear Regulatory Commission. Title 10, Chapter 1, *Code of Federal Regulations–Energy, Part 35, medical use of by-product material.* Washington, DC: Government Printing Office, 2003.

55. van der Laarse R. Optimization of high dose rate brachytherapy. *Act—Selectron User's Newsl* 1989;2:14–15.

56. Van der Laarse R, Edmundson GK, Luthmann RW, et al. Optimization of HDR brachytherapy dose distributions. *Act—Selectron User's Newsl* 1991;5:94–101.

57. Van't Riet A, Mak A, Moerland M, et al. A conformation number to quantify the degree of conformality in brachytherapy and external beam irradiation: application to the prostate. *Int J Radiat Oncol Biol Phys* 1997;37:731–736.

58. Williamson J, Ezzel G, Olch A, et al. Quality assurance for high dose rate brachytherapy. In Nag S, ed. *Textbook and high dose rate brachytherapy.* Armonk, NY: Futura Publishing Co, 1994: 147–212.

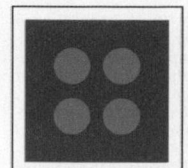

Chapter 22
Clinical Aspects and Applications of High–Dose-Rate Brachytherapy

Subir Nag, Granger R. Scruggs

Brachytherapy has the advantage of delivering a high dose to the tumor while sparing the surrounding normal tissues. Brachytherapy procedures were previously performed by inserting the radioactive material directly into the tumor ("hot" loading), thereby giving high radiation exposure to the physicians performing the procedure. Manually afterloaded techniques were introduced to increase accuracy and reduce the radiation hazards. In afterloaded techniques, hollow needles, catheters, or applicators are first inserted into the tumor then loaded with radioactive materials. The introduction of remote-controlled insertion of sources eliminated radiation exposure to visitors and medical personnel (60,113,156,201,234,236,237). In this technique, the patient is housed in a shielded room and the radiation therapist controls the treatment from outside the room. Hollow applicators, needles, or catheters are inserted into the tumor and connected by transfer tubes to the radioactive material, which is stored in a shielded safe within the high–dose-rate afterloader. The radiation source is driven through the transfer tubes and into the tumor by remote control.

Remote-controlled brachytherapy can be performed using low–dose-rate (LDR), medium–dose-rate (MDR), or high–dose-rate (HDR) techniques. Although, the International Commission on Radiation Units and Measurements (ICRU) definition No. 38 of HDR is >12 Gy/h (68), the usual dose rate employed in current HDR brachytherapy units is about 100 to 300 Gy/h. HDR has the added advantage that the treatments take only a few minutes, which can be given on an outpatient basis with minimal risk of applicator movement and minimal patient discomfort. Additionally, use of a single-stepping source, as used in most modern HDR afterloaders, allows optimization of dose distribution by varying the dwell time at each dwell position. However, it should be emphasized that while optimization can improve the dose distribution, it should not be used to substitute for a poorly placed implant. Nag and Samsami (138) have provided examples of inappropriate optimization strategies that can lead to suboptimal dosimetry plans and clinical problems. HDR is normally given as a course of a number of fractionated HDR treatments, although it can be given as a single treatment, as in intraoperative HDR brachytherapy, if doses to the normal tissues can be sufficiently reduced by displacement or shielding. The advantages and disadvantages of HDR in comparison to LDR are enumerated in Table 22.1.

The advantages listed above have led to increased use of HDR worldwide; however, training and expertise is required for proper administration of these treatments. Guidelines and recommendations for the use of HDR at various sites have been published (9,121,122,128,130,135,140,147,185), much of which is summarized in this chapter. The reader should refer to these publications for details, and controlled clinical trials are needed to critically evaluate the efficacy of these procedures.

Radiobiological Principles of High–Dose-Rate Brachytherapy

Most radiation oncologists are familiar with LDR brachytherapy. LDR (at 30 to 50 cGy/h) can be added to external beam radiation therapy (EBRT) doses (at 2 Gy/d) to obtain equivalent total doses. HDR brachytherapy is a relatively new modality that is distinct from LDR brachytherapy, and radiation oncologists who are accustomed to LDR techniques must realize that experience in LDR cannot be automatically translated into expertise in HDR. It is important to review the current literature and survey the experiences of centers that have been performing HDR. When converting from LDR to HDR, one must keep the other parameters (chemotherapy, EBRT field/dose, dose-specification point, applicators, patient population, and so forth) the same, changing only the LDR to HDR.

Fractionation schemes for HDR are widely variable, and many radiation oncologists are not very familiar with the resultant biological effects. Empirical methods such as the NSD (nominal standard dose), TDF (time-dose factor), or a dose reduction factor of 0.6 have been used in the past to convert HDR doses to LDR equivalent doses. The linear-quadratic (LQ) equation can be used to guide development of HDR doses and fractionation schedules (12). However, the LQ mathematical calculations are tedious and may not be practical on a day-to-day basis. Hence, a simplified computer program was developed by Nag and Gupta (126) to obtain the isoeffective doses to be used for HDR. The clinician needs only to enter the EBRT total dose and dose/fraction, HDR dose, and the number of HDR fractions. The computer program will automatically calculate the isoeffective doses for tumor and normal tissue effects. Isoeffective doses are expressed in clinically familiar terms (as if given at 2 Gy per fraction) rather than as biologically equivalent doses (BED), which are unfamiliar to clinicians. Furthermore, a dose-modifying factor (DMF) is applied to the normal tissues to account for the fact that doses to normal tissues are different from the doses to the tumor, thus providing a more realistic equivalent normal tissue effect. This program can be used to determine HDR doses that are equivalent to LDR brachytherapy doses (isoeffective dose) used to treat various cancers. Alternatively, the program may be used to express the isoeffective dose of different HDR dose-fractionation regimes as shown for cervical cancer in Table 22.2. It is remarkable that the isoeffective doses for tumor effects for the various fractionation regimes used for early stage cervical cancers are so similar, ranging from 82 to 85 Gy, while those used for advanced cancers are about 90 Gy (see Table 22.2). The isoeffective dose for normal tissue late effects depends on the assumed DMF (0.6, 0.7, or 0.9). For the fractionation scheme shown in Table 22.2, row 1, the equivalent late effect on normal tissue (bladder or rectum) would be 59.5, 71, or 98 Gy, respectively if the doses to normal tissues were 60%, 70%, or 90% of the prescribed dose to point A.

Although the LQ biomathematical model can be helpful in determining isoeffective doses, it has many limitations that must be kept in mind when using the program. The LQ model accounts for the repair of sublethal damage but it does not account for reoxygenation of hypoxic cells, reassortment within the cell cycle, or repopulation of tumor cells. These factors are generally small under normal circumstances. However, large doses per fraction do not allow reoxygenation of hypoxic tumor cells or reassortment of tumors from radioresistant S phase. Hence, a large radiation dose will preferentially kill radiosensitive cells,

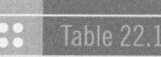 Table 22.1   **ADVANTAGES AND DISADVANTAGES OF HIGH–DOSE-RATE COMPARED WITH LOW–DOSE-RATE BRACHYTHERAPY.**

Advantages	Disadvantages
1. Radiation protection • HDR eliminates radiation exposure hazard for care givers and visitors. Care givers are able to provide optimal patient care without fear of radiation exposure. • HDR eliminates source preparation and transportation. • Since there is only one source, there is minimal risk of losing a radioactive source. 2. Allows shorter treatment times • There is less patient discomfort since prolonged bed rest is eliminated. • It is possible to treat patients who may not tolerate long periods of isolation and those who are at high risk for pulmonary embolism due to prolonged bed rest. • There is less risk of applicator movement during therapy. • There are reduced hospitalization costs since outpatient therapy is possible. • HDR may allow greater displacement of nearby normal tissues (by packing or retraction) which could potentially reduce morbidity. • It is possible to treat a larger number of patients in institutions that have a high volume of brachytherapy patients but insufficient inpatient facilities (e.g., in some developing countries). • Allow intraoperative treatments, which are completed while patient is still in the operating room. 3. HDR sources are of smaller diameter than the cesium sources that are used for intracavitary LDR • This reduces the need for dilatation of the cervix and therefore reduces the need for heavy sedation or general anesthesia. • High-risk patients who are unable to tolerate general anesthesia can be more safely treated. • HDR allows for interstitial, intraluminal, and percutaneous insertions. 4. HDR makes treatment dose distribution optimization possible • Variations of the dwell times of a single stepping source allow an almost infinite variation of the effective source strengths, and the source position allows for greater control of the dose distribution and potentially less morbidity.	1. Radiobiological • The short treatment times do not allow for the repair of sublethal damage in normal tissue or the redistribution of cells within the cell cycle or reoxygenation of the tumor cells; hence, multiple treatments are required. 2. Limited experience • Few centers in the United States have long-term (>20 years) experience. • Until recently, standardized treatment guidelines were not available; however, the American Brachytherapy Society (ABS) has recently provided guidelines for HDR at various sites (121,122,128,130,135,147,185). 3. The economic disadvantage • The use of HDR brachytherapy as compared to manual afterloading techniques requires a large initial capital expenditure since the remote afterloaders cost about $300,000. • There are additional costs for a shielded room and personnel costs are higher as the procedures are more labor intensive. 4. Greater potential risks • Since a high activity source is used, there is greater potential harm if the machine malfunctions or if there is a calculation error. The short treatment times, compared to LDR, allow much less time to detect and correct errors.

HDR, high–dose-rate; LDR, low–dose-rate

leaving a high number of hypoxic, radioresistant cells. Therefore, the computer program will overestimate the tumor effect of a single large dose per fraction (unless a resensitization factor is introduced).

The LQ equation does not take into account the proliferation of tumor cells. This factor is small if the treatments are performed over a short duration. However, if the treatments are highly protracted (e.g., there is a long time interval between EBRT and HDR), or in cases of tumors with high proliferation rates, the LQ model will overestimate the actual tumor effect. It also must be noted that individual α/β values are very variable. The α/β values for early reactions vary from 6 to 13 (the default in the program is set at 10); the α/β values for late reactions vary from 1 to 7 (default being set at 3), while α/β values for tumors vary from 0.4 to 13 (the default being set at 10). However, α/β values for a particular patient are not known and may vary even within the same tissue. The isoeffective doses obtained will therefore depend on the α/β values used for that

Table 22.2   **AMERICAN BRACHYTHERAPY SOCIETY SUGGESTED DOSES OF EXTERNAL-BEAM RADIATION THERAPY AND HIGH–DOSE-RATE BRACHYTHERAPY TO BE USED IN TREATING EARLY AND ADVANCED CERVICAL CANCER**

Total EBRT Dose (Gy) at 1.8 Gy/Fraction	No. of HDR Fractions	HDR per Fraction (Gy)	Isoeffective Dose (Gy) for Tumor Effects[a]	Isoeffective Dose (Gy) for Late Effects with DMF = 0.6[b]	Isoeffective Dose (Gy) for Late Effects with DMF = 0.7[b]	Isoeffective Dose (Gy) for Late Effects with DMF = 0.9[b]
Early cervical cancer						
19.8	6	7.5	85.1	59.5	71.0	98.0
19.8	7	6.5	82.0	56.7	67.1	91.5
19.8	8	6.0	83.5	57.0	67.4	91.6
45	5	6.0	84.3	67.0	73.4	88.6
45	6	5.3	84.8	66.8	73.1	87.7
Advanced cervical cancer						
45	5	6.5	88.9	70.1	77.6	95.0
45	6	5.8	90.1	70.3	77.6	94.7
50.4	4	7.0	89.2	72.6	79.4	95.3
50.4	5	6.0	89.6	72.1	78.6	93.7
50.4	6	5.3	90.1	72.0	78.3	92.9

DMF, dose modifying factor; EBRT, external beam radiation therapy; HDR, high dose rate
[a]α/β ratio assumed for tumor = 10
[b]α/β ratio assumed for normal tissue late effects = 3.

Techniques, Modalities, and Modifiers in Radiation Oncology

particular calculation. The LQ model assumes complete repair between fractions. If the time interval between fractions is too short (<6 hours) or the half-time of repair is very long, the repair of normal tissues will be incomplete, and the LQ formula will underestimate the biological effect. Hence, it is important to have sufficient time interval (at least 6 hours) between treatment fractions.

The infinite variation of the dwell times that is possible with HDR (or pulsed–dose rate) allows better optimization of the doses than can be achieved with LDR. Better packing or retraction of normal tissues is possible with HDR, due to the short treatment duration. This factor is not usually taken into account in the LQ model (unless the DMF is altered). Another difference not accounted for in the LQ model is that the dose stated in brachytherapy is generally the minimum tumor dose. The doses within the tumor are much higher. Hence, the effective dose (for tumor control probability) is much higher for brachytherapy than for EBRT.

In view of the many limitations of the LQ model, it must be stressed that, as with any mathematical model, the LQ model should be used judiciously only as a guide and should always be correlated with clinical judgment and outcome results. Caution is especially warranted whenever large fraction sizes are used, since their clinical results have not been well studied (25).

Common Uses of High–Dose-Rate Brachytherapy

Although HDR brachytherapy has been used in almost every site in the body, it is most commonly used to treat cancers of the cervix, endometrium, lung, and esophagus (136). Less common treated sites for HDR include the prostate, bile duct, breast, brain, rectum, head and neck, skin, soft tissues, and blood vessels (coronary and peripheral arteries). HDR is generally used as a component of multimodality treatment that includes EBRT and/or chemotherapy and surgery. A summary of the clinical uses of HDR is included in this chapter, while the details of the physics and radiobiology of HDR are provided in another chapter.

Carcinoma of the Cervix

Cervical carcinoma is treated by a combination of pelvic EBRT and brachytherapy. It is emphasized that brachytherapy is a necessary component in the curative treatment of cervical cancers (135,136). Traditionally, cervical carcinoma has been treated using LDR brachytherapy. HDR has gained popularity in the United States over the past decade due to the advantages alluded to earlier, specifically the possibility of therapy on an outpatient basis, avoidance of long-term bed rest, and avoidance of cervical dilation. Additionally, greater sparing of the rectum and bladder by temporary retraction, dose optimization, and integration with EBRT to the pelvis are possible (157). These advantages must be counterbalanced with the greater number of treatments required (typically four to six treatments, lasting approximately 10 to 15 minutes each).

The American Brachytherapy Society (ABS) recommends keeping the total duration of treatment (EBRT and HDR) to <8 weeks since prolongation adversely affects local control and survival (135). Because the overall treatment duration would be unduly prolonged if HDR treatments were started after completion of EBRT, the HDR is interdigitated during the course of EBRT. However, it should be noted that EBRT is not given on the day of a HDR treatment. Typically, if the vaginal geometry is optimal, HDR brachytherapy begins after 2 weeks of starting EBRT; HDR is continued one time per week with the EBRT given on the other 4 days of the week. If large tumor volume requires delaying the start of HDR brachytherapy, it may be necessary to perform two implants per week after the EBRT has been completed to keep the total treatment duration to <8 weeks.

The insertion of the applicator is usually performed under intravenous sedation. Because the cervix need not be dilated, general or spinal anesthesia is not required. It is sometimes mistakenly assumed that bladder and rectal retraction is not required due to the short duration of treatment. It should be emphasized that rectal and bladder retraction (by the use of packing or retractors) is essential in HDR as it is for LDR. Some centers prefer to use an external immobilization device (EID) to fix the position of the applicators, but this is not essential. Various types of applicators (Fletcher and Ring being the most common) have been used and depend on the preference of the radiation oncologist.

The HDR dose is generally prescribed to an applicator-based definition of point A (119,135). In the treatment of cervical carcinoma, the combined EBRT and HDR dose to point A is an LDR equivalent of 80 to 85 Gy for early stage disease and 85 to 90 Gy for advanced stage (135). Early disease is defined as nonbulky stage I or II <4 cm in diameter; advanced diseased is defined as stage I or II >4 cm in diameter or stage IIIB. The total pelvic sidewall dose recommendations are 50 to 55 Gy for smaller lesions and 55 to 60 Gy for larger ones. The ratio of EBRT to brachytherapy is dependent on the stage, with a larger EBRT dose used for the more advanced stages. Although there is marked variation in the dose and fractionation employed for cervical HDR (42,148), most centers use a schedule of about 6 to 8 Gy per fraction in four to six fractions (a smaller number of fractions is used by those using larger doses per fraction) (42,157). The HDR dose is also dependent on the stage of the disease and the dose of pelvic EBRT.

HDR doses can be obtained from the LDR equivalent using the LQ equation (12). Because of the dose-rate effect in HDR, the total physical dose will be lower for HDR than for LDR brachytherapy. Because conversion of HDR doses to LDR equivalent doses mathematically may not be practical on a day-to-day basis, a simplified computer program can be used to obtain the isoeffective dose (126). Although recognizing that many efficacious HDR fractionation schedules exist, the ABS suggestions are given in Table 22.2 as a guide. The recommended HDR dose per fraction may vary by ±0.25 Gy. It is emphasized that extra care must be taken to ensure adequate bladder and rectal packing if high dose (>7 Gy) per fraction is used.

In certain clinical situations (e.g., a narrow fibrotic vagina, bulky tumors, the inability to enter the cervical os, extension to the lateral parametria or pelvic sidewall, lower vaginal extension, and suboptimal applicator placement), the normal tissue tolerance may be exceeded if the above doses are used. In these situations, a repacking should be attempted. If this fails to reduce the normal tissue doses, the HDR fraction size can be decreased (which requires an increase in the fraction number), or the EBRT dose increased while decreasing the HDR total dose. Alternatively, an interstitial implant (either LDR or HDR) may be used instead. In the event of reduced vaginal capacity and if an interstitial technique is not available, Sharma et al. (198) have described an intracavitary technique that utilizes a central tandem with a single ovoid alternating with the contralateral ovoid with subsequent insertions.

Results

LDR brachytherapy has been used with good results in carcinoma of the cervix for almost 100 years. Hence, it is important to critically analyze whether the results obtained with HDR brachytherapy, which has a much shorter history, compare with those obtained with LDR. Unfortunately, most of the published reports have been nonrandomized studies. The earlier studies showed good local control and survival rates that compared well to those obtained with LDR; however, initially some increased late complications were noted (73). Subsequent studies, which used lower dose per fraction and a greater number of fractions, demonstrated good control comparable to LDR without

Table 22.3 SUMMARY OF RETROSPECTIVE ANALYSIS OF HIGH–DOSE-RATE BRACHYTHERAPY IN THE TREATMENT OF CERVICAL CANCER

Author (Reference)	Stage	No. of Patients	EBRT (Gy)	HDR (Gy × Fractions)	Local Control	Survival	Late Complications
Lorvidhaya et al. (92)	I–III	1992	30–50	7–7.5 × 4 5.5–6 × 6	75.2%	68.2% (5 y)	4.8% Gr 3,4 Bowel 3.5% Gr 3,4 Bladder
Potter et al. (176)	I–IV	189	48.6–50	7 × 3–6	77.6% (3 y)	58.2% (3 y)	6% Gr 3,4 Rectal 4% Gr 3,4 Bowel 2.9% Gr 3,4 Bladder
Toita et al. (231)	I–III	88	50	6 × 3	82% (3 y)	77% (3 y)	12% Proctitis 11% Cystitis 14% Enterocolitis
Sood et al. (204)	I–III	49	45 9 Gy boost	9–9.4 × 2	77% w/o chemo 88% w/ chemo (3 y)	78% (5 y)	4.1% ≥Gr 2
Patel et al. (158)	II–III	121	Gr 1: 40 Gy (CS) Gr 2: 46 Gy	9 × 5 9 × 2	87.5% (5 y) 71.1% (5 y)	–	None ≥Gr 3 Rectal 1.7% ≥Gr 3 Bladder
Ferrigno et al. (36)	I–III	118	40–50	6 × 4	65% (5 y)	55% (5 y)	6% Rectal 6% Small bowel 1.7% Urinary tract
Souhami et al. (209)	I–IVA	282	45	8 × 3	75% (15 y)	57% (5 y)	6.3% Gr 3,4 Bowel 3.5% Gr 3,4 Bladder

CS, central shielding; EBRT, external beam radiation therapy; Gr, grade; HDR, high–dose-rate

increased morbidity (1,7,8,19,36,92,158,167,176,192,204,209, 231). Table 22.3 summarizes the HDR fractionation and results of the most recently published retrospective literature.

Meta-analyses and published literature reviews have compared HDR with LDR brachytherapy. Orton et al. (157) published an analysis of data comparing HDR and LDR obtained from a survey of 56 institutions treating 17,068 patients with HDR and 5,666 patients with LDR. Five-year survival data were available for 6,939 HDR patients and 3,365 LDR patients and was 82.7% versus 82.4% for stage I, 66.6% versus 66.8% for stage II, and 47.2% versus 42.6% for stage III, respectively. Fu and Phillips (42) reached a similar conclusion in their worldwide review. In 1999 Petereit and Peracey (166) published a literature review that included 5,619 patients treated with HDR brachytherapy and demonstrated 5-year pelvic control rates of 91%, 82%, and 71% in stage I, II, and III patients, respectively. Five-year overall survival by stage and complication rates was similar to previous meta-analyses. Statistically quantifiable conclusions cannot be drawn from comparisons of the results of

uncontrolled studies using different methodologies from various centers; however, this anecdotal evidence suggests that the results of HDR are at least as good as those achieved by LDR brachytherapy. Table 22.4 summarizes the HDR fractionation and results by stage of the meta-analyses and review literature.

Four randomized studies have compared the use of HDR with the use of LDR brachytherapy in carcinoma of the cervix (57,88,159,199). Shigematsu et al. (199) reported on 143 patients treated with HDR brachytherapy compared to 106 patients treated with LDR for stage IIB and III disease. Although the randomization technique was suboptimal (i.e., some patients who were randomized to LDR were actually treated with HDR because of limited LDR availability), the HDR arm achieved superior local control with no difference in survival as compared to the LDR arm. In a randomized study of LDR versus HDR brachytherapy reported from India, there was no difference in local control, survival, or severe complications between the two treatment modalities in 482 patients (159). However, there was

Table 22.4 SUMMARY OF META-ANALYSIS AND REVIEW LITERATURE OF HIGH–DOSE-RATE VS. LOW–DOSE-RATE BRACHYTHERAPY IN CERVICAL CANCER

Author (Reference)	Stage	No. of HDR Patients	No. of LDR Patients	HDR (Gy × Fractions)	5-Year Control (HDR Only)	5-Year Survival HDR	5-Year Survival LDR	Late Complications
Fu and Phillips (42)	I	668	297	3–14 × 2–13	—	71%–100%	74%–89%	0.7%–36% Rectal
	II	1,387	719			40%–76%	53%–76%	0.3%–9.2% Bladder
	III	1,378	850			27%–62%	24%–49%	
Orton et al. (157)	I	1,327	630	7.5 × 5	—	82.7%	82.4%	9.05%
	II	2,891	1,271			66.6%	66.8%	(Moderate + Severe)
	III	2,721	1,464			47.2%	42.6%	
Petereit and Peracey (166)	I	1,048	—	7 × 4	91%	85%	—	5% Overall
	II	1,995	—		82%	68%	—	
	III	2,576	—		71%	47%	—	

HDR, high–dose-rate; LDR, low–dose-rate

Table 22.5 SUMMARY OF RESULTS OF RANDOMIZED TRIALS OF HIGH–DOSE-RATE VS. LOW–DOSE-RATE BRACHYTHERAPY IN CERVICAL CANCER

Author (Reference)	Stage	EBRT (Gy)	No. of Patients		Local Control		5-Year Survival	
			LDR	HDR	LDR (%)	HDR (%)	LDR (%)	HDR (%)
Shigematsu et al. (199)	IIB-III	40	106	143	77	90	55	55
Teshima et al. (230)[a]	I	40	171	259	73	76	89	66
	II						73	61
	III						45	47
Patel et al. (159)	I–III	35–45	246	236	80	76	58	58
Hareyama et al. (57)	II	50	71	61	—	—	87[b]	69[b]
	III						60[b]	51[b]
Lertsanguansinchai et al. (88)	I–III	40–54	109	112	89	86	71[c]	68[c]

EBRT, external beam radiation therapy; HDR, high–dose-rate; LDR, low–dose-rate
[a]Update of Shigematsu et al.
[b]Disease specific survival.
[c]Three-year survival

a statistical difference in rectal complications, with a 20% rate in the LDR group and only a 6% rate in the HDR group. In 2002, Hareyama et al. (57) reported their results of 132 patients with stage II and IIIB cervical carcinoma. The 5-year disease-specific survival of LDR versus HDR for stage II was 87% versus 69% respectively and for stage IIIB 60% versus 51%, respectively. The difference between survival rates was not statistically significant. The most recent randomized study was reported from Thailand in 2004 (88). In this trial, 237 patients were evaluated and there was no difference in overall survival, relapse-free survival, or pelvic control between LDR and HDR brachytherapy. In addition there was no statistical difference in complication rates for the rectum, bladder, or small bowel. Tables 22.5 and 22.6 summarize the results and complications respectively of the available randomized studies.

In summary, the available data from randomized trials, retrospective analyses, and meta-analyses suggest that survival and local control of HDR treatments are probably equivalent to that of LDR, with similar or lower morbidity.

Image-based Treatment Planning

Recently there has been interest regarding image-based treatment planning in brachytherapy for carcinoma of the cervix. It is well established that magnetic resonance imaging (MRI) is superior to other current imaging modalities in delineating gross tumor involving the cervix and adjacent normal tissues

(64,78,220). The underlying principle for using modern radiographic imaging techniques such as MRI is simply to potentially better delineate the target volume, which could allow dose escalation for better tumor control and simultaneously limit dose to normal tissues. Historically, prescription doses are referenced to point A, which unfortunately does not necessarily reflect the dose to the tumor. The ICRU has recommended determining the tissue volume encompassed by the 60 Gy reference isodose surface (reference volume) to compare intracavitary treatments performed in different institutions regardless of the applicator system, insertion technique, method of treatment, and prescription used (68). However, this dose determination is made only infrequently in gynecological intracavitary brachytherapy specifications (51,178).

A gynecological working group was formed by the Groupe European de Curietherapie and European Society for Therapeutic Radiology and Oncology (GEC-ESTRO) in 2000 to formulate and describe new terminology regarding three-dimensional (3D) image-based treatment planning in cervical cancer brachytherapy. Their recommendations were published in March 2005 and are summarized in Table 22.7 (56). This working group recognized that most patients with cervical cancer are treated with combined modality therapy including external radiotherapy, chemotherapy, and brachytherapy and that there is significant change of gross tumor during such treatment. Because of this, a fluid description of treatment volumes during the course of treatment is required to have a better

Table 22.6 SUMMARY OF COMPLICATIONS OF RANDOMIZED TRIALS OF HIGH–DOSE-RATE VS. LOW–DOSE-RATE BRACHYTHERAPY IN CERVICAL CANCER

Author (Reference)	Bladder				Rectum			
	Grade 1+2		Grade 3+4		Grade 1+2		Grade 3+4	
	LDR (%)	HDR (%)	LDR (%)	HDR (%)	LDR (%)	HDR (%)	LDR (%)	HDR (%)
Shigematsu et al. (199)	—	—	—	—	—	—	—	—
Teshima et al. (230)	—	3[a]	—	—	3[a]	4[a]	—	—
Patel et al. (159)	3.7	3.8	—	—	17.5	5.9	2.4	0.4
Hareyama et al. (57)	—	—	7.5	4	—	—	8.7	3.5
Lertsanguansinchai et al. (88)	21	14	2.7	0.9	31	15	0.9	4.5

HDR, high–dose-rate; LDR, low–dose-rate
[a]Includes grade 2 and 3.

Table 22.7	GEC-ESTRO IMAGE-BASED PLANNING VOLUME DEFINITIONS FOR CERVICAL CANCER	
Volume		**Description**
GTV_D	GTV at diagnosis	Macroscopic tumor extension at diagnosis as detected by clinical examination and visualized on MRI
$GTV_{B1,B2,B3...}$	GTV at each BT procedure	Macroscopic tumor extension at time of brachytherapy as detected by clinical examination and as visualized on MRI
$HR\ CTV_{B1,B2,B3...}$	High-risk CTV at each BT procedure	Includes $GTV_{B1,B2...}$, the whole cervix and presumed extracervical tumor extension at time of brachytherapy by means of clinical examination and by MRI
$IR\ CTV_{B1,B2,B3...}$	Intermediate risk CTV at each BT procedure	Encompasses high-risk CTV with a safety margin of 5 to 15 mm (safety margin is chosen according to tumor size and location, potential tumor spread, tumor regression, and treatment strategy). The IR CTV is never less than GTV_D

BT, brachytherapy; CTV, clinical target volume; GEC-ESTRO, Groupe European de Curietherapie and European Society for Therapeutic Radiology and Oncology; GTV, gross tumor volume; HR, high risk; IR, intermediate risk; MRI, magnetic resonance imaging

understanding of dose-to-volume relationships throughout treatment and to more accurately compare treatments between institutions and patients. They devised definitions of gross tumor volume (GTV) at diagnosis and at each brachytherapy procedure as well as high-risk and intermediate-risk clinical target volumes (CTV). Each of these volumes would be determined via clinical examination and MRI (preferably T2 weighted) at their respective times during the course of treatment. The CTVs are based on tumor load and represent risk of recurrence. Thus "high risk" is that which includes macroscopic tumor, "intermediate risk" is that which includes significant microscopic disease, and "low risk" is that which includes potential microscopic tumor spread. It is assumed that the low risk region is successfully treated with surgery and/or external beam radiotherapy. In early 2006 the working group released an update to their original recommendations to include descriptions of dose-volume parameters for organs at risk and a step-wise procedure for transition from the traditional dose prescription to the 3D image-based volume prescription (175). The group recommended for organs at risk that the minimum dose in the most irradiated tissue volumes of 0.1 cm^3, 1 cm^3, and 3 cm^3 be reported. Ultimately, it is their intention not to alter current clinical and dosimetric reporting, but to assess the feasibility, value, and reproducibility of such volumes. If it is found to be feasible and of value there would be potential to alter dose recommendations and possibly improve clinical outcomes.

Similarly, in November 2004 the U.S.-based Image Guided Brachytherapy Working Group consisting of members from Gynecology Oncology Group (GOG), Radiologic Physics Center, ABS, American College of Radiology, American College of Radiology Imaging Network, American Association of Physicists in Medicine, and Radiation Therapy Oncology Group published similar guidelines (117). In addition to proposing definitions of GTV and CTV, the committee devised guidelines for contouring organs at risk and recommended which dose volume parameters should be reported in conjunction with the standard dose prescription methods (i.e., point A).

There was some initial confusion immediately after the publication of the two main reports, since there were some differences in definition/nomenclature by the two working groups (174). However, a closer examination showed more similarities than differences (118). It was obvious that the two groups needed to work together to further image-based cervical cancer brachytherapy (118,174). At a recent transatlantic workshop on image-based cervical cancer brachytherapy (Chicago, July 28, 2005), it was suggested that since the recommendations are so similar and to prevent confusion, the nomenclature suggested by the European Group be adopted and future joint contouring workshops be organized to facilitate image-based cervical cancer brachytherapy (115).

Appropriate concerns to the feasibility of 3D image-based treatment planning for brachytherapy includes the increased cost of obtaining serial MRIs during a course of treatment (on average at least four to six during a normal course of treatment) and the limited availability and high cost of MRI-compatible applicator instrumentation for brachytherapy procedures. This increase in cost will need to be offset by a significant improvement in treatment result and quality of life for patients with cervical carcinoma.

Carcinoma of the Endometrium

HDR brachytherapy is commonly used for adjuvant treatment of the vaginal cuff after hysterectomy in patients with an intermediate or high risk for vaginal recurrence (high-grade, deep myometrial invasion or advanced stage). Additionally, brachytherapy may be used for primary treatment in inoperable endometrial carcinoma and for treatment of recurrences after hysterectomy.

Vaginal Cuff Irradiation

The standard management for operable carcinoma of the endometrium is total abdominal hysterectomy with bilateral salpingo-oophorectomy (TAH-BSO). Patients at high risk for vaginal recurrences (deep myometrial invasion, high histologic grade and stage, lymphovascular invasion, cervical or extrauterine spread, squamous cell or papillary histology) should receive radiation therapy. Since the last published edition, two significant randomized trials have been published demonstrating the benefit of postoperative pelvic radiation therapy for patients with early stage endometrial carcinoma and intermediate to high risk features for recurrence (23,76,194). The Post Operative Radiation Therapy in Endometrial Carcinoma (PORTEC) 1 (23,194) study and the GOG-99 (76) study are discussed in detail in the chapter on endometrial cancer. Both trials utilized external beam radiation therapy only, and both demonstrated a significant improvement in local control with radiation therapy with no difference in overall survival. However, the best method of delivering postoperative radiation therapy, either via pelvic EBRT, vaginal vault brachytherapy, or a combination, remains unanswered. EBRT has the advantage of irradiating the pelvic lymph nodes, but takes about 5 weeks to perform and has some morbidity. Brachytherapy is more convenient, has low morbidity, but does not treat the lymph nodes. Hence, some centers combine both EBRT and brachytherapy, although it has not been proven that the combination yields any superior results. Others prefer "watchful waiting" and use salvage irradiation if there is a recurrence, since the final survival rate is not compromised. However, in cases of recurrence, a combination of pelvic EBRT and brachytherapy is required.

If pelvic EBRT is used in combination with brachytherapy, the EBRT dose is usually 40 to 45 Gy in 20 to 25 treatments with midline shielding after about 40 Gy (122). A vaginal cylinder is commonly used to deliver HDR brachytherapy. The largest diameter cylinder that comfortably fits the vagina should be used to increase the depth dose. The length of vaginal vault treated varies. Some treat the superior 3 or 5 cm, while others treat the superior half or two thirds of the vagina (3,4,6,17,96,99,122, 164,168,183,208,217,239). For serous and clear cell histologies, treatment of the entire vaginal canal should be considered. The use of a single-line iridium 192 (^{192}Ir) source creates a dose inhomogeneity at the vaginal apex due to source anisotropy. However, the clinical significance of source anisotropy is debatable. The use of ovoids, circular rings, or an angled source may reduce the dose inhomogeneity at the apex created by the ^{192}Ir source anisotropy (122). The applicator should be placed in the midline, as horizontal as possible and parallel to the longitudinal axis of the body for appropriate dose distribution. Placement of a radio-opaque seed or clip at the vaginal apex helps to verify that the applicator is in contact with the vaginal apex on fluoroscopy or radiographs. However, these clips or seeds can sometimes fall off or migrate deep to the mucosa and, therefore, may not always indicate the position of the apex. Some centers prefer to use an external immobilization device to minimize movement; however, this is not mandatory.

The dose distribution should be optimized to deliver the prescribed dose either at the vaginal surface or at 0.5 cm depth, depending on the institutional policy. It is important to place dose optimization points not only along the lateral aspect of the vaginal wall but also at specified points about the dome of the vaginal cylinder to avoid higher vaginal apex doses, which can lead to vaginal vault necrosis (138). Regardless of the prescription method, doses to both the vaginal surface and at 0.5 cm depth should be reported (122).

The dose per fraction used has varied from 4.5 Gy to 16 Gy, and the number of fractions has varied from two to seven with the interval between fractions of 1 to 2 weeks (3,4,6,17,63,96, 98,99,164,168,183,208,217,239). The lower doses per fraction are usually given using either a larger number of fractions or in combination with EBRT to the pelvis. Sorbe et al. (207) evaluated two fractionation schemes (2.5 Gy × 6 vs. 5 Gy × 6) in a randomized trial and found no difference in locoregional recurrence rates, but an increase in vaginal shortening, mucosal atrophy, and bleeding in the 5 Gy per fraction arm. The ABS dose suggestions (122) for HDR alone or in combination with 45 Gy EBRT are given in Table 22.8. Since some institutions specify the dose to the vaginal surface and others specify the dose at 0.5-cm depth, suggested HDR doses have been given for both specification methods.

From retrospective analysis, the 5-year survival rates of HDR therapy vary from 72% to 97%, depending on the stage, grade, and depth of myometrial invasion (3,4,6,17,63,96,98,99,164, 168,182,183,188,208,239). A recent retrospective analysis by Jolly et al. (72) of 243 patients delivering 30 Gy in six fractions demonstrated a 4-year overall survival of 97% with a local

recurrence rate of 4%. The severe (grade III or IV) late complication rate is usually <2% and depends on the dose per fraction (3,4,6,63,99,168,188,203,208,239). The incidence of vaginal shortening is also very much dose dependent, reportedly as high as 70% when 9 Gy per fraction was prescribed at 1-cm depth to 31% when the dose was reduced to 4.5 Gy per fraction (208). Other factors that increase morbidity include the use of a small (2 cm) diameter vaginal cylinder, the addition of pelvic external beam radiation, and a dose specification point beyond 0.5 cm (99).

Pearcey and Petereit (160) published a literature review analyzing 1,800 cases of post-operative HDR brachytherapy alone in patients with low to intermediate risk endometrial cancer. They found an overall vaginal control rate of 99.3%. Late morbidity was significantly higher with isoeffective doses for late responding tissues exceeding 100 Gy.

Currently, the PORTEC-2 trial is accruing and randomizing patients postoperatively to either pelvic EBRT alone or vaginal brachytherapy alone. Eligible patients include patient's age 60 or older with stage 1C and histologic grade 1 or 2 or stage 1B with histologic grade 3. Those with stage 2A grade 1 or 2 histology, or stage 2A, grade 3 histology, and <50% myometrial invasion of any age are also eligible. Vaginal brachytherapy will be delivered via a vaginal cylinder covering the proximal half of the vagina and will be prescribed to a point at 5-mm distance from the surface of the cylinder. LDR, MDR, and HDR treatments are allowable and left to the discretion of the treating physician. The HDR schedule involves three fractions of 7 Gy each 1 week apart. The results of the PORTEC-2 trial is not yet published.

Treatment of Recurrences at the Vaginal Cuff

A combination of pelvic EBRT and brachytherapy is generally used to treat recurrences at the vaginal cuff. With distal vaginal recurrences, the entire vagina and medial inguinal nodes are included in the EBRT field. Intracavitary vaginal brachytherapy should be used only for nonbulky recurrences (thickness <5 mm after the completion of EBRT) (122). Interstitial brachytherapy is to be used for bulky recurrences (thickness >5 mm after the completion of EBRT) and for previously irradiated patients. Apical recurrences are often more extensive superiorly than can be judged on physical examination, thus favoring the use of interstitial brachytherapy. These patients are best treated at centers with considerable experience in interstitial brachytherapy. Radio-opaque marker seeds or surgical clips should be placed at the margins of gross disease to delineate disease extent. If the relapse is limited to one wall of the vagina, consideration should be given to limiting the dose to the opposite wall. The

Table 22.8	AMERICAN BRACHYTHERAPY SOCIETY SUGGESTED DOSES OF HIGH–DOSE-RATE BRACHYTHERAPY ALONE OR IN COMBINATION WITH PELVIC EXTERNAL-BEAM RADIATION THERAPY TO BE USED FOR ADJUVANT TREATMENT OF POSTOPERATIVE ENDOMETRIAL CANCER		
EBRT (Gy) at 1.8 Gy/Fraction	**No. of HDR Fractions**	**HDR per Fraction (Gy)**	**Dose Specification Point**
0	3	7.0	0.5 cm depth
0	4	5.5	0.5 cm depth
0	5	4.7	0.5 cm depth
0	3	10.5	vaginal surface
0	4	8.8	vaginal surface
0	5	7.5	vaginal surface
45	2	5.5	0.5 cm depth
45	3	4.0	0.5 cm depth
45	2	8.0	vaginal surface
45	3	6.0	vaginal surface

EBRT, external beam radiation therapy; HDR, high–dose-rate

Table 22.9	AMERICAN BRACHYTHERAPY SOCIETY SUGGESTED DOSES OF HIGH–DOSE-RATE BRACHYTHERAPY TO BE USED IN COMBINATION WITH PELVIC EXTERNAL-BEAM RADIATION THERAPY FOR TREATING VAGINAL CUFF RECURRENCES FROM ENDOMETRIAL CANCER		
EBRT (Gy) at 1.8 Gy/Fraction	No. of HDR Fractions	HDR per Fraction (Gy)	Dose Specification
45	3	7.0	0.5 cm depth
45	4	6.0	0.5 cm depth
45	5	6.0	vaginal surface
45	4	7.0	vaginal surface

EBRT, external beam radiation therapy; HDR, high–dose-rate

ABS suggested doses for HDR brachytherapy (in combination with 45 Gy EBRT) are provided in Table 22.9 (122).

Inoperable Endometrial Carcinoma

Patients with adenocarcinoma of the endometrium who are not candidates for surgery because of severe medical problems are treated with radiation therapy. A combination of pelvic EBRT and brachytherapy is preferred whenever possible. However, many of the conditions that do not allow surgery in these cases are also relative contraindications for EBRT and for LDR brachytherapy. In such cases, these patients may be treated with HDR alone.

Numerous applicators can be used for treatment of primary endometrial cancer. A tandem and colpostat are often used; however, these applicators will not irradiate the uterine fundus homogeneously. Others have used a curved tandem, turning it to the left and right in alternate insertions. A Y-shaped applicator irradiates the fundus more evenly. Other possibilities include modified Heyman capsules or multiple tandems. The dose is commonly specified at 2 cm from the source, although CT-based treatment planning to ensure a more homogeneous dose to the entire myometrium is preferred. The dose per fraction has ranged from 5 to 12 Gy, and three to six fractions are commonly employed (80,83,84,116,151,152,188,202,205,216, 217,229). The dose and/or the dose per fraction is reduced if EBRT can be added. The ABS suggested doses for HDR brachytherapy alone or in combination with 45 Gy EBRT are given in Table 22.10 (122). The survival at 5 years for stage I is about 70% to 80%, which is slightly lower than that obtained by surgery. The toxicity is higher (about 7%) when patients are treated with high doses per fraction (84,205,206).

Endobronchial Radiation

The use of HDR brachytherapy is well established for palliation of cough, dyspnea, pain, and hemoptysis in patients with advanced or metastatic lung cancer. The use of brachytherapy as a boost to EBRT in curative cases should be restricted to a select group of patients who have predominantly endobronchial disease, are medically inoperable, or have small/occult carcinomas of the lung.

An initial bronchoscopy is performed to evaluate the airway and locate the site of obstruction. Either a 5- or 6-French (Fr) catheter (inserted through the brush channel of the bronchoscope) can be used to deliver the brachytherapy. Use of a 6-Fr catheter allows the HDR source to negotiate tight curves, which is not possible with the 5-Fr catheter. If a 6-Fr catheter is used, a large bronchoscope (with brush channel diameter of at least 2.2 mm) is required. The bronchoscope can be connected to a teaching head or a video monitor so that the radiation oncologist can also visualize the lesion and the catheter. It is extremely important to note the distances between the proximal extent of the tumor and fixed structures such as the carina. The catheter is inserted through the brush channel of the bronchoscope, passed through the tumor, and lodged in one of the smaller bronchi. Fluoroscopic confirmation of the catheter's position is desirable. The radiation oncologist then pushes the afterloading catheter in while the pulmonologist slowly withdraws the bronchoscope. The use of fluoroscopy assists in keeping the catheter in place during this push-pull technique of bronchoscope removal. The catheter is then secured with tape at the nose, and its position is marked in ink to alert the radiation oncologist in case of displacement. As an additional precautionary measure, the external length of the catheter from the tip of the nostril is noted. If multiple catheters are to be used, the procedure is repeated, taking care to clearly label each catheter. Localization x-rays with radio-opaque dummy wires in the catheter are then obtained. The location of the obstruction and the target length are marked on the x-rays to determine the length to be irradiated and the initial dwell position.

The dose has been prescribed at various points from 0.5 to 2 cm, although 1 cm from the source is commonly used (128,213). The length to be irradiated usually includes the endobronchial tumor and 1.0- to 2.0-cm proximal and distal margins. If a single catheter is used and there is minimal curvature of the catheter

Table 22.10	AMERICAN BRACHYTHERAPY SOCIETY SUGGESTED DOSES OF HIGH–DOSE-RATE BRACHYTHERAPY ALONE OR IN COMBINATION WITH EXTERNAL-BEAM RADIATION THERAPY FOR TREATMENT OF INOPERABLE PRIMARY ENDOMETRIAL CANCER	
EBRT (Gy) at 1.8 Gy/Fraction	No. of HDR Fractions	HDR per Fraction (Gy)[a]
45	2	8.5
45	3	6.3
45	4	5.2
0	4	8.5
0	5	7.3
0	6	6.4
0	7	5.7

EBRT, external beam radiation therapy; HDR, high–dose-rate
[a]HDR doses are specified at 2 cm from the midpoint of the intrauterine sources.

Techniques, Modalities, and Modifiers in Radiation Oncology

in the area to be irradiated, it is possible to minimize the treatment planning time by using preplanned dosimetry. For example, Ohio State University has precalculated treatment plans for 3-, 5-, 7-, and 10-cm lengths to be irradiated to 5 or 7.5 Gy at 1 cm from the source using equal dwell times. This allows the treatment to be performed without any delay if standard lengths and doses are used. Individualized image-based treatment planning must be performed if multiple catheters are used.

Palliative Endobronchial Brachytherapy

Candidates for palliative endobronchial brachytherapy include (47,108,110,128,212):

1. Patients with a significant endobronchial tumor component that causes symptoms such as shortness of breath, hemoptysis, persistent cough, and other signs of postobstructive pneumonitis. Tumors with a predominantly endobronchial component are considered suitable, as opposed to extrinsic tumors that compress the bronchus or the trachea. Endobronchial brachytherapy can generally give quicker palliation of obstruction than EBRT. Furthermore, brachytherapy can be more convenient than 2 to 3 weeks of daily EBRT.
2. Patients who are unable to tolerate any EBRT because of poor lung function.
3. Patients with previous EBRT of sufficient total dose to preclude further EBRT.

A variety of doses have been successfully used by various centers. Total doses ranging from 15 Gy to 47 Gy HDR in one to five fractions calculated at 1 cm have been reported (47,110). The ABS suggests using three weekly fractions of 7.5 Gy each or two fractions of 10 Gy each or four fractions of 6 Gy each prescribed at 1 cm when HDR is used as the sole modality for palliation (128). These fractionation regimes have similar radiobiological equivalence using the linear quadratic model (126), and there is no evidence of superiority for one regime over the other. The benefits of fewer bronchoscopic applications should be weighed against the risks of higher dose per fraction. Additional treatments or doses higher than those suggested can

be considered for nonirradiated patients or those who have received limited radiation. When HDR is used as a planned boost to supplement palliative EBRT of 30 Gy in 10 to 12 fractions, the ABS suggests using two fractions of 7.5 Gy each or three fractions of 5 Gy each or four fractions of 4 Gy each (prescribed at 1 cm) in patients with no previous history of thoracic irradiation (128). The interval between fractions is generally 1 to 2 weeks. The brachytherapy dose should be reduced when aggressive chemotherapy is given. Concomitant chemotherapy should be avoided during brachytherapy, unless it is in the context of a clinical trial.

The results from various centers (summarized in Table 22.11) show clinical improvement from 50% to 100% and bronchoscopy response from 59% to 100% (11,13,15,16,18,34,75, 97,109,112,210,218,226,244). Comparison of these results is difficult because of the differences in patient population and the variability in dose and fractionation employed. Radiation bronchitis and stenosis may occur after endobronchial brachytherapy (214), necessitating close follow-up.

Another more serious complication is fatal hemoptysis. The hemoptysis could be a radiation therapy complication resulting from the high dose delivered to the area of the pulmonary artery, or it could represent the failure of treatment due to the progression of disease (211). Multiple courses of brachytherapy, a high previous external beam radiation dose, a left upper lobe location, or long irradiated segments increases the rate of hemoptysis (13,77). Incidence of fatal hemoptysis varies from 0% to 50% with a median value of 8% (110).

Curative Endobronchial Brachytherapy

The standard, definitive therapy for unresectable lung cancer is a combination of chemotherapy and EBRT. Select patients (i.e., those with predominantly endobronchial tumor) may benefit from endobronchial brachytherapy, either alone or as a boost to EBRT. The ideal patients for curative endobronchial radiation alone are those with occult carcinomas of the lung confined to the bronchus or trachea. Preliminary results of the few reported series are encouraging (43,163,191,227,232). See Table 22.12.

				Percentage Improved		
Author (Reference)	No. of Patients	HDR per Fraction (Gy)[a]	No. of Fractions	Symptoms	X-Ray	Bronchoscopy
Burt et al. (15)	50	15–20	1	50–86	46	88
Miller et al. (112)	88	10	3	NA	NA	80
Stout et al. (218)	100	15–20	1	50–86	46	NA
Aygun et al. (11)	62	5	3–5	NA	36	76
Bedwinek et al. (13)	38	6	3	76	64	82
Mehta et al. (109)	31	4	4+	88	71–100	85
Sutedja et al. (226)	31	10	3	82	NA	NA
Speiser and Spratling (210)	144	10	3	85–99	NA	80
	151	7.5	3			
Zajac et al. (244)	82	10–47	1–5	82	NA	74
Chang et al. (18)	76	7	3	79–95	NA	87
Macha et al. (97)	365	5	3–4	66	NA	NA
Kelly et al. (75)	175	15	1–2	66	88	78
Celebioglu et al. (16)	95	7.5–10	2–3	100	NA	100
Escobar-Sacristan et al. (34)	81	5[b]	4	85	NA	97
Totals	1,569		1–4	50%–100%	36%–100%	74%–100%

Table 22.11 | SUMMARY OF HIGH–DOSE-RATE ENDOBRONCHIAL BRACHYTHERAPY FOR PALLIATION

HDR, high–dose-rate; NA, not available
[a]Dose prescribed at 1 cm.
[b]Dose prescribed at 0.5 to 1 cm.

Table 22.12	SUMMARY OF ENDOBRONCHIAL BRACHYTHERAPY WITH OR WITHOUT EXTERNAL-BEAM RADIATION THERAPY FOR OCCULT CARCINOMAS OF THE LUNG								
Author (Reference)	No. of Patients	EBRT (Gy)	HDR per Fraction (Gy)	Prescription Depth (cm)	No. of Fractions	Total HDR (Gy)	Cause Specific Survival (%)	Mean Follow-Up (mo)	Complications
Sutedja et al. (227)	2	No	10	1	3	30	100	40	NA
Perol et al. (163)	19	No	7	1	3–5	35	78	28	NA
Furuta et al. (43)	5	40	6	0.2–1	3	18	100	30	S
Tredaniel et al. (232)	29	Yes	7	1	6	42	NA	23	1 FH, 2 MB, 3 RB

EBRT, external beam radiation therapy; FH, fatal hemoptysis; HDR, high–dose-rate; MB, massive bronchorrhea; NA, not available; RB, radiation bronchitis; S, stenosis

Endobronchial brachytherapy can be used in combination with EBRT for selected patients with inoperable non–small-cell lung carcinoma (Table 22.13) (5,11,18,22,66,109,114,180). In cases of postobstructive pneumonia or lung collapse, brachytherapy can be used to open the bronchus and aerate the lung such that the tumor volume is better defined. This allows some sparing of normal lung from the EBRT field. Muto et al. (114) performed a nonrandomized prospective study evaluating three endobronchial brachytherapy schemes concomitantly with EBRT on 320 patients with advanced inoperable non–small-cell lung cancer. Endobronchial brachytherapy consisted of either 10 Gy in one fraction, 14 Gy in two fractions, or 21 Gy in three fractions. Median survival for all patients was 11.1 months with a symptomatic response rate ranging from 82% to 94%. Complications were the least in the group of patient's receiving 21 Gy in three fractions.

Endobronchial brachytherapy with curative intent is indicated in early stage patients who are medically inoperable because of decreased pulmonary function, advanced age, or refusal of surgery. Marsiglia et al. (101) reported a survival rate of 78% with a median follow-up of 2 years in 34 patients treated with an HDR dose of 30 Gy in six fractions (5 Gy fractions given once a week).

Endobronchial brachytherapy can be used as adjuvant treatment in cases with minimal residual disease after surgical resection. Macha et al. (97) reported tumor-free survival up to 4 years in 19 patients with doses of 20 Gy delivered in four fractions at 1 cm from the source axis.

The ABS suggests an HDR dose of three 5 Gy fractions or two 7.5 Gy fractions as a boost to EBRT (either 60 Gy in 30 fractions or 45 Gy in 15 fractions) (128). The HDR dose should be prescribed at a distance of 1 cm from the central axis of the catheter and given weekly. If endobronchial brachytherapy is used alone (in previously nonirradiated patients), HDR doses of five 5-Gy fractions or three 7.5-Gy fractions prescribed to 1 cm may be used.

Cancer of the Esophagus

The results of treatment for advanced cancer of the esophagus are dismal (5-year survival is 6%); hence, treatment is essentially palliative. HDR brachytherapy can be used for the treatment of esophageal cancer either alone or in combination with EBRT (38,39,48,62,189,221–225,246). Brachytherapy is relatively simple to perform, since a single catheter is used for the treatment. A nasogastric tube or a specially designed esophageal applicator is used to deliver the treatments. The largest diameter applicator that can be inserted easily (either intraorally or intranasally) should be used to minimize the mucosal dose relative to the dose at depth. The site to be irradiated, which includes the tumor and a margin of 2 to 5 cm, can be confirmed by fluoroscopy or endoscopy. The ABS recommends an HDR dose of 10 Gy in two fractions, prescribed at 1 cm from the source, to boost 50 Gy EBRT (48). HDR brachytherapy can be given before, concurrently with, or after EBRT. The advantage of giving brachytherapy after EBRT is that a more uniform dose can be delivered to the residual tumor after it has been reduced by EBRT. Brachytherapy given initially provides rapid relief of dysphagia. HDR brachytherapy at doses of 16 Gy in two fractions or 18 Gy in three fractions have been used without additional EBRT to palliate esophageal cancers (222,224).

A few randomized studies have evaluated esophageal HDR brachytherapy and are summarized in Table 22.14. Zhao et al. (246) from Shanxi Cancer Hospital, have shown in a

Table 22.13	SUMMARY OF ENDOBRONCHIAL HIGH–DOSE-RATE BRACHYTHERAPY WITH SUPPLEMENTARY EXTERNAL-BEAM RADIATION THERAPY FOR CURATIVE THERAPY IN LOCALLY ADVANCED LUNG CANCER						
Author (Reference)	No. of Patients	EBRT (Gy)	Dose per Fraction/ Depth (Gy/cm)	No. of Fractions	Total HDR (Gy)	Median Survival (mo)	Complications
Reddi and Marbach (180)	32	60	7.5/1	3	22.5	8	NA
Aygun et al. (11)	62	50–60	5.0/1	3–5	15.0–25.0	13	9 FH, S
Mehta et al. (109)	22	60	4.0/2	2	16.0	8.5	NA
Chang et al. (18)	54	20–70	7.0/1	3	21.0	NA	2 FH
Cotter et al. (22)	65	55–66	2.7–10.0/1	2–4	6.0–35.0	8	9 N, 4 S, 1 FH, 3 TEF
Huber et al. (66)	56	60	4.8/1	2	9.6	10	11 FH
Muto et al. (114)	84		10.0/1	1	10		
	47	60	7.0/1	2	14	11.1	10 FH, 3 BEF, 51 S
	50		5.0/1	3	15		
	139		5.0/0.5	3	15		
Anacak et al. (5)	30	60	5/1	3	15	11	6 S, 2 FH

BEF, bronchoesophageal fistula; EBRT, external beam radiation therapy; FH, fatal hemoptysis; HDR, high–dose-rate; N, necrosis; NA, not available; S, stenosis; TEF, tracheoesophageal fistula

| Table 22.14 | SUMMARY OF ESOPHAGEAL HIGH–DOSE-RATE BRACHYTHERAPY |

Author (Reference)	No. of Patients	EBRT Dose (Gy)	No. of HDR Fractions	HDR per Fraction (Gy)	Relief of Dysphagia at 6 Months (%)	Relief of Dysphagia at 1 Year (%)	Survival at 1 Year
Definitive							
Zhao et al. (246)	100	70	—	—	—	—	56%
Zhao et al. (246)	100	50	3–4	6.54	—	—	78%
Sur et al. (225)	25	55	—	—	53.5	37.5	44%
	25	35	2	6	90.5	70.6	78%
Palliation							
Sur et al. (223)	25	35	—	—	12.5	—	16%
	25	35	2	6	84.2	58.3	69%
Sur et al. (224)	112	—	3	6	~75	~75	~25%
	120	—	2	8	~75	~60	~25%
Sur et al. (221)	30	—	2	8	>50	—	7.2 months[a]
	30	30	2	8	>50%	—	7.5 months[a]

EBRT, external beam radiation therapy; HDR, high–dose-rate
[a]Median survival.

randomized trial that results of EBRT combined with brachytherapy were better than those of EBRT alone in cancer of the esophagus. One hundred patients were treated in the EBRT-alone arm and given 70 Gy in 35 fractions over a period of 7 weeks. One hundred patients in the second arm received EBRT of 50 Gy in 25 fractions followed by HDR brachytherapy of 6.54 Gy per week for three or four applications using cesium 137 (^{137}Cs). EBRT combined with brachytherapy gave survival results of 78%, 31%, and 17% at 1, 3, and 5 years respectively, compared to 56%, 19%, and 10% for EBRT alone in the same time frames. The improvements were statistically significant for 1- and 3-year survival data, but not for 5-year survival data.

In 1992 Sur et al. (225) reported a randomized trial of 50 patients with squamous cell carcinoma of the esophagus. The group receiving EBRT alone (55 Gy in 25 treatments) had a 12-month survival of 44% compared to 78% in the group receiving 35 Gy EBRT followed by HDR brachytherapy of 12 Gy in two fractions. There was a statistical improvement in the relief of dysphagia with the addition of HDR brachytherapy at 3 months (60% vs. 87.5%) and at 6 months (53.5% vs. 90.5%).

Sur et al. (223) reported another randomized trial of 50 patients with squamous cell carcinoma of the esophagus, again comparing EBRT alone versus EBRT plus HDR brachytherapy; however, in this trial the EBRT dose was 35 Gy in 15 treatments in both arms. The group receiving EBRT alone had a 12 month survival of 16% compared to 69% in the group receiving 35 Gy EBRT followed by 12 Gy in two fractions of HDR brachytherapy. There was a statistical improvement in the relief of dysphagia with the addition of HDR brachytherapy at 3 months (24% vs. 82%), and at 6 months (13% vs. 84%).

A multicenter, prospective randomized study conducted under the auspices of the International Atomic Energy Agency (IAEA) evaluated two HDR regimens in 232 patients (224). Patients were randomized to receive 18 Gy in three fractions/alternate days (Group [Gr] A—112 patients) or 16 Gy in two fractions/alternate days (Gr B—120 patients). The HDR dose was prescribed at 1 cm from the center of the source axis. The dysphagia-free survival for the whole group was 7.1 months (Gr A = 7.8 months, Gr B = 6.3 months; p >0.05). The overall survival was 7.9 months for the whole group (Gr A = 9.1 months, Gr B = 6.9 months; p >0.05). The incidence of strictures (Gr A = 12, Gr B = 13; p >0.05) and fistulae (Gr A = 11, Gr B = 12; p >0.05) was similar in both groups. The authors concluded that dose fractions of 6 Gy × 3 and 8 Gy × 2 within 1 week gave similar results for dysphagia-free survival, overall survival, and incidence of strictures and fistulae.

Sur et al. (221) recently reported on a randomized trial of 60 patients comparing HDR brachytherapy alone versus HDR brachytherapy plus EBRT for palliative treatment of advanced esophageal cancer. All patients received 16 Gy in two fractions over a 3-day period and then randomized to observation (Group A) versus EBRT (Group B) of 30 Gy in 10 fractions. At 12 months there was no difference in dysphagia-free survival or overall survival for the two groups. In addition the incidence of strictures (Group A = 7, Group B = 4; p >0.05) and fistulas (Group A = 3, Group B = 1; p >0.05) was similar in both groups.

Hishikawa et al. (62), in a nonrandomized trial, found that patients treated with EBRT plus HDR brachytherapy had better survival than those treated with EBRT alone (28% 2-year survival compared to 4%). The local control rate was also higher (63% vs. 20%). The high dose delivered to the esophageal mucosa resulted in a high incidence of esophageal ulcers, fistulae, and strictures.

In summary, retrospective studies as well as prospective, randomized clinical trials show that there is improved local control and survival when HDR brachytherapy is added to EBRT and that HDR brachytherapy alone can be used for palliation of advanced esophageal cancers. Since a high dose is delivered to the esophageal mucosa, side effects may include ulcerations, fistulae, and esophageal strictures.

Carcinoma of the Prostate

Currently, permanent implantation of iodine 125 (^{125}I) or palladium 103 (^{103}Pd) seeds is the most common type of prostate brachytherapy. However, several centers have used HDR brachytherapy as a boost to EBRT (10,26,27,44,45,65,70,103, 106,107,215) for the treatment of prostate cancer with encouraging results (Table 22.15). Galalae et al. (45) reported the results of 611 patients (some of which are included in Table 22.15) treated at three institutions (Kiel, Germany; William Beaumont Hospital; Seattle Prostate Institute) with EBRT and HDR brachytherapy for localized prostate cancer. Different fractionation schemes were used as seen in Table 22.15. Five-year biochemical control for low-risk, intermediate-risk, and high-risk patients was 96%, 88%, and 69%, respectively. One of the major advantages of HDR is that the dose distribution can be intraoperatively optimized by varying the dwell times at various dwell positions (33), potentially allowing reliable and reproducible delivery of the prescribed dose to the target volume while keeping the doses to normal structures (i.e., rectum, bladder, and urethra), within acceptable limits. Another potential

Table 22.15	RESULTS OF TREATMENT WITH INTERSTITIAL HIGH–DOSE-RATE BRACHYTHERAPY AS A BOOST TO EXTERNAL-BEAM RADIATION THERAPY FOR PROSTATE CANCER				
Author (Reference)	No. of Patients	EBRT Dose (Gy)	HDR (Gy × Fractions)	5-Year % bNED	% Complications Grade 3 (GU/GI)
Astrom et al. (10)	214	50	10 × 2	92 (low risk) 87 (int. risk) 56 (high risk)	10/0
Demanes et al. (27)	209	36	5.5–6 × 4	90 (low risk)[a] 87 (int. risk)[a] 69 (high risk)[a]	6.7/0
Deger et al. (26)	442	40–50.4	9–10 × 2	81 (low risk) 65 (int. risk) 59 (high risk)	11
Hsu et al. (65)	64	45	6 × 3	93.8[b]	0/1.6
Jo et al. (70)	98	36.8–45	5.5–6 × 3–4	92.9	8.1/0
Stevens et al. (215)	82	45	5.5 × 3	91[c]	6/1
Martinez et al. (103)	149 58	46	8.25–11.5 × 2 5.5–6.5 × 3	87 52	8/1
Galalae et al. (44)	144	40–50	15 × 2	72.9[d]	2.3/4.1
Eulau (35) Mate et al. (107)	104	50.4	3–4 × 4	91 (PSA <10)[a] 65 (PSA 10–20)[a] 59 (PSA ≥20)[a]	8.7/2

bNED, biologically without evidence of recurrence; EBRT, external beam radiation therapy; GU/GI, genitourinary/gastrointestinal; HDR, high–dose-rate; Int, Intermediate; NS, not stated; PSA, prostate-specific antigen
[a]Ten-year bNED.
[b]Median follow-up of 50 months.
[c]Three-year bNED.
[d]Eight-year bNED.

advantage of HDR brachytherapy in prostate cancer is the theoretical consideration that prostate cancer cells behave more like late-reacting tissue with a low α/β ratio and they should, therefore, respond more favorably to higher-dose fractions rather than to the lower-dose rate delivered in LDR brachytherapy (32,41).

Patients with stages T1b to T3b prostate cancers without evidence of distant metastases are candidates for HDR brachytherapy as a boost to EBRT. Patients with distant metastases, a life expectancy of <5 years, or those who are medically unfit for anesthesia or in whom it is technically not feasible to implant the entire prostate should be excluded. Relative contraindications include large gland size (>80 cc), recent transurethral resection of the prostate (TURP) within the last 6 months or large TURP defects, all of which increase the risk of urinary morbidity.

Standard fractionation EBRT (39.6 to 50.4 Gy) is given before, concurrently with, or after HDR brachytherapy. The minimum volume treated should include the entire prostate and seminal vesicles with a margin, with or without pelvic lymph nodes. The HDR dose is given in multiple fractions in one or two implant procedures. A variety of dose and fractionation schemes may be appropriate for same-stage disease as shown in Table 22.16 (10,44,103,106,107). The HDR fractions are generally given twice a day with a minimum of 6 hours between fractions. The most commonly encountered acute genitourinary (GU) morbidities include urinary irritative symptoms, hematuria, hematospermia, and/or urinary retention, similar to LDR permanent implants.

HDR brachytherapy is also being used as monotherapy in a few centers, but long-term results are still forthcoming (Table 22.17) (52,102,186,242). HDR doses of 38 Gy delivered in four fractions, two times daily over 2 days or 54 Gy in nine fractions given twice a day over 5 days have been reported (52,104,241,242). Grills et al. (52) compared 149 patients with localized prostate cancer treated with interstitial HDR brachytherapy versus permanent implant in a retrospective analysis. HDR brachytherapy was delivered in four fractions for a total dose of 38 Gy. Biochemical evidence of no disease at 3 years was 98% and 97% for HDR and permanent implant, respectively. In those patients treated with HDR, they

Table 22.16	DOSE FRACTIONATION AND ISOEFFECTIVE DOSES (AS IF GIVEN AT 2 GY/FRACTION) OF COMMON COMBINED EXTERNAL-BEAM RADIATION THERAPY AND HIGH–DOSE-RATE BRACHYTHERAPY DOSES USED FOR PROSTATE CANCER					
EBRT Dose (Gy)	Total HDR (Gy)	HDR per Fraction (Gy)	No. of HDR Fractions	Isoeffective Dose (Gy) ($\alpha/\beta = 1.5$)	Isoeffective Dose (Gy) ($\alpha/\beta = 5$)	Isoeffective Dose (Gy) ($\alpha/\beta = 10$)
39.6	22	5.5	4	81	72	67
45	18	6	3	81	72	68
39.6	26	6.5	4	97	81	75
50.4	19.5	6.5	3	92	81	76
46	19	9.5	2	106	85	77

EBRT, external beam radiation therapy; HDR, high–dose-rate

Table 22.17 **RESULTS OF TREATMENT WITH INTERSTITIAL HIGH–DOSE-RATE BRACHYTHERAPY AS MONOTHERAPY FOR PROSTATE CANCER**

Author (Reference)	No. of Patients	T Stage	HDR (Gy × Fractions)	Total HDR (Gy)	3 Year % bNED	% Late Complications Grade 3 (GU/GI)
Grills et al. (52)	84	1–2	9.5 × 4	38	98	3/0
Martin et al. (102)	52	1–2	9.5 × 4	38	NS	3.8/0 (acute)
Rodriguez et al. (186)	35	1–2	6.75–7 × 6	40.5–42	97	0/0
Yoshioka et al. (242)	43	1–4	6 × 9	54	55	0/0

bNED, biologically without evidence of recurrence; GU/GI, genitourinary/gastrointestinal; HDR, high dose rate; NS, not stated

noted statistically significant decreased rates of acute Radiation Therapy Oncology Group (RTOG) grade 1 to 3 dysuria, urinary frequency/urgency, and rectal pain, as well as chronic urinary frequency. There was no difference in chronic dysuria, urinary incontinence, retention, or hematuria between the two groups. The 3-year impotence rate was less for patients treated with HDR (16% vs. 45%). Urinary stricture rates were higher in patients treated with HDR; however, this was not statistically significant. Rodriguez et al. (186) reported preliminary results of 35 patients with low- to intermediate-risk prostate cancer treated with HDR monotherapy delivering six fractions of 6.75 to 7 Gy per fraction. Three-year prostate specific antigen (PSA) progression-free survival was 97% with no chronic RTOG grade 3 or 4 lower gastrointestinal (GI) or GU morbidity.

Neihoff et al. (153) have recently reported their results of using HDR brachytherapy along with EBRT as salvage treatment for local recurrences after radical prostatectomy. Thirty-five patients were treated with either 30 or 40 Gy EBRT plus a HDR brachytherapy dose of 15 Gy in two fractions. Thirty-four patients had a decrease in PSA and at a mean follow-up of 27 months 91% were alive. Mean duration of biochemical nonevidence of disease was 12 months, and there were no reported RTOG grade III or IV side effects.

HDR brachytherapy as a boost to EBRT for localized prostate cancer has been well defined and is being used more commonly. Its use as monotherapy is emerging, and initial results are promising. For recurrent disease after radical prostatectomy, further studies are needed to more clearly define the role of HDR brachytherapy.

Biliary Cancers

Tumors of the bile duct are often unresectable and are treated palliatively by biliary drainage and EBRT. The biliary drainage tube can be accessed to provide brachytherapy to the area of obstruction either by LDR, ^{192}Ir brachytherapy (61,141) or by HDR brachytherapy (93,154,193,200,233) alone or in combination with EBRT. Although brachytherapy is commonly delivered through a transhepatic cholangiogram catheter (55), it has also been delivered using an endoscopic retrograde technique (233). A size 12-Fr biliary drainage catheter is required to accommodate a 6-Fr HDR brachytherapy catheter. Therefore, the in-dwelling biliary drainage catheter is upsized to a size 12-Fr biliary drainage catheter, if required. Under fluoroscopy, the brachytherapy catheter is inserted into the biliary drainage catheter and advanced past the area of obstruction. A Tuohy-Borst (Y-shaped) adapter attached to the end of the biliary catheter allows concurrent external biliary drainage while holding the HDR catheter in place. The area of the obstruction is irradiated along with 1- to 2-cm proximal and distal margins. The dose per fraction delivered is variable, but about 5 Gy per fraction at a distance of 1 cm from the source is commonly used for three or four fractions (15 to 20 Gy total) to boost 45 Gy EBRT (154). If EBRT is not delivered, a palliative dose of 30 Gy

in six fractions can be used (154). Concurrent chemotherapy (5-FU) is often added. It is important to leave the biliary drainage catheter in place after therapy to minimize biliary stricture.

Head and Neck Cancers

Brachytherapy, especially using manually afterloaded ^{192}Ir, has been widely used to treat head and neck cancers. HDR brachytherapy has been used in selected cases to reduce radiation exposure and permit optimization as summarized in Table 22.18 (28,30,53,67,87,89,94,129,143,147,150,155,243). However, these advantages are offset by the need for multiple fractionation since the head and neck area does not tolerate high doses per fraction. The nasopharynx is a site within the head and neck area that is easily accessed by an intracavitary HDR applicator (46,90). Doses of 18 Gy in six fractions are delivered by a special nasopharynx applicator to boost 46 to 60 Gy of EBRT (90).

The use of HDR brachytherapy catheters incorporated in removable dental molds allows repeated, highly reproducible, fractionated outpatient brachytherapy of superficial (<0.5-cm thick) tumors without requiring repeated catheter insertion into the tumor (71). Suitable sites for mold therapy include the scalp, face, pinna, lip, buccal mucosa, maxillary antrum, hard palate, oral cavity, external auditory canal, and the orbital cavity after exenteration. HDR can be used as the sole modality or in conjunction with EBRT. A total HDR dose equivalent to about 60 Gy LDR (prescribed at 0.5-cm depth) is recommended when used as the sole modality (147). The HDR can also be used as a boost to 45 to 50 Gy EBRT, in which case the HDR doses are appropriately reduced to LDR equivalent doses of 15 to 30 Gy. The actual HDR dose per fraction and number of fractions can be varied to suit individual situations (including site and treatment volume). Biomathematical (LQ) modeling can be used to assist in the conversion of LDR to HDR (126).

Another innovative approach is the use of intraoperative HDR brachytherapy, which permits normal tissues to be retracted or shielded during brachytherapy. Intraoperative HDR brachytherapy can reach many sites in the head and neck area that are difficult to treat or are inaccessible by either LDR brachytherapy or intraoperative electron beam radiation. The catheters are removed immediately after the single dose of radiation, hence, minimizing inconvenience and permitting the use of brachytherapy in areas such as the base of skull (139,143). Doses of 7.5 to 15 Gy are given when EBRT of 45 to 50 Gy can be added. In recurrent tumors where no further EBRT can be given, a single intraoperative dose of 15 to 20 Gy can be given (129,143).

Soft Tissue Sarcomas

Excellent results are obtained with a combination of wide excision of the tumor and adjuvant EBRT. However, irradiation of large volumes after surgery gives rise to morbidity, especially

Table 22.18	HIGH–DOSE-RATE BRACHYTHERAPY FOR HEAD AND NECK CANCERS						
Author (Reference)	Site	EBRT Dose (Gy)	HDR per Fraction (Gy)	No. of Fractions	Isoeffective Dose (Gy)[a]	No. of Patients	5-Year Local Control (%)
Donath et al. (30)	Various	0	4.5–5	10	54–63	13	77[b]
Lau et al. (87)	Tongue	0	6.5	7	63	27	53
Dixit et al. (28)	Various	0	3	20	65	3	—
Inoue et al. (67)	Tongue	0	6	10	80	25	87
Leung et al. (89)	Tongue	0	4.5–6.3	10	54–86	19	95[c]
Guinot et al. (53)	Lip	0	4.5–5.5	8–10	54–57	39[d]	88[e]
Yu et al. (243)	Various	50	2.7	6	67	12	79[f]
Dixit et al. (28)	Various	40–48	3	7	63–71	18	80[g]
Nag et al. (143)	Sinus	45–50	10–12.5	1	66–68	27	65
		45–63	15–20	1	94–95	7	
Lu et al. (94)	Nasopharynx	66	5	2	79	33	94[e]
Nose et al. (155)	Oropharynx	0	6	8–9	64–72	14	82
		14.4–66.6	6	3–6	62–90	68	
Ng et al. (150)	Nasopharynx	43.2–70.4	2.5–3	2–7	65–79	38	96
Nag et al. (129)	Various	45–50	7.5–20	1	61–95	65	59

EBRT, external beam radiation therapy; HDR, high–dose-rate.
[a]Isoeffective dose for tumor effects as if given at 2 Gy/day using the linear quadratic model with an α/β ratio of 10.
[b]Median follow-up of 9 months.
[c]Four-year local control.
[d]One patient received 50 Gy EBRT with 3.5 Gy × 6 HDR.
[e]Three-year local control.
[f]Two-year local control.
[g]Median follow-up of 14 months.

normal tissue fibrosis. To minimize morbidity, a few centers have used LDR brachytherapy, either alone (58) or with EBRT (195). A prospective randomized trial showed superior local control (80% at 5 years) in the group receiving brachytherapy versus 62% in the group not receiving brachytherapy (58). The major problem with LDR brachytherapy of large volumes is the radiation exposure involved. Hence, a few centers are investigating the use of HDR brachytherapy for soft tissue sarcomas (2,24,29,81,190,240). HDR brachytherapy catheters are implanted along the tumor bed and radio-opaque clips indicate the margins. A 2- to 5-cm margin proximally and distally is used after gross excision of tumor. Optimized treatment planning can be used to deliver a more homogeneous dose. Doses of 40 to 50 Gy are given in 12 to 15 fractions if the HDR is given alone (2,29). If EBRT (45 to 50 Gy) is added, the brachytherapy dose is limited to 18 to 25 Gy in four to seven fractions (137). It is important to delay the start of brachytherapy for about 4 to 7 days after surgery to allow for wound healing (140). Nerve tolerance to high-dose per fraction is poor, and HDR should be used with caution when catheters have to be placed in contact with neurovascular structures. The ABS suggests the following interventions to minimize morbidity in soft tissue sarcomas (140):

1. When brachytherapy is used as adjuvant monotherapy, the source loading should start no sooner than 5 to 6 days after wound closure. However, the radioactive sources may be loaded earlier (as soon as 2 to 3 days after surgery) if doses of <20 Gy are given with brachytherapy as a supplement to EBRT.
2. Minimize dose to normal tissues (e.g., gonads, breasts, thyroid, skin) whenever possible, especially in children and patients of childbearing age.
3. Limit the allowable skin dose—the 40 Gy isodose line (LDR) to <25 cm² and the 25 Gy isodose line to <100 cm².

Outcome of nonrandomized studies using HDR doses in the range of 2 to 9 Gy per fraction given once or twice daily or single fraction intraoperative HDR brachytherapy are outlined in Table 22.19 (2,20,24,29,81,82,165,179,190,240).

Pediatric Tumors

LDR brachytherapy has been used in children to reduce the deleterious effects of EBRT (37,40,49). However, LDR brachytherapy is difficult to perform in young children and infants because they require prolonged sedation and immobilization with close monitoring, which increases the risk of radiation exposure to nursing staff and parents. HDR is therefore very appealing in infants and younger children and has undergone trials at Ohio State University (123,124,133,142,145). The recommended dose for HDR as monotherapy is 36 Gy in 12 fractions given at 3 Gy per fraction (prescribed at 0.5 cm) twice a day (123,140,142). The interval between fractions is at least 6 hours. There are no published data giving any dose recommendations for HDR as boost to EBRT. The linear-quadratic model (126) can be used to calculate a fractionation scheme equivalent to that of an LDR implant boost dose of 15 to 25 Gy (prescribed at 0.5 cm). The recommended dose for intraoperative HDR brachytherapy as a boost to EBRT is 10 to 15 Gy (prescribed at 0.5 cm), depending on the extent of residual disease (111,144,177,196,245). According to the Inter-group Rhabdomyosarcoma Study (IRS) the standard EBRT dose for pediatric soft tissue sarcomas is 40 Gy for microscopic disease and 50 Gy for gross disease. Intraoperative HDR allows reduction in the dose of EBRT to 27 to 30 Gy so that concerns for impaired growth and organ function is greatly reduced (123,132,144). The results of HDR brachytherapy in the treatment of pediatric tumors are summarized in Table 22.20 (50,105,144–146,149,196). Although the long-term morbidity of HDR brachytherapy in young children is not fully known, one may expect preservation of organ functions similar to that seen with LDR brachytherapy (37). Due to the complexities involved in pediatric HDR brachytherapy, it is recommended that

Table 22.19 OUTCOME OF NONRANDOMIZED STUDIES OF HIGH–DOSE-RATE BRACHYTHERAPY USED FOR PRIMARY SOFT TISSUE SARCOMAS

Author (Reference)	No. of Patients	Median Follow-Up (mo)	Local Control (%)	Complications (%)
Donath et al. (29)	19	12	70	16
Alekhteyar et al. (2)	13	16	77	NS
Ryan et al. (190)	32	50	82	48
Yoshida et al. (240)	13	24	72	8
Crownover et al. (24)	10	12	100	0
Koizumi et al. (81)	16	30	50	6
Chun et al. (20)	11	31	100	9
Rachbauer et al. (179)[a]	39	26	100	28
Petera et al. (165)	10	20	100	20
Kretzler et al. (82)[a]	11	51[b]	91	—

HDR, high dose rate; NS, not stated
[a]Intraoperative single fraction HDR.
[b]Mean follow-up.

the use of HDR brachytherapy in pediatric tumors be limited to centers that have experience with pediatric implants (140).

Breast

EBRT is the standard radiation modality used after lumpectomy in the conservative management of breast cancer. Recently there has been interest in using brachytherapy as the sole modality of treatment (86,171,197,219) to decrease the 6-week treatment duration required for a course of EBRT to about 5 days. Table 22.21 lists the patients in whom an accelerated (4 to 5 days) brachytherapy treatment course can be an attractive alternative to 6 weeks of EBRT (130). The ABS recommends a total dose of 34 Gy in 10 fractions to the CTV when HDR brachytherapy is used as the sole modality (130). The HDR treatments of 3.4 Gy are generally given at two fractions per day separated by at least 6 hours. This was also the dose used in a phase II RTOG trial (85). The results of HDR brachytherapy as the sole modality are included in Table 22.22 (14,21,74,79,86,161,162,170–172,219,235,238). Depending on the selection criteria, final pathologic assessment is necessary to completely evaluate a patient for partial breast brachytherapy, and, therefore, the ABS does not advocate intraoperative treatment delivery at this time (9). The use of a single channel MammoSite applicator has simplified the brachytherapy procedure (197). Keisch et al. (74) reported a good to excellent cosmetic result of 84% and no local recurrences at a median follow-up of 29 months in 43 patients treated with the MammoSite applicator (Cytyc Corporation, Marlborough, MA). In addition, a multi-institutional registry trial performed by the American Society of Breast Surgeons

to evaluate the clinical use of the MammoSite applicator recently reported an early first analysis of a good to excellent cosmetic result of 95% (1,030 of 1,084 patients) and one local recurrence at a median follow-up of 5 months in 1,237 patients (235).

In March 2005 the RTOG, in conjunction with the National Surgical Adjuvant Breast and Bowel Project (NSABP), opened a phase III randomized study (NSABP B-39) investigating standard whole breast radiotherapy versus partial breast radiotherapy after lumpectomy for women with early stage breast cancer. The partial breast treatment arm consists of three therapeutic options which are intensity-modulated radiation therapy (IMRT), HDR brachytherapy via MammoSite, and HDR brachytherapy via a multicatheter interstitial implant. The required dose for the brachytherapy treatment is 34 Gy given in 10 fractions over 5 days. Target accrual is 3,000 patients over 29 months, and it is hoped that over time the data will shed some light on the usefulness of partial breast irradiation and brachytherapy as a sole modality of treatment. Further clinical studies are required to define the most appropriate candidates for breast brachytherapy as a sole modality treatment and to determine the best delivery method of brachytherapy (multicatheter interstitial implant vs. balloon brachytherapy) in such patients.

Brachytherapy has been used to boost the EBRT dose in select high-risk patients (100,173,187). Data on the use of HDR as a boost are limited (see Table 22.22) (59,100,169,181). Polgar et al. (169) reported the results of a randomized trial involving 207 women with stage I or II breast cancer treated with breast-conserving surgery and whole breast radiotherapy and subsequently randomized to either no further therapy or radiation

Table 22.20 RESULTS OF HIGH–DOSE-RATE BRACHYTHERAPY USED FOR TREATMENT OF PEDIATRIC TUMORS

Author (Reference)	No. of Patients	Brachytherapy	HDR (Gy)	EBRT Dose (Gy)	Median Follow-Up (mo)	Local Control (%)	Late Toxicity (%)
Nag et al. (145)	15	F-HDR	36 (3 Gy ×12)	0	120	80	20
Martinez-Monge et al. (105)	5	F-HDR	24 (4 Gy × 6)	27–45	27	100	0
Nakamura et al. (149)	16	F-HDR	10 (5 Gy × 2)	45–55	54	94	—
Schuck et al. (196)	20	IOHDR	10	45–55	24	65	40 (postop)
Nag et al. (144)	13	IOHDR	10–15	27–30	47	95	23
Goodman et al. (50)	66	IOHDR	4–15	0–56	12	56	12
Nag et al. (146)	13	IOERT	10–15	0–50.4	42	72	31

EBRT, external beam radiation therapy; F-HDR, fractionated high dose rate (given twice a day); IOERT, intraoperative electron beam radiation therapy; IOHDR, intraoperative high dose rate

Table 22.21	BRACHYTHERAPY IN THE CONSERVATIVE MANAGEMENT OF BREAST CANCER

Indications for Brachytherapy as the Sole Modality	Selection Criteria for Brachytherapy as the Sole Modality	Indications for Brachytherapy as a Boost to EBRT
1. The patient lives a long distance from radiation oncology treatment facilities.	1. All patients should be appropriate candidates for standard breast conservation therapy	1. For patients with close, positive, or unknown margins
2. The patient lacks transportation.	2. Unifocal, invasive ductal carcinoma	2. For patients with EIC
3. The patient is a professional whose schedule will not accommodate a 6-week course of therapy.	3. <3 cm in size	3. For younger patients
4. The patient is elderly, frail, or in poor health and therefore unable to travel for a prolonged course of daily treatment.	4. Negative microscopic surgical margins of excision	4. For deep tumor location in a large breast
5. The patient's breasts are sufficiently large that they may have unacceptable toxicity with EBRT.	5. Axillary node negative by level I/II axillary dissection or sentinel node evaluation	5. For CTV of irregular thickness

CTV, clinical target volume; EBRT, external beam radiation therapy; EIC, extensive intraductal component

boost to the tumor bed. The radiation boost consisted of either 16 Gy of electron irradiation or 12 to 14.5 Gy fractionated HDR brachytherapy. Fifty-two patients were treated with HDR brachytherapy and the 5-year local tumor control rate was 91.4%. Excellent to good cosmesis was reported in 88.5% of patients. Similar results were noted in the group of patients receiving an electron irradiation boost. Because brachytherapy is an invasive procedure, it should be used selectively as a boosting technique. Situations in which brachytherapy may be advantageous as a boost are listed in Table 22.21. The brachytherapy boost can be given before or after EBRT, usually with a 1-to 2-week gap between EBRT and brachytherapy. The ABS recommends a dose fractionation scheme that yields early and late

effects approximately equivalent to those of 10 to 20 Gy LDR following 45 to 50 Gy EBRT (130). Biomathematical models are often used to estimate equivalent HDR regimens (12,126). For example, an HDR regimen of five fractions of 310 cGy per fraction should approximate the early and late effects of 20 Gy LDR delivered at 0.5 Gy/h. Although biomathematical models can be used to estimate the appropriate dose, there is no standardized HDR fractionation schedule that can be recommended for the use of HDR as a boost. Controlled clinical studies are required to further define the most appropriate doses to be used for boost treatment.

Use of interstitial HDR brachytherapy as neoadjuvant treatment in select patients not amenable to breast conserving

Table 22.22	RESULTS OF BREAST-CONSERVING THERAPY WITH LUMPECTOMY PLUS HIGH–DOSE-RATE BRACHYTHERAPY OR AS A BOOST TO EXTERNAL-BEAM RADIATION THERAPY

Author (Reference)	No. of Patients	HDR (Gy × Fractions)	Total Dose (Gy)	Median Follow-Up (mo)	Local Recurrence (%)	Good/Excellent Cosmetic Results (%)
HDR Alone						
Clarke et al. (21)	45	10 × 2	20	18	8.8	95
		7 × 4	28			
		6 × 6	36			
Perera et al. (161,162)	39	3.72 × 10	37.2	20	2.6	Not stated
Kuske et al. (79,86)	26	4 × 8	32	75	2[a]	67[b]
Polgar et al. (172)	46	5.2 × 7	36.4	30	0	Not stated
Polgar et al. (171)	37	5.2 × 7	36.4	81	6.7	84.4
	8	4.33 × 7	30.3			
Wazer et al. (238)	32	3.4 × 10	34	33	3	88
Benitez et al. (14)	79	4 × 8	32	45.6	1.5	95–99[c]
		3.4 × 10	34			
Strnad et al. (219)	176	4 × 8	32	12	0	93.7 (doctor's opinion)
		PDR 0.6 Gy	49.8			91.6 (patient's opinion)
Keisch et al. (74)[d]	43	3.4 × 10	34	29	0	84
Vicini et al. (235)[d]	1237	3.4 × 10	34	5	0.1	95
HDR Boost						
Hennequin et al. (59)	106	5 × 2	55	45	5.1	63
Manning et al. (100)	18	2.5 × 6	65	50	0	68
Polgar et al. (169)	19	4 × 3	12	63.6	7.7	88.5
	33	4.75 × 3	14.25			
Resch et al. (181)	274	7–12 × 1	7–12	104 (Mean)	1.5	38

EBRT, external beam radiation therapy; HDR, high–dose-rate; LDR, low–dose-rate; PDR, pulsed–dose-rate.
[a]Percentage of local recurrence of 51 patients treated either by LDR or HDR.
[b]Twenty months' follow-up.
[c]Includes patients treated with LDR.
[d]HDR via MammoSite.

Techniques, Modalities, and Modifiers in Radiation Oncology

surgery at presentation has recently been reported by Roddiger et al. (184). Fifty-three patients who were unable to undergo breast conserving surgery either because of initial tumor size or an unfavorable breast–tumor ratio were treated with systemic chemotherapy and HDR brachytherapy with 5 Gy twice per day for 3 days (total dose 30 Gy). Of these patients 56.6% went on to receive breast conserving surgery, and with a median follow-up of 56 months the local recurrence rate was 2%. Further studies are needed to fully define the roll of interstitial HDR brachytherapy as neoadjuvant treatment, but these results are encouraging.

Skin Cancer

The widespread availability of HDR remote afterloading brachytherapy units allows the use of surface molds as an alternative to electron beam and for cases where surface irregularity, proximity to bone, or poor intrinsic tolerance of tissues do not allow for satisfactory treatment by electron beam. For most cases, a satisfactory mold can be made from 5-mm thick sheets of wax with the HDR catheters spaced 1-cm apart. A simpler alternative is to use commercially available surface template applicators (e.g., Freiburg flab from Nucletron Corp, Columbia, MD and HAM applicator from Mick Radionuclear Instruments Inc, Bronx, NY) that are used for intraoperative HDR brachytherapy (54,125,228).

There is a wide range of recommended doses and fractionation schemes for treating skin cancer. Doses in the range of 3,500 cGy in five fractions to 5,000 cGy in 10 fractions have been used with success in HDR molds. Standard, more prolonged fractionation schemes with 180 to 200 cGy daily or twice daily fractions can also be used. The linear quadratic radiobiological model can be used to determine the total dose for a given fractionation scheme (12,126)

Intraoperative High–Dose-Rate Brachytherapy

Intraoperative high–dose-rate brachytherapy (IOHDR) is an extreme example of reduced fractionation in that only a single HDR brachytherapy dose is applied (31,95,125,131,134). This results in an inherent radiobiological disadvantage since the advantages of fractionation (repair of normal tissue damage, reoxygenation of hypoxic tumor cells, and movement of tumor cells from the radioresistant S phase to the more radiosensi-

tive mitotic phase of the cell cycle) are lost. LQ model calculations show that there has to be a dose reduction of 20% to 25% to the late reacting normal tissues for isoeffect. However, the dose reduction achieved by 1- to 4-cm displacement of normal tissue is much more (closer to 60% to 90% reduction) (134). Hence, HDR in these situations becomes advantageous. However, if such a dose reduction cannot be achieved in normal tissues, HDR brachytherapy becomes disadvantageous. Intraoperative HDR brachytherapy also has the advantage that normal tissues can be displaced and/or partially shielded during irradiation.

In IOHDR, the surgery is performed in a shielded operating room with remote anesthesia and a video monitoring system. Maximum surgical debulking is attempted whenever possible. Then the tumor bed is irradiated using special intraoperative applicators containing HDR catheters that are 1-cm apart and parallel to each other. The use of a fixed geometry applicator allows the patient to be treated without delay using preplanned dosimetry for the selected applicator. Normal tissues are either retracted from the high-dose area or shielded. Doses of 10 to 20 Gy are usually given as a single fraction over 10 to 30 minutes (131). The advantages of IOHDR brachytherapy over perioperative brachytherapy or electron beam intraoperative radiation therapy (IORT) are listed in Table 22.23. Unfortunately, the relative scarcity of shielded operating rooms has currently limited its availability to just a few centers (31,95,111,125,127,131,245).

Reduction of Brachytherapy Errors

The International Commission on Radiological Protection (ICRP) (69) released Publication 97 in November 2005 which outlines quality assurance (QA) procedures necessary to prevent accidents with HDR brachytherapy. The ICRP gave general and specific recommendations for HDR brachytherapy programs which are summarized in Tables 22.24 and 22.25. The general recommendations include establishing a written comprehensive QA program, formation of a hospital radiation safety committee, external auditing of procedures, peer reviewing of each case, and reporting of every incident or accident. The specific recommendations cover a broad range of topics. Training in HDR brachytherapy should commence prior to acquisition of machines, follow a team approach, and should be sequential in the introduction of techniques with simpler techniques first followed by more complex treatments. For example, multiple plane flexible implants should not be attempted first. Transport

| Table 22.23 | ADVANTAGES OF SURGICAL DEBULKING WITH INTRAOPERATIVE HIGH–DOSE-RATE BRACHYTHERAPY OVER PERIOPERATIVE BRACHYTHERAPY OR ELECTRON BEAM INTRAOPERATIVE RADIATION THERAPY |

Advantages over Perioperative Brachytherapy	Advantages over Electron Beam IORT
1. It is possible to use retraction or shielding to reduce the dose to normal tissues.	1. Electron beam IORT can only be delivered to areas accessible to the electron cone and, therefore, cannot treat steeply sloping surfaces, narrow cavities, or areas such as the diaphragm, pubis, and anterior abdominal wall. Intraoperative HDR brachytherapy has less anatomical constraints than electron beam IORT.
2. Normal structures can be temporarily moved while the radiation is given and then replaced in their normal position. For example, to access the base of skull, the maxilla can be removed and later regrafted. Ureters can be severed and then reimplanted into the bladder. During liver transplantation procedures, the liver hilum can be irradiated during the interval between the removal of the host liver and reimplantation of the donor liver.	2. The HDR machine costs less than an electron beam linear accelerator.
3. The process is rapid. Using a surface applicator eliminates the needs to individually suture the catheters to the tumor bed.	3. Since the HDR afterloader can be transported between the radiation department and the operating room, dedicated equipment is not required.
4. HDR allows the treatment to be delivered at sites into which catheters cannot be sutured.	
5. Since catheters are not left in the patient, there is no risk of catheter displacement, extrusion, or infection.	

HDR, high–dose-rate brachytherapy; IORT, intraoperative radiation therapy

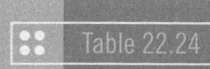

Table 22.24	INTERNATIONAL COMMISSION ON RADIOLOGICAL PROTECTION PUBLICATION 97—PREVENTION OF HIGH–DOSE-RATE BRACHYTHERAPY ACCIDENTS—GENERAL RECOMMENDATIONS

1. Written comprehensive QA program.
2. Compliance to QA procedures will contribute to minimizing the occurrence of errors, both in number and magnitude.
3. Hospital Radiation Safety committee (QA committee) needs to exist and interact with regulatory and health authorities.
4. Maintenance is an indispensable component of QA.
5. External audits of procedures reinforce good and safe practice and identify potential causes of errors.
6. Peer review of each case improves quality.
7. Every incident or accident should be reported as required to the appropriate authority.

QA, quality assurance

regulations of sources should be adhered to and performed by a factory trained and certified operator. In addition new sources should be measured in a calibrated well chamber to verify reported activity, at which time it is advisable to do a full commissioning including physics and mechanical QA checks. It is recommended that all systems of delivery (i.e., catheters) be close ended, that the step size at a particular center be constant (i.e., 5 mm) for all treatments, and that a dedicated self-contained brachytherapy suite exist to house all equipment. Prior to initiating treatment with the HDR machine a few standard procedures should be employed. These include manual insertion of a test wire to verify programmed treatment length and identify any kinks or obstructions, verifying applicator position with an appropriate imaging modality (i.e., fluoroscopy), and ensuring that all tubes outside the patient's body are as far away as possible to minimize unintended doses. Following treatment a survey of the patient by a portable radiation monitor is essential. Finally, emergency plans and security procedures should be in place and strictly adhered to. "False alarms" and "interlock failures" should be thoroughly investigated, and persons responsible for emergency procedures should remain in the vicinity

of the brachytherapy suite during the entire treatment. In some countries it is a requirement that both the clinician and physicist remain in the vicinity of the HDR suite. The possibility of theft of an HDR source for use as a weapon for nuclear terrorism is real, and the machine and source should be kept secure at all times. Particular attention should be paid if the facility or machine is decommissioned. It is believed that if a HDR brachytherapy center follows these general and specific recommendations, errors and accidents will be minimized.

High–Dose-Rate Brachytherapy in Developing Countries

HDR brachytherapy has special relevance for developing countries where resources may be scarce. In this regard, the IAEA has issued recommendations for the use of HDR brachytherapy in the developing countries (120). A brief summary is given here; however, readers interested in the details are referred to the original article. An HDR treatment system should be purchased as a complete unit that includes the ^{192}Ir radioactive

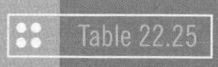

Table 22.25	INTERNATIONAL COMMISSION ON RADIOLOGICAL PROTECTION PUBLICATION 97—PREVENTION OF HIGH–DOSE-RATE BRACHYTHERAPY ACCIDENTS—SPECIFIC RECOMMENDATIONS

1. Training in an HDR center should commence prior to machine acquisition and should include the specific techniques to be used.
2. Training should be directed toward ensuring a team approach involving clinician, physicist, technician, and nurse.
3. Training and introduction of techniques should be sequential, commencing with simpler techniques before attempting more complex activities. Fixed geometry applicators and implants are less likely to result in errors.
4. Transport regulations should be adhered to and performed by a factory-trained and certified operator. This includes on-site container inspection for damage, removal of the old source and its transfer to the container, and installation of the new one into the safe.
5. New sources should be measured in a calibrated well chamber to verify the manufacturers reported activity and the results entered immediately into the software. At this time it is advisable to do a full commissioning (physics and mechanical QA checks).
6. All systems of delivery must be closed ended (catheters, needles, and fine tubes).
7. Manual insertion of a test wire (check cable) clearly marked at the programmed treatment length before each treatment to ensure that the total length of the transfer tube plus applicator equals the programmed treatment length. A manual check cable also helps to identify any kinks or obstruction in the catheter or transfer tube.
8. The step size in a particular center should be kept constant (e.g., 5 mm) for all treatments to avoid errors of using incorrect step size.
9. Keeping all tubes outside of the body as far distant as possible from the patient's skin will help to minimize unintended doses.
10. Dedicated self-contained brachytherapy suite with adequate shielding housing all requirements is highly advisable.
11. Applicator positioning should be verified before each treatment.
12. So-called false alarms and interlock failures should be thoroughly investigated and appropriated action taken and repaired.
13. Survey of patient by portable radiation monitor after each treatment.
14. An emergency plan should be prepared and practiced with commencement of operations.
15. The person responsible for performing an emergency procedure should remain in the brachytherapy suite during the entire treatment.
16. The HDR machine and source should be kept secure at all times.

HDR, high–dose-rate; QA, quality assurance

Table 22.26	COMPARISON OF DIFFERENT BRACHYTHERAPY TECHNIQUES					
	LDR ^{192}Ir	LDR Remote	MDR	PDR	HDR	IOHDR
Dose rate	Low	Low	Medium	High	High	High
Duration of each treatment	2–6 days	2–4 days	1 day	Minutes	Minutes	Minutes
Overall duration of treatment	2–6 days	2–4 days	1 day	2–4 days	3–5 weeks	Minutes
Radiation hazards	High	Small	Small	Small	Small	Small
Availability (worldwide)	++	—	—	—	+	—
Ease of optimization	—	—	—	+	+	+
Dose as sole modality (Gy)	60	60	40	60	30–40	15–20
Dose as boost to EBRT (Gy)	20–40	20–40	20–30	20–40	20–30	10–15

EBRT, external beam radiation therapy; HDR, high–dose-rate; IOHDR, intraoperative high–dose-rate; LDR, low–dose-rate; MDR, medium–dose-rate; PDR, pulsed–dose-rate.

source, source loading unit, applicators, treatment planning system, and control console. Infrastructure support may require additional or improved buildings and procurement of or access to new imaging facilities. A supportive budget is needed for quarterly source replacement and the annual maintenance necessary to keep the system operational. The radiation oncologist, medical physicist, and technologist should be specially trained before HDR can be introduced. Training for the oncologist and medical physicist is an ongoing process as new techniques or sites of treatment are introduced. Procedures for QA of patient treatment and the planning system must be introduced. Emergency procedures with adequate training of all associated personnel must be in place. The decision to select HDR in preference to alternate methods of brachytherapy is influenced by the ability of the machine to treat a wide variety of clinical sites. In departments with personnel and budgetary resources to support this equipment appropriately, economic advantage becomes evident only if large numbers of patients are treated. With HDR it is possible to treat a large number of patients in institutions that have a high volume of brachytherapy patients but insufficient in-patient facilities for LDR brachytherapy or insufficient finances for the purchase of ^{125}I or ^{103}Pd seeds for permanent implants. Intangible benefits of source safety, personnel safety, and easy adaptation to fluctuating demand for treatments also require consideration when evaluating the need to introduce this treatment system.

Summary

Although brachytherapy is a very effective modality, case selection and proper patient evaluation are essential. If the tumor is very large or widely metastatic, one is doomed to fail due to the physics of dose distribution in the former case and due to the biology of the tumor in the latter case. There are some differences between various brachytherapy modalities (Table 22.26). These differences should be kept in mind when selecting the brachytherapy modality in a particular situation. When HDR brachytherapy is used, the treatments must be executed carefully because the short treatment times do not allow any time for correction of errors, and mistakes can result in harm to patients. Hence, it is very important that all personnel involved in HDR brachytherapy be well trained and constantly alert. However, with proper case selection and delivery technique, HDR brachytherapy has great promise and convenience because of avoidance of radiation exposure, short treatment times, and outpatient therapy.

It is expected that the use of HDR brachytherapy will greatly expand over the next decade and that refinements will occur primarily in the integration of imaging (computed tomography, magnetic resonance imaging, intraoperative ultrasonography), and optimization of dose distribution (56,91,117). It is antici-

pated that better tumor localization and normal tissue definition will help to optimize dose distribution to the tumor and reduce normal tissue exposure (117). The development of well-controlled randomized trials addressing issues of efficacy, toxicity, quality of life, and costs versus benefits will ultimately define the role of HDR brachytherapy in the therapeutic armamentarium.

References

1. Akine Y, Arimoto H, Ogino T, et al. High-dose-rate intracavitary irradiation in the treatment of carcinoma of the uterine cervix: Early experience with 84 patients. *Int J Radiat Oncol Biol Phys* 1988;14:893–898.
2. Alekhteyar KM, Porter AT, Herskovic AM, et al. Preliminary results of hyperfractionated high dose rate brachytherapy in soft tissue sarcoma. *Endocuriether Hypertherm Oncol* 1994;10:179–184.
3. Alektiar KM, McKee A, Venkatraman E, et al. Intravaginal high-dose-rate brachytherapy for stage IB (FIGO grade 1,2) endometrial cancer. *Int J Radiat Oncol Biol Phys* 2002;53:707–713.
4. Alektiar KM, Venkatraman E, Chi DS, et al. Intravaginal brachytherapy alone for intermediate-risk endometrial cancer. *Int J Radiat Oncol Biol Phys* 2005;62:111–117.
5. Anacak Y, Mogulkoc N, Ozkok S, et al. High dose rate endobronchial brachytherapy in combination with external beam radiotherapy for stage III non-small cell lung cancer. *Lung Cancer* 2001;34:253–259.
6. Anderson JM, Stea B, Hallum AV, et al. High-dose-rate postoperative vaginal cuff irradiation alone for stage IB and IC endometrial cancer. *Int J Radiat Oncol Biol Phys* 2000;46:417–425.
7. Arai T, Morita S, Kutsutani Y, et al. Relationships between total iso-effect dose and number of fractions for the treatment of uterine cervical carcinoma by high dose-rate intracavitary irradiation. *Br J Radiol* 1980;17[Suppl 17]:89–92.
8. Arai T, Nakano T, Morita S, et al. High-dose-rate remote afterloading intracavitary radiation therapy for cancer of the uterine cervix: A 20-year experience. *Cancer* 1992;69:175–180.
9. Arthur DW, Vicini F, Kuske RR, et al. Accelerated partial breast irradiation: An updated report from the American Brachytherapy Society. *Brachytherapy* 2003;2:124–130.
10. Astrom L, Pedersen D, Mercke C, et al. Long-term outcome of high dose rate brachytherapy in radiotherapy for localised prostate cancer. *Radiother Oncol* 2005;74:157–161.
11. Aygun C, Weiner S, Scariato A, et al. Treatment of non-small cell lung cancer with external beam radiotherapy and high dose rate brachytherapy. *Int J Radiat Oncol Biol Phys* 1992;23:127–132.
12. Barendsen GW. Dose fractionation, dose rate, and iso-effect relationships for normal tissue responses. *Int J Radiat Oncol Biol Phys* 1982;8:1981–1997.
13. Bedwinek J, Petty A, Bruton C, et al. The use of high dose rate endobronchial brachytherapy to palliate symptomatic endobronchial recurrence of previously irradiated bronchogenic carcinoma. *Int J Radiat Oncol Biol Phys* 1992;22:23–30.
14. Benitez PR, Chen PY, Vicini FA, et al. Partial breast irradiation in breast-conserving therapy by way of interstitial brachytherapy. *Am J Surg* 2004;188:355–364.
15. Burt PA, O'Driscoll BR, Notley HM, et al. Intraluminal irradiation for the palliation of lung cancer with high dose rate microSelectron. *Thorax* 1990;45:765–768.
16. Celebioglu B, Gurkan OU, Erdogan S, et al. High dose rate endobronchial brachytherapy effectively palliates symptoms due to inoperable lung cancer. *Jpn J Clin Oncol* 2002;32:443–448.
17. Chadha M, Nanavati PJ, Liu P, et al. Patterns of failure in endometrial carcinoma stage IB grade 3 and IC patients treated with postoperative vaginal vault brachytherapy. *Gynecol Oncol* 1999;75:103–107.
18. Chang LFL, Horvath J, Peyton W. High dose rate afterloading intraluminal brachytherapy in malignant airway obstruction of lung cancer. *Int J Radiat Oncol Biol Phys* 1994;28:589–596.
19. Chen MS, Lin FJ, Hong CH, et al. High-dose-rate afterloading technique in the radiation treatment of uterine cervical cancer: 399 cases and 9 years experience in Taiwan. *Int J Radiat Oncol Biol Phys* 1991;20:915–919.
20. Chun M, Kang S, Kim BS, et al. High dose rate interstitial brachytherapy in soft tissue sarcoma: Technical aspects and results. *Jpn J Clin Oncol* 2001;31:279–283.
21. Clarke DH, Vincini F, Jacobs H, et al. High dose brachytherapy for breast cancer. In: Nag S, ed. *High dose rate brachytherapy: A textbook*. Armonk, NY: Futura Publishing Co, 1994;321–329.

22. Cotter GW, Craig L, Ellingwood KE, et al. Inoperable endobronchial obstructing lung cancer treated with combined endobronchial and external beam irradiation: A dosimetric analysis. *Int J Radiat Oncol Biol Phys* 1993;27:531–535.
23. Creutzberg CL, Van Putten WLJ, Koper PCM, et al. Surgery and postoperative radiotherapy versus surgery alone for patients with stage-1 endometrial carcinoma: Multicentre randomised trial. *Lancet* 2000;355:1404–1411.
24. Crownover RL, Marks KE, Zehr RJ. Initial results with high dose rate brachytherapy for soft-tissue sarcomas. *Sarcoma* 1997;1:196–205.
25. Dale RG. The use of small fraction numbers in high dose-rate gynecological afterloading: Some radiobiological considerations. *Br J Radiol* 1990;63:290–294.
26. Deger S, Boehmer D, Roigas J, et al. High dose rate (HDR) brachytherapy with conformal radiation therapy for localized prostate cancer. *Eur Urology* 2005;47:441–448.
27. Demanes DJ, Rodriguez RR, Schour L, et al. High-dose-rate intensity-modulated brachytherapy with external beam radiotherapy for prostate cancer: California endocurietherapy's 10-year results. *Int J Radiat Oncol Biol Phys* 2005;61:1306–1316.
28. Dixit S, Baboo HA, Rakesh V, et al. Interstitial high dose rate brachytherapy in head and neck cancers: Preliminary results. *J Brachyther Int* 1997;13:363–370.
29. Donath D, Clark C, Kaufmann MD, et al. Postoperative adjuvant high dose rate brachytherapy in the treatment of poor-prognosis soft-tissue sarcoma. *Endocuriether Hypertherm Oncol* 1993;9:48(abstr).
30. Donath D, Vuong T, Shnouda G, et al. The potential uses of high-dose-rate brachytherapy in patients with head and neck cancer. *Eur Arch Otorhinolaryngol* 1995;252:321–354.
31. Dritschilo A, Harter KW, Thomas D, et al. Intraoperative radiation therapy of hepatic metastases: Technical aspects and report of a pilot study. *Int J Radiat Oncol Biol Phys* 1988;14:1007–1011.
32. Duchesne GM, Peters LJ. What is the α/β ratio for prostate cancer? Rationale for hypofractionated high-dose-rate brachytherapy. *Int J Radiat Oncol Biol Phys* 1999;44:747–748.
33. Edmundson GK, Yan D, Martinez A. Intraoperative optimization of needle placement and dwell times for conformal prostate brachytherapy. *Int J Radiat Oncol Biol Phys* 1995;33:1257–1264.
34. Escobar-Sacristan JA, Granda-Orive JI, Gutierrez JT, et al. Endobronchial brachytherapy in the treatment of malignant lung tumors. *Eur Respir J* 2004; 24:348–352.
35. Eulau S, van Hollebeke L, Cavanagh W, et al. High dose rate iridium 192 brachytherapy in localized prostate cancer: Results and toxicity with maximum follow-up of 10 years. *Int J Radiat Oncol Biol Phys* 2000;48[Suppl]:149(abstr).
36. Ferrigno R, Nishimoto IN, dos Santos Novaes PER, et al. Comparison of low and high dose rate brachytherapy in the treatment of uterine cervix cancer. Retrospective analysis of two sequential series. *Int J Radiat Oncol Biol Phys* 2005;62:1108–1116.
37. Flamant F, Gerbaulet A, Nihoul-Fekete C, et al. Long-term sequelae of conservative treatment by surgery brachytherapy and chemotherapy for vulval and vaginal rhabdomyosarcoma in children. *J Clin Oncol* 1990;8:1847–1853.
38. Flores A, Nelems B, Evans K, et al. The impact of new radiotherapy modalities on the surgical management of cancer of the esophagus and cardia. *Int J Radiat Oncol Biol Phys* 1989;17:937–944.
39. Flores AD, Rowland CG, Yin WB. High dose rate brachytherapy of carcinoma of the esophagus. In: Nag S, ed. *High dose rate brachytherapy: A textbook*. Armonk, NY: Futura Publishing Co, 1994;275–294.
40. Fontanesi J, Kun L, Pao W, et al. Brachytherapy as primary or "boost" irradiation in 18 children with solid tumors. *Endocuriether Hypertherm Oncol* 1991;7:195–200.
41. Fowler J, Chappel R, Ritter M. Is α/β for prostate tumors really low? *Int J Radiat Oncol Biol Phys* 2001;50:1021–1031.
42. Fu K, Phillips T. High-dose-rate versus low-dose-rate intracavitary brachytherapy for carcinoma of the cervix. *Int J Radiat Oncol Biol Phys* 1990;19:791–796.
43. Furuta M, Tsukiyama I, Ohno T, et al. Radiation therapy for roentogenographically occult lung cancer by external beam irradiation and endobronchial high dose rate brachytherapy. *Lung Cancer* 1999;25:183–189.
44. Galalae RM, Kovacs G, Schultze J, et al. Long-term outcome after elective irradiation of the pelvic lymphatics and local dose escalation using high-dose-rate brachytherapy for locally advanced prostate cancer. *Int J Radiat Oncol Biol Phys* 2002;52:81–90.
45. Galalae RM, Martinez A, Mate T, et al. Long-term outcome by risk factors using conformal high-dose-rate brachytherapy (HDR-BT) boost with or without neoadjuvant androgen suppression for localized prostate cancer. *Int J Radiat Oncol Biol Phys* 2004;58:1048–1055.
46. Gao Li, Xu Guo-zhen, Yin Wei-bo, et al. Preliminary experience in HDR brachytherapy for 72 nasopharyngeal carcinoma patients. In: Mould RF, ed. *Brachytherapy in the Peoples Republic of China*. Kowloon, China: Nucletron Far East, 1992;E76–E81.
47. Gaspar LE. Brachytherapy in lung cancer. *J Surg Oncol* 1998;67(1):60–70.
48. Gaspar LE, Nag S, Herskovic A, et al. American Brachytherapy Society (ABS) consensus guidelines for brachytherapy of esophageal cancer. *Int J Radiat Oncol Biol Phys* 1997;38:127–132.
49. Gerbaulet AP, Esche BA, Hail CM, et al. Conservative treatment for lower gynecological tract malignancies in children and adolescents: The Institut Gustave-Roussy Experience. *Int J Radiat Oncol Biol Phys* 1989;16:655–658.
50. Goodman KA, Wolden SL, LaQuaglia MP, et al. Intraoperative high-dose-rate brachytherapy for pediatric solid tumors: A 10-year experience. *Brachytherapy* 2003;2:139–146.
51. Grigsby PW, Williamson JF, Clifford Chao KS, et al. Cervical tumor control evaluated with ICRU 38 reference volumes and integrated reference air kerma. *Radiother Oncol* 2001;58:19–23.
52. Grills IS, Martinez AA, Hollander M, et al. High-dose rate brachytherapy as prostate cancer monotherapy reduces toxicity compared to low dose rate palladium seeds. *J Urology* 2004;171:1098–1104.
53. Guinot JL, Arribas L, Chust ML, et al. Lip cancer treatment with high dose rate brachytherapy. *Radiother Oncol* 2003;69:113–115.
54. Guix B, Finestres F, Tello J, et al. Treatment of skin carcinomas of the face by high-dose-rate brachytherapy and custom-made surface molds. *Int J Radiat Oncol Biol Phys* 2000;47:95–102.
55. Haffty BG, Mate TP, Greenwood LH, et al. Malignant biliary obstruction: Intracavitary treatment with a high-dose-rate remote afterloading device. *Radiology* 1987;164:574–576.
56. Haie-Meder C, Potter R, Van Limbergen E, et al. Recommendations from Gynaecological (GYN) GEC-ESTRO Working Group (I): Concepts and terms in 3D image based 3D treatment planning in cervix cancer brachytherapy with emphasis on MRI assessment of GTV and CTV. *Radiother Oncol* 2005;74:235–245.
57. Hareyama M, Sakata K, Oouchi A, et al. High-dose rate and low-dose rate intracavitary therapy for carcinoma of the uterine cervix: A randomized trial. *Cancer* 2002;94:117–124.
58. Harrison LB, Franzese F, Gaynor JJ, et al. Long-term results of a prospective randomized trial of adjuvant brachytherapy in the management of completely resected soft tissue sarcomas of the extremity and superficial trunk. *Int J Radiat Oncol Biol Phys* 1992;27:259–265.
59. Hennequin C, Durdux C, Espie M, et al. High-dose-rate brachytherapy for early breast cancer: An ambulatory technique. *Int J Radiat Oncol Biol Phys* 1999;45:85–90.
60. Henschke UK, Hilaris BS, Mahan GD. Remote afterloading with intracavitary applicators. *Radiology* 1964;83:344–345.
61. Herskovic A, Heaston D, Engler MG, et al. Irradiation of biliary carcinoma. *Radiology* 1981;139:219–222.
62. Hishikawa Y, Kamikonya N, Tanaka S, et al. Radiotherapy or esophageal carcinoma; role of high dose rate intracavitary irradiation. *Radiother Oncol* 1987;9:13–20.
63. Horowitz NS, Peters WA, Smith MR, et al. Adjuvant high dose rate vaginal brachytherapy as treatment of stage I and II endometrial carcinoma. *Obstet Gynecol* 2002;99:235–240.
64. Hricak H, Yu K. Radiology in invasive cervical cancer. *AJR AM J Roentgenol* 1996;167:1101–1108.
65. Hsu ICJ, Cabrera AR, Weinberg V, et al. Combined modality treatment with high-dose-rate brachytherapy boost for locally advanced prostate cancer. *Brachytherapy* 2005;4:202–206.
66. Huber RM, Fischer R, Haútmann H, et al. Does additional brachytherapy improve the effect of external irradiation? A prospective, randomized study in central lung tumors. *Int J Radiat Oncol Biol Phys* 1997;38:533–540.
67. Inoue T, Inoue T, Yoshida K, et al. Phase III trial of high– vs. low–dose-rate interstitial radiotherapy for early mobile tongue cancer. *Int J Radiat Oncol Biol Phys* 2001;51:171–175.
68. International Commission on Radiation Units and Measurements. *ICRU Report 38: Dose and volume specification for reporting intracavitary therapy in gynecology*. Bethesda, MD: International Commission on Radiation Units and Measurements, 1985.
69. International Commission on Radiological Protection 2001–2005. ICRP Publication 97: Prevention of high-dose-rate brachytherapy accidents. *Ann ICRP* 2005;35(2):1–51.
70. Jo Y, Hiratsuka J, Fujii T, et al. High-dose-rate iridium-192 afterloading therapy combined with external beam radiotherapy for T1c-T3bN0M0 prostate cancer. *Urology* 2004;64:556–560.
71. Jolly DE, Nag S. Technique for construction of dental molds for high-dose-rate remote brachytherapy. *Special Care Dent* 1992;12:219–224.
72. Jolly S, Vargas C, Kumar T, et al. Vaginal brachytherapy alone: An alternative to adjuvant whole pelvis radiation for early stage endometrial cancer. *Gynecol Oncol* 2005;97:887–892.
73. Joslin CA. The Cathetron as part of the radical management of cervix cancer. *Br J Radiol* 1980;17[Suppl 17]:11–16.
74. Keisch M, Vicini F, Scroggins T, et al. Thirty month results with the MammoSite breast brachytherapy applicator: Cosmesis, toxicity, and local control in partial breast irradiation. *Int J Radiat Oncol Biol Phys* 2004;60[Suppl]:272.
75. Kelly JF, Delclos ME, Morice C, et al. High-dose-rate endobronchial brachytherapy effectively palliates symptoms due to airway tumors: The 10-year M.D. Anderson Cancer Center experience. *Int J Radiat Oncol Biol Phys* 2000;48:697–702.
76. Keys HM, Roberts JA, Brunetto VL, et al. A phase III trial of surgery with or without adjunctive external pelvic radiation therapy in intermediate risk endometrial adenocarcinoma: A Gynecologic Oncology Group study. *Gynecol Oncol* 2004;92:744–751.
77. Khanavkar B, Stern P, Alberti W, et al. Complications associated with brachytherapy alone or with laser in lung cancer. *Chest* 1991;99:1062–1065.
78. Kim SH, Choi BI, Lee HP, et al. Uterine cervical carcinoma: Comparison of CT and MRI findings. *Radiology* 1990;175:45–51.
79. King TA, Bolton JS, Kuske RR, et al. Long-term results of wide-field brachytherapy as the sole method of radiation therapy after segmental mastectomy for Tis,1,2 breast cancer. *Am J Surg* 2000;180:299–304.
80. Knocke TH, Kucera H, Weidinger B, et al. Primary treatment of endometrial carcinoma with high-dose-rate brachytherapy: Results of 12 years of experience with 280 patients. *Int J Radiat Oncol Biol Phys* 1997;37:359–365.
81. Koizumi M, Inoue T, Yamazaki H, et al. Perioperative fractionated high-dose rate brachytherapy for malignant bone and soft tissue tumors. *Int J Radiat Oncol Biol Phys* 1999;43:989–993.
82. Kretzler A, Molls M, Gradinger R, et al. Intraoperative radiotherapy of soft tissue sarcoma of the extremity. *Strahlenther Onkol* 2004;180:365–370.
83. Kucera H, Knocke TH, Potter R. Treatment of endometrial carcinoma with high-dose-rate brachytherapy alone in medically inoperable stage I patients. *Acta Obstet Gynecol Scand* 1998;77:1008–1012.
84. Kucera H, Weghaupt K. Treatment of inoperable endometrial carcinoma with intracavitary high dose rate iridium irradiation. *Strahlenther Onkol* 1986;9:508–514.
85. Kuske RR, Bolton JS, Harrison W. *RTOG 95–17. A phase I/II trial to evaluate brachytherapy as the sole method of radiation therapy for stage I and II breast carcinoma*. Philadelphia, PA: Radiation Therapy Oncology Group, 1998.
86. Kuske RR, Bolton JS, Wilenzick RM, et al. Brachytherapy as the sole method of breast irradiation in TIS, T1, T2, N0–1 breast cancer. *Int J Radiat Oncol Biol Phys* 1994;30[Suppl 1]:245.
87. Lau HY, Hay JH, Flores AD, et al. Seven fractions of twice daily high–dose-rate brachytherapy for node-negative carcinoma of the mobile tongue results in loss of therapeutic ratio. *Radiother Oncol* 1996;39:15–18.
88. Lertsanguansinchai P, Lertbutsayanukul C, Shotelersuk K, et al. Phase III randomized trial comparing LDR and HDR brachytherapy in treatment of cervical carcinoma. *Int J Radiat Oncol Biol Phys* 2004;59:1424–1431.

89. Leung TW, Wong VYW, Kwan KH, et al. High–dose-rate brachytherapy for early stage oral tongue cancer. *Head Neck* 2002;24:274–281.

90. Levendag PC, Vikram B, Flores AD, et al. High–dose-rate brachytherapy for cancer of the head and neck. In: Nag S, ed. *High dose rate brachytherapy: A textbook.* Armonk, NY: Futura Publishing Co, 1994;237–273.

91. Li S, Frassica D, DeWeese T. A real-time image-guided intraoperative high-dose-rate brachytherapy system. *Brachytherapy* 2003;2:5–16.

92. Lorvidhaya V, Tonusin A, Changwiwit W, et al. High-dose-rate afterloading brachytherapy in carcinoma of the cervix: And experience of 1992 patients. *Int J Radiat Oncol Biol Phys* 2000;46:1185–1191.

93. Lu JJ, Bains YS, Abdel-Wahab M, et al. High-dose-rate remote afterloading intracavitary brachytherapy for the treatment of extrahepatic biliary duct carcinoma. *Cancer J* 2002;8:74–78.

94. Lu JJ, Shakespeare TP, Tan LKS, et al. Adjuvant fractionated high-dose-rate intracavitary brachytherapy after external beam radiotherapy in T1 and T2 nasopharyngeal carcinoma. *Head Neck* 2004;26:389–395.

95. Lukas P, Kneschaurek P, Ries G, et al. A new modality for intraoperative radiotherapy using a high dose rate afterloading unit. In: ed. *Proceedings of Sixth International High Dose Rate Remote Afterloading Conference, Budapest, Hungary, May 2–4.* 1991;62–66.

96. Lybert MLM, van Putten WLJ, Ribot JG, et al. Endometrial carcinoma: High dose rate brachytherapy in combination with external irradiation–a multivariate analysis of relapses. *Radiother Oncol* 1989;16:245–252.

97. Macha HN, Wahlers B, Reichle C, et al. Endobronchial radiation therapy for obstructing malignancies: Ten years' experience with iridium-192 high-dose radiation brachytherapy afterloading technique in 365 patients. *Lung* 1995;173:271–280.

98. Macleod C, Fowler A, Duval P, et al. Adjuvant high-dose-rate brachytherapy with or without external beam radiotherapy post-hysterectomy for endometrial cancer. *Int J Gynecol Cancer* 1999;9:247–255.

99. Mandell LM, Nori D, Anderson LL, et al. Postoperative vaginal radiation in endometrial cancer using a remote afterloading technique. *Int J Radiat Oncol Biol Phys* 1985;11:473–478.

100. Manning MA, Arthur DW, Schmidt-Ullrich RK, et al. Interstitial high dose rate brachytherapy boost: The feasibility and cosmetic outcome of a fractionated outpatient delivery scheme. *Int J Radiat Oncol Biol Phys* 2000;48:1301–1306.

101. Marsiglia H, Baldeyrou P, Lartigau E, et al. High-dose-rate brachytherapy as a sole modality for early-stage endobronchial carcinoma. *Int J Radiat Oncol Biol Phys* 2000;47:665–672.

102. Martin T, Baltas D, Kurek R, et al. 3-D conformal HDR brachytherapy as monotherapy for localized prostate cancer. *Strahlenther Onkol* 2004;180:225–232.

103. Martinez AA, Gustafsom G, Gonzalez J, et al. Dose escalation using conformal high-dose-rate brachytherapy improves outcome in unfavorable prostate cancer. *Int J Radiat Oncol Biol Phys* 2002;53:316–327.

104. Martinez A, Pataki I, Edmundson G, et al. Phase II prospective study of the use of conformal high-dose rate brachytherapy as monotherapy for the treatment of favorable stage prostate cancer: A feasibility report. *Int J Radiat Oncol Biol Phys* 2001;49:61–69.

105. Martinez-Monge R, Garran C, Cambeiro M, et al. Feasibility report of conservative surgery, perioperative high-dose-rate brachytherapy (PHDRB), and low-to-moderate dose external beam radiation therapy (EBRT) in pediatric sarcomas. *Brachytherapy* 2004;3:196–200.

106. Mate T, Kovacs G, Martinez A. High dose rate brachytherapy of the prostate. In: Nag S, ed. *High dose rate brachytherapy: A textbook.* Armonk, NY: Futura Publishing Co, 1994;355–371.

107. Mate TP, Gottesman JE, Hatton J, et al. High dose-rate afterloading iridium-192 prostate brachytherapy: Feasibility report. *Int J Radiat Oncol Biol Phys* 1998;41:525–533.

108. Mehta MP, Lamond JP, Nori D, et al. Brachytherapy of lung cancer. In: Nag S, ed. *Principles and practice of brachytherapy.* Armonk, NY: Futura Publishing Co, 1997;323–349.

109. Mehta MP, Petereit DG, Chosy L, et al. Sequential comparison of low dose rate and hyperfractionated high dose rate endobronchial radiation for malignant airway occlusion. *Int J Radiat Oncol Biol Phys* 1992;23:133–139.

110. Mehta MP, Speiser BL, Macha HN. High dose rate brachytherapy for lung cancer. In: Nag S, ed. *High dose rate brachytherapy: A textbook.* Armonk, NY: Futura Publishing Co, 1994;295–319.

111. Merchant TE, Zelefsky MJ, Sheldon JM, et al. High-dose rate intraoperative radiation therapy for pediatric solid tumors. *Med Ped Oncol* 1998;30:34–39.

112. Miller JI Jr, Phillips TW. Neodymium: YAG laser and brachytherapy in the management of inoperable bronchogenic carcinoma. *Ann Thorac Surg* 1990;50:190–196.

113. Mundinger F, Sauerwein K. Gamma Med: Ein Gerat zur Bestrahlung von Himgeschwulsten mit Radioisotopen. *Acta Radiol* 1966;5:48–52.

114. Muto P, Ravo V, Panelli G, et al. High-dose rate brachytherapy of bronchial cancer: Treatment optimization using three schemes of therapy. *Oncologist* 2000;5:209–214.

115. Nag S. Controversies and new developments in gynecologic brachytherapy–image-based intracavitary brachytherapy for cervical carcinoma. *Sem Radiat Oncol* 2006;16:164–167.

116. Nag S. Modern techniques of radiation therapy for endometrial cancer. *Clin Obstet Gynecol* 1996;39:728–744.

117. Nag S, Cardenes H, Chang S, et al. Proposed guidelines for image-based intracavitary brachytherapy for cervical carcinoma: Report from Image-Guided Brachytherapy Working Group. *Int J Radiat Oncol Biol Phys* 2004;60:1160–1172.

118. Nag S, Cardenes H, Chang S, et al. In response to Dr. Potter et al: Recommendation for image-based intracavitary brachytherapy of cervical cancer: The Gyn GEC ESTRO Working Group point of view. *Int J Radiat Oncol Biol Phys* 2005;62:295–296(letter).

119. Nag S, Chao C, Erickson B, et al. The American Brachytherapy Society recommendations for low-dose-rate brachytherapy for carcinoma of the cervix. *Int J Radiat Oncol Biol Phys* 2002;52:33–48.

120. Nag S, Dally M, De la Torre M, et al. Recommendations for implementation of high dose rate 192-Ir brachytherapy in developing countries by the Advisory Group of International Atomic Energy Agency. *Radiother Oncol* 2002;64:297–308.

121. Nag S, Dobelbower R, Glasgow G, et al. Inter-society standards for brachytherapy: A joint report from AAPM, ABS, ACMP, and ACRO. *Crit Rev Oncol Hematol* 2003;48:1–17.

122. Nag S, Erickson B, Parikh S, et al. The American Brachytherapy Society recommendations for HDR brachytherapy for carcinoma of the endometrium. *Int J Radiat Oncol Biol Phys* 2000;48:779–790.

123. Nag S, Fernandes PS, Martínez-Monge R, et al. Use of brachytherapy to preserve function in children with soft-tissue sarcomas. *Oncology* 1999;13:361–374.

124. Nag S, Grecula JC, Ruymann F. Aggressive chemotherapy, organ preserving surgery, and high dose rate remote brachytherapy in the treatment of rhabdomyosarcoma in infants and young children. *Cancer* 1993;72:2769–2776.

125. Nag S, Gunderson L, Harrison L. Techniques of intraoperative radiation therapy vs. intraoperative high dose rate brachytherapy. In: Gunderson LL, Willet CG, Harrison LV, et al., eds. *Intraoperative irradiation: Techniques and results.* Totowa, NJ: Humana Press, 1999;111–130.

126. Nag S, Gupta N. A simple method of obtaining equivalent doses for use in HDR brachytherapy. *Int J Radiat Oncol Biol Phys* 2000;46:507–513.

127. Nag S, Hu K. Intraoperative high dose rate brachytherapy. *Surg Oncol Clin North Am* 2003;12:1079–1097.

128. Nag S, Kelly JF, Horton JL, et al. The American Brachytherapy Society recommendations for HDR brachytherapy for carcinoma of the lung. *Oncology* 2001;15:371–381.

129. Nag S, Koc M, Schuller D, et al. Intraoperative single fraction high dose rate brachytherapy for head and neck cancers. *Brachytherapy* 2005;4:217–223.

130. Nag S, Kuske RR, Vicini F, et al. The American Brachytherapy Society recommendations for brachytherapy for carcinoma of the breast. *Oncology* 2001;15:195–207.

131. Nag S, Martínez-Monge R, Gupta N. Intraoperative radiation therapy using electron-beam and high-dose-rate brachytherapy. *Cancer J* 1997;10:94–101.

132. Nag S, Martínez-Monge R, Ruymann FB, et al. Feasibility of intraoperative high-dose rate brachytherapy to boost low dose external beam radiation therapy to treat pediatric soft tissue sarcomas. *Med Ped Oncol* 1998;31:79–85.

133. Nag S, Olson T, Ruymann F, et al. High dose rate brachytherapy in childhood sarcomas: A local control strategy preserving bone growth and function. *Med Ped Oncol* 1995;25:463–469.

134. Nag S, Orton C. Development of intraoperative high dose rate brachytherapy for treatment of resected tumor beds in anesthetized patients. *Endocuriether Hypertherm Oncol* 1993;9:187–193.

135. Nag S, Orton C, Petereit DG, et al. The American Brachytherapy Society recommendations for HDR brachytherapy of the cervix. *Int J Radiat Oncol Biol Phys* 2000;48:201–211.

136. Nag S, Owen J, Pajak T, et al. Survey of brachytherapy practice in the U.S.: A report of the Clinical Research Committee of The American Endocurietherapy Society. *Int J Radiat Oncol Biol Phys* 1995;31:103–107.

137. Nag S, Porter AT, Donath D. The role of high dose rate brachytherapy in the management of adult soft tissue sarcomas. In: Nag S, ed. *High dose rate brachytherapy: A textbook.* Armonk, NY: Futura Publishing Co, 1994;393–398.

138. Nag S, Samsami N. Pitfalls of inappropriate optimization. *J Brachyther Int* 2000;16:187–198.

139. Nag S, Schuller D, Pak V, et al. Pilot study of intraoperative high dose rate brachytherapy for head and neck cancer. *Radiother Oncol* 1996;41:125–130.

140. Nag S, Shasha D, Janjan N, et al. The American Brachytherapy Society recommendations for brachytherapy of soft tissue sarcomas. *Int J Radiat Oncol Biol Phys* 2001;49:1033–1043.

141. Nag S, Tai DL, Gold RE. Biliary tract neoplasms: A simple management technique. *South Med J* 1984;77:593–595.

142. Nag S, Tippin D. Brachytherapy for pediatric tumors. *Brachytherapy* 2003;2:131–138.

143. Nag S, Tippin D, Grecula J, et al. Intraoperative high dose rate brachytherapy for paranasal sinus tumors. *Int J Radiat Oncol Biol Phys* 2004;58:155–160.

144. Nag S, Tippin D, Ruymann FB. Intraoperative high-dose-rate brachytherapy for the treatment of pediatric soft tissue sarcomas. *Int J Radiat Oncol Biol Phys* 2001;51:729–735.

145. Nag S, Tippin D, Ruymann FB. Long-term morbidity in children treated with fractionated high-dose-rate brachytherapy for soft tissue sarcomas. *J Pediatric Hematol Oncol* 2003;25:448–452.

146. Nag S, Tippin D, Smith S, et al. Intraoperative electron beam treatment for pediatric malignancies: The Ohio State University experience. *Med Ped Oncol* 2003;40:360–366.

147. Nag S, Vikram B, Demanes JD, et al. The American Brachytherapy Society recommendations for HDR brachytherapy for head and neck carcinoma. *Int J Radiat Oncol Biol Phys* 2001;50:1190–1198.

148. Nag S, Young D, Orton C, et al. Survey of the brachytherapy practice for carcinoma of the cervix: A report of the Clinical Research Committee of the American Brachytherapy Society. *Gynecol Oncol* 1999;73:111–118.

149. Nakamura RA, Dos Santos Novaes PER, Antoneli CBG, et al. High-dose-rate brachytherapy as part of a multidisciplinary treatment of nasopharyngeal lymphoepithelioma in childhood. *Cancer* 2005;104:525–531.

150. Ng T, Richards GM, Emery RS, et al. Customized conformal high-dose-rate brachytherapy boost for limited-volume nasopharyngeal cancer. *Int J Radiat Oncol Biol Phys* 2005;61:754–761.

151. Nguyen T, Petereit DG. High-dose-rate brachytherapy for medically inoperable stage I endometrial cancer. *Gynecol Oncol* 1998;71:196–203.

152. Niazi TM, Souhami L, Portelance L, et al. Long-term results of high-dose-rate brachytherapy in the primary treatment of medically inoperable stage I-II endometrial carcinoma. *Int J Radiat Oncol Biol Phys* 2005;63:1108–1113.

153. Niehoff P, Loch T, Nurnberg N, et al. Feasibility and preliminary outcome of salvage combined HDR brachytherapy and external beam radiotherapy (EBRT) for local recurrences after radical prostatectomy. *Brachytherapy* 2005;4:141–145.

154. Nori D, Nag S, Rogers D, et al. Remote afterloading high dose rate brachytherapy for carcinoma of the bile duct. In: Nag S, ed. *High dose rate brachytherapy: A textbook.* Armonk, NY: Futura Publishing Co, 1994;331–338.

155. Nose T, Koizumi M, Nishiyama K. High-dose-rate interstitial brachytherapy for oropharyngeal carcinoma: Results of 83 lesions in 82 patients. *Int J Radiat Oncol Biol Phys* 2004;59:983–991.

156. O'Connell D, Howard N, Joslin CA, et al. A remotely-controlled unit for the treatment of uterine carcinoma. *Lancet* 1965;2:570.

157. Orton CG, Seyedsadr M, Somnay A. Comparison of high and low dose rate remote afterloading for cervix cancer and the importance of fractionation. *Int J Radiat Oncol Biol Phys* 1991;21:1425–1434.

158. Patel FD, Rai B, Mallick I, et al. High-dose-rate brachytherapy in uterine cervical carcinoma. *Int J Radiat Oncol Biol Phys* 2005;62:125–130.

159. Patel FD, Sharma SC, Pritam SN, et al. Low dose rate versus high dose rate brachytherapy in the treatment of carcinoma of the uterine cervix: A clinical trial. *Int J Radiat Oncol Biol Phys* 1994;28:335–341.
160. Pearcey RG, Petereit DG. Post-operative high dose rate brachytherapy in patients with low to intermediate risk endometrial cancer. *Radiother Oncol* 2000;56:17–22.
161. Perera F, Chisela F, Engel J, et al. Method of localization and implantation of the lumpectomy site for high dose rate brachytherapy after conservative surgery for T1 and T2 breast cancer. *Int J Radiat Oncol Biol Phys* 1995;31:959–965.
162. Perera F, Engel J, Holliday R, et al. Local resection and brachytherapy confined to the lumpectomy site for early breast cancer: A pilot study. *J Surg Oncol* 1997;65:263–267.
163. Perol M, Caliandro R, Pommier P, et al. Curative irradiation of limited endobronchial carcinomas with high-dose-rate brachytherapy. Results of a pilot study. *Chest* 1997;111:1417–1423.
164. Peschel RE, Healey G, Smith RJ. High dose rate remote afterloading for endometrial cancer. *Endocuriether Hypertherm Oncol* 1989;5:209–214.
165. Petera J, Neumanova R, Odrazka K, et al. Perioperative fractionated high-dose rate brachytherapy in the treatment of soft tissue sarcomas. *Neoplasma* 2004;51:59–63.
166. Petereit D, Peracey R. Literature analysis of high dose rate brachytherapy fractionation schedules in the treatment of cervical cancer: Is there an optimal fractionation schedule? *Int J Radiat Oncol Biol Phys* 1999;43:359–366.
167. Petereit DG, Sarkaria JN, Potter DM, et al. High-dose-rate versus low-dose-rate brachytherapy in the treatment of cervical cancer: Analysis of tumor recurrence–the University of Wisconsin experience. *Int J Radiat Oncol Biol Phys* 1999;45:1267–1274.
168. Petereit DG, Tannehill SP, Grosen EA, et al. Outpatient vaginal cuff brachytherapy for endometrial cancer. *Int J Gynecol Cancer* 1999;9:456–462.
169. Polgar C, Fodor J, Orosz Z, et al. Electron and high-dose-rate brachytherapy boost in the conservative treatment of stage I-II breast cancer. *Strahlenther Onkol* 2002;178:615–623.
170. Polgar C, Major T, Somogyi A, et al. Brachytherapy of the tumor bed after breast conserving surgery: New radiotherapeutic option in the management of early breast cancer. *Orv Hetil* 1999;140:1461–1466.
171. Polgar C, Major T, Somogyi A, et al. High-dose-rate brachytherapy alone versus whole breast radiotherapy with or without tumor bed boost after breast-conserving surgery: Seven-year results of a comparative study. *Int J Radiat Oncol Biol Phys* 2004;60:1173–1181.
172. Polgar C, Sulok Z, Fodor J, et al. Sole brachytherapy of the tumor bed after conservative surgery for T1 breast cancer: Five-year results of a phase I–II study and initial findings of a randomized phase III trial. *J Surg Oncol* 2002;80:121–128.
173. Poortmans P, Bartelink H, Horiot JC, et al. The influence of the boost technique on local control in breast conserving treatment in the EORTC "boost versus no boost" randomised trial. *Radiother Oncol* 2004;72:25–33.
174. Potter R, Dimopoulos J, Kirisits C, et al. Recommendations for image-based intracavitary brachytherapy of cervix cancer: The Gyn GEC ESTRO Working Group point of view. *Int J Radiat Oncol Biol Phys* 2005;62:293295 (letter).
175. Potter R, Haie-Meder C, Van Limbergen E, et al. Recommendations from gynaecological GEC ESTRO working group (II): Concepts and terms in 3D image-based treatment planning in cervix cancer brachytherapy—3D dose volume parameters and aspects of 3D image-based anatomy, radiation physics, radiobiology. *Radiother Oncol* 2006;78:67–77.
176. Potter R, Knocke TH, Fellner C, et al. Definitive radiotherapy based on HDR brachytherapy with iridium 192 in uterine cervix carcinoma: Report of the Vienna University Hospital findings (1993–1997) compared to the preceding period in the context of ICRU 38 recommendations. *Cancer Radiother* 2000;4:159–172.
177. Potter R, Knocke TH, Kovacs G, et al. Brachytherapy in the combined modality treatment of pediatric malignancies. principles and preliminary experience with treatment of soft tissue sarcoma (recurrence) and Ewing's sarcoma. *Klin Padiatr* 1995;207:164–173.
178. Potter R, Van Limbergen E, Gerstner N, et al. Survey of the use of the ICRU 38 in recording and reporting cervical cancer brachytherapy. *Radiother Oncol* 2001;58:11–18.
179. Rachbauer F, Sztankay A, Kreczy A, et al. High-dose-rate intraoperative brachytherapy (IOHDR) using flab technique in the treatment of soft tissue sarcomas. *Strahlenther Onkol* 2003;179:480–485.
180. Reddi RP, Marbach JC. HDR remote afterloading brachytherapy of carcinoma of the lung. *Selectron Brachyther J* 1992;6:21–23.
181. Resch A, Potter R, van Limbergen E, et al. Long-term results (10 years) of intensive breast conserving therapy including a high-dose and large-volume interstitial brachytherapy boost (LDR/HDR) for T1/T2 breast cancer. *Radiother Oncol* 2002;63:47–58.
182. Rippa P, Seppo K, Kauppila MD. Comparison of Heyman packing and Cathetron afterloading methods in the treatment of endometrial cancer. *Br J Radiol* 1985;58:437–441.
183. Rittenberg PVC, Lotocki RJ, Heywood MS, et al. High-risk surgical stage I endometrial cancer: Outcomes with vault brachytherapy alone. *Gynecol Oncol* 2003;89:288–294.
184. Roddiger SJ, Kolotas C, Filipowicz I, et al. Neoadjuvant interstitial high-dose-rate (HDR) brachytherapy combined with systemic chemotherapy in patients with breast cancer. *Strahlenther Onkol* 2006;182:22–29.
185. Rodriguez R, Nag S, Mate T, et al. High dose rate brachytherapy for prostate cancer: Assessment of current clinical practice and recommendations of the American Brachytherapy Society. *J Brachyther Int* 2001;17:265–282.
186. Rodriguez RR, Demanes DJ, Altieri GA, et al. High-dose-rate (HDR) monotherapy for early stage prostate cancer: Preliminary results. *Brachytherapy* 2003;2:62.(Abstract)
187. Romestaing P, Lehingue Y, Carrie C, et al. Role of a 10 Gy boost in the conservative treatment of early breast cancer: Results of a randomized clinical trial in Lyon, France. *J Clin Oncol* 1997;15:963–968.
188. Rotte K. Technique and results of HDR afterloading in cancer of the endometrium. In: Martinez AA, Orton CG, Mould RF, eds. *Brachytherapy HDR and LDR*. Columbia, MD: Nucletron, 1990;68–79.
189. Rowland CG, Pagliero KM. Intracavitary irradiation in palliation of carcinoma of the esophagus and cardia. *Lancet* 1985;2:981–983.
190. Ryan J, Chuba R, Ben-Josef EB, et al. Adjuvant brachytherapy for primary and recurrent soft tissue sarcoma at WSU. *Radiother Oncol* 1996;39[Suppl 1:S4(abstr).
191. Saito M, Yokoyama A, Kurita Y, et al. Treatment of roentgenographically occult endobronchial with external beam radiotherapy and intraluminal low dose rate brachytherapy: Second report. *Int J Radiat Oncol Biol Phys* 2000;47:673–680.
192. Sato S, Yajima A, Suzuki M. Therapeutic results using high-dose-rate intracavitary irradiation in cases of cervical cancer. *Gynecol Oncol* 1984;19:143–147.
193. Schleicher UM, Staatz G, Alzen G, et al. Combined external beam and intraluminal radiotherapy for irresectable Klatskin tumors. *Strahlenther Onkol* 2002;178:682–687.
194. Scholten AN, van Putten WLJ, Beerman H, et al. Postoperative radiotherapy for stage I endometrial carcinoma: Long-term outcome of the randomized PORTEC trial with central pathology review. *Int J Radiat Oncol Biol Phys* 2005;63:834–838.
195. Schray MF, Gunderson LL, Sim FH, et al. Soft tissue sarcoma. Integration of brachytherapy, resection, and external irradiation. *Cancer* 1990;66:451–456.
196. Schuck A, Willich N, Rube C, et al. Intraoperative high-dose-rate brachytherapy after preoperative radiochemotherapy in the treatment of Ewing's sarcoma. *Front Radiat Ther Oncol* 1997;31:153–157.
197. Shah NM, Tenenholz T, Arthur D, et al. MammoSite and interstitial brachytherapy for accelerated partial breast irradiation: Factors that affect toxicity and cosmesis. *Cancer* 2004;101:727–734.
198. Sharma V, Mahantshetty U, Menon V, et al. A modified technique for high-dose-rate intracavitary brachytherapy in advanced cancer of the cervix. *Brachytherapy* 2003;2:246–248.
199. Shigematsu Y, Nishiyama K, Masaki N, et al. Treatment of carcinoma of the uterine cervix y remotely controlled afterloading intracavitary radiotherapy with high-does rate: A comparative study with a low-dose rate system. *Int J Radiat Oncol Biol Phys* 1983;9:351–356.
200. Shin HS, Seong J, Kim WC, et al. Combination of external beam irradiation and high-dose-rate intraluminal brachytherapy for inoperable carcinoma of the extra-hepatic bile ducts. *Int J Radiat Oncol Biol Phys* 2003;57:105–112.
201. Sievert RM. Two arrangements for reducing dangers in teleradium treatment. *Acta Radiol* 1937;18:157–162.
202. Sipila R, Kauppila A. Intracavitary irradiation of endometrial carcinoma using a high intensity Co-60 afterloading method. *Acta Radiol* 1989;28:601–605.
203. Solhjem MC, Petersen IV, Haddock MG. Vaginal brachytherapy alone is sufficient adjuvant treatment of surgical stage I endometrial cancer. *Int J Radiat Oncol Biol Phys* 2005;62:1379–1384.
204. Sood BM, Gorla G, Gupta S, et al. Two fractions of high-dose-rate brachytherapy in the management of cervix cancer: Clinical experience with and without chemotherapy. *Int J Radiat Oncol Biol Phys* 2002;53:702–706.
205. Sorbe B, Frankendal B. Intracavitary irradiation of endometrial carcinoma stage I by a high dose rate afterloading technique. *Gynecol Oncol* 1989;33:135–145.
206. Sorbe B, Kjelligren O, Stenson S. Prognosis of endometrial carcinoma stage I in two Swedish regions. A study with special regard to the effects of intracavitary irradiation with high dose rate afterloading technique. *Acta Radiol* 1990;29:29–37.
207. Sorbe B, Straumits A, Karlsson L. Intravaginal high-dose-rate brachytherapy for stage I endometrial cancer: A randomized study of two dose-per-fraction levels. *Int J Radiat Oncol Biol Phys* 2005;62:1385–1389.
208. Sorbe BG, Smeds AC. Postoperative vaginal irradiation with high dose rate afterloading technique in endometrial carcinoma stage I. *Int J Radiat Oncol Biol Phys* 1990;18:305–314.
209. Souhami L, Corns R, Duclos M, et al. Long-term results of high dose rate brachytherapy in cervix cancer using a small number of fractions. *Gynecol Oncol* 2005;97:508–513.
210. Speiser B, Spratling L. Intermediate dose rate remote afterloading brachytherapy for intraluminal control of bronchogenic carcinoma. *Int J Radiat Oncol Biol Phys* 1990;18:1443–1448.
211. Speiser B, Spratling L. Fatal hemoptysis: Complication or failure of treatment. *Int J Radiat Oncol Biol Phys* 1993;25:925.
212. Speiser BL. Brachytherapy in the treatment of thoracic tumors: Lung and esophageal. *Hematol Oncol Clin North Am* 1999;13:609–634.
213. Speiser BL. High dose-rate endobronchial brachytherapy: Whither goest thou? *Int J Radiat Oncol Biol Phys* 1992;23:250.
214. Speiser BL, Spratling L. Radiation bronchitis and stenosis secondary to high dose rate endobronchial irradiation. *Int J Radiat Oncol Biol Phys* 1993;25:589–597.
215. Stevens MJ, Stricker PD, Saalfeld J, et al. Treatment of localized prostate cancer using a combination of high dose rate iridium-192 brachytherapy and external beam irradiation: Initial Australian experience. *Austral Radio* 2003;47:152–160.
216. Stitt JA. Dose specification for inoperable endometrial carcinoma: The Madison system. *Act/Int Selectron Brachyther J* 1991;[Suppl 2]:32–34.
217. Stitt JA. High dose rate intracavitary brachytherapy for gynecologic malignancies. *Oncology* 1992;6:59–79.
218. Stout R, Barber PV, Burt PA, et al. Intraluminal brachytherapy in bronchial carcinoma. *Br J Radiol* 1990;63:16(abstr).
219. Strnad V, Ott O, Potter R, et al. Interstitial brachytherapy alone after breast conserving surgery: Interim results of a German-Austrian multicenter phase II trial. *Brachytherapy* 2004;3:115–119.
220. Subak L, Hricak H, Powell B, et al. Cervical carcinoma: Computed tomography and magnetic resonance imaging for pre-operative staging. *Obstet Gynecol* 1995;86:43–50.
221. Sur R, Donde B, Falkson C, et al. Randomized prospective study comparing high-dose-rate intraluminal brachytherapy (HDRILBT) alone with HDRILBT and external beam radiotherapy in the palliation of advanced esophageal cancer. *Brachytherapy* 2004;3:191–195.
222. Sur RK, Donde B, Levin CV, et al. Fractionated high dose rate intraluminal brachytherapy in palliation of advanced esophageal cancer. *Int J Radiat Oncol Biol Phys* 1998;40:447–453.
223. Sur RK, Kochar R, Negi PS, et al. High dose rate intraluminal brachytherapy in palliation of esophageal carcinoma. *Endocuriether Hypertherm Oncol* 1994;10:25–29.
224. Sur RK, Levin CV, Donde B, et al. Prospective randomized trial of HDR brachytherapy as a sole modality in palliation of advanced esophageal carcinoma: An International Atomic Energy Agency study. *Int J Radiat Oncol Biol Phys* 2002;53:127–133.
225. Sur RK, Singh DP, Sharma SC, et al. Radiation therapy of esophageal cancer: Role

of high dose rate brachytherapy. *Int J Radiat Oncol Biol Phys* 1992;22:1043–1046.

226. Sutedja G, Baris G, Schaake-Koning C, et al. High dose rate brachytherapy in patients with local recurrence after radiotherapy of non-small cell lung cancer. *Int J Radiat Oncol Biol Phys* 1992;24:551–553.

227. Sutedja G, Baris G, van Zandwijk N. High dose rate brachytherapy has a curative potential in patients with intraluminal squamous cell lung cancer. *Respiration* 1994;61:167–168.

228. Svoboda VH, Koyarik J, Morris F. High dose-rate microSelectron molds in the treatment of skin tumors. *Int J Radiat Oncol Biol Phys* 1995;31:967–972.

229. Taina E. High versus low dose rate intracavitary radiotherapy in the treatment of carcinoma of the uterus. *Acta Obstet Gynecol Scand Suppl* 1981;103:1–17.

230. Teshima T, Inoue T, Ikeda H, et al. High-dose rate and low-dose rate intracavitary therapy for carcinoma of the uterine cervix: Final results of Osaka University Hospital. *Cancer* 1993;72:2409–2414.

231. Toita T, Kakinohana Y, Ogawa K, et al. Combination external beam radiotherapy and high-dose-rate intracavitary brachytherapy for uterine cervical cancer: Analysis of doses and fractionation schedule. *Int J Radiat Oncol Biol Phys* 2003;56:1344–1353.

232. Tredaniel J, Hennequin C, Zalcman G, et al. Prolonged survival after high dose rate endobronchial radiation for malignant airway obstruction. *Chest* 1994;105:767–772.

233. Urban MS, Siegel JH, Pavlou W. Treatment of malignant biliary obstruction with a high-dose rate remote afterloading device using a 10F nasobiliary tube. *Gastrointest Endosc* 1990;36:292–296.

234. Van't Hooft E. The Selectron. In: Shearer DR, ed. *Recent advances in brachytherapy physics*. PM Monograph No. 7, New York: American Institute of Physics, 1981;167–177.

235. Vicini F, Beitsch P, Quiet C, et al. First analysis of patient demographics, technical reproducibility, cosmesis, and early toxicity: Results of the American Society of Breast Surgeons MammoSite breast brachytherapy registry trial. *Cancer* 2005;104:1138–1148.

236. Wakabayashi M, Ohsawa T, Mitsuhashi H, et al. High dose rate intracavitary radiotherapy using the Ralstron. Introduction and Part I. (Treatment of carcinoma of the uterine cervix). *Nippon Acta Radiol* 1971;31:340–378.

237. Walstam R. Studies on therapeutic short-distance and intracavitary gamma beam techniques. *Acta Radiol Suppl* 1965;236:1–129.

238. Wazer DE, Berle L, Graham R, et al. Preliminary results of a phase I/II study of HDR brachytherapy alone for T1/T2 breast cancer. *Int J Radiat Oncol Biol Phys* 2002;53:889–897.

239. Weiss E, Hirnle P, Arnold-Bofinger H, et al. Adjuvant vaginal high-dose-rate afterloading alone in endometrial carcinoma: Patterns of relapse and side effects following low-dose therapy. *Gynecol Oncol* 1998;71:72–76.

240. Yoshida K, Inoue T, Kuizumi M, et al. Perioperative high dose rate brachytherapy for bone and soft tissue tumors. *Nippon Igaku Hoshasen Gakkai Zasshi* 1996;41:1635–1641.

241. Yoshioka Y, Nose T, Yoshida K, et al. High-dose rate interstitial brachytherapy as a monotherapy for localized prostate cancer: Treatment description and preliminary results of a phase I/II clinical trial. *Int J Radiat Oncol Biol Phys* 2000;48:675–681.

242. Yoshioka Y, Nose T, Yoshida K, et al. High-dose rate brachytherapy as monotherapy for localized prostate cancer: A retrospective analysis with special focus on tolerance and chronic toxicity. *Int J Radiat Oncol Biol Phys* 2003;56:213–220.

243. Yu L, Vikram B, Chadha M, et al. High dose rate interstitial brachytherapy in patients with cancers of the head and neck. *Endocuriether Hypertherm Oncol* 1996;12:1–6.

244. Zajac AJ, Kohn ML, Heiser D, et al. High dose rate intraluminal brachytherapy in the treatment of endobronchial malignancy. *Radiology* 1993;187:571–575.

245. Zelefsky MJ, LaQuaglia MP, Ghavimi F, et al. Preliminary results of phase I/II study of high-dose rate intraoperative radiation therapy for pediatric tumors. *J Surg Oncol* 1996;62:267–272.

246. Zhao R-F, et al. Combination of external irradiation and intracavitary cesium-137 radiotherapy for esopharyngeal carcinoma. *Chin J Radiat Oncol Phys Biol* 1990;2:85–87.

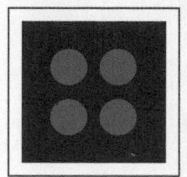

Chapter 23
Radioimmunoglobulins and Nonsealed Radionuclide Therapy

Reiner Class, Monika Jost, Stephan Mose, Hans-Walter Weber, Luther W. Brady

Radioimmunoglobulins

Basic Cancer Biology and Immunology

The immune system constantly screens the body for newly formed tumor cells and eliminates those as soon as potentially dangerous signals are detected. As a consequence, tumor cells are exposed to constant immune-selective pressure. Because most tumor cells are genetically instable, this pressure can lead to the generation of a new cell population capable of escaping recognition by the immune system (70). Several clinically relevant tumor cell evasion strategies have been described: Down-regulation of human lymphocyte antigen-I (HLA-I), breakdown of the antigen-processing machinery, suppression of natural killer cell activity, interference with apoptotic pathways, shedding and modification of antigens, release of immunosuppressive cytokines, lack of costimulation, and escape from cell cycle control (71).

For years, scientists have tried to overcome the immune system's tolerance of cancer cells by vaccination protocols intended to teach the immune system to rerecognize and subsequently eliminate those previously undetected cancer cells. However, most vaccinations were administered in late stages of the disease, at which time patients are often immunosuppressed or not very responsive to immunizations. It is therefore not surprising that vaccination-based immunotherapy regimens have not been more successful in the clinical setting. One important goal of antibody-based cancer therapy is to bypass the immune system's tolerance of autologous cancer cells. Some of these clinically relevant immune escape strategies will be described here.

Down-Regulation of HLA-I

The immune system is constantly surveying the body for "danger" signals. One such signal is the presentation of tumor-associated antigens (TAA) in context with the HLA-I and the recognition of this complex by regulatory T cells. The latter recognize the TAA/HLA-I complex and initiate a cascade of cellular events, ultimately resulting in the destruction of the respective cancer cell by highly potent cytotoxic T cells (CTLs). Some cancer cells acquire the ability to down-regulate the HLA portion of the complex and prohibit the presentation of TAA on their surface. Even if highly potent TAA-primed CTLs are present, they cannot recognize, bind to, and destroy the cancer cells. The "stealth" cancer cell evades recognition and keeps proliferating past the point at which CTLs could have controlled the tumor mass.

Breakdown of the Antigen-Processing Machinery

CTLs are the major effector cells that control tumor growth in humans (125). They recognize TAA in association with HLA-I only after those antigens have been processed by the antigen-processing machinery (APM). There is convincing evidence that deregulation of the APM leads to loss of CTL recognition, which is linked to malignant transformation of cells. Because the APM contains a multitude of different components, impairment of just one can prevent presentation of TAA-derived peptides to CTL, thereby providing tumor cells with a way to avoid recognition by the immune system (72).

Suppression of Natural Killer (NK) Cell Activity

The choice between stimulating or inhibitory activity is determined by the type and quality of the receptor-ligand interaction between NK and tumor cells. Recent evidence suggests that tumor cells can shift this balance toward inhibition by expression of nonclassic HLA molecules (e.g., E, F, and G). Impaired NK cell function has been described in many tumors including breast (59) and ovarian carcinoma (69), and melanoma (93).

Interference with Apoptosis Machinery

Apoptosis is one of the most important mechanisms by which unwanted cells, such as tumor cells, are eliminated from the body. Enhancing proapoptotic and inhibiting antiapoptotic pathways shifts the balance between cell death and survival toward tumor growth. It has been shown that in certain B-cell leukemias and lymphomas, the bcl-2 gene locus on chromosome 18 has been translocated to chromosome 14 in close proximity to an antibody heavy chain enhancer locus (16). As a consequence, the Bcl-2 protein is overexpressed, enhancing cell survival and allowing the cells to proliferate. Some melanoma cells can avoid apoptotic cell death by suppression of another proapoptotic gene, apaf-1. Other antiapoptotic escape mechanisms include killing of regulatory T cells by expression of Fas-Ligand (46) and blocking of apoptosis by expression of decoy receptors and secretion of soluble receptors (95).

Shedding and Modification of Antigens

Tumor cells shed TAA in large quantities, thereby overloading the immune system. As a consequence, T- and B-cell populations, initially directed against the tumor cells, become tolerant, so that an effective anticancer immune response is not initiated. Furthermore, TAA can also be withdrawn from the surface or even altered to evade recognition by T cells.

Antigenic Targets on Tumor Cells

The first attempts to direct the immune system against tumor cells were undertaken in the late 1800s by W. Coley, who observed that microbe-induced immune stimulation or, perhaps, the induced fever, resulted in the regression of tumors in a patient (44). Later, it was recognized that antibodies can be used as customizable weapons in the fight against cancer. Through the hybridoma technology developed by Köhler and Milstein (50), antibodies became readily available for clinical use in large quantities. Today's monoclonal antibodies (mAb) are used either "naked" or bound to a second component such as a toxin (i.e., immunotoxin) or a radionuclide (i.e., radioimmunoglobulin). The premise underlying cancer radioimmunotherapy (RIT) is that radionuclide-conjugated antibodies bind to their specific

| Table 23.1 | TUMOR-ASSOCIATED ANTIGENS AS TARGETS FOR ANTIBODY THERAPY |

Target	Cellular Expression	Biologic Functions	Oncology Indication
17-1A	Epithelial cells	Cell adhesion	Colorectal carcinoma
CEA	During fetal development only	Cell adhesion	Colorectal, non–small cell lung and breast carcinoma
CD20	B cells	Unknown	NHL
CD33	Myeloid progenitor cells, monocytes	Regulation of proliferation, differentiation and apoptosis	AML
CD52	Thymocytes, T cells, B cells (not plasma cells), monocytes, granulocytes	Unknown	B-CLL
EGFR (HER1, erbB-1)	Epidermis	Proliferation, antiapoptotic, angiogenesis, dedifferentiation, migration	Colorectal, head and neck cancer, lung
GD2	T-cell subset	Neuron function	Neuroectodermal (e.g., brain tumors, melanoma), epithelial cancers (small cell lung cancer)
GD3	T-cell subset	Neuron function	Neuroectodermal (e.g., brain tumors, melanoma), epithelial cancers (small cell lung cancer)
HER2 (erbB-2)	Epidermis	Proliferation, differentiation, survival	Breast carcinoma
MUC-1	Secretory epithelial cells	Cell protection	Epithelial tumors
VEGF	Epithelial cells	Proangiogenic	Solid tumors

CEA, carcinoembryonic antigen; NHL, non-Hodgkin's lymphoma; AML, acute myelogenous leukemia; B-CLL, B-cell chronic lymphocytic leukemia; EGFR, epidermal growth factor receptor; MUC1, mucine 1; VEGF, vascular endothelial growth factor receptor.

antigen on the tumor cell surface, thereby accumulating on the target cell and delivering cytotoxic doses of radiation to the tumor.

In order to channel the therapeutic potential of antibodies toward the tumor site and to prevent unwanted side effects toward normal tissue, antibodies need to be directed against antigens that are preferentially expressed on tumor cells. Those antigens have been termed *tumor-associated antigens (TAAs)* because they can be found in association with tumor cells, although not exclusively (Table 23.1). More recently, a specific type of TAA, the cancer/testis antigens, has been discovered as novel and promising targets. Cancer/testis antigens are normally expressed in healthy testicular tissue but become highly immunogenic in cancer patients (119). Because their expression is tissue-restricted, they represent an interesting target for antibody-based immunotherapy.

In the past decades, a large variety of TAA-specific mAbs have been raised. Today, they represent the largest class of biotechnological protein therapeutics: As of 2005, 18 different mAbs have been approved by the U.S. Federal Food and Drug Administration (FDA), 8 are used against cancer and 2 are used for RIT (Table 23.2).

Use of Monoclonal Antibodies in the Treatment of Cancer

Cancer cells often evade recognition and destruction by the immune system. Antibody-based therapeutics are designed to counteract these various evasion strategies. They release their antineoplastic potential in different ways: Some deliver the lethal hit directly to the tumor cell; others work indirectly through the initiation of secondary mechanisms, largely depending on the type of antibody employed.

We can discriminate four main classes of antibody-based therapeutics: Naked antibodies, conjugated antibodies, im-

munoliposomes, and antibody-cytokine fusion proteins. Naked antibodies are unmodified immunoglobulin molecules, whereas conjugated antibodies are attached to other agents (drugs, toxins, or radionuclides).

Naked Antibodies

Naked antibodies mimic naturally occurring antibodies and restore or support the immune response against cancer cells, affecting tumor cell growth and survival in different ways. Some flag the tumor cell for subsequent destruction by specialized components of the immune system, whereas others block stimulation by growth and survival factors through competitive binding to growth factor receptors on the cell surface. Antibody-dependent cell–mediated cytotoxicity and, less importantly, complement-dependent cytotoxicity, are the predominant mode of action for the anticancer effect of mAb (47). Although several naked antibodies (e.g., Herceptin, rituximab) have been used successfully in certain types of cancer, greater efficiency can be achieved by using the mAb to deliver a toxic payload to the tumor cell.

Antibody-drug conjugates combine the TAA-targeting properties of an antibody with the tumoricidal effects of a chemotherapeutic drug. The tandem is capable of delivering chemotherapeutic drugs directly to the tumor cell (121). Several standard chemotherapeutic agents, including antifolates, vinca alkaloids, and anthracyclines, have been linked to mAb and introduced into clinical development (reviewed in [121]). However, most proved to be inefficient because therapeutic drug concentrations were not achievable. To date, only one mAb-drug conjugate, Mylotarg (gemtuzumab ozogamicin), has been approved by the FDA for the treatment of cancer. The antibody moiety of Mylotarg is directed against the CD33 antigen, which is expressed on the majority of acute myeloid leukemia (AML) cells. The antibody is fused to ozogamicin, a highly toxic chemotherapeutic agent. Mylotarg is approved for the treatment of elderly

mAb Name	Trade Name	Company	Approval Year	Target Antigen	Indication	Antibody Type	Label
Rituximab	Rituxan	Genentech IDEC	US 1997 EU 1998	CD20	NHL	Chimeric	None
Trastuzumab	Herceptin	Genentech Hoffmann-La Roche	US 1998 EU 2001	HER2	Breast carcinoma	Humanized	None
Gemtuzumab ozogamicin	Mylotarg	Celltech Group Wyeth-Ayerst	US 2000	CD33	AML	Humanized	Drug
Alemtuzumab	Campath	Millenium/ILEX	US 2001 EU 2001	CD52	CLL	Humanized	None
Ibritumomab tiuxetan	Zevalin	Biogen IDEC Genentech Hoffmann-La Roche	US 2002	CD20	NHL	Murine	Radioisotope
Tositumo mab	Bexxar	Corixa Corp GlaxoSmithKline	US 2003	CD20	NHL	Murine	Radioisotope
Cetuximab	Erbitux	ImClone Merck	US 2004	EGFR	Colorectal carcinoma	Chimeric	None
Bevacizumab	Avastin	Genentech	US 2004	VEGF	Colorectal carcinoma	Humanized	None

Table 23.2 ANTIBODIES APPROVED BY THE FOOD AND DRUG ADMINISTRATION FOR THERAPEUTIC USE

US, United States; NHL, non-Hodgkin's lymphoma; EU, Europe; AML, acute myelogenous leukemia; CLL, chronic lymphocytic leukemia; EGFR, epidermal growth factor receptor; VEGF, vascular endothelial growth factor receptor.

patients with CD33-positive AML in their first relapse if they are not eligible for other chemotherapies.

Immunotoxins

Immunotoxins are conjugates in which the mAb is linked to a toxin. In contrast to low-molecular mass chemotherapeutic drugs, toxins are naturally occurring poisonous substances, usually peptides or proteins. The biggest advantage of toxins over chemotherapeutic drugs is that as little as one single toxin molecule is usually sufficient to induce tumor cell death, whereas chemotherapeutic agents have to reach high intracellular concentrations.

Radioimmunoglobulins

Radioimmunoglobulins combine the natural properties of an antibody with the physical effects of a radionuclide to efficiently seek and destroy cancer cells. One of the most promising approaches is to use mAb that recognize and/or antagonize growth receptors (e.g., epidermal growth factor receptor {EGFR}) as carriers for radioactivity. In doing so, several advantages can be combined to obtain maximal therapeutic effect: The antigen-specific mAb specifically seeks out cancer cells distributed throughout the entire body (including micrometastases), the binding of the mAb to growth factor receptors blocks growth- and survival-promoting signals (e.g., epidermal growth factor) and the radioactive payload delivers a potentially lethal dose of radiation directly to the tumor cell. It is therefore not surprising that many mAb successfully used as cancer therapeutics are directed against molecules involved in the regulation of proliferation or apoptosis (e.g., CD33, CEA, Her2, EGFR, VEGF).

As of 2006, two radiolabeled antibodies have been approved in the United States for the treatment of cancer: Zevalin (90Y-ibritumomab, tiuxetan; Biogen IDEC Corporation, San Diego, CA) and Bexxar (131I-tositumomab; Glaxo-Smith-Kline, Philadelphia, PA). Both mAb target the CD20-antigen, a pan B-lymphocyte marker expressed on both healthy and malignant B cells

Immunoliposomes and Radioimmunoliposomes

Immunoliposomes are vesicles composed of a phospholipid bilayer with a toxic component encapsulated in their core and mAb bound to their surface. Attachment of the antibody moiety is achieved either by coupling mAb directly to the lipid bilayer or to PEG (polyethylene glycol) chains that are attached to the liposomal surface. The antibody secures the targeted delivery of the liposome together with its toxic content to the tumor cell surface antigens where the toxic load is released (141). The idea of targeting liposomes to specific cells by coupling mAbs to the liposome surface was born more than 25 years ago (42,60). Since then, the technology has undergone many improvements to overcome problems with stability, immunogenicity, and rapid elimination from the circulation by the reticuloendothelial system (51). One of the major advancements was stabilization of liposomes by coating with PEG (stealth liposomes). Immunoliposomes are especially attractive for treatment of intraperitoneal tumors because of their high retention time in the intraperitoneal cavity compared with antibody molecules, which tend to escape and, thus, are taken up by other tissues (139). Despite the fact that promising results have already been obtained *in vitro* (39) as well as in animal models (66), immunoliposomes have not been widely introduced into the clinical setting. A few formulations of liposomally delivered cytotoxic drugs have been approved for cancer treatment, such as anti-Her2 Doxil (ALZA Corp., Mountain View, CA) and doxorubicin-loaded sterically stabilized anti-Her2 immunoliposomes (92).

So far, clinical applications of radiolabeled liposomes have been limited to diagnostic imaging; however, their potential for radionuclide therapy is currently being explored by several groups. A study in Greece, in which patients with glioblastoma (GBM) or brain metastases were infused with ^{99}mTc-diethylenetriaminepentaacetic acid (DTPA)-Caelyx (doxorubicin PEG liposomes), demonstrated that radiolabeled liposomes can cross

Techniques, Modalities, and Modifiers in Radiation Oncology

the blood–brain barrier (53). The liposomes accumulated in brain tumors with a high tumor-to-normal brain ratio. A more complex multistep approach for radioliposomal treatment was explored by Xiao et al. (146) *in vitro*. They used a combination of anti-CA-125 and antibiotin bispecific Ab and biotinylated liposomes loaded with surface-bound ^{188}Re and showed specific binding and slow internalization of liposomes without significant shedding. Sapra and Allen (115) compared the efficacy of targeting an internalizing antigen (CD19) versus a noninternalizing antigen (CD20) toward a namalwa B-cell lymphoma xenograft. Efficacy was increased when both liposomes were combined, which was confirmed by another study (57). The emerging nanotechnology is making an impact in this field in the shape of shell-crosslinked nanoparticles (SCKs) for targeting cancer cells. A group at Washington University studied folate- and unconjugated SCKs in KB cell xenografts (114). The nanospheres were labeled with ^{64}Cu for imaging and therapy. Despite high uptake into the reticuloendothelial system, SCKs exhibited long circulation in blood and were able to passively accumulate in tumors. In small-sized tumors, interaction with the folate receptor could be demonstrated.

Antibody-Cytokine Fusion Proteins

Antibody-cytokine fusion proteins are composed of a single amino acid chain tandem of an anti-TAA mAb and a cytokine. The goal is to use the TAA-specific mAb to deliver the cytokine to the immediate vicinity of the tumor and, in doing so, to directly enhance the therapeutic effect of the antibody and/or augment the host's immune response against the tumor. Cytokines used as fusion partner include, but are not limited to, interleukin (IL)-2, IL-12, and GM-CSF. Initial preclinical results are encouraging (94), but no clinical data are available yet.

Monoclonal Antibodies

Development of Monoclonal Antibodies

The clinical development of mAbs was largely hampered by the patients' immune response against the "foreign" murine part of the mAb. This "human antimouse antibody" (HAMA) response results in neutralization of the biologic effects of mAb and their quick removal from the circulation. Advances in antibody production technology led to the development of antibodies in which the potentially antigenic mouse portion of the mAb—the constant (Fc) domain—was replaced with a much less antigenic human Fc part. It was now possible to genetically engineer chimeric, humanized, and fully human antibodies in which the mouse component could be decreased by ~67%, 90% to 95%, or 100%, respectively. The residual "original" murine portion in fully humanized mAb hides within the highly variable, antigen-binding domain of the complementary determining regions. The first humanized mAb was the anti-CD52 mAb Campath. Although humanized and fully human antibodies are a major improvement over murine mAb, they still are foreign proteins that can trigger the generation of potentially neutralizing human antihuman antibodies (HAHA). A special type of HAMA is the so-called anti-idiotypic antibody that mimics the "internal image" of the antigen recognized by the therapeutic antibody. Despite the neutralizing effect, an anti-idiotypic immune response has been associated with improved outcome in many patients (79).

Antibodies often cannot penetrate larger tumor masses because of their relatively large size (~170 kDa). One approach to overcome this limitation was to reduce their size by eliminating parts of the constant region that is not required for antigen binding (Fig. 23.1). Single-chain variable fragments antibodies (scFvs) are still capable of antigen-binding but are reduced to

the hypervariable region of the antibody. Unavoidably, biologic effects associated with other constant regions of mAb, such as the Fc portion, will be lost in the process. Although smaller antibody fragments have better tumor penetration, especially into poorly vascularized regions, their reduced size can result in much faster clearance from the circulation and reduced retention at the tumor site (85).

In oncology, antibodies were initially used exclusively as diagnostic tools up to the late 1980s. In 1995, the first mAb was approved in Germany for adjuvant treatment of patients with colorectal carcinoma (CRC). Panorex was raised against the CRC-associated TAA 17-1A that is highly expressed on most colon carcinoma cells. A clinical study conducted by Riethmüller et al. (105) demonstrated that the mAb reduced metastasis in one third of the patients after curative resection of stage III CRC (Dukes' C) paired with improved survival. However, larger studies failed to show an improvement over standard care, and Panorex was withdrawn from the market in 2001.

The Choice of Isotopes

The rationale behind therapeutic use of radioimmunoglobulins is the targeted delivery of a specific radiation dose to a tumor cell while reducing unwanted exposure of the surrounding normal tissue. Several radionuclides have been studied in clinical settings (Table 23.3). Isotopes emitting mainly β-radiation are preferably used for therapeutic approaches, whereas γ-emitters are favored for imaging purposes. Yttrium-90 (^{90}Y) and iodine-131 (^{131}I) are the most widely used radionuclides for RIT. The choice of radioisotope for a particular application depends on factors such as tumor penetration, simplicity of labeling, stability of isotope-antibody complex, toxicity, half-life, cost of production, and radiation exposure of health care personnel. Furthermore, the particular features of the mAb must be considered. If the antibody-antigen complex is internalized on binding, one might select an isotope with high linear energy transfer (LET) and low γ-component (e.g., ^{90}Y) to deliver a high radiation dose to the nucleus with very little effect on neighboring cells. If an effect on neighboring cells is desirable (bystander effect), an isotope with a high γ-component (e.g., ^{131}I) might be the more appropriate choice, whereas an antibody that is deposited in close proximity to the nucleus should be labeled with an isotope decaying by electron capture, thus emitting very high LET Auger electrons (e.g., ^{125}I). The choice of radionuclide and administration scheme (single bolus vs. fractionation vs. infusion) further depends on the tumor type and size. Smaller tumors should be treated with a single dose of a radionuclide emitting short-range radiation, and for larger tumor masses, fractionated application of a long-range radiation emitter is indicated (86). Regardless of the isotope used, the total dose of radiation deposited on the tumor cell has to overcome sublethal DNA damage repair and must prevent proliferation or even induce cell death (27).

RIT Toxicity

In general, RIT is well tolerated compared with other standard treatment regimens. Toxicities observed for radiolabeled mAb used in therapy are primarily hematologic. Patients treated with the FDA-approved mAb Bexxar and Zevalin required supportive measures with platelet transfusions (22% and 15%, respectively), erythropoietin or epoetin alfa (8% and 7%, respectively) or filgrastim (13% and 12%, respectively) (128). The radiation-emitting component is a significant source of toxicity. Radionuclides with a pathlength of several millimeters (e.g., ^{131}I) can cause collateral damage to the surrounding normal tissue (e.g., bone marrow), especially at higher tumor burden, causing myelosuppression and subsequent loss of mature cells, which can be fatal. In contrast to chemotherapy, nadir counts

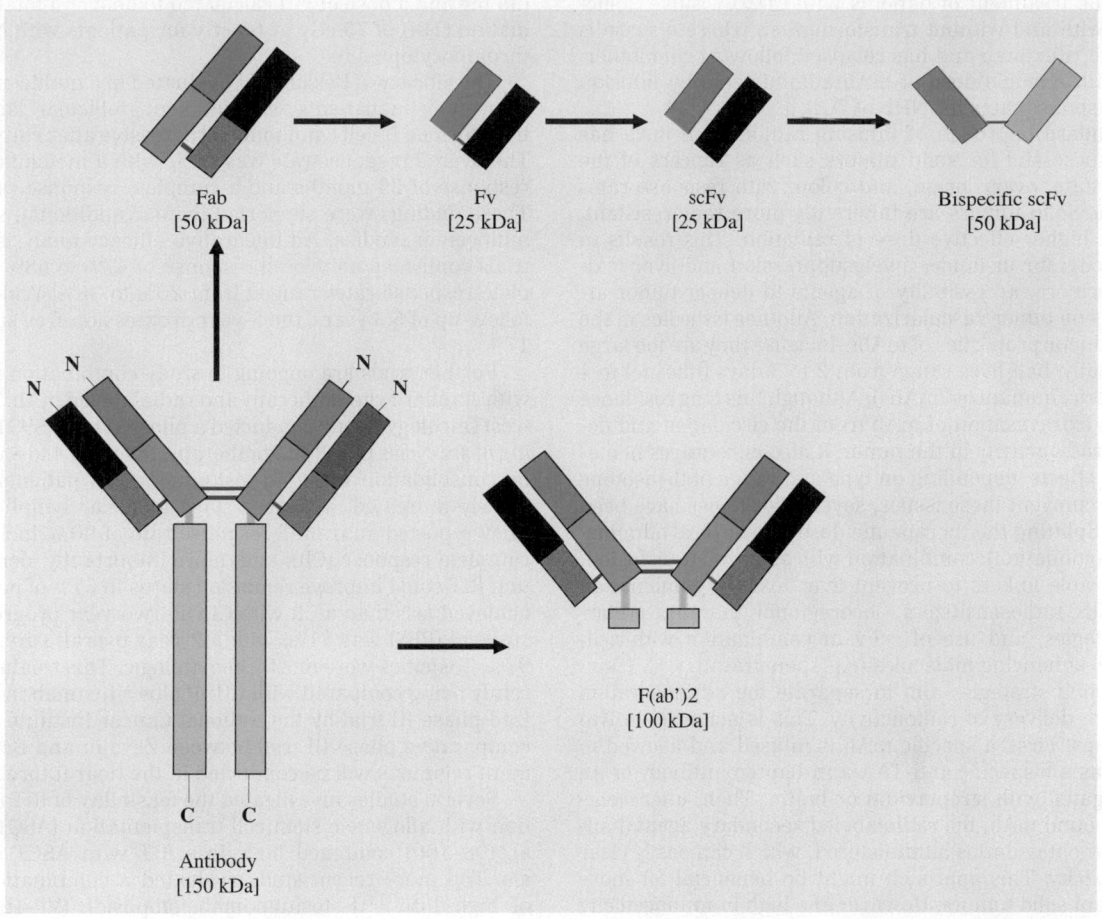

FIGURE 23.1. Schematic representation of an antibody (IgG) and its smaller fragments used for clinical purposes. Fab, antigen-binding fragment; Fv, variable fragment; scFv, single-chain variable fragment

in patients treated with RIT often occur several weeks later (18). Another source of toxicity are immune responses against the antibody component such as HAHA, but those are infrequent (<2%). Serious adverse events are rare (36). Nevertheless, even minor changes in a patient's response to antibody binding have the potential to impair downstream processes, which can cause severe side effects and even death. The most common nonhematologic toxicities include nausea, chills, fever, muscle cramps, and abdominal pain, which are subsumed as "cytokine release symptom/acute infusion reaction" and represent a separate category of symptoms in the FDA Common Toxicity Criteria (14). Those symptoms are mostly transient in nature and can be managed with medication.

Clinical Results

The biggest progress so far has been achieved in RIT of hematopoietic cancers. Leukemias and lymphomas are attractive targets for RIT because of their radiosensitivity and good accessibility of the malignant cells to circulating radiolabeled antibodies. Two anti-CD20 antibodies for RIT in lymphoma are approved in the United States: Zevalin (^{90}Y-ibritumomab) and Bexxar (^{131}I-tositumomab) for the treatment of non-Hodgkin's lymphoma (NHL). Zevalin was approved in the United States and Europe for the treatment of relapsed or refractory follicular/low-grade or transformed NHL, including rituximab-refractory follicular NHL. Bexxar was approved in the United

| Table 23.3 | RADIONUCLIDES USED IN RADIOIMMUNOTHERAPY AND THEIR CHARACTERISTICS |

Characteristic	^{67}Cu	^{125}I	^{131}I	^{186}Re	^{188}Re	^{90}Y
Chemical name	Copper	Iodine	Iodine	Rhenium	Rhenium	Yttrium
Principal radiation emitted	β	EC,γ	β,γ	β,γ	β,γ	β
α-Energy (MeV)	0	0	0	0	0	0
β-Energy (MeV)	0.40	0	0.606	1.07	0.12	2.25
γ-Energy (MeV)	0	0.036	0.364	0	0	0
Mean β-path length (nm)	0.3	n/a	0.4	0.9	2.4	2.5
$t_{1/2}$ (days)	2.5	59.4	8.04	3.7	0.7	2.7
Auger electrons	No	Yes	No	No	No	No

EC, electronic capture.

States for the treatment of patients with CD20-positive, follicular NHL, with and without transformation, whose disease is refractory to rituximab and has relapsed following chemotherapy. RIT with a single dose of mAb administered by infusion achieved response rates for NHL of 70% to 80%.

The standard approach of infusing radiolabeled mAb has been less successful for solid tumors such as cancers of the breast, prostate, ovary, brain, and colon, with response rates often <10%. Solid tumors are inherently more radioresistant, requiring a higher effective dose of radiation. This results in higher toxicity; for instance, myelosuppression and liver toxicity. Furthermore, accessibility of agents to deeper tumor areas depends on tumor vascularization. Another issue lies in the pharmacokinetic properties of mAbs. Because they are too large to clear readily, half-lives range from 2 to 3 days (murine) to 4 days (chimeric, humanized mAbs). Although this long residence time allows extravasation of mAb from the circulation and deposition of radioactivity in the tumor, it also encourages hematologic side effects, depending on type and range of the isotope used. To circumvent these issues, several strategies have been developed: Splitting the therapeutic dose into several administrations (fractionation), combination with stem cell transfusion, use of cleavable linkers to prevent liver toxicity, combination therapy with radiosensitizers, locoregional therapy, pretargeting strategies, and use of scFv in combination with cell-penetration–enhancing molecules (e.g., penetratin).

Pretargeting strategies aim to separate the administration of mAb from delivery of radioactivity. This is achieved in two or more steps. First, a specific mAb is infused and allowed to bind, such as a bispecific anti-TAA/anti-hapten antibody or an mAb conjugated with streptavidin or biotin. Then, after clearance of unbound mAb, the radiolabeled secondary agent (hapten/biotin/streptavidin) is administered, which can easily clear to avoid toxicity. This approach might be beneficial for more radioresistant solid tumors. However, the high immunogenicity of streptavidin and biotin limits their application to one single injection.

Radioimmunoglobulin Therapy in Leukemia and Lymphoma

Zevalin, one of two radiolabeled mAbs approved for oncology, is a conjugate of mAb (ibritumomab) covalently attached to the linker-chelator tiuxetan and bound to ^{90}Y. The antibody is a murine immununoglobulin-G ($IgG_1\kappa$) recognizing the CD20 antigen on the surface of normal and malignant B lymphocytes. CD20 is expressed on >90% of NHL B cells. ^{90}Y emits β-particles with a range of up to 5 mm, which makes this isotope useful even for large tumor masses. Cell damage is caused by radiation-induced formation of free (oxygen) radicals in the target and neighboring tumor cells (cross-fire or bystander effect). Zevalin-RIT is a two-step regimen in which 250 mg/m^2 rituximab with a fixed dose of 5 mCi (1.6 mg total antibody dose) of ^{111}In-ibritumomab is first infused, followed 7 to 9 days later by a second therapeutic dose of 250 mg/m^2 of rituximab with 0.4 mCi/kg of ^{90}Y-ibritumomab. A randomized controlled trial demonstrated that Zevalin-RIT is more effective than rituximab for patients with relapsed indolent NHL, achieving an overall response rate of 80% compared with 56% in the rituximab group (144).

Bexxar is a conjugate of mAb (tositumomab) covalently attached to ^{131}I. The antibody is a murine IgG$_2\lambda$, recognizing the CD20 antigen. Similar to Zevalin-RIT, the lethal cell damage is caused by cross-fire effect. Bexxar-RIT is also a multistep treatment. For dosimetry, 5 mCi ^{131}I and tositumomab (35 mg) are infused with 450 mg unlabeled tositumomab. The therapeutic phase starts 7 to 14 days later and consists of sequential infusions of unlabeled tositumomab (450 mg), followed by Bexxar

(35 mg and a dose of ^{131}I calculated to deliver a total body irradiation (TBI) of 75 cGy or 65 cGy for patients with NCI grade I thrombocytopenia).

The efficacy of Bexxar was evaluated in a multicenter, single-arm study in patients with indolent, follicular large-cell, or transformed B-cell lymphoma, progressive after rituximab (45). The overall response rate was 63%, with a median duration of response of 25 months and a complete response rate of 29%. These findings were supported by four additional, single-arm, multicenter studies. An integrative efficacy analysis of all five trials confirmed an overall response of 47% to 68% (34). Complete response rates ranged from 20% to 38%. With a median follow-up of 5.3 years, the 5-year progression-free survival was 17%.

Further trials are ongoing to study combination treatments with standard chemotherapy and radiolabeled mAb. The Southwest Oncology Group conducted a phase II trial (S9911) consisting of six cycles CHOP chemotherapy, followed 4 to 8 weeks later by consolidation with ^{131}I-tositumomab in patients with previously untreated, advanced-stage follicular lymphoma (100). They reported an overall response rate of 90%, including 67% complete response (CR), and, more importantly, demonstrated that RIT could improve remission status in 57% of patients who achieved less than a CR with CHOP. Two-year progression-free survival (PFS) was 81%, with a 2-year overall survival (OS) of 97%. Toxicities were mostly hematologic. This treatment is currently being compared with CHOP plus rituximab in a randomized phase III trial by the National Cancer Institute (S0016). A comparative phase III trial between Zevalin and Bexxar treatment regimens will be conducted in the near future (21).

Several studies investigated the feasibility of RIT in conjunction with allogeneic stem cell transplantation (ASCT). Press et al. (98–100) combined high-dose RIT with ASCT in two trials. The more recent study evaluated a combination therapy of high-dose ^{131}I- tositumomab, etoposide (VP-16), and cyclophosphamide with ASCT in patients with NHL and demonstrated favorable outcome compared with patients treated with chemotherapy and TBI. A similar phase I/II study demonstrated feasibility of high-dose ^{90}Y-ibritumomab tiuxetan in combination with high-dose VP-16 and cyclophosphamide followed by ASCT in patients with CD20$^+$ NHL without additional toxicity (83). Recently, Fietz et al. (32) reported good engraftment in a study combining ^{90}Y-tositumomab, rituximab, and fludarabine/cyclophosphamide with ASCT. Thus, RIT can be safely incorporated into regimens using ASCT.

The CD45 antigen has been targeted to improve outcome in bone marrow transplants (BMTs). CD45 is a cell-surface glycoprotein broadly expressed by all circulating leukocytes and lymphocytes and by approximately 70% of nucleated cells in normal marrow, but not by cells outside the lymphoid and hematopoietic lineages. Mathews et al. (73) showed that it is possible to deliver two to four times more radiation to the target organs (marrow and spleen) without excessive toxicity by using the ^{131}I-labeled anti-CD45 mAb BC-8 to specifically target the bone marrow in a cyclophosphamide/TBI BMT protocol in AML and acute lymphocytic leukemia. In a follow-up study (74), biodistribution and toxicity of escalating doses of ^{131}I-labeled anti-CD45 mAb in combination with 120 mg/kg cyclophosphamide and 12 Gy TBI prior to BMT were investigated in patients with advanced acute leukemias (AML, acute myelogenous leukemia) or myelodysplastic syndrome (MDS). Favorable distribution to the bone marrow was confirmed. Maximum tolerated dose (MTD) was reached at 10.5 Gy delivered to the liver.

BMT is still problematic in older patients. CD66, a marker of early normal granulopoietic cells, was targeted by RIT to replace TBI in this patient population. Bunjes et al. (11,12) attempted to intensify the conditioning regimen using ^{188}Re-labeled anti-CD66 mAb. They could deliver a mean dose of 15.5 Gy to the red marrow without increasing acute organ toxicity. The dose-limiting organ was the kidney, with 11% of patients developing late radiation nephropathy due to *in vivo* instability of [188]Re-conjugates. In a follow-up study (106), [188]Re or ^{90}Y-labeled anti-CD66 mAb were used as part of a dose-reduced conditioning regimen followed by a T-cell–depleted graft for patients with AML and MDS ≥55 years of age. Dosimetry was favorable in all patients, allowing them to proceed to transplant, indicating feasibility of this regimen. RIT provided a mean dose of 21.9(± 8.4) Gy to the bone marrow with a significantly higher dose when ^{90}Y was used instead of [188]Re.

Several RIT studies targeted the CD33 antigen as conditioning treatment for allogeneic BMT. CD33 is expressed by myeloid progenitors and monocytes. Initial studies demonstrated localization to the bone marrow and internalization of ^{131}I-labeled anti-CD33 M195 mAb (120). A recent phase I study (13) investigated the safety of combining ^{131}I-labeled anti-CD33-mAb M195 or its humanized version, HuM195 (122 to 437 mCi), with busulfan and cyclophosphamide as conditioning treatment for allogeneic BMT in patients with AML, chronic myelogenous leukemia, or MDS. They demonstrated absorption of radioactivity to the target organs and showed feasibility of this approach. Hyperbilirubinemia was the most common extramedullary toxicity. Sgouros et al. (127) evaluated HuM195, labeled with the short-lived alpha emitter [213]Bi, for pharmacokinetics and dosimetry. Patients in this phase I trial received a dose of 0.6 to 1.6 GBq and were imaged immediately after injection. The [213]Bi-labeled mAb was proven suitable for imaging. The absorbed dose ratio between target organs and the whole body for [213]Bi-HuM195 was 1,000-fold greater than that commonly observed with β-emitting radionuclides used for RIT.

Epratuzumab (Immunomedics, Morris Plains, NJ) is the humanized version of the LL2 mAb, which targets CD22 on B-cell lymphoma (132). CD22 is a B-cell–restricted, lineage-dependent antigen that has been suggested to play a role as component of the B-cell activation complex (117) and as an adhesion molecule (29). Linden et al. (65) initiated a phase I/II trial for B-cell NHL with fractionated dosing of unlabeled and ^{90}Y-labeled epratuzumab. Patients received 2 to 4 weekly administrations of 185 MBq/m^2 (5 mCi/m^2) ^{90}Y-epratuzumab coinfused with unconjugated mAb at 1.5 mg/kg/wk. Dosimetry was performed by coinfusion of 180 MBq/m^2 [111]I-epratuzumab at first dosing. This treatment achieved an objective response in 62% of patients (25% complete response) and 14 to 41 months of event-free survival. Response correlated with CD22 expression. Hematologic toxicity was moderate, and dose-limiting hematologic toxicity was not encountered until the fourth weekly dose. No HAHA response was observed.

The IL-2Rα is a target for RIT in adult T-cell lymphocytic leukemia, a very aggressive form of leukemia induced by human T-cell lymphotropic retrovirus I. The receptor is not expressed on resting T cells, B cells, or monocytes, but on populations of malignant T cells in certain forms of lymphoma and leukemia. Waldmann et al. (143) performed successive trials with ^{90}Y-labeled anti-tac, a mouse monoclonal IgG$_{2a}$ antibody that targets the IL-2Rα in adult T-cell lymphocytic leukemia. After demonstrating safety, they administered a uniform dose of ^{90}Y-anti-tac. At the 5 to 15 mCi doses, 9 of 16 evaluable patients responded with a partial response (PR) (7 patients) or CR (2 patients). Toxicity was largely limited to the hematopoietic system.

Radioimmunoglobulin Therapy in Solid Tumors

EGFR (ErbB-1) overexpression occurs in many solid tumors of epithelial origin, including head and neck, breast, and colon carcinomas and often correlates with unfavorable outcome. The EGFR is also overexpressed in GBM, the most common and fatal primary brain tumor in adults. Our own group at Drexel University College of Medicine is conducting a phase I/II trial to assess the efficacy of adjuvant treatment with ^{125}I-labeled anti–EGF-R mAb 425 in patients with astrocytoma with anaplastic foci (AAF) and GBM. The mAb 425, a murine IgG$_{2a}$ antibody, was raised against the EGFR-overexpressing A431 epidermoid carcinoma cell line and binds to the external domain of the human EGFR, thereby inhibiting ligand binding, stimulating receptor internalization and down-regulation of the EGFR without stimulation of tyrosine kinase activity (111). After surgical debulking and radiation therapy, patients in this trial (>180 patients with AAF and GMB) received a fractionated treatment regimen of three infusions of ^{125}I-labeled mAb 425 to deliver a cumulative mean dose of 140 mCi (5.2 GBq) while avoiding myelosuppression. With surgery and radiation therapy alone, median survival of GBM patients is about 12.1 months. Adjuvant therapy with ^{125}I-mAb 425 increased overall median survival to 13.4 for GBM and 50.9 months for AAF (28). HAMA responses or acute toxicities were rarely observed. Recently, temozolomide (Temodal; Schering-Plough, Kenilworth, NJ) has been approved for adjuvant chemotherapy in GBM and AAF and is now part of the current standard of care for GBM (surgical resection, followed by adjuvant radiotherapy and adjuvant chemotherapy with temozolomide). Low-dose chemotherapy with temozolomide used concurrently with radiation followed by an additional 6 months of adjuvant temozolomide showed a statistically significant increase of median survival to 14.6 months in GBM (19). We are currently investigating whether adding adjuvant treatment with ^{125}I-mAb 425 to this regimen will offer an additional advantage.

The TAA carcinoembryonic antigen (CEA) is expressed in various types of solid malignancies, including colorectal, small cell lung, and thyroid cancer. Wong et al. (145) evaluated ^{90}Y-radiolabeled anti-CEA chimeric antibody T84.66 in a phase I trial in patients with CEA-expressing malignancies. Chimeric T84.66 (cT84.66) is a high-affinity anti-CEA IgG$_1$. After imaging with [111]I-labeled T84.66, a single therapeutic dose of ^{90}Y-labeled mAb was given 1 to 2 weeks later and clearing agent DTPA was infused for the following 3 days. CEA-antibody complexes were detected in the serum of all three patients treated, but a therapeutic dose was not reached, and two patients developed HACA response. Mittal et al. (80) combined ^{131}I anti-CEA mAb IMMU-4 mAb, (Immunomedics) with hyperthermia in a phase I/II trial in patients with advanced CRC. Patients who tested positive for tumor uptake received 30 or 60 mCi/m^2 mAb and hyperthermia. Although treatment was well tolerated, no beneficial effect was observed. Vuillez et al. (142) used a pretargeting approach in a phase I/II trial in patients with small cell lung cancer. Patients were first injected with a bispecific anti-CEA/anti-DTPA antibody and 4 days later with di-(In-DTPA)-tyrosyl-lysine hapten labeled with 1.48–6.66 GBq (40 to 180 mCi) of [131]I. Of 12 patients evaluated, 9 showed tumor progression, 2 had partial responses, and 1 had stable disease of more than 24 months. Efficiency and toxicity were dose-related. The maximal tolerable dose without hematologic rescue was 150 mCi. In a parallel phase I/II trial, a similar approach was tested in 26 patients with recurrent medullary thyroid cancer. Patients were injected with anti-CEA/N alpha-(diethylenetriamine-N,N,N′,N″-tetraacetic acid)-In bispecific Ab, F6-734, and 40 to 100 mCi of ^{131}I-hapten 4 days apart (54). Of 17 evaluable patients, 4 cases of pain relief, 5 minor tumor responses, and 4 biologic responses of thyrocalcitonin decrease were reported. Nine patients developed HAMA. Dose-limiting toxicity was hematologic with an MTD of 48 mCi/m^2. Therapeutic responses occurred mainly in patients with small tumor burden, suggesting an application for the treatment of minimal residual disease. To reduce immunogenicity, a ^{131}I-labeled humanized version of the bispecific antibody, composed of humanized anti-CEA antibody hMN14 (labetuzumab; Immunomedics, Morris Plains, NJ) and the murine antihapten mAb m734, were developed by the same group (55) and studied in 22 patients with various solid tumors (56). Patients received two doses of chimeric bispecific Ab, followed by infusion with escalating doses of ^{131}I-hapten 5 days later. In 9 of 22 patients, stable disease was achieved, correlating with antibody dose. These studies demonstrate the importance of the timing of immune agent administration and radioactivity dose carried by the hapten.

High-dose ^{90}Y-labeled humanized labetuzumab was combined in another phase I clinical trial with doxorubicin and peripheral blood stem cell rescue in patients with advanced medullary thyroid cancer (128). After complexing circulating CEA with unlabeled mAb, treatment was escalated from 740 to 1,850 MBq/m^2. Antibody infusion was followed by bolus administration of doxorubicin (60 mg/m^2) 1 day later. Tumor targeting with the antibody was excellent; however, overall response was low. ^{131}I-labetuzumab was used in a phase II trial in patients after salvage resection of colorectal metastases in the liver (64). A total of 23 patients received doses of 40 to 60 mCi/m^2 of ^{131}I-labetuzumab and showed improved median survival of 68 months compared to 28 to 40 months (historical data) or 31 months for contemporaneous controls.

Another attractive target molecule for RIT in solid tumors is tenascin-C, an extracellular matrix glycoprotein, which is abundantly expressed in the stroma of several solid tumors (67,84). Tenascin is a hexameric glycoprotein that can undergo alternative splicing, resulting in large (up to 320 kDa monomer) or small (220 kDa monomer) isoforms. The large variant, which is preferentially expressed in malignant tissues, has been shown to facilitate metastasis through its antiadhesive effects (35,48). This variant is ubiquitously expressed in high-grade gliomas, but not in normal brain, and plays a significant role in a variety of cellular processes that facilitate astrocytic tumor cell invasion and migration, endothelial cell spreading, adhesion, and proliferation. Tenascin-C expression was exploited in several clinical trials in patients with GBM. In trials performed at Duke University, a ^{131}I-labeled murine antitenascin mAb (^{131}I-mu81C6) was used for locoregional treatment of patients with GBM. The 81C6-antitenascin mAb (IgG$_{2b}$) binds to an epitope within the alternatively spliced fibronectin type III region of tenascin-C (TN-C). In a phase I trial, 3,700 MBq in recurrent tumors and 4,400 MBq in primary treatment injected directly into the surgical cavity were established as MTD (20). In follow-up trials, efficacy of intratumoral injection (120 mCi) was demonstrated by increase of median survival in patients with newly diagnosed or recurrent glioma (102,103). Newly diagnosed patients received a single injection of labeled antibody (120 mCi, 4,400 MBq), followed by conventional external-beam radiotherapy and chemotherapy, and had an overall median survival of 87 (all patients) and 79 weeks (GBM). Patients with recurrent primary or metastatic malignant brain tumors were treated with 100 mCi (3,700 MBq) locoregionally into the surgical cavity, followed by chemotherapy. Median survival was greater than that of historical controls treated with surgery plus ^{125}I brachytherapy; 79% of patients developed HAMA. The authors conclude that the optimal dose to the surgical resection cavity margin is 44 Gy and propose future studies with an initial dosimetry step to optimize the dose for the individual patient.

Application of antitenascin mAb is not limited to solid tumors. A group at Duke University observed involvement of tenascin in NHL. Tenascin-C expression is increased in the tumor stroma and correlates with increased resistance and disease progression (109). In a phase I trial, ^{131}I-labeled chimeric 81C6 mAb was administered intravenously to patients with NHL. Activity was escalated down from 1,480 MBq (4 mCi) to 1,110 MBq (30 mCi) because of hematologic toxicity. Of nine patients treated, one had a complete and one had a partial re-

sponse. No HACA response was elicited. Other antitenascin antibodies (e.g., BC-2 and BC-4) were also studied. In a trial in Italy by Riva et al. (107), more than 100 patients with high-grade malignant glioma were treated locoregionally with up to six courses of ^{131}I-BC-2 and BC-4 (1,809.3 MBq per cycle). They conclude that outcomes were more favorable in with small tumor burden (22 of 62 evaluable patients) compared with patients with macroscopic disease (22 of 62 evaluable patients), both in terms of median survival (27 vs. 17 months) and response rate (70% vs. 17%). The same group also performed a phase I study with ^{90}Y-labeled mAb with similar median survival for GBM (108).

TAG-72 antigen is a high-molecular-weight glycoprotein expressed on adenocarcinomas of the breast (68), colon (133), and lung (134). It is recognized by the murine mAb CC49 (Dow Chemical Company, Midland, MI). Divgi et al. (26) treated patients with TAG-72-expressing metastatic colon carcinoma with ^{131}I-labeled in a clinical phase I trial and established an MTD of 75 mCi/m^2, confirming a previous trial by Murray et al. (82). Interferon (IFN)-α and IFN-γ have been shown to enhance expression of TAG-72 tumor antigen and improve localization of radiolabeled antibody to tumor cells (81,113). This was exploited in a clinical trial targeting hormone refractory prostate cancer (130), in which patients were pretreated with IFN-γ 7 days prior to ^{131}I-CC49 infusion. All 14 patients (of 16) who responded with up-regulation of TAG-72 were treated with the radiolabeled mAb at 75 mCi/m^2. Although local uptake of ^{131}I-CC49 was demonstrated, no response was achieved, but the dose may have been subtherapeutic according to dosimetry calculations. Meredith et al. (78) treated ovarian cancer patients with IFN and ^{77}Lu-labeled CC49 in a phase I study and studied combination treatment of ^{90}Y-CC49 with IFN and chemotherapy (2). In both studies, the mAb was applied into the peritoneal cavity; IFN-α 2b was given subcutaneously and paclitaxel was given intraperitoneally. The MTD for ^{90}Y-CC49 (intraperitoneally) was reached at 24 mCi/m^2. In two of nine patients with measurable disease, a partial response was achieved. The group plans on using a humanized genetically engineered version of CC49 in future trials.

Another epitope expressed on epithelial tumors (lung, colon, breast, prostate, and ovary) as well as some normal tissues including gastrointestinal epithelium (87), Ep-CAM, was targeted in clinical trials using pretargeting techniques with the murine mAb NR-LU-10. After optimization in a phase I trial (9), patients with metastatic colon cancer were treated with a three-step procedure in a phase II trial (49). Patients received sequential infusions of NR-LU-10/streptavidin on day 1, clearing agent (biotin-galactose-human serum albumin) on day 2, and biotin-DOTA-labeled with 110 mCi/m^2 ^{90}Y (^{90}Y-tetra-azacyclododecanetetra-acetic acid-biotin) on day 3. Patients experienced both hematologic and nonhematologic toxicities, mostly severe gastrointestinal toxicity. Therapeutic response was very limited (8% overall response rate).

RIT is not limited to using a single antibody molecule. A group in Italy (37) treated patients with metastatic ovarian cancer with cocktail of antibodies in a three-step phase I protocol. First, a mix of three mAb-recognizing epithelial tumor markers (anti-CEA, B72.3, and antifolate receptor MoV18) were injected intraperitoneally, followed by intraperitoneal injection of native avidin as clearing agent and, lastly, injection of ^{90}Y-labeled biotin (10 to 100 mCi) intraperitoneally or, when contraindicated, intravenously. Radioactivity was well tolerated. Of 38 patients, 3 had a partial response and 12 showed stable disease.

The MUC-1 glycoprotein is a heavily glycosylated transmembrane member of the mucin family localized at the apical surface of normal epithelial cells of the breast, salivary glands, and lung. Virtually all invasive breast carcinomas overexpress an underglycosylated form of MUC-1. In a phase I trial for breast and prostate carcinoma, Richman et al. (104) combined a radiolabeled mAb against the MUC-1 antigen (m170) with a radiosensitizer (paclitaxel) and linked the radiometal (^{90}Y or ^{111}I) to the macrocyclic chelate of the radiometal, DOTA, via a cleavable linker (Gly3Phe). This linker has been shown to be susceptible to the endopeptidase activity of intrahepatic cathepsins *in vitro* (62), thereby facilitating clearance and reducing liver toxicity. Cyclosporine was given to suppress HAMA response. A total of 16 patients were first injected with the ^{111}I-labeled antibody (^{111}I-DOTA-pep-m170) for dosimetry, then with a therapeutic dose of ^{90}Y-DOTA-pep-m170 (12 to 22 mCi/m^2). Paclitaxel was given 2 days after the therapeutic dose. The cleavable linker significantly reduced liver toxicity without effecting tumor binding. Nevertheless, an effective dose was not achieved, and further modification may be necessary. Many patients required stem cell transfusions because of myelosuppression.

The A33 antigen, a 43 kDa glycoprotein with homology to the immunoglobulin superfamily, is a promising target for the treatment of colon cancer (15,41). The antigen is homogeneously expressed by >95% of colon cancers and in normal intestinal mucosa but not in other epithelial tissues. Scott et al. (124) conducted a phase I trial with a humanized anti-A33-mAb, labeled with ^{131}I in patients with CRC. Twelve patients were treated with 400 MBq (10 mCi) ^{131}I-huA33 and 40 MBq 125-1 mCi) I-huA33 1 week before surgery in a single dose. No dose-limiting toxicities were observed, and excellent tumor uptake was demonstrated.

Renal carcinoma was targeted with a chimeric antibody recognizing carbonic anhydrase IX (cG250) by Divgi et al. (25) in a phase I study. In order to achieve a therapeutic dose, dosing was fractionated according to a radiation-absorbed dose schema. After infusing an initial dose of 5 mg ^{131}I-labeled cG250 ab (5 mCi), pharmacokinetic data were recorded and used to calculate the required activity. The therapeutic dose was administered in a fractionated pattern with a 2- to 3-day time interval and was escalated from a whole-body absorbed dose of 0.50 Gy (1,110 MBq, 30 mCi) in 0.25-Gy increments. The MTD was reached at 0.75 Gy. Two of 15 patients reacted with HACA. Despite tumor targeting, no clinical response was observed.

Tumor necrosis therapy targets necrotic regions that are found in tumors but are absent from normal tissues and organs. In contrast to classic antibody targeting approaches that use mAb binding cell surface antigens expressed on viable tumor cells, tumor necrosis therapy antibodies recognize nonviable zones found primarily in hypoxic areas of the tumor, representing between 30% and 80% of the tumor mass (30). In a multicenter phase I trial in China, Chen et al. (17) treated patients with lung cancer with a chimeric antitumor-necrosis antibody (^{131}I-chTNT) now approved in China. The labeled mAb was administered either intravenously at 0.8 mCi/kg body weight or intratumorally at 0.8 mCi/m3 tumor volume, two doses 2 to 4 weeks apart. For the 10 patients with small cell lung cancer, the overall response rate was 50%, with one CR and four PR. For the 97 patients with non–small cell lung cancer, the overall response rate was 33%, with three CR and 29 PR. No effect on OS was observed. Both routes of administration achieved mAb retention of the tumor and comparable overall response, but hematologic toxicity was lower for intratumoral administration. No HACA response was elicited. In a follow-up trial, the optimal route of administration of ^{131}I-chTNT was investigated in 43 patients with advanced lung cancer (147): Two doses administered either intravenously (n = 22) or by intratumoral injection using a computed tomography-guided catheter (n = 16), or a combination of both (n = 5). Partial responses were observed in all groups, but complete responses only in intratumorally injected patients (with or without intravenous injection).

Prostate cancer cells express antigens attractive for treatment, for example, PMSA, a membrane protein. This protein was targeted in a phase I trial using ^{177}Lu-labeled J591 in pa-

tients with androgen-independent prostate cancer (4). Myelosuppression was the major rate-limiting factor in treatment. In this study, only 4 of 35 patients experienced a prostate-specific antigen (PSA) decline of greater than 50% lasting from 3 to 8 months, and no patient had an objective measurable disease response.

A phase I/II clinical trial by Zeng et al. (148) evaluated whether long-term survival of unresectable hepatocellular carcinoma (HCC) could be improved by intrahepatic arterial infusion of ^{131}I-anti-HCC (hepama-1) mAb. Thirty-two patients with inoperable HCC received one, two, or three doses of the labeled mAb (0.93 to 4 GBq). Compared to control groups of 33 patients with intrahepatic chemotherapy, 5-year survival could be improved significantly (28.1% vs. 9.1%).

Head and neck carcinoma was targeted in a phase I study with the ^{186}Re-labeled mAb BIWA-4 (bivatuzumab) (8). This humanized antibody was developed from the mouse mAb BIWA-1. It recognizes CD44 splice variants containing the v6 domain. Expression of v6-containing CD44 variants has been related to aggressive behavior of various tumor types and was found to be particularly high and homogeneous on the outer cell surface of HNSCC (43). RIT with ^{186}Re-BIWA 4 was shown to be safe with a MTD of 50 mCi/m^2; at that dose, disease stabilization was observed in three of six patients. A similar study used ^{186}Re-BIWA-4 in patients with early-stage breast cancer (52). Although treatment was safe, tumor-to-nontumor ratios were unfavorable, with no apparent correlation with CD44v6 expression, tumor-cell cellularity, or tumor diameter. BIWA 4, therefore, appears to have limitations as a vehicle for RIT in patients with breast cancer.

⠿ | Nonsealed Radionuclide Therapy

Systemic nonsealed radionuclide therapy is a crucial treatment tool for many patients with benign or malignant disease for cure or effective palliation. It consists of oral, intravenous, or intracavitary administration of nonsealed sources. To deliver a therapeutic radiation dose, the substance has to accumulate in a site for sufficient time (high LET) while sparing the remainder of the body (high target/nontarget ratio) (24). Because most therapeutic radionuclides additionally emit γ-radiation detectable by gamma cameras, dosimetry and therapy response can be evaluated. This chapter will discuss biophysical properties of the most commonly used radiopharmaceuticals, their most important indications in malignant disease, clinical results, and toxicity of treatment as well as some directions regarding quality assurance.

Biophysical Properties

Iodine-131

^{131}I emits β-particles and decays to stable xenon-131. These particles do not penetrate deeply into tissue (mean range, 0.5 mm; maximum, 2 mm). Furthermore, ^{131}I decays by emitting γ-radiation (364 and 637 keV). Iodine uptake is heterogeneous in both normal and neoplastic thyroid tissue because of differential expression of the sodium-iodide symporter (NIS) (75,110).

Strontium-89

^{89}Sr is a pure β-emitting isotope (maximum energy, 1.46 MeV; half-life, 50.5 days) and is incorporated into the inorganic matrix of bone. Its distribution is identical to technetium bone-scanning agents with an uptake proportional to the degree of osteoblastic activity. Whereas 30% to 35% of ^{89}Sr remains in healthy bone for 10 to 14 days with 20% retention after

3 months, 80% to 90% of activity administered is retained in metastatic sites. Because of its low mean range (2.4 mm; maximum range, 7 mm), activity is focused on the tumor lesions, whereas bone marrow toxicity is limited. With at least 50% of the dose localized in the skeleton, ^{89}Sr is cleared rapidly from the blood through the kidneys (80%) and intestines (20%) (33,76,129).

Samarium-153

[153]Sm (maximum energy, 0.81 MeV; mean β-energy, 0.58 MeV; γ-radiation, 103 keV; half-life, 1.9 days; mean range, 0.6 mm; maximum range, 2.5 mm) has an affinity to areas with high bone turnover and accumulates on the endosteal surface of the bone. Bone metastases retain about five times more [153]Sm than healthy bone. To obtain the optimal combination of high bone uptake, rapid blood clearance, and renal excretion, [153]Sm is chelated with ethylene-diamine-tetramethylene-phosphonate (EDTMP). This complex selectively accumulates in skeletal tissue in association with hydroxyapatite (50% to 66% of the activity within 2 to 3 hours); $\leq$1% of the dose remains in circulation 1 hour after administration. [153]Sm not localized to bone is excreted by the kidneys within 6 to 8 hours (7,33,76).

Rhenium-186/-188

[186]Re has a maximum β-energy of 1.07 MeV (mean energy, 0.34; half-life, 3.8 days) with low γ-radiation (0.137 MeV). It is complexed with 1-1-hydroethylidene diphosphate (HEDP) with high affinity to osteoclastic cells (mean range, 1.1 mm; maximum range, 4.5 mm). Approximately 50% is deposited in the bone. Within 24 hours, about 70% of the radioisotope is excreted in the urine. [188]Re (maximum β-energy, 2.12 MeV; mean β-energy, 0.73 MeV; γ-radiation, 0.155 MeV; maximum range, 11 mm; mean range, 2.7 mm) can also be complexed with diphosphate ligands (i.e., HEDP). The half-life in bone is about 16 hours, in the whole body about 12 to 13 hours. Within 8 hours, about 40% of the activity is cleared by renal excretion. Radiochemistry of rhenium isotopes is similar to that of technetium, which makes them suitable for labeling similar compounds. This includes diphosphonates as well as a variety of peptides and proteins used for RIT (33,76,129).

Phosphorus-32

[32]P is a pure high-energy β-particle emitter (maximum energy, 1.71 MeV; mean, 0.69 MeV; half-life, 14.3 days) with deep tissue penetration (maximum, 8 mm; average, 1 to 4 mm). Within bone, ^{32}P sodium phosphate is bound to the hydroxyapatite matrix (85%), whereas within soft tissue and bone marrow, it predominantly distributes to the cells. After administration, uptake of orthophosphate by the skeletal system exceeds that by muscles, fat, or skin by a factor of 4 to 6 at day 1 and 6 to 10 at day 2. Excretion is mainly renal (20% to 50% within a week) whereas <2% are excreted in the feces. Only few data are available with regard to exact dosimetry; the average skeletal dose is $\leq$15 cGy after administration of 37 MBq. [32]P chromic phosphate is a radiocolloid with biokinetics and dosimetry different from those of ^{32}P sodium phosphate. It can be used for intracavitary instillation. Its distribution pattern stabilizes within 24 hours after injection and can be imaged with a high-energy collimator using the bremsstrahlung of [32]P (3,76).

Clinical Results

Iodine-131

Thyroid Malignancies

[131]I is standard therapy after thyroidectomy (1.11 to 5.5 GBq [30 to 150 mCi]), in local recurrences (3.7 to 5.5 GBq [100

to 150 mCi]) as well as metastatic disease (3.7 to 11.1 GBq [100 to 300 mCi]) of differentiated cancer of the thyroid. In general, the indication is accepted for any patient with a solitary carcinoma >1 cm (largest diameter) or with a cancer of any size with apparent lymph node involvement, extrathyroidal expansion of cancer, or multicentricity. Furthermore, therapy with ^{131}I is also recommended for all patients with incomplete surgical resection (primary or recurrent tumor as well as—if possible—metastases) (58,75,77,110,118). Following surgery, the patient should not receive thyroxin replacement for 4 to 6 weeks to increase endogenous thyroid-stimulating hormone secretion (above 25 to 30 mU/L) or should be given recombinant human thyroid-stimulating hormone to consequently ensure an adequate iodine uptake in thyroid cells. Based on a diagnostic scan, the uptake in the thyroid bed is determined to prescribe the optimal activity of [131]I. However, specific dosimetry studies regarding the optimal prescription are difficult to perform. Up to now, it could not be demonstrated that an individualized approach is more effective than standard treatment with fixed activities (58,75,110). [131]I is usually given orally in capsules or as a liquid solution; the intravenous route will be chosen in patients unable to ingest the oral medication. Prior to treatment, several relevant issues have to be considered: Absence of iodine-containing medications, iodinated contrast-agents, exogenous thyroid hormone, and antithyroid medications (24).

Further details of ^{131}I treatment of thyroid cancer are reviewed in Chapter 47.

Strontium-89

General Considerations Regarding the Use of Radioisotopes in Osseous Metastases

Most studies evaluating radioisotopes in the treatment of bone metastases were performed with hormone-refractory prostate cancer patients (80% to 90%); some other trials additionally included metastatic breast cancer patients (<5% to 10%) as well as metastatic bronchial carcinoma patients (5% to 10%); other tumor types were rarely reported. The cumulative data recommend the use of radioisotopes as effective treatment for selected patients with widespread bone metastases and diffuse pain for whom hormone therapy and/or chemotherapy are not sufficiently effective, unavailable, and for whom localized radiotherapy is not indicated (Table 23.4). Pain relief is reported in 40% to 95% of patients with 20% to 30% complete responses. Pain reduction starts 1 to 4 weeks after the beginning of therapy and lasts up to 17 months. This is commonly associated with reduced intake of analgesic medication and with low and reversible, mainly hematologic, toxicity in most patients. Repeated doses given after a 3-month interval confirm the efficacy in most patients who already initially responded to treatment. Additionally, some data suggest a possible tumoricidal effect, which may be effected by the mean path of the β-particles in the bone marrow; however, there is conflicting evidence. Up to now, significant differences regarding a consistent dose-response relationship, response rate, toxicity, and improved survival favoring one radioisotope (^{89}Sr, [153]Sm, ^{32}P, [186]Re, [188]Re) over another were not found (6,33,76,129).

In a retrospective study, with data from 44 patients, Liepe et al. (63) reported pain relief in 81%, 77%, and 80% of patients treated with [188]Re, [186]Re, and ^{89}Sr, respectively. However, a significant increase in terms of the performance status was observed in [188]Re patients. A randomized trial with 50 women suffering from breast cancer-induced bone metastases was performed by Sciuto et al. (122). The overall response rate was 84% in ^{89}Sr-treated patients and 92% in [186]Re-treated patients. Whereas the duration of response tended to be improved by [89]Sr (range, 2 to 15 months vs. 1 to 12 months), pain reduction started earlier in the [186]Re group (4 vs. 21 days). The mechanisms leading to pain relief in cancer-induced bone

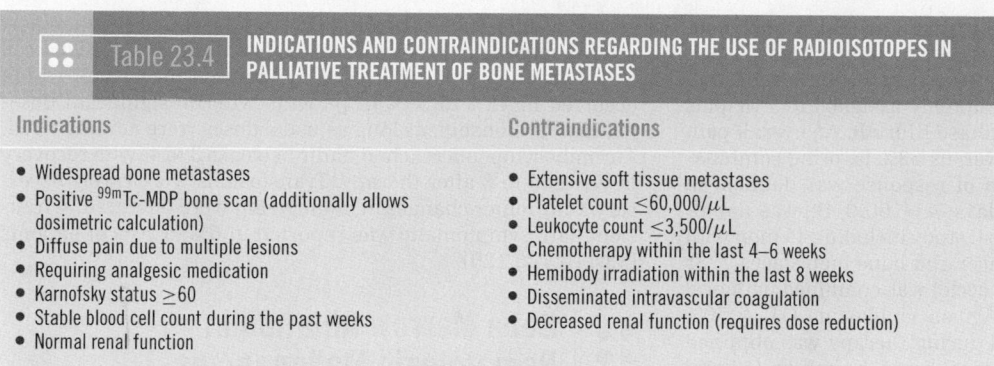

Indications	Contraindications
• Widespread bone metastases	• Extensive soft tissue metastases
• Positive ^{99m}Tc-MDP bone scan (additionally allows dosimetric calculation)	• Platelet count $\leq$60,000/μL
• Diffuse pain due to multiple lesions	• Leukocyte count $\leq$3,500/μL
• Requiring analgesic medication	• Chemotherapy within the last 4–6 weeks
• Karnofsky status $\geq$60	• Hemibody irradiation within the last 8 weeks
• Stable blood cell count during the past weeks	• Disseminated intravascular coagulation
• Normal renal function	• Decreased renal function (requires dose reduction)

pain are not yet fully understood. Presumably, the cytocidal effect of β-particles on radiosensitive cells such as lymphocytes, which are probably responsible for producing cytokines and, thus, for modulating of pain response, could lead to a reduction in cytokine-induced pain (91,138). Furthermore, there are some important variables affecting the results in pain relief (Table 23.5). Also, the different methods for pain measurement as well as time of follow-up in those studies have to be taken into consideration, and the results may be affected by the histology of the underlying tumor and the low number of patients in some studies. Therefore, future studies should attempt to obtain sufficient information about the changes in analgesic use, to decrease the variability in pain response assessment, to increase the sample size of carefully selected patients, to yield new data about combined treatments (bisphosphonates, chemotherapy, external radiotherapy), and to explore the economic benefit of the use of radioisotopes (6,33,129).

Bone Metastases

Although several dose-finding studies could not assess a dose-response relationship, ^{89}Sr (1.5 to 2.2 MBq/kg) is found to be very effective in palliation of osseous metastases with an overall pain relief in 65% to 90% and complete responses in 5% to 32% of patients. The effect starts 4 to 28 days after initiation of therapy and lasts for up to 15 months with a reduction of analgesic intake in 71% to 81% of patients (33,129). Up to 70% of patients demonstrate a reduction of hot spots on bone scans. This and other data showing decreasing PSA levels after therapy in prostate cancer patients, support the assumption that the treatment with ^{89}Sr will probably have a tumoricidal effect, which is currently controversially discussed in the literature (22,131,137). Patients with limited bone involvement and higher Karnofsky performance status achieve better results than patients with multiple sites and lower scores. In those patients who initially respond, a second therapy seems to be appropriate (22,33,129).

Several randomized trials were performed with the aim to evaluate the efficacy of ^{89}Sr. In patients with hormone-refractory prostate cancer, Lewington et al. (61) demonstrated that ^{89}Sr was significantly more effective than nonradioactive, stable ^{88}Sr. In a double-blind, randomized trial by Porter and McEwan (96), 126 patients with hormone-refractory prostate cancer were treated with local radiotherapy and either ^{89}Sr (399.6 MBq) or placebo. At 3 months, 40% of ^{89}Sr-treated patients were pain-free versus 23% in the placebo group; the median time to additional radiotherapy was 35 weeks (^{89}Sr) compared to 20 weeks (placebo group). Furthermore, the incidence of new painful metastases was lower in the treatment group, which was additionally confirmed by an improved benefit on pain and physical activity. In contrast, Smeland et al. (131) were unable to confirm these results. In their double-blind study, 93 eligible patients with locally irradiated bone metastases were randomized to receive either a standard dose of 150 MBq ^{89}Sr or placebo. At 3 months, no differences were found in terms of progression and survival, although progression-free survival was marginally improved in ^{89}Sr-treated prostate cancer patients. Quilty et al. (101) described results in 152 men with metastatic, hormone-refractory prostate cancer stratified to local or hemibody irradiation and then randomized to irradiation or ^{89}Sr (200 MBq). Partial and complete pain relief was reported in 65% to 70% of ^{89}Sr-treated men compared with 67% of external beam-irradiated patients. However, fewer new metastatic sites were registered in patients who received ^{89}Sr (64% and 73% vs. 42% after local radiotherapy, and 51% after hemibody irradiation, respectively). In a phase III study of the European Organisation for Research and Treatment of Cancer, 203 men with hormone-resistant prostate cancer were randomized to ^{89}Sr (150 MBq) and to local radiotherapy (89). The authors found a marginally statistically significant difference in median OS and 1-year-survival favoring the radiotherapy group (11 vs. 7.2 months; 45% vs. 34%). Time to progression as well as assessment of pain demonstrated no differences (radiotherapy, 33%; ^{89}Sr, 35%).

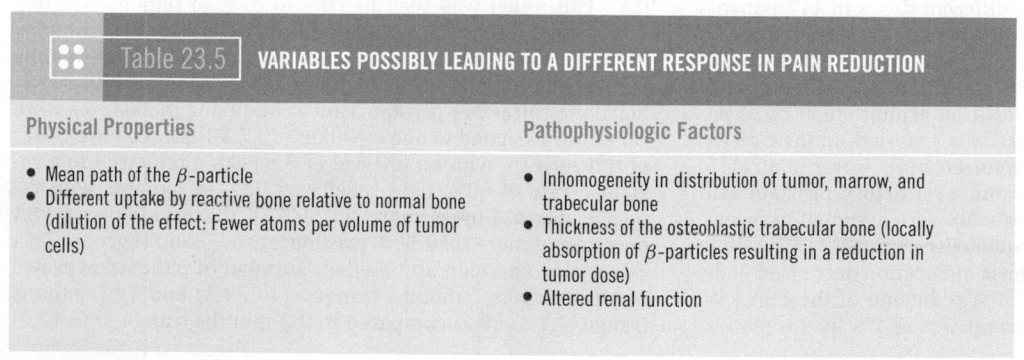

Physical Properties	Pathophysiologic Factors
• Mean path of the β-particle	• Inhomogeneity in distribution of tumor, marrow, and trabecular bone
• Different uptake by reactive bone relative to normal bone (dilution of the effect: Fewer atoms per volume of tumor cells)	• Thickness of the osteoblastic trabecular bone (locally absorption of β-particles resulting in a reduction in tumor dose)
	• Altered renal function

Another interesting strategy in treating selected hormone-refractory prostate cancer patients with bone metastases is the combination of ^{89}Sr and chemotherapy. In 2002, Sciuto et al. (123) reported on 70 patients randomly assigned to ^{89}Sr plus cisplatin and ^{89}Sr plus placebo (phase III trial). An overall pain reduction was obtained in 91% versus 63% favoring combination treatment. Median duration of response was doubled in these patients (120 days vs. 60 days; $p = .002$), OS was not affected (9 vs. 6 months). In a phase II study including 44 men with hormone-refractory prostate cancer and bone metastases, [89]Sr (2.2 MBq/kg, day 1 of a 12-week cycle) was combined with oral estramustine and intravenously given vinblastine (1). A 50% or greater decrease of PSA level during therapy was obtained in 48% of patients. Median survival was 13 months (1- and 2-year survival, 55% and 25%, respectively). In another phase II trial, 72 patients were randomized to receive doxorubicin with or without ^{89}Sr after response to intensive chemotherapy (136). The results suggested an improved time to progression (13.9 vs. 7 months) and OS (28 vs. 17 months) in favor of the patients additionally treated with [89]Sr. This procedure had no adverse effect on delivery of subsequent cycles of chemotherapy or other additional therapies (7,135). After treatment with ^{89}Sr, hematologic toxicity is most commonly observed (nadir, week 5 to 8), returning to normal values within 10 to 16 weeks without intervention in most patients. White blood cells are reduced to 11% to 65% from baseline in 12% to 80% of patients and platelets to 24% to 70% in 29% to 80% of patients, respectively, whereas changes of red cells rarely occur. In studies where higher activities or combined protocols were used, hematologic side-effects grade III to IV occurred in 3% to 32% of patients (1,96,101,123,136). Flare is reported in 15% of patients (33,129).

Samarium-153

Bone Metastases

[153]Sm-EDTMP is approved in the United States and in Europe for palliative therapy of skeletal metastases. The standard dose intravenously administered is 37 MBq/kg. Pain relief starts within 5 to 10 days in 55% to 95% of patients and is independent of the dose given. Reduction of pain continues up to 11 months; however, repeated doses can improve the duration of pain response in up to 50% of patients. Conflicting results are reported regarding the reduction of hot spots on bone scans (33,129). Three prospective, randomized phase III trials have been performed with [153]Sm-EDTMP in palliation of pain with bone metastases. Serafini et al. (126) assessed the effectiveness of two different doses (18.5 and 37 MBq) versus placebo in 118 patients with osseous metastases. A significant higher complete pain relief (31%) was achieved in patients with the highest dose compared with the low-dose group (28%) and placebo group (14%). Pain relief started as early as 1 week after injection. In 57% of patients initially receiving placebo, pain relief occurred after treatment with 37 MBq. [153]Sm-EDTMP. Olea et al. (88) compared three different doses in 417 patients with metastatic cancer: 18.5 MBq versus 37 MBq versus 55 MBq. An overall pain response rate independent of activity administered was observed in 73% at 4 months without providing exact data according to the three groups. In 60% of patients, a reduced analgesic intake was reported. In their recent prospective, double-blind, randomized trial, Sartor et al. (116) reported on 152 men with hormone-refractory prostate cancer and painful bone metastases who were assigned to receive 37 MBq [153]Sm-EDTMP or nonradioactive [153]Sm-EDTMP. Within 3 to 4 weeks, the need for analgesic medication decreased in the verum group. Furthermore, a 50% reduction of the PSA level was measured in the verum group versus 2% in the placebo

group. A difference regarding OS was not found (median survival, 7 months). The major toxic effects were white blood cell and platelet count decreases. Dose-limiting myelosuppression occurred in 45% to 59% of patients with no significant dose-toxicity relationship, as long as usual doses were administered. Thrombocytopenia reached nadir in weeks 3 to 4, with recovery in weeks 5 to 8 after therapy. Transfusions were rarely necessary. Only minor changes in hemoglobin were observed. A transient flare symptomatic was reported in 6% to 20% of patients (33,116,126,129).

Bone Marrow Ablation in Hematologic Malignancies

Using bone-seeking agent labeled with [153]Sm to deliver an ablative radiation dose to the bone marrow and to minimize nonhematologic toxicity could be an alternative approach to myeloablative chemoradiotherapy and subsequent rescue by stem cell transplantation. Bartlett et al. (5) performed a dosimetry and toxicity study in 42 patients prior to stem cell reinfusion and stated that, although administration of [153]Sm is unlikely to cause effective myelosuppression, [153]Sm may be a candidate for inclusion in BMT protocols. Comparable recommendations were given by Rodriguez et al. (112).

Rhenium-186

Bone Metastases

Like other bone-seeking radioisotopes, [186]Re-HEDP is only effective in those patients in whom ^{99m}Tc-scintigraphy demonstrate pathological bone uptake. [186]Re as well as [188]Re are unavailable in the United States, whereas they are widely used in Europe. Numerous prospective phase I and II trials were conducted suggesting a role of [186]Re-HEDP in palliation of bone metastases. Pain relief was observed in 38% to 92% of patients without a clear dose-response relationship (1,110 to 2,590 MBq). The maximum tolerated activity is 2,960 MBq for osseous metastases caused by prostate cancer and 2,405 MBq for metastases caused by breast cancer. Duration of pain relief is 5 to 12 months, with results likely to be improved after repeated injections; the effect starts 1 to 3 weeks after treatment (6,38,129). Major side effects are hematologic changes (white blood count, platelets) and are rarely clinically important. A rise in pain intensity is observed in <10% to 42% of patients (6,33,129).

Rhenium-188

Bone Metastases

[188]Re-HEDP is still investigational in palliative treatment. In a recent review, only four studies including 135 patients with mixed tumor types and used doses (1.1 to 6.9 GBq) were found (33). Pain relief was seen in 76% to 87% of patients starting 1 to 8 weeks after administration and lasted up to 3 months. Recently, one randomized phase II trial has been published by Palmedo et al. (90). In their study, 64 men with progressive, hormone-refractory prostate cancer and bone metastases were randomly assigned to one injection (40.7 MBq/kg) or two doses of [188]Re-HEDP with an interval of 8 weeks. Compared to a response rate of 60%, pain relief was 92% in patients with repeated doses. Furthermore, in 39% of these patients, a PSA decrease of more than 50% was measured (control group, 7%). Time to progression and median survival of patients with two treatments was 7 months (range, 0 to 24.1) and 12.7 months (range, 4.1 to 32.2) compared to 2.3 months (range, 0 to 12.2)

and 7 months (range, 1.3 to 36.7) in the other patients with one injection ($p = .0013$ and .04), respectively. In 0% to 25% (average, 17%), a decrease of platelets and in 16% to 30% (average, 24%) a decrease of leucocyte counts were seen, respectively. Within 4 to 12 weeks, the values returned to baseline. The reduction of blood cell count appears to be dose-dependent. Pain flare was reported in about 20% of patients (33,90).

Phosphorus-32

Malignant Ascites and Pleural Effusion

^{32}P chromic phosphate (370 to 740 MBq) may be used for intraperitoneal therapy of malignant ascites to disseminate the radioisotope throughout the abdominal cavity similar to the spread of exfoliated or ruptured tumor cells or in the primary management of ovarian cancer (see Chapter 68). Presupposition is the ability of the radioisotope to spread uniformly, which should be determined by the abdominal instillation of ^{99m}Tc colloid (75). Possible complications are generally short-lived and include nausea, fleeting abdominal pain, vomiting, diarrhea, and low-grade fever in 22% of patients. Bowel perforation requiring surgical intervention was observed in 1.5% of patients and has been reported in association with external irradiation (3,75). Furthermore, in contrast to several modalities to treat malignant pericardial effusion with an overall response rate of 75%, intrapericardial ^{32}P-colloid installation (185 to 370 MBq) is a simple and reliable therapy with a complete response rate of 94% (23). If other treatment options failed, ^{32}P chromic phosphate may also be discussed to treat malignant pleural effusions (222 to 444 MBq).

Malignant Cysts of the CNS

The use of colloidal ^{32}P has been reported in patients with cystic CNS tumors. Using stereotactic treatment planning and application system, 189 to 250 Gy were applied to the inner surface of the cyst wall. A cyst regression was reported in 70% to 88% of selected patients with cystic craniopharyngiomas demonstrating the effectiveness for the control of tumor cysts but not of solid tumor components (40,140). Voges et al. (140), who used ^{90}Yttrium or ^{32}P in 62 patients, observed a mean survival of 9 ± 0.9 years (median follow-up, 11.9 years) after intracavitary irradiation. After a mean follow-up of 7 years after diagnosis and 4 years after ^{32}P treatment, the survival rates were 90% at 5 years and 80% at 10 years after diagnosis in 49 patients reported by Hasegawa et al. (40). Visual deficits had improved in 48% to 60% of patients; in 10% to 12%, complications occurred (blindness, third nerve palsy, diabetes insipidus, panhypopituitarism) (40,140).

Bone Metastases

During many years, ^{32}P has shown its effectiveness in reducing pain caused by osseous metastases, although the optimum activity for administration is still unknown. Single and repeated injections of ^{32}P-orthophosphate with 185 to 444 MBq up to 888 MBq (5 to 24 mCi) were recommended. The overall response rate is approximately 85%; the mean duration of pain relief is 5.1 ± 2.6 months, although in some series pain reduction could be achieved in up to 17 months. The most common side effect is pancytopenia, which was more severe compared with other radioisotopes used; however, cell counts return to normal within 8 weeks after therapy. An increase in bone pain was observed in up to 50% of patients. The leukemogenic effect of ^{32}P does not principally exclude administration of ^{32}P in metastatic patients, although it fell out of routine widespread use because of perceived significantly increased side effects (31,76,129).

Radiation Safety and Quality Assurance

The administration of nonsealed radioisotopes has to be done in accordance with the American College of Radiology Practice Guideline for the Performance of Therapy with Unsealed Radiopharmaceutical Sources (see later discussion).

Close cooperation between physicians responsible for clinical management and administration of the radioisotope as well as hospital staff is mandatory. As required by the Nuclear Regulatory Commission or state regulations, a quality management program is necessary to ensure secure handling of radioisotopes in terms of efficacy, and to protect the patients, the staff, and the public from side effects, complications, and unintended exposure. Three modes of exposure have to be differentiated: External exposure, internal exposure due to contamination, and environmental pathways. It is mandatory that radioisotopes are given by a physician who is trained in nonsealed radionuclide therapy. Important radiation precautions and patient release criteria are described in the Nuclear Regulatory Commission Regulatory Guide 8.39, in the federal Code 10 CFR 35.75, as well as in NUREG-1556 "Program-Specific Guidance about Medical Use Licenses" (10). For treatment outside the United States, regulations of corresponding national regulatory bodies are put in place. Quality assurance for the handling of radioactive as well as for dealing with spillages should therefore be developed by each institution:

Quality Management in Therapy with Unsealed Sources (in Accordance with the American College of Radiology Guidelines)

- Written directives signed and dated by the authorized user
- Duplicative procedures for identifying the patients and documentation of signed informed consent
- Careful record keeping to ensure correct administered activity
  - Appropriate protection in opening delivered radioisotopes
  - Measurement by a radionuclide dose calibrator immediately before administration
- In case of intravenously given radioisotopes, reducing possibility of infiltration (i.e., use of a flexible indwelling catheter)
- Procedures for minimizing radiation exposure or radiopharmaceutical contamination of the hospital staff, relatives, and the public
  Medical staff
  - Protective shoe covers, gloves, and apron
  - Established, quick, and efficiently done work
  - Greatest distance as justifiable with care of the patient
  - Notification of rules for handling blood and urine
  - Leaving soiled items in the patient's area for disposal
  - Washing hands after leaving the patient
  Patient
  - Proper use of flushable toilet (flushing toilet twice, cleanness of the toilet regarding any spilled urine)
  - Washing hands after using the toilet
  - Washing of soiled cloths immediately and separately
  - Washing away spilled blood from cuts
  Procedures for containment of radioactivity
  - Routine blood work and laboratory specimens should be obtained prior to therapy
  - Limitation of the patient's access to personnel and visitors

Techniques, Modalities, and Modifiers in Radiation Oncology

- Monitoring and storing of all trash and residual nondisposable items after the patient's release until radiation levels are acceptable low to allow disposal or reuse
- Monitoring the contamination of the room until radiation level is sufficiently low to permit its general use
- Audit mechanism to ensure the compliance with the program

Whereas radioisotopes are generally given on an outpatient basis in some countries, radiation precautions require the patient to be admitted to the hospital because of γ-emitting radiopharmaceuticals. In contrast to β-particles, γ-rays can pass the patient's body, leading to an external risk for others. [131]I leads to the largest exposure. Therefore, in many countries, patients are hospitalized for administration of >0.7 to 1 GBq (20 to 30 mCi). According to Nuclear Regulatory Commission regulations and based on dose calculations as prescribed in NUREG-1556, a patient may be released 2 to 3 days after administration if the total activity equivalent to any other adult, who is exposed to the patient, is not likely to exceed 5 mSv (500 mrem). In other countries, regulations are even more restrictive. Generally, it has to be ensured especially that female patients are not pregnant or breast-feeding at the time of treatment. After treatment with ^{131}I, no further breast-feeding is recommended until the next pregnancy, which should be avoided during the following 12 months. Furthermore, it is important to avoid the contamination of children (e.g., by saliva), which could result in significant doses to the child's thyroid (24).

References

1. Akerley W, Butera J, Wehbe T, et al. A multiinstitutional, concurrent chemoradiation trial of strontium-89, estramustine, and vinblastine for hormone refractory prostate carcinoma involving bone. *Cancer* 2002;94:1654–1660.
2. Alvarez RD, Huh WK, Khazaeli MB, et al. A phase I study of combined modality (90)yttrium-CC49 intraperitoneal radioimmunotherapy for ovarian cancer. *Clin Cancer Res* 2002;8:2806–2811.
3. Balink H, Sijmons EA, Zonnenberg BA, et al. Repetitive phosphorus-32 peritoneal instillations in a patient with malignant ascites. *Clin Nucl Med* 2003;28:545–547.
4. Bander NH, Milowsky MI, Nanus DM, et al. Phase I trial of 177 lutetium-labeled J591, a monoclonal antibody to prostate-specific membrane antigen, in patients with androgen-independent prostate cancer. *J Clin Oncol* 2005;23:4591–4601.
5. Bartlett ML, Webb M, Durrant S, et al. Dosimetry and toxicity of quadramet for bone marrow ablation in multiple myeloma and other haematological malignancies. *Eur J Nucl Med Mol Imaging* 2002;29:1470–1477.
6. Bauman G, Charette M, Reid R, et al. Radiopharmaceuticals for the palliation of painful bone metastasis-a systemic review. *Radiother Oncol* 2005;75:258–270.
7. Ben-Yosef R, Pelled O, Marko R, et al. Establishing schedules for repeated doses of strontium and for concurrent chemotherapy in hormone-resistant patients with prostate cancer: Measurement of blood and urine strontium levels. *Am J Clin Oncol* 2005;28:138–142.
8. Borjesson PK, Postema EJ, Roos JC, et al. Phase I therapy study with (186)re-labeled humanized monoclonal antibody BIWA 4 (bivatuzumab) in patients with head and neck squamous cell carcinoma. *Clin Cancer Res* 2003;9:3961S–3972S.
9. Breitz HB, Weiden PL, Beaumier PL, et al. Clinical optimization of pretargeted radioimmunotherapy with antibody-streptavidin conjugate and 90Y-DOTA-biotin. *J Nucl Med* 2000;41:131–140.
10. Broseus RW, Bhalla, Lanzisera PA, et al. Program-specific guidance about medical use licenses: Final report. *U.S. Nuclear Regulatory Commission 1556.* Washington, DC: U.S. Nuclear Regulatory Commission; 2005;9.
11. Bunjes D, Buchmann I, Duncker C, et al. Rhenium 188-labeled anti-CD66 (a, b, c, e) monoclonal antibody to intensify the conditioning regimen prior to stem cell transplantation for patients with high-risk acute myeloid leukemia or myelodysplastic syndrome: Results of a phase I-II study. *Blood* 2001;98:565–572.
12. Bunjes D. 188 Re-labeled anti-CD66 monoclonal antibody in stem cell transplantation for patients with high-risk acute myeloid leukemia. *Leuk Lymphoma* 2002;43:2125–2131.
13. Burke JM, Caron PC, Papadopoulos EB, et al. Cytoreduction with iodine-131-anti-CD33 antibodies before bone marrow transplantation for advanced myeloid leukemias. *Bone Marrow Transplant* 2003;32:549–556.
14. Cancer therapy evaluation program, common terminology criteria for adverse events, version 3.0, DCTD, NCI, NIH, DHHS. Available at: http://ctep.cancer.gov. Accessed April 2006.
15. Catimel B, Ritter G, Welt S, et al. Purification and characterization of a novel restricted antigen expressed by normal and transformed human colonic epithelium. *J Biol Chem* 1996;271:25664–25670.
16. Chao DT, Korsmeyer SJ. BCL-2 family: Regulators of cell death. *Annu Rev Immunol* 1998;16:395–419.
17. Chen S, Yu L, Jiang C, et al. Pivotal study of iodine-131-labeled chimeric tumor necrosis treatment radioimmunotherapy in patients with advanced lung cancer. *J Clin Oncol* 2005;23:1538–1547.
18. Cheson BD. Radioimmunotherapy of non-Hodgkin lymphomas. *Blood* 2003;101:391–398.
19. Cohen MH, Johnson JR, Pazdur R. Food and drug administration drug approval summary: Temozolomide plus radiation therapy for the treatment of newly diagnosed glioblastoma multiforme. *Clin Cancer Res* 2005;11:6767–6771.
20. Cokgor I, Akabani G, Kuan CT, et al. Phase I trial results of iodine-131-labeled antitenascin monoclonal antibody 81C6 treatment of patients with newly diagnosed malignant gliomas. *J Clin Oncol* 2000;18:3862–3872.
21. Comparative trial between Bexxar and Zevalin. Available at: ClinicalTrials.gov identifier: NCT00078676. Accessed April 2006.
22. Dafermou A, Colamussi P, Giganti M, et al. A multicentre observational study of radionuclide therapy in patients with painful bone metastases of prostate cancer. *Eur J Nucl Med* 2001;28:788–798.
23. Dempke W, Firusian N. Treatment of malignant pericardial effusion with 32P-colloid. *Br J Cancer* 1999;80:1955–1957.
24. Dillehay GL, Ellerbroek NA, Balon H, et al. Practice guideline for the performance of therapy with unsealed radiopharmaceutical sources. *Int J Radiat Oncol Biol Phys* 2006;64:1299–1307.
25. Divgi CR, O'Donoghue JA, Welt S, et al. Phase I clinical trial with fractionated radioimmunotherapy using 131I-labeled chimeric G250 in metastatic renal cancer. *J Nucl Med* 2004;45:1412–1421.
26. Divgi CR, Scott AM, Dantis L, et al. Phase I radioimmunotherapy trial with iodine-131-CC49 in metastatic colon carcinoma. *J Nucl Med* 1995;36:586–592.
27. Dixon KL. The radiation biology of radioimmunotherapy. *Nucl Med Commun* 2003;24:951–957.
28. Emrich JG, Brady LW, Quang TS, et al. Radioiodinated (I-125) monoclonal antibody 425 in the treatment of high grade glioma patients: Ten-year synopsis of a novel treatment. *Am J Clin Oncol* 2002;25:541–546.
29. Engel P, Nojima Y, Rothstein D, et al. The same epitope on CD22 of B lymphocytes mediates the adhesion of erythrocytes, T and B lymphocytes, neutrophils, and monocytes. *J Immunol* 1993;150:4719–4732.
30. Epstein AL, Chen FM, Taylor CR. A novel method for the detection of necrotic lesions in human cancers. *Cancer Res* 1988;48:5842–5848.
31. Fettich J, Padhy A, Nair N. Comparative clinical efficacy and safety of phosphorus-32 and strontium-89 in the palliative treatment of metastatic bone pain: Results of an IAEA coordinated research project. *World J Nucl Med* 2003;2:226–231.
32. Fietz T, Uharek L, Gentilini C, et al. Allogeneic hematopoietic cell transplantation following conditioning with 90Y-ibritumomab-tiuxetan. *Leuk Lymphoma* 2006;47:59–63.
33. Finlay IG, Mason MD, Shelley M. Radioisotopes for the palliation of metastatic bone cancer: A systematic review. *Lancet Oncol* 2005;6:392–400.
34. Fisher RI, Kaminski MS, Wahl RL, et al. Tositumomab and iodine-131 tositumomab produces durable complete remissions in a subset of heavily pretreated patients with low-grade and transformed non-Hodgkin's lymphomas. *J Clin Oncol* 2005;23:7565–7573.
35. Ghert MA, Jung ST, Qi W, et al. The clinical significance of tenascin-C splice variant expression in chondrosarcoma. *Oncology* 2001;61:306–314.
36. Gordon LI, White CA, Leonard JP, et al. Radioimmunotherapy is associated with a low incidence of human-anti mouse antibody (HAMA) and human anti-rituxan ®antibody (HACA) response. *Blood* 2001;98:228b228b(abstr 4632).
37. Grana C, Bartolomei M, Handkiewicz D, et al. Radioimmunotherapy in advanced ovarian cancer: Is there a role for pre-targeting with (90)Y-biotin? *Gynecol Oncol* 2004;93:691–698.
38. Han SH, de Klerk JM, Tan S, et al. The PLACORHEN study: A double-blind, placebo-controlled, randomized radionuclide study with (186)re-etidronate in hormone-resistant prostate cancer patients with painful bone metastases. Placebo controlled rhenium study. *J Nucl Med* 2002;43:1150–1156.
39. Hansen CB, Kao GY, Moase EH, et al. Attachment of antibodies to sterically stabilized liposomes: Evaluation, comparison and optimization of coupling procedures. *Biochim Biophys Acta* 1995;1239:133–144.
40. Hasegawa T, Kondziolka D, Hadjipanayis CG, et al. Management of cystic craniopharyngiomas with phosphorus-32 intracavitary irradiation. *Neurosurgery* 2004;54:813–822.
41. Heath JK, White SJ, Johnstone CN, et al. The human A33 antigen is a transmembrane glycoprotein and a novel member of the immunoglobulin superfamily. *Proc Natl Acad Sci U S A* 1997;94:469–474.
42. Heath TD, Fraley RT, Papahdjopoulos D. Antibody targeting of liposomes: Cell specificity obtained by conjugation of F(ab)2 to vesicle surface. *Science* 1980;210:539–541.
43. Heider KH, Sproll M, Susani S, et al. Characterization of a high-affinity monoclonal antibody specific for CD44v6 as candidate for immunotherapy of squamous cell carcinomas. *Cancer Immunol Immunother* 1996;43:245–253.
44. Hoption Cann SA, van Netten JP, van Netten C. Dr William Coley and tumour regression: A place in history or in the future. *Postgrad Med J* 2003;79:672–680.
45. Horning SJ, Younes A, Jain V, et al. Efficacy and safety of tositumomab and iodine-131 tositumomab (Bexxar) in B-cell lymphoma, progressive after rituximab. *J Clin Oncol* 2005;23:712–719.
46. Hug H. Fas-mediated apoptosis in tumor formation and defense. *Biol Chem* 1997;378:1405–1412.
47. Iannello A, Ahmad A. Role of antibody-dependent cell-mediated cytotoxicity in the efficacy of therapeutic anti-cancer monoclonal antibodies. *Cancer Metastasis Rev* 2005;24:487–499.
48. Jahkola T, Toivonen T, Virtanen I, et al. Tenascin-C expression in invasion border of early breast cancer: A predictor of local and distant recurrence. *Br J Cancer* 1998;78:1507–1513.
49. Knox SJ, Goris ML, Tempero M, et al. Phase II trial of yttrium-90-DOTA-biotin pretargeted by NR-LU-10 antibody/streptavidin in patients with metastatic colon cancer. *Clin Cancer Res* 2000;6:406–414.
50. Köhler G, Milstein C. Continuous cultures of fused cells secreting antibody of predefined specificity. *Nature* 1975;256:495–497.
51. Kontermann RE. Immunoliposomes for cancer therapy. *Curr Opin Mol Ther* 2006;8:39–45.
52. Koppe M, Schaijk F, Roos J, et al. Safety, pharmacokinetics, immunogenicity, and biodistribution of (186)re-labeled humanized monoclonal antibody BIWA 4 (bivatuzumab) in patients with early-stage breast cancer. *Cancer Biother Radiopharm* 2004;19:720–729.

53. Koukourakis MI, Koukouraki S, Fezoulidis I, et al. High intratumoural accumulation of stealth liposomal doxorubicin (caelyx) in glioblastomas and in metastatic brain tumours. *Br J Cancer* 2000;83:1281–1286.

54. Kraeber-Bodere F, Bardet S, Hoefnagel CA, et al. Radioimmunotherapy in medullary thyroid cancer using bispecific antibody and iodine 131-labeled bivalent hapten: Preliminary results of a phase I/II clinical trial. *Clin Cancer Res* 1999;5:3190s–3198s.

55. Kraeber-Bodere F, Faivre-Chauvet A, Ferrer L, et al. Pharmacokinetics and dosimetry studies for optimization of anti-carcinoembryonic antigen x anti-hapten bispecific antibody-mediated pretargeting of iodine-131-labeled hapten in a phase I radioimmunotherapy trial. *Clin Cancer Res* 2003;9:3973S–81S.

56. Kraeber-Bodere F, Rousseau C, Bodet-Milin C, et al. Targeting, toxicity, and efficacy of 2-step, pretargeted radioimmunotherapy using a chimeric bispecific antibody and 131I-labeled bivalent hapten in a phase I optimization clinical trial. *J Nucl Med* 2006;47:247–255.

57. Laginha K, Mumbengegwi D, Allen T. Liposomes targeted via two different antibodies: Assay, B-cell binding and cytotoxicity. *Biochim Biophys Acta* 2005;1711:25–32.

58. Lamonica D. Iodine 131 ((131)I) as adjuvant therapy of differentiated thyroid cancer. *Surg Oncol Clin North Am* 2004;13:129–149.

59. Lefebvre S, Antoine M, Uzan S, et al. Specific activation of the non-classical class I histocompatibility HLA-G antigen and expression of the ILT2 inhibitory receptor in human breast cancer. *J Pathol* 2002;196:266–274.

60. Leserman LD, Barbet J, Kourilsky F, et al. Targeting to cells of fluorescent liposomes covalently coupled with monoclonal antibody or protein A. *Nature* 1980;288:602–604.

61. Lewington VJ, McEwan AJ, Ackery DM, et al. A prospective, randomised double-blind crossover study to examine the efficacy of strontium-89 in pain palliation in patients with advanced prostate cancer metastatic to bone. *Eur J Cancer* 1991;27:954–958.

62. Li M, Meares CF. Synthesis, metal chelate stability studies, and enzyme digestion of a peptide-linked DOTA derivative and its corresponding radiolabeled immunoconjugates. *Bioconjug Chem* 1993;4:275–283.

63. Liepe K, Franke WG, Kropp J, et al. Comparison of rhenium-188, rhenium-186-HEDP and strontium-89 in palliation of painful bone metastases. *Nuklearmedizin* 2000;39:146–151.

64. Liersch T, Meller J, Kulle B, et al. Phase II trial of carcinoembryonic antigen radioimmunotherapy with 131I-labetuzumab after salvage resection of colorectal metastases in the liver: Five-year safety and efficacy results. *J Clin Oncol* 2005;23:6763–6770.

65. Linden O, Hindorf C, Cavallin-Stahl E, et al. Dose-fractionated radioimmunotherapy in non-hodgkin's lymphoma using DOTA-conjugated, 90Y-radiolabeled, humanized anti-CD22 monoclonal antibody, epratuzumab. *Clin Cancer Res* 2005;11:5215–5222.

66. Lopes de Menezes DE, Pilarski LM, et al. In vitro and in vivo targeting of immunoliposomal doxorubicin to human B-cell lymphoma. *Cancer Res* 1998;58:3320–3330.

67. Mackie EJ. Molecules in focus: Tenascin-C. *Int J Biochem Cell Biol* 1997;29:1133–1137.

68. MacLean GD, Reddish M, Koganty RR, et al. Immunization of breast cancer patients using a synthetic sialyl-tn glycoconjugate plus detox adjuvant. *Cancer Immunol Immunother* 1993;36:215–222.

69. Malmberg KJ, Levitsky V, Norell H, et al. IFN-gamma protects short-term ovarian carcinoma cell lines from CTL lysis via a CD94/NKG2A-dependent mechanism. *J Clin Invest* 2002;110:1515–1523.

70. Malmberg KJ. Effective immunotherapy against cancer: A question of overcoming immune suppression and immune escape? *Cancer Immunol Immunother* 2004;53:879–892.

71. Mapara MY, Sykes M. Tolerance and cancer: Mechanisms of tumor evasion and strategies for breaking tolerance. *J Clin Oncol* 2004;22:1136–1151.

72. Marincola FM, Jaffee EM, Hicklin DJ, et al. Escape of human solid tumors from T-cell recognition: Molecular mechanisms and functional significance. *Adv Immunol* 2000;74:181–273.

73. Matthews DC, Appelbaum FR, Eary JF, et al. Development of a marrow transplant regimen for acute leukemia using targeted hematopoietic irradiation delivered by 131I-labeled anti-CD45 antibody, combined with cyclophosphamide and total body irradiation. *Blood* 1995;85:1122–1131.

74. Matthews DC, Appelbaum FR, Eary JF, et al. Phase I study of (131)I-anti-CD45 antibody plus cyclophosphamide and total body irradiation for advanced acute leukemia and myelodysplastic syndrome. *Blood* 1999;94:1237–1247.

75. McDougall IR. Systemic radiation therapy with unsealed radionuclides. *Semin Radiat Oncol* 2000;10:94–102.

76. McEwan AJ. Use of radionuclides for the palliation of bone metastases. *Semin Radiat Oncol* 2000;10:103–114.

77. Menzel C, Grunwald F, Schomburg A, et al. "High-dose" radioiodine therapy in advanced differentiated thyroid carcinoma. *J Nucl Med* 1996;37:1496–1503.

78. Meredith RF, Alvarez RD, Partridge EE, et al. Intraperitoneal radioimmunochemotherapy of ovarian cancer: A phase I study. *Cancer Biother Radiopharm* 2001;16:305–315.

79. Mirick GR, Bradt BM, Denardo SJ, et al. A review of human anti-globulin antibody (HAGA, HAMA, HACA, HAHA) responses to monoclonal antibodies. not four letter words. *Q J Nucl Med Mol Imaging* 2004;48:251–257.

80. Mittal BB, Zimmer MA, Sathiaseelan V, et al. Phase I/II trial of combined 131I anti-CEA monoclonal antibody and hyperthermia in patients with advanced colorectal adenocarcinoma. *Cancer* 1996;78:1861–1870.

81. Murray JL, Macey DJ, Grant EJ, et al. Enhanced TAG-72 expression and tumor uptake of radiolabeled monoclonal antibody CC49 in metastatic breast cancer patients following alpha-interferon treatment. *Cancer Res* 1995;55:5925s–5928s.

82. Murray JL, Macey DJ, Kasi LP, et al. Phase II radioimmunotherapy trial with 131I-CC49 in colorectal cancer. *Cancer* 1994;73:1057–1066.

83. Nademanee A, Forman S, Molina A, et al. A phase 1/2 trial of high-dose yttrium-90-ibritumomab tiuxetan in combination with high-dose etoposide and cyclophosphamide followed by autologous stem cell transplantation in patients with poor-risk or relapsed non-Hodgkin lymphoma. *Blood* 2005;106:2896–2902.

84. Natali PG, Nicotra MR, Bigotti A, et al. Comparative analysis of the expression of the extracellular matrix protein tenascin in normal human fetal, adult and tumor tissues. *Int J Cancer* 1991;47:811–816.

85. Nielsen UB, Adams GP, Weiner LM, et al. Targeting of bivalent anti-ErbB2 diabody antibody fragments to tumor cells is independent of the intrinsic antibody affinity. *Cancer Res* 2000;60:6434–6440.

86. O'Donoghue JA, Sgouros G, Divgi CR, et al. Single-dose versus fractionated radioimmunotherapy: Model comparisons for uniform tumor dosimetry. *J Nucl Med* 2000;41:538–547.

87. Okabe T, Kaizu T, Fujisawa M, et al. Monoclonal antibodies to surface antigens of small cell carcinoma of the lung. *Cancer Res* 1984;44:5273–5278.

88. Olea E, Riccabona G, Tian J, et al. Efficacy and toxicity of 153Sm EDTMP in the palliative treatment of painful skeleton metastases: Results of an IAEA international multicenter study. *J Nucl Med.* 2000;51:146 P.

89. Oosterhof GO, Roberts JT, de Reijke TM, et al. Strontium(89) chloride versus palliative local field radiotherapy in patients with hormonal escaped prostate cancer: A phase III study of the European Organisation for Research and Treatment of Cancer, genitourinary group. *Eur Urol* 2003;44:519–526.

90. Palmedo H, Manka-Waluch A, Albers P, et al. Repeated bone-targeted therapy for hormone-refractory prostate carcinoma: Randomized phase II trial with the new, high-energy radiopharmaceutical rhenium-188 hydroxyethylidenediphosphonate. *J Clin Oncol* 2003;21:2869–2875.

91. Pandit-Taskar N, Batraki M, Divgi CR. Radiopharmaceutical therapy for palliation of bone pain from osseous metastases. *J Nucl Med* 2004;45:1358–1365.

92. Park JW, Kirpotin DB, Hong K, et al. Tumor targeting using anti-her2 immunoliposomes. *J Control Release* 2001;74:95–113.

93. Paul P, Cabestre FA, Le Gal FA, et al. Heterogeneity of HLA-G gene transcription and protein expression in malignant melanoma biopsies. *Cancer Res* 1999;59:1954–1960.

94. Penichet ML, Morrison SL. Antibody-cytokine fusion proteins for the therapy of cancer. *J Immunol Methods* 2001;248:91–101.

95. Pitti RM, Marsters SA, Lawrence DA, et al. Genomic amplification of a decoy receptor for fas ligand in lung and colon cancer. *Nature* 1998;396:699–703.

96. Porter AT, McEwan AJ. Strontium-89 as an adjuvant to external beam radiation improves pain relief and delays disease progression in advanced prostate cancer: Results of a randomized controlled trial. *Semin Oncol* 1993;20:38–43.

97. Press OW, Eary JF, Appelbaum FR, et al. Radiolabeled-antibody therapy of B-cell lymphoma with autologous bone marrow support. *N Engl J Med* 1993;329:1219–1224.

98. Press OW, Eary JF, Badger CC, et al. High-dose radioimmunotherapy of B cell lymphomas. *Front Radiat Ther Oncol* 1990;24:204–227.

99. Press OW, Eary JF, Gooley T, et al. A phase I/II trial of iodine-131-tositumomab (anti-CD20), etoposide, cyclophosphamide, and autologous stem cell transplantation for relapsed B-cell lymphomas. *Blood* 2000;96:2934–2942.

100. Press OW, Unger JM, Braziel RM, et al. A phase 2 trial of CHOP chemotherapy followed by tositumomab/iodine I 131 tositumomab for previously untreated follicular non-Hodgkin lymphoma: Southwest Oncology Group protocol S9911. *Blood* 2003;102:1606–1612.

101. Quilty PM, Kirk D, Bolger JJ, et al. A comparison of the palliative effects of strontium-89 and external beam radiotherapy in metastatic prostate cancer. *Radiother Oncol* 1994;31:33–40.

102. Reardon DA, Akabani G, Coleman RE, et al. Phase II trial of murine (131)I-labeled antitenascin monoclonal antibody 81C6 administered into surgically created resection cavities of patients with newly diagnosed malignant gliomas. *J Clin Oncol* 2002;20:1389–1397.

103. Reardon DA, Akabani G, Coleman RE, et al. Salvage radioimmunotherapy with murine iodine-131-labeled antitenascin monoclonal antibody 81C6 for patients with recurrent primary and metastatic malignant brain tumors: Phase II study results. *J Clin Oncol* 2006;24:115–122.

104. Richman CM, Denardo SJ, O'Donnell RT, et al. High-dose radioimmunotherapy combined with fixed, low-dose paclitaxel in metastatic prostate and breast cancer by using a MUC-1 monoclonal antibody, m170, linked to indium-111/yttrium-90 via a cathepsin cleavable linker with cyclosporine to prevent human anti-mouse antibody. *Clin Cancer Res* 2005;11:5920–5927.

105. Riethmüller G, Holz E, Schlimok G, et al. Monoclonal antibody therapy for resected dukes' C colorectal cancer: Seven-year outcome of a multicenter randomized trial. *J Clin Oncol* 1998;16:1788–1794.

106. Ringhoffer M, Blumstein N, Neumaier B, et al. 188Re or 90Y-labelled anti-CD66 antibody as part of a dose-reduced conditioning regimen for patients with acute leukaemia or myelodysplastic syndrome over the age of 55: Results of a phase I-II study. *Br J Haematol* 2005;130:604–613.

107. Riva P, Franceschi G, Arista A, et al. Local application of radiolabeled monoclonal antibodies in the treatment of high grade malignant gliomas: A six-year clinical experience. *Cancer* 1997;80:2733–2742.

108. Riva P, Franceschi G, Frattarelli M, et al. Loco-regional radioimmunotherapy of high-grade malignant gliomas using specific monoclonal antibodies labeled with 90Y: A phase I study. *Clin Cancer Res* 1999;5:3275s–3280s.

109. Rizzieri DA, Akabani G, Zalutsky MR, et al. Phase 1 trial study of 131I-labeled chimeric 81C6 monoclonal antibody for the treatment of patients with non-Hodgkin lymphoma. *Blood* 2004;104:642–648.

110. Robbins RJ, Schlumberger MJ. The evolving role of (131)I for the treatment of differentiated thyroid carcinoma. *J Nucl Med* 2005;46[Suppl 1]:28S–37S.

111. Rodeck U, Herlyn M, Herlyn D, et al. Tumor growth modulation by a monoclonal antibody to the epidermal growth factor receptor: Immunologically mediated and effector cell-independent effects. *Cancer Res* 1987;47:3692–3696.

112. Rodriguez V, Erlandson L, Arndt CA, et al. Low toxicity and efficacy of (153)samarium-EDTMP and melphalan as a conditioning regimen for secondary acute myelogenous leukemia. *Pediatr Transplant* 2005;9:122–126.

113. Roselli M, Guadagni F, Buonomo O, et al. Systemic administration of recombinant interferon alfa in carcinoma patients upregulates the expression of the carcinoma-associated antigens tumor-associated glycoprotein-72 and carcinoembryonic antigen. *J Clin Oncol* 1996;14:2031–2042.

114. Rossin R, Pan D, Qi K, et al. 64Cu-labeled folate-conjugated shell cross-linked nanoparticles for tumor imaging and radiotherapy: Synthesis, radiolabeling, and biologic evaluation. *J Nucl Med* 2005;46:1210–1218.

115. Sapra P, Allen TM. Improved outcome when B-cell lymphoma is treated with combinations of immunoliposomal anticancer drugs targeted to both the CD19 and CD20 epitopes. *Clin Cancer Res* 2004;10:2530–2537.

116. Sartor O, Reid RH, Hoskin PJ, et al. Samarium-153-lexidronam complex for treatment of painful bone metastases in hormone-refractory prostate cancer. *Urology* 2004;63:940–945.

117. Sato S, Tuscano JM, Inaoki M, et al. CD22 negatively and positively regulates signal transduction through the B lymphocyte antigen receptor. *Semin Immunol* 1998;10:287–297.

118. Sawka AM, Thephamongkhol K, Brouwers M, et al. Clinical review 170: A systematic review and metaanalysis of the effectiveness of radioactive iodine remnant ablation for well-differentiated thyroid cancer. *J Clin Endocrinol Metab* 2004;89:3668–3676.

119. Scanlan MJ, Simpson AJ, Old LJ. The cancer/testis genes: Review, standardization, and commentary. *Cancer Immunol* 2004;4:1.

120. Scheinberg DA, Lovett D, Divgi CR, et al. A phase I trial of monoclonal antibody M195 in acute myelogenous leukemia: Specific bone marrow targeting and internalization of radionuclide. *J Clin Oncol* 1991;9:478–490.

121. Schrama D, Reisfeld RA, Becker JC. Antibody targeted drugs as cancer therapeutics. *Nat Rev Drug Discov* 2006;5:147–159.

122. Sciuto R, Festa A, Pasqualoni R, et al. Metastatic bone pain palliation with 89-sr and 186-re-HEDP in breast cancer patients. *Breast Cancer Res Treat* 2001;66:101–109.

123. Sciuto R, Festa A, Rea S, et al. Effects of low-dose cisplatin on 89Sr therapy for painful bone metastases from prostate cancer: A randomized clinical trial. *J Nucl Med* 2002;43:79–86.

124. Scott AM, Lee FT, Jones R, et al. A phase I trial of humanized monoclonal antibody A33 in patients with colorectal carcinoma: Biodistribution, pharmacokinetics, and quantitative tumor uptake. *Clin Cancer Res* 2005;11:4810–4817.

125. Seliger B, Maeurer MJ, Ferrone S. Antigen-processing machinery breakdown and tumor growth. *Immunol Today* 2000;21:455–464.

126. Serafini AN, Houston SJ, Resche I, et al. Palliation of pain associated with metastatic bone cancer using samarium-153 lexidronam: A double-blind placebo-controlled clinical trial. *J Clin Oncol* 1998;16:1574–1581.

127. Sgouros G, Ballangrud AM, Jurcic JG, et al. Pharmacokinetics and dosimetry of an alpha-particle emitter labeled antibody: 213Bi-HuM195 (anti-CD33) in patients with leukemia. *J Nucl Med* 1999;40:1935–1946.

128. Sharkey RM, Hajjar G, Yeldell D, et al. A phase I trial combining high-dose 90Y-labeled humanized anti-CEA monoclonal antibody with doxorubicin and peripheral blood stem cell rescue in advanced medullary thyroid cancer. *J Nucl Med* 2005;46:620–633.

129. Silberstein EB. Teletherapy and radiopharmaceutical therapy of painful bone metastases. *Semin Nucl Med* 2005;35:152–158.

130. Slovin SF, Scher HI, Divgi CR, et al. Interferon-gamma and monoclonal antibody 131I-labeled CC49: Outcomes in patients with androgen-independent prostate cancer. *Clin Cancer Res* 1998;4:643–651.

131. Smeland S, Erikstein B, Aas M, et al. Role of strontium-89 as adjuvant to palliative external beam radiotherapy is questionable: Results of a double-blind randomized study. *Int J Radiat Oncol Biol Phys* 2003;56:1397–1404.

132. Stein R, Belisle E, Hansen HJ, et al. Epitope specificity of the anti-(B cell lymphoma) monoclonal antibody, LL2. *Cancer Immunol Immunother* 1993;37:293–298.

133. Stramignoni D, Bowen R, Atkinson BF, et al. Differential reactivity of monoclonal antibodies with human colon adenocarcinomas and adenomas. *Int J Cancer* 1983;31:543–552.

134. Szpak CA, Johnston WW, Roggli V, et al. The diagnostic distinction between malignant mesothelioma of the pleura and adenocarcinoma of the lung as defined by a monoclonal antibody (B72.3). *Am J Pathol* 1986;122:252–260.

135. Tu SM, Kim J, Pagliaro LC, et al. Therapy tolerance in selected patients with androgen-independent prostate cancer following strontium-89 combined with chemotherapy. *J Clin Oncol* 2005;23:7904–7910.

136. Tu SM, Millikan RE, Mengistu B, et al. Bone-targeted therapy for advanced androgen-independent carcinoma of the prostate: A randomised phase II trial. *Lancet* 2001;357:336–341.

137. Turner SL, Gruenewald S, Spry N, et al, Metastron Users Group. Less pain does equal better quality of life following strontium-89 therapy for metastatic prostate cancer. *Br J Cancer* 2001;84:297–302.

138. Urch C. The pathophysiology of cancer-induced bone pain: Current understanding. *Palliat Med* 2004;18:267–274.

139. Vergote I, Larsen RH, De Vos L, et al. Distribution of intraperitoneally injected microspheres labeled with the alpha-emitter astatine (211At) compared with phosphorus (32P) and yttrium (90Y) colloids in mice. *Gynecol Oncol* 1992;47:358–365.

140. Voges J, Sturm V, Lehrke R, et al. Cystic craniopharyngioma: Long-term results after intracavitary irradiation with stereotactically applied colloidal beta-emitting radioactive sources. *Neurosurgery* 1997;40:263–270.

141. Voinea M, Simionescu M. Designing of 'intelligent' liposomes for efficient delivery of drugs. *J Cell Mol Med* 2002;6:465–474.

142. Vuillez JP, Kraeber-Bodere F, Moro D, et al. Radioimmunotherapy of small cell lung carcinoma with the two-step method using a bispecific anti-carcinoembryonic antigen/anti-diethylenetriaminepentaacetic acid (DTPA) antibody and iodine-131 di-DTPA hapten: Results of a phase I/II trial. *Clin Cancer Res* 1999;5:3259s–3267s.

143. Waldmann TA, White JD, Carrasquillo JA, et al. Radioimmunotherapy of interleukin-2R alpha-expressing adult T-cell leukemia with yttrium-90-labeled anti-tac. *Blood* 1995;86:4063–4075.

144. Witzig TE, Gordon LI, Cabanillas F, et al. Randomized controlled trial of yttrium-90-labeled ibritumomab tiuxetan radioimmunotherapy versus rituximab immunotherapy for patients with relapsed or refractory low-grade, follicular, or transformed B-cell non-Hodgkin's lymphoma. *J Clin Oncol* 2002;20:2453–2463.

145. Wong JY, Williams LE, Yamauchi DM, et al. Initial experience evaluating 90yttrium-radiolabeled anti-carcinoembryonic antigen chimeric T84.66 in a phase I radioimmunotherapy trial. *Cancer Res* 1995;55:5929s–5934s.

146. Xiao Z, McQuarrie SA, Suresh MR, et al. A three-step strategy for targeting drug carriers to human ovarian carcinoma cells in vitro. *J Biotechnol* 2002;94:171–184.

147. Yu L, Ju DW, Chen W, et al. 131I-chTNT radioimmunotherapy of 43 patients with advanced lung cancer. *Cancer Biother Radiopharm* 2006;21:5–14.

148. Zeng ZC, Tang ZY, Liu KD, et al. Improved long-term survival for unresectable hepatocellular carcinoma (HCC) with a combination of surgery and intrahepatic arterial infusion of 131I-anti-HCC mAb. Phase I/II clinical trials. *J Cancer Res Clin Oncol* 1998;124:275–280.

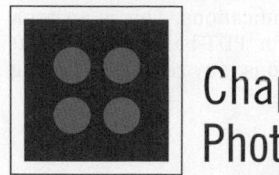

Chapter 24
Photodynamic Therapy

Ron R. Allison, Claudio H. Sibata

The medicinal properties of light have been appreciated for centuries with no less than Hippocrates a practitioner of this art (6). Photodynamic therapy (PDT) was serendipitously discovered, at the turn of the past century, by a medical student, Oscar Raab. Working in conjunction with his professor, Von Tappeiner who coined the term, the mechanism of action was elucidated and excellent clinical outcomes were obtained. This culminated in a textbook of principles and practice published in 1907. Despite these promising findings and several subsequent rebirths, it was not until the late 1970s with Thomas Dougherty's rediscovery of PDT that a commercially viable therapeutic intervention again emerged to the clinical arena.

Photodynamic Therapy Components

PDT involves application of a photosensitizing agent, which when selectively activated by light leads to the production of singlet oxygen (34). This reactive species induces necrosis, apoptosis, or a combination thereof. Clinically, vascular shut down also occurs with selective destruction of the lesion and minimal permanent damage to surrounding normal tissue.

Photosensitizer

As in photosynthesis, photosensitizers are substances that when activated by light transform light energy into chemical energy. Many structures have this ability; however, very few photosensitizers have made it through clinical trials and even fewer are commercially available (Table 24.1). The characteristics of a clinically successful photosensitizer will vary but overall should include some of the following (5): nontoxic and toxic-free byproducts, nonmutagenic, reliable activation at clinically useful wavelengths of light, production of clinically relevant amounts of singlet oxygen, concentration in tumor or rapidly proliferating tissue, clear normal tissue, pain-free therapy, and versatile administration—either topically, orally, or intravenously. The ideal photosensitizer would have the ability to be employed in myriad indications and offer selective destruction of the lesion without undue normal tissue toxicity. This transparency is far from what is presently clinically available, yet, despite multiple limitations, currently available photosensitizers can offer excellent outcomes.

The original photosensitizers were dyes, with ink being a potent member of this family. These platforms generally have prolonged tissue half-lives, particularly with skin retention. This results in unintentional PDT to sunlight-exposed skin many months after photosensitizer administration, a serious clinical drawback.

The porphyrin family, which not coincidentally forms the backbone of hemoglobin and chlorophyll, is a major source of viable photosensitizers. They also may have radiation sensitizing properties and may enhance diagnostic imaging, impressive, but so far clinically underutilized capabilities. Porfimer sodium, a hematoporphyrin derivative (HpD), was the first commercially available photosensitizer. This proprietary complex of monomers, dimmers, and oligomers has been employed in thousands of patients over many decades and has brought PDT to a worldwide audience. Porfimer sodium concentrates in rapidly proliferating tissue and is also cleared from normal tissue to allow for a clinically exploitable differential. Although nontoxic, reliable, and offering pain-free therapy, it is not very efficient; Therefore, illumination times can be relatively prolonged. Further, as this is a large chemical, it can only be intravenously introduced. Some porfimer sodium will be retained in normal skin, so 4 to 6 weeks of skin sunlight photosensitivity is expected.

Based on porfimer sodium's pioneering success, numerous "second generation" photosensitizers were developed that minimize some of these drawbacks or offer enhanced response. Temoporfin, a chlorine derivative, is significantly more active so treatment time is measured in seconds. Systemic application results in 2 weeks of skin photosensitivity. In contrast to porfimer sodium, this photosensitizer is so reactive that patients must be kept in dim light for about 24 hours postinfusion. Treatment initiates 96 hours postinfusion, so scheduling can be an issue. Benzoporphyrin derivative (BPD), verteporfin, accumulates rapidly in neovasculature and also clears within 24 hours from normal tissues, including skin, despite its intravenous introduction. Therapy can be initiated as soon as 30 minutes postinfusion, a very convenient schedule. Mono-L-aspartyl chlorin e6 (NPe6), a member of the chlorine family, conveniently allows treatment shortly after intravenous injection. An interesting chlorine-based intravenous photosensitizer, hpph 2-1-hexyloxyethyl-2-devinyl pyropheophorbide-a (HPPH), still in clinical trials, has excellent activity, rapid pain-free treatment, and a short window of cutaneous photosensitivity of 24 to 48 hours.

Another approach to photosensitizer application is by topical application. This has particular relevance for cutaneous PDT as this obviates the potential for a generalized cutaneous photosensitivity reaction. So far the only commercially available and successful topical photosensitizer is based on aminolevulinic acid (ALA). This is a prodrug that is enzymatically converted in the heme synthetic pathway to protoporphyrin IX, a potent photosensitizer. When topically applied only this region becomes photosensitized. In contrast, when ALA is introduced orally or systemically, skin photosensitivity of 24 to 48 hours is expected. A methylated form of ALA (M-ALA) may enhance concentration within neoplastic and dysplastic tissue. Conveniently, illumination can occur several hours after topical administration. Two major shortcomings of ALA PDT are that the illumination can be painful and, more significantly, topical application allows for only a few millimeters of tissue penetration, thus limiting indications amenable to therapy.

Illumination

The goal of illumination is to successfully activate the photosensitizer within the lesion (24). Each photosensitizer has its own characteristic wavelength(s) and intensity of light required. In general, clinically successful photosensitizers are limited to activation wavelengths between approximately 400 to 800 nm (therapeutic window). Below these wavelengths the penetration is minimal and above, water preferentially absorbs light energy preventing significant photosensitizer activation. Light

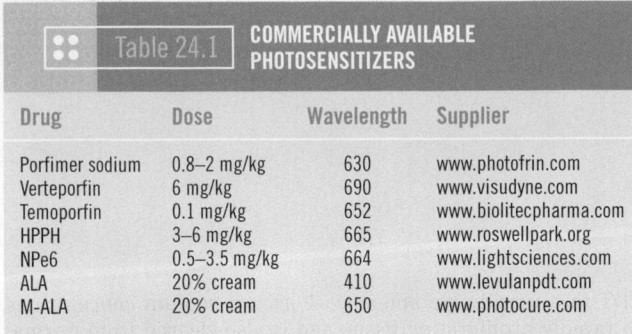

Table 24.1	**COMMERCIALLY AVAILABLE PHOTOSENSITIZERS**		
Drug	Dose	Wavelength	Supplier
Porfimer sodium	0.8–2 mg/kg	630	www.photofrin.com
Verteporfin	6 mg/kg	690	www.visudyne.com
Temoporfin	0.1 mg/kg	652	www.biolitecpharma.com
HPPH	3–6 mg/kg	665	www.roswellpark.org
NPe6	0.5–3.5 mg/kg	664	www.lightsciences.com
ALA	20% cream	410	www.levulanpdt.com
M-ALA	20% cream	650	www.photocure.com

of 400 nm (blue) penetrates tissues only several millimeters while longer wavelengths such as 630 nm (red) may penetrate about a centimeter. Thus, in addition to only illuminating the region at risk, choosing the appropriate wavelength of activation is a means to control depth and location of PDT. Sunlight is a very potent, broad spectrum source of illumination that can easily activate all current photosensitizers. Thus unintentional PDT can occur to sun-exposed body parts. This is why sunlight precautions are critical. Classically, to achieve the activation wavelength and light intensity for a particular photosensitizer, lamps with filters and lasers were employed. Recently, cost-effective light emitting diodes (LED) were introduced. For most cutaneous treatments, standard or fluorescent bulbs with filters to achieve the indicated wavelength can also be employed. Fiber optics, either attached to a laser or generated with LEDs, allow for highly versatile illumination. These components can be shaped to deliver illumination in one direction like a flashlight (microlens) or circumferentially (diffuser). They can be manufactured to fit endoscopes and are sturdy enough for interstitial implantation. In particular, interstitial illumination allows for therapy of lesions larger than those that ordinarily could be treated by surface illumination. Like brachytherapy, this also is an excellent means to deliver a localized treatment. It should be emphasized that PDT illumination is nonthermal in nature. Miniature illumination devices can be implanted to allow for prolonged or metronomic therapy.

Photodynamic Reaction

Once light successfully activates the photosensitizer, a photodynamic reaction (PDR) occurs (15). A photosensitizer, originally in the ground state, absorbs a photon and is excited to one of several higher-energy singlet states. The photosensitizer can readily undergo decay back to the ground state characterized by the emission of energy as fluorescence (visible light) or heat. Alternatively, a spin inversion followed by intersystem crossing can generate the longer-lived excited triplet state of the photosensitizer. In the triplet state, the photosensitizer can undergo two types of reaction with surrounding molecules: an electron transfer process (type I reaction) producing free radicals or an energy transfer to ground-state molecular oxygen (type II reaction). In the type II reaction (PDR), the product is the excited $^1O_2$, the major cytotoxic species responsible for the damaging effects of PDT.

As photosensitizer concentrates in cell membranes, this is generally where the PDR occurs, explaining its noncarcinogenic profile. As photosensitizer does not routinely concentrate in connective tissue, healing without fibrosis is common. Originally, PDT was felt to be a local phenomenon. However, necrosis of cells and vasculature release myriad cytokines, which may up-regulate the immune system. The release of these proteins and chemicals may be bypassed by the apoptotic pathway. Thus, pushing PDT in one direction to necrosis or in another di-

rection to apoptosis has clinical ramifications. This is an area of active investigation particularly for PDT-based vaccines. It may also explain why untreated lesions may regress following PDT (2).

Dosimetry

PDT dosimetry and physics are nowhere near the level of availability and relevance found in radiation oncology (37). Yet despite these limitations, reproducible clinical success is possible. Certainly, PDT will be improved by enhanced use of real-time dosimetry and treatment planning as is done in radiation oncology. Complicating factors for real-time dosimetry include the additional cascading issues of oxygen, photosensitizer concentration, and light distribution measurements. Without real-time dosimetry, overdosage of therapy to normal tissue and underdosage to tumor beds are possible. To minimize this clinicians employ a system using photosensitizer dose (mg/kg of body weight), light dose (usually prescribed but not measured), and drug infusion to light interval (DLI). These parameters are not individualized for each patient and may explain some of the variability in PDT outcomes. Each photosensitizer has its own characteristic parameters based on clinical data to guide success. By minimizing drug dose and maximizing illumination, a phenomena known as photobleaching can be exploited but is underutilized clinically. Photosensitizer concentrates preferentially in tumor over normal tissue. Using a clinically determined minimal amount of photosensitizer, one can retain enough photosensitizer in tumor to have, during illumination, a clinically significant PDR. The surrounding normal tissue will have less photosensitizer and be below threshold for a PDR to occur. Therefore, tumor can be ablated without damage of normal tissue by a selective response. Phototransformation can be used as a dosimetric parameter, correlated to PDT outcome (37). Fluorescence can intentionally be used to define PDT fields. Fluorescence can also be used for photodiagnosis (PD), sometimes termed *optical biopsy*, as normal tissue and tumors have differential optical characteristic. This may assist or replace histological evaluation in the future.

Clinical Photodynamic Therapy

Treatment simplicity has made PDT an attractive therapy. The fact that this therapy does not require huge investments in infrastructure, such as a sterile operating suite or linac vault, has expanded PDT to a worldwide audience (8). Further, PDT can offer a function sparing and cosmetically pleasing oncological intervention. This type of treatment paradigm may be common in countries with advanced medical systems but is certainly not the norm in developing countries. Therefore, PDT may have its greatest success in these arenas. Originally, patients with massive symptomatic failure, not an ideal population for local therapy, complicated by technical difficulties in terms of illumination were treated. However, as success was achieved, paradigms were refined and devices improved, culminating in Food and Drug Administration (FDA) or equivalent approval worldwide for various indications (Table 24.2).

Skin

The first clinical report from Dougherty showed impressive tumor control rates for recalcitrant primary and metastatic cutaneous malignancies of various histologies with porfimer PDT (16). Subsequent reports evaluating several thousand basal cell and in situ squamous cell tumors treatments with 1 mg/kg porfimer and 200 J/cm² illumination at 48 hours revealed complete response (CR) rates of >90% with a single session (11). Similar response was noted for basal cell nevus syndrome, where

Table 24.2 | SELECT PHOTODYNAMIC THERAPY TRIALS

Anatomy	Drug	Indication	Trial	Outcome	Ref
Skin	ALA	Actinic keratosis	PDT vs. placebo	72% vs. 20% CR	(29)
Skin	ALA	Actinic keratosis	PDT vs. placebo	89% vs. 13% CR	(32)
Skin	M-ALA	Basal cell cancer	PDT vs. cryotherapy	8% vs. 16% LF	(9)
Skin	M-ALA	Actinic keratosis	PDT vs. cryotherapy	LC equal, PDT better cosmesis	(35)
Skin	Porfimer sodium	Bowen/basal cell cancer	PDT first treatment	92% LC	(38)
Skin	ALA	Bowen	PDT vs. 5FU	LC equal, PDT better cosmesis	(33)
Breast	Porfimer sodium	Chest wall recurrence	PDT salvage	92% CR, 7% PR	(1)
Breast	Porfimer sodium	Chest wall recurrence	PDT salvage	91% CR, 8% PR	(13)
Brain	Porfimer sodium	Recurrence	Intraoperative surgery	Increase LC and survival	(26)
Eye	Verteporfin	WMD	PDT vs. placebo	Slows disease progression	(19)
Head and neck	Temoporfin	Oral cavity-incurable	PDT salvage	17% CR	(14)
Head and neck	Temoporfin	Oral cavity-recurrent	PDT salvage	58% CR	(36)
Head and neck	Temoporfin	Oral cavity-primary	T_1/T_2 lesions	82% CR	(23a)
Head and neck	Porfimer sodium	Larynx	Primary and recurrent	89% CR	(10)
Head and neck	Porfimer sodium	In situ	Diffuse and recurrent	98% CR and PR	(3)
Lung	Porfimer sodium	Endobronchial recurrent	PDT salvage	Palliation in 90% of patients	(25)
Lung	Porfimer sodium	Endobronchial primary	Tis/T_1	85% CR	(20)
Lung	NPe6	Parenchymal lung	T_1N_0	90% CR	(21)
Esophagus	Porfimer sodium	Obstruction	PDT vs. YAG laser	32% vs. 20% CR	(23)
Esophagus	Porfimer sodium	Barrett's	PDT vs. conventional	78% vs. 38% CR	(31)
Biliary	Porfimer sodium	Obstruction	PDT/stent vs. stent	PDT increased survival	(30)
Liver	LSII	Primary, mets	Interstitial	40% CR/PR	(12)
Bladder	Porfimer sodium	Recurrent CIS	PDT salvage	High LC, high fibrosis	(28)
Prostate	Temoporfin	Recurrent	Interstitial	Morbid	(27)

CIS, carcinoma in situ; CR, complete response; LC, local control; LF, local failure; PDT, photodynamic therapy; PR, partial response; YAG, yttrium-aluminum-garnet

multiple waves of tumors develop beginning at an early age. In contrast to a surgical approach, PDT allows for excellent cosmesis, an important consideration, particularly for young individuals.

As they avoid systemic photosensitization, topical ALA-based photosensitizers have been brought to the forefront of treatment to primary cutaneous lesions. In multiple, well-designed, randomized trials both ALA and M-ALA were able to reproducibly offer >90% CR for actinic keratosis and basal cell lesions. These results are equal or superior to cryotherapy, 5 FU cream, or curettage, and PDT offers better cosmesis. Lesion selection is critical as ALA will only penetrate 2 mm on topical application.

Cutaneous T-cell lymphoma, Kaposi's sarcoma, and other cutaneous histologies have been successfully eliminated with a number of photosensitizers. As PDT is a local treatment, cutaneous lesions with risk for nodal spread require a multimodality approach. Although PDT can eradicate isolated melanomatous lesions, its role here is not defined.

Breast

With the large number of breast cancers diagnosed, even low local failure rates translate into a large recurrence patient population. Porfimer PDT, as salvage for surgical and radiation failures, is possible (7). Various drug and light dose combinations on over a thousand lesions have been reported. It appears that a low dose of porfimer sodium (0.8 mg/kg) in combination with a high light dose (135 to 150 J/cm^2) can offer greater than a 90% rate of lesion control with good wound healing. Further, the treatment can take place with minimal discomfort in an outpatient setting. Similar excellent local control and wound healing were found in clinical trial with rostaporfin (SnET2), a chlorine-based photosensitizer. Temoporfin PDT offered excellent lesion control, but high normal tissue toxicity, showing the critical need for better dosimetry. PDT to downstage or as

local treatment for primary breast cancer is an interesting but unexplored potential indication. Breast conservation treatment strategies rely on postlumpectomy radiation therapy, which is not routinely available worldwide. This implies an important role for PDT in the future.

Ophthalmic/Neurologic

Ophthalmic treatment of wet macular degeneration (WMD) with verteporfin PDT is an approved indication worldwide (20). This disease leads to blindness by leaky neovasculature. As verteporfin accumulates in these vessels, a true niche for this photosensitizer was found. In well-designed clinical trials, PDT slows disease progression. Within 30 minutes of infusion, illumination by a highly accurate, commercially available ophthalmic laser is undertaken in an outpatient setting.

Well-designed randomized studies of porfimer PDT following resection of primary high-grade central nervous system recurrence have been published (26). Prior to surgery the photosensitizer is infused and after resection, intraoperatively, illumination via balloon catheter of the resection bed occurs. This has resulted in improved local control and progression-free survival. As photosensitizer accumulates in central nervous system tumors, the tumor fluorescence has been used to assist in surgical resection.

Head and Neck

PDT is an ideal local treatment for select head and neck tumors to allow for local control with minimal functional and cosmetic loss (3,19). However, as a local treatment, patients at risk for nodal metastasis may not be best served by PDT alone. In a prospective study for patients with locally advanced recurrence who had failed radiation and surgery, temoporfin PDT achieved a 50% palliation rate and a 17% durable CR. Patients with a more limited recurrence could achieve a durable

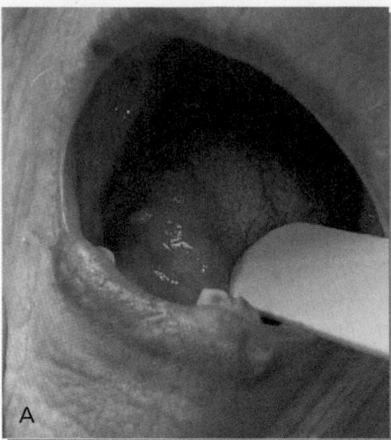 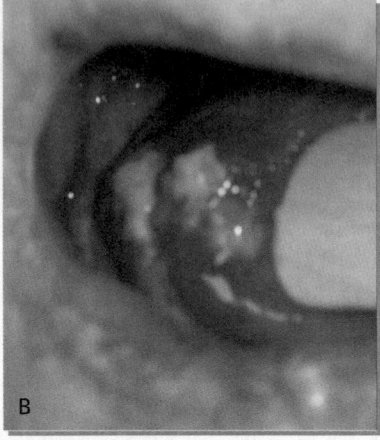 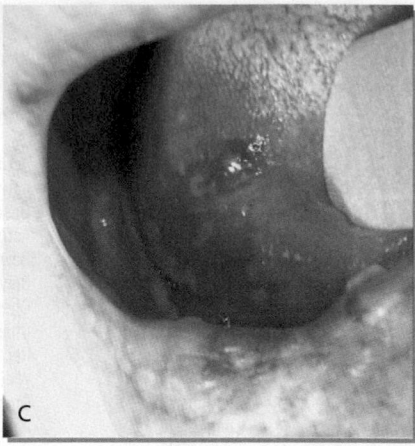

FIGURE 24.1. Low dose porfimer sodium photodynamic therapy to multifocal in situ squamous cell cancer. **A:** Pretreatment. **B:** 7 days posttreatment (note selective response). **C:** 14 days posttreatment (excellent healing, biopsy no evidence of disease).

58% CR. Temoporfin PDT to individuals with primary T_1/T_2 oral cavity squamous cell cancers achieved a durable 75% CR, with failures salvaged by surgery or radiation. Primary squamous cell tumors of the lip achieved a 92% durable CR. Particularly well suited for PDT are true larynx lesions, as they have a low incidence of nodal spread. Employing porfimer to patients with primary or locally recurrent larynx cancer achieved a 89% CR with excellent voice preservation following a single outpatient PDT session (10). In situ disease of the oral cavity and pharynx also responds well with function and cosmesis maintained. This is an attractive option, particularly for patients who experience multiple lesions, progression, or recurrence (Fig. 24.1).

Lung

Advanced lung cancer often has a component of endobronchial spread. PDT is an accepted, on label option to palliate these individuals. In a randomized trial comparing endoscopic PDT to yttrium-aluminum-garnet (YAG) laser, PDT offered significantly prolonged palliation (25). A review and meta-analysis by Moghissi and Dixon (25) of 636 patients with symptomatic endobronchial progression found virtually all patients had clinically significant pulmonary palliation, minimal morbidity, and cost-effective therapy with PDT. PDT can also be safely combined with stenting and high dose rate brachytherapy (HDR) to offer enhanced pulmonary palliation for these individuals. At the other end of the spectrum, ablation of early invasive and in situ endobronchial tumors with minimal pulmonary toxicity is possible. Patients have equal local control rates with far less morbidity when compared to resection. Recently, interstitial fiber placement via computed tomography (CT) scan to treat early invasive parenchymal lesions using MACE PDT had an 85% CR. PDT has also been employed as an adjunct to resection of advanced mesothelioma (5). Although technically challenging, enhanced local control was reported with both porfimer and temoporfin.

Esophagus/Gastrointestinal

Advanced, obstructing esophageal cancer is an on-label indication for porfimer PDT. In a multicenter randomized trial, endoesophageal porfimer PDT outperformed laser ablation in terms of palliation rates and duration of response (23). Porfimer also has FDA approval for the treatment of Barrett's esophagus with randomized data showing an 80% CR rate (31). Rather than esophagectomy, an outpatient illumination procedure can be undertaken. As illumination to these circumferential lesions is also circumferential, stricture is the most common morbidity. This can be relieved by dilation with functional retention. Trials with ALA-based PDT, with its limited depth penetration, have been explored to minimize stricture. However, deeper pockets of submucosal disease are a concern.

A randomized trial for symptomatic locally advanced cholangiocarcinoma, comparing the combination of PDT with stenting to PDT alone revealed a 1-year survival advantage when PDT was employed (2). Pilot studies of interstitial PDT to pancreatic and liver cancers have been successful. These studies show the versatility of PDT as well as the development of flexible tools to allow for placement of illumination devices in deep-seated anatomy (2).

Gynecological

In Japan and Europe, PDT has been employed to achieve destruction of both carcinoma in situ of the cervix (CIN) and vagina (VIN) (4). Both topical ALA-based treatment and porfimer sodium have been used with most series showing high local control rates and functional retention, an important consideration in gynecological intervention. Vaginal vault tumors that recur after surgery and radiation may be salvaged with PDT. Intraperitoneal PDT for ovarian metastasis has been attempted. The large volume and inhomogeneous illumination have so far been a problem.

Genitourinary

The original approval for porfimer PDT was achieved in Canada for in situ carcinoma of the bladder (15). Extremely high clearance rates with bladder preservation were possible. However, the irregular shape of the bladder led to an inability to homogeneously illuminate this site, resulting in excessive fibrosis and bladder capacity loss. Much interest has recently been generated by intravesicular or oral application of ALA for both photodiagnosis and PDT. ALA does not appear to penetrate deeply into the bladder muscular layers, thus diminishing fibrosis.

PDT has also been applied by interstitial transperineal placement of illumination catheters for locally recurrent prostate cancer. Although feasible, dosimetry is extremely complicated and results appear with excess morbidity. An elegant treatment of benign prostatic hyperplasia (BPH) with transurethral photosensitizer infusion and illumination in a outpatient basis have been described (2). Preliminary results are excellent and form the basis for a randomized trial. This may also be an approach for PDT to prostate cancer.

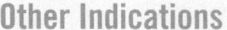

Other Indications

PDT can occur wherever photosensitizer accumulates. Treatment of infection, wounds, dental disease, and regenerative medicine have been reported (2). Of particular interest is cutaneous rejuvenation of skin (17), a new application.

Morbidity

The potential for PDT morbidity starts when the photosensitizer is applied. Sunlight precautions are critical as unintentional illumination of appropriate wavelength and strength can activate the photosensitizer, leading to burns. For most photosensitizers, except for temoporfin, room light is of no consequence. Generally, the illumination session is without discomfort with the exception of ALA. Topical anesthesia is not enough to eliminate the pain; however, narcotics can mitigate pain as can a judiciously placed ice pack.

Following illumination a relatively rapid reaction occurs in the treated region. Tumor will often appear hypovascular and necrotic. Normal illuminated tissue may be with edema and erythema. Too much drug or light may result in nonselective normal tissue destruction. If edema is expected or occurs in a critical region, steroids may be used. In the airway, a planned surveillance procedure will be undertaken generally 24 to 48 hours post-PDT to ensure that any necrotic tumor is cleared to prevent obstruction. In rare instances, a temporary tracheotomy may be planned for head and neck therapy. What PDT will essentially produce is the replacement of a growing tumor with a healing wound. Superficial lesions clear in days; deeper lesions may take several weeks or even months. Ideally, this time frame will be made clear to the patient. Sunlight exposure and wound healing issues are the major sources of morbidity with PDT. Fortunately, they respond well to antibiotics, steroids, and pain control.

Future Directions

The simplicity of PDT combined with its ability to preserve function and offer excellent cosmesis has been a growth engine for this therapy. This cost-effective intervention, even under relatively primitive conditions, offers cancer treatments to patients who might not otherwise obtain therapy.

Continued improvement in dosimetry and photosensitizers may be able to predict and enhance outcome, while technological advances create progressively more flexible illumination devices able to reach all anatomy. This has allowed for prolonged and deep-seated illumination as well as serial intermittent (metronomic) protocols that were not feasible even a few years ago.

This paradigm shift will bring new success but also new challenges. Viewing PDT as a complimentary therapeutic intervention rather than as competition will only help patients as well as those involved in cancer care.

References

1. Allison R, Mang T, Hewson G, et al. Photodynamic therapy for chest wall progression from breast carcinoma is an underutilized treatment modality. *Cancer* 2001;91:1–8.

2. Allison RR, Bagnato VS, Cuenca R, et al. The future of photodynamic therapy in oncology. *Future Oncol* 2006;2:53–71.
3. Allison RR, Cuenca R, Downie GH, et al. Clinical photodynamic therapy of head and neck cancers—a review of applications and outcomes. *Photodiagnosis Photodynamic Ther* 2005;2:205–222.
4. Allison RR, Cuenca R, Downie GH, et al. PD/PDT for gynecological disease: A clinical review. *Photodiagnosis Photodynamic Ther* 2005;2:51–63.
5. Allison RR, Downie GH, Cuenca R, et al. Photosensitizers in clinical PDT. *Photodiagnosis Photodynamic Ther* 2004;1:27–42.
6. Allison RR, Mota HC, Sibata CH. Clinical PD/PDT in North America: An historical review. *Photodiagnosis Photodynamic Ther* 2004;1:263–277.
7. Allison RR, Sibata C, Mang TS, et al. Photodynamic therapy for chest wall recurrence from breast cancer. *Photodiagnosis Photodynamic Ther* 2004;1:157–171.
8. Bagnato VS, Kurachi C, Ferreira J, et al. PDT experience in Brazil: A regional profile. *Photodiagnosis Photodynamic Ther* 2005;2:107–118.
9. Basset-Seguin N, Ibbotson S, Emtestam L. Photodynamic therapy using Metvix is as efficacious as cryotherapy in BCC, with better cosmetic results. *J Eur Acad Dermatol Venereol* 2001;15:226.
10. Biel MA. Photodynamic therapy in head and neck cancer. *Curr Oncol Rep* 2002;4:87–96.
11. Brown SB, Brown EA, Walker I. The present and future role of photodynamic therapy in cancer treatment. *Lancet Oncol* 2004;5:497–508.
12. Chen J, Keltner L, Christophersen J, et al. New technology for deep light distribution in tissue for phototherapy. *Cancer J* 2002;8:154–163.
13. Cuenca RE, Allison RR, Sibata C, et al. Breast cancer with chest wall progression: treatment with photodynamic therapy. *Ann Surg Oncol* 2004;11:322–327.
14. D'Cruz AK, Robinson MH, Biel MA. mTHPC-mediated photodynamic therapy in patients with advanced, incurable head and neck cancer: A multicenter study of 128 patients. *Head Neck* 2004;26:232–240.
15. Dougherty TJ, Gomer CJ, Henderson BW, et al. Photodynamic therapy. *J Natl Cancer Inst* 1998;90:889–905.
16. Dougherty TJ, Kaufman JE, Goldfarb A, et al. Photoradiation therapy for the treatment of malignant tumors. *Cancer Res* 1978;38:2628–2635.
17. Goldman MP, Dover JS, Alam M, eds. *Photodynamic therapy*. 1st ed. Procedures in Cosmetic Dermatology series. Philadelphia: Elsevier Saunders, 2005.
18. Hopper C. Photodynamic therapy: A clinical reality in the treatment of cancer. *Lancet Oncol* 2000;1:212–219.
19. Houle JM, Strong A. Clinical pharmacokinetics of verteporfin. *J Clin Pharmacol* 2002;42:547–557.
20. Kato H. Photodynamic therapy for lung cancer—A review of 19 years' experience. *J Photochem Photobiol B* 1998;42:96–99.
21. Kato H, Furukawa K, Sato M, et al. Phase II clinical study of photodynamic therapy using mono-L-aspartyl chlorin e6 and diode laser for early superficial squamous cell carcinoma of the lung. *Lung Cancer* 2003;42:103–111.
22. Lou PJ, Jones L, Hoper C. Clinical outcomes of photodynamic therapy for head-and-neck cancer. *Tech. in Cancer Res and Treatment*, 2003:311–317.
23. Lightdale CJ. Role of photodynamic therapy in the management of advanced esophageal cancer. *Gastrointest Endosc Clin North Am* 2000;10:397–408.
24. Mang, T. Lasers and light sources for PDT: Past, present and future. *Photodiagnosis Photodynamic Ther* 2004;1:43–48.
25. Moghissi K, Dixon K. Is bronchoscopic photodynamic therapy a therapeutic option in lung cancer? *Eur Respir J* 2003;22:535–541.
26. Muller PJ, Wilson BC. Photodynamic therapy for malignant newly diagnosed supratentorial gliomas. *J Clin Laser Med Surg* 1996;14:263–270.
27. Nathan TR, Whitelaw DE, Chang SC, et al. Photodynamic therapy for prostate cancer recurrence after radiotherapy: A phase I study. *J Urol* 2002;168:1427–1432.
28. Nseyo UO, DeHaven J, Dougherty TJ, et al. Photodynamic therapy (PDT) in the treatment of patients with resistant superficial bladder cancer: A long-term experience. *J Clin Laser Med Surg* 1998;16:61–68.
29. Ormrod D, Jarvis B. Topical aminolevulinic acid HCl photodynamic therapy. *Am J Clin Dermatol* 2000;1:133–139; Discussion 140–141.
30. Ortner MA. Photodynamic therapy in cholangiocarcinomas. *Best Pract Res Clin Gastroenterol* 2004;18:147–154.
31. Overholt BF, Lightdale CJ, Wang K, et al. International, multicenter, partially blinded, randomised study of the efficacy of photodynamic therapy (PDT) using porfimer sodium (POR) for the ablation of high-grade dysplasia (HGD) in Barrett's esophagus (BE): Results of 24-month follow-up. *Gastroenterology* 2003;124:A20.
32. Piacquadio DJ, Chen DM, Farber HF, et al. Photodynamic therapy with aminolevulinic acid topical solution and visible blue light in the treatment of multiple actinic keratoses of the face and scalp: Investigator-blinded, phase 3, multicenter trials. *Arch Dermatol* 2004;140:41–46.
33. Salim A, Leman JA, McColl JH, et al. Randomized comparison of photodynamic therapy with topical 5-fluorouracil in Bowen's disease. *Br J Dermatol* 2003;148:539–543.
34. Sibata CH, Colussi VC, Oleinick NL, et al. Photodynamic therapy in oncology. *Expert Opin Pharmacother* 2001;2:917–927.
35. Szeimies RM, Karrer S, Radakovic-Fijan S, et al. Photodynamic therapy using topical methyl 5-aminolevulinate compared with cryotherapy for actinic keratosis: A prospective, randomized study. *J Am Acad Dermatol* 2002;47:258–262.
36. Tan B. Foscan mediated photodynamic therapy in recurrent and second primary oral cavity cancers. *Laryngo-Rhino-Otology* 2000;79:318.
37. Wilson BC, Patterson MS, Lilge L. Implicit and explicit dosimetry in photodynamic therapy: A new paradigm. *Lasers Med Sci* 1997;12:182–199.
38. Zeitouni NC, Shieh S, Oseroff AR. Laser and photodynamic therapy in the management of cutaneous malignancies. *Clin Dermatol* 2001;19:328–338.

Techniques, Modalities, and Modifiers in Radiation Oncology

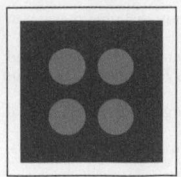

Chapter 25
Radiation Oncology in the Developing World

Timothy P. Hanna

One of the great challenges facing the international radiation oncology community is the increasing need for cancer prevention, early detection, treatment, and palliation in low- and middle-income countries. Low-income countries have a per capita gross national income of less than US $875, and for middle-income countries the range is US $876 to $10,725 (80). Nations falling into these income groups are often described as developing countries.

Global Burden of Disease

In 2005 cancer comprised 13% of all deaths worldwide (86). In 2000, Parkin et al. (53) performed projections to assess the future global burden of cancer. In 2000, there were an estimated 6.2 million deaths from cancer and 10.1 million new cases. In 2020, 9.8 million people are projected to die of cancer and 15.4 million new cases of cancer will be diagnosed (10,53). In many developing countries, cancer tends to present in predominantly advanced stages, partly because of lack of comprehensive screening and poor access to effective treatments (34). As a result, the age-adjusted survival for breast and cervix cancer is estimated overall to be 57% and 41% in developing countries, respectively, compared with 73% and 61% in developed countries (52). By 2020, 61% of all incident cancer cases are projected to be in developing countries. This is largely because, in all economic groups, the life expectancy of the world population is increasing while fertility rates are declining most in developed countries (74,75). In 2004, 60% of people ≥65 years of age lived in developing countries, and this is expected to rise to 80% by 2050 (75).

In comparison to the worldwide burden of cancer, cardiovascular disease is responsible for 30% of deaths and other chronic conditions and injuries kill 18% and 9%, respectively. Communicable diseases, maternal and perinatal conditions, and nutritional deficiencies comprise 30% of deaths (86). In total, 60% of mortality worldwide today is the result of chronic disease (6). This burden of chronic disease is not limited to developed countries (68,84). Results from the Global Burden of Disease study indicate that in 2001, in low- and middle-income countries, cancer was among the top five most common causes of death in five of the six world regions (42). The exception was sub-Saharan Africa, where a large proportion of mortality is due to human immunodeficiency virus/acquired immunodeficiency syndrome (HIV/AIDS) (42). In low-income countries, where death from communicable disease and other related causes are still common, chronic disease accounts for almost as many deaths as these causes and is expected to surpass them by 2015 (68). This growing burden of chronic disease represents a significant epidemiologic transition for developing countries and a dual challenge for disease control efforts in this setting (12).

Epidemiology of Cancer Worldwide

Worldwide, lung cancer is the most common incident cancer and cause of cancer death, with an estimated 1.35 million new cases and 1.18 million deaths in 2002 (Fig. 25.1) (52). Gastric cancer and liver cancer are the second and third most common causes, respectively, of cancer death. Breast cancer is the second most common cause of cancer (1.15 million). Prostate and breast cancer are both more common in developed countries (Fig 25.2) (52). Although cervix cancer is the seventh most commonly diagnosed cancer among women in developed countries, it is the second most common cancer among women after breast cancer in developing nations due to a lack of sufficient screening programs (61). Cervix cancer is extremely common in Latin America, sub-Saharan Africa, and parts of Asia such as India (30). Gastric cancer and hepatocellular carcinoma are also far more common in developing countries, with 42% of all cases of gastric cancer in the world in China alone (30). Kaposi's sarcoma is extremely common in sub-Saharan Africa because of the AIDS epidemic, and esophageal cancer has the highest incidence rates worldwide in regions of Asia and Africa. Oral cancer is the most commonly diagnosed cancer among men in India (30).

Among nine common modifiable risk factors for cancer, tobacco smoking is associated with the largest proportion of attributable risk (18). In the developing world, an estimated 49% of men and 8% of women were current smokers in 1995 (31). With their large populations and high smoking rates in China and smoked and smokeless tobacco use in India, tobacco is an extremely important risk factor for cancer in Asia (33,64). In general, many low- and middle-income countries have shown rising trends in tobacco use during the past 3 decades, with peak use in the mid-1980s and early 1990s (24,64). History has shown a 30- to 40-year delay between the peak in smoking rates in a population and the peak in tobacco-related mortality (41). Thus, an increasing rate of tobacco-related malignancies is expected in low- and middle-income countries such as China during the next half century (48,87).

Twenty-six percent of cancers in the low- and middle-income countries are attributed to infectious causes (51). Hepatitis B and C are the major risk factors for hepatocellular carcinoma in developing countries and aflatoxin produced from *Aspergillus* in certain poorly preserved foods has also been implicated in liver carcinogenesis (28,54). Human papillomavirus and *Helicobacter pylori* are also important etiologic agents, and there are numerous other infectious agents relevant to cancer in the developing world including the Epstein-Barr virus, HIV, schistosomiasis, human T-cell leukemia virus type 1, (HTLV-1) and human herpesvirus 8 (HHV-8) (29,51).

Among cancers common to the developed world, diet plays a role in the cause of colorectal cancer and obesity is a risk factor for endometrial cancer and renal cell cancer (16,35). Although plausible, a link between diet and breast cancer has not been clearly established (35). The impact of genetic polymorphisms on patterns of global cancer incidence has not been fully elucidated but there is some suggestion of their relevance (9,39).

Global Status of Access to Radiation Therapy

Access to radiation therapy is a multifactorial issue. Not only does one need to consider machine supply, but there are also

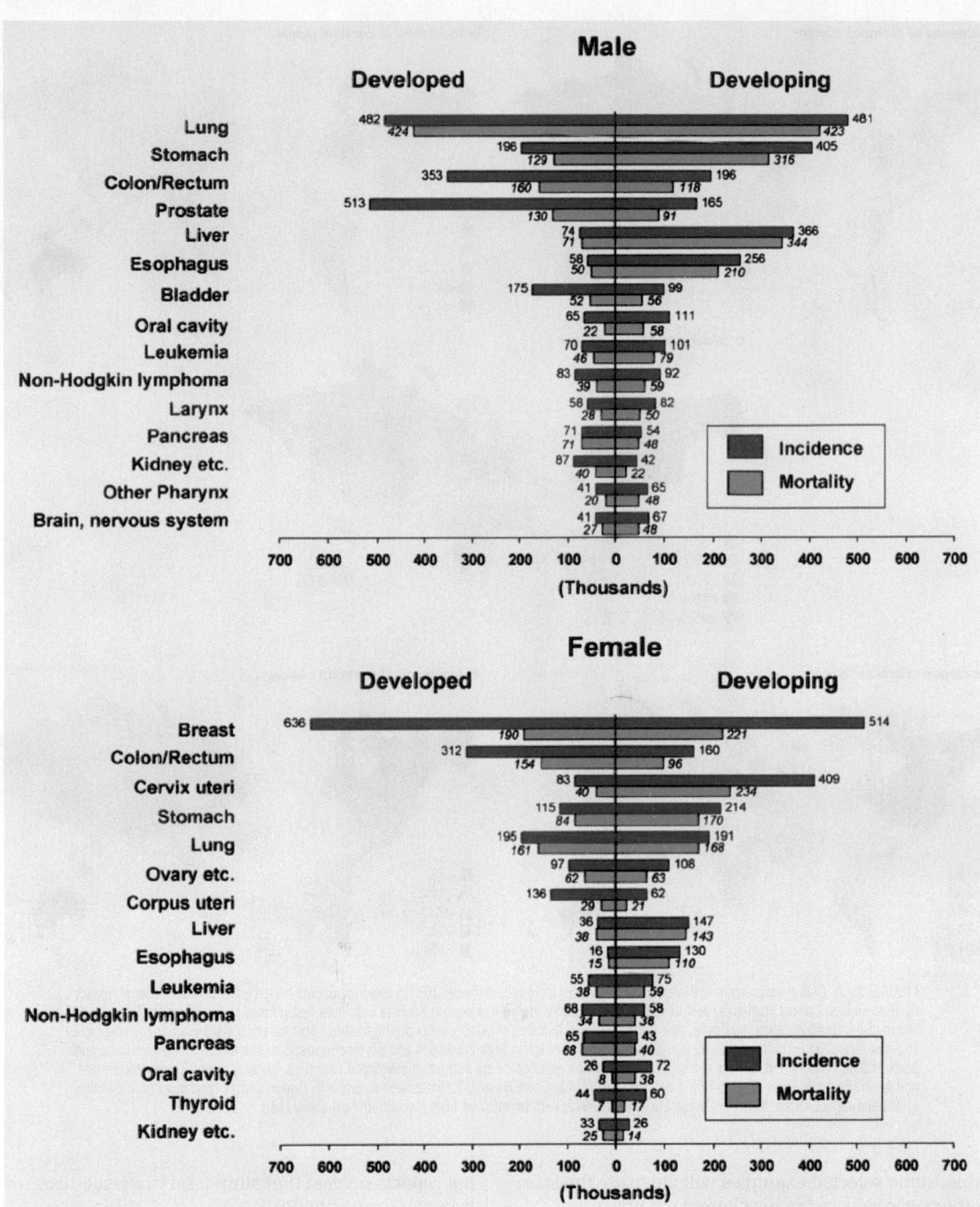

FIGURE 25.1. Estimated numbers of new cancer cases (incidence) and deaths (mortality) worldwide in 2002. Data are shown in thousands for developing and developed countries by cancer site and sex. (Reproduced from Parkin DM, Bray F, Ferlay J, et al. Global cancer statistics, 2002. *CA Cancer J Clin* 2005;55:74–108, with permission.)

many other considerations, including workforce, geographic distribution of equipment, access to surgery and other multidisciplinary care, availability of technical support and a reliable power supply, as well as the financial capacity of patients in countries with little or no health insurance. With cervical cancer being so common in developing countries and the high frequency of late-stage presentations requiring palliation, radiation therapy has an important role in developing countries. One indicator of access to radiation therapy is the number of megavoltage machines per million population (MV/million). In the United States, Japan, France, and Australia there are estimated to be 10.2, 6.4, 5.9, and 5.0 MV/million, respectively (50,59,66,74,79). The European Society for Therapeutic Radiology and Oncology (ESTRO) Quantification of Radiation Ther-

apy Infrastructure and Staffing Needs (QUARTS) projects estimated that the actual need for radiation therapy varied in a sample of 25 European Union countries between 4.0 and 8.1 MV/million (8).

Estimating the required number of radiation machines to fully satisfy need depends on the incidence rate of cancer, the types of incident cancers, the accepted radiation therapy indications for these, patient preference, and the workload seen per machine (21). For these reasons, one cannot simply take radiation therapy rates from high-income countries and apply them to low- and middle-income countries. For instance, many megavoltage machines in China have been reported to be working at more than twice the patient load per day seen in Western settings (40). Although systematic information for all countries

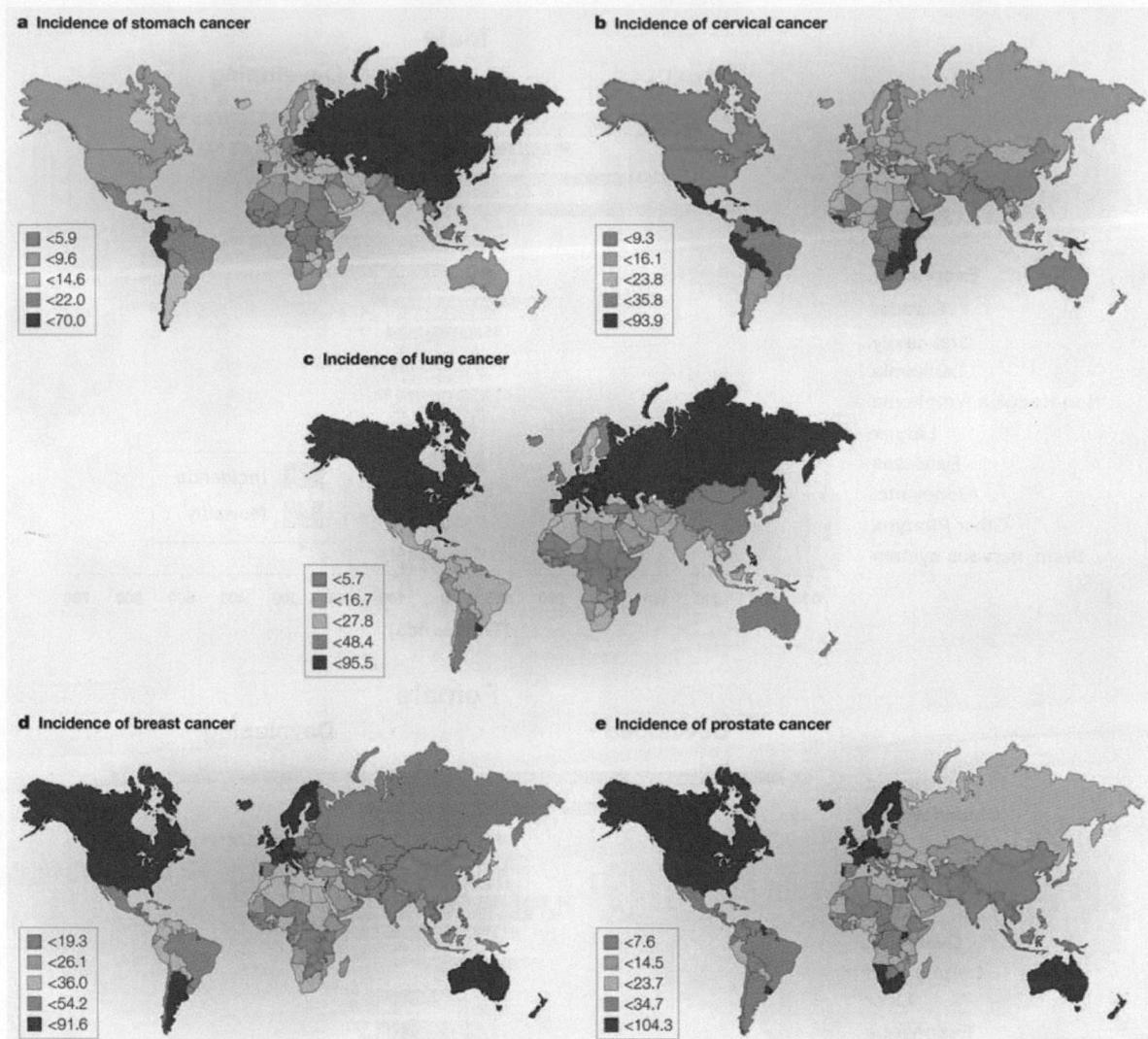

FIGURE 25.2. Global variation in age-standardized cancer incidence rates per 10^5 for specific cancers based on 2002 International Agency for Research on Cancer statistics. **a:** Rates of stomach cancer are high in regions such as East Asia, Latin America, and Eastern Europe and low in India, North America, Australia, and parts of Africa. **b:** Rates of cervix cancer are highest in Latin America, Africa, and southeast and south central Asia including India. **c:** Lung cancer rates are high in both developed and developing parts of the world, including China and parts of South America. **d, e:** Breast cancer and prostate cancer rates are highest in developed countries, notably in North America, Europe, and Australia, with lower rates in China and parts of Africa. (From Rastogi T, Hildesheim A, Sinha R. Opportunities for cancer epidemiology in developing countries. *Nat Rev Cancer* 2004;4:909–917, with permission from Macmillan Publishers Ltd.)

is not available, some selected examples will illustrate the state of radiation therapy resources in developing countries.

Africa

In 1999, Levin et al. (37) documented the availability and distribution of radiation therapy equipment in Africa. Only 22 of 56 countries in Africa were confidently known to have megavoltage radiation therapy facilities. The population in countries without any known access to radiation therapy was more than 176 million people and, including these, more than 400 million Africans have effectively no access to radiation therapy. A total of 155 megavoltage machines were identified in Africa, although 53 of these were in Egypt and 40 were in South Africa. Sixty percent of machines in Africa were cobalt-60. The availability of remote afterloading brachytherapy devices for treating gynecologic cancer has not yet been fully reported. The number of individuals served by each radiation machine varied from 0.01 to 1.7 MV/million, with only Mauritius having >1 MV/million and most countries with radiation therapy having <0.1 MV/million. The state of repair of most of these machines is not known,

but reports suggest that simple service issues can severely stifle treatment capacity (20).

Asia and Pacific Region

A number of country-specific reports on the status of radiation therapy exist as well as a comprehensive survey of 17 countries in the region (13,15,19,70,78). Tatsuzaki and Levin (70) found an 82-fold variation in the number of megavoltage machines per million population (Table 25.1); 45% were cobalt machines. The variation in supply of megavoltage machines correlated well with national economic status (Fig. 25.3). This emphasizes the importance of national economic status as a determinant of health (38). China and India, representing almost 40% of the world's population, had an estimated 0.53 and 0.30 MV/million, respectively (70,74). Excluding high-income countries, many radiation facilities did not have a simulator in 2001. Workforce resources varied considerably between countries, and most countries had less than two radiation oncologists per 1,000 cancer patients annually.

| | | MEGAVOLTAGE MACHINE SUPPLY IN ASIA PACIFIC COUNTRIES BY PER CAPITA GROSS NATIONAL INCOME | | |
| Table 25.1 | | | | |

Country	Per Capita Gross National Income ($US)	Population (millions)	Megavoltage (MV) Machines Total	MV/Million
Myanmar	n.a.	44.5	7	0.16
Vietnam	380	77.6	11	0.14
Bangladesh	390	124.8	11	0.09
Mongolia	400	2.4	2	0.83
India	450	970.9	291	0.30
Pakistan	480	130.6	34	0.26
Indonesia	590	204.4	24	0.12
Sri Lanka	810	18.8	7	0.37
China	930	1255.7	667	0.53
Philippines	1040	75.2	17	0.23
Thailand	1990	61.2	50	0.82
Malaysia	3430	21.0	26	1.24
Korea, Republic	9790	46.4	69	1.49
New Zealand	13680	3.8	28	7.39
Australia	20060	18.8	90	4.80
Singapore	23030	3.9	10	2.58
Japan	35140	126.4	816	6.46
Total		3186.4	2160	0.68

n.a., not available.
Year 2000 gross national income information provided by the World Bank Group: World development indicators 2006 data query. http://devdata.worldbank.org/data-query. Population and machine information from Tatsuzaki H, Levin CV. Quantitative status of resources for radiation therapy in Asia and Pacific region. *Radiother Oncol* 2001;60:81–89, with permission from Elsevier.

Reports from individual countries in the Asia-Pacific region support the findings from the regional survey. In 1996, Liu (40) reported that in China, workloads of 100 patients per machine per day were common at some sites. Only about 50% of radiation therapy departments had simulators. More recent reports from China highlight the rapid growth of radiation therapy capacity between 1986 and 2001 (13,78). Even so, Cao et al. (13) comment on the lack of sufficient radiation therapy equipment to treat patients. A shortage of physicists has been a major problem in China, with a current physicist-to-radiation oncologist ratio of 1:8 (13). In India, radiation oncology faces many challenges, including poor supply of radiation oncologists, physicists, and therapists, few treatment facilities, limited access for rural populations, an estimated 80% rate of advanced locore-

gional disease (T3/4), a high burden of acute and chronic non-malignant disease, as well as adherence issues with therapy and loss to follow-up (19).

Latin America

In Latin America, there are significant shortfalls in radiation therapy equipment and human resources. In 2004, Zubizarreta et al. (89) reported that 7 of 19 countries in the region had <1 MV/million. The range of equipment supply was 0.19 MV/million in Nicaragua to 4.12 MV/million for Uruguay; 56% of machines were cobalt-60. Supply of equipment varied according to per capita gross national income as in other regions. Only 19% of centers had simulators. In the 12 countries that reported

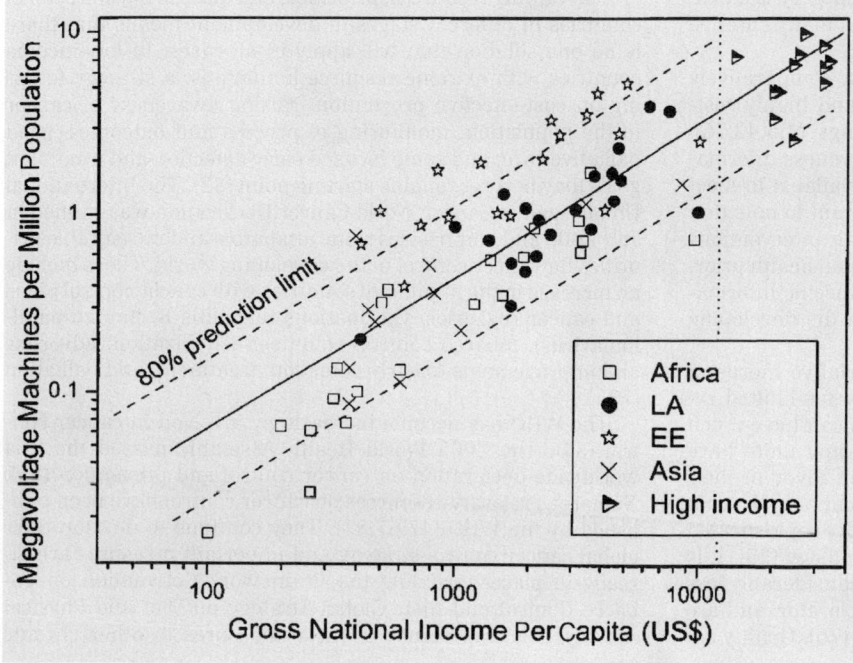

FIGURE 25.3. Megavoltage machines per million population versus gross national income per capita on a log-log scale. Countries are divided into incomes more than US $12,000 (high income) and then by region: Africa, Latin America (LA), Eastern Europe (EE), and Asia. The *solid line* is a linear regression line and *dotted lines* are the 80% confidence limit. The *vertical dotted line* represents the cutoff for high income. (From Levin V, Tatsuzaki H. Radiotherapy services in countries in transition: Gross national income per capita as a significant factor. *Radiother Oncol* 2002;63:147–150, with permission from Elsevier.)

Techniques, Modalities, and Modifiers in Radiation Oncology

on brachytherapy resources, there were 397 documented sets of brachytherapy equipment, the majority of which were manual afterloading cesium. Zubizarreta et al. identified lack of trained human resources as the greatest barrier to patient service in Latin America. In 2003, 69% more radiation oncologists were estimated to be needed (642), as well as 176% more physicists (627) and 109% more radiation technologists (2,500).

Eastern Europe and the Middle East

There has not been a formal survey of Eastern Europe, although Barton et al. (3) reported on rates of megavoltage machines ranging from 0.26 MV/million in Albania to 5.24 MV/million in the Czech Republic. Thirteen of 22 countries in the region had <2 MV/million. There has not been a formal survey of radiation therapy resources in low- and middle-income countries of the Middle East outside Africa, although data from the International Atomic Energy Agency (IAEA) *Directory of Radiotherapy Centers* suggests significant variation in access to radiation therapy in this region (26).

Considerations in Delivery of Radiation Therapy in Low- and Middle-Income Countries

Despite having 80% of the world's population, the IAEA estimates that developing countries only have about 40% of the world's radiation therapy facilities (60). The IAEA estimated in 1998 that a total of 2,500 teletherapy machines existed in developing countries with a total need of close to 5,000 (27). With the expected 75% increase of cancer incidence in the developing world between 2000 and 2020, the number of needed machines would increase accordingly (53). The estimates of the IAEA assume each machine treats 500 patients a year, which may be an underestimate of capacity given the high rate of palliative indications. A second important consideration is the effect of daily patient throughput. Extended working hours can potentially have a large impact on machine number required to meet national demand.

Providing radiation therapy in limited resource settings is far more complicated than equipment availability. Culturally appropriate plans sensitive to a region's social and political concerns are needed. Access to multidisciplinary care, including surgery, pathology, chemotherapy, rehabilitation, and palliative care are important considerations (7,62). The need for surgery is an especially notable problem given its importance in many curative situations such as with breast or gastric cancer.

Radiation therapy has been shown to be a comparatively cheap cancer therapy in developing settings and highly cost-effective in numerous developed world settings (4,5,43,76). Even so, it cannot be forgotten that cost-effectiveness information is context-specific and funding must be available to meet the opportunity cost (69). Moreover, it is important to note that there are numerous highly cost-effective health interventions that policy makers must balance in setting national health priorities, and unfortunately there is little context-specific information available on most cancer interventions in the developing setting to aid in decision-making (11,23).

There has been some debate about the relative merits of cobalt-60 versus linear accelerator technology for limited resource settings (19,56,76). Linear accelerators can have much appeal, especially as standard cobalt teletherapy units have been all but abandoned by richer countries in favor of their newer counterparts. At the same time, cobalt technology has not been optimized. For instance, it is capable of more sophisticated collimation including multileaf collimator technology (55). It is useful to remember that cobalt machines are considerably less expensive than even an entry-level linear accelerator, and are generally more reliable, requiring less service (76). Quality assurance and maintenance costs are estimated to be seven times less expensive than for linear accelerators (76). In a time when much attention has been given to new and expensive radiation therapy technologies requiring a high level of technical support and quality assurance that may not be immediately achievable in many developing settings, it is worth remembering that cobalt-60 machines have been shown to produce satisfactory treatment results in many settings and save lives (32,49,72).

Challenges to delivering cancer control and radiation therapy in limited-resource settings may include insufficient priority of cancer control among some governments and donor agencies with many competing priorities and problems, political or social instability, conflict, corruption, fragmented and underfinanced health care systems not equipped to manage chronic disease, lack of cancer awareness and knowledge among health care workers and the public, lack of diagnostic and treatment equipment and infrastructure, limitations in referral systems, challenges due to geography and population distribution, and inadequate cancer registry data (56,58,62). Often there can be a mismatch between resources and need, and the nature of this varies. For instance, there may be insufficient human resources but fair equipment supply, or adequate brachytherapy equipment but inadequate supply of teletherapy equipment (70,89). In addition, there is an overall shortage of health care workers in many countries in the developing world that limit available trainees for radiation oncology and other specialties. The World Health Organization (WHO) estimated that in 1993 there were 287 physicians per 100,000 population in developed countries versus 77 per 100,000 in developing countries (83).

Translating Knowledge into Action

What can be done? In the face of seemingly impossible odds, it may be encouraging to first highlight the progress that has already been made in increasing radiation therapy capacity in many developing countries. Between 1991 and 1998, machine supply more than doubled in Africa (37). Between 1989 and 2003, the number of linear accelerators in selected Latin American countries tripled overall (71,89). In the Asia-Pacific region there has been a threefold increase in the number of megavoltage machines between 1976 and 1999, and China's supply has more than doubled between 1994 and 2001 (13,70).

The varying resources, priorities, and disease burden seen in countries in different stages of development means that there is no one solution that will apply in all cases. In low-income countries with extreme resource limitations, a strategy focusing on cost-effective prevention, raising awareness of cancer in the population, monitoring of process and outcomes, good palliative care, and some focused early detection and treatment goals may be a reasonable starting point (82). The International Union Against Cancer World Cancer Declaration was ratified in July 2006 and emphasizes some attainable and measurable priorities for cancer control in the developing world. These include an increase in the number of countries with cancer control plans and cancer registries, vaccinations (hepatitis B, human papillomavirus), tobacco control, volunteer mobilization, advocacy and improvements to early detection, treatment, and palliation (73).

The WHO has become increasingly involved in cancer control (84). The 2005 World Health Assembly passed the first worldwide declaration on cancer control and prevention (85). Numerous relevant resources on cancer control have been published by the WHO (47,67,81). They continue to develop their global cancer control strategy and important measures are already in place, including the Framework Convention on Tobacco Control and their Global Strategy on Diet and Physical Activity. The importance of these measures to other chronic diseases illustrates the synergy of addressing multiple risks in tackling a broad spectrum of health problems.

The IAEA plays an important role in quality assurance, safety standards, and dose calibration of radiation therapy equipment internationally and has been involved in a number of technical cooperation projects in developing countries (60). In 2004, the IAEA launched the Program of Action for Cancer Treatment (PACT) in order to widen the scope of their work in radiation therapy capacity building. Their wide-ranging plan starts with the development of sustainable demonstration radiation treatment sites in six countries throughout the developing world. The PACT program situates the delivery of radiation therapy within a comprehensive framework including prevention, early detection, treatment, and palliation. Plans sensitive to the target country's social and political situation are under development through local and international partnerships. Development of the first demonstration center in Tanzania is well under way.

ESTRO has been extensively involved in numerous training courses and conferences in developing countries. The American Society for Therapeutic Radiology and Oncology has also been involved in organizing radiation oncology training courses in developing countries as well as supporting other educational and collaborative activities. Similarly, the Royal College of Radiology supports traveling professorships to developing countries, and the European School of Oncology has also been involved in training courses. In addition to seminars, the International Campaign for Establishment and Development of Oncology Centers has been involved in consultations in the developing world (45). Breast cancer treatment guidelines stratified by availability of resources have been developed through the Breast Health Global Initiative (1).

The importance of improving learning resources cannot be overstated given the global workforce shortage of radiation treatment professionals. Some initial efforts have been made at developing curriculum and educational approaches (2,17,55,65). Designing educational programs within developing countries themselves using equipment similar to what the trainee will ultimately use are important and are probably more likely to retain staff in developing countries than comprehensive training programs based solely in developed countries. The issue of loss of trained staff from developing to developed countries is a notable one (25).

Many developing countries have quite advanced resources to sustain research activities, for instance, the Advanced Center for Treatment Research and Education in Cancer (ACTREC), part of the Tata Memorial Center in India. Also, a number of research/teaching partnerships between developed and developing countries have been reported in the literature, particularly in pediatric oncology, providing some general principles for those considering collaboration (44,45,77). Supporting research on cancer by clinicians in the developing world is important as it can build local capacity. There are many fundamental questions that remain unanswered. For instance, it cannot be assumed that approaches to treating cancer from developed settings will produce the same results when applied in limited resource settings or to genetically distinct populations (14,22,57,88). There are many unknowns in cancer epidemiology and basic science. Also, more health services research is needed; as mentioned, little is known about cost-effectiveness of cancer treatments offered in developing settings (9). The International Network for Cancer Treatment and Research has been involved in designing clinical trials relevant to developing world situations, and the U.S. National Cancer Institute has been involved with numerous international collaborations.

Undoubtedly, industry and development will play an important role in improving access to quality radiation therapy equipment. Cheaper, more durable, more reliable equipment is needed. Creative public-private partnerships and alternative financing solutions will be important. Perhaps lessons can be learned from the determined work of those who have fought to deliver treatment for HIV/AIDS and multidrug resistant tuberculosis in the developing world, previously treatments so expensive as to be unattainable by most in need (36). Additionally, creativity in equipment design will be important. This has been exemplified by a group in Canada that has pioneered cobalt-60 tomotherapy (63). Telemedicine may improve access to care and allow for sharing of limited resources in some settings.

Lastly, a society's perceptions or beliefs about determinants of health play a role in their setting of private and public health policies (46). Increased global public awareness of the role that chronic diseases like cancer play in the health of individuals in developing countries will be critical. Given the shortage of national funding for cancer care in poorer countries, international private and public donor support will be of considerable importance.

Conclusion

Cancer in the developing world is an urgent problem, reaching critical proportion. By 2020, more than 60% of all cancer cases will be diagnosed in the developing world. Most individuals in developing countries have either limited access or no access to radiation therapy. At a time when new gains in oncology outcomes in the developed world are incremental, oncologists have the chance to introduce absolute survival gains in the developing world of potentially 15% to 30% or more through early detection and treatment. In addition, the potential for health care gains through cancer prevention and the relief of suffering through palliative care are enormous. The poor deserve fair access to quality cancer care. The challenge will now be to deliver this in a thoughtful and contextually appropriate way.

References

1. Anderson BO, Shyyan R, Eniu A, et al. Breast cancer in limited-resource countries: An overview of the breast health global initiative 2005 guidelines. *Breast J* 2006;12[Suppl 1]:S3–15.
2. Barton MB, Bell P, Sabesan S, et al. What should doctors know about cancer? Undergraduate medical education from a societal perspective. *Lancet Oncol* 2006;7:596–601.
3. Barton MB, Frommer M, Shafiq J. Role of radiotherapy in cancer control in low-income and middle-income countries. *Lancet Oncol* 2006;7:584–595.
4. Barton MB, Gebski V, Manderson C, et al. Radiation therapy: Are we getting value for money? *Clin Oncol (R Coll Radiol)* 1995;7:287–292.
5. Barton MB, Jacob SA, Gebsky V. Utility-adjusted analysis of the cost of palliative radiotherapy for bone metastases. *Australas Radiol* 2003;47:274–278.
6. Beaglehole R, Yach D. Globalisation and the prevention and control of non-communicable disease: The neglected chronic diseases of adults. *Lancet* 2003; 362:903–908.
7. Behera D. Managing lung cancer in developing countries: Difficulties and solutions. *Indian J Chest Dis Allied Sci* 2006;48:243–244.
8. Bentzen SM, Heeren G, Cottier B, et al. Towards evidence-based guidelines for radiotherapy infrastructure and staffing needs in Europe: The ESTRO QUARTS project. *Radiother Oncol* 2005;75:355–365.
9. Bono AV. The global state of prostate cancer: epidemiology and screening in the second millennium. *BJU Int* 2004;94[Suppl 3]:1–2.
10. Bray F, Moller B. Predicting the future burden of cancer. *Nat Rev Cancer* 2006;6:63–74.
11. Brown ML, Goldie SJ, Draisma G, et al. Health service interventions for cancer control in developing countries. In: Jamison DT, Breman JG, Measham AR, et al, eds. *Disease control priorities in developing countries*. Washington, DC: World Bank and Oxford University Press, 2006:569–589.
12. Bulatao RA. Mortality by cause, 1970–2015. In: Gribble JN, Preston SH, eds. *The epidemiological transition. Policy and planning for developing countries*. Washington, DC: National Academy Press, 1993:42–68.
13. Cao J, Zhou J, Zhou X, et al. Status of radiotherapy in China. *Radiat Med* 2004;22: 9–11.
14. Carles J, Monzo M, Amat M, et al. Single-nucleotide polymorphisms in base excision repair, nucleotide excision repair, and double strand break genes as markers for response to radiotherapy in patients with stage I and II head-and-neck cancer. *Int J Radiat Oncol Biol Phys* 2006;66:1022–1030.
15. Chansilpa Y, Petsuksiri J. Current status of radiation therapy in Thailand. *Radiat Med* 2004;22:6–7
16. Chow WH, Gridley G, Fraumeni JF, et al. Obesity, hypertension, and the risk of kidney cancer in men. *N Engl J Med* 2000;343:1305–1311.
17. Coffey M, Engel-Hills P, El-Gantiry M, et al. A core curriculum for RTTs (radiation therapists/radiotherapy radiographers) designed for developing countries under the auspices of the International Atomic Energy Agency (IAEA). *Radiother Oncol* 2006;81:324–325.

18. Danaei G, Vander Hoorn S, Lopez AD, et al. Causes of cancer in the world: comparative risk assessment of nine behavioural and environmental risk factors. *Lancet* 2005;366:1784–1793.

19. Dinshaw KA. Radiation oncology: The Indian scenario. *Int J Radiat Oncol Biol Phys* 1996;36:941–943.

20. Durosinmi-Etti FA. An overview of cancer management by radiotherapy in anglophone West Africa. *Int J Radiat Oncol Biol Phys* 1990;19:1263–1266.

21. Esco R, Palacios A, Pardo J, et al. Infrastructure of radiotherapy in Spain: A minimal standard of radiotherapy resources. *Int J Radiat Oncol Biol Phys* 2003;56:319–327.

22. Grau C, Prakash Agarwal J, Jabeen K, et al. Radiotherapy with or without mitomycin C in the treatment of locally advanced head and neck cancer: Results of the IAEA multicentre randomised trial. *Radiother Oncol* 2003;67:17–26.

23. Groot MT, Baltussen R, Uyl-de Groot CA, et al. Costs and health effects of breast cancer interventions in epidemiologically different regions of Africa, North America, and Asia. *Breast J* 2006;12[Suppl 1]:S81–90.

24. Guindon GE, Boisclair D. Past, current and future trends in tobacco use. In: de Beyer J, Guindon E, Yurekli A, eds. *Economics of tobacco control*. Washington, DC: World Bank, 2003.

25. Hongoro C, McPake B. How to bridge the gap in human resources for health. *Lancet* 2004;364:1451–1456.

26. IAEA. *Directory of radiotherapy centers (DIRAC)*. Available at: http://www-naweb.iaea.org/nahu/dirac/default.shtm. Accessed December 16, 2006.

27. IAEA. *Design and implementation of a radiotherapy programme: Clinical, medical physics, radiation protection and safety aspects (TECDOC 1040)*. Vienna: IAEA, 1998.

28. IARC. *IARC monographs on the evaluation of carcinogenic risks to humans: Some naturally occurring substances: food items and constituents, heterocyclic aromatic amines and mycotoxins*. Vol 56. Lyon, France: World Health Organization, 1993.

29. IARC. *IARC monographs on the evaluation of carcinogenic risks to humans: Schistosomes, liver flukes and Helicobacter pylori*. Lyon, France: World Health Organization, 1994.

30. IARC. *GLOBOCAN 2002 database*. Available at: http://www-dep.iarc.fr/. Accessed December 21, 2006.

31. Jha P, Ranson MK, Nguyen SN, et al. Estimates of global and regional smoking prevalence in 1995, by age and sex. *Am J Public Health* 2002;92:1002–1006.

32. Jimenez J, Alert J, Beldarrain L, et al. Carcinoma of the uterine cervix. Results of treatment in 2248 cases. *Acta Radiol Oncol Radiat Phys Biol* 1979;18:465–469.

33. John RM. Tobacco consumption patterns and its health implications in India. *Health Policy* 2005;71:213–222.

34. Kanavos P. The rising burden of cancer in the developing world. *Ann Oncol* 2006;17[Suppl 8]:viii, 15–23.

35. Key TJ, Schatzkin A, Willett WC, et al. Diet, nutrition and the prevention of cancer. *Public Health Nutr* 2004;7:187–200.

36. Kidder T. *Mountains beyond mountains*. New York: Random House, 2004.

37. Levin CV, El Gueddari B, Meghzifene A. Radiation therapy in Africa: Distribution and equipment. *Radiother Oncol* 1999;52:79–84.

38. Levin V, Tatsuzaki H. Radiotherapy services in countries in transition: Gross national income per capita as a significant factor. *Radiother Oncol* 2002;63:147–150.

39. Liede A, Narod SA. Hereditary breast and ovarian cancer in Asia: Genetic epidemiology of BRCA1 and BRCA2. *Hum Mutat* 2002;20:413–424.

40. Liu TF. History and heritage: Development of radiation oncology in China. *Int J Radiat Oncol Biol Phys* 1996;36:1267–1270.

41. Lopez AD, Collishaw NE, Piha T. A descriptive model of the cigarette epidemic in developed countries. *Tobacco Control* 1994;3:242–247.

42. Lopez AD, Mathers CD, Ezzati M, et al. Global and regional burden of disease and risk factors, 2001: Systematic analysis of population health data. *Lancet* 2006;367:1747–1757.

43. Marks LB, Hardenbergh PH, Winer ET, et al. Assessing the cost-effectiveness of postmastectomy radiation therapy. *Int J Radiat Oncol Biol Phys* 1999;44:91–98.

44. Masera G, Baez F, Biondi A, et al. North-south twinning in paediatric haemato-oncology: The La Mascota programme, Nicaragua. *Lancet* 1998;352:1923–1926.

45. Mellstedt H. Cancer initiatives in developing countries. *Ann Oncol* 2006;17[Suppl 8]:24–31.

46. Mustard JF. Health and social capital. In: Blane D, Brunner E, Wilkinson R, eds. *Health and social organization*. New York: Routledge, 1996:303–313.

47. Ngoma T. World Health Organization cancer priorities in developing countries. *Ann Oncol* 2006;17[Suppl 8]:9–14.

48. Niu SR, Yang GH, Chen ZM, et al. Emerging tobacco hazards in China: 2. Early mortality results from a prospective study. *BMJ* 1998;317:1423–1424.

49. Nordman EM, Kytta JT. Five-year survival of patients with larynx carcinoma treated with irradiation. *Strahlentherapie* 1978;154:245–248.

50. Owen JB, Coia LR, Hanks GE. The structure of radiation oncology in the United States in 1994. *Int J Radiat Oncol Biol Phys* 1997;39:179–185.

51. Parkin DM. The global health burden of infection-associated cancers in the year 2002. *Int J Cancer* 2006;118:3030–3044.

52. Parkin DM, Bray F, Ferlay J, et al. Global cancer statistics, 2002. *CA Cancer J Clin* 2005;55:74–108.

53. Parkin DM, Bray FI, Devesa SS. Cancer burden in the year 2000. The global picture. *Eur J Cancer* 2001;37[Suppl]:S4–66.

54. Pisani P, Parkin DM, Munoz N, et al. Cancer and infection: Estimates of the attributable fraction in 1990. *Cancer Epidemiol Biomarkers Prev* 1997;6:387–400.

55. Podgorsak EB, ed. *Radiation oncology physics: A handbook for teachers and students*. Vienna: IAEA; 2005.

56. Porter A, Aref A, Chodounsky Z, et al. A global strategy for radiotherapy: a WHO consultation. *Clin Oncol (R Coll Radiol)* 1999;11:368–370.

57. Pullarkat ST, Stoehlmacher J, Ghaderi V, et al. Thymidylate synthase gene polymorphism determines response and toxicity of 5-FU chemotherapy. *Pharmacogenomics J* 2001;1:65–70.

58. Reeler AV, Mellstedt H. Cancer in developing countries: Challenges and solutions. *Ann Oncol* 2006;17 Suppl 8:viii, 7–8.

59. Ruggieri-Pignon S, Pignon T, Marty M, et al. Infrastructure of radiation oncology in France: A large survey of evolution of external beam radiotherapy practice. *Int J Radiat Oncol Biol Phys* 2005;61:507–516.

60. Salminen E, Izewska J, Andreo P. IAEA's role in the global management of cancer-focus on upgrading radiotherapy services. *Acta Oncol* 2005;44:816–824.

61. Sankaranarayanan R, Ferlay J. Worldwide burden of gynaecological cancer: The size of the problem. *Best Pract Res Clin Obstet Gynaecol* 2006;20:207–225.

62. Schraub S. *Personal communication*. November 26, 2006.

63. Schreiner LJ, Kerr A, Salomons G, et al. The potential for image guided radiation therapy with cobalt-60 tomotherapy. In: Ellis RE, Peters TM, eds. *Lecture notes in computer science: Proceedings of the 6th annual international conference on medical image computing and computer assisted intervention (MICCAI)*. Heidelberg: Springer-Verlag, 2003:449–456.

64. Shafey O, Dolwick S, Guindon GE, eds. *Tobacco control country profiles*, 2nd ed. Atlanta, GA: American Cancer Society; 2003.

65. Shakespeare TP, Back MF, Lu JJ, et al. External audit of clinical practice and medical decision making in a new Asian oncology center: Results and implications for both developing and developed nations. *Int J Radiat Oncol Biol Phys* 2006;64:941–947.

66. Shibuya H, Tsujii H. The structural characteristics of radiation oncology in Japan in 2003. *Int J Radiat Oncol Biol Phys* 2005;62:1472–1476.

67. Stewart BW, Kleihues P, eds. *World cancer report*. Lyon: IARC Press, 2003.

68. Strong K, Mathers C, Leeder S, et al. Preventing chronic diseases: How many lives can we save? *Lancet* 2005;366:1578–1582.

69. Tan Torres Edejer T, Baltussen R, Adam T, et al. eds. *Making choices in health: WHO guide to cost-effectiveness analysis*. Geneva: World Health Organization, 2003.

70. Tatsuzaki H, Levin CV. Quantitative status of resources for radiation therapy in Asia and Pacific region. *Radiother Oncol* 2001;60:81–89.

71. Teixeira LC. Situation of radiotherapy in Latin America. *Int J Radiat Oncol Biol Phys* 1990;19:1267–1270.

72. Thomas G. Cervical cancer: Treatment challenges in the developing world. *Radiother Oncol* 2006;79:139–141.

73. UICC: *World cancer declaration*. Washington, DC, July 2006.

74. United Nations. *World population prospects: The 2004 revision population database, 2004*. Available at: http://esa.un.org/unpp/index.asp?panel = 1. Accessed December 15, 2006.

75. United Nations. *World population prospects: The 2004 revision. Volume III analytical report*. New York: United Nations, 2006.

76. Van Der Giessen PH, Alert J, Badri C, et al. Multinational assessment of some operational costs of teletherapy. *Radiother Oncol* 2004;71:347–355.

77. Veerman AJ, Sutaryo, Sumadiono. Twinning: A rewarding scenario for development of oncology services in transitional countries. *Pediatr Blood Cancer* 2005;45:103–106.

78. Weibo Y, Fenghua T, Xianzhi G. Radiation oncology in China: The third survey of personnel and equipment in radiation oncology. *Int J Radiat Oncol Biol Phys* 1999;44:239–241.

79. Wigg DR, Morgan GW. Radiation oncology in Australia: Workforce, workloads and equipment 1986–1999. *Australas Radiol* 2001;45:146–169.

80. World Bank. World Bank list of economies (July 2006). Available at: www.worldbank.org. Accessed December 15, 2006.

81. World Health Organization. *Cancer control: Knowledge into action: WHO guide for effective programmes module 1*. Geneva: World Health Organization, 2006.

82. World Health Organization. *National cancer control programmes: Policies and managerial guidelines*. Geneva: World Health Organization, 2002.

83. World Health Organization. *The world health report 1997: Conquering suffering, enriching humanity*. Geneva: World Health Organization; 1997.

84. World Health Organization. *Preventing chronic disease: A vital investment*. Geneva: World Health Organization; 2005.

85. World Health Organization. *The fifty-eighth World Health Assembly, resolution on cancer prevention and control*. (WHA 58.22) Geneva: World Health Organization, 2005.

86. World Health Organization. *World health statistics 2006*. France: World Health Organization, 2006.

87. World Health Organization and Center for Disease Control. Tobacco or health: a global status report. Available at: http://www.cdc.gov/tobacco/who/index.htm. Accessed December 2, 2006.

88. Wu X, Gu J, Wu TT, et al. Genetic variations in radiation and chemotherapy drug action pathways predict clinical outcomes in esophageal cancer. *J Clin Oncol* 2006;24:3789–3798.

89. Zubizarreta EH, Poitevin A, Levin CV. Overview of radiotherapy resources in Latin America: A survey by the International Atomic Energy Agency (IAEA). *Radiother Oncol* 2004;73:97–100.

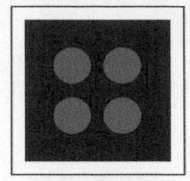

Chapter 26
Chemical Modifiers of Radiation Response

David M. Brizel

Chemical agents have been administered in conjunction with radiotherapy (RT) for both the enhancement of antitumor therapeutic efficacy and the amelioration of treatment-induced toxicity. Two concepts are fundamental to understanding the rationale for chemical modification of radiation response and to interpreting the studies that have addressed this issue. The first is the therapeutic ratio (TR), which is defined as the TCP/NTCP where TCP is the tumor control probability and NTCP is the normal tissue complication probability. Both of these parameters have sigmoid dose-response curves (Fig. 26.1). The horizontal separation between these two curves for any given treatment will often determine the overall utility of that treatment. As the separation between these curves increases, the likelihood increases that treatment will be effective and not cause an unacceptable level of morbidity. Conversely, the closer together these two curves are, the less the likelihood is that treatment will be effective without causing an unacceptable level of morbidity.

The second concept is the efficacy/toxicity profile of the putative chemical modifier, which can directly affect the TR. A radiosensitizing agent that exacerbates toxicity to the same extent that it improves efficacy (tumor and normal tissue dose-response curves moving to the left) may leave the TR unchanged or worsened and not be clinically practical. Conversely, a radioprotective agent that also reduces RT efficacy against the tumor (tumor and normal tissue dose-response curves moving to the right) also may not affect or may reduce the TR. The intrinsic toxicity of a radioprotector must also be considered when reduction of NTCP is the primary goal of a given chemical modification strategy. A compound that causes significant side effects of its own may render it unsuitable even if it can reduce the radiotherapeutic toxicity in question. This chapter will explore chemical radiosensitization and radioprotective strategies. The primary focus will be on treatments that have been clinically tested in head and neck cancer in order to amplify these concepts.

Chemical Radiosensitization

The Oxygen Effect

Tumor cell killing is produced by direct ionizations within critical cellular targets as well as by the indirect effect of energy deposited in other cellular molecules including water. Ionizing radiation generates free radicals, which can lead to cellular death via the creation of single strand and double strand breaks in DNA. This damage can be fixed or repaired by the chemical processes of oxidation and reduction, respectively (28). The addition of molecular oxygen to target free radicals produces altered chemical structures that are potentially lethal. Tumor hypoxia reduces radiosensitivity *in vitro* and *in vivo* (41,85). Well-oxygenated cells (partial pressure of oxygen or Po_2 >10 mm Hg) are approximately 2.5 times more sensitive to a given dose of ionizing radiation than their hypoxic counterparts.

Clinical data clearly demonstrate the existence of tumor hypoxia in head and neck cancer (5,10) and extremely strong correlations between hypoxia and both in-field treatment failure and overall survival (Figs. 26.2 and 26.3) (1,16). This effect is independent of presenting stage of disease (64). Tumor hypoxia has also been correlated with local and distant recurrence in carcinoma of the cervix treated with surgery (3,46) or radiotherapy (39) and with distant failure in soft tissue sarcomas treated with surgery and adjuvant radiotherapy (17).

Augmentation of Tumor Oxygenation

Therapeutic attempts to overcome the deleterious effect of tumor hypoxia can be classified into three basic lines of investigation: overcoming hypoxia by eliminating it with treatment that increases delivery of oxygen to the tumor, administration of oxygen mimetic agents that preferentially sensitize hypoxic cells to radiation, or administration of agents that are preferentially cytotoxic to hypoxic tumor cells. Hemoglobin concentration is the major determinant of the oxygen delivery capability of blood to tissue. Hemoglobin oxygen saturation exceeds 90% when the arterial Po_2 is >70 mm Hg. Oxygen is relatively insoluble in plasma under normobaric conditions, but under hyperbaric conditions, considerable quantities of oxygen can be dissolved into plasma and thus be potentially available for delivery to hypoxic tissues.

Clinical trials of hyperbaric oxygen (HBO) and radiotherapy were conducted from the 1950s to the 1970s. Trials conducted in patients with cancer of the central nervous system (27), lung (25), bladder (24), and skin (78) showed no benefit from the addition of HBO. Randomized trials conducted in carcinoma of the cervix (94), and head and neck (43,44) did, however, show improvements in locoregional control and overall survival. The cumbersome logistics associated with the delivery of HBO in conjunction with radiotherapy necessitated the utilization of nonconventional hypofractionated treatment regimens. This reality has prevented HBO from becoming adopted into routine clinical use.

The utilization of carbogen (95% O_2/5% CO_2) breathing with or without the concurrent administration of nicotinamide, a derivative of vitamin B, has been utilized to attempt to augment tumor oxygenation in order to enhance the response to radiotherapy. The rationale for the addition of the CO_2 to the gas breathing mixture is that the addition of a mild acidosis will right shift the oxyhemoglobin association curve and thereby facilitate unloading of oxygen into the most hypoxic tissues. The rationale for the administration of nicotinamide is based on preclinical studies showing that it enhances tumor blood flow (47,48).

Polarographic electrode assessments in cervix and head and neck cancer have demonstrated that carbogen breathing and nicotinamide administration improve tumor oxygenation in some patients (9,36,55). The use of ARCON (accelerated radiotherapy with carbogen and nicotinamide) has been tested in a phase II trial of 215 head and neck cancer patients (51). Ninety-seven percent of these patients had stage III or IV disease, and the primary tumor site was laryngeal in 46%, hypopharyngeal in 23%, and oropharyngeal in 23%. Nicotinamide was administered 1 to 1.5 hours prior to radiotherapy at 60 to 80 mg/kg. Full compliance with carbogen breathing during radiotherapy was obtained in 88% of patients. Nicotinamide-induced nausea

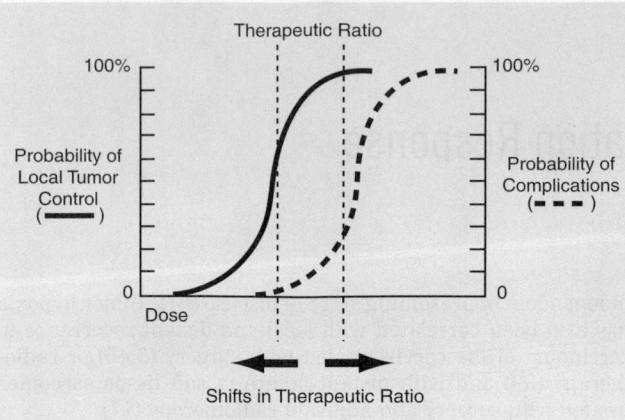

FIGURE 26.1. A graphic representation of the therapeutic index (TI). The tumor control probability (TCP) is to the left of the normal tissue complication probability (NTCP) and both are displayed as sigmoid dose-response curves. Larger separations are indicative of higher TIs. Ideally, normal tissue protection strategies would move the NTCP curve to the right without compromising TCP (moving the TCP curve to the right). Ideal therapeutic intensification strategies would move the TCP curve to the left without worsening NTCP (moving the NTCP curve to the left).

and vomiting necessitated discontinuation of the drug in 10% of patients receiving it at the lower dose and 31% of the patients receiving the higher dose. Three-year locoregional control rates were 69% for the hypopharynx primaries and 88% for the larynx and oropharynx primaries.

A randomized trial of hyperfractionated irradiation in patients with T_2 to T_4 squamous carcinoma of the oropharynx, larynx, and hypopharynx was conducted at the University of Florida from 1996 to 2002 (60). The intent of this trial was to detect a 20% improvement in 2-year local control in the carbogen arm relative to the RT alone arm and a 15% improvement in 4-year cause-specific survival. Virtually all enrolled patients in both arms of the trial completed their prescribed courses of treatment. The addition of carbogen to radiotherapy did not appear to improve any of the planned end points of this trial. Most important, however, was the fact that while the design of this trial called for the enrollment of 675 patients, only 101 were entered over a 5-year period. The trial was therefore significantly underpowered in terms of its ability to detect the desired treatment effect. The inability to accrue patients, however, calls into question the overall viability of strategies utilizing carbogen.

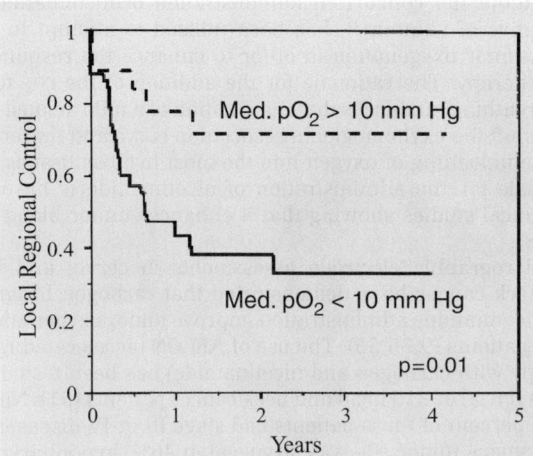

FIGURE 26.2. The correlation between pretreatment head and neck tumor oxygenation and local-regional disease control after RT with or without concurrent chemotherapy. Dashed line represents tumor median Po_2 >10 mm Hg. Solid line represents tumor median Po_2 <10 mm Hg.

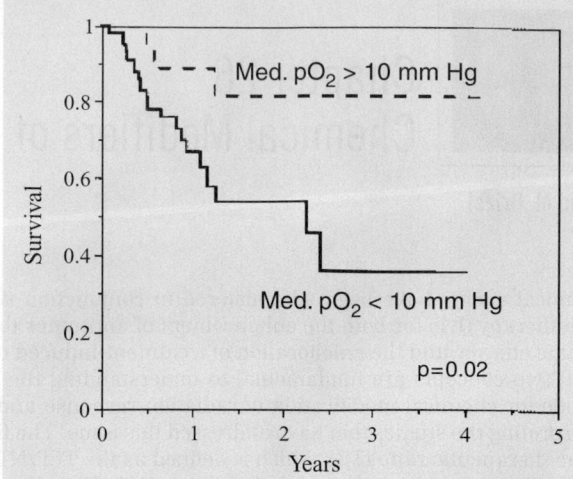

FIGURE 26.3. The correlation between pretreatment head and neck tumor oxygenation and local-regional disease control after RT with or without concurrent chemotherapy. Dashed line represents tumor median Po_2 >10 mm Hg.

Allosteric modifiers of hemoglobin structure that shift the oxyhemoglobin dissociation curve to the right and thus increase O_2 delivery to hypoxic tissues have been identified (84). One of these, RSR-13 (efaproxiral) was tested in animal models and shown to improve tumor oxygenation (49) and enhance the effectiveness of radiotherapy (52). A phase III open label trial of whole brain radiotherapy and oxygen breathing with or without daily infusion of efaproxiral was conducted in 538 patients with brain metastases (83). Overall, no improvement in survival was detected. Fifty-four percent of the patients on this trial had metastatic non–small-cell lung cancer and 20% had metastatic breast cancer. A retrospective subset analysis suggested a significant improvement in median survival time in breast patients who had levels of efaproxiral in their erythrocytes. A phase III trial of efaproxiral and oxygen breathing as an adjunct to radiotherapy in patients with breast cancer metastatic to brain is now being conducted.

Anemia is a very powerful adverse prognostic factor in patients with carcinoma of the lung (75), cervix (23,34), and head and neck amongst others (37,56,70). Polarographic electrode oxygen measurements in head and neck cancer have demonstrated that anemic patients are significantly more likely to have poorly oxygenated tumors than nonanemic patients, but significant tumor hypoxia has also been detected in patients who are not anemic (11,16). A 351 patient double-blind, placebo-controlled randomized trial of radiotherapy with or without administration of erythropoietin was conducted in order to test the hypothesis that correction or prevention of anemia during head and neck radiotherapy would significantly improve treatment outcome (45). The primary end point of this trial was local-regional progression-free survival. Eighty-two percent of patients who received erythropoietin maintained (54) >14 g/dL (women) or 15 g/dL (men), while only 15% patients in the placebo arm attained this benchmark. The relative risk of local regional progression, however, was 1.62 compared to the placebo patients, however ($p = 0.0008$). Similarly, survival was worse in the patients who received erythropoietin (relative risk 1.39; $p = 0.02$). To date, there is no level 1 evidence that correction of anemia improves radiotherapeutic outcome; current data suggest the contrary in fact.

Sensitization of Hypoxic Cells

Electron-affinic compounds can oxidize radiation-induced free radical damage in the cell to produce increased kill (6). The use of these agents would be particularly attractive in the hypoxic tumor microenvironment where low oxygen concentrations impair the effectiveness of radiotherapy. The 2-nitroimidazoles are one such class of compounds that are metabolized into their active form under hypoxic conditions. Misonidazole, the prototype 2-nitroimidazole, was tested in two randomized trials. The Danish Head and Neck Cancer Study 2 (DAHANCA 2) performed a double-blind randomized trial evaluating the effect of misonidazole given in two drug schedules with split-course irradiation in the treatment of carcinoma of the larynx and pharynx (67). Patients were stratified according to tumor site (larynx versus pharynx), nodal status, and institution. The total misonidazole dose was 11 g/m^2. The study accessed 626 patients. Overall, the misonidazole-treated group did not have a significantly better local tumor control than the placebo group. Serious peripheral neuropathy, the dose-limiting toxicity of all nitroimidazoles, occurred in 26% of patients receiving misonidazole. The European Organization for Research and Treatment of Cancer (EORTC) conducted a randomized trial of modified fractionation radiation with or without misonidazole versus conventionally fractionated irradiation in advanced head and neck cancer with no difference seen in treatment outcome. Again, no benefit was observed from the use of this drug (88).

Etanidazole (SR2508) is an analog of misonidazole with lower lipid solubility that had less neurotoxicity in phase II studies in head and neck cancer (93). A Radiation Therapy Oncology Group (RTOG) phase III study with etanidazole in head and neck tumors entered 521 patients who received conventionally fractionated irradiation with or without etanidazole 2 mg/m^2 three times per week. Of those on the etanidazole arm, 77% received at least 14 doses of the drug. No grade III or IV central nervous system or peripheral neuropathy was observed. The 2-year actuarial local tumor control was 40% in each arm, and the survival was 41% and 43%, respectively, in the irradiation alone and the irradiation plus etanidazole arms. A similar study of 374 patients performed in Europe did not show any overall benefit to treatment with etanidazole but did demonstrate increased neurotoxicity in the patients who received the drug (35).

Nimorazole is a 5-nitroimidazole of the same structural class as metronidazole (65). Its dose-limiting toxicity is nausea and vomiting; however, the drug can be administered with each radiation treatment. DAHANCA conducted a phase III trial of nimorazole (1.2 g/m^2 vs. placebo) for squamous cell cancer of the larynx and pharynx (66). There was a statistically significant improvement in locoregional tumor control (52% vs. 33% at 4 years; $p = 0.006$) but not for survival, which is consistent with the DAHANCA misonidazole trial. The use of nimorazole has become the standard of care in Denmark but has not been adopted in other countries.

Pharmacologic Targeting of Hypoxic Cells

Mitomycin C is an alkylating agent that is metabolized in regions of low oxygen concentration and preferentially cytotoxic to hypoxic cells. Yale University investigators designed their treatment strategy around this principle. They treated 195 patients in two randomized trials with mitomycin C (MMC). The Yale treatment program consisted of 68 Gy with or without MMC on days 1 and 43 of RT. Local control was improved with the addition of MMC from 54% to 76% ($p = 0.003$). Survival improved from 42% to 48%, but this was not statistically significant. The majority of patients in these trials received adjuvant postoperative or preoperative irradiation. Only 74 (38%) received definitive, primary RT, and the benefit from the addition of MMC in this subset is unclear. Mitomycin C plays an important role in conjunction with radiotherapy and 5FU (fluorouracil), the definitive, nonsurgical management squamous carcinoma of the anus (30).

A three-armed randomized trial conducted by the University of Vienna compared conventionally fractionated (CF) RT (2 Gy daily to 70 Gy) against continuous hyperfractionated accelerated RT with or without mitomycin C (V-CHART + MMC and V-CHART, respectively) (31). RT was given as an initial 2.5-Gy fraction followed by 1.65 Gy twice a day to a total dose of 55.3 Gy in 17 days. MMC was given as a 20 mg/m^2 bolus on day 5 of RT. Of the 239 patients enrolled, 85% had T3 or T4 primaries and 79% had nodal involvement. Three-year actuarial locoregional control was 48% for V-CHART + MMC versus 32% for V-CHART and 31% for CF ($p = 0.05$ and 0.03, respectively). Survival including death from all causes was also improved to 41% in the V-CHART + MMC arm as compared with 31% for V-CHART and 24% for CF ($p = 0.03$).

The incidence of confluent mucositis was 90% in both experimental arms as compared with 33% in the CF arm. The median time to complete resolution of mucositis was 6 to 7 weeks in all three arms. Grade –3 or 4 hematologic toxicity, primarily thrombocytopenia, developed in 18% of the V-CHART + MMC patients.

Porfiromycin, which is a derivative of mitomycin C, provides greater differential cytotoxicity between hypoxic and oxygenated cells in vitro (76). The Yale investigators also studied porfiromycin in a phase III study that compared patients treated with conventionally fractionated radiation plus mitomycin C versus radiation plus porfiromycin (42). Hematologic and nonhematologic toxicity was equivalent in the two treatment arms. The median follow-up is >6 years. Mitomycin C was superior to porfiromycin with respect to 5-year local relapse-free survival (91.6% vs. 72.7%; $p = 0.01$), local-regional relapse-free survival (82% vs. 65.3%; $p = 0.05$), and disease-free survival (72.8% vs. 52.9%; $p = 0.03$). There were no significant differences between the two arms with respect to overall survival (49% vs. 54%) or distant metastasis-free rate (80% vs. 76%). Their data supported the continuing use of mitomycin C as an adjunct to radiation therapy in advanced head and neck cancer and will become the control arm for future studies.

Tirapazamine (also known as SR-4233; WIN 59075; 3-amino-1,2,4-benzotriazine 1,4-dioxide) is a bioreductive agent preferentially cytotoxic to hypoxic cells *in vitro*. Twenty five to 200 times more drug is required to produce the same level of cell killing in aerobic compared to anaerobic conditions (96,98). A free radical 1-electron reduction product (97) formed rapidly under hypoxic conditions and believed to be the toxic species induces DNA strand breaks resulting from oxidative damage to pyrimidines (91). Analysis of DNA and chromosomal breaks after hypoxic exposure to tirapazamine suggests that DNA double-strand breaks are the primary lesion causing cell death (91).

This bioreductive agent differs from oxygen-mimetic sensitizers, such as the nitroimidazoles, in that it is itself cytotoxic to hypoxic tissues. Unlike the oxygen-mimetic sensitizers, tirapazamine-mediated therapeutic enhancement occurs both when the drug is given before or after irradiation (19,20). In fractionated radiation therapy of murine tumors, tirapazamine is as effective as if not superior to etanidazole (19). The efficacy of this radiation modifier depends on the number of "effective doses" that can be administered during a course of radiation therapy and the presence of hypoxic tumor cells (21). Tirapazamine can also enhance the cytotoxicity of cisplatin (40).

Rischin et al. (72,73) have investigated the use of concurrent tirapazamine, cisplatin, and radiotherapy in advanced head and neck cancer in a series of phase I and phase II trials. The phase I trial established the dosing schedule for tirapazamine given with radiation and cisplatin. The phase II trial compared the combination of RT, cisplatin, and tirapazamine against RT and concurrent cisplatin/5FU and found that the former was more effective than the latter (3-year local regional failure-free survival 84% vs. 66%; $p = 0.07$).

Tumor hypoxia assessment with ^{18}F-misonidazole PET scanning was performed in 45 of the patients on these studies (71). Hypoxia was identified in primary or nodal sites in 71% of the patients. Eight of 13 (62%) patients with hypoxic tumors who received platinum/5FU experienced subsequent local-regional failure as opposed to only one of 19 (5%) patients with hypoxic tumors who received tirapazamine (HR = 15; $p = 0.001$). Only 1/10 of patients with nonhypoxic tumors who received platinum/5FU had a local-regional failure. The findings in this trial strongly suggest that the benefit of tirapazamine resulted from improved treatment efficacy against tumor hypoxia.

A phase III trial has been conducted to validate the concept of targeting of hypoxic cells in head and neck cancer. Concurrent chemoradiation with standard fractionation RT (70 Gy) and tirapazamine/cisplatin was tested against conventional chemoradiation with standard single agent cisplatin. This trial enrolled 880 patients and is in a follow-up phase. A confirmatory trial with a planned enrollment of 550 patients is ongoing.

Biologic Modifiers of Radiation Response

Overexpression of the epidermal growth factor receptor (EGFR-1) is associated with an adverse outcome in squamous head and neck cancer (HNC) (7). Cetuximab (C225) is a chimeric monoclonal antibody to EGFR. Preclinical studies have demonstrated that cetuximab sensitizes cells to the cytotoxic effects of ionizing irradiation (4,50,77). Preliminary studies demonstrated that this drug could be safely administered in conjunction with a course of radiotherapy for head and neck cancer (74). An open label, phase III trial tested the impact of weekly injections of cetuximab added to a course of radiotherapy alone. Most patients received accelerated fractionation with concomitant boost, although hyperfractionation and standard fractionation schemes were also permitted. Oral cavity primary tumors were ineligible for enrollment. Two-year local regional increased from 48% with RT to 56% with RT and cetuximab ($p = 0.02$). Three-year survival was similarly increased from 44% with RT alone to 57% with the addition of cetuximab ($p = 0.02$) (14).

This trial provides an important proof of principle that adding a biologically targeted agent to a physically targeted modality improves therapeutic outcome. One third of the patients enrolled had stage III disease, however, and thus had less advanced disease with more favorable prognoses than a significant proportion of patients undergoing chemoradiotherapy (CRT). Whether RT with C225 is more effective than CRT remains unknown. RTOG Trial 0522 will address this question by randomizing patients with locally advanced disease to receive radiation and concurrent cisplatin with or without cetuximab.

EGFR inhibition is presently a very active area of investigation in head and neck cancer. Agents currently in clinical trial include fully humanized monoclonal antibodies to the EGFR-1 receptor. Orally administered small molecules that inhibit the tyrosine kinase domains of EGFR-1 or EGFR-1 and EGFR-2 (HER-2) simultaneously are also being studied.

Chemical Radioprotection

The protection of normal tissues from the deleterious effects of radiation is a critical component in the development of a comprehensive treatment plan. Strategies for the accomplishment of this aim include the physical manipulation of the beam, modification of the fractionation schedule, and pharmacologic manipulation of the radiation response. Physical radiation protection rests on the principle of exclusion of normal tissue from the high dose region and may be accomplished by contouring the shape with the radiation beam, the use of multiple treatment fields, the use of different beam energies, and modulation of the dose delivery from each beam (intensity-modulated

radiation therapy [IMRT]). Modified fractionation typically uses multiple fractions of treatment per day as opposed to the conventional once daily paradigm in order to exploit the differing radiation repair capabilities of normal tissues as opposed to tumors. Physical modification of the treatment beam and altered fractionation are discussed elsewhere.

Protection

Pharmacologic radioprotection itself can be classified into three categories: protection, mitigation, and treatment. The direct cytotoxicity of ionizing irradiation results from the generation of free radicals that cause DNA strand breaks and lead to a mycotic cell death. Amifostine (WR2721; Ethyol, Medimmune Inc, Gaithersburg, MD) is the prototype pharmacologic radioprotector that functions via free radical scavenging. Amifostine is a thiol containing pro drug that preferentially accumulates in the kidneys and salivary glands where it is metabolized to its active moiety, WR1065 (95).

An open label phase III randomized trial was conducted from 1995 to 1997 to assess the ability of this drug to reduce the incidence of grade ≥ 2 acute and late xerostomia and grade ≥ 3 acute mucositis (18). Patients enrolled on this trial received curative intent or adjuvant postoperative irradiation. All treatment was delivered with conventional once daily fractionation of 1.8 to 2.0 Gy. Curative intent delivery consisted of 66 to 70 Gy total dose, and postoperative irradiation was delivered at 50 to 60 Gy total dose depending on the patient's assessed risk for recurrence. IMRT was not utilized and inclusion of >75% of both parotid glands was required for inclusion on the study. Those patients who were randomized to receive amifostine were given a daily dose of 200 mg/m^2 intravenously 15 to 30 minutes every day prior to each fraction of radiotherapy.

Three hundred three patients were enrolled in this trial, and minimum follow-up is 2 years. Amifostine did not reduce the incidence of grade 3 mucositis but it did significantly reduce the incidence of acute and long-term grade >2 xerostomia. One-year post-RT the incidence was 34% versus 56% for patients who received amifostine versus those who did not ($p = 0.002$). Unstimulated saliva production >0.1 g was also more common in patients who received amifostine (72% vs. 49%; $p = 0.003$). Two years post-RT, amifostine use was still associated with a significantly lower incidence of xerostomia, although the magnitude of benefit was lower (19% vs. 36%; $p = 0.05$). The lower incidences in both groups of patients also suggest some late recovery of salivary function. Reinforcing this idea of late recovery of salivary function is the fact that the percentage of patients who did not receive amifostine but who could exceed the >0.1 g of unstimulated saliva threshold had increased to 57% (92).

Severe toxicity (CTC grade >3) attributable to amifostine occurred in <10% of patients on this trial and consisted of nausea and vomiting and transient hypotension. Nearly two thirds of the patients had less severe grades of these side effects. Drug-related toxicity did cause approximately 20% of patients to discontinue amifostine prior to completing radiotherapy. Subcutaneous administration of the drug causes less nausea, vomiting, and hypotension than intravenous dosing but is associated with an increased risk of cutaneous toxicity, which again causes 15% to 20% of patients to not complete a full course of amifostine in conjunction with their radiation (53). The incidence of severe cutaneous toxicity including erythema multiforme, Stevens-Johnson syndrome, and toxic epidermal necrolysis is 6 to 9/100,000 (13).

Some have argued that the size of this trial made it underpowered to detect a very small compromise in survival caused by amifostine (tumor protection) (57). This argument is technically correct but overlooks the reality that absolute refutation of a small compromise of antitumor efficacy attributable to amifostine would have required an equivalence trial. Demonstration that amifostine reduced survival from a hypothetical 45% to 40% ($p = 0.05$; 80% power) would have necessitated >1,200 patients per study arm (80). Such a large study cannot be performed in head and neck cancer. Patient resources are too scarce. The largest randomized head and neck trial ever conducted, RTOG 90-03, required 8 years to enroll 1,113 patients into four treatment arms (38). A meta-analysis of all randomized trials of RT plus amifostine is ongoing to further address the tumor protection issue. Preliminary data show no evidence of amifostine-mediated compromise of the effectiveness of RT (15).

The potential of amifostine as a protector against radiation-induced esophagitis during the treatment of non–small-cell lung cancer was studied in a randomized trial conducted by the RTOG (62,63). No reduction in the incidence of grade 3 esophagitis was observed, although less swallowing dysfunction was observed in the patients who received amifostine. Part of the explanation for this absence may be attributable to the study design, which utilized a hyperfractionated radiation schedule 5 days per week (69.6 Gy total dose) and concurrent carboplatin/paclitaxel. Amifostine 500 mg intravenous was delivered 4 days per week prior to the afternoon fraction only. Moreover, 28% of the patients did not complete the full course of the drug either because of toxicity or refusal. Consequently, approximately 50% of the radiotherapy was delivered in the absence of the radioprotective drug in those patients who were randomized to receive it. Preclinical study of amifostine delivered daily in conjunction with fractionated lung and esophageal irradiation has demonstrated morphologic and immunohistochemical evidence of radioprotection (86,89,90).

The U.S. Food and Drug Administration–approved xerostomia indication for amifostine is in the setting of radiotherapy alone. The majority of both curative intent and adjuvant postoperative RT for head and neck cancer that requires the treatment of large target volumes that put the parotid glands at risk is now delivered in conjunction with concurrent chemotherapy. Small phase II and III trials suggest that amifostine has a cytoprotective benefit in the chemoradiation setting, but level-1 evidence is lacking (8,22). Similarly, IMRT, which is a very effective means to achieve parotid gland sparing, has become widespread in its usage. The utility of amifostine in conjunction with IMRT is unknown and the subject of current investigation.

Mitigation

Administration of compounds that mitigate damage caused by previous radiation exposure constitutes a different approach to the management of radiation-induced toxicity. This strategy contrasts to the classical free radical scavenging radioprotective mechanism of drugs such as amifostine. The leading drug under development in this category is palifermin. Palifermin is a recombinant human keratinocyte growth factor that belongs to the fibroblast growth factor family of cytokines (FGF-7). It stimulates cellular proliferation and differentiation in a variety of epithelial tissues including mucosa throughout the alimentary tract, salivary glands, and type II pneumocytes. Palifermin also regulates intrinsic glutathione-mediated cytoprotective mechanisms. Administration of palifermin in preclinical rodent models leads to a significant thickening of oral tongue mucosa (69). Preclinical studies of fractionated radiotherapy have revealed that the administration of palifermin leads to increases in the dose of radiotherapy necessary to induce ulcerative mucositis and to reductions in the duration of this ulceration when it does occur (32,33). Parotid gland production of saliva is also preserved when palifermin is administered in the setting of radiotherapy in preclinical systems. Preclinical evaluation of palifermin in a rodent model has also demonstrated that administration of a single dose of this drug after completion of a course of fractionated thoracic irradiation significantly reduces the sever-

ity and duration of pneumonitis and the severity of pulmonary fibrosis (Fig. 26.4) (29).

The ability of palifermin to reduce mucositis in a clinical setting has been tested in a pivotal phase III double-blind placebo-controlled trial of patients with non-Hodgkin's lymphoma undergoing bone marrow transplantation (82). The bone marrow ablative regimen consisted of 1,200 cGy of total-body irradiation (TBI) given at 150 cGy twice a day. Thereafter, VP-16 and cyclophosphamide were administered. Palifermin was delivered prior to the initiation of TBI and again after the completion of chemotherapy, which also corresponded to 5 days after the completion of TBI. The dose schedule of palifermin was 60 mcg/kg per day three times for both administrations. This trial enrolled 212 patients who were equally divided between the placebo and palifermin arms. The WHO scoring system was used. The incidence of grade 3 or 4 mucositis approached 90% in the placebo arm as opposed to approximately 60% in the palifermin arm. For those patients who developed this level of toxicity, the duration was significantly reduced from 10.4 days in the placebo arm to 3.7 days in the palifermin arm (p <0.001). Grade IV mucositis developed in 62% of the placebo arm patients and only 20% of the palifermin arm patients (p >0.001). Mean duration of grade IV mucositis was reduced from 6.2 days to 3.3 days with the use of this drug (p <0.001).

The clinical experience with palifermin in head and neck cancer is limited to one phase I and one phase II trials. Both of these trials integrated palifermin into regimens of radiation and concurrent CDDP/5FU chemotherapy for patients with American Joint Commission for Cancers (AJCC) stages III or IV nonmetastatic squamous carcinoma of the head and neck. Both trials utilized a dose of palifermin prior to the initiation of chemoradiation and then delivered an additional dose at the end of each week of radiotherapy. The primary end point of the phase I trial was safety and tolerability of the drug. The dose of palifermin was escalated from 20 to 80 mcg/kg. The most common toxicity of the drug was erythema of the face, which occurred in 9 of 60 patients (50%) and was a nondose-limiting toxicity. Hypersalivation occurred as a dose-limiting toxicity in one patient. Transient, asymptomatic elevations of amylase and lipase were observed. The maximum tolerated dose was not determined in the dose schedule tested in this trial. There was a 3:1 randomization to palifermin and placebo in this trial and no evidence of compromise of treatment outcome in patients receiving palifermin.

A phase II trial was subsequently performed in which the same type of patient population received concurrent chemoradiation. Patients were randomized 2:1 between palifermin and placebo. Institutions had the discretion to deliver radiotherapy via conventional once-daily 2 Gy fractions or with an accelerated hyperfractionated regimen of 1.25 Gy twice daily. One hundred patients were enrolled on this trial, of whom 34 received accelerated hyperfractionation and the remainder received standard fractionation. Palifermin was delivered at a dose of 60 mcg/kg.

Again, the first dose was delivered prior to the initiation of CRT and then every Friday afternoon after the last fraction of radiation. Two additional doses of palifermin were given 1 and 2 weeks after the completion of radiotherapy for a total of 10 doses of the drug. Palifermin did not reduce the incidence or duration of mucosal or salivary gland toxicity. The subset of patients receiving hyperfractionated radiation, however, showed significant improvements in the duration and severity of mucositis (Fig. 26.5). They also had improved swallowing function and less salivary gland toxicity relative to patients who received placebo.

The relative lack of success of palifermin in the head and neck setting as opposed to the transplant context may be multifactorial. The dose intensity of palifermin relative to the total dose of irradiation delivered was significantly greater in the

H and E   ## Masson's Trichrome

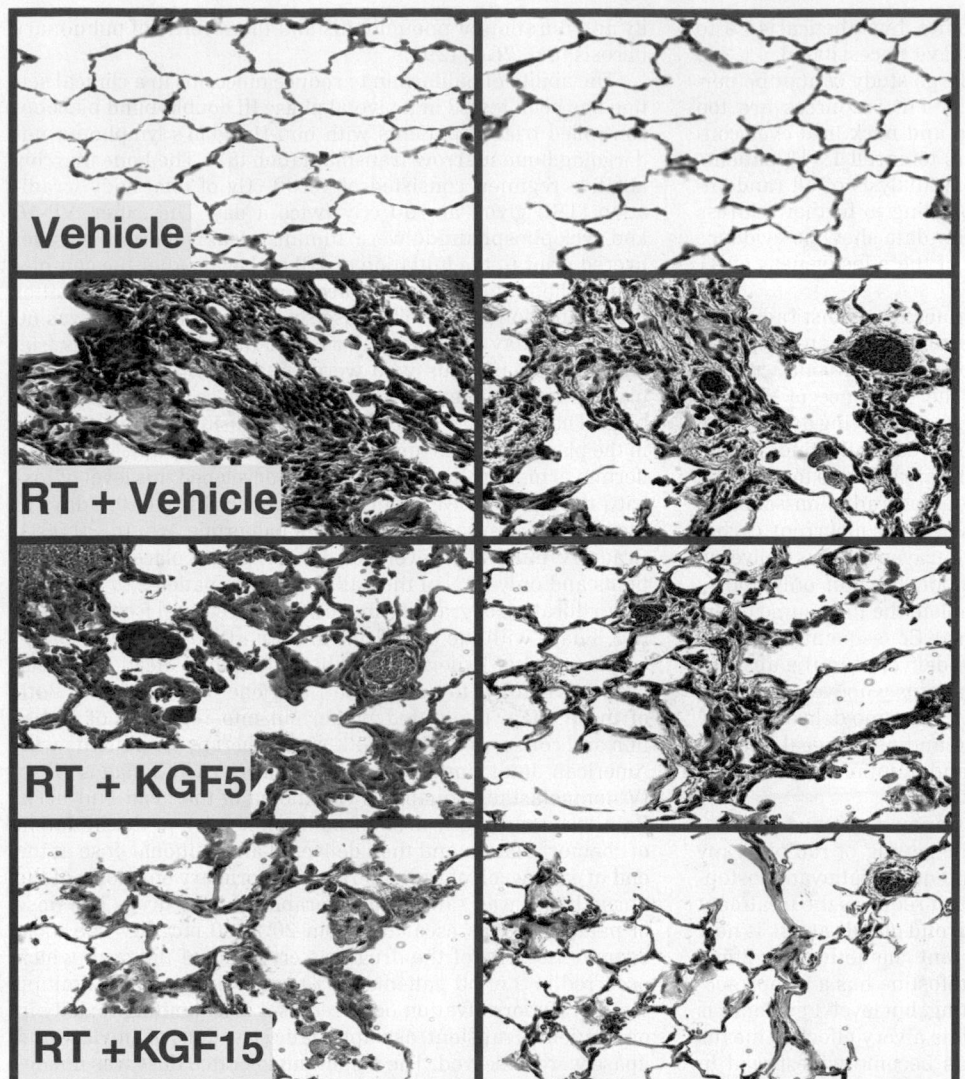

Vehicle

RT + Vehicle

RT + KGF5

RT + KGF15

FIGURE 26.4. Mitigation of radiation induced fibrosis attributable to single dose of recombinant human keratinocyte growth factor (KGF) administered after a course of fractionated hemi-thorax irradiation. The H and E slides show the morphologic changes in the alveoli induced by irradiation including the inflammatory infiltrate and alveolar wall thickening. The Masson's trichrome panels show the collagen deposition that is characteristic of fibrosis. KGF was given either at 5 mg/kg or 15 mg/kg. Less injury is seen with the higher dose of KGF, suggesting that a dose response effect exists.

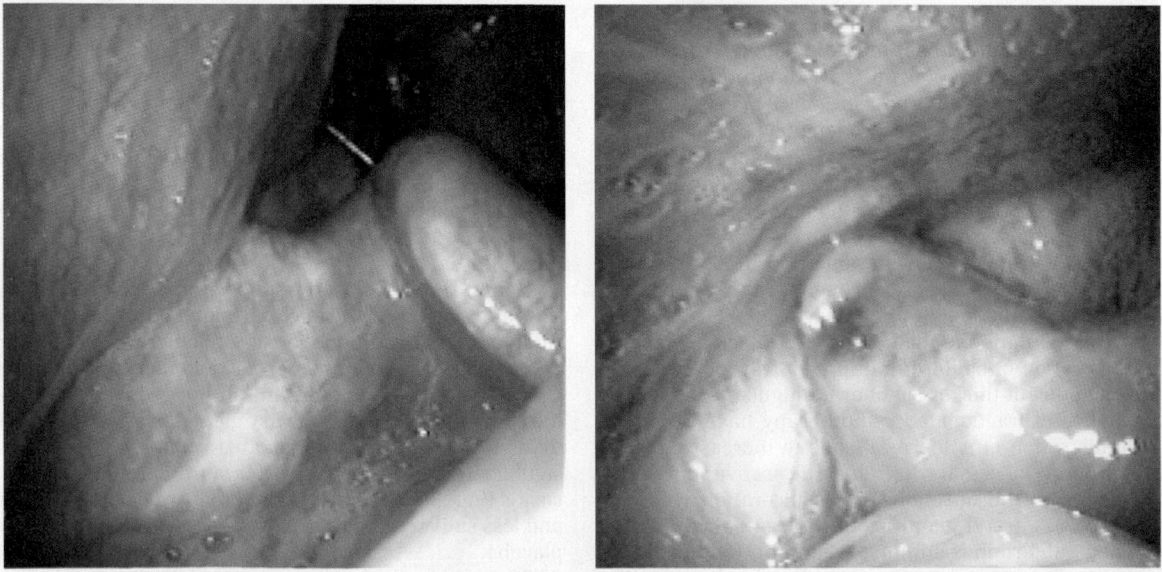

A   B

FIGURE 26.5. Confluent mucositis induced by concurrent chemoradiation in the base of tongue and supraglottic larynx regions. **A:** Demonstrates normal mucosa prior to the initiation of treatment. **B:** Demonstrates the pseudomembranous exudate, hemorrhage, and edema that are characteristic of this condition.

transplant trial than in the head and neck studies. Cumulative doses of 180 mcg/kg were sandwiched around a total dose of 1,200 cGy of radiotherapy. This contrasts with doses of 60 to 80 mcg/kg that were sandwiched around weekly doses of 1,000 to 1,200 cGy delivered to a cumulative dose of 7,000 cGy in the head and neck studies. The effect of this lesser dose intensity of palifermin would then have been amplified by the significantly larger doses of mucosal irradiation that are delivered for head and neck cancer as opposed to bone marrow transplant conditioning. Normal volunteer studies conducted after the completion of the phase I and II head and neck trials further demonstrated that administration of palifermin in single doses of 120 to 180 mcg/kg were considerably more effective in stimulating mucosal proliferation than doses of 60 to 80 mcg/kg (Amgen; unpublished data). Lastly, the head and neck trials used the RTOG/CTC version 2.0 scale which mandated a cutoff of assessment 90 days after the initiation of therapy. Mucositis after concurrent CRT for head and neck cancer commonly persists for >6 weeks beyond the completion of treatment, the implication of which is that mucositis is often still present at the end of the 90-day cutoff date. Consequently, the scoring system used in these trials was insensitive in terms of distinguishing a difference between a patient whose mucositis resolved 91 days after the initiation of therapy versus 120 days after the completion of therapy. Such patients would both be censored from analysis at 90 days.

Presently investigation of palifermin in conjunction with concurrent chemoradiation for head and neck cancer is ongoing, both in the definitive and adjuvant postoperative settings. These studies are investigating the utility of doses of 180 mcg/kg administered both during and after the completion of chemoradiation.

Treatment

Radioprotectors and radiation mitigators are both designed with the intent of minimizing the risk of clonogenic death of normal cells and subsequent disruption of the protective mucosal barrier. Head and neck radiotherapy also initiates a local cytokine cascade, which includes interleukin-1, and -6, and tumor necrosis factor (TNF)-α. An inflammatory response results, which contributes to the ultimate anatomic disruption of the mucosa. Secondary bacterial and fungal overgrowth are thought to exacerbate the local pathophysiology.

Sucralfate, a basic aluminum salt of sucrose, is used in the treatment of peptic ulcer disease. It provides a protective coating to ulcerated tissue by means of binding to exposed proteins in damaged cells (59). It also stimulates mucus production, mitosis, and surface migration of cells. Sucralfate has been tested in several double-blind placebo-controlled randomized trials. Despite the attractive conceptual nature of using it to ameliorate mucositis, the clinical data do not show any benefit from sucralfate (26,58,61,68).

Benzydamine HCl is a nonsteroidal anti-inflammatory drug that also possesses antimicrobial activity (79). It is a potent inhibitor of TNF-α (81). Expression of this proinflammatory cytokine is upregulated in mucosal tissue of the head and neck regions, with peak levels typically peak at approximately 2,000 cGy (conventionally fractionated) just prior to the first signs of mucosal ulceration. The ability of benzydamine to reduce mucositis during head and neck radiotherapy was tested in a randomized double-blind placebo-controlled trial (32). The primary end point of this trial was the area under the curve for the mean mucositis score over a cumulative radiotherapy dose up to a total dose of 5,000 cGy. Secondary end points included use of concomitant pain medication, oral pain at rest and with eating, body weight, and the use of enteral nutritional support.

Benzydamine therapy resulted in a 30% reduction in mucosal erythema and ulceration. Most of this benefit was observed once doses >2,500 cGy had been delivered. One third of the benzydamine patients did not develop any mucosal ulceration at all, compared with only 18% of the placebo-treated patients ($p = 0.04$). There was a nonsignificant trend toward reduction in mouth pain at rest for the patients who received benzydamine. Importantly, benzydamine was no more effective than placebo with respect to the reduction of pain during meals. Cumulative weight loss during radiotherapy was equivalent in the two treatment groups. There was no difference in the proportion of patients who required enteral nutritional support between the two treatment arms.

The data from the benzydamine trials suggest that this agent is active against mucositis but are inconclusive regarding whether or not it has any clinical role in treating this condition. There was no significant benefit regarding the functional sequelae of mucositis. Mucosal assessment was not performed beyond 5,000 cGy, and most patients received radiotherapy doses of 6,400 to 7,400 cGy. The study design may thus explain the discordance between the improvement in the anatomic assessment of mucosal integrity associated with benzydamine and the lack of any functional benefit, as the latter parameters were assessed throughout a patient's entire course of radiotherapy. The most severe mucositis during a course of head and neck radiotherapy occurs beyond the 5,000 cGy level. Fewer than 10% of the patients enrolled in this trial received concurrent chemotherapy, even though most of them had stage III or IV disease. Concurrent CRT has become the standard of care for most patients with this extent of disease. Consequently, the clinical value of benzydamine has not been proved for patients receiving high-dose radiotherapy with or without concurrent chemotherapy.

Endogenous oral flora may exacerbate the mucosal inflammatory process once the mucosal integrity is disrupted. Secondary infections may prolong the course of mucositis and compromise overall patient well-being. Protegrins are naturally occurring peptides that have broad-spectrum antimicrobial activity (12). Iseganan is a synthetic analog of this class of compounds. A placebo-controlled trial in patients receiving chemotherapy suggested that iseganan reduced the incidence of ulcerative stomatitis and decreased both mouth pain and swallowing difficulty.

A phase III double-blind, placebo-controlled trial was subsequently conducted to test this concept in patients receiving head and neck radiotherapy (87). This trial mandated that a minimum dose of 6,000 cGy be delivered but allowed different fractionation schemes. Forty percent of the patients enrolled received concurrent chemotherapy. The study contained three treatment arms: iseganan plus standard oral care, placebo plus standard oral care, and supportive oral care (SOC) only. Iseganan and placebo were equivalent to one another with respect to all end points in the trial. Interestingly, iseganan and placebo were both superior to standard oral care. Two thirds of the patients in both arms had confluent mucositis compared with 79% in the supportive oral care arm ($p = 0.02$). Only 2% of the SOC patients had no mucosal ulceration versus 9% in both the iseganan and placebo arms ($p = 0.04$). Peak mouth pain and difficulty swallowing were also significantly worse for the patients assigned to supportive oral care. Radiotherapy dose reductions were also significantly more common in the supportive oral care patients.

The iseganan trial showed no benefit from the administration of the study drug. It did, however, reveal the importance of adherence to a strict regimen of oral hygiene during head and neck radiotherapy. Patients on both the drug and placebo arms were instructed to swish and gargle prior to each administration of study drug. They also maintained study diaries to help ensure adequate compliance with administration of the study drug. These interventions were not performed in the patients assigned to supportive oral care. This trial provides an important foundation in the evaluation of new therapies for mucositis through its demonstration of the value of organized and systematic attention to the maintenance of good oral hygiene throughout a course of head and neck CRT.

Summary

The chemical modification of radiation response both for enhancing treatment efficacy and reducing therapy-induced toxicity is an area of active investigation. Attempts to improve outcome by augmenting tumor oxygen delivery have a mixed record of success. The use of drugs that are preferentially cytotoxic to hypoxic cells holds promise. Proof of principle for chemical radioprotection has been established in salivary glands but not elsewhere and is associated with significant toxicity in its own right. The use of growth factors has been established as a means for protecting the mucosa from low total doses of irradiation in the bone marrow transplant setting. The efficacy of this strategy is being explored in the context of high-dose treatment for solid tumors.

References

1. Adams GE. Hypoxia-mediated drugs for radiation and chemotherapy. *Cancer* 1981;48:696–707.
2. Ang KK, Berkey BA, Tu X, et al. Impact of epidermal growth factor receptor expression on survival and pattern of relapse in patients with advanced head and neck carcinoma. *Cancer Res* 2002;62:7350–7356.
3. Antonadou D, Pepelassi M, Synodinou M, et al: Prophylactic use of amifostine to prevent radiochemotherapy-induced mucositis and xerostomia in head-and-neck cancer. *Int J Radiat Oncol Biol Phys* 2002;52:739–747.
4. Aquino-Parsons C, Lim P, Green A, et al. Carbogen inhalation in cervical cancer: assessment of oxygenation change. *Gynecol Oncol* 1999;74:259–264.
5. Becker A, Hansgen G, Bloching M, et al. Oxygenation of squamous cell carcinoma of the head and neck: comparison of primary tumors, neck node metastases, and normal tissue. *Int J Radiat Oncol Biol Phys* 1998;42:35–41.
6. Becker A, Stadler P, Lavey RS, et al. Severe anemia is associated with poor tumor oxygenation in head and neck squamous cell carcinomas. *Int J Radiat Oncol Biol Phys* 2000;46:459–466.
7. Bellm L, Lehrer RI, Ganz T: Protegrins: new antibiotics of mammalian origin. *Expert Opin Investig Drugs* 2000;9:1731–1742.
8. Boccia R, Anne PR, Bourhis J, et al. Assessment and management of cutaneous reactions with amifostine administration: findings of the ethyol (amifostine) cutaneous treatment advisory panel (ECTAP). *Int J Radiat Oncol Biol Phys* 2004;60:302–309.
9. Bonner JA, Harari PM, Giralt J, et al. Radiotherapy plus cetuximab for squamous-cell carcinoma of the head and neck. *N Engl J Med* 2006;354:567–578.
10. Bourhis J TH, Brizel DM, Movsas B, et al. Meta-analysis of amifostine in radiotherapy (MAART): preliminary analysis of 11 randomized clinical trials including 1,014 patients. *Int J Radiat Oncol Biol Phys* 2006;66:S67.
11. Brizel DM, Dodge RK, Clough RW, et al: Oxygenation of head and neck cancer: changes during radiotherapy and impact on treatment outcome. *Radiother Oncol* 1999;53:113–117.
12. Brizel DM, Rosner GL, Prosnitz LR, et al. Patterns and variability of tumor oxygenation in human soft tissue sarcomas, cervical carcinomas, and lymph node metastases. *Int J Radiat Oncol Biol Phys* 1995;32:1121–1125.
13. Brizel DM, Scully SP, Harrelson JM, et al: Tumor oxygenation predicts for the likelihood of distant metastases in human soft tissue sarcoma. *Cancer Res* 1996;56:941–943.
14. Brizel DM, Sibley GS, Prosnitz LR, et al: Tumor hypoxia adversely affects the prognosis of carcinoma of the head and neck. *Int J Radiat Oncol Biol Phys* 1997;38:285–289.
15. Brizel DM, Wasserman TH, Henke M, et al. Phase III randomized trial of amifostine as a radioprotector in head and neck cancer. *J Clin Oncol* 2000;18:3339–3345.
16. Brown JM, Lemmon MJ. Potentiation by the hypoxic cytotoxin SR 4233 of cell killing produced by fractionated irradiation of mouse tumors. *Cancer Res* 1990;50:7745–7749.
17. Brown JM, Lemmon MJ. SR 4233: a tumor specific radiosensitizer active in fractionated radiation regimes. *Radiother Oncol* 1991;20[Suppl 1]:151–156.
18. Brown JM. Therapeutic targets in radiotherapy. *Int J Radiat Oncol Biol Phys* 2001;49:319–326.
19. Buntzel J, Glatzel M, Kuttner K, et al. Amifostine in simultaneous radiochemotherapy of advanced head and neck cancer. *Semin Radiat Oncol* 2002;12:4–13.
20. Bush RS, Jenkin RD, Allt WE, et al. Definitive evidence for hypoxic cells influencing cure in cancer therapy. *Br J Cancer Suppl* 1978;3:302–306.
21. Cade IS, McEwen JB, Dische S, et al. Hyperbaric oxygen and radiotherapy: a Medical Research Council trial in carcinoma of the bladder. *Br J Radiol* 1978;51:876–868.
22. Cade IS, McEwen JB. Clinical trials of radiotherapy in hyperbaric oxygen at Portsmouth, 1964–1976. *Clin Radiol* 1978;29:333–338.
23. Carter DL, Hebert ME, Smink K, et al. Double blind randomized trial of sucralfate vs placebo during radical radiotherapy for head and neck cancers. *Head Neck* 1999;21:760–766.
24. Chang CH. Hyperbaric oxygen and radiation therapy in the management of glioblastoma. *Natl Cancer Inst Monogr* 1977;46:163–169.
25. Chapman JD, Reuvers AP, Borsa J, et al. Chemical radioprotection and radiosensitization of mammalian cells growing in vitro. *Radiat Res* 1973;56:291–306.
26. Chen L, Brizel DM, Rabbani ZN, et al. The protective effect of recombinant human keratinocyte growth factor on radiation-induced pulmonary toxicity in rats. *Int J Radiat Oncol Biol Phys* 2004;60:1520–1529.
27. Cummings BJ, Keane TJ, O'Sullivan B, et al. Epidermoid anal cancer: treatment by radiation alone or by radiation and 5-fluorouracil with and without mitomycin C. *Int J Radiat Oncol Biol Phys* 1991;21:1115–1125.
28. Dobrowsky W, Naude J. Continuous hyperfractionated accelerated radiotherapy with/without mitomycin C in head and neck cancers. *Radiother Oncol* 2000;57:119–124.
29. Dorr W, Spekl K, Farrell CL. Amelioration of acute oral mucositis by keratinocyte growth factor: fractionated irradiation. *Int J Radiat Oncol Biol Phys* 2002;54:245–251.
30. Dorr W, Spekl K, Farrell CL. The effect of keratinocyte growth factor on healing of manifest radiation ulcers in mouse tongue epithelium. *Cell Prolif* 2002;35[Suppl 1]:86–92.
31. Dunst J, Kuhnt T, Strauss HG, et al. Anemia in cervical cancers: impact on survival, patterns of relapse, and association with hypoxia and angiogenesis. *Int J Radiat Oncol Biol Phys* 2003;56:778–787.
32. Epstein JB, Silverman S Jr, Paggiarino DA, et al. Benzydamine HCl for prophylaxis of radiation-induced oral mucositis: results from a multicenter, randomized, double-blind, placebo-controlled clinical trial. *Cancer* 2001;92:875–885.
33. Eschwege F, Sancho-Garnier H, Chassagne D, et al. Results of a European randomized trial of etanidazole combined with radiotherapy in head and neck carcinomas. *Int J Radiat Oncol Biol Phys* 1997;39:275–281.
34. Falk SJ, Ward R, Bleehen NM. The influence of carbogen breathing on tumour tissue oxygenation in man evaluated by computerised p02 histography. *Br J Cancer* 1992;66:919–924.
35. Frommhold H, Guttenberger R, Henke M. The impact of blood hemoglobin content on the outcome of radiotherapy. The Freiburg experience. *Strahlenther Onkol* 1998; 174[Suppl 4]:31–34.
36. Fu KK, Pajak TF, Trotti A, et al. A Radiation Therapy Oncology Group (RTOG) phase III randomized study to compare hyperfractionation and two variants of accelerated fractionation to standard fractionation radiotherapy for head and neck squamous cell carcinomas: first report of RTOG 9003. *Int J Radiat Oncol Biol Phys* 2000;48: 7–16.
37. Fyles AW, Milosevic M, Wong R, et al. Oxygenation predicts radiation response and survival in patients with cervix cancer. *Radiother Oncol* 1998;48:149–156.
38. Goldberg Z, Evans J, Birrell G, et al. An investigation of the molecular basis for the synergistic interaction of tirapazamine and cisplatin. *Int J Radiat Oncol Biol Phys* 2001;49:175–182.
39. Gray LH, Conger AD, Ebert M, et al. The concentration of oxygen dissolved in tissues at the time of irradiation as a factor in radiotherapy. *Br J Radiol* 1953;26:638–648.
40. Haffty BG, Wilson LD, Son YH, et al. Concurrent chemo-radiotherapy with mitomycin C compared with porfiromycin in squamous cell cancer of the head and neck: final results of a randomized clinical trial. *Int J Radiat Oncol Biol Phys* 2005;61:119–128.
41. Henk JM, Kunkler PB, Smith CW. Radiotherapy and hyperbaric oxygen in head and neck cancer. Final report of first controlled clinical trial. *Lancet* 1977;2:101–103.
42. Henk JM. Late results of a trial of hyperbaric oxygen and radiotherapy in head and neck cancer: a rationale for hypoxic cell sensitizers? *Int J Radiat Oncol Biol Phys* 1986;12:1339–1341.
43. Henke M, Laszig R, Rube C, et al. Erythropoietin to treat head and neck cancer patients with anaemia undergoing radiotherapy: randomised, double-blind, placebo-controlled trial. *Lancet* 2003;362:1255–1260.
44. Hockel M, Knoop C, Schlenger K, et al. Intratumoral Po_2 predicts survival in advanced cancer of the uterine cervix. *Radiother Oncol* 1993;26:45–50.
45. Hockel M, Schlenger K, Aral B, et al. Association between tumor hypoxia and malignant progression in advanced cancer of the uterine cervix. *Cancer Res* 1996;56: 4509–4515.
46. Horsman MR, Brown JM, Hirst VK, et al. Mechanism of action of the selective tumor radiosensitizer nicotinamide. *Int J Radiat Oncol Biol Phys* 1988;15:685–690.
47. Horsman MR, Overgaard J, Christensen KL, et al. Mechanism for the reduction of tumour hypoxia by nicotinamide and the clinical relevance for radiotherapy. *Biomed Biochim Acta* 1989;48:S251–S254.
48. Hou H, Khan N, O'Hara JA, et al. Effect of RSR13, an allosteric hemoglobin modifier, on oxygenation in murine tumors: an *in vivo* electron paramagnetic resonance oximetry and bold MRI study. *Int J Radiat Oncol Biol Phys* 2004;59:834–843.
49. Huang SM, Bock JM, Harari PM. Epidermal growth factor receptor blockade with C225 modulates proliferation, apoptosis, and radiosensitivity in squamous cell carcinomas of the head and neck. *Cancer Res* 1999;59:1935–1940.
50. Huang SM, Harari PM. Modulation of radiation response after epidermal growth factor receptor blockade in squamous cell carcinomas: inhibition of damage repair, cell cycle kinetics, and tumor angiogenesis. *Clin Cancer Res* 2000;6:2166–2174.
51. Kaanders JH, Pop LA, Marres HA, et al. ARCON: experience in 215 patients with advanced head-and-neck cancer. *Int J Radiat Oncol Biol Phys* 2002;52:769–778.
52. Khandelwal SR, Kavanagh BD, Lin PS, et al. RSR13, an allosteric effector of haemoglobin, and carbogen radiosensitize FSAII and SCCVII tumours in C3H mice. *Br J Cancer* 1999;79:814–820.
53. Koukourakis MI, Kyrias G, Kakolyris S, et al. Subcutaneous administration of amifostine during fractionated radiotherapy: a randomized phase II study. *J Clin Oncol* 2000;18:2226–2233.
54. Laramore GE, Scott CB, al-Sarraf M, et al. Adjuvant chemotherapy for resectable squamous cell carcinomas of the head and neck: report on Intergroup Study 0034. *Int J Radiat Oncol Biol Phys* 1992;23:705–713.
55. Laurence V, Ward R, Dennis I, et al. Carbogen breathing with nicotinamide improves the oxygen state of tumours in patients. *Br J Cancer* 1995;72:198–205.
56. Lee WR, Berkey B, Marcial V, et al. Anemia is associated with decreased survival and increased locoregional failure in patients with locally advanced head and neck carcinoma: a secondary analysis of RTOG 85-27. *Int J Radiat Oncol Biol Phys* 1998;42:1069–1075.
57. Lindegaard JC, Grau C. Has the outlook improved for amifostine as a clinical radioprotector? *Radiother Oncol* 2000;57:113–118.
58. Makkonen TA, Bostrom P, Vilja P, et al. Sucralfate mouth washing in the prevention of radiation-induced mucositis: a placebo-controlled double-blind randomized study. *Int J Radiat Oncol Biol Phys* 1994;30:177–182.
59. Martin F, Farley A, Gagnon M, et al. Comparison of the healing capacities of sucralfate and cimetidine in the short-term treatment of duodenal ulcer: a double-blind randomized trial. *Gastroenterology* 1982;82:401–405.

60. Mendenhall WM, Morris CG, Amdur RJ, et al. Radiotherapy alone or combined with carbogen breathing for squamous cell carcinoma of the head and neck: a prospective, randomized trial. *Cancer* 2005;104:332–337.

61. Meredith R, Salter M, Kim R, et al. Sucralfate for radiation mucositis: results of a double-blind randomized trial. *Int J Radiat Oncol Biol Phys* 1997;37:275–279.

62. Movsas B, Scott C, Langer C, et al. Randomized trial of amifostine in locally advanced non-small-cell lung cancer patients receiving chemotherapy and hyperfractionated radiation: radiation therapy oncology group trial 98-01. *J Clin Oncol* 2005;23:2145–2154.

63. Movsas B. Exploring the role of the radioprotector amifostine in locally advanced non-small cell lung cancer: Radiation Therapy Oncology Group trial 98-01. *Semin Radiat Oncol* 2002;12:40–45.

64. Nordsmark M, Bentzen SM, Rudat V, et al. Prognostic value of tumor oxygenation in 397 head and neck tumors after primary radiation therapy. An international multi-center study. *Radiother Oncol* 2005;77:18–24.

65. Overgaard J, Hansen HS, Andersen AP, et al. Misonidazole combined with split-course radiotherapy in the treatment of invasive carcinoma of larynx and pharynx: report from the DAHANCA 2 study. *Int J Radiat Oncol Biol Phys* 1989;16:1065–1068.

66. Overgaard J, Hansen HS, Overgaard M, et al. A randomized double-blind phase III study of nimorazole as a hypoxic radiosensitizer of primary radiotherapy in supraglottic larynx and pharynx carcinoma. Results of the Danish Head and Neck Cancer Study (DAHANCA) Protocol 5-85. *Radiother Oncol* 1998;46:135–146.

67. Overgaard J, Overgaard M, Nielsen OS, et al. A comparative investigation of nimorazole and misonidazole as hypoxic radiosensitizers in a C3H mammary carcinoma in vivo. *Br J Cancer* 1982;46:904–911.

68. Pfeiffer P, Madsen EL, Hansen O, et al. Effect of prophylactic sucralfate suspension on stomatitis induced by cancer chemotherapy. A randomized, double-blind cross-over study. *Acta Oncol* 1990;29:171–173.

69. Potten CS, O'Shea JA, Farrell CL, et al. The effects of repeated doses of keratinocyte growth factor on cell proliferation in the cellular hierarchy of the crypts of the murine small intestine. *Cell Growth Differ* 2001;12:265–275.

70. Prosnitz RG, Yao B, Farrell CL, et al. Pretreatment anemia is correlated with the reduced effectiveness of radiation and concurrent chemotherapy in advanced head and neck cancer. *Int J Radiat Oncol Biol Phys* 2005;61:1087–1095.

71. Rischin D, Hicks RJ, Fisher R, et al. Prognostic significance of [18F]-misonidazole positron emission tomography-detected tumor hypoxia in patients with advanced head and neck cancer randomly assigned to chemoradiation with or without tirapazamine: a substudy of Trans-Tasman Radiation Oncology Group Study 98.02 *J Clin Oncol* 2006;24:2098–2104.

72. Rischin D, Peters L, Fisher R, et al. Tirapazamine, cisplatin, and radiation versus fluorouracil, cisplatin, and radiation in patients with locally advanced head and neck cancer: a randomized phase II trial of the Trans-Tasman Radiation Oncology Group (TROG 98.02). *J Clin Oncol* 2005;23:79–87.

73. Rischin D, Peters L, Hicks R, et al. Phase I trial of concurrent tirapazamine, cisplatin, and radiotherapy in patients with advanced head and neck cancer. *J Clin Oncol* 2001;19:535–542.

74. Robert F, Ezekiel MP, Spencer SA, et al. Phase I study of anti-epidermal growth factor receptor antibody cetuximab in combination with radiation therapy in patients with advanced head and neck cancer. *J Clin Oncol* 2001;19:3234–3243.

75. Robnett TJ, Machtay M, Hahn SM, et al. Pathological response to preoperative chemoradiation worsens with anemia in non-small cell lung cancer patients. *Cancer J* 2002;8:263–267.

76. Rockwell S, Hughes CS. Effects of mitomycin C and porfiromycin on exponentially growing and plateau phase cultures. *Cell Prolif* 1994;27:153–163.

77. Saleh MN, Raisch KP, Stackhouse MA, et al. Combined modality therapy of A431 human epidermoid cancer using anti-EGFr antibody C225 and radiation. *Cancer Biother Radiopharm* 1999;14:451–463.

78. Sealy A, Hockly J, Shepstone B. The treatment of malignant melanoma with cobalt and hyperbaric oxygen. *Clin Radiol* 1974;25:211–215.

79. Segre G, Hammarstrom S. Aspects of the mechanisms of action of benzydamine. *Int J Tissue React* 1985;7:187–193.

80. Simon RM. Clinical trials in cancer. In· DeVita V, Rosenberg S, eds. *Cancer principles and practice of oncology.* Philadelphia: Lippincott-Raven, 1997;520–521.

81. Sironi M, Pozzi P, Polentarutti N, et al. Inhibition of inflammatory cytokine production and protection against endotoxin toxicity by benzydamine. *Cytokine* 1996;8:710–716.

82. Spielberger R, Stiff P, Bensinger W, et al. Palifermin for oral mucositis after intensive therapy for hematologic cancers. *N Engl J Med* 2004;351:2590–2598.

83. Stea B, Shaw E, Pinter T, et al. Efaproxiral red blood cell concentration predicts efficacy in patients with brain metastases. *Br J Cancer* 2006;94:1777–1784.

84. Teicher BA, Wong JS, Takeuchi H, et al. Allosteric effectors of hemoglobin as modulators of chemotherapy and radiation therapy in vitro and in vivo. *Cancer Chemother Pharmacol* 1998;42:24–30.

85. Thomlinson RH, Gray LH. The histological structure of some human lung cancers and the possible implications for radiotherapy. *Br J Cancer* 1955;9:539–549.

86. Thrasher B BM, Vujaskovic Z, Brizel D. Preclinical evaluation of amifostine mediated esophageal radioprotection in a rodent model. *Int J Radiat Oncol Biol Phys* 2006;66:S556–S557.

87. Trotti A, Garden A, Warde P, et al. A multinational, randomized phase III trial of iseganan HCl oral solution for reducing the severity of oral mucositis in patients receiving radiotherapy for head-and-neck malignancy. *Int J Radiat Oncol Biol Phys* 2004;58:674–681.

88. Van den Bogaert W, van der Schueren E, Horiot JC, et al. The EORTC randomized trial on three fractions per day and misonidazole in advanced head and neck cancer: prognostic factors. *Radiother Oncol* 1995;35:100–106.

89. Vujaskovic Z, Feng QF, Rabbani ZN, et al. Assessment of the protective effect of amifostine on radiation-induced pulmonary toxicity. *Exp Lung Res* 2002;28:577–590.

90. Vujaskovic Z, Feng QF, Rabbani ZN, et al. Radioprotection of lungs by amifostine is associated with reduction in profibrogenic cytokine activity. *Radiat Res* 2002;157:656–660.

91. Wang J, Biedermann KA, Brown JM. Repair of DNA and chromosome breaks in cells exposed to SR 4233 under hypoxia or to ionizing radiation. *Cancer Res* 1992;52:4473–4477.

92. Wasserman TH, Brizel DM, Henke M, et al. Influence of intravenous amifostine on xerostomia, tumor control, and survival after radiotherapy for head-and- neck cancer: 2-year follow-up of a prospective, randomized, phase III trial. *Int J Radiat Oncol Biol Phys* 2005;63:985–990.

93. Wasserman TH, Lee DJ, Cosmatos D, et al. Clinical trials with etanidazole (SR-2508) by the Radiation Therapy Oncology Group (RTOG). *Radiother Oncol* 1991;20[Suppl 1]:129–135.

94. Watson ER, Halnan KE, Dische S, et al. Hyperbaric oxygen and radiotherapy: a Medical Research Council trial in carcinoma of the cervix. *Br J Radiol* 1978;51:879–887.

95. Yuhas JM, Spellman JM, Culo F. The role of WR-2721 in radiotherapy and/or chemotherapy. *Cancer Clin Trials* 1980;3:211–216.

96. Zeman EM, Brown JM, Lemmon MJ, et al. SR-4233: a new bioreductive agent with high selective toxicity for hypoxic mammalian cells. *Int J Radiat Oncol Biol Phys* 1986;12:1239–1242.

97. Zeman EM, Brown JM. Pre- and post-irradiation radiosensitization by SR 4233. *Int J Radiat Oncol Biol Phys* 1989;16:967–971.

98. Zeman EM, Hirst VK, Lemmon MJ, et al. Enhancement of radiation-induced tumor cell killing by the hypoxic cell toxin SR 4233. *Radiother Oncol* 1988;12:209–218.

Techniques, Modalities, and Modifiers in Radiation Oncology

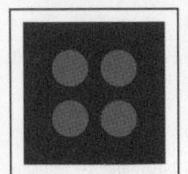

Chapter 27
Oncologic Imaging/Oncologic Anatomy

Chris R. Kelsey, Lawrence B. Marks

This chapter addresses two related topics central to the radiotherapeutic management of patients with cancer. Oncologic imaging is discussed first, including illustrations to underscore the advantages of various imaging modalities. A discussion on oncologic anatomy follows. A sound understanding of anatomy, especially pertaining to malignant processes, facilitates interpretation of imaging studies. Likewise, understanding the advantages and limitations of individual imaging modalities assists in defining rational clinical target volumes that maximize the therapeutic ratio.

▪▪ | Oncologic Imaging

Radiologic imaging is an integral component of the overall management of patients with cancer. Initially, imaging is utilized in the workup and clinical staging. In radiation oncology, imaging is also used for treatment planning, for both external beam radiation therapy and brachytherapy. Following a course of treatment, depending on the primary site, imaging is performed at regular intervals to assess for recurrence or second primary malignancies.

Radiation oncologists must become familiar with the various imaging modalities utilized in daily practice and understand the accuracy and limitations of each. In particular, having a general sense of the sensitivity, specificity, and positive and negative predictive values of imaging studies helps the clinician assimilate and interpret information that is sometimes contradictory. As a detailed study of each imaging modality is far beyond the scope of this chapter, the imaging modalities utilized most frequently in clinical practice are focused on, with special emphasis on underlying anatomy.

Computed Tomography

The computed tomography (CT) system was developed by Godfrey Newbold Hounsfield in 1972, for which he received the Nobel Prize in Medicine in 1979. The fundamental principles of CT are as follows. An x-ray source rotates around the patient with sensors located on the opposite side from the source. As the patient is passed through the gantry, data from multiple projections are obtained. Axial images from the raw data are created using a mathematical process, termed tomographic reconstruction. CT technology is continually improving. Spiral (helical) and multidetector CT units have replaced conventional (incremental) units. Spiral CT more readily allows for multiplanar and three-dimensional reconstructions. Multiple detector rows allow for faster acquisition, higher spatial resolution, and the ability to retrospectively choose scan thickness. Rapid data acquisition, with minimization of respiratory and swallowing artifacts, allows for clear multiplanar reconstructions that rivals direct magnetic resonance imaging (MRI).

Contrast agents help visualize organs of interest, tumors, and/or blood vessels. Contrast is usually delivered by three routes—intravenous, oral, and rectal. Intravenous (IV) contrast, typically utilizing iodinated compounds that absorb x-rays, is used most frequently. IV contrast helps identify vascular spaces and changes in organ perfusion patterns, which may be indicative of disease. For example, contrast can evaluate perfusion in the lung for diagnosis of pulmonary embolus, or liver and brain for diagnosis of hemangiomas and metastases. Abnormal vasculature within tumors often leads to leakage of contrast into the parenchyma and is seen as "enhancement" on CT. Since the contrast is excreted in the kidney, the integrity of the urinary collecting system can be assessed with IV contrast. Iodinated contrast is generally well tolerated, although some patients may develop flushing, pruritis, or a metallic taste in the mouth. Anaphylactic reactions are uncommon. In patients with a known allergy to iodinated contrast (often associated with an allergy to shellfish), noniodinated contrast agents are available.

Oral and rectal contrast is used to highlight the internal cavities of the gastrointestinal tract. The most commonly used substances are barium sulfate and Gastrograffin. Gastrograffin can cause chemical pneumonitis and should be used with caution if a tracheoesophageal fistula is suspected. The major contraindication to the use of barium is radiographic or clinical suspicion of perforation since barium can result in peritonitis. The primary side effect of both Gastrografin and barium is constipation. Gastrointestinal (GI) contrast is widely used during radiation therapy (RT) planning, for example, to identify the esophagus during treatment planning for esophageal or lung tumors, or to identify the stomach and intestines during planning for abdominal/pelvic tumors.

The CT numbers for each pixel are used during radiation treatment planning dose calculation, and thus, contrast can affect these calculations. If indicated, the CT number within a structure that is enhancing with the contrast agent (i.e., the bladder when planning for prostate cancer) can be set to an alternate value prior to planning.

CT has become the core modality for oncologic imaging due to its relatively low cost, widespread availability, and versatility. CT also plays a primary role in RT treatment planning. More accurate target delineation is achieved with CT-based planning, as compared with conventional simulation, allowing for tighter margins and less normal tissue irradiation. In addition, unconventional beam arrangements are more easily employed using three-dimensional treatment planning. CT-based planning also allows for dose calculations based on tissue density.

CT is the cornerstone of oncologic imaging and is employed for a wide spectrum of malignancies. The following examples highlight the utility of CT imaging.

Laryngeal Cancer

The *mucosal* extent of most head and neck cancers can be assessed with direct fiberoptic laryngoscopy. Imaging may better elucidate the extent of *submucosal* extension. CT is the standard modality to stage most head and neck cancers, including laryngeal cancer (Fig. 27.1). A thin-section CT examination with images obtained parallel to the plane of the true vocal cords, with reformatted images in the sagittal plane, is used to evaluate for early cartilage invasion, anterior and/or posterior commissure involvement, subglottic extension, and invasion of the pre-epiglottic and paraglottic space.

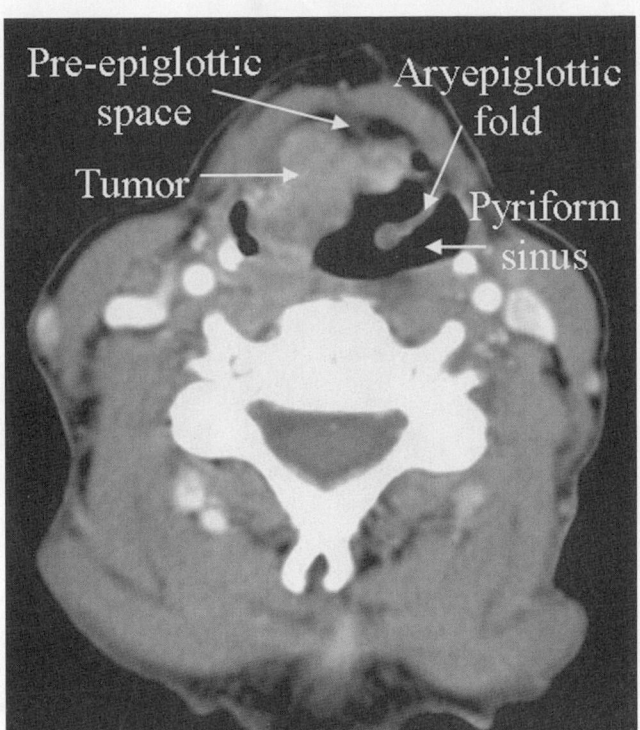

FIGURE 27.1. Axial computed tomography image demonstrating a squamous cell carcinoma involving the right aryepiglottic fold with anterior extension into the pre-epiglottic space.

Pancreatic Cancer

Adenocarcinoma of the pancreas most frequently arises in the head of the gland, to the right of the superior mesenteric/portal vein. It usually appears as a hypodense mass relative to the normally enhancing pancreas. Surgical resection typically pro-

vides the only chance of cure, and high-speed helical CT with thin sections and IV contrast enhancement is an important modality to assess resectability. Encasement of the superior mesenteric artery (SMA) or celiac trunk defines an unresectable T4 tumor. On the other hand, the presence of a fat plane around the celiac trunk and SMA, along with a patent superior mesenteric/portal vein, defines potentially resectable disease. Borderline cases include those with tumor abutment on the SMA (Fig. 27.2), severe unilateral SMV/portal vein impingement, or adjacent organ invasion. CT does not, however, detect small volume peritoneal or surface liver metastases that can be identified with laparoscopy.

Magnetic Resonance Imaging

The basic principles of MRI are as follows. A magnet generates a strong magnetic field (up to 3 T for clinical systems), aligning the nuclei of hydrogen atoms within the patient. Shim coils function to make the magnetic field as homogenous as possible. Radiofrequency (RF) excitation pulses transmitted by antennae or coils perturb this alignment. When the RF pulse is removed the nuclei realign with the magnetic field, emitting a transient radio signal in the process. A receiver coil detects these radio signals that are known as a *spin echo*, or more frequently, an *echo*. If the echo is detected in the presence of a magnetic field gradient, spatial information is encoded in the measured signal. A computer reconstructs the images from the echoes. The computer programs used to control the RF and gradient pulses are called *pulse sequences*. MRI can be manipulated by varying pulse sequence parameters like the repetition time (TR) and the echo time (TE). The TR is the time between RF excitation pulses in the pulse sequence. The TE is the time between the center of the RF excitation pulse and the center of the echo. Image contrast is affected by TR and TE times. T1-weighted images use intermediate TR values (400 to 3,000 ms) and short TE values (<30 ms), while T2-weighted images use long TR values (>3,000 ms) and intermediate TE values (50 to 120 ms).

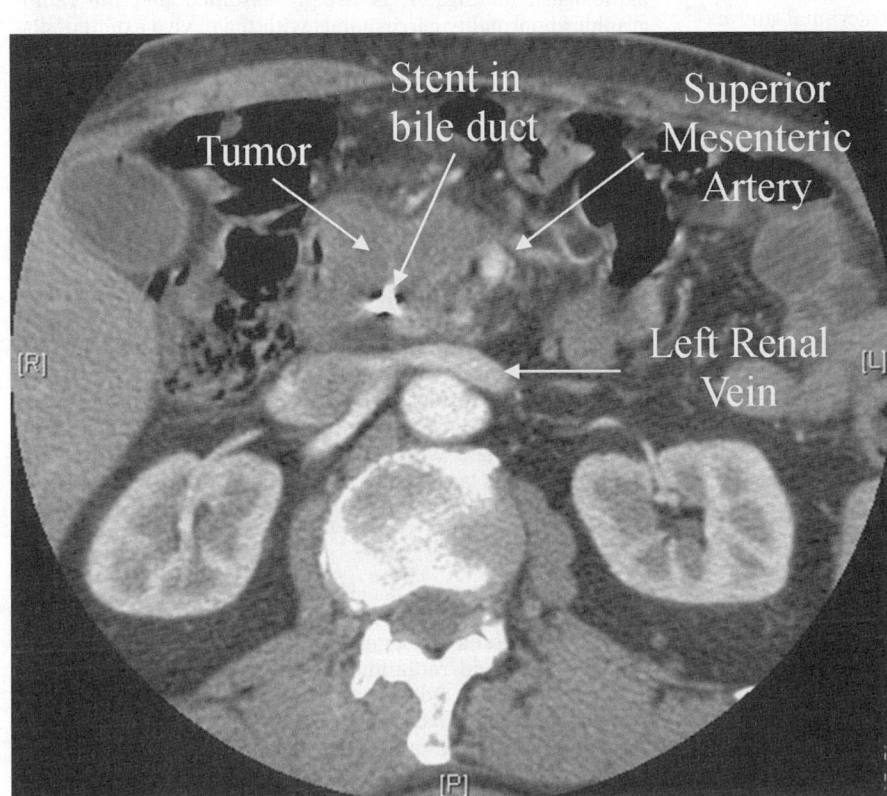

FIGURE 27.2. Axial computed tomography image demonstrating an adenocarcinoma of the pancreatic head with tumor abutting the superior mesenteric artery.

Table 27.1	MAGNETIC RESONANCE IMAGING SIGNAL INTENSITIES (SPIN-ECHO IMAGING)		
	T1WI	T2WI	FLAIR
Cerebrospinal fluid	Dark	Bright	Dark
Fat[a]	Bright	Dark	Bright
Solid mass (tumor)	Dark	Bright	Bright
Cyst	Dark	Bright	Dark

Bright—hyperintense; dark—hypointense; T1—T1-weighted image; T2—T2-weighted image
[a]Fat is bright on T2 that is fast spin echo (FSE) or gradient echo.

The FLAIR pulse sequence produces T2-weighted images with suppression of the cerebral spinal fluid (CSF) signal to facilitate imaging lesions adjacent to the ventricles or cisterns (Table 27.1).

Due to excellent soft tissue contrast and ability to directly image in multiple planes, MRI is the preferred imaging modality for most intracranial and spinal tumors as well as many extracranial tumors. Furthermore, MRI may be superior to CT when imaging regions surrounded by bone, such as the temporal lobes and posterior fossa, since there may be artifacts associated with dense bone on CT. Most intracranial neoplasms are hypointense on T1-weighted images and hyperintense on T2-weighted images. However, other processes (infarcts, demyelinating diseases, and inflammatory lesions) can have a similar appearance, thus limiting the specificity of MRI.

The most commonly used MR contrast agent is gadolinium. Gadolinium is impermeable to an intact blood–brain barrier (BBB). Some intracranial sites, such as the pituitary gland, pineal gland, choroid plexus, and dura, will enhance normally. Malignant neoplasms with adherent vasculature will allow gadolinium to pass into the brain parenchyma, leading to enhancement. In general, high-grade lesions enhance more frequently than low grade neoplasms, but this is not always the case. A notable exception is pilocytic astrocytomas.

A few of the commonly encountered intracranial and extracranial tumors for which MRI is utilized are reviewed below.

Brain Metastases

The most sensitive imaging study to detect intracranial metastases is contrast-enhanced MRI (76). For patients with a single brain metastasis detected with a conventional single-dose MRI contrasted study, triple-dose studies will depict additional metastases in up to 25% of patients (75) and is an active area of investigation. Most metastases gain access to the brain through the vasculature and typically arise at the junction of the gray and white matter (16), presumably because the caliber of blood vessels decreases at this point, acting as a trap for tumor emboli. Approximately 80% of brain metastases are found in the cerebral hemispheres, with less frequent involvement of the cerebellum (15%) and brainstem (5%), reflecting their smaller volume and blood flow. Brain metastases are typically well circumscribed, briskly enhance, and are associated with a disproportionate amount of surrounding edema (Fig. 27.3). The detection of multiple lesions helps to distinguish metastases from primary brain tumors and guides the appropriate treatment for patients with brain metastases.

Glioblastoma Multiforme

In adults, glioblastoma multiforme (GBM) usually arises in the cerebral hemispheres, while in children, GBMs commonly arise in the posterior fossa. GBMs are characterized by an iso- to hypointense mass with irregular gadolinium enhancement, often

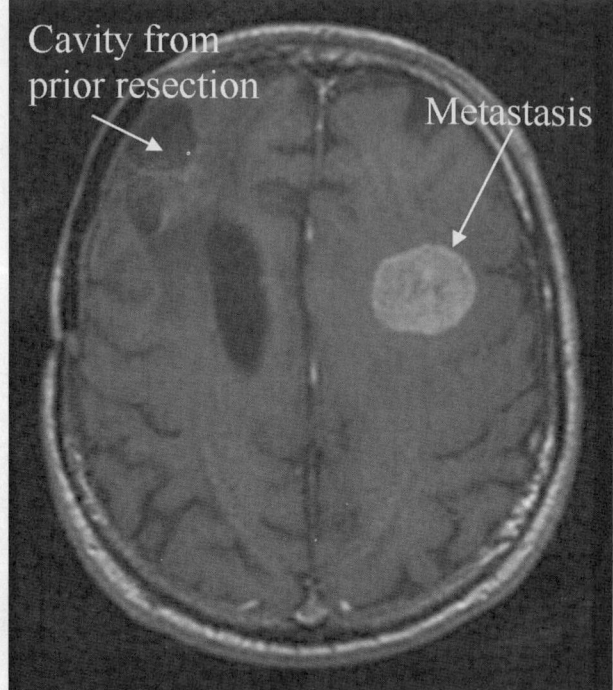

FIGURE 27.3. Axial T1 magnetic resonance image with contrast demonstrating a 2.5 cm melanoma brain metastasis in the left frontal lobe. Note the prior resection cavity in the right frontal lobe.

with central necrosis. T2-weighted imaging shows a heterogeneous, hyperintense mass with surrounding T2-signal abnormality corresponding to edema, in which malignant cells are known to frequently reside (33).

Few clinicopathologic studies have systematically correlated the location and size of tumors visualized radiologically to pathological findings. It is usually assumed that the radiographic abnormality corresponds with the in vivo extent of disease, but this may or may not always be the case. In a pathologic study of adults who died with GBM, Burger et al. (11) demonstrated that infiltrating margins of tumor often extend into regions of brain appearing normal on CT. Conversely, regions appearing abnormal on CT did not always contain tumor. This study should be a reminder that there are limitations to all imaging modalities, and a knowledge concerning the patterns of spread of each malignancy facilitates rational RT treatment planning.

GBM most commonly grows along white matter tracts and does not typically involve the dura or skull. Other potential routes of spread, including subependymal extension with CSF contamination or hematogenous dissemination, are possible but unusual. Compared with CT, MRI is more accurate in delineating the local gross extent of primary brain tumors. In a series of 52 patients with primary brain tumors, the MRI signal abnormality was larger than the CT abnormality in 62% of patients. Furthermore, 10 patients with equivocal CT scans had clear abnormalities on MRI (37).

Nasopharyngeal Cancer

Multiple studies have suggested that MRI may be superior to CT for staging and radiation treatment planning of nasopharyngeal carcinoma (NPC) (14,48). In a series of 67 patients, MRI was more sensitive than CT in detecting skull-base involvement, intracranial extension, and retropharyngeal adenopathy. T-stage was changed in 27% of cases (15/18 upstaged, 3/18 downstaged) (48). Involvement of the skull base occurs in three

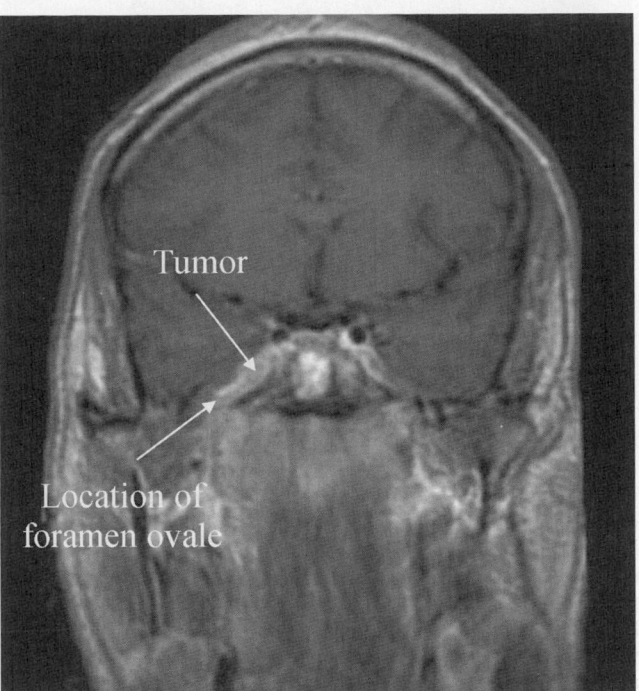

FIGURE 27.4. Coronal T1 magnetic resonance image with contrast demonstrating nasopharyngeal carcinoma extending through foramen ovale into Meckel's cave.

primary patterns (53). First, widening of the petroclival fissure, indicating early involvement of the skull base, is visualized well with CT or MRI. Second, direct infiltration by NPC into bone can occur. Contrary to common belief, MRI is actually more sensitive than CT in detecting bone involvement. MRI can often detect cancellous bone involvement before cortical destruction takes place (48). Finally, NPC can invade through the foramina in the base of the skull (foramen lacerum, foramen ovale, and so forth), gaining access to the middle cranial fossa and cavernous sinus (Fig. 27.4). Dural thickening along the floor of the middle cranial fossa is suspicious for early intracranial extension.

Superior Sulcus Tumors

Similar to the nasopharynx, the superior sulcus of the lung is surrounded by multiple critical structures. The subclavian artery and vein pass anterior to the lung apex, the brachial plexus and its branches cross over the apex of the lung toward the arm, and the stellate ganglia lie posteriorly alongside the exiting nerve roots of the lower cervical and upper thoracic spine. Other structures that can be involved by superior sulcus tumors are the vertebral bodies, trachea, and esophagus. Compared with CT, MRI more accurately depicts the anatomy of the superior sulcus (28) and may be helpful in determining resectability. Sagittal imaging to assess for vascular involvement is particularly helpful.

Positron Emission Tomography

Positron emission tomography (PET), utilizing the radiopharmaceutical fluorodeoxyglucose (FDG), is a functional imaging modality that discriminates malignant cells from nonmalignant ones on the basis of their increased metabolic rate. Neoplastic cells are more reliant on glycolysis than normal cells and are characterized by increased levels of glucose transporters and hexokinase and decreased levels of glucose-6-phosphatase (71). Furthermore, the metabolism of FDG differs from native glucose. After FDG is phosphorylated, it is not further metabolized

and remains trapped within the cell (except in the liver where the large concentration of phosphatase enzymes results in dephosphorylation). These metabolic differences between normal cells and cancer cells, and between glucose and FDG, are exploited by PET scanning.

The radionuclides used for PET imaging are positron emitters. The emitted positron ($\beta+$) travels at most a few millimeters in tissue before combining with an electron ($\beta-$) with subsequent annihilation of both particles. The mass of the two particles is converted into two 511 keV photons emitted simultaneously at approximately 180 degrees to each other. Since the two photons are generated simultaneously, detection of both photons within a limited time window is the principle underlying PET image acquisition. The radionuclide used most frequently in clinical practice is fluorine 18 (^{18}F), which has a half-life of approximately 110 minutes.

PET scans are being utilized more frequently in clinical practice for a wide range of malignancies and clinical scenarios. More recently, PET scanners have been combined with CT scanners. These scanners provide high-resolution anatomic information combined with metabolic information. A few of the most notable indications receive further discussion below.

Non–Small Cell Lung Cancer

Treatment decisions are often predicated on the status of the mediastinum in patients with operable non–small cell lung cancer (NSCLC). Patients without mediastinal disease generally proceed directly to resection, while those with mediastinal spread often receive induction therapy or definitive chemoradiotherapy. The standard noninvasive staging tool has been CT. In general, the sensitivity and specificity of CT is less than optimal (17,23,80) (Table 27.2). Thus, mediastinoscopy is often utilized to pathologically stage the mediastinum. Mediastinoscopy is associated with a low rate of morbidity. Nevertheless, if noninvasive studies proved highly accurate, this procedure might be avoided in many patients.

Table 27.2	"ACCURACY" OF COMPUTED TOMOGRAPHY AND POSITRON EMISSION TOMOGRAPHY FOR MEDIASTINAL STAGING OF NON–SMALL CELL LUNG CANCER		
End Point	**Toloza et al.**[a]	**Gould et al.**[b]	**Dwamena et al.**[c]
Computed Tomography			
Sensitivity	0.57	0.61	0.60
Specificity	0.82	0.79	0.77
Positive predictive value	0.56	ns	0.50
Negative predictive value	0.83	ns	0.85
Positron Emission Tomography			
Sensitivity	0.84	0.85	0.79
Specificity	0.89	0.90	0.91
Positive predictive value	0.79	ns	0.90
Negative predictive value	0.93	ns	0.93

ns, not stated
[a]Toloza EM, Harpole L, McCrory DC. Noninvasive staging of non-small cell lung cancer: A review of the current evidence. *Chest* 2003;123:137S–146S.
[b]Gould MK, Kuschner WG, Rydzak CE, et al. Test performance of positron emission tomography and computed tomography for mediastinal staging in patients with non-small-cell lung cancer: A meta-analysis. *Ann Intern Med* 2003;139:879–892.
[c]Dwamena BA, Sonnad SS, Angobaldo JO, et al. Metastases from non-small cell lung cancer: Mediastinal staging in the 1990s—meta-analytic comparison of PET and CT. *Radiology* 1999;213:530–536.

Numerous studies and meta-analyses (17,23,80) have assessed the ability of CT and PET to accurately stage the mediastinum in patients with NSCLC (Table 27.2). Although significant heterogeneity exists among the individual studies, several conclusions can be drawn. First, the positive predictive value of CT is poor (~50%). PET is somewhat better (80% to 90%). Still, 10% to 20% of patients with PET abnormalities in the mediastinum will have no evidence of disease at mediastinoscopy (though insufficient sampling may be explanatory in some cases). Therefore, many still advocate mediastinoscopy in the setting of a positive PET. The negative predictive value of PET appears to be better (93% to 98%), especially when there are no enlarged lymph nodes on CT (60). Immediate thoracotomy, bypassing staging mediastinoscopy, may be reasonable in patients with negative PET imaging of the mediastinum, given its high negative predictive value.

Hodgkin's and Non-Hodgkin's Lymphoma

PET imaging is routinely obtained in patients with Hodgkin's disease (HD) and non-Hodgkin's lymphoma (NHL) (Fig. 27.5). Along with other diagnostic tests, PET is used to determine the initial extent of disease (stage), evaluate the response to treatment (in particular the status of residual masses), and assess for relapse after treatment is complete. Evaluating the accuracy of PET in lymphoma staging is problematic, as the disease is not typically managed surgically. Thus, pathologic information is not typically available to confirm presence or absence of disease, hindering the assessment of sensitivity, specificity, and so forth. Most publications assessing the accuracy of PET in lymphoma staging compare PET to CT and other conventional imaging studies. Despite this major limitation, PET appears to be a more sensitive staging tool than CT (68). In addition, multiple studies have shown that residual PET abnormalities after chemotherapy for aggressive NHL and HD predict for future relapse (31,46,72) (Fig. 27.5). Mikhaeel et al. (46) showed that posttreatment PET scans predicted outcome better than posttreatment CT scans. Of 45 patients with aggressive NHL, the relapse rate was 100% (9/9) for patients with abnormal post-

treatment PET scans versus 17% (4/36) for patients with negative posttreatment PET scans. Of these 45 patients, 33 also had posttreatment CT imaging. Only 41% of patients with abnormal CT imaging failed, while 25% of patients with negative CT scans eventually relapsed.

Esophageal Cancer

The most commonly used staging tools are barium swallow, endoscopic ultrasound (EUS), CT, and PET. EUS, discussed later in this chapter, is the most accurate modality to assess depth of invasion (T stage), but is less accurate assessing nodal involvement (N stage). The ability to perform fine needle aspiration biopsies of suspicious nodes, primarily disease in the celiac axis, has increased the ability of EUS to stage regional nodes. The reported accuracy of EUS for T and N stage is approximately 85% to 90% and 75%, respectively (39,65). CT is primarily used to assess for metastatic disease. It is fairly unreliable in predicting T or N stage. The optimal role of PET in esophageal cancer staging is undefined, but it is generally used to evaluate for local/regional nodal disease and distant metastases. However, the sensitivity of PET for local/regional nodal disease does not appear to be superior to EUS (84). It may be most helpful in detecting distant metastases and differentiating patients who have residual disease after neoadjuvant chemoradiotherapy, requiring surgical resection, from those who are complete responders and may be spared the morbidity of surgery (86).

Radionuclide Bone Scan and Bone Metastases

Normal bone undergoes continuous remodeling, maintaining a delicate balance between osteoblastic and osteoclastic activity. Most bone metastases originate as intramedullary lesions, having gained access to the bone through the vasculature. As the lesions enlarge, reactive osteoblastic and osteoclastic changes result in characteristic radiographic changes indicative of bone metastases (sclerotic, lytic, or mixed lesions). Rapidly growing metastases tend to produce lytic lesions, while more slowly

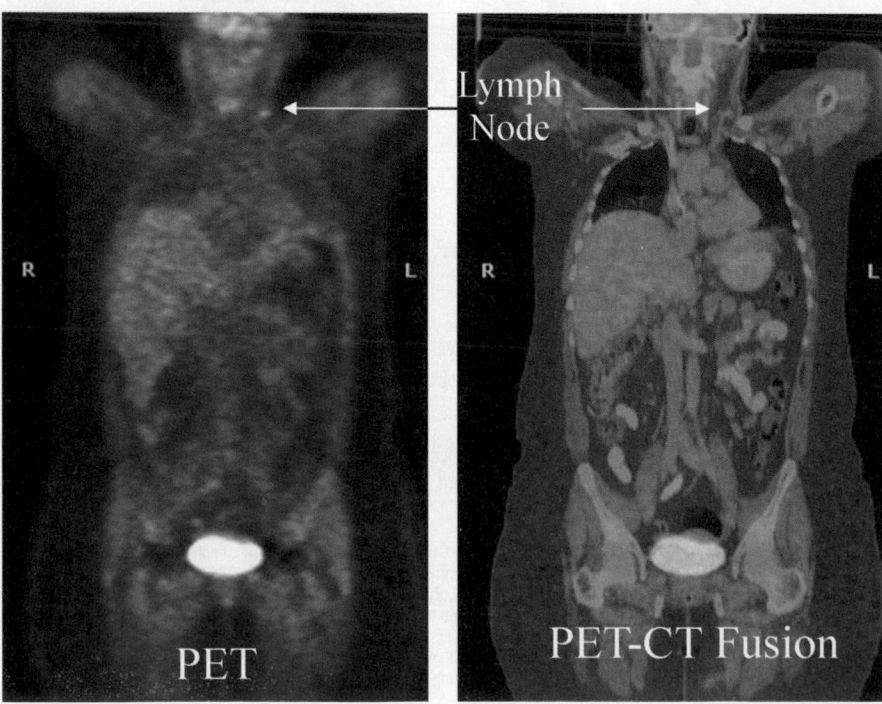

FIGURE 27.5. Postchemotherapy coronal positron emission tomography scan images of a patient with IVa Hodgkin's disease demonstrating a hypermetabolic left supraclavicular lymph node. The lymph node was <1 cm on CT, and would not be considered suspicious. Biopsy confirmed persistent disease. (*Left*) PET image. (*Right*) PET/CT fusion image. (Image courtesy of Dr. Edward Coleman.)

growing metastases typically produce sclerotic (or blastic) lesions. Metastases from multiple myeloma, thyroid cancer, and renal cell carcinoma are predominantly lytic, while blastic lesions are associated with breast and prostate cancer.

Detection of skeletal metastases is the primary indication for radioisotope bone scans. The most commonly used tracer is technetium-99m bound to methylene diphosphonate (^{99m}Tc-MDP), which is not a tumor-specific tracer. ^{99m}Tc-MDP is absorbed onto bone surface in the presence of increased skeletal metabolic activity and skeletal vascularity. Pure lytic lesions, especially with rapid growth, are often "cold" on bone scan and may be overlooked. Although 30% to 50% reduction in bone density must occur before bone metastases are detected on plan x-rays, as little as 5% to 10% change is required to detect such on a bone scan (9,19). Furthermore, bone scans are relatively inexpensive, convenient, and visualize the entire skeleton, including sites that are difficult to assess on plain films (e.g., ribs, sternum, scapula, sacrum). Reported sensitivities range from 62% to 100% with similar specificity rates (78% to 100%) (25). Rapid/pure lytic progression is the main cause for false-negative findings, while false-positive findings can be related to trauma, healing, benign bone tumors, or arthritic changes. Although studies have shown that MRI may be more sensitive than bone scans, especially for vertebral metastases, bone scans are considered sufficiently sensitive that MRI should be reserved for equivocal bone scans in the context of high clinical suspicion or for patients with positive bone scans but low clinical suspicion.

Bone metastases are considered "nonmeasurable" using the Response Evaluation Criteria in Solid Tumors criteria (79). Although a decrease in the intensity of radionuclide uptake is often ascribed to a response to treatment and an increase is attributed to progressive disease, several points must be considered. First, tumor response may cause a "flare phenomenon," resulting from increased activity secondary to new osteoblastic activity concomitant with new bone formation. This may be falsely attributed to progressive disease. Similarly, lytic lesions that were previously "cold" on bone scan can transform into hot spots after treatment. Second, rapidly progressive osseous disease with overwhelming bone destruction without new bone formation can be misinterpreted as stable disease on bone scan.

Many patients are at low risk of harboring occult metastatic disease and, in the absence of symptoms, a bone scan can be omitted from the staging workup. In prostate cancer, only ~1% of patients with a prostate-specific antigen (PSA) <10 will have a positive bone scan (22,35). Patients with a Gleason sum ≤7 and PSA 10 to 20 have a similar low risk of bone metastases (54). In these patients, a bone scan should be omitted in the absence of symptoms. Similarly, a bone scan may be omitted in asymptomatic patients with node-negative breast cancer and lung cancer. The use of bone scan may be declining as PET is being more commonly used, since whole body PET also images the skeleton. In a study comparing PET to bone scan for skeletal staging, both were found to be equally sensitive (90%). However, bone scan had many more false positives (e.g., due to degenerative disease), leading to a specificity and positive predictive values of 61% and 35%, respectively (vs. 98% and 90% for PET) (12).

Endoscopic Ultrasonography

Endoscopic ultrasonography was introduced in the early 1980s and has become an important staging tool for multiple gastrointestinal malignancies, most commonly esophageal and rectal cancer. A standard 5 to 12 MHz probe identifies five layers within the wall of the gastrointestinal tract (Table 27.3 and Fig. 27.6) (29). Higher frequency probes can identify additional layers, such as the muscularis mucosa and lamina propria. Normal lymph nodes are usually oval, <1 cm in size, and can have an isoechoic, hyperechoic, or hypoechoic echo texture. Suspicious

Table 27.3	**ENDOSCOPIC ULTRASOUND WALL LAYERS**		
Layer	**EUS Characteristic**	**Histologic Layer**	**AJCC T Stage**
1	Hyperechoic	Superficial mucosa	T1*m*
2	Hypoechoic	Deep mucosa	T1*m*
3	Hyperechoic	Submucosa	T1*sm*
4	Hypoechoic	Muscularis propria	T2
5	Hyperechoic	Subserosa, serosa, adventitia	T3

AJCC, American Joint Committee on Cancer Staging; EUS, endoscopic ultrasound; *m*, mucosa; *sm*, submucosa

lymph nodes are typically >1 cm, round with distinct borders, and/or have a hypoechoic medulla (Fig. 27.7). Interobserver variability and overlap in the features of benign and malignant lymph nodes limit the accuracy of EUS for nodal staging. The prefix *u* should be used to denote staging utilizing EUS (e.g., uT3N1). The ability of EUS to predict T stage is generally superior to its ability to predict N stage, although suspicious lymph nodes can often be biopsied through the echoendoscope. One exception is peritumoral lymph nodes, which are not accessible without passing through the primary lesion.

The accuracy of T staging for esophageal cancer is 85% to 90% (65) and increases with higher stage (>90% for T3 disease) (39). Nodal staging is less accurate, in the range of 75%, but significantly better than CT. Although peritumoral lymph nodes are not typically biopsied, abnormal celiac lymph nodes are accessible. This is particularly important for proximal esophageal lesions, as celiac involvement is a sign of metastatic spread. EUS is less helpful after neoadjuvant chemoradiotherapy, presumably because treatment-induced fibrosis and inflammation are indistinguishable from residual tumor.

Rectal cancer is one of the most common indications for EUS. Although surgery alone is sufficient for patients with stage I disease, surgery and chemoradiotherapy is indicated for patients with stage II or III tumors. The German Rectal Cancer Study Group showed that preoperative chemoradiotherapy is associated with improved local control with less acute and late toxicity than postoperative chemoradiotherapy (67). Accurate preoperative staging ensures that neoadjuvant treatment is appropriately applied to patients with stage II or III disease. The accuracy of EUS for rectal cancer is similar to esophageal cancer (~85% for T stage and ~75% for N stage) (58,78). In the German study, 18% of patients in the immediate surgery group, believed to have stage II or III disease by EUS, were found to have stage I disease after surgical resection (67). Thus, further improvements in preoperative staging are needed to appropriately select patients for neoadjuvant therapy.

Mammography/Ultrasonography

Multiple randomized trials have shown that screening mammography reduces the risk of breast cancer mortality by 20% to 35% in women aged 50 to 69 (2,3,47,52,77). The efficacy of screening in younger women (ages 40 to 49) and elderly women (age ≥70) is less certain. Most published guidelines suggest initiating screening at age 40. Screening mammography includes two standard views of each breast: A craniocaudal (CC) view and a mediolateral oblique (MLO) view. These images are taken at ~45 degree angulation to each other (i.e., they are not orthogonal). Although the CC view is oriented in the long axis of the patient (i.e., superior/inferior), the MLO is oriented in the medial-superior/lateral-inferior direction. The MLO view increases visualization of the upper outer quadrant and tail of the breast, while the CC view ensures adequate visualization of the

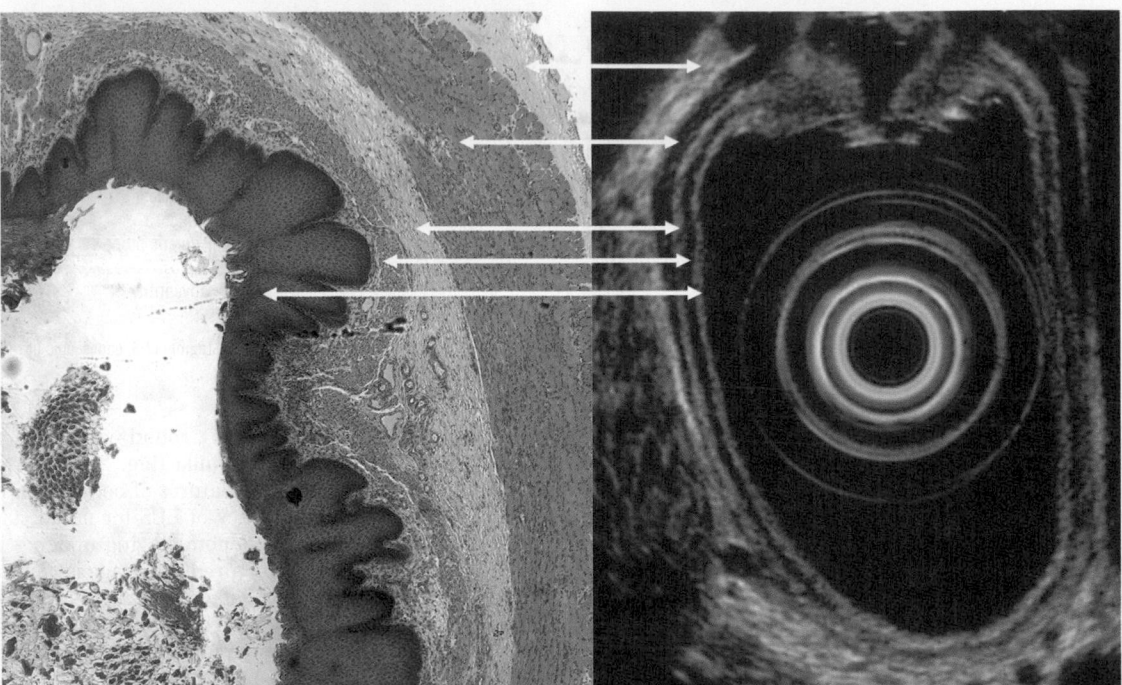

FIGURE 27.6. Axial endoscopic ultrasound image (*right*) and histologic specimen (*left*) from a normal esophagus. The endoscopic ultrasound layers and histologic layers of the esophagus are correlated (see Table 27.3). (Endoscopic ultrasound image courtesy of Dr. Frank Gress. Histologic image courtesy of Dr. Daniel Goodenough.)

inferior and medial aspects of the breast. Additional views can be utilized to further evaluate suspicious lesions.

It is important to realize that the majority of women (~95%) with abnormalities on a screening mammogram do not have breast cancer. Thus, the positive predictive value is low. The sensitivity and specificity varies with age and breast density. Overall, sensitivity of screening mammography is approx-

imately 75% (i.e., 25% of women diagnosed with breast cancer have a history of a normal mammogram 12 to 24 months prior to diagnosis [15]). The sensitivity of mammography in women with extremely dense breasts is approximately 63% compared with 87% in women with almost entirely fatty breasts. The specificity of mammography is approximately 92%, approaching 97% in women with fatty breasts (13). Guidelines for quality assurance of screening mammography have been developed in the United States. These guidelines, the Breast Imaging Reporting and Data System (BI-RADS), are shown in Table 27.4.

Mammographic abnormalities on screening studies are often nonspecific and prompt further diagnostic imaging or biopsy. An irregular mass, with spiculated borders, is highly suggestive of malignancy and appears spiculated due to invasion into, or reactive changes within, the surrounding breast parenchyma. However, spiculated masses can also be secondary to fat necrosis, postoperative scarring, or other nonmalignant processes. Round, well-circumscribed lesions are more often benign. Calcifications associated with ductal carcinoma *in situ* or invasive carcinoma are typically pleomorphic (heterogeneous) in appearance and grouped in a localized area. Linear, branching patterns are suggestive of intraductal carcinoma.

Ultrasonography is often used in conjunction with diagnostic mammography when evaluating a suspicious mass. It is most helpful in differentiating fluid-filled cysts from solid tumors. Calcifications, readily apparent on mammography, are not well visualized on ultrasonography. Ultrasound is currently under investigation as a screening tool but is not currently approved by the Food and Drug Administration for this indication.

Imaging of Normal Tissue

There is growing interest in combining functional imaging with anatomical imaging in RT treatment planning. For example, conventional CT imaging of the thorax can adequately visualize the normal lung. However, each portion of the lung may not be of equal functional importance. In an otherwise healthy individual,

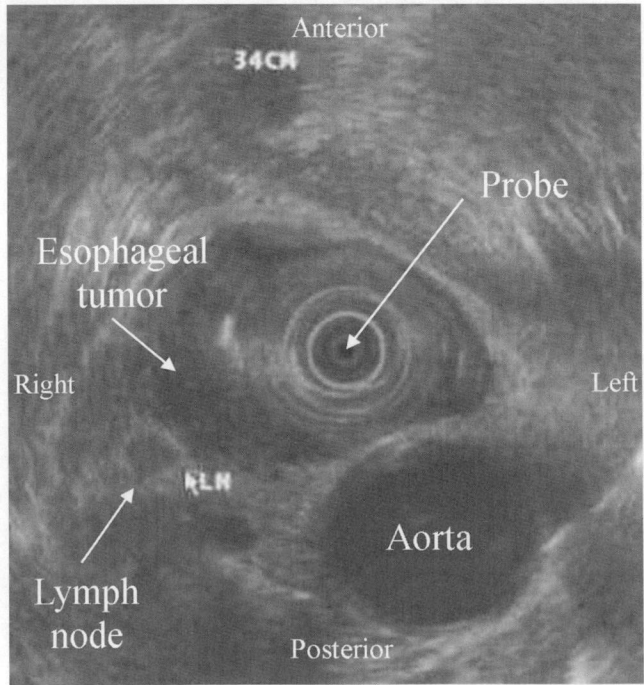

FIGURE 27.7. Endoscopic ultrasound image demonstrating a T3 esophageal tumor with an abnormal peritumoral lymph node. (Image courtesy of Dr. Frank Gress.)

	BREAST IMAGING REPORTING AND DATA SYSTEM (BIRADS) CATEGORIES USED FOR MAMMOGRAPHY EXAMINATIONS AND RISK OF MALIGNANCY		
Table 27.4			
Assessment Category	**Assessment**	**Definition**	**Risk of Malignancy**
0	Need additional imaging evaluation	A lesion is noted for which additional imaging is needed	N/A
1	Negative	Breasts appear normal	<0.1%
2	Benign finding	A negative mammogram result but the radiologist wishes to describe a finding	<0.1%
3	Probably benign finding; short-interval follow-up suggested	Lesion with a high probability of being benign	<2%
4	Suspicious abnormality—biopsy should be considered	A lesion is noted for which the radiologist has sufficient concern to recommend a biopsy	25%–50%
5	Highly suggestive of malignancy	A lesion is noted that has a high probability of being cancer	75%–99%

Adapted from Elmore JG, Armstrong K, Lehman CD, et al. Screening for breast cancer. *JAMA* 2005;293:1245–1256.

function may be relatively uniform throughout the lung. On the other hand, distribution of function is likely to be nonuniform in a patient with a prior history of tobacco use, chronic obstructive pulmonary disease (COPD), and lung cancer.

Single photon emission computed tomography (SPECT) imaging provides a three-dimensional map of functioning alveolar-capillary units. This information may be useful during the treatment planning process. For example, when selecting beam orientations for a patient with an intrathoracic tumor, one can orient the beam such that it preferentially passes through hypoperfused regions of the lung (43). Similarly, the quantitative functional information from SPECT can be used to define dose/volume constraints for intensity-modulated radiation therapy (IMRT) planning (45) (Fig. 27.8). These data are probably most helpful in patients with compromised pulmonary function. This approach assumes that hypoperfused regions of the lung are permanently nonfunctioning. If hypoperfusion is caused by tumor, then it may be temporary and may *improve*

with tumor shrinkage. Posttreatment reperfusion of previously hypoperfused areas has been reported (43,69). In general, this reperfusion is only seen in the regions of lung that are *adjacent* to a central tumor mass. Presumably, the tumor is compressing regional blood vessels, leading to reductions in regional perfusion. Similar reperfusion has *not* been observed in regions of hypoperfusion that are "apart" from the tumor mass. These latter areas are likely permanently hypoperfused, perhaps due to COPD. Thus, when we use pre-RT perfusion maps to plan RT beams, we consider the hypoperfused regions "adjacent" and "apart" from the tumor separately.

Similarly, functional imaging of the kidney is currently used to assist in radiotherapy treatment design. For many patients with intra-abdominal tumors, incidental irradiation of the kidney is common. It is usually necessary to assess the degree of function of each kidney to ensure that adequate renal reserve will exist after radiotherapy. Conventional renal scans provide this type of quantitative information. Similar functional

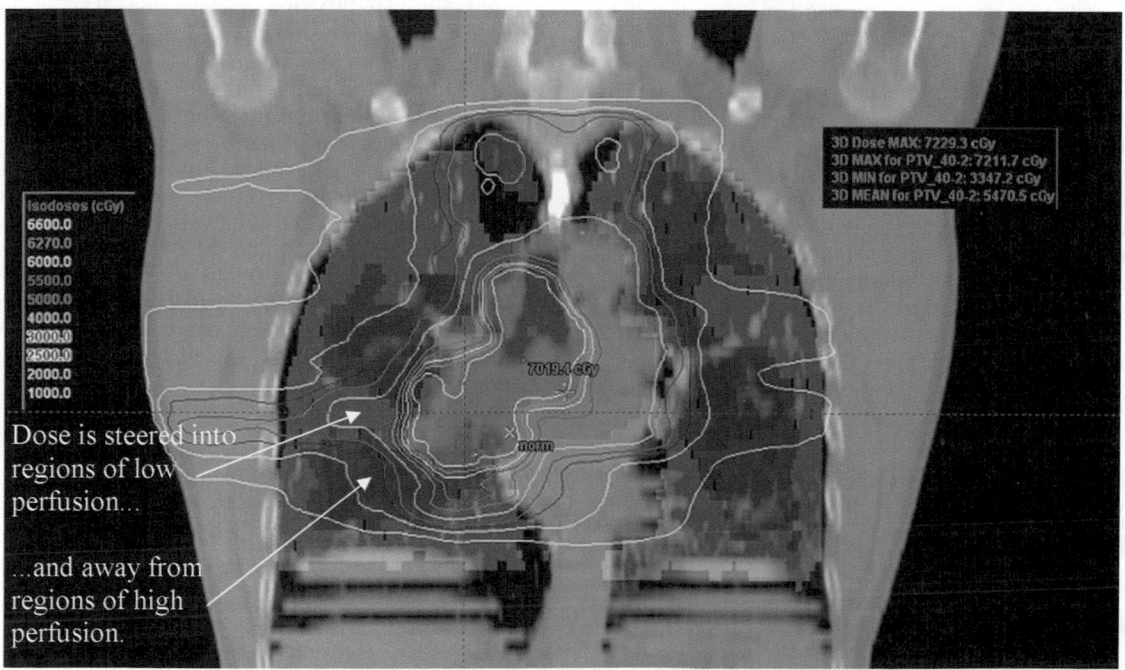

FIGURE 27.8. Intensity-modulated radiation therapy plan for lung cancer where the functional information from single photon emission computed tomography (SPECT) was used during the beam intensity optimization process (McGuire S, Zhou S, Marks L, et al. Using SPECT-guidance to reduce intensity modulated radiation therapy [IMRT] dose to functioning lung. In: 48th Annual Meeting of the American Association of Physicists in Medicine; 2006; Abstract). The segmented SPECT lung regions, in order of most to least functional, are red, orange, yellow, and green. Image courtesy of Dr. Shiva Das.

information may be provided by bone scan, PET, contrasted CT, and intravenous pyelogram.

Oncologic Anatomy

The term *onco-anatomy* describes the fusion of clinical oncology and anatomy. The successful practice of radiation oncology requires a comprehensive understanding of anatomy. A cornerstone of radiation therapy is the delivery of therapeutic doses of radiation to the target, while minimizing incidental irradiation of surrounding normal tissues. Advances in diagnostic imaging have increased our ability to visualize macroscopic disease, referred to as gross tumor volume (GTV). Imaging is currently unable to identify microscopic tumor extension around a primary tumor or occult nodal involvement. A clinical target volume (CTV) is created to account for both of these uncertainties. A rationale definition of the CTV should reflect the clinician's knowledge regarding the patterns of spread for each particular cancer. This involves both local spread around the primary site and patterns of lymphatic drainage. Appropriate expansion of a GTV to a CTV minimizes the risk of local failure (i.e., marginal miss), while reducing the risk of complications by avoiding structures at low risk of involvement (Table 27.5).

Radiation treatment planning has undergone considerable evolution during the past 20 years. With conventional planning, the physician conceives of a beam orientation and aperture shape based on the interpretation of available clinical and diagnostic information, including three-dimensional (3D) imaging data such as CT or MRI. The beam is then applied to the patient using a fluoroscopy-based conventional simulator. With conventional simulation, physicians rely on their knowledge of tumor and normal tissue anatomy, and its association with fluoroscopic bony anatomy and surface anatomy, to design treatment beams. Beam orientations are essentially limited to those where the physician can visualize and understand the underlying anatomical associations, either clinically or via fluoroscopy. Beam apertures are used that include a relatively generous margin to account for the inherent uncertainties of the process.

With 3D treatment planning, 3D anatomic information, typically from CT images, is transferred to a computer. The images are segmented to define the tumor and normal tissues. Software allows this 3D information to be displayed and viewed from any orientation. Beam orientation and shape are chosen to encompass the target, yet minimize, as much as possible, normal tissue exposure. Thus, 3D planning tools allow the 3D anatomy to be more accurately incorporated into the planning process than with conventional techniques. The computer allows the planner to use beam orientations that are nonstandard (e.g., nonaxial beams). Beam apertures are typically smaller than with conventional simulation due to reduced uncertainty in the entire process. Current technology also allows data from other imaging modalities (MRI, PET, and so forth) to be fused with the planning CT data set and hence considered in the planning process. It is advantageous to position the patient similarly during the imaging and treatment planning scans to facilitate accurate image correlation.

With 3D treatment planning, the entire target is encompassed within each of the treatment beams. Further, each RT beam typically delivers a relatively homogeneous dose to each part of the target. Thus, a significant RT dose is typically received by all tissues in the shadow of the target as seen in the beam's eye view. Thus, selection of the beam orientation is critical with 3D planning. Compensators, such as wedges, can be added to the beam to modify the intensity profile of the beam. However, such compensators are relatively simple and provide only uniform and monotonic modulation of the beam's intensity (e.g., the entire anterior part of a lateral photon beam is given less intensity than the posterior aspect of the field).

With IMRT, each portion of the beam, or beamlet, is modulated to provide a unique intensity. Thus, each beam can deliver highly variable doses to each region of the tumor. The purposefully nonuniform doses from several beam orientations are combined to deliver the desired dose in 3D space. Normal tissues in the shadow of the target seen in the beam's eye view do not necessarily receive a significant dose of RT, and thus the selection of beam orientation is less critical with IMRT than with 3D planning. It is typically not practical for a planner to "forwardly design" the necessary nonuniform intensity profiles that will yield the desired dose distribution. Rather, the physician defines the desired 3D dose distribution, and software is used to compute a set of beam intensity profiles. Since this process of defining the desired doses and then the beam intensities is the reverse order from conventional planning, this process has been termed *inverse planning*. In many instances, IMRT is replacing conventional RT techniques due to its capability to generate more customized dose distributions. IMRT requires the clinician to explicitly delineate target volumes, including elective nodal basins, as well as avoidance structures. This is not necessary when conventional shrinking lateral fields are used, for example, in head and neck cancer. Arguably, conventional simulation techniques require less 3D anatomic expertise. The introduction of IMRT has revolutionized radiation treatment planning, and in the process, has required clinicians to become more proficient in 3D anatomy. Several groups have published guidelines demarcating elective nodal stations on axial CT images, especially for head and neck cancer (24,87) and lung cancer (15). These stations are somewhat artificial but facilitate rationale demarcation of nodal stations at risk, reporting of patterns of spread and failure, and communication with surgical colleagues.

One of the risks of 3D and IMRT is a false sense of security in the accuracy of imaging to portray the *in vivo* extent of disease. Modern imaging tools are not perfect. A sound understanding of malignant patterns of spread is still needed in the treatment planning process. This is illustrated in the following examples.

Table 27.5 | **VOLUME DEFINITIONS FOR RADIATION THERAPY PLANNING**

Structure	Defined	Method of Assessment
Gross tumor volume	Palpable or visible disease	Physical examination, radiographs
Clinical target volume	GTV + expansion for microscopic spread	Knowledge of patterns of spread (onco-anatomy)
Planning target volume	CTV + expansion for margin—set up error and organ motion	Imaging studies (fluoroscopy or 4D CT to define degree of motion) and reproducibility/stability of mobilization/localization systems

4D, four dimensional; CT, computed tomography; CTV, clinical target volume; GTV, gross tumor volume

Anatomical Illustrations

The Nasopharynx and the Cranial Nerves

Most malignancies of the nasopharynx are carcinomas, though lymphomas, angiofibromas, and plasmacytomas are sometimes encountered. Specific symptoms and signs result from local invasion and regional dissemination (see Chapter 38). The cranial nerves should be considered when evaluating a patient with NPC.

One-fifth of patients with NPC present with symptoms of cranial nerve involvement (Table 27.6). The most commonly involved cranial nerves are the abducent nerve (CN VI) and the trigeminal nerve (CN V). CN VI originates in the ventral aspect of the brainstem, ascends on the clivus, and crosses the internal carotid artery near the superior aspect of foramen lacerum before entering the cavernous sinus. It then exits the skull through the superior orbital fissure. The motor and sensory nerve roots of CN V exit the pons, pass underneath the free edge of the tentorium cerebelli into Meckel's cave, forming the trigeminal (Gasserian) ganglion. From the ganglion, V_1 and V_2 enter the cavernous sinus and subsequently exit the skull through the superior orbital fissure and foramen rotundum, respectively. V_3 exits the skull through foramen ovale.

The nasopharynx is in close proximity to foramen lacerum, rotundum, and ovale, explaining the frequent tumor involvement of CN V and VI. Invasion of foramen lacerum and involvement of the trigeminal ganglion could lead to dysfunction in all three branches of CN V. In fact, most patients with NPC and CN V involvement have isolated deficits of V_2 or V_3. This occurs due to extension into foramen rotundum and ovale, respectively (see Fig. 27.4). After gaining access to the middle cranial fossa, NPC may extend superiorly into the cavernous sinus. Four cranial nerves, including two branches of CN V, pass through the cavernous sinus. Within the sinus, the oculomotor nerve (CN III) is located most superiorly, while the maxillary nerve (CN V_2) is located most inferiorly. One would suspect that cranial nerves located more superiorly in the cavernous sinus would be involved less frequently than those located closer to the base of skull. This is consistent with what is observed clinically (see Table 27.6).

Lower cranial nerve involvement can occur without intracranial extension. The fossa of Rosenmüller is the most common site of origin of NPC. The lateral border of the fossa of Rosenmüller is the pharyngeal space. Direct tumor extension laterally into the parapharyngeal space or lymphatic metastases to high parapharyngeal lymph nodes can affect the cranial nerves exiting the jugular foramen (CN IX, X, and XI), and hypoglossal canal (CN XII). This may result in loss of the gag reflex (CN IX), hoarseness or dysphagia (CN X), atrophy/paralysis of trapezius and sternocleidomastoid (CN XI), as well as tongue deviation (CN XII).

Based on the patterns of spread of NPC, a careful inquiry into possible cranial nerve involvement through history, physical examination, and review of imaging is imperative. When using opposed lateral fields, the entire skull base is usually considered part of the initial CTV to allow coverage of potential routes of intracranial spread. Three-dimensional, and in

| Table 27.6 | MAJOR FORAMINA AND OTHER APERTURES IN THE CRANIAL FOSSAE AND THEIR PRIMARY CONTENTS |

Foramina/Opening	Contents	Frequency of Involvement by NPC[a] (%)
Anterior Cranial Fossa		
Foramina in cribriform plate	Axons of olfactory cells (CN I)	0
Middle Cranial Fossa		
Optic canal	Optic nerve (CN II)	6
	Ophthalmic artery	
Superior orbital fissure	Oculomotor nerve (CN III)	9
	Trochlear nerve (CN IV)	17
	Abducent nerve (CN VI)	44
	Ophthalmic nerve (CN V_1)	45
Foramen rotundum	Maxillary nerve (CN V_2)	67
Foramen ovale	Mandibular nerve (CN V_3)	48
Foramen spinosum	Meningeal branch of CN V_3	14
	Middle meningeal artery/vein	
Foramen lacerum	Internal carotid artery[b]	
Petrous Portion of the Temporal Bone		
Internal acoustic meatus	Facial nerve (CN VII)[c]	9
	Vestibulocochlear nerve (CN VIII)	0
	Labyrinthine artery	
Posterior Cranial Fossa		
Jugular foramen	Glossopharyngeal nerve (CN IX)	20
	Vagus nerve (CN X)	20
	Spinal accessory nerve (CN XI)	14
	Internal jugular vein (superior bulb)	
Foramen magnum	Spinal roots of spinal accessory nerve (CN XI)	14
	Medulla	
	Vertebral artery	
	Anterior/posterior spinal artery	
Hypoglossal canal	Hypoglossal nerve (CN XII)	24

NPC, nasopharyngeal carcinoma
[a]From Leung SF, Tsao SY, Teo P, et al. Cranial nerve involvement by nasopharyngeal carcinoma: Response to treatment and clinical significance. *Clin Oncol (R Coll Radiol)* 1990;2:138–141.
[b]After entering the skull through the carotid canal.
[c]The facial nerve exits the skull through the stylomastoid foramen.

Techniques, Modalities, and Modifiers in Radiation Oncology

particular IMRT techniques, require explicit delineation of the CTV. It may be not sufficient to identify the GTV on diagnostic imaging and then uniformly expand this to define the CTV. Rather, the GTV should be explicitly enlarged to appropriately cover specific microscopic areas at risk. An understanding of the anatomy of the base of skull, together with the clinical presentation, facilitates rational and individualized CTV definition for patients with NPC.

With 3D and IMRT, the concepts of GTV, CTV, and PTV (planning target volume) have become more widely used. Uniform expansion of the GTV to define the CTV does *not* consider the biologic/anatomic characteristics of tumors, as noted above for NPC. An analogous discussion applies to acoustic neuromas and meningiomas. These tumors tend to track along the course of the eighth cranial nerve and meninges, respectively, rather than into the surrounding brain. The use of a uniform margin to define CTVs in these settings may also be illogical.

Malignant Pleural Mesothelioma and the Pleural Recesses

Malignant pleural mesothelioma is an aggressive malignancy, arising from the pleural lining of the lung. The visceral pleura is adherent to all of the surfaces of the lung, while the parietal pleura is adherent to the thoracic wall, diaphragm, and pericardium. The pleural recesses are potential spaces where portions of opposed parietal pleura are in contact during quiet respiration (Fig. 27.9). The inferior extension of the costodiaphragmatic recess can be easily underestimated, as can the medial extent of the costomediastinal recess (Fig. 27.10). The inferior aspect of the costodiaphragmatic recess often extends to the level of the mid-kidney. The posteromedial extent of the pleura often wraps anteriorly over the descending aorta.

Treatment of mesothelioma has challenged radiation oncologists for decades. Local disease progression is the primary obstacle to cure. Tumor can spread anywhere within the pleural space, including the fissures, diaphragmatic and pericardial surfaces, and the pleural recesses. In addition, lymphatics exist within the pleura draining to mediastinal, internal mammary, diaphragmatic, and intercostal lymph node regions. Historically, radiation therapy techniques were suboptimal to fully encompass sites at risk while respecting normal tissue tolerance. IMRT is particularly useful for targets with irregular shapes and concavities. Investigators at M.D. Anderson Cancer Center have

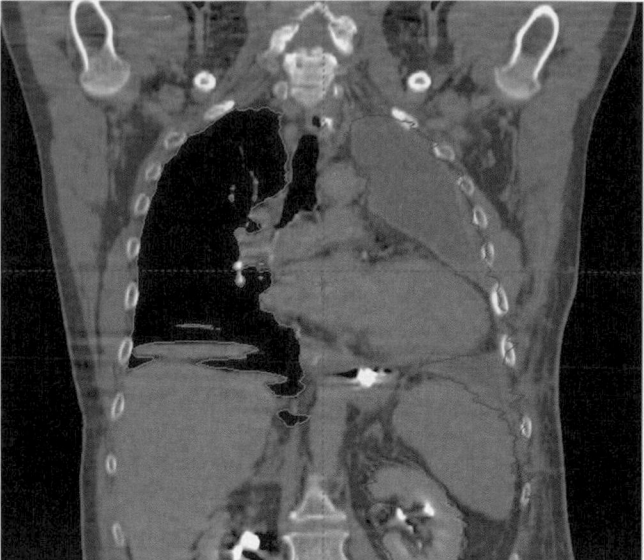

FIGURE 27.10. Digitally reconstructed coronal image from a treatment planning computed tomography scan illustrating the inferior extent of the costodiaphragmatic recess, which extends to the level of the mid-kidney. The patient had previously undergone an extrapleural pneumonectomy at which time metallic clips were placed, demarcating the inferior extent of the recess. The clinical target volume is illustrated in red.

systematically defined the tissues at risk for these patients and exploited IMRT techniques to more effectively irradiate the entire clinical target volume while minimizing dose to surrounding structures (1). Following extrapleural pneumonectomy, postoperative radiation therapy using IMRT was administered to large, irregularly shaped clinical target volumes. Demarcation of the boundaries of the pleural space by the thoracic surgeon using metallic clips facilitated radiation treatment planning. Of 62 patients treated, there was one in-field recurrence and three marginal recurrences, after a median follow-up of 13 months (74).

Breast Cancer and the Internal Mammary Nodes

Elective treatment of internal mammary nodes (IMNs) is controversial. Proponents of such argue that the surgical literature

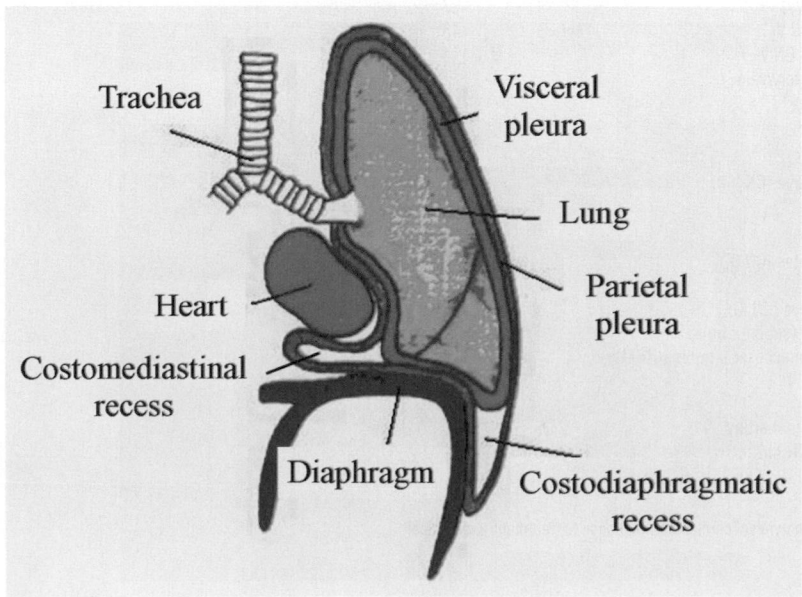

FIGURE 27.9. The extent of the pleura is illustrated. Note the inferior extension of the costodiaphragmatic recess and the medial extension of the costomediastinal recesses. (Image courtesy of the University of Bristol, Department of Anatomy.)

clearly demonstrates that the risk of occult disease in IMNs, in the setting of positive axillary lymph nodes, is high enough to warrant elective treatment (40,49,50,82). In addition, recent landmark trials showing a benefit for postmastectomy RT included elective treatment of the IMNs (55,56,62). Opponents contend that clinical IMN failures are uncommon and the value of elective RT to the IMNs has never been demonstrated in controlled trials. Furthermore, elective treatment of the IMNs increases dose to the lungs and heart. Randomized trials are under way to assess the role of elective nodal irradiation. An active National Cancer Institute of Canada study randomizes node-positive patients to adjuvant radiotherapy to the breast with or without treatment of supraclavicular and IMN lymph nodes. A similar study was conducted by the European Organization of Radiation Treatment Centers, but it also included node-negative patients with medial/central tumors. This trial is closed but results have not yet been reported.

Until results of these trials are available, and likely even thereafter, anatomic principles can be applied to reach a reasonable compromise in this debate. First, the probability of internal mammary node involvement depends on the number of involved axillary lymph nodes as well as the location of the primary tumor (Table 27.7). When the axilla is negative, the risk of IMN involvement, as assessed by surgical series utilizing extended radical mastectomy, is 5% to 15% (40,50,82), somewhat less with outer quadrant tumors as compared to medial/central tumors. The risk rises when axillary lymph nodes are involved (23% to 55%), especially with medial/central tumors. In addition, the risk of IMN involvement rises with increasing axillary disease burden. Second, the probability of IMN involvement depends on the intercostal level. Noguchi et al. (50) reported that when IMNs were pathologically involved, the first, second, third, and fourth intercostal levels contained disease in 80%, 75%, 40%, and 5% of patients, respectively. The observation that the superior three intercostal spaces are most likely to contain nodal disease has been confirmed by others (40,82). Furthermore, Urban and Marjani (82) reported that involved lymph nodes were found equally often medial or lateral to the vessels.

Therefore, treatment of the IMN regions does not need to be "all or nothing." One can selectively irradiated the superior IMNs without the inferior levels in patients at high risk of IMN involvement, primarily those with involved axillary lymph nodes. This dramatically improves the dose distribution to the heart for patients with left-sided tumors, since the heart is situated in the inferior aspect of the chest. At Duke, we have been using partly wide tangential fields to selectively irradiate the superior IMNs for many years (42).

Non–Small Cell Lung Cancer and Postoperative Radiation Therapy

Local or regional recurrence of NSCLC after surgical resection occurs in ~20% of patients with stage I disease (26,81) and in up to 50% of patients with stage III disease (8,57,66,73). Postoperative RT (PORT) has been shown in multiple randomized trials to improve local and regional control, even for pathologic stage I disease (41,44,73,83). However, the enthusiasm for PORT waned after the 1998 meta-analysis demonstrated a 7% absolute *increase* in mortality associated with PORT (59). The incongruity between an improvement in local control and detriment in survival may have been secondary to RT-induced cardiopulmonary complications. The studies in the PORT meta-analysis used relatively large RT fields with coverage of the bronchial stump, ipsilateral hilum, entire mediastinum, and sometimes the supraclavicular fossae. These fields are fairly standard in modern practice and essentially encompass *all* sites of possible involvement within the thorax. This strategy, based on the findings of the PORT meta-analysis, appears to be suboptimal. It is logical to believe that smaller RT fields, encompassing only those sites *most likely* to contain microscopic disease, would be associated with less toxicity. Theoretically, this might improve the therapeutic ratio. Both anatomical (27,64) and clinical (4,27,30,51,85) inquiries have investigated routes of spread of bronchogenic cancers as well as patterns of failure. Generalizations from these studies can help clinicians design tailored radiation fields.

First, both anatomical and clinical studies have shown that bronchogenic tumors frequently spread directly into mediastinal lymph nodes, bypassing intrapulmonary and hilar lymph nodes. This phenomenon appears to occur more frequently for upper lobe tumors (64). For right-sided tumors, these pathways most frequently lead to ipsilateral paratracheal and subcarinal lymph node stations. For left-sided tumors, direct spread to anterior mediastinal lymph node stations (prevascular, paraaortic, and aortopulmonary [AP] window) is more common than to other mediastinal nodal stations. Second, right lung segments drain predominantly into the ipsilateral mediastinum. Conversely, left lung tumors commonly spread to both sides of the mediastinum (27,51). Third, direct passageways to the supraclavicular fossa exist but are rare. Clinically, supraclavicular

	RISK OF INTERNAL MAMMARY LYMPH NODE INVOLVEMENT BASED ON STATUS OF AXILLA AND LOCATION WITHIN THE BREAST		
Table 27.7			
Scenario	Livingston and Arlen[a] (%)	Urban and Marjani[b] (%)	Noguchi et al.[c] (%)
Negative Axilla	8	8	5
Outer quadrant primary	5	10	ns
Medial/central primary	14	16	ns
Positive Axilla	33	52	35
Outer quadrant primary	23	43	ns
Medial/central primary	48	55	ns
1–3 + axillary nodes	ns	ns	20
≥4 + axillary nodes	ns	ns	52

ns, not stated
[a]Livingston SF, Arlen M. The extended extrapleural radical mastectomy: Its role in the treatment of carcinoma of the breast. *Ann Surg* 1974;179:260–265.
[b]Urban JA, Marjani MA. Significance of internal mammary lymph node metastases in breast cancer. *Am J Roentgenol Radium Ther Nucl Med* 1971;111:130–136.
[c]Noguchi M, Ohta N, Koyasaki N, et al. Reappraisal of internal mammary node metastases as a prognostic factor in patients with breast cancer. *Cancer* 1991;68:1918–1925.

Techniques, Modalities, and Modifiers in Radiation Oncology

failures are uncommon and are usually associated with failure in upper paratracheal lymph node stations (34). Fourth, most clinical studies have shown that subcarinal lymph nodes are frequently involved by both upper and lower lobe tumors. Finally, we showed that the bronchial stump/wedge resection line is the most common site of failure and occurs more frequently after less radical surgery (e.g., wedge resection vs. lobectomy or pneumonectomy) (34). This is consistent with the randomized trial of lobectomy versus wedge resection for stage I NSCLC (20), which demonstrated local failure rates of 17% and 6% following wedge resection and lobectomy, respectively.

The risk of local or regional recurrence after resection of NSCLC is not trivial, even for stage I disease. Systemic therapy for NSCLC is improving. With improved systemic control, attention will be redirected to sites of intrathoracic recurrence. There is emerging evidence that PORT, using modern treatment planning and delivery, may be beneficial. In a recent study from Italy, not included in the 1998 meta-analysis, the utility of PORT directed to small volumes was assessed (81). Patients with *pathologic stage I disease* were randomized to receive or not to receive PORT (50.4 Gy) to the bronchial stump and ipsilateral hilum using 3D treatment planning (the lower ipsilateral mediastinum was incidentally treated). In this modest-size study of 104 patients, there was a statistically significant improvement in local control (98% vs. 77%; $p < 0.01$) *and* overall survival at 5 years (67% vs. 58%; $p = 0.048$). The small fields used in this study encompassed the sites most at risk for harboring residual disease based on the anatomical and clinical studies cited (Fig. 27.11), and equally important, seemed to be associated with far less toxicity than is typically ascribed to PORT.

The White Matter Tracts, the Brainstem, and Diffuse Pontine Gliomas

Brainstem gliomas comprise ~10% of intracranial tumors in children. They can arise anywhere within the brainstem, and are described as focal or diffuse, depending on their appearance on MRI. Most brainstem gliomas diffusely infiltrate the pons and are associated with a poor long-term survival. The most common presenting symptoms are ataxia, motor weakness, and cranial nerve deficits. The cranial nerves most frequently involved are those arising in the pons (CN V to VIII), especially the abducent nerve (CN VI) and facial nerve (CN VII). Cranial nerves arising with the medulla (CN IX to XII) and midbrain (CN III to IV) are less frequently affected.

The pyramidal tracts consist of neurons controlling voluntary motor movement for lower motor neurons in the brainstem and spinal cord. Its two major divisions are the corticospinal tracts (spinal nerves) and corticobulbar tracts (cranial nerves). The pyramidal tracts course from the cerebral cortex, through the posterior limb (corticospinal) or genu (corticobulbar) of the internal capsule, and subsequently enter the ventral aspect of the brainstem. The corticospinal tracts cross at the pyramids in the lower medulla. The spinal nerves receive innervation from contralateral neurons within the corticospinal tract above the pyramids. On the contrary, most cranial nerves receive innervation from both sides of the corticobulbar tracts. The two notable exceptions being the hypoglossal nerve (CN XII) and inferior branches of the facial nerve (CN VII). Detailed knowledge of these neuronal pathways helps correlate patient's symptoms and physical examination findings to what is observed radiographically.

The classic presenting symptoms of diffuse pontine gliomas can be explained by the anatomy of the pons. A unilateral lesion in the ventral pons with involvement of the pyramidal tracts (upper motor neurons) might cause contralateral motor weakness in the arms or legs. In addition, cranial nerves within the pons might also be affected (e.g., CN VI), unilaterally, without com-

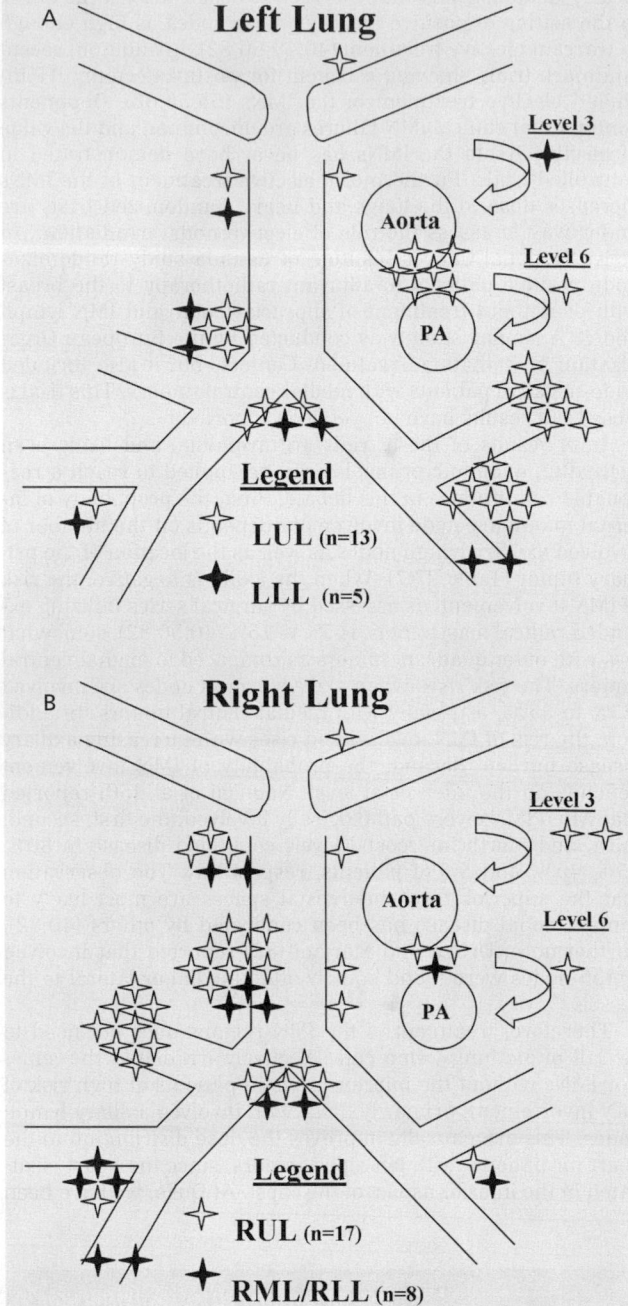

FIGURE 27.11. Diagrams illustrating sites of local/regional recurrence of non–small cell lung cancer after resection of stage I disease. **A:** Patterns of failure for left lung tumors. **B:** The same for right lung tumors. LUL, left upper lobe; LLL, left lower lobe; RLL, right lower lobe; RML, right middle lobe; RUL, right upper lobe; PA, pulmonary artery. (Adapted from Kelsey C, Light K, Marks L. Patterns of failure after resection of non-small cell lung cancer: Implications for postoperative RT volumes. *Int J Radiat Oncol Biol Phys* 2006;65:1097–1105.)

plete paralysis because of bilateral innervation of the cranial nerves by fibers in the corticobulbar tracts. Ataxia, denoting impairment of coordination without weakness, can be caused by involvement of fibers projecting from the pons to the cerebellum within the middle cerebellar peduncle. Through this pathway, the cerebellum receives a copy of the information for muscle movement that the corticospinal tracts relay to lower motor neurons, facilitating the complicated act of coordination.

Gliomas, including pontine gliomas, preferentially spread along nerve tracts. Thus, patients with pontine gliomas are at risk for harboring disease in the neighboring medulla and midbrain. Deficits in cranial nerves arising within the medulla and mid-brain suggest local extension of disease, and the radiation fields should be enlarged accordingly. For gliomas in general, the expansion of the GTV to define the CTV should not necessarily be uniform, in recognition of their propensity to spread along nerves and not, for example, into the surrounding skull. Currently, most malignant gliomas recur in the high-dose region and not, for example, near the beam edge (marginal miss). Nevertheless, an understanding of patterns of spread together with central nervous system anatomy facilitates the design of rationale target volumes that will maximize the chance of tumor control while minimizing treatment-related toxicity.

Cervical Cancer and the Uterosacral Ligaments

Four major paired ligaments anchor the uterus/cervix in place within the pelvis. The broad ligament extends laterally from the uterus to the pelvic sidewall. The round ligaments (ligamentum teres uteri) extend anterolaterally from the uterus toward the pelvic sidewall. They then pass through the inguinal canal and blend with the connective tissue of the labia majora. The transverse cervical ligaments (cardinal ligaments) secure the cervix to the pelvic sidewall. Finally, the sacrouterine ligaments attach the cervix to the sacrum, inserting primarily into S1 to S3 (10).

Cervical cancer most commonly spreads via direct extension into paracervical tissues and through the lymphatic system. The uterosacral ligaments are situated in the posterior parametrium and contain lymphatic channels and lymph nodes (6,7). Thus, involvement of this ligament can arise by both direct extension (36) or through lymphatic metastases (6). Surgical series have shown, at least for early stage cervical cancer, that posterior extension with involvement of presacral lymph nodes and the uterosacral ligament is less common than anterior and lateral routes of spread (7,21). However, involvement of parametrial lymph nodes in general increases with increasing stage (21). Thus, for advanced cervical cancer managed with radiation therapy and chemotherapy, posterior involvement to presacral nodes and the uterosacral ligament needs to be considered. One should be cautious when shielding the rectum on the lateral portals, as this will also shield potential sites of disease. Although special attention is often paid to the lateral parametrium, posterior spread along the uterosacral ligament can be easily overlooked.

Hodgkin's Disease and the Spleen

Most patients with early stage HD are treated with combination chemotherapy followed by involved-field radiation therapy. In current practice, few patients are treated with radiation therapy alone. However, many of the principles learned in the era when radiation therapy was the customary therapy for early stage HD can guide the clinician managing contemporary patients, as well as patients with chemotherapy-refractory disease undergoing salvage radiation therapy. An example of this is the spleen.

Clinical staging of the spleen has always been fraught with difficulty. Hence, staging laparotomy typically included splenectomy with careful examination of histologic sections to establish splenic involvement. Although preliminary reports suggest that PET is superior to conventional imaging studies (63), few data exist comparing PET results with pathologic findings at laparotomy. However, data from Stanford collected when staging laparotomy was routine show that the incidence of splenic involvement is very high when para-aortic lymph nodes are involved (~86%). Conversely, only ~5% of patients without pathologic evidence of splenic involvement have involved para-aortic lymph nodes (32). Thus, when involved-field radiation therapy is undertaken for involved para-aortic lymph nodes, one should strongly consider inclusion of the spleen, irrespective of its radiographic appearance prior to treatment. This does, of course, increase the volume of left kidney in the treatment field as the spleen is located immediately superior and anterior to the left kidney.

Elective Nodal Irradiation and Modern Treatment Planning

The enthusiasm for elective nodal irradiation (ENI) has waxed and waned over the years. Its value is currently being questioned for multiple malignancies, including NSCLC. Photon beams (and proton beams, perhaps to a lesser degree) unavoidably result in normal tissue irradiation. With the sophisticated treatment planning tools that are now available, such as 3D and IMRT, the clinician has increased discretion on where to "deposit" incidental irradiation. These tools allow us to essentially redistribute the incidental photons, but not eliminate them (70). It seems prudent to deliver, to the degree possible, the incidental photons to regions of likely microscopic tumor spread.

Treatment of NSCLC provides a good case study for this. As noted previously, surgical series have also shown that NSCLC spreads in a fairly predictable pattern. This anatomic knowledge can be used to more rationally define targets and beam orientations. For example, incidental radiation to nontarget tissues can be minimized by orienting the radiation beam such that it is as parallel as possible to the long access of the target (61). In this manner, the cross-section of the target, as seen in the beams eye view, will be reduced. Lower lobe lung cancers present a good opportunity to exploit this treatment planning and anatomic principle. For example, a right lower lobe tumor with hilar lymphadenopathy can be included within an AP field as shown in Figure 27.12A. Alternatively, one can orient that radiation beam such that it enters from the anterior-left-superior direction and exits in the posterior-right-inferior orientation, as show in Figure 27.12B. In this manner, the beam is oriented along the long axis of the target. Further, there is added benefit of including the lymph nodes located in the ipsilateral lower mediastinum. Again, knowledge of the likely patterns of spread and a more rational definition of clinical target volumes can alter, and hopefully improve, beam selection. Further, nonaxial beams may be less sensitive to respiratory motion than AP/PA (posteroanterior) beams. Appropriate use of ENI requires detailed anatomic knowledge of the nodal patterns of spread for each tumor site.

These concepts are addressed specifically for several tumor sites elsewhere. For example, tumors of the lower vagina, vulva, and distal anal canal often drain into inguinal nodes. On the other hand, tumors of the upper vagina and rectum more commonly drain into pelvic nodes. The left testicle drains into the region of the left renal hilum, while the right testicle drains into aortocaval lymph nodes adjacent to the inferior vena cava; both nodal drainage patterns follow their venous pathways. Therefore, RT fields for seminoma of the left testicle should cover the ipsilateral renal hilum, while this may be unnecessary for a right-sided testicular tumors. Further, patterns of metastatic/hematologic spread can be better understood in the context of normal anatomy. Batson (5) described an often-forgotten system of veins that provide a route of spread from the prostate to the lumbar spine; the breast to the scapula, clavicle, and cervical spine; and the lung to the brain. These anatomic connections may explain the metastatic patterns observed clinically.

Summary

The Educational Role of the Oncologist

The term *onco-anatomy* describes the fusion of clinical oncology and anatomy, for the betterment of both. The successful

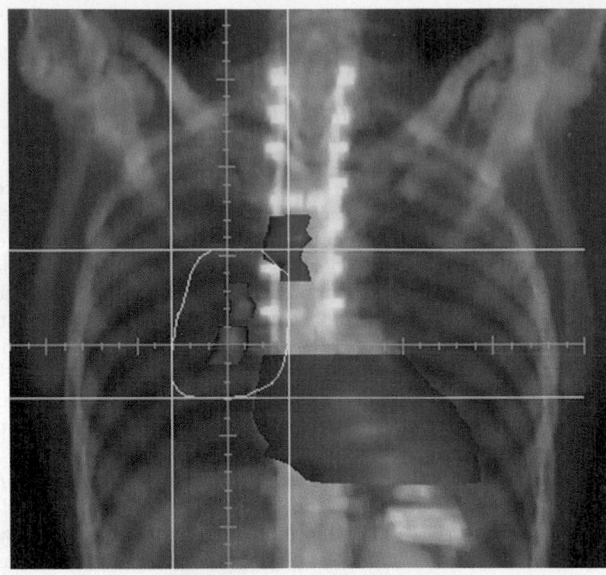
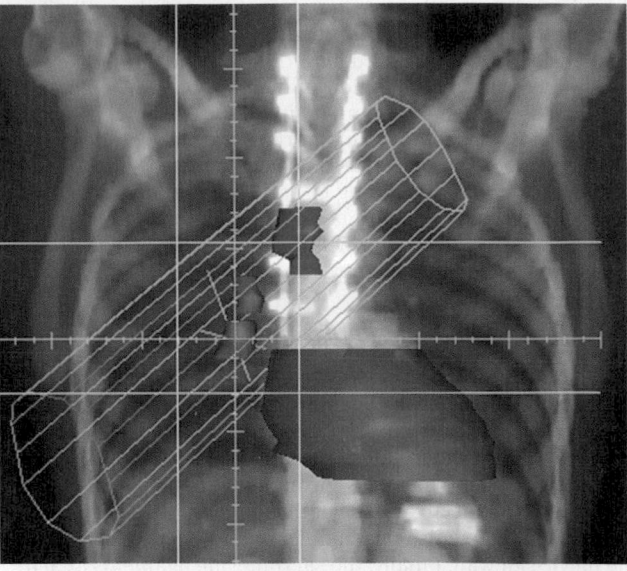

FIGURE 27.12. A: A right middle lobe tumor with hilar adenopathy (pink) can be treated with an anteroposterior field. **B:** A nonaxial beam orientation (left anterior superior oblique) can be utilized, which incidentally includes the lower ipsilateral paratracheal lymph node station (blue). The heart is shown in red.

practice of radiation oncology requires a thorough understanding of anatomy. Likewise, the study of malignancy and observations regarding spread of malignant tumors aids in the understanding and instruction of anatomy. Radiation oncologists have a unique opportunity to assist in the instruction of anatomy. For most medical students, gross anatomy is an early first-year course before significant clinical experience is obtained. Over the ensuing years of medical school and residency, much of this knowledge is lost as it is not routinely applied during clinical practice. It is incumbent on those who seek advanced training in fields such as surgery, radiology, and radiation oncology to again become students of anatomy, as the successful practice of such disciplines requires an in-depth understanding of anatomical principles. Practitioners in these fields have the opportunity to assist in the education of medical and other allied-health stu-

dents. For several decades at the University of Rochester, Dr. Philip Rubin and John Hansen and colleagues taught an elective course on onco-anatomy. The patterns of spread of malignant tumors were used to reinforce anatomic principles (25a).

At Duke University Medical Center, a course has been designed termed Onco-Anatomy. This consists of a monthly conference where the anatomy of a particular disease site is reviewed, along with pertinent clinical implications. Following this didactic session, the presentation continues in the gross anatomy suite where members from the Department of Biological Anthropology and Anatomy demonstrate the anatomy on prosections (Fig. 27.13). This course is attended by medical students, residents, and faculty members from multiple disciplines. The expertise of all involved contributes to a valuable educational environment.

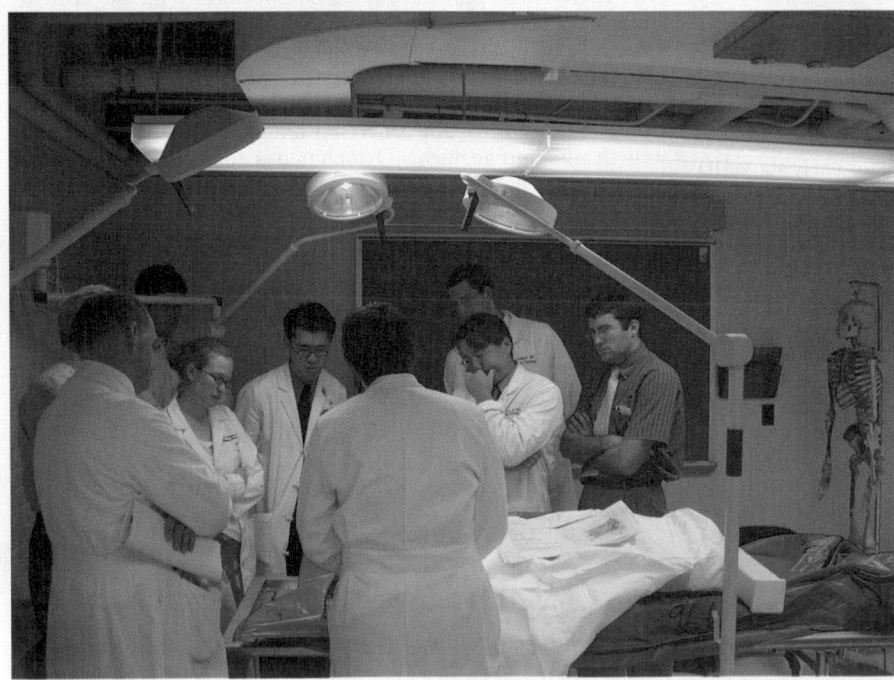

FIGURE 27.13. Residents and students gather around a cadaver with an anatomist during the Onco-Anatomy class at Duke. (Image courtesy of Dr. Alexander van Nievelt.)

Acknowledgment

Special thanks to Drs. Srinivasan Mukundan, Frank Gress, Mary Scott Soo, Leonard Prosnitz, David Brizel, Thomas Raidy, Edward Coleman, Ann Zumwalt, and Bridget Koontz for their expertise and assistance in preparing the manuscript. Thanks to Dr. Philip Ruben and Edward Halperin for their encouragement and guidance.

References

1. Ahamad A, Stevens CW, Smythe WR, et al. Intensity-modulated radiation therapy: A novel approach to the management of malignant pleural mesothelioma. *Int J Radiat Oncol Biol Phys* 2003;55:768–775.
2. Alexander FE, Anderson TJ, Brown HK, et al. 14 years of follow-up from the Edinburgh randomised trial of breast-cancer screening. *Lancet* 1999;353:1903–1908.
3. Andersson I, Janzon L. Reduced breast cancer mortality in women under age 50: Updated results from the Malmo Mammographic Screening Program. *J Natl Cancer Inst Monogr* 1997;22:63–67.
4. Asamura H, Nakayama H, Kondo H, et al. Lobe-specific extent of systematic lymph node dissection for non-small cell lung carcinomas according to a retrospective study of metastasis and prognosis. *J Thorac Cardiovasc Surg* 1999;117:1102–1111.
5. Batson O. The function of the vertebral veins and their role in the spread of metastases. *Ann Surg* 1940;112:138–141.
6. Benedetti-Panici P, Maneschi F, D'Andrea G, et al. Early cervical carcinoma: The natural history of lymph node involvement redefined on the basis of thorough parametrectomy and giant section study. *Cancer* 2000;88:2267–2274.
7. Benedetti-Panici P, Maneschi F, Scambia G, et al. Lymphatic spread of cervical cancer: An anatomical and pathological study based on 225 radical hysterectomies with systematic pelvic and aortic lymphadenectomy. *Gynecol Oncol* 1996;62:19–24.
8. Betticher DC, Hsu Schmitz SF, Totsch M, et al. Mediastinal lymph node clearance after docetaxel-cisplatin neoadjuvant chemotherapy is prognostic of survival in patients with stage IIIA pN2 non-small-cell lung cancer: A multicenter phase II trial. *J Clin Oncol* 2003;21:1752–1759.
9. Blake GM, Park-Holohan SJ, Cook GJ, et al. Quantitative studies of bone with the use of 18F-fluoride and 99mTc-methylene diphosphonate. *Semin Nucl Med* 2001;31:28–49.
10. Buller JL, Thompson JR, Cundiff GW, et al. Uterosacral ligament: Description of anatomic relationships to optimize surgical safety. *Obstet Gynecol* 2001;97:873–879.
11. Burger PC, Heinz ER, Shibata T, et al. Topographic anatomy and CT correlations in the untreated glioblastoma multiforme. *J Neurosurg* 1988;68:698–704.
12. Bury T, Barreto A, Daenen F, et al. Fluorine-18 deoxyglucose positron emission tomography for the detection of bone metastases in patients with non-small cell lung cancer. *Eur J Nucl Med* 1998;25:1244–1247.
13. Carney PA, Miglioretti DL, Yankaskas BC, et al. Individual and combined effects of age, breast density, and hormone replacement therapy use on the accuracy of screening mammography. *Ann Intern Med* 2003;138:168–175.
14. Chang JT, Lin CY, Chen TM, et al. Nasopharyngeal carcinoma with cranial nerve palsy: The importance of MRI for radiotherapy. *Int J Radiat Oncol Biol Phys* 2005;63:1354–1360.
15. Chapet O, Kong FM, Quint LE, et al. CT-based definition of thoracic lymph node stations: An atlas from the University of Michigan. *Int J Radiat Oncol Biol Phys* 2005;63:170–178.
16. Delattre JY, Krol G, Thaler HT, et al. Distribution of brain metastases. *Arch Neurol* 1988;45:741–744.
17. Dwamena BA, Sonnad SS, Angobaldo JO, et al. Metastases from non-small cell lung cancer: Mediastinal staging in the 1990s—meta-analytic comparison of PET and CT. *Radiology* 1999;213:530–536.
18. Elmore JG, Armstrong K, Lehman CD, et al. Screening for breast cancer. *JAMA* 2005;293:1245–1256.
19. Even-Sapir E. Imaging of malignant bone involvement by morphologic, scintigraphic, and hybrid modalities. *J Nucl Med* 2005;46:1356–1367.
20. Ginsberg RJ, Rubinstein LV. Randomized trial of lobectomy versus limited resection for T1 N0 non-small cell lung cancer. Lung Cancer Study Group. *Ann Thorac Surg* 1995;60:615–622; discussion 622–623.
21. Girardi F, Lichtenegger W, Tamussino K, et al. The importance of parametrial lymph nodes in the treatment of cervical cancer. *Gynecol Oncol* 1989;34:206–211.
22. Gleave ME, Coupland D, Drachenberg D, et al. Ability of serum prostate-specific antigen levels to predict normal bone scans in patients with newly diagnosed prostate cancer. *Urology* 1996;47:708–712.
23. Gould MK, Kuschner WG, Rydzak CE, et al. Test performance of positron emission tomography and computed tomography for mediastinal staging in patients with non-small-cell lung cancer: A meta-analysis. *Ann Intern Med* 2003;139:879–892.
24. Gregoire V, Levendag P, Ang KK, et al. CT-based delineation of lymph node levels and related CTVs in the node-negative neck: DAHANCA, EORTC, GORTEC, NCIC, RTOG consensus guidelines. *Radiother Oncol* 2003;69:227–236.
25. Hamaoka T, Madewell JE, Podoloff DA, et al. Bone imaging in metastatic breast cancer. *J Clin Oncol* 2004;22:2942–2953.
25a. Hansen JT, Rubin P. Clinical anatomy in the oncology patient: A preclinical elective that reinforces cross-sectional anatomy using examples of cancer spread. *Clin Anat* 1998;11:95–99.
26. Harpole DH Jr, Herndon JE 2nd, Young WG Jr, et al. Stage I non–small-cell lung cancer. A multivariate analysis of treatment methods and patterns of recurrence. *Cancer* 1995;76:787–796.
27. Hata E, Hayakawa K, Miyamoto H, et al. Rationale for extended lymphadenectomy for lung cancer. *Theor Surg* 1990;5:19–25.
28. Heelan RT, Demas BE, Caravelli JF, et al. Superior sulcus tumors: CT and MR imaging. *Radiology* 1989;170:637–641.
29. Ingram M, Arregui ME. Endoscopic ultrasonography. *Surg Clin North Am* 2004;84:10351059, vi.
30. Ishida T, Yano T, Maeda K, et al. Strategy for lymphadenectomy in lung cancer three centimeters or less in diameter. *Ann Thorac Surg* 1990;50:708–713.
31. Jerusalem G, Beguin Y, Fassotte MF, et al. Whole-body positron emission tomography using 18F-fluorodeoxyglucose for posttreatment evaluation in Hodgkin's disease and non-Hodgkin's lymphoma has higher diagnostic and prognostic value than classical computed tomography scan imaging. *Blood* 1999;94:429–433.
32. Kaplan H. Patterns of anatomic distribution. In: *Hodgkin's disease*, 2nd ed. Cambridge, MA: Harvard University Press, 1980; .
33. Kelly PJ, Daumas-Duport C, Kispert DB, et al. Imaging-based stereotaxic serial biopsies in untreated intracranial glial neoplasms. *J Neurosurg* 1987;66:865–874.
34. Kelsey C, Light K, Marks L. Patterns of failure after resection of non-small cell lung cancer: Implications for postoperative RT volumes. *Int J Radiat Oncol Biol Phys* 2006;65:1097–1105.
35. Kosuda S, Yoshimura I, Aizawa T, et al. Can initial prostate specific antigen determinations eliminate the need for bone scans in patients with newly diagnosed prostate carcinoma? A multicenter retrospective study in Japan. *Cancer* 2002;94:964–972.
36. Landoni F, Bocciolone L, Perego P, et al. Cancer of the cervix, FIGO stages IB and IIA: Patterns of local growth and paracervical extension. *Int J Gynecol Cancer* 1995;5:329–334.
37. Lee BC, Kneeland JB, Cahill PT, et al. MR recognition of supratentorial tumors. *AJNR Am J Neuroradiol* 1985;6:871–878.
38. Leung SF, Tsao SY, Teo P, et al. Cranial nerve involvement by nasopharyngeal carcinoma: Response to treatment and clinical significance. *Clin Oncol (R Coll Radiol)* 1990;2:138–141.
39. Lightdale CJ, Kulkarni KG. Role of endoscopic ultrasonography in the staging and follow-up of esophageal cancer. *J Clin Oncol* 2005;23:4483–4489.
40. Livingston SF, Arlen M. The extended extrapleural radical mastectomy: Its role in the treatment of carcinoma of the breast. *Ann Surg* 1974;179:260–265.
41. Lung Cancer Study Group. Effects of postoperative mediastinal radiation on completely resected stage II and stage III epidermoid cancer of the lung. *N Engl J Med* 1986;315:1377–1381.
42. Marks LB, Hebert ME, Bentel G, et al. To treat or not to treat the internal mammary nodes: A possible compromise. *Int J Radiat Oncol Biol Phys* 1994;29:903–909.
43. Marks LB, Spencer DP, Sherouse GW, et al. The role of three dimensional functional lung imaging in radiation treatment planning: The functional dose-volume histogram. *Int J Radiat Oncol Biol Phys* 1995;33:65–75.
44. Mayer R, Smolle-Juettner FM, Szolar D, et al. Postoperative radiotherapy in radically resected non-small cell lung cancer. *Chest* 1997;112:954–959.
45. McGuire S, Zhou S, Marks L, et al. A methodology for using SPECT to reduce intensity-modulated radiation therapy (IMRT) dose to functioning lung. *Int J Radiat Oncol Biol Phys* 2006;66:1543–1552.
46. Mikhaeel NG, Timothy AR, O'Doherty MJ, et al. 18-FDG-PET as a prognostic indicator in the treatment of aggressive non-Hodgkin's lymphoma-comparison with CT. *Leuk Lymphoma* 2000;39:543–553.
47. Miller AB, To T, Baines CJ, et al. Canadian National Breast Screening Study-2: 13-year results of a randomized trial in women aged 50–59 years. *J Natl Cancer Inst* 2000;92:1490–1499.
48. Ng SH, Chang TC, Ko SF, et al. Nasopharyngeal carcinoma: MRI and CT assessment. *Neuroradiology* 1997;39:741–746.
49. Noguchi M, Ohta N, Koyasaki N, et al. Reappraisal of internal mammary node metastases as a prognostic factor in patients with breast cancer. *Cancer* 1991;68:1918–1925.
50. Noguchi M, Taniya T, Koyasaki N, et al. A multivariate analysis of en bloc extended radical mastectomy versus conventional radical mastectomy in operable breast cancer. *Int Surg* 1992;77:48–54.
51. Nohl-Oser HC. An investigation of the anatomy of the lymphatic drainage of the lungs as shown by the lymphatic spread of bronchial carcinoma. *Ann R Coll Surg Engl* 1972;51:157–176.
52. Nystrom L, Andersson I, Bjurstam N, et al. Long-term effects of mammography screening: Updated overview of the Swedish randomised trials. *Lancet* 2002;359:909–919.
53. O'Malley B, Mukherji S. Cancer of the nasopharynx: Radiologic imaging concerns. In: Harrison L, Sessions R, Hong W (eds.) *Head and neck cancer*. Philadelphia: Lippincott Williams & Wilkins, 2004;544–545.
54. O'Sullivan JM, Norman AR, Cook GJ, et al. Broadening the criteria for avoiding staging bone scans in prostate cancer: A retrospective study of patients at the Royal Marsden Hospital. *BJU Int* 2003;92:685–689.
55. Overgaard M, Hansen PS, Overgaard J, et al. Postoperative radiotherapy in high-risk premenopausal women with breast cancer who receive adjuvant chemotherapy. Danish Breast Cancer Cooperative Group 82b Trial. *N Engl J Med* 1997;337:949–955.
56. Overgaard M, Jensen MB, Overgaard J, et al. Postoperative radiotherapy in high-risk postmenopausal breast-cancer patients given adjuvant tamoxifen: Danish Breast Cancer Cooperative Group DBCG 82c randomised trial. *Lancet* 1999;353:1641–1648.
57. Pass HI, Pogrebniak HW, Steinberg SM, et al. Randomized trial of neoadjuvant therapy for lung cancer: Interim analysis. *Ann Thorac Surg* 1992;53:992–928.
58. Pijl ME, Chaoui AS, Wahl RL, et al. Radiology of colorectal cancer. *Eur J Cancer* 2002;38:887–898.
59. PORT Meta-analysis Trialists Group. Postoperative radiotherapy in non-small-cell lung cancer: Systematic review and meta-analysis of individual patient data from nine randomised controlled trials. *Lancet* 1998;352:257–263.
60. Pozo-Rodriguez F, Martin de Nicolas JL, Sanchez-Nistal MA, et al. Accuracy of helical computed tomography and [18F] fluorodeoxyglucose positron emission tomography for identifying lymph node mediastinal metastases in potentially resectable non-small-cell lung cancer. *J Clin Oncol* 2005;23:8348–8356.
61. Quaranta B, Light K, Das S, et al. Utility of non-axial beams for treatment of lower lobe lung cancers. Presented at: ASTRO 44th Annual Meeting, New Orleans, LA; October 6–10, 2002. *Int J Radiat Oncol Biol Phys* 2002;54(2)[Suppl]:(abstr 2216).
62. Ragaz J, Jackson SM, Le N, et al. Adjuvant radiotherapy and chemotherapy in node-positive premenopausal women with breast cancer. *N Engl J Med* 1997;337:956–962.

63. Rini JN, Leonidas JC, Tomas MB, et al. 18F-FDG PET versus CT for evaluating the spleen during initial staging of lymphoma. *J Nucl Med* 2003;44:1072–1074.

64. Riquet M, Hidden G, Debesse B. Direct lymphatic drainage of lung segments to the mediastinal nodes. An anatomic study on 260 adults. *J Thorac Cardiovasc Surg* 1989;97:623–632.

65. Rosch T. Endosonographic staging of esophageal cancer: A review of literature results. *Gastrointest Endosc Clin North Am* 1995;5:537–547.

66. Rosell R, Gomez-Codina J, Camps C, et al. A randomized trial comparing preoperative chemotherapy plus surgery with surgery alone in patients with non-small-cell lung cancer. *N Engl J Med* 1994;330:153–158.

67. Sauer R, Becker H, Hohenberger W, et al. Preoperative versus postoperative chemoradiotherapy for rectal cancer. *N Engl J Med* 2004;351:1731–1740.

68. Schiepers C, Filmont JE, Czernin J. PET for staging of Hodgkin's disease and non-Hodgkin's lymphoma. *Eur J Nucl Med Mol Imaging* 2003;30[Suppl 1]:S82–S88.

69. Seppenwoolde Y, Muller SH, Theuws JC, et al. Radiation dose-effect relations and local recovery in perfusion for patients with non-small-cell lung cancer. *Int J Radiat Oncol Biol Phys* 2000;47:681–690.

70. Shafman T, Marks L, Das S, et al. Conservation of integral-dose within, and dose-gradient between, shells surrounding targets: Physical realities and clinical consequences. Presented at: ASTRO 44th Annual Meeting, New Orleans, LA, October 6–10, 2002. *Int J Radiat Oncol Biol Phys* 2002;54(2):(abstr 2215).

71. Smith TA. FDG uptake, tumour characteristics and response to therapy: A review. *Nucl Med Commun* 1998;19:97–105.

72. Spaepen K, Stroobants S, Dupont P, et al. Prognostic value of positron emission tomography (PET) with fluorine-18 fluorodeoxyglucose ([18F]FDG) after first-line chemotherapy in non-Hodgkin's lymphoma: Is [18F]FDG-PET a valid alternative to conventional diagnostic methods? *J Clin Oncol* 2001;19:414–419.

73. Stephens RJ, Girling DJ, Bleehen NM, et al. The role of post-operative radiotherapy in non-small-cell lung cancer: A multicentre randomised trial in patients with pathologically staged T1–2, N1–2, M0 disease. Medical Research Council Lung Cancer Working Party. *Br J Cancer* 1996;74:632–639.

74. Stevens C, Forster K, Zhu X, et al. Excellent local control and survival after extrapleural pneumonectomy and IMRT for mesothelioma. *Proc ASTRO* 2005; 63:S103.

75. Sze G, Johnson C, Kawamura Y, et al. Comparison of single- and triple-dose contrast material in the MR screening of brain metastases. *AJNR Am J Neuroradiol* 1998;19:821–828.

76. Sze G, Milano E, Johnson C, et al. Detection of brain metastases: Comparison of contrast-enhanced MR with unenhanced MR and enhanced CT. *AJNR Am J Neuroradiol* 1990;11:785–791.

77. Tabar L, Fagerberg G, Chen HH, et al. Efficacy of breast cancer screening by age. New results from the Swedish Two-County Trial. *Cancer* 1995;75:2507–2517.

78. Tamerisa R, Irisawa A, Bhutani MS. Endoscopic ultrasound in the diagnosis, staging, and management of gastrointestinal and adjacent malignancies. *Med Clin North Am* 2005;89:139158, viii.

79. Therasse P, Arbuck SG, Eisenhauer EA, et al. New guidelines to evaluate the response to treatment in solid tumors. European Organization for Research and Treatment of Cancer, National Cancer Institute of the United States, National Cancer Institute of Canada. *J Natl Cancer Inst* 2000;92:205–216.

80. Toloza EM, Harpole L, McCrory DC. Noninvasive staging of non-small cell lung cancer: A review of the current evidence. *Chest* 2003;123:137S–146S.

81. Trodella L, Granone P, Valente S, et al. Adjuvant radiotherapy in non-small cell lung cancer with pathological stage I: Definitive results of a phase III randomized trial. *Radiother Oncol* 2002;62:11–19.

82. Urban JA, Marjani MA. Significance of internal mammary lymph node metastases in breast cancer. *Am J Roentgenol Radium Ther Nucl Med* 1971;111:130–136.

83. Van Houtte P, Rocmans P, Smets P, et al. Postoperative radiation therapy in lung cancer: A controlled trial after resection of curative design. *Int J Radiat Oncol Biol Phys* 1980;6:983–986.

84. Van Westreenen HL, Westerterp M, Bossuyt PM, et al. Systematic review of the staging performance of 18F-fluorodeoxyglucose positron emission tomography in esophageal cancer. *J Clin Oncol* 2004;22:3805–3812.

85. Watanabe Y, Shimizu J, Tsubota M, et al. Mediastinal spread of metastatic lymph nodes in bronchogenic carcinoma. Mediastinal nodal metastases in lung cancer. *Chest* 1990;97:1059–1065.

86. Westerterp M, van Westreenen HL, Reitsma JB, et al. Esophageal cancer: CT, endoscopic US, and FDG PET for assessment of response to neoadjuvant therapy—systematic review. *Radiology* 2005;236:841–851.

87. Wijers OB, Levendag PC, Tan T, et al. A simplified CT-based definition of the lymph node levels in the node negative neck. *Radiother Oncol* 1999;52:35–42.

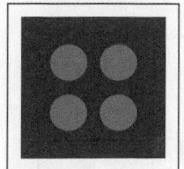

Chapter 28
Hyperthermia as a Treatment Modality

Ellen L. Jones, Thaddeus V. Samulski, Zeljko Vujaskovic, Leonard R. Prosnitz, Mark W. Dewhirst

The rationale for combining hyperthermia with radiation rests on several mechanisms. Hyperthermia is known to cause direct cytotoxicity and also acts as a radiosensitizer. Studies performed in vitro yield a pattern of survival curves similar to radiation survival curves. The mechanisms of action of hyperthermia appear to be complementary to the effects of radiation with regard to inhibition of potentially lethal damage and sublethal damage repair, cell cycle sensitivity, and effects of hypoxia and nutrient deprivation. In addition, hyperthermia has effects on blood flow and tumor physiology, which may be of particular interest with regard to tumor oxygenation and combination therapy with liposomal agents. Recent developments in the field of gene therapy may also establish a role for hyperthermia as a strategy for targeted, localized induction of gene therapy using the heat shock protein (HSP) 70 promoter.

Implementation of hyperthermia in the clinic presents significant challenges. Several approaches have been taken to deliver locoregional hyperthermia, and the challenge remains to heat tumor tissue volumes with uniformity and precision. Techniques for measuring temperature and the actual definition and calculation of thermal dose are nontrivial.

The biologic rationale for hyperthermia is strongly compelling and is founded on principles of classic radiobiology, molecular biology, and tumor physiology. Further improvements in technologies to deliver hyperthermia and measure thermal dose remain crucial. Moreover, there are now 17 randomized trials of hyperthermia in human cancer patients, the majority of which have demonstrated a local control and/or survival advantage with the addition of hyperthermia to standard therapy.

The Biology of Hyperthermia

Definition of Hyperthermia

Hyperthermia means elevation of temperature to a supraphysiological level. When cells or tumor tissues are subjected to elevated temperatures a number of events follow that have important biological consequences for cancer therapy. Hyperthermia can kill cells in its own right, but perhaps more importantly, it can sensitize tumor cells to other forms of therapy, including radiation and chemotherapy. Some of the physiologic consequences have implications for radiotherapy as well, such as thermally induced reoxygenation. Changes induced in microvessel pore size can lead to increased delivery of liposomally encapsulated drugs (96–99) as well as macromolecular therapeutic agents, such as monoclonal antibodies (71) or drug-carrying polymers (121). The adaptive response to hyperthermic exposure (thermotolerance) may augment host immune responses against tumor cells (8). This chapter will not deal directly with the use of whole body hyperthermia, since it has not been combined with radiation therapy.

Effects of Hyperthermia on Cell Survival

Hyperthermia kills cells in a log-linear fashion depending on the time at a defined temperature (Fig. 28.1A). Resulting survival curves typically have an initial shoulder region, followed by an exponential portion. The initial shoulder region indicates that damage has to accumulate to a certain level before cells begin to die. This is somewhat analogous to the sublethal damage that is seen with ionizing radiation, except that the shoulder region may not return to the same level for a subsequent heat fraction, depending on whether thermotolerance (heat-induced thermal resistance, as described in more detail below) is induced and still present from the initial heat fraction. At lower temperatures, a resistant tail may appear at the end of the heating period. This resistant tail is not a resistant subpopulation, as might be seen for radiation therapy when there is a hypoxic subfraction. The appearance of the resistant tail is also due to the induction of thermotolerance, which develops during the heating period. At temperatures above 43°C the tail does not develop, because temperatures in this range are nonpermissive for development of thermotolerance during heating. More details on the mechanism of thermotolerance and its potential clinical significance are discussed below. There is good evidence to suggest that human cells are more thermally resistant than rodent cells. As an example, Fig. 28.1B demonstrates that for a given time–temperature combination, relatively more human melanoma cells survive as compared with the Chinese hamster ovary (CHO) cell line.

The Arrhenius Relationship and Thermal Isoeffect Dose

Arrhenius found that the temperature dependence of the rate of hydrolysis of sucrose in the presence of various acids was too great to be accounted for in terms of the kinetic energy of the molecules. He found that the difference in rates at two temperatures was a logarithmic function of the absolute temperatures at which the two reactions were conducted (6). These observations have physiologic relevance. For example, the rate of cellular metabolism increases as temperature rises in cells or tissues, up to a point where thermal damage is created (202).

In the case of therapeutic levels of hyperthermia, the Arrhenius relationship is used to define the rate of cell killing to temperature. This is done by plotting the log of the slope (1/Do) of cell survival curves as a function of temperature (Fig. 28.2). Typically, Arrhenius plots have a biphasic curve and the point at which the slope changes is referred to as a "break point." Above the breakpoint for nearly all cell types, a change in temperature of 1°C will double the rate of cell killing. Below the breakpoint, the rate of cell killing drops by a factor of 4 to 8 for every drop in temperature of 1°C. The change in slope below the breakpoint is due to the development of thermotolerance during heating.

Arrhenius plots have been made for normal tissue and tumor. Although there are variations in the absolute thermal sensitivity of these tissues, the slopes of the Arrhenius plots are virtually identical to those that are derived from in vitro studies (54). This provides a strong rationale for using the Arrhenius relationship as a basis for thermal dosimetry.

The recognition that there is a definable relationship between the rate of cell killing and temperature led Sapareto

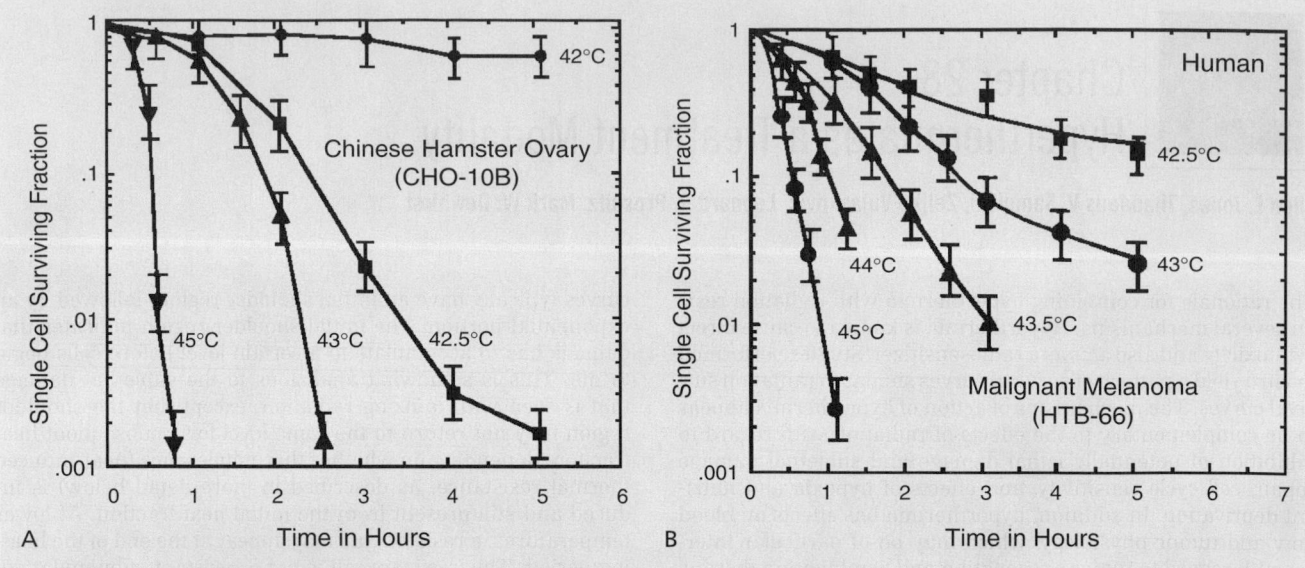

FIGURE 28.1. A: Cell survival curves for the CHO (Chinese hamster ovary) cell line, plotted as a log of surviving fraction as a function of time of heating at a defined temperature. Note that the rate of cell killing is highly temperature dependent. For example, 5 hours of heating at 42°C kills very few cells, while 5 hours of heating at 0.5°C higher (42.5°C) results in nearly three logs of cell killing. **B:** Cell survival curves for a human melanoma cell line. Note that this human cell line appears to be more thermally resistant than the CHO line (i.e., for a given temperature–time combination, a greater proportion of human cells survive as compared with the CHO cell line. This difference in thermal sensitivity has important clinical implications that will be discussed under the section on thermal dosimetry. (From Roizin-Towle L, Pirro JP. The response of human and rodent cells to hyperthermia. *Int J Radiat Oncol Biol Phys* 1991;20:751–756, with permission.)

and Dewey (177) to propose using this relationship to normalize thermal data from hyperthermia treatments. The rationale came from the observations that time–temperature histories vary from patient to patient and that temperatures within tumors were almost always nonuniform, thereby preventing the goal of reaching a uniform target temperature–time combination for therapy. The formulation for this relationship is quite

straightforward and takes the following form:

$$CEM\,43°C = tR^{(43-T)} \tag{1}$$

where CEM 43°C is the cumulative equivalent minutes at 43°C (the temperature suggested for normalization), t is the time of treatment, T is this average temperature during desired interval

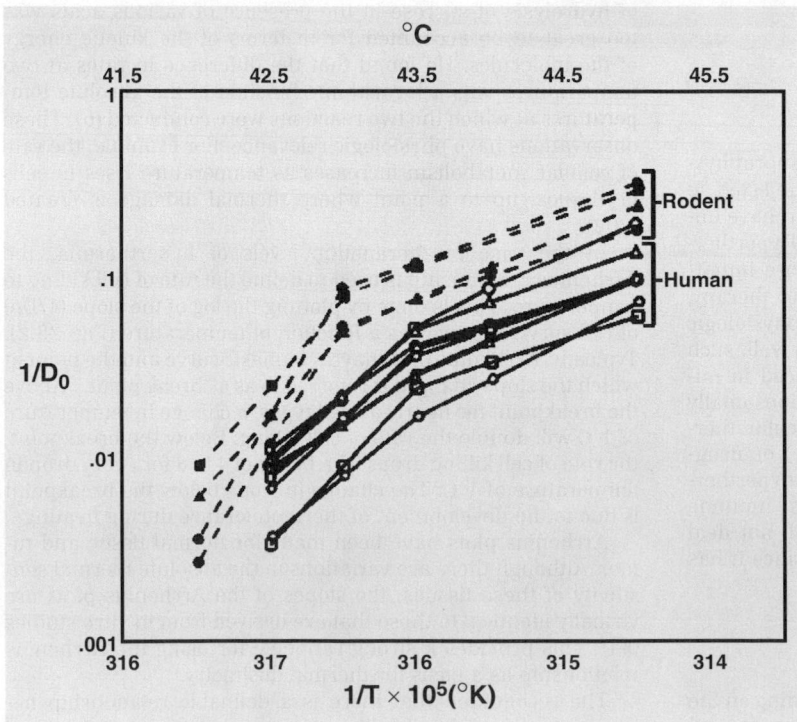

FIGURE 28.2. Arrhenius plots for a variety of rodent and human tumor cell lines, as assessed in vitro. Note that all human cells are below and to the right of the rodent cell lines. This means that for a given temperature, the slope of the cell-killing curve is less steep for human than rodent cells. Additionally, the breakpoint of the Arrhenius plot appears to be about 0.5°C higher for human than rodent cells. These observations mean that human cells are more thermally resistant than rodent cells. (From Roizin-Towle L, Pirro JP. The response of human and rodent cells to hyperthermia. *Int J Radiat Oncol Biol Phys* 1991;20:751–756, with permission.)

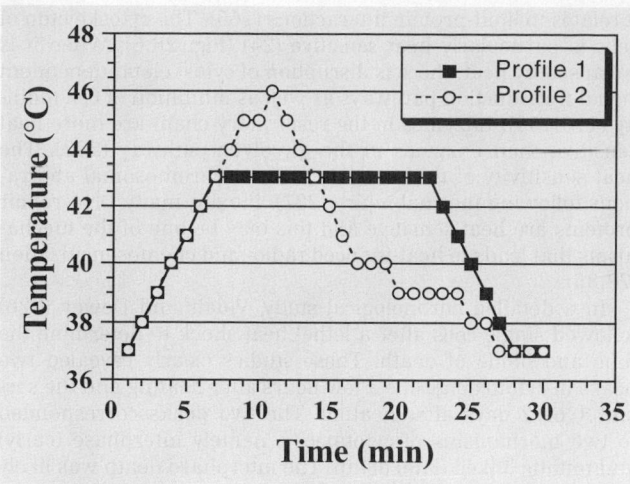

FIGURE 28.3. Comparison of CEM 43°C for two different time–temperature histories. The text discusses which profile yields the greatest degree of cell killing.

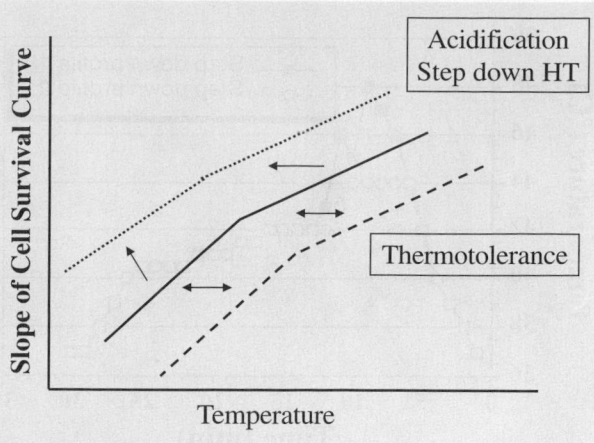

FIGURE 28.4. Comparison of the effects of modifiers of the Arrhenius relationship. Thermotolerance reduces the slope for cell killing by hyperthermia, thereby making hyperthermia less effective at killing cells at a defined temperature. Step down heating and acute acidification do the opposite. Both effects are transient, and surviving cells will recover back toward baseline thermal sensitivity.

Techniques, Modalities, and Modifiers in Radiation Oncology

of heating, and R is a constant. When above the breakpoint, which is usually assumed to be 43°C, R = 0.5. When below the breakpoint, R = 0.25.

For a complex time–temperature history, the heating profile is broken into intervals of time (t) length, where the temperature remains relatively constant. CEM 43°C is calculated using the average T (T_{avg}) for each interval, and the resultant data are summed to give a final CEM 43°C for the entire heating regimen.

$$\text{CEM } 43°C = \sum tR^{(43-Tavg)} \tag{2}$$

To illustrate the importance of using this relationship for temperature normalization, two time–temperature profiles are compared with respect to the relative efficacies for killing (Fig. 28.3). In profile 1, the temperature increases monotonically and plateaus at 43°C for 16 minutes and then declines back to baseline by the end of a 30-minute heating period. In the second profile, temperature also increases monotonically, but reaches a peak value of 46°C before trending downward to reach 37°C at the end of the heating period. In this second example, temperatures exceed the maximum value for profile 1 for a total of 5 minutes and they are beneath profile 1 temperatures for an additional 13 minutes. One might guess that profile 1 would be more effective at killing cells, but in fact profile 2 is predicted to be more effective by 60%. The CEM 43°C for profile 1 is 17 minutes and for profile 2 it is 27 minutes. The reason for this difference is due to the short period of time when the cells were at temperatures above 43°C. In contrast, 1 minute at 46°C is equal to 8 minutes at 43°C.

The CEM 43°C (thermal isoeffect dose) formulation has been used extensively and successfully in clinical trials to assess the efficacy of heating as is discussed in the clinical section of this chapter. The issue becomes somewhat more complex when one is dealing with nonuniform temperature fields, however. In this situation, which temperature does one use to depict the thermal history of the whole tumor? As will be discussed in detail in the clinical section, this has been handled primarily by using an analogy drawn from radiation therapy, namely to use a descriptor of the low end of the temperature distribution.

Modifiers of Thermal Isoeffect Dose

There are factors that are known to affect the position and slopes of the Arrhenius plot. Currently, these are not taken into account in routine clinical practice (Fig. 28.4).

Thermotolerance is defined as a transient adaptation to thermal stress that renders surviving heated cells more resistant to additional heat stress. Thermotolerance tends to shift the Arrhenius plot to the right and downward, reflecting greater thermal resistance to heat killing. The maximum degree of shift is known to be equivalent to about 1°C. Thus, the breakpoint will be shifted upward by 1°C, and the time of heating to achieve an isoeffect would need to be doubled, as compared with nonthermally tolerant cells. Generally speaking, the way this is handled clinically is to use long intervals between hyperthermia treatments to allow for decay of thermotolerance. Typically, this is 2 to 3 days. More details on the kinetics of thermotolerance induction and decay are discussed in the section on thermotolerance.

Acute acidification will sensitize cells to killing in two ways. The Arrhenius plot is shifted to the left and the R-value below the breakpoint approaches 0.5 (the slope above the breakpoint) because thermotolerance induction is at least partially inhibited. This phenomenon does not normally occur spontaneously. However, achieving acute acidification for thermal sensitization has been studied extensively in preclinical models and in humans (58,59,107,131,192,231). More detail on how this is done is provided in the section on hyperthermia and physiology. If pH reduction is developed to the point that it can be done successfully, this effect could be accounted for by correcting the CEM 43°C, or it could simply be used as a covariate in clinical trial design or interpretation of outcome.

Step down heating occurs when temperatures rise above the breakpoint and then drop below the breakpoint for the remainder of a treatment (37). This occurs clinically in two circumstances: When power is turned down after heating has started in response to pain or excessively high normal tissue temperatures or when perfusion is increased in response to increased temperatures. When step down heating occurs, thermotolerance induction is prevented for a period of time that is sufficient to stop it for the duration of the rest of the heating session, which typically lasts 1 to 2 hours. The net effect of step down heating may or may not be important in terms of accumulating thermal isoeffect dose. Two examples are provided in Figure 28.5. In the first example, temperatures rise quickly to reach a maximum of 48°C and then drop below 43°C 3 to 4 minutes later. In the second example, the profile is similar, but peak temperatures do not exceed 44°C. In both cases thermotolerance is prevented from occurring, but in the first example the effect is negligible.

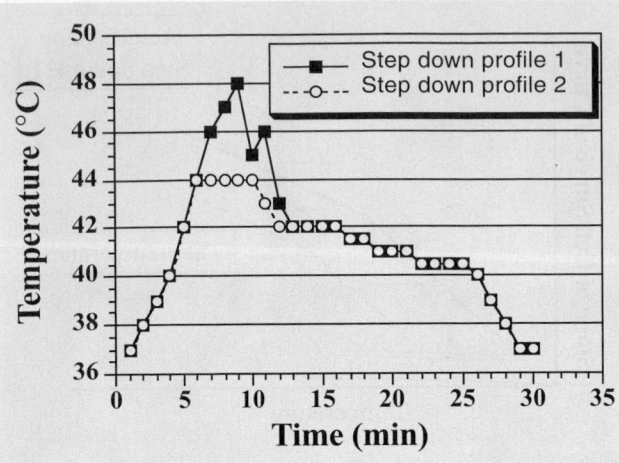

FIGURE 28.5. Temperature–time profiles for examining effects of step down heating on thermal cytotoxicity. The profile with maximum temperature of 44°C (profile 2) is affected more by step down heating than the profile with a maximum temperature of 48°C (profile 1).

This is because the peak temperature at 48°C provides so much additional dose that step down heating effects are small. The CEM 43°C assuming step down heating is 76 minutes and that assuming no step down heating is 73 minutes. The difference between these two is only 3%. In the second example, the effect of step down heating is more obvious because peak temperatures are lower, thereby contributing less to the overall CEM 43°C. Correcting for step down heating, the CEM 43°C is 16 minutes and without this correction it is 13 minutes, a difference of 23%. It is not known if making these corrections would be useful in the clinical setting when using CEM 43°C for correlation with tumor response. To our knowledge, it has never been tested.

Mechanisms of Hyperthermic Cytotoxicity

Cellular and Tissue Responses to Hyperthermia: Targets for Hyperthermic Cytotoxicity

When cells are exposed to elevated temperatures ($\geq 41°C$), damage is inflicted in multiple sites, but the predominant molecular target appears to be protein (165). Evidence for protein as a target comes from Arrhenius analysis of rates of cell killing versus temperature. This type of analysis allows one to derive the heat of inactivation, based on thermodynamic principles (35). For many cells and tissues (both tumor and normal), the heat of inactivation for cell killing is in the range of that necessary for protein denaturation (130–170 kcal/mole). Additional evidence for proteins being the primary target for cell killing is the importance of heat shock proteins in protecting cells from thermal damage. When cells are exposed to heat shock the synthesis of nearly all proteins is stopped with the exception of heat shock proteins, the synthesis of which is up-regulated (126). One of the primary functions of heat shock proteins is to refold other proteins that have been denatured or damaged (127). There does not seem to be a counterpart to the heat shock protein for specific repair of lipids or DNA, which are the other two primary components of cells. Heat shock proteins do play a role in the repair or protection of other specialized DNA repair proteins (85), and they are known to be the mediators of thermotolerance (109).

Some cellular organelles are especially important in controlling the thermal response. For example, modification of cellular membrane lipid content or use of membrane active agents, such as alcohols, can sensitize cells to heat killing, but the sensitization is probably related to destabilization of the membrane as it relates to lipid-protein interactions (165). The cytoskeleton of cells is particularly heat sensitive (24) (Fig. 28.6). When it is collapsed by heat, there is disruption of cytoskeletal-dependent signal transduction pathways as well as inhibition of cell motility (110,159). Enzymes in the respiratory chain are more heat sensitive than enzymes in the glycolytic pathway (202). The heat sensitivity of the centriole leads to chromosomal aberrations following thermal injury (227). Finally, many DNA repair proteins are heat sensitive and this may be one of the mechanisms that leads to heat-induced radio- and chemosensitization (73,85).

In a detailed chronological study, Vidair and Dewey (226) followed single cells after a lethal heat shock to determine the time and mode of death. These studies clearly revealed two peaks in cytotoxicity, one a few hours after heating and the second 1 or 2 days after heating. The two peaks corresponded to two mechanisms of cytotoxicity, namely interphase (early) and mitotic linked (late) death. The interphase death was likely apoptosis.

Interphase death after heat shock has been associated with both apoptosis and necrosis in in vivo studies. The difference between which of the two develops depends on the severity of the thermal injury. Greater thermal injury leads to a larger degree of protein denaturation, thereby increasing the likelihood of necrosis. Sakaguchi et al. (176) studied apoptosis in normal and tumor tissues of rats following total body hyperthermia at a temperature of 41.5°C for periods up to 1 to 2 hours. Evidence for apoptosis was found as early as 4 hours post-hyperthermia. In normal tissues (gut, bone marrow, lymph nodes) apoptosis declined after the early peak at 4 hours. In contrast, the apoptotic index reached a much higher level in tumors and persisted longer than in normal tissues (176).

McRae et al. (119) utilized electrical impedance measurements to noninvasively monitor changes in tissue characteristics after local hyperthermia at temperatures between 44°C and 45°C. In this case, cell swelling and membrane breakdown were observed during and after heating, consistent with a necrosis. Little information is available from human tumors to know what proportion of cells is killed with heat alone or what the underlying mechanisms of cell death might be. Such information may be important with respect to reoxygenation, which has been seen in rodent, canine, and human tumors (193) after hyperthermia. Induction of apoptosis could lead to reoxygenation following heating as a result of reduced oxygen consumption, which could in turn increase radiation sensitivity. Alternatively, induction of necrosis is not likely to affect hypoxia, since both vessels and tumor cells would be killed in the process.

Thermotolerance

Thermotolerance is defined as a transient adaptation to thermal stress that renders surviving heated cells more resistant to additional heat stress. Whether or not a cell dies as a result of thermal insult is dependent on the net balance between how much protein is damaged and how much is protected and repaired via thermotolerance. Thermotolerance can develop either during or after heat stress and can persist for several days. If cells are not exposed to thermal stress again, the thermotolerance will decay. The time of peak thermal resistance and the time of decay are positively correlated with the severity of the heat shock, however. In other words, the larger the initial heat shock, the longer it takes for the thermotolerance of surviving cells to be induced and to decay (20) (Fig. 28.7). Concerns over the persistence of thermotolerance after hyperthermia treatment has had significant impact on the design of many clinical trials of thermoradiotherapy. In most trials, a minimum of 48 hours has been suggested between hyperthermia fractions in order to avoid retreatment during thermotolerance. Because of this, it has not been possible to design clinical trials to maximize the

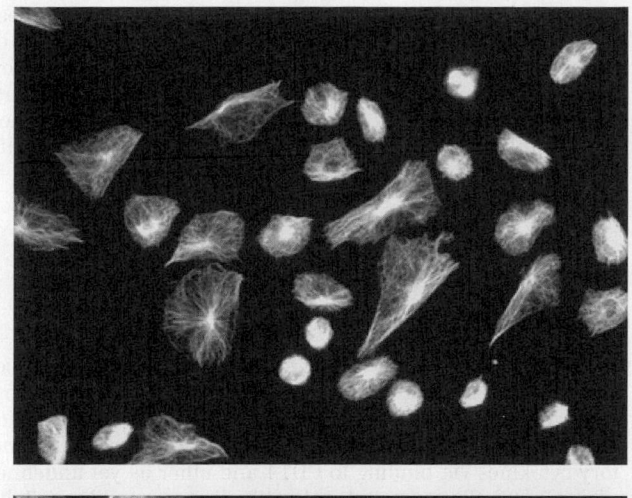

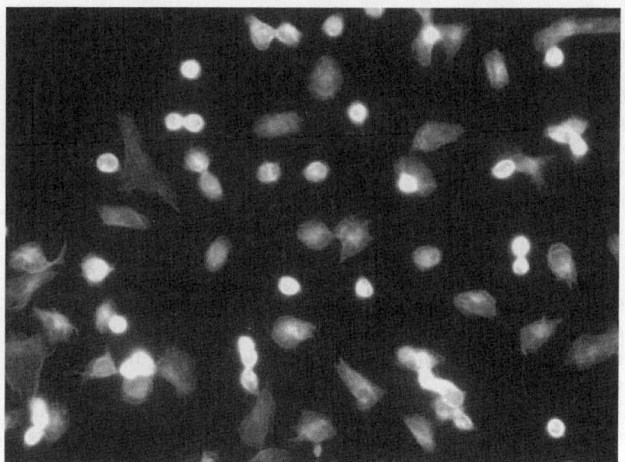

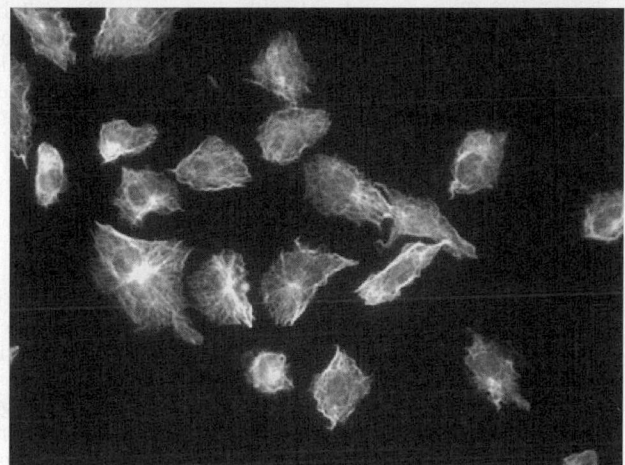

FIGURE 28.6. Appearance of cytoskeleton of Chinese hamster ovary (CHO) cells in tissue culture grown at: **(A)** 37°C, pH 7.3; **(B)** heated at 42°C for 6 hours, pH 7.3; **(C)** heated at 42°C, pH 6.7, but grown at pH 6.77. Collapse of the cytoskeleton is seen with heating at 42°C, when cells are cultured at normal pH (A, B). When cells are chronically grown at a low pH and heated, there is protection against cytoskeletal collapse (C). (Figure kindly provided by Dr. Ronald Coss.)

interactions between hyperthermia and conventionally fractionated radiation, as might be achieved by using hyperthermia every day with radiation therapy. In order to circumvent this limitation many early trials utilized radiation fractionation schemes with relatively large doses per fraction (e.g., 4 Gy per fraction, 2 to 3 times per week) (151,155,225). With this type of schedule it is possible to combine the hyperthermia with every radiation fraction, but the nonstandard radiation fractionation scheme is readily open to criticism because of concerns over normal tissue tolerance and limitations on the total dose that can be delivered with such scheduling. Under such circumstances, one could argue that the same effect might be achieved

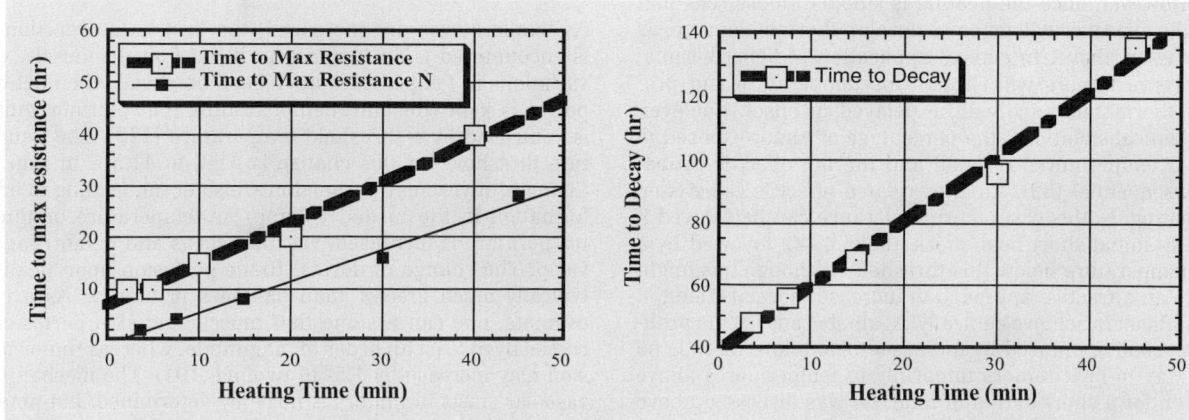

FIGURE 28.7. Kinetics of thermotolerance induction to (*left*) maximum level and (*right*) decay back to baseline after a heat shock of 43.5°C. Growth delay time of a C3H mammary tumour following split dose heat treatment is the parameter used for induction and decay. (Data abstracted from Nielsen OS, Overgaard J. Importance of preheating temperature and time for the induction of thermotolerance in a solid tumour in vivo. *Br J Cancer* 1982;46:894–903.) Additional data for mouse ear skin necrosis (N) are provided with reference to time to induction. (Data abstracted from Nielsen OS, Overgaard J. Importance of preheating temperature and time for the induction of thermotolerance in a solid tumour in vivo. *Br J Cancer* 1982;46:894–903.)

if more radiation dose were delivered using conventional radiation fractionation schedules.

Alternatively, some investigators have suggested that one should take advantage of heat radiosensitization, rather than hyperthermic cytotoxicity, and ignore the issue of thermotolerance. The degree of hyperthermia-mediated cytotoxicity may be low with hyperthermia as it is currently practiced because temperatures achieved are largely below that needed for direct cell killing. Further, heat radiosensitization is relatively unaffected by thermotolerance (5).

Most of the early hyperthermia research was done on rodent cell lines, which are more prone to develop thermotolerance in the clinically relevant temperature range compared to human cells (4,174). If this paradigm is true for most human tumors, then it may be possible to administer hyperthermia fractions more frequently without incurring the risk of inducing thermotolerance during heating. Unfortunately, virtually no human clinical data are available in which the thermotolerance response has been evaluated.

Evaluation of the development of thermotolerance after heating has been attempted in a pilot clinical project. A systematic evaluation of heat shock protein synthesis was made in a small group of human patients ($n = 23$) with chest wall recurrences of breast cancer who underwent radiotherapy with or without hyperthermia. Elevated levels of heat shock proteins in biopsy specimens after treatment correlated with lower probability of attaining a complete response (111). In another study of patients treated with 5FU (fluorouracil) plus thermoradiotherapy for colorectal cancer, no correlation between HSP27 or HSP70 levels, either before or after treatment, and outcome was seen (169). Interpretation of clinical studies is complicated by the fact that heat shock protein expression is frequently up-regulated in tumors, in the absence of heat stress (126). Stresses other than hyperthermia, such as hypoxia and hypoxia-reoxygenation injury, which occur with high frequency in tumors as a result of poor oxygen transport coupled with unstable blood flow (16,38,64) and acidosis (92,230), can cause elevations in heat shock protein levels. This generalized stress response may lead to treatment resistance to therapies other than hyperthermia. Elevated HSP27 or HSP70 has been tied to poorer survival in cancers of the breast, ovary, bone, liver, and prostate (7,23,95,218,224).

Modifiers of the Thermotolerance Response

There are circumstances where thermotolerance can theoretically be avoided, at least during heating. If the thermal exposure is above 43°C, thermotolerance during the heating is prevented. However, once the heating is stopped, those cells that survive the exposure will go on to develop thermotolerance, as was discussed above. In clinical application of hyperthermia, some parts of tumors will exceed this temperature and presumably thermotolerance will be delayed in onset. However, in most clinical situations, the percentage of tumor exposed to such high temperatures is small and the net effect is probably inconsequential (39). Another related effect is called step down heating. In this case, thermotolerance can be delayed if there is an initial short heat shock above 43°C, followed by a drop in temperature below this threshold. Although this might seem like an attractive approach to increase thermal killing, it is quite difficult to achieve clinically. Again, because of the problems with cooling induced by increased blood flow, there is no reliable way to heat tumors uniformly to temperatures above 43°C, even for a short period of time. As was discussed above in the section on modifiers of thermal isoeffect dose, induction of step down heating is not likely to have a large effect on CEM 43°C, so efforts to deliberately induce it are probably not worth the effort.

It has also been shown that acute reduction in pH, of even a few tenths of a pH unit, can delay the onset of thermotol-

erance (59). Methods to achieve this effect clinically have been tested and are discussed below in the section Hyperthermia and Physiology. This latter method holds some promise for achieving thermal sensitization as well as avoiding thermotolerance during heating. Pharmacologic means to block the onset of thermotolerance are being investigated and could represent fertile ground for manipulation of thermal response (190,243).

Immunological Implications of the Heat Shock Response

Heat shock proteins have been shown to be expressed on cell surfaces after hyperthermia (132) and may be involved in antigen presentation to dendritic cells (195). HSP70 may function as a cytokine in signaling monocytes to produce proinflammatory cytokines via binding to CD14 and other as yet undefined receptors (8). Since monoclonal antibodies are readily available to such proteins, it may be possible to use radiolabeled antibodies to monitor cell surface expression of these proteins noninvasively. This would certainly be preferable to biopsy methods, which are fraught with issues of sampling error and uncertainties about thermal history (238).

Hyperthermia and Physiology

Tumor blood flow and metabolism have important influences on the efficacy of hyperthermia, and, conversely, the physiologic consequences of hyperthermia can influence the efficacy of other treatments the patient may receive. For example, changes in blood flow induced by hyperthermia could affect radiation response by altering tumor oxygenation, and changes in perfusion and permeability could affect drug delivery. On the other hand, human tumors with acidotic extracellular pH are more sensitive to damage by hyperthermia than tumors with a more normal pH (51). In this section, we will discuss what is known about the physiologic consequences of hyperthermia and will then discuss how physiology can be manipulated to enhance the efficacy of hyperthermic treatment.

Physiologic Response to Hyperthermia

As temperatures are increased, the first tissue reaction that is encountered is an increase in blood flow. In muscle, cyclic variations in temperature have been observed when delivered power is kept constant, demonstrating that thermoregulation is controlled by a threshold temperature (173). The temperature threshold for this change is 41°C to 41.5°C in skin (42). Changes in vascular permeability also occur, leading to edema formation in the heated volume. As temperature or time-at-temperature is increased, vascular stasis and hemorrhage develop. The change in normal tissue perfusion upon heating is typically much greater than one sees in tumors. As a rough estimate, one can assume that muscle and skin perfusion increase by at least an order of magnitude, whereas tumor perfusion may increase by 1.5- to twofold (191). The mechanism of vascular stasis in tumors is not fully determined, but potential sources include arteriovenous shunting, thrombus formation, and leukocyte plugging (171). Hemorrhage probably occurs as a result of enlarged endothelial cell gaps or loss of endothelial cell and basement membrane integrity along the vessel wall. The temperature threshold for such damage in human tumors appears to be higher than in murine tumors (234).

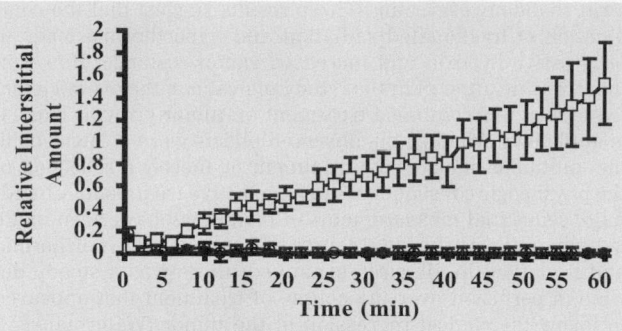

FIGURE 28.8. Effects of 42°C hyperthermia on 100nm liposomal extravasation from microvessels of SKOV3 human ovarian carcinoma xenografts. Microvessels of this tumor are refractory to extravasation of liposomes at 34°C (normal skin temperature), but permit extravasation at 42°C. (Data replotted from Kong G, Braun RD, Dewhirst MW. Hyperthermia enables tumor-specific nanoparticle delivery: Effect of particle size. *Cancer Res* 2000;60:4440–4445.)

Taking Advantage of Physiological Response to Hyperthermia

We have recently evaluated the effects of hyperthermia on liposomal extravasation from vessels into tumor parenchyma, using the SKOV3 human ovarian carcinoma xenograft line that is relatively impermeable to liposomes under normothermic conditions. A liposome is a small lipid vesicle ($\approx$100 nm diameter) that contains water or saline in the center. Drugs can be loaded into liposomes at high concentration.

Albumin extravasates from these vessels at normothermia, but heating at 42°C increases the rate by 25%. Liposomes that are 100 nm in diameter do not extravasate at normothermia (34°C for mouse skin), but extravasate well at 42°C (Fig. 28.8). The amount of extravasation of 100 nm liposomes during heating is equivalent to that of albumin. Extravasation of 200 and 400 nm liposomes was also seen at 42°C, but to a lesser extent (97). These results suggest that 42°C hyperthermia increases microvessel pore size to sizes between 100 to 400 nm. In contrast, there was no effect of hyperthermia on 100 nm liposomal extravasation from normal vessels. The threshold for increased liposomal extravasation from tumor vessels was 40°C, and the rate of extravasation increased by a factor of 2 for every degree temperature rise to a maximum of 42°C (Fig. 28.9). Heating >42°C in this model created vascular stasis and hemorrhage,

thus reducing liposomal extravasation. These results are consistent with the hypothesis that the increase in extravasation is due to cytoskeletal collapse in the vessel wall (endothelial cell). Further evidence for protein as being the target comes from evaluation of split dose heating (98). When the tissues were heated during liposome administration 8 hours after an initial heating, extravasation was blocked completely. If heating was administered and liposomal extravasation was examined 2 to 6 hours later after returning to normothermia, liposomal extravasation gradually returned to baseline. These results suggest that thermotolerance protects against changes in protein structure responsible for increased pore size. The increase in liposomal extravasation can be exploited as a drug delivery vehicle, particularly since the effect appears to be preferential to tumors. Many investigators have shown that hyperthermia increases liposomal drug accumulation in tumors, leading to enhanced antitumor efficacy of a variety of drugs, compared with liposome administration alone or free drug administered with hyperthermia (99). When temperature-sensitive liposomes are used, even better antitumor effects can be achieved, particularly using burst release–type liposomes that have been described recently (138). The improved effectiveness of these drugs when combined with hyperthermia is directly related to the increase in drug delivery.

Although the changes in perfusion in tumors are relatively small in comparison with normal tissues, there have been a number of efforts to exploit them as a means to augment drug delivery to tumors. For relatively small agents, such as most chemotherapeutic drugs, there is no real advantage to using heat to augment delivery, although increased cellular uptake has been seen with a number of drugs (28). For drugs with molecular weight <1,000, the primary mechanism that governs drug transport is diffusion, which is controlled by the concentration gradient across the vascular wall (26). The temperature dependence of diffusion is not large, so hyperthermia has relatively little effect. However, for molecules >1,000 molecular weight, the primary driving force for transport is convection, which is controlled by the pressure gradient across the wall. Accordingly, it has been shown that hyperthermia can augment the transvascular delivery of agents such as monoclonal antibodies (71) and polymeric peptides that can carry drugs or radioisotopes (121).

Effects of Hyperthermia on Tumor Metabolism and Oxygenation

The effects of heat on energy metabolism demonstrated that enzymes for aerobic metabolism were more heat sensitive than those involved in anaerobic metabolism (202). The net result of this difference in heat sensitivity is that nutrient stores are more rapidly depleted during heat shock, leading to a reduction in adenosine triphosphate (ATP) and buildup of lactic acid. A number of rodent studies have demonstrated changes in energy balance and pH after heating. For example, Kelleher et al. (90) reported decreases in ATP and increases in lactate concentration occurring concomitantly with reduction in tumor blood flow after heating. In a series of human patients with soft tissue sarcomas who were treated preoperatively with hyperthermia and radiation therapy, a reduction in magnetic resonance spectroscopy ATP/Pi (Pi, inorganic phosphate) was significantly correlated with a higher probability for tumor sterilization (161). These results are consistent with the theory that a reduction in tumor respiration occurs after hyperthermia treatment, but independent measurement of perfusion and oxygenation changes after hyperthermia in human patients would need to be made to validate the mechanism.

A shift toward anaerobic metabolism would decrease oxygen consumption rates, which could lead to improvement in

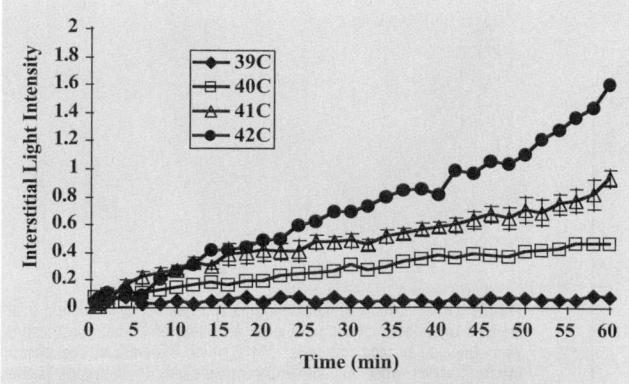

FIGURE 28.9. Effects of temperature on liposomal extravasation from microvessels of SKOV3 ovarian carcinoma xenografts. The temperature threshold for increased liposomal extravasation is 40°C. ◆; 39°C, □; 40°C, △; 41°C, ●; 42°C. (Kong G, Braun RD, Dewhirst MW. Characterization of the effect of hyperthermia on nanoparticle extravasation from tumor vasculature. *Cancer Res* 2001;61:3027–3032.)

tumor oxygenation. We theoretically considered the relative contributions that perfusion and consumption make on tumor oxygenation (181). This simulation was done using vascular geometries obtained from tumors, combined with other experimentally derived data, such as baseline oxygen consumption rates, microvessel perfusion rates, and hematocrits. The simulation predicted that elimination of hypoxia would require a three- to fourfold increase in perfusion versus a 30% reduction in oxygen consumption rate. Thus, even a small decrease in respiration (oxygen consumption) could lead to profound changes in tumor oxygenation.

Oleson (143) suggested that some of the benefits of hyperthermia in the clinical setting (other than its cytotoxic and radiosensitizing effects) may result from improvements in oxygenation. Results from several studies in rodent tumors and human tumor xenografts support the notion that an overall improvement in tumor oxygenation can result from time–temperature combinations below those which cause vascular damage (e.g., 41°C to 41.5°C, 60 minutes). Higher thermal doses that cause vascular damage (e.g., >43°C, 60 minutes) lead to decreases in tumor oxygenation (193).

It has been reported that hyperthermia improves tumor oxygenation in canine and human soft tissue sarcomas (19,229). In the human study, failure to reoxygenate after the first hyperthermia fraction led to a significantly lower probability to achieve pathologic complete response at the time of surgery (19). Of note, most of these patients had several fractions of radiation therapy before the first hyperthermia treatment. There was no significant change in oxygenation during that interval, compared with baseline measurements taken before therapy initiation. In the canine soft tissue sarcoma study, a median temperature >44°C resulted in a decrease in perfusion and tumor oxygenation (Fig. 28.10). This threshold temperature for vascular damage resulting in a decline in tumor perfusion and Po_2 (partial pressure of oxygen) is higher in canine than in rodent tumors. In humans, the threshold for thermal damage leading to vascular stasis is also higher than in rodents (234), but the thermal doses required to achieve vascular damage are not well defined. Achieving a median temperature >44°C is difficult in human tumors where patients are typically awake during treatment. For example, in the soft tissue sarcoma study reported by Brizel et al. (19) only 4/39 patients achieved median temperatures exceeding that value (19). It is important to note that thresholds for thermal vascular damage may be quite different for different tumor types.

Zywietz et al. (244) reported that twice weekly heating to 43°C for 60 minutes in combination with 60 Gy delivered in 20 fractions over 4 weeks resulted in a steady decline in Po_2 of a rat rhabdomyosarcoma. These results suggest that the combination of fractionated radiation and hyperthermia leads to progressive hypoxia and increased radioresistance. However, there was no attempt in that study to evaluate the overall effectiveness of this combined treatment on tumor growth. Thus, it is not known whether the observed effects were deleterious to the antitumor effect of the treatment or merely a reflection of the physiologic consequences of an effective treatment. A handful of sequential measurements of blood flow have been made in human tumors during a course of fractionated hyperthermia and radiation. In all cases examined, there was a steady decline in perfusion over the course of treatment that appeared to follow the clinical regression of the tumor (Waterman FM, personal communication, June, 2003). Thus, it may be that perfusion and oxygenation of tumors decrease concomitantly with increased cytotoxicity. Additional work needs to be done in the context of fractionated thermoradiotherapy to assess this issue in more detail.

Song et al. (193) have found that fractionated hyperthermia (42.5°C for 60-minute conditioning dose followed by 44.5°C for up to 90 minutes) can lead to vascular thermotolerance. This means that the likelihood of vascular damage decreases if a second hyperthermia treatment is given within 1 to 2 days after the first treatment, at a time when thermotolerance may still be present. These results may at first seem at odds with the results of Zywietz et al. (244). However, in the latter case the time between fractions of hyperthermia was ≥72 hours, which likely allowed for nearly complete decay of thermotolerance between the two treatments. It is not known whether vascular thermotolerance occurs in human tumors.

Tissue Damage from Hyperthermia

Thermal damage to tissues follows a predictable pathologic course. Within a few hours to days there is an inflammatory reaction, with edema, focal hemorrhage, and granulocytic infiltrates (53). Chronic changes, seen after a few weeks, include fibrosis, parenchymal necrosis (death of tissue cells), and lymphohistiocytic infiltration. Depending on the tissue, it is also possible to see parenchymal regeneration.

There has been speculation as to whether tumor tissues might be more sensitive to thermal damage than normal tissues. Many studies have compared tumor to normal cells in vitro. There is no inherent difference in the thermal sensitivity. However, the microenvironment of tumors, which is often acidotic and nutritionally deprived, leads to an increase in thermal sensitivity (50). Clinically it has been reported that tumors with lowered pretreatment extracellular pH are more sensitive

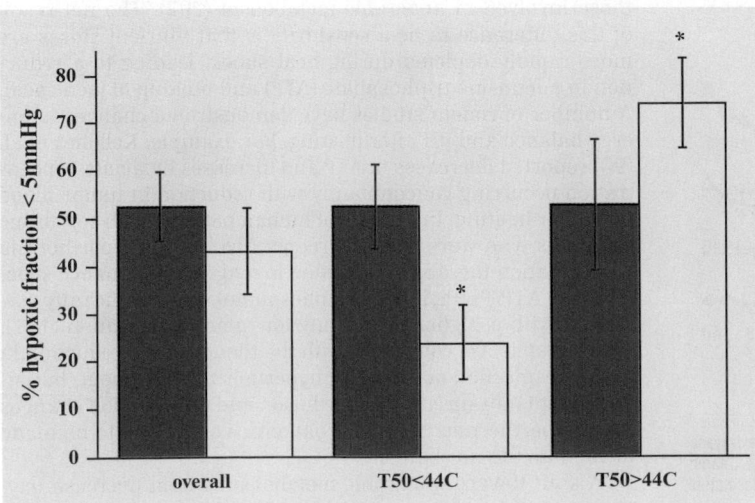

FIGURE 28.10. Effects of median temperature during hyperthermia treatment on oxygenation of canine tumors, as measured 24-hour postheating. When the median temperature is <44°C, there is significant reduction in hypoxic fraction. When median temperature exceeds 44°C, hypoxic fraction increases. Closed bar indicates measurements taken before hyperthermia and open bar indicates measurements taken 24 hours after hyperthermia treatment. (Data replotted from Vujaskovic Z, Poulson J, Gaskin A, et al. Temperature dependent changes in physiologic parameters of spontaneous canine soft tissue sarcomas after combined radiotherapy and hyperthermia. *Int J Radiat Oncol Biol Phys* 1999;46(1):179–185.)

to thermoradiotherapy (51). Interestingly, the opposite trend is seen if one examines the relationship between intracellular pH (as measured by magnetic resonance spectroscopy) and therapy outcome. In a series of 20 human and 10 canine soft tissue sarcomas, the likelihood of achieving a positive response to thermoradiotherapy was improved when intracellular pH was in the basic to normal range as compared with more acidic tumors (194). Although the results of these two studies may at first seem at odds with each other, in fact they may be similar. This is because of the effort that cells undertake to maintain a neutral pH when exposed to an acidic environment. In such instances, hydrogen ion pumps are up-regulated to maintain a normal intracellular pH (152,192). Thus, in circumstances where extracellular pH is low, one is most likely to observe relatively high intracellular pH. The mechanism underlying the increase in thermal sensitivity with low extracellular pH is not well defined, because in tissue culture, cells that are chronically conditioned to a low pH environment are no more sensitive to thermal damage than cells grown at normal pH (65). In vivo there may be a reversal of the pH gradient after hyperthermia, which may contribute to enhanced cytotoxicity under lowered extracellular pH conditions (80).

It has also been suggested that tumor cells might be more sensitive to heat killing because of depleted energy stores. Studies in vitro and in rodent models have supported this theory (94,100). However, studies of thermal sensitivity of human and canine soft tissue sarcomas, relative to energy status as delineated by 31-P magnetic resonance spectroscopy, found no relationship between energy status and treatment outcome (194).

Physiologic Approaches to Enhance Thermal Cytotoxicity pH Modification

Although cells that are chronically grown at low extracellular pH are no more sensitive to thermal cytotoxicity than cells grown at normal pH, it is well established that an acute reduction in extracellular pH can greatly enhance sensitivity to hyperthermia. It is also known that the reason for this is that cells adapted to grow at low pH have little reserve to further increase proton pumping, and it is the reduction in intracellular pH that is actually responsible for the increase in cytotoxicity (231). The potential degree of enhancement in killing is substantial and as a result considerable effort has been made to accomplish this feat in vivo. The most widely studied method has been induction of hyperglycemia. The logic behind this approach is that excess glucose load to the tumor will push it toward glycolysis and lactic acid production, since most tumors have a limited oxygen supply and also have defects in respiratory pathways. Induction of a hyperglycemic state may also reduce blood flow by increasing blood viscosity. Reduced perfusion could compromise heat exchange capacity, thereby increasing temperatures in tumor during heating. Many early studies in rodents focused on administering glucose intraperitoneally and led to hypovolemia as a result of shifts in water balance to offset the hyperosmotic state in the peritoneal cavity. The resultant shifts in tumor pH were dramatic, but not clinically relevant (233). When hyperglycemia has been administered intravenously, there has been less of an effect on perfusion, but changes in extracellular pH have still been observed (107,189). Effects on perfusion, however, may be glucose-dose dependent. In a recent study, it was shown that 1 g/kg glucose had no effect on perfusion, while 4 g/kg showed transient reduction in perfusion by 30% (189). In this case, the changes in perfusion are likely attributable to changes in red cell deformability created by the hyperglycemic condition (214).

In humans, the induction of hyperglycemia has been accomplished by either oral or intravenous glucose administration.

Results using this approach have been mixed. On average, the drop in extracellular pH is about 0.17 pH units, which is near the goal of 0.2 pH units (107). However, there is considerable variation from one patient to the next in terms of how effective this approach is. Furthermore, in prediabetic patients, the trend is toward an increase in pH rather than a decrease. In canine patients with soft tissue sarcomas, induction of hyperglycemia via intravenous administration did not result in any significant change in either intracellular or extracellular pH (160).

The use of hyperglycemia has resulted in improved response to thermochemotherapy and thermoradiotherapy in rodents (117,221). It is not known whether the degree of pH reduction resulting from a pH manipulation strategy in human tumors correlates with an improvement in response to thermoradiotherapy. One human study in a limited number of patients suggested improvement in response with the use of hyperglycemia combined with thermoradiotherapy (134). However, pH was not measured, and the study was not randomized.

The addition of agents that can selectively drive down tumor intracellular pH, such as glucose combined with the respiratory inhibitor MIBG (metaiodobenzylguanidine), has the potential to further enhance hyperthermic cytotoxicity selectively in tumor tissues (Fig. 28.11) (12,242). Some groups have also focused on the use of pharmacologic agents that block the extrusion of hydrogen ions from cells, which is normally accomplished via membrane bound pumps. Utilization of such agents, in combination with acidification of the extracellular space, can lead to enhanced hyperthermic cell killing both in vitro and in vivo (192).

Blood Flow Manipulation

There is no question that blood perfusion is a major impediment to effective heating. This is because perfusion is the primary mechanism for conducting heat. Thus, if tumor blood flow can be effectively reduced, temperatures in the tumor will increase. A number of vasoactive agents have been shown to reduce tumor blood flow, including those that are normally considered to be vasodilators. The reason for this paradoxic effect in tumors relates to several factors:

1. The relative lack of arteriolar input to tumors,
2. Pre-existing vasodilation in the few arterioles that tumors have, and
3. The presence of relatively high flow resistance, which is exacerbated when blood pressure is reduced as is frequently encountered with the use of vasodilators (82,183,184).

Many studies have been conducted in murine models with agents such as hydralazine (82). Although use of such agents can quite effectively decrease tumor blood flow, they may not be easily implemented clinically because of the attendant risks of creating hypotension. In human clinical studies, reduction in tumor blood flow following hydralazine administration does not occur in the absence of hypotension (41). Continuous administration of nitroprusside to a dose that decreases mean arterial pressure by 40% will lead to significant improvement in tumor temperatures, but the attendant risk to the patient makes this approach unfeasible (162). Hypertensive agents, such as angiotensin II, will not work because, although they cause vasoconstriction, they also cause hypertension. Thus, the net effect on tumor blood flow is unpredictable and heterogeneous (11,213).

Another approach would be to use agents that cause peripheral vasoconstriction, such as nitric oxide synthase inhibitors. Whereas such approaches are effective means to reduce tumor perfusion (123,212) and Po2 in preclinical models (66), they have not been tested clinically. This method was attempted in a pilot study in dogs. When the nitric oxide synthase inhibitor L-NAME was administered to normal beagles undergoing local

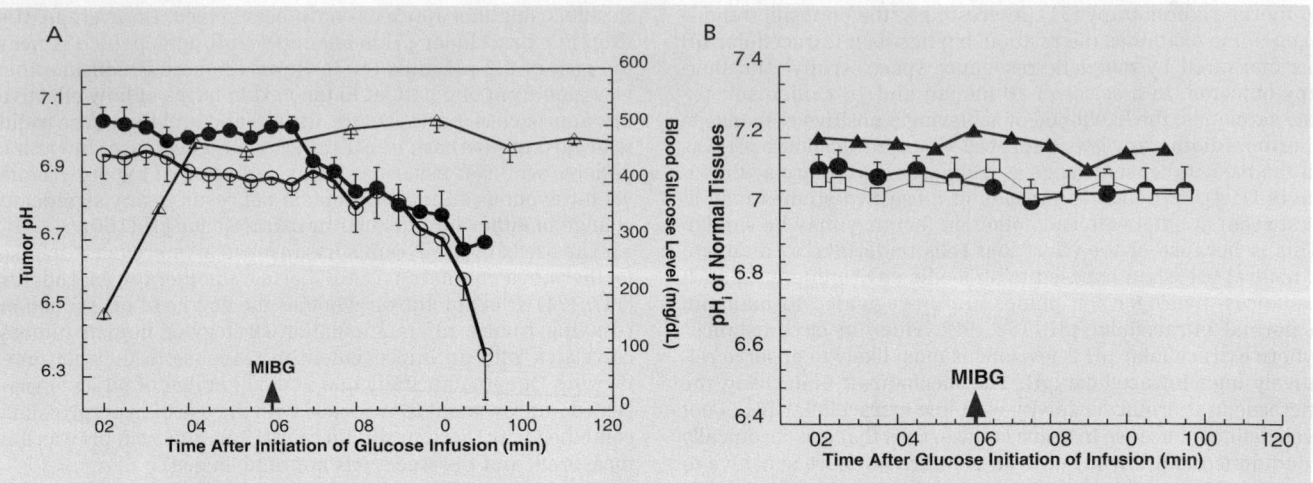

FIGURE 28.11. A: The pH profile of human melanoma xenografts (≤ 8 mm; $n = 7$) in response to hyperglycemia and metaiodobenzylguanidine (MIBG) (30 mg/kg, i.p.). ●, pH_i O, pH_e. The profile of blood glucose levels (△) during intravenous infusion of glucose without MIBG was obtained from weight- and age-matched cohorts ($n = 9$), which were not used in MRI experiments. Points are mean ± SEM. **B:** The pH_i profile of normal tissues (liver, muscle, and brain) in response to hyperglycemia (475 mg/dL) and MIBG (30 mg/kg); ●, liver ($n = 3$); □, muscle ($n = 1$); σ, brain ($n = 1$). Points are mean ± SEM. Note that the combination of hyperglycemia and MIBG causes selective acidification of tumor, with little effect on normal tissues. (From Zhou R, Bansal N, Leeper DB, et al. Intracellular acidification of human melanoma xenografts by the respiratory inhibitor m-iodobenzylguanidine plus hyperglycemia: A 31P magnetic resonance spectroscopy study. *Cancer Res* 2000;60:3532–3536, with permission.)

hyperthermia to the thigh, slight hypertension occurred, but there were no substantive toxicities after treatment. The treatment was effective in reducing muscle perfusion, because temperatures in the heated volume increased after L-NAME administration. In two older animals with spontaneous soft tissue sarcomas, however, pancreatitis developed posttreatment (158). Careful examination of the histories of these two animals suggested that they had comorbid conditions that predisposed them toward developing pancreatitis. This may explain why the younger and healthier beagles did not develop this side effect. There is still merit in this approach in humans, since nitric oxide synthase inhibitors have been administered for treatment of other conditions such as septic shock (180). Pancreatitis has not been reported as a side effect in humans.

Clearly it makes sense to consider combinations of approaches that can reduce both tumor blood flow and pH. The dual combination of both approaches could lead to improved temperature distributions as well as heat sensitization. A pioneer in the application of this general approach was Manfredd von Ardenne, who coined the term *cancer multistep therapy*, when he combined hyperglycemia, nitroprusside, and hyperthermia (199,228).

Hyperthermia and Metastases

Hyperthermia causes abrupt changes in tumor microvascular function, including increased perfusion, and changes in endothelial gap size (97,171). Such changes suggest that there might be opportunity for enhanced tumor cell shedding. One series of papers examined this question in the B16 melanoma model and found that local hyperthermia enhanced the metastatic rate when tumor was grown in the foot pad (136, 137). Two other studies with different tumor models showed either a reduction in metastases following local hyperthermia (2) or no effect on the incidence of metastases, relative to controls (10).

The question of whether local hyperthermia increases the risk for metastasis is difficult to answer in clinical trials unless the primary therapy has high probability for local control. In a phase III trial of canine patients with primary malignant melanomas treated with the combination of hyperthermia and

radiation or radiation alone, we found that there was no difference in the likelihood for metastasis between the two groups (44). However, local recurrence was a common event, and its onset was frequently followed by appearance of distant metastases. In a recently completed phase III randomized trial of human melanomas treated in a similarly designed trial, there was significant improvement in the likelihood for survival when the local tumor was controlled. Since the use of hyperthermia in that trial resulted in improved local control, the implication is that the combination therapy reduced the probability for metastases in this setting (150,151). Gillette et al. (62) conducted a randomized phase II study comparing graded doses of radiation with or without hyperthermia for treatment of canine soft tissue sarcomas. Higher normal tissue temperatures in the region of the tumor were positively correlated with a lower likelihood for distant metastases.

In a randomized phase II study, dogs received radiation therapy in combination with local hyperthermia alone or local hyperthermia plus whole body hyperthermia (209). There was no improvement in duration of local control with the combination of local and whole body hyperthermia. Of more concern, perhaps, was the observation that the addition of whole body hyperthermia increased the likelihood for distant metastases. In a separate study, Lord et al. (114) reported alteration in the location of metastases of dogs with osteosarcoma that were treated with whole body hyperthermia. Kapp and Lawrence (88) also performed a retrospective study of patients who had received brachytherapy for carcinoma of the cervix and found an increased risk for developing distant metastases in the group of women who developed fever during the period of the brachytherapy.

The question of enhanced metastases with hyperthermia has rarely been examined carefully in other human clinical trials where local or regional hyperthermia has been used, however, because many patients in such series already had metastatic disease or had tumors with high likelihood for development of them anyway. Perhaps one exception to this rule has been an extensive series of patients with previously untreated high-grade soft tissue sarcomas who were treated preoperatively with hyperthermia and radiation. A recent update on this series of nearly 100 patients indicates that the local control rate is near 90%, but about 50% have gone on to develop distant metastases

(163). This rate of metastasis is nearly identical to that seen with preoperative radiotherapy alone in other patient series.

The conclusion that can be drawn regarding this issue is that with the exception of one study with the B16 melanoma, there is no evidence that local-regional hyperthermia causes an increase in metastases. When whole body hyperthermia is used, the issue is not resolved.

Radiation and Hyperthermia

Rationale for Combining Hyperthermia with Radiotherapy

When radiation is combined with hyperthermia, complementary effects occur. Cells in the S-phase of the cell cycle are relatively radioresistant. In the case of hyperthermia, these cells are most sensitive. Hypoxic cells are known to be three times more resistant to radiation, as compared with aerobic cells. With hyperthermia, there is no difference in sensitivity between aerobic and hypoxic cells. There is good evidence in one human tumor (soft tissue sarcoma) and in some rodent models that hyperthermia can lead to reoxygenation, which will further improve radiation response (19,193,229). Finally, hyperthermia inhibits the repair of both sublethal and potentially lethal damage via its effects in inactivating crucial DNA repair pathways (125,167,168).

Factors to Consider When Combining Hyperthermia with Radiotherapy

The interaction between radiation and hyperthermia is described by the *thermal enhancement ratio* (TER), which is analogous to a dose-modifying factor for any adjuvant to radiation. When examining paired radiation survival curves, the TER is equal to the ratio of doses to achieve an isosurvival. Alternatively, it can be defined as a ratio of doses to achieve an isoeffect, such as the dose to achieve 50% probability for tumor control. A number of murine studies compared TERs for tumor and normal tissues, and in some cases it was possible to demonstrate therapeutic gain. However, the methods used for induction of hyperthermia in rodent studies (usually waterbath) resulted in equivalent heating in both the normal tissue and tumor (148). Although this approach probably resulted in defining the limiting case for normal tissue tolerance, it was not analogous to the clinical setting where it is relatively difficult to heat normal tissue as effectively as tumor because of differences in perfusion response to heating. In spite of these limitations of waterbath heating, many authors have demonstrated therapeutic gains for thermoradiotherapy compared with either treatment alone in a variety of preclinical models.

The most typical normal tissue end point has been moist desquamation. For this end point, the sequence between irradiation and hyperthermia has been critical, with simultaneous application of the two treatments not yielding any evidence for a therapeutic gain. The goal to achieve a therapeutic gain would be to have the $TER_{tumor} > TER_{normal}$. The best therapeutic gains were seen when 3 or 4 hours were allowed to elapse between administration of radiation and hyperthermia (146–148,208).

Since moist desquamation is rarely dose limiting in radiotherapy, it is not a very relevant clinical end point. Urano et al. (219) reported that the TERs for late tissue complications in the feet of mice that received combinations of hyperthermia and radiation were lower than TERs for moist desquamation. Similar results were reported by Stone (200), using leg contracture as an end point for normal tissue damage. Sminia et al. (187) examined the effects of hyperthermia combined with radiation in the lumbosacral region. With 41.1°C heating for 30 minutes following irradiation of single doses of 20 to 32 Gy, the TER was between 1.24 and 1.32 and the time to paralysis was shortened from 359 to 214 days. Of perhaps equal importance was the observation that tumorigenesis was significantly enhanced with this protocol. The incidence of tumors in the group of animals treated with radiation alone was 17% and the incidence was doubled when hyperthermia was added (33%). Other papers by this same author demonstrated a similar effect in animals treated in the cervical spine region (187), and Urano et al. (219) have reported similar results for the combination of heat and radiation therapy on mouse feet. Most of the tumors were sarcomas, and in the study by Sminia et al. (187) there were no tumors of the spinal cord or associated adventitia. It is important to consider the fact that the rodent lines used by these investigators are particularly tumor prone. Other studies done in mice, with long-term follow-up following thermoradiotherapy applied to limbs have not reported any data relating to tumor induction (200). Additionally, to date there have been no clinical reports of tumorigenesis in sites previously treated with thermoradiotherapy, even with long-term follow-up. Thus, it is not known whether this observation has clinical relevance.

Thermal enhancement ratios for local control have been estimated for a number of human tumors using historical control data for radiation alone (149). In most tumor types examined, these ratios were >1 for tumor control. Assessment of normal tissue TER has not been attempted except in a few cases. For those examples, TER values for normal tissue damage have been less than those for tumor in the same patient population, suggesting potential for therapeutic gain for thermoradiotherapy compared with radiotherapy alone (149). Prospective randomized trials in dogs with spontaneous tumors have also shown evidence for therapeutic gain with hyperthermia (61,62). In one prospective randomized study in dogs with oral squamous cell carcinomas, the TER for bone necrosis was not >1, whereas the TER for tumor control was approximately 1.2, demonstrating that a modest therapeutic gain was achieved (61). In a second study involving dogs with soft tissue sarcomas, a radiation-dose effect relationship was not identified, and, therefore, it was not possible to determine a TER (62). This may have been attributable to the fact that a large degree of heterogeneity existed with respect to other prognostically important variables, including thermal doses achieved within the tumors, tumor size, and variation in grade. In another prospective randomized study involving cats and dogs with a variety of tumors that were treated with radiotherapy with or without hyperthermia, there was no difference in the incidence of late normal tissue complications between the two arms. This trial was done using a single radiation dose fractionation scheme, so calculation of a TER would not be possible. However, the fact that there was no difference in late complications for this single dose suggests that the TER was likely near a value of 1 (43).

The greatest degree of interaction between hyperthermia and radiation occurs when the two treatments are administered simultaneously. Until recently, it was not technically feasible to perform simultaneous treatment when external beam irradiation was used, but methodologies to achieve this effect are currently under development and clinical evaluation (128,133,201). The rationale for doing simultaneous treatment comes from the fact that normal tissue is rarely heated as well as tumor. This is partly because of differences in heat transfer capacity of tumors versus normal tissues. In addition, usually power is deposited preferentially into tumor, either because of the physical setup of applicators for treatment of superficial tumors or interstitial applications, or adjustment of phase and amplitude of phased array devices for treatment of deep-seated tumors. When the two modalities are separated by more than 30 to 60 minutes, the interaction is dominated by additive effects. Hyperthermia has also been shown to eliminate the radiation dose-rate effect in situations where it is administered continuously or intermittently with brachytherapy (232).

In summary, most available data from preclinical and clinical studies indicate that therapeutic gain is achievable for the combination of hyperthermia with radiotherapy. There is very little evidence to suggest that hyperthermia enhances the incidence or severity of late normal tissue complications, particularly when temperatures in surrounding normal tissue tend to be less than tumor. The reports by Sminia et al. (187) indicating the possibility for enhanced damage to spinal cord following thermoradiotherapy provide a cautionary note for using heating methods that might heat the cord, if this is done in conjunction with doses of radiation near the cord that are within 30% of tolerance.

Hyperthermia and Chemotherapy

Rationale for Using Hyperthermia with Chemotherapy

Many chemotherapeutic agents have demonstrated synergism with hyperthermia including cisplatin and related compounds, melphalan, cyclophosphamide, nitrogen mustards, anthracyclines, nitrosoureas, bleomycin, mitomycin C, and hypoxic cell sensitizers (69). The mechanisms that underlie the synergy may include (a) increased cellular uptake of drug, (b) increased oxygen radical production, and (c) increased DNA damage and inhibition of repair (28). Hypoxia and pH appear important in the thermochemotherapeutic response.

Factors to Consider When Combining Hyperthermia with Radiotherapy

An important factor in the potential use of hyperthermia with many drugs is its ability to reverse, at least partially, drug resistance. Examples of drugs for which this has been shown include cisplatin (31,74), melphalan (153), nitrosoureas (27), and doxorubicin, when combined with the MDR inhibitor, verapamil (9). The mechanisms underlying the reversal of drug resistance are not well defined and are not always the obvious target. For example, reversal of drug resistance has been seen in vivo for melphalan-resistant human rhabdomyosarcoma xenografts, but this could not be explained by alterations in cellular glutathione levels, although this is a known resistance mechanism for melphalan (103).

Combinations of camptothecins with hyperthermia have not shown consistent results in vitro. The interaction between these agents and hyperthermia is schedule and temperature dependent (89,139). In one report, temperatures up to 41.8°C increased the activity of topoisomerase II, which may be the explanation for the increased activity of these drugs at elevated temperatures (89). Enhancement of drug activity has been seen in vivo (207).

Tubulin binding agents, such as taxol, show no evidence for interaction in vitro (105), but studies in combination with radiation therapy in vivo are more encouraging (22). There may be physiologic consequences of the combination of taxol and hyperthermia that make the combination work better than predicted from in vitro studies. As was discussed above, clinically relevant temperature–time combinations can lead to reoxygenation. Taxanes can do the same thing via induction of apoptosis (124). Although it has not been studied directly, one can speculate that the combination of these two treatments may improve tumor oxygenation better than either one alone.

Generally speaking, most antimetabolites do not interact with hyperthermia when given concomitantly (28). However,

it is important to consider issues such as time of drug exposure and temperature, both of which may be important in determining where and when to expect a positive interaction. When 5FU has been given simultaneously with hyperthermia, there have been only additive effects (141). However, 5FU has been shown to interact supra-additively with hyperthermia under specific conditions. Heating to 39°C to 41°C can lead to enhanced conversion to active metabolites, thereby increasing drug cytotoxicity. In addition, continuous infusion protocols with this drug may lead to cell cycle block in S phase, a relatively sensitive part of the cell cycle to hyperthermia (93).

For most drugs (excluding 5FU and perhaps other antimetabolites), the optimal sequence between heat and drug is to administer them simultaneously or to give the drug immediately before the onset of heating. For platinum containing drugs, the tissue extraction rate of drug may be increased with hyperthermia, further substantiating the rationale for use of this sequence (220).

The degree of interaction between drugs and hyperthermia is temperature and cell line dependent (28). There are certain drugs that are not particularly active at normothermia but become very cytotoxic at elevated temperatures. Such drugs have not been investigated extensively, but if this feature could be exploited further, it could be a means to protect critical non-heated normal tissues from chemotherapeutic damage. One such drug is the free radical generator, AAPH (2,2'-azobis [2-amidinopropane] dihydrochloride). Under normothermic conditions, this agent is minimally cytotoxic to CHO cells in vitro. However, when the temperature is increased to 42°C, several logs of cell killing can be seen for 60-minute heating (101).

There are also some classes of drugs for which there has been no demonstrated synergistic interaction. Interactions with etoposide have been unpredictable, and current recommendations are that one cannot expect synergistic interactions with it (28). There is also no evidence for synergistic interaction between vinca alkaloids and hyperthermia.

In the case of hyperthermia, the term *trimodality* has been used to describe combination therapy of hyperthermia, drugs, and radiation. It has been studied in in vitro and in vivo models (72). Limited, but encouraging pilot human data, based on the combination of the hypoxic cell sensitizer, etanidazole, radiation, and hyperthermia, have been reported (14). The combination of 5FU, hyperthermia, and radiation therapy has yielded favorable responses in patients with locally advanced colorectal cancer in a phase II study (170), which has led to the current conduct of a randomized phase III trial of 5FU with radiation with or without hyperthermia.

Hyperthermia and Liposomally Encapsulated Drugs

In a classic paper, Yatvin et al. (240) suggested that a temperature-sensitive liposome could be used to selectively deliver drug to tumors. Several subsequent papers have described the potential of using hyperthermia to augment liposomal drug delivery to tumors (52,76,93,132). These studies have involved use of thermally sensitive liposomes as well as more traditional liposomal formulations, with or without PEGylation of the lipid to extend circulation time. In general, it can be stated that the combination of hyperthermia with such drug carriers has increased drug delivery and drug efficacy as compared with using drug carrier alone or free drug with hyperthermia (99). Studies in cats with spontaneous vaccine-associated soft tissue sarcomas demonstrated a two- to 16-fold increase in liposomal delivery to tumors when hyperthermia was used (118). Until recently, there had been no systematic comparison of hyperthermia with free drug, nonthermally sensitive liposomes and thermally sensitive liposomes. This comparison has now

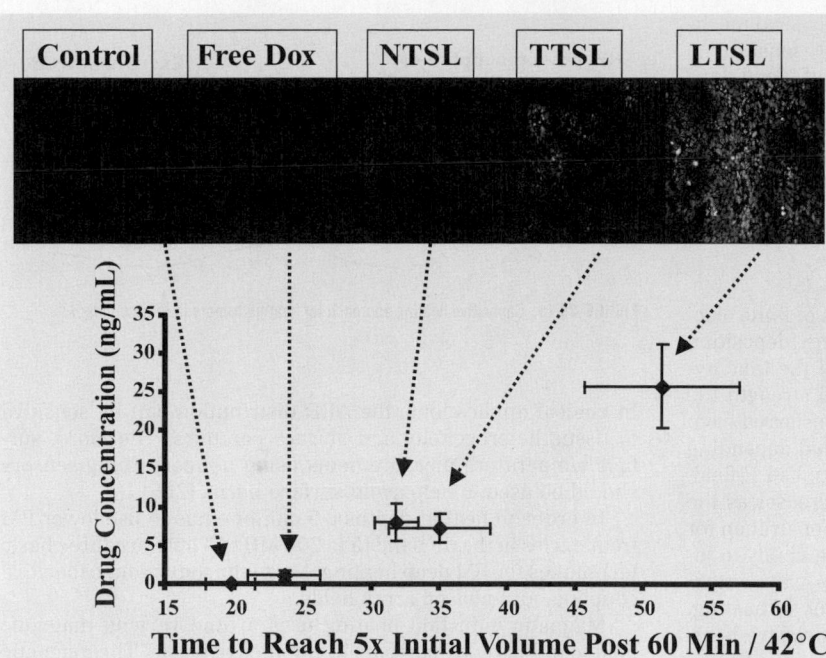

FIGURE 28.12. Relationship between the amount of drug delivered, as measured directly in tumor tissue and growth delay in FaDu human tumor xenograft line for a variety of doxorubicin containing liposome formulations. Top panel depicts fluorescence micrographs of frozen sections. Since doxorubicin is fluorescent, it provides a visual comparison of the amount of drug in each type of tumor. Actual concentrations of drug were measured using standard extraction and HPLC methods. In the LTSL group, 17/20 animals were tumor free at 60 days post-treatment (end of experiment), so follow-up time was set to 60 days. All data in this figure represent animals that received local heating of the tumor-bearing limb (42°C for 60 minutes). Control, heat only; free Dox, free drug plus heat; NTSL, nonthermally sensitive PEGylated (long circulating) liposome plus heat; TTSL, thermally sensitive PEGylated liposome formulation developed by Gaber (Gaber MH, Wu NZ, Hong K, et al. Thermosensitive liposomes: Extravasation and release of contents in tumor microvascular networks. *Int J Radiat Oncol Biol Phys* 1996;36:1177–1187) that releases contents at about 42.5°C to 43°C; LTSL, low temperature sensitive liposome that releases contents at 39.5°C to 40.0°C. (Data replotted from Kong G, Anyarambhatla G, Petros WP, et al. Efficacy of liposomes and hyperthermia in a human tumor xenograft model: Importance of triggered drug release. *Cancer Res* 2000;60:6950–6957.)

been made, using doxorubicin-containing liposomes, including a novel low temperature sensitive formulation that exhibits very rapid release of drug (50% release when reaching its release temperature of 40°C) (138). The low-temperature–sensitive liposome was clearly more effective than any other formulation as assessed using tumor growth delay as an end point. The difference in effectiveness was demonstrated to be related to a significant improvement in drug delivery to tumor as well as increased drug binding to DNA (96) (Fig. 28.12).

Hyperthermia and Gene Therapy

Several investigators have exploited the heat shock response as a means to perform gene therapy. The heat shock promoter is highly inducible and relatively quiescent under normothermic conditions. For example, heating to 42°C for 30 minutes in a cell line that has been stably transduced with green fluorescence protein, under control of the HSP70 promoter, yields several hundred-fold induction of reporter protein expression (76). GFP expression as assessed by fluorescence, under normothermic conditions, is indistinguishable from nontransduced cells. Cell lines transduced with interleukin 12 (IL-12) under control of the same promoter yielded over a 13,000-fold induction of protein expression following 30 minutes heating at 42°C. Levels of expression in vivo were over 30-fold induced following intratumoral injection of adenovirus containing the HSP70-IL12 gene. Therapeutic studies with this approach yielded several important observations:

1. The gene therapy plus hyperthermia induced tumor growth delay in the B16 melanoma model was superior to heat alone or gene therapy alone,
2. When radiation therapy was added, superior results were obtained, relative to all controls (112) (Fig. 28.13),
3. Following intratumoral injection of adenovirus, gene expression could be localized to heated tumor only for the heat inducible promoter, whereas spurious expression patterns were seen when a constitutive promoter was used (113).

Other investigators have sought to further increase transgene expression by combining the HSP70 promoter with a con-

stitutive promoter (57). Additional approaches that have been investigated include use of the HSP70 promoter to drive suicide gene therapy mediated by thymidine kinase conversion of the prodrug gancyclovir to a toxic chemotherapeutic agent (13,15), other cytokines such as tumor necrosis factor-α (TNF-α) (79) and restoration of wild-type P53 to induce apoptosis (142,164).

Hyperthermia Physics

Clinical hyperthermia is usually achieved by exposing tissues to conductive heat sources or nonionizing radiation (e.g., electromagnetic [EM] or ultrasonic [US] fields). Although these

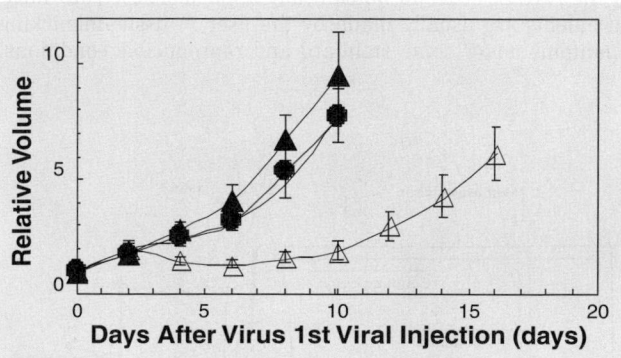

FIGURE 28.13. Adenovirus-mediated, heat-regulated gene therapy in a mouse melanoma model. The HSP70 promoter was used to drive gene expression of interleukin-12 (IL-12). Experimental tumors were established in syngeneic C57BL6 black mice by implanting 10^6 tissue cultured B16F10 melanoma cells. Viral injections were carried out 1 week later when tumors grew to sizes of 5 to 7 mm in diameter. Mice were injected intratumorally with adenoviruses encoding (a) a heat inducible EGFP gene alone (●); (b) a heat inducible EGFP gene with heat treatment (□); (c) the murine IL-12 gene (σ) alone; and (d) the murine IL-12 gene with heat treatment (△). There were 10 animals in each group. The error bars for all the data points represent the standard error of the mean. (Data replotted from Huang Q, Hu JK, Lohr F, et al. Heat-induced gene expression as a novel targeted cancer gene therapy strategy. *Cancer Res* 2000;60:3435–3439.)

modalities deposit energy in tissue by different physical mechanisms, they have general similarities. They are sensitive to the heterogeneity of tissue properties, geometry of blood flow, and the practical problems of coupling the energy source into tissue. Conductive heating is largely restricted to interstitial applications because of the close source-tissue proximity. For the physical fields (EM or US), energy transfer can be delivered either invasively or noninvasively.

Electromagnetic Heating

When an electric field (E-field) exists in materials of finite electrical conductivity resistant heating occurs. Energy deposition is proportional to conductivity and the square of the time average magnitude of the E-field. For a given field strength the conductivity determine the amount of energy transferred from the EM field into tissue. Conductivity varies 50-fold depending on the type of tissue and the frequency of the applied E-field. For all tissue types the electrical conductivity increases as the EM frequency increases. This implies, improved penetration for low frequency or long wavelengths. However, the ability to localize EM energy deposition is dependent on the wavelength. The longer the wavelength, the broader the focus of heating. Thus, there is a fundamental constraint on noninvasive heating by EM techniques that does not allow localized heating at depths >2 to 5 cm. Deep penetration implies regional energy deposition involving substantial volumes of normal tissue.

Electromagnetic Heating Devices

A range of EM heating devices have been developed for external applications of hyperthermia. These devices can be separated into two categories: Superficial applicators with effective penetration into tissue in the range of 2 to 5 cm and deep heating devices that have effective penetration >5 cm. The superficial devices include waveguides, microstrip or patch antennas that operate in the microwave band typically at 433, 915, or 2,450 MHz (Fig. 28.14) (36). More sophisticated array applicators are also available, such as multielement arrays and mechanically scanned antennas. These devices provide local control of the energy absorption rate distribution (ARD) to prevent hot and cold regions in the tissue (67,106,196). All of these devices are usually coupled into tissue through a deionized water bolus. This bolus is usually temperature controlled to maintain the skin temperature below 43°C. These devices require measurements of the ARD in order to be clinically applied. These ARD measurements are usually made by the user in tissue-mimicking phantoms under some standard and reproducible conditions.

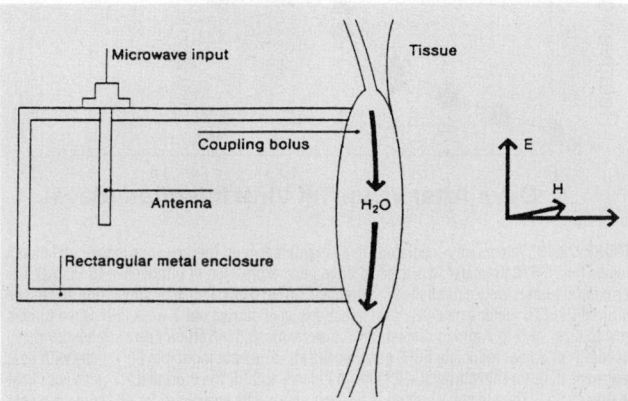

FIGURE 28.14. Generic schematic of the microwave waveguide device used for superficial tumors.

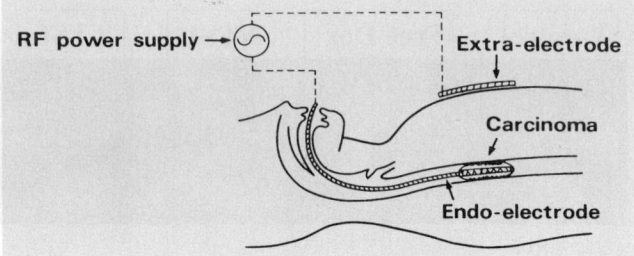

FIGURE 28.15. Capacitive heating approach for heating tumors in the esophagus.

In clinical applications, the ARD distribution can be sensitive to tissue heterogeneity and surface contours. Therefore, surface temperature measurements using nonperturbing sensors should be used to help avoid surface burns (236).

In order to heat at depths >5 cm, one has to use lower EM frequencies in the RF band (5 to 200 MHz). There are three basic techniques for EM deep heating: Magnetic induction, capacitive coupling, and phased array fields.

Magnetic induction heating uses a time varying magnetic field to induce eddy currents in conductive tissue. The magnetic susceptibly for all tissues is essentially equal to 1. Therefore, the magnetic field distribution is not sensitive to tissue type and is consistently predictable. However, the eddy current distribution is governed by paths of least resistance and will be affected by tissue conductivity. In addition, for static induction coils there are null regions in the ARD.

Deep heating using the capacitive technique uses RF field in the frequency range of 5 to 30 MHz. Ion currents are driven between two or more conductive electrodes. With this technique the heating tends to be concentrated at the electrodes. Therefore, the electrodes make contact through a saline pad or bolus. The saline can be temperature controlled to prevent hot spots on the skin surface and superficial fat. Varying the size of the respective electrodes can shift the current distribution toward or away from the respective electrode. An extreme application of this is to use a needle electrode with a large surface return electrode to do thermal ablation in tissue. Similarly, this can be done with a balloon electrode for intracavitary applications (e.g., esophagus) (Fig. 28.15) (116).

The third option for noninvasive deep heating is the RF phased array technique (216). These devices consist of an array of RF antennas arranged in a geometric pattern that is conducive to the body region that is to be heated (Fig. 28.16) (36). The antennas are driven from a common RF source (i.e., coherently). This means that at any time there is fixed phase relationship among the antennas. This allows the RF fields from the antennas to add together in a way to form a null or a focus. In the latter case, one can achieve better ARD penetration into tissue than what one would achieve by operating the antennas independently (i.e., driving the antennas incoherently).

For phase array applications in the abdomen and pelvis, the antennas are arranged circumferentially to allow the RF E-fields parallel to the fat–muscle interface (see Fig. 28.16) (36). This configuration reduces the risk of hot spots in the superficial fat. In general, the phased array technique has more flexibility for controlling the ARD than magnetic induction and capacitive techniques.

Ultrasound Heating

Energy transfer from the acoustic field is associated with viscous friction. Energy absorption is characterized by the acoustic absorption coefficient, which increases with frequency. Therefore, the penetration of US field decreases with frequency.

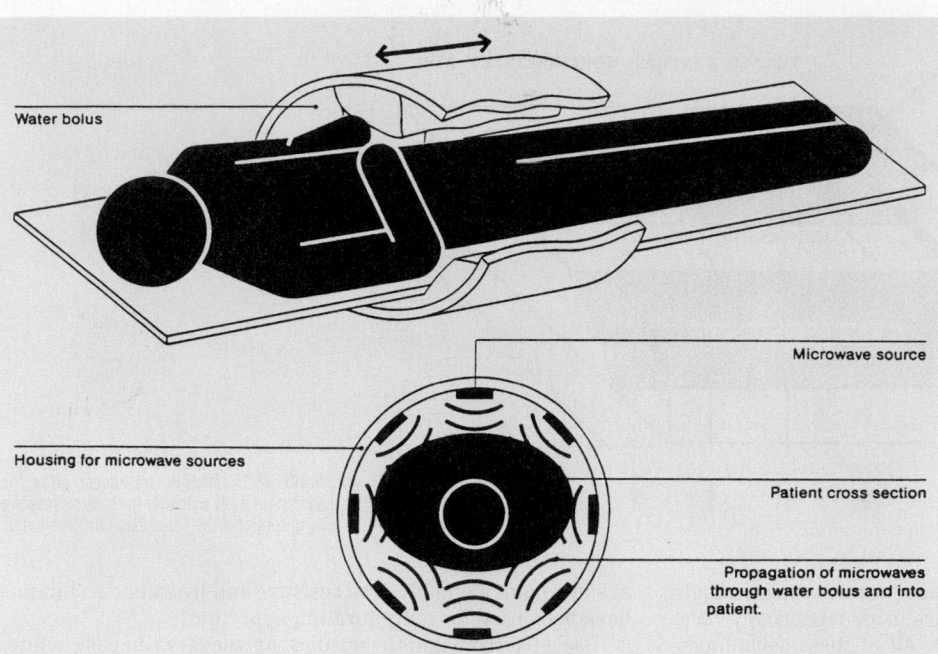

FIGURE 28.16. Generic schematic of the electromagnetic-phased array device for heating the lower abdomen and pelvis.

However, because the wavelength of an US field is several orders of magnitude smaller than that of an equipenetrant EM field, the problems of applicator size and focusing of US field energy in deeper tissues are greatly reduced. However, as previously noted, anatomic geometry and tissue heterogeneity (air reflects, bone preferentially absorbs) severely limit the utility of US. The availability of an adequate "acoustic window" (a path unobstructed by bone or air proximal and distal to the target) is often a problem in clinical applications. The size of entry window for the US beam will determine the size and depth of the target volume that a focused beam can effectively heat.

Ultrasound Heating Devices

As with the EM device, there are parallel sets of devices using US radiation. These include single transducers and multiple transducer devices for superficial tumors (2 to 5 cm) heating (Fig. 28.17) (36). These devices operative in the 1 to 3 MHz range (Fig. 28.18) (128,129,217). These devices are also coupled into tissue using a water bolus. The water in the bolus is temperature controlled to control surface temperatures. Since US cannot propagate in air, the bolus water has to be degassed (i.e., air has to be removed). This can be done by boiling the water or using vacuum techniques. If the water is not degassed the high intensity of the US field can form small air bubbles in the bolus water and thus scatter and reflect the US energy. Additionally, care has to be taken at the bolus and body surface interface to ensure energy transfer into tumor. Good surface contact is achieved by using a coupling gel.

Deep heating using US is accomplished by using scanned focused transducer, phased arrays, or multiple scanned focused transducers (Fig. 28.19) (36). US frequency for deep heating are in the 500 kHz to 2 MHz range. At these frequencies the penetration in soft tissue is substantial, and this can cause problems with bony structures both in front and behind the target volume. Care has to be taken if the beam path both enters and exits the body. In this situation, the exit surface will reflect the beam at the body air interface. This can cause an exit surface burn. An additional water bolus at the exit surface will prevent the burn.

Interstitial Hyperthermia

Interstitial heating has the same characteristics as interstitial radiation: A highly localized and inhomogeneous dose, invasiveness, and sensitivity to technique. It is usually combined with brachytherapy where one can make double use of the implant for both hyperthermia and radiation. Some techniques permit simultaneous delivery, but most clinical experience has been with sequential heat and radiation.

Several techniques have been proposed for utilizing conductive heat sources. These include electrical resistive heating

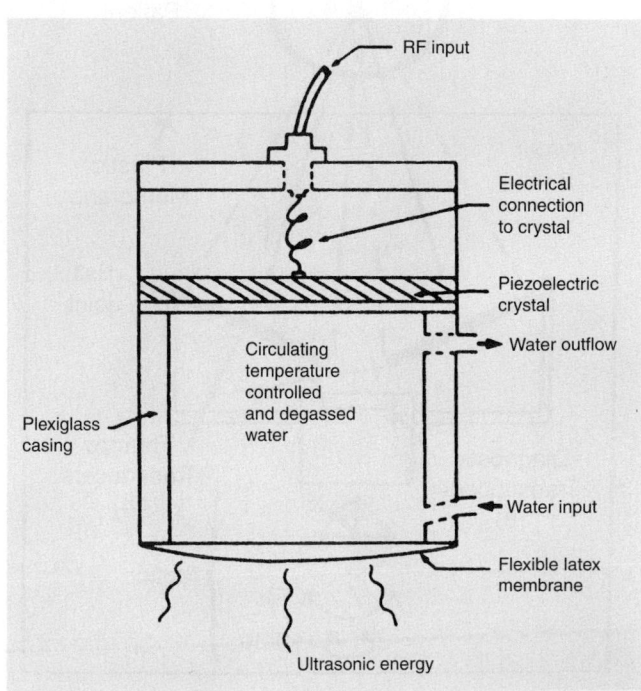

FIGURE 28.17. Generic schematic of the single transducer ultrasound applicator for use in superficial hyperthermia.

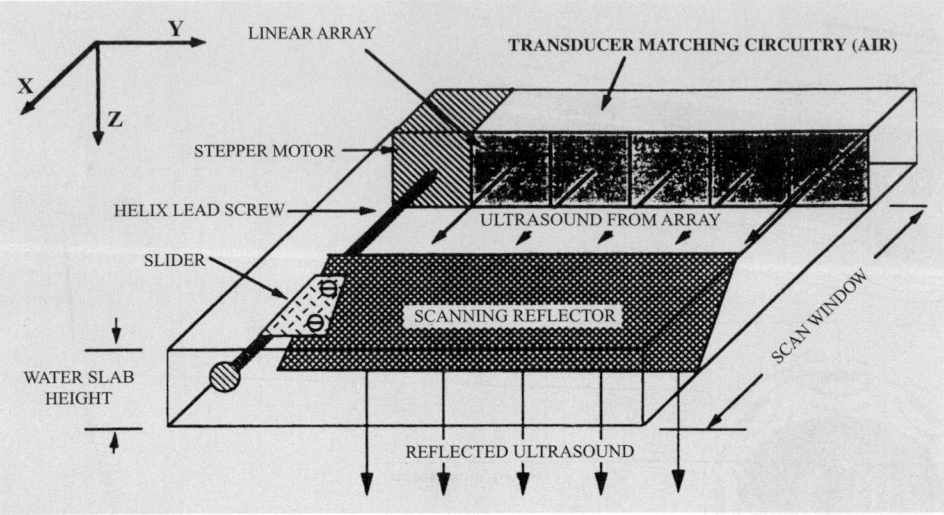

FIGURE 28.18. Multiple transducer array that can mechanically scan over the body surface providing control of the absorption rate distribution.

elements, hydraulic systems that circulate heated water through tubes, and ferromagnetic seeds that are heated externally via a time-varying magnetic field (17,197). All of these techniques require relatively dense implant spacing (<1.0 cm between sources) because the heat transfer is through thermal conduction. Additionally, the uniformity of the temperature is very sensitive to blood flow cooling.

The hydraulic technique is conceptually simple but requires control of fluid flow through manifolds to multiple small diameter tubes. For resistive heating, an electrical resister and temperature sensor are included in a metallic implant needle (32), allowing control of the temperature of each needle (at least

at some point along it). Both resistive and hydraulic techniques have been used for long-duration hyperthermia.

Use of ferromagnetic needles or seeds with well-defined Curie points offer the possibility of intrinsic thermal regulation. By positioning the implant in a low frequency (~ 100 kHz) external magnetic field, the ferromagnetic material is heated by induced eddy currents (18,197). When the seeds heat above the Curie temperature, the alloy undergoes reversible phase transition from high to low magnetic susceptibility, energy absorption decreases, and the seed temperature becomes self-regulating at the Curie point. Although an elegant idea, the use of ferromagnetic seeds has had limited success in clinical applications (211) in part due to the failure of the developed alloys to perform as ideal ferromagnetics. Recent advances may solve this problem (120).

The most common interstitial heating techniques have used low frequency (0.2 to 30 MHz) RF or MW fields (198). With the former, two or more implanted needle electrode pairs are connected to an RF generator and RF current (predominantly mobile ions) flows between oppositely polarized electrodes (Fig. 28.20) (25). Direct contact between the metal electrodes and tissue is required, but insulation can be used to prevent heating along selected regions of the electrodes (e.g., at the skin puncture site). This technique suffers from the concentration of current density around the electrodes, thus requiring close electrode spacing (1 to 1.5 cm) and regular geometry. Heating near electrodes often causes treatment-limiting pain. Electrode cooling with air or water is advantageous but has not been routinely employed. Heterogeneous tissue conductivity or nonparallel electrodes can further compromise temperature uniformity. Recent devices have incorporated sequential electrodes that allow for more control of the temperature distributions (Fig. 28.21) (222).

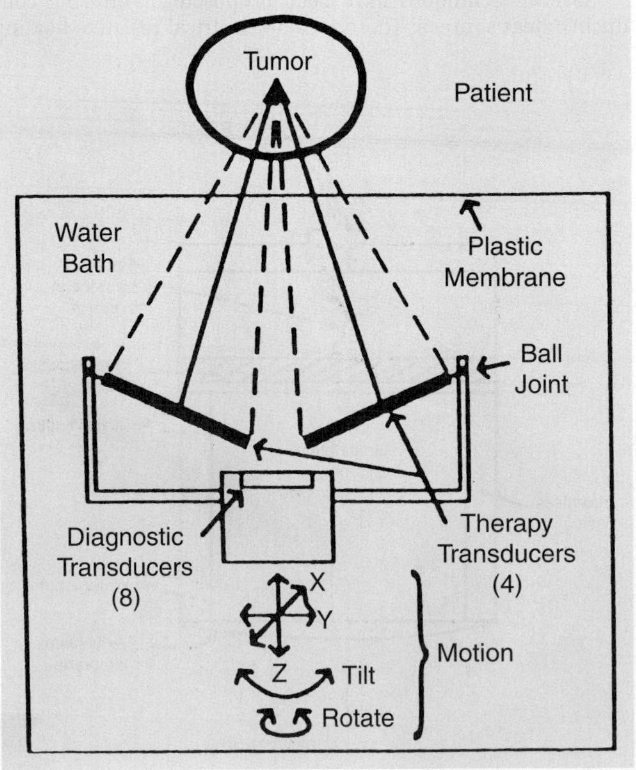

FIGURE 28.19. Schematic of mechanically scanned focused ultrasound transducers for deep heating.

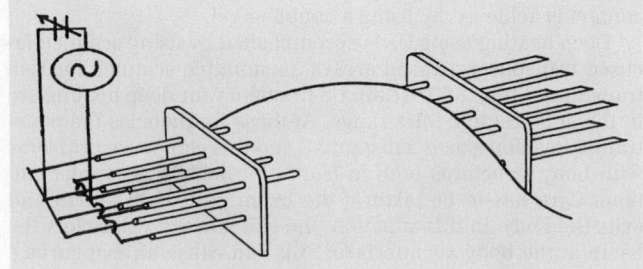

FIGURE 28.20. Schematic of the radiofrequency interstitial implant.

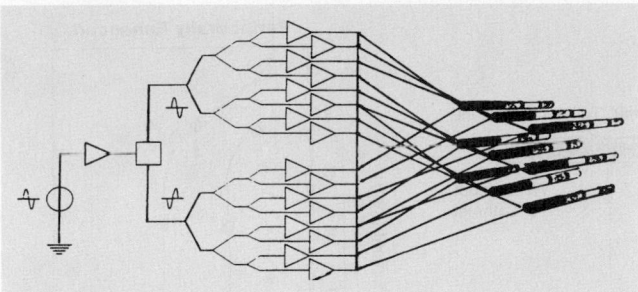

FIGURE 28.21. Schematic of radiofrequency implants having segmented electrodes that provide more control over the heating distribution.

For MW interstitial heating (204), the EM wavelength in tissue is on the order of a few centimeters. Therefore, the length of a single implanted electrode is about equal to the EM wavelength so it is not an equipotential surface and heating is intrinsically nonuniform along its length. In addition, insulation has little effect because in this frequency range, current induction is predominantly capacitive (due to molecular polarization) instead of conductive (due to free ion drift).

Interstitial MW antennae are usually designed as a coaxial transmission line having outer and inner conducting elements separated by a low-loss insulating layer. If the outer conductor is interrupted, the EM field leaks or radiates into the space around the interruption. Various designs for terminating the coaxial line have been used to allow this region to efficiently radiate EM energy into the surrounding tissue. One method is to remove a specified length (e.g., one quarter wavelength) of the outer conductor at the end of the coaxial line. A specific antenna will operate efficiently only in a narrow frequency band, and the radiation field pattern can depend on the antenna's insertion depth into tissue. The radiation field along a specific antenna cannot be adjusted to accommodate varying tumor dimensions. In practice, different antennae operating at different frequencies are required. The frequencies most commonly employed are 433, 915, and 2,450 MHz. These frequencies are appropriate for heating linear tissue dimensions of 10, 5, and 3 cm, respectively.

Another problem with interstitial MW antennae is that the field at the tip of the insertion end is generally significantly less than the field a quarter wavelength removed from the antenna end. Because of this "cold tip," the antenna must extend beyond the margins of the target tissue (not always clinically permissible). Variations in antenna design can somewhat reduce this effect (179).

Although heating along the length of interstitial antennae has fundamental problems, the radial energy deposition pattern is less concentrated around a MW antenna than an RF electrode, particularly when antenna arrays are employed which permit larger spaces between the array elements (e.g., 2 cm). In addition, EM fields from adjacent coherently phased antennae can interact constructively, allowing advantageous energy distributions, resulting in maximum temperature in the center of the array rather than around each antenna. Controlling the field and heating pattern by dynamically changing the relative phases of antennae in an array is another possibility (215,241).

Ultrasonic elements for interstitial heating have been developed (46,78). Small cylindrical piezoelectric elements are aligned in a linear array with lengths on the order of several centimeters (45) (Fig. 28.22A,B). The elements radiate US in the frequency range of 3 to 6 MHz. Penetration at these frequencies permits implant spacing of 2 cm with better temperature uniformity than MW. A further advantage of this approach is the stacked-array structure that can provide longitudinal control along the implant (46). This differs from the segmented low frequency electrode since each array element can be independently controlled.

Thermal Dosimetry

Cell death and tissue damage associated with hyperthermia are dependent on the magnitude and duration of temperature elevation. For several in vivo and ex vivo systems the damage has been characterized by an Arrhenius response. For in vitro cell lines, the Arrhenius relation can be used to derive an isoeffect for cell kill. One commonly used isoeffect for hyperthermia cytotoxicity is that of Sapareto and Dewey (177), which characterizes the CHO cell line:

$$t_{43} = \int_{t=0}^{f} R^{[43° - T(t)]} dt \tag{3}$$

$$\sim \sum_{n=1}^{N} R^{(43° - T_n)} \Delta t_n \tag{4}$$

where t_{43} is the time at 43°C that produces the same cell kill as the temperature–time history indicated in the integral or summation. The coefficient R is a compilation of various activation energies associated with biological effects, some destructive and some protective for cell life. Thus it is observed that R takes on different values for temperatures above and below 42.5°C:

$$R = \begin{cases} \frac{1}{2} \text{ for } T \geq 42.5° \\ \frac{1}{4} \text{ for } T \leq 42.5° \end{cases} \tag{5}$$

This temperature is referred to as the break point. It may have different values for different cell types (166). Nonetheless, the concept of equivalent minutes at 43°C has been used as a basic unit in hyperthermia. Measured dose using equivalent minutes has been shown to correlate with clinical outcome (69,86,145,186).

Bioheat Transfer

To appreciate this problem of quantitative dosimetry for thermal therapies consider the process of bioheat transfer in tissue. A bioheat differential equation can be written:

$$\rho_t c_t \frac{\partial T}{\partial t}(\vec{R}, t) = \dot{Q}_0(\vec{R}, t) + \nabla \cdot [\bar{k}_t \vec{R}] \cdot \nabla T(\vec{R}, t)] + \dot{Q}_b(\vec{R}, t)\vec{R} \tag{6}$$

where $\rho_t, c_t, \bar{k}_t, (\vec{R})$ are the density, specific heat and thermal conductivity of tissue, respectively. The term on the left side of the equation represents the rate of gain or loss of thermal energy in a given differential volume ΔV. The right side of this equation is separated into several terms that represent the rates of heat production associated with metabolic processes, $\dot{Q}_m$, energy absorption due to external or nonmetabolic internal sources, $\dot{Q}_0$, energy transfer by thermal conduction, $\nabla \cdot [\bar{k}_t(\vec{R}) \cdot \nabla T(\vec{R})]$, and blood flow, $\dot{Q}_b$. At normal resting temperatures an equilibrium state exists:

$$0 = \dot{Q}_m(\vec{R}) + \nabla \cdot [\bar{k}_t(\vec{R}) \nabla T(\vec{R})] + \dot{Q}_b(\vec{R}) \tag{7}$$

This equation indicates a condition where thermal energy generated from the metabolic processes is exactly balanced by the transfer in and out of a given volume by thermal conduction and blood flow. In attempts to produce local or regional hyperthermia, an additional energy source term, $\dot{Q}_0$, is introduced. This energy source is usually derived from a device (such as an electromagnetic or ultrasound radiator) that directly transfers energy into tissue. The addition of energy to tissue temporarily induces a rise in tissue temperature (i.e., $\frac{\partial T(\vec{R}, t)}{\partial t} \geq 0$) until a new state of equilibrium is achieved:

$$0 = \dot{Q}_m(\vec{R}) + \dot{Q}_0(\vec{R}) + \nabla[\bar{k}_t(\vec{R}) \cdot \nabla T'(\vec{R})] + \dot{Q}_b(\vec{R}) \tag{8}$$

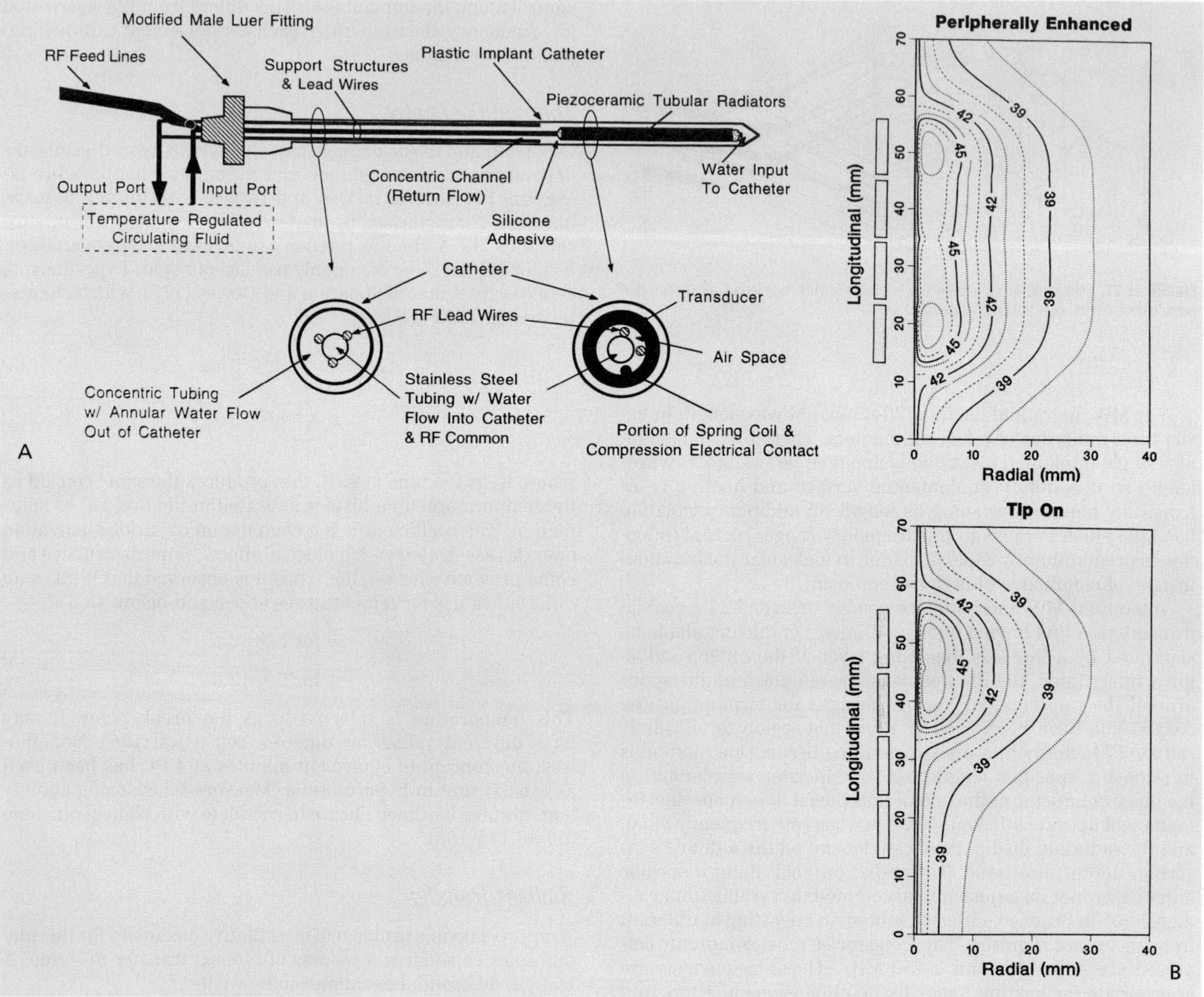

FIGURE 28.22. A: Schematic of the segmented ultrasound interstitial needles. **B:** Demonstration of absorption rate distribution control with the segmented ultrasound implant needles.

This added energy source plus the original metabolic source is again counter balanced by thermal conduction and blood flow. However, the new equilibrium state is at a higher absolute temperature, $T'(\bar{R})$, than that found originally. When the external energy source is removed the tissue temperature returns to its original level. This time–temperature history is illustrated in Figure 28.23 (172).

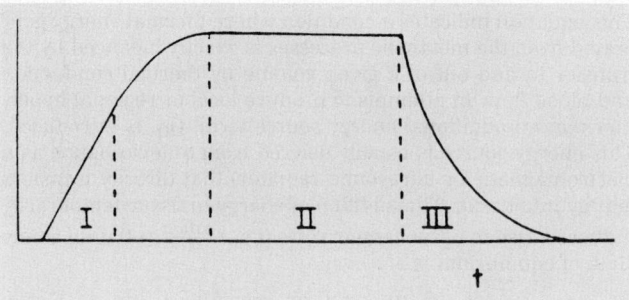

FIGURE 28.23. Time versus temperature plot for hyperthermia treatments.

The objective of conventional local or regional hyperthermia therapy is to achieve an equilibrium state in which temperatures are nominally in the range of 40°C to 45°C, and maintain this elevated temperature condition for a time period on the order of an hour. Uniform dose requires the construction of the term, $\dot{Q}_o(\bar{R}, t)$ with sufficient magnitude, spatial, and temporal variation in order to balance the thermal conduction and blood flow heat transfer processes in the target volume. This power density distribution (W/m³) when divided by the respective tissue density ($\dot{Q}_o/\rho$) is referred to as the specific absorption rate (SAR) and has units of watts/kg.

The conductive and blood flow processes of heat transfer associated with in vivo systems are complex, and achieving the desired state of clinical hyperthermia is difficult. There is an indication of this in the specific terms of equation 6. For example, thermal conduction is a well-understood process of heat transfer, but in the clinical applications the thermal conductivity, $\bar{k}_t(\bar{R})$, is dependent on tissue type. This is additionally complicated by the irregularities of tissue geometry and interfaces. Second, heat transfer by blood flow is a complex phenomenon. It depends on the vascular architecture and has its own temperature-dependent dynamics, both of which are not subject to generalization in that they depend on the particular clinical problem (i.e., differs for each patient). Therefore,

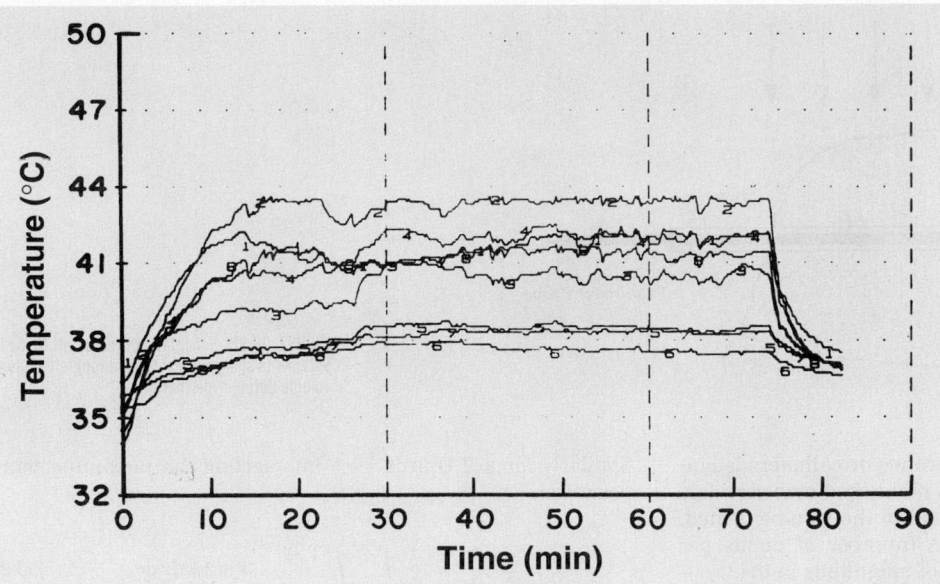

FIGURE 28.24. Typical temperature data acquired during a hyperthermia treatment.

even if it were technically possible to produce SAR with arbitrary control, additional knowledge of tissue thermal properties, geometry, and blood flow are needed in order to obtain temperature uniformity in a given local or regional target volume. The practical consequence of this is that temperature heterogeneity is the rule in the current state of the art for clinical local/regional hyperthermia (Fig. 28.24). Also, since real-time heat transfer calculations are not feasible, temperature has to be measured invasively during the treatment. Needless to say, such measurements are severely limited and estimations of thermal dose delivery are suspect.

If one considers the thermal isoeffect relation equation 3, it predicts that a very high temperature for a short time period will produce the same thermal damage as a long time period at low temperature. For example, a given volume of tissue heated to 60°C for 5 to 10 seconds will produce cell kill that is equivalent to a 43°C exposure for ~182 hours. Tissue exposed to such a temperature will be totally destroyed. When the thermal dose is delivered in a short time period compared to the characteristic times associated with thermal conduction and blood flow heat transfer, the temperature distribution is closely approximated by the SAR distribution. This short duration, high temperature thermal dose delivery provides a way to reduce the temperature heterogeneity encountered in low temperature, long duration hyperthermia. Thus, for rapid hyperthermia, the main consideration required to characterize the thermal dose distribution is absorbed power distribution. (Note there can still be dose heterogeneity associated with power absorption in different tissue types.) Provided the power device is not limited, a thermal exposure based on a minimum dose can be delivered to completely destroy tissues in some predefined volume. This type of therapy is referred to as thermal ablation.

Thermal tissue ablation has a long history in therapeutics. The use of RF currents to cauterize tissue to prevent bleeding during surgery is one example. Recently, there has been considerable interest in the idea of noninvasive tissue ablation using RF probes and ultrasound radiation. This idea also is not new (55), but there is a resurgence of interest because of the feasibility of combining real-time imaging to guide the positioning of an externally focused US beam (78). In particular, the use of thermally sensitive magnetic resonance imaging (MRI) techniques presents a variety of potential ablation applications for benign as well as malignant conditions. Image guided thermal ablation is in clinical testing.

Invasive Thermometry

Dosimetry in hyperthermic oncology is limited with respect to quantifying temperatures achieved in tissue. Typical temperature distributions are highly nonuniform and this lack of uniformity is not predictable based on the present applications of bioheat transfer modeling. The latter is true because the approximations used in the theoretical formulations of bioheat transfer equations do not produce solutions that model realistic clinical situations. Furthermore, empirical determinations of complete temperature distributions are not yet technically feasible, and resorting to a limited number of invasive temperature measurements seems an inadequate characterization in raw form.

A number of clinical reports correlate some temperature-related parameters (based on invasive sampling) to effective response (86,145). However, this effort has not been definitive with respect to defining prospectively the delivery of hyperthermia in a quantitative manner. Minimum temperature has been one of the more often-quoted prognostic temperature descriptors (69, 86,145). Biologically, it appears reasonable that treatment success is associated with the minimum achieved temperature. However, the determination of the true minimum temperature by sparse invasive sampling necessarily includes a large amount of sampling noise. This naturally leads toward testing measures of low temperatures that might be less sensitive to the variations associated with measurement of the extremes (i.e., maximum and minimum temperature). For example, the temperature denoting the lowest tenth percentile of measured temperatures may prove to be a more reliable predictor for prescribing effective hyperthermia prospectively (82,108). Further, one might assume that if complete knowledge of clinical temperature distributions were available, an association of clinical response with the fraction of target volume $(\frac{V_T}{V})$ achieving temperatures greater than some minimum value (T) would be a strongly predictive index.

Current clinical treatments are characterized by sampling several points within the volume during heating. In more aggressive situations, 15 to 30 spatial points are sampled using multiple sensor probes or by mechanically translating temperature probes through invasively placed catheters (thermal mapping) (60,77) (Fig. 28.25). Thermal mapping or its equivalent is now a quality assurance requirement in the delivery of hyperthermia in multi-institutional trials (40).

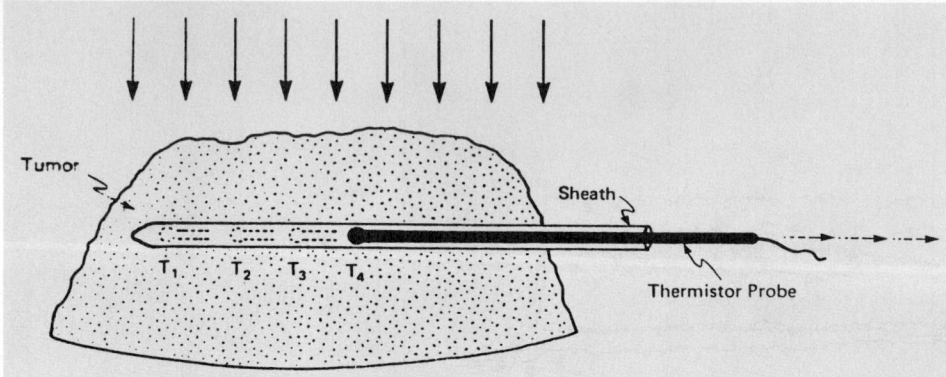

FIGURE 28.25. Schematic of temperature measurements along a linear track through the tumor volume during hyperthermia.

Because the number of invasive probes or catheters is limited in practice, the number of points monitored may correlate with but is not necessarily proportional to the volume heated. Thus, the density of sampled points (number of points per heated volume) can vary by an order of magnitude in the treatment of small tumors (<3 cm in diameter) compared to large tumors (>10 cm in diameter). Similarly, strategies for choosing sampled points (e.g., volume center vs. edge) are highly variable. Therefore, the value of sparse invasive temperature sampling for quantitatively characterizing hyperthermia treatments under such circumstances is suspect.

The possibility of estimating thermal descriptors such as $(\frac{V_T}{V})$ using measured data alone without explicit knowledge of bioheat transfer parameters such as blood flow, absorbed power density, and other relevant thermal tissue properties have been investigated (48). In particular, these prior results indicated the types of measurement bias that result from estimating $(\frac{V_T}{V})$ from linear temperature maps that might be routinely obtained in the clinic. It can be shown that in cases where nested geometry is associated with the isothermal distribution, a judicious choice of catheter placement would lend itself to making reasonable approximations of $(\frac{V_T}{V})$ using linear mapped data (48).

There is evidence that nested isotherms exist in tissue during hyperthermia, particularly for the low temperature isotherms (Fig. 28.26). A distribution of nested strictly increasing isotherms can be expressed in spherical coordinates as:

$$T_{(r,\theta,\phi)} = f\left[1 - \frac{r}{R(\theta,\phi)}\right] \tag{9}$$

where r, θ, ϕ are the spherical conduits, and $T(r, \theta, \phi)$ is the temperature for a point located at (r, θ, ϕ). The angular function $R(\theta, \phi)$ describes the general boundary shape of all isotherms f(0) yields the minimum tumor isotherm and f(1) gives the maximum tumor temperature. Since f(r) is a strictly increasing function, an inverse exists and the radial dependence of a given isotherm can be determined:

$$r = \alpha_T R(\theta, \phi) \tag{10}$$

where $\alpha_T = [1 - f^{-1}(T)]$, and T is the temperature of the isotherm.

This type of nested distribution allows a simple evaluation of the descriptor $\frac{V_T}{V}$:

$$\frac{V_T}{V} = \frac{1}{V} \int_0^\pi \int_0^\pi \int_0^{\alpha_T R(\theta,\phi)} r^2 \sin\phi \, dr \, d\theta \, d\phi \tag{11}$$
$$= (\alpha_T)^3$$

Similarly for a 2-D area slice intersecting the maximum temperature:

$$\frac{A_T}{A} = \frac{1}{A} \int_0^{2\pi} \int_0^{\alpha_T R(\theta,\phi')} r \sin\theta \, dr \, d\theta \tag{12}$$
$$= (\alpha_T)^2$$

where A is the area of the slice defined by ϕ' and $\frac{A_T}{A}$ is the fraction of this area that is at or greater than temperature T. Finally, for a linear track that intersects the maximum temperature

$$\frac{L_T}{L} = \frac{1}{L} \int_0^{\alpha_T R(\theta'',\phi'')} dr \tag{13}$$
$$= \alpha_T$$

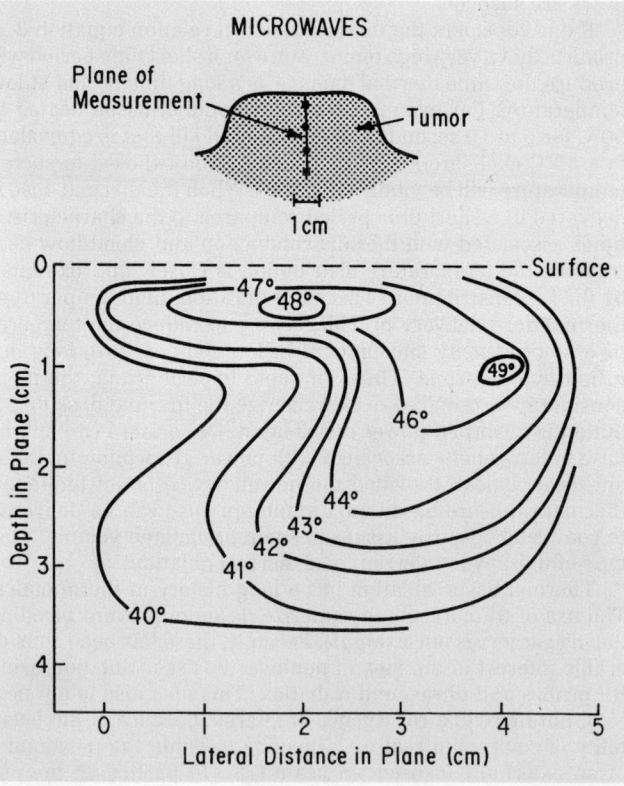

FIGURE 28.26. A reconstruction of temperature isotherms based on measurements using linear maps. These isotherms have nested isotherms particularly for the lower temperature values.

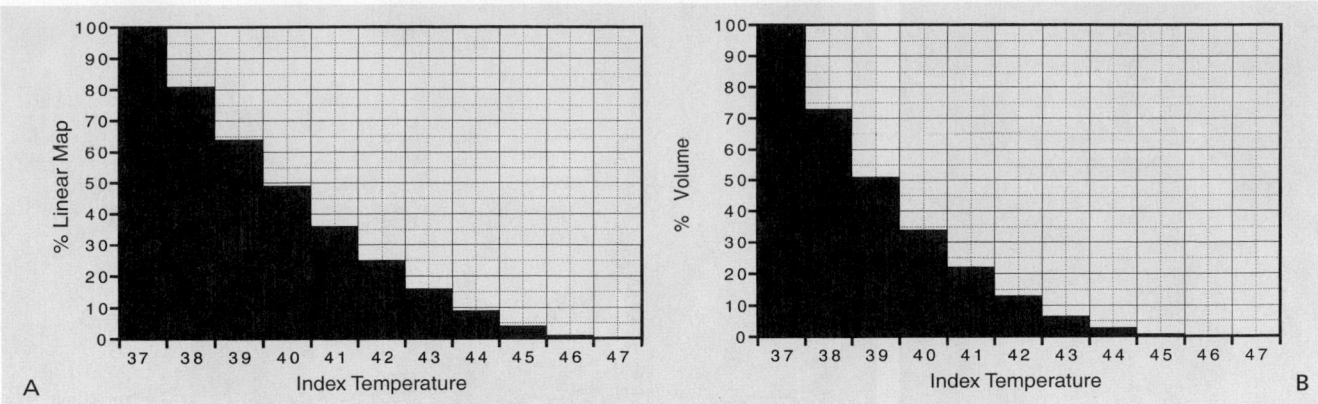

FIGURE 28.27. A: The distribution based on linear maps of the percentage of temperatures greater than a given index temperature. **B:** The distribution of the percentage of volume above a given index temperature derived from the linear map distribution of (A).

where L is the length of a linear track in the tumor at orientation defined by the angles (θ'', ϕ''), and $\frac{L_T}{L}$ is the fraction of that track at or above temperature T. Thus, the existence of nested isotherms points to a simple relationship whereby measured linear map data can be used to estimate αT and thereby estimates of $\frac{L_T}{L}$, $\frac{A_T}{A}$, and $\frac{V_T}{V}$. For the set of two-dimensional and three-dimensional temperature distributions, the linear temperature profiles obtained can be used to estimate αT and then, by squaring and cubing αT, estimates of $\frac{A_T}{A}$, and $\frac{V_T}{V}$. Thus, in clinical practice careful linear mapping of temperature distribution can provide volumetric estimate of the tumor dose (Fig. 28.27A,B).

Noninvasive Measurements of Thermal Dose

Progress in two areas, numerical modeling and MRI thermometry, have opened the door to noninvasive assessments of thermal dose. The development of finite element (FE) and finite difference (FD) models for calculating the SAR for specific heating devices allow for patient treatment planning and treatment optimization (29,210). These models are based on patient-specific anatomy derived from computed tomography (CT) or MRI scans. This geometry is segmented with respect to tissue type in order to assign appropriate material properties (e.g., thermal conduc-

tivity, electrical conductivity, dielectric constant) and assigned to each voxel of the FE or FD calculation (Fig. 28.28) (154). Depending on the grid resolution and numerical algorithms, SAR calculations can be carried out in a matter of hours (Fig. 28.29) (237). Verification of SAR calculations in vivo is difficult because of the limitation of invasive measurements. Nonetheless, there are several reports that indicate invasive measurement trend with the SAR calculations (29,210). More extensive verifications have been reported in phantom models (81).

The limitation of invasive techniques for characterizing temperature distributions has stimulated the development of noninvasive thermometry techniques. MRI is currently the preferred technology. Several MRI parameters are temperature sensitive including the relaxation time T_1, T_2, bulk magnetization and the proton resonance frequency shift (PRFS). The latter has shown to provide the best temperature sensitivity and is most commonly used (115,239).

Noninvasive temperature measurements using MRI has been shown to be useful for measuring SAR distribution in phantoms (30) with results of 0.3°C to 0.5°C. Reports in vivo have produced results of 0.5°C to 1°C with similar spatial resolution (21).

It is not clear at this time that MRI thermometry can be used to monitor and control thermal therapies in general. It has been

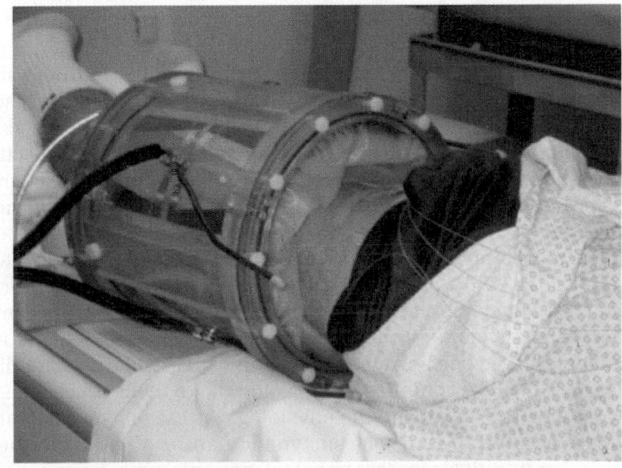
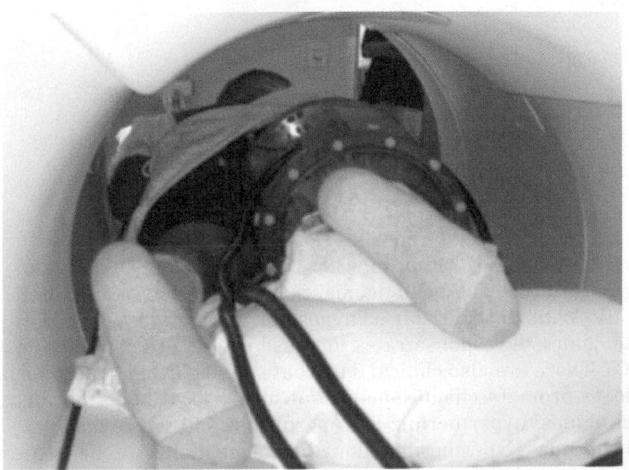

FIGURE 28.28. View of soft tissue extremity applicator **(A)** and patient positioning **(B)** in magnet for real-time noninvasive thermometry.

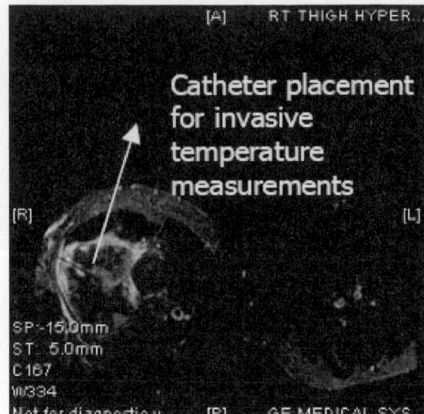
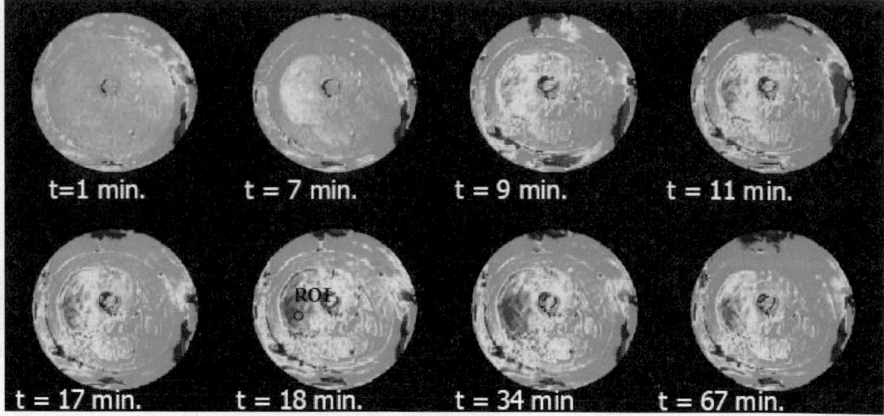

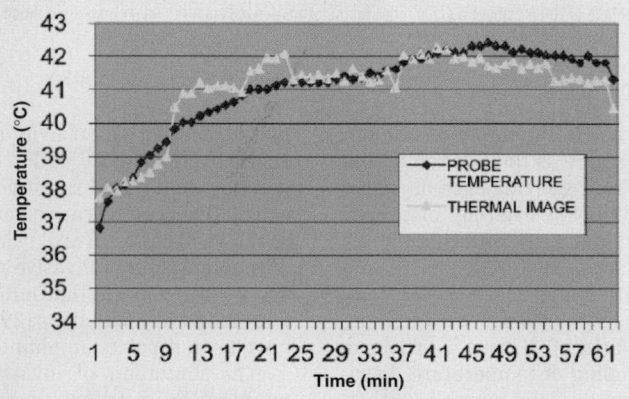

FIGURE 28.29. Magnetic resonance imaging localization of thermometry catheter (*top left*), thermal images taken during a treatment (*top right*), and comparison of the measured probe temperature and thermal images (*bottom*).

shown that this is feasible in specific applications such as thermal ablation with high intensity US for target volumes on the order of 3 to 4 cm^3. It has also shown that real-time control in MRI thermometry is possible for an intracavitary US device for heating the prostate. Other applications have been shown for tumors in the lower extremity (21). A role for MRI thermometry in large tumors in the lower abdomen and pelvis has yet to be demonstrated.

One can anticipate in the future that MRI and noninvasive MRI thermometry will be used to help verify the accuracy of numerical calculations of in vivo temperature distributions. An example of this is illustrated in Figure 28.30. These images represent the major achievement for this area of study.

Clinical Hyperthermia

General Considerations

There are numerous reports of hyperthermia combined with radiation, demonstrating superior complete response rates and significant thermal enhancement as compared to radiation alone. With the addition of hyperthermia to radiation, absolute complete response rates increase on the order of 20% to 30%. There are also clinical data that support using hyperthermia to promote chemosensitization using local hyperthermia techniques, hyperthermic limb perfusion, and whole body hyperthermia. Hyperthermia alone has been studied in the treatment of superficial tumors (122). Although an occasional response may rarely be noted, duration of response is short and

no long-term tumor control has been described with the use of hyperthermia as a sole treatment modality.

Clinical circumstances that may warrant the addition of hyperthermia to radiation or chemotherapy would include tumors that are locally advanced and unresectable such as bulky advanced cervix cancer. In addition, hyperthermia may be of benefit in neoadjuvant and adjuvant regimens to increase local control or decrease extent of surgery as for esophageal tumors, rectal cancer, or soft tissue sarcomas. Hyperthermia may be used for palliation of metastatic disease, particularly in situations where retreatment doses of radiotherapy may be limited due to prior treatment. There may also be a unique benefit to the addition of hyperthermia to radiation for melanoma, due to radiobiologic qualities of a broad shoulder on the radiation cell survival curve that may be obliterated with the addition of hyperthermia.

Overall, hyperthermia is quite well tolerated and does not significantly increase the toxicity of radiation or combined modality therapy. The most common side effect is superficial or subcutaneous tissue burn, first or second degree, which occurs in approximately 5% of all hyperthermia treatment sessions. There are potential medical contraindications to hyperthermia treatment that are related to the hyperthermia itself and effects of treatment devices. Regional deep hyperthermia is often associated with a physiologic stress similar to an exercise workout. Patients exhibit increased heart rate and blood pressure; vital signs should be monitored every 5 minutes. Patients ineligible for hyperthermia have significant cardiovascular disease or medical conditions that would make them vulnerable to complications related to the physiologic stress of hyperthermia. Also, because of the electromagnetic nature of the hyperthermia heating devices, treatment of patients with large metallic implants such as orthopedic rods and plates is not feasible.

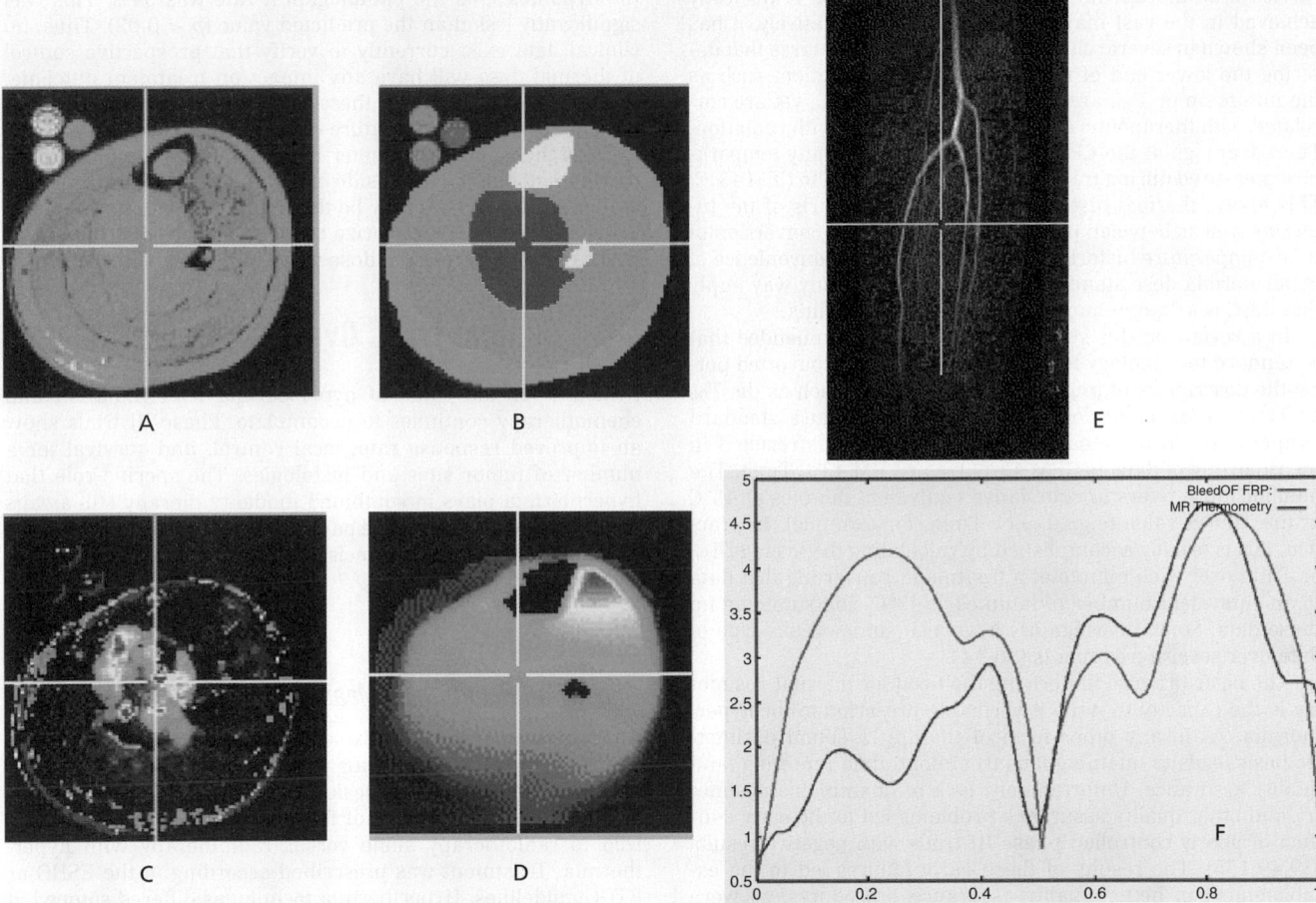

FIGURE 28.30. A: Magnetic resonance (MR) imaging is used to define the normal anatomy and tumor. **B:** Dynamic contrast studies with MR gives information associated with tissue perfusion. **C:** MR angiogram provides spatial locations of large vasculature. **D:** The SAR calculation is combined with the heat transfer equation solved with appropriate boundary conditions to obtain a temperature distribution. **E:** During the treatment MR thermometry data are acquired and compared with the numerical result. **F:** This combination of numerical prediction and MR measurement can be used to confirm the calculated distributions including the heat transfer dynamics.

Patients with pacemakers are not suitable hyperthermia treatment candidates.

Principles of Thermal Dosimetry

Currently, thermometry in the clinic is dependent on measurement of a fixed number of points, usually obtained via indwelling catheters. Successful implementation of thermal dosimetry requires three steps: (a) standardization of thermometric data acquisition, (b) standardization of data reporting, and (c) conversion of time–temperature data to units that have biologic and clinical meaning.

Data acquisition standards have previously been set by both the RTOG (Radiation Therapy Oncology Group) (40,178) and ESHO (European Society of Hyperthermic Oncology) (68,102). Standards for data reporting have not been established, but most parameters that have been described are based on simple descriptions of the multipoint thermometry, such as minimum temperature, average temperature, and so forth. A parameter that has proven useful for describing temperature distributions is the 10th percentile of the temperature distribution, which is commonly referred to as the T_{90} (90% of measured points exceed this value).

It is well established that the rate of cell killing is exponential and dependent on the temperature achieved. Roughly speaking, over the clinically relevant range of temperatures (39.5°C to 50°C), the rate of cell killing doubles for every degree increase in temperature. If thermotolerance is present at temperatures below 43°C, then the rate of cell killing changes by a factor of 4 for every degree decrease in temperature (37). This well-characterized relationship between temperature and rate of cell killing facilitated the development of a method for converting any time–temperature history into an equivalent number of minutes at a standard temperature, such as 43°C (177) (commonly referred to as CEM 43°C). There was slow acceptance of this dosimetric concept, largely because of early concerns about factors that could alter the rate of cell killing (such as thermotolerance). However, the value of this method of dosimetry for prediction of tumor response and duration of local control has now been established in a number of clinical trials (37), and early concerns about the validity of the concept have largely been dispelled (34).

One disservice that the CEM 43°C concept did for the hyperthermia community, however, was to foster the view that 43°C was a treatment goal, and that inability to achieve this temperature during treatment meant that the treatment had failed. Evaluation of many published clinical series state that the target treatment temperature was 43°C, and the primary design goal for many hyperthermia devices has been to achieve this temperature (203). In point of fact, temperatures during hyperthermia are never spatially uniform and frequently range between 39°C and 50°C during a single treatment. Some small zone within a tumor may reach the target of 43°C, but most temperatures are lower. Thus, a prescription based on a single target temperature carries little therapeutic meaning and cannot be realistically achieved in the vast majority of patients. Alternatively, it has been shown in several clinical series that temperatures that describe the lower end of the temperature distribution, such as the minimum or T_{90}, are usually well below 43°C, yet are correlated with therapeutic effects when combined with radiation. The advantage of the CEM 43°C concept is that any temperature measured during treatment can be converted to CEM 43°C. This allows thermal histories within different parts of the tumor as well as between patients to be made. The conversion of time–temperature histories to CEM 43°C for the convenience of hyperthermia dose standardization does not in any way imply that 43°C is a "target temperature" for hyperthermia.

In a review on this subject, Dewey (33) recommended that a standard terminology be implemented, which converted percentile descriptors of multipoint thermal data, such as the T_{90} or Tmin, to an equivalent number of minutes at a standard temperature. In the most common form, this has resulted in the reporting of data as CEM 43°C T_{90} or CEM 43°C Tmin. The nomenclature refers to cumulative equivalent minutes at 43°C at the Tindex value (e.g., T_{90} or Tmin, for example). In practice, this is usually accomplished by calculating the average T_{90} or Tmin over each minute of a treatment, converting that data to an equivalent number of minutes at 43°C, and summing up those data. Some investigators have also summed this type of data over several treatments (86,144).

The basic premise underlying the need for thermal dosimetry is the capacity to write a verifiable prescription for hyperthermia. As in any other form of therapy, a sound dosimetric basis leads to unambiguous treatment, data reporting, and quality assurance. Unfortunately, lack of quantifiable dosimetry and other quality assurance problems led to the early conduct of poorly controlled phase III trials with negative results (39,49,155). The results of these early failures led to the establishment of better quality assurance procedures, as were adopted by European, Asian, and North American investigators (37).

Many trials have shown positive relationships between measures of thermal dosimetry and treatment outcome (37,182). In all of these studies, thermal analysis was performed retrospectively. Two studies were published that compared various numbers of heat treatments, given in combination with fractionated radiotherapy (52,86), using the assumption that more treatments would yield greater thermal dose. Neither of these papers showed any benefit with higher numbers of hyperthermia fractions, which could in part be due to the fact that there was considerable overlap in thermal doses. Temperature is a stronger determinant of thermal dose than time-at-temperature because dose is an exponential function of temperature.

Thrall et al. (209) tested the hypothesis that radiation therapy combined with whole body hyperthermia plus local hyperthermia would yield greater CEM 43°C T_{90} than local hyperthermia alone and superior local control rates in dogs with soft tissue sarcomas. This study failed to show any advantage for combining the two heating methods in spite of the fact that the thermal doses were higher in the whole body plus local hyperthermia arm. One potential explanation for the lack of improvement in local control might have been the induction of thermotolerance during the whole body hyperthermia phase, which was administered prior to application of local heating.

Based on retrospective analysis of thermal dosimetry results from an earlier phase II trial examining the value of preoperative thermoradiotherapy for soft tissue sarcomas (144), we designed a prospective thermal dose prescription trial. The dose prescription was to achieve a cumulative thermal dose between 10 and 100 CEM 43°C T_{90}. The outcome variable was pathologic complete response (CR) rate assessed at the time of surgery. Based on our historical data, we predicted that the CR rate should be >75%. In a recent report, we were unable to prove

the hypothesis, as the pathologic CR rate was 54%. This was significantly less than the predicted value ($p < 0.02$). Thus, no clinical data exist currently to verify that prospective control of thermal dose will have any impact on treatment outcome. One explanation for why these trials have been negative relates to the sparse temperature sampling that is used. Typically, a single thermometry catheter is placed in the tumor, and the thermometer is moved inside the catheter to obtain multiple temperature points. It may be that more detailed thermometry is needed to fully characterize the temperature distribution as well as to control thermal dose more uniformly.

Clinical Trials Overview

Evidence for the value of hyperthermia with radiation and chemotherapy continues to accumulate. Phase III trials show an improved response rate, local control, and survival for a number of tumor sites and histologies. The specific role that hyperthermia plays in combined modality therapy still awaits further refinements, in large part due to the technical challenges of heating tumors and imprecise knowledge of thermal dosimetry.

Breast Cancer

Chest Wall Recurrence: Measurable Disease

An international collaborative effort combined the results from five randomized control trials with individual patient data for measurable breast cancer lesions where local therapy was indicated and surgery was not feasible. Patients were randomized to radiotherapy alone versus radiotherapy with hyperthermia. Treatment was prescribed according to the ESHO or RTOG guidelines. Hyperthermia techniques differed somewhat between the various studies but details of technique and thermometry are thoroughly documented. Figure 28.31 shows the odds ratio for a complete response for each individual trial as well as for the combined individual data. Overall, the odds ratio shows a benefit to the addition of hyperthermia (odds ratio 2.3 with a 95% confidence interval 1.4 to 3.8).

There are several potential shortcomings of this study, some of which are inherent to the meta-analysis process. There is significant heterogeneity in the patient selection criteria and treatment parameters. In addition, the use of concurrent systemic chemotherapy was employed in a nonrandomized manner. This is a reflection of the necessary medical management in this population of patients with high risk for systemic relapse and/or already existing distant metastases. Nonetheless, this is a very important collaborative study that helps to define the role of hyperthermia in breast cancer chest wall recurrence.

Two papers were published on thermal dose response in the combined radiotherapy and hyperthermia arms of the previous five randomized trials. Five thermal parameters were tested in one of these analyses, and all of these parameters were associated with the low regions of the measured temperature distributions. Two of five thermal parameters were found to have a significant association with the complete response rates: Max (TDmin) and Sum (TDmin). TDmin is the lowest thermal dose recorded at any measurement point during a treatment. (TDmin) is equivalent to the parameter equivalent minutes EQMIN T_{100} 43°C introduced by Oleson et al. (145). The Max (TDmin) is the maximum of these TDmin values over a series of treatment for a particular patient. Sum (TDmin) is the TDmin values summed over a series of treatments for a particular patient.

Using a categorical relationship with a cut off of 10 minutes for Sum (TDmin), the complete response rate was 77% for Sum (TDmin) >10 minutes and 43% for Sum (TDmin) ≤10 minutes ($p = 0.022$, adjusted for study center and significant clinical

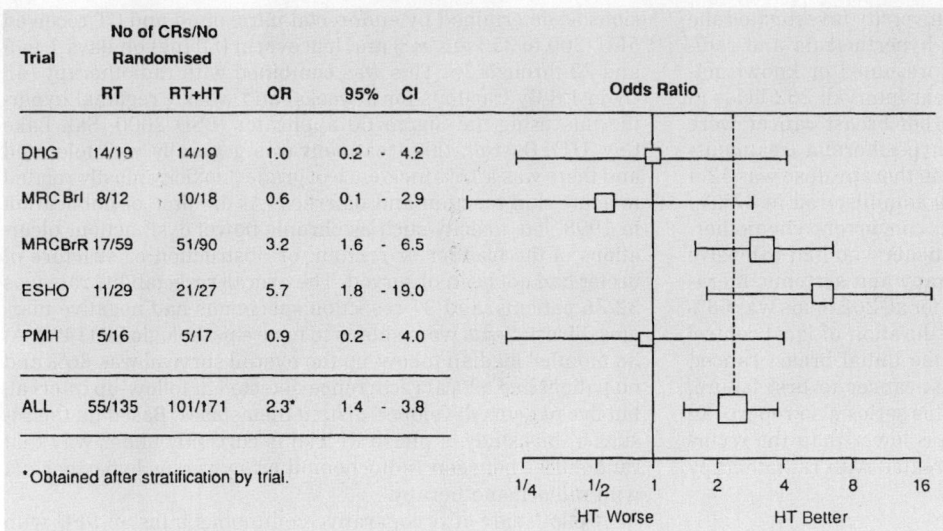

Trial	No of CRs/No Randomised		OR	95% CI	
	RT	RT+HT			
DHG	14/19	14/19	1.0	0.2 - 4.2	
MRC BrI	8/12	10/18	0.6	0.1 - 2.9	
MRCBrR	17/59	51/90	3.2	1.6 - 6.5	
ESHO	11/29	21/27	5.7	1.8 - 19.0	
PMH	5/16	5/17	0.9	0.2 - 4.0	
ALL	55/135	101/171	2.3*	1.4 - 3.8	

*Obtained after stratification by trial.

FIGURE 28.31. Odds ratio for a complete response by trial, with associated 95% confidence intervals. The trials were performed by four collaborating groups: Dutch Hyperthermia Group (DHG), Medical Research Council (MRC) at Hammersmith Hospital (trials MRC BrI and BrR); the European Society of Hyperthermic Oncology (ESHO), and the hyperthermia group at Princess Margaret Hospital (PMH). (From Vernon CC, Hand JW, Field SB, et al. Radiotherapy with or without hyperthermia in the treatment of superficial localized breast cancer: Results from five randomized controlled trials. International Collaborative Hyperthermia Group. *Int J Radiat Oncol Biol Phys* 1996;35:731–744.)

factors). The overall complete response rate for the hyperthermia and radiation was 61% in these studies compared to 41% for radiation alone. Either Max (TDmin) or Sum (TDmin) was also associated with local disease-free survival, time to local failure, and overall survival. Similar analysis of the thermal parameters from the LLBrR and BrI trials were also published. This revealed that the cumulative minimal thermal isoeffective dose (equivalent minutes at 43°C accrued over the first and second, and first, second, and third treatment sessions) was the only treatment parameter that exhibited a consistent association with complete response.

An interesting finding from this analysis of dose response is that although the addition of hyperthermia to radiation was not associated with a change in overall survival compared to the radiation alone, there was an apparent survival benefit if hyperthermia treatments were classified according to the "quality" of treatment. In multivariate analysis, the Sum (TDmin) was significantly correlated with overall survival with poorer hyperthermia treatments associated with worse overall survival. This association between the quality of hyperthermia and overall survival raises several hypotheses. Is the quality of the hyperthermia having a direct effect on the outcome, or alternatively, is it merely an indicator for some other clinical characteristic? For example, patients with more advanced disease may be in a less adequate general physical condition to be able to tolerate multiple hyperthermia sessions. In this case, poor hyperthermia would be associated with poor response, not necessarily because of a direct effect of hyperthermia treatment. Alternatively, the inability to heat effectively may be indicative of increased tumor vascularity, which may be associated with a more malignant phenotype of disease. Again, the quality of the hyperthermia in this scenario may be influenced by the inherent tumor physiology.

To further address whether there may be some bias introduced to these findings on the basis of a patient's overall condition, an additional analysis was performed that divided the patients into two groups: Those with and those without systemic disease at entry. Systemic disease was felt to be an indicator of general disease advancement and, therefore, prospects for an unfavorable outcome. For those patients with systemic disease at entry, none of the thermal parameters was significantly associated with any of the outcomes studied. In addition, patients with systemic disease at entry were more likely to receive poor hyperthermia and only 41% of this cohort achieved Sum (TDmin) >10 minutes, whereas for patients without systemic disease 62% achieved Sum (TDmin) >10 minutes.

These findings suggest a selection effect is occurring in that the poorer response for patients receiving less hyperthermia dose may be related to the fact that a large proportion of these patients had systemic disease. For patients with no systemic disease at entry, a significant association was noted between hyperthermia quality and overall survival.

A prospective randomized trial was recently completed at Duke University, which involved the randomization of patients with superficial tumors (<3 cm in thickness) between two hyperthermia arms, one of which delivers <1 minute of hyperthermia CEM 43°C T_{90} versus ≥10 minutes CEM 43°C T_{90} (84). This trial employed rigorous thermal dose prescription and administration and was designed to test whether a thermal dose of more than 10 CEM 43°C T_{90} results in improved complete response and duration of local control compared with a thermal dose of ≤1 CEM 43°C T_{90}. Patients received a test dose of HT ≤CEM 43°C T_{90}, and tumors deemed heatable were randomly assigned to additional HT versus no additional IIT. IIT was given using microwave spiral strip applicators operating at 433 MHz. One hundred twenty-two patients were enrolled; 109 (89%) were deemed heatable and were randomly assigned. The complete response rate was 66.1% in the HT arm and 42.3% in the no-HT arm. The odds ratio for complete response was 2.7 (95% CI, 1.2 to 5.8; $p = 0.02$). Previously irradiated patients had the greatest incremental gain in complete response: 23.5% in the no-HT arm versus 68.2% in the HT arm. No overall survival benefit was seen. However, adjuvant hyperthermia with a thermal dose more than 10 CEM 43°C T_{90} confers a significant local control benefit in patients with superficial tumors receiving radiation.

Chest Wall Recurrence: Microscopic Disease

The treatment of a local-regional recurrence of breast cancer following mastectomy remains a clinically challenging problem. Often these patients have received radiotherapy and chemotherapy. Although high complete response rates have been reported following radiation therapy for treatment of isolated local-regional recurrence of breast cancer after mastectomy (1), approximately half of these patients who achieve an initial complete response will subsequently have a recurrence within or adjacent to the treated fields. Thus, long-term local control rates of only 40% to 50% are obtained. Even if a local recurrence is amenable to resection, risks remain high for a recurrence.

A phase I or II study at Stanford University investigated the efficacy and side effects of combined hyperthermia and radiation therapy in the management of presumed or known microscopic residual tumors. Over a 6-year interval, 262 fields in 89 patients with local-regional recurrent breast cancer were treated. All fields received one to six hyperthermia treatments (average 1.74) and the average radiation therapy dose was 42.4 Gy; concurrent hormonal therapy was administered in 37% of the treatments and no fields received concurrent chemotherapy. The majority of fields were in patients who had extensive prior therapy including radiation therapy and systemic therapies. The 3-year actuarial local control for all 262 fields was 68% (87). Parameters that correlated with duration of local control included estrogen receptor status of the initial breast cancer, initial T stage, time from initial breast cancer to first failure, age, and concurrent radiation dose. This series also reports an infield recurrence rate of 15%, which is lower than the recurrence rate of 29% reported for fields treated with radiotherapy alone.

Other Superficial Tumors

The RTOG conducted a randomized phase III study of irradiation and hyperthermia versus radiation alone in superficial measurable tumors (RTOG 8104) (156). A total of 307 patients with superficial measurable tumors were treated either with radiation alone or radiation followed immediately by hyperthermia (prescribed 42.5°C for 45 to 60 minutes). The complete response rate observed was 30% versus 32% in those receiving combined treatment. Patients consisted mostly of head and neck or breast chest wall recurrences. In tumors <3 cm located in the breast, trunk, or extremities, a better CR rate was noted with radiation and heat (62%) than with radiation alone (40%). Also in lesions <3 cm there was an improved local control. For lesions >3 cm there was no difference in local control between these two arms. It was postulated that the higher response rate in patients with smaller lesions was related to the fact that these tumors received an adequate thermal dose.

This theme of technical constraints limiting the clinical outcomes for hyperthermia is also reflected in the RTOG trial, which randomized interstitial thermoradiotherapy compared with interstitial radiotherapy alone in the treatment of recurrent or persistent tumors. In this trial, 184 patients with persistent or recurrent tumors after previous radiotherapy and/or surgery were randomized to interstitial radiation alone versus interstitial radiotherapy and interstitial hyperthermia. There was no overall difference in any of the study end points between the two arms. Complete response rate was 53% and 55% in both arms, and 2-year survival was 34% and 35%, respectively. The patient population was quite heterogeneous and consisted of primarily head and neck and pelvic tumors, the majority of which were ≥4 cm. A set of minimal adequacy criteria for the delivery of hyperthermia was developed. This included specifications with regard to the volume of implant, number of temperature sensors, and minimum intratumoral temperature, minimum average, and maximum intratumoral temperatures. Also specifications were made with regard to spacing between heat sources. When these criteria were applied, only one patient in the entire group of 184 had an adequate hyperthermia session. This experience highlights the importance of quality assurance procedures and detailed reporting of thermal dosimetry as a crucial component of hyperthermia clinical trials.

Rectal Cancer

A prospective phase II study for locally advanced rectal cancer was undertaken at the Humboldt University of Berlin with preoperative regional hyperthermia combined with radiochemotherapy (170). Thirty-seven patients with T3 or T4 lesions as determined by endorectal ultrasound and CT received 5FU (300 to 350 mg/m²) and leucovorin (50 mg) on days 1 to 5 and 22 through 26. This was combined with radiotherapy (45 Gy in 1.8 Gy fractions for 5 weeks) and weekly regional hyperthermia using the Sigma 60 applicator (BSD 2000, Salt Lake City, UT). Overall, this treatment was generally well tolerated and there was a 16% incidence of grade 3 toxicity mostly related to acute skin reaction and diarrhea. At the time of publication in 1998, late toxicity such as chronic bowel dysfunction, ulcerations of the bladder or rectum, or obstruction or stricture of ureter had not been observed. The overall resectability rate was 32/36 patients, and 31 resection specimens had negative margins. Five patients were shown to have a pathologic CR (14%). At 38 months' median follow-up the overall survival was 86% and no patient had a local recurrence detected at follow-up interval, but five patients developed distant metastases. Based on the results of this study, a phase III trial is currently under way that randomizes between radiochemotherapy versus hyperthermia with radiochemotherapy.

A pilot study of preoperative continuous infusion 5FU with external beam radiotherapy and hyperthermia was performed for locally advanced unresectable or recurrent rectal cancer at Duke University. From July 1995 through February 1999, 15 patients were enrolled in the study. Chemotherapy consisted of 5FU 250 mg/m² per day with 4,500 cGy whole pelvis radiotherapy and weekly hyperthermia. All patients completed the chemoradiotherapy portion of the protocol and 11/15 patients completed all five hyperthermia treatments. Five of 15 patients required treatment interruption due to toxicity ≥grade 3. Of the 14 patients in whom surgery was planned, 11 were resectable and there was one pathologic complete response (3).

Ultimately, the role of hyperthermia in the neoadjuvant treatment of rectal cancer will be better defined by phase III protocols such as the ongoing German phase III protocol. Should this prove a benefit to the addition of hyperthermia, it would be reasonable to consider a phase III study using continuous infusion 5FU as the systemic regimen.

Sarcoma

A series of 97 sarcoma patients were treated with preoperative hyperthermia and radiotherapy from 1984 to 1996 at Duke University. The majority of these patients had extremity sarcoma (78/97). All tumors were high grade, 44 >10 cm in size (maximum tumor diameter), 43 were 5 to 10 cm in size, and 10 were <5 cm. The 10-year actuarial overall survival, cause-specific survival, and relapse-free survival are 50%, 47%, and 47%, respectively. The 10-year actuarial local control was 94%. The predominant pattern of failure was pulmonary metastasis (163).

In these same patients, in vivo tumor physiology studies using Eppendorf measurement of Po_2 demonstrated the prognostic significance of tumor hypoxia as a predictor for distant metastases (19). Furthermore, it was shown that hyperthermia achieved an improvement in tumor oxygenation, which persisted for at least 24 hours after treatment. The magnitude of improvement in tumor oxygenation after the first hyperthermia fraction relative to the pretreatment baseline was positively correlated with the amount of necrosis seen in the resection specimen. Thus, the potential role of hyperthermia as a modulator of oxygenation and tumor physiology has been demonstrated in human patients and raises other possible mechanisms of improved radiosensitization by decreasing tumor hypoxia.

There are two phase II European studies of high-risk soft tissue sarcomas. The first (RHT-91) was a combination of neoadjuvant EIA chemotherapy (etoposide, ifosfamide, and doxorubicin) combined with regional hyperthermia followed by surgical resection and additional adjuvant treatment. At the time of surgery, a pathologic CR occurred in 6/59 patients. Patients entered the trial either with primary tumors of size >8 cm and/or extracompartmental location (31 patients) or with local recurrence of tumor tumors bearing these characteristics (28 patients). In 31 nonextremity soft tissue sarcomas, tumors were located in the trunk or within the abdomen and the pelvis. Local recurrence occurred in 33 patients (56%), and overall survival did not differ between extremity versus nonextremity sarcomas.

In a follow-up study (RHT-95), 54 patients were treated prospectively with four cycles of EIA chemotherapy with regional hyperthermia followed by surgery, another four cycles of EIA without hyperthermia, followed by external beam radiation. The 4-year overall survival was 40% and local control was 59% (234a). The major distinction between these two studies was that RHT-91 had hyperthermia only in the preoperative setting, while RHT-95 employed hyperthermia in the preoperative and postoperative chemotherapy regimens. The group without postsurgery thermochemotherapy (RHT-91) showed an inferior local failure-free survival, but this did not effect the distant metastasis-free survival or overall survival. Thus, it was felt that the postsurgical thermochemotherapy seemed important for local control without impacting on survival. Based on these studies, an EORTC phase III protocol is under way testing the overall benefit of the addition of hyperthermia to the neoadjuvant and adjuvant chemotherapy regimens.

Head and Neck Cancers

There are two randomized series demonstrating an advantage to hyperthermia combined with radiotherapy. The first study conducted in New Delhi, India, randomized 65 patients to radiation alone versus radiotherapy and heat (30a). Radiotherapy doses consisted of 50 Gy in 5 weeks to the primary site and regional lymphatics followed by a further dose of 10 to 15 Gy given to the site of gross disease in fractions of 2 Gy. Hyperthermia was given twice a week with a period of 72 hours between each session. Concomitant use of local hyperthermia with radiotherapy did not impact the response in patients with early stage disease. For patients in this subgroup (13 total), all but one had a complete response by the 8-week follow-up posttreatment. By contrast, the complete response reserved for stage III patients was 20% in the radiotherapy alone group versus 58% in the radiation and heat group. Likewise, stage IV patients also demonstrated a better complete response rate when treated with combined therapy compared to radiotherapy alone (38% vs. 7%, respectively). Another randomized study for head and neck cancers evaluated the role of hyperthermia for N_3 metastatic squamous cell cervical lymph nodes treated with conventional fractionated radiotherapy versus radiotherapy plus twice a week hyperthermia. The two major end points were local control rates at 3 months and incidence of acute local toxicity. A planned interim analysis had revealed a statistically significant difference and complete response rates in favor of the combined arm, which demonstrated a complete response rate of 82.3% (14/17) versus 36.8% (7/19) for the control radiation alone arm. Acute local toxicities were similar in both groups and only skin burn was observed. One patient in the combined heat and radiotherapy arm died 2 months after completion of therapy with a carotid rupture, which may have been associated with extensive tumor necrosis. In a report of the long-term follow-up of this series, 5-year follow-up confirmed the efficacy and absence of severe toxicity (242b). The improved early response in favor of the combined treatment arm resulted in an improved 5-year actuarial nodal control and an improved overall survival at 5 years ($p = 0.02$).

Esophagus

Two randomized studies demonstrated an advantage to the addition of hyperthermia to chemoradiotherapy or chemother-

apy alone in the neoadjuvant treatment of esophagus cancer. In the first study, 53 patients with squamous cell carcinoma of the thoracic esophagus underwent surgery after combined hyperthermia and chemoradiotherapy versus chemoradiotherapy alone. Chemotherapy consisted of bleomycin (5 mg) given intravenously concurrent with hyperthermia (42.5 to 44 cGy for 30 minutes) given 1 hour before radiation. This was given in a 3-week regimen for an average total dose of 31.8 Gy. The clinical response as well as the pathologic response was significantly improved in the trimodality arm with a "markedly effective" microscopic response in 25.9% of combined modality versus 7.7% of chemoradiotherapy alone (205).

In a follow-up study, 40 patients with squamous cell carcinoma of the thoracic esophagus received preoperative chemotherapy (bleomycin and CDDP) given either combined with or without hyperthermia. Again, an improvement in the histopathologic response was noted favoring the hyperthermia group (18.8% vs. 41.2%). The bleomycin chemotherapy in this trial consisted of a paced suspension that was applied directly over the ulcerated tumor region. This was given concurrently with an intravenous infusion of cisplatin. Local hyperthermia was given concurrently with the local applications of bleomycin and this was given six times over the 3-week preoperative interval, while platinum at 15 mg/m² was given once a week during that same time. Although treatment in the control arm would not be considered standard therapy, a benefit to the addition of hyperthermia was clearly demonstrated in both of these studies (206).

Malignant Melanoma

Seventy patients with 134 metastatic or recurrent malignant melanoma lesions were randomized to receive radiotherapy (three fractions of 8 or 9 Gy in 8 days alone) or radiotherapy followed by hyperthermia (43°C for 60 minutes). Hyperthermia was well tolerated but because of technical difficulties only 14% of treatments achieved the protocol objective of a minimum tumor temperature of 43°C within 30 minutes. Despite these constraints, there was a beneficial effect to the addition of hyperthermia (radiation alone 28% actuarial local control vs. 46% with combined radiotherapy and hyperthermia). A difference in the complete response and 2-year control rates were also seen between the 8 Gy per fraction versus 9 Gy per fraction arm. No difference was seen in the response rate, and 2-year control based on size ≥/<4 cm (151).

Glioblastoma Multiforme

Over a 5-year interval, 112 patients were entered into a randomized trial of brachytherapy boost with or without hyperthermia for adult patients with newly diagnosed focal supratentorial glioblastoma multiforme ≤5 cm in diameter. Hyperthermia treatments were given for 30 minutes immediately before and after brachytherapy. Time to progression and survival from date of diagnosis were estimated, demonstrating an improvement in time to progression and survival with the addition of hyperthermia (Fig. 28.32).

In this trial, hyperthermia was delivered via an interstitial technique with helical coiled microwave antennas implanted within the target volume. Thermal dose calculations were performed and the median CEM 43°C T_{90} in this trial was 14.1. No thermal dose–response relationship was found. However, the number of patients evaluated was relatively small, and the trial was not designed to look for thermal dose–response relationship. This was a landmark trial that represents the first prospective randomized trial in North America to show a local control and survival benefit for hyperthermia. The influence of heat on survival was even more significant in the multivariate analysis adjusting for age and Karnofsky performance status.

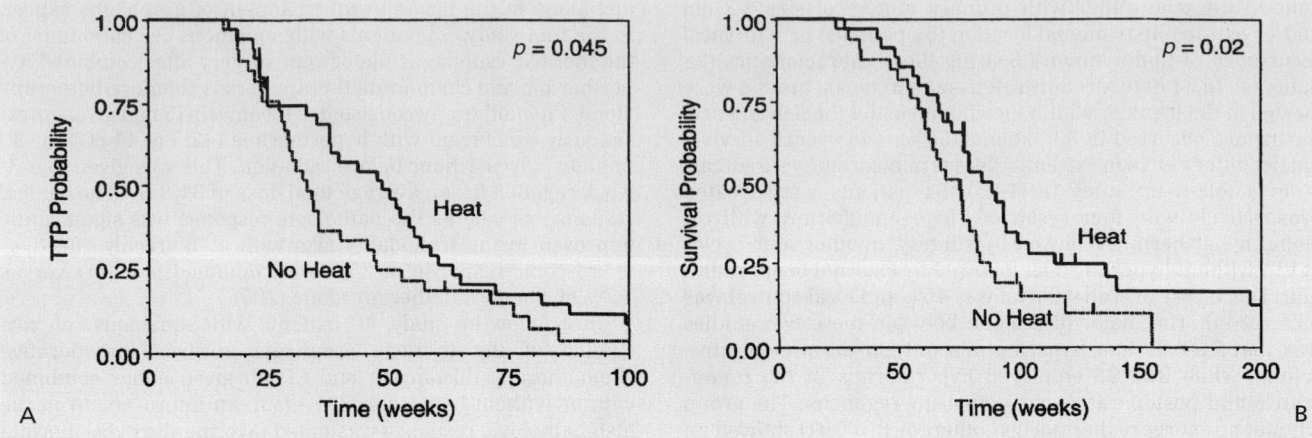

FIGURE 28.32. A: Results for patients with glioblastoma multiforme treated with radiation with or without hyperthermia. Kaplan-Meier time to progression (TTP) curves for evaluable patients who actually had brachytherapy boost comparing 33 no heat patients to 35 heat patients (log rank *p* = 0.045). The median TTP was 33 weeks for the no heat group versus 49 weeks for the heat group. **B:** Kaplan-Meier survival curves for evaluable patients who actually had brachytherapy boost, comparing 33 no heat patients to 35 heat patients (log rank *p* = 0.02). The median survival was 76 weeks for no heat patients versus 85 weeks for heat patients with 2-year survival probabilities of 15% versus 31%, respectively. (From Sneed PK, Stauffer PR, McDermott MW, et al. Survival benefit of hyperthermia in a prospective randomized trial of brachytherapy boost +/− hyperthermia for glioblastoma multiforme. *Int J Radiat Oncol Biol Phys* 1988;40:287–295, with permission.)

Salvage therapies were well balanced between the two arms and were not felt to be a factor explaining the survival difference (188).

Cervical Cancer

Results from five prospective randomized trials including almost 1,900 women with locally advanced cervix carcinoma showed an overall survival advantage for cisplatin-based chemotherapy given concurrently with radiation, compared with radiation alone or radiation and noncisplatin chemotherapy (91,130,157,175,235). The patient populations included were women with FIGO stages IIb or IVa and certain women with stage I or IIa with poor prognostic factors found at the time of primary surgery (metastatic disease, pelvic nodes, parametrial disease, or positive surgical margins). The addition of concurrent cisplatin reduced the risk of death from cervical cancer by 30% to 50%. A meta-analysis of combined modality therapy for cervix cancer demonstrated the absolute benefit in progression-free and overall survival was 16% (95% CI 13/19) and 12% (8/16), respectively. A significant benefit of chemoradiation on both local (odds ratio 0.61; *p* < 0.0001) and distant recurrence (0.57; *p* < 0.0001) was also noted (63).

The Dutch Hyperthermia Group trial of RT alone compared with RT plus HT in locally advanced pelvic tumors (223). This study, initiated in 1990 and completed in 1996, entered patients with locally advanced tumors of the bladder, rectum, and 114 patients with cervical cancer. The cervical cancer patients had bulky stage IB, IIB, to IVA disease. In contrast to the chemotherapy trials described above, negative para-aortic nodes were not required for entry. There was a very significant benefit for the addition of HT to RT. The complete response rate improved from 57% to 87% (*p* = 0.003). Three-year overall survival was 51% in the RT plus heat group compared with 27% in the RT alone group (*p* = 0.009). There were no particular differences with regard to toxicity, particularly late toxicity. Approximately 11% of the hyperthermia patients sustained subcutaneous or skin burns, but these were small, and healed readily with conservative treatment. There are two other phase II trials of RT and HT for cervical cancer, and two additional smaller phase III trials, all showing an advantage to thermoradiotherapy (Fig. 28.33) (47,70,75,185).

Two other randomized trials of radiation with or without hyperthermia for cervix cancer also demonstrated positive results (70,185). Fifty patients with stages II and III carcinoma of the cervix were entered into this prospective randomized study. Twenty-five cases (group I) were treated only by radical radiation, whereas the remaining 25 cases (group II) received local hyperthermia in addition to radical radiation. Hyperthermia was delivered by intracavitary brachyhyperthermia approach using an Endotrac applicator. Both the groups were followed up for a minimum period of 18 months. Group II patients achieved better local control (14/20 evaluable cases) than the group I patients (11/22 evaluable cases).

In another small series from Japan, 40 patients with stage IIIB uterine cervix carcinoma were treated with external beam irradiation to the pelvis, combined with iridium-192 high-dose–rate intracavitary brachytherapy. All patients were divided randomly into the following two groups: Radiotherapy (RT) (*n* = 20) and thermoradiotherapy (TRT) (*n* = 20). Thermoradiotherapy patients underwent three sessions of hyperthermia in addition

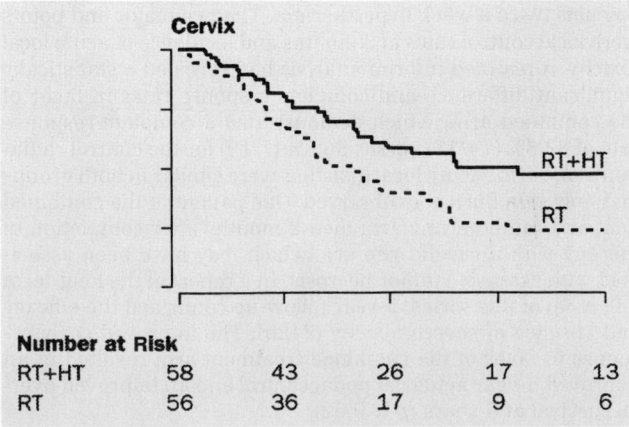

FIGURE 28.33. Overall survival for cervix patients treated with radiation and hyperthermia versus hyperthermia alone in the phase III Dutch deep hyperthermia trial (From van der Zee J, Gonzalez Gonzalez D, van Rhoon GC, et al. Comparison of radiotherapy alone with radiotherapy plus hyperthermia in locally advanced pelvic tumours: A prospective, randomised, multicentre trial. Dutch Deep Hyperthermia Group. *Lancet* 2000;355:1119–1125, with permission.)

to radiotherapy. The primary end point of this study was local complete response and survival. A complete response was achieved in 50% (10/20) in the RT group versus 80% (16/20) in the TRT group ($p = 0.048$). The 3-year overall survival and disease-free survival of the patients who were treated with TRT (58.2% and 63.6%, respectively) were better than those of the patients treated with RT (48.1% and 45%, respectively), but these differences were not statistically significant. The 3-year local relapse-free survival of the patients who were treated with TRT (79.7%) was significantly better than that of the patients treated with RT (48.5%) ($p = 0.048$). TRT, as delivered in this trial, was well tolerated and did not significantly add to either the relevant clinical acute or long-term toxicity over radiation alone. TRT resulted in a better treatment response and 3-year local relapse-free survival rate than radiotherapy alone for patients with FIGO stage IIIB cervical carcinoma (70).

A pilot study of combined hyperthermia, radiation therapy, and concurrent weekly cisplatin chemotherapy has been conducted at Duke University (83). From August 1998 through December 2000, 12 patients with locally advanced cervical cancer or locally recurrent cervical cancer following hysterectomy were enrolled on a pilot study combining weekly cisplatin, hyperthermia, and radiotherapy. Ten patients were treated at initial diagnosis. All had clinical complete response and durable local control. Two of these 10 failed outside the pelvis, one with pulmonary metastasis and one with isolated para-aortic nodal involvement. The latter patient was rendered disease free with further radiotherapy and cisplatin and remained without disease at 20 months' follow-up. Two patients treated for locally recurrent cervical cancer had local and systemic progression and died of disease within 6 months. In this small series, trimodality therapy resulted in an excellent clinical response and was well tolerated. The addition of hyperthermia to chemoradiotherapy represents a promising new strategy that merits multi-institutional collaborative efforts for phase III confirmation.

References

1. Aberizk W, Silver B, Henderson I, et al. The use of radiotherapy for treatment of isolated locoregional recurrence of breast carcinoma after mastectomy. *Cancer* 1986;58:1214–1218.
2. Ando K, Urano M, Kenton L, et al. Effect of thermochemotherapy on the development of spontaneous lung metastases. *Int J Hyperthermia* 1987;3:453–458.
3. Anscher MS, Lee C, Hurwitz H, et al. A pilot study of preoperative continuous infusion 5-fluorouracil, external microwave hyperthermia, and external beam radiotherapy for treatment of locally advanced, unresectable, or recurrent rectal cancer. *Int J Radiat Oncol Biol Phys* 2000;47:719–724.
4. Armour EP, McEachern D, Wang Z, et al. Sensitivity of human cells to mild hyperthermia. *Cancer Res* 1993;53:2740–2744.
5. Armour EP, Wang ZH, Corry PM, et al. Sensitization of rat 9L gliosarcoma cells to low dose rate irradiation by long duration 41 degrees C hyperthermia. *Cancer Res* 1991;51:3088–3095.
6. Arrhenius S. Uber die reaktionsgeschwindigkeit bei der inversion von rohrzucker durch Sauren. *Zeitschr Physik Chem* 1889;4:226–248.
7. Arts HJ, Hollema H, Lemstra W, et al. Heat-shock-protein-27 (hsp27) expression in ovarian carcinoma: Relation in response to chemotherapy and prognosis. *Int J Cancer* 1999;84:234–238.
8. Asea A, Kraeft SK, Kurt-Jones EA, et al. HSP70 stimulates cytokine production through a CD14-dependant pathway, demonstrating its dual role as a chaperone and cytokine. *Nat Med* 2000;6:435–442.
9. Averill DA, Su C. Sensitization to the cytotoxicity of adriamycin by verapamil and heat in multidrug-resistant Chinese hamster ovary cells. *Radiat Res* 1999;151:694–702.
10. Bataille N, Vallancien G, Chopin D. Antitumoral local effect and metastatic risk of focused extracorporeal pyrotherapy on Dunning R-3327 tumors. *Eur Urol* 1996;29:72–77.
11. Bell KM, Prise VE, Shaffi KM, et al. A comparative study of tumour blood flow modification in two rat tumour systems using endothelin-1 and angiotensin II: Influence of tumour size on angiotensin II response. *Int J Cancer* 1996;67:730–738.
12. Biaglow JE, Manevich Y, Leeper D, et al. MIBG inhibits respiration: Potential for radio- and hyperthermic sensitization. *Int J Radiat Oncol Biol Phys* 1998;42:871–876.
13. Blackburn RV, Galoforo SS, Corry PM, et al. Adenoviral-mediated transfer of a heat-inducible double suicide gene into prostate carcinoma cells. *Cancer Res* 1998;58:1358–1362.
14. Bornstein BA, Herman TS, Hansen JL, et al. Pilot study of local hyperthermia, radiation therapy, etanidazole, and cisplatin for advanced superficial tumours. *Int J Hyperthermia* 1995;11:489–499.
15. Braiden V, Ohtsuru A, Kawashita Y, et al. Eradication of breast cancer xenografts by hyperthermic suicide gene therapy under the control of the heat shock protein promoter. *Hum Gene Ther* 2000;11:2453–2463.
16. Braun RD, Lanzen JL, Dewhirst MW. Fourier analysis of fluctuations of oxygen tension and blood flow in R3230Ac tumors and muscle in rats. *Am J Physiol* 1999;277:H551–H568.
17. Brezovich IA, Atkinson WJ, Lilly MB. Local hyperthermia with interstitial techniques. *Cancer Res* 1984;44:4752S–4756S.
18. Brezovich IA, Meredith RF. Practical aspects of ferromagnetic thermoseed hyperthermia. *Radiol Clin North Am* 1989;27:589–602.
19. Brizel DM, Scully SP, Harrelson JM, et al. Radiation therapy and hyperthermia improve the oxygenation of human soft tissue sarcomas. *Cancer Res* 1996;56:5347–5350.
20. Burgman P, Nussensweig A, Li G. Thermotolerance. In: Seegenschmiedt M, Fessenden P, Vernon C, eds. *Thermoradiotherapy and thermochemotherapy.* Berlin: Springer-Verlag, 1995;75–84.
21. Carter DL, MacFall JR, Clegg ST, et al. Magnetic resonance thermometry during hyperthermia for human high-grade sarcoma. *Int J Radiat Oncol Biol Phys* 1998;40:815–822.
22. Cividalli A, Cruciani G, Livdi E, et al. Hyperthermia enhances the response of paclitaxel and radiation in a mouse adenocarcinoma. *Int J Radiat Oncol Biol Phys* 1999;44:407–412.
23. Cornford PA, Dodson AR, Parsons KF, et al. Heat shock protein expression independently predicts clinical outcome in prostate cancer. *Cancer Res* 2000;60:7099–7105.
24. Coss RA, Linnemans WA. The effects of hyperthermia on the cytoskeleton: A review. *Int J Hyperthermia* 1996;12:173–196.
25. Cossett JM. *Interstitial, endocavitary, and perfusional hyperthermia.* Berlin: Springer Verlag, 1990.
26. Curry FE. Determinants of capillary permeability: A review of mechanisms based on single capillary studies in the frog. *Circ Res* 1986;59:367–380.
27. Da Silva VF, Feeley M, Raaphorst GP. Hyperthermic potentiation of BCNU toxicity in BCNU-resistant human glioma cells. *J Neurooncol* 1991;11:37–41.
28. Dahl O. Interaction of heat and drugs in vitro and in vivo. In: Seegenschmiedt M, Fessenden P, Vernon C, eds. *Thermoradiotherapy and thermochemotherapy.* Berlin: Springer Verlag, 1995;103–155.
29. Das SK, Clegg ST, Anscher MS, et al. Simulation of electromagnetically induced hyperthermia: A finite element gridding method. *Int J Hyperthermia* 1995;11:797–808.
30. Das SK, Jones EA, Samulski TV. A method of MRI-based thermal modelling for a RF phased array. *Int J Hyperthermia* 2001;17:465–482.
30a. Datta NR, Bose AK, Kapoor HK, et al. Head and neck cancers: results of thermoradiotherapy versus radiotherapy. *Int J Hyperthermia* 1990;6(3):479–486.
31. de Graeff A, Slebos RJ, Rodenhuis S. Resistance to cisplatin and analogues: Mechanisms and potential clinical implications. *Cancer Chemother Pharmacol* 1988;22:325–332.
32. DeFord JA, Babbs CF, Patel UH, et al. Accuracy and precision of computer-simulated tissue temperatures in individual human intracranial tumours treated with interstitial hyperthermia. *Int J Hyperthermia* 1990;6:755–769.
33. Dewey WC. Interaction of heat with radiation and chemotherapy. *Cancer Res* 1984;44:4714S–4720S.
34. Dewey WC. Arrhenius relationships from the molecule and cell to the clinic. *Int J Hyperthermia* 1994;10:457–483.
35. Dewey WC, Hopwood LE, Sapareto SA, et al. Cellular responses to combinations of hyperthermia and radiation. *Radiology* 1977;123:463–474.
36. Dewhirst MaS T. *Hyperthermia in the treatment of cancer.* Kalamazoo, MI: Upjohn, 1988.
37. Dewhirst MW. Thermal dosimetry. In: Seegenschmiedt M, Fessenden P, Vernon CC, eds. *Thermoradiotherapy and thermochemotherapy.* Berlin: Springer Verlag, 1995;123–128.
38. Dewhirst MW. Concepts of oxygen transport at the microcirculatory level. *Semin Radiat Oncol* 1998;8:143–150.
39. Dewhirst MW, Griffin TW, Smith AR, et al. Intersociety Council on Radiation Oncology essay on the introduction of new medical treatments into practice. *J Natl Cancer Inst* 1993;85:951–957.
40. Dewhirst MW, Phillips TL, Samulski TV, et al. RTOG quality assurance guidelines for clinical trials using hyperthermia. *Int J Radiat Oncol Biol Phys* 1990;18:1249–1259.
41. Dewhirst MW, Prescott DM, Clegg S, et al. The use of hydralazine to manipulate tumour temperatures during hyperthermia. *Int J Hyperthermia* 1990;6:971–983.
42. Dewhirst MW, Sim D, Gross J, et al. Effects of heating rate on normal and tumor microcirculatory function. In: Diller K, Roemer RB, eds. *Heat and mass transfer in the microcirculation of thermally significant vessels.* Anaheim, CA: ASME, 1986;75–80.
43. Dewhirst MW, Sim DA. The utility of thermal dose as a predictor of tumor and normal tissue responses to combined radiation and hyperthermia. *Cancer Res* 1984;44:4772S–4780S.
44. Dewhirst MW, Sim DA, Forsyth K, et al. Local control and distant metastases in primary canine malignant melanomas treated with hyperthermia and/or radiotherapy. *Int J Hyperthermia* 1985;1:219–234.
45. Diederich CJ. Interstitial ultrasound applicators are practical from an engineering perspective for treating large tumours. *Int J Hyperthermia* 1996;12:305–306.
46. Diederich CJ. Ultrasound applicators with integrated catheter-cooling for interstitial hyperthermia: Theory and preliminary experiments. *Int J Hyperthermia* 1996;12:279–297; discussion 299–300.
47. Dinges S, Harder C, Wurm R, et al. Combined treatment of inoperable carcinomas of the uterine cervix with radiotherapy and regional hyperthermia. Results of a phase II trial. *Strahlenther Onkol* 1998;174:517–521.
48. Edelstein-Keshet L, Dewhirst MW, Oleson JR, et al. Characterization of tumour temperature distributions in hyperthermia based on assumed mathematical forms. *Int J Hyperthermia* 1989;5:757–777.
49. Emami B, Scott C, Perez CA, et al. Phase III study of interstitial thermoradiotherapy compared with interstitial radiotherapy alone in the treatment of recurrent or persistent human tumors. A prospectively controlled randomized study by the Radiation Therapy Group. *Int J Radiat Oncol Biol Phys* 1996;34:1097–1104.
50. Engin K. Biological rationale for hyperthermia in cancer treatment (II). *Neoplasma* 1994;41:277–283.

51. Engin K, Leeper D, Thistlethwaite A, et al. Tumor extracellular pH as a prognostic factor in thermoradiotherapy. *Int J Radiat Oncol Biol Phys* 1994;29:125–132.
52. Engin K, Tupchong L, Moylan DJ, et al. Randomized trial of one versus two adjuvant hyperthermia treatments per week in patients with superficial tumours. *Int J Hyperthermia* 1993;9:327–340.
53. Fajardo LF. Pathological effects of hyperthermia in normal tissues. *Cancer Res* 1984;44:4826S–4835S.
54. Field SB, Morris CC. The relationship between heating time and temperature: Its relevance to clinical hyperthermia. *Radiother Oncol* 1983;1:179–186.
55. Fry FJ, Johnson LK. Tumor irradiation with intense ultrasound. *Ultrasound Med Biol* 1978;4:337–341.
56. Gaber MH, Wu NZ, Hong K, et al. Thermosensitive liposomes: Extravasation and release of contents in tumor microvascular networks. *Int J Radiat Oncol Biol Phys* 1996;36:1177–1187.
57. Gerner EW, Hersh EM, Pennington M, et al. Heat-inducible vectors for use in gene therapy. *Int J Hyperthermia* 2000;16:171–181.
58. Gerweck L. Modification of cell lethality at elevated temperatures. The pH effect. *Radiat Res* 1977;70:224–235.
59. Gerweck LE, Richards B, Michaels HB. Influence of low pH on the development and decay of 42 degrees C thermotolerance in CHO cells. *Int J Radiat Oncol Biol Phys* 1982;8:1935–1941.
60. Gibbs FA Jr. "Thermal mapping" in experimental cancer treatment with hyperthermia: Description and use of a semi-automatic system. *Int J Radiat Oncol Biol Phys* 1983;9:1057–1063.
61. Gillette EL, McChesney SL, Dewhirst MW, et al. Response of canine oral carcinomas to heat and radiation. *Int J Radiat Oncol Biol Phys* 1987;13:1861–1867.
62. Gillette SM, Dewhirst MW, Gillette EL, et al. Response of canine soft tissue sarcomas to radiation or radiation plus hyperthermia: A randomized phase II study. *Int J Hyperthermia* 1992;8:309–320.
63. Green JA, Kirwan JM, Tierney JF, et al. Survival and recurrence after concomitant chemotherapy and radiotherapy for cancer of the uterine cervix: A systematic review and meta-analysis. *Lancet* 2001;358:781–786.
64. Gulledge CJ, Dewhirst MW. Tumor oxygenation: A matter of supply and demand. *Anticancer Res* 1996;16:741–749.
65. Hahn GM, Shiu EC. Adaptation to low pH modifies thermal and thermo-chemical responses of mammalian cells. *Int J Hyperthermia* 1986;2:379–387.
66. Hahn JS, Braun RD, Dewhirst MW, et al. Stroma-free human hemoglobin A decreases R3230Ac rat mammary adenocarcinoma blood flow and oxygen partial pressure. *Radiat Res* 1997;147:185–194.
67. Hand JaJ JR. *Physical techniques in clinical hyperthermia*. New York: John Wiley and Sons, 1986.
68. Hand JW, Lagendijk JJ, Bach Andersen J, et al. Quality assurance guidelines for ESHO protocols. *Int J Hyperthermia* 1989;5:421–428.
69. Hand JW, Machin D, Vernon CC, et al. Analysis of thermal parameters obtained during phase III trials of hyperthermia as an adjunct to radiotherapy in the treatment of breast carcinoma. *Int J Hyperthermia* 1997;13:343–364.
70. Harima Y, Nagata K, Harima K, et al. A randomized clinical trial of radiation therapy versus thermoradiotherapy in stage IIIB cervical carcinoma. *Int J Hyperthermia* 2001;17:97–105.
71. Hauck M, Zalutsky M, Dewhirst MW. Enhancement of radiolabeled monoclonal antibody uptake in tumors with local hyperthermia. In: Torchilin V, ed. *Targeted delivery of imaging agents*. Boca Raton, FL: CRC Press, 1995;335–361.
72. Herman TS, Teicher BA. Sequencing of trimodality therapy [cis- diamminedichloroplatinum(II)/hyperthermia/radiation] as determined by tumor growth delay and tumor cell survival in the FSaIIC fibrosarcoma. *Cancer Res* 1988;48:2693–2697.
73. Herman TS, Teicher BA, Chan V, et al. Effect of heat on the cytotoxicity and interaction with DNA of a series of platinum complexes. *Int J Radiat Oncol Biol Phys* 1989;16:443–449.
74. Hettinga JV, Konings AW, Kampinga HH. Reduction of cellular cisplatin resistance by hyperthermia—a review. *Int J Hyperthermia* 1997;13:439–457.
75. Hornback NB, Shupe RE, Shidnia H, et al. Advanced stage IIIB cancer of the cervix treatment by hyperthermia and radiation. *Gynecol Oncol* 1986;23:160–167.
76. Huang Q, Hu JK, Lohr F, et al. Heat-induced gene expression as a novel targeted cancer gene therapy strategy. *Cancer Res* 2000;60:3435–3439.
77. Hynynen K, Colucci V, Chung A, et al. Noninvasive arterial occlusion using MRI-guided focused ultrasound. *Ultrasound Med Biol* 1996;22:1071–1077.
78. Hynynen K, Davis KL. Small cylindrical ultrasound sources for induction of hyperthermia via body cavities or interstitial implants. *Int J Hyperthermia* 1993;9:263–274.
79. Ito A, Shinkai M, Honda H, et al. Heat-inducible TNF-alpha gene therapy combined with hyperthermia using magnetic nanoparticles as a novel tumor-targeted therapy. *Cancer Gene Ther* 2001;8:649–654.
80. Jayasundar R, Honess D, Hall LD, et al. Simultaneous evaluation of the effects of RF hyperthermia on the intra- and extracellular tumor pH. *Magn Reson Med* 2000;43:1-8.
81. Jia X, Paulsen KD, Buechler DN, et al. Finite element simulation of Sigma 60 heating in the Utah phantom: Computed and measured data compared. *Int J Hyperthermia* 1994;10:755–774.
82. Jirtle RL. Chemical modification of tumour blood flow. *Int J Hyperthermia* 1988;4:355–371.
83. Jones EL, Brizel DM, Samulski TV, et al. A pilot phase I/II trial of concurrent radiotherapy, chemotherapy, and hyperthermia for locally advanced cervix carcinoma. 2003;98(2):277–282.
84. Jones EL, Samulski TV, Dewhirst MW, et al. A pilot phase II trial of concurrent radiotherapy, chemotherapy, and hyperthermia for locally advanced cervical carcinoma. *Cancer* 2003;98:277–282.
85. Kampinga HH, Dikomey E. Hyperthermic radiosensitization: Mode of action and clinical relevance. *Int J Radiat Biol* 2001;77:399–408.
86. Kapp DS, Cox RS. Thermal treatment parameters are most predictive of outcome in patients with single tumor nodules per treatment field in recurrent adenocarcinoma of the breast. *Int J Radiat Oncol Biol Phys* 1995;33:887–899.
87. Kapp DS, Cox RS, Barnett TA, et al. Thermoradiotherapy for residual microscopic cancer: Elective or post-excisional hyperthermia and radiation therapy in the management of local-regional recurrent breast cancer. *Int J Radiat Oncol Biol Phys* 1992;24:261–277.
88. Kapp DS, Lawrence R. Temperature elevation during brachytherapy for carcinoma of the uterine cervix: Adverse effect on survival and enhancement of distant metastasis. *Int J Radiat Oncol Biol Phys* 1984;10:2281–2292.
89. Katschinski DM, Robins HI. Hyperthermic modulation of SN-38-induced topoisomerase I DNA cross- linking and SN-38 cytotoxicity through altered topoisomerase I activity. *Int J Cancer* 1999;80:104–109.
90. Kelleher DK, Engel T, Vaupel PW. Changes in microregional perfusion, oxygenation, ATP and lactate distribution in subcutaneous rat tumours upon water-filtered IR-A hyperthermia. *Int J Hyperthermia* 1995;11:241–255.
91. Keys HM, Bundy BN, Stehman FB, et al. Cisplatin, radiation, and adjuvant hysterectomy compared with radiation and adjuvant hysterectomy for bulky stage IB cervical carcinoma. *N Engl J Med* 1999;340:1154–1161.
92. Kiang JG, Tsokos GC. Heat shock protein 70 kDa: Molecular biology, biochemistry, and physiology. *Pharmacol Ther* 1998;80:183–201.
93. Kido Y, Kuwano H, Maehara Y, et al. Increased cytotoxicity of low-dose, long-duration exposure to 5- fluorouracil of V-79 cells with hyperthermia. *Cancer Chemother Pharmacol* 1991;28:251–254.
94. Kim JH, Kim SH, Dutta P, et al. Preferential killing of glucose-depleted HeLa cells by menadione and hyperthermia. *Int J Hyperthermia* 1992;8:139–146.
95. King KL, Li AF, Chau GY, et al. Prognostic significance of heat shock protein-27 expression in hepatocellular carcinoma and its relation to histologic grading and survival. *Cancer* 2000;88:2464–2470.
96. Kong G, Anyarambhatla G, Petros WP, et al. Efficacy of liposomes and hyperthermia in a human tumor xenograft model: Importance of triggered drug release. *Cancer Res* 2000;60:6950–6957.
97. Kong G, Braun RD, Dewhirst MW. Hyperthermia enables tumor-specific nanoparticle delivery: Effect of particle size. *Cancer Res* 2000;60:4440–4445.
98. Kong G, Braun RD, Dewhirst MW. Characterization of the effect of hyperthermia on nanoparticle extravasation from tumor vasculature. *Cancer Res* 2001;61:3027–3032.
99. Kong G, Dewhirst MW. Hyperthermia and liposomes. *Int J Hyperthermia* 1999;15:345–370.
100. Koutcher JA, Barnett D, Kornblith AB, et al. Relationship of changes in pH and energy status to hypoxic cell fraction and hyperthermia sensitivity. *Int J Radiat Oncol Biol Phys* 1990;18:1429–1435.
101. Krishna MC, Dewhirst MW, Friedman HS, et al. Hyperthermic sensitization by the radical initiator 2,2'-azobis (2-amidinopropane) dihydrochloride (AAPH). I. In vitro studies. *Int J Hyperthermia* 1994;10:271–281.
102. Lagendijk JJ, Van Rhoon GC, Hornsleth SN, et al. ESHO quality assurance guidelines for regional hyperthermia. *Int J Hyperthermia* 1998;14:125–133.
103. Laskowitz DT, Elion GB, Dewhirst MW, et al. Hyperthermia-induced enhancement of melphalan activity against a melphalan-resistant human rhabdomyosarcoma xenograft. *Radiat Res* 1992;129:218–223.
104. Law MP. Induced thermal resistance in the mouse ear: The relationship between heating time and temperature. *Int J Radiat Biol* 1979;35:481–485.
105. Leal BZ, Meltz ML, Mohan N, et al. Interaction of hyperthermia with Taxol in human MCF-7 breast adenocarcinoma cells. *Int J Hyperthermia* 1999;15:225–236.
106. Lee ER, Wilsey TR, Tarczy-Hornoch P, et al. Body conformable 915 MHz microstrip array applicators for large surface area hyperthermia. *IEEE Trans Biomed Eng* 1992;39:470–483.
107. Leeper DB, Engin K, Thistlethwaite AJ, et al. Human tumor extracellular pH as a function of blood glucose concentration. *Int J Radiat Oncol Biol Phys* 1994;28:935–943.
108. Leopold KA, Dewhirst MW, Samulski TV, et al. Cumulative minutes with T_{90} greater than Tempindex is predictive of response of superficial malignancies to hyperthermia and radiation. *Int J Radiat Oncol Biol Phys* 1993;25:841–847.
109. Li GC, Mivechi NF, Weitzel G. Heat shock proteins, thermotolerance, and their relevance to clinical hyperthermia. *Int J Hyperthermia* 1995;11:459–488.
110. Liang P, MacRae TH. Molecular chaperones and the cytoskeleton. *J Cell Sci* 1997;110:1431–1440.
111. Liu FF, Miller N, Levin W, et al. The potential role of HSP70 as an indicator of response to radiation and hyperthermia treatments for recurrent breast cancer. *Int J Hyperthermia* 1996;12:197–208; discussion 209–110.
112. Lohr F, Hu K, Huang Q, et al. Enhancement of radiotherapy by hyperthermia-regulated gene therapy. *Int J Radiat Oncol Biol Phys* 2000;48:1513–1518.
113. Lohr F, Huang Q, Hu K, et al. Systemic vector leakage and transgene expression by intratumorally injected recombinant adenovirus vectors. *Clin Cancer Res* 2001;7:3625–3628.
114. Lord PF, Kapp DS, Morrow D. Increased skeletal metastases of spontaneous canine osteosarcoma after fractionated systemic hyperthermia and local X-irradiation. *Cancer Res* 1981;41:4331–4334.
115. MacFall J, Prescott DM, Fullar E, et al. Temperature dependence of canine brain tissue diffusion coefficient measured in vivo with magnetic resonance echo-planar imaging. *Int J Hyperthermia* 1995;11:73–86.
116. Maehara Y, Kuwano H, Kitamura K, et al. Hyperthermochemoradiotherapy for esophageal cancer [Review]. *Anticancer Res* 1992;12:805–810.
117. Matsushita S, Reynolds R, Urano M. Synergism between alkylating agent and cisplatin with moderate local hyperthermia: The effect of multidrug chemotherapy in an animal system. *Int J Hyperthermia* 1993;9:285–296.
118. Matteucci ML, Anyarambhatla G, Rosner G, et al. Hyperthermia increases accumulation of technetium-99m-labeled liposomes in feline sarcomas [In Process Citation]. *Clin Cancer Res* 2000;6:3748–3755.
119. McRae DA, Esrick MA, Mueller SC. Non-invasive, in-vivo electrical impedance of EMT-6 tumours during hyperthermia: Correlation with morphology and tumour-growth-delay. *Int J Hyperthermia* 1997;13:1–20.
120. Meijer JG, van Wieringen N, Koedooder C, et al. The development of PdNi thermoseeds for interstitial hyperthermia. *Med Phys* 1995;22:101–104.
121. Meyer DE, Kong GA, Dewhirst MW, et al. Targeting a genetically engineered elastin-like polypeptide to solid tumors by local hyperthermia. *Cancer Res* 2001;61:1548–1554.
122. Meyer JL. The clinical efficacy of localized hyperthermia. *Cancer Res* 1984;44:4745S–4751S.
123. Meyer RE, Shan S, DeAngelo J, et al. Nitric oxide synthase inhibition irreversibly decreases perfusion in the R3230Ac rat mammary adenocarcinoma. *Br J Cancer* 1995;71:1169–1174.

124. Milas L, Hunter NR, Mason KA, et al. Role of reoxygenation in induction of enhancement of tumor radioresponse by paclitaxel. *Cancer Res* 1995;55:3564–3568.
125. Mivechi NF, Dewey WC. DNA polymerase alpha and beta activities during the cell cycle and their role in heat radiosensitization in Chinese hamster ovary cells. *Radiat Res* 1985;103:337–350.
126. Morano KA, Thiele DJ. Heat shock factor function and regulation in response to cellular stress, growth, and differentiation signals. *Gene Expr* 1999;7:271–282.
127. Morimoto RI, Kroeger PE, Cotto JJ. The transcriptional regulation of heat shock genes: A plethora of heat shock factors and regulatory conditions. *EXS* 1996;77:139–163.
128. Moros EG, Straube WL, Klein EE, et al. Simultaneous delivery of electron beam therapy and ultrasound hyperthermia using scanning reflectors: A feasibility study. *Int J Radiat Oncol Biol Phys* 1995;31:893–904.
129. Moros EG, Straube WL, Myerson RJ. Potential for power deposition conformability using reflected-scanned planar ultrasound. *Int J Hyperthermia* 1996;12:723–736.
130. Morris M, Eifel PJ, Lu J, et al. Pelvic radiation with concurrent chemotherapy compared with pelvic and para-aortic radiation for high-risk cervical cancer. *N Engl J Med* 1999;340:1137–1143.
131. Mueller-Klieser W, Walenta S, Kelleher DK, et al. Tumour-growth inhibition by induced hyperglycaemia/hyperlactacidaemia and localized hyperthermia. *Int J Hyperthermia* 1996;12:501–511.
132. Multhoff G, Botzler C, Wiesnet M, et al. A stress-inducible 72-kDa heat-shock protein (HSP72) is expressed on the surface of human tumor cells, but not on normal cells. *Int J Cancer* 1995;61:272–279.
133. Myerson RJ, Straube WL, Moros EG, et al. Simultaneous superficial hyperthermia and external radiotherapy: Report of thermal dosimetry and tolerance to treatment. *Int J Hyperthermia* 1999;15:251–266.
134. Nagata K, Murata T, Shiga T, et al. Enhancement of thermoradiotherapy by glucose administration for superficial malignant tumours. *Int J Hyperthermia* 1998;14:157–167.
135. Nah BS, Choi IB, Oh WY, et al. Vascular thermal adaptation in tumors and normal tissue in rats. *Int J Radiat Oncol Biol Phys* 1996;35:95–101.
136. Nathanson SD, Cerra RF, Hetzel FW, et al. Changes associated with metastasis in B16-F1 melanoma cells surviving heat. *Arch Surg* 1990;125:216–219.
137. Nathanson SD, Nelson L, Anaya P, et al. Development of lymph node and pulmonary metastases after local irradiation and hyperthermia of footpad melanomas. *Clin Exp Metastasis* 1991;9:377–392.
138. Needham D, Anyarambhatla G, Kong G, et al. A new temperature-sensitive liposome for use with mild hyperthermia: Characterization and testing in a human tumor xenograft model. *Cancer Res* 2000;60:1197–1201.
139. Ng CE, Bussey AM, Raaphorst GP. Sequence of treatment is important in the modification of camptothecin induced cell killing by hyperthermia. *Int J Hyperthermia* 1996;12:663–678; discussion 679–680.
140. Nielsen OS, Overgaard J. Importance of preheating temperature and time for the induction of thermotolerance in a solid tumour in vivo. *Br J Cancer* 1982;46:894–903.
141. Ning SC, Hahn GM. Combination therapy: Lonidamine, hyperthermia, and chemotherapy against the RIF-1 tumor in vivo. *Cancer Res* 1991;51:5910–5914.
142. Okamoto K, Shinoura N, Egawa N, et al. Adenovirus-mediated transfer of p53 augments hyperthermia-induced apoptosis in U251 glioma cells. *Int J Radiat Oncol Biol Phys* 2001;50:525–531.
143. Oleson JR. Eugene Robertson Special Lecture. Hyperthermia from the clinic to the laboratory: A hypothesis. *Int J Hyperthermia* 1995;11:315–322.
144. Oleson JR, Dewhirst MW, Harrelson JM, et al. Tumor temperature distributions predict hyperthermia effect. *Int J Radiat Oncol Biol Phys* 1989;16:559–570.
145. Oleson JR, Samulski TV, Leopold KA, et al. Sensitivity of hyperthermia trial outcomes to temperature and time: Implications for thermal goals of treatment. *Int J Radiat Oncol Biol Phys* 1993;25:289–297.
146. Overgaard J. Simultaneous and sequential hyperthermia and radiation treatment of an experimental tumor and its surrounding normal tissue in vivo. *Int J Radiat Oncol Biol Phys* 1980;6:1507–1517.
147. Overgaard J. Fractionated radiation and hyperthermia: Experimental and clinical studies. *Cancer* 1981;48:1116–1123.
148. Overgaard J. Influence of sequence and interval on the biological response to combined hyperthermia and radiation. *Natl Cancer Inst Monogr* 1982;61:325–332.
149. Overgaard J. The current and potential role of hyperthermia in radiotherapy. *Int J Radiat Oncol Biol Phys* 1989;16:535–549.
150. Overgaard J, Gonzalez Gonzalez D, Hulshof MC, et al. Randomised trial of hyperthermia as adjuvant to radiotherapy for recurrent or metastatic malignant melanoma. European Society for Hyperthermic Oncology. *Lancet* 1995;345:540–543.
151. Overgaard J, Gonzalez Gonzalez D, Hulshof MC, et al. Hyperthermia as an adjuvant to radiation therapy of recurrent or metastatic malignant melanoma. A multicentre randomized trial by the European Society for Hyperthermic Oncology. *Int J Hyperthermia* 1996;12:3–20.
152. Owen CS, Pooler PM, Wahl ML, et al. Altered proton extrusion in cells adapted to growth at low extracellular pH. *J Cell Physiol* 1997;173:397–405.
153. Parsons PG. Dependence on treatment time of melphalan resistance and DNA cross-linking in human melanoma cell lines. *Cancer Res* 1984;44:2773–2778.
154. Paulsen KD, Geimer S, Tang J, et al. Optimization of pelvic heating rate distributions with electromagnetic phased arrays. *Int J Hyperthermia* 1999;15:157–186.
155. Perez CA, Gillespie B, Pajak T, et al. Quality assurance problems in clinical hyperthermia and their impact on therapeutic outcome: A report by the Radiation Therapy Oncology Group. *Int J Radiat Oncol Biol Phys* 1989;16:551–558.
156. Perez CA, Pajak T, Emami B, et al. Randomized phase III study comparing irradiation and hyperthermia with irradiation alone in superficial measurable tumors. Final report by the Radiation Therapy Oncology Group. *Am J Clin Oncol* 1991;14:133–141.
157. Peters WA 3rd, Liu PY, Barrett RJ 2nd, et al. Concurrent chemotherapy and pelvic radiation therapy compared with pelvic radiation therapy alone as adjuvant therapy after radical surgery in high-risk early-stage cancer of the cervix. *J Clin Oncol* 2000;18:1606–1613.
158. Poulson JM, Dewhirst MW, Gaskin AA, et al. Acute pancreatitis associated with administration of a nitric oxide synthase inhibitor in tumor-bearing dogs. *In Vivo* 2000;14:709–714.

159. Pratt WB, Silverstein AM, Galigniana MD. A model for the cytoplasmic trafficking of signalling proteins involving the hsp90-binding immunophilins and p50cdc37. *Cell Signal* 1999;11:839–851.
160. Prescott DM, Charles HC, Sostman HD, et al. Manipulation of intra- and extracellular pH in spontaneous canine tumours by use of hyperglycaemia. *Int J Hyperthermia* 1993;9:745–754.
161. Prescott DM, Charles HC, Sostman HD, et al. Therapy monitoring in human and canine soft tissue sarcomas using magnetic resonance imaging and spectroscopy. *Int J Radiat Oncol Biol Phys* 1994;28:415–423.
162. Prescott DM, Samulski TV, Dewhirst MW, et al. Use of nitroprusside to increase tissue temperature during local hyperthermia in normal and tumor-bearing dogs. *Int J Radiat Oncol Biol Phys* 1992;23:377–385.
163. Prosnitz LR, Maguire P, Anderson JM, et al. The treatment of high-grade soft tissue sarcomas with preoperative thermoradiotherapy. *Int J Radiat Oncol Biol Phys* 1999;45:941–949.
164. Qi V, Weinrib L, Ma N, et al. Adenoviral p53 gene therapy promotes heat-induced apoptosis in a nasopharyngeal carcinoma cell line. *Int J Hyperthermia* 2001;17:38–47.
165. Raaphorst G. Fundamental aspects of hyperthermic biology. In: Field S, Hand J, eds. *An introduction to the practical aspects of clinical hyperthermia.* London: Taylor and Francis, 1990;10–54.
166. Raaphorst GP. *Hyperthermia.* London: Taylor and Francis, 1990.
167. Raaphorst GP, Ng CE, Yang DP. Thermal radiosensitization and repair inhibition in human melanoma cells: a comparison of survival and DNA double strand breaks. *Int J Hyperthermia* 1999;15:17–27.
168. Raaphorst GP, Yang DP, Ng CE. Effect of protracted mild hyperthermia on polymerase activity in a human melanoma cell line. *Int J Hyperthermia* 1994;10:827–834.
169. Rau B, Gaestel M, Wust P, et al. Preoperative treatment of rectal cancer with radiation, chemotherapy and hyperthermia: Analysis of treatment efficacy and heat-shock response. *Radiat Res* 1999;151:479–488.
170. Rau B, Wust P, Gellermann J, et al. [Phase II study on preoperative radio-chemo-thermotherapy in locally advanced rectal carcinoma]. *Strahlenther Onkol* 1998;174:556–565.
171. Reinhold HS. Physiological effects of hyperthermia. *Recent Results Cancer Res* 1988;107:32–43.
172. Roemer RB, Fletcher AM, Cetas TC. Obtaining local SAR and blood perfusion data from temperature measurements: Steady state and transient techniques compared. *Int J Radiat Oncol Biol Phys* 1985;11:1539–1550.
173. Roemer RB, Oleson JR, Cetas TC. Oscillatory temperature response to constant power applied to canine muscle. *Am J Physiol* 1985;249:R153–R158.
174. Roizin-Towle L, Pirro JP. The response of human and rodent cells to hyperthermia. *Int J Radiat Oncol Biol Phys* 1991;20:751–756.
175. Rose PG, Bundy BN, Watkins EB, et al. Concurrent cisplatin-based radiotherapy and chemotherapy for locally advanced cervical cancer. *N Engl J Med* 1999;340:1144–1153.
176. Sakaguchi Y, Stephens LC, Makino M, et al. Apoptosis in tumors and normal tissues induced by whole body hyperthermia in rats. *Cancer Res* 1995;55:5459–5464.
177. Sapareto SA, Dewey WC. Thermal dose determination in cancer therapy. *Int J Radiat Oncol Biol Phys* 1984;10:787–800.
178. Sapozink MD, Corry PM, Kapp DS, et al. RTOG quality assurance guidelines for clinical trials using hyperthermia for deep-seated malignancy. *Int J Radiat Oncol Biol Phys* 1991;20:1109–1115.
179. Satoh T, Stauffer PR. Implantable helical coil microwave antenna for interstitial hyperthermia. *Int J Hyperthermia* 1988;4:497–512.
180. Schoonover LL, Stewart AS, Clifton GD. Hemodynamic and cardiovascular effects of nitric oxide modulation in the therapy of septic shock. *Pharmacotherapy* 2000;20:1184–1197.
181. Secomb TW, Hsu R, Braun RD, et al. Theoretical simulation of oxygen transport to tumors by three-dimensional networks of microvessels. *Adv Exp Med Biol* 1998;454:629–634.
182. Seegenschmiedt MH, Feldmann HJ, Molls M. Hyperthermia—its actual role in radiation oncology. Part II: Clinical fundamentals and results in superficial tumors. *Strahlenther Onkol* 1993;169:635–654.
183. Sevick EM, Jain RK. Geometric resistance to blood flow in solid tumors perfused ex vivo: Effects of tumor size and perfusion pressure. *Cancer Res* 1989;49:3506–3512.
184. Sevick EM, Jain RK. Viscous resistance to blood flow in solid tumors: Effect of hematocrit on intratumor blood viscosity. *Cancer Res* 1989;49:3513–3519.
185. Sharma S, Sandhu AP, Patel FD, et al. Side-effects of local hyperthermia: Results of a prospectively randomized clinical study. *Int J Hyperthermia* 1990;6:279–285.
186. Sherar M, Liu FF, Pintilie M, et al. Relationship between thermal dose and outcome in thermoradiotherapy treatments for superficial recurrences of breast cancer: Data from a phase III trial. *Int J Radiat Oncol Biol Phys* 1997;39:371–380.
187. Sminia P, Jansen W, Haveman J, et al. Incidence of tumours in the cervical region of the rat after treatment with radiation and hyperthermia. *Int J Radiat Biol* 1990;57:425–436.
188. Sneed PK, Stauffer PR, McDermott MW, et al. Survival benefit of hyperthermia in a prospective randomized trial of brachytherapy boost +/− hyperthermia for glioblastoma multiforme. *Int J Radiat Oncol Biol Phys* 1998;40:287–295.
189. Snyder SA, Lanzen JL, Braun RD, et al. Simultaneous administration of glucose and hyperoxic gas achieves greater improvement in tumor oxygenation than hyperoxic gas alone. *Int J Radiat Oncol Biol Phys* 2001;51:494–506.
190. Soncin F, Calderwood SK. Reciprocal effects of pro-inflammatory stimuli and anti-inflammatory drugs on the activity of heat shock factor-1 in human monocytes. *Biochem Biophys Res Commun* 1996;229:479–484.
191. Song CW. Effect of local hyperthermia on blood flow and microenvironment: A review. *Cancer Res* 1984;44:4721S–4730S.
192. Song CW, Kim GE, Lyons JC, et al. Thermosensitization by increasing intracellular acidity with amiloride and its analogs. *Int J Radiat Oncol Biol Phys* 1994;30:1161–1169.
193. Song CW, Park H, Griffin RJ. Improvement of tumor oxygenation by mild hyperthermia. *Radiat Res* 2001;155:515–528.
194. Sostman HD, Prescott DM, Dewhirst MW, et al. MR imaging and spectroscopy for prognostic evaluation in soft-tissue sarcomas. *Radiology* 1994;190:269–275.
195. Srivastava PK, Amato RJ. Heat shock proteins: The "Swiss Army Knife" vaccines against cancers and infectious agents. *Vaccine* 2001;19:2590–2597.

196. Stauffer P, Manfrini V, Leoncini M, et al. *Hyperthermic oncology.* Rome: Editorgrafica, 1996.

197. Stauffer PR, Cetas TC, Fletcher AM, et al. Observations on the use of ferromagnetic implants for inducing hyperthermia. *IEEE Trans Biomed Eng* 1984;31:76–90.

198. Stauffer PR, Sneed PK, Suen SA, et al. Comparative thermal dosimetry of interstitial microwave and radiofrequency-LCF hyperthermia. *Int J Hyperthermia* 1989;5:307–318.

199. Steinhausen D, Mayer WK, von Ardenne M. [Evaluation of systemic tolerance of 42.0 degrees C infrared-A whole-body hyperthermia in combination with hyperglycemia and hyperoxemia. A Phase-I study.] *Strahlenther Onkol* 1994;170:322–334.

200. Stone HB. Thermal enhancement of radiation-induced leg contracture. *Int J Radiat Oncol Biol Phys* 1990;18:595–602.

201. Straube WL, Klein EE, Moros EG, et al. Dosimetry and techniques for simultaneous hyperthermia and external beam radiation therapy. *Int J Hyperthermia* 2001;17:48–62.

202. Streffer C. Metabolic changes during and after hyperthermia. *Int J Hyperthermia* 1985;1:305–319.

203. Strohbehn JW. Hyperthermia equipment evaluation. *Int J Hyperthermia* 1994;10:429–432.

204. Strohbehn JW, Bowers ED, Walsh JE, et al. An invasive microwave antenna for locally-induced hyperthermia for cancer therapy. *J Microw Power* 1979;14:339–350.

205. Sugimachi K, Kitamura K, Baba K, et al. Hyperthermia combined with chemotherapy and irradiation for patients with carcinoma of the oesophagus—a prospective randomized trial. *Int J Hyperthermia* 1992;8:289–295.

206. Sugimachi K, Kuwano H, Ide H, et al. Chemotherapy combined with or without hyperthermia for patients with oesophageal carcinoma: A prospective randomized trial. *Int J Hyperthermia* 1994;10:485–493.

207. Teicher BA, Holden SA, Khandakar V, et al. Addition of a topoisomerase I inhibitor to trimodality therapy [cis-diamminedichloroplatinum(II)/heat/radiation] in a murine tumor. *J Cancer Res Clin Oncol* 1993;119:645–651.

208. Thrall DE, Gillette EL, Dewey WC. Effect of heat and ionizing radiation on normal and neoplastic tissue of the C3H mouse. *Radiat Res* 1975;63:363–377.

209. Thrall DE, Prescott DM, Samulski TV, et al. Radiation plus local hyperthermia versus radiation plus the combination of local and whole-body hyperthermia in canine sarcomas. *Int J Radiat Oncol Biol Phys* 1996;34:1087–1096.

210. Tilly W, Wust P, Rau B, et al. Temperature data and specific absorption rates in pelvic tumours: Predictive factors and correlations. *Int J Hyperthermia* 2001;17:172–188.

211. Tohnai I, Hayashi Y, Mitsudo K, et al. Thermochemotherapy for cancer of the tongue using magnetic induction hyperthermia (implant heating system: IHS). *Nagoya J Med Sci* 1996;59:49–54.

212. Tozer GM, Prise VE, Bell KM, et al. Reduced capacity of tumour blood vessels to produce endothelium-derived relaxing factor: Significance for blood flow modification. *Br J Cancer* 1996;74:1955–1960.

213. Tozer GM, Shaffi KM, Prise VE, et al. Spatial heterogeneity of tumour blood flow modification induced by angiotensin II: Relationship to receptor distribution. *Int J Cancer* 1996;65:658–663.

214. Traykov TT, Jain RK. Effect of glucose and galactose on red blood cell membrane deformability. *Int J Microcirc Clin Exp* 1987;6:35–44.

215. Trembly BS, Douple EB, Ryan TP, et al. Effect of phase modulation on the temperature distribution of a microwave hyperthermia antenna array in vivo. *Int J Hyperthermia* 1994;10:691–705.

216. Turner PF. Regional hyperthermia with an annular phased array. *IEEE Trans Biomed Eng* 1984;31:106–114.

217. Underwood HR, Burdette EC, Ocheltree KB, et al. A multi-element ultrasonic hyperthermia applicator with independent element control. *Int J Hyperthermia* 1987;3:257–267.

218. Uozaki H, Ishida T, Kakiuchi C, et al. Expression of heat shock proteins in osteosarcoma and its relationship to prognosis. *Pathol Res Pract* 2000;196:665–673.

219. Urano M, Kenton LA, Kahn J. The effect of hyperthermia on the early and late appearing mouse foot reactions and on the radiation carcinogenesis: Effect on the early and late appearing reactions. *Int J Radiat Oncol Biol Phys* 1988;15:159–166.

220. Vaden SL, Page RL, Williams PL, et al. Effect of hyperthermia on cisplatin and carboplatin disposition in the isolated, perfused tumour and skin flap. *Int J Hyperthermia* 1994;10:563–572.

220a. Valdagni R, Amichetti M, Pani G. Radical radiation alone versus radical radiation plus microwave hyperthermia for N3 (TNM-UICC) neck nodes: a prospective randomized clinical trial. *Int J Radiat Oncol Biol Phys* 1988;15(1):13–24.

220b. Valdagni R, Amichetti M. Report of long-term follow-up in a randomized trial comparing radiation therapy and radiation therapy plus hyperthermia to metastatic lymph nodes in stage IV head and neck patients. *Int J Radiat Oncol Biol Phys* 1994;28(1):163–169.

221. Van Den Berg AP, Van Den Berg-Blok AE, Kal HB, et al. A moderate elevation of blood glucose level increases the effectiveness of thermoradiotherapy in a rat tumor model II. Improved tumor control at clinically achievable temperatures. *Int J Radiat Oncol Biol Phys* 2001;50:793–801.

222. Van Der Koijk JF, Crezee J, van Leeuwen GM, et al. Dose uniformity in MECS interstitial hyperthermia: The impact of longitudinal control in model anatomies. *Phys Med Biol* 1996;41:429–444.

223. Van Der Zee J, Gonzalez Gonzalez D, van Rhoon GC, et al. Comparison of radiotherapy alone with radiotherapy plus hyperthermia in locally advanced pelvic tumours: A prospective, randomised, multicentre trial. Dutch Deep Hyperthermia Group. *Lancet* 2000;355:1119–1125.

224. Vargas-Roig LM, Gago FE, Tello O, et al. Heat shock protein expression and drug resistance in breast cancer patients treated with induction chemotherapy. *Int J Cancer* 1998;79:468–475.

225. Vernon CC, Hand JW, Field SB, et al. Radiotherapy with or without hyperthermia in the treatment of superficial localized breast cancer: Results from five randomized controlled trials. International Collaborative Hyperthermia Group. *Int J Radiat Oncol Biol Phys* 1996;35:731–744.

226. Vidair CA, Dewey WC. Division-associated and division-independent hyperthermic cell death: Comparison with other cytotoxic agents. *Int J Hyperthermia* 1991;7:51–60.

227. Vidair CA, Doxsey SJ, Dewey WC. Heat shock alters centrosome organization leading to mitotic dysfunction and cell death. *J Cell Physiol* 1993;154:443–455.

228. von Ardenne M. Principles and concept 1993 of the Systemic Cancer Multistep Therapy (sCMT). Extreme whole-body hyperthermia using the infrared-A technique IRATHERM 2000—selective thermosensitisation by hyperglycemia—circulatory back-up by adapted hyperoxemia. *Strahlenther Onkol* 1994;170:581–589.

229. Vujaskovic Z, Poulson J, Gaskin A, et al. Temperature dependent changes in physiologic parameters of spontaneous canine soft tissue sarcomas after combined radiotherapy and hyperthermia. *Int J Radiat Oncol Biol Phys* 2000;46(1):179–185.

230. Wachsberger PR, Landry J, Storck C, et al. Mammalian cells adapted to growth at pH 6.7 have elevated HSP27 levels and are resistant to cisplatin. *Int J Hyperthermia* 1997;13:251–255; discussion 257–259.

231. Wahl ML, Bobyock SB, Leeper DB, et al. Effects of 42 degrees C hyperthermia on intracellular pH in ovarian carcinoma cells during acute or chronic exposure to low extracellular pH. *Int J Radiat Oncol Biol Phys* 1997;39:205–212.

232. Wang Z, Armour EP, Corry PM, et al. Elimination of dose-rate effects by mild hyperthermia. *Int J Radiat Oncol Biol Phys* 1992;24:965–973.

233. Ward KA, DiPette DJ, Held TN, et al. Effect of intravenous versus intraperitoneal glucose injection on systemic hemodynamics and blood flow rate in normal and tumor tissues in rats. *Cancer Res* 1991;51:3612–3616.

234. Waterman FM, Tupchong L, Liu CR. Modified thermal clearance technique for determination of blood flow during local hyperthermia. *Int J Hyperthermia* 1991;7:719–733.

234a. Wendtner C, Abdel-Rahman S, Baumert J, et al. Treatment of primary, recurrent or inadequately resected high-risk soft-tissue sarcomas (STS) of adults: results of a Phase II pilot study (RHT-95) of neoadjuvant chemotherapy combined with regional hyperthermia. *Eur J Cancer* 2001;37(13):1609–1616.

235. Whitney CW, Sause W, Bundy BN, et al. Randomized comparison of fluorouracil plus cisplatin versus hydroxyurea as an adjunct to radiation therapy in stage IIB-IVA carcinoma of the cervix with negative para-aortic lymph nodes: A Gynecologic Oncology Group and Southwest Oncology Group study. *J Clin Oncol* 1999;17:1339–1348.

236. Wickersheim KA, Alves RV. Fluoroptic thermometry: A new RF-immune technology. *Prog Clin Biol Res* 1982;107:547–554.

237. Wlodarczyk W, Hentschel M, Wust P, et al. Comparison of four magnetic resonance methods for mapping small temperature changes. *Phys Med Biol* 1999;44:607–624.

238. Woo SY, Anderson RL, Kapp DS, et al. Heterogeneity of heat response in murine, canine and human tumors: Influence on predictive assays. *Int J Radiat Oncol Biol Phys* 1991;20:479–488.

239. Wust P, Nadobny J, Felix R, et al. Strategies for optimized application of annular-phased-array systems in clinical hyperthermia. *Int J Hyperthermia* 1991;7:157–173.

240. Yatvin MB, Weinstein JN, Dennis WH, et al. Design of liposomes for enhanced local release of drugs by hyperthermia. *Science* 1978;202:1290–1293.

241. Zhang Y, Joines WT, Oleson JR. Heating patterns generated by phase modulation of a hexagonal array of interstitial antennas. *IEEE Trans Biomed Eng* 1991;38:92–97.

242. Zhou R, Bansal N, Leeper DB, et al. Intracellular acidification of human melanoma xenografts by the respiratory inhibitor m-iodobenzylguanidine plus hyperglycemia: A 31P magnetic resonance spectroscopy study. *Cancer Res* 2000;60:3532–3536.

243. Zhou R, Bansal N, Leeper DB, et al. Enhancement of hyperglycemia-induced acidification of human melanoma xenografts with inhibitors of respiration and ion transport. *Acad Radiol* 2001;8:571–582.

244. Zywietz F, Reeker W, Kochs E. Changes in tumor oxygenation during a combined treatment with fractionated irradiation and hyperthermia: An experimental study. *Int J Radiat Oncol Biol Phys* 1997;37:155–162.

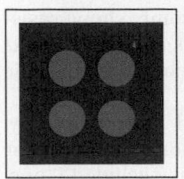

Chapter 29
Basic Concepts of Chemotherapy and Irradiation Interaction

Hak Choy, Rob MacRae, Michael Story

For decades, radiation therapy has been a major treatment modality for locally or regionally confined cancers. The rate of treatment failure is still high, particularly for large tumors or advanced disease, which lowers the overall cure rate and the length of patient survival. Improvements in radiation therapy have continuously been made both in the arena of technological innovations that allow delivery of higher radiation doses to the tumor or lower doses to normal tissues, and in the implementation of strategies that modulate the biologic response of tumors or normal tissues to radiation. These strategies include altered fractionation scheduling, combined modality treatments using chemical or biologic agents, and, more recently, targeting molecular processes and signaling pathways that have become dysregulated in cancer cells.

Among all these strategies to improve therapy, the combining of chemotherapeutic drugs with radiation has perhaps had the strongest impact on current cancer radiation therapy practice. This combination has been in use for many decades but has now become a common treatment option in many clinical settings. This is particularly true for concurrent chemoradiation therapy, which in many recent clinical trials has been shown to be superior to radiation therapy alone in controlling locoregional disease and in improving patient survival. Combining chemotherapeutic drugs with radiation therapy has a strong biologic rationale. Such agents reduce the number of cells in tumors undergoing radiation therapy by their independent cytotoxic action and by rendering tumor cells more susceptible to killing by ionizing radiation. An additional benefit of combined treatment is that chemotherapeutic drugs, by virtue of their systemic activity, may also act on metastatic disease. Most drugs have been chosen for combination with radiation therapy based on their known clinical activity in particular disease sites. Alternatively, agents that are effective in overcoming resistance mechanisms associated with radiation therapy could be chosen. There have been recent clinical successes of concurrent chemoradiation therapy using traditional drugs, such as cisplatin and 5-fluorouracil (5-FU), but these studies have led to extensive research on exploring newer chemotherapeutic agents for their interactions with radiation. A number of new potent chemotherapeutic agents, including taxanes, nucleoside analogs, and topoisomerase inhibitors, have entered clinical trials or practice. Preclinical testing has shown that they are potent enhancers of radiation response and thus might further improve the therapeutic outcome of chemoradiation therapy. Also, there are rapidly emerging molecular targeting strategies aimed at improving the efficacy of chemoradiation therapy (see Chapter 23).

This chapter reviews the biologic rationale and principles fundamental to the use of chemoradiation therapy and discusses mechanistic interactions between drugs and radiation, the knowledge of which is essential in developing the optimal treatment strategies. As well, it overviews current treatment applications and advances in the clinic. Owing to limited space, this review is far from comprehensive; additional information can be found in other reviews on this subject (100,102, 189)

Therapeutic Index

Both radiation and chemotherapeutic drugs are cytotoxic to tumor and normal tissue cells. This lack of specificity is a major limitation in their use when applied either as individual treatments or in combination. Radiation inflicts damage to tumor and normal tissues in the radiation treatment field, whereas drugs, because of their systemic action, can affect any tissue in the body. Damage is often accentuated when the two agents are combined and when they affect the same tissue. In general, both the antitumor effectiveness and the severity of normal tissue damage produced by either radiation or drugs are increased as their dose is increased. This dose-effect relationship is sigmoidal and enables estimation of the therapeutic index (ratio), which is defined as the ratio between the doses (radiation, drug) that produce the same level (probability) of antitumor efficacy and normal tissue damage. To be therapeutically beneficial, the therapeutic ratio must be positive (>1); that is, individual agents or their combination must be more effective against tumors than normal tissues. To define therapeutic benefit in clinical settings, many factors must be taken into account, such as whether the treatment is curative or palliative, which tissues are dose-limiting (critical tissues), what degree of tissue damage is acceptable, and so forth. The balance between a given level of antitumor efficacy and acceptable normal tissue complications gives a measure of the therapeutic ratio of a treatment.

Exploitable Strategies in Chemoradiation Therapy

The goals of combining chemotherapeutic drugs with radiation therapy are to increase patient survival by improving locoregional tumor control, decreasing or eliminating distant metastases, or both, while preserving organ and tissue integrity and function. Combined-modality treatment can further improve positive therapeutic outcome of individual treatments through a number of specific strategies, which Steel and Peckham (219) classified into four groups: "spatial cooperation," independent toxicity, enhancement of tumor response, and protection of normal tissues.

Spatial cooperation was the initial rationale for combining chemotherapy with radiation therapy, in which the action of radiation and chemotherapeutic drugs is directed toward different anatomic sites. Localized tumors would be the domain of radiation therapy because large doses of radiation can be given. On the other hand, chemotherapeutic drugs are likely to be more effective in eliminating disseminated micrometastases than in eradicating larger primary tumors. Thus, the cooperation between radiation and chemotherapy is achieved through the independent action of two agents. Spatial cooperation is the basis for adjuvant chemoradiation therapy, in which radiation is given first to control the primary tumor, and chemotherapy is given later to cope with micrometastases. The concept of spatial cooperation is also applied in the treatment of hematologic malignancies that have spread to "sanctuary" sites, such as the brain. These sites are poorly accessible to chemotherapeutic agents, and thus they are more appropriately treated with radiation therapy.

Independent toxicity is another important strategy for increasing the therapeutic ratio of chemoradiation therapy. Normal tissue toxicity is the main dose-limiting factor for both chemotherapy and radiation therapy. Therefore, combinations of radiation and drugs would be better tolerated if drugs were selected such that toxicities to specific cell types and tissues do not overlap with, or minimally add to, radiation-induced toxicities. This strategy requires a thorough knowledge of drug toxicity, underlying mechanisms, and drug pharmacokinetics. Careful drug selection based on these mechanisms may minimize normal tissue damage while retaining antitumor efficacy when combined with radiation therapy.

Another strategy in chemoradiation therapy is to exploit the ability of chemotherapeutic agents to enhance tumor radioresponse. The enhancement denotes the existence of some type of interaction between drugs and radiation at the molecular, cellular, or pathophysiologic (microenvironmental, metabolic) level, resulting in an antitumor effect greater than would be expected on the basis of additive actions. Many mechanisms may be involved in drug–radiation interactions leading to tumor radio enhancement, and some of them are elaborated on further in the text. The enhancement must be selective or preferential to tumors compared with critical normal tissues to achieve therapeutic gain. The ability of chemotherapeutic agents to enhance tumor radioresponse by counteracting determinants associated with tumor radioresistance is a major rationale for concurrent radiation therapy.

An additional strategy is to protect normal tissues so that higher doses of radiation can be delivered to the tumor. This can be achieved through technical improvements in radiation delivery or administration of chemical or biologic agents that selectively or preferentially protect normal tissues against the damage by radiation or drugs. A separate section in this chapter discusses radioprotectors in more detail.

Assessment of Drug–Radiation Interaction

Any drug considered for use in combination with radiation therapy needs to undergo preclinical evaluation for its interaction with radiation both in *in vitro* cell culture systems and *in vivo*, with the aim of assessing antitumor activity and normal tissue toxicity. The interaction between two agents is more easily defined and quantified *in vitro* because complete cell survival curves are readily obtained. The *in vitro* cell survival assay measures the ability of cells to produce colonies of a defined minimum size. A variety of *in vitro* established cell culture lines are available for this testing, or cells can be freshly derived from tumors. Cell survival is determined after treatment with a drug or radiation alone, given at different doses, or after treatment with both agents, in which case the cells are exposed to the drug before, during, or after irradiation. Survival curves are usually plots of the surviving fraction of cells on a logarithmic scale and the dose of radiation or drugs on a linear scale.

The cell survival curve after irradiation characteristically has a "shoulder" of varying width at lower doses of radiation followed by an exponential portion that appears at higher doses of radiation. The shoulder denotes the capacity of cells to repair radiation damage. The curves that describe survival after chemotherapeutic agents show much more variation both in absolute sensitivity to drugs and their shape than those after radiation, all depending on the drug tested. Some curves

possess shoulders, some lack them, and some show resistant "tails" at higher drug doses. The tails denote the existence of cell subpopulations resistant to chemotherapeutic agents.

To assess the effect of the drug on cell radiosensitivity, the combined drug–radiation curve is commonly plotted after the cytotoxicity produced by the drug alone is excluded ("normalized"). The radiation cell survival curve is not changed if the drug does not influence cell radiosensitivity regardless of whether the drug is cytotoxic on its own. In this case, the cytotoxicity of the drug contributes only to the overall cell killing by the combined treatment (*additive effect*) of both agents. Chemotherapeutic agents may interact with radiation by altering cell radiosensitivity such that the combination results in a *supraadditive* or *subadditive effect,* depending on whether the cell killing is greater or smaller than the sum of cell killings produced by individual agents. Drugs may eliminate the shoulder on the radiation survival curve, implying that drugs can inhibit cell repair from radiation damage, or they may change the slope of the exponential portion of the survival curve. A steeper slope indicates increased sensitization to radiation, whereas a shallower slope indicates protection.

Because of nonlinear dose-related characteristics in cell killing by both chemotherapeutic agents and radiation, the effects of the combined treatment are best assessed using the "isobologram," an isoeffect plot for the dose response to the combination of two agents (219) (Fig. 29.1). Dose–response curves are determined for each agent to generate the isobologram, an envelope of additivity, which denotes expected additive response over a range of doses of the agents used. If the interaction between drugs and radiation is supraadditive or synergistic (i.e., the effect is caused by lower doses of the two agents than the envelope of additivity would predict), the effect is shown at the left side of the envelope. In contrast, the effect of the subadditive or antagonistic interaction is shown to the right of the envelope: The effect required higher doses of the two agents than predicted. The width of the envelope of additivity depends on the degree of the nonlinearity in the dose response

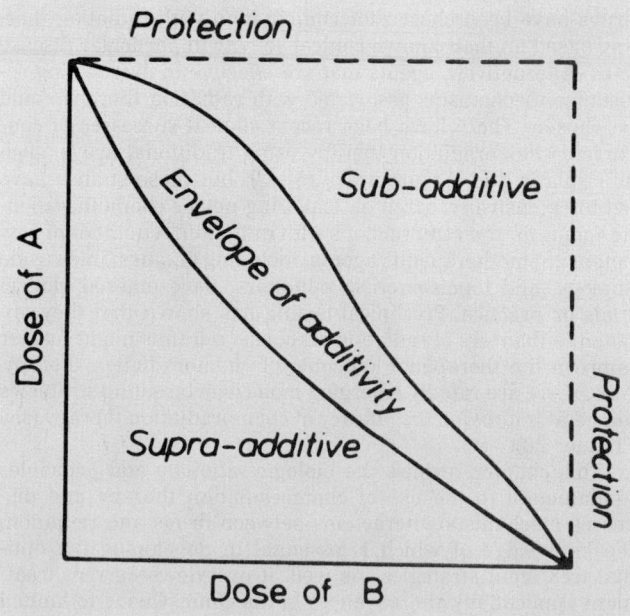

FIGURE 29.1. An isobologram for two agents when their dose–response curves are nonlinear. The isobologram shows the envelope of additivity and regions of supraadditivity and subadditivity. (Modified from Steel GG, Peckham MJ. Exploitable mechanisms in combined radiotherapy-chemotherapy: The concept of additivity. *Int J Radiat Oncol Biol Phys* 1979;5:85–91, with permission. Copyright 1979 by Elsevier Science, Inc.)

to individual agents. The envelope is wider as the degree of nonlinearity increases. In the case of a linear dose–response relationship for each agent, which is rare, the isobologram is also linear, represented by a single straight line.

In vitro testing is often followed by *in vivo* exploration of drug–radiation interactions, which allows assessment of the combined treatment on both tumors and normal tissues. This is essential for determination of therapeutic gain, as discussed earlier in this chapter. Syngeneic animal tumors or human tumor xenografts in nude mice are most often used for this purpose. The efficacy of the treatment is determined by the extent of tumor growth delay or the rate of tumor cure. In normal tissues, the effect of chemotherapeutic drugs on radiation response of acutely and late-responding tissues can be assessed using a variety of available assays. Some of these assays are clonogenic, such as the jejunal crypt assay, where the end point depends directly on the reproductive integrity of individual cells. More frequently, however, dose–response relationships for normal tissues are based on functional end points (such as breathing rate in lung damage and paralysis in spinal cord damage). These end points tend to reflect the minimum number of functional cells remaining in tissues or organs and not the proportion of cells retaining reproductive integrity.

Mechanistic Considerations in Drug–Radiation Interactions

Increasing Initial Radiation Damage

Radiation induces many different lesions in the DNA molecule, which is the critical target for radiation damage. The lesions consist of single-strand breaks (SSBs), double-strand breaks (DSBs), base damage, DNA–DNA and DNA–protein cross-links, and so forth. DSBs and chromosome aberrations that occur in association with or as a consequence of DSBs are usually considered to be the principal damage that results in cell death (198). Any agent that makes DNA more susceptible to radiation damage may enhance cell killing. Certain drugs, such as halogenated pyrimidines, incorporate into DNA and make it more susceptible to radiation damage (122).

Inhibition of Cellular Repair

Both sublethal (73) and potentially lethal (113,137) damage inflicted by radiation can be repaired. Although sublethal damage repair (SLDR) denotes the increase in cell survival when the radiation dose is split into two fractions of radiation separated by a time interval, potentially lethal damage repair (PLDR) designates the increase in cell survival as the result of postirradiation environmental conditions. SLDR is rapid, with a half-time of approximately 1 hour, and is complete within 4 to 6 hours after irradiation. This time between two radiation fractions allows radiation-induced DSBs in DNA to rejoin and repair. SLDR is expressed as the restitution of the shoulder on the cell survival curve for the second dose. PLDR occurs when environmental conditions prevent cells from dividing for several hours, such as keeping *in vitro* growing cells in plateau phase after irradiation. Preventing cells from division allows the completion of repair of DNA lesions that would have been lethal had DNA undergone replication within several hours after irradiation. PLDR is considered to be a major determinant responsible for radioresistance in some tumor types, such as melanomas. The repair can be achieved through restoration of damaged molecules by reducing species that donate electrons to oxidized substrates or through involvement of enzymes mediating homologous and nonhomologous recombination repair of DNA DSBs, base

excision repair of base damage, and nucleotide excision repair of DNA–protein cross-links.

Many chemotherapeutic agents used in chemoradiation therapy interact with cellular repair mechanisms and inhibit repair, and hence may enhance cell or tissue response to radiation. The aforementioned halogenated pyrimidines enhance cell radiosensitivity not only through increasing initial radiation damage but by inhibiting cellular repair (122,248). Nucleoside analogs, such as gemcitabine, are a class of chemotherapeutic agents potent in inhibiting the repair of radiation-induced DNA and chromosome damage (93,130,192). They have been shown strongly to enhance tumor radioresponse in preclinical studies and are being extensively investigated for such activity in patients with cancer (85,160).

Cell Cycle Redistribution

Both chemotherapeutic agents and radiation are more effective against proliferating than nonproliferating cells. Their cytotoxic action further depends on the position of cells in the cell cycle. Cell cycle dependency in response to radiation was first reported almost 35 years ago (234). Terasima and Tolmach (234) reported that the sensitivity of the cell response to radiation varied widely depending on which phase of the cell cycle the cells were in at the time of irradiation, and that cells in the G_2 and M cell cycle phases were approximately three times more sensitive than cells in the S phase. The exact reason for this variability is still unknown.

The influence of cell cycle on cell response to cytotoxic agents can be therapeutically exploited in chemoradiation therapy using cell cycle redistribution strategies. For example, some chemotherapeutic drugs, such as taxanes, can block transition of cells through mitosis, with the result that cells accumulate in the radiosensitive G_2 and M phases of the cell cycle. Radiation delivered at the time of significant accumulation of cells in both the G_2 and M phases results in enhanced radioresponse of cells *in vitro* (48,237) and of tumors *in vivo* (162,165). However, this cell cycle mechanism of taxane-induced enhancement of tumor radioresponse is dominant only in tumors that are resistant to paclitaxel or docetaxel as a single treatment. Although tumor growth in taxane-resistant tumors is not substantially affected by the drug, tumors do exhibit significant transient accumulation of cells in mitosis 6 to 12 hours after the treatment (165). Taxanes also enhance the radioresponse of tumors that respond by significant tumor growth delay to taxanes given as a single treatment modality, but a major mechanism for radio enhancement in such tumors is reoxygenation of radioresistant hypoxic cells, as discussed later (162).

Elimination of the radioresistant S-phase cells by the chemotherapeutic agents may be another cell cycle redistribution strategy in chemoradiation therapy. Nucleoside analogs, such as fludarabine or gemcitabine, are good examples of the agents that become incorporated into S-phase cells and eliminate them by inducing apoptosis (93,160). In addition to purging S-phase cells, the analogs induce the surviving cells to undergo parasynchronous movement to accumulate in the G_2 and M phases of the cell cycle between 1 and 2 days after drug administration, a time when the highest enhancement of tumor radioresponse was observed (160).

Tumors with a high cell growth fraction are likely to respond better to the cell cycle redistribution strategy in chemoradiation therapy than tumors with a low cell growth fraction.

Counteracting Hypoxia-Associated Tumor Radioresistance

Solid malignant tumors usually are characterized by defective vascularization, both in the number of blood vessels and vessel function. Because of this, blood supply to tumor cells is inadequate, cells lack oxygen and nutrients, and multiple tumor microregions become hypoxic, acidic, and eventually necrotic. Hypoxia occurs at distances from blood vessels larger than 100 to 150 μm. The hypoxic cell content in tumors varies widely and can be more than 50%. The presence of hypoxia makes tumors more aggressive (hypoxia is conducive to the emergence of more virulent tumor cell variants and stimulates metastatic spread [36,39]) and more resistant to radiation as well as most chemotherapeutic agents. Hypoxic cells are 2.5 to 3 times more resistant to radiation than well-oxygenated cells. The fact that hypoxia may be a cure-limiting factor in radiation therapy, at least in some clinical situations, is suggested by the findings that reduced hemoglobin levels (41) and low tumor Po_2 (103,178) are associated with higher treatment failure rates. Also, there are reports showing that local tumor control by radiation therapy can be improved by the use of hypoxic cell radiosensitizers (67) or hyperbaric oxygen (98). With respect to the effects of chemotherapy, hypoxic regions are less accessible to chemotherapeutic drugs; in addition, hypoxic tumor cells are either nonproliferating or they proliferate poorly, and as such do not respond well to drugs.

Combining chemotherapeutic agents with radiation therapy can reduce or eliminate hypoxia or its negative influence on tumor radioresponse. Most chemotherapeutic drugs preferentially kill proliferating cells, which are primarily found in well-oxygenated regions of the tumor. Because these regions are located close to blood vessels, they are easily accessible to chemotherapeutic agents. Destruction of tumor cells in these areas leads to an increased oxygen supply to hypoxic regions, and hence reoxygenates hypoxic tumor cells. Massive loss of cells after chemotherapy lowers the interstitial pressure, which then allows the reopening of previously closed capillaries and the reestablishment of blood supply. It also causes tumor shrinkage so that previously hypoxic areas are closer to capillaries and thus accessible to oxygen. Finally, by eliminating oxygenated cells, more oxygen becomes available to cells that survived chemotherapy. It was recently shown that tumor reoxygenation is a major mechanism underlying the enhancement of tumor radioresponse induced by taxanes in tumors sensitive to these drugs (162).

Another approach to counteract the negative impact of hypoxia is selective killing of hypoxic cells through bioreductive drugs, such as tirapazamine (36), which undergo reductive activation in a hypoxic milieu, rendering them cytotoxic. A related possibility is to exploit the acidic state (low pH) of tumors, which develops as a result of hypoxia-driven anaerobic metabolism that produces lactic acid (243), through the use of drugs that selectively accumulate in acidic environments or become activated by a low pH (228).

The use of agents that selectively radiosensitize hypoxic cells to reduce their negative impact has been considered and tested in clinical trials for some time (see Chapter 22). These drugs increase radiation damage by mimicking the effect of oxygen. Many clinical trials have tested these drugs, particularly misonidazole, in combination with radiation therapy, but few of them have shown an improved treatment outcome. Neurotoxicity associated with the administration of hypoxic cell radiosensitizers was the major limitation that prevented the delivery of clinically effective doses of these agents.

Inhibition of Tumor Cell Repopulation

The constant balance between cell production and cell loss maintains the integrity of normal tissues. When this balance is perturbed by cytotoxic action of chemotherapeutic drugs or radiation, the integrity of tissues is reestablished by an increased rate of cell production. The cell loss after each fraction of radiation during radiation therapy induces compensatory cell re-

generation (repopulation), the extent of which determines tissue tolerance to radiation therapy. In contrast to normal tissues, malignant tumors are characterized by an imbalance between cell production and cell loss in favor of cell production. As with normal tissues, tumors also respond to radiation- or drug-induced cell loss with a compensatory regenerative response. Preclinical studies provided ample evidence demonstrating that the rate of cell proliferation in tumors treated by radiation or chemotherapeutic drugs is higher than that in untreated tumors (99,166,221). This increased rate of treatment-induced cell proliferation is commonly termed *accelerated repopulation*. Accelerated repopulation of tumor clonogens has been shown to occur during clinical radiation therapy as well. Withers et al. (252) showed that the total dose of radiation needed to control 50% of head and neck carcinomas progressively increased with time whenever radiation therapy treatment was prolonged beyond 1 month. This increase in radiation dose required to achieve tumor control was greater than what would be anticipated based on the pretreatment tumor volume doubling time of approximately 60 days for head and neck tumors. The increase was attributed to accelerated repopulation, and it was estimated to average approximately 0.6 Gy/day (252), but may be as high as 1 Gy/day (230).

Although accelerated cell proliferation is beneficial for normal tissues because it spares them from radiation damage, it has an adverse impact on tumor control by radiation therapy or chemotherapy. Therefore, any approach that reduces or eliminates accelerated clonogen repopulation in tumors would improve radiation therapy. Chemotherapeutic drugs, because of their cytotoxic or cytostatic activity, can reduce the rate of proliferation when given concurrently with radiation therapy, and hence increase the effectiveness of the treatment. Caution must be taken to select drugs that preferentially affect rapidly proliferating cells and preferentially localize in malignant tumors. However, the main limitation of concurrent chemoradiation therapy is the enhanced toxicity of rapidly dividing normal tissues because most available chemotherapeutic agents show poor tumor selectivity. Moreover, accelerated repopulation induced by chemotherapeutic drugs may have a negative influence on the outcome of tumor response to radiation when drugs are used in induction or neoadjuvant chemotherapy protocols. In this strategy, chemotherapy precedes radiation therapy. Treatment outcomes after induction chemotherapy followed by radiation therapy have not been overly encouraging in terms of both local tumor control and patient survival, even if a large proportion of tumors initially responded with total or partial clinical regression by the time of radiation therapy implementation. Some experimental evidence suggests that the drug-induced accelerated cell repopulation can actually make the tumor more difficult to control with radiation (166,221).

Timing of Drug Administration in Relation to Radiation Therapy

Most clinical chemoradiation therapy regimens evolved empirically: Drugs known to be active against a tumor type were combined with radiation, and the doses of both agents and their administration schedules were selected for safety. Increasingly, however, information from preclinical studies is being considered in planning the optimal timing of drug administration in relation to radiation therapy. Depending on the principal aim of the therapy, drugs are administered before (*induction* or *neoadjuvant chemotherapy*), during (*concurrent* or *concomitant chemotherapy*), or after (*adjuvant chemotherapy*) the course of radiation therapy. The advantages and disadvantages of each approach are summarized in Table 29.1.

Table 29.1	ADVANTAGES AND DISADVANTAGES OF DIFFERENT CHEMORADIATION SEQUENCING STRATEGIES	
Strategy	**Advantages**	**Disadvantages**
Sequential chemoradiation	• Least toxic • Maximizes systemic therapy • Smaller radiation fields if induction shrinks tumor	• Increased treatment time • Lack of local synergy
Concurrent chemoradiation	• Shorter treatment time • Radiation enhancement	• Compromised systemic therapy • Increased toxicity • No cytoreduction of tumor
Concurrent chemoradiation and adjuvant chemotherapy	• Maximizes systemic therapy • Radiation enhancement • Both local and distant therapy delivered upfront	• Increased toxicity • Increased treatment time • Difficult to complete chemotherapy after chemoradiation
Induction chemotherapy and concurrent chemoradiation	• Maximizes systemic therapy • Radiation enhancement	• Increased toxicity • Increased treatment time • Difficult to complete chemoradiation after induction therapy

Induction chemotherapy is aimed at both the disseminated disease and the primary tumor. It is initiated soon after tumor diagnosis to cope with metastatic foci while they still contain a small number of tumor cells. In regard to the primary tumor, induction chemotherapy may reduce the number of clonogenic cells and cause the reoxygenation of the surviving hypoxic cells, both of which render tumors more controllable by radiation. In addition, chemotherapy-induced tumor shrinkage may allow the use of smaller radiation fields, in which case less normal tissue is exposed and damaged by radiation. This treatment approach is often used in the therapy of solid tumors in children and of lymphomas. Induction chemotherapy precedes radiation therapy for a few weeks to a few months, which improves tolerability of the combined treatment.

Induction chemotherapy has resulted in therapeutic improvement in a number of clinical trials compared with radiation therapy, but in general the therapeutic benefits are below expectations. A number of factors could account for this, including accelerated proliferation of tumor cell clonogens and selection or induction of drug-resistant cells that are cross-resistant to radiation. The preclinical findings provide solid evidence for the existence of accelerated repopulation in tumors treated with chemotherapeutic agents. On the other hand, although development of drug resistance is a significant problem in chemotherapy, the evidence that cells that acquire drug resistance are also resistant to radiation is not convincing.

The treatment approach in which chemotherapeutic agents are given during a course of radiation therapy is referred to as *concurrent chemotherapy*. This form of treatment is intended to cope with both disseminated lesions and the primary tumor, but it takes advantage of drug–radiation interactions to maximize tumor radioresponse. The drug scheduling in relation to individual radiation fractions is highly important, and the selection of optimal timing of drug administration must be based on mechanisms of tumor radio enhancement by a given drug, the drug's normal tissue toxicity, and the conditions under which the highest enhancement is achieved. The data from preclinical studies can greatly contribute to the selection of the most optimal schedules. For example, it has been demonstrated that murine tumors sensitive to taxanes show enhanced radioresponse, but the best effect is achieved if drug treatment precedes radiation by 1 to 3 days (162). A major mechanism for tumor radio enhancement was reoxygenation of hypoxic cells. Based on this preclinical information, one would anticipate

that in clinical protocols such tumors would best respond to a bolus of a taxane given once or twice weekly during radiation therapy. In contrast, tumors resistant to taxanes on their own would call for daily administration of a taxane because they show accumulation of radiosensitive G_2- and M-phase cells 6 to 12 hours after drug administration. If the objective is to counteract rapid repopulation of tumor cell clonogens induced by radiation, then administration of cell cycle-specific chemotherapeutic agents during the second half of radiation therapy, when accelerated repopulation is more expressed, might be more effective. Optimal scheduling is essential in concurrent chemotherapy not only to maximize tumor radioresponse but to minimize increases in toxicity to critical normal tissues. At present, the enhancement in normal tissue complications remains the major limitation of concurrently combining chemotherapy with radiation therapy. Nevertheless, as is made evident later in the text, concurrent chemoradiation therapy has provided better clinical results both in terms of local tumor control and patient survival than have other modes of chemoradiation therapy combinations (170,172).

Adjuvant chemotherapy designates a treatment modality in which chemotherapeutic drugs are given some time after completion or radiation therapy. The primary objective is to eradicate disseminated disease; however, the control of the primary tumor may also be improved by the ability of drugs to deal with tumor cells that survived radiation.

Emerging Strategies for Improvement in Chemoradiation Therapy

In spite of increasing therapeutic achievements of chemoradiation therapy, the use of this form of therapy is still very much restricted by its narrow therapeutic index. The available agents are either insufficiently effective on their own or in combination with radiation against tumors, or normal tissue toxicity prevents the use of effective doses of drugs or radiation. Significant research efforts, both preclinical and clinical, have been undertaken to improve chemoradiation therapy. They include development of more selective and more effective chemotherapeutic agents and incorporating additional agents into chemoradiation therapy that either protect normal tissues from injury by drugs or radiation or selectively target molecular processes responsible for tumor radioresistance or chemoresistance.

Increasing Antitumor Efficacy of Chemotherapeutic Drugs

A number of newer chemotherapeutic agents are highly effective against common cancers in humans and are potent enhancers of tumor radioresponse. Among these are taxanes, nucleoside analogs, and topoisomerase inhibitors. However, normal tissue toxicity is still a major limitation for the effective use of these agents, especially when combined concurrently with radiation. One approach to make current chemotherapeutic drugs more effective against tumors and at the same time less toxic to normal tissues is to conjugate them with water-soluble polymeric drugs, such as polyglutamic acid. These conjugates accumulate in tumors and release the active drug into the tumor in high concentrations and for a longer time. The enhancement in uptake by and prolongation of drug release in tumors are thought to be due to the enhanced permeability and retention effect of macromolecular compounds in solid tumors (135,145). The abnormal vasculature in tumors is porous to macromolecules, but high concentrations of drug can build up in tumors owing to inadequate lymphatic drainage, whereas polymer–drug conjugates are confined to the bloodstream in normal tissue (145). A highly promising polyglutamic acid–paclitaxel conjugate was recently developed. It is less toxic, more effective against tumors, and more enhancing of tumor radioresponse in preclinical studies than unconjugated paclitaxel (134,135).

Incorporation of Molecular Targeting

Recent discoveries in molecular biology have identified a number of receptors, enzymes, or growth factors that may be responsible for resistance of cancer cells to radiation or other cytotoxic agents, and as such may serve as targets for augmentation of radioresponse or chemoresponse. Among this expanding list of determinant proteins are epidermal growth factor receptor (EGFR); cyclooxygenase-2 (COX-2) enzyme; mutated *ras*; cell cycle checkpoint control proteins such as CHK1; a number of the DNA repair enzymes including DNA-PK, ATM, RAD51, as examples; the proteosome; angiogenic molecules, and various other molecules that regulate different steps in their signal transduction pathways (150). Some are potentially single pathway targets and others are able to target multiple molecular signaling pathways. Some newly emerging molecular strategies to improve chemoradiation therapy are shown in Table 29.2.

EGFR is probably the paradigm for the combination of small molecular therapy and radiation. EGFR is also known as ErbB1, a member of the ErbB family of receptor tyrosine kinases which also includes ErbB2 (HER2/neu). EGFR is a 170-kD transmembrane glycoprotein with an intracellular domain possessing intrinsic tyrosine kinase activity. On binding to a ligand, such as epidermal growth factor (EGF) or transforming growth factor-α, EGFR undergoes autophosphorylation and initiates transduction signals regulating cell division, proliferation, differentiation, vascularization, and death (Fig. 29.2). EGFR plays an important role in tumor growth and response to cytotoxic agents, including ionizing radiation. The receptor is frequently expressed in high levels in many types of cancer, which is often associated with more aggressive tumors, poor patient prognosis, and tumor resistance to treatment with cytotoxic agents including radiation (22,112,136,158,214). *In vitro* experimental studies have provided solid evidence linking EGFR with resistance to cytotoxic drugs. Although transfection of EGFR into tumor cells increases their resistance to drugs (65), the blockade of the EGFR-mediated signaling pathway with antibodies to EGFR enhances the sensitivity of tumor cells to drugs (158) and ionizing radiation (110). *In vivo* studies have shown that blockade of EGFR, such as with C225 anti-EGFR monoclonal antibody, or interference with its downstream signaling processes can improve tumor treatment with both chemotherapeutic agents and radiation (111,164). Indeed, three drugs have Food and Drug Administration approval for use as a chemotherapeutic agent, each targeting the activity of EGFR in different ways. Cetuximab targets the extracellular binding domain inhibiting dimer formation, gefitinib targets the intracellular tyrosine kinase domain, and erlotinib also targets the activity of the tyrosine kinase domain. However, the activity of EGFR is complicated by the signal diversity due to the formation of homo- and heterodimers with other members of the ErbB family and by the specific autophosphorylation patterns within each ErbB family member. This is further compounded by the recent identification of specific mutations within EGFR that confer sensitivity to certain EGFR inhibitors. The approach of combining an anti-EGFR antibody with cytotoxic agents in the treatment of patients with cancer is being tested (18,97,204,239) as are new agents such as AEE788, which targets EGFR, ErbB2, and vascular endothelial growth factor (VEGF) simultaneously (238).

COX-2, another potential molecular target, is an inducible gene that catalyzes the synthesis of prostaglandins from arachidonic acid. Prostaglandins possess diverse biologic activities, including vasoconstriction, vasodilatation, stimulation or inhibition of platelet aggregation, and immunomodulation (primarily immunosuppression). They are also implicated in the promotion of development and growth of malignant tumors, as well as in the response of tumor and normal tissues to cytotoxic agents, including radiation (124,161,167). Two COX enzymes, COX-1 and COX-2, mediate production of prostaglandins. Whereas COX-1 is constitutively expressed and ubiquitous, with physiologic roles in maintaining homeostasis, such as the integrity of gastric mucosa, normal platelet function, and regulation of renal blood flow, COX-2 is nonphysiologic and induced by diverse inflammatory stimuli, mitogens, and carcinogens. Increasing evidence shows that COX-2 expression is up-regulated in many human tumors, including colon, pancreatic, prostate, gastric, and head and neck cancers, where it is associated with more aggressive tumor behavior with decreased apoptosis, angiogenesis, and poor patient prognosis (81,120,121,139,148,177,195,202,216). COX-2 is also implicated as a causative factor in colorectal tumorigenesis (124,220).

This selective or preferential expression of COX-2 in tumors makes this enzyme a potential target for cancer therapy. Selective COX-2 inhibitors such as celecoxib or rofecoxib are reported to enhance tumor response to chemotherapeutic drugs or radiation in human colon, breast, lung, and prostate cancers (124,163,167,210). The mechanisms of the enhancement seem to be multiple, including increases in induction of apoptosis via the down-regulation of bcl-2 or the inactivation of Akt, and the inhibition of tumor neoangiogenesis (109,140,163,197). The action correlates with a reduction in prostaglandin production in tumors.

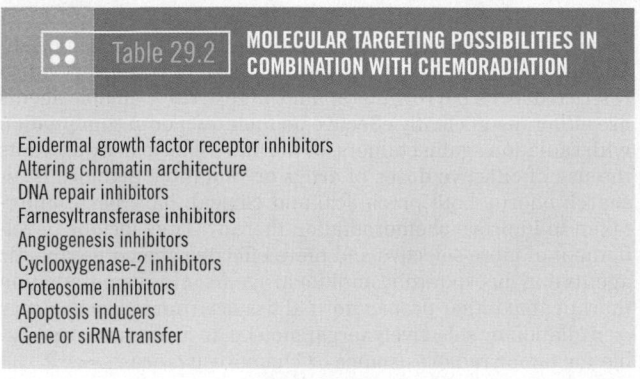

Table 29.2	MOLECULAR TARGETING POSSIBILITIES IN COMBINATION WITH CHEMORADIATION

Epidermal growth factor receptor inhibitors
Altering chromatin architecture
DNA repair inhibitors
Farnesyltransferase inhibitors
Angiogenesis inhibitors
Cyclooxygenase-2 inhibitors
Proteosome inhibitors
Apoptosis inducers
Gene or siRNA transfer

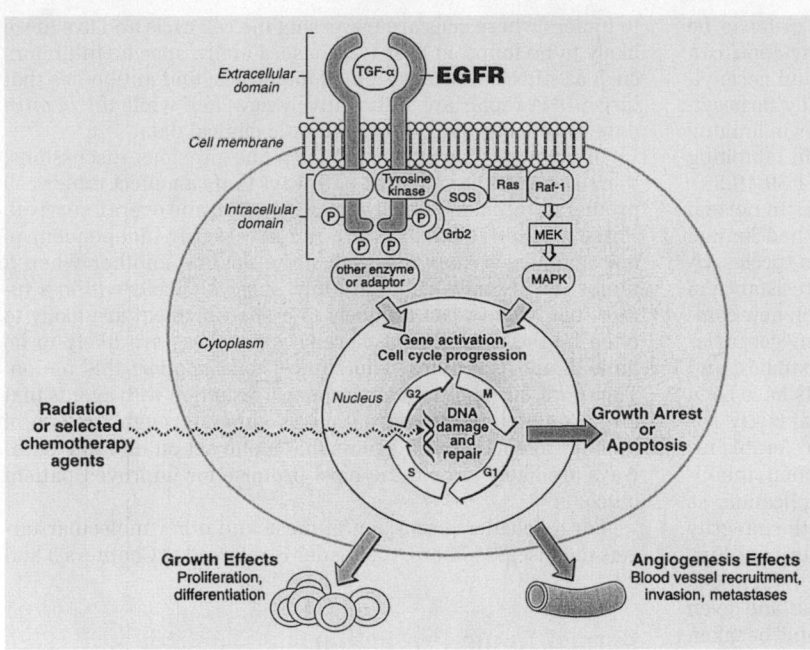

FIGURE 29.2. The cellular influence of the epidermal growth factor receptor (EGFR) illustrating the potential benefits of blocking the EGFR. (From Harari PM, Huang SM. Modulation of molecular targets to enhance radiation. *Clin Cancer Res* 2000;6:323–325, with permission from the American Association for Cancer Research, Inc.)

Recently, in a group of patients with prostate-specific antigen recurrent prostate cancer after either definitive radiotherapy or radical prostatectomy, celecoxib administration was shown to limit prostate-specific antigen increase during the study period in an androgen-independent manner (195). In this case, celecoxib may have delayed or prevented tumor progression. Although it ultimately came to similar conclusions, a similar study (217) was stopped after the information on cardiovascular toxicity and COX-2 inhibitors was released (196,242). Although long-term administration of COX-2 inhibitors may need to be evaluated for risk for cardiovascular toxicity when given as a chemopreventive agent, there is no evidence for enhanced risk for short-term exposures. As such, there is a therapeutic rationale for the use of COX-2 inhibitors in settings in which COX-2 is overexpressed. This is particularly true for radiotherapy because COX-2 inhibition does not effect the production of prostaglandins in normal tissues, thus limiting the probability of normal tissue toxicity.

Perhaps no molecular targets have been investigated for possible tumor treatment strategies more than inhibitors of tumor angiogenesis or agents that act on the resting vasculature. The formation of tumor vasculature, which is a prerequisite for progressive tumor growth, is initiated and sustained by angiogenic mediators secreted by tumor cells and cells from the surrounding stroma. Many different angiogenic factors have been identified, including vascular endothelial growth factor/vascular permeability factor, members of the fibroblast growth factor family, platelet-derived growth factor, interleukin-8, and prostaglandins. In addition to angiogenic factors, tumors secrete substances that inhibit angiogenesis, such as angiostatin, endostatin, thrombospondin-1, and interferons, so that the final outcome of angiogenesis (and hence tumor growth) depends on the balance between proangiogenic and antiangiogenic activities.

Inhibitors of angiogenesis have undergone extensive preclinical testing, with some agents moving into clinical trials. However, as monotherapeutic agents, the early agents, such as angiostatin and endostatin have not been as promising as their preclinical evaluations had suggested (182). High doses and longevity of treatment have hindered their utility, and they tend not to eradicate disease because tumor growth can resume after the removal of therapy. Even though it was assumed

that an antiangiogenic agent would impair the efficacy of radiotherapy via the enhancement of hypoxia, early evidence for radiotherapy in combination with angiostatin showed both improved oxygenation and reduced oxygenation (144,173,232). However, the first clinical trial with a specific inhibitor of angiogenesis, angiostatin, showed a synergistic effect (152). Since then, the role of specific factors in vascular growth and maintenance has become clearer. VEGF receptors, in particular, play a critical role in vascular integrity, including angiogenesis and endothelial cell survival via their tyrosine kinase activities (187). VEGF expression induces endothelial cell proliferation by creating a vascular sprout that subsequently organizes into a capillary tube (128,185). VEGF also promotes angiogenesis through the formation of a hyperpermeable immature vascular network (19). VEGF expression is enhanced following radiation, which is likely a survival response for vascular endothelial cells, ultimately in support of tumor survival. Receptor tyrosine kinases, EGFR in particular, up-regulate VEGF, and COX-2 inhibitors limit the up-regulation of VEGF by prostaglandins.

Because radiation can limit the mobilization of angiogenesis inhibitors such as angiostatin, combining radiation with agents that inhibit vascularization seems prudent. Indeed, new agents that target VEGF signaling are undergoing preclinical and clinical evaluations. Compounds such as ZD6474 (AstraZeneca), whose preclinical evaluations show an inhibition of VEGF signaling and angiogenesis with oral administration in an animal model (1), has entered into clinical trials. Other compounds such as SU5416 and SU6668 (SUGEN, Inc.) are being used in combination with radiation and with radiation and chemotherapy as triple therapy in preclinical studies in which enhanced apoptosis in endothelial cells, reduced migration and invasion of vascular, an inhibition of tumor proliferation is evident (1,28,215).

Activating mutations in the ras oncogene are found in many tumors including lung, colon, head and neck, glioblastoma, and others. The overall rate of ras mutations in human cancers is 25% to 30%, but for some cancers the mutation rate can be quite high. For instance, in pancreatic cancer the rate of activating mutations is approximately 90%, and in colon cancer it is approximately 45%. These activating mutations drive key intracellular signaling pathways that confer proliferative and survival advantages to tumors cells, including radioresistance, through the chronic activation of the PI3K and the Ras/MAP kinase pathways (24,44,247). Ras must be prenylated in order to be membrane-bound, where it becomes active. Prenylation can occur by two enzymatic processes, farnesylation and geranyl-geranylation. Inhibitors of farnesylation, specifically farnesyl-trasnferase inhibitors (FTIs), have had some success in limiting the negative impact of ras activation, particularly in inhibiting tumor cell radioresistance *in vitro* and *in vivo* (23,24,39,49,50). FTIs selectively affect tumors because the *ras* genes in normal tissues are not mutated. The activity of FTIs has had limited success, partly due to the activity against a given ras species, H-ras versus n-Ras or K-ras, and because of the FTI resistance of geranylgeranylated K-ras (23,24,154–156). However, new compounds that target both farnesylation as well as geranylgeranylation have been shown to be effective in preclinical studies, and new molecular targets for radiosensitization by FTIs have been identified (38,247) which may enhance their clinical utility.

Many therapy agents target the DNA of cells, preferably tumor cells. This can be through DNA damage induction, inhibition of cell cycle traversal, or inhibition of DNA replication, as examples, and targeting the enzymes that manage the integrity of the DNA of cells represents a sound therapeutic strategy. Furthermore, differences between tumor and normal cells in cell cycle checkpoint controls, DNA repair capabilities, and even chromatin architecture, have been identified that could be taken advantage of by combined therapies. As an example, inhibitors of histone deacetylase relax chromatin structure. This can lead to increased radiosensitivity through enhanced DNA damage (42,141). However, some histone deacetylase inhibitors have also been shown to down-regulate the expression of both EGFR and ErbB2 and to inhibit PI3K and AKT signaling (46,86,256), all strong potentiators of tumor cell survival and modulators of DNA DSB repair (59). This combination of DNA damage enhancement, inhibition of DNA repair, and down-regulation of strong survival signals highlights the utility of agents that attack multiple signaling pathways.

There are multiple strategies to targeting DNA repair pathways with drugs or small molecules. First, DNA damage must be sensed, and there are several key enzymes that are considered damage sensors. The most established sensors are TRF2, the MRN complex, and ATM (32,143). These proteins set off the cascade of events that alter chromatin, recruit repair enzymes to the break site, and initiate cell cycle checkpoint control following DNA damage. Key regulatory proteins within each of these areas are being successfully targeted in preclinical studies. Examples include a specific inhibitor of ATM, Ku55933, which has shown enhanced radiosensitivity in *in vitro* experiments (101); small molecules that reconstitute wild type p53 protein structure in mutant p53 molecules (56); and radiotherapy combined with adenoviral WTp53 delivered *in vivo* by liposomal carriers in clinical trials for lung cancer (225). Preclinical evaluations of compounds that target DNA repair components directly, particularly when combined with radiation and radiosensitizing compounds such as cisplatin or gemcitabine, are ongoing. Inhibitors of DNAPKcs, a critical enzyme in hon-homolous end joining, have been successful in preclinical studies on tumor cell lines; however, a treatment advantage for normal tissue may provide a challenge (47,71,184,208,244,251).

There are novel therapeutic targets within the DNA repair pathway known as *homologous recombination* (HR). For instance, RAD51 and BRCA1/2 defective cell lines are radiosensitive, and antisense strategies against RAD51 have been used against a number of cancer cell lines. Interestingly, targeting HR may have a distinct advantage over the NHEJ pathway. NHEJ occurs throughout the cell cycle, whereas HR is considered to be a dominant repair pathways during S and G2 phases of the cell cycle because of the need for a template strand of DNA. This implies that for most normal tissues, where there is little to no cellular turnover and where NHEJ is the dominant DNA repair pathway, there would be a survival advantage compared to tumors where cells are traversing the cell cycle and are more likely to be found in S or G2 phase. Finally, specific inhibitors such as siRNA, antisense, small molecules, and antibodies that target DNA repair are still relatively new, and while the *in vitro* data are encouraging, there are little clinical data.

In summary, as suggested from the previous discussions, there are multiple signaling pathways that can effect tumor cell proliferation, chemo- and radio-resistance, and overall survival. These signaling pathways are not necessarily independent of one another, or they may substitute for one another when a tumor cell is challenged. Certainly, subsets of cells within a tumor that would react uniquely to a specific agent are likely to often be the case. Single-therapy approaches are likely to be limited, and preclinical and clinical data support this notion. Therefore, strategies that incorporate radiation with agents that target multiple signaling pathways either through the use of multiple agents or with agents that alone act on multiple pathways are likely to hold the most promise for improved patient outcome.

For a broader discussion of these and other molecular targets not discussed here, the reader is referred to Chapters 3 and 23.

Normal Tissue Protection

Because normal tissue toxicity represents a major limitation of concurrent chemoradiation therapy, every effort must be taken to prevent or minimize complications. This could be achieved through the incorporation into the treatment of radioprotective or chemoprotective agents or through improvements of radiation delivery. A number of chemical and biologic compounds are available that exhibited either selective or preferential protection of normal tissues in preclinical *in vivo* testing (68,95,138,161,257). In addition, there are many candidate compounds, particularly extracts from plants used in traditional medicine settings, that are undergoing *in vitro* evaluation (11–13). Most commonly tested radioprotectors are thiol compounds, such as WR-2721 (amifostine), a prodrug that must be converted *in vivo* to its active metabolite WR-1065. Amifostine is currently the only Food and Drug Administration-approved radioprotector. The principal mechanisms of protection by these agents include scavenging of free radicals generated by ionizing radiation and some chemotherapy agents, such as alkylating agents, and donating hydrogen atoms to facilitate direct chemical repair of DNA damage. However, amifostine modulates transcriptional regulation of genes involved in apoptosis, cell cycle regulation, and DNA repair as well (119). The protector is taken up preferentially by normal tissues, where the entry into cells is accomplished by active transport. In contrast, the drug diffuses passively into tumors, where its availability is also reduced by deficient tumor vasculature. Amifostine has been shown to reduce normal tissue toxicity in a number of clinical settings, including protection of salivary glands in head and neck radiation therapy (34,35), prevention of acute and late normal tissue toxicities from chemoradiation in cancers of the head and neck (10) and the esophagus in chemoradiation therapy of lung cancer (125), without adversely affecting tumor response to treatment. The drug significantly protects against cisplatin-induced nephrotoxicity, ototoxicity, and neuropathy.

Growth factors, particularly hematopoietic growth factors, may be especially useful in amelioration of toxicities resulting from chemotherapeutic drugs (188). A number of them are used clinically relatively often, including granulocyte colony-stimulating factor, granulocyte–macrophage colony-stimulating factor, and erythropoietin. A higher degree of hematopoietic protection against the damage induced by radiation or chemotherapeutic agents can be achieved by combining granulocyte colony-stimulating factor with WR-2721 than when individual protectors are used.

Technical improvements in radiation therapy, such as three-dimensional treatment planning, conformational radiation therapy, or the use of protons or hadrons, are other approaches likely to minimize the toxicity and, consequently, enhance the effectiveness of chemoradiation. The use of either radioprotective compounds or the implementation of technical advances may enable administration of higher doses of radiation, chemotherapeutic drugs, or both, which may result in superior treatment outcome. For more detailed discussion on radioprotective and chemoprotective agents, see Chapter 22.

Interaction of Specific Chemotherapies and Radiation in the Treatment of Cancer

This section provides an overview of the evidence that exists for combining particular chemotherapies with radiation. In many cases, the level of support that exists for combined therapy mirrors the age of the drug. However, as would be expected, newer drugs have generally been subject to more rigorous preclinical assessment of their efficacy before their introduction into the clinical setting (Table 29.3). Although the pinnacle of this strategy of preclinical assessment has yet to be attained, the incorporation of new, targeted biologic agents, which are less toxic than conventional chemotherapy, into combination therapies holds the promise of increased tumor selectivity in radiation-based treatments.

Platinum-Based Drugs

This group of compounds, distinguished from most others by its metallic element base, has come to be recognized as one of the most potent chemotherapies available to date. Cisplatin (*cis*-diamminedichloroplatinum II), which is the prototype drug, has been acknowledged to be a potent radiosensitizer for many years. Preclinical work done using murine models by Rosenberg et al. (206) in the late 1960s showed that cisplatin is an effective antitumor chemotherapy. Subsequent efforts have shown that its primary mechanism of inhibition of tumor growth appears to involve the inhibition of DNA synthesis (106,229). Another

secondary mechanism includes the inhibition of transcription elongation by DNA interstrand cross-links (54).

Work on nonmammalian systems first demonstrated the radiosensitizing abilities of platinum-based compounds (200,201, 259). This was confirmed in several mammalian systems as well (69,226,253). This makes inherent sense because these platinum compounds have a high electron affinity and react preferentially with hydrated electrons. The exact mechanism for the increased cell death seen with combinations of ionizing radiation and platinum drugs is not known for certain; however, the evidence would seem to point to the inhibition of PLDR (43) and to the radiosensitization of hypoxic tumor cells (222). Cisplatin free radical–mediated sensitization may involve the ability to scavenge free electrons formed by the interaction between radiation and DNA. The reduction of the platinum moiety may serve to stabilize DNA damage that would otherwise be repairable (63). Greater than additive effects of cisplatin and radiation are seen in tumor models most reliably when the drug is administered with fractionated radiation (63), explained by its inhibition of SLDR.

Carboplatin, a new second-generation platinum compound with a different toxicity profile, has also been studied as a radiosensitizer (21,180). Its potential efficacy as a radiosensitizer has allowed for its incorporation into regimens used in several randomized trials. Interest exists in the combination of radiation with other platinum analogs, including oxaliplatin (83) as well as orally administered compounds like JM-216 (6).

Taxanes

The radiosensitizing properties of a relatively new group of plant-derived chemotherapeutic agents, the taxanes, have been studied extensively in both preclinical models and in clinical trials. Paclitaxel (Taxol) and docetaxel (Taxotere) act as mitotic spindle inhibitors through their promotion of microtubule assembly and inhibition of disaggregation (207). Both taxanes bind to the *N*-terminal 31–amino-acid sequence of the β-tubulin subunit of cellular tubulin polymers, stabilizing the polymers by shifting the dynamic equilibrium that exists between tubulin dimers and microtubules in favor of the polymerized state (146,199). Although there is preclinical evidence that docetaxel has both a higher affinity for the tubulin-binding site and greater *in vitro* cytotoxicity than paclitaxel, this has not necessarily

Table 29.3	MECHANISMS OF CHEMOTHERAPY-INDUCED RADIATION SENSITIZATION	
Class of Compound	**Mechanism of Radiosensitization**	**References**
Platinum-based compounds	Inhibition of DNA synthesis	23,45,71,180
	Inhibition of transcription elongation by DNA interstrand cross-links	
	Inhibition of repair of radiation-induced DNA damage	
Taxanes	Cellular arrest in the G_2M phase of the cell cycle	8,150,162,163
	Induction of apoptosis	
	Reoxygenation of tumor cells	
Topoisomerase I inhibitors	Inhibition of repair of radiation-induced DNA strand breaks	10,47,182
	Redistribution into G_2 phase of the cell cycle	
	Conversion of radiation-induced single-strand breaks into double-strand breaks	
Hypoxic cell cytotoxins	Complementary cytotoxicity with radiation on euoxic and hypoxic tumor cells	38,93
Antimetabolites	Nucleotide pool perturbation	95,130,131,151
	Lowering apoptotic threshold	
	Cell cycle redistribution	
	Tumor cell reoxygenation	

translated into greater clinical efficacy because the toxicity profiles of the two drugs also differ (64,203).

The administration of a taxane leads to cellular arrest in the G_2/M phase of the cell cycle, which is the precise point associated with increased sensitivity to the lethal effects of ionizing radiation (96). Early laboratory studies with a human lung cancer cell line (48) and human astrocytoma cells (237) bore out the prospect of significant radiosensitization, with relative enhancement ratios in the 1.48 to 1.8 range when paclitaxel was administered before irradiation.

The exact conditions used in various studies appear to determine the strength of the interaction between radiation and paclitaxel because subadditive effects have been seen in addition to the more widely reported additive and supraadditive effects (165). In general, enhancement of radiation effects is seen when proliferating cells have been incubated with moderate concentrations of paclitaxel for 24 hours before irradiation. Conditions leading to a less-than-optimal response include paclitaxel-mediated G_1 arrest, wherein a more resistant cell subpopulation counteracts the effects of a G_2/M block; paclitaxel-induced cell cycle effects such as the G_2/M block in cells destined to die before irradiation; and incubation conditions insufficient to exert cellular effects. The fact that nonproliferating cells are also sensitized to the effects of radiation by the use of paclitaxel suggests that mechanisms other than the cell cycle arrest in G_2/M phase underlie paclitaxel's sensitizing abilities.

Paclitaxel also acts to induce programmed cell death; work from the M. D. Anderson Cancer Center (165) has examined the relationship between mitotic arrest, apoptosis, and the antineoplastic activity of paclitaxel in 16 murine tumors. Single-dose paclitaxel (40 mg/kg) induced mitotic arrest to varying degrees in all tumors; however, apoptosis was induced in only 50% of tumors. This study also revealed that pretreatment levels of apoptosis correlated with both paclitaxel-induced apoptosis and tumor growth delay. Therefore, both pretreatment apoptotic rate and paclitaxel-induced apoptotic rate could potentially act as predictors of the response to paclitaxel.

Reoxygenation is also thought to play a substantial role in the potentiation of tumor radioresponse. Preferential killing of those oxygenated cells located close to blood vessels is possible with both radiation and chemotherapy. Milas et al. (165) summarized observations that showed (a) massive loss of tumor cells though the apoptotic pathway was restricted to the perivascular region, and (b) radio enhancement occurring during this period of cell loss became even more impressive when apoptotic cells were removed from the tumor. Experiments in which tumor xenografts were treated with paclitaxel and exposed to radiation under hypoxic or air-ambient conditions were pursued (162). It was found that the creation of hypoxic conditions greatly reduced the efficacy of paclitaxel in its enhancement of radioresponse. Measurements of tumor oxygenation using Eppendorf histographs confirmed that the median tumor PO_2 increased from the control value of 6.8 to 10.5 mm Hg at 24 hours to 31.2 mm Hg at 48 hours after paclitaxel treatment. The percentage of hypoxic cells decreased from 32% in untreated tumors to 4%, 2%, and 1% at 9, 24, and 48 hours, respectively, after drug administration. It appears that a combination of cell cycle effects, drug-induced reoxygenation, and drug-induced apoptosis underlies paclitaxel's radiosensitizing abilities.

Docetaxel has also been found to be a respectable radiosensitizer in both *in vitro* (7) and *in vivo* models (149). Radiation response in the presence of docetaxel was examined in three different cell lines that have widely different responses to radiation alone (55). Their findings suggest that the p53 status of tumor cells may have a profound effect on the radiosensitizing effects of a taxane. Other novel taxanes or taxane analogs that continue to attract the interest of investigators for their poten-

tial to enhance radiation effects include taxoltere metro (255), the epothilones (5), and orally available taxanes (174).

Mitomycin C

The rationale for the use of mitomycin C in combined-modality therapy is based on its ability to target hypoxic cells that are known to be relatively radiation-resistant (33). There is preclinical evidence to suggest that mitomycin C administered before irradiation leads to a supraadditive interaction (92). Given that normal tissues are not hypoxic, the selective targeting of this cell population with mitomycin C has the potential to improve cures without compromising normal tissue complication rates. The use of mitomycin C is also limited by its hematologic toxicities; however, investigators have pursued a similar strategy as outlined previously with the development of tirapazamine, another hypoxic cell cytotoxin (36,37). Brown (37) has discovered that tirapazamine, which is a benzotriazine di-*N*-oxide, is toxic to hypoxic cells at concentrations much lower than what is needed to radiosensitize cells. It has the greatest differential toxicity known between hypoxic and well-oxygenated cells. Essentially, this drug functions through its intracellular reduction to form a highly reactive radical capable of causing both SSBs and DSBs (142). In the presence of oxygen, this free electron is absorbed, and the compound is back-oxidized to the parent compound with the concomitant release of a superoxide radical, which is much less cytotoxic than the tirapazamine radical. Clinical trials are ongoing in multiple tumor sites.

Antimetabolites

The radiosensitizing properties of 5-FU have been known for years (16). Several mechanisms have been proposed for the cytotoxicity of this drug:

(a) Its incorporation into RNA, which leads to a disruption of RNA function;
(b) Inhibition of thymidylate synthetase function and subsequently of DNA synthesis; and
(c) Direct incorporation of the drug into DNA.

It is believed that a combination of these effects underlies its radiosensitizing properties (40). Optimization of its schedule of delivery is crucial to obtaining an effect with this combination, and it is accepted that cytotoxic doses of 5-FU are needed to obtain a radiosensitizing effect. In general, it is thought that a continuous infusion of the drug is needed to obtain the desired drug levels after irradiation (153). Long-standing clinical experience with this drug bears out much of the laboratory studies of its effectiveness as a radiation sensitizer.

Gemcitabine is another nucleoside analog that acts as a very potent radiosensitizer. The biologic action of gemcitabine is due almost completely to its effects on DNA metabolism. Early studies of this drug in leukemic cell lines found that notable decreases in cellular deoxynucleotide triphosphates occurred with the use of the drug. These decreases were most impressive in terms of the levels of deoxycytidine triphosphate; however, deoxyadenosine triphosphate and deoxyguanosine triphosphate were also affected (192). Direct incorporation of the drug into DNA as well as drug-induced apoptosis are also thought to underlie its cytotoxicity (193). The metabolism of gemcitabine in the cell is complex, and it is able to potentiate its cytotoxicity as a sole therapy (193). Depending on the cell line tested, the drug concentration, the schedule of administration, as well as the cell proliferative status (e.g., plateau vs. exponential growth), relative enhancement ratios in the range of 1.1 to 2.5 have been reported.

Gemcitabine is S-phase–specific and as such should be selectively toxic to proliferating cells (94), decreasing the amount of proliferation that can occur during fractionated radiation therapy. In addition, cell cycle redistribution induced by these agents may improve cell kill by allowing more cells to be treated in the more sensitive parts of the cell cycle (163). As DNA synthesis inhibitors, these drugs may act to inhibit the repair of radiation-induced DNA damage (93). Finally, as DNA chain terminators, they may serve to trigger the apoptotic response (130).

There is strong preclinical evidence to suggest that the radiosensitizing abilities of gemcitabine are intimately linked to cellular deoxyadenosine triphosphate levels (130). Interesting results from Latz et al. (129) show quite clearly that cells that are pretreated with gemcitabine no longer show a progressive increase in radioresistance as they progress toward DNA replication, and sensitization, therefore, appears to be greatest in the S phase.

Milas et al. (160) found the largest enhancement of growth delay when gemcitabine was delivered 24 to 60 hours before irradiation in a murine sarcoma tumor model. Interestingly, the use of gemcitabine in combination with radiation also decreased the risk for development of lung metastases in those mice that attained durable local control (73% in the radiation-alone group vs. 40% in the combined-modality group). This observation has been confirmed in a second study with a larger number of mice (151). This preclinical work is supportive of the principles of combined-modality therapy in that better local control translated into decreased systemic spread of tumor cells in a significant percentage of study animals.

The same authors also report a dose-dependent increase in the apoptotic rate after the administration of gemcitabine (163), which they believe correlates with the elimination of the more radioresistant S-phase population of cells and a redistribution of the remaining cells into more radiosensitive parts of the cell cycle. They also report that reoxygenation of the resistant hypoxic fraction of tumor cells is a mechanism for the radiosensitizing action of gemcitabine (151).

In summary, the preclinical evidence suggests that gemcitabine acts through several mechanisms (nucleotide pool perturbation, lowering of the apoptotic threshold, cell cycle redistribution, and tumor cell reoxygenation) to enhance the effect of ionizing radiation on tumors. Clinical experience has shown that this drug is indeed a potent sensitizer with the potential for significant toxicity (212) as well as improvement in tumor control when combined with radiation.

Topoisomerase I Inhibitors

The camptothecins are potent radiation sensitizers that are still in their infancy in clinical studies. Camptothecin is a plant alkaloid obtained from the *Camptotheca acuminata* tree. Its initial clinical evaluation in the 1960s and 1970s was abandoned because of severe and unpredictable hemorrhagic cystitis (169,171). Camptothecin and its derivatives (e.g., irinotecan, topotecan, 9-aminocamptothecin, SN-38) target DNA topoisomerase I (9,107,108). This enzyme relaxes both positively and negatively supercoiled DNA and allows for diverse essential cellular processes, including replication and transcription, to proceed. In the presence of camptothecin, a camptothecin–topoisomerase I–DNA complex becomes stabilized with the 5'-phosphoryl terminus of the enzyme-catalyzed DNA SSB bound covalently to a tyrosine residue of topoisomerase I. These stabilized cleavable complexes interact with the advancing replication fork during the S phase or during unscheduled DNA replication after genomic stress and cause the conversion of SSBs into irreversible DNA DSBs, resulting in cell death (103).

Several investigators have reported that camptothecin enhances the cytotoxic effect of radiation *in vitro* and *in vivo* (45,181). Chen et al. (45) showed that cells exposed to 20(S)-10,11 methylenedioxycamptothecin before or during radiation had sensitization ratios of 1.6, whereas those treated with

the drug after radiation had substantially less enhancement of radiation-induced DNA damage. There are several hypotheses regarding the mechanism of interaction between radiation and irinotecan, which is perhaps the best-studied of the camptothecin derivatives. The first hypothesis suggests that inhibition of topoisomerase I by irinotecan leads to inhibition of repair of radiation-induced DNA strand breaks. The second hypothesis suggests that irinotecan causes a redistribution of the cells into the more radiosensitive G_2 phase of the cell cycle. The third hypothesis is that topoisomerase I–DNA adducts are trapped by irinotecan at the sites of radiation-induced SSBs, leading to their conversion into DSBs (8). The primary mechanism involved with radiosensitization may depend on which camptothecin derivative is being used; there is currently insufficient evidence to identify the underlying mechanism with certainty.

Data from *in vivo* experiments demonstrate that combination 9-aminocamptothecin and irradiation is more effective when fractionated, compared with single doses (123). There is also evidence for circadian-dependent cytotoxicity and radiation sensitization when camptothecin derivatives like 9-aminocamptothecin are used as radiation sensitizers (123).

The integration of this group of drugs into clinical treatments with radiation is ongoing. Much of the current experience with irinotecan has been accumulated in non–small cell lung cancer (NSCLC) (227), whereas much of the experience with topotecan has occurred in brain tumors (78,91).

The Clinical Experience with Chemoradiation in Cancer Therapy

The level of clinical experience with the combination of radiation and chemotherapy has increased dramatically during the years. In several tumor types, the sequencing and method of administration of the combination have been very important in attaining improved outcomes seen in randomized trials. Improved local control and better overall survival rates have resulted from combination therapy in a number of diseases, including rectal cancer, limited-stage small cell lung cancer, locally advanced NSCLC, esophageal cancer, anaplastic astrocytomas, cervical cancer, and rhabdomyosarcomas. Equally important are the successes seen in the realm of organ preservation in sarcomas of the extremity, bladder cancers, carcinomas of the anal canal, head and neck cancers, and breast cancer. Sadly, there are many tumor types for which ineffective therapies have not been able to improve outcomes in a tangible fashion for patients. Ongoing studies that incorporate novel combinations of drugs with radiation do, however, hold hope for the future in that they may provide superior survival rates with less toxicity and a better overall quality of life for patients.

As outcomes in each of the solid tumors improve with concurrent therapy, we need to become cognizant of the potential for significant long-term toxicity from combination chemoradiation and do our best to minimize the risks that these side effects pose to patient survival and quality of life. Several well-documented chemoradiation-imposed late effects are summarized in Table 29.4.

Lung

Small Cell Carcinoma

Although the natural history of this malignancy involves early seeding of distant metastases, patients diagnosed with localized or limited-stage tumors are potentially curable. Chemotherapy remains the mainstay of therapy; however, up to 80% of patients treated with chemotherapy alone relapse in the chest, some of whom have no noted distant disease (249).

	Table 29.4	**THE LONG-TERM TOXICITY OF COMBINED CHEMORADIATION THERAPY**		
Agent	**Toxicity**	**Mechanism**		**References**
Bleomycin	Pneumonitis/pulmonary fibrosis	Undefined but related to total drug dose and effects on pulmonary macrophages, type I and II alveolar cells; effects/lethality exacerbated by the administration of radiation.		53,147,209
Actinomycin D	Hepatopathy	Altered liver function postradiation leads to decreased metabolism of agents, including actinomycin, which in turn worsens the hepatopathy.		157,231
Doxorubicin	Cardiomyopathy	There is an additive interaction between doxorubicin and radiation with recall of radiation effects occurring. Primary radiation effect is on the endothelial cell, whereas doxorubicin affects the connective tissue stroma of the myocardium.		29,77,127,159
Methotrexate	Leukoencephalopathy	Methotrexate may cause this syndrome on its own. Radiation effects on the blood–brain barrier and the choroid plexus can alter methotrexate clearance, leading to higher levels in the brain. Effects are increased when both modalities are used.		6,116,221,236

Meta-analyses that examined the value of thoracic radiation in the limited stage of this disease performed by both Warde and Payne (249) and Pignon et al. (190) demonstrated an improvement in 2- to 3-year survival rates of 5%. The analysis of Warde and Payne showed that thoracic irradiation improved local control by 25%. The use of cisplatin and etoposide in concurrent therapy is generally accepted because these drugs lack many of the toxicities caused when the cyclophosphamide–doxorubicin–vincristine (CAV) regimen is delivered with radiation therapy. The intergroup randomized trial that examined the benefit of delivering hyperfractionated irradiation with the first cycle of chemotherapy found that the 2- and 5-year survival rates with the hyperfractionated regimen were 47% and 26%, respectively, compared with only 41% and 21% with the once-daily regimen (240). On further analysis, it was found that not only was the local control improved in the group that received hyperfractionated irradiation, but that there was a decreased incidence of simultaneous local and distant failure. This suggests that improved local control may lead to improved survival even with a malignancy that tends to disseminate systemically.

Two recent systematic reviews have raised the suggestion that not only is early concurrent radiation with cisplatin-based treatment important in achieving optimal outcomes but that the overall time of delivery of the chemoradiation package is also significant (61,84). DeRuysscher et al. (61) put forward that when the time between the start of chemotherapy and the last day of radiation is less than 30 days, the 5-year survival is greater than 20% (relative risk = 0.62; 95% confidence interval = 0.49–0.80; $p = 0.0003$) (84). These results seemingly imply that accelerated repopulation of clonagens during prolonged overall treatment times account for poorer outcomes with those strategies and that the overall treatment time needs to be considered in future trial development.

The principle of spatial cooperation enters the treatment realm in this disease, wherein the practice of prophylactic cranial irradiation is associated with a decrease in the incidence of brain metastases. This decreased incidence of brain metastases is associated with an increased survival rate in patients with limited-stage disease who have had a complete response to therapy (17,126). As such, prophylactic cranial irradiation forms a standard part of the treatment of limited-stage small cell lung cancer.

Non–Small Cell Carcinoma

There are multiple trials that have compared the delivery of standard irradiation to chemoradiation therapy in NSCLC (66,132,211,213). The median survival improvement from 9.6

months with irradiation therapy alone to 13.7 months with sequential chemoradiation in the original study by Dillman et al. (66) illustrates the benefit of the addition of chemotherapy. A meta-analysis confirms that cisplatin-based chemotherapy in combination with irradiation does improve outcome compared with radiation therapy alone in NSCLC, at the expense of increased toxicity (194).

Two more phase III trials have moved the paradigm one step further in that they both found a benefit to delivering radiation and chemotherapy concurrently. Furuse et al. (87) have presented the results of their Japanese trial that administered MVP (mitomycin C, vindesine, and cisplatin) with 56 Gy in both sequential and concurrent fashions. There was an improved median survival of 16.5 versus 13.3 months with the concurrent therapy. The concurrent therapy was also well tolerated because the radiation therapy was delivered in a split-course fashion, with comparable rates of esophagitis in both treatment arms. The Radiation Therapy Oncology Group (RTOG) 9410 randomized phase III experience has confirmed the benefit to concurrent therapy (58). This trial used cisplatin-based therapy delivered in one of three fashions:

(a) Sequentially with vinblastine followed by radiation therapy,
(b) Concurrently with vinblastine and once-daily radiation therapy, and
(c) Concurrently with etoposide and twice-daily hyperfractionated radiation therapy.

Arm B, in which the chemotherapy was delivered concurrently with once-daily irradiation, has revealed a statistical benefit over the sequential administration of chemotherapy and radiation therapy, with a median survival of 17 months versus 14.6 months ($p = 0.038$).

Multiple randomized phase II studies that integrate newer chemotherapeutic agents have been undertaken and their results published (22,82,245,258). They seem to yield similar results to the Furuse et al. (87) and RTOG (58) trials with median survivals of about 17 months and 2-year survivals in the range of 35%. At present, it would seem that concurrent delivery of therapy is the most important determinant of outcome, although results from the trial published by Belani et al. (224) would suggest that optimal therapy involves upfront concurrent chemoradiation (82,245,258). As such, most ongoing trials have incorporated this sequence. Strategies seeking to maximize radiation dose with the delivery of high-dose conformal therapy remain investigational, as do efforts to integrate newer targeted drugs. No trials demonstrate a substantial survival benefit to postoperative therapy (60,117). The improvement in patient outcome

Table 29.5 **OUTCOME OF TREATMENT IN LOCALLY ADVANCED NON–SMALL CELL LUNG CANCER**

Treatment	Study Authors	Design	No. of Patients	RT (Gy) and CT Treatment	Median Survival (mo)	2- to 5-year Survival (%)
RT alone	Dillman et al. (66)	Phase III	77	60 Gy	9.6	13/3
	Sause et al. (211)	Phase III	152	60 Gy	11.4	21/5
	Sause et al. (211)	Phase III	154	69.6 Gy	12	24/6
CT	Dillman et al. (66)	Phase III	78	Cis + Vlb → 60 Gy	13.2	26/10
↓	Sause et al. (211)	Phase III	152	Cis + Vlb → 60 Gy	13.8	32/8
RT	Furuse et al. (87)	Phase III	158	MVCis → 56 Gy	13.3	27.4/8.9
	Curran et al. (58)	Phase III	200	Cis + Vlb → 60 Gy	14.6	—/—
CT/RT	Curran et al. (58)	Phase III	200	Cis + Vlb/60 Gy	17	—/—
	Furuse et al. (87)	Phase III	156	MVCis/56 Gy	16.5	34.6/15.8
	Belani et al. (22)	Phase II	92	Weekly P+C + 63 Gy→P+C	16.3	31/—
	Zatloukal et al. (258)	Phase II	52	Cis + N/60 Gy	16.6	34.2/—

RT, radiation therapy; CT, chemotherapy; Cis, cisplatin; Vlb, vinblastine; M, mitomycin C; V, vindesine; P, paclitaxel; C, carboplatin; N, vinorelbine.

with the integration of concurrent chemoradiation therapy is illustrated in Table 29.5.

Head and Neck

Traditional management of locally advanced squamous cell cancers of the head and neck has involved a combination of surgery and radiation therapy in most cases. Despite aggressive therapy with significant morbidity, treatment often yields poor long-term survival rates when there is unresectable disease, with 5-year survival rates in the range of 30%. Alternative fractionation schemes that exploit the differential ability of cells to repair radiation-induced damage and allow for delivery of a higher tumor dose, or those that attempt to deliver therapy in a shorter overall treatment time to combat accelerated repopulation of tumors, have become more popular therapies because some trials have suggested a benefit (85,104).

Approximately 70 randomized trials have been performed to examine the contribution of combined chemoradiation therapy on local control and overall survival. Many studies have been small, with inadequate power to detect a significant benefit in the addition of chemotherapy to radiation therapy in a heterogeneous population of tumors. As such, several meta-analyses have been undertaken to assess a larger patient population and help determine the absolute benefits of the addition of chemotherapy (31,74,172,191).

The MACH-NC study, which evaluated 63 trials and a total of 10,741 patients, is the largest of the meta-analyses (191). Individual data rather than literature-based data, with the inclusion of updated data and unpublished trials, were assessed, including individual data updated in 66% of the trials for as long as a median follow-up of 6.8 years. Subcategorization into locoregional treatment with and without concomitant chemotherapy, induction/adjuvant chemotherapy, and laryngeal preservation with induction chemotherapy, rather than definitive treatment for laryngeal and hypopharyngeal tumors, was reported. No benefit was detected for neoadjuvant or adjuvant chemotherapy, whereas a trend toward a statistically significant benefit (4%) was reported for concurrent or alternating chemoradiation therapy (p = .23).

Munro (172) performed a meta-analysis of 54 trials, including those before 1965. Two of these trials addressed maxillary sinus carcinoma and nasopharyngeal carcinoma specifically, and the Veteran's Affairs Laryngeal Cancer study was also included. Munro found an overall benefit to adding chemotherapy of 6.5% (3.7% for induction, 12.1% for concomitant; adjuvant chemotherapy was not assessed). Finally, the review by El-Sayed and Nelson (74) of 42 trials, including 6 trials published before 1965, revealed that the addition of chemotherapy to locoregional treatment added an absolute benefit of 4%; absolute benefits of concomitant chemotherapy were 8% (neoadjuvant and adjuvant chemotherapy was not assessed). These data suggest a small but real benefit to combined-modality therapy with "older" drugs at the expense of increased toxicity. There are no current randomized studies that confirm if newer chemotherapies like paclitaxel or docetaxel are associated with improved outcome.

The literature does justify the use of neoadjuvant chemotherapy in the setting of advanced laryngeal or hypopharyngeal primaries with the dual goals of organ preservation and the treatment of micrometastatic disease. Induction chemotherapy has been considered appropriate in this setting because it does improve laryngeal preservation without compromising overall survival. The landmark Veteran's Affairs Laryngeal Study randomized patients into two arms: induction cisplatin/5-FU for three cycles followed by radiation, or laryngectomy followed by radiation; 332 patients were entered (114). An evaluation occurred after two cycles of chemotherapy. Patients with a partial response received a third cycle of chemotherapy followed by radiation therapy. Those patients without an initial response to induction chemotherapy received a laryngectomy followed by radiation therapy. Patients with residual disease after the completion of radiation therapy underwent surgical resection. With a median follow-up of 33 months, an estimated 2-year survival rate of 68% in both groups failed to demonstrate a difference in overall survival (p = .9846), although a majority of patients (64%) were able to preserve function of the larynx. Recurrences differed between the two groups, with increased locoregional control (p = .0005) and decreased metastases (p = .016) in the induction chemotherapy group. Given that there was no compromise of overall survival, induction therapy is thought to be feasible in the setting of laryngeal carcinoma to allow organ preservation without compromise of overall survival. These results have been confirmed by the European Organization for the Research and Treatment of Cancer (EORTC) (133).

However, the results of the Intergroup trial R91-11 add to the picture (80). Five hundred forty-seven patients with stage III and IV potentially resectable carcinoma of the larynx were randomized to receive one of three treatments. Arm A used induction cisplatin 100 mg/m^2 and continuous-infusion 5-FU 1,000 mg/m^2/day for three cycles, followed by 70 Gy of radiation therapy in responding patients, whereas arm B used concurrent cisplatin at 100 mg/m^2 on days 1, 22, and 43, with 70 Gy, and arm C patients received radiation therapy alone. At 2 years, the locoregional control rates for the treatments were A, 61%; B, 78%; and C, 56%. Locoregional control was significantly better for those patients who received concurrent chemoradiotherapy than among those who received either of the other therapies (A vs. B, $p = 0.004$; B vs. C, $p \leq 0.001$). Although there was no difference in the 2- and 5-year overall survival figures, patients who received chemotherapy had improved disease-free survival compared to those who were treated with radiation alone. This would confirm that concurrent chemoradiation therapy is the preferred therapy for this population when organ preservation is desired.

In addition, there are now other studies that justify the use of concurrent chemotherapy in the head and neck. Denis et al. (62) have updated the results of the French Head and Neck Oncology and Radiotherapy Group randomized trial in advanced stage oropharyngeal cancer to 5 years. In this trial, patients with stage III and IV oropharyngeal cancers with good performance status were randomized to treatment with 70 Gy of radiation alone or to receive concurrent carboplatin and infusional 5-FU for three cycles. The 5-year overall survival, disease-free survival, and locoregional control were 22% and 16% ($p = 0.05$), 27% and 15% ($p = 0.01$), and 48% and 25% ($p = 0.002$), respectively. Although there was no statistical difference in late toxicity between the arms, there was a trend to concurrent treatment causing more late grade 3 or 4 effects (56% vs. 30%). In other studies that have used different radiation fractionation schemes or different chemotherapy regimens (88,112), better disease-related outcomes are also seen; however, all of these trials of concurrent therapy have the significant trade-off of significant increased acute and late toxicity. Garden et al. (88) report that 30% of patients had prophylactic feeding tubes placed and up to 56% of additional patients required them during therapy, underscoring the toxicity of the therapy.

Both the RTOG and the EORTC have described the results of their randomized trials of concurrent chemoradiation in the postoperative setting (26,52). In the RTOG trial (52), 459 patients were randomized to receive either 60 to 66 Gy to the head and neck alone, or with three cycles of cisplatin at 100 mg/m² on days 1, 22, and 43. Local control was improved from 72% to 82% in the combined therapy arm, which was associated with improved disease-free survival, but no overall survival benefit. Combined therapy was once again associated with significant increased acute toxicity, with 34% versus 77% of patients experiencing a grade 3 or 4 toxicity ($p < 0.001$). Four patients died in the combined arm of a protocol-related adverse event, whereas none died in the radiation alone arm. The population treated in the EORTC postoperative randomized trial was slightly different, but similar improvements in local control were seen and the survival benefit reached statistical significance, with 5-year Kaplan-Meir estimates of overall survival of 53% versus 40%. In an analysis of pooled data from both trials, the presence of extracapsular extension and/or involved surgical margins were the only risk factors for which the impact of concurrent therapy was significant in both trials (25). With all the caveats attached to retrospective analyses, these patients appear to derive the greatest benefit from chemoradiation.

Although the previously described trials have established a new standard for treatment of head and neck cancer, they come with a significant cost of increased acute morbidity and long-term problems with swallowing. As such, the trial reported by Bonner et al. (29) is remarkable in that it is the first trial to show a substantial survival benefit with the addition of the molecularly targeted agent, cetuximab, which is a humanized monoclonal antibody directed against the EGFR. In this trial patients with nonmetastatic stage III or IV carcinoma of the pharynx, hypopharynx, or larynx were randomized to receive radiation delivered with curative intent or radiation plus intravenous cetuximab starting at 400 mg/m² the week before radiotherapy and continuing weekly at 250 mg/m² for the duration of the therapy. Remarkably, there was no difference with compliance with therapy, and aside from increased acneform rash and transfusion reactions, there were no increased serious toxicities associated with the combined treatment. Additionally, there are real and sustained improved outcomes with a median follow-up of 54 months in the report. Local control was improved with 47% in the experimental arm at 3 years compared to 34% with radiation alone ($p < 0.01$). This translates into a median survival of 49 months for combined therapy compared to only 29.3 months for radiotherapy alone ($p = 0.03$). The question as to whether the benefit from concurrent chemoradiation with its increased toxicities is comparable to the benefit of concurrent cetuximab remains unanswered. This trial represents one of the first triumphs in the translation of our knowledge of molecularly targeted agents impacting on patients with potentially curable malignancies.

Al-Sarraf et al. (3) have performed a large randomized, prospective, phase III Intergroup trial of 185 patients randomized to radiation therapy alone or concomitant chemoradiation therapy in locally advanced nasopharyngeal cancer. All patients received 35 to 39 fractions of daily irradiation and were randomized to receive concomitant cisplatin (100 mg/m² on days 1, 22, and 43) followed by three cycles of adjuvant cisplatin (80 mg/m², day 1) and continuous-infusion 5-FU (1,000 mg/m², days 1 to 4) every 28 days. The superiority of combined treatment was seen in the concomitant chemoradiation therapy arm, with a 3-year progression-free survival rate of 69% versus 24% ($p < 0.001$) and a 3-year overall survival rate of 78% versus 47% ($p = .005$). Hence, the recommended standard of care in treating patients with more advanced nasopharyngeal carcinoma has become concomitant chemoradiation therapy.

In the last few years there have been a number of modern trials that have reported improved outcomes with concurrent chemoradiation with or without an altered fractionation scheme of radiation delivery. The improved outcome has come at the price of significantly increased acute and late toxicity that has an impact on overall quality of life for these patients.

Uterine Cervix

Although the exact indications and the regimen of choice remain controversial, there is convincing evidence from recent studies that concurrent chemotherapy can improve outcome in patients requiring radiation for locally advanced cervical cancer (235). Although several studies with debatable results have been conducted using hydroxyurea and 5-FU, the weight of the data suggests that a cisplatin-containing concurrent regimen is now the treatment of choice for many patients. There is no evidence to support the use of neoadjuvant or adjuvant chemotherapy at present (250).

A Gynecologic Oncology Group trial in which patients with locally advanced disease who had negative para-aortic nodes at lymphadenectomy were randomized to receive concurrent hydroxyurea plus radiation therapy versus concurrent cisplatin and 5-FU plus radiation therapy has been completed and has shown a benefit for the cisplatin-containing arm (205). In a second trial, two more aggressive cisplatin-containing chemotherapy regimens showed benefit over a hydroxyurea and radiation regimen (235). Both cisplatin-containing treatments yielded dramatic, highly significant improvements in local disease control and survival.

During the same period, the RTOG designed a trial comparing a combination of cisplatin, 5-FU, and pelvic irradiation with extended-field irradiation alone in RTOG 90-01 (170). Patients were required to have negative para-aortic lymph nodes based on a lymphangiogram or retroperitoneal lymph node dissection. The radiation-alone arm was based on a previous study that found a survival benefit when prophylactic para-aortic irradiation was added to standard pelvic irradiation. This trial was published early when an interim analysis revealed a highly significant improvement in overall survival, disease-free survival, local disease control, and rate of freedom from distant metastases in the combined-modality arm.

Two further trials (118,186) have demonstrated a survival benefit when cisplatin is added to radiation therapy in the setting of earlier-stage disease followed by an extrafascial hysterectomy, or when cisplatin is added to pelvic radiation in those patients who have already undergone a radical hysterectomy.

Of the recent trials looking at the addition of cisplatin-based chemotherapy, only the National Cancer Institute of Canada (NCI Canada) trial has not demonstrated a survival benefit with the addition of concurrent chemotherapy (183). However, the authors of this study maintain that the optimization of radiation therapy as it was delivered in their trial may account for the lack of benefit. The issues of how best to integrate newer chemotherapies like the taxanes, which have considerable radiation-sensitization properties, targeted biologic agents, and agents that may optimize the oxygenation status of the tumors are still under investigation.

Urinary Bladder

The natural history of muscle-invasive bladder cancer is much more aggressive than superficial disease, with a 5-year survival rate of only 50%. The strategy of using radiation therapy, chemotherapy, or a maximal transurethral resection of a bladder tumor in isolation to achieve lasting pelvic control pales in comparison with the modern radical cystectomy. This surgical therapy yields local control in better than 90% of all cases. Issues related to overall survival benefits as well as quality-of-life end points have led to the pursuit of a combined-modality strategy that incorporates all elements of therapy in an attempt to preserve organ function.

The only randomized trial to show a benefit to the addition of concurrent chemotherapy in the definitive treatment of bladder cancer is that of the NCI Canada, which showed a significant improvement in local control ($p = .036$) and suggested a survival difference (47% vs. 33%, $p = .34$) with the addition of concurrent cisplatin to local therapy (53). This study was unfortunately small and not adequately powered to show a survival benefit.

In 1993, investigators at the Massachusetts General Hospital published the results of a single-arm institutional study that has become the model for several subsequent trials (115). Fifty-three patients underwent maximal transurethral resection of a bladder tumor, followed by two cycles of cisplatin, methotrexate, and vinblastine (CMV), followed by 40 Gy with two cycles of concurrent single-agent cisplatin. At this point, they underwent endoscopic re-evaluation, and if they had an incomplete response to therapy, they underwent a cystectomy, if medically feasible; whereas complete responders were consolidated with an additional 24.8 Gy and an additional cycle of cisplatin. A total of 42 patients completed therapy; there was no chemotherapy-related mortality. Radical cystectomy was required in a total of 15 patients, including 3 who had a salvage surgery. After 48 months of follow-up, 53% of the patients were alive and 42% had no evidence of disease. An updated report on 106 patients found that 34% of the patients ultimately required a salvage cystectomy, with 49% of patients alive, and 43% alive with their native bladders intact (115).

Eapen et al. (72) have also published their experience with novel administration of concurrent cisplatin during bladder radiation with three doses of intra-arterial chemotherapy delivered in an attempt to improve local control. They have reported on 200 patients treated during a 15-year period. At follow-up cystoscopy there was a 90% complete response rate in evaluable patients, which has translated into a 75% bladder preservation rate, and survivals were slightly lower but comparable to surgical treatment with cystectomy. This therapy has been

complicated by significant sensory neuropathy, the severity and duration of which has been improved by decreasing the dose of cisplatin to 90 mg/m^2.

Series from several other centers or groups (70,105,226) have tested bladder-conservation strategies with reasonable results and far more patients failing with distant disease than local-only failures. Although there is not likely to be a definitive randomized trial comparing a bladder-conservation approach with radical cystectomy, it would appear that combined-modality therapy is not an unreasonable option for patients. Ongoing studies are looking at integrating the taxanes and other biologic agents into therapy to improve outcome.

Anus

In the case of tumors originating in the anus, the early experience of Nigro et al. (175) suggested that there may not be a need to perform surgery as part of the initial therapy of this cancer, reserving the abdominoperineal resection for local recurrence. Three patients treated with preoperative radiation, 5-FU, and mitomycin C were found to have had a complete pathologic response at the time of their surgery. This work has been expanded by Cummings et al. (57) in their series of patients who were treated by various concurrent regimens over time, and by several large Intergroup studies (75,79) that have demonstrated the value of concurrent chemoradiation therapy in this disease.

The United Kingdom Coordinating Committee on Cancer Research trial showed that the combined-modality arm improved 3-year actuarial local control rates from 29% to 61% and was significant (75). This trial did not show a survival benefit with the addition of chemotherapy, and the combined arm had more early grade 4 toxicity. Similar benefit in terms of local control was also seen in the EORTC trial with the addition of 5-FU and mitomycin C (5-year colostomy-free survival rate, 72% vs. 40%) (17). However, once again a survival benefit was not seen. The Intergroup trial, which randomized patients to treatment with or without mitomycin C, confirmed its benefit to therapy with a higher complete response rate (92% vs. 85%) and a significantly lower colostomy rate (9% vs. 22%) (79). However, there was no significant survival benefit. The results of the completed RTOG 98-11 trial examining the benefit of two cycles of induction 5-FU and cisplatin are pending.

Esophagus

Although the ideal approach to the management of locally advanced disease is controversial, the evidence from several randomized trials shows that chemoradiation is associated with an improved survival rate compared with radiation alone (4,218). The Intergroup trial RTOG 85-01 has had a profound influence on patterns of practice (4). In this phase III study, patients were randomized to treatments consisting of 5-FU (1,000 mg/m^2/day for 96 hours), cisplatin (75 mg/m^2, day 1), and 50 Gy in 25 fractions of daily irradiation starting on the first day of chemotherapy or 64 Gy of daily radiation in 2-Gy fractions. This chemotherapy was administered every 4 weeks during radiation and every 3 weeks after its completion. Concurrent therapy was associated with significant benefits in terms of 5-year overall survival rates (26% vs. 0%; $p < .0001$) as well as decreased local failure (45% vs. 68%; $p = .0123$). Concurrent therapy, as delivered in this trial, is associated with significant toxicity (i.e., 20% grade 4 toxicity and one treatment-related death). Based on these studies, concurrent chemoradiation therapy has become the standard of care for the nonsurgical management of esophageal cancer, whereas radiation alone is reserved for those patients who are unable to tolerate the addition of chemotherapy. Intensifying the radiation to deliver a dose of 64.8 Gy was more recently tested in a phase III Intergroup study

(INT 0123/RTOG 94-05) with the intent of further improving local control and, potentially, survival. Results revealed no significant difference with the intensified radiation therapy in median survival (12.9 vs. 17.6 months), the 2-year survival rate (29% vs. 38%), or the locoregional failure rate (59% vs. 52%). After the first interim analysis, the trial was closed (168). Efforts to improve primary chemoradiation therapy through the incorporation of novel radiosensitizing chemotherapies continue.

The realm of treating resectable esophageal cancer is far less clear. Although several randomized studies have been completed comparing neoadjuvant chemoradiation followed by esophagectomy versus surgery alone, they have been underpowered, have used unconventional fractionation schemes or split-course radiation, and may have had unbalanced treatment arms (30,241,246). What may have been the more definitive trial (Cancer and Leukemia Group B 9781) was closed because of poor accrual. Because the evidence from these randomized trials is plagued by design-related issues and conflicting results, the literature does not clearly support the use of preoperative chemoradiation outside a clinical trial. Efforts to incorporate new agents, including the taxanes, UFT (uracil/tegafur), and irinotecan, are ongoing.

Rectum

The location of the rectum in the confines of the bony pelvis and its intimate relationships with adjacent organs make resection of these tumors with wide radial margins difficult unless a total mesorectal excision is undertaken. Tumors originating in the rectum are often associated with a higher risk of local failure compared with extrapelvic colon cancers on a stage-by-stage basis. Neoadjuvant therapies are often given in an effort to improve the resectability of tumors and in the hope of increasing sphincter preservation rates. The value of adjuvant therapy with chemoradiation to improve local control as well as overall survival is well recognized.

The Gastrointestinal Tumor Study Group has performed a four-arm randomized trial looking at the benefit of adjuvant therapies with patients allocated to surgery alone, postoperative pelvic irradiation, postoperative chemotherapy, or postoperative chemoradiation therapy in patients with stage B2 or C disease (89). The local recurrence rate was reduced in the chemoradiation therapy arm from 25% to 11%, and overall survival was improved by 14% to 56%. Confirmation of these results was found with the National Surgical Adjuvant Breast and Bowel Project R-01 trial (77); consequently, the National Institutes of Health issued a clinical announcement recommending adjuvant 5-FU–based chemotherapy and concurrent radiation therapy for patients with stage B2, B3, and C rectal cancer (176). Although these initial trials included semustine, several randomized studies examined the value of adding this drug to therapy, and their results have led to the dropping of semustine from adjuvant treatment because it was not associated with a significant benefit (90,179,233,254).

The most recent Intergroup trial (INT-0114) randomized patients to pelvic irradiation and 6 months of bolus 5-FU versus bolus 5-FU and levamisole, leucovorin, or both (199). A preliminary analysis revealed no significant difference in disease-free survival or overall survival rates (78% to 80%) among the four treatment arms and, as expected, toxicity was greatest with the three-drug regimen. Efforts to further refine the delivery of 5-FU–based therapy are ongoing and include the use of a prolonged venous infusion, which is associated with less myelosuppression but more diarrhea.

The benefits of preoperative therapy are well recognized and include sphincter preservation, less bowel-related toxicity at the expense of possible overtreatment, and increased wound healing. A German trial randomized patients staged by endoscopic ultrasonography to preoperative or postoperative irradiation

with concurrent 5-FU by prolonged venous infusion for two cycles followed by maintenance 5-FU (210). The reported analysis of toxicity showed significantly fewer grade 3 and 4 complications with preoperative chemoradiation therapy (27% vs. 40%; $p = 0.001$). In addition pro-operative therapy was associated with less long-term complications and improved local control with only 5-year cumulative incidence of local failure of 6 versus 13% ($p = 0.006$). No difference in overall survival was seen. This trial may provide some guidance on whether preoperative or postoperative adjuvant therapy is advantageous.

The question of how to incorporate newer chemotherapies, including paclitaxel, irinotecan, oxaliplatin, and the taxanes, into therapy of rectal cancers remains investigational.

Glioblastoma Multiforme

Until recently, the options for treatment of this tumor have been limited at best with combinations of surgery and radiation. Chemotherapies delivered either concurrently or at relapse seemed to have modest activity. A contemporary randomized trial conducted by the EORTC and NCI Canada has demonstrated that the early concurrent addition of temozolamide to cranial radiation prolongs the survival of patients with glioblastome multiforme (224). This trial enrolled 573 patients from August 2000 to March 2002. Both groups received 60 Gy of radiation to the primary tumor. Those patients in the experimental arm also received 75 mg/m^2 for 7 weeks and then 4 weeks later began up to six adjuvant cycles of the drug at 150 to 200 mg/m^2. Results demonstrated a median survival benefit of 2.5 months from 12.1 months with radiation alone to 14.6 months with combined treatment. In addition, the 2-year survival rate was improved to 26.5% compared to only 10.1% with radiation alone. A phase II study from Greece would seem to confirm these results (14). An ongoing international trial will examine the benefits of increasing the dose intensity of the temozolamide delivery as well as examine the prognostic value of methylguanine methyltransferase excision repair enzyme (MGMT) status. Of the patients in the EORTC/NCI Canada trial who were able to be analyzed, 45% had a methylated MGMT promoter and these patients had a superior survival of 46% at 2 years and a median survival of 22 months (223). The international trial will be able to confirm or refute the value of MGMT status. Current research efforts are trying to incorporate novel targeted agents into the temozolamide-radiotherapy paradigm.

▪▪ | Concluding Remarks

The combination of chemotherapy and radiation therapy has become a common strategic practice in the therapy of locally advanced cancers, with recent emphasis on the concurrent delivery of both modalities. Improvements in treatment outcome in terms of both local control and patient survival have been achieved with traditional chemotherapeutic agents such as cisplatin and 5-FU. Nonetheless, the cure rates of the majority of solid tumors remain poor, and the addition of combined treatments is frequently associated with increased normal tissue toxicity. Thus, there is considerable room for improvement of the combined treatment strategies. However, selection of the most effective drug or the optimal treatment approach remains a significant challenge.

Newer chemotherapies—such as the taxanes, nucleoside analogs, and topoisomerase inhibitors, which interfere with one or more tumor radioresistance mechanisms—are becoming available at an increasing rate. These agents have high potential for increasing the therapeutic effectiveness of radiation therapy, and therefore their evaluation—both in the laboratory and in the clinic, in combination with radiation therapy—is essential for improvement of cancer treatment. Preclinical studies provide not only a biologic rationale for the use of a given drug with radiation but are able to generate information that is critical to the design of effective treatment schedules in clinical settings. Studies of the mechanisms of chemotherapy–radiation therapy interaction at the genetic–molecular, cellular, and tumor (or normal tissue) microenvironmental levels are essential for obtaining clear insight into the radiomodulating potential of chemotherapeutic agents and their ability to increase radiotherapeutic effects.

Significant progress has been made in our understanding of the basic mechanisms of radiation injury, as well as of the injury inflicted by chemotherapeutic agents and the cellular processing of these injuries in both normal and malignant cells. Recent advances in molecular biology have exposed many potential targets for augmentation of radioresponse or chemoresponse, including EGFR, COX-2, angiogenic molecules, and various components of the signal transduction pathways that these molecules initiate. It has become possible to intervene actively in some molecular pathways to improve the therapeutic ratio, and the incorporation of molecular targeting strategies into chemoradiation therapy is being increasingly used for therapeutic intervention in many types of human cancer.

References

1. Abdollahi A, Lipson KE, Han X, et al. SU5416 and SU6668 attenuate the angiogenic effects of radiation-induced tumor cell growth factor production and amplify the direct anti-endothelial action of radiation in vitro. *Cancer Res* 2003;63:3755–3763.
2. Allen JC, Thaler HT, Deck MD, et al. Leukoencephalopathy following high-dose intravenous methotrexate chemotherapy: Quantitative assessment of white matter attenuation using computed tomography. *Neuroradiology* 1978;16:44–47.
3. Al-Sarraf M, LeBlanc M, Giri PG, et al. Chemoradiotherapy versus radiotherapy in patients with advanced nasopharyngeal cancer: Phase III randomized Intergroup study 0099. *J Clin Oncol* 1998;16:1310–1317.
4. Al-Sarraf M, Martz K, Herskovic A, et al. Progress report of combined chemoradiotherapy versus radiotherapy alone in patients with esophageal cancer: An intergroup study. *J Clin Oncol* 1997;15:277–284.
5. Altmann KH, Wartmann M, O'Reilly T. Epothilones and related structures—a new class of microtubule inhibitors with potent in vivo antitumor activity. *Biochim Biophys Acta* 2000;1470:M79–91.
6. Amorino GP, Freeman ML, Carbone DP, et al. Radiopotentiation by the oral platinum agent, JM216: Role of repair inhibition. *Int J Radiat Oncol Biol Phys* 1999;44:399–405.
7. Amorino GP, Hamilton VM, Choy H. Enhancement of radiation effects by combined docetaxel and carboplatin treatment in vitro. *Radiat Oncol Investig* 1999;7:343–352.
8. Amorino GP, Hercules SK, Mohr PJ, et al. Preclinical evaluation of the orally active camptothecin analog, RFS-2000 (9-nitro-20(S)-camptothecin) as a radiation enhancer. *Int J Radiat Oncol Biol Phys* 2000;47:503–509.
9. Andoh T, Ishii K, Suzuki Y, et al. Characterization of a mammalian mutant with a camptothecin-resistant DNA topoisomerase I. *Proc Natl Acad Sci U S A* 1987;84:5565–5569.
10. Antonadou D, Pepelassi M, Synodinou M, et al. Prophylactic use of amifostine to prevent radiochemotherapy-induced mucositis and xerostomia in head-and-neck cancer. *Int J Radiat Oncol Biol Phys* 2002;52:739–747.
11. Arora R, Chawla R, Puri SC, et al. Radioprotective and antioxidant properties of low-altitude Podophyllum hexandrum (LAPH). *J Environ Pathol Toxicol Oncol* 2005;24:299–314.
12. Arora R, Chawla R, Sagar R, et al. Evaluation of radioprotective activities Rhodiola imbricata Edgew—a high altitude plant. *Molecular and cellular biochemistry* 2005;273:209–223.
13. Arora R, Gupta D, Chawla R, et al. Radioprotection by plant products: Present status and future prospects. *Phytother Res* 2005;19:1–22.
14. Athanassiou H, Synodinou M, Maragoudakis E, et al. Randomized phase II study of temozolomide and radiotherapy compared with radiotherapy alone in newly diagnosed glioblastoma multiforme. *J Clin Oncol* 2005;23:2372–2377.
15. Auperin A, Arriagada R, Pignon JP, et al. Prophylactic cranial irradiation for patients with small-cell lung cancer in complete remission. Prophylactic Cranial Irradiation Overview Collaborative Group. *N Engl J Med* 1999;341:476–484.
16. Bagshaw MA. Possible role of potentiators in radiation therapy. *Am J Roentgenol Radium Ther Nucl Med* 1961;85:822–833.
17. Bartelink H, Roelofsen F, Eschwege F, et al. Concomitant radiotherapy and chemotherapy is superior to radiotherapy alone in the treatment of locally advanced anal cancer: Results of a phase III randomized trial of the European Organization for Research and Treatment of Cancer Radiotherapy and Gastrointestinal Cooperative Groups. *J Clin Oncol* 1997;15:2040–2049.
18. Baselga J, Pfister D, Cooper MR, et al. Phase I studies of anti-epidermal growth factor receptor chimeric antibody C225 alone and in combination with cisplatin. *J Clin Oncol* 2000;18:904–914.
19. Bates DO, Heald RI, Curry FE, et al. Vascular endothelial growth factor increases Rana vascular permeability and compliance by different signalling pathways. *J Physiol* 2001;533:263–272.
20. Baumann M, Krause M. Targeting the epidermal growth factor receptor in radiotherapy: Radiobiological mechanisms, preclinical and clinical results. *Radiother Oncol* 2004;72:257–266.
21. Begg AC, van der Kolk PJ, Emondt J, et al. Radiosensitization in vitro by cis-diammine (1,1-cyclobutanedicarboxylato) platinum(II) (carboplatin, JM8) and ethylenediammine-malonatoplatinum(II) (JM40). *Radiother Oncol* 1987;9:157–165.
22. Belani CP, Choy H, Bonomi P, et al. Combined chemoradiotherapy regimens of paclitaxel and carboplatin for locally advanced non-small-cell lung cancer: A randomized phase II locally advanced multi-modality protocol. *J Clin Oncol* 2005;23:5883–5891.
23. Bernhard EJ, McKenna WG, Hamilton AD, et al. Inhibiting Ras prenylation increases the radiosensitivity of human tumor cell lines with activating mutations of ras oncogenes. *Cancer Res* 1998;58:1754–1761.
24. Bernhard EJ, Stanbridge EJ, Gupta S, et al. Direct evidence for the contribution of activated N-ras and K-ras oncogenes to increased intrinsic radiation resistance in human tumor cell lines. *Cancer Res* 2000;60:6597–6600.
25. Bernier J, Cooper JS, Pajak TF, et al. Defining risk levels in locally advanced head and neck cancers: A comparative analysis of concurrent postoperative radiation plus chemotherapy trials of the EORTC (#22931) and RTOG (#9501). *Head Neck* 2005;27:843–850.
26. Bernier J, Domenge C, Ozsahin M, et al. Postoperative irradiation with or without concomitant chemotherapy for locally advanced head and neck cancer. *N Engl J Med* 2004;350:1945–1952.
27. Billingham ME, Bristow MR, Glatstein E, et al. Adriamycin cardiotoxicity: Endomyocardial biopsy evidence of enhancement by irradiation. *Am J Surg Pathol* 1977;1:17–23.
28. Bischof M, Abdollahi A, Gong P, et al. Triple combination of irradiation, chemotherapy (pemetrexed), and VEGFR inhibition (SU5416) in human endothelial and tumor cells. *Int J Radiat Oncol Biol Phys* 2004;60:1220–1232.
29. Bonner JA, Harari PM, Giralt J, et al. Radiotherapy plus cetuximab for squamous-cell carcinoma of the head and neck. *N Engl J Med* 2006;354:567–578.
30. Bosset JF, Gignoux M, Triboulet JP, et al. Chemoradiotherapy followed by surgery compared with surgery alone in squamous-cell cancer of the esophagus. *N Engl J Med* 1997;337:161–167.
31. Bourhis J, Pignon JP. Meta-analyses in head and neck squamous cell carcinoma. What is the role of chemotherapy? *Hematol Oncol Clin North Am* 1999;13:769–775.
32. Bradshaw PS, Stavropoulos DJ, Meyn MS. Human telomeric protein TRF2 associates with genomic double-strand breaks as an early response to DNA damage. *Nat Genet* 2005;37:193–197.
33. Bristow RG HR. Molecular and cellular basis of radiotherapy. In: Tannock IF HR, eds. *The basic science of oncology,* 3rd ed. Montreal: McGraw-Hill, 1998:295–321.
34. Brizel DWT, Strnad V, et al. Final Report of a phase III randomized trial of amifostine as a radioprotetant in head and neck cancer. *Int J Radiat Oncol Biol Phys* 1999;45[Suppl 3]:147–148.
35. Brizel DM, Wasserman TH, Henke M, et al. Phase III randomized trial of amifostine as a radioprotector in head and neck cancer. *J Clin Oncol* 2000;18:3339–3345.
36. Brown JM, Giaccia AJ. The unique physiology of solid tumors: Opportunities (and problems) for cancer therapy. *Cancer Res* 1998;58:1408–1416.
37. Brown JM. The hypoxic cell: A target for selective cancer therapy—eighteenth Bruce F. Cain Memorial Award lecture. *Cancer Res* 1999;59:5863–5870.
38. Brunner TB, Cengel KA, Hahn SM, et al. Pancreatic cancer cell radiation survival and prenyltransferase inhibition: The role of K-Ras. *Cancer Res* 2005;65:8433–8441.
39. Brunner TB, Gupta AK, Shi Y, et al. Farnesyltransferase inhibitors as radiation sensitizers. *Int J Radiat Biol* 2003;79:569–576.
40. Buchholz DJ, Lepek KJ, Rich TA, et al. 5-Fluorouracil-radiation interactions in human colon adenocarcinoma cells. *Int J Radiat Oncol Biol Phys* 1995;32:1053–1058.
41. Bush RS, Jenkin RD, Allt WE, et al. Definitive evidence for hypoxic cells influencing cure in cancer therapy. *Br J Cancer Suppl* 1978;37:302–306.
42. Camphausen K, Scott T, Sproull M, et al. Enhancement of xenograft tumor radiosensitivity by the histone deacetylase inhibitor MS-275 and correlation with histone hyperacetylation. *Clin Cancer Res* 2004;10:6066–6071.
43. Carde P, Laval F. Effect of cis-dichlorodiammine platinum II and X rays on mammalian cell survival. *Int J Radiat Oncol Biol Phys* 1981;7:929–933.
44. Chakravarti A, Dicker A, Mehta M. The contribution of epidermal growth factor receptor (EGFR) signaling pathway to radioresistance in human gliomas: A review of preclinical and correlative clinical data. *Int J Radiat Oncol Biol Phys* 2004;58:927–931.
45. Chen AY, Okunieff P, Pommier Y, et al. Mammalian DNA topoisomerase I mediates the enhancement of radiation cytotoxicity by camptothecin derivatives. *Cancer Res* 1997;57:1529–1536.
46. Chinnaiyan P, Vallabhaneni G, Armstrong E, et al. Modulation of radiation response by histone deacetylase inhibition. *Int J Radiat Oncol Biol Phys* 2005;62:223–229.
47. Choudhury A, Cuddihy A, Bristow RG. Radiation and new molecular agents part I: Targeting ATM-ATR checkpoints, DNA repair, and the proteasome. *Semin Radiat Oncol* 2006;16:51–58.
48. Choy H, Rodriguez FF, Koester S, et al. Investigation of taxol as a potential radiation sensitizer. *Cancer* 1993;71:3774–3778.
49. Cohen-Jonathan E, Evans SM, Koch CJ, et al. The farnesyltransferase inhibitor L744,832 reduces hypoxia in tumors expressing activated H-ras. *Cancer Res* 2001;61:2289–2293.
50. Cohen-Jonathan E, Muschel RJ, Gillies McKenna W, et al. Farnesyltransferase inhibitors potentiate the antitumor effect of radiation on a human tumor xenograft expressing activated HRAS. *Radiat Res* 2000;154:125–132.
51. Comis RL. Bleomycin pulmonary toxicity: Current status and future directions. *Semin Oncol* 1992;19:64–70.
52. Cooper JS, Pajak TF, Forastiere AA, et al. Postoperative concurrent radiotherapy and chemotherapy for high-risk squamous-cell carcinoma of the head and neck. *N Engl J Med* 2004;350:1937–1944.
53. Coppin CM, Gospodarowicz MK, James K, et al. Improved local control of invasive bladder cancer by concurrent cisplatin and preoperative or definitive radiation. The National Cancer Institute of Canada Clinical Trials Group. *J Clin Oncol* 1996;14:2901–2907.
54. Corda Y, Job C, Anin MF, et al. Transcription by eucaryotic and procaryotic RNA polymerases of DNA modified at a d(GG) or a d(AG) site by the antitumor drug cis-diamminedichloroplatinum(II). *Biochemistry* 1991;30:222–230.

55. Creane M, Seymour CB, Colucci S, et al. Radiobiological effects of docetaxel (Taxotere): A potential radiation sensitizer. *Int J Radiat Biol* 1999;75:731–737.
56. Cuddihy AR, Bristow RG. The p53 protein family and radiation sensitivity: Yes or no? *Cancer Metastasis Rev* 2004;23:237–257.
57. Cummings BJ, Keane TJ, O'Sullivan B, et al. Epidermoid anal cancer: Treatment by radiation alone or by radiation and 5-fluorouracil with and without mitomycin C. *Int J Radiat Oncol Biol Phys* 1991;21:1115–1125.
58. Curran WSC, Langer C, et al. Phase III comparison of sequential vs. concurrent chemoradiation for patients with unresected stage III non-small cell lung cancer (NSCLC): Report of Radiation Therapy Oncology Group (RTOG) 9410 (abstract303). *Lung Cancer* 2000;29[Suppl 1]:93(abstr).
59. Das A, Sato M, Story MD, et al. Non-small cell lung cancers with kinase domain mutations inthe epidermal growth factor receptor are sensitive to lonizing radiation. *Cancer Res* 2006;66:9601–9608.
60. Dautzenberg B, Arriagada R, Chammard AB, et al. A controlled study of postoperative radiotherapy for patients with completely resected nonsmall cell lung carcinoma. Groupe d'Etude et de Traitement des Cancers Bronchiques. *Cancer* 1999;86:265–273.
61. De Ruysscher D P-JM, Bentzen SM, et al. Time between the first day of chemotherapy and the last day of chest radiation is the most important predictor of survival in limited-disease small cell lung cancer. *J Clin Oncol* 2006;24:1057–1063.
62. Denis F, Garaud P, Bardet E, et al. Final results of the 94-01 French Head and Neck Oncology and Radiotherapy Group randomized trial comparing radiotherapy alone with concomitant radiochemotherapy in advanced-stage oropharynx carcinoma. *J Clin Oncol* 2004;22:69–76.
63. Dewit L. Combined treatment of radiation and cisdiamminedichloroplatinum (II): A review of experimental and clinical data. *Int J Radiat Oncol Biol Phys* 1987;13:403–426.
64. Diaz JF, Andreu JM. Assembly of purified GDP-tubulin into microtubules induced by taxol and taxotere: Reversibility, ligand stoichiometry, and competition. *Biochemistry* 1993;32:2747–2755.
65. Dickstein BM, Wosikowski K, Bates SE. Increased resistance to cytotoxic agents in ZR75B human breast cancer cells transfected with epidermal growth factor receptor. *Mol Cell Endocrinol* 1995;110:205–211.
66. Dillman RO, Herndon J, Seagren SL, et al. Improved survival in stage III non-small-cell lung cancer: Seven-year follow-up of cancer and leukemia group B (CALGB) 8433 trial. *J Natl Cancer Inst* 1996;88:1210–1215.
67. Dische S. Modifying radiosensitivity to improve clinical radiotherapy. Progress in radio-oncology, IV. Vienna: International Club of Radio-Oncology; 1988.
68. Dittmann K, Toulany M, Classen J, et al. Selective Radioprotection of Normal Tissues by Bowman-Birk Proteinase Inhibitor (BBI) in Mice. *Strahlenther Onkol* 2005;181:191–196.
69. Douple EBRR, Logan ME. Therapeutic potentiation in a mouse mammary tumour and an intracerebral rat brain tumour by combined treatment with cis-dichlorodiammineplatinum (II) and radiation. *J Clin Hematol Oncol* 1977;30:585–603.
70. Dunst J, Sauer R, Schrott KM, et al. Organ-sparing treatment of advanced bladder cancer: A 10-year experience. *Int J Radiat Oncol Biol Phys* 1994;30:261–266.
71. Durant S, Karran P. Vanillins—a novel family of DNA-PK inhibitors. *Nucleic Acids Res* 2003;31:5501–5512.
72. Eapen L, Stewart D, Collins J, et al. Effective bladder sparing therapy with intra-arterial cisplatin and radiotherapy for localized bladder cancer. *J Urol* 2004;172:1276–1280.
73. Elkind MM, Sutton H. X-ray damage and recovery in mammalian cells in culture. *Nature* 1959;184:1293–1295.
74. El-Sayed S, Nelson N. Adjuvant and adjunctive chemotherapy in the management of squamous cell carcinoma of the head and neck region. A meta-analysis of prospective and randomized trials. *J Clin Oncol* 1996;14:838–847.
75. Epidermoid anal cancer: Results from the UKCCCR randomised trial of radiotherapy alone versus radiotherapy, 5-fluorouracil, and mitomycin. UKCCCR Anal Cancer Trial Working Party. UK Co-ordinating Committee on Cancer Research. *Lancet* 1996;348:1049–1054.
76. Fajardo LF, Eltringham JR, Steward JR. Combined cardiotoxicity of adriamycin and x-radiation. *Lab Invest* 1976;34:86–96.
77. Fisher B, Wolmark N, Rockette H, et al. Postoperative adjuvant chemotherapy or radiation therapy for rectal cancer: Results from NSABP protocol R-01. *J Natl Cancer Inst* 1988;80:21–29.
78. Fisher BJ, Scott C, Macdonald DR, et al. Phase I study of topotecan plus cranial radiation for glioblastoma multiforme: Results of Radiation Therapy Oncology Group Trial 9507. *J Clin Oncol* 2001;19:1111–1117.
79. Flam M, John M, Pajak TF, et al. Role of mitomycin in combination with fluorouracil and radiotherapy, and of salvage chemoradiation in the definitive nonsurgical treatment of epidermoid carcinoma of the anal canal: Results of a phase III randomized intergroup study. *J Clin Oncol* 1996;14:2527–2539.
80. Forestier AGH, Maor M, et al. Concurrent chemotherapy and radiotherapy for organ presercation in advanced laryngeal cancer. *N Engl J Med* 2003;349:2091–8.
81. Fosslien E. Molecular pathology of cyclooxygenase-2 in neoplasia. *Ann Clin Lab Sci* 2000;30:3–21.
82. Fournel P, Robinet G, Thomas P, et al. Randomized phase III trial of sequential chemoradiotherapy compared with concurrent chemoradiotherapy in locally advanced non-small-cell lung cancer: Groupe Lyon-Saint-Etienne d'Oncologie Thoracique-Groupe Francais de Pneumo-Cancerologie NPC 95-01 Study. *J Clin Oncol* 2005;23:5910–5917.
83. Freyer G, Bossard N, Romestaing P, et al. Addition of oxaliplatin to continuous fluorouracil, l-folinic acid, and concomitant radiotherapy in rectal cancer: The Lyon R 97-03 phase I trial. *J Clin Oncol* 2001;19:2433–2438.
84. Fried DB, Morris DE, Poole C, et al. Systematic review evaluating the timing of thoracic radiation therapy in combined modality therapy for limited-stage small-cell lung cancer. *J Clin Oncol* 2004;22:4837–4845.
85. Fu KK, Pajak TF, Trotti A, et al. A Radiation Therapy Oncology Group (RTOG) phase III randomized study to compare hyperfractionation and two variants of accelerated fractionation to standard fractionation radiotherapy for head and neck squamous cell carcinomas: First report of RTOG 9003. *Int J Radiat Oncol Biol Phys* 2000;48:7–16.
86. Fuino L, Bali P, Wittmann S, et al. Histone deacetylase inhibitor LAQ824 down-regulates Her-2 and sensitizes human breast cancer cells to trastuzumab, taxotere, gemcitabine, and epothilone B. *Mol Cancer Ther* 2003;2:971–984.
87. Furuse K, Fukuoka M, Kawahara M, et al. Phase III study of concurrent versus sequential thoracic radiotherapy in combination with mitomycin, vindesine, and cisplatin in unresectable stage III non-small-cell lung cancer. *J Clin Oncol* 1999;17:2692–2699.
88. Garden AS, Harris J, Vokes EE, et al. Preliminary results of Radiation Therapy Oncology Group 97-03: A randomized phase ii trial of concurrent radiation and chemotherapy for advanced squamous cell carcinomas of the head and neck. *J Clin Oncol* 2004;22:2856–2864.
89. Gastrointestinal Tumor Study Group. Prolongation of the disease-free interval in surgically treated rectal carcinoma. *N Engl J Med* 1985;312:1465–1472.
90. Gastrointestinal Tumor Study Group. Radiation therapy and fluorouracil with or without sumustine for the treatment of patients with surgical adjuvant adencarcinoma or the rectum. *J Clin Oncol* 1992;10:549–557.
91. Grabenbauer GG, Buchfelder M, Schrell U, et al. Topotecan as a 21-day continuous infusion with accelerated 3D-conformal radiation therapy for patients with glioblastoma. *Front Radiat Ther Oncol* 1999;33:364–368.
92. Grau C, Overgaard J. Radiosensitizing and cytotoxic properties of mitomycin C in a C3H mouse mammary carcinoma in vivo. *Int J Radiat Oncol Biol Phys* 1991;20:265–269.
93. Gregoire V, Beauduin M, Bruniaux M, et al. Radiosensitization of mouse sarcoma cells by fludarabine (F-ara-A) or gemcitabine (dFdC), two nucleoside analogues, is not mediated by an increased induction or a repair inhibition of DNA double-strand breaks as measured by pulsed-field gel electrophoresis. *Int J Radiat Biol* 1998;73:511–520.
94. Gregoire V, Hittelman WN, Rosier JF, et al. Chemo-radiotherapy: Radiosensitizing nucleoside analogues (review). *Oncol Rep* 1999;6:949–957.
95. Hahn SM, Krishna CM, Samuni A, et al. Potential use of nitroxides in radiation oncology. *Cancer Res* 1994;54:2006s–2010s.
96. Hall EJ. *Radiobiology for the radiologist,* 4th ed. Philadelphia: JB Lippincott, 1994.
97. Harari PM, Huang S. Radiation combined with EGFR signal inhibitors: Head and neck cancer focus. *Semin Radiat Oncol* 2006;16:38–44.
98. Henk JM, Smith CW. Radiotherapy and hyperbaric oxygen in head and neck cancer. Interim report of second clinical trial. *Lancet* 1977;2:104–105.
99. Hermens AF, Barendsen GW. The proliferative status and clonogenic capacity of tumour cells in a transplantable rhabdomyosarcoma of the rat before and after irradiation with 800 rad of X-rays. *Cell Tissue Kinet* 1978;11:83–100.
100. Herscher LL, Cook JA, Pacelli R, et al. Principles of chemoradiation: Theoretical and practical considerations. *Oncology (Williston Park)* 1999;13:11–22.
101. Hickson I, Zhao Y, Richardson CJ, et al. Identification and characterization of a novel and specific inhibitor of the ataxia-telangiectasia mutated kinase ATM. *Cancer Res* 2004;64:9152–9159.
102. Hill B, Bellamy A. *Antitumor drug-radiation interactions*. Boca Raton, FL: CRC Press, 1990.
103. Hockel M, Knoop C, Schlenger K, et al. Intratumoral pO2 predicts survival in advanced cancer of the uterine cervix. *Radiother Oncol* 1993;26:45–50.
104. Horiot JC, Le Fur R, N'Guyen T, et al. Hyperfractionation versus conventional fractionation in oropharyngeal carcinoma: Final analysis of a randomized trial of the EORTC cooperative group of radiotherapy. *Radiother Oncol* 1992;25:231–241.
105. Housset M, Maulard C, Chretien Y, et al. Combined radiation and chemotherapy for invasive transitional-cell carcinoma of the bladder: A prospective study. *J Clin Oncol* 1993;11:2150–2157.
106. Howle JA, Gale GR. Cis-dichlorodiammineplatinum (II). Persistent and selective inhibition of deoxyribonucleic acid synthesis in vivo. *Biochem Pharmacol* 1970; 19:2757–2762.
107. Hsiang YH, Hertzberg R, Hecht S, et al. Camptothecin induces protein-linked DNA breaks via mammalian DNA topoisomerase I. *J Biol Chem* 1985;260:14873–14878.
108. Hsiang YH, Liu LF. Identification of mammalian DNA topoisomerase I as an intracellular target of the anticancer drug camptothecin. *Cancer Res* 1988;48:1722–1726.
109. Hsu AL, Ching TT, Wang DS, et al. The cyclooxygenase-2 inhibitor celecoxib induces apoptosis by blocking Akt activation in human prostate cancer cells independently of Bcl-2. *J Biol Chem* 2000;275:11397–11403.
110. Huang SM, Bock JM, Harari PM. Epidermal growth factor receptor blockade with C225 modulates proliferation, apoptosis, and radiosensitivity in squamous cell carcinomas of the head and neck. *Cancer Res* 1999;59:1935–1940.
111. Huang SM, Harari PM. Modulation of radiation response after epidermal growth factor receptor blockade in squamous cell carcinomas: Inhibition of damage repair, cell cycle kinetics, and tumor angiogenesis. *Clin Cancer Res* 2000;6:2166–2174.
112. Huguenin P, Beer KT, Allal A, et al. Concomitant cisplatin significantly improves locoregional control in advanced head and neck cancers treated with hyperfractionated radiotherapy. *J Clin Oncol* 2004;22:4665–4673.
113. Iliakis G. Radiation-induced potentially lethal damage: DNA lesions susceptible to fixation. *Int J Radiat Biol Relat Stud Phys Chem Med* 1988;53:541–584.
114. Induction chemotherapy plus radiation compared with surgery plus radiation in patients with advanced laryngeal cancer. The Department of Veterans Affairs Laryngeal Cancer Study Group. *N Engl J Med* 1991;324:1685–1690.
115. Kaufman DS, Shipley WU, Griffin PP, et al. Selective bladder preservation by combination treatment of invasive bladder cancer. *N Engl J Med* 1993;329:1377–1382.
116. Keime-Guibert F, Napolitano M, Delattre JY. Neurological complications of radiotherapy and chemotherapy. *J Neurol* 1998;245:695–708.
117. Keller SM, Adak S, Wagner H, et al. A randomized trial of postoperative adjuvant therapy in patients with completely resected stage II or IIIA non-small-cell lung cancer. Eastern Cooperative Oncology Group. *N Engl J Med* 2000;343:1217–1222.
118. Keys HM, Bundy BN, Stehman FB, et al. Cisplatin, radiation, and adjuvant hysterectomy compared with radiation and adjuvant hysterectomy for bulky stage IB cervical carcinoma. *N Engl J Med* 1999;340:1154–1161.
119. Khodarev NN, Kataoka Y, Murley JS, et al. Interaction of amifostine and ionizing radiation on transcriptional patterns of apoptotic genes expressed in human microvascular endothelial cells (HMEC). *Int J Radiat Oncol Biol Phys* 2004;60:553–563.
120. Kim YB, Kim GE, Cho NH, et al. Overexpression of cyclooxygenase-2 is associated with a poor prognosis in patients with squamous cell carcinoma of the uterine cervix treated with radiation and concurrent chemotherapy. *Cancer* 2002;95:531–539.
121. Kim YB, Kim GE, Pyo HR, et al. Differential cyclooxygenase-2 expression in

squamous cell carcinoma and adenocarcinoma of the uterine cervix. *Int J Radiat Oncol Biol Phys* 2004;60:822–829.
122. Kinsella TJ, Dobson PP, Mitchell JB, et al. Enhancement of X ray induced DNA damage by pre-treatment with halogenated pyrimidine analogs. *Int J Radiat Oncol Biol Phys* 1987;13:733–739.
123. Kirichenko AV, Rich TA. Radiation enhancement by 9-aminocamptothecin: The effect of fractionation and timing of administration. *Int J Radiat Oncol Biol Phys* 1999;44:659–664.
124. Koki AT, Leahy KM, Masferrer JL. Potential utility of COX-2 inhibitors in chemo-prevention and chemotherapy. *Expert Opin Investig Drugs* 1999;8:1623–1638.
125. Komaki R, Leahy KM, Curran W, et al. Sequential vs. concurrent chemotherapy and radiation therapy for inoperable phase III study (RTOG 9410). *Int J Radiat Oncol Biol Phys* 2000;48:113.
126. Kotalik J, Yu E, Markman BR, et al. Practice guideline on prophylactic cranial irradiation in small-cell lung cancer. *Int J Radiat Oncol Biol Phys* 2001;50:309–316.
127. LaMonte CS, Yeh SD, Straus DJ. Long-term follow-up of cardiac function in patients with Hodgkin's disease treated with mediastinal irradiation and combination chemotherapy including doxorubicin. *Cancer Treat Rep* 1986;70:439–444.
128. Lamoreaux WJ, Fitzgerald ME, Reiner A, et al. Vascular endothelial growth factor increases release of gelatinase A and decreases release of tissue inhibitor of metalloproteinases by microvascular endothelial cells in vitro. *Microvasc Res* 1998;55:29–42.
129. Latz D, Fleckenstein K, Eble M, et al. Radiosensitizing potential of gemcitabine (2′,2′-difluoro-2′-deoxycytidine) within the cell cycle in vitro. *Int J Radiat Oncol Biol Phys* 1998;41:875–882.
130. Lawrence TS, Chang EY, Hahń TM, et al. Radiosensitization of pancreatic cancer cells by 2′,2′-difluoro-2′-deoxycytidine. *Int J Radiat Oncol Biol Phys* 1996;34: 867–872.
131. Lawrence TS, Eisbruch A, Shewach DS. Gemcitabine-mediated radiosensitization. *Semin Oncol* 1997;24:S7–S24.
132. Le Chevalier T, Arriagada R, Quoix E, et al. Radiotherapy alone versus combined chemotherapy and radiotherapy in nonresectable non-small-cell lung cancer: First analysis of a randomized trial in 353 patients. *J Natl Cancer Inst* 1991;83:417–423.
133. Lefebvre JL, Chevalier D, Luboinski B, et al. Larynx preservation in pyriform sinus cancer: Preliminary results of a European Organization for Research and Treatment of Cancer phase III trial. EORTC Head and Neck Cancer Cooperative Group. *J Natl Cancer Inst* 1996;88:890–899.
134. Li C, Ke S, Wu QP, et al. Potentiation of ovarian OCa-1 tumor radioresponse by poly (L-glutamic acid)-paclitaxel conjugate. *Int J Radiat Oncol Biol Phys* 2000;48:1119–1126.
135. Li C, Ke S, Wu QP, et al. Tumor irradiation enhances the tumor-specific distribution of poly(L-glutamic acid)-conjugated paclitaxel and its antitumor efficacy. *Clin Cancer Res* 2000;6:2829–2834.
136. Liang K, Ang KK, Milas L, et al. The epidermal growth factor receptor mediates radioresistance. *Int J Radiat Oncol Biol Phys* 2003;57:246–254.
137. Little JB, Hahn GM, Frindel E, et al. Repair of potentially lethal radiation damage in vitro and in vivo. *Radiology* 1973;106:689–694.
138. Liu B, Zhao L, Yu X, et al. Live attenuated Salmonella carrying platelet factor 4 cDNAs as radioprotectors. *Radiat Res* 2006;166:352–359.
139. Liu XH, Kirschenbaum A, Yao S, et al. Inhibition of cyclooxygenase-2 suppresses angiogenesis and the growth of prostate cancer in vivo. *J Urol* 2000;164:820–825.
140. Liu XH, Yao S, Kirschenbaum A, et al. NS398, a selective cyclooxygenase-2 inhibitor, induces apoptosis and down-regulates bcl-2 expression in LNCaP cells. *Cancer Res* 1998;58:4245–4249.
141. Ljungman M. The influence of chromatin structure on the frequency of radiation-induced DNA strand breaks: A study using nuclear and nucleoid monolayers. *Radiat Res* 1991;126:58–64.
142. Lloyd RV, Duling DR, Rumyantseva GV, et al. Microsomal reduction of 3-amino-1,2,4-benzotriazine 1,4-dioxide to a free radical. *Mol Pharmacol* 1991;40:440–445.
143. Lukas J, Lukas C, Bartek J. Mammalian cell cycle checkpoints: Signalling pathways and their organization in space and time. *DNA Repair (Amst)* 2004;3:997–1007.
144. Lund EL, Bastholm L, Kristjansen PE. Therapeutic synergy of TNP-470 and ionizing radiation: Effects on tumor growth, vessel morphology, and angiogenesis in human glioblastoma multiforme xenografts. *Clin Cancer Res* 2000;6:971–978.
145. Maeda H, Seymour LW, Miyamoto Y. Conjugates of anticancer agents and polymers: Advantages of macromolecular therapeutics in vivo. *Bioconjug Chem* 1992;3:351–362.
146. Manfredi JJ, Horwitz SB. Taxol: An antimitotic agent with a new mechanism of action. *Pharmacol Ther* 1984;25:83–125.
147. Mansfield CM, Kimler BF, Henderson SD, et al. Development of normal tissue damage in the rat subsequent to thoracic irradiation and prior treatment with cancer chemotherapeutic agents. *Am J Clin Oncol* 1984;7:425–430.
148. Masferrer JL, Leahy KM, Koki AT, et al. Antiangiogenic and antitumor activities of cyclooxygenase-2 inhibitors. *Cancer Res* 2000;60:1306–1311.
149. Mason KA, Kishi K, Hunter N, et al. Effect of docetaxel on the therapeutic ratio of fractionated radiotherapy in vivo. *Clin Cancer Res* 1999;5:4191–4198.
150. Mason KA, Komaki R, Cox JD, et al. Biology-based combined-modality radiotherapy: Workshop report. *Int J Radiat Oncol Biol Phys* 2001;50:1079–1089.
151. Mason KA, Milas L, Hunter NR, et al. Maximizing therapeutic gain with gemcitabine and fractionated radiation. *Int J Radiat Oncol Biol Phys* 1999;44:1125–1135.
152. Mauceri HJ, Hanna NN, Beckett MA, et al. Combined effects of angiostatin and ionizing radiation in antitumour therapy. *Nature* 1998;394:287–291.
153. McGinn CJ, Kinsella TJ. The experimental and clinical rationale for the use of S-phase-specific radiosensitizers to overcome tumor cell repopulation. *Semin Oncol* 1992;19:21–8.
154. McKenna WG, Bernhard EJ, Markiewicz DA, et al. Regulation of radiation-induced apoptosis in oncogene-transfected fibroblasts: Influence of H-ras on the G2 delay. *Oncogene* 1996;12:237–245.
155. McKenna WG, Weiss MC, Bakanauskas VJ, et al. The role of the H-ras oncogene in radiation resistance and metastasis. *Int J Radiat Oncol Biol Phys* 1990;18:849–859.
156. McKenna WG, Weiss MC, Endlich B, et al. Synergistic effect of the v-myc oncogene with H-ras on radioresistance. *Cancer Res* 1990;50:97–102.
157. McVeagh P, Ekert H. Hepatotoxicity of chemotherapy following nephrectomy and radiation therapy for right-sided Wilms tumor. *J Pediatr* 1975;87:627–628.
158. Mendelsohn J, Fan Z. Epidermal growth factor receptor family and chemosensitization. *J Natl Cancer Inst* 1997;89:341–343.
159. Merrill J, Greco FA, Zimbler H, et al. Adriamycin and radiation: Synegistic cardiotoxicity. *Ann Intern Med* 1975;82:122–123.
160. Milas L, Fujii T, Hunter N, et al. Enhancement of tumor radioresponse in vivo by gemcitabine. *Cancer Res* 1999;59:107–114.
161. Milas L, Hanson WR. Eicosanoids and radiation. *Eur J Cancer* 1995;31A:1580–1585.
162. Milas L, Hunter NR, Mason KA, et al. Role of reoxygenation in induction of enhancement of tumor radioresponse by paclitaxel. *Cancer Res* 1995;55:3564–3568.
163. Milas L, Kishi K, Hunter N, et al. Enhancement of tumor response to gamma-radiation by an inhibitor of cyclooxygenase-2 enzyme. *J Natl Cancer Inst* 1999;91:1501–1504.
164. Milas L, Mason K, Hunter N, et al. In vivo enhancement of tumor radioresponse by C225 antiepidermal growth factor receptor antibody. *Clin Cancer Res* 2000;6:701–708.
165. Milas L, Milas MM, Mason KA. Combination of taxanes with radiation: Preclinical studies. *Semin Radiat Oncol* 1999;9:12–26.
166. Milas L, Nakayama T, Hunter N, et al. Dynamics of tumor cell clonogen repopulation in a murine sarcoma treated with cyclophosphamide. *Radiother Oncol* 1994;30:247–253.
167. Milas L. Cyclooxygenase-2 (COX-2) enzyme inhibitors as potential enhancers of tumor radioresponse. *Semin Radiat Oncol* 2001;11:290–299.
168. Minsky BD, Pajak TF, Ginsberg RJ, et al. INT 0123 (Radiation Therapy Oncology Group 94-05) phase III trial of combined-modality therapy for esophageal cancer: High-dose versus standard-dose radiation therapy. *J Clin Oncol* 2002;20:1167–1174.
169. Moertel CG, Schutt AJ, Reitemeier RJ, et al. Phase II study of camptothecin (NSC-100880) in the treatment of advanced gastrointestinal cancer. *Cancer Chemother Rep* 1972;56:95–101.
170. Morris M, Eifel PJ, Lu J, et al. Pelvic radiation with concurrent chemotherapy compared with pelvic and para-aortic radiation for high-risk cervical cancer. *N Engl J Med* 1999;340:1137–1143.
171. Muggia FM, Creaven PJ, Hansen HH, et al. Phase I clinical trial of weekly and daily treatment with camptothecin (NSC-100880): Correlation with preclinical studies. *Cancer Chemother Rep* 1972;56:515–521.
172. Munro AJ. An overview of randomised controlled trials of adjuvant chemotherapy in head and neck cancer. *Br J Cancer* 1995;71:83–91.
173. Murata R, Nishimura Y, Hiraoka M. An antiangiogenic agent (TNP-470) inhibited reoxygenation during fractionated radiotherapy of murine mammary carcinoma. *Int J Radiat Oncol Biol Phys* 1997;37:1107–1113.
174. Nicoletti MI, Colombo T, Rossi C, et al. IDN5109, a taxane with oral bioavailability and potent antitumor activity. *Cancer Res* 2000;60:842–846.
175. Nigro ND, Vaitkevicius VK, Considine B Jr. Combined therapy for cancer of the anal canal: A preliminary report. *Dis Colon Rectum* 1974;17:354–356.
176. NIH Consensus Conference. Adjuvant therapy for patients with colon rectal cancer. *JAMA* 1990;264:1444–1450.
177. Nix P, Lind M, Greenman J, Stafford N, et al. Expression of Cox-2 protein in radioresistant laryngeal cancer. *Ann Oncol* 2004;15:797–801.
178. Nordsmark M, Overgaard M, Overgaard J. Pretreatment oxygenation predicts radiation response in advanced squamous cell carcinoma of the head and neck. *Radiother Oncol* 1996;41:31–39.
179. O'Connell MJ, Martenson JA, Wieand HS, et al. Improving adjuvant therapy for rectal cancer by combining protracted-infusion fluorouracil with radiation therapy after curative surgery. *N Engl J Med* 1994;331:502–507.
180. O'Hara JA, Douple EB, Richmond RC. Enhancement of radiation-induced cell kill by platinum complexes (carboplatin and iproplatin) in V79 cells. *Int J Radiat Oncol Biol Phys* 1986;12:1419–1422.
181. Omura M, Torigoe S, Kubota N. SN-38, a metabolite of the camptothecin derivative CPT-11, potentiates the cytotoxic effect of radiation in human colon adenocarcinoma cells grown as spheroids. *Radiother Oncol* 1997;43:197–201.
182. O'Reilly MS. Radiation combined with antiangiogenic and antivascular agents. *Semin Radiat Oncol* 2006;16:45–50.
183. Pearcey R, Brundage M, Drouin P, et al. Phase III trial comparing radical radiotherapy with and without cisplatin chemotherapy in patients with advanced squamous cell cancer of the cervix. *J Clin Oncol* 2002;20:966–972.
184. Peng Y, Woods RG, Beamish H, et al. Deficiency in the catalytic subunit of DNA-dependent protein kinase causes down-regulation of ATM. *Cancer Res* 2005;65:1670–1677.
185. Pepper MS, Montesano R, Mandriota SJ, et al. Angiogenesis: A paradigm for balanced extracellular proteolysis during cell migration and morphogenesis. *Enzyme Protein* 1996;49:138–162.
186. Peters WA, 3rd, Liu PY, Barrett RJ 2nd, et al. Concurrent chemotherapy and pelvic radiation therapy compared with pelvic radiation therapy alone as adjuvant therapy after radical surgery in high-risk early-stage cancer of the cervix. *J Clin Oncol* 2000;18:1606–1613.
187. Petrova TV, Makinen T, Alitalo K. Signaling via vascular endothelial growth factor receptors. *Exp Cell Res* 1999;253:117–130.
188. Phillips KA, Tannock IF. Design and interpretation of clinical trials that evaluate agents that may offer protection from the toxic effects of cancer chemotherapy. *J Clin Oncol* 1998;16:3179–3190.
189. Phillips T. Radiation-chemotherapy interactions. In: Pass HI, MJ, Johnson DH, et al., eds. *Lung cancer: Principles and practice.* Philadelphia: Lippincott-Raven; 1996.
190. Pignon JP, Arriagada R, Ihde DC, et al. A meta-analysis of thoracic radiotherapy for small-cell lung cancer. *N Engl J Med* 1992;327:1618–1624.
191. Pignon JP, Bourhis J, Domenge C, et al. Chemotherapy added to locoregional treatment for head and neck squamous-cell carcinoma: Three meta-analyses of updated individual data. MACH-NC Collaborative Group. Meta-Analysis of Chemotherapy on Head and Neck Cancer. *Lancet* 2000;355:949–955.
192. Plunkett WGV, Chubb S, et al. 2′,2′-Diflurodeoxycytidine metabolism and mechanis of action in human lukemia cells. *Nucleosides Nucleotides* 1989;8:775–785.
193. Plunkett W, Huang P, Xu YZ, et al. Gemcitabine: Metabolism, mechanisms of action, and self-potentiation. *Semin Oncol* 1995;22:3–10.
194. Pritchard RS, Anthony SP. Chemotherapy plus radiotherapy compared with

radiotherapy alone in the treatment of locally advanced, unresectable, non-small-cell lung cancer. A meta-analysis. *Ann Intern Med* 1996;125:723–729.
195. Pruthi RS, Derksen JE, Moore D, et al. Phase II trial of celecoxib in prostate-specific antigen recurrent prostate cancer after definitive radiation therapy or radical prostatectomy. *Clin Cancer Res* 2006;12:2172–2177.
196. Pruthi RS, Derksen JE, Moore D. A pilot study of use of the cyclooxygenase-2 inhibitor celecoxib in recurrent prostate cancer after definitive radiation therapy or radical prostatectomy. *BJU Int* 2004;93:275–278.
197. Pyo H, Choy H, Amorino GP, et al. A selective cyclooxygenase-2 inhibitor, NS-398, enhances the effect of radiation in vitro and in vivo preferentially on the cells that express cyclooxygenase-2. *Clin Cancer Res* 2001;7:2998–3005.
198. Radford IR. Evidence for a general relationship between the induced level of DNA double-strand breakage and cell-killing after X-irradiation of mammalian cells. *Int J Radiat Biol Relat Stud Phys Chem Med* 1986;49:611–620.
199. Rao S, Krauss NE, Heerding JM, et al. 3′-(p-azidobenzamido)taxol photolabels the N-terminal 31 amino acids of beta-tubulin. *J Biol Chem* 1994;269:3132–3134.
200. Richmond RC, Powers EL. Radiation sensitization of bacterial spores by cis-dichlorodiammineplatinum(II). *Radiat Res* 1976;68:251–257.
201. Richmond RC, Zimbrick JD, Hykes DL. Radiation-induced DNA damage and lethality in E. coli as modified by the antitumor agent cis-dichlorodiammineplatinum (II). *Radiat Res* 1977;71:447–460.
202. Richter M, Weiss M, Weinberger I, et al. Growth inhibition and induction of apoptosis in colorectal tumor cells by cyclooxygenase inhibitors. *Carcinogenesis* 2001;22:17–25.
203. Ringel I, Horwitz SB. Studies with RP 56976 (taxotere): A semisynthetic analogue of taxol. *J Natl Cancer Inst* 1991;83:288–291.
204. Robert F, Ezekiel MP, Spencer SA, et al. Phase I study of anti—epidermal growth factor receptor antibody cetuximab in combination with radiation therapy in patients with advanced head and neck cancer. *J Clin Oncol* 2001;19:3234–3243.
205. Rose PG, Bundy BN, Watkins EB, et al. Concurrent cisplatin-based radiotherapy and chemotherapy for locally advanced cervical cancer. *N Engl J Med* 1999;340:1144–1153.
206. Rosenberg B, VanCamp L, Trosko JE, et al. Platinum compounds: A new class of potent antitumour agents. *Nature* 1969;222:385–386.
207. Rowinsky EK. The development and clinical utility of the taxane class of antimicrotubule chemotherapy agents. *Annu Rev Med* 1997;48:353–74.
208. Salles B, Calsou P, Frit P, et al. The DNA repair complex DNA-PK, a pharmacological target in cancer chemotherapy and radiotherapy. *Pathol Biol (Paris)* 2006;54:185–193.
209. Samuels ML, Johnson DE, Holoye PY, et al. Large-dose bleomycin therapy and pulmonary toxicity. A possible role of prior radiotherapy. *JAMA* 1976;235:1117–1120.
210. Sauer R, Becker H, Hohenberger W, et al. Preoperative versus postoperative chemoradiotherapy for rectal cancer. *N Engl J Med* 2004;351:1731–1740.
211. Sause W, Kolesar P, Taylor SI, et al. Final results of phase III trial in regionally advanced unresectable non-small cell lung cancer: Radiation Therapy Oncology Group, Eastern Cooperative Oncology Group, and Southwest Oncology Group. *Chest* 2000;117:358–364.
212. Scalliet PGC, Galdermans D, et al. Gemzar(Gemcitabine) with thoracic radiotherapy: A phase II pilot study in chemonaice patients with advanced nonsmall cell lung cancer (NSCLC). *Proc Am Soc Clin Oncol* 1998;17:499a(abst).
213. Schaake-Koning C, van den Bogaert W, Dalesio O, et al. Effects of concomitant cisplatin and radiotherapy on inoperable non-small-cell lung cancer. *N Engl J Med* 1992;326:524–530.
214. Schmidt-Ullrich RK, Dent P, Grant S, et al. Signal transduction and cellular radiation responses. *Radiat Res* 2000;153:245–257.
215. Schuuring J, Bussink J, Bernsen HJ, et al. Irradiation combined with SU5416: Microvascular changes and growth delay in a human xenograft glioblastoma tumor line. *Int J Radiat Oncol Biol Phys* 2005;61:529–534.
216. Smith FM, Reynolds JV, Kay EW, et al. COX-2 overexpression in pretreatment biopsies predicts response of rectal cancers to neoadjuvant radiochemotherapy. *Int J Radiat Oncol Biol Phys* 2006;64:466–472.
217. Smith MR, Manola J, Kaufman DS, et al. Celecoxib versus placebo for men with prostate cancer and a rising serum prostate-specific antigen after radical prostatectomy and/or radiation therapy. *J Clin Oncol* 2006;24:2723–2728.
218. Smith TJ, Ryan LM, Douglass HO Jr, et al. Combined chemoradiotherapy vs. radiotherapy alone for early stage squamous cell carcinoma of the esophagus: A study of the Eastern Cooperative Oncology Group. *Int J Radiat Oncol Biol Phys* 1998;42:269–276.
219. Steel GG, Peckham MJ. Exploitable mechanisms in combined radiotherapy-chemotherapy: The concept of additivity. *Int J Radiat Oncol Biol Phys* 1979;5:85–91.
220. Steinbach G, Lynch PM, Phillips RK, et al. The effect of celecoxib, a cyclooxygenase-2 inhibitor, in familial adenomatous polyposis. *N Engl J Med* 2000;342:1946–1952.
221. Stephens TJ SG. Regeneration of tumors after cytotxic treatment. In: Meyn R WH, eds. *Radiation biology in cancer research.* New York: Raven Press; 1980: 385–395.
222. Stratford IJ, Williamson C, Adams GE. Combination studies with misonidazole and a cis-platinum complex: Cytotoxicity and radiosensitization in vitro. *Br J Cancer* 1980;41:517–522.
223. Stupp R, Hegi ME, van den Bent MJ, et al. Changing paradigms—an update on the multidisciplinary management of malignant glioma. *Oncologist* 2006;11:165–180.
224. Stupp R, Mason WP, van den Bent MJ, et al. Radiotherapy plus concomitant and adjuvant temozolomide for glioblastoma. *N Engl J Med* 2005;352:987–996.
225. Swisher SG, Roth JA, Komaki R, et al. Induction of p53-regulated genes and tumor regression in lung cancer patients after intratumoral delivery of adenoviral p53 (INGN 201) and radiation therapy. *Clin Cancer Res* 2003;9:93–101.
226. Szumiel I, Nias AH. The effect of combined treatment with a platinum complex and ionizing radiation on chinese hamster ovary cells in vitro. *Br J Cancer* 1976;33:450–458.
227. Takeda K, Negoro S, Kudoh S, et al. Phase I/II study of weekly irinotecan and concurrent radiation therapy for locally advanced non-small cell lung cancer. *Br J Cancer* 1999;79:1462–1467.
228. Tannock IF, Rotin D. Acid pH in tumors and its potential for therapeutic exploitation. *Cancer Res* 1989;49:4373–4384.
229. Taylor DM, Tew KD, Jones JD. Effects of cis-dichlorodiammine platinum (II) on DNA synthesis in kidney and other tissues of normal and tumour-bearing rats. *Eur J Cancer* 1976;12:249–254.
230. Taylor JMWH, Mendenhal WM,. Dose-time cosiderations of head and neck squamous cell carcinomas treated with irradiation. *Radiother Oncol* 1990;17:95–102.
231. Tefft M, Lattin PB, Jereb B, et al. Acute and late effects on normal tissues following combined chemo- and radiotherapy for childhood rhabdomyosarcoma and Ewing's sarcoma. *Cancer* 1976;37:1201–1217.
232. Teicher BADN, Kusomoto T, et al. Antiangiogenic agents can increase tumor oxygenation and response to radiation therapy. *Radiat Oncol Invest* 1997;2:269–276.
233. Tepper JE, O'Connell MJ, Petroni GR, et al. Adjuvant postoperative fluorouracil-modulated chemotherapy combined with pelvic radiation therapy for rectal cancer: Initial results of intergroup 0114. *J Clin Oncol* 1997;15:2030–2039.
234. Terasima T, Tolmach LJ. Variations in several responses of HeLa cells to x-irradiation during the division cycle. *Biophys J* 1963;3:11–33.
235. Thomas GM. Improved treatment for cervical cancer—concurrent chemotherapy and radiotherapy. *N Engl J Med* 1999;340:1198–1200.
236. Thompson CB, Sanders JE, Flournoy N, Buckner CD, Thomas ED. The risks of central nervous system relapse and leukoencephalopathy in patients receiving marrow transplants for acute leukemia. *Blood* 1986;67:195–199.
237. Tishler RB, Geard CR, Hall EJ, et al. Taxol sensitizes human astrocytoma cells to radiation. *Cancer Res* 1992;52:3495–3497.
238. Traxler P, Allegrini PR, Brandt R, et al. AEE788: A dual family epidermal growth factor receptor/ErbB2 and vascular endothelial growth factor receptor tyrosine kinase inhibitor with antitumor and antiangiogenic activity. *Cancer Res* 2004;64:4931–4941.
239. Tuccillo C, Romano M, Troiani T, et al. Antitumor activity of ZD6474, a vascular endothelial growth factor-2 and epidermal growth factor receptor small molecule tyrosine kinase inhibitor, in combination with SC-236, a cyclooxygenase-2 inhibitor. *Clin Cancer Res* 2005;11:1268–1276.
240. Turrisi AT, 3rd, Kim K, Blum R, et al. Twice-daily compared with once-daily thoracic radiotherapy in limited small-cell lung cancer treated concurrently with cisplatin and etoposide. *N Engl J Med* 1999;340:265–271.
241. Urba SG, Orringer MB, Turrisi A, et al. Randomized trial of preoperative chemoradiation versus surgery alone in patients with locoregional esophageal carcinoma. *J Clin Oncol* 2001;19:305–313.
242. US Food and Drug Administration. FDA Public Health Advisory: FDA Announces Important Changes and Additional Warnings for COX-2 Selective and Non-Selective Non-Steroidal Anti-Inflammatory Drugs (NSAIDs). Available at http://www.fda.gov/cder/drug/advisory/COX2.htm. Accessed April, 2005.
243. Vaupel P, Kallinowski F, Okunieff P. Blood flow, oxygen and nutrient supply, and metabolic microenvironment of human tumors: A review. *Cancer Res* 1989;49:6449–6564.
244. Veuger SJ, Curtin NJ, Richardson CJ, et al. Radiosensitization and DNA repair inhibition by the combined use of novel inhibitors of DNA-dependent protein kinase and poly(ADP-ribose) polymerase-1. *Cancer Res* 2003;63:6008–6015.
245. Vokes EE, Herndon JE 2nd, Crawford J, et al. Randomized phase II study of cisplatin with gemcitabine or paclitaxel or vinorelbine as induction chemotherapy followed by concomitant chemoradiotherapy for stage IIIB non-small-cell lung cancer: Cancer and leukemia group B study 9431. *J Clin Oncol* 2002;20:4191–4198.
246. Walsh TN, Noonan N, Hollywood D, et al. A comparison of multimodal therapy and surgery for esophageal adenocarcinoma. *N Engl J Med* 1996;335:462–467.
247. Wang CC, Liao YP, Mischel PS, et al. HDJ-2 as a target for radiosensitization of glioblastoma multiforme cells by the farnesyltransferase inhibitor R115777 and the role of the p53/p21 pathway. *Cancer Res* 2006;66:6756–6762.
248. Wang Y, Pantelias GE, Iliakis G. Mechanism of radiosensitization by halogenated pyrimidines: The contribution of excess DNA and chromosome damage in BrdU radiosensitization may be minimal in plateau-phase cells. *Int J Radiat Biol* 1994;66:133–142.
249. Warde P, Payne D. Does thoracic irradiation improve survival and local control in limited-stage small-cell carcinoma of the lung? A meta-analysis. *J Clin Oncol* 1992;10:890–895.
250. Whitney CW, Sause W, Bundy BN, et al. Randomized comparison of fluorouracil plus cisplatin versus hydroxyurea as an adjunct to radiation therapy in stage IIB-IVA carcinoma of the cervix with negative para-aortic lymph nodes: A Gynecologic Oncology Group and Southwest Oncology Group study. *J Clin Oncol* 1999;17:1339–1348.
251. Willmore E, de Caux S, Sunter NJ, et al. A novel DNA-dependent protein kinase inhibitor, NU7026, potentiates the cytotoxicity of topoisomerase II poisons used in the treatment of leukemia. *Blood* 2004;103:4659–4665.
252. Withers HR, Taylor JM, Maciejewski B. The hazard of accelerated tumor clonogen repopulation during radiotherapy. *Acta Oncol* 1988;27:131–146.
253. Wodinsky I, Swiniarski J, Kensler CJ, et al. Combination radiotherapy and chemotherapy for P388 lymphocytic leukemia in vivo. *Cancer Chemother Rep 2* 1974;4:73–97.
254. Wolmark N, Wieand HS, Hyams DM, et al. Randomized trial of postoperative adjuvant chemotherapy with or without radiotherapy for carcinoma of the rectum: National Surgical Adjuvant Breast and Bowel Project Protocol R-02. *J Natl Cancer Inst* 2000;92:388–396.
255. Yang LX, Wang HJ, Holton RA. In vitro efficacy of a novel chemoradiopotentiator–taxoltere metro. *Int J Radiat Oncol Biol Phys* 2000;46:159–163.
256. Yu X, Guo ZS, Marcu MG, et al. Modulation of p53, ErbB1, ErbB2, and Raf-1 expression in lung cancer cells by depsipeptide FR901228. *J Natl Cancer Inst* 2002;94:504–513.
257. Yuhas JM, Storer JB. Differential chemoprotection of normal and malignant tissues. *J Natl Cancer Inst* 1969;42:331–335.
258. Zatloukal P, Petruzelka L, Zemanova M, et al. Concurrent versus sequential chemoradiotherapy with cisplatin and vinorelbine in locally advanced non-small cell lung cancer: A randomized study. *Lung Cancer* 2004;46:87–98.
259. Zimbrick JD, Sukrochana A, Richmond RC. Studies on radiosensitization of *Escherichia coli* cells by cis-platinum complexes. *Int J Radiat Oncol Biol Phys* 1979;5:1351–1354.

Section III | Clinical Radiation Oncology

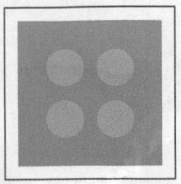

Chapter 30
Skin

Merrill J. Solan, Luther W. Brady

Anatomy of the Skin

The three layers comprising the skin include the outer epidermis followed by dermis and subcutis. The avascular epidermis contains stratified squamous cells and varies in thickness from about 0.05 mm on the eyelids to 0.15 mm on palms and soles. Outer surface cells are chronically shed and replaced by mitotic cells from the basal layer; as cells migrate from basal to outer epidermis, they lose their nuclei and ability to replicate. The 1- to 2-mm thick dermis consists of a papillary layer adjacent to the epidermis basement membrane and a deeper reticular layer. Connective tissue stroma of collagen and elastin fibers gives the skin structural integrity and contains nerves, blood and lymphatic vessels, and adnexal structures. The subcutis has the most variable thickness and contains connective tissue and fat supporting larger nerves and vessels.

Epidemiology and Etiology of Skin Cancer

Nonmelanoma skin cancer (NMSC) is the most common of all cancers, with over one million cases yearly in the United States (36). Basal cell carcinoma (BCC) comprises about 80% and squamous cell carcinoma (SCC) 20% of NMSC (Figs. 30.1 and 30.2). Rare tumors include Merkel cell carcinoma (MCC), cutaneous connective tissue tumors such as dermatofibrosarcoma protuberans (DFSP), and tumors of skin adnexa including eccrine and apocrine sweat gland and sebaceous carcinomas. Melanoma comprises only 3% of all skin cancers but accounts for about 75% of skin cancer mortality (Fig. 30.3).

Exposure to ultraviolet solar radiation, especially ultraviolet B (UVB; 290 to 320 nm), is the most common cause of skin cancer and the most preventable. Carcinogenesis results from ultraviolet solar radiation-induced DNA mutations in the *p53* tumor suppressor gene and induction of immunologic changes that inhibit immune response against the tumor. Painful sunburn before age 20 is related to later development of premalignant lesions as well as NMSC and melanoma (37). Cumulative lifetime sun exposure is related to increased risk of SCC and BCC.

Host risk factors include blonde or red hair, fair complexion, blue eyes, and tendency to burn rather than tan. Genetic predisposition occurs with xeroderma pigmentosum, basal cell nevus (Gorlin's) syndrome, epidermodysplasia verruciformis, Muir-Torre syndrome, porokeratosis, Bazex syndrome, Rombo syndrome, albinism, and phenylketonuria. An association exists between cutaneous SCC and human papillomavirus. Transplant recipients on immunosuppressive therapy and patients with acquired immunodeficiency syndrome, multiple myeloma, leukemia, and lymphoma also are at increased risk. Skin cancers are more frequent and aggressive in areas of chronic skin damage such as ulcers, osteomyelitis, sinus tracts and burn (Marjolin's ulcer), or vaccination scars. Areas of chronic skin inflammation such as discoid lupus erythematosus, lichen sclerosus, lichen planus, dystrophic epidermolysis bullosa, and lupus vulgaris also are predisposed to develop skin cancers.

Exposure to ionizing radiation is a risk factor for both BCC and SCC, especially in those people with sun-sensitive phenotype and younger age at exposure (2,39). Lesions develop within the radiated area with latency periods of 20 to 40 years (39), and risk is directly related to cumulative radiation dose (2). Increased incidence of NMSC also occurs with chronic radiation dermatitis following therapeutic radiation. Chemical skin cancer carcinogens include arsenic, soot, and polycyclic aromatic hydrocarbons from coal tar, cutting oils, and pitch (2). An association exists between cigarette or pipe smoking and cutaneous SCC, with risk proportional to the number of cigarettes or pipes smoked daily and higher in current rather than former smokers (24).

Sun-related skin cancer in blacks is rare, but skin cancer occurs with equal frequency in blacks and whites in areas of chronic dermatitis or scars. Mortality is higher in blacks because of tendency to present with more advanced disease, preponderance of aggressive lesions unrelated to sun exposure, and higher incidence of SCC over the more favorable BCC histology.

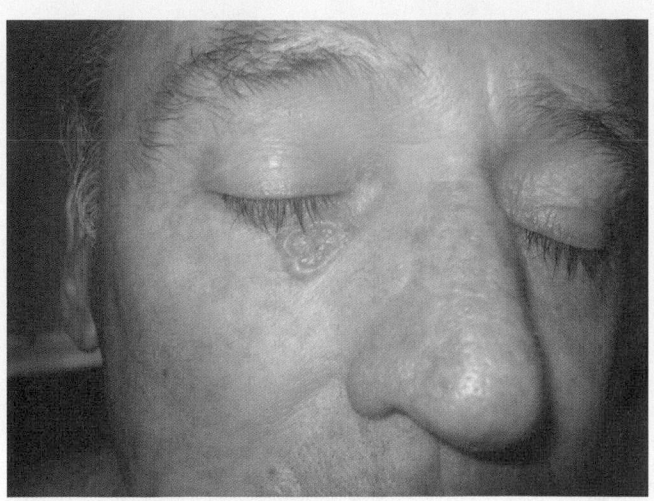

FIGURE 30.1. Basal cell carcinoma of the skin. (Courtesy of Professor Russell P. Hall, Duke University, Durham, NC.)

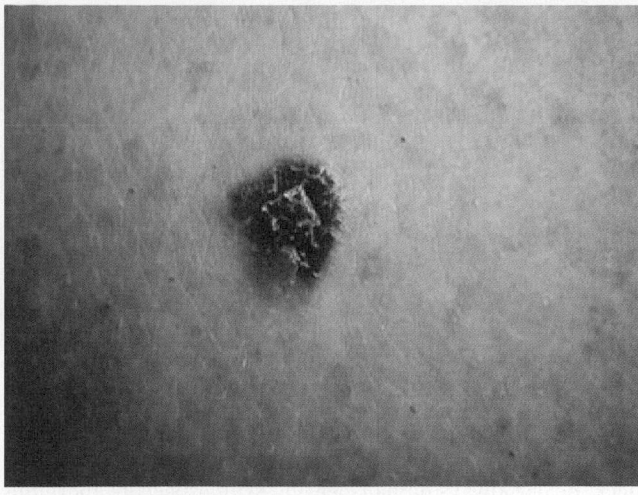

FIGURE 30.3. Malignant melanoma. (Courtesy of Professor Russell P. Hall, Duke University, Durham, NC.)

Premalignant Skin Lesions

Actinic (Solar) Keratoses

Actinic keratoses tend to be multiple and located on sun-exposed body areas as hyperkeratotic, erythematous patches. Malignant transformation to SCC occurs in about 1% of le-

sions, with cumulative lifetime risk 6% to 10% depending on number and length of time lesions are present (2). Treatment options include excision, cryotherapy, desiccation and curettage, dermabrasion, topical chemotherapy, and laser resurfacing.

Bowen's Disease

Bowen's disease, or SCC *in situ*, appears as a velvety red, keratotic plaque or nodule. Lesions typically occur in sun-damaged skin, may be single or multiple, sharply demarcated, and covered by a variable thickness scale. Progression to invasive SCC occurs in 5% to 20% of cases. Surgical excision is usually preferred; however, radiation therapy may be considered as an alternative. Time-dose-fractionation (TDF) values of 92 to 108 are recommended with schedules of 45 to 50 Gy at 2.5 to 3.5 Gy per fraction commonly employed. Facial lesions require 56 Gy at 2.0 Gy per fraction for improved cosmesis. Radiation therapy may be contraindicated for lower extremity lesions, as chronic, nonhealing ulcers are reported (27). Local recurrence was rare in a recent series of 42 patients treated with radiation. The authors recommend 25 Gy in 10 fractions and avoidance of fractions >4 Gy to reduce toxicity (43).

Keratoacanthoma

Keratoacanthomas usually are benign, self-healing lesions; however, they have the potential to destroy large volumes of tissue and may be associated with SCC. Lesions can be treated with radiation, particularly when biopsy reveals coexisting SCC. Doses of 35 Gy in 12 to 14 fractions or 45 Gy in 15 to 20 fractions have been used. The rare variant, aggressive giant keratoacanthoma, grows rapidly, frequently involves the face, and may cause severe cosmetic deformity. Radiation therapy is effective using 2.5 to 3 Gy fractions for large lesions and 4 to 5 Gy fractions for smaller lesions to total doses of 40 to 60 Gy.

Lentigo Maligna

Lentigo maligna is a pigmented patch containing abnormal melanocytes that may progress to melanoma. It is commonly found in the elderly on exposed surfaces of the body, particularly the face. Treatment is by surgical excision or cryotherapy. Radiation therapy may be employed primarily or as an adjuvant to surgery with doses of 45 to 50 Gy in 15 to 20 fractions (59).

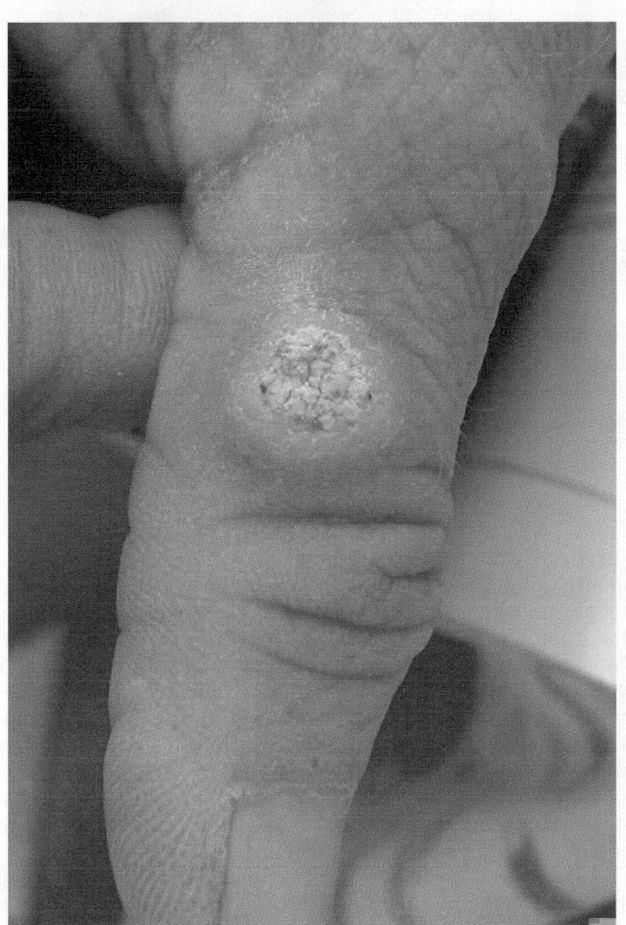

FIGURE 30.2. Squamous cell carcinoma of the skin. (Courtesy of Professor Russell P. Hall, Duke University, Durham, NC.)

Nevi

Dysplastic and congenital nevi are believed to be precursor lesions for melanoma and strong markers for melanoma risk. Up to 10% of all melanoma lesions are associated with a familial dysplastic nevus syndrome. Congenital nevi >2 cm have up to 20% risk of malignant degeneration and should be excised.

Nonmelanoma Skin Cancer

Basal Cell Carcinoma

BCC represents about 80% of all NMSC. There is no precursor lesion, and tumors are associated with mutations in the tumor suppressor gene on chromosome *9q* and *p53* (23). Untreated, these "rodent ulcers" burrow deeply, infiltrate vital areas, and cause marked deformity. Most tumors occur on the head and neck, nearly always on hair-bearing skin, especially above the line joining the earlobe to the angle of the mouth. BCC may infiltrate more deeply at embryologic junctional areas; tumors rarely metastasize, do not develop on mucous membranes, and are rare on palms and soles. Subtypes of BCC are nodular, superficial, pigmented, micronodular, and morpheaform (infiltrating, sclerosing, or desmoplastic) (69).

A typical BCC is a smooth nodule with central depression secondary to necrosis, surrounded by raised pearly or translucent borders. Telangiectatic vessels often are present in or around the lesion, and bleeding with minor trauma is common. The sclerosing morphea subtype shows deep, diffuse dermal infiltration, sparing the skin surface. Risk factors for BCC recurrence after treatment include location and size of the primary lesion, poor border definition, recurrent tumor, immunosuppression, site of prior radiation therapy, aggressive histology (morpheaform, sclerosing, infiltrative, micronodular), multifocality, and perineural involvement (69). The majority of recurrences occur within 3 years of treatment, and metastases are rare.

Squamous Cell Carcinoma

SCC is a tumor of keratinizing cells of the epidermis that has invaded beyond the dermal-epidermal junction, commonly associated with mutations in the *p53* tumor suppressor gene. Typical lesions are round-to-irregular, plaquelike or nodular, and overlaid with a warty keratotic scale or conical keratinized cutaneous horn. Surrounding erythema may be present, and bleeding results from minimal trauma. Although usually superficial, invasion of the subcutis does occur with muscle invasion and extension along periosteal, perineural, and angiolymphatic channels. Tumors arising from actinic keratoses are slow-growing and rarely metastasize; those arising from burn scars and areas of chronic inflammation or developing *de novo* are more aggressive. Nodal and distant metastases occur in approximately 10% of all cases, and although death from NMSC is rare, the usual cause is SCC. Clayman et al. (19) related mortality risk to tumor size ≥4 cm, perineural invasion, and invasion beyond the subcutis. In their analysis of 210 SCC patients, 3-year disease-specific survival was 100% without and 70% with at least one risk factor.

Recurrence risk factors for SCC include tumor size and location, poor border definition, recurrent tumor, immunosuppression, and site of prior radiation. Additional risk factors include site of a chronic inflammatory process; rapid tumor growth; neurologic symptoms; moderate-to-poorly differentiated adenoid (acantholytic), adenosquamous (with mucin production), or desmoplastic histology; Clark level IV to V (deep reticular dermis to subcutaneous fat) or thickness ≥4 mm; and perineural or vascular invasion (69).

Table 30.1	AMERICAN JOINT COMMITTEE STAGING SYSTEM FOR NONMELANOMA SKIN CANCER		
Primary tumor (T)			
TX	Primary tumor cannot be assessed		
T0	No evidence of primary tumor		
Tis	Carcinoma *in situ*		
T1	Tumor ≤2 cm in greatest dimension		
T2	Tumor >2 cm but not >5 cm in greatest dimension		
T3	Tumor >5 cm in greatest dimension		
T4	Tumor invades deep extradermal structures (i.e., cartilage, skeletal muscle, or bone)		
Regional lymph nodes (N)			
NX	Regional lymph nodes cannot be assessed		
N0	No regional lymph node metastasis		
N1	Regional lymph node metastasis		
Distant metastasis (M)			
MX	Presence of distant metastasis cannot be assessed		
M0	No distant metastasis		
M1	Distant metastasis		
Stage grouping			
Stage 0	Tis	N0	M0
Stage I	T1	N0	M0
Stage II	T2-3	N0	M0
Stage III	T4	N0	M0
	Any T	N1	M0
Stage IV	Any T	Any N	M1

From Green FL, Page DL, Fleming ID, et al., eds. *AJCC cancer staging manual*, 6th ed. New York: Springer-Verlag; 2002, with permission.

Staging of Nonmelanoma Skin Cancer

The staging system for NMSC appears in Table 30.1.

General Management of Nonmelanoma Skin Cancer

For most BCC or SCC lesions, surgical treatments or radiation therapy offer equivalent excellent cure rates of 90% to 95%. However, treatment approach must be individualized based on specific risk factors and patient characteristics for the most acceptable cosmetic and functional outcome.

Surgery

Curettage with electrodesiccation and cryosurgery can treat small, well-defined tumors <1.5 cm but are contraindicated in deeply infiltrating lesions. Wound contracture may cause tissue distortion and impaired cosmesis. Cryosurgery is better suited for actinic keratoses or Bowen's disease and rarely employed for BCC or SCC. Mohs' micrographic surgery involves fixation of tumor to enable tumor mapping and surgical excision with multiple frozen sections taken until microscopically clear. Cosmesis, often poor just after the procedure, improves with time. This technique is employed for BCC and SCC in embryonic fusion zones, recurrent or deeply invasive lesions, and tumors with potential for diffuse lateral spread or perineural invasion.

Surgical excision of NMSC is an expedient treatment offering the advantage of pathologic margin assessment and potential concurrent management of lymph nodes. Surgery is preferred for scalp tumors and for lesions <3 cm that can be removed with little cosmetic or functional impairment. Surgery is excellent for small tumors on the head and neck, trunk, extremity, shin, and dorsum of the hands or feet, and is recommended in areas of burns, scarring, chronic dermatitis, or prior irradiation and in patients with collagen vascular disease.

Radiation Therapy

Radiation therapy is an important management option in selected NMSC patients, offering an advantage in treating large lesions with deep tissue infiltration, and alone or combined with surgery for tumors along embryonic fusion planes (75). Treatment margins may be as wide as necessary for facial tumors, obviating the need for extensive surgical reconstruction. Radiation may be preferred for elderly, debilitated, or medically inoperable patients as anesthesia is not necessary, and when cosmesis is not a factor, fractionation can minimize the number of treatments (52).

Skin cancers with perineural invasion are particularly difficult to control, and salvage after surgical recurrence is unlikely. In reported series, asymptomatic patients with microscopic, incidental, perineural invasion receiving postoperative irradiation had 78% local control versus 50% for patients with neurologic symptoms or gross perineural extension (44,45). Magnetic resonance imaging (MRI) documents gross perineural spread and facilitates radiation planning. Treatment fields encompass the nerve at risk to the base of skull with postoperative radiation to 60 Gy to the tumor bed, 50 Gy to the proximal involved nerve with negative surgical margins, and 66 to 70 Gy for microscopic or gross positive margins (51).

Radiation fields can encompass multiple lesions or regional nodes. Although lymph node metastases are rare for BCC, they are seen in 5% to 10% of cutaneous SCC. Parotid area nodes, most commonly involved for cancers of the face, scalp, and ear, are particularly suited to treatment with radiation as definitive management or after surgical resection with prophylactic treatment of the ipsilateral neck.

Radiation therapy may be contraindicated in young patients because of potential carcinogenesis and tendency toward cosmetic deterioration over time (51). Contrary to early reports that involvement of bone or cartilage is a contraindication to radiation therapy, excellent control rates with good cosmesis, function preservation, and rare complications are achieved with modern techniques and equipment (51,75).

Postoperative radiation therapy may be employed after incomplete surgical resection. Although the 10-year actuarial probability of local control is excellent for patients with BCC treated either immediately after surgery for positive margins (92%) or at time of recurrence (90%) (40), this is not true for patients with SCC in whom local control and survival are improved when they receive radiation immediately after incomplete excision. Perez (54) found 87% tumor control and 10% to 15% nodal metastases in initially treated patients versus 65% tumor control and 39% nodal metastases in patients treated for salvage.

Follow-Up and Prevention of Nonmelanoma Skin Cancer

Patients with NMSC have a 30% to 50% risk of developing a second skin cancer within 5 years of treatment and are at risk for both NMSC and melanoma (2,69). Follow-up includes reinforcement of principles of sun protection and avoidance, self-examination, aggressive management of precancerous lesions, and total-body skin surveillance every 3 to 6 months for 1 year and every 6 months thereafter (2,69).

Considerable evidence suggests that high sun protection factor sunscreens are effective in preventing UVB-induced im-

munosuppression, and that regular use can induce actinic keratoses remission and prevent development of actinic keratoses and SCC (23). It is particularly important to encourage use of high sun protection factor sunscreens in children and adolescents to reduce lifetime skin cancer risk; frequent reapplication during sun exposure should also be encouraged (30). Sunscreens containing avobenzone (Parsol 1789), zinc oxide, or titanium dioxide offer the best protection against both UVA and UVB radiation (23).

Radiation Therapy Techniques

Many specialized radiation therapy techniques are used to treat skin cancer, depending on the size, depth, and anatomic location of the lesion. Quality of radiation is selected based on the best ratio between surface dose and ideal treatment depth. Field size is determined by lesion size and histopathology. TDF schedule depends on cosmetic and functional considerations balanced against desire for expedient, less costly treatment.

Quality of Radiation

Most skin cancers can be treated with superficial or orthovoltage x-rays; however, superficial x-ray units are no longer widely available in the United States. Although superficial x-rays deposit a maximum dose (D_{max}) at the skin surface, the exponential decrease in dose at depth results in greater dosage to deeper structures as treatment depth increases. Megavoltage electrons and photons generated by linear accelerators are now generally employed in NMSC management.

Modern linear accelerators produce a variety of electron energies from 6 to 20 MeV, offering the advantage of rapid falloff of depth dose to enable sparing of underlying normal tissues. Typical electron beam depth-dose profiles appear in Table 30.2; however, dose profiles are less accurate for small field sizes, and direct measurement of actual dose delivered is necessary for the small fields used to treat most skin tumors.

Depth of tissue covered is a function of electron beam energy. Electrons are "skin-sparing," with buildup to D_{max} below the surface so that modifications are necessary to increase surface dose when electrons are employed (51,52,75). The most frequent modification is placement of "tissue-equivalent" material (bolus) directly on the skin surface. Bolus effectively draws the beam isodose lines upward toward the skin surface, and bolus thickness must be considered in the selection of beam energy. Generally, the electron energy chosen is the lowest energy requiring the least bolus thickness to place D_{max} at the skin surface and the 90% depth at the desired treatment depth in the patient. Electron beam perturbation increases with beam obliquity, affecting dose profile. When treating skin cancers with electrons, the gantry must be rotated so that the surface to be treated is perpendicular to the beam axis to minimize sloping surface effect on tumor coverage (51,52,75).

Table 30.2	DEPTH-DOSE CHARACTERISTICS FOR ELECTRON BEAM ENERGIES USED IN THE TREATMENT OF SKIN CANCER				
Energy (MeV)	Surface (%)	D90 (cm)	D_{max} (cm)	D90 (cm)	D10 (cm)
6	82.3	.6	1.4	2.0	3.4
8	84.3	.6	1.8	2.5	4.2
10	84.7	.7	2.3	3.1	5.1
12	—	—	2.5	4.0	5.6
15	90.6	—	3.0	4.7	7.6

Beyond a depth of 5 to 6 cm, photon beam irradiation with surface bolus must be employed in conjunction with electrons for uniform coverage of both deep and superficial tumor extension. Photon-electron mixed-beam combinations delivering optimal depth-dose characteristics are readily selected employing modern three-dimensional conformal planning.

Customized surface molds employing afterloading ^{192}Ir or high-dose-rate brachytherapy sources are useful when protracted daily treatment fractionation is inconvenient or for treatment of lesions on the shin or dorsum of the hand, where conventional radiation therapy is poorly tolerated (34,68). Low-dose-rate interstitial brachytherapy can treat periorificial tumors of embryonic fusion regions of the face. Excellent disease control (92.5%) and cosmesis are reported with doses of 55 to 65 Gy at dose-rates ≤ 2 Gy/hr with low risk of late complications (56).

Field Size

Field size depends on lesion size, site treated, and quality of radiation employed. Choo et al. (18) assessed resection margins in 71 NMSC lesions excised by Mohs' technique. Microscopic tumor extension varied from 1 to 15 mm (mean, 5.2 mm). The authors determined a margin of 10 mm around gross tumor was necessary for 95% likelihood of margin negativity and that larger tumors were associated with greater microscopic extension. Geographic or marginal miss is a common cause of failure of NMSC, and generous margins should be employed in the presence of high histologic grade, recurrent tumor, indistinct borders, and sclerosing BCC histology (52). Although a tight field margin may be theoretically sufficient for small, low-grade tumors, marginal miss is more likely with extremely small field sizes because of daily setup variability.

Low-energy electron beam dosimetry requires larger lateral field margins for small fields because of constriction of high isodose lines at depth, and a wider field margin is required for electron beam than superficial or orthovoltage fields. Megavoltage photon beams have better flatness and sharper penumbra than electron beams. Photon margins of 0.5 to 1 cm and electron margins of 1 to 1.5 cm are employed for tumors up to 2 cm and photon margins of 1.5 to 2 cm and electron margins of 2 to 2.5 cm for tumors >2 to 7 cm (51,52).

As with lateral margins, depth of tumor extension often is underestimated, and computed tomography (CT) and MRI are helpful in assessing deep tissue penetration. For lesions of the eyelid, pinna, or nasal ala where tissue thickness is readily measured, full-thickness treatment is recommended. For tumors up to 4 cm, treatment depth should be about 5 mm below the expected tumor depth and is typically at least 1 cm. Larger, recurrent, and high-grade lesions, especially if located along embryonic fusion planes, have higher risk of occult deep extension, and treatment depths of at least 2 cm are required.

Time-Dose Fractionation

Similar total doses and fractionation regimens are employed for BCC and SCC of similar size and depth, although some authors advocate higher doses for SCC than BCC (42). Higher doses per fraction cause greater late effects and worse cosmesis, so concern about cosmesis and late tissue damage must be weighed against considerations of patient age and comorbidity.

The relative biologic effectiveness (RBE) is 10% to 20% less for megavoltage than for superficial or orthovoltage beams; therefore, treatment with megavoltage photons or electrons requires 10% to 20% dose increase for similar biologic effect. Dose adjustment for RBE entails either prescription to the 80% to 90% depth or dose increase of 10% to 20% and prescription to D_{max} for megavoltage treatment when converting from orthovoltage schedules. When comparing treatment schedules, it is helpful to

Table 30.3 — COMPARISON OF DIFFERENT TIME-DOSE-FRACTIONATION (TDF) SCHEDULES FOR MANAGEMENT OF NONMELANOMA SKIN CANCER

Tumor Characteristics	Dose Fractionation	TDF
MGH (75)[a]		
<1 cm tumor; debilitated patient	20–24 Gy in 1 fraction	—
<2 cm tumor	45 Gy in 5–9 fractions	122—131
2–4 cm or cosmetic concerns	52 Gy in 13 fractions	125
>4 cm tumor	60 Gy in 20 fractions	123
	64 Gy in 25 fractions	116
MDACC (51)[b]		
≤1 cm; elderly patient	40 Gy in 8 fractions	125
>1–2 cm in elderly or ≤2 cm in young patient	50 Gy in 15–20 fractions	108–127
Large fields needing good cosmesis	60 Gy in 30 fractions	115
Large, infiltrating tumors	64 to 66 Gy in 32–33 fractions	122–126
University of Florida (49)[b]		
Large, untreated + bone/cartilage invasion or large, recurrent	65 Gy in 35 fractions	115
Large, untreated + minimal or suspected bone/cartilage invasion	60 Gy in 34 fractions	112
Moderate-to-large inner canthus, eyelid, nasal, pinna (20–30 cm^2)	55 Gy in 30 fractions	99
Small, thin (<1.5 cm) eye, nose, ear (10 cm^2)	50 Gy in 20 fractions	108
Moderate or postoperative cut-through on free skin	45 Gy in 15 fractions	107
Small (1 cm) on free skin	40 Gy in 10 fractions	111
	30 Gy in 5 fractions	103
Cosmesis not important	40 Gy in 10 fractions	111
	30 Gy in 5 fractions	89
	20 Gy in 1 fractions	

MGH, Massachusetts General Hospital; MDACC, M.D. Anderson Cancer Center.
[a]Megavoltage.
[b]Orthovoltage doses. For megavoltage, prescribe dose to D90% or add 10% to total dose and prescribe to D_{max}.

consider isobioeffect TDF values. Table 30.3 compares recommended fractionation schedules and corresponding TDF values from Massachusetts General Hospital, M.D. Anderson Cancer Center (MDACC), and the University of Florida.

Patient Setup and Shielding

The region treated is immobilized to achieve stability and maximize setup reproducibility. The machine gantry is angled so the treated surface is perpendicular to the beam axis when using electrons. Shielding of surrounding normal tissues and critical structures is particularly important in the treatment of skin cancers involving head and neck regions. When treating with electrons, the thickness of lead in millimeters required to reduce transmission to <5% of maximum is approximately E/2, where E is electron beam energy. A lead cut-out placed in the head of the machine cone avoids a high-dose zone under the shield edge when treating with high-energy electrons; however, this is not a concern with the low-energy electron beams usually employed to treat skin cancers. Secondary beam collimation with a lead cut-out placed directly on the skin surface generally is preferred because the dose at the beam margins is lower than at the center (51).

Special shielding devices are required when treating lesions involving the eye, nose, mouth, and ear. The dose threshold for cataract formation is 5 to 10 Gy, and a tungsten eye shield placed daily directly under the eyelids is required for protection of the superficial structures of the eye and lens. Tungsten shields reduce the ocular dose to <5% from electron energies up to 9 MeV (62). An alternative method involves rotation of the lens and cornea out of the beam by having the patient stare away from the beam source during treatment; however, daily reproducibility is difficult, and the maneuver may result in greater exposure to the retina. Topical anesthetic facilitates shield placement, and antibiotic ointment is recommended after removal. It is preferable to use the largest eye shield that can be placed comfortably.

Exit beam blocking is necessary when treating tumors involving the nose, mouth, or ear. The nasal septum and canal are shielded by lead strips coated with either wax or dental acrylic placed directly in the nose. The coating absorbs electron backscatter from the lead. Similar shields are placed under the lip when treating tumors around the mouth to protect the gingiva and oral mucosa. An exit beam shield can be placed at the junction of the posterior surface of the pinna with the scalp over the mastoid to treat auricle lesions (52).

Treatment by Specific Anatomic Site

Eyelid

Surgery usually is the preferred treatment for eyelid tumors <0.5 cm or for salvage of radiation failures, and modern oculoplastic techniques usually result in excellent outcome. Radiation therapy is employed after surgical recurrence or incomplete resection and for large carcinomas of the eyelids and canthi where good surgical margins cannot be obtained. Eyelid tumors may appear superficial but actually penetrate deeply into the globe. CT is essential for accurate determination of tumor extent. Failure at the field margin is not uncommon, and care must be taken to ensure adequate field size and treatment depth.

Because the eyelid dermis is extremely thin, protracted fractionation schemes at relatively small daily doses usually result in the best cosmetic and functional results, especially for large, infiltrating lesions. If possible, when treating upper eyelid tumors the lacrimal gland should be shielded to avoid late keratoconjunctivitis due to dry eye. Similarly, protection of the lacrimal duct is desirable in treatment of lower lid lesions to avoid late stricture and overflow tearing. Large cancers involving the medial canthus may develop ectropion and epiphora because of inability to shield the lacrimal drainage system, but these complications are rare. In all cases, shielding should be withheld rather than blocking tumor because complications often can be treated with minor surgical procedures. Epilation of the eyelashes always occurs with techniques and doses necessary to control skin cancers, and wherever possible, the uninvolved eyelid should be shielded.

Ear

In most instances, electron beam radiation offers cosmetic advantages over surgery for skin cancers of the external ear. Extensive, deeply infiltrating tumors with bone or cartilage involvement require megavoltage techniques and more protracted fractionation. Techniques to minimize dose inhomogeneities due to the irregular contours are described including use of a scatter plate to flatten the ear and water in the concha and external auditory canal (51,52). Silva et al. (63) reported the Princess Margaret Hospital experience treating 334 cancers of the pinna. Statistical predictors of local failure were T size >2 cm, low biologic effective dose, high T stage, cartilage necrosis, recurrent lesions, field size >6 cm, and protracted treatment time.

Nose

Because of the sloping surface of the nose, a wax or tissue-equivalent block may be necessary to ensure homogeneous dose distribution at depth, and photons may be required to reach deeply infiltrating tumors with bone or cartilage invasion. Lesions of the nasal vestibule require special consideration as histology at this location is more often SCC than BCC; approximately 10% of these lesions present with lymph node involvement and another 10% to 15% subsequently fail in regional nodes, usually submandibular, unless treated electively.

Lip

NMSC of the lip shows regional node involvement in up to 7% of cases and 3% tumor-related mortality. Most tumors involve the lower lip. Large upper lip lesions commonly extend up to the ala nasi and columella nasi. Treatment techniques include interstitial implant, external-beam irradiation with low-energy electrons, or both in combination. The incidence of subclinical node involvement with SCC is highly dependent on tumor grade; however, because of low overall incidence, prophylactic neck irradiation usually is not recommended.

Dorsum of the Hand

SCC is the most common skin cancer to involve the dorsum of the hand. In general, tumors in this location are best treated by surgical excision. Treatment by radiation therapy usually is with surface molds containing afterloading catheters or high-dose-rate microselectron molds (68). Lesions in the thumb web space, interdigital clefts, or proximal phalanges often are aggressive and prone to recurrence, lymph node metastases, and radionecrosis. External-beam radiation techniques are discouraged because of paucity of subcutaneous tissue and high incidence of complications such as radionecrosis and loss of function.

Results of Irradiation of Nonmelanoma Skin Cancer

Locke et al. (42) published an update of treatment results for 339 cutaneous SCC and BCC lesions. Contrary to earlier reports, the authors found similar control rates with electron beam and superficial or orthovoltage x-ray treatment. The study found histologic type a risk factor for recurrence, with local tumor control of 92% for BCC and 80% for SCC. As in previous series, control rates were better for previously untreated lesions (94% for BCC and 89% for SCC), and importance of early treatment to maximize control and cosmesis is stressed.

Melanoma

The cell of origin for malignant melanoma is the melanocyte, present in all areas of the epidermis and in parts of the eye and upper respiratory, gastrointestinal, and genitourinary tracts. The incidence of melanoma in the United States has risen at the rate of 6% per year, and 59,580 new cases of melanoma and 7,770 deaths were estimated in 2005 (36). Mortality has decreased from a 5-year relative survival of 80% in cases diagnosed between 1974 and 1976 to 91% between 1995 and 2000 (36), largely because of heightened awareness and screening programs resulting in earlier detection. Melanoma is the fourth leading cancer type in men and the fifth in women in the United States, representing 5% and 4% of 2005 new cancer diagnoses, respectively (36). Lesions occur most frequently in white adults, with peak incidence in the fourth and fifth decades. Melanoma tends to involve the extremities in women and the head and neck or trunk in men, and women have an apparent survival advantage.

Cho et al. (17) examined risk factors in three cohort studies that included 535 cases of invasive melanoma in whites to devise a statistical model for calculating a melanoma risk score. The study identified older age, male sex, family history of melanoma, high number of nevi >3 mm on arms or lower legs, history of severe sunburn, and light hair color as significant risk factors. Melanoma is rare in dark-skinned races, and when found usually involves palms and soles. Although most melanomas are believed to arise *de novo*, they also may develop from pre-existing benign nevi, especially those subject to repeated trauma and irritation.

Superficial spreading melanoma (SSM) accounts for about 70% of cases and displays a radial growth pattern in the epidermis and invasion into papillary dermis. SSM is associated with intermittent recreational sun exposure, is most common on the trunk and extremities, and often develops from precursor nevi. Radial growth over many years has a 5% metastatic potential, and vertical growth that follows is rapid and carries a 35% to 80% metastatic risk. Nodular melanoma represents 30% of cases and is the most malignant form. Nodular melanoma has a 2:1 male-to-female ratio and occurs at a median age of 50 years. It is characterized by vertical growth only during several months to a year on trunk or head and neck sites and arises *de novo*. Lentigo maligna melanoma (LMM), representing 4% to 15% of all melanomas and having the most benign behavior, is associated with occupational exposure and involvement of the head and neck and dorsum of the hands. LMM is a disease of the elderly and is not associated with pre-existing nevi. Acral lentiginous melanoma (ALM) accounts for 2% to 8% of melanomas overall but 35% to 90% of melanomas in blacks, Asians, and Hispanics. ALM involves the palms and soles or subungual regions, usually is seen in the sixth decade, and commonly metastasizes. LLM, SSM, and ALM are most curable during the indolent, radial growth phase. Vertical growth signals rapid progression with deeper penetration and increased metastatic potential. Desmoplastic melanoma (DM) is an uncommon variant occurring in only 1% to 3% of cases (41). DM is characterized by pronounced neurotropism and infiltrative growth resulting in locally aggressive behavior and frequent local recurrence, although lymphatic and distant metastases are uncommon (4,41). These tumors are often amelanotic, and skip lesions in the perineural space are common in spite of negative resection margins (4). Case-matched comparison found that while DM patients tend to present with thicker tumors, their overall, cause-specific, and disease-free survival are similar to matched melanoma controls of similar thickness (41).

Staging of Melanoma

The revised melanoma staging system shown in Table 30.4 was adopted by the American Joint Committee on Cancer in 2002 and is the result of a prognostic factors analysis of 17,600 patients in prospective melanoma databases (6). Staging incorporates information obtained from sentinel lymph node (SLN) mapping. This technique has evolved as perhaps the single most important prognostic factor (71) and results in considerable stage migration of patients who previously would have been staged node-negative by clinical criteria.

General Management of Melanoma

Surgery

Current recommendations for primary melanoma excision margins are 0.5 cm for *in situ* melanoma, 1 cm for lesions up to 1 cm

Table 30.4	AMERICAN JOINT COMMISSION ON CANCER STAGING SYSTEM FOR MELANOMA OF THE SKIN
Tumor (T)	
TX	Primary tumor cannot be assessed (e.g., shave biopsy or regressed)
T0	No evidence of primary tumor
Tis	Melanoma *in situ*
T1	≤1 mm in thickness (a. without ulceration or b. with ulceration or level IV or V)
T2	1.01–2 mm in thickness (a. without or b. with ulceration)
T3	2.01–4 mm in thickness (a. without or b. with ulceration)
T4	>4 mm in thickness (a. without or b. with ulceration)
Nodes (N)	
NX	Regional lymph node metastases cannot be assessed
N0	No regional lymph node metastases
N1	1 lymph node (a. micrometastasis[a] or b. macrometastasis[b])
N2	2–3 lymph nodes (a. micrometastasis[a] or b. macrometastasis) c. Satellite or in-transit metastasis *without* nodal metastasis
N3	≥4 nodes; matted nodes; or in-transit metastasis or satellites *with* metastasis in regional node(s)
Metastasis (M)	
MX	Distant metastasis cannot be assessed
M0	No distant metastasis
M1a	Skin, subcutaneous tissues, or distant nodes
M1b	Lung
M1c	All other visceral or any distant metastasis with elevated LDH

LDH, lactate dehydrogenase.
[a]Micrometastases are diagnosed after elective or sentinal lymphadenectomy.
[b]Macrometastases are clinically detectable lymph node metastases confirmed by therapeutic lymphadenectomy or any lymph node with gross extracapsular extension.
Modified from Green FL, Page DL, Fleming ID, et al., eds. *AJCC cancer staging manual*, 6th ed. New York: Springer-Verlag; 2002.

in size and ≤1 mm thick, and 2 cm for lesions >1 cm in size or 1 to 4 mm thick (55,73). Elective lymph node dissection has been abandoned in favor of observation or SLN biopsy. With risk of occult node involvement <5%, observation alone has been recommended for lesions up to 1 mm thick. As risk of occult node involvement rises to 15% to 25% for lesions 1 to 4 mm thick and 35% for lesions >4 mm thick, SLN biopsy is recommended (55). Patients with SLN biopsies revealing metastasis go on to therapeutic dissection of the involved nodal basin.

Surgery also may be considered for patients with solitary metastasis to subcutaneous tissue, lung, nonregional lymph nodes, and brain for both palliation and prolongation of progression-free survival. This is especially pertinent for patients with long disease-free interval after primary management.

Radiation Therapy

Radiation therapy can play several important roles in the management of melanoma: adjuvant treatment after resection of the primary lesion or metastatic regional nodes, elective treatment of regional nodes at high risk for subclinical disease, palliative treatment of distant metastatic lesions and local recurrences, and, rarely, definitive treatment of primary lesions. In spite of recent estimates that radiation therapy is indicated in at least 23% of all melanoma patients, actual utilization rates range only from 1% to 13% (25). The long-held belief that melanoma was a radioresistant tumor was resolved by *in vitro* studies demonstrating a wide shoulder on the cell survival curve for melanoma cell lines, suggesting large capacity for repair of sublethal damage and the possible therapeutic advantage of hypofractionated treatment regimens. Potential enhancement of cell kill using high-dose fractionation must be weighed against potential increases in late normal tissue complications.

Clinical Radiation Oncology

Adjuvant Radiation Therapy of the Primary Lesion and/or Regional Lymph Nodes

In spite of the <5% overall local recurrence after excision of primary melanoma lesions, certain factors carry increased recurrence risk. Published reports indicate recurrence risk of 6% to 14% for tumor thickness ≥4 mm, 5% to 17% for head and neck primary locations, 10% to 17% in the presence of ulceration, 14% to 16% with satellite lesions, and 23% to 48% for the desmoplastic histologic (DM) variant (4,8,66). In view of these data, indications for adjuvant radiation therapy to the primary tumor site at MDACC include DM histology, tumor thickness >4 mm with either ulceration or satellite lesions, positive resection margins, and either as primary or adjuvant treatment of locally recurrent disease (8).

Therapeutic resection of clinically involved lymph nodes in melanoma results in 85% control of nodal disease (8). However, 30% to 50% risk of nodal recurrence after therapeutic resection is reported in conjunction with extracapsular extension, four or more involved nodes, lymph node size >3 cm, cervical node location, and recurrent nodal disease after initial resection (8,12,38). Morris et al. (50) reported their experience using hypofractionated adjuvant irradiation after surgical debulking of nodal or subcutaneous melanoma deposits in 41 patients. In-field failure occurred in only two patients (4.8%), and treatment morbidity was minor. Stevens et al. (66) employed adjuvant hypofractionated radiation therapy to the primary site in 35 patients and to regional nodes in 139 patients at high risk based on similar criteria. In this series, in-field recurrence occurred in 11% of patients (vs. 50% in surgery-only series) and was the only predictive factor for decreased survival with median survival of 13 months with and 35 months without infield recurrence (66).

Data from MDACC revealed a regional control rate of 87% in the axilla after adjuvant radiation therapy for one or more high-risk features (9). In spite of a 43% overall incidence of mild-to-moderate arm edema at 5 years, symptoms, if any, were minor. In contrast, in the Australian series reported by Stevens et al. (66), in spite of excellent local control, symptomatic arm edema occurred in 58% of 2-year survivors irradiated after axillary dissection. Caution is recommended in the consideration of adjuvant radiation therapy after dissection of involved inguinal nodes because of the propensity for clinically significant lymphedema in this cohort. These concerns have prompted MDACC recommendations for adjuvant radiation therapy to inguinal lymph nodes only when two or more high-risk features are present (10).

Elective Radiation Therapy of Clinically Negative Regional Lymphatics

The risk of subclinical involvement of regional lymph nodes is directly related to the depth of the primary lesion: <5% for lesions ≤0.75 mm, 10% for lesions 0.76 to 1.50 mm, 20% for lesions 1.51 to 4 mm, and 30% to 50% for lesions >4 mm (8). At MDACC, elective node irradiation in head and neck melanomas of ≥1.50 mm or Clark level ≥IV (involvement of reticular dermis or subcutis) achieved 89% actuarial local control at 5 and 10 years (14). Overall, multiple studies report improvement in locoregional control from about 50% with surgery alone to 82% to 95% with adjuvant irradiation in high-risk patients in spite of similar survival of 38% to 50% (12).

Definitive Primary Radiation Therapy

Radiation therapy as a definitive treatment approach remains an option for large LMM lesions of the face and for inoperable patients. Probability of control with radiation is related to lesion size, and regimens of 3 to 8 Gy per fraction are employed (21). Schmid-Wendtner et al. (59) achieved local control in 20 of 22 LMM patients treated by excision of the nodular portion of the lesion followed by 100 Gy in 10-Gy fractions five times per week using superficial radiation. Lesions all were located on the head and neck in patients who were considered unsuitable for surgery.

Palliative Radiation Therapy

Median survival for patients with stage IV melanoma is 6 to 10 months, and 5-year survival is <5% (73). Palliative radiation therapy is widely used for unresectable locoregional disease and distant metastases.

Dermal, subcutaneous, and lymph node metastases are palliated by radiation therapy in about two-thirds of patients. A hypofractionated regimen of 5 to 6 fractions of 6 Gy delivered twice weekly generally is preferred, although more conservative fractionation of 50 Gy in daily 2.0- to 2.5-Gy fractions may be appropriate for patients with inguinal or axillary nodal disease to reduce risk of lymphedema and/or neuropathy (7). Response decreases with increasing lesion size, and radiation should be initiated early.

Brain metastases are a clinical problem in 10% to 40% of melanoma patients and are detected in up to 75% in autopsy series (5). Whole-brain irradiation (WBRT) is effective in palliating symptoms of brain metastases, with 60% to 70% of patients showing improvement by 1 to 2 months (7). However, response duration usually is short and neurologic progression the usual cause of death. Fife et al. (29) reported outcome for 646 melanoma patients treated for brain metastasis at the Sydney melanoma unit between 1985 and 2000. Median survival was 8.9 months for surgery and postoperative irradiation, 8.7 months for surgery alone, 3.4 months for radiation therapy alone, and 2.1 months for supportive care. Factors associated with improved survival were surgery, absence of extracerebral metastasis, younger age, and longer disease-free interval, prompting the suggestion that patients with these favorable characteristics be selected for aggressive management.

Radiotherapy after resection of a solitary brain metastasis has shown a more durable response with improvement in both median survival and time to recurrence (21), and in this situation, consideration of 35 Gy in 14 fractions by shrinking field technique in the absence of extracranial metastasis has been recommended (7). Recent reviews favor treatment selection based on size, location, and number of metastatic lesions and patient prognostic grouping: surgery and WBRT for patients with solitary brain metastasis, limited or absent extracranial disease, and good performance status; radiosurgery as an alternative to resection for solitary brain metastasis ≤3 cm or up to six lesions when surgically inaccessible or poor performance status followed by WBRT; or WBRT alone, with or without chemotherapy, for patients with single brain metastasis not amenable to resection or radiosurgery and patients with active systemic disease, multiple brain metastases, and poor performance status (5,46).

About 80% of patients with painful bone metastases from melanoma achieve relief from palliative radiation therapy (7). Frequently employed regimens deliver 20 Gy in five fractions during 1 week or 30 Gy in 10 fractions during 2 weeks. Impending or actual pathologic fracture of long bones is managed by surgical stabilization prior to irradiation. In this situation, Ballo and Ang (7) recommend 36 Gy in 6 fractions for higher RBE. In the presence of spinal cord compression, laminectomy and surgical debulking is recommended prior to radiation therapy. Standard fractionation regimens of 30 Gy in 10 fractions usually are recommended; however, more durable response may be obtained in patients without evidence of other metastatic disease employing 45 to 50 Gy in 2.5-Gy fractions (7).

Radiation Time-Dose-Fractionation Schedules and Treatment Techniques

TDF schedules recommended for melanoma vary widely and are the subject of considerable controversy. The Radiation Therapy Oncology Group compared 8 Gy delivered in four weekly fractions to 32 and 2.5 Gy daily, 5 days per week for 20 fractions, to 50 Gy and found no significant difference between the regimens in terms of complete response or partial response (58).

In spite of the Radiation Therapy Oncology Group findings, the recommended dose-fractionation schedule at MDACC is 30 Gy in 5 fractions of 6 Gy per fraction during 2.5 weeks with treatment on either a Monday/Thursday or Tuesday/Friday schedule (8). The brain, brainstem, spinal cord, and small bowel are limited to 24 Gy by this schedule, or conventional fractionation is employed. Adjuvant treatment of the primary tumor bed employs 2- to 4-cm margins using electron beam with appropriate bolus. Irradiation for a head and neck primary consists of comprehensive electron beam coverage of the primary site and ipsilateral neck, including supraclavicular nodes. Electron energies are determined by CT-guided treatment planning and appropriate bolus employed for prescription to D_{max} with field junctions moved twice during treatment. Axillary nodal irradiation includes ipsilateral low cervical, supraclavicular, and axillary levels I through III with shaped anterior and posterior fields containing wedges or compensating filters. Inguinal lymph node treatment is delivered to involved nodes only, without prophylaxis of external or common iliac nodes, in an attempt to avoid late lymphedema (10).

Follow-Up of Patients With Melanoma

Surveillance, Epidemiology and End Results (SEER) database analysis indicates the risk of developing a subsequent melanoma to be 10 times the rate of a first melanoma among the general SEER population (73), with the highest risk in the first 2 years after treatment (32) and a lifetime risk of 4% to 6% (71). Melanoma patients also are at increased risk for NMSC. The National Comprehensive Cancer Network recommends life-long surveillance with frequency dependent on individual risk factors (family history, skin type, presence of dysplastic nevi, and/or NMSC) and stage (71).

Merkel Cell Carcinoma

MCC, or neuroendocrine carcinoma of the skin, is a rare primary dermal tumor, and only about 470 cases of MCC are anticipated yearly in the United States (31). These tumors are recognized for their aggressive and potentially lethal behavior. They are characterized by local recurrence after surgical excision (25% to 75%), frequent involvement of regional lymph nodes (30% to 80%), and distant metastatic spread (20% to 75%). The most common metastatic sites are skin, lung, central nervous system, and bone. Mortality rates of 20% to 55% are reported (1,13,31,33,47).

The Merkel cell described in the basal layer of the epidermis and in hair follicles are of epidermal origin and believed to function in neurotactile sensation. Dense core granules on electron microscopy and immunohistochemical characteristics of both epithelial and neuroendocrine cells suggest that MCC tumors are of epithelial origin and have undergone neuroendocrine differentiation. Three histologic subtypes are described—trabecular, intermediate, and small cell—but prognosis and treatment approach are similar (13).

MCC usually presents in the sixth and seventh decades and involves sun-exposed areas of the head and neck (50% to 75%), extremities (20% to 40%), or trunk (<10%) (1,31,77). More than 90% of MCCs occur in whites, and sun exposure, long-term psoralen and UVA therapy (PUVA), and immuosuppression have been implicated as causative factors (13,31,33,47,77). MCC usually presents as a ≤2 cm, painless, firm, pink-red to violaceous-blue solitary nodule with intact epidermis. Vascular and lymphatic permeation is common and mitotic index is high. Electron microscopy and immunohistochemical analysis help distinguish these tumors from metastatic small cell lung cancer, lymphoma, or other small cell tumors (13,77).

Treatment of Merkel Cell Carcinoma

Surgery

The initial treatment for MCC is excision of the primary tumor with 2- to 3-cm lateral and deep margins extending down to the fascia or periosteum and therapeutic dissection of pathologically involved regional nodes (13,31). Mohs' surgery may be an alternative to wide excision (31) and used in addition or alternative to adjuvant radiation therapy if complete histologic margin control is attained (33).

Controversy exists over the management of clinically uninvolved regional nodes. MCC is believed to spread in a manner similar to melanoma, with orderly progression to regional nodes before distant spread, prompting many authors to recommend surgical evaluation or prophylactic treatment of clinically uninvolved regional nodes (63,72). SLN biopsy may be applied to patients with MCC as an alternative to prophylactic node dissection or radiation therapy in SLN-negative patients (31,47,72).

Radiation Therapy

Radiation sensitivity of MCC is well documented, and the >50% rate of locoregional recurrence after surgical resection is thought by many investigators to warrant the routine use of adjuvant radiation therapy (47,72). Generous 3- to 5-cm field margins are recommended because of propensity for in-transit metastasis and marginal recurrence. Surgical resection should be followed by wide-field irradiation to the primary tumor site, surgical bed and scar, and draining lymphatics. For head and neck primaries, the entire ipsilateral neck is irradiated in all cases, and the contralateral neck is included for bilateral or midline lesions. Recommended doses are similar to those employed for SCC (47). The primary tumor site receives 56 to 60 Gy for subclinical disease with negative margins, 60 to 66 Gy for microscopically positive margins, and 66 to 70 Gy for gross residual disease at conventional fractionation. Nodal doses of 46 to 50 Gy are employed for prophylaxis of subclinical disease and 56 to 60 Gy for gross disease (13,47).

A recent publication by Allen et al. (3) challenged the routine use of adjuvant radiation therapy after resection of MCC. The authors reviewed 251 cases of MCC treated at Memorial Sloan-Kettering Cancer Center during a 32-year period. Only 8% of patients resected with negative margins recurred locally and only 14% of patients who underwent lymph node dissection suffered nodal recurrence, even without adjuvant radiotherapy. With 5-year disease-specific survival of 64%, stage at presentation, and not use of adjuvant therapy, predicted survival. The authors stress the importance of wide excision of the primary and surgical staging of the nodal basin in all patients. At Memorial Sloan-Kettering Cancer Center, adjuvant radiation therapy is recommended only for patients at high locoregional recurrence risk as with positive excision margins, multiple positive nodes, or extranodal tumor extension.

For medically or surgically inoperable patients, radiation therapy can be employed in a definitive attempt with elective treatment of clinically uninvolved nodes. There is evidence that salvage surgery and radiation for recurrent locoregional disease and the addition of chemotherapy in the presence of distant metastasis can improve survival (28); however, this aggressive, potentially toxic approach may have limited applicability in this elderly population.

Prognosis of Merkel Cell Carcinoma

The most important prognostic factor for MCC is extent of tumor at diagnosis, and the most commonly used staging system divides patients by the absence (stage I) or presence (stage II) of regional nodal metastasis or by the presence (stage III) of distant metastasis. Regional lymph nodes are clinically involved in 20% to 30% of patients at presentation, and nodal relapse occurs in >50% of untreated clinically node-negative patients. Fewer than 5% of patients have distant metastasis at presentation (31,47,77). Overall survival at 3 years is reported at 31% to 62% (13,77). Most recurrences occur within 6 to 12 months of initial treatment (28,31,64,77) with a mean time of 8 months for locoregional and 18 months for distant failure. Follow-up is therefore recommended every 1 to 3 months for the first 2 years, every 3 to 6 months the third year, and then yearly after initial treatment (72).

Rare Cutaneous Tumors

Dermatofibrosarcoma Protuberans

DFSP is a monoclonal dermal sarcoma of fibroblast origin with an incidence of 0.8 cases per million people per year (70). Lesions typically are low grade and characterized by indolent growth, frequent local recurrence, and rare lymphatic or hematogenous metastasis (11,70). The 10% to 15% of DFSP lesions with high-grade fibrosarcoma elements may exhibit more aggressive behavior (22,48). Delayed diagnosis is common, and lesions may reach substantial size prior to biopsy. DFSP typically appears as a painless pink or red dermal plaque on the trunk, head and neck, or proximal extremities. Incidence is higher in men, and presentation is usually in the fourth decade. A horizontal dermal growth pattern may persist for months or years before nodular growth with deep extension and fixation to the subcutis.

Work-up for DFSP includes core needle or incisional biopsy. MRI helps assess depth of invasion. Enlarged regional nodes should be biopsied. Chest x-ray or CT is employed to rule out pulmonary metastasis, especially for recurrent or high-grade tumors. Occasionally, the pathologic diagnosis is unclear and immunohistochemistry is helpful in distinguishing DFSP from benign dermatofibroma or fibrous histiocytoma (48). DFSP is staged according to American Musculoskeletal Tumor Society guidelines as IA, low-grade without extension beyond the subcutaneous compartment, or IB, low-grade with involvement of fascia or muscle (48).

Surgery is the mainstay of treatment, and clear resection margins of 3 cm down to and including muscle or fascia result in a local recurrence rate <10% (15,26,48). Because of the propensity for irregular shape and wide peripheral microscopic infiltration, careful assessment of histologic borders is essential (26,70). Late recurrences during 5 years after initial resection are not uncommon, and long-term follow-up is advised.

Preoperative irradiation should be considered for patients at high risk for positive resection margins based on large tumor size or location where critical structures preclude optimal re-section. Postoperative irradiation is advised for close or positive margins because of recurrence risk >50%. Dose recommendations for microscopic disease range from 59.4 to 65 Gy employing daily (1.8 to 2 Gy) or twice-daily (1.2-Gy) fractionation (22). Anecdotal reports of radiation therapy alone for DFSP indicate that these tumors require doses of 65 to 75 Gy. Ballo et al. (11) achieved 95% actuarial local control at 10 years in 16 DFSP patients treated with postoperative irradiation after conservation surgery. Similarly, Sun et al. (67) reported 37.5% local recurrence in 24 patients treated with surgery alone versus 10% in 10 patients treated with surgery and adjuvant radiation for 7-year overall actuarial local control of 28% versus 80%, respectively.

Based on these results, we recommend preoperative radiation therapy to 50 Gy to palpable tumor with a 3- to 5-cm margin in all directions for DFSP patients whose tumors otherwise would require extensive resection with compromised cosmesis or function followed by surgery in 4 to 6 weeks. Postoperative radiation therapy is recommended for patients with close resection margins to 60 Gy, microscopic positive margins to 60 to 65 Gy, and gross residual disease to 65 to 75 Gy with field reductions after 50 Gy. Similarly, adjuvant radiation therapy should be considered for all recurrent or high-grade lesions regardless of margin status.

Carcinoma of the Skin Adnexa

Carcinomas of the skin adnexa arising from eccrine and apocrine sweat glands, hair follicles, and sebaceous glands comprise about 0.2% of skin cancers. These tumors are characterized by propensity for aggressive biologic behavior and local recurrence. Diagnosis often is delayed because of benign clinical appearance, and misdiagnosis even after excision is common. Histopathologic diagnosis may require the use of immunohistochemical markers (57,74).

Malignant Sweat Gland Carcinoma

Eccrine sweat glands function primarily in the regulation of body temperature and are distributed widely except on the lips and genitalia. Apocrine sweat glands are distributed in the axilla, anogenital region, areola and nipple, and in modified form in the external ear and eyelids in association with hair follicles. Sweat gland carcinomas comprise about 1 in 20,000 skin malignancies (74). The head and neck, trunk, and extremities are the most common sites for eccrine carcinomas and the axilla for apocrine carcinomas. Tumors often exhibit long periods of indolent growth followed by rapid progression with deep infiltration, the development of satellite lesions, lymph node metastasis, and finally, distant visceral metastasis.

In spite of multiple histologic subtypes of malignant eccrine carcinoma, including microcystic adnexal carcinoma, primary mucinous carcinoma of the skin, and clear cell eccrine carcinoma, biologic behavior is similar. Chronic radiation dermatitis and UV exposure have been implicated as possible causative factors for microcystic adnexal carcinoma (60), and it has been suggested that use of therapeutic radiation in the management of these lesions may induce more aggressive behavior (65).

Although surgical excision is the treatment of choice, several authors have suggested a role for adjuvant radiation therapy (16,35). Harari et al. (35) recommend radiation therapy in the presence of dermal lymphatic invasion, nerve-sheath involvement, deep structure infiltration, positive resection margins, high-grade, and extracapsular node extension. The authors recommend ≥70 Gy to the surgical bed and 50 Gy to lymph node chains at risk by combination of photon and electron beam. Lymph node dissection followed by adjuvant radiation is recommended for node-positive disease and either elective lymph node dissection or radiation of clinically uninvolved primary drainage sites. Adjuvant radiation therapy after resection of apocrine carcinomas is advocated in the presence of high-risk features of tumor size >5 cm, close (<1 cm) or positive margins, high-grade, and vascular or lymphatic invasion. Irradiation of the draining nodal basin may be indicated postoperatively in cases of extensive (≥4) node involvement or extracapsular node extension (16) or if resection is limited by anatomic constraints.

Sebaceous Carcinoma

Sebaceous carcinomas typically present on the upper eyelid, scalp, or face in the seventh decade, and are more common in women. Sebaceous carcinoma accounts for <5% of all malignant eyelid tumors overall, but this incidence may approach 30% in the Asian population and 40% to 60% in the Indian population (15,61). The parotid gland is the most common extraocular site for sebaceous carcinoma. The development of sebaceous carcinoma has been linked to prior radiation exposure of ocular adnexa as well as UV light exposure, chronic inflammatory conditions of the eyelid, and immunosuppression (15,61). Sebaceous carcinomas of the eyelid are aggressive tumors characterized by orbital invasion, visceral spread, and 25% mortality (15). In extraocular locations, behavior may be less aggressive. Initial spread to regional nodes occurs in about 30% of cases (61). Upper eyelid tumors spread primarily to preauricular and parotid nodes, and lower eyelid tumors spread to submandibular and cervical nodes.

The treatment of choice for sebaceous carcinoma is surgical excision or Mohs' surgery, with radiation therapy reserved for unresectable lesions. However, complete surgical removal is often difficult because of anatomic constraints and the propensity for multicentricity and intraepithelial pagetoid spread along the tarsal plate, lacrimal apparatus, and conjunctiva (15,61,76). Reports of radiotherapy in the management of sebaceous carcinoma are sporadic and anecdotal (20,53,76). Although these tumors appear to be radiosensitive, the potential for late damage to ocular structures must be considered. Pardo et al. (53) report four patients treated with definitive irradiation to 45 to 63 Gy and six treated postoperatively with 90% local control after 2- to 10-year follow-up and overall disease-specific actuarial survival of 96% at 5 years. Moderate-dose radiation therapy (50 Gy) may be helpful as an adjuvant to surgical resection in the setting of high-risk features such as positive excision margins or extensive nodal involvement. Definitive irradiation to doses >55 Gy may be considered as an alternative to extensive surgery in the elderly or infirm (76).

Sequelae of Skin Irradiation

Treatment of most skin cancers requires doses and fractionation schemes that destroy the basal layers of the epidermis but spare the underlying dermis. Erythema is the earliest noticeable radiation effect; its appearance depends on dose, field size, fractionation regimen, and beam quality. Dry desquamation, or peeling, occurs at intermediate dose levels. Moist desquamation is expected at doses required to control skin cancers. The eradication of all basal cells of the epidermis results in exposure of the dermis and serous oozing from the surface. Epidermal regrowth occurs from the field periphery and from more resistant epithelial cells around hair follicles in the field.

Management of acute radiation reactions includes avoidance of trauma to the skin, such as shaving, scratching, or sun exposure. The skin should be cleansed with mild soap and patted dry. Application of creams, cosmetics, or harsh cleansers, especially those containing alcohol, should be avoided. A mild steroid cream such as 1% hydrocortisone or 0.025% triamcinolone treats skin erythema and dry desquamation and relieves pruritis. Moist reactions may be treated with dilute hydrogen peroxide or 1% aqueous gentian violet to dry the lesion and prevent infection. Silver sulfadiazine 1% cream also is commonly used to treat moist desquamation and promote healing.

The new skin formed after irradiation is thin and atrophic and easily injured by mechanical trauma, chemical or sun exposure, or reirradiation. Capillaries are reduced in number and dilated, resulting in telangiectasia formation. Whereas irradiation initially may cause hyperpigmentation by melanocyte stimulation, cancerocidal doses result in permanent hypopigmentation from melanocyte destruction. Permanent hair loss is dose-dependent and usually follows radiation therapy for skin cancer. Deeper-penetrating, skin-sparing megavoltage irradiation often results in subcutaneous fibrosis. Sebaceous and sweat glands show decreased or absent function in the treated area after therapy for skin cancer.

References

1. Akhtar S, Oza KK, Wright J. Merkel cell carcinoma: report of 10 cases and review of the literature. *J Am Acad Dermatol* 2000;43:755–767.
2. Alam M, Ratner D. Cutaneous squamous-cell carcinoma. *N Engl J Med* 2001;344:975–983.
3. Allen PJ, Bowne WB, Jaques DP, et al. Merkel cell carcinoma: prognosis and treatment of patients from a single institution. *J Clin Oncol* 2005;23:2300–2309.
4. Anderson TD, Weber RS, Guerry D, et al. Desmoplastic neurotropic melanoma of the head and neck: the role of radiation therapy. *Head Neck* 2002;24:1068–1071.
5. Bafaloukos D, Gogas H. The treatment of brain metastases in melanoma patients. *Cancer Treat Rev* 2004;30:515–520.
6. Balch CM, Soong S-J, Atkins MB, et al. An evidence-based staging system for cutaneous melanoma. *CA Cancer J Clin* 2004;54:131–149.
7. Ballo MT, Ang KK. Radiation therapy for malignant melanoma. *Surg Clin North Am* 2003;83:323–342.
8. Ballo MT, Ang KK. Radiotherapy for cutaneous malignant melanoma: rationale and Indications. *Oncology* 2004;18:99–107.
9. Ballo MT, Strom EA, Zagars GK, et al. Adjuvant irradiation for axillary metastases from malignant melanoma. *Int J Radiat Oncol Biol Phys* 2002;52:964–972.
10. Ballo MT, Zagars GK, Gershenwald JE, et al. A critical assessment of adjuvant radiotherapy for inguinal lymph node metastases from melanoma. *Ann Surg Oncol* 2004;11:1079–1084.
11. Ballo MT, Zagars GK, Pisters P, et al. The role of radiation therapy in the management of dermatofibrosarcoma protuberans. *Int J Radiat Oncol Biol Phys* 1998;40:823–827.
12. Bastiaannet E, Beukema JC, Hoekstra HJ. Radiation therapy following lymph node dissection in melanoma patients: treatment, outcome and complications. *Cancer Treat Rev* 2005;31:18–26.
13. Beenken SW, Urist MM. Treatment options for Merkel cell carcinoma. *J Natl Compr Canc Netw* 2004;2:89–92.
14. Bonnen MD, Ballo MT, Myers JN, et al. Elective radiotherapy provides regional control for patients with cutaneous melanoma of the head and neck. *Cancer* 2004;100:383–389.
15. Brown MD. Recognition and management of unusual cutaneous tumors. *Dermatol Clin* 2000;18:543–551.
16. Chamberlain RS, Huber K, White JC, et al. Apocrine gland carcinoma of the axilla: Review of the literature and recommendations for treatment. *Am J Clin Oncol* 1999;22:131–135.
17. Cho E, Rosner BA, Feskanich D, et al. Risk factors and individual probabilities of melanoma for whites. *J Clin Oncol* 2005;23:2669–2675.
18. Choo R, Woo T, Assaad D, et al. What is the microscopic tumor extent beyond clinically delineated gross tumor boundary in nonmelanoma skin cancers? *Int J Radiat Oncol Biol Phys* 2005;62:1096–1099.
19. Clayman GL, Lee JJ, Holsinger FC, et al. Mortality risk from squamous cell skin cancer. *J Clin Oncol* 2005;23:759–765.
20. Conill C, Toscas I, Morilla I, et al. Radiation therapy as a curative treatment in extraocular sebaceous carcinoma. *Br J Dermatol* 2003;149:441–442.
21. Cooper JS. Radiation therapy of malignant melanoma. *Dermatol Clin* 2002;20:713–716.
22. Dogan R, Morris C, Zlotecki, et al. Radiotherapy in the treatment of dermatofibrosarcoma protuberans. *Am J Clin Oncol* 2005;28:537–539.
23. DeBuys HV, Levy SB, Murray JC, et al. Modern approaches to photoprotection. *Dermatol Clin* 2000;18:577–590.
24. De Hertog SAE, Wensveen CAH, Bastiaens MT, et al. Relation between smoking and skin cancer. *J Clin Oncol* 2001;19:231–238.
25. Delaney G, Barton M, Jacob S. Estimation of an optimal radiotherapy utilization rate for melanoma: a review of the evidence. *Cancer* 2004;100:1293–1301.
26. DuBay D, Cimmino V, Lowe L, et al. Low recurrence rate after surgery for dermatofibrosarcoma protuberans: A multidisciplinary approach from a single institution. *Cancer* 2004;100:1008–1016.
27. Dupree MT, Kiteley RA, Weismantle K, et al. Radiation therapy for Bowen's disease: Lessons for lesions of the lower extremity. *J Am Acad Dermatol* 2001;45:401–404.
28. Eng TY, Gaguib M, Fuller CD, et al. Treatment of recurrent merkel cell carcinoma: an analysis of 46 cases. *Am J Clin Oncol* 2004;27:576–583.
29. Fife KM, Colman MH, Stevens GN, et al. Determinants of outcome in melanoma patients with cerebral metastases. *J Clin Oncol* 2004;22:1293–1300.
30. Gallagher RP. Sunscreens in melanoma and skin cancer prevention. *J Can Med Assoc* 2005;173:244–245.
31. Goessling W, McKee PH, Mayer RJ. Merkel cell carcinoma. *J Clin Oncol* 2002;20:588–598.
32. Goggins WB, Tsao H. A population-based analysis of risk factors for a second primary cutaneous melanoma among melanoma survivors. *Cancer* 2003;97:639–643.

33. Gollard R, Weber R, Kosty MP, et al. Merkel cell carcinoma: review of 22 cases with surgical, pathologic, and therapeutic considerations. *Cancer* 2000;88:1842–1851.

34. Guix B, Finestres F, Tello JI, et al. Treatment of skin carcinomas of the face by high-dose-rate brachytherapy and custom-made surface molds. *Int J Radiat Biol Phys* 2000;47:95–102.

35. Harari PM, Shimm DS, Bangert JL, et al. The role of radiotherapy in the treatment of malignant sweat gland neoplasms. *Cancer* 1990;65:1737–1740.

36. Jemal A, Murray T, Ward E, et al. Cancer statistics 2005. *CA Cancer J Clin* 2005; 55:10–30.

37. Kennedy C, Bajdik CD, Willemze R, et al. The influence of painful sunburns and lifetime sun exposure on the risk of actinic keratoses, seborrheic warts, melanocytic nevi, atypical nevi, and skin cancer. *J Invest Dermatol* 2003;120:1087–1093.

38. Lee RJ, Gibbs JF, Proulx GM, et al. Nodal basin recurrence following lymph node dissection for melanoma: implications for adjuvant radiotherapy. *Int J Radiat Oncol Biol Phys* 2000;46:467–474.

39. Lichter AD, Karagas MR, Mott LA, et al. Therapeutic ionizing radiation and the incidence of basal cell carcinoma and squamous cell carcinoma. *Arch Dermatol* 2000;136:1007–1011.

40. Liu FF, Maki E, Warde P, et al. A management approach to incompletely excised basal cell carcinomas of skin. *Int J Radiat Oncol Biol Phys* 1991;20:423–429.

41. Livestro DP, Muzikansky A, Kaine EM, et al. Biology of desmoplastic melanoma: a case-control comparison with other melanomas. *J Clin Oncol* 2005;23:6739–6746.

42. Locke J, Karimpour S, Young G, et al. Radiotherapy for epithelial skin cancer. *Int J Radiat Oncol Biol Phys* 2001;51:748–755.

43. Lukas VanderSpek LAL, Pond GR, Wells W, et al. Radiation therapy for Bowen's disease of the skin. *Int J Radiat Oncol Biol Phys* 2005;63:505–510.

44. McCord MW, Mendenhall WM, Parsons JT, et al. Skin cancer of the head and neck with clinical perineural invasion. *Int J Radiat Oncol Biol Phys* 2000;47:89–93.

45. McCord MW, Mendenhall WM, Parsons JT, et al. Skin cancer of the head and neck with incidental microscopic perineural invasion. *Int J Radiat Oncol Biol Phys* 1999;43:591–595.

46. McWilliams RR, Brown PD, Buckner JC, et al. Treatment of brain metastases from melanoma. *Mayo Clin Proc* 2003;78:1529–1536.

47. Mendenhall WM, Mendenhall CM, Mendenhall NP. Merkel cell carcinoma. *Laryngoscope* 2004;114:906–910.

48. Mendenhall WM, Ziotecki RA, Scarborough MT. Dermatofibrosarcoma protuberans. *Cancer* 2004;101:2503–2508.

49. Million RR, Cassisi NJ. *Management of head and neck cancer,* 2nd ed. Philadelphia: JB Lippincott; 1994: 672.

50. Morris KT, Marquez CM, Holland JM, et al. Prevention of local recurrence after surgical debulking of nodal and subcutaneous melanoma deposits by hypofractionated radiation. *Ann Surg Oncol* 2000;7:680–684.

51. Morrison WH, Garden AS, Ang KK. Radiation therapy for nonmelanoma skin carcinoma. *Clin Plast Surg* 1997;24:719–729.

52. Moss WT, Stevens KR, Garcia R. Skin cancer in treatment planning. In: Khan FM, Potish RA, eds. *Radiation oncology.* Baltimore, MD: Williams & Wilkins, 1998: 449–458.

53. Pardo FS, Wang CC, Albert D, et al. Sebaceous carcinoma of the ocular adnexa: radiotherapeutic management. *Int J Radiat Oncol Biol Phys* 1989;17: 643–647.

54. Perez CA. Management of incompletely excised carcinoma of the skin. *Int J Radiat Oncol Biol Phys* 1991;20:903–904.

55. Reeves ME, Coit DG. Melanoma: a multidisciplinary approach for the general surgeon. *Surg Clin North Am* 2000;80:581–601.

56. Rio E, Bardet E, Ferron C, et al. Interstitial brachytherapy of periorificial skin carcinomas of the face: a retrospective study of 97 cases. *Int J Radiat Oncol Biol Phys* 2005;63:753–757.

57. Saga, K. Histochemical and immunohistochemical markers for human eccrine and apocrine sweat glands: an aid for histopathologic differentiation for sweat gland tumors. *J Investigative Dermatol* 2001;6:49–53.

58. Sause WT, Cooper JS, Rush S, et al: Fraction size in external beam radiation therapy in the treatment of melanoma. *Int J Radiat Oncol Biol Phys* 1991;20:429–432.

59. Schmid-Wendtner MH, Brunner B, Konz B, et al. Fractionated radiotherapy of lentigo maligna and lentigo maligna melanoma in 64 patients. *J Am Acad Dermatol* 2000;43:477–482.

60. Schwarze HP, Loche F, Lamant L, et al. Microcystic adnexal carcinoma induced by multiple radiation therapy. *Int J Dermatol* 2000;39:363–382.

61. Shields JA, Demirci H, Marr BP, et al. Sebaceous carcinoma of the ocular region: a review. *Surv Opthalmol* 2005;50:103–122.

62. Shiu AS, Tung SG, Gastorf RJ, et al. Dosimetric evaluation of lead and tungsten eye shields in electron beam treatment. *Int J Radiat Oncol Biol Phys* 1996;35:599–604.

63. Silva JJ, Tsang RW, Panzarella T, et al. Results of radiotherapy for epithelial skin cancer of the pinna: the Princess Margaret Hospital experience, 1983-1993. *Int J Radiat Oncol Biol Phys* 2000;47:451–459.

64. Smith DE, Messina JI, Perrott R, et al. Clinical approach to neuroendocrine carcinoma of the skin (Merkel cell carcinoma). *Cancer Control* 2000;7:72–83.

65. Stein JM, Ormsby A, Esclamado R, et al. The effect of radiation therapy on microcystic adnexal carcinoma: a case report. *Head Neck* 2003;25(3):251–254.

66. Stevens G, Thompson JF, Firth I, et al. Locally advanced melanoma: results of postoperative hypofractionated radiation therapy. *Cancer* 2000;88:88–94.

67. Sun LM, Wang CJ, Huang CC, et al. Dermatofibrosarcoma protuberans: treatment results of 35 cases. *Radiother Oncol* 2000;57:175–181.

68. Svoboda VH, Kovarik J, Morris F. High dose-rate microselectron molds in the treatment of skin tumors. *Int J Radiat Oncol Biol Phys* 1995;31:967–972.

69. The NCCN basal cell and squamous cell skin cancers clinical practice guidelines in oncology. *J Natl Compr Canc Netw* 2004;2:6–27.

70. The NCCN dermatofibrosarcoma protuberans clinical practice guidelines in oncology. *J Natl Compr Canc Netw* 2004;74–78.

71. The NCCN melanoma clinical practice guidelines in oncology. *J Natl Compr Canc Netw* 2004;2:46–60.

72. The NCCN Merkel cell carcinoma clinical practice guidelines in oncology. *J Natl Compr Canc Netw* 2004: 80–87.

73. Tsao H, Atkins MB, Sober AJ. Management of cutaneous melanoma. *New Engl J Med* 2004;351:998–1012.

74. Voutsadakis IA, Bruckner HW. Eccrine sweat gland carcinoma: a case report and review of diagnosis and treatment. *Conn Med* 2000;64:263–266.

75. Wong JR, Wang CC. Radiation therapy in the management of cutaneous malignancies. *Clin Dermatol* 2001;19:348–353.

76. Yen MT, Tse DT, Wu X, et al. Radiation therapy for local control of eyelid sebaceous cell carcinoma: report of two cases and review of the literature. *Ophthal Plast Reconstr Surg* 2000;16:211–215.

77. Youker SR. Merkel cell carcinoma. *Adv Dermatol* 2003;19:185–205.

Clinical Radiation Oncology

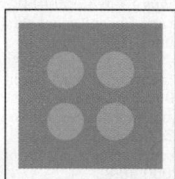

Chapter 31
Malignant Neoplasms Associated with the Acquired Immunodeficiency Syndrome

Bernadine R. Donahue, Jay S. Cooper

We cannot deal with AIDS by making moral judgments or refusing to face unpleasant facts, and still less by stigmatizing those who are infected.

—Kofi Annan, U. N. Secretary General

HIV Infection

One of the greatest public health challenges of the last half of the 20th century was the emergence of the human immunodeficiency virus (HIV). Although the biology of the virus has been elucidated, diagnostic tests have been created, and effective drugs and care systems have been established, HIV remains an epidemic in the 21st century, particularly in the developing world. HIV infection, immunosuppression, and enhanced tumor growth characterize the acquired immunodeficiency syndrome (AIDS). In 1981, a lead article in the *New England Journal of Medicine* described the unexpected occurrence of *Pneumocystis jiroveci* pneumonia in previously healthy homosexual men (80), and soon the medical establishment, as well as society as a whole, was forced to react to the protean consequences of HIV infection. At that time, a diagnosis of (what was later to be named) AIDS was tantamount to a rapidly imposed death sentence. Twenty years later, medical progress yielded another lead article in the same journal that reported the feasibility of discontinuing prophylaxis against *Pneumocystis jiroveci* in patients who already had AIDS, if they received the newly developed, so-called highly active antiretroviral therapy (HAART) (112).

Modification of high-risk behaviors, HIV screening, early diagnosis, institution of HAART, and the development of effective treatments for HIV-associated infections and malignancies have reduced the number of deaths from AIDS in the United States by 70% since 1995 (34). Despite this progress, AIDS remains a "worldwide health catastrophe" (151). Over 20 million people have died of AIDS since 1981 (166). At the start of the current millennium, over 90% of HIV-infected individuals worldwide had little or no access to life-sustaining antiretroviral and protease inhibitor "triple-drug" combinations (81).

It has been estimated that, despite the reduction in HIV-related mortality and morbidity with HAART as proven in randomized trials, only 1 million of the estimated 40 million people infected with HIV worldwide are receiving this treatment (148). In December 2003, the World Health Organization and the United Nations launched the "3 by 5" global target to provide antiretroviral treatment to 3 million people living with HIV/AIDS in developing countries by the end of 2005. This was a vital step toward the ultimate goal of providing universal access of integrated HIV/AIDS services to all who need them (162). The problem, however, is daunting. It is estimated that 40 million people currently are infected (167). Sub-Saharan Africa has just over 10% of the world's population, but is home to more than 60% of all people living with HIV. In 2005, some 8.3 million people were living with HIV in Asia. Worldwide, almost 5 million people became infected with HIV in 2005 (167). Without a major change, they too will soon be dead of AIDS.

Although the toll of HIV infection in the United States can be viewed as relatively small in comparison to Africa, the statistics are nevertheless devastating in absolute terms. As of 2005, more than half a million Americans have died of AIDS (68). Furthermore, recent data suggest a resurgence of HIV infection in young urban homosexuals in the United States (33). The estimated number of people living with HIV in the United States at the end of 2003 exceeded 1 million for the first time (167). Particularly worrisome are estimates that suggest that up to half of all HIV-infected persons in the United States currently are not receiving optimal care (24). For some, the monetary cost of HAART is prohibitive, while for others, the toxicity associated with HAART is unbearable. More deaths are therefore likely.

If there is "good news" it is that where comprehensive medical care is available and when the side effects of HAART are tolerable, the picture has become brighter. In such settings, AIDS has become *almost* a chronic condition. The development of progressively more effective triple-drug antiretroviral therapies, including protease inhibitors, has dramatically influenced the replication of HIV (often decreasing the viral load to undetectable levels) and slowed the progression of AIDS (130). Highly active antiretroviral therapy has also produced a marked decrease in AIDS-related infectious complications and resultant mortality. Unfortunately, initial hopes that HAART could eradicate HIV infection have not been realized, and cure remains only a hope (153). Even in patients whose blood appears to be free of HIV for more than 2 years, uniformly rapid reappearance of virus occurs after HAART is discontinued. Thus our progress has not rendered HIV medically unimportant even for those victims who can afford and tolerate HAART.

HIV infection therefore needs to be addressed in two substantially different clinical scenarios: a more virulent illness without HAART and a more chronic one with HAART. Consequently, to provide a more complete picture of AIDS-associated neoplasms throughout this chapter, we will attempt to discuss the issues relevant, and therapies available, to HIV-infected individuals in both circumstances. This chapter represents the current state-of-the-art. As evidenced by developments over the past 25 years, it must be remembered that AIDS is not a static disease and that both its associated morbidities as well as treatments evolve over time. However, many of the basic principles of its management remain steadfast.

HIV-Associated Malignancies

Two decades after the initial descriptions of AIDS, the manifestations of infection with and treatment of the human immunodeficiency virus continue to evolve. Although the most common source of morbidity and mortality from AIDS has been opportunistic infections, AIDS-associated malignancy is a well-recognized, not-infrequent, and potentially lethal consequence of the disease.

Early in the epidemic, three types of malignancies showed a sufficiently increased incidence that they qualified as AIDS-defining conditions when they occurred in conjunction with HIV infection: Kaposi's sarcoma (KS), non-Hodgkin's lymphoma (NHL), and carcinoma of the uterine cervix. In 1981, the appearance of Kaposi's sarcoma in young homosexual men heralded the association tumors and HIV infection (29). Intermediate- or high-grade B-cell lymphomas in HIV-infected individuals were classified as AIDS-defining events in 1985 (31). Cervical carcinoma was recognized in 1993 as an AIDS-defining illness for HIV-infected women (32). The incidence of Hodgkin's disease and anal carcinomas has been thought by some to be increased in HIV-infected people (88), as have unusual pediatric age malignancies in HIV-infected children (15). Data reported from the AIDS-Cancer Match Registry Study (including more than 300,000 adult persons with HIV/AIDS) demonstrated the expected increased relative risks of developing the three AIDS-defining tumors (69). In addition, the data suggested an increase in Hodgkin's disease, particularly mixed cellularity and lymphocyte depletion subtypes, and to a lesser degree squamous cell lip cancer and testicular seminoma. Some other tumors were also more frequent than expected; however, these increases might be explicable by other factors (lung cancer by smoking; penile cancer by frequent exposure to human papillomavirus (HPV); soft tissue malignancies by miscoding of Kaposi's sarcoma). A study of non–AIDS-defining cancers in a cohort of 4,144 HIV-infected U.S. Department of Defense beneficiaries, revealed higher rates of skin cancers (melanoma and squamous and basal cell carcinomas), prostate and anal carcinomas, and Hodgkin's disease among the HIV-infected cohort as compared with age-adjusted rates for the general U.S. population (25).

We have chosen to include Hodgkin's disease, anal carcinoma, and unusual pediatric-age malignancies in this chapter, if for no other reason than the behavior of these diseases in association with AIDS warrants comment, realizing that they currently are not strictly defined as AIDS-related tumors.

AIDS-Defining Malignancies in the HAART Era

HAART was introduced in the last half of the 1990s and had a profound effect on the prognosis of HIV-infected individuals. Currently, HAART usually consists of a two-drug nucleoside analog backbone administered with either a protease inhibitor or a nonnucleoside reverse transcriptase inhibitor.

HAART has exerted an uneven effect on the development of malignancies. The incidence of Kaposi's sarcoma and non-Hodgkin's lymphoma has declined substantially since the development of HAART, but, thus far, there has been no major change in the incidence of cervical cancer or Hodgkin's disease (89). In fact, there is a suggestion that the numbers of non–AIDS-defining cancers are increasing (19).

This chapter is subsequently organized by histologic type of HIV-associated malignancy. Epidemiology, patterns of disease, pathology, diagnostic evaluation, treatment, and prognosis are included. The use of radiation as it relates specifically to each malignancy in the setting of HIV is discussed. For additional details regarding the *delivery* of radiation, the specific chapters within this volume addressing each neoplasm should be consulted.

Lymphoma

The incidence of lymphoma in association with HIV infection is approximately 60 to 100 times greater than expected in the general population (10,16). Although primary central nervous system lymphoma (PCNSL) was one of the initial Centers for Disease Control–approved criteria for a diagnosis of AIDS (30), the inclusion of systemic high-grade B-cell lymphoma did not occur until 1985 (31). Epstein-Barr virus (EBV) was implicated in its etiology by the finding of anti-EBV immunoglobulins and circulating EBV-infected B cells in the setting of HIV (99). However, additional factors probably need to be present to cause malignant transformation of B cells, such as c-myc gene rearrangements (101). Where available, HAART appears to have decreased the incidence of non-Hodgkin's lymphoma. The overall adjusted incidence per 1,000 person-years in the HIV seropositive population decreased from 6.2 from 1992 through 1996 to 3.6 from 1997 through 1999 (89). However, unlike the effect on Kaposi's sarcoma, it is not clear if HAART has improved the outcome of therapy of patients who develop AIDS-NHL (106,117).

Primary Central Nervous System Non-Hodgkin's Lymphoma

Epidemiology and Risk Factors

The incidence of PCNSL increased steadily after the onset of the AIDS epidemic. At its height, the incidence of non-Hodgkin's lymphomas originating in the brain without evidence of systemic involvement in persons with AIDS was 3,600-fold higher than in the general population (53). It appears that HAART has decreased the high risk of developing this disorder in persons who are infected with HIV. One series from an urban medical center reported a 67% decline in biopsy proven central nervous system (CNS) lymphoma between 1995 and 1997, corresponding with the introduction of HAART (145). Another series showed that, among persons living with AIDS, the average annual incidence of PCNSL decreased from 8.4 per 1,000 person-years pre-HAART to 1.1 per 1,000 person-years post-HAART (56).

Patterns of Disease

In most patients who have HIV-associated PCNSL, the diagnosis is suggested by the onset of headaches or a change in mental status (59). In our series, 25% presented with headaches and more than half the patients presented with change in mental status (57). Nearly one-third had motor or sensory abnormalities. Unfortunately, PCNSL can be clinically and radiographically indistinguishable from other pathologic processes (most notably toxoplasmosis) in HIV-infected patients. In general, the typical radiographic findings are that of multiple contrast-enhancing lesions, often, but not exclusively, in a periventricular location (Fig. 31.1).

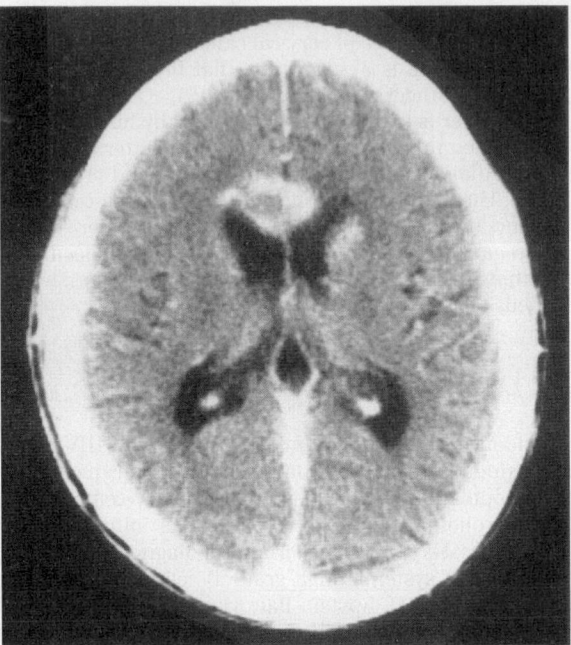

FIGURE 31.1. Example of periventricular location of human immunodeficiency virus–associated primary central nervous system lymphoma.

Diagnostic Work-Up

Prior to HAART, it was common for an HIV-infected patient to present with a clinical and radiographic picture that could be consistent with either toxoplasmosis or PCNSL. A "negative" toxoplasmosis titer did not eliminate the diagnosis of toxoplasmosis, and similarly a "positive" toxoplasmosis titer did not preclude the presence of PCNSL (113,136). Because there was a high incidence of toxoplasmosis in the HIV-infected population, the standard first-line treatment for an HIV-infected patient who developed a neurologic abnormality and had a radiographically visible brain lesion consistent with either toxoplasmosis or CNS lymphoma was the institution of antitoxoplasmosis antibiotics. During the first decade of the epidemic, it was common to administer *empiric* cranial radiation therapy in patients who did not manifest clinical or radiographic improvement by the second or third week of antitoxoplasmosis treatment. However, as our knowledge of the myriad HIV-related opportunistic infections expanded and the poor outcome with this empiric approach was recognized, the emphasis shifted to recommending biopsy (stereotactically if necessary) for definitive diagnosis (52).

Standardized guidelines for the baseline evaluation and response assessment of PCNSL have been established by the International PCNSL Collaborative Group. Extent-of-disease evaluation should include gadolinium-enhanced MRI, lumbar puncture for cerebrospinal fluid (CSF) cytology, unless medically contraindicated, detailed ophthalmological examination, computed tomography (CT) scans of the chest, abdomen, and pelvis, bone marrow biopsy with aspirate, and consideration of testicular ultrasound (1).

Pathology and Prognostic Factors

The majority of primary CNS lymphomas are B-cell large immunoblastic types, and EBV DNA is identifiable in nearly all cases (85). Polymerase chain reaction amplification of EBV DNA in the CSF is usually positive in these patients and may become negative following treatment.[3] In general, PCNSL is seen later in the course of HIV infection than is systemic non-Hodgkin's lymphoma. Patients usually have CD4 counts <50 cells per cubic millimeter before PCNSL becomes evident (103). Although the overall median survival of these patients is poor, patients no older than 35 years who have Karnofsky performance scores of at least 80% tend to survive 5 to 6 months, rather than the 2 months typically observed in less favorable subgroups (50).

General Management

Radiation therapy of the brain and meninges has been the mainstay of treatment for HIV-associated PCNSL. It has been suggested that the institution of HAART may result in regression of existing PCNSL, but to date scant evidence exists to support this claim (23,49,119).

Methotrexate-based chemotherapy has been shown to prolong the median survival in immunocompetent patients who have PCNSL (2), however, many HIV-infected patients who are sufficiently immunosuppressed to develop PCNSL may be unable to tolerate this approach. In the pre-HAART era, Jacomet et al. (90) reported a trial of high-dose methotrexate in patients with AIDS; median survival (in the 10 patients with biopsy-proven PCNSL) was 2.5 months. This is markedly different from the median survival of 41 months reported in immunocompetent patients treated with methotrexate-based chemotherapy (2). Newer agents such as temozolomide, an alkylating agent, and rituximab, a human-mouse chimeric anti-CD20 antibody, are being studied by the RTOG for the treatment of PCNSL in immunocompetent patients (RTOG 0227), but these agents have not yet been tested on a large scale for HIV–associated PCNSL.

Radiation

Various regimens of radiotherapy have been employed, and there is unquestionable clinical and radiographic evidence of tumor response (Fig. 31.2A,B). However, regardless of the nature of the course of radiation therapy delivered (a short palliative-intent course of 3,000 cGy in 10 fractions over 2 weeks versus a more definitive-intent course of 5,000 cGy, delivered in 180 to 200 cGy per fraction over 5 to 6 weeks), mean overall survival has been in the range of 2 to 5 months (3,8,50,57,67,79,95,111,139). Therefore, brief regimens such as 3,000 cGy in 10 fractions or 3,500 cGy in 15 fractions continue to be used widely (51). The irradiated volume typically includes the cranial meninges and posterior orbits.

Results of treatment of HIV-associated PCNSL from multiple series uniformly are poor (Table 31.1). The strategy of up-front chemotherapy that has proven successful in immunocompetent patients has not been shown to produce comparable benefit in this setting. In 1994 the Eastern Cooperative Oncology Group, the Radiation Therapy Oncology Group (RTOG), the Cancer and Acute Leukemia Group B, and the AIDS Clinical Trials Group jointly embarked on a prospective phase II trial utilizing CHOD (cyclophosphamide, doxorubicin, vincristine, and dexamethasone) for one cycle followed by 3,000 cGy in 12 fractions to the whole brain plus 1,000 cGy in four fractions to the radiographically evident lesion(s) plus a margin. Median survival was 2.4 months in 34 patients, with seven patients dying prior to completion of radiotherapy (3).

The majority of these series predate the use of HAART, and it remains to be determined what the precise influence of aggressive antiretroviral treatment will be on the outcome of patients with this diagnosis. There are anecdotal reports of regression of PCNSL with the institution of HAART (23,49,119). However, to date, this remains the exception and not the rule. Nevertheless, there is a suggestion that the addition of HAART to radiation therapy may improve outcome. Cohort data from Australia showed that in a subset analysis of 47 patients with biopsy-proven PCNSL, antiretroviral therapy with at least two

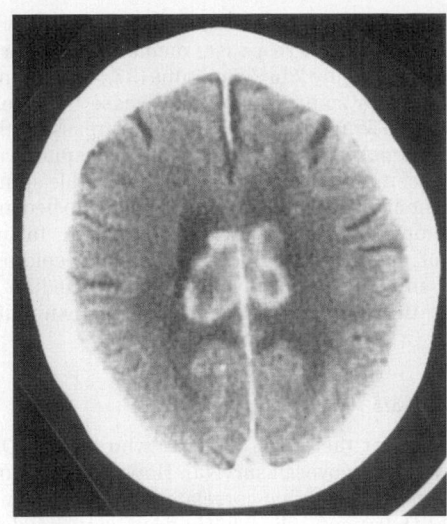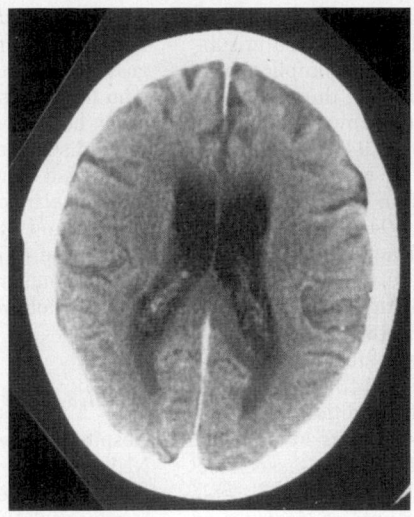

FIGURE 31.2. Example of human immunodeficiency virus–associated primary central nervous system lymphoma before (**A**) and after (**B**) cranial radiation.

agents along with radiation therapy were associated with better survival (125).

Additionally, it is possible that the improved immune function that results from HAART may allow for more aggressive treatment of PCNSL. A review of registry data from San Diego showed that 9% of these patients received chemotherapy in the pre-HAART era compared with 18% post-HAART (56). In essence, HAART appears to have decreased the incidence of HIV-associated PCNSL; however, its effect on the outcome of the disease that does occur is uncertain.

Systemic Non-Hodgkin's Lymphoma

Epidemiology and Risk Factor

Although lymphoma has been the initial AIDS-defining illness in 3% of HIV-infected persons, it is the cause of death in 16% to 20% of these patients (107). Multivariate analysis has shown an increased risk of lymphoma correlating with the duration of immunosuppression, CD4 count 1 year prior to the diagnosis of NHL, and B-cell stimulation (83). The observed fall in the incidence of NHL with the introduction of HAART appears to be secondary to an overall decrease in the proportion of patients with low CD4 counts. In a study using a French hospital database, the incidence decreased from 8.6 per 1,000 person-years in the pre-HAART era to 4.3 per 1,000 person-years post-HAART; however, there was no change in the incidence within strata of

patients with similar CD4 counts during these two time periods (14). Furthermore, it appears that non-nucleoside transcriptase inhibitor-based HAART is as protective as protease inhibitor-based HAART, and more protective than nucleoside analogues alone (20,149).

Diagnosis

Rapidly developing adenopathy and/or constitutional B symptoms (fevers, unexplained weight loss, night sweats) are the most common presentations of HIV-associated systemic NHL. Nearly 75% of all patients will present with advanced-stage disease (stage III or IV) and most will manifest B symptomatology (141). Diagnosis generally is obtained from the biopsy of a clinically suspicious peripheral lymph node. The most common histologic subtypes are high-grade B-cell lymphoma or Burkitt's lymphoma; however, intermediate-grade (diffuse large cell type) lymphomas are not uncommon. As patients who have AIDS NHL frequently have extranodal involvement, staging evaluation should include chest, abdomen, and pelvic computerized tomograms, bone marrow biopsy, and CSF analysis.

Treatment

Early in the AIDS epidemic, treatment for AIDS-NHL lymphoma was based on high-dose chemotherapy regimens that

			OUTCOME OF TREATMENT IN HIV-ASSOCIATED PRIMARY CENTRAL NERVOUS SYSTEM LYMPHOMA		
Series (Reference)	**Number of Patients/ All Biopsied?**	**Chemotherapy**	**Median Radiation Dose (cGy)/ Number of Fractions**	**Percentage with Clinical Response**	**Median Survival (months)**
New York University (57)	20/no	no	3,000/10	73	2.1
New York University (59)	32/no	no	3,000/10	50	2.1
University of California San Francisco (111)	41/no	no	4,000/15	71	3.2
Montefiore-Einstein (79)	17/yes	no	3,500/10	60	2.4
University of Southern California (67)	10/yes	IT MTX (1 patient) Post RT BACOD (1 pt)	4,200/21	70	5.5
Multi-institution (51)	163/no	no	3,000/10	53	—
Intergroup (3)	34/yes	Pre RT CHOD	4,000/16	—	2.4
Multi-institution (125)	111/no	no	range <3,000 to >3,000	—	1.6

BACOD, bleomycin, doxorubicin, cyclophosphamide, vincristine and dexamethasone; CHOD, cyclophosphamide, doxorubicin, vincristine, dexamethasone; IT MTX,; RT, radiation therapy

had been developed for non-AIDS-related lymphomas (74,92). These treatments were not well tolerated and resulted in substantial toxicity, as well as high rates of infectious complications, both opportunistic and bacterial. Subsequently, therapy relied on attenuated doses of cytotoxic chemotherapy or standard-dose chemotherapy plus cytokine support (11,94,104,108,109). Most studies reported complete remission rates of approximately 50%, but median survivals of only 6 to 7 months and 1-year survivals of approximately 25% (94). Further study helped to define a regimen with high efficacy with acceptable toxicity using infusional cyclophosphamide, doxorubicin, and etoposide (CDE). A multicenter trial employing this regimen has shown that the median 1-year survival of 48% achieved with CDE is approximately twice as high as was achievable with previously standard regimens (e. g., m-BACOD) (146).

Some retrospective data suggest that the addition of HAART to cytotoxic chemotherapy significantly lengthens overall survival (by a factor of 10) for patients who have AIDS-associated NHL (17). However, other data are contradictory (117), and further study will be needed to clarify the precise influence of HAART on HIV-associated systemic NHL.

CNS prophylaxis with intrathecal chemotherapy has been controversial in the setting of high grade NHL and HIV infection, but frequently was used, especially in patients with extranodal disease. However, it appears that patients who do not have EBV-infected tumors may not require such prophylaxis. In one Italian study of 50 patients who had newly diagnosed AIDS-associated NHL, all patients with CNS involvement had EBV-infected tumors, and all but one had EBV DNA in the CSF (41). The risk of CNS involvement was 10 times higher in patients who were EBV positive, as compared with those who were EBV negative. It may be that prophylaxis can be reserved for a select subset of patients. The sustained-release formulation of intrathecal cytarabine may have an increasingly important role to play in both the prophylaxis and treatment of CNS meningeal involvement (118).

A previously unrecognized form of lymphoma, called primary effusion or body cavity lymphoma, has been identified in HIV-infected patients (5). It accounts for approximately 4% of AIDS-related NHL (143). There appears to be an association with human herpesvirus 8 (HHV-8) (91). Typically, such patients present with an effusion in a body cavity, in the absence of widespread lymphadenopathy. The effusion contains numerous atypical lymphoid cells with a plasmacytoid appearance and an indeterminate (non-B or T cell) immunophenotype and clonal immunoglobulin heavy- and light-chain gene rearrangements. MUM/IRF4 (multiple myeloma 1/interferon regulatory factor 4) protein expression can be used to differentiate primary effusion lymphoma from other lymphomas (27). Survival of patients who have primary effusion lymphoma remains very short, on the order of 2 to 5 months, even with aggressive therapy.

Radiation Therapy

The role of consolidative radiation therapy following systemic treatment in AIDS patients who have NHL has not been evaluated methodically. It has been suggested that radiation should be used as a consolidative boost in patients with bulky disease who have demonstrated slow or partial response to chemotherapy (45,155). More obviously, radiation also is indicated for palliation of bulky lesions.

Radiation therapy is also used to provide palliative therapy for patients who develop lymphomatous meningitis. The majority of these patients have far-advanced AIDS and to minimize further bone marrow suppression (in these already very compromised patients), treatment usually is limited to cranial radiation (not craniospinal) and intrathecal chemotherapy in an attempt to clear the cerebrospinal fluid of malignant cells.

Although this approach has been shown to result in a 60% to 70% clinical and/or cytological response, median time to progression is on the order of only 2 to 2.5 months (37,58). Patients who have grossly evident spinal meningeal disease have generally been treated to a limited volume only encompassing the gross disease and a small margin. Unfortunately, despite brief survival, it is not uncommon for previously undetectable spinal meningeal involvement outside the irradiated volume to become evident and symptomatic prior to the patient's death. In our experience, 40% of patients developed symptomatic epidural spinal metastases either concurrently with, or at a median of 1 month following, the diagnosis of lymphomatous meningitis (58).

Results and Prognosis

Despite our best current therapies, patients who have AIDS-NHL generally have a poor overall survival. However, prognostic factors have been identified that correlate with the length of survival (98,105,114). Patients who have bone marrow involvement, low Karnofsky performance status at diagnosis (<70%), low CD4 counts, and/or a prior diagnosis of AIDS have a median survival on the order of 4 months. Those without these adverse features have a median survival of 11 months. Rossi et al. (140) reported that the International Prognostic Index (IPI), a model designed to predict the outcome of NHL in general, is a reliable prognostic indicator of outcome of patients who have AIDS-related NHL. Both the likelihood of complete response and median survival after treatment correlated appropriately with IPI score. Moreover, the IPI score correlated with the CD4 cell count, suggesting that the degree of immunodeficiency imparted by HIV infection influenced the aggressiveness of non-Hodgkin's lymphomas. More recently, a prognostic model for systemic AIDS-related NHL treated in the era of highly active antiretroviral therapy has been established based solely on the IPI and the CD4 count (20).

NHL remain an important cause of morbidity and mortality in AIDS patients. Registry data from San Diego suggest an improvement in median survival for these patients from approximately 4 months to 9 months after the introduction of HAART (56). There is hope that newer targeted agents, such as rituximab, which has shown an improvement in survival for patients with non HIV-associated NHL, will improve the outcome in HIV-associated NHL. An AIDS Malignancies Consortium phase III trial that randomized patients to CHOP versus CHOP plus rituximab (R-CHOP) showed a higher complete response rate (57%) in the R-CHOP arm as compared with CHOP alone (47%); this, however, was not statistically significant and there was an increased risk of death from infection in the R-CHOP arm (93). To evaluate the efficacy and safety of rituximab for HIV-associated NHL further, an ongoing AIDS Malignancies Consortium (AMC 034) trial is randomizing patients to EPOCH (etoposide, prednisone, vincristine, cyclophosphamide, and doxorubicin) with concurrent rituximab versus EPOCH followed sequentially by rituximab (163).

Hodgkin's Lymphoma

The relationship between Hodgkin's disease and HIV infection is not clearly understood (86). Although there may be an increased risk of Hodgkin's disease in patients who are infected with HIV, this increase is difficult to measure because both illnesses typically occur in the same age population. One Italian study suggested that the incidence of Hodgkin's disease is increasing in HIV-infected persons in the era of HAART (137). A joint Danish and U.S. study of 302,824 HIV-infected (including AIDS) patients between the ages of 15 and 69 years showed a relative risk of 11.5 of developing Hodgkin's disease in HIV-infected individuals (159). Although the precise association of

HIV and Hodgkin's remains to be defined, it is already clear that when Hodgkin's disease occurs in patients who are HIV-infected, it tends to be advanced, associated with B symptoms, and is not likely to be cured (64). Importantly, Hodgkin's disease in HIV-infected individuals can present with unusual manifestations, such as presentation with a gastric or intracranial mass (60,65).

In the past, only 50% of patients had a complete response following combination chemotherapy (4,132). However, more recent data suggest that the outcome may be improving. A phase II study in 59 patients with HIV and Hodgkin's disease (52 of whom also received concurrent HAART) resulted in a complete response rate of 81% with the Stanford V regimen, although 3-year overall survival was only 51% (147). A report from the M.D. Anderson Cancer Center suggests that radiation therapy is appropriate for approximately 50% of HIV-associated Hodgkin's disease, usually in combination with chemotherapy; in that series (with a median follow-up of 64 months) 5-year overall survival was 54% (156).

Kaposi's Sarcoma

Epidemiology and Risk Factors

At the start of the epidemic, AIDS often was identified by the diagnosis of KS, and KS in this setting became known as epidemic Kaposi's sarcoma (EKS). People infected with HIV had at least a 20,000 times greater risk of developing KS than uninfected individuals (9). The discovery that HIV-infected gay or bisexual men were more likely than HIV-infected heterosexual men to develop KS was one of the first clues that KS or its etiologic agent might somehow be sexually transmitted. The hypothesis was later reinforced by the finding that women who acquired HIV infection from bisexual men had an approximately fourfold greater risk of developing KS than women who contracted the virus from either exclusively heterosexual men or intravenous drug users (9).

With the introduction of progressively more effective antiretroviral therapies, the incidence of KS in the United States, as a component of AIDS, has diminished over time. In the early 1980s, approximately 50% of HIV-infected patients were diagnosed as having AIDS on the basis of KS (55). By the early 1990s the incidence of KS as an AIDS-defining illness had fallen to 14% (71,89,102), and the CDC dropped the requirement of KS or other overt illnesses for a diagnosis of AIDS (the most recent definition of AIDS, formulated in 1993, includes HIV-infected persons who have no overt illness but are immunosuppressed to the point of being at risk for an AIDS-defining illness with CD4 <200 cells/uL or <14%) (32). The explanations for this decline in KS incidence include the recognition of other risk groups (e.g., intravenous drug users), changes in the definition of AIDS, and changes in sexual transmission of HIV since the gay community became active in advocating safe-sex practices. However, the decline is most likely attributable to the institution of HAART. A report from the International Collaboration on HIV and Cancer evaluating the cancer incidence from 23 prospective studies that included 47,936 HIV-seropositive individuals from North America, Europe, and Australia showed that the adjusted incidence rate for KS declined from 15.2 in the period of time from 1992 through 1996 to 4.9 between 1997 and 1999 (89). A report from the Swiss HIV Cohort Study showed that the risk of developing KS declined by 66% during the 15 months after HAART was initiated ($p = .001$), as compared to the pre-HAART era (102).

In December 1994, a herpes virus that appeared to be associated with the etiology of KS was identified (38). This was termed human herpesvirus 8 and was also known as KS-associated herpesvirus (KSHV). The virus was detected in both the epidemic (AIDS-related) and endemic (previously typical African) forms of KS, as well as classic (elderly men of Eastern European or Mediterranean ancestry) KS. In a 1996 report from the Multicenter AIDS Cohort Study, antibodies to HHV-8 were detected in 80% of HIV-infected men who subsequently went on to develop KS (72). The antibodies to HHV-8 were identified at a median of 2.5 years prior to any clinical sign of disease. The virus was identified in only 18% of the men who never developed KS. This suggested that KS resulted from infection with HHV-8, rather than being a direct result of HIV itself or to cytokines induced by the HIV virus. It now appears that the high incidence of KS in the early years of the AIDS epidemic was a result of coinfection with both HIV and HHV-8 in the homosexual and bisexual population; HIV produced the immunosuppression that facilitated HHV-8 expression as KS. HHV-8 has a large number of genes that can encode homologues of host genes, many of which are involved in angiogenesis and the cell cycle. Additionally, increased levels of interleukin-6 (IL-6), which is thought to be an important growth factor in HHV-8–associated neoplasms, have been found in tissues affected by HHV-8 (26).

Patterns of Disease

KS is characterized by purplish lesions on the skin or mucosal surfaces. This is a vascular tumor and a number of angiogenic growth factors are produced by KS tumor cells and/or the surrounding supportive network of stromal cells and extracellular matrix. The lesions can be macular, plaquelike, or nodular, with or without associated lymphadenopathy and/or lymphedema (Figs. 31.3–31.12). At presentation, skin lesions can be either single or multiple and may cause pain, bleeding, or disfigurement. As involvement of lymph nodes and lymphatic spaces occurs, progressive edema can result. This is seen most commonly in lesions involving the lower extremity, the inguinal regions, the genitalia, and the face. Visceral KS typically involves the aerodigestive tracts. Oropharyngeal lesions can result in life-threatening airway obstruction. Pulmonary involvement can result in life-threatening respiratory failure. Although we generally advocate biopsy confirmation prior to the initiation of therapy, this is most feasible with skin lesions. Biopsy of visceral lesions may be contraindicated because of the risk of hemorrhage, and in these settings characteristic endoscopic and radiographic findings should be used to establish the diagnosis.

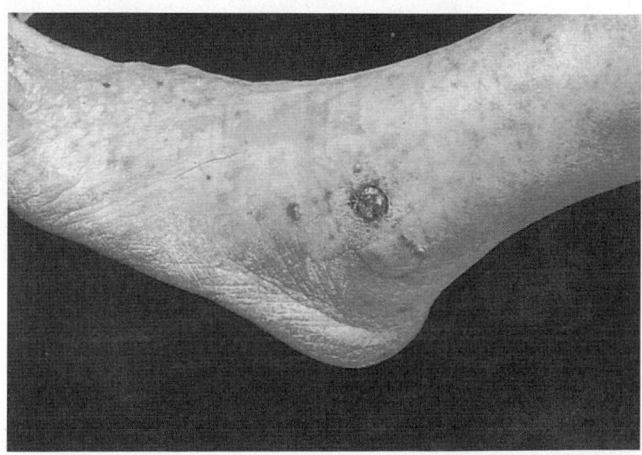

FIGURE 31.3. Purple, 1.5-cm nodular classic Kaposi's sarcoma on the ankle of an elderly man. (From Krigel RL, Friedman-Kien AE. Kaposi's sarcoma of AIDS: diagnosis and treatment. In: DeVita VT Jr., Hellman S, Rosenberg SA, eds. *AIDS: etiology, diagnosis, treatment, and prevention*, 2nd ed. Philadelphia: J.B. Lippincott, 1988, with permission.)

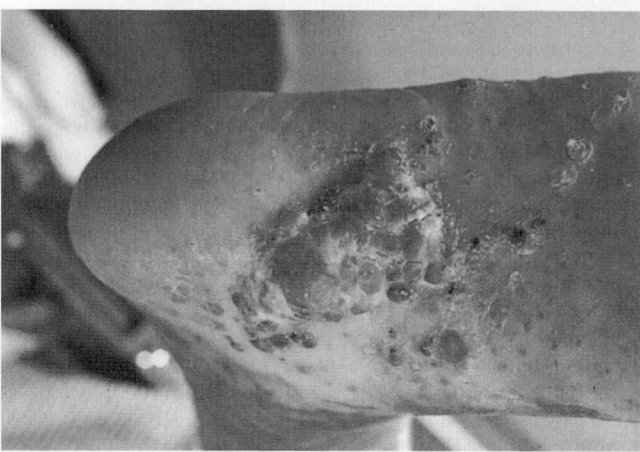

FIGURE 31.4. Classic Kaposi's sarcoma. Multiple red to purple papules on the sole of the foot. (From Krigel RL, Friedman-Kien AE. Kaposi's sarcoma of AIDS: diagnosis and treatment. In: DeVita VT Jr., Hellman S, Rosenberg SA, eds. *AIDS: etiology, diagnosis, treatment, and prevention*, 2nd ed. Philadelphia: J.B. Lippincott, 1988, with permission.)

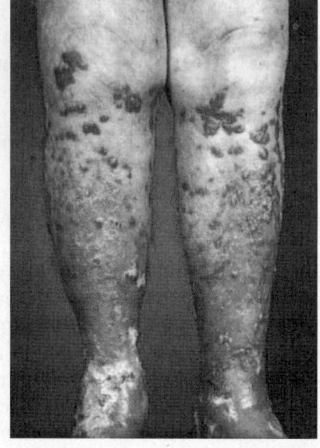

FIGURE 31.6. Extensive superficial and deep Kaposi's sarcoma producing lymphedema. (From Krigel RL, Friedman-Kien AE. Kaposi's sarcoma of AIDS: diagnosis and treatment. In: DeVita VT Jr., Hellman S, Rosenberg SA, eds. *AIDS: etiology, diagnosis, treatment, and prevention*, 2nd ed. Philadelphia: J.B. Lippincott, 1988, with permission.)

Diagnostic Work-Up

In addition to inspection of all visible skin and mucosal surfaces, the likelihood of visceral KS is sufficiently high that endoscopic evaluation of the gastrointestinal tract is appropriate for any patient with gastrointestinal symptoms. In any patient who develops KS as the first sign of AIDS, a more comprehensive work-up for HIV should be undertaken: complete physical examination, blood count and chemistries including CD4 lymphocyte count and viral load, chest x-ray, tuberculin test, anergy screen, and screen for sexually transmitted diseases.

Pathology

It is generally agreed that KS is a neoplasm of mesenchymal origin, and the histologic diagnosis of KS requires the identification of both spindle cell and vascular elements within the lesion. The spindle-shaped cells look much like fibroblasts and are generally considered the neoplastic element. Overall, the appearance often is suggestive of slitlike embryonic vascular channels filled with red blood cells; however, red cells characteristically are also found mixed within the spindle cell framework of the tumor.

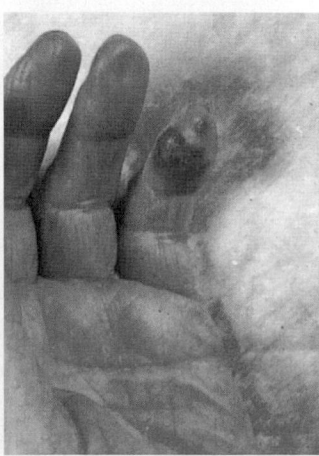

FIGURE 31.5. Nodular purple classic Kaposi's sarcoma near the tip of the patient's fifth finger. (From Krigel RL, Friedman-Kien AE. Kaposi's sarcoma of AIDS: diagnosis and treatment. In: DeVita VT Jr., Hellman S, Rosenberg SA, eds. *AIDS: etiology, diagnosis, treatment, and prevention*, 2nd ed. Philadelphia: J.B. Lippincott, 1988, with permission.)

Treatment: Options to or In Association with Radiation Therapy

EKS typically exhibits multifocal distribution at the time of presentation and, as such, generally requires a systemic approach. Early in the HAART era it was observed that the introduction of protease inhibitors in some patients who had KS resulted not only in stabilization of existing lesions and slowing of the progression of the disease, but brought about measurable regression of existing lesions (155). The role of HAART is now well established and appears to result in durable clinical response rates of over 60% of patients (6). It is important to recognize, however, that a small subset of patients may experience a worsening of symptoms when HAART is instituted. Bower et al. (22) have reported that after commencing HAART, 6.6% of patients with HIV-associated KS developed progressive immune reconstitution inflammatory syndrome-KS, that is, a worsening in their clinical status (despite control of virologic and immunologic parameters), felt to be secondary to an immune response against a pre-existing pathogen. Despite this, the patients successfully continued on HAART, although half required chemotherapy or radiation therapy within 1 year for treatment of their KS.

Systemic chemotherapy has been used for patients with advanced disease. A concern had been that cytotoxic chemotherapy potentially could further compromise the immune system and accelerate the effects of HIV infection. Also, the standard doses of chemotherapy used for solid tumors often resulted in unacceptable morbidity for these patients (73,100). Consequently, treatment protocols were developed with low-dose chemotherapy to which epidemic KS was responsive (75). The regimen of doxorubicin, bleomycin, and vincristine (ABV) became the "gold" standard in the 1990s.

Liposomal daunorubicin and doxorubicin were subsequently approved by the Food and Drug Administration for the treatment of EKS. Randomized studies comparing these drugs with the standard ABV showed at least comparable activity with a more favorable toxicity profile (78,127), and the liposomal drugs are generally now used as first-line therapy. Response rates of 25% with a median duration of 4 months can be expected (78,127).

Paclitaxel is also approved for treatment. Toxicity is mild except for myelosuppression, which can be dealt with by growth factors when necessary (76,77). Gill et al. (76) reported a 60% response rate (nearly all partial responses) with a 10-month median duration of response in one phase II trial. Even though

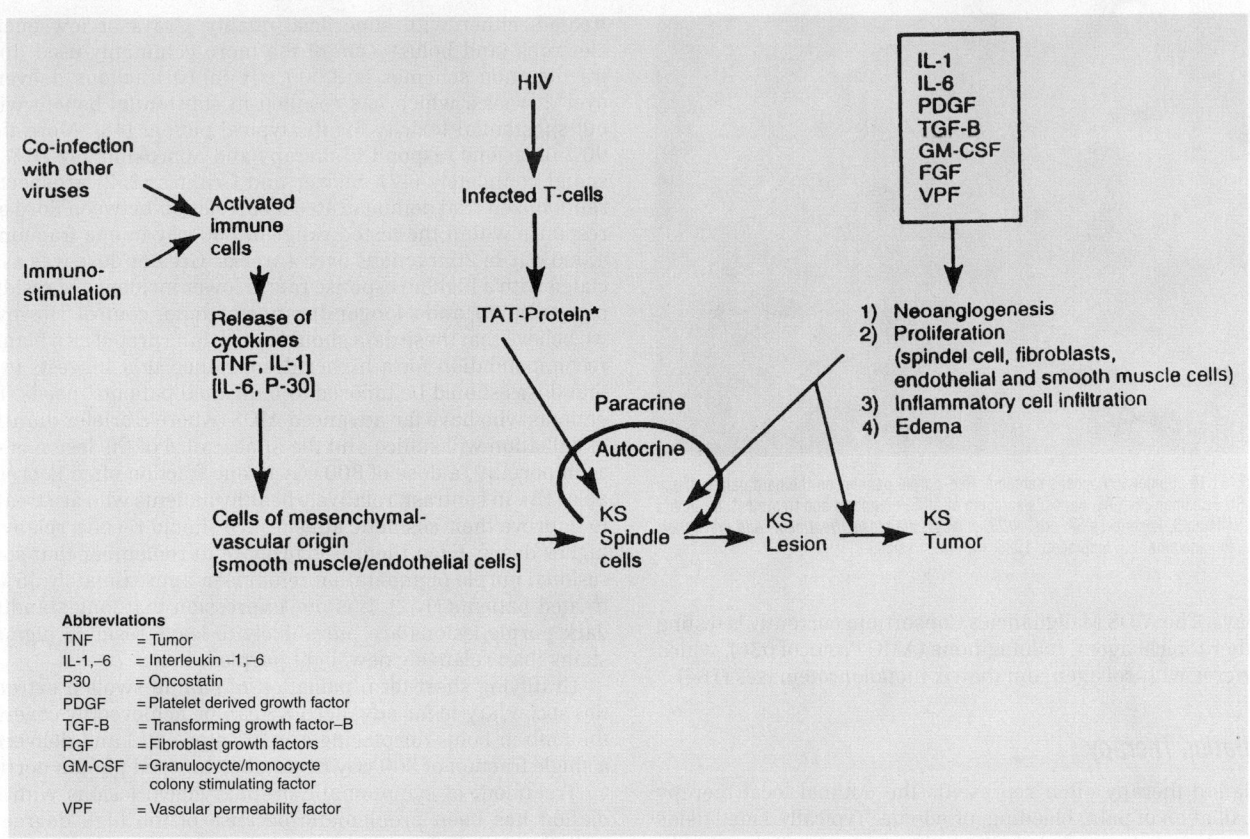

FIGURE 31.7. A schematic model for the pathogenesis of acquired immunodeficiency syndrome–associated Kaposi's sarcoma. (From Stein M, Spencer D, Kuten A, et al. AIDS-related Kaposi's sarcoma: a review. *Isr J Med Sci* 1994;30:298–305, with permission.)

there are other active drugs available, such as VP-16, paclitaxel has become a common second- or third-line drug following the liposomal agents, due to its activity and acceptable toxicity.

Without HAART, patients often require ongoing therapy to control symptomatic KS. However, when HAART is available and decreases HIV RNA to undetectable levels, chronic chemotherapy frequently can be discontinued (158).

All of the above treatments attempt to decrease the burden of disease and palliate distressing signs and symptoms for the duration of a patient's remaining lifespan. In some settings, however, patients do not require systemic therapy. Rarely, palliation can be obtained by surgically excising lesions. Cryotherapy (with liquid nitrogen) also offers a rapid option for small lesions; however, caution must be exercised when treating deeply pigmented areas, as the healed site often will be noticeably hypopigmented. Intralesional injections of vinblastine induce tumor regression in approximately 80% of treated lesions, but have a slower onset of action and generally require repeated injections (18). Alitretinoin gel has provided a noninvasive alternative. In one prospective, randomized, multicenter trial, response to topical application occurred in 27% overall, and was 38% in the subgroup of patients who were also taking protease inhibitors (62). The median time to the onset of response was 33 days and the best response occurred at 43 days. Unfortunately, 45% of initially responding lesions relapsed at a median of

FIGURE 31.8. Epidemic Kaposi's sarcoma. Red-purple macule near the tip of the patient's nose. (From Krigel RL, Friedman-Kien AE. Kaposi's sarcoma of AIDS: diagnosis and treatment. In: DeVita VT Jr., Hellman S, Rosenberg SA, eds. *AIDS: etiology, diagnosis, treatment, and prevention*, 2nd ed. Philadelphia: J.B. Lippincott, 1988, with permission.)

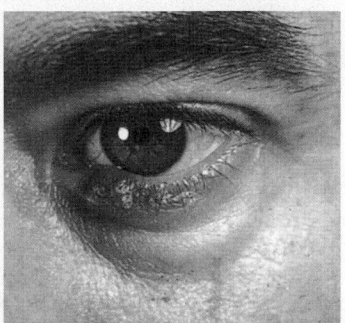

FIGURE 31.9. Nodular purple epidemic Kaposi's sarcoma on the patient's lower eyelid. (From Krigel RL, Friedman-Kien AE. Kaposi's sarcoma of AIDS: diagnosis and treatment. In: DeVita VT Jr., Hellman S, Rosenberg SA, eds. *AIDS: etiology, diagnosis, treatment, and prevention*, 2nd ed. Philadelphia: J.B. Lippincott, 1988, with permission.)

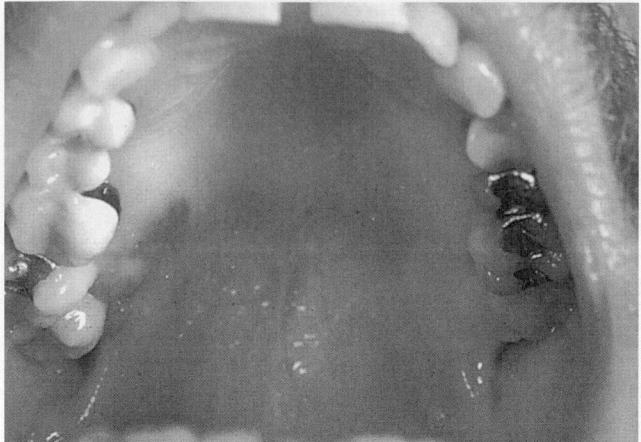

FIGURE 31.10. Epidemic Kaposi's sarcoma. Red-purple papules on the hard palate. (From Krigel RL, Friedman-Kien AE. Kaposi's sarcoma of AIDS: diagnosis and treatment. In: DeVita VT Jr., Hellman S, Rosenberg SA, eds. *AIDS: etiology, diagnosis, treatment, and prevention*, 2nd ed. Philadelphia: J.B. Lippincott, 1988, with permission.)

98 days. The AIDS Malignancies Consortium currently is testing another topical agent, halofuginone (AMC Protocol 036), which interferes with collagen and matrix metalloproteinases (164).

Radiation Therapy

Radiation therapy often represents the optimal local therapy for palliation of pain, bleeding, or edema. Typically, small fields that include only the distressing lesion and a small margin are treated, either with superficial quality x-rays or low energy electrons (and bolus). One of the more commonly used dose-fractionation schemes is 3,000 cGy in 10 fractions delivered over 2 weeks, which has resulted in substantial benefit without substantial toxicity for the typical patient (48). More than 90% of lesions respond to therapy and approximately 70% respond completely (47). Stelzer and Griffin's (152) prospective randomized trial demonstrated a correlation between dose and response within the tested range of 800 cGy in one fraction to 4,000 cGy in 20 fractions over 4 weeks. Greater dose was associated with a higher response rate, a lower incidence of residual pigmentation, and a longer duration of tumor control. However, we believe that these data should not be interpreted as a blanket recommendation for a higher dose; rather, this suggests to us that doses should be tailored to individual patients' needs. For patients who have far-advanced AIDS (where a briefer duration of palliation will suffice and the appearance of the lesion is not as important), a dose of 800 cGy in one fraction often is preferable (13). In contrast, relatively healthy patients who are treated to improve their cosmetic appearance should receive relatively higher doses. Even then, it is prudent to remember that some residual purple pigmentation remains in approximately 55% of treated patients (152). It is our impression that long-standing, dark purple lesions are more likely to leave residual pigment stains than relatively new, light purple lesions.

Gratifying short-term palliation of painful swollen extremities secondary to far advanced KS can be achieved by covering the limb in bolus (or placing it in a water-bath) and delivering a single fraction of 800 cGy by parallel opposed photon portals.

Treatment of symptomatic oropharyngeal lesions with radiation has been problematic because of the high degree of radiation-induced mucositis that these patients develop even

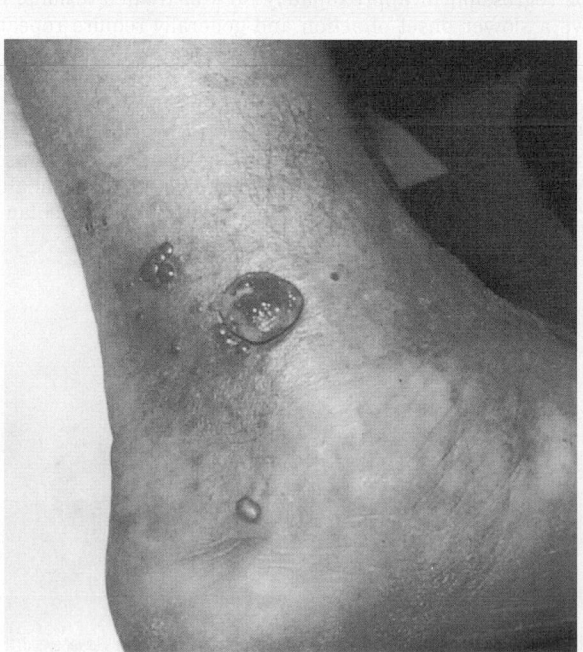

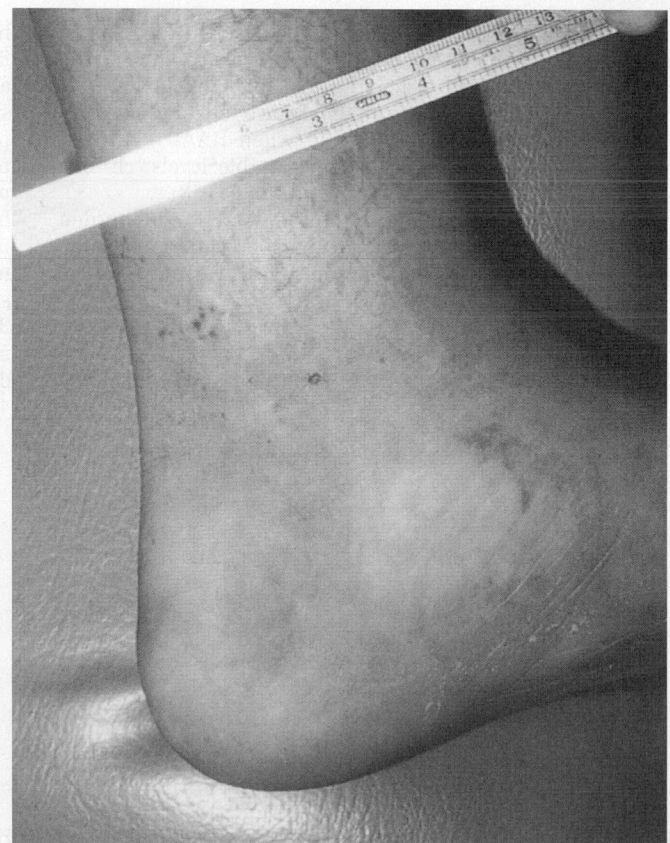

FIGURE 31.11. A: Epidemic Kaposi's sarcoma of the foot before treatment. **B:** Same patient approximately 1.5 years after 30 Gy was delivered in 10 fractions over 2 weeks by 6-MeV electron beam therapy (with bolus).

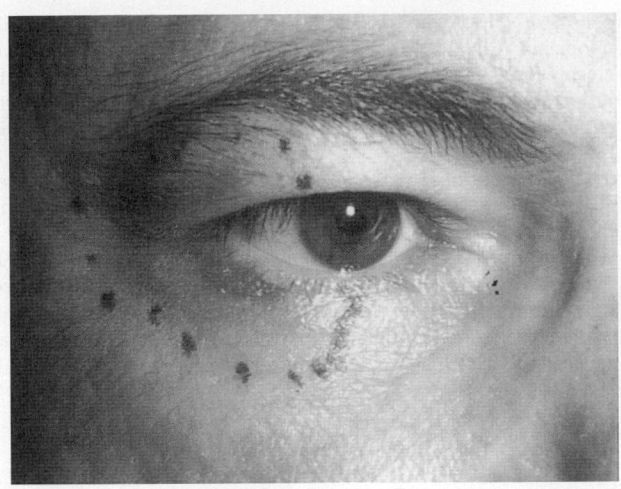
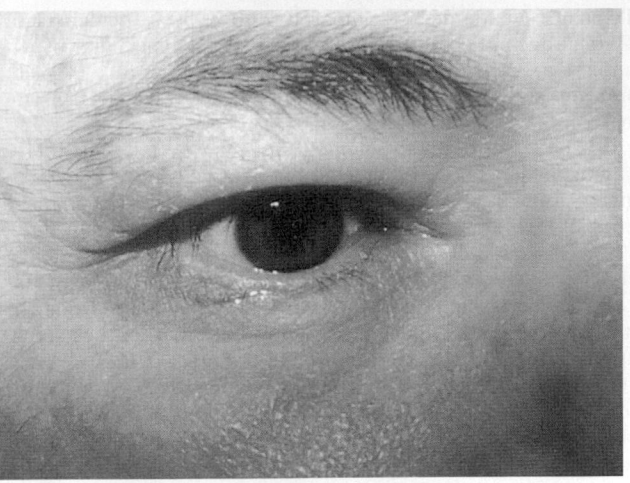

FIGURE 31.12. A: Epidemic Kaposi's sarcoma of the upper and lower lateral eyelids before treatment. **B:** Same patient approximately 1 month after 30 Gy was delivered in 10 fractions over 2 weeks by kilovoltage x-rays. An eye shield was used to protect the lens of the eye. Residual pigmentation is visible.

following low-dose radiation therapy (46). Palliation of symptomatic visceral or mucosal disease nearly always should first be attempted with chemotherapy and HAART. However, there are rare instances in which a patient's lesions have failed to respond to systemic chemotherapy or in which patients are unable to tolerate systemic chemotherapy. These patients may benefit from attenuated doses of local radiation to palliate bleeding or obstructive lesions. Piedbois et al. (134) have reported 88% objective response and "good palliation of symptoms" following 1,000 to 2,000 cGy (250 cGy per fraction, four fractions per week) for delicate anatomic sites, such as the penis, the palms, oral mucosa, or the conjunctivae. In one report of 25 patients who had pulmonary lesions treated with radiation therapy (1,050 to 1,500 cGy at 150 cGy per fraction), subjective improvement was observed in nearly 90% of patients, although only one third of patients survived for 3 months (122).

:: | Anal Carcinoma

The incidence of anal carcinoma in the general population has increased in the past several years (121), and according to the U.S. National Cancer Institute approximately 4,000 cases were diagnosed in 2004 (165). Although there may be an association of anal carcinomas with condylomata and/or male homosexual contact, it is unclear if the increase in anal cancer is directly linked to HIV. Additionally, although HIV infection has been implicated as an independent risk factor for anal cancer (120), studies of homosexual men in New York City and San Francisco have shown a greater increase in the incidence of anal cancer in HIV-seronegative men than in HIV-seropositive men (28).

Anal carcinomas, like cervical carcinomas, appear to be related to sexually transmitted HPV (primarily HPV-16), with anal intercourse being a risk factor (70). HIV-infected homosexual men have increased serum HPV DNA as compared with HIV-seronegative homosexual men (128). In one study, more than 60% of HIV-infected men with abnormal anogenital examinations were found to have squamous intraepithelial lesions on biopsy (124). As with cervical carcinoma, the key to diagnosis is rigorous surveillance for anal intraepithelial neoplasia in the population at risk, with anal cytology and anoscopy (129). Similarly as with cervical carcinoma, the impending licensure of a vaccine against HPV potentially would represent a major public health advance against anal cancer (150).

It is unclear how HAART impacts the development of anal intraepithelial neoplasia and the subsequent development of invasive anal cancer. Some authors have reported that antiretroviral treatment does not protect against the development of premalignant or malignant lesions (12). Others have reported that HAART can decrease the prevalence of anal intraepithelial neoplasia in men with persistent HPV but does not affect the HPV (160).

At present, it appears that HAART does not diminish the excess risk of anal cancer in the HIV-positive population.

Carcinoma *in situ* frequently can be approached with measures employed for the treatment of genital warts (i.e., topical podophyllin, topical 5-fluorouacil [5-FU], and laser therapy). In patients with low-grade, early stage lesions (T1 and possibly some T2) without any evidence of nodal involvement, local excision with wide margins may be acceptable if the sphincter function is preserved. However, the majority of patients with HIV anal carcinoma present with more advanced T stages and/or nodal involvement, and, if treatment is to be definitive, chemoradiation is the treatment of choice. Both the European Organisation for Research and Treatment of Cancer (EORTC) phase III randomized trial showing the benefit of the addition of chemotherapy to radiation and the RTOG phase III randomized trial showing the benefit of adding mitomycin to 5-FU/radiation have led to the general acceptance of 5-FU/mitomycin-C and radiation therapy as the standard of care in patients not infected with HIV (7,66). This treatment should be offered to HIV-infected patients with appropriately staged anal carcinoma if possible. However, consideration should be given to withholding mitomycin in patients with advanced HIV due to the potential for severe myelosuppression and hemolytic uremic syndrome. Although the RTOG data has shown a higher incidence of recurrence and need for colostomy in patients with breaks >10 days during the course of treatment, radiation administered in conjunction with chemotherapy for anal cancer frequently results in marked moist desquamation, necessitating temporary interruption of therapy. There is evidence that patients with HIV infection require longer breaks from chemoradiation because of severe skin reactions and almost uniformly require chemotherapy dose reductions because of neutropenia (87).

In our experience, 79% of patients required treatment breaks, mostly because of grade 3 skin toxicity; 36% experienced grade 3 or 4 hematologic toxicity (40). Other series as well have reported an 80% incidence of acute toxicities in

HIV-positive patients as compared with a 30% incidence in HIV-negative patients (97). There is anecdotal experience using amifostine, a radioprotector, to increase the tolerance of such compromised individuals, including patients with AIDS, to treatment (126).

As compared with the non-HIV-infected population, there is a suggestion that HIV-infected patients who have anal carcinoma appear to have a shorter survival and a higher incidence of local failure. Kim et al. (97) reported a median time to cancer-related death of 1.4 years in HIV-positive individuals versus 5.3 years in HIV-negative individuals with anal cancer. In another series, four of the seven HIV-positive patients died, at a mean of 8 months, following therapy, and three of these four experienced local recurrence prior to their death (155). However, eight HIV-infected patients treated with chemotherapy and reduced-dose radiation (3,000 cGy in 15 fractions) in one series achieved complete response (131). At a median follow-up of 38 months, four patients were alive and free of disease. The remaining four were dead of AIDS-related causes, but they remained free of anal cancer until death. In our experience of utilizing chemoradiation in 14 patients with HIV-associated anal carcinoma, nearly 80% of patients remain free of disease at a median follow-up of 10 months (40). The variable outcomes in these series is probably due to multiple factors, including the heterogeneity of patients, the extent of their immunosuppression, and length of follow-up. Newer strategies employing targeted agents, such as in an AIDS Malignancy Consortium phase II study employing cetuximab in addition to 5-FU, cisplatin, and radiation (180 cGy per fraction to a total of 4,500 cGy without a planned break) may improve the outcome of HIV-associated anal carcinoma (138).

Cervical Carcinoma

Epidemiology

Cervical carcinoma in the presence of HIV infection has been accepted by the CDC as an AIDS-defining illness (32). In a retrospective study of women registered from 1987 through 1995 by the New York City Department of Health and institutional tumor registries, cervical cancer was the sixth most common initial AIDS-defining illness in women (115). For women, cervical cancer was the most common AIDS-related malignancy (55% of the cases), followed by lymphoma (29%) and Kaposi's sarcoma (16%). As is true in HIV-uninfected populations, cervical dysplasia appears to be a precursor to cervical malignancies, and cervical dysplasia occurs in 40% of HIV-infected women (142). The association between HIV and cervical cancer is complex and, although it has been clearly demonstrated that there is an increased incidence of preinvasive lesions in HIV-infected women, it is not clear that there is a substantially higher incidence of invasive disease (39). Some authors have argued that since the introduction of HAART, there is little evidence to support the continued status of cervical cancer as an AIDS-defining illness, since cervical cancer does not appear to have a strong relationship to immune function as determined by CD4 count or responsiveness to HAART (21).

There appears to be an association between HPV infection and risk for cervical epithelial abnormalities in HIV-infected women (161).

Specifically, as compared to HIV-seronegative women, HIV-infected women have a higher rate of persistent infection with HPV-16 or HPV-18, the viral types that are most strongly associated with cervical carcinoma (154). Moreover, the frequency and severity of dysplasia appear to correlate inversely with CD4 counts, thus implying a link to immunosuppression (157); 20% of HIV-infected women who have screening CD4 lymphocyte counts of $\leq$500 cells/mm^3 will manifest cervical intraepithelial neoplasia (CIN), a forerunner of invasive disease, if followed closely for 1 year. This compares with a rate of ~5% in similar uninfected women. Women who are coinfected with HPV, principally high and intermediate risk types, are at particular risk (42,61).

The benefit of HAART on HIV-associated CIN is not entirely clear, although there are data suggesting that HAART may induce regression of CIN in HIV positive women. In a study of women with AIDS, the prevalence of CIN fell from 66% to 49% 5 months after the institution of HAART (84). One study showed that, after adjustment for CD4 count and Pap smear status, women receiving HAART were 40% more likely to demonstrate regression, and less likely to demonstrate progression of CIN lesions (123).

Diagnosis

Routine gynecological evaluation, including Pap smears (and colposcopy when warranted), is the most successful means of detecting the dysplastic and *in situ* lesions (CIN) that give rise to invasive lesions. Unfortunately, to date, HIV-infected women most often present with advanced-stage disease. Up to 50% of HIV-infected women had stage III or IV disease when they first sought care, as compared to approximately 20% of noninfected women (116).

Treatment

Treatment should be dictated by the extent of disease, taking into account the patient's history of opportunistic infections and overall medical status. The small proportion of patients who have early stage, nonbulky disease are usually treated with a radical hysterectomy and pelvic lymph node dissection. Patients who have more advanced local-regional disease should be treated, we believe, in the same fashion as their non-HIV-infected counterparts. Although previously this would have been radiation therapy alone, in one series of patients treated by radiation alone for advanced disease, 50% had no or minimal response to treatment, and at a median follow-up of 3 months all had progression of disease (35). The current standard of care for advanced cervical cancer is a combination of radiation therapy and cisplatin-based chemotherapy (133). At present there are insufficient data to demonstrate the routine feasibility and/or efficacy of this approach in the setting of AIDS. However, based on the tolerability of combined modality approaches in AIDS-related lymphomas and the evidence of improved outcome in advanced cervical cancer in the general population, we believe that advanced cervical cancers in women who do not have a specific contraindication for chemotherapy should receive concurrent chemotherapy, external-beam radiotherapy, and an intracavitary boost. Patients who have hematogenously borne metastatic disease may benefit from palliative chemotherapy or radiation therapy in an effort to reduce symptoms such as pain and bleeding.

Results and Prognosis

Although there initially was concern over the ability to deliver "standard" treatment to HIV-infected patients with cervical carcinoma, available data suggest treatment can be delivered, albeit with a higher risk of complications (35). HIV-infected women treated with laser/cone or cryotherapy for CIN have an increased risk of excessive bleeding or infection as compared with uninfected patients (54). Unfortunately, as is true of other malignancies, cervical carcinoma appears to be more aggressive in the HIV-infected population than in the immunocompetent population. This may reflect the more aggressive biology of the disease in these patients and/or the more advanced stage with which they present. In one study of 16 HIV-infected women who had cervical carcinoma, nine died of cervical cancer at a mean interval of only 9.2 months from diagnosis (35).

Early diagnosis of cervical abnormalities prior to the development of invasive cancer appears to be critical if we are to hope for increased cure rates. As there appears to be a 10% to 20% progression rate from CIN-1 to CIN-2 or -3 over 1 to 2 years in the HIV population (115), it is imperative that close surveillance with gynecological evaluations, including PAP smears and colposcopy, be offered to all HIV-infected women. The development of a vaccine targeting HPV-16 and HPV-18 now offers hope. In a phase III trial researchers demonstrated a lower incidence in the development of CIN-2 and -3 in a cohort of vaccinated women as compared to women vaccinated with placebo (0/5301 vs. 21/5258) (144). The Food and Drug Administration has now approved a recombinant vaccine that is given as three injections over a 6-month period.

Pediatric Malignancies

Where available, the use of antiretroviral drugs in HIV-infected pregnant women and their infants has resulted in a dramatic decline in perinatally acquired HIV infection (43). However, maternal-infant transmission remains widespread in many parts of the world where the cost of antiretroviral drugs is prohibitive. Children who go on to develop AIDS appear to be at increased risk of developing tumors of the same types as adults, particularly non-Hodgkin's lymphomas (63), but also appear to be at risk of developing leiomyosarcomas (36,82). In one review of 11 cancer registries and AIDS databases, Biggar et al. (15) found a 2.5% incidence of cancer in 4,954 children, aged 14 and under, who had AIDS (15). NHL was approximately 600 times more common than would be expected in an uninfected population and was diagnosed at a median of 14 months after the onset of AIDS. Burkitt lymphomas accounted for the most common histologic subtype; however, primary CNS lymphomas were overrepresented at approximately 7,000 times their expected incidence. KS was diagnosed exclusively within 2 years of the diagnosis of AIDS, whereas leiomyosarcoma tended to be found several years after the onset of AIDS.

In an analysis of 2,969 infected children followed by the Pediatric AIDS Clinical Trials Group, 37 cancers were diagnosed in the cohort from 1993 through 2003. Compared with uninfected children, the standardized incidence ratio was 10.08, and in multivariate regression, the cancer rate was 3.09 times higher in children with 2 or fewer years of HAART than in children with more than 2 years of HAART (96).

A multicenter case-control study of children with HIV at 26 institutions participating in the Pediatric Oncology Group reported 28 non-Hodgkin lymphomas, four B-cell acute lymphoblastic leukemias, one Hodgkin's disease, eight leiomyosarcomas, one hepatoblastoma, and one schwannoma. High EBV burden was associated with the development of malignancy in HIV-infected children, although the effect was modified by CD4 cell count (135).

Summary

HIV infection fosters immunosuppression, and immunosuppression fosters the appearance of malignancies. Thus, the explosive appearance of KS, in epidemic proportions, was an early clue to the epidemiology of AIDS, even before HIV was discovered. Soon after, other malignancies began to occur with greater than expected frequency in association with HIV infection: non-Hodgkin's lymphoma and cervical cancer. Possibly, other malignancies (Hodgkin's, anal cancer, pediatric leiomyosarcomas) are also promoted by HIV infection. Fur-

thermore, the extent of disease seen at presentation is more advanced than in typical uninfected populations, again suggesting a clinically relevant, immunosuppression-mediated, process. Remembering that (even in uninfected patients) radiotherapy and/or chemotherapy rarely is thought to eradicate the last malignant cell, in the face of such immunosuppression it is remarkable that they have reasonable efficacy. Progress requires therapies that counteract the immunosuppression associated with HIV infection.

Influence of HAART on HIV-Associated Neoplasms

HAART appears to be a major step in the right direction. Often, HAART can suppress viral levels to currently undetectable levels and thereby help improve the immune status of the host. In consequence, infected individuals should be less prone to develop malignancies and potentially would have improved outcomes when they do manifest malignancies. However, the data at this point in time remain contradictory (44). HAART appears to have decreased the incidence of KS (89,102) and PCNSL (106); however, there may be an increased incidence of Hodgkin's disease in HIV-infected persons in the era of HAART (137). Data regarding the influence of HAART on prognosis of malignancies remain difficult to interpret, with some studies claiming improved survival for patients with systemic NHL (17), while others claim no influence (117). Furthermore, even in areas where HAART is widely available, individual patients may not access or comply with treatment, and, if general adherence to or effectiveness of therapy is poor, the overall immune status of the population will remain low, and, consequently, there will be no decline in the incidence of HIV-associated malignancies (110). Although HAART has dramatically changed the face of AIDS, major challenges, not the least of which is the emergence of viral resistance, unfortunately ensure that improvements in the treatment of AIDS-associated malignancies will continue be needed. Ultimately, the key to eradicating AIDS-associated malignancies will lie in the prevention of HIV transmission.

References

1. Abrey LE, Batchelor TT, Ferreri AJM, et al. Report of an international workshop to standardize baseline evaluation and response criteria for primary CNS lymphoma. *J Clin Oncol* 2005;23(22):1–10.
2. Abrey LE, Yahalom J, DeAngelis LM. Treatment for primary CNS lymphoma: the next step. *J Clin Oncol* 2000;18:3144–3150.
3. Ambinder RF, Lee S, Curran WJ, et al. Phase II intergroup trial of sequential chemotherapy and radiotherapy for AIDS-related primary central nervous system lymphoma. *Cancer Ther* 2003;1:215–221.
4. Ames ED, Conjalka MS, Goldberg AF, et al. Hodgkin's disease and AIDS: twenty-three new cases and a review of the literature. *Hematol Oncol Clin North Am* 1991;5:343–356.
5. Ansari MQ, Dawson DB, Nadon R, et al. Primary body cavity-based AIDS-related lymphomas. *Am J Clin Pathol* 1996;105:221–229.
6. Aversa SM, Cattelan AM, Salvango L, et al. Treatments of AIDS-related Kaposi's sarcoma. *Crit Rev Oncol Hematol* 2005;53:253–265.
7. Bartelink H, Roelofsen F, Eschwege F, et al. Concomitant radiotherapy and chemotherapy is superior to radiotherapy alone in the treatment of locally advanced anal cancer: results of a phase III randomized trial of the European Organization for Research and Treatment of Cancer Radiotherapy and Gastrointestinal Cooperative Groups. *J Clin Oncol* 1997;15:2040–2049.
8. Baumgartner JE, Rachlin JR, Beckstead JH, et al. Primary central nervous system lymphomas: natural history: response to radiation therapy in 55 patients with acquired immunodeficiency syndrome. *J Neurosurg* 1990;73:206–211.
9. Beral V, Peterman TA, Berkelman RL, et al. Kaposi's sarcoma among persons with AIDS: a sexually transmitted infection? *Lancet* 1990;335:123–128.
10. Beral V, Peterman T, Berkelman R, et al. AIDS-associated non-Hodgkin's lymphoma. *Lancet* 1991;337:805–809.
11. Bermudez AM, Grant K, Rodvien R, et al. Non-Hodgkin's lymphoma in a population with or at risk for acquired immunodeficiency syndrome: indications for intensive chemotherapy. *Am J Med* 1989;86:71–76.
12. Berry JM, Palefsky JM, Welton ML. Anal cancer and its precursors in HIV-positive patients: perspectives and management. *Surg Oncol Clin North Am* 2004;13:355–373.
13. Berson AM, Quivey JM, Harris JW, et al. Radiation therapy for AIDS-related Kaposi's sarcoma. *Int J Radiat Oncol Biol Phys* 1990;19:569–575.
14. Besson C, Goubar A, Gabarre J, et al. Changes in AIDS-related lymphomas since the era of highly active antiretroviral therapy. *Blood* 2001;98:2339–2344.

15. Biggar RJ, Frisch M, Goedert JJ. AIDS-Cancer Match Registry Group. Risk of cancer in children with AIDS. *JAMA* 2000;284:205–209.
16. Biggar RJ, Rabkin CS. The epidemiology of acquired immunodeficiency syndrome-related lymphomas. *Curr Opin Oncol* 1992;4:883–893.
17. Blay J-Y, Bouhour D, Brachet L, et al. Highly active antiretroviral therapy (HAART) is an independent prognostic factor for progression free survival (PFS) in patients (PTS) with HIV+NHL: a retrospective study (abstr 584). Proceedings of the American Society of Hematology 42nd Annual Meeting and Exposition. December 2000.
18. Boudreaux AA, Smith LL, Cosby CD, et al. Intralesional vinblastine for cutaneous Kaposi's sarcoma associated with acquired immunodeficiency syndrome. A clinical trial to evaluate efficacy and discomfort associated with injection. *J Am Acad Dermatol* 1993;28(1):61–65.
19. Bower M. AIDS-related malignancies: changing epidemiology and the impact of highly active antiretroviral therapy. *Curr Opin Infect Dis* 2006;19(1):14–19.
20. Bower M, Gazzard B, Mandalia S, et al. A prognostic index for systemic AIDS-related non-Hodgkin lymphoma treated in the era of highly active antiretroviral therapy. *Ann Intern Med* 2005;143:265–273.
21. Bower M, Mazhar D, Stebbing J. Should cervical cancer be an acquired immunodeficiency syndrome-defining cancer? *J Clin Oncol* 2006;24(16):2417–2419.
22. Bower M, Nelson M, Young AM, et al. Immune reconstitution inflammatory syndrome associated with Kaposi's sarcoma. *J Clin Oncol* 2005;23:5224–5228.
23. Boyle B, Merrick S, Jacobs J. Primary CNS lymphoma and HAART. *Int Conf AIDS* 1998;12:854(abstr 42404).
24. Bozzette SA, Berry SH, Duan N, et al. The HIV cost and services utilization study consortium. The care of HIV-infected adults in the United States. *N Engl J Med* 1998;339:1897–1904.
25. Burgi S, Brodine S, Wegner S, et al. Incidence and risk factors for the occurrence of non-AIDS-defining cancers among human immunodeficiency virus-infected individuals. *Cancer* 2005;104:1505–1511.
26. Cannon M, Cesarman E. Kaposi's sarcoma-associated herpes virus and acquired immunodeficiency-related malignancy. *Semin Oncol* 2000;27:409–419.
27. Carbone A, Gloghini A, Cozzi MR, et al. Expression of MUM/IRF4 selectively clusters with primary effusion lymphoma among lymphomatous effusions: implications for disease histogenesis and pathogenesis. *Br J Haemetol* 2000;111:247–257.
28. Carlson RH. Increase in anal cancer rates not due to AIDS. *Oncology Times* Oct. 1996.
29. Centers for Disease Control. Kaposi's sarcoma and pneumocystis pneumonia among homosexual men—New York City and California. *Morb Mortal Wkly Rep* 1981;30:305–308.
30. Centers for Disease Control. Update on acquired immune deficiency syndrome (AIDS)—United States. *Morb Mortal Wkly Rep* 1981;31:507–514.
31. Centers for Disease Control. Revision of the case definition of acquired immunodeficiency syndrome for national [sic] reported: United States. *Ann Intern Med* 1985;103:402–403.
32. Centers for Disease Control. 1993 revised classification system for HIV infection and expanded surveillance case definition for AIDS among adolescents and adults. *JAMA* 1993;269:729–730
33. Centers for Disease Control. HIV incidence among young men who have sex with men-seven U.S. Cities 1994–2000. *Morb Mort Wkly Rep* 2001;50(21):440–444.
34. Centers for Disease Control. Advancing HIV prevention: new strategies for a changing epidemic—United States, 2003. *Morb Mortal Wkly Rep* 2003;52:329–332.
35. Chadha M, Sood B, Stanson R. Patients with human immunodeficiency virus (HIV): Infections and cervical neophasia. *Int J Rad Oncol Biol Phys* 1984; 30(S1):284.
36. Chadwick EG, Connor EJ, Hanson IC, et al. Tumors of smooth-muscle origin in HIV-infected children. *JAMA* 1990;263:3182–3184.
37. Chamberlain MC, Dirr L. Involved-field radiotherapy and intra-ommaya methotrexate/cytarabine in patients with AIDS-related lymphomatous meningitis. *J Clin Oncol* 1993;11:1978–1984.
38. Chang Y, Cesarman E, Pessin MS, et al. Identification of herpesvirus-like DNA sequences in AIDS-associated Kaposi's sarcoma. *Science* 1994;266:1865–1869.
39. Chirenje ZM. HIV and cancer of the cervix. *Best Pract Res Clin Obstet Gynaecol.* 2005;19(2):269–276.
40. Cho DS, Shieh G, Kuber N, et al. Definitive radiotherapy in the combined modality treatment of HIV anal carcinoma. *Proc ASCO* 2001;20:150b(abstr 2350).
41. Cingolani A, Gastaldi R, Fassone L, et al. Epstein-Barr virus infection is predictive of CNS involvement in systemic AIDS-related non-Hodgkin's lymphoma. *J Clin Oncol* 2000;18:3325–3330.
42. Cohn JA, Gagnon S, Spence MR, et al. The role of human papillomavirus deoxyribonucleic acid assay and repeated cervical cytologic examination in the detection of cervical intraepithelial neoplasia among human immunodeficiency virus–infected women. *Am J Obstet Gynecol* 2001;184:322–330.
43. Connor EM, Sperling RS, Gelber R, et al. Reduction of maternal-infant transmission of human immunodeficiency virus type 1 with zidovudine treatment. *N Engl J Med* 1994;331:1173–1180.
44. Conti S, Masocco M, Pezzotti P, et al. Differential impact of combined antiretroviral therapy on the survival of Italian patients with specific AIDS-defining illnesses. *J Acquir Immune Defic Syndr* 2000;25:451–458.
45. Cooper JS, Donahue BR. The Swift article reviewed (editorial). *Oncology* 1997;11:697–702.
46. Cooper JS, Fried PR. Toxicity of oral radiotherapy in patients having AIDS. *Arch Otolaryngology* 1987;113:327–328.
47. Cooper J, Steinfeld A, Lerch, I. Intentions and outcomes in the radiotherapeutic management of epidemic Kaposi's sarcoma. *Int J Radiat Oncol Biol Phys* 1991;20:419–422.
48. Cooper JS, Steinfeld AS, Lerch IA. The prognostic significance of residual pigmentation following radiotherapy of epidemic Kaposi's sarcoma. *J Clin Oncol* 1989;7:619–621.
49. Corales R, Taege A, Rehm S, et al. Regression of AIDS-related CNS lymphoma with HAART (abstr MoPpB1086). Program and abstracts of the XIII International AIDS Conference. Durban, South Africa; July 9–14, 2000.
50. Corn B, Donahue B, Rosenstock J, et al. Performance status and age as independent predictors of survival among AIDS patients with primary CNS lymphoma: a multivariate analysis of a multi-institutional experience. *Cancer J Sci Am* 1997;3:52–56.
51. Corn BW, Donahue BR, Rosenstock JG, et al. Palliation of AIDS-related primary lymphoma of the brain: observations from a multi-institutional database. *Int J Rad Oncol Biol Phys* 1997;38:601–605.
52. Corn BW, Trock BJ, Curran WJ. Management of primary central nervous system lymphoma for the patient with acquired immunodeficiency syndrome. *Cancer* 1995;76:163–166.
53. Cote TR, Manns A, Hardy CR, et al. Epidemiology of brain lymphoma among people with or without acquired immunodeficiency syndrome. *J Natl Cancer Inst* 1996;88:675–679.
54. Cuthill S, Maiman M, Fruchter RG. Complications after treatment of cervical intraepithelial neoplasia in women infected with the human immunodeficiency virus. *J Reprod Med* 1995;40(12):823–828.
55. De Jarlais DC, Marmor M, Thomas P, et al. Kaposi's sarcoma among four different AIDS risk groups. *N Engl J Med* 1984;310:1119.
56. Diamond C, Taylor TH, Aboumrad T, et al. Changes in acquired immunodeficiency syndrome-related non-Hodgkin lymphoma in the era of highly active antiretroviral therapy. *Cancer* 2006;106:128–135.
57. Donahue B, Cooper J, Rush S, et al. Results of empiric radiotherapy for HIV associated primary CNS lymphomas. *Int J Rad Oncol Biol Phys* 1989;17:223.
58. Donahue B, Steinfeld AD, Torrey MJ, et al. Lymphomatous meningitis in HIV-associated non-Hodgkin's lymphoma: an unexpected pattern of relapse. Proceedings of the Ninth International Congress on Anti-cancer Treatment. Paris; January 1999.
59. Donahue BR, Sullivan JW, Cooper JS. Additional experience with empiric radiotherapy for HIV-associated primary CNS lymphoma. *Cancer* 1995;76:328–332.
60. Doweiko J, Dezube BJ, Pantanowitz L. Unusual sites of Hodgkin's lymphoma: case 1. HIV-associated Hodgkin's lymphoma of the stomach. *J Clin Oncol* 2004;22(20):4227–4228.
61. Duerr A, Kieke B, Warren D, et al. Human papillomavirus–associated cervical cytologic abnormalities among women with or at risk of infection with human immunodeficiency virus. *Am J Obstet Gynecol* 2001;184:584–590.
62. Duvic M, Friedman-Kien AE, Looney DJ, et al. Topical treatment of cutaneous lesions of acquired immunodeficiency syndrome-related Kaposi sarcoma using alitretinoin gel: results of phase 1 and 2 trials. *Arch Dermatol* 2000;136(12):1461–1469.
63. Epstein LG, DiCarlo FJ, Joshi VV, et al. Primary lymphomas of the central nervous system in two children with acquired immunodeficiency syndrome. *Ann J Clin Pathol* 1990;94:722–728.
64. Errante D, Zaganel V, Vaccher E, et al. Hodgkin's disease in patients with HIV infection and in the general population: comparison of clinicopathologic features and survival. *Ann Oncol* 1994;2:37–40.
65. Figueroa BE, Brown JR, Nascimento A, et al. Unusual sites of Hodgkin's lymphoma: case 2. Hodgkin's lymphoma of the CNS masquerading as a meningioma. *J Clin Oncol* 2004;22(20):4228–4230.
66. Flam M, John M, Pajak TF, et al. Role of mitomycin in combination with fluorouracil and radiotherapy, and of salvage chemoradiation in the definitive nonsurgical treatment of epidermoid carcinoma of the anal canal: results of a phase III randomized intergroup study. *J Clin Oncol* 1996;14:2527–2539.
67. Formenti SC, Gill PS, Lean E, et al. Primary central nervous system lymphoma in AIDS—results of radiation therapy. *Cancer* 1989;63:1101–1107.
68. Frieden TR, Das-Douglas M, Kellerman SE, et al. Applying public health principles to the HIV epidemic. *N Engl J Med* 2005;353(22):2397–2402.
69. Frisch M, Biggar RJ, Engels EA, et al. Association of cancer with AIDS-related immunosuppression in adults. *JAMA* 2001;85:1736–1745.
70. Frisch M, Glimelius B, Van Der Brule AJC, et al. Sexually transmitted infection as a cause of anal cancer. *New Engl J Med* 1997;337:1350–1358.
71. Gallant JE, Moore RD, Richman DD, et al. Risk factors for Kaposi's sarcoma in patients with advanced human immunodeficiency virus disease treated with zidovudine: Zidovudine Epidemiology Study Group. *Arch Intern Med* 1994;154: 566–572.
72. Gao SJ, Kingsley L, Hoover DR, et al. Seroconversion to antibodies against Kaposi's sarcoma—associated herpesvirus-related latent nuclear antigens before the development of Kaposi's sarcoma. *N Engl J Med* 1996;335:233–241.
73. Gelmann E, Longo D, Lane H, et al. Combination chemotherapy of disseminated Kaposi's sarcoma in patients with the acquired immune deficiency syndrome. *Am J Med* 1987;82:456–461.
74. Gill PS, Levine AM, Krailo M, et al. AIDS-related malignant lymphoma: results of prospective treatment trials. *J Clin Oncol* 1987;5:1322–1328.
75. Gill PS, Rarick MU, McCutchan JA, et al. Systemic treatment of AIDS-related Kaposi's sarcoma: results of a randomized trial. *Am J Med* 1991;90:427–433.
76. Gill PS, Tulpule A, Espina BM, et al. Paclitaxel is safe and effective in the treatment of advanced AIDS-related Kaposi's sarcoma. *J Clin Oncol* 1999;17:1876–1883.
77. Gill PS, Tulpule A, Reynolds T, et al. Paclitaxel (Taxol) in the treatment of relapsed or refractory advanced AIDS-related Kaposi's sarcoma. *Proc ASCO* 1996;15:A854.
78. Gill PS, Wernz J, Scadden D, et al. Randomized phase III trial of liposomal daunorubicin versus doxorubicin, bleomycin, and vincristine in AIDS-realated Kaposi's sarcoma. *J Clin Oncol* 1996;14:2353–2364.
79. Goldstein JD, Dickson DW, Moser FG, et al. Primary central nervous system lymphoma in acquired immune deficiency syndrome—a clinical and pathologic study with results of treatment with radiation. *Cancer* 1991;67:2756–2765.
80. Gottlieb MS, Schroff R, Schanker HM, et al. *Pneumocystis carinii* pneumonia and mucosal candidiasis in previously healthy homosexual men: evidence of a new acquired cellular immunodeficiency. *N Engl J Med* 1981;305:1425–1431.
81. Gould AB. Post mortem of the international AIDS conference. Available at: http://www.rnw.nl/science/html/aids000718.html. Accessed July 18, 2000.
82. Granovsky MO, Mueller BU, Nicholson HS, et al. Cancer in human immunodeficiency virus infected children: a case series from the Children's Cancer Group and the National Cancer Institute. *J Clin Oncol* 1988;16:1729–1735.
83. Grulich AE, Wan X, Law MG, et al. B-cell stimulation and prolonged immune deficiency are risk factors for non-Hodgkin's lymphoma in people with AIDS. *AIDS* 2000;14:133–140.
84. Heard I, Schmitz V, Costagliola D, et al. Early regression of cervical lesions in HIV-seropositive women receiving highly active antiretroviral therapy. *AIDS* 1998;12:1459–1464.
85. Herndier BG, Kaplan LD, McGrath MS. Pathogenesis of AIDS lymphomas. *AIDS* 1994;8:1025–1049.
86. Hessol NA, Katz MH, Liu JY, et al. Increased incidence of Hodgkin's disease in homosexual men with HIV infection. *Ann Intern Med* 1992;117:309–311.

87. Holland JM, Swift PS. Tolerance of patients with human immunodeficiency virus and anal carcinoma to treatment with combined chemotherapy and radiation therapy. *Radiology* 1994;193:251–254.

88. IARC Monograph on the Evaluation of Carcinogenic Risks to Humans. *Human immunodeficiency viruses and T-cell lymphotropic viruses*, Vol. 67. Lyon, France: IARC, 1996.

89. International Collaboration on HIV and Cancer. Highly active antiretroviral therapy and incidence of cancer in human immunodeficiency virus-infected adults. *JNCI* 2000;92:1823–1830.

90. Jacomet C, Girard PM, Lebrette MG, et al. Intravenous methotrexate for primary central nervous system non-Hodgkin's lymphoma in AIDS. *AIDS* 1997;11(14):1725–1730.

91. Jaffe ES. Primary body cavity-based AIDS-related lymphomas. Evolution of a new disease entity. *Am J Clin Pathol* 1996;105:141–143.

92. Kaplan LD, Abrams DI, Feigel E, et al. AIDS-associated non-Hodgkin's lymphomas in San Francisco. *JAMA* 1989;261:719–724.

93. Kaplan LD, Lee JY, Ambinder RF, et al. Rituximab does not improve clinical outcome in a randomized phase 3 trial of CHOP with or without rituximab in patients with HIV-associated non-Hodgkin lymphoma: AIDS-Malignancies Consortium Trial 010. *Blood* 2005;106(5):1538–43.

94. Kaplan LD, Straus DJ, Testa MA, et al. Low-dose compared with standard-dose m-BACOD chemotherapy for non-Hodgkin's lymphoma associated with human immunodeficiency virus infection. *N Engl J Med* 1997;336:1641–1648.

95. Kasamon YL, Ambinder RF. AIDS-related primary central nervous system lymphoma. *Hematol Oncol Clin North Am* 2005;19:665–687.

96. Kest H, Brogly S, McSherry G, et al. Malignancy in perinatally human immunodeficiency virus-infected children in the United States. *Pediatr Infect Dis J* 2005;24(3):237–242.

97. Kim JH, Sarani B, Orkin BA, et al. HIV-positive patients with anal carcinoma have poorer treatment tolerance and outcome than HIV-negative patients. *Dis Colon Rectum* 2001;44(10):1496–1502.

98. Knowles DM, Chemulak GA, Subar M, et al. Lymphoid neoplasia associated with the acquired immunodeficiency syndrome (AIDS). *Ann Int Med* 1988;108:744–753.

99. Lane HC, Fauci AS. Immunologic abnormalities in the acquired immunodeficiency syndrome. *Ann Rev Immunol* 1985;3:477–500.

100. Laubenstein LJ, Krigel RL, Odajnky CM, et al. Treatment of epidemic Kaposi's sarcoma with etoposide or a combination of doxorubicin, bleomycin, and vincristine. *J Clin Oncol* 1984;2:1115–1120.

101. Laurence J, Astrin SM. Human immunodeficiency virus induction of malignant transformation in human B lymphocytes. *Proc Nat Acad Sci U S A* 1991;88:7635–7639.

102. Ledergerber B, Egger M, Erard V, et al. AIDS-related opportunistic illnesses occurring after initiation of potent antiretroviral therapy: the Swiss Cohort Study. *JAMA* 1999;282:2220–2226.

103. Levine AM. AIDS-associated malignant lymphoma. *Med Clin North Am* 1992;76:253–268.

104. Levine AM, Espina BE, Tulpule A, et al. Low dose mBACOD with concomitant dideoxycytidine (ddC): an effective regimen in AIDS-related lymphoma. *Blood* 1993;82[Suppl 1):A1531.

105. Levine AM, Gill PS, Meyer PR, et al. Retrovirus and malignant lymphoma in homosexual men. *JAMA* 1985;254:1921–1925.

106. Levine AM, Seneviratne L, Espina BM, et al. Evolving Characteristics of AIDS-related Lymphoma. *Blood* 2000;96:4084–4090.

107. Levine AM, Seneviratne L, Tulpule A. Incidence and management of AIDS-related lymphoma. *Oncology* 2001;15(5):629–639.

108. Levine AM, Sullivan-Halley J, Pike MC, et al. Human immunodeficiency virus-related lymphoma. Prognostic factors predictive of survival. *Cancer* 1991;68:2466–2472.

109. Levine AM, Wernz JC, Kaplan L, et al. Low dose chemotherapy with central nervous system prophylaxis and zidovudine maintenance in AIDS-related lymphoma. *JAMA* 1991;226:84–88.

110. Lim ST, Levine A. Recent advances in acquired immunodeficiency syndrome (AIDS)–related lymphoma. *CA Cancer J Clin* 2005;55:229–241.

111. Ling SM, Roach M, Larson DA, et al. Radiotherapy of primary central nervous system lymphoma in patients with and without human immunodeficiency virus—ten years of treatment experience at the University of California San Francisco. *Cancer* 1994;73:2570–2582.

112. Lopez Bernaldo de Quiros JC, Miro JM, Peña JM, et al. A randomized trial of the discontinuation of primary and secondary prophylaxis against *Pneumocystosis carinii* pneumonia after highly active antiretroviral therapy in patients with HIV infection. *N Engl J Med* 2001;344(3):159–167.

113. Loureiro C, Gill PS, Meyer PR, et al. Autopsy findings in AIDS-related lymphoma. *Cancer* 1988;62:735–739.

114. Lowenthal DA, Strauss DJ, Campbell SW, et al. AIDS-related lymphoid neoplasia: the Memorial Hospital experience. *Cancer* 1988;61:2325–2337.

115. Maiman M, Fruchter RG, Clark M, et al. Cervical cancer as an AIDS-defining illness. *Obsts Gynecol* 1997;89:76–80.

116. Maiman M, Fruchter RG, Guy L, et al. Human immunodeficiency virus infection and invasive cervical carcinoma. *Cancer* 1993;71:402–406.

117. Matthews GV, Bower M, Mandalia S, et al. Changes in acquired immunodeficiency syndrome-related lymphoma since the introduction of highly active antiretroviral therapy. *Blood* 2000;96:2730–2734.

118. Mazhar D, Stebbing J, Bower M. Non-Hodgkin's lymphoma and the CNS: prophylaxis and therapy in immunocompetent and HIV-positive individuals. *Expert Rev Anticancer Ther* 2006;6(3):335–341.

119. McGowan JP, Shah S. Long-term remission of AIDS-related primary central nervous system lymphoma associated with highly active antiretroviral therapy. *AIDS* 1998;12:952–954.

120. Melbye M, Cote TR, Kessler L. High incidence of anal cancer among AIDS patients. *Lancet* 1994;343:636–639.

121. Melbye M, Rabkin CS, Frisch M, et al. Changing patterns of anal cancer incidence in the United States, 1946–1989. *Am J Epidemiol* 1994;139:772–780.

122. Meyer JL. Whole lung irradiation for Kaposi's sarcoma. *Ann J Clin Oncol* 1993;16:372–376.

123. Minkoff H, Ahdieh L, Massa LS, et al. The effect of highly active antiretroviral therapy on cervical cytologic changes associated with oncogenic HPV among HIV-infected women. *AIDS* 2001;15:2157–2164.

124. Muldrow ME, Orr LK, Douglas JM, et al. Intraepithelial neoplasia of the anogenital area in HIV infected homosexual men. *J Acquir Immune Defic Syndr Hum Retrovirol* 1997;14(4):A18(abstr 10).

125. Newell ME, Hoy JF, Cooper SG, et al. Human immunodeficiency virus-related primary central nervous system lymphoma: factors influencing survival in 111 patients. *Cancer* 2004;100:2627–2636.

126. Nguyen NP, B Levinson, Dutta S, et al. Amifostine and curative intent chemoradiation for compromised cancer patients. *Anticancer Res* 2003;23(2C):1649–1656.

127. Northfelt D, Stewart S. DOXIL (pegylated liposomal doxorubicin) as first-line therapy of AIDS-related Kaposi's sarcoma (KS): integrated efficacy and safety results from two comparative trials. *Abstracts of the 4th Conference on Retroviruses and Opportunistic Infections* 1997;736:200.

128. Northfelt DW, Swift PS, Palefsky JM. Anal dysplasia: Pathogenesis, diagnosis and management. In: Krown SE, von Roenn JH, eds. *Hematologic and oncologic aspects of HIV infection, Hematology Oncology Clinics of North America.* Philadelphia: W.B. Saunders, 1996;117–1188.

129. Palefsky JM, Holly EA, Hogeboom CJ. Anal cytology as a screening tool for anal squamous intraepithelial lesions. *J Acquir Immune Defic Syndr Hum Retrovirol* 1997;14:415–422.

130. Palella FJ Jr, Delaney KM, Moorman AC, et al. Declining morbidity and mortality among patients with advanced human immunodeficiency virus infection. *N Engl J Med* 1998;338:853–860.

131. Peddada AV, Smith PE, Rao AR. Chemotherapy and low-dose radiotherapy in the treatment of HIV-infected patients with carcinoma of the anal canal. *Int J Radiat Oncol Biol Phys* 1997;37:1101–1105.

132. Pelstring RJ, Zellmer RB, Sulak LE, et al. Hodgkin's disease in association with human immunodeficiency virus infection: pathologic and immunologic features. *Cancer* 1991;67:1865–1873.

133. Perez CA, Kavanagh BD. Uterine cervix. In: Perez CA, Brady LW, Halperin EC, et al., eds. *Principles and practice of radiation oncology,* 4th ed. Philadelphia: Lippincott Williams & Wilkins, 2003;1800–1915.

134. Piedbois P, Frikha H, Martin L, et al. Radiotherapy in the management of epidemic Kaposi's sarcoma. *Int J Radiat Oncol Biol Phys* 1994;30(5):1207–1211.

135. Pollock BH, Jenson HB, Leach CT, et al. Risk factors for pediatric human immunodeficiency virus-related malignancy. *JAMA* 2003;289(18):2393–2399.

136. Porter SB, Sarde MA. Toxoplasmosis of the central nervous system in the acquired immunodeficiency syndrome. *N Engl J Med* 1992;327:1640–1643.

137. Re A, Casari S, Stellini R, et al. Increased incidence in HIV-associated Hodgkin disease (HD) in the era of highly active antiretroviral therapy (HAART) (abstr 3586). *Proceedings of the American Society of Hematology 42nd Annual Meeting and Exposition.* December 2000.

138. Remick SC. Commentary on the "Management of anal cancer in the HIV-positive population." *Oncology* 2005;19(12):1645–1648.

139. Remick SC, Diamond C, Migliozzi JA, et al. Primary central nervous system lymphoma in patients with and without the acquired immunodeficiency syndrome—a retrospective analysis and review of the literature. *Medicine* 1990;69:345–360.

140. Rossi G, Donisi A, Casari S, et al. The international prognostic index can be used as a guide to treatment decisions regarding patients with human immunodeficiency virus-related systemic non-Hodgkin lymphoma. *Cancer* 1999;86:2391–2397.

141. Safai B, Diaz B, Schwartz J. Malignant neoplasms associated with human immunodeficiency virus infection. *CA-A Cancer J Clin* 1996;42:74–90.

142. Schafer A, Friedman W, Mielke M, et al. The increased frequency of cervical dysplasia-neoplasia in women infected with the human immunodeficiency virus is related to the degree of immunosuppression. *Am J Obstet Gynecol* 1991;164:593–599.

143. Simonelli C, Spina M, Cinella R, et al. Clinical features and outcome of primary effusion lymphoma in HIV-infected patients: a single-institution study. *J Clin Oncol* 2003;21:3948–3954.

144. Skjeldestad FE. Future II Steering Committee. Prophylactic quadrivalent human papillomavirus (HPV) (types 6, 11, 16, 18) L1 virus-like particle (VLP) vaccine (Gardasil) reduces cervical intraepithelial neoplasia (CIN) 2/3 risk (abstr LB-8a). Paper presented at: 43rd Annual Meeting of the Infectious Diseases Society of America. 2005.

145. Sparano JA, Anand K, Desai J. Effect of highly active antiretroviral therapy on the incidence of HIV-associated malignancies at an urban medical center. *J Acquir Immune Defic Syndr* 1999;21[Suppl 1]:S18–22.

146. Sparano JA, Lee S, Chen M, et al. Phase II Trial of infusional cyclophosphamide, doxorubicin and etoposide (CDE) in HIV-associated non-Hodgkin's lymphoma: an Eastern Cooperative Oncology Group Trial (E1494) 3rd AIDS Malignancy Conference, Bethesda, MD, 1999. *J Acquir Imune Defic Syndr* 1999;21:A39(abstr 120).

147. Spina M, Gabarre J, Rossi G, et al. Stanford V regimen and concomitant HAART in 59 patients with Hodgkin disease and HIV infection. *Blood* 2002;100:1984–1988.

148. Stebbing J, Gazzard B. Stemming the epidemic: prevention and therapy go hand-in-hand. *J HIV Ther* 2003;8:51–55.

149. Stebbing J, Gazzard B, Mandalia S, et al. Antiretroviral treatment regimens and immune parameters in the prevention of systemic AIDS-related non-Hodgkin's lymphoma. *J Clin Oncol* 2004;22:2177–2183.

150. Steinbrook R. The potential of human papillomavirus vaccines. *N Engl J Med* 2006;354(11):1109–1112.

151. Steinbrook R, Drazen JM. AIDS-Will the next 20 years be different? (editorial) *N Engl J Med* 2001;344:1781–1782.

152. Stelzer KJ, Griffin TW. A randomized prospective trial of radiation therapy for AIDS-associated Kaposi's sarcoma. *Int J Radiat Oncol Biol Phys* 1993;27(5):1057–1061.

153. Stephenson J. Hopes for HIV eradication dim as stopping HAART allows resurgence. *JAMA* 1999;282:1317–1318.

154. Sun XW, Kuhn L, Ellenbrock TV, et al. Human papillomavirus infection in women infected with the human immunodeficiency virus. *New Engl J Med* 1997;337:1343–1349.

155. Swift PS. Radiation therapy for malignancies in the setting of HIV disease. *Oncology* 1997;11:683–694.

156. Tsimberidou AM, Sarris AH, Medeiros LJ, et al. Hodgkin's disease in patients infected with human immunodeficiency virus: frequency, presentation and clinical outcome. *Leuk Lymphoma* 2001;41(5–6):535–544.

157. Varmuad SH, Kelley KF, Klein RS, et al. High risk of human papilloma virus infection and cervical squamous intraepithelial lesions among women with symptomatic human immunodeficiency virus infection. *Am J Obstet Gynecol* 1991;165:392–400.
158. Volm M, Wernz J. Patients with advanced AIDS-related Kaposi's sarcoma (EKS) no longer require systemic chemotherapy after introduction of effective antiretroviral therapy. *Proc ASCO* 1997;16:A46.
159. Watson J. Investigation reveals Hodgkin's disease might be an AIDS-defining condition. *Hem/Onc Today* 2001;2:6.
160. Wilkin TJ, Palmer S, Brudney KF, et al. Anal intraepithelial neoplasia in heterosexual and homosexual HIV-positive men with access to antiretroviral therapy. *J Infect Dis* 2004;190:1685–1691.
161. Williams B, Darragh TM, Vranizar K, et al. Analysis of cervical human papilloma virus infection and risk of anal and cervical epithelial abnormalities in human immunodeficiency virus-infected women. *Obstet Gynecol* 1994;83: 205–211.
162. AIDS Media Center. Available at: www.aidsmedia.org.
163. AIDS Malignancy Consortium. Available at: www.amc.uab.edu/trials.htm.
164. AIDS Malignancy Consortium. Available at: www.amc.uab.edu/036des.htm.
165. U.S. Nation Cancer Institute. Available at: www.cancer.gov.
166. Joint United Nations Programme on AIDS. 2004 Report on the Global AIDS Epidemic. Available at: www.unaids.org/en.
167. Joint United Nations Programme on AIDS. UNAIDS/WHO AIDS epidemic update: December 2005. Available at: www.unaids.org/epi/2005/doc/report_pdf.asp.

Part C Central Nervous System Tumors

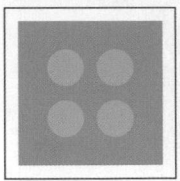

Chapter 32
Primary Intracranial Neoplasms

Malika L. Siker, Bernadine R. Donahue, Michael A. Vogelbaum, Wolfgang A. Tome,
Mark R. Gilbert, Minesh P. Mehta

Anatomy

The central nervous system (CNS) is enveloped by three layers of tissues called the meninges. The *dura mater* (also known as the pachymeninges) is a tough, fibrous tissue that comprises the most external meningeal layer. The much thinner *pia mater* is the innermost layer, which folds into the sulci, indentations, and irregularities of the CNS surface. Between them is the *arachnoid mater*, a webbed structure that is attached to the pia mater. These two layers (pia-arachnoid) are also referred to at the leptomeninges, and within them is the subarachnoid space, which is filled with cerebrospinal fluid (CSF). Within the cranial cavity, dural folds separate the two hemispheres of the cerebrum (falx cerebri) and the cerebrum from the cerebellum and brainstem (tentorium).

The brain measures, on average, 16 cm anteroposteriorly, 14 cm transversely, and 12 cm superoinferiorly. Brain volume is approximately 1,300 cm³; its surface area is approximately 2,000 cm², and it weighs approximately 1,300 g (range 800 to 2,000 g). The average thickness of the cerebral cortex is 2.5 mm (194). The CNS is composed of white matter (60%) and gray matter (40%).

The frontal and parietal lobes are separated by a well-defined sulcus ("central sulcus"). The frontal and temporal lobes are separated by the Sylvian fissure, while the parietal and occipital lobes are separated by the calcarine sulcus (Figs. 32.1–32.3). Functionally, the brain can be separated into anatomically defined regions that have clearly associated neurological functions and other regions that perform higher level processing but are less well defined anatomically. In the cerebrum, the primary motor and sensory areas are located in front of and behind the central sulcus, respectively, and collectively this region is referred to as the Rolandic cortex. The pre- and postcentral gyri control body and face motor and sensory functions and are organized so that the face is represented laterally and the legs mesially (the representation is called *homunculus*). Speech and language functions are controlled primarily by two regions in the frontal and temporal lobes. The motor–speech area of Broca is located in the dominant frontal lobe just above the Sylvian fissure; damage to this area causes expressive aphasia. Sensory, or receptive, aphasia (Wernicke's) results from dam-age to the dominant superior temporal gyrus at the posterior end of the Sylvian fissure. The mesial part of the temporal lobe (hippocampus and fornix) is associated with short-term memory. The primary visual cortex is represented on the medial and inferior surface at the occipital pole.

The diencephalon consists of the thalamus and the pineal region and is situated between the cerebrum and the mesencephalon, adjacent to the third ventricle. The thalamus is involved primarily in the integration of sensory functions. Lateral to the thalamus is the internal capsule, which carries the motor fibers (upper motor neurons) from the cortex en route to the brainstem and spinal cord.

At the tentorial notch, the mesencephalon rides on the upper part of the clivus. Its interior, the tectum, is partially occupied by cranial nerve nuclei (for the oculomotor, trochlear, and proprioceptive portions of the trigeminal nerves). The dorsal plate houses the superior and inferior colliculi, which regulate eye movements and hearing impulses, respectively. The trochlear nerve is the only cranial nerve that exits from this dorsal location.

The pons relays information between the two cerebellar hemispheres and from the spinal cord to the cerebellum, carries the major ascending and descending pathways between the mesencephalon and the medulla oblongata, and contains the major motor and tactile sensory nuclei for the trigeminal nerve, which emerges from its lateral surface. The border between the pons and the medulla oblongata is noteworthy for the emergence of the abducens, facial, and vestibulocochlear (acoustic) cranial nerves.

The cerebellum develops laterally and posteriorly from the pons and differentiates into the median vermis cerebelli and the bilateral hemispheres, which are flattened by the sloping tentorium on both sides. Anteriorly, the cerebellum faces the dorsal aspects of the pons and the medulla oblongata (the floor of the fourth ventricle).

The medulla oblongata forms the link between the pons, the spinal cord, and the cerebellum. It houses the majority of the cranial nerve nuclei (abducens, facial, vestibulocochlear, glossopharyngeal, vagal, accessory, and hypoglossal).

The brain receives its arterial supply from the internal carotid arteries (anterior circulation) and the vertebral vessels, which join to form the basilar artery (posterior circulation).

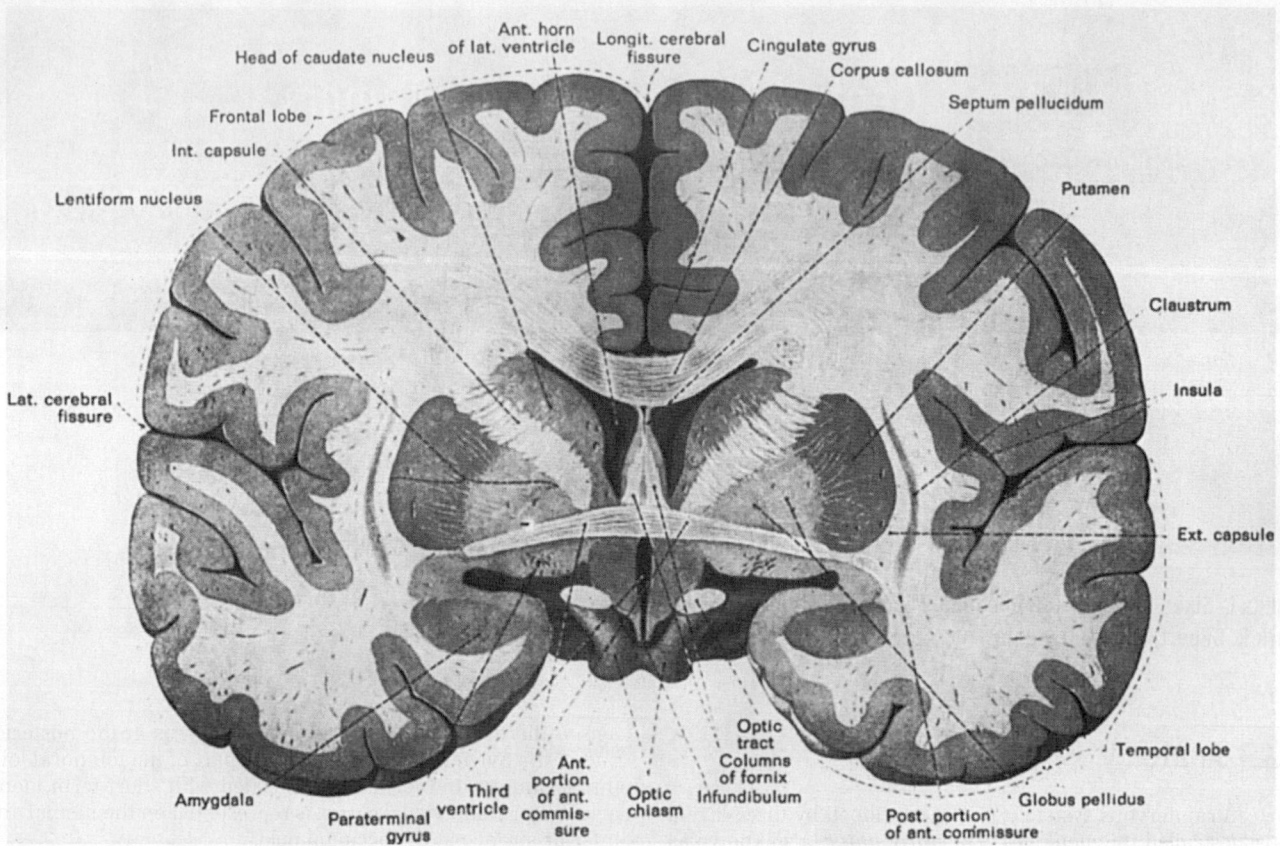

FIGURE 32.1. Frontal section through the telencephalon at the plane of the anterior commissure. (From *Sobotta/Figge atlas of human anatomy*, Vol. 2, 9th ed. Munich: Urban & Schwartzenberg, 1977, with permission.)

Several anastomotic vessels (one anterior communicating artery and two posterior communicating arteries) produce communication between the anterior and posterior circulations and form the so-called circle of Willis. Although the degree of formation of a complete circle of Willis varies among individuals, this anatomic ring allows for bilaterally uninterrupted oxygen supply in case of local vascular obstruction.

The arterial supply to the lateral surface of the brain is dominated by the middle cerebral artery, which emerges anteriorly in the Sylvian fissure as the major branch from the internal carotid artery. Most of the mesial interhemispheric surface is supplied by the anterior cerebral artery. The parietal and occipital lobes are served by the posterior cerebral artery, which is a terminal branch of the basilar artery.

The ventricular system develops by ballooning from the primitive neural canal. It is lined with a specialized form of glia, referred to as ependyma. CSF is produced by the choroid plexus, which lies in the roofs of the fourth and third ventricles as well as in the medial walls of the central body and inferior horns of the lateral ventricles. The foramina of Munro transmit CSF between the third and lateral ventricles at the superolateral corners of the third ventricle. The aqueduct of Sylvius in the midbrain transmits CSF from the third to the fourth ventricles. It is the narrowest canal of the intracranial nervous system and is therefore the most common location of obstruction of flow by compression or tumor deposits, resulting in noncommunicating hydrocephalus.

CSF in the fourth ventricle flows out of the ventricular system through the midline foramen of Magendie and the two lateral foramina of Luschka to the subarachnoid space. All three foramina are located in the roof and lateral corners of the fourth ventricle at the level of the medulla oblongata. The subarachnoid space widens into several cisterns, the largest of which are the cisterna magna (posterior to the medulla oblongata at the foramen magnum), the cistern of the lateral sulcus bilaterally at the base of the brain, and the ambient cistern posterior to the midbrain. CSF resorption back into the venous system occurs at arachnoid (or Pacconian) granulations, special outpouching structures from the arachnoid membrane that enhance fluid movement from the CSF space into the venous sinus system. Scarring from infection or inflammation or clogging of the arachnoid granulations causes increased pressure in the CSF space and communication hydrocephalus.

Epidemiology

In 2005 there were an estimated 20,000 new cases of primary CNS tumors in the United States and 13,000 deaths (34), for an incidence of approximately 7.4 per 100,000 persons. The incidence of brain tumors increases with age to reach 50 per 100,000 at ages >75 years (34).

The majority of CNS tumors in adults arise in the supratentorial compartment. Most arise in the parenchyma and the majority of these are high-grade gliomas (34). There is a male preponderance for most brain tumor types except neurinomas and meningiomas; for the latter, the female to male ratio is approximately 2:1 (34). During the 1990s, an increase in tumors among older patients was noted, independent of the increasing percentage of older individuals in our society. This may have been partly due to better detection after the introduction of magnetic resonance imaging (MRI). An increase in incidence of primary CNS lymphoma is most likely due to the increasing numbers of immunosuppressed patients in the setting of human immunodeficiency virus (HIV) and posttransplant use of immunosuppressants (47).

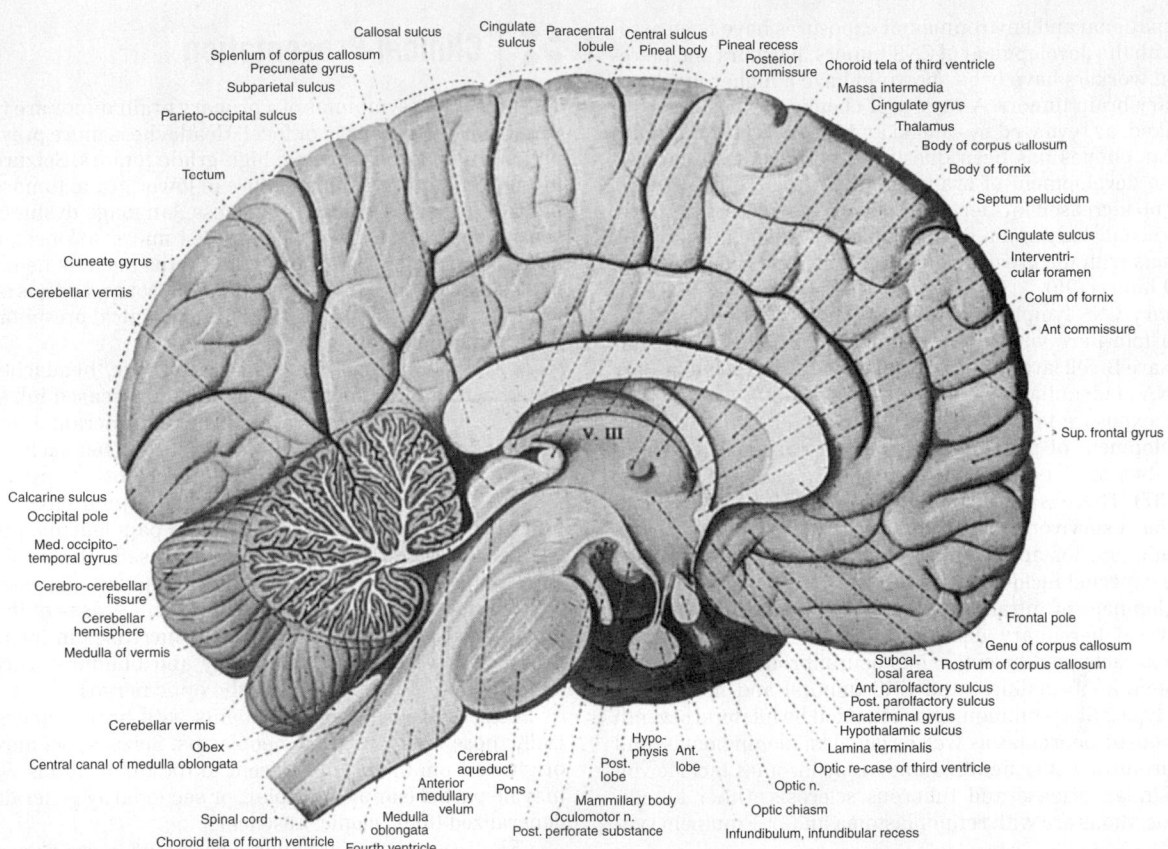

FIGURE 32.2. The supratentorial parts of the central nervous system (CNS) include the telencephalon (cerebral hemispheres with frontal, parietal, occipital, and temporal lobes) and the diencephalon, with the dominant thalamus nucleus, the hypothalamus, the pituitary stalk, and the neurohypophysis inferoanteriorly and the pineal body posteriorly, which represent the midline central structures of the supratentorial CNS. (From *Sobotta/Figge atlas of human anatomy,* Vol. 2, 9th ed. Munich: Urban & Schwartzenberg, 1977, with permission.)

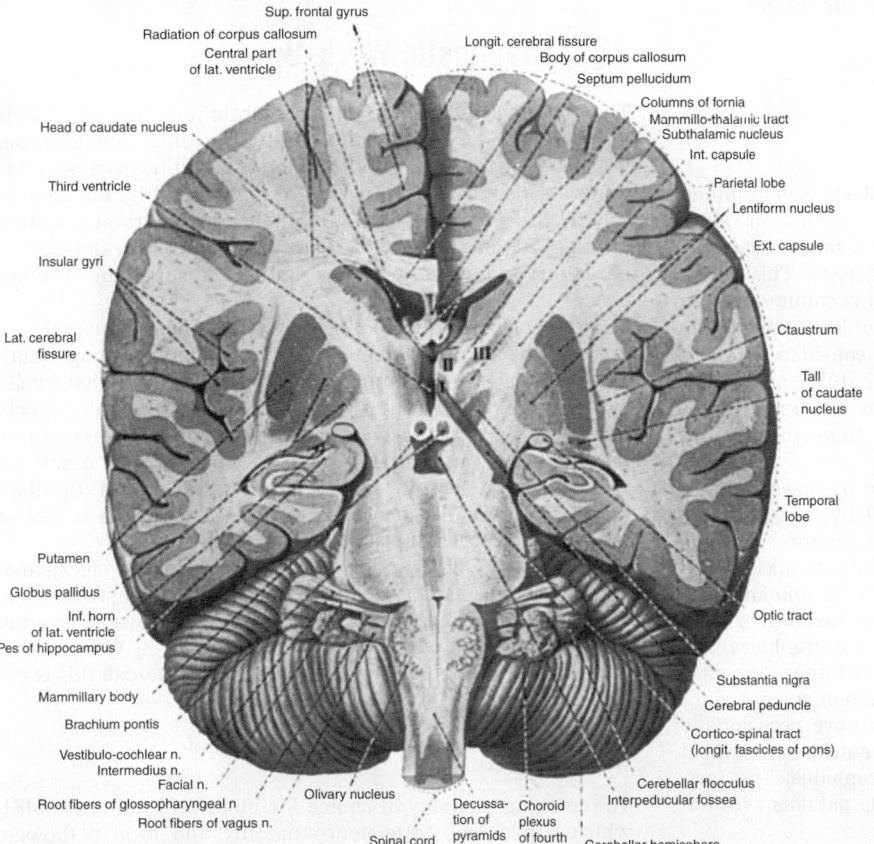

FIGURE 32.3. Section through telencephalon and brainstem parallel with the cerebral peduncles. View of the posterior surface of the plane of sectioning. On the right side of the figure, the section reaches back to approximately the middle of the cerebral peduncle (oblique section). I to III indicate thalamic nuclei: I, medial nucleus; II, anterior nucleus; III, lateral nucleus. (From *Sobotta/Figge atlas of human anatomy,* Vol. 2, 9th ed. Munich: Urban & Schwartzenberg, 1977, with permission.)

Occupational and environmental exposures have been associated with the development of CNS tumors. Farmers and petrochemical workers have been shown to have a higher incidence of primary brain tumors. A variety of chemical exposures have been linked, as reviewed by Ohgaki and Kleihues (165). The use of cellular phones has been questioned as a contributing factor to the development of brain tumors. Although two studies showed no increased incidence in cellular phone users (99,106), a more recent study found the overall odds ratio highest among individuals with the greatest cumulative lifetime cell phone use (>2,000 hours) (95).

Primary CNS lymphoma has been shown to be associated with Epstein-Barr virus. The majority of primary CNS lymphomas are B-cell large immunoblastic types, and Epstein-Barr virus DNA is identifiable in nearly all cases (100).

Prior exposure to ionizing radiation is a known risk factor for development of primary CNS tumors, particularly meningiomas, but also astrocytomas, sarcomas, and other tumor types (137). There is a 2.3% incidence of primary brain tumors in long-term survivors among children given prophylactic cranial irradiation for acute leukemia; this is a 22-fold increase over the expected incidence (5,157).

Development of intracranial malignancy is also associated with several hereditary diseases such as neurofibromatosis type 1 (characterized by cutaneous neurofibromas, café au lait spots, bone abnormalities, and CNS tumors) and neurofibromatosis type 2 (less common, characterized by bilateral seventh nerve acoustic neuromas as well as gliomas, meningiomas, and neurofibromas). Other neurocutaneous syndromes include von Hippel-Lindau disease and tuberous sclerosis. Other hereditary associations are with retinoblastoma and Li-Fraumeni syndrome.

Although the exact nature of the carcinogenic events leading to brain tumor induction is not known, experimental evidence suggests an accumulation of genetic alterations that lead to the acquisition of a malignant phenotype through activation of cellular oncogenes and loss of cellular tumor suppressor genes (164,165).

Natural History

The natural history of a primary brain neoplasm is determined by its histology, grade, and location. The majority of adult gliomas spread invasively without forming a natural capsule. They frequently cause edema in surrounding tissue. This edema may be vasogenic, ischemic, or cytotoxic. It is commonly seen on T2-weighted MRI and is responsible for at least some of the clinical symptoms and signs. The edema is considered to be a consequence of altered blood–brain barrier (BBB) permeability. Different tumors cause varying amounts of edema (in descending order: metastases, astrocytomas, meningiomas, and oligodendrogliomas).

Some high-grade neoplasms metastasize by "seeding" into the subarachnoid and ventricular spaces and, by gravity or flow, cause metastatic deposits in the spinal canal. Tumors that have a propensity for CSF spread include medulloblastomas, primitive neuroectodermal tumors (PNET), and CNS lymphoma. The exact frequency of CSF spread among other histologies (e.g., germ cell tumors, ependymomas) is debated in the literature. Extracranial metastases from primary brain tumors are rare but can occur with medulloblastomas, germinomas, and high-grade astrocytomas. Peritoneal metastases have occasionally been noted in patients who have had a ventriculoperitoneal shunt placed to relieve obstructive hydrocephalus. The incidence is low and does not preclude shunting patients with obstruction.

Clinical Presentation

The presenting symptoms of a primary brain tumor are typically classified as generalized or focal. Headache is more prevalent in patients with faster growing, high-grade tumors. Seizures are a more common presenting feature in lower grade tumors. Focal neurologic deficits such as weakness, language dysfunction, or sensory loss are seen with low-grade tumors, a consequence of their slower rate of growth. Acute events such as hemorrhage markedly alter the tempo of symptom onset regardless of tumor grade. Table 32.1 summarizes common clinical presentations of the more common CNS tumors.

Because brain parenchyma is anesthetic, headaches associated with brain tumors may be due to increased intracranial pressure or to local pressure on sensitive intracranial structures (mainly dura and vessels). Characteristically headaches associated with increased intracranial pressure occur in the morning. Associated findings may include focal neurologic deficits, motor deficits, behavioral changes, and papilledema. Cushing's triad is classically associated with increased intracranial pressure, but the full triad (hypertension, bradycardia, respiratory irregularity) is seen in only one third of the cases of increased intracranial pressure. Long-standing increases in intracranial pressure may lead to optic atrophy and blindness because of transmission of the pressure to the optic nerves.

Seizures are common in patients with brain tumors, especially those with low-grade neoplasms. Seizure foci most likely originate from the brain adjacent to the tumor nidus. Seizures may be partial (simple, complex, or secondarily generalized) or generalized (tonic clonic, absence).

CSF dissemination of tumor cells should be suspected in patients with neurologic deficits that cannot be attributed to the primary tumor. Lumbar back pain or bowel or bladder dysfunction, for example, may suggest CSF metastasis in the lumbar cistern with involvement of the cauda equina.

Diagnostic Work-Up

The initial work-up of patients with brain tumors must include a complete history and general physical examination. Information obtained from relatives and friends is helpful because many tumors cause mental changes not appreciated by the patient. Inherited diseases associated with brain tumors and history of infections may be indicators of etiology and in the case of hereditary syndromes increase vigilance in surveying for other cancers.

Neurologic examination includes assessment of mental condition (behavior, mood, sensorium, intelligence, thought content, language, insight into own disease), coordination (walking, balance, alternating movement), sensation (pain, touch, vibration, position sense, stereognosis, point discrimination), reflexes (deep, superficial, clonus), motor (strength, tonus, resistance to passive movement), and cranial nerves. Ophthalmoscopy is performed to check for papilledema as a sign of increased intracranial pressure.

In patients with symptoms, signs, or imaging suggestive of systemic involvement, biopsy confirmation of at least one of the metastatic sites is recommended. Solitary brain lesions in adult patients with systemic cancer are far more likely to be a cerebral metastasis than a primary CNS tumor, although this is not always the case.

Imaging Studies

The imaging modality of choice for most CNS tumors is MRI, which can demonstrate neuroanatomy and local pathologic

Table 32.1 | SYMPTOMS, SIGNS, AND DIAGNOSTIC CHARACTERISTICS OF VARIOUS INTRACRANIAL TUMORS

Tumor	Common Symptoms	Common Signs	Imaging Characteristics
Glioblastoma multiforme	Headache, seizure, unilateral weakness, mental changes	Focal presentation related to tumor location	Enhancing MRI or CT lesion, hypodense interior, often with associated edema
Meningioma	Localized headache	Focal presentation related to tumor location	Enhancing MRI or CT lesion associated with dura
Astrocytoma	Headache, seizure, unilateral weakness, mental changes	Focal presentation related to tumor location	May not enhance on CT or MRI
Cerebral	Headache, seizure, unilateral weakness, mental changes	Focal presentation related to tumor location	
Cerebellar	Occipital headache	Increased intracranial pressure (i.e., papilledema), abducens and oculomotor nerve deficits; coordination	
Brainstem or thalamus	Nausea, vomiting, ataxia	Increased intracranial pressure (i.e., papilledema), abducens and oculomotor nerve deficits; ataxia	May be seen only on MRI
Optic nerve	Ocular changes	Ocular changes	Uniform enhancement on MRI or CT scan
Medulloblastoma	Morning headaches, nausea, vomiting	Coordination, increased intracranial pressure (i.e., papilledema), abducens and oculomotor nerve deficits	Heterogeneously enhancing on MRI or CT, typical lateral location in adults
Ependymoma	Morning headaches, nausea, vomiting	Coordination, increased intracranial pressure (i.e., papilledema), abducens and oculomotor nerve deficits	Heterogeneous enhancement on MRI or CT with or without calcification
Neurilemoma, schwannoma, neurinomas	Unilateral deafness, vertigo	Ipsilateral acoustic and facial or trigeminal nerve deficits	Homogenous enhancing mass on MRI or CT, arising from cranial nerve
Oligodendroglioma	Insidious headache, mental changes	Focal presentation related to tumor location	Heterogeneous lesion that may or may not enhance on MRI or CT, frequently with calcification, cystic regions, or hemorrhage
Lymphoma	Focal presentation related to tumor location	Focal presentation related to tumor location	Homogeneous, intense enhancement on MRI, may have a diffuse or "cotton wool" appearance
Craniopharyngioma	Headache, mental changes, hemiplegia, seizure, vomiting, visual impairment	Cranial nerve deficits (II–VII)	Mixed cystic, calcified lesion on MRI and CT, arising from suprasellar region

CT, computed tomography; MRI, magnetic resonance imaging

Clinical Radiation Oncology

processes in exquisite detail. Computed tomography (CT) is generally reserved for those unable (implanted pacemaker, metal fragment, paramagnetic surgical clips) or unwilling because of claustrophobia to undergo MRI.

Magnetic Resonance Imaging

The most useful imaging studies are T1-weighted sagittal images, gadolinium (Gd)-enhanced and unenhanced T1 axial images, and T2-weighted axial images. As with CT contrast, the gadolinium leaks into parenchyma in areas with BBB breakdown, and the paramagnetic properties of gadolinium generate increased signal on T1 scans. T1 images usually are better at demonstrating anatomy and areas of contrast enhancement. T2 and FLAIR (fluid-attenuated inversion recovery) images are more sensitive for detecting edema.

Tumor appearance on T1-weighted MRI is similar to that on CT, as are the contrast enhancement patterns. The anatomic definition and image resolution are much better with MRI, however, and tumor volumes are better delineated than with CT, particularly with low-grade neoplasms that do not enhance with the administration of contrast material (Fig. 32.4). Tumor and edema demonstrate increased signal on T2-weighted MRI. The area of increased T2 signal on MRI usually includes the hypodense area on CT, but the MRI typically identifies a larger edema volume than the corresponding CT scan. Although both edema and tumor can be seen to extend along white matter tracts,

T2 signal tracking across the corpus callosum is more commonly due to tumor involvement than edema.

Neuraxis Imaging

For neoplasms at high risk of spread to the CSF, staging of the neuraxis is essential. Gd-enhanced MRI of the spine has replaced myelography as the imaging modality of choice. Ideally, neuraxis imaging should be performed before surgery. In the immediate postoperative period, spinal MRI scans may be difficult to interpret because arachnoiditis and blood products in the CSF can mimic leptomeningeal metastasis. Delayed spinal MRI (>3 weeks after surgery), combined with an increased dose of intravenous gadolinium, is a sensitive imaging study for leptomeningeal disease.

Newer Imaging Modalities

Improved MRI technology permits extremely rapid acquisition of sequential MRIs, allowing detailed imaging of tumor perfusion and cerebral blood flow to help clarify tumor architecture. Functional mapping of the cerebral cortex may be possible through measurements of local changes in oxygen consumption with specific tasks. This anatomic identification of functionally eloquent regions of brain parenchyma permits more extensive surgical resection while avoiding injury to these critical areas. Positron emission tomography (PET) also can give information on metabolic and BBB function (Fig. 32.5). MR-spectroscopy

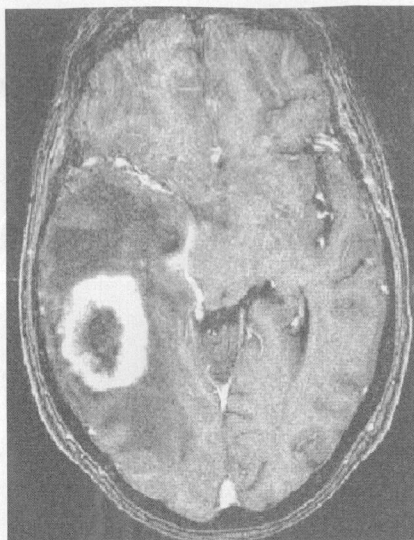
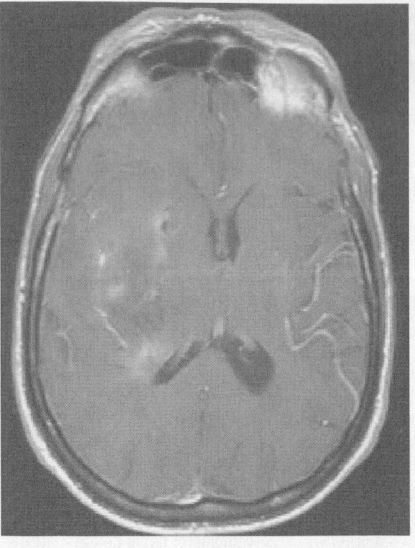

A

B

FIGURE 32.4. Magnetic resonance image of brain showing (**A**) glioblastoma, demonstrating a contrast-enhancing lesion with central necrosis and vasogenic edema; and (**B**) low-grade glioma, illustrating a nonenhancing lesion difficult to delineate from normal parenchyma.

may better delineate infiltrating tumor from peritumoral edema in the nonenhancing region surrounding the tumor mass. In the future, incorporation of three-dimensional (3D) MRI reconstructions, functional imaging, and metabolic maps may allow a comprehensive assessment of tumor volume and its relationship to the functional normal brain. Such information should facilitate surgical resection and radiotherapy planning. Integration of metabolic scans into posttreatment follow-up may help distinguish between tumor recurrence and treatment-related changes, although most modalities have a relatively high false negative rate (i.e., scan suggests treatment-related changes, but active tumor is actually present).

Histologic Confirmation of Diagnosis

Tissue diagnosis is required for most brain tumors. The morbidity of biopsy has decreased significantly with improvements in operative technique and anesthesia, as well as the availability of stereotactic biopsy techniques. Exception might be made in selected patients, for example, patients with known active systemic cancer and multiple lesions that are radiographically consistent with brain metastases, patients with typical clinical and MRI findings of a brainstem glioma or optic nerve meningioma, or HIV-positive patients with CT or MRI findings consistent with primary CNS lymphoma.

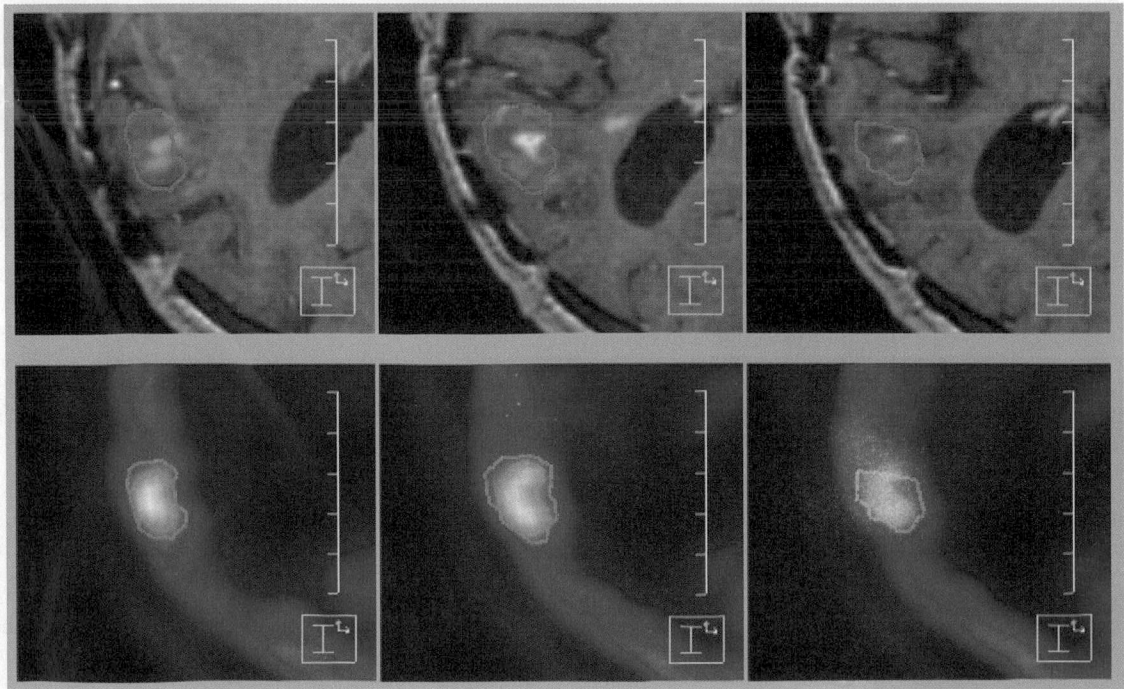

FIGURE 32.5. Oligodendroglioma imaged using an anatomical imaging technique, contrast enhanced 3D-SPGR T1-w MRI (*top image panel*), and a functional imaging technique, FDG PET (*bottom image panel*). The red contour delineates the extent of increased metabolic activity seen using functional imaging. Looking at the top panel, one can appreciate the fact that if the anatomical image set alone would be used for target definition it would yield a gross underestimation of the target volume as compared with the functional imaging technique.

Table 32.2	DIFFERENTIAL DIAGNOSIS OF SPACE-OCCUPYING LESIONS ON COMPUTED TOMOGRAPHY OR MAGNETIC RESONANCE IMAGING
Pathology	**Features on CT or MRI**
Neoplasm	
Primary	Solitary, no prior cancer, thick nodular CE
Metastatic	Multiple, prior cancer, ++edema, located at gray/white junction
Infectious	
Abscess	Fever, acutely ill, ± systemic infection, cyst cavity with smooth thin walls and CE
Cerebritis	Fever, acutely ill, ± systemic infection, diffuse T2 change, no CE mass
Meningitis	Diffuse enhancement of meninges on T1-weighted imaging (may simulate leptomeningeal metastases)
Vascular	
Infarct	Gray and white matter involvement, wedgelike vascular distribution
Bleeding	Homogenous, clears quickly, residual hemosiderin ring
Treatment-related necrosis	Central hypodensity, ring CE, edema, >6 mo after radiation therapy or chemotherapy, metabolic scan shows low activity

CE, contrast enhancement; CT, computed tomography; MRI, magnetic resonance imaging

Cerebrospinal Fluid Cytology

CSF cytology is essential for staging tumors with a propensity for CSF spread (e.g., medulloblastoma, PNET, germ cell tumors, CNS lymphoma). Sampling of the CSF in the immediate postoperative period may lead to false-positive results, however, and is best done before surgery or more than 3 weeks after surgery, as long as there is no uncontrolled raised intracranial pressure.

CSF spread of tumor may be associated with several abnormal findings by CSF examination. These include CSF pressure above 150 mm H_2O at the lumbar level in a laterally positioned patient, elevated protein level, typically >40 mg/dL, a reduced glucose level (below 50 mg/mL), and the finding of tumor cells by cytologic examination. Tumor markers in the CSF may help in making the diagnosis.

Differential Diagnosis

Most adults with new or persistent neurologic findings (focal deficit, increased intracranial pressure, seizures, altered mentation) are investigated using CT or MRI. Thus, the differential diagnosis of brain tumors usually is reduced to the differential diagnosis of space-occupying lesions (Table 32.2).

⠿ Pathology

Primary intracranial tumors are of ectodermal and mesodermal origin and arise from the brain, cranial nerves, meninges, pituitary, pineal, and vascular elements. The nomenclature of brain tumors has changed over time. The most widely used classification system at the present time is that of the World Health Organization (WHO). The WHO classification of primary CNS tumors lists approximately 100 distinct pathologic subtypes of CNS malignancies in 12 broad categories (Table 32.3) (117). Guidelines for assigning grade of malignancy are provided, where applicable.

⠿ Molecular Genetics

Gliomagenesis, or the genetic alterations that characterize the malignant transformation of normal glial cells (astrocytes or oligodendroglial cells) into tumor cells, is an area of active investigation. Although still incompletely understood, most of the efforts have focused on astrocytic tumors. These studies demonstrate that astrocytes undergo transformation with the loss of

tumor suppressor genes critical for cell growth, differentiation, and function. These genes are TP53, the retinoblastoma (RB) gene, the INK4a (inhibitor of cyclin-dependent kinase 4) gene, and the PTEN gene. In low-grade astrocytomas TP53 is rendered inactive by gene mutation or gene deletion. This critical step in transformation is found in approximately 60% of low-grade gliomas. The progression into anaplastic astrocytoma and glioblastoma multiforme (GBM), here secondary GBM, is accompanied by RB and PTEN mutations with cell aneuploidy and overexpression of cyclin-dependent kinase 4 (CDK4). Most series report that 40% of GBM are secondary GBM and that the average patient age is younger. Some studies report a favorable prognosis for patients with secondary GBM, although this may be related to the impact of younger age and better performance

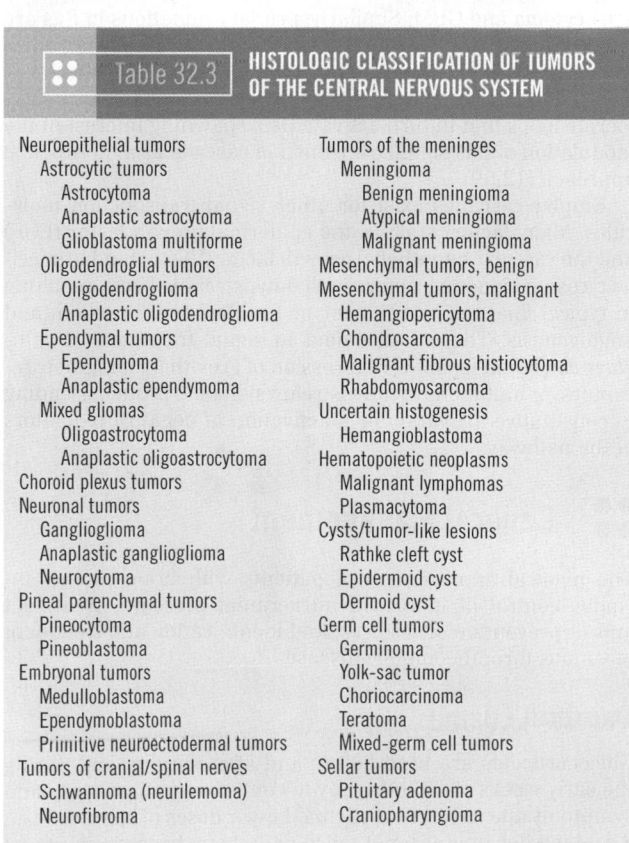

Table 32.3	HISTOLOGIC CLASSIFICATION OF TUMORS OF THE CENTRAL NERVOUS SYSTEM
Neuroepithelial tumors	Tumors of the meninges
Astrocytic tumors	Meningioma
Astrocytoma	Benign meningioma
Anaplastic astrocytoma	Atypical meningioma
Glioblastoma multiforme	Malignant meningioma
Oligodendroglial tumors	Mesenchymal tumors, benign
Oligodendroglioma	Mesenchymal tumors, malignant
Anaplastic oligodendroglioma	Hemangiopericytoma
Ependymal tumors	Chondrosarcoma
Ependymoma	Malignant fibrous histiocytoma
Anaplastic ependymoma	Rhabdomyosarcoma
Mixed gliomas	Uncertain histogenesis
Oligoastrocytoma	Hemangioblastoma
Anaplastic oligoastrocytoma	Hematopoietic neoplasms
Choroid plexus tumors	Malignant lymphomas
Neuronal tumors	Plasmacytoma
Ganglioglioma	Cysts/tumor-like lesions
Anaplastic ganglioglioma	Rathke cleft cyst
Neurocytoma	Epidermoid cyst
Pineal parenchymal tumors	Dermoid cyst
Pineocytoma	Germ cell tumors
Pineoblastoma	Germinoma
Embryonal tumors	Yolk-sac tumor
Medulloblastoma	Choriocarcinoma
Ependymoblastoma	Teratoma
Primitive neuroectodermal tumors	Mixed-germ cell tumors
Tumors of cranial/spinal nerves	Sellar tumors
Schwannoma (neurilemoma)	Pituitary adenoma
Neurofibroma	Craniopharyngioma

status of this group compared with patients with *de novo* (primary) GBM. Emerging data suggest that promoter methylation of the PTEN gene in low-grade gliomas may be causally linked to secondary malignant transformation to GBM.

In *de novo* (primary) GBM, the sequence of genetic changes is different, although the phenotype by routine histopathology is indistinguishable. In addition, recent studies suggest that there are major differences in gene expression profiles between primary and secondary GBM with the former demonstrating a mesenchymal or stromal pattern, whereas the secondary genotype is characterized by abnormalities in cell cycle components (250). Primary GBM often (60%) show amplification of the epidermal growth factor receptor (EGFR) with or without expression of the EGFR deletion mutant variant III, deletions in the INK4a gene with loss of p14 and p16, and diploid cells. In addition, PTEN mutation is far more common in primary GBM compared with secondary GBM, approximately 25% versus 4% (164). The loss of heterozygosity in chromosome 10q causes inactivation of PTEN, a gene downstream of focal adhesion kinase (Fak) that controls cell migration and invasiveness. This effect is mediated by activating Akt, a serine/threonine (ser/thr) kinase involved in cell proliferation and survival (138,238). The loss of heterozygosity of chromosome 10 has been shown in several studies to have a highly significant and independent impact on prognosis (164,235,244).

The protein encoded by the RB gene (pRb) regulates the cell cycle by inhibiting progression beyond the G1/S restriction point. Mitogenic signals activate a molecular cascade known as Ras-mitogen activated protein kinase (Ras/MAPK). MAPK inhibits pRb, activates the transcriptional factor E2 F, and cells enter the S phase. The INK4a gene converges on the Rb pathway by activating three cyclin kinase inhibitors (CKIs): p15, p16, and p19. These CKIs inhibit a family of kinases known as cyclin-dependent kinases (CDKs) 2, 4, and 6, triggering cell cycle progression by inhibiting pRb. Thus, although mutation or deletion of the Rb gene is uncommon, alterations in the control of the Rb pathway play a major role in the phenotype of anaplastic astrocytoma and GBM. Similarly, primary mutations in Ras are less common or absent in glial tumors compared with other cancers. However, there is overexpression or constitutive activation of other receptor tyrosine kinases (RTKs) as well as autocrine loops that in turn activate Ras, spawning interest in the modulation of Ras signal transduction cascade as a therapeutic approach (12,59).

Similar cascades exist for other signal transduction molecules. Many factors such as the epidermal growth factor (EGF) and the vascular endothelial growth factor (VEGF) bind to specific tyrosine kinase receptors with downstream effects, resulting in typical final tumor behavior or proliferation, invasion, and angiogenesis. The enhancement in signal transduction pathways can result from overexpression of growth factors, their receptors, or mutations in downstream signaling proteins, leading to constitutive activation or inactivation of negative regulators of the pathway.

General Management

The medical management of patients with brain tumors includes control of increased intracranial pressure, treatment and/or prevention of seizures, and identification and treatment of venous thromboembolic disease.

Cerebral Edema

Glucocorticoids are used before and after surgery and during the early weeks of radiotherapy to control neurologic signs and symptoms due to cerebral edema. Lower doses of steroids (e.g., 2 to 4 mg dexamethasone) twice daily have been shown to be as effective as higher doses. Prolonged steroid use is associated with a number of significant medical problems, such that this medication should be tapered to the lowest dose necessary to control symptoms and discontinued if possible. Dexamethasone is the most common corticosteroid used because of lesser mineral-corticoid effects. As with all corticosteroids, a slow taper is mandatory to prevent a rebound in cerebral edema. The taper may require several weeks, and adrenal function tests may be necessary to determine if physiologic steroid replacement is required.

Seizures

Patients with seizures due to tumor or to treatment-associated necrosis or gliosis require treatment with anticonvulsants. Since first-generation anticonvulsants such as carbamazepine, phenobarbital, and valproate have been shown to induce hepatic cytochrome P450 isoenzymes, markedly increasing the metabolism and clearance of several cancer chemotherapy agents such as paclitaxel and irinotecan (68,78), newer generation anticonvulsants, such as levetiracetam, lamotrigine, and pregabalin that do not affect cytochrome P450 activity are now preferred.

Prophylactic anticonvulsant use remains controversial, although the American Academy of Neurology has concluded that data supporting the use of prophylactic anticonvulsant use do not exist (80).

Surgery

In general terms, surgical procedures can be summarized as biopsy for diagnosis only, surgical resection for cure, surgical debulking for management of mass effect related symptoms, or CSF diversion procedures to relieve acute symptoms caused by increased intracranial pressure or hydrocephalus. Complete resection of tumor is associated with a survival advantage for most tumor types (123,258). However, for some radio- and/or chemosensitive malignancies such as primary CNS lymphoma, aggressive resection is unnecessary, and the surgeon's role is limited to providing diagnostic material.

Operative Technique

CT- and MRI-guidance systems provide surgeons with intraoperative navigation based upon preoperative and/or intraoperative imaging studies. In general, these systems consist of a computer workstation operated by the surgeon into which the relevant imaging studies have been loaded, together with infrared or ultrasound detectors that recognize the 3D orientation and position in space of various tools. Once the patient is registered, the tumor's margins are "visualized" below the scalp so that the surgeon can plan the smallest and safest approach. Resection is assisted by use of the intraoperative microscope and guided by the appearance and consistency of tumor tissue compared with surrounding normal brain. Intraoperative CT, MRI, or ultrasonography can be used to evaluate the completeness of tumor resection. In the case of lesions that are in or near suspected functional cortex, cortical mapping can be performed to localize areas that are critical for motor or speech function. Endoscopy can be used to minimize access for resection of intraventricular lesions or pituitary tumors, as well as for re-establishing pathways of CSF flow, for example, in cases of tumors that have obstructed the cerebral aqueduct, thereby avoiding the need for a CSF shunt.

Stereotactic biopsy is performed by applying the same general principles. With either a stereotactic frame or surface applied scalp fiducials in place, a CT or MRI is performed and the imaging data loaded into an image guidance system. A target and entry points are selected and the trajectory is visualized on the computer workstation. The entry point is located on the patient's scalp and a small burr hole or twist drill hole is made. The biopsy needle is oriented using the image guidance system, passed to the appropriate depth, and tissue samples are obtained. Multiple tissue samples may be obtained along the needle tract, until the pathologist can provide intraoperative frozen-section confirmation that adequate tissue has been obtained. The volume of tissue removed during stereotactic biopsy is insufficient to relieve mass effect, and patients who are symptomatic due to mass effect are better treated by craniotomy and resection.

Radiotherapy

Radiobiological Considerations Underlying Tissue Injury

The process of radiation injury in the brain is highly complex and dependent on a variety of factors including dose, volume, fraction size, and the specific target cell population, as well as secondary mechanisms of expression of injury such as vascular leak causing edema, vascular endothelial loss resulting in hypoxic injury, and reactive gliosis. Some structures (e.g., the hypothalamus) appear to be substantially more sensitive to radiation than others (151). Even focal lesions may result in widespread radiographic and/or functional perturbations. The time course for the manifestation of injury can be highly variable and the clinical picture easily confounded with tumor progression. The effect on endothelial cells often becomes manifest as an early T2 signal abnormality on MRI, possibly due to disruption of the BBB and edema formation. Metabolic perturbations observed with PET may reflect demyelination of oligodendroglial cells. Further vascular perturbation and regeneration in response to injury results in an enhancing lesion on imaging. Delayed effects include white matter necrosis and vascular obliteration. The time course can be shortened from several months to a few weeks by increasing the volume of brain irradiated or increasing the fraction size or total dose.

Historically, late injury from radiotherapy has been reported as the "tolerance" dose at either the 5% or 50% risk level at 5 years (TD 5/5 or TD 50/5). The values for whole-brain fractionated radiotherapy at 2 Gy per fraction are 60 Gy and 70 Gy, respectively. With partial brain irradiation, the corresponding values are 70 Gy and 80 Gy, respectively. Recent studies that have modeled the effect of increasing fraction size on cell survival in late-responding normal tissues suggest that when only a small volume of normal tissue is included in high isodose lines (as in high precision small field radiotherapy), the use of a hypofractionated regimen may be biologically sound, given the advantage of larger fraction sizes in terms of tumor cell kill.

Treatment Delivery

Conventional External-Beam Radiotherapy

Conventional external-beam radiotherapy commonly is started 2 to 4 weeks after surgery to allow for wound healing. Typically a dose of 45 to 60 Gy is delivered in 25 to 30 fractions over a period of 5 to 6 weeks. Fraction sizes >2 Gy generally are avoided because of the higher risk of late CNS toxicity.

The volume of normal brain irradiated to high doses must be minimized. For a small lesion, multiple noncoplanar treatment fields that have unique entrance and exit pathways can be used. The use of intensity-modulated radiotherapy (IMRT) may yield even more conformal dose distributions and better avoidance of organs at risk (226). For larger lesions a vertex field in combination with two wedged lateral fields or a wedge pair to stay off the contralateral hemisphere typically is employed. Patient immobilization devices that limit inter- and intrafraction patient motion as well as daily online imaging, using orthogonal x-ray imaging systems, cone beam CT, or megavoltage CT, all permit use of smaller margins and thereby contribute to limiting the amount of normal brain irradiated (249). Radiotherapy techniques are described in detail below.

Stereotactic Radiosurgery

Stereotactic radiosurgery (SRS) requires a team comprised at a minimum of a neurosurgeon, radiation oncologist, and radiation oncology physicist. SRS can be delivered using a linear accelerator (LINAC) system or a Gamma Knife (Elekta Corp, Stockholm). In LINAC radiosurgery circular collimators ranging from 4 to 40 mm are used to collimate the treatment beam into a circular pencil beam, and treatment is delivered using multiple noncoplanar arcs that intersect at a single point to treat an approximately spherical target of <4 cm in diameter. Newer miniaturized multileaf collimators allow beam shaping. The Gamma Knife is a fixed beam multisource radiation unit containing 201 cobalt-60 (^{60}Co) sources that are collimated using a helmet with circular apertures ranging from 4 to 18 mm that are focused onto a single target point. For irregularly shaped lesions, treatments delivered using either noncoplanar arcs delivered through a single circular collimator or a single collimator helmet lead to the inclusion of a large amount of normal brain and yield inferior conformality. In these cases it is advantageous to use multiple circular collimators or collimator helmets placed on different target points.

Radiation Therapy Oncology Group (RTOG) study 90-05 established the maximum tolerated dose of single faction SRS to be 24 Gy, 18 Gy, and 15 Gy for tumors ≤20 mm, 21–30 mm, and 31–40 mm in maximum diameter, respectively (213).

Fractionated Stereotactic Radiotherapy

For lesions larger than 4 cm and/or located in critical regions, the delivery of a single large fraction treatment as in SRS is not desirable because of a high risk of CNS toxicity. Fractionated stereotactic radiotherapy (FSRT) is a hybrid between conventionally fractionated radiotherapy and SRS that combines fractionation with stereotactic localization and targeting techniques. Various systems for FSRT have been developed, with a reported accuracy between 1 and 3 mm (16,146,269). As for SRS, the use of multiple arcs and circular collimators for irregularly shaped lesions leads to the inclusion of a large amount of normal tissue, and the use of multiple noncoplanar fixed fields each having a unique entrance and exit pathway will be preferable because of better conformality (248,249).

Heavy Charged Particles

Heavy charged particle beams deposit their dose at a depth that depends on their energy over a distance of few millimeters when the heavy charged particles come to rest, the so-called Bragg peak. In order to cover a larger volume, the particle beam can be modulated, in effect adding up multiple Bragg peaks. The very sharp dose gradient at the distal edge permits the use of high-dose radiotherapy for tumors in critical locations, such as at the clivus and base of skull, and provides better normal tissue sparing in other situations, especially, for example, in craniospinal irradiation (116).

Brachytherapy and Radiocolloid Solutions

Selection criteria for brachytherapy include tumor confined to one hemisphere, no transcallosal or subependymal spread, small size (<5 to 6 cm), well circumscribed on CT or MRI, and accessible location for the implant. A balloon-based system placed into the cavity at the time of surgery has been employed in the treatment of recurrent malignant gliomas whose largest spatial dimension is <4 cm and are roughly spherical (240). After treatment planning the balloon is filled with a liquid that contains organically bound iodine-125 (^{125}I) and treatment is completed within 3 to 7 days. Direct infusion of radioimmunoglobulins has been used in primary and recurrent brain gliomas (199).

Radiotherapy Techniques

The radiotherapy techniques most commonly employed in the management of CNS tumors are craniospinal irradiation (CSI), whole brain radiotherapy (WBRT), and partial brain irradiation. The indications for each of these techniques are discussed under the sections on the individual tumor types. CSI is a complex technique that requires considerable expertise. It is more frequently used in management of pediatric CNS tumors and is discussed in detail in Chapter 82. Partial brain irradiation is the technique most commonly used for the treatment of adult CNS tumors.

General Concepts

Pertinent Anatomic Landmarks

The skull contains radiographic and surface topographic reference points for appreciation of beam-to-head projection geometry. The external auditory meatus participate in the definition of anatomic reference planes in the head (e.g., Reid's baseline and the Frankfort horizontal plane, connecting points in the two external auditory meatus and one anterior infraorbital edge). Unless marked at simulation, the external auditory meatus may be difficult to see on lateral projections because of the overlying temporal bone structures. The two lateral parts of the anterior cranial fossa, the two anterior parts of the middle cranial fossa floors, and the two mandibular angle points, with their lateral locations, represent appropriate reference points.

In a lateral radiograph, the sella turcica is centrally located and marks the lower border of the median telencephalon and diencephalon. The hypothalamic structures are located an additional 1 cm superior to the sellar floor, and the optic canal runs at most 1 cm superior and 1 cm anterior to that point. The pineal body (or the tentorial notch) usually sits approximately 1 cm posterior and 3 cm superior to the external auditory meatus.

The cribriform plate is the most inferior part of the anterior cranial fossa; it is an important reference point for the inferior border of whole-brain irradiation fields. In most patients, little distance is found between the lateral projections of the lens and the most inferior part of the cribriform plate.

The temporal lobes are situated in the middle cranial fossae, the floor of which is easily identified on lateral radiographs. Individualized blocks should always be used to delineate the field inferior border for WBRT.

On an anteroposterior radiograph with a Frankfort horizontal plane (ear markers and one inferior orbital edge in a horizontal plane), the temporal bones (pyramids) project in the orbits. This implies that the ethmoid sinuses and the sphenoid sinus will project between the orbits, the sella just above these air cavities, and the foramen magnum just below the connection line between the inferior orbital edges. The frontal and occipital lobes therefore project above the orbits, and the temporal lobes and cerebellum in and somewhat below the orbits.

Treatment Setup

The head should be positioned so that its major axes are parallel with and perpendicular to the central axis incident beam and the treatment table. It may be preferable to fully flex or extend the neck in some patients depending on tumor location and choice of beams, although the use of noncoplanar fields and IMRT techniques makes this less necessary.

Reproducibility of head positioning is achieved by using a fixation device. Many commercial and home-built devices are available for this purpose, with a precision ranging from 1 to 5 mm. With the advent of image-guided radiation therapy (IGRT) and intrafraction motion detection, unprecedented accuracy can be achieved in delivering radiotherapy. This permits substantial reduction in margins for setup variability (249).

Target Volume Definition

Two major factors drive margin selection: the inaccuracy of estimating the clinical target volume (CTV) and the specific dosimetric and setup variability components that are institution-specific and determine the planning target volume (PTV). In general, for benign tumors such as meningioma, the gross target volume (GTV) estimate relatively accurately reflects the CTV, and only a minor margin expansion of a few millimeters is necessary, with particular attention to the region referred to as the "tail," where the distinction between tumor and vasculature can be difficult. For nonenhancing glial neoplasms, WHO grade II and III tumors, the use of FLAIR or T2 abnormality plus a 1 to 2 cm margin is commonly employed for CTV definition. For enhancing high-grade gliomas, a shrinking field approach is utilized: the initial CTV includes the enhancing tumor plus FLAIR or T2 abnormality plus approximately 2 cm, and the boost field the enhancing tumor only plus 2 cm.

Common sense and practice dictates that these CTV expansion margins should not traverse anatomically discontiguous structures or include areas unlikely to be infiltrated by tumor. Inclusion of the bony skull is unnecessary unless direct tumor extension is suspected. With some exceptions, "compartmental crossing" to the contralateral hemisphere or, for example, into the posterior fossa or the brainstem for a supratentorial cortical tumor, is not necessary.

Ten Haken et al. (243) compared volumetric reconstructions of target volumes with CT or MRI data for 3D treatment planning and concluded that MRI defined larger volumes; on average, increases in block margin were approximately 0.5 cm. Interobserver variation in volume definition was on the order of magnitude of the differences between the CT and MRI. The CT scan defined abnormalities were not always perceptible on the MRI studies, confirming the need for integration of MRI and CT scan data for optimal 3D treatment planning for CNS tumors.

Treatment Techniques

Partial Brain Irradiation

Precise immobilization, employing a mask or other fixation system, is routine. Treatment planning CT scans are used for dose-calculation purposes, but since the majority of CNS tumors are best visualized using MRI, CT-MRI coregistration is performed to enable contouring using the MRI data sets. Most modern treatment planning software allows for CT-MRI coregistration, but physics expertise is required to ensure that the MRI studies are obtained in a controlled and reproducible environment so as not to degrade the anatomic fidelity of the images. The 3D contrast-enhanced STEALTH (Medtronic, Louisville, Co) sequence acquisitions that are commonly employed for intraoperative planning serve well for radiotherapy planning as well. For nonenhancing tumors, especially glial neoplasms, the FLAIR sequence and T2 sequences are best for the definition of tumor extent. Such sequences are also helpful for patients with GBM treated with partial brain irradiation since they best demonstrate the extent of any so-called edema. MRI-based planning also permits more accurate identification and contouring of normal dose-sensitive structures, which can be avoided using IMRT or conformal avoidance techniques. The unique and irregular tumor shapes and surrounding normal structures preclude the use of "prescriptive fields." Multiple field arrangements, using 3D planning sometimes including noncoplanar beam arrangements and IMRT, are recommended.

Three-dimensional conformal therapy is increasingly used in the treatment of both primary and metastatic brain tumors. Significant sparing of normal brain can be achieved using conformal irradiation rather than conventional treatment (246). In the University of Michigan study, a 3D treatment plan reduced the volume encompassed by the 95% isodose by over 50% compared with conventional lateral opposed partial-brain fields. A small series of patients with conformally planned fields to doses of more than 70 Gy have been treated without significant increase in morbidity (132).

The RTOG has recently completed a large trial (RTOG 9803) employing 3D techniques for GBM. Patients (n = 104) were treated with 3D conformal radiotherapy to an initial clinical target volume defined by the resection cavity, residual gross tumor and a margin of 1.5 cm, and 0.3 cm for setup error. The resection cavity, residual gross tumor volume plus 0.3 cm was boosted to a total of 66 or 72 Gy. Grade 3 or greater late radiotherapy toxicity was seen in only three patients: two developed grade 3 brain toxicity after 66 Gy and one had grade 4 brain toxicity after 72 Gy. The 78-Gy dose level is currently being analyzed.

Multiple planar and noncoplanar fields (minimum five to six) encompassing the tumor and surrounding edema with an appropriate margin (PTV), sometimes with the use of static or dynamic wedges and multileaf collimation, can be used to deliver 60 to 64.8 Gy in 1.8-Gy fractions (Fig. 32.6A,B). Marks et al. (140) described some of these techniques and suggested that noncoplanar beams were preferable to coplanar beams when the target was located in the central regions of the head. Soisson et al. (226) analyzed coplanar IMRT versus noncoplanar beams, further validating the value of noncoplanarity for skull base tumors. Three-dimensional and IMRT techniques are especially helpful for cochlear sparing (21).

Whole Brain Irradiation

WBRT is used most often for patients with brain metastases, but also for patients with primary CNS lymphomas and glioblastomatosis cerebrii, and as a component of CSI.

Whole-brain irradiation is administered through parallel-opposed lateral portals. The inferior field border should be inferior to the cribriform plate, the middle cranial fossa, and the foramen magnum, all of which should be distinguishable on simulation or portal localization radiographs (Fig. 32.7). The safety margin depends on penumbra width, head fixation, and anatomic factors, but should be at least 1 cm, even under optimal conditions. A special problem arises anteriorly because sparing of the ocular lenses may require blocking with <5-mm margins at the cribriform plate.

The anterior border of the field must be approximately 3 cm posterior to the ipsilateral eyelid for the diverging beam to exclude the contralateral lens. However, this results in only approximately 40% of the prescribed dose to the posterior eye. A better alternative is to angle the beam approximately 3 degrees or more (100- or 80-cm source-to-axis distance midline, but also field size dependent) against the frontal plane so that the

anterior beam border traverses posterior to the lenses (approximately 2 cm posterior to eyelid markers). Placing a radiopaque marker on both lateral canthi and aligning the markers permits individualization in terms of the couch angle. This arrangement provides full dose to the posterior eyes. However, the eyelid-to-lens and -retina topography is individually more constant than the canthus, and lateral beam eye shielding is better individualized with the aid of CT or MRI scans (112). When in doubt about tumor coverage or lens sparing for tumors in a subfrontal or middle cranial fossa location, CT-based contouring and planning should be considered.

With attention to the margin below the cribriform plate, the middle cranial fossa, and the posterior fossa and blocking the eyes, no substantial clinical problems with cataract development, lacrimal gland injury, or isolated relapses at the cribriform plate or in the posterior fossa have been reported.

Craniospinal Irradiation

Traditional CSI techniques utilize opposed lateral cranial fields and one or more posterior spinal fields depending on patient size. The junctioning of noncoplanar fields in the cervical region is potentially hazardous because of the risk of overlap resulting in radiation myelitis. Consequently, great attention needs to be paid to precise immobilization, and a variety of immobilization devices are available for this purpose. Image guidance during radiotherapy can help in ensuring day-to-day reproducibility. The prone position permits direct visualization of the light field from the linear accelerator on the patient thereby allowing daily adjustments of the junctions. However, if anesthesia or sedation are required as may be the case with young children, a supine setup may be considered safer (245). To avoid the risk of dose overlap, two techniques (with numerous variations) are used. In the first, a gap is employed between abutting fields such that the beam edges intersect deep to the spinal cord. This gap could result in a cold spot in a small segment of the spinal cord. If the beam intersection point were raised dorsally, a hot spot would result. The second technique attempts to avoid this problem by using a half-beam technique in which the caudal edge of the brain is matched precisely with the cephalad edge of the abutting spine field without cold or hot spots. This requires collimator angulation and sometimes a couch rotation as well. For both techniques, the use of moving junctions (known as "feathering") smooths out any dose inhomogeneity (115). Several studies have demonstrated that adequate coverage of the subfrontal region, posterior fossa, and depth assessment of the cord requires CT-based planning. Given the complexity of CSI, we recommend that it be delivered at centers with adequate staff, experience, and expertise.

With sophisticated techniques such as tomotherapy, it is possible to treat the entire neuraxis in a single setup (7). In recent years, protons as well as IMRT techniques have been used for CSI.

▪▪ | Chemotherapy and Targeted Agents

Conventional Chemotherapy

Many conventional chemotherapy agents do not adequately penetrate brain, while some drugs, despite having a molecular weight and chemical structure that make them appear capable of crossing the BBB, are p-glycoprotein substrates that are actively prevented from crossing into brain parenchyma. Even when drug delivery is adequate, most CNS tumors have proven to be quite resistant to most chemotherapeutic agents. Alkylating agents have been most widely studied, beginning with

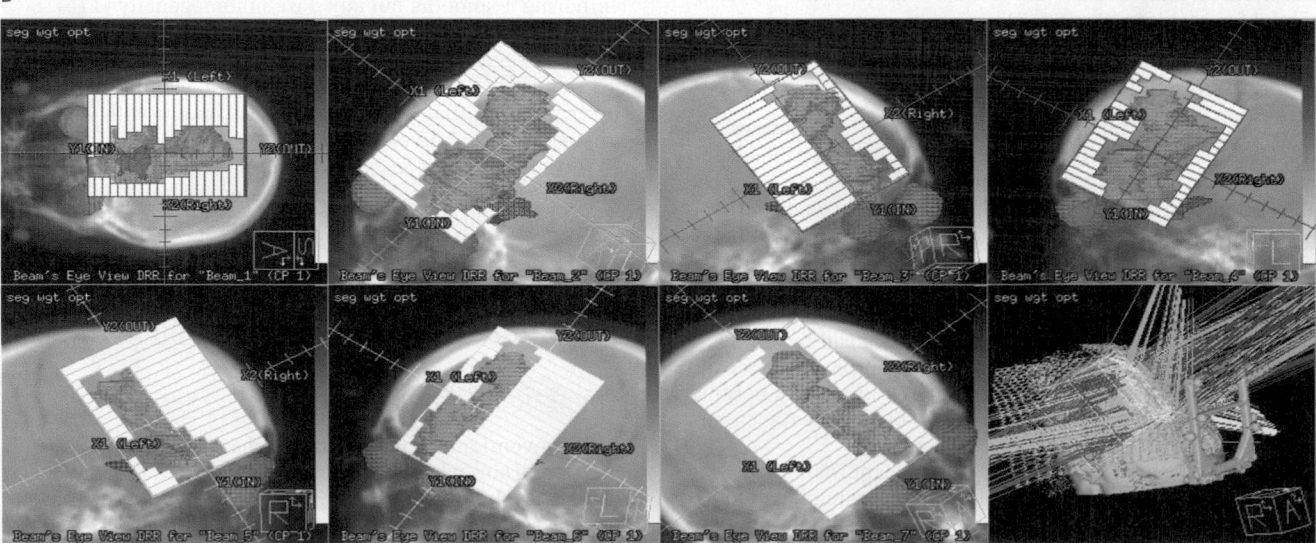

FIGURE 32.6. **A:** Intensity-modulated radiotherapy treatment (IMRT) plan of a right-sided residual oligodendroglioma (*orange*) demonstrating tight target coverage and excellent conformal avoidance of critical structures, optic chiasm (*red*), and pituitary (*purple*), as evidenced by the dose volume histogram. **B:** IMRT beam arrangement employed in the IMRT plan shown in (A). Surface renderings of the right-sided residual oligodendroglioma (*orange*), the optic chiasm (*red*), the pituitary (*purple*), and the eyes are shown. The beam arrangement clearly illustrates the principles of geometric avoidance of critical structures.

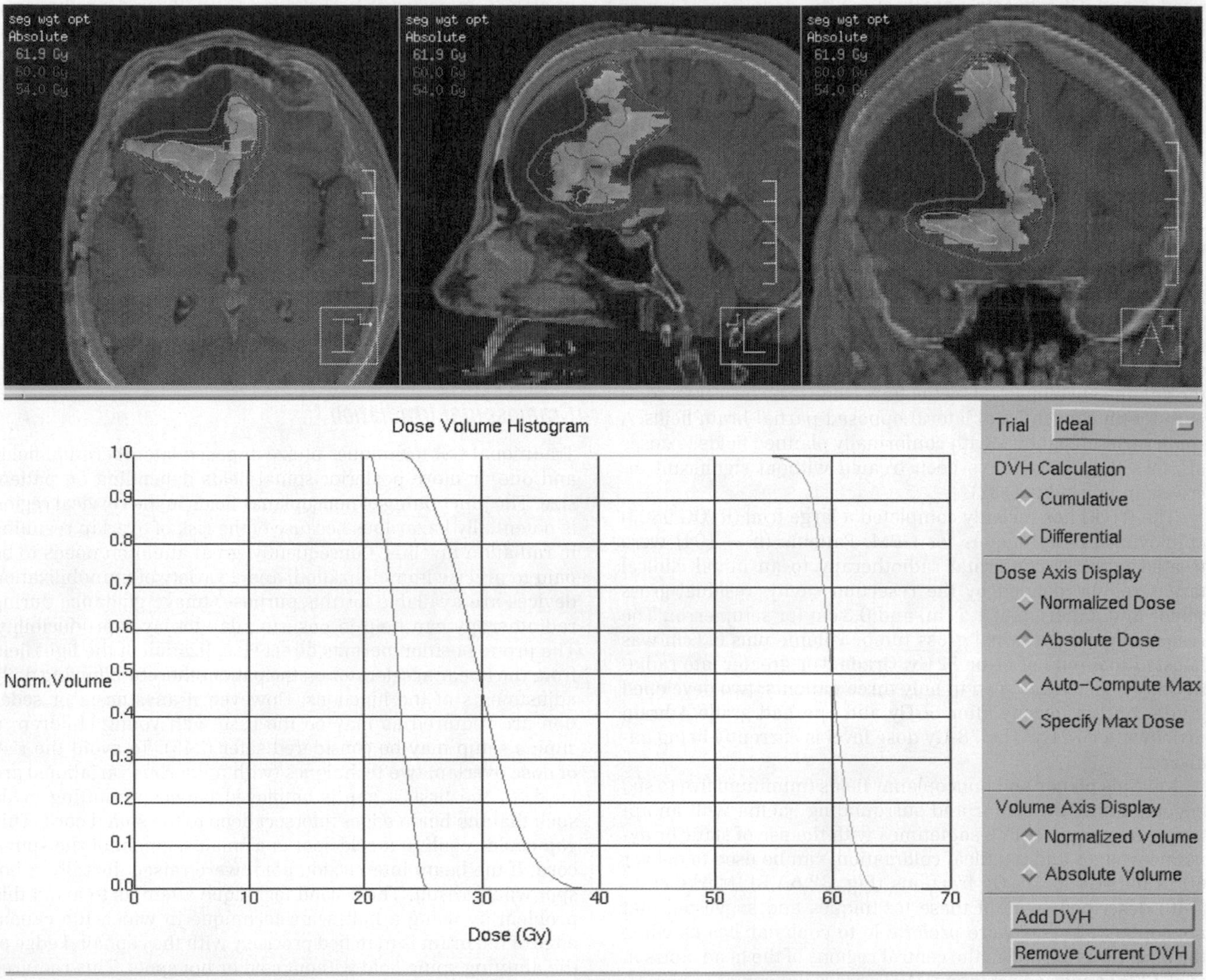

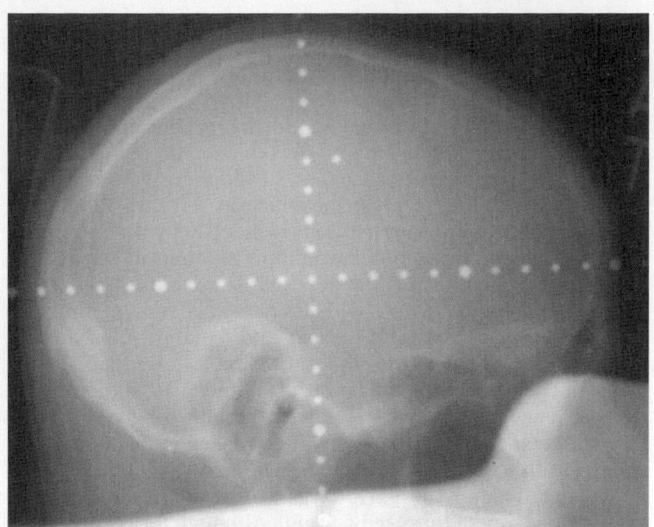

FIGURE 32.7. Lateral portal localization film of whole brain illustrating adequate inclusion of the cribriform plate and the anterior and middle cranial fossae.

early clinical trials that used the nitrosoureas, BCNU (carmustine) and CCNU (lomustine). These drugs cross the BBB, but prolonged use is difficult because of cumulative myelotoxicity and the dose-related risk of pulmonary fibrosis. Despite response in 15% to 40% of patients, the impact on survival has been modest at best. Procarbazine has similar efficacy but is better tolerated. Cisplatin and carboplatin have been used as either single agents or in combination regimens. Response rates have been modest and, as with other alkylating agents, their impact on survival is unclear. Topoisomerase I (CPT-11, irinotecan) and topoisomerase II inhibitors (etoposide) have shown only modest activity. Taxanes, such as paclitaxel, have not demonstrated activity as single agents. Temozolomide is a recent addition that is administered orally with excellent bioavailability and a good toxicity profile and has been shown to provide a survival benefit for some glial tumors.

Combination regimens, such as BCNU and temozolomide, have not been shown to be more efficacious (190). This disappointing result is likely the consequence of needing to reduce the dose of each agent because of overlapping myelotoxicity.

Convection-Enhanced Delivery

Methods for circumventing the BBB include intrathecal injection of chemotherapy agents into the CSF space, implantation of slow-release chemotherapy wafers into a tumor resection cavity (22,268), chemotherapy along with pharmacologic or osmotic BBB disruption (60,121), and convection enhanced drug delivery (CED). CED involves the use of intracerebrally implanted catheters to deliver a drug of interest into the brain parenchyma or tumor, at a slow but continuous rate of flow. Unlike diffusion, in which a drug distributes along an exponentially decaying concentration gradient and which is highly dependent upon the size of the drug molecules, drug distribution by CED is less size dependent, occurs over a much larger volume of brain tissue, and results in a more uniform drug concentration (87). Drugs and agents that do not normally cross the BBB are not substrates for the active transporters that constitute the BBB. These are large and/or hydrophilic and are ideal candidates for delivery via CED. Examples of drugs and agents that have been studied for CED include viruses (92), paclitaxel (133), topotecan (110), and a variety of toxins. These toxins are engineered to include a targeting ligand (e.g., interleukin-4 [IL-4], IL-13, tumor growth factor-α [TGF-α], transferrin) and a genetically altered bacte-

rial toxin that is effective only when internalized by a cell that expresses the target of the ligand (113,202,265,266). Combinations of these agents with chemotherapy and radiotherapy are in early stages of investigation.

Polymer Delivery

BCNU impregnated in a polymer and made into a wafer has been used for local delivery, placed on the walls of the resection cavity at the time of surgery. The wafer slowly undergoes biodegradation, releasing the active drug. This local delivery system has the advantages of minimal systemic toxicity, no limitation posed by the BBB, and delivery of very high local concentrations of chemotherapy. Initial studies in GBM have been promising (22,268).

Targeted Agents

The molecular changes seen in gliomas offer opportunities for targeted therapies. Signal transduction pathways, for example, are often markedly enhanced and may contribute to the cancer phenotypic and biologic changes, and new molecules that block signal transduction pathways are undergoing extensive investigation (197). These include drugs that block angiogenesis (vascular endothelial growth factor receptor [VEGFR]); proliferation, tumor cell invasion, and survival (EGFR); cell survival (platelet-derived growth factor receptor [PDGFR]); as well as inhibitors of downstream signaling molecules such as AKT, Ras, Raf kinase, and mTOR. To date, single agent strategies have shown minimal efficacy, and, since in the molecularly complex situation that characterizes high-grade glioma modulation of a single pathway is unlikely to result in meaningful or durable tumor responses, clinical trials are now focusing on combination regimens (197).

⠿ | Follow-Up

The follow up schedule for the patient with a brain tumor must be frequent enough to check on side effects and to taper steroids shortly after completion of treatment. Periodic CT scans or MRIs are used to detect early evidence of tumor recurrence at a stage when further therapy may be contemplated. Assessment of intellectual functioning and quality of life is important, and patients must be monitored for neuroendocrine and ophthalmologic side effects.

⠿ | Sequelae of Treatment

Surgery

With appropriate patient selection, diligent surgical technique and use of surgical adjuncts such as speech and/or motor mapping, the rate of complications can be minimized. Even in the best of hands new temporary neurological deficits can be seen in 15% or more of patients, although the rate of permanent new deficits is typically now <5% (242). The incidence and types of deficits seen following surgery depend upon the location of the tumor and the deficits present preoperatively. The most common complications associated with surgery are bleeding and infection, particular in the case of reoperation in a patient who has received prior radiotherapy and/or chemotherapy or when chemotherapy wafers are placed into a resection cavity (142). It has been suggested that the use of linear incisions (as opposed to U-shaped flaps) can help reduce the incidence of incision-related complications, such as infection (42). Posterior fossa resections, particularly in children with medulloblastoma, may be associated with posterior fossa syndrome (mutism plus bulbar symptoms). Transient perioperative edema, within about 48 hours of surgery, may be responsible for early postoperative neurologic worsening and can often be mitigated with the use of a short course of high-dose steroid therapy.

Patients with postoperative neurologic deterioration require careful clinical assessment, and in most cases a CT or MRI is required to determine the cause of the deterioration. MRI diffusion weighted sequences can be used to detect the presence of a new infarct. A high index of suspicion should be maintained for postoperative infection because symptoms may be masked by perioperative steroid use, and the headache and fever associated with craniotomy may obscure the classic signs of meningitis.

Radiotherapy

The response of intracranial tissues to radiation has been classically divided into three phases based on the timing of onset of symptoms: acute, subacute, and late.

Acute Toxicity

Transient worsening of pretreatment deficits may develop during the course of treatment, and further acute toxicities may manifest up to 6 weeks following completion of irradiation. These symptoms are believed to be the consequence of a transient peritumoral edema and usually respond to a short-term increase or the institution of corticosteroids. Persistent or refractory symptoms may be caused by tumor progression, and repeat imaging while under treatment may be indicated if the clinical condition worsens despite steroids.

General symptoms such as fatigue, headache, and drowsiness may be seen, especially in individuals treated with large brain fields or with CSI. A mild dermatitis that develops in irradiated areas may be treated with topical agents if necessary. Alopecia within the irradiated areas is common and may be permanent with higher total doses. Nausea and vomiting independent of changes in intracranial pressure may occur, particularly with posterior fossa or brainstem irradiation. Otitis externa can be seen if the ear is included in the irradiation fields, and serous otitis media also may occur. Patients treated with CSI with photons are at risk for mucositis and esophagitis because of the exit dose from the spinal fields through the oropharynx and mediastinum. Hematologic toxicity may also be seen in these patients due to irradiation of the vertebral bodies, a major depot of bone marrow in adults.

Subacute Toxicity

Subacute or "early delayed" toxicity that develops during the 6-week to 6-month period following irradiation is attributed to changes in capillary permeability as well as transient demyelination due to damage to oligodendroglial cells. Symptoms, which include headache, somnolence, fatigability, and deterioration of pre-existing deficits, usually respond to steroids. The main challenge is to distinguish the clinical and imaging findings from tumor recurrence.

Late Sequelae

Late sequelae of radiotherapy appear from 6 months to many years following treatment and are usually irreversible and progressive. They are thought to be due to white matter damage from vascular injury, demyelination, and necrosis. The pathophysiology of radiation induced neurocognitive damage is complex and involves inter- and intracellular interactions between vasculature and parenchymal cells, particularly oligodendrocytes, which are important for myelination. Oligodendrocyte

death occurs either due to direct p53 dependent radiation apoptosis or due to exposure to radiation induced TNF-α (29,43). Postradiation injury to the vasculature involves damage to the endothelium leading to platelet aggregation and thrombus formation, followed by abnormal endothelial proliferation and intraluminal collagen deposition (49).

The most serious late reaction to radiotherapy is radiation necrosis, which has a peak incidence at 3 years. Radiation necrosis can mimic recurrent tumor clinically by the reappearance and worsening of initial symptoms and neurologic deficits and radiographically with the development of a progressive, irreversible, enhancing mass with associated edema on imaging. PET, MR-spectroscopy, and nuclear and dynamic CT scanning procedures may aid in the differentiation of radiation necrosis from recurrent tumor. The best treatment for symptomatic necrosis is control of symptoms with steroids followed by surgical debulking, although even after resection necrosis may progress. Other measures include use of corticosteroids with anticoagulation or hyperbaric oxygen, although randomized trials have not shown these to be useful. Although focal necrosis is usually due to radiotherapy alone, diffuse leukoencephalopathy is more commonly associated with the combination of radiotherapy and chemotherapy, particularly methotrexate.

Inclusion of the middle ear may result in high-tone hearing loss and vestibular damage, especially in patients who receive cisplatin. Retinopathy or cataract formation may be seen if the eye is in the radiation field. Optic chiasm and nerve injury may manifest as a decrease in visual acuity, visual field changes, or blindness at doses >54 to 60 Gy. Onset of hormone insufficiency from irradiation of the hypothalamic–pituitary axis is variable but may be seen with doses as low as 20 Gy.

Cranial irradiation can produce neuropsychological changes and neurocognitive impairment; other factors such as tumor-related morbidity, as well as the effects of surgery and chemotherapy, may also contribute (49,127). These changes are thought to be due to interactions between the vasculature and parenchymal cells. Hippocampal-dependent functions of new learning, memory, and spatial information processing appear to be most affected (151). Doses as low as 2 Gy can induce apoptosis in the proliferating cells in the hippocampus (173). Agents such as methylphenidate and memantine may improve neurocognitive function (148).

Management of Individual Tumors

Malignant Glioma

Malignant or high-grade gliomas account for approximately half of all primary brain tumors in adults. They are rapidly growing tumors that directly invade the brain parenchyma but only rarely metastasize outside the CNS. They may occur in any age group, but most often present in late adulthood. Malignant gliomas correspond to anaplastic gliomas (WHO grade III) and GBM (WHO grade IV). Molecular genetics and results from clinical series have shown these to be two distinct diseases with unique behavior, response to treatment, and prognosis. Historical trials that included grade III and IV gliomas are described in the section on GBM, as patients with GBM comprised the majority of subjects, while anaplastic gliomas are discussed in further detail in the following section.

Glioblastoma Multiforme

GBM accounts for approximately 75% of all high-grade gliomas. The histopathologic features of GBM include nuclear atypia, mitotic activity, vascular proliferation, and necrosis, and any three of these suffice to make the diagnosis. GBM is typically diffusely infiltrative, involving large portions of the brain. MRI characteristically shows vasogenic edema and ring enhancement around central necrotic regions.

The prognosis for patients with GBM is poor with a median survival time of only approximately 1 year. Pretreatment patient and tumor characteristics such as age at diagnosis, tumor histology, and Karnofsky performance status (KPS) are the best predictors of outcome. As well, Simpson et al. (223) found tumor location to be a significant prognostic factor in patients with frontal lobe tumors having improved survival compared to those with parietal or temporal lobe lesions (median survival 11.4 vs. 9.6 vs. 9.1 months; $p = .01$). Extent of surgical resection, duration of neurologic symptoms, and radiographic response to treatment have also been suggested as predictors of survival.

Using nonparametric recursive partitioning analysis (RPA), a statistical tool that allows for the identification of significant prognostic factors and subsequent classification of patients into groups with similar outcomes, to analyze data from three RTOG trials that included 1,578 patients with malignant gliomas, Curran et al. (50) showed that age was the most important predictor of survival, with patients <50 years faring better than older patients. KPS (KPS ≥70 more favorable than <70) was the next most significant prognostic factor in patients with GBM. Taking into account these and other variables, patients could be divided into groups with similar outcomes with 2-year overall survival ranging from 4% to 76% and median survival ranging from 2.7 to 58.6 months (Table 32.4).

Treatment

Historically, standard treatment of patients with GBM consisted of surgical resection followed by adjuvant radiotherapy. Recent evidence suggests improved survival for patients with GBM treated with maximal surgical resection followed by radiotherapy with concomitant and adjuvant temozolomide, and this is the new standard of care. Other approaches including alterations in the delivery of radiotherapy, newer chemotherapeutic agents, and radiosensitizers, and other agents are the subject of ongoing research.

Radiotherapy Target Volume

Randomized trials have demonstrated a clear survival benefit to the use of radiotherapy after surgery (259). Localized irradiation volumes are recommended despite evidence from several sources that GBM may be more widely disseminated. Dandy (51), for example, identified recurrences in the contralateral

hemisphere even after hemispherectomy, showing the phenomenal capability of malignant gliomas to spread along white matter tracts. Such findings as well as autopsy studies (25,120,141) led to recommendations that the entire intracranial contents should be irradiated. However, Hochberg and Pruitt (104) reported that in 35 patients who had a CT scan within 2 months prior to autopsy, 78% of recurrences of GBM were within 2 cm of the margin of the initial tumor bed and 56% were within 1 cm or less of the volume outlined by the CT scan. These findings were confirmed by Wallner KE, et al. (262) who showed that 78% of unifocal tumors (25/32) recurred within 2 cm of the initial tumor volume, defined as the enhancing edge of the tumor on CT scan, and 56% of tumors (18/32) recurred within 1 cm of the initial tumor margin. No unifocal tumor recurred as a multifocal lesion, and large tumors were not more likely to recur farther from the initial tumor margin than smaller tumors. These results were supported by a study by Oppitz et al. (168) who found that 33/34 patients with CT-confirmed recurrent GBM had regrowth within the original 90% isodose on 3D review. In an analysis of patterns of failure in 34 patients with malignant gliomas treated with 3D conformal radiotherapy with small margins to 90 Gy, Chan et al. (39) showed that 23/34 patients (68%) recurred in the high-dose region.

In a correlative study, Halperin et al. (94) reviewed CT scans and multiple pathologic sections of 15 brains of patients with GBM who received minimal or no radiotherapy. If radiation treatment portals had been designed to cover the contrast-enhancing volume along and peritumoral edema with a 1-cm margin, the portals would have covered histologically identified tumor in only 6/11 cases. On the other hand, treatment of the contrast-enhancing area and all surrounding edema with a 3-cm margin around the edema would have covered all histologically identified tumors in all cases.

Kelly et al. (114) reported on 40 patients with intracranial glial neoplasms who underwent CT- and MRI-guided stereotactic serial biopsies. Histologic analysis of 195 biopsy specimens showed that contrast enhancement most often corresponded to tumor tissue without intervening parenchyma and hypodensity to parenchyma infiltrated by isolated tumor cells, to tumor in low-grade gliomas, or to edema. Isolated tumor cell infiltration extended at least as far as T2 changes on MRI. T2-weighted MRI revealed much larger volumes of infiltrated parenchyma than shown by low attenuation on CT scans.

Therefore, inclusion of all radiographic evidence of tumor and associated edema with generous margins is the rule in the design of treatment portals. With advances in MRI technology, the definition of tumor margins may change. For example, Pirzkall et al. (181) showed metabolically active tumor extending outside the region defined on T2-weighted MRI in 88% of patients. PET imaging with methionine and/or thymidine may also prove useful.

Radiotherapy Dose

Standard therapy currently is a total dose of 60 Gy in 30 to 33 fractions. Walker et al. (261) reported a dose–response analysis using data from 420 patients treated on Brain Tumor Cooperative Group protocols. Doses ranged from <45 to 60 Gy using daily fractions of 1.7 to 2 Gy; only one third of the patients received <60 Gy. A significant improvement in median survival from 28 to 42 weeks in the groups treated with doses of 50 to 60 Gy was found. A Medical Research Council study of 443 patients also showed a significant survival advantage in patients who received 60 Gy compared to those who received 45 Gy (12 vs. 9 months; $p = .007$) (14).

For patients with poor pretreatment prognostic factors and a limited expected survival who are not able to tolerate conventional treatment, a shorter course of treatment may provide good palliation. Older patients (>65 years), especially those

Class	Patient Characteristics	Median Survival (mo)
	RADIATION THERAPY ONCOLOGY GROUP **RECURSIVE PARTITIONING ANALYSIS OF MALIGNANT GLIOMA** Table 32.4	
I, II	Anaplastic astrocytoma Age ≤50 y, normal mental status or age >50 y, KPS >70, symptoms >3 mo	40–60
III, IV	Anaplastic astrocytoma Age ≤50 y, abnormal mental status Age >50 y, symptoms <3 mo Glioblastoma Age <50 Age >50 y, KPS ≥70	11–18
V, VI	Glioblastoma Age >50 y, KPS <70 or abnormal mental status	5–9

KPS, Karnofsky performance status.

Clinical Radiation Oncology

with poor performance status, have been shown to have limited posttreatment improvement or rapid neurological deterioration following conventional radiotherapy (152). Phillips et al. (178) randomized 68 such patients to standard radiotherapy to 60 Gy in 30 fractions or a shorter course to 35 Gy in 10 fractions. There was no significant survival difference between the two arms. In another prospective trial, Roa et al. (200) randomized 100 patients with GBM over 60 years to receive standard radiotherapy of 60 Gy in 30 fractions or an shorter course of 40 Gy in 15 fractions. Overall survival between the two arms was not significantly different.

Dose Escalation and Altered Fractionation

With the vast majority of tumor recurrences occurring within the previous irradiation field and the poor outcomes associated with standard therapy, regimens designed to deliver a larger dose have been attempted to improve local control and enhance survival.

A benefit for doses >60 Gy using conventional treatment has not been demonstrated. The RTOG and Eastern Cooperative Oncology Group (ECOG) randomized 253 patients to either whole-brain irradiation to 60 Gy given in 6 to 7 weeks or 60 Gy plus a 10-Gy boost to a limited volume given in 7 to 8 weeks (159). There was no benefit for the higher irradiation dose. Median survival was 9.3 months for patients receiving 60 Gy and 8.2 months for those receiving 70 Gy.

Dose intensification using 3D conformal radiotherapy or IMRT also has not consistently shown to improve clinical outcome. Chan et al. (39) published the results of 34 patients with high-grade gliomas treated using 3D conformal IMRT to a dose of 90 Gy. At median follow-up of 11.7 months, median survival was found to be 11.7 months and 1- and 2-year survivals of 47.1% and 12.9%, respectively, comparable to historical controls. In contrast, a retrospective study by Tanaka et al. (239) suggested a survival advantage for patients treated with high-dose conformal radiotherapy. Ninety patients with malignant glioma (29 with anaplastic astrocytoma and 61 with GBM) treated with conformal radiotherapy at 80 to 90 Gy were compared to a group of 94 patients (34 with anaplastic astrocytoma and 60 with GBM) treated with conventional radiotherapy at 60 Gy. There was a significant improvement in survival for patients with GBM ($p = .014$) as well as those with anaplastic astrocytoma ($p = .011$) treated with the higher doses. Median survival for patients with GBM was 16.2 months in the higher dose group compared to 12.4 months in the lower dose group. Although increased toxicity was associated with the group receiving higher doses, this did not result in increased disability. Although 3D conformal radiotherapy or IMRT may allow a delivery of a higher dose without increased risk to surrounding structures the value of dose escalation using these approaches remains unproven, and they should be used with caution, especially given the additional cost.

Several groups have used hyperfractionated or accelerated regimens as a means to escalate dose, using twice daily, three times daily, and even four times daily fractionation (54,171,220). Only the study of Shin et al. (220) showed an improvement in survival using multiple daily fractionation. In this study, 81 patients were randomized to 61.4 Gy in 69 fractions of 0.89 Gy given three times daily over 4.5 weeks or conventional fractionation to 58 Gy in 30 fractions given once daily over 6 weeks. Median survival in the two groups was 39 and 27 weeks, respectively, and the 1-year survival rates were 41% and 20%, respectively ($p < .001$).

Others have failed to confirm these results. In a prospective, randomized phase I/II trial, RTOG 83-02 examined dose escalation using twice daily fractionation in patients with malignant gliomas. Hyperfractionated regimens studied were 64.8, 72.0, 76.8, and 81.6 Gy given in 1.2 Gy fractions twice daily, and accelerated hyperfractionated regimens were 48 and 54.4 Gy given in 1.6 Gy twice daily fractions. Patients also received chemotherapy with BCNU. An early report from this trial suggested optimal survival for those in the 72-Gy arm at the cost of increased toxicity with higher doses (158). In a follow-up report, quality-adjusted survival was found to be significantly improved in the 72 Gy group (153). In the final report on all 747 patients, there were no significant differences between the treatment arms with regard to median survival time (267). Late toxicities were slightly increased with higher doses. The results of this trial led to a phase III trial comparing conventional radiotherapy to 60 Gy in 30 daily fractions to hyperfractionated radiotherapy to 72 Gy in 60 fractions of 1.2 Gy given twice daily (209). No difference in survival was found. Several other accelerated hyperfractionation regimens to doses over 70 Gy have been investigated, also without significant improvement in survival (48,188).

Dose Escalation Using Radiosurgery and FSRT

A radiosurgical boost was reported as effective in patients with newly diagnosed malignant glioma in a retrospective analysis of 115 patients treated at three institutions (75 from the Joint Center for Radiation Therapy, 30 from the University of Wisconsin, and 10 from the University of Florida) with a combination of surgery, external-beam radiotherapy, and LINAC-based radiosurgery on similar institutional protocols (205). Patients were stratified into six prognostic classes (classes 1 to 6) based on the RTOG RPA analysis. The actuarial 2-year and median survival for all patients was 45% and 96 weeks, respectively. In comparison to results for 1,578 patients treated on three RTOG external-beam radiotherapy protocols from 1974 to 1989, patients treated with radiosurgery had significantly improved 2-year and median survival ($p = .01$), corresponding with a standardized mortality risk ratio of 0.51 (95% confidence interval, 0.31 to 0.85). This improvement in survival was seen predominantly for the worse prognostic classes (RPA classes 3 to 6): 2-year survival for the patients treated with radiosurgery was 81% versus 76% for conventionally treated patients RPA classes 1 and 2, 75% versus 35% for RPA class 3, 34% versus 15% for RPA class 4, and 21% versus 6% for RPA classes 5 and 6. Patient selection may in part account for these results: it has been estimated that selection criteria limit the application of radiosurgery to approximately only 20% to 30% of patients with GBM.

In a prospective randomized trial, Souhami et al. (227) compared conventional radiotherapy (60 Gy) plus adjuvant BCNU with and without radiosurgery in 203 patients with GBM. The radiosurgery dose varied depending on tumor size, ranging from 15 to 24 Gy. At a median follow-up of 61 months, a significant improvement in median survival was not found (13.5 vs. 13.6 months). There was no difference in failure pattern between the two groups, and measurements of quality of life and cognitive decline were found to be comparable as well.

The use of a boost using FSRT was tested prospectively in RTOG 0023. Seventy-six patients with GBM with postoperative residual tumor plus tumor cavity diameter <60 mm were treated with 50 Gy standard radiotherapy in daily 2 Gy fractions, plus four FSRT treatments given once weekly during weeks 3 to 6 of radiotherapy. The FSRT dose was either 5 Gy or 7 Gy per fraction for a cumulative dose of 70 or 78 Gy in 29 treatments over 6 weeks. Significant toxicity included three patients with acute grade 4 toxicity (neurologic, constitutional, metabolic) and one with grade 3 late necrosis. The median survival time was 12.5 months. Overall, no survival advantage was seen when compared to the RTOG historical database. However, subset analysis showed that patients who had undergone gross total resection had a median survival time of 16.6 compared with 12.0 months for historic controls ($p = .14$), suggesting that patients with minimal disease burden may benefit from this form of treatment (30).

Dose Escalation Using Brachytherapy

Laperriere et al. (125) used brachytherapy as a boost to conventional radiotherapy in patients with malignant gliomas. Patients were randomized to external-beam radiotherapy (50 Gy in 25 fractions) alone (n = 69) or external-beam radiotherapy plus a temporary stereotactic ^{125}I implant delivering a minimum peripheral tumor dose of 60 Gy (n = 71). Median survival was not significantly different between the two arms (13.8 vs. 13.2 months; $p = .49$). Univariate analysis identified age ≤ 50 years, KPS ≥ 90, and chemotherapy or surgical resection at recurrence as predictors of survival.

The results of the Brain Tumor Cooperative Group National Institutes of Health Trial 87-01 reported by Selker et al. (210) support these findings. In this randomized, prospective trial, 299 patients with newly diagnosed malignant glioma received surgery, external-beam radiotherapy, and BCNU with or without an interstitial radiotherapy boost with ^{125}I. Treatment with an interstitial boost did not prolong life as compared to conventional treatment. Median survival was 68.1 versus 58.8 weeks ($p = .101$), respectively. Age, KPS, and pathology were found to be important prognostic factors.

Radiotherapy delivered by an inflatable balloon catheter is a new approach to brachytherapy. Tatter et al. (240) evaluated the safety and performance of one such device (GliaSite Radiation Therapy System, Cytyc, Marlborough, MA). Twenty-one patients with recurrent malignant gliomas underwent surgical resection and implantation of a subcutaneous port. At 1 to 2 weeks following implantation, the catheter was filled with an aqueous solution of organically bound ^{125}I for delivering a minimum of 40 to 60 Gy over 3 to 6 days, with subsequent removal of the device. This treatment was well tolerated with no serious adverse effects. Median survival was 12.7 months. Prospective, randomized trials are needed for further evaluation.

Radiosensitizers

Studies using radiation modifiers in conjunction with radiotherapy to overcome the hypoxia present in malignant gliomas have generally shown disappointing results. Chang (40) reported on 38 patients treated with hyperbaric oxygen and irradiation using fractionation schedules ranging from 36 Gy given in 3 weeks to 60 Gy given in 6 to 7 weeks and compared them with 42 patients treated with radiotherapy alone. An improvement in 18-month survival rate from 10% to 28% and an increase of median survival from 31 to 38 weeks was noted. The increased cost and difficulty of the widespread application of this treatment make this approach impractical. Perfluorocarbon emulsions, such as Fluosol, Green Cross, Osaka, Japan, which have enormous oxygen carrying capacity, have been tested as hypoxic sensitizers without significant benefit (63). Randomized studies reported by several groups failed to show significant improvement with the addition of the hypoxic cell sensitizer misonidazole (15,54,160).

Miralbell et al. (150) reported the results of a European Organisation for Research and Treatment of Cancer (EORTC) trial examining the addition of carbogen and nicotinamide to overcome the effects of proliferation and hypoxia presumed responsible for radioresistance in GBM. In this prospective phase I and II trial, 107 eligible patients received radiotherapy (60 Gy) with carbogen breathing during each treatment session (n = 23) or a daily oral dose of nicotinamide (n = 28), or both (n = 56). Patients receiving nicotinamide had higher rates of acute toxicity. Overall survival was similar in all three groups (median survival 10.1 vs. 9.7 vs. 11.1 months) and did not differ from results of series using radiotherapy alone.

Although previous trials were unable to demonstrate an improved clinical outcome with radiosensitizers, interest in radiosensitizers has increased with the development of motexafin gadolinium (MGd). The agent has been shown to be a promising sensitizer for both radiotherapy and chemotherapy. It is a redox active drug that selectively accumulates in tumor cells. It is thought to sensitize tumors through the production of reactive oxygen species that destabilize cellular metabolism. In a phase I clinical trial, MGd was shown to be a radiosensitizer for

patients with GBM (74). A phase II trial, RTOG 05–13, will assess overall survival in patients with newly diagnosed GBM treated with MGd and conventional therapy.

Chemotherapy

Although currently the standard of care, numerous earlier retrospective and prospective trials failed to show a clinical benefit in patients with GBM treated with chemotherapy regimens following surgery and radiotherapy (54,130,143).

Adjuvant treatment with nitrosoureas has been justified by trials showing a small long-term survival benefit in patients with GBM treated with surgery followed by nitrosoureas plus radiotherapy compared to surgery followed by radiotherapy alone (260). A systematic review and meta-analysis using updated data on individual patients from all available randomized trials that compared radiotherapy alone with radiotherapy plus chemotherapy in high-grade gliomas showed a small improvement in survival with the addition of chemotherapy (231). This effect was equivalent to an absolute increase in the 1-year survival rate of 6%, from 40% to 46%, and a 2-month increase in median survival time. There was no evidence that the effect of chemotherapy differed in any group of patients defined by age, sex, histology, performance status, or extent of resection. Treatment with these agents is associated with increased toxicity.

The role of chemotherapy in GBM has been redefined on the basis of a phase III cooperative group trial published by Stupp et al. (233) conducted by the EORTC Brain and Radiotherapy Groups and National Cancer Institute of Canada (NCIC), EORTC 22981/26981, NCIC CE.3. This trial showed a significant survival benefit in patients with GBM treated with concomitant and adjuvant temozolomide, an oral alkylating agent that is able to cross the BBB. In this trial, 573 patients were randomized to receive either standard radiotherapy alone (total dose of 60 Gy given as 2 Gy fractions 5 days per week over 6 weeks) or concomitant daily temozolomide (75 mg/m^2/day) with standard radiotherapy followed by up to six cycles of maintenance temozolomide (150 to 200 mg/m^2/day on days 1 to 5 every 28 days). The group receiving chemoradiotherapy experienced improved survival compared to the group receiving radiotherapy alone, with improved median survival and 2-year survival rates of 26% and 10%, respectively ($p < .0001$). Toxicity with chemoradiotherapy was acceptable with 7% grade 3 or 4 hematologic toxicity, compared to none in the group treated with radiotherapy alone.

The results of this trial are supported by the results of a more recent Greek trial. Athanassiou et al. (3) randomized 130 patients to receive either concomitant daily temozolomide at 75 mg/m^2/day with standard radiotherapy followed by adjuvant temozolomide at 150 mg/m^2 on days 1 to 5 and 15 to 19 every 28 days for six cycles or standard radiotherapy alone. Patients treated with chemoradiotherapy had superior survival compared to patients treated with radiotherapy alone (median survival 13.4 vs. 7.7 months; 1-year survival 56 vs. 16%). Toxicity was mainly hematologic and reversible with the exception of one patient with grade 4 myelotoxicity who died of sepsis.

Although the findings of these trials show improved survival in patients receiving concomitant and adjuvant temozolomide, a large proportion of patients benefited only marginally from this regimen. Different levels of expression of O^6-methylguanine-DNA methyltransferase (MGMT), an enzyme responsible for DNA repair, have been proposed as a possible explanation for differing responses to chemoradiotherapy. With temozolomide, methylation of the O^6 position of guanine has been identified as key to its cytotoxic effect. MGMT is a "suicide enzyme" that removes methyl groups from the O^6 position of guanine, thus allowing the cell to avoid apoptosis; in the process, MGMT itself becomes irreversibly methylated. MGMT is therefore consumed and must be regenerated for further activity.

The gene that encodes for MGMT is located on chromosome 10q26. The loss of function of this gene is most often due to epigenetic changes, specifically promoter-region methylation, leading to lack of MGMT expression. Epigenetic silencing of the MGMT gene through promoter methylation has been found to lead to increased overall survival and better response to treatment with temozolomide and BCNU in patients with gliomas (62,97,172).

To determine if MGMT gene promoter methylation status had an impact on survival in the patients enrolled in the EORTC/NCIC study, Hegi et al. (98) evaluated the methylation status of the MGMT gene promoter region in patients with available and adequate specimens. Methylation status was assessed for 206/573 original patients (36%) through methylation-specific polymerase chain reaction. MGMT promoter methylation was found in 45% of assessable patients. Median overall survival, irrespective of treatment assignment, was increased in patients with methylated MGMT promoter regions compared to those with unmethylated MGMT promoter regions (18.2 months and 12.2 months, respectively; $p < .001$). When treatment assignment was considered with MGMT promoter methylation status, a survival benefit from the addition of temozolomide to radiotherapy was seen only in patients with MGMT promoter methylation. In this subgroup, median overall survival was 21.7 months in patients treated with radiotherapy plus temozolomide in contrast to 15.3 months in patients treated with radiotherapy alone ($p = .007$). In patients without MGMT promoter methylation, the difference in the median overall survival in patients treated with radiotherapy plus temozolomide and radiotherapy alone was not found to be statistically significant, 12.7 months and 11.8 months, respectively.

Other chemotherapeutic regimens, such as the combination of CPT-11 and temozolomide, have shown promising results in a phase II trial with an objective response rate of 25% and 6-month progression-free rate of 38% (77). Conventional cytotoxic chemotherapeutic agents have also been combined with agents designed to modulate tumor biology. These combinations, such as temozolomide with cis-retinoic acid (isotretinoin), are well tolerated because of the absence of overlapping toxicities. Although some look promising, confirmation will require randomized phase III trials.

Investigational Approaches

Radioimmunotherapy

Radioimmunotherapy using monoclonal antibodies against EGFR tagged with ^{125}I has been evaluated in the treatment of high-grade gliomas. In a phase II trial by Brady et al. (19), 25 patients with malignant gliomas (10 with anaplastic astrocytoma and 15 with GBM) were treated with surgical resection or biopsy followed by definitive external-beam radiotherapy and one or multiple doses (35 to 90 mCi per intravenous or intra-arterial infusion) of ^{125}I-labeled monoclonal antibody-425. The total cumulative dose ranged from 40 to 224 mCi. At 1 year, 60% of patients were alive, and the median survival was 15.6 months. In an updated report of this study that included a total of 180 patients with a minimum follow-up of 5 years, median survival was 13.4 months for those with GBM (61).

Another potential target is tenascin, an extracellular protein overexpressed in malignant gliomas but not found in normal tissue. Radiolabeled monoclonal antibodies to tenascin have been evaluated in phase I or II trials showing activity against newly diagnosed and recurrent malignant gliomas (195,196). In a phase II trial by Reardon et al. (195), ^{131}I-labeled murine antitenascin monoclonal antibody was injected directly into the surgical resection cavity in 33 patients with untreated malignant glioma. Patients were subsequently treated with external-beam radiotherapy and 1 year of alkylator-based chemotherapy. Even after accounting for prognostic factors, median survival (86.7

weeks) was longer than that of historical controls. Treatment-related toxicities were mild; only one patient required reoperation for radionecrosis.

Particle Therapy

Alternate radiation modalities used in the treatment of gliomas include neutrons, protons, helium ions, other heavy nuclei, negative pi-mesons, and thermal neutrons in conjunction with boronated compounds (boron neutron capture therapy). To date, most studies have been phase I or II to determine optimal dose scheduling, efficacy, and safety. Despite theoretical advantages with respect to dose distribution and/or radiobiologic effect, most trials have failed to demonstrate improved survival.

In a controlled pilot study, Catterall et al. (33) did not find a difference in survival in patients treated with fast neutrons to 14 Gy versus photon therapy with external-beam to 50 Gy in patients with malignant gliomas. In an RTOG study, 166 patients with GBM were randomized to receive a neutron boost or a photon boost after 50 Gy photon external-beam radiotherapy (86). Although autopsies showed persistent tumor in all photon-treated patients and none in the majority of neutron-treated patients, no significant difference was found in median survival (9.8 vs. 8.6 months). A randomized neutron dose searching study was performed by the RTOG testing the efficacy of neutron boost following whole-brain photon irradiation in patients with malignant glioma (126). There was no difference in overall survival in the groups tested.

Trials examining other charged particles in the treatment of malignant gliomas have similarly not found a survival benefit when compared to convention photons (32,179) with the exception of one study by Fitzek et al. (70) that suggested a role for proton/photon irradiation. In this prospective phase II trial, 23 patients with GBM were treated with 90 cobalt Gy equivalent with conformal protons and photons. Median survival was 20 months, which represented a 5- to 11-month increase when compared to conventionally treated patients. Tumor recurrence was prevented centrally in most cases.

Targeted Therapies

EGFR gene amplification is seen in approximately 40% to 50% of patients with GBM. EGFR is associated with control of cell growth through autocrine and peregrine effects of growth factors. Inhibitors of EGFR tyrosine kinase such as gefitinib and erlotinib and EGFR antibodies have shown activity against GBM in early clinical trials (198,257). However, in a study by Chakravarti et al. (36), EGFR levels as measured by quantitative immunohistochemistry were not of prognostic value for patients with newly diagnosed GBM. Response to gefitinib did not correlate with tumor EGFR status in a study by Uhm et al. (251). The presence of an EGFR deletion mutant variant III, leading to a constitutively active variant of a key cell survival pathway, and the presence of intact PTEN, a downstream inhibitor of this signaling pathway, have been found to be significantly associated to clinical response to EGFR kinase inhibitors in patients with GBM (145). Further studies are needed to define the significance of EGFR mutations and downstream regulators of associated pathways.

Mutations and loss of the PTEN gene are encountered in approximately 70% of patients with GBM. PTEN inhibits signaling through the PI3-kinase and AKT signaling pathway. Loss of PTEN results in loss of effectiveness of EGFR inhibitors, probably due to constitutive signaling through PI3-kinase, which bypasses any upstream EGFR inhibitor effect. Specific inhibitors such as CCI-779, RAD 001, and rapamycin are in clinical testing. Preclinical experiments suggest that these agents are potential radiosensitizers (193).

Neovascularization is a major feature of GBM, and many studies demonstrate that GBM secrete VEGF in abundance. The supporting endothelium strongly express receptors for VEGF. Strategies inhibiting angiogenesis are under active investigation and include agents such as bevacizumab, an antibody to VEGF. In a recent report of 10 patients with recurrent GBM, four achieved an objective response within a few days (as early as 18 days) of administering bevacizumab (185). In particular, the "fluffy" enhancing areas responded best, but nodular tumors responded less well. There was striking reduction in peritumoral edema, implying that bevacizumab has considerable effect on restoring the BBB, which could prove to have therapeutic value. Initial trials with other agents such as enzastaurin, which inhibits VEGF signaling by inhibiting protein kinase $c\beta2$, have been tested with encouraging response rates (69), but follow-up trials failed to yield the expected results and further development of this agent was terminated; nevertheless, interest in inhibitors of angiogenesis remains high, especially with early promising results using bevacizumab which is currently being actively investigated.

Treatment at Recurrence

Although several therapeutic options have been considered for patients with recurrent GBM, none are curative and therefore the management goals should be palliative. Hospice referral for palliative care is reasonable for many patients. Medical management consists of appropriate use of steroids and anticonvulsants. Palliative debulking may help selected patients by relieving mass effect, but survival following a second resection is usually very short. The use of polymer-based local chemotherapy (carmustine wafers) has been tested in a randomized trial that included 222 patients with recurrent glioma (mostly GBM); survival increased from 44% to 64% at 6 months ($p = .02$) for patients with GBM, and median survival from 23 to 31 weeks (23). Systemic chemotherapeutic agents have been tested mostly in the context of clinical trials and have been uniformly disappointing (102), as have targeted agents with the notable exception of EGFR tyrosine kinase inhibitors in patients with recurrent GBM expressing wild type PTEN and mutant EGFR (145). Of 37 patients with recurrent GBM treated with EGFR tyrosine kinase inhibitors at UCLA there were seven responders, while 19 had early progression. Coexpression of mutant EGFR and wild type PTEN had 86% sensitivity, 89% specificity, and a positive predictive value of 75% for response.

Repeat radiotherapy using one of several different methods (including radiosurgery, brachytherapy, GliaSite balloon brachytherapy, and even repeat external beam radiotherapy) may be considered for carefully selected patients (203).

Evidence-Based Treatment Summary

1. Maximal surgical resection, although not tested in a prospective trial, is generally associated with more favorable outcome and is recommended whenever feasible.
2. Postoperative radiotherapy has been shown to provide a survival advantage in several clinical trials. The typical radiotherapy dose is 60 Gy in 6 weeks; dose escalation strategies have generally failed. Although there is much interest in incorporating advanced imaging in treatment planning and using newer treatment modalities, their benefits in GBM remain to be demonstrated.
3. Temozolomide, given during and after radiotherapy, provides a significant survival advantage that is greatest in patients with methylation of the promoter region of the MGMT gene.

Anaplastic Glioma

Anaplastic gliomas constitute approximately 25% of high-grade gliomas in adults. They generally occur during young to middle adulthood. Anaplastic gliomas, comprising anaplastic astrocytomas, anaplastic oligodendrogliomas, and anaplastic mixed oligoastrocytomas, correspond to WHO grade III. Histologically, these tumors have nuclear atypia and mitotic activity, without necrosis or neovascularization. On imaging, anaplastic gliomas may show enhancement and necrosis similar to GBM or appear nonenhancing like grade II gliomas. They display clinical and biologic heterogeneity.

Overall, patients with anaplastic astrocytoma have a median survival of approximately 3 years following diagnosis. Prognostic factors include age at diagnosis, mental status, and performance status (see Table 32.4). Patients with anaplastic oligodendroglioma have a better prognosis, particularly those with tumor containing the chromosome changes characterized by loss of heterozygosity of 1p and 19q for whom median survival is approximately 5 to 7 years (27,254). The prognosis for patients with a mixed tumor, anaplastic oligoastrocytoma, varies depending on the dominant histological cell type (55).

Molecular Genetics

Allelic loss of 1p and 19q is thought to be an early genetic alteration in the transformation and progression of oligodendrogliomas. Combined 1p and 19q deletions have been found in 63% of patients with anaplastic oligodendroglioma and 52% of patients with mixed anaplastic oligoastrocytoma, whereas astrocytic tumors have a low incidence (8% to 11%) of combined 1p and 19q deletions (224). Deletions in 1p and 19p have been associated with longer progression-free survival and chemo- and radiosensitivity (8,28,224).

This has been confirmed in two recent phase III trials. RTOG 94-02 assessed 1p and 19q status in 206/289 enrolled patients (71%) with anaplastic oligodendroglioma/oligoastrocytoma randomized to receive chemotherapy with procarbazine, CCNU, and vincristine (PCV) followed by radiotherapy or radiotherapy alone (27). Combined loss of 1p and 19q was present in 43% of patients in the PCV plus radiotherapy arm and 50% in the radiotherapy alone arm. Combined loss of 1p and 19q resulted in a longer median survival time of >7 years versus 2.8 years ($p < .001$). There was no effect of tumor genotype on overall survival by treatment. The addition of PCV to radiotherapy did not improve survival for any patient subgroup. However, there was a lower risk of progression in patients with 1p and 19q deletions after treatment with PCV plus radiotherapy, providing indirect evidence that allelic loss of 1p and 19q may be predictive for chemotherapy response.

In EORTC 26951 368 patients with anaplastic oligodendroglioma/oligoastrocytoma were randomized to receive radiotherapy followed by PCV or radiotherapy alone (254). Patients with codeletions of 1p and 19q had significantly longer overall survival irrespective of treatment, but in contrast to the RTOG trial, the addition of PCV did not result in a better outcome compared to radiotherapy alone. Presence of 1p or 19q loss was found to be the most important predictor of outcome, with a hazard ratio of 0.27, confirming that patients with loss of 1p or 19q represent a unique biologic subset.

Treatment

The current standard of care for patients with anaplastic gliomas is maximal surgical resection followed by postoperative radiotherapy (259). The radiotherapy target volume and dose are the same as for GBM.

Chemotherapy

Adjuvant chemotherapy has been justified on the basis of prospective trials and a meta-analysis showing a small long-term survival benefit in patients with anaplastic glioma treated with alkylating agents (231,259). However, because treatment is associated with significant toxicity and because of the marginal survival benefit, the use of chemotherapy has not been universally adopted.

Anaplastic Astrocytoma

Levin et al. (130) randomized patients with anaplastic gliomas or GBM to receive radiotherapy with adjuvant BCNU or PCV. The use of PCV was found to be associated with an improved outcome in patients with anaplastic glioma. In contrast, a retrospective review of 432 patients with newly diagnosed anaplastic astrocytoma treated with BCNU or PCV on RTOG studies showed no improvement in survival with chemotherapy (186).

A prospective phase III trial by the United Kingdom Medical Research Council randomized 674 patients of whom 117 (17%) had anaplastic astrocytoma after surgery to radiotherapy alone or radiotherapy followed by PCV (143). There was no advantage for adjuvant PCV in any subgroup. The median survival of patients with anaplastic astrocytoma, 13 to 15 months, was substantially lower than the median survival of 2 to 3 years reported in previous trials, which has led to debate over the applicability of these results.

The addition of difluoromethylornithine (DFMO), an inhibitor of ornithine decarboxylase, to PCV in adjuvant treatment of anaplastic gliomas was evaluated in a phase III trial by Levin et al. (129). Patients were randomized to PCV alone or PCV plus DFMO, following radiotherapy. Of the 228 evaluable patients, the majority had anaplastic astrocytoma (69.3% and 78.1%, respectively). Although the hazard function showed a significant difference in survival over the first 2 years of the study (hazard ratio 0.53; $p = .02$), this did not continue after 2 years (hazard ratio 1.06; $p = .84$). Differences in overall survival and progression-free survival were not significant.

A phase II trial by Levin et al. (131) investigated the safety of accelerated fractionated radiotherapy combined with carboplatin followed by PCV in patients with anaplastic gliomas. A total of 90 patients (76.7% with anaplastic astrocytoma) were enrolled. Median survival for anaplastic glioma patients was 28.7 months. Neurologic deterioration and/or dementia were seen in 10% of patients. The authors concluded that while excessive CNS toxicity from this intense regimen may have been a major contributing factor to the inferior median survival found in patients in this study, patients with treatment-induced necrosis had a significantly longer survival compared to those without any radiologic or histologic evidence of necrosis.

Temozolomide has shown activity in patients with recurrent anaplastic astrocytoma. In a phase II trial by Yung et al. (270), 162 patients with anaplastic astrocytoma were treated with temozolomide (150–200 mg/m^2/day on days 1–5 every 28 days) at first relapse. The 6-month progression-free survival was 46% and overall survival was 13.6 months. The objective response rate was 35% (complete response 8%, partial response 27%). The agent was well tolerated, with mild to moderate hematologic toxicity in <10% of patients. The results of this trial suggest that temozolomide has antitumor activity with an acceptable safety profile for anaplastic astrocytoma.

Anaplastic Oligodendroglioma/Oligoastrocytoma

Anaplastic oligodendroglioma and oligoastrocytoma are generally thought of as chemosensitive primarily based on high response rates to PCV in several studies. However, two large randomized trials investigating the use of sequential chemoradiotherapy in patients with anaplastic oligodendroglioma and oligoastrocytoma failed to show any survival advantage over radiotherapy alone with chemotherapy reserved for salvage (27,254). In one, RTOG 94–02, reported by Cairncross et al. (27) 289 patients with newly diagnosed anaplastic oligodendroglioma and oligoastrocytoma were randomized to either radiotherapy alone or neoadjuvant PCV (CCNU 130 mg/m^2 day 1, procarbazine 75 mg/m^2 days 8 to 21, vincristine 1.4 mg/m^2 days 8 and 29, every 6 weeks for up to four cycles) followed by

radiotherapy. With 3-year follow-up on all patients, no difference in survival was found. Median survival was 4.9 years after PCV plus radiotherapy and 4.7 years after radiotherapy alone ($p = .26$). Progression-free survival was better in the group treated with PCV followed by radiotherapy, 2.6 years versus 1.7 years for radiotherapy alone ($p = .008$). However, grade 3 or 4 toxicity was observed much more frequently, occurring in 65% of patients treated with PCV and resulting in one death.

The second study, EORTC 26951, assessed radiotherapy followed by adjuvant PCV chemotherapy. In this trial, reported by van den Bent et al. (254), 368 patients were randomized to receive either radiotherapy alone or radiotherapy followed by up to six cycles of adjuvant PCV. At a median follow-up of 5 years, median progression-free survival was 23 months in the group receiving radiotherapy plus adjuvant PCV compared to 13.2 months in the group receiving radiotherapy alone ($p = .0018$). Median survival was 40.3 months and 30.6 months, respectively ($p = .23$).

The effect of salvage therapy in patients treated on the radiotherapy alone arms of the RTOG 94-02 and EORTC 26951 trials has been offered as a possible explanation for the lack of benefit observed in these trials. In RTOG 94-02, 57% of patients treated with radiotherapy alone received salvage chemotherapy with PCV or temozolomide at recurrence. As well, 43% of patients treated with radiotherapy alone were treated with second surgery at recurrence compared to 20% in the PCV plus radiotherapy arm. In EORTC 26951, salvage PCV was given at recurrence to 65% of patients in the radiotherapy only arm and to 11% of patients in the radiotherapy and adjuvant PCV arm. Salvage with any type of chemotherapy was used in 82% of patients in the radiotherapy alone arm, compared to 55% of patients in the radiotherapy plus PCV arm. Given the high percentage of patients receiving salvage therapy, these trials may be interpreted as assessing the benefit of early or delayed chemotherapy.

Temozolomide has produced high response rates in patients with anaplastic oligodendroglioma. Chinot et al. (41) administered temozolomide to 48 patients with anaplastic oligodendroglioma/oligoastrocytoma who had previously failed PCV chemotherapy. The objective response rate was 43.8% (complete response 16.7%, partial response 27.1%). Grade 3 thrombocytopenia occurred in 6.3% patients. Vogelbaum et al. (256) reported the results of RTOG 01-31, a phase II trial in which temozolomide was given preradiotherapy to newly diagnosed patients with anaplastic oligodendroglioma/oligoastrocytoma. In the 27 patients available for review, the objective response rate was 33.3% (complete response 3.7%, partial response 29.6%). The 6-month-progression rate was 10.3%. Toxicity was acceptable. Response to temozolomide has also been shown to be significantly associated with loss of 1p in a small retrospective study (35).

Radiosensitizers

Prados et al. (187) randomized patients with anaplastic astrocytomas to receive conventional radiotherapy with or without bromodeoxyuridine (BUdR) given as an infusion during each week of radiotherapy plus adjuvant PCV. The study was closed before full accrual based on an interim analysis that predicted no survival advantage for the bromodeoxyuridine (BUdR) arm. In the 190 patients who were eligible for analysis, there was no survival benefit found with the addition of BUdR.

Evidence-Based Treatment Summary

1. Maximal surgical resection, although not tested in a prospective trial, is generally associated with more favorable outcome and is recommended whenever feasible.
2. Postoperative radiotherapy has been shown to provide a survival advantage in several clinical trials. These trials included

patients with WHO grade III and IV tumors; no trial for only grade III tumors has been conducted. The standard of care is as for GBM in terms of radiotherapy target volume and dose, typically 60 Gy in 6 weeks.

3. The role of chemotherapy remains undefined. The most widely tested agent, BCNU, and combination, PCV, have no definite survival benefit. Temozolomide is active in recurrent anaplastic astrocytoma and is currently being tested in the up-front setting.

4. Patients with codeletions of 1p and 19q have a more favorable prognosis and respond better to both chemotherapy and radiotherapy, but even in this subset, chemoradiotherapy does not have proven survival advantage over radiotherapy alone.

Low-Grade Glioma

Low-grade gliomas are slow-growing tumors accounting for approximately 20% of patients with gliomas and approximately 10% of all primary intracranial tumors in adults. They are divided into pilocytic and nonpilocytic subtypes.

Pilocytic Astrocytoma

Pilocytic astrocytoma, also known as juvenile pilocytic astrocytoma, corresponds to WHO grade I treatment. They are more common in children. On imaging, they are well circumscribed enhancing lesions, often with a cystic component.

Treatment

Pilocytic astrocytomas are more amenable to total resection than other low-grade gliomas. Fenestration of the cyst and resection of the mural nodule are usually curative. In tumors in which the wall of the cyst enhances, cystic degeneration of a larger tumor is more likely, and resection of the entire cyst is necessary.

Complete resection of pilocytic astrocytomas is associated with excellent survival, with the majority (>90%) of patients cured of the tumor. No adjuvant therapy is necessary.

Incomplete resection is associated with long-term survival rates of 70% to 80% at 10 years. The benefit of postoperative radiotherapy is unclear. Although the usual recommendation is for close follow-up, there is evidence of improved progression-free survival in this situation (216), and immediate postoperative irradiation may be appropriate in some cases, depending on the location of the tumor, the extent of residual disease, the feasibility of repeated surgical excision, and availability for follow-up. If radiotherapy is indicated, the dose is typically 50 to 55 Gy (1.8 to 2 Gy fractions).

Evidence-Based Treatment Summary

1. Maximal surgical resection, although not tested in a prospective trial, is associated with more favorable outcome and is recommended whenever feasible.
2. Postoperative radiotherapy may be considered in patients with incompletely resected tumors.
3. Chemotherapy does not have an established role in pilocytic astrocytoma in adults.

Nonpilocytic/Diffusely Infiltrating Gliomas

Nonpilocytic or diffusely infiltrating low-grade gliomas are classified as WHO grade II tumors. They may arise from astrocytic, oligodendrocytic, or mixed lineage. Presentation usually occurs in the third or fourth decade of life. CT typically demonstrates an ill-defined, diffuse, nonenhancing low-density region, often in the frontal or temporal lobes. Calcifications are commonly seen with oligodendrogliomas. MRI is more sensitive in detecting and defining these lesions which are hypointense and nonenhancing on T1-weighted images and hyperintense on T2-weighted images.

Histologically, these tumors are well differentiated and lack mitoses, nuclear pleomorphism, anaplasia, vascular proliferation, and necrosis. Differentiation from reactive gliosis can be difficult. Histologic subtypes are often identified in low-grade astrocytomas. Fibrillary and protoplasmic subtypes convey no specific prognostic information. Gemistocytic subtypes behave in a fashion more consistent with a malignant glioma.

Factors associated with improved outcome include young age, good neurologic status, oligodendroglial subtype, and low proliferation indices. Median survival is approximately 5 years for patients with astrocytoma and approximately 10 years for patients with oligodendroglioma (214). The 5-year survival rate is 37% for patients with astrocytoma, 56% for mixed oligoastrocytoma, and 70% for oligodendroglioma (34). A Ki-67 (MIB-I) index >3% has been shown to correlate with a worse prognosis (96). Malignant transformation portends a poor outcome.

Molecular Diagnosis

Smith et al. (224) found loss of 1p and 19q in 44% of 52 patients with oligodendrogliomas, of which 34 (65%) were low grade. Combined loss of 1p and 19q was associated with an improved probability of survival, independent of other factors such as age. Fallon et al. (65) examined 139 tumor samples from 80 patients with primary and recurrent oligodendrogliomas of which 74% were grade II at initial diagnosis. Combined loss of 1p and 19q occurred in 71% of patients, more commonly in pure oligodendrogliomas (75%) than in mixed oligoastrocytomas (39%). Patients with combined loss of 1p and 19q had an overall median survival of 14.9 years compared to 4.7 years for those without 1p and 19q deletions.

Okamota et al. (166) found a similar frequency of loss of 1p and 19q of 70% in patients with low-grade oligodendrogliomas in a population-based study. In a review of 44 cases of low-grade oligodendrocytic tumors, Sasaki et al. (206) considered half of the cases classical oligodendroglioma and the remainder nonclassical oligodendroglioma with more astrocytic features on histopathology. Deletion of 1p was detected in 86% and 27% of these groups, respectively. Response to chemotherapy was assessed at time of recurrence in 13 patients. Of the 11 who responded to chemotherapy, 10 had loss of 1p. Both of the nonresponders were found not to have loss of 1p. A small prospective trial by Hoang-Xuan et al. (103) found a similar trend. Loss of 1p with or without loss of 19q, which was detected in 12/26 patients with low-grade oligodendrocytic tumors treated with temozolomide, was found to have a significant association with response to chemotherapy ($p < .004$). Other small studies have not shown an association between molecular findings and chemosensitivity (24,230).

Prognostic Variables

In addition to histology and molecular characteristics, several clinical variables have been found to be of prognostic importance. Pignatti et al. (180) performed the most comprehensive of these analyses and constructed a scoring system to identify patients at low and high risk. This trial was based on data from two large European phase III trials for low-grade glioma designed to examine the dose and timing of postoperative radiotherapy, EORTC 22844 and 22845. Cox regression analysis was used to identify prognostic variables from 322 patients from EORTC 22844 and then validated on 288 patients from EORTC 22845. Multivariate analysis showed that age 40 or older, astrocytoma histology, maximum diameter 6 cm or greater, tumor crossing the midline, and presence of neurologic deficits negatively impacted survival. A prognostic scoring system was derived: patients with up to two of these factors were considered low risk (median survival 7.7 years) and patients with three or more, high risk (median survival 3.2 years).

Treatment

Treatment, in particular the timing of intervention, for patients with diffusely infiltrative low-grade tumors remains controversial. The clinical course is variable with some patients having long survival even without treatment and others suffering from progressive deterioration despite treatment. In general, early intervention is indicated for patients with increasing symptoms, radiographic progression, and high-risk features suggestive of transformation to a higher-grade tumor. Adequate tissue sampling is critical to ensure accurate diagnosis, and maximal surgical resection in this context may be advisable in appropriately selected patients. In younger patients (<40 years) who have undergone complete resection, observation with serial imaging are options. In those who have undergone a subtotal resection or those with high-risk features, postoperative radiotherapy may be recommended, typically 50 Gy in 1.8 Gy fractions. Recent evidence suggests that chemotherapy may have a role, particularly in patients with loss of 1p and 19q. Accrual of patients into well-designed clinical trials is imperative to define optimal treatment.

Surgery

Although surgery is considered an integral part of treatment, the goal of surgery and its timing are still debated. In practice, most patients undergo surgery at presentation in order to establish the diagnosis and to determine histology, grade, and molecular characteristics that affect treatment. However, even under the best circumstances, total resection with an adequate margin is rarely achieved due to the diffusely infiltrative nature of these tumors and involvement of eloquent regions (44). Although controversial, most studies have found total or subtotal (>90%) resection to be associated with improved outcome (10,44,128). Moreover, with the advent of imaging to assist in identifying critical areas of the brain, resection may be achieved with less morbidity and mortality than in the past. Proponents of aggressive resection are also supported by studies that suggest that radical surgery results in more accurate histopathologic diagnosis (107). However, surgical resection is unlikely to be curative. In RTOG 98-02 median time to progression in 111 good risk patients, defined as patient age <40 and gross total tumor resection, was 5 years (215).

Radiotherapy

Three recent phase III trials provide the best evidence with respect to the indications for radiotherapy as well as the dose (Table 32.5).

Patients considered favorable by the scoring system introduced by Pignatti et al. (180) are typically observed postoperatively and given radiotherapy at disease progression or recurrence. This practice is based on the results of a phase III trial by van den Bent et al. (253) in EORTC 22845. In this multi-institutional trial, 314 patients with low-grade gliomas were randomized to receive postoperative radiotherapy to 54 Gy in fractions of 1.8 Gy (n = 157) or radiotherapy at progression (n = 157). A significant improvement in median progression-free survival was found with early radiotherapy, 5.3 versus 3.4 years (p <.0001), but there was no difference in median survival, 7.4 versus 7.2 years (p = .872). It is of note that only 65% the patients in the delayed radiotherapy group received radiotherapy at progression. Malignant transformation occurred in 65% to 72% of patients with no difference between the two groups. Although seizure control was superior in the early radiotherapy group, adequate data on quality of life were not obtained. The authors concluded that while early radiotherapy may be appropriate in some situations, for example, patients with symptomatic lesions, withholding radiotherapy until tumor progression does not jeopardize survival.

Table 32.5	PHASE III TRIALS OF PATIENTS WITH LOW-GRADE GLIOMA TREATED WITH RADIOTHERAPY		
Study (Reference)	Treatment Arm	N	5-Year Survival (%)
EORTC 22845	Observation[a]	157	66
	54 Gy (30 fractions)	157	68
EORTC 22844	45 Gy (25 fractions)	171	58
	59.4 Gy (33 fractions)	172	59
NCCTG	50.4 (28 fractions)	101	72
	64.8 (36 fractions)	102	64

EORTC, European Organization for Research and Treatment of Cancer; N, number of patients; NCCTG, North Central Cancer Treatment Group
[a]Treatment with radiotherapy at progression.

For patients given radiotherapy postoperatively, the dose has been established by 2 phase III trials. In EORTC 22844 379 patients were randomized to receive 45 Gy in 5 weeks or 59.4 Gy in 6.6 weeks postoperatively (111). With a median follow-up of 74 months, overall survival (58% vs. 59%) and progression-free survival (47% vs. 50%) were similar in both arms.

In a joint North Central Cancer Treatment Group (NCCTG), RTOG, and ECOG study, 203 patients were randomized to low-dose radiotherapy to 50.4 Gy in 28 fractions (n = 101) or high-dose radiotherapy to 64.8 Gy in 36 fractions (212). There was no significant difference in progression-free survival or overall survival. Survival at 2 and 5 years was 94% and 72%, respectively, with low-dose radiotherapy and 85% and 64% with high-dose radiotherapy. Grade 3 to 5 neurotoxicity occurred in 5% of patients in the high-dose cohort and 2.5% of patients in the low-dose cohort.

Consequently low-dose radiotherapy, 50 Gy in 1.8 Gy fractions, is the standard of care for patients with low-grade gliomas. The target volume is local, with a margin of 2 cm beyond changes demonstrated on traditional MRI sequences. Using FLAIR images, which usually show abnormality beyond any enhancing or nonenhancing tumor, a smaller margin of 0.8 to 1 cm may be used.

Chemotherapy

There is no established role for chemotherapy in adult patients with low-grade gliomas. A Southwest Oncology Group (SWOG) study by Eyre et al. (64) randomly assigned 60 patients with incompletely excised low-grade gliomas to receive radiotherapy alone (55 Gy in 6.5 to 7 weeks) or radiotherapy plus CCNU. Median survival was 4.5 years for radiotherapy alone and 7.4 years for radiotherapy plus CCNU (p = .7). This trial was closed early due to slow accrual. It has been argued that continued enrollment may have led to a significant difference in survival considering the large difference between the two arms (252).

Multiagent chemotherapy, in particular PCV, appeared promising with response rates ranging from 50% to 80% in recurrent and newly diagnosed tumors (24,230) but proved no better than radiotherapy alone in RTOG 98-02 (215). In this phase III trial, 251 unfavorable patients (age 40 or greater with subtotal resection or biopsy) were randomized to receive radiotherapy alone to 54 Gy in 30 fractions or radiotherapy followed by six cycles of standard dose PCV. With a median follow-up of 4 years, overall survival at 2 and 5 years was 87% and 61%, respectively, in those treated with radiotherapy alone and 86% and 70%, respectively, in those treated with radiotherapy plus PCV. Progression-free survival was not different between the two arms. Moreover, acute grade 3 or 4 toxicity occurred in 67% who received radiotherapy plus PCV as compared with 9% of patients who received radiotherapy alone.

Temozolomide has been shown to have activity in phase II trials in newly diagnosed and recurrent low-grade gliomas

(18,103,191,255). The EORTC is currently conducting a phase III trial (EORTC 22041) comparing radiotherapy to 50.4 Gy and temozolomide with stratification of 1p and 19q allele status.

Evidence-Based Treatment Summary

1. Maximal surgical resection, although not tested in a prospective trial, is generally associated with more favorable outcome and is recommended whenever feasible.
2. Postoperative radiotherapy has not been shown to provide a survival advantage in the only clinical trial testing this question, although progression-free survival and seizure control were superior. The typical radiotherapy dose is 45 to 54 Gy; randomized trials do not show a survival advantage with higher doses.
3. CCNU and PCV do not provide a survival advantage over radiotherapy alone. Temozolomide has not been tested in a phase III trial.

Gliomatosis Cerebri

Gliomatosis cerebri is a rare condition with diffuse involvement of multiple parts of the brain (greater than two lobes), sparing neurons and normal structures. On MRI, there is typically diffuse increased signal on T2-weighted and FLAIR images and low or absent signal in the affected areas on T1-weighted images. Treatment remains undefined. Perkins et al. (175) reviewed the treatment outcomes of 30 patients with gliomatosis cerebri treated with radiotherapy at M.D. Anderson Hospital. Transient radiographic improvement or disease stabilization was achieved in 87% of patients with clinical improvement observed in 70%. Patients younger than 40 and those with nonglioblastoma histology had significantly improved overall survival.

In a French trial, 63 patients with gliomatosis cerebri were treated initially with PCV or temozolomide (204). Objective responses were observed in 33% of patients and radiologic responses in 26% with no significant difference between the two regimens. Median progression-free survival and overall survival were 16 and 29 months, respectively. Regardless of regimen, patients with an oligodendroglial component had significantly better outcomes in terms of progression-free and overall survival.

A retrospective review of 296 patients with gliomatosis cerebri from the literature (n = 206) and the Association des Neuro-Oncologues d'Expression Francaise (ANOCEF) network (n = 90) was recently published (237). Median survival was 14.5 months. Patients younger than 42, with better KPS, low-grade histology, or oligodendroglial subtype, had better outcomes. The impact on survival of radiotherapy remained unclear.

Evidence-Based Treatment Summary

1. Maximal surgical resection is not an achievable goal.
2. Radiotherapy is considered the standard, but no trials have validated its role.
3. The role of chemotherapy remains ill defined.

Adult Brainstem Glioma

Brainstem gliomas account for 15% of all pediatric brain tumors (225) but are rare in adults. They can be divided into several distinct types. The diffuse intrinsic pontine tumors are generally high-grade astrocytomas, either anaplastic astrocytomas or GBM, while focal, dorsally exophytic or cervicomedullary are usually low grade and have a much better prognosis. Although rare, other aggressive tumors such as PNETs and atypical teratoid-rhabdoid tumors also occur in the brainstem (26,271). Nonneoplastic processes that may be confused with a primary

brainstem tumor include neurofibromatosis, demyelinating diseases, arteriovenous malformations, abscess, and encephalitis.

Diffuse intrinsic pontine glioma remains one of the most challenging brain tumors. Even biopsy is restricted because of the substantial risk of morbidity and mortality. This appears to be as true in the adult population as in children (154). The diagnosis is usually based on a short history of rapidly developing neurologic findings of multiple cranial nerve palsies (most commonly VI and VII), hemiparesis, and ataxia, in combination with the classic MRI finding of diffuse enlargement of the pons with poorly marginated T2 signal involving 50% or greater of the pons (57). Most are nonenhancing. Enhancement, particularly in a focal lesion, may suggest a juvenile pilocytic astrocytoma rather than a high-grade glioma; these lesions should be biopsied.

Treatment

Corticosteroids may be necessary to manage neurologic symptoms until treatment is instituted. Patients with hydrocephalus may require placement of a ventriculoperitoneal shunt. The approach to treatment should be based on the type of brainstem glioma as determined by both the clinical presentation and radiographic findings. Surgery is the treatment of choice for operable lesions (i.e., accessible focal tumors, dorsally exophytic and cervicomedullary tumors). For low-grade tumors amenable to surgical resection, as in other low-grade gliomas, the role of postoperative radiotherapy is controversial and many would advocate close observation. For unresectable low-grade tumors radiotherapy should be delivered using volumes and doses as for low-grade gliomas in other locations.

Involved field radiotherapy is the primary treatment for infiltrating pontine gliomas. The GTV is usually best defined using T2-weighted or FLAIR MRI. A margin of 1 to 1.5 cm is added to create a CTV and further expanded by 0.3 to 0.5 cm to create a PTV. Margins may not need to be uniform in all directions, particularly where bone limits tumor extension. These lesions should be treated with doses on the order of 55.8 to 60 Gy using daily fractions of 1.8 to 2.0 Gy per day. Although radiotherapy provides short-term benefits, long-term results remain dismal. There is no advantage to the use of higher doses given using hyperfractionation. Chemotherapy has no established role. Chapter 82 provides more details as most data on intrinsic pontine gliomas come from pediatric trials.

Fewer data exist with respect to brainstem glioma in adults, but there is some evidence that these tumors may be less aggressive in adults, with overall survival that ranges from 45% to 66% at 2 to 5 years (Table 32.6), perhaps because of a greater frequency of more favorable tumor types (211). In the series from ANOCEF, 48 adult patients with brainstem gliomas were grouped on the basis of their clinical, radiological, and histologic features (89). Nearly half had nonenhancing diffusely infiltrative tumors and had symptoms that were present for more than 3 months. Eleven of these 22 patients underwent biopsy, and nine had low-grade histology. Nearly all underwent radiotherapy and had a median survival of 7.3 years. A second group of 15 patients who had presented with rapid progression of symptoms and had contrast enhancement on MRI were described. Fourteen of these patients underwent biopsy and anaplasia was identified in all 14 specimens. Despite radiotherapy, the median survival in this group was 11.2 months, which approximates the survival in pediatric series.

Evidence-Based Treatment Summary

1. Surgical resection is indicated for patients with favorable tumor types but is not an achievable goal in patients with intrinsic pontine gliomas.
2. For intrinsic pontine tumors, radiotherapy is considered the standard. Dose-escalation strategies have been ineffective.

Table 32.6	ADULT BRAINSTEM GLIOMA TREATED WITH RADIOTHERAPY			
Authors (Reference)	Adult Patients (Total Patients)	RT Dose (Gy)	RT Dose per Fraction	Overall Survival
Shrieve et al. (222)	19 (60)	66–78	1 Gy b.i.d.	53% (2 y)
Guiney et al. (90)	21 (53)	44–55	1.67–2.25 Gy daily	49% (3 y)
Linstadt et al. (135)	14	66–78	1 Gy b.i.d.	59% (3 y)
Landolfi et al. (124)	19	59.4–72	1.8 daily or 1 Gy b.i.d.	45% (5 y)
Guillamo et al. (89)	48	52–68 (mean dose)	1.8–2.0 Gy daily or 1–1.2 Gy b.i.d.	66% (2 y)

RT, radiotherapy; b.i.d., twice daily

Ependymoma

Ependymoma accounts for only 1.8% of all adult brain tumors (34). Rosette formation is a hallmark of ependymoma on pathological examination. The presence of increased cellularity, cytologic atypia, and microvascular proliferation suggests a diagnosis of anaplastic ependymoma. Ependymomas may expand locally, extend along ependymal spaces, and occasionally disseminate through the CSF. However, the predominant pattern of relapse is local, even when anaplasia is present (84,147,201,247,263).

Treatment

Maximal surgical resection, including second surgery if necessary, is the initial treatment for ependymoma. Surgery alone may be sufficient in selected patients based on the results of pediatric series described in Chapter 82. However, the standard of care for most adults is postoperative irradiation. There appears to be a radiation dose response with improved tumor control with doses >50 Gy and doses of 54 to 59.4 Gy are typically prescribed.

Historically, for posterior fossa tumors, the entire posterior fossa has been irradiated. However, Paulino (170) has shown that the pattern of failure to be "local", i.e., within the tumor bed itself. In nine patients who received radiation therapy to the tumor bed plus a 2 cm margin, the two failures in this group were within the tumor bed (i.e., there were no failures within the posterior fossa outside the tumor bed). For most patients, a more usual volume now consists of the tumor bed and any residual disease (GTV) plus an anatomically defined margin of 1 to 1.5 cm to create a CTV. Larger margins may be required in areas of infiltration, and special attention must be paid to areas of spread along the cervical spine since 10% to 30% of fourth ventricular tumors extend down through the foramen magnum to the upper cervical spine (217,263).

In the past, craniospinal irradiation was recommended for patients with high-grade and infratentorial tumors who were believed to be at an increased risk of CSF spread (201). Modern series document that local recurrence is the primary pattern of failure, and that the incidence of isolated spinal relapses is low even among the highest-risk patients, with the majority of spinal failures associated with local recurrences (84,247). As a result, the current recommendation for patients with ependymomas is limited-field radiation if the spinal MRI scan and CSF cytology are negative. Patients with neuraxis spread (positive MRI or positive CSF cytology) should receive craniospinal irradiation (40 to 45 Gy) with boosts to the areas of gross disease and to the primary tumor to total doses of 50 to 54 Gy.

Chemotherapy has not been proven useful in ependymoma. However, a regimen consisting of preirradiation cyclophosphamide, vincristine, cisplatin, and etoposide used in a recent Children's Cancer Group study (CCG-9942) for patients with residual ependymoma appears more promising than agents and regimens used in the past. Additionally, cisplatin-based chemotherapy has shown some activity in recurrent ependymoma in adults (20).

Results of Treatment

In modern series that utilized mostly local fields for patients with nondisseminated disease 5-year survival is on the order of 70% (56,66,76,201,208,217). Several authors have attempted to identify variables associated with improved outcome in adults. Ferrante et al. (66) analyzed 20 patients with fourth ventricle ependymomas. The 5-year survival rate in patients older than 16 years was 60%. The use of postoperative irradiation was associated with a markedly improved 5-year survival of 68% versus 18% without radiotherapy ($p = .011$).

A retrospective study of 23 adult patients with supratentorial ependymomas treated at Columbia-Presbyterian Medical Center with a variety of radiotherapy field sizes and doses (including stereotactic radiosurgery) showed a 5-year survival rate of 100% for hemispheric tumors and 73% for third ventricular tumors (208). Of interest, six patients with low-grade tumors did not receive postoperative irradiation. Five remained free of recurrence during a mean follow-up period of 69 months.

Five-year survival was 62% for a French series of 34 adult patients with ependymoma, 17 of whom had anaplastic histology (91). Gross total resection was performed in 27 patients. Half of the 34 patients were irradiated; 13 of these received local fields to a mean dose of 56 Gy. Univariate analysis showed that anaplasia and location in the brain parenchyma predicted for poor outcome.

Evidence-Based Treatment Summary

1. Maximal surgical resection should be performed when feasible.
2. Postoperative radiotherapy is considered the standard, but no prospective trials have validated its role. Craniospinal irradiation is used only in patients with disseminated disease.
3. The role of chemotherapy remains to be defined.

Medulloblastoma

Medulloblastoma is a relatively rare tumor in adults with an incidence of 0.5 per 100,000 (31,34). The majority arise in the 20- to 40-year age group. Adult medulloblastomas are more frequently located laterally than those in childhood (50% vs. 10%), and are more frequently desmoplastic (189). Medulloblastoma is a densely cellular tumor with small, darkly staining ovoid cells with hyperchromatic nuclei and frequent mitoses. Homer-Wright rosettes (clustered cells surrounding a central eosinophilic core) are characteristic. CSF dissemination may manifest as positive cytology or macroscopic seeding of the subarachnoid space and is not uncommon. Systemic spread is seen in approximately 5% of patients, mostly to bone and bone marrow. Shunt procedures have been suggested as a cause, although modern series dispute this (9).

In children, adverse prognostic factors include male gender and age <3 years (169). Patients with total or near-total resections fare better than those with subtotal resection or biopsy only, and residual tumor >1.5 cm^2 on postoperative scans is an adverse prognostic factor. Patients with CSF spread have a worse prognosis. Patients are classified as "average risk" if there is <1.5 cm^2 residual tumor and no dissemination; patients with >1.5 cm^2 residual and/or dissemination are considered "high risk."

Treatment

All patients with nondisseminated medulloblastoma should undergo complete resection if feasible. In some cases, extension into the brainstem precludes complete resection without significant morbidity.

Although it is not clear if the biology of adult medulloblastoma is different from pediatric medulloblastoma, long-term survival seems comparable, and in general the treatment guidelines for pediatric medulloblastoma detailed in Chapter 82 should probably be followed. Postoperative radiotherapy should begin within 28 to 30 days following surgical resection whenever possible. Radiotherapy is delivered to the entire craniospinal axis. This is followed by a boost to the entire posterior fossa using parallel-opposed portals or more commonly now posterior oblique fields or other multifield techniques to spare the cochlea. Although there may be less concern over long-term toxicity of full-dose CSI in adults as compared with children, adults treated for medulloblastoma with a mean dose to the whole brain of 35 Gy have been shown to have long-term cognitive deficits (119). It may be reasonable to extrapolate from the pediatric experience and to treat healthy young adults with average risk disease with reduced dose CSI (23.4 Gy) as long as appropriate chemotherapy is administered. The total dose to the posterior fossa should be 54 to 55.8 Gy. However, a note of caution is advised. Many adult patients, particularly those who are "older" or who have comorbidities, may not tolerate the postradiation chemotherapy as well as their pediatric counterparts, and the long-term outcome in adults treated with reduced-dose craniospinal irradiation and chemotherapy is not known. Full-dose CSI (36 Gy) should be delivered in the setting of high-risk disease. This is then followed by a boost to the posterior fossa as for average-risk disease. Intracranial and spinal metastases should be boosted as well to total doses on the order of 45 to 50 Gy for spinal metastases and 50 to 54 Gy for intracranial metastases. Treatment is usually delivered at 1.8 Gy per day.

The role of adjuvant chemotherapy in children with medulloblastoma is well established but remains unclear in adults. A series of 32 adults with medulloblastoma from Germany has shown a nonsignificant trend to prolonged survival with adjuvant chemotherapy (101). In general treatment in adults should probably parallel that in children, even though as noted treatment may be compromised by poorer tolerance to chemotherapy.

Results of Treatment

The group from University of California–San Francisco reported their experience of adult patients with medulloblastoma between 1975 and 1991 (189). Twenty patients had complete resection, 23 had subtotal resection, and four had biopsy alone. Thirteen patients had dissemination of disease. All patients received CSI and 32 received chemotherapy. The 5-year overall survival rate was 60%. Survival was significantly associated with extent of disease: it was 81% for patients with average-risk disease and 54% for those with high-risk disease. Male patients and those who required a shunt fared worst; longer survival was associated with the use of adjuvant chemotherapy. The majority of relapses, 16/28, had a posterior fossa component.

Frost et al. (75) reviewed 48 patients over the age of 16 years (36 men and 12 women). Complete macroscopic removal was achieved in 22 patients, subtotal removal in 23, and biopsy only in three; 46 patients received CSI and two were treated with local irradiation only. The 5- and 10-year overall survival rates were 62% and 41%, respectively. Significant factors for disease-free survival were stage, functional status at the time of radiotherapy, and absence or presence of hydrocephalus before surgery. Recurrent disease developed in 24 patients, 14 of whom relapsed first in the posterior fossa. Subtotal tumor removal was the only factor predictive of posterior fossa relapse.

Giordana et al. (79) reported on 44 patients older than 18 years of age with medulloblastoma. The overall 5- and 10-year survival rates were 40% and 35.6%, respectively. Factors that predicted a longer survival were age younger than 37 years, decade of diagnosis (1977 to 1990), radiotherapy (50 to 55 Gy to the posterior fossa and 30 to 35 Gy to the spinal canal), and nuclear isomorphism.

A retrospective review of 32 patients 16 years of age or older was reported from Harvard (38). The tumors were located laterally in 19 patients and in the midline in 13. Eight patients had evidence of CSF dissemination. All patients received CSI with a median dose of 36 Gy to the craniospinal axis and 55 Gy to the posterior fossa. Additionally, 24 patients received chemotherapy. The disease-free survival at 5 years was 57%, but importantly, nearly 30% all relapses occurred more than 5 years after treatment. Another interesting finding in this series was the unusual pattern of bone as the only site of relapse in three of eight average risk patients who had received radiotherapy alone. This mirrors an experience from Memorial Sloan-Kettering Cancer Center in which nine recurrences in 45 adults with medulloblastoma involved extraneural sites (177).

The largest series to date of adult medulloblastoma is a retrospective review of 253 patients over the age of 18 treated at thirteen different French institutions between 1975 and 2004. The median follow-up in this series was seven years. On multivariate analysis, brainstem involvement, fourth ventricular floor involvement, and posterior fossa radiation dose <50 Gy were negative prognostic factors. Overall survival was 72% at 5 years and 55% at 10 years. One hundred and twenty-four patients were classified as having average risk disease, and 67 of these received chemotherapy along with CSI. Overall survival was not different between patients treated with full-dose CSI alone and patients treated with CSI doses <34 Gy in combination with chemotherapy. However, it should be noted that this was a heterogenous group of patients, and only 12 of these patients received a spinal dose ≤29 Gy. Thus, long-term outcome of adults treated with reduced-dose CSI to 23.4 Gy and chemotherapy is still unknown (169a).

Evidence-Based Treatment Summary

1. There are no prospective randomized trials evaluating major therapeutic issues in this disease in adults.
2. Maximal surgical resection should be performed, where feasible.
3. Standard treatment consists of postoperative radiotherapy to the craniospinal axis followed by a boost to the posterior fossa.
4. The use of chemotherapy generally follows the pediatric indications and guidelines.

Primary Central Nervous System Lymphoma

CNS lymphomas comprise <3% of primary intracranial malignancies. Immunodeficiency, either congenital or acquired (organ transplant or HIV disease), is the only known risk factor for the development of primary CNS lymphoma. Nonimmunosuppressed patients present typically in the sixth and seventh decades of life, whereas immunosuppressed individuals more commonly present in the third and fourth decades of life. Since the early 1990s, there has been a large increase in the incidence of primary CNS lymphoma, primarily due to patients with acquired immunodeficiency syndrome (AIDS). In patients with a diagnosis of HIV infection surviving longer than 4 years, the frequency may be as high as 10% to 20%, although with the introduction of effective antiviral regimens the incidence of primary CNS lymphoma is decreasing.

The majority of primary CNS lymphomas are B-cell lymphomas of intermediate or high grade. The diagnosis is made after no systemic involvement has found. They typically develop as solitary or multiple periventricular masses in the cerebral hemispheres, although they can also arise in the meninges or the vitreous/retina. They are intensely enhancing on MRI and may have a diffuse or "cotton wool" appearance on imaging. Although on CT or MRI they appear focal, diffuse involvement of the parenchyma is invariably present. Primary CNS lymphomas frequently seed the CSF space either at presentation (16% to 47% reported) or at relapse. Involvement of the vitreous and retina is seen in 15% to 20% of patients. Primary intraocular lymphoma is associated with the subsequent development of CNS lymphoma in up to 80% of patients.

The symptoms and signs of CNS lymphoma are those of any intracranial mass lesions, and the CT or MRI appearance usually suggests the diagnosis. Tissue diagnosis with open or stereotactic biopsy is necessary to rule out other primary or metastatic tumors. Immunohistochemical analysis should be performed to confirm monoclonality and B- versus T-cell type. Staging investigations should include an ophthalmologic assessment to rule out ocular involvement, CSF cytology, complete blood count, Epstein-Barr virus, and HIV serology. Systemic staging (CT of chest and abdomen, bone marrow biopsy) is rarely positive in patients with typical findings of CNS lymphoma, but should be performed if systemic symptoms are present (weight loss, night sweats, fever).

Treatment

The role of surgery is limited to establishing the tissue diagnosis. This is best achieved by stereotactic biopsy; extensive tumor resection offers no survival benefit. Since primary CNS lymphoma often responds dramatically to corticosteroid therapy, corticosteroids should be avoided if possible until after tissue is obtained.

The optimal treatment for primary CNS lymphoma remains controversial. Early reports focused on radiotherapy and given the widespread involvement, whole-brain radiotherapy is required. Median survival with radiotherapy is approximately 18 months (219). RTOG 83-15 reported a local control rate of only 39% with whole-brain irradiation to 40 Gy plus a 20-Gy boost to primary tumor site (46). Unlike non-CNS lymphoma there appears to be a dose response with a threshold between 30 and 50 Gy, with a median of 40 Gy. A study by Bessell et al. (11) comparing two different radiotherapy schedules in patients who had complete response to chemotherapy with CHOD/BVAM (cyclophosphamide, doxorubicin, vincristine, and dexamethasone/BCNU, vincristine, methotrexate, and cytarabine) showed a higher relapse rate and reduced survival rate in patients who received 30.6 versus 45 Gy. This was significant for patients younger than 60.

The combination of radiation and chemotherapy may be superior to radiation alone; 5-year survival rates are 22% to 40% compared with 3% to 26% with radiotherapy alone. Systemic high-dose methotrexate seems to be the most effective agent, with a response rate (partial and complete) of >50% and a 2-year survival rate when combined with radiotherapy of 43% to 73% (184). High-dose methotrexate regimens produce adequate levels of drug in the CSF so that direct instillation of

chemotherapy (e.g., using an Ommaya reservoir) into the CSF is not necessary (81).

The commonly used schedule for primary CNS lymphoma in nonimmunosuppressed patients is 40 to 45 Gy to the whole brain. The posterior orbits should be included in the whole-brain fields. In patients with ocular involvement, the whole eye should be treated to 30 to 40 Gy, with shielding of the anterior chamber and lacrimal apparatus after this dose. The frequent association of ocular lymphoma with synchronous or metachronous CNS lymphoma has led to the recommendation of prophylactic brain irradiation in all patients by some investigators. Others recommend only ocular irradiation in the absence of demonstrable CNS disease. CSI has been advocated for patients with documented CSF involvement. However, intrathecal chemotherapy may be equally efficacious and less toxic, with less impact on bone marrow reserve.

For immunosuppressed patients with primary CNS lymphoma, modification of the irradiation dose and schedule may be necessary. Patients with poor prognostic features (low KPS, CD4 counts <200, advanced AIDS) may be treated with an abbreviated course of radiotherapy (e.g., 36 to 40 Gy).

Results of Treatment

Corticosteroids and radiotherapy produce clinical improvement in most patients, but there are few long-term survivors. In a prospective RTOG study in which patients were treated with 40 Gy to the whole brain with a local boost to 60 Gy (161), local control and survival were not significantly improved over previous reports of whole-brain doses of 45 to 50 Gy, suggesting a plateau in radiation response. As in the earlier study, the pattern of failure was predominantly local (60%), with isolated spinal relapse being very uncommon (<5%). Younger age (<60 years vs. >60 years) and higher pretreatment performance status (KPS ≥70 vs. KPS <70) were associated with longer survivals (20 to 24 months vs. 4 to 6 months). Overall median survival was 11.6 months, with a 2-year survival rate of 28%.

Long-term results with intravenous and intrathecal methotrexate, cranial radiotherapy, and intravenous cytarabine are encouraging, especially in patients younger than 50 years (5-year survival rate of 60%). In older patients (>50 years), results are poor (5-year survival of rate of <10%) and toxicity is greater with dementia and ataxia in a substantial proportion of patients (67).

Chemotherapy has also been used without radiotherapy or as a means of delaying radiotherapy particularly in patients over age 60 because of the substantial risk of neurologic toxicity associated with the use of combined modality treatment in this patient population (13). Complete responses are typically seen in over 50% of patients. Single agent methotrexate using a dose of 8 g/m² had a high response rate, but responses were of a relatively short duration with a median progression-free survival of approximately 1 year (6). An intensive combination regimen using methotrexate, cytarabine, a vinca alkaloid and cyclophosphamide, and ifosfamide together with intrathecal chemotherapy resulted in complete response in approximately 60% of patients and median progression-free survival of 21 months. There was a 9% treatment-related death rate (174). High-dose chemotherapy with stem cell rescue has also been tested in patients with newly diagnosed primary CNS lymphoma. An initial report describes 14 patients who responded to initial induction chemotherapy then received intensive chemotherapy with stem cell rescue (1). Progression-free survival was only 9 months.

In patients with immunosuppression and primary CNS lymphoma, results are discouraging, although selected patients (non-HIV immunosuppression, favorable-prognosis patients with AIDS) may have survival comparable with that of nonimmunosuppressed populations when treated in a standard fashion (52).

Evidence-Based Treatment Summary

1. Surgical resection is not necessary.
2. For most patients, whole-brain radiotherapy is considered the standard to a volume that includes the posterior orbits.
3. High-dose methotrexate-based regimens, generally used in preradiotherapy, have become widely accepted in patients fit enough to tolerate them and appear to be associated with improved survival.
4. Chemotherapy alone with deferred radiotherapy may be preferred in elderly patients because of substantial risk of neurotoxicity associated with combined chemotherapy-radiotherapy regimens.

Meningioma

Meningiomas account for approximately 30% of primary intracranial neoplasms and are the most common benign intracranial tumor in adults (34). The peak age incidence is in the sixth and seventh decades, although they may be seen at any age. They are more common in women. Typical locations for meningiomas include the cerebral convexities, falx cerebri, tentorium cerebelli, cerebellopontine angle, and sphenoid ridge. Malignant varieties with invasive growth and aggressive behavior occasionally occur.

Grossly, meningiomas are well-circumscribed firm, tan, or grayish lesions arising from the meninges. Hyperostosis of adjacent bone may be present. Microscopically benign meningiomas usually have a bland whorled appearance with little anaplasia or mitotic activity. Psammoma bodies may be present. Histologic variants (e.g., fibrous, transitional, angiomatous) can be identified but are of little prognostic significance. Malignant varieties are identified on the basis of clinical behavior (rapid growth or recurrence, invasiveness) or pathologic features such as microscopic features of malignancy (cellular or nuclear anaplasia, mitotic figures) or specific histologic type (rhabdoid, papillary, anaplastic). In the WHO grading system (136), benign meningiomas (~90% all) are classified as WHO grade I and associated with slower growth and lower risk of recurrence, atypical meningiomas (5% to 7%) WHO grade II with an increased likelihood of aggressive behavior, and anaplastic or malignant gliomas (3% to 5%) WHO grade III, which are highly invasive and carry the worst prognosis.

Meningiomas are known to be induced by ionizing radiation, with an average interval to diagnosis of 19 to 35 years, depending on the dose of radiation. They may be multiple particularly in patients with neurofibromatosis type 2 (NF2) and in non-NF2 families with a hereditary predisposition to meningioma.

The most common cytogenetic alteration in meningiomas involves a deletion of chromosome 22. Molecular genetics findings indicate that approximately 50% of meningiomas have allelic losses that involve band q12 on chromosome 22. Allelic losses of chromosomal arms 6q, 9p, 10q, and 14q are seen in both atypical and anaplastic meningiomas. Genetic and cytogenetic alterations accumulate with progression from WHO grade I to WHO grade III lesions. Mutations in the NF2 gene have been detected in 60% of sporadic meningiomas.

The incidental finding of a meningioma on CT or MRI is not uncommon, particularly in older people. Many patients with meningiomas are asymptomatic and may remain so for a long time (82,167). Lesions in the cerebellopontine angle commonly present with symptoms of cranial neuropathy. Cerebral convexity meningioma may present with symptoms of headache or a seizure. Meningiomas of the sphenoid wing or optic nerve may be associated with visual loss. The differential diagnosis of meningioma in the base of the skull or spine includes bone metastasis or primary bone tumors (chondrosarcoma, chordoma, osteosarcoma). In the cerebellopontine angle, acoustic neuromas may resemble meningiomas in location and in CT or MRI appearance.

Meningiomas typically grow slowly. In 47 asymptomatic patients with meningioma diagnosed incidentally by MRI, Nakamura et al. (156) reported a mean annual growth measured using serial MRI of 14.6% and a mean tumor doubling time of 21.6 years. Higher annual growth rates were seen in young patients and lower annual growth rates in patients with calcification and hypointense or isointense T2 signals on MRI. The location of the lesion, extent of surgical resection, and histopathologic features of the tumor (benign or malignant) are the most important determinants of prognosis (73).

After surgery, the average time to recurrence is approximately 4 years. In a review of 38 patients who underwent subtotal resection, the mean diameter increase was 0.37 cm/year and mean tumor doubling time was 8 years (109).

Treatment

Grade I Meningioma

Patients with asymptomatic lesions may be observed and followed with serial imaging. The treatment of choice for symptomatic or progressive benign meningiomas is complete surgical resection if it can be accomplished with acceptable morbidity. Resection of these typically vascular tumors may be facilitated by preoperative angiography with or without embolization. Even after complete resection, 7% to 12% of these tumors recur at 5 years and 20% to 25% recur at 10 years (45,228) so that follow-up with serial imaging is necessary.

Complete resection may be difficult without significant morbidity in the base of the skull, cerebellopontine angle, or cavernous sinus meningiomas. Subtotal resections are associated with higher relapse rates of 39% to 47% at 5 years and 60% to 61% at 10 years without adjuvant therapy (45,228). For these patients, conservative subtotal resection followed by postoperative irradiation may give good local control with less morbidity than an aggressive base of skull resection. An alternative approach for patients who have undergone subtotal resection is follow up with further surgery, if feasible, and radiotherapy delayed to time of recurrence.

In patients with subtotally excised unresectable or recurrent meningiomas the typical radiotherapy dose is 50 to 54 Gy in 25 to 30 fractions over 5 to 6 weeks. The target volume for radiotherapy is defined by CT or MRI scan and modified according to the neurosurgeon's description of the location of residual tumor. The margin expansion for meningiomas is based on the knowledge of direction of spread, especially through neural foramina, bony invasion, dural tails, and so forth. The GTV is the enhancing abnormality on contrast-enhanced MRI. Margin expansions then incorporate setup errors and block margins; these can vary from 0.5 to 1 cm in total depending on the precision of the immobilization and delivery systems. Multiple fields with wedges or rotational fields and 3D conformal techniques are used for maximal sparing of normal brain tissue. IMRT may be helpful in avoiding adjacent surrounding structures.

Postoperative irradiation after less than complete resection improves local control, prolongs the interval to recurrence, and improves survival. Barbaro et al. (4) retrospectively compared 54 patients who had subtotal resection and radiotherapy with a control group of 30 patients who underwent subtotal resection alone; 60% of the nonirradiated patients had recurrence, in contrast to 32% of patients who received radiotherapy. The median time to recurrence in the irradiated group was 125 months compared with 66 months in the nonirradiated group ($p < .05$). No complications were reported with irradiation. Taylor et al. (241) also found that only 15% of patients treated with subtotal excision and postoperative irradiation had recurrences as compared with 69% after subtotal excision alone ($p = .01$). The actuarial determinate 10-year survival rate was 81% for patients who received combined treatment and 49% for nonirradiated patients. The actuarial probability of local tumor control achieved with radiotherapy after subtotal resection was similar to that observed for total excision. In series by Condra et al. (45), subtotal resection with postoperative irradiation had a local control rate of 87% at 15 years compared to 76% following total excision and 30% after subtotal excision ($p = .0001$). In modern series using MRI and CT localization 5-year local control is reported to be >90% (83).

Radiosurgery as the sole modality or as postoperative adjuvant therapy may be of interest for selected patients, generally those with smaller tumors. In recent series 5-year progression-free survival rates are >80% (53,93,162,183,229). EORTC 26021-22021 is an important phase III trial that will randomize patients to observation, conformal external-beam radiotherapy, or radiosurgery following subtotal resection or biopsy.

Chemotherapy has not been useful in the treatment of benign meningiomas. Given the high estrogen and progesterone receptor expression on meningiomas, progesterone receptor antagonists have been tested but have not been found beneficial.

Grade II and III Meningioma

For atypical or malignant meningiomas, the recurrence rate after surgery alone is high (41% to 100% at 5 years), even after complete surgical resection (58,176), and postoperative irradiation after maximal resection is recommended for all patients. The target volume is more generous than that used for benign meningiomas. The GTV is typically expanded by 1.5 to 2 cm around the contrast-enhancing visible tumor to account for microscopic invasion of brain parenchyma. The recommended dose is on the order of 60 Gy in 30 to 33 fractions, although some have reported improved local control with higher doses (105).

In a review of 38 patients with malignant meningiomas by Dziuk et al. (58), complete use of postoperative radiotherapy resulted in superior local control. At 5 years, irradiation following initial resection improved 5-year disease-free survival from 15% to 80% ($p = .002$). Progression-free survival was 57% in patients treated with total resection and radiotherapy compared to 28% in patients treated with total resection alone.

Systemic therapy has no defined role. Combined chemotherapy with vincristine, adriamycin, and cyclophosphamide has shown some efficacy in patients with malignant meningiomas (37). Targeted agents represent an area of active research in the treatment of high-grade meningiomas. Increased expression of cyclooxygenase-2 (COX-2) has been shown to be associated with more aggressive phenotypes (134). Additionally, malignant meningiomas have recently been shown to have increased EGFR staining, suggesting another investigational treatment strategy.

Unresectable or Recurrent Meningioma

In patients in whom aggressive surgery is not an option, radiotherapy may relieve symptoms and decrease the rate of tumor progression.

Radiotherapy may be useful in the treatment of recurrent meningioma. In a review by Miralbell et al. (149), progression-free survival at 8 years for patients treated with subtotal resection and radiotherapy at first recurrence was 78% compared to 11% in patients treated with resection alone ($p = .001$).

Various chemotherapy treatments that have been used in patients with recurrent meningiomas include combined doxorubicin and dacarbazine or ifosfamide and mesna (122). Long-term low-dose daily hydroxyurea may have some activity (207).

Hormonal manipulation, including tamoxifen and the antiprogesterone drug RU486, showed some activity in a SWOG phase II evaluation of tamoxifen in unresectable or refractory

meningiomas. Partial response or prolonged tumor stabilization was seen in 47% of patients (85). However, a subsequent SWOG phase III, double-blind, randomized, placebo-controlled study of mifepristone for the treatment of unresectable meningioma was negative. Median freedom from progression was 10 months for mifepristone and 12 months for placebo ($p = .44$) (88).

Evidence-Based Treatment Summary

1. Small asymptomatic meningiomas in noncritical locations, especially in the elderly or in patients with other comorbidities can be observed.
2. The goal of surgery is to completely resect the meningioma, with negative margins as patients with WHO grades I and II completely resected meningiomas have low rates of relapse and can be observed postoperatively.
3. For subtotally resected or unresectable progressive meningioma radiotherapy is frequently used but has not been tested in a prospective clinical trial. Local control appears to be improved with postoperative radiotherapy. Both radiosurgery and radiotherapy have been used in this context, but have not been directly compared.
4. For high-grade and especially malignant meningioma postoperative radiotherapy is routinely recommended.
5. Primary radiotherapy or radiosurgery could be used for unresectable, progressive meningiomas.
6. Systemic therapy does not have a defined role in meningioma.

Craniopharyngioma

Craniopharyngiomas arise from epithelial remnants of the Rathke pouch and are typically found in the suprasellar region in children or adolescents. They account for <5% of all CNS neoplasms in adults. They are slowly growing tumors that often have solid and cystic components, the latter filled with lipoid, cholesterol-laden ("crankcase oil") fluid. Although appearing well encapsulated, craniopharyngiomas typically demonstrate invaginations into adjacent brain and may provoke a vigorous glial reaction.

The cystic nature of craniopharyngiomas is usually evident on CT and MRI and helps distinguish these tumors from other base of skull lesions and pituitary adenomas. The solid portion is often calcified and enhancing, whereas the cystic portion typically demonstrates a thin rim of enhancement. The finding of multiple cysts of varying intensity on T1- and T2-weighted MRI is characteristic of craniopharyngioma.

Intrasellar lesions may compress the pituitary and hypothalamus, producing hormonal abnormalities, especially antidiuretic and growth hormone deficits. Prechiasmal lesions may compress the optic pathway, leading to visual field cuts or decreased central visual acuity. Retrochiasmal lesions may grow into the third ventricle and cause hydrocephalus or compress the optic tracts. Craniopharyngiomas can occasionally reach enormous size and produce neurologic impairment by direct impingement on brain parenchyma. Surgical decompression is the optimal treatment for rapid symptom relief. However, the location, proximity, and adhesiveness of the tumor to adjacent structures often preclude complete resection.

Treatment

A discussion of craniopharyngioma in the pediatric context is provided in Chapter 82. Management options include complete resection, subtotal resection alone, or subtotal resection or biopsy followed by postoperative radiotherapy.

Complete surgical resection, which is applicable only to a minority of patients, is associated with local control and long-term survival in 70% to 90% of patients (17). However, aggressive resection may be associated with significant morbidity, with up to a 10% incidence of perioperative mortality and up to 30% severe morbidity, especially diabetes insipidus or other endocrine deficits, visual impairment, obesity, and memory impairment.

Partial resection or cyst aspiration and biopsy rapidly relieve local compressive symptoms and have less operative morbidity but are associated with eventual tumor progression in most cases. Long-term survival and local control are achieved only in approximately 30% of patients. In contrast to aggressive resections, subtotal resections carry a mortality of about 1%.

With a limited surgical procedure (partial resection or cyst aspiration plus biopsy) followed by radiotherapy local control and survival rates are nearly equivalent to those achieved with complete resection, with survival rates of 89% and 77% at 5 and 10 years, respectively, as compared with 53% to 37% for patients who have had subtotal resection alone. Typically, doses of 50 to 54 Gy in 25 to 30 fractions (1.8 Gy) over 6 weeks are delivered to the preoperative tumor volume with a 1- to 1.5-cm margin depending on the accuracy of the imaging used for planning and the reproducibility of the treatment setup. In patients with compressive symptoms, surgical decompression before irradiation is essential because the tumor typically responds slowly to radiotherapy, and radiation-induced edema may worsen compressive symptoms.

With these dose recommendations (i.e., 1.8-Gy fractions to 50 to 54 Gy), the risk of visual impairment is very low (1% and 1.5%). In a retrospective analysis of patients treated with 51.3 to 70 Gy, a higher incidence of radiation-related complications was seen in those who received more than 60 Gy (with an actuarial incidence of optic neuropathy of 30% and brain necrosis of 12.5%), without any concomitant improvement in tumor control (72).

Radiotherapy may be given as salvage rather than immediately after subtotal resection. In a series of 76 patients treated at the University of Pennsylvania, long-term survival rates were equivalent (232). In another series radiotherapy given at recurrence yielded a 10-year progression-free survival rate of >70% (108). Recurrences occur from 3 to 192 months (median 12 months) after subtotal resection so that close surveillance is necessary during the first years following incomplete resection.

Other modalities used in the treatment of craniopharyngioma have included intralesional bleomycin and radioactive colloid instillations for cystic tumors. Radiosurgery may be useful in ablating small residual or recurrent tumors (118).

Evidence-Based Treatment Summary

1. Surgical resection is recommended, when feasible.
2. The use of postoperative radiotherapy has not been tested in prospective trials, but reduces the risk of recurrence and improves survival in incompletely resected tumors. Cyst decompression and biopsy followed by radiotherapy may be an acceptable treatment for patients for whom resection is not considered feasible.
3. Intracavitary bleomycin or radiocolloids may be useful in cystic tumors.

Vestibular Schwannoma and Neurofibroma

Neurilemomas, also known as schwannomas and neurinomas, arise from the Schwann cells of the myelin sheath of the peripheral nerves. When occurring close to the eighth cranial nerve, they are also called vestibular schwannomas or acoustic neuromas. These tumors account for approximately 6% of CNS neoplasms in adults. They may be sporadic or associated with NF2, with bilateral vestibular schwannomas being pathognomonic of this disease. The majority of sporadic vestibular schwannomas are unilateral and occur in the fourth and fifth decades of life. Those arising in patients with NF2 tend to occur in the second or third decades. These tumors grow slowly

in a well-circumscribed, expansile fashion, displacing adjacent nerves rather than invading them. The majority arise from cranial nerve VIII in the medial internal auditory canal. Less commonly, they may arise from other cranial nerves, the trigeminal nerve being the most common alternate site.

Growth in the internal auditory canal gives rise to vestibular and hearing abnormalities in up to 95% of patients. A progressive unilateral sensorineural hearing loss is characteristic. Expansion into the cerebellopontine angle may lead to trigeminal symptoms, and a unilateral absent corneal reflex is an early sign of trigeminal involvement. Large tumors may impinge on the cerebellum and brainstem, leading to ataxia and long tract signs as well as involvement of cranial nerves IX, X, XI, and XII.

Pure tone and speech audiometry are the most useful screening tests. Selective loss of speech discrimination in excess of pure tone loss is particularly suggestive of vestibular schwannoma. Brainstem auditory evoked responses typically demonstrate a slowing of conduction, and electronystagmography may detect a decrease in caloric response on the ipsilateral side. Thin-slice Gd-enhanced MRI through the cerebellopontine angle is the imaging modality of choice for suspected vestibular schwannoma. Thin-slice, contrast-enhanced, high-resolution CT scan is an acceptable alternative when MRI is not obtainable. An intensely enhancing lesion close to the internal auditory canal is highly suggestive of this diagnosis. Patients with suspected neurofibromatosis should have complete imaging of the craniospinal axis to document other neurilemomas, neurofibromas, and meningiomas that may be present.

Neurofibromas differ from neurilemomas in their cellular composition and growth pattern. Although neurofibromas also arise from peripheral nerves, they are most commonly multiple and associated with NF1. Neurofibromas expand rather than displace the nerve of origin. Histologically, neurofibromas are composed of a hypertrophied mass of fibroblasts and Schwann cells through which run normal neurons. Symptoms are caused primarily through compression of the involved or adjacent nerves.

Treatment

Treatment should offer a high chance of local control as well as preservation of cranial nerve function. Observation alone may be appropriate in patients willing to undergo regular clinical and imaging follow-up and may allow treatment to be deferred for some time. The mainstay of treatment has been microsurgical resection. Retrosigmoid (suboccipital) middle fossa and translabyrinthine approaches offer the possibility of hearing preservation but are associated with higher incidences of seventh nerve damage and postoperative complications. The translabyrinthine approach is associated with low operative morbidity and mortality but sacrifices hearing. At centers with expertise in microsurgical resection, total or near-total resection rates of 90% are routinely obtained with a surgical mortality rate of <2%. Anatomic preservation of the facial nerve may be achieved in 90% of patients and functional preservation in more than two-thirds. Preservation of useful hearing is reported in 30% to 50%. In patients in whom a near-total or total resection is achieved, the tumor recurrence rate is <10%. In patients in whom a subtotal resection is achieved, tumor recurrence may occur in one-third to one-half. Adjuvant radiotherapy may reduce the rate of recurrence to that of complete resection.

At the University of California–San Francisco, the percentage of tumors that are totally resected has increased from 50% to over 80% in the past three decades (262). Only 2/63 patients who had total resection recurred. Patients who underwent near-total resection (defined as removal of 90% to 99% of the tumor, as judged by the surgeon at the time of operation) had a recurrence rate of only 7% compared with 46% (6/13) in patients who underwent subtotal resection (<90% of the tumor resected), with an actuarial recurrence rate of 59% at

15 years. Patients who received postoperative irradiation after subtotal resection had an actuarial recurrence rate of only 6% at 15 years ($p = .01$). Three patients treated with radiotherapy after biopsy alone were without disease progression at 7 to 14 years after therapy. All recurrences were in the tumor bed.

In patients with a medical contraindication to surgery, treatment with external beam irradiation alone is an option. A dose of 50 to 55 Gy in 25 to 30 fractions over 5 to 6 weeks is recommended. Maire et al. (139) evaluated 24 patients with stage III and IV cerebellopontine angle schwannomas treated with external irradiation; seven had phacomatosis. Indications for radiotherapy were poor general condition or old age contraindicating surgery in 14 cases, hearing preservation in bilateral neurinomas after contralateral tumor removal in five cases, partial resection or high risk of recurrence after subsequent surgery for relapse in four cases, and nonsurgical relapse in two cases. Mean doses were 51 Gy in fractions of 1.8 Gy. With median follow-up of 60 months, there was an 88% tumor control rate with no injuries to the cranial nerve V or VIII.

Radiosurgery may be an alternative to microsurgical resection. The well-circumscribed nature of these tumors, coupled with their typical intense enhancement on MRI, facilitates their localization and treatment using stereotactic techniques. The progression-free survival rate with radiosurgery is nearly 90% at 20 years. Radiosurgical treatment with higher doses yielded high rates of tumor growth arrest (>80%) and tumor shrinkage in up to two thirds of patients, although facial or trigeminal neuropathy develops in nearly one third of patients as long as 2 years after therapy. The volume of the lesion is a significant risk factor for complications involving cranial nerve V, VII, or VIII. Temporary enlargement may occur up to 2 years following radiosurgery (155).

Noren (163) reviewed the results of 669 patients with vestibular schwannoma treated with Gamma Knife radiosurgery between 1969 and 1997. Long-term growth control was achieved in 95%. Facial weakness and/or numbness occurred in approximately one third of patients during the 1970s but in <2% in the 1990s. Hearing was preserved in 65% to 70% of patients, although tinnitus was rarely changed by treatment. With dose reduction to 12 to 13 Gy, high rates of tumor control and cranial nerve preservation may be achieved. Flickinger et al. (71) reported the results of 313 patients treated with radiosurgery to median dose of 13 Gy. The actuarial 6-year tumor control rate was 98.6%. The actuarial 6-year rates for preservation of seventh nerve function, normal fifth nerve function, unchanged hearing level, and useful hearing were 100%, 95.6%, 70.3%, and 78.6%, respectively.

Radiosurgery provides similar local control with less morbidity than surgery for small (<3 cm) unilateral tumors. In a series from the University of Pittsburgh, radiosurgery was found to have improved preservation of facial function ($p < .05$) and hearing ($p < .03$) with decreased associated morbidity ($p < .01$) when compared to surgical resection (182). Postoperative functional outcomes and patient satisfaction were greater after radiosurgery, although this did not reach statistical significance. Return to independent functioning occurred earlier ($p < .001$), and hospital stay was shorter ($p < .001$) after radiosurgery, suggesting that radiosurgery may be an equally effective and less costly management strategy than surgical resection for small tumors.

FSRT has been shown to give local control rates of 91% to 97% with similar effects on cranial nerves V and VII (2,144, 221,234). However, in one series FSRT resulted in 2.5-fold greater preservation of hearing compared to radiosurgery (2).

For neurofibromas, treatment is usually complete resection of compressive lesions with expectant observation of any asymptomatic synchronous lesions. Treatment of neurofibromas is associated with a high rate of local control (>90%) when complete excision is possible. For subtotally excised lesions, ad-

juvant radiotherapy (50 to 55 Gy) may decrease the risk of local recurrence.

Evidence-Based Treatment Summary

1. Small nonprogressive tumors can be observed.
2. Surgical resection is generally considered the standard of care for symptomatic lesions.
3. Radiosurgery produces outcomes equivalent to surgery, although these modalities have not been prospectively compared.
4. Fractionated stereotactic radiotherapy is being increasingly employed, with institutional reports suggesting a lower incidence of cranial neuropathies than radiosurgery, but this has not been prospectively validated.

Hemangioblastoma and Hemangiopericytoma

Hemangioblastomas are benign vascular tumors that present during the third and fourth decades of life. They account for 1% to 2% of primary CNS tumors in adults. Most arise in the cerebellum, constituting the most common primary cerebellar tumors in adults. An association with von Hippel-Lindau disease is noted in 10% of patients. Histologically, the tumor consists of closely packed, thin-walled blood vessels in a stroma of large, oval foamy cells. The lesions are intensely enhancing on CT and MRI, and angiography confirms the vascular nature of the lesion. Imaging of the craniospinal axis often documents multiple lesions in patients with von Hippel-Lindau disease. Treatment is surgical and complete resection is curative. Radiosurgery has also been shown to be useful in patients with unresectable disease but is associated with higher rates of recurrence (192,236,264).

Hemangiopericytoma is a sarcomatous lesion developing from smooth muscle in blood vessels usually along the base of the skull, although intraparenchymal lesions may be seen. In contrast to other primary CNS tumors, hemangiopericytomas commonly develop systemic metastases. There is a 90% 9-year actuarial risk for local failure following surgical resection only. Postoperative radiotherapy to total doses of 50 to 60 Gy reduces the risk of recurrence rate and improves overall survival. Tumor control is dose dependent, with doses >50 Gy associated with superior outcomes. Radiographic response is slow. Radiosurgery has been used for recurrent hemangiopericytomas, with reported local control rates of approximately 80% following treatment (218).

Evidence-Based Treatment Summary

1. Surgical resection is recommended, when feasible, for both of these diseases.
2. Radiotherapy is generally reserved for subtotally resected progressive hemangioblastoma, but there are no prospective data.
3. Postoperative radiotherapy is recommended for subtotally resected hemangiopericytoma, but there are no prospective data.
4. Radiotherapy or radiosurgery may be considered for unresectable tumors.

References

1. Abrey LE, Moskowitz CH, Mason WP, et al. Intensive methotrexate and cytarabine followed by high-dose chemotherapy with autologous stem-cell rescue in patients with newly diagnosed primary CNS lymphoma: an intent-to-treat analysis. *J Clin Oncol* 2003;21(22):4151–4156.
2. Andrews DW, Suarez O, Goldman HW, et al. Stereotactic radiosurgery and fractionated stereotactic radiotherapy for the treatment of acoustic schwannomas: comparative observations of 125 patients treated at one institution. *Int J Radiat Oncol Biol Phys* 2001;50(5):1265–1278.

3. Athanassiou H, Synodinou M, Maragoudakis E, et al. Randomized phase II study of temozolomide and radiotherapy compared with radiotherapy alone in newly diagnosed glioblastoma multiforme. *J Clin Oncol* 2005;23(10):2372–2377.

4. Barbaro NM, Gutin PH, Wilson CB, et al. Radiation therapy in the treatment of partially resected meningiomas. *Neurosurgery* 1987;20(4):525–528.

5. Bassal M, Mertens AC, Taylor L, et al. Risk of selected subsequent carcinomas in survivors of childhood cancer: a report from the Childhood Cancer Survivor Study. *J Clin Oncol* 2006;24(3):476–483.

6. Batchelor T, Carson K, O'Neill A, et al. Treatment of primary CNS lymphoma with methotrexate and deferred radiotherapy: a report of NABTT 96-07. *J Clin Oncol* 2003;21(6):1044–1049.

7. Bauman G, Yartsev S, Coad T, et al. Helical tomotherapy for craniospinal radiation. *Br J Radiol* 2005;78(930):548–552.

8. Bauman GS, Ino Y, Ueki K, et al. Allelic loss of chromosome 1p and radiotherapy plus chemotherapy in patients with oligodendrogliomas. *Int J Radiat Oncol Biol Phys* 2000;48(3):825–830.

9. Berger MS, Baumeister B, Geyer JR, et al. The risks of metastases from shunting in children with primary central nervous system tumors. *J Neurosurg* 1991;74(6):872–877.

10. Berger MS, Deliganis AV, Dobbins J, et al. The effect of extent of resection on recurrence in patients with low grade cerebral hemisphere gliomas. *Cancer* 1994;74(6):1784–1791.

11. Bessell EM, Lopez-Guillermo A, Villa S, et al. Importance of radiotherapy in the outcome of patients with primary CNS lymphoma: an analysis of the CHOD/BVAM regimen followed by two different radiotherapy treatments. *J Clin Oncol* 2002;20(1):231–236.

12. Besson A, Yong VW. Mitogenic signaling and the relationship to cell cycle regulation in astrocytomas. *J Neurooncol* 2001;51(3):245–264.

13. Blay JY, Conroy T, Chevreau C, et al. High-dose methotrexate for the treatment of primary cerebral lymphomas: analysis of survival and late neurologic toxicity in a retrospective series. *J Clin Oncol* 1998;16(3):864–871.

14. Bleehen NM, Stenning SP. A Medical Research Council trial of two radiotherapy doses in the treatment of grades 3 and 4 astrocytoma. The Medical Research Council Brain Tumour Working Party. *Br J Cancer* 1991;64(4):769–774.

15. Bleehen NM, Wiltshire CR, Plowman PN, et al. A randomized study of misonidazole and radiotherapy for grade 3 and 4 cerebral astrocytoma. *Br J Cancer* 1981;43(4):436–442.

16. Bova FJ, Buatti JM, Friedman WA, et al. The University of Florida frameless high-precision stereotactic radiotherapy system. *Int J Radiat Oncol Biol Phys* 1997;38(4):875–882.

17. Brada M, Thomas DG. Craniopharyngioma revisited. *Int J Radiat Oncol Biol Phys* 1993;27(2):471–475.

18. Brada M, Viviers L, Abson C, et al. Phase II study of primary temozolomide chemotherapy in patients with WHO grade II gliomas. *Ann Oncol* 2003;14(12):1715–1721.

19. Brady LW, Markoe AM, Woo DV, et al. Iodine125 labeled anti-epidermal growth factor receptor-425 in the treatment of malignant astrocytomas. A pilot study. *J Neurosurg Sci* 1990;34(3–4):243–249.

20. Brandes AA, Cavallo G, Reni M, et al. A multicenter retrospective study of chemotherapy for recurrent intracranial ependymal tumors in adults by the Gruppo Italiano Cooperativo di Neuro-Oncologia. *Cancer* 2005;104(1):143–148.

21. Breen SL, Kehagioglou P, Usher C, et al. A comparison of conventional, conformal and intensity-modulated coplanar radiotherapy plans for posterior fossa treatment. *Br J Radiol* 2004;77(921):768–774.

22. Brem H, Ewend MG, Piantadosi S, et al. The safety of interstitial chemotherapy with BCNU-loaded polymer followed by radiation therapy in the treatment of newly diagnosed malignant gliomas: phase I trial. *J Neurooncol* 1995;26(2):111–123.

23. Brem H, Piantadosi S, Burger PC, et al. Placebo-controlled trial of safety and efficacy of intraoperative controlled delivery by biodegradable polymers of chemotherapy for recurrent gliomas. The Polymer-brain Tumor Treatment Group. *Lancet* 1995;345(8956):1008–1012.

24. Buckner JC, Gesme D Jr., O'Fallon JR, et al. Phase II trial of procarbazine, lomustine, and vincristine as initial therapy for patients with low-grade oligodendroglioma or oligoastrocytoma: efficacy and associations with chromosomal abnormalities. *J Clin Oncol* 2003;21(2):251–255.

25. Bull JWD, Rovit RL. The radiographic localization of intracerebral gliomata. *J Fac Radiol Lond* 1957;8:147–157.

26. Burger PC, Yu IT, Tihan T, et al. Atypical teratoid/rhabdoid tumor of the central nervous system: a highly malignant tumor of infancy and childhood frequently mistaken for medulloblastoma: a Pediatric Oncology Group study. *Am J Surg Pathol* 1998;22(9):1083–1092.

27. Cairncross G, Berkey B, Shaw E, et al. Phase III trial of chemotherapy plus radiotherapy compared with radiotherapy alone for pure and mixed anaplastic oligodendrogliomas: Intergroup Radiation Therapy Oncology Group 9402. *J Clin Oncol* 2006;24(18):2707–2714.

28. Cairncross JG, Ueki K, Zlatescu MC, et al. Specific genetic predictors of chemotherapeutic response and survival in patients with anaplastic oligodendrogliomas. *J Natl Cancer Inst* 1998;90(19):1473–1479.

29. Cammer W. Effects of TNF-alpha on immature and mature oligodendrocytes and their progenitors in vitro. *Brain Res* 2000;864(2):213–219.

30. Cardinale R, Won M, Choucair A, et al. A phase II trial of accelerated radiotherapy using weekly stereotactic conformal boost for supratentorial glioblastoma multiforme: RTOG 0023. *Int J Radiat Oncol Biol Phys* 2006;65(5):1422–1428.

31. Carrie C, Lasset C, Blay JY, et al. Medulloblastoma in adults: survival and prognostic factors. *Radiother Oncol* 1993;29(3):301–307.

32. Castro JR, Saunders WM, Austin-Seymour MM, et al. A phase I-II trial of heavy charged particle irradiation of malignant glioma of the brain: a Northern California Oncology Group Study. *Int J Radiat Oncol Biol Phys* 1985;11(10):1795–1800.

33. Catterall M, Bloom HJ, Ash DV, et al. Fast neutrons compared with megavoltage x-rays in the treatment of patients with supratentorial glioblastoma: a controlled pilot study. *Int J Radiat Oncol Biol Phys* 1980;6(3):261–266.

34. www.CBTRUS.org. Statistical report: Primary brain tumors in the United States, 1998–2002 Central Brain Tumor Registry of the United States 2005. www.cbtns.org/reports/reports.html June 14, 2006.

35. Chahlavi A, Kanner A, Peereboom D, et al. Impact of chromosome 1p status in response of oligodendroglioma to temozolomide: preliminary results. *J Neurooncol* 2003;61(3):267–273.

36. Chakravarti A, Seiferheld W, Tu X, et al. Immunohistochemically determined total epidermal growth factor receptor levels not of prognostic value in newly diagnosed glioblastoma multiforme: report from the Radiation Therapy Oncology Group. *Int J Radiat Oncol Biol Phys* 2005;62(2):318–327.

37. Chamberlain MC. Adjuvant combined modality therapy for malignant meningiomas. *J Neurosurg* 1996;84(5):733–736.

38. Chan AW, Tarbell NJ, Black PM, et al. Adult medulloblastoma: prognostic factors and patterns of relapse. *Neurosurgery* 2000;47(3):623–631; discussion 31–32.

39. Chan JL, Lee SW, Fraass BA, et al. Survival and failure patterns of high-grade gliomas after three-dimensional conformal radiotherapy. *J Clin Oncol* 2002;20(6):1635–1642.

40. Chang CH. Hyperbaric oxygen and radiation therapy in the management of glioblastoma. *Natl Cancer Inst Monogr* 1977;46:163–139.

41. Chinot OL, Honore S, Dufour H, et al. Safety and efficacy of temozolomide in patients with recurrent anaplastic oligodendrogliomas after standard radiotherapy and chemotherapy. *J Clin Oncol* 2001;19(9):2449–2455.

42. Cho J, Harrop J, Veznadaroglu E, et al. Concomitant use of computer image guidance, linear or sigmoid incisions after minimal shave, and liquid wound dressing with 2-octyl cyanoacrylate for tumor craniotomy or craniectomy: analysis of 225 consecutive surgical cases with antecedent historical control at one institution. *Neurosurgery* 2003;52(4):832–840; discussion 40–41.

43. Chow BM, Li YQ, Wong CS. Radiation-induced apoptosis in the adult central nervous system is p53-dependent. *Cell Death Differ* 2000;7(8):712–720.

44. Claus EB, Horlacher A, Hsu L, et al. Survival rates in patients with low-grade glioma after intraoperative magnetic resonance image guidance. *Cancer* 2005;103(6):1227–1233.

45. Condra KS, Buatti JM, Mendenhall WM, et al. Benign meningiomas: primary treatment selection affects survival. *Int J Radiat Oncol Biol Phys* 1997;39(2):427–436.

46. Corn BW, Dolinskas C, Scott C, et al. Strong correlation between imaging response and survival among patients with primary central nervous system lymphoma: a secondary analysis of RTOG studies 83-15 and 88-06. *Int J Radiat Oncol Biol Phys* 2000;47(2):299–303.

47. Cote TR, Manns A, Hardy CR, et al. Epidemiology of brain lymphoma among people with or without acquired immunodeficiency syndrome. AIDS/Cancer Study Group. *J Natl Cancer Inst* 1996;88(10):675–679.

48. Coughlin C, Scott C, Langer C, et al. Phase II, two-arm RTOG trial (94-11) of bischloroethyl-nitrosourea plus accelerated hyperfractionated radiotherapy (64.0 or 70.4 Gy) based on tumor volume (>20 or ≤20 cm[2], respectively) in the treatment of newly-diagnosed radiosurgery-ineligible glioblastoma multiforme patients. *Int J Radiat Oncol Biol Phys* 2000;48(5):1351–1358.

49. Crossen JR, Garwood D, Glatstein E, et al. Neurobehavioral sequelae of cranial irradiation in adults: a review of radiation-induced encephalopathy. *J Clin Oncol* 1994;12(3):627–642.

50. Curran WJ Jr. , Scott CB, Horton J, et al. Recursive partitioning analysis of prognostic factors in three Radiation Therapy Oncology Group malignant glioma trials. *J Natl Cancer Inst* 1993;85(9):704–710.

51. Dandy WE. Removal of right cerebral hemisphere for certain tumors with hemiplegia. *JAMA* 1928;90:823–825.

52. Deangelis LM. Current management of primary central nervous system lymphoma. *Oncology (Williston Park)* 1995;9(1):63–671; discussion, 5–6, 8.

53. Debus J, Wuendrich M, Pirzkall A, et al. High efficacy of fractionated stereotactic radiotherapy of large base-of-skull meningiomas: long-term results. *J Clin Oncol* 2001;19(15):3547–3553.

54. Deutsch M, Green SB, Strike TA, et al. Results of a randomized trial comparing BCNU plus radiotherapy, streptozotocin plus radiotherapy, BCNU plus hyperfractionated radiotherapy, and BCNU following misonidazole plus radiotherapy in the postoperative treatment of malignant glioma. *Int J Radiat Oncol Biol Phys* 1989;16(6):1389–1396.

55. Donahue B, Scott CB, Nelson JS, et al. Influence of an oligodendroglial component on the survival of patients with anaplastic astrocytomas: a report of Radiation Therapy Oncology Group 83-02. *Int J Radiat Oncol Biol Phys* 1997;38(5):911–914.

56. Donahue B, Steinfeld A. Intracranial ependymoma in the adult patient: successful treatment with surgery and radiotherapy. *J Neurooncol* 1998;37(2):131–133.

57. Donaldson SS, Laningham F, Fisher PG. Advances toward an understanding of brainstem gliomas. *J Clin Oncol* 2006;24(8):1266–1272.

58. Dziuk TW, Woo S, Butler EB, et al. Malignant meningioma: an indication for initial aggressive surgery and adjuvant radiotherapy. *J Neurooncol* 1998;37(2):177–188.

59. Elsayed YA, Sausville EA. Selected novel anticancer treatments targeting cell signaling proteins. *Oncologist* 2001;6(6):517–537.

60. Emerich DF, Dean RL, Osborn C, et al. The development of the bradykinin agonist labradimil as a means to increase the permeability of the blood-brain barrier: from concept to clinical evaluation. *Clin Pharmacokinet* 2001;40(2):105–123.

61. Emrich JG, Brady LW, Quang TS, et al. Radioiodinated (I-125) monoclonal antibody 425 in the treatment of high grade glioma patients: ten-year synopsis of a novel treatment. *Am J Clin Oncol* 2002;25(6):541–546.

62. Esteller M, Garcia-Foncillas J, Andion E, et al. Inactivation of the DNA-repair gene MGMT and the clinical response of gliomas to alkylating agents. *N Engl J Med* 2000;343(19):1350–1354.

63. Evans RG, Kimler BF, Morantz RA, et al. Lack of complications in long-term survivors after treatment with Fluosol and oxygen as an adjuvant to radiation therapy for high-grade brain tumors. *Int J Radiat Oncol Biol Phys* 1993;26(4):649–652.

64. Eyre HJ, Crowley JJ, Townsend JJ, et al. A randomized trial of radiotherapy versus radiotherapy plus CCNU for incompletely resected low-grade gliomas: a Southwest Oncology Group study. *J Neurosurg* 1993;78(6):909–914.

65. Fallon KB, Palmer CA, Roth KA, et al. Prognostic value of 1p, 19q, 9p, 10q, and EGFR-FISH analyses in recurrent oligodendrogliomas. *J Neuropathol Exp Neurol* 2004;63(4):314–322.

66. Ferrante L, Mastronardi L, Schettini G, et al. Fourth ventricle ependymomas. A study of 20 cases with survival analysis. *Acta Neurochir (Wien)* 1994;131(1-2):67–74.

67. Ferreri AJ, Abrey LE, Blay JY, et al. Summary statement on primary central nervous system lymphomas from the Eighth International Conference on Malignant Lymphoma, Lugano, Switzerland, June 12 to 15, 2002. *J Clin Oncol* 2003;21(12):2407–2414.

68. Fetell MR, Grossman SA, Fisher JD, et al. Preirradiation paclitaxel in glioblastoma multiforme: efficacy, pharmacology, and drug interactions. New Approaches

to Brain Tumor Therapy Central Nervous System Consortium. *J Clin Oncol* 1997;15(9):3121–3128.
69. Fine HA, Kim L, Royce C, et al. Results from phase II trial of Enzastaurin (LY317615) in patients with recurrent high grade gliomas. 2005 ASCO Annual Meeting Proceedings. *J Clin Oncol* 2005;23–16S):1504.
70. Fitzek MM, Thornton AF, Rabinov JD, et al. Accelerated fractionated proton/photon irradiation to 90 cobalt gray equivalent for glioblastoma multiforme: results of a phase II prospective trial. *J Neurosurg* 1999;91(2):251–260.
71. Flickinger JC, Kondziolka D, Niranjan A, et al. Acoustic neuroma radiosurgery with marginal tumor doses of 12 to 13 Gy. *Int J Radiat Oncol Biol Phys* 2004;60(1):225–230.
72. Flickinger JC, Lunsford LD, Singer J, et al. Megavoltage external beam irradiation of craniopharyngiomas: analysis of tumor control and morbidity. *Int J Radiat Oncol Biol Phys* 1990;19(1):117–122.
73. Forbes AR, Goldberg ID. Radiation therapy in the treatment of meningioma: the Joint Center for Radiation Therapy experience 1970 to 1982. *J Clin Oncol* 1984;2(10):1139–1143.
74. Ford JM, Seiferheld W, Mehta M, et al. Comparison of survival of patients in the phase I study of Motexafin Gadolinium (MGd) with radiation therapy (RT) for glioblastoma multiforme (GBM), with a matched cohort of patients from the RTOG RPA glioma database. *Proc Am Soc Clin Oncol* 2003;22:106.
75. Frost PJ, Laperriere NJ, Wong CS, et al. Medulloblastoma in adults. *Int J Radiat Oncol Biol Phys* 1995;32(4):951–957.
76. Garrett PG, Simpson WJ. Ependymomas: results of radiation treatment. *Int J Radiat Oncol Biol Phys* 1983;9(8):1121–1124.
77. Gilbert M, Kuhn J, Lamborn K, et al. Phase I/II study of combination temozolomide (TMZ) and irinotecan (CPT-11) for recurrent malignant gliomas: a North American Brain Tumor Consortium (NABTC) study. *Proc Am Soc Clin Oncol* 2003;22:103.
78. Gilbert MR, Supko JG, Batchelor T, et al. Phase I clinical and pharmacokinetic study of irinotecan in adults with recurrent malignant glioma. *Clin Cancer Res* 2003;9(8):2940–2949.
79. Giordana MT, Cavalla P, Chio A, et al. Prognostic factors in adult medulloblastoma. A clinico-pathologic study. *Tumori* 1995;81(5):338–346.
80. Glantz MJ, Cole BF, Forsyth PA, et al. Practice parameter: anticonvulsant prophylaxis in patients with newly diagnosed brain tumors. Report of the Quality Standards Subcommittee of the American Academy of Neurology. *Neurology* 2000; 54(10):1886–1893.
81. Glantz MJ, Cole BF, Recht L, et al. High-dose intravenous methotrexate for patients with nonleukemic leptomeningeal cancer: is intrathecal chemotherapy necessary? *J Clin Oncol* 1998;16(4):1561–1567.
82. Go RS, Taylor BV, Kimmel DW. The natural history of asymptomatic meningiomas in Olmsted County, Minnesota. *Neurology* 1998;51(6):1718–1720.
83. Goldsmith BJ, Wara WM, Wilson CB, et al. Postoperative irradiation for subtotally resected meningiomas. *A retrospective analysis of 140 patients treated from 1967 to 1990. J Neurosurg* 1994;80(2):195–201.
84. Goldwein JW, Corn BW, Finlay JL, et al. Is craniospinal irradiation required to cure children with malignant (anaplastic) intracranial ependymomas? *Cancer* 1991;67(11):2766–2771.
85. Goodwin JW, Crowley J, Eyre HJ, et al. A phase II evaluation of tamoxifen in unresectable or refractory meningiomas: a Southwest Oncology Group study. *J Neurooncol* 1993;15(1):75–77.
86. Griffin TW, Davis R, Laramore G, et al. Fast neutron radiation therapy for glioblastoma multiforme. Results of an RTOG study. *Am J Clin Oncol* 1983;6(6): 661–667.
87. Groothuis DR. The blood-brain and blood-tumor barriers: a review of strategies for increasing drug delivery. *Neuro-oncol* 2000;2(1):45–59.
88. Grunberg SM, Rankin C, Townsend J, et al. Phase III double-blind randomized placebo-controlled study of mifepristone (RU) for the treatment of unresectable meningioma. *Proc Am Soc Clin Oncol* 2001;20:56.
89. Guillamo JS, Monjour A, Taillandier L, et al. Brainstem gliomas in adults: prognostic factors and classification. *Brain* 2001;124(Pt 12):2528–2539.
90. Guiney MJ, Smith JG, Hughes P, et al. Contemporary management of adult and pediatric brain stem gliomas. *Int J Radiat Oncol Biol Phys* 1993;25(2):235–241.
91. Guyotat J, Signorelli F, Desme S, et al. Intracranial ependymomas in adult patients: analyses of prognostic factors. *J Neurooncol* 2002;60(3):255–268.
92. Hadaczek P, Mirek H, Berger MS, et al. Limited efficacy of gene transfer in herpes simplex virus-thymidine kinase/ganciclovir gene therapy for brain tumors. *J Neurosurg* 2005;102(2):328–335.
93. Hakim R, Alexander E 3rd, Loeffler JS, et al. Results of linear accelerator-based radiosurgery for intracranial meningiomas. *Neurosurgery* 1998;42(3):446–453; discussion 53–54.
94. Halperin EC, Burger PC, Bullard DE. The fallacy of the localized supratentorial malignant glioma. *Int J Radiat Oncol Biol Phys* 1988;15(2):505–509.
95. Hardell L, Carlberg M, Hansson Mild K. Pooled analysis of two case-control studies on use of cellular and cordless telephones and the risk for malignant brain tumours diagnosed in 1997–2003. *Int Arch Occup Environ Health* 2006;79(8):630–639.
96. Heegaard S, Sommer HM, Broholm H, et al. Proliferating cell nuclear antigen and Ki-67 immunohistochemistry of oligodendrogliomas with special reference to prognosis. *Cancer* 1995;76(10):1809–1813.
97. Hegi ME, Diserens AC, Godard S, et al. Clinical trial substantiates the predictive value of O-6-methylguanine-DNA methyltransferase promoter methylation in glioblastoma patients treated with temozolomide. *Clin Cancer Res* 2004;10(6):1871–1874.
98. Hegi ME, Diserens AC, Gorlia T, et al. MGMT gene silencing and benefit from temozolomide in glioblastoma. *N Engl J Med* 2005;352(10):997–1003.
99. Hepworth SJ, Schoemaker MJ, Muir KR, et al. Mobile phone use and risk of glioma in adults: case-control study. *BMJ* 2006;332(7546):883–887.
100. Herndier BG, Kaplan LD, McGrath MS. Pathogenesis of AIDS lymphomas. *AIDS* 1994;8(8):1025–1049.
101. Herrlinger U, Steinbrecher A, Rieger J, et al. Adult medulloblastoma: prognostic factors and response to therapy at diagnosis and at relapse. *J Neurol* 2005;252(3):291–299.
102. Hess KR, Wong ET, Jaeckle KA, et al. Response and progression in recurrent malignant glioma. *Neuro-oncol* 1999;1(4):282–288.
103. Hoang-Xuan K, Capelle L, Kujas M, et al. Temozolomide as initial treatment for adults with low-grade oligodendrogliomas or oligoastrocytomas and correlation with chromosome 1p deletions. *J Clin Oncol* 2004;22(15):3133–3138.
104. Hochberg FH, Pruitt A. Assumptions in the radiotherapy of glioblastoma. *Neurology* 1980;30(9):907–911.
105. Hug EB, Devries A, Thornton AF, et al. Management of atypical and malignant meningiomas: role of high-dose, 3D-conformal radiation therapy. *J Neurooncol* 2000;48(2):151–160.
106. Inskip PD, Tarone RE, Hatch EE, et al. Cellular-telephone use and brain tumors. *N Engl J Med* 2001;344(2):79–86.
107. Jackson RJ, Fuller GN, Abi-Said D, et al. Limitations of stereotactic biopsy in the initial management of gliomas. *Neuro-oncol* 2001;3(3):193–200.
108. Jose CC, Rajan B, Ashley S, et al. Radiotherapy for the treatment of recurrent craniopharyngioma. *Clin Oncol (R Coll Radiol)* 1992;4(5):287–289.
109. Jung HW, Yoo H, Paek SH, et al. Long-term outcome and growth rate of subtotally resected petroclival meningiomas: experience with 38 cases. *Neurosurgery* 2000;46(3):567–574; discussion 74–75.
110. Kaiser MG, Parsa AT, Fine RL, et al. Tissue distribution and antitumor activity of topotecan delivered by intracerebral clysis in a rat glioma model. *Neurosurgery* 2000;47(6):1391–1398; discussion 8–9.
111. Karim AB, Maat B, Hatlevoll R, et al. A randomized trial on dose-response in radiation therapy of low-grade cerebral glioma: European Organization for Research and Treatment of Cancer (EORTC) Study 22844. *Int J Radiat Oncol Biol Phys* 1996;36(3):549–556.
112. Karlsson U, Kirby T, Orrison W, et al. Ocular globe topography in radiotherapy. *Int J Radiat Oncol Biol Phys* 1995;33(3):705–712.
113. Kawakami K, Kawakami M, Liu Q, et al. Combined effects of radiation and interleukin-13 receptor-targeted cytotoxin on glioblastoma cell lines. *Int J Radiat Oncol Biol Phys* 2005;63(1):230–237.
114. Kelly PJ, Daumas-Duport C, Scheithauer BW, et al. Stereotactic histologic correlations of computed tomography- and magnetic resonance imaging-defined abnormalities in patients with glial neoplasms. *Mayo Clin Proc* 1987;62(6): 450–459.
115. Kiltie AE, Povall JM, Taylor RE. The need for the moving junction in craniospinal irradiation. *Br J Radiol* 2000;73(870):650–654.
116. Kirsch DG, Tarbell NJ. Conformal radiation therapy for childhood CNS tumors. *Oncologist* 2004;9(4):442–450.
117. Kleihues P, Scheithauer BW. *Histological typing of tumors of the central nervous system.* 2nd ed. Berlin: Springer-Verlag, 1993.
118. Kobayashi T, Kida Y, Mori Y, et al. Long-term results of gamma knife surgery for the treatment of craniopharyngioma in 98 consecutive cases. *J Neurosurg* 2005;103[6 Suppl]:482–488.
119. Kramer JH, Crowe AB, Larson DA, et al. Neuropsychological sequelae of medulloblastoma in adults. *Int J Radiat Oncol Biol Phys* 1997;38(1):21–26.
120. Kramer S. Tumor extent as a determining factor in radiotherapy of glioblastomas. *Acta Radiol Ther Phys Biol* 1969;8(1):111–117.
121. Kroll RA, Neuwelt EA. Outwitting the blood-brain barrier for therapeutic purposes: osmotic opening and other means. *Neurosurgery* 1998;42(5):1083–1099; discussion 99–100.
122. Kyritsis AP. Chemotherapy for meningiomas. *J Neurooncol* 1996;29(3):269–272.
123. Lacroix M, Abi-Said D, Fourney DR, et al. A multivariate analysis of 416 patients with glioblastoma multiforme: prognosis, extent of resection, and survival. *J Neurosurg* 2001;95(2):190–198.
124. Landolfi JC, Thaler HT, DeAngelis LM. Adult brainstem gliomas. *Neurology* 1998;51(4):1136–1139.
125. Laperriere NJ, Leung PM, McKenzie S, et al. Randomized study of brachytherapy in the initial management of patients with malignant astrocytoma. *Int J Radiat Oncol Biol Phys* 1998;41(5):1005–1011.
126. Laramore GE, Diener-West M, Griffin TW, et al. Randomized neutron dose searching study for malignant gliomas of the brain: results of an RTOG study. Radiation Therapy Oncology Group. *Int J Radiat Oncol Biol Phys* 1988;14(6):1093–1102.
127. Lee AW, Kwong DL, Leung SF, et al. Factors affecting risk of symptomatic temporal lobe necrosis: significance of fractional dose and treatment time. *Int J Radiat Oncol Biol Phys* 2002;53(1):75–85.
128. Leighton C, Fisher B, Bauman G, et al. Supratentorial low-grade glioma in adults: an analysis of prognostic factors and timing of radiation. *J Clin Oncol* 1997;15(4):1294–1301.
129. Levin VA, Hess KR, Choucair A, et al. Phase III randomized study of postradiotherapy chemotherapy with combination alpha-difluoromethylornithine-PCV versus PCV for anaplastic gliomas. *Clin Cancer Res* 2003;9(3):981–990.
130. Levin VA, Silver P, Hannigan J, et al. Superiority of post-radiotherapy adjuvant chemotherapy with CCNU, procarbazine, and vincristine (PCV) over BCNU for anaplastic gliomas: NCOG 6G61 final report. *Int J Radiat Oncol Biol Phys* 1990;18(2):321–324.
131. Levin VA, Yung WK, Bruner J, et al. Phase II study of accelerated fractionation radiation therapy with carboplatin followed by PCV chemotherapy for the treatment of anaplastic gliomas. *Int J Radiat Oncol Biol Phys* 2002;53(1):58–66.
132. Lichter AS, Sandler HM, Robertson JM, et al. Clinical experience with three-dimensional treatment planning. *Semin Radiat Oncol* 1992;2(4):257–266.
133. Lidar Z, Mardor Y, Jonas T, et al. Convection-enhanced delivery of paclitaxel for the treatment of recurrent malignant glioma: a phase I/II clinical study. *J Neurosurg* 2004;100(3):472–479.
134. Lin CC, Kenyon L, Hyslop T, et al. Cyclooxygenase-2 (COX-2) expression in human meningioma as a function of tumor grade. *Am J Clin Oncol* 2003;26(4): S98–102.
135. Linstadt DE, Edwards MS, Prados M, et al. Hyperfractionated irradiation for adults with brainstem gliomas. *Int J Radiat Oncol Biol Phys* 1991;20(4): 757–760.
136. Louis DN, Scheithauer BW, Budka H, et al. *Meningiomas.* In: Kleihues P, Cavenee WK, eds. *WHO classification of tumors.* Lyon: IARC Press, 2000;176–184.
137. Mack EE, Wilson CB. Meningiomas induced by high-dose cranial irradiation. *J Neurosurg* 1993;79(1):28–31.
138. Maher EA, Furnari FB, Bachoo RM, et al. Malignant glioma: genetics and biology of a grave matter. *Genes Dev* 2001;15(11):1311–1133.
139. Maire JP, Caudry M, Darrouzet V, et al. Fractionated radiation therapy in the treatment of stage III and IV cerebello-pontine angle neurinomas: long-term results in 24 cases. *Int J Radiat Oncol Biol Phys* 1995;32(4):1137–1143.
140. Marks LB, Sherouse GW, Das S, et al. Conformal radiation therapy with fixed shaped coplanar or noncoplanar radiation beam bouquets: a possible alternative to radiosurgery. *Int J Radiat Oncol Biol Phys* 1995;33(5):1209–1219.
141. Matsukado Y, Maccarty CS, Kernohan JW. The growth of glioblastoma

multiforme (astrocytomas, grades 3 and 4) in neurosurgical practice. *J Neurosurg* 1961;18:636–644.
142. McGovern PC, Lautenbach E, Brennan PJ, et al. Risk factors for postcraniotomy surgical site infection after 1,3-bis (2-chloroethyl)-1-nitrosourea (Gliadel) wafer placement. *Clin Infect Dis* 2003;36(6):759–765.
143. Medical Research Council Brain Tumor Working Party. Randomized trial of procarbazine, lomustine, and vincristine in the adjuvant treatment of high-grade astrocytoma: a Medical Research Council trial. *J Clin Oncol* 2001;19(2):509–518.
144. Meijer OW, Vandertop WP, Baayen JC, et al. Single-fraction vs. fractionated LINAC-based stereotactic radiosurgery for vestibular schwannoma: a single-institution study. *Int J Radiat Oncol Biol Phys* 2003;56(5):1390–1396.
145. Mellinghoff IK, Wang MY, Vivanco I, et al. Molecular determinants of the response of glioblastomas to EGFR kinase inhibitors. *N Engl J Med* 2005;353(19):2012–2024.
146. Menke M, Hirschfeld F, Mack T, et al. Photogrammetric accuracy measurements of head holder systems used for fractionated radiotherapy. *Int J Radiat Oncol Biol Phys* 1994;29(5):1147–1155.
147. Merchant TE, Jenkins JJ, Burger PC, et al. Influence of tumor grade on time to progression after irradiation for localized ependymoma in children. *Int J Radiat Oncol Biol Phys* 2002;53(1):52–57.
148. Meyers CA, Weitzner MA, Valentine AD, et al. Methylphenidate therapy improves cognition, mood, and function of brain tumor patients. *J Clin Oncol* 1998;16(7):2522–2527.
149. Miralbell R, Linggood RM, de la Monte S, et al. The role of radiotherapy in the treatment of subtotally resected benign meningiomas. *J Neurooncol* 1992;13(2):157–164.
150. Miralbell R, Mornex F, Greiner R, et al. Accelerated radiotherapy, carbogen, and nicotinamide in glioblastoma multiforme: report of European Organization for Research and Treatment of Cancer trial 22933. *J Clin Oncol* 1999;17(10):3143–3149.
151. Monje ML, Palmer T. Radiation injury and neurogenesis. *Curr Opin Neurol* 2003;16(2):129–134.
152. Muacevic A, Kreth FW. Quality-adjusted survival after tumor resection and/or radiation therapy for elderly patients with glioblastoma multiforme. *J Neurol* 2003;250(5):561–568.
153. Murray KJ, Nelson DF, Scott C, et al. Quality-adjusted survival analysis of malignant glioma. Patients treated with twice-daily radiation (RT) and carmustine: a report of Radiation Therapy Oncology Group (RTOG) 83-02. *Int J Radiat Oncol Biol Phys* 1995;31(3):453–459.
154. Mursch K, Halatsch ME, Markakis E, et al. Intrinsic brainstem tumours in adults: results of microneurosurgical treatment of 16 consecutive patients. *Br J Neurosurg* 2005;19(2):128–136.
155. Nakamura H, Jokura H, Takahashi K, et al. Serial follow-up MR imaging after gamma knife radiosurgery for vestibular schwannoma. *AJNR Am J Neuroradiol* 2000;21(8):1540–1546.
156. Nakamura M, Roser F, Michel J, et al. The natural history of incidental meningiomas. *Neurosurgery* 2003;53(1):62–70.
157. Neglia JP, Meadows AT, Robison LL, et al. Second neoplasms after acute lymphoblastic leukemia in childhood. *N Engl J Med* 1991;325(19):1330–1336.
158. Nelson DF, Curran WJ Jr. , Scott C, et al. Hyperfractionated radiation therapy and bis-chlorethyl nitrosourea in the treatment of malignant glioma—possible advantage observed at 72.0 Gy in 1.2 Gy b.i.d. fractions: report of the Radiation Therapy Oncology Group Protocol 8302. *Int J Radiat Oncol Biol Phys* 1993;25(2): 193–207.
159. Nelson DF, Diener-West M, Horton J, et al. Combined modality approach to treatment of malignant gliomas—re-evaluation of RTOG 7401/ECOG 1374 with long-term follow-up: a joint study of the Radiation Therapy Oncology Group and the Eastern Cooperative Oncology Group. *NCI Monogr* 1988;(6):279–284.
160. Nelson DF, Diener-West M, Weinstein AS, et al. A randomized comparison of misonidazole sensitized radiotherapy plus BCNU and radiotherapy plus BCNU for treatment of malignant glioma after surgery: final report of an RTOG study. *Int J Radiat Oncol Biol Phys* 1986;12(10):1793–1800.
161. Nelson DF, Martz KL, Bonner H, et al. Non-Hodgkin's lymphoma of the brain: can high dose, large volume radiation therapy improve survival? Report on a prospective trial by the Radiation Therapy Oncology Group (RTOG): RTOG 8315. *Int J Radiat Oncol Biol Phys* 1992;23(1):9–17.
162. Nicolato A, Foroni R, Alessandrini F, et al. Radiosurgical treatment of cavernous sinus meningiomas: experience with 122 treated patients. *Neurosurgery* 2002;51(5):1153–1159.
163. Noren G. Long-term complications following gamma knife radiosurgery of vestibular schwannomas. *Stereotact Funct Neurosurg* 1998;70[Suppl 1]:65–73.
164. Ohgaki H, Dessen P, Jourde B, et al. Genetic pathways to glioblastoma: a population-based study. *Cancer Res* 2004;64(19):6892–6899.
165. Ohgaki H, Kleihues P. Epidemiology and etiology of gliomas. *Acta Neuropathol (Berl)* 2005;109(1):93–108.
166. Okamoto Y, Di Patre PL, Burkhard C, et al. Population-based study on incidence, survival rates, and genetic alterations of low-grade diffuse astrocytomas and oligodendrogliomas. *Acta Neuropathol (Berl)* 2004;108(1):49–56.
167. Olivero WC, Lister JR, Elwood PW. The natural history and growth rate of asymptomatic meningiomas: a review of 60 patients. *J Neurosurg* 1995;83(2):222–224.
168. Oppitz U, Maessen D, Zunterer H, et al. 3D-recurrence-patterns of glioblastomas after CT-planned postoperative irradiation. *Radiother Oncol* 1999;53(1):53–57.
169. Packer RJ, Rood BR, MacDonald TJ. Medulloblastoma: present concepts of stratification into risk groups. *Pediatr Neurosurg* 2003;39(2):60–67.
170. Paulino AC. The local field in infratentorial ependymoma: does the entire posterior fossa need to be treated? *Int J Radiat Oncol Biol Phys* 2001;49(3):757–761.
171. Payne DG, Simpson WJ, Keen C, et al. Malignant astrocytoma: hyperfractionated and standard radiotherapy with chemotherapy in a randomized prospective clinical trial. *Cancer* 1982;50(11):2301–2306.
172. Paz MF, Yaya-Tur R, Rojas-Marcos I, et al. CpG island hypermethylation of the DNA repair enzyme methyltransferase predicts response to temozolomide in primary gliomas. *Clin Cancer Res* 2004;10(15):4933–4938.
173. Peissner W, Kocher M, Treuer H, et al. Ionizing radiation-induced apoptosis of proliferating stem cells in the dentate gyrus of the adult rat hippocampus. *Brain Res Mol Brain Res* 1999;71(1):61–78.
174. Pels H, Schmidt-Wolf IG, Glasmacher A, et al. Primary central nervous system lymphoma: results of a pilot and phase II study of systemic and intraventricular chemotherapy with deferred radiotherapy. *J Clin Oncol* 2003;21(24):4489–4495.
175. Perkins GH, Schomer DF, Fuller GN, et al. Gliomatosis cerebri: improved outcome with radiotherapy. *Int J Radiat Oncol Biol Phys* 2003;56(4):1137–1146.
176. Perry A, Stafford SL, Scheithauer BW, et al. Meningioma grading: an analysis of histologic parameters. *Am J Surg Pathol* 1997;21(12):1455–1465.
177. Peterson K, Walker RW. Medulloblastoma/primitive neuroectodermal tumor in 45 adults. *Neurology* 1995;45(3 Pt 1):440–442.
178. Phillips C, Guiney M, Smith J, et al. A randomized trial comparing 35 Gy in ten fractions with 60 Gy in 30 fractions of cerebral irradiation for glioblastoma multiforme and older patients with anaplastic astrocytoma. *Radiother Oncol* 2003;68(1):23–26.
179. Pickles T, Goodman GB, Rheaume DE, et al. Pion radiation for high grade astrocytoma: results of a randomized study. *Int J Radiat Oncol Biol Phys* 1997;37(3):491–497.
180. Pignatti F, van den Bent M, Curran D, et al. Prognostic factors for survival in adult patients with cerebral low-grade glioma. *J Clin Oncol* 2002;20(8):2076–2084.
181. Pirzkall A, McKnight TR, Graves EE, et al. MR-spectroscopy guided target delineation for high-grade gliomas. *Int J Radiat Oncol Biol Phys* 2001;50(4): 915–928.
182. Pollock BE, Lunsford LD, Kondziolka D, et al. Outcome analysis of acoustic neuroma management: a comparison of microsurgery and stereotactic radiosurgery. *Neurosurgery* 1995;36(1):215–224; discussion 24–29.
183. Pollock BE, Stafford SL. Results of stereotactic radiosurgery for patients with imaging defined cavernous sinus meningiomas. *Int J Radiat Oncol Biol Phys* 2005;62(5):1427–1431.
184. Poortmans PM, Kluin-Nelemans HC, Haaxma-Reiche H, et al. High-dose methotrexate-based chemotherapy followed by consolidating radiotherapy in non-AIDS-related primary central nervous system lymphoma: European Organization for Research and Treatment of Cancer Lymphoma Group Phase II Trial 20962. *J Clin Oncol* 2003;21(24):4483–4488.
185. Pope WB, Lai A, Nghiemphu P, et al. MRI in patients with high-grade gliomas treated with bevacizumab and chemotherapy. *Neurology* 2006;66(8):1258–1560.
186. Prados MD, Scott C, Curran WJ Jr. , et al. Procarbazine, lomustine, and vincristine (PCV) chemotherapy for anaplastic astrocytoma: a retrospective review of radiation therapy oncology group protocols comparing survival with carmustine or PCV adjuvant chemotherapy. *J Clin Oncol* 1999;17(11):3389–3395.
187. Prados MD, Seiferheld W, Sandler HM, et al. Phase III randomized study of radiotherapy plus procarbazine, lomustine, and vincristine with or without BUdR for treatment of anaplastic astrocytoma: final report of RTOG 9404. *Int J Radiat Oncol Biol Phys* 2004;58(4):1147–1152.
188. Prados MD, Wara WM, Sneed PK, et al. Phase III trial of accelerated hyperfractionation with or without difluoromethylornithine (DFMO) versus standard fractionated radiotherapy with or without DFMO for newly diagnosed patients with glioblastoma multiforme. *Int J Radiat Oncol Biol Phys* 2001;49(1):71–77.
189. Prados MD, Warnick RE, Wara WM, et al. Medulloblastoma in adults. *Int J Radiat Oncol Biol Phys* 1995;32(4):1145–1152.
190. Prados MD, Yung WK, Fine HA, et al. Phase 2 study of BCNU and temozolomide for recurrent glioblastoma multiforme: North American Brain Tumor Consortium study. *Neuro-oncol* 2004;6(1):33–37.
191. Quinn JA, Reardon DA, Friedman AH, et al. Phase II trial of temozolomide in patients with progressive low-grade glioma. *J Clin Oncol* 2003;21(4):646–651.
192. Rajaraman C, Rowe JG, Walton L, et al. Treatment options for von Hippel-Lindau's haemangioblastomatosis: the role of gamma knife stereotactic radiosurgery. *Br J Neurosurg* 2004;18(4):338–342.
193. Rao RD, Buckner JC, Sarkaria JN. Mammalian target of rapamycin (mTOR) inhibitors as anti-cancer agents. *Curr Cancer Drug Targets* 2004;4(8):621–635.
194. Rauber K. *Lehrbuch und Atlas der Anatomie des Menschen.* 19th ed. Stuttgart: Georg Thieme-Verlag, 1955.
195. Reardon DA, Akabani G, Coleman RE, et al. Phase II trial of murine (131)I-labeled antitenascin monoclonal antibody 81C6 administered into surgically created resection cavities of patients with newly diagnosed malignant gliomas. *J Clin Oncol* 2002;20(5):1389–1397.
196. Reardon DA, Akabani G, Coleman RE, et al. Salvage radioimmunotherapy with murine iodine-131-labeled antitenascin monoclonal antibody 81C6 for patients with recurrent primary and metastatic malignant brain tumors: phase II study results. *J Clin Oncol* 2006;24(1):115–122.
197. Reardon DA, Wen PY. Therapeutic advances in the treatment of glioblastoma: rationale and potential role of targeted agents. *Oncologist* 2006;11(2):152–164.
198. Rich JN, Reardon DA, Peery T, et al. Phase II trial of gefitinib in recurrent glioblastoma. *J Clin Oncol* 2004;22(1):133–142.
199. Riva P, Arista A, Franceschi G, et al. Local treatment of malignant gliomas by direct infusion of specific monoclonal antibodies labeled with 131I: comparison of the results obtained in recurrent and newly diagnosed tumors. *Cancer Res* 1995;55[23 Suppl]:5952S–5956S.
200. Roa W, Brasher PM, Bauman G, et al. Abbreviated course of radiation therapy in older patients with glioblastoma multiforme: a prospective randomized clinical trial. *J Clin Oncol* 2004;22(9):1583–1588.
201. Salazar OM, Castro-Vita H, VanHoutte P, et al. Improved survival in cases of intracranial ependymoma after radiation therapy. Late report and recommendations. *J Neurosurg* 1983;59(4):652–659.
202. Sampson JH, Akabani G, Archer GE, et al. Progress report of a phase I study of the intracerebral microinfusion of a recombinant chimeric protein composed of transforming growth factor (TGF)-alpha and a mutated form of the Pseudomonas exotoxin termed PE-38 (TP-38) for the treatment of malignant brain tumors. *J Neurooncol* 2003;65(1):27–35.
203. Sanghavi S, Skrupsky R, Badie B, et al. Recurrent malignant gliomas treated with radiosurgery. *J Radiosurgery* 1999;2:119–125.
204. Sanson M, Cartalat-Carel S, Taillibert S, et al. Initial chemotherapy in gliomatosis cerebri. *Neurology* 2004;63(2):270–275.
205. Sarkaria JN, Mehta MP, Loeffler JS, et al. Radiosurgery in the initial management of malignant gliomas: survival comparison with the RTOG recursive partitioning analysis. Radiation Therapy Oncology Group. *Int J Radiat Oncol Biol Phys* 1995;32(4):931–941.
206. Sasaki H, Zlatescu MC, Betensky RA, et al. Histopathological-molecular genetic correlations in referral pathologist-diagnosed low-grade "oligodendroglioma." *J Neuropathol Exp Neurol* 2002;61(1):58–63.
207. Schrell UM, Rittig MG, Anders M, et al. Hydroxyurea for treatment of unresectable and recurrent meningiomas. II. Decrease in the size of meningiomas in patients treated with hydroxyurea. *J Neurosurg* 1997;86(5):840–844.

208. Schwartz TH, Kim S, Glick RS, et al. Supratentorial ependymomas in adult patients. *Neurosurgery* 1999;44(4):721–731.

209. Scott C, Curran W, Yung W, et al. Long term results of RTOG 9006: a randomized trial of hyperfractionated radiotherapy (RT) to 72.0 Gy and carmustine vs. standard RT and carmustine for malignant glioma patients with emphasis on anaplastic astrocytoma (AA) patients.*Proc Am Soc Clin Oncol* 1998;16:384.

210. Selker RG, Shapiro WR, Burger P, et al. The Brain Tumor Cooperative Group NIH Trial 87-01: a randomized comparison of surgery, external radiotherapy, and carmustine versus surgery, interstitial radiotherapy boost, external radiation therapy, and carmustine. *Neurosurgery* 2002;51(2):343–355; discussion 55–57.

211. Selvapandian S, Rajshekhar V, Chandy MJ. Brainstem glioma: comparative study of clinico-radiological presentation, pathology and outcome in children and adults. *Acta Neurochir (Wien)* 1999;141(7):721–726 discussion 6-7.

212. Shaw E, Arusell R, Scheithauer B, et al. Prospective randomized trial of low-versus high-dose radiation therapy in adults with supratentorial low-grade glioma: initial report of a North Central Cancer Treatment Group/Radiation Therapy Oncology Group/Eastern Cooperative Oncology Group study. *J Clin Oncol* 2002;20(9):2267–2276.

213. Shaw E, Scott C, Souhami L, et al. Single dose radiosurgical treatment of recurrent previously irradiated primary brain tumors and brain metastases: final report of RTOG protocol 90-05. *Int J Radiat Oncol Biol Phys* 2000;47(2):291–298.

214. Shaw EG, et al. Astrocytomas, oligoastrocytomas, and oligodendrogliomas: a comparative survival study. *Neurology* 1992;42[Suppl 3]:342.

215. Shaw EG, Berkey BA, Coons SW, et al. Initial report of Radiation Therapy Oncology Group (RTOG) 9802: prospective studies in adult low-grade glioma (LGG). *Proc Am Soc Clin Oncol* 2006;24:1500.

216. Shaw EG, Daumas-Duport C, Scheithauer BW, et al. Radiation therapy in the management of low-grade supratentorial astrocytomas. *J Neurosurg* 1989;70(6):853–861.

217. Shaw EG, Evans RG, Scheithauer BW, et al. Postoperative radiotherapy of intracranial ependymoma in pediatric and adult patients. *Int J Radiat Oncol Biol Phys* 1987;13(10):1457–1462.

218. Sheehan J, Kondziolka D, Flickinger J, et al. Radiosurgery for treatment of recurrent intracranial hemangiopericytomas. *Neurosurgery* 2002;51(4):905–910; discussion 10–11.

219. Shibamoto Y, Ogino H, Hasegawa M, et al. Results of radiation monotherapy for primary central nervous system lymphoma in the 1990s. *Int J Radiat Oncol Biol Phys* 2005;62(3):809–813.

220. Shin KH, Urtasun RC, Fulton D, et al. Multiple daily fractionated radiation therapy and misonidazole in the management of malignant astrocytoma. A preliminary report. *Cancer* 1985;56(4):758–760.

221. Shirato H, Sakamoto T, Takeichi N, et al. Fractionated stereotactic radiotherapy for vestibular schwannoma (VS): comparison between cystic-type and solid-type VS. *Int J Radiat Oncol Biol Phys* 2000;48(5):1395–1401.

222. Shrieve DC, Wara WM, Edwards MS, et al. Hyperfractionated radiation therapy for gliomas of the brainstem in children and in adults. *Int J Radiat Oncol Biol Phys* 1992;24(4):599–610.

223. Simpson JR, Horton J, Scott C, et al. Influence of location and extent of surgical resection on survival of patients with glioblastoma multiforme: results of three consecutive Radiation Therapy Oncology Group (RTOG) clinical trials. *Int J Radiat Oncol Biol Phys* 1993;26(2):239–244.

224. Smith JS, Perry A, Borell TJ, et al. Alterations of chromosome arms 1p and 19q as predictors of survival in oligodendrogliomas, astrocytomas, and mixed oligoastrocytomas. *J Clin Oncol* 2000;18(3):636–645.

225. Smith MA, Freidlin B, Ries LA, et al. Trends in reported incidence of primary malignant brain tumors in children in the United States. *J Natl Cancer Inst* 1998;90(17):1269–1277.

226. Soisson ET, Tome WA, Richards GM, et al. Comparison of LINAC based fractionated stereotactic radiotherapy and tomotherapy treatment plans for skull-base tumors. *Radiother Oncol* 2006;78(3):313–321.

227. Souhami L, Seiferheld W, Brachman D, et al. Randomized comparison of stereotactic radiosurgery followed by conventional radiotherapy with carmustine to conventional radiotherapy with carmustine for patients with glioblastoma multiforme: report of Radiation Therapy Oncology Group 93-05 protocol. *Int J Radiat Oncol Biol Phys* 2004;60(3):853–860.

228. Stafford SL, Perry A, Suman VJ, et al. Primarily resected meningiomas: outcome and prognostic factors in 581 Mayo Clinic patients, 1978 through 1988. *Mayo Clin Proc* 1998;73(10):936–942.

229. Stafford SL, Pollock BE, Foote RL, et al. Meningioma radiosurgery: tumor control, outcomes, and complications among 190 consecutive patients. *Neurosurgery* 2001;49(5):1029–1037; discussion 37–38.

230. Stege EM, Kros JM, de Bruin HG, et al. Successful treatment of low-grade oligodendroglial tumors with a chemotherapy regimen of procarbazine, lomustine, and vincristine. *Cancer* 2005;103(4):802–809.

231. Stewart LA. Chemotherapy in adult high-grade glioma: a systematic review and meta-analysis of individual patient data from 12 randomised trials. *Lancet* 2002;359(9311):1011–1018.

232. Stripp DC, Maity A, Janss AJ, et al. Surgery with or without radiation therapy in the management of craniopharyngiomas in children and young adults. *Int J Radiat Oncol Biol Phys* 2004;58(3):714–720.

233. Stupp R, Mason WP, van den Bent MJ, et al. Radiotherapy plus concomitant and adjuvant temozolomide for glioblastoma. *N Engl J Med* 2005;352(10):987–996.

234. Szumacher E, Schwartz ML, Tsao M, et al. Fractionated stereotactic radiotherapy for the treatment of vestibular schwannomas: combined experience of the Toronto-Sunnybrook Regional Cancer Centre and the Princess Margaret Hospital. *Int J Radiat Oncol Biol Phys* 2002;53(4):987–991.

235. Tada K, Shiraishi S, Kamiryo T, et al. Analysis of loss of heterozygosity on chromosome 10 in patients with malignant astrocytic tumors: correlation with patient age and survival. *J Neurosurg* 2001;95(4):651–659.

236. Tago M, Terahara A, Shin M, et al. Gamma Knife surgery for hemangioblastomas. *J Neurosurg* 2005;102[Suppl]:171–174.

237. Taillibert S, Chodkiewicz C, Laigle-Donadey F, et al. Gliomatosis cerebri: a review of 296 cases from the ANOCEF database and the literature. *J Neurooncol* 2006;76(2):201–205.

238. Tamura M, Gu J, Tran H, et al. PTEN gene and integrin signaling in cancer. *J Natl Cancer Inst* 1999;91(21):1820–1828.

239. Tanaka M, Ino Y, Nakagawa K, et al. High-dose conformal radiotherapy for supratentorial malignant glioma: a historical comparison. *Lancet Oncol* 2005;6(12):953–960.

240. Tatter SB, Shaw EG, Rosenblum ML, et al. An inflatable balloon catheter and liquid ^{125}I radiation source (GliaSite Radiation Therapy System) for treatment of recurrent malignant glioma: multicenter safety and feasibility trial. *J Neurosurg* 2003;99(2):297–303.

241. Taylor BW Jr., Marcus RB Jr., Friedman WA, et al. The meningioma controversy: postoperative radiation therapy. *Int J Radiat Oncol Biol Phys* 1988;15(2):299–304.

242. Taylor MD, Bernstein M. Awake craniotomy with brain mapping as the routine surgical approach to treating patients with supratentorial intra-axial tumors: a prospective trial of 200 cases. *J Neurosurg* 1999;90(1):35–41.

243. Ten Haken RK, Thornton AF Jr., Sandler HM, et al. A quantitative assessment of the addition of MRI to CT-based, 3-D treatment planning of brain tumors. *Radiother Oncol* 1992;25(2):121–133.

244. Terada K, Tamiya T, Daido S, et al. Prognostic value of loss of heterozygosity around three candidate tumor suppressor genes on chromosome 10q in astrocytomas. *J Neurooncol* 2002;58(2):107–114.

245. Thomadsen B, Mehta M, Howard S, et al. Craniospinal treatment with the patient supine. *Med Dosim* 2003;28(1):35–38.

246. Thornton AF Jr., Hegarty TJ, Ten Haken RK, et al. Three-dimensional treatment planning of astrocytomas: a dosimetric study of cerebral irradiation. *Int J Radiat Oncol Biol Phys* 1991;20(6):1309–1315.

247. Timmermann B, Kortmann RD, Kuhl J, et al. Combined postoperative irradiation and chemotherapy for anaplastic ependymomas in childhood: results of the German prospective trials HIT 88/89 and HIT 91. *Int J Radiat Oncol Biol Phys* 2000;46(2):287–295.

248. Tome WA, Meeks SL, Buatti JM, et al. A high-precision system for conformal intracranial radiotherapy. *Int J Radiat Oncol Biol Phys* 2000;47(4):1137–1143.

249. Tome WA, Meeks SL, McNutt TR, et al. Optically guided intensity modulated radiotherapy. *Radiother Oncol* 2001;61(1):33–44.

250. Tso CL, Freije WA, Day A, et al. Distinct transcription profiles of primary and secondary glioblastoma subgroups. *Cancer Res* 2006;66(1):159–167.

251. Uhm JH, Ballman KV, Giannini C, et al. Phase II study of ZD1839 in patients with newly diagnosed grade 4 astrocytoma. *Proc Am Soc Clin Oncol* 2004;22[14 Suppl]:1505.

252. van den Bent MJ. Can chemotherapy replace radiotherapy in low-grade gliomas? Time for randomized studies. *Semin Oncol* 2003;30[6 Suppl 19]:39–44.

253. van den Bent MJ, Afra D, de Witte O, et al. Long-term efficacy of early versus delayed radiotherapy for low-grade astrocytoma and oligodendroglioma in adults: the EORTC 22845 randomised trial. *Lancet* 2005;366(9490):985–990.

254. van den Bent MJ, Carpentier AF, Brandes AA, et al. Adjuvant procarbazine, lomustine, and vincristine improves progression-free survival but not overall survival in newly diagnosed anaplastic oligodendrogliomas and oligoastrocytomas: a randomized European Organization for Research and Treatment of Cancer phase III trial. *J Clin Oncol* 2006;24(18):2715–2722.

255. van den Bent MJ, Chinot O, Boogerd W, et al. Second-line chemotherapy with temozolomide in recurrent oligodendroglioma after PCV (procarbazine, lomustine and vincristine) chemotherapy: EORTC Brain Tumor Group phase II study 26972. *Ann Oncol* 2003;14(4):599–602.

256. Vogelbaum MA, Berkey B, Peereboom D, et al. RTOG 0131: Phase II trial of pre-irradiation and concurrent temozolomide in patients with newly diagnosed anaplastic oligodendrogliomas and mixed anaplastic oligodendrogliomas. *Proc Am Soc Clin Oncol* 2005;23(16S):1520.

257. Vogelbaum MA, Peereboom D, Stevens GH, et al. Phase II study of single agent therapy with the EGFR tyrosine kinase inhibitor erlotinib in recurrent glioblastoma multiforme. *Ann Oncol* 2004;15(3):iii206.

258. Vuorinen V, Hinkka S, Farkkila M, et al. Debulking or biopsy of malignant glioma in elderly people—a randomised study. *Acta Neurochir (Wien)* 2003;145(1):5–10.

259. Walker MD, Alexander E, Jr., Hunt WE, et al. Evaluation of BCNU and/or radiotherapy in the treatment of anaplastic gliomas. A cooperative clinical trial. *J Neurosurg* 1978;49(3):333–343.

260. Walker MD, Green SB, Byar DP, et al. Randomized comparisons of radiotherapy and nitrosoureas for the treatment of malignant glioma after surgery. *N Engl J Med* 1980;303(23):1323–1329.

261. Walker MD, Strike TA, Sheline GE. An analysis of dose-effect relationship in the radiotherapy of malignant gliomas. *Int J Radiat Oncol Biol Phys* 1979;5(10):1725–1731.

262. Wallner KE, Sheline GE, Pitts LH, et al. Efficacy of irradiation for incompletely excised acoustic neurilemomas. *J Neurosurg* 1987;67(6):858–863.

263. Wallner KE, Wara WM, Sheline GE, et al. Intracranial ependymomas: results of treatment with partial or whole brain irradiation without spinal irradiation. *Int J Radiat Oncol Biol Phys* 1986;12(11):1937–1941.

264. Wang EM, Pan L, Wang BJ, et al. The long-term results of gamma knife radiosurgery for hemangioblastomas of the brain. *J Neurosurg* 2005;102[Suppl]:225–229.

265. Weaver M, Laske DW. Transferrin receptor ligand-targeted toxin conjugate (Tf-CRM107) for therapy of malignant gliomas. *J Neurooncol* 2003;65(1):3–13.

266. Weber FW, Floeth F, Asher A, et al. Local convection enhanced delivery of IL4-Pseudomonas exotoxin (NBI-3001) for treatment of patients with recurrent malignant glioma. *Acta Neurochir Suppl* 2003;88:93–103.

267. Werner-Wasik M, Scott CB, Nelson DF, et al. Final report of a phase I/II trial of hyperfractionated and accelerated hyperfractionated radiation therapy with carmustine for adults with supratentorial malignant gliomas. Radiation Therapy Oncology Group Study 83-02. *Cancer* 1996;77(8):1535–1543.

268. Westphal M, Lamszus K, Hilt D. Intracavitary chemotherapy for glioblastoma: present status and future directions. *Acta Neurochir Suppl* 2003;88:61–67.

269. Yeung D, Palta J, Fontanesi J, et al. Systematic analysis of errors in target localization and treatment delivery in stereotactic radiosurgery (SRS). *Int J Radiat Oncol Biol Phys* 1994;28(2):493–498.

270. Yung WK, Prados MD, Yaya-Tur R, et al. Multicenter phase II trial of temozolomide in patients with anaplastic astrocytoma or anaplastic oligoastrocytoma at first relapse. Temodal Brain Tumor Group. *J Clin Oncol* 1999;17(9):2762–2771.

271. Zagzag D, Miller DC, Knopp E, et al. Primitive neuroectodermal tumors of the brainstem: investigation of seven cases. *Pediatrics* 2000;106(5):1045–1053.

Chapter 33
Pituitary

David Roberge, George Shenouda, Luis Souhami

Anatomy and Physiology

Anatomically, the pituitary gland is a midline structure measuring approximately 15 mm in the anteroposterior, and 12 mm in the superoinferior axis. The pituitary gland occupies a cavity of the sphenoid bone, called the *sella turcica* (Fig. 33.1). The diaphragm sellae, an extension of the dura, separates the pituitary gland from the structures lying above it, namely the optic chiasm, the chiasmatic cisterns, the anterior cerebral arteries, the hypothalamus, and the floor of the third ventricle. The diaphragm sellae is traversed by the pituitary stalk, which connects the median eminence of the pituitary to the hypothalamus. The posterior border of the sella is formed by the dorsum sellae, which is a thin structure with two prominences: the posterior clinoids. The tuberculum sellae lies anteriorly in the floor of the sella turcica, and projects laterally as the anterior clinoid processes. Lateral to the sella are the cavernous sinuses, which include the internal carotid arteries surrounded by a plexus of sympathetic nerves, the second, third, fourth, and sixth cranial nerves as well as the ophthalmic and maxillary divisions of the fifth cranial nerve.

The pituitary gland has two components of distinct embryologic origins. The anterior and intermediate lobes of the pituitary gland arise from Rathke's pouch, which is an evagination of ectodermal tissue from the roof of the oral cavity. The posterior lobe (or neurohypophysis) and stalk arise from a downpocketing of the third ventricle. The posterior lobe contains terminal axons from neurons originating in the hypothalamus. Secretory granules are synthesized in the supraoptic and paraventricular nuclei and transported along the stalk to the posterior lobe, where they are released as the posterior pituitary hormones oxytocin and vasopressin. Secretion of anterior pituitary hormones is controlled by hypothalamic hormones carried by the hypothalamic-hypophyseal portal system. There are eight known releasing or inhibiting hormones: corticotropin-releasing hormone, thyrotropin-releasing hormone, growth hormone-releasing hormone, growth hormone-inhibiting hormone or somatostatin, follicle-stimulating hormone-releasing hormone, luteinizing hormone-releasing hormone, prolactin-releasing hormone, and prolactin-inhibiting hormone. These hypothalamic hormones in turn control the production and release of six anterior pituitary hormones: adrenocorticotropic hormone (ACTH), thyroid-stimulating hormone (TSH), growth hormone (GH), follicle-stimulating hormone (FSH), luteinizing hormone (LH), and prolactin.

The output of hypothalamic hormones is controlled by a combination of feedback of endocrine products and direct neural impulses. In the case of thyroxine, feedback is provided directly to the pituitary gland.

Epidemiology

Approximately 10% of the healthy adult population has pituitary abnormalities detectable by magnetic resonance imaging (MRI). In autopsy series, adenomas are identified in 3% to 25% of pituitary glands (94). Pituitary neoplasms account for 10% to 15% of diagnosed primary intracranial neoplasms. Approximately 70% are endocrinologically active. The incidence of macroadenomas is similar between males and females. However, clinical manifestations of microadenomas are more frequent in women. Seventy percent of adenomas present between the ages of 30 and 50.

The etiology of most pituitary adenomas is unknown. A genetic predisposition to develop pituitary adenomas has been described in multiple endocrine neoplasia (MEN) 1 syndrome, the Carney complex, and in isolated familial somatotropinomas (IFS) (20). Patients affected by MEN type-1 have an autosomal dominant condition characterized by the development of tumors of the pituitary, parathyroid glands, and pancreatic islet cells. Pituitary adenomas develop in 25% of patients with MEN type-1. The Carney complex is a rare inherited condition characterized by spotty skin pigmentation, myxomas, endocrine overactivity, and schwannomas. IFS is the rarest of the three syndromes and is defined by the occurrence of two or more cases of acromegaly in a family in the absence of MEN or the Carney complex.

Natural History

When small, pituitary adenomas tend to be smooth, round tumors. Microadenomas may cause focal anterior bulging, asymmetry, or sloping of the sella floor. As size increases, macroadenomas often become irregular, with nodular extensions. Their local invasive properties are well known, but malignant behavior with distant metastases is very rare.

Pituitary tumors usually have a long natural history with an insidious onset of symptoms. Symptoms are commonly present for years prior to diagnosis.

There are few data on the natural history of symptomatic tumors postdiagnosis. Of 43 patients followed untreated with symptomatic (galactorrhea, amenorrhea) prolactinomas for as long as 20 years, only two patients showed radiologic tumor progression. Spontaneous clinical regression with resumption of normal menses was even seen in three patients (87). Roth et al. (86) followed seven untreated acromegalic patients; only five showed an increase in plasma GH level over a period of 1 to 4 years. In a series of 50 patients followed for a minimum of 2 years for nonfunctioning adenomas incidentally detected on imaging, only one of 31 microadenomas enlarged, and 5 of 19 macroadenomas progressed (29).

Clinical Presentation and Diagnostic Work-Up

Pituitary adenomas can present with symptoms of hormonal malfunction or of local tumor growth with pressure effects (Fig. 33.2). The procedures used for diagnosis are outlined in Table 33.1.

Endocrine abnormalities may be a consequence of hyper- or hyposecretion of anterior pituitary hormones. Some of these changes, such as loss of libido or lethargy, can be subtle. Clinical

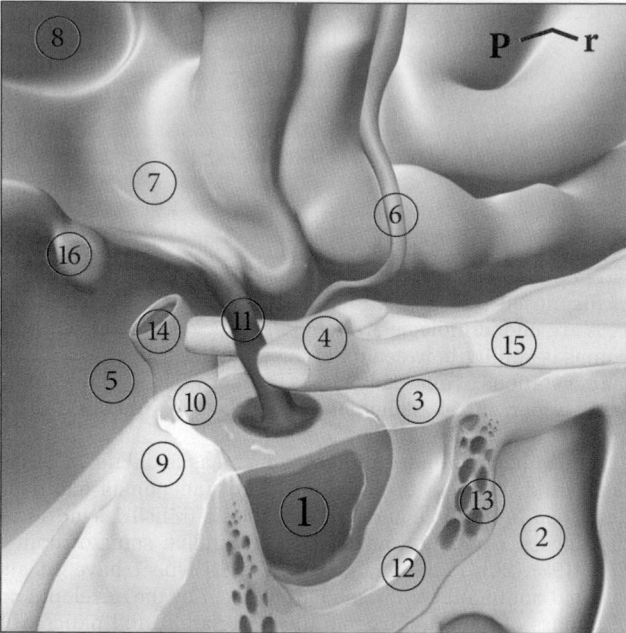

FIGURE 33.1. Posterolateral view of the pituitary gland. P, posterior; r, right. 1, Pituitary gland; 2, sphenoid sinus; 3, diaphragm sellae; 4, optic chiasm; 5, chiasmatic cistern; 6, anterior cerebral artery; 7, hypothalamus; 8, third ventricle; 9, dorsum sellae; 10, posterior clinoid; 11, pituitary stalk; 12, sella turcica; 13, cavernous sinus; 14, internal carotid artery; 15, right optic nerve; 16, mamillary body.

Table 33.1	DIAGNOSTIC WORK-UP FOR PITUITARY TUMORS

General
   History and physical examination
   Neurologic examination with special attention to cranial nerves
Special tests
   Formal testing of visual fields
Imaging studies
   MRI
   Skeletal survey (for acromegaly)
   Computed tomography (if MRI unavailable)
Laboratory studies
   Complete blood count, blood chemistry, urinalysis
   Endocrine evaluation of abnormal secretion:
      Prolactin hypersecretion: prolactin
      Growth hormone hypersecretion: basal growth hormone, IGF-I, glucose suppression, insulin tolerance, thyrotropin-releasing hormone stimulation
      ACTH hypersecretion: serum ACTH, 24-h urine for 17-hydroxy-corticosteroids and free cortisol, dexamethasone suppressed corticotropin-releasing hormone test
      In Cushing's disease with negative neuroimaging studies: selective bilateral simultaneous venous sampling of ACTH from inferior petrosal sinuses
Evaluation of normal endocrine function
   Gonadal function: FSH, LH, estradiol, testosterone
   Thyroid function: thyroxine, free thyroxine index, TSH
   Adrenal function: basal plasma or urinary steroids; cortisol response to insulin-induced hypoglycemia and plasma ACTH response to metyrapone administration

MRI, magnetic resonance imaging; IGF-I, insulin growth factor-I; ACTH, adrenocorticotropic hormone; FSH, follicle-stimulating hormone; LH, luteinizing hormone; TSH, thyroid-stimulating hormone.

manifestations of common hypersecreting pituitary tumors are summarized in Table 33.2.

Patients may be asymptomatic but have significant visual field defects. The most common field defects are bitemporal hemianopic and superior temporal deficits, homonymous hemianopsia, central scotoma, and inferior temporal field defects. Visual field testing at the time of diagnosis is necessary to establish a baseline and assist in the treatment decision-making process.

Pituitary apoplexy is a rare clinical syndrome resulting from acute hemorrhage or infarction of the pituitary gland. It can occur at presentation or during follow-up of a patient with a pituitary adenoma. It can be characterized by headache, nausea, photophobia, hypopituitarism, visual defects, or ocular palsy. Apoplexy can lead to altered consciousness and require urgent surgical decompression of the pituitary fossa.

The diagnosis of a secreting pituitary adenoma can be made on the basis of MRI findings and biochemical evidence of hypersecretion. In the case of a nonsecreting lesion, a biopsy is often necessary as the differential diagnosis of a sellar lesion includes craniopharyngioma, lymphoma, chordoma, germ cell tumor, meningioma, metastatic tumor, cysts, and inflammatory lesions.

Staging

Pituitary tumors are classified according to both endocrine function and anatomic extent. When classifying tumors by clinical/endocrine presentation, they are broadly categorized as either functional or nonfunctional based on their secretory activity. Although the 2004 World Health Organization classification recognizes tumors with elevated serum FSH or LH as functional, these tumors are almost always included in reports of clinically nonfunctional tumors. Hardy and Vezina (42) developed an imaging/surgical classification system that has gained only partial acceptance. Tumors are separated into microadenomas (size ≤1 cm) and macroadenomas (size >1 cm) and classified into five grades according to the extent of expansion or erosion of the sella:

- Grade 0: Intrapituitary microadenoma with normal sellar appearance
- Grade I: Normal-sized sella (15 × 12 mm) with asymmetry of the floor

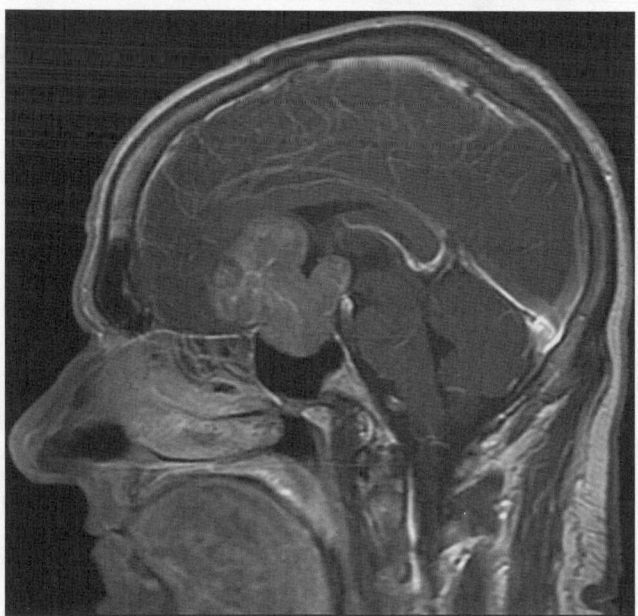

FIGURE 33.2. Saggital T1-weighted, contrast-enhanced magnetic resonance image of a nonfunctional pituitary adenoma with massive suprasellar extension.

Table 33.2	CLINICAL MANIFESTATIONS OF HORMONAL EXCESS		
Disease	**Clinical Manifestations**		**Diagnosis**
Acromegaly	Changes in skull, facial features, jaws, hands, feet; hyperhidrosis; heat intolerance; fatigue; weight gain; paresthesias; arthralgias; glucose intolerance (50% of patients); hypogonadism (>50% of patients); rarely, hypoadrenalism or hypothyroidism		Elevated basal state serum growth hormone (in excess of 10 ng/mL in 90% of patients); if normal or borderline, nonsuppressibility with hyperglycemia establishes diagnosis; elevated IGF-I
Hyperprolactinemia	Amenorrhea, oligomenorrhea, or infertility in women; decreased libido or impotence in men; galactorrhea (mild, transient, if present); osteoporosis; hypopituitarism (more common with large tumors and sellar enlargement)		Basal serum prolactin level >100 ng/mL (normal, 5–20 ng/mL); range of 30–100 mg/mL may indicate microadenoma or loss of suppression; hyperprolactinemia with demonstration of pituitary tumor on imaging confirms diagnosis
Cushing's disease	Obesity (central distribution); hypertension; glucose intolerance; hirsutism; easy bruising; striae; osteoporosis; psychological changes; hypogonadism; rarely hypopituitarism		Plasma cortisol >10 μg/mL 8–9 h after 1 mg dexamethasone is diagnostic in 95% of cases; UFC of >10 μg/24 h; plasma ACTH often normal to moderately elevated.

IGF-I, insulin growth factor-I; UFC, urinary free cortisol; ACTH, adrenocorticotropic hormone.

- Grade II: Enlarged sella with an intact floor
- Grade III: Localized erosion or destruction of the sellar floor
- Grade IV: Diffusely eroded or destroyed floor

In the Hardy and Vezina system, suprasellar extension requires a secondary designation by type: from A (bulging into the chiasmatic cistern) to D (extension into the temporal or frontal fossae). This system assigns a lesser degree of importance to involvement of brain, cavernous sinus, or optic apparatus, which all have a significant impact on both selection and effectiveness of therapy. To further describe large tumors, some authors have variably defined the entity of *giant adenoma* by tumor size (>40 mm) (93) or extension (beyond the sella and suprasellar space) (54).

Pathologic Classification

Tumors arising from the neural components of the posterior pituitary gland (pituicytomas, gangliogliomas, or choristomas) are rare. The focus of this chapter is the anterior pituitary. Histopathologic features of pituitary adenomas often do not correlate with tumor behavior, and the clinical relevance of classifying them into typical and atypical adenomas (60) (based, in part, on labeling index and nuclear staining for p53) is unclear.

When classic fixation, staining, and light microscopy had to be relied on, pituitary tumors were designated as chromophobic, basophilic, or acidophilic. Acidophilic tumors were thought to be associated with acromegaly, basophilic tumors with Cushing's disease, and chromophobic tumors with nonfunction. However, these tinctorial properties may not correlate with clinical or immunohistochemical findings and are now only of historical interest. Newer methods of fixation and staining, electron microscopy, and immunohistochemical procedures can identify cells secreting GH, ACTH, TSH, and prolactin. Hormonally inactive adenomas referred to as *null cell adenomas*, are now often pathologically classified as members of the gonadotroph family. Table 33.3 shows the World Health Organization classification of pituitary adenomas by cytodifferentiation (3).

General Management

Input regarding management options should come from the disciplines of neuroradiology, neuroophthalmology, endocrinology, neurosurgery, radiation oncology, and pathology. The goals are to define tumor extent, remove or control tumor masses, control hypersecretion, and correct endocrine deficiencies while minimizing the risk of hypopituitarism or injury to adjacent structures. If an asymptomatic pituitary tumor is not treated, imaging must be performed at least yearly for the duration of the patient's life. Observation is an option for nonsecreting microadenomas and small asymptomatic prolactinomas (Fig. 33.3). Tumor growth on imaging, symptoms of hypersecretion, and/or development of visual field deficits are all indications for intervention.

The choice of treatment modality is determined by factors including the need for rapid relief of mass effect or symptoms related to hormonal abnormalities, the need for histologic confirmation of the diagnosis, and the potential morbidity of a given therapy.

Comorbidities associated with alterations in hormonal levels, including hypertension, osteopenia, diabetes, electrolyte imbalance, and dyslipidemia, are managed as in the general population.

Table 33.3	WORLD HEALTH ORGANIZATION CLASSIFICATION OF PITUITARY ADENOMAS BY CYTODIFFERENTIATION
Tumor Type	**Hormones**
Somatotroph adenoma	
Densely granulated somatotroph adenoma	GH
Sparsely granulated somatotroph adenoma	GH
Mammosomatotroph/mixed adenoma	GH, PRL
Lactotroph adenoma	
Sparsely granulated lactotroph adenoma	PRL
Densely granulated lactotroph adenoma	PRL
Acidophil stem cell adenoma	β-TSH
Thyrotroph adenoma	PRL
Plurihormonal adenoma	ACTH
ACTH family	
Corticotroph adenoma	GH, PRL, β-TSH
Gonadotropin family	
Gonadotroph adenoma	β-FSH, β-LH
Unclassified adenoma	
Hormone-negative/null cell adenoma	None
Plurihormonal adenoma	Multiple

GH, growth hormone; PRL, prolactin; TSH, thyroid-stimulating hormone; ACTH, adrenocorticotropic hormone; LH, luteinizing hormone.

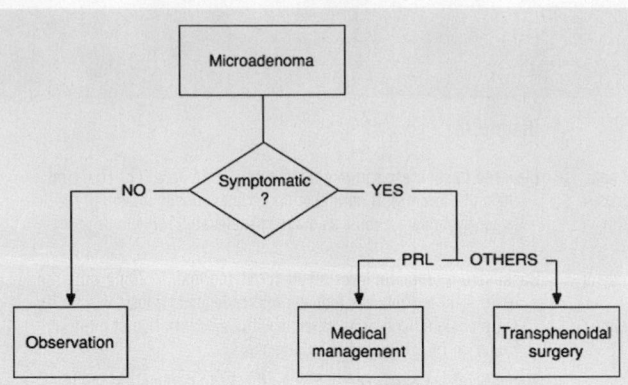

FIGURE 33.3. Management scheme for pituitary microadenomas. PRL, prolactinoma.

Medical Management

Medical management is the modality of choice for most prolactinomas and can play an important role in the suppression of hormonal hypersection associated with the other secreting adenomas. The drugs used are dopamine agonists, somatostatin analogues, and pegvisomant, a GH receptor antagonist. New drugs are under investigation and in the future may play a more significant role in the management of these disorders (30,43). Reports of the use of cytotoxic chemotherapy for locally aggressive or metastatic tumors are anecdotal (48). Responses rates are disappointing and outcomes for chemotherapy-treated patients are poor.

Surgical Management

The standard surgery for most tumors is transsphenoidal microsurgery, which accounts for more than 95% of procedures. Transsphenoidal microsurgery is particularly effective in selective removal of microadenomas, but it also is used for adenomas that extend outside the sella. The procedure is relatively safe with a mortality rate of approximately 0.5% (6,19). Major complications, including meningitis, cerebrospinal fluid leak, hemorrhage, stroke, or visual loss, occur in approximately 1.5% of the procedures. Contraindications to the transsphenoidal approach include sphenoid sinusitis, ectatic midline carotid arteries, and significant lateral suprasellar extent. A transcranial approach is preferred in the latter situations.

Radiation Therapy

The choice of radiation modality for the treatment of pituitary adenoma often depends more on availability, physician preference, and perceived differences in toxicity rather than any convincing difference in reported outcomes.

Conventional External-Beam Radiation Therapy

Radiation therapy can be effective in control of hypersecretion and mass effects due to large or recurrent tumors. External-beam radiation therapy controls hypersecretion in approximately 80% of patients with acromegaly, in 50% to 80% of those with Cushing's disease, and in approximately one-third of those with hyperprolactinemia. Reirradiation is sometimes employed for postradiotherapy recurrences, although stereotactic radiosurgery is usually preferred (89).

Radiosurgery

In a recent review of the literature (9), 29 retrospective studies were identified involving 1,153 patients. These series are generally limited by short, inconsistent, and incomplete follow-up. With few exceptions (28,81), outcomes and complications are not reported actuarially. Despite these caveats, the literature does suggest a high freedom from local tumor progression and variable biochemical cure rates. Whether radiosurgery leads to faster decline in pathologic hormone production is a matter of controversy (9). Few series compare time to hormone normalization. Some retrospective data suggest that time to hormone normalization is shorter with radiosurgery (67) but these data must be viewed with much caution as time to normalization depends on several factors, including initial hormone levels and length of follow-up.

Radiosurgery remains an accepted and appropriate treatment for selected cases: specifically, the smaller, radiologically well-defined tumors located at a distance (3 to 5 mm) from the optic apparatus sufficient to limit the dose to the optic chiasm and optic nerves to <8 to 10 Gy.

Fractionated Stereotactic Radiation Therapy (FSRT)

FSRT is the application of the dose conformality and precise patient localization of radiosurgery to fractionated radiotherapy. The technique is still new; its popularity is growing with advances in noninvasive immobilization, radiation delivery, and image guidance. As of March 2006, there were fewer than 500 cases of pituitary adenomas in published series (Table 33.4). Most series have limited follow-up and contain a mix of secreting and nonsecreting lesions. Early results with respect to tumor control compare favorably with those reported for conformal radiation therapy. The data are insufficient to draw conclusions on hormonal response. No neurocognitive changes, second malignancies, brain necrosis, or cerebrovascular events have been reported. However, these toxicities are rare and, with the exception of necrosis, require long follow-up.

FSRT is widely applicable, even to large tumors in intimate relationship with the optic apparatus. It is our current institutional bias to offer this form of radiation to virtually all previously unirradiated patients because of its favorable safety and efficacy profile.

Charged Particle Therapy

Protons have been used to deliver either single fractions (proton radiosurgery) or fractionated conformal therapy. When first proposed in 1946 (107), high-energy protons presented a significant dosimetric advantage over supervoltage x-rays. With advances in the delivery of megavoltage photons, the dosimetric differences have become subtle. There is limited published experience in the treatment of pituitary adenoma. Recent updates from the Massachusetts General Hospital (77) and the Loma Linda University Center (85) have reported the outcomes of 61 and 47 patients, respectively. Tumor control (100%), hormonal cure (38% to 52%), and induced hypopituitarism (22% to 44%) are not different than those with photon therapy. In contrast to protons, heavier charged particles differ radiobiologically from photons. It remains to be seen if this translates into an improvement in the therapeutic ratio. A 1991 review summarized the treatment of 810 patients with helium ion beam therapy (56). More than 40% of these patients were irradiated to cause hypopituitarism as treatment for selected systemic diseases. In the patients with adenomas, high hormonal cure and tumor control rates are reported with acceptable toxicity. Clinical experience with these modalities is expected to grow as they become more widely available.

Table 33.4 RESULTS OF FRACTIONATED STEREOTACTIC RADIATION THERAPY

Authors	Year	No. of Patients	Tumor Type	Median Dose (or range)	Median Daily Dose (or range)	Median Follow-Up (mo)	Local Control	Hormonal Cure (%)	Complications
Mitsumori et al. (67)	1998	30	18 funct, 12 nonF	45	1.8	34	85% 3-y actuarial	39	3-y 20.1% hypopituitarism
Milker-Zabel et al. (63)	2001	62	20 funct, 42 nonF	50.4–52.2	1.8–2	38.7[a]	93% 5-y actuarial	20	5% hypopituitarism, 7% decrease visual acuity
Voduc et al. (104)	2002	37	17 funct, 20 nonF	50.4	1.8	19.1	100%	30	2-y actuarial hypopituitarism 20%
Milker-Zabel et al. (64)	2004	20	20 GH	52.2 (41.4–55.8)	1.8	61.3	100%	80	1 trigeminal hypoesthesia, 1 visual, 3/18 hypopituitarism
Kajiwara et al. (47)	2005	20	6 funct, 14 nonF	nonF 12.6[a,b], funct 17.5[a,b]	NR (2–5 fractions)	35[a]	95%	33	10% hypopituitarism
Paek et al. (73)	2005	68	68 nonF	46–50.4	1.8–2	30	98% 5-y actuarial	NR	2/68 optic neuropathy, 5-y actuarial hypopituitarism 10%
Colin et al. (17)	2005	110	47 funct, 63 nonF	50.4	1.8	80	99%	43	36.7% new hormone replacement, 2 visual losses not ascribed to FSRT
Minniti et al. (65)	2006	92	25 funct, 68 nonF	45	1.8	32	98% 5-y actuarial	38	22% new hormone deficit

funct, functional; nonF, nonfunctioning; GH, growth hormone; NR, not reported; FSRT, fractionated stereotactic radiation therapy.
[a]Mean.
[b]"Single-fraction equivalent."

Intensity Modulated Radiation Therapy (IMRT)

Pituitary adenoma targets generally do not present significant concave surfaces. They are small and do not require differential dosing. Consequently, pituitary adenomas are not ideal targets for inverse-planned IMRT. This is borne out by dosimetric studies in which IMRT shows similar conformality and sparing when compared to noncoplanar conformal therapy. The use of IMRT is thus limited to the occasional large, irregular tumor.

Posttherapy Evaluations

Contrast-enhanced MRI is the imaging modality of choice. It should be obtained at least yearly. Monitoring of hormonal response does not replace tumor imaging as the two parameters can be dissociated. In acromegaly, despite a recent consensus statement suggesting the use of a nadir level below 0.4 μg/L (62), the most commonly used criterion for hormonal control is a posttreatment GH value of less than 1 μg/L. Both insulin growth factor-I (somatomedin-C or IGF-I) and GH levels should be followed. In prolactin-secreting tumors, the therapeutic objective is to lower the prolactin level into the normal range. Evaluation of the response to therapy in Cushing's disease requires measurement of plasma and urine steroids and plasma ACTH levels. Periodic assessment of gonadal, thyroid, and adrenal function is necessary as hypopituitarism may develop years after treatment. Finally, regular formal visual field testing should be performed following radiotherapy.

Treatment Results

Nonfunctioning Pituitary Tumors

Management of these tumors is first directed toward relief of any mass effect (Fig. 33.4). If the tumor cannot be resected com-

pletely, decompression of the chiasm (if indicated) followed by radiation provides excellent long-term results. In a series of 252 patients treated with radiation therapy at the Royal Marsden Hospital, the actuarial 20-year progression-free survival rate following definitive irradiation was 94%, which was not significantly different from the 91% progression-free survival seen following combined debulking and adjuvant irradiation (11). Although this suggests that tumors without significant mass effect can be reasonably managed with primary radiation, surgery remains the backbone of standard treatment. It is quite clear from retrospective data that the use of adjuvant radiotherapy significantly reduces local recurrence; it is not as clear what is gained or lost by reserving radiotherapy for progression. Although local invasion, suprasellar extent, and residual tumor on postoperative imaging are known risk factors for recurrence (37), the identification of patients at low risk for recurrence can be difficult. In a series from the Princess Margaret Hospital, 21 of 65 patients selected for low risk of recurrence eventually had tumor regrowth (99). More recent series suggest that, for what is often a minority of patients with MRI-confirmed complete resection, the low recurrence rate (0% to 20% at 5 years) may justify observation without radiation (22,37). These data must be interpreted with caution as recurrences continue to occur 10 to 20 years following surgery. For patients with invasive tumors, especially those with baseline hypopituarism, adjuvant radiotherapy can still be considered. For all patients observed, it is important to ensure long-term imaging follow-up to avoid symptomatic recurrences, visual loss and need for repeat surgery.

Fractionated External-Beam Radiation Therapy and Radiosurgery

Park et al. (75) reported on 258 patients operated for nonfunctioning adenomas. Seventy patients were treated with immediate postoperative radiotherapy. The remaining 168 were followed with serial imaging studies—80% of these patients had been assigned to observation based on total or near-total tumor resection. The 10-year recurrence rate was 2.3% in irradiated patients and 50.5% in those observed. Symptomatic recurrences were limited to patients lost to follow-up. These findings are corroborated by a series of 126 patients from Gittoes et al. (34) in which the 15-year recurrence rate was 7% with adjuvant radiotherapy and 67% following surgery alone.

The retrospective series of radiosurgery for nonfunctioning tumors are small, selected, and heterogeneous. However, the available data suggest a high probability of local control, similar to that provided by fractionated radiation. Series of 20 patients or more are presented in Table 33.5.

Functioning Pituitary Tumors

The goals of radiation for functioning pituitary tumors are similar across tumor types: arrest tumor progression and suppress hormone secretion. Radiation is generally used as an adjuvant or salvage to other failed or incompletely effective therapies. Control of mass effect is more readily achieved than cure, as defined by suppression of inappropriate hormone secretion. This is illustrated by a large series of hormonally active tumors treated at the Princess Margaret Hospital (100) in which 145 patients received 50 Gy of conventionally fractionated external-beam radiation therapy. The local control rate was 96%, with a 10-year disease-specific survival rate of 97%. However, the hormonal cure rate at 10 years was only 39% without the addition of medical therapies.

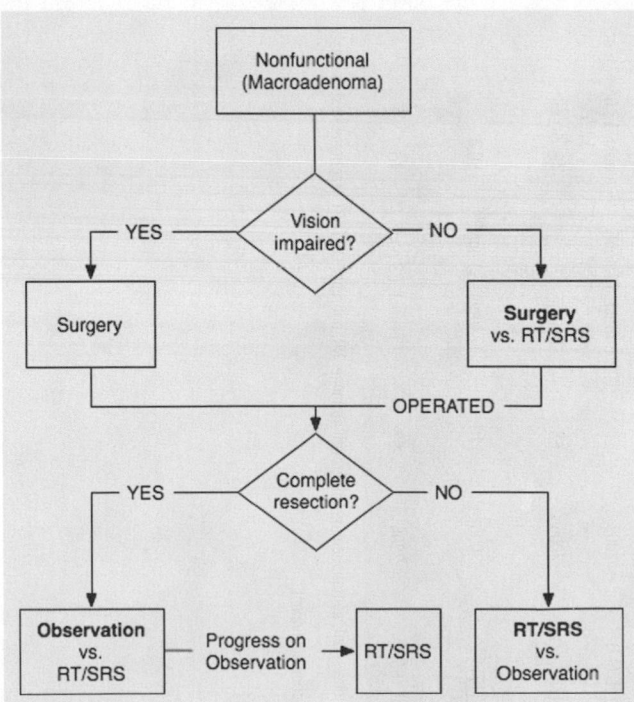

FIGURE 33.4. Management scheme for nonfunctioning pituitary tumors (with preferred approach in **bold**). RT/SRS

Table 33.5	SELECTED SERIES OF RADIOSURGERY FOR NONFUNCTIONING PITUITARY ADENOMAS					
Authors	Year	No. of Patients	Mean Follow-Up (months)	Mean Dose (Gy)	Tumor Control (crude)	Induced Hypopituitarism
Mokry et al. (68)	1999	31	21	13.8	97%	2 patients
Izawa et al. (45)	2000	23	30.1	19.5	95.6%	None
Sheehan et al. (90)	2002	42	31.2	16	98%	None
Feigl et al. (28)	2002	61	55.2[a]	15[a]	94%[a]	100% 8-y actuarial[a]
Petrovich et al. (78)	2003	56	41	15	100%	4%[a]
Pollock and Carpenter (81)	2003	33	Median 43	Median 16	97%	41% 5-y actuarial
Muacevic et al. (70)	2004	51	Median 21.7	Median 16.5	90% 5-y actuarial	2 patients
Picozzi et al. (79)	2005	51	40.6	16.5	89.8% 5-y actuarial	Not reported

[a]Of a larger series including functioning adenomas.

Growth Hormone–Secreting Tumors

Excess circulating levels of GH and IGF-I are responsible for multiple metabolic disturbances, cardiovascular and respiratory comorbidities, which explain the increased mortality rates seen in acromegaly (109). The reduction of circulating hormone levels is thus as important as reversal of mass effect. Surgical intervention alone provides the most rapid means of achieving both goals. Radiation therapy and radiosurgery are appropriate adjuvant therapies for patients with residual tumor and persistently elevated GH levels after surgery, and are radical alternatives for medically inoperable patients (Fig. 33.5). Pharmacological therapy is useful following failure of local therapies or while awaiting the typically slow response to radiation.

Medical Therapy

Three pharmacologic alternatives are available: somatostatin analogs, dopamine agonists, and a GH receptor antagonist. The somatostatin analogs (octreotide and lanreotide) reduce GH and IGF-I levels in 50% to 60% of patients who have failed surgery, and they have been the medical therapy of choice (33). Tumor shrinkage occurs in 30% to 45% of patients. The most common side effects are gastrointestinal and include transient abdominal cramps, malabsorptive diarrhea, and nausea of mild-to-moderate intensity. Gallbladder sludge or stones may develop in 15% of patients but in most cases remains asymptomatic. Dopamine agonists are considerably less effective. Pegvisomant, a genetically engineered GH receptor antagonist, has been shown to be effective in reducing serum IGF-I concentrations and improving clinical conditions in a placebo-controlled randomized trial (97). Daily injections of pegvisomant resulted in normalization of IGF-I in 89% of patients. The most common toxicities of pegvisomant include diarrhea, nausea, flu syndrome, and abnormal liver function tests. Because pegvisomant does not inhibit GH secretion or tumor growth, it is generally reserved for patients failing other therapies.

Transsphenoidal Resection

Changes in criteria for biochemical cure make comparison of surgical series difficult. In one of the largest published series (32), biochemical cure rate (defined with GH <5 μg/L) was 68%, 54%, and 20% for patients with microadenomas, macroadenomas, and giant adenomas, respectively. Davis et al. (21) reported on 175 evaluable patients who underwent surgery as their initial treatment. The criterion used to define surgical success was either a postoperative fasting or glucose-suppressed GH level ≤2 ng/mL. Actuarial 1-year remission rate, representing primarily the effects of surgery, was 49%. The probability of a recurrence after achieving a remission was 31% at 5 years. In another series with long-term follow-up for 129 patients in postsurgical remission (GH level <5 ng/mL), only 7% had disease recurrence (1). Most importantly, the mortality rate among the patients in remission was similar to the general population, while it was significantly increased for patients with persistent disease. Although tumor size, preoperative GH level, and tumor extension may predict a higher risk of recurrence, these are not considered indications for adjuvant treatment.

Even in patients for whom complete resection is not possible, surgical debulking may improve biochemical cure and local control over definitive radiotherapy alone (13).

Radiation Therapy and Radiosurgery

Modern series have shown the efficacy of radiation therapy in both the definitive and adjuvant setting. In radiotherapy-treated patients, the most significant predictive factors are tumor size

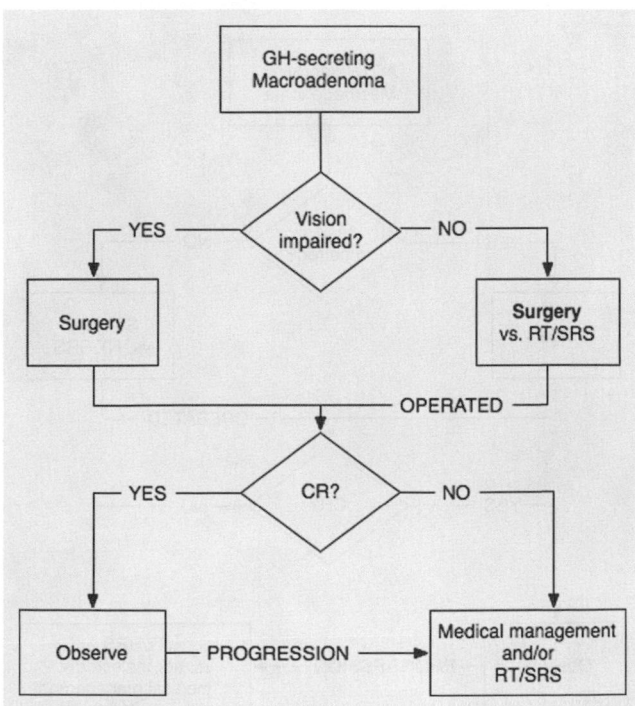

FIGURE 33.5. Management scheme for growth hormone (GH)-secreting macroadenomas (with preferred approach in **bold**). RT/SRS; CR

Table 33.6   SELECTED SERIES OF RADIOSURGERY FOR GROWTH HORMONE (GH)-SECRETING TUMORS

Authors	Year	No. of Patients	Mean Follow-Up (mo)	Tumor Control (crude)	Hormonally Controlled (%)	Criteria for Control	Induced Hypopituitarism (%)
Thoren et al. (95)	1991	21	65	NR (≥2 failures)	30	GH ≤2.2 for women, ≤1.9 U/mL for men	24
Lim et al. (57)	1998	20	25.5[a]	100%	38	GH ≤2.0 ng/mL	6
Witt (108)	1998	20	NR	100%	20	Normal IGF-I	NR
Laws and Vance (53)	1999	36	Minimum 6	NR	25	Normal IGF-I	NR
Izawa et al. (45)	2000	29	26.4[a]	100%	41	NR	None
Zhang et al. (110)	2000	68	34	100%	96 (at 24 mo)	GH <12 μg/L	None
Vladyka et al. (103)	2000	91	Median 24	100%	43	Normal IGF-I and GH ≤2 μg/L	4.4
Pollock et al. (82)	2002	26	42.4[a]	100%	42	Normal IGF-I and GH <2 ng/mL	16
Attanasio et al. (5)	2003	30	Median 46	100%	23	Normal IGF-I	7
Kobayashi et al. (51)	2005	67	32.5	100%	4.8	GH <1.0 ng/mL	14.6
Castinetti et al. (14)	2005	82	49.5	NR	17	Normal IGF-I and GH <2 ng/mL	17

NR, not reported; IGF-I, insulin growth factor-I.
[a]Of a larger series.

and pretreatment GH levels. Long-term follow-up is required because GH levels decrease over a period of several years. Typically, by 10 years after radiation therapy, 60% to 100% of patients have GH levels <10 ng/mL (27,61,91). Continued response can be seen even past 10 years: in a series from Eastman et al. (24,25), GH levels were below 10 ng/mL in 83% of patients at 15 years and 92% of those followed for more than 15 years. The posttreatment *half-life* of serum GH could better characterize response as it may be independent of pre-treatment GH levels. A 50% reduction in serum GH is expected after approximately 2 years (2).

Radiosurgery series of 20 patients of more are presented in Table 33.6. The majority of patients in these series were treated following transsphenoidal surgery. Local control is excellent. Hormonal control depends on the criteria used with biochemical cure rates of 5% to 40%.

Cushing's Disease

Medical Therapy

Medical management of patients with Cushing's disease is reserved for patients who fail either surgery or radiotherapy (Fig. 33.6). Medical therapy is lifelong and associated with important side effects. Two types of compounds are used: agents that modulate pituitary ACTH release and agents that inhibit steroidogenesis. Compounds that act on corticotropin-releasing hormone or ACTH synthesis/release, including cyproheptadine, bromocriptine, somatostatin, and valproic acid provide poor response rates with only modest effect. Ketoconazole, mitotane, trilostane, aminoglutethimide, and metyrapone inhibit steroidogenesis, with important side effects and limited efficacy.

Surgical Management

Selective transsphenoidal removal of the ACTH-secreting adenoma remains the standard of care for patients with Cushing's disease. Hormonal cure rates range from 57% to 90%, with the highest success rates seen in patients harboring well-defined microadenomas. Variable criteria used to define hormonal cure may partly explain the range of results. The mortality rate for patients achieving remission is similar to that of the normal

population. Recurrence rates after achieving surgical remission range from 2% to 25% (4).

Bilateral adrenalectomy is reserved for patients who have failed other treatment modalities. The procedure, which can now be performed laparoscopically, induces a predictable and rapid hormonal response. However, patients subsequently require lifelong treatment with glucocorticoids and mineralocorticoids. Bilateral adrenalectomy can also result in the development of Nelson's syndrome: local progression of the pituitary tumor with characteristic skin pigmentation resulting from the high concentrations of corticotropin.

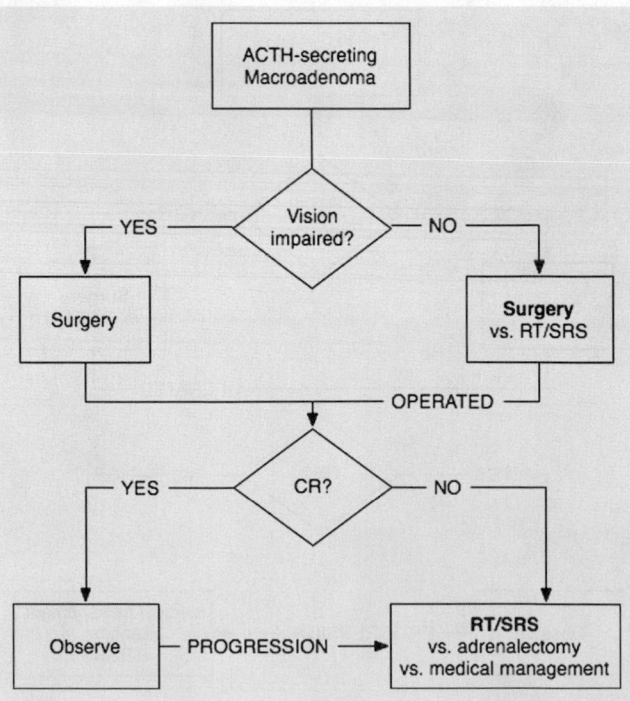

FIGURE 33.6. Management scheme for adrenocorticotropic hormone (ACTH)-secreting macroadenomas (with preferred approach in **bold**). RT/SRS; CR, complete resection; RT/SRS, radiotherapy or radiosurgery.

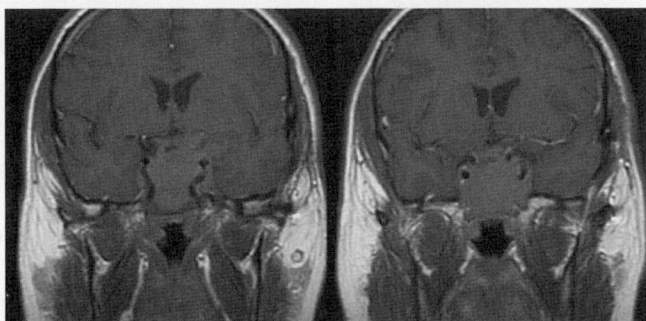
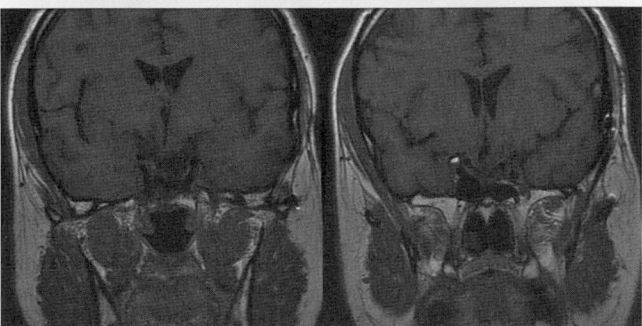

FIGURE 33.7. Coronal T1-weighted magnetic resonance images prior to (top) and 68 months following (*bottom*) fractionated external beam radiotherapy for a large, recurrent adrenocorticotropic hormone-secreting pituitary adenoma. Complete tumor response was accompanied by hormonal cure.

Radiation Therapy and Radiosurgery

Historically, adjuvant or definitive radiotherapy with doses of 35 to 50 Gy have provided hormonal control rates of 50% to 100% (39,72) (Fig. 33.7), with better results at doses ≥50 Gy (8,59).

Estrada et al. (26) reported a series of 30 patients treated with radiation therapy following failure of transsphenoidal surgery. Patients received a mean dose of 50 Gy delivered through lateral opposed fields. Patients had a 3-year actuarial cure rate of 83% with most remissions achieved in the first 2 years. As is typical of these series, no tumor progression was seen. In a series of 51 patients treated with definitive radiotherapy, Orth and Liddle (72), using strict biochemical criteria (urinary 17-hydroxycorticosteroid, <7 mg/g creatinine and mean plasma cortisol, <10 g/dL), reported a cure rate of 23%. Another 30% of patients improved to the point that further therapy was unnecessary.

In a series of 25 patients treated with a median of 50 Gy, Tsang et al. (100) have reported a 53% normalization of urinary free cortisol at 10 years (with further responses in subsequent years). Other authors report similar cure rates with or without the addition of medical management (44,59).

Radiosurgery has been mainly used as salvage therapy after failed or incomplete transsphenoidal surgery. Devin et al. (23) reported the outcomes of 35 patients treated with linear accelerator-based radiosurgery—mainly after failed transsphenoidal surgery. Forty-nine percent of patients normalized their cortisol level at a median of 7.5 months following radiosurgery. One patient had tumor progression and three patients had recurrent hypercortisolemia at a median of 30.5 months following radiosurgery, possibly representing a trend for late recurrences in up to 20% of patients treated with radiosurgery (102). A summary of series of 20 patients or more is presented in Table 33.7.

Prolactin-Secreting Adenomas

Once other causes of increased prolactin are ruled out, treatment options include observation, surgery, medical therapy, and radiotherapy (Figs. 33.3 and 33.8). The decision to treat is based principally on tumor size and symptoms. Even for small asymptomatic tumors, an argument for treatment can be made because of the risk of osteoporosis related to prolonged hyperprolactinemia.

Medical Therapy

It is now generally accepted that the therapy of choice for most prolactinomas is a dopamine agonist. Bromocriptine and cabergoline are approved in North America for the treatment of prolactinomas. Bromocriptine results in rapid normalization of prolactin levels in 80% to 90% of patients (69). Bromocriptine can also reduce tumor size in about 80% of cases, although size reduction can be modest (69). Long-term therapy appears to be required, although the dose may be reduced considerably once a response is obtained. Complete discontinuation of bromocriptine results in recurrent hyperprolactinemia in 80% to 90% of patients, but tumor enlargement is observed in only 10% to 20% (101). The most common side effects are transient nausea and vomiting. Orthostatic hypotension may also occur at the initiation of therapy.

Cabergoline is at least as effective as bromocriptine in lowering prolactin levels and reducing tumor size but has a better toxicity profile. In a randomized comparison, cabergoline was significantly more effective in normalizing prolactin levels and led to fewer patients stopping treatment because of drug intolerance (106). Colao et al. (16) reported on 200 patients treated with cabergoline in which withdrawal of the drug was allowed if they had a normal serum prolactin level and a partial or complete response by imaging. Biochemical recurrence rates 2 to 5 years after withdrawal were 31% in patients with microprolactinomas and 36% in macroprolactinomas. Renewed tumor growth did not occur in any patient.

Transsphenoidal Resection

Indications for surgery include rapidly progressive vision loss, increase in adenoma size despite dopamine agonists, and intolerance or inadequate hormonal response to medical therapy. Molitch (69) compiled the results of 34 surgical series and reported that, in 74% of microprolactinomas and 32% of macroadenomas, prolactin levels normalize 1 to 12 weeks postsurgery. However 20% of patients present a biochemical recurrence within 1 year. Thus, using a normal prolactin level as the sole criterion for cure, the overall long-term surgical cure rate is about 50% to 60% and 25% for microadenomas and macroadenomas, respectively. Patients with large tumors (>2 cm in diameter) or prolactin levels above 20 ng/mL typically fare worse (41).

Radiation Therapy

Older series by Grigsby et al. (38), Gomez et al. (35), and Sheline (92) showed that mean prolactin levels after radiation ranged from 25% to 50% of the pretreatment levels, with few patients achieving normal values. More recent reports with long-term follow-up show biochemical cure rates of 25% to 50% (98,100).

Long-term follow-up with appropriate concomitant medical management is important as biochemical response is slow. Tsagarakis et al. (98) reported the results of 36 women with prolactin-secreting macroadenomas treated to 45 Gy in 25 fractions. At a mean follow-up of 8.7 years, 50% of patients had normal prolactin levels and 61% of patients had resumed normal menses. The mean time required to reach normal prolactin levels was 7.3 years.

Landolt and Lomax (52) reported their experience with radiosurgery for prolactinomas. With a median follow-up of

Table 33.7   SELECTED SERIES OF RADIOSURGERY FOR CUSHING'S DISEASE

Authors	Year	No. of Patients	Mean Follow-Up (mo)	Tumor Control (crude)	Hormonally Controlled (%)	Criteria for Control	Induced Hypopituitarism (%)
Rähn et al. (83)	1991	59	2-y minimum	100%	82[a]	"Clinical remission"	20
Witt (108)	1998	29	20	NR	52	Normal 24-h UFC *or* A.M. cortisol *or* serum ACTH	NR
Sheehan et al. (88)	2000	43	39.1	100%	63	Normal 24-h UFC	16
Kobayashi et al. (51)	2002	25	64.1	100%	35	ACTH <50 pg/mL, cortisol <10 μg/dL	NR
Devin et al. (23)	2004	35	42	91%	49	Normal 24-h UFC	40

NR, not reported; UFC, urinary free cortisol; AM; ACTH, adrenocorticotropic hormone.
[a]Includes patients with more than one radiosurgical procedure.

29 months, 25% of patients experienced hormonal cure, whereas another 55% showed improvement of hormone levels. Patients receiving dopamine agonists at the time of radiosurgical treatment had a significantly worse outcome compared with those who were not. A 2-month break between medical therapy and radiosurgery was thus suggested. In a large series of 128 patients, Pan et al. (74) reported that biochemical cure may be improved with marginal doses >30 Gy. Further radiosurgical series are presented in Table 33.8.

Thyrotropin-Secreting Adenomas

Thyrotropin-secreting tumors are rare, representing 1% of pituitary adenomas (60). They have historically presented principally as macroadenomas (12) although there is a trend, with ultrasensitive TSH measurements, toward earlier diagnosis (93). Initial treatment for these tumors will generally be transsphenoidal resection, although surgical failures are common. These tumors are responsive to somatostatin analogues (93). Radiotherapy may control tumors that have failed other treatment modalities. In a large review of TSH-secreting adenomas, thyroid hormone levels were normalized in two-thirds of 27 patients treated with adjuvant or definitive radiation (7).

Pituitary Carcinomas

Pituitary carcinomas are composed of adenohypophysial cells and their malignant nature cannot be clearly identified by their microscopic appearance (76). The diagnosis of pituitary carcinoma is thus clinical. It is based on the finding of a pituitary tumor with subarachnoid, parenchymal brain, or systemic metastases (60). This is rare, seen in 0.2% of pituitary tumors. The majority of pituitary carcinomas were initially diagnosed as invasive macroadenomas (49). Clinical features are similar to those of pituitary adenomas, with the majority being hormonally active (most often ACTH or prolactin-secreting). Even with aggressive treatment, the prognosis is poor with only a handful of patients experiencing long-term survival.

Radiation Therapy Techniques

Image-based treatment planning using a three-dimensional technique is the standard of care, but in countries where access to computed tomography (CT) or MRI-based treatment planning is limited, the moderate doses used and the relationship of pituitary tumors to the bony anatomy of the skull base make adequate two-dimensional treatment planning possible.

Conventional Radiation Therapy

All diagnostic evidence, but particularly MRI and CT, as well as clinical and surgical findings, should be used to define the tumor volume. CT simulation assists in defining treatment volumes and provides the information on electron density used in the production of digitally reconstructed radiographs. Registration of a contrast-enhanced MRI scan with the treatment CT scan allows for optimum definition of the tumor and the optic apparatus. The gross tumor volume (GTV) is the pituitary adenoma, including any extension into adjacent anatomic regions. In cases in which a recent MRI with a clearly defined tumor is available for registration, a clinical target volume (CTV) limited to a 5-mm margin around the tumor is adequate. With invasive tumors, such as those involving the sphenoid sinus, cavernous sinus, or other intracranial structures, there is greater uncertainty that must be considered in determining the volume to be included. Often, the entire contents of the sella and, if appropriate, the entire cavernous sinus are included in the CTV. The largest planning target volume (PTV) component is uncertainty in daily patient setup. Standard thermoplastic masks are associated with setup variability of the order of 3 to 4 mm. A total PTV margin of 5 mm is usually reasonable.

Simulation

For two-dimensional planning in which an eye-sparing anterior or vertex beam will be used, the patient is positioned supine with neck flexed and the head at a 45-degree angle. Otherwise, the patient is generally positioned with the head and neck in a neutral position. Immobilization will generally be performed with a thermoplastic mask. In two-dimensional planning, open

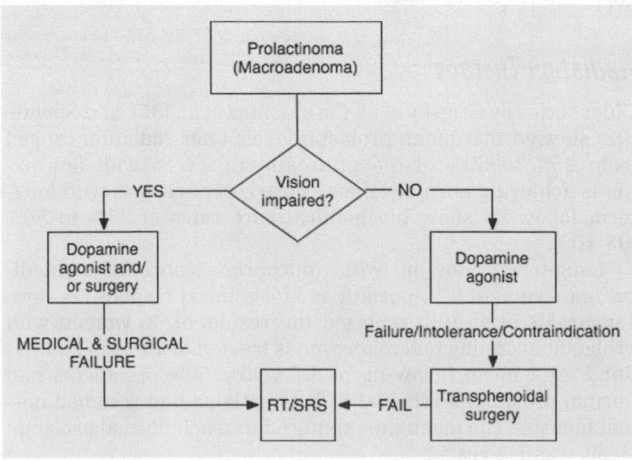

FIGURE 33.8. Management scheme for prolactin-secreting macroadenomas. RT/SRS, radiotherapy or radiosurgery.

| Table 33.8 | SELECTED SERIES OF RADIOSURGERY FOR PROLACTINOMAS |

Authors	Year	No. of Patients	Mean Follow-Up (mo)	Tumor Control (crude)	Hormonally Controlled (%)	Criteria for Control	Induced Hypopituitarism
Mokry et al. (68)	1999	21	31	100%	21	"Could discontinue bromocriptine"	3 cases
Landolt and Lomax (52)	2000	20	28.6	NR	25	<19 ng/mL for women, <16 ng/mL for men	NR
Pan et al. (74)	2000	128	33.2	98%	13	Normal prolactin level without a dopamine agonist	NR
Choi et al. (15)	2003	21	42.5[a]	100%	24	<20 ng/mL	None
Wang et al. (105)[b]	2003	61	38.4[a]	97%	54	"Normal" prolactin and resolution of symptoms	NR

NR, not reported.
[a]Of a larger series.
[b]All microadenomas.

or shaped fields will be centered on the sella during fluoroscopic simulation. For three-dimensional simulation, a contrast-enhanced planning CT scan is obtained. When possible, a thin-slice T1-weighted contrast-enhanced MRI should be registered to the planning CT scan. The volumes described previously are then defined on the MRI but reviewed on the CT. Normal structures to be contoured include, as a minimum, the eyes (lenses), optic nerves, optic chiasm, brainstem, and temporal lobes.

Several treatment techniques have been described. The use of two lateral opposed portals should be avoided in order to decrease the dose to the temporal lobes. A simple technique is to use three static shaped beams: wedged opposed laterals and an anterior or vertex beam that enters above the eyes (Fig. 33.9). Alternatively, two 110-degree arcs rotating in a coronal plane at the level of the ears have been used. Typically, a 30-degree wedge is used and flipped between arcs. When complex treatment planning is available, five noncoplanar beams present a good solution. This allows custom beam shaping and optimal normal structure sparing. The beams are hemispherically distributed, avoiding entry or exit through the eyes. All three-dimensional plans should be assessed by using dose-volume histograms.

Photons in the megavoltage range should be used to spare surrounding structures, most notably the temporal lobes. Energy selection is a compromise between depth dose and penumbra width. Six- to 10-MV photons generally provide an acceptable balance between these competing concerns.

After completion of treatment planning, initial verification films can be taken on a conventional simulator or at the treatment unit; these should include orthogonal radiographs to verify the isocenter and films of any poured blocks or multileaf collimation used. Portal films are obtained during treatment to verify accuracy of the treatment setup.

Dose and Fractionation Schedule

Pituitary adenomas show dose-response rates that depend on tumor type (38). Nonfunctioning tumors are usually controlled with 45 to 50.4 Gy using daily fractions of 1.8 Gy. Functioning tumors require slightly higher doses, typically 50.4 to 54 Gy (Table 33.9).

Fractionated Stereotactic Radiation Therapy

FSRT is characterized by improved patient localization, tighter volume definition, and more conformal isodose distributions. FSRT often involves a formal stereotactic reference space, noncoplanar beam delivery, and increased target dose heterogeneity.

Immobilization

Immobilization for FSRT should aim to achieve a patient positioning error of less than 3 mm. This can be achieved by

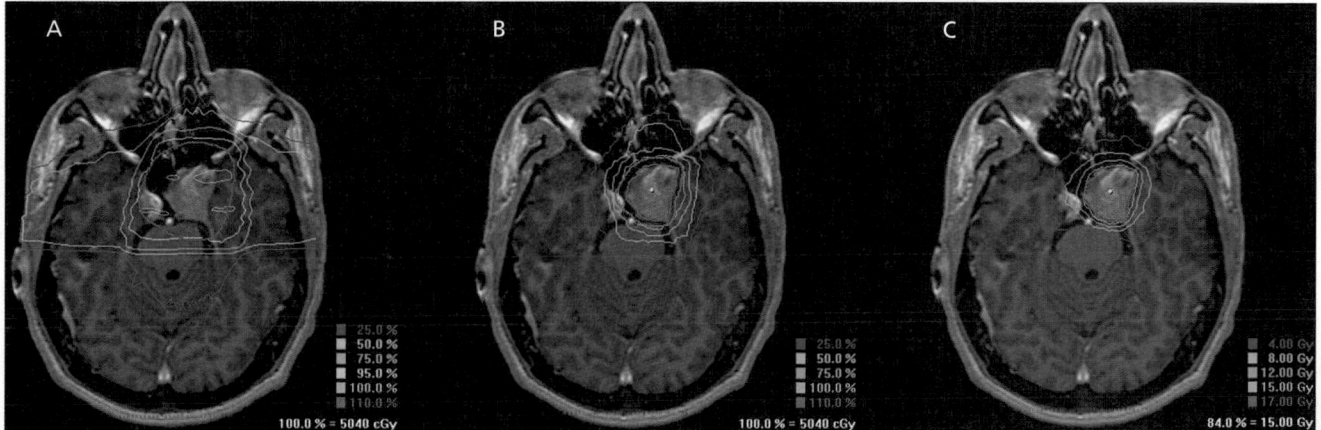

FIGURE 33.9. Comparison of isodose curves for varying treatment plans. **A:** Conventional radiation therapy with a 10-mm margin on the gross tumor volume. **B:** Fractionated stereotactic radiation therapy with a 2-mm margin. **C:** Linear accelerator stereotactic radiosurgery with no planning margin.

Table 33.9	RADIATION THERAPY DOSING GUIDELINES

Tumor Type	External-Beam Radiation Therapy or FSRT (1.8 Gy/Fraction)	Stereotactic Radiosurgery (Optic Chiasm Dose ≤9 Gy)
Nonfunctioning	50.4 (45–50.4) Gy[a]	15 (12–20) Gy to tumor margin
Functioning	50.4 (50.4–54) Gy[a]	25 (15–30) Gy to tumor margin

FSRT, fractionated stereotactic radiation therapy.
[a]Conventional radiotherapy prescribed to isocenter; FSRT prescribed to isocenter or 90%–95% surface isodose.

physical means, which have ranged from the use of an invasive halo-ring, a radiocamera bite block, various noninvasive head frames, to improved thermoplastic masks. The desired level of accuracy can also be achieved through image-guidance techniques, such as those coupled with robotic linear accelerators.

Simulation

FSRT is always a three-dimensional treatment modality. Patients are imaged with thin-slice (≤2.0 mm) contrast-enhanced CT in the immobilization system (which may include an external fiducial system, depending on the delivery system). A thin-slice (≤2.0 mm) MRI is performed to help in volume definition. These imaging studies are then coregistered.

Target Volume Definition

The GTV is designed with the help of all available clinical information, principally MRI. The help of a neuroradiologist should be enlisted and any ambiguous area (e.g., difficulties in discriminating tumor from postsurgical changes or precisely defining the extent of cavernous sinus invasion) should be included in the target volume. No additional margin is added for a CTV. In growing the GTV to a PTV, the main source of error is patient positioning. With the relocatable system used at our institution (Brainlab, Heimstetten, Germany), a 2- to 3-mm margin is used. Normal structures are identified as for conventional radiotherapy.

Treatment Planning

Planning is highly dependent on the delivery system. Options include fixed portals, multiple spherical "shots," dynamic conformal arcs, and nonisocentric robotic delivery. At McGill, our preference is for a limited number of noncoplanar fields (typically 5). This arrangement presents a good balance of simplicity, normal tissue-sparing, and conformality.

Dose Prescription

There is no standardization in the prescription or reporting of FRST doses. The way FSRT is prescribed can reflect the equipment used or the expectations an institution has for the technique. An example of a prescription favoring normal tissue protection is one in which the dose is prescribed at the isocenter with the 90% isodose surface covering the periphery of the PTV (63). At the other end of the spectrum are prescriptions to a relatively low marginal dose (80% to 83%) (18,73), thus favoring dose intensity. A dose of 50.4 Gy in 28 daily fractions of 1.8 Gy prescribed to the isocenter or a high peripheral isodose (90% to 95%) is a reasonable prescription for all adenomas.

Radiosurgery

Radiosurgery is contraindicated if the optic chiasm is closer than 3 to 5 mm to the tumor. For cases selected for radiosurgery, delivery options include various linear accelerator–based techniques and Gamma Knife (Elekta Instrument, Stockholm, Sweden) radiosurgery. After fixation of the appropriate stereotactic head frame, a high-resolution imaging study is obtained. In the case of the Gamma Knife, this is typically an MRI; for linear accelerator–based radiosurgery, a stereotactic CT scan is often registered to a high-resolution MRI. When Gamma Knife radiosurgery is used, the smallest collimators and maximum number of isocenters should be employed to produce an isodose surface (typically 50%) that matches the borders of the GTV. Linear accelerator radiosurgery planning will vary depending on whether a cone-based, micromultileaf, or nonisocentric robotic system is used. Whichever device is used, the dose to the optic chiasm must be kept <8 to 9 Gy. In the case of the Gamma Knife, this may require custom blocking of individual sources (31). A variety of conformality indices can be used to assist in determining appropriate coverage of the tumor (80), although none of these replace careful visual inspection of the isodose lines on axial imaging. The dose prescribed to the tumor margin will be 12 to 20 Gy for nonfunctioning tumors and 15 to 30 Gy for functioning adenomas.

Whether medical management should be withheld in the periradiosurgical period is debatable. It is prudent—after conferring with the patient's endocrinologist—to temporarily discontinue medical therapy prior to radiosurgery. If nothing else, this will permit a final baseline assessment of hypersecretion prior to treatment (14).

Sequelae of Treatment

The acute complications of conventional radiation therapy for pituitary tumors include fatigue, focal alopecia, and otitis (when the treatment fields enter/exit through the ears).

Noad et al. (71) performed a retrospective comparison between two groups of patients with pituitary tumors; one group had undergone transsphenoidal surgery and radiotherapy and the other group had transsphenoidal surgery alone. A decrease in cognitive function was observed regardless of treatment allocation, with a greater decrease in the radiotherapy group. Grattan-Smith et al. (36) reported on the neuropsychological assessment of 65 patients with pituitary tumors. There was an impairment of memory and executive functions that did not appear related to the use of radiotherapy or surgery, raising the possibility that the pituitary and/or hypothalamic hormones have a role in the modulation of memory and behavioral pathways.

Treatment will commonly induce pituitary hypofunction. In general, microsurgery carries the lowest risk for hypopituitarism, followed by radical radiation therapy, with the highest risk seen following combined modality therapy. The speed of onset appears to be related to the total dose and dose per fraction of radiotherapy (58,99). GH production is most sensitive to the effects of radiation (84). Estimates of the risk of hypopituitarism can be found in Table 33.10.

Brada et al. (10) studied 334 patients treated at the Royal Marsden Hospital between 1962 and 1986 with surgery and postoperative radiotherapy. There were 33 cerebrovascular deaths compared to 8.04 expected with a relative risk of 4.11. The cerebrovascular death rate was higher in women, and in patients who had debulking surgery as compared with no surgery or biopsy. Age at time of radiotherapy had no impact. Suggested risk factors for increased cerebrovascular mortality were hypopituitarism, radiotherapy, and extent of surgery.

With conventionally fractionated radiation therapy, damage to the optic apparatus is rare. Most cases reported are in

Risk	Conventional Radiotherapy (%)	Radiosurgery (%)	Fractionated Stereotactic Radiotherapy (%)
Hypopituitarism	25–80	5–40[a]	10–40[a]
Injury of vision	1–2	1–2[b]	1–2
Brain necrosis	<1	<1	<1
Second malignancy	2	Unlikely[a]	≤1[a]

Table 33.10 ESTIMATES OF RISKS AND TOXICITIES FOR PATIENTS TREATED WITH PITUITARY ADENOMAS

[a]Limited data.
[b]If dose to chiasm is <9 Gy.

patients treated with doses in excess of 50 Gy or daily fractions greater than 2 Gy (50).

With single-fraction radiosurgery, injury to the optic apparatus is highly dose-dependent. There is a steep dose response, with a 27% incidence of optic neuropathy at doses between 10 and 15 Gy, 78% above 14 Gy, and only rare cases below 10 Gy (55). Prior external-beam radiotherapy to the optic apparatus is a significant risk factor and must always be taken into account. In contrast to the optic apparatus, the third through sixth cranial nerves traversing the cavernous sinus are relatively tolerant to large doses of ionizing radiation (96).

Minniti et al. (66) reported an increased risk of second brain tumors in a cohort of 426 patients treated with conservative surgery and external beam radiotherapy. The cumulative risk of second brain tumors (mainly meningiomas and high-grade astrocytomas) was 2.4% at 20 years. In contrast, in a series of 332 cases treated with a uniform megavoltage technique at St. Bartholomew's Hospital and followed for a median of 11 years, no excess intracranial malignancies were seen (46).

Finally, brain necrosis is very rare in patients irradiated for pituitary tumors, with a risk of approximately 0.04% at doses between 45 and 50.4 Gy (32,40).

References

1. Abosch A, Tyrrell JB, Lamborn KR, et al. Transsphenoidal microsurgery for growth hormone-secreting pituitary adenomas: initial outcome and long-term results. *J Clin Endocrinol Metab* 1998;83:3411–3418.
2. af Trampe EA, Lundell G, Lax I, et al. External irradiation of growth hormone producing pituitary adenomas: prolactin as a marker of hypothalamic and pituitary effects. *Int J Radiat Oncol Biol Phys* 1991;20:655–660.
3. Al-Shraim M, Asa SL. The 2004 World Health Organization classification of pituitary tumors: what is new? *Acta Neuropathol (Berl)* 2006;111:1–7.
4. Atkinson AB, Kennedy A, Wiggam MI, et al. Long-term remission rates after pituitary surgery for Cushing's disease: the need for long-term surveillance. *Clin Endocrinol (Oxf)* 2005;63:549–559.
5. Attanasio R, Epaminonda P, Motti E, et al. Gamma-knife radiosurgery in acromegaly: a 4-year follow-up study. *J Clin Endocrinol Metab* 2003;88:3105–3112.
6. Barker FG 2nd, Klibanski A, Swearingen B. Transsphenoidal surgery for pituitary tumors in the United States, 1996–2000: mortality, morbidity, and the effects of hospital and surgeon volume. *J Clin Endocrinol Metab* 2003;88:4709–4719.
7. Beck-Peccoz P, Brucker-Davis F, Persani L, et al. Thyrotropin-secreting pituitary tumors. *Endocr Rev* 1996;17:610–638.
8. Boucot N, Dohan FC, Raventos A, et al. Roentgen therapy in Cushing's syndrome without adrenocortical tumor. *J Clin Endocrinol Metab* 1957;17:8–32.
9. Brada M, Ajithkumar TV, Minniti G. Radiosurgery for pituitary adenomas. *Clin Endocrinol (Oxf)* 2004;61:531–543.
10. Brada M, Ashley S, Ford D, et al. Cerebrovascular mortality in patients with pituitary adenoma. *Clin Endocrinol (Oxf)* 2002;57:713–717.
11. Brada M, Rajan B, Traish D, et al. The long-term efficacy of conservative surgery and radiotherapy in the control of pituitary adenomas. *Clin Endocrinol (Oxf)* 1993;38:571–578.
12. Brucker-Davis F, Oldfield EH, Skarulis MC, et al. Thyrotropin-secreting pituitary tumors: diagnostic criteria, thyroid hormone sensitivity, and treatment outcome in 25 patients followed at the National Institutes of Health. *J Clin Endocrinol Metab* 1999;84:476–486.
13. Caruso M, Shaw E, Davis D. Radiation treatment of growth hormone secreting pituitary adenomas. *Int J Radiat Oncol Biol Phys* 1991;21[Suppl]:121–122.
14. Castinetti F, Taieb D, Kuhn JM, et al. Outcome of gamma knife radiosurgery in 82 patients with acromegaly: correlation with initial hypersecretion. *J Clin Endocrinol Metab* 2005;90:4483–4488.
15. Choi JY, Chang JH, Chang JW, et al. Radiological and hormonal responses of functioning pituitary adenomas after gamma knife radiosurgery. *Yonsei Med J* 2003;44:602–607.
16. Colao A, Di Sarno A, Cappabianca P, et al. Withdrawal of long-term cabergoline therapy for tumoral and nontumoral hyperprolactinemia. *N Engl J Med* 2003;349:2023–2033.
17. Colin P, Jovenin N, Delemer B, et al. Treatment of pituitary adenomas by fractionated stereotactic radiotherapy: a prospective study of 110 patients. *Int J Radiat Oncol Biol Phys* 2005;62:333–341.
18. Colin P, Scavarda D, Delemer B, et al. [Fractionated stereotactic radiotherapy: results in hypophyseal adenomas, acoustic neurinomas, and meningiomas of the cavernous sinus]. *Cancer Radiother* 1998;2:207–214.
19. Couldwell WT. Transsphenoidal and transcranial surgery for pituitary adenomas. *J Neurooncol* 2004;69:237–256.
20. Daly AF, Jaffrain-Rea ML, Beckers A. Clinical and genetic features of familial pituitary adenomas. *Horm Metab Res* 2005;37:347–354.
21. Davis DH, Laws ER Jr., Ilstrup DM, et al. Results of surgical treatment for growth hormone-secreting pituitary adenomas. *J Neurosurg* 1993;79:70–75.
22. Dekkers OM, Pereira AM, Roelfsema F, et al. Observation alone after transsphenoidal surgery for non-functioning pituitary macroadenoma. *J Clin Endocrinol Metab* 2006.
23. Devin JK, Allen GS, Cmelak AJ, et al. The efficacy of linear accelerator radiosurgery in the management of patients with Cushing's disease. *Stereotact Funct Neurosurg* 2004;82:254–262.
24. Eastman RC, Gorden P, Glatstein E, et al. Radiation therapy of acromegaly. *Endocrinol Metab Clin North Am* 1992;21:693–712.
25. Eastman RC, Gorden P, Roth J. Conventional supervoltage irradiation is an effective treatment for acromegaly. *J Clin Endocrinol Metab* 1979;48:931–940.
26. Estrada J, Boronat M, Mielgo M, et al. The long-term outcome of pituitary irradiation after unsuccessful transsphenoidal surgery in Cushing's disease. *N Engl J Med* 1997;336:172–177.
27. Feek CM, McLelland J, Seth J, et al. How effective is external pituitary irradiation for growth hormone-secreting pituitary tumors? *Clin Endocrinol (Oxf)* 1984;20:401–408.
28. Feigl GC, Bonelli CM, Berghold A, et al. Effects of gamma knife radiosurgery of pituitary adenomas on pituitary function. *J Neurosurg* 2002;97:415–421.
29. Feldkamp J, Santen R, Harms E, et al. Incidentally discovered pituitary lesions: high frequency of macroadenomas and hormone-secreting adenomas—results of a prospective study. *Clin Endocrinol (Oxf)* 1999;51:109–113.
30. Fernando MA, Heaney AP. Alpha1-adrenergic receptor antagonists: novel therapy for pituitary adenomas. *Mol Endocrinol* 2005;19:3085–3096.
31. Flickinger JC, Maitz A, Kalend A, et al. Treatment volume shaping with selective beam blocking using the Leksell gamma unit. *Int J Radiat Oncol Biol Phys* 1990;19:783–789.
32. Flickinger JC, Nelson PB, Taylor FH, et al. Incidence of cerebral infarction after radiotherapy for pituitary adenoma. *Cancer* 1989;63:2404–2408.
33. Freda PU. Somatostatin analogs in acromegaly. *J Clin Endocrinol Metab* 2002;87:3013–3018.
34. Gittoes NJ, Bates AS, Tse W. Radiation therapy for non-functioning pituitary tumors. *Clin Endocrinol* 1998;48:331–337.
35. Gomez F, Reyes FI, Faiman C. Nonpuerperal galactorrhea and hyperprolactinemia. Clinical findings, endocrine features and therapeutic responses in 56 cases. *Am J Med* 1977;62:648–660.
36. Grattan-Smith PJ, Morris JG, Shores EA, et al. Neuropsychological abnormalities in patients with pituitary tumours. *Acta Neurol Scand* 1992;86:626–631.
37. Greenman Y, Ouaknine G, Veshchev I, et al. Postoperative surveillance of clinically nonfunctioning pituitary macroadenomas: markers of tumour quiescence and regrowth. *Clin Endocrinol (Oxf)* 2003;58:763–769.
38. Grigsby PW, Simpson JR, Emami BN, et al. Prognostic factors and results of surgery and postoperative irradiation in the management of pituitary adenomas. *Int J Radiat Oncol Biol Phys* 1989;16:1411–1417.
39. Grigsby PW, Simpson JR, Stokes S, et al. Results of surgery and irradiation or irradiation alone for pituitary adenomas. *J Neurooncol* 1988;6:129–134.
40. Grigsby PW, Stokes S, Marks JE, et al. Prognostic factors and results of radiotherapy alone in the management of pituitary adenomas. *Int J Radiat Oncol Biol Phys* 1988;15:1103–1110.
41. Halberg FE, Sheline GE. Radiation therapy of pituitary tumors. *Endocrinol Metab Clin* 1997;16:667–684.
42. Hardy J, Vezina JL. Transsphenoidal neurosurgery of intracranial neoplasm. *Adv Neurol* 1976;15:261–273.
43. Heaney AP, Fernando M, Melmed S. PPAR-gamma receptor ligands: novel therapy for pituitary adenomas. *J Clin Invest* 2003;111:1381–1388.
44. Imaki T, Tsushima T, Hizuka N, et al. Postoperative plasma cortisol levels predict long-term outcome in patients with Cushing's disease and determine which patients should be treated with pituitary irradiation after surgery. *Endocr J* 2001;48:53–62.
45. Izawa M, Hayashi M, Nakaya K, et al. Gamma knife radiosurgery for pituitary adenomas. *J Neurosurg* 2000;93[Suppl 3]:19–22.
46. Jones A. Radiation oncogenesis in relation to the treatment of pituitary tumours. *Clin Endocrinol (Oxf)* 1991;35:379–397.
47. Kajiwara K, Saito K, Yoshikawa K, et al. Image-guided stereotactic radiosurgery with the CyberKnife for pituitary adenomas. *Minim Invasive Neurosurg* 2005;48:91–96.
48. Kaltsas GA, Mukherjee JJ, Plowman PN, et al. The role of cytotoxic chemotherapy in the management of aggressive and malignant pituitary tumors. *J Clin Endocrinol Metab* 1998;83:4233–4238.
49. Kaltsas GA, Nomikos P, Kontogeorgos G, et al. Clinical review: diagnosis and management of pituitary carcinomas. *J Clin Endocrinol Metab* 2005;90:3089–3099.
50. Khaouam L, Souhami L, Albuloushi A, et al. Review of the results of patients treated with radiotherapy for pituitary macroadenomas between 1992 and 2003 at McGill University. *Radiother Oncol* 2004;71[Suppl]:S37–38.
51. Kobayashi T, Kida Y, Mori Y. Gamma knife radiosurgery in the treatment of Cushing disease: long-term results. *J Neurosurg* 2002;97:422–428.
52. Landolt AM, Lomax N. Gamma knife radiosurgery for prolactinomas. *J Neurosurg* 2000;93[Suppl 3]:14–18.
53. Laws ER Jr, Vance ML. Radiosurgery for pituitary tumors and craniopharyngiomas. *Neurosurg Clin North Am* 1999;10:327–336.

Clinical Radiation Oncology

54. Laws ER, Jane JA Jr. Neurosurgical approach to treating pituitary adenomas. *Growth Horm IGF Res* 2005;15[Suppl A]:S36–41.

55. Leber KA, Bergloff J, Pendl G. Dose-response tolerance of the visual pathways and cranial nerves of the cavernous sinus to stereotactic radiosurgery. *J Neurosurg* 1998;88:43–50.

56. Levy RP, Fabrikant JI, Frankel KA, et al. Heavy-charged-particle radiosurgery of the pituitary gland: clinical results of 840 patients. *Stereotact Funct Neurosurg* 1991;57:22–35.

57. Lim YL, Leem W, Kim TS, et al. Four years' experiences in the treatment of pituitary adenomas with gamma knife radiosurgery. *Stereotact Funct Neurosurg* 1998;70[Suppl 1]:95–109.

58. Littley MD, Shalet SM, Beardwell CG, et al. Hypopituitarism following external radiotherapy for pituitary tumours in adults. *Q J Med* 1989;70:145–160.

59. Littley MD, Shalet SM, Beardwell CG, et al. Long-term follow-up of low-dose external pituitary irradiation for Cushing's disease. *Clin Endocrinol (Oxf)* 1990;33:445–455.

60. Lloyd RV, Kovacs K, Young WFJ, et al. In: DeLellis RA, Lloyd RV, Heitz PU, et al., eds. *Pathology and genetics. Tumours of the pituitary gland*. IARC, Lyon, France: IARC, 2004:9–48.

61. Macleod AF, Clarke DG, Pambakian H, et al. Treatment of acromegaly by external irradiation. *Clin Endocrinol (Oxf)* 1989;30:303–314.

62. Melmed S, Casanueva F, Cavagnini F, et al. Consensus statement: medical management of acromegaly. *Eur J Endocrinol* 2005;153:737–740.

63. Milker-Zabel S, Debus J, Thilmann C, et al. Fractionated stereotactically guided radiotherapy and radiosurgery in the treatment of functional and nonfunctional adenomas of the pituitary gland. *Int J Radiat Oncol Biol Phys* 2001;50:1279–1286.

64. Milker-Zabel S, Zabel A, Huber P, et al. Stereotactic conformal radiotherapy in patients with growth hormone-secreting pituitary adenoma. *Int J Radiat Oncol Biol Phys* 2004;59:1088–1096.

65. Minniti G, Traish D, Ashley S, et al. Fractionated stereotactic conformal radiotherapy for secreting and nonsecreting pituitary adenomas. *Clin Endocrinol (Oxf)* 2006;64:542–548.

66. Minniti G, Traish D, Ashley S, et al. Risk of second brain tumor after conservative surgery and radiotherapy for pituitary adenoma: update after an additional 10 years. *J Clin Endocrinol Metab* 2005;90:800–804.

67. Mitsumori M, Shrieve DC, Alexander E 3rd, et al. Initial clinical results of LINAC-based stereotactic radiosurgery and stereotactic radiotherapy for pituitary adenomas. *Int J Radiat Oncol Biol Phys* 1998;42:573–580.

68. Mokry M, Ramschak-Schwarzer S, Simbrunner J, et al. A six year experience with the postoperative radiosurgical management of pituitary adenomas. *Stereotact Funct Neurosurg* 1999;72[Suppl 1]:88–100.

69. Molitch ME. In: Melmed S, ed. *The pituitary Prolactinoma*. Malden, MA: Blackwell Publishing; 2002: 455–495.

70. Muacevic A, Uhl E, Wowra B. Gamma knife radiosurgery for nonfunctioning pituitary adenomas. *Acta Neurochir Suppl* 2004;91:51–54.

71. Noad R, Narayanan KR, Howlett T, et al. Evaluation of the effect of radiotherapy for pituitary tumours on cognitive function and quality of life. *Clin Oncol (R Coll Radiol)* 2004;16:233–237.

72. Orth DN, Liddle GW. Results of treatment in 108 patients with Cushing's syndrome. *N Engl J Med* 1971;285:243–247.

73. Paek SH, Downes MB, Bednarz G, et al. Integration of surgery with fractionated stereotactic radiotherapy for treatment of nonfunctioning pituitary macroadenomas. *Int J Radiat Oncol Biol Phys* 2005;61:795–808.

74. Pan L, Zhang N, Wang EM, et al. Gamma knife radiosurgery as a primary treatment for prolactinomas. *J Neurosurg* 2000;93[Suppl 3]:10–13.

75. Park P, Chandler WF, Barkan AL, et al. The role of radiation therapy after surgical resection of nonfunctional pituitary macroadenomas. *Neurosurgery* 2004;55:100–107.

76. Pernicone PJ, Scheithauer BW, Sebo TJ, et al. Pituitary carcinoma: a clinicopathologic study of 15 cases. *Cancer* 1997;79:804–812.

77. Petit JH, Coon J, Yock T, et al. 2004. Proton radiosurgery in the management of functioning and non-functioning pituitary adenomas: a 10-year experience at the Massachusetts General Hospital. Abstr 1094. 46th Annual Meeting of the American Society for Therapeutic Radiology and Oncology, October 3–7, 2004, Atlanta, GA.

78. Petrovich Z, Yu C, Giannotta SL, et al. Gamma knife radiosurgery for pituitary adenoma: early results. *Neurosurgery* 2003;53:51–61.

79. Picozzi P, Losa M, Mortini P, et al. Radiosurgery and the prevention of regrowth of incompletely removed nonfunctioning pituitary adenomas. *J Neurosurg* 2005;102[Suppl]:71–74.

80. Podgorsak E, Podgorsak M. In: Van Dyk J, ed. *The modern technology of radiation oncology: Stereotactic irradiation*. Madison, WI: Medical Physics Publishing, 1999:589–639.

81. Pollock BE, Carpenter PC. Stereotactic radiosurgery as an alternative to fractionated radiotherapy for patients with recurrent or residual nonfunctioning pituitary adenomas. *Neurosurgery* 2003;53:1084–1091.

82. Pollock BE, Nippoldt TB, Stafford SL, et al. Results of stereotactic radiosurgery in patients with hormone-producing pituitary adenomas: factors associated with endocrine normalization. *J Neurosurg* 2002;97:525–530.

83. Rähn T, Thorén M, Werner S. In: Faglia G, Beck-Peccoz P, Ambrosi B, et al., eds. *Pituitary adenomas: New trends in basic and clinical research*. Proceedings of the 5th European Workshop on Pituitary Adenomas; March 7–20, 1991, Venice, Italy. Amsterdam: Elsevier Science Publishers, 1991:303–312.

84. Richards GE, Wara WM, Grumbach MM, et al. Delayed onset of hypopituitarism: sequelae of therapeutic irradiation of central nervous system, eye, and middle ear tumors. *J Pediatr* 1976;89:553–559.

85. Ronson BB, Schulte RW, Han KP, et al. Fractionated proton beam irradiation of pituitary adenomas. *Int J Radiat Oncol Biol Phys* 2006;64:425–434.

86. Roth J, Gorden P, Brace K. Efficacy of conventional pituitary irradiation in acromegaly. *N Engl J Med* 1970;282:1385–1391.

87. Selman WR, Laws ER Jr, Scheithauer BW, et al. The occurrence of dural invasion in pituitary adenomas. *J Neurosurg* 1986;64:402–407.

88. Sheehan JM, Vance ML, Sheehan JP, et al. Radiosurgery for Cushing's disease after failed transsphenoidal surgery. *J Neurosurg* 2000;93:738–742.

89. Sheehan JP, Kondziolka D, Flickinger J, et al. Radiosurgery for residual or recurrent nonfunctioning pituitary adenoma. *J Neurosurg* 2002;97:408–414.

90. Sheehan JP, Niranjan A, Sheehan JM, et al. Stereotactic radiosurgery for pituitary adenomas: an intermediate review of its safety, efficacy, and role in the neurosurgical treatment armamentarium. *J Neurosurg* 2005;102:678–691.

91. Sheline GE, Wara WM. In: Seydel HG, ed. *Tumors of the central nervous system: Radiation therapy of acromegaly and non-secretory chromophobe adenomas*. New York, NY: Wiley; 1983: 119–131.

92. Sheline GE. In: Linfoot JA, ed. *Recent advances in the diagnosis and treatment of pituitary tumors: The role of conventional radiation therapy in the treatment of functional pituitary tumors*. New York, NY: Raven Press, 1979:289–313.

93. Socin HV, Chanson P, Delemer B, et al. The changing spectrum of TSH-secreting pituitary adenomas: diagnosis and management in 43 patients. *Eur J Endocrinol* 2003;148:433–442.

94. Teramoto A, Hirakawa K, Sanno N, et al. Incidental pituitary lesions in 1,000 unselected autopsy specimens. *Radiology* 1994;193:161–164.

95. Thoren M, Rahn T, Guo WY, et al. Stereotactic radiosurgery with the cobalt-60 gamma unit in the treatment of growth hormone-producing pituitary tumors. *Neurosurgery* 1991;29:663–668.

96. Tishler RB, Loeffler JS, Lunsford LD, et al. Tolerance of cranial nerves of the cavernous sinus to radiosurgery. *Int J Radiat Oncol Biol Phys* 1993;27:215–221.

97. Trainer PJ, Drake WM, Katznelson L, et al. Treatment of acromegaly with the growth hormone-receptor antagonist pegvisomant. *N Engl J Med* 2000;342:1171–1177.

98. Tsagarakis S, Grossman A, Plowman PN, et al. Megavoltage pituitary irradiation in the management of prolactinomas: long-term follow-up. *Clin Endocrinol (Oxf)* 1991;34:399–406.

99. Tsang RW, Brierley JD, Panzarella T, et al. Radiation therapy for pituitary adenoma: treatment outcome and prognostic factors. *Int J Radiat Oncol Biol Phys* 1994;30:557–565.

100. Tsang RW, Brierley JD, Panzarella T, et al. Role of radiation therapy in clinical hormonally-active pituitary adenomas. *Radiother Oncol* 1996;41:45–53.

101. van't Verlaat JW, Croughs RJ. Withdrawal of bromocriptine after long-term therapy for macroprolactinomas; effect on plasma prolactin and tumour size. *Clin Endocrinol (Oxf)* 1991;34:175–178.

102. Vance ML, Chernavvsky DR, Steiner L, et al. Relapse of Cushing's disease after successful gamma knife treatment, pp. OR9–4. 87th annual meeting Endocrine Society. June 4–7, 2005. San Diego, CA.

103. Vladyka V, Liscak R, Simonova G, et al. [Radiosurgical treatment of hypophyseal adenomas with the gamma knife: results in a group of 163 patients during a 5-year period]. *Cas Lek Cesk* 2000;139:757–766.

104. Voduc KD, Ma R, McKenzie M. Fractionated steretactic radiotherapy (SRT) for pituitary adenomas. *J Clin Oncol* 2005;23: Abstract 1543.

105. Wang LG, Guo Y, Zhang X, et al. [Analysis of the results of 143 cases of pituitary micro-adenoma treated by Linac X-Knife stereotactic radioneurosurgery]. *Ai Zheng* 2003;22:510–513.

106. Webster J, Piscitelli G, Polli A, et al. A comparison of cabergoline and bromocriptine in the treatment of hyperprolactinemic amenorrhea. Cabergoline Comparative Study Group. *N Engl J Med* 1994;331:904–909.

107. Wilson RR. Radiological uses of fast protons. *Radiology* 1946;47:487–491.

108. Witt TC. Stereotactic radiosurgery for pituitary tumors. *Neurosurg Focus* 2003;14::e10.

109. Wright AD, Hill DM, Lowy C, et al. Mortality in acromegaly. *Q J Med* 1970;39:1–16.

110. Zhang N, Pan L, Wang EM, et al. Radiosurgery for growth hormone-producing pituitary adenomas. *J Neurosurg* 2000;93[Suppl 3]:6–9.

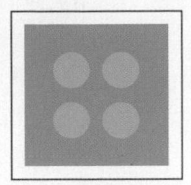

Chapter 34
Spinal Canal

Jeff M. Michalski

Tumors of the spinal cord and cauda equina account for 4% of all central nervous system (CNS) tumors overall and for 6% of CNS tumors in children (9). They are classified by their location relative to the protective layers of the spinal cord (Fig. 34.1). Intramedullary lesions arise from the intrinsic substance of the spinal cord. The histopathology of intramedullary spinal cord neoplasms includes gliomas such as astrocytomas, ependymomas, and oligodendrogliomas. Intradural–extramedullary tumors arise from the connective tissues, blood vessels, or coverings adjacent to the cord or cauda equina. Common histologies include ependymoma, nerve sheath tumors, meningioma, and vascular tumors. Finally, some tumors are extradural; they are commonly metastatic, although primary tumors in this compartment may occur. Primary extradural tumors may arise from the vertebral bodies and include benign or malignant bone tumors. Nonmetastatic tumors arising in an extradural spinal location include epidural hemangiomas, lipomas, extradural meningiomas, nerve sheath tumors, and lymphomas.

Radiation therapy is an important modality in the management of both primary and metastatic tumors involving the spinal canal. This chapter focuses on the management of primary spinal cord tumors. Primary extradural tumors are usually managed in a manner similar to tumors arising at other locations and will not be discussed here.

Anatomy of the Spinal Cord

The spinal cord is a slender cylinder composed of functional segments corresponding to 31 pairs of spinal nerves: Eight cervical, 12 thoracic, five lumbar, five sacral, and one coccygeal. Unlike the brain, the white matter of the spinal cord is located in the periphery and surrounds the central gray matter. The gray matter contains the cell bodies of sensory, motor, and autonomic neurons. On cross-section, the gray matter is a butterfly-shaped region with anterior horns controlling motor function, lateral horns (in the thoracic and upper lumbar region) controlling autonomic functions, and posterior horns involved in sensation. The white matter contains the axonal elements of neurons that transmit impulses to and from the brain. As in the brain, the axons of the spinal cord white matter possess a myelin sheath formed by the cytoplasmic extension of glial cells. Schwann cells sheath the spinal nerves that enter and exit the spinal cord. The spinal cord is organized into somatotopically distinct regions (Fig. 34.2). The lateral and anterior spinal cord white matter contains the nerve tracts that are involved with fine motor control and tone, including the corticospinal tracts. The spinocerebellar tracts transmit muscle stretch and tone sensation from the extremities to the cerebellum. The lateral spinal thalamic tract is located laterally near the spinal cord surface and carries ascending crossed pain fibers to the thalamus. The dorsal columns transmit fine touch and positional sensation from the extremities to the brain. Because of its serial organization, injury to the spinal cord results in characteristic neurologic findings that depend on the location of the insult.

The spinal cord is surrounded by the meninges, the innermost of which is the pia mater that covers the spinal cord and its blood vessels. This layer condenses laterally into approximately 20 pair of dentate ligaments, which suspend the cord to the dura mater.

The dura mater forms a dense, fibrous barrier between the bony spinal canal and the spinal cord. The dura ends inferiorly at the level of the second sacral vertebra but continues with the filum terminale down to the coccyx. The arachnoid mater resides between the dura mater and the pia mater.

The arachnoid encloses the subarachnoid space filled with cerebrospinal fluid (CSF). The subarachnoid space follows the arachnoid down to the end of the dural sac. At each spinal ganglion and nerve, there is a subarachnoid space sleeve. CSF pressure depends on body position. With a person in a horizontal position, normal CSF pressure is 70 to 200 mm H_2O, increasing to 100 to 300 mm H_2O in an erect position (measured in the lumbar region) (85). The amount of CSF is normally 150 mL, with a turnover of 300 mL each 24 hours.

The growth of the vertebral column takes place at a rate and to an extent greater than that of the spinal cord. By adulthood, the spinal cord is nearly 25 cm shorter than the vertebral column and ends near the level of the L1 vertebral body. Because of this differential growth, the exit level of each pair of spinal nerves in the spinal cord is usually higher than the corresponding vertebral body level. In the adult, the C8 nerve root leaves the cord at the C6 vertebral body, the T6 nerve at the T3 vertebral level, and the T12 nerve at the T9 vertebral level. All of the lumbar nerves exit the spinal cord from vertebral levels T10 through T12, and all of the sacral nerves exit the spinal cord near the L1 vertebral level. The lower lumbar, sacral, and coccygeal nerves form the cauda equina, the collection of nerves that fills the thecal sac below L1. At its most caudal extent, the cord tapers to a thin segment, the conus medullaris. It is tethered to the coccyx by the filum terminale, a dense thread of pia mater.

Spinal Canal

The posterior body surfaces and arches of the vertebrae form the spinal canal. It is triangular in the lumbar and cervical regions, where the cord is mostly mobile, and round in the thoracic region.

The spinal canal is lined with ligaments, including the posterior longitudinal ligament on its anterior wall, the flaval ligaments between adjacent arches, and the interspinous ligaments between the spinous processes.

Blood Supply

Two posterolateral arteries and one anterior longitudinal artery, formed by radicular arteries that enter through the intervertebral foramina, supply the spinal cord. The vertebral artery supplies the cervical and upper thoracic segments. The mid thoracic region is supplied from the radicular artery at approximately T7, and the thoracolumbar region is supplied from the lower thoracic radicular artery. The venous drainage for the cord and the spine is more extensive. Intradural and extradural

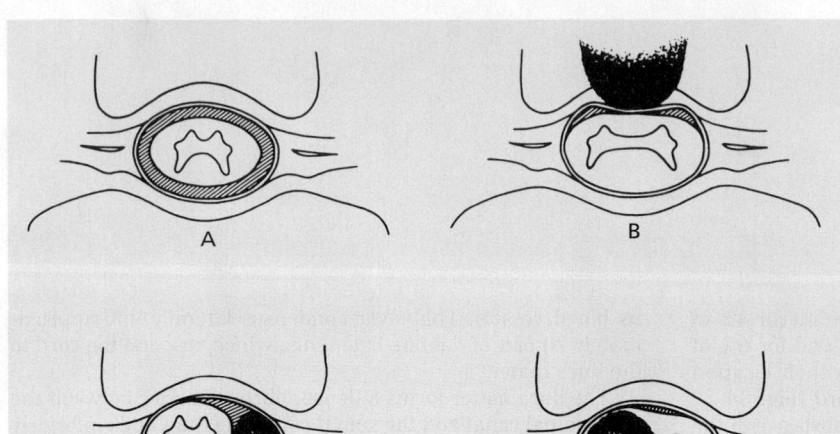

FIGURE 34.1. Neoplasms affecting the spinal cord. **A:** Normal transverse spine. The spinal cord is enveloped by the pia, arachnoid, and dura mater, which are housed in the spinal canal and surrounded by ligaments supporting the vertebral bony structures. The subarachnoid space contains cerebrospinal fluid (*striped*). **B:** Transverse spine with extradural mass. An extradural mass (e.g., metastasis) from the vertebral body is compressing the dural sac and the spinal cord from the anterior direction. The subarachnoid space becomes obliterated at that level, causing a myelographic block. **C:** Transverse spine with an intradural–extramedullary mass. The mass, typically a meningioma or nerve sheath tumor, is compressing the spinal cord and roots in the dural sac, causing a myelographic block with a laterally displaced cord and, at times, producing a capping contour of contrast border. **D:** Transverse spine with intramedullary mass. An intramedullary mass (astrocytoma or ependymoma) is infiltrating and expanding the spinal cord within the dural sac, causing a myelographic block.

venous plexuses communicate with each other and with intervertebral veins through the vertebral foramina (85).

Epidemiology

Primary spinal canal tumors comprise 4% to 6% of all primary CNS tumors (56). True primary spinal cord neoplasms are relatively rare and typically intradural in location. In adults, nearly two-thirds of all intradural tumors are extramedullary and are typically nerve sheath tumors, meningiomas, or ependymomas. The other third of intradural tumors are intramedullary, with the most common histologies being astrocytoma and ependymoma, followed by hemangioblastoma and other tumor types (Table 34.1). Extramedullary nerve sheath tumors and meningiomas represent the most common spinal canal neoplasms, followed by intramedullary ependymomas and astrocytomas. The spine is frequently involved by metastatic cancer. Metastatic tumors can invade the vertebral bones, epidural soft tissues, or even the spinal cord itself.

Primary tumors of the spinal canal are relatively more frequent in children (33,91), and more than 50% of pediatric patients are younger than 10 years of age (14,18). In a review of 872 children with intraspinal tumors, 36% had intramedullary tumors, 27% had intradural extramedullary tumors, and 24% had extradural tumors (13% were unclassified) (14). Nearly 75% of pediatric intramedullary tumors were astrocytomas or gangliogliomas, and few were ependymomas. Approximately 25% of the intradural–extramedullary tumors were ependymomas, followed in incidence by dermoids (23%), teratomas (16%), nerve sheath tumors (14%), lipomas (13%), and meningiomas (9%) (14). In adults, extramedullary nerve sheath tumors and meningiomas represent the most common spinal canal neoplasms, followed by intramedullary ependymomas and astrocytomas.

Natural History

Most primary tumors of the spinal canal are histologically benign. Despite this, they are often the cause of significant disability because they compress or invade the spinal cord and interfere with neurologic function. Intramedullary tumors produce neurologic damage by local invasion or cystic compression

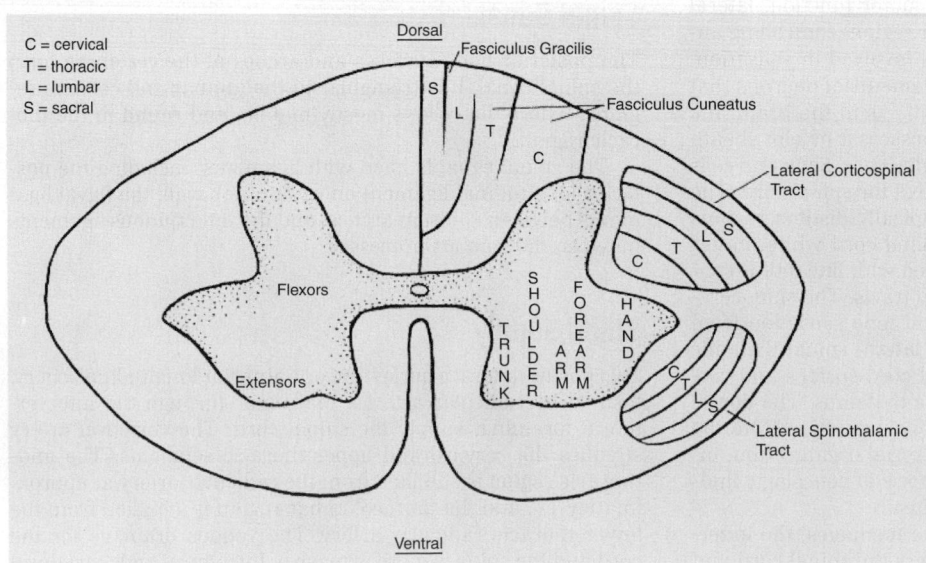

FIGURE 34.2. Somatotopic organization of the cervical spinal cord in transection. (From Devinsky O, Feldman E. *Examination of the cranial and peripheral nerves.* Philadelphia: Churchill Livingstone, 1988, with permission.)

Table 34.1	PRIMARY SPINAL CANAL TUMORS: LOCATIONS, TYPES, AND FREQUENCIES

Location	Frequency (%)	Type	Comments
Extradural	Few	Meningioma	~10% of spinal meningiomas
Intradural–extramedullary	70	Nerve sheath tumor	45% of primary tumors in this location, thoracic preference
		Meningioma	<40% of primary tumors at this location, thoracic preference
		Ependymoma in cauda	60% of all spinal ependymomas
		Vascular malformations	<10% of primary tumors at this location
		Teratoma, dermoid, squamous cell neoplasia	10% of primary tumors at this location, sacrococcygeal preference
		Lipoma	Few, subpial
Intradural–intramedullary	30	Ependymoma in cord	<40% of all spinal canal ependymomas
		Astrocytoma	<45% of primary tumors at this location
		Vascular malformations	Rare
		Oligodendroglioma	~15% of primary tumors at this location
		Teratoma	Rare
		Hemangioma	Rare

of the cord, whereas extramedullary lesions compress, stretch, or distort the cord or the spinal nerves. Primary spinal cord tumors may be focal or relatively localized in some patients but may involve nearly the entire length of the cord in others. In one report, 73% of affected children presented with widening of the entire spinal cord from the medulla or cervical medullary junction to the conus medullaris (20). These "holocord" tumors typically consist of a discrete solid mass and associated cystic component or syrinx that extends over a significant length of the spinal cord. Local tumor progression is the dominant form of treatment failure of spinal cord tumors. CSF seeding is possible but is uncommon (33,41,50,85). The major causes of death in patients with spinal canal tumors are complications of paraplegia or quadriplegia such as infection or respiratory compromise. Because the CNS has no lymphatics, spread to lymph nodes is not seen with spinal canal tumors. Likewise, hematogenous spread is extremely rare.

Clinical Presentation

Pain is the presenting symptom in nearly 75% of patients. Often the pain is localized to the region of involvement and may be present for a long time before the patient manifests localizing neurologic signs. Radicular pain, a result of pressure on nerve roots, reflects the distribution of the involved root and indicates that conduction is intact. Extramedullary tumors can cause distention of the dura with pain severe in the region of the tumor that is characteristically aggravated by recumbency because of venous congestion. Thus, pain is often worse at night (20). Movement or the Valsalva maneuver also may worsen pain. Less commonly, pain is characterized as a burning sensation in one or more extremities. Numbness replacing pain is a more advanced sign that indicates compromise of spinal nerve or nerve tract conduction.

Other symptoms of CNS involvement include weakness (75% of patients), sensory changes (65%), and sphincter dysfunction (15%) (33). Low-grade tumors in general have a more prolonged duration of symptoms than high-grade tumors. Bladder and bowel dysfunction as presenting symptoms are relatively uncommon except for tumors that involve the conus medullaris and filum terminale.

Lower extremity weakness often manifests as a disturbance in gait. In young children, there may be a history of failure to achieve milestones, such as ambulation and voluntary control of bladder and bowel, or of regression of already acquired skills. With tumors of the cervical region, torticollis may occur in chil-

dren, but adult patients usually complain of nuchal pain and stiffness.

Tumors involving the lumbosacral spine present with a cauda equina nerve root compression syndrome. Patients may have radicular pain in the anterior (L4), lateral (L5), or posterior (S1) thigh with corresponding paresthesias followed by muscle wasting of the glutei, hamstrings, or tibialis anterior muscles. Saddle anesthesia, absent ankle reflexes (S1), or plantar (S2) responses may be present. Impotence and loss of anal or bulbar cavernous reflexes also may occur.

Diagnostic Work-Up

History and Physical Findings

Table 34.2 shows the diagnostic work-up for primary tumors of the spinal cord. The need for a meticulous and accurate patient history and physical examination cannot be overemphasized. The differential diagnosis of a patient with a spinal cord tumor may include syringomyelia, multiple sclerosis, amyotrophic lateral sclerosis, diabetic neuropathy, viral myelitis, or paraneoplastic syndromes. The neurologic examination should concentrate on testing motor and sensory functions and reflexes.

A cutaneous sensory level may be definable, although the level of cord compression is a few segments higher than the

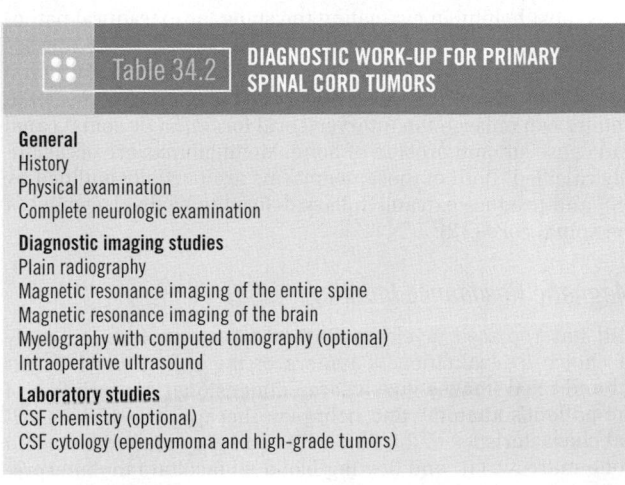

Table 34.2	DIAGNOSTIC WORK-UP FOR PRIMARY SPINAL CORD TUMORS

General
History
Physical examination
Complete neurologic examination

Diagnostic imaging studies
Plain radiography
Magnetic resonance imaging of the entire spine
Magnetic resonance imaging of the brain
Myelography with computed tomography (optional)
Intraoperative ultrasound

Laboratory studies
CSF chemistry (optional)
CSF cytology (ependymoma and high-grade tumors)

CSF, cerebrospinal fluid.

superior level of sensory loss because of pathway crossing characteristics. Loss of pain, heat, and cold sensation below a specific dermatomal level indicates compromise of the spinothalamic pathway in the lateral columns. Impaired posture, gait, and coordination and loss of vibration sense indicate compromise of the posterior spinocerebellar pathways or the posterior columns.

At the level of the lesion, flaccid weakness and loss of tendon reflexes may occur. Below the lesion, the same signs are noticed in acute stages, but spastic plegia and hyperactive tendon reflexes plus an upward Babinski's toe sign ensue in subacute and chronic stages. These findings are consistent with lower and upper motor neuron involvement, respectively. The signs and symptoms of neurologic dysfunction may be asymmetric. In some cases, a classic Brown-Séquard syndrome may be present with ipsilateral loss of motor function and fine touch sensation and contralateral loss of pain and temperature sensation below the level of the lesion.

Autonomic reflexes (e.g., sweating) frequently are increased below the level of the lesion and may encompass the whole body if the lesion is cervical (6). Sweating disappears at the level of the compressed cord. Disruption of urinary and bowel function usually occurs later than sensory and motor dysfunction. Early loss of bladder function, saddle anesthesia, and later pain characterize neoplasms of the conus medullaris and filum terminale.

Radiographic Studies

Abnormalities detected on plain films that are caused by increased intracanal pressure include erosion of vertebral pedicles, enlargement of the anteroposterior diameter of the bony canal, or scalloping of the posterior wall of the vertebral bodies. Overall, plain radiographs of the spine show abnormalities in approximately 50% of patients with primary spinal canal neoplasms (7,35,68,83). Changes are more likely to be detected on plain radiographs in children than in adults (14,18,21,37).

Calcification may be seen in extramedullary tumors, especially meningiomas, and less frequently in nerve sheath tumors. Spinal canal tumors also may be associated with scoliosis or kyphoscoliosis, especially in children (21).

Myelography, once considered the standard examination in evaluation of the spinal cord and canal, is now used only in patients who are unable to undergo magnetic resonance imaging (MRI) because of the presence of implanted ferromagnetic materials. In this situation, computed tomography (CT) scanning combined with myelography will give better spatial resolution.

Computed Tomography

CT is most helpful in evaluating the spine for extradural pathologic processes. Bone tumors or paraspinal soft tissue masses that secondarily involve the spinal cord (e.g., dumbbell tumors) can be imaged with contrast-enhanced CT scans. Nerve sheath tumors can enlarge the intervertebral foramina or spinal canal and cause smooth erosion of bone. Meningiomas are occasionally calcified. Both of these neoplasms are partially outlined by CSF and produce extramedullary deformity by displacement of the spinal cord (32).

Magnetic Resonance Imaging

MRI has replaced myelography and CT as the imaging study of choice in evaluation of tumors of the spinal canal. Sagittal and axial images give a three-dimensional appreciation of the patient's anatomy and help plan therapy. The various signal characteristics of the CSF, white and gray matter, bone and bone marrow, fat, and flowing blood all facilitate the interpretation of the study. Some cystic tumors, vascular lesions, or lipomas can be diagnosed based on their characteristic signals on T1- and T2-weighted images without contrast injection. Intravenous gadolinium-diethylenetriamine pentaacetic acid (Gd-DTPA) administration improves the sensitivity of MRI by enhancing the solid component of intramedullary tumors and differentiating them from surrounding edema or syrinx cavities (Figs. 34.3 and 34.4). Unlike low-grade gliomas in the brain, nearly all spinal cord gliomas, regardless of grade, enhance with Gd-DTPA (84). Sagittal T1-weighted images usually localize intramedullary mass neoplasms along with adjacent cysts. Intradural–extramedullary lesions also show enhancement on T1-weighted images after administration of Gd-DTPA. The use of Gd-DTPA increases the sensitivity of detecting leptomeningeal metastases (84).

MRI of the brain should be done in patients with ependymoma or anaplastic ependymoma to exclude the possibility of neuraxis seeding or the presence of an intracranial primary tumor.

Cerebrospinal Fluid

A patient suspected of having a spinal canal neoplasm should not be subjected to a lumbar puncture before MRI. Symptoms may be exacerbated after a spinal tap because of shifting of the spinal cord and incarceration before the tumor can be localized adequately (37). The CSF usually has increased protein levels and may exhibit xanthochromia, especially with extradural compression conditions, but lower values can be found in cases of intramedullary disease and with compression in the cervical region (6).

Cytological examination of the cerebrospinal fluid should be done in patients with ependymoma, anaplastic ependymoma, or high-grade glioma.

Tissue Diagnosis

Suspected primary tumors of the spinal cord and spinal canal must be pathologically confirmed in all circumstances. Strong consideration should be given to biopsy of any presumed metastatic tumors if they are the first site of disease recurrence after successful management of a previous malignant primary tumor. Percutaneous needle biopsy under fluoroscopic or CT guidance may be sufficient to establish the diagnosis of metastatic extradural or epidural tumor. In patients presenting with spinal cord compression without a prior diagnosis of cancer, a surgical decompression by laminectomy or anterior corpectomy may confirm the diagnosis and provide immediate relief of the presenting neurologic deficit. In rare circumstances in which emergency radiation therapy is indicated to relieve spinal cord compression in the absence of a confirmed cancer diagnosis, a patient should be made aware of the consequences of treatment in the absence of a definitive diagnosis, including the delay of appropriate treatment for nonmalignant etiologies.

■■ | Pathologic Classification

Intramedullary Tumors

Most intramedullary tumors of the spinal cord are glial in origin, with astrocytomas and ependymomas accounting for the majority.

Astrocytomas are the most common intramedullary spinal cord tumors, comprising 40% to 45% of all reported cases in adults. In children, 75% to 90% of intramedullary spinal cord tumors are astrocytomas, and approximately 85% of these are low-grade, fibrillary, or juvenile pilocytic astrocytomas

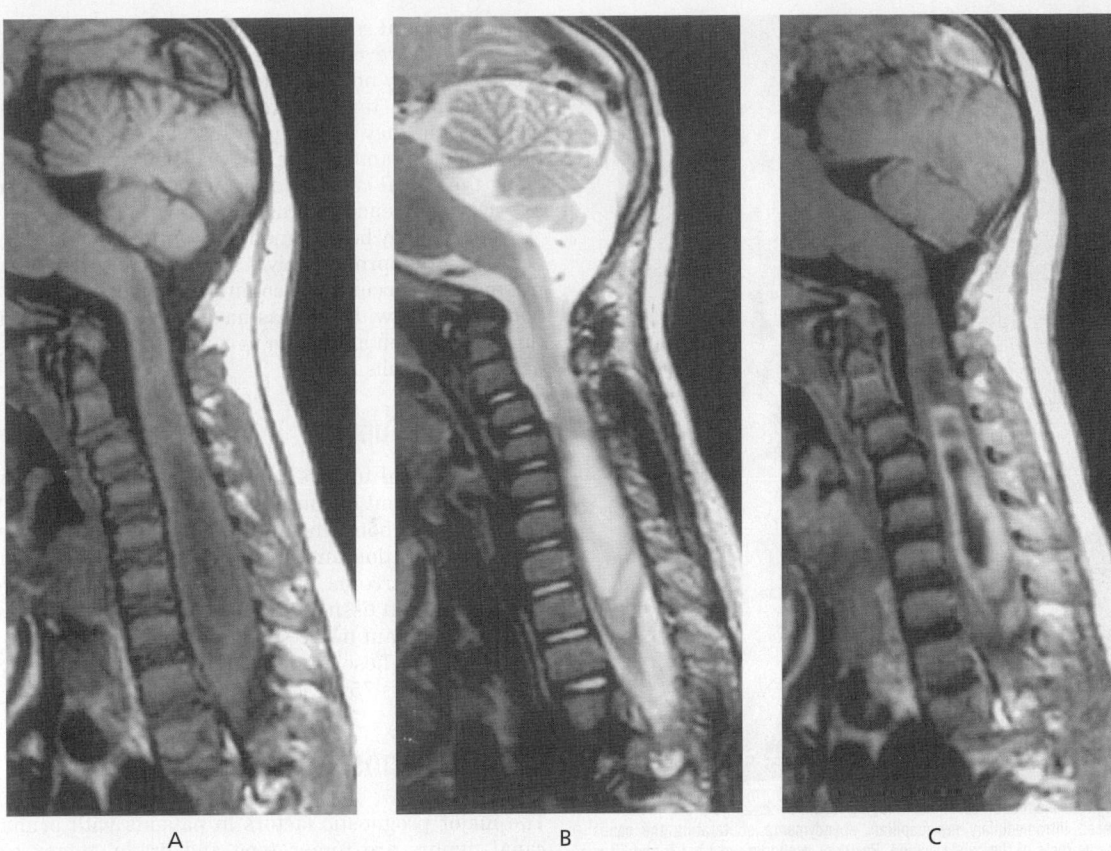

FIGURE 34.3. Sagittal magnetic resonance imaging scans of a child with a cystic astrocytoma involving the cervical spine. **A:** T1-weighted image demonstrates cystic expansion of the cervical cord. **B:** T2-weighted image demonstrates rostral and caudal extent of bright signal from tumor with narrowing of the subarachnoid space. **C:** Gadolinium enhancement suggests the neoplastic nature of the spinal cord lesion. (Courtesy of Ben Lee, M.D., Mallinckrodt Institute of Radiology, St. Louis, MO.)

(22,55,56). The latter in particular, as in other locations in the CNS, are not infiltrative in nature and recognition of this feature, along with advances in surgical techniques and intraoperative monitoring, has led neurosurgeons to manage these tumors with more radical resections (3,21,23,72). However, many fibrillary astrocytomas as well as anaplastic astrocytomas and glioblastoma multiforme are infiltrative, and complete resection carries a significant risk of neurologic disability. In these cases, a subtotal resection or biopsy may be the only safe surgical option. Less than 10% of pediatric and 25% of adult spinal cord astrocytomas are malignant (22,55).

Astrocytomas are more likely to occur in the cervical and thoracic regions than ependymomas. Astrocytomas are frequently associated with cysts that can extend rostrally or caudally for a significant distance. The cystic component of a holocord astrocytoma can contribute to a neurologic deficit.

Ependymomas are derived from glial cells similar to those lining the ventricular system. Several histologic types have been reported and include cellular, epithelial, tanycytic, subependymoma, myxopapillary, or mixed types. Ependymomas more often affect the lumbar spinal cord and cauda equina. All varieties are usually histologically benign, and they may have a long and often indolent course. Primary anaplastic ependymomas of the spinal cord are rare. Rostral tumors are more frequently cellular variants, whereas distal tumors (including those of the cauda equina) are more commonly the myxopapillary variant (12,69,75,79,82).

Approximately two-thirds of all spinal canal ependymomas occur in the lumbosacral region, and 40% arise from within the filum terminale. Most intradural–extramedullary ependymomas in the lumbosacral spine are of the myxopapillary type

(12,69,75,79,82). They frequently can be completely excised. In many circumstances, however, these tumors tightly envelope the nerve roots of the cauda equina, making en bloc excision difficult. Gross total resection of these tumors often requires piecemeal removal. The myxopapillary variant may be biologically less aggressive than the cellular variant, but late recurrences can occur even after complete gross excision; therefore, long-term follow-up of these patients is required (10,61,71,78,82).

Vascular Malformations

A variety of vascular neoplasms can arise from within the spinal cord, including arteriovenous malformations, hemangiomas, and hemangioblastomas. They frequently are associated with von Hippel-Lindau disease (55). These are benign neoplasms that are usually well circumscribed and amenable to surgery.

Intradural–Extramedullary Tumors

Most intradural–extramedullary neoplasms are meningiomas, nerve sheath tumors, or myxopapillary ependymomas. They usually are amenable to complete surgical excision.

Meningiomas are usually benign, well-encapsulated neoplasms that are easily separated from the spinal cord; most can be completely excised, and they rarely recur. They may arise anywhere within the intradural space but are found in the thoracic region in approximately 80% of patients (49,64,81). Meningiomas are uncommon in the lumbar region and rare in the sacrum. At least 80% of meningiomas occur in women 40 years of age or older (49,64).

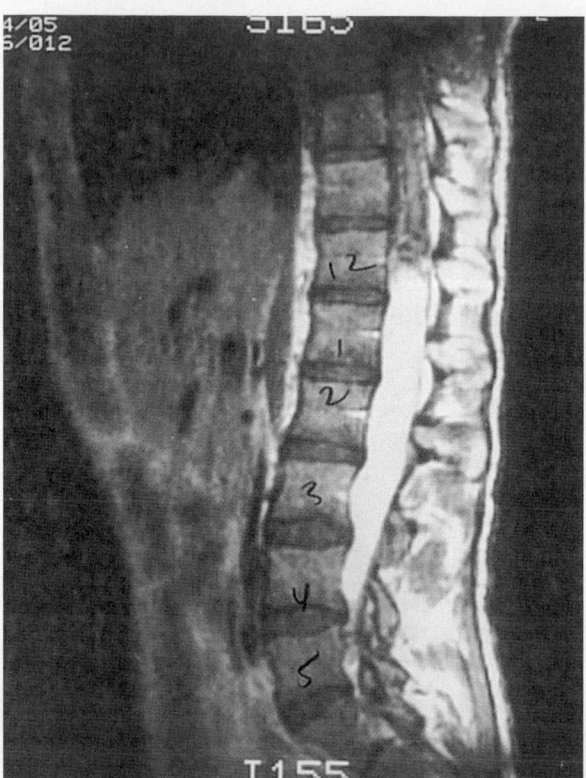

FIGURE 34.4. Sagittal magnetic resonance imaging scan of a 21-year-old man with a contrast-enhanced intramedullary myxopapillary ependymoma obliterating the conus medullaris and nerve roots of the cauda equina. Posterior scalloping of L1, L2, and L3 is demonstrated.

Nerve sheath tumors arise from the Schwann cell, the cell responsible for insulating peripheral nerves and contributing to impulse conduction. Nerve sheath tumors have been called, *neurofibroma, schwannoma, neuroma,* and *neurilemoma* in the past. More recently, a distinction between neurofibroma and schwannoma has been made. Although both tumors arise from Schwann cells, certain gross, microscopic, and clinical features help distinguish the two (56). Neurofibromas produce plexiform enlargements of the involved spinal nerve that make distinguishing the nerve from the tumor tissue impossible. Schwannomas, in contrast, are globoid and eccentrically attached to a nerve. The plexiform neurofibroma is associated with type 1 neurofibromatosis, and the presence of multiple tumors helps establish the diagnosis of this genetic condition. Nerve sheath tumors usually are solitary and may occur in any section of the spinal canal. They are evenly distributed in the cervical, thoracic, and lumbar regions; they are least common in the sacrum. They occur in men and women with equal frequency and are most commonly diagnosed in the fourth through sixth decades of life. Most of these tumors are completely intradural, although 10% to 15% may have an extradural component as well (so-called dumbbell tumors). Most nerve sheath tumors are benign, well-encapsulated lesions that are amenable to total surgical excision. The rare malignant nerve sheath tumors have a natural history similar to soft tissue sarcomas, and they should be treated as such (87).

Miscellaneous Neoplasms

Unusual intradural–extramedullary tumors include lipomas, dermoids, and epidermoid tumors.

Dermoids are so rare that their incidence is not easily assessed. There is a slight male predominance, and most occur in the lumbosacral region (73). If incompletely excised, dermoids can recur. However, their growth is slow, and clinical signs of recurrence may not be evident for many years.

Epidermoid tumors are more common in men than in women, and they are usually discovered in patients between the ages of 20 and 50 years (73). They can be seen anywhere along the spinal canal and are usually benign. If incompletely excised, recurrences are usually slow.

Lipomas may be intramedullary or extramedullary, and they account for approximately 1% of spinal canal primary neoplasms. They occur more commonly in men than in women (5). Some patients with lipomas have congenital anomalies. Small tumors are often amenable to complete removal with excellent neurologic results (17).

Extradural Tumors

Most extradural tumors are metastatic, and the presentation and management of these is discussed in Chapter 91. A variety of primary bone and soft tissue tumors may arise from an extradural location and involve the spinal canal. Bone tumors include osteosarcoma, chondrosarcoma, Ewing's sarcoma, and chordomas. Soft tissue tumors include soft tissue sarcomas, including malignant nerve sheath tumors, lymphomas, and neuroblastomas. These tumors and their management are discussed Chapters 75, 81, and 84 respectively.

Prognostic Factors

The major prognostic factors in patients with primary spinal canal tumors are tumor type and grade, tumor extent and location, patient age, and presenting neurologic function. Treatment-related factors that influence the outcome include tumor resectability and the use of radiation therapy for certain tumor types. Many of these factors are interdependent. For example, ependymomas occur most frequently in the distal spinal canal and are more often resectable than astrocytic tumors. In general, patients with ependymomas survive longer without recurrence than patients with astrocytomas (11,16,38, 40,42,47,50,80).

Several investigators have reported that patients with rostral tumors have a worse survival and neurologic outcome than patients with more caudal tumors (11,29,33,38). Guidetti et al. (38) stated that patients with cervical lesions had a higher surgical risk and complication rate, which made thorough resection of tumors in this location difficult and sometimes inadvisable. In a series of 62 patients with exclusively intramedullary ependymomas, patients with high cervical presentations (above C5) accounted for 4/6 postoperative deaths because of apneic respiratory complications (29). In the Mallinckrodt Institute of Radiology experience, Garcia (33) reported that the primary tumor location was the most important prognostic feature. It was suggested that a greater concentration of function per unit volume of the upper spinal cord compared with that of the cauda equina accounted for the worst neurologic outcome and survival in patients with rostral tumors. Chun et al. (11), from the Medical College of Virginia, also reported that patients with cervical lesions had significantly worse outcomes than patients with tumors in other sites. In both the Mallinckrodt Institute of Radiology and the Medical College of Virginia experiences, tumors affecting the rostral or cervical spinal cord were more likely to be astrocytomas, and tumors in the caudal spinal cord, filum terminale, or cauda equina were more likely to be ependymomas. The anatomic dependence of various tumor types may contribute to the better prognosis seen in patients with tumors of the lower spinal canal.

High histopathologic tumor grade is associated with a high rate of disability and death. The median survival of patients with malignant astrocytomas is <6 months, with few patients living >1 year (13). Most series report no survivors of adult patients with malignant spinal cord astrocytomas (23,46,50). Radiographic or autopsy evidence of tumor dissemination is seen in as many as 58% of patients with malignant astrocytomas (13). In a pooled series from six institutions, Abdel-Wahab et al. (3) reported a twofold increased rate of tumor progression in 57 patients with high-grade astrocytomas. Patients with high-grade astrocytomas also had a significantly worse overall survival than patients with low- to moderate-grade tumors. Anaplastic ependymomas are associated with an increased recurrence rate and risk of death (86,90).

Extensive involvement of the spinal cord with an ependymoma is associated with a worse outcome. Linstadt et al. (50) reported a 93% 10-year disease-specific survival rate with localized ependymoma compared with 50% for patients with diffuse tumors. Extensive tumors have a 50% local failure rate after surgery and radiation therapy, compared with only 20% for limited disease (one to three vertebral body segments) (79). Extent of disease has not been a prognostic factor in other series (36). Myxopapillary ependymomas that most commonly involve the cauda equina are felt to be less aggressive than other ependymomas (10,61,82), but they have been reported to seed the CSF (26,58). Encapsulated myxopapillary tumors of the cauda equina are frequently amenable to complete en bloc excision, and the recurrence rate is very low. Unencapsulated or adherent tumors often are removed piecemeal and are associated with a high local recurrence rate after surgery alone (71,79,82,89).

Neurologic function at diagnosis is an important clinical prognostic factor. In general, the fewer the symptoms and the better the neurologic function at presentation, the greater the likelihood that the tumor will be controlled with fewer long-term adverse neurologic sequelae (23,29,33,34,38). Poor neurologic function in patients with spinal cord tumors is often attributable to the disease process and a prolonged delay in diagnosis rather than the effect of surgery or radiation therapy (18,22,27,52,55,63).

As is true for low-grade astrocytomas in general, younger age is associated with a better than 5-year recurrence-free survival rate (23,74). In a pooled series of 126 patients with ependymoma from six institutions, Abdel-Wahab et al. (3) reported a 27% lower risk of disease progression for every 10 years' increase in age. Most other series of spinal cord ependymoma do not report an association between age and prognosis (29,34, 79,90).

Surgical Management

Intradural–Extramedullary Tumors

The treatment of choice for most tumors in this location is as complete a surgical excision as possible consistent with preservation of neurologic function. Most benign nerve sheath tumors and meningiomas can be completely resected using a posterior approach with a standard posterior laminectomy (56). Nerve sheath tumors rarely recur after satisfactory surgical removal. In contrast, as much as 15% of spinal meningiomas recur as late as 10 years after gross total or near total removal (60). Piecemeal resection of ependymomas of the filum terminale can be accomplished with little neurologic disability; however, the risk of recurrence in these patients is significant, and adjuvant radiation therapy is warranted (79,80,82,89).

In young children, posterior laminectomy is being abandoned and replaced with posterior laminotomy. Replacing the posterior bony elements of the spinal canal is less likely to cause significant kyphotic deformity and affords better protection of the spinal cord (1,43).

Intramedullary Tumors

Intramedullary tumors, 95% of which are astrocytomas and ependymomas, present a challenge. Complete surgical excision is the treatment of choice if it can be achieved without compromising neurologic function. Complete excision of intramedullary tumors with preservation of neurologic function was not possible until 1940, when Greenwood (37) introduced the bipolar coagulation forceps. Radical, total gross resection of intramedullary tumors has been facilitated by microsurgical techniques and recently by the use of the Cavitron ultrasonic surgical aspirator (CUSA) and the carbon dioxide laser.

Intraoperative ultrasonography has become indispensable in the surgical management of intramedullary spinal cord neoplasms. After the posterior spinal bony elements have been cleared, this real-time imaging tool is used to localize the lesion, define its extent, and characterize the tumor as cystic or solid. Ultrasonography facilitates placement of a myelotomy incision and initiation of tumor resection. The ultrasound scan helps the surgeon assess the progress of tumor resection and adjacent cyst drainage with internal spinal cord decompression (25). Modern surgical techniques have increased the complete resectability of both ependymomas and astrocytomas (23,24,39,57). Ependymomas are more frequently amenable to gross total excision than are astrocytomas (3,38,47). Resection of astrocytic tumors begins from within the tumor at the initial midline myelotomy. Removal proceeds until the interface between the tumor and the normal spinal cord is evident by changes in tissue color and consistency (22,55). The CUSA allows aspiration of tissue fragments from within 1 mm of the vibrating tip, permitting dissection immediately adjacent to vital neural tissue. The carbon dioxide laser vaporizes remaining fragments with little risk of injury (22,55). Resection of tumors that have progressed or are recurrent after radiation therapy is more difficult, either because the tumor in these situations is more infiltrative or because of radiation-induced changes in the spinal cord.

If complete excision of spinal cord tumors is achieved, no postoperative therapy is necessary because the local recurrence rate is low and prognosis is excellent. In patients who recur, tumor regrowth is often slow, and second resection may be possible (8,16,24). Delaying the use of adjuvant radiation therapy is particularly important in children because of the effects on vertebral body growth (see later). Constantini et al. (15) updated the series from Beth Israel Medical Center. In their series of 164 patients younger than 21 years of age, they achieved a gross total resection or subtotal resection in 77% and 20% of patients, respectively. The 3-month neurologic function was 60% stable, 16% improved, and 24% deteriorated compared with preoperative function. The 5-year progression-free survival rate for low-grade and high-grade tumors was 78% and 30%, respectively.

If complete surgical excision is not feasible without sacrificing neurologic function, a subtotal excision should be performed. Often a subtotal excision is sufficient to relieve the neurologic dysfunction caused by the intramedullary tumor. In many cases of incomplete tumor excision, postoperative radiation therapy is indicated to prevent or delay tumor regrowth. The benefits of postoperative radiation therapy need to be weighed against the possible late sequelae. Because of the low growth rate of many of these tumors, the initiation of radiation therapy can sometimes be delayed until the time of tumor regrowth.

Chemotherapy

In an effort to delay or eliminate radiation therapy and its significant deleterious late effects in young children, some have advocated the use of chemotherapy in these patients. Although it is widely accepted that there is an important need for effective and nontoxic therapy for spinal cord tumors, chemotherapy is not yet of established value for either ependymoma or low-grade astrocytoma.

There are two prospective cooperative group trials that have included children with primary spinal cord astrocytomas. In one clinical trial conducted by the French Society of Pediatric Oncology, eight children with unresectable or recurrent intramedullary low-grade gliomas were treated with a planned 16-month course of carboplatin, procarbazine, vincristine, cyclophosphamide, etoposide, and cisplatin. Seven of the patients had a clinical or radiographic response to the chemotherapy. Five of the patients remained progression free with follow-up ranging from 16 to 59 months (19). In the Children's Cancer Group 945 trial, 13 children with high-grade astrocytic spinal cord neoplasms were assigned to receive two cycles of "8-drugs-in-1-day" chemotherapy before radiation therapy, then eight additional cycles thereafter. At 5 years, 46% of the children had no progression and 54% were alive. The authors argued that more intensive therapy was necessary (4). Continued investigation remains a priority in patients with high-grade spinal cord gliomas. Children with high-grade astrocytomas of the spinal cord are currently eligible to enroll on a Children's Oncology Group clinical trial of radiation with temozolomide and lomustine chemotherapy for high-grade gliomas.

:: | Radiation Therapy

Radiation therapy is not indicated for patients with intramedullary astrocytomas and ependymomas who have undergone complete resection; the prognosis is excellent with no additional therapy. For tumors that are incompletely excised, strong consideration should be given to the administration of adjuvant radiation therapy in an effort to provide durable local control and improve survival. Uncontrolled local tumor is the major cause of death in patients with spinal cord gliomas.

Nonetheless, there are clinical circumstances in which careful follow-up after surgery is appropriate, with a second surgery and/or radiation therapy considered at the time of progression or recurrence. For example, young children who are diagnosed before their pubertal growth spurt are at significant risk for development of radiation-induced bone growth delay with kyphoscoliosis or short stature, especially affecting their sitting height. This radiation-induced deformity is most severe in patients who have extensive tumors or holocord involvement of the spine. In these young children, if their neurologic function is good or improved after a subtotal resection, close follow-up is not an unreasonable course of action. Most spinal cord tumors in young children are either low-grade astrocytomas or well-differentiated ependymomas that have a very low growth rate. Delaying radiation therapy until recurrence or tumor progression may allow the child to grow at a normal rate for several years before receiving radiation therapy. Even at the time of recurrence the patient may be a candidate for reresection. If this can be accomplished with minimal injury, the patient may be observed again without adjuvant therapy until progressive neurologic signs or symptoms appear or if radiographic evidence of inoperable tumor appears.

In contrast, evidence supports the use of postoperative radiation therapy in patients with ependymoma after incomplete or piecemeal excision. Guidetti et al. (38) first reported a beneficial outcome in patients receiving radiation therapy after an incomplete excision of an ependymoma. Some radiation therapy series have demonstrated that increasing doses of irradiation are associated with better tumor control in patients with ependymoma (33,47,79). Shaw et al. (79) reported that the local failure

rate was 35% in patients receiving ≤50 Gy compared with only 20% in patients receiving >50 Gy.

The data supporting the routine use of adjuvant radiation therapy in subtotally resected astrocytic tumors of the spinal cord are less conclusive. The prolonged natural history and slow growth of these neoplasms make it difficult to prove that radiation therapy is beneficial. In their multi-institutional series, Abdel-Wahab et al. (3) reported that radiation significantly improved progression-free survival in the 40 patients with low- and intermediate-grade astrocytomas. Most clinicians argue that the beneficial effects of radiation therapy in the management of subtotally resected astrocytomas of the cerebrum present reasonable evidence that these tumors are radioresponsive (33). However, the spinal cord is more radiosensitive, and even when using irradiation doses that are at or above the tolerance of the spinal cord, local recurrence remains the predominant pattern of treatment failure. This pattern of treatment failure has led some investigators to treat spinal cord tumors beyond the tolerance of the spinal cord when the tumor was so advanced that no meaningful functional recovery could be expected with treatment of the tumor. In these few cases of "radiocordectomy," some patients have achieved control over their disease, albeit sustaining permanent disability (80). Although such an aggressive approach may be considered in situations of tumor progression following prior radiation therapy (e.g., reirradiation), it is not advisable in patients who have never been irradiated or those who have good neurologic function.

Abdel-Wahab et al. (3) reported the outcome of 242 patients from six institutions, only 183 of whom had sufficient treatment data on follow-up to be included in the analysis. The overall survival for the 126 patients with ependymoma was 91%, 84%, and 75% at 5, 10, and 15 years, respectively. Survival was favorably influenced by complete resection and older age. Progression-free survival in the ependymoma patients was adversely influenced by use of radiation, nonwhite race, younger age, higher tumor grade, and incomplete resection. It is likely that patients who received radiation therapy had other adverse risk factors that caused them to have a higher rate of progressive disease than patients who had not received postoperative adjuvant therapy, and in multivariate analysis only age was a significant factor for progression-free survival. In the 57 patients with spinal cord astrocytoma, the overall survival was 59%, 53%, and 32% at 5, 10, and 15 years, respectively. Tumor grade had a significant effect on overall survival in their multivariate analysis. Progression-free survival of patients with astrocytoma was 42%, 29%, and 15% at 5, 10, and 15 years, respectively. Postoperative radiation therapy significantly reduced the risk of progression with low- and intermediate-grade tumors.

Patients who have had complete tumor excision of either astrocytoma (21,23,56,70,72) or ependymoma (8,24,30,57,67) have an excellent local control rate without additional therapy. Patients who have undergone complete excision of a cauda equina ependymoma by piecemeal removal have a local failure rate that ranges from 20% to 43% (79,82,89). The addition of radiation therapy in patients who have undergone piecemeal excision of a cauda equina ependymoma produces a local recurrence rate equal to that of patients undergoing gross total resection (79,80,89).

Nadkarni and Rekate (62) reviewed the available published literature on the topic of surgical and adjuvant therapy in the management of patients with intramedullary spinal cord gliomas. There exist no class I (randomized, controlled) data on the topic of spinal cord tumors. The majority of published data falls into class II (prospective reviews or retrospective data comparing two definable groups) or class III (everything else). Nadkarni and Rekate's treatment recommendations for astrocytomas and ependymomas are summarized in Tables 34.3 and 34.4, respectively.

	SUMMARY OF NADKARNI'S TREATMENT RECOMMENDATIONS FOR PEDIATRIC SPINAL CORD ASTROCYTOMA
Table 34.3	

Level of Recommendation	Treatment Recommendation
Standard Guidelines	No standards exist Withhold radiation therapy if radical or total resection of low-grade astrocytoma is achieved Monitor somatosensory evoked potentials to improve safety of surgery Treat malignant astrocytomas with postoperative irradiation
Options	Use ultrasonic aspirator as surgical adjunct Monitor motor-evoked potentials to improve safety of surgery Withhold radiation therapy for low-grade astrocytomas before tumor progression occurs Use osteoplastic laminotomy to decrease postoperative deformity

Modified from Nadkarni TD, Rekate HL. Pediatric intramedullary spinal cord tumors. *Childs Nerv Syst* 1999;15:17–28, with permission.

Radiation Therapy Techniques

Target Volume

Historically, it had been recommended that superior and inferior field borders encompass two vertebral bodies above and below a tumor defined by myelography. Today, more accurate definition of the gross tumor with MRI allows for a more appropriate gross tumor volume (GTV) consisting of the preoperative tumor plus a clinical target volume (CTV) margin of 0.5 to 1 cm for low-grade astrocytoma or ependymoma. The CTV should encompass the preoperative GTV plus any associated intratumoral cysts. It is not necessary to include an intramedullary syrinx that extends above or below the primary tumor unless there is radiographic or surgical evidence of tumor extension to these regions. Merchant et al. (59) described a diffuse failure pattern in children with high-grade gliomas shortly after com-

	SUMMARY OF REKATE'S TREATMENT RECOMMENDATIONS FOR PEDIATRIC SPINAL CORD EPENDYMOMA
Table 34.4	

Level of Recommendation	Treatment Recommendation
Standard	Resect totally Reoperate if postoperative magnetic resonance imaging shows unexpected residual tumor Withhold radiation therapy if gross total resection achieved
Guidelines	Follow extent of resection with intraoperative ultrasonography Monitor somatosensory evoked potentials to improve safety of surgery
Options	Attempt total resection if cleavage plane exists Reoperate for recurrences in ambulatory patients Use ultrasonic aspirator as surgical adjunct Monitor motor-evoked potentials to improve safety of surgery Use osteoplastic laminotomy to decrease postoperative deformity

Modified from Nadkarni TD, Rekate HL. Pediatric intramedullary spinal cord tumors. *Childs Nerv Syst* 1999;15:17–28, with permission.

pleting radiation therapy, suggesting that the tumor was not adequately covered in the irradiated volume, confirming the need for larger CTV margins of 1.5 cm craniocaudally for high-grade astrocytoma or anaplastic ependymoma. The clinical target volume should encompass the intervertebral foramina if tumor extension is suspected.

For myxopapillary ependymomas involving the conus, a 1.5-cm CTV margin cephalad and caudad to the GTV is used. If the cauda equina is involved, the CTV should extend inferiorly to encompass the entire thecal sac with the volume widened at the sacroiliac joints to ensure adequate coverage of the meningeal sleeves in the intervertebral foramina. Failure adequately to encompass the thecal sac has been associated with an increased rate of treatment failure (89).

Craniospinal or spinal axis irradiation usually is not indicated in the treatment of spinal cord tumors; local failure accounts for most tumor recurrences (3,33,50,70,74,79). However, neuraxis dissemination may be seen in patients with anaplastic ependymomas (90), malignant gliomas (13,46), and myxopapillary ependymomas. Craniospinal irradiation may be considered in this situation.

Technique

Primary tumors of the spinal canal are easily treated with a direct posterior field. The width of posterior fields should encompass the spinal canal with a 1- to 1.5-cm margin. Fields as small as 5 cm may be considered for young children. Some tumors of the lumbar region, including tumors of the cauda equina, may require opposed anteroposterior–posteroanterior portals because of the lumbar lordosis and the deep location of the vertebral canal near the midline of the trunk. Other techniques in the treatment of spinal canal tumors have been described and should be considered when exit dose to the anterior midline structures of the trunk would otherwise be excessive (Fig. 34.5). Tumors exclusively involving the cervical spine may be treated with opposed lateral fields to avoid incidental irradiation of the hypopharynx and oral cavity. Similarly, tumors involving the thoracic and lumbar spinal canal can be treated with a paired set of oblique-wedged fields to get a superior dose distribution compared with a single posterior field. The oblique-paired field plan, although more complex, treats the midline structures anterior to the spinal column to a lower cumulative irradiation dose. Administration of a high dose to the subcutaneous tissues delivered by a single posteroanterior field is also avoided. In some parts of the trunk, care is necessary to avoid excessive dose to the lungs or kidneys with paired oblique fields, and a posteroanterior treatment technique either exclusively or in combination with the oblique fields may be a better approach. In female patients requiring treatment to the lumbosacral spine for cauda equina tumors, a lateral technique may be used to avoid exit irradiation to the ovaries and uterus (Fig. 34.6). Wedges may be required on these lateral lumbosacral fields to provide a homogeneous dose distribution. Care should be taken to avoid irradiating the kidneys at the L1 through L3 levels with this technique. Arms should be positioned appropriately to avoid entrance or exit irradiation from the lateral beams.

The depth of the vertebral surface of the cord beneath the skin surface is determined from CT or MRI, and for short field lengths this depth is used for dose prescription. The depth also can be determined by obtaining a lateral radiograph of the spine on the simulator, using a wire on the skin surface and measuring the distance to the posterior aspect of the vertebral bodies using the magnification factor used for the film.

If large segments of the spinal cord are irradiated, it is necessary to compute the spinal cord dose at multiple points because of the variation in curvature of the spine and depth of the spinal cord and the different source–skin distances below and above the central axis of the beam. A transverse and sagittal treatment

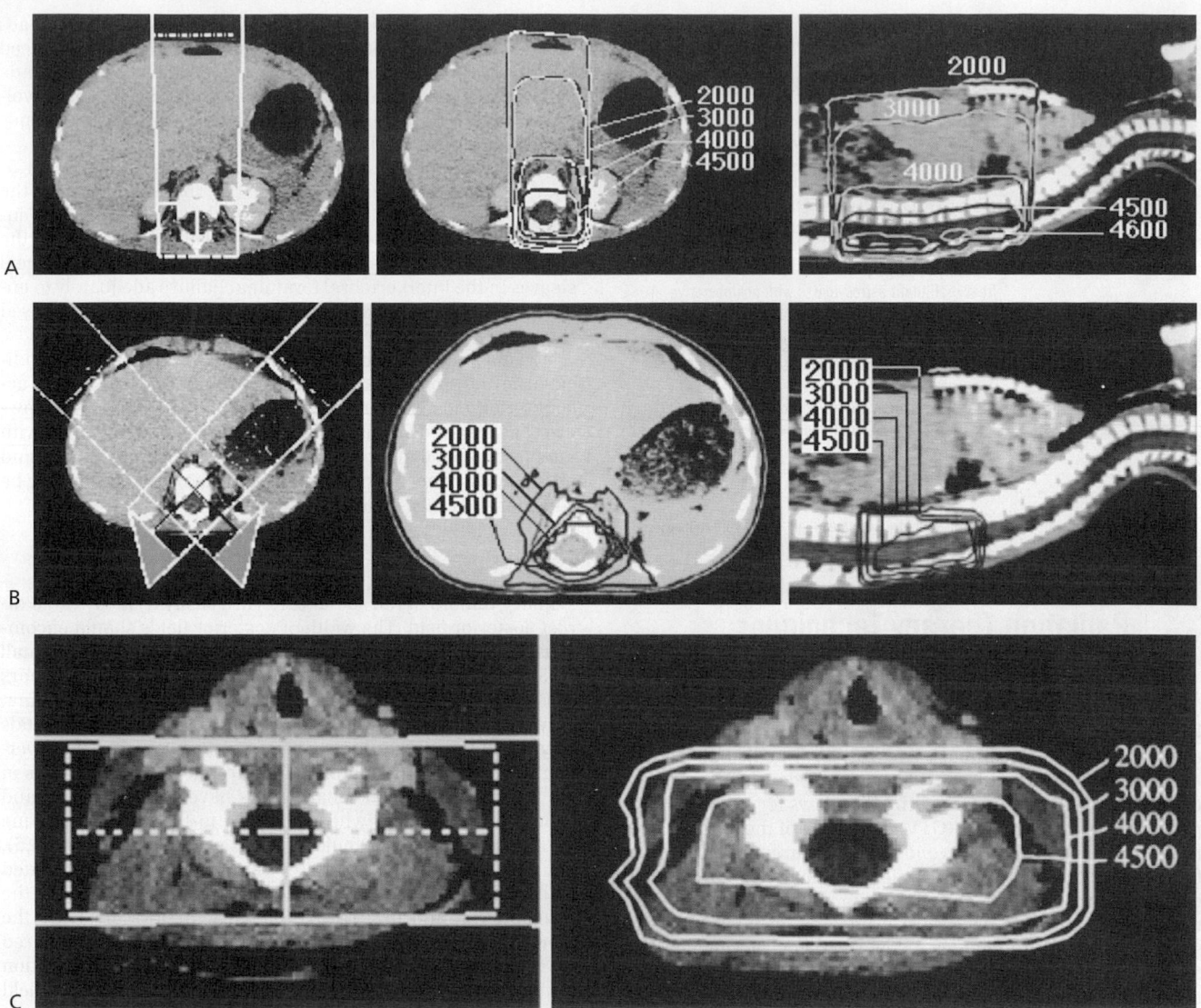

FIGURE 34.5. Treatment planning for spinal cord tumors. **A:** A single posteroanterior field. The advantages of this beam arrangement include simplicity and near-universal applicability in most spinal cord radiation therapy treatments. One disadvantage of this field arrangement is the large volume of tissue that receives a significant exit dose. The axial and sagittal isodose displays reflect a 6-MV x-ray beam treated to a 4-cm depth. **B:** Paired posterior oblique wedge fields. The advantage of this technique is a decrease in high exit-dose irradiation to anterior tissues with a more conformal irradiation dose distribution near the target volume. Disadvantages include more complicated treatment setup and verification. The axial and sagittal isodose displays reflect a 45-degree wedged pair of 6-MV x-ray beams treated to the center of the spinal cord volume with a 90-degree hinge angle. **C:** Opposed lateral fields. An advantage is a homogeneous dose distribution in the target volume with sparing of anterior structures from significant irradiation dose. A disadvantage is limited applicability in cervical and lower lumbosacral sites. Exclusive use of this field arrangement in the thorax and upper abdomen is inappropriate because of limited lung and kidney tolerance. The axial isodose display reflects a pair of laterally directed 6-MV x-ray fields treated to the midplane of the cervical spine.

plan using the CT and MRI scan should be performed (see Fig. 34.5). A sagittal treatment plan can be prepared from a lateral spine radiograph with the midline skin wired and documentation of the magnification factor of the film. Similarly, a sagittal reconstruction or MRI scan can be used for planning purposes (see Fig. 34.5).

The treatment plan should provide a homogeneous dose distribution. For small lesions of the cervical spinal cord, where lateral fields will be used, radiation beam energies of 4- to 6-MV photons achieve a homogeneous dose distribution. Lesions involving the thoracic and lumbar spine often require combinations of low-energy (4 to 6 MV) and high-energy (18 to 25 MV) photons to achieve a homogeneous dose distribution when posterior fields are used. Attention to the exit dose delivered to anterior anatomical structures needs to be considered against dose heterogeneity in the target volume. Parallel-opposed pos-

terior and anterior fields or paired oblique wedge fields can give homogeneous dose distributions with x-ray energies as low as 4 or 6 MV. It has been suggested that conformal or intensity-modulated radiation therapy (IMRT) methods may reduce some of the risk of late effects that frequently follow the radiation treatment of these patients (58). If IMRT is being considered for tumors of the spinal canal, the volume of normal tissue receiving a low to moderate radiation dose needs to be closely evaluated. IMRT may deliver a substantial integral dose that may have clinical consequences in radiation sensitive structures in the thorax or abdomen.

Radiation Dose

Intramedullary ependymomas and astrocytomas should be irradiated to a total dose of 50.4 Gy, given in 1.8 Gy daily fractions.

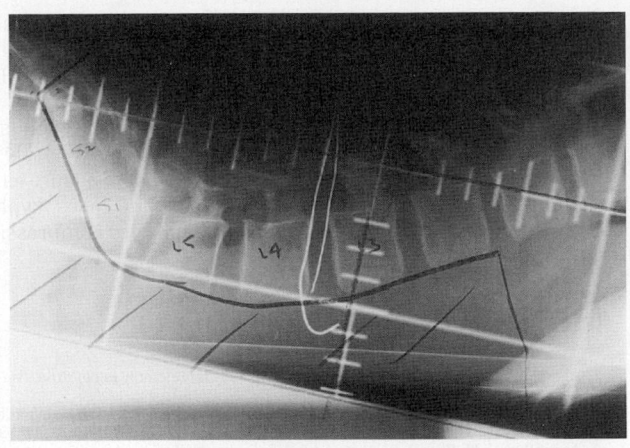
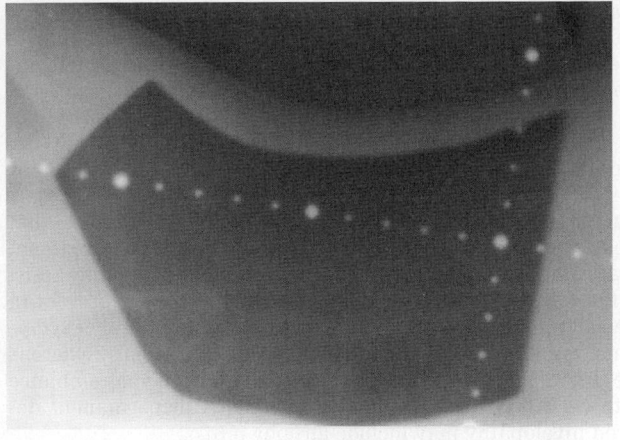

FIGURE 34.6. Simulation **(A)** and portal **(B)** films of lateral field technique for lumbosacral spine. This technique prevents the anterior pelvic structures from receiving significant irradiation dose, which is desirable in young women and girls to minimize incidental irradiation of the ovaries. The superior aspect of this field can be matched to the divergence of a superior posteroanterior field in a fashion similar to the junction of a cranial portal to a spinal portal in craniospinal irradiation. Beam modifiers such as wedges or tissue compensators may be required with this lateral beam arrangement.

Although the target volume is larger for high-grade astrocytoma, the dose is the same as for low-grade tumors in order to avoid the higher risks of morbidity with doses >50.4 Gy.

Results of Radiation Therapy

Analysis of the results of therapy is complicated by the various natural histories and heterogeneity of the tumor types that affect the spinal canal. Furthermore, the rarity of even the more common histologic types leaves even the largest experiences with small numbers of patients affected by a single tumor type. As well, many of these series have spanned several decades, during which time the imaging, surgical, and radiation therapy disciplines have undergone tremendous evolution. For surgery, the introduction of the operating microscope, CUSA, intraoperative ultrasonography, laser coagulation, and evoked potential monitoring has made complete resection of many low-grade astrocytomas and ependymomas more likely and less risky. Radiation therapy, likewise, has evolved over the past decades. Better pretreatment imaging studies, such as MRI, have improved treatment targeting. Megavoltage linear accelerators have improved the radiation dose distribution and subsequently decreased the likelihood of severe or late sequelae. One of the most important factors that has contributed to the improved outcome of patients diagnosed with spinal cord tumors is the advancement of our knowledge regarding the natural histories of these tumors after various surgical procedures. We can now better select the group of patients who are most likely to benefit from radiation therapy and avoid or delay the use of this modality in many of these patients.

Intramedullary Tumors

Since 1990, the 5- and 10-year overall survival rates of patients treated for primary spinal cord astrocytoma range from 57% to 100% and 40% to 75%, respectively (2,3,11,42,45,70,74,80). In the largest published series from a six-institution consortium, the 5- and 10-year overall survival was 50% and 53%, respectively. In their series of 57 patients with astrocytoma there were 24 deaths. Of the 24 deaths, five occurred in patients treated with surgery alone and 19 in patients who received radiation therapy. Only two of 19 had a complete resection, whereas nine had partial resection and eight had biopsy only.

During the same time period, the 5- and 10-year overall survival rates of patients treated for primary spinal cord ependymoma range from 66% to 100% and 62% to 91%, respectively (2,3,11,12,39–42,80–86,89,90). In the same multi-institutional experience reported by Abdel-Wahab et al. (3), the 5- and 10-year overall survival rates were 91% and 84%, respectively. In the 126 patients with ependymoma, there were 15 deaths. Three of the deaths occurred in the group of 64 patients treated with surgery only. Twelve of the 62 patients receiving postoperative radiation died. Only one of those patients had a complete resection, eight had partial resections, and three had a biopsy only.

Intradural–Extramedullary Tumors

The prognosis is excellent for most patients with intradural–extramedullary tumors, which rarely recur after total excision. However, subtotally resected meningiomas may recur late after surgery (60). Some investigators have suggested a benefit to postoperative radiation therapy in this circumstance because of the favorable outcome reported in patients with intracranial presentations of similar histologies (48). Radiation therapy is beneficial to patients undergoing subtotal resection or piecemeal excision of intradural–extramedullary ependymomas (50,79,82,89). Data supporting the routine use of radiation therapy in the management of patients with nerve sheath tumors, vascular malformations, lipomas, hemangiomas, teratomas, and dermoids are nonexistent.

Sequelae of Radiation Therapy

Spinal Cord Tolerance

A reversible myelopathy can manifest itself within 2 to 6 months after radiation therapy. L'Hermitte's sign, characterized by shocklike sensations radiating to the hands and feet when the neck is flexed, is the classic finding. It is believed that this phenomenon is related to transient demyelination of the treated length of the spinal cord (28,44). This syndrome usually lasts a few weeks, and no therapy is required. It is not associated with chronic progressive myelitis.

Chronic, progressive, or delayed myelopathy can occur months to years after radiation therapy. The latency period of chronic myelopathy has been reported to be bimodal with peaks of incidence occurring at 13 and 29 months (76). The early peak may correspond to white matter injury with subsequent demyelination, and the latter peak may correspond to microvascular injury (76). Permanent myelopathy is characterized by progressive motor weakness, paresthesias, and loss of pain or temperature sensation. Patients ultimately lose bowel and bladder control and experience complete sensory and motor function loss. A Brown-Séquard syndrome or complete transection may occur. Diagnosis of radiation myelopathy requires that the dominant neurologic abnormality be localized to a segment irradiated and other causes have been ruled out. MRI may assist in the diagnosis, with cord edema frequently being present in the early delayed phase. Within 8 months of the onset of symptoms, the T1-weighted image may show low intensity, whereas the T2 image shows high intensity. The lesion may enhance with Gd-DTPA. Late changes in patients with permanent delayed myelopathy may include atrophy (66).

The occurrence of chronic progressive myelopathy depends on total dose, fraction size, volume, and region irradiated (48,65,88). Historically, radiation oncologists have limited the spinal cord dose to 45 to 50 Gy with fractionation schedules of 1.8 to 2 Gy per day. These estimates came from an era of inexact dose estimation with a bias toward reporting injury in highly selected populations. More recently, data have been published from institutions that have treated large groups of patients in systematic and reliable fashion. Marcus and Million (53) analyzed outcome in 1,112 patients treated to the head and neck with doses >30 Gy. They saw only two cases of myelopathy in patients receiving <50 Gy. They argued that the onset of permanent myelopathy in patients receiving <50 Gy was idiosyncratic (53). The actual incidence of myelopathy with these conventionally fractionated doses is estimated to be <0.2% to 0.5% after 50 Gy and 1% to 5% after 60 Gy (53,77). The dose required to cause a 50% rate of myelopathy is in the range of 68 to 73 Gy (77). The linear-quadratic model of radiation effects has been applied to radiation myelopathy with a α/β estimate of 2 giving a good fit to clinical observation (31,51). As the dose per daily fraction increases, the maximum tolerated dose decreases. The cervical spinal cord may tolerate slightly higher doses of irradiation than the thoracic or lumbar spinal cord.

When treating a patient with a spinal cord tumor, the radiation oncologist must weigh the risk of causing myelopathy after radiation therapy against the risk of progressive tumor resulting in severe neurologic dysfunction. Indeed, after radiation therapy for spinal cord tumor it is often difficult to determine if progressive neurologic symptoms are related to tumor progression or radiation-induced myelopathy.

Late Effects in Children

Children diagnosed and treated for primary tumors of the spinal canal present special prognostic concerns and apprehensions because of the increased potential for treatment-induced morbidity. The spinal cord in children and adolescents may have a lower tolerance to irradiation.

Radiation therapy of the spine in a child may produce a spinal deformity (i.e., scoliosis or kyphosis) because of retardation of bone growth from damage to epiphyseal plates of the vertebral bodies as well as soft tissue fibrosis and contracture (54). Other organs that may receive a significant irradiation dose include the thyroid, heart, bowel, and ovaries. Irradiation dose to these organs may be minimized by modifying the treatment technique, as described in previous sections. Children should be followed for the long term for the development of any late radiation-induced sequelae.

Children are at greater risk than adults for development of complications after surgery. Extensive laminectomy can produce severe kyphosis and scoliosis, which are typically accentuated during the adolescent growth spurt. The spinal deformity is more severe when it involves the higher vertebral levels or many levels or after radiation therapy. An osteoplastic laminotomy may be associated with a lower risk of spinal deformity (1). Reconstructive procedures, such as Harrington rod or Cotrel-Dubousset system placement, may be necessary to prevent significant damage, and children must be followed very closely by the neurosurgeon and by a pediatric orthopedist to ensure early treatment of skeletal abnormalities (14). In some cases, kyphosis can be of such severity that it causes spinal cord compression and myelopathy (14).

References

1. Abbott R, Feldstein N, Wisoff JH, et al. Osteoplastic laminotomy in children. *Pediatr Neurosurg* 1992;18:153–156.
2. Abdel-Wahab M, Corn B, Wolfson A, et al. Prognostic factors and survival in patients with spinal cord gliomas after radiation therapy. *Am J Clin Oncol* 1999;22:344–351.
3. Abdel-Wahab M, Etuk B, Palermo J, et al. Spinal cord gliomas: A multi-institutional retrospective analysis. *Int J Radiat Oncol Biol Phys* 2006;64:1060–1071.
4. Allen JC, Aviner S, Yates AJ, et al. Treatment of high-grade spinal cord astrocytoma of childhood with "8-in-1" chemotherapy and radiotherapy: A pilot study of CCG-945. Children's Cancer Group. *J Neurosurg* 1998;88:215–220.
5. Ammerman BJ, Henry JM, De Girolami U, et al. Intradural lipomas of the spinal cord. A clinicopathological correlation. *J Neurosurg* 1976;44:331–336.
6. Bannister R. Disorders of the spinal cord. In: Brain WR, Bannister R, eds. *Clinical neurology.* London: Oxford University Press, 1985; .
7. Barone BM, Elvidge AR. Ependymomas. A clinical survey. *J Neurosurg* 1970;33:428–438.
8. Brotchi J, Fischer G. Spinal cord ependymomas. *Neurosurg Focus* 1998; .
9. CBTRUS. *Statistical Report: Primary Brain Tumors in the United States, 1998–2002.* : Central Brain Tumor Registry of the United States, 2005:17–26.
10. Chan HS, Becker LE, Hoffman HJ, et al. Myxopapillary ependymoma of the filum terminale and cauda equina in childhood: Report of seven cases and review of the literature. *Neurosurgery* 1984;14:204–210.
11. Chun HC, Schmidt-Ullrich RK, Wolfson A, et al. External beam radiotherapy for primary spinal cord tumors. *J Neurooncol* 1990;9:211–217.
12. Clover LL, Hazuka MB, Kinzie JJ. Spinal cord ependymomas treated with surgery and radiation therapy. A review of 11 cases. *Am J Clin Oncol* 1993;16:350–353.
13. Cohen AR, Wisoff JH, Allen JC, et al. Malignant astrocytomas of the spinal cord. *J Neurosurg* 1989;70:50–54.
14. Constantini S, Epstein FJ. Intraspinal tumors in infants and children. In: Youman JR, ed. *Neurological surgery.* Philadelphia: W.B. Saunders, 1996; .
15. Constantini S, Miller DC, Allen JC, et al. Radical excision of intramedullary spinal cord tumors: Surgical morbidity and long-term follow-up evaluation in 164 children and young adults. *J Neurosurg* 2000;93:183–193.
16. Cooper PR. Outcome after operative treatment of intramedullary spinal cord tumors in adults: Intermediate and long-term results in 51 patients. *Neurosurgery* 1989;25:855–859.
17. de Divitiis E, Cerillo A, Carlomagno S. Subpial spinal Lipomas. *Neurochirurgia (Stuttg)* 1982;25:14–18.
18. DeSousa AL, Kalsbeck JE, Mealey J Jr, et al. Intraspinal tumors in children. A review of 81 cases. *J Neurosurg* 1979;51:437–445.
19. Doireau V, Grill J, Zerah M, et al. Chemotherapy for unresectable and recurrent intramedullary glial tumours in children. Brain Tumours Subcommittee of the French Society of Paediatric Oncology (SFOP). *Br J Cancer* 1999;81:835–840.
20. Epstein F. Spinal cord astrocytomas of childhood. *Adv Tech Stand Neurosurg* 1986;13:135–169.
21. Epstein F, Epstein N. Surgical treatment of spinal cord astrocytomas of childhood. A series of 19 patients. *J Neurosurg* 1982;57:685–689.
22. Epstein FJ, Farmer JP. Pediatric spinal cord tumor surgery. *Neurosurg Clin North Am* 1990;1:569–590.
23. Epstein FJ, Farmer JP, Freed D. Adult intramedullary astrocytomas of the spinal cord. *J Neurosurg* 1992;77:355–359.
24. Epstein FJ, Farmer JP, Freed D. Adult intramedullary spinal cord ependymomas: The result of surgery in 38 patients. *J Neurosurg* 1993;79:204–209.
25. Epstein FJ, Farmer JP, Schneider SJ. Intraoperative ultrasonography: An important surgical adjunct for intramedullary tumors. *J Neurosurg* 1991;74:729–733.
26. Fassett DR, Pingree J, Kestle JR. The high incidence of tumor dissemination in myxopapillary ependymoma in pediatric patients. Report of five cases and review of the literature. *J Neurosurg* 2005;102:59–64.
27. Fearnside MR, Adams CB. Tumours of the cauda equina. *J Neurol Neurosurg Psychiatry* 1978;41:24–31.
28. Fein DA, Marcus RB Jr, Parsons JT, et al. Lhermitte's sign: Incidence and treatment variables influencing risk after irradiation of the cervical spinal cord. *Int J Radiat Oncol Biol Phys* 1993;27:1029–1033.
29. Ferrante L, Mastronardi L, Celli P, et al. Intramedullary spinal cord ependymomas—a study of 45 cases with long-term follow-up. *Acta Neurochir (Wien)* 1992;119:74–79.
30. Fischer G, Mansuy L. Total removal of intramedullary ependymomas: Follow-up study of 16 cases. *Surg Neurol* 1980;14:243–249.
31. Fowler JF. The linear quadratic formula and progress in fractionated radiotherapy. *Br J Radiol* 1989;62:6679–6694.
32. Gado M, Sartor K, Hodges F. The spine. In: Lee JK, Sagel SS, Stanley RJ, eds. *Computed body tomography.* New York: Raven Press, 1989.
33. Garcia DM. Primary spinal cord tumors treated with surgery and postoperative irradiation. *Int J Radiat Oncol Biol Phys* 1985;11:1933–1939.
34. Garrett PG, Simpson JR. Ependymomas: Results of radiation treatment. *Int J Radiat Oncol Biol Phys* 1983;9:1121–1124.
35. Giuffre R, Di Lorenzo N, Fortuna A. Primary spinal tumors in infancy and childhood. *Zentralbl Neurochir* 1981;42:87–95.
36. Goh KY, Velasquez L, Epstein FJ. Pediatric intramedullary spinal cord tumors: Is surgery alone enough? *Pediatr Neurosurg* 1997;27:34–39.

37. Greenwood J. Spinal cord tumors. In: Youman JR, ed. *Neurological surgery*. Philadelphia: W.B. Saunders, 1982.
38. Guidetti B, Mercuri S, Vagnozzi R. Long-term results of the surgical treatment of 129 intramedullary spinal gliomas. *J Neurosurg* 1981;54:323–330.
39. Hanbali F, Fourney DR, Marmor E, et al. Spinal cord ependymoma: Radical surgical resection and outcome. *Neurosurgery* 2002;51:1162–1172; discussion 1172–1174.
40. Hardison HH, Packer RJ, Rorke LB, et al. Outcome of children with primary intramedullary spinal cord tumors. *Childs Nerv Syst* 1987;3:89–92.
41. Hely M, Fryer J, Selby G. Intramedullary spinal cord glioma with intracranial seeding. *J Neurol Neurosurg Psychiatry* 1985;48:302–309.
42. Hulshof MC, Menten J, Dito JJ, et al. Treatment results in primary intraspinal gliomas. *Radiother Oncol* 1993;29:294–300.
43. Inoue A, Ikata T, Katoh S. Spinal deformity following surgery for spinal cord tumors and tumorous lesions: Analysis based on an assessment of the spinal functional curve. *Spinal Cord* 1996;34:536–542.
44. Jones A. Transient radiation myelopathy (with reference to Lhermitte's sign of electrical paraesthesia). *Br J Radiol* 1964;37:727–744.
45. Jyothirmayi R, Madhavan J, Nair MK, et al. Conservative surgery and radiotherapy in the treatment of spinal cord astrocytoma. *J Neuro-Oncol* 1997;33:205–211.
46. Kopelson G, Linggood RM. Intramedullary spinal cord astrocytoma versus glioblastoma: The prognostic importance of histologic grade. *Cancer* 1982;50:732–735.
47. Kopelson G, Linggood RM, Kleinman GM, et al. Management of intramedullary spinal cord tumors. *Radiology* 1980;135:473–479.
48. Larson DA. Radiation therapy of tumors of the spine. In: Youman JR, ed. *Neurological surgery*. Philadelphia: W.B. Saunders, 1996.
49. Levy WJ Jr, Bay J, Dohn D. Spinal cord meningioma. *J Neurosurg* 1982;57:804–812.
50. Linstadt DE, Wara WM, Leibel SA, et al. Postoperative radiotherapy of primary spinal cord tumors. *Int J Radiat Oncol Biol Phys* 1989;16:1397–1403.
51. Macbeth FR, Wheldon TE, Girling DJ, et al. Radiation myelopathy: Estimates of risk in 1048 patients in three randomized trials of palliative radiotherapy for non-small cell lung cancer. The Medical Research Council Lung Cancer Working Party. *Clin Oncol (R Coll Radiol)* 1996;8:176–181.
52. Malis LI. Intramedullary spinal cord tumors. *Clin Neurosurg* 1978;25:512–539.
53. Marcus RB Jr, Million RR. The incidence of myelitis after irradiation of the cervical spinal cord. *Int J Radiat Oncol Biol Phys* 1990;19:3–8.
54. Mayfield JK. Postradiation spinal deformity. *Orthop Clin North Am* 1979;10:829–844.
55. McCormick PC, Stein BM. Intramedullary tumors in adults. *Neurosurg Clin North Am* 1990;1:609–630.
56. McCormick PC, Stein BM. Spinal cord tumors in adults. In: Youman Jr, ed. *Neurological surgery*. Philadelphia: W.B. Saunders, 1996.
57. McCormick PC, Torres R, Post KD, et al. Intramedullary ependymoma of the spinal cord. *J Neurosurg* 1990;72:523–532.
58. Merchant TE, Kiehna EN, Thompson SJ, et al. Pediatric low-grade and ependymal spinal cord tumors. *Pediatr Neurosurg* 2000;32:30–36.
59. Merchant TE, Nguyen D, Thompson SJ, et al. High-grade pediatric spinal cord tumors. *Pediatr Neurosurg* 1999;39:1–5.
60. Mirimanoff RO, Dosoretz DE, Linggood RM, et al. Meningioma: Analysis of recurrence and progression following neurosurgical resection. *J Neurosurg* 1985;62:18–24.
61. Mork SJ, Loken AC. Ependymoma: A follow-up study of 101 cases. *Cancer* 1977;40:907–915.
62. Nadkarni TD, Rekate HL. Pediatric intramedullary spinal cord tumors. Critical review of the literature. *Childs Nerv Syst* 1999;15:17–28.
63. Nishio S, Morioka T, Fujii K, et al. Spinal cord gliomas: Management and outcome with reference to adjuvant therapy. *J Clin Neurosci* 2000;7:20–23.
64. Onofrio BM. Intradural extramedullary spinal cord tumors. *Clin Neurosurg* 1978;25:540–555.
65. Phillips TL, Buschke F. Radiation tolerance of the thoracic spinal cord. *Am J Roentgenol Radium Ther Nucl Med* 1969;105:659–664.
66. Rampling R, Symonds P. Radiation myelopathy. *Curr Opin Neurol* 1998;11:627–632.
67. Rawlings CE. 3rd, Giangaspero F, Burger PC, et al. Ependymomas: A clinicopathologic study. *Surg Neurol* 1988;29:271–281.
68. Reimer R, Onofrio BM. Astrocytomas of the spinal cord in children and adolescents. *J Neurosurg* 1985;63:669–675.
69. Rivierez M, Oueslati S, Philippon J, et al. [Ependymoma of the intradural filum terminale in adults. 20 cases]. *Neurochirurgie* 1990;36:96–107.
70. Robinson CG, Prayson RA, Hahn JF, et al. Long-term survival and functional status of patients with low-grade astrocytoma of spinal cord. *Int J Radiat Oncol Biol Phys* 2005;63:91–100.
71. Ross DA, McKeever PE, Sandler HM, et al. Myxopapillary ependymoma. Results of nucleolar organizing region staining. *Cancer* 1993;71:3114–3118.
72. Rossitch E Jr, Zeidman SM, Burger PC, et al. Clinical and pathological analysis of spinal cord astrocytomas in children. *Neurosurgery* 1990;27:193–196.
73. Russell DC, Rubenstein LJ. *Pathology of tumours of the nervous system*. Baltimore: Williams & Wilkins, 1977.
74. Sandler HM, Papadopoulos SM, Thornton AF.Jr, et al. Spinal cord astrocytomas: Results of therapy. *Neurosurgery* 1992;30:490–493.
75. Schiffer D, Chio A, Giordana MT, et al. Histologic prognostic factors in ependymoma. *Childs Nerv Syst* 1991;7:177–182.
76. Schultheiss TE, Higgins EM, El-Mahdi AM. The latent period in clinical radiation myelopathy. *Int J Radiat Oncol Biol Phys* 1984;10:1109–1115.
77. Schultheiss TE, Stephens LC, Jiang GL, et al. Radiation myelopathy in primates treated with conventional fractionation. *Int J Radiat Oncol Biol Phys* 1990;19:935–940.
78. Schweitzer JS, Batzdorf U. Ependymoma of the cauda equina region: Diagnosis, treatment, and outcome in 15 patients. *Neurosurgery* 1992;30:202–207.
79. Shaw EG, Evans RG, Scheithauer BW, et al. Radiotherapeutic management of adult intraspinal ependymomas. *Int J Radiat Oncol Biol Phys* 1986;12:323–327.
80. Shirato H, Kamada T, Hida K, et al. The role of radiotherapy in the management of spinal cord glioma. *Int J Radiat Oncol Biol Phys* 1995;33:323–328.
81. Simeone FA. Intradural tumors. In: Rothman RH, Simeone FA, eds. *The spine*. Philadelphia: W.B. Saunders, 1992.
82. Sonneland PR, Scheithauer BW, Onofrio BM. Myxopapillary ependymoma. A clinicopathologic and immunocytochemical study of 77 cases. *Cancer* 1985;56:883–893.
83. Stein BM. Intramedullary spinal cord tumors. *Clin Neurosurg* 1983;30:717–741.
84. Sze G. Neoplastic disease of the spine and spinal cord. In: Atlas SW, ed. *Magnetic resonance imaging of the brain and spine*. Philadelphia: Lippincott-Raven, 1996.
85. Vakili H. *Spinal cord*. New York: Intercontinental Medical Book Corporation, 1967.
86. Waldron JN, Laperriere NJ, Jaakkimainen L, et al. Spinal cord ependymomas: A retrospective analysis of 59 cases. *Int J Radiat Oncol Biol Phys* 1993;27:223–229.
87. Wanebo JE, Malik JM, VandenBerg SR, et al. Malignant peripheral nerve sheath tumors. A clinicopathologic study of 28 cases. *Cancer* 1993;71:1247–1253.
88. Wara WM, Phillips TL, Sheline GE, et al. Radiation tolerance of the spinal cord. *Cancer* 1975;35:1558–1562.
89. Wen BC, Hussey DH, Hitchon PW, et al. The role of radiation therapy in the management of ependymomas of the spinal cord. *Int J Radiat Oncol Biol Phys* 1991;20:781–786.
90. Whitaker SJ, Bessell EM, Ashley SE, et al. Postoperative radiotherapy in the management of spinal cord ependymoma. *J Neurosurg* 1991;74:720–728.
91. Wood EH, Berne AS, Taveras JM. The value of radiation therapy in the management of intrinsic tumors of the spinal cord. *Radiology* 1954;63:11–24.

Clinical Radiation Oncology

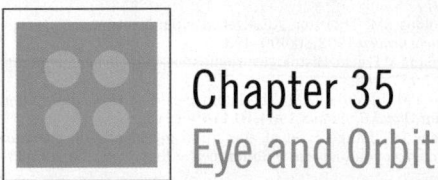

Chapter 35
Eye and Orbit

Jorge E. Freire, Michelle M. Kolton, Luther W. Brady, Jerry A. Shields, Carol L. Shields

Intraocular and orbital tumors, although rare, represent an important entity in the field of oncology. The American Cancer Society estimated approximately 2,360 new diagnoses of ocular and orbital tumors in the United States during the year 2006 and 230 deaths from ocular and orbital tumors during the same period (3). Of these, 75% are choroidal or uveal melanomas, with lymphomas being the next most common. Retinoblastoma, predominately a pediatric tumor, makes up approximately 20% of new ocular tumor diagnoses. The remainder of the subtypes includes orbital tumors such as rhabdomyosarcoma, optic nerve glioma, conjunctival tumors, and eyelid carcinomas, as well as metastatic tumors to the eye.

Radiation, either as external beam or brachytherapy, remains an effective therapeutic option and has been exhaustively studied by a several centers. Satisfactory results have been observed in the management of both intraocular and orbital tumors when radiotherapy is used as primary or adjuvant therapy along with surgery, chemotherapy, thermotherapy, immunotherapy, cryotherapy, photocoagulation, and other treatments still under investigation.

This chapter will outline the most relevant aspects of different malignant and benign neoplasia with emphasis on irradiation.

:: | Anatomy

The ocular adnexa consist of structures including the eyelids, cilia, lacrimal glands, lacrimal drainage apparatus, and conjunctiva. The eyeball, or globe, is a spherical organ composed of three tunicae (Fig. 35.1). The outer coat consists of the clear cornea on the front and the sclera, a fibrous hypocellular layer that occupies 90% of the posterior aspect of the globe. The uvea, or middle coat, is formed by the choroid, ciliary body, and iris, all of which contain a high concentration of melanocytes as well as vessels. The innermost and sensory layer is the retina and its analogs. This coat extends from the ora serrata retinae anteriorly to the optic nerve posteriorly.

The vascular supply to the posterior half of the retina derives from the central retinal artery, which enters the globe through the optic nerve. The choroid is split into anterior ciliary and posterior ciliary arteries. The lens is suspended from the ciliary body and is located posterior to the iris. The orbit is composed of seven bones: frontal, maxilla, lacrimal, palatine, ethmoid, sphenoid and zygomatic. The bony orbit encloses the ocular globe, vessels, nerves, orbital fat, lacrimal gland, and ocular muscles: superior, inferior, medial, and lateral recti as well as superior and inferior oblique muscles that are inserted on the sclera.

:: | Benign Ocular Diseases

A variety of diseases are categorized as benign or malignant ophthalmic tumors (Table 35.1) (52,162). Radiation therapy is most commonly used for the treatment of malignant tumors, however for many years it has been applied to the eye globe or the orbit with the purpose of achieving control of selective benign processes.

Pterygium

Pterygium is a benign ocular growth of fibrovascular tissue on the conjunctiva. Although benign, they can cause irritation, erythema of the cornea, may obstruct vision, and become of cosmetic concern for a patient. Pterygium most often occur in patients 20 to 50 years of age, and more frequently in dry, dusty, and hot conditions. These conditions cause trauma to the corneal stem cells and cause slow decay of these cells, which in turn allows overgrowth of thickened fibrovascular tissue at the limbus and onto the cornea. The loss of corneal stem cells is most apparent at the horizontal limbal region where exposure to the environment is greatest. It is also theorized that ultraviolet light exposure may increase the risk of development of pterygium (71). They develop most frequently in the medial/nasal aspect of the conjunctiva.

The primary treatment for pterygium is surgery. Complete surgical excision and replacement of lost stem cells by autograft is the surgery of choice; however, depending on the location and extent of disease, other surgical procedures can be considered. Recurrence rates of pterygium after surgery alone are in the range of 20% to 68% (35). Adjuvant treatment for pterygium can involve radiation therapy or topical chemotherapeutic agents to minimize regrowth of fibrovascular tissue.

In a prospective randomized study, 96 eyes with primary pterygium were operated on and received β-radiation with a

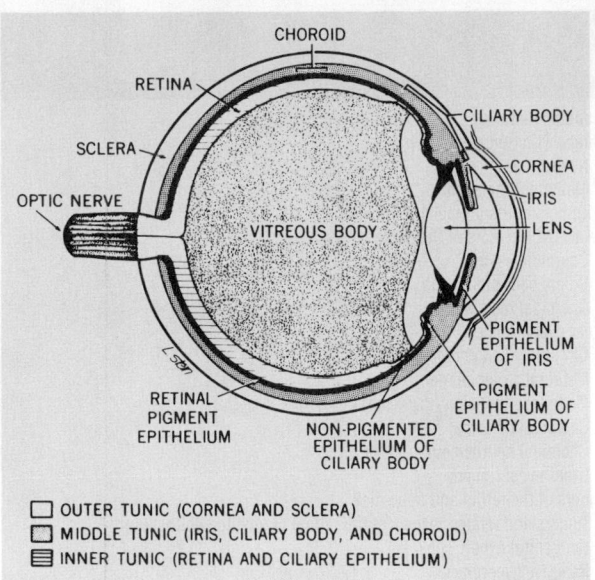

FIGURE 35.1. Various ocular relationships. (Courtesy of Drs. Carol and Jerry Shields, Wills Eye Hospital, Philadelphia, Pennsylvania.)

strontium-90 (^{90}Sr) eye applicator, or sham radiation within 24 hours of surgery. Control rates were approximately 93.2% for the β-radiation group verses 33.3% for the sham radiation group. Single dose β-radiation after surgery proved to be a simple, safe, and effective treatment to reduce the risk of pterygium recurrence (71). Current surgical techniques have made the use of irradiation for pterygium sporadic and is only employed in selected cases.

Choroidal Hemangiomas

Choroidal hemangiomas are rare, congenital, benign vascular tumors of the choroid that have a wide range of symptomatology, signs, associated systemic features, clinical course, and treatment options.

There are two types of choroidal hemangiomas: circumscribed and diffuse (Fig. 35.2). Circumscribed choroidal hemangiomas are usually small with a mean diameter of 7 mm, located in the posterior choroid within 3 mm of the foveola and occasionally in the subfoveal region. The subfoveal tumors tend to cause visual loss early in life due to the anterior displacement of the retina by the underlying tumor. Patients with parafoveal tumors remain asymptomatic until the third or fourth decade of life. External ocular examination in these patients is usually unremarkable.

In contrast to circumscribed choroidal hemangiomas, the diffuse variety is large, often extends anterior to the equator, and is typically associated with facial nevus flammeus or other manifestations of the Sturge-Weber syndrome (SWS). Diffuse tumors are usually diagnosed in young patients either due to examination of the fundus prompted by a facial hemangioma or due to visual impairment secondary to serous retinal detachment or hyperopic amblyopia.

Choroidal hemangiomas do not transform into malignant tumors. Therefore, the indication for treatment is loss of visual acuity, although treatment may be indicated for extensive retinal detachment and for associated glaucoma. Treatment alternatives include laser photocoagulation, thermotherapy, photodynamic therapy, and radiotherapy. Radiotherapy is typically reserved for eyes with extensive subretinal fluid.

Favorable responses of choroidal hemangiomas to low dose radiation therapy in the form of fractionated, lens-sparing lin-

ear accelerator therapy, episcleral plaque therapy, proton beam therapy, and stereotactic radiotherapy have been reported. Based on current literature, a total dose of 18 to 30 Gy delivered in 10 to 18 fractions of external beam photon radiation therapy seems to be effective for both circumscribed and diffuse choroidal hemangiomas.

Patients have generally shown at least partial flattening of the hemangioma, complete resorption of subretinal fluid, and reattachment of the retina within 6 to 12 months (61,76). Furthermore, at a mean follow-up of 3.6 years no recurrence of subretinal fluid was noted in one series (61). At 66 months, subretinal fluid had reaccumulated in only 1/12 patients treated. This patient with a diffuse choroidal hemangioma was treated by a second course of linear accelerator (LINAC)-based therapy (20 Gy in 10 fractions) and showed prompt response (76). In very advanced cases with retinal detachment, the authors have prescribed 36 Gy in fractions of 1.8 Gy in two cases, which appears to be efficacious; however, this theory should be proved with a larger number of cases in a controlled study (61,76).

Potential short- and long-term side effects of irradiation include retinopathy and papillopathy. These side effects have not been observed after <40 Gy of lens-sparing LINAC-based irradiation.

Lens-sparing techniques advocate prevention of cataract formation; however, backscatter radiation to the lens exceeds the tolerance and subsequently cloudiness of the lens is manifested in several months or years after treatment. In cases of diffuse choroidal hemangioma, such as in SWS, a noncoplanar without bolus, three-dimensional (3D) conformal technique has been implemented by Freire and Brady (56) and used by other authors (192).

Brachytherapy via iodine-125 (^{125}I), ruthenium-106 (^{106}Ru), and cobalt-60 (^{60}Co) for the treatment of mostly circumscribed choroid hemangiomas have been reported. All these studies showed excellent results, most importantly, complete and permanent resolution of subretinal fluid and reattachment of the retina with at least preservation of pretreatment visual acuity. The dose at the apex and base of the study using ^{60}Co was 40 to 60 Gy and 90 to 240 Gy, respectively (90). The apex and base doses in the studies using ^{125}I or ^{106}Ru were 26 to 50 Gy and 85 to 237.5 Gy, respectively. The plaque sizes varied between 10 and 18 mm in these studies (61,76,90). Currently, ^{125}I plaque applicators are most commonly used for brachytherapy, particularly in the United States, whereas ^{106}Ru is popular in Europe and could be round or notched.

Capillary Hemangioma

Although capillary hemangiomas usually occur elsewhere in the body, they present unique problems when they occur on the eyelids and may represent a component of the von Hippel-Lindau syndrome (VHL) or the Sturge-Weber syndrome.

The natural history of the lesion is spontaneous regression over 3 to 4 years. Therefore, a conservative approach of observation is the treatment of choice (94). Occasionally, however, the lesion may be large enough to obstruct the child's vision, and amblyopia may occur. The lid may ulcerate because of tumor compression of the vascular supply. Intervention is then accomplished by the cautious use of steroids.

Low-energy photons or electron-beam therapy have been used historically, 5 to 7.5 Gy in two or three fractions (41,66) or a total dose of 16 to 20 Gy

However, at present, laser photocoagulation, cryotherapy, or photodynamic therapy are somewhat effective and should be attempted first. The use of irradiation must be reserved for select cases that have failed to current therapies.

Clinical Radiation Oncology

Table 35.1   CATEGORIES OF ORBITAL AND OCULAR TUMORS

Eyelids and lacrimal drainage systems
Benign tumors of the surface epithelium of eyelids
  Papilloma
  Keratoacanthoma
  Seborrheic keratosis
Premalignant and malignant tumors of surface epithelium of eyelids
  Senile (actinic) keratosis
  Basal cell epithelioma
  Nevoid basal cell carcinoma syndrome
  Squamous cell carcinoma
Glandular and adnexal tumors of eyelids
  Sebaceous gland carcinoma
  Sweat gland and hair follicle tumors
Melanocytic tumors of eyelids
  Nevus
  Malignant melanoma
  Congenital melanocytosis
Neurogenic tumors of eyelids
  Neurofibroma
  Neurilemoma
Vascular tumors of eyelids
  Capillary hemangiomas
  Port-wine stain
Xanthomatous tumors of eyelids
  Xanthelasma
  Metastatic tumors to eyelids
  Tumors of lacrimal drainage system

Conjunctiva
Congenital tumors
  Dermoid
Benign tumors of surface epithelium
  Papilloma
  Benign hereditary intraepithelial dyskeratosis
Premalignant/malignant lesions of surface epithelium
  Dysplasia
  Carcinoma *in situ*
  Invasive squamous cell carcinoma
Melanocytic tumors
  Nevus
  Benign acquired melanomas
  Malignant melanoma
Other conjunctival tumors

Systemic hamartomatoses
Tuberous sclerosis
Neurofibromatosis
Retinocerebellar capillary hemangiomatosis (von Hippel-Lindau
  syndrome)
Encephalofacial cavernous hemangiomatosis (Sturge-Weber syndrome)
Racemose hemangiomatosis (Wyburn-Mason syndrome)
Retinal cavernous hemangiomatosis with cutaneous and central nervous system
  involvement

Intraocular tumors
Melanocytic tumors of the iris
  Nevus
  Malignant melanoma
  Tumors of iris pigment epithelium
Melanocytic tumors of the posterior uvea
  Choroidal nevus
  Ciliary body melanoma
  Choroidal melanoma
Other uveal tumors
  Circumscribed choroidal hemangioma
  Metastatic carcinoma
  Medulloepithelioma (diktyoma)
  Choroidal osteoma
  Choroidal neurilemoma
  Other uveal tumors
Tumors of the retina and optic disk
  Tumors and related lesions of the retinal pigmented epithelium
  Congenital hypertrophy
  Reactive hyperplasia
  Combined hamartoma
  Adenoma and adenocarcinoma
Retinoblastoma
Vascular tumors of retina and optic disk
  Capillary hemangioma
  Cavernous hemangioma
  Racemose hemangioma
  Acquired nonfamilial retinal hemangioma
  Glial tumors of retina and optic disk
  Massive gliosis
  Astrocytoma
Melanocytoma of optic nerve
Intraocular lymphoid tumors and leukemias
  Histiocytic lymphoma (reticulum cell sarcoma)
  Leukemias
  Reactive lymphoid hyperplasia of uvea

Orbital tumors
Dermoid cyst
Mucocele
Capillary hemangioma
Cavernous hemangioma
Lymphangioma
Juvenile pilocytic astrocytoma
Meningioma
Fibrous histiocytoma
Fibroosseous tumors
  Fibrous dysplasia
  Juvenile ossifying fibroma
Peripheral nerve tumors
  Neurofibroma
  Neurilemoma
Rhabdomyosarcoma
Lymphoid tumors
Leukemia
Metastatic tumors to orbit
Lacrimal gland tumors

Orbital Pseudolymphoma, Lymphoid Hyperplasia, and Lymphoma

Benign primary lymphoreticular tumors, if localized to the orbit, have a good prognosis with a 5-year survival rate of 70% (54). Approximately 20% to 25% of cases of apparent pseudolymphoma can convert to malignant lymphoma (118). However, it is often difficult to differentiate between pseudolymphoma and true lymphoma by biopsy specimens, and additional studies like immunophenotypic and molecular genetic analysis are necessary in some cases.

Steroids can be effective, but radiation therapy appears to be more effective and can control cases that have been refractory to steroids (8). In our experience, surgical excision of localized pseudolymphomas has been associated with the least chance of control. Radiation therapy may consist of a single exposure of 8 Gy directed through an anterior portal (7,8,54,59). However, in our department at Drexel University College of Medicine,

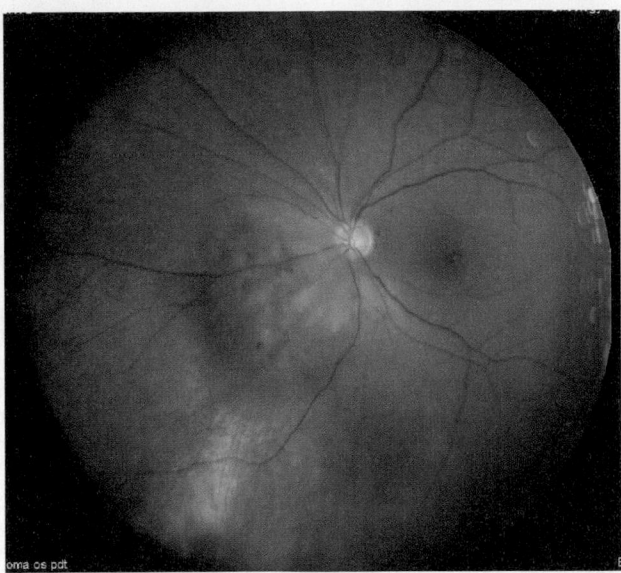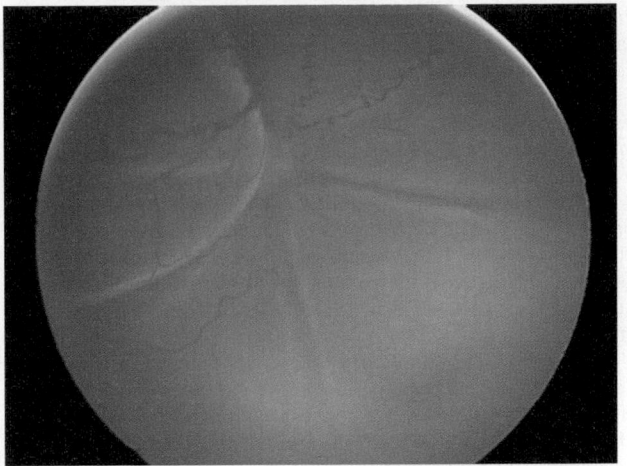

FIGURE 35.2. A: Circumscribed choroidal hemangioma. **B:** Diffuse choroidal hemangioma in a Sturge-Weber syndrome patient with complete retinal detachment and subretinal fluid.

Hahnemann University Hospital, we elect to treat with 20 to 25 Gy given in fractions of 180 to 200 cGy a day, which can cause the condition to dramatically resolve along with reabsorption of subretinal fluid.

Anterior, lateral, or oblique portals similar to those used in the therapy of malignant lymphoma of the orbit, ^{60}Co, 4- to 6-MV photons, or 15- to 16-MeV electron beams are used for treatment of these lesions. Orbital pseudolymphoma associated with angiitis is refractory to this therapy, but inflammatory lymphocytic infiltration responds dramatically (7).

Graves' Ophthalmopathy

In some patients with hyperthyroidism, exophthalmos may occur. The primary tissues involved are the intraocular muscles. They become thickened as a result of lymphocytic infiltration and edema, which subsequently causes the eye globe to protrude forward. Retrobulbar fat is also increased in Graves' disease. Indications for therapy include corneal exposure, which may cause corneal ulceration and can progress to cause scarring and compression of the optic nerve, thus rendering partial or permanent visual loss. The diagnosis is aided by computed tomography (CT) imaging, which may demonstrate thickened muscles.

Steroid therapy or orbital decompression are considered the first-line treatment, and steroids are administered during a minimum of 2 to 8 weeks, but radiation therapy can be beneficial if these treatments fail. Radiation treatment can be delivered by a single lateral portal excluding the ipsilateral lens. A dose of 20 Gy in 10 fractions is usually sufficient to alleviate symptoms. Electrons, usually 12 to 15 MeV, are ideal for the treatment of these patients. At Hahnemann University Hospital, for bilateral disease we recommend two lateral opposing fields encompassing the muscles up to the insertion at the orbital apex, designed through CT planning with an anterior edge just posterior to the lens. We recommend using a dose of 20 Gy in 2-Gy fractions.

In a series of 35 patients with thyroid ophthalmopathy, Sandler et al. (133) reported that 71% of patients receiving 20 Gy in 2-Gy fractions required no further steroid therapy or surgical decompression. Of the failures, 7/21 patients (33%) had failed prior steroid therapy; two of the seven patients (28%) had failed prior surgical decompression; and only one of seven patients

(14%) had no prior treatment. The main prognostic factor for failure was an interval of <6 months between eye disease and radiation therapy. In a series of over 300 patients, Peterson et al. (112) showed that 20 Gy in 10 fractions gave identical results to 30 Gy in 15 fractions, and that as many as 76% of treated patients responded positively to treatment.

Ocular and Orbital Malignant Tumors

Clinical Presentation, Diagnosis, and Staging

Symptoms and findings of malignant ocular and orbital neoplasia are varied and, along with diagnostic work-up, will be covered in the respective anatomic subsections of this chapter. The *American Joint Committee Manual for Staging of Cancer* has outlined the staging systems for many of these tumors. Because of the volume of material, the reader is referred to the original publication (58).

Intraocular Tumors

Metastatic Carcinoma to the Posterior Uvea

Tumor metastases to the uvea were once considered rare events (152). However, it is now recognized that metastatic carcinoma is probably the most common malignant disease involving the eye (47). Metastatic uveal lesions arise as precocious metastases in approximately 15% of cases, as synchronous metastases in approximately 4% of cases, and as metachronous metastases in most of the remaining cases, except in 8% for which the appropriate parameters cannot be established (18).

Uveal metastases most commonly originate from primary breast and lung cancers in women, and lung and gastrointestinal tract cancers in men (18,47,152,172). In an autopsy series of patients with breast cancer, a third of the cases included uveal metastases (15). Uveal metastases are often unifocal but may be multifocal within the eye or may be bilateral (152,166). Shields et al. (152) published an analysis of 520 eyes containing 950 uveal metastatic tumors and found 88% in the posterior uvea, 9% in the iris, and 2% in the ciliary body.

The aim of therapy is to return visual function to the patient, although survival time may be limited to several months after the diagnosis of uveal metastases. Observation for small lesions may be appropriate if the patient is receiving an effective regimen of systemic chemotherapeutic management, which can stabilize or regress metastatic intraocular tumors, thus reserving irradiation for failure.

The treatment of uveal metastasis depends largely on the systemic condition of the patient. If the patient has visual symptoms, treatment should be offered as soon as possible in order to maintain and, in many cases, improve visual acuity.

Chemotherapy or hormonal therapy is used to manage disseminated systemic disease, when indicated, while the eye is monitored (38,79). If there is no evidence of systemic metastatic disease or if the uveal metastasis does not respond to systemic therapy, external beam or brachytherapy to the eye is often performed.

Almost 90% of patients have positive objective responses to therapy (18). For patients with uveal metastases and active systemic disease, palliative response is achieved by delivering a 30 to 40 Gy over 3 to 4 weeks to the entire ocular structure. In the absence of active systemic disease, precocious metastases and in patients with breast or colon cancer, in whom the potential for long-term survival is greater, a more aggressive approach is taken. In such cases, brachytherapy with ^{125}I plaque and a prescribed dose of 40 Gy to the tumor apex is recommended.

Rappaport et al. (119) reported globe preservation of 98% of 188 patients and 43% experienced improvement in visual acuity. For many years, different techniques have been described and included lateral portals and shielding of the lens and cornea, but it may produce underdosing of metastases located on the anterior aspect of the choroid or uvea. Electrons in the range of 15 to 18 MeV may be used, although 6 MV photon beam is commonly used.

In general, cataract formation usually takes 2 to 3 years, and many of these patients present with partially controlled disease outside the eye globe, consequently a good palliation is achieved when the lens is not considered a limiting factor and a more uniform, homogeneous distribution is obtained by irradiating the globe up to the posterior chamber.

With the current availability of 3D conformal radiotherapy (Fig. 35.3) or intensity-modulated radiation therapy (IMRT) planning, it is possible to adequately treat the uveal lesions, minimizing dose to surrounding tissues.

Currently, hypofractionated CyberKnife (Accuray, Sunnyvale, CA) radiosurgery is being explored for the treatment of uveal metastasis, although no dose recommendations are available at the time of this publication, until Institutional Review Board (IRB) protocols are complete.

Brachytherapy, or plaque radiation therapy, has been used as the only treatment modality for single uveal metastases or those failing external beam irradiation. In a series of 36 patients with uveal metastasis treated with plaque radiation therapy, the mean time for treatment was 86 hours, and the mean therapeutic dose was 68.8 Gy to the tumor apex and 235.6 to the tumor base (151). Regression of the uveal metastasis was documented in 94% of cases. Plaque irradiation salvaged five of six eyes that had failed prior external beam radiation therapy.

At Wills Eye Hospital and the Department of Radiation Oncology, Hahnemann University Hospital, 40 Gy to the tumor apex is prescribed, delivered over 4 to 5 days, depending on tumor thickness.

Malignant Melanoma of the Posterior Uvea

The most common primary intraocular tumor in adults is the uveal melanoma. The incidence in the United States is approximately six cases per million per year, or about 2,000 new cases in the United States per year (92). Uveal melanoma affects both sexes with a slight predominance in males. The disease is found in all ages; however, the mean age at diagnosis is in the mid-50s (92). Uveal melanoma has one tenth the incidence of cutaneous melanomas. In a case-controlled study, risk factors for developing uveal melanoma were characterized including family history of uveal melanoma or personal history of cutaneous melanoma (109). Protective factors in the same study were olive or black skin, dark iris color, high resistance to sunburn, and wearing prescription glasses.

The diagnosis of malignant uveal melanoma has become easier and more accurate with a variety of techniques, reducing the risk of unnecessary enucleation (158). Diagnostic

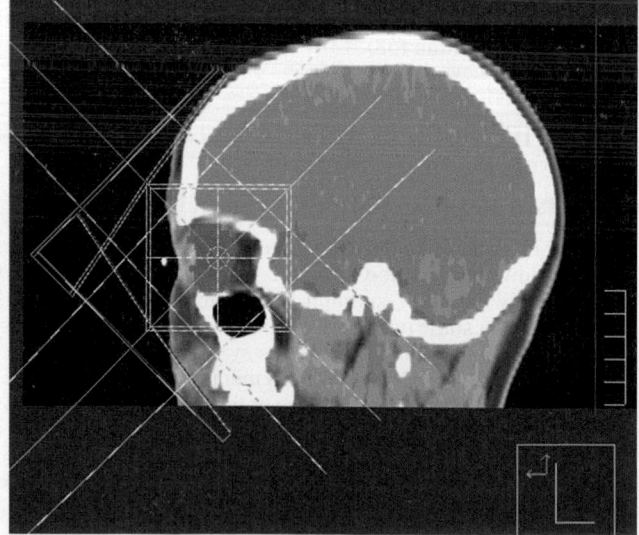
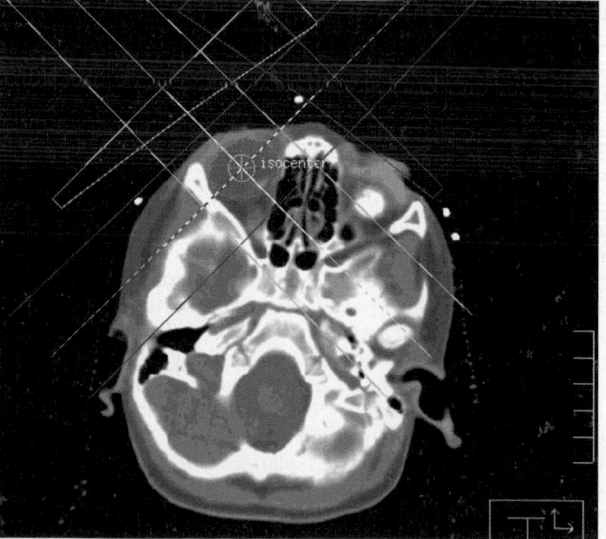

FIGURE 35.3. Three-dimensional computed tomography scan reconstruction image showing beam arrangement for unilateral retinoblastoma cases: anterior medial and lateral fields **(A)**, anterior superior and inferior fields **(B)**, sagittal view of composite isodose distribution **(C)**, and axial transverse view of isodose distribution **(D)**. Note that the tumor volume includes a minimum of 5 mm of proximal optic nerve, which is convered by the 95% line. The 50% line is barely outside the orbital cavity, with a significant dose drop to the chiasm, brainstem, and the like. For bilateral cases, six fields are used **(E)**: two lateral opposing fields plus two anterosuperior and anteroinferior fields as shown on **(A)** for each eye. Composite isodose distribution that shows a uniform coverage with the 95% line to each eye globe and proximal optic nerve **(F)**. (*continued*)

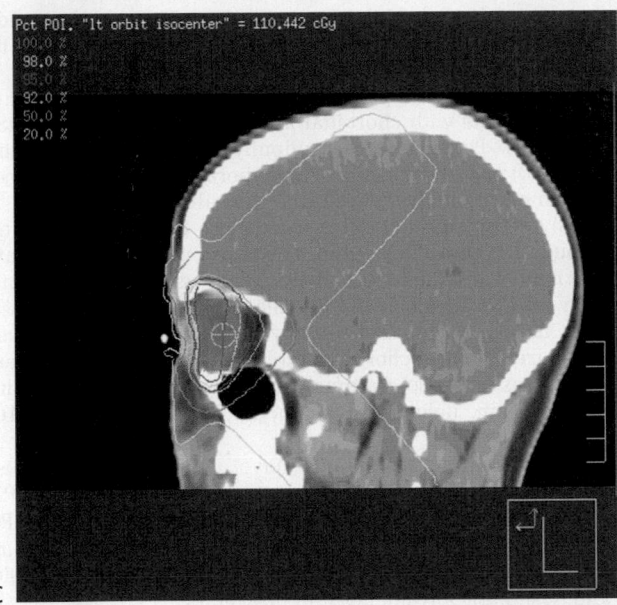

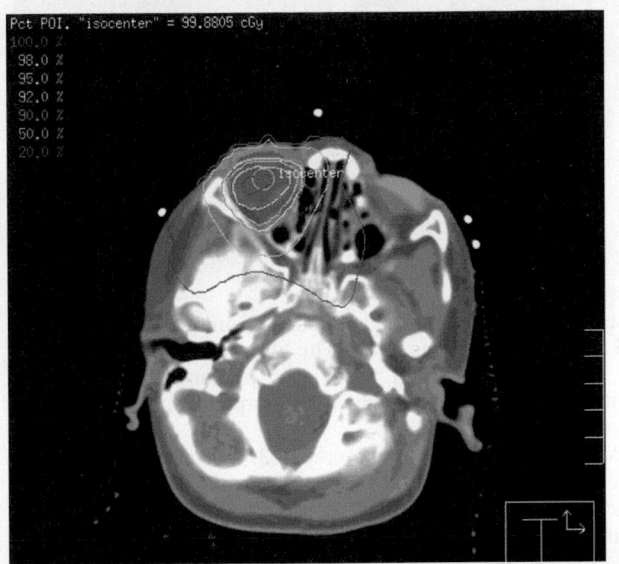

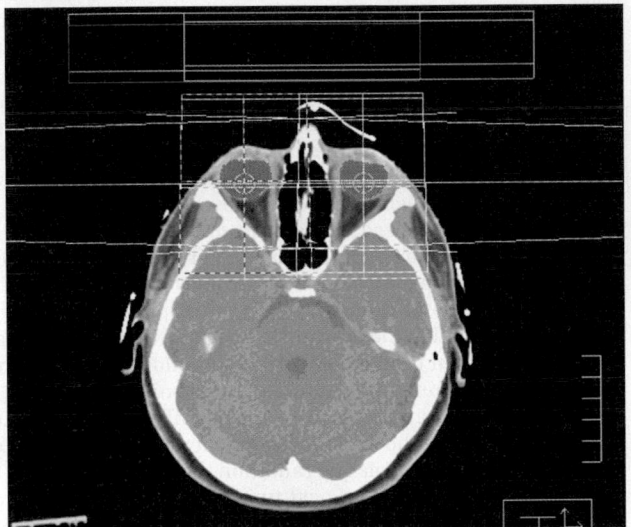

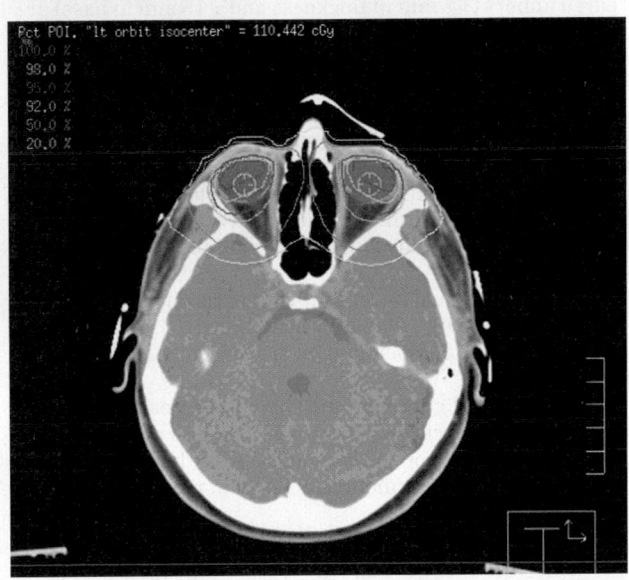

FIGURE 35.3. (continued)

procedures include indirect ophthalmoscopy, fundus photography, autofluorescence photography, fluorescein and indocyanine angiography, ultrasound (both A and B modes), optical coherence tomography (OCT), magnetic resonance imaging (MRI), and CT scan.

By far the most important means of diagnosis is the detection of the clinical features of the tumor, observed during an ophthalmoscopic examination, where orange pigment is found on the surface of the tumor along with a history of a nevus that showed signs of growth over time.

From the histopathological point of view, Callender in 1942, proposed a classification of uveal melanomas based on cell type and other histological characteristics including pigment content, tumor necrosis, argyrophilic fibers (Table 35.2). This was subsequently modified by McLean in 1983 that correlated between cell type and mortality.

Management of uveal melanoma continues to be controversial. Several options for management have been advocated, including periodic observation, laser photocoagulation, thermotherapy, plaque brachytherapy, charged particle radiotherapy, local resection, and enucleation (92,152,160, 164).

Several considerations influence the therapeutic options in the management of uveal melanoma and include tumor size, activity, location, growth pattern, patient's general health, age, and status of opposite eye. All of these factors should be analyzed collectively when making a decision for treatment. In those cases where there is hope for useful vision, every attempt should be done with an organ-conserving procedure, however, if chances for functional visual acuity are minimal or intraocular pressure is elevated, enucleation is warranted (196).

Tumor size and stage become determining factors for treatment modalities (Tables 35.3 and 35.4). Small melanomas (<10 mm in diameter and <3 mm thickness) are usually

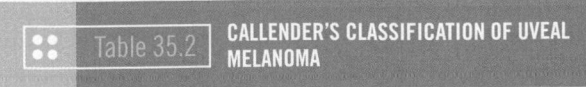

| Table 35.2 | CALLENDER'S CLASSIFICATION OF UVEAL MELANOMA |

1. Spindle A cell (the most benign, <5% 5-y mortality rate)
2. Spindle B cell (mortality rate 40% in 5 y)
3. Pure epithelioid cell (most aggressive, mortality rate 69% in 5 y)
4. Mixed cell (mortality rate 51% in 5 y)

Table 35.3	TNM CLASSIFICATION OF UVEAL MELANOMA (INTERNATIONAL UNION AGAINST CANCER UICC)
T1	<10 mm greatest dimension, <3 mm thickness
T1 A	<8 mm greatest dimension, <2 mm thickness
T1 B	>8 to 10 mm greatest dimension, >2–3 mm thickness
T2	10–15 mm greatest dimension, 3–5 mm thickness
T3	>15 mm greatest dimension, >5 mm thickness
T4	Extraocular extension
N1	All sites, regional
M	Metastasis

observed, with exception of a subset of tumors that show clinical risks for metastasis (143). The high-risk small melanomas are commonly managed with laser photocoagulation, thermotherapy, charged particle radiotherapy, plaque brachytherapy, and/or local resection.

Medium-size uveal melanomas (3 to 8 mm in thickness and 10 to 15 mm in diameter) can be managed with plaque brachytherapy, charged particle radiotherapy, local resection, or enucleation depending on particular factors. At present these are usually treated with plaque radiotherapy.

Large tumors (>8 mm in thickness and >15 mm in base) are managed with local resection or plaque brachytherapy. Enucleation is preferred due to ocular intolerance to conservative methods (196).

Uveal melanoma with involvement of the iris, ciliary body, or the posterior choroid and are managed accordingly. Tumors that are diffuse, display a relatively fast growth pattern, and have extrascleral extension are amenable to be treated with enucleation; however, if there is less extensive disease, radiotherapy should be employed in the form of plaque brachytherapy (Fig. 35.4).

Iris melanoma could be treated with excision (186,187), full radial or "boomerang" plaque brachytherapy (Figs. 35.5 and 35.6), or enucleation depending on size and other characteristics (183,186).

Ciliary body and choroidal melanoma are treated by either brachytherapy or excision. With regard to brachytherapy, the closer the tumor to the optic disc and fovea, the higher the risk of irreversible visual impairment as a result of radioactive plaque brachytherapy (39,40).

Posterior uveal melanoma has traditionally been treated by enucleation of the affected eye globe, although the concept of enucleation has been questioned (159,161,164,191). In assessing the outcome of enucleation by actuarial survival tables, Zimmerman and McLean (191) suggested that the prognosis after enucleation may be worse than for an untreated patient. Some investigators have postulated that tumor seeding is affected by the manipulation of the globe during the surgical procedure and advocate a "no-touch" approach to enucleation (55). Another suggestion is that radical reduction of tumor burden by enucleation alters the immune surveillance capacity, and distant micrometastases begin to grow (46).

In the United States and Canada, the melanoma treatment controversy has led to the development of the Collaborative Ocular Melanoma Study (COMS) (32,92,173). COMS is a prospec-

tive randomized study that, among other aims, was designed to compare survival in patients treated with either brachytherapy or enucleation.

COMS report 28, published in December 2006, evaluated 1,317 patients with choroidal melanoma accrued from 1987–1998 (32). Patients were randomly assigned to enucleation (n = 660) or to ^{125}I plaque brachytherapy (n = 657). The conclusion of this study showed that mortality rates following ^{125}I brachytherapy did not differ from those following enucleation through 12 years of follow-up. The power of this study indicated that neither treatment was likely to increase nor decrease mortality rates by as much as 25% relative to the other.

A variety of radiation therapy approaches have been used in the treatment of choroidal melanoma (105). External beam techniques use ^{60}Co, Gamma Knife (Elekta Corp., Stockholm), proton beam, helium ion beam (24,25,31,34,75,86,102,103, 117,135,138).

Brachytherapy techniques have used a variety of isotopes as ophthalmic applicators, such as ^{60}Co, [106]Ru/[106]Rh (rhodium-106), radon-222 ([222]Rn), palladium-103 ([103]Pd), ^{125}I, gold-198 ([198]Au) and tantalum-182 ([182]Ta) (10,26,73,81, 83,89,93,101,107,170,171). Each isotope can provide physical and dosimetric advantages and downfalls.

At present, ^{125}I is predominantly used in the United States, Canada, and the United Kingdom (11), whereas [106]Ru is quite popular in Germany. The current relative indications for treating a posterior uveal melanoma with plaque radiation therapy are generally as follows: (a) selected small melanomas that are documented to be growing or that show clear-cut signs of activity on the first visit, (b) most medium-sized and some large choroidal and ciliary body melanomas in an eye with potential salvageable vision, or (c) almost all actively growing melanomas that occur in the patient's only useful eye.

If a melanoma exceeds 15 mm in diameter and 10 mm in thickness, one should anticipate visual morbidity from radiation therapy, and enucleation should be strongly advised (160). The surgical technique of radioactive plaque application has been described in detail in the literature. Specially designed notched plaques have been used effectively to surround the optic nerve and irradiate tumors in a juxtapapillary location (40).

There does not appear to be a major difference in local tumor control among the various brachytherapy techniques. Local tumor relapse after plaque radiation therapy occurs in up to 16% of cases (40,84,125). Local tumor recurrence constitutes an important posttreatment clinical indicator of the tumor's great malignant potential and the patient's increased risk of melanoma-specific mortality (179). In two series of 93 patients with juxtapapillary choroidal melanoma managed by plaque irradiation, local tumor recurrence was documented in 14 cases (15%) (40,84). The younger age of the patient (<35 years) and the superior and inferior location of the tumor were predictive for local tumor recurrence (40).

In an analysis of 270 patients with choroidal melanoma treated with custom-designed plaque radiotherapy combined with transpupillary thermotherapy, long-term tumor control was achieved in 97% of eyes. The excellent control in this series was attributed to the custom design of the plaque by the radiation oncology team and precision of plaque placement by the surgical ocular oncology team. In fact, patients with juxtapapillary choroidal melanoma, the most difficult location for therapy due to the proximity to the optic nerve, achieved 95% long-term control in this series (141).

The visual outcome of an eye treatment with brachytherapy depends mainly on tumor size and location as well as on the development of radiation retinopathy and papillopathy (108,125). Patients with tumors located near the fovea or optic disc and those with larger tumors have the worst visual outcome (108,125). In their series of 77 patients with posterior uveal melanoma managed by ^{60}Co plaque irradiation, Cruess et al. (33) found that eyes receiving a radiation dose in excess

Table 35.4	AMERICAN JOINT COMMITTEE ON CANCER (AJCC) STAGE GROUPING FOR UVEAL MELANOMA		
Stage IA	T1A	N0	M0
Stage IB	T1B	N0	M0
Stage II	T2	N0	M0
Stage III	T3	N0	M0
Stage IVA	T4	N0	M0
Stage IVB	Any T	N1	M0
	Any T	Any N	M1

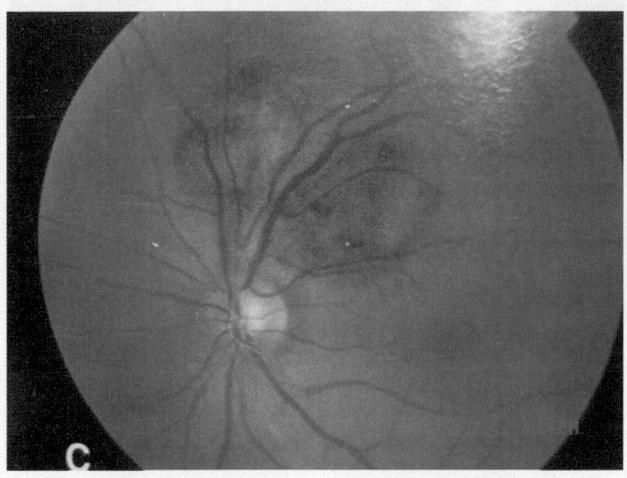 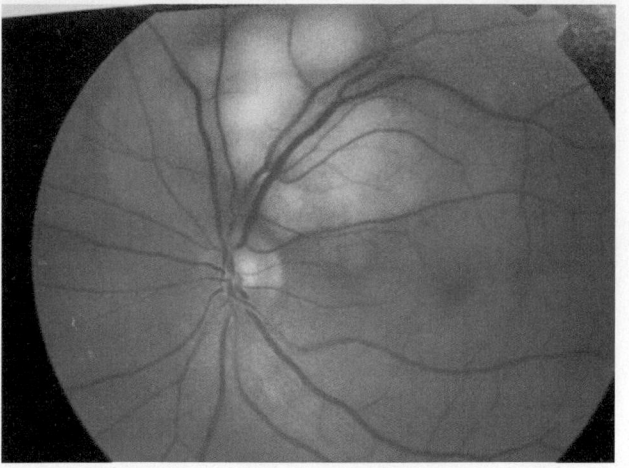

FIGURE 35.4. Choroidal melanoma: **(A)** before and **(B)** after iodine-125 plaque brachytherapy.

of 50 Gy to the fovea and/or optic disc commonly lost a substantial amount of vision within 2 to 3 years.

In a more recent series of 93 patients with choroidal melanoma touching the optic disc, DePotter et al. (40) from Wills Eye Hospital found an 87% incidence of retinopathy and 52% incidence of radiation papillopathy after a mean interval of 21 and 27 months, respectively, after plaque therapy. When life-table analysis was used, the proportion of patients who experienced a decrement of at least three lines of vision was 0% by 0 to 20 months, 22% by 20 to 30 months, 45% by 30 to 40 months, and 72% by 50 to 60 months. These results also were confirmed in a series by Lommatzsch et al. (84) after use of ^{106}Ru/^{106}Rh plaques for juxtapapillary choroidal melanomas.

Shields et al. (147) provided long-term analysis of visual acuity following plaque radiotherapy for choroidal melanoma in 1,106 patients. In this group, poor visual acuity of 20/200 to no light perception was found in 34% at 5 years and 68% at 10 years follow-up. From multivariable analysis, the group of clinical factors that best predicted poor visual acuity was tumor thickness (increasing) ($p = .0001$), proximity to foveola (<5 mm) ($p = .0001$), plaque shape (notched) ($p = .0001$), tumor recurrence ($p = .0001$), patient age ($\geq$60 years) ($p = .0006$), subretinal fluid ($p = .002$), isotope (cobalt [$p = .006$], ruthenium [$p = .02$], iridium [$p = .03$]), anterior tumor margin (posterior to equator) ($p = .01$), and initial visual acuity (worse) ($p = .03$). The mean percentage of patients with poor visual acuity at 5 years was

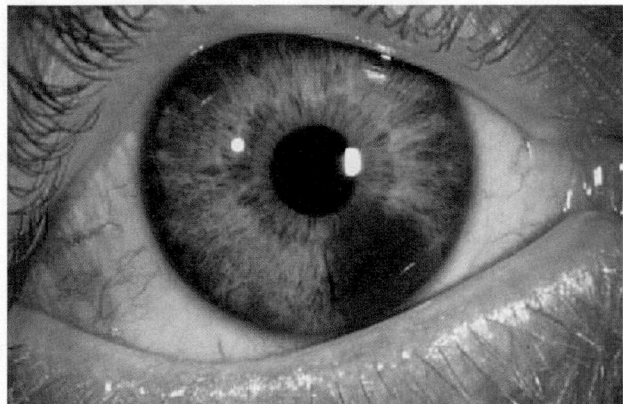 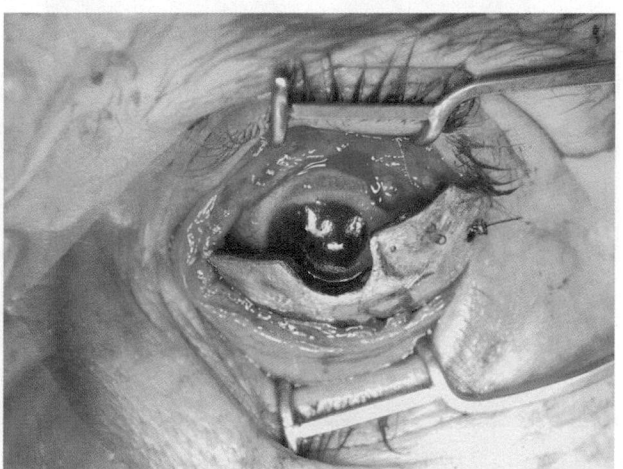

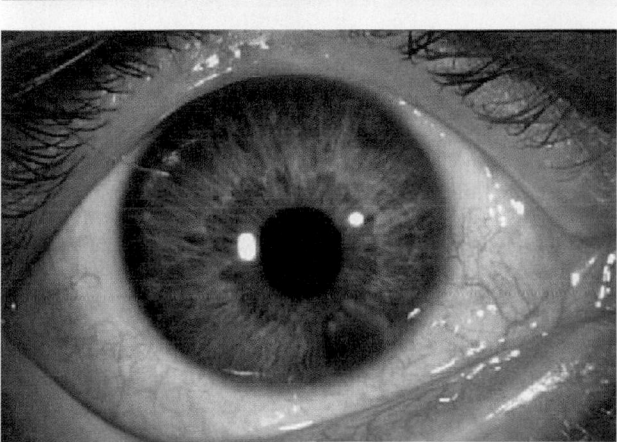

FIGURE 35.5. Localized iris melanoma: **(A)** before, **(B)** partial "boomerang" plaque application, and **(C)** 6 months after iodine-125 plaque brachytherapy.

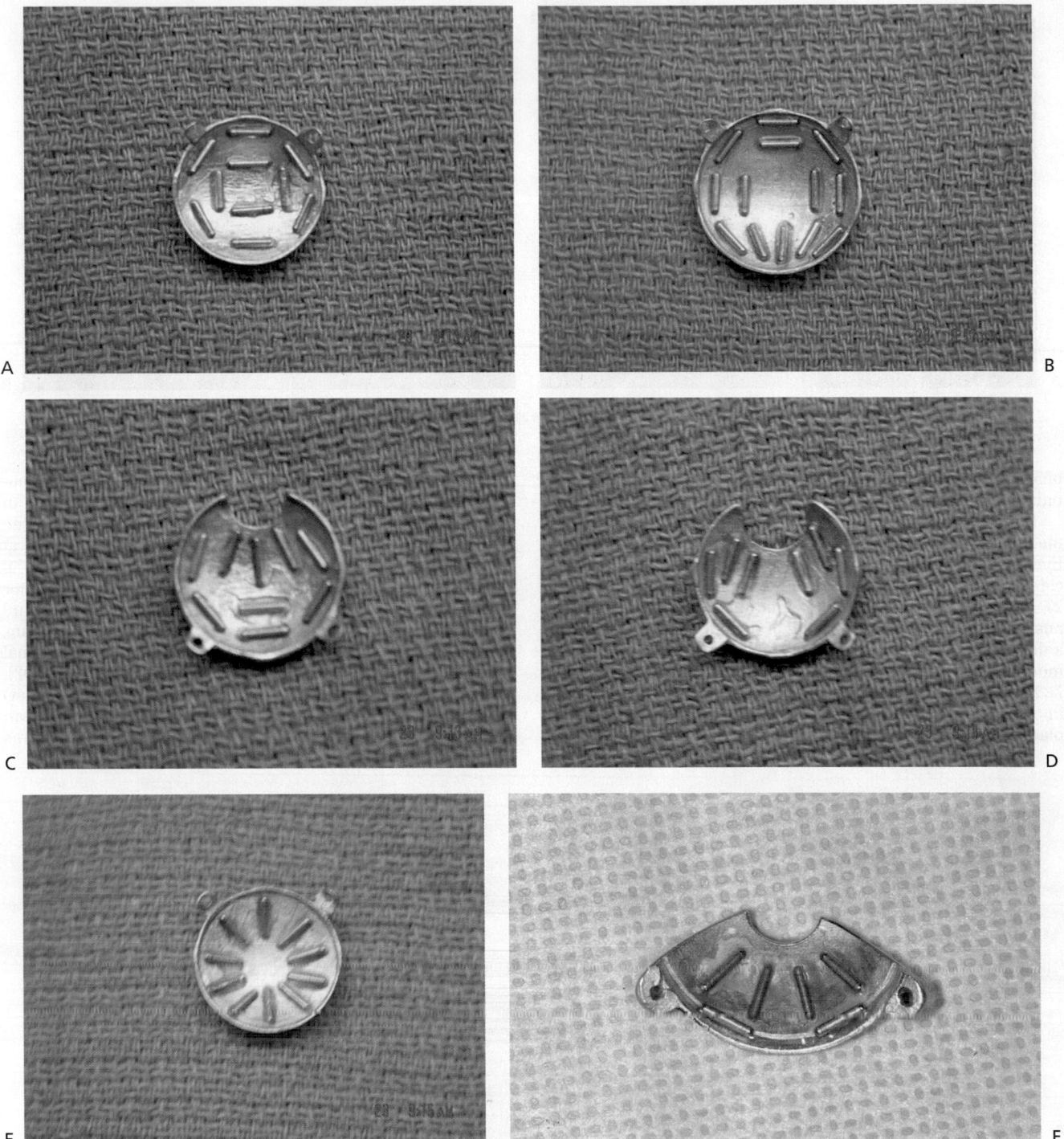

FIGURE 35.6. Iodine-125 plaques: **(A)** round standard, **(B)** round customized, **(C)** notched regular, **(D)** deep notched, **(E)** radial for diffused iris melanoma, and **(F)** partial "boomerang" for localized iris or ciliary body melanoma.

19% with no clinical risk factors, 39% with one risk factor, 49% with two risk factors, and 58% with three or more risk factors.

Combined plaque irradiation and laser photocoagulation or thermotherapy have been used recently to increase the likelihood of complete local tumor destruction, particularly in patients with tumor adjacent to the optic disc (6). Shields et al. published in 1998 the results of a 100 patients treated with plaque and transpupillary thermotherapy and found a recurrence rate of 3% in 8 years.

Particle-beam therapy has been reported to yield higher local control rates than common brachytherapy techniques. The Harvard group reported an estimated 5-year probability of local tumor control of 96.3% (10). The absolute local recurrence rate after helium ion therapy in patients observed for more than 5 years after treatment was given as only <3% (75). However, it was unclear whether all tumors were included or only those of the posterior uvea. The more anterior tumors, especially ciliary body tumors, are associated with a high enucleation rate (34). There does not appear to be any dose–response correlation for helium ion therapy from 5,000 to 8,000 cGyE (i.e., centigray equivalent, which is equal to the physical dose in cGy multiplied by the relative biologic effectiveness factor of 1.3). A similar result with proton-beam therapy, which uses a relative biologic effectiveness factor of 1.1, has not been reported. Survival, complications, and visual acuity also did not show any dose–response association with helium ion therapy (19,75).

It is generally agreed that very large ocular melanomas and cases of extrascleral extension of tumor at diagnosis are not readily amenable to radiation treatment. These eyes should be enucleated. However, the arguments of Zimmerman and McLean (191) that the process of enucleation may worsen the prognosis of these patients and the fact that survival of patients with very large intraocular tumors has been only about 50% in classic series have led to the investigation of preoperative radiation therapy as a means of improving survival in these patients. The adopted schema has been 20 Gy delivered to the globe and proximal optic nerve, including the major draining vessels from the posterior uveal tract, in five fractions over 5 to 7 days, with enucleation within 24 to 48 hours of the last treatment fraction. Eyes thus treated have been enucleated and cells harvested for tissue culture analysis. The irradiated cells did not grow and did not attach to culture vessels, demonstrating that irradiation can alter the *in vitro* growth of human ocular melanomas (74). Unfortunately, the initial clinical report, using nonrandomized techniques, has suggested a significantly lower survival in 41 patients receiving preoperative irradiation compared with the survival of 31 patients treated by enucleation alone (25). However, there were significant differences between the two groups, and the results must be interpreted cautiously. We have conducted a prospective, statistically matched study with 29 patients in each group and have shown no survival differences between preoperative radiation therapy and enucleation alone over a 5-year follow-up interval. In a recent study, no long-term beneficial effect on survival of patients with uveal melanoma could be found after 8-Gy pre-enucleation irradiation (87).

Custom-designed plaque irradiation appears to be an effective alternative method of controlling nonresectable diffuse iris melanoma. In the series of Shields et al. (150), 14 patients with nonresectable iris melanoma were treated with ^{125}I plaque irradiation. The mean length of treatment was 96 hours to give a mean dose of 293 Gy to the base (corneal endothelium) and 106 Gy to the apex of the iris melanoma. Tumor control was achieved in 93% of patients. Despite the large dose of irradiation given transcorneally, the cornea tolerated it very well without corneal melting. Cataract developed in six patients. All patients except one had tumor control and retention of the eye. Further analysis of this technique in 38 patients showed continued excellent tumor control with recurrence at approximately 5% of eyes. Secondary glaucoma remains a long-term concern.

A retrospective analysis of ocular melanoma patients treated with ^{125}I plaque brachytherapy was performed by Jensen et al. (69) at the Mayo Clinic. In that study, 156 patients were treated with episcleral plaques in concordance with COMS design. Excellent tumor control was observed with 5-year overall survival of 83% and 5-year disease-specific survival of 91%. They observed that dose rates >90 to 100 cGy/hour were associated with increased systemic control but worse radiation toxicity.

Retinal Tumors

Retinoblastoma

Retinoblastoma is the most common intraocular malignancy of childhood, making up approximately 4% of pediatric malignancies (146). The incidence is approximately one in 15,000 to 18,000 live births, and 250 to 300 new cases per year in the United States (43,146,156). It is seen infrequently in routine ophthalmologic practice. The disease is bilateral in 20% to

30% of patients (43). Of newly diagnosed children, 10% have a family history of retinoblastoma, and these are always heritable cases (42,43). The remaining 90% are sporadic, of which 20% to 30% are bilateral, and these are heritable cases. Of the remaining 70% to 80% of apparent unilateral, sporadic cases, 10% to 12% are heritable (42). Therefore, of all cases diagnosed in the United States annually, approximately 40% to 50% are heritable. Retinoblastoma can arise in hereditary, nonhereditary, and chromosome-deletion forms, the latter occurring on the long arm of chromosome 13 (13q) (42,43).

In general, the hereditary form is diagnosed earlier than the nonhereditary form of the disease, carries a risk of other malignancies, and can affect the offspring of the affected individual. The disease may be bilateral or unilateral. The chromosomal abnormality can result from a germinal mutation or may be inherited.

The nonhereditary form is unilateral; the children of the affected individual are normal, and this form of the disease is not associated with an increased risk of other malignancies (42,43). The chromosomal abnormality is from a somatic mutation (43).

As a result of molecular genetic studies, it is now understood that the 13q14 mutation takes place on the long arm of chromosome 13, locus 14, which is a tumor suppressor gene termed the RB gene.

The RB gene is a large gene of about 200,000 base pairs that encodes a protein the inhibitory function of which is thought to be on cell growth. When the function is lost, there is increased cellular growth unopposed by any inhibitory signal. Loss of the entire RB gene, a portion of it, or a point mutation within it leading to a subtle change in the encoded protein may lead to a lack of inhibitory function. Because there are two copies of each gene, one on each of the paternally and maternally derived chromosomes, if one copy is defective or missing, the other copy is still capable of producing sufficient regulatory protein to prevent uncontrolled growth.

In the hereditary form of retinoblastoma, the mutation is thought to be in the germ cell; therefore, every cell in the body of the offspring will contain the defective gene copy. Either through spontaneous mutation or under the influence of some event (biologic, physical, chemical) that increases the probability of mutation, the normal gene copy may be sufficiently damaged in the offspring during retinal development to allow for the complete inhibition of the regulatory protein, leading to the development of retinoblastoma. Whether the defective allele is inherited from an affected parent or arises as a new mutation in a parental germ cell, the end result is identical. There is a high possibility in this inherited form of the disease for bilateralism as well as multifocality. Because the child has inherited only one defective allele in the germ cell, there is a 50% probability of transmission of this allele to any offspring.

The true sporadic disease is postulated to arise from two separate mutations, each in a separate copy of the RB gene within the same somatic cell. This form of the disease is not heritable because the germ cells are not involved, and not all cells in the body are affected. Therefore, there is a low probability for multifocality and bilaterality.

The conventional wisdom in the molecular genetics of cancer is that, besides inactivation of suppressor genes, such as the RB gene, activation of at least one oncogene may be required. The oncogene for retinoblastoma has not been identified, but it is known that the growth promotion of the myc oncogene can be modulated by a protein encoded by the RB gene (182).

Although the disease may be present at birth, most children with retinoblastoma are diagnosed before age 3 or 4 years, and rarely beyond the age of 6 years (42). The most common presenting signs and symptoms are leukokoria, strabismus, or a mass in the fundus noticed during ocular examination (156). Accurate diagnosis is paramount because several nonmalignant conditions can present similarly. In a series of 136 children

Clinical Radiation Oncology

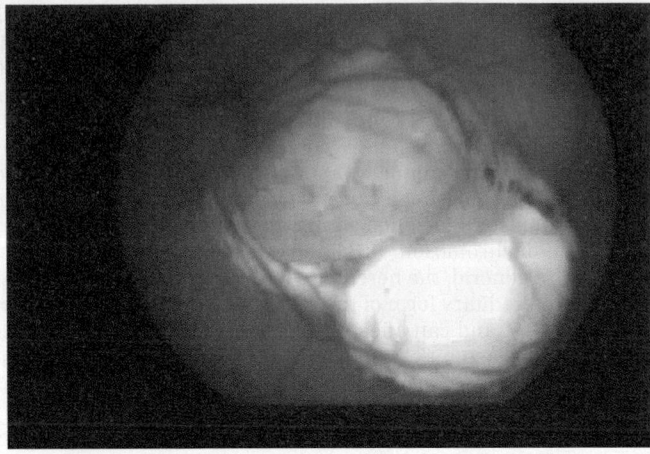
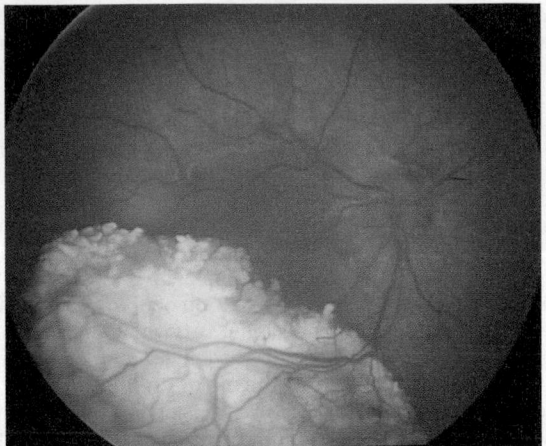

A   B

FIGURE 35.7. Fundoscopy in a patient with bilateral retinoblastoma. Whitish color due to tumor high calcium content that reflects the light and "white pupil" or leukokoria.

referred for evaluation, only 44% had retinoblastoma and the remainder had pseudoretinoblastoma (155). Shields and Shields published in 1999 a concise review on the recent developments in the management of retinoblastoma, which explains the different treatment modalities being used.

Evaluation begins with an accurate history that emphasizes prenatal and parturition information, prematurity, oxygen therapy, whether leukokoria was present at birth or was noticed later, whether the child has had contact with puppies or other animals, and whether anyone in the family has had retinoblastoma.

Children with retinoblastoma rarely have leukokoria or strabismus at birth, but this sign is usually noticed at 6 to 24 months of age. It is frequent for the parents or other relatives of the child to notice a whitish papillary reflex at a certain angle and light intensity or to observe a "white eye" instead of the usual "red eye" in photographs, which raises the suspicion of something wrong in the child's eye that prompts the parents to seek medical attention.

A careful ophthalmologic examination of the child must be performed to rule out other diagnoses compatible with pseudoretinoblastoma. Slit-lamp biomicroscopy with the pupils dilated may reveal congenital cataract or a retrolental membrane, suggesting diagnoses other than retinoblastoma in which the lens and anterior chamber usually remain clear (Fig. 35.7). Binocular indirect ophthalmoscopy seeking characteristic ophthalmic features of retinoblastoma or spontaneously regressed retinoblastoma remains the most important diagnostic tool (166).

Retinoblastoma exhibits certain ultrasonographic features that are typical but not pathognomonic. On A-mode ultrasonography, the detection of very intense reflections from calcium deposits is very suggestive of retinoblastoma. B-mode ultrasonography shows a heterogenous acoustic solidity with highly reflective intrinsic echoes within the tumor and attenuation of orbital pattern (36). On CT scan, retinoblastoma usually appears as a dense heterogenous lesion with hyperdense foci corresponding to calcification. CT is valuable for assessing extraocular extension and invasion of the optic nerve (36). Because of its soft tissue definition and multiplanar capability, MRI appears to be most helpful in differentiating retinoblastoma from simulating lesions such as Coats disease, retinal detachment, retinopathy of prematurity, and persistent hyperplastic primary vitreous. Involvement of the optic nerve, extraocular extension, and intracranial midline neoplasm in trilateral retinoblastoma are best detected by contrast-enhanced MRI studies (36).

The final ophthalmologic procedure is accurate mapping and sizing of tumor deposits in both eyes, which is best accom-

plished by indirect bilateral ophthalmoscopy with the child under general anesthesia. Mapping and sizing permit visual prognostic classification using the system of Reese and Ellsworth (122). In 2003, a new classification of retinoblastoma was introduced and is referred to as the International Classification of Retinoblastoma (Table 35.5). More recently, two staging systems, the American Joint Committee on Cancer (AJCC) (Table 35.6) and the St. Jude's System (Table 35.7), have been developed to include extraocular extension and metastasis, which determine survival after treatment.

Table 35.5	INTERNATIONAL CLASSIFICATION OF RETINOBLASTOMA		
Group	**Quick Reference**	**Specific Features**
A	Small tumor	Retinoblastoma ≤3 mm[a]
B	Larger tumor	Retinoblastoma >3 mm[a] or
	Macula	Macular retinoblastoma location (≤3 mm to foveola)
	Juxtapupillary	Juxtapupillary retinoblastoma location (≤1.5 mm to disc)
	Subretinal fluid	Additional subretinal fluid (≤3 mm from margin)
C	Focal seeds	Retinoblastoma with:
		Subretinal seeds ≤3 mm from retinoblastoma
		Vitreous seeds ≤3 mm from retinoblastoma
		Both subretinal and vitreous seeds ≤3 mm from retinoblastoma
D	Diffuse seeds	Retinoblastoma with:
		Subretinal seeds >3 mm from retinoblastoma
		Vitreous seeds >3 mm from retinoblastoma
		Both subretinal and vitreous seeds 3 mm from retinoblastoma
E	Extensive retinoblastoma	Extensive retinoblastoma occupying >50% globe or
		Neovascular glaucoma
		Opaque media from hemorrhage in anterior chamber, vitreous, or subretinal space
		Invasion of postlaminar optic nerve, choroid (>2 mm), sclera, orbit, anterior chamber

[a]Refers to 3 mm in basal dimension or thickness.

Table 35.6	AMERICAN JOINT COMMITTEE ON CANCER TUMOR STAGING SYSTEM FOR RB
T1/p1	<25% of retina
T2/pT2	>25–50% of retina
T3/Pt3	>50% of retina and/or intraocular beyond retina
T3a/pT3a	>50% of retina and/or cells in vitreous
T3B	Optic disk
pT3b	Optic nerve up to lamina cribrosa
T3c	Anterior chamber and/or uvea
pT3c	Anterior chamber and/or uvea and/or intrascleral
T4/pT4	Extraocular
T4a	Optic nerve
pT4a	Beyond lamina cribrosa, not at resection line
T4b	Other extraocular
pT4b	Other extraocular and/or at resection line
N1/pN1	Regional
MI	Distant metastases

Final staging studies, usually performed by the pediatric oncologist, consist of lumbar puncture with cytospin analysis of the cerebrospinal fluid for malignant cells and a bone scan if these studies are indicated, based on clinical findings. The siblings of the affected child and the child's parents also should undergo bilateral indirect ophthalmoscopy to detect disease or regressed disease.

Enucleation of the involved globe has been the traditional method of therapy for unilateral disease, and early enucleation after diagnosis has been given as the main reason for the marked improvement in survival during the past half century (155). The fellow eye, although apparently normal at diagnosis, remains at risk and must be examined at frequent intervals until the child is at least of school age.

The therapy of bilateral disease is more complex and traditionally has consisted of enucleation of the eye with more advanced disease and radiation therapy for the less involved eye. Tragically, in some cases, both eyes contain advanced tumors, and there is no hope of retaining useful vision. In such cases, bilateral enucleation has been traditionally recommended. Fortunately, there is often asymmetric development of the dis-

ease, and one of the eyes may be salvageable by radiation therapy. Even if the most advanced eye has more than half of the retina spared or a potential for retention of useful vision, an attempt may be made to salvage both eyes by radiation therapy, reserving enucleation for salvage of failures (155).

Management of Reese-Ellsworth group I to IV has recently changed to the use of chemoreduction, and external beam radiotherapy is reserved for selected group V cases. Nonetheless, favorable cases group I or II with solitary tumors close to the fovea can be treated with external beam radiation therapy.

Group III and IV tumors can be treated by external beam irradiation or complex plaque techniques. Because of the severe nature of the disease in group V, there is frequent failure of radiation therapy, and enucleation may be the final outcome.

Recent developments with chemotherapy regimens have allowed dramatic control of intraocular retinoblastoma, and chemoreduction plays an important role in the initial management of patients. Shields et al. use carboplatin, etoposide, and vincristine as initial chemotherapy agents for adequate tumor reduction and allow for more focused, less damaging therapeutic measures such as laser photocoagulation, cryotherapy, thermotherapy or plaque brachytherapy. The goals of chemoreduction are to avoid enucleation and external beam irradiation. After 2 months of chemoreduction, there was a mean of 35% decrease in tumor base and nearly 50% decrease in tumor thickness. Focal treatment was mandatory to completely eradicate the residual tumor. Currently, six cycles of chemotherapy are administered before evaluation and recommendation of adjuvant therapies is made. According to the International Classification or Retinoblastoma, successful treatment with chemoreduction was achieved in 100% of group A, 93% of group B, 90% of group C, and 47% of group D eyes. Group E retinoblastoma is generally treated with enucleation (143).

External Beam Techniques for Retinoblastoma

The first successful treatment of retinoblastoma by x-rays was reported by Hilgartner (63) in 1903. External beam irradiation is used if preservation of sight is possible and the tumor is not thought to be life threatening. Armstrong (5) and Weiss et al. (184) described various techniques including the classic single temporal portal and modifications that allowed retinal irradiation and shielding of the lens and anterior chamber. This technique, however, results in underdosing the anterior and posterior chamber, which increases the risk for anterior recurrences and treatment failures and makes additional therapies more complex to apply. In addition, the rate of cataract formation remains quite significant.

The modified technique uses a lateral portal with the anterior beam edge at the equator of the globe and an anterior portal containing a 7-mm diameter central divergent block hung in a pendulum fashion along the central axis of the beam to protect the lens (184). Donaldson and Egbert (42) recommended the use of the Comberg contact lens with the field edge at the ora serrata. This technique was also associated with recurrences in ciliary body recesses and can be difficult to control.

At Hahnemann University Hospital we have discouraged lens-sparing techniques for external beam irradiation of retinoblastoma. We attempted uniform treatment of the entire retina using a hinged wedge technique, accepting the potential for ultimate cataract formation. Other radiation oncologists have confirmed this philosophy.

McCormick et al. (95) compared a lens-sparing technique with a modified lateral technique designed to reduce the lens dose to 50% of the volume dose to the globe. The lens-sparing technique was associated with relapse in about two thirds of the treated eyes compared with 17% with the modified lateral technique. Chin et al. (28) used three pairs of noncoplanar arcs

Table 35.7	ST. JUDE'S TUMOR STAGING SYSTEM

Stage I: Tumor (unifocal or multifocal) confined to retina
   a. Occupying one quadrant or less
   b. Occupying two quadrants or less
   c. Occupying more than 50% of retinal surface

Stage II: Tumor (unifocal or multifocal) confined to globe
   a. With vitreous seeding
   b. Extending to optic nerve head
   c. Extending to choroid
   d. Extending to choroid and optic nerve head
   e. Extending to emissaries

Stage III: Extraocular extension of tumor
   a. Extending beyond cut end of optic nerve (including subarachnoid extension)
   b. Extending through sclera into orbital contents
   c. Extending to choroid and beyond cut end of optic nerve (including subarachnoid extension)
   d. Extending through sclera into orbital contents and beyond cut end of optic nerve (including subarachnoid extension)

Stage IV: Distant metastases
   a. Extending through optic nerve to brain
   b. Blood-borne metastases to soft tissue(s) and bone(s)
   c. Bone marrow metastases

to treat the globe and expose the lens to 30% to 35% of the target dose. No patient data were given. Foote et al. (51) reported that treatment of retinoblastoma by anterior segment–sparing techniques resulted in 10/14 treated eyes requiring further treatment. When an anterior approach with no attempt at lens sparing was used, only 4/11 treated eyes required further treatment. Three of these four eyes required additional treatment for tumors in the posterior pole.

The whole-eye and lens-sparing techniques were reviewed by the group at St. Bartholomew's Hospital in London (65,176). They found that the eye-preservation rate has improved markedly from those of older series, and that the rate of ocular salvage depended on the stage of the disease (Reese-Ellsworth group) at the time of the treatment as well as the availability of focal therapy for limited recurrences. Among 175 eyes treated with whole-eye radiation therapy alone, the overall ocular rate was 57%, although with salvage therapy 80% of the eyes could be preserved (65). Among the 67 eyes subjected to lens-sparing irradiation with prior adjuvant treatment of anterior tumors, the overall ocular rate was 72%, and with salvage therapy 93% of the eyes could be preserved (176). These results compare favorably with those of the whole-eye technique.

Schipper (136) described various techniques for the treatment of retinoblastoma with lateral or oblique portals, depending on whether the contra lateral eye was to be spared.

3D Conformal Radiotherapy Technique

Freire et al., at Hahnemann University Hospital, in cooperation with Wills Eye Hospital, have developed and used a technique based on 3D conformal radiotherapy in several patients with diagnosis of either unilateral or bilateral retinoblastoma (see Fig. 35.3).

This technique was implemented based on the concern that the ophthalmologists, pediatricians, and radiation oncologists had with regard to short- and long-term side effects associated with irradiation, such as orbital bone hypoplasia characterized by a cosmetical defect that required, in some cases, reconstructive plastic surgery. Those patients had been treated in the 1950s or earlier with orthovoltage machines. At that level of energy the predominant mode of radiation absorption by the different tissues is the photoelectric effect, which is dependent on the atomic number (Z), consequently, the high calcium content in the bone absorbed most of the energy and was the determining factor for stunned bone growth. The same effect is obtained with the use of electrons. However, photons of 4 or 6 MV lack this property, for the predominant absorption mechanism is the Compton effect and independent of the atomic number; therefore, it is expected that the orbital hypoplasia will be significantly less. A prospective study will be able to confirm the accuracy of this proposed beneficial outcome.

Treatment of unilateral retinoblastoma cases consists of four noncoplanar fields that are employed based on a 3D planning. All fields are anterior oblique: superior, inferior, medial, and lateral. Depending on the stage and anatomy, a 0.5 cm bolus can be used. Extreme caution must be taken to minimize the dose to critical structures such as fellow eye, chiasm, pituitary gland, brainstem, posterior-most upper teeth, and upper cervical spine. The entire retina should be treated, including 5 to 8 mm of proximal optic nerve. With this technique, the tumor volume is treated approximately to the 98% line, whereas the 50% line encompasses the orbit with the above-mentioned organs and tissues receiving significantly less dose.

For patients with bilateral disease that require treatment to both eyes, six noncoplanar fields are used: two lateral opposing and two anterior oblique fields to each eye following the same criteria described above. The authors recommend a dose of 42 to 44 Gy in daily fractions of 1.8 or 2.0 Gy over a period of 4.5 to 5 weeks.

Since 70% to 80% of patients are 3 years or younger, conscious sedation applied by an anesthesiologist during the CT scan for treatment planning, simulation, and on a daily basis for treatments may be necessary. Both the induction and recovery of sedation is fast and safe under the team supervision and greatly improves accuracy of treatment as well as patient comfort.

Brachytherapy for Retinoblastoma

In 1929, Foster-Moore and Scott reported their experience with radon seed implantation of retinoblastoma. Stallard (169) described his development of the radium applicator in 1948, which was later replaced by the ^{60}Co plaque. Our past techniques using cobalt episcleral applicators consisted of delivering 40 Gy to the tumor apex.

Plaque radiation therapy can be used as primary or secondary treatment. Amendola et al. (2) reported their experience with 20 patients treated with brachytherapy as a boost after external beam therapy for very large or locally recurring tumors. Sixteen of 20 patients (80%) had tumor control; the remaining four patients (20%) required enucleation for failure. In fact, in 70% of cases plaque radiation therapy is used as secondary treatment to salvage a globe after prior failed treatment, usually external beam irradiation (62,148). In the series of Shields et al. (164), solitary plaque radiation therapy was used in 91 cases of recurrent or residual retinoblastoma in which the only other option was enucleation. Tumor control and globe salvage were achieved in 89% of cases with plaque irradiation (mean dose to tumor apex, 41 Gy) during a mean follow-up of 52 months. In another series of 103 tumors treated with solitary plaque irradiation, there was 87% tumor control rate with one application of plaque radiation therapy (154). Carefully selected retinoblastomas, even juxtapapillary and macular tumors, can be successfully treated with plaque radiation therapy. Visual outcome varies with tumor size and location, as well as with radiation and the complications of retinopathy and papillopathy (148). In a series of 103 eyes managed with plaque therapy (initial or secondary treatment, mean apical dose of 42.27 Gy), the visual outcome was good in 62% and poor in 29%; enucleation was required in 9%. The poor vision was due to foveal retinoblastoma.

Chemoreduction has been implemented for retinoblastoma, and if they recur, ^{125}I plaque radiotherapy has been successfully used. In a series by Shields et al. (143), 84 cases of recurrent retinoblastoma in children were reviewed. All underwent chemoreduction prior to recurrence. With the use of ^{125}I plaque brachytherapy, tumor control was achieved in 95% of eyes. Anticipated complications including radiation retinopathy and mild vitreous hemorrhage occurred at acceptable rates.

Sequential paired opposed plaque technique (SPOP) has been used as primary or secondary treatment (2,157). Preliminary results were encouraging, however, this technique should be explored further to evaluate its impact on controlling retinoblastoma and related significant toxicity.

The Hahnemann/Wills Eye Hospital team prescribe a dose of 40 Gy to the apex delivered over 4 days. Plaques of different size, shape, and seed distribution are used for the treatment of retinoblastoma (see Fig. 35.6).

Second Malignancies in Retinoblastoma

Trilateral retinoblastoma describes the association of bilateral and/or familial retinoblastoma and neuroblastic tumors in the pineal gland or other midline structures. In series by DePotter et al. (37), the incidence of trilateral retinoblastoma was 8% of all bilateral familial retinoblastomas and 5% of all sporadic retinoblastomas. The tumor usually occurs in children at a mean age of 23 months. The disease is highly fatal despite aggressive treatment with chemotherapy, radiation therapy, Gamma Knife therapy, and others. Trilateral retinoblastoma is a major cause of mortality in children within the first 5 years after the diagnosis of retinoblastoma. Longer survival has been correlated with earlier tumor diagnosis in asymptomatic patients with routine CT or MRI studies of the brain, which should be performed until the age of 4.5 years (37). Shields et al. (144) have observed that the rate of pinealoblastoma development has significantly declined in the era of chemoreduction. They attribute the reduction to chemoprevention.

There has been extensive evaluation of second malignancies in retinoblastoma. Smith et al. (167) reviewed 55 patients seen at Stanford University Medical Center between 1954 and 1986. Of 53 available patients, eight developed 11 second primary tumors, with all occurring in patients with the hereditary form of the disease. Three of the 11 second primary tumors were outside the area treated for the primary retinoblastoma. The actuarial incidence of development of second primary malignancies was 4.4% to 6% at 10 years after treatment for retinoblastoma, and the rate increased to 26% to 38% at 30 years (124,167). The latent period from primary therapy to development of the second primary tumor ranged from 5.2 to 36.2 years, with a median of 16 years. Aggressive multimodal treatment of the second primary disease in five of eight patients was associated with 80% survival without evidence of disease at 22 to 72 months after treatment. Seven of 11 second primary tumors were osteogenic sarcomas. Overall, the cumulative probability of death from second primary neoplasms was 26% at 40 years after bilateral retinoblastoma diagnosis (45).

Loss or mutation of both copies of the growth-control genes on chromosome 13 is also associated with the development of osteogenic sarcoma and other types of mesenchymal tumors (137). Schwarz et al. (137) report that the second malignant tumors arising after treatment for retinoblastoma consist of osteogenic sarcoma (58%), fibrosarcoma (21%), and other sarcomas (21%). They propose a strong role for radiation induction based on the increased number of sarcomas arising in the previously irradiated field, prolonged latency periods (12.4 years), and predominant sites for these secondary sarcomas, which are not characteristic of spontaneously occurring primary sarcomas.

Hawkins et al. (60) reported observing 30-fold more second primary tumors and over 400-fold more osteogenic sarcomas than would be expected in the general population after the diagnosis of retinoblastoma. In the absence of radiation therapy or chemotherapy, the inherent risk of second primary tumors after primary genetic retinoblastoma was 13-fold greater than the expected number and over 200-fold greater than the expected number of osteogenic sarcomas.

Leukemic Retinopathy

Retinal hemorrhage and infiltration of the optic nerve and retina are both manifestations of childhood leukemia that may cause permanent visual damage. Treatment consists of low-dose irradiation of 10 to 15 Gy fractionated over 4 to 5 days to the eye and retrobulbar region (123).

Intraocular Lymphomas

Primary intraocular lymphoma is a rare disease that can involve the retina, vitreous, or optic nerve with or without extension to the central nervous system (27). Histologically, they are most commonly diffuse large B-cell lymphomas; however, rarely they can be T-cell lymphomas. The initial manifestation is usually blurred vision or floaters resulting from a cellular infiltration of the vitreous cavity. In many cases, there appears to be no systemic manifestation, and the diagnosis is made either by enucleation or by vitreous biopsy (99).

For intraocular lymphomas, radiation therapy was once considered the treatment of choice (27). Michels et al. (98) treated two cases of intraocular lymphoma with 30 Gy external beam irradiation directed through lateral portals.

At Hahnemann University Hospital, ocular lymphoma patients are being treated with 3D conformal radiotherapy using four oblique fields, delivering a tumor dose of 36 Gy with 1.8 to 2.0 Gy fractions over approximately 4 weeks. However, more recently, it is believed that chemotherapy is the first-line treatment. The regimen of choice is methotrexate and cytosine arabinoside, which are able to cross the blood–ocular barrier (9,27).

Optic Glioma

Optic (nerve) glioma is most common in children under 15 years of age (189). The name is justified by the mixture of astrocytic-dominant (129) and oligodendroglial cell lines. The incidence is about 1% of all central nervous system tumors. A significant number of patients with neurofibromatosis contract this tumor. A slight female preponderance has been noted. A genetic factor has been implicated (67).

Optic glioma grows slowly. Symptoms often predate diagnosis by about 2 years (13). Tumors often engage the optic chiasm (more than 50% of cases), and some exhibit extension into the hypothalamus.

Unilateral proptosis and vision defects indicate chiasmal involvement and the possibility of hypothalamic symptoms (endocrine defects and increased intracranial pressure) (4). Optic atrophy or nystagmus can be a presenting symptom (4).

CT and MRI offer excellent evidence for an anatomic diagnosis (85). Visual acuity and field examinations indicate severity and progress of defects. Tumor extension into the hypothalamus may cause enlargement of the sella. A histopathologic analysis of resected tumor or biopsy is preferred for treatment evaluation. The adult type tends to show malignant features (1).

In children, the similarity of many anterior optic glioma tumors to pilocytic astrocytoma and meningioma has caused this tumor to be regarded as benign and resectable (180). Progressive symptoms and the prevalence of intracranial tumor extensions have justified an attitudinal change toward postoperative adjuvant therapy, which is assuming a more prominent role in management.

Completeness of surgical excision correlates with survival, but intracranial surgery alone exhibits low survival figures (128,175). Radiation therapy is indicated when intracranial or progressive symptoms are evident (64,100,162). Bilateral temporal or multiportal beam arrangements are preferred for lesions involving both the posterior optic nerve and chiasm. A wedged-beam pair could be appropriate for intraorbital lesions. A dose of 50 Gy in 1.8- to 2-Gy fractions five times per week is generally recommended for adults and 45 Gy in 1.6- to 1.8-Gy daily fractions for children <15 years of age.

The majority of patients with optic pathway tumors have stable disease whether they receive radiation therapy or chemotherapy. This is an indolent tumor, and for the most part it is not life threatening. Because of this, issues regarding appropriate therapeutic approaches have yet to be resolved. Most agree that in patients with progressive visual loss and tumor limited to the orbit, surgery can be associated with a cure. The downside is the loss of vision associated with surgical extirpation. Radiation therapy rather than surgery has been the mainstay of treatment for intracranial tumors of the optic pathway. To eliminate side effects associated with radiation therapy in the young child, chemotherapy may be an alternative (29).

Numerous reports document the value of radiation therapy for patients with optic glioma (50,64,114,185). Long-term survival rates range from 80% to 100%. Improvement or stabilization of symptoms can be expected in a majority of patients. Radiation therapy complications (calcification, necrosis, and chiasmal damage) are rare except for endocrine disorders in children (114,120). Reirradiation for recurrent disease may be advantageous (49,185). Chemotherapy is evolving as an alternative in young children (126).

Jenkin et al. (68) reported on 87 children with optic glioma. Overall 10-year survival, relapse-free survival, and freedom from second relapse were 84%, 68%, and 85%, respectively; 27 patients relapsed or progressed, and 40% were free of a second relapse 10 years after the first relapse. The 35 patients with anteriorly located tumors, involving the optic nerve or chiasm and optic nerves, fared better than the 52 patients with posteriorly located tumors with spread beyond the chiasm. The 10-year survival rates were 95% and 76%, respectively ($p = .02$), and the 10-year relapse-free survival rates were 80% and 59%, respectively ($p = .02$). For posterior tumors, primary irradiation was more effective than primary subtotal resection for prevention of relapse; the 10-year relapse-free survival rates were 75% and 41%, respectively ($p = .02$), but salvage therapy was, in part, successful. Multivariate analysis of prognostic factors influencing survival for posterior tumors indicated that neither primary resection nor irradiation was a significant factor. For first relapse, primary irradiation and the presence of neurofibromatosis were significant favorable factors. Since 1977, subtotal resection or surveillance was used in 21/29 patients (72%) with posterior optic glioma compared with 4/23 (17%) previously. The 10-year survival rates before and after 1977 were 78% and 67%, and the 10-year relapse-free survival rates were 64% and 56%, respectively.

Gould et al. (57) reported on 25 children with optic gliomas evaluated by sequential computed axial tomography; 20 patients received radiation therapy. Of these, 10 patients had tumor regression, nine were stable, and one was worse. This result contrasts with five untreated patients, four of whom had tumor progression and one who was stable ($p < .001$). Of the 18 treated patients who could be tested reliably, visual function or regression occurred in seven children. None of the untreated patients improved. There were no definite complications of radiation therapy.

Kovalic et al. (77) described results in 33 patients with optic glioma: five patients (15%) had tumor confined to the optic nerve, eight (24%) had optic nerve and chiasmal involvement, and the remaining 20 patients (61%) had invasion of contiguous structures as well as chiasmal involvement. Eleven patients (33%) had a history of neurofibromatosis. Two thirds of the patients had either biopsy or partial resection of the tumor, with the remaining one-third being clinically diagnosed. All patients received irradiation to local fields; the median dose was 50.4 Gy in 1.6-Gy fractions. With a median follow-up of 12.3 years, the 5-, 10-, and 15-year overall actuarial survivals were 94%, 81%, and 74%, respectively. Extension of the primary lesion to the optic chiasm and age of 15 years or younger were the only variables to have statistically significant inferior 15-year progression-free survival on multivariate analysis. Eighteen patients (55%) had treatment-related complications, with most involving pituitary gland function.

At the University of Pittsburgh, 36 patients were treated for glioma of the optic nerve and/or chiasm (50). Median follow-up was 10.2 years. Pathologic verification was obtained in 32 patients. Tumor initially confined to the optic nerve recurred in one of five patients after complete resection. The actuarial survival rates for 25 patients irradiated for biopsy-proven glioma of the optic chiasm were 96%, 90%, and 90% at 5, 10, and 15 years, respectively, and the progression-free survival rate was 87% at 5, 10, and 15 years. Vision stabilized or improved in 86% of patients after radiation therapy.

Wong et al. (188) reviewed 38 cases of optic glioma; two patients died in the postoperative period and were excluded from analysis. Twenty-nine cases (76%) involved the optic chiasm, and nine cases (24%) were confined to one optic nerve. Most tumors were slow growing and progressive, although there were three cases of adult chiasmal gliomas that exhibited unusually aggressive behavior. With a mean follow-up of 9.4 years, the 10-year overall actuarial survival rate was 87%, and the relapse-free survival rate was 55%. Chiasmal tumors had a poorer prognosis than did optic nerve tumors, with 56% of chiasmal tumors recurring versus 22% of optic nerve tumors. Radiation therapy was beneficial in chiasmal gliomas, initially improving vision in 35% (6/17) and decreasing recurrence from 86% (six of seven) without radiation therapy to 45% (9/20) with irradiation.

The association between neurofibromatosis and visual pathway gliomas is well documented. Lesions tend to be more extensive in patients with neurofibromatosis, and the clinical course is more variable. Twelve of 24 patients with neurofibromatosis had symptoms of progressive disease at the time of diagnosis and underwent treatment with variable results; 12 children with neurofibromatosis and visual pathway lesions had static lesions at the time of diagnosis, and to date, three have developed progressive disease (106). Concerning the management of children with neurofibromatosis and visual pathway gliomas, many questions remain unanswered.

Optic gliomas in 29 patients, including 14 with von Recklinghausen neurofibromatosis (NF1), were treated with x-ray therapy (44). The projected 20-year survival rate was 92%. Among NF1 patients, 86% were stabilized or improved, whereas among non-NF1 patients, only 47% were stabilized or improved.

At present the use of fractionated stereotactic radiotherapy, as described in the pertinent chapter in this volume, is an excellent manner to address this issue for its ability to accurately focus on the tumor and minimizing irradiation to the surrounding tissues. The tumor volume includes a tight margin of 1 or 2 mm, two or three isocenters, and several arcs to deliver the prescribed dose of radiation.

In selected cases, fractionated stereotactic radiotherapy is indicated. This technique requires the use of a dedicated LINAC machine, also called X-knife, for daily treatments similar to conventional radiotherapy. Combs et al. (30) describe fractionated stereotactic radiotherapy as safe and well tolerated in 15 patients treated for optic pathway gliomas to a median dose of 52.2 Gy in five fractions of 1.8 Gy weekly. Progression-free rates at 3 and 5 years were 92% and 72%, respectively, and the 5-year survival rate was 90%. Stereotactic radiosurgery with X-knife or Gamma Knife is rarely indicated due to the fact that it consists of a single high-dose treatment that can be associated with higher incidence of side effects.

CyberKnife radiosurgery could be an alternative to be explored using hypofractionation for the treatment of optic gliomas; however, there is no dose recommendation as yet and more studies are needed.

Orbital Tumors

Primary malignant tumors of the orbit are rare. Among them we must include tumors arising from the eyelids, conjunctiva, Meibomian gland carcinomas, malignant lymphoma, rhabdomyosarcoma, and lacrimal gland tumors account for most cases. Of these, rhabdomyosarcoma has generated the most interest.

Eyelid Basal and Squamous Cell Carcinomas

In the treatment of basal cell and squamous cell carcinomas of the eyelids, radiation therapy can achieve an overall 90% to 95% cure rate. After the diagnosis is confirmed by biopsy, 50 to 60 Gy (depending on histology and size of the tumor) can be delivered by photon or electron-beam techniques. An internal

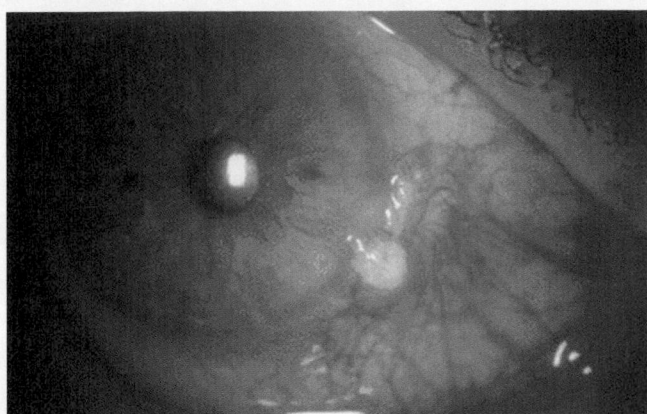

FIGURE 35.8. Conjunctival squamous cell carcinoma.

eye shield may be used to protect the globe. Although surgery is the treatment of choice, radiation therapy may be able to provide more acceptable cosmetic outcome in selected cases while providing similar cure rates.

Conjunctival Tumors

The conjunctiva can be the site of squamous cell carcinoma (Fig. 35.8), melanoma, or lymphomas. Squamous cell carcinomas arise in most cases at the inner canthus and can infiltrate to the eyelids, lacrimal duct, and cornea. Treatment of choice is surgical resection followed by cryotherapy to the surrounding healthy conjunctiva, and radiation is selected in refractory or recurrent tumors. Brachytherapy after resection and cryotherapy may be used by the authors, with episcleral plaque applied weekly in order to deliver 10 Gy at 1-mm depth for a total dose of 50 Gy in 5 weeks, but longer follow-up results are pending at present. Preliminary response is satisfactory.

Conjunctival melanoma in general is surgically resected similar to squamous cell carcinoma, cryotherapy, and weekly plaque therapy for 6 weeks for a total dose of 60 Gy in fractions of 10 Gy. Fractionated plaque brachytherapy results in high tumor control and low risk of complications compared to single application with a high dose of radiation.

Conjunctival lymphoma is occasionally observed to present as an isolated site in 2% of patients with extranodal non-Hodgkin's lymphoma (Fig. 35.9). It has been found that approximately 24% to 48% of lymphomas are extranodal and involve the stomach, intestine, or mucosalassociated lymphoma tumors

(MALT); tonsils or adenoids; and skin. Some of these tumors respond to a short course of antibiotics against *Chlamydia trachomatis* or *Helicobacter pilorii*, but most often they require systemic chemotherapy and/or local treatment with irradiation in the form of 3D conformal external beam or electron therapy with a dose of 30 to 36 Gy.

Sebaceous Carcinoma

Meibomian gland (sebaceous) carcinomas make up 1% to 5.5% of eye malignancies and have a mortality rate of 30% (22,104). Surgery is considered the first treatment option followed by radiation for partial resection or positive margins. These tumors can be multicentric, which may lead to local recurrences. Radiation therapy may be used for the treatment of these tumors in selected cases, particularly if surgery would not provide acceptable cosmesis or if the disease recurs after surgery. In our experience, high doses of irradiation (60 to 65 Gy in 6 to 7 weeks) are required.

Pardo et al. (110) reported a series of 30 patients with sebaceous carcinoma, 10 of whom received radiation therapy. Four were treated with curative intent, and the other six were treated postoperatively for parotid metastases after initial surgery. Doses ranged from 45 to 63 Gy, but the irradiation schema varied from 45 Gy in four fractions over 5 days to 60 Gy delivered in 2-Gy fractions over 51 days. The four patients treated definitively were free of disease at 36 to 117 months, and the patients treated in the adjuvant setting for metastatic disease were free of disease at 24 to 84 months.

Rhabdomyosarcoma

Rhabdomyosarcoma (RMS) is the most common soft tissue sarcoma in children with an incidence of 50% to 60% of all soft tissue sarcomas. Each year, approximately 350 cases of rhabdomyosarcoma are diagnosed in the United States with about 35 of those being orbital RMS (72).

There are three main histological types: embryonal, alveolar, and botryoid. The former is frequently found in the head and neck area, either in the orbit or as parameningeal tumor (163). Alveolar and botryoid types are most commonly seen in the genitourinary system and extremities.

Rhabdomyosarcoma of the orbit is most often seen in young children and carries a favorable prognosis. It has a rapid onset with marked proptosis and swelling of the adnexal tissue. Previously, the recommended treatment was orbital exenteration because many ophthalmologists thought that the tumor was radioresistant (20,70,117). The current recommendations are for combined radiation therapy and chemotherapy as the initial management, limiting surgical intervention to biopsy or local excision (80,130).

Lederman (78) provided the foundations for integrated management with surgery and radiation therapy and developed guidelines for the radiation therapy technique and dosage. Sagerman et al. (132) suggested the necessity of higher radiation doses. A minimum tumor dose of 45 to 50 Gy should be delivered by megavoltage equipment over 5 to 7 weeks, with some protection of sensitive ocular structures. All long-term survivors exhibit late radiation effects ranging from minimal change to phthisis bulbi, requiring enucleation.

According to the most recent recommendations of the International Rhabdomyosarcoma Group (IRSG), the IRS-IV trial for orbital RMS was reported to be superior to IRS-III, where the former had 100% successful outcome compared to 83% in the latter, according to Wharam et al. (181), which was thought to be explained by the use of a radiation dose of 50.4 Gy or higher and chemotherapy comprising vincristine and actinomycin-D without cyclophosphamide.

Forstner et al. (53) performed a retrospective review of patients with orbital RMS treated with multidisciplinary

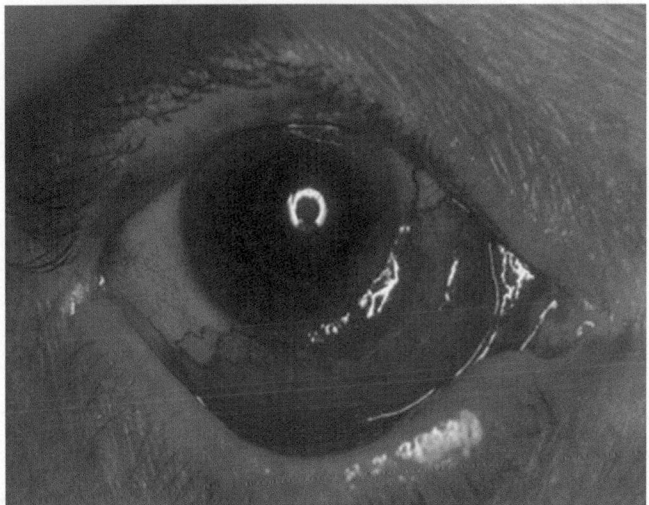

FIGURE 35.9. Conjunctival lymphoma. Typical "salmon" fleshy coloration.

treatment, revealing overall survival of 80% in a mean follow-up of 8 years. Although high cure rates were observed, toxicity including facial bone hypoplasia, cataract formation, and growth hormone deficiency was observed. They emphasize the importance of implementing modern radiation techniques to target therapy as best possible. With regard to irradiation, we advocate the use of 3D conformal radiotherapy or IMRT whenever possible to properly treat the tumor volume with an adequate margin.

Malignant Lymphoma of the Orbit

Although clear pathologic criteria for malignant lymphomas of the orbit differentiate them from pseudolymphomas, the diagnosis is not always clear (119). Malignant lymphomas are characterized by diffuse or nodular lymphoid infiltrates, and they frequently exhibit atypical cells, mitoses, and invasion of adjacent tissues in contrast to pseudotumors, which are characterized by a polymorphic admixture of cells including mature lymphocytes organized in reactive germinal centers with inflammatory changes. Surface markers may indicate a specific cell type.

Rao et al. (118) and Mittal et al. reported 23 and 22 patients, respectively, treated for malignant or indeterminate lymphomas of the orbit. Treatment was given with anterior or lateral portals covering the entire orbit and using ^{60}Co, 4- to 6-MV photons, or 15- to 16-MeV electrons. Control of the orbital tumor was achieved in 20/23 of the patients in the study by Rao et al., with doses of 30 to 40 Gy. The few patients who failed to respond received doses below 20 Gy.

Fitzpatrick and Macko (48) observed tumor control in 100% of 19 patients with malignant lymphoma confined to the orbit after delivery of doses ranging from 25 Gy in 10 fractions to 45 Gy in 15 fractions. Austin-Seymour et al. (7) had comparable results in 24 patients with benign lymphomatous conditions and eight patients with malignant lymphomas of the orbit treated with mean doses of 23.6 Gy and 36.25 Gy, respectively.

Reddy et al. (121) reported 17 patients with primary orbital lymphoma. Fourteen of these had 18 eyes treated by radiation therapy, and four patients were treated for local recurrence after surgery. Local control was achieved in 100%. Three patients died of systemic progression of lymphoma, 11 died of unrelated causes, and three patients remain alive without evidence of disease.

In a smaller series of patients with primary lymphoma of the orbit, Makepeace et al. (91) reported 100% local regression after radiation therapy. However, a third of their patients developed recurrent disease. The 5-year overall survival rate was 89%.

Bessell et al. (12) treated 115 patients with orbital lymphoid tumors; 18 had high-grade and 43 had low-grade malignant lymphomas; the remainder (47%) were considered to have indeterminate lymphocytic lesions. Survival of patients presenting with stage I low-grade malignant lymphoma and indeterminate lymphocytic lesions was similar to that of a normal population of the same age. However, the clinical features and dissemination patterns of the indeterminate lymphoid lesions were identical to those for low-grade malignant lesions. This suggested that most, if not all, lymphoid masses presenting in the orbit are neoplastic rather than reactive, and that patients should be as completely staged as those with lymphomas arising in other primary sites.

Radiation therapy is now considered the treatment of choice for localized primary orbital lymphomas (121). The suggested irradiation dose is 36 to 40 Gy administered in conventional fractionation schedules.

We have treated, at present, 15 patients with orbital lymphoma using CyberKnife robotic radiosurgery using hypofractionation scheme delivered in five fractions for a total dose of 16 Gy, which is equivalent to a standard dose of 36 Gy by employing the biologic effective dose (BED) equation. Longer follow-up and IRB qualified protocols are needed to conclude on the total dose and fraction size, and this analysis will be published in the future.

The new CyberKnife radiosurgery allows surgeons to spare healthy tissues, whenever possible, due to the accurate conformality of the dosimetric distribution and hypofractionation, achieving fast response, like the case illustrated in Fig. 35.10; a patient with stage IIIA non-Hodgkin's lymphoma and exophthalmus of the right eye who responded in 5 days of treatment. Follow-up in 6 months did not show local recurrent tumor. Longer follow-up is needed.

Lacrimal Gland Tumors

The aggressiveness of lacrimal gland tumors, the most prevalent being adenoid cystic carcinoma, is a challenge to control properly, partially caused by the difficulty of the surgical approach and the tendency of these tumors to infiltrate the orbital nerves and travel along to the base of the skull. Although relatively radioresistant, lacrimal gland tumors should routinely be irradiated after surgery to reduce postoperative recurrences (48). Tumor doses of 50 to 60 Gy are necessary, depending on the size of the lesion or, preferably, after surgical resection and/or enucleation in cases where there is compromise of the optic nerve by tumor wrapping around the nerve extending to the orbital apex and beyond.

We have attempted to control microscopic adenoid cystic carcinoma postenucleation in a 16-year-old boy who had failed the first tumor resection and later showed regrowth. The technique used was CyberKnife robotic radiosurgery in five fractions of 6 Gy each and a total dose of 30 Gy, a BED equivalent to 72 Gy external beam or IMRT standard fractionation. Eight months posttreatment, MRI showed no evidence of orbital or intracranial tumor activity (Fig. 35.11).

Metastatic Orbital Tumors

Metastatic tumors to the orbit may be treated with 40 Gy fractionated over 4 weeks. The treatment design depends on the location and extent of tumor within the orbit. Again, we advocate 3D conformal treatment to treat the tumor with a margin and attempt to decrease normal tissue toxicity. Orbital metastasis are also amenable to be treated with the current robotic CyberKnife radiosurgery. Further research with this technique is necessary on an IRB-approved protocol.

⠒ Sequelae of Therapy

Skin and Adnexa

Skin changes resulting from radiation therapy may include erythema, hyperpigmentation, depigmentation, atrophy, telangiectasia, and ectropion or entropion of the eyelid. Although conjunctival changes are usually insignificant, a corneal abrasion may result from the formation of a keratotic plaque in a radiation-injured conjunctiva.

Loss of the cilia from the scalp, eyebrow, or eyelid may occur after radiation therapy to the ocular area. Hair loss from the scalp may occur at an exit area of an external beam portal. Eyebrow loss occasionally occurs when a ^{60}Co plaque has been used anteriorly and superiorly to treat choroidal malignant melanoma (10). The loss of eyelashes that may accompany the use of x-ray therapy in the treatment of basal cell carcinoma is usually permanent. Similar lash loss may follow radioactive plaque therapy of ciliochoroidal melanomas.

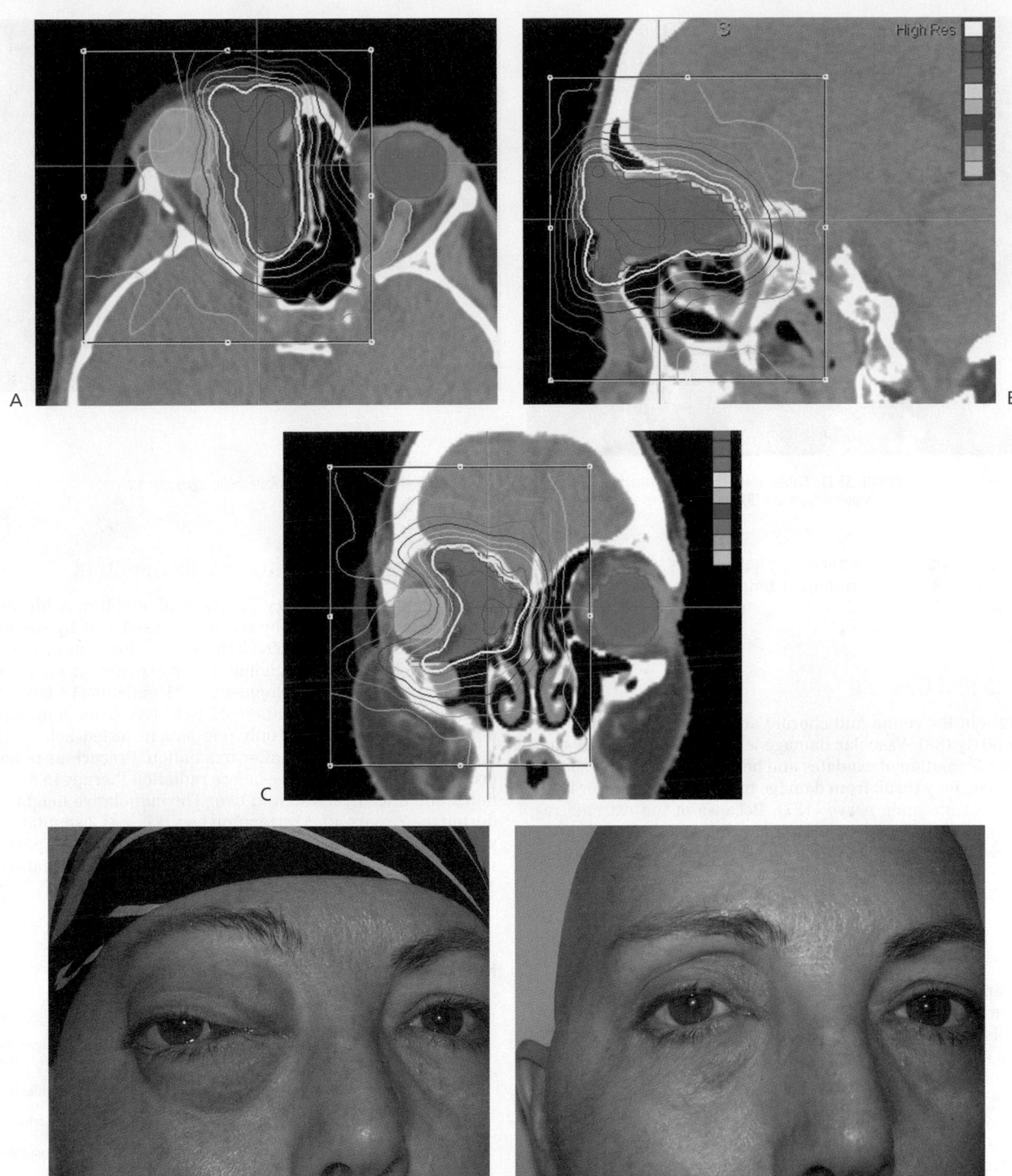

FIGURE 35.10. Right orbital lymphoma causing exophthalmus in a patient with stage IIIA non-Hodgkin's lymphoma: **(A)** before and **(B)** after 5 days of treatment with CyberKnife robotic radiosurgery. Axial **(C)**, sagittal **(D)**, and coronal **(E)** isodose plan views showing a conformal coverage of tumor and significant sparing of surrounding tissues.

Cornea

Direct corneal injury may result from irradiation of ocular and adjacent structures (16,17). Blodi (16) classified this damage as purely epithelial with a good prognosis for recovery or stromal with a poor prognosis. Experiments indicate that 72 Gy fractionated over 8 days leads to corneal perforation, but 48 Gy fractionated over the same time produces mostly reversible epithelial changes with minimal stromal damage.

Lens

A great concern in the treatment of ocular disease is the risk of radiation-induced cataract. Merriam and Focht (96) have shown that as little as 2 Gy in a single fraction or 8 Gy fractionated delivered at the level of the lens can significantly elevate the incidence of cataract development. At higher doses, the percentage of lenses that develop cataracts increases to 100% (see Fig. 35.6). With the use of improved shielding, beam-control

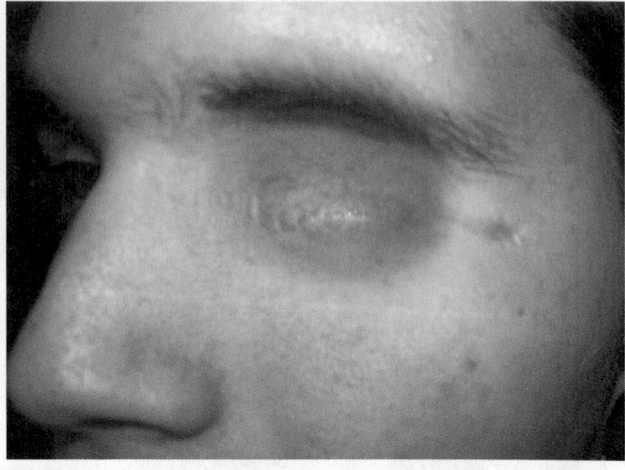

FIGURE 35.11. Sixteen-year-old boy with adenoid cystic carcinoma of the left eye s/p excenteration: **(A)** CyberKnife radiosurgery plan for microscopic disease and **(B)** patient 2 months after five fractions.

techniques, and more inherently sharp beams, an 80% reduction in the incidence of radiation-induced cataracts is expected (63,96).

Retina and Choroid

Changes in the retina and choroid are observed after doses of 45 to 60 Gy (88). Vascular damage leads to infarction of tissue with the formation of exudates and hemorrhages. Decreased visual acuity may result from damage to the retinal tissue or from atrophy of the optic nerve (127). Because of the extreme radioresistance of the sclera, which may tolerate doses to 750 Gy or more, only a few cases of scleral necrosis have been reported (21).

Lacrimal Gland and Bony Orbit

Radiation damage to the lacrimal gland may decrease tear production and produce irreversible corneal changes. A particularly distinctive and disfiguring orbital change that sometimes occurs in children irradiated for ocular or orbital tumors is the arrested development of the lateral orbital wall growth center, leading to subsequent temporal osteomalacia. Another rare, but disastrous, complication is the development of osteogenic sarcoma of the orbit, which was fatal in 100% of the reported cases (52,116,131,139,168,174,190). However, Smith et al. (167) report two of four patients with malignant osteogenic sarcoma surviving without disease more than 3 years after aggressive multimodal therapy.

Optic Nerve

Parsons et al. (111) described retrobulbar optic neuropathy in 12 nerves in 131 patients at mean and median times of 47 and 28 months, respectively. No injuries were observed in 106 optic nerves that received a total dose of <59 Gy. Among nerves that received doses of 60 Gy or higher, the 15-year actuarial risk of optic neuropathy was 11% when treatment was administered in fraction sizes <1.9 Gy compared with 47% when given in larger fractions.

Hypothalamus and Pituitary Dysfunction

Hypothalamus or pituitary function in children with optic glioma may be impaired by the tumor itself and by the high cranial irradiation doses used in treatment. Brauner et al. evaluated the effect of optic glioma and its treatment on patient growth and pubertal development in 21 patients (13 boys and 8 girls) treated with irradiation (45 to 55 Gy). Growth hormone deficiency was present in only one patient tested before irradiation and in all patients after irradiation. Precocious puberty occurred in seven patients—before radiation therapy in five patients and after irradiation in two. The cumulative height loss during the 2 years after irradiation was 0.2 ± 0.2 standard deviation (mean ± standard error of the mean) in seven patients with precocious puberty and 1.1 ± 0.2 standard deviation in 14 prepubertal patients (p <.01).

References

1. Alvord EC, Lofton S. Gliomas of the optic nerve and chiasm: outcome by patient's age, tumor site, and treatment. *J Neurosurg* 1988;68:85.
2. Amendola BE, Markoe AM, Augsburger JJ, et al. Analysis of treatment results in 36 children with retinoblastoma treated by scleral plaque irradiation. *Int J Radiat Oncol Biol Phys* 1989;17:63.
3. American Cancer Society. Detailed guide: eye cancer. Available at: www.cancer.gov, 2007.
4. Appleton RE, Jan JE. Delayed diagnosis of optic nerve glioma: a preventable cause of visual loss. *Pediatr Neurol* 1989;5:226–228.
5. Armstrong DI. The use of 4-6 MeV electrons for the conservative treatment of retinoblastoma. *Br J Radiol* 1974;47:326.
6. Augsburger JJ, Mullen D, Kleineidan M. Planned combined I-125 plaque irradiation and indirect ophthalmoscope laser therapy for choroidal melanoma. *Ophthalmol Surg* 1993;24:76–81.
7. Austin-Seymour MM, Donaldson SS, Egbert PR, et al. Radiotherapy of lymphoid diseases of the orbit. *Int J Radiat Oncol Biol Phys* 1985;1:371.
8. Barthold HJ, Harvey A, Markoe AM, et al. Treatment of orbital pseudo tumor and lymphoma. *Am J Clin Oncol* 1986;9:527.
9. Bauman MA, Ritch PS, Hande KR, et al. Treatment of intraocular lymphoma with high dose Ara-C. *Cancer* 1986;57:1273–1275.
10. Bedford MA, Bedotto C, MacFaul PA. Radiation retinopathy after application of a cobalt plaque: report of three cases. *Br J Ophthalmol* 1970;54:505.
11. Bell DJ, Wilson MW. Choroidal melanoma: natural history and management options. *Cancer Control* 2004;11:296.
12. Bessell EM, Henk JM, Wright JE, et al. Orbital and conjunctival lymphoma treatment and prognosis. *Radiother Oncol* 1988;13:237.
13. Bilgic S, Erbengi A, Tinaztepe B, et al. Optic glioma of childhood: clinical, histopathological, and histochemical observations. *Br J Ophthalmol* 1989;72:832–837.
14. Blahut RJ, Beierwaltes WH, Lampe I. Exophthalmos response during roentgen therapy. *Am J Roentgenol Radium Ther Nucl Med* 1963;90:261.
15. Bloch RS, Gartner S. The incidence of ocular metastatic carcinoma. *Arch Ophthalmol* 1971;85:673.

16. Blodi FC. The late effects of x-irradiation on the cornea. *Trans Am Ophthalmol Soc* 1958;56:413.
17. Blodi FC. The effects of experimental x-radiation on the cornea. *Arch Ophthalmol* 1960;63:44.
18. Brady LW, Shields JA, Augsburger JJ, et al. Malignant intraocular tumors. *Cancer* 1982;49:578.
19. Brady LW, Shields JA, Augsburger JJ, et al. Posterior uveal melanomas. In: Phillips TL, Pistenmaa DA, eds. *Radiation oncology annual,* Vol. 1. New York: Raven, 1984;:233–245.
20. Calhoun FP, Reese AB. Rhabdomyosarcoma of the orbit. *Arch Ophthalmol* 1982;27:558.
21. Cappin JM. Radiation scleral necrosis simulating early scleromalacia perforans. *Br J Ophthalmol* 1973;57:4525.
22. Cavanagh HO, Gren WR Goldberg HK. Multicentric sebaceous adenocarcinomas of the meibomian gland. *Am J Ophthalmol* 1974;77:326.
23. Char DH, Castro JR. Helium ion therapy for choroidal melanoma. *Arch Ophthalmol* 1982;100:935.
24. Char DH, Castro JR, Quivey JM. Helium ion charged particle therapy for choroidal melanoma. *Ophthalmology* 1982;87:565.
25. Char DH, Phillips TL, Andejeski Y, et al. Failure of pre-enucleation radiation to decrease uveal melanoma mortality. *Am J Ophthalmol* 1988;106:21.
26. Chenery SG, Fitzpatrick PJ, Japp B, et al. Treatment of choroidal melanoma with radioisotopes. Paper presented at: American Society of Therapeutic Radiology Meeting, Los Angeles; 1978.
27. Chi-Chao C, Wallace DJ. Intraocular lymphoma: update on diagnosis and management. *Cancer Control* 2004;11:285.
28. Chin LM, Harter KW, Svansson GK, et al. An external-beam treatment technique for retinoblastoma. *Int J Radiat Oncol Biol Phys* 1988;15:455.
29. Cohen ME, Duffner PK. Optic pathway tumors [review]. *Neurol Clin* 1991;9:467–477.
30. Combs SE, Schulz-Ertner D, Moschos D, et al. Fractionated stereotactic radiotherapy of optic pathway gliomas: tolerance and long-term outcome. *Int J Radiation Oncol Biol Phys* 2005;62:814.
31. Constable IJ. Proton irradiation therapy for ocular melanoma. *Trans Ophthalmol Soc UK* 1977;97:430.
32. Collaborative Ocular Melanoma Study Group. COMS Report 28. *Arch Ophthalmol* 2006;124:1684–1693.
33. Cruess AF, Augsburger JJ, Shields JA, et al. Visual results following cobalt plaque radiotherapy for posterior uveal melanoma. *Ophthalmology* 1984;91:131–136.
34. Decker MM, Castro JR, Linstadt DE, et al. Ciliary body melanoma treated with helium particle irradiation. Paper presented at: 31st Annual ASTRO Meeting, San Francisco; 1989.
35. de Keizer RJ, Swart-van-den-Berg M, Baartse WJ. Results of pterygium excision with Sr-90 irradiation, lamellar keratoplasty and conjunctival flaps. *Doc Ophthalmol* 1987;67:33(abstr).
36. DePotter P, Gonzalez CF, Flanders AE, et al. Imaging studies of intraocular tumors. In: Alberti WE, Sagerman RH, eds. *Medical radiology: radiotherapy of intraocular and orbital tumors.* Berlin: Springer-Verlag, 1993:295–309.
37. DePotter P, Shields CL, Shields JA. Clinical variation of trilateral retinoblastoma: a report of 13 cases. *J Pediatr Ophthalmol Strab* 1994;31:26–31.
38. DePotter P, Shields CL, Shields JA, et al. Uveal metastasis from prostate carcinoma. *Cancer* 1993;71:2791–2796.
39. DePotter P, Shields CL, Shields JA, et al. Impact of enucleation versus plaque radiotherapy in the management of juxtapapillary choroidal melanoma on patient survival. *Br J Ophthalmol* 1994;78:109–114.
40. DePotter P, Shields CL, Shields JA, et al. Plaque radiotherapy for juxtapapillary choroidal melanoma: visual acuity and survival outcome. *Arch Ophthalmol* 1996; 114:1357–1365.
41. de Venecia G, Lobek CC. Successful treatment of eyelid hemangioma with prednisone. *Arch Ophthalmol* 1970;84:98.
42. Donaldson SS, Egbert PR. Retinoblastoma. In: Pizzo P, Poplack D, eds. *Principles and practice of pediatric oncology.* Philadelphia: J.B. Lippincott, 1989;.
43. Donaldson SS, Smith LA. Retinoblastoma: biology, presentation and current management. *Oncology* 1989;3:45.
44. Easley JD, Scharf L, Chou JL, et al. Controversy in the management of optic pathway gliomas: 29 patients treated with radiation therapy at Baylor College of Medicine from 1967 through 1987. *Neurofibromatosis* 1988;1:248–251.
45. Eng C, Li FP, Abramson DH, et al. Mortality from second tumors among long-term survivors of retinoblastoma. *J Natl Cancer Inst* 1993;85:1121–1128.
46. Federman JL, Lewis MG, Clark WH, et al. Tumor-associated antibodies in the serum of ocular melanoma patients. *Trans Am Acad Ophthalmol Otolaryngol* 1974;78:784.
47. Ferry AP, Font RL. Carcinoma metastatic to the eye and orbit. *I. A clinicopathologic study of 227 cases. Arch Ophthalmol* 1974;92:276.
48. Fitzpatrick PJ, Macko S. Lymphoreticular tumors of the orbit. *Int J Radiat Oncol Biol Phys* 1984;10:333.
49. Flickinger JC, Deutsch M, Lunsford LD. Repeat megavoltage irradiation of pituitary and suprasellar tumors. *Int J Radiat Oncol Biol Phys* 1989;17:171–175.
50. Flickinger JC, Torres C, Deutsch M. Management of low-grade gliomas of the optic nerve and chiasm. *Cancer* 1988;61:635–642.
51. Foote RL, Garretson BR, Schomberg PJ, et al. External-beam irradiation for retinoblastoma: patterns of failure and dose-response analysis. *Int J Radiat Oncol Biol Phys* 1989;16:823.
52. Forrest AW. Tumors following radiation about the eye. *Trans Am Acad Ophthalmol Otolaryngol* 1961;65:694.
53. Forstner D, Borg M, Saxon B. Orbital rhabdomyosarcoma: multidisciplinary treatment experience. *Australas Radiol* 2006;50:41.
54. Franklin CIV. Primary lymphoreticular tumors in the orbit. *Clin Radiol* 1975;26: 137.
55. Fraunfelder FT, Boozman FW 3rd, Wilson DS, et al. "No-touch" technique for intraocular malignant melanomas. *Arch Ophthalmol* 1977;95:1616.
56. Freire JE, Brady LW, et al. Brachytherapy in primary ocular tumors. *Semin Surg Oncol* 1997;13:167–176.
57. Gould RJ, Hilal SK, Chutorian AM. Efficacy of radiotherapy in optic gliomas. *Pediatr Neurol* 1987;3:29–32.
58. Green FL, Paige DL, Fleming ID, et al, eds. *American Joint Committee on Cancer: manual for staging of cancer,* 6th ed. Philadelphia: J.B. Lippincott, 2002.
59. Halnan KS. Tumors of the eye treated by radiotherapy. *Clin Radiol* 1962;13:19.
60. Hawkins MM, Draper GJ, Kingston JE. Incidence of second primary tumors among childhood cancer survivors. *Br J Cancer* 1987;56:339.
61. Heimann H, Bornfeld N, Vij O, et al. Vasoproliferative tumours of the retina. *Br J Ophthalmol* 2000;84:1162–1169.
62. Hernandez JC, Brady LW, Shields CL, et al. Conservative treatment of retinoblastoma: the use of plaque brachytherapy. *Am J Clin Oncol* 1993;16:397–401.
63. Hilgartner HL. Report of a case of double glioma treated with x-ray. *Tex Med J* 1903;18:322.
64. Horwich A, Bloom HJ. Optic gliomas: radiation therapy and prognosis. *Int J Radiat Oncol Biol Phys* 1985;11:1067–1079.
65. Hungerford JL, Toma NMG, Plowman PN, et al. External beam radiotherapy for retinoblastoma. *I. Whole eye technique. Br J Ophthalmol* 1995;79:109–111.
66. Jacobiec FA, Jones IS. Vascular tumors, malformations and degenerations. In: Duane TD, ed. *Clinical ophthalmology,* Vol. 2. Hagerstown, MD: Harper & Row, 1976;1–40.
67. Janisch JW, Schneider M, Gerlach H. Role of genetic factors in the pathogenesis of optic nerve glioma. *Neurochirurgie* 1976;37:169–176.
68. Jenkin D, Angyalfi S, Becker L, et al. Optic glioma in children: surveillance, resection, or irradiation? *Int J Radiat Oncol Biol Phys* 1993;25:215–225.
69. Jensen AW, Peterson IA, Kline RW, et al. Radiation complications and tumor control after ^{125}I plaque brachytherapy for ocular melanoma. *Int J Radiation Oncol Biol Phys* 2005;63:101.
70. Jones IS, Reese AB, Krout J. Orbital rhabdomyosarcoma: an analysis of 62 cases. *Trans Am Ophthalmol Soc* 1965;63:223.
71. Jurgenliemk-Schulz IM, Hartman LJ, Roesink JM, et al. Prevention of pterygium recurrence by postoperative single-dose beta-irradiation: a prospective randomized clinical double-blind trial. *Int J Radiat Oncol Biol Phys* 2004;59(4):1138–1147.
72. Karcioglu, ZA, Hadjistilianou, D, Rozans M. Orbital rhabdomyosarcoma. *Cancer Control* 2004;11:328.
73. Karlsson UL, Augsburger JJ, Shields JA, et al. Recurrence of posterior uveal melanoma after ^{60}Co episcleral plaque therapy. *Ophthalmology* 1989;96:382.
74. Kenneally CL, Farber MG, Smith ME, et al. In vitro melanoma cell growth after pre-enucleation radiation therapy. *Arch Ophthalmol* 1988;106:223.
75. Kindy-Degnan NA, Char DH, Castro JR, et al. Effect of various doses of radiation for uveal melanoma on regression, visual acuity, complications, and survival. *Am J Ophthalmol* 1989;107:114.
76. Kivela T, Tenhunen M, Joensuu T, et al. Stereotactic radiotherapy of symptomatic circumscribed choroidal hemangiomas. *Opthalmology* 2003;110:1977–1982.
77. Kovalic JJ, Grigsby PW, Shepard MJ, et al. Radiation therapy for gliomas of the optic nerve and chiasm. *Int J Radiat Oncol Biol Phys* 1990;18:927–932.
78. Lederman M. Radiotherapy in treatment of orbital tumors. *Br J Ophthalmol* 1956; 40:592.
79. Letson AD, Davidorf FH, Bruce RA Jr. Chemotherapy for treatment of choroidal metastases from breast carcinoma. *Am J Ophthalmol* 1982;93:102–106.
80. Liebner EJ. Embryonal rhabdomyosarcoma of head and neck in children: correlation of stage, radiation dose, local control and survival. *Cancer* 1976;37:2777.
81. Lommatzsch P. Treatment of choroidal melanomas with ^{106}Rh beta-ray applicators. *Surv Ophthalmol* 1974;19:85.
82. Lommatzsch P. Beta-irradiation of retinoblastoma with ^{106}Ru/^{106}Rh applicators. *Mod Probl Ophthalmol* 1977;18:128.
83. Lommatzsch PK. Beta irradiation with ^{106}Ru/^{106}Rh applicators of choroidal melanomas: sixteen years' experience. In: Lommatzsch PK, Blodi FC, eds. *Intraocular tumors.* Berlin: Academie-Verlag, 1983;290–301.
84. Lommatzsch PK, Alberti W, Lommatzsch, et al. Radiation effects on the optic nerve observed after brachytherapy of choroidal melanomas with ^{106}Ru/^{106}Rh plaques. *Graefes Arch Clin Exp Ophthalmol* 1994;232:482–487.
85. Lufkin R, Flannigan BD, Bentson JR, et al. Magnetic resonance imaging of the brainstem and cranial nerves. *Surg Radiol Anat* 1986;8:49–66.
86. Lunstadt D, Char DH, Castro JR, et al. Vision following helium ion radiotherapy of uveal melanoma: a Northern California Oncology Group study. *Int J Radiat Oncol Biol Phys* 1988;15:347.
87. Luyten GP, Mooy CM, Eijkenboom WMH, et al. No demonstrated effect of pre-enucleation irradiation on survival of patients with uveal melanoma. *Am J Ophthalmol* 1995;119:786–791.
88. MacFaul PA, Bedford MA. Ocular complications after therapeutic irradiation. *Br J Ophthalmol* 1970;54:237.
89. MacFaul PA, Morgan G. Histopathological changes in malignant melanomas of the choroid after cobalt plaque therapy. *Br J Ophthalmol* 1977;61:221.
90. MacLean AL, Maumenee AE. Hemangioma of the choroid. *Am J Opthalmol* 1960; 55:3–26.
91. Makepeace AR, Fermont DC, Bennett MH. Primary non-Hodgkin's lymphoma of the orbit. *J R Soc Med* 1988;81:640.
92. Margo CE. The collaborative ocular melanoma study: an overview. *Cancer Control* 2004;11:304.
93. Markoe AM, Brady LW, Shields JA, et al. Radioactive eye-plaque therapy versus enucleation for the treatment of posterior uveal malignant melanoma. *Radiology* 1985;156:801.
94. Marquileth A, Museles M. Cutaneous hemangiomas in children: diagnosis and conservative management. *JAMA* 1965;1974:523.
95. McCormick B, Ellsworth R, Abramson D, et al. Radiation therapy for retinoblastoma: comparison of results with lens-sparing versus lateral beam techniques. *Int J Radiat Oncol Biol Phys* 1988;15:567.
96. Merriam GR, Focht E. A clinical study of radiation cataracts and their relationship to dose. *Am J Roentgenol Radium Ther Nucl Med* 1957;77:759.
97. Meyer-Schwickerath G. Further progress in the field of light coagulation. *Trans Ophthalmol Soc UK* 1957;77:421.
98. Michels RC, Knox DL, Erozan YS, et al. Intraocular reticulum cell sarcoma: diagnosis by pars plana vitrectomy. *Arch Ophthalmol* 1975;93:1331.
99. Minckler DS, Font RL, Zimmerman LE. Uveitis and reticulum cell sarcoma of brain with bilateral neoplastic seeding of vitreous without retinal or uveal involvement. *Am J Ophthalmol* 1975;80:433.
100. Montgomery AB, Griffin T, Parker RG. Optic nerve glioma: the role of radiation therapy. *Cancer* 1977;40:2079.
101. Muller RP, Busse H, Potter R, et al. Results of high dose 106 ruthenium irradiation of choroidal melanomas. *Int J Radiat Oncol Biol Phys* 1986;12:1749.
102. Munzenrider JE, Gragoudas ES, Seddon JM, et al. Conservative treatment of uveal

melanoma: probability of eye retention after proton treatment. *Int J Radiat Oncol Biol Phys* 1988;15:553.
103. Munzenrider JE, Verhey LS, Gragoudas ES, et al. Conservative treatment of uveal melanoma: local recurrence after proton beam therapy. *Int J Radiat Oncol Biol Phys* 1989;17:493.
104. Nelson BR, Hamlet KR, Gillard M, et al. Sebaceous carcinoma. *J Am Acad Dermatol* 1995;33:1.
105. Newman GH, Davidorf FH, Havener WH, et al. Conservative management of malignant melanoma. *I. Irradiation as a method of treatment for malignant melanoma of the choroid. Arch Ophthalmol* 1970;83:21.
106. Packer RJ, Bilaniuk LT, Cohen BH, et al. Intracranial visual pathway gliomas in children with neurofibromatosis. *Neurofibromatosis* 1988;1:212–222.
107. Packer S. Iodine 125 radiation of posterior uveal melanoma. *Ophthalmology* 1987;94:1621.
108. Packer S, Stoller S, Lesser ML, et al. Long term results of Iodine 125 irradiation of uveal melanoma. *Ophthalmology* 1992;99:767–774.
109. Pane AR, Hirst LW. Ultraviolet light exposure as a risk for ocular melanoma in Queensland, Australia. *Ophthalmic Epidemiol* 2000;7:159.
110. Pardo FS, Wang CC, Albert D, et al. Sebaceous carcinoma of the ocular adnexa: radiotherapeutic management. *Int J Radiat Oncol Biol Phys* 1989;17:643.
111. Parsons JT, Bova FJ, Fitzgerald CR, et al. Radiation optic neuropathy after megavoltage external-beam irradiation: analysis of time-dose factors. *Int J Radiat Oncol Biol Phys* 1994;30:755–763.
112. Peterson IA, Donaldson SS, McDougall MB, et al. Prognostic factors in the radiotherapy of Grave's ophthalmopathy. Paper presented at: 31st Annual ASTRO Meeting, San Francisco; 1989.
113. Peyman GA, Apple DJ. Local excision of a choroidal malignant melanoma: full thickness eye wall resection. *Arch Ophthalmol* 1974;92:216.
114. Pierce SM, Barnes PD, Loeffler JS, et al. Definitive radiation therapy in the management of symptomatic patients with optic glioma: survival and long-term effects. *Cancer* 1990;65:45–52.
115. Porterfield JF, Zimmerman LE. Rhabdomyosarcoma of the orbit: a clinicopathologic study of 55 cases. *Virchows Arch [A]* 1962;335:329.
116. Raivio I, Tarkkanen A. Sarcoma following radiation for retinoblastoma. *Acta Ophthalmol (Copenh)* 1965;43:428.
117. Rand RW, Khonsary A, Brown WJ, et al. Leksell stereotactic radiosurgery in the treatment of eye melanoma. *Neurol Res* 1987;9:142.
118. Rao DV, Smith M, Griffith R, et al. Orbital lymphomas and pseudolymphomas. *Int J Radiat Oncol Biol Phys* 1982;8:114.
119. Rappaport H, Winter WJ, Hicks EB. Follicular lymphoma: based on a survey of 253 cases. *Cancer* 1956;9:792.
120. Rappaport R, Brauner R. Growth and endocrine disorders secondary to cranial irradiation [review]. *Pediatr Res* 1989;25:561–567.
121. Reddy BK, Bhatia P, Evans RG. Primary orbital lymphomas. *Int J Radiat Oncol Biol Phys* 1988;15:1239.
122. Reese AB, Ellsworth RM. The evaluation and current concept of retinoblastoma therapy. *Trans Am Acad Ophthalmol Otolaryngol* 1963;67:164.
123. Ridgeway WE, Jaffe N, Walton DS. Leukemic ophthalmopathy in children. *Cancer* 1976;38:1744.
124. Roarty JD, McLean IW, Zimmerman CE. Incidence of second neoplasms in patients with bilateral retinoblastoma. *Ophthalmology* 1988;95:1583.
125. Robertson DM, Earle J, Kline RW. Brachytherapy for choroidal melanoma. In: Ryan SJ, ed. Retina 2nd ed. St. Louis, MO: C.V. Mosby, 1994;773–784.
126. Rosenstock JG, Packer RJ, Bilaniuk L, et al. Chiasmatic optic glioma treated with chemotherapy: a preliminary report. *J Neurosurg* 1985;63:862–866.
127. Ross H, Rosenberg S, Friedman AH. Delayed radiation necrosis of the optic nerve. *Am J Ophthalmol* 1973;76:683.
128. Rush JA, Younge BR, Campbell RJ, et al. Optic glioma: long-term follow-up of 85 histopathologically verified cases. *Ophthalmology* 1982;89:1213–1219.
129. Russell DS, Rubinstein LJ. Gliomas of the optic nerve and chiasm. In: Russell DS, Rubinstein LJ, eds. *Pathology of the nervous system*, 5th ed. Baltimore: Williams & Wilkins, 1989;370–376.
130. Sagerman RH, Cassady JR, Tretter P. Radiation therapy for rhabdomyosarcoma of the orbit. *Trans Am Acad Ophthalmol Otolaryngol* 1968;72:849.
131. Sagerman RH, Cassady JR, Tretter P, et al. Radiation-induced neoplasm following external beam therapy for children with retinoblastoma. *Am J Roentgenol Radium Ther Nucl Med* 1969;105:529.
132. Sagerman RH, Tretter P, Ellsworth RM. The treatment of orbital rhabdomyosarcoma of children with primary radiation therapy. *Am J Roentgenol Radium Ther Nucl Med* 1972;114:31.
133. Sandler HM, Rubenstein JH, Fowble BL, et al. Results of radiotherapy for thyroid ophthalmopathy. *Int J Radiat Oncol Biol Phys* 1989;17:823.
134. Sauer R. Optic gliomas. In: Jellinger K, ed. Therapy of malignant brain tumors. Wien: Springer-Verlag, 1987;242–245.
135. Saunders WM, Char DH, Quivey JM, et al. Precision high dose radiotherapy: helium ion treatment of uveal melanoma. *Int J Radiat Oncol Biol Phys* 1985;11:227.
136. Schipper J. An accurate and simple method for megavoltage radiation therapy of retinoblastoma. *Radiother Oncol* 1983;1:31.
137. Schwarz MB, Burgess LP, Fee WE Jr., et al. Postirradiation sarcoma in retinoblastoma: Induction or predisposition. *Arch Otolaryngol Head Neck Surg* 1988;114:640.
138. Seddon JM, Gragoudas ES, Egan KA, et al. Uveal melanomas near the optic disc or fovea: visual results after proton beam irradiation. *Ophthalmology* 1987;94:354.
139. Shah IC, Arlen M, Miller T. Osteogenic sarcoma developing after radiotherapy for retinoblastoma. *Am Surg* 1974;40:485.
140. Singh AD, Shields CL, Shields JA. Prognostic factors in uveal melanoma. *Melanoma Res* 2001;11:1–9.
141. Shields CL, Cater J, Shields JA, et al. Combined plaque radiotherapy and transpupillary thermotherapy for choroidal melanoma in 270 consecutive patients. *Arch Ophthalmol* 2002;120:933–940.
142. Shields CL, DePotter P, Himmelstein B, et al. Chemoreduction in the initial management of intraocular retinoblastoma. *Arch Ophthalmol* 1996;114:1330–1338.
143. Shields CL, Mashayekhi A, Au AK, et al. The International Classification of Retinoblastoma predicts chemoreduction success. *Ophthalmology* 2006;113:2276–2280.
144. Shields CL, Meadows AT, Shields JA, et al. Chemoreduction for retinoblastoma may prevent intracranial neuroblastic malignancy (trilateral retinoblastoma). *Arch Ophthalmol* 2001;119:1269–1272.
145. Shields CL, Naseripour M, Shields JA, et al. Custom designed plaque radiotherapy for non-resectable iris melanoma in 38 patients. *Tumor control and ocular complications. Am J Ophthalmol* 2003;135:648–656.
146. Shields CL, Shields JA. Diagnosis and management of retinoblastoma. *Cancer Control* 2004;11:317.
147. Shields CL, Shields JA, Cater J, et al. Plaque radiotherapy for uveal melanoma. Long-term visual outcome in 1,106 patients. *Arch Ophthalmol* 2000;118:1219–1228.
148. Shields CL, Shields JA, DePotter P, et al. Plaque radiotherapy in the management of retinoblastoma: use as a primary and secondary treatment. *Ophthalmology* 1993;100:216–224.
149. Shields CL, Shields JA, DePotter P, et al. Transpupillary thermotherapy in the management of choroidal melanoma. *Ophthalmology* 1996;103(10):1642–1650.
150. Shields CL, Shields JA, DePotter P, et al. Treatment of non-resectable malignant iris tumors with custom designed plaque radiotherapy. *Br J Ophthalmol* 1995;79:306–312.
151. Shields CL, Shields JA, DePotter P, et al. Short-term plaque radiotherapy for treatment of choroidal metastasis. Proceedings of the 99th Annual Meeting of American Academy of Ophthalmology, Atlanta, GA; October 29–November 2, 1995.
152. Shields CL, Shields JA, Gross N, et al. Survey of 520 eyes with uveal metastases. *Ophthalmology* 1997;104:1265–1276.
153. Shields CL, Shields JA, Honavar SG, et al. The clinical spectrum of primary ophthalmic rhabdomyosarcoma. *Ophthalmology* 2001;108:2284–2292.
154. Shields CL, Shields JA, Minelli S, et al. Regression of retinoblastoma after plaque radiotherapy. *Am J Ophthalmol* 1993;115:181–187.
155. Shields JA. Modern techniques in the management of retinoblastoma. *Trans Pacific Coast Otolaryngol Ophthalmol Soc* 1979;60:235.
156. Shields JA, Augsburger JJ. Current approaches to the diagnosis and management of retinoblastoma. *Surv Ophthalmol* 1981;25:347.
157. Shields JA, Giblin ME, Shields CL, et al. Episcleral plaque radiotherapy for retinoblastoma. *Ophthalmology* 1989;96:530.
158. Shields JA, McDonald PR. Improvement in the diagnosis of posterior uveal melanomas. *Arch Ophthalmol* 1974;91:259.
159. Shields JA, Shields CL. *Atlas of eyelid and conjunctival tumors.* Philadelphia: Lippincott Williams & Wilkins, 1999.
160. Shields JA, Shields CL. *Atlas of intraocular tumors.* Philadelphia: Lippincott Williams & Wilkins, 1999.
161. Shields JA, Shields CL. *Atlas of orbital tumors.* Philadelphia: Lippincott Williams & Wilkins, 1999.
162. Shields JA, Shields CL. Management of posterior uveal melanoma. In: Shields JA, Shields CL, eds. *Intraocular tumors: a textbook and atlas.* Philadelphia: W.B. Saunders, 1992;171–205.
163. Shields JA, Shields CL. Rhabdomyosarcoma: review for the ophthalmologist. *Surv Ophthalmol* 2003;48:39–57.
164. Shields JA, Shields CL, DePotter P, et al. Plaque radiotherapy for residual or recurrent retinoblastoma in 91 cases. *J Pediatr Ophthamol Strab* 1994;31:242–245.
165. Shields JA, Shields CL, Donoso LD. Management of posterior uveal melanoma. *Surv Ophthalmol* 1991;36:161–195.
166. Shields JA, Stephens RA, Augsburger JJ. Metastatic tumor to the uveal tract. In: Lommatzsch PK, Blodi FC, eds. *Intraocular tumors.* Berlin: Akademie-Verlag, 1983;433–444.
167. Smith LM, Donaldson SS, Egbert PR, et al. Aggressive management of second primary tumors in survivors of hereditary retinoblastoma. *Int J Radiat Oncol Biol Phys* 1989;17:499.
168. Soloway HB. Radiation-induced neoplasms following curative therapy for retinoblastoma. *Cancer* 1966;19:1984.
169. Stallard HB. Radiotherapy of malignant intraocular neoplasms. *Br J Ophthalmol* 1948;32:618.
170. Stallard HB. Malignant melanoma of the choroid treated with radioactive applicators. *Trans Ophthalmol Soc UK* 1959;79:373.
171. Stallard HB. Partial choroidectomy. *Br J Ophthalmol* 1966;50:660.
172. Stephens RF, Shields JA. Diagnosis and management of cancer metastatic to the uvea: a study of 70 cases. *Ophthalmology* 1979;86:1336.
173. Straatsma BR, Fine SL, Earle JD, et al. The Collaborative Ocular Melanoma Study Research Group: enucleation versus plaque irradiation for choroidal melanoma. *Ophthalmology* 1988;95:1000–1004.
174. Tebbet RD, Vickery RD. Osteogenic sarcoma following irradiation for retinoblastoma. *Am J Ophthalmol* 1952;3:811.
175. Tenny RT, Laws ER, Younge BR, et al. The neurosurgical management of optic gliomas: results in 104 patients. *J Neurosurg* 1982;57:452–458.
176. Toma NMG, Hungerford JL, Plowman PN, et al. External beam radiotherapy for retinoblastoma. II. Lens sparing technique. *Br J Ophthalmol* 1995;79:112–117.
177. Van Den Brenk HAA. Results of prophylactic postoperative irradiation in 1,300 cases of pterygium. *Am J Roentgenol Radiat Ther Nucl Med* 1968;103:723.
178. Vogel MH. Treatment of malignant choroidal melanoma with photocoagulation: evaluation of 10-year follow-up data. *Am J Ophthalmol* 1972;74:1.
179. Vrabec TR, Augsburger JJ, Gamel JW, et al. Impact of local tumor relapse on patient's survival after cobalt 60 plaque radiotherapy. *Ophthalmology* 1991;98:984–988.
180. Walter GF. Cerebellar astrocytoma and optic glioma: a comparative ultrastructural study. *Virchows Arch [A]* 1978;380:59–79.
181. Wharam M, Anderson J, Laurie F, et al. Failure-free survival for orbit rhabdomyosarcoma patients on Intergroup Rhabdomyosarcoma Study IV (IRS IV) is improved compared to IRS III. In: *IRSG Abstracts from American Society of Clinical Oncology (ASCO).* 1997;9–121(abstr).
182. Weinberg RA. Integration of molecular genetics into cancer management. Keynote presentation at National Conference on Integration of Molecular Genetics into Cancer Management. Miami, FL; April 10-12, 1991.
183. Weiss AH, Karr DJ, Kalina RE, et al. Visual outcomes of macular retinoblastoma after external beam radiation therapy. *Ophthalmology* 1994;101:1244–1249.
184. Weiss DR, Cassady JR, Petersen R. Retinoblastoma: a modification in radiation therapy technique. *Radiology* 1975;114:705.
185. Weiss L, Sagerman RH, King GA, et al. Controversy in the management of optic nerve glioma. *Cancer* 1987;59:1000–1004.

186. Winter FC. Surgical excision of tumors of the ciliary body and iris. *Arch Ophthalmol* 1963;70:19.

187. Winter FC. Iridocyclectomy for malignant melanoma of the iris and ciliary body. In: Boniuk M, ed. *Ocular and adnexal tumors: new and controversial aspects*. St. Louis, MO: C.V. Mosby, 1964;341–352.

188. Wong JY, Ulh V, Wara WM, et al. Optic gliomas: a reanalysis of the University of California, San Francisco experience. *Cancer* 1987;60:1847–1855.

189. Yanoff M, Davis RL, Zimmerman LE. Juvenile pilocytic astrocytoma ("glioma") of optic nerve: clinicopathological study of 63 cases. In: Jakobiek FA, ed. Ocular and adnexas tumors. Birmingham, AL: Aesculapius, 1978;685.

190. Yoneyama T, Greenlaw RH. Osteogenic sarcoma following radiotherapy for retinoblastoma. *Radiology* 1969;93:1185.

191. Zimmerman LE, McLean IW. Changing concepts concerning the malignancy of ocular tumors. *Arch Ophthalmol* 1975;78:487.

192. Zografos L, Gailloud C, Bercher L. Irradiation treatment of choroidal hemangiomas. *Fr Opthalmol* 1989;12:797–807.

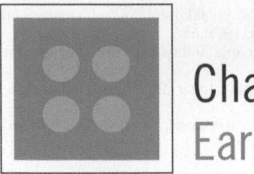

Chapter 36
Ear

K. S. Clifford Chao, V. Rao Devineni

:: | Anatomy

The external, middle, and inner components of the ear develop from the three embryonic layers: ectoderm, mesoderm, and endoderm.

The external ear consists of the auricle or pinna, the external auditory meatus (canal), and the tympanic membrane (Fig. 36.1). The auricle is composed of elastic cartilage covered with skin. The external auditory meatus connects the tympanic membrane to the exterior and is approximately 2.4 cm long. The outer third is cartilaginous, and the inner two-thirds is bony and slightly narrower. The external auditory canal is related anteriorly to the parotid gland at the temporomandibular joint. Inferiorly, it lies near the jugular bulb and the facial nerve as it descends through the stylomastoid foramen. The skin lining the auditory canal is continuous with that of the auricle, and in the outer third of the canal, it contains hair follicles and sebaceous and ceruminous glands. The tympanic membrane, which is made of multiple layers of squamous epithelium, separates the auditory canal from the middle ear.

The tympanic, or middle ear, cavity houses the auditory ossicles and opens into the eustachian tube to communicate with the pharynx. The middle ear cavity is lined with a mucoperiosteal membrane, and the eustachian tube is lined with stratified columnar epithelium and has numerous mucous glands in the two-thirds of the tube closer to the pharynx. The overall length of the eustachian tube is 3.5 cm (22).

The inner or internal ear lies in the petrous portion of the temporal bone and consists of the bony labyrinth and the membranous labyrinth. The membranous labyrinth, which holds the organ of hearing, is housed in the bony labyrinth.

Blood supply to the auricle and the external auditory canal is from branches of the posterior auricular artery and the superficial temporal artery, which arise from the external carotid artery. Blood is supplied to the middle ear region from branches of ascending pharyngeal and middle meningeal arteries and from the artery of the pterygoid canal. The inner ear is supplied by the internal auditory artery, which is a branch of the basilar artery, and from the anterior inferior cerebellar artery.

The nerves innervating the ear include cranial nerves V, VIII, IX, and X. The VIII or acoustic nerve, which arises at the lateral termination of the internal acoustic meatus and ends in the brainstem between the pons and the medulla, is responsible for auditory and vestibular function.

Lymphatic vessels of the tragus and anterior external portion of the auricle drain into the superficial parotid lymph nodes. Those of the posterior external and whole cranial aspect of the auricle drain into the retroauricular lymph nodes, and those of the lobule drain in the superficial cervical group of lymph nodes. Lymphatics from the middle ear and the mastoid antrum pass into the parotid nodes and into the upper deep cervical lymph nodes. The lymphatics in the middle ear and eustachian tube are rather sparse, and the inner ear has no lymphatics.

:: | Epidemiology

Malignant disease of the ear is rare (22). Chronic otitis media was a predisposing factor in the past, but it is now an infrequent catalyst (7,23). Tumors of the external ear are most often cutaneous malignancies and may have some correlation to solar exposure. Other predisposing factors described, although their significance is in question, are otorrhea, chronic eczema, chronic dermatologic conditions, and chronic ulcerations from trauma (32).

Tumors of the external ear most commonly occur in patients 50 to 80 years of age; tumors of the middle ear and the mastoid are more common in patients 40 to 60 years of age. More women than men have middle ear tumors, but more men have tumors of the external ear (23,37).

:: | Clinical Presentation

External Ear

Basal cell carcinomas are more common than squamous cell carcinomas in the external ear. They present as small ulcerations, mostly on the helix (1,3). Although metastasis to the lymphatics is possible, it is seen in less than 15% of patients (34,37).

External Auditory Canal

Most patients present with symptomatic lesions of the external canal. Pruritus and pain are common. Swelling behind the ear, decreased hearing, and facial paralysis are seen in advanced cases. Spread of the tumor into the lymphatic areas is more common than to other areas of the ear. Tumors arising in the cartilaginous portion of the canal invade the cartilaginous walls and spread into the bony canal areas. However, those arising in the bony canal have a more effective barrier (preventing spread) and therefore progress predominantly along the main axis of the canal, eventually invading the middle ear or the cartilaginous part of the canal. Distant metastases are rarely seen with these tumors.

:: | Diagnostic Work-Up

Table 36.1 summarizes diagnostic procedures. Plain radiography and computed tomography (CT) have now been replaced by high-resolution CT (6,32,45) (Fig. 36.2). The CT scan shows abnormal soft tissue, soft tissue enhancement, distortion of the normal tissue planes, and bone destruction. All areas of the temporal bone, infratemporal fossa, and base of the skull can be adequately evaluated using CT (4). High-resolution CT scanning can help in determining the operability of tumors (28). Sometimes magnetic resonance imaging can provide excellent

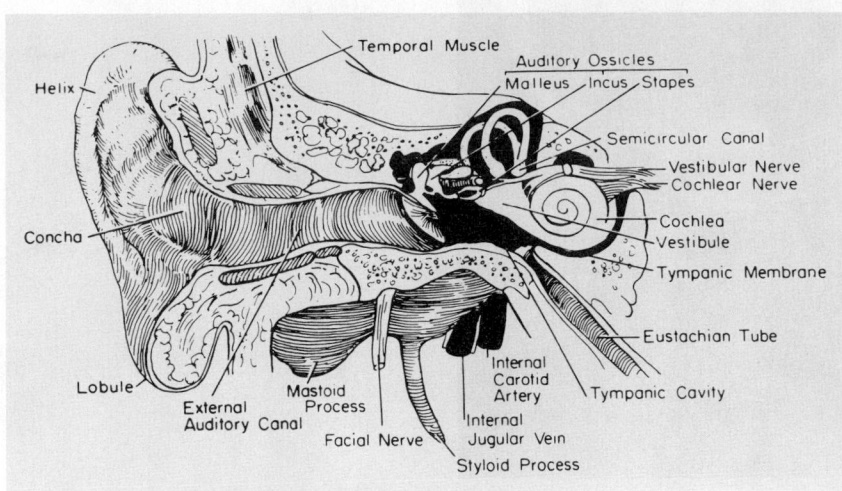

FIGURE 36.1. Anatomy of the ear. (From Million RR, Cassisi NJ, eds. *Management of head and neck cancer: a multidisciplinary approach.* Philadelphia: JB Lippincott, 1984.)

delineation of soft tissue tumor margins, muscle infiltration, intracranial extension, and vessel encasement (9,16). Except in selected cases, angiography and jugular venography have also been abandoned in favor of CT.

Diagnosis is always established by biopsy and occasionally by aspiration of the exudative material or by surgical exploration. A bone scan may be done to determine the changes in the temporal bone around the tumor, but it provides very nonspecific information and is not a recommended method of evaluation.

Pathologic Classification

Approximately 85% of the tumors involving the auditory canal, middle ear, and mastoid area are squamous cell carcinomas. Infrequently, basal cell carcinomas, adenocarcinomas, adenoid cystic carcinomas, and melanomas are seen (20). Even rarer are sarcomas, specifically embryonic rhabdomyosarcomas. Ceruminous gland tumors and papillomas rarely arise in the auditory canal (20,27,32,33). Only five cases of carcinoid tumor of the middle ear have been reported (42). Certain groups of benign adenomas of the middle ear are now called *aggressive*

papillary middle ear tumors. They are distinct clinicopathologically and are characterized by slow growth but extensive local invasion and bone destruction (12).

Prognostic Factors

Lesions of the external ear are usually more easily controlled than are lesions of the middle ear or mastoid. External ear lesions are usually diagnosed earlier; they are mostly cutaneous, and adequate surgery or radiation therapy is usually effective (3). Large lesions involving the middle ear and those with extension into the temporal bone are usually the most difficult to treat. There does not appear to be a correlation between degree of tumor differentiation and survival, although it may serve as a predictor for local control in tumors involving the petrous temporal bone (14,25). Seventh nerve palsy associated with middle ear tumors indicates poor local control (5,25). Spread of tumors to the lymph nodes usually indicates a poor prognosis because this is often a late event in the natural history of the disease (34).

Staging

Neither the American Joint Committee on Cancer (AJCC) nor the International Union Against Cancer (UICC) has a staging system for tumors of the ear. Stell and McCormick (43) have proposed a staging system using the UICC guidelines. In their study of 47 patients, they were able to correlate significant predictors with the proposed staging system (Table 36.2).

General Management

External Ear

Tumors of the external ear are most often treated with limited surgery or external radiation therapy. Treatment in early stages with irradiation is usually in the form of orthovoltage or electron beam therapy (17). Most techniques have been fairly successful in the treatment of lesions in this area. Surgery is beneficial if the lesion has invaded the cartilage of the ear or extends medially into the auditory canal. If squamous cell carcinoma of the external ear is treated with surgery alone, there is a

Table 36.1	**DIAGNOSTIC EVALUATION FOR CARCINOMA OF THE EAR**

History

Physical examination
  Otoscopy
  Careful assessment of regional lymph nodes

Laboratory tests
  Complete blood count
  Blood chemistry

Radiographic studies
  High-resolution computed tomography (standard)
  Magnetic resonance imaging (selected patients)
  Arteriography (optional)

Biopsy

Other studies
  Audiology testing

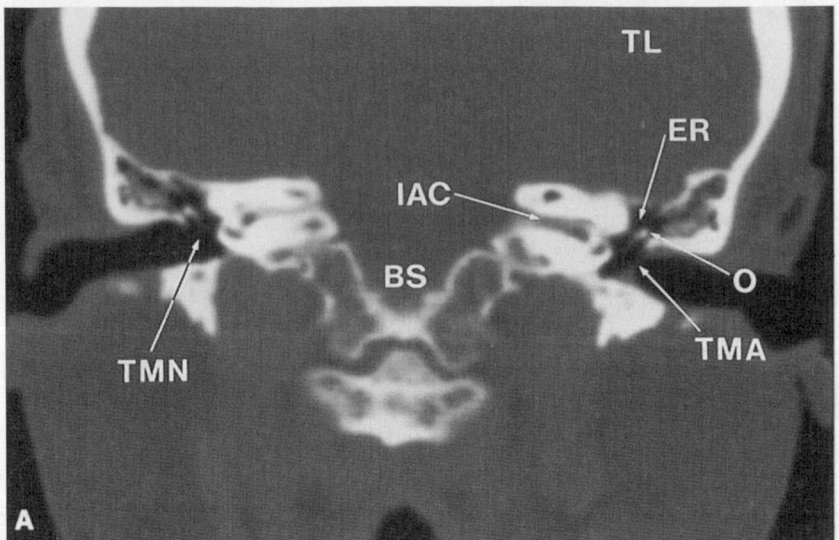

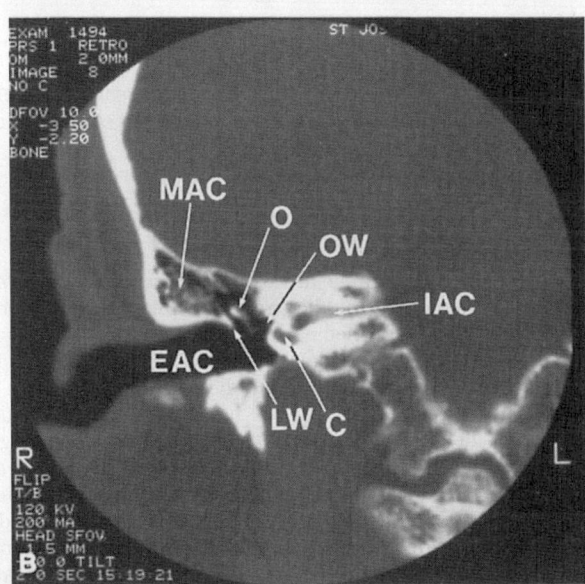

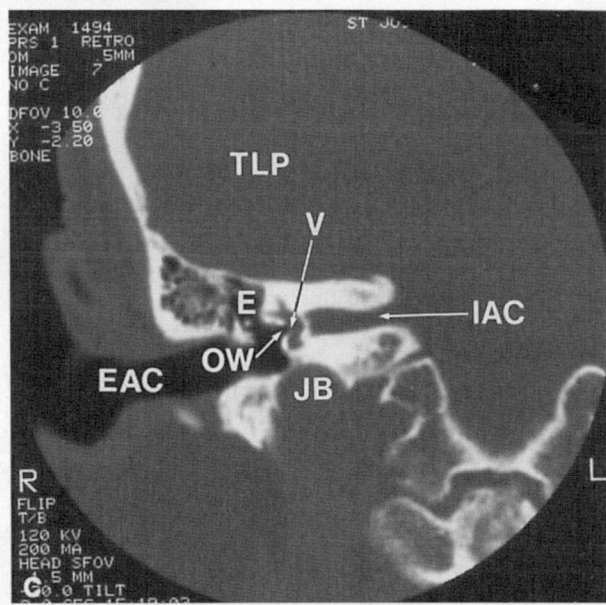

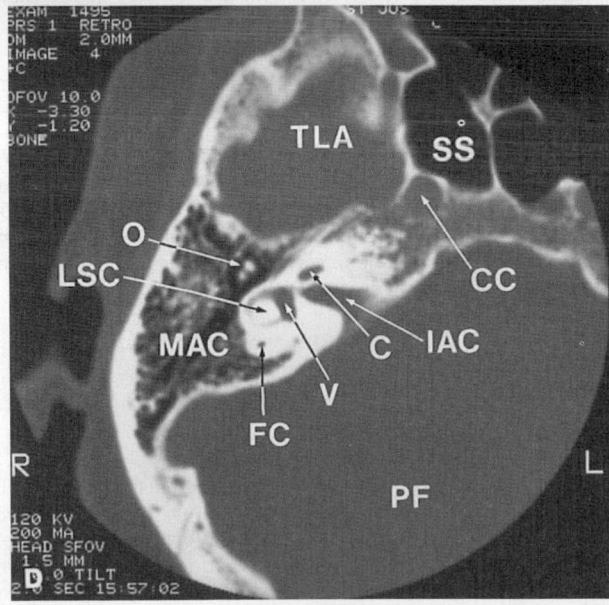

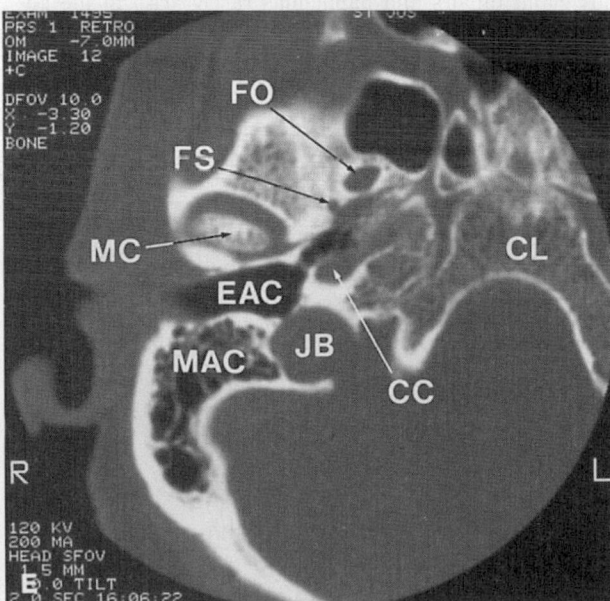

FIGURE 36.2. Normal anatomy of the ear. **A–C:** Coronal sections. **D, E:** Transverse sections. BS, brainstem; C, cochlea; CC, carotid canal; CL, clivus; E, epitympanum; EAC, external auditory canal; ER, epitympanic recess; FC, facial canal; FO, foramen ovale; FS, foramen spinosum; IAC, internal auditory canal; JB, jugular bulb; LSC, lateral semicircular canal; LW, lateral wall, epitympanic recess (scutum); MAC, mastoid air cells; MC, mandibular condyle; OS, ossicles; OW, oval window; PF, posterior fossa; TLA, temporal lobe, anterior portion; TLP, temporal lobe, posterior portion; TMN, tympanic membrane, normal appearance; TMA, tympanic membrane, abnormally thickened; SS, sphenoid sinus; V, vestibule. (CT scans and text courtesy of Robert Gresick, MD, DePaul Health Center, St. Louis, MO.)

	PROPOSED STAGING SYSTEM FOR TUMORS OF THE EAR
Table 36.2	
T1	Tumor limited to site of origin, with no facial nerve paralysis and no bone destruction detected radiographically
T2	Tumor extending beyond the site of origin indicated by facial paralysis or radiographic evidence of bone destruction, but no extension beyond the organ of origin
T3	Clinical or radiographic evidence of extension to surrounding structures (e.g., dura, base of skull, parotid gland, temporomandibular joint)
Tx	Insufficient data for classification, including patients previously seen and treated elsewhere

From Stell PM, McCormick MS. Carcinoma of the external auditory meatus and middle ear: prognostic factors and a suggested staging system. *J Laryngol Otol* 1985;99:847, with permission.

recurrence rate of 19% (38). Advanced lesions involving a significant portion of the ear canal are managed with a combination of irradiation and surgery. Palmer and Snell (30) describe the use of radical soft tissue and subtotal temporal bone excision with deltopectoral flap coverage for extensive tumors of the auricular area.

Treatment of draining lymphatics is normally not required for early stages of external ear tumors (3). Afzelius and Gunnarsson (1) indicate that lesions over 4 cm and those with cartilage invasion have an increased risk of nodal spread; they recommend prophylactic neck dissection (2). Most investigators do not agree with this approach because the overall chance of lymph node involvement in tumors of the external ear is only 16%.

Interstitial irradiation using afterloading ^{192}Ir, particularly for tumors smaller than 4 cm, is also an effective method of treatment, affording excellent local control with good cosmesis (15,26) (Table 36.3).

Radical surgery and postoperative radiation therapy are the accepted methods of treatment for more advanced lesions of the external auditory canal and lesions in the middle ear and mastoid (8,14,18,47). Except in tumors that are detected early, neither modality is considered optimal, and a combination of the two produces the best results.

Lesions of the outer part of the auditory canal require local excision with at least a 1-cm margin between the lesion and the tympanic membrane if there is no radiographic evidence of invasion of the mastoid. Surgery for tumors of the auditory canal is performed through a "U"-shaped incision with elevation of the flap from below. A split-thickness skin graft is usually required to cover the deficit along the auditory canal.

	TREATMENT OF CARCINOMA OF THE EXTERNAL EAR
Table 36.3	

	Modality	
Result[a]	Surgery	Irradiation
Local control (3)	49/50 (98%)[b]	42/45 (93%)
Cure at 3 y (34)	330/358 (92%)	141/174 (81%)
Local control at 2 y (17)		35/43 (81%)
Local control at 4 y (26)		60/61 (99%)

[a]Reference to study given in parentheses.
[b]Results given as number of successful outcomes/patients population.

When the tumor involves the bony auditory canal and impinges on the tympanic membrane but does not involve the middle ear or the mastoid, a partial temporal bone resection may be necessary; in this procedure, the auditory canal, tympanic membrane, malleus, and incus are removed along with the temporomandibular joint, and the defect is grafted with a split-thickness skin graft.

Middle Ear and Temporal Bone

In management of temporal bone tumors originating from the middle ear and mastoid area, surgeons have extended their abilities to resect tumors in these areas owing to advances in surgical techniques, modern neurosurgical anesthesia, intensive care, microsurgery, and cranial base reconstruction with microvascular flaps (2,11,13,35). Depending on the tumor extent, the surgical options are mastoidectomy, lateral temporal bone resection, subtotal temporal bone resection, and total temporal bone resection. Postoperative radiation therapy is essential to increase the chance of local tumor control (8,14,39,46). In studies that suggest limited benefit of postoperative irradiation, the results may be related to the extent of the tumor (31). Some investigators favor only limited surgery and postoperative irradiation (36). Chemotherapy has not been beneficial in tumors of the ear.

Radiation Therapy Techniques

Tumors involving the pinna can be treated with electrons or with superficial or orthovoltage irradiation. The fields can be round or polygonal, drawn around the tumor to spare surrounding normal tissues. For small superficial tumors, margins of 1 cm are adequate. However, more extensive lesions require large portals, which may encompass the entire pinna or external canal and require 2- to 3-cm margins around the clinically apparent tumor (Fig. 36.3). Lesions involving the pinna must be treated with slow fractionation (1.8 to 2 Gy daily) to prevent cartilage necrosis. Doses of 65 Gy over a period of 6.5 weeks are required to achieve adequate tumor control.

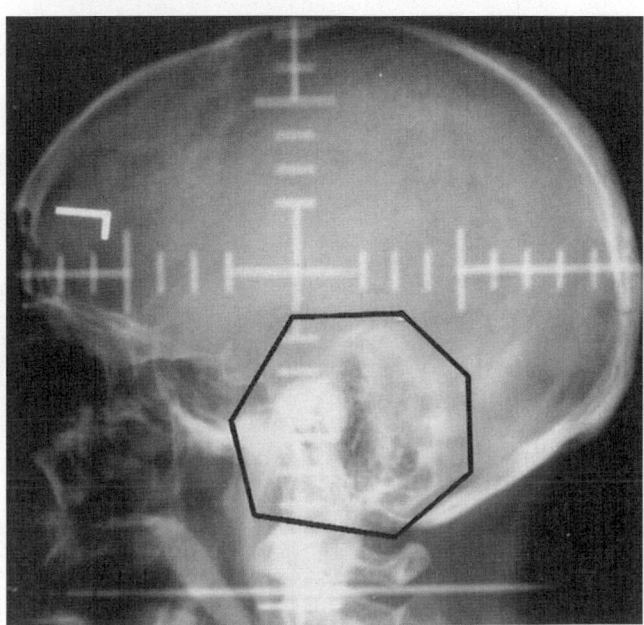

FIGURE 36.3. Example of treatment portal for tumor of the middle ear involving the petrous bone. The mastoid is included in irradiated volume.

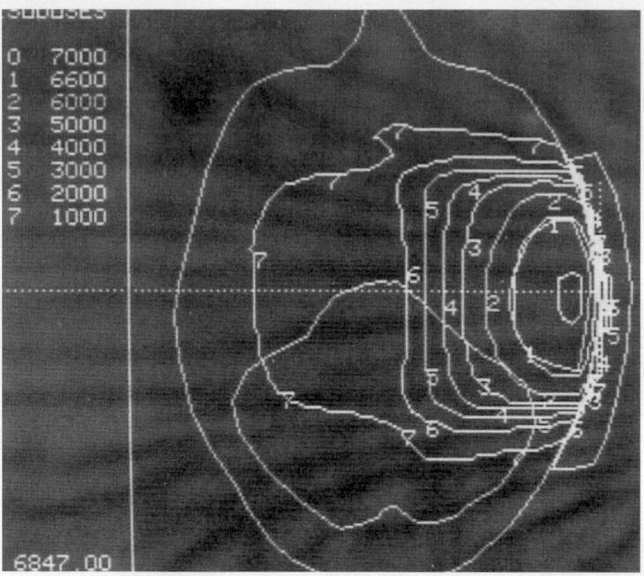

FIGURE 36.4. Computerized isodose distribution for treatment of a middle ear tumor using a combination of 4-MV photons (20%) and 16-MeV electrons (80%).

Large lesions of the external auditory canal are treated with irradiation alone or combined with surgery; the portals should encompass the entire ear and temporal bone with an adequate margin (3 cm). The volume treated should include the ipsilateral preauricular, postauricular, and subdigastric lymph nodes. Treating lymphatics beyond the jugulodigastric area is usually not necessary.

Extremely advanced tumors that are unresectable should be treated with high-energy ipsilateral electron beam therapy (16 to 20 MeV) alone or mixed with photons (4 to 6 MV) or with wedge pair (superior inferiorly angled beams) techniques using low-energy photons. Doses of 60 to 70 Gy over 6 to 7 weeks are required. Doses higher than this may produce osteoradionecrosis of the temporal bone. If various types of radiation therapy beams are available, individualized treatment plans should be devised (Fig. 36.4). Most patients receiving radiation therapy

to the middle ear and temporal bone regions benefit from immobilization devices such as the Aquaplast system. When electron beam radiation therapy is used, use of water bolus in the external auditory canal and concha may reduce the auricular complications. It is possible that as more experience is gained, three-dimensional conformal radiation therapy may become a valuable technique in the treatment of these tumors.

Palliative Radiation Therapy

Radiation therapy offers significant palliation in recurrent or advanced disease. Pain relief is reported in 61% of patients with tumors of the auditory canal and middle ear (29). Recurrences developing after previous irradiation may be retreated with low-dose radiation therapy and hope for control of tumor in approximately 20% of patients (10). When a small-volume local recurrence occurs after previous radiation therapy, fractionated high–dose-rate treatment may be considered.

Results of Therapy

The series of patients reported from several institutions are small. Results of treatment with various modalities are shown in Tables 36.4 and 36.5. In more extensive lesions, combinations of surgery and irradiation have yielded satisfactory results. Overall 5-year survival rates with combination therapy for tumors involving the middle ear and external auditory canal range from 40% to 60%, with patients with earlier-stage tumors achieving a 70% survival rate at 5 years with no evidence of disease.

Data from Washington University (Fig. 36.5) indicate that there is a negative effect of extent of disease on survival without evidence of tumor; these data also provide evidence of the success of combined surgery and postoperative irradiation for malignancies of the temporal bone (15,21,41).

Sequelae of Treatment

Possible sequelae with surgery are hemorrhage, infection, loss of facial nerve function, and, rarely, carotid artery thrombosis.

Table 36.4   TREATMENT OF CARCINOMA OF THE MIDDLE EAR AND TEMPORAL BONE

| Investigators | Modality | | |
	Surgery	Radiation Therapy	Surgery and Radiation Therapy
Sinha and Aziz (39)		1/7 (14%)	6/15 (40%)
Lewis (24)	8/28 (28.5%)[a]		18/73 (25%) preoperative
			11/31 (35.5%) postoperative
Lederman (20)		12/39 (31%)	
Wang (47)			11/23 (48%)
Sorensen (40)			5/11 (45%)
Hahn et al. (14)			6/14 (43%)[b]
Spector (41)			26/34 (76%)[c]
Birzgalis et al. (5)		8/10 (80%) early	
		10/39 (26%) advanced	
Liu et al. (25)		3/13 (23%)	8/15 (54%)

[a]Results given as patients surviving 5 years/patient population.
[b]The rate of response becomes 55.6% if petrous bone was not involved.
[c]Three-year disease-free survival.

Table 36.5 | TREATMENT OF CARCINOMA OF THE EXTERNAL AUDITORY CANAL

Investigator	Survival (y)	Surgery	Modality Radiation Therapy	Surgery and Radiation Therapy
Crabtree et al. (8)	5			9/21 (43%) E 2/14 (14%) A
Johns & Headington (18)	5			5/10 (50%) E 1/10 (10%) A
Hahn et al. (14)	5	3/4 (75%) E[a]		1/1 (100%) E
Lewis (23)	3	5/6 (83%) E 11/13 (85%) A		
Lederman (20)	5		6/25 (24%)	
Million & Cassisi (27)	2		4/5 (80%)	
Gabriele et al. (10)	5		9/15 (60%)	9/11 (82%)
Korzeniowski & Pszon (19)	5			18/29 (53%)[b]
Tiwari et al. (44)	3			10/23 (41%)

E, early stage; A, advanced stage.
[a]Results are given as patients surviving/patient population.
[b]Some patients had biopsy only.

Occasionally, vertigo is reported after temporal bone resection. Vertigo may last for 2 weeks, and a period of unsteadiness may last for a few months. Permanent deafness usually occurs on the operated side.

Radiation therapy sequelae include cartilage necrosis of the external auditory canal and osteoradionecrosis of temporal bone (3,48). Very rarely, secondary infection and meningitis are reported (23). Because of the proximity of the brainstem and medulla oblongata, it is extremely difficult to deliver a high dose of irradiation to the temporal bone without a significant risk of injury to these structures. An overall 10% incidence of bone necrosis can be expected after administration of 60 to 65 Gy. After external ear lesions are treated with interstitial irradiation, there is a 4% incidence of late cutaneous and cartilage necrosis. Risk of necrosis increases for lesions over 4 cm (26).

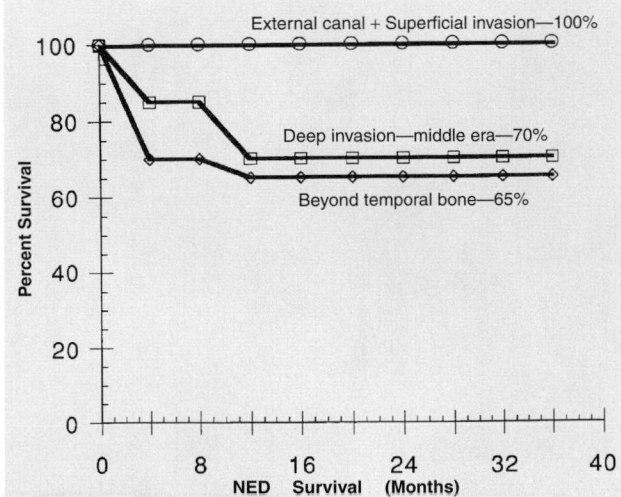

FIGURE 36.5. Data from patients with tumors of middle ear and external auditory canal from Washington University demonstrate the association between survival with no evidence of disease and original extent of disease. (From Spector G. Management of temporal bone carcinomas. *Otolaryngol Head Neck Surg* 1991;104:58, with permission.)

References

1. Afzelius L-E, Gunnarsson MHN. Guidelines for prophylactic radical lymph node dissection in cases of carcinoma of the external ear. *Arch Otolaryngol Head Neck Surg* 1980;2:361.
2. Ariyan S, Sasaki C, Spencer D. Radical en bloc resection of the temporal bone. *Am J Surg* 1981;142:443.
3. Avila J, Bosch A, Aristizabal S, et al. Carcinoma of the pinna. *Cancer* 1977;40:2891.
4. Bird C, Hasso A, Stewart C, et al. Malignant primary neoplasms of the ear and temporal bone studied by high-resolution computed tomography. *Radiology* 1983;149:171.
5. Birzgalis A, Keith A, Farrington W. Radiotherapy in the treatment of middle ear and mastoid carcinoma. *Clin Otolaryngol* 1992;17:113.
6. Chakeres D, Spiegel P. A systematic technique for comprehensive evaluation of the temporal bone by computed tomography. *Radiology* 1983;146:97.
7. Conley J, Schuller D. Malignancies of the ear. *Laryngoscope* 1976;86:1147.
8. Crabtree J, Britton B, Pierce M. Carcinoma of the external auditory canal. *Laryngoscope* 1976;86:405.
9. Friedman D, Rao V. MR and CT of squamous cell carcinoma of the middle ear and mastoid complex. *AJNR Am J Neuroradiol* 1991;12:872.
10. Gabriele P, Magnano M, Albera R. Carcinoma of the external auditory meatus and middle ear: results of the treatment of 28 cases. *Tumori* 1994;80:40.
11. Gacek R, Goodman M. Management of malignancy of the temporal bone. *Laryngoscope* 1977;87:1622.
12. Gaffey M, Mills S, Fechner R, et al. Aggressive papillary middle-ear tumor: a clinicopathologic entity distinct from middle-ear adenoma. *Am J Surg Pathol* 1988;12:790.
13. Graham M, Sataloff R, Kemink J, et al. Total en bloc resection of the temporal bone and carotid artery for malignant tumors of the ear and temporal bone. *Laryngoscope* 1984;94:528.
14. Hahn S, Kim J, Goodchild N, et al. Carcinoma of the middle ear and external auditory canal. *Int J Radiat Oncol Biol Phys* 1983;9:1003.
15. Hammer J, Eckmayr A, Zoidl J, et al. Case report: Salvage fractionated high dose rate after-loading brachytherapy in the treatment of recurrent tumor in the middle ear. *Br J Radiol* 1994;67:504.
16. Horowitz S, Leonetti J, Azar-Kia B. CT and MR of temporal bone malignancies primary and secondary to parotid carcinoma. *AJNR Am J Neuroradiol* 1994;15:755.
17. Hunter R, Pereira D, Pointon R. Megavoltage electron beam therapy in the treatment of basal and squamous cell carcinomata of the pinna. *Clin Radiol* 1982;33:341.
18. Johns M, Headington J. Squamous cell carcinoma of the external auditory canal: a clinicopathologic study of 20 cases. *Arch Otolaryngol* 1974;100:45.
19. Korzeniowski S, Pszon J. The results of radiotherapy of cancer of the middle ear. *Int J Radiat Oncol Biol Phys* 1990;18:631.
20. Lederman M. Malignant tumors of the ear. *J Laryngol Otol* 1965;79:85.
21. Lesser R, Spector G, Devineni V. Malignant tumors of the middle ear and external auditory canal: a 20-year review. *Arch Otolaryngol Head Neck Surg* 1987;96:43.
22. Lewis J. Cancer of the external auditory canal, middle ear, and mastoid. In: Suen J, Myers E, eds. *Cancer of the head and neck.* New York: Churchill Livingstone, 1981: 557–575.
23. Lewis J. A guide to cancer of the ear. *Cancer* 1977;27:42.
24. Lewis J. Surgical management of tumors of the middle ear and mastoid. *J Laryngol Otol* 1983;97:299.
25. Liu F, Keane T, Davidson J. Primary carcinoma involving the petrous bone. *Head Neck* 1993;15:39.
26. Mazeron J-J, Ghalie R, Zoller J, et al. Radiation therapy for carcinoma of the pinna using iridium 192 wires: a series of 70 patients. *Int J Radiat Oncol Biol Phys* 1986; 12:1757.
27. Million R, Cassisi N, eds. *Management of head and neck cancer: a multidisciplinary approach.* Philadelphia: JB Lippincott, 1984.
28. Olsen K, Desanto L, Forbes G. Radiographic assessment of squamous cell carcinoma of the temporal bone. *Laryngoscope* 1983;93:1162.

29. Paaske P, Witten J, Schwer S, et al. Results in treatment of carcinoma of the external auditory canal and middle ear. *Cancer* 1987;59:156.

30. Palmer J, Snell G. Surgical treatment of extensive tumors of the lateral face and auricular areas by radical soft tissue and subtotal temporal bone excision with deltopectoral flap coverage. *J Otolaryngol* 1979;8:531.

31. Prasad S, Janecka I. Efficacy of surgical treatments for squamous cell carcinoma of the temporal bone: a literature review. *Otolaryngol Head Neck Surg* 1994;110:270.

32. Pulec J. Glandular tumors of the external auditory canal. *Laryngoscopy* 1977;87: 1601.

33. Rogers K, Snow J. Squamous cell papilloma of the external auditory canal and middle ear treated with radiation therapy. *Laryngoscope* 1968;78:2183.

34. Schewe E, Pappalardo C. Cancer of the external ear. *Am J Surg* 1962;104:753.

35. Sekhar L, Pomeranz S, Janecka I, et al. Temporal bone neoplasms: a report on 20 surgically treated cases. *J Neurosurg* 1992;76:578.

36. Shaheen O. The management of tumours of the middle ear. *J Laryngol Otol* 1983; 97:313.

37. Shiffman N. Squamous cell carcinomas of the skin of the pinna. *Can J Surg* 1975; 18:279.

38. Shockley W, Stucker F. Squamous cell carcinoma of the external ear: a review of 75 cases. *Arch Otolaryngol Head Neck Surg* 1987;97:308.

39. Sinha P, Aziz H. Treatment of carcinoma of the middle ear. *Radiology* 1978;126: 485.

40. Sorensen H. Cancer of the middle ear and mastoid. *Acta Radiol* 1960;54:460.

41. Spector G. Management of temporal bone carcinomas. *Otolaryngol Head Neck Surg* 1991;104:58.

42. Stanley M, Horwitz C, Levinson R, et al. Carcinoid tumors of the middle ear. *Am J Clin Pathol* 1987;87:592.

43. Stell P, McCormick M. Carcinoma of the external auditory meatus and middle ear: prognostic factors and a suggested staging system. *J Laryngol Otol* 1985;99: 847.

44. Tiwari R, Feenstra L, Karim A. Temporal bone resections for carcinoma of the middle ear and the external ear canal. *Am J Surg* 1992;164:648.

45. Valvassori G, Mafee M, Dobben G. Computerized tomography of the temporal bone. *Laryngoscopy* 1982;92:562.

46. Wagenfeld D, Keane T, Van Nostrand A, et al. Primary carcinoma involving the temporal bone: analysis of 25 cases. *Laryngoscope* 1980;90:912.

47. Wang C. Radiation therapy in the management of carcinoma of the external auditory canal, middle ear, or mastoid. *Radiology* 1975;116:713.

48. Wang C, Doppke K. Osteoradionecrosis of the temporal bone: consideration of nominal standard dose. *Int J Radiat Oncol Biol Phys* 1976;1:881.

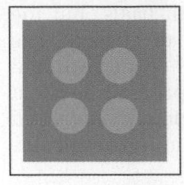

Chapter 37

The Role of Combined Radiotherapy and Chemotherapy in the Management of Locally Advanced Squamous Carcinoma of the Head and Neck

David M. Brizel

Approximately 40,000 patients are newly diagnosed annually with squamous cell carcinoma of the head and neck in the United States. Worldwide, approximately 600,000 patients are afflicted. Nearly 60% of this population presents with locally advanced, but nonmetastatic disease. Locoregional failure constitutes the predominant recurrence pattern, and most fatalities result from uncontrolled local and/or regional disease.

Radiotherapy (RT) alone has long been the standard nonsurgical therapy for locally advanced disease. The state of the art regarding radiation dose fractionation has evolved from once-daily treatment to hyperfractionation and accelerated fractionation (34,47,48,65). These newer strategies lead to a 7% to 10% improvement in locoregional control relative to once-daily treatment schemes. Nonetheless, even the most effective RT regimens result in local control rates of 50% to 70% and disease-free survivals (DFSs) of 30% to 40%. This circumstance has stimulated the investigation of treatments combining RT and chemotherapy. Recent review articles explore the different chemotherapeutic agents and RT schemes of these treatment programs (36,56).

Most reported trials have used sequential or neoadjuvant (induction) chemotherapy followed by RT. Randomized trials of induction cisplatin and 5-fluorouracil ( ) chemotherapy followed by standard fractionation versus laryngectomy and postoperative RT in advanced larynx and hypopharynx cancer performed by the Veterans Administration Cooperative Group and the European Organization for the Research and Treatment of Cancer (EORTC), respectively, initially showed that larynx preservation could be achieved without compromising overall survival.

Most randomized clinical trials show the superiority of combined radiotherapy (RT) and chemotherapy to RT alone for the treatment of locally advanced, nonmetastatic squamous carcinoma of the head and neck (HNC). A meta-analysis of individual patient data from >10,000 participants in 63 trials conducted prior to 1993 (Meta-Analysis of Chemotherapy on Head and Neck Cancer [MACH-NC]) demonstrated that adding chemotherapy to RT in both definitive and adjuvant postoperative settings resulted in a 12% reduction in the risk of death from HNC corresponding to an absolute improvement of 4% in 5-year survival (69). An update that included an additional 24 trials revealed that the majority of this benefit resulted from the use of concurrent chemotherapy, a 19% reduction in the risk of death, and an overall 8% improvement in 5-year survival compared to treatment with RT alone (p <.0001) (68). The 2% survival improvement attributable to induction chemotherapy was not statistically significant.

Randomized comparisons of concurrent chemoradiation versus induction chemotherapy followed by radiotherapy alone are few but confirm that the former strategy is superior (32,75). The Radiation Therapy Oncology Group (RTOG) conducted a three-arm trial of radiation alone versus radiation and concurrent cisplatin versus induction cisplatin followed by irradiation in larynx carcinoma. Concurrent therapy clearly constituted the most effective means of larynx preservation and provided the best disease control, albeit without a statistically significant survival benefit (32). Neoadjuvant chemotherapy followed by RT was no more efficacious than RT alone. Despite the lack of evidence supporting sequential chemoradiation strategies, this strategy was the most common method of integrating the two modalities in the community practice setting until recently (44). A recent survey demonstrates that concurrent RT and chemotherapy is now used more frequently (43).

RT and concurrent chemotherapy represents a more attractive strategy because some chemotherapeutic agents may both radiosensitize cells and provide additive cytotoxicity. The superiority of this type of nonsurgical strategy relative to RT alone has been demonstrated in randomized trials in squamous cell carcinoma of other anatomic sites including the esophagus and uterine cervix (25,72,76).

Certain issues must be considered when evaluating the role of RT and concurrent chemotherapy for advanced head and neck cancer. The first consideration relates to the effectiveness of the RT-alone control arm. Specifically, does the RT as delivered represent optimal single modality treatment? If the concurrent regimen is more effective than radiation alone but the radiation is suboptimal, then it is difficult to accurately gauge whether or not the combined modality regimen represents a true improvement in therapy. The second consideration is the toxicity of radiation and concurrent chemotherapy. Typically, the acute mucositis arising from these regimens is greater than that seen with RT alone. It is the most significant impediment to the timely delivery of concurrent therapy. Because prolongation of total treatment time adversely affects the success of RT in HNC (27,66,82), a major challenge has been the development of treatment schedules that integrate RT and chemotherapy and yet do not excessively increase total treatment time. A thorough understanding of toxicity is mandatory as avoidance of the functional morbidity associated with surgery in advanced head and neck cancer is one of the main reasons for the utilization of concurrent therapy in the first place.

Efficacy of Radiation and Concurrent Chemotherapy

The MACH-NC meta-analysis included 3,727 patients treated on 26 different trials of concurrent RT and chemotherapy. It showed an absolute survival advantage of 8% at 5 years favoring those patients who received combined modality treatment. This benefit was more pronounced in patients receiving multiagent chemotherapy as opposed to single agent. Analysis of the design and outcome of several of the trials that were examined in this meta-analysis will illustrate these points.

Radiotherapy and chemotherapy may be integrated in synchronous or alternating schemes. Synchronous administration results in the delivery of RT and CT on the same days. Typically, chemotherapy will be given for 1 or more days at the initiation of RT and then repeated in the same fashion several weeks later. Alternating regimens usually sandwich RT and CT around one another. Radiation and drugs are therefore not necessarily given on the same days. In such a scheme, CT would be given during the first week of treatment with RT following in subsequent week(s) before CT is given again.

Synchronous Radiation and Single-agent Chemotherapy

Synchronous treatment is completed more quickly than alternating treatment. It is therefore preferable from a theoretical standpoint in terms of addressing the issue of accelerated repopulation, albeit at the expense of increased acute side effects. Early randomized trials of conventionally fractionated RT and CT used single-agent chemotherapy. These studies are summarized in Table 37.1. The RTOG 90-03 and EORTC 22791 trials are included in the table to provide a basis for comparing the efficacy of the combined modality arms of these trials against what can now be considered state-of-the-art single modality irradiation. Both the Northern California Oncology Group (NCOG) and the EORTC tested radiation and synchronous bleomycin against radiation therapy alone (31,35). Acute toxicity was

worse in the combined modality arm in both trials, but the outcomes were quite different with respect to efficacy. The EORTC trial showed no improvement in DFS or survival and the RT/bleomycin combination in the NCOG program led to a statistically significant doubling of both locoregional control and DFS, as well as a near-significant improvement in overall survival from 24% to 43%.

Differences in study design and execution may explain the discrepancy between outcomes in the EORTC and NCOG trials. Fractionation was similar in the two studies, but patients in the EORTC trial received 15 mg of bleomycin twice weekly during the first 5 weeks of RT for a total dose of 150 mg, whereas the NCOG patients received 5 mg twice weekly for a total dose of 70 mg. Acute mucosal and skin toxicity was worse in the RT/bleomycin arm in both trials. Toxicity significantly prolonged the RT delivery time in 30% of the combined modality patients in the EORTC trial but not in any of the RT-alone patients. This prolongation of treatment time in such a large

Table 37.1 RANDOMIZED TRIALS OF ONCE-DAILY IRRADIATION AND CONCURRENT CHEMOTHERAPY IN ADVANCED HEAD AND NECK CANCER

Institution	N	Radiotherapy	Chemotherapy	Outcome RT RT/CCT p Value	Comments
RTOG 90-03 Accelerated fractionation and conc. Boost	268	72 Gy/42 d 1.8 Gy q d and 1.5 Gy concurrent boost	None	LC: 54% DFS: 39% S: 51%	
RTOG 90-03 Hyperfractionation	263	81 Gy/49d 1.2 Gy b.i.d.	None	LC: 54% DFS: 38%, S: 54%	
NCOG	104	70 Gy (1.8 Gy/d)	Bleo 5 mg ^{2} × /wk Weeks 1–7; Synchronous	LC: 35% 70% 0.001 DFS: 15% 31% 0.04 S: 24% 43% 0.11	RT/CCT → ↑acute toxicity, but RT not delayed
EORTC	224	64 Gy (1.8–2.0 Gy/d)	Bleo 15 mg ^{2} × /wk Wk 1–5; synchronous	DFS: 22% 23% NS S: 23% 22% NS	RT/CCT → ↑acute toxicity with RT delayed in 30%
Christie Hospital	313	50–55 Gy (3.3 Gy/d)	MTX 100 mg/m ^{2} Days 0, 14; synchronous	LC: 50% 70% 0.02 S: 37% 47% 0.07	Statistically significant benefit in LC & S for oropharynx
NCI Canada	175	66 Gy (2.0 Gy/d)	5-FU 1,200 mg/m ^{2} Days 1–3; 15–17 synchronous	DFS: 30% 50% 0.06 S: 50% 63% 0.08	Placebo-controlled trial
Yale University	195	68 Gy (1.8–2.0 Gy/d)	MM C 15 mg/m ^{2} Days 5, 43; synchronous	LC: 54% 76% 0.003 S: 42% 48% NS	Predominantly postop series. 1° RT in 74 patients. Benefit unclear in this patient group.
Cleveland Clinic	100	66–72 Gy (1.8–2.0 Gy/d)	5 FU 1,000 mg/m ^{2} CI CDDP 20 mg/m ^{2} CI Days 1–4, 22–25; synchronous	LC: 35% 55% 0.02 DFS: 52% 67% 0.03 S: 58% 58% NS	RT/CCT ↑ toxicity but RT not delayed. LC means survival with 1° site organ preservation
Princess Margaret Hospital	209	50 Gy (2.5 Gy/d)	MMC 10 mg/m ^{2} 5-FU 1,000 mg/m ^{2} CI synchronous	LC: ~40% ~40% S: ~40% ~40%	RT only: continuous course RT/CT: 4-week break after 25 Gy
NICR Italy	157	RT/CCT: 60 Gy RT: 66 Gy	5-FU 200 mg/m ^{2} bolus CDDP 20 mg/m ^{2} bolus Days 1–5, 22–26, 43–47, 64–68; alternating	LC: 32% 64% 0.04 DFS: 9% 21% 0.008 S: 10% 24% 0.01	Unresectable disease RT/CCT : RT on weeks 2,3,5,6,8,9 RT only: ≥2 week delay in >30%
GORTEC 94-01	226	70 Gy (2 Gy/d)	CBDCA 70 mg/m ^{2} 5-FU 600 mg/m²/d CI	LC: 25% 48% 0.002 DFS: 15% 27% 0.01 S: 16% 23% 0.05	Significantly increased acute and late toxicity with RT/CCT
Intergroup Nasopharynx	193	70 Gy (2 Gy/d)	CDDP 100 mg/m² Days 1,22,43 Post-RT CDDP/5-FU	DFS: 24% 69% <0.001 S: 47% 78% 0.005	Early trial closure

RT/CCT, radiotherapy and concurrent chemotherapy; RTOG, Radiation Therapy Oncology Group; LC, local control; DFS, disease-free survival; S, survival; b.i.d, twice daily; Bleo, bleomycin; EORTC, European Organization for the Research and Treatment of Cancer; NS, not significant; MTX, methotrexate; MMC, mitomycin C; NCI, National Cancer Institute; 5-FU, 5-fluorouracil; CDDP, cisplatin; CI, continuous infusion; NICR, National Institute for Cancer Research.

proportion of patients may have negated any benefit accrued from the use of concurrent therapy. There were no differences in overall treatment time between the two treatment arms in the NCOG trial. One can infer from these two studies that in some instances, lower doses of a given drug may improve the therapeutic ratio more effectively than higher doses as it is less likely that drug-related toxicity will disrupt the delivery of RT.

The Christie Hospital in Great Britain evaluated RT and 100 mg/m^2 of single-agent methotrexate (MTX) given at the commencement of and after 2 weeks of a 3-week course of treatment (41). Most of the 313 patients in this protocol received 50 to 55 Gy in 15 or 16 fractions. Mucositis was significantly greater in the patients receiving MTX, but there was no difference in long-term toxicity. The addition of MTX increased local control from 50% to 70% ($p = .02$) and survival from 37% to 47% ($p = .07$). The greatest benefit was seen in patients with oropharyngeal primaries who constituted one third of the study population. Local control with RT/MTX was 78% versus 38% with RT alone ($p = .002$) in this patient subset. Survival was 25% with RT alone and 50% with RT/MTX ($p = .009$). Unfortunately, the data from this trial are not generally applicable to current clinical practice because of the large radiation fraction sizes that were used.

5-FU has been used in conjunction with RT more frequently than any other chemotherapeutic agent. Lo et al. (58) originally reported a significant improvement in local control and survival with the addition of 5-FU to RT in squamous carcinoma of the oral cavity. The chemotherapy was given via bolus injection. It is now generally accepted that continuous infusion is a superior mode of 5-FU administration in concurrent RT and chemotherapy regimens.

Browman et al. (20) compared RT and continuous infusion 5-FU against RT alone in a placebo-controlled randomized trial sponsored by the National Cancer Institute of Canada. All 175 patients received 66 Gy in 2 Gy fractions. 5-FU was given in a dose of 1,200 mg/m^2/day for the first 3 days of the first and third weeks of irradiation. Confluent mucositis was more frequent in the 5-FU arm than in the placebo arm (32% vs. 11%; $p = .001$) as was weight loss >15% from pretreatment baseline (41% vs. 11%; $p < .0001$). This increased acute toxicity did not prolong the delivery of RT in the RT/5-FU arm relative to the RT/placebo arm. Two-year DFS and survival were 30% and 50% for RT/placebo patients and 50% and 63% for RT/5-FU patients ($p = .06$ and .08, respectively).

The relative radioresistance of hypoxic cells *in vitro* is well understood (40). Recently, the existence of hypoxia both in head and neck primary tumors and metastatic lymph nodes has been described, and its adverse impact on the prognosis of patients treated with RT has been demonstrated (16,64). Investigators from Yale University designed their treatment strategy around this principle. They treated 195 patients in two randomized trials with mitomycin C (MMC). This agent is predominantly metabolized in and preferentially cytotoxic to hypoxic cells. The Yale treatment program consisted of 68 Gy ± MMC on days 1 and 43 of RT. Local control was improved with the addition of MMC from 54% to 76% ($p = .003$). Survival improved from 42% to 48%, but this was not statistically significant. The majority of patients in these trials received adjuvant postoperative or preoperative irradiation, however. Only 74 (38%) received definitive, primary RT, and the benefit from the addition of MMC in this subset is unclear (42).

Synchronous Radiation and Multiagent Chemotherapy

Like 5-FU, cisplatin (CDDP) is a radiosensitizer (8). The combination of CCDP and 5-FU is also one of the most active cytotoxic drug combinations against SCCHN. Consequently, investigators have incorporated both of these drugs into a variety of concurrent treatment strategies. A randomized trial from the Cleveland Clinic assigned patients to receive 66 to 72 Gy ± two cycles of

synchronous CDDP (20 mg/m^2/day × 4) and infusional 5-FU (1,000 mg/m^2/d × 4) during weeks 1 and 4 of RT (1). The main objective of this study was primary site organ preservation. Surgical salvage was allowed for patients with persistent disease. Acute toxicity was significantly greater in the combined modality treatment arm, especially with respect to weight loss. Mucosal recovery usually required 8 to 12 weeks after completion of RT and chemotherapy. There were no differences in the total time required for RT delivery, however. Three-year DFS was significantly better for the patients receiving chemoradiotherapy (67% vs. 52%; $p = .03$). Three-year survival with primary site preservation was also higher in the combined modality group (57% vs. 35%, $p = .02$), although there was no significant difference in overall survival.

MMC and 5-FU were used together in a trial of 209 patients conducted at the Princess Margaret Hospital (51). Patients were treated with continuous course RT alone at 2.5 Gy/day to 50 Gy in 28 days. Patients randomized to receive RT/chemotherapy received the same dose fractionation scheme as those receiving RT alone but over a total time of 56 days due to a planned 4-week treatment interruption after 25 Gy. Bolus MMC (10 mg/m^2) was given on days 1 and 43. Two cycles of continuous infusion 5-FU (1,000 mg/m^2/day) were given on days 1 to 4 and 43 to 46. The intent of the treatment break was to maintain comparable levels of acute toxicity in the two treatment arms. Acute toxicity was, in fact, equivalent in the two groups. Unfortunately, however, there was no difference in 4-year local control (~40%) or survival (~40%).

The Princess Margaret trial raises an important question: can one quantify the contribution provided by concurrent chemotherapy in terms of the delivery of an equivalent dose of irradiation? Analysis of the study design provides some insight. Approximately 0.6 Gy/day is necessary to compensate for the tumor repopulation that transpires with each day of prolongation of standard course RT (82). Thus, the total dose in the Princess Margaret Hospital RT/chemotherapy arm would have to have been about 67 Gy [(2.5 Gy × 20) + (0.6 Gy/day × 28 days)] in order to have been isoeffective with the 50-Gy regimen in the RT-alone arm. The equivalent efficacy of the two treatments in this trial therefore suggests that the 5-FU/MMC chemotherapy compensated for the tumor repopulation that occurred during the treatment break. Stated differently, one could argue that the chemotherapy was equivalent to approximately 17 Gy of additional irradiation. There can be no doubt as to the inferiority of the split-course fractionation scheme in this trial had it been delivered without chemotherapy and compared head-to-head against the continuous-course RT regimen. Conversely, if the combined modality treatment had been given with continuous-course RT, it would quite probably have been more efficacious than the RT-only regimen.

A Spanish three-arm randomized trial (N = 859) provides additional information that is pertinent to the estimation of the radiotherapeutic dose equivalent provided by the delivery of concurrent chemotherapy. Patients were assigned to receive one of the following regimens:

(a) 2 Gy/day to 60 Gy/42 days,
(b) 1.1 Gy twice daily to 70.4 Gy/44 days, or
(c) 2 Gy/day to 60 Gy/42 days with concurrent bolus 5-FU 250 mg/m^2 given every other day (73).

Progression-free survival and overall survival were significantly worse in arm A as compared with arms B and C, as one would expect. Arms B and C were equally efficacious. Not accounting for the different fractionation in arms B and C and the unconventional administration of chemotherapy, it is still clear that the addition of 5-FU was comparable to dose escalation of approximately 10 Gy.

Neither the Princess Margaret nor the Spanish trial delivered maximally intensive radiotherapy in their respective control arms. In such a context, the rationale for treatment intensification with the addition of concurrent chemotherapy as opposed to simple RT dose escalation is weak. The situation may be dramatically different, however, when the RT-alone arm is maximally intensive such as in RTOG 90-03 or EORTC 22791. Dose escalations of 10 to 15 Gy are not possible with accelerated regimens that already deliver 72 Gy during 6 weeks or with hyperfractionated regimens delivering 79 Gy in 7 weeks. Concurrent chemotherapy, however, can be added to modified fractionation regimens $\geq$70 Gy (*vide infra*).

Alternating Radiotherapy and Chemotherapy

Alternating therapy produces less acute mucosal toxicity than synchronous therapy but may prolong the overall treatment time by as much as several weeks. Although longer treatment times adversely affect efficacy in programs of standard RT-alone due to tumor repopulation, the significance of overall treatment time (for RT) in a continuous course of alternating RT and chemotherapy is controversial. Some investigators have suggested that the usual time-dose relationships do not apply (83).

The National Institute for Cancer Research in Italy conducted a phase III trial that compared RT with a regimen of alternating RT and chemotherapy in 157 patients with unresectable head and neck cancer (59,60). The RT arm was designed to give 70 Gy/7 weeks via standard fractionation. The combined therapy arm scheduled chemotherapy on weeks 1, 4, 7, and 10 and radiation (60 Gy) on weeks 2 to 3, 5 to 6, and 8 to 9. Each 2-week cycle of radiation consisted of 20 Gy/10 fractions. Each cycle of chemotherapy included 5 days of bolus CDDP (20 mg/m^2/day) and bolus 5-FU (200 mg/m^2/day). The incidence of grade 3/4 mucositis (18% to 19%) was the same in both treatment groups. However, RT treatment delays occurred more often in the RT-alone patients: 32% with a 1-week prolongation and 25% with a $\geq$2-week prolongation. Corresponding delays in the combined modality treatment group were 11% and 15%, respectively. The median dose of RT delivered in the combined modality treatment group matched the planned dose of 60 Gy, but it was only 62 Gy in the RT-alone group. Five-year actuarial survival was significantly better in the combined modality treatment patients (24% vs. 10%; $p = .01$), as were DFS (21% vs. 9%; $p = .008$) and local control (64% vs. 32%; $p = .04$).

Given the similar levels of acute toxicity, it is unclear why treatment times were prolonged and total doses reduced so extensively in the RT-only patients. Better protocol compliance in the control arm might well have changed the outcome of this trial. There are no other randomized trials of RT and alternating chemotherapy. Further randomized trials of alternating therapy will be necessary to determine its true value because the deficiencies of the National Institute for Cancer Research study prevent definitive conclusions.

Despite its drawbacks, the Italian study, like the Princess Margaret Hospital trial, strongly reinforces the idea that in some settings, chemotherapy counteracts tumor repopulation during treatment. The total RT treatment time was prolonged in the combined modality arms in both studies. The fundamental difference between these two trials is that patients received no treatment during the RT break in the Princess Margaret Hospital trial and the patients in the Italian trial received chemotherapy during each interruption of RT.

Modern Era Randomized Trials of RT and Concurrent Chemotherapy

Curative Intent Treatment

The MACH-NC meta-analysis reviewed patients who were enrolled in trials conducted between 1965 and 1993. Many of these trials used RT and chemotherapy regimens that would now be considered suboptimal. Moreover, this work did not address any of the toxicity issues associated with concurrent therapy. Since 1993, several large, well-executed randomized trials, not included in the original meta-analysis and with an aggregate accrual >2,200 patients, have been performed to further evaluate the issue of radiation and concurrent chemotherapy versus RT alone in advanced head and neck cancer. These trials employed viable radiation dose fractionation schemes, appropriate chemotherapeutic agents, and demonstrated in different clinical contexts the superiority of radiation and concurrent chemotherapy.

The multi-institutional French trial, GORTEC 94-01, was performed with patients who had stage 3/4 oropharyngeal carcinoma (23,28). Radiotherapy was delivered in both arms via conventional 2 Gy, once daily fractions to a total dose of 70 Gy. Patients on the combined modality arm also received three cycles of concurrent carboplatin (70 mg/m^2) and continuous infusion 5-FU (600 mg/m^2/day × 4 days). Two hundred twenty-six patients were enrolled in the trial, and the median follow-up exceeds 4 years. Combined modality treatment resulted in significant improvement in 5-year locoregional control (48% vs. 25%; $p = .002$) DFS (27% vs. 15%; $p = .01$) and survival (23% vs. 16%; $p = .05$) (Fig. 37.1). This improvement in efficacy was accompanied by a significant increase in acute mucositis (grade $\geq$2) from 39% to 71% ($p = .005$). Severe acute cutaneous and hematologic toxicity and worse nutritional status were also significantly more prevalent in the patients who received combined modality therapy. Severe late toxicity, primarily cervical fibrosis, occurred in 27% of the combined modality patients and in 12% of those treated with RT alone ($p = .04$). Severe dental complications were twice as frequent in the combined modality patients (37% vs. 18%; $p = .01$).

Wendt et al. (81) conducted a multi-institutional trial that evaluated radiochemotherapy versus RT alone for patients with unresectable stage 3/4 head and neck cancer (81). In this trial, patients randomized to concurrent chemotherapy received three cycles of cisplatin, 5-FU, and leucovorin during a 7-week period. Cisplatin was given as a 60 mg/m^2 bolus. 5-FU was given as an initial 350 mg/m^2 bolus followed by a 4-day continuous infusion of 350 mg/m^2/day. Leucovorin was also given for 4 days at 100 mg/m^2/day. Radiotherapy was given in a cyclical fashion in both treatment arms. It coincided with the chemotherapy on the combined modality arms. Each cycle consisted of 23.4 Gy given with a 1.8-Gy bid fractionation. Treatment breaks were intentionally placed between the cycles of treatment to ameliorate treatment-induced mucositis. The cumulative dose of radiation therapy in both treatment arms was 70.2 Gy in 7 weeks.

One third of the 270 patient population had an oropharyngeal primary site. The minimum follow-up is greater than 3 years. Again, combined modality treatment doubled both 3-year local control (35% vs. 17%; $p < .004$) and survival (49% vs. 24%; $p < .003$) (Fig. 37.2). In a fashion similar to the GORTEC 94-01 oropharyngeal trial, confluent mucositis was significantly higher (38% vs. 16%; $p < .001$) with the use of combined modality therapy.

Treatment of advanced nasopharynx carcinoma with radiation and concurrent chemotherapy was the subject of an intergroup study in which patients in both arms received conventionally fractionated RT (1.8 to 2.0 Gy/day) to a total dose of 70 Gy (5). Those patients who were randomized to concurrent chemotherapy also received three cycles of cisplatin during RT at a dose of 100 mg/m^2. After the completion of RT, they received an additional three cycles of cisplatin at 80 mg/m^2 as well as 4-day continuous infusions of 5-FU at 1,000 mg/m^2/day. All patients had stage 3/4, M0 disease. In spite of the initial plan of enrolling 270 patients, the trial was terminated early when an interim analysis demonstrated the superiority of the

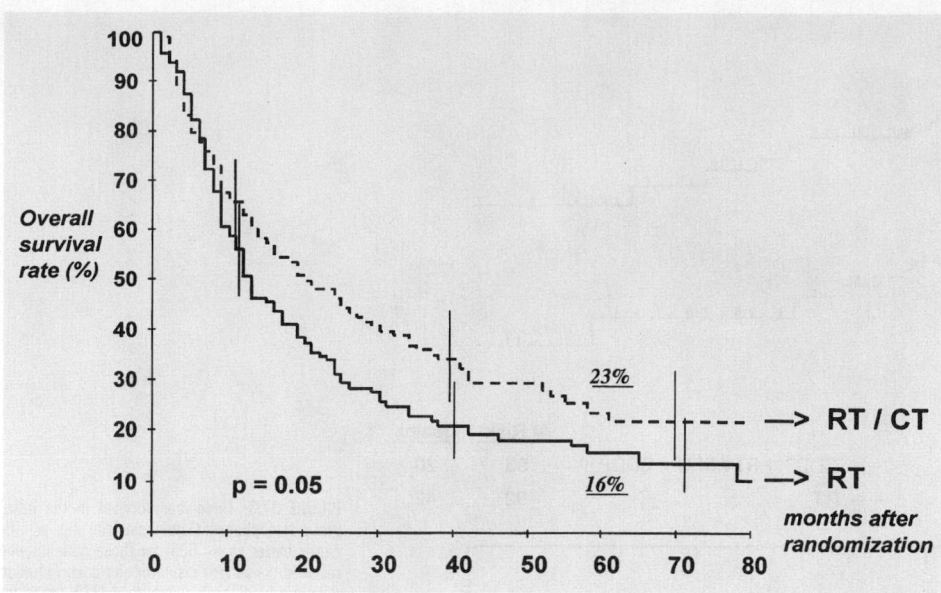

FIGURE 37.1. Five-year survival in the GORTEC 94-01 trial of conventional radiotherapy ± concurrent carboplatin and 5-fluorouracil for the treatment of stage 3/4 oropharyngeal carcinoma. Patients who received combined modality treatment had a better outcome ($p = .05$).

combined modality regimen. One hundred ninety-three patients were enrolled, and the median follow-up is 2.7 years. Three-year progression-free survival favored the combined modality patients (69% vs. 24%; $p < .001$). Similarly, 3-year survival was 78% versus 47% ($p = .005$) in favor of the patients who received concurrent chemotherapy (Fig. 37.3). Table 37.1 summarizes the data from the trials of conventionally fractionated irradiation and concurrent chemotherapy.

The fractionation schemes of the control arms of the previous three trials varied, but they all delivered 70 Gy in 7 weeks, making them comparable from a time-dose standpoint. The RTOG 90-03 trial compared conventionally fractionated 70 Gy in 7 weeks with three different accelerated fractionation or hyperfractionation schemes. Two of these schedules, namely concurrent boost (acceleration) and hyperfractionation, provided significantly better locoregional control than standard fraction-

ation (34). This trial reinforced earlier randomized studies from the EORTC, which demonstrated the benefits of modified daily fractionation (47,48). Recently, a meta-analysis of 15 randomized clinical trials (>6,500 patients total) confirmed that hyperfractionation also led to a modest but significant 4% improvement in overall survival compared to conventional fractionation (14).

Consequently, one must ask not only whether RT and concurrent chemotherapy is more effective than conventionally fractionated RT alone, but also whether it is superior to single-modality hyperfractionated or accelerated fractionation irradiation. A prospective randomized trial from Duke University provides some insight into this issue (15). Patients with locally advanced head and neck cancer were randomized to hyperfractionated irradiation alone versus split course hyperfractionation with concurrent CDDP/5-FU chemotherapy. Patients in the

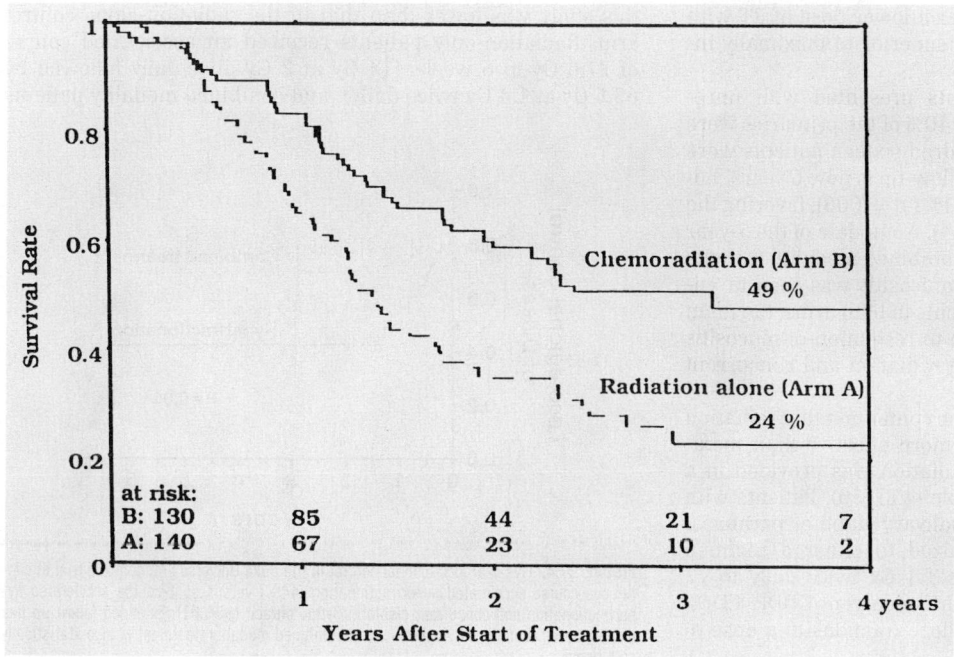

FIGURE 37.2. Three-year survival in the German trial of split-course accelerated fractionation radiotherapy ± concurrent 5-fluorouracil, leucovorin, and cisplatin for unresectable head and neck carcinoma. Combined modality treatment resulted in better survival ($p < .0003$).

Clinical Radiation Oncology

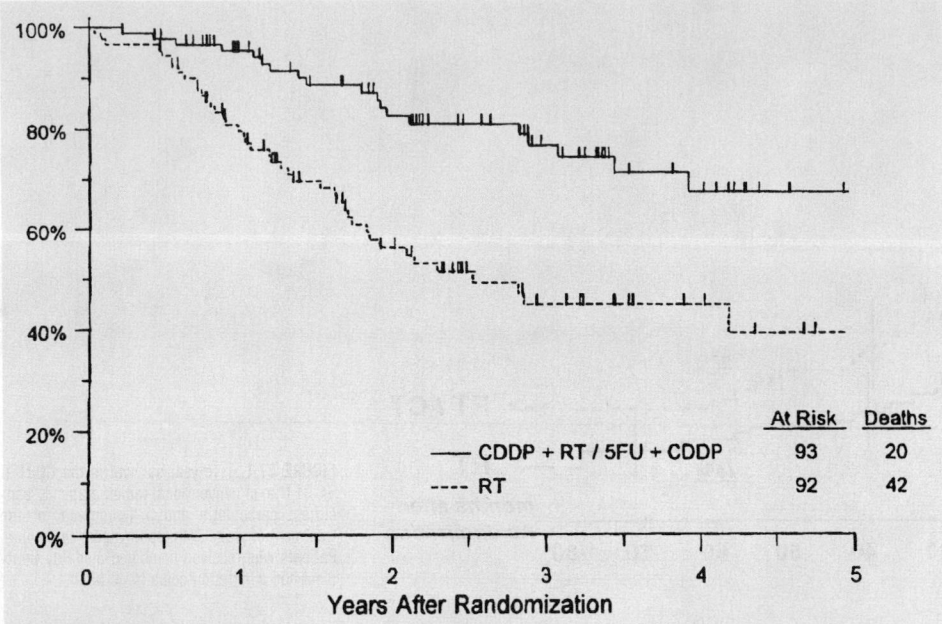

FIGURE 37.3. Three-year survival in the Intergroup Nasopharynx Carcinoma Trial was significantly better ($p = .005$) for those patients who received concurrent cisplatin and postirradiation adjuvant cisplatin/5-fluorouracil (78%) than for those who received radiotherapy alone (47%). These results led to early trial closure.

RT-alone arm received 1.25 Gy twice daily continuous course to 75 Gy in 6 weeks, whereas those patients on the combined modality arm received 1.25 Gy twice daily split course to 70 Gy in 7 weeks. Chemotherapy was given during weeks 1 and 6 of irradiation (CDDP 12 mg/m^2/d × 5 days; 5 FU continuous infusion was 600 mg/m^2/d × 5 days).

The time-dose aspects of the RT in the combined modality arm are similar to those of the previously discussed trials. The time-dose characteristics of the RT in the control arm were similar to certain aspects of both the concurrent boost arm (total dose and treatment time) and the hyperfractionation arm (daily fractionation) of RTOG 90-03. Furthermore, the RT in the control arm of the Duke University study was more intensive than that in the combined modality arm, both with respect to the total dose delivered (higher) and the total treatment time (shorter). This study design was intentional because a primary objective of the trial was to determine whether a lower dose of RT with concurrent chemotherapy would be superior to maximally intensive/effective RT alone.

Fifty-four percent of the patients presented with unresectable disease, and approximately 40% of the primaries were located in the oropharynx. One hundred sixteen patients were enrolled, and the updated median follow-up is now 5 years. Locoregional control was 70% versus 44% ($p = .006$), favoring the combined modality patients (Fig. 37.4). An update of the 5-year survival revealed superiority in the combined modality patients (42% vs. 27%; $p = .04$). Confluent mucositis was seen in approximately three fourths of the patients in both arms, the main difference being that the mean time to resolution of mucositis was longer in the patients receiving radiation and concurrent chemotherapy (6 vs. 4 weeks).

Additional evidence supporting the contention that radiation and concurrent chemotherapy are more effective than maximally intensive single modality irradiation was provided in a Yugoslavian trial reported by Jeremic et al (50). Patients with stage 3 or 4 disease, not including salivary gland or paranasal sinus primary sites, were randomized to either a regimen of pure hyperfractionation given as 1.1 Gy twice daily to 77 Gy in 7 weeks or the same RT with concurrent CDDP. CDDP was given daily between radiation dose fractions at a dose of 6 mg/m^2.

One hundred thirty patients were enrolled; primary tumors originated in the oropharynx in approximately one-third the group. Fifty-nine percent presented with T3 or T4 primaries, and 80% had nodal involvement. The median follow-up is 6.5 years. Five-year locoregional control (50% vs. 36%; $p = .04$), progression-free survival (46% vs. 25%; $p = .007$), and overall survival (46% vs. 25%; $p = .007$) (Fig. 37.5) were all significantly improved with the addition of concurrent chemotherapy. Of note, the distant metastasis-free survival was also improved in the concurrent therapy patients (86% vs. 57%; $p = .01$).

A German multicenter trial further supports the notion that concurrent therapy is superior to maximally intensive single-modality irradiation. Three hundred eighty-four patients, 93% of whom had either stage 3 or 4 oropharyngeal or hypopharyngeal primaries, were enrolled. As in the Duke University trial, the total dose of RT delivered in the concurrent arm of this study was lower than that in the radiation-alone control arm. Radiation-only patients received an accelerated course of 77.6 Gy in 6 weeks (14 Gy at 2 Gy once daily followed by 63.6 Gy at 1.4 Gy twice daily), and combined modality patients

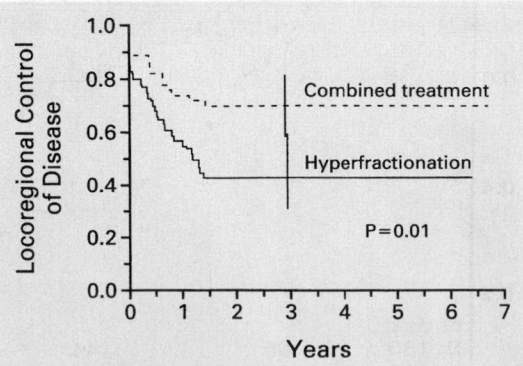

FIGURE 37.4. Five-year locoregional control in the Duke University randomized trial of continuous course accelerated hyperfractionation (44%) versus split-course accelerated hyperfractionation and concurrent cisplatin/5-fluorouracil ($p = .01$). Extended follow-up has demonstrated that the survival benefit of combined modality treatment is also statistically significant.

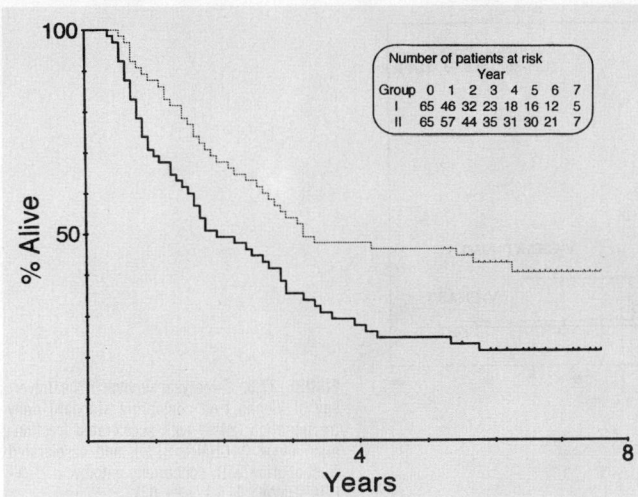

FIGURE 37.5. Five-year survival in the Yugoslavian trial of hyperfractionated irradiation alone (25%) or with daily low dose concurrent cisplatin (46%) ($p = .007$).

received 70.6 Gy during 6 weeks (30 Gy at 2 Gy per day followed by 40.6 Gy at 1.4 Gy twice daily). Chemotherapy consisted of mitomycin C (10 mg/m^2) on days 5 and 35 and 5-FU given as a single bolus of 350 mg/m^2 and a 5-day continuous infusion of 600 mg/m^2/day. Two-year survival was significantly better in the combined modality arm (54% vs. 45%; $p = .05$), as was locoregional control (61% vs. 45%; $p = .001$). Acute and chronic toxicity were equivalent in the two treatment populations.

A French cooperative group (FNLCC-GORTEC) tested a related concept in 163 patients with technically unresectable carcinomas of the oropharynx and hypopharynx (10). RT was administered at 1.2 Gy twice daily to a total dose of 80.4 Gy/46 days to oropharyngeal primaries and 75.6 Gy/44 days to hypopharyngeal primaries. The experimental arm received the same RT and concurrent CDDP (100 mg/m^2) on days 1, 22, and 43 of RT. Three 5-day cycles of continuous infusion 5-FU were also administered. The first cycle was 750 mg/m^2/day and the second and third cycles were 430 mg/m^2/day. Three-year DFS favored the concurrent chemoradiation arm (48% vs. 25%; $p = .002$) as did overall survival (38% versus 20%; $p = .04$). Post-hoc subset analyses demonstrated that the larger (and statistically significant) benefit was confined to the patients with oropharyngeal carcinomas. However, the trial was not designed to compare treatment efficacy in these two different primary sites of origin.

A three-armed randomized trial from the University of Vienna compared conventionally fractionated RT (2 Gy daily to 70 Gy) against continuous hyperfractionated accelerated RT with/without mitomycin C (V-CHART + MMC and V-CHART, respectively). Radiotherapy was given as an initial 2.5-Gy fraction followed by 1.65 Gy twice daily to a total dose of 55.3 Gy in 17 days. MMC was given as a 20 mg/m^2 bolus on day 5 of RT. Of the 239 patients enrolled, 85% had T3-4 primaries, and 79% had nodal involvement (29).

Three-year actuarial locoregional control was 48% for V-CHART + MMC versus 32% for V-CHART and 31% for conventional fractionation (CF) ($p = .05$ and .03, respectively). Survival including death from all causes (Fig. 37.6) was also improved to 41% in the V-CHART + MMC arm as compared with 31% for V-CHART and 24% for CF ($p = .03$).

The incidence of confluent mucositis was 90% in both experimental arms as compared with 33% in the CF arm. The median time to complete resolution of mucositis was 6 to 7 weeks in all

three arms. Grade 3/4 hematologic toxicity, primarily thrombocytopenia, developed in 18% of the V-CHART + MMC patients. Table 37.2 summarizes the data from the trials that used modified fractionation and concurrent chemotherapy and includes the RTOG 90-03 and EORTC 22791 data as a point of reference for optimally delivered RT alone.

Adjuvant Postoperative Irradiation

The role of chemotherapy for patients receiving primary resection and postoperative irradiation has been studied less extensively than in the definitive irradiation setting. The National Cancer Institute Head and Neck Contracts Program (4) conducted a three-arm trial that evaluated the addition of one cycle of preoperative cisplatin and bleomycin with or without six cycles of sequential cisplatin (80 mg/m^2) maintenance chemotherapy after surgery and postoperative irradiation. The control arm consisted of surgery and postoperative irradiation alone. This trial enrolled 443 patients and demonstrated no benefit with respect to locoregional control or survival from the addition of chemotherapy. Nearly half of the patients who were randomized to receive maintenance chemotherapy never received it. Despite this flaw in study execution, the incidence of distant metastases as site of first relapse was 9% in the patients assigned to maintenance chemotherapy as opposed to 19% in those who were not ($p = .02$).

Intergroup Study 0034 readdressed the issue of postoperative chemotherapy in a trial that randomized patients after surgery to three 21-day cycles of sequential cisplatin (100 mg/m^2) and infusion 5-FU (1,000 mg/m^2/day for 5 days) followed by 50 to 60 Gy versus 50 to 60 Gy alone with no chemotherapy (57). Again, there was no significant improvement in locoregional control or overall survival associated with the use of chemotherapy, but the incidence of distant metastases was reduced from 30% to 20% ($p = .02$).

In contrast to the use of sequential postoperative RT and chemotherapy, the EORTC conducted a randomized trial in which patients were given either postoperative RT alone (2 Gy daily to 66 Gy) or the same RT with three cycles of cisplatin (100 mg/m^2) on days 1, 22, and 43 of irradiation (11). Three hundred thirty-four patients were enrolled. Two thirds of patients on the combined modality arm received all three cycles of chemotherapy. The median followup is 5 years. Three-year DFS was increased from 41% to 59% ($p = .001$), and 3-year survival was increased from 49% to 65% ($p = .006$) in favor of the group of patients receiving concurrent therapy. Acute mucosal toxicity grade >3 was significantly higher in the concurrent treatment arm (41% vs. 21%; $p = .001$).

The RTOG lead an intergroup trial that randomized 459 high risk postoperative patients to receive 60 to 66 Gy with or without concurrent CDDP in the same dose and schedule as in the EORTC study (26). Sixty-one percent of patients on the concurrent therapy arm received all three cycles of CDDP. The median follow-up for this study is 4 years; 2-year actuarial local regional control favored the combined modality arm by 82% versus 72% (hazard ratio [HR], 0.61; $p = .61$) with only eight local or regional recurrences occurring beyond the 2-year point. DFS also favor concurrent therapy (HR, 0.78; $p = .04$). There was no statistically significant difference in survival (HR, 0.84; $p = .19$). Acute toxicity grade $\geq$3 was higher in the concurrent therapy patients (77% vs. 34%; $p < .001$), but late toxicity was similar (21% vs. 17%).

Principles for the Choice of Concurrent Treatment Regimens

Three general statements can summarize the previously reviewed randomized trials:

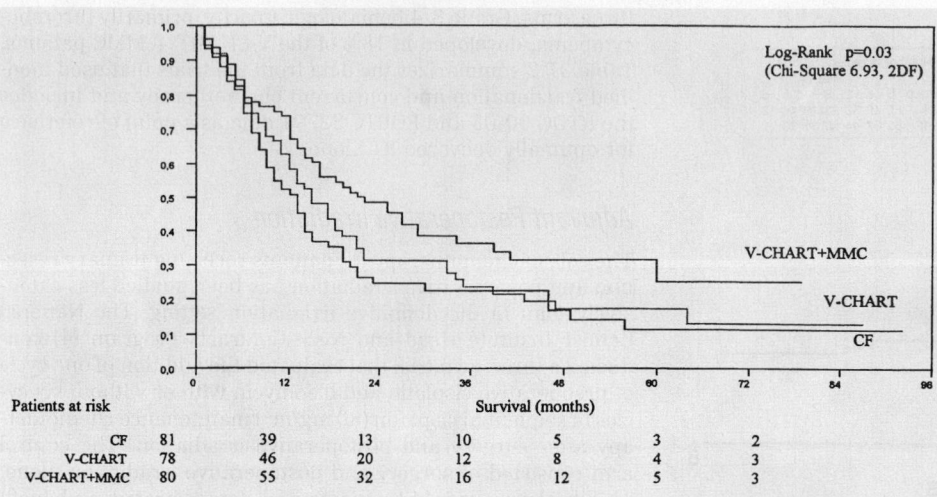

Patients at risk

CF	81	39	13	10	5	3	2
V-CHART	78	46	20	12	8	4	3
V-CHART+MMC	80	55	32	16	12	5	3

FIGURE 37.6. Three-year survival in the University of Vienna trial comparing standard daily fractionation (24%) with accelerated fractionation alone (V-CHART: 31%), and accelerated fractionation with concurrent mitomycin C (V-CHART/MMC: 41%) ($p = .03$).

(a) RT with concurrent chemotherapy is more efficacious than conventionally fractionated RT alone in advanced head and neck cancer;

(b) Concurrent therapy appears to be more effective than maximally intensive single-modality RT administered via a modified fractionation regimen; and

(c) Acute and late toxicity are increased with the use of concurrent chemotherapy.

No consensus exists, however, regarding either the optimal radiation dose fractionation scheme or the optimal scheduling of chemotherapy in these concurrent regimens. These controversies pose a decision-making dilemma to the physician when

---

Table 37.2   RANDOMIZED TRIALS OF ACCELERATED OR HYPERFRACTIONATED RADIOTHERAPY AND CONCURRENT CHEMOTHERAPY IN ADVANCED HEAD AND NECK CANCER

Institution	N	Radiotherapy	Chemotherapy	Outcome RT RT/ CCT p value	Comments
RTOG 90-03 Accelerated fractionation and conc. boost	268	72 Gy/42 d 1.8 Gy q day and 1.5 Gy concurrent boost	None	LC: 54% DFS: 39% S: 51%	
RTOG 90-03 Hyperfractionation	263	81 Gy/49 d 1.2 Gy b.i.d.	None	LC: 54% DFS: 38%, S: 54%	
University of Munich	308	70.2 Gy/51 d 1.8 Gy b.i.d. in both arms 23.4 Gy × 3 cycles 10-d split between cycles	5-FU 350 mg/m² bolus d 2 5-FU 350 mg/m²/d × 4 CI Leucovorin 50 mg/m²/d × 4 CDDP 60 mg/m² × 1 Days 1–4, 22–25, 42–45	LC: 17% 34% 0.01 S: 24% 48% <0.0003	Unresectable disease Toxicity not reported
University of Vienna	239	55 Gy/2.5 weeks for V-CHART + MMC 70 Gy/7 weeks CF control	MMC 20 mg/m² on d 5	LC: 32% 48% 0.05 S: 31% 49% 0.03	V-CHART vs. V-CHART/MMC
Yugoslavian Cooperative	130	77 Gy/49 d in both arms 1.1 Gy b.i.d.	CDDP 6 mg/m²/d	LC: 36% 50% 0.04 DFS: 25% 46% 0.007 S: 25% 46% 0.007	Daily chemotherapy
Charite' University, Berlin	384	RT/CT: 70.6 Gy/ 6 wk RT: 77.6 Gy/6 wk	MMC 10 mg/m² d 5/35 5-FU 350 mg/m² bolus 5-FU 600 mg/m² 5 d CI	LC: 45% 61% 0.001 S: 24% 29% 0.009	
Duke University	116	RT/CCT: 70 Gy/48 d (1 week break @40 Gy) RT: 74 Gy/42 d (Continuous course) 1.25 Gy b.i.d. both arms	5-FU 600 mg/m2/d CI CDDP 12 mg/m²/d bolus Days 1–5; 36–40	LC: 44% 70% 0.007 DFS: 41% 61% 0.06 S: 34% 55% 0.04	Acute and chronic toxicity comparable between RT and RT/CCT
FNLCC-GORTEC	163	80 Gy/47 d (oropharynx) 76 Gy/44 d (hypopharynx)	80 Gy/47 d CDDP 100 mg/m² on days 1, 22, 43 5-FU 750 mg/m² × 5 d cycle 1 and 430 mg/m² × 5 d cycles 2 and 3	LC: DFS: 25% 48% 0.002 S: 20% 38% 0.04	All patients with unresectable disease
Swiss Cooperative Group	224	74.4 Gy/44 d 1.2 Gy b.i.d.	74 Gy/40 d 1.2 Gy b.i.d. CDDP 20 mg/m²/d Two 5-d cycles	LC: 33% 51% 0.04 DFS: 24% 27 >0.10 S: 32% 46% 0.15	

RT/CCT, radiotherapy and concurrent chemotherapy; RTOG, Radiation Therapy Oncology Group; LC, local controls; DFS, disease-free survival; S, survival; b.i.d., twice daily; 5-FU, 5-fluorouacil; CI, continuous infusion; CDDP, cisplatin; V-CHART, Vienna-Continuous Hyperfractionated Acclerated Radiation Therapy; MMC, mitomycin C; CF, conventional fractionation.

it is time to devise a treatment plan. The application of certain principles may serve as a guide in this selection process, though. The radiochemotherapy regimen should be more effective than maximally effective single modality radiation. The use of an RT/chemotherapy regimen, which is superior to a suboptimal RT-alone regimen, does not offer the potential for a therapeutic gain to the patient (73).

One rational approach to the choice of a radiation dose fractionation scheme within the context of concurrent chemotherapy would start with the selection of an optimal single modality therapy and a definition of both its clinical efficacy and toxicity. Different dose-fractionation schemes in concurrent treatment programs could then be normalized to one another using the biologically equivalent dose (BED) concept (33). The BED = nd[1 + d/(α/β)], where n = the number of fractions delivered, d = the dose per fraction, and α/β = 10 for tumors and acute responding normal tissues and 2 for late-responding tissues. The intent of this normalization process is to allow a comparison of these different treatment programs in order to identify those having a favorable profile in terms of maximizing the probability of tumor control while minimizing the risk of late toxicity.

An example of an optimal, maximally intensive single modality regimen would be that used in EORTC 22791, which compared pure hyperfractionation (115 cGy twice daily to 8050 cGy in 7 weeks) with CF (200 cGy daily to 7000 cGy in 7 weeks) in oropharyngeal cancer. Five-year locoregional control was significantly higher in the hyperfractionation arm than in the CF arm (59% vs. 40%; p = .02). Grade-3 mucositis was also increased to 67% (48).

The concurrent boost arm of RTOG 90-03, which used an accelerated fractionation scheme to deliver 72 Gy in 6 weeks, is another example of an optimal single-modality treatment (34).

Patients on the control arm received 70 Gy/7 weeks. Five-year locoregional control was increased from 45% to 54% (p = .03), but at the expense of significant increases in both acute (59% vs. 36%) and late (37% vs. 26%) grade-3 toxicity (p = .01).

A third iteration of optimal RT alone is the DAHANCA trial, which tested an acceleration of 70 Gy/6 weeks against 70 Gy/7 weeks. Two-Gy fractions were given six times per week in the experimental arm (65). Local-regional control increased from 60% with CF to 70% with acceleration (p = .0005). The incidence of acute grade 3 mucositis was higher in the accelerated arm (53% vs. 33%; p <.0001). No differences in chronic morbidity were observed, and overall survival was not influenced by the fractionation regimen.

Table 37.3 lists the RT of the previously discussed modern era randomized trials and provides the linear-quadratic dose normalization both for acute toxicity/efficacy and late toxicity of the different regimens. The RTOG 90-03 and EORTC 22791 and DAHANCA trials are again included as optimal radiation-alone benchmarks in order to facilitate the assessment of the adequacy of the RT component of these chemoradiation trials. One limitation of this method is that is does not account for the differences in overall treatment time of the different fractionation schemes. Consequently, the V-CHART trial cannot be evaluated within this framework because the total treatment times of the experimental arms differ significantly from those in the other chemoradiation trials. Another limitation is that it does not address the likelihood that different levels of radiosensitization are associated with differing doses of various chemotherapeutic agents.

If one compares these combined modality regimens against the RT-alone standards of the RTOG and EORTC from an efficacy standpoint, the least intensive regimen was only 12% less so

Table 37.3	BIOLOGICALLY EQUIVALENT DOSE NORMALIZATION OF DIFFERENT DOSE FRACTIONATION SCHEMES USED IN THE TREATMENT OF ADVANCED HEAD AND NECK CANCER		
Study	**Prescribed Dose (Gy)**	**Efficacy/Acute Toxicity** $\alpha/\beta = 2$	**Late Toxicity** $\alpha/\beta = 2$
RTOG 90-03			
Concurrent boost	72 Gy/6 weeks	84 Gy$_{10}$	132 Gy$_2$
Hyperfractionation	79 Gy/7 weeks	89 Gy$_{10}$	127 Gy$_2$
EORTC 22791	80 Gy/7 weeks	90 Gy$_{10}$	127 Gy$_2$
DAHANCA	70 Gy/6 weeks	84 Gy$_{10}$	140 Gy$_2$
GORTEC[a]	70 Gy/7weeks	84 Gy$_{10}$	140 Gy$_2$
Munich University[b]	70 Gy/7weeks	83 Gy$_{10}$	133 Gy$_2$
Yugoslavia[c]	77 Gy/7 weeks	85 Gy$_{10}$	119 Gy$_2$
Duke University			
RT + chemotherapy	70 Gy/7 weeks	79 Gy$_{10}$	114 Gy$_2$
RT alone	75 Gy/6 weeks	84 Gy$_{10}$	121 Gy$_2$
Charite' University, Berlin			
RT + chemotherapy	70 Gy/6 weeks		
RT alone	77 Gy/6 weeks		
		82 Gy$_{10}$	129 Gy$_2$
		89 Gy$_{10}$	155 Gy$_2$
Swiss Cooperative	74 Gy/6 weeks	83 Gy$_{10}$	119 Gy$_2$
FNLCC-GORTEC	80 Gy/6.5 weeks	90 Gy$_{10}$	129 Gy$_2$
	75 Gy/6 weeks	85 Gy$_{10}$	121 Gy$_2$
Intergroup Nasopharynx[a]	70 Gy/7weeks	90 Gy$_{10}$	140 Gy$_2$
University of Vienna[d]	65 Gy/7weeks	65 Gy$_{10}$	102 Gy$_2$
V-CHART/MMC	55 Gy/2.5 weeks	65 Gy$_{10}$	102 Gy$_2$
V-CHART	55 Gy/2.5 weeks	84 Gy$_{10}$	140 Gy$_2$
RT alone	70 Gy/7 weeks		

RTOG, Radiation Therapy Oncology Group; LC, local control; EORTC, European Organization for the Research and Treatment of Cancer; RT, radiotherapy; V-CHART,
[a]2 Gy/d continuous course for RT and RT/chemotherapy (CT) arms.
[b]1.8 Gy b.i.d. (twice daily) with two 10-day breaks for RT and RT/CT arms.
[c]1.1 Gy b.i.d. continuous course for RT and RT/CT arms.
[d]1.65 Gy b.i.d. for V-CHART ± MMC.

Clinical Radiation Oncology

($79 \text{ Gy}_{10}/90 \text{ Gy}_{10}$); some of them were equally intensive. This relative parity in dose intensity occurred within the context of simultaneous administration of two to three cycles of single-agent or multiagent chemotherapy.

Conversely, from the standpoint of late toxicity risk, the RTOG concurrent boost arm is 16% more intensive than that of the RT in the least intensive chemoradiation regimen ($132 \text{ Gy}_2/114 \text{ Gy}_2$). A direct comparison of the chemoradiation regimens themselves demonstrates that again there is only a 12% difference in intensity between the least and most intensive with respect to efficacy (Duke 79 Gy_{10} vs. Intergroup nasopharynx 90 Gy_{10}). Late toxicity risk is likely to be higher with the Intergroup program as it is 23% more intensive (140 Gy_2 vs. 114 Gy_2).

An unresolved question is whether modified fractionation irradiation and concurrent chemotherapy is superior to conventionally fractionated irradiation and concurrent chemotherapy. RTOG 0129 was designed to address this issue. Patients (N = 720) were randomized to receive accelerated fractionation/concomitant boost to 72 Gy/6 weeks as per RTOG 90-03 and two cycles of concurrent bolus cisplatin (100 mg/m^2) or conventionally fractionated RT 70 Gy/7 weeks and three cycles of concurrent bolus cisplatin (100 mg/m^2). Accrual is complete, but the outcome is pending.

Both RT and chemotherapy constitute experimental variables in this trial. Accelerated fractionation and two cycles of chemotherapy are being compared against standard fractionation and three cycles of chemotherapy. This trial will answer the fractionation question if the results favor the accelerated concomitant boost arm. It will be inconclusive, however, if no difference is observed because the third cycle of chemotherapy in the control arm may serve to compensate for the inferiority of its RT dose-fractionation scheme relative to the investigational arm.

Many investigators refer to 100 mg/m^2 bolus dosing of CDDP on days 1, 22, and 43 of RT as standard. This schedule was originally developed for use in clinical trials of induction chemotherapy and later incorporated into Chemoradiotherapy (CRT) regimens. This traditional cyclical approach to delivery of concurrent CDDP has not been compared directly with schedules that use smaller, more frequent doses. In fact, randomized clinical trials comparing so-called nonstandard schedules of platinum-based CRT against RT alone (12,15,49,81) have treated equivalent numbers of patients as those that have compared bolus CDDP CRT against RT alone (2,5,32).

It is clear that schedules that deliver drug in smaller doses on a more frequent basis are also quite effective in improving outcome. Given the efficacy of these nonstandard platinum schedules, they may be preferable to cyclical bolus administration on two counts. More frequent administration could provide radiosensitizing chemotherapy during a larger proportion of the course of RT. Smaller individual doses of drug may lead to less chemotherapy-induced morbidity without compromise of efficacy (55,63). Concurrent CRT using such schedules has proven very effective and become the standard of care in squamous carcinoma of the uterine cervix (62,67,72,76).

Compliance is a significant problem with the standard three-cycle concurrent CDDP paradigm. Nearly one third of patients do not receive all cycles, and subset analyses suggest that two cycles are as effective as three (10,11,26,32). Schedules that administer chemotherapy throughout the course of RT deliver approximately the same cumulative dose as would result from two cycles of bolus CDDP. A common thread with respect to chemotherapy delivery in all of the successful RT/concurrent single-agent cisplatin schedules, both "standard" and otherwise is the delivery of a minimum cumulative dose of 200 mg/m^2 during the course of irradiation. The data suggest that this dose may be necessary to attain efficacy (7) with treatment-related morbidity being the outcome that is most affected by drug schedule.

Developmental Aspects of Combined Modality Therapy

Sequential Chemoradiation

Induction or neoadjuvant chemotherapy followed by RT essentially failed to meet its expectations. Two significant aspects of the unsuccessful trials that tested the induction concept are worth discussion before completely dismissing the value of this strategy. First, the most active and frequently used induction regimen was the platinum-5-FU (PF) combination. Second, conventionally fractionated RT only was used for subsequent definitive therapy. It is now clear that conventionally fractionated irradiation alone is inferior to concurrent chemoradiation for definitive treatment of locally advanced head and neck cancer.

Recent phase III trials have demonstrated that adding a taxane to PF induction chemotherapy leads to significant improvements in overall survival with less toxicity than PF only. EORTC 24971 treated 358 patients with four cycles of induction chemotherapy consisting of either docetaxel (75 mg/m^2), platinum (75 mg/m^2), 5-FU ($750 \text{ mg/m}^2 \times 5$ days), or platinum (100 mg/m^2) and 5-FU alone ($1,000 \text{ mg/m}^2 \times 5$ days) followed by RT alone. Three fourths of all patients received conventionally fractionated RT. Overall median survival increased from 14.5 months with PF to 18.5 months with TPF (HR, 0.73; $p = .02$). The TPF regimen was also less toxic than PF[57]. A Spanish multicenter trial randomized 382 patients to three cycles of the same PF induction regimen versus paclitaxel (175 mg/m^2), cisplatin (100 mg/m^2), and 5-FU ($500 \text{ mg/m}^2 \times 5$ days). Subsequently, all patients received conventionally fractionated irradiation (70 Gy) with concurrent CDDP (100 mg/m^2 on days 1, 22, and 43). The primary study end point, CR rate, was significantly higher in the PCF arm (33% vs. 14%; $p < .001$). Two-year survival was 66% versus 54% in favor of the PCF arm ($p = .06$). Overall, PCF also caused less serious toxicity (45).

The problem of distant metastatic failure persists despite the improvements in local regional control and survival attributable to the addition of concurrent chemotherapy. Proponents of induction chemotherapy argue that concurrent chemotherapy provides local radiosensitization but no systemic adjuvant effect. They contend that the more intensive induction regimens are necessary to achieve this aim. The issue is controversial, however. It should be noted that the incidence of distant failure in the Spanish trial was not affected by the induction regimen (45).

The improvements in induction chemotherapy and the ascent of concurrent therapy as standard definitive treatment have spawned a new generation of clinical studies. These trials are testing the concept of sequential chemoradiation, that is, induction chemotherapy followed by concurrent chemoradiotherapy. Several phase III investigations are currently being conducted under the auspices of National Cancer Institute cooperative groups and ad hoc single institution directed cooperative groups.

Biologically Targeted Therapy

Overexpression of the epidermal growth factor receptor (EGFR-1) is associated with an adverse outcome in squamous HNC (6). An open label, phase III trial tested the impact of weekly injections of cetuximab (C225), a chimeric monoclonal antibody to EGFR, added to a course of radiotherapy alone (13). Oral cavity primary tumors were ineligible for enrollment. Two-year local regional increased from 48% with RT to 56% with RT/cetuximab ($p = .02$). Three-year survival was similarly increased from 44% with RT alone to 57% with the addition of cetuximab ($p = .02$).

This trial provides an important proof of principle that adding a biologically targeted agent to a physically targeted modality improves therapeutic outcome. One third of the patients enrolled had stage III disease, however, and thus had less advanced disease with more favorable prognoses than a significant proportion of patients undergoing CRT. Whether RT/C225 is more effective than CRT remains unknown. RTOG trial 0522 will address this question by randomizing patients with locally advanced disease to receive radiation and concurrent cisplatin ± cetuximab.

EGFR inhibition is presently a very active area of investigation in head and neck cancer. Agents currently in clinical trial include fully humanized monoclonal antibodies to the EGFR-1 receptor. Orally administered small molecules that inhibit the tyrosine kinase domains of EGFR-1 or EGFR-1 and EGFR-2 (HER-2) simultaneously are also being studied.

Hypoxia is one of the most important characteristics of the aggressive malignant phenotype (39,53,61). Poorly oxygenated tumors are less likely to respond to surgery (46), radiotherapy (9,16,18,37,54), and chemotherapy. Hypoxic primary tumors are more likely to develop distant metastases after treatment (17). A recent review of nearly 400 HNC patients who underwent tumor oxygenation measurement demonstrated that hypoxia was strongly associated with treatment failure independently of stage and therapeutic modality (64).

Tirapazamine, a bioreductively activated compound, is one to two orders of magnitude more cytotoxic to hypoxic cells than well-oxygenated cells and also potentiates the activity of cisplatin (0). Phase I/II studies in advanced squamous HNC have demonstrated efficacy with acceptable toxicity when this drug is incorporated into cisplatin containing CRT regimens (70,71). Two phase III trials are being conducted to determine whether targeting of hypoxic cells with tirapazamine/cisplatin CRT is superior to cisplatin CRT. The first trial (HEADSTART) enrolled 880 patients and is currently in follow-up. A confirmatory trial, TRACE, with a planned enrollment of 550 patients is ongoing.

Toxicity Management Strategies

The most common and clinically significant toxicities arising from head and neck irradiation are acute and chronic xerostomia and acute mucositis. Radiotherapy and concurrent chemotherapy cause a high incidence and prolonged duration of acute mucositis (2,3,11,15,21,26). Mucositis necessitated a compromise in the RT delivery; that is, a treatment interruption, in some of the previously discussed trials, which attempted to use a modified fractionation scheme. The net effect was that the multiple fractions per day may simply have offset tumor repopulation (82) that occurred during the break. The ability to ameliorate mucositis such that modified fractionation irradiation and concurrent chemotherapy can be given without a treatment break would be ideal and would actually represent a dose intensification relative to those regimens now in use.

Xerostomia develops as an acute side effect early in the course of head and neck RT and may persist as a lifelong consequential late effect. It disrupts normal activities including eating and speaking, and may lead to sequelae including dental caries and tooth loss with the secondary risk of osteonecrosis.

The radioprotective potential of thiol-containing compounds has been recognized for decades (84). Amifostine (WR-2721, Ethyol, Medimmune Corp., Gaithersburg, MD) and its active metabolite, WR-1065, accumulate in many epithelial tissues with the highest concentrations found in the salivary glands and kidneys. Its putative mechanism of radioprotection is through the scavenging of radiation-induced free radicals.

A prospective randomized trial was conducted in which squamous carcinoma head and neck patients received curative intent or postoperative irradiation with or without intravenous amifostine (200 mg/m^2) each day 15 to 30 minutes preceding RT (19,80). Patients with primary tumors arising in the salivary glands were ineligible for enrollment. Radiotherapy was delivered 1.8 to 2.0 Gy/day to 50 to 70 Gy total. Doses were prescribed according to definitive or postoperative status.

The primary study end points included the incidence of grade ≥ 2 acute and late xerostomia and grade ≥ 3 acute mucositis. Secondary, confirmatory end points included the quantitation of whole saliva production and patient self-assessment of benefit.

Two thirds of the patients received postoperative treatment. The median total dose of RT delivered was 65 Gy in both treatment arms. The incidence of acute grade ≥ 2 xerostomia was 51% in the patients who received amifostine plus irradiation versus 78% in those patients who received RT alone ($p < .0001$). One year postirradiation, 57% of the RT-alone patients had grade ≥ 2 xerostomia compared with 34% of the patients treated in the amifostine plus RT group ($p = .002$). At 2 years postirradiation, the figures were 36% and 19%, respectively ($p = .05$). The reduction in xerostomia corresponded with an increase in the quantity of unstimulated saliva that patients could produce. The median quantity of saliva produced by patients receiving amifostine was 0.26 g, but only 0.10 g for patients who did not receive amifostine ($p = .04$). Patients who received amifostine had significantly less difficulty with activities such as eating, speaking, and swallowing throughout the posttreatment follow-up period (79).

Amifostine did not reduce the incidence of grade ≥ 3 mucositis in this trial. A post-hoc subset analysis suggested significantly less mucositis for those patients with smaller treatment fields who also received amifostine. Larger doses of amifostine may be necessary for mucosal protection as opposed to salivary gland protection (22). Based on the original trial design, however, one must conclude that mucosal protection with amifostine has not been definitively demonstrated and requires further investigation. There was no evidence that amifostine compromised efficacy of RT in this trial. A meta-analysis is being conducted to evaluate this issue in greater detail.

Compounds such as recombinant human keratinocyte growth factor, rHuKGF (palifermin, Kepivance Amgen, Thousand Oaks, CA) represent an approach to toxicity reduction differing from the classic radioprotection provided by amifostine. When administered after RT in a preclinical setting, a rapid increase in basal cell proliferation is seen. Radiotherapy and chemotherapy-induced injury to oral and gastrointestinal tract mucosa and pulmonary alveoli is significantly ameliorated with rHuKGF (24,30,74). Use of palifermin in conjunction with total body irradiation in the bone marrow transplant setting significantly reduces the duration and severity of mucositis and the requirement for narcotic analgesics. The drug was also well tolerated (74). The RTOG has just opened a phase III trial to evaluate palifermin-mediated mucosal protection in patients undergoing concurrent RT and cisplatin for advanced head and neck cancer. Potential tumor protection will need to be carefully evaluated in all trials using this drug.

∷ | Summary

The use of modified daily fractionation as opposed to conventional once daily fractionation improves the prognosis of patients who receive curative intent RT for advanced head and neck cancer. Radiation therapy and concurrent chemotherapy in turn are superior to both single-modality conventional and modified fractionation radiation therapy in the nonsurgical management of advanced head and neck cancer. Anti-EGFR targeted therapy also enhances the effectiveness of RT. The role of EGFR inhibition in a chemoradiation setting is under investigation. Likewise, the benefit of adding induction chemotherapy to a platform of chemoradiation is being tested.

The increased acute and late toxicity that results from combining these multiple modalities poses immediate challenges. These include the need to develop criteria for *a priori* selection of those patients with advanced stage disease who can still be adequately treated with radiotherapy alone and the need to create effective strategies for toxicity prophylaxis and management. These efforts will allow for the optimal integration of radiotherapy, chemotherapy, and biologically targeted therapy for those patients requiring combined modality therapy.

References

1. Adelstein DJ, Lavertu P, Saxton JP, et al. Mature results of a phase III randomized trial comparing concurrent chemoradiotherapy with radiation therapy alone in patients with stage III and IV squamous cell carcinoma of the head and neck. *Cancer* 2000;88:876–883.
2. Adelstein DJ, Li Y, Adams GL, et al. An intergroup phase III comparison of standard radiation therapy and two schedules of concurrent chemoradiotherapy in patients with unresectable squamous cell head and neck cancer. *J Clin Oncol* 2003;21:92–98.
3. Adelstein DJ, Saxton JP, Rybicki LA, et al. Multiagent concurrent chemoradiotherapy for locoregionally advanced squamous cell head and neck cancer: Mature results from a single institution. *J Clin Oncol* 2006;24:1064–1071.
4. Adjuvant chemotherapy for advanced head and neck squamous carcinoma. Final report of the Head and Neck Contracts Program. *Cancer* 1987;60:301–311.
5. Al-Sarraf M, LeBlanc M, Giri PG, et al. Chemoradiotherapy versus radiotherapy in patients with advanced nasopharyngeal cancer: Phase III randomized Intergroup study 0099. *J Clin Oncol* 1998;16:1310–1317.
6. Ang KK, Berkey BA, Tu X, et al. Impact of epidermal growth factor receptor expression on survival and pattern of relapse in patients with advanced head and neck carcinoma. *Cancer Res* 2002;62:7350–7356.
7. Ang KK. Concurrent radiation chemotherapy for locally advanced head and neck carcinoma: Are we addressing burning subjects? *J Clin Oncol* 2004;22:4657–4659.
8. Bartelink H, Kallman RF, Rapacchietta D, et al. Therapeutic enhancement in mice by clinically relevant dose and fractionation schedules of cis-diamminedichloroplatinum (II) and irradiation. *Radiother Oncol* 1986;6:61–74.
9. Becker A, Hansgen G, Bloching M, et al. Oxygenation of squamous cell carcinoma of the head and neck: Comparison of primary tumors, neck node metastases, and normal tissue. *Int J Radiat Oncol Biol Phys* 1998;42:35–41.
10. Bensadoun RJ, Benezery K, Dassonville O, et al. French multicenter phase III randomized study testing concurrent twice-a-day radiotherapy and cisplatin/5-fluorouracil chemotherapy (BiRCF) in unresectable pharyngeal carcinoma: Results at 2 years (FNCLCC-GORTEC). *Int J Radiat Oncol Biol Phys* 2006;64:983–994.
11. Bernier J, Domenge C, Ozsahin M, et al. Postoperative irradiation with or without concomitant chemotherapy for locally advanced head and neck cancer. *N Engl J Med* 2004;350:1945–1952.
12. Bernier J. Alteration of radiotherapy fractionation and concurrent chemotherapy: A new frontier in head and neck oncology? *Nat Clin Pract Oncol* 2005;2:305–314.
13. Bonner JA, Harari PM, Giralt J, et al. Radiotherapy plus cetuximab for squamous-cell carcinoma of the head and neck. *N Engl J Med* 2006;354:567–578.
14. Bourhis J, Overgaard J, Audry H, et al. Hyperfractionated or accelerated radiotherapy in head and neck cancer: A meta-analysis. *Lancet* 2006;368:843–854.
15. Brizel DM, Albers ME, Fisher SR, et al. Hyperfractionated irradiation with or without concurrent chemotherapy for locally advanced head and neck cancer. *N Engl J Med* 1998;338:1798–1804.
16. Brizel DM, Dodge RK, Clough RW, et al. Oxygenation of head and neck cancer: Changes during radiotherapy and impact on treatment outcome. *Radiother Oncol* 1999;53:113–117.
17. Brizel DM, Scully SP, Harrelson JM, et al. Tumor oxygenation predicts for the likelihood of distant metastases in human soft tissue sarcoma. *Cancer Res* 1996;56:941–943.
18. Brizel DM, Sibley GS, Prosnitz LR, et al. Tumor hypoxia adversely affects the prognosis of carcinoma of the head and neck. *Int J Radiat Oncol Biol Phys* 1997;38:285–289.
19. Brizel DM, Wasserman TH, Henke M, et al. Phase III randomized trial of amifostine as a radioprotector in head and neck cancer. *J Clin Oncol* 2000;18:3339–3345.
20. Browman GP, Cripps C, Hodson DI, et al. Placebo-controlled randomized trial of infusional fluorouracil during standard radiotherapy in locally advanced head and neck cancer. *J Clin Oncol* 1994;12:2648–2653.
21. Budach V, Stuschke M, Budach W, et al. Hyperfractionated accelerated chemoradiation with concurrent fluorouracil-mitomycin is more effective than dose-escalated hyperfractionated accelerated radiation therapy alone in locally advanced head and neck cancer: Final results of the radiotherapy cooperative clinical trials group of the German Cancer Society 95–06 Prospective Randomized Trial. *J Clin Oncol* 2005;23:1125–1135.
22. Buntzel J, Kuttner K, Frohlich D, et al. Selective cytoprotection with amifostine in concurrent radiochemotherapy for head and neck cancer. *Ann Oncol* 1998;9:505–509.
23. Calais G, Alfonsi M, Bardet E, et al. Randomized trial of radiation therapy versus concomitant chemotherapy and radiation therapy for advanced-stage oropharynx carcinoma. *J Natl Cancer Inst* 1999;91:2081–2086.
24. Chen L, Brizel DM, Rabbani ZN, et al. The protective effect of recombinant human keratinocyte growth factor on radiation-induced pulmonary toxicity in rats. *Int J Radiat Oncol Biol Phys* 2004;60:1520–1529.
25. Cooper JS, Guo MD, Herskovic A, et al. Chemoradiotherapy of locally advanced esophageal cancer: Long-term follow-up of a prospective randomized trial (RTOG 85–01). *Radiation Therapy Oncology Group. Jama* 1999;281:1623–1627.
26. Cooper JS, Pajak TF, Forastiere AA, et al. Postoperative concurrent radiotherapy and chemotherapy for high-risk squamous-cell carcinoma of the head and neck. *N Engl J Med* 2004;350:1937–1944.
27. Cox JD, Pajak TF, Marcial VA, et al. Interruptions adversely affect local control and survival with hyperfractionated radiation therapy of carcinomas of the upper respiratory and digestive tracts. New evidence for accelerated proliferation from Radiation Therapy Oncology Group Protocol 8313. *Cancer* 1992;69:2744–2748.
28. Denis F, Garaud P, Bardet E, et al. Final results of the 94–01 French Head and Neck Oncology and Radiotherapy Group randomized trial comparing radiotherapy alone with concomitant radiochemotherapy in advanced-stage oropharynx carcinoma. *J Clin Oncol* 2004;22:69–76.
29. Dobrowsky W, Naude J. Continuous hyperfractionated accelerated radiotherapy with/without mitomycin C in head and neck cancers. *Radiother Oncol* 2000;57:119–124.
30. Dorr W, Noack R, Spekl K, et al. Modification of oral mucositis by keratinocyte growth factor: Single radiation exposure. *Int J Radiat Biol* 2001;77:341–347.
31. Eschwege F, Sancho-Garnier H, Gerard JP, et al. Ten-year results of randomized trial comparing radiotherapy and concomitant bleomycin to radiotherapy alone in epidermoid carcinomas of the oropharynx: Experience of the European Organization for Research and Treatment of Cancer. 1988; NCI Monogr:275–278.
32. Forastiere AA, Goepfert H, Maor M, et al. Concurrent chemotherapy and radiotherapy for organ preservation in advanced laryngeal cancer. *N Engl J Med* 2003;349:2091–2098.
33. Fowler JF. Modelling altered fractionation schedules. *BJR Suppl* 1992;24:187–192.
34. Fu KK, Pajak TF, Trotti A, et al. A Radiation Therapy Oncology Group (RTOG) phase III randomized study to compare hyperfractionation and two variants of accelerated fractionation to standard fractionation radiotherapy for head and neck squamous cell carcinomas: First report of RTOG 9003. *Int J Radiat Oncol Biol Phys* 2000;48:7–16.
35. Fu KK, Phillips TL, Silverberg IJ, et al. Combined radiotherapy and chemotherapy with bleomycin and methotrexate for advanced inoperable head and neck cancer: Update of a Northern California Oncology Group randomized trial. *J Clin Oncol* 1987;5:1410–1418.
36. Fu KK. Combined-modality therapy for head and neck cancer. *Oncology* (Williston Park) 11:1781–90, 1796; discussion 1796, 179, 1997.
37. Fyles AW, Milosevic M, Wong R, et al. Oxygenation predicts radiation response and survival in patients with cervix cancer. *Radiother Oncol* 1998;48:149–156.
38. Gatzemeier U, Rodriguez G, Treat J, et al. Tirapazamine-cisplatin: The synergy. *Br J Cancer* 1998;77[Suppl 4]:15–17.
39. Graeber TG, Osmanian C, Jacks T, et al. Hypoxia-mediated selection of cells with diminished apoptotic potential in solid tumours. *Nature* 1996;379:88–91.
40. Gray LH, Conger AD, Ebert M, et al. The concentration of oxygen dissolved in tissues at the time of irradiation as a factor in radiotherapy. *Br J Radiol* 1953;26:638–648.
41. Gupta NK, Pointon RC, Wilkinson PM. A randomised clinical trial to contrast radiotherapy with radiotherapy and methotrexate given synchronously in head and neck cancer. *Clin Radiol* 1987;38:575–581.
42. Haffty BG, Son YH, Papac R, et al. Chemotherapy as an adjunct to radiation in the treatment of squamous cell carcinoma of the head and neck: results of the Yale Mitomycin Randomized Trials. *J Clin Oncol* 1997;15:268–276.
43. Harari PM, Cleary JF, Hartig GK. Evolving patterns of practice regarding the use of chemoradiation for advanced head and neck cancer patients. *Proceedings ASCO* 2001;20:226a.
44. Harari PM. Why has induction chemotherapy for advanced head and neck cancer become a United States community standard of practice? *J Clin Oncol* 1997;15:2050–2055.
45. Hitt R, Lopez-Pousa A, Martinez-Trufero J, et al. Phase III study comparing cisplatin plus fluorouracil to paclitaxel, cisplatin, and fluorouracil induction chemotherapy followed by chemoradiotherapy in locally advanced head and neck cancer. *J Clin Oncol* 2005;23:8636–8645.
46. Hockel M, Schlenger K, Aral B, et al. Association between tumor hypoxia and malignant progression in advanced cancer of the uterine cervix. *Cancer Res* 1996;56:4509–4515.
47. Horiot JC, Bontemps P, van den Bogaert W, et al. Accelerated fractionation (AF) compared to conventional fractionation (CF) improves loco-regional control in the radiotherapy of advanced head and neck cancers: Results of the EORTC 22851 randomized trial. *Radiother Oncol* 1997;44:111–121.
48. Horiot JC, Le Fur R, N'Guyen T, et al. Hyperfractionation versus conventional fractionation in oropharyngeal carcinoma: Final analysis of a randomized trial of the EORTC cooperative group of radiotherapy. *Radiother Oncol* 1992;25:231–241.
49. Huguenin P, Beer KT, Allal A, et al. Concomitant cisplatin significantly improves locoregional control in advanced head and neck cancers treated with hyperfractionated radiotherapy. *J Clin Oncol* 2004;22:4665–4673.
50. Jeremic B, Shibamoto Y, Milicic B, et al. Hyperfractionated radiation therapy with or without concurrent low-dose daily cisplatin in locally advanced squamous cell carcinoma of the head and neck: A prospective randomized trial. *J Clin Oncol* 2000;18:1458–1464.
51. Keane TJ, Cummings BJ, O'Sullivan B, et al. A randomized trial of radiation therapy compared to split course radiation therapy combined with mitomycin C and 5 fluorouracil as initial treatment for advanced laryngeal and hypopharyngeal squamous carcinoma. *Int J Radiat Oncol Biol Phys* 1993;25:613–618.
52. Koch CJ. Unusual oxygen concentration dependence of toxicity of SR-4233, a hypoxic cell toxin. *Cancer Res* 1993;53:3992–3997.
53. Koukourakis MI, Giatromanolaki A, Sivridis E, et al. Hypoxia-inducible factor (HIF1A and HIF2A), angiogenesis, and chemoradiotherapy outcome of squamous cell head-and-neck cancer. *Int J Radiat Oncol Biol Phys* 2002;53:1192–1202.
54. Koukourakis MI, Giatromanolaki A, Sivridis E, et al. Hypoxia-regulated carbonic anhydrase-9 (CA9) relates to poor vascularization and resistance of squamous cell head and neck cancer to chemoradiotherapy. *Clin Cancer Res* 2001;7:3399–3403.
55. Kurihara N, Kubota T, Hoshiya Y, et al. Pharmacokinetics of cis-diamminedichloroplatinum (II) given as low-dose and high-dose infusions. *J Surg Oncol* 1996;62:135–138.
56. Lamont EB, Vokes EE. Chemotherapy in the management of squamous-cell carcinoma of the head and neck. *Lancet Oncol* 2001;2:261–269.
57. Laramore GE, Scott CB, al-Sarraf M, et al. Adjuvant chemotherapy for resectable squamous cell carcinomas of the head and neck: Report on Intergroup Study 0034. *Int J Radiat Oncol Biol Phys* 1992;23:705–713.
58. Lo TC, Wiley AL, Jr., Ansfield FJ, et al. Combined radiation therapy and 5-fluorouracil for advanced squamous cell carcinoma of the oral cavity and oropharynx: A randomized study. *AJR Am J Roentgenol* 1976;126:229–235.
59. Merlano M, Benasso M, Corvo R, et al. Five-year update of a randomized trial of alternating radiotherapy and chemotherapy compared with radiotherapy alone in treatment of unresectable squamous cell carcinoma of the head and neck. *J Natl Cancer Inst* 1996;88:583–589.

60. Merlano M, Vitale V, Rosso R, et al. Treatment of advanced squamous-cell carcinoma of the head and neck with alternating chemotherapy and radiotherapy. *N Engl J Med* 1992;327:1115–1121.

61. Moeller BJ, Cao Y, Li CY, et al. Radiation activates HIF-1 to regulate vascular radiosensitivity in tumors: Role of reoxygenation, free radicals, and stress granules. *Cancer Cell* 2004;5:429–441.

62. Morris M, Eifel PJ, Lu J, et al. Pelvic radiation with concurrent chemotherapy compared with pelvic and para-aortic radiation for high-risk cervical cancer. *N Engl J Med* 1999;340:1137–1143.

63. Nagai N, Ogata H. Quantitative relationship between pharmacokinetics of unchanged cisplatin and nephrotoxicity in rats: Importance of area under the concentration-time curve (AUC) as the major toxicodynamic determinant in vivo. *Cancer Chemother Pharmacol* 1997;40:11–18.

64. Nordsmark M, Bentzen SM, Rudat V, et al. Prognostic value of tumor oxygenation in 397 head and neck tumors after primary radiation therapy. An international multi-center study. *Radiother Oncol* 2005;77:18–24.

65. Overgaard J, Hansen HS, Specht L, et al. Five compared with six fractions per week of conventional radiotherapy of squamous-cell carcinoma of head and neck: DAHANCA 6 and 7 randomised controlled trial. *Lancet* 2003;362:933–940.

66. Overgaard J, Hjelm-Hansen M, Johansen LV, et al. Comparison of conventional and split-course radiotherapy as primary treatment in carcinoma of the larynx. *Acta Oncol* 1988;27:147–152.

67. Peters WA 3rd, Liu PY, Barrett RJ 2nd, et al. Concurrent chemotherapy and pelvic radiation therapy compared with pelvic radiation therapy alone as adjuvant therapy after radical surgery in high-risk early-stage cancer of the cervix. *J Clin Oncol* 2000;18:1606–1613.

68. Pignon JP, Baujat B, Bourhis J. Individual patient data meta-analyses in head and neck carcinoma: What have we learnt?]. *Cancer Radiother* 2005;9:31–36.

69. Pignon JP, Bourhis J, Domenge C, et al. Chemotherapy added to locoregional treatment for head and neck squamous-cell carcinoma: Three meta-analyses of updated individual data. MACH-NC Collaborative Group. Meta-Analysis of Chemotherapy on Head and Neck Cancer. *Lancet* 2000;355:949–955.

70. Rischin D, Peters L, Fisher R, et al. Tirapazamine, Cisplatin, and Radiation versus Fluorouracil, Cisplatin, and Radiation in patients with locally advanced head and neck cancer: A randomized phase II trial of the Trans-Tasman Radiation Oncology Group (TROG 98.02). *J Clin Oncol* 2005;23:79–87.

71. Rischin D, Peters L, Hicks R, et al. Phase I trial of concurrent tirapazamine, cisplatin, and radiotherapy in patients with advanced head and neck cancer. *J Clin Oncol* 2001;19:535–542.

72. Rose PG, Bundy BN, Watkins EB, et al. Concurrent cisplatin-based radiotherapy and chemotherapy for locally advanced cervical cancer. *N Engl J Med* 1999;340:1144–1153

73. Sanchiz F, Milla A, Torner J, et al. Single fraction per day versus two fractions per day versus radiochemotherapy in the treatment of head and neck cancer. *Int J Radiat Oncol Biol Phys* 1990;19:1347–1350.

74. Spielberger R, Stiff P, Bensinger W, et al. Palifermin for oral mucositis after intensive therapy for hematologic cancers. *N Engl J Med* 2004;351:2590–2598.

75. Taylor SGt, Murthy AK, Vannetzel JM, et al. Randomized comparison of neoadjuvant cisplatin and fluorouracil infusion followed by radiation versus concomitant treatment in advanced head and neck cancer. *J Clin Oncol* 1994;12:385–395.

76. Thomas GM. Improved treatment for cervical cancer–concurrent chemotherapy and radiotherapy. *N Engl J Med* 1999;340:1198–1200.

77. Tuttle SW, Hazard L, Koch CJ, et al. Bioreductive metabolism of SR-4233 (WIN 59075) by whole cell suspensions under aerobic and hypoxic conditions: Role of the pentose cycle and implications for the mechanism of cytotoxicity observed in air. *Int J Radiat Oncol Biol Phys* 1994;29:357–362.

78. Vermorken JB, Remenar E, van Herpen C, et al. Standard cisplatin/infusional 5-fluorouracil (PF) vs docetaxel (T) plus PF (TPF) as neoadjuvant chemotherapy for nonresectable locally advanced squamous cell carcinoma of the head and neck (LA-SCCHN): A phase III trial of the EORTC Head and Neck Cancer Group (EORTC #24971). *J Clin Oncol* (Meeting Abstracts) 2004;22:5508.

79. Wasserman T, Mackowiak JI, Brizel DM, et al. Effect of amifostine on patient assessed clinical benefit in irradiated head and neck cancer. *Int J Radiat Oncol Biol Phys* 2000;48:1035–1039.

80. Wasserman TH, Brizel DM, Henke M, et al. Influence of intravenous amifostine on xerostomia, tumor control, and survival after radiotherapy for head-and-neck cancer: 2-year follow-up of a prospective, randomized, phase III trial. *Int J Radiat Oncol Biol Phys* 2005;63:985–990.

81. Wendt TG, Grabenbauer GG, Rodel CM, et al. Simultaneous radiochemotherapy versus radiotherapy alone in advanced head and neck cancer: A randomized multicenter study. *J Clin Oncol* 1998;16:1318–1324.

82. Withers HR, Taylor JM, Maciejewski B. The hazard of accelerated tumor clonogen repopulation during radiotherapy. *Acta Oncol* 1988;27:131–146.

83. Wong WW, Mick R, Haraf DJ, et al. Time-dose relationship for local tumor control following alternate week concomitant radiation and chemotherapy of advanced head and neck cancer. *Int J Radiat Oncol Biol Phys* 1994;29:153–162.

84. Yuhas JM, Spellman JM, Culo F. The role of WR-2721 in radiotherapy and/or chemotherapy. *Cancer Clin Trials* 1980;3:211–216.

Chapter 38
Nasopharynx

Anne W. M. Lee, Carlos A. Perez, Stephen C. K. Law, Daniel T. T. Chua, William I. Wei, Vincent Chong

Anatomy

The nasopharynx is a cuboidal open chamber that begins at the posterior choana and slopes downward along the airway to the level of the free border of the uvula. Anteriorly it communicates with the nasal cavity via the choana, and inferiorly it continues into the oropharynx via the pharyngeal isthmus. The roof and the posterior wall are formed by the basisphenoid, the clivus, and the first cervical vertebra. The floor is the superior surface of the soft palate. The eustachian tube opens into the lateral wall of the nasopharynx. The posterior portion of the eustachian tube is cartilaginous and protrudes into the nasopharynx, making a ridge called the *torus tubarius*. Posterior to the torus is a recess called the *fossa of Rosenmüller*. The lateral and posterior walls of the nasopharynx are supported by the pharyngobasilar fascia, which is attached to the base of the skull (Fig. 38.1).

A number of foramina and fissures located in the base of the skull are important routes by which nasopharyngeal carcinoma (NPC) can extend intracranially and involve various cranial nerves (Fig. 38.2 and Table 38.1). The most important are the foramen lacerum and the foramen ovale, which are in close anatomic relationship with the cavernous sinus and hence cranial nerves III to VI (Fig. 38.3).

Histologically, the nasopharyngeal mucosa is covered by respiratory-type ciliated epithelium, but variable degrees of squamous metaplasia are common. The stroma is rich in lymphatic plexus and lymphoid tissue that often includes reactive lymphoid follicles; the epithelium is commonly infiltrated by many small lymphoid cells.

The lymphatics of the nasopharynx have three major pathways (63) (Fig. 38.4). One pathway drains into a small group of nodes that lies in the parapharyngeal space, in close proximity to cranial nerves IX to XII. The uppermost node is the retropharyngeal node called the *node of Rouviere* (Fig. 38.5). Another lymphatic pathway drains into the jugular chain to involve the jugulodigastric and deep jugular nodes. The third pathway drains into the spinal accessory chain; the uppermost node lies beneath the sternomastoid muscle at the tip of the mastoid process.

Epidemiology

NPC shows a distinct racial and geographical distribution. As reported by the International Agency for Research on Cancer (181), the annual incidence rate (per 100,000 per year) in 1988–1992 ranged from <1 among whites to >20 among Southern Chinese male populations. According to the Surveillance, Epidemiology, and End Results Cancer Statistics Review, the incidence rate of NPC in the United States during 1996–2000 was 1.1 for men and 0.4 for women.

In low-risk populations, a bimodal age distribution is observed. The first peak incidence occurs at 15 to 25 and the second peak at 50 to 59 years of age. In contrast, the incidence in high-risk populations rises after 30 years of age, peaks at 40 to 60 years, and declines thereafter (59). The age distribution is similar in both genders. The incidence rates in male populations are commonly two to threefold that of female populations.

Descendants from Chinese who have migrated to Western countries show progressively lower risk, but their incidence remains higher than the indigenous populations (8,93). The study by Dickson and Flores (55) reported that the incidence rate in Chinese who were born in the Orient was 20.5, compared with 1.3 for Chinese and 0.2 for white people born in Canada. Buell (8) reported that among Chinese in the United States, the American-born second generation had a lower risk than the Asian-born first generation, while California whites born in Southeast Asia had an increased risk compared with their American-born counterparts.

Furthermore, familial aggregation of NPC has been reported in diverse populations. In a study of Southern Chinese by Yu et al. (245), NPC was detected in 6% of first-degree relatives of NPC patients as compared with 1% of first-degree relatives of controls in the same neighborhood.

These epidemiologic observations suggest a multifactorial cause that includes both inherited genetic predisposition and environmental factors. The near constant association of Epstein-Barr virus (EBV) with nonkeratinizing NPC, irrespective of ethnic background, indicates a probable oncogenic role in the carcinogenesis (15). Supporting evidences include presence of EBV-DNA or RNA in nearly all tumor cells, its presence in a clonal episomal form indicating that the virus has entered the tumor cell before clonal expansion, and its presence in the precursor lesion of NPC, but not in normal nasopharyngeal epithelium (188). Exposure to carcinogens in traditional southern Chinese food (volatile nitrosamines in preserved salted fish, in particular) have been incriminated (75,184). Cigarette smoking, previous irradiation, occupational exposure to dust, smoke, and chemical fumes has also been implicated, but definitive conclusion is difficult.

Table 38.2 shows the changing epidemiology in different ethnic groups during different periods. The study by Lee et al. (120) of 21,768 new cases of NPC and 8664 related deaths registered in Hong Kong showed steady reduction in the age-standardized incidence rate (per 100,000 per year) from 28.5 in 1980–1984 to 20.2 in 1995–1999 for men, and from 11.2 to 7.8 for women. The total decrease thus amounted to 30% for both genders during this 20-year period (Fig. 38.6). Furthermore, the age-standardized mortality/incidence ratio decreased from 0.48 to 0.39 for men, and from 0.40 to 0.29 for women in the corresponding periods. As there was no substantial change in the proportion of Chinese in the community, the genetic background was relatively stable; the declining incidence was probably attributed to changing environmental risk factors as the lifestyle for most citizens changed progressively to a more Western style, particularly in terms of diets. Interestingly, review of the incidence in other representative communities during the same period shows that Hong Kong was thus far the only place where such encouraging reduction was achieved.

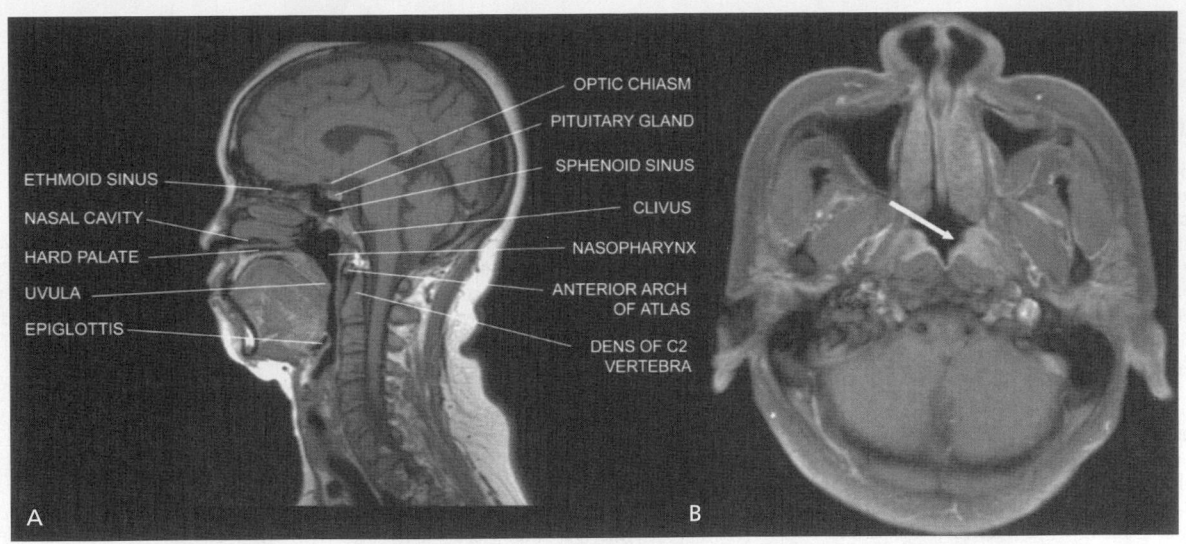

FIGURE 38.1. A: Midsagittal magnetic resonance image (MRI) of the head, showing the nasopharynx and related structures. **B:** Axial contrast-enhanced MR image showing a small tumor in the left fossa of Rosenmüller (arrow) and normal structures in the rest of the nasopharynx.

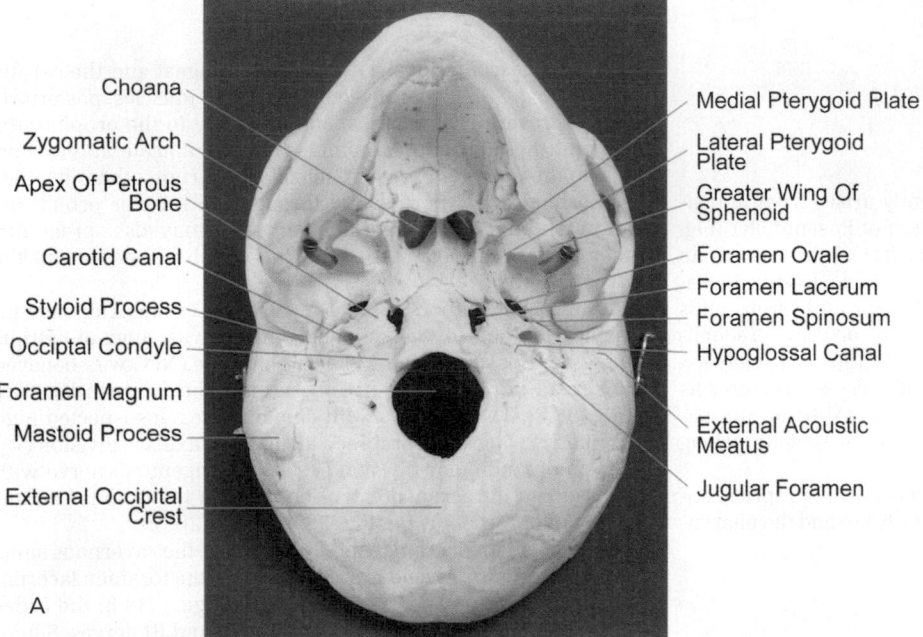

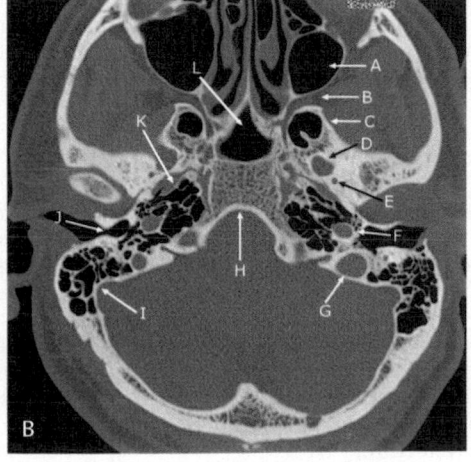

(A)- Maxillary Sinus
(B)- Pterygopalatine Fossa
(C)- Pneumatized Pterygoid Process
(D)- Foramen Ovale
(E)- Foramen Spinosum
(F)- Carotid Canal
(G)- Jugular Bulb
(H)- Clivus
(I)- Mastoid Cells
(J)- External Auditory Canal
(K)- Pneumatized Petrous Apex
(L)- Sphenoid Sinus

FIGURE 38.2. A: Basal view of skull illustrating the foramina of the base of the skull and the occupying structures. **B:** Axial computed tomography scan illustrating the bony anatomy.

Table 38.1	FORAMINA OF THE BASE OF THE SKULL AND ASSOCIATED ANATOMIC STRUCTURES

Foramen/Fissure	Cranial Nerve	Other Structures
Cribriform plate	Olfactory nerve (I)	Anterior ethmoidal nerve
Optic foramen	Optic nerve (II)	Ophthalmic artery
Superior orbital fissure	Oculomotor (III), trochlear (IV), ophthalmic division of trigeminal (V_1) nerve, abducent (VI) nerves	Ophthalmic vein, orbital branch of middle meningeal and recurrent branch of lacrimal arteries, sympathetic plexus, filaments from carotid plexus
Foramen rotundum	Maxillary division of trigeminal (V_2) nerve	
Foramen ovale	Mandibular division of trigeminal (V_3) nerve	Accessory meningeal artery, lesser superficial petrosal nerve
Foramen lacerum		Internal carotid, sympathetic carotid plexus; vidian nerve, meningeal branch of ascending pharyngeal artery, emissary vein
Foramen spinosum	Recurrent branch of V_3 nerve	Middle meningeal artery and vein
Stylomastoid foramen	Facial (VII) nerve	
Internal acoustic meatus	Auditory (VIII) nerve	Internal auditory artery
Jugular foramen	Glossopharyngeal (IX), vagus (X), spinal accessory (XI) nerves	Inferior petrosal sinus; transverse sinus, meningeal branches from occipital and ascending pharyngeal arteries
Hypoglossal canal	Hypoglossal (XII) nerve	Meningeal branch of ascending pharyngeal artery
Foramen magnum		Spinal cord, spinal accessory nerve, vertebral vessels, anterior and posterior spinal vessels

Natural History

Local Extension

Carcinoma of the nasopharynx frequently arises from the lateral wall, with a predilection for the fossa of Rosenmüller (Fig. 38.1B). The tumor may obstruct the orifice of the eustachian tube or infiltrate the levator veli palatine muscle, leading to disequilibrium of air pressure in the middle ear and serous otitis media. The tumor may involve the mucosa or grow predominantly in the submucosa (197). Local infiltration is usually extensive; the frequency of involvement of various structures as shown by the magnetic resonance imaging (MRI) of 308 patients from Pamela Youde Nethersole Eastern Hospital (Hong Kong) (15) is summarized in Table 38.3.

Adjacent soft tissues are first infiltrated as tumors spread anteriorly into the nasal fossa, posterolaterally beyond the pharyn-

gobasilar fascia to involve the parapharyngeal and the carotid spaces (Fig. 38.7), laterally to the pterygoid muscles, posteriorly to the prevertebral muscles, and inferiorly to the oropharynx. Beyond these structures, tumors further infiltrate anterolaterally to the pterygoid process, maxillary antrum, ethmoid sinus, the orbital apex (particularly through the inferior orbital fissure), and the infratemporal fossa; tumor may also spread further posteroinferiorly to involve the vertebral bodies and the hypopharynx.

Superiorly, tumors cause bony erosion of the skull base involving the floor of the sphenoid sinus, clivus, apex of petrous bone, and basal foramina. For a long time, NPC was believed to spread intracranially, mainly through the foramen lacerum (Fig. 38.8). The advent of MRI demonstrates unsuspected high frequency of perineural spread along the maxillary division (V_2) and the mandibular division (V_3) of the trigeminal nerve with subsequent intracranial extension through the foramen rotundum and foramen ovale (Fig. 38.9) (34,36,203).

Involvement of cranial nerves III to VI at the cavernous sinus occurs as tumors extend intracranially via the foramen lacerum and/or foramen ovale. As illustrated in Figure 38.3, the order of involvement is V and VI, followed by IV and III nerves. Sometimes the V_3 nerve is involved at the gasserian ganglion. In advanced cases, tumors involve the hypoglossal canal and jugular foramen. The IX to XII nerves are infiltrated at these regions or in the parapharyngeal space as they emerge from the base of the skull (33). Compression of the cervical sympathetic nerve may rarely occur.

Lymphatic Spread

As the nasopharynx has a rich submucosal lymphatic network, gross cervical lymphadenopathy is present in more than 70% of NPC patients at presentation (118). There is an orderly pattern of lymph node involvement from upper to lower neck (Fig. 38.10). King et al. (91) reported that the frequency of retropharyngeal nodes abnormality was as high as 94%, internal jugular nodes 72%, and spinal accessory nodes 57%, while submandibular (3%) and parotid (2%) involvements were rare. Other series showed that the jugulodigastric nodes are the most frequently involved (196).

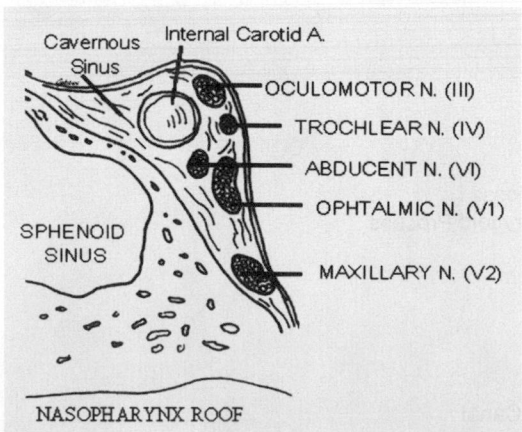

FIGURE 38.3. Coronal section through the sphenoid sinus and roof of the nasopharynx showing the relative positions of the cranial nerves III to VI. (Modified from Chao KSC. *Practical essentials of intensity-modulated radiation therapy.* Philadelphia: Lippincott Williams & Wilkins; 2005:138, with permission.)

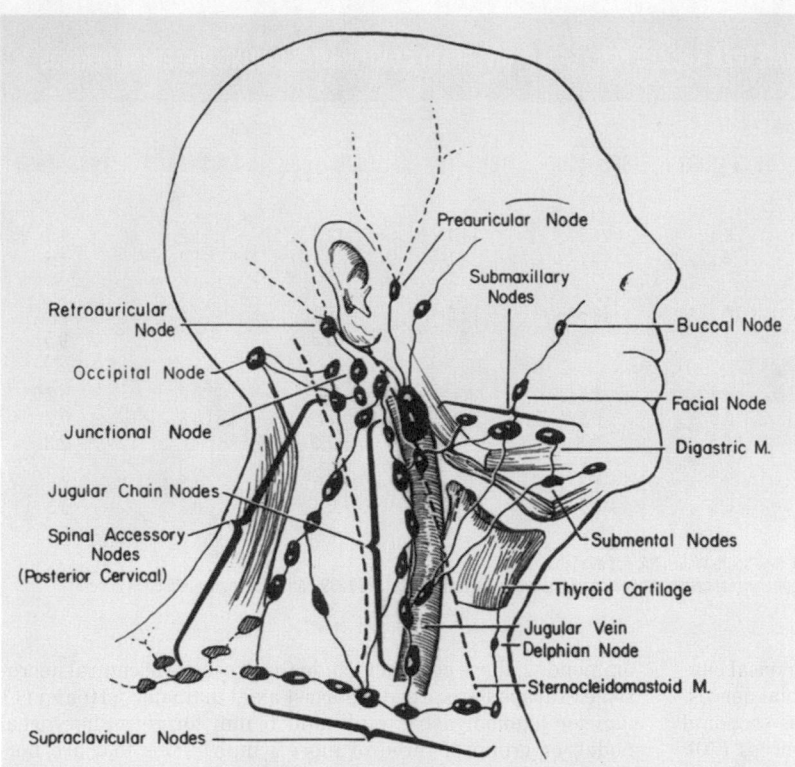

FIGURE 38.4. Pathways for lymphatic spread of nasopharyngeal carcinoma. (Redrawn from Rouviere H. *Anatomy of the human lymphatic system.* Ann Arbor, MI: Edward Brothers; 1938:27, with permission.)

The study by Ng et al. (171) on the pattern of nodal involvement by radiologic levels based on MRI showed that the incidences in order of frequency were 94% at level II, 85% at level III, 80% retropharyngeal node, 46% V_A, 19% IV, 17% V_B, and 17% at level I (Fig. 38.11).

Hematogenous Dissemination

NPC is notorious for its predilection for hematogenous dissemination. Both the N-category and the T-category are the main risk-determining factors (112,117). Patients with lymphatic spread down to the supraclavicular fossa have an especially high risk of distant metastasis.

Gross evidence of distant metastases is uncommon at presentation (6%), but more than 30% of patients with advanced locoregional disease eventually died of distant failure (129). A study by Hui et al. (79) showed that the commonest metastatic site was bone, followed closely by liver and lung. Lung metastasis was associated with better prognosis than other sites; the median overall survival (OS) was 3.9 years. Brain and skin metastases are extremely rare (156,172).

Clinical Presentation

The frequency of different presenting symptoms and signs is summarized in Table 38.4. Both the studies by Chao and Perez (19) and Lee et al. (118) showed that painless enlargement of upper neck nodes was the most common presenting feature, followed by nasal symptoms and aural problems. About 20% of patients had signs of cranial nerve palsy at diagnosis. The V and VI nerves were the commonest involved, whereas I, VII, and VIII nerves were rarely affected (Table 38.5).

Lee et al. (122) further showed that there was significant association between the duration of symptoms before diagnosis and the presenting stage, which in turn affected survival. Increased awareness by both the public and the primary care doctors are necessary to minimize delay in diagnosis.

One special feature calling for increased awareness is that NPC is the commonest malignancy associated with dermatomyositis in endemic areas (137). Teo et al. (211) reported that 0.9% (10/1,154) NPC patients suffered from dermatomyositis.

Diagnostic and Staging Work-Up

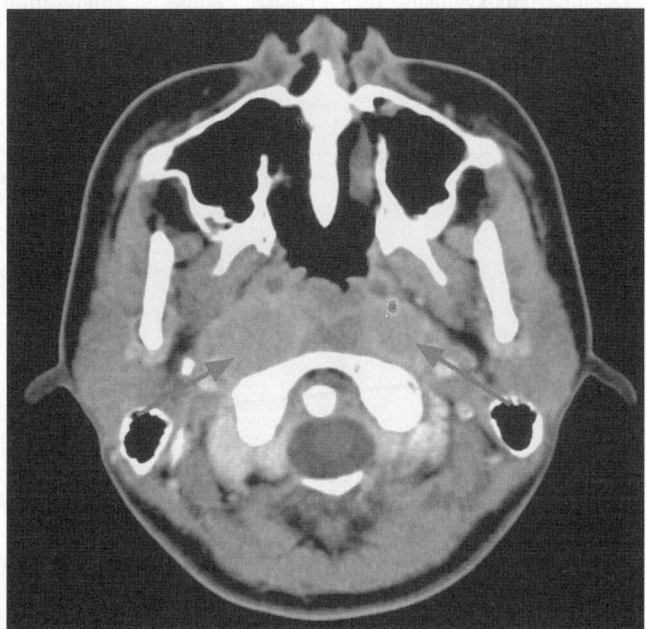

FIGURE 38.5. Axial contrast-enhanced computed tomography scan showing involvement of bilateral retropharyngeal lymph nodes (arrows) by nasopharyngeal carcinoma.

Table 38.6 lists the diagnostic and staging procedures generally recommended for NPC. Detailed evaluation of locoregional

| Table 38.2 | AGE-STANDARDIZED INCIDENCE RATE (PER 100,000 PER YEAR) IN DIFFERENT COMMUNITIES DURING DIFFERENT PERIODS |

	Male				Female			
Year	1973–1977	1978–1982	1983–1987	1988–1992	1973–1977	1978–1982	1983–1987	1988–1992
China								
Hong Kong	32.9	30	28.5	24.3	14.4	12.9	11.2	9.5
Shanghai	5.6	4.4	4	4.5	2.5	2	1.9	1.8
Singapore								
Chinese	19.4	18.1	18.1	18.5	7.5	7.9	7.4	7.3
Indian	0.9	0.3	1	0.5	0	1.3	0.2	0.5
United States								
SEER: White	NA	NA	0.5	0.5	NA	NA	0.2	0.2
SEER: Black	NA	NA	0.8	0.9	NA	NA	0.3	0.2
LA: Chinese	7.1	9.9	6.5	9.8	4	7.3	3	2.8
England and Wales	NA	0.4	0.4	0.4	NA	0.2	0.2	0.2
Australia: NSW	0.6	0.8	0.8	0.9	0.3	0.3	0.2	0.3

SEER, Surveillance, Epidemiology, and End-Results; LA, Los Angeles; NSW, New South Wales. NA, not available.
Modified from Lee A, Foo W, Mang O, et al. Changing epidemiology of nasopharyngeal carcinoma in Hong Kong over a 20-year period (1980–99): An encouraging reduction in both incidence and mortality. *Int J Cancer*, 2003;103:680–685.

extent should include endoscopic examination of the nasal cavities and whole pharynx, thorough testing of all cranial nerves, and assessment of neck node involvement. Cross-sectional imaging is mandatory to complete the staging process (70). MRI is the study of choice because of its superior sensitivity (36,169,173); computed tomography (CT) with axial and coronal cut with contrast is accepted as an alternative.

Ng et al. (169) compared the assessment by MRI versus CT: A significantly higher detection rate by MRI was observed for intracranial extension (57% vs. 36%), skull base involvement (60% vs. 40%), retropharyngeal node (58% vs. 21%), and prevertebral muscle infiltration (51% vs. 22%). Using MRI, the T-category was upstaged in 22% and down-staged in 4%; MRI missed none of the patients with bony erosion on CT. Another study by Nishioka et al. (173) similarly showed that MRI was superior in early detection of skull base involvement, resulting in 38% upstaged from T1-2 to T3-4.

The radiologic criteria advocated by Van den Brekel et al. (215) for defining a lymph node as metastatic are commonly rec-

ommended; these criteria include the presence of central necrosis, extracapsular spread, shortest axial diameter ≥10 mm (11 mm for jugulodigastric node and 5 mm for retropharyngeal node), or group of three of more lymph nodes that are borderline in size.

Detailed assessment of nodal enlargement by palpation and imaging should include the size and location of enlarged node, unilateral/bilateral involvement, and whether the lowest extent has reached the supraclavicular fossa (Fig. 38.11). A study by Lee et al. (121) of 5,020 patients showed that fixation (movable vs. fixed to skin and underlying structures) was also a strongly significant prognostic factor (*p* <.01). However, this is not included as an N-staging criterion because determination of fixation is subjective and varies with the examiner.

Comprehensive search for distant metastases is indicated for patients with advanced locoregional disease (particularly N3), and those with suspicious clinical or laboratory abnormalities. A comparative study by Chang et al. (16) showed that [18 F]fluorodeoxyglucose (FDG) positron emission tomography

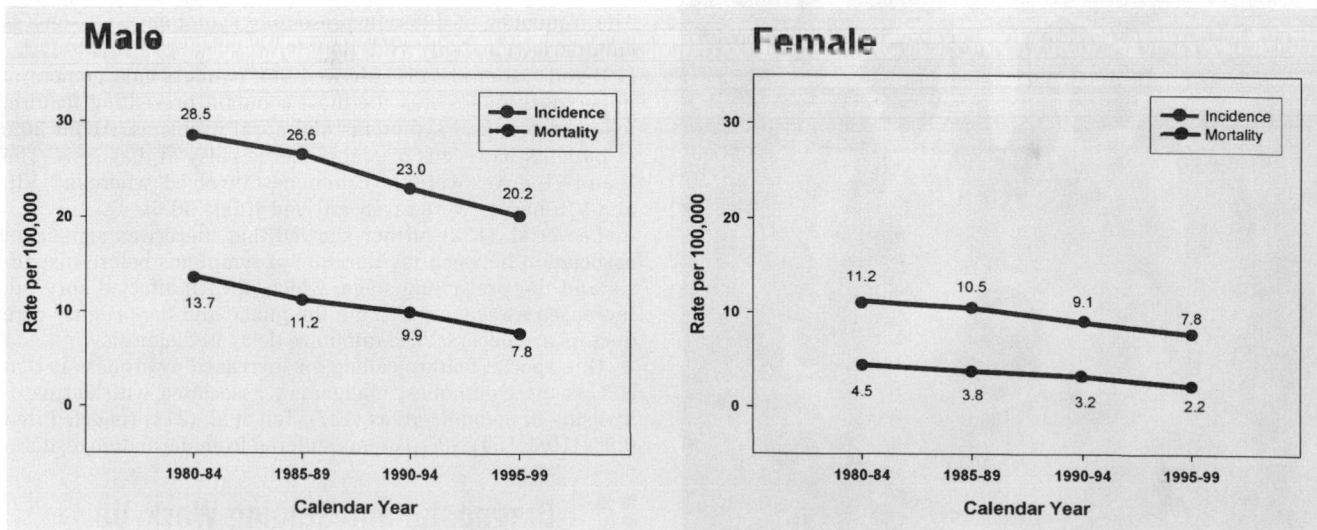

FIGURE 38.6. Changing epidemiology of nasopharyngeal carcinoma in Hong Kong from 1980 to 1999. (Modified from Lee A, Foo W, Mang O, et al. Changing epidemiology of nasopharyngeal carcinoma in Hong Kong over a 20-year period (1980–99): An encouraging reduction in both incidence and mortality. *Int J Cancer* 2003;103:680–685.)

Table 38.3	STRUCTURES LOCALLY INFILTRATED BY NASOPHARYNGEAL CARCINOMA AT DIAGNOSIS[a]	
Structures Involved		**Frequency (%)**
Adjacent soft tissue		
Nasal cavity		87
Parapharyngeal space, carotid space		68
Pterygoid muscle (medial, lateral)		48
Oropharyngeal wall, soft palate		21
Prevertebral muscle		19
Bony erosion/paranasal sinus		
Clivus		41
Sphenoid bone, foramina lacerum, ovale, rotundum		38
Pterygoid plate(s), pterygomaxillary fissure, pterygopalatine fossa		27
Petrous bone, petro-occipital fissure		19
Ethmoid sinus		6
Maxillary antrum		4
Jugular foramen, hypoglossal canal		4
Pituitary fossa/gland		3
Extensive/intracranial extension		
Cavernous sinus		16
Infratemporal fossa		9
Orbit, orbital fissure(s)		4
Cerebrum, meninges, cisterns		4
Hypopharynx		2

[a]Based on magnetic resonance imaging of 308 patients from Pamela Youde Nethersole Eastern Hospital, Hong Kong.
Modified from Chan J, Bray F, McCarron P, et al. Nasopharyngeal carcinoma. In: *Pathology and Genetics of Head and Neck Tumours.* World Health Organization Classification of Tumours. Lyon, France: IARC Press; 2005.

(PET) was superior to conventional work-up (using chest radiograph, isotope bone scan, and abdominal ultrasonography) in detection of distant metastases: 12% of patients were upstaged to stage IVC by PET. N-category was the most significant factor for predicting distant metastases ($p < .01$); the incidence was as high as 56% (9/16) in patients with N3 disease. Hence, PET coupled with CT (Fig. 38.12) is the investigation of choice, if resource allows.

Staging System

An accurate staging system is crucial not only for predicting prognosis, but also for guiding treatment strategy for different risk groups, and facilitating exchange of experience between oncology centers. An international consensus was finally reached in 1997 that a customized system is required for NPC (61,200) because the natural behavior and therapeutic considerations are uniquely different from other head and neck cancers.

Table 38.7 shows the staging criteria and groupings of the current sixth edition of the staging system jointly used by the American Joint Committee on Cancer (70), and International Union Against Cancer (199) (AJCC/UICC). Figure 38.11 illustrates the anatomic boundaries used for defining the supraclavicular fossa.

The definition of masticator space (one of the staging criteria for T4) used in the staging handbook should be noted (70): "Extension of tumor beyond the anterior surface of the lateral pterygoid muscle, or lateral extension beyond the posterolateral wall of the maxillary antrum, and the pterygomaxillary fissure," is meant to be the same as that used for infratemporal fossa. Unfortunately, different definitions are used by radiologists (201), and this may lead to unnecessary confusion.

Although there is little controversy that the current AJCC/UICC system is superior to the past systems, assessment for continual suitability with changing investigation and treatment methods is needed. A recent study by the Hong Kong Nasopharyngeal Cancer Study Group (HKNPCSG) of 2,687 patients staged by CT and/or MRI during 1996–2000 (112) supports that the current system is overall a good system with fairly even distribution and accurate prognostication for all major end points. However, modifications by down-staging of T2a to T1, N3a to N2, and subgroup T2N0 to stage I, could result in more orderly increase in the hazard ratio (HR) of cancer-specific deaths (from 1 for stage I to 1.98 for II, 3.5 for III, 6.08 for IVA, and 8.62 for IVB), and better hazard consistency among subgroups of the same stage.

Retrospective application of these suggested criteria to 677 patients by Low et al. (153) from Singapore showed similar improvements. Further validation of this proposal with series

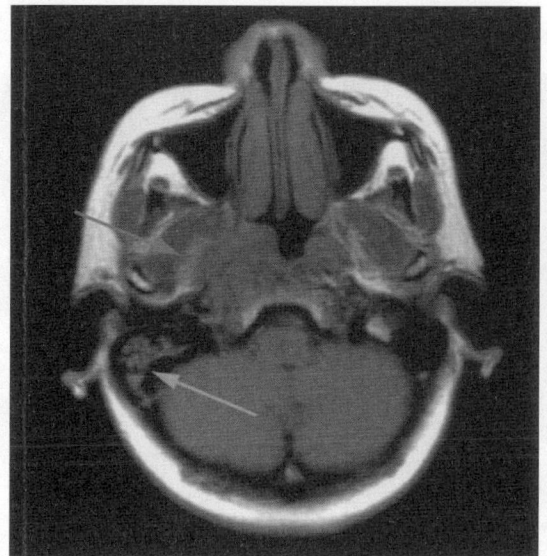
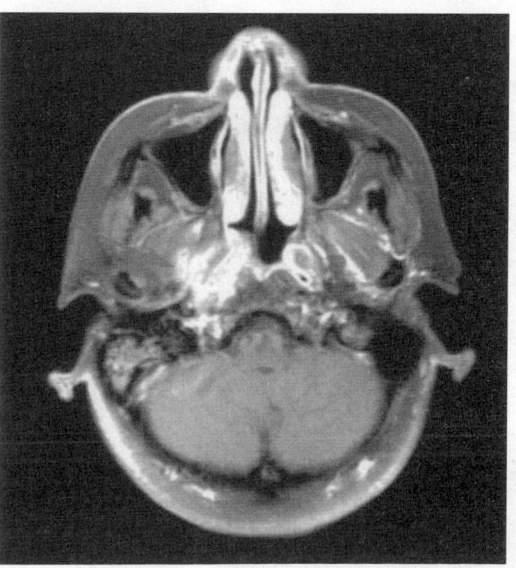

FIGURE 38.7. A: Axial T1-weighted magnetic resonance image (MRI) showing tumor infiltration of the right parapharyngeal space *(red arrow)*. Note the resultant serous otitis media *(blue arrow)*. **B**: Axial contrast-enhanced MRI showing enhanced tumor involving the parapharyngeal space and medial pterygoid muscles *(red arrow)*.

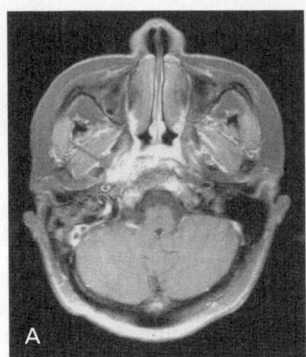 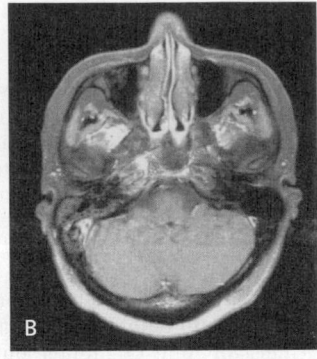 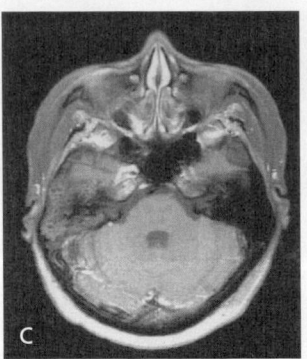 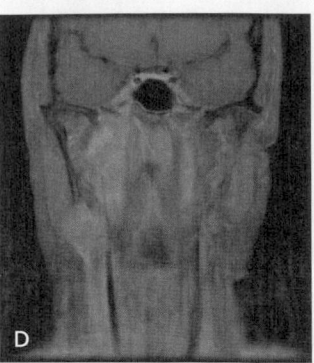

FIGURE 38.8. A: Axial contrast-enhanced magnetic resonance image (MRI) showing tumor in the right fossa of Rosenmüller *(arrow).* **B:** Axial contrast-enhanced MRI showing tumor invading the foramen lacerum *(arrow).* **C:** Axial contrast-enhanced MRI showing tumor encasing the intracranial internal carotid artery *(arrow).* **D:** Coronal contrast-enhanced MRI showing tumor invading the right foramen lacerum with encasement of the carotid artery *(arrow).*

staged by MRI and data from nonendemic countries are needed before universal recommendations can be made.

Pathologic Classification

Most malignant tumors arising in the nasopharynx are carcinoma, which is divided into three types (Fig. 38.13) according to the World Health Organization Classification, 2005 edition (15). Keratinizing squamous cell carcinoma (type 1) is characterized by the formation of keratin pearls or intracellular keratin.

Nonkeratinizing carcinoma (type 2), characterized by total absence of keratin formation, is further subdivided into differentiated (type 2.1) and undifferentiated subtypes (type 2.2). Although still widely quoted in the literature, the use of the numerical designation of types I, II, and III according to the original 1978 edition should be replaced by the current system. Lymphoepithelioma is considered as a morphologic variant of undifferentiated carcinoma. The third type of NPC is basaloid squamous cell carcinoma, which consists of closely packed small tumor cells forming a lobular and sometimes pallisading pattern, with focal squamous carcinoma components. This type is very rare; the frequency is less than 0.2% (15).

There are marked differences in histologic pattern among different ethnic groups (Table 38.8). The frequency of nonkeratinizing carcinoma ranged from 99% in Hong Kong to 75% in the United States (15). Pure nasopharyngeal carcinoma *in situ* is an extremely rare entity. Two of the three cases described by Pak et al. (179) transformed into invasive NPC in 40 to 48 months.

Other malignant tumors of the nasopharynx include nasopharyngeal papillary adenocarcinoma, plasmacytoma, minor salivary gland tumors, melanoma, rhabdomyosarcoma, and chordoma. The majority of lymphoma of the nasopharynx is non-Hodgkin's lymphoma, diffuse large B cell type.

Prognostic Factors

The extent of local infiltration and lymphatic extension, as reflected by the TNM staging, is the most important prognostic factor. In general, advanced T-category is associated with worse local control and survival; advanced N-category is associated with increased risk of distant failure and worse survival. The patterns of failure and survival rate for different stages are summarized in the section Results of Treatment.

The significance of parapharyngeal extension is controversial. The study by Chua et al. (45) showed that extension to the

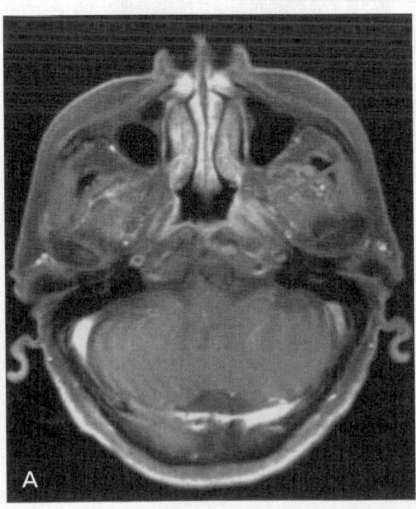 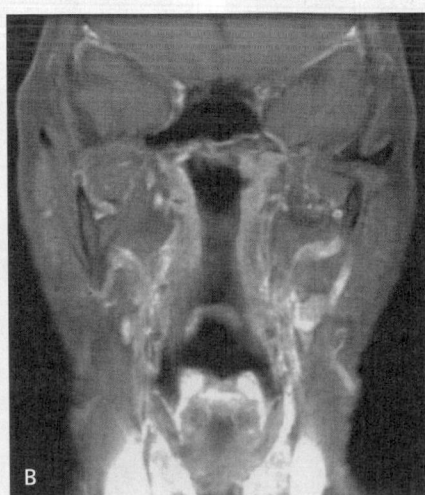 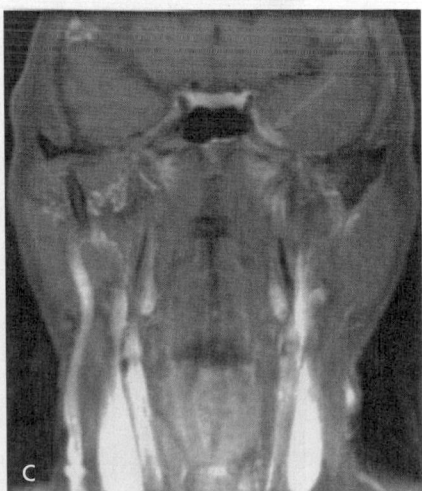

FIGURE 38.9. A: Axial contrast-enhanced magnetic resonance image (MRI) showing a low-volume tumor in the left fossa of Rosenmüller *(arrow).* **B:** Coronal contrast-enhanced MRI showing intracranial tumor extension through the left foramen ovale *(arrow).* **C:** Coronal contrast-enhanced MRI showing tumor involvement of the cavernous sinus *(arrow).*

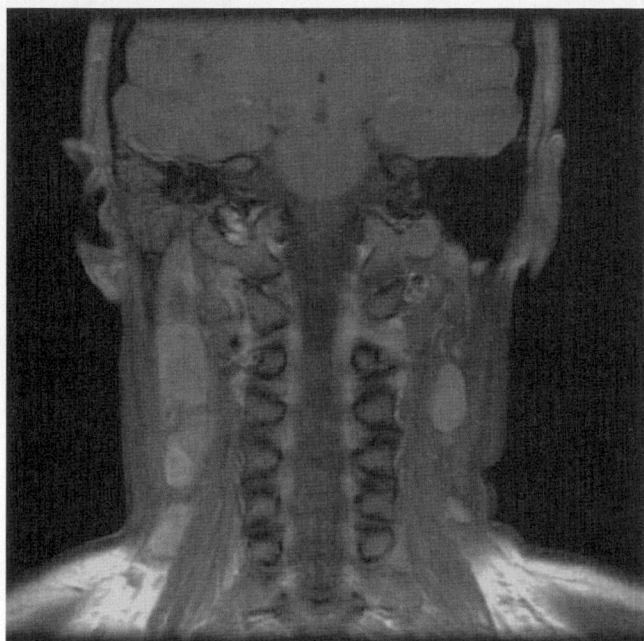

FIGURE 38.10. Coronal contrast-enhanced magnetic resonance image (MRI) showing bilateral cervical lymphadenopathy. There is orderly downward lymphatic spread toward the supraclavicular fossa.

prestyloid space or the anterior portion of the masticator space was associated with lower 5-year local failure-free rate (L-FFR; 72% vs. 86%) and distant failure-free rate (D-FFR; 68% vs. 87%), when compared with those with no or minimal parapharyngeal involvement. Similar findings of significance were reported by other investigators (74,159,194).

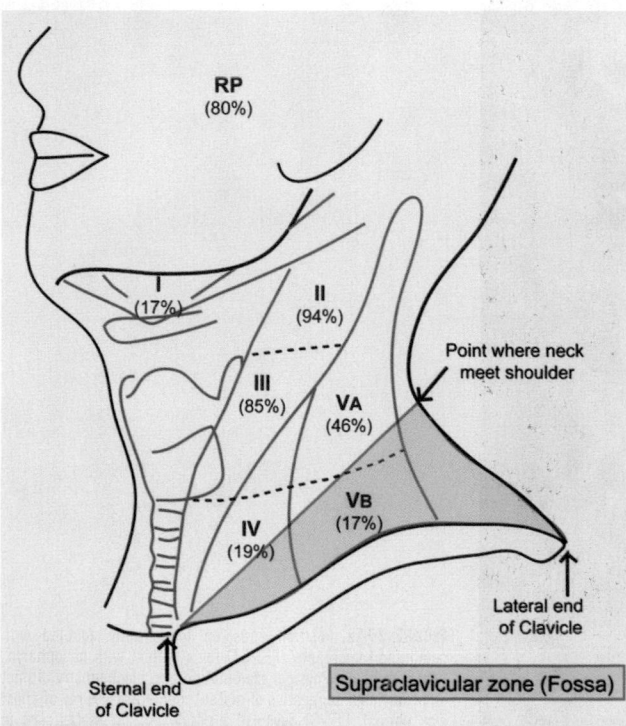

FIGURE 38.11. Distribution of positive nodes at different radiologic levels based on magnetic resonance imaging of 202 patients with nasopharyngeal carcinoma treated at Pamela Youde Nethersole Eastern Hospital (Hong Kong). Note the anatomic boundaries of the supraclavicular fossa as defined by the AJCC/UICC staging system.

	Table 38.4	SYMPTOMS AND PHYSICAL SIGNS OF NASOPHARYNGEAL CARCINOMA AT PRESENTATION	
Symptom/Sign		Chao and Perez[a] (N = 164) (%)	Lee et al.[b] (N = 4,768) (%)
Neck mass		66	76
Nasal (discharge, bleeding, obstruction)		>37	73
Aural (tinnitus, hearing loss, pain, discharge)		41	62
Headache		40	35
Cranial nerve palsy		23	20
Neurologic symptoms			
Ophthalmic (diplopia, squint)			11
Facial numbness			8
Slurring of speech			2
Sore throat		16	
Weight loss			7
Trismus			3
Distant metastases			3
Dermatomyositis			1

[a]Chao KS, Perez CA. Nasopharynx. *Principles and Practice of Radiation Oncology, 4th ed.* Philadelphia: Lippincott Williams & Wilkins, 1997:918–961.
[b]Lee AWM, Foo W, Law SC, et al. Nasopharyngeal carcinoma: Presenting symptoms and duration before diagnosis. *Hong Kong Med J* 1997;3:355–361.

However, Teo et al. (210), who first reported on possible significance of parapharyngeal extension, did not find any significant impact in a subsequent study of 903 patients (213). The study by Au et al. (4) of 1,294 patients, using the AJCC/UICC definition of extension beyond the pharyngobasilar fascia, also showed that parapharyngeal extension was not a significant factor on multivariate analysis. These differences might be related to the various definitions of parapharyngeal space used by different authors, suboptimal detection by CT, and mixing with retropharyngeal node metastases.

Although there is significant overall correlation between T-category and the gross volume of the primary tumor (GTV-P), there is considerable variability in tumor volume within the same stage (23,38,46,205) (Fig. 38.14). There is increasing evidence that tumor volume is an independent significant

	Table 38.5	INCIDENCE OF CRANIAL NERVE INVOLVEMENT AT DIAGNOSIS OF NASOPHARYNGEAL CARCINOMA	
Cranial Nerve		Chao and Perez[a] (N = 164) (%)	Lee et al.[b] (N = 722) (%)
I		—	—
II		1.3	0.8
III		3.5	1.3
IV		2.4	0.6
V		7.8	V_1, 3.5; V_2, 5.8%; V_3, 3.9
VI		13.3	5.1
VII		3.6	0.1
VIII		4.8	—
IX–XII		IX, 2; X, 5.4; XI, 1.3; XII, 4.8	2.4

[a]Chao KS, Perez CA. Nasopharynx. *Principles and Practice of Radiation Oncology, 4th ed.* Philadelphia: Lippincott Williams & Wilkins, 1997:918–961.
[b]Chan J, Bray F, McCarron P, et al. Nasopharyngeal carcinoma. In: *Pathology and Genetics of Head and Neck Tumors. World Health Classfication of Tumors.* IARC Press, Lyon, France, 2005:85–97.

Table 38.6	DIAGNOSTIC AND STAGING WORK-UP FOR NASOPHARYNGEAL CARCINOMA

General
Medical history
Physical examination:
Palpation of neck node (record size, laterality and lowest extent of enlarged nodes)
Testing of cranial nerve (including assessment of vision and hearing functions)
Exclusion of gross signs of distant metastases

Endoscopic examination
Nasopharyngoscopy and biopsies
± Panendoscopy

Otologic assessment
Inspection of tympanic membranes (as clinically indicated)
Baseline audiologic testing (preferable)

Laboratory studies
Complete blood picture
Liver function studies
± Baseline hormonal profile

Radiographic studies

Assessment of locoregional extent
Magnetic resonance imaging (study of choice)
Computed tomography (acceptable alternative)

Chest radiograph

Additional metastatic work-up if clinically indicated or N3 disease
Positron-emission tomography (study of choice)
Computed tomography of thorax and upper abdomen, or ultrasound of liver, and bone scan (acceptable alternative)

factor that can give better prediction of prognosis than T-category by the system of Ho (46) or AJCC/UICC fifth edition (23, 205).

In 308 patients staged with MRI, Sze et al. (205) showed that patients with GTV-P <15 mL had significantly higher L-FFR than those ≥15 mL (97% vs. 82% at 3 years; p <.01). Multivariate analysis showed that GTV-P was a strongly significant factor independent of T-category by AJCC/UICC fifth edition; the risk of local failure increased by 1% for every 1 mL increase in volume. With increasing ease of calculation by computer software, further refinement of prognostication by incorporation of tumor volume as a staging criterion should be explored.

Although some series have not found age and gender to be of prognostic significance for NPC, most have reported significantly better prognosis for female and younger patients. Perez et al. (182) reported a 5-year survival rate of 45% in patients younger than 50 years of age in contrast with ≤27% in older patients. The study by Sham and Choy (193) also showed a higher 5-year survival rate in those younger than 40 years compared with older patients (50% vs. 40%), and female compared with male patients (45% vs. 28%). The study by Au et al. (4) similarly showed poorer survival in male patients (HR = 1.28) and patients older than 50 years (HR = 1.79).

Data on the prognostic significance of histologic types is difficult to interpret. Studies on Chinese patients showed no prognostic difference between the different histologic types (13), but histologies other than nonkeratinizing carcinoma were distinctly uncommon. Many studies from nonendemic regions showed that patients with keratinizing squamous cell carcinoma had a worse prognosis than those with nonkeratinizing carcinoma (66,88,163), but others did not find histology to be an independent prognostic factor (183). A study by Corry et al.

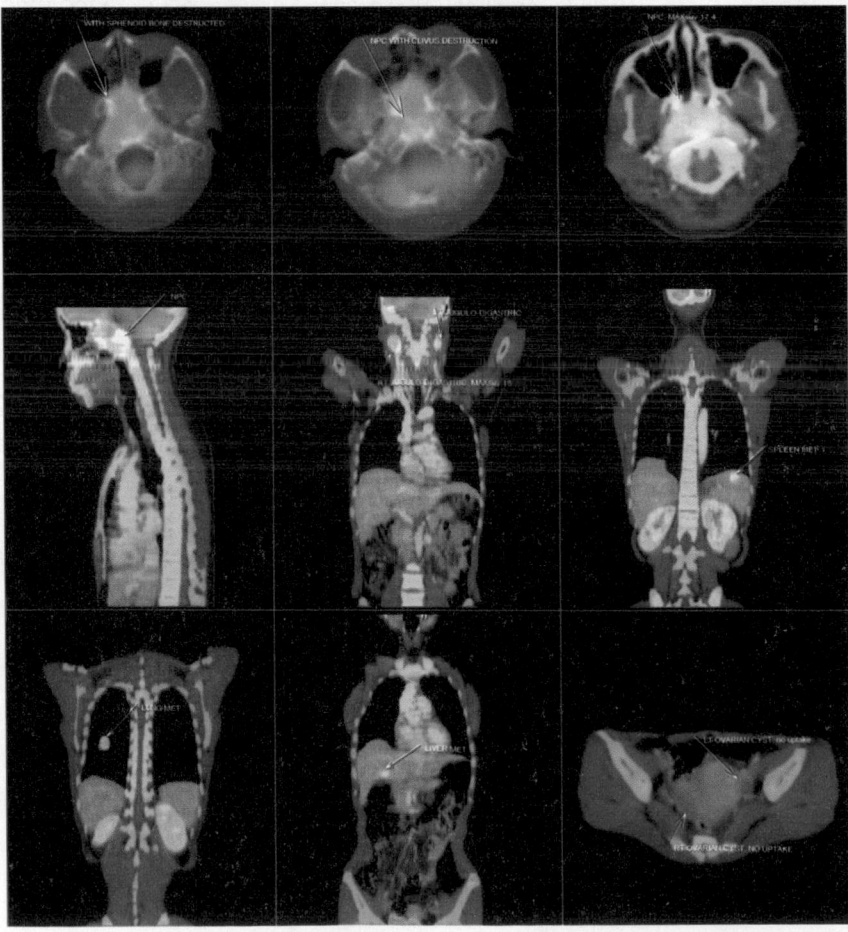

FIGURE 38.12. Positron emission tomography coupled with computed tomography (PET-CT) for a patient with nasopharyngeal carcinoma. Physical examination and biochemistry did not show any sign suggestive of distant metastases. X-ray of chest was normal. PET-CT revealed multiple distant metastases in lung, liver, and spleen, in addition to extensive local infiltration and bilateral cervical lymph nodes. (From Chan J, Bray F, McCarron P, et al. Nasopharyngeal carcinoma. In: *Pathology and genetics of head and neck tumours*. World Health Organization Classification of Tumours. Lyon, France: IARC Press; 2005.)

Clinical Radiation Oncology

| Table 38.7 | THE AMERICAN JOINT COMMITTEE ON CANCER AND INTERNATIONAL UNION AGAINST CANCER STAGING SYSTEM |

Stage	Staging Criteria		
T-category			
TX	Primary tumor cannot be assessed		
T0	No evidence of primary tumor		
Tis	Carcinoma *in situ*		
T1	Tumor confined to the nasopharynx		
T2	Tumor extends to adjacent soft tissues: Nasal cavity,[a] oropharynx[b]		
	T2 a. Tumor without parapharyngeal extension[c]		
	T2b. Tumor with parapharyngeal extension		
T3	Tumor involves bony structures and/or paranasal sinuses		
T4	Tumor with intracranial extension, involvement of cranial nerves, hypopharynx, orbit, infratemporal fossa,[d] or masticator space[d]		
N-category			
NX	Regional lymph nodes cannot be assessed		
N0	No regional lymph node metastasis		
N1	Unilateral metastasis in lymph node(s), $\leq$6 cm in greatest dimension, above the supraclavicular fossa		
N2	Bilateral metastasis in lymph node(s), $\leq$6 cm in greatest dimension, above the supraclavicular fossa		
N3	Metastasis in lymph node(s)		
	N3 a. >6 cm in dimension		
	N3b. Extension to the supraclavicular fossa[e]		
M-category			
MX	Distant metastasis cannot be assessed		
M0	No distant metastasis		
M1	Distant metastasis		
Stage grouping			
0	Tis	N0	M0
I	T1	N0	M0
IIA	T2a	N0	M0
IIB	T1	N1	M0
	T2a	N1	M0
	T2b	N0	M0
	T2b	N1	M0
III	T1	N2	M0
	T2a	N2	M0
	T2b	N2	M0
	T3	N0	M0
	T3	N1	M0
	T3	N2	M0
Stage IVA	T4	N0	M0
	T4	N1	M0
	T4	N2	M0
Stage IVB	Any T	N3	M0
Stage IVC	Any T	Any N	M1

[a]Nasal cavity: Anterior extension beyond the posterior margins of the choanal orifices.
[b]Oropharynx: Inferior extension beyond the level of the free border of the soft palate. The junction at C1/C2 level is recommended as a more consistent radiologic landmark (37).
[c]Parapharyngeal extension: Posterolateral infiltration beyond the pharyngobasilar fascia.
[d]Masticator space and infratemporal fossa: Extension beyond the anterior surface of the lateral pterygoid muscle, or lateral extension beyond the posterolateral wall of the maxillary antrum, and the pterygomaxillary fissure.
[e]Supraclavicular fossa: Triangular region defined by the superior margin of the sternal end of the clavicle, the superior margin of the lateral end of the clavicle, and the point where the neck meets the shoulder.
From Greene F, Page D, Fleming I, eds. *AJCC cancer staging manual*, 6th ed. New York: Springer-Verlag; 2002; and Sobin L. International Union Against Cancer (UICC): *TNM classification of malignant tumours*, 6th ed. New York: Wiley-Liss; 2002.

(52) showed that within nonkeratinizing carcinoma, there is no prognostic difference between ethnic Asian and non-Asian patients.

Preliminary data suggest that circulating cell-free DNA of EBV is a useful prognostic marker. Studies by Lo et al. (152) and Lin et al. (148) showed that high pretreatment titers were associated with advanced stages and poor prognosis. A study focused on patients with stage I-II NPC by Leung et al. (138) showed that pretreatment plasma EBV-DNA concentration >4000 copies/mL was associated with a higher risk of dis-

tant failure. If confirmed, this will be useful for tailoring appropriate treatment for high-risk patients.

However, a report by Le et al. (110) showed no correlation between pretreatment EBV-DNA levels and survival, whereas the posttreatment titers were strongly significant predictor of outcome. The 2-year OS for patients with undetectable posttreatment EBV-DNA was significantly higher than for those having detectable titer: 94% versus 55% ($p = .002$).

The prognostic significance of posttreatment titers was also reported by Lo et al. (150) and Chan et al. (12). In a study of

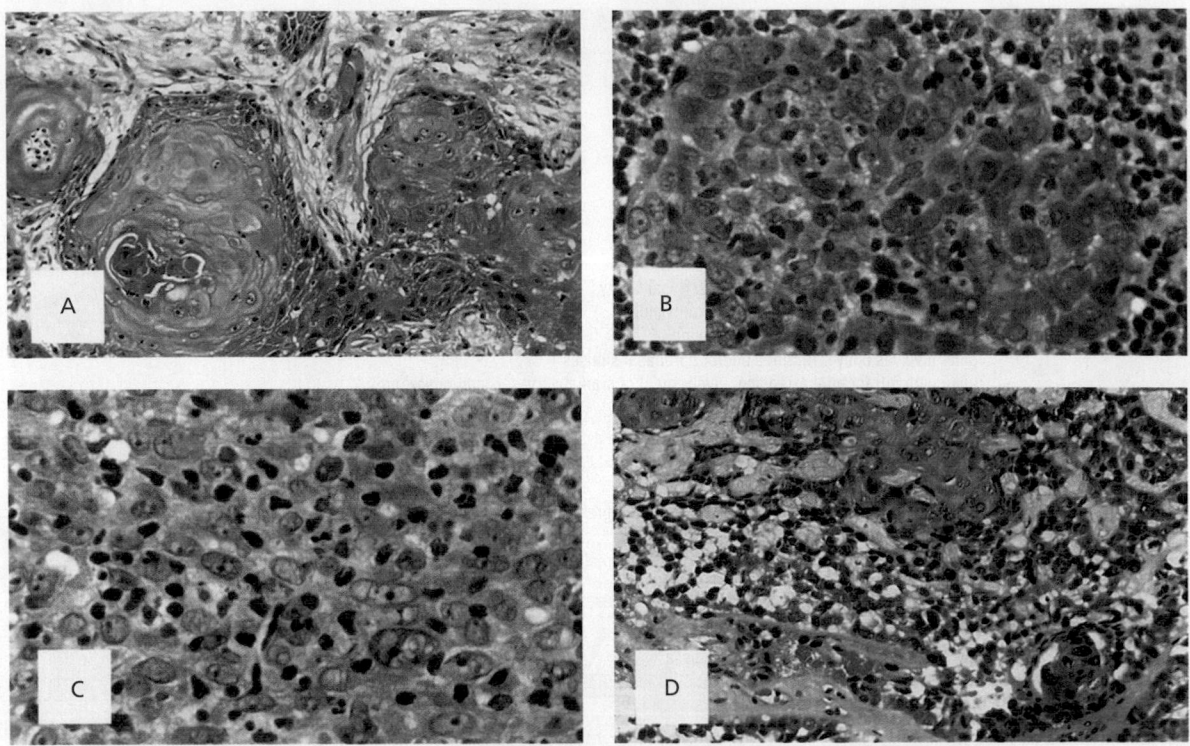

FIGURE 38.13. Photomicrographs of nasopharyngeal carcinoma. **A:** Keratinizing squamous cell carcinoma. **B:** Nonkeratinizing carcinoma, differentiated subtype. **C:** Nonkeratinizing carcinoma, undifferentiated subtype. **D:** Basaloid squamous cell carcinoma. (From Chan J, Bray F, McCarron P, et al. Nasopharyngeal carcinoma. In: *Pathology and genetics of head and neck tumours*. World Health Organization Classification of Tumours. Lyon, France: IARC Press; 2005.)

31 patients treated with induction chemotherapy followed by concurrent chemoradiotherapy, Chan et al. (12) showed that all patients who remained disease-free had plasma EBV-DNA ≤500 copies/mL, whereas 8 of 9 patients with treatment failure had titer increased to >500 copies/mL 2 to 16 months before clinical evidence of disease progression. More clinical data are awaited to determine the consistency and reliability of this test before recommendation for routine use.

Similar to other head and neck squamous cell carcinomas, epidermal growth factor receptor (EGFR) expression is common in NPC. Chua et al. (41) found expression of EGFR in 89% of NPC patients, and showed that overexpression was associated with a significantly poorer treatment outcome: The 5-year disease-specific survival for those with EGFR extent ≥25% was 48%

compared to 86% for those with extent <25%. Ma et al. (158) studied several biomarkers (including p53, HER2, Ki67 antigen, microvessel density, and EGFR) in 78 patients, and showed that EGFR expression only was an independent prognostic factor.

The study by Hui et al. (78) showed that 58% of NPC patients had expression of hypoxia-inducible factor 1α and 57% had carbonic anhydrase IX; those with high expression of both markers had a worse progression-free survival.

Other biologic factors that might have prognostic significance include E-cadherin and β-catenin (248), tumor proliferative fractions or aneuploid status (242), c-erbB2 (191), p53 (164), nm23-HI (72), interleukin-10 (65), and vascular endothelial growth factor (187). However, clinical data are still scanty, and further validation is needed.

Table 38.8   **FREQUENCY OF DIFFERENT HISTOLOGIC SUBTYPES OF NASOPHARYNGEAL CARCINOMA**

	High Incidence Population (%)	Intermediate Population (%)	Low Incidence Population (%)
	Hong Kong	Singapore	Tunisia
Squamous cell carcinoma	1	17	8
Nonkeratinizing carcinoma	99	83	82
Undifferentiated	(92)	(42)	(76)
Differentiated	(7)	(41)	(16)
Basaloid-squamous carcinoma	<0.2	NA	NA

NA, not available.
Modified from Chan J, Bray F, McCarron P, et al. Nasopharyngeal carcinoma. In: *Pathology and Genetics of Head and Neck Tumours*. World Health Organization Classification of Tumours, Lyon, France: IARC Press; 2005, with permission.

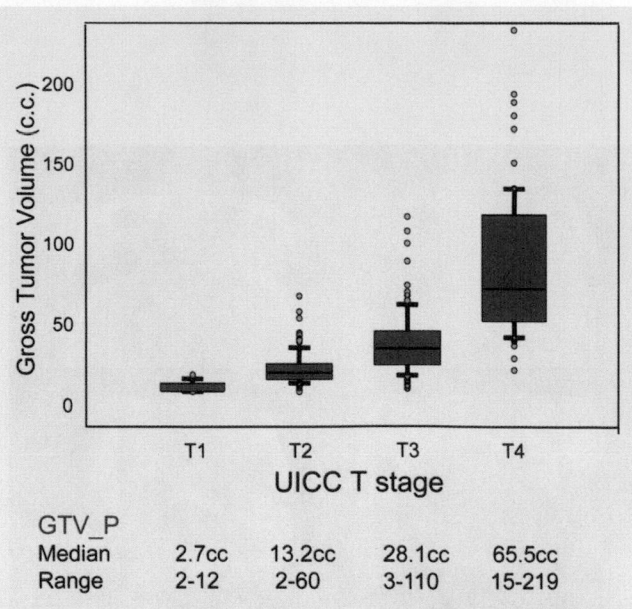

FIGURE 38.14. The correlation between T-category and gross volume of primary tumor (GTV-P). UICC, International Union Against Cancer. (Modified from Sze W, Lee A, Yau T, et al. Primary tumor volume of nasopharyngeal carcinoma: Prognostic significance for local control. *Int J Radiat Oncol Biol Phys* 2004;59:21–27.)

Treatment Strategy

Because of the deep-seated location of the nasopharynx and the anatomic proximity to critical structures, radical surgical resection is very difficult. The role of surgery is limited to biopsy for histologic confirmation and salvage of persistent or recurrent disease.

Treatment strategy should be tailored to the specific pattern of failure for different risk groups. Historically, megavoltage radiation therapy (RT) has been the mainstay of treatment. Although excellent results have been achieved with early stages disease, the results are less satisfactory for advanced diseases. Numerous trials have studied the therapeutic gain by adding chemotherapy at different sequences. The current data essentially show that concurrent chemotherapy is the only sequence of combination with significant survival benefit.

Hence, the current recommendation is to treat patients with stage I-II disease with RT alone, and those with stage III-IVB (± bulky IIB) disease with concurrent chemoradiotherapy (CRT). Whether induction or adjuvant chemotherapy adds further benefit to concurrent CRT remains to be demonstrated.

Radiation Therapy

To achieve the best therapeutic ratio, every single step in the RT procedures (immobilization, localization of gross tumor and target volumes, optimization of dose fractionation, determination of treatment techniques, and precision in RT delivery) is important.

Treatment Preparation

All patients should have dental evaluation and dietitian consultation prior to commencement of RT. Patients should be advised to abstain from smoking and drinking alcohol. The patient is set up in a supine position with head extended. A customized thermoplastic mask covering the head to shoulder region is made to immobilize the patient (Fig. 38.15).

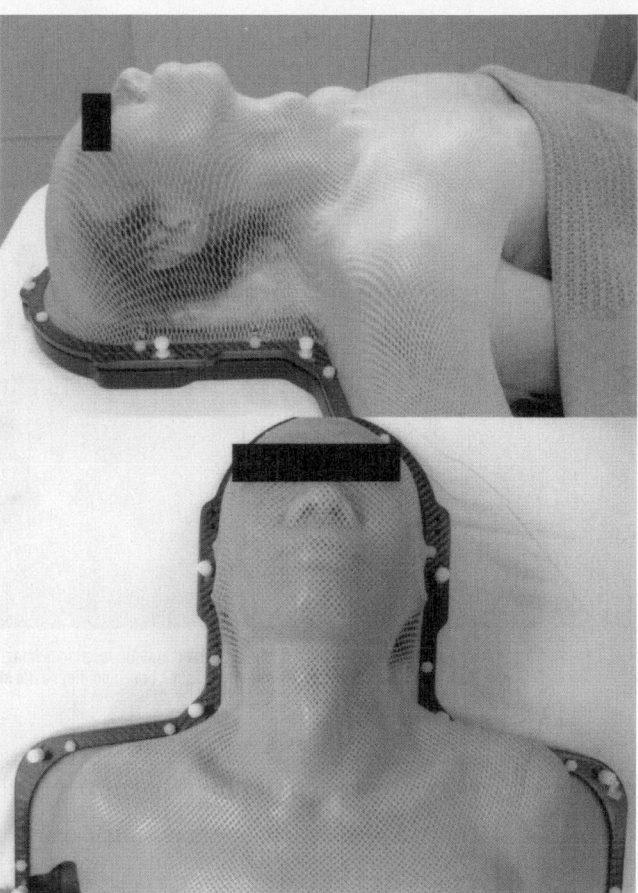

FIGURE 38.15. Immobilization of patient in a customized thermoplastic mask covering the whole head-to-shoulder region.

Computerized planning for intensity-modulated radiotherapy (IMRT) is recommended as far as resources allow. Planning CT covering from skull vertex to 2 cm below clavicles, with 3-mm slice thickness at gross tumor regions, is performed. Fusion of diagnostic MRI with planning CT is useful for more accurate delineation of tumor targets and critical structures (56) (Fig. 38.16).

For patients to be treated by conventional two-dimensional (2D) technique, mouth bite is useful to minimize the dose to the oral cavity and enlarged neck nodes are marked with wire before taking simulation films.

Dose, Time, and Fractionation

The majority of retrospective studies, based on patients irradiated with 2D techniques, have shown a significant dose-response. Both Marks et al. (162) and Vikram et al. (217) showed that local tumor control was significantly improved in patients who received >67 Gy to the tumor target. Perez et al. (183) reported that for patients with T1-2 tumors, the local tumor control rate was 100% for those given >70 Gy, compared with 80% for those given 66 to 70 Gy. However, local control for patients with T3-4 tumors did not rise above 55%, even with total dose >70 Gy. Similar findings were reported by Mesic et al. (165); better local control for T1-2 tumors was achieved with ≥70 Gy when compared with 60 Gy (94% vs. 76%), but no significant impact of higher doses or larger fields was noted in T3-4 tumors. These observations suggest that, in addition to consideration of prescribed dose, the problem of adequate coverage has to be overcome for advanced tumors.

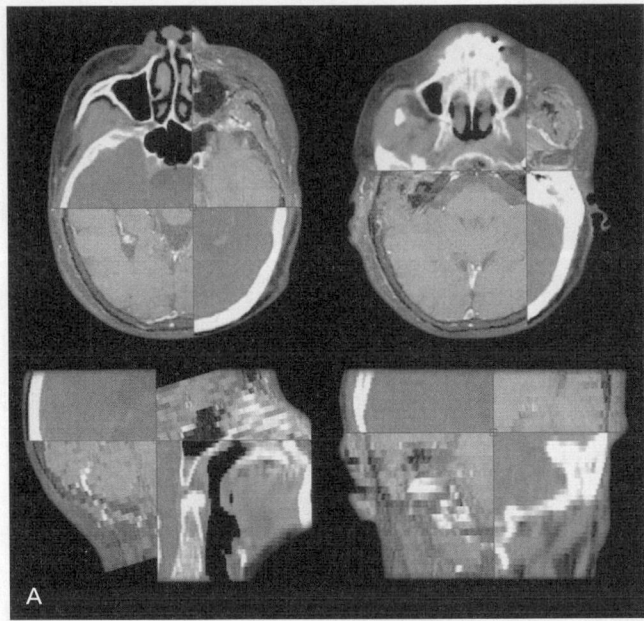

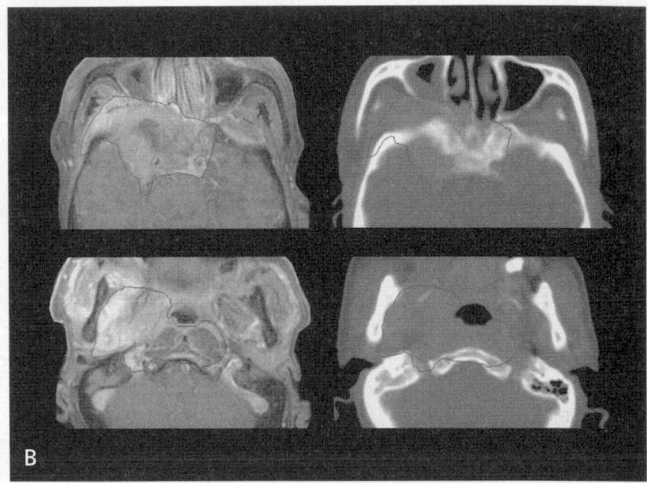

FIGURE 38.16. A: Fusion of diagnostic magnetic resonance imaging (MRI) and planning computed tomography (CT) for computerized planning. **B:** Delineation of gross tumor volume based on diagnostic MRI (left) transferred to planning CT (right) for more accurate localization.

A study by Lee et al. (113) of 1,008 patients with T1 tumors irradiated by four different fractionation schedules showed that total dose was the most important radiation factor ($p = .01$). The hazard of local failure decreased by 8% per additional Gy. Fractional dose did not affect local control, but it was a significant risk factor for temporal lobe necrosis (115,123). Dose per fraction >2 Gy should be avoided (see section Sequelae of Treatment).

The impact of the time factor is more controversial. A randomized study by Marcial et al. (161) in which 62 patients were treated with split-course irradiation (30 Gy in 10 fractions in 2 weeks, a 3-week rest period, and then another 30 Gy in 10 fractions) and 59 patients with 66 Gy in 33 fractions in 6.5 to 7 weeks, showed no significant difference in 5-year local control (86% vs. 80%), nodal control (86% vs. 78%), or disease-free survival (40% vs. 30%).

However, Vikram et al. (217) observed that local tumor control in patients with interruption of RT for ≥21 days was significantly poorer than those without interruptions (34% vs. 67%). A study by Luo et al. (157) of 1,446 patients also showed similar findings for patients with advanced disease. Kwong et al. (99), in a study of 1,301 patients with T1-4 tumors, supported the significance of the time factor with the hazard of local failure increasing by 3% per additional day of prolongation. The general consensus is that prolongation is likely to be detrimental, even for nonkeratinizing NPC, but whether modest acceleration can achieve significant benefit has yet to be confirmed.

Hence, the prescription generally recommended for NPC is a total dose of about 70 Gy during 7 weeks to the gross tumor, and 50 to 60 Gy for elective treatment of potential risk sites.

Tumor Target Volumes

The GTV includes the primary nasopharyngeal tumor and involved lymph nodes as shown by clinical, endoscopic, and radiologic examinations. For patients given induction chemotherapy, it is recommended that the targets be based on the prechemotherapy extent.

Elective irradiation of bilateral cervical lymphatics is recommended in N0 patients. A study by Lee et al. (129) of patients with clinically negative findings in necks showed that patients with elective neck irradiation had significantly lower nodal re-

lapse rate than those untreated (40% vs. 11%). Furthermore, despite successful salvage by subsequent treatment, patients with nodal relapse had a significantly higher incidence of distant metastases than those without relapse (21% vs. 6%).

The clinical target volume (CTV) covers the GTV, microscopic infiltration and anatomic structures at risk. Different centers may have different philosophies in defining the margins and dose level. For example, Table 38.9 shows the delineation criteria for different CTV currently used at Pamela Youde Nethersole Eastern Hospital. The CTV aimed at 70 Gy (CTV_70) includes the GTV with a 5 to 10 mm margin (if possible) and the whole nasopharynx. The CTV aimed at 60 Gy (CTV_60) covers high-risk local structures (including the parapharyngeal spaces, posterior third of nasal cavities and maxillary sinuses, pterygoid processes, base of skull, lower half of sphenoid sinus, anterior half of the clivus, and petrous tips), and lymphatic regions (including bilateral retropharyngeal nodes, levels II, III and V_A). The CTV aimed at 50 Gy (CTV_50) covers the remaining levels IV to V_B. The level I nodes can be spared for patients with N0 disease.

The planning target volume (PTV) covers the CTV and the margin needed for systemic and random setup variations. Different centers should gauge the range of variations in their actual practice for determining this margin. With proper immobilization and meticulous care in setup, an expansion margin of 2 mm was used at Pamela Youde Nethersole Eastern Hospital for delineating PTV.

Conventional 2D Treatment Techniques

The classic 2D technique used in Hong Kong is that of Ho (76), which composes two phases. Phase I consists of lateral-opposed facial-cervical fields for the primary tumor and enlarged neck nodes, together with a lower anterior cervical field for the lower cervical lymphatics. Phase II is used after 40 Gy to avoid the spinal cord. This consists of three fields (lateral-opposed plus anterior facial fields) for the nasopharyngeal region and an anterior cervical field for the whole neck. Typical radiologic landmarks and treatment portals are shown in Fig. 38.17. Shrinking field arrangement with cone-down after 50 to 60 Gy should be made whenever possible to maximize protection of critical structures.

	Table 38.9	**EXAMPLE OF GUIDELINE ON ANATOMIC STRUCTURES/BOUNDARIES FOR DELINEATING CLINICAL TARGET VOLUMES (CTV) FOR INTENSITY-MODULATED RADIATION THERAPY**[a]

	Delineation of CTV	
CTV	**Structures**	**Anatomic Boundaries**
CTV_70	• GTV + 5–10 mm margin (2 mm if abut neurological structures)	
	• Whole nasopharynx	5–10 mm from mucosal surface of nasopharynx Anterior: Junction with nasal choana Lateral: Medial border of parapharyngeal space Caudal: Caudal border of C1 vertebra
CTV_61.25	• CTV_70 + 5 mm margin (2 mm if abut neurologic or bony structures)	
	• Posterior nasal cavity	Anterior: Posterior third of nasal cavity
	• Posterior maxillary sinuses	Anterior: Posterior third of maxillary sinuses
	• Pterygoid fossae	
	• Parapharyngeal spaces	Lateral: Lateral border of styloid processes
	• Lower sphenoid sinus	Cranial: Lower half of sphenoid sinus
	• Base of skull	Posterior: Anterior half of clivus if no gross invasion, whole clivus if invasion detected Lateral: Lateral border of foramen ovale
	• Elective nodal levels	All: Bilateral retropharyngeal, level II, III, V$_A$ If node-positive: Add level I$_B$ Caudal: 15 mm below CTV_70 for enlarged node
CTV_52.5	• Upper sphenoid sinus (if sphenoid involved)	Part of sphenoid sinus at and above the level of optic chiasma
	• Elective nodal levels	Bilateral levels IV and V$_B$

GTV, Gross primary tumor and involved lymph nodes.
[a]Based on guideline currently used at Pamela Youde Nethersole Eastern Hospital (Hong Kong).
Planning target value = CTV + 2-mm margin.
Total dose prescription at
PTV_70: 70 Gy in 35 fractions (2 Gy per fraction)
PTV_61.25: 61.25 Gy in 35 fractions (1.75 Gy per fraction)—equivalent to 60 Gy at 2 Gy per fraction.
PTV_52.5: 52.5 Gy in 30 fractions (1.75 per fraction)—equivalent to 50 Gy at 2 Gy per fraction.
Note: Spare ≥3 mm dermal tissues if no skin involvement.

The advantage of the three-field technique in phase II is to minimize the dose to bilateral temporal lobes and temporomandibular joints. However, coverage may be inadequate for tumors with extensive posterolateral extension to the parapharyngeal spaces or caudal extension to oropharynx; supplementary dose via a posterolateral field with avoidance of neurologic structures is given to rectify this deficit (212).

Another 2D technique widely used in other centers is to use lateral-opposed portals throughout. The typical field arrangement used at Mallinckrodt Institute of Radiology (United States) is shown as an example (19) (Fig. 38.18A). Phase I consists of lateral-opposed fields that are angled posteriorly 5 degrees to ensure adequate coverage of the posterior wall of the nasopharynx, while reducing the dose to the contralateral lens and avoiding direct irradiation to the ipsilateral external and middle ear.

The posterior borders of the lateral fields are displaced anteriorly after about 43 Gy to shield the spinal cord. High-energy photons (18 MV) are used in phase II to deliver the last 20 to 25 Gy while diminishing the dose to the mandible and temporomandibular joints. With the shrinking field method, a boost of 5 to 10 Gy is delivered to the nasopharynx through reduced lateral portals for patients with T4 tumors.

The lower neck and supraclavicular fossa are treated with a single anterior field at 2-Gy daily fractions to 50 Gy given dose (Fig. 38.18B). Posterior neck nodes are given a supplementary dose of 5 to 15 Gy with 9-MeV electrons through small lateral fields.

Other options for phase II include arc rotation technique as designed by Wang (219) and the anterior infraorbital oblique fields technique of Fletcher (62).

Three-Dimensional (3D) Conformal Treatment Techniques

Development of computerized 3D treatment plans is an important technical advance for NPC with its typically concave tumor volumes. Several investigators have designed innovative multifield conformal plans; for example, the seven-field technique used at Memorial Sloan-Kettering Cancer Center (United States) (231) and the "Boomerang" technique (Fig. 38.19) used at Peter MacCallum Cancer Institute (Australia) (53). All of the evaluation studies showed better tumor dose coverage while reducing normal tissue dose in comparison with conventional 2D plans (20,95,218).

Leibel et al. (136) from Memorial Sloan-Kettering Cancer Center showed that the target volume underdosed at the 95% isodose level was reduced with 3D plans when compared with 2D plans (7% vs. 22%). With the mean tumor dose increased by an average of 13%, it was estimated that the probability of uncomplicated tumor control would increase by 15%.

However, subsequent analysis of 68 patients for whom this technique was used to deliver a boost of 20 to 26 Gy following phase I conventional 2D treatment for 50 Gy did not show significant improvement; the 5-year L-FFR was 77% and late toxicity grade ≥3 was 25% (231).

More encouraging results were achieved by Jen et al. (85), who retrospectively compared 72 patients treated with 3D conformal technique throughout with 108 patients treated with 2D technique. They reported significant improvement in 3-year L-FFR for T4 (86% vs. 47%), and event-free survival for both stage III (80% vs. 56%) and stage IV (82% vs. 33%). In addition, the

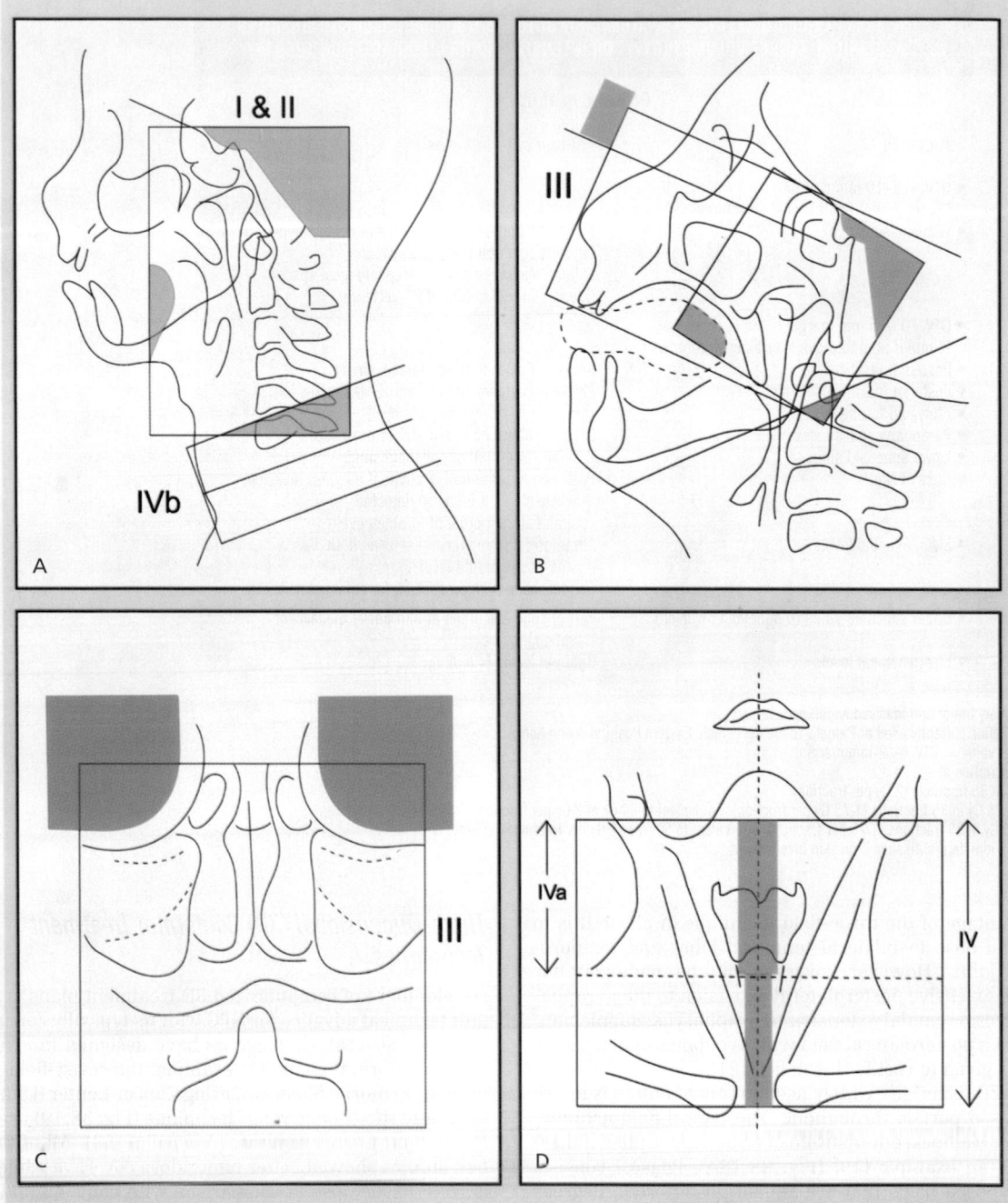

FIGURE 38.17. Conventional two-dimensional radiotherapy using Ho's technique. **A:** Phase I, lateral-opposed faciocervical fields (I–II) and lower anterior cervical field (IVb). **B:** Phase II, sagittal view showing lateral-opposed facial fields and noncoplanar anterior facial field (III). **C:** Coronal view of anterior facial field (III). **D:** Anterior cervical field for whole neck (IV).

incidence of xerostomia at 3 years was significantly reduced, although there were little differences for most other late toxicities.

IMRT Techniques

With the clear advantages of sculpting the high-dose volume with tight dose gradients around the targets, dosimetric studies from different centers all show that IMRT techniques can further improve the conformity of dose distribution for NPC (24,80,89,234). There is little controversy that this technique is advocated for treating NPC if resources permit. With the tight margin now employed, precision in target localization and RT

delivery become even more important; all the precautions in treatment preparation and quality control must be strictly followed.

Another potential of interest is the possibility of biologic enhancement by simultaneous modulated accelerated-radiation therapy (SMART) as a new way of delivering accelerated fractionation (AF) schedule, a concept that was first reported by Butler et al. (9) for the treatment of other head and neck cancers with IMRT.

Various methods and dose fractionation schemes for IMRT are being explored by different investigators; Table 38.10 summarizes the key features and the results achieved. Most of the patients treated in these series also received additional

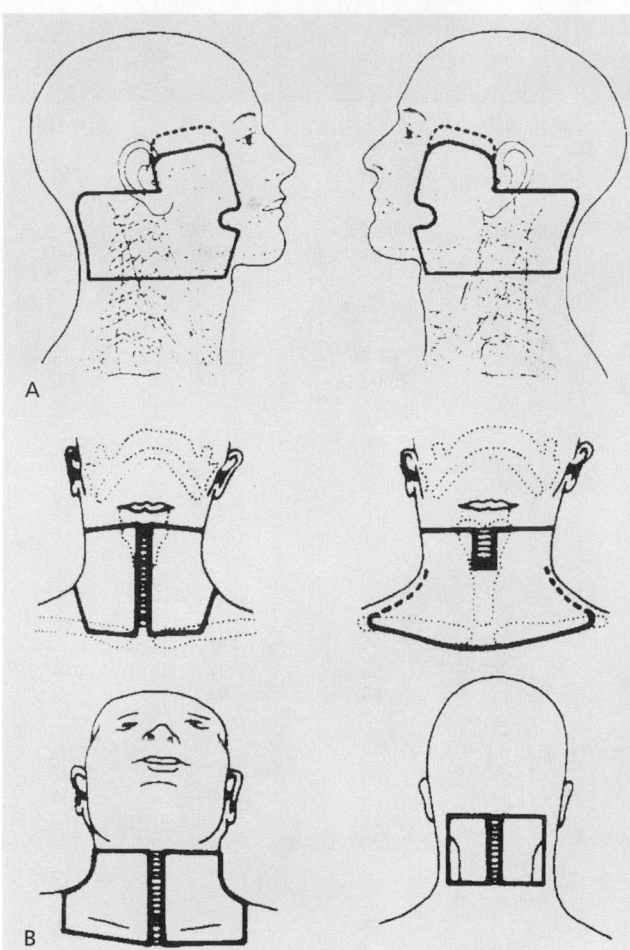

FIGURE 38.18. Conventional two-dimensional technique used at Mallinckrodt Institute of Radiology. **A:** Diagrams of external portals. **B:** Various types of portals used for treatment of the lower neck lymphatics, depending on whether clinically positive nodes are present (larger fields) or only elective irradiation is administered (smaller fields). If electron beam is not available, a posterior portal blocking the midline may be used to treat the posterior cervical lymph nodes with ^{60}Co or 4- to 6-MV photons.

chemotherapy and/or enhanced RT with boosts or AF. All reported most encouraging early results with local control in excess of 90% at 2 to 4 years.

At the University of California, San Francisco, conventional once-daily fraction was used for all patients. A total dose of 70 Gy at 2.12 Gy/fraction was given to the gross tumor, while the CTV (that included both potential microscopic infiltration and margin for setup error) received 60 Gy at 1.8 Gy/fraction, and the neck with clinically negative findings received 54 Gy at 1.65 Gy/fraction (7,135). Updated results of 118 patients by Bucci et al. (7) confirmed excellent locoregional control of 96%. However, distant failure was still high (28%) despite extensive use of concurrent-adjuvant CRT, the OS was 74% at 4 years. One patient died of torrential epistaxis without tumor recurrence was reported by Lee et al. (135).

At Memorial Sloan-Kettering Cancer Center, treatment was delivered with dynamic multileaf collimation, using seven coplanar 6-MV intensity-modulated fields, positioned every 30 degrees from the posterior and lateral directions. Wolden et al. (230) reported their experience on 74 patients: 59 were treated with AF using the concomitant boost method and 15 by the SMART method. For the latter group, a total dose of 70.2 Gy at 2.34 Gy/fraction was given to the gross tumor, and the "microscopic" PTV received 54 Gy at 1.8 Gy/fraction. The 3-year L-FFR was better than for patients treated by 3D conformal boost (91% vs. 79%), although the difference was not statistically significant.

Further dose escalation with SMART boost in 50 patients with T3 to 4 tumors was reported by Kwong et al. (100) from Queen Mary Hospital (Hong Kong). Their goal was to deliver a total dose of 76 Gy at 2.17 Gy/fraction to the gross tumor. Although the early result for locoregional control was excellent (96% at 2 years), there were serious concerns about late toxicities because 4% of patients had life-threatening bleeding from carotid artery pseudoaneurysm, and another 4% developed temporal lobe necrosis at a median follow-up of 2.1 years.

Kam et al. (90) from Prince of Wales Hospital (Hong Kong) prescribed a total dose of only 66 Gy at 2 Gy/fraction to the gross tumor, but supplemented this with an additional boost to 56% of patients. The 3-year L-FFR for their series of 63 patients was 92%; the incidence of xerostomia (grade 2) was only 23% and hearing loss (grade 3) was 13%. However, other serious late toxicities were substantial; 2% developed osteonecrosis of C1 and C2 vertebrae requiring surgical restoration, 3% developed temporal lobe necrosis, and 23% had endocrine dysfunction.

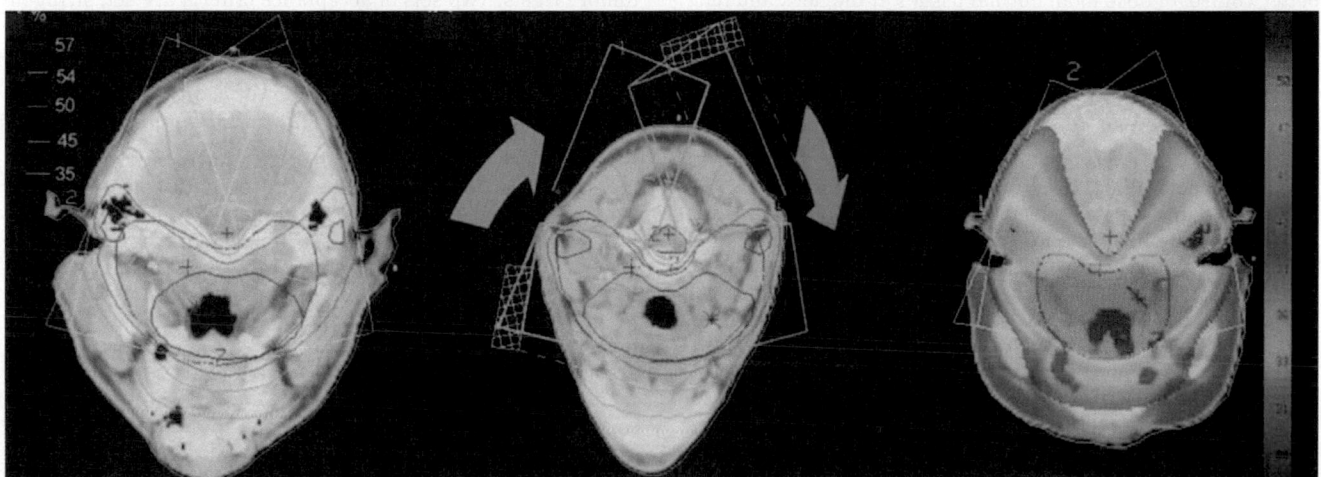

FIGURE 38.19. The three-dimensional conformal technique used at Peter MacCallum Cancer Institute: The "Boomerang" technique. (From Corry J, Hornby C, Fisher R, et al. 'Boomerang' technique: An improved method for conformal treatment of locally advanced nasopharyngeal cancer. *Australas Radiol* 2004;48:170–180, with permission.)

Table 38.10 INTENSITY-MODULATED RADIATION THERAPY FOR NASOPHARYNGEAL CARCINOMA: METHODS AND RESULTS BY DIFFERENT CENTERS

	UCSF (7,135)	MSKCC (230)	PWH (90)	SYS (39)	QMH (97)	QMH (100)
No. of patients	118	74	63	104	50	50
Patient characteristics						
Treatment period	1995–2003	1998–2004	2000–2002	2001–2004	2000–2002	2000–2004
T-category	All	All	All	All	T1–T2	T3–T4
Intensity-modulated RT						
PTV-G						
Margin around GTV (mm)	—	5–10	2	—	—	—
Total dose (Gy)	70	70.2	66	64–70	68–70	76
Dose per fraction (Gy)	2.12	2.34	2	2.33–2.56	2–2.06	2.17
Additional treatment						
Accelerated fractionation	—	80%	—	—	—	—
Boost	22% ICB		32% ICB 24% 3D	—	—	—
Chemotherapy (%)	90	93	30	23	0	68
Median follow-up (mo)	30	35	29	19	14	25
Tumor control						
Time point (y)	4	3	3	3	2	2
Local-FFR (%)	96	91	92	99	100	96
Nodal-FFR (%)	98	93	98	99	94	—
Distant-FFR (%)	72	78	79	88	94	94
Overall survival (%)	74	83	90	86	NR	92
Late toxicities						
Xerostomia (grade ≥2) (%)	2[a] (2 y)	32 (1 y)	23 (2 y)	—	—	—
Deafness (grade >2) (%)	7[a]	>15	15	—	—	42
Fibrosis (grade >2) (%)	—	—	11	—	—	14
Dysphagia (grade >2) (%)	1[a]	—	5	—	—	—
Hypopituitarism (%)	—	0	23	—	—	—
Osteonecrosis (%)	0.8	0	2	—	—	—
Temporal lobe necrosis (%)	0.8	0	3	—	—	4
Carotid pseudoaneurysm/epistaxis (%)	0.8[a]	—	—	—	—	4

UCSF, University of California, San Francisco (United States); MSKCC, Memorial Sloan Kettering Cancer Center (United States); PWH, Prince of Wales Hospital (Hong Kong); SYS, Sun Yat-sen Cancer Center (China); QMH, Queen Mary Hospital (Hong Kong); RT, radiation therapy; PTV-G, planning target volume for gross tumor; GTV, gross tumor volume; ICB, intracavitary brachytherapy; 3D, three-dimensional conformal boost; FFR, failure-free rate; NR, not reported.

[a]Based on data reported by Lee et al. at 2002 (135).

Different centers have to work out what is their best affordable technique. Some centers only treat the primary tumor and upper neck with IMRT, while the lower neck is treated with a matching field. However, to avoid dose uncertainty at the match line due to the potential angles of IMRT beams, and to attain better control of dose to all normal tissues at the neck and lung apex, whole-volume IMRT technique is the preferred option.

Figure 38.20 shows the delineation of targets and the technique with nine coplanar beams (6-MV photon) covering the entire region that is currently used at Pamela Youde Nethersole Eastern Hospital. A total dose of 70 Gy at 2 Gy/fraction was given to the PTV for gross tumor, while the PTV for high-risk structures received 61.25 Gy at 1.75 Gy/fraction and the PTV for low-risk structures received 52.5 Gy also at 1.75 Gy/fraction by reducing the field size for the last five fractions. Instead of using SMART, patients with T3-4 tumors are treated with a moderate AF schedule of 2 Gy/fraction, six daily fractions per week (see section Dose Escalation and Altered Fractionation). Figures 38.21 and 38.22 illustrate the tumor targets and dose-distribution plan for patients with early and advanced disease, respectively.

Skillful specification of dose constraints is important for inverse planning. Different dose constraint templates have been designed (80,235). Overstringent control of normal tissue constraints might result in inadequate coverage of tumor targets; optimal balance is critical. An example of dose-constraint guidelines is provided in Table 38.11, which shows the guidelines cur-

rently used at Pamela Youde Nethersole Eastern Hospital. Top priority is given to critical neurologic structures, followed by tumor targets, organs with intermediate importance, and finally those with lesser importance. Doses to parotids and cochlea are reduced as much as possible, but without sacrificing coverage of tumor targets. Two sets of acceptance criteria are set, stringent ideals are attempted as far as possible, but safe compromise within tolerance will have to be considered for difficult cases.

Dose Escalation and Altered Fractionation

Excellent local tumor control has also been reported by giving additional boost to patients with early disease treated by conventional 2D technique. The most widely used method is brachytherapy. Different types of applicators have been designed for intracavitary brachytherapy and various isotopes have been used for interstitial treatment. Vikram (216) used permanent implantation with iodine-125. Wang (220) used low dose-rate brachytherapy with cesium sources, while most others used high dose-rate with the advent of after-loading equipment (Fig 38.23).

Table 38.12 summarizes reports on the use of brachytherapy as a boost for dose escalation. Most studies demonstrated that local control up to 90% to 95% could be achieved for T1-2 tumors without excessive late damages. The retrospective comparison by Wang (219) from Massachusetts General Hospital (United States) showed that patients given an

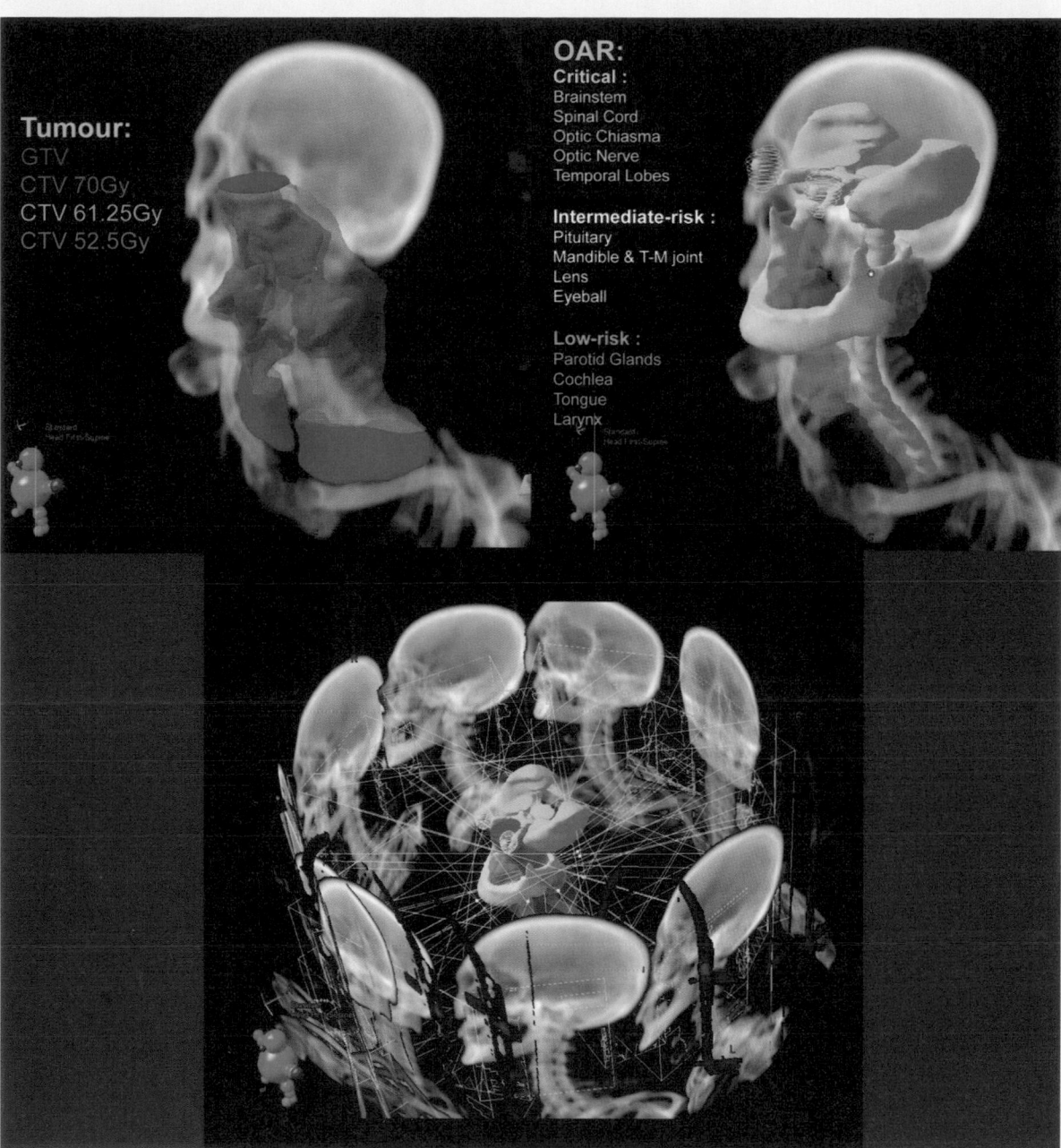

FIGURE 38.20. The intensity-modulated radiation therapy technique used at Pamela Youde Nethersole Eastern Hospital: Nine coplanar beams cover the whole volume of nasopharyngeal and cervical targets.

additional 7 to 10 Gy boost by low dose-rate brachytherapy following 60 to 64 Gy by external beam radiation (EBRT) had significantly higher 5-year L-FFR than those treated by EBRT alone (91% vs. 60%; p <.01). A similar retrospective comparison by Teo et al. (209) showed excellent 5-year L-FFR of 95% in patients given an additional 18 to 24 Gy in three fractions by high dose-rate brachytherapy, but the gain over the group without boost was not statistically significant (95% vs. 90%; p = .17). In addition, the comparison by Ozyar et al. (177) of 106 patients with T1-4 tumors did not show any improvement (86% vs. 94%; p = .23). The exact benefit of dose escalation has yet to be addressed in prospective randomized studies.

One major limitation of brachytherapy is that the dose delivered is adequate only for superficial nonbulky tumors. Furthermore, optimal positioning of the applicators depends both on the individual clinician's skill and the patient's anatomic features. The advent of stereotactic radiosurgery or fractionated

radiotherapy, enabling precise delivery of highly conformal RT with rapid dose falloff (Fig. 38.24), provides a valuable alternative for dose escalation. In the update from Stanford University Medical Center by Le et al. (111), excellent 3-year L-FFR of 100% was achieved in 45 patients with T1-4 tumors given a median SRT boost of 12 Gy following conventional RT to 66 Gy. However, despite the addition of CRT in 80% of the patients, the distant failure rate was 31% and OS was 75%. With a median follow-up of 31 months, 7% of patients developed asymptomatic temporal lobe necrosis, 2% developed retinopathy, and 9% developed cranial nerve paresis. The risk was especially high in patients with T4 tumors; late toxicity is a major concern.

Randomized trials on other head and neck cancers have confirmed that altered fractionation is an effective option for improving local control, but data that are specific for NPC are very scant. Separate evaluation is needed because acceleration may not be able to achieve similarly significant benefit for poorly

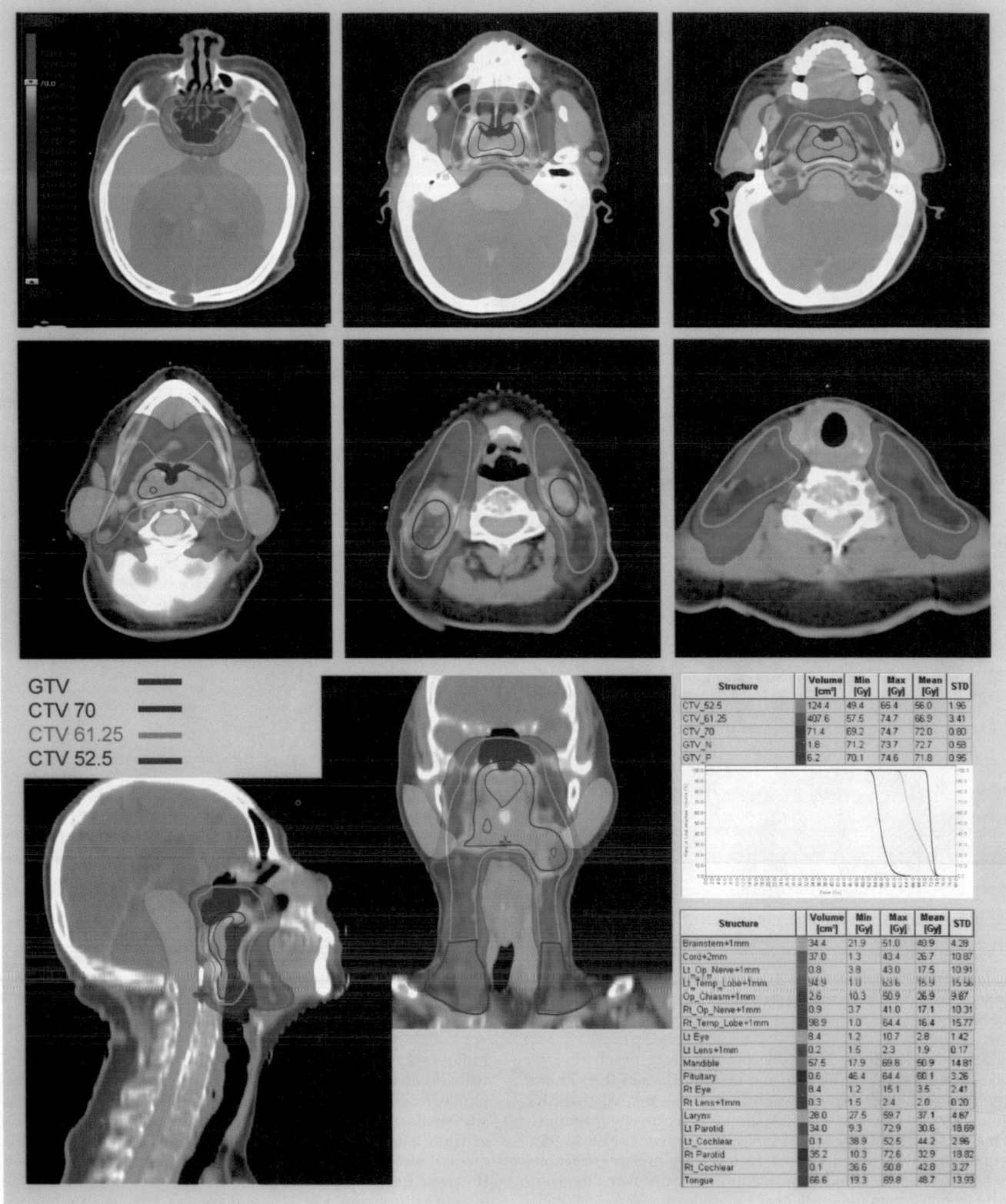

GTV
CTV 70
CTV 61.25
CTV 52.5

Structure	Volume [cm³]	Min [Gy]	Max [Gy]	Mean [Gy]	STD
CTV_52.5	124.4	49.4	65.4	56.0	1.96
CTV_61.25	407.6	57.5	74.7	66.9	3.41
CTV_70	71.4	69.2	74.7	72.0	0.80
GTV_N	1.6	71.2	73.7	72.7	0.58
GTV_P	6.2	70.1	74.6	71.8	0.95

Structure	Volume [cm³]	Min [Gy]	Max [Gy]	Mean [Gy]	STD
Brainstem+1mm	34.4	21.9	51.0	40.9	4.29
Cord+2mm	37.0	1.3	43.4	26.7	10.87
Lt_Op_Nerve+1mm	0.8	3.8	43.0	17.5	10.91
Lt_Temp_Lobe+1mm	94.9	1.0	63.6	16.9	15.56
Op_Chiasm+1mm	2.6	10.3	50.9	26.9	9.87
Rt_Op_Nerve+1mm	0.9	3.7	41.0	17.1	10.31
Rt_Temp_Lobe+1mm	98.9	1.0	64.4	16.4	15.77
Lt Eye	8.4	1.2	10.7	2.8	1.42
Lt Lens+1mm	0.2	1.5	2.3	1.9	0.17
Mandible	57.5	17.9	69.8	50.9	14.81
Pituitary	0.6	46.4	64.4	60.1	3.26
Rt Eye	8.4	1.2	15.1	3.5	2.41
Rt Lens+1mm	0.3	1.5	2.4	2.0	0.20
Larynx	28.0	27.5	59.7	37.1	4.87
Lt Parotid	34.0	9.3	72.9	30.6	18.69
Lt_Cochlear	0.1	38.9	52.5	44.2	2.96
Rt Parotid	35.2	10.3	72.6	32.9	18.82
Rt_Cochlear	0.1	36.6	50.8	42.8	3.27
Tongue	66.6	19.3	69.8	48.7	13.93

FIGURE 38.21. Intensity-modulated radiation therapy for a patient with T2bN2M0 nasopharyngeal carcinoma treated at Pamela Youde Nethersole Eastern Hospital, showing delineation of gross tumor targets (GTV) and clinical target volumes (CTV) for 70 Gy, 61.25 Gy, and 52.5 Gy, the dose distribution, and the dose volume histogram (DVH) for tumor targets and organs at risk.

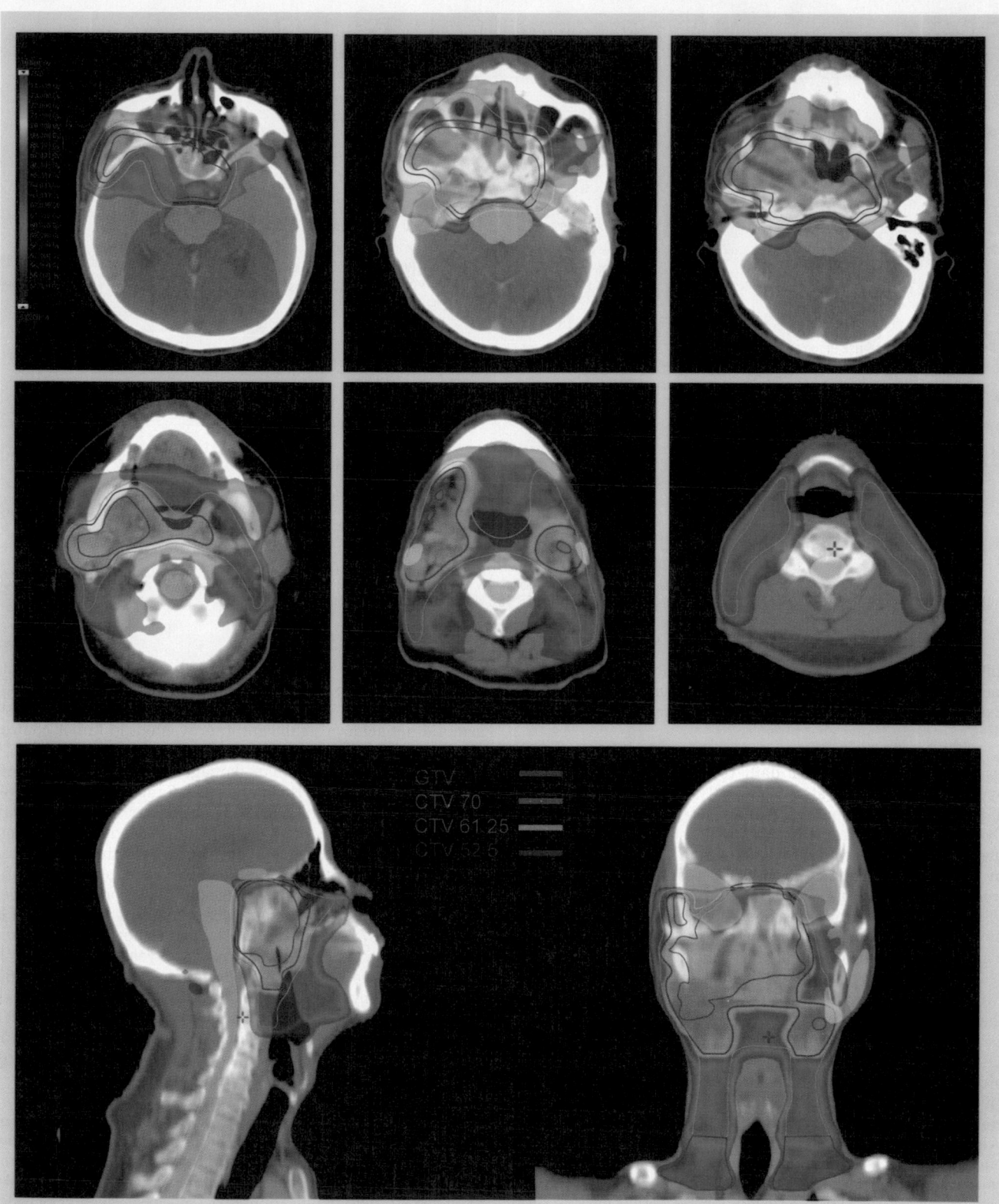

GTV
CTV 70
CTV 61.25
CTV 52.5

FIGURE 38.22. Intensity-modulated radiation therapy for a patient with T4N2M0 nasopharyngeal carcinoma treated at Pamela Youde Nethersole Eastern Hospital, showing delineation of gross tumor (GTV) and clinical target volumes (CTV) for 70 Gy, 61.25 Gy, and 52.5 Gy, the dose distribution.

Table 38.11	INTENSITY-MODULATED RADIATION THERAPY FOR NASOPHARYNGEAL CARCINOMA: AN EXAMPLE OF SPECIFICATION ON DOSE CONSTRAINTS[a]	
	First Criteria: Ideal	**Second Criteria: Acceptable**
Priority 1: Critical organ at risk		
Brainstem	Point <54 Gy	Point & 1% volume <60 Gy
Spinal cord	Point <45 Gy	Point & 1 mL volume <50 Gy
Optic chiasma	Point <54 Gy	Point & 1% volume <60 Gy
Optic nerve	Point <54 Gy	Point & 1% volume <60 Gy
Temporal lobes	Point <65 Gy & 1% volume <60 Gy	Point <70 Gy & 1% volume <65 Gy
Priority 2: Tumor targets		
GTV	≥98% dose to 100% GTV	<1% GTV receive <95% dose
PTV_70, 61.25, 52.5	≥95% dose to 100% PTV	<5% PTV receive <100% dose
		<1% PTV receive <93% dose
	<10% PTV_70 receive ≥107% dose	<20% PTV_70 receive ≥110% dose
Priority 3: Intermediate-risk Organ at Risk		
Pituitary	Point <60 Gy	1% volume <65 Gy
Mandible/TMJ	1% volume <70 Gy	1% volume <75 Gy
Lens	Point <6 Gy	Point & 1% volume <10 Gy
Eyeball	Point <50 Gy	Mean <35 Gy
Priority 4: Low-risk Organ at Risk		
Parotid glands	Mean <26 Gy (at least 1 gland)	50% volume <30 Gy (1 gland)
Cochlea	Mean <50 Gy	-
Tongue	1% volume <70 Gy	Mean dose <55 Gy
Larynx	Mean <30 Gy	Mean <45 Gy
Nonspecified tissues	<1% volume ≥75 Gy	<5% volume ≥70 Gy

[a]Based on guideline currently used at Pamela Youde Nethersole Eastern Hospital (Hong Kong).
GTV, gross tumor volume; PTV_70, 61.25, 52.5, planning target volume aimed at 70, 61.25, 52.5 Gy, respectively; TMJ, temporomandibular joint.

differentiated carcinoma, and the risk of late toxicity may be more serious because of the proximity of neurologic structures. Extra caution is needed in designing fractionation schedules for NPC.

The use of AF for NPC was first reported by Wang (219). Using 1.6 Gy/fraction twice daily (BID), phase I with lateral-opposed fields was treated to 38.4 Gy, followed by 10 to 14 days rest, and then phase II with arc rotation for another 31.6 Gy with or without a brachytherapy boost of 7 Gy. Retrospective comparison showed that patients with T2-4 tumors treated by AF achieved significantly better 5-year results than those treated by conventional fractionation (CF), both in terms of L-FFR (65% vs. 47%) and disease-specific survival (DSS; 70% vs. 35%), but the benefits for T1 tumors were statistically insignificant. No excessive late damage was incurred.

However, using a similar schedule of 1.6 Gy/fraction BID (with a 4 hour interval) to 67 Gy, Leung et al. (139) observed that the incidence of temporal lobe necrosis was as high as 24% (4/17), compared to none (0/15) in patients treated with CF. In the study by Jen et al. (83) using conventional 2D technique and BID fractions with a 6-hour interval, 76 patients were given 1.2 Gy/fraction to a median dose of 80 Gy, and 12 patients were given AF at 1.6 Gy/fraction to a median dose of 70 Gy. When compared with 134 patients treated with conventional once-daily (QD) fractionation, there was no statistically significant difference in 5-year L-FFR (T1-3 tumors, 93% vs. 86%; T4 tumors, 44% vs. 37%). The results for T4 were especially disappointing. Although the 1.2 Gy/fraction schedule did not incur excessive toxicity, the incidence of symptomatic temporal lobe necrosis was as high as 27% in patients treated with the 1.6 Gy/fraction schedule (82). See section Sequelae of Treatment for further information on the influence of dose fractionation for brain necrosis.

The first randomized trial on AF for NPC by Teo et al. (208) used an uncommon schedule of 2.5 Gy/fraction QD for 8 fractions before randomization to an experimental arm using 1.6 Gy BID for another 32 fractions versus a control arm using 2.5 Gy

QD for another 16 fractions. The trial was prematurely terminated because of excessive neurologic toxicities (49% vs. 23%). For this series of 159 patients (62% with T1-2 tumors), the AF arm did not achieve significant improvement in tumor control (5-year L-FFR, 89% vs. 85%).

To minimize the risk of late damage, the more moderate AF schedule of the Danish Head and Neck Cancer Study Group 6–7 Trials using 2 Gy/fraction, 6 fractions per week (175) was tested for NPC by Lee et al. (131). A retrospective comparison of patients irradiated to a total dose of 66 Gy with 2D technique showed that those treated with this AF schedule had significantly higher L-FFR than those treated with conventional five fractions per week. The benefit was significant particularly for T3-4 tumors (87% vs. 62%; $p < .01$). Furthermore, no significant increase in late toxicity was observed at 3 years (20% vs. 15%).

This schedule was hence used in the subsequent NPC-9902 Trial initiated by the HKNPCSG (132), which aimed to assess the therapeutic benefit by AF and/or concurrent-adjuvant CRT using the Intergroup-0099 regimen for patients with T3-4N0-1M0 nonkeratinizing carcinoma. The trial was stopped early because of slow accrual, but the 189 patients randomized were basically balanced in patient characteristics except for unfavorable gender distribution in the AF-alone arm (90% men). Preliminary results at 3 years showed that AF per se did not show significant improvement in event-free survival (EFS) when compared with CF alone (63% vs. 70%), but AF combined with CRT achieved strongly significant improvement (see section New Attempts with Concurrent Chemoradiotherapy).

Chemotherapy

Effective systemic therapy is needed for patients with advanced locoregional disease because of the notorious predilection for hematogenous dissemination and the need for further improvement of local control. Although NPC is well known for its

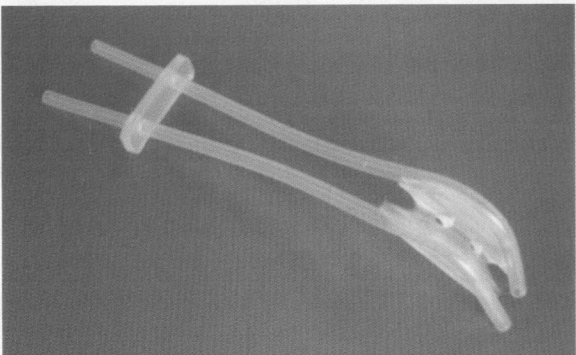

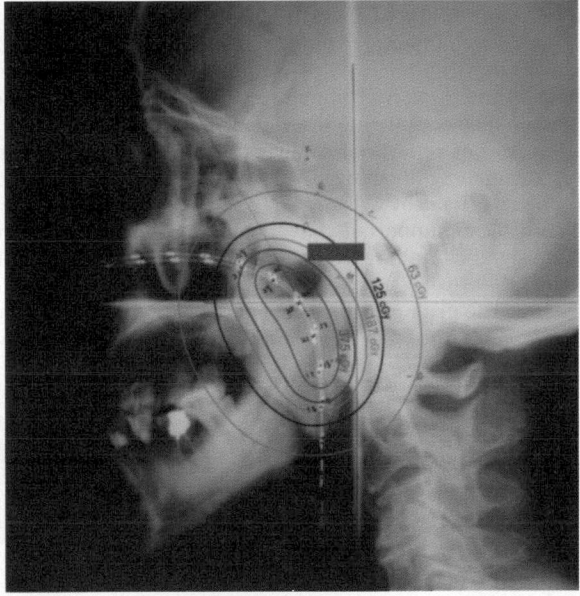

FIGURE 38.23. Endocavitary brachytherapy for nasopharyngeal carcinoma. *Upper:* The Rotterdam nasopharyngeal applicator. *Lower:* The simulator check-film showing the position of the radioactive sources and the dose distribution.

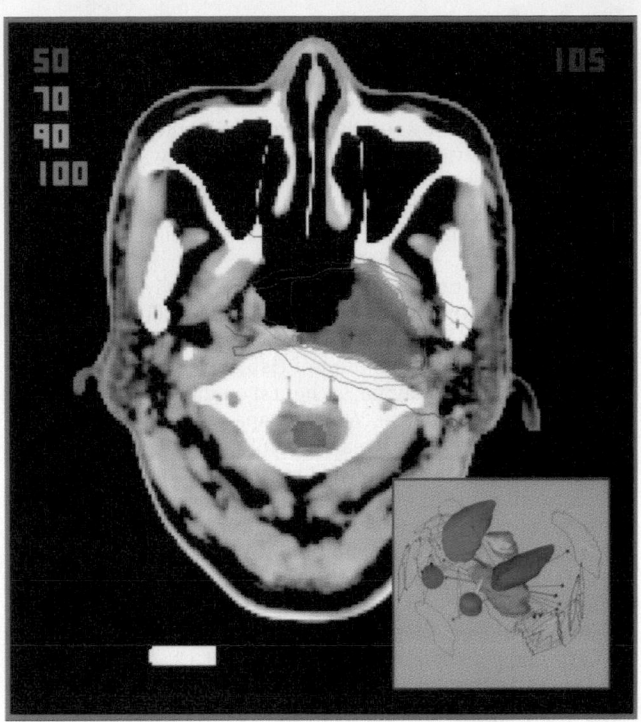

FIGURE 38.24. Stereotactic radiotherapy for nasopharyngeal carcinoma with bulky persistent tumor, showing the dose distribution and the beams arrangement.

chemoresponsiveness, review of the clinical trials on the value of chemotherapy shows contradictory results.

Up to the year 2004, there were 11 randomized trials comparing combined treatment versus RT alone published in the English literature. All except the one by Rossi et al. (190) used cisplatin-based regimens; the studied populations included patients with stages II-IVB by the current criteria of the AJCC/UICC Staging System (sixth edition); all patients were treated with conventional RT using 2D technique and CF.

Table 38.12   ADJUVANT BRACHYTHERAPY BOOST FOR PRIMARY TREATMENT OF NASOPHARYNGEAL CARCINOMA

Author	T-Category	External RT Dose (Gy)	Brachytherapy Modality	Dose (Gy)	Fraction	Day	Local Control Year	Rate (%)
Chang et al. (18)	T1	65–68	HDR-ICB	5–11	1–2	1–8	5	94
		65–68	HDR-ICB	15–16.5	3	15		80 vs. 74
		68–72	Control	—				(p = .01)
Lee et al. (134)	T1-3	54–72	HDR-ICB or LDR-ICB	5–7 10–54	2	1	5	89
Levendag et al. (144)	T1-2a	60	HDR-ICB	15	5	3	5	92
	T2b	70	HDR-ICB	11	3	2		
Lu et al. (154)	T1-2	66	HDR-ICB	10	2	8	2	94
Ng et al. (170)	T1-4	43–70	HDR-ICB	6–15	2–5	2–5	5	96
Ozyar et al. (177)	T1-4	59–71	HDR-ICB	12	3	3	5	86 vs. 94
		59–74	Control	—				(p = .23)
Syed et al. (204)	T1-4	50–60	ICB + interstitial	33–37	1	3	5	93
Teo et al. (209)	T1-2a	60–71	HDR-ICB	18–24	3	15	5	95 vs. 90
		60–71	Control	—				(p = .17)
Vikram (216)	T1-4	60–66	Interstitial	160 in 1 yr			5	96
Wang (220)	T1-2	60–64	LDR-ICB	7–10	1	1	5	91 vs. 60
		65–70	Control	—				(p <.01)

HDR, high-dose-rate; ICB, intracavitary brachytherapy; LDR, low-dose-rate; NR, not reported.

Of the five trials on induction chemotherapy (14,43,73,81, 160), only the trial by the International Nasopharynx Cancer Study Group (81) using cisplatin, epirubicin, and bleomycin achieved significant improvement in EFS (58% vs. 35% at 3 years; p <.01). However, treatment mortality was substantially higher (8% vs. 1%), and no benefit in OS was shown even with longer follow-up (40% vs. 46% at 5 years) (71). The results of adjuvant chemotherapy have been even more disappointing; none of the three trials (32,98,190) achieved significant benefit in any end points.

The first trial that achieved significant survival benefit was the Intergroup-0099 Study (2), using cisplatin (100 mg/m^2) on days 1, 22, and 43 in concurrence with RT (70 Gy in 35 fractions) followed by combination of cisplatin (80 mg/m^2) and 5-fluorouracil (1 g/m^2/day for 96 hours) on days 71, 99, and 127 during the post-RT phase. When compared with RT alone, significant benefit in both 3-year EFS (69% vs. 24%; p <.01) and OS (78% vs. 47%; p = .01) was first reported in 1996, and further confirmed with subsequent update (OS: 67% vs. 37% at 5 years; p <.01) (3). However, controversies remain, particularly regarding the actual magnitude of benefit, because the results of the RT-alone arm were grossly inferior to those achieved by most centers.

The trials on concurrent *with or without* adjuvant chemotherapy are summarized in Table 38.13. Among the subsequent trials, that by Lin et al. (146) using concurrent cisplatin and 5-fluorouracil, also achieved significant benefit in both EFS and OS, the gain in 5-year survival was 18% (OS: 72% vs. 54%;

p = .002). However, in a subsequent reanalysis (147) with retrospective restaging of the accrued patients and more accurate segregation into different risk groups, the benefit was insignificant for the high-risk group.

Two other trials from Hong Kong, that by Chan et al. (11) using concurrent cisplatin and that by Kwong et al. (98) using concurrent uracil and tegafur *with or without* adjuvant cisplatin-combination, both showed borderline improvement in OS, with survival gain of around 10% ($p \geq .06$), but no corresponding improvement in EFS (p >.14).

A meta-analysis by Baujat et al. (5), based on updated patient data of 1,753 patients from eight accepted trials (2,11,14,32,43,73,81,98), showed a small but significant benefit by adding chemotherapy: The absolute gain for 5-year EFS was 10% (52% vs. 42%) and for OS it was 6% (62% vs. 56%). The reduction in the pooled HR of death was significant: 0.82, 95% confidence interval (CI): 0.71–0.94; p = .006 (Fig. 38.25). However, the treatment effect was heterogeneous because of significant interaction of timing (p = .03); the survival benefit was essentially confined to the concurrent subset.

More recent reports of confirmatory trials using the Intergroup regimen again showed varying conclusions (Fig. 38.26). The SQNP01 Trial by Wee et al. (222) of patients with stages III-IVB disease supported that the Intergroup regimen could achieve significant improvement in both EFS and OS for Asian patients; the 3-year survival gain was 15% (OS: 80% vs. 65%; p = .006). The preliminary results of the NPC-9901 Trial of patients with N2-3 diseases by the HKNPCSG (124) also showed

							NPC-9902 (132)	
	IGS-0099 (2,3)	Lin et al. (146)	Chan et al. (11)	Kwong et al. (98)	Wee (222)	NPC-9901 (124)	CF	AF
Patient characteristics								
No. enrolled	193	284	350	222[a]	221	348	189	
Treatment period	1989–1995	1993–1999	1994–1997	1995–2001	1997–2003	1999–2004	1999–2004	
Stage equivalent by AJCC-6	II-IVB	II-IVB	II-IVB	II-IVB	III-IVB	III-IVB	III-IVA	
Histology: WHO II (%)	78 vs. 72	98 vs. 96	99 vs. 100	99 vs. 99	All	All	All	
Radiotherapy								
Fractionation	CF	CF	CF	CF	CF	CF	CF	AF
Total dose (Gy)	70	70–74	66	62.5–68	70	mean 68	mean 69	
Chemotherapy								
Concurrent								
No. of cycles	3	2	6–8	6–7 wk	3	3	3	2–3
Cisplatin dose (mg/m^2)	100 q3wk	80 q4wk	40 q1wk	—	25 (D1–4) q3wk	100 q3wk	100 q3wk	
Other drugs		F		U				
Adjuvant								
No. of cycles	3	—	—	3 / 3	3	3	3	3–4
Cisplatin dose (mg/m^2)	80 q4wk	—	—	100 q6wk	20 (D1–4) q4wk	80 q4wk	80 q4wk	
Other drugs	F	—	—	F/VBM	F	F	F	
Tumor control (%)								
Time point (year)	5	5	5	3	3	3	3	
Locoregional control		L: 89 vs. 73		80 vs. 72	NR	92 vs. 82	81 vs. 85	94 vs. 85
		S	NS	NS		p = 0.01	NS	NS
Distant control		79 vs. 70		85 vs. 71	87 vs. 70 (2y)[b]	76 vs. 73	89 vs. 81	97 vs. 81
		S	NS	p = 0.03	p <.01	NS	NS	p = 0.03
		(p = 0.06)						
Event-free survival	58 vs. 29[c]	72 vs. 53	60 vs. 52	69 vs. 58	72 vs. 53[c]	72 vs. 62	74 vs. 70	94 vs. 70
	p <0.01	p = 0.01	NS	NS	p = 0.01	p = 0.03	NS	p = 0.01
Overall survival	67 vs. 37	72 vs. 54	70 vs. 59	87 vs. 77	80 vs. 65	78 vs. 78	87 vs. 83	88 vs. 83
	p <0.01	p <0.01	(p = 0.07)	(p = 0.06)	p = 0.01	NS	NS	NS

Table 38.13   RANDOMIZED TRIALS COMPARING CONCURRENT CHEMORADIOTHERAPY VS. RADIOTHERAPY ALONE FOR NASOPHARYNGEAL CARCINOMA

CF, conventional fractionation; AF, accelerated fractionation; AJCC-6, American Joint Committee on Cancer, 6th edition; WHO II, nonkeratinizing/undifferentiated carcinoma; F, 5-fluorouracil; U, uracil and tegafur; VBM, vincristine, bleomycin, and methotrexate; L, local; NR, not reported; S, significant but no detailed data; NS, no statistical significance (p >.1).
[a] 2 × 2 factorial trial.
[b] Two-year incidence of freedom from distant failure as the first site of failure.
[c] Defining events included both failures and death.

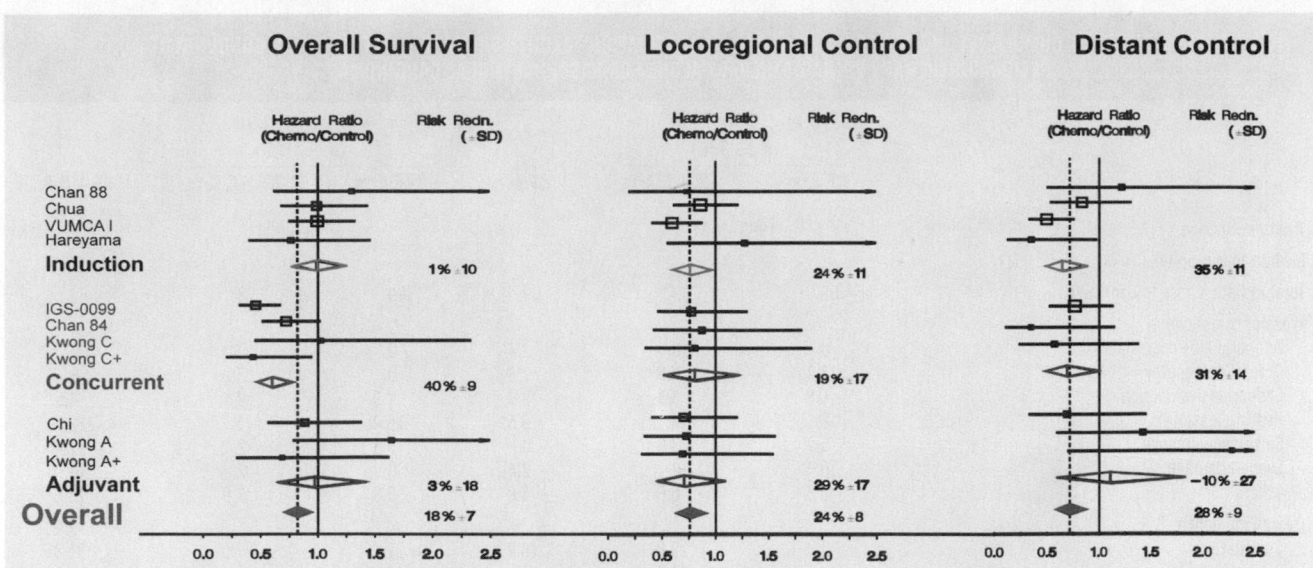

FIGURE 38.25. Meta-analyses on chemoradiotherapy versus radiotherapy alone for nasopharyngeal carcinoma: Overall survival, locoregional control, and distant control. (From Baujat B, Audry H, Bourhis J, et al. Chemotherapy in locally advanced nasopharyngeal carcinoma: An individual patient data meta-analysis of eight randomized trials and 1753 patients. *Int J Radiat Oncol Biol Phys* 2006;64:47–56, with permission.)

significant improvement in 3-year EFS (72% vs. 62%; $p = .027$). However, with the favorable results by RT alone and aggressive salvage of treatment failures, no corresponding survival benefit was yet observed (78% vs. 78%), although the improvement in tumor control might translate into significant survival benefit with longer follow-up.

One serious concern about the Intergroup regimen is its efficacy for distant control. Preliminary results of the NPC-9901 Trial (124) showed that the improvement in D-FFR for patients with N2-3 disease was minimal (76% vs. 73%; $p = .47$). Further-

more, both the series treated by IMRT from University of California, San Francisco (7,135) and that by stereotactic boost from Stanford University Medical Center (111) showed disappointingly high incidence of distant failure ($\geq$25%), despite achievement of excellent locoregional control ($\geq$93%) and extensive use of the Intergroup regimen ($\geq$75% of patients).

Another concern about CRT is tolerance and the risk of toxicities. No treatment-related mortality was observed in the Intergroup-0099 Trial, but both Asian confirmatory trials (124,222) reported 1% mortality by the same regimen. The

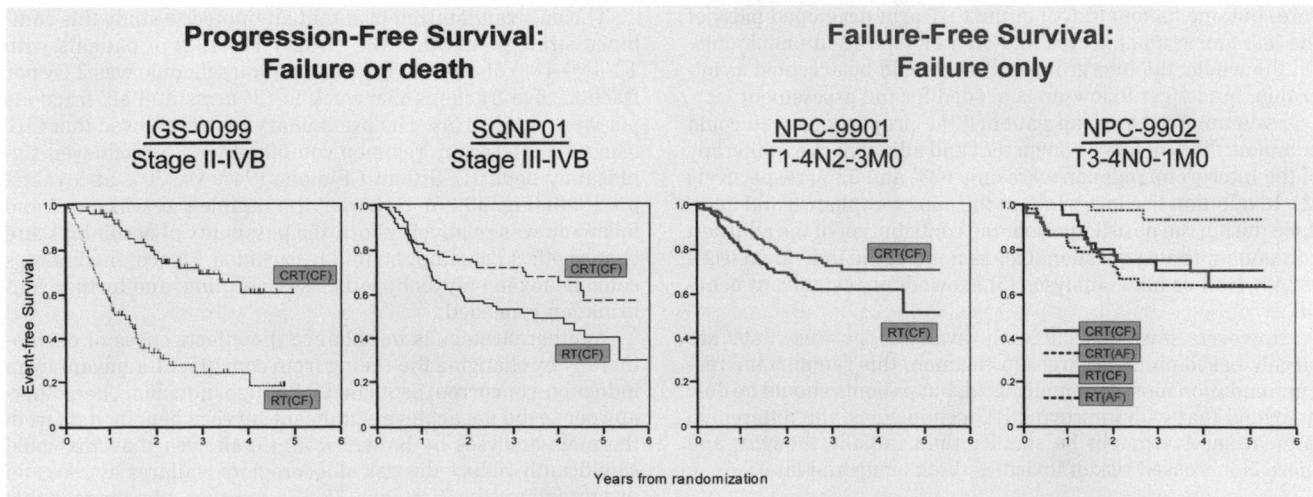

FIGURE 38.26. Randomized trials comparing concurrent-adjuvant chemoradiotherapy using the Intergroup-0099 regimen versus radiotherapy alone for nasopharyngeal carcinoma. End point used in the Intergroup-0099 trial and SQNP01 trial by Wee et al: Progression-free survival (defining events include both failures and deaths); end point used in NPC-9901 and NPC-9902: Failure-free survival (defining events include failures only). (Modified from Al-Sarraf M, LeBlanc M, Giri PG, et al. Chemoradiotherapy versus radiotherapy in patients with advanced nasopharyngeal cancer: Phase III randomized Intergroup study 0099. *J Clin Oncol* 1998;16:1310–1317, with permission; Wee J, Tan EH, Tai BC. Randomized trial of radiotherapy versus concurrent chemoradiotherapy followed by adjuvant chemotherapy in patients with American Joint Committee on Cancer/International Union Against Cancer Stage III and IV nasopharyngeal cancer of the endemic variety. *J Clin Oncol* 2005;23:6730–6738, with permission; Lee AWM, Lau WH, Tung SY, et al. Preliminary results of a randomized study on therapeutic gain by concurrent chemotherapy for regionally-advanced nasopharyngeal carcinoma: NPC-9901 Trial by the Hong Kong Nasopharyngeal Cancer Study Group. *J Clin Oncol* 2005;23:6966–6975; Lee AWM, Tung SY, Chan AT, et al. Preliminary results of a randomized study (NPC-9902 Trial) on therapeutic gain by concurrent chemotherapy and/or accelerated fractionation for locally-advanced nasopharyngeal carcinoma. *Int J Radiat Oncol Biol Phys* 2006;66:142–151.)

Table 38.14	**CUMULATIVE INCIDENCE RATE (%) OF LATE IRRADIATION TOXICITIES (GRADE ≥3) FOLLOWING CONCURRENT CHEMORADIOTHERAPY VS. RADIOTHERAPY ALONE FOR NASOPHARYNGEAL CARCINOMA**

	NPC-9901 Trial[a] (N = 348)		NPC-9902 Trial[b] (N = 189)			
	CF Arm	CF+C Arm	CF Arm	AF Arm	CF+C Arm	AF+C Arm
Treatment period	1999–2004		1999–2004			
Median follow-up (y)	2.3		2.9			
Total radiation dose (mean) (Gy)	68	69	69	69	68	69
Types of complication						
Temporal lobe necrosis	0	0	2.4	0	0	0
Cranial neuropathy	1.1	0.6	2.4	0	3.9	0
Endocrine dysfunction	0.6	3.5	2.4	1.9	2	4.5
Hearing loss/otitis	8	14.1	9.5	15.4	15.7	22.7
Soft tissue damage	1.7	3.6	0	3.8	2	11.4
Eyeball damage	0	0	2.4	0	2	0
Others	0.6	0.6	4.8	5.8	3.9	13.6
Overall incidence						
Cumulative	11.4	19.8	16.7	21.2	27.5	31.8
3-year actuarial rate	13	28	14	22	31	34
Comparisons with CF	—	$p = .024$	—	$p = .37$	$p = .13$	$p = .05$
Mortality	0	0.6	0	0	0	0

CF, conventional fractionation (2 Gy/fraction five fractions per week); +C, with the Intergroup-0099 regimen of concurrent cisplatin and adjuvant cisplatin + 5-fluoruracil; AF, accelerated fractionation (2 Gy/fraction six fractions per week).
[a]Lee AWM, Lau WH, Tung SY, et al. Preliminary results of a randomized study on therapeutic gain by concurrent chemotherapy for regionally-advanced nasopharyngeal carcinoma: NPC-9901 Trial by the Hong Kong Nasopharyngeal Cancer Study Group. *J Clin Oncol* 2005;23:6966–6975.
[b]Lee AWM, Tung SY, Chan AT, et al. Preliminary results of a randomized study (NPC-9902 Trial) on therapeutic gain by concurrent chemotherapy and/or accelerated fractionation for locally-advanced nasopharyngeal carcinoma. *Int J Radiat Oncol Biol Phys* 2006;66:142–151.

NPC-9901 Trial (124) is the first trial that assesses the impact on late toxicity. Besides the expected increase in acute toxicities (84% vs. 53%; p <.01), the CRT arm also had significantly higher incidence of major late toxicities (28% vs. 13% at 3 years; p = .02) (Table 38.14). This was mostly due to increased otologic toxicities (14% vs. 8%), peripheral neuropathy (2% vs. 0%), and endocrine dysfunction (4% vs. 1%). The majority of toxicities were grade 3 in severity. Damages to neurologic structures were rare, but one patient (0.6%) in the CRT arm developed palsy of the last four cranial nerves and died of aspiration pneumonia. On the whole, the Intergroup regimen could be accepted as tolerable, but longer follow-up is needed for full assessment.

Even among American patients, the proportions who could complete the scheduled concurrent and adjuvant chemotherapy of the Intergroup regimen were only 63% and 55%, respectively (2). In addition to concern about the poor compliance and tolerance during the post-RT period, the contribution of the adjuvant component is also questionable, as none of the individual trials (32,98,190) or meta-analyses (5) showed any significant benefits.

However, since the currently available positive data are largely based on the Intergroup regimen, this remains the recommendation most commonly used; but patients should be duly informed that with improving RT technologies, the differential gain in survival might be smaller than initially thought, and there is increased risk of toxicities (both acute and late).

New Attempts with Concurrent Chemoradiotherapy

Building on the current achievement by concurrent CRT, different approaches for further improvement of treatment results have been explored (Table 38.15).

One strategy is to enhance the effectiveness of RT by changing the fractionation from CF to AF. Retrospective studies combining AF with concurrent-adjuvant CRT had shown reasonable tolerability and encouraging preliminary results (86,145,232).

In a series of 50 patients (44% stage IVA-B) treated at Memorial Sloan-Kettering Cancer Center using the concomitant boost schedule to deliver 70 Gy in 6 weeks combined with the Intergroup regimen, Wolden et al. (232) showed that 3-year L-FFR of 89% and OS of 84% could be achieved. The study by Jian et al. (86) using a hyperfractionation schedule of 1.2 Gy BID to 74.4 Gy combined with CRT, achieved 3-year OS of 100% for T3 and 63% for T4.

The only randomized trial that attempted to study this combined strategy was the NPC-9902 Trial (132) of patients with T3-4N0-1M0 diseases. The fractionation schedule was 2 Gy per fraction, five fractions per week in CF arms and six fractions per week in AF arms. The preliminary results showed that CRT using the Intergroup regimen combined with AF achieved significantly better EFS than CF alone (94% vs. 70% at 3 years; p = .008) (Fig. 38.26). However, the sample size was small and follow-up was relatively short; the possibility of occult bias and chance effect could not be totally excluded. Hence, the findings could be taken only as hypothesis-generating, and further confirmation is needed.

Another strategy is to enhance the effectiveness of chemotherapy by changing the timing from concurrent-adjuvant to an induction-concurrent sequence. Although induction chemotherapy per se did not achieve significant survival benefit, data from the meta-analyses by Baujat et al. (5) showed that this could significantly reduce the risk of locoregional failures by 24% and distant failures by 35% (Fig. 38.25). Another advantage is that patients' compliance and tolerance are substantially better during the induction phase than the adjuvant phase (133). This early use of potent combinations of cytotoxic drugs at full dose might be particularly advantageous for NPC with extensive locoregional infiltration, as this could shrink the primary tumor to give wider margin for irradiation (Fig. 38.27).

All five phase II studies using induction-concurrent CRT with CF reported encouraging preliminary results (1,12,87, 174,189). Using a combination of cisplatin, 5-fluoruracil, and

Table 38.15	NEW ATTEMPTS WITH CONCURRENT CHEMORADIOTHERAPY FOR NASOPHARYNGEAL CARCINOMA

		Stage IV	Radiotherapy		Chemotherapy					Tumor Control (%)			
Author	N	(%)	Dose (Gy)	Time (wk)	Induction	Concurrent	Adjuvant	Time (y)	OS	EFS	LR-FFR	D-FFR
Concurrent-adjuvant chemoradiotherapy with accelerated fractionation												
Wolden et al. (232)	50	44	70	6	—	P	PF	3	84	66	89 (L)	79
Jian et al. (86)	48	>77	74	7	—	P	PF	3	72	71	91 (L)	NR
Lin et al. (145)	63	NR	72–74	6	—	PF	± PF	3	74	64	89 (L)	74
Induction-concurrent chemoradiotherapy with conventional fractionation												
Rischin et al. (189)	35	40	60	6	PEF	P	—	4	90	81	97 (L)	94
Oh et al. (174)	27	NR	70	14[a]	PFI	HF	—	5	77	86[b]	93	92
Johnson et al. (87)	44	NR	70	7	PF	PF	—	3	78	69	75 (C)	89 (C)
								5	66	55		
Al-Amro et al. (1)	110	74	66	6.5	PE	P	—	3	71	53	68	74
Chan et al. (12)	31	39	66	6.5	TJ	P	—	2	92	79	90 (C)	81 (C)
Induction-concurrent chemoradiotherapy with accelerated fractionation												
Lee et al. (133)	49	100	70	6	PF	P	—	3	71	61	77	75
Yau et al. (238)	37	100	70	6	PG	P	—	3	76	63	78	76

OS, overall survival; EFS, event-free survival; LR-FFR, locoregional failure-free rate; D-FFR, distant failure-free rate; P, cisplatin; F, 5-fluorouracil; L, local failure-free rate alone; NR, not reported; E, epirubicin; I, interferon-α; H, hydroxyurea; C, crude incidence; T, paclitaxel; J, carboplatin; G, gemcitabine.
[a]Split fractionation (2 Gy/fraction daily × five fraction, q2wk).
[b]Defining events included both failures and treatment-related death.

epirubicin as induction chemotherapy and cisplatin in concurrence with RT to 60 Gy, Rischin et al. (189) achieved excellent 4-year results in 35 patients (40% stage IV) with OS of 90%, distant control of 94%, and locoregional control of 97%.

For the most difficult stage IV patients with locoregional disease infiltrating or abutting neurologic structures, a more aggressive approach combining induction-concurrent CRT with AF has been explored at Pamela Youde Nethersole Eastern Hospital. Two different induction regimen have been tested:

Pre-Treatment

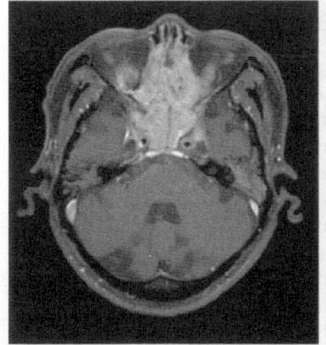 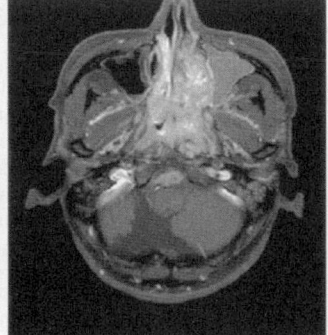 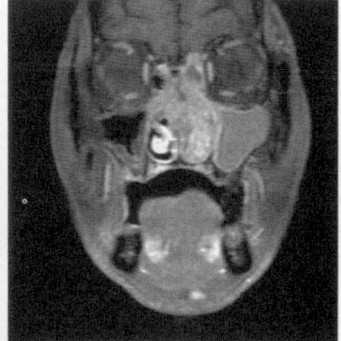 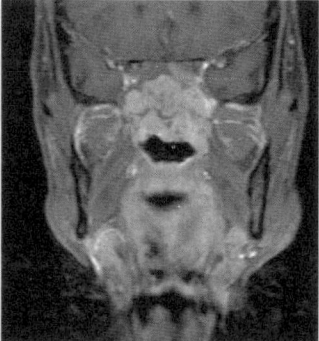

After 3 cycles of induction chemotherapy

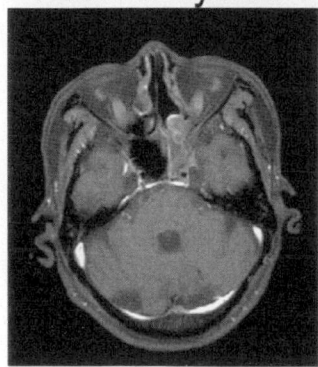 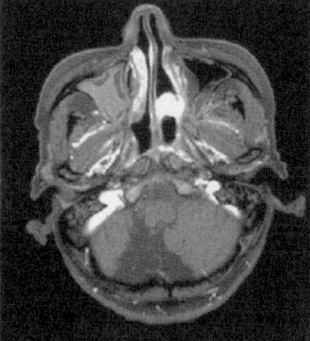 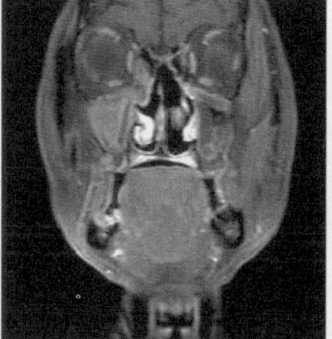 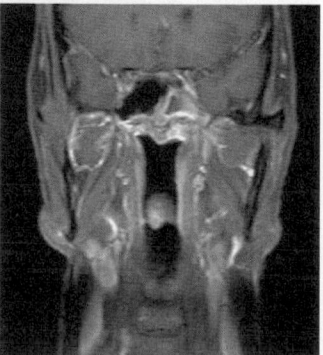

FIGURE 38.27. Magnetic resonance imaging showing shrinkage of primary tumor by induction chemotherapy using cisplatin and 5-fluorouracil before proceeding to concurrent cisplatin and radiotherapy. (From Lee A, Yau T, Wong D, et al. Treatment of stage IV (A–B) nasopharyngeal carcinoma by induction-concurrent chemoradiotherapy and accelerated fractionation. *Int J Radiat Oncol Biol Phys* 2005;63:1331–1338.)

Cisplatin and 5-fluoruracil was used in the first pilot study by Lee et al. (133), and a newer combination of cisplatin and gemcitabine was used by Yau et al. (238). These were then followed by cisplatin in concurrence with RT to 70 Gy using the six fractions per week AF schedule. Given the grave prognosis of this notorious group in the past, 3-year OS of 71% (133) and 76% (238), respectively achieved in the two studies, were very encouraging. Further confirmation of efficacy is warranted.

Persistent/Recurrent NPC

Early Detection and Diagnosis

Despite improving control rate with primary treatment for NPC, local failure remains a problem for patients with advanced T-category. Distinction should be made between persistent disease (tumors that do not completely regress following primary treatment) and recurrent disease (tumors that re-emerge after initial complete regression) because the therapeutic considerations and prognosis are different.

As it takes time for tumors to regress following RT, one difficult decision is when to consider residual tumors as genuine persistence and proceed with salvage treatment. Kwong et al. (96) performed serial biopsies from the nasopharynx in 617 patients and showed that the percentage of positive biopsies dropped spontaneously from 29% in the first week after completion of RT to 12% by the ninth week and then rose again. The 5-year L-FFR was 82% for patients who achieved early histologic remission (<5 weeks), 77% for those with delayed remission (5 to <12 weeks), but only 54% for those with persistent tumors at 12 weeks, despite subsequent salvage treatment. The optimal time for intervention remains uncertain; avoidance of unnecessary overtreatment and excessive delay in treatment are both important, and an observation period of 8 weeks is a reasonable balance commonly used.

Early detection of locoregional failure is crucial for a better chance of salvage. However, both CT and MRI have relatively low sensitivity and specificity in detection of persistent/recurrent disease. Generally, MRI is superior to CT. Gong et al. (68) showed that recurrent tumor exhibited higher signal intensity on T1-weighted spin-echo images, whereas radiation fibrosis showed low or medium intensity in T1 and T2 images. The high-intensity feature, however, is not specific for tumor, and may be seen with radiation edema or infection. Technetium-99 m MIBI SPECT may be a useful tool. Kostakoglu

et al. (94) showed that this was superior to MRI performed at 3 to 6 months post-RT in diagnosing complete response. The advent of FDG-PET is a valuable development. Yen et al. (241) compared FDG-PET and MRI in 67 NPC patients 4 to 70 months after completion of RT and showed that FDG-PET was superior to MRI in all aspects, including sensitivity (100% vs. 62%) and specificity (93% vs. 44%).

Preliminary data suggest that circulating cell-free DNA of EBV may be another useful tool for early detection of treatment failure. A longitudinal study by Lo et al. (151) showed that elevation of EBV-DNA titer was noted in patients with relapse up to 6 months before detectable clinical disease. However, this measurement is more sensitive for distant metastases than locoregional recurrence; up to one third of patients with locoregional recurrence did not show elevated EBV-DNA copies (229).

Additional Radiation for Persistent Disease

Brachytherapy has been widely used for locally persistent disease after a full course of EBRT (Table 38.16, part A). Excellent results with 5-year L-FFR in the range of 87% to 95% for patients with initial T1-2 a tumors have been reported (101,109,140,209,246). There is preliminary evidence suggesting that patients with initial T2b tumors could also be effectively treated by brachytherapy (143).

Stereotactic RT is a valuable advance for delivering additional EBRT. Yau et al. (239) studied 755 patients with T1-4 tumors and showed that 7% had positive biopsies 8 weeks after completion of primary RT. The 21 patients treated with fractionated stereotactic RT to a median dose of 15 Gy achieved a 3-year L-FFR of 82%, a result that was very close to corresponding L-FFR of 86% in the contemporary cohort with complete remission, and was substantially better than corresponding L-FFR of 71% in 24 patients treated with high dose-rate brachytherapy to a median dose of 20 Gy.

Reirradiation for Recurrent Disease

Aggressive salvage treatment should be attempted because long-term survival can be achieved for a substantial proportion of patients with early locoregional recurrence and useful palliation for those with extensive disease. However, there is a high risk of normal tissue damage. It is crucial to restrict the irradiation of normal tissue to a minimum.

The most important prognostic factor is the TNM stage of the tumor at the time of recurrence. Thorough restaging,

Table 38.16	**RESULTS OF LOCALLY PERSISTENT/RECURRENT NASOPHARYNGEAL CARCINOMA TREATED WITH BRACHYTHERAPY**							
			Brachytherapy				**Local Control**	
Author	T-Category	Modality	Dose (Gy)	Fraction	Day	Time (y)	Rate (%)
Part A. Local persistence							
Kwong et al. (101)	T1	Interstitial gold grain	60			5	87
Law et al. (109)	T1–2a	Iridium mold	40			5	90
Leung et al. (140)	T1–2	HDR-ICB	22.5–24	3	15	5	95
Leung et al. (143)	T2b	HDR-ICB	22.5–24	3	15	5	97
Zheng et al. (246)	T1	HDR-ICB	15–30	5–6	15–18	5	100
	T2	HDR-ICB	15–30	5–6	15–18		90
Part B. Local recurrence							
Kwong et al. (101)	rT1	Interstitial gold grain	60			5	63
Law et al. (109)	rT1–2a	Iridium mold	50–55[a]			5	89
Leung et al. (141)	rT1–2	EBRT + HDR-ICB	50 + 14.8[a]	3	15	3	72

HDR-ICB, high-dose-rate intracavitary brachytherapy; EBRT, external beam radiotherapy.
[a]Median dose

including metastatic work-up, is needed. A study of 891 patients with local recurrence by Lee et al. (125) showed that 54% of patients also developed regional and/or distant failures. Another significant factor is reirradiation dose: Most series using EBRT with conventional 2D technique showed that doses ≥ 60 Gy were associated with better outcome (119,186,221).

A retrospective comparison by Lee et al. (116) of the symptomatic late toxicity rate in 487 patients with two courses of EBRT versus 3,635 patients with one course showed that the summated total biologic dose tolerated (BED-Σ) was higher than that expected with a single-course treatment (BED-1), suggesting partial recovery of normal tissues (particularly for patients with reirradiation after an interval >2 years). Assuming an α/β ratio of 3 Gy, the BED-Σ that incurred 20% toxicity at 5 years was 129% that of BED-1.

Brachytherapy has been widely used for treatment of recurrent NPC (Table 38.16, part B). Early-stage recurrent NPC could be effectively salvaged by brachytherapy alone (101,109). Kwong et al. (101), using interstitial implants with radioactive gold grains, reported a 5-year L-FFR of 63%; complications included headache (28%), palatal fistula (19%), and mucosal necrosis (16%). Law et al. (109), using iridium mold, achieved excellent local salvage up to 89%, but the complication rate was 53%.

The combination of brachytherapy and EBRT is useful, particularly when conventional 2D technique is used. Lee et al. (119) showed that patients reirradiated by combined modes had higher salvage rate than those by EBRT or brachytherapy alone: The 5-year L-FFR was 45%, 32%, and 29%, respectively. Simi-

lar pattern of superiority by combined method was reported by other investigators (64,141,186,219,221).

Stereotactic radiosurgery or fractionated stereotactic radiotherapy is another useful tool for retreatment of local recurrence. Control rates ranging from 53% to 86% have been reported (22,44,50,178). For advanced recurrence with extension beyond the nasopharynx, this method will give better dose coverage than brachytherapy. A higher salvage rate by adding stereotactic radiation (17,44,236) as a boost after EBRT has been reported. Although most series reported a low risk of complications, massive hemorrhage with potential fatal outcome has been described (44). To minimize this risk, radiosurgery should be avoided when there is direct tumor encasement of the carotid artery or when a high cumulative dose has already been delivered.

Table 38.17 summarizes the treatment outcome and severe late complications by external reirradiation. Past series using 2D technique achieved 5-year survival rates in the range of 21% to 41%, and the incidence of temporal lobe necrosis ranged from 2% to 27%. The use of 3D conformal radiotherapy showed improving results. Chang et al. (17) showed that none of the patients reirradiated by 3D technique developed temporal lobe necrosis compared with 14% in those reirradiated by 2D technique. Zheng et al. (247), reported a very encouraging 5-year local salvage rate of 71%, but the actuarial rate of late toxicities (grade 4) was still as high as 49%.

Preliminary reports using IMRT for reirradiation show encouraging short-term results. Using IMRT to deliver 68–70 Gy, Lu et al. (155) reported 100% salvage rate without any

Table 38.17 RESULTS ON REIRRADIATION FOR LOCAL RECURRENCE OF NASOPHARYNGEAL CARCINOMA

Author	N	Reirradiation Technique	Time (y)	Treatment Outcome (Actuarial Rate) Local Control (%)	Survival (%)	Major Late Toxicity (Cumulative Incidence) Overall (%)	Brain Necrosis (%)
Teo et al. (207)	123	All 2D	5	rT1: 43 rT2: 31 rT3-4: 16	rT1: 63 rT2: 48 rT3-4: 31	NR	20
Lee et al. (119)	654	All 2D	5	rT1: 35 rT2: 28 rT3-4: 11	16	26	3
Fu et al. (64)	39	All 2D	5	26	41	23	NR
Wang (221)	51	All 2D	5	NR	33	6	2
Pryzant et al. (186)	53	All 2D	5	35	18	NR	NR
Yan et al. (237)	219[a]	All 2D	5	NR	18	>29	>12
Chua et al. (47)	97	All 2D	5	NR	rT1-2: 57 rT3: 42 rT4: 17	NR	16
Leung et al. (141)	91	All 2D	5	38	30	57	27
Chang et al. (17)	186	81% 2D, 19% 3D	3	NR	rT1: 39 rT2: 24 rT3: 28 rT4: 4	2D: 23 3D: 9	2D: 14 3D: 0
Zheng et al. (247)	86	All 3D	5	rT1: 92 rT2: 81 rT3: 68 rT4: 41	rT1: 70 rT2: 52 rT3: 32 rT4: 10	49	16
Lu et al. (155)	49	IMRT	3/4	100	NR	NR	NR
Chua et al. (48)	31	IMRT	1	rT1-3: 10% rT4: 35	63	19	7

2D, conventional two-dimensional external radiotherapy and/or brachytherapy; 3D, three-dimensional conformal radiotherapy; IMRT, intensity-modulated radiotherapy.
[a]Patients with regional relapse included.

severe late complications in a series of 49 patients with a median follow-up of 9 months. Using IMRT to a median dose of 54 Gy in 31 patients (with or without induction chemotherapy and stereotactic boost), Chua et al. (48) reported a locoregional salvage rate of 56% and late complications (grade 3) of 25% at 1 year. Longer follow-up is clearly needed.

Chemoradiotherapy may also improve treatment outcome for recurrent NPC. Using gemcitabine and cisplatin as induction chemotherapy followed by reirradiation with IMRT in 20 patients (95% rT3-4), Chua et al. (42) reported a 1-year local salvage rate of 75%. In a study of 35 patients (66% rT3-4), Poon et al. (185) reported a 1-year EFS of 42% by concurrent cisplatin followed by adjuvant chemotherapy with cisplatin and 5-fluorouracil.

Surgical Treatment

For patients who develop local or nodal persistent/recurrent disease without distant metastasis, surgical salvage is an important option to consider. For patients with nodal failure following RT, lymph node involvement is often extensive, Radical neck dissection is the recommended salvage procedure (224). A study by Wei et al. (226) showed that salvage with radical neck dissection could achieve a 5-year nodal control rate of 66% and a disease-free survival of 37%. For those with tumor extending beyond the lymph node confines and involving nearby structures, addition of after-loading brachytherapy to the tumor bed following radical neck dissection might be useful (225).

For selected patients with persistent/recurrent disease localized in the nasopharynx, surgical salvage by nasopharyngectomy is an option. As the nasopharynx is located in the center of the head, adequate exposure for oncologic extirpation of the tumor is a great challenge. A number of approaches have been employed. These include an infratemporal approach from the lateral aspect (60), transpalatal, transmaxillary and transcervical approaches from the inferior aspect (58,166), and an anterolateral approach (227). As all the patients concerned have undergone prior radical RT, the associated morbidities of trismus and palatal fistula are common, but the mortalities associated with these surgical procedures have been low.

Recurrent NPC is frequently located in the pharyngeal recess on the lateral wall. Direct access to this region is essential for complete tumor extirpation. Wei and Sham (228) advocated the anterolateral approach or the maxillary swing approach for surgical salvage of localized failure in the nasopharynx. Following facial incisions and the appropriate osteotomies, the maxilla bone is swung laterally while attached to the anterior cheek flap as one osteocutaneous unit (Figs. 38.28 and 38.29). The nasopharynx with the persistent/recurrent tumor and its vicinity including the paranasopharyngeal region are then widely exposed for oncologic resection. At completion of nasopharyn-

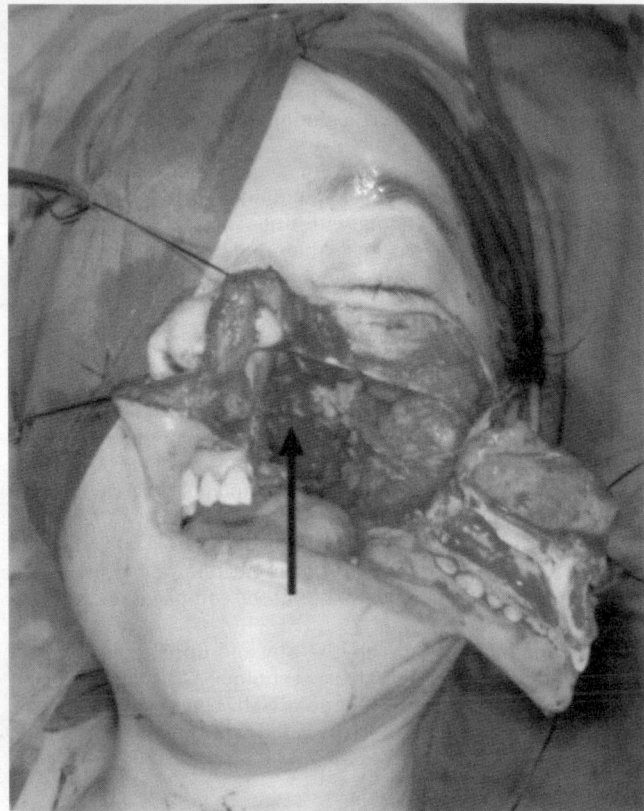

FIGURE 38.29. The left maxilla is swung laterally, exposing the nasopharynx *(arrow)*.

gectomy, the maxilla is returned and fixed to the rest of the facial skeleton with miniplates.

Wei et al. (228) studied 161 patients with salvage nasopharyngectomy using this approach performed at Queen Mary Hospital (Hong Kong) for recurrent NPC following primary treatment by radical RT. Twelve patients also had prior brachytherapy as a salvage procedure. Preoperative assessment showed the tumors of all patients were recurrent stage T1. Negative tumor resection margins, confirmed by frozen section, were achieved in 78% of patients, and the remaining patients had microscopic tumor at the internal carotid artery or the skull base detected during surgery, making further resection impossible. All patients recovered from this anterolateral approach nasopharyngectomy and were discharged. Associated morbidities included trismus of different degrees in 60% and palatal fistula in 25% of patients. Recent modification of the palatal incision has eliminated the problem of palatal fistula (168). In concurrence with other reports, satisfactory long-term results could be achieved for persistent/recurrent tumor that can be completely removed surgically. The 5-year local salvage rate was around 65% and disease-free survival was 54% (57,223).

Results of Treatment

The specific results of various new treatments have been summarized in the preceding respective sections. This section focuses on the overall results in major series of patients treated in the past two decades (Table 38.18).

Two of the representative series from the past, 5,037 patients treated at Queen Elizabeth Hospital (Hong Kong) during 1976–1985 (129) and 378 patients treated at M.D. Anderson Cancer Center (United States) during 1954–1992 (67,192), both reported very similar results with DSS of around 50% at 5 years

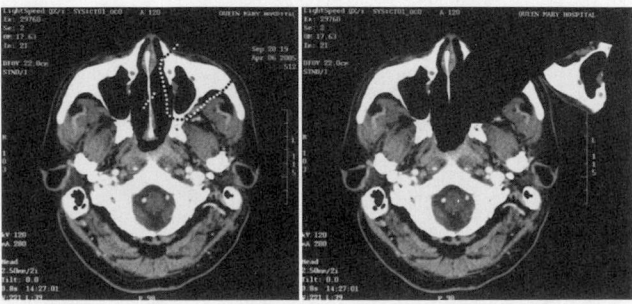

FIGURE 38.28. *Left:* Computed tomography shows planned osteotomies of the maxilla and the posterior part of the nasal septum *(broken line)*. *Right:* The maxilla is swung laterally while still attached to the anterior cheek flap.

	Table 38.18	**TREATMENT RESULTS FOR DIFFERENT STAGES BY AMERICAN JOINT COMMITTEE ON CANCER AND INTERNATIONAL UNION AGAINST CANCER STAGING SYSTEM**

Author	Treatment Period	N	RT Special (%)	Chemotherapy (%)	Time (y)	Control Rate (%) Local	Nodal	Distant	End Point	Survival (%) I	IIA-B	III	IVA-B	All
Geara et al. (67) and	1954–1992	378	8 AF	None	5	71	84	70	DSS					53
Sanguineti et al. (192)					10	66	83	68						45
Casanova et al. (10)	1965–1999	54	—	?	5				OS		82	60	39	
Wang (219)	1970–1994	259	52 AF	None	5	65	NR	81	DSS					59
Cooper et al. (51)	1971–1994	107	—	None	5				OS	71	50	55	30	
									DSS	75	50	58	40	
Lee et al. (117,129)	1976–1985	5037	—	9	5	66	67	62	DSS					52
					10	61	64	59		77	65	54	29	43
Yeh et al. (240)	1983–1998	849	—	None	5	78	94	75	OS					59
Corry et al. (52)	1985–1999	86[a]	20 3D	70	5	74			OS					75
		72[b]	22 3D	71		82								63
Hong et al. (77)	1987–1988	411	—	None	5	74		78	DSS	96	73	50	24	
Au et al. (4)	1987–1990	1294	—	20	5	76	85	75	DSS	82	80–72	69	39	69
Chua et al. (49)	1989–1991	324	—	16	5	98–69	98–75	98–71	OS	98	79	80	60	
Leung et al. (142)	1990–1998	1070	—	20	5	81	93	77	OS	91	92–78	62	44–43	71
									DSS	85	95–82	67	50–46	67
Palazzi et al. (180)	1990–1999	171	—	62	5	84	80	83	OS					72
									DSS					74
Heng et al. (74)	1992–1994	677	—	None	5				OS	88	75–74	60	35–28	57
Ma et al. (159)	1993–1994	621	—	None	5	75		77	OS	89	70	53	37	
Ozyar et al. (176)	1993–1997	90	—	66	3	88–85		100–57	OS	100	72	65	55	65
Lee et al. (112,130)	1996–2000	2687	10 3D	23	5	85	94	81	OS	90	84	76	52	75
									DSS	92	87	81	60	80

RT, radiation therapy; AF, accelerated fractionation; DSS, disease-specific survival; OS, overall survival; NR, not reported; 3D, three-dimensional.
[a]Asian patients.
[b]Non-Asian patients.

and 45% at 10 years. The risk of delayed "relapse" is another feature of NPC that is distinct from other head and neck cancers; long-term follow-up is needed.

Almost all retrospective analyses have demonstrated steady improvement in treatment results when compared with historical data at the same institution. Taking the series that includes only patients treated from 1985 onward as contemporary series, the average 5-year survival now achieved is up to 70% (range in OS, 57% to 75%; DSS, 67% to 80%). Such encouraging results were reported not only from Asia (4,130,142), but also from Europe (180) and Australia (52).

Retrospective analyses by Su and Wang (202) of patients with NPC of different histologic types treated at Massachusetts General Hospital (United States) during 1979–1996 showed that Chinese race per se was not a significant prognostic factor. The 5-year OS for Chinese versus non-Chinese patients was 49% versus 56%. The study by Corry et al. (52) of patients with nonkeratinizing NPC treated at Peter MacCallum Cancer Institute (Australia) during 1985–1999 also showed that race had no significant impact. The 5-year OS for Asian versus non-Asian patients was 75% versus 63%.

A representative contemporary series reported by the HKNPCSG (130) of 2,687 patients treated in all public centers in Hong Kong during 1996–2000, with 53% of patients staged III-IVB by the current AJCC/UICC system, showed that a 5-year OS of 75% and DSS of 80% could now be achieved. Figure 38.30 shows the OS achieved for different stages during this era. Treatments during this period were not state of the art because of resource constraints; only 32% of the series were staged by MRI (the rest by CT), 90% were irradiated with conventional 2D technique to a median total dose of 66 Gy, and

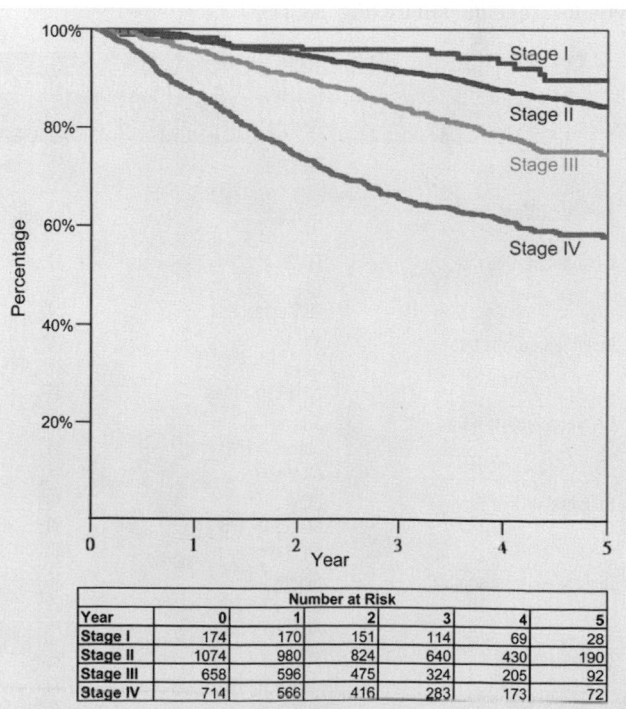

FIGURE 38.30. Overall survival achieved for different stages of nasopharyngeal carcinoma in a series 2,687 patients treated in public centers in Hong Kong during 1996–2000. (From Lee A, Sze W, Au J, et al. Treatment results for nasopharyngeal carcinoma in the modern era: The Hong Kong experience. *Int J Radiat Oncol Biol Phys* 2005;61:1107–1116.)

Number at Risk						
Year	0	1	2	3	4	5
Stage I	174	170	151	114	69	28
Stage II	1074	980	824	640	430	190
Stage III	658	596	475	324	205	92
Stage IV	714	566	416	283	173	72

Clinical Radiation Oncology

only 14% had additional treatment with concurrent chemotherapy and 9% sequential chemotherapy. Hence, similar, if not better, results should be achievable at least for nonkeratinizing NPC.

Review of contemporary series (Tables 38.18) shows that the average 5-year L-FFR was 80% (range, 74% to 85%), nodal-FFR was 90% (range, 80% to 94%), and D-FFR was 77% (range, 75% to 83%).

Excellent nodal control can usually be achieved. Based on the contemporary series with detailed results for different N-categories (130,142), the average 5-year nodal-FFR was 97% for N0, 95% for N1, 90% for N2, and 75% for N3. Routine surgery is not indicated; radical neck dissection should be reserved for those with nodal persistence or recurrence after RT.

T category is the most important prognostic factor for local control. Based on the contemporary series treated mostly by conventional 2D technique (4,130,142,158,159), the average 5-year L-FFR varied from 90% (range, 82% to 93%) for T1, 82% (range, 77% to 87%) for T2, 70% (range, 69% to 80%) for T3, to 68% (range, 58% to 77%) for T4 tumors. With all the technological development, dose escalation, and/or addition of concurrent chemotherapy, 3-year local control close to 100% has been reported (7,111,189).

Distant failure remains the most challenging problem. The risk correlates significantly with both T and N category, but N category is by far the most significant predicting factor. The study from the HKNPCSG (112) showed that the HR of distant failure in patients with N3b disease was as high as 6.26 (95% CI: 4.42 to 8.88) when compared with N0.

Based on the contemporary series with detailed results for different stages (49,130,142), the average 5-year D-FFR varied from 93% for stage I, 85% for stage II, 78% for stage III, to 60% for stage IVA-B. A study of 2,070 patients treated by RT alone in the HKNPCSG series (130) showed that both the presenting stage and achievement of locoregional control were significant predictors for distant failure. The 5-year D-FFR for stages I-IIB versus stages III-IVB were 90% versus 75% for patients who achieved locoregional control, but 81% versus 65% for those with locoregional failure (Fig. 38.31).

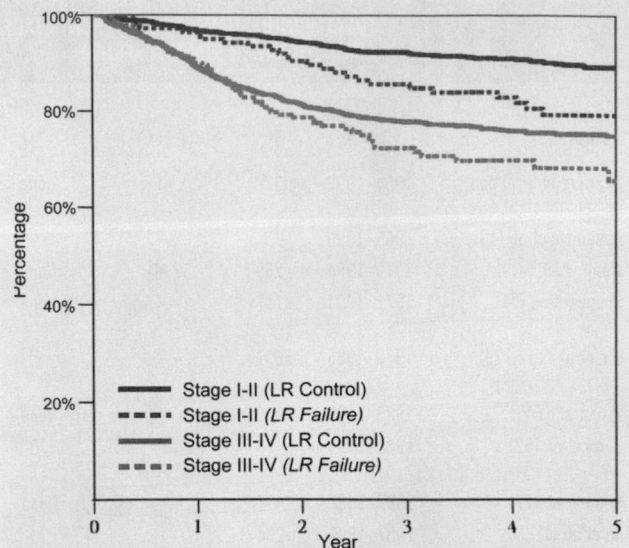

FIGURE 38.31. Distant failure-free rates for 2,070 patients treated by radiotherapy alone showing the significance of presenting stage and locoregional control status. (From Lee A, Sze W, Au J, et al. Treatment results for nasopharyngeal carcinoma in the modern era: The Hong Kong experience. *Int J Radiat Oncol Biol Phys* 2005;61:1107–1116.)

One difficulty in the interpretation of treatment results for different stages is that the phenomenon of stage migration inevitably occurs with changing investigation methods. Detailed analyses of the HKNPCSG series (130) showed that, together with simultaneous changes in treatment provisions, the MRI-staged patients achieved significantly better results for corresponding stages than those who were CT-staged. The treatment results of different stages in the two differently staged groups are shown in Table 38.19 as a reference for contemporary results.

Table 38.19	**TREATMENT RESULTS FOR NASOPHARYNGEAL CARCINOMA ACHIEVED IN HONG KONG (1996–2000)**			
		Groups		**Whole Series**
Results (% at 5 y)	**Stages**	**CT-Staged**	**MRI-Staged**	
Local failure-free rate	T1–2	87	91	88
	T3–4	76	83	79
	All T-categories	84	88	85
Nodal failure-free rate	N0–1	96	97	96
	N2–3	87	91	89
	All N-categories	94	95	94
Distant failure-free rate	Stages I–II	87	90	88
	Stages III–IVB	74	74	74
	All stages	81	79	81
Progression-free survival	Stages I–II	73	79	74
	Stages III–IVB	50	58	53
	All stages	62	66	63
Disease-specific survival	Stages I–II	86	94	88
	Stages III–IVB	69	77	72
	All stages	79	83	80
Overall survival	Stages I–II	83	93	85
	Stages III–IVB	63	72	66
	All stages	74	80	75

CT, computed tomography; MRI, magnetic resonance imaging.
From Lee AWM, Sze WM, Au JSK, et al. Treatment results for nasopharyngeal carcinoma in the modern era: The Hong Kong experience. *Int J Radiat Oncol Biol Phys* 2005;61:1107–1116.

Sequelae of Treatment

Overall Incidence and Types

With the anatomic proximity to critical structures, the need for high radiation doses and adequate field coverage, the risks of radiation-induced toxicities are substantial. The diagnosis of irradiation injury can be difficult. A high degree of awareness is demanded and every effort must be made to exclude other possible causes (tumor recurrence in particular).

Table 38.20 lists the incidence of late toxicities following radical RT with conventional technique (without any concurrent chemotherapy) in five representative series with long-term follow-up. Both the studies on patients treated by RT alone at M.D. Anderson Cancer Center during 1954–1992 (192) and those treated at Mallinckrodt Institute of Radiology during 1956–1991 (19) showed an overall treatment mortality rate of 3%. Both showed encouraging reduction of severe toxicity in later years, even with the use of higher radiation doses. Sanguineti et al. (192) reported that the 10-year actuarial rate of severe toxicity (grade 4–5) decreased from 14% in 1954–1971 to 5% in 1983–1992. Chao and Perez (19) reported a similar reduction rate of toxicity (grade ≥3) from 17% in 1956–1965 to 4% in 1986–1991.

To minimize the risk of late damage, the importance of maximum conformity and precision in RT delivery cannot be overemphasized. The advent of IMRT enhances the feasibility of protecting normal tissues. All the studies using this technique have shown substantial sparing of parotid glands (90,97,135). However, it should be cautioned that attempts at dose escalation together with concurrent chemotherapy might lead to severe toxicities (100).

The extensive use of concurrent CRT increases the risk of toxicities. Preliminary data from NPC-9901 and NPC-9902 trials (124,132) showed significant increase in toxicities (grade ≥3) when patients treated with CRT using the Intergroup regimen were compared with those with RT alone (Table 38.14). Hearing loss is the most common problem with cisplatin-based regimens; RT technique with sparing of cochlea should be attempted as far as possible.

Temporal Lobe Necrosis

Temporal lobe necrosis (TLN) is the most worrisome complication; the study by Lee et al. (126) of 4,527 patients treated during 1976–1985 showed that this accounted for 65% (40/62) of all irradiation-induced deaths. In a study of 1,008 patients with T1 tumors, Lee et al. (115) showed that the 10-year actuarial incidence of TLN ranged from 4.6% to 18.6% for schedules

Table 38.20 INCIDENCE OF LATE TOXICITY FOLLOWING RADIATION WITH CONVENTIONAL TECHNIQUE (WITHOUT CONCURRENT CHEMOTHERAPY) FOR NASOPHARYNGEAL CARCINOMA

Severe Late Complication	Sanguineti et al. (192) (N = 378)	Chao and Perez (19) (N = 164)	Lee et al. (126) (N = 4527)	Yeh et al. (240) (N = 849)	Leung et al. (142) (N = 880)[a]
Period	1954–1992	1956–1991	1976–1985	1983–1998	1990–1998
Radiotherapy					
Total dose (Gy)	61–70	56–69	65[b]	68–76	62.5–66[b]
Dose per fraction (Gy)	NR	1.8–2	2.5–4.2	1.8	2–2.5
Altered fractionation (%)	8	Nil	Nil	Nil	Nil
Sequential chemotherapy (%)	Nil	Nil	8	Nil	20
Overall incidence (%)					
Grading of toxicity	≥3	≥3	≥2	≥1	?
Crude rate	30.4	14	30.8	NR	16.5
Actuarial rate	19 (10-y)	NR	60 (10 y)	NR	14 (5 y)
Treatment mortality	3.2	3	1.4	NR	0.9
Types of complications					
Temporal-lobe necrosis	1.1	1.2	3	6[c]	1.1
Brainstem encephalopathy/ myelopathy	2.4		1		
Cranial neuropathy	4.5		5.3	3.3	6.8
Endocrine dysfunction	7.9		3.5		8.6
Severe epistaxis		1.2	0.6		0.3
Carotid rupture		0.6			
Hearing loss	2.6		8.2	54[c]	
Persistent otitis			2.5	32[c]	
Trismus	2.9	0.6	5.1	12[c]	0.7
Bone damage[d]	2.6	2.4	0.4		
Eyeball damage[e]			0.2		
Soft-tissue necrosis/fistula	1.1	1.8	0.4		0.5
Pharynx stricture/dysphagia		4.2		6[c]	
Soft-tissue fibrosis	4.2		15.9	25[c]	1.4
Persistent lymphedema	0.5	0.6	0.1		
Radiation-induced malignancy			<0.1		

NR, not reported.
[a] Patients with one course of radiotherapy.
[b] Median dose equivalent to 2 Gy/fraction.
[c] Five-year actuarial rate.
[d] Bone necrosis, fracture, or osteomyelitis.
[e] Cataract, retinitis, corneal ulcer.

with fraction sizes of 2.5 to 4.2 Gy. The fractional effect is the most significant risk factor.

In a subsequent study of 1,032 patients with T1-2 tumors treated with conventional 2D technique during 1990–1995, Lee et al. (123) showed that the incidence of symptomatic TLN ranged from 0% (with 2 Gy/fraction, five fractions/week, for 33 fractions) to 24% (3.5 Gy/fraction, three fractions/week, for 17 fractions), and 33% for an altered fractionation schedule (71.2 Gy in 5 weeks). Besides fractional effect, overall treatment time was also found to be a significant factor. Overacceleration and fractional dose >2 Gy should be avoided.

The presenting features in 102 patients with TLN were summarized by Lee et al. (127). Thirty-nine percent presented with vague symptoms (dizziness, poor memory, or behavioral changes); hence, diagnosis was often delayed. Only 31% had classic temporal lobe epilepsy with absence attacks, hallucinations, or déjà vu, and 14% had symptoms of headache, confusion, convulsion, or hemiparesis. Sixteen percent were asymptomatic.

The early classic radiologic feature is fingerlike white matter edema confined to the inferomedial part of the temporal lobes, followed by contrast-enhancing necrosis involving the grey matter (35) (Fig 38.32). Some lesions may resolve spontaneously; others remain stationary or progress to massive edema, cyst formation (Fig 38.33), acute hemorrhage (26), or develop brain abscess (27).

Control of temporal lobe epilepsy by anticonvulsants and close monitoring of symptoms or signs of increased intracranial pressure are the main treatments. Early promising results with high-dose steroids for more than 4 months were hampered with severe and sometimes fatal infection (127), and the apparent high remission rate shown on CT was not confirmed with MRI (114). Hence, intervention with steroids and/or surgery is usually reserved for markedly symptomatic patients.

The possible risk of Kluver-Bucy syndrome is a serious concern when considering bilateral temporal lobectomy (128). A study in Queen Elizabeth Hospital of 520 patients with TLN showed that 9% (49 patients) had temporal lobe surgery performed, and their postsurgery 5-year OS was 32%. Among the six patients who had bilateral lobectomy, none have had Kluver-Bucy syndrome thus far (S. C. K. Law, unpublished data, 2006).

The degree of cognitive dysfunction with TLN correlates with the volume and site of radionecrosis (31). Lesions predominantly in the right and the left side are associated with loss of visual and verbal memory, respectively. General intelligence is usually intact (30).

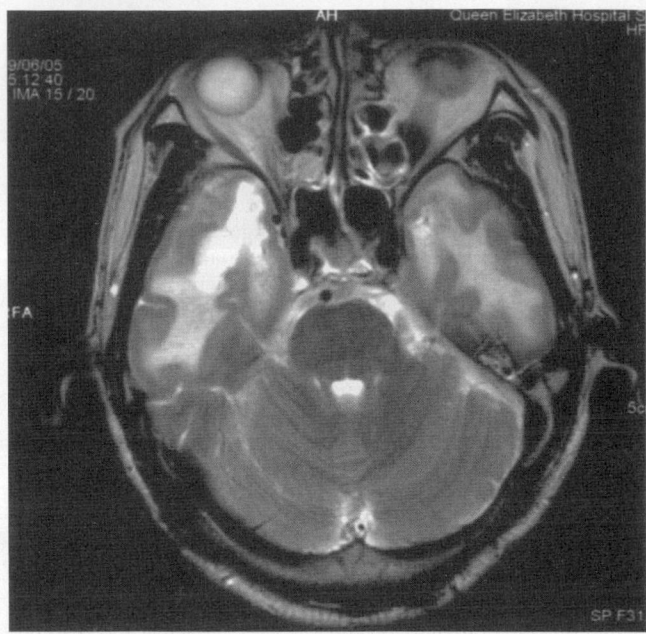

FIGURE 38.33. Early cyst formation at right temporal lobe with bilateral fingerlike edema (T2-weighted axial image).

Brainstem Encephalopathy/Cervical Spinal Cord Myelopathy

In the past, this was a common neurologic sequelae leading to spastic paraparesis or quadriparesis. In the study by Lee et al. (126), 59% of the 44 affected patients progressed rapidly to a debilitated state and 34% died. There was no effective treatment to arrest this pathologic process. Fortunately, this sequela has become rare with improving RT technique and accuracy in delivery. Lee et al. (126) showed that all affected patients were treated before 1983.

Cranial Neuropathy

The last four cranial nerves, especially the twelfth, are the most frequently injured (126,142,149). This is related to marked fibrosis, particularly among patients with an additional boost

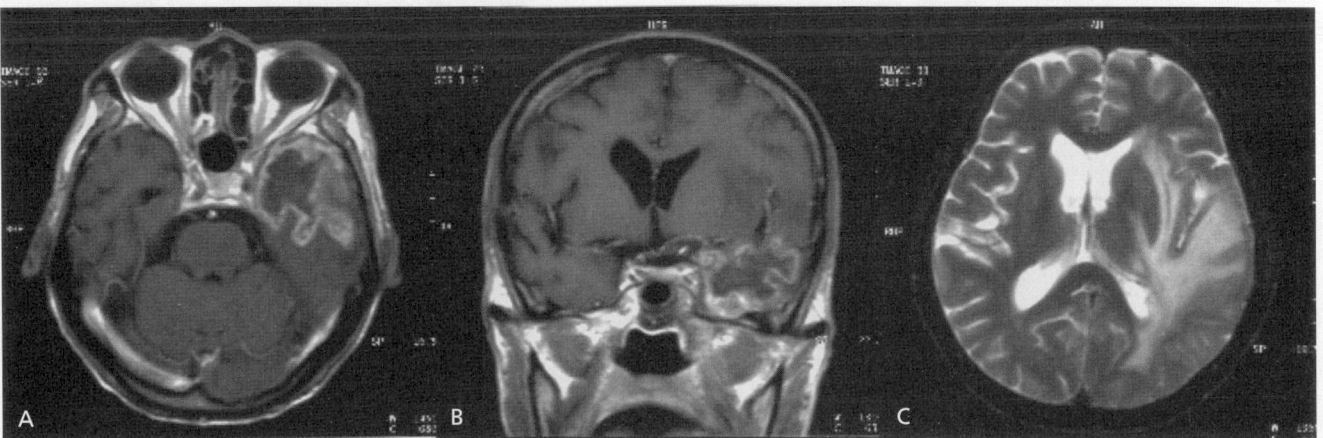

FIGURE 38.32. Temporal lobe necrosis with irregular contrast-enhancing rim and adjacent white matter edema extending to parietal lobe, forming typical fingerlike appearance. **A:** T1-weighted axial image with contrast; **B:** T1-weighted coronal image with contrast; **C:** T2-weighted axial image.

dose to parapharyngeal space. Affected patients usually present with slurring of speech, twitching of neck muscles, and/or swallowing difficulties that can lead to fatal aspiration pneumonia. Wu et al. (233) studied 31 patients with post-RT dysphagia in NPC and found that 77% aspirated after the act of swallowing.

The sixth nerve is another commonly affected nerve, and is frequently associated with TLN (126). Isolated palsy of branches of the fifth nerve is less common, and optic neuropathy is rare with careful attention to the RT technique. Intracranial recurrence must be excluded before making a clinical diagnosis of radiation injury.

Endocrine Dysfunction

Amenorrhea and/or galactorrhea from hyperprolactinemia in female patients are the commonest presenting feature(s), followed by hypothyroidism and hypoadrenalism. Very few male patients complain of impotence or decreased libido.

Symptomatic hypothalamic-pituitary dysfunction was clinically observed in 5% of patients after a median latency of 5 years in the series reported by Lee et al. (126). However, detailed endocrine assessment and longitudinal study by Lam et al. (105) showed that biochemical dysfunction might be detected as early as 1 year after RT, and the 5-year incidence was up to 62% (104). The deficiency of releasing or inhibitory factors suggests that the main damage occurs at the hypothalamus (103,106). Deficiencies in growth hormone, gonadotropins, corticotrophin, and thyrotropin were found, in decreasing order of frequency.

Sham et al. (195), in a randomized trial of 152 patients treated with 2D technique using a hypofractionation schedule (3.5 Gy/fraction, three daily fractions/week, for 17 fractions), showed that additional shielding could significantly reduce the incidence of symptomatic endocrine dysfunction from 11% to 0%, and TLN from 21% to 0%. The importance of maximum conformity for protection of normal tissues cannot be overemphasized.

Aural Toxicity

Hearing loss is a common sequela, particularly for patients treated with concurrent CRT using cisplatin-based regimens. Kwong et al. (102) followed 132 NPC patients with serial audiograms for a median period of 30 months after RT, showed that 24% of patients developed sensorineural deafness (mainly affecting the high-frequency range). Grau et al. (69) further showed significant correlation between hearing loss and the cochlear dose. It should be noted that sudden deafness with late onset (more than 5 years) might result from vascular insufficiency and recover after treatment with a vascular expander like dextran 40 (243).

Another major mechanism of ear complications is dysfunction of eustachian tube (244), causing otitis media with effusion. Lau et al. (108) showed that tinnitus developed in 49% of patients, and persisted in 29% at 1 year. The benefit of prophylactic insertion of ventilation tubes is controversial. Chowdhury et al. (40) showed that patients with tubes inserted had less conductive hearing loss, tinnitus, and/or otitis. However, Skinner et al. (198) showed that this did not lead to long-term benefit for hearing. Chen et al. (21) showed that this might even worsen postirradiation otitis media, with increased risk of ascending infection from all adjacent irradiated areas.

Oral Complications

Xerostomia is almost universal with conventional RT using 2D technique. Jen et al. (84) showed that the salivary flow dropped by half after dose of 7.2 Gy, reached the nadir after 36 Gy, and then further dropped after completion of RT without recovery during the following 2 years. However, with parotid sparing by IMRT (mean parotid dose, 34 Gy), Lee et al. (135) from University of California, San Francisco, reported marked recovery, with grade 2 xerostomia decreasing from 64% at 3 months to 2.4% at 2 years.

Dental decay is commonly associated with xerostomia. Appropriate dental care with prophylactic fluoride treatment and extractions of decayed teeth prior to commencement of RT can help to reduce the risk of dental sequelae (6). Cheng et al. (28) showed that 2.7% of 1,758 patients developed osteoradionecrosis at the maxilla and 1.7% developed it at the mandible. They found no difference in the risk of oesteonecrosis between extractions performed before and after RT. Tong et al. (214) reported that the incidence of complications following post-RT extraction of posterior maxillary teeth could be as high as 29%, with 10.5% developing osteonecrosis.

Carotid Artery Injury/Epistaxis

Stenosis of the extracranial and pseudoaneurysm of the intracranial portion of carotid arteries are two potentially fatal complications. Cheng et al. (29) studied 96 patients with a mean follow-up of 6.7 years after RT for NPC and 96 healthy controls by color flow duplex ultrasonography. Severe stenosis with ≥70% occlusion at the internal or the common carotid artery was found in 16% of patients, but none among the controls. Ultrasound screening of carotids for high-risk patients (age more than 60 years, history of smoking, heart disease, cerebrovascular symptoms) was advocated.

Lam et al. (107) also detected carotid stenosis with ≥50% occlusion in 24 (30%) of 80 patients, 9 of whom had a history of stroke or transient ischemic attack. A high index of suspicion is required. Carotid endarterectomy or endoplasty may be needed for severe cases.

Ruptured pseudoaneurysm presents acutely with massive epistaxis/hemoptysis or severe otalgia, often with a catastrophic outcome (25). This has been reported following IMRT with dose escalation (100) and reirradiation for local recurrence (25). It usually affects the heavily irradiated petrous portion of the internal carotid artery. Urgent diagnosis with angiography and emergency intervention by endovascular occlusion or stenting could be life-saving.

Other causes of intractable epistaxis include severe telangiectasia and hypervascularization in the internal maxillary artery territory. Emergency embolization may also be considered.

Second Malignancies

Radiation-induced malignancy is a rare sequela. In one study, the incidence was 0.04% and the latency was more than 10 years (126). Maxillary osteosarcoma (54) and soft tissue sarcoma (92) are the usual histologic types. Surgery is the only chance of cure, but the prognosis is often poor. A second primary head and neck cancer is relatively uncommon for NPC patients, but Teo et al. (206) reported an excessive risk of tongue cancer at 0.13% per patient-year. The possibility of radiation carcinogenesis cannot be excluded.

▪▪ | Final Remarks

In summary, the current standard recommendation for NPC is RT alone for stages I-II, combined RT and concurrent chemotherapy for stages III-IVB (± bulky stage IIB). Intensity-modulated RT technique is preferred if resources allow. A total dose of about 70 Gy is generally recommended. The Intergroup-0099 regimen of cisplatin-based concurrent and adjuvant chemotherapy with RT at conventional fractionation remains the chemoradiotherapy regimen with the most supporting data. Further enhancement of efficacy by using accelerated fractionation for T3-4 tumors and/or changing the timing of chemotherapy to induction-concurrent sequence for stage IV is worth considering. Verification of these new strategies by randomized trials is awaited.

Patients should be duly informed that, with improving results achievable by modern RT techniques, the absolute magnitude of survival benefits by adding chemotherapy might not be large and that the new treatments do incur higher risk of toxicities. Yet the prognosis for patients with relapse is so gloomy that achieving radical eradication of the cancer by best-quality primary treatment is crucially important. Patients should be encouraged to consider the treatment option that could maximize the chance of tumor control. More accurate prognostication is needed for further refinement of treatment strategies tailored to individual risk patterns.

Medical progress in the battle against NPC is one of the most gratifying successes. This peculiar cancer was invariably lethal before the advent of megavoltage RT, and it was not until the mid-1960s that we saw the first reports showing 25% of patients alive at 5 years (167). Contemporary results show that 5-year overall survival 75% and above can be achieved. Furthermore, the age-standardized incidence rate (per 100,000 male populations) in Hong Kong (one of the most prevalent sites) has steadily decreased from the peak of 40 in 1978 to 16 in 2003. With concerted efforts by all, we are highly optimistic that even greater global success in reducing the health burden by this notorious cancer can be achieved in the near future.

Acknowledgment

The authors thank Doctors W.T. Ng, T.W. Leung, S.K. Au, and T.K. Yau; Mr. Albert Hung, Mr. Michael Lee, Mr. Samuel Leung, Ms. Connie Chan, Ms. Ellie Pang, Ms. K.L. Yuen, and Ms. A. Choi for their collaboration in the preparation of this chapter.

References

1. Al-Amro A, Al-Rajhi N, Khafaga Y, et al. Neoadjuvant chemotherapy followed by concurrent chemo-radiation therapy in locally advanced nasopharyngeal carcinoma. *Int J Radiat Oncol Biol Phys* 2005;62:508–513.
2. Al-Sarraf M, LeBlanc M, Giri PG, et al. Chemoradiotherapy versus radiotherapy in patients with advanced nasopharyngeal cancer: Phase III randomized Intergroup study 0099. *J Clin Oncol* 1998;16:1310–1317.
3. Al-Sarraf M, LeBlanc M, Giri PG, et al. Chemoradiotherapy (CT-RT) vs radiotherapy (RT) in patients (PTS) with advanced nasopharyngeal cancer (NPC). Intergroup (0099) (SWOG8892, RTOG8817, ECOG2388) Phase III Study: Progress report. *J Clin Oncol* 1998;17:385(abstr1483).
4. Au JS, Law CK, Foo W, et al. In-depth evaluation of the AJCC/UICC 1997 staging system of nasopharyngeal carcinoma: Prognostic homogeneity and proposed refinements. *Int J Radiat Oncol Biol Phys* 2003;56:413–426.
5. Baujat B, Audry H, Bourhis J, et al. Chemotherapy in locally advanced nasopharyngeal carcinoma: An individual patient data meta-analysis of eight randomized trials and 1753 patients. *Int J Radiat Oncol Biol Phys* 2006;64:47–56.
6. Bedwinek JM, Shukovsky LJ, Fletcher GH, et al. Osteonecrosis in patients treated with definitive radiotherapy for squamous cell carcinomas of the oral cavity and naso-and oropharynx. *Radiology* 1976;119:665–667.
7. Bucci M, Xia P, Lee N, et al. Intensity modulated radiation therapy for carcinoma of the nasopharynx: An update of the UCSF experience. *Int J Radiat Oncol Biol Phys* 2004;60:S317–318.
8. Buell P. Race and place in the etiology of nasopharyngeal cancer: A study based on California death certificates. *Int J Cancer* 1973;11:268–272.
9. Butler EB, Teh BS, Grant WH, et al. SMART (simultaneous modulated accelerated radiation therapy) boost: A new accelerated fractionation schedule for the treatment of head and neck cancer with intensity modulated radiotherapy. *Int J Radiat Oncol Biol Phys* 1999;45:21–32.
10. Casanova M, Ferrari A, Gandola L, et al. Undifferentiated nasopharyngeal carcinoma in children and adolescents: Comparison between staging systems. *Ann Oncol* 2001;12:1157–1162.
11. Chan AT, Leung SF, Ngan RK, et al. Overall survival after concurrent cisplatin-radiotherapy compared with radiotherapy alone in locoregionally advanced nasopharyngeal carcinoma. *J Natl Cancer Inst* 2005;97:536–539.
12. Chan AT, Ma BB, Lo YM, et al. Phase II study of neoadjuvant carboplatin and paclitaxel followed by radiotherapy and concurrent cisplatin in patients with locoregionally advanced nasopharyngeal carcinoma: Therapeutic monitoring with plasma Epstein-Barr virus DNA. *J Clin Oncol* 2004;22:3053–3060.
13. Chan AT, Teo ML, Lee WY, et al. The significance of keratinizing squamous cell histology in Chinese patients with nasopharyngeal carcinoma. *Clin Oncol (R Coll Radiol)* 1998;10:161–164.
14. Chan AT, Teo PM, Leung TW, et al. A prospective randomized study of chemotherapy adjunctive to definitive radiotherapy in advanced nasopharyngeal carcinoma. *Int J Radiat Oncol Biol Phys* 1995;33:569–577.
15. Chan J, Bray F, McCarron P, et al. Nasopharyngeal carcinoma. In: *Pathology and genetics of head and neck tumours. World Health Organization classification of tumours*. Lyon, France: IARC Press; 2005:85–97.
16. Chang JT, Chan SC, Yen TC, et al. Nasopharyngeal carcinoma staging by (18)F-fluorodeoxyglucose positron emission tomography. *Int J Radiat Oncol Biol Phys* 2005;62:501–507.
17. Chang JT, See LC, Liao CT, et al. Locally recurrent nasopharyngeal carcinoma. *Radiother Oncol* 2000;54:135–142.
18. Chang JT, See LC, Tang SG, et al. The role of brachytherapy in early-stage nasopharyngeal carcinoma. *Int J Radiat Oncol Biol Phys* 1996;36:1019–1024.
19. Chao KS, Perez CA. Nasopharynx. *Principles and practice of radiation oncology*, 4th ed. Philadelphia: Lippincott Williams & Wilkins; 1997:941–961.
20. Chau RM, Teo PM, Choi PH, et al. Three-dimensional dosimetric evaluation of a conventional radiotherapy technique for treatment of nasopharyngeal carcinoma. *Radiother Oncol* 2001;58:143–153.
21. Chen CY, Young YH, Hsu WC, et al. Failure of grommet insertion in post-irradiation otitis media with effusion. *Ann Otol Rhinol Laryngol* 2001;110:746–748.
22. Chen HJ, Leung SW, Su CY. Linear accelerator based radiosurgery as a salvage treatment for skull base and intracranial invasion of recurrent nasopharyngeal carcinomas. *Am J Clin Oncol* 2001;24:255–258.
23. Chen MK, Chen TH, Liu JP, et al. Better prediction of prognosis for patients with nasopharyngeal carcinoma using primary tumor volume. *Cancer* 2004;100:2160–2166.
24. Cheng JC, Chao KS, Low D. Comparison of intensity modulated radiation therapy (IMRT) treatment techniques for nasopharyngeal carcinoma. *Int J Cancer* 2001;96:126–132.
25. Cheng KM, Chan CM, Cheung YL, et al. Endovascular treatment of radiation-induced petrous internal carotid artery aneurysm presenting with acute haemorrhage. A report of two cases. *Acta Neurochir (Wien)* 2001;143:351–355.
26. Cheng KM, Chan CM, Fu YT, et al. Acute hemorrhage in late radiation necrosis of the temporal lobe: Report of five cases and review of the literature. *J Neurooncol* 2001;51:143–150.
27. Cheng KM, Chan CM, Fu YT, et al. Brain abscess formation in radiation necrosis of the temporal lobe following radiation therapy for nasopharyngeal carcinoma. *Acta Neurochir (Wien)* 2000;142:435–440.
28. Cheng SJ, Lee JJ, Ting LL, et al. A clinical staging system and treatment guidelines for maxillary osteoradionecrosis in irradiated nasopharyngeal carcinoma patients. *Int J Radiat Oncol Biol Phys* 2006;64:90–97.
29. Cheng SW, Ting AC, Lam LK, et al. Carotid stenosis after radiotherapy for nasopharyngeal carcinoma. *Arch Otolaryngol Head Neck Surg* 2000;126:517–521.
30. Cheung MC, Chan AS, Law SC, et al. Cognitive function of patients with nasopharyngeal carcinoma with and without temporal lobe radionecrosis. *Arch Neurol* 2000;57:1347–1352.
31. Cheung MC, Chan AS, Law SC, et al. Impact of radionecrosis on cognitive dysfunction in patients after radiotherapy for nasopharyngeal carcinoma. *Cancer* 2003;97:2019–2026.
32. Chi KH, Chang YC, Guo WY, et al. A phase III study of adjuvant chemotherapy in advanced nasopharyngeal carcinoma patients. *Int J Radiat Oncol Biol Phys* 2002;52:1238–1244.
33. Chong VF, Fan YF. Hypoglossal nerve palsy in nasopharyngeal carcinoma. *Eur Radiol* 1998;8:939–945.
34. Chong VF, Fan YF. Pterygopalatine fossa and maxillary nerve infiltration in nasopharyngeal carcinoma. *Head Neck* 1997;19:121–125.
35. Chong VF, Fan YF, Chan LL. Temporal lobe necrosis in nasopharyngeal carcinoma: Pictorial essay. *Australas Radiol* 1997;41:392–397.
36. Chong VF, Fan YF, Khoo JB. Nasopharyngeal carcinoma with intracranial spread: CT and MR characteristics. *J Comput Assist Tomogr* 1996;20:563–569.
37. Chong VF, Mukherji SK, Ng SH, et al. Nasopharyngeal carcinoma: Review of how imaging affects staging. *J Comput Assist Tomogr* 1999;23:984–993.
38. Chong VF, Zhou JY, Khoo JB, et al. Correlation between MR imaging-derived nasopharyngeal carcinoma tumor volume and TNM system. *Int J Radiat Oncol Biol Phys* 2006;64:72–76.
39. Chong Z. Improved local control with intensity modulated radiation therapy in patients with nasopharyngeal carcinoma. *Int J Radiat Oncol Biol Phys* 2004;60:S317 (abstr 1102).
40. Chowdhury CR, Ho JH, Wright A, et al. Prospective study of the effects of ventilation tubes on hearing after radiotherapy for carcinoma of nasopharynx. *Ann Otol Rhinol Laryngol* 1988;97[2 Pt 1]:142–145.
41. Chua DT, Nicholls JM, Sham JS, et al. Prognostic value of epidermal growth factor receptor expression in patients with advanced stage nasopharyngeal carcinoma treated with induction chemotherapy and radiotherapy. *Int J Radiat Oncol Biol Phys* 2004;59:11–20.
42. Chua DT, Sham JS, Au GK. Induction chemotherapy with cisplatin and gemcitabine followed by reirradiation for locally recurrent nasopharyngeal carcinoma. *Am J Clin Oncol* 2005;28:464–471.
43. Chua DT, Sham JS, Choy D, et al. Preliminary report of the Asian-Oceanian Clinical Oncology Association randomized trial comparing cisplatin and epirubicin followed by radiotherapy versus radiotherapy alone in the treatment of patients with locoregionally advanced nasopharyngeal carcinoma. Asian-Oceanian Clinical Oncology Association Nasopharynx Cancer Study Group. *Cancer* 1998;83:2270–2283.
44. Chua DT, Sham JS, Hung KN, et al. Stereotactic radiosurgery as a salvage treatment for locally persistent and recurrent nasopharyngeal carcinoma. *Head Neck* 1999;21:620–626.
45. Chua DT, Sham JS, Kwong DL, et al. Prognostic value of paranasopharyngeal extension of nasopharyngeal carcinoma. A significant factor in local control and distant metastasis. *Cancer* 1996;78:202–210.
46. Chua DT, Sham JS, Kwong DL, et al. Volumetric analysis of tumor extent in nasopharyngeal carcinoma and correlation with treatment outcome. *Int J Radiat Oncol Biol Phys* 1997;39:711–719.
47. Chua DT, Sham JS, Kwong DL, et al. Locally recurrent nasopharyngeal carcinoma: Treatment results for patients with computed tomography assessment. *Int J Radiat Oncol Biol Phys* 1998;41:379–386.
48. Chua DT, Sham JS, Leung LH, et al. Re-irradiation of nasopharyngeal carcinoma with intensity-modulated radiotherapy. *Radiother Oncol* 2005;77:290–294.

49. Chua DT, Sham JS, Wei WI, et al. The predictive value of the 1997 American Joint Committee on Cancer stage classification in determining failure patterns in nasopharyngeal carcinoma. *Cancer* 2001;92:2845–2855.
50. Cmelak AJ, Cox RS, Adler JR, et al. Radiosurgery for skull base malignancies and nasopharyngeal carcinoma. *Int J Radiat Oncol Biol Phys* 1997;37:997–1003.
51. Cooper JS, Cohen R, Stevens RE. A comparison of staging systems for nasopharyngeal carcinoma. *Cancer* 1998;83:213–219.
52. Corry J, Fisher R, Rischin D, et al. Relapse patterns in WHO 2/3 nasopharyngeal cancer: Is there a difference between ethnic Asian vs. non-Asian patients? *Int J Radiat Oncol Biol Phys* 2006;64:63–71.
53. Corry J, Hornby C, Fisher R, et al. "Boomerang" technique': An improved method for conformal treatment of locally advanced nasopharyngeal cancer. *Australas Radiol* 2004;48:170–180.
54. Dickens P, Wei WI, Sham JS. Osteosarcoma of the maxilla in Hong Kong Chinese postirradiation for nasopharyngeal carcinoma. A report of four cases. *Cancer* 1990;66:1924–1926.
55. Dickson RI, Flores AD. Nasopharyngeal carcinoma: An evaluation of 134 patients treated between 1971–1980. *Laryngoscope* 1985;95:276–283.
56. Emami B, Sethi A, Petruzzelli GJ. Influence of MRI on target volume delineation and IMRT planning in nasopharyngeal carcinoma. *Int J Radiat Oncol Biol Phys* 2003;57:481–488.
57. Fee WE Jr, Moir MS, Choi EC, et al. Nasopharyngectomy for recurrent nasopharyngeal cancer: A 2- to 17-year follow-up. *Arch Otolaryngol Head Neck Surg* 2002;128:280–284.
58. Fee WE Jr, Roberson JB Jr, Goffinet DR. Long term survival after surgical resection for recurrent nasopharyngeal cancer after radiotherapy failure. *Arch Otolaryngol Head Neck Surg* 1991;117:1233–1236.
59. Ferlay J, Bray F, Pisani P, et al. Globocan 2000: Cancer incidence, mortality and prevalence worldwide. 10th ed. Lyon, France. IARC Press, 2001.
60. Fisch U. The infratemporal fossa approach for nasopharyngeal tumors. *Laryngoscope* 1983;93:36–44.
61. Fleming I, Cooper J, Henson D.American Joint Committee on Cancer: *AJCC cancer staging manual*, 5th ed. Philadelphia: Lippincott-Raven; 1997:31–39.
62. Fletcher GH. *Textbook of radiotherapy*, 3rd ed. Philadelphia: Lea & Febiger; 1980:322.
63. Fletcher GH, Healey JJ, McGraw J, et al. Nasopharyngeal. In: MacComb W, Fletcher G, eds. *Cancer of the head and neck*. Baltimore, MD: Williams & Wilkins; 1967:152–178
64. Fu KK, Newman H, Phillips TL. Treatment of locally recurrent carcinoma of the nasopharynx. *Radiology* 1975;117:425–431.
65. Fujieda S, Lee K, Sunaga H, et al. Staining of interleukin-10 predicts clinical outcome in patients with nasopharyngeal carcinoma. *Cancer* 1999;85:1439–1445.
66. Gallo O, Bianchi S, Giannini A, et al. Correlations between histopathological and biological findings in nasopharyngeal carcinoma and its prognostic significance. *Laryngoscope* 1991;101:487–493.
67. Geara FB, Sanguineti G, Tucker SL, et al. Carcinoma of the nasopharynx treated by radiotherapy alone: Determinants of distant metastasis and survival. *Radiother Oncol* 1997;43:53–61.
68. Gong QY, Zheng GL, Zhu HY. MRI differentiation of recurrent nasopharyngeal carcinoma from postradiation fibrosis. *Comput Med Imaging Graph* 1991;15:423–429.
69. Grau C, Moller K, Overgaard M, et al. Sensori-neural hearing loss in patients treated with irradiation for nasopharyngeal carcinoma. *Int J Radiat Oncol Biol Phys* 1991;21:723–728.
70. Greene F, Page D, Fleming I, eds. *AJCC cancer staging manual*, 6th ed. New York: Springer-Verlag; 2002.
71. Gueddari BE on behalf of International Nasopharynx Cancer Study Group. Final results of the VUMCA I randomized trial comparing neoadjuvant chemotherapy (CT) (BEC) plus radiotherapy (RT) to RT alone in undifferentiated nasopharyngeal carcinoma (UCNT). *J Clin Oncol* 1998;17:385(abstr1482).
72. Guo X, Lui WO, Qian CN, et al. Identifying cancer-related genes in nasopharyngeal carcinoma cell lines using DNA and mRNA expression profiling analyses. *Int J Oncol* 2002;21:1197–1204.
73. Hareyama M, Sakata K, Shirato H, et al. A prospective, randomized trial comparing neoadjuvant chemotherapy with radiotherapy alone in patients with advanced nasopharyngeal carcinoma. *Cancer* 2002;94:2217–2223.
74. Heng DM, Wee J, Fong KW, et al. Prognostic factors in 677 patients in Singapore with nondisseminated nasopharyngeal carcinoma. *Cancer* 1999;86:1912–1920.
75. Ho JHC. An epidemiologic and clinical study of nasopharyngeal carcinoma. *Int J Radiat Oncol Biol Phys* 1978;4:182–198.
76. Ho JHC. Nasopharynx In: Halnan KE, ed. *Treatment of Cancer.* London: Chapman and Hall; 1982:249–268.
77. Hong MH, Mai HQ, Min HQ, et al. A comparison of the Chinese 1992 and fifth-edition International Union Against Cancer staging systems for staging nasopharyngeal carcinoma. *Cancer* 2000;89:242–247.
78. Hui EP, Chan AT, Pezzella F, et al. Coexpression of hypoxia-inducible factors 1alpha and 2alpha, carbonic anhydrase IX, and vascular endothelial growth factor in nasopharyngeal carcinoma and relationship to survival. *Clin Cancer Res* 2002;8:2595–2604.
79. Hui EP, Leung SF, Au JS, et al. Lung metastasis alone in nasopharyngeal carcinoma: A relatively favorable prognostic group. A study by the Hong Kong Nasopharyngeal Carcinoma Study Group. *Cancer* 2004;101:300–306.
80. Hunt MA, Zelefsky MJ, Wolden S, et al. Treatment planning and delivery of intensity-modulated radiation therapy for primary nasopharynx cancer. *Int J Radiat Oncol Biol Phys* 2001;49:623–632.
81. International Nasopharynx Cancer Study Group: VUMCA I Trial. Preliminary results of a randomized trial comparing neoadjuvant chemotherapy (cisplatin, epirubicin, bleomycin) plus radiotherapy vs. radiotherapy alone in stage IV (> or = N2, M0) undifferentiated nasopharyngeal carcinoma: A positive effect on progression-free survival. International Nasopharynx Cancer Study Group. VUMCA I trial. *Int J Radiat Oncol Biol Phys* 1996;35:463–469.
82. Jen YM, Hsu WL, Chen CY, et al. Different risks of symptomatic brain necrosis in NPC patients treated with different altered fractionated radiotherapy techniques. *Int J Radiat Oncol Biol Phys* 2001;51:344–348.
83. Jen YM, Lin YS, Su WF, et al. Dose escalation using twice-daily radiotherapy for nasopharyngeal carcinoma: Does heavier dosing result in a happier ending? *Int J Radiat Oncol Biol Phys* 2002;54:14–22.
84. Jen YM, Lin YC, Wang YB. Dramatic and prolonged decrease of whole salivary secretion in nasopharyngeal carcinoma patients treated with radiotherapy. *Oral Surg Oral Med Oral Pathol Oral Radiol Endod* 2006;101:332–337.
85. Jen YM, Shih R, Lin YS. Parotid gland-sparing 3-dimensional conformal radiotherapy results in less severe dry mouth in nasopharyngeal cancer patients: A dosimetric and clinical comparison with conventional radiotherapy. *Radiother Oncol* 2005;75:204–209.
86. Jian JJ, Cheng SH, Tsai SY, et al. Improvement of local control of T3 and T4 nasopharyngeal carcinoma by hyperfractionated radiotherapy and concomitant chemotherapy. *Int J Radiat Oncol Biol Phys* 2002;53:344–352.
87. Johnson FM, Garden AS, Palmer JL, et al. A phase I/II study of neoadjuvant chemotherapy followed by radiation with boost chemotherapy for advanced T-stage nasopharyngeal carcinoma. *Int J Radiat Oncol Biol Phys* 2005;63:717–724.
88. Kaasa S, Kragh-Jensen E, Bjordal K, et al. Prognostic factors in patients with nasopharyngeal carcinoma. *Acta Oncol* 1993;32:531–536.
89. Kam MK, Chau RM, Suen J, et al. Intensity-modulated radiotherapy in nasopharyngeal carcinoma: Dosimetric advantage over conventional plans and feasibility of dose escalation. *Int J Radiat Oncol Biol Phys* 2003;56:145–157.
90. Kam MK, Teo PM, Chau RM, et al. Treatment of nasopharyngeal carcinoma with intensity-modulated radiotherapy: The Hong Kong experience. *Int J Radiat Oncol Biol Phys* 2004;60:1440–1450.
91. King AD, Ahuja AT, Leung SF, et al. Neck node metastases from nasopharyngeal carcinoma: MR imaging of patterns of disease. *Head Neck* 2000;22:275–281.
92. King AD, Ahuja AT, Teo PM, et al. Radiation induced sarcomas of the head and neck following radiotherapy for nasopharyngeal carcinoma. *Clin Radiol* 2000;55:684–689.
93. King H, Haenszel K. Cancer mortality among foreign and naive-born Chinese in the United States. *J Chron Dis* 1972;26:623–646.
94. Kostakoglu L, Uysal U, Ozyar E, et al. Monitoring response to therapy with thallium-201 and technetium-99m-sestamibi SPECT in nasopharyngeal carcinoma. *J Nucl Med* 1997;38:1009–1014.
95. Kutcher GJ, Fuks Z, Brenner H, et al. Three-dimensional photon treatment planning for carcinoma of the nasopharynx. *Int J Radiat Oncol Biol Phys* 1991;21:169–182.
96. Kwong DL, Nicholls J, Wei WI, et al. The time course of histologic remission after treatment of patients with nasopharyngeal carcinoma. *Cancer* 1999;85:1446–1453.
97. Kwong DL, Pow EH, Sham JS, et al. Intensity-modulated radiotherapy for early-stage nasopharyngeal carcinoma: A prospective study on disease control and preservation of salivary function. *Cancer* 2004;101:1584–1593.
98. Kwong DL, Sham JS, Au GK, et al. Concurrent and adjuvant chemotherapy for nasopharyngeal carcinoma: A factorial study. *J Clin Oncol* 2004;22:2643–2653.
99. Kwong DL, Sham JS, Chua DT, et al. The effect of interruptions and prolonged treatment time in radiotherapy for nasopharyngeal carcinoma. *Int J Radiat Oncol Biol Phys* 1997;39:703–710.
100. Kwong DL, Sham JS, Leung LH, et al. Preliminary results of radiation dose escalation for locally advanced nasopharyngeal carcinoma. *Int J Radiat Oncol Biol Phys* 2006;64:374–381.
101. Kwong DL, Wei WI, Cheng AC, et al. Long term results of radioactive gold grain implantation for the treatment of persistent and recurrent nasopharyngeal carcinoma. *Cancer* 2001;91:1105–1113.
102. Kwong DL, Wei WI, Sham JS, et al. Sensorineural hearing loss in patients treated for nasopharyngeal carcinoma: A prospective study of the effect of radiation and cisplatin treatment. *Int J Radiat Oncol Biol Phys* 1996;36:281–289.
103. Lam KS, Ho JH, Lee AWM, et al. Symptomatic hypothalamic-pituitary dysfunction in nasopharyngeal carcinoma patients following radiation therapy: A retrospective study. *Int J Radiat Oncol Biol Phys* 1987;13:1343–1350.
104. Lam KS, Tse VK, Wang CC, et al. Effects of cranial irradiation on hypothalamic-pituitary function-a 5-year longitudinal study in patients with nasopharyngeal carcinoma. *Q J Med* 1991;78:165–176.
105. Lam KS, Tse VK, Wang CC, et al. Early effects of cranial irradiation on hypothalamic-pituitary function. *J Clin Endocrinol Metab* 1987;64:418–424.
106. Lam KS, Wang CC, Yeung RT, et al. Hypothalamic hypopituitarism following cranial irradiation for nasopharyngeal carcinoma. *Clin Endocrinol (Oxf)* 1986;24:643–651.
107. Lam WW, Yuen HY, Wong KS, et al. Clinically underdetected asymptomatic and symptomatic carotid stenosis as a late complication of radiotherapy in Chinese nasopharyngeal carcinoma patients. *Head Neck* 2001;23:780–784.
108. Lau SK, Wei WI, Sham JS, et al. Early changes of auditory brain stem evoked response after radiotherapy for nasopharyngeal carcinoma—a prospective study. *J Laryngol Otol* 1992;106:887–892.
109. Law SC, Lam WK, Ng MF, et al. Reirradiation of nasopharyngeal carcinoma with intracavitary mold brachytherapy: An effective means of local salvage. *Int J Radiat Oncol Biol Phys* 2002;54:1095–1113.
110. Le QT, Jones CD, Yau TK, et al. A comparison study of different PCR assays in measuring circulating plasma Epstein-Barr virus DNA levels in patients with nasopharyngeal carcinoma. *Clin Cancer Res* 2005;11:5700–5707.
111. Le QT, Tate D, Koong A, et al. Improved local control with stereotactic radiosurgical boost in patients with nasopharyngeal carcinoma. *Int J Radiat Oncol Biol Phys* 2003;56:1046–1054.
112. Lee AWM, Au JS, Teo PM, et al. Staging of nasopharyngeal carcinoma: Suggestions for improving the current UICC/AJCC Staging System. *Clin Oncol (R Coll Radiol)* 2004;16:269–276.
113. Lee AWM, Chan DK, Fowler JF, et al. Effect of time, dose and fractionation on local control of nasopharyngeal carcinoma. *Radiother Oncol* 1995;36:24–31.
114. Lee AWM, Cheng LO, Ng SH, et al. Magnetic resonance imaging in the clinical diagnosis of late temporal lobe necrosis following radiotherapy for nasopharyngeal carcinoma. *Clin Radiol* 1990;42:24–31.
115. Lee AWM, Foo W, Chappell R, et al. Effect of time, dose, and fractionation on temporal lobe necrosis following radiotherapy for nasopharyngeal carcinoma. *Int J Radiat Oncol Biol Phys* 1998;40:35–42.
116. Lee AWM, Foo W, Law SC, et al. Total biological effect on late reactive tissues following reirradiation for recurrent nasopharyngeal carcinoma. *Int J Radiat Oncol Biol Phys* 2000;46:865–872.
117. Lee AWM, Foo W, Law SC, et al. Staging of nasopharyngeal carcinoma: From Ho's to the new UICC system. *Int J Cancer* 1999;84:179–187.
118. Lee AWM, Foo W, Law SC, et al. Nasopharyngeal carcinoma: Presenting symptoms and duration before diagnosis. *Hong Kong Med J* 1997;3:355–361.

119. Lee AWM, Foo W, Law SC, et al. Reirradiation for recurrent nasopharyngeal carcinoma: Factors affecting the therapeutic ratio and ways for improvement. *Int J Radiat Oncol Biol Phys* 1997;38:43–52.
120. Lee AWM, Foo W, Mang O, et al. Changing epidemiology of nasopharyngeal carcinoma in Hong Kong over a 20-year period (1980–99): An encouraging reduction in both incidence and mortality. *Int J Cancer* 2003;103:680–685.
121. Lee AWM, Foo W, Poon YF, et al. Staging of nasopharyngeal carcinoma: Evaluation of N-staging by Ho and UICC/AJCC systems. Union Internationale Contre le Cancer. American Joint Committee for Cancer. *Clin Oncol (R Coll Radiol)* 1996;8:146–154.
122. Lee AWM, Ko WM, Foo W, et al. Nasopharyngeal carcinoma—time lapse before diagnosis and treatment. *Hong Kong Med J* 1998;4:132–136.
123. Lee AWM, Kwong DL, Leung SF, et al. Factors affecting risk of symptomatic temporal lobe necrosis: Significance of fractional dose and treatment time. *Int J Radiat Oncol Biol Phys* 2002;53:75–85.
124. Lee AWM, Lau WH, Tung SY, et al. Preliminary results of a randomized study on therapeutic gain by concurrent chemotherapy for regionally-advanced nasopharyngeal carcinoma: NPC-9901 Trial by the Hong Kong Nasopharyngeal Cancer Study Group. *J Clin Oncol* 2005;23:6966–6975.
125. Lee AWM, Law SC, Foo W, et al. Retrospective analysis of patients with nasopharyngeal carcinoma treated during 1976–1985: Survival after local recurrence. *Int J Radiat Oncol Biol Phys* 1993;26:773–782.
126. Lee AWM, Law SC, Ng SH, et al. Retrospective analysis of nasopharyngeal carcinoma treated during 1976–1985: Late complications following megavoltage irradiation. *Br J Radiol* 1992;65:918–928.
127. Lee AWM, Ng SH, Ho JH, et al. Clinical diagnosis of late temporal lobe necrosis following radiation therapy for nasopharyngeal carcinoma. *Cancer* 1988;61:1535–1542.
128. Lee AWM, Ng SH, Tse VK, et al. Bilateral temporal lobectomy for necrosis induced by radiotherapy for nasopharyngeal carcinoma. *Acta Oncol* 1993;32:343–344.
129. Lee AWM, Poon YF, Foo W, et al. Retrospective analysis of 5037 patients with nasopharyngeal carcinoma treated during 1976–1985: Overall survival and patterns of failure. *Int J Radiat Oncol Biol Phys* 1992;23:261–270.
130. Lee AWM, Sze WM, Au JS, et al. Treatment results for nasopharyngeal carcinoma in the modern era: The Hong Kong experience. *Int J Radiat Oncol Biol Phys* 2005;61:1107–1116.
131. Lee AWM, Sze WM, Yau TK, et al. Retrospective analysis on treating nasopharyngeal carcinoma with accelerated fractionation (6 fractions per week) in comparison with conventional fractionation (5 fractions per week): Report on 3-year tumor control and normal tissue toxicity. *Radiother Oncol* 2001;58:121–130.
132. Lee AWM, Tung SY, Chan AT, et al. Preliminary results of a randomized study (NPC-9902 Trial) on therapeutic gain by concurrent chemotherapy and/or accelerated fractionation for locally-advanced nasopharyngeal carcinoma. *Int J Radiat Oncol Biol Phys* 2006;66:142–151.
133. Lee AWM, Yau TK, Wong DH, et al. Treatment of stage IV(A-B) nasopharyngeal carcinoma by induction-concurrent chemoradiotherapy and accelerated fractionation. *Int J Radiat Oncol Biol Phys* 2005;63:1331–1338.
134. Lee N, Hoffman R, Phillips TL, et al. Managing nasopharyngeal carcinoma with intracavitary brachytherapy: One institution's 45-year experience. *Brachytherapy* 2002;1:74–82.
135. Lee N, Xia P, Quivey JM, et al. Intensity-modulated radiotherapy in the treatment of nasopharyngeal carcinoma: An update of the UCSF experience. *Int J Radiat Oncol Biol Phys* 2002;53:12–22.
136. Leibel SA, Kutcher GJ, Harrison LB, et al. Improved dose distributions for 3D conformal boost treatments in carcinoma of the nasopharynx. *Int J Radiat Oncol Biol Phys* 1991;20:823–833.
137. Leow YH, Goh CL. Malignancy in adult dermatomyositis. *Int J Dermatol* 1997;36:904–907.
138. Leung SF, Chan AT, Zee B, et al. Pretherapy quantitative measurement of circulating Epstein-Barr virus DNA is predictive of posttherapy distant failure in patients with early-stage nasopharyngeal carcinoma of undifferentiated type. *Cancer* 2003;98:288–291.
139. Leung SF, Kreel L, Tsao SY. Asymptomatic temporal lobe injury after radiotherapy for nasopharyngeal carcinoma: Incidence and determinants. *Br J Radiol* 1992;65:710–714.
140. Leung TW, Tung SY, Sze WK, et al. Salvage brachytherapy for patients with locally persistent nasopharyngeal carcinoma. *Int J Radiat Oncol Biol Phys* 2000;47:405–412.
141. Leung TW, Tung SY, Sze WK, et al. Salvage radiation therapy for locally recurrent nasopharyngeal carcinoma. *Int J Radiat Oncol Biol Phys* 2000;48:1331–1338.
142. Leung TW, Tung SY, Sze WK, et al. Treatment results of 1070 patients with nasopharyngeal carcinoma: An analysis of survival and failure patterns. *Head Neck* 2005;27:555–565.
143. Leung TW, Tung SY, Wong VY, et al. Nasopharyngeal intracavitary brachytherapy: The controversy of T2b disease. *Cancer* 2005;104:1648–1655.
144. Levendag PC, Lagerwaard FJ, Noever I, et al. Role of endocavitary brachytherapy with or without chemotherapy in cancer of the nasopharynx. *Int J Radiat Oncol Biol Phys* 2002;52:755–768.
145. Lin JC, Chen KY, Jan JS, et al. Partially hyperfractionated accelerated radiotherapy and concurrent chemotherapy for advanced nasopharyngeal carcinoma. *Int J Radiat Oncol Biol Phys* 1996;36:1127–1136.
146. Lin JC, Jan JS, Hsu CY. Concurrent chemoradiotherapy versus radiotherapy alone for advanced nasopharyngeal carcinoma: Positive effect on overall and progression-free survival. *J Clin Oncol* 2003;21:637–637.
147. Lin JC, Liang WM, Jan JS, et al. Another way to estimate outcome of advanced nasopharyngeal carcinoma-is concurrent chemoradiotherapy adequate? *Int J Radiat Oncol Biol Phys* 2004;60:156–164.
148. Lin JC, Wang WY, Chen KY, et al. Quantification of plasma Epstein-Barr virus DNA in patients with advanced nasopharyngeal carcinoma. *N Engl J Med* 2004;350:2461–2470.
149. Lin YS, Jen YM, Lin JC. Radiation-related cranial nerve palsy in patients with nasopharyngeal carcinoma. *Cancer* 2002;95:404–409.
150. Lo YM, Chan AT, Chan LY, et al. Molecular prognostication of nasopharyngeal carcinoma by quantitative analysis of circulating Epstein-Barr virus DNA. *Cancer Res* 2000;60:6878–6881.
151. Lo YM, Chan LY, Chan AT, et al. Quantitative and temporal correlation between circulating cell-free Epstein-Barr virus DNA and tumor recurrence in nasopharyngeal carcinoma. *Cancer Res* 1999;59:5452–5455.
152. Lo YM, Chan LY, Lo KW, et al. Quantitative analysis of cell-free Epstein-Barr virus DNA in plasma of patients with nasopharyngeal carcinoma. *Cancer Res* 1999;59:1188–1191.
153. Low JS, Heng DM, Wee JT. The question of T2a and N3a in the UICC/AJCC (1997) staging system for nasopharyngeal carcinoma. *Clin Oncol (R Coll Radiol)* 2004;16:581–583.
154. Lu JJ, Shakespeare TP, Tan LK, et al. Adjuvant fractionated high-dose-rate intracavitary brachytherapy after external beam radiotherapy in Tl and T2 nasopharyngeal carcinoma. *Head Neck* 2004;26:389–395.
155. Lu TX, Mai WY, Teh BS, et al. Initial experience using intensity-modulated radiotherapy for recurrent nasopharyngeal carcinoma. *Int J Radiat Oncol Biol Phys* 2004;58:682–687.
156. Luk NM, Yu KH, Choi CL, et al. Skin metastasis from nasopharyngeal carcinoma in four Chinese patients. *Clin Exp Dermatol* 2004;29:28–31.
157. Luo RX, Tang QX, Guo KP, et al. Comparison of continuous and split-course radiotherapy for nasopharyngeal carcinoma-an analysis of 1446 cases with squamous cell carcinoma grade 3. *Int J Radiat Oncol Biol Phys* 1994;30:1107–1109.
158. Ma BB, Poon TC, To KF, et al. Prognostic significance of tumor angiogenesis, Ki 67, p53 oncoprotein, epidermal growth factor receptor and HER2 receptor protein expression in undifferentiated nasopharyngeal carcinoma-a prospective study. *Head Neck* 2003;25:864–872.
159. Ma J, Mai HQ, Hong MH, et al. Is the 1997 AJCC staging system for nasopharyngeal carcinoma prognostically useful for Chinese patient populations? *Int J Radiat Oncol Biol Phys* 2001;50:1181–1189.
160. Ma J, Mai HQ, Hong MH, et al. Results of a prospective randomized trial comparing neoadjuvant chemotherapy plus radiotherapy with radiotherapy alone in patients with locoregionally advanced nasopharyngeal carcinoma. *J Clin Oncol* 2001;19:1350–1357.
161. Marcial VA, Hanley JA, Chang C, et al. Split-course radiation therapy of carcinoma of the nasopharynx: Results of a national collaborative clinical trial of the Radiation Therapy Oncology Group. *Int J Radiat Oncol Biol Phys* 1980;6:409–414.
162. Marks JE, Bedwinek JM, Lee F, et al. Dose-response analysis for nasopharyngeal carcinoma: An historical perspective. *Cancer* 1982;50:1042–1050.
163. Marks JE, Phillips JL,Menck HR. The National Cancer Data Base report on the relationship of race and national origin to the histology of nasopharyngeal carcinoma. *Cancer* 1998;83:582–588.
164. Masuda M, Shinokuma A, Hirakawa N, et al. Expression of bcl-2-, p53, and Ki-67 and outcome of patients with primary nasopharyngeal carcinomas following DNA-damaging treatment. *Head Neck* 1998;20:640–644.
165. Mesic JB, Fletcher GH, Goepfert H. Megavoltage irradiation of epithelial tumors of the nasopharynx. *Int J Radiat Oncol Biol Phys* 1981;7:447–453.
166. Morton RP, Liavaag PG, McLean M, et al. Transcervico-mandibulo-palatal approach for surgical salvage of recurrent nasopharyngeal cancer. *Head Neck* 1996;18:352–358.
167. Moss WT. *Therapeutic radiology*, 2nd ed. St Louis, MO: Mosby; 1965:142–180.
168. Ng RW, Wei WI. Elimination of palatal fistula after the maxillary swing procedure. *Head Neck* 2005;27:608–612.
169. Ng SH, Chang TC, Ko SF, et al. Nasopharyngeal carcinoma: MRI and CT assessment. *Neuroradiology* 1997;39:741–746.
170. Ng T, Richards GM, Emery RS, et al. Customized conformal high-dose-rate brachytherapy boost for limited-volume nasopharyngeal cancer. *Int J Radiat Oncol Biol Phys* 2005;61:754–761.
171. Ng WT, Lee AWM, Kan WK, et al. Pattern of nodal involvement in patients with nasopharyngeal carcinoma and possibility of re-defining N3 category by magnetic resonance imaging. East-West Symposium on Nasopharyngeal Cancer; June 16–18, 2005; Toronto, Canada.
172. Ngan RK, Yiu HH, Cheng HK, et al. Central nervous system metastasis from nasopharyngeal carcinoma: A report of two patients and a review of the literature. *Cancer* 2002;94:398–405.
173. Nishioka T, Shirato H, Kagei K, et al. Skull-base invasion of nasopharyngeal carcinoma: Magnetic resonance imaging findings and therapeutic implications. *Int J Radiat Oncol Biol Phys* 2000;47:395–400.
174. Oh JL, Vokes EE, Kies MS, et al. Induction chemotherapy followed by concomitant chemoradiotherapy in the treatment of locoregionally advanced nasopharyngeal cancer. *Ann Oncol* 2003;14:564–569.
175. Overgaard J, Hansen HS, Specht L, et al. Five compared with six fractions per week of conventional radiotherapy of squamous-cell carcinoma of head and neck: DAHANCA 6 and 7 randomised controlled trial. *Lancet* 2003;362:933–940.
176. Ozyar E, Yildiz F, Akyol FH, et al. Comparison of AJCC 1988 and 1997 classifications for nasopharyngeal carcinoma. American Joint Committee on Cancer. *Int J Radiat Oncol Biol Phys* 1999;44:1079–1087.
177. Ozyar E, Yildiz F, Akyol FH, et al. Adjuvant high-dose-rate brachytherapy after external beam radiotherapy in nasopharyngeal carcinoma. *Int J Radiat Oncol Biol Phys* 2002;52:101–108.
178. Pai PC, Chuang CC, Wei KC, et al. Stereotactic radiosurgery for locally recurrent nasopharyngeal carcinoma. *Head Neck* 2002;24:748–753.
179. Pak MW, To KF, Lo YM, et al. Nasopharyngeal carcinoma in situ (NPCIS)—pathologic and clinical perspectives. *Head Neck* 2002;24:989–995.
180. Palazzi M, Guzzo M, Tomatis S, et al. Improved outcome of nasopharyngeal carcinoma treated with conventional radiotherapy. *Int J Radiat Oncol Biol Phys* 2004;60:1451–1458.
181. Parkin DM, Whelan SL, Ferlay J, et al., eds. *Cancer incidence in five continents*, vol. VII. IRAC Scientific Publications Number 143. Lyon, France: IRAC; 1997:334–337.
182. Perez CA, Ackerman LV, Mill WB, et al. Cancer of the nasopharynx. Factors influencing prognosis. *Cancer* 1969;24:1–17.
183. Perez CA, Devineni VR, Marcial-Vega V, et al. Carcinoma of the nasopharynx: Factors affecting prognosis. *Int J Radiat Oncol Biol Phys* 1992;23:271–280.
184. Poirier S, Ohshima H, de-The G, et al. Volatile nitrosamine levels in common foods from Tunisia, south China and Greenland, high-risk areas for nasopharyngeal carcinoma (NPC). *Int J Cancer* 1987;39:293–296.
185. Poon D, Yap SP, Wong ZW, et al. Concurrent chemoradiotherapy in locoregionally recurrent nasopharyngeal carcinoma. *Int J Radiat Oncol Biol Phys* 2004;59:1312–1318.
186. Pryzant RM, Wendt CD, Delclos L, et al. Re-treatment of nasopharyngeal carcinoma in 53 patients. *Int J Radiat Oncol Biol Phys* 1992;22:941–947.
187. Qian CN, Zhang CQ, Guo X, et al. Elevation of serum vascular endothelial growth factor in male patients with metastatic nasopharyngeal carcinoma. *Cancer* 2000;88:255–261.

188. Raab-Traub N. Epstein-Barr virus in the pathogenesis of NPC. *Semin Cancer Biol* 2002;12:431–441.
189. Rischin D, Corry J, Smith J. Excellent disease control and survival in patients with advanced nasopharyngeal cancer treated with chemoradiation. *J Clin Oncol* 2002;20:1845–1852.
190. Rossi A, Molinari R, Boracchi P, et al. Adjuvant chemotherapy with vincristine, cyclophosphamide, and doxorubicin after radiotherapy in local-regional nasopharyngeal cancer: Results of a 4-year multicenter randomized study. *J Clin Oncol* 1988;6:1401–1410.
191. Roychowdhury DF, Tseng A Jr, Fu KK, et al. New prognostic factors in nasopharyngeal carcinoma. Tumor angiogenesis and C-erbB2 expression. *Cancer* 1996;77:1419–1426.
192. Sanguineti G, Geara FB, Garden AS, et al. Carcinoma of the nasopharynx treated by radiotherapy alone: Determinants of local and regional control. *Int J Radiat Oncol Biol Phys* 1997;37:985–996.
193. Sham JS, Choy D. Prognostic factors of nasopharyngeal carcinoma: A review of 759 patients. *Br J Radiol* 1990;63:51–58.
194. Sham JS, Choy D. Prognostic value of paranasopharyngeal extension of nasopharyngeal carcinoma on local control and short-term survival. *Head Neck* 1991;13:298–310.
195. Sham JS, Choy D, Kwong PW, et al. Radiotherapy for nasopharyngeal carcinoma: Shielding the pituitary may improve therapeutic ratio. *Int J Radiat Oncol Biol Phys* 1994;29:699–704.
196. Sham JS, Choy D, Wei WI. Nasopharyngeal carcinoma: Orderly neck node spread. *Int J Radiat Oncol Biol Phys* 1990;19:929–933.
197. Sham JS, Wei WI, Nicholls J, et al. Extent of nasopharyngeal carcinoma involvement inside the nasopharynx. Lack of prognostic value on local control. *Cancer* 1992;69:854–859.
198. Skinner D, Lesser T, Richard S. A 15-year follow-up of a controlled trial of the use of grommets in glue ear. *Clin Otolaryngol* 1988;13:341–346.
199. Sobin L. International Union Against Cancer (UICC): *TNM classification of malignant tumours*, 6th ed. New York: Wiley-Liss; 2002.
200. Sobin L, Wittekind C. International Union Against Cancer (UICC): *TNM classification of malignant tumours*, 5th ed. New York: Wiley-Liss; 1997.
201. Som PM, Curtin HD. *Head and neck imaging*, 3rd ed. St Louis, MO: Mosby, 1999.
202. Su CK, Wang CC. Prognostic value of Chinese race in nasopharyngeal cancer. *Int J Radiat Oncol Biol Phys* 2002;54:752–758.
203. Su CY, Lui CC. Perineural invasion of the trigeminal nerve in patients with nasopharyngeal carcinoma. Imaging and clinical correlations. *Cancer* 1996;78:2063–2069.
204. Syed AM, Puthawala AA, Damore SJ, et al. Brachytherapy for primary and recurrent nasopharyngeal carcinoma: 20 years' experience at Long Beach Memorial. *Int J Radiat Oncol Biol Phys* 2000;47:1311–1321.
205. Sze WM, Lee AWM, Yau TK, et al. Primary tumor volume of nasopharyngeal carcinoma: Prognostic significance for local control. *Int J Radiat Oncol Biol Phys* 2004;59:21–27.
206. Teo PM, Chan AT, Leung SF, et al. Increased incidence of tongue cancer after primary radiotherapy for nasopharyngeal carcinoma-the possibility of radiation carcinogenesis. *Eur J Cancer* 1999;35:219–225.
207. Teo PM, Kwan WH, Chan AT, et al. How successful is high-dose (> or = 60 Gy) reirradiation using mainly external beams in salvaging local failures of nasopharyngeal carcinoma? *Int J Radiat Oncol Biol Phys* 1998;40:897–913.
208. Teo PM, Leung SF, Chan AT, et al. Final report of a randomized trial on altered-fractionated radiotherapy in nasopharyngeal carcinoma prematurely terminated by significant increase in neurologic complications. *Int J Radiat Oncol Biol Phys* 2000;48:1311–1322.
209. Teo PM, Leung SF, Lee WY, et al. Intracavitary brachytherapy significantly enhances local control of early T-stage nasopharyngeal carcinoma: The existence of a dose-tumor-control relationship above conventional tumoricidal dose. *Int J Radiat Oncol Biol Phys* 2000;46:445–458.
210. Teo PM, Shiu W, Leung SF, et al. Prognostic factors in nasopharyngeal carcinoma investigated by computer tomography—an analysis of 659 patients. *Radiother Oncol* 1992;23:79–93.
211. Teo PM, Tai TH, Choy D. Nasopharyngeal carcinoma with dermatomyositis. *Int J Radiat Oncol Biol Phys* 1989;16:471–474.
212. Teo PM, Tsao SY, Shiu W, et al. A clinical study of 407 cases of nasopharyngeal carcinoma in Hong Kong. *Int J Radiat Oncol Biol Phys* 1989;17:515–530.
213. Teo PM, Yu P, Lee WY, et al. Significant prognosticators after primary radiotherapy in 903 nondisseminated nasopharyngeal carcinoma evaluated by computer tomography. *Int J Radiat Oncol Biol Phys* 1996;36:291–304.
214. Tong AC, Leung AC, Cheng JC, et al. Incidence of complicated healing and osteoradionecrosis following tooth extraction in patients receiving radiotherapy for treatment of nasopharyngeal carcinoma. *Aust Dent J* 1999;44:187–194.
215. Van Den Brekel MWM, Stel HV, Castelijns JA. Cervical lymph node metastasis: Assessment of radiologic criteria. *Radiology* 1990;177:379–384.
216. Vikram B, Mishra S. Permanent iodine-125 (I-125) boost implants after external radiation therapy in nasopharyngeal cancer. *Int J Radiat Oncol Biol Phys* 1994;28:699–701.
217. Vikram B, Mishra UB, Strong EW, et al. Patterns of failure in carcinoma of the nasopharynx: I. Failure at the primary site. *Int J Radiat Oncol Biol Phys* 1985;11:1455–1459.
218. Waldron J, Tin MM, Keller A, et al. Limitation of conventional two dimensional radiation therapy planning in nasopharyngeal carcinoma. *Radiother Oncol* 2003;68:153–161.
219. Wang CC. Carcinoma of the nasopharynx. In: Wang CC. *Radiation therapy for head and neck neoplasms*, 3rd ed. New York: Wiley-Liss; 1997:265.
220. Wang CC. Improved local control of nasopharyngeal carcinoma after intracavitary brachytherapy boost. *Am J Clin Oncol* 1991;14:5–8.
221. Wang CC. Re-irradiation of recurrent nasopharyngeal carcinoma-treatment techniques and results. *Int J Radiat Oncol Biol Phys* 1987;13:953–956.
222. Wee J, Tan EH, Tai BC. Randomized trial of radiotherapy versus concurrent chemoradiotherapy followed by adjuvant chemotherapy in patients with American Joint Committee on Cancer/International Union Against Cancer Stage III and IV nasopharyngeal cancer of the endemic variety. *J Clin Oncol* 2005;23:6730–6738.
223. Wei WI. Cancer of the nasopharynx: Functional surgical salvage. *World J Surg* 2003;27:844–848.
224. Wei WI, Ho CM, Wong MP, et al. Pathological basis of surgery in the management of postradiotherapy cervical metastasis in nasopharyngeal carcinoma. *Arch Otolaryngol Head Neck Surg* 1992;118:923–929.
225. Wei WI, Ho WK, Cheng AC, et al. Management of extensive cervical nodal metastasis in nasopharyngeal carcinoma after radiotherapy: A clinicopathological study. *Arch Otolaryngol Head Neck Surg* 2001;127:1457–1462.
226. Wei WI, Lam KH, Ho CM, et al. Efficacy of radical neck dissection for the control of cervical metastasis after radiotherapy for nasopharyngeal carcinoma. *Am J Surg* 1990;160:439–442.
227. Wei WI, Lam KH, Sham JS. New approach to the nasopharynx: The maxillary swing approach. *Head Neck* 1991;13:200–207.
228. Wei WI, Sham JS. Nasopharyngeal carcinoma. *Lancet* 2005;365:2041–2054.
229. Wei WI, Yuen AP, Ng RW, et al. Quantitative analysis of plasma cell-free Epstein-Barr virus DNA in nasopharyngeal carcinoma after salvage nasopharyngectomy: A prospective study. *Head Neck* 2004;26:878–883.
230. Wolden SL, Chen WC, Pfister DG, et al. Intensity-modulated radiation therapy (IMRT) for nasopharyngeal carcinoma: Update of the Memorial Sloan-Kettering experience. *Int J Radiat Oncol Biol Phys* 2006;64:57–62.
231. Wolden SL, Zelefsky MJ, Hunt MA, et al. Failure of a 3D conformal boost to improve radiotherapy for nasopharyngeal carcinoma. *Int J Radiat Oncol Biol Phys* 2001;49:1229–1234.
232. Wolden SL, Zelefsky MJ, Kraus DH, et al. Accelerated concomitant boost radiotherapy and chemotherapy for advanced nasopharyngeal carcinoma. *J Clin Oncol* 2001;19:1105–1110.
233. Wu CH, Hsiao TY, Ko JY, et al. Dysphagia after radiotherapy: Endoscopic examination of swallowing in patients with nasopharyngeal carcinoma. *Ann Otol Rhinol Laryngol* 2000;109:320–325.
234. Xia P, Fu KK, Wong GW, et al. Comparison of treatment plans involving intensity-modulated radiotherapy for nasopharyngeal carcinoma. *Int J Radiat Oncol Biol Phys* 2000;48:329–337.
235. Xia P, Lee N, Liu YM, et al. A study of planning dose constraints for treatment of nasopharyngeal carcinoma using a commercial inverse treatment planning system. *Int J Radiat Oncol Biol Phys* 2004;59:886–896.
236. Xiao J, Xu G, Miao Y. Fractionated stereotactic radiosurgery for 50 patients with recurrent or residual nasopharyngeal carcinoma. *Int J Radiat Oncol Biol Phys* 2001;51:164–170.
237. Yan JH, Hu YH, Gu XZ. Radiation therapy of recurrent nasopharyngeal carcinoma. Report on 219 patients. *Acta Radiol Oncol* 1983;22:23–28.
238. Yau TK, Lee AWM, Wong DHM. Induction chemotherapy with Cisplatin and Gemcitabine followed by accelerated radiotherapy and concurrent cisplatin in patients with stage IV(A-B) nasopharyngeal carcinoma. *Head Neck* 2006;28:880–887.
239. Yau TK, Sze WM, Lee WM, et al. Effectiveness of brachytherapy and fractionated stereotactic radiotherapy boost for persistent nasopharyngeal carcinoma. *Head Neck* 2004;26:1024–1030.
240. Yeh SA, Tang Y, Lui CC, et al. Treatment outcomes and late complications of 849 patients with nasopharyngeal carcinoma treated with radiotherapy alone. *Int J Radiat Oncol Biol Phys* 2005;62:672–679.
241. Yen RF, Hung RL, Pan MH, et al. 18 Fluoro-2-deoxyglucose positron emission tomography in detecting residual/recurrent nasopharyngeal carcinomas and comparison with magnetic resonance imaging. *Cancer* 2003;98:283–287.
242. Yip TT, Ngan RK, Lau WH, et al. A possible prognostic role of immunoglobulin-G antibody against recombinant Epstein-Barr virus BZLF-1 transactivator protein ZEBRA in patients with nasopharyngeal carcinoma. *Cancer* 1994;74:2414–2424.
243. Young YH, Lou PJ. Post-irradiation sudden deafness. *J Laryngol Otol* 1999;113:815–817.
244. Young YH, Lu YC. Mechanism of hearing loss in irradiated ears: A long-term longitudinal study. *Ann Otol Rhinol Laryngol* 2001;110:904–906.
245. Yu MC, Garabrant DH, Huang TB, et al. Occupational and other non-dietary risk factors for nasopharyngeal carcinoma in Guangzhou, China. *Int J Cancer* 1990;45:1033–1039.
246. Zheng XK, Chen LH, Chen YQ, et al. Three-dimensional conformal radiotherapy versus intracavitary brachytherapy for salvage treatment of locally persistent nasopharyngeal carcinoma. *Int J Radiat Oncol Biol Phys* 2004;60:165–170.
247. Zheng XK, Ma J, Chen LH, et al. Dosimetric and clinical results of three-dimensional conformal radiotherapy for locally recurrent nasopharyngeal carcinoma. *Radiother Oncol* 2005;75:197–203.
248. Zheng Z, Pan J, Chu B, et al. Downregulation and abnormal expression of E-cadherin and beta-catenin in nasopharyngeal carcinoma: Close association with advanced disease stage and lymph node metastasis. *Hum Pathol* 1999;30:458–466.

Clinical Radiation Oncology

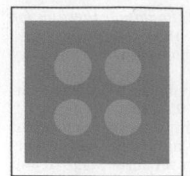

Chapter 39
Nasal Cavity and Paranasal Sinuses

Anesa Ahamad, K. Kian Ang

Anatomy

Nasal Vestibule

The nasal vestibule is the triangular-shaped space located inside the aperture of the nostril as a slight dilatation that extends as a small recess toward the apex of the nose. It is defined laterally by the alae, medially by the membranous septum, the distal end of the cartilaginous septum and columella, and inferiorly by the adjacent floor of the nasal cavity. It is lined by skin containing hairs and sebaceous glands; therefore, tumors at this location are those that frequently arise from the skin, usually squamous cell cancers (23) but may occasionally be basal cell carcinoma (43), sebaceous carcinoma (50), melanoma (57), non-Hodgkin's lymphoma (66).

Nasal Cavity

The nasal cavity extends from the hard palate inferiorly to the base of skull superiorly. It is above and behind the vestibule and is defined anteriorly by the transition from skin to mucous membrane and posteriorly by the choanae, which open directly into the nasopharynx (12). The lateral walls correspond with the medial walls of the maxillary sinuses and consist of thin bony structures that have three shell-shaped projections (superior, middle, and inferior conchae or turbinates) into the nasal cavity. The septum divides the nasal cavity into right and left halves.

Each nasal cavity contains an olfactory region, consisting of the superior nasal concha and the opposed part of the septum, and a respiratory region, which comprises the rest of the cavity. Within the olfactory region, the olfactory nerves from the superior nasal concha and the upper third of the septum penetrate the roof of the nasal cavity and exit through the cribriform plate. The respiratory region comprises the remaining part of the nasal cavity and contains orifices connecting the nasal cavity with the paranasal sinuses. The superior meatus connects the nasal cavity with the posterior ethmoid cells, the middle meatus with the anterior and middle ethmoid cells and the frontal and maxillary sinuses, and the inferior meatus with the nasolacrimal duct. The sphenoid sinus drains into the nasal cavity through an opening in the anterior wall.

Ethmoid Sinuses

The ethmoid sinuses are composed of several small cavities, the ethmoid air cells, within the ethmoid labyrinth located below the anterior cranial fossa and between the nasal cavity and the orbit. They are separated from the orbital cavity by a thin, porous bone, the *lamina papyracea*, and from the anterior cranial fossa by a portion of the frontal bone, the *fovea ethmoidalis*. They are in close proximity to the optic nerves laterally and the optic chiasm posteriorly. The ethmoid sinuses are divided into anterior, middle, and posterior groups of air cells. The middle ethmoid cells open directly into the middle meatus. The anterior cells may drain indirectly into the middle meatus via the infundibulum. The posterior cells open directly into the superior meatus.

Maxillary Sinuses

The maxillary sinuses are the largest of the paranasal sinuses. They are pyramid-shaped cavities located in the maxillae. The lateral walls of the nasal cavity form the base and the roofs correspond to the orbital floors, which contain the infraorbital canals. The floors of the maxillary sinuses are composed of the alveolar processes. The apices extend toward and frequently into the zygomatic bones. Secretions drain by mucociliary action into the middle meatus via the hiatus semilunaris through an aperture near the roof of the maxillary sinus. Ohngren's line is a theoretic plane dividing each maxillary sinus into the suprastructure and infrastructure; it is defined by connecting the medial canthus with the angle of the mandible.

Sphenoid Sinus and Frontal Sinuses

The sphenoid bone forms a midline inner cavity that communicates with the nasal cavity through an aperture in its anterior wall. It is directly apposed superiorly to the pituitary gland and optic chiasm, laterally to the cavernous sinuses, anteriorly to the ethmoid sinuses and nasal cavity, and inferiorly to the nasopharynx. The paired, typically asymmetric frontal sinuses are located between the inner and outer tables of the frontal bone. They are anterior to the anterior cranial fossa, superior to the sphenoid and ethmoid sinuses, and superomedial to the orbits. They usually communicate with the middle meatus of the nasal cavity.

Epidemiology

Cancers of the nasal cavity and paranasal sinuses are relatively uncommon. Fewer than 4,500 patients are diagnosed with these neoplasms each year in the United States, an incidence of 0.75 per 100,000 (59). Cancers of the maxillary sinus are twice as frequent as those of the nasal cavity; cancers of the ethmoid, frontal, and sphenoid sinuses are extremely rare. They generally develop after the age of 40 years, except for esthesioneuroblastoma (ENB), which has a unique bimodal age distribution (20), and occur twice as frequently in men than in women (38). These tumors are more common in Japan and South Africa.

The etiologic factors vary by tumor type and location. Adenocarcinomas of the nasal cavity and ethmoid sinus have been reported to occur more frequently in carpenters and sawmill workers who are exposed to wood dust (1,2,32). Synthetic wood, binding agents, and glues may also be involved as co-carcinogens (61). Squamous cell carcinomas of the nasal cavity have been seen more often in nickel workers (67). Maxillary sinus carcinomas have been associated with radioactive thorium-containing contrast material (Thorotrast) used for radiographic study of the maxillary sinuses in the past. Occupational exposure in the production of chromium, mustard gas, isopropyl alcohol, and radium also may increase the risk for sinonasal carcinomas.

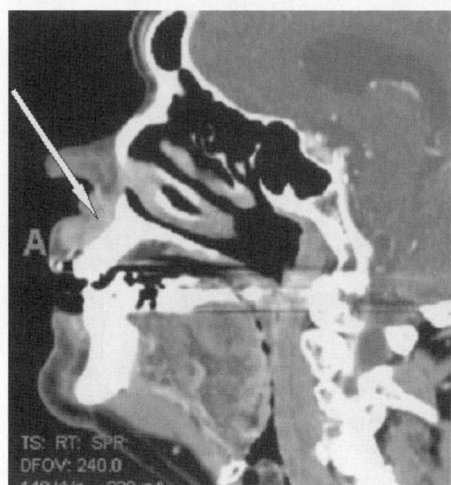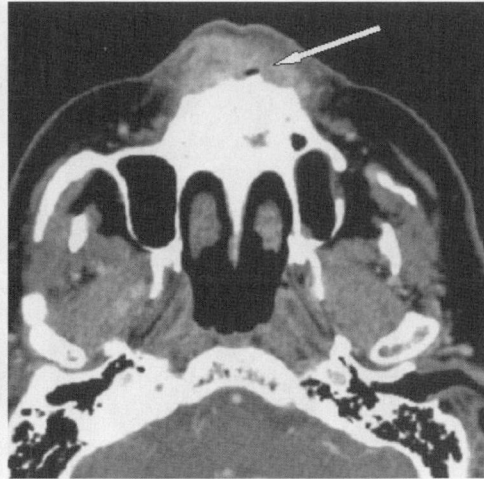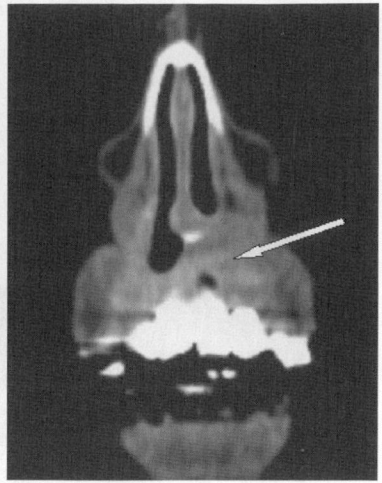

FIGURE 39.1. Computed tomography scan of a nasal vestibule squamous cell carcinoma that has spread by direct invasion of the upper lip (*arrow* in anel **A**) and gingivolabial sulcus and premaxilla (*arrow* in panels **B** and **C**).

Cigarette smoking is reported to increase the risk of nasal cancer, with a doubling of risk among heavy or long-term smokers and a reduction in risk after long-term cessation. After adjustment for smoking, a significant dose-response relation has also been noted between alcohol drinking and risk of nasal cancer (72).

Natural History

Nasal Vestibule

Nasal vestibule carcinomas can spread by direct invasion of the upper lip, gingivolabial sulcus, premaxilla (early events), or nasal cavity (late event) as shown in Figure 39.1. Vertical invasion may result in septal (membranous or cartilaginous) perforation or alar cartilage destruction. Lymphatic spread from nasal vestibule carcinomas is usually to the ipsilateral facial (buccinator and mandibular) and submandibular nodes. Large lesions extending across midline may spread to the contralateral facial or submandibular nodes. The incidence of nodal metastasis at diagnosis is approximately 5% (6,45,70). Without elective nodal treatment, approximately 15% of patients develop nodal relapse. Hematogenous metastases are rare.

Nasal Cavity and Ethmoid Sinuses

The pattern of contiguous spread of carcinomas varies with the location of the primary lesion. Tumors arising in the upper nasal cavity and ethmoid cells can extend to the orbit through the thin lamina papyracea and to the anterior cranial fossa via the cribriform plate, or they may grow through the nasal bone to the subcutaneous tissue and skin. Lateral wall primaries invade the maxillary antrum, ethmoid cells, orbit, pterygopalatine fossa, and nasopharynx. Primaries of the floor and lower septum may invade the palate and maxillary antrum. Perineural extension (typically involving branches of the trigeminal nerve) is seen most frequently with adenoid cystic carcinomas.

Lymphatic spread of nasal cavity primaries is uncommon, although spread to retropharyngeal and cervical lymph nodes is possible. In The University of Texas M. D. Anderson Cancer Center (MDACC) series of 51 patients, only 1 had palpable subdigastric nodes at diagnosis. Of the 36 patients who did not receive elective lymphatic irradiation, 2 (6%) experienced subdigastric nodal relapse (4). Hematogenous dissemination is rare. In the

MDACC series, for example, distant metastasis to bone, brain, or liver occurred in 4 of 51 patients (4).

The olfactory region is the site of origin of ENB and, occasionally, adenocarcinomas. Esthesioneuroblastoma is a tumor of neural crest origin first reported by Berger and Luc in 1924 as esthesioneuroepithelioma olfactif (7). Other names include *olfactory neuroblastoma* and *esthesioneurocytoma*. Esthesioneuroblastoma constitutes approximately only 3% of all intranasal neoplasms. About 250 cases were reported in the literature between 1924 and 1990 (24). The tumor typically is composed of round, oval, or fusiform cells containing neurofibrils with pseudorosette formation and diffusely increased microvascularity (30). Esthesioneuroblastoma may be mistaken for any other "small round-cell tumor," that is, a group of aggressive malignant tumors composed of small and monotonous undifferentiated cells that includes Ewing's sarcoma, peripheral primitive neuroectodermal tumor (also known as *extraskeletal Ewing's*), rhabdomyosarcoma, lymphoma, small cell carcinoma (undifferentiated or neuroendocrine), and mesenchymal chondrosarcoma. The clinical presentations of these entities often overlap, but clinicopathologic features and immunohistochemistry may help in differentiation.

The route of contiguous spread of ENBs is similar to that of ethmoid carcinomas. Lymph node involvement and distant metastasis are infrequent at diagnosis (11% and 1%, respectively [8]).

Maxillary Sinuses

The pattern of spread of maxillary sinus cancers varies with the site of origin. Suprastructure tumors extend into the nasal cavity, ethmoid cells, orbit, pterygopalatine fossa, infratemporal fossa, and base of skull (Fig. 39.2, A through C). Invasion of these structures gives lesions of the suprastructure a poorer prognosis. As well, treatment is associated with greater morbidity as a consequence of craniofacial resection or radiation of intracranial and ocular structures. Infrastructure tumors often infiltrate the palate, alveolar process, gingivobuccal sulcus, soft tissue of the cheek, nasal cavity, masseter muscle, pterygopalatine space, and pterygoid fossa (Fig. 39.2, D through J).

The maxillary sinuses are believed to have a limited lymphatic supply (60), and there is a correspondingly low incidence of lymphadenopathy at diagnosis (37,55). Only 6 of the 73 patients (8%) in the MDACC series had palpable lymphadenopathy at diagnosis. The incidence of nodal spread, however, varies with the histologic type (17%, or 5/29, for patients with

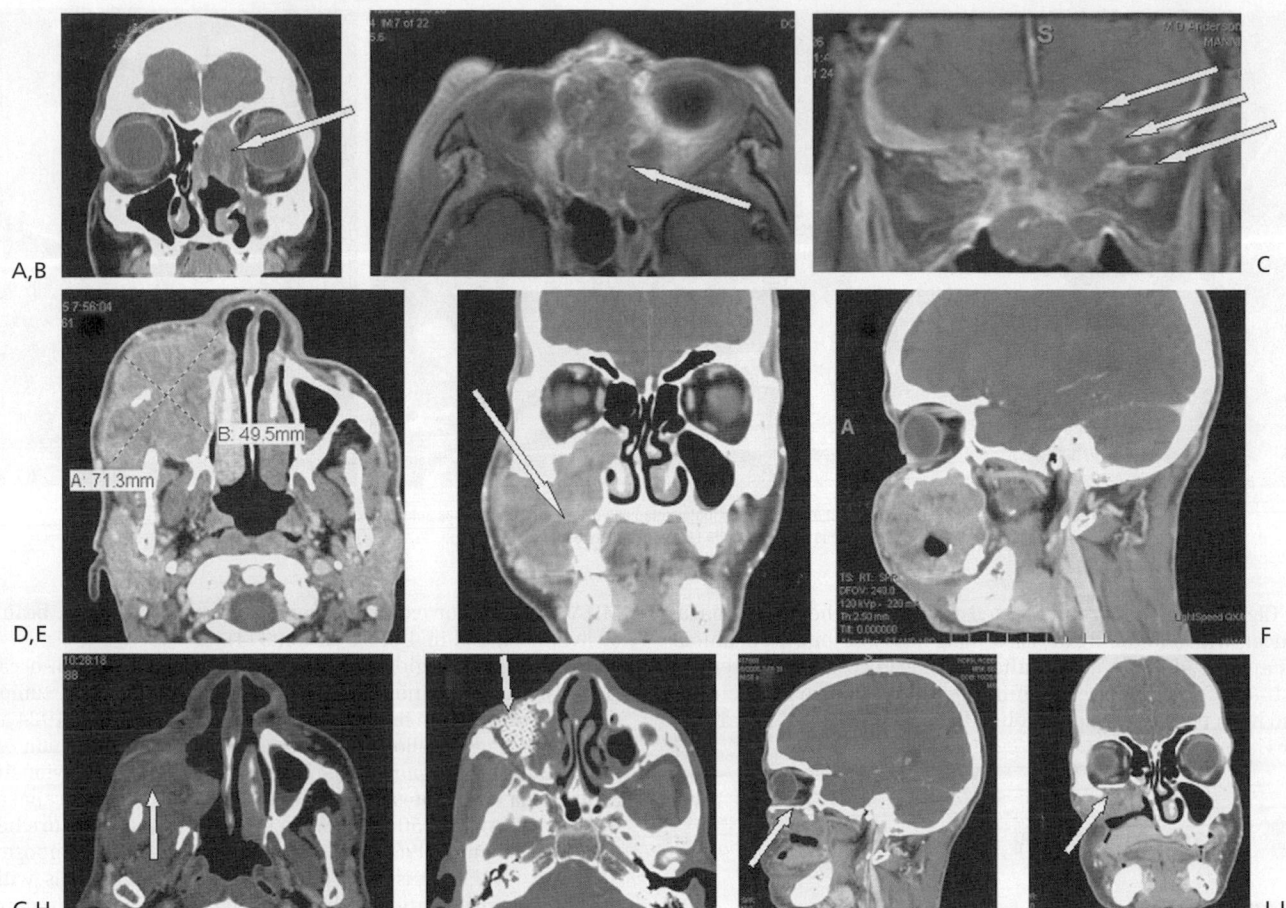

FIGURE 39.2. The pattern of spread of maxillary sinus cancers. Suprastructure tumors are shown in panels **A** through **C** with arrows indicating the involvement of the nasal cavity and ethmoid cells in panel A, the orbit in panel B, and the base of skull in panel C. Advanced tumor shown in panels **D** through **J** with arrows indicating alveolar process destruction with loosening of a tooth in panel E and abutment of the orbital floor without frank intraorbital invasion in panel F. The patient had a maxillectomy and orbital floor resection with an anterolateral thigh (ALT) flap marked by an arrow in panel G, and titanium mesh reconstuction of the orbital floor shown in panels H, I, and J.

squamous cell and poorly differentiated carcinomas versus 4%, or 1/27, for patients with adenocarcinoma, adenoid cystic carcinoma, and mucoepidermoid carcinoma). The incidence of subclinical disease as reflected in the rate of nodal relapse in patients who did not receive elective neck treatment also varies with histologic type (38%, or 9/24, for patients with squamous cell and poorly differentiated carcinomas versus 8%, or 2/26, for patients with adenocarcinoma, adenoid cystic carcinoma, and mucoepidermoid carcinoma). The cumulative incidence of nodal involvement (gross and microscopic) for patients with squamous cell and poorly differentiated carcinomas is about 30%. The risk of regional recurrence after treatment is 20% to 30% or higher, depending on the extent of disease and elective neck treatment (46). Ipsilateral subdigastric and submandibular nodes are involved most frequently. Hematogenous spread is uncommon.

Clinical Presentation

Nasal Vestibule

Carcinomas of the nasal vestibule usually present as asymptomatic plaques or nodules, often with crusting and scabbing. Advanced lesions may extend beyond the vestibule and may cause pain, bleeding, or ulceration. Large ulcerated lesions may become infected, leading to severe tenderness that requires anesthesia for complete clinical assessment.

Nasal Cavity

Nasal cavity tumors present with symptoms and signs of nasal polyps (e.g., chronic unilateral discharge, ulcer, obstruction, anterior headache, and intermittent epistaxis), hence delaying the diagnosis. Additional symptoms and signs develop as the lesion enlarges: medial orbital mass, proptosis, expansion of the nasal bridge, diplopia resulting from invasion of the orbit, epiphora due to obstruction of the nasolacrimal duct, anomaly of smell or anosmia from involvement of the olfactory region, or frontal headache due to extension through the cribriform plate.

The common presenting symptoms of ENBs are nasal obstruction and epistaxis. Spaulding et al. (64) found that anosmia could precede diagnosis by many years. Other symptoms are related to contiguous disease extension into the orbit (proptosis, visual-field defects, orbital pain, epiphora), paranasal sinuses (medial canthus mass, facial swelling), anterior cranial fossa (headache), or are due to inappropriate antidiuretic hormone secretion (64).

Ethmoid Sinuses

The presenting symptoms and signs are central/facial headaches and referred pain to the nasal or retrobulbar region, a subcutaneous mass at the inner canthus, nasal obstruction and discharge, diplopia, and proptosis. Of the 34 patients with ethmoid sinus cancers treated at MDACC between 1969 and 1993, nasal cavity symptoms (nasal obstruction, epistaxis, discharge) were reported in 25 patients (74%), orbital symptoms (diplopia, orbital pain, vision loss, proptosis, inner canthus mass, tearing) in 12 (35%), headache in 6 (18%), and hyposmia or anosmia in 5 (15%) (28).

Maxillary Sinuses

Maxillary sinus cancers usually are diagnosed at advanced stages. Symptoms and signs are facial swelling, pain, or paresthesia of the cheek induced by disease extension to the premaxillary region, epistaxis, nasal discharge and obstruction related to tumor spread to the nasal cavity, ill-fitting denture, alveolar or palatal mass, unhealed tooth socket after extraction from spread to the oral cavity, and proptosis, diplopia, impaired vision, or orbital pain due to orbital invasion (27).

Diagnostic Work-Up

The recommended pretreatment physical, diagnostic, and staging evaluations are listed in Table 39.1.

Physical Examination

Inspection and palpation of the orbits, nasal and oral cavities, and nasopharynx provide preliminary determination of tumor extent. Bimanual palpation is important in assessing contiguous extension of nasal vestibule lesions and in identifying buccinator and submandibular nodal involvement. Careful examination of cranial nerves is required. Fiberoptic nasal endoscopy after mucosal decongestion and topical analgesia allows assessment of local extent and facilitates biopsy of tumor involving the nasal cavity or nasopharynx.

Radiographic Evaluation

Imaging plays a crucial role in the staging of sinonasal tumors. Magnetic resonance imaging (MRI) and computed tomography (CT) (33) scans are complementary. MRI is superior at detecting direct intracranial or perineural or leptomeningeal spread (62). T2-weighted MRI can be helpful in differentiating tumor (low signal) from obstructed secretions (bright) (63). CT is superior for detecting early cortical bone erosion or extension through the cribriform plate or orbital walls.

Certain features provide clues as to the nature of the tumors in this region. Slowly progressive lesions tend to deform instead of destroy bony structures. Intermediate-grade tumors can cause sclerosis of adjacent bone. Lymphomas tend to permeate bone without frank destruction, and carcinomas and sarcomas infiltrate and destroy adjacent bone.

Table 39.1	PRETREATMENT EVALUATION FOR TUMORS OF THE NASAL CAVITY AND PARANASAL SINUSES
General	Complete history and physical examination
	Fiberoptic endoscopic examination with biopsies
Radiographic	Computed tomography/magnetic resonance imaging of the primary site and neck
	Chest x-ray; computed tomography of thorax if adenoid cystic or neuroendocrine carcinoma
Laboratory	Complete blood count
Other	Dental evaluation with extractions/restorations as needed
	Baseline ophthalmologic examination
	Baseline speech and swallowing assessment if surgery is planned

Biopsy

Transnasal biopsy is preferred for tumors arising from or extending into the nasal cavity or nasopharynx. Some paranasal sinus tumors may be more easily sampled using transoral procedures or an open Caldwell-Luc approach.

Laboratory Studies

Complete blood counts and serum chemistries provide screening for distant metastases. Abnormalities of these tests can be further investigated as necessary.

Staging

The 6th edition of the American Joint Committee on Cancer (AJCC) TNM classification includes staging for cancers of the maxillary sinus, ethmoid sinus, and the nasal cavity (25). Significant updates in the 6th edition are:

(a) The nasoethmoid complex is divided into two regions: the nasal cavity proper and the ethmoid sinuses.
(b) The nasal cavity is divided into four subsites (vestibule, septum, floor, and lateral wall) and the ethmoid sinuses into two subsites (right and left).
(c) Descriptions of the T staging of ethmoid tumors was added.
(d) T4 maxillary sinus tumors are divided into T4a (resectable) and T4b (unresectable).

There was no official AJCC staging for nasal carcinomas before the publication of the 6th edition of the AJCC *Cancer Staging Manual* (25). Table 39.2 summarizes the University of Florida (UF) nasal tumor staging system (54) and the Kadish staging system for ENB (34) used in the past. Tumors of the sphenoid and frontal sinuses are rare, and no specific staging system is available.

Pathologic Classification

Most nasal vestibule cancers are squamous cell carcinomas; the remaining are basal cell or adnexal carcinomas. The majority of cancers of the nasal cavity and paranasal sinuses are also squamous cell carcinomas, although minor salivary gland neoplasms (adenocarcinoma, adenoid cystic carcinoma, and

Table 39.2	PREVIOUSLY USED STAGING SYSTEMS FOR NASAL CAVITY NEOPLASMS
A. University of Florida system for nasal cavity[a]	
Stage I	Tumor limited to the nasal fossa
Stage II	Tumor extends beyond the nasal fossa to involve adjacent sites (paranasal sinuses, skin, orbit, pterygomaxillary fossa, nasopharynx)
Stage II	Tumor with local extension beyond structures designated in stage II
B. Kadish system for esthesioneuroblastoma[b]	
Stage A	Tumor confined to the nasal cavity
Stage B	Tumor confined to the nasal cavity and one or more paranasal sinuses
Stage C	Tumor extending beyond the nasal cavity and paranasal sinuses (includes orbit, base of skull, or intracranial cavity, cervical lymph nodes, and distant metastases)

[a]Parsons JT, Mendenhall WM, Mancuso AA, et al. Malignant tumors of the nasal cavity and ethmoid and sphenoid sinuses. *Int J Radiat Oncol Biol Phys* 1988;14:11–22.
[b]Kadish S, Goodman M, Wine CC. Olfactory neuroblastoma: a clinical analysis of 17 cases. *Cancer* 1976;37:1571–1576.

mucoepidermoid carcinoma) account for 10% to 15% of lesions in these locations. Melanoma accounts for 5% to 10% of nasal cavity malignancies but is rare in the paranasal sinuses. Neuroendocrine carcinomas of the sinonasal region (including small cell carcinoma, ENB, and sinonasal undifferentiated carcinoma), lymphomas, sarcomas, and plasmacytomas are even less common.

Prognostic Factors

Patient-specific factors (primarily prognostic for survival) include age and performance status. Disease-specific factors (primarily prognostic for locoregional control) include location, histology, and locoregional extent (reflected in TNM stage), and perineural invasion. Extensive local disease involving the nasopharynx, base of skull, or cavernous sinuses markedly increases surgical morbidity as well as the risk of subtotal surgical excision. Tumor extension into the orbit may require enucleation but minimal invasion of the floor or medial wall may be dealt with by resection and reconstruction, sparing the globe.

General Management

Nasal Vestibule

Primary radiotherapy may be preferable for nasal vestibule carcinoma for better cosmetic outcome, although surgery can yield a high control rate with excellent cosmetic results in selected small superficial tumors. Depending on the location and size of the primary tumor, radiation treatment can be delivered by external-beam irradiation, brachytherapy, or a combination of both. Cartilage invasion is not a contraindication for radiation therapy because the risk for necrosis is low with fractionated treatment (48). Rare cases of large primary disease with extensive tissue destruction and distortion are best managed by surgical resection in combination with pre- or postoperative radiotherapy, although there are proponents of primary radiotherapy with salvage surgery in this situation (44). Experienced prosthodontists can design aesthetically satisfactory nasal prostheses after radical surgery.

Nasal Cavity and Ethmoid Sinuses

Radiotherapy and surgery are equally effective in curing early lesions of the respiratory region. The choice of therapy, therefore, depends on the size and location of the tumor and the anticipated cosmetic outcome. Posterior nasal septum lesions generally are treated by surgery, but small anterior-inferior septal lesions (≤1.5 cm) can be treated effectively with interstitial brachytherapy (^{192}Ir implant). For cosmetic considerations, it is usually preferable to treat lateral wall lesions extending to the ala nasi with external irradiation. Locally advanced lesions of the respiratory region (stages II-IVa) are best treated with surgery, with or without postoperative irradiation.

A single modality treatment, either surgery or radiotherapy, yields >90% ultimate locoregional control for early ENBs (Kadish stage A) (20). The optimal therapy for stage B disease is unclear, partly because this group is heterogeneous; a combination of surgery and radiotherapy may have a slight advantage. For patients with stage C lesions, evidence suggests better results with the combination of surgery and radiotherapy. The available data do not justify routine elective nodal treatment because the incidence of isolated nodal relapse is <15%.

Ethmoid sinus carcinomas traditionally have been managed with surgery and postoperative radiotherapy. Selected cases may be treated with radiation alone or with radiotherapy and concurrent chemotherapy to avoid structural or functional deficits (69). Surgery generally involves medial maxillectomy and *en bloc* ethmoidectomy; a craniofacial approach is required if tumor extends superiorly to the ethmoid roof or olfactory region (11,41).

Maxillary Sinuses

Surgery alone can yield a high control rate in patients presenting with T1 or T2 tumors of the infrastructure. The combination of surgery and postoperative radiotherapy is the treatment of choice for patients with more advanced but resectable disease who are medically fit to undergo resection. Radical maxillectomy with or without orbital exenteration may be necessary, and a craniofacial approach is used if the tumor extends superiorly to the ethmoid roof or olfactory region. Definitive radiotherapy generally is recommended only for patients who are medically inoperable or who refuse radical surgery.

Chemotherapy—Neoadjuvant and Concomitant

Neoadjuvant chemotherapy is sometimes offered in order to reduce tumor volume, which may permit removal of tumor with a less morbid resection or facilitate radiotherapy planning if shrinkage pulls away tumor from critical structures such as brain, optic nerve, or chiasm. Alternatively, chemotherapy may be given concurrent with radiotherapy in the management of inoperable tumors on the basis of improved results in more frequent head and neck carcinomas. The sequence and agents used vary with the tumor type, tumor extent, and medical comorbidities. In general, the data suggest that concurrent chemotherapy is more effective than neoadjuvant chemotherapy with respect to local control.

Chemotherapy is not routinely for patients with ENB. Although responses to chemotherapy have been reported, they are usually of limited duration (68). Overall, local therapy with surgery and postoperative radiotherapy (58) yield excellent results at 5 years with regard to both overall survival (93.1%) and local control (96.2%). Concurrent chemotherapy during radiation may be considered in inoperable cases.

Palliation

Symptoms of incurable sinonasal cancer are particularly distressing. Multidisciplinary input is required even with very advanced cases as palliation may involve limited surgery, radiotherapy, chemotherapy, investigational studies, or best supportive care. The morbidity of each modality has to be balanced with the benefit to symptom control and improvement in quality of life. Attention is required to address in particular:

- the control of pain and discomfort as a first priority, and
- the impact of disfigurement and dysfunction, which is frequently present.

Chemotherapy may be given as single agent in investigational setting. If radiotherapy is given, larger dose per fraction is the usual practice in order to reduce the duration of treatment. However, if concurrent chemotherapy is added, consideration should be given to treating at 2 Gy per fraction to avoid severe acute effects. Treatment with radiotherapy or chemotherapy is often effective in reducing tumor bulk and providing relief of symptoms such as disfiguring masses, proptosis, discomfort or neuropathic pain, headache, epistaxis or other bleeding, nasal obstruction or discharge, and trismus.

Radiation Therapy Techniques

Nasal Vestibule

Target Volumes

For small, well-differentiated lesions measuring ≤1.5 cm, small fields with a 1- to 2-cm margin are appropriate. The initial target volume for all poorly differentiated tumors and well-differentiated primaries of >1.5 cm without palpable lymphadenopathy includes both nasal vestibules with at least 2- to 3-cm margins around the primary tumor (wider margins for infiltrative tumor) as well as bilateral facial, submandibular, and subdigastric nodes. When lymph node involvement is present at diagnosis, the lower neck is also irradiated.

For postoperative radiotherapy, the initial target volume includes the operative bed plus a 1- to 1.5-cm margin and the elective nodal regions. The volume is reduced off the undissected nodal regions after 50 Gy (25 fractions) to deliver an additional 6 Gy to the surgical bed. At 56 Gy, a final cone down is done to include the preoperative tumor bed to administer 4 Gy for a total dose of 60 Gy. If there are positive margins or if only a limited excision was done, this final cone down is given 10 Gy (total dose, 66 Gy).

Treatment Techniques

External Beam

External-beam radiotherapy may be delivered using either superficial or orthovoltage x-rays for very thin lesions or electrons for thicker lesions. A technique for external-beam irradiation using electrons is illustrated in Figure 39.3. The patient lies supine, immobilized with the neck slightly flexed using a custom mask to align the anterior surface of the maxilla parallel with the top of the couch. This setup allows irradiation of the primary lesion through a vertical appositional field, usually with a combination of electrons and photons in a ratio of 4:1. Skin collimation is used to minimize scatter irradiation to the eye and reduce the penumbra of the beam and reduce the field size required. Custom beeswax bolus material (Fig. 39.3, D through F) is prepared to allow a relatively flat surface contour onto which the electron beam is incident, avoiding inhomogeneity due to oblique incidence and surface irregularity. Bolus is also used to fill the nares to avoid the dose perturbation due to the air cavity with electron beams. Bolus is removed for photon treatments for skin-sparing, unless there is involvement of the overlying skin. An intraoral Cerrobend-containing stent is used to displace the tongue posteriorly and partially shield the upper alveolar ridge.

When indicated, the right and left facial lymphatics are irradiated with appositional fields; these require an approximately

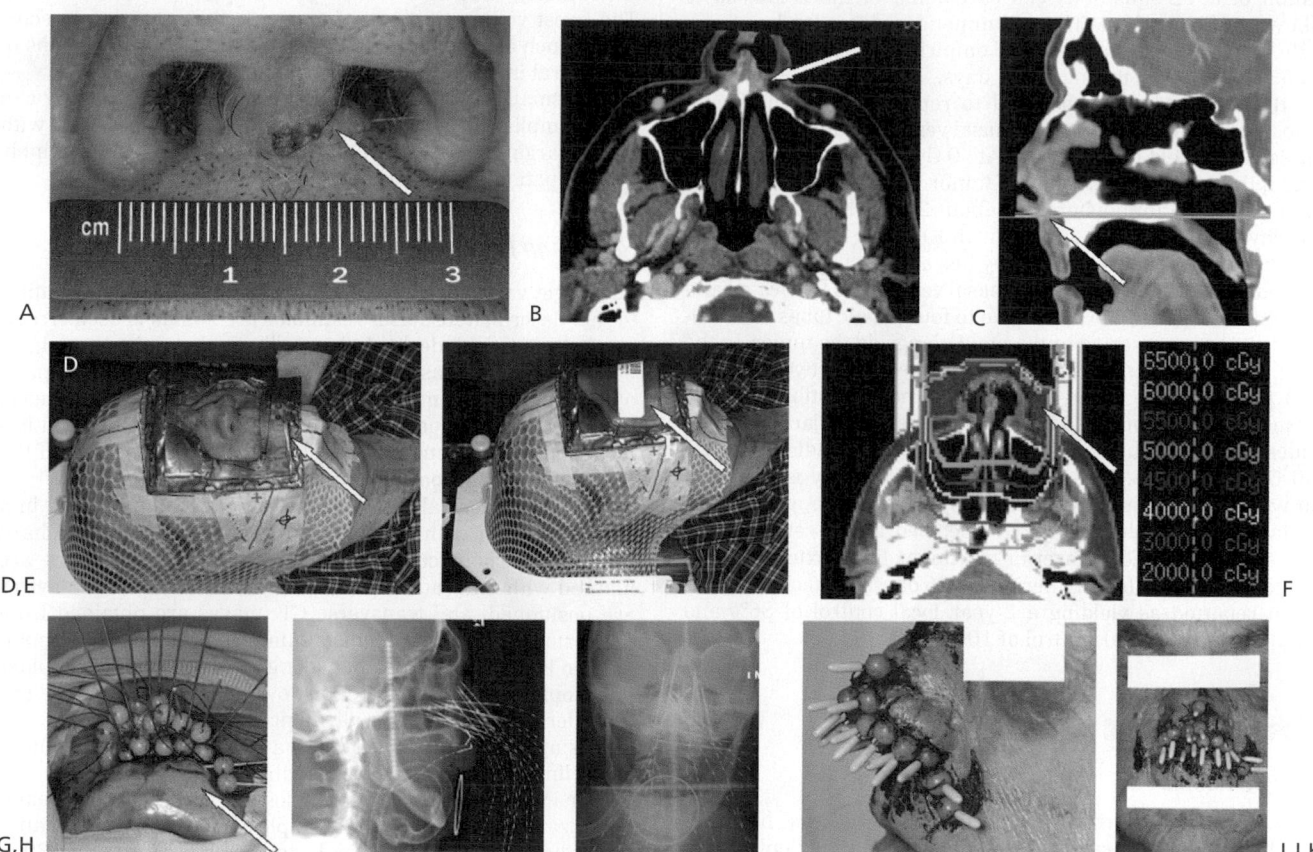

FIGURE 39.3. Nasal vestibule squamous cell carcinoma. Arrows in panel **A** indicate tumor expanding the columella. Arrows in panels **B** and **C** indicate invasion downward into the upper gingivobuccal sulcus on computed tomography (CT) imaging. Arrow in panel **D** shows setup for electron-beam phase of therapy with custom lead skin collimation *in situ*. Arrow in panel **E** shows the beeswax bolus *in situ*. Panel **F** shows the dosimetry to 50 Gy resulting from an appositional electron beam with beeswax bolus (*arrow*) to compensate for surface obliquity. The primary tumor, facial, and level II nodes were treated to 50 Gy. This was followed by 25 Gy administered by an interstitial low-dose-rate iridium needle implant at 55 cGy per hour. Panel **G** shows the dummy wires inserted into each hollow tubes. Each needles tube has a ball anchor at the distal end of the needles, which is pushed snugly against the skin and sutured to the skin. Note the placement of transverse "moustache" needles. Panels **H** and **I** show the orthogonal x-ray (anteroposterior, lateral) films that were taken to document the placement of the needles. CT-based planning was performed. Panels **J** and **K** show the live sources *in situ*.

15-degree gantry rotation to the respective side, each abutting the appositional primary lesion portal and the upper neck fields. The junctions are moved twice during the course of treatment to reduce dose heterogeneity. The submandibular and subdigastric nodes are treated with lateral parallel-opposed photon fields. In patients with involved nodes, these upper neck fields are matched inferiorly to an anterior portal treating the middle and lower neck nodes.

The external-beam radiation schedule for lesions up to 1.5 cm using a combination of electrons and photons is typically 50 Gy in 25 fractions followed by a boost of 10 to 16 Gy in 5 to 8 fractions (prescribed at 90% isodose line). Larger lesions to be treated by external-beam radiation alone receive 50 Gy in 25 fractions plus a boost of 16 to 20 Gy in 8 to 10 fractions. The schedule for elective nodal irradiation is 50 Gy in 25 fractions. Palpable nodes are given a boost to a total dose of 66 to 70 Gy in 33 to 35 fractions, depending on the size.

Brachytherapy

Brachytherapy for small lesions is accomplished using a ^{192}Ir wire implant or, in selected cases, by intracavitary ^{192}Ir mold. Hollow needles for afterloading are inserted under general anesthesia, which allows good exposure of the tumor as well as protection of the airway in the event of bleeding from the vascular Kiesselbach's plexus on the anterior nasal septum or from posterior hemorrhages originating from larger vessels near the sphenopalatine artery, behind the middle turbinate. Implantation of a T2 squamous cell carcinoma of the columella is shown in Figure 39.3. The recommended doses for low-dose-rate brachytherapy have evolved empirically and range from 60 to 65 Gy delivered during 5 to 7 days.

Brachytherapy may be used to replace an external-beam boost in patients with T1 or T2 nasal vestibule tumors following initial larger field radiotherapy. At 50 Gy, the patient is assessed and if there is good reduction of tumor volume, a boost of 20 to 25 Gy may be administered in about 2 days by low-dose-rate brachytherapy (Fig. 39.3, G through K).

High-dose-rate brachytherapy has also been used to deliver the boost. A custom mold of the nasal vestibule is fabricated and tumor is marked in the mold. Two to four plastic tubes with 1.0-cm spacing are inserted in the mold alongside the tumor. In the case of tumors of the lateral part of the vestibule, two catheters are placed on the inner aspect of the nasal vestibule. In the case of medially localized tumors, catheters are placed on both sides of the vestibule. Following external-beam radiotherapy to 50 Gy in 5 weeks, high-dose-rate brachytherapy is delivered in week 6. The dose is typically 3 Gy per fraction, given twice a day, to a total dose of 18 Gy specified at the center of the tumor. With a median overall treatment time (external-beam radiotherapy plus brachytherapy) of 36 days, this technique has been reported as yielding a 2-year local control of 86% and ultimate locoregional control of 100% (34).

Nasal Cavity and Ethmoid Sinuses

Target Volume

The technique for primary or postoperative external-beam radiotherapy of nasal cavity tumors depends on the depth of the neoplasm. For tumors located <3.5 to 4.0 cm from the skin of the apex of the nose, electrons may be used as 20 MeV electrons will provide coverage up to 5 cm in depth. A margin of at least 1 cm deep to the posterior edge has to be included in the full-dose volume. The technique is as previously described for nasal vestibule carcinoma. CT-based treatment planning is necessary for accurate target localization and dose calculation.

Intensity-modulated radiotherapy (IMRT) is recommended for tumors of the nasal cavity in which the target volume extends >5 cm depth or for tumors of the ethmoid sinus (Fig. 39.4). This technique delivers the desired dose to the target volume while minimizing the dose to critical organs such as cornea, lens, lacrimal glands, retina, optic nerve, optic chiasm, brain, and brainstem. For postoperative radiotherapy, the primary clinical target volume (CTV) descriptions are given in Table 39.3. The CTV_1 consists of the primary tumor bed with a 1.0- to 1.5-cm margin. A boost subvolume consisting of high-risk regions (sites of positive margins, gross macroscopic residual tumor) to be treated to higher dose may be outlined. The CTV_2 includes the entire operative bed. For ethmoid sinus tumors, this might include the frontal sinus, maxillary sinus, and sphenoid sinus. The bony orbit is part of the operative bed when orbital exenteration is performed because of tumor invasion. For lesions involving the ethmoid sinuses or olfactory region, the CTV should also include the cribriform plate. A third CTV may be delineated to encompass the tract of cranial nerve V2 to the foramen rotundum if there is perineural invasion. For primary radiotherapy using IMRT, the CTV_1, consisting of the gross tumor volume plus a margin of 1 to 2 cm, receives the full dose of 66 to 70 Gy. In patients receiving neoadjuvant chemotherapy, target volume definition is based on the extent of disease before chemotherapy.

For three-dimensional (3D) conformal radiotherapy, the initial target volume for postoperative radiotherapy consists of the surgical bed with 1- or 2-cm margins, depending on the surgical pathology findings and the proximity of critical structures. The boost volume consists of areas at greatest risk for recurrence, such as close or positive resection margins or regions of perineural invasion, with 1- to 2-cm margins.

For small anteroinferior septal lesions, brachytherapy can be accomplished by a single-plane implant of the lesion with 2-cm margins. Elective neck irradiation is not given routinely even in patients with large tumors or ENB.

Setup and Field Arrangement

For target volumes <5 cm deep, an electron technique similar to that described for nasal vestibule carcinomas is used. Treatment devices include lead skin collimation to obtain a sharp penumbra as well as bolus material in the nasal cavity, postoperative defects, and on skin scars. An intraoral stent is used to depress the tongue, provide a patent airway, and aid in immobilization. Tungsten internal eye shields may be used if the target volume approaches the orbits (Fig. 39.3).

For 3D conformal or IMRT, the patient is immobilized in a supine position with the head positioned such that the hard palate is perpendicular to the treatment couch. Scars are marked with thin radio-opaque wires, bolus and other devices are positioned, and transverse CT images are obtained from the vertex to the upper mediastinum. For IMRT, rigid immobilization is necessary, including using special head and shoulder thermoplastic masks that extend down to the upper thorax. The shoulders may be additionally depressed and fixed, for example, using wrist straps tethered to a footboard. Target volumes are delineated as previously described.

For IMRT, multiple gantry angles are used based on beam-optimization algorithms. An example of a 10-field noncoplanar arrangement with two vertex beams is shown in Figure 39.4. The beam angle selections are based on the same principles as for 3D conformal therapy:

(a) Preference for the shortest path to the target;
(b) Avoidance of direct irradiation of the critical structures (e.g., avoid beam entry through the contralateral eye after ipsilateral exenteration); and
(c) Use of as large beam separation as possible.

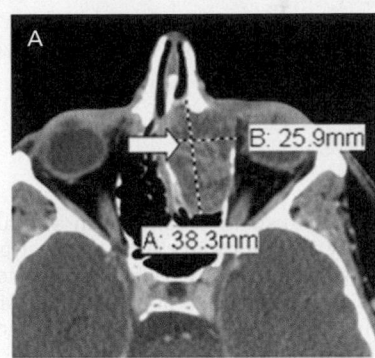
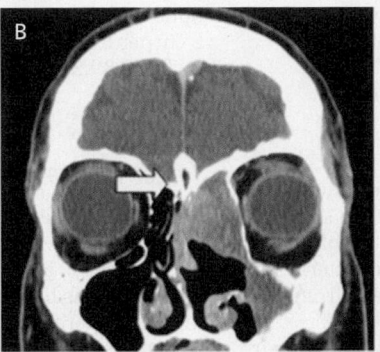
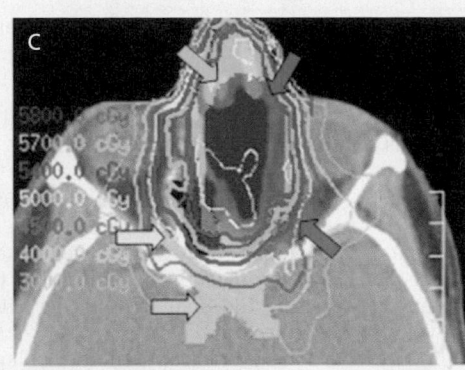

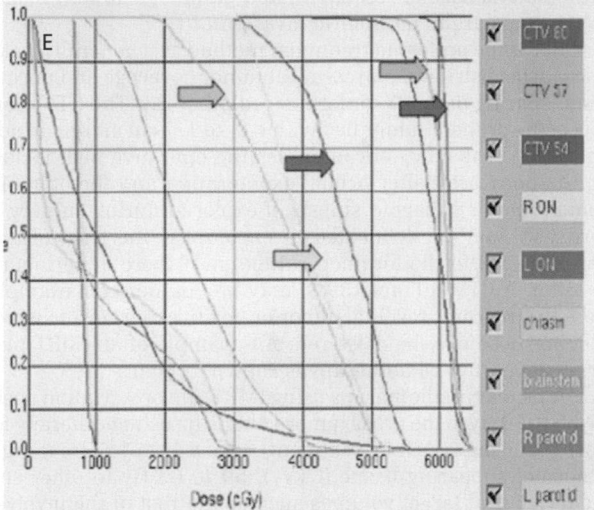
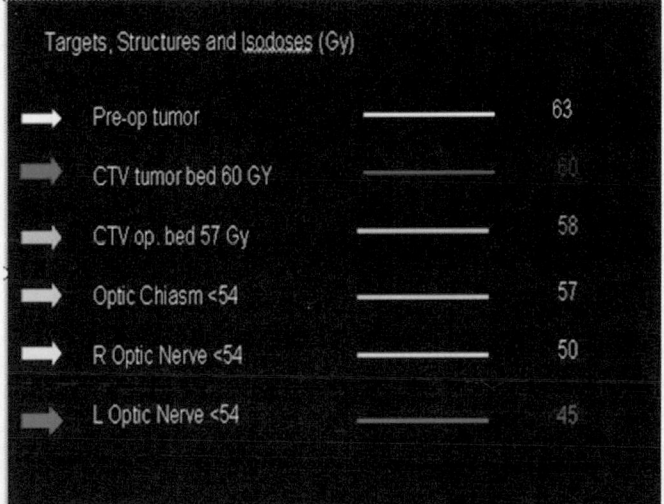

FIGURE 39.4. Intensity-modulated radiotherapy for adjuvant radiotherapy for an adenoid cystic carcinoma of the ethmoid sinus, anterior skull base, nasal cavity, and medial orbit following endoscopic anteroposterior ethmoidectomy with resection of tumor, left maxillary antrostomy with disease removal, bilateral sphenoidotomy, and frontal sinusotomy with anterior approach to the anterior skull base including a left lateral rhinotomy and medial maxillectomy and extradural resection of anterior cranial base. **A,B:** preoperative computed tomography scan with tumor indicated by white arrow. **C:** Transverse section at the level of the orbit that shows sharp dose gradient at the interface of the clinical target volume and the optic nerves and chiasm. **E:** Cumulative dose volume (y-axis) histogram.

Table 39.3	**TARGET VOLUMES FOR RADIOTHERAPY OF SINONASAL CANCERS USING INTENSITY-MODULATED RADIOTHERAPY**	

Target	Description	Dose (33–35 fractions) (Gy)
	Primary radiotherapy	
GTV	GTV (= prechemotherapy volume)	66–70
CTV$_1$ (primary CTV)	GTV + 1.0–1.5 cm	66–70
CTV$_2$ (intermediate-dose CTV)	Primary CTV + 1.0–1.5 cm	59–63
CTV$_3$ (elective CTV)	Nodal volumes, nerve tract, and base of skull margin	54–57

Target	Description	Dose (30 fractions) (Gy)
	Postoperative radiotherapy	
CTV$_{HR}$ (high-risk CTV)	Sites of suspected positive margins, gross macroscopic residual tumor, extracapsular nodal disease	66–70[a]
CTV$_1$ (primary CTV)	Primary tumor bed with 1.0–1.5 cm margin	60
CTV$_2$ (intermediate dose CTV)	Surgical bed	57
CTV$_3$ (low-dose CTV)	Trigeminal nerve if there is perineural invasion, additional skull base margin, elective nodal volume if indicated	54

GTV, gross tumor volume; CTV, clinical target volume.
[a]70 Gy may be given by adding a second boost plan or increasing the number of fractions to 35.

Inverse planning is usually done and multiple iterations may be necessary to ensure that the following are accomplished:

(a) Targets are covered;
(b) Normal tissue constraints are respected; and
(c) Dose is relatively homogenous.

Dose calculations should include heterogeneity corrections because of the significant amount of air and bone of the sinuses. The radiation oncologist must work closely with the physicist and dosimetrist. It is important to realize that the criteria for accepting or rejecting the plan may not be evident from the dose-volume histogram.

For 3D conformal radiotherapy, anterior oblique wedge-pair photon fields are appropriate for lesions located in the anterior lower half of the nasal cavity. Opposed-lateral fields may be used to treat tumors at the posterior part of the nasal fossa, provided the ethmoid cells are not involved. The optic pathway can be excluded from the radiation fields with this setup. For primaries of the upper nasal cavity and ethmoidal air cells, a three-field setup allows coverage of the ethmoid cells while sparing the optic apparatus. CT-based treatment planning is necessary to select beam and wedge angles (usually 45 to 60 degrees) and the relative loading of the fields, as well as to evaluate the dose to critical structures such as brain, brainstem, and optic structures.

Dose Fractionation Schedule

The dose schedule for low dose rate brachytherapy is 60 to 65 Gy during 5 to 7 days. The external-beam regimen for primary radiotherapy is 50 Gy in 25 fractions followed by a boost of 16 to 20 Gy in 8 to 10 fractions, depending on the size of the lesion. Postoperative radiotherapy consists of 50 Gy to elective tissue, 56 Gy to the operative bed, and 60 Gy to the tumor bed, with an optional boost to close or positive surgical margins, all given at 2 Gy per fraction. The dose regimens for IMRT are summarized in Table 39.3.

Maxillary Sinuses

Target Volume

Because maxillary cancers are usually diagnosed in a locally advanced stage and surgery is the primary therapy, most patients receive postoperative radiotherapy. Delineation of target volumes is based physical examination, pretreatment imaging, intraoperative findings (tumor extension relative to critical structures such as orbital wall, cribriform plate, cranial nerve foramina,and ease of resection), and pathologic findings (such as positive margin, perineural invasion).

IMRT is the preferred treatment method as it generally yields better dose distribution in terms of tumor coverage and normal tissue-sparing than 3D conformal radiotherapy. The CTV_1 consists of the primary tumor bed with 1.0- to 1.5-cm margin of normal tissue. The CTV_2 encompasses the operative bed, including the bony orbit after orbital exenteration and the ethmoid, frontal, and/or sphenoid sinuses if explored during surgery. A third CTV may be delineated to encompass the tract of cranial nerve V2 to the foramen rotundum if there is perineural invasion. A CTV_{HR} (Table 39.3) may be outlined; for example, gross macroscopic residual tumor or positive margins, to which a higher dose may be delivered. An example of an IMRT plan for postoperative radiotherapy is shown in Figure 39.5.

For primary radiotherapy using IMRT, the prescription doses are 66 to 70 Gy to the gross tumor volume (prechemotherapy for those receiving systemic treatment), plus a 1- to 1.5-cm margin of normal-appearing tissue (CTV_1), 59 to 63 Gy to other secondary clinical target volumes such as the rest of the involved sinus and wider region around the primary target, and 56 to

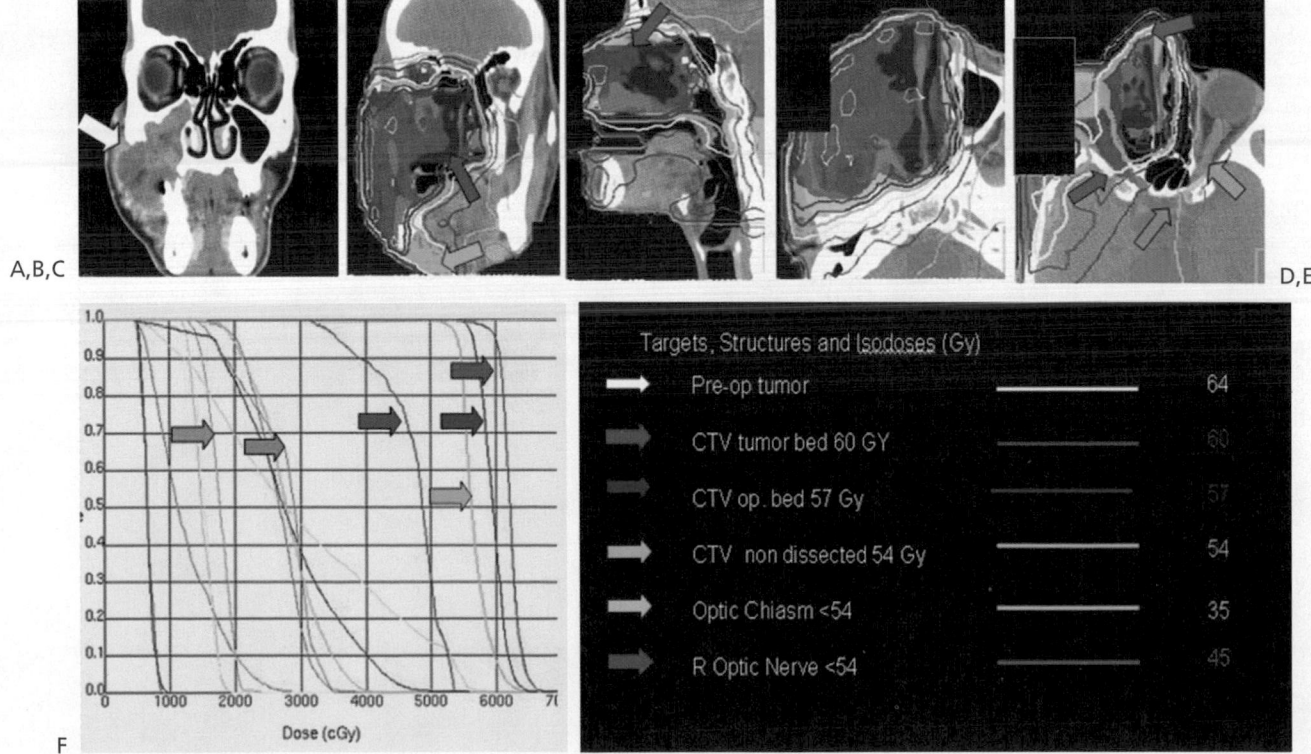

FIGURE 39.5. Intensity-modulated radiotherapy for adjvant radiotherapy for a squamous cell carcinoma post maxillectomy and orbital floor resection with an anterolateral thigh (ALT) and titanium mesh reconstuction of the orbital floor. **A:** Preoperative computed tomography scan with tumor indicated by white arrow. **B–E:** Sections showing coverage of the target volumes and avoidance of the optic nerves, chiasm, brain, and brainstem. **F:** Cumulative dose-volume histogram.

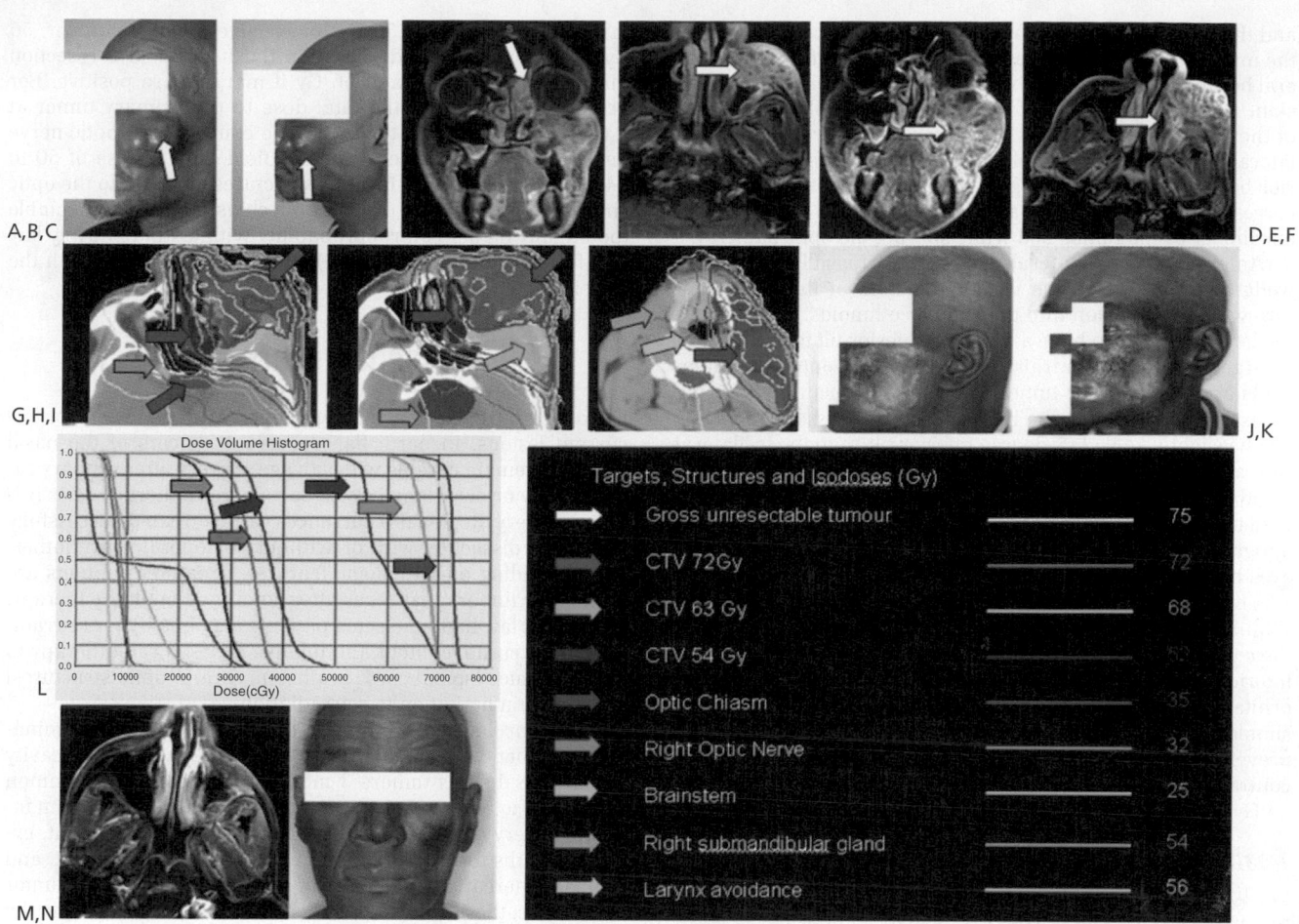

FIGURE 39.6. Intensity-modulated radiotherapy (IMRT) for definitive radiotherapy for T4N0 squamous cell carcinoma of the maxillary sinus. **A,B:** Pretreatment photographs showing skin of cheek involvement. **C,D:** Magnetic resonance imaging (MRI) scan with tumor indicated by white arrow. **E,F:** MRI following induction chemotherapy showed progressive disease involving left maxilla, left nasoethmoid region, extending inferiorly into the premaxillary soft tissues. **G—I:** IMRT plan with sections showing coverage of the target volumes. The patient was treated using concomitant boost fractionation. The primary plan delivered 57 Gy and a concomitant boost plan administered an additional 15 Gy. Sections G and H also show avoidance of the normal tissues as listed in the key and illustrated further in the cumulative dose-volume histogram in panel **L**. **J,K:** The skin reaction during final week of radiotherapy. **M,N:** The MRI and patient photo at follow-up, showing healed skin with hyperpigmentation. The tumor was in complete remission at the last visit 7 months after therapy.

Clinical Radiation Oncology

57 Gy to the tracts of nerves if there is perineural invasion and to elective nodal regions. An example of an IMRT plan for primary definitive radiotherapy of a T4N0 squamous cell carcinoma is shown in Figure 39.6.

For postoperative radiotherapy using a 3D conformal technique, the initial target volume consists of the operative bed with 1- to 2-cm margins. The boost field consists of the primary tumor bed and areas at higher risk for recurrence such as positive resection margins or perineural invasion. Radiation is administered to the neck following node dissection if multiple nodes are involved and/or there is presence of extracapsular extension. Elective radiation of ipsilateral submandibular and subdigastric nodes is given in patients with squamous cell or poorly differentiated carcinoma.

Setup and Field Arrangement

The patient is immobilized in a supine position with the head slightly hyperextended to bring the floor of the orbit parallel to the axis of the anterior field. An intraoral stent is used to open the mouth and depress the tongue out of the radiation field. Following palatectomy, the stent can be designed to hold a water-filled balloon to obliterate the large air cavity in the surgical defect in order to improve dose homogeneity. An orbital exenteration defect can also be filled directly with a water-filled balloon to decrease the dose delivered to the temporal lobe. Marking of the lateral canthi, oral commissures, external auditory canals, and external scars facilitates target volume delineation. The planning CT scan should include the entire head in order to allow the use of vertex beams. The principles of target delineation and plan evaluation for IMRT of the maxillary sinus cancer are the same as those described for nasal cavity and ethmoid tumors.

For 3D conformal radiotherapy, a three-field technique consisting of an anterior and right and left lateral fields is used for tumors involving the suprastructure or extending to the roof of the nasal cavity and ethmoid cells. The lateral fields may have a 5-degree posterior tilt and 60-degree wedges. The relative loading varies from 1:0.15:0.15 to 1:0.07:0.07 depending on the tumor location and photon energy. For the initial target volume, the superior border of the anterior portal is above the crista galli to encompass the ethmoids and, in the absence of orbital invasion, at the lower edge of the cornea to cover the orbital floor. The inferior border is 1 cm below the floor of the sinus and the medial border is 1 to 2 cm (or more if necessary) across the midline to cover contralateral ethmoidal extension. The lateral border is 1 cm beyond the apex of the sinus or falling off the skin. The superior border of the lateral portals follows the floor of the anterior cranial fossa, the anterior border is behind the lateral bony canthus parallel to the slope of the face, the posterior border covers the pterygoid plates, and the inferior border corresponds to that of the anterior portal. The boost volume encompasses the tumor bed while sparing the optic pathway.

Anterior and ipsilateral wedge-pair (usually 45-degree wedges) photon fields are used for tumors of the infrastructure with no extension into the orbit or ethmoids. If necessary, the lateral portal can have a 5-degree inferior tilt to avoid beam divergence into the contralateral eye. Lateral-opposed photon fields are preferred for tumors of the infrastructure spreading across midline through the hard palate. If necessary, the fields can be slightly angled (5-degree inferior tilt from the ipsilateral side and 5-degree superior tilt from the contralateral side) to avoid irradiating the contralateral eye. The use of a half-beam with the isocenter placed at the level of the orbital floor and the upper half of the fields shielded further reduces exposure of the eyes by beam divergence.

The eyes and the optic pathway are of particular concern. With 3D conformal techniques, it is generally possible to shield the cornea in patients with limited involvement of the medial or inferior orbital wall to avoid keratitis. If the tumor invades the orbital cavity without necessitating orbital exenteration, care should be taken to avoid irradiation of the lacrimal gland to prevent xerophthalmia. It is important to keep the dose to the contralateral optic nerve as well as the optic chiasm below 54 Gy in 27 fractions to prevent bilateral blindness.

Treatment of the Neck

For squamous and undifferentiated carcinoma, elective neck irradiation is recommended (13). Ipsilateral upper neck treatment is delivered using a lateral appositional electron field (usually 12 MeV). With conventional radiotherapy, careful matching is required to prevent hot or cold spots. The superior border of the field slopes up from the horizontal ramus of the mandible anteriorly to match the inferior border of the primary portal posteriorly, leaving a small triangle over the cheek untreated. The anterior border is just behind the oral commissure, the posterior border is at the mastoid process, and the inferior border is at the thyroid notch (above the arytenoids). The nodal volume can also be covered using IMRT with sparing of the parotid gland. Alternatively, the primary tumor bed and the upper neck can be treated with IMRT with the isocenter above the arytenoids and matched to a separate unmodulated lower neck field. This allows sparing of the laryngeal structures using a larynx block.

If the maxillary sinus is being treated with conventional radiotherapy (non-IMRT), the central axes of the primary (sinus) fields and the opposed-lateral upper neck fields all are placed in the plane of the inferior border of the maxillary fields (i.e., usually 1 cm below the floor of the maxillary sinus). An independent collimator jaw is used to shield the caudal half of the maxillary fields and the cephalad half of the neck field. The junction between the primary and the neck fields can be moved during the course of treatment to reduce dose heterogeneity in this region. Portal reduction is made after 42 Gy and treatment to the posterior neck continues with abutting electron fields to the desired dose. The middle and lower neck is irradiated with an anterior appositional photon field matched to the inferior border of the opposed-lateral upper neck fields.

Dose Fractionation Schedule

Table 39.3 summarizes the dose regimens for IMRT. With 3D conformal techniques, the dose for postoperative radiotherapy at 2 Gy per fraction is 50 Gy for elective nodal treatment, 56 Gy to the operative bed, 60 Gy to the tumor bed if resection margins are negative, and 66 Gy if margins are positive. For primary radiotherapy, the total dose to the primary tumor at 2 Gy per fraction is 66 to 70 Gy. The contralateral optic nerve and chiasm are excluded from the field after a dose of 50 to 54 Gy. When the tumor invades structures adjacent to the optic chiasm, a dose of up to 60 Gy to the chiasm may be acceptable (potentially higher control probability with a still relatively low risk for visual impairment [44]) after clear discussion with the patient.

Follow-Up and Recurrences

Salvage is possible for some patients with persistent or recurrent lesions. In particular, recurrent cancers of the nasal vestibule remain curable with salvage surgery after primary radiotherapy or occasionally with salvage radiotherapy after primary surgery. Regional recurrences can be treated successfully with neck dissection with or without postoperative radiotherapy depending on pathologic features. Treatment options are limited for tumors that recur after combined modality therapy, although a few highly selected patients may qualify for reirradiation with curative intent. Cumulative doses of radiotherapy to neural tissues (spinal cord, brainstem, brain, optic structures) are the main limitation to reirradiation.

Most oncologists recommend a baseline physical examination together with CT or MRI for patients with nasal cavity or paranasal sinus tumors 3 months posttreatment. Common practice is to repeat clinical examination and imaging when indicated every 4 months for the first 3 years posttreatment, every 6 months for the fourth and fifth years posttreatment, and annually thereafter. In addition to evaluating for possible tumor recurrence, these follow-up visits are critical with respect to the identification and management of side effects of treatment.

Results of Treatment

The results of treatment have improved during the past 4 decades, with overall survival increasing progressively from 33% ± 18% in the 1960s, to 42% ± 15% in the 1970s, 54% ± 15% in the 1980s, and 56% ± 13% in the 1990s ($p < .001$) (17). In a systematic review of published series spanning 40 years, Dulguerov et al. (17) demonstrated a progressive improvement in outcome for all treatment modalities (surgery, surgery + radiotherapy, and radiotherapy).

Nasal Vestibule

Table 39.4 summarizes the results of six series of patients treated by brachytherapy, external-beam irradiation, or both, modalities (18,34,37,46,47). Either brachytherapy or external-beam radiotherapy cures up to 95% to 100% of small (up to 2 cm) tumors. When adequate doses of radiation are used, 70% to 80% of lesions >2 cm can be controlled. Although as many as 40% of patients with larger lesions who do not receive elective nodal irradiation will fail in the neck, most can be salvaged and ultimate regional control is excellent. Proper selection of radiation technique, dose, and fractionation results in a low rate of severe late complications.

An excellent analysis was conducted by the Groupe Europeen de Curietherapie (43). Of 1,676 carcinomas of the skin of the nose and nasal vestibule treated by brachytherapy or external-beam irradiation, the overall local control rate was 93%. Local control was dependent on tumor size (<2 cm, 96%; 2 to 3.9 cm, 88%; ≥4 cm, 81%), site (external surface, 94%; vestibule, 75%), as well as new versus recurrent tumors (95% vs.

| Table 39.4 | LOCAL AND REGIONAL CONTROL RATES OF NASAL VESTIBULE CARCINOMAS TREATED BY DEFINITIVE RADIOTHERAPY |

Series	Patients	Local Control	Regional Control	Comments/Complications
U. of Florida (47) 1970–1995	56	RT alone: T1–2: 94% (5-yr); T3–4: 71% (5 -yr)	Clinically N0, no ENI: 39/46 controlled	23% complication rate: majority had transient soft-tissue necrosis; 1 cataract.
	4	Surgery + RT: T4: 100% (5-yr)	Clinically N0, ENI: 7/7 controlled	
M. D. Anderson (15) 1967–1984	32	BT: 11/11 controlled EB: 20/21 (95%) controlled	Small lesions, no ENI: 11/11 Large lesions, no ENI: 5/9 (56%) Large lesions, ENI: 12/12 (100%)	Osteonecrosis, epistaxis: 1 patient each
PMH (70) 1958–1983	54	EB: T1: 97% (5-yr) ; >T1[a]: 57% (5-yr); Dose <55 Gy: 30%; Dose >55 Gy: 82%	No ENI: 51/54 (94%)	Osteonecrosis: 2 patients; nasal stenosis: 2 patients; massive epistaxis: 1 patient
Rotterdam (42) 1968–1978	32	EB: <1.5 cm: 72% (5-yr) ; >1.5 cm: 50% (5-yr) Dose <54 Gy: 37% ; >54 Gy: 82%	Data not available	External-beam radiotherapy was hypofractionated (2.5–3 Gy/fraction)
VU University, Amsterdam (34)	56	Overall: 79% (ultimate LC : 95%) <1.5 cm (n = 32): 83% (ultimate: 94%) ≥1.5 cm (n = 24): 74% (ultimate: 96%)	Routine ENI to the mustache region 2-yr control rate: 87% (6 of 7 neck relapses were salvaged). 5-yr Ultimate control rate: 97%	Rhinorrhea: 45%; nasal dryness 39%; epistaxis 15%; adhesions 4%. Skin necrosis: 3 patients (all in IDR BT group) Sarcoma in the nasal vestibule: 1 patient.
French Groupe Europeen de Curietherapie (43)	1676	Skin of nose and nasal vestibule carcinoma treated by BT or EB (ortho- or megavoltage). Overall LC = 93% (FU ≥2 yr); < 2 cm: 96%; 2–3.9 cm; 88%; >4 cm: 81%. LC of nose skin: 94%; vestibule: 75%. LC for previously untreated: 95% vs. 88% for recurrent tumors.		

RT, radiotherapy; ENI, elective nodal irradiation; BT, brachytherapy; EB, external beam; PMH, Princess Margaret Hospital; VU, LC, local control; IDR, FU, follow-up.

88%). Local control was independent of histology for tumors <4 cm, but for those >4 cm, basal cell carcinomas were more frequently controlled than were squamous cell carcinomas. There were few complications (necrosis, 2%). The local control rate with surgery was approximately 90%.

Nasal Cavity and Ethmoid Sinuses

Table 39.5 summarizes the results of relatively large series focusing on nasal cavity and ethmoid sinus tumors. Overall local control rates range from 60% to 80% (4,5,10). Results are best for patients with lesions confined to the nasal septum that are generally small and well controlled with primary radiotherapy. Interstitial brachytherapy alone may be the treatment of choice for such patients. Regional failure rates are low. In the MDACC series, nodal recurrence was approximately 5% in patients with nasal cavity tumors who did not receive elective nodal treatment. Complications such as soft tissue necrosis, nasal stenosis, and visual impairment are seen in 5% to 11% of patients.

The data on 783 of a total of 981 patients with nasal cavity cancer included in the Surveillance, Epidemiology, and End Results (SEER) database from 1988 through 1998 were recently analyzed (9). Squamous cell carcinoma was the most common tumor type (49.3%), followed by ENB (13.2%). More than half of the cases presented with a small primary tumor (T1), and only 5% had positive nodes at diagnosis. Overall mean (median) survival was 76 months and overall 5-year survival 56.7%. On multivariate analysis, male gender, increasing age, T stage, N stage, and poorer tumor grade adversely affected survival (p <.05). Radiotherapy was administered in 50.5% of patients, and also independently predicted poorer survival (p =.03), likely due to selection of patients with poor prognostic features such as per-

ineural invasion, positive margins, or poor performance status (medically unfit for surgery) for radiotherapy. Five-year survival by tumor type, T stage, and N stage is shown in Table 39.6 (9). Five-year survival also correlates with tumor dedifferentiation: 75.3%, 61.9%, 47.6%, and 36.8% for well-, moderately, poorly, and undifferentiated cancers, respectively.

Esthesioneuroblastoma

Among the 783 cases of nasal cavity cancer extracted from the SEER database, 103 (13.2%) were ENB. Median survival was 88 months and overall 5-year survival 63.6% (9). Tables 39.7 and 39.8 summarize the results of treatment. The prognosis of patients with stage A disease is excellent. Overall, 30% of patients with stage B tumor died of the disease. About 60% of patients with stage C tumors died of the disease, primarily because of failure to control the primary tumor. Distant metastasis is uncommon (10%) even in locoregionally advanced disease.

Spaulding et al. (64) reported results for 25 patients treated at the University of Virginia Medical Center from 1959 through 1986 and followed for 2 years after therapy. There had been a gradual evolution of treatment with progressive introduction of craniofacial resections, complex field megavoltage radiation, and, for stage C disease, the addition of chemotherapy. Therefore, patients were divided into two groups, based on treatment era, for comparative analysis. Although the series is relatively small, it revealed two interesting findings for this rare disease: (a) extensive craniofacial resection does not appear to confer a major advantage over wide local excision for patients with stage B lesions, and (b) the addition of chemotherapy to craniofacial resection and radiotherapy for patients with stage C tumors may yield a higher disease-specific survival.

Table 39.5   LOCAL AND REGIONAL CONTROL RATES OF NASAL CAVITY AND ETHMOID SINUS CANCERS, EXCLUDING ESTHESIONEUROBLASTOMA

Series	Patients	Local Control	Regional Control and Survival	Complications
U. of Florida (31) 1964–1998 Nasal cavity, ethmoid, sphenoid, and frontal sinuses	78	Overall 60% (5-yr) Stage I: 86%; II: 65%; III: 34% RT alone: 49% Surgery + RT: 79%	Clinically N0, no ENI: 33/39 (85%) controlled Clinically N0, ENI: 25/28 (89%) controlled 5-yr CSS: 56% (all patients) 5-yr OS: 50% (all patients)	Osteonecrosis/bone exposure, hypopituitarism, and 5% unanticipated bilateral blindness (RT alone).
M. D. Anderson (28) 1969–1993 Ethmoid sinuses only	34	Overall 71% (5-yr) RT alone: 64% Surgery + RT: 74% Median time to relapse: 9 months.	Clinically N0, no ENI: 28/31 (90%) controlled Clinically N0, ENI: 2/2 controlled 5-yr CSS: 63% (all patients) 5-yr OS: 55% (all patients)	Osteonecrosis/bone exposure,[a] hypopituitarism, 6% brain necrosis, 3% unanticipated bilateral blindness (RT alone).
Princess Margaret Hospital (69) 1976–1994 Ethmoid sinuses only	29	RT alone: 41% (5-yr)	Overall: 24/29 (83%) controlled Clinically N0 patients did not receive ENI. 5-yr CSS: 58% (all patients) 5-yr OS: 39% (all patients)	3% brain necrosis, 3% unanticipated bilateral blindness (RT alone).
M. D. Anderson (4) 1969–1985 Nasal cavity only	45	Overall: 33/45 (73%) Septum: 12/14 (86%) Lateral wall/floor lesions: 21/31 (68%) controlled	Clinically N0, ENI: 6/6 controlled Septum: Clinically N0, no ENI: 2/8 controlled Lateral wall/floor: all controlled 5-yr CSS: 83% (all patients) 5-yr OS: 75% (all patients)	Osteonecrosis/bone exposure, nasal stenosis, 4% unanticipated bilateral blindness (RT alone).
Mallinckrodt (26) 1969–1984 Nasal cavity (includes 6 nasal vestibule lesions)	62	Overall: 44/62 (71%) RT alone: 16/28 (49%) Surgery + RT: 28/34 (82%)	Overall: 50/62 (81%) Clinically N0 patients did not receive ENI 5-yr RFS: 47% (all patients) 5-yr OS: 52% (all patients)	Severe complications: 11% (osteonecrosis/bone exposure, nasal stenosis, brain necrosis, optic neuropathy).

RT, radiation therapy; N0: clinically lymph-node negative; ENI, elective nodal irradiation; CSS, cause-specific survival; OS, overall survival; 5-yr-RFS, relapse-free survival at 5 years.
[a]All severe complications occurred in patients treated prior to 1964.

An analysis of 72 sinonasal neuroendocrine tumors treated at MDACC between 1982 and 2002 included a spectrum of histologies: ENB (31 patients), sinonasal undifferentiated carcinoma (SNUC, 16 patients), neuroendocrine carcinoma (NEC, 18 patients), and small cell carcinoma (7 patients). The overall survival at 5 years was 93.1% for patients with ENB, 62.5% for SNUC, 64.2% for NEC, and 28.6% for small cell carcinoma ($p = .0029$; log rank test). The local control rate at 5 years also was superior for patients with ENB (96.2%) compared with patients who had SNUC (78.6%), NEC (72.6%), or small cell carcinoma (66.7%) ($p = .04$). The regional failure rate at 5 years was 8.7% for patients with ENB, 15.6% for SNUC, 12.9% for NEC, and 44.4% for small cell carcinoma. The corresponding distant metastasis rates were 0% for ENB, 25.4% for SNUC, 14.1% for NEC, and 75.0% small cell carcinoma. ENB had excellent local

and distant control rates with local therapy alone (58). Eight patients with ENB were treated at MDACC during the past 3.5 years with surgery and adjuvant radiotherapy using IMRT to 60 Gy. One patient had stage B disease and seven had stage C, of whom five had intracranial extension. There were no local recurrences and one nodal recurrence was salvaged surgically. All eight patients were alive with no evidence of disease at the last follow-up.

Maxillary Sinuses

For patients with carcinoma of the maxillary sinuses, the combination of surgery and radiation yields 5-year local control and survival rates of 44% to 80% (Table 39.9). These rates are better than those achieved with either surgery or radiotherapy alone.

Table 39.6   TREATMENT RESULTS FOR NASAL CAVITY CANCER FROM THE SURVEILLANCE, EPIDEMIOLOGY AND END RESULTS DATABASE FOR 1988 THROUGH 1998[a]

Tumor Type	5-Yr Survival (%)	T Classification	5-Yr Survival (%)
Adenocarcinoma	49.0	T1	66.4
Adenoid cystic carcinoma	59.1	T2	51.8
Melanoma	22.1	T3	45.6
Other tumors	59.5	T4	40.2
Sarcoma	78.0	Overall	56.7
Squamous cell carcinoma	61.6	N Classification	5-yr Survival (%)
Esthesioneuroblastoma	63.6	N0	62.3
SNUC	49.5	N+	28.4

SNUC, sinonasal undifferentiated carcinomas.
[a]Results are shown by tumor type and by T and N stage. Because of rounding, percentages may not total 100.
From Bhattacharyya N. Cancer of the nasal cavity: survival and factors influencing prognosis. *Arch Otolaryngol* 2002;128:1079–1083.

Table 39.7 OVERALL TREATMENT RESULTS OF ESTHESIONEUROBLASTOMA

Series	Patients	Local Control	Regional Control and Survival	Comments/Complications
M. D. Anderson (58) 1982–2002	31	5-yr: 96.2%	5-yr: 91.3% 5-yr OS: 93.1%.;DM: 0%	
UCLA (17) 1970–1990	26	Overall: 18/26 (69%) S alone: 1/7 (14%) RT alone: 2/5 (40%) S + RT: 10/12 (83%)	4/26 (15%) patients had nodal disease (at presentation or after initial therapy) 5-yr CSS: 74%. 5-yr RFS: 58%	Postoperative cerebrospinal fluid leak, epiphora, radiation retinopathy (3/17 patients)
Mayo Clinic (22) 1951–1990	49	5-yr: 65% (all patients) S alone: 73% S + RT: 86%	3/49 (6%) had N1 at presentation and 8/46 (17%) had regional relapse (7/8 with concurrent local failure). 5-yr DFS and OS: 55% & 69% (all patients)	Osteonecrosis of trephine bone plate (4 patients)
U. of Virginia (19) 1959–1991	40	Overall: 30/40 (75%) controlled	4/40 (10%) clinically N1 at presentation and 4/36 (11%) developed regional relapse. 5-yr OS: 78%	—
U. of Virginia Health System, 1976–2004 treated with a standardized protocol[a] (40)	50	17 patients (34%) developed recurrent disease, which was locoregional in 12 patients	5-yr DFS: 86.5% Possibility for surgical salvage.	—
Hospital do Cancer Instituto Nacional de Cancer, Rio de Janeiro, Brazil (16) 1983–2000	36	S + RT: 18; RT only: 14; S only: 1 RT and chemotherapy: 2	5- and 10-yr DFS: 46% and 24% 5- and 10-yr OS: 55% and 46% N+ and DM adversely affected prognosis ($p < .001$ and $p = .01$, respectively).	Kadish classification best predicted disease-free survival

OS, absolute overall survival; DM, distant metastases; S, surgery; RT, radiation therapy; CSS, cause-specific survival; RFS, relapse-free survival; DFS, disease-free survival.
[a]Kadish A or B received preoperative RT followed by craniofacial resection; Kadish stage C disease was treated with preoperative chemotherapy and RT followed by a craniofacial resection.

For radiotherapy alone, the 5-year local control rate ranges from 22% to 39% and the 5-year overall survival rate is 22% to 40%.

Sequelae of Treatment

Soft Tissue and Bone

The formation of nasal cavity synechiae (fibrous mucosal bands causing airway stenosis) can be prevented by intermittent dila- tion of the nasal passages with a petroleum-coated cotton swab until mucositis has resolved. Dry mucous membranes can be managed symptomatically with saline nasal spray. Soft-tissue or cartilage necrosis is uncommon after therapy with an esti- mated incidence of 5% to 10% (19,35,52,53).

Eyes and Optic Pathway

Chronic keratitis and iritis ("dry-eye syndrome") can develop after radiotherapy if tumor extension to the orbital cavity man- dates irradiation of the lacrimal gland to doses of more than 30

Table 39.8 PATTERN OF FAILURE AND RESULTS OF SALVAGE TREATMENT OF ESTHESIONEUROBLASTOMA BY STAGE AND TREATMENT

Kadish Stage	Therapy	Local Control	Nodal Relapse	Salvage by Subsequent RT or S	Distant Metastasis	Died of Disease
A (n = 24)	RT	3/5	1/5	3/3	0/5	0/5
	S	5/9	1/9	4/4	0/9	0/9
	S + RT	9/10	2/10	2/2	1/10	1/10
	All	17/24 (71%)	4/24 (17%)	9/9	1/24 (4%)	1/24 (4%)
B (n = 33)	RT	6/7	2/7	0/1	0/7	3/7
	S	3/6	0/6	1/2	0/6	2/6
	S + RT	15/20	1/20	3/4	3/20	5/20
	All	24/33 (73%)	3/33 (9%)	4/7	3/33 (9%)	10/33 (30%)
C (n = 21)	RT	2/5	2/7	0/0	1/5	4/5
	S	1/1	0/6	0/0	0/1	0/1
	S + RT	9/15	1/20	1/1	1/15	8/15
	All	12/21 (57%)	3/33 (9%)	1/1	2/21 (10%)	12/21 (57%)

RT, radiotherapy; S, surgery.
Modified from Elkon D, Hightower SI, Lim ML, et al. Esthesioneuroblastoma. *Cancer* 1979;44:1087–1094.

Table 39.9 OUTCOME OF PATIENTS WITH LOCALLY ADVANCED CANCER OF THE PARANASAL SINUSES TREATED WITH COMBINED SURGERY AND RADIOTHERAPY

Study	Year	Patients	5-yr Survival (%)	Local Recurrence (%)	Distant Metastasis (%)
A. Results from surgery and conventional radiation therapy					
Lavertu et al. (35)	1989	54	38	52	—
Spiro et al. (65)	1989	105	38	49	15
Zaharia et al. (71)	1989	149	36	43	—
Paulino et al. (56)	1998	48	47	46	17
Le et al. (36)	1999	97	34	54	34
Myers et al. (51)	2002	141	52	56	33
Jiang, et al. (27)	1991	67[a]	53[b]	24	27
Katz et al. (31)	2002	31		21	
Bristol ASTRO (13)	2005	56	62%	30	12

Study	Year	Patients	Survival (%)	Local Recurrence (%)	Distant Metastasis (%)
B. Results from surgery and intensity-modulated radiation therapy					
Duthoy et al. (18) 1998 and 2003	2005	39	2-yr OS 68% / 4-yr OS 59%	2-yr 27 / 4-yr 32	—
Ahamad et al.[c] (3)	2005	53	Crude: 88.6%	Crude: 15.1 / 2-yr 20; 4-yr 25	20.7

C: Side effects of a combination of surgery and radiotherapy in patients with paranasal sinus cancers

Vetibulo-cochlear	Vestibular dysfunction, persistent otitis, tinnitus, hearing impairment.
Opthalmologic (lacriamal gland, eyes, lens, optic nerves and chiasm)	Retinopathy, xerophthalmia, keratopathy, cataracts, visual impairment
Neurologic (brain, brainstem, spinal cord, temporal lobe)	Neurocognitive impairment, cranial neuropathy, myelopathy, brain necrosis
Endocrine (pituitary gland, hypothalamus, thyroid gland if neck irradiated)	Multiple endocrine dysfunction: hyperprolactinemia, syndromes associated with decreased GH, FSH, LH, T4, TSH, ACTH, and their downsteam hormones.
Oral (major salivary glands, oral mucosa, mandible and temporomandibular joint)	Xerostomia, dental caries, dysguesia, mandible exposure, and necrosis, trismus.
Connective tissue complications (oral cavity, soft palate musculature, pharynx, larynx, skin and subcutaneous tissues, skull bones)	Soft tissue necrosis, skin changes, persistent lymphedema, subcutaneous fibrosis, cartilage necrosis, nasal dryness, choanal stenosis, swallowing and voice dysfunction, bone necrosis

OS, overall survival; GH, growth hormone; FSH, follicle-stimulating hormone; LH, luteinizing hormone; TSH, thyroid-stimulating hormone; ACTH, adrenocorticotropic hormone.
[a]Node-negative patients.
[b]Five-year relapse-free survival.
[c]M. D. Anderson Cancer Center data using intensity-modulated radiation therapy.

to 40 Gy (53). Without lacrimal irradiation, fewer than 20% of patients treated with up to 55 Gy to the cornea develop chronic corneal injury (29). There is an approximately 5% risk (at 5 years) of cataract formation after doses of up to 10 Gy to the lenses using conventional fractionation; this risk increases to 50% at 5 years after 18 Gy (21).

Radiation retinopathy is rare after doses of less than 45 Gy, but the incidence increases to about 50% after doses of 45 to 55 Gy (52). The reported incidence of optic neuropathy is <5% after 50 to 60 Gy but increases to around 30% for doses of 61 to 78 Gy. The parameters that influence the risk of radiation-induced optic neuropathy were recently analyzed in 273 patients treated between 1964 and 2000 in whom the radiation fields included the optic nerves and/or chiasm (46). The likelihood of developing optic neuropathy was primarily influenced by the total dose, but fraction size was marginally significant. The 5-year rates of freedom from optic neuropathy were 95% for doses ≤63 Gy treated once daily, 98% for doses ≤63 Gy treated twice daily, 78% for doses >63 Gy treated once daily, and 91% for doses >63 Gy treated twice daily. On multivariate analysis, the risk of optic neuropathy was correlated with increasing total dose ($p = .0047$). A trend was seen with increasing patient age ($p = .091$), once daily versus twice-daily fractionation ($p = .068$), and overall treatment time ($p = .097$). When the target volumes include the optic pathway, special attention must be paid to hot spots and dose per fraction.

References

1. Acheson ED, Cowdell RH, Hadfield E, et al. Nasal cancer in woodworkers in the furniture industry. *Br Med J* 1968;2:587–596.
2. Acheson ED, Hadfield EH, Macbeth RG. Carcinoma of the nasal cavity and accessory sinuses in woodworkers. *Lancet* 1967;1:311–312.
3. Ahamad A, Garden AS, Morrison WH, et al. 4 Year experience of intensity modulated radiotherapy (imrt) for tumors of the nasal cavity, paranasal sinuses and orbit. In: Proceedings of the American Society for Therapeutic Radiology and Oncology Annual Meeting; 2005; Denver, CO.
4. Ang KK, Jiang G-L, Frankenthaler RA, et al. Carcinomas of the nasal cavity. *Radiother Oncol* 1992;24:163–168.
5. Badib AO, Kurohara SS, Webster JH, et al. Treatment of cancer of the nasal cavity. *Am J Roentgenol Radium Ther Nucl Med* 1969;106:824–830.
6. Bars G, Visser AG, Van Andel JG. The treatment of squamous cell carcinoma of the nasal vestibule with interstitial iridium implantation. *Radiother Oncol* 1985;4:121–125.
7. Beitler JJ, Fass DE, Brenner HA, et al. Esthesioneuroblastoma: is there a role for elective neck treatment? *Head Neck* 1991;13:321–326.
8. Bhandare N, Monroe AT, Morris CG, et al. Does altered fractionation influence the risk of radiation-induced optic neuropathy? *Int J Radiat Oncol Biol Phys* 2005;62:1070–1077.
9. Bhattacharyya N. Cancer of the nasal cavity: survival and factors influencing prognosis. *Arch Otolaryngol* 2002;128:1079–1083.
10. Bosch A, Vallecillo L, Frias Z. Cancer of the nasal cavity. *Cancer* 1976;37:1458–1463.
11. Bridger GP, Kwok B, Baldwin M. Craniofacial resection for paranasal sinus cancers. *Head Neck* 2000;22:772–780.

12. Bridger MW, van Nostrand AW. The nose and paranasal sinuses—applied surgical anatomy. A histologic study of whole organ sections in three planes. *J Otolaryngol* 1978;7:1–33.

13. Bristol IJ, Ahamad A, Ang KK. Post-operative radiation for maxillary sinus carcinoma: does elective nodal irradiation affect regional control? In: Proceedings of the American Society for Therapeutic Radiology and Oncology Annual Meeting; 2005; Denver, CO.

14. Bush SE, Bagshaw MA. Carcinoma of the paranasal sinuses. *Cancer* 1982;50:154–158.

15. Chobe R, McNeese M, Weber R, et al. Radiation therapy for carcinoma of the nasal vestibule. *Otolaryngol Head Neck Surg* 1988;98:67–71.

16. Dias FL, Sa GM, Lima RA, et al. Patterns of failure and outcome in esthesioneuroblastoma. *Arch Otolaryngol* 2003;129:1186–1192.

17. Dulguerov P, Jacobsen MS, Allal AS. Nasal and paranasal sinus carcinoma: are we making progress? *Cancer* 2001;92:3012–3029.

18. Duthoy W, Boterberg T, Claus F, et al. Postoperative intensity-modulated radiotherapy in sinonasal carcinoma. *Cancer* 2005;104:71–82.

19. Eden BV, Debo RF, Larner JM, et al. Esthesioneuroblastoma. Long-term outcome and patterns of failure—the University of Virginia experience. *Cancer* 1994;73:255–2562.

20. Elkon D, Hightower SI, Lim ML, et al. Esthesioneuroblastoma. *Cancer* 1979;44:1087–1094.

21. Emami B, Lyman J, Brown A, et al. Tolerance of normal tissue to therapeutic irradiation. *Int J Radiat Oncol Biol Phys* 1991;21:109–122.

22. Foote RL, Morita A, Ebersold MJ, et al. Esthesioneuroblastoma: the role of adjuvant radiation therapy. *Int J Radiat Oncol Biol Phys* 1993;27:835–842.

23. Goepfert H, Guillamondegui OM, Jesse RH, et al. Squamous cell carcinoma of nasal vestibule. *Arch Otolaryngol* 1974;100:8–10.

24. Goldsweig HG, Sundaresan N. Chemotherapy of recurrent esthesioneuroblastoma. Case report and review of the literature. *Am J Clin Oncol* 1990;13:139–143.

25. Greene FL, Page DL, Fleming ID. *AJCC cancer staging manual.* New York: Springer-Verlag; 2002.

26. Hawkins RB, Wynstra JH, Pilepich MV, et al. Carcinoma of the nasal cavity–results of primary and adjuvant radiotherapy. *Int J Radiat Oncol Biol Phys* 1988;15:1129–1133.

27. Jiang GL, Ang KK, Peters LJ, et al. Maxillary sinus carcinomas: natural history and results of postoperative radiotherapy. *Radiother Oncol* 1991;21:193–200.

28. Jiang G-L, Morrison WH, Garden AS, et al. Ethmoid sinus carcinomas: natural history and treatment results. *Radiother Oncol* 1998;49:21–27.

29. Jiang GL, Tucker SL, Guttenberger R, et al. Radiation-induced injury to the visual pathway. *Radiother Oncol* 1994;30:17–25.

30. Kadish S, Goodman M, Wang CC. Olfactory neuroblastoma. A clinical analysis of 17 cases. *Cancer* 1976;37:1571–1576.

31. Katz TS, Mendenhall WM, Morris GC, et al. Malignant tumors of the nasal cavity and paranasal sinuses. *Head Neck* 2002;24:821–829.

32. Klintenberg C, Olofsson J, Hellquist H, et al. Adenocarcinoma of the ethmoid sinuses. A review of 28 cases with special reference to wood dust exposure. *Cancer* 1984;54:482–488.

33. Kondo M, Horiuchi M, Inuyama Y, et al. Value of computed tomography for radiation therapy of tumors of the nasal cavity and paranasal sinuses. *Acta Radiol Oncol Radiat Phys Biol* 1983;22:3–7.

34. Langendijk JA, Poorter R, Leemans CR, et al. Radiotherapy of squamous cell carcinoma of the nasal vestibule. *Int J Radiat Oncol Biol Phys* 2004;59:1319–1325.

35. Lavertu P, Roberts JK, Kraus DH, et al. Squamous cell carcinoma of the paranasal sinuses: the Cleveland Clinic experience 1977–1986. *Laryngoscope* 1989;99:1130–1136.

36. Le QT, Fu KK, Kaplan M, et al. Treatment of maxillary sinus carcinoma: a comparison of the 1997 and 1977 American Joint Committee on cancer staging systems. *Cancer* 1999;86:1700–1711.

37. Le Q-T, Fu KK, Kaplan MJ, et al. Lymph node metastasis in maxillary sinus carcinoma. *Int J Radiat Oncol Biol Phys* 2000;46:541–549.

38. Lewis JS, Castro EB. Cancer of the nasal cavity and paranasal sinuses. *J Laryngol Otol* 1972;86:255–262.

39. Logue JP, Slevin NJ. Carcinoma of the nasal cavity and paranasal sinuses: an analysis of radical radiotherapy. *Clin Oncol (R Coll Radiol)* 1991;3:84–89.

40. Loy AH, Reibel JF, Read PW, et al. Esthesioneuroblastoma: continued follow-up of a single institution's experience. *Arch Otolaryngol* 2006;132:134–138.

41. Lund VJ, Howard DJ, Wei WI, et al. Craniofacial resection for tumors of the nasal cavity and paranasal sinuses. A 17-year experience. *Head Neck* 1998;20:97–105.

42. Mak AC, Van Andel JG, van Woerkom-Eijkenboom WM. Radiation therapy of carcinoma of the nasal vestibule. *Eur J Cancer* 1980;16:81–85.

43. Mazeron JJ, Chassagne D, Crook J, et al. Radiation therapy of carcinomas of the skin of nose and nasal vestibule: a report of 1676 cases by the Groupe Europeen de Curietherapie. *Radiother Oncol* 1988;13:165–173.

44. McCollough WM, Mendenhall NP, Parsons JT, et al. Radiotherapy alone for squamous cell carcinoma of the nasal vestibule: management of the primary site and regional lymphatics. *Int J Radiat Oncol Biol Phys* 1993;26:73–79.

45. McNeese MD, Chobe R, Weber RS. Carcinoma of the nasal vestibule: treatment with radiotherapy. *Cancer Bull* 1989;41:84–87.

46. Mendenhall WM, Mendenhall CM, Riggs CEJ, et al. Sinonasal undifferentiated carcinoma. *Am J Clin Oncol* 2006;29:27–31.

47. Mendenhall WM, Stringer SP, Cassisi NJ, et al. Squamous cell carcinoma of the nasal vestibule. *Head Neck* 1999;21:385–393.

48. Million RR. The myth regarding bone or cartilage involvement by cancer and the likelihood of cure by radiotherapy. *Head Neck* 1989;11:30–40.

49. Miyamoto RC, Gleich LL, Biddinger PW, et al. Esthesioneuroblastoma and sinonasal undifferentiated carcinoma: impact of histological grading and clinical staging on survival and prognosis. *Laryngoscope* 2000;110:1262–1265.

50. Murphy J, Bleach NR, Thyveetil M. Sebaceous carcinoma of the nose: multi-focal presentation?. *J Laryngol Otol* 2004;118:374–376.

51. Myers LLN, Bradford B, Teknos CR, et al. Paranasal sinus malignancies: an 18-year single institution experience. *Laryngoscope* 2002;112:1964–1969.

52. Parsons JT, Bova FJ, Fitzgerald CR, et al. Radiation retinopathy after external-beam irradiation: analysis of time-dose factors. *Int J Radiat Oncol Biol Phys* 1994;30:765–773.

53. Parsons JT, Bova FJ, Fitzgerald CR, et al. Severe dry-eye syndrome following external beam irradiation. *Int J Radiat Oncol Biol Phys* 1994;30:775–780.

54. Parsons JT, Mendenhall WM, Mancuso AA, et al. Malignant tumors of the nasal cavity and ethmoid and sphenoid sinuses. *Int J Radiat Oncol Biol Phys* 1988;14:11–22.

55. Paulino AC, Fisher SG, Marks JE. Is prophylactic neck irradiation indicated in patients with squamous cell carcinoma of the maxillary sinus?. *Int J Radiat Oncol Biol Phys* 1997;39:283–289.

56. Paulino AC, Marks JE, Bricker P, et al. Results of treatment of patients with maxillary sinus carcinoma. *Cancer* 1998;83:457–465.

57. Prasad ML, Patel SG, Busam KJ. Primary mucosal desmoplastic melanoma of the head and neck. *Head Neck* 2004;26:373–377.

58. Rosenthal DI, Barker JLJ, El-Naggar AK, et al. Sinonasal malignancies with neuroendocrine differentiation. *Cancer* 2004;101:2567–2573.

59. Roush G. Epidemiology of cancer of the nose and paranasal sinuses: current concepts. *Head Neck Surg* 1979;2:3–11.

60. Rouviere H, Tobias MJ. *Anatomy of the human lymphatic system.* Ann Arbor, MI: Edwards Bros; 1938.

61. Schwaab G, Julieron M, Janot F. Epidemiology of cancers of the nasal cavities and paranasal sinuses. *Neurochirurgie* 1997.

62. Shapiro MD, Som PM. MRI of the paranasal sinuses and nasal cavity. *Radiol Clin North Am* 1989;27:447–475.

63. Som PM, Shapiro MD, Biller HF, et al. Sinonasal tumors and inflammatory tissues: differentiation with MR imaging. *Radiology* 1988;167:803–808.

64. Spaulding CA, Kranyak MS, Constable WC, et al. Esthesioneuroblastoma: a comparison of two treatment eras. *Int J Radiat Oncol Biol Phys* 1988;15:581–590.

65. Spiro JD, Soo KC, Spiro RH. Squamous carcinoma of the nasal cavity and paranasal sinuses. *Am J Surg* 1989;158:328–332.

66. Su K, Xu J, Qiao M, et al. CT characters of primary nasal non-Hodgkin lymphoma. *J Clin Otorhinolaryngol* 2003;17:261–263.

67. Torjussen W, Solberg LA, Hogetveit AC. Histopathological changes of the nasal mucosa in active and retired nickel workers. *Br J cancer* 1979;40:568–580.

68. Wade PMJ, Smith RE, Johns ME. Response of esthesioneuroblastoma to chemotherapy. Report of five cases and review of the literature. *Cancer Bull* 1984;53:1036–1041.

69. Waldron JN, rsquo, Sullivan B, et al. Ethmoid Sinus Cancer: Twenty-nine Cases Managed With Primary Radiation Therapy. *Int J Radiat Oncol Biol Phys* 1998;41:361–369.

70. Wong CS, Cummings BJ, Elhakim T, et al. External irradiation for squamous cell carcinoma of the nasal vestibule. *Int J Radiat Oncol Biol Phys* 1986;12:1943–1946.

71. Zaharia M, Salem LE, Travezan R, et al. Postoperative radiotherapy in the management of cancer of the maxillary sinus. *Int J Radiat Oncol Biol Phys* 1989;17:967–971.

72. Zheng W, McLaughlin JK, Chow WH, et al. Risk factors for cancers of the nasal cavity and paranasal sinuses among white men in the United States. *Am J Epidemiol* 1993;43:61–63.

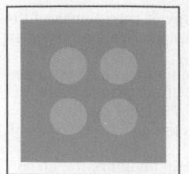

Chapter 40
Salivary Glands

Chris H. J. Terhaard

The salivary glands consist of the three large, paired major glands—parotid, submandibular, and sublingual (Fig. 40.1)—and many smaller, minor glands located throughout the upper aerodigestive tract. Salivary gland malignancies make up only approximately 0.4% of all cancers, and account for less than 5% of the annual incidence of head and neck malignancies in the United States. The international variation in the incidence is between 0.4 and 2.6/100 per year (72), with a mean of approximately 1/100. No significant change in incidence has been shown in the past decades in the United States and Sweden (72,97).

:: | Anatomy

Major Salivary Glands

Parotid Gland

The parotid gland is located superficial to and partly behind the ramus of the mandible and covers the masseter muscle. Superficially, it overlaps the posterior part of the muscle and largely fills the space between the ramus of the mandible and the anterior border of the sternocleidomastoid muscle. One or more isthmi that wrap around the branches of the facial nerve connect the superficial and deep lobes of the gland. The nerve enters the deep surface of the gland as a single trunk, passing posterolateral to the styloid process. It usually leaves the gland as five or more branches, emerging at the anterior, upper, and lower borders of the gland. The facial nerve runs superficial to the main blood vessels that traverse the gland but is interwoven within the glandular tissue and its ducts. Thus, removal of all or part of the parotid gland demands meticulous dissection if the nerve is to be spared.

The parotid gland contains an extensive lymphatic capillary plexus, many aggregates of lymphocytic cells, and numerous intraglandular lymph nodes in the superficial lobe. Lymphatics drain from more lateral areas on the face, including parts of the eyelids, diagonally downward and posteriorly toward the parotid gland, as do the lymphatics from the frontal region of the scalp. Associated with the gland, both superficially and more deeply, are parotid nodes. These drain downward along the retromandibular vein to empty in part into the superficial lymphatics and nodes along the outer surface of the sternocleidomastoid muscle and in part into upper nodes of the deep cervical chain. Lymphatics from the parietal region of the scalp drain partly to the parotid nodes in front of the ear and partly to the retroauricular nodes in back of the ear, which, in turn, drain into upper deep cervical nodes (46) (Fig. 40.2).

Submandibular Gland

The submandibular gland largely fills the triangle between the two bellies of the digastric and the lower border of the mandible and extends upward deep to the mandible. It lies partly on the lower surface of the mylohyoid and partly behind the muscle against the lateral surface of the muscle of the tongue, the hypoglossus. The submandibular gland has a larger superficial part, or body, and a smaller deep process. The inferior surface is adjacent to the submandibular lymph nodes, and the deep process of the submandibular gland lies between the mylohyoid laterally and the hyoglossus medially, and between the lingual nerve above and the hypoglossal nerve below (7). Bimanual palpation with one finger in the floor of the mouth and one under the edge of the mandible facilitates clinical detection of masses in this gland.

A rich lymphatic capillary network lies in the interstitial spaces of the gland. From the lateral and superior portions of the gland, lymph flows to the prevascular or preglandular submandibular lymph nodes. The posterior portion of the gland gives rise to one or two lymphatic trunks, which follow the facial artery and go directly to the anterior subdigastric nodes of the internal jugular chain (40,43). The nodes overlying the submandibular gland, followed by the subdigastric and high midjugular lymph nodes, are those involved in nodal metastases.

Sublingual Gland

This smallest of the three major salivary glands, along with many minor salivary glands, lies between the mucous membrane of the floor of the mouth above and the mylohyoid muscle below, the mandible laterally, and the genioglossus muscles of the tongue medially (Fig. 40.1). This is a rare site for malignant neoplasms; they are difficult to distinguish from cancer of the floor of the mouth accounting for fewer than 2% of all reported cases of salivary gland tumors (72,93). The sublingual gland drains either to the submandibular lymph nodes or more posteriorly into the deep internal jugular chain between the digastric and omohyoid muscles. Rarely, the lymphatics of the sublingual gland drain into a submental node or supraomohyoid jugular node (40).

Minor Salivary Glands

Minor salivary glands are widely distributed in the upper aerodigestive tract, palate, buccal mucosa, base of tongue, pharynx, trachea, cheek, lip, gingiva, floor of mouth, tonsil, paranasal sinuses, nasal cavity, and nasopharynx.

:: | Epidemiology

Seventy percent of all salivary tumors arise in the parotid gland, 8% in the submandibular gland, and 22% in the minor salivary glands (93). The proportion of malignant tumors increases from parotid (25%) to submandibular (43%) to minor salivary glands (65%) (57,93). There is a preponderance of benign tumors in women; malignant tumors exhibit an equal sex distribution. Patients with benign tumors are younger (mean age, 46 years) compared with those with malignant tumors (mean age, 54 years), with a trend to an older age for submandibular and minor salivary gland locations (93). Two percent to 3% of salivary neoplasms occur in children, in whom half of the tumors are malignant (21). The majority of cancers are located in

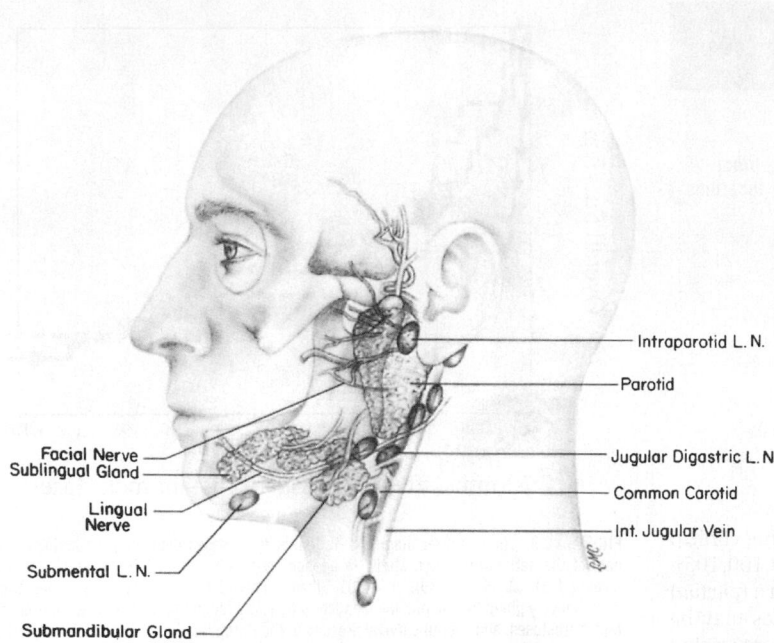
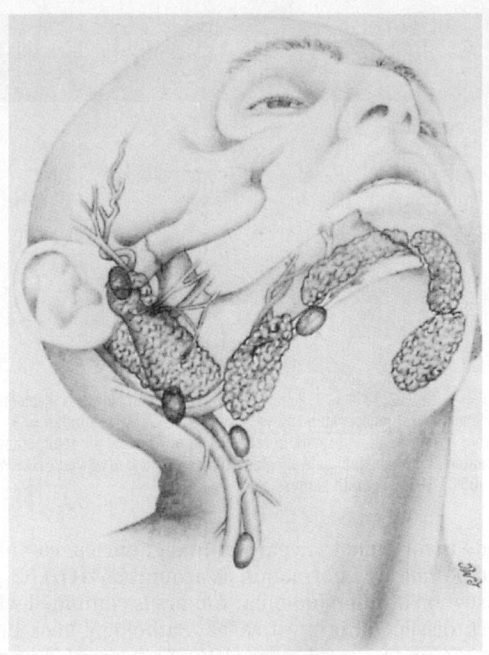

Intraparotid L. N.

Parotid

Facial Nerve
Sublingual Gland

Jugular Digastric L. N.

Common Carotid

Lingual
Nerve

Int. Jugular Vein

Submental L. N.

Submandibular Gland

FIGURE 40.1. Anatomy of salivary glands.

the parotid gland, with mucoepidermoid cancers predominating (88).

Etiologic factors are not clearly defined. Nutrition may be a factor because Eskimos in the Arctic, who have low intake of vitamins A and C, have a high incidence (56). Cigarette smoking and alcohol consumption is in general not related with salivary gland cancer (68), although cigarette consumption more than 80 pack-years may contribute to salivary gland cancer (98). Irradiation can also be a cause, as evidenced by the increased incidence in survivors of the atomic bombs dropped on Hiroshima and Nagasaki, and in those irradiated to the head and neck for benign conditions during childhood (67,83,84,111). Saku et al. (83) studied salivary gland tumors in atomic bomb survivors of Hiroshima and Nakasaki. Two-thirds of all cases were parotid, and the remainder was equally distributed between submandibular and minor salivary glands. Mucoepidermoid cancer and Warthin's tumor (benign) were particularly elevated compared with nonexposed persons, and disproportionately high at high radiation doses. Modan et al. (67) found

a clear dose-response effect in a matched control study of patients who had low-dose head–neck irradiation in childhood; there was a 2.6-fold increase of benign tumors and a 4.5-fold increase of cancer. The majority of these tumors are mucoepidermoid cancers (84,111); however, less than 1% of salivary gland tumors may be caused by former irradiation (8).

Workers in various occupations experience an increased risk of salivary gland cancer (47). For women employed as hairdressers or working in beauty shops, a significant elevated risk was observed in a study by Swanson and Burns (98). A correlation of incidence with ultraviolet exposure remains controversial (97,98).

Women with salivary gland cancer may have a 2.5 elevated breast cancer risk (50), probably confined to women with salivary gland cancer before age 35 (97). After treatment for salivary gland cancer, an increased risk for subsequent oropharyngeal, thyroid, and lung cancer is noted (97).

Natural History

Local invasion is the initial route of spread of malignant tumors of the salivary glands, depending on location and histologic type. For parotid tumors, this may result in fixation to structures in around 20% of cases (75). Skin invasion is more often seen in parotid tumors (10%), compared with submandibular tumors (3%) (101).

Approximately 25% of patients with a malignant parotid salivary gland tumor present with facial palsy from cranial nerve invasion (31,75,93,100,105).

A detailed study of the Dutch Head and Neck Oncology Group (NWHHT) concerning patients with a salivary gland malignancy found an overall incidence of clinically positive nodes of 14% and clinically occult, pathologically positive nodes in an additional 11% of patients (101). This percentage depends on the number of neck dissections performed, the tumor location, histology, and T-stage. The number of elective neck dissections performed varies between the tumor locations. Stennert et al. (94) performed a neck dissection in all malignant parotid tumors and found 53% unilateral positive nodes and 0% contralateral nodes. In selected patients in other studies, the percentage positive nodes varied between 20% (115) and 38% (100). Lymph

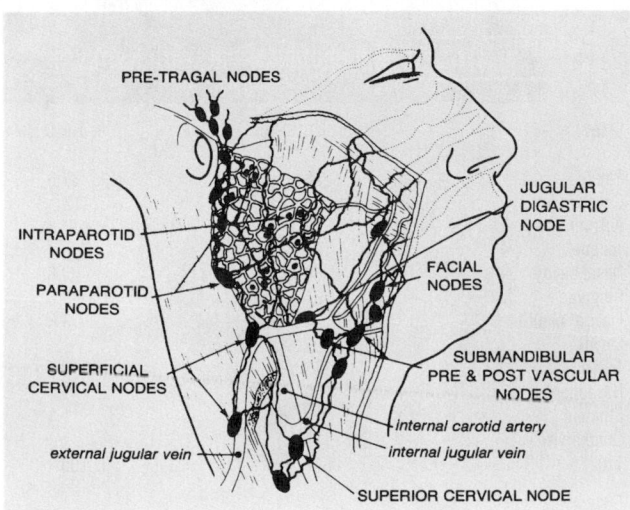

PRE-TRAGAL NODES

INTRAPAROTID
NODES

PARAPAROTID
NODES

SUPERFICIAL
CERVICAL NODES

external jugular vein

JUGULAR
DIGASTRIC
NODE

FACIAL
NODES

SUBMANDIBULAR
PRE & POST VASCULAR
NODES

internal carotid artery
internal jugular vein

SUPERIOR CERVICAL NODE

FIGURE 40.2. Lymph node distribution in and around the parotid gland.

Table 40.1	**RISK ESTIMATION (%) FOR POSITIVE NECK NODES**			
Summation: T Score + Histologic Type Score	**Parotid Gland**	**Submandibular Gland**	**Oral Cavity**	**Other locations**
2	4	0	4	0
3	12	33	13	29
4	25	57	19	56
5	33	60	—	—
6	38	50	—	—

T1 = 1, T2 = 2, T3-4 = 3; acinic/adenoid cystic/carcinoma ex pleomorphic adenoma = 1, mucoepidermoid = 2, squamous/undifferentiated = 3.
From Terhaard CHJ, Lubsen H, Rasch CRN, et al. The role of radiotherapy in the treatment of malignant salivary gland tumors. *Int J Radiat Oncol Biol Phys* 2005;61:103–111, with permission.

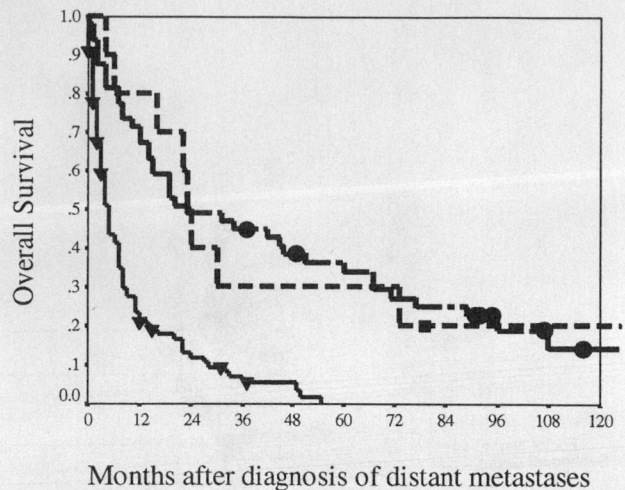

Months after diagnosis of distant metastases

FIGURE 40.3. Survival after diagnosis of distant metastases depending on histology, update of the nationwide Dutch study. ● adenoid cystic carcinoma (49); ■ acinic cell carcinoma (11); ▲ others (99); *p* <.001. (From Terhaard CHJ, Lubsen H, Van der Tweel, et al. Salivary gland carcinoma: Independent prognostic factors for locoregional control, distant metastases, and overall survival: Results of the Dutch Head and Neck Oncology Cooperative Group. *Head Neck* 2004; August: 26(8):681–693, with permission.)

node involvement for parotid malignancies, combining clinical and pathologic information, is around 25% (10,62,79,100,105). Resection of submandibular tumors is combined with a (partial) neck dissection in most cases. Pathologic neck nodes may be seen in up to 42% of cases (100). Salivary gland tumors arising in the oral cavity produce an incidence of cervical node metastases of less than 10% (57,65,74,100). Nasopharyngeal salivary gland tumors have a high risk of occult metastases (50%) (85). The risk of positive findings in the neck may be based on a combination of T-stage and histology (79,100). The highest risk is seen for squamous cell, undifferentiated cancer, and salivary duct cancer (79,100). There is an intermediate risk for mucoepidermoid cancer and a low risk for acinic cell, adenoid cystic carcinoma, and carcinoma ex pleomorph adenoma (100). A 15% risk is found for T1 tumors, 26% for T2, and 33% for T3–4 (100). An example of a rating scale to estimate the risk of positive neck nodes, based on tumor location, T-stage, and histologic type, is shown in Table 40.1.

Distant metastases overall are encountered in 3% of patients at presentation and in 33% after 10 years (101). They are fairly common with adenoid cystic, salivary duct, squamous cell, and undifferentiated carcinomas; in the case of adenoid cystic carcinomas, they may occur quite late in the course of the disease, without recurrence of the primary tumor (42,52,74,92,101). Distant metastases are primarily to lung, bone, and occasionally to the liver (101). Reported incidence of distant metastases in patients with adenoid cystic carcinoma after 10 years of follow-up is around 40% (64,92,101). Five years after diagnosis of distant metastases of adenoid cystic carcinoma, more than one third of the patients are still alive; 10% are alive after 10 years. An update of the survival data of the NWHHT study after diagnosis of distant metastases of salivary gland cancer is shown in Figure 40.3.

Clinical Presentation

Three of four parotid masses are benign (93). Patients most often have a painless, rapidly enlarging mass, often present for years before a sudden change in its indolent growth pattern prompts the patient to seek medical attention. Duration of clinical symptoms before diagnosis may last more than 10 years (93,101). For malignant tumors, the median duration of clinical symptoms generally is shorter (3 to 6 months) (9,101) compared to that of benign tumors, although for some minor salivary gland tumors, median periods of 2 year have been reported (65,85).

Pain is more frequently associated with malignant disease (93). Although as many as one third of parotid cancers may have facial nerve involvement, only 10% to 20% of patients complain of pain (75,93,101). Pain may appear with involvement of

deeper structures (masseter, temporal, and pterygoid muscles). Rarely, tumors of the parotid may involve the base of skull and cause intractable pain and paralysis of various cranial nerves.

The signs and symptoms associated with tumors of the minor salivary glands vary because of their diverse locations. The distribution of presenting sites for 492 cases of minor salivary gland tumors, 88% of which were malignant, is shown in Table 40.2 (93). Most are intraoral, and a painless lump is the most common presenting symptom. For tumors arising in the nasal cavity or sinuses, facial pain is the most common presenting symptom, followed by nasal obstruction. Laryngeal primary tumors most frequently cause hoarseness or voice change.

Clinical features suggesting a malignant salivary gland tumor are rapid growth rate, pain, facial nerve palsy, childhood occurrence, skin involvement, and cervical adenopathy.

Diagnostic Work-Up and Staging

Major Salivary Glands

The diagnostic work-up of major salivary gland tumors includes a careful history and physical examination, with particular

Table 40.2	**DISTRIBUTION OF PRESENTING SITES**	
Site	**No. of Patients**	**Percentage**
Palate	228	37.5
Cheek or lips	73	12
Antrum	72	11.8
Tongue	63	10.4
Nasal cavity	60	9.8
Gingivae	34	5.6
Floor of mouth	22	3.6
Larynx	21	3.5
Tonsil	13	2
Nasopharynx	9	1.4
Ethmoid	9	1.4
Oropharynx	3	1
Total	607	100

From Spiro RH. Salivary neoplasms: Overview of a 35-year experience with 2,807 patients. *Head Neck Surg* 1986;8:177–184 with permission.

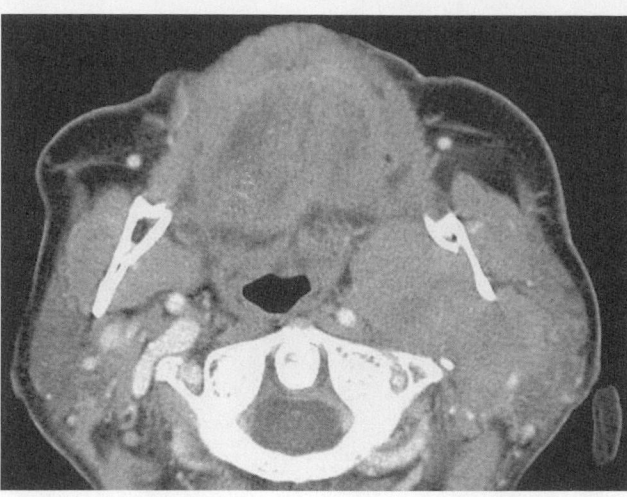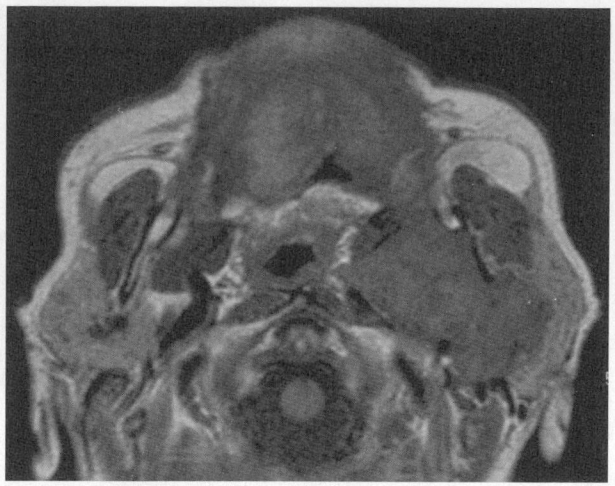

A   B

FIGURE 40.4. A patient with acinic cell cancer of the left parotid gland. A: Axial contrast-enhanced computed tomography image. B: T1-weighted magnetic resonance image. Both images show an infiltrating soft tissue mass involving the deep and superficial lobe. The tumor has widened the left pterygoid musculature. The left internal carotid artery is displaced medially. (Courtesy of Dr. F.A. Pameyer, radiologist, University Medical Center Utrecht.)

attention to signs of local fixation or regional adenopathy. Computed tomography (CT) scans are useful in evaluating the extent of lesions involving the parotid gland, especially the deep lobe. Magnetic resonance imaging (MRI) is superior to other modalities, especially when malignancy is suspected (Fig. 40.4). T1-weighted images are excellent to assess the margins, deep extent, and patterns of infiltration because the (fatty) background of the gland is hyperintense. In general, benign tumors are hyperintense, and malignant tumors are intermediate or low intensity at T2-weighted MR images (73,114). The MRI has a sensitivity of 87% and a specificity of 94% (73). Perineural invasion of adenoid cystic carcinoma may be evaluated with both CT (foraminal enlargement) and MRI (fat-suppressed T1-weighted images). Such findings may well change the surgical approach and treatment regimen (15,114).

Fine-needle aspiration in the diagnosis of parotid and submandibular salivary gland tumors is a reliable procedure. The sensitivity for malignancy varies between 80% and 90%; the specificity is more than 90% (20,73,76,95). The negative predictive value for malignancy, however, is around 70% to 75% (20,73). False-negative findings may be seen as result of lack of representative material or a cyst. In these cases, ultrasound fine-needle aspiration is advised (76). The relative low negative predictive value of fine-needle aspiration will be improved if MRI and fine-needle aspiration are combined (74). Fine-needle aspiration has been quite accurate in the diagnosis of benign salivary gland tumors (20,95).

The sixth edition of the manual of the American Joint Committee on Cancer (2) and the sixth edition of the classification system of the International Union Against Cancer (90) are identical for major salivary glands (Table 40.3). They are based on size, extension, and nodal involvement. Relative survival rates for major salivary gland cancer according to stage are shown in Figure 40.5.

Minor Salivary Glands

Various radiographic studies may be used, including plain films, to ascertain bone erosion in advanced lesions, and CT and MRI scans may be used to evaluate depth and contiguous involvement. The definitive diagnostic procedure is an excisional biopsy, particularly if malignancy is clinically expected. Unplanned incisional biopsies should be avoided, and fine-needle biopsies are impractical because of the polymorphism of most malignant salivary gland tumors.

A formal staging system has not been developed for minor gland tumors. The same staging system for minor salivary glands as for squamous cell carcinoma in sites other than the parotid or submandibular glands may be used. The American Joint Committee on Cancer and International Union Against Cancer classification and stage regrouping system has been reported to be a major long-term outcome predictor in minor salivary gland carcinoma (104).

Pathologic Classification

The histologic classification of salivary gland neoplasia is very demanding for the head and neck pathologist. In 1991 the World Health Organization classification for salivary gland tumors was expanded. Various types of carcinomas were distinguished based on recognition, prognosis, and treatment, discussed more in detail by Seifert and Sobin (87) (Table 40.4). Classification may be difficult, as shown in a re-evaluation of 101 intraoral salivary gland tumors by experienced pathologists; major disagreement was seen in 8 and there was minor disagreement in 33 (103).

Neoplastically transformed myoepithelial cells play a role in the development of monomorphic and pleomorphic adenomas, adenoid cystic carcinomas, mucoepidermoid carcinomas, and the rare myoepitheliomas (7). The reserve cell system of the intercalated and excretory duct is thought to be the site of origin of most neoplasms (7).

Salivary gland carcinomas may be graded as low and high malignant, particularly for mucoepidermoid tumors. However, there is a disparity for grading, even among experienced pathologists (13). Low-grade mucoepidermoid, polymorphous low-grade adenocarcinoma (PLGA), epithelial-myoepithelial, and acinic cell carcinomas comprise a group of low-to-moderate malignancy; high-grade mucoepidermoid, malignant mixed, adenoid cystic, squamous, undifferentiated, and salivary duct carcinomas represent more high-grade malignancies (105). The percentage of the histologic subtypes varies from series to series, and from the localization of the tumor (Fig. 40.6). In parotid tumors in children and adults, the most common malignant subtype is the mucoepidermoid (10,21,37,88,91,108). Acinic cell cancer derives from cells of the terminal ducts and intercalated ducts. Grading for acinic cell cancer is controversial (45). Most tumors (86%) are located in the parotid gland (Fig 40.6) (45). Adenoid cystic carcinoma is most common in minor salivary glands (Fig. 40.7) (57,74,101,104), followed by

Table 40.3   AMERICAN JOINT COMMITTEE ON CANCER STAGING SYSTEM FOR MAJOR SALIVARY GLAND CANCER (PAROTID, SUBMANDIBULAR, SUBLINGUAL)

Primary tumor (T)

TX	Primary tumor cannot be assessed
T0	No evidence of primary tumor
T1	Tumor ≤2 cm in greatest dimension without extraparenchymal extension[a]
T2	Tumor >2 cm to ≤4 cm in greatest dimension, without extraparenchymal extension[a]
T3	Tumor >4 cm and/or tumor having extraparenchymal extension[a]
T4a	Tumor invades skin, mandible, ear canal, and/or facial nerve
T4b	Tumor invades skull base and/or pterygoid plates and/or encases carotid artery

Regional lymph nodes (N)

NX	Regional lymph nodes cannot be assessed
N0	No regional lymph node metastasis
N1	Metastasis in a single ipsilateral lymph node, ≤3 cm in greatest dimension
N2	Metastasis in a single ipsilateral lymph node, >3 cm but not >6 cm in greatest dimension, or in multiple ipsilateral or bilateral or contralateral lymph nodes, none >6 cm in greatest dimension
N2a	Metastasis in a single ipsilateral lymph node >3 cm but <6 cm in greatest dimension
N2b	Metastasis in multiple ipsilateral lymph nodes, none >6 cm in greatest dimension
N2c	Metastasis in bilateral or contralateral lymph nodes, none >6 cm in greatest dimension
N3	Metastasis in a lymph node >6 cm in greatest dimension

Distant metastases (M)

MX	Presence of distant metastasis cannot be assessed
M0	No distant metastasis
M1	Distant metastasis

Stage grouping

I	T1	N0	M0
II	T2	N0	M0
III	T3	N0	M0
	T1, T2, T3	N1	M0
IVA	T1, T2, T3	N2	M0
	T4a	N0, N1, N2	M0
IVB	T4b	Any N	M0
	Any T	N3	M0
IVC	Any T	Any N	M1

[a]Extraparenchymal extension is clinical or macroscopic evidence of invasion of soft tissues or nerve, except those listed under T4a and 4b. Microscopic evidence alone does not constitute extraparenchymal extension for classification purposes.
From *American Joint Committee of Cancer: Manual for staging of cancer,* 6th ed. Philadelphia: JB Lippincott; 2002, with permission.

the submandibular gland (Fig. 40.6) (11,96,101,108). Perineural invasion is common in adenoid cystic carcinoma (107). The adenoid cystic variety has a tubular pattern that has been associated with the best prognosis, a cribriform pattern with an intermediate prognosis, and a solid pattern with the worst prognosis (28). The PLGA and salivary duct carcinomas are the most common new subtypes of the World Health Organization 1991 classification. PLGA is a solid, ovoid, nonencapsulated mass with a highly variable growth pattern (Fig. 40.8). Most are located in the palate, and the prognosis generally is good (17,29). Salivary duct carcinoma resembles ductal breast cancer morphologically (Fig. 40.8). They derive from excretory duct cells. They are usually located in the parotid gland and are highly aggressive (42,48,52). There is also a low-grade subtype (23).

Prognostic Factors

A number of prognostic variables have been studied in the management of salivary gland cancer. In these studies, multivariate analyses have been performed consider-

ing locoregional control, distant metastases, and survival. Results of studies with sufficient number of patients and follow-up have been summarized in Table 40.5. Local control and overall survival is influenced by site, favoring tumors of the oral cavity (101,102). T- and N-stages are independent variables for locoregional control, distant metastases, and survival, regardless of site (10,37,57,58,62,65,66,74,75,92, 101,102,105). In the NWHHT study, histologic type was an independent prognostic factor for distant metastases (101).

Oncogene expression has been evaluated in the search for additional prognostic factors. Expression of the oncoprotein p53 was found in an Italian study to be higher in malignant tumors than in benign tumors (35). Furthermore, tumors with moderate-to-high expression of p53 were more frequently associated with regional and distant metastasis and a lower disease-free and overall actuarial survival rate, compared with patients with no p53 expression. Univariate and multivariate analyses confirmed the independent prognostic value of p53 expression. Vascular endothelial growth factor significantly correlates with p53 expression and is an independent prognostic factor

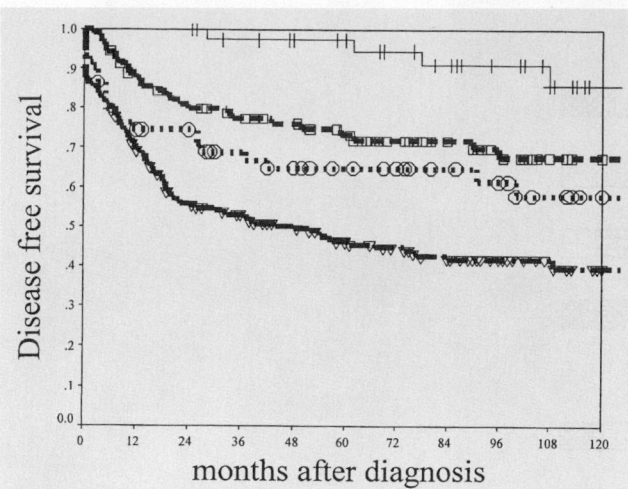

FIGURE 40.5. Disease-free survival for major salivary glands according to the 2002 classification of the American Joint Committee on Cancer. Results of the nationwide Dutch study: +, stage I; □, stage II; ○, stage III; ▽, stage IV.

for survival for salivary gland cancer (61). Overexpression of HER-2/neu was seen in approximately one third of mucoepidermoid carcinomas in a series of 50 parotid gland cancers studied at the University of Southern California (78) and in 20% in a series of 50 salivary duct carcinomas in a study from Germany (52). Overexpression was seen and appeared to be an independent marker of poor prognosis. It also has been similarly associated with poor prognosis in carcinomas of the breast, ovary, and endometrium. Another molecular feature studied in relationship to prognosis was the DNA content in adenoid cystic carcinomas. DNA aneuploidy is correlated with the solid type, and thus with poor prognosis (28). Franzen et al. (32) found a correlation of grade with aneuploidy as well as stage.

Major Salivary Glands

The survival of patients with submandibular cancers is inferior to that of parotid cancers according to a study by Spiro et al. (91). Extraglandular extension (10,37) and skin invasion (70,101,105) in parotid cancers results in decreased disease-free survival. More advanced age was found to be a negative prognostic factor for locoregional control in some studies (58,75,79) and for disease-free and overall survival in most studies (10,58,62,75,91,105,106). Impairment of function of the facial nerve is a known prognostic factor, not only influencing locoregional control (37,70,101), but also disease-free survival (36,62,70,105). Pain at presentation may be associated with reduced disease-free survival (105). Perineural invasion and pain are closely related: not pain, but perineural growth, in some studies, is an independent prognostic factor for distant metastases (101) or disease-free survival (37,44).

The importance of histologic subtype for major salivary gland cancer varies in published studies. In most studies, histologic types are subdivided into low and high grade. The main prognostic significance of grading relates to disease-free survival (10,62), although grade was not a prognostic factor in most studies. The best prognosis is seen for acinic cell and (low-grade) mucoepidermoid cancer (91,101), the worst for undifferentiated (70,101) and squamous cell cancer (91,101). At the Netherlands Cancer Institute, a prognostic score for patients with parotid carcinoma was developed and validated adequately with the NWHHT database (105,106). The preoperative prognostic score was based on a weighted combination of prognostic factors (age, pain, clinical T- and N-stages, skin invasion, and facial nerve dysfunction); histology and grading were not incorporated. Four subgroups were formed with markedly differ-

| Table 40.4 | HISTOLOGIC CLASSIFICATION OF SALIVARY GLAND TUMORS |

	Tumor Type	ICD-O and SNOMED Code[a]
1	Adenomas	
1.1	Pleomorphic adenoma	8940/0
1.2	Myoepithelioma (myoepithelial adenoma)	8982/0
1.3	Basal cell adenoma	8147/0
1.4	Warthin tumor (adenolymphoma)	8561/0
1.5	Oncocytoma (oncocytic adenoma)	8290/0
1.6	Canalicular adenoma	
1.7	Sebaceous adenoma	8410/0
1.8	Ductal papilloma	8503/0
1.8.1	Inverted ductal papilloma	8053/0
1.8.2	Intraductal papilloma	8503/0
1.8.3	Sialadenoma papilliferum	8260/0
1.9	Cystadenoma	8440/0
1.9.1	Papillary cystadenoma	8450/0
1.9.2	Mucinous cystadenoma	8470/0
2	Carcinomas	
2.1	Acinic cell carcinoma	8550/3
2.2	Mucoepidermoid carcinoma	8430/3
2.3	Adenoid cystic carcinoma	8200/3
2.4	Polymorphous low-grade adenocarcinoma (terminal ductal adenocarcinoma)	
2.5	Epithelial-myoepithelial carcinoma	
2.6	Basal cell adenocarcinoma	8147/3
2.7	Sebaceous carcinoma	8140/3
2.8	Papillary cystadenocarcinoma	8450/3
2.9	Mucinous adenocarcinoma	8480/3
2.10	Oncocytic carcinoma	8290/3
2.11	Salivary duct carcinoma	8500/3
2.12	Adenocarcinoma	8140/3
2.13	Malignant myoepithelioma (myoepithelial carcinoma)	8982/3
2.14	Carcinoma in pleomorphic adenoma (malignant mixed tumor)	8941/3
2.15	Squamous cell carcinoma	8070/3
2.16	Small cell carcinoma	8041/3
2.17	Undifferentiated carcinoma	8020/3
2.18	Other carcinomas	
3	Nonepithelial tumors	
4	Malignant lymphomas	
5	Secondary tumors	
6	Unclassified tumors	
7	Tumorlike lesions	
7.1	Sialadenosis	71000
7.2	Oncocytosis	73050
7.3	Necrotizing sialometaplasia (salivary gland infarction)	73220
7.4	Benign lymphoepithelial lesion	72240
7.5	Salivary gland cysts	33400
7.6	Chronic sclerosing sialadenitis of submandibular gland (Küttner tumor)	45000
7.7	Cystic lymphoid hyperplasia in AIDS	

AIDS, acquired immunodeficiency syndrome.
[a]Morphology code of the International Classification of Diseases for Oncology (ICD-O) and the Systematized Nomenclature of Medicine (SNOMED).
From Seifert G, Sobin LH. The World Health Organization's histological classification of salivary gland tumors. *Cancer* 1992;70:379–385, with permission.

ent prognoses. In the postoperative score, perineural invasion and positive surgical margins were also included. Positive or close surgical margins result in an increase in local recurrence rate (77,96,101,102). Radiation therapy in addition to surgery improves locoregional control in patients with adverse prognostic factors (70,75,81,100,102). Improvement of survival has only been shown in two studies (11,70), and for stage III and IV major salivary glands in a matched-pair analysis (4).

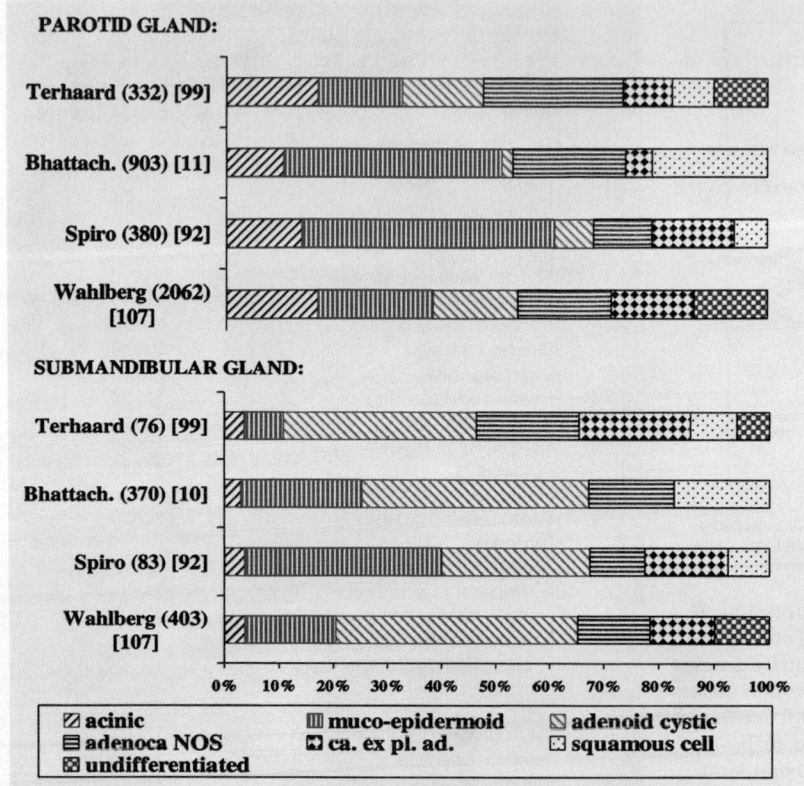

FIGURE 40.6. Major salivary gland malignancies: Distribution of cell types in various series (name of first author provided from study). NOS, not otherwise specified; ca.ex pl. ad., carcinoma ex pleomorphic adenoma.

Minor Salivary Glands

The poorest prognosis is associated with adenoid cystic carcinoma (9,65). Stage, base of skull involvement, and bone invasion are risk factors for locoregional recurrence and survival in minor salivary gland cancers (9,24,25,57,65,77). Locoregional control may be improved by adding postoperative radiotherapy (74).

General Management

The general management of salivary gland malignancies in most patients includes surgical excision followed by radiation therapy for unfavorable prognostic factors (Table 40.5) (3). Postoperative radiotherapy to enhance local control is recommended for T3–4 tumors, close or incomplete resection, bone involvement, perineural invasion, high-grade cancer, and

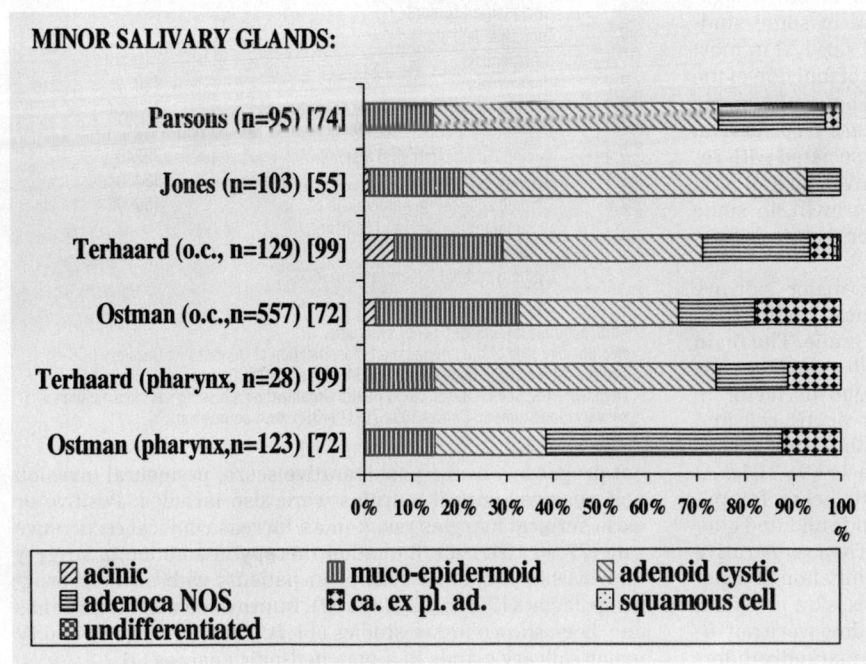

FIGURE 40.7. Minor salivary gland malignancies: Distribution of cell types in various series (name of first author provided from study). o.c., oral cavity; NOS, not otherwise specified; ca.ex pl.ad., carcinoma ex pleomorphic adenoma.

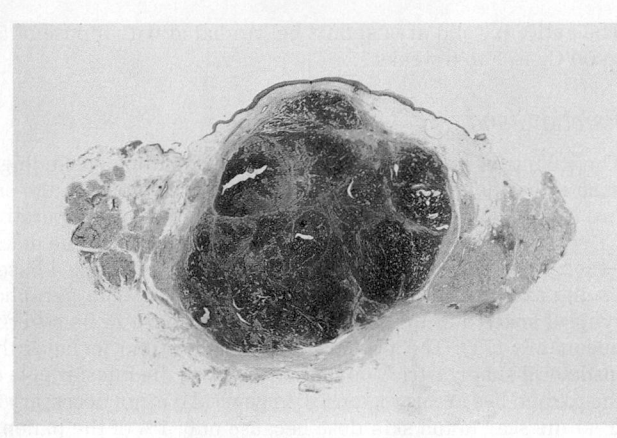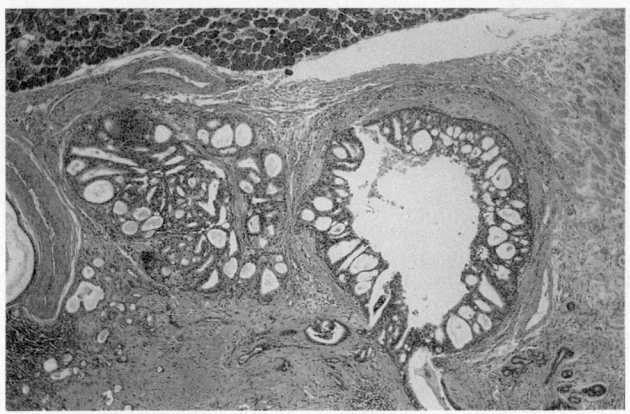

A   B

FIGURE 40.8. Examples of polymorphous low-grade adenocarcinoma (A) and salivary duct carcinoma (B). (Courtesy of Prof. Dr. P. Slootweg, pathologist, Radboud University Medical Center Nijmegen.)

recurrent cancer (9,37,58,70,96,101). To date, adjuvant chemotherapy has not been considered efficacious. For advanced, inoperable, and recurrent salivary gland cancers, primary neutron therapy may lead to superior local control rates, compared with primary photon therapy, without evidence of improved survival rates (24,49,60). The use of conventional radiation therapy along with hyperthermia has been reported to have similar efficacy in this patient population (34).

Major Salivary Glands

Surgical technique depends on location and extent of primary disease and regional adenopathy. Preservation of the facial nerve, at least partially, followed by postoperative radiotherapy is the preferable treatment unless the facial nerve is involved by tumor (6). Aggressive surgery does not improve disease-free survival. A decrease in extended surgery, resulting in a decrease of sacrifice of the facial nerve, has been shown in the course of years (91). Cable facial nerve grafting with the greater auricular or sural nerve graft decreases the incidence of facial palsy postoperatively, especially if branches and not the main trunk are involved (14,56). Adjuvant postoperative radiotherapy has no negative effect on facial nerve function (14).

Surgical treatment includes neck dissection in cases of clinically positive nodes, followed by postoperative radiotherapy (100). The risk of occult nodal disease depends on T-stage and histologic type. As shown in the scoring system in Table 40.1, the decision to treat the neck for parotid tumors will be indicated by a score of at least 4 (100). When local prognostic factors indicate postoperative radiotherapy, no elective neck dissection has to be performed; the neck nodes will also be irradiated (30,94). Parotid tumors with facial nerve weakness are associated with

| Table 40.5 | PROGNOSTIC FACTORS FOR SALIVARY GLAND CANCER—SELECTION OF MULTIVARIATE ANALYZED STUDIES |

Study (by Name of First Author)	No.	Locoregional Control	Distant Meta-Analyses	Survival
General		L: T, site, bone+	Sex, T, N, skin, histology,	OS: Sex, age, T, skin+, bone invasion
Terhaard (101)	565	R : N VII dysfunction, N	Perineural+	
		L + R: Margin, therapy[a]		
Therskilden (102)	251	L: Histology, site, N, margin, therapy		CS: Histology, stage, margin
Mendenhall (66)	224	L: T	Stage	CS: Stage
Parotid				OS: Stage, age, histology, site
Spiro (91)	470			
Bhattacharryya (10)	903			OS: Age, T, N, extraglandular extension
Poulsen (77)	209	L: Age, N, margin, grade		
Garden (39)	166	L: N VII dysfunction, N		DS: >4 nodes, sex, named nerve+, extraglandular extension
Submandibular				OS: Age, grade,
Bhattachatyya (11)	370			
Storey (96)	83	Grade, histology, margin, early years		DS: Early years
Minor		L: T, N		OS: T, general condition
Jones (57)	103	R: Stage		
Lopes (65)	103	N, histology, bone invasion		CS: Stage, therapy[b]
Beckhardt (9)	116	Histology		DS: Grade, T, margin
Parsons (74)	95	L: Stage, therapy[a]		CS: Stage, therapy[a]

L, local; R, regional; OS, overall survival; CS, cause-specific survival; DS, disease-free survival.
[a]S + RT > S.
[b]S + RT > RT.

frequent occult neck nodes; elective treatment is also indicated (30). In most cases, elective neck dissection of level I-III combined with a local resection is performed for submandibular tumors. There is no indication for neck dissection for T1 acinic or T1 adenoid cystic tumors (Table 40.1) (96,100).

Minor Salivary Glands

The treatment of minor salivary gland tumors varies with location but usually involves an attempt at adequate surgical excision first. Irradiation has been used in surgically inaccessible sites or combined with surgery because of locally aggressive tumor behavior and the occurrence of incomplete resection (9,38,74,101). For tumors arising in the palate, tongue, floor of the mouth, oral cavity, or oropharynx, surgical exposure is readily available, and resection usually can be accomplished with acceptable morbidity. Tumors arising in the posterior nasal cavity, nasopharynx, or sphenoid region, however, are relatively inaccessible and are mostly treated with radiation therapy (38). Elective neck treatment is usually not indicated (38,74,100), except for tumors of the floor of mouth, oral tongue, pharynx, and larynx (74,85,115). Surgery alone may be used to treat early-stage hard palate lesions without evidence of positive margins, perineural spread, or bone invasion; simple excision must be avoided (9). Patients with adenoid cystic carcinoma can have a long natural history with late recurrences (38), and consideration should be given to careful surgical reconstruction and rehabilitation because even patients who are not cured can live many years before dying of disease (Fig. 40.3) (101). Occasionally, a patient may present after simple excision (shelling out) of a lesion and the pathologic examination shows adenoid cystic carcinoma. If re-excision would cause significant functional or cosmetic sequelae, irradiation alone may be used (74). However, simple excision is not recommended as the initial management of these tumors because of the potential for a significant volume of residual disease.

Radiation Therapy Techniques

Pleomorphic Adenoma

The pleomorphic adenoma (benign mixed tumor) is histologically benign, occurs frequently in a relatively young population, and comprises 65% to 75% of all parotid epithelial tumors (57,91). Standard therapy has been conservative (superficial) parotidectomy, with recurrence rates of about 0% to 5% (112). Simple excision results in a high recurrence rate of around 25% as focal capsular exposure occurs in virtually all cases (112). In the past at some institutions, local excision and radiation therapy have been used to lower the frequency of facial nerve injury and Frey's syndrome (22). Dawson and Orr (22) reported results for 311 patients. They found a 2.5% recurrence rate at 10 years and an additional 5.5% by 20 years. None of the patients had malignant recurrences at 10 years, 0.5% had such recurrences at 15 years, and 3% had recurrences at 20 years. The later recurrences were more likely to show malignant transformation. The authors concluded that the primary treatment should be surgery because of the patient's young age, benign histology, and the remote possibility of subsequent radiation-induced malignancy. However, certain patients may be referred for radiation therapy (63). Indications for postoperative irradiation may include recurrent disease; microscopically positive margins after surgical resection; and large, deep-seated lesions that may not allow complete surgical excision with adequate margins or would require sacrificing the facial nerve (16,22,63,80). Radiotherapy may decrease the risk of a second recurrence in case of multinodular recurrence only, not for uninodular disease (81).

The entire parotid area should be irradiated with a dose of 50 to 60 Gy in 5 to 6 weeks.

Parotid Gland

The volume of irradiation is determined by pathologic findings, such as perineural invasion of a major nerve. Typically, the entire ipsilateral parotid gland is delineated on the postoperative CT scan performed in a stabilization device (37,71). The delineation of the clinical target volume will be individualized based on the extent of the disease and surgery (37). The parapharyngeal space and the infratemporal fossa have to be covered adequately (71). The primary treatment volume includes the ipsilateral subdigastric nodal areas because the inferior pole of the parotid lies in this region (3). In general it is not necessary to treat the scar to full skin dose because only 1% of the patients have a scar failure (58). For very superficial localized tumors and in case of skin invasion, a bolus over the scar is required. In tumors with named perineural invasion (e.g., adenoid cystic carcinoma), it is important to cover the cranial nerve pathways from the parotid up to the base of the skull (39,96). Focal perineural invasion only is not an indication for routine inclusion of the nerve pathways (39). No clear relationship between dose and local control has been found. In general, a dose of at least 60 Gy postexcision is recommended (39,71,100), and at least 66 Gy (33 fractions) for positive margins (37,39).

The ipsilateral neck is treated after a neck dissection has been performed for positive nodes; level I-V should be included (100). There is no indication for bilateral elective neck treatment (94). The recommended postoperative dose for positive nodes is at least 60 Gy (30 fractions) (100). Elective irradiation of the neck should be considered for advanced T-stage, certain histologic subtypes (Table 40.1), facial nerve dysfunction at presentation, and recurrent disease. At least level Ib, II, and III should be included (5,30,100). A dose of around 46 to 50 Gy is recommended (3,37,100).

Three basic radiation therapy approaches are used, depending on available equipment: Conventional, three-dimensional conformal radiation therapy (3DCRT) planning procedure, and intensity-modulated radiation therapy (IMRT) planning. The first involves unilateral anterior and posterior wedged pair fields using ^{60}Co or 4- to 6-MV photons (Fig. 40.9A). A slight inferior angulation of the beams avoids an exit dose through the contralateral eye. A simpler technique uses homolateral fields with 12- to 16-MeV electrons in combination with photons (37,41,113). Usually, 80% of the dose is delivered with electrons and 20% with ^{60}Co or 4- to 6-MV photons to spare the opposite salivary gland, reduce mucositis, and decrease the skin reaction produced by electrons (Fig. 40.9B). Yaparpalvi et al. (113) compared nine conventional treatment techniques. Ipsilateral wedge pair technique with 6-MV photons, wedged anteroposterior and posteroanterior and lateral technique with 6-MV photons, and mixed beam using 6-MV photons and 16-MeV electrons (1:4 weighted) were most optimal, considering dose homogeneity within the target and dose to normal tissues. Electron beam (9 to 12 MeV) and tangential photon fields are effective conventional techniques for sparing the underlying spinal cord (from doses more than 45 Gy) and the opposite parotid gland in elective neck irradiation. Conventional techniques do not allow for tissue heterogeneity (air cavity, dense bones, and tissues); underdose and overdose may be seen.

After outlining of the target volumes and critical normal tissues on the planning CT scan, a more conformal 3DCRT plan by the use of geometrically shaped beams of uniform intensity may be reached (71). More normal tissue may be spared with this technique (71). Probably the most conformal radiation technique is IMRT. It can produce convex dose distributions and steep dose gradients. Five- to seven-field inverse IMRT allows excellent coverage of the tumor with sparing of mandible,

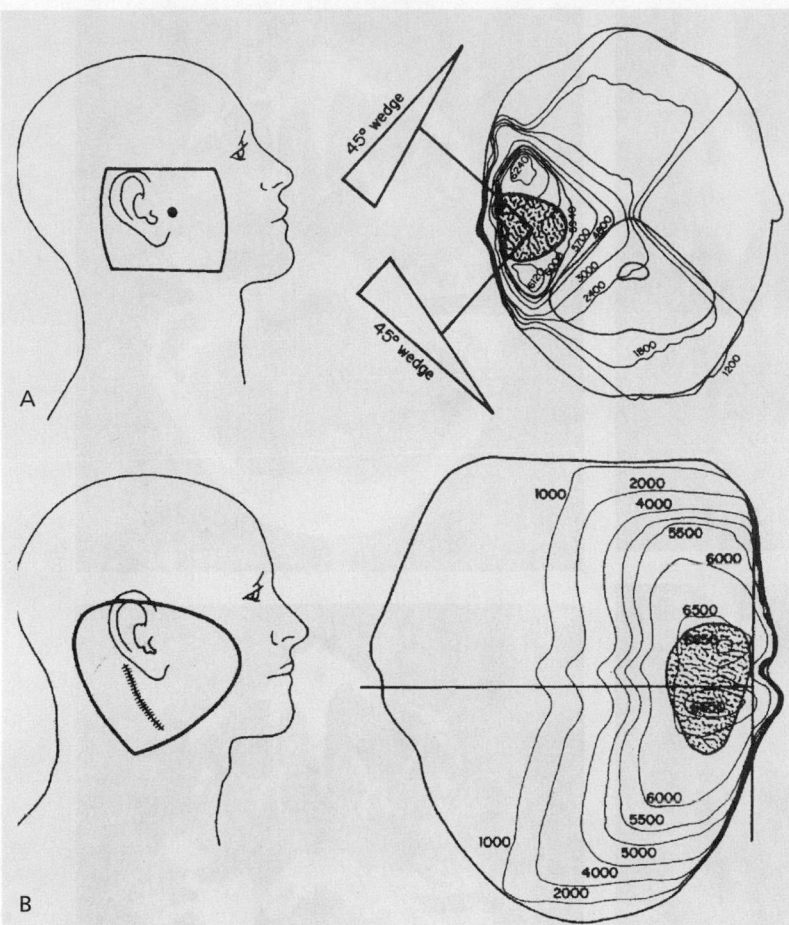

FIGURE 40.9. Conventional radiotherapy for parotid cancer. **A:** Unilateral wedge arrangement and isodose distribution using wedged pair. **B:** Ipsilateral 16-MeV electrons plus ^{60}Co (4:1) electron beam field.

cochlea, spinal cord, brain, and oropharynx (12,71), compared with conformal 3DCRT. Figure 40.10 shows a comparison of 3DCRT and IMRT planning for a postoperative radiotherapy plan for a parotid cancer treated with a dose of 66 Gy. The mean dose to the mastoid, meatus acusticus externus, and contralateral parotid gland was 53 and 43 Gy, 57 and 51 Gy, 1 and 9 Gy, for 3DCRT and IMRT, respectively. The maximum dose to the cochlea was 39 and 32 Gy, respectively.

Submandibular Gland

Except for small acinic cell and adenoid cystic cancer (Table 40.1), the neck nodes level I–IV (5) should be irradiated electively, following the indications outlined for parotid tumors; technical considerations are similar. Bilateral fields may be required for tumor extension toward the midline. If there is no gross residual tumor or perineural invasion, 50 Gy in 5 weeks should be adequate for microscopic disease. If there is named perineural invasion of a major nerve, a tumor dose of 60 to 66 Gy in 6 to 6.5 weeks is recommended, and the nerve path to the base of skull should be treated, preferably by 3DCRT or IMRT. For an adenoid cystic carcinoma of the submandibular gland with only focal perineural invasion, an attempt to encompass the base of the skull would require a significant change in the treatment volume and may not be warranted because of potential morbidity and the low rate of relapse at that site (38). An example of 3DCRT for a T2 adenoid cystic carcinoma of the submandibular gland is shown in Figure 40.11.

Minor Salivary Glands

The radiation therapy technique for treating minor salivary gland tumors depends on the area involved and is similar to the treatment for squamous cell carcinomas in these areas, with two significant exceptions. First, when a named branch of a cranial nerve is involved by adenoid cystic carcinoma, the nerve pathways to the base of the skull should be electively treated. When only focal perineural invasion of small unnamed nerves is present, treatment of the base of the skull depends on the site. Second, for tumors of the palate or paranasal sinuses, the base of the skull is included because of its proximity to the tumor bed. In case of an adenoid cystic carcinoma with perineural invasion, IMRT may reduce the high-dose volume, compared to conventional bilateral opposed fields; Figure 40.12 shows an example for a patient with a minor salivary gland cancer of the palate. IMRT is a useful strategy for irradiating minor salivary gland sites such as the ethmoid sinuses while sparing the optic pathways (19).

Also, because the incidence of lymph node metastases is usually lower than that for squamous cell carcinomas of similar size, the radiation therapy fields are rarely extended to cover such areas if there are no palpable lymph node metastases. Indications for treating the neck are a primary tumor that arose in the tongue, floor of the mouth, pharynx, or larynx (74), and the neck was not dissected, or after resection of metastatic neck lymphadenopathy.

For patients receiving postoperative irradiation after surgical resection, a dose of 60 Gy is given for negative margins and 66 Gy for microscopically positive margins. For gross residual disease after surgery or for lesions treated with irradiation

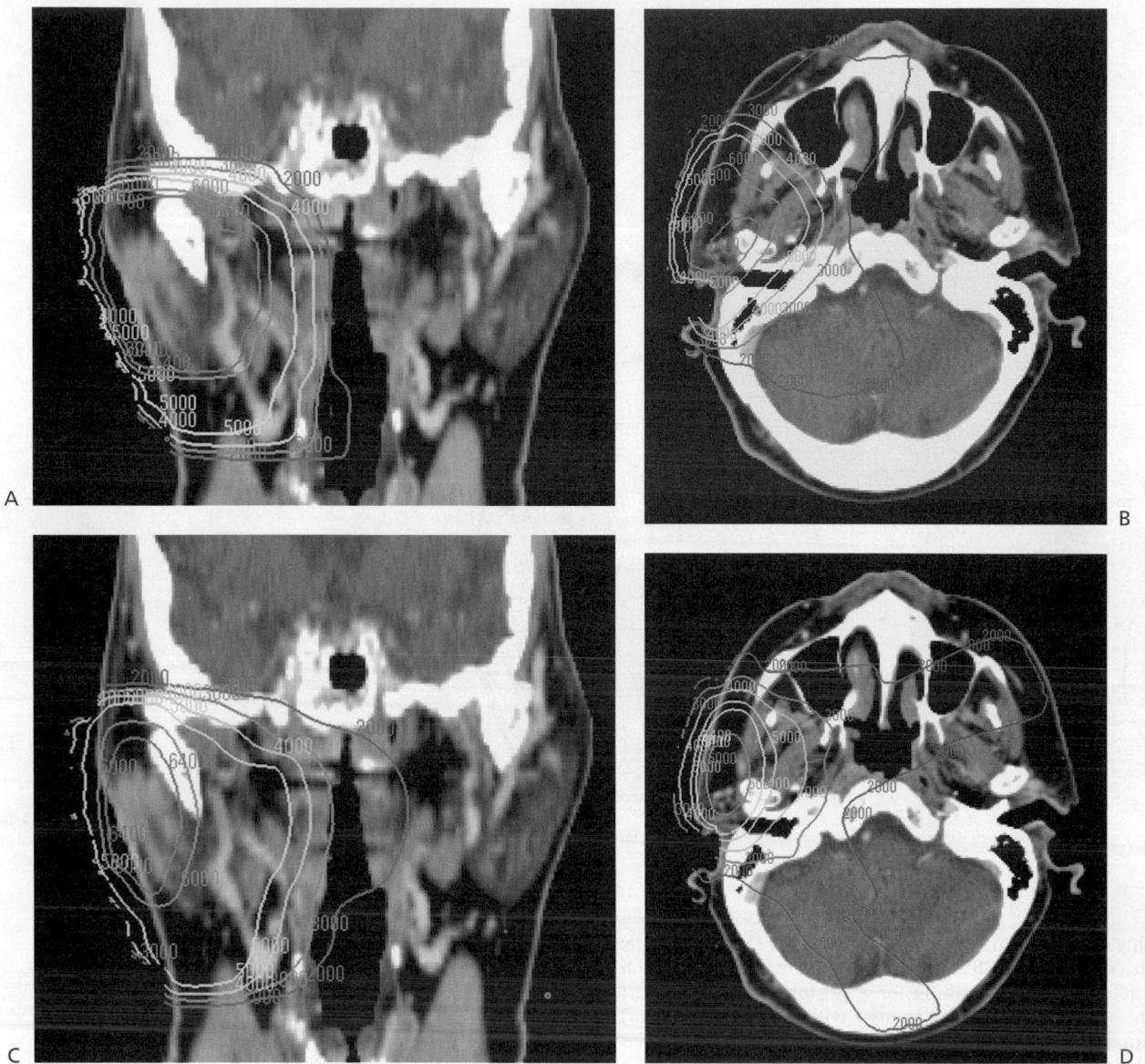

FIGURE 40.10.   Postoperative radiation therapy of a parotid cancer, microscopically incomplete resected. Coronal **(A,C)** and transversal **(B,D)** dose distribution for three-dimensional conformal radiation therapy (25 × 2 Gy primary field, 8 × 2 Gy boost) **(A,B)** and intensity-modulated radiation therapy (inverse, 7 fields and 39 segments; simultaneously moderated accelerated radiotherapy (SMART): 33 × 1.6 Gy primary field, 33 × 2 Gy boost) **(C,D)**.

alone, a total dose of 70 Gy is recommended at 2 Gy per fraction.

Results of Therapy

Surgery Plus or Minus Postoperative Radiotherapy

Tables 40.6 through 40.8 list local control rates and 5- and 10-year survival rates for several series reporting the surgical, irradiation, and combination treatment of carcinomas of the major and minor salivary glands. Little adverse effect of delay between surgery and radiotherapy may be predicted for what are, in general, slow-growing salivary gland cancers. In only two studies, one concerning submandibular cancer (96) and another for minor salivary gland (38), impaired locoregional control rates were seen for a delay of more than 6 weeks, which was not confirmed in the Dutch study (100). The prognosis for children with a malignant salivary gland cancer (mostly mucoepidermoid cancer of the parotid gland) is excellent, with a 10 year overall sur-

vival of more than 90% (88). Most are treated with surgery alone because of the possible risk on radiation-induced malignancies.

Long-term follow-up is recommended because failures may appear after 5 years, especially for minor salivary gland tumors (17,29,57,101). Recurrent tumors in general are more difficult to control than are primary ones, so high initial locoregional control rates should be the goal (101). Because of high rates of local failure of approximately 40% for parotid, 60% for submandibular, and 65% for minor salivary glands with surgery alone in the past (93), many institutions have advocated postoperative irradiation especially to reduce the incidence of local failure. Local tumor control appears to be improved by the combination of surgery and irradiation, although randomized, controlled trials have not been performed. Evidence of a positive role of postoperative radiotherapy is based on retrospective studies and a matched-pair analysis. In the study by Armstrong et al. (4), postoperative radiotherapy significantly improved locoregional control (from 17% to 51% for stage III-IV), not for stage I and II major salivary gland cancer. Locoregional control for patients with positive nodes increased from 40% to

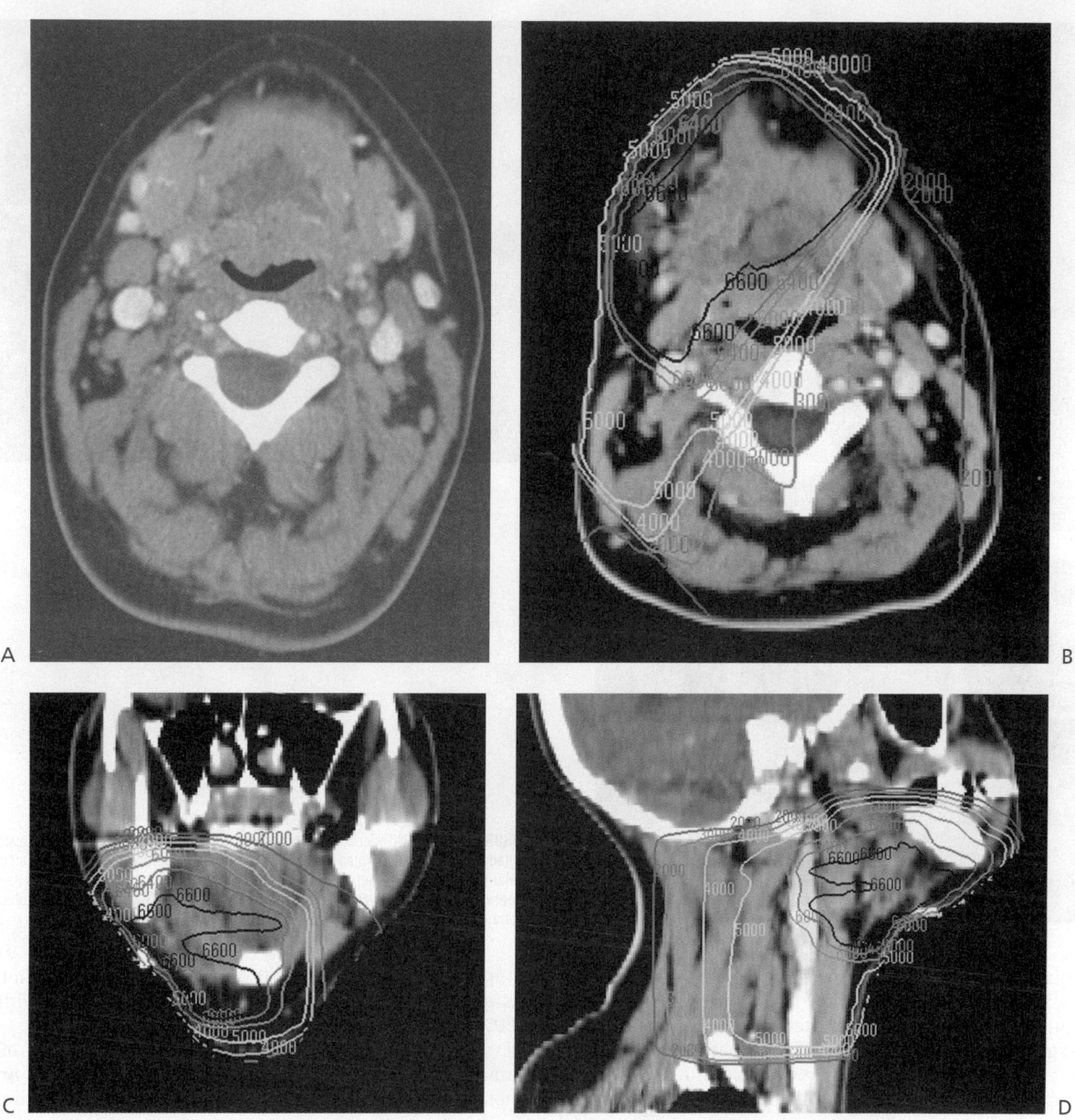

FIGURE 40.11. Dose distribution for a T2 N0 adenoid cystic cancer of the right submandibular gland. Computed tomography performed before microscopically incomplete local excision **(A)**. Three-dimensional conformal radiation therapy, three fields (one right and two left oblique): 25 × 2 Gy, 5 × weekly primary tumor and level I-III nodes, 8 × 2 Gy boost; transversal **(B)**, coronal **(C)**, and sagittal **(D)** planes. Mean dose to contralateral submandibular gland is 27 Gy.

69%. In most studies, an imbalance in prognostic factors is seen comparing surgery alone with combined therapy, favoring surgery alone. Despite this imbalance, locoregional control with combined surgery and postoperative radiotherapy is superior to surgery alone for patients with negative prognostic factors, irrespective of site (33,66,100–102). In the nationwide Dutch study, the relative risk for surgery alone, compared with combined treatment, was 9.7 for local recurrence and 2.3 for regional recurrence (100). In a study from Denmark, the relative risk of no radiotherapy versus radiotherapy was 4.7 for locoregional control (102). Postoperative radiotherapy is particularly effective if there are close and microscopic positive resection margins, enhancing local control from around 50% to 80% to 95% (33,41,77,100,102). Comparable results are noted for T3-T4 tumors and pathologically confirmed bone and perineural invasion (66,100). However, for a T1 or T2 tumor that was completely resected with no bone or perineural invasion, surgery alone will result in more than 90% 10-year local control rate, and radiotherapy is not indicated (100).

Treatment results also may depend on histopathologic status. However, after review, histologic type may change, even among experienced pathologists. In general, the best prognosis is shown for acinic cell and mucoepidemoid cancer, with a 15% risk of distant metastases after 10 years and a 10-year locoregional control rate of around 85%. Ten-year overall survival is around 80% and 65%, respectively (11,45,93,101). In one of three patients, postoperative radiotherapy is indicated (45,101). Squamous cell and undifferentiated tumors have been associated with a 10-year overall survival of 35% or less, caused by a high risk of distant metastases (35% and 50%, respectively) and locoregional recurrence (77,93,101). Postoperative radiotherapy is indicated in all cases to improve locoregional control. The intermediate-risk group consists of adenoid cystic cancer and cancer ex pleomorphic adenoma. Distant failure after 10 years is around 35% (39,92,101). Although the risk of nodal recurrence is low (5% to 10%), local recurrence is diagnosed more often (20% to 30%). A precipitous decrease in relapse-free survival is noted among 5 (around 70%), 10 (around 50%),

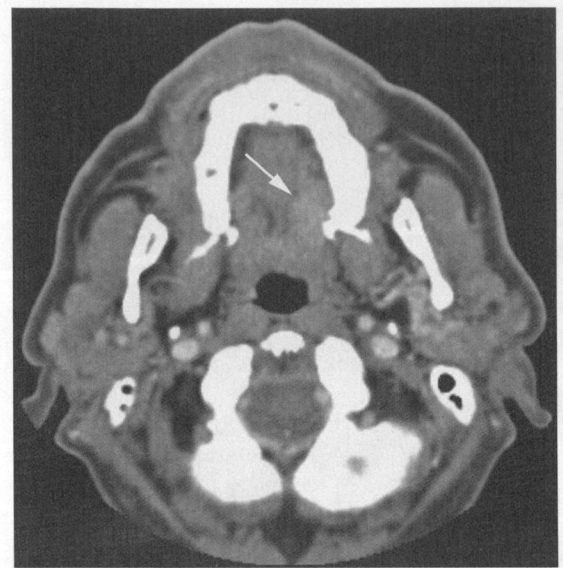

A

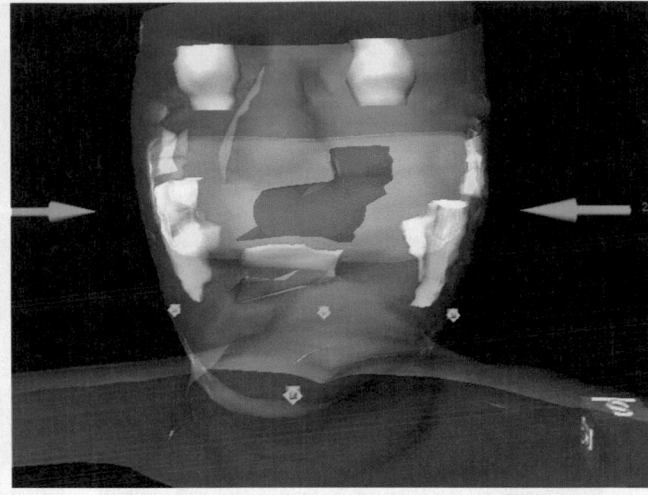

B

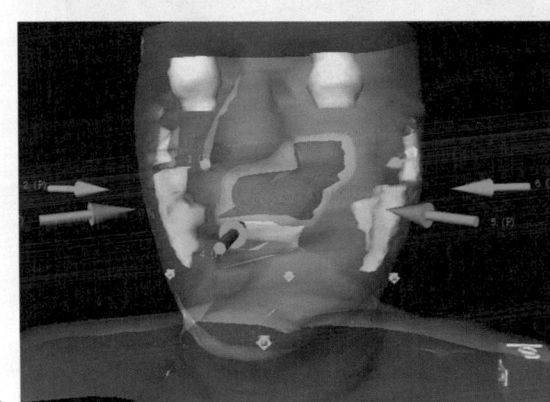

C

FIGURE 40.12. T2N0 adenoid cystic cancer of the palate with major perineural invasion. Computed tomography performed before local excision (**A**, *arrow:* Tumor); target includes right palatinus major nerve until base of skull. Dose distribution (25 × 2 Gy primary field) in transversal planes; conventional bilateral opposed fields (**B**); intensity-modulated radiation therapy (7 fields, 40 segments) (**C**); 95% isodose of 50 Gy in red.

and 15 years (around 45%) for patients with adenoid cystic carcinomas, which are well known for late recurrences (39,101). Significant improvement was reported in local control for adenoid cystic cancer with combined surgery and irradiation in several studies (33,39,81,89,96), regardless of site. Local tumor control rates with combined modality therapy for these tumors

approach 85% to 90% at 10 years. Postoperative radiotherapy is also able to improve locoregional control rates with about 20% for high-grade tumors (62,81,96).

In the World Health Organization classification of 1991, among others, two new subtypes were described that are diagnosed relatively frequently. PLGA is situated solely in the palate.

Table 40.6   RESULTS OF STANDARD THERAPY FOR CANCER OF THE PAROTID

Study (by Name of First Author)	No. of Patients	Treatment	% 5-Year Survival	% 10-Year Survival	% Local Control
Fu (33)	63	S, S + R, R	68	54	73
Bhattacharyya (10)	903	S ± R	67	50	NA
Spiro (93)	623	S	55	47	61
Terhaard (101)	37	S	67	61	51 (10 yr)
	254	S + R	65	51	88 (10 yr)
Garden (37)	166	S + R	78	60	90 (10 yr)
North (70)	19	S	59	na	74
	50	S + R	75	na	98
Poulsen (77)	209	S + R	71	65	76
Renehan (81)	37	S	77	63	57 (locoreg.)
	66	S + R	78	67	85 (locoreg.)
Pohar (75)	56	S	65	50	63 (locoreg.)
	91	S + R	55	40	89 (locoreg.)

S, surgery; R, irradiation; NA, not available; locoreg., locoregional.

Table 40.7	RESULTS OF STANDARD THERAPY FOR CANCER OF THE SUBMANDIBULAR GLANDS				
Study (by Name of First Author)	No. of Patients	Treatment	% 5-Year Survival	% 10-Year Survival	% Local Control
Spiro (93)	129	S	31	22	40 (locoreg.)
Terhaard (101)	68	S + R	57	45	91 (10 yr)
Storey (96)	83	S + R	60 (DFS)	53 (DFS)	88 (locoreg.)
Bhattacharyya (11)	370	S ± R	60	NA	NA

S, surgery; locoreg., locoregional: R, irradiation; DFS, disease-free survival; NA, not available.

Treatment consists of wide local excision. In a report by Castle et al. (17), treatment results of 164 tumors were analyzed, with 90% treated with surgery alone. Local control was 90%, with only few patients dying from PLGA. However, local failures may be seen even after long follow-up. In a series from Evans and Luna (29) of 40 patients with PLGA, local recurrence was seen in 43% of patients treated with surgery alone, mainly because of close and microscopic positive resection margins. No recurrence was seen in the nine patients treated with postoperative radiotherapy.

Salivary duct carcinoma is a very aggressive disease, and postoperative locoregional radiotherapy is indicated in all cases. Most patients die of disease, despite often successful locoregional combined therapy. Because of a high percentage of distant metastases, 5-year survival is only around 10% to 15% (42,52). The prognosis correlates with HER-2/*neu* receptor status; 3-year survival is 56% and 17% for (+)HER-2/*neu* and (+ + +)HER-2/*neu*, respectively (52).

Minor salivary gland tumors of the oral cavity have a more favorable prognosis than paranasal sinus tumors (maxillary and ethmoid sinus and nasal cavity) (38). Patients with hard palate lesions tend to be diagnosed when they have small asymptomatic lumps, which are easily detected on physical examination. On the other hand, paranasal sinus tumors usually do not cause symptoms until they are locally advanced. The surgical approach for these tumors is more difficult, with a greater chance for leaving behind residual disease, leading to high recurrence rates. A combined approach with surgery and postoperative irradiation is recommended.

Primary Radiotherapy

The poor results for salivary gland cancer with irradiation alone in several series have been attributed to the use of primary radiotherapy for patients with locally advanced lesions or distant metastases at presentation, who were essentially treated for palliation. Locoregional control rates after conventional photon or electron therapy are around 25% (49,60,66). For treatment with photons with curative intent, a clear dose-response relationship has been described (100). A dose of 66 to 70 Gy may result in 50% 5-year local control. Wang and Goodman (109) reported local control as high as 85% with accelerated hyperfractionated photon therapy. The follow-up was rather short, and the results have not been updated (109). The generally slow rate of regression of advanced salivary gland tumors have made them a logical target for alternative radiation therapy approaches, such as fast neutrons.

Neutron Therapy

Patients with inoperable primary or recurrent major or minor salivary glands were included in the RTOG-MRC randomized phase III clinical trial. Patients were randomized between 70 Gy for 7.5 weeks or 55 Gy for 4 weeks photon therapy and neutron

Table 40.8	RESULTS OF STANDARD THERAPY FOR MINOR SALIVARY GLANDS				
Study (by Name of First Author)/Site	No. of Patients	Treatment	% 5-Year Survival	% 10-Year Survival	% Local Control
Fu (33)	30	S, S + R, R	70	61	63
Spiro (93)	526	S	48	37	35 (locoreg.)
Simpson (89) (adenoid cystic)	71	S + R	65	36	83
Garden (38)	160	S + R	81	65	88 (15 yr)
Terhaard (101) (oral cavity)	67	S	87	76	91
	54	S + R	85	72	98
Lopes (65) (oral cavity)	59	S	86	83	90 (locoreg.)
	32	S + R	88	56	78 (locoreg.)
	15	R	46	—	13 (locoreg.)
Beckhardt (9) (palate)	79	S	90 (DSS)	80 (DSS)	NA
	35	S + R	87 (DSS)	83 (DSS)	NA
Vander Poorten (104)	55	S ± R	66	57	76 (locoreg.)
Schramm (85), (nasopharynx)	23	S + R	67 (DSS)	48 (DSS)	77 (5 year)

S, surgery; R, irradiation; locoreg., locoregional; DSS, disease-specific survival,; NA, not available.

therapy. The study had to be stopped because of a statistically significant difference in 2-year locoregional control, after inclusion of only 32 patients. The 10-year locoregional control probability was 17% after photon therapy, and 56% after neutron therapy (60). However, survival was identical. Late morbidity was somewhat higher for neutron therapy. Douglas et al. (24) of the University of Washington have published results of 279 patients treated with neutrons. Almost all patients had evidence of gross residual disease. Major and minor salivary gland sites were equally distributed. Total dose, administered with neutrons, varied from 17.4 to 20.7 Gy. The 6-year locoregional control and cause-specific survival were 59% and 49%, respectively, conforming to the results of most studies. Locoregional control was only 19% for base of skull involvement and 67% for no involvement. Locoregional control was 72% for minor sites and 61% for major sites. The 6-year actuarial grade 3 and 4 toxicity was 10%. Less severe late morbidity may occur if neutron therapy is combined with photons. A study from Heidelberg for advanced, inoperable, recurrent, or incompletely resected adenoid cystic carcinoma compared results of treatment with neutrons, photons, or mixed beam (49). Severe late grade 3 and 4 toxicity was 19% with neutrons, compared to 10% with mixed beam and 4% with photon therapy. The 5-year local control was 75% for neutrons and 32% for mixed beams and photons; survival was identical.

In an effort to improve poor results for tumors invading the base of skull, several new techniques have been developed. A combination of neutron therapy with, after a 4-week split, a Gamma Knife stereotactic radiosurgical boost has been used for tumors invading the base of skull (26). Local control of eight patients treated with this technique looks promising; however, follow-up was only 2 years. Another option is a combination of photons (54 Gy) and carbon ions (18 Gy) radiotherapy (86). In a series of 16 patients with adenoid cystic cancer invading the base of skull, the 3-year local control was 65%, without late effects exceeding grade 2. Longer follow-up results of these new techniques are awaited.

In conclusion, neutron beam therapy seems to be the treatment of choice for unresectable, residual, or recurrent salivary gland tumors. Despite high locoregional control, survival is not improved and late toxicity is of concern.

Systemic Therapy

The rarity of these neoplasms and their localized nature provide limited opportunities for trials with chemotherapy. In a review by Lalami et al. (59), they stated that chemotherapy has to be considered as palliative treatment and should only be given for disease-related symptoms and rapidly progressive disease. Cisplatin as monotherapy shows a 20% response rate for locoregional disease and only 7% for distant failures, with a duration of 6 to 9 months. A combination of 5-fluorouacil, cyclophosphamide, cisplatin, and doxorubicin gives a response rate of 50% (59).

Carcinoma ex pleomorphic adenomas and salivary duct carcinomas express androgen receptors in a high frequency (69). There may be a possible role for antiandrogen therapy, combined with other treatment modalities. However, the efficacy of this treatment option for some salivary gland cancers still has to be proven.

Expression of vascular endothelial growth factor is seen frequently in salivary gland cancer and is related with poor prognosis. Overexpression of HER-2/neu also correlates with poor prognosis, and a great variety between histologic types has been demonstrated (59). In the future, the role of molecular-targeted therapy for these salivary gland cancers has to be established.

Sequelae of Treatment

The most notable complication of treatment of parotid malignancies is facial nerve paralysis, which is often caused by the initial or a repeated surgical procedure. However, various series have shown that facial nerve sacrifice is rarely necessary, unless the nerve is directly involved by tumor, particularly when postoperative irradiation is given (33,77,91). When facial nerve sacrifice is required, facial nerve grafting and postoperative radiation therapy achieve comparable facial nerve function compared with unirradiated graft despite more negative prognostic factors (14). Other postoperative sequelae, such as salivary fistulae and neuromas of the greater auricular nerve, are sometimes seen. Frey's syndrome (i.e., gustatory sweating) may occur in a few patients after parotid surgery, but it is rarely bothersome (58).

Partial xerostomia after irradiation of the parotid gland is frequently observed and may be permanent. Trismus may result from radiation-induced fibrosis of the temporomandibular joint or the masseter muscles. It usually occurs when there is extensive tumor infiltration of the masseter muscle and high doses are given. Data on dose-response relationship for radiation-induced hearing impairments are sparse. In a study by Chen et al. (18), with 21 patients treated for malignant parotid tumors, a significant hearing loss was noted after a cochlear dose of ≥60 Gy in 60%, and in no patient after a dose <60 Gy. Conductive hearing loss was caused by serous effusion in the middle ear and/or obstruction of the tuba Eustachius. In general, a dose as low as possible (<30 Gy) should be attempted (53).

Garden et al. (38) reported complications of irradiation in 51 of 160 patients receiving postoperative irradiation for minor salivary gland tumors. The most common complication was decreased hearing in 26 patients, 20 of whom had myringotomies or myringotomy tubes placed for serous otitis media. Bone necrosis or exposure was observed in several patients; however, this complication has been seen infrequently during the past decade with improved radiation therapy techniques and treatment of multiple, as opposed to single, fields per day. Complications to the eyes or optic pathways were most common in patients with paranasal sinus primary tumors. At least six cases of contralateral optic atrophy occurred. Other eye complications included dry eye syndrome, nasolacrimal duct obstruction, cataract, retinopathy, and perforated globe. To reduce the incidence of bilateral blindness, the dose to the optic chiasm and contralateral optic nerve is limited to 54 Gy. In patients with extensive tumor involvement of the orbit it may be preferable to remove the eye surgically rather than to subject the entire orbit to high doses. Radiation-induced injury to the visual pathway is dose-dependent. None of the patients receiving a dose of less than 50 Gy develop optic neuropathy or chiasm injury, whereas the 10-year actuarial incidences of optic nerve chiasm injury is 5% and 30% for patients receiving 50 to 60 Gy and 61 to 78 Gy, respectively (54).

Radiotherapy of tumors of the pharynx, and less frequently the oral cavity, may result in permanent complaints of xerostomia. The mean dose to the parotid glands that relates to 1-year xerostomia may range from 26 Gy (27) to 39 Gy (82). This serious late complication may be significantly reduced by the use of IMRT (51,99). For those patients with a dose to both parotid glands that exceeds at least 39 Gy, amifostine administration during head and neck radiotherapy will reduce the severity and duration of xerostomia 2 years after radiotherapy (110), without compromising locoregional control.

Treatment of Recurrence

Retreatment usually involves additional surgery, if feasible, and postoperative irradiation in previously unirradiated patients (Fig. 40.13). In the retreatment of parotid neoplasms,

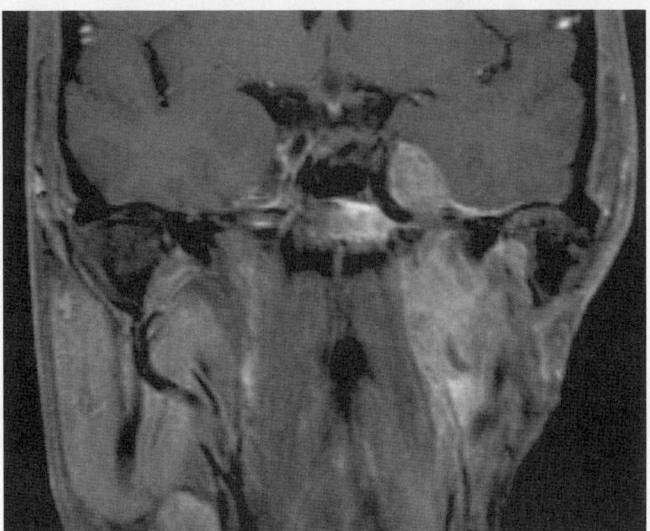

FIGURE 40.13. Coronal fat-suppressed contrast-enhanced magnetic resonance image shows a recurrence of squamous cell cancer of the parotid gland after total parotidectomy. The tumor is centered in the left articulator space with perineural spread along the nV3. Retrograde perineural spread of tumor through foramen ovale on the left side. (Courtesy of Dr. F.A. Pameyer, radiologist, University Medical Center Utrecht)

preserving facial nerve function and obtaining local control are more difficult than for the initial tumor. Therapy consisting of surgery with postoperative irradiation has demonstrated enhanced local control, and facial nerve sacrifice may be necessary less often if this combination is used. In certain histologic subtypes (e.g., adenoid cystic carcinoma), retreatment of locally recurrent disease yields prolonged survival (89). Aggressive local therapy for recurrent disease is indicated if the probability of long-term survival is high.

Chemotherapy also has been used for recurrent disease. Polychemotherapy for recurrent high-grade disease may result in around 45% response rate, with a median duration of 7.5 months (1). However, in view of its significant toxicity and modest response rates in a population that may have recurrent yet indolent progressive disease, trials of aggressive cytotoxic therapy are recommended only on carefully drafted protocols. In the future, molecular target agents may be tested in selected recurrent salivary gland cancers.

References

1. Airoldi M, Cortesina G, Giordanao C, et al. Update and perspectives on non-surgical treatment of salivary gland malignancies. *Acta Otorhinolaryngol Ital* 2003;23:368–376.
2. American Joint Committee on Cancer Staging. *Manual for staging of cancer*, 6th ed. Philadelphia: J.B. Lippincott; 2002.
3. Ang KK, Kaanders JHAM, Peters LJ. *Radiotherapy for head and neck cancers: Indications and techniques*. Philadelphia: Lea & Febiger; 1994:109–118.
4. Armstrong JG, Harrison LB, Spiro RH, et al. Malignant tumors of major salivary gland origin. *Arch Otolaryngol Head Neck Surg* 1990;116:290–293.
5. Armstrong JG, Harrison LB, Thaler HT, et al. The indications for elective treatment of the neck in cancer of the major salivary glands. *Cancer* 1992;69:615–619.
6. Ball ABS, Fish S, Thomas JM. Malignant epithelial parotid tumours: A rational treatment policy. *Br J Surg* 1995;82:621–623.
7. Batsakis JC. Tumors of the major salivary glands and neoplasms of the minor and "lesser" major salivary glands. In: Batsakis JC, ed. *Tumors of the head and neck: Clinical and pathological considerations*, 2nd ed. Baltimore: Williams & Wilkins; 1979.
8. Beal KP, Singh B, Kraus D, et al. Radiation-induced salivary gland tumors: A report of 18 cases and a review of the literature. *Cancer J* 2003;9:467–471.
9. Beckhardt RN, Weber RS, Zane R, et al. Minor salivary gland tumors of the palate: Clinical and pathologic correlates of outcome. *Laryngoscope* 1995;105:1155–1160.
10. Bhattacharyya N, Fried MP. Determinants of survival in parotid gland carcinoma: A population-based study. *Am J Otolaryngol-Head Neck Med Surg* 2005;26:39–44.
11. Bhattacharyya N. Survival and prognosis for cancer of the submandibular gland. *J Oral Maxillofac Surg* 2004;62:427–430.
12. Bragg CM, Conway J, Robinson MH. The role of intensity-modulated radiotherapy in the treatment of parotid tumors. *Int J Radiat Oncol Biol Phys* 2002;52:729–738.
13. Brandwein MS, Ivanov K, Wallace DI, et al. Mucoepidermoid carcinoma: A clinicopathologic study of 80 patients with special reference to histological grading. *Am J Surg Pathol* 2001;25:835–845.
14. Brown PD, Eshleman JS, Foote RL, et al. An analysis of facial nerve function in irradiated and unirradiated facial nerve grafts. *Int J Radiat Oncol Biol Phys* 2000;48:737–743.
15. Caldemeyer KS, Mathews VP, Righi PD, et al. Imaging features and clinical significance of perineural spread or extension of head and neck tumors. *Radiographics* 1998;18:97–110.
16. Carew JF, Spiro RH, Singh B, et al. Treatment of recurrent pleomorphic adenomas of the parotid gland. *Otolaryngol Head Neck Surg* 1999;121:539–542.
17. Castle JT, Thompson LDR, Frommelt RA, et al. Polymorphous low grade adenocarcinoma. A clinicopathologic study of 164 cases. *Cancer* 1999;86:207–219.
18. Chen WC, Liao CT, Tsai HC, et al. Radiation-induced hearing impairment in patients treated for malignant parotid tumor. *Ann Otol Rhinol Laryngol* 1999;108:1159–1164.
19. Claus F, De Gersem W, De Wagter C, et al. An implementation of strategy for IMRT of ethmoid sinus cancer with bilateral sparing of the optic pathways. *Int J Radiat Oncol Biol Phys* 2001;51:18–31.
20. Cohen EG, Patel SG, Lin O, et al. Fine-needle aspiration biopsy of salivary gland lesions in a selected patient population. *Arch Otolaryngol Head Neck Surg* 2004;130:773–778.
21. da Cruz Perez DE, Pires FR, Alves FA, et al. Salivary gland tumors in children and adolescents: A clinicopathologic and immunohistochemical study of fifty-three cases. *Int J Pediatr Otorhinolaryngol* 2004;68:895–902.
22. Dawson AK, Orr JA. Long-term results of local excision and radiotherapy in pleomorphic adenoma of the parotid. *Int J Radiat Oncol Biol Phys* 1985;11:451–455.
23. Delgado R, Klimstra D, Albores-Saavedra J. Low grade salivary duct carcinoma. A distinctive variant with a low grade histology and a predominant intraductal growth pattern. *Cancer* 1996;78:958–967.
24. Douglas JG, Koh W, Austin-Seymour M, et al. Treatment of salivary gland neoplasms with fast neutron radiotherapy. *Arch Otolaryngol Head Neck Surg.* 2003;129:944–948.
25. Douglas JG, Lee S, Laramore GE, et al. Neutron radiotherapy for the treatment of locally advanced major salivary gland tumors. *Head Neck* 1999;21:255–263.
26. Douglas JG, Silbergeld DL, Laramore GE. Gamma Knife stereotactic radiosurgical boost for patients treated primarily with neutron radiotherapy for salivary gland neoplasms. *Stereotact Funct Neurosurg* 2004;82:84–89.
27. Eisbruch A, ten Haken RK, Kim HM, et al. Dose, volume, and function relationships in parotid salivary glands following conformal and intensity-modulated irradiation of head-and-neck cancer. *Int J Radiat Oncol Biol Phys* 1999;45:577–587.
28. Enamorado I, Lakhani R, Korkmaz H, et al. Correlation of histopathological variants, cellular DNA content, and clinical outcome in adenoid cystic carcinoma of the salivary glands. *Otolaryngol Head Neck Surg* 2004;131:646–650.
29. Evans HL, Luna MA. Polymorphous low-grade adenocarcinoma. A study of 40 cases with long-term follow up and an evaluation of the importance of papillary areas. *Am J Surg Pathol* 2000;24:1319–1328.
30. Ferlito A, Pellitteri PK, Robbins T, et al. Management of the neck in cancer of the major salivary glands, thyroid and parathroid glands. *Acta Otolaryngol* 2002;122:673–678.
31. Frankenthaler RA, Luna MA, Lee SS, et al. Prognostic variables in parotid gland cancer. *Arch Otolaryngol Head Neck Surg* 1991;117:1251–1256.
32. Franzen G, Nordgard S, Boysenn M, et al. DNA content in adenoid cystic carcinomas. *Head Neck* 1995;17:49–55.
33. Fu KK, Leibel SA, Levine ML, et al. Carcinoma of the major and minor salivary glands. Analysis of treatment results and sites and causes of failures. *Cancer* 1977;40:2882–2890.
34. Gabriele P, Amichetti M, Orecchia R, et al. Hyperthermia and radiation therapy for inoperable or recurrent parotid carcinoma. *Cancer* 1995;75:908–913.
35. Gallo O, Franchi A, Bianchi S, et al. P53 oncoprotein expression in parotid gland carcinoma is associated with clinical outcome. *Cancer* 1995;75:2037–2044.
36. Gallo O, Franchi A, Vittorio Bottai G, et al. Risk factors for distant metastases from carcinoma of the parotid gland. *Cancer* 1997;80:844–851.
37. Garden AS, el-Naggar AK, Morrison WH, et al. Postoperative radiotherapy for malignant tumors of the parotid gland. *Int J Radiat Oncol Biol Phys* 1997;79–85.
38. Garden AS, Weber RS, Ang KK, et al. Postoperative radiation therapy for malignant tumors of minor salivary glands. Outcome and patterns of failure. *Cancer* 1994;73:2563–2569.
39. Garden AS, Weber RS, Morrison WH, et al. The influence of positive margins and nerve invasion in adenoid cystic carcinoma of the head and neck treated with surgery and radiation. *Int J Radiat Oncol Biol Phys* 1995;32:619–626.
40. Gardner E, Gray DJ, O'Rahily R, eds. *Anatomy: A regional study of human structure*, 3rd ed. Philadelphia: WB Saunders; 1969.
41. Guillamondegui O, Byers RM, Tapley NdV. Malignant tumors of salivary glands. In: Fletcher GH, ed. *Textbook of radiotherapy*, 3rd ed. Philadelphia: Lea & Febiger; 1980.
42. Guzzo M, di Palma S, Grandi C, et al. Salivary duct carcinoma: Clinical characteristics and treatment strategies. *Head Neck* 1997;19:126–133.
43. Haagensen CD, Feind CR, Herter FP. *The lymphatics in cancer*. Philadelphia: WB Saunders; 1972.
44. Hocwald E, Korkmaz H, Yoo GH, et al. Prognostic factors in major salivary gland cancer. *Laryngoscope* 2001;111:1434–1439.
45. Hoffman HT, Karnell LH, Robinson RA, et al. National cancer database report on cancer of the head and neck: Acinic cell carcinoma. *Head Neck* 1999;21:297–309.
46. Hollingshed WH, Cornelius R. *Textbook of anatomy*, 4th ed. Philadelphia: Harper & Row; 1985.
47. Horn-Ross PL, Ljung BM, Morrow M. Environmental factors and the risk of salivary gland cancer. *Epidemiology* 1997;10:414–419.
48. Hosal AS, Fan C, Barnes L, et al. Salivary duct carcinoma. *Otolaryngol Head Neck Surg* 2003;129:720–725.
49. Huber PE, Debus J, Latz D, et al. Radiotherapy for advanced adenoid cystic carcinoma: Neutrons, photons or mixed beam? *Radiother Oncol* 2001;59:161–167.
50. In der Maur CD, Klokman WJ, Van Leeuwen FE, et al. Increased risk of breast cancer development after diagnosis of salivary gland tumour. *Eur J Cancer* 2005;41:1311–1315.
51. Jabbari S, Kim HM, Feng M, et al. Matched case-control study of quality of life and xerostomia after intensity-modulated radiotherapy or standard radiotherapy for

head-and-neck cancer: Initial report. *Int J Radiat Oncol Biol Phys* 2005;63:725–731.

52. Jaehne M, Roeser K, Jaekel T, et al. Clinical and immunohistologic typing of salivary duct carcinoma. A report of 50 cases. *Cancer* 2005;103:2526–2533.

53. Jereczek-Fossa BA, Zarowski A, Milani F et al. Treatment induced complications. Radiotherapy-induced ear toxicity. *Cancer Treatment Reviews* 2003;29:417–430.

54. Jiang GL, Tucker SL, Guttenberger R, et al. Radiation-induced injury to the visual pathway. *Radiother Oncol* 1994;30:17–25.

55. Johns ME, Goldsmith MM. Current management of salivary gland tumors. *Oncology* 1989;3:85.

56. Johns ME, Kaplan MJ. Surgical therapy of tumors of the salivary glands. In: Thawley SE, Panje W, Batsakis J, et al., eds. *Comprehensive management of head and neck tumors*. Philadelphia: WB Saunders; 1986.

57. Jones AS, Beasley NJP, Houghton DJ, et al. Tumours of the minor salivary glands. *Clin Otolaryngol* 1998;23:27–33.

58. Kirkbride P, Liu FF, O'Sullivan B, et al. Outcome of curative management of malignant tumors of the parotid gland. *J Otolaryngol* 2001;30:271–279.

59. Lalami Y, Vereecken P, Dequanter D, et al. Salivary gland carcinomas, paranasal sinus cancers and melanoma of the head and neck: An update about rare but challenging tumors. *Curr Opinion Oncol* 2006;18:258–265.

60. Laramore GE, Krall JM, Griffin TW, et al. Neutron versus photon irradiation for unresectable salivary gland tumors: Final report of an RTOG-MRC randomized clinical trial. *Int J Radiat Oncol Biol Phys* 1993;27:235–240.

61. Lim JJ, Kang S, Lee MR, et al. Expression of vascular endothelial growth factor in salivary gland carcinomas and its relation to p53, Ki-67 and prognosis. *J Oral Pathol Med* 2003;32:552–561.

62. Lima RA, Tavares MR, Dias FL, et al. Clinical prognostic factors in malignant parotid gland tumors. *Otolaryngol Head Neck Surg* 2005;133:702–708.

63. Liu F-F, Rotstein L, Davison AJ, et al. Benign parotid adenomas: A review of the Princess Margaret Hospital experience. *Head Neck* 1995;17:177–183.

64. Locati LD, Guzzo M, Bossi P, et al. Lung metastasectomy in adenoid cystic carcinoma (ACC) of salivary gland. *Oral Oncol* 2005;41:890–894.

65. Lopes MA, Santos GC, Kowalski LP. Multivariate survival analysis of 128 cases of oral cavity minor salivary gland carcinomas. *Head Neck* 1998;20:699–706.

66. Mendenhall WM, Morris CG, Amdur RJ, et al. Radiotherapy alone or combined with surgery for salivary gland carcinoma. *Cancer* 2005;103:2544–2550.

67. Modan B, Alfandary E, Tamir A, et al. Increased risk of salivary gland tumors after low-dose irradiation. *Laryngoscope* 1998;108:1095–1097.

68. Muscatt JE, Wynder EL. A case/control study of risk factors for major salivary gland cancer. *Otolaryngol Head Neck Surg* 1998;118:195–198.

69. Nasser SM, Faquin WC, Dayal Y. Expression of androgen, estrogen, and progesterone receptors in salivary gland tumors. Frequent expression of androgen receptor in a subset of malignant salivary gland tumors. *Am J Clin Pathol* 2003;119:801–806.

70. North CA, Lee DJ, Piantadosi S, et al. Carcinoma of the major salivary glands treated by surgery or surgery plus postoperative radiotherapy. *Int J Radiat Oncol Biol Phys* 1990;18:1319–1326.

71. Nutting CM, Rowbottom CG, Cosgrove VP, et al. Optimisation of radiotherapy for carcinoma of the parotid gland: A comparison of conventional, three-dimensional conformal, and intensity-modulated techniques. *Radiother Oncol* 2001;60:163–172.

72. Östman J, Anneroth G, Gustafsson H, et al. Malignant salivary gland tumours in Sweden 1960–1989. An epidemiological study. *Oral Oncol* 1997;33:169–176.

73. Paris J, Facon F, Pascal T, et al. Preoperative diagnostic values of fine-needle cytology and MRI in parotid gland tumors. *Eur Arch Otorhinolaryngol* 2005;262:27–31.

74. Parsons JT, Mendenhall WM, Stringer SP, et al. Management of minor salivary gland carcinomas. *Int J Radiat Oncol Biol Phys* 1996;35:443–454.

75. Pohar S, Gay H, Rosenbaum P, et al. Malignant parotid tumors: Presentation, clinical/pathologic prognostic factors, and treatment outcomes. *Int J Radiat Oncol Biol Phys* 2005;61:112–118.

76. Postema RJ, Van Velthuysen MLF, Van Den Brekel, et al. Accuracy of fine-needle aspiration cytology of salivary gland lesions in the Netherlands cancer institute. *Head Neck* 2004;26:418–424.

77. Poulsen MG, Pratt GR, Kynaston B, et al. Prognostic variables in malignant epithelial tumors of the parotid. *Int J Radiat Oncol Biol Phys* 1992;23:327–330.

78. Press MF, Pike MC, Hung G, et al. Amplification and overexpression of HER-2/neu in carcinomas of the salivary gland: Correlation with poor prognosis. *Cancer Res* 1994;54:5675–5682.

79. Régis de Brito Santos I, Kowalski LP, Cavalcante de Araujo V, et al. Multivariate analysis of risk factors for neck metastases in surgically treated parotid carcinoma. *Arch Otolaryngol Head Neck Surg* 2001;127:46–60.

80. Renehan A, Gleave EN, Mc Gurk M. An analysis of the treatment of 114 patients with recurrent pleomorphic adenomas of the parotid gland. *Am J Surg* 1996;172:710–714.

81. Renehan AG, Gleave EN, Slevin NJ, et al. Clinico-pathological and treatment-related factors influencing survival in parotid cancer. *Br J Cancer* 1999;80:1296–1300.

82. Roesink JM, Moerland MA, Battermann JJ, et al. Quantative dose volume response analysis in parotid gland function after radiotherapy in the head and neck region. *Int J Radiat Oncol Biol Phys* 2001;51:938–946.

83. Saku T, Hayashi Y, Takahara O, et al. Salivary gland tumors among atomic bomb survivors, 1950–1987. *Cancer* 1997;79:1465–1475.

84. Schneider AB, Lubin J, Ron E, et al. Salivary gland tumors after childhood radiation treatment for benign conditions of the head and neck: Dose-response relationship. *Radiat Res* 1998;149:625–630.

85. Schramm VL, Imola MJ. Management of nasopharyngeal salivary gland malignancy. *Laryngoscope* 2001;111:1533–1544.

86. Schulz-Ertner D, Nikoghosyan A, Jäkel, et al. Feasibility and toxicity of combined photon and carbon ion radiotherapy for locally advanced adenoid cystic carcinomas. *Int J Radiat Oncol Biol* 2003;56:391–398.

87. Seifert G, Sobin LH. The World Health Organization's histological classification of salivary gland tumors. *Cancer* 1992;70:379–385.

88. Shapiro NL, Bhattacharyya N. Clinical characteristics and survival for major salivary gland malignancies in children. *Otolaryngol Head Neck Surg* 2006;134:631–634.

89. Simpson JR, Thawley SE, Matsuba HM. Adenoid cystic salivary gland carcinoma: Treatment with irradiation and surgery. *Radiology* 1984;151:509.

90. Sobin LH, Wittekind Ch. *TNM Classification of malignant tumors*, 6th ed. New York: Wiley-Liss; 2002.

91. Spiro RH, Armstrong J, Harrison L, et al. Carcinoma of major salivary glands. *Arch Otolaryngol Head Neck Surg* 1989;115:316–321.

92. Spiro RH. Distant metastasis in adenoid cystic carcinoma of salivary origin. *Am J Surg* 1997;174:495–498.

93. Spiro RH. Salivary neoplasms: Overview of a 35-year experience with 2,807 patients. *Head Neck Surg* 1986;8:177–184.

94. Stennert E, Kisner D, Jungehuelsing M, et al. High incidence of lymph node metastasis in major salivary gland cancer. *Arch Otolaryngol Head Neck Surg* 2003;129:720–723.

95. Stewart CJR, MacKenzie K, McGarry GW, et al. Fine-needle aspiration cytology of salivary gland: A review of 341 cases. *Diagn Cytopathol* 2000;22:139–146.

96. Storey MR, Garden AS, Morrison WH, et al. Postoperative radiotherapy for malignant tumors of the submandibular gland. *Int J Radiat Oncol Biol Phys* 2001;51:952–958.

97. Sun EC, Curtis R, Melbye M, et al. Salivary gland cancer in the United States. *Cancer EpidemiolBiomarkers Prev* 1999;8:1095–1100.

98. Swanson GM, Burns PB. Cancers of the salivary gland: Workplace risk among women and men. *Ann Epidemiol* 1997;7:639–374.

99. Braam PM, Terhaard CHJ, Roesink JM, et al. Intensity-modulated radiotherapy significantly reduces xerostomia compared with conventional radiotherapy. *Int J Radiat Oncol Biol Phys* 2006;66:975–980.

100. Terhaard CHJ, Lubsen H, Rasch CRN, et al. The role of radiotherapy in the treatment of malignant salivary gland tumors. *Int J Radiat Oncol Biol Phys* 2005;61:103–111.

101. Terhaard CHJ, Lubsen H, Van Der Tweel, et al. Salivary gland carcinoma: Indopendent prognostic factors for locoregional control, distant metastases, and overall survival: Results of the Dutch Head and Neck Oncology Cooperative Group. *Head Neck* 2004; August: 681–693.

102. Therkildsen MH, Christensen M, Andersen LJ, et al. Salivary gland carcinomas-prognostic factors. *Acta Oncol* 1998;37:701–713.

103. Van Der Wal JE, Carter RL, Klijanienko J, et al. Histological re-evaluation of 101 intraoral salivary gland tumors by an EORTC-study group. *J Oral Pathol Med* 1993;22:21–22.

104. Vander Poorten VL, Balm AJ, Hilgers FJ, et al. Stage as major long term outcome predictor in minor salivary gland carcinoma. *Cancer* 2000;89:1195.

105. Vander Poorten VL, Balm AJM, Hilgers FJM, et al. The development of a prognostic score for patients with parotid carcinoma. *Cancer* 1999;85:2057–2067.

106. Vander Poorten VLM, Hart AAM, Van Der Laan BFAM, et al. Prognostic index for patients with parotid carcinoma. External validation using the nationwide 1985—1994 Dutch Head and Neck Oncology Cooperative Group Database. *Cancer* 2003;97:1453–1463.

107. Vrielinck LJG, Ostyn F, Van Damme B, et al. The significance of perineural spread in adenoid cystic carcinoma of the major and minor salivary glands. *Int J Oral Maxillofac* 1998;17:190–193.

108. Wahlberg P, Anderson H, Björklund A, et al. Carcinoma of the parotid and submandibular glands—a study of survival in 2465 patients. *Oral Oncol* 2002;38:706–713.

109. Wang CC, Goodman M. Photon irradiation of unresectable carcinomas of salivary glands. *Int J Radiat Oncol Biol Phys* 1991;21:569–576.

110. Wasserman Th, Brizel DM, Henke M, et al. Influence of intravenous amifostine on xerostomia, tumor control, and survival after radiotherapy for head and neck cancer: 2-year follow-up of a prospective, randomized, phase III trial. *Int J Radiat Oncol Biol Phys* 2005;6:985–990.

111. Whatley WS, Thompson JW, Rao B. Salivary gland tumors in survivors of childhood cancer. *Otolaryngol Head Neck Surg* 2006;134:385–388.

112. Witt RL. The significance of the margin in parotid surgery for pleomorphic adenoma. *Laryngoscope* 2002;112:2141–2154.

113. Yaparpalvi R, Fontenla DP, Tyerech SK, et al. Parotid gland tumors: A comparison of postoperative radiotherapy techniques using three dimensional (3D) dose distributions and dose-volume histograms (DVHS). *Int J Radiat Oncol Biol Phys* 1998;40:43–49.

114. Yousem DM, Kraut MA, Chalian AA. Major salivary gland imaging. *Radiology* 2000;216:19–29.

115. Zbären P, Schüpbach J, Nuyens M, et al. Elective neck dissection versus observation in primary parotid carcinoma. *Otolaryngol Head Neck Surg* 2005;132:387–391.

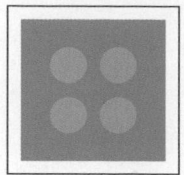

Chapter 41
Oral Cavity Cancer

Rafael R. Mañon, Jeffrey N. Myers, Deepak Khuntia, Paul M. Harari

The oral cavity consists of the lips, oral tongue, floor of mouth, retromolar trigone, alveolar ridge, buccal mucosa, and hard palate (Figs. 41.1–41.3). Cancer of the oral cavity comprises approximately 30% of head and neck region tumors and 3% of all cancers in the United States (46). On the order of 31,000 new cases of oral cavity and oropharynx cancer were diagnosed in the United States in 2006 (104). Worldwide, head and neck cancer is the sixth most common malignancy, with over 274,000 new oral cavity cancers diagnosed annually (104). For all stages combined, the 5-year relative survival rate is 59% and the 10-year survival rate is 44% (104). Mortality rates for oral and pharyngeal cancers have shown a gradual decrease in the United States since the 1980s based on data from the World Health Organization (WHO) (111). One of the major prognostic factors for oral cavity cancer is the presence of lymph node metastases. The 5-year cancer-specific survival can be as high as 70% to 90% for patients without lymph node metastasis but drops by half for patients with node-positive disease (52). Worldwide, oral cancer is a substantial public health problem as one of the leading causes of cancer death in parts of Asia and Europe.

In the United States oral cavity cancer is predominantly a disease of older males. The disease is associated with the consumption of tobacco and alcohol (30). However, this trend is evolving as the prevalence of tobacco use in women increases (20). Recently, there has been some increase in the incidence of tongue carcinoma in younger nonsmokers and nondrinkers in the United States. The squamous lining of the oral cavity is composed of relatively thick mucosa with a keratin layer. However, the floor of mouth and ventral and lateral tongue possess a thinner mucosa with less surface keratin, potentially contributing to the higher incidence of cancer in these subsites (73).

A variety of distinct histologic types of cancer can arise in the oral cavity. The majority of these (95%) are squamous-cell carcinomas (45). The second most common histologic type derives from minor salivary gland rests. Other nonepithelial tumors such as melanoma, lymphoma, sarcoma, and ameloblastoma may also arise in the oral cavity, but are relatively uncommon in absolute numbers. Classification of tumors by subsite is useful because patterns of spread and clinical outcomes vary by specific subsite, partly reflecting the variable risk of nodal spread by anatomic site of presentation.

Anatomy

Lip

The lips begin at the junction of the vermilion border with the skin and form the anterior aspect of the oral vestibule. The lips are comprised of the vermilion surface, which is the portion of the lip that comes in contact with the opposing lip. The lips are well defined into an upper and lower. The primary motor control of the lips is provided by the buccal and mandibular branches of the facial nerve.

Oral Tongue

The anterior two thirds of the tongue is mobile and considered part of the oral cavity. The oral tongue extends anteriorly from the circumvallate papillae to the undersurface of the tongue at the junction of the floor of mouth. The fibrous septum divides the tongue into right and left halves. The oral tongue can be demarcated into four anatomic areas: the tip, lateral borders, dorsal surface, and undersurface (ventral surface). There are six pairs of muscles that form the oral tongue. Three of these muscles are extrinsic, while the other three are intrinsic. The extrinsic muscles include the genioglossus, hyoglossus, and styloglossus. The intrinsic muscles include the lingual, vertical, and transverse muscles. The former primarily move the body of the tongue, while the latter alter the shape and conformation of the tongue during speech and swallowing. The blood supply to the tongue is primarily via the lingual artery, tonsillar branch of the facial artery, and the ascending pharyngeal artery with primary drainage by the internal jugular vein. General sensation of the anterior two thirds of the tongue is supplied by the lingual nerve. Excluding the circumvallate papillae, taste fibers from the anterior two thirds of the tongue run in the chorda tympani branch of the facial nerve; the glossopharyngeal nerve provides sensation and taste to the posterior third of the tongue and circumvallate papillae.

Floor of the Mouth

The floor of the mouth is a semilunar space extending from the lower alveolar ridge to the undersurface of the tongue. The floor of the mouth overlies the mylohyoid and hyoglossus muscles. The posterior boundary of the floor of the mouth is the base of the anterior tonsillar pillar. This region is divided into right and left by the frenulum of the tongue and contains the ostia of the submandibular and sublingual salivary glands. A sling formed by the mylohyoid muscles medially supports the anterior floor of the mouth, and the hyoglossus supports the posterior floor of the mouth. The lingual and hypoglossal nerves are lateral to the hyoglossus, while the lingual artery is medial to the hyoglossus. Innervation of the floor of the mouth is provided by the lingual nerve.

Hard Palate

The hard palate extends from the inner surface of the superior alveolar ridge to the posterior edge of the palatine bone. This is a semilunar area between the superior alveolar ridge and the mucous membrane covering the palatine process of the maxillary palatine bones.

Alveolar Ridge

The alveolar ridges include the alveolar processes of the maxilla and mandible and the overlying mucosa. The mucosal covering of the lower alveolar ridge extends from the line of attachment of mucosa in the buccal gutter to the line of free mucosa of the

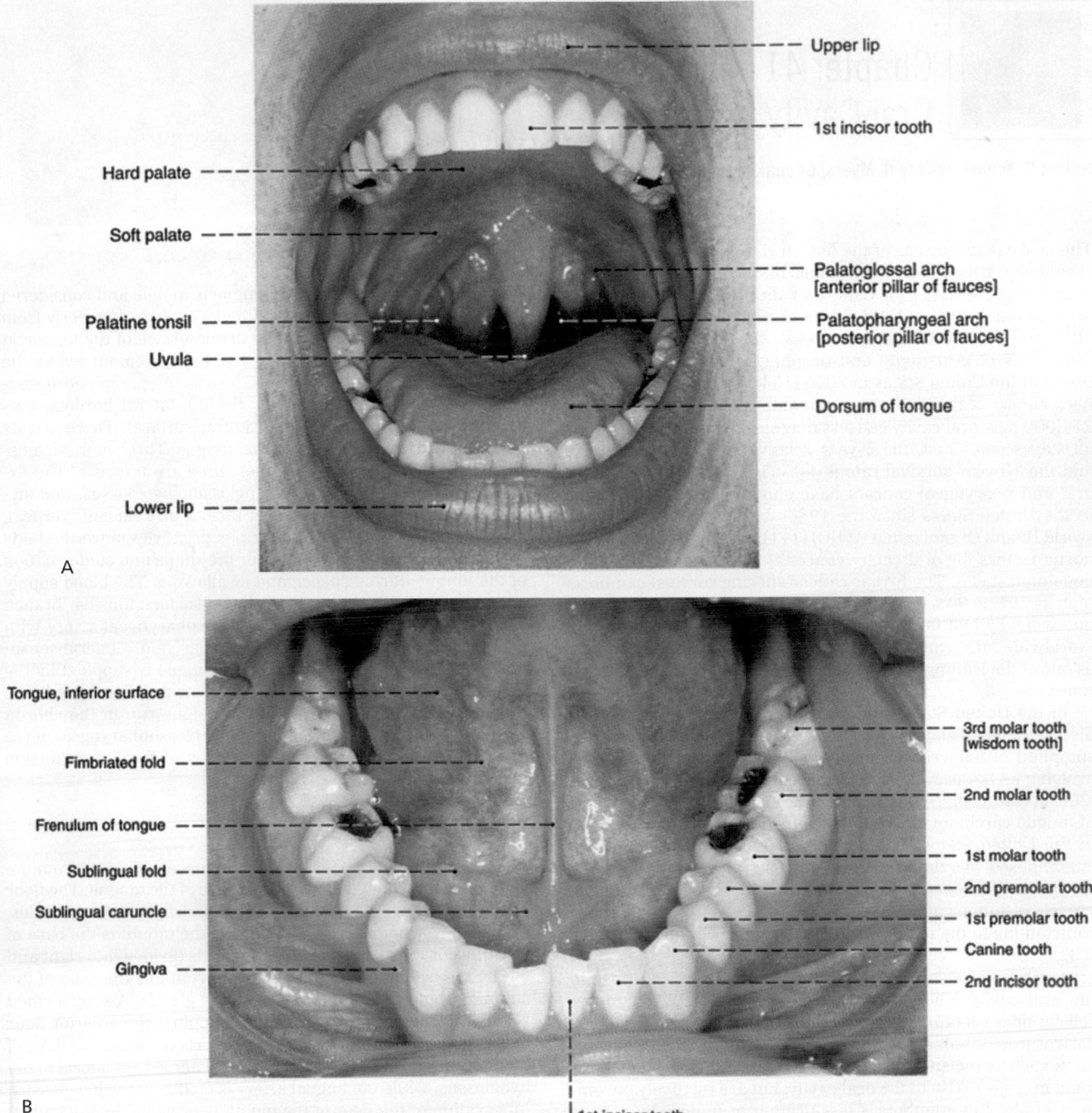

FIGURE 41.1. A: Oral cavity surface anatomy. **B:** Floor of mouth surface anatomy. (From Sobotta J. *Atlas of human anatomy*, vol. 1. Munich: Lippincott Williams & Wilkins, 2001, with permission.)

floor of mouth. The lower alveolar ridge extends to the ascending ramus of the mandible posteriorly. The superior alveolar ridge mucosa extends from the line of attachment of mucosa in the upper gingival buccal gutter to the junction of the hard palate. The posterior margin is the upper end of the pterygopalatine arch.

Retromolar Trigone

The retromolar trigone is the triangular area overlying the ascending ramus of the mandible. The base of the triangle is formed by the posterior most molar, and the apex lies at the maxillary tuberosity.

Buccal Mucosa

The buccal mucosa includes the mucosal surfaces of the cheek and lips from the line of contact of the opposing lips to the pterygomandibular raphe posteriorly. This extends to the line of attachment of the mucosa of the upper and lower alveolar ridge superiorly and inferiorly. Innervation is supplied by the buccal nerve, a branch of the mandibular nerve.

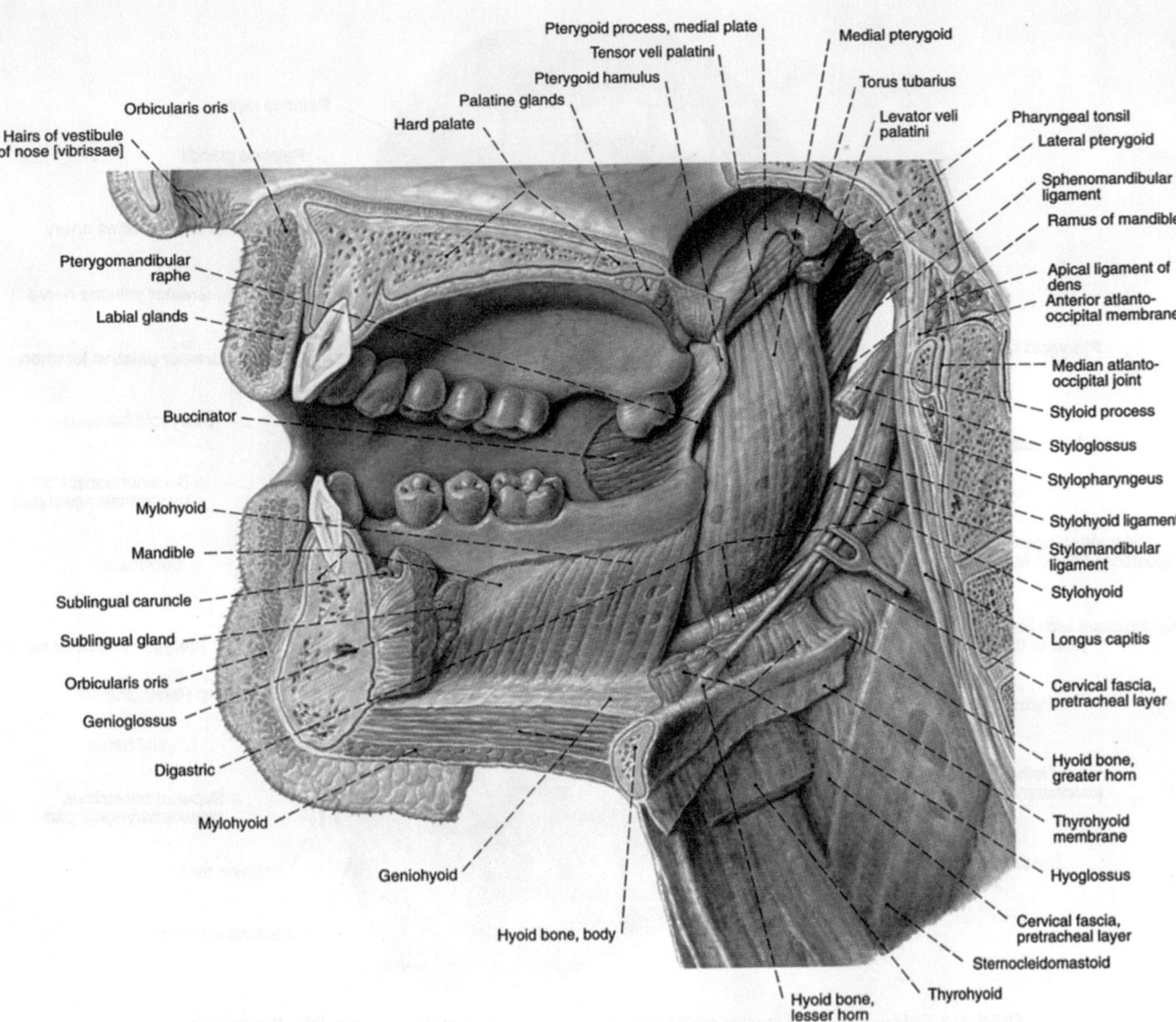

FIGURE 41.2. Oral cavity; paramedian section depicting regional anatomy. (From Sobotta J, *Atlas of human anatomy*, Vol 1. Munich: Lippincott Williams & Wilkins, 2001, with permission.)

Epidemiology

Oral cavity tumors comprise roughly 30% of all head and neck cancers. The epidemiology of oral cancer strongly reflects exposure to certain environmental agents, particularly tobacco and alcohol. Worldwide, the incidence of oral cancer varies considerably. The age-adjusted world incidence for cancer of the oral cavity and pharynx is 8.3 per 100,000, but varies greatly with respect to age and sex (17). In Western Europe and Australia the incidence of oral cavity cancer closely approximates that of the United States. The incidence of cancer among males is highest in northern France, southern India, a few regions of central and Eastern Europe, and Latin America (69). Among women, the highest incidence is observed in India (40). The elevated rates of oral cavity cancer in France and Eastern Europe have been linked to the high rates of alcohol consumption in these countries.

A review of studies conducted between 1994 and 2001 indicates a strong causal relationship between smoking and cancer of the oral cavity (9,56,65). Smoking is identified as an independent risk factor in 80% to 90% of patients who present with cancer of the oral cavity (9,56,65). Cessation of smoking is associated with a decline in the risk of cancer of the oral cavity. Abstaining from the use of cigarettes resulted in a 30% reduction in the risk of cancer in those quitting from 1 to 9 years and a 50% reduction in those who quit for more than 9 years (65). In India the habit of chewing betel nut leaves rolled with lime and tobacco (mixture known as "pan"), which results in prolonged carcinogen exposure to the oral mucosa, is thought to be the leading cause of oral cancer (82,98). The practice of "reverse smoking" (smoking with the lighted end of the cigar in the mouth, also known as Chutta), peculiar to certain parts of India, is associated with increase in cancer of the hard palate (89). Although alcohol and tobacco have a synergistic effect on carcinogenesis, alcohol consumption may be an independent factor in the etiology of oral cavity cancer. Surveys of census-based population data in England and Wales suggest that the association between alcohol consumption and oral cavity cancer in males may be greater than that observed for cigarette smoking (49).

In the United States, cancer of the oral cavity afflicts older patients more than younger patients, and is three times more frequent in men than women (18). The incidence and mortality

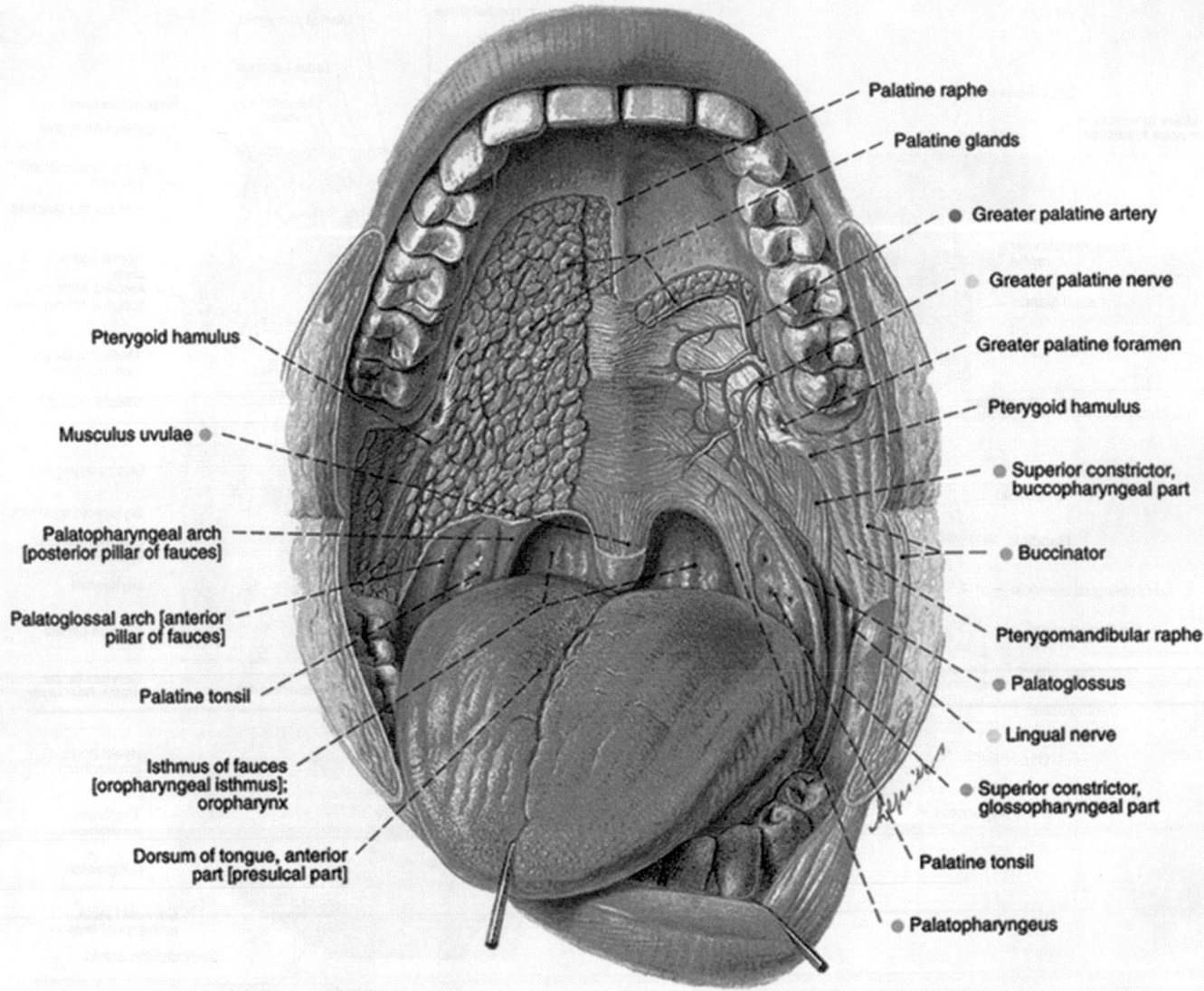

Palatine raphe

Palatine glands

Greater palatine artery

Greater palatine nerve

Greater palatine foramen

Pterygoid hamulus

Superior constrictor, buccopharyngeal part

Buccinator

Pterygomandibular raphe

Palatoglossus

Lingual nerve

Superior constrictor, glossopharyngeal part

Palatine tonsil

Palatopharyngeus

Pterygoid hamulus

Musculus uvulae

Palatopharyngeal arch [posterior pillar of fauces]

Palatoglossal arch [anterior pillar of fauces]

Palatine tonsil

Isthmus of fauces [oropharyngeal isthmus]; oropharynx

Dorsum of tongue, anterior part [presulcal part]

FIGURE 41.3. Oral cavity illustration depicting regional anatomy. (From Sobotta J, *Atlas of human anatomy*, Vol 1. Munich: Lippincott Williams & Wilkins, 2001, with permission.)

rates are higher for African American men (99). The mortality rates for African American males with oral or pharyngeal cancer is 7.5/100,000, nearly double that of Caucasians (3.9/100,000) (104). The survival rates are 61% in whites versus 39% in African Americans. Recent studies suggest that there may be a rising incidence in cancer of the tongue and mouth in young adults (80). Studies reveal that 4% to 6% of oral cancers now occur at ages younger than 40 years (63). Reports examining risk factors for oral cancer in the young provide evidence that many younger patients have never smoked or consumed alcohol; predisposition to genetic instability has been hypothesized as a causative factor (63).

Ultraviolet radiation has been associated with carcinoma of the lip. In geographic regions where there are long daily periods of sun exposure, cancer of the lip may represent up to 60% of all cancers of the oral cavity (4). Herpes simplex virus (HSV) and human papilloma virus (HPV) have also been implicated in the etiology of oral cavity cancer. The former has been shown to act as a cocarcinogen with tobacco and ultraviolet light in animal models (12,57). HPV-6 and -16 are the most common types of HPV associated with cancer of the oral cavity (79). HPV-16 is found two and five times more likely in precancerous oral mucosa and cancer in the oral cavity respectively, compared to normal mucosa (72). In males, HPV-16 confers a threefold

risk of developing oral cavity cancer (66). Despite the fact that studies have detected high-risk HPV in nearly 50% of cases of oral cavity cancer, it is still uncertain whether infection with the virus is sufficient to promote development of oral cavity cancer (79).

Certain syndromes such as Plummer-Vinson (characterized by iron-deficiency anemia, hypopharyngeal webs, weight loss, and dysphagia) have been associated with oral cavity cancer. However, Plummer-Vinson syndrome is rare and accounts for a small number of cancers of the oral cavity. Disorders such as xeroderma pigmentosum, ataxia telangiectasia, Bloom syndrome, and Fanconi's anemia are a result of defective "caretaker" genes. Because such defects result in genetic instability, an increased incidence of second primary malignancies, including oral cancer, has been reported (88). By contrast, with the exception of Li Fraumeni syndrome, abnormalities in "gatekeeper" genes, which inhibit cell proliferation and/or promote cell death, do not appear to predispose to oral cancer. However, despite such reports, the genetics of oral cavity cancer have not been well delineated (18).

In patients with cancer of the oral cavity the risk of developing a second primary cancer is well recognized. The concept of field cancerization described by Slaughter and Smejkal (102) in 1953 and Day et al. (25) may explain the significantly higher rate of second malignancy in patients with head and neck cancers compared to the general population. In an analysis of 851 patients with squamous cell carcinoma of the head and neck, 19% of the study population developed a secondary head and neck carcinoma 5 years after undergoing initial therapy (95). The probability of developing a second metachronous malignancy at 5 years was 22% (18% for the subset of patients with oral cavity cancer) (95). Day and Blot (24) evaluated the risks of subsequent malignancies in 21,371 patients with oral and pharyngeal cancers between 1973 and 1987. The rate of development of second tumors was 3.7% per year. The risk of second primary cancer was 2.8 times greater than expected, with 20-fold increases of oral or esophageal cancers and fourfold to sevenfold increases of respiratory cancers. Crosher and McIlroy (22), in an analysis of the Scottish Cancer registry, found the overall risk of second cancers in patients with carcinoma of the oral cavity was 2.03 (95% confidence intervals 1.8 to 2.4) times greater than expected in the general population. In a meta-analysis patients with carcinoma of the oral cavity had the highest rate of second primaries, most of which occurred in the upper aerodigestive tract (51). Second primary cancers have an adverse effect on prognosis and are the major cause of treatment failure in patients with early stage disease (62,95).

Molecular Biology

In parallel to the Fearon and Vogelstein (37) model describing the genetic basis of colon cancer, there are a series of specific genetic events that precede the development of oral squamous cell carcinoma (16,47). Cancer progression models describe several steps that occur during tumor development: oncogenes become activated and tumor suppressor genes become deactivated and a series of these alterations are required for carcinogenesis. In the oral mucosa this genetic progression is reflected histologically by the transformation from normal mucosa to dysplastic epithelium and ultimately to a frankly invasive squamous-cell carcinoma. Data to support this model come from studies that reveal genetic alterations in histologically normal tissues and in premalignant lesions, including loss of heterozygosity at chromosomes 3p14 and 9p21. Furthermore, mutations in the region of chromosome 17p13, which encompass the tumor suppressor gene p53, are among the early events that contribute to malignant transformation. Indeed, biopsies of normal mucosa from patients with upper aerodigestive tract carcinomas frequently harbor p53 mutations. The accumulation of specific mutations contribute to changes in critical cellular processes that regulate growth, survival, immortality, tissue invasion, and new blood vessel formation, leading to changes in the biology of epithelial cells to the point where they acquire distinct histological characteristics. Why the same environmental exposure leads to tumor development in some individuals and not others may be explained in part by genetic susceptibility to tobacco carcinogens (59). This susceptibility has been linked to the ability to metabolize and break down carcinogens and/or repair damage to their DNA caused by the mutagens in tobacco.

Natural History and Patterns of Spread

Premalignant Lesions

Leukoplakia

Leukoplakia and erythroplakia are gross clinical descriptors that do not always correspond directly to specific pathologic entities (18,77). The WHO defines leukoplakia as a white patch or plaque that cannot be rubbed off or characterized clinically or pathologically as any other disease (77) (Fig. 41.4). Leukoplakia is not related to the presence or absence of dysplasia; however, it is the most common precursor of cancer of the oral cavity. Leukoplakia has a varied clinical appearance, and its appearance frequently changes over time. This is primarily a clinical entity, with certain key pathologic features. These features include hyperkeratosis and acanthosis. Leukoplakias begin as thin gray or gray/white plaques that may appear somewhat translucent, are sometimes fissured or wrinkled, and are typically soft and flat. They frequently have sharply demarcated borders but occasionally blend gradually into normal surrounding mucosa.

Homogenous leukoplakia is a uniform white lesion that is prevalent in the buccal mucosa. These lesions represent the most common variety of leukoplakia and have a low malignant potential. Conversely, high-risk oral leukoplakia demonstrates abnormal orientation of cells, nuclear hyperchromatism, increased mitosis, and nuclear cytoplasmic ratio (18). Clinically these lesions are nonhomogenous, nodular, speckled, or verrucous, with central ulceration or erosion (77,79). Follow-up studies demonstrate that between <1% to 18% of oral leukoplakias develop into oral cancer, with the latter clinical subtype conferring a higher risk of malignant transformation (54,90).

The natural history of leukoplakia is variable. Leukoplakia may regress spontaneously without therapy. A baseline biopsy can be performed to establish diagnosis and rule-out malignant transformation. Leukoplakia with clinically or histologically aggressive features, demonstrating dysplasia, should be excised.

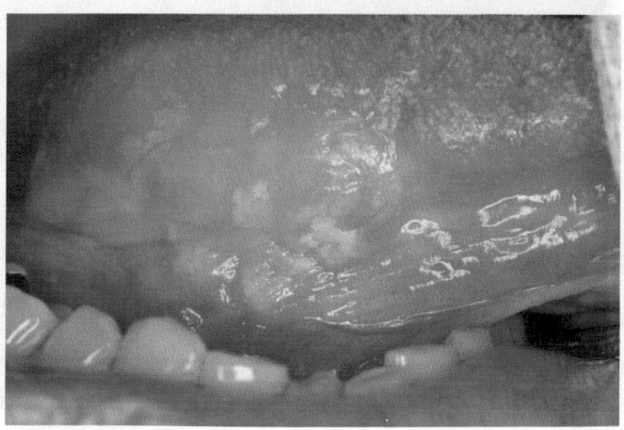
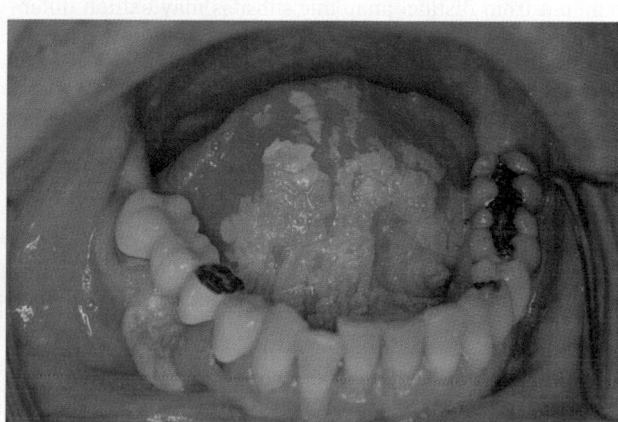

FIGURE 41.4. A: Superficial patches of leukoplakia involving the lateral and ventral surface of the oral tongue. **B:** Extensive leukoplakia involving the ventral oral tongue, floor of mouth, and mandibular alveolus.

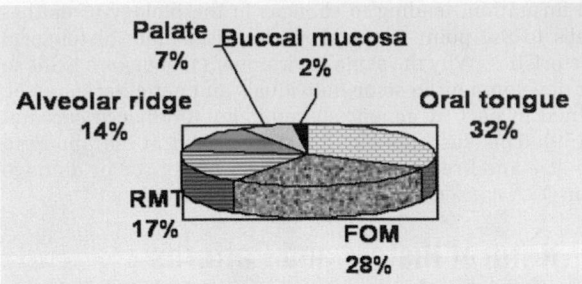
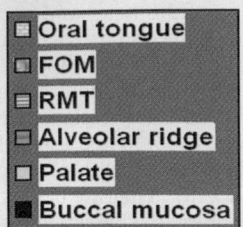

FIGURE 41.5. Subsite distribution of 3308 de novo cancers of the oral cavity treated at the University of Texas M.D. Anderson Cancer Center from 1970–1999. FOM, floor of mouth; RMT, retromolar trigone (From Chen AY, Myers JN. Pathogenesis and progression of squamous cell carcinoma of the oral cavity. *Dis Mon* 2001;47:275–361, with permission.)

Erythroplakia

The term erythroplakia describes a chronic, red, generally asymptomatic lesion or patch on the mucosal surface that cannot be attributed to a traumatic, vascular, or inflammatory cause. Erythroplakia, like leukoplakia, is a clinical diagnosis of exclusion that requires the clinician to rule out all other erythematous oral lesions (96). However, erythroplakia is associated with a higher risk of malignant transformation than leukoplakia. Transformation rates are considered to be the highest among all precancerous oral lesions and conditions (91). Histopathologically it has been documented that in homogenous oral erythroplakia, 51% showed invasive carcinoma, 40% carcinoma *in situ*, and 9% mild or moderate dysplasia (91). The treatment of choice for erythroplakia is surgical excision.

Oral Cavity Cancer

Relative Distribution

The most common subsite for squamous-cell carcinoma of the oral cavity (excluding the lip) is the oral tongue (Fig. 41.5). In a review of 3,308 cases of oral cavity cancer treated at the University of Texas M.D. Anderson Cancer Center between 1970 and 1999, 32% were located in the oral tongue (18). The floor of the mouth is the second most common subsite where oral cavity carcinomas may arise. Carcinoma of the alveolar ridge accounts for approximately 10% of oral cavity carcinomas. Squamous-cell carcinoma of the retromolar trigone and hard palate is rare. Similarly, carcinoma of the buccal mucosa is rare in the United States, but is the most common carcinoma of the oral cavity in Southeast Asia because of the widespread use of betel nut (18).

Patterns of Spread

Local Spread

Carcinoma from distinct anatomic subsites may exhibit different tendencies for spread based on natural anatomic barriers and location. For instance, the majority of lip cancers are local growths that do not invade deeply into the tissues of the oral cavity or mandible (121). However, a select few lip carcinomas may be deeply invasive with perineural involvement, posterior spread to involve cortical bone, extension to the inferior alveolar nerve, or spread to the skin of the face (Fig. 41.6). Squamous-cell carcinoma of the floor of the mouth can secondarily involve the ventral tongue, extend along the lingual nerve, submandibular duct, or invade the cortex of the mandible. Tumors in this location can invade deeply, involving the muscles of the floor of the mouth. There is an anatomical gap between the mylohyoid and hyoglossus muscles through which a carcinoma can gain access to submandibular and sublingual areas. Carcinomas of the alveolar ridge and retromolar trigone tend to invade bone early. Tumors of the inferior alveolar ridge may access the mandibular canal and the inferior alveolar nerve, while tumors of the superior alveolar ridge may pass into the maxillary

antrum or floor of the nose. Infiltrating lesions of the buccal mucosa can invade the buccinator muscle, extend to the buccal fat pad, and invade the subcutaneous tissue. The hard palate has a relatively dense mucoperiosteum that is relatively resistant to tumor invasion. However, the primary and secondary palates are fused at the incisive fossa, where tumors can gain access into the nasal cavity. The greater palatine foramina can allow tumors to spread posteriorly and enter the pterygopalatine fossa and skull base.

Lymphatic Metastases

For the purpose of staging and treatment planning, the neck is generally divided into five primary levels. Level I includes the submental and submandibular triangles. Level II includes the upper jugular chain lymph nodes from the base of skull to the carotid bifurcation and from the sternohyoid muscle anteriorly to the posterior border of the sternocleidomastoid posteriorly. Level III includes the mid-jugular nodes, which extend from the carotid bifurcation to the omohyoid muscle inferiorly, the sternohyoid medially, and the posterior aspect of the sternocleidomastoid posteriorly. Level IV includes the inferior jugular nodes, bounded by the omohyoid muscle superiorly, the clavicle inferiorly, and the posterior aspect of the sternocleidomastoid posteriorly. Level V includes nodes in the posterior triangle, bordered by the base of the skull superiorly, clavicle inferiorly, and posterior aspect of the sternocleidomastoid anteriorly.

The oral cavity has an extensive group of lymphatics that manifest a fairly predictable lymph node drainage pattern based on location (subsite) within the oral cavity (14) (Table 41.1). The upper and lower lip demonstrate distinct patterns of lymphatic drainage. The principal lymphatic drainage of the upper lip is to preauricular, periparotid, submental, and submandibular

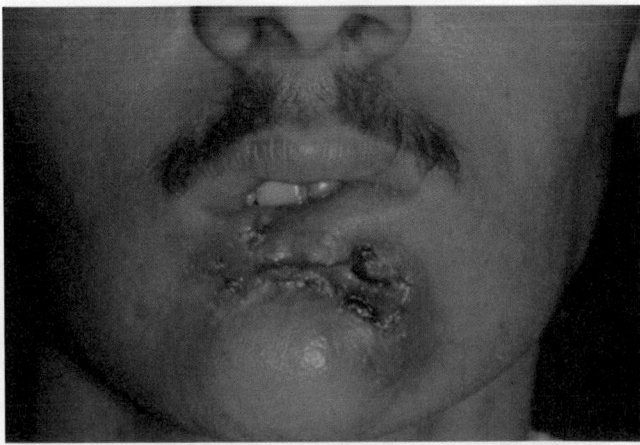

FIGURE 41.6. Advanced, destructive, ulcerative squamous-cell carcinoma involving the lower lip, buccogingival soft tissues, and skin in a patient with long-term habit of tobacco chewing.

Table 41.1	RELATIVE INVOLVEMENT OF LYMPH NODE REGIONS BY ORAL CAVITY SUBSITE			
	Percentage Involved			
	Submaxillary	Submental	Upper Jugular	Mid-Jugular
Oral tongue	18	9	73	18
FOM	64	7	43	0
RMT	25	0	63	12.5

FOM, floor of mouth; RMT, retromolar trigone
From Byers RM, Wolf PF, Ballantyne AJ. Rationale for elective modified neck dissection. *Head Neck Surg* 1988;10:160–167.

lymph nodes (level I), which secondarily drain to deep jugular lymph nodes. The medial portion of the lower lip drains primarily to the submental lymph nodes (level Ia), while the lateral portion drains to the submandibular triangle (level Ib).

A classical study by Lindberg (61) demonstrated that the superior deep jugular nodes are most frequently involved by cancers of the oral cavity. The oral tongue has an extensive lymphatic drainage. The anterior portion of the tongue drains to the submental nodes, and the lateral portion drains to the submandibular and deep jugular nodes (level Ia/Ib and level II). The posterior oral tongue drains into the upper jugulodigastric group of lymph nodes (level II). The lymphatics of the oral tongue also have extensive communication across midline; thus carcinomas of the oral tongue can metastasize bilaterally. Studies suggest that some carcinomas of the lateral oral tongue may metastasize to level IV lymph nodes without involving levels I, II, or III (13). This implies that there may be separate lymphatic channels draining from the oral tongue directly to level IV nodes, allowing for apparent "skip metastases."

Dye injection studies have shown that the floor of the mouth has superficial and deep lymphatic drainage systems (13). The superficial system crosses randomly in the midline and drains into both the ipsilateral and contralateral submandibular lymph nodes (level I). The deep lymphatic system is thought to penetrate the periosteum and drains into the submandibular and upper jugular lymph nodes. Lymphatics from the buccal mucosa drain into the periparotid, submental, and submandibular nodes (level I). Tumors of the alveolar ridge may drain into the submental and submandibular triangles, upper deep jugular, and retropharyngeal lymph nodes. Tumors of the inferior alveolus are more likely to metastasize to the neck than tumors of the superior alveolus. The main lymphatic drainage from the retromolar trigone is into the superior-deep jugular lymph nodes (level II); however, there may be some drainage into periparotid and retropharyngeal lymph nodes. Lymphatics in the hard palate are few, but drainage is into submandibular (level I), superior deep jugular (level II), and retropharyngeal nodes.

The risk of neck metastases depends on several factors including site and size of the primary tumor. Overall, for patients with squamous-cell carcinoma of the oral cavity, cervical metastases occur in approximately 30% of cases (79). The rate of neck metastases for carcinoma of the lip is nearly 10% (79). Squamous-cell cancer of the oral tongue carries the highest risk of nodal metastases. The frequency of neck metastases can range from 15% to 75%, depending on the size of the primary lesion (61,109). Approximately 25% of patients with carcinoma of the oral cavity will have occult nodal metastases, and 3% of patients will have contralateral metastases (61,109). Contralateral metastases are more common in tumors that approach or cross the midline. Early tumors of the floor of the mouth have approximately a 12% to 30% incidence of occult nodal metastases depending on the thickness of the lesion, while larger lesions

can have an incidence of nearly 50% (106). Approximately 15% to 20% of upper alveolar ridge tumors will involve the neck at presentation; the risk of occult metastases in a clinically negative neck is approximately 15% to 20% (61). The incidence of neck metastases in lower alveolar ridge tumors is higher than for tumors of the upper alveolar ridge (61). For cancers of the buccal mucosa, the incidence of positive cervical lymph nodes at diagnosis is 10% to 30%; the incidence of pathologically positive nodes in a clinically negative neck is about 15%. Similar rates of occult metastases occur for squamous-cell carcinoma of the retromolar trigone; however, patients tend to present with more advanced disease, resulting in a somewhat higher rate of regional metastases (79). The incidence of lymph node involvement from carcinoma of the hard palate is low, approximately 15% (100,121).

Distant Metastases

The majority of oral cavity cancers present as localized disease and remain localized until late in the course of their development. Distant metastasis occurs in approximately 15% to 20% of patients who eventually die of their disease (79). The risk of distant metastases increases with the degree of lymph node involvement. Patients with recurrent disease are also at higher risk for distant metastases (70). Patients without clinically appreciable neck disease rarely fail distantly after treatment. In general terms with respect to head and neck cancer, 66% of distant metastasis are to the lungs, 22% to the bones, and 9.5% to the liver (38). On rare occasion, the oral cavity will serve as a site for distant metastasis from another anatomic primary tumor site (Fig. 41.7).

Pathologic Classification

The predominant histopathologic type of cancer in the oral cavity is squamous-cell carcinoma. There are several variants of squamous-cell carcinoma, including basaloid squamous-cell carcinoma and verrucous squamous-cell carcinoma. Basaloid squamous-cell carcinoma is believed to have a worse prognosis than traditional squamous-cell carcinoma. In a retrospective comparison between basaloid squamous-cell carcinoma and traditional poorly differentiated squamous-cell carcinoma, the former had a higher incidence of advanced disease at presentation, distant metastases, and poorer overall survival rate (128). Verrucous carcinoma is an uncommon variant of squamous-cell carcinoma. It is generally considered a low-grade malignancy

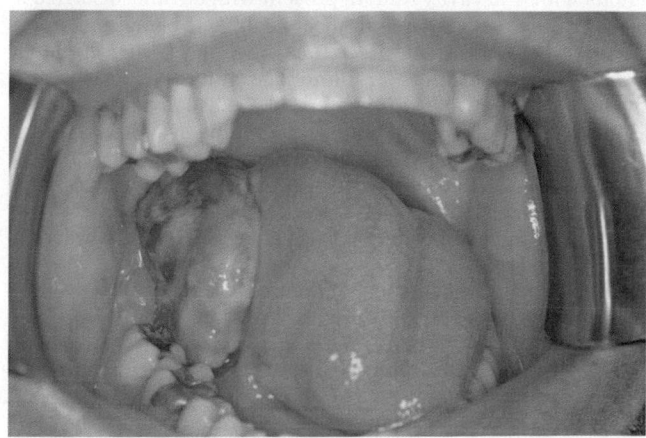

FIGURE 41.7. Unusual oral cavity metastasis in a patient with known renal-cell carcinoma. This advanced, hemorrhagic metastasis showed identical pathology to the patient's known renal-cell carcinoma.

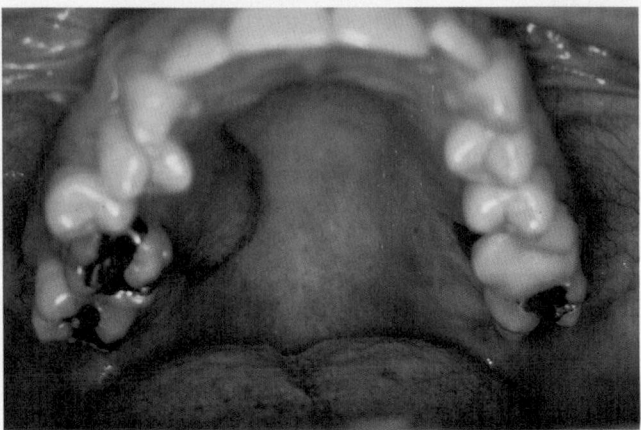

FIGURE 41.8. Kaposi's sarcoma involving the hard palate and maxillary alveolus in a patient with human immunodeficiency virus.

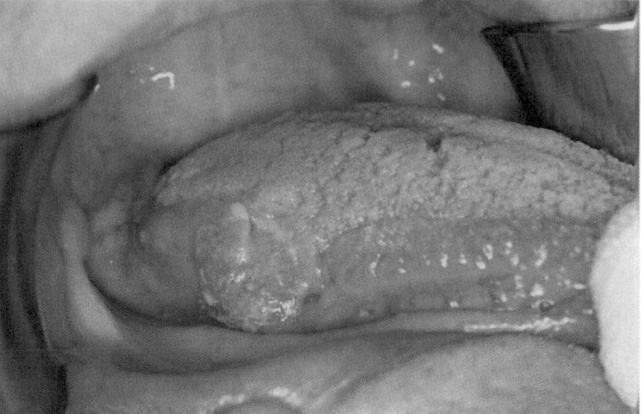

FIGURE 41.9. T2N0M0 squamous-cell carcinoma involving the right lateral oral tongue.

with low metastatic potential and good overall prognosis (18). For these reasons adjuvant radiation and elective neck dissection are often not indicated. Sarcomatoid carcinomas can be found in the oral cavity and larynx. This variant of squamous-cell carcinoma carries a poor prognosis with a mean survival of approximately 2 years (33).

Less than 10% of neoplasms of the oral cavity have nonsquamous histology. Most of these are minor salivary gland tumors, which tend to arise in the hard palate. Adenoid cystic carcinoma accounts for approximately 30% to 40% of minor salivary gland cancers of the oral cavity (126). Other histologies that can occur in the oral cavity include adenocarcinomas, melanoma, ameloblastoma, lymphoma, and Kaposi's sarcoma (Fig. 41.8). Approximately 50% of acquired immunodefiency syndrome–related cases of Kaposi's sarcoma have oral cavity involvement (79). Most lymphomas in the head and neck arise in Waldeyer's ring (tonsil, base of tongue, and nasopharynx). Only 2% of all lymphomas are found in the oral cavity (41). Fortunately, melanoma of the oral cavity is very rare and represents only 0.2% to 8% of all melanomas (103). Mucosal melanomas generally have a worse prognosis than cutaneous melanomas.

Clinical Presentation

The oral cavity is an anatomic region that is readily accessible to visual inspection and palpation. Despite this fact, many patients with oral cavity tumors present with advanced stage disease as initial symptoms may be vague and painless. Tumors of the oral tongue often present as small ulcers and gradually invade the musculature of the tongue. Advanced lesions may be either ulcerative or exophytic and are usually quite evident. Some cancers of the oral tongue are painful even in their early stages. Cervical metastases occur early in the natural history of the disease, with 30% to 40% of patients harboring cervical lymph node metastases at diagnosis. Squamous-cell carcinomas of the oral tongue most often arise along the lateral borders of the tongue (18) (Fig. 41.9).

Lesions of the floor of the mouth are often infiltrative and may invade bone, the muscles of the floor of the mouth, and the tongue. The frenulum is frequently a site of involvement. Clinical fixation of the tumor to the mandible suggests periosteal involvement, which may occur early.

Tumors of the alveolar ridge may present with pain while chewing, loose teeth, or ill-fitting dentures in edentulous patients. These cancers often arise in edentulous areas or along the free margin of the mandibular alveolus (Figs. 41.10 and

41.11). Anesthesia of the lower lip and teeth may indicate involvement of the mandibular canal and inferior alveolar nerve.

Tumors involving the retromolar trigone region may present with an exophytic growth pattern and limited involvement of underlying bone (Fig. 41.12), or they may infiltrate cortical bone and spread along regional tissue planes to involve the pterygoid complex and parapharyngeal space. These latter lesions often induce trismus early in the clinical course.

Carcinoma of the buccal mucosa is rarely symptomatic early in its course. Lesions may be papillary or erosive and located near the dental occlusal line. These tumors are often relatively asymptotic and therefore seldom come to medical attention as T1 lesions. Often, these tumors manifest associated leukoplakia. Multiple primary sites and local recurrence are also common. These tumors most frequently arise adjacent to the lower molars along the occlusal line of the teeth.

Carcinoma of the hard palate is often painless, and the sole presenting symptom may be an irregularity in the mucosa or ill-fitting dentures. Other presenting symptoms include nonhealing ulcers of the hard palate, intermittent bleeding, and pain.

Diagnostic Evaluation

Patients with oral cavity cancer should undergo a comprehensive history and physical examination. Detailed examination is particularly important for oral cavity tumors in that much

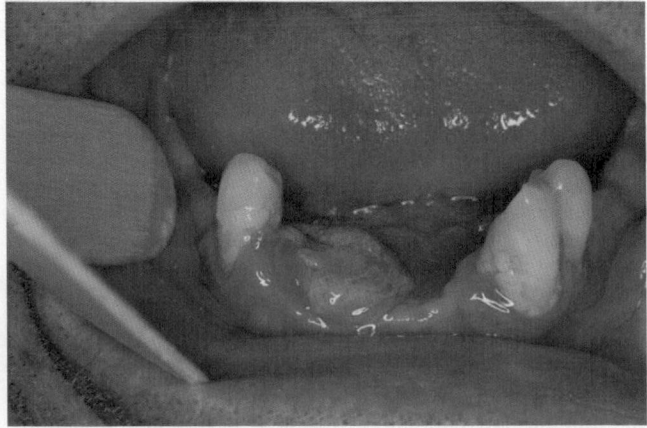

FIGURE 41.10. T1N0M0 squamous-cell carcinoma of the mandibular alveolus. No evidence of bone invasion identified on panorex or computed tomography imaging.

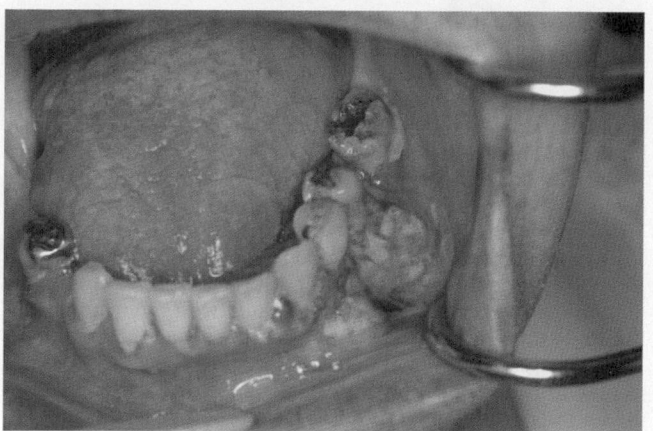

FIGURE 41.11. Squamous-cell carcinoma involving the mandibular alveolus and buccogingival space.

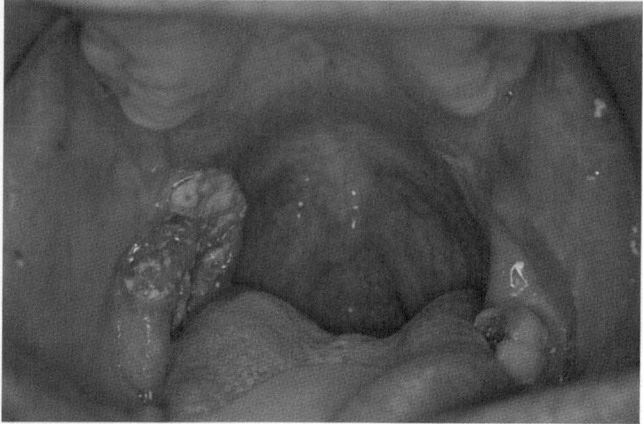

FIGURE 41.12. Exophytic T3 carcinoma involving the right retromolar trigone, anterior tonsillar pillar, and proximal soft palate with minimal infiltration into the right base of tongue.

can be learned about cancers that afford opportunity for direct visual inspection and digital palpation. A biopsy of lesions in question should be obtained as well as a thorough dental assessment. Computed tomography (CT) scans, panoramic radiographs, magnetic resonance imaging (MRI), and other imaging studies may also be important for accurate staging of the tumor and in treatment planning.

The history of present illness should address the following issues: tobacco and alcohol use; dysphagia; odynophagia; pain; trismus; difficulties with speech; hoarseness; loose teeth; ill-fitting dentures; hypoesthesia in the lips or mandible; weight loss; and malnutrition. Otalgia suggests involvement of the ninth or tenth cranial nerve. Hypoesthesia usually results from perineural invasion, often from penetration of the mandible and perineural spread along the inferior alveolar nerve. The presence of trismus may indicate extension into the pterygoid musculature, signifying locally advanced disease. Other symptoms include a persistent ulcer, bleeding, drooling, or respiratory distress. A patient's comorbid illnesses must also be taken into account in the treatment plan.

A detailed examination of the head and neck should be performed, with particular focus on the oral cavity and oropharynx.

This usually begins with a full inspection of the oral cavity, including thorough inspection of the teeth. Palpation of the oral cavity can help assess bony involvement, tongue fixation, and depth of involvement. Deviation or fixation of the tongue suggests involvement of extrinsic muscles of the tongue. Bimanual palpation can help assess the depth of tumor invasion into musculature of the tongue and floor of the mouth. A thorough palpation of the neck is important to assess regional nodal disease.

Imaging can complement the physical examination in determining the extent of disease. A chest x-ray should be performed to exclude lung metastases or a second primary cancer. CT is the modality most commonly used to determine the extent of soft tissue and bony involvement and occult disease in the neck (Fig. 41.13). CT may be used to determine the extent of invasion into the deep musculature of the tongue and adjacent structures. Moreover, CT is a valuable modality for visualizing invasion of the mandible, palate, and pterygopalatine fossa. If CT scanning is not available, then panoramic radiographs can be used to demonstrate mandibular invasion. MRI may be used in case of contrast allergy or a lesion that is not well visualized on CT. For instance, MRI may be used if a patient has significant dental

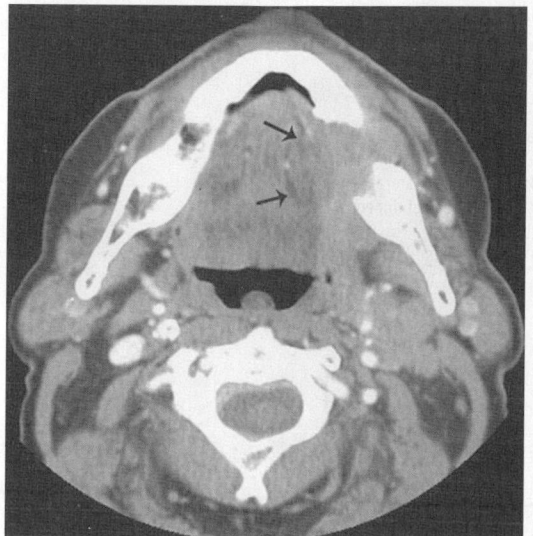

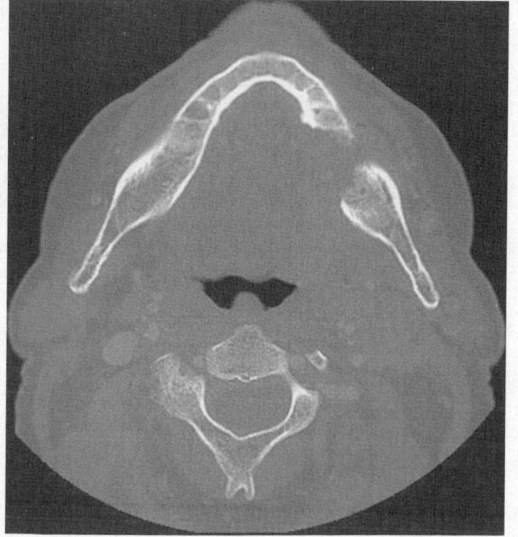

FIGURE 41.13. A: Transverse computed tomography image with contrast depicting infiltrative squamous-cell carcinoma of the left lateral oral tongue and floor of the mouth with associated bone destruction. There is posterior tumor extension to involve the retromolar trigone and tonsillar complex. **B:** Corresponding computed tomography bone window views demonstrating destruction of the mandibular body.

artifact that obscures visualization of the primary tumor on CT. MRI provides excellent definition of tumor involving the tongue and is a good modality for evaluating the possibility of perineural spread. Ultrasound may be used to screen for enlarged lymph nodes that are not clinically detectable. In experienced hands, the accuracy of ultrasound when combined with fine needle aspiration may be superior to CT or MRI for staging the neck (118). Positron emission tomography (PET) and CT/PET are emerging technologies. Their greatest utility in head and neck cancer to date appears to be in identifying distant metastases and detecting persistent or recurrent disease. Reports have indicated that the overall sensitivity and specificity of PET may be equivalent or superior to CT and MRI for evaluating persistent or recurrent disease, particularly in patients who have received previous radiotherapy (5,36). PET/CT may improve the anatomic localization of abnormalities identified on PET and decrease the number of equivocal PET findings (94).

Clinical Staging

The American Joint Committee on Cancer has established a staging system for cancer of the oral cavity (Table 41.2). The staging guidelines apply to all forms of carcinoma (45). Nonepithelial malignancies are not included in the staging system.

General Management

Surgical resection, radiation, chemotherapy, or combined modality approaches are classical treatment options for patients with cancers of the oral cavity. The choice of treatment modality, either singly or in combination, depends on the stage and size of the tumor and relevant patient factors such as toxicity, performance status, comorbid disease, and convenience. Broadly speaking, single modality treatment (i.e., surgery or radiation) is preferred for early stage, T1 or T2 lesions. The control rates are generally the same for early stage lesions with either modality alone. For more advanced lesions a combined modality treatment approach is preferred.

In general, the choice for initial treatment of early stage oral cavity cancer is surgical resection. Surgical resection is expeditious, convenient, and often associated with modest morbidity. Radiation therapy may require both external beam and interstitial treatment for optimal therapeutic effect. A course of radiation can require several weeks of daily therapy followed by an interstitial implant. Moreover, the risk of associated xerostomia, osteoradionecrosis, and need for fluoride treatment may render radiation therapy a less attractive choice for single modality therapy. Nevertheless, for patients who are at significant surgical risk or in whom surgical resection would result in significant functional loss, radiation therapy offers a good alternative for definitive treatment.

For patients with advanced lesions of the oral cavity a combined modality approach is generally recommended. The timing of radiation, before or after surgery, has been a matter of some debate. There are advantages and disadvantages to either approach. The preponderance of data and practice pattern suggests that postoperative radiation is usually preferred. Further, there is emerging data that for selected patients with high-risk pathologic features, the addition of concurrent chemotherapy during the postoperative radiation treatment course may

Table 41.2	STAGING OF ORAL CAVITY CARCINOMA		
A			
Tis	Carcinoma *in situ*		
T1	Tumor ≤2 cm in greatest dimension		
T2	Tumor >2 cm in greatest dimension, but ≤4 cm		
T3	Tumor >4 cm in greatest dimension		
T4 (lip)	Tumor invades through cortical bone, inferior alveolar nerve, floor of mouth, or skin of face (i.e., chin or nose).		
T4a (oral cavity)	Tumor invades adjacent structures (e.g., through cortical bone, into deep [extrinsic] muscles of the tongue, maxillary sinus, skin of face)		
T4b	Tumor invades masticator space, pterygoid plates, or skull base and/or encases carotid artery		
B			
Nx	Regional lymph nodes cannot be assessed		
N0	No regional lymph nodes		
N1	Metastases in a single ipsilateral lymph node ≤3 cm in greatest dimension		
N2	Metastases in a single ipsilateral lymph node >3 cm, but <6 cm in greatest dimension; or in multiple lymph nodes none >6 cm in greatest dimension; or in bilateral or contralateral lymph nodes		
N2a	Metastases in a single ipsilateral lymph node >3 cm, but ≤6 cm in greatest dimension		
N2b	Metastases in multiple lymph nodes none ≤6 cm in greatest dimension		
N2c	Metastases in bilateral or contralateral lymph nodes, none 6 cm in greatest dimension		
N3	Metastases in a lymph node >6 cm in greatest dimension		
C			
Stage 0	Tis	N0	M0
Stage I	T1	N0	M0
Stage II	T2	N0	M0
Stage III	T3	N0	M0
	T1-3	N1	M0
Stage IVA	T4a	N0	M0
	T4a	N1	M0
	T1-4a	N2	M0
Stage IVB	Any T	N3	M0
	T4a	Any N	M0
Stage IVC	Any T	Any N	M1

From Green FL PD, Fleming ID, et al. *AJCC cancer staging manual.* New York: Springer, 2002, with permission.

further augment tumor control rates provided the chemotherapy can be tolerated (7,21,26). High-risk features commonly include advanced T stage, multiple positive nodes, extracapsular tumor spread, positive resection margins, and perineural invasion (7,21).

Surgical Management

Cancer of the oral cavity is most commonly treated surgically when the disease is in its early stages (18). Since successful treatment of oral cavity carcinoma relies on effective management of the regional lymphatics as well as the primary cancer, the neck should be addressed in treatment planning. Elective neck treatment is often used for management of the clinically node negative patient with oral cancer, and therapeutic neck dissections are performed for patients with clinically apparent nodal disease. Postoperative radiation or chemoradiation is administered to those patients with pathologic evidence of extensive nodal disease and/or extracapsular spread. Because of the high occult metastatic rate for many cancers, elective neck treatment is encouraged in all but the earliest stages of primary site disease.

Surgical approaches to cancers of the oral cavity may either be transoral, transcervical (pull-through), or alternatively, via mandibulectomy, which is sometimes necessary to obtain the exposure required to achieve adequate margins. In cases where the mental or alveolar nerve is involved with tumor, the nerve should be proximally resected and analyzed microscopically. A tracheotomy is often necessary to maintain a patent airway because of the large amount of oral edema resulting from extensive resection and placement of myocutaneous flaps in the oral cavity.

Tumors that approximate the gingiva should be resected with the gingiva and periosteum as an additional deep margin, while those that appear to involve the periosteum should be resected with an additional deep margin of bone. This last procedure is termed a marginal mandibulectomy. Depending on the extent of tumor involvement, this may involve resection of a bicortical rim of bone at the upper aspect of the alveolus (rim mandibulectomy), or alternatively selective removal of the inner cortex using a vertical or oblique resection (sagittal mandibulectomy). It is commonly recommended to leave at least a 1-cm thick segment of bone inferiorly following a rim mandibulectomy to reduce the risk of pathologic fracture. Those lesions that directly invade bone should be resected with a segment of bone. This often requires soft-tissue or osseous reconstruction of the resected bone segment.

Regarding reconstruction after tumor resection, small surgical defects may not require reconstruction and therefore are often allowed to heal by secondary intention. Larger defects may be reconstructed by primary closure, skin graft, regional flap, or free tissue transfer from different sites. Goals of reconstruction are to replicate the function and appearance of the resected tissue. Urken et al. (115) have developed a systematic approach to functional reconstruction of the oral cavity. Their approach to reconstruction is based on the extent and functional status of the residual tongue and the presence or absence of an associated mandibulectomy.

Split thickness skin grafts are often used for reconstruction and are usually most expedient and efficacious for small defects. Larger defects may require a local or regional flap. Small intraoral defects can be reconstructed effectively with palatal, tongue, and buccal mucosa flaps but usually at the cost of decreased function. Regional flaps that are used in the reconstruction of the oral cavity include the pectoralis major flap, trapezius flap, and latissimus dorsi flap. Continuing developments in microvascular surgery have allowed for head and neck reconstructive surgeons to perform free tissue transfer to reconstruct oral cavity defects. Disadvantages of this procedure include the complexity of the technique and the increased surgical time. The free flaps most commonly utilized in the oral cavity are the radial forearm flap, the anterolateral thigh flap, the rectus abdominis flap, and the fibula flap.

Total glossectomy defects are well suited for free flap reconstruction. Reconstruction of the mandible often requires free flaps that contain bone and soft tissue such as the fibula flap, the iliac crest flap, and the scapular flap. Compared to reconstruction plates free flaps also allow the potential for a sensate flap through neural anastomosis. A sensate flap may result in improved swallowing and speech function, but few studies have unequivocally demonstrated an improvement in these functional outcomes (6,112–114,116,117).

Radiation Therapy

General Principles

For early lip, oral tongue, and floor of the mouth tumors, radiation therapy is an effective means of securing tumor control (50). Acceptable control rates have been achieved with brachytherapy alone or with a combination of brachytherapy and external beam radiation. Early work indicates that the success rate of radiotherapy is higher if some or all of the treatment is administered with brachytherapy (42,44). Decroix and Ghossein (28) reported outcomes in 602 patients with cancer of the oral tongue treated with radium implantation or implantation plus external beam radiation. In this series, recurrence at the primary site or at the primary site and neck was 14% and 22% for T1 and T2 lesions, respectively. The Royal Marsden Hospital reported local control rates of 90% at 5 years for T1 and T2 tumors treated with interstitial radiation with or without external beam radiation (27). Pernot et al. (84) reported local control rates of 96% for T1, 85% for T2, and 64% for T3 lesions of the oral cavity treated with brachytherapy and neck dissection. In this series, local regional control rates were 83%, 70%, and 44%, respectively. Retrospective studies suggest that control rates at the primary site of early oral cavity lesions treated with brachytherapy alone or a combination of brachytherapy plus external beam radiation range from approximately 70% to >95% (27,28,83,84). Involvement of the mandible is a contraindication to definitive radiotherapy because it compromises control and increases the risk of osteoradionecrosis.

Intraoral cone, like interstitial brachytherapy, is a localized radiation therapy technique that has been used to boost the dose to the primary tumor in the oral cavity. Institutions with significant experience with this technique have reported results that rival those obtained by interstitial brachytherapy (122,123). Either technique for boosting the primary tumor has resulted in improved outcomes compared to high-dose radiation therapy alone (34,125). In general, external beam radiation therapy followed by either technique is preferable over radiation therapy alone. As with all specialized procedures, the skill and experience of the radiation oncologist is of critical importance to the successful delivery and outcome of interstitial radiation or intraoral cone therapy.

The outcomes for advanced lesions of the oral cavity (T3 and T4) are less than satisfactory with either surgery or radiation alone. In most advanced stage cancers single modality therapy is inferior to combined modality therapy (44,97,119). Adjuvant radiation therapy can be delivered preoperatively or postoperatively (97,122). Although each strategy has potential advantages and disadvantages, postoperative radiation therapy is generally preferred. Notable disadvantages of preoperative radiation therapy include a delay in definitive surgical treatment and limitations on the dose of radiation that can be delivered due to the risk of wound complications after surgery. Postoperative radiation treatment carries the advantage of no dose limitation, no delay in the implementation of surgical resection, and complete pathologic staging of the tumor. However, it must be borne in mind that postoperative wound complications may delay the implementation of postoperative radiation, and the regional hypoxia that can accompany the postoperative state may diminish the effectiveness of radiation compared to that achievable under conditions of full oxygenation.

Adjuvant Radiation

Although surgery has emerged as the preferred initial treatment approach for the majority of patients with tumors of the oral cavity, adjuvant radiation is commonly recommended to enhance the likelihood of locoregional tumor control. Robertson et al. (92) conducted a phase III study in the United Kingdom of 350 patients with T2-4/N0-2 oral cavity or oropharyngeal cancers comparing surgery and postoperative radiation versus radiation alone. Because a difference in survival was identified, the study was closed early. The authors found that after 23 months, overall survival, cause-specific survival, and local control were all improved on the surgery plus radiation arm. Indications for postoperative radiation therapy include multiple cervical metastases, positive or close margins, extracapsular extension, perineural invasion, advanced T stage, and suspicion of mandibular cortical involvement. In regards to buccal mucosa cancers, Mishra et al. (74) conducted a prospective randomized trial of surgery with or without adjuvant radiation 6 weeks after surgery. They reported a 30% absolute improvement in disease-free survival, although there was no difference in overall survival with the use of adjuvant radiation therapy.

Recently, there has been interest in the evaluation of postoperative chemoradiation for patients with high-risk pathologic features. The results of two randomized trials suggest that postoperative chemoradiation may be beneficial for improving local–regional control and disease-free survival among selected patients with specific high-risk features (7,21).

Neoadjuvant Therapy

At the current time, neoadjuvant radiation and chemotherapy remain largely experimental for cancer of the oral cavity. The use of preoperative chemotherapy has been studied in at least two randomized trials. Licitra et al. (60) conducted a phase III study of 195 patients with T2-4 (>3 cm) N0-2 squamous-cell carcinoma of the oral cavity and randomized patients to surgery alone versus three cycles of cisplatin and 5-fluorouracil (5-FU) followed by surgery. The authors found no difference in overall survival but did comment on the possibility of neoadjuvant chemotherapy as potentially improving resectability and reducing the need for adjuvant radiation therapy. In a similarly designed trial, Volling et al. (120) also reported no difference in overall survival with the use of neoadjuvant chemotherapy, although there was an improvement in disease-free survival.

Preoperative chemoradiation has been studied prospectively by Mohr et al. (76). The authors randomized 268 patients with T2-4/N0-3 oral cavity and oropharyngeal cancers to either preoperative chemoradiation with cisplatin versus surgery alone. Results of this study revealed an improvement in overall survival and local control with the use of preoperative therapy. This regimen, however, has not shown common adoption in other centers around the world.

Radiation Techniques

Carcinoma of the oral cavity has traditionally been treated with opposed lateral fields, using either two-dimensional or three-dimensional CT-based techniques. During simulation and treatment patients are commonly immobilized with a thermoplastic mask. Patients are placed in supine position with a bite block (for oral tongue and floor of mouth cases) to depress the tongue away from the palate (Fig. 41.14); some institutions use a cork and tongue blade for this purpose. For patients with a short neck, the shoulders are depressed by having the patient pull on a tensioning device looped beneath the feet. Generally, the oral cavity tumor bed and upper echelon lymph nodes are included within the initial lateral fields (Fig. 41.15). The upper border of the field is positioned to provide a 1.5- to 2-cm border on the tumor bed in an attempt to partially spare parotid glands and hard palate if possible without compromising coverage of the tumor bed and regional lymphatics. The inferior border of the field resides at approximately the thyroid notch, just above the true vocal cords. The posterior border is set at the mid-vertebral body level if level V nodal coverage is not required. The nodal volume should include level Ia-Ib, II, and III. For patients with more advanced neck disease or neck risk or positive level V lymph nodes, where the posterior chain requires radiation, the initial fields should be set behind the C1 vertebral body spinous process. The portals are then reduced at approximately 45 Gy to spare high dose to the spinal cord. If patients harbor cervical lymph node metastases, or high-risk disease, then the lower neck will also be treated. In this case, a single half-beam-blocked anteroposterior field is matched to the inferior border of the opposed lateral fields at the level of the thyroid notch (Fig. 41.16). An anterior larynx block is used, which protects not only the central larynx from unnecessary radiation dose, but also protects against spinal cord overdose due to three-field overlap.

Megavoltage beams with an energy range between 4 and 6 MV are most suitable for treatment of cancers involving the oral cavity. Cobalt-60 (similar average energy to that from 4 MV linear accelerators) remains a very acceptable radiation delivery unit for cancers in this region owing to the small lateral separation distances in the head and neck area. When higher energy beams are used, bolus material may be necessary to bring dose to the surface as required for tumors that extend to the skin. This is particularly important in patients with large volume nodal disease or extracapsular extension where particular attention should be paid to adequate dosing of superficial tissues. Tissue compensating filters should be used with opposed lateral fields when the variation of the separation is >3 cm. All fields should be treated daily and at least 5 treatment days per week.

In recent years, there has been increasing use of intensity-modulated radiation therapy (IMRT) for the treatment of head

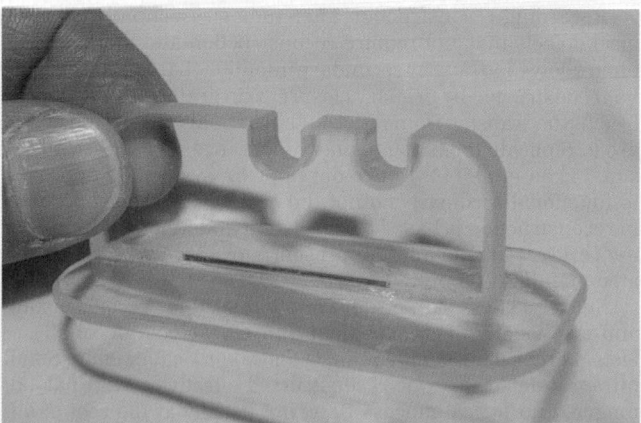

FIGURE 41.14. Lucite oral cavity mouthpiece fabricated at the University of Wisconsin for patients with oral cavity carcinomas. Upper dentition or maxillary alveolus links to u-shaped notch and tongue rests beneath smooth undersurface of mouthpiece. Note embedded solder wire in mouthpiece floor to facilitate visualization of tongue positioning at the time of simulation and beam design.

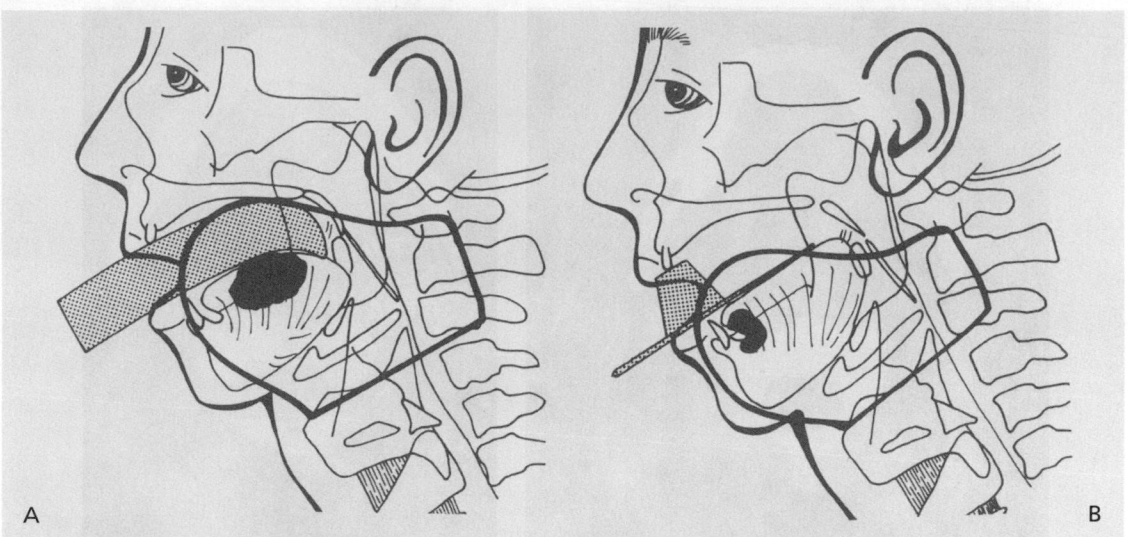

FIGURE 41.15. **A:** Illustration of field design for treatment of carcinoma of the oral tongue with an N0 neck. **B:** Illustration of field design for treatment of carcinoma of the floor of mouth with an N0 neck (From Million RR, Cassisi NJ, eds. *Management of head and neck cancer: a multidisciplinary approach*, 2nd ed. Philadelphia: Lippincott, 1994, with permission.)

and neck region tumors (Fig. 41.17). With regard to oral cavity cancer, IMRT offers the opportunity to diminish normal tissue toxicities, including damage to major salivary glands (xerostomia) and to the mandible (osteoradionecrosis) (23,110,129). Dosimetric analysis of radiation dose to the parotid glands with evaluation of resultant salivary function suggests that limiting mean parotid dose to <26 Gy is associated with improved postradiation salivary function (31). Ideal candidates for IMRT include patients with T1-3 primary lesions with ≤N2b neck disease. In light of the steep dose gradients that often accompany IMRT plans, successful delivery is dependent on accurate and reproducible localization and immobilization. At several centers, an optically guided localization system is used to

enhance daily treatment precision for IMRT delivery. Tomotherapy, which involves the helical delivery of intensity modulated radiation, enables a high degree of target conformality coupled with the capacity for diagnostic CT scanning, thereby allowing image guidance for adaptive radiotherapy and daily setup verification (39,48,101).

Dose and Fractionation

When postoperative radiation is used for oral cavity cancer, the most common dose fractionation in the United States is 1.8 to 2.0 Gy per day. Dissected tissues that harbored the original tumor should generally receive on the order of 60 Gy. However,

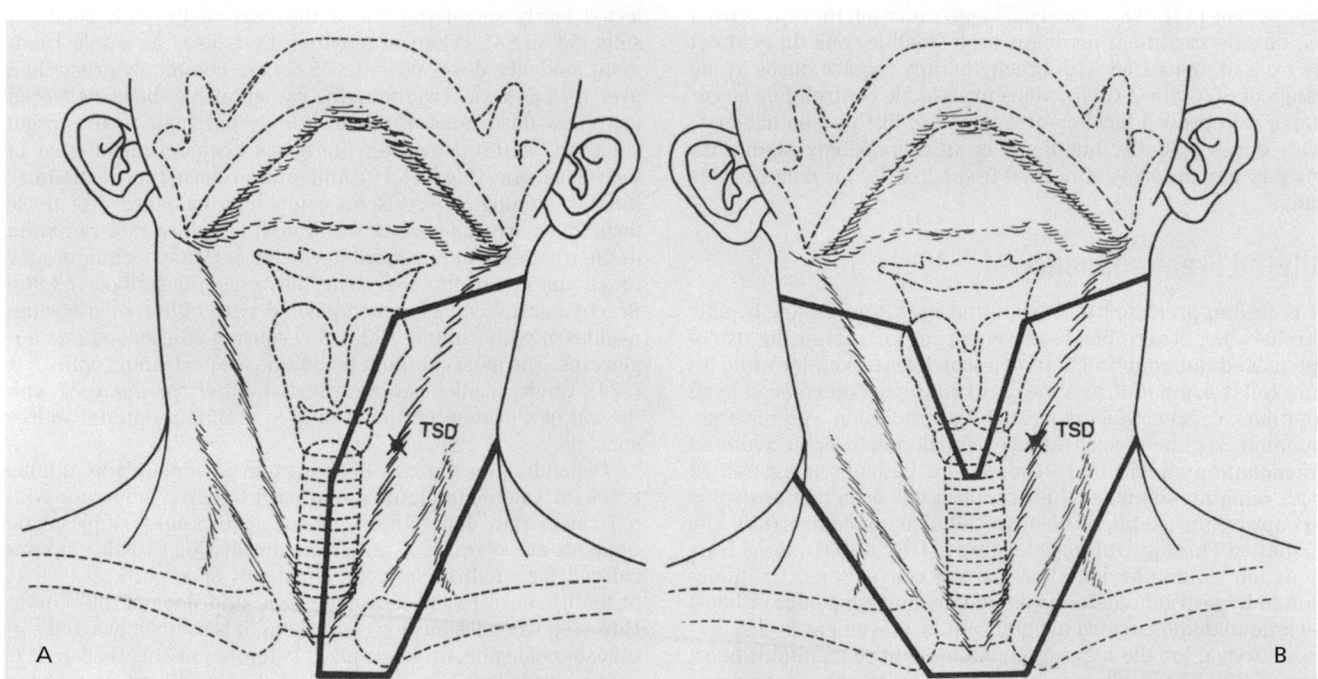

FIGURE 41.16. Illustration of field design for treatment of the neck. **A:** Well-lateralized lesion with clinically negative neck. **B:** Elective bilateral neck irradiation. (From Million RR, Cassisi NJ, eds. *Management of head and neck cancer: a multidisciplinary approach*, 2nd ed. Philadelphia: Lippincott, 1994, with permission.)

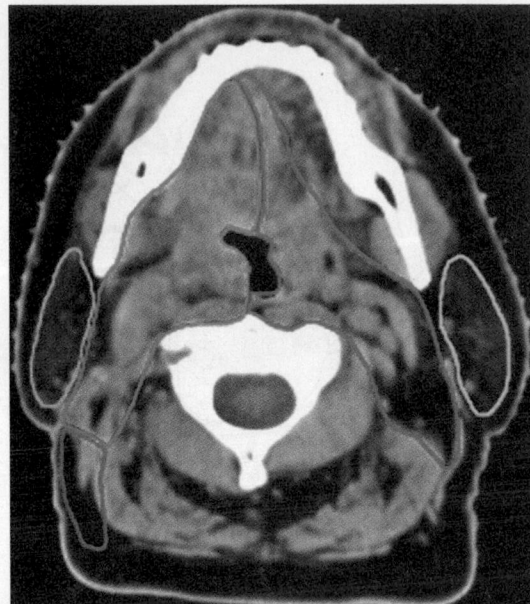
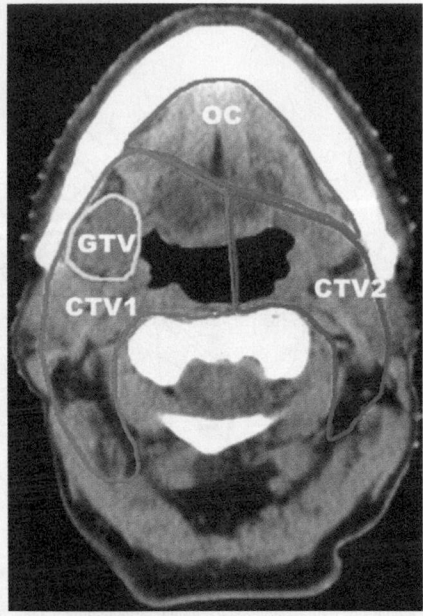

FIGURE 41.17. A: Clinical target volume (CTV) delineation for patient with T2-N2b oral tongue carcinoma receiving postoperative intensity-modulated radiation therapy (IMRT). CTV1 (*red line*), CTV2 (*dark blue line*), and parotid glands also noted. **B:** CTV delineation for patient with T3-N2b retromolar trigone carcinoma receiving definitive IMRT. Gross tumor volume (GTV) (*yellow line*), CTV1 (*red line*), CTV2 (*dark blue line*), and oral cavity (*magenta line*) are shown. (From Chao KS, Ozyigit, G, eds. *Intensity modulated radiation therapy for H&N cancer.* Philadelphia: Lippincott Williams & Wilkins, 2003, with permission.)

for close or positive microscopic margins or extracapsular nodal extension, a 4- to 6-Gy localized boost should be considered. If there is gross residual disease, either further surgical resection or focal boosting up to 70 Gy is advisable. Regions of somewhat lesser risk (i.e., clinically or pathologically uninvolved necks) should receive on the order of 50 to 54 Gy.

When definitive radiation is used for oral cavity cancer, boosting the primary tumor with either interstitial implantation, submental, or intraoral cone therapy can result in increased tumor control and decreased complications, particularly osteoradionecrosis (34). When external beam radiation therapy is used as the sole treatment modality, even small lesions that cannot be excised or treated with brachytherapy require doses in the range of 66 Gy in 2-Gy fractions for reliable control. For larger tumors, improved local control rates are likely to be achieved with doses ≥70 Gy, but there is an increasingly significant price to pay in terms of normal tissue toxicity for doses in this range.

Altered Fractionation

It is well appreciated that head and neck tumors are rapidly proliferating. There has been significant interest in the use of intensified radiation fractionation schedules to counter rapid tumor cell repopulation as a means of improving outcome in head and neck cancer patients treated with radiation. Altered fractionation regimens such as hyperfractionation or accelerated fractionation should be considered for patients being treated with radiation alone, as this approach has been demonstrated to improve the likelihood of locoregional tumor control (85). The Radiation Therapy Oncology Group's (RTOG 90-03) altered fractionation randomized trial comparing conventional fractionation to hyperfractionation, split-course, and concomitant boost technique demonstrated a significant improvement in disease-free survival for the hyperfractionation and concomitant boost arms (43). These altered fractionation regimens were associated with higher incidence of grade 3 or worse acute mucosal toxicity, but no significant difference in overall toxicity at 2 years following completion of treatment. However, oral

cavity carcinoma constituted a minority of cases enrolled in these studies.

Brachytherapy

Historically, brachytherapy has played an important role in the treatment of oral cavity carcinoma. Brachytherapy has been used to boost the primary site in the oral cavity before or following external beam radiation (Fig. 41.18). This technique has also been used as a sole modality in the treatment of selected (early stage) tumors of the oral cavity with good results (58,83,84). When brachytherapy is used as a sole treatment modality, doses of 65 to 75 Gy are commonly prescribed over 6 to 7 days. Traditionally, radiation has been delivered using low-dose rates of 0.4 to 0.6 Gy per hour to the target volume (75,108). However, there has been recent interest in high-dose rate (Fig. 41.19) and pulsed-dose rate techniques (68,93), although there is no compelling evidence that these techniques are superior to traditional low-dose rate radiation in the treatment of head and neck cancer. Many techniques for brachytherapy in the oral cavity have been described (73,86). Brachytherapy can be accomplished with either rigid cesium needles or with iridium-192 (^{192}Ir) sources afterloaded into angiocaths. The most common technique is afterloading with ^{192}Ir (124). Guide needles can be inserted either free-hand or with the aid of a custom template to help maintain optimal source spacing.

Depending on the size of the lesion a single plane, double plane, or volume implant can be used to cover the tumor with a 1-cm margin. For tumors <1 cm in thickness, single plane implants are adequate. Surface mold radiation can also be considered for small tumors <1 cm depth or superficial lesions of the lip, hard palate, lower gingiva, and floor of the mouth. However, when lesions exceed 2.5 cm, it is difficult to avoid significant cold spots in the implant volume. For this reason, it is recommended that for lesions larger than 2.5 cm part of the treatment be given with external beam radiation to supplement the dose to the cold spots. In this setting, a combined treatment plan typically gives 50 Gy over 5 weeks with external beam

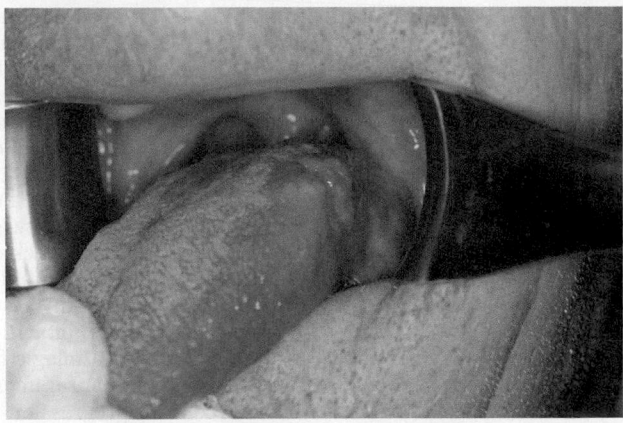

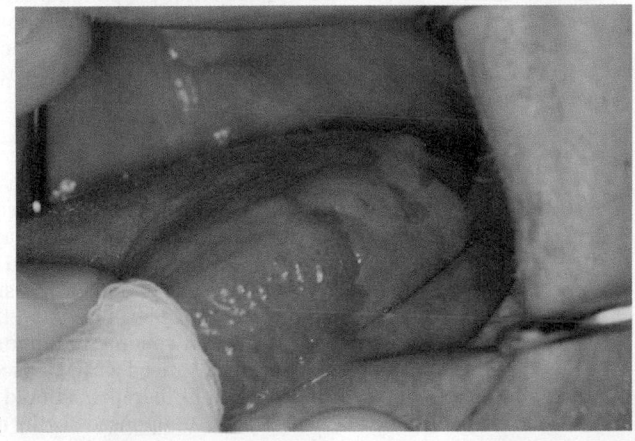

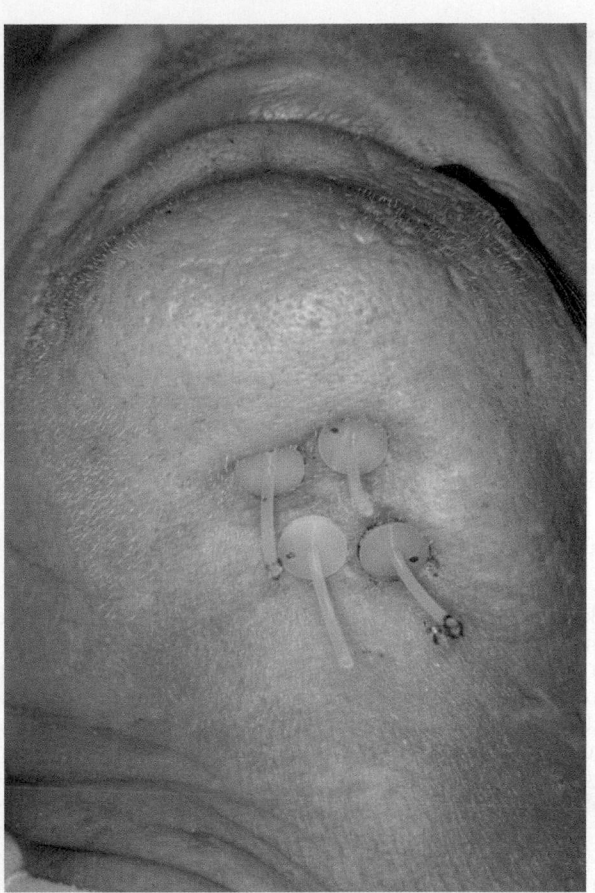

FIGURE 41.18. A: T2/N0/M0 squamous-cell carcinoma involving the left lateral oral tongue. **B:** Submental view of interstitial implantation catheters housing ^{192}Ir seeds for delivery of 25-Gy tumor boost following external beam radiation of 50 Gy. **C:** Implantation bed mucositis conforming to the tumor distribution seven days following 25-Gy implant boost.

radiation followed by 30 Gy with a brachytherapy implant. What must be borne in mind is that as tumors get too close to the mandible or are large in volume, the risk of osteoradionecrosis increases (64).

Over the past decade or more, stepwise improvements in reconstructive surgery techniques have diminished the practice frequency of brachytherapy in the treatment of oral cavity carcinoma. In addition, a diminishing percentage of radiation oncologists remain highly skilled and experienced with the requisite implant techniques. Finally, the steady advancement of highly

conformal external beam techniques (IMRT, tomotherapy) has contributed to less frequent practice of brachytherapy in head and neck cancer overall. The identical comments parallel the use of intraoral cone radiation treatment described further in the section below.

Intraoral Cone

The intraoral cone is another delivery tool to enable boosting of radiation dose to sites within the oral cavity while avoiding

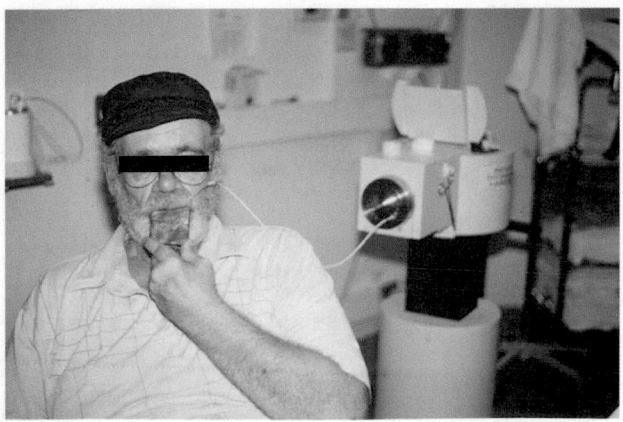

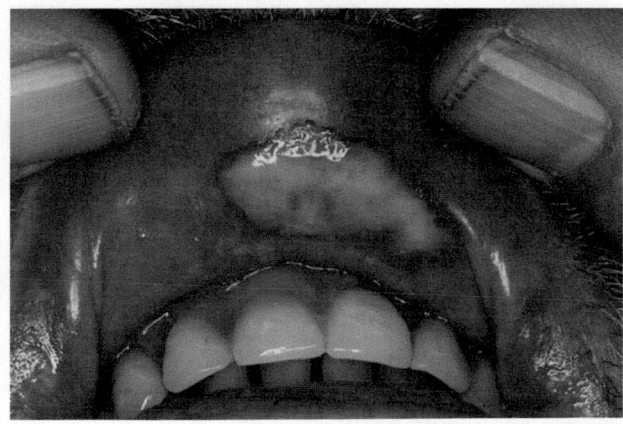

FIGURE 41.19. A: Patient undergoing high–dose rate (HDR) brachytherapy for superficial T1 upper lip squamous-cell carcinoma (buccal surface) using a single interstitial catheter for source delivery. **B:** Focal mucositis 1 week following completion of HDR brachytherapy treatment course.

direct dose to the mandible (Fig. 41.20). This technique is generally best suited for anterior oral cavity lesions in edentulous patients. However, palatal arch sites can be targeted with the intraoral cone as well. Treatment with intraoral cone involves either 100 to 250 kilovolt (peak) (kvp) x-rays or electron beams in the 6 to 12 MeV range (73,122,123). Lesions up to 3 cm are amenable to treatment with intraoral cone as long as they are accessible. Intraoral cone therapy requires careful daily positioning and verification by the physician. For this purpose the device is equipped with a periscope to visualize the lesion. The cone abuts the mucosa and is centered directly over the lesion. Intraoral cone treatment should take place prior to external beam radiation so that the lesion can be adequately visualized. A major advantage of cone therapy is that it is highly focal to the tumor bed but noninvasive. Hence, when available, for suitable lesions, it may be preferred over brachytherapy. However, as noted for brachytherapy delivery, operator experience and dedication are essential to optimize outcome.

Chemotherapy and Radiation

The application of chemotherapy to the treatment of head and neck cancer dates back to the 1960s. Over the decades the role of chemotherapy has advanced from initial use only in the recurrent or metastatic setting to active current use in the definitive treatment setting. There are a number of studies that demonstrate a benefit of concurrent chemotherapy administration in the definitive treatment of head and neck cancer with radiation (1,10,15,29,71,107,127). Although these trials vary with respect to radiation dose, fractionation schedule, and chemotherapy regimen, they have in common a randomized comparison between radiotherapy and radiotherapy plus chemotherapy. The advantage of concurrent chemotherapy with radiation has been further examined in the context of several meta-analyses (11,32,78,87). These meta-analyses generally identify a small overall survival benefit for the use of chemotherapy on the order of 1% to 8% (49). Summary analyses suggest no significant survival benefit for the use of neoadjuvant and adjuvant chemotherapy, but do suggest a clear benefit for the use of concurrent chemoradiation. However, in many of the randomized studies comparing radiation alone to chemoradiation, oral cavity patients are either excluded or make up only a small proportion of the study population.

Several recent studies have focused on the use of chemoradiation in patients with high-risk pathologic features following initial surgery. Cooper et al. (21) reported the results of a randomized study in North America comparing radiation alone (60 to 66 Gy) to chemoradiation (same radiation dose plus three cycles of 100 mg/m² cisplatin) in patients with head and neck carcinoma demonstrating high-risk features after gross total resection. High-risk disease was defined as any or all of the following: two or more involved lymph nodes, extracapsular extension of nodal disease, and microscopically involved resection margins. This study demonstrated a benefit in local–regional control and disease-free survival for the chemoradiation arm, but no overall survival benefit was appreciated. A parallel study in Europe by Bernier et al. (7) randomized patients to essentially equivalent treatment arms following head and neck cancer surgery. Eligibility criteria included patients with pathologic T3 or T4 disease (except T3/N0), or patients with any T-stage disease with two or more involved lymph nodes, or patients with T1-2 and N0-1 disease with unfavorable pathologic findings (extranodal spread, positive margins, perineural involvement, or vascular embolism). Local control, progression-free survival, and overall survival were superior for patients on the chemoradiation arm. These studies suggest that the addition of chemoradiation following surgery may be beneficial in selected patients with high-risk head and neck cancer, although with increased toxicity profiles.

Dental Care

Prior to the initiation of head and neck radiation a careful oral and dental evaluation, including a panoramic radiograph, should be performed. Dentition in poor condition should be identified and considered for extraction to minimize the subsequent risk of osteoradionecrosis. Specifically, those teeth that will reside within the high-dose radiation volume that demonstrate significant periodontal disease, advanced caries, abscess formation, or are otherwise in a state of disrepair should be extracted. In addition, impacted teeth, unopposed teeth, and teeth that could potentially oppose a segment of a resected jawbone should be considered for extraction if they are anticipated to reside within the high-dose radiation treatment volume. Extraction of marginal teeth should also be considered in patients who are deemed unable to maintain adequate oral hygiene.

Radiation can induce several chronic effects in the oral cavity that warrant routine surveillance. Radiation can impair bone healing and diminish the capacity for successful recovery following trauma or oral surgery. For this reason, elective oral surgical procedures including extractions must be very carefully considered after radiation. Escalation of dental caries deriving from xerostomia following radiation is well recognized (Fig. 41.21). Radiation of the major salivary glands changes the nature of salivary secretions (121), which can increase the

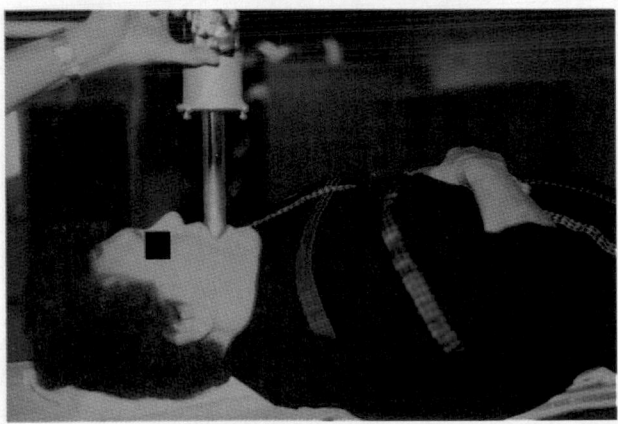
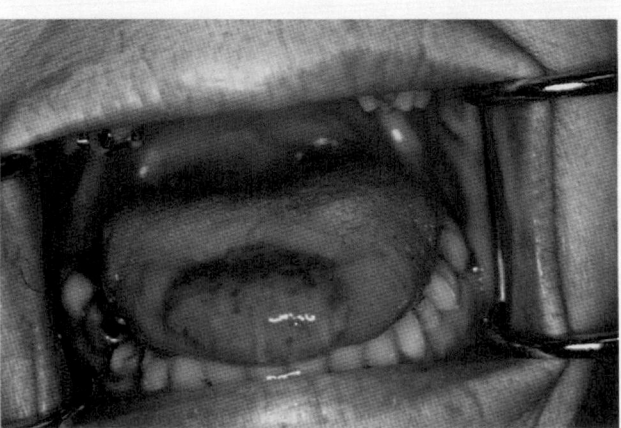

A   B

FIGURE 41.20. A: Intraoral cone boost technique at the University of Wisconsin for focal delivery of electron beam radiation. The electron cone is mounted directly to the accelerator gantry with a side view periscope enabling direct vision and positioning for daily treatment. **B:** Focal mucositis involving the distal oral tongue following treatment of a 1-cm tumor in this location with intraoral cone technique.

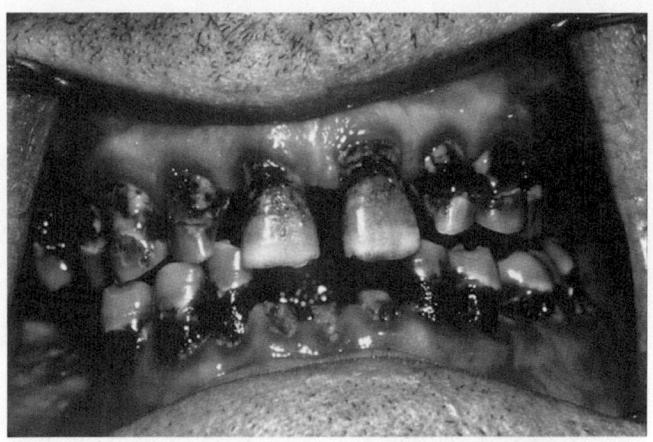

FIGURE 41.21. Advanced dental caries in a patient with profound radiation xerostomia and lack of attention to dental hygiene over many years following treatment.

accumulation of plaque and debris, reduce salivary pH, and reduce the buffering ability of saliva (55). This creates an environment in the oral cavity, which predisposes patients to caries. During a course of radiation to the oral cavity, simple techniques such as the use of custom molds to absorb electron backscatter can diminish hot-spot mucositis from dental fillings and improve treatment tolerance (Fig. 41.22). Attention to oral hygiene with frequent dental follow-up examinations and cleanings, daily fluoride therapy (Fig. 41.23), flossing, and brushing

should be an integral component of the education and postradiation care of patients who undergo radiation to the oral cavity.

Prognostic and Predictive Factors

The most significant prognostic factor for outcome in oral cavity carcinoma is the presence of cervical metastases (81). In patients with positive cervical metastases the 5-year survival is reduced by approximately 50% from that in the absence of metastases (53). The prognosis diminishes further when patients harbor multiple levels of nodal involvement or extracapsular extension (ECE). In a retrospective review, Myers et al. (81) found that 5-year disease-specific and overall survival rates for pathologically N0 patients were 88% and 75%, respectively; these decreased to 65% and 50%, respectively, if patients were node positive but without evidence of ECE. Patients who were node positive with evidence of ECE had 5-year disease-specific and overall survival rates of 48% and 30%, respectively.

Several histopathologic factors in the primary lesion are associated with adverse prognosis. Tumor thickness and depth of invasion have been shown to confer a higher risk of regional metastases (18). Perineural invasion has been correlated with cervical lymph node metastases, extracapsular extension, and diminished survival (8,35,105). Microvascular invasion has also been correlated significantly with cervical lymph node metastases (19,67). However, lymphatic invasion has not been correlated significantly with cervical lymph node invasion (18). The

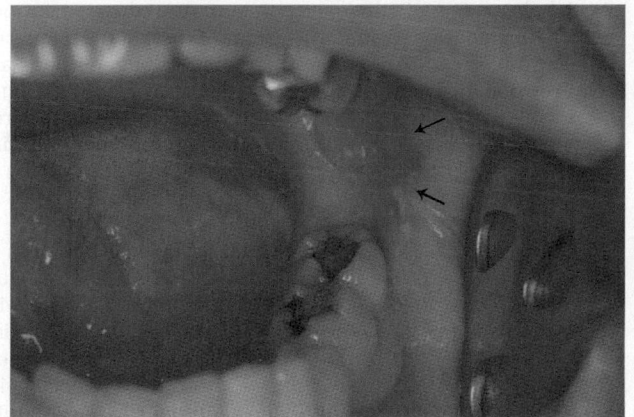

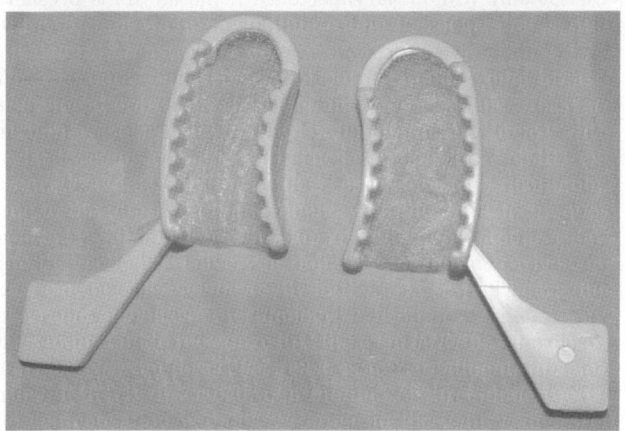

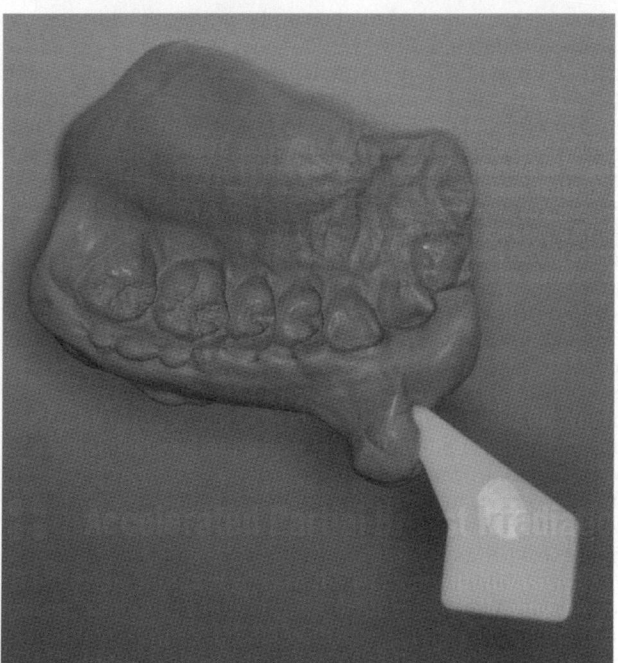

FIGURE 41.22. A: Focal patches of mucositis from electron backscatter secondary to dense molar fillings early in a course of external beam radiation. **B:** Plastic bitewing dental tray to support custom mold impression to absorb electron backscatter adjacent to metallic dental fillings. **C:** Completed dental impression for daily insertion during treatment to absorb electron backscatter within mold thereby avoiding hot-spot mucositis.

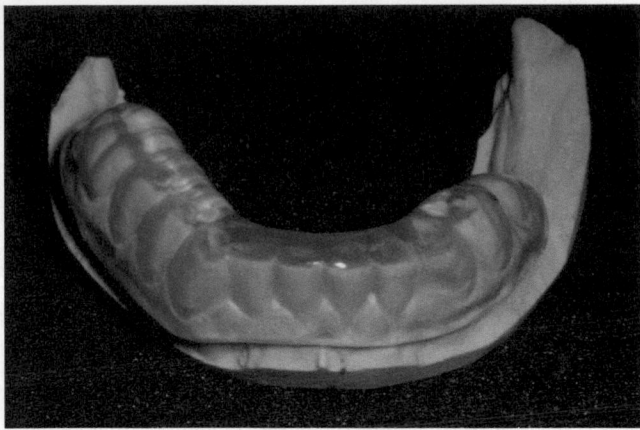

FIGURE 41.23. Custom designed fluoride carrier trays to facilitate daily fluoride application to existing dentition.

prognostic significance of grade has also been evaluated (3). Because of the wide variation in pathologic interpretation, it is difficult to discern the independent value of histologic grading as a prognostic or predictive value (18).

Subsite-Specific Treatment and Results

Lip

Early stage carcinoma of the lip can be managed with surgery or radiation therapy. However, surgery is generally preferred for small tumors (<2 cm). Although the local control of T1 and T2 squamous cancers of the lip is excellent with surgical resection, disruption of the oral sphincter provided by the orbicularis muscle can lead to oral incompetence if not properly reconstructed. Therefore, a number of reconstructive methods have been developed to help preserve oral sphincteric function even following large excisions for T3 and T4 lesions. For these larger lesions, surgery followed by radiotherapy remains a standard therapy.

When primary radiotherapy is used to treat lip cancer, the target volume should include the primary tumor plus a 1.5- to 2-cm margin. For early stage lesions, photons in the orthovoltage range (100 to 200 keV) or electrons may be used. The electron energy should be chosen based on the thickness of the lesion (commonly 6 to 9 MeV). Effort should be made to shield the underlying gum, dentition, and mandible as appropriate. This can be accomplished with the use of oral shields or cerrobend stents. The recommended dose is 50 Gy in 4.5 to 5 weeks for smaller lesions and 60 Gy in 5 to 6 weeks for larger lesions. Some institutions have used an approach where external beam radiation is given to approximately 40 to 50 Gy followed by a brachytherapy boost, or smaller lesions are treated by primary brachytherapy alone. An important consideration in managing lip cancer is the risk of regional metastatic disease. Generally, the risk of regional lymph node metastatic disease for T1 and T2 cancers of the lip is lower than for stage-matched tumors of other oral cavity sites. Thus, elective neck dissection is recommended for patients with T3 and T4 carcinomas of the lip; however, it may not be warranted for all T1 and T2 lesions. Some institutions have used a "moustache field" for elective irradiation of the perifacial lymphatics (approximately 50 Gy) for more advanced upper lip lesions (2). Sentinel lymph node biopsy may prove to be useful in the management of patients of node-negative lip cancers, but further clinical investigation in this area is needed.

Oral Tongue

Although primary radiation therapy and surgery are potential treatment options for carcinoma of the oral tongue, most oral tongue cancers in the United States are treated surgically (18). Surgical resection and reconstruction as appropriate is generally preferred for medically operable patients. Postoperative radiation therapy is recommended for patients with large primary tumors (T3, T4), close or positive surgical margins, evidence of perineural spread, multiple positive nodes, or extracapsular extension (2). Postoperative chemoradiation should be considered for patients with adverse risk factors who are able to tolerate combined modality treatment (7,21). Primary radiotherapy techniques can be used for patients who refuse or are unable to tolerate surgery.

Superficial T1 lesions can be treated with brachytherapy alone. Commonly, ^{192}Ir temporary implants are used to deliver 50 to 60 Gy with dose rates of 40 to 60 cGy per hour. For infiltrating T1 or T2 lesions, a combined approach using external beam and a brachytherapy or intraoral cone boost should be considered. More advanced lesions should be treated with an approach combining surgery and radiation therapy. Postoperative treatment should include the site of primary tumor, dissected neck, and draining lymphatics. Opposing lateral fields are used to encompass the tongue and upper neck bilaterally, and this volume should be treated to 50 to 54 Gy (see Fig. 41.12A and Table 41.1). High-risk areas (primary surgical bed, positive/close margins, extracapsular extension, perineural spread) should receive additional boost treatment up to 60 to 66 Gy.

Surgical approaches to oral tongue cancers can either be transoral, transcervical, or alternatively via mandibulectomy to obtain the exposure necessary to achieve adequate margins. Partial glossectomy is the most common procedure performed for oral tongue cancers, and the extent of resection depends on the size and growth pattern of the tumor, as some lesions are relatively infiltrative while others may be more exophytic. Since the tongue is essentially comprised of skeletal muscle covered by mucosa, the tissue is extremely elastic, and wide margins are encouraged at the onset of resection to avoid retraction of muscle fibers with microscopic tumor cells that could serve as a source of local recurrence.

Total glossectomy may be indicated for extensive tumors or those that involve the intrinsic tongue musculature. Total glossectomy, even with reconstruction, can result in difficulty with deglutition and maintenance of an adequate airway. Aspiration may be a chronic problem, and, thus, laryngectomy may be necessary in some cases. However, properly selected patients with adequate postoperative rehabilitation can be treated with total glossectomy without laryngectomy. If the larynx is preserved, laryngeal suspension and palatal augmentation may help with the rehabilitative efforts.

Tumor size and depth of invasion are currently the most reliable indicators for predicting cervical metastases in patients with oral tongue squamous-cell carcinoma. Because of the high risk of nodal metastases the neck should be addressed either with surgery or radiation in all but the earliest tumors of the oral tongue. Patients with small oral tongue cancers should be considered for neck therapy, particularly if the primary tumor exhibits extension onto the floor of mouth or there is increased tumor thickness. Treatment of the clinically negative neck is most often accomplished by supraomohyoid neck dissection. Elective neck dissection appears to result in better overall cancer outcome than observation. Potential pitfalls of observation include a salvage rate of only one-third for patients who do not undergo elective neck dissection along with resection of the oral cavity primary. For patients with a clinically and radiographically N0 neck, with well-lateralized disease, or those who do not undergo neck dissection, 50 to 54 Gy should be considered to the ipsilateral neck as elective nodal irradiation (Fig. 41.16).

Patients with advanced lesions and high-risk disease (particularly with multiple positive nodes) should receive radiation treatment to the bilateral neck.

Floor of the Mouth

Early stage floor of the mouth cancer can be treated effectively by radiation therapy or surgery. However, surgery is usually preferred in patients who are medically operable because proximity of the tumor to the mandible confers a significant risk of radiation-induced ulceration and osteoradionecrosis. Small lesions of the floor of the mouth are most commonly resected transorally. The surgical defect can be left to heal by granulation or reconstructed with a split thickness skin graft or local flap. Advanced stage floor of the mouth cancers are usually managed by a combination of surgery and radiation or chemoradiation.

Small (T1 and T2) lesions may be treated with a combination of external beam radiation and boost with interstitial implant or intraoral cone. For lesions that are very close to the mandible, brachytherapy is contraindicated because of the risk of osteoradionecrosis. Infiltrative lesions that are tethered to the mandible and advanced lesions following surgical resection should receive postoperative radiation. Portals for postoperative treatment are similar to that for oral tongue carcinoma. Opposing lateral fields are used to encompass the oral cavity tumor bed and upper neck bilaterally, and this volume is commonly treated to 50 to 54 Gy. High-risk areas (primary surgical bed, positive/close margins, extracapsular extension, perineural spread) may receive additional boost treatment up to 60 to 66 Gy.

In the surgical management of floor of the mouth cancer, special attention should be paid to mandibular invasion. A cancer that appears to involve only the periosteum or that only superficially invades the mandible can be removed via a transoral or transcervical approach in which a marginal mandibulectomy is performed. However, segmental mandibulectomy may be necessary for patients with a limited mandibular height when there is no direct bone invasion, because marginal mandibulectomy may leave these patients with insufficient bone, placing them at high risk for radionecrosis or pathologic fracture. A full thickness segmental resection may be necessary if there is frank bone invasion. For advanced cancers, resection of the anterior arch of the mandible may be necessary. Defects of the anterior segment of the mandible require reconstruction with bone, usually with a free fibular or iliac crest graft.

Management of the neck is similar to that for other tumors of the oral cavity. Patients with lesions <2-mm thick with no adverse pathologic factors and a clinically and radiographically negative neck may be observed after primary resection and observation. Otherwise most N0 patients should receive either selective neck dissection or radiation therapy. Patients with advanced lesions and high-risk disease (particularly with multiple positive nodes) should receive radiation treatment to bilateral necks.

Hard Palate and Upper Alveolar Ridge

Tumors of the hard palate are quite rare, accounting for only 0.5% of all oral cancers in the United States. Most carcinomas manifest as a granular superficial ulceration of the hard palate. Initial growth tends to be superficial, although these tumors can extend through the periosteum of bone into regions adjacent to the oral cavity, such as the paranasal sinuses and floor of the nose. Although radiation can be used to treat carcinomas of this site, surgery is preferred. Postoperative radiation therapy should be delivered when there are adverse features; that is, close/positive margins, perineural extension, vascular invasion, high-grade histology, multiple positive nodes, or extracapsular extension. The radiation field should encompass the entire surgical bed. In most cases it is necessary to treat with opposed lateral fields to cover the volume at risk. However, for well-lateralized lesions of the upper alveolar ridge, ipsilateral radiation with a wedge pair may be adequate. Conformal treatment techniques can also be used to tailor the radiation coverage to the high-risk tissue bed and draining lymphatics as appropriate.

Wide local excision may be adequate to obtain surgical margins. However, infrastructure maxillectomy may in some cases be necessary. For tumors that extensively involve the adjacent bony and soft tissue structures a total maxillectomy, with or without orbital exenteration, may be required. A defect in the maxilla results in lack of oral/nasal separation that can impair the ability to speak and swallow effectively. An obturator with or without a skin graft is the most common method used to restore oral/nasal separation. The obturator is commonly fabricated from a synthetic polymer and provides oronasal separation that can yield improved speech and swallowing function. Regional pedicled flaps and free-tissue transfers may provide alternatives to obturation. However, their use is somewhat controversial for reconstruction of palatal defects since these nonremovable flaps may mask local recurrences that can be more readily identified in patients whose defects are obturated.

Elective treatment of the neck is controversial for hard palate region tumors. Although some series have shown lower rates of occult metastases for palatal tumors when compared to other oral cavity sites, preoperative imaging should be performed to evaluate for the presence of metastases to the retropharyngeal nodes since these are difficult to evaluate on clinical examination and are at some risk for spread from primary palatal tumors.

Retromolar Trigone

Squamous-cell carcinoma of the retromolar trigone is uncommon, and the true incidence is difficult to determine since these cancers often involve both the retromolar trigone and adjacent sites, thereby making it difficult in some cases to identify the original tumor epicenter. Cancers of the retromolar trigone may be advanced at presentation because only a thin layer of soft tissue overlies the bone in this region and invasion of the underlying bone may occur early. In addition, there are multiple pathways for spread from this site including the buccal mucosa, tonsillar fossa, glossopharyngeal sulcus, floor of the mouth, base of the tongue, hard and soft palate, masticator space, and maxillary tuberosity. As patients tend to present with advanced disease of the retromolar trigone, many have regional metastases at the time of presentation.

Early stage T1 and T2 cancers can be treated equally effectively with surgery or radiation with primary control rates for T1 and T2 tumors of 92% and 88%, respectively. For more extensive superficial lesions that extend to involve the soft palate or tonsillar complex but do not invade bone, radiotherapy may be a better treatment option, since broad resection of the palate can result in poor speech and swallow outcomes. Well-lateralized lesions of the retromolar trigone can be treated by ipsilateral mixed beam techniques or angled wedge techniques.

Stage III and IV lesions commonly require combined surgery and radiation. The resection of advanced cancer of the retromolar trigone usually requires a composite resection of soft tissue and bone. A limiting factor for the achievement of adequate surgical resection margins for tumors in this area includes extension of tumor posterosuperiorly into the pterygopalatine fossa and into the base of skull.

Buccal Mucosa

Verrucous carcinoma accounts for <5% of all oral cavity carcinomas, occurs most often in the buccal mucosa, has a more favorable prognosis, and is considered a low-grade malignancy. Surgical resection remains the preferred mode of treatment for primary lesions of the buccal mucosa. Adjuvant radiation treatment is usually not indicated. Since verrucous carcinomas rarely metastasize, elective neck dissection is often not indicated for patients with this disease. Careful pathology review with clinical correlation is important in the categorization of verrucous carcinomas, as this diagnosis can influence subsequent treatment recommendations.

Squamous-cell carcinoma of the buccal mucosa can be an especially aggressive cancer of the oral cavity, as buccal cancers have multiple potential routes of spread to adjacent areas in the head and neck. Posteriorly, they can extend to involve the pterygoid muscles, and superiorly, they can grow to involve the alveolar ridge, palate, or maxillary sinus. The majority of patients have cancer that extends beyond the buccal mucosa. Metastasis to the cervical lymph nodes most commonly affects the submandibular nodes.

T1 and T2 tumors of the buccal mucosa can be managed with equal effectiveness by either surgery or radiation. Transoral resection is preferred and is most convenient for small lesions. Tumors approximating the gingiva should be resected with the gingiva and periosteum as an additional deep margin, while those that involve the periosteum should be resected with an additional deep margin of bone. Cancers that directly invade bone should be resected with a segment of bone. Larger tumors (T3 or T4) may require surgery combined with radiation therapy.

Management of Recurrent Disease

The appropriate management of recurrent oral cavity cancer depends largely on the extent of disease, the prior therapy administered, and whether the recurrences are local, regional, or both. Obviously, if there is distant disease recurrence, systemic therapy approaches will likely assume primary importance. In the case of small recurrences at the primary site for patients treated with primary excision only, further excision with or without postoperative radiotherapy is often recommended. For larger recurrences in patients who received radiation as part of their initial management, the rate of surgical salvage is quite low. In some cases, further resection may be considered for palliation or curative treatment attempt, particularly in the setting of a clinical trial. Systemic therapy, reirradiation, and palliative care are other options for this group of patients, and the risks and benefits of each should be discussed with the individual patient.

References

1. Adelstein DJ, Li Y, Adams GL, et al. An intergroup phase III comparison of standard radiation therapy and two schedules of concurrent chemoradiotherapy in patients with unresectable squamous cell head and neck cancer. *J Clin Oncol* 2003;21:92–98.
2. Ang KK, Garden AS. *Radiotherapy for head and neck cancers: indications and techniques*. Philadelphia: Lippincott Williams & Wilkins, 2006.
3. Anneroth G, Batsakis J, Luna M. Review of the literature and a recommended system of malignancy grading in oral squamous cell carcinomas. *Scand J Dent Res* 1987;95:229–249.
4. Antoniades DZ, Styanidis K, Papanayotou P, et al. Squamous cell carcinoma of the lips in a northern Greek population. Evaluation of prognostic factors on 5-year survival rate—I. *Eur J Cancer B Oral Oncol* 1995;31B:333–339.
5. Anzai Y, Carroll WR, Quint DJ, et al. Recurrence of head and neck cancer after surgery or irradiation: prospective comparison of 2-deoxy-2-[F-18]fluoro-D-glucose PET and MR imaging diagnoses. *Radiology* 1996;200:135–141.
6. Aviv JE, Hecht C, Weinberg H, et al. Surface sensibility of the floor of the mouth and tongue in healthy controls and in radiated patients. *Otolaryngol Head Neck Surg* 1992;107:418–423.
7. Bernier J, Domenge C, Ozsahin M, et al. Postoperative irradiation with or without concomitant chemotherapy for locally advanced head and neck cancer. *N Engl J Med* 2004;350:1945–1952.
8. Borges AM, Shrikhande SS, Ganesh B. Surgical pathology of squamous carcinoma of the oral cavity: its impact on management. *Semin Surg Oncol* 1989;5:310–317.
9. Boyle P, Macfarlane GJ, Scully C. Oral cancer: necessity for prevention strategies. *Lancet* 1993;342:1129.
10. Brizel DM, Albers ME, Fisher SR, et al. Hyperfractionated irradiation with or without concurrent chemotherapy for locally advanced head and neck cancer. *N Engl J Med* 1998;338:1798–1804.
11. Browman GP, Hodson DI, Mackenzie RJ, et al. Choosing a concomitant chemotherapy and radiotherapy regimen for squamous cell head and neck cancer: a systematic review of the published literature with subgroup analysis. *Head Neck* 2001;23:579–589.
12. Burns JC, Murray BK. Conversion of herpetic lesions to malignancy by ultraviolet exposure and promoter application. *J Gen Virol* 1981;55:305–313.
13. Byers RM, Weber RS, Andrews T, et al. Frequency and therapeutic implications of "skip metastases" in the neck from squamous carcinoma of the oral tongue. *Head Neck* 1997;19:14–19.
14. Byers RM, Wolf PF, Ballantyne AJ. Rationale for elective modified neck dissection. *Head Neck Surg* 1988;10:160–167.
15. Calais G, Alfonsi M, Bardet E, et al. Randomized trial of radiation therapy versus concomitant chemotherapy and radiation therapy for advanced-stage oropharynx carcinoma. *J Natl Cancer Inst* 1999;91:2081–2086.
16. Califano J, van der Riet P, Westra W, et al. Genetic progression model for head and neck cancer: implications for field cancerization. *Cancer Res* 1996;56:2488–2492.
17. Canto MT, Devesa SS. Oral cavity and pharynx cancer incidence rates in the United States, 1975–1998. *Oral Oncol* 2002;38:610–617.
18. Chen AY, Myers JN. Cancer of the oral cavity. *Dis Mon* 2001;47:275–361.
19. Close LG, Burns DK, Reisch J, et al. Microvascular invasion in cancer of the oral cavity and oropharynx. *Arch Otolaryngol Head Neck Surg* 1987;113:1191–1195.
20. Constantinides MS, Rothstein SG, Persky MS. Squamous cell carcinoma in older patients without risk factors. *Otolaryngol Head Neck Surg* 1992;106:275–277.
21. Cooper JS, Pajak TF, Forastiere AA, et al. Postoperative concurrent radiotherapy and chemotherapy for high-risk squamous-cell carcinoma of the head and neck. *N Engl J Med* 2004;350:1937–1944.
22. Crosher R, McIlroy R. The incidence of other primary tumours in patients with oral cancer in Scotland. *Br J Oral Maxillofac Surg* 1998;36:58–62.
23. Daly ME, Lieskovsky Y, Pawlicki T, et al. Evaluation of patterns of failure and subjective salivary function in patients treated with intensity modulated radiotherapy for head and neck squamous cell carcinoma. *Head and Neck* 2007;29:211–220.
24. Day GL, Blot WJ. Second primary tumors in patients with oral cancer. *Cancer* 1992;70:14–19.
25. Day GL, Blot WJ, Shore RE, et al. Second cancers following oral and pharyngeal cancers: role of tobacco and alcohol. *J Natl Cancer Inst* 1994;86:131–137.
26. Day TA, Davis BK, Gillespie MB, et al. Oral cancer treatment. *Curr Treat Options Oncol* 2003;4:27–41.
27. Dearnaley DP, Dardoufas C, A'Hearn RP, et al. Interstitial irradiation for carcinoma of the tongue and floor of mouth: Royal Marsden Hospital Experience 1970 1986. *Radiother Oncol* 1991;21:183–192.
28. Decroix Y, Ghossein NA. Experience of the Curie Institute in treatment of cancer of the mobile tongue: I. Treatment policies and result. *Cancer* 1981;47:496–502.
29. Denis F, Garaud P, Bardet E, et al. Final results of the 94-01 French Head and Neck Oncology and Radiotherapy Group randomized trial comparing radiotherapy alone with concomitant radiochemotherapy in advanced-stage oropharynx carcinoma. *J Clin Oncol* 2004;22:69–76.
30. Dobrossy L. Epidemiology of head and neck cancer: magnitude of the problem. *Cancer Metastasis Rev* 2005;24:9–17.
31. Eisbruch A, Ship JA, Dawson LA, et al. Salivary gland sparing and improved target irradiation by conformal and intensity modulated irradiation of head and neck cancer. *World J Surg* 2003;27:832–837.
32. El-Sayed S, Nelson N. Adjuvant and adjunctive chemotherapy in the management of squamous cell carcinoma of the head and neck region. A meta-analysis of prospective and randomized trials. *J Clin Oncol* 1996;14:838–847.
33. Ellis GL, Corio RL. Spindle cell carcinoma of the oral cavity. A clinicopathologic assessment of fifty-nine cases. *Oral Surg Oral Med Oral Pathol* 1980;50:523–533.
34. Emami B. *Oral cavity*. Philadelphia: Lippincott William & Wilkins, 2004.
35. Fagan JJ, Collins B, Barnes L, et al. Perineural invasion in squamous cell carcinoma of the head and neck. *Arch Otolaryngol Head Neck Surg* 1998;124:637–640.
36. Farber LA, Benard F, Machtay M, et al. Detection of recurrent head and neck squamous cell carcinomas after radiation therapy with 2-18F-fluoro-2-deoxy-D-glucose positron emission tomography. *Laryngoscope* 1999;109:970–975.
37. Fearon ER, Vogelstein B. A genetic model for colorectal tumorigenesis. *Cell* 1990;61:759–767.
38. Ferlito A, Shaha AR, Silver CE, et al. Incidence and sites of distant metastases from head and neck cancer. *ORL J Otorhinolaryngol Relat Spec* 2001;63:202–207.
39. Fiorino C, Dell Oca I, Pierelli A, et al. Significant improvement in normal tissue sparing and target coverage for head and neck cancer by means of helical tomotherapy. *Radiother Oncol* 2006;78:276–282.
40. Franceschi S, Bidoli E, Herrero R, et al. Comparison of cancers of the oral cavity and pharynx worldwide: etiological clues. *Oral Oncol* 2000;36:106–115.
41. Freeman C, Berg JW, Cutler SJ. Occurrence and prognosis of extranodal lymphomas. *Cancer* 1972;29:252–260.
42. Fu KK, Chan EK, Phillips TL, et al. Time, dose and volume factors in interstitial Radium implants of carcinoma of the oral tongue. *Radiology* 1976;119:209–213.
43. Fu KK, Pajak TF, Trotti A, et al. A Radiation Therapy Oncology Group (RTOG) phase III randomized study to compare hyperfractionation and two variants of accelerated fractionation to standard fractionation radiotherapy for head and neck squamous cell carcinomas: first report of RTOG 9003. *Int J Radiat Oncol Biol Phys* 2000;48:7–16.
44. Fu KK, Ray JW, Chan EK, et al. External and interstitial radiation therapy of carcinoma of the oral tongue. A review of 32 years' experience. *AJR Am J Roentgenol* 1976;126:107–115.
45. Green FL PD, Fleming ID, et al. *AJCC cancer staging manual*. New York: Springer, 2002.
46. Greenlee RT, Murray T, Bolden S, et al. Cancer statistics, 2000. *CA Cancer J Clin* 2000;50:7–33.
47. Ha PK, Benoit NE, Yochem R, et al. A transcriptional progression model for head and neck cancer. *Clin Cancer Res* 2003;9:3058–3064.
48. Harari PM, Jaradat HA, Connor NP, et al. Refining target coverage and normal tissue avoidance with helical tomotherapy vs linac-based IMRT for oropharyngeal cancer. *Int J Radiat Oncol Biol Phys* 2004;60:S160.
49. Harari PM, Mehta MP, Ritter MA, et al. Clinical promise tempered by reality in the delivery of combined chemoradiation for common solid tumors. *Semin Radiat Oncol* 2003;13:3–12.

50. Harrison LB, Fass DE. Radiation therapy for oral cavity cancer. *Dent Clin North Am* 1990;34:205–222.
51. Haughey BH, Gates GA, Arfken CL, et al. Meta-analysis of second malignant tumors in head and neck cancer: the case for an endoscopic screening protocol. *Ann Otol Rhinol Laryngol* 1992;101:105–112.
52. Hiratsuka H, Miyakawa A, Nakamori K, et al. Multivariate analysis of occult lymph node metastasis as a prognostic indicator for patients with squamous cell carcinoma of the oral cavity. *Cancer* 1997;80:351–356.
53. Johnson JT, Barnes EL, Myers EN, et al. The extracapsular spread of tumors in cervical node metastasis. *Arch Otolaryngol* 1981;107:725–729.
54. Kannan S, Balaram P, Pillai MR, et al. Ultrastructural variations and assessment of malignant transformation risk in oral leukoplakia. *Pathol Res Pract* 1993;189:1169–1180.
55. Keene HJ, Fleming TJ. Prevalence of caries-associated microflora after radiotherapy in patients with cancer of the head and neck. *Oral Surg Oral Med Oral Pathol* 1987;64:421–426.
56. Kurumatani N, Kirita T, Zheng Y, et al. Time trends in the mortality rates for tobacco- and alcohol-related cancers within the oral cavity and pharynx in Japan, 1950–94. *J Epidemiol* 1999;9:46–52.
57. Larsson PA, Johansson SL, Vahlne A, et al. Snuff tumorigenesis: effects of long-term snuff administration after initiation with 4-nitroquinoline-N-oxide and herpes simplex virus type 1. *J Oral Pathol Med* 1989;18:187–192.
58. Lefebvre JL, Coche-Dequeant B, Buisset E, et al. Management of early oral cavity cancer. Experience of Centre Oscar Lambret. *Eur J Cancer B Oral Oncol* 1994;30B:216–220.
59. Lentsch EJ, Myers JN. *Pathogenesis and progression of squamous cell carcinoma of the head and neck*, 4th ed. Philadelphia: W.B. Saunders, 2004.
60. Licitra L, Grandi C, Guzzo M, et al. Primary chemotherapy in resectable oral cavity squamous cell cancer: a randomized controlled trial. *J Clin Oncol* 2003;21:327–333.
61. Lindberg R. Distribution of cervical lymph node metastases from squamous cell carcinoma of the upper respiratory and digestive tracts. *Cancer* 1972;29:1446–1449.
62. Lippman SM, Hong WK. Second malignant tumors in head and neck squamous cell carcinoma: the overshadowing threat for patients with early-stage disease. *Int J Radiat Oncol Biol Phys* 1989;17:691–694.
63. Llewellyn CD, Johnson NW, Warnakulasuriya KA. Risk factors for squamous cell carcinoma of the oral cavity in young people—a comprehensive literature review. *Oral Oncol* 2001;37:401–418.
64. Lozza L, Cerrotta A, Gardani G, et al. Analysis of risk factors for mandibular bone radionecrosis after exclusive low dose-rate brachytherapy for oral cancer. *Radiother Oncol* 1997;44:143–147.
65. Macfarlane GJ, Zheng T, Marshall JR, et al. Alcohol, tobacco, diet and the risk of oral cancer: a pooled analysis of three case-control studies. *Eur J Cancer B Oral Oncol* 1995;31B:181–187.
66. Maden C, Beckmann AM, Thomas DB, et al. Human papillomaviruses, herpes simplex viruses, and the risk of oral cancer in men. *Am J Epidemiol* 1992;135:1093–1102.
67. Martinez-Gimeno C, Rodriguez EM, Vila CN, et al. Squamous cell carcinoma of the oral cavity: a clinicopathologic scoring system for evaluating risk of cervical lymph node metastasis. *Laryngoscope* 1995;105:728–733.
68. Mazeron JJ, Noel G, Simon JM, et al. Brachytherapy in head and neck cancers. *Cancer Radiother* 2003;7:62–72.
69. Menegoz F, Black RJ, Arveux P, et al. Cancer incidence and mortality in France in 1975–95. *Eur J Cancer Prev* 1997;6:442–466.
70. Merino OR, Lindberg RD, Fletcher GH. An analysis of distant metastases from squamous cell carcinoma of the upper respiratory and digestive tracts. *Cancer* 1977;40:145–151.
71. Merlano M, Benasso M, Corvo R, et al. Five-year update of a randomized trial of alternating radiotherapy and chemotherapy compared with radiotherapy alone in treatment of unresectable squamous cell carcinoma of the head and neck. *J Natl Cancer Inst* 1996;88:583–589.
72. Miller CS, Johnstone BM. Human papillomavirus as a risk factor for oral squamous carcinoma: a meta-analysys 1982–1997. *Oral Surg Oral Med Oral Pathol Oral Radiol* 2001;91:622–635.
73. Million RCN, Mancuso A. *Oral cavity*. Philadelphia: J.B. Lippincott, 1994.
74. Mishra RC, Singh DN, Mishra TK. Post-operative radiotherapy in carcinoma of buccal mucosa, a prospective randomized trial. *Eur J Surg Oncol* 1996;22:502–504.
75. Mohanti BK, Bansal M, Bahadur S, et al. Interstitial brachytherapy with or without external beam irradiation in head and neck cancer: Institute Rotary Cancer Hospital experience. *Clin Oncol (R Coll Radiol)* 2001;13:345–352.
76. Mohr C, Bohndorf W, Carstens J, et al. Preoperative radiochemotherapy and radical surgery in comparison with radical surgery alone. A prospective, multicentric, randomized DOSAK study of advanced squamous cell carcinoma of the oral cavity and the oropharynx (a 3-year follow-up). *Int J Oral Maxillofac Surg* 1994;23:140–148.
77. Monteil RA. Oral leukoplakia: clinical or histologic entity? *Ann Pathol* 1983;3:257–261.
78. Munro AJ. An overview of randomised controlled trials of adjuvant chemotherapy in head and neck cancer. *Br J Cancer* 1995;71:83–91.
79. Myers E. *Cancer of the head and neck*. Philadelphia: Saunders, 2003.
80. Myers JN, Elkins T, Roberts D, et al. Squamous cell carcinoma of the tongue in young adults: increasing incidence and factors that predict treatment outcomes. *Otolaryngol Head Neck Surg* 2000;122:44–51.
81. Myers JN, Greenberg JS, Mo V, et al. Extracapsular spread. A significant predictor of treatment failure in patients with squamous cell carcinoma of the tongue. *Cancer* 2001;92:3030–3036.
82. Pande P, Soni S, Chakravarti N, et al. Prognostic impact of ETS-1 overexpression in betel and tobacco related oral cancer. *Cancer Detect Prev* 2001;25:496–501.
83. Pernot M, Hoffstetter S, Peiffert D, et al. Epidermoid carcinomas of the floor of mouth treated by exclusive irradiation: statistical study of a series of 207 cases. *Radiother Oncol* 1995;35:177–185.
84. Pernot M, Verhaeghe JL, Guillemin F, et al. Evaluation of the importance of systematic neck dissection in carcinoma of the oral cavity treated by brachytherapy alone for the primary lesion (apropos of a series of 346 patients). *Bull Cancer Radiother* 1995;82:311–317.
85. Peters LJ, Ang KK, Thames HD Jr. Accelerated fractionation in the radiation treatment of head and neck cancer. A critical comparison of different strategies. *Acta Oncol* 1988;27:185–194.
86. Pierquin B, Wilson JF, Chassagne D. *Basic techniques for endocurietherapy*. New York: Masson, 1987.
87. Pignon JP, Bourhis J, Domenge C, et al. Chemotherapy added to locoregional treatment for head and neck squamous-cell carcinoma: three meta-analyses of updated individual data. MACH-NC Collaborative Group. Meta-analysis of chemotherapy on head and neck cancer. *Lancet* 2000;355:949–955.
88. Prime SS, Thakker NS, Pring M, et al. A review of inherited cancer syndromes and their relevance to oral squamous cell carcinoma. *Oral Oncol* 2001;37:1–16.
89. Reddy CR, Kumari KR. Microinvasive carcinoma of hard palate in reverse smoking females. *Indian J Cancer* 1974;11:386–393.
90. Reibel J. Prognosis of oral pre-malignant lesions: significance of clinical, histopathological, and molecular biological characteristics. *Crit Rev Oral Biol Med* 2003;14:47–62.
91. Reichart PA, Philipsen HP. Oral erythroplakia—a review. *Oral Oncol* 2005;41:551–561.
92. Robertson AG, Soutar DS, Paul J, et al. Early closure of a randomized trial: surgery and postoperative radiotherapy versus radiotherapy in the management of intra-oral tumours. *Clin Oncol (R Coll Radiol)* 1998;10:155–160.
93. Rudoltz MS, Perkins RS, Luthmann RW, et al. High-dose-rate brachytherapy for primary carcinomas of the oral cavity and oropharynx. *Laryngoscope* 1999;109:1967–1973.
94. Schoder H, Yeung HW, Gonen M, et al. Head and neck cancer: clinical usefulness and accuracy of PET/CT image fusion. *Radiology* 2004;231:65–72.
95. Schwartz LH, Ozsahin M, Zhang GN, et al. Synchronous and metachronous head and neck carcinomas. *Cancer* 1994;74:1933–1938.
96. Shafer WG, Waldron CA. Erythroplakia of the oral cavity. *Cancer* 1975;36:1021–1028.
97. Shah JP, Lydiatt W. Treatment of cancer of the head and neck. *CA Cancer J Clin* 1995;45:352–368.
98. Sharma DC. Betel quid and areca nut are carcinogenic without tobacco. *Lancet Oncol* 2003;4:587.
99. Shavers VL, Harlan LC, Winn D, et al. Racial/ethnic patterns of care for cancers of the oral cavity, pharynx, larynx, sinuses, and salivary glands. *Cancer Metastasis Rev* 2003;22:25–38.
100. Shear M, Hawkins DM, Farr HW. The prediction of lymph node metastases from oral squamous carcinoma. *Cancer* 1976;37:1901–1907.
101. Sheng K, Molloy JA, Read PW. Intensity-modulated radiation therapy (IMRT) dosimetry of the head and neck: a comparison of treatment plans using linear accelerator-based IMRT and helical tomotherapy. *Int J Radiat Oncol Biol Phys* 2006;65:917–923.
102. Slaughter DP SH, Smejkal W. Field cancerization in oral cavity stratified squamous epithelium: clinical implications and multicentric origin. *Cancer* 1953;6:963–968.
103. Smyth AG, Ward-Booth RP, Avery BS, et al. Malignant melanoma of the oral cavity—an increasing clinical diagnosis? *Br J Oral Maxillofac Surg* 1993;31:230–235.
104. Society AC. Cancer statistics. American Cancer Society. Cancer Facts and Figures 2006. *www.caner.org*
105. Soo KC, Carter RL, O'Brien CJ, et al. Prognostic implications of perineural spread in squamous carcinomas of the head and neck. *Laryngoscope* 1986;96:1145–1148.
106. Spiro RH, Huvos AG, Wong GY, et al. Predictive value of tumor thickness in squamous carcinoma confined to the tongue and floor of the mouth. *Am J Surg* 1986;152:345–350.
107. Staar S, Rudat V, Stuetzer H, et al. Intensified hyperfractionated accelerated radiotherapy limits the additional benefit of simultaneous chemotherapy—results of a multicentric randomized German trial in advanced head-and-neck cancer. *Int J Radiat Oncol Biol Phys* 2001;50:1161–1171.
108. Strnad V. Treatment of oral cavity and oropharyngeal cancer. Indications, technical aspects, and results of interstitial brachytherapy. *Strahlenther Onkol* 2004;180:710–717.
109. Strong EW. Carcinoma of the tongue. *Otolaryngol Clin North Am* 1979;12:107–114.
110. Studer G, Studer SP, Zwahlen RA, et al. Osteoradionecrosis of the mandible: minimized risk profile following intensity-modulated radiation therapy (IMRT). *Strahlenther Onkol* 2006;182:283–288.
111. Tanaka S, Sobue T. Comparison of oral and pharyngeal cancer mortality in five countries: France, Italy, Japan, UK and USA from the WHO Mortality Database (1960–2000). *Jpn J Clin Oncol* 2005;35:488–491.
112. Urken ML. Composite free flaps in oromandibular reconstruction. Review of the literature. *Arch Otolaryngol Head Neck Surg* 1991;117:724–732.
113. Urken ML. Advances in head and neck reconstruction. *Laryngoscope* 2003;113:1473–1476.
114. Urken ML, Bridger AG, Zur KB, et al. The scapular osteofasciocutaneous flap: a 12-year experience. *Arch Otolaryngol Head Neck Surg* 2001;127:862–869.
115. Urken ML, Moscoso JF, Lawson W, et al. A systematic approach to functional reconstruction of the oral cavity following partial and total glossectomy. *Arch Otolaryngol Head Neck Surg* 1994;120:589–601.
116. Urken ML, Weinberg H, Buchbinder D, et al. Microvascular free flaps in head and neck reconstruction. Report of 200 cases and review of complications. *Arch Otolaryngol Head Neck Surg* 1994;120:633–640.
117. Urken ML, Weinberg H, Vickery C, et al. Oromandibular reconstruction using microvascular composite free flaps. Report of 71 cases and a new classification scheme for bony, soft-tissue, and neurologic defects. *Arch Otolaryngol Head Neck Surg* 1991;117:733–744.
118. van den Brekel MW, Castelijns JA, Stel HV, et al. Modern imaging techniques and ultrasound-guided aspiration cytology for the assessment of neck node metastases: a prospective comparative study. *Eur Arch Otorhinolaryngol* 1993;250:11–17.
119. Vikram B, Strong EW, Shah J, et al. Elective postoperative radiation therapy in stages III and IV epidermoid carcinoma of the head and neck. *Am J Surg* 1980;140:580–584.
120. Volling P, Schroder M, Eckel H, et al. Results of a prospective randomized trial with induction chemotherapy for cancer of the oral cavity and tonsils. *HNO* 1999;47:899–906.

121. Wang C. *Radiation therapy for head and neck neoplasms*. New York: Wiley-Liss, 1997.

122. Wang CC. Radiotherapeutic management and results of T1N0, T2N0 carcinoma of the oral tongue: evaluation of boost techniques. *Int J Radiat Oncol Biol Phys* 1989;17:287–291.

123. Wang CC. Intraoral cone for carcinoma of the oral cavity. *Front Radiat Ther Oncol* 1991;25:128–131.

124. Wang CC, Boyer A, Mendiondo O. Afterloading interstitial radiation therapy. *Int J Radiat Oncol Biol Phys* 1976;1:365–368.

125. Wang CC, Doppke KP, Biggs PJ. Intra-oral cone radiation therapy for selected carcinomas of the oral cavity. *Int J Radiat Oncol Biol Phys* 1983;9:1185–1189.

126. Weber RS, Palmer JM, el-Naggar A, et al. Minor salivary gland tumors of the lip and buccal mucosa. *Laryngoscope* 1989;99:6–9.

127. Wendt TG, Grabenbauer GG, Rodel CM, et al. Simultaneous radiochemotherapy versus radiotherapy alone in advanced head and neck cancer: a randomized multicenter study. *J Clin Oncol* 1998;16:1318–1324.

128. Winzenburg SM, Niehans GA, George E, et al. Basaloid squamous carcinoma: a clinical comparison of two histologic types with poorly differentiated squamous cell carcinoma. *Otolaryngol Head Neck Surg* 1998;119:471–475.

129. Yao M, Dornfeld KJ, Buatti JM, et al. Intensity-modulated radiation treatment for head-and-neck squamous cell carcinoma— the University of Iowa experience. *Int J Radiat Oncol Biol Phys* 2005;63:410–421.

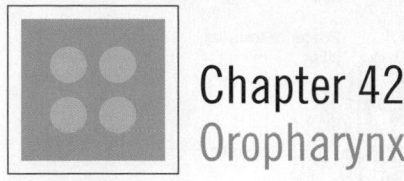

Chapter 42
Oropharynx

Peter C. Levendag, David N. Teguh, Ben J. Heijmen

Epidemiology

The oropharynx is the posterior continuation of the oral cavity and connects with the nasopharynx (above) and laryngopharynx (below). It is located between the soft palate superiorly, and the hyoid bone inferiorly. The main sites of the oropharynx consist of the posterior and lateral pharyngeal wall, faucial arches, tonsillar fossa (TF), soft palate (SP), and the base of tongue (BOT). These structures play a crucial role in swallowing and speech. By obstructing the "air space" or by infiltrating muscles or nerves, locally advanced oropharyngeal tumors can significantly impede these functions. The same holds for intensive treatment regimen: it can cause deformities and/or impairment of particular functional (sub) units, resulting eventually in severe (late) side effects. It has long been known that patients with a history of smoking or excessive consumption of alcohol are believed to be at increased risk for developing cancer in the oropharynx (31,37). Overall these cancers comprise less than 0.5% of all cancers in men in the United States, which amounts to approximately 5000 new cases each year (319). According to the Surveillance, Epidemiology, and End Results report of the National Cancer Institute, in 2001 the age-adjusted incidence was 1.5 per 100,000 white men and 3.2 per 100,000 black men (271). These cancers more often afflict men (4:1); they are diagnosed most frequently in the sixth and seventh decades of life. Oropharyngeal cancers are readily accessible to clinical examination and staging. Historically, in the early stage and in the moderately advanced tumors, radiation therapy (RT) has been the preferred therapy mode because of its organ function-preservation properties (300,321). Most (±95%) oropharyngeal cancers are squamous cell carcinomas (SCC). Although reports can be found of other histologic subtypes (1,14,72,93,158), such as minor salivary gland tumors, lymphoepitheliomas, malignant lymphomas, mesenchymal tumors, or metastases from other extracranial tumor sites, these will not be discussed in great detail as they are considered beyond the scope of the present chapter.

Anatomy

The SP, anterior faucial pillar, and the retromolar trigone are embryologically connected to the oral cavity. However, because of their clinical behavior, tumors of these structures are preferably classified with oropharyngeal malignancies. The inferior part of the TF is referred to as the *glossopalatine sulcus* (Fig. 42.1). The lateral border of the retromolar trigone extends upward into the buccal mucosa, medially it blends with the anterior tonsillar pillar. Its base is formed by the last lower molar and the adjacent gingivolingual surface. The lateral walls of the oropharynx are limited posteriorly by the TF proper and the posterior tonsillar pillar. The anterior and posterior tonsillar pillars are the folds of mucous membrane that cover the underlying glossopalatine and pharyngopalatine muscles, respectively. Deep to the lateral wall of the TF are major vessels (Figs. 42.2 and 42.3) and muscular components such as the superior constrictor muscle, the upper fibers of the middle constrictor

muscle, the pharyngeus and stylopharyngeus muscles, and the glossopalatine and pharyngopalatine muscles. Stratified squamous epithelium covers all of these structures. The tonsil has a heavy lymphoid network. The pharyngeal wall is related to the second and third cervical vertebrae. Nerve supply is from the cranial nerves IX and X. The BOT lies posterior and inferior to the palatoglossal arch. It is bounded anteriorly by the circumvallate papillae, laterally by the glossopharyngeal sulci and oropharyngeal walls, and inferiorly by the valleculae and the pharyngoepiglottic fold. Embryologically, its epithelium is derived from the entoderm, unlike that from the oral tongue (ectoderm). The body of the BOT is formed by thick muscles, the genioglossus, styloglossus, palatoglossus, and hypoglossus muscles. The muscles originate from the margins of the mandible and are attached to the hyoid bone. The blood supply and the innervation are by the lingual arteries and hypoglossal nerve, respectively.

Natural History

In general, tumors of the anterior tonsillar pillar and soft palate are better differentiated and biologically less aggressive than those of the TF. For example, 50% to 60% of patients with primary tumors in the anterior tonsillar pillar, retromolar trigone, and SP had necks with clinically negative findings, in contrast to only 24% of those with TF primaries (149). Lesions of the TF (231), retromolar trigone (39), and BOT tend to grow more extensively. Perez et al. (234) observed that the primary tumor was confined to the TF in only 5.4%. Byers et al. (171) described 14% mandibular invasion in carcinomas of the retromolar trigone. At diagnosis, 75% of BOT cancers have invaded adjacent structures, including the glossopharyngeal sulcus, pharyngeal wall, larynx, and/or faucial arches. The most common complaint at presentation of tumors in the oropharynx is pain; this pain is either attributed to (severe) mucositis, deep infiltration of the tumor or is referred (Fig. 42.4). However, patients with primary tumors of the oropharynx can also be asymptomatic or have only vague discomfort at presentation. BOT tumors, for example, typically grow insidiously. Because the BOT is devoid of pain fibers, they are mostly asymptomatic until they have progressed significantly. With local advancement and/or with infiltration of the pterygoid muscles, patients can experience trismus and, ultimately, bleeding or swallowing problems, or can have difficulty with speech.

Diagnosis is typically established by clinical examination in the outpatient clinic and/or examination under general anesthesia, including morphologic confirmation (biopsy) of the lesion and tattooing of the clinical target volume (CTV). In the Erasmus Medical Center—Daniel den Hoed, Rotterdam (Erasmus MC), at the time of diagnosis/staging, with the patient still under general anesthesia, the lesion is frequently marked with marker seeds. This enables the extensions of the lesion to be visualized on x-ray films. From a series of patients implanted with platinum markers, we found, for example, that the TF significantly moves during swallowing and even in rest (because of respiration). Maximum excursions in rest were found to be 3.6 mm. This type of information contributes to a more

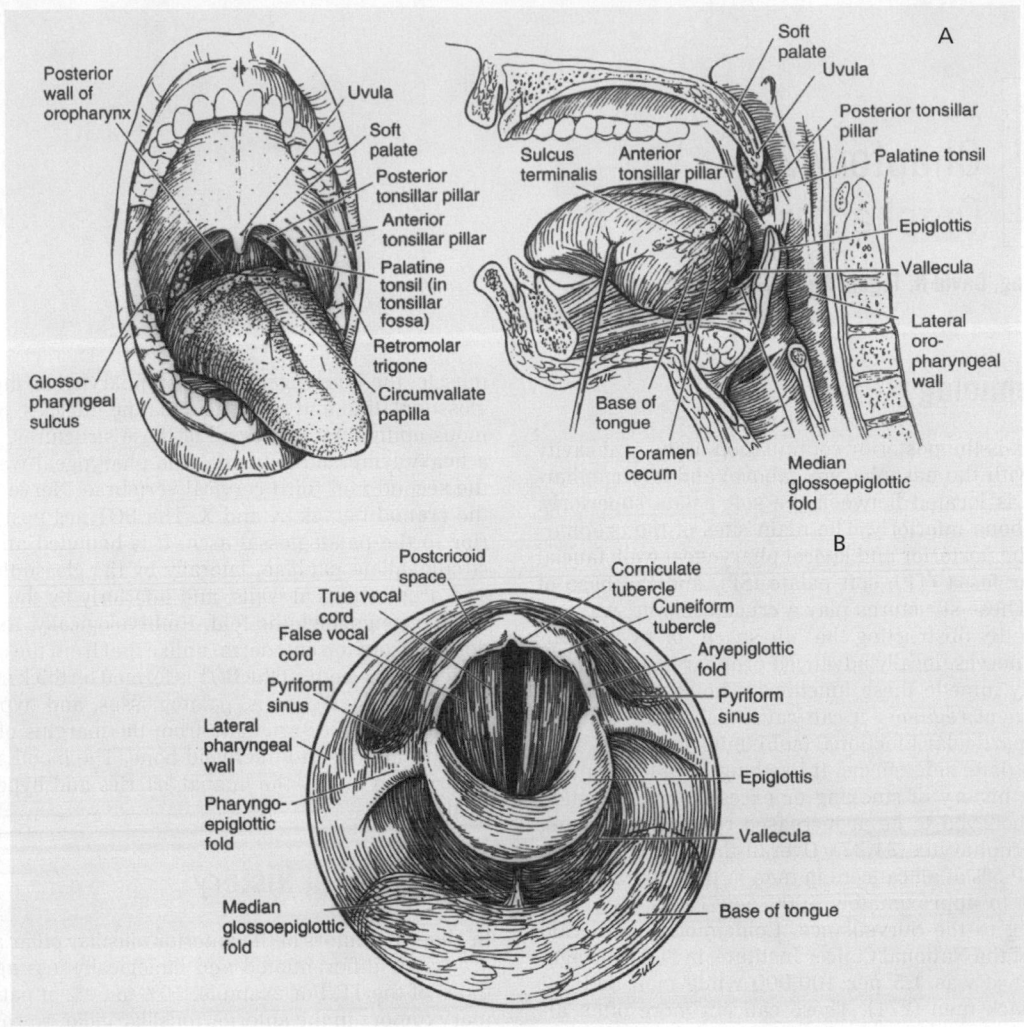

FIGURE 42.1. Anatomy oropharynx. **A:** Sagittal view showing the oral cavity, hard palate, mobile tongue and posterior part of the oropharynx. **B:** Axial cut looking from above at the caudal level of the oropharynx, that is viewing structures such as the entrance of the larynx (epiglottis and vocal cords), the piriform sinus on both sides, and the base of the tongue and vallecula. (From Cox JD, Ang KK. *Radiation oncology: rationale, technique, results,* 8th ed. St Louis, MO: Mosby; 2003:196–218.)

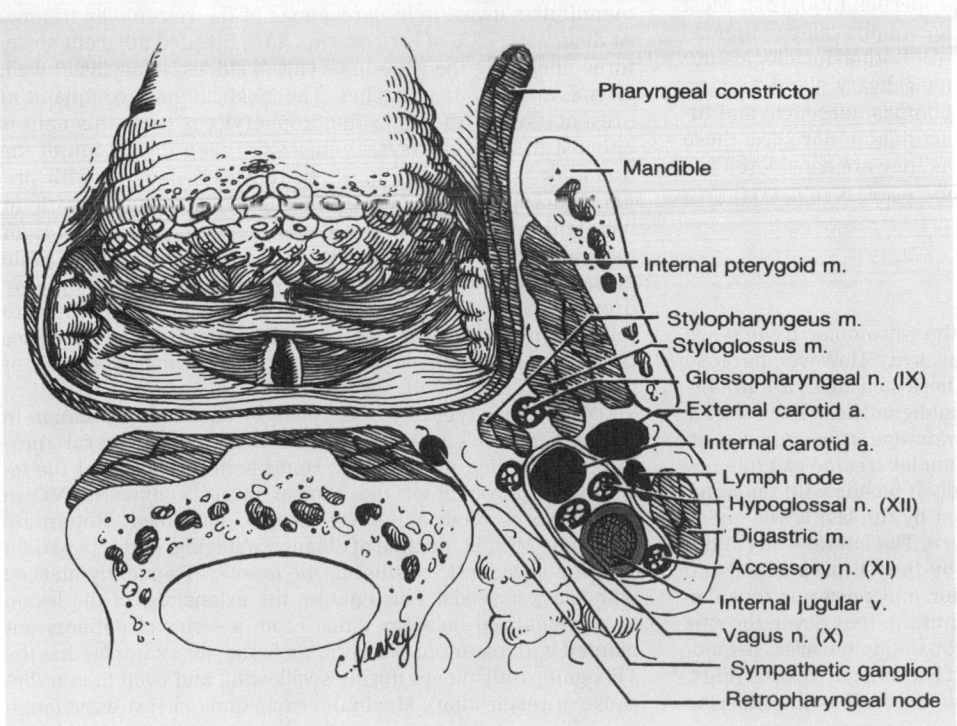

FIGURE 42.2. Cross-section midoropharynx. (From Million RR, Cassisi NJ. *Management of head and neck cancer: a multidisciplinary approach,* 2nd ed. Philadelphia: JB Lippincott; 1994: 401–429.)

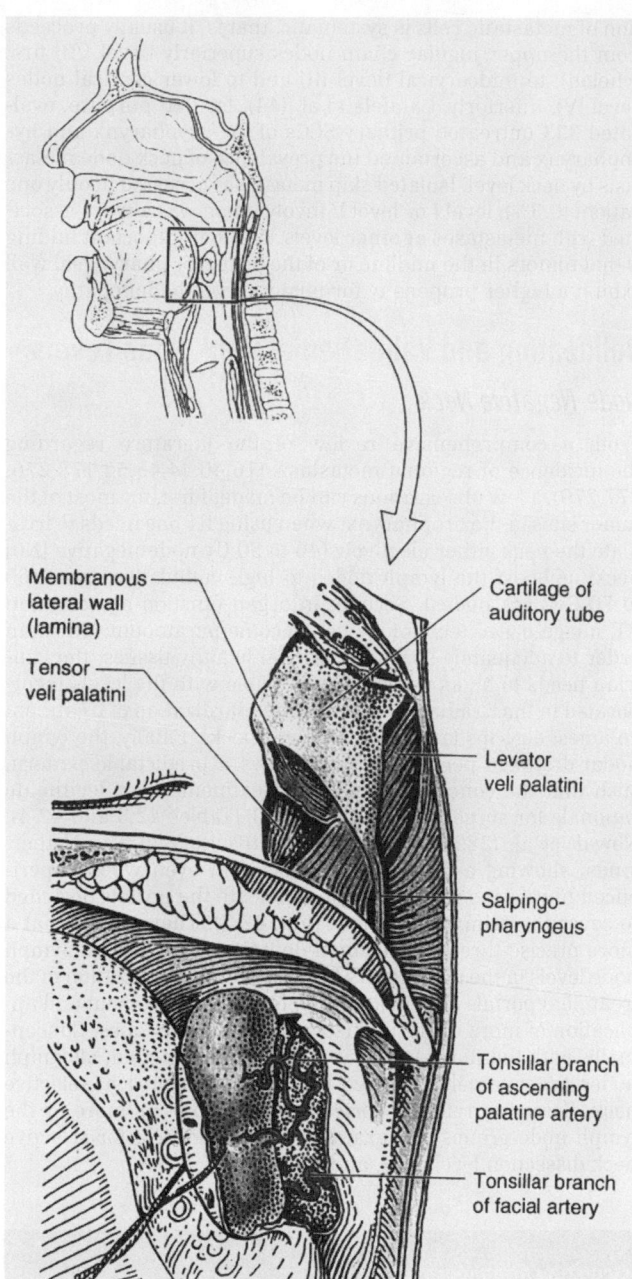

FIGURE 42.3.   Inside view of lateral oropharangeal wall. Note major vessels in parapharyngeal space. (From Moore KL, Dalley, II, AF. *Clinically oriented anatomy*, 4th ed. Paul J. Kelly, ed. Baltimore: Lippincott Williams & Wilkins; 1999.)

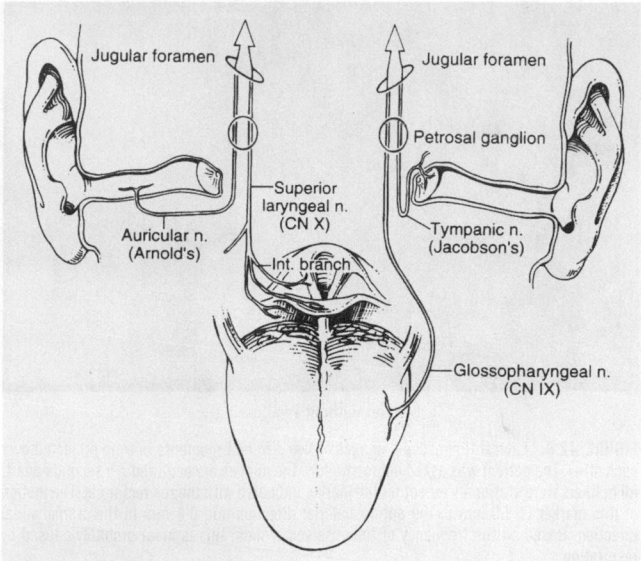

FIGURE 42.4.   Neural pathways of referred otalgia. (From Leibel SA, Philips T. Textbook of Radiation Oncology, 2nd ed. Section on Clinical Radiation Oncology, Part 2, Chapter 28: Saunders, Elsevier, Inc. 2004.)

infiltration. CT combined with positron emission tomography scanning seems an extremely promising, powerful tool for diagnostic and simulation purposes, but is not yet available in every institution. Several textbooks contain helpful overviews (8,59,123,171,208,232).

Tumors are staged according to the American Joint Committee on Cancer classification system (Table 42.1) (6). Dentulous patients are at increased risk for caries and osteoradionecrosis from the reduction and qualitative change of salivary flow, change in pH, and proliferation of bacteria believed to be responsible for caries. Panorex x-ray films, identification of nonrestorable teeth for pretreatment extraction, dental trays for fluoride rinse, protection against scatter radiation, as well as education about long-term oral hygiene, should be engaged before RT and/or chemotherapy (CHT) is applied. In fact, the quite common development of osteoradionecrosis in the past (17) should be prevented by adequate measures. Finally, given the complexity of head and neck tumors, all patients should be

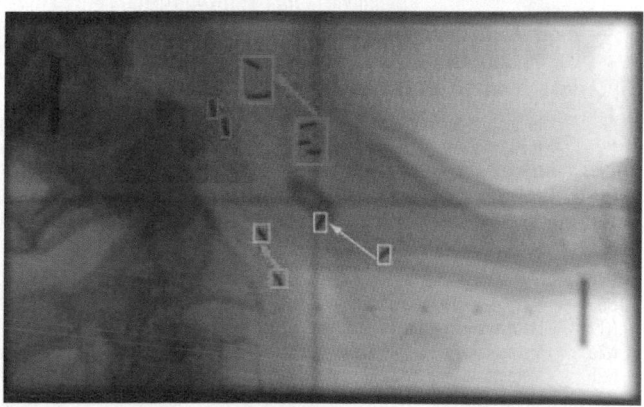

Motion_swallowing

FIGURE 42.5.   Lateral fluoroscopic images of two different moments in time projected over each other. The patient was instructed to swallow. The images are acquired 0.5 seconds apart. The colored rectangles indicate the motion of the markers. The arrow indicates the direction of movement (from equilibrium to extreme position during swallowing). For the yellow, green, and red markers, the amplitude in the lateral view was 13.4, 9.3, and 2.4 mm, respectively. For the markers in the blue rectangle, the amplitude of the most cranial marker was 15.6 mm.

accurate determination of the planning target volume (PTV) margin (Figs. 42.5 and 42.6). Conventionally, platinum (Pt) or gold (Au) marker seeds were used, particularly for those patients to be boosted by brachytherapy (BT) (175). Because of significant scattering properties on computed tomography (CT), nonmetallic seeds are being tested. Panendoscopy can reveal synchronous second primaries. Ultrasound fine-needle aspiration biopsy has become an indispensable tool for pro diagnosis and for staging, especially where it concerns the lymph nodes. Multislice CT and magnetic resonance imaging (MRI) scans are now obligatory imaging tools. CT scanning with contrast enhancement using 2-mm slices is better for detecting lymph nodes and for bone detail. MRI is preferred for the evaluation of the parapharyngeal space. Axial slices are usually sufficient; sagittal MRI is helpful for detecting early pre-epiglottic space

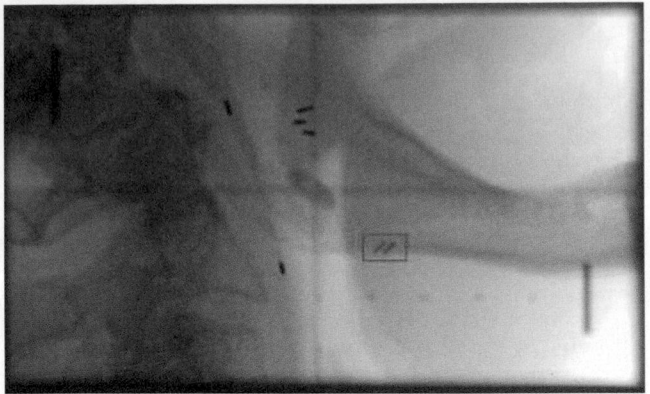

Motion without swallowing

FIGURE 42.6. Lateral fluoroscopic images of two different moments in time projected over each other. The patient was asked not to swallow. The images are acquired 7.5 seconds apart. All markers were stationary except for the marker indicated with the red rectangle. The motion of this marker is 2.0 mm in the anteroposterior direction and 0.4 mm in the craniocaudal direction. Based on the frequency of the observed motion, this is most probably caused by respiration.

formally discussed in a head and neck tumor board, with or without the patient being present, before the initiation of any treatment.

Lymphatics of the Oropharynx

The lymphatic drainage of the oropharynx and the neck was first described by Rouviere (262) in 1938 and has been refined since by others (113,149). The nodal groups in the neck were originally described along the lines of lymph node chains, located in particular anatomic regions and draining specific (sub) sites. Instead of using the term *jugular chain nodes*, Robbins et al. (255,256,254) proposed the "level system" for classifying the location of lymph nodes in the neck relative to surgical-anatomic landmarks (Table 42.2). The level classification (levels I to VI) was recently refined with the addition of sublevels (Ia/Ib, IIa/IIb, and Va/Vb), also using some of the radiologically defined landmarks as proposed by Som et al. (283). The probability of lymphatic (regional) metastasis is related to size and location of the primary site within the oropharynx. The order of progres-

sion of metastatic cells is systematic, that is, it usually proceeds from the upper jugular chain nodes superiorly (level I/II; first echelon), to midcervical (level III) and to lower cervical nodes (level IV), inferiorly. Candela et al. (44), for that purpose, evaluated 333 untreated primary SCCs of the oropharynx and hypopharynx and ascertained the prevalence of neck node metastasis by neck level. Isolated skip metastases occurred in only one patient (0.3%); level I or level V involvement was always associated with metastases at other levels. Another important finding is that tumors in the midline or of the posterior pharyngeal wall exhibit a higher propensity for bilateral lymphadenopathy.

Delineating and Validation of Neck Node Levels

Node-Negative Neck

From a comprehensive review of the literature regarding the incidence of regional metastasis (16,40,44,45,52,178,276, 277,279), a few observations can be made. First, for most of the tumor sites in the oropharynx, when using RT one needs to irradiate the neck either electively (46 to 50 Gy node-negative [N0] neck) or boost the lymph nodes to high cumulative doses (60 to 70 Gy neck nodes). Second, in organ function-preservation RT, image-based technology has become paramount. Third, in order to adequately spare the critical healthy tissues, the clinician needs to be as selective as possible with the levels incorporated in the irradiated volumes (standardization of treatment volumes; e.g., ipsilateral vs. bilateral neck). Finally, the lymph nodal drainage per tumor site follows a predictable pattern, such that the concept of selective treatment has a legitimate rationale for surgery as well as for RT (Tables 42.3 and 42.4). Nowak et al. (222) reported on an inventory in The Netherlands, showing a lack of standardization even when experienced physicians were asked to delineate the portals designed to cover the primary and neck (Fig. 42.7). They argued that a more precise three-dimensional definition on CT of the lymph node levels in the neck allows for a better standardization of the treatment portals and, in addition, for the development and application of more conformal (selective) RT techniques. Conceptually, with the radical and modified neck dissection, all lymph nodes are routinely removed (255,256). In contrast, selective neck dissection refers to preservation of one or more of the lymph node groups (for example, see Table 42.2 for selective neck dissection levels I, II, and III).

Table 42.1 | **2002 AMERICAN JOINT COMMITTEE ON CANCER CLASSIFICATION OF OROPHARYNGEAL CANCER**

Primary Tumor (T)		Stage			
T1	Tumor ≤2 cm in greatest dimension	Stage 0	Tis	N0	M0
T2	Tumor >2 cm but not >4 cm in greatest dimension	Stage I	T1	N0	M0
T3	Tumor >4 cm in greatest dimension	Stage II	T2	N0	M0
T4a	Tumor invades the larynx, deep/extrinsic muscle of the tongue, medial pterygoid, hard palate, or mandible				
T4b	Tumor invades lateral pterygoid muscle, pterygoid plates, lateral nasopharynx, or skull base or encases carotid artery				
Regional lymph nodes (N)					
		Stage III	T3	N0	M0
N0	No regional lymph node metastasis				
N1	Metastasis in a single ipsilateral node, ≤3 cm		T1-3	N1	M0
N2a	Metastasis in a single ipsilateral node, >3 cm but <6 cm	Stage IVa	T4a	N0	M0
N2b	Metastasis in multiple ipsilateral nodes, >3 cm but <6 cm		T4a	N1	M0
N2c	Metastasis in bilateral or contralateral lymph nodes, none >6 cm		T1-3	N2	M0
N3	Metastasis in a lymph node >6 cm		T4b	Any N	M0
Distant metastasis (M)					
M0	No distant metastasis present	Stage IVb	Any T	N3	M0
M1	Distant metastasis present	Stage IVc	Any T	Any N	M1

(From: Greene F, Page D, Fleming I, et al. AJCC cancer staging manual, 6th ed. New York; Springer-Verlag, 2002).

Table 42.2	ANATOMICAL STRUCTURES DEFINING SURGICAL LEVELS			
Levels	**Cranial**	**Caudal**	**Anterior (Medial)**	**Posterior (Lateral)**
Ia	Symphysis of Mandible	Body Hyoid	Anterior Belly CL Digastric M	Anterior Belly Digastric M
Ib	Body of Mandible	Posterior belly Digastric muscle	Anterior Belly Digastric M	Stylohoid M
IIa	Base of Skull	Inferior Body of Hyoid	Stylohyoid M	SAN
IIb	Base of Skull	Inferior Body of Hyoid	SAN	Lateral Border SCMM
III	Inferior Body of Hyoid	Inferior Cricoid	Lateral Border Sternohyoid M	Lateral Border SCMM
IV	Inferior Body of Hyoid	Clavicle	Lateral Border Sternohyoid M	Lateral Border SCMM
Va	Apex Convergence SCMM and Trapezius M	Inferior Cricoid	Posterior Edge SCMM	Anterior Border Trapezius M
Vb	Lower Border Cricoid	Clavicle	Posterior Edge SCMM	Anterior Border Trapezius M
VI	Hyoid Bone	Suprasternal	Common Carotid Artery	Common Carotid Artery

(Modified after Robbins, 2002. see also references Robbins et al., 1991, 1999). [SCMM] Sterno-Cleido Mastoid Muscle; [SCJ] Sterno Clavicular Joint; [M] Muscle; [SAN] Spinal Accessory Nerve; [RPh] Retropharyngeal; [RSS] Retro-Styloid Space; [SCF] Sub-Clavicular Fossa) See also references Robbins et al., 1991, 1999, 2002

Table 42.3	INCIDENCE AND DISTRIBUTION OF REGIONAL METASTASIS FOR LEVELS I-V FOR CLINICALLY N0 NECK.				
	Levels Involved (%)				
Tumor Site	I	II	III	IV	V
Oral cavity	20	17	9	3	0.5
Oropharynx	2	25	19	8	2
Hypopharynx	0	13	13	0	0
Larynx	5	19	20	9	2.5

(See references: Bataini, Byers, Candela Chao, Lindberg, Shah, Shah). Gregoire V, Couche E, Cosnard et al, Radiotherapy and Oncology, 2000;56 (2):135–150.

In order to be as selective as with surgery, first the clinical (research) groups of Rotterdam and Brussels have translated the surgical-anatomy boundaries (Table 42.2) to corresponding borders on CT (108,223). The Rotterdam guidelines have further evolved into a "simplified version" for routine clinical practice (Fig. 42.8) (318). In fact, the proposed simplified delineation guidelines were based on easy-to-identify anatomic landmarks on CT, leading to a simple-to-execute delineation procedure ("learning curve"). Besides the Rotterdam system being more generous, the comparison with the Brussels guidelines revealed small but essential discrepancies (Fig. 42.9). After adjustments, a common set of recommendations for the delineation of neck node levels for the N0 neck was proposed (110). This proposal was discussed with major cooperative groups in Europe (DAHANCA, EORTC, GORTEC, NCIC, RTOG) and after some minor modifications, it was fully endorsed (Table 42.5, Fig. 42.10).

Finally, a series of clinical experiments was performed to validate the "international consensus guidelines" on the delineation of the CT-based lymph node levels (174,173). In the first experiment, the superior border of the N0 neck (cranial border level II) was determined. In 10 consecutive patients, clips were placed at the most cranial border of the neck at the time of a neck dissection. Anteroposterior and lateral x-ray films were obtained intraoperatively. The clips lined up at the caudal part of the transverse process of C1 (Fig, 42.11). Thus, the cranial border is situated much lower than the base of skull. From the position of the parotid gland, one can appreciate that this is of great importance when sparing the major salivary gland. In a second series of experiments, the neck levels I-VI in three patients first were contoured on preoperative contrast-enhanced CT scans according to the international consensus guidelines. Of each of those three patients, after placing clips at relevant surgical-anatomic–based level boundaries, an intraop-

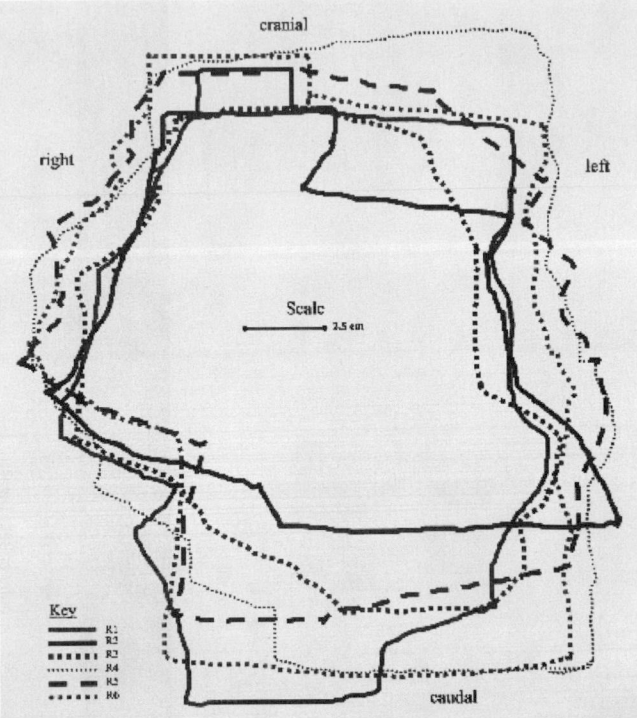

FIGURE 42.7. Variations found for same clinical indication by radiation oncologists of different institutions due to lack of standardization in radiation therapy portals, as depicted on lateral x-ray films. (Nowak P, van Dieren E, van Sörnsen de Koste J, et al. Treatment portals for elective radiotherapy of the neck: an inventory in the Netherlands. *Radiotherapy and Oncology* 1997;43:81–86.)

erative CT scan was also obtained. The preoperative (CT-based delineated boundaries) and intraoperative (surgical-anatomic defined level boundaries) CT scans were then fused. The caudal border of level IV can be identified by the clips positioned next to traverse cervical artery (Fig. 42.12). The posterior border of level IV and Vb is determined by a virtual line drawn between the heads of the trapezius muscle (Fig. 42.12). The posterior border of surgical level IIa (spinal accessory nerve) did not fully match with posterior border of CT-based level IIa (internal jugular vein); the other surgical boundaries and CT-based contours were in perfect agreement (Fig. 42.13).

This second series of experiments was also designed to examine whether the subdivision into sublevels IIa and IIb, as suggested by Robbins (256), is of any benefit in selective RT. It can be argued that because of the heavy infestation of occult metastatic cells in the lymph channels around the IJV and carotid artery, the division of level II into radiologic sublevels IIa and IIb may not be relevant and may even be risky (174) (Figs. 42.14 and 42.15). In contrast to CT-based contoured sublevels in cases of selective RT, the division into surgical sublevels IIa/IIb makes sense as this could reduce serious morbidity, that is, could prevent potential damage to the spinal accessory nerve (174).

Node-Positive Neck

Retrospective intensity-modulated radiation therapy (IMRT) series have reported marginal recurrences in the neck of node-positive (N+) patients treated primarily or postoperatively with radiotherapy. Eisbruch et al. (74) reported a series of 135 patients treated bilaterally from 1994 to 2002 with three-dimensional conformal radiation therapy or IMRT for primary tumors located mainly in the oropharynx. With a median

Table 42.4	INCIDENCE AND DISTRIBUTION OF REGIONAL METASTASIS FOR LEVELS I-V FOR CLINICALLY N+ NECK.				
	Levels Involved (%)				
Tumor Site	I	II	III	IV	V
Oral cavity	48	39	31	15	4
Oropharynx	15	71	42	27	9
Hypopharynx	10	75	72	45	11
Larynx	6	61	54	30	6
Nasopharynx	13	95	60	21	44

(See references: Bataini, Byers, Candela Chao, Lindberg,, Shah, Shah, Sham). Gregoire V, Coche E, Cosnard et al, Radiother and Oncology, 2000;56 (2): 135–150.

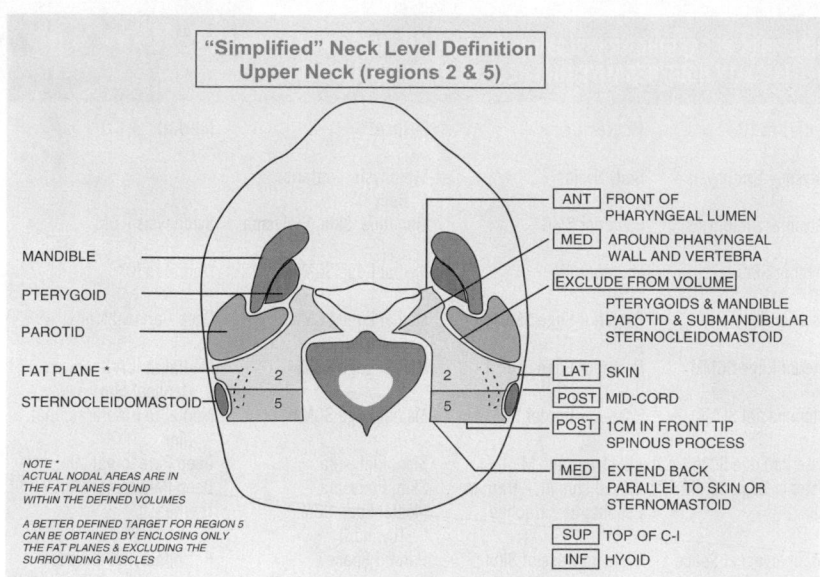

FIGURE 42.8. Simplified computed tomography-based definition of the lymph node levels in the superior part of the node-negative Neck. Middle and inferior part neck not shown. ANT, anterior; MED, medial; LAT, lateral; POST, posterior; SUP, superior; INF, inferior. (Wÿers OB, Levendag PC, Tan T, et al. A simplified CT-based definition of the lymph node level in the node-negative neck. *Radiotherapy and Oncology* 1999;1:35–42.)

follow-up of 32 months, 21 patients had a locoregional recurrence, 4 of which were marginal. Some of the marginal recurrences were observed near the base of skull above the upper limit of the delineated level II. Thus, it seems reasonable, as a first modification in case of infiltration of the upper part of level II, to include in the CTV the fatty space around the internal jugular vein and internal carotid artery up to the jugular foramen (base of skull) in the N+ neck (109). From an anatomic point of view, this space belongs to the upper most part of the retrostyloid space (Fig. 42.16). Also included are the tumor-infiltrated nonlymphoid structures. As a third modification with

respect to the N+ neck, the guidelines for the caudal limits were modified. For the N+ neck, the caudal border was modified basically by lowering it down to the sternoclavicular joint. For a boost volume, the involved level and the directly surrounding uninvolved neck node levels are used (109). The optimal management of cervical metastases is still subject to considerable debate. For example, Roy et al. (263) reported on patients with TF/SP and BOT tumors and N2 neck disease. After a full course of RT, 65% of these patients still had pathologically confirmed disease in cases of clinical and/or CT-based evidence of persistent disease. For those patients with no evidence of residual disease, 33% still had remaining disease in the neck dissection specimen. Their data lend support to a planned neck dissection. In contrast, Su et al. (291) argued that for patients with oropharyngeal tumors, a neck dissection only improves regional control for those patients with a complete clinical response. In fact, a close follow-up is advocated for this category.

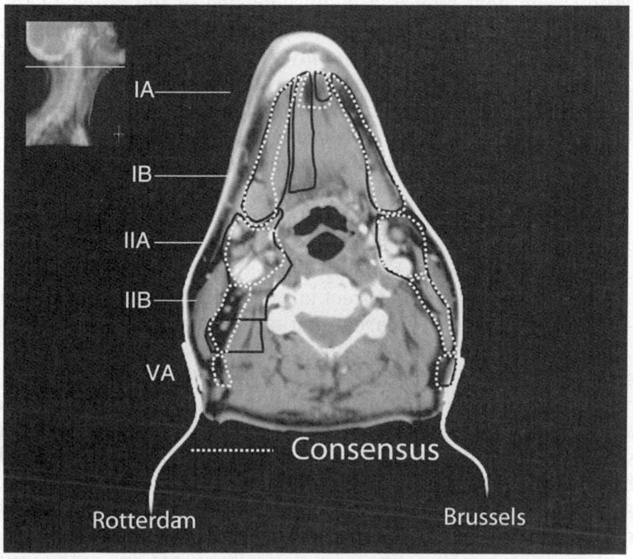

Postoperative Neck

In cases of postoperative RT (PORT), one relies on the long-established institutional guidelines (24,109). As an example, the routine clinical criterion for PORT as used in the Erasmus MC, Rotterdam, and those established by the University of Texas, M.D. Anderson Cancer Center, Houston, are summarized in Table 42.6. Basically, with regard to the tumor bed, if feasible, in PORT one tries to mirror the contralateral noninvolved neck. Finally, the previously discussed consensus guidelines established for the N0 neck will remain the foundation for PORT (and N+ neck).

Clinical Presentation

Patients with carcinoma of the oropharynx present most frequently with a sore throat. They also may complain of difficulty swallowing or pain in the ear, which is related to the anastomotic–tympanic nerve of Jacobson. Carcinomas of the tonsil usually are ulcerated and sometimes exophytic. They infiltrate the glossopharyngeal sulcus and BOT, many times with little or no mucosal involvement. Trismus may be a late manifestation of the disease if the masseter or pterygoid muscle is involved.

FIGURE 42.9. Axial computed tomography slice, upper neck region, with levels Ia, Ib, II, and V (*solid black lines*) contoured according to Rotterdam (right neck) and Brussels (left neck) delineation protocols. Rotterdam and Brussels delineation protocols were meticulously compared and adapted to surgical level definitions as defined by 2002 AAO-HNS classification. International consensus was reached. Stipulated white lines (both necks) demarcate contours of levels and sublevels as defined by international consensus protocol. This figure illustrates contours of levels Ia, Ib, IIa, IIb, and Va (middle and inferior neck guidelines not shown). (Levendag P, Braaksma M, Coche E. Rotterdam and Brussels CT-based neck nodal delineation compared to the surgical levels as defined by the American Academy of Otolaryngology—Head and Neck Surgery 2004;58:1:113–123.)

Table 42.5   INTERNATIONAL CONSENSUS GUIDELINES REGARDING TRANSLATION OF SURGICAL-ANATOMY BOUNDARIES OF LYMPHNODAL LEVELS I–VI IN CLINICALLY NODE NEGATIVE (N0) NECK TO CT-BASED BORDERS.

Levels	Cranial	Caudal	Medial to ICA	Posterior	Lateral	Medial
Ia	Caudal Mandible	Body Hyoid	Platysma, Symphysis	Body Hyoid	Symphysis - Anterior Belly DM	
Ib	Cranial SMG, Mylohyoid M	Central Hoid Bone	Platysma, Symphysis	Posterior SMG	Mandible, Skin, Platysma	Symphysis - DM
IIa	Transverse Process C-I (caudal Border)	Caudal Border Hyoid	Posterior SMG	Posterior IJV	Medial Edge SCMM	Medial to ICA
IIb	Transverse Process C-I (caudal Border)	Caudal Border Hyoid	Posterior IJV	Posterior Edge SMCM	Medial Edge SCMM	Deep Cervical Mm
III	Inferior Hyoid	Inferior Cricoid	Anterior Edge SCMM	Posterior Edge SCMM	Medial Edge SCMM	Medial to ICA Deep Cervical Mm
IV	Inferior Cricoid	2 cm Superior SCJ	Anteromedial SCMM	Posterior Border SCMM	Medial Edge SCMM	Medial to ICA Paraspinal Mm
Va	Cranial Hyoid	Inferior Cricoid	Posterior Edge SCMM	AL - Trapezius M	Skin, Platysma	Deep Paraspinal Mm
Vb	Inferior Cricoid	Transverse Cerv. a.	Posterior Edge SCMM	Virtual Line AL - Trap. M	Skin, Platysma	Deep Paraspinal Mm
VI	Caudal Thyroid	Sternal Manubrium	Skin	Esophagus / Trachea	Medial Edge SCMM, Thyroid G	Trachea
RSS	Base of Skull (jugular foramen)	Upper Limit Level II	Parapharyngeal Space	Vertebra Base of Skul	Parotid Space	Retropharyngeal Nodes
SCF	Lower border IV/Vb	Sternoclavicular joint	SCMM, Skin, Clavicle	Anterior border Posterior Scalenus M	Lateral edge Posterior Scalenus M	Trachea/Thyroid
RPhs	Base of Skull	Cranial Edge Hyoid	Fascia Pharynx Mucosa	Longus Colli/Capitus M	Medial Edge Internal carotid A	Midline

Also depicted are retrostyloid space, subclavicular fossa and retropharyngeal space (see text). ([SCMM] Sterno-Cleido Mastoid Muscle; [SCJ] Sterno Clavicular Joint; [RPhS] Retropharyngeal Space; [RSS] Retro-Styloid Space; [SCF] Sub-Clavicular Fossa; [C-I] Vertebra Corpus C-I; [SMG] Sub-Mandibular Gland; [IJV] Internal Jugular Vein; [Mm] Muscles; [a] artery; [AL-Trap.M] Antero Lateral Edge Trapezius Muscle; [G] Gland.

Cancers of the BOT, unlike those of the oral tongue, rarely are visualized by the patient and may grow to a large size before detection. The patient usually can point to the site of pain and the location of the tumor. Difficulty in swallowing because of pain is common, but dysphagia and impaired deglutition caused by massive infiltration of the tongue by tumor are less so. In advanced tumors that fix the root of the tongue, poor articulation is caused by impaired tongue mobility.

It is common for patients with oropharyngeal cancer to notice a mass in the cervical region, usually subdigastric (jugulodi-gastric), as the first manifestation of disease. Initially, distant metastases are extremely rare.

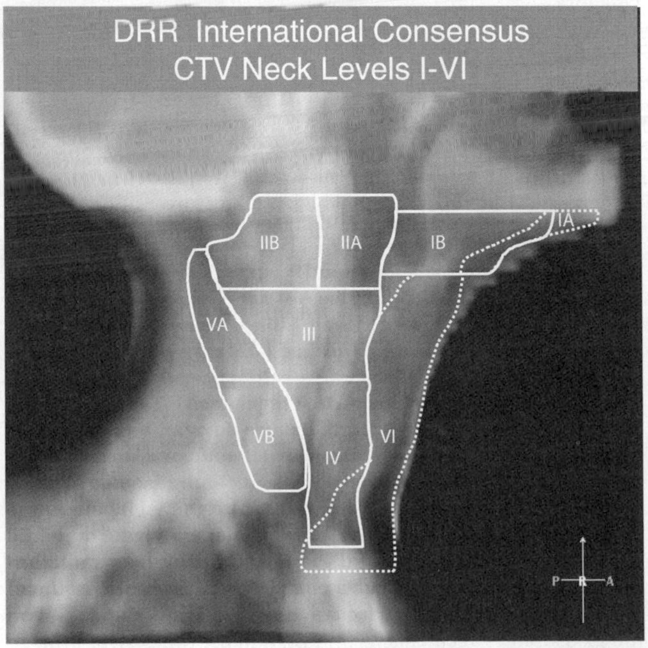

Diagnostic Work-Up

The evaluation of patients with carcinoma of the oropharynx always begins with a complete history and physical examination. The next step is a comprehensive examination of the head and neck, including oral cavity, oropharynx, nasopharynx, hypopharynx, and larynx. Mirror or fiberoptic examination of the nasopharynx, hypopharynx, and larynx always should be performed to detect any tumor extension or associated pathology. In many centers, panendoscopy has become a routine procedure because of the risk of second primaries in the upper digestive tract.

After indirect laryngoscopy, careful digital examination with a gloved finger should evaluate submucosal involvement of the glossopalatine sulcus, base of the tongue, buccal mucosa, or lateral pharyngeal wall. Direct laryngoscopy under anesthesia seldom is required for carcinoma of the faucial arch, but it is very useful to evaluate patients with larger tonsillar or BOT lesions.

Physical examination should include a thorough evaluation of the neck for detection of metastatic lymph nodes as well as a search for distant metastases. Examination of the neck should be done with the physician standing behind the seated patient. Anatomic position, size, consistency, tenderness, and mobility of palpable cervical lymph nodes should be recorded.

Histologic confirmation of a clinically suspicious malignant lesion always must be obtained, and biopsies should be performed, preferably at the margins of the tumor. Incisional or punch forceps biopsies can be performed with local anesthesia on an outpatient basis. When a lymphoma is suspected, the lesion may be submucosal; a large amount of tissue may be required for electron microscopy and immunologic typing of the tumor. Fine-needle aspiration biopsy of suspicious palpable neck nodes may be used to make the initial diagnosis.

DRR International Consensus CTV Neck Levels I-VI

FIGURE 42.10. Digital reconstructed radiograph (DRR) levels I–VI. CTV, clinical target volume.

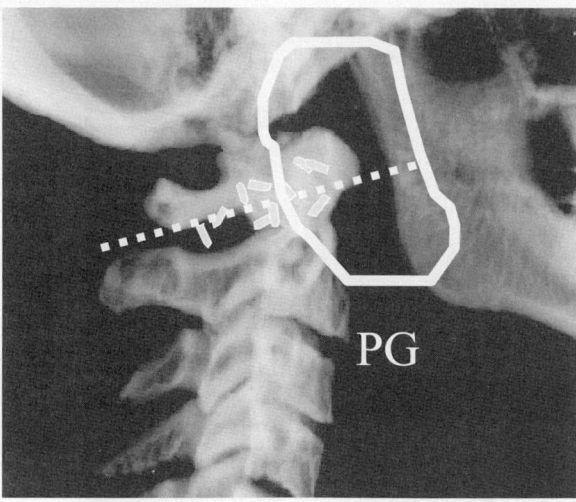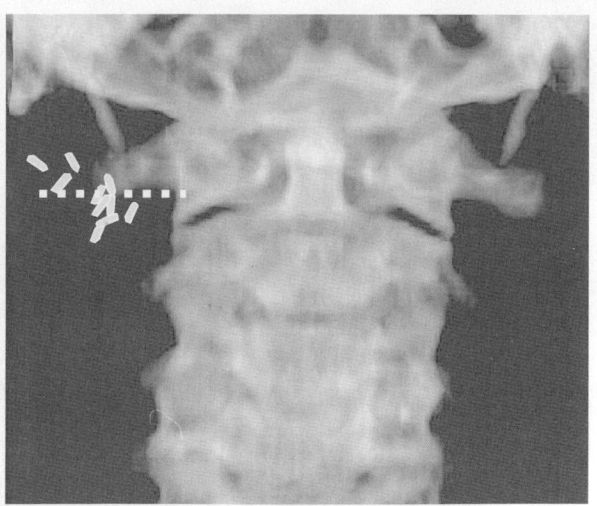

FIGURE 42.11. Projection of clips (anteroposterior and lateral x-ray films) placed intraoperatively at cranial border node-negative neck. Clips cluster around caudal border transverse process corpus vertebra C1. See also the projection of circumference of parotid gland (PG) as determined by computed tomography.

Complete blood counts, chemistry profiles, and urinalysis should be obtained.

Plain films of the soft tissues of the neck or mandible may show involvement of soft tissues or bony structures. CT with contrast has become standard in delineating the extent of tumor and evaluating involvement of the mandible or extension into the base of the skull. MRI scans and positron emission tomography with their superior soft tissue contrast can be quite sensitive in detecting tumor extension and lymph node distributions (232). Criteria used for tumor involvement are abnormal contrast enhancement, soft tissue thickening, presence of a bulky mass, infiltration of lymphatic tissues (even without distortion of surrounding tissues), or a combination of these. Neck lymph nodes are considered pathologic when the smallest diameter is greater than 1 cm. In other studies, the presence of hypodense areas in more than 33% of the lymph nodes has been defined as *nodal necrosis*. Extracapsular extension is thought to be present when the nodal margin appears irregular, without clear distinction with the surrounding fat or when there is thickening of surrounding fibroadipose tissue or muscle.

Chest x-ray films should be routine. Bone scans should be requested only if bone involvement is suspected. X-ray films of the skeleton may be required in patients with positive findings on bone scans or clinical suspicion of bony lesions.

Follow-Up

Patients with oropharyngeal cancer usually are followed up with careful physical and indirect laryngoscopic examination as well as thorough cervical lymph node evaluation on a monthly basis for the first 6 months after therapy, every 3 months in years 2 and 3, every 6 months from year 3 to 5, and yearly thereafter. A recent report on 46 patients treated with irradiation showed that postirradiation CT scans may not add incremental information to the clinical examination for predicting local tumor control. Diffuse and symmetric changes of the soft tissue or asymmetry without detectable mass or less than 10 mm was associated with primary tumor control (174).

Staging

In staging oropharyngeal tumors, it is extremely important to include both the ulcerated and infiltrating components of the tumor and all of its submucosal extensions. Because of a tendency to overestimate the size of oropharyngeal tumors, a ruler or caliper must be used to measure the diameter of the lesion (160). Visual, palpatory, and radiographic findings are critical in accurate staging. The usual staging classification for carcinoma of the oropharynx, including lymph node involvement, is that of the International Union Against Cancer or the American Joint Committee on Cancer (Table 42.1) (6). A criticism of this staging system is that it is largely two-dimensional and does not take into account the third dimension, which determines tumor bulk and morphology (e.g., endophytic or exophytic lesions of similar size, which respond differently to similar treatment) (232).

Pathologic Classification

These tumors have characteristic features, including keratin in many cases, although some are nonkeratinizing; the tumors are

Definition Caudal & Posterior Boundary Level Vb

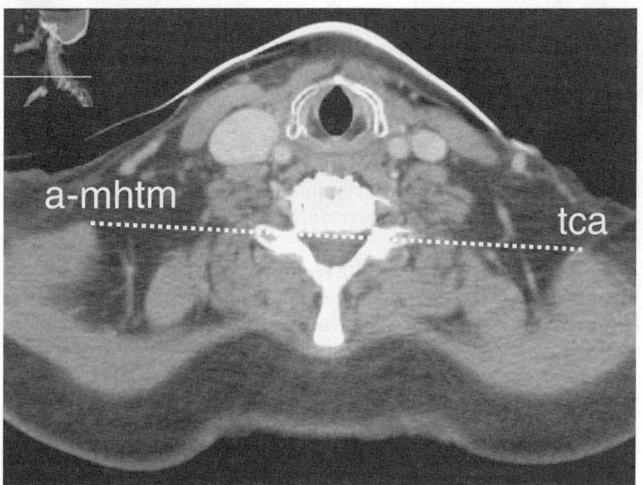

FIGURE 42.12. Caudal border level IV; computed tomography slice at the level of transverse cervical artery (tca). Posterior border level IV and Vb; virtual line, anterior medial heads of trapezius muscle (a-mhtm).

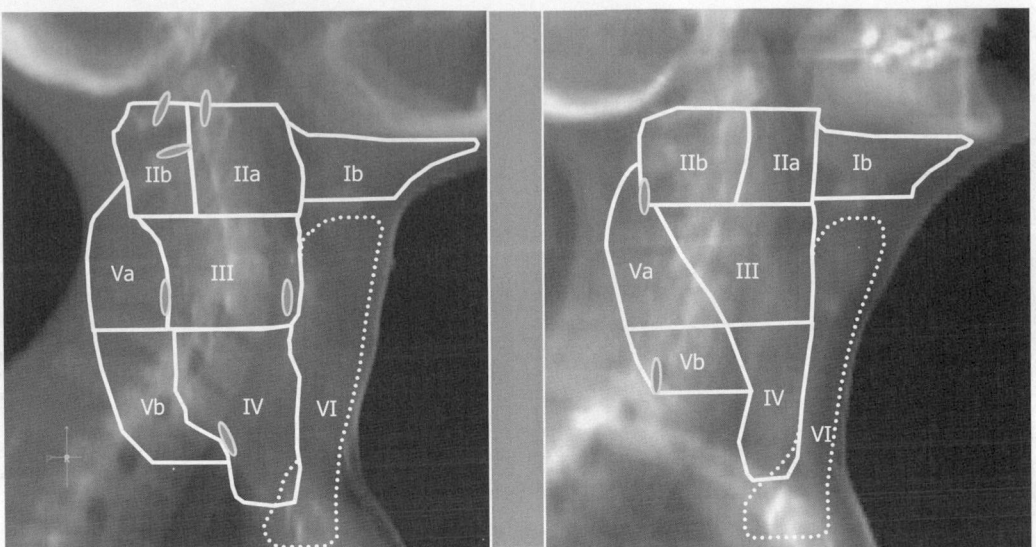

FIGURE 42.13. Digitally reconstructed radiographs validated the position of clips at cranial border IIa, IIb, and boundaries level III, Va, and IV, Vb **(left panel)**. Digitally reconstructed radiographs validated the position of intraoperatively defined clips, demarcating boundaries of levels IIb, Va, and Vb, as they were in good agreement with previously contoured (and matched) computed tomography-based boundaries **(right panel)** (Levendag P, Grégoire V, et al. Intraoperative validation of CT-based lymphnodal levels, sublevels IIA/IIB: is it of clinical relevance in selective radiation therapy? *Int J Radiat Oncol Biol Phys* 2005;62:3:690–699.)

graded I to IV, depending on the degree of differentiation. Carcinomas that arise in the faucial arch, usually of the squamous cell type, tend to be keratinizing and more differentiated than tumors that arise from the TF.

SCCs, often poorly differentiated, account for more than 90% of cancers of the BOT. Although it has been suggested that keratinizing, more differentiated tumors have a somewhat better prognosis than others, no definite correlation between histologic type and pattern of behavior or response to therapy has been reported (232).

Lymphoepithelioma is much rarer in the tonsil or BOT (less than 1.5%) than in the nasopharynx. Most pathologists agree that lymphoepithelioma represents a poorly differenti-

ated, nonkeratinizing SCC with a profuse lymphoid infiltration (232).

Other cell types include mucoepidermoid, adenocarcinoma, and adenoid cystic, which appear to behave more like salivary gland tumors of similar histology in other sites rather than like SCCs of similar size. Tumors of the salivary gland type are uncommon in the tonsil or faucial arch. Malignant melanomas of the TF are also rare (232).

Primary small cell carcinoma of the tonsil, with neurosecretory granules demonstrated by electron microscopy, have been infrequently described. As in other locations, this tumor has a high propensity for regional, nodal, and distant metastatic spread with a very poor prognosis.

Malignant lymphomas, usually non-Hodgkin's type, constitute 10% to 15% of malignant tumors of the tonsil and 1% to 2% of the BOT. They tend to grow submucosally and may reach large size without significant mucosal ulceration. The surface of the tumor is covered by the same mucous membrane that covers the soft palate. Primary Hodgkin's disease in the tonsil is extremely rare.

Metastatic carcinoma to the tonsil is rare, with only 98 cases reported in the world literature (232).

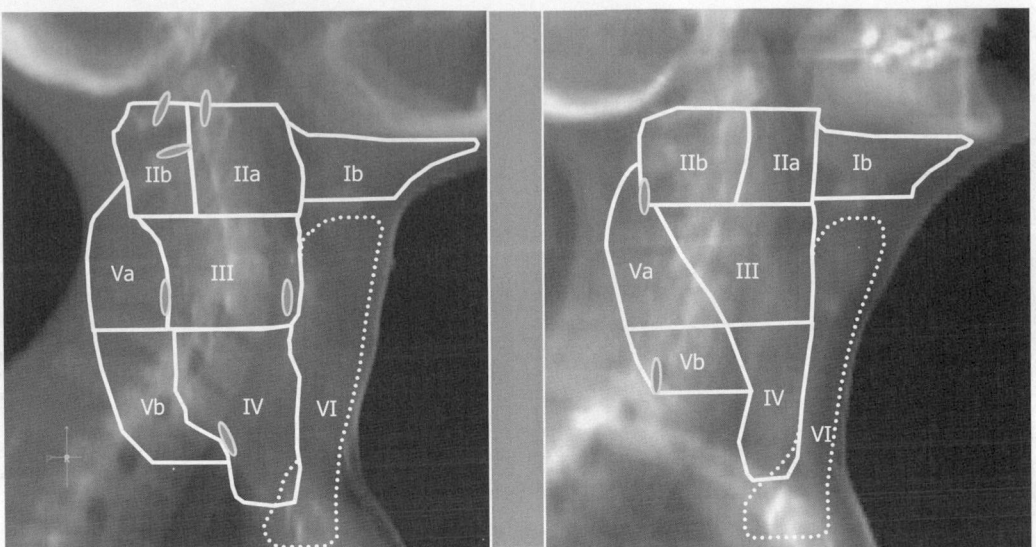

FIGURE 42.14. Photograph and schematic drawing of right upper-neck region in patient with right radical neck dissection. In schematic diagram symbols I–IV denote neck nodal levels. Radiopaque surgical clips positioned at the most cranial part of the neck, anterior (143) and posterior (247) to the internal jugular vein (IJV). Also seen is a clip (1) at the site where the spinal accessory nerve (SAN) enters the sternocleidomastoid muscle (SCMM). The triangular area, denoted as "no-man's land," belongs to either the posterior part of surgical level IIa or the ventral (anterior) part of computed tomography-based level IIb. The triangular area is formed by SAN, clips 2 and 3, the posterior boundary of the IJV, and part of the hyoid line. (Levendag P, Grégoire V, et al. Intraoperative validation of CT-based lymphnodal levels, sublevels IIA/IIB: is it of clinical relevance in selective radiation therapy? *Int J Radiat Oncol Biol Phys* 2005;62:3:690–699.)

Prognostic Factors

Host and tumor factors have been correlated with survival but not consistently with primary, nodal, and distant relapses. Age and gender are *host characteristics* that may have prognostic significance (232).

In some reports, women have shown a better prognosis than men, possibly because of earlier detection of tumors in women although other authors observed no significant survival difference between the genders. Significant differences in survival based on age (e.g., patients younger or older than 40 years) have not been established in sufficiently large and uniform patient cohorts and need to be stratified by disease stage and performance status (232).

Tumor characteristics that have prognostic significance include tumor size and extension (stage); presence of palpable lymph nodes; and location, number, and size of involved lymph nodes. Tumor regression during radiation therapy and

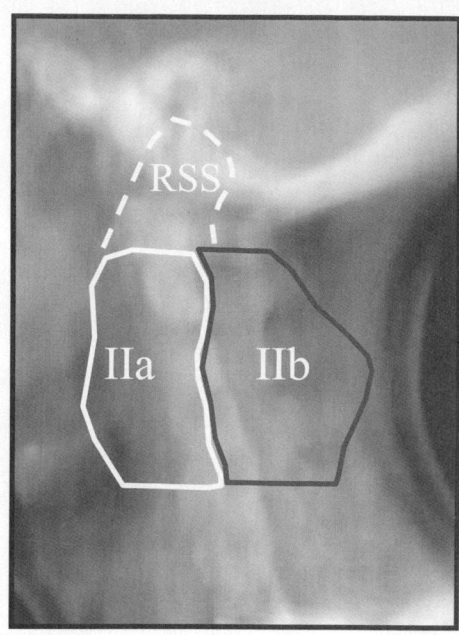
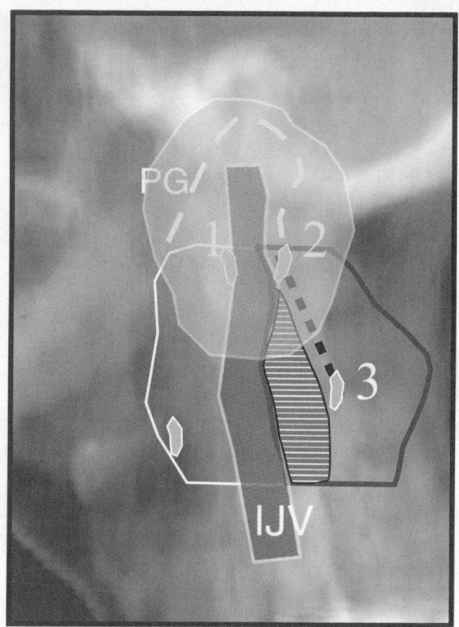

FIGURE 42.15. Digitally reconstructed radiograph **(left panel)** is shown of the computed tomography-based contoured sublevels IIa and IIb and the retrostyloid space (RSS). **Right panel:** superimposed on the delineated sublevels, the contoured internal jugular vein (IJV) and the clips positioned intraoperatively at the relevant surgical boundaries of sublevels IIa/IIb and the hyoid (clips 1, 2, 3, 5). The stipulated line demarcates the position of the boundary between the surgically defined sublevels IIa and IIb. The "no-man's land" zone is the triangularly shaped, cross-hatched area between the posterior border of the surgically defined sublevel IIa (SAN: spinal accessory nerve. The SAN is represented by the stipulated line 2–3 in the right panel) and the posterior border of the CT-based level IIa (posterior boundary of the IJV). RT, radiation therapy. (Levendag P, Grégoire V, et al. Intraoperative validation of CT-based lymphnodal levels, sublevels IIA/IIB: is it of clinical relevance in selective radiation therapy? *Int J Radiat Oncol Biol Phys* 2005;62:3:690–699.)

histologic differentiation are additional prognostic factors reported. P53 and epidermal growth factor receptor overexpression has been associated with increased survival (232).

A significant correlation has been found between the stage of the primary tumor, the presence of involved cervical lymph nodes, and 5-year survival (234). Tonsil tumor extension into the base of the tongue is associated with decreased survival (232).

There is no definite correlation between histologic type or degree of tumor differentiation and patient survival. In patients treated surgically after irradiation, more than 90% with negative histologic specimens survived for 5 years compared with only 30% of patients with persistent tumor (232).

Overall, BOT cancers have a worse prognosis than do their oral tongue or tonsil counterparts because of greater size at diagnosis, more frequent spread to adjacent structures, and higher rates of lymphatic spread. However, stage for stage, they may have similar prognoses as oral tongue cancers. Small exophytic tumors (i.e., superficial surface lesions) have higher rates of local tumor control by surgery or irradiation and a better prognosis than infiltrating or large tumors. Patients with tumors confined to the BOT survive longer than those with tumors that extend to the faucial arch, oral cavity, or larynx and hypopharynx (232). The prognosis is better for patients without palpable lymph nodes (N0) and for those with small, ipsilateral, mobile lymph nodes rather than those with large, fixed, contralateral, or bilateral nodes (234).

Management Strategies, Results, and Outcomes

Lymphoepithelioma, representing a poorly differentiated, non-keratinizing SCC with a profuse lymphoid infiltration, is rare (less than 1.5%) in the TF/SP and BOT. Mucoepidermoid, adenocarcinoma, and adenocystic carcinomas behave more or less like "salivary gland type of tumors" of similar histology in other sites of the head and neck, rather than like SCC. Moreover, these salivary glandlike tumors are particularly uncommon in the faucial arch and TF (287). Koss et al. (159) and Abedi and Sismanis (1) found only a few cases of small cell carcinomas of the tonsil. Malignant lymphomas, mostly of the non-Hodgkin's type, constitute 10% to 15% of the TF and 1% to 2% of the BOT tumors. In contrast to non-Hodgkin's lymphoma, primary Hodgkin's disease in the oropharynx is extremely rare (14). Metastatic lesions to the TF/SP and BOT are exceptionally rare as well. Oreggia et al. (224) found women to have a better prognosis than men (at 5-year overall survival [OS], 40% vs. 9%). In contrast, Vallis et al. (301) observed no significant difference between genders. Similarly, young age has not proven to be of prognostic significance (150).

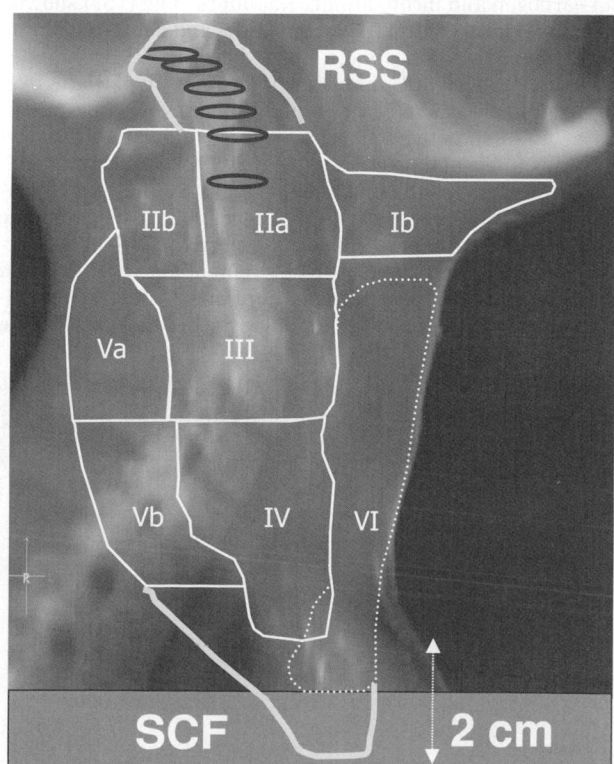

FIGURE 42.16. Digital reconstructed radiograph with levels Ib-VI, including delineation of the retrostyloid space (RSS) and subclavicular fossa (SCF).

| Table 42.6 | INDICATIONS FOR POSTOPERATIVE RADIATION THERAPY (PORT) |

PORT: Risk Groups

Hard criteria: Irradical resection Lymph node metastases with ECE two or more nodes Soft criteria: Perineural growth Close margins T3-T4	High risk Intermediate risk	**66 Gy** (66 Gy EQD2,33) 6 fx/week **60 Gy** (60 Gy EQD2,33) 6 fx/week
No risk factors:	Low risk	**No PORT**

PORT: Risk Groups

Hard-risk group: >= 2 factors Oral cavity primary Mucosal margins close or positive Nerve invasion Largest node > 3 cm ≥2 Positive lymph nodes Treatment delay greater than 6 weeks Zubrod performance status >= 2	**63 Gy** 7 fx/week (53.2 Gy EQD2,33) **63 Gy** 5 fx/week (63 Gy EQD2,33) 3 weeks 1 fx/day - 2 wks 2 fx/day
Intermediate-risk: 1 *Adverse feature other than ECE*	**57.6 Gy** 5 fx/week (61.8 Gy EQD2,33)

Criteria used in Erasmus MC—Daniel den Hoed Cancer Center, Rotterdam. (upper panel) and University of Texas, MD Anderson Cancer Center, Houston (lower panel).

Tumor characteristics like tumor size, stage, lymph nodal status, and tumor regression during therapy have been found to be of some prognostic significance. No definite correlation has been observed between histologic type, tumor differentiation, and patient survival (250,301). In contrast, p53 overexpression and targeting the epidermal growth factor receptor family do seem to be of prognostic value (267). For the more advanced tumors, there is a need for improvement, and the jury is still out on which treatment approach offers better tumor control and fewer side effects at the same time. One approach addressing the problem of improving the locoregional control in advanced tumors is reported by Hoogsteen et al. (136). They tried to modify the response of malignant cells to radiation by overcoming tumor hypoxia. The Head and Neck Oncology group of the department of Radiotherapy of the St. Radbond University Hospital in Nijmegen argued that this can be done in several ways including, for example, hyperbaric oxygen, carbogen breathing combined with nicotinamide, hypoxic cell sensitizers, and erythropoietin. There is now compelling evidence that shows that low hemoglobin levels before and during treatment are associated with reduced tumor control and decreased survival. The authors investigated the impact of low hemoglobin levels on locoregional control in patients who have been treated with accelerated radiotherapy with carbogen and nicotinamide. This is another example of good local tumor control and survival by modulating tumor cell biology (e.g., hypoxia) (Tables 42.7 and 42.8). For BOT tumors treated with accelerated radiotherapy with carbogen and nicotinamide, Kaanders et al. (153) showed an actuarial local control (LC) rate of 84% and actuarial OS rate of 50%. Similar findings were observed for TF/SP tumors at 5 years: LC rate of 86% and OS rate of 33%. Hyperbaric oxygen as adjunctive therapy, although never proven in a randomized setting, is another effective way of modulating the oxygen status of normal tissues beneficially (92). In Erasmus MC, such a trial is currently ongoing. To measure the oxygen status of the tissues of those patients, a novel optical spectroscopic technique is used; this so called differential path-length spectroscopy allows for the *in vivo* measurement of hypoxia-related parameters such as blood oxygenation, blood content, and microvessel size in the most superficial layer of tissue (5). For the

| Table 42.7 | COMPARISON OF RADIATION THERAPY SCHEDULES FOR TREATMENT OF CARCINOMA OF THE TONSILLAR FOSSA/SOFT PALATE AND BASE OF TONGUE: 5 YEARS ACTUARIAL LOCAL CONTROL |

	Therapy	T1 # of Pat (%)	T2 # of Pat (%)	T3 # of Pat (%)	T4 # of Pat (%)
MD Anderson[1]					
TF/SP	Concomitant Boost	5 (100%)	29 (96%)	41 (78%)	4 (50%)
BOT	Concomitant Boost	4 (100%)	27 (96%)	22 (70%)	1 (NE)
Erasmus MC[2]					
TF/SP	EBRT 6 fr./week + HDR/IRT	13 (100%)	65 (89%)	24 (91%)	1 (100%)
TF/SP	EBRT 6 fr./week + S+PORT	5 (100%)	22 (95%)	58 (85%)	8 (69%)
BOT	EBRT 6 fr./week + HDR/IRT	9 (100%)	13 (84%)	9 (56%)	10 (89%)
BOT	EBRT 6 fr./week + S+PORT	0	1 (100%)	10 (100%)	6 (100%)
KUN[3]					
TF/SP	ARCON	0	3 (100%)	17 (100%)	8 (53%)
BOT	ARCON	1 (100%)	4 (100%)	4 (100%)	15 (76%)

Data obtained from references (1) Gwozdz et al., and Mak et al., (2) Levendag et al., (3) Kaanders et al. See also bibliography.

	Therapy	T1 # of Pat (%)	T2 # of Pat (%)	T3 # of Pat (%)	T4 # of Pat (%)
COMPARISON OF RADIATION THERAPY SCHEDULES FOR TREATMENT OF CARCINOMA OF THE TONSILLAR FOSSA/SOFT PALATE AND BASE OF TONGUE: 5 YEARS ACTUARIAL OVERALL SURVIVAL — Table 42.8					
MD Anderson[1]					
TF/SP	Concomitant Boost	5	29 (64%)	41 (63%)	4 (58%)
BOT	Concomitant Boost	4	27 (80%)	22 (57%)	1 (55%)
Erasmus MC[2]					
TF/SP	EBRT 6 fr./week + HDR/IRT	13 (77%)	65 (68%)	24 (66%)	1 (100%)
TF/SP	EBRT 6 fr./week + S+PORT	5 (67%)	22 (72%)	58 (50%)	8 (38%)
BOT	EBRT 6 fr./week + HDR/IRT	9 (67%)	13 (54%)	9 (53%)	10 (40%)
BOT	EBRT 6 fr./week + S+PORT	0	1 (0%)	10 (27%)	6 (67%)
KUN[3]					
TF/SP	ARCON	0	3 (33%)	17 (38%)	8 (25%)
BOT	ARCON	1 (100%)	4 (50%)	4 (50%)	15 (47%)

Data obtained from references (1) Gwozdz et al. and Mak et al., (2) Levendag et al., (3) Kaanders et al. See also bibliography.

advanced oropharyngeal tumors, there are many more innovative approaches feasible. For example, Suntharalingam (292) reviewed the beneficial effect of systemic and/or intra-arterial CHT as organ-preservation therapy. The author argued that the real focus in the treatment approach of the tumor, however, should be on newer biologic agents targeting cellular protein receptors. For more details one is referred to XII.

Tumors of the Tonsillar Fossa and/or Soft Palate

For general reading on TF and/or SP tumors treated by external beam RT (EBRT) and/or surgery, one is referred to the literature search as referenced in this section (3,7,14,15, 18,51,66,70,87,96,97,101,102,138,145,164,170,175,189,190, 193,196,203,209,225,226,233,234,246,250,268,273,301,313, 316,322,320,323). The TF and/or SP tumors are also typically tumor sites very suitable for BT. For an overview on the techniques and results obtained with BT, see the following references for example (71,80,81,176,178,199–202,230,236,237, 246,327). Perez et al. (234) addressed the important issue of ipsilateral and/or contralateral neck failure in a series of 384 patients treated in a single institution (Washington University, St. Louis, MO) (Fig. 42.17). A similar type of analysis was done for the 254 patients with TF and/or SP tumors treated at Erasmus MC, Rotterdam (Fig. 42.18). Interestingly, in the Erasmus MC series, 37 patients received no treatment to the contralateral clinically N0 neck; only 1 patient (3%) had a recurrence in the neck. Based on these findings, in recent years one has become more selective in treating the contralateral neck. That is, according to treatment protocol in Erasmus MC, the contralateral neck is only treated if the CTV is crossing the midline, or when dealing with N2c,3 disease, or if the TF tumor is infiltrating the glossopalatine sulcus and/or the BOT (175).

Clinical Radiation Oncology

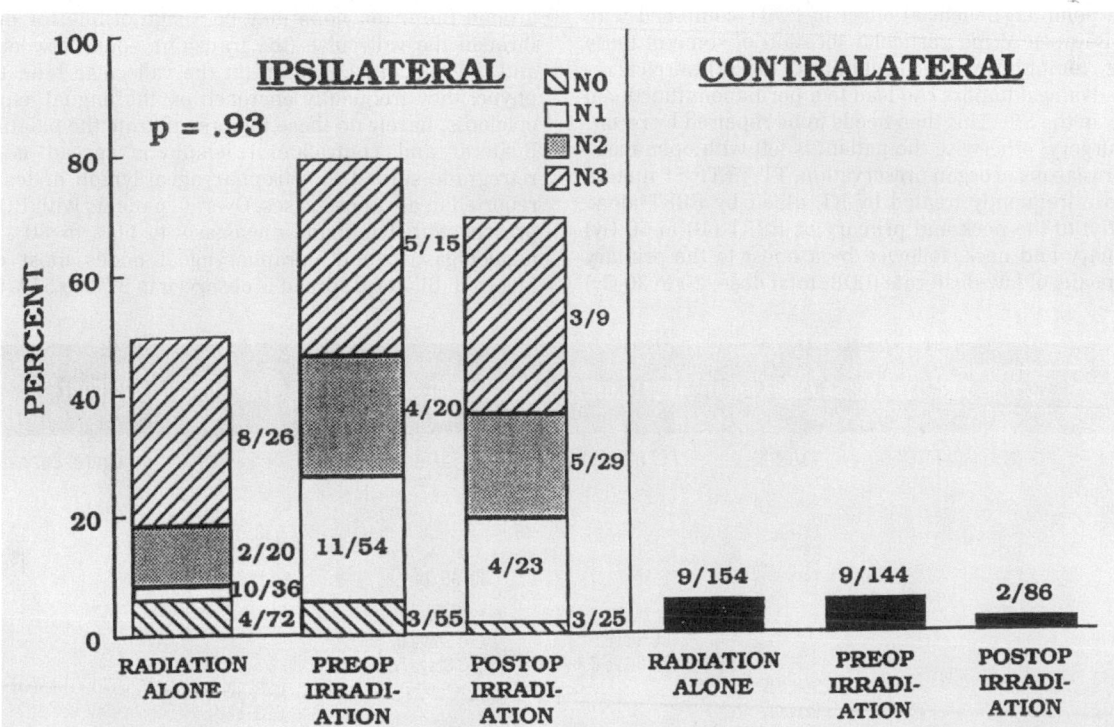

FIGURE 42.17. Carcinoma of the tonsil. Incidence of ipsilateral and contralateral neck recurrence in 384 patients treated with irradiation alone or combined with surgery at Mallinckrodt Institute of Radiology, Washington University. (From Perez CA, Brady LW, Halperon EG, et al. *Principles and practice of radiation oncology.* Philadelphia: Lippincott Williams & Wilkins; 2004:1031.)

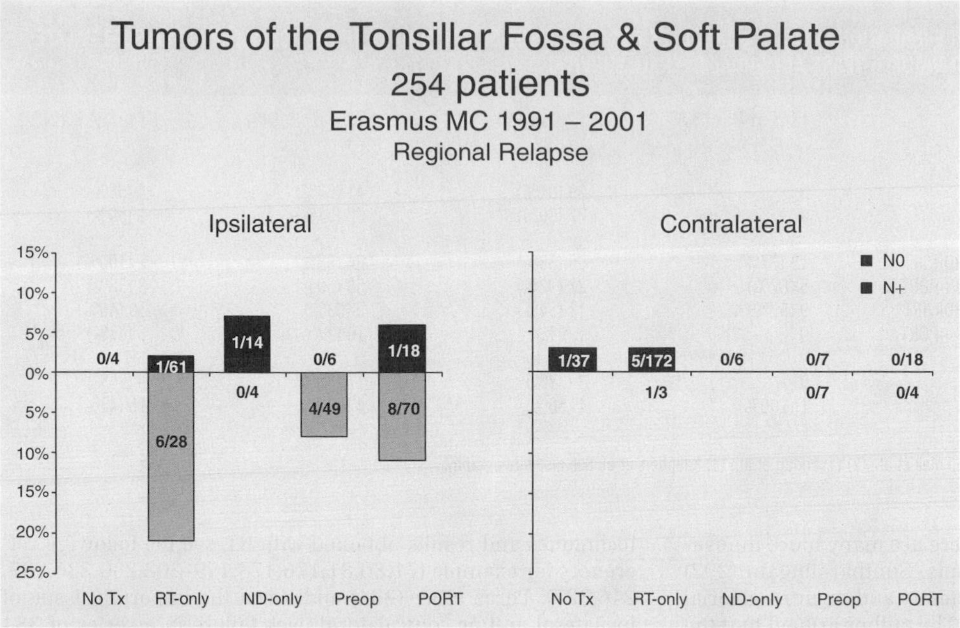

Tumors of the Tonsillar Fossa & Soft Palate
254 patients
Erasmus MC 1991 – 2001
Regional Relapse

FIGURE 42.18. Tumors of the tonsillar fossa and soft palate. No Tx, no treatment; RT-only, radiation therapy as a single modality; ND-only, neck was treated by neck dissection alone; Preop, neck treated by neck dissection and preoperative irradiation, 46 Gy; PORT, neck dissection and postoperative radiation therapy.

Treatment Results

T1 lesions less than 1 cm can be treated with surgical resection or irradiation to the primary only to a dose of 65 to 70 Gy in 7 weeks. The majority of T1 or T2 tumors of the TF and/or SP are treated by irradiation, the ipsilateral neck inclusive, be it electively or because of N+ disease (see previous section). For T3 and T4 tumors, surgery of the primary is often advocated; it can require removal of the primary tumor, partial removal of the mandible in combination with an ipsilateral neck dissection (combined resection). Because of the high incidence of a recurrence with surgery as a single modality (86), surgery is to be followed by PORT (23). Recent insights have demonstrated the potential beneficial effect of PORT combined with CHT (56). Because of the particular location of some of these tumors (e.g., tumor growth in the midline of the SP), surgical resection of advanced tumors can lead to a permanent functional defect (e.g., in the SP). This then needs to be repaired by reconstructive surgery; otherwise the patient is left with open nasal speech. For reasons of organ preservation, T1-T3 TF/SP tumors are therefore frequently treated by RT, albeit by EBRT alone (70 to 75 Gy) to the neck and primary or EBRT (40 to 50 Gy) to the primary and neck, followed by a boost to the primary tumor by means of low dose rate (LDR, total dose, 20 to 30 Gy)

or high-dose-rate (fractionated HDR; total dose, 20 to 25 Gy) BT (for details on BT, see Clinical Section on Tonsillar Fossa and/or Soft Palate and Tumors of the Base of Tongue). For the advanced cases, EBRT is combined with concomitant CHT (22). Data from the literature on the surgical, EBRT only, and EBRT plus IRT results with regard to LC and survival are summarized in Tables 42.9, 42.10, and 42.11, respectively.

Tumors of the Base of Tongue

SCCs, often poorly differentiated, account for more than 90% of cancers of the BOT. It is often difficult to estimate exact tumor extension by clinical examination. Fullness in the soft tissue around the hyoid bone may be a sign of inferior penetration through the valleculae (the transition zone between the BOT and the epiglottis). Tumors in the valleculae tend to be exophytic; they frequently encroach on the lingual aspect of the epiglottis. Rarely do these tumors infiltrate the palatine tonsils. Bilateral and contralateral lymphatic spread is common; retrograde spread to retropharyngeal lymph nodes has been reported in advanced cases. Overall, patients with BOT cancers present with lymphatic metastasis in 50% to 80%, with the jugulodigastric and parapharyngeal nodes most commonly involved. Bilateral spread is observed in 37% to 55% (179,227).

Table 42.9		**TONSILLAR FOSSA / SOFT PALATE: LOCAL CONTROL AND SURVIVAL ACCORDING TO STAGE SURGERY AND PORT**					

First Author	N	T1/T2 %	T3/T4 %	LCT1/T2 5-Yrs %	LC T3/T4 5-Yrs %	DFS 5-Yrs %	Overall Survival 5-Yrs %
Mizono, 1986	40			LRC: 73			
Parsons, 2002	406		12(T4)	76		CSS: 57	47
Perez, 1991	127		69	41 3-yrs			39
Perez, 1998	230		14	T1: 80, T2: 71	T3: 65, T4: 58		
Foote, 1994	72		3	T1: 78, T2: 76	T3: 4, T4: 0/2		
				LRC Stage I: 73	LRC Stage III: 53		
				LRC Stage II: 69	LRC Stage IV: 56		
Schuller, 1979	20		Stage IV: 20			CSS: 20	
Rabuzzi, 1982	47		Stage IV: 45			CSS: 57	
Givens, 1981	37		Stage IV: 51			CSS: 54	
Gluckman, 1985	82		Stage IV: 39			CSS: 56	

LC, local control; LRC, local regional control; CSS, cause specific survival.

Table 42.10	TONSILLAR FOSSA / SOFT PALATE: LOCAL CONTROL AND SURVIVAL ACCORDING TO STAGE EXTERNAL BEAM RADIOTHERAPY

First Author	N	T1/T2 %	T3/T4 %	LCT1/T2 5-Yrs %	LC T3/T4 5-Yrs %	DFS 5-Yrs %	Overal Survival 5-Yrs %
Jackson, 1999	170		63	DSS: 76.2		DSS 61	55.7
Marcial, 1993	137		92				24
Horiot, 1992	325		56			35	
O'Sullivan, 1997	229						
Bataini, 1989	465		35	T1: 90, T2: 84	T3: 64, T4: 47		

LC, local control; LRC, local regional control; CSS, cause specific survival; DFS, disease free survival; TF, tonsillar fossa; SP, soft palate.

The incidence of pathologic lymph nodes (pN+) in the ipsilateral clinical N0 neck is estimated to be 22% to 33%. Contralateral lymphatic metastasis at presentation is observed in 37%, albeit by RT or surgery. These data testify to the fact that in BOT cancer, the neck should be treated electively bilaterally (N0; levels II-IV), or therapeutically (N+; levels I-V). An overview of the pertinent literature on BOT cancer can be obtained from references 15,44,66,87,101,119,123,124,127–129,135,136,141, 143,148,155,163,168,169,184,189,192,193,205,241,245,249, 274,281,284,292,298,311.

Treatment Results

With regard to the management of BOT tumors, in short, the primary tumor in early-stage oropharyngeal cancers can be treated by either EBRT or IRT or surgery, whereas more advanced lesions often are treated by surgery plus PORT. Also EBRT, followed by a boost by IRT or intraoral cone and/or concomitant CHT for the more advanced cases, is frequently used. In the majority of institutions, however, RT is the preferred definitive treatment mode for T1, T2, and some of the exophytic T3, N0, N1 cancers. In general, a neck dissection is warranted only in these early cancer stages in patients treated by RT and experiencing a residual regional mass 6 weeks after completion of the therapy. In this respect, Doweck et al. (71) discussed the controversial role of selective neck dissection after definitive RT. For N1–3 disease, some protocols have successfully used routine neck dissections after preoperative RT (46 Gy), with excellent control rates. For the more advanced (endophytic) T3 lesions, as well as for the T4 tumors with significant extension into normal surrounding tissues, organ/normal tissue deformities are frequently the cause of clinical problems, for example, resulting in swallowing disability and trismus. For this category of patients, the treatment is frequently "tailor made" and

surgery followed by PORT might sometimes be a more sensible option (299).

Reviewing the literature, however, the implementation of concomitant CHT has also been shown to be a highly effective treatment combination. BOT tumors may be resected transorally or via mandibulotomy; the last approach is frequently combined with reconstruction by tissue grafting (272). Patients with advanced tumors may require a glossectomy. In these cases, a tracheotomy (to avoid aspiration) with placement of a speech button and a percutaneous endoscopic gastrostomy to circumvent swallowing dysfunction (thus to secure adequate food intake during treatment and immediate follow-up) is often performed at the time of surgery. The relevant data taken from the literature with regard to locoregional tumor control and survival has been summarized in Table 42.12 (for surgery), Table 42.13 (for EBRT), and Table 42.14 (for EBRT combined with a BT boost).

Finally, two typical protocols, exemplified by Figures 42.19 and 42.20, illustrate different treatment approaches, but similar (good) LC and survival for oropharyngeal tumors. Figure 42.19 represents the oropharynx protocol of Erasmus MC, with emphasis on organ function-preserving properties by using accelerated fractionation during the first series of IMRT (6 fractions per week) and HDR-BT, or Cyber Knife as a boost technique. Figure 42.20 illustrates the protocol of the M.D. Anderson Cancer Center, with the main focus on the concomitant boost (altered fractionation) technique.

Tumors of the Lateral and Posterior Pharyngeal Walls

These tumors are less frequently reported in the literature and generally do not do so well with either RT or surgery

Table 42.11	TONSILLAR FOSSA / SOFT PALATE: LOCAL CONTROL AND SURVIVAL ACCORDING TO STAGE BRACHYTHERAPY BOOST

First Author	N	T1/T2 %	T3/T4 %	LC T1/T2 5-Yrs %	LC T3/T4 5-Yrs %	DFS 5-Yrs %	Overall Survival 5-Yrs %
Pernot, 1992	277		57	76 5-yrs			51
Puthawala, 1985	80		24	84			
				LRC Stage I: 3/3	LRC Stage III: 85		
				LRC Stage II: 100	LRC Stage IV: 56		
Pernot, 1994	361		1	T1:80, T2:71	T3: 65, T4: 58	CSS: 63	53
				LRC: 75			
Levendag, 2004	104	77			T1-T3: 88	57	67
Esche, 1988	43	T1: 34/43			92	CSS: 64	37
Mazeron, 1993		100		94		71	53
Peiffert, 1994	73	65/73	2/73	T: 80, T2:67		CSS: 64	30

LC, local control; LRC, local regional control; CSS, cause specific survival; DFS, disease free survival.

Clinical Radiation Oncology

Table 42.12   BASE OF TONGUE: LOCAL CONTROL AND SURVIVAL ACCORDING TO STAGE SURGERY AND PORT

First Author	N	T1/T2 %	T3/T4 %	N0 %	LC T1/T2 5-Yrs %	LC T3/T4 5-Yrs %	DFS 5-Yrs %	Overall Survival 5-Yrs %
Pol, 2004	58		26 (T4)	18	91		55	40
Foote, 1993	55			49	LRC: 48			55
Kraus, 1993	100			38	LRC: 72		DSS 61	55
Malone, 2004	40		70	25	LRC: 100 2-yrs		DSS 93.6	74.7
Parsons, 2002	390		13(T4)		76		CSS: 62	49
Sessions, 2003	262		19	45	LRC: 74		CSS: 49.6	42.4

LC, local control; LRC, local regional control; CSS, cause specific survival.

Table 42.13   BASE OF TONGUE: LOCAL CONTROL AND SURVIVAL ACCORDING TO STAGE EXTERNAL BEAM RADIOTHERAPY

First Author	N	T1/T2 %	T3/T4 %	N0 %	LC T1/T2 5-Yrs %	LC T3/T4 5-Yrs %	DFS 5-Yrs %	Overall Survival 5-Yrs %
Selek, 2004	40	100		100			76	83
Spanos, 1976	174		37		T1: 91, T2: 71	T3: 78, T4: 52		
Jaulerry, 1991	166		59	30	69	32		27
Mendenhall, 2000	217		19 (T4)		T1: 96, T2: 91	T3: 81. T4: 38	CSS: 50	64
Mak, 1995	54			17	LRC T1/T2: 85 LRC T3: 67			59
Hinerman, 1994	47 qd			18	LRC: 70			44
	90 bid							
Marcial, 1983	141			25	LRC: 31			15
Housset, 1987	29	100		0	T1: 100, T2: 74			52
Wang, 1991	79 qd	T1-T3-Conventional			T1/T2: 79	T3:24		T1/T2: 65, T3: 14
	90 bid	T1-T3 bid			T1/T2: 85			T1/T2: 76, T3: 53
Chao, 2004	18				LRC: 88		80 4-yrs	

LC, local control; LRC, local regional control; CSS, cause specific survival; DFS, disease free survival; bid, twice daily; qd, one fraction per day.

Table 42.14   BASE OF TONGUE: LOCAL CONTROL AND SURVIVAL ACCORDING TO STAGE BRACHYTHERAPY BOOST

First Author	N	T1/T2 %	T3/T4 %	N0 %	LC T1/T2 5-Yrs %	LC T3/T4 5-Yrs %	DFS 5-Yrs %	Overall Survival 5-Yrs %
Harrison, 1997	68		3(T4)		T1:87, T2:93	T3: 82, T4: 100	T1: 88, T2: 93, T3: 82	87
Puthawala, 1988	70		17 (T4)		T1: 100, T2:88	T3: 75, T4: 67	67	35
Barrett, 2004	20		35	10	2-yrs		33	
Takacsi-Nagy, 2004	37		81	19	100	60	52	46
Karakoyun-Celik, 2005	40		54	30	LC: T1-4: 78		54	62
Pol, 2004	30		67 (T4)	30	LC 63		45	40
Gibs, 2003	41		49	32	14	20	79	66
Brunin, 1999	216		61	30	T1:93, T2:66	T3:45. T4: 18	CSS I-IV: 63-23	27
Crook, 1988	48	100			T1:85, T2:71		50	
Hoffstetter, 1996	136	55/136		N0/N1 81	T1: 86,T2: 69	T3:64		
Horwitz, 1996	20	11/20	9/20		10/11	T4: 8/9		72
Housset, 1987	29	100			T1:6/6, T2:74			30.5
Lusinchi, 1989	108	57/108	T3:51/108		T1:85, T2: 50	T3: 69		26

LC, local control; CSS, cause specific survival; DFS, disease free survival.

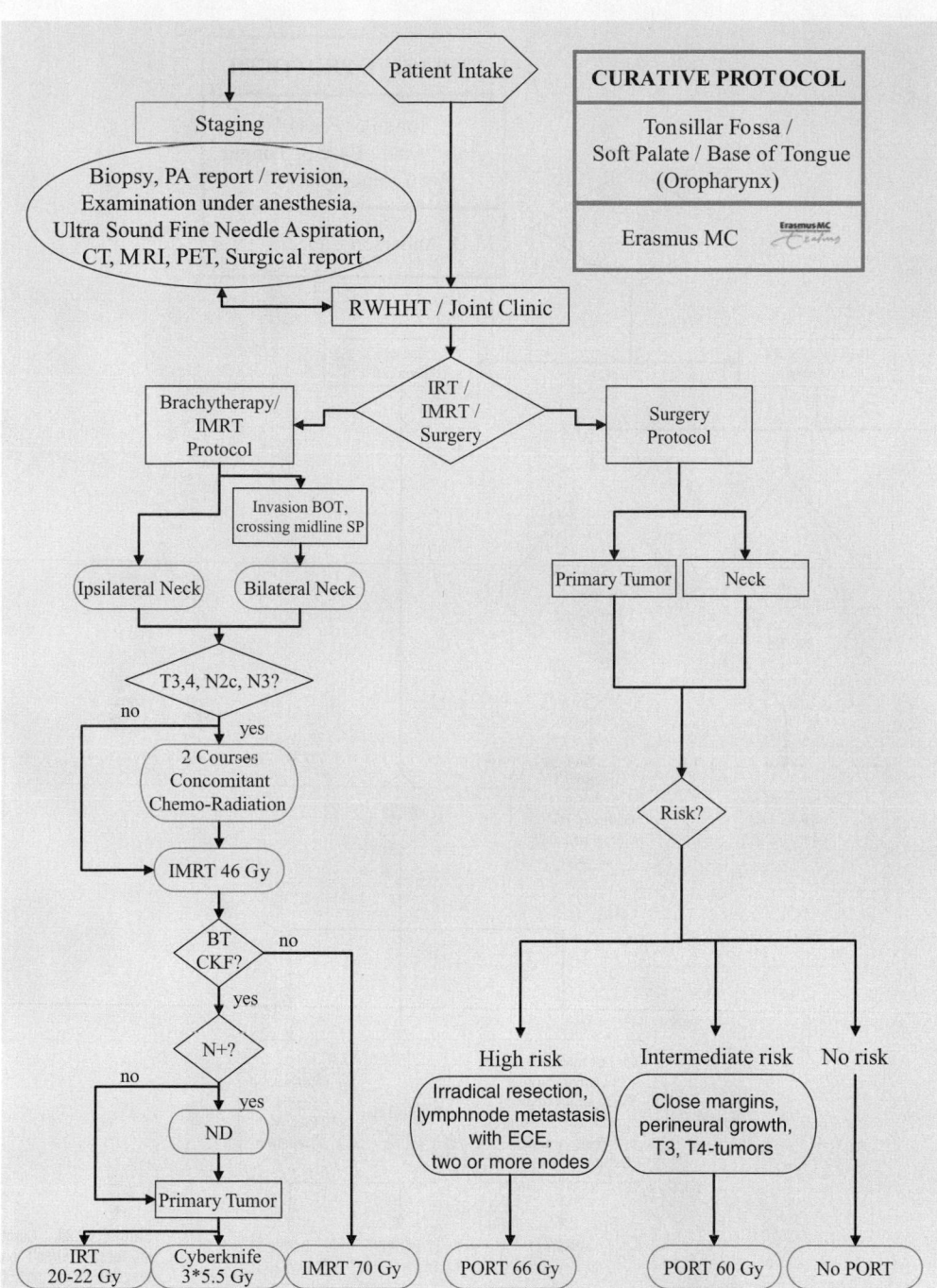

FIGURE 42.19. All curative cases at Erasmus MC are treated by six fractions per week. PORT, postoperative radiation therapy; RWHHT, Rotterdam working party on head and neck tumors; IRT, interstitial radiation therapy; IMRT, intensity modulated radiotherapy; BOT, base of tongue; BT, brachytherapy.

as opposed to the TF and/or SP tumors or the tumors of the BOT. For a short bibliography see references 53,59,63, 83,144,152,191,206,208,242,285,293,295,326.

Treatment Results

Guillamondequi et al. (112) found 28% recurrences after surgery, with salvage in less than one third of the patients. Fein et al. (81) at the University of Florida compared retrospectively once-daily versus twice-daily fractionation. The observed LC rates were 100% versus 100% for the T1 category, 67% versus 92% for the T2 tumors, 43% versus 80% for T3 tumors, and 17% versus 50% for T4 tumors. Meoz-Mendez et al. (207) reported

on a mixed group of patients with hypopharyngeal and pharyngeal wall carcinomas treated in the M.D. Anderson Cancer Center: the LC for T1 was 91%; for T2, 73%; for T3, 61%; and for T4, 37%. Those treated with surgery and PORT or preoperative RT fared better (LC, 75%) as opposed to RT alone (LC, 51%). A study by Marks et al. (194,195) compared preoperative RT with definitive RT. There was no difference in LC, but significantly more grade III/IV complications in the surgery group. Spiro et al. (286), from Memorial Sloan Kettering Cancer Center in New York, reported on 78 patients with posterior wall carcinomas. The cumulative 5-year survival was poor: 32%. Good results, albeit in a small selected series of patients, were obtained with an I125 or Ir192 implant; there was an LC rate of 82% at 5 years

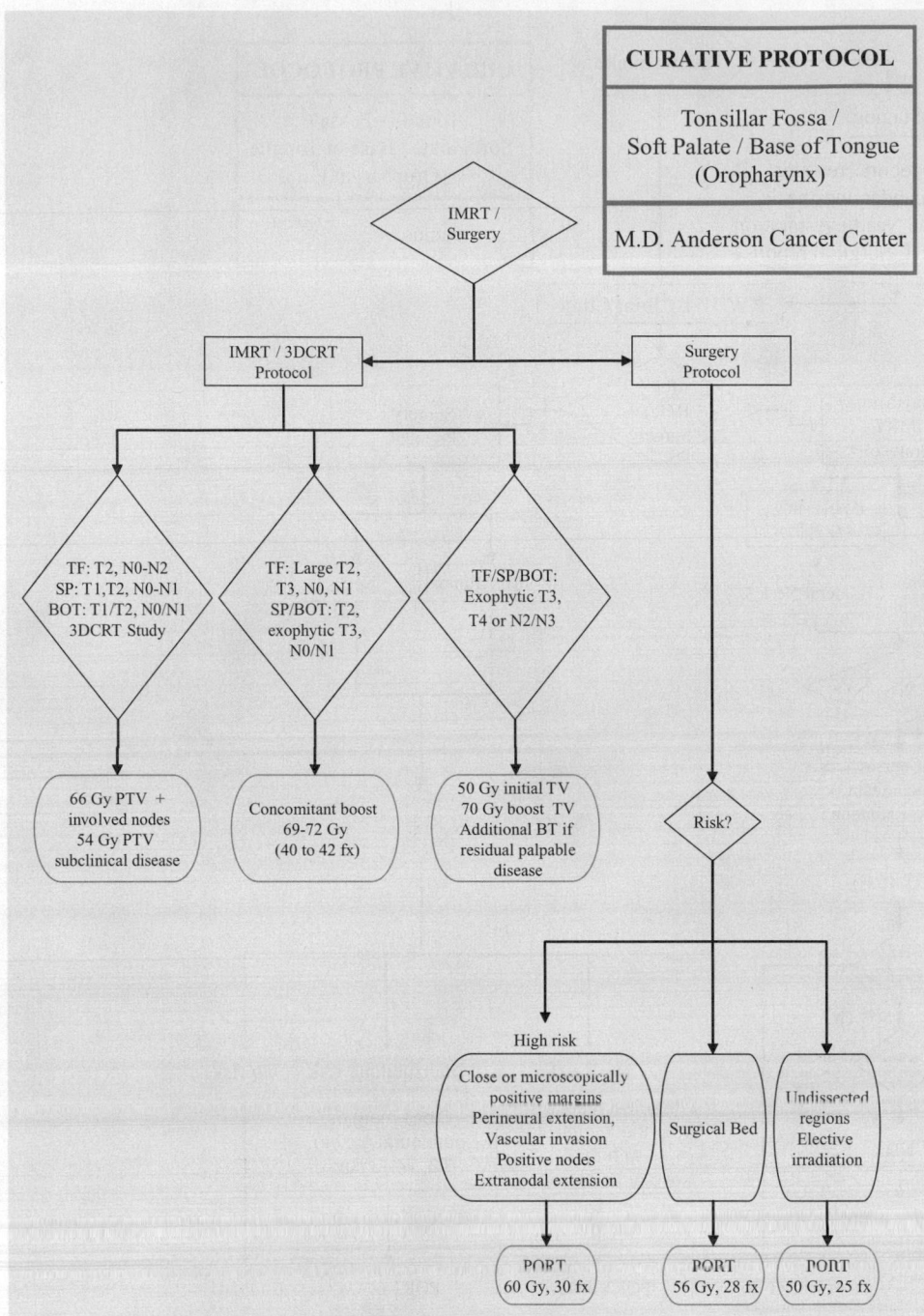

CURATIVE PROTOCOL

Tonsillar Fossa /
Soft Palate / Base of Tongue
(Oropharynx)

M.D. Anderson Cancer Center

IMRT /
Surgery

IMRT / 3DCRT
Protocol

Surgery
Protocol

TF: T2, N0-N2
SP: T1,T2, N0-N1
BOT: T1/T2, N0/N1
3DCRT Study

TF: Large T2,
T3, N0, N1
SP/BOT: T2,
exophytic T3,
N0/N1

TF/SP/BOT:
Exophytic T3,
T4 or N2/N3

66 Gy PTV +
involved nodes
54 Gy PTV
subclinical disease

Concomitant boost
69-72 Gy
(40 to 42 fx)

50 Gy initial TV
70 Gy boost TV
Additional BT if
residual palpable
disease

Risk?

High risk

Close or microscopically
positive margins
Perineural extension,
Vascular invasion
Positive nodes
Extranodal extension

Surgical Bed

Undissected
regions
Elective
irradiation

PORT
60 Gy, 30 fx

PORT
56 Gy, 28 fx

PORT
50 Gy, 25 fx

FIGURE 42.20. Curative protocol for tonsillar fossa (TF)/soft palate (SP) and base of tongue (BOT) in the M.D. Anderson Cancer Center, Houston.

(284). In general, the locoregional outcome and survival is significantly better for the early T1, T2, and T3N0,1 carcinomas as opposed to the (endophytic) T3,T4 and N2,3 tumors. Although RT alone most likely confers less functional impairment than is the case with surgery, surgery followed by PORT remains a valuable treatment option for advanced tumors.

Different surgical approaches have been proposed for the primary tumor (see Chapter 17 in Harrison et al. [126]). A (bilateral) modified neck dissection is also included in the treatment approach of these difficult-to-manage malignant tumors. Posterior pharyngeal wall tumors in particular pose a technical problem when one needs to deliver high doses of definitive radiation to the primary tumor because of the proximity of the spinal cord. Grimard et al. (111) described an

elegant technique for radiating these tumors without compromising the spinal cord tolerance by using two posterior arcs with closure of one jaw beyond the central axis. The initial target volume encompasses the primary tumor and the bilateral neck levels II-V, with the parapharyngeal and retropharyngeal lymphatics inclusive. Finally, results in terms of tumor control, survival, and (severe) complications are summarized in Table 42.15.

Recurrent Disease and Salvage

The management of a locoregional failure in the head and neck remains a formidable challenge. Most recurrences (80%) manifest in the first 2 years following primary treatment. At least 50%

Table 42.15 PHARYNGEAL WALL

First Author	N	Modality	T1/T2 %	T3/T4 %	N0 %	LC T1/T2 5-Yrs %	LC T3/T4 5-Yrs %	DFS 5-Yrs %	Overal S. 5-Yrs %	Severe Complications
Pommier, 1997	14	Brachytherapy	55					37	21	None
Chenal, 1996	55	Radiotherapy/Surgery							38, mean 23 months	
Fein, 1993	9	Radiotherapy				T1:100, T2:92 2 daily fx, 2-yrs	T3:80, T4:50		67	
Mak-Kregar, 1994	8	Radiotherapy/Surgery		100					38	
Spiro, 1990	78	Radiotherapy/Surgery					50		32	
Mendenhall, 1988	75	Radiotherapy/Brachytherapy				T1: 75, T2: 57	T3: 44, T4: 20		II:44, III:19, IVA: 0, IVB: 8	I: 0/2, II:1/16, III:2/22, IVA: 2/14, IVB: 3/20
Hull, 2003	148	Radiotherapy/Surgery	40	59	36	T1:93, T2:82	T3: 59, T4: 50	I: 89, II:88, III: 44, IV: 34	I: 56, II: 52, III: 24, IV: 22	16
Julieron, 2001	77	Surgery+PORT				Local Failure: 11			35	General postoperative: 22
Chang, 1996	74	Radiotherapy				2-yrs; T1:100, T2: 55	2-yrs; T3:31, T4:29	2-yrs; I: 100, II: 85, III: 58, IV: 40	2-yrs; I:75, II: 67, III: 33, IV: 30	
Cooper, 2000	22	Radiotherapy					3-yrs; 73	CSS: 48	3-yrs: 5	
Yoshida, 2004	51	Radiotherapy/Surgery					56			
Meoz-Mendez, 1978	164	Radiotheray	13/56	53/108	69/164	1-yrs; T1: 91, T2: 73	1-yrs; T3: 61, T4: 37			I: 0, II:7, III:15, IV:17

Local control for posterior pharyngeal wall tumors after treatment by radiation therapy and/or surgery.

of patients who die from uncontrolled disease have local and/or regional disease as their sole site of failure. Moreover, the majority (80%) of those who develop distant metastases also have local and/or regional failure. Another, related clinical entity is the management of second primary tumors (about 3% per year [161,220]) occurring in previously irradiated regions. Selected patients with locoregional recurrences can be successfully salvaged with surgery and/or RT. Treatment options are more limited if initial treatment consists of surgery combined with RT or high-dose RT. The average cure rate of these patients has been reported to vary between 30% and 40%, and most failures are due to locoregional relapses. The use of surgery alone as a salvage procedure in case of recurrent BOT cancer was reported by Pradhan et al. (242). In approximately one third of the patients, LC was achieved for the duration of 1 year. Thirty-five patients required a total glossectomy. The role of RT is not widely appreciated as yet, mainly because of concerns about the tolerance of local tissues to reirradiation. In this regard, BT plays a crucial role (high-dose, small volume, rapid dose fall-off) (140,165,197). An equivalent EBRT dose of 60/2 Gy by five fractions per week

is being applied mostly as the reirradiation dose schedule. An important prognostic factor favoring long-term LC is an interval of more than 1 year between the radiation courses. Langlois et al. (165), for example, report on 123 patients treated for recurrent cancer or a new cancer of the tongue or oropharynx, arising in previously irradiated volumes. The actuarial LC rate was 67% at 2 years and 59% at 5 years. Levendag et al. (176) analyzed a 13-year experience with reirradiation. An improvement in LC was observed (50% vs. 29%) for the EBRT plus IRT as opposed to the EBRT-alone series. The improvement in LC was typically not reflected in a survival benefit; that is, an actuarial OS of 20% at 5 years was observed in both series. Mazeron et al. (200) had similar results: actuarial LC was 72% at 2 years and 69% at 4 years. Although LC of the tumor was achieved in the majority of these patients, only 14% remained alive at 5 years. Best results were achieved in lesions of the faucial arch and posterior pharyngeal wall (LC, 100%).

Other ways of applying reirradiation is in an intraoperative setting for residual microscopic disease by means of a silicone flexible intraoperative template (Fig. 42.21). After the dose of 10 Gy (prescribed mostly at 1 cm from the afterloading catheter

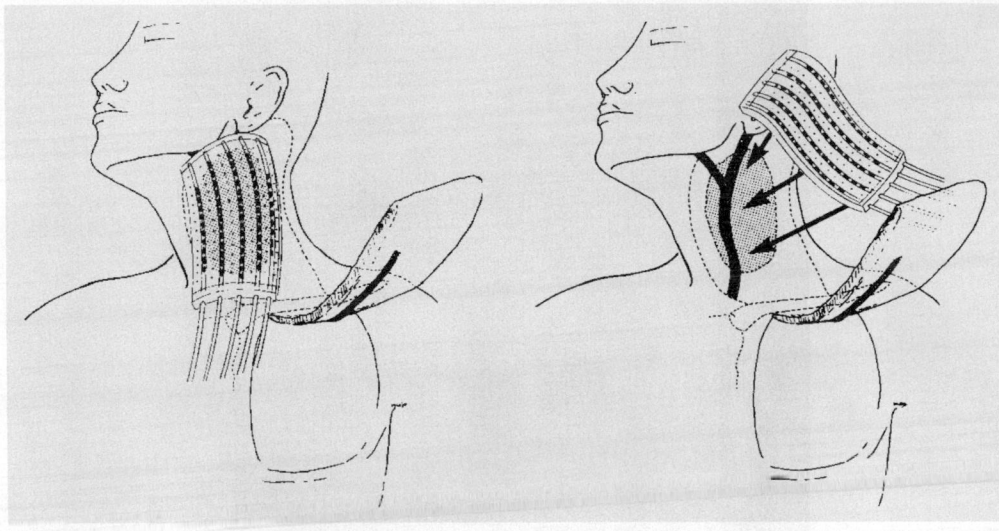

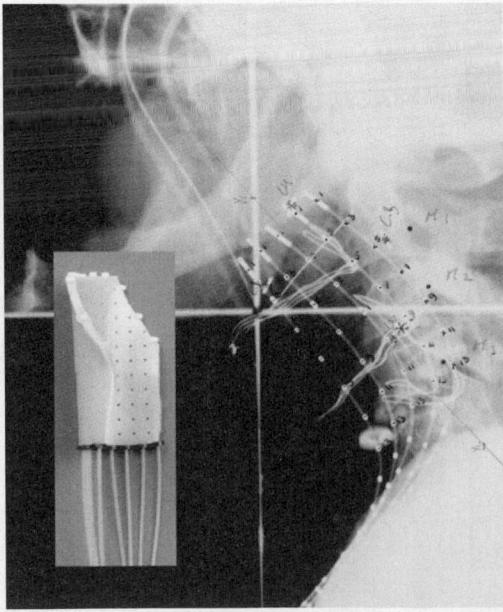

FIGURE 42.21. Top: Drawing showing flexible intraoperative template (FIT) positioned on the tumor bed and a deltopectoral flap used to close the skin defect. **Bottom:** the simulation radiograph of the FIT *in situ* (neck).

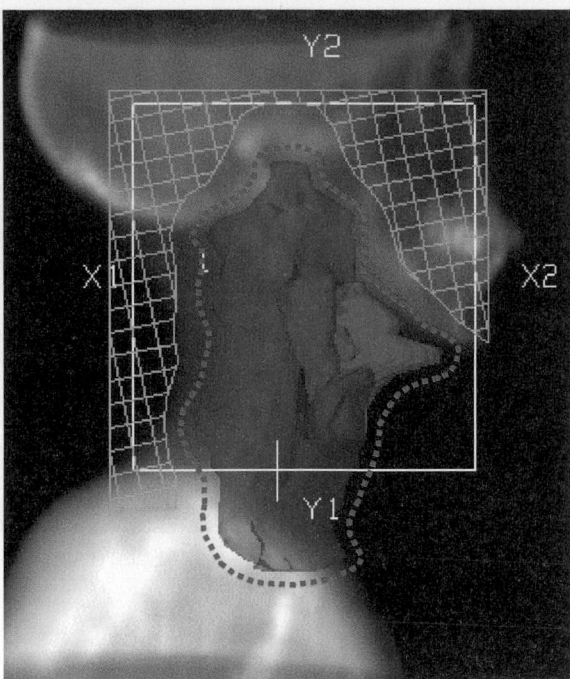 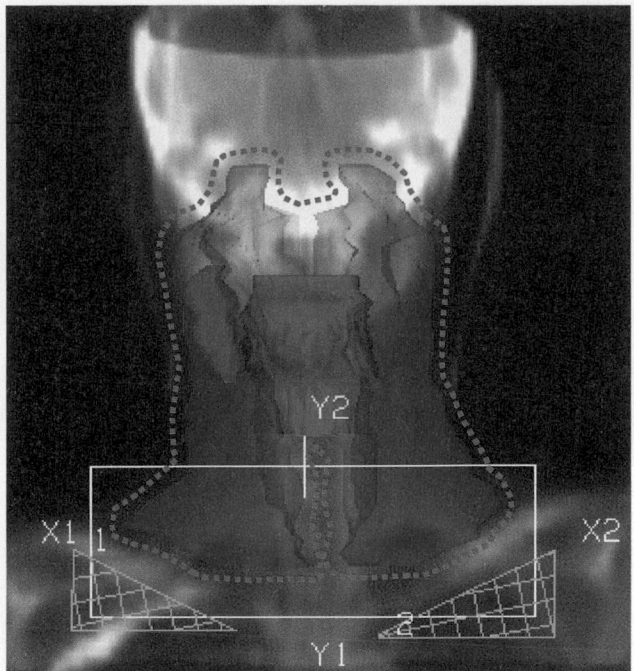

FIGURE 42.22.   Base of tongue tumor, staged T2N2b. Beam's-eye view of conventional parallel-opposed fields of the upper neck. Red dotted line, planning target volume; blue volume, clinical target volume, neck; red volume, primary tumor; magenta volume, lymph nodal volume, levels II and III.

in the flexible intraoperative template) has been delivered, the surgical defect can be closed by a reconstructive procedure using "fresh," that is, donor tissue (e.g., deltopectoral flap) that has not been previously irradiated. The dose is mostly prescribed to a distance of 1 cm (157); subsequently, a course of fractionated EBRT is applied as an outpatient procedure (e.g., 26 × 1.8 Gy). As with any retreatment situation, the complication rate is substantially higher than with primary therapy.

Radiation Therapy Techniques

Conventional Radiation Therapy

Irradiation portals for oropharyngeal cancers should encompass the primary tumor and its local and regional "extensions,"

with a margin for the CTV (approximately 0.7 cm) and for the PTV (approximately 0.5 cm). The concept of regional coverage has been eluded to before extensively. Patients are generally treated in the supine position with bite-block and thermoplastic mask immobilization, with daily treatment of all fields. Neck portals should extend superiorly until C1 for N0, and the base of skull (retrostyloid space) in case of N+ disease. Patient examples (T2N2b BOT tumor and T2N2b TF/SP tumor) with regard to the geometry of portals, treatment techniques used, and dose distributions are shown in Figures 42.22 through 42.33. In the examples presented in Figures 42.22 through 42.26, the primary tumor and both sides of the upper neck are irradiated using a conventional lateral parallel-opposed technique for the upper neck in case of a T2N2b BOT tumor. Both sides of the lower neck are generally irradiated through a single anteroposterior field, sometimes with a midline block. In order to prevent overdose

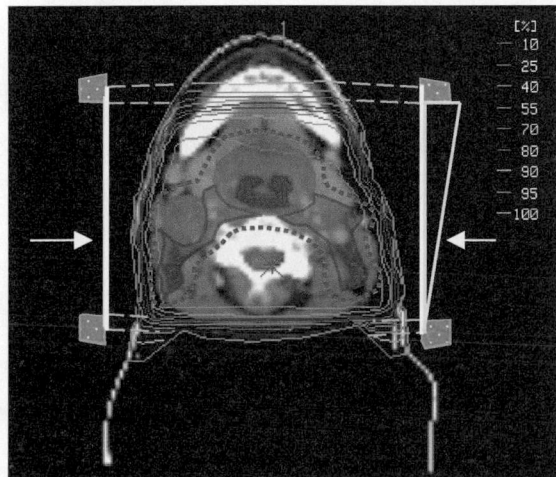 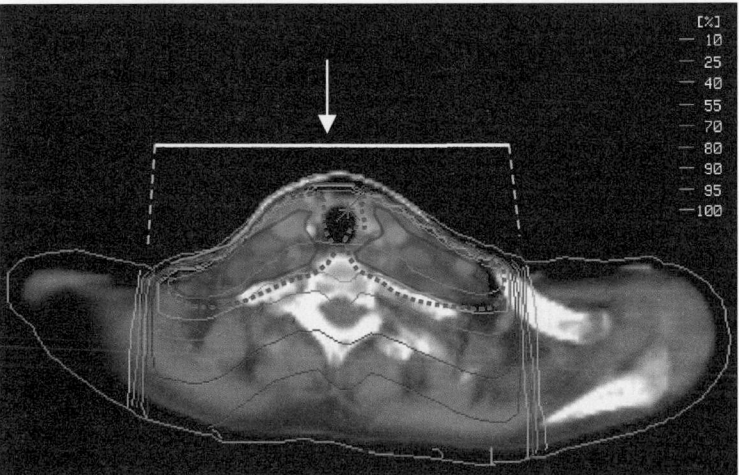

FIGURE 42.23.   See legend for Fig. 42.20. Dose (46/2 Gy) distribution axial computed tomography slice, upper neck and low anterior neck. Dose generally prescribed at 3-cm depth or at a particular point of interest (e.g., in cases of lymph nodes in lower neck). Note that there is no midline block because of potential shielding of tumor extensions.

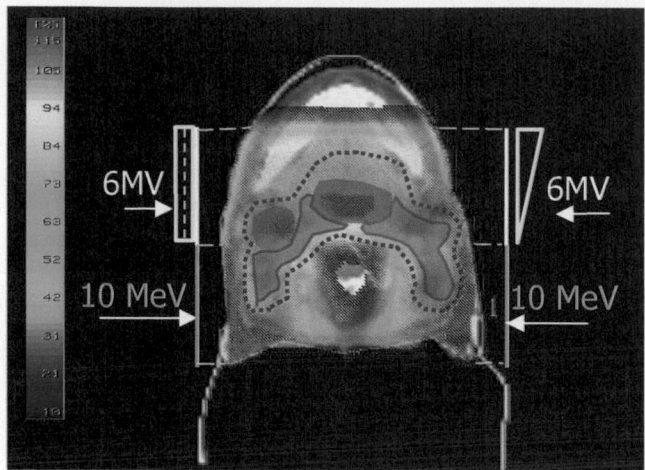

FIGURE 42.24. See legend Figure 42.20. Field configuration and dose distribution boost to primary tumor to total dose of 24/2 Gy using parallel-opposed fields. Note shielding posterior neck (cord); dose in shielded area supplemented by abutted high-energy electron fields (10 MeV).

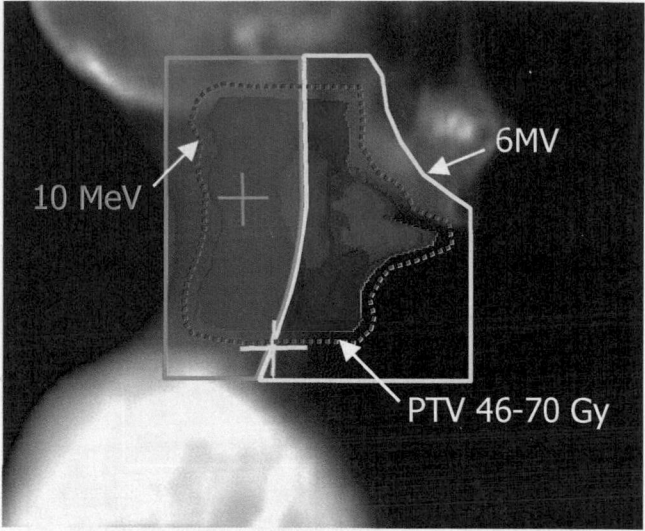

FIGURE 42.25. See legend Figure 42.20. Beam's-eye view treatment of primary tumor and neck node levels II and III (boost). PTV, planning target volume.

at the junction line, a junction zone of 1 cm between the lateral fields and the anteroposterior portals is treated daily in Erasmus MC with maximum or minimum field sizes (the so called slip zone). If appropriate, the midline block shields the larynx and spinal cord. The spinal cord is shielded after administration of 46/2 to 50/2 Gy and if indicated, the posterior cervical triangles are boosted with 10-MeV electrons, therewith sparing the spinal cord. Tissue compensators (wedges) are used to ensure dose homogeneity in the lateral portals and to prevent excessive dose to the supraglottic larynx. After 46/2 Gy with 4- to 6-MV photon beams has been applied, the remaining dose can be delivered with high-energy photons (15 to 18 MV) in order to reduce the dose to the parotids, the mandible, and/or the temporomandibular joints (buildup). The middle ear and inner ear should be carefully shielded posteriorly. Small tumors of the TF, anterior tonsillar pillar, and retromolar trigone can be treated by ipsilateral wedged anterior and posterior fields or with BT.

With the wedge technique, the dose to the mandible is high, and a greater incidence of complications (e.g., soft tissue necrosis and osteonecrosis of the mandible) can be anticipated. Limiting irradiation to the ipsilateral neck reduces the probability of xerostomia (18). This approach was confirmed by O'Sullivan and Grice (225), who reported a 3-year tumor control rate of 77% and cause-specific survival rate of 76% in 228 patients with carcinoma of the tonsillar region treated with ipsilateral-only RT techniques (oblique wedge pair arrangement). Contralateral neck failure was observed in only eight patients (3.5%). Levendag et al. had similar observations (Fig. 42.18). Contralateral failure in the untreated neck was only 3% (175).

The intraoral cone technique, using orthovoltage or electrons, has been used selectively in the treatment of patients with small lesions. Adequate tumor coverage is aided by CT-based treatment planning (with or without MRI fusion); moreover,

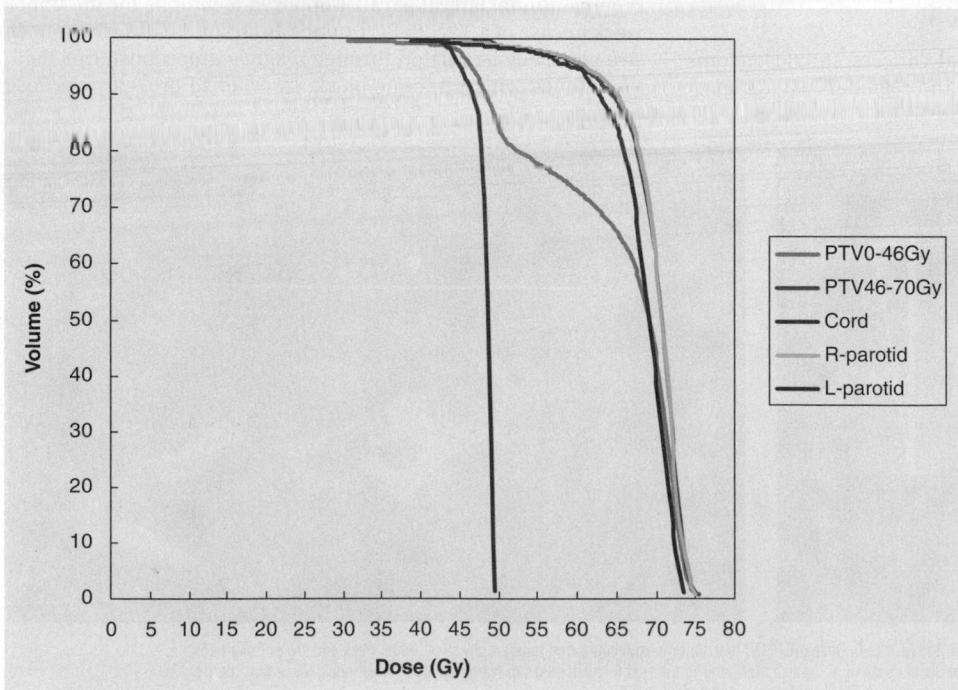

FIGURE 42.26. Cumulative dose volume histograms of base of tongue tumor treated to a cumulative dose of 70/2 Gy. See also legend for Figures 42.20 and 42.23. PTV, planning target volume.

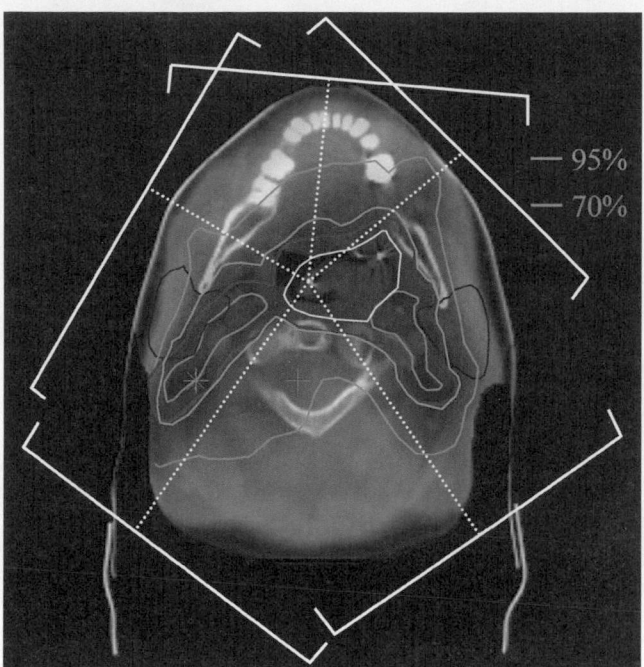

FIGURE 42.27. Dose distribution (color wash) tonsillar fossa and soft palate tumor, staged to T2N2b for first series of radiation therapy (46/2 Gy). Upper neck and primary tumor irradiated using a five-field intensity-modulated radiation therapy (IMRT) technique. Clinical target volume consists of primary tumor and neck levels I–V (ipsilateral, left) and neck levels II–IV (contralateral, right). Dose prescribed according International Commission on Radiation Units and Measurements Report 50 guidelines. Field configuration: upper neck IMRT (this figure), lower neck anteroposterior portal (Fig. 42.33). Equal sparing of both parotid glands was achieved.

at the present time it is reasonable to consider CT-based treatment planning for head and neck cancer more or less obligatory. Many of the previously described techniques have therefore substantially changed since the introduction of new and innovative technology, such as IMRT, three-dimensional confor-

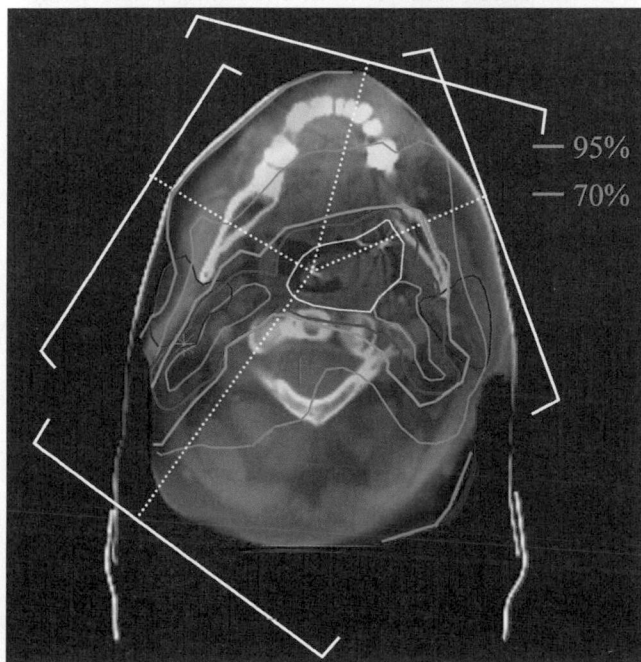

FIGURE 42.28. See legend for Figure 42.27. In order to better spare the contralateral parotid gland, relaxation of the ipsilateral parotid constraint is pursued and an asymmetric four-field intensity-modulated radiation therapy technique was implemented. Dose is prescribed to International Commission on Radiation Units and Measurements Report 50 guidelines. For abutted low anterior neck portal, see Figure 42.33.

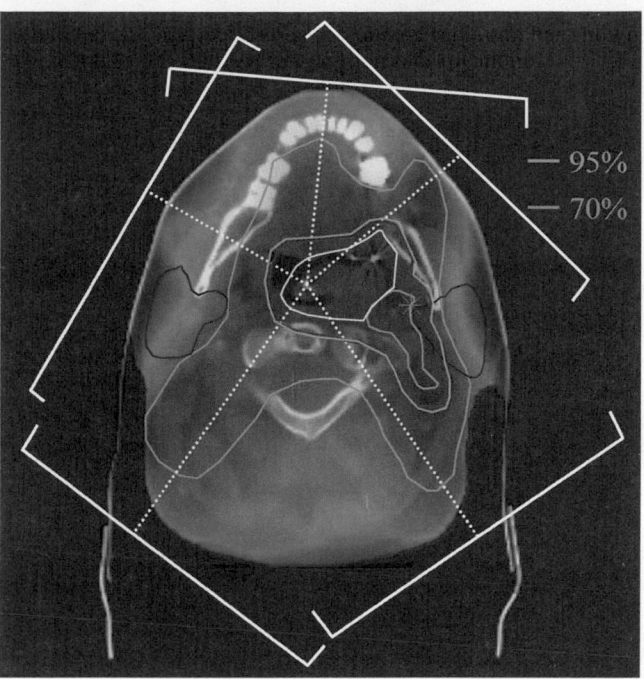

FIGURE 42.29. See legend for Figure 42.27. In order to improve sparing of contralateral parotid gland, contralateral cranial border of upper neck (level II) is lowered by 1 cm. A five-field intensity-modulated radiation therapy technique was used. For abutted low anterior neck portal, see Figure 42.33.

mal radiation therapy, and cone beam CT (see also dedicated section XIII on IMRT). Figures 42.27 through 42.33 represent a TF and SP tumor treated by IMRT techniques. The figures depict adequate target coverage and maximum effort to spare major salivary glands. We have compared, for bilateral irradiation, bilateral sparing of parotid glands (Fig. 42.27), as opposed to maximum sparing of contralateral parotid glands (Fig. 42.28), or reducing CTV contralateral side (Fig. 42.29). The corresponding dose-volume histograms are depicted in Figures 42.30 to 42.32. Also, using this technology, new concepts can be incorporated in future treatment protocols. For example, Thorstad et al. (298) from M.D. Anderson Cancer Center, report favorable results for SCC of the oropharynx treated with IMRT. Multivariate analysis showed that the GTV (primary tumor $\pm$ nodes) became an independent risk factor determining locoregional control (GTV <50 mL LC $\pm$ 90% vs. GTV >50 mL LC $\pm$ 20%; p <.0001). From this type of data, the authors concluded that selecting "high-volume" patients for aggressive treatment protocols might be warranted. For more details, see IMRT section.

Dose and Fractionation Primary Sites in Oropharynx

In general for T1–2 lesions, doses of 66 to 70 Gy in 6.5 to 7 weeks with conventional fractionation (1.8 to 2.0 Gy per fraction daily, six fractions per week) are recommended for definitive radiotherapy. However, for T3–4 oropharyngeal cancers, several studies have demonstrated better locoregional control when either accelerated or hyperfractionated regimens are used with concurrent CHT (41,88,91,155). (For details on altered fractionation, see section Chemotherapy, Targeted Therapy, and Altered Fractionation Regimens). For locally advanced lesions in the head and neck, in recent years the addition of concurrent CHT to either conventional or altered fractionated radiation has shown to be beneficial compared to radiation therapy alone.

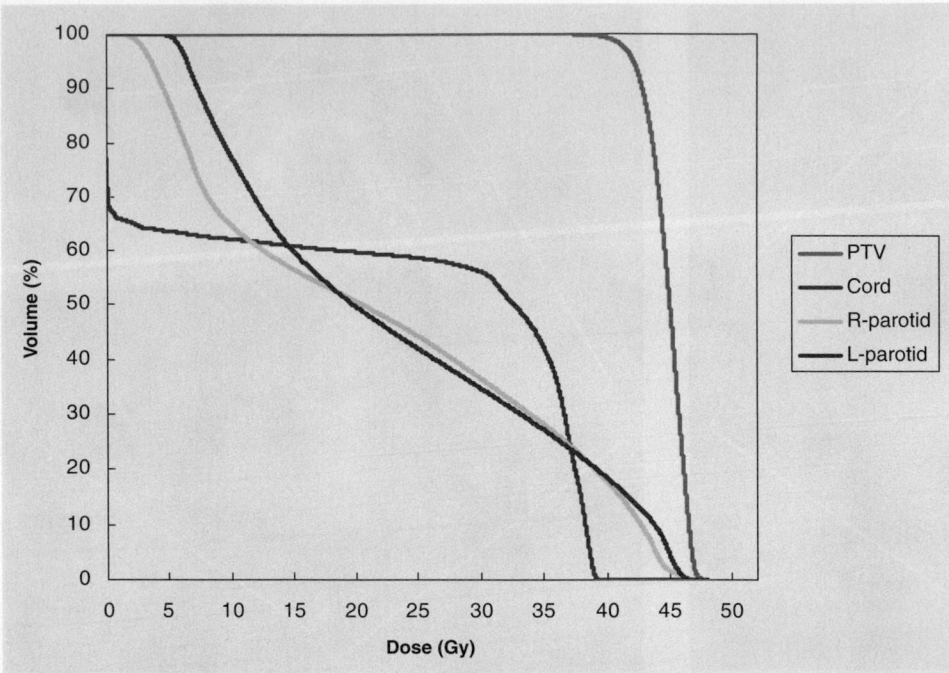

FIGURE 42.30. Dose-volume histograms corresponding to Figure 42.27. Note: mean dose left parotid gland, 23.2 Gy; mean dose right parotid gland, 22.0 Gy. PTV, planning target volume.

Side Effects of Conventional Treatment Techniques

Normal Tissue Toxicity Profile—Acute Effects

The major sequelae of RT can be divided into acute and chronic side effects. They are multifactorial. The potential acute effects on the oral cavity and pharynx after approximately 1 to 3 weeks of RT include mucositis (ulcer), sore throat, loss of taste, and xerostomia (if any of the major salivary glands are in the treatment portal). Approximately 5% of patients develop sialadenitis within 24 hours of the first irradiation treatment, but this usu-

ally resolves within 24 to 48 hours. The skin experiences erythema, peeling, and pigmentation. If the capacity of the basal cell layer to repopulate the epidermis is overwhelmed, the result is moist desquamation. Likewise, epilation of hair-bearing areas with accompanying loss of sweat and sebaceous gland function occurs.

Normal Tissue Toxicity Profile—Late Effects

The late effects after definitive RT can include xerostomia, dental caries, altered sense of taste, swallowing problems, dysphagia, altered quality of voice, lymphedema, hypothyroidism,

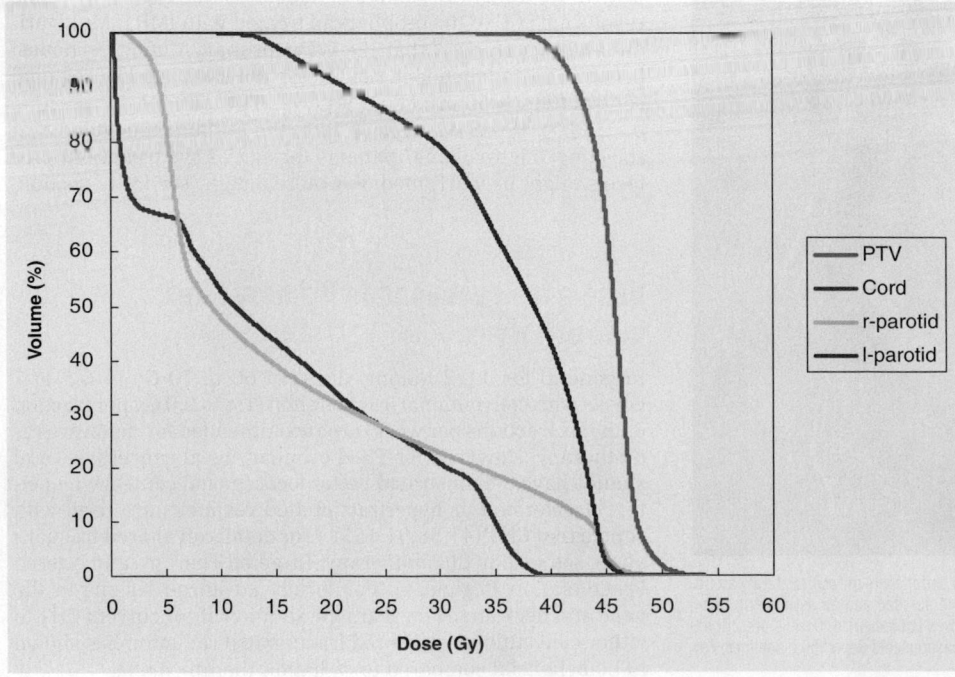

FIGURE 42.31. Dose-volume histograms corresponding to Figure 42.28. Note: mean dose left parotid gland, 34.8 Gy; however, mean dose right (contralateral) parotid gland (16.9 Gy) improved by about 5 Gy. PTV, planning target volume.

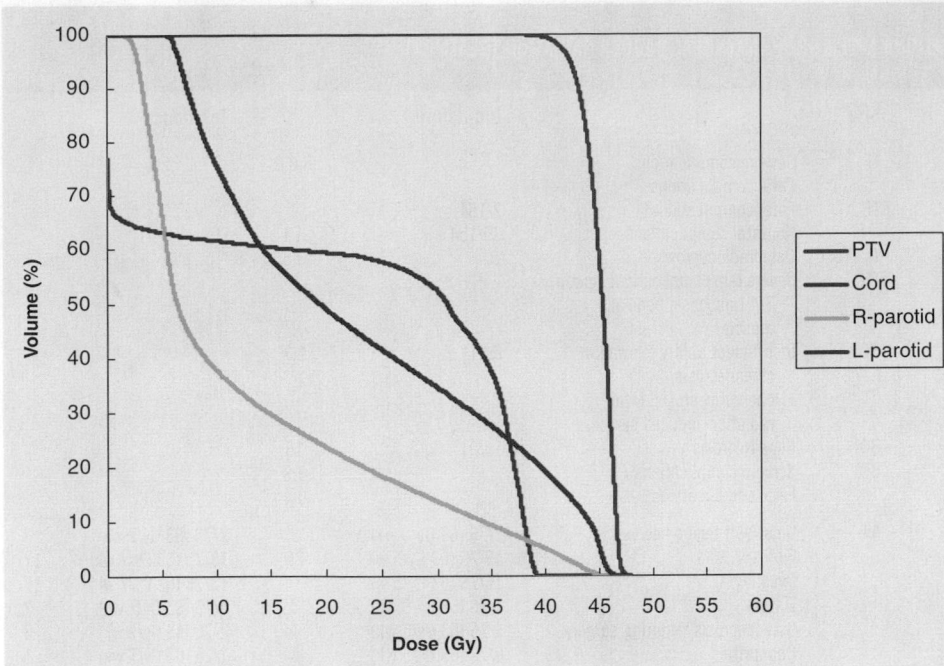

Clinical Radiation Oncology

FIGURE 42.32. Dose-volume histograms corresponding to Figure 42.29. Note: mean dose left parotid gland, 23.0 Gy; mean dose right (contralateral) parotid gland, 12.7 Gy. A significant amount of sparing was obtained by lowering the cranial border of the right neck. PTV, planning target volume.

epilation, trismus, cervical fibrosis, atrophy of the mucosa and skin, as well as soft tissue and bone necrosis. In a Rotterdam series on oropharyngeal tumors 25% grade III/IV mucositis ("pinpoint ulcer," 47/190) and 10% trismus (19/190) were reported. In the process of osteoradionecrosis, radiation is believed to exert an avascular effect on tissues and epithelia that are thinner and more susceptible to injury. The process usually starts with ulceration of soft tissues, which can progress to bone exposure. For refractory cases, hyperbaric oxygen treatment has been advocated. Factors that can influence osteoradionecrosis include elective dental extraction after RT and treatment of tumors near bone. In the modern era, osteonecrosis should be an uncommon event (<5%) (17). Technique could also play a role, the BT nonlooping technique being associated with a higher reported injury rate than the looping technique (124,191). Of these late side effects, xerostomia is the most prominent (317), and will be discussed in more detail in the next paragraph. Dysphagia and trismus, although clinically important to prevent, are still somewhat underscored. These are given a prominent place in the discussion involving quality of life (QOL) in the section Performance Status Scale, Socioeconomic Outcomes, and Quality of Life. Finally, clinical reports on late side effects are summarized data in Table 42.16 (9,99,121,145,175,184,203,226,227,234,285,320).

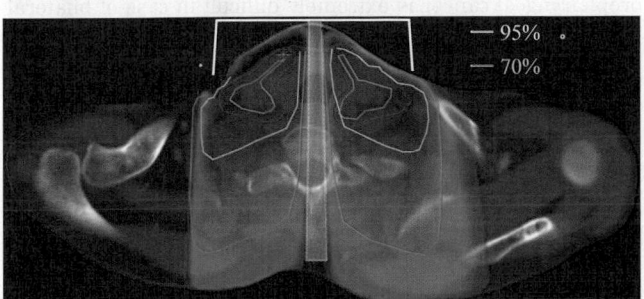

FIGURE 42.33. Low anterior neck dose distribution; dose generally prescribed at 3-cm depth or at a particular point of interest in the neck (e.g., in cases of lymph nodes in lower neck). Note: midline block sparing (e.g., larynx).

Xerostomia

Given the way most patients were treated in the (recent) past, frequently using nonsparing parallel-opposed techniques, xerostomia seems to be the overriding side effect. Roesink, et al. from the Utrecht Medical Center reported important observations on the dry mouth syndrome, in particular related to the dose-effect relationship of the major salivary glands (Fig. 42.34). Irradiation of the salivary glands is obviously associated with loss of function, quantitatively and qualitatively, thus among other things resulting in a reduction in salivary flow and consequently dryness of the mouth. Moderate-to-severe xerostomia occurs in more than 75% of patients treated with conventional lateral beam arrangements. The best definition for objective parotid gland toxicity appeared to be reduction of stimulated output to <25% of the preradiotherapy output (260). Two dose-response curves for stimulated parotid saliva flow rates obtained from relatively large patient groups are available (76,259) (Fig. 42.34). Both studies conclude that the mean dose to the parotid gland best predicts its function after radiotherapy. The steepness of the dose-response curve and the TD$_{50}$ value at 1 year after irradiation differ. However, we can conclude from these studies that it is rather safe, in terms of preservation of stimulated parotid gland function, to have a mean parotid gland dose of less than 25 Gy. When a mean dose is reached above 50 Gy, nearly all patients will have a severe decrease in parotid flow rate.

It is generally accepted that IMRT is a valuable tool for reducing the dose to the parotid gland. Several studies report on salivary flow after IMRT for oropharyngeal tumors. However, clinical studies that objectively demonstrate and quantify the advantages of IMRT compared with conventional beam arrangements are scarce. Chao et al. (49) found a correlation of the parotid flow ratio with the mean parotid dose, and a lower mean parotid dose in 27 IMRT patients compared with 14 patients treated conventionally. IMRT versus conventional treatment, however, did not independently influence the functional outcome of the salivary glands in this study. Roesink (259,260) and Terhaard et al. (297) prospectively evaluated a total of 56 patients with oropharyngeal cancer. Of these, 26 received conventional radiotherapy and 30 patients were treated with IMRT. The mean dose to the parotid glands was 48.1 Gy for

Table 42.16 LATE COMPLICATIONS AFTER OROPHARYNGEAL CANCER RADIATION TREATMENT

	N	First Author	Site		Incidence	%	Incidence	%
External Beam Radiotherapy	2308	Parsons, 2002	TF	Servere complications Fatal complications		6 0.8		
	154	Perez, 1998	TF	Fatal complications	2/154	1		
				Nonfatal complications	30/154	19		
	178	Jackson, 1999	TF	Osteoradionecrosis		3.5		
	676	Withers, 1995	TF	Severe late complications, grade 3/4 (mucossa, bone and muscle)				
	217	Mendenhall, 2000	BOT	Insufficient ability to swallow, osteonecrosis, chondronecrosis, fatal radiation-induced sarcoma	8/217	3.7		
	91	Spanos, 1976	BOT	Bone Necrosis	15/91	16		
	842	Parsons, 2002	BOT	Servere complications Fatal complications		3.8 0.4		
Surgery + PORT	151	Ang et al, 2001	All	Ulcer/soft tissue necrosis	2/76 (63 Gy/5 wk)	3	2/75 (63 Gy/7 wk)	3
				Fibrosis	19/76 (63 Gy/5 wk)	25	13/75 (63 Gy/7 wk)	17
				Dysphagia	16/76 (63 Gy/5 wk)	21	13/75 (63 Gy/7 wk)	17
				Fistula	2/76 (63 Gy/5 wk)	3	5/75 (63 Gy/7 wk)	7
				Osteonecrosis requiring surgery	1/76 (63 Gy/5 wk)	1	2/75 (63 Gy/7 wk)	3
				Chondritis	0/76 (63 Gy/5 wk)	0	1/75 (63 Gy/7 wk)	1
	86	Levendag, 2004	All	Late effect: Mucosa	6/86	7		
				Late effect: Salivary glands	2/86	2		
				Late effect: Dysphagia	14/86	16		
				Late effect: Pain	9/86	10		
				Late effect: Trismus	18/86	21		
	616	Parsons, 2002	TF	Servere complications		23		
				Fatal complications		3.2		
	86	Perez, 1998	TF	Fatal complications	2/86	2		
				Nonfatal complications	46/86	53		
	17	Machtay, 1997	BOT	Gastrostomy and/or tracheostomy	5/17	29.4		
				Osteoradionerosis/soft-tissue necrosis	0/17	0		
				Grade 3 trismus	1/17	5.9		
				Facial edema	1/17	5.9		
	407	Parsons, 2002	BOT	Severe complications		32		
				Fatal complications		3.5		
Brachytherapy	104	Levendag, 2004	All	Late effect: Mucosa	41/104	39		
				Late effect: Salivary glands	6/104	6		
				Late effect: Dysphagia	21/104	20		
				Late effect: Pain	21/104	20		
				Late effect: Trismus	1/104	1		
	68	Harrison, 1998	BOT	Fatal complications		3		
	41	Gibbs, 2003	BOT	Soft-tissue necrosis/ulceration	3/41	7.3		
				Osteoradionecrosis	2/41	4.8		
				Gastrostomy	1/41	2.4		
				Sarcoma	1/41	2.4		

the conventional treatment and 33.7 Gy for IMRT. As a result, 6 weeks after treatment the number of parotid complications was significantly lower after IMRT (55%) than after conventional radiotherapy (87%).

There are several studies using toxicity scoring systems instead of saliva measurements. Eisbruch et al. report on parotid function after conformal radiotherapy and IMRT (76). In a matched case control study with a low number of patients treated with standard radiotherapy, the QOL scores of patients treated with IMRT improved over time after irradiation, and no improvement was seen in patients treated with standard radiotherapy (144). In the studies of Chao et al. (50), the dosimetric advantage of IMRT compared with conventional techniques did translate into a significant reduction of late salivary toxicity in patients with oropharyngeal carcinoma. One has to keep in mind that the submandibular glands also play a major role in producing saliva: in resting state, 70% of the saliva production is believed to be generated by the submandibular glands. The submandibular glands as well as the minor salivary glands are

given more attention in clinical research at the present time, but much research on role of these structures still has to be performed. However, sparing of the submandibular gland in oropharyngeal cancer is extremely difficult in case of bilateral treatment of the neck. One possible future avenue is to routinely transfer the submandibular gland ventrally in the contralateral node-negative neck.

Performance Scale Status, Socioeconomic Outcomes, and Quality of Life

Performance Status Scale and Socioeconomic Outcome

A great deal of clinical interest and research is devoted at the present time to (functional) QOL issues, in particular after

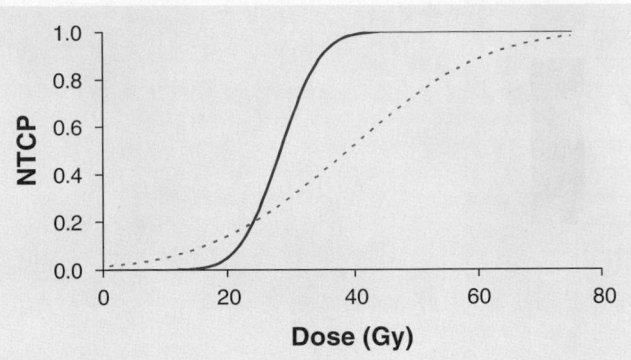

FIGURE 42.34. Dose-effect relationship, xerostomia from observations by Roesink et al. (See text for details.) NTCP, normal tissue control probability.

treatment with interstitial RT (237,258). This seems relevant, in particular because of the great variation in treatment modalities and treatment schemes used in head and neck cancer with otherwise similar tumor control and survival outcome (253). The acute toxicity of concurrent chemoradiation is significant. However, because of organ preservation, according to an article by Nguyen et al. (217), patients may achieve a better QOL after chemoradiation compared with conventional use of surgery and PORT. Measurement instruments, such as validated questionnaires for QOL, are still evolving but are becoming a routine part of (clinical) research protocols. One such set of evaluation tools frequently used in head and neck cancer is the Performance Status Scale (PSS), as designed by List et al. (179,180). The system yields scores reflecting patients' ability to eat in public, understandability of patient's speech, and normalcy of diet. The scale has been validated; the best possible score is 100 (normal). Harrison et al. (125) retrospectively examined patients with SCC of the BOT who were treated with RT or surgery, comparing QOL and functional outcome using PSS. Patients treated with RT had consistently better performance status and QOL scores and no difference was observed in all three functional PSS (eat in public, understandability of patient's speech, and normalcy of diet) scores, for early and for the more locally advanced tumors (p = .84). For surgery, the PSS deteriorated significantly when comparing T1 and T2 versus T3 and T4 (p = 0.0014). Pol et al. (240) studied retrospectively similar type of patients; that is, locally advanced T3/T4 BOT cancer treated by surgery plus PORT or EBRT plus HDR-IRT. The authors concluded that for all PSS, the patients scored better in functional QOL when treated by RT as opposed to surgery (p = N.S.). The difference in functional outcome could help clinical investigators in the future as to which treatment is to be preferred per tumor site. In fact, the findings also illustrate the preference of patients for organ-preservation therapy in general. Harrison et al. (123) also reported that at a median follow-up of 5 years, patients' annual incomes were similar to those at presentation, and the great majority of patients were still in full-time work. Nijdam and Levendag (218) studied the total hospital costs of TF and/or SP tumors treated by either IMRT plus BT boost with or without neck dissection versus surgery plus PORT (IMRT). Excellent locoregional tumor control (at 5 years, ±85%) was observed for either combined modality approach. Of particular interest is that the weighted mean cost for BT was significantly less as opposed to surgery: $18,001 versus $28,130. The main denominator in the excessive costs for surgery in this protocol is the number of days of clinical admission to the hospital. Table 42.17 summarizes the costs for the different treatment options in the current Erasmus MC protocol.

Health-Related Quality of Life

Several questionnaires have been developed to assess health-related quality of life (HRQOL) for head and neck cancer patients (27,30,46,314). Each of the side effects can have a different impact on the HRQOL (28,29,105,106,115,116), varying from changes of speech and voice quality to impact on well-being and HRQOL in a broader sense. Interestingly, Nordgren et al. (220,221) evaluated the HRQOL of patients with pharyngeal carcinoma at diagnosis and after 1 and 5 years in a prospective multicenter study. Again, the HRQOL at diagnosis seems to be an important factor for the prognosis of both HRQOL over time and survival.

Trismus and Quality of Life

Trismus, severely restricted mouth opening, is a common problem in head and neck oncology. According to Dijkstra et al. (67,68), it is present at the time of diagnosis in approximately 2% of patients due to tumor growth; in tumors originating from or in the parapharyngeal space it is even more frequent (55%). Additionally, another 8% increase in trismus is due to treatment per se, be it surgery or RT (312). One of the reasons for this variation in reporting is the lack of uniform criteria. Dijkstra et al. proposed to use as a cut-off point for mouth opening 35 mm, irrespective of dental status, but they acknowledge that differences per subgroup may exist. The paired mastication apparatus facilitates opening of the mouth; it consists of the processes coronoideus and the condyle of the mandible, as well as the muscles responsible for jaw movement. The functionality of this muscular compartment (95) can be summarized as follows: *depression* (lateral pterygoid, gravity), *elevation* (temporalis, masseter and medial pterygoid), *protrusion* (lateral pterygoid, masseter, temporalis), *retraction* (posterior fibers temporalis, deep fibers masseter), and *lateral* movement (contralateral lateral pterygoid, bilateral temporalis). Surgery and RT may induce trismus by causing fibrosis of one of the aforementioned muscles. Fibrosis might significantly impact QOL of the patient

Table 42:17	COSTS OF DIFFERENT TREATMENT MODALITIES USED ACCORDING TO ERASMUS MC PROTOCOL FOR OROPHARYNGEAL CANCER		
	Mean Costs BT (weighted # patients)	**Mean Costs S** (weighted # patients)	**Mean Costs EBRT** (weighted # patients)
Treatment	$13,466	$24,219	$12,502
Follow-up	$649	$607	$482
(Treatment of) Relapse and/or Metastases	$2,848	$1,897	$4,577
Complications	$1,038	$1,407	$3,582[a]
Mean costs total group	$18,001	$28,130	$21,143

Mean costs all groups, weighted for by number of patients
[a]Only two patients with significant late side effects needing long lasting treatments.

Right temporalis muscle		Left Coronoid process	
Left temporalis muscle		Right Mandibular condyl	
Right lateral pterygoid muscle		Left Mandibular condyl	
Right medial pterygoid muscle		Right parotid gland superficial lobe	
Left lateral pterygoid muscle		Left parotid gland superficial lobe	
Left medial pterygoid muscle		Right parotid gland deep lobe	
Right masseter muscle		Left parotid gland deep lobe	
Left masseter muscle		Oral mucosa	
Right Coronoid process			

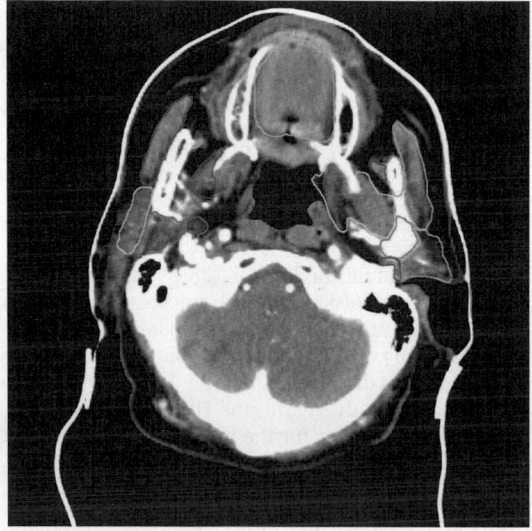

FIGURE 42.35. Paired mastication apparatus with structures of relevance depicted on axial computed tomography slice. See text for details.

as it can affect the *phonation, nutritional status*, and *dental hygiene* of the patient (248). The development of some of these late effects typically depend on factors like previous treatment, total dose, fractionation, irradiated volume, and treatment techniques. Dijkstra reported mandibular function impairments in 18% of 89 patients with cancers in the oral cavity and oropharynx. In the Rotterdam series, the incidence was only 1% for the treatment group EBRT plus BT; for the surgery plus PORT series it amounted to 21% (67).

Ways to counteract this often long-lasting problem of trismus are mechanical appliances to reduce the severity of fibrosis (161), hyperbaric oxygen (156), pentoxifylline (54,312), surgical corrective measures (48), and IMRT. Figure 42.35 depicts an axial CT slice on which the relevant muscles for jaw movement are delineated, the processes coronoideus and condyle of the mandible inclusive. One may decrease the dose to the masseter muscle significantly with IMRT by putting a constraint on the masseter muscle (Fig. 42.36).

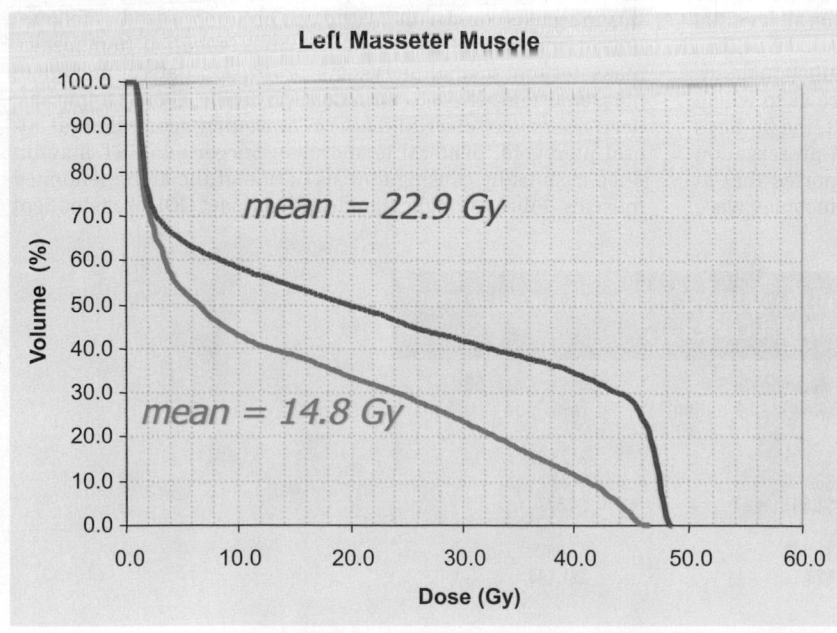

FIGURE 42.36. Dose-volume histograms showing reduction in mean dose to masseter muscle, with or without constraint (in masseter muscle), when using intensity-modulated radiation therapy techniques.

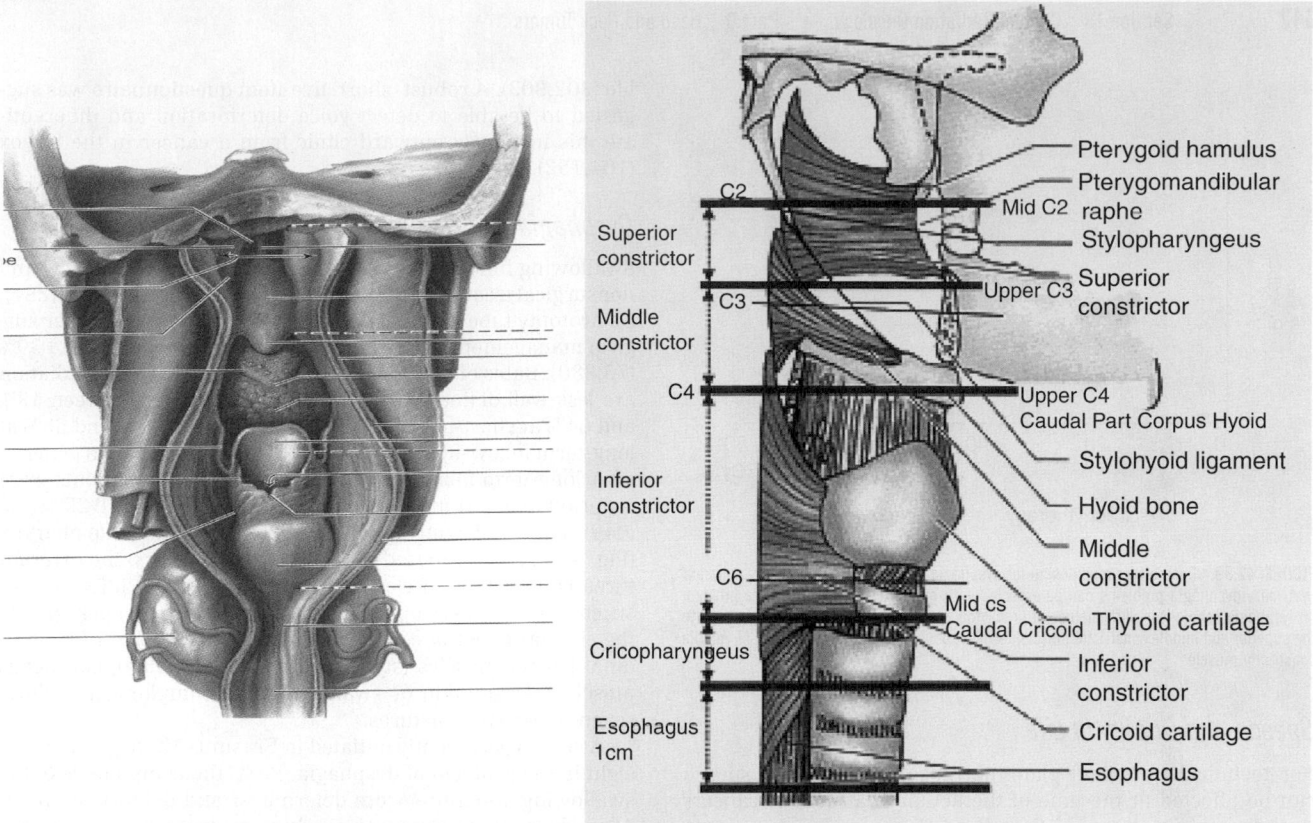

FIGURE 42.37. Anatomy of swallowing apparatus. See text for details on dysphagia. (From Moore KL, Dalley AF. *Clinically oriented anatomy,* 4th ed. Iphia: Lippincott Williams & Wilkins; 1999:1051.)

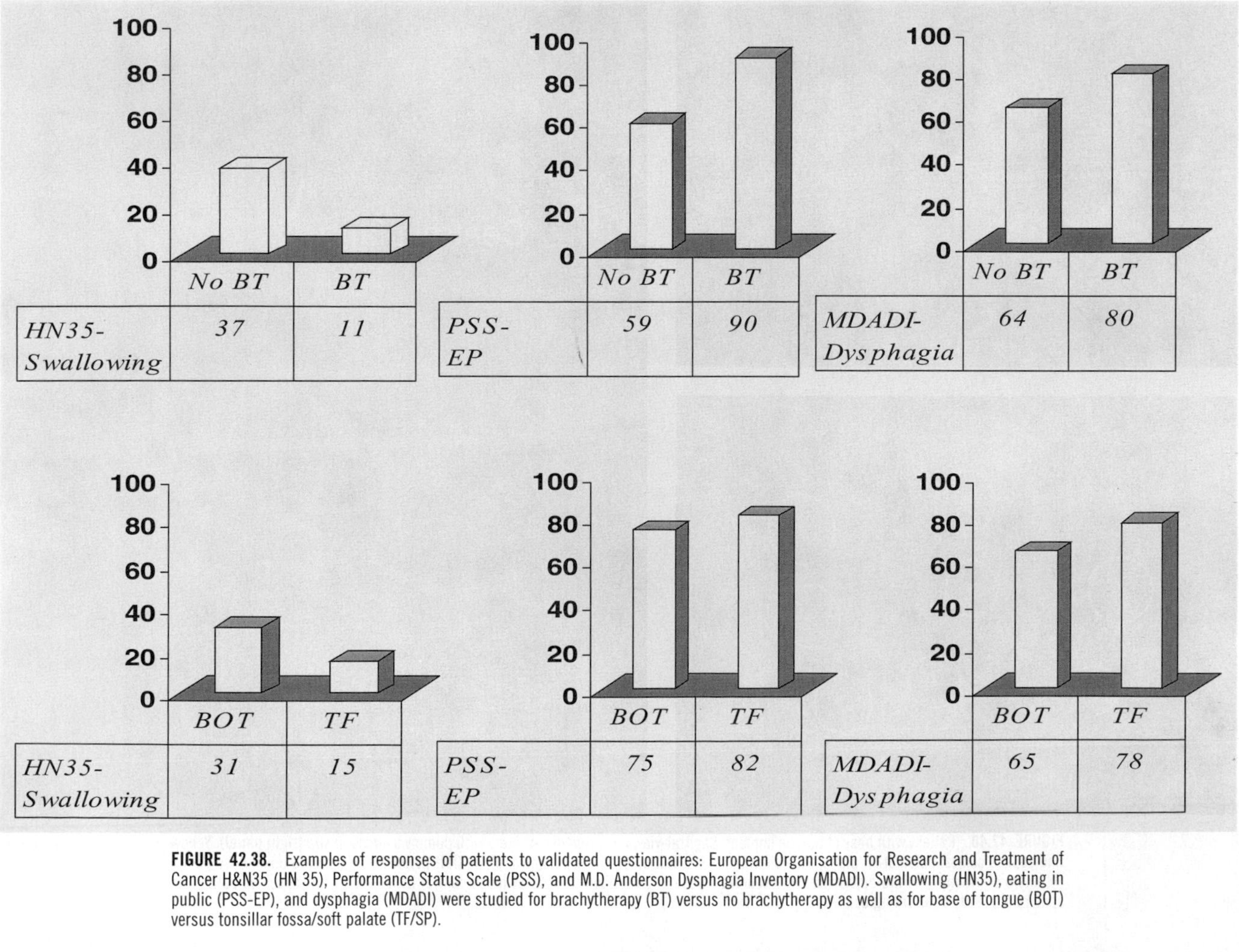

	No BT	BT
HN35-Swallowing	37	11

	No BT	BT
PSS-EP	59	90

	No BT	BT
MDADI-Dysphagia	64	80

	BOT	TF
HN35-Swallowing	31	15

	BOT	TF
PSS-EP	75	82

	BOT	TF
MDADI-Dysphagia	65	78

FIGURE 42.38. Examples of responses of patients to validated questionnaires: European Organisation for Research and Treatment of Cancer H&N35 (HN 35), Performance Status Scale (PSS), and M.D. Anderson Dysphagia Inventory (MDADI). Swallowing (HN35), eating in public (PSS-EP), and dysphagia (MDADI) were studied for brachytherapy (BT) versus no brachytherapy as well as for base of tongue (BOT) versus tonsillar fossa/soft palate (TF/SP).

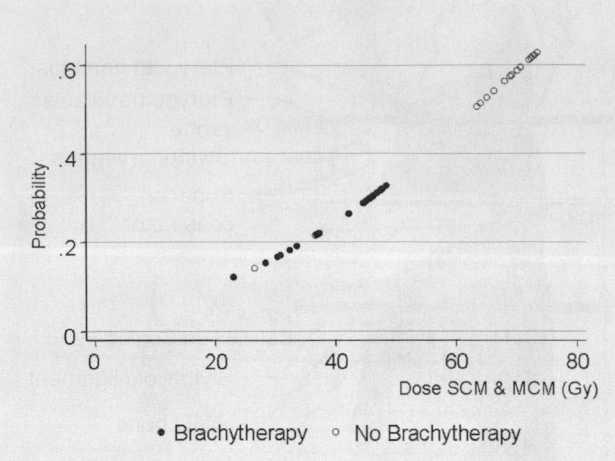

FIGURE 42.39. Dose-effect relationship for dysphagia. From the figure it seems apparent that more dysphagia problems can be expected with higher doses. Moreover, the problem of dysphagia seems less with the use of brachytherapy as a boost technique (less dose to the superior and middle constrictor muscle). SCM, superior constrictor muscle; MCM, middle constrictor muscle.

Speech and Quality of Life

For technical treatment planning reasons, voice, and speech can be affected at the time of the actual treatment of cancers in the oropharynx and during the follow-up period. In a recent article by van Gogh et al. (104), the authors also concluded that deviant voice quality can also lead to limitations in social life (302,303). A robust, short, five-item questionnaire was suggested to be able to detect voice deterioration and differentiate this in a busy outward clinic from a cancer in the larynx (104,152).

Dysphagia and Quality of Life

Swallowing function may be affected adversely by surgical and nonsurgical treatment of advanced oropharyngeal cancer (281). Gastrotomy tube (G-tube) dependence 6 to12 months after surgical management varies in the literature between 6% and 39% (75,280). Rates of swallowing dysfunction after chemoradiation are less well defined; G-tube dependence varies between 13% and 64% at short-term follow-up and between 13% and 33% at long-term follow-up (94,107,185,215,216,221,265). In general, after long-term follow-up (>1 year), one third of patients were reported to be G-tube–dependent (BOT 67% vs. TF/SP 25%; *p* = .049). The swallowing apparatus, being the wall of the pharynx (Fig. 42.37), is composed of two layers of muscles: the *external* three constrictor muscles (superior, middle, and inferior constrictor [with its cricopharyngeal and thyropharyngeal part]), the circular fibers of esophagus inlet, and the *internal* longitudinal levator muscles (stylopharyngeus and palatopharyngeus muscles). Deglutition or swallowing is a complex act of these seven muscular structures.

A study was recently initiated in Erasmus MC to get more insight in the problem of dysphagia. First, the components of the swallowing apparatus were determined and delineated on CT. After delineation, dose-volume histograms were constructed and mean doses calculated for every muscular structure. Fifty-five patients with cancer in the oropharynx who were treated

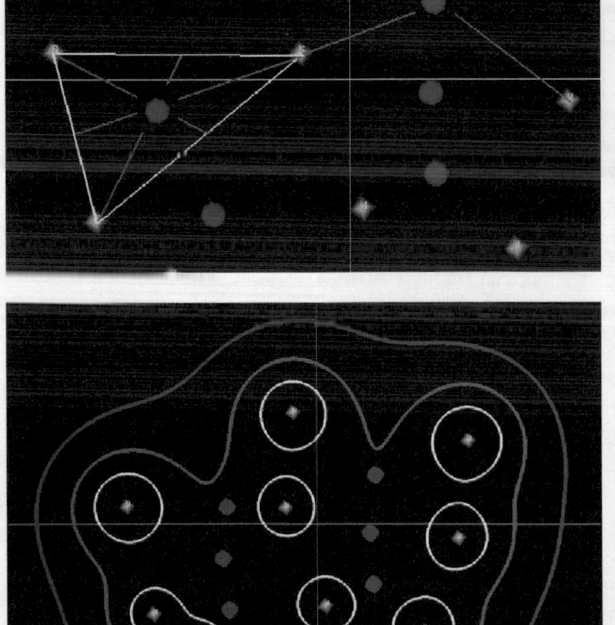

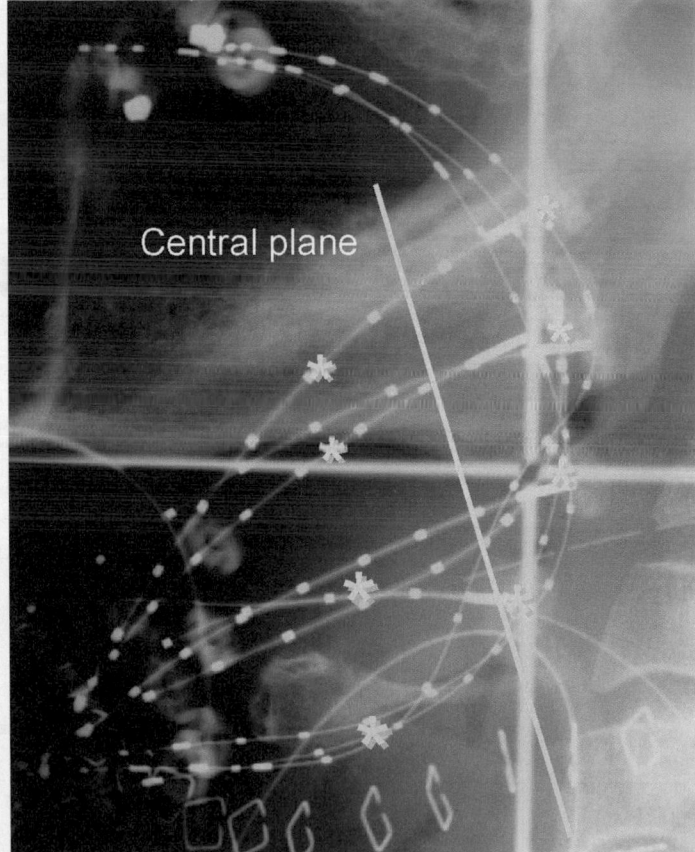

FIGURE 42.40. Patient with base of tongue implant. Sagittal-view x-ray film of catheters with dummy sources *in situ* (**right panel**). Yellow line depicts central calculation plane. Also shown is cross-section of tumor in central plane (**left panel**). Blue dots are basal dose points ("centers of gravity"). White dots represent "sources." Dose is prescribed to 85% of mean central dose (average of doses calculated in centers of gravity of all triangles).

Brachytherapy Boost PDR 22 Gy Total Dose

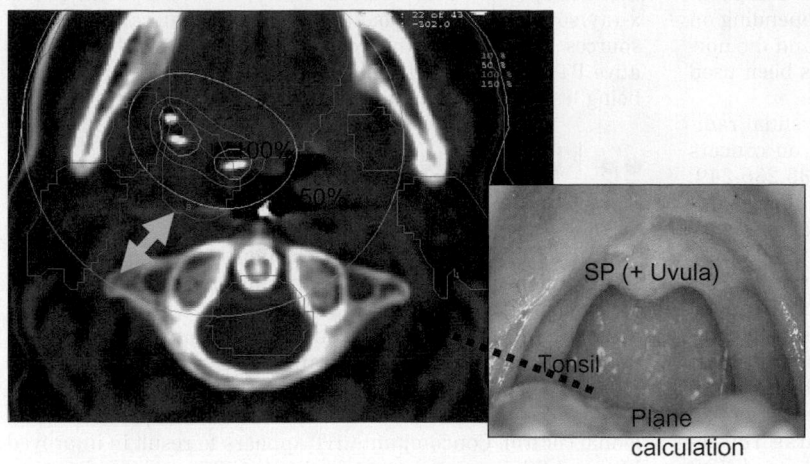

FIGURE 42.41. Tonsillar fossa and soft palate implant. Dose distribution, central plane. Dose prescribed to 0.5 cm after geometric optimization. PDR, pulsed dose rate.

Clinical Radiation Oncology

between 2000 and 2005 in Erasmus MC were used to study the problem of dysphagia in more detail. All patients were asked to respond to validated questionnaires PSS, EORTC H&N35, and the M.D. Anderson Dysphagia Inventory (Fig. 42.38). Using a univariate ordered logistic regression analysis technique, it was found that the probability for having serious complaints with swallowing increases significantly with dose (Fig. 42.39), but interestingly, this was significant for the superior and middle constrictor muscles. A multivariate analysis showed that the only significant factor was BT (dose). However, given the tight enveloping nature of the deglutition musculature, it needs very sophisticated three-dimensional treatment planning to spare the constrictor muscles without compromising on the dose to the primary tumor.

Brachytherapy

The history of BT dates back to the beginning of the 20th century, when the first BT procedures were performed using Radium-226 needles. Brachytherapy ("*brachy*" = Greek for "short") is a treatment modality in which the tumor is irradiated by positioning the radioactive sources very close to (mould or endocavitary techniques) or even inside the tumor volume (interstitial implant), either by permanent (seed) implant or by temporarily inserted applicators or afterloading catheters. In principle, BT is a conformal type of radiation therapy technique. In recent years, artificial radionuclides such as Cs^{137}, Co^{60}, I^{125}, and Ir^{192} have become available. Manual afterloading of the sources into applicators or afterloading tubes replaced direct loading of sources into the patient. The French developed the so-called "Paris system" for low-dose-rate dosimetry purposes; that is, for parallel-equidistant sources, the system suggests specifying the dose of the implant as being 85% of the average dose in the basal dose points (local minima). A similar type of dose prescription is used for HDR BT (Figs. 42.40 and 42.41). Also, computer-controlled afterloading devices, supported by sophisticated treatment planning software with optimization capabilities, became available. The BOT implant consists of afterloading catheters after the percutaneous introduction of trocars in a submental or submandibular approach (Fig. 42.42) (103). For patients with disease extension toward the pharyngoepiglottic fold, lateral loops are added. The spacing between each end of the "looping" catheters running over the dorsum of the tongue is ±1 cm. As a safety precaution, when removing the implant, a temporary tracheostomy is sometimes performed in patients immediately before the implantation. A typical case for fractionated HDR TF and SP implant is depicted in Figure 42.41. In the majority of cases, two to three catheters are implanted in TF and faucial arches (Fig. 42.41, inset). A temporary nasogastric feeding tube is placed at the completion of most of our BT procedures. The development

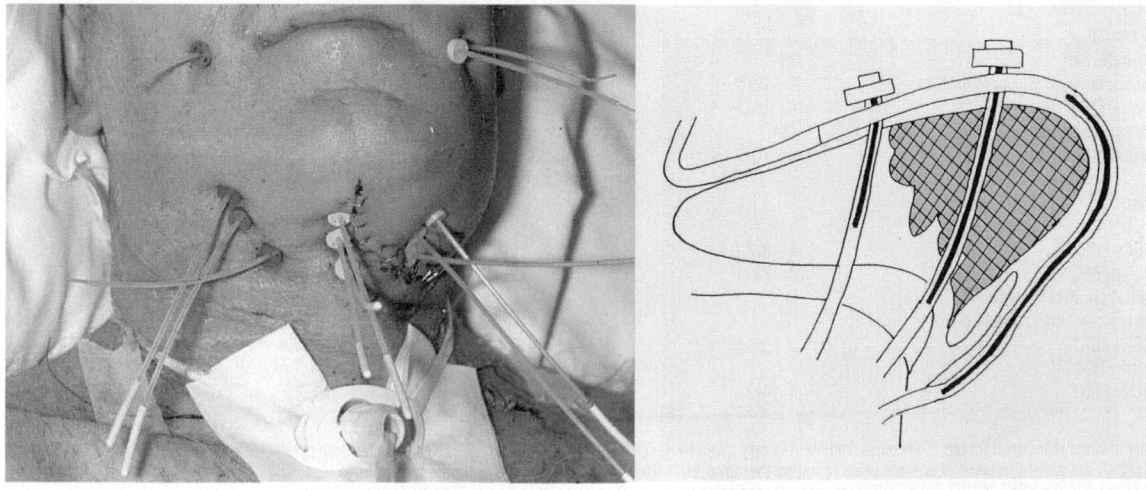

FIGURE 42.42. Patient with catheter configuration for base of tongue implant.

of radiobiologic models enables one to predict to a certain extent the tumor control probability and normal tissue complication probability after the application of BT, much depending on factors such as fraction size, dose rate, the tumor, and the normal tissues one is dealing with. Temporary BT has been used with several dose-rate categories.

The French have published extensively on interstitial radiation therapy of TF and/or SP tumors, as well as on cancers of the BOT (32,60,69,79,86,98,139,175,201,229,235,236,249, 274,327); most of these data regard LDR implants. For example, Mazeron et al. (199) report on a subset of patients with early-stage (T1, T2) tumors of the TF and/or SP, with a LC rate of approximately 85%, that is, a regional control rate of 97% for N0, and 88% N1–3 disease. Patients were typically treated by 45 Gy EBRT and a 30 Gy LDR Ir^{192} boost. Soft tissue ulceration occurred in 17 patients. Similar locoregional control rates were reported by Pernot et al. (235,236) (LC LDR boost TF/SP T1,T2N0 tumors 90% vs. T1,T2N1–3 86%) and Levendag et al. (175,177) (TF and/or SP tumors LRC 87% at 5 years). The series of patients in Rotterdam were treated by fractionated HDR BT (daytime regimen) or PDR (24 hours regime) (Table 42.18). Esche et al. (79) described 43 patients with carcinoma of the SP and uvula with LC rate of 92%. Overall survival was 60% at 3 years and 37% at 5 years. The cause-specific survivals were 81% and 64%, respectively. The leading cause of death was other aerodigestive cancers (these cancers occur with an actuarial rate of 3% per year posttreatment). The "BT school" of Memorial Sloan Kettering Cancer Center in New York pioneered large-volume implants in particular for cancer of the BOT, a technique initially designed by Vikram and Hilaris (307) and Vikram et al. (308). Harrison et al. (120,121,125,127) elaborated on cancer of the BOT and also related outcomes to QOL. Some of the control rates with IRT can be taken from Table 42.11 (TF/SP) and Table 42.14 (BOT). In skillful, well-trained, hands, BT remains an extremely gratifying technique for applying high doses of radiation for small-volume disease located in the midline (e.g., SP tumors) with (in case of fractionated HDR) highly conformal and accelerated properties.

Finally, IRT can also be a very rewarding technique, given the high doses in small-volume disease and the rapid dose falloff in the treatment of recurrent cancers and/or in case of reirradiation (58). For the future, image-guided BT will become routine; summation of dose distributions of BT and EBRT will become mandatory (Fig. 42.43). Moreover, by the development of soft x-ray sources and afterloading machines that carry multiple sources and have multiple drives, the flexibility of intraoperative BT has increased. One of these sources that is currently being tested is yyterbium (169).

Chemotherapy Targeted Therapy, and Altered Fractionation Regimes

Concurrent CHT and altered fractionated irradiation have shown independently to improve the outcome for head and neck cancer patients. The combination maximizes the chance for preservation of organ function and has the potential to improve the results even more by integration with new biologic agents (10,36,187,206,261,264,288). Many of the hyperfractionated and/or accelerated schedules have resulted in improved locoregional control. Concomitant CHT appears to result in improved LRC and OS, in contrast to neoadjuvant CHT and maintenance CHT (22,42,217). Not infrequently, these treatment regimes increase toxicity as well. Finally, the role of intra-arterial CHT (206,213,257) as well as the benefit of induction (neoadjuvant) and adjuvant CHT remains to be determined. In their concise review on randomized trials concerning multimodality treatment approaches, Bernier and Bentzen (22) emphasized that, to maximize outcome, each of the components of a particular treatment regime needs to be optimized separately. Importantly, Benasso et al. (20) and Taylor et al. (295) conducted multivariate analyses of patients treated in chemoradiotherapy head and neck trials, and pointed out that the second most important prognostic factor is the experience of the Center.

Regarding the effects on OS and locoregional control by altered fractionation and/or concomitant CHT, in 2004 Rosenthal and Kian (261) made some recommendations for treatment selection: conventional fractionation (and dose) for T1 and favorable T2N0,1 tumors, altered fractionation for unfavorable T2 or exophytic T3N0,1 (with or without neck dissection in case of N2,3 disease), and concurrent CHT for the more advanced cancers. Meanwhile, toxicity amelioration and identification of predictive biomarkers and effective molecularly targeted therapy should be pursued (261,292). Salama et al. (264)

Table 42.18   TABLE OF REFERENCE (IN GY) FOR FRACTIONATED HDR (FR. HDR) AND PDR BRACHYTHERAPY AS OF 2001.

Tumor Site	fr.HDR	PDR	SRT
BT as full course:			
Nasal vestibule, Skin, Lip	4+12x3+4		
One-plane implant: microscopic disease	4+12x3+4	2.5+29x1.5+2.5	
Any other site T1-4	4+16x3+4	2.5+38x1.5+2.5	6x6
Re-irradiation nasopharynx	15x3		
Re-irradiation other tumors	4+15x3+4	2.5+35x1.5+2.5 (preference)	
BT as boost:			
Nasopharynx			
After 60Gy EBRT	4+3x3+4		
After 70Gy EBRT	4+3+4		4x2.8
Re-irradiation after 46 Gy EBRT	6x3		
One-plane implant: microscopic disease			
After 46Gy EBRT	4+3+4	2+8x1+2	
Any other site T1-4			
After 46Gy EBRT	4+4x3+4	2+18x1+2	3x5.5

Total number of brachytherapy fractions. Full course: radiation is only given by means of brachytherapy. In the case of booster doses, generally 46/2 Gy are given by means of external beam radiation therapy (EBRT). The booster dose for cancer in the nasopharynx is given after either 60/2 Gy EBRT or 70/2 Gy EBRT. SRT (stereotactic radiation therapy) means a booster dose by Cyberknife (as of 2005). Fractionation schedules for "fractionated HDR", "PDR" and SRT (Cyberknife) used in the Erasmus MC-DDHCC.

Adding 3D dose distribution of External Beam Radiotherapy and Brachytherapy

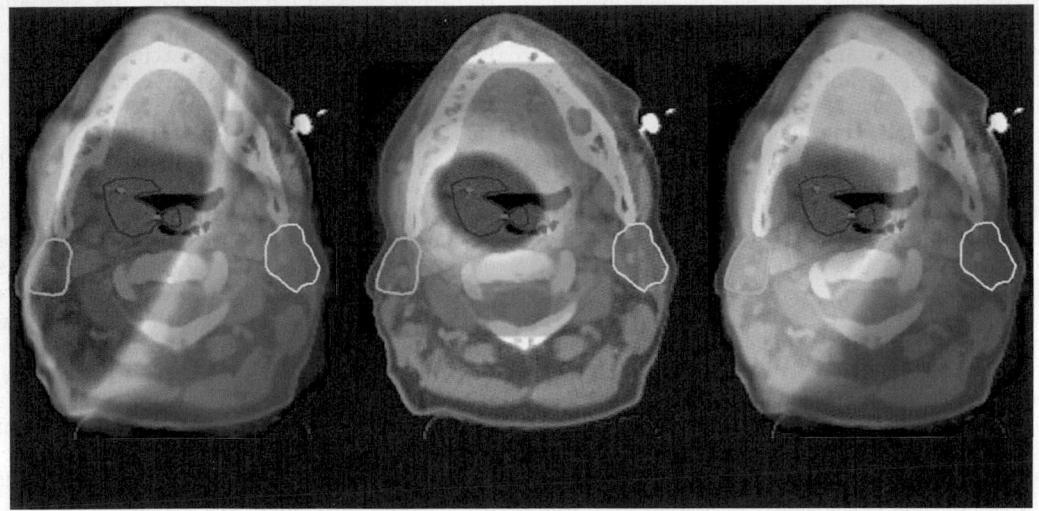

FIGURE 42.43. Treatment-planning software is currently being developed in Erasmus MC to summate intensity-modulated radiation therapy doses with brachytherapy (BT) doses, taking into account deformation of the target volume and normal tissues during treatment. EBRT, external beam radiation therapy.

published on aggressive trimodality treatment for the subset of patients with recurrent and/or second primary cancers in the head and neck. They evaluated 115 patients treated with a median lifetime radiation dose of 131 Gy. The locoregional control, OS, and freedom from distant metastasis rate at 3 years were 22%, 51%, and 61%, respectively. However, of note is that 19 patients died of treatment-related toxicity, 5 of these because of carotid blow-out. Suntharalingam (292) reviewed the early trials in 2003. Recognizing the mostly nonspecific nature of the toxicities of healthy tissues consequential to combined modality therapy, he argued that the real focus should be on researching newer biologic agents, targeting cellular protein receptors. Epidermal growth factor receptor is one of these receptors critical to cellular proliferation, differentiation, and survival. As it has been shown to be widely expressed in SCC cells of the head and neck, it was suggested that anti–epidermal growth factor receptor therapy could become a powerful agent in combined modality therapy in the future.

Nonrandomized Studies

Some of the studies reviewed in this section are designed to treat advanced cancers in the head and neck in general and not focused solely on tumors in the oropharynx. As has been shown by the meta-analyses, concomitant CHT and/or altered fractionation result in improved locoregional control and OS, but also a substantial amount of toxicity has been observed (35,238). In fact, with regard to concomitant CHT, Pignon and Bourhis (238) showed at 5 years an 8% increase in OS and a hazard ratio of 2.17 for overall toxicity. Harrison (128) published the results of a phase II trial treating 82 patients with unresectable head and neck cancer using the delayed concomitant boost technique with concurrent cisplatin. The 3-year LC for oropharynx cancers was 64%. Twenty-four percent of patients required a treatment break. Two deaths due to sepsis occurred during treatment. Severe chronic toxicity occurred in three patients: one osteoradionecrosis, one frontal lobe necrosis, and one case of lung toxicity secondary to adjuvant CHT. Bieri (25) reported on delayed concomitant boost radiation in which a planned total dose of 69.6 Gy was given in 5.5 weeks; one third of the

patients received concurrent cisplatin-based CHT. Among the 55 patients with oropharynx carcinoma, LRC at 3 years was 69.5%. Eighty-two percent experienced grade 3 and 4 mucositis. Patients receiving CHT had more grade 3 dysphagia (68% vs. 25%; $p = .003$), hospitalization (37% vs. 14%; $p = .08$), and a need for nasogastric tube (68% vs. 22%; $p = .001$). Nathu (214) published the results of induction CHT followed by RT for patients with oropharyngeal carcinomas treated at the University of Florida. Neoadjuvant CHT consisted of cisplatinum (100 mg/m^2) and 5-fluorouracil (1.0 mg/m^2/day × 5 days) for three cycles, and was followed by definitive RT (83% received hyperfractionated RT from 74.4 to 81.75 Gy). Outcome was compared with oropharyngeal tumors treated with a similar radiation regimen, but without CHT. Multivariate analysis showed no difference in local failure or distant failure. However, disease-specific survival and OS were improved in those who received induction CHT (58% vs. 27% and 42% vs. 17%, respectively). Because of the nonrandomized nature of the study and the lack of statistically significant improvement in parameters of tumor control, the authors cautioned against any conclusions regarding the benefit of induction chemotherapy.

A phase II study on 61 patients with advanced oropharyngeal carcinoma using induction chemotherapy followed by concurrent chemoradiation was reported by Vokes (309). Neck dissections (n = 35) were performed for N2 to N3 disease. At a median follow-up of 39 months (68 months among survivors), LRC was 70%, distant metastasis-free survival was 89%, disease-free survival was 64%, and OS was 51%. Acute toxicity was substantial, with severe or life-threatening mucositis and leukopenia during the induction phase, whereas 81% had grade 3 or 4 mucositis during the concurrent chemoradiotherapy. The authors concluded that the treatment sequence of induction chemotherapy followed by concurrent chemoradiotherapy and optional organ-preservation surgery is promising but that less toxic regimens need to be identified. Bensadoun (21) reported on 54 patients with unresectable oropharynx and hypopharynx carcinoma treated with concomitant hyperfractionated radiation (75.6 to 80.4 Gy) and three cycles of 5-FU/cisplatin in weeks 1, 4, and 7. Four percent mortality was observed from treatment related septicemia, 86% grade 3/4 mucositis but no patient required a treatment break greater than 4 days because of mucositis. Grade 2 xerostomia was observed in 70% of the patients and grade 2 cervical fibrosis in 45% of the patients. At a median follow-up of 16 months, disease-specific survival was 72%.

There are many other examples of chemoradiotherapy regimen for oropharyngeal carcinomas with encouraging LRC rates, but with short-term follow-up and/or too small patient numbers (10,100,187). A promising approach was presented by the Memorial Sloan Kettering Cancer Center. Arruda et al. (62) studied 50 patients treated by IMRT in conjunction with concurrent CHT (86%). At 2 years, local progression-free OS and distant metastases-free survival is 98%, 98%, and 84%, respectively. Six of 42 patients remained with their percutaneous endoscopic gastrostomy until the time of analysis.

Randomized Trials

A prime example of a multinational, randomized trial of molecularly targeted therapy is the study by Bonner et al. (33) that was recently published in the *New England Journal of Medicine*. It compares patients with advanced cancers in the head and neck treated with high-dose RT alone (n = 213) or with RT plus weekly cetuximab, a monoclonal antibody against epidermal growth factor. The outcome of the study showed a significant improvement of locoregional control (hazard ratio locoregional progression or death 0.68; $p = .005$) and OS (49 months for combined therapy vs. 29.3 months for RT alone [hazard ratio for death, 0.74; $p = 0.03$]). It reduced mortality without increasing the common side effects of radiation. Studies for future targeted therapies combining cetuximab with chemotherapeutic agents such as Taxotere, cisplatin, and 5FU are now underway. Concurrent CHT with hyperfractionated radiation was explored by Brizel (36) in a phase III randomized trial. One hundred sixteen patients with advanced head and neck cancer were randomized to hyperfractionated radiation alone treated with 1.25 Gy twice daily 5 days per week to 75 Gy during a 6-week period versus a concurrent CHT arm consisting of 5-FU/CDDP given on weeks 1 and 6 of split-course hyperfractionated radiation. Both groups received two adjuvant courses of 5-FU/CDDP after completion of radiation. At a median follow-up of 41 months, the concurrent CHT showed improved LRC (70% vs. 44%; $p = .01$) and a trend toward improved 3-year OS (55% vs. 34%; $p = .07$) and relapse-free survival (61% vs. 41%; $p = .08$). However, patients in the chemoradiotherapy arm developed more acute toxicity, including the requirement for more feeding tubes (44% vs. 29%) and worse hematologic suppression. Chronic toxicity was no different, with about a 10% incidence of necrosis of the skin or bone in both arms. The trial has been criticized, not only for the added toxicity, but also because of the imbalance in the proportion of advanced neck disease (44% vs. 63%) treated in the concurrent chemoradiotherapy, which may have accounted for the difference in LRC. Jeremic (148) reported a phase III randomized study testing whether daily low-dose cisplatin improved outcome for patients undergoing hyperfractionation radiation compared with those treated with the same hyperfractionated radiation alone in locally advanced head and neck cancers (37% were oropharynx). One hundred thirty patients with stage III or IV disease were randomized to 1.1 Gy twice daily to 77 Gy per 7 weeks with or without cisplatin (6 mg/m^2/day). At a median follow-up of 79 months, the investigational arm showed improved LRC (50% vs. 36% at 5 years; $p = .041$), progression-free survival (46% vs. 25% at 5 years; $p = .0068$), and OS (46% vs. 25% at 5 years; $p = .0075$), and fewer distant metastases (14% vs. 43% at 5 years; $p = .0013$). Daily concurrent CHT was well tolerated, with no increase in acute grade 3 mucositis and esophagitis. There were no increases in late skin or severe effects to bone or salivary gland. A multicenter randomized trial reported by Staar (288) tested whether the combination of hyperfractionated accelerated

radiation (69.9 Gy/5 × 5.5 weeks) with carboplatin (70 mg/m^2) and 5-FU (600 mg/m^2/day × 5 days) on weeks 1 and 5 of RT improved outcome compared with the same radiation regimen alone. At a median follow-up of 22 months, the 1- and 2-year respective rates of LRC were 69% and 52% after chemotherapy/RT compared with 58% and 45% after RT alone ($p = .14$). Patients with oropharyngeal carcinomas had a trend toward improved 2-year LRC with chemoradiotherapy compared with RT alone (51% vs. 42%; $p = .07$).

Another German multicenter randomized trial compared hyperfractionated accelerated radiotherapy alone (77.6 Gy) with hyperfractionated accelerated radiochemotherapy (70.6 Gy) using mitomycin C and 5-FU (130). For patients treated inside the trial, no significant difference in survival was observed. A randomized phase II EORTC trial explored the feasibility of concomitant cisplatin and RT with conventional fractionation or multiple fractions per day (MFD). The MFD schedule was designed to achieve higher tumor concentrations of cisplatin at the time of irradiation by reducing the number of radiation treatment weeks from 7 to 3. No difference in acute and late side effects in both treatment arms while better tumor response was obtained with MFD. It is argued that the better tumor response in the MFD might be due to a (67%) higher daily dose of cisplatin concomitant with RT being given in a 3-week period (13). Hao et al. (119) updated the meta-analyses outcome of concomitant CHT trials to date in SCC of the head and neck. They confirmed an 8% benefit in 5-year absolute survival. Toxicity in general seems to be more pronounced with combined modality regimens using hyperfractionated RT or when the concomitant CHT regimen included carboplatin plus 5-FU. Several other randomized studies (e.g., Horiot et al. [139] or Fu et al. [93]) have demonstrated the beneficial effect of hyperfractionation and/or accelerated fractionation over standard fractionation. Also, Calais (42,43) demonstrated better locoregional control when altered fractionation is used with concurrent CHT. According to Hao et al. (119), the current state of the evidence supports strongly to offer platinum-based concurrent CHT with conventional fractionated RT as a treatment option for patients with advanced head and neck cancers treated outside a clinical trial.

⣿ | Three-Dimensional Conformal RTIMRT

The introduction of the multileaf collimator and three-dimensional treatment planning systems (TPS) in the 1990s has been instrumental for the development and application of three-dimensional conformal radiation therapy and IMRT. The major advantages of IMRT for irradiation of the complex head and neck anatomy are now generally recognized. The possibility of tightly shaping the higher isodose surfaces around the often concave target volumes allows for substantial sparing of critical structures. The use of electrons for irradiating the posterior neck, without exceeding the cord dose, has become almost obsolete. In this section, procedures are described for a safe and beneficial application of this powerful tool with focus on the IMRT techniques as used in the Erasmus MC.

IMRT

Treatment Planning

In the Erasmus MC, in case of radical radiation therapy of oropharyngeal cancer, IMRT is used to deliver a total dose of 46 Gy, 2 Gy per fraction, 6 fractions per week, to the primary tumor and neck, generally followed by a BT- or CyberKnife boost (Fig. 42.19). In line with the International Commission on Radiation Units and Measurements criteria for dose homogeneity in the PTV, it is generally required that 100% of the PTV must

Table 42.19	DOSE CONSTRAINTS FOR THE CRITICAL STRUCTURES ACCORDING TO THE RADIATION THERAPY ONCOLOGY GROUP (RTOG) PROTOCOL H-0022, AND AS APPLIED IN IMRT TECHNIQUES AS USED IN THE ERASMUS MC	
	ERASMUS MC	**RTOG Protocol H-0022**
Spinal cord	$D_{max} < 50$ Gy	$D_{max} < 45$Gy
Mandible		$D_{max} < 70$Gy
Glottic Larynx	(1)	2/3 below 50 Gy
Brainstem	$D_{max} < 50$ Gy	$D_{max} < 54$ Gy
Parotid gland	$D_{mean} < 26$ Gy	$D_{mean} < 26$ Gy[a]
Oral cavity	$D_{mean} < 26$ Gy	

[a]At least 50% of either parotid gland receives < 30 Gy, or at least 20 cc of the combined volume of both parotid glands receives < 20 Gy.

obtain more than 95% of the prescribed dose (143), although small underdosages (e.g., around the salivary glands) are acceptable in specific cases. Tolerating minor PTV underdosages has also been described by Fogliata et al. (83) and Wu et al. (325). Recently, we have studied this trade-off between full PTV coverage and sparing of the parotid glands, using a model for calculation of the subclinical disease control probability (163). For the patients in the study, the mean parotid gland dose decreased by more than 10 Gy by allowing for a small underdosage in the PTV, corresponding with a reduction in the calculated subclinical disease control probability of typically 1% and a little higher.

The applied planning constraints for the critical structures for IMRT as used in Erasmus MC are presented in Table 42.19 and compared with the RTOG H-0022 protocol (247). For plan design, the constraints for the cord and the PTV are overriding, and the criteria for the parotids and oral cavity are planning objectives rather than hard constraints. To create a safety margin, the cord constraint is set for the spinal canal, rather than for the cord per se.

Depending on the patient geometry, different planning strategies are used. The most favorable strategy is to spare both parotid glands. This is done using a nonequiangular, five-field technique, with gantry angles of 0 degrees, ±60 degrees and ±140 degrees (optimized for each individual patient), using 6-MV beams. Especially when the boost is also delivered with IMRT, significant sparing of both parotids is frequently not feasible. It may then be decided to largely relax the constraint for the ipsilateral parotid gland and to focus on sparing of the contralateral gland. Generally, a nonsymmetrical four-field technique is then applied, with two parallel-opposed beams at gantry angles of around 350 degrees and 160 degrees (or 10 degrees and 200 degrees, depending on tumor position). With such an approach, that is, sparing of a single parotid gland structure Eisbruch et al. (73) observed a salivary flow increase after 2 years.

In the absence of positive nodes, the lower neck region is treated with two non-IMRT anterior fields, positioned on either side of the cord with sparing of the larynx (midline block) (Fig. 42.33). The International Commission on Radiation Units and Measurements dose homogeneity criterion is then less strictly enforced. Another technique to cover the lower neck region is to extend the upper IMRT fields.

Figures 42.27 and 42.30 show a five-field technique (0 to 46 Gy) for a patient with a TF tumor (T2N1) to be treated by RT to the primary and bilateral neck. For this bilateral parotid sparing treatment plan, mean doses to the parotids are 22 and 23 Gy, respectively. For comparison purposes, Figures 42.28 and 42.31 show a treatment plan with focus on maximum sparing of the contralateral parotid, yielding mean doses of 17 Gy (contralateral parotid gland) and 30 Gy (ipsilateral parotid gland).

Patient Setup Verification, Correction, and PTV-Margins

IMRT is most effective when used in combination with narrow PTV margins that have to be in line with the geometrical uncertainties for the patient involved. This implies a proper knowledge of the setup variations. Each patient has a setup error that occurs during all fractions (the systematic or mean error) and day-to-day variations around this mean setup error (the random errors) (26,278). By its nature, the systematic error of an individual patient can be obtained only from measurements during each fraction, and is therefore not known at the time of treatment planning. The setup uncertainties are generally quantified by three standard deviations Σ_x, Σ_y, and Σ_z, describing the distribution of systematic setup errors in the patient group, and the standard deviations σ_x, σ_y, and σ_z that represent the day-to-day variations. For head and neck cancer patients, these standard deviations are mostly derived from measurements with electronic portal imaging devices (EPIDs). Stroom et al. (289,290), from our institution, derived for each direction, i, the required PTV margin, M_i, given by:

$$M_i = 0.7 \cdot \sigma_i + 2 \cdot \Sigma_i.$$

In this approach, the PTV margin of each new patient is fully based on setup measurements performed for previously treated patients. The formula reflects the idea that systematic errors, potentially leading to an underdosage of a specific part of the tumor in all fractions, are more severe than random errors. The equation was confirmed by the work of van Herk et al. (132). Setup errors can be minimized using EPID measurements and a correction protocol. Deviations in the patient setup are then quantified by comparison of the EPID images with digitally reconstructed radiographs derived from the planning CT scan. It is essential that the demarcations on the patient's skin or mask, used for setup at the linac, are in exact agreement with the isocenter of the planning CT scan. These demarcations should not be adjusted in a session at a conventional simulator, neither should verification be based on acquired simulator images (19). In an online protocol, the patient setup error is assessed in each fraction using a few monitor units (MUs), followed by a subsequent correction and delivery of the remainder of the MUs. With such a protocol, both the systematic error and the random component can be substantially reduced. However, a disadvantage of online protocols is the involved workload at the treatment unit and the unavoidable increase of the fraction time. For this reason, so-called off-line protocols are more often applied than online protocols. In an off-line protocol, EPID images are only acquired in a limited number of fractions, and all image analyses are performed off-line, that is, not during the time of the delivery of the fractions. The latter excludes the possibility of reduction of random errors, which is

Table 42.20

SET-UP ERRORS AND CALCULATED MARGINS (IN MM) FOR H&N CANCER PATIENTS TREATED IN THE ERASMUS MC WITH IMRT

	LR	CC	AP
σ	1.6	1.6	1.4
Σ_{init}	2.3	1.6	2.1
M_{init}	6	5	6
Σ_{NAL}	0.9	0.9	0.8
M_{NAL}	3	3	3

Left-right (LR), cranio-caudal (CC), anterior-posterior (AP) directions. Standard deviations σ (distributions of random errors), Σ_{NAL} (residual systematic errors with the clinically applied NAL set-up correction protocol), Σ_{init} (systematic errors that would have occurred without NAL), M_{NAL}, and M_{init} are margins calculated with the equation in the text.

of lesser relevance for the determination of the required margin (equation). Instead, the aim of an off-line protocol is to reduce the more important systematic patient setup errors by estimating the optimal *a priori* setup correction for subsequent fractions.

In the Erasmus MC we have developed and implemented the no-action level (NAL) protocol for off-line corrections (63), which is now applied for most patient groups, including those with oropharyngeal cancer. For each patient, the protocol starts with acquisition of EPID images during the first N_m fractions (Erasmus MC $N_m = 2$ for head and neck sites), without applying any setup corrections. The involved systematic setup error for the complete fractionated treatment is then estimated by calculation of the mean setup error in these first N_m fractions. In the remainder of the fractions, the patient is first set up using the (original) marks on the patient mask. Then, prior to dose delivery, an *a priori* setup correction is performed as prescribed by minus the (estimated systematic error), followed by irradiation; no images are acquired. The first application of the NAL

protocol for head and neck cancer was described by de Boer et al. (65). The patients in this study were treated with parallel-opposed laterals, and the NAL protocol was therefore only applied in two directions. Table 42.20 shows the setup errors for IMRT patients, as derived in a recent analysis (not published). As previously outlined, for each patient, the setup correction is based on an estimate of the systematic setup error, derived from measurements in only two fractions. As a consequence, application of the NAL protocol will diminish the systematic errors, but not cancel them out. In Table 42.20, both the distribution of the residual systematic errors, Σ_{NAL}, and the distribution of (calculated) initial systematic errors, Σ_{init}, that would have occurred without application of NAL, are presented. The presented margins are calculated with the equation provided. In clinical practice, margins of 5 mm are used for all directions, leaving some room for delineation uncertainty. Recently, the NAL protocol has been extended (eNAL) to systematically update setup corrections based on weekly follow-up measurements (64).

Dosimetric Quality Assurance

In our institution, IMRT is delivered with dynamic multileaf collimation (DMLC), using the sliding window technique. Because of the complexity, a dedicated quality assurance (QA) protocol is instituted, supplementing the QA procedures for non-IMRT treatments. All involved dosimetric measurements for IMRT are performed with EPIDs (Fig. 42.44) (89,90,131). For daily linac QA, the sliding-gap method as proposed by LoSasso et al. (181), measuring the leaf positioning accuracy with an ionization chamber for a single leaf pair, has been extended to two-dimensional, using the EPID (305). The measurements take 3 minutes, including the analyses. Errors in leaf positioning as small as 0.1 to 0.2 mm can be detected. Apart from the daily verification of the leaf motions, QA procedures are performed for each individual IMRT patient (228,304,306,328,329). These procedures aim at (a) verification of the final TPS dose calculation for the optimized treatment parameters such as the leaf

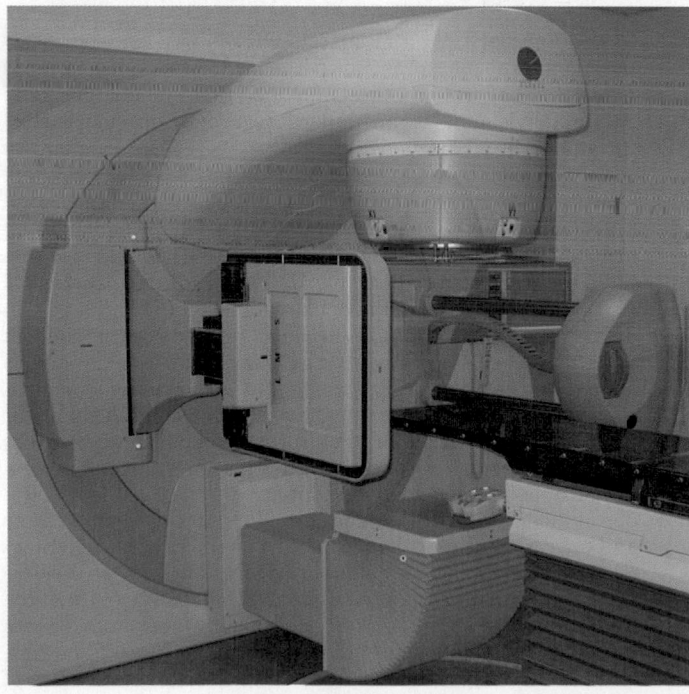
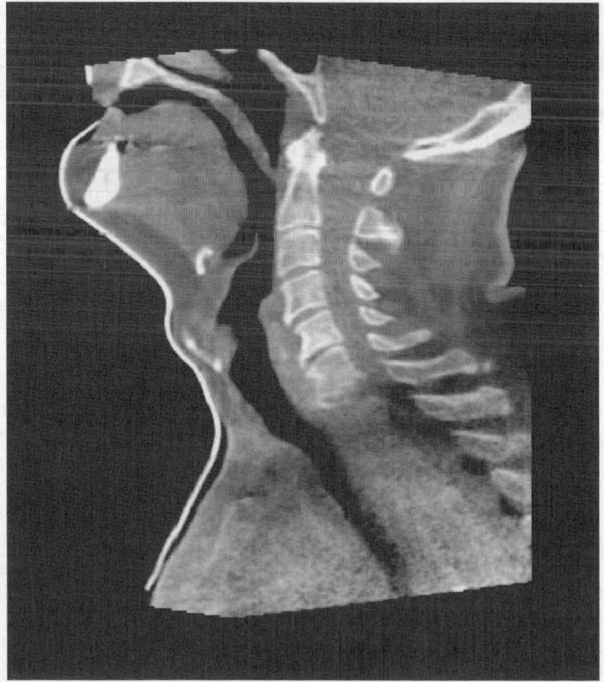

FIGURE 42.44. Left panel: the Elekta Synergy system with an additional kV tube and two-dimensional detector for acquisition of cone-beam computed tomography (CT) scans, and the Theraview NT electronic portal imaging device (Theraview NT, Cablon Medical, The Netherlands) for setup verification and dosimetric quality assurance. **Right panel:** sagittal cone beam CT slice for a head and neck cancer patient.

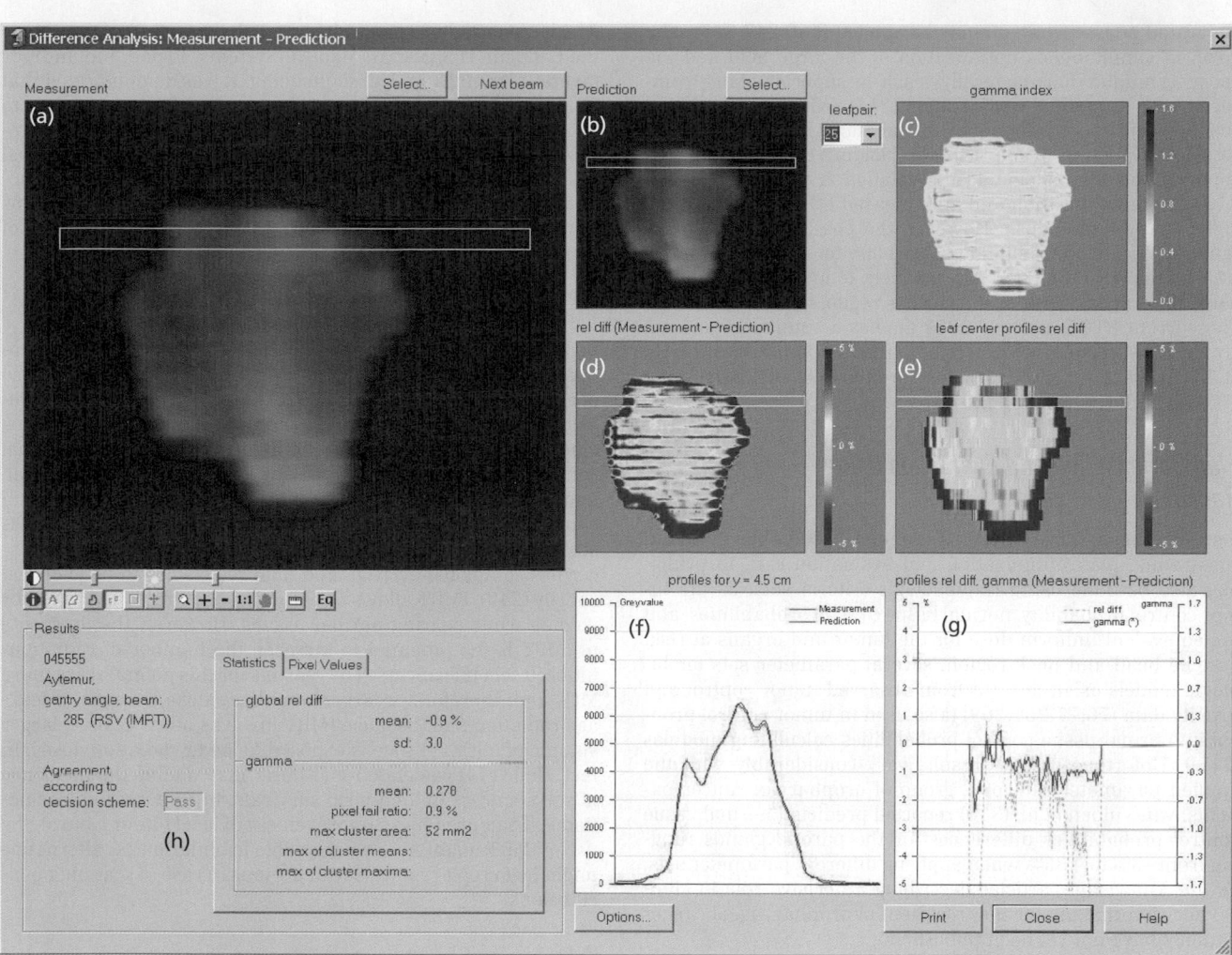

FIGURE 42.45. Screen shot for dosimetric intensity-modulated radiation therapy verification with an electronic portal imaging device. Portal dose images (PDIs) measured prior to the start of the first treatment fraction, compared with predictions. **(a)** measured PDI; **(b)** predicted PDI; **(c)** PDI comparison using the γ-index; **(d)** PDI difference image; **(e)** PDI difference image, excluding the tongue-and-groove areas; **(f)** profile comparison for the leaf pair marked with a yellow line in (a) through (e); **(g)** dose and γ-index differences for this leaf pair; and **(h)** result of the automated test for two-dimensional image comparison (pass, in this case).

trajectories, and (b) verification of the correct execution of the plan at the linac. Currently, the TPS dose is only verified by an independent dose calculation for a single or few points in the center of the tumor. A fully three-dimensional procedure is being developed. For verification of the correct fluence delivery at the linac, EPID dose measurements are performed both prior to the first treatment fraction (pretreatment verification [229,306]), and during treatment ("*in vivo*" verification [305]). For pretreatment verification, portal dose images (a two-dimensional dose distribution in the plane of the fluorescent screen of the EPID) measured with the EPID are compared with predictions. Differences point at errors in leaf sequencing, data transfer from the TPS to the linac, or to dosimetric/mechanical linac performance problems. Presently, portal dose image comparison (Fig. 42.45) has been fully integrated in the applied EPID software (Theraview NT, Cablon Medical, Heusden, The Netherlands); a method for automated image analysis also has been implemented. Images are only reviewed by a physicist in case of a failure to pass the automated test. Because of the high spatial resolution, EPIDs are suited for detection of tongue-and-groove underdosage effects. For a group of 270 IMRT patients, the pretreatment procedure has revealed four serious errors prior to the start of treatment (329). Recently, methods have been developed for back-projection of fluence profiles, measured with the

EPID, in the planning CT scan or in an in-room acquired cone beam CT scan, allowing full three-dimensional analyses (328).

Deviations in *in vivo* measured PDIs may be due to errors in fluence delivery, but may also be caused by changes in patient anatomy or variations in patient setup. To discriminate between the two, the split IMRT field technique (305) has been developed, which is now routinely applied for all head and neck cancer patients.

Alternative IMRT Approaches

Beam Orientations

Instead of dedicated orientations, often a relatively large number of equiangular beams are used. Whereas some articles report techniques with seven equiangular beams for oropharynx tumors (62,239), others advocate nine beams (324). Generally, an odd number is used to avoid opposing beams.

Simultaneous Integrated Boost

For oropharyngeal cancer patients treated in the Erasmus MC, the boost is generally delivered with BT or the CyberKnife after 46 Gy. When using IMRT for full-dose delivery, a simultaneous integrated boost technique may be applied (166,247,325). The involved simultaneous optimization of the large field and the boost technique does generally result in superior plans, compared with sequential optimization (211). With the simultaneous integrated boost technique, an enhanced fraction dose may be selected for the primary tumor, yielding two simultaneous opportunities for biologic dose escalation: a shortening of the total treatment duration and an increased LC as a result of the higher daily tumor dose. However, the possibilities for application of escalated fraction doses are limited by the risk of increased toxicity (166,325). Alternatively, to minimize complications, the fraction dose in the elective regions may be reduced. The current RTOG study H-0022 applies a simultaneous integrated boost technique, prescribing a GTV total dose of 66 Gy at 2.2 Gy/fraction, and a dose for the subclinical disease region of 54 Gy (1.8 Gy/fraction) (247).

Plan Optimization and Evaluation Using Radiobiologic Models

Instead of using dose- and dose-volume–based objectives and constraints, plan optimization and evaluation can, in principle, also be done using radiobiologic criteria such as the tumor control probability, normal tissue control probabilities, and the equivalent uniform dose for the tumor and organs at risk. For the head and neck region, several parameter sets for biologic models exist, derived from observed tumor control and toxicity data (76,77,259,269) (also used in tumor control probability/normal tissue control probabilities calculating modules [315]). Unfortunately, the results vary considerably with the applied parameter set: for a group of oropharynx cancer patients, van Vulpen et al. (310) reported predicted normal tissue control probabilities differences for the parotid glands ranging from –3% to +35% when applying different parameter sets. To our knowledge, articles describing a decisive role in clinical decision-making for the treatment of oropharyngeal cancer patients have not yet been published.

Step-and-Shoot or Segmental IMRT (SMLC)

Apart from the DMLC technique, intensity modulated profiles can also be generated by sequential delivery of static field segments, with a variable shape and number of monitor units (SMLC). In the transition period from end of delivery of one segment to shaping of the next segment, the beam is switched off. DMLC allows for more precise realization of the optimized fluence profiles. However, some studies have concluded that the differences are of minor clinical importance (4,55,83). It has also been reported that DMLC treatments require more MUs and SMLC treatments take more time.

A leaf-sequencing algorithm for DMLC has been developed that fully prevents the occurrence of tongue-and-groove under-

dosage reported by van Santvoort et al. (266). Currently, we use the Cadplan TPS (Varian Medical Systems, Espoo, Finland) for inverse planning and leaf sequencing. It was demonstrated that for extreme profiles, tongue-and-groove underdosage of up to 30% may occur with this TPS (80). However, the protocol for pretreatment verification of the fluence profiles of each individual IMRT patient has never revealed a clinically relevant tongue-and-groove error. Also for SMLC, leaf-sequencing algorithms have been developed that reduce or prevent the occurrence of tongue-and-groove underdosage (61,182).

Clinical Results

Some of the clinical results are presented in the section Xerostomia. Excellent reviews are presented by Puri et al. (243) and Lee et al. (168). Table 42.21 summarizes the preliminary clinical results of several studies of IMRT treatment for oropharyngeal carcinoma. The studies confirm the high rates for (loco-) regional control, distant metastases-free survival, disease-free survival, and OS in combination with reduced toxicity in comparison to conventional radiotherapy. Finally the multi-institutional RTOG study (H-0022) using IMRT for early-stage oropharyngeal cancer has completed accrual, and final results are to be expected shortly (247). IMRT allows dose to be concentrated in the tumor volume while sparing normal tissues. However, the downside to IMRT is the potential to increase the number of radiation-induced second cancers. The reasons for this potential are more MUs and, therefore, a larger total-body dose because of leakage radiation and, because IMRT involves more fields, a larger volume of normal tissue is exposed to lower radiation doses. In fact, Hall (114) calculated that IMRT may double the incidence of solid cancers in long-term survivals. In contrast to older patients, if balanced by an improvement of local tumor control, the use of IMRT might not be acceptable in children. An alternative might be to replace x-rays with protons in case of scanning pencil beams.

Alternative External Beam Approaches

Helical Tomotherapy

Apart from IMRT with linear accelerators, helical tomotherapy (186) (HiArt, TomoTherapy Inc., Madison, WI) can also be used for highly conformal dose delivery. Several articles report on dose distributions for head and neck cancer patients that might be superior to those obtained with linacs, regarding sparing of critical structures (82,230,310). Long-term clinical evaluations are not available as yet. Compared to linac-based IMRT, tomotherapy requires more MUs to deliver the same target dose, because of the applied fan-beam (212). This increases the whole-body dose equivalent, which may increase the risk for radiation-induced secondary malignancies (84). The clinical

		Median	LRC	DFS	DMFS	OS	Acute Xerostomia	Acute Mucositis	Late Xerostomia	Late Mucositis
Study	N	FU	(%)	(%)	(%)	(%)	≥gr2 (%)	≥gr2 (%)	≥gr2 (%)	≥gr3 (%)
Chao 2005	74	33 mo	78	66	84	87		41	12	
Garden 2004	80	17 mo	94							
Huang 2003	41	14 mo	89	91		89				
De Arruda 2006	50	18 mo	86		84	98	60	38	33	
Yao 2005	56	18 mo	98							
Chao 2001	26	47 mo	88	80				42	30	10

Table 42.21 OVERVIEW OF REPORTED TREATMENT RESULTS OF OROPHARYNGEAL CANCER USING IMRT

Toxicity scored according to RTOG criteria. LRC: local-regional control. DFS: disease free survival. DMFS: distant metastases free survival. OS: overall survival.

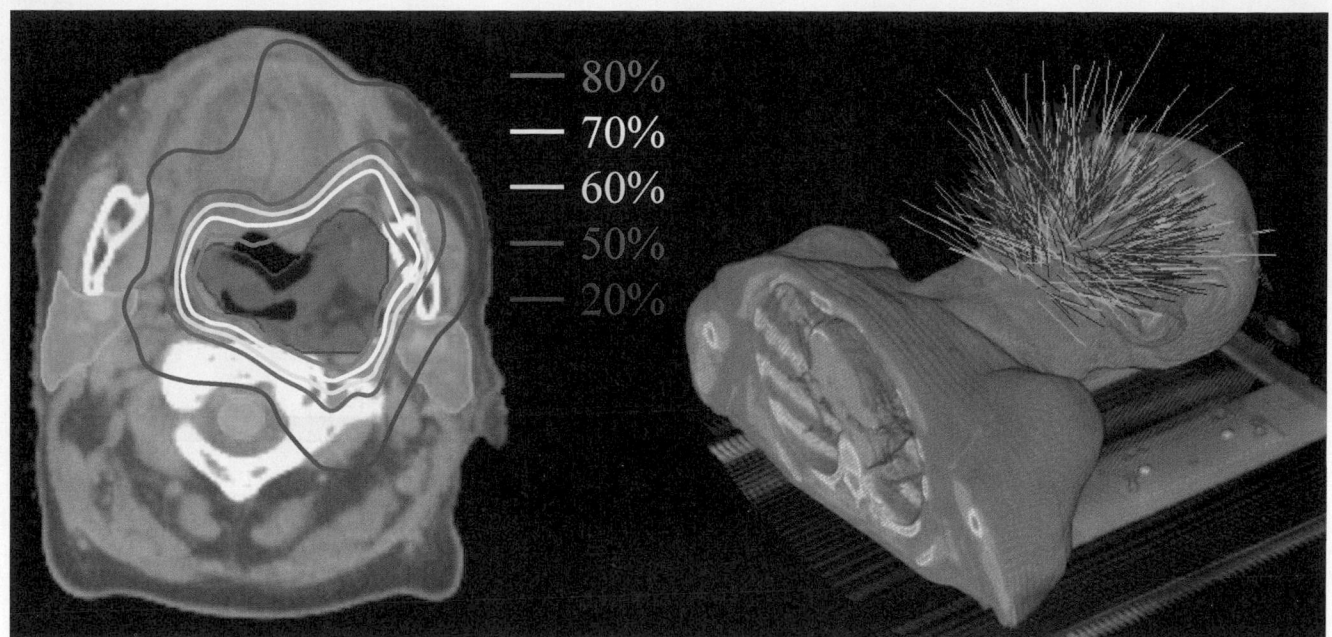

FIGURE 42.46. Left Panel: CyberKnife boost dose distribution of a patient with a tonsillar fossa tumor. **Right panel:** The applied beam setup. The light blue rods represent the beam directions that were actually used for treatment, with lengths proportional to the beam weight. The beams marked with the dark blue rods were available for treatment planning, but were not selected in the final plan.

implications of irradiating larger volumes to lower doses with tomotherapy, compared with smaller volumes with intermediate doses in linac IMRT, are unknown.

CyberKnife

The robotic CyberKnife system (Accuray Inc., Sunnyvale, CA) is another means of applying high dose of radiation with high accuracy (2). Some preliminary experience with the CyberKnife is available from the Erasmus MC for cancer in the oropharynx (Fig. 42.19 shows the protocol). This regards the delivery of a boost treatment of three fractions of 5.5 Gy on each consecutive day, prescribed at the 80% isodose. Patients are immobilized with the regular thermoplastic mask with a three-point fixation. Highly conformal plans with steep dose gradients are generated using 100 to 200 noncoplanar and nonisocentric coned beams. Figure 42.46 shows a typical dose distribution for a CyberKnife boost with the applied beam orientations. The CyberKnife image-guidance system and the patient skull are used for frequent measurement of the patient setup during treatment. Observed translations and rotations are used for immediate correction of the position and direction of the next beams. Because of these continuous adjustments, a PTV margin of only 2 mm was applied originally. Recently, the images obtained with the CyberKnife image-guidance system have been retrospectively analyzed, to quantify patient motion during delivery of a treatment fraction (135). For head and neck cancer and brain cancer patients, the maximum observed displacement in a 2-minute period was 2.8 mm in a single direction; a maximum rotation of 2.3 degrees was observed after 3 minutes. The overall systematic and random three-dimensional errors after 15 minutes are 1.3 and 1.2 mm (2 SD), respectively. With the CyberKnife image-guidance system, these in-fraction patient movements are automatically compensated using the robotic manipulator.

Cone-Beam CT

An important next step in image-guided RT for head and neck tumors may be the use of the recently introduced cone-beam CT scanners, integrated in linacs (Fig. 42.44) (146,172,202). In contrast to EPIDs, these systems allow for visualization of soft tissues. So far, the image quality is not as good as for modern diagnostic scanners. During the fractionated head and neck treatment, various processes may result in a gradual change of the patient anatomy, such as postoperative changes/edema, weight loss, and shrinking of the primary tumor and/or nodal masses (11,118). Large changes in the size of the GTV and the size and position of the parotid glands have been observed. These changes may result in suboptimal treatment as the dose delivery in all fractions is usually based on a treatment plan that is designed for the patient anatomy in the planning CT scan, which is acquired prior to the start of treatment. Studies have been performed to investigate the impact of replanning based on, or triggered by, anatomy changes observed in acquired cone beam CT scans (118,210). A major clinical question to be answered is the target definition in case of a shrunken gross target volume.

As part of the IMRT QA protocol, cone-beam CT scans may also be used to assess the "dose of the day" (328).

Future Technical Developments

Dose-Calculation Algorithms

It is well known that, especially in the presence of low-density inhomogeneities, significant dose-calculation errors may occur for single beams, even when using a modern commercial TPS. Such errors have also been observed for clinical, multibeam head and neck treatment plans (34,251,270). Improved accuracies can be obtained with Monte Carlo dose-calculation algorithms, and vendors of TPSs have started to offer this tool (129,251). However, to obtain clinically acceptable calculation times, approximations and simplifications are often used that could jeopardize the potential advantages of the full Monte Carlo technique. A comprehensive overview is provided by Reynaert et al. (252).

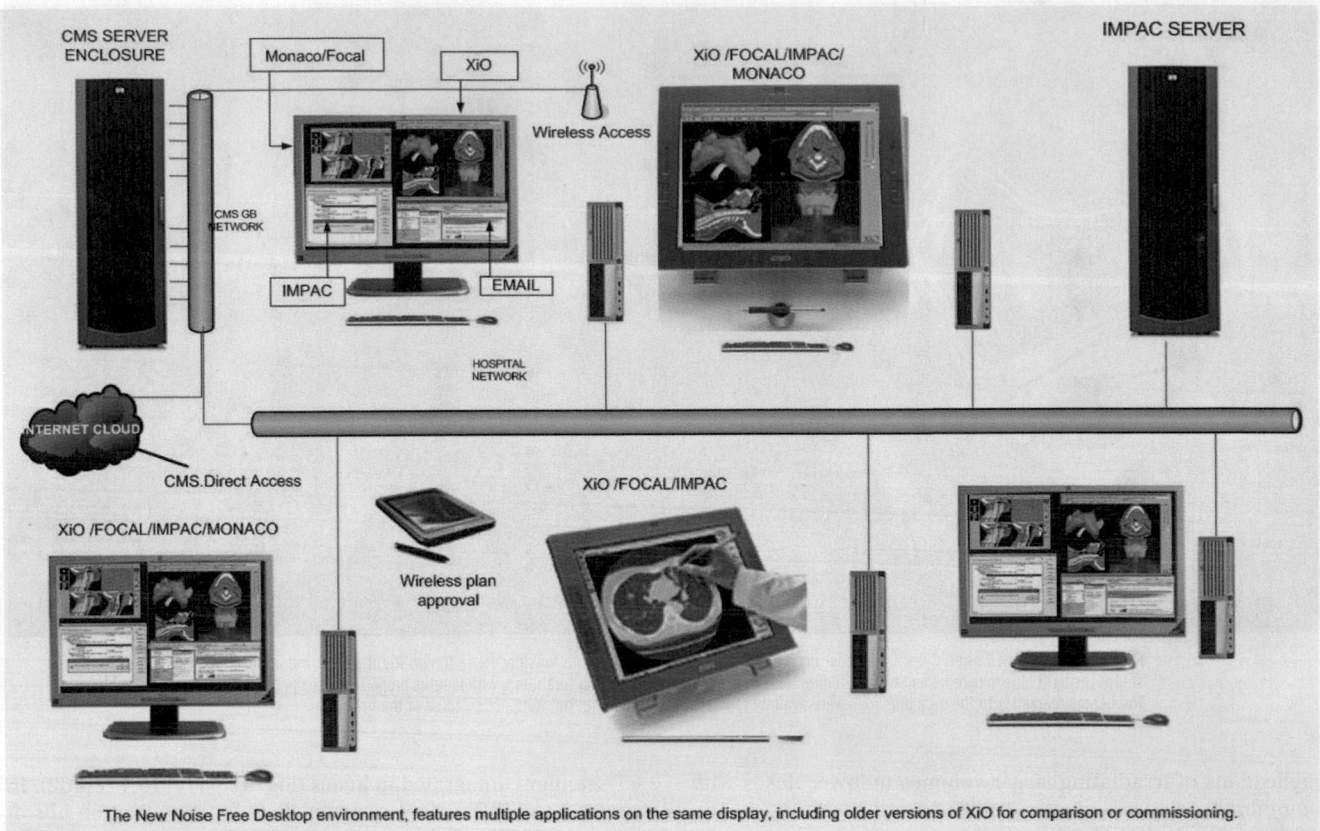

The New Noise Free Desktop environment, features multiple applications on the same display, including older versions of XiO for comparison or commissioning.

FIGURE 42.47.   Various applications are consolidated in a vendor's independent workspace: flexibility and freedom of access to any application are available with a click of a button in a truly paperless office.

Paperless Electronic Records

In the previous section one is confronted with innovative, highly technological care, but also with clinical research regarding QOL issues. These processes will undoubtedly go on with virtually no limitations. From the organizational (data-retrieval) point of view, one could envisage that most departments of radiation oncology will eventually be structured as a "paperless office" (Fig. 42.47). Direct architecture changes the conventional workflow into a productive workspace environment; that is, with a click of a button it combines the ease of the use of Windows with access to all types of vendor applications, including record and verify, e-mail, IMRT-QA, and office applications. This server client architecture gives users the freedom to access their applications anywhere in the hospital or in the world for collaboration, consultation, or to access particular applications for personal use. Features like pen-enabled computing, centralized storage, and secure remote access of the applications via broadband are not new in the information technology arena, but definitely are not routine to radiation therapy. It is setting a stage for any type of new application to fit into the existing infrastructure without adding new workstations or PCs in the already fully taken workspace. The future generation of connectivity between radiotherapy applications is true flexibility at the physician's desk, a solution without constraints.

Acknowledgments

The authors of this chapter are greatly indebted to the scientific work of the many authors of referenced articles (well over 300 references), as well as to the many coworkers of the Department of Radiation Oncology of the Erasmus MC, Rotterdam, for their enthusiastic and skillful support. In particular, we would like to mention the laborious effort to help revise and to provide new information by Inge Noever, Peter Voet, Henrie van der Est, Erik Franken, Mischa Hoogeman, Eric van 't Hooft, Johan Pöll, Peter van Rooij, Eliana Vásquez Osorio, Jeanette Bruinsma-v.d Hill, Jeanette Schilperoord, Schandra Manusama, and Marlies de Gelder.

References

1. Abedi E, Sismanis A. Extrapulmonary oat-cell carcinoma of the tonsil. *Ear Nose Throat J* 66:112–115.
2. Adler J Jr, Chang S, Murphy M, et al. The Cyberknife. a frameless robotic system for radiosurgery. *Stereotact Funct Neurosurg* 1997;69:124–128.
3. al-Abdulwahed S, Kudryk W, al Rajhi N, et al. Carcinoma of the tonsil: prognostic factors. *J Otolaryngol* 1997;26:296–299.
4. Alaei P, Higgins P, Weaver R, et al. Comparison of dynamic and step-and-shoot intensity-modulated radiation therapy planning and delivery. *Med Dosim* 2004;29:1–6.
5. Amelink A, Bard MPL, Burgers JA, et al. In vivo measurement of the local optical properties of tissue using differential pathlength spectroscopy. *Opt Lett* 2004;29:1087–1089.
6. American Joint Committee on Cancer. *Manual for Staging of Cancer*. 6th ed. New York: Springer-Verlag 2002.
7. Amornmarn R, Prempee T, Jaiwatana J. Radiation manangement of carcinoma of the tonsillar region. *Cancer* 1984;54:1293–1299.
8. Ang K, Garden AS. Radiotherapy for Head and Neck Cancers: indications and techniques. Lippincott Williams & Wilkins, 3rd ed Oropharynx 88–117.
9. Ang KK, Trotti A, et al. Randomized trial addressing risk features and time factors of surgery plus radiotherapy in advanced head-and-neck cancer. *Int J Radiat Oncol Biol Phys* 2001;51:571–578.
10. Arcangeli G, Saracino B, Tirindelli D. Accelerated hyperfractionated radiotherapy and concurrent protracted venous infusion chemotherapy in locally advanced head and neck cancer. *Am J Clin Oncol* 2002;25:431–437.
11. Barker JJ, Garden AS, Ang K, et al. Quantification of volumetric and geometric changes occurring during fractionated radiotherapy for head-and-neck cancer using an integrated CT/linear accelerator system. *Int J Radiat Oncol Biol Phys* 2004;59:960–970.
12. Barrett WL, Gluckman JL, Wilson KM, et al. A comparison of treatments of

squamous cell carcinoma of the base of tongue: surgical resection combined with external radiation therapy, external radiation therapy alone, and external radiation therapy combined with interstitial radiation. *Brachytherapy* 2004;3:240–245.
13. Bartelink H, Van Den BW, Horiot J-C. Concomitant cisplatin and radiotherapy in a conventional and modified fractionation schedule in locally advanced head and neck cancer: a randomised phase II EORTC trial. *Eur J Cancer* 2002;38:667–673.
14. Barton JH, Osborne BM, Butler JJ. Non-Hodgkin's lymphoma of the tonsil: a clinicopathologic study of 65 cases. *Cancer* 1984;53:86–95.
15. Bataini JP, Asselain B, Jaulerry C, et al. A multivariate primary tumour control analysis in 465 patients treated by radical radiotherapy for cancer of the tonsillar region: clinical and treatment parameters as prognostic factors. *Radiother Oncol* 1989;14:265–277.
16. Bataini JP, Bernier J, Bernier J. Natural history of neck disease in patients with squamous cell carcinoma. *Radiother Oncol* 1985;3:245–255.
17. Bedwinek JM, Shukovsky LJ, Fletcher GH, et al. Osteonecrosis in patients treated with definitive radiotherapy for squamous cell carcinomas of the oral cavity and naso- and oropharynx. *Radiology* 1976;119:665.
18. Beitler J. Is ipsilateral radiation for tonsil cancer with limited tongue extension or T2N1 tonsil cancer without tongue involvement appropriate? *Int J Radiat Oncol Biol Phys* 2002;154:301.
19. Bel A, Bartelink H, Vijlbrief R, et al. Transfer errors of planning CT to simulator: a possible source of setup inaccuracies? *Radiother Oncol* 1994;31:176–180.
20. Benasso M, Bonelli L, Numico G. Treatment with cisplatin and fluoruracil alternating with radiation favour prognosis of inoperable squamous cell carcinoma of he head and neck: a multivariate analysis on 273 patients. *Am Oncol* 1997;8:773–779.
21. Bensadoun RJ. Concomitant b.i.d. radiotherapy and chemotherapy with cisplatin and 5-fluorouracil in unresectable squamous-cell carcinoma of the pharynx: clinical and pharmacological data of a French multicenter phase II study. *Int J Radiat Oncol Biol Phys* 1998;42:237–245.
22. Bernier J, Bentzen SM. Altered fractionation and combined radio-chemotherapy approaches: pioneering new opportunities in head and neck oncology. *Eur J Cancer* 2003;39:560–571.
23. Bernier J, Cooper JS, Pajak TF, et al. Defining risk levels in locally advanced head and neck cancers: a comparative analysis of concurrent postoperative radiation plus chemotherapy trials of the EORTC (#22931) and RTOG (#9501). EORTC (#22931), RTOG (#9501) .
24. Bernier J, Cooper JS. Chemoradiation after surgery for high risk head and neck cancer patients: how strong is the evidence? *Oncologist* 2005;10:215–224.
25. Bieri S. Concomitant boost radiotherapy in oropharynx carcinomas. *Acta Oncol* 1998;37:687–691.
26. Bijhold J, Lebesque J, Hart A, et al. Maximizing setup accuracy using portal images as applied to a conformal boost technique for prostatic cancer. *Radiother Oncol* 1992;24:261–271.
27. Bjordal K, Graeff dA, Fayers PM. A 12-country field study of the EORTC QLQ-C30 (version 3.0) and the head and neck cancer specific module (EORTC QLQ-H&N35) in head and neck patients. *Eur J Cancer* 2000;36:1796–1807.
28. Bjordal K, Kaasa S, Mastekaasa A. Quality of life in patients treated for head and neck cancer: a follow-up study 7 to 11 years after radiotherapy. *Int J Radiat Oncol Biol Phys* 1994;28:847–856.
29. Bjordal K, Kaasa S. Psychological distress in head and neck cancer patients 7-11 years after curative treatment. *Br J Cancer* 1995;71:592–597.
30. Boer dM, McCormick LK, Pruyn JF. Physical and psychosocial correlates of head and neck cancer: a review of the literature. *Otolaryngol Head Neck Surg* 1999;120:427–436.
31. Boffeta P, Mashberg A, Winkelmann R. Carcinogenic effect of tobacco smoking and alcohol drinking on anatomic sites of oral cavity and oropharynx. *Int J Cancer* 1992;52:530–533.
32. Bolner A, Mussari S, Fellin G, et al. The role of brachytherapy in the management of oropharyngeal carcinomas: the Trento experience. *Tumori* 2002;88:137–141.
33. Bonner JA, Harari PM, Giralt J, et al. Radiotherapy plus cetuximab for squamous-cell carcinoma of the head and neck. *N Engl J Med* 2006;354:567–578.
34. Boudreau C, Heath E, Seuntjens J, et al. IMRT head and neck treatment planning with a commercially available Monte Carlo based planning system. *Phys Med Biol* 2005:50, 879–890.
35. Bourhis J, Syz N, Overgaard J. Conventional versus modified fractionated radiotherapy: meta-analysis based on individual data of patients with head and neck squamous cell carcinoma (HNSCC) ESTRO Conference, Prague, September 17–21, 2002. *Radiother Oncol* 2002;64[Suppl 1]. (abstr).
36. Brizel DM. Hyperfractionated irradiation with or without concurrent chemotherapy for locally advanced head and neck cancer. *N Engl J Med* 1998;338:1798–1804.
37. Brownian GP, Wong G, Hodson I. Influence of cigarette smoking on the efficacy of radiation therapy in head and neck cancer. *N Engl J Med* 1993;328:159.
38. Brunin F, Mosseri V, Jaulerry C, et al. Cancer of the base of the tongue: past and future. *Head Neck* 1999;21:751–759.
39. Byers RM, Anderson B, Schwarz EA. Treatment of squamous carcinoma of the retro molar trigone. *Am J Clin Oncol* 1984;7:647–652.
40. Byers RM, Wolf PF, Ballantyne AJ. Rationale for elective modified neck dissection. *Head Neck Surg* 1988;10:160–167.
41. Calais G. Radiation (RT) alone versus RT with concomitant chemotherapy (CT) in stages III and IV oropharynx carcinoma. Final results of the 94—01 GORTEC randomized study. *Int J Radiat Biol Phys* 2001;51[3 Suppl 1]:1.
42. Calais G. Randomized trial of radiation therapy versus concomitant chemotherapy and radiation therapy for advanced-stage oropharynx carcinoma. *J Natl Cancer Inst* 1999;91:2081–2016.
43. Calais G. Stage III and IV cancers of the oropharynx: results of a randomized study of Gortec comparing radiotherapy alone with concomitant chemotherapy. *Bull Cancer* 2000;87:48–53.
44. Candela FC, Kothari K, Shah JP. Patterns of cervical node metastases from squamous carcinoma of the oropharynx and hypopharynx. *Head Neck* 1990;12:197–203.
45. Candela FC, Shah J, Jaques DP. Patterns of cervical node metastases from squamous carcinoma of the larynx. *Arch Otolaryngol Head Neck Surg* 1990;116:116–432.
46. Cella DF, Tulsky DS, Gray G. The functional assessment of cancer therapy scale: development and validation of the general measure. *J Clin Oncol* 1993;11:570–579.
47. Chang L, Stevens KR, Moss WT. Squamous cell carcinoma of the pharyngeal walls treated with radiotherapy. *Int J Radiat Oncol Biol Phys* 1996;35:477–483.
48. Chang YM, Tsai CY, Kildal M. Importance of coronoidotomy and masticatory muscle myotomy in surgical release of trismus caused by submucous fibrosis. *Plast Reconstr Surg* 2004;13:1949–1954.
49. Chao KS, Deasy JO, Markman J, et al. A prospective study of salivary function sparing in patients with head-and-neck cancers receiving intensity-modulated or three-dimensional radiation therapy: initial results. *Int J Radiat Oncol Biol Phys* 2001;49:907–916.
50. Chao KS, Majhail N, Huang CJ, et al. Intensity-modulated radiation therapy reduces late salivary toxicity without compromising tumor control in patients with oropharyngeal carcinoma: a comparison with conventional techniques. *Radiother Oncol* 2001;61:275–280.
51. Chao KS, Ozyigit G, Blanco AI, et al. Intensity-modulated radiation therapy for oropharyngeal carcinoma: impact of tumor volume. *Int J Radiat Oncol Biol Phys* 2004;59:43–50.
52. Chao KSC, Wippold FJ, Ozyigit G. Determination and delineation of nodal target volumes for head and neck cancer based on patterns of failure in patients receiving definitive and postoperative IMRT. *Int J Radiat Oncol Biol Phys* 2002;53:1174–1184.
53. Chenal C, Julienne V, Fleury F. Radiotherapy and curietherapy of squamous cell carcinoma of the posterior pharyngeal wall (excluding the nasopharynx). *Bull Cancer Radiother.* 1996;83:54–59.
54. Chua DTT, Lo CEN, Yuen JNS, et al. A pilot study of pentoxifylline in the treatment of radiation-induced trismus. *Am J Clin Oncol* 2001;24:366–369.
55. Chui C, Chan M, Yorke E, et al. Delivery of intensity-modulated radiation therapy with a conventional multileaf collimator: comparison of dynamic and segmental methods. *Med Phys.* 2001;28:2441–2449.
56. Cooper JS, Pajak TF, Forastiere AA. Postoperative concurrent radiotherapy and chemotherapy for high-risk squamous-cell carcinoma of the head and neck. *N Engl J Med* 2004;350:1937–1944.
57. Cooper RA, Slevin NJ, Carringron BM. Radiotherapy for carcinoma of the posterior pharyngeal wall. *Int J Oncol* 2000;16:611–615.
58. Cornes PG, Cox HJ, Rhys-Evans PR. Salvage treatment for inoperable neck nodes in head and neck cancer using combined iridium-192 brachytherapy and surgical reconstruction. *Br J Surg* 1996;83:1620–1622.
59. Cox JD, Ang KK. *Radiation oncology: rationale, technique, results*, 8th ed. St Louis, MO: Mosby; 2003:196–218.
60. Crook J, Mazeron JJ, Marinello G. Combined external and interstitial implantation for T1 and T2 epidermoid carcinoma of base of tongue: the Creteil experience. *Int J Radiat Oncol Biol Phys* 1988;15:105–114.
61. Dai J, Que W. Simultaneous minimization of leaf travel distance and tongue-and-groove effect for segmental intensity-modulated radiation therapy. *Phys Med Biol.* 2004;49:5319–31.
62. de Arruda F, Puri D, Zhung J, et al. Intensity-modulated radiation therapy for the treatment of oropharyngeal carcinoma: the Memorial Sloan-Kettering Cancer Center experience. *Int J Rad Oncol Biol Phys* 2006;64:363–373.
63. de Boer J, Heijmen B. A protocol for the reduction of systematic patient setup errors with minimal portal imaging workload. *Int J Radiat Oncol Biol Phys* 2001;50:1350–1365.
64. de Boer J, Heijmen B. eNAL: an extension of the NAL set-up correction protocol for effective use of weekly measurements. *Int J Radiat Oncol Biol Phys* 2007;67:1586–1595.
65. de Boer J, van Sörnsen de Koste J, Creutzberg C. Electronic portal image assisted reduction of systematic set-up errors in head and neck irradiation. *Radiother Oncol* 2001;61:299–308.
66. Di Marco A, Rizzotti A, Grandinetti A, et al. External radiotherapy in the treatment of tonsillar carcinomas. Analysis of 183 cases. *Tumori* 1990;76:244–249.
67. Dijkstra PU, Huisman PM, Roodenburg JLN. Criteria for trismus in head and neck oncology. *Int J Oral Maxillofacial Surg* 2006;35:337–342.
68. Dijkstra PU, Kalk WWI, Roodenburg JLN. Trismus in head and neck oncology: a systematic review. *Oral Oncology* 2004;40:879–889.
69. Dixit S, Babbo HA, Rakesh V, et al. Interstitial high dose rate brachytherapy in head and neck cancers: preliminary results. *J Brachyther Int* 1997;13:363–10.
70. Douglas WG, Rigual NR, Giese W, et al. Advanced soft palate cancer: the clinical importance of the parapharyngeal space. *Otolaryngol Head Neck Surg* 2005;133:66–69.
71. Doweck I, Robbins KT, Mendenhall WM, et al. Neck level-specific nodal metastases in oropharyngeal cancer: is there a role for selective neck dissection after definitive radiation therapy? *Head Neck* 2003;25:960–967.
72. Dubey P, Ha C, Ang KK. Nonnasopharyngeal lymphoeitheliomas of the head and neck. *Cancer* 1998;82:1556–1562.
73. Eisbruch A, Kim HM, Terrell JE, et al. Xerostomia and its predictors following parotid-sparing irradiation of head-and-neck cancer. *Int J Radiat Oncol Biol Phys* 2001;50:695–704.
74. Eisbruch A, Marsh LH, Dawson LA, et al. Recurrences near base of skull after IMRT for head-and neck cancer: implications for target delineation in high neck and for parotid gland sparing. *Int J Radiat Oncol Biol Phys.* 2004;59:28–42.
75. Eisbruch A, Schwartz M, Rasch C, et al. Dysphagia and aspiration after chemoradiotherapy for head-and-neck cancer: which anatomic structures are affected and can they be spared by IMRT? *Int J Radiat Onco Biol Phys* 2004;60:1425–1439.
76. Eisbruch A, Ten Haken RK, Kim HM. Dose, volume, and function relationships in parotid salivary glands following conformal and intensity-modulated irradiation of head and neck cancer. *Int J Radiat Oncol Biol Phys* 1999;45:577–587.
77. Emami B, Lyman J, Brown A, et al. Tolerance of normal tissue to therapeutic irradiation. *Int J Radiat Oncol Biol Phys* 1991;21:109–122.
78. Erkal HS, Serin M, Amdur RJ, et al. Squamous cell carcinomas of the soft palate treated with radiation therapy alone or followed by planned neck dissection. *Int J Radiat Oncol Biol Phys* 2001;50:359–366.
79. Esche BA, Haie CM, Gerbaulet AP, et al. Interstitial and external radiotherapy in carcinoma of the soft palate and uvula. *Int J Radiat Oncol Biol Phys.* 1988;15:619–625.
80. Essers M, Langen de M, Dirkx M, et al. Commissioning of a commercially available system for intensity-modulated radiotherapy dose delivery with dynamic multileaf collimation. *Radiother Oncol.* 2001;60:215–24.
81. Fein DA, Mendenhall WM, Parsons JT. Pharyngeal wall carcinoma treated with

radiotherapy: impact of treatment technique and fractionation. *Int J Radiat Oncol Biol Phys* 1993;26:751–757.
82. Fiorino C, Dell'Oca I, Pierelli A, et al. Significant improvement in normal tissue sparing and target coverage for head and neck cancer by means of helical tomotherapy. *Radiother Oncol* 2006;78:276–282.
83. Fogliata A, Bolsi A, Cozzi L. Comparative analysis of intensity modulation inverse planning modules of three commercial treatment planning systems applied to head and neck tumour model. *Radiother Oncol.* 2003;66:29–40.
84. Followill D, Geis P, Boyer A. Estimates of whole-body dose equivalent produced by beam intensity modulated conformal therapy. *Int J Radiat Oncol Biol Phys.* 1997;38:667–72.
85. Foote RL, Olfsen KD, Davis DL. Base of tongue carcinoma: patterns of failure and predictors of recurrence after surgery alone. *Head Neck* 1993;15:300–307.
86. Foote RL, Parsons JT, Mendenhall WM. Is interstitial implantation essential for successful treatment of base of tongue carcinoma? *Int J Radiat Oncol Bol Phys* 1990;18:1293–1298.
87. Foote RL, Schild SE, Thompson WM. Tonsil cancer: patterns of failure after surgery, combined with postoperative radiation therapy. *Cancer* 1994;73:2638–2647.
88. Forastiere AA. Phase III trial to preserve the larynx: induction chemotherapy and radiotherapy versus concomitant chemoradiotherapy versus radiotherapy alone, Intergroup Trial R91-11. Proceedings of the ASCO 2001:20.
89. Franken E, de Boer J, Barnhoorn J, et al. Characteristics relevant to portal dosimetry of a cooled CCD camera-based EPID. *Med Phys.* 2004;31:2549–51.
90. Franken E, de Boer J, Heijmen B. A novel approach to accurate portal dosimetry using CCD-camera based EPIDs. *Med Phys.* 2006;33:888–903.
91. Fu KK, Pajak TF, Trotti A. A Radiation Therapy Oncology Group (RTOG) phase III randomized study to compare hyperfractionation and two variants of accelerated fractionation to standard fractionation for head and neck squamous cell carcinomas: First report of RTOG 9003. *Int J Radiat Oncol Biol Phys* 2000;48:7–16.
92. Gal TJ, Yueh B, Futran ND. Influence of prior hyperbaric oxygen therapy in complications following microvascular reconstruction for advanced osteoradionecrosis. *Arch Otolaryngol Head Neck Surg* 2003;129:72–76.
93. Garden AS, Weber RS, Ang KK. Postoperative radiation therapy for malignant tumors of minor salivary glands. *Cancer* 1994;73:2563–2569.
94. Gardner E, Gray DJ, O'Rahilly R. *A regional study of human structure*, 2nd ed. Philadelphia: WB Saunders;1963:937–946.
95. Gardner E, Gray DJ, O'Rahily R. *Anatomy. Muscles of mastication*, 2nd ed. Philadelphia: WB Saunders;1963:839–845.
96. Garret PG, Beale FA, Cummings BJ, et al. Carcinoma of the tonsil: the effect of dose-time-volume factors on local control. *Int J Radiat Oncol Biol Phys* 1985;11:703–706.
97. Genden EM, Ferlito A, Scully C, et al. Current management of tonsillar cancer. *Oral Oncol.* 2003;39:337–342.
98. Gerbaulet A, P"tter R, Mazeron JJ. *The GEC ESTRO handbook of brachytherapy*. 2002.
99. Gibbs I.C, Quynh-Thu, L, Shah, R.D, et al. Long-term outcomes after external beam irradiation and brachytherapy boost for base-of-tongue cancers. *Int J Radiat Oncol Biol Phys* 2003;57:489–494.
100. Giralt JL. Preoperative induction chemotherapy followed by concurrent chemoradiotherapy in advanced carcinoma of the oral cavity and oropharynx. *Cancer* 2000;89:939–945.
101. Givens CD Jr, Johns ME, Cantrell RW. Carcinoma of the tonsil. Analysis of 162 cases. *Arch Otolaryngol.* 1981;107:730–734.
102. Gluckman JL, Black RJ, Crissman JD. Cancer of the oropharynx. *Otolaryngol Clin North Am.* 1985;18:451–459.
103. Goffinet DR, Fee WE.Jr, Wells J. 192 Ir pharyngoepiglottic fold interstitial implants. The key to successful treatment of base tongue carcinoma by radiation therapy. *Cancer* 1985;55:941–948.
104 Gogh vC, Verdonck-de Leeuw IM, Boon-Kamma BA, et al. A screening questionnaire for voice problems after treatment of early glottic cancer. *Int J Radiat Oncol Biol Phys* 2005;63:700–705.
105. Graeff dA, Leeuw d Jr, Ros WJ, et al. Long-term quality of life patients with head and neck cancer. *Laryngoscope* 2000;110:98–106.
106. Graeff dA, Leeuw dR, Ros WJ, et al. A prospective study on quality of life of laryngeal cancer patients treated with radiotherapy. *Head Neck* 1999;21:291–296.
107. Graner DE, Foote RL, Kasperbauer JL. Swallow function in patients before and after intra-arterial chemoradiation. *Laryngoscope* 2003;113:573–579.
108. Gregoire V, Coche E, Cosnard G, et al. Selection and delineation of lymph node target volumes in head and neck conformal radiotherapy. Proposal for standardizing terminology and procedure based on the surgical experience. *Radiother Oncol* 2000;56:135–150.
109. Gregoire V, Eisbruch A, Levendag P. Proposal for the delineation of the nodal CTV in the node-positive and the post-operative neck. *Radiother Oncol* 2006;79:15–20.
110. Gregoire V, Levendag P, Ang KK, et al. CT-based delineation of lymphnode levels and related CTV's in the node-negative neck: DAHANCA, EORTC, GORTEC, NCIC, RTOG consensus guidelines. 69:227-236. *Radiother Oncol* 2003;69:227–236.
111. Grimard L, Szanto J, Girard A. Asymmetric Arch Technique for posterior pharyngeal wall and retro pharyngeal space tumors. *Int J Radiat Oncol Biol Phys* 1995;31:611–615.
112. Guillamondegui OM, Meoz R, Jess RE. Surgical treatment of squamous cell carcinoma of the pharyngeal wall. *Am J Surg* 1978;136:474–476.
113. Haagensen C. *The lymphatics in cancer*. Philadelphia: Saunders; 1972.
114. Hall EJ. Intensity-modulated radiation therapy, protons, and the risk of second cancers. *Int J Rad Oncol Biol Phys* 2006;56; 1:1–7.
115. Hammerlid E, Bjordal K, Ahlner-Elmqvist M. Prospective, longitudinal quality-of-life study of patients with head and neck cancer. A feasibility study: including the EORTC QLQ-C30. *Otolaryngol Head Neck Surg* 1997;116[6 Pt 1]:666–673.
116. Hammerlid E, Silander E, Hornestam L. Health-related quality of life three years after diagnosis of head and neck cancer—a longitudinal study. *Head Neck* 2001;23:113–125.
117. Han P, Hu K, Frank DK, et al. Management of cancer of the base of tongue. *Otolaryngol Clin North Am* 2005;38:75–85.
118. Hansen E, Bucci M, Quivey J, et al. Repeat CT imaging and replanning during the course of IMRT for head-and-neck cancer. *Int J Radiat Oncol Biol Phys.* 2006, 64:355–62.
119. Hao D, Ritter M, Oliver T. Platinum-based concurrent chemoradiotherapy for tumor of the head and neck and the esophagus. *Semin Radiat Oncol* 2005;16:10–19.
120. Harrison LB, Ferlito A, Ashok R. Current philosophy on the management of cancer of the base of the tongue. *Oral Oncology* 2003;101–105.
121. Harrison LB, Lee HJ, Pfister DG, et al. Long term results of primary radiotherapy with/without neck dissection for squamous cell cancer of the base of tongue. *Head Neck*. 1998;20:668–673.
122. Harrison LB, Lee HJ, Pfister DG. Long term result of primary radiotherapy with/without neck dissection for squamous cell cancer of the base of tongue. *Head Neck* 1992;14:99–101.
123. Harrison LB, Sessions RB, Hong WK. *Head and neck cancer: a multidisciplinary approach*. Philadelphia: Lippincott Williams & Wilkins; 2004:306–351.
124. Harrison LB, Sessions RB, Strong EW. Brachytherapy as part of the definitive management of squamous cancer of the base of tongue. *Int J Radiat Oncol Biol Phys* 1989;17:1309–1312.
125. Harrison LB, Zelefsky MJ, Armstrong JG. Performance status after treatment for squamous cell cancer of the base of tongue - a comparison of primary radiation therapy versus primary surgery. *Int J Radiat Oncol Biol Phys* 1994;30:953–957.
126. Harrison LB, Zelefsky MJ, Pfister D. Detailed quality of life assessment in patients treated with primary radiotherapy for squamous cell cancer of the base of tongue. *Head Neck* 1997;19:169–175.
127. Harrison LB, Zelefsky MJ, Pfister D. Detailed quality of life assessment on long term survivors of primary radiation therapy for cancer of the base of tongue. *Head Neck* 1997;19:169–175.
128. Harrison LB. A prospective phase II trial of concomitant chemotherapy and radiotherapy with delayed accelerated fractionation in unresectable tumors of the head and neck. *Head Neck* 1998;20:497–503.
129. Heath E, Seuntjens J, Sheikh-Bagheri D. Dosimetric evaluation of the clinical implementation of the first commercial IMRT Monte Carlo treatment planning system at 6MV. *Med Phys.* 2004: 31, 2771–2779.
130. Hehr T, Classen J, Schreck U. Hyperfractionated accelerated radiotherapy alone and with concomitant chemotherapy to the head and neck: treated within and outside of randomized clinical trials. *Int J Rad Oncol Biol Phys* 2004;58:1424–1430.
131. Heijmen B, Pasma K, Kroonwijk M, et al. Portal dose measurement in radiotherapy using an electronic portal imaging device. *Phys Med Biol.* 1995;40:1943–1955.
132. Herk van M, Remeijer P, Rasch C, et al. The probability of correct target dosage: dose-population histograms for deriving treatment margins in radiotherapy. *Int J Radiat Oncol Biol Phys* 2000;47:1121–1135.
133. Hinerman RW, Parsons JT, Mendenhall WM. External beam irradiation alone or combined with neck dissection for base of tongue carcinoma: An alternative to primary surgery. *Laryngosope* 1994;104:1466.
134. Hoffstetter S, Malissard L, Pernot M. Retrospective study of a series of 136 carcinomas of the base of tongue treated in Centre Alexis Vautrin. *Bull Cancer Radiother* 1996;83:90–96.
135. Hoogeman M, Nuyttens J, Levendag P, et al. Intra-fraction motion of immobilized intra-cranial and extra-cranial patients assessed by the CyberKnife image-guidance system. 2006, submitted.
136. Hoogsteen I, Pop AM, Marres HAM. Oxygen-modifying treatment with ARCON reduces the prognostic significance of hemoglobin in squamous cell carcinoma of the Head and Neck. *Int J Radiation Oncology Biol Phys.* 2006;64:83–89.
137. Horiot JC, Bontemps P, Van Den BW. Accelareted fracionation (AF) compared to conventional fracionation (CF) improves loco-regional control in the radiotherapy of advanced head and neck cancers: results of the EORTC 22851 randomized trial. *Radiother Oncol* 1997;44;111–121.
138. Horiot JC, Le Fur R, N'Guyen T, et al. Hyperfractionation versus conventional fractionation in oropharyngeal carcinoma: final analysis of a randomized trial of the EORTC cooperative group of radiotherapy. *Radiother Oncol* 1992;25:231–241.
139. Horwitz EM, Frazier AJ, Martinez AA. Excellent functional outcome in patients with squamous cell carcinoma of the base of the tongue treated with external irradiation and interstitial iodine 125 boost. *Cancer* 1996;78:948–957.
140. Housset M, Baillet F, Delanian S. Split course interstitial brachytherapy with a source shift: the results of a new iridium implant technique versus single course implants for salvage irradiation of base of tongue cancers in 55 patients. *Int J Radiat Oncol Biol Phys* 1991;20:965–971.
141. Housset M, Baillet F, Dessard-Diana B. A retrospective study of three treatment techniques for T1-2 base of tongue lesions: surgery plus postoperative irradiation, external irradiation plus interstitial implantation and external irradiation alone. *Int J Radiat Oncol Biol Phys* 1987;13:511–516.
142. Hull MC, Morris CG, Tannehill SP. Definitive radiotherapy alone or combined with a planned neck dissection for squamous cell carcinoma of the pharyngeal wall. *Cancer* 2003;98:2224–2232.
143. International Commission on Radiations Units and Measurements. Prescribing, recording, and reporting photon beam therapy (supplement to ICRU report 50). ICRU Report 62. Bethesda, MD: International Commission on Radiation Units and Measurements; 1999.
144. Jabbari S, Kim HM, Feng M, et al. Matched case-control study of quality of life and xerostomia after intensity-modulated radiotherapy or standard radiotherapy for head-and-neck cancer: initial report. *Int J Radiat Oncol Biol Phys* 2005;63:725–731.
145. Jackson SM, Hay JH, Flores AD, et al. Cancer of the tonsil: the results of ipsilateral radiation treatment. *Radiother Oncol* 1999;51:123–128.
146. Jaffray D, Drake D, Moreau M, et al. A radiographic and tomographic imaging system integrated into a medical linear accelerator for localization of bone and soft-tissue targets. *Int J Radiat Oncol Biol Phys.* 1999;45:773–89.
147. Jaulerry C, Rodriguez J, Brunin F. Results of radiation therapy in carcinoma of the base of the tongue. *Cancer* 1991;67:1532.
148. Jeremic B. Hyperfractonated radiation therapy with or without conccurrent low-dose daily cisplatin in locally squamous cell carcinoma of the head and neck: a prospective randomized trial. *J Clin Oncol* 2000;18:1458–1464.
149. Jesse RH Jr, Fletcher GH. Metastases in cervical lymph nodes from oropharyngeal carcinoma: treatment and results. *Am J Roentgenol* 1963;90:990–996.
150. Johnston WD, Byers RM. Squamous cell carcinoma of the tonsil in young adults. *Cancer* 1977;39:633–636.
151. Julieron M, Kolk F, Schwaab G. Surgical management of posterior pharyngeal wall carcinomas: functional and oncologic results. *Head Neck* 2001;23:80–86.
152. Kaanders JHAM, Hordijk GJ. Carcinoma of the larynx: The Dutch national

guideline for diagnostics, treatment, supportive care and rehabilitation. *Radiother Oncol* 2002;63:299–307.

153. Kaanders JHAM, Pop LAM, Marres HAM, et al. ARCON: Experience in 215 patients with advanced head and neck cancer. *Int J Radiat Oncol Phys* 2002;52:769–781.

154. Karakoyun-Celik O, Norris CM, Tishler R. Definitive radiotherapy with interstitial implant boost for squamous cell carcinoma of the tongue base. *Head Neck* 2005;353–361.

155. Kies MS. Induction chemotherapy followed by concurrent chemoradiation for advanced head and neck cancer: improved disease control and survival. *J Clin Oncol* 1998;16:2715–2721.

156. King GE, Scheetz J, Jacob RF. Electrotherapy and hyperbaric oxygen: promising treatments for postradiation complications. *J Prosthet Dent.* 1989;62:331–458.

157. Kolkman-Deurloo IK, Nuyttens JJ, Hanssens PEJ. Intraoperative HDR brachytherapy for rectal cancer using a flexible intraoperative template: standard plans versus individual planning. *Rad Oncol* 2004;70:75–79.

158. Kong JS, Fuller LM, Butler JJ. Stages I and II non-Hodgkin's lymphomas of Waldeyer's ring and the neck. *Am J Clin Oncol* 1984;7:629–639.

159. Koss L, Shapiro R, Jahdu S. Small cell (oat cell) carcinoma of minor salivary gland origin. origin. *Cancer* 1972;30:737–741.

160. Kotwall C, Sako K, Razack MS. Metastatic patterns in squamous cell cancer of the head and neck. *Am J Surg* 1987;154:439–442.

161. Kouyoumdjian JH, Chalian VA, Hutton C. An intraoral positive-Arch pressure device for treatment of trismus. *Oral Surg Oral Med Oral Pathol.* 1986;61:456–458.

162. Kraus DH, Vastola P, Huvos AG. Surgical management of squamous cell carcinoma of the base of the tongue. *Am J Surg* 1993;166:384–388.

163. Kruijff de W, Heijmen B, Voet P, et al. Proceedings of the 23rd ESTRO meeting, Amsterdam, 2004. *Radiother Oncol.* 73, S89.

164. Laccourreye O, Hans S, Menard M, et al. Transoral lateral oropharyngectomy for squamous cell carcinoma of the tonsillar region: II. An analysis of the incidence, related variables, and consequences of local recurrence. *Arch Otolaryngol Head Neck Surg* 2005;131:592–599.

165. Langlois D, Hoffsteitter S, Malissard L. Salvage irradiation of oropharynx and mobile tongue about iridium brachytherapy in Centre Alexis Vautrin. *Int J Radiat Oncol Biol Phys* 1988;14:849–853.

166. Lauve A, Morris M, Schmidt-Ullrich R, et al. Simultaneous integrated boost intensity-modulated radiotherapy for locally advanced head-and-neck squamous cell carcinomas: II-clinical results. *Int J Radiat Oncol Biol Phys.* 2004;60:374–87.

167. Lee HJ, Zelefsky MJ, Kraus DH, et al. Long-term regional control after radiation therapy and neck dissection for base of tongue carcinoma. *Int J Radiat Oncol Biol Phys* 1997;15 38:995–1000.

168. Lee N, Puri D, Blanco A, et al. Intensity-modulated radiation therapy in head and neck cancers: an update. *Head Neck.* 2007;29:387–400.

169. Lee N. Counterpoint: brachytherapy versus intensity-modulated radiation therapy in the management of base of tongue cancers. *Brachytherapy* 2005;4:1–4.

170. Leemans CR, Engelbrecht WJ, Tiwari RM. Carcinoma of the soft palate and anterior tonsillar pillar. *Laryngoscope* 1994;104:1477–1481.

171. Leibel S, Phillips T. *Textbook of radiation oncology*, 2nd ed.

172. Letourneau D, Wong J, Oldham M, et al. Cone-beam-CT guided radiation therapy: technical implementation. *Radiother Oncol.* 2005;75:279–86.

173. Levendag P, Braaksma M, Coche E. Rotterdam and Brussels CT-based neck nodal delineation compared to the surgical levels as defined by the American Academy of Otolaryngology—Head Neck Surgery. *Int J Radiat Oncol Biol Phys* 2004;58:1:113–123.

174. Levendag P, Gregoire V, et al. Intraoperative validation of CT-based lymph nodal levels, sublevels IIA and IIB: is it of clinical relevance in selective radiation therapy? *Int J Radiat Oncol Biol Phys* 2005;62:690–699.

175. Levendag P, Nijdam W, Noever I, et al. Brachytherapy versus surgery in carcinoma of tonsillar fossa and/or soft palate: late adverse sequelae and performance status: can we be more selective and obtain better tissue sparing? *Int J Radiat Oncol Biol Phys* 2004;59:713–724.

176. Levendag PC, Meeuwis CA, Visser AG. Reirradiation of recurrent head and neck cancers: external and/or interstitial radiation therapy. *Radiother Oncol.* 1992;23:6–15.

177. Levendag PC, Schmitz PIIM, Jansen PP. Fractionated high-dose-rate and pulsed-dose-rate brachytherapy: first clinical experience in squamous cell carcinoma of the tonsillar fossa and soft palate. *Int J Radiat Oncol Biol Phys* 1997;38:497–506.

178. Lindberg R. Distribution of cervical lymph node metastases from squamous cell carcinoma of the upper respiratory and digestive tracts. *Cancer* 1992;29:1446–1449.

179. List M, Ritter-Ster C, Lansky S. A performance status scale for head and neck cancer patients. *Cancer* 1990;66:564–569.

180. List MA, Stracks J, Colangelo L. How do head and neck cancer patients prioritize treatment outcomes before initiating treatment. *J Clin Oncol* 2000;18:877–884.

181. LoSasso T, Chui C, Ling C. Physical and dosimetric aspects of a multileaf collimation system used in dynamic mode for implementing intensity modulated radiotherapy. *Med. Phys.* 1998;25:1919–1927.

182. Luan S, Wang C, Chen D, et al. An improved MLC segmentation algorithm and software for step-and-shoot IMRT delivery without tongue-and-groove error. *Med Phys* 2006;33:1199–1212.

183. Lusinchi A, Eskandari J, Son Y, et al. External Irradiation plus curietherapy boost in 108 base of tongue carcinoma. *Int J Rad Oncol Biol Phys* 1989;17:1191–1197.

184. Machtay M, Perch S, Markiewicz D, et al. Combined surgery and postoperative radiotherapy for carcinoma of the base of radiotherapy for carcinoma of the base of tongue: analysis of treatment outcome and prognostic value of margin status. *Head Neck.* 1997;19:494–499.

185. Machtay M, Rosenthal DI, Hershock D. Organ preservation therapy using induction plus concurrent chemoradiation for advanced resectable oropharyngeal carcinoma: a University of Pennsylvania Phase II trial. *J Clin Oncol* 2002;20:3964–3971.

186. Mackie T, Holmes T, Swerdloff S, et al. Tomotherapy: a new concept for the delivery of dynamic conformal radiotherapy. *Med Phys* 1993;20:1709–1719.

187. Maguire PD, Meyerson MD, Neal CR. Toxic cure: hyperfrationated radiotherapy with concurrent cisplatin and fluorouracil for stage III and IVA head-and-neck cancer in the community. *Int J Radiation Oncology Biol Phys.* 2004;28:689–704.

188. Mak AC, Morrison WH, Garden AS. Base of tongue carcinoma: Treatment results using concomitant boost radiotherapy. *Int J Radiat Oncol Biol Phys* 1995;33:289–296.

189. Mak-Kregar S, Baris G, Lebesque JV, et al. Radiotherapy of tonsillar and base of tongue carcinoma. Prediction of local control. *Oral Oncol Eur J Cancer* 1993;29B:119–125.

190. Mak-Kregar S, Keus RB, Balm AJ, et al. Carcinoma of the soft palate and the posterior oropharyngeal wall. *Clin Otolaryngol Allied Sci.* 1994;19:22–27.

191. Malone JP, Stephens JA, Grecula JC, et al. Disease control, survival, and functional outcome after multimodal treatment for advanced-stage tongue base cancer. *Head Neck* 2004;26:561–572.

192. Marcial VA, Hanley JA, Hendrickson F, et al. Split-course radiation therapy of carcinoma of the base of the tongue: results of a prospective national collaborative clinical trial conducted by the Radiation Therapy Oncology Group. *Int J Radiat Oncol Biol Phys.* 1983;9:437–443.

193. Marcial VA, Pajak TF, Rotman M, et al. "Compensated" split-course versus continuous radiation therapy of carcinoma of the tonsillar fossa. Final results of a prospective randomized clinical trial of the Radiation Therapy Oncology Group. *Am J Clin Oncol.* 1993;16:389–396.

194. Marks JE, Freeman RB, Lee F. Pharyngeal wall cancer: an analysis of treatment results, complications, and patterns of failure. *Int J Radiat Oncol Biol Phys* 1978;4:587–593.

195. Marks JE, Smith PG, Sessions DG. Pharyngeal wall cancer: a reappraisal after comparison of treatment methods. *Arch Otolaryngol* 1985;111:79–85.

196. Mau T, Oh Y, Bucci MK, et al. Management of cervical metastases in advanced squamous cell carcinoma of the tonsillar fossa following radiotherapy. *Arch Otolaryngol Head Neck Surg* 2005;131:600–604.

197. Maulard C, Housset M, Delanian S. Salvage split course brachytherapy for tonsil and soft palate carcinoma: treatment techniques and results. *Laryngoscope* 1994;104:359–363.

198. Mazeron JJ, Belkacemi Y, Simon JM. Place of iridium 192 implantation in definitive irradiation of faucial arch squamous cell carcinomas. *Int J Radiat Oncol Biol Phys* 1993;27:251–257.

199. Mazeron JJ, Crook J, Martin M. Iridium 192 implantation of squamous cell carcinomas of the oropharynx. *Am J Otolaryngol* 1989;10:317–321.

200. Mazeron JJ, Langlois D, Glaubiger D. Salvage irradiaton of oropharyngeal cancers using Iridium 192 wire implants: 5-year results of 70 cases. *Int J Radiat Oncol Biol Phys* 1987;13:957–962.

201. Mazeron JJ, Marinello G, Crook J. Definitive radiation treatment for early stage carcinoma of the soft palate and uvula: the indication for iridium 192 implantation. *Int J Radiat Oncol Biol Phys* 1987;13:1829–1837.

202. McBain CA, Henry AM, Sykes J, et al. X-ray volumetric imaging in image-guided radiotherapy: the new standard in on-treatment imaging. *Int J Radiat Oncol Biol Phys.* 2006;64:625–34.

203. Mendenhall WM, Amdur RJ, Stringer SP, et al. Radiation therapy for squamous cell carcinoma of the tonsillar region: a preferred alternative to surgery? *J Clin Oncol* 2000;18:2219–2225.

204. Mendenhall WM, Morris CG, Amdur RJ. Definitive Radiotherapy for Squamous Cell Carcinoma of the Base of the Tongue. *Am J Clin Oncol* 2006;29:32–39.

205. Mendenhall WM, Parsons JT, Mancuso AA. Squamous cell carcinoma of the pharyngeal wall treated with irradiation. *Radiother Oncol* 1988;11:205–212.

206. Mendenhall WM, Riggs CE, Amdur RJ. Altered Fractionation and/or Adjuvant Chemotherapy in Definitive Irradiation of Squamous Cell Carcinoma of the Head and Neck. *Laryngoscope* 2003;113:546–551.

207. Meoz-Mendez RT, Fletcher GH, Guillamondegui OM. Analysis of the results of irradiation in the treatment of squamous cell carcinomas of the pharyngeal walls. *Int J Radiat Oncol Biol Phys* 1978;4:579–585.

208. Million RR, Cassisi NJ. *Management of head and neck cancer: a multidisciplinary approach*, 2nd ed. Philadelphia: JB Lippincott;1994:401–429.

209. Mizono GS, Diaz RF, Fu KK, et al. Carcinoma of the tonsillar region. *Laryngoscope.* 1986;96:240–244.

210. Mohan, R, Zhang, X, Wang, H, et al. Use of deformed intensity distributions for on-line modification of image-guided IMRT to account for interfractional anatomic changes. *Int J Radiat Oncol Biol Phys.* 2005;61:1258–66.

211. Mundt A, Roeske J. Intensity modulated radiation therapy, a clinical perspective. Hamilton: BC Decker;2005. 7 Simultaneous integrated boost, Wu Q and Mohan R.

212. Mutic S, Low D. Whole-body dose from tomotherapy delivery. *Int J Radiat Oncol Biol Phys.* 1998;42:229–32.

213. Naidu SI, Vieira F, Samant S, et al. Target intra-arterial chemoradiation for advanced tonsil cancer. *Otolaryngol Head Neck Surg.* 2005;133:882–887.

214. Nathu RM. Induction chemotherapy and radiation therapy for T4 oropharyngeal carcinoma. *Radiat Oncol Invest* 1999;7:98–105.

215. Newman LA, Robbins KT, Logemann JA. Swallowing and speech ability after treatment for head and neck cancer with targeted intraarterial versus intravenous chemoradiation. *Head Neck* 2002;24:68–77.

216. Newman LA, Vieira F, Schwiezer V. Eating and weight changes following chemoradiation therapy for advanced head and neck cancer. *Arch Otolaryngol Head Neck Surg* 1998;124:589–592.

217. Nguyen NP, Sallah S, Karlsson U. Combined chemotherapy and radiation therapy for head and neck malignancies. *Cancer* 2002;94:1131–1141.

218. Nijdam WM, Levendag PCN. Cost analysis comparing brachytherapy versus surgery for primary carcinoma of the tonsillar fossa and/or soft palate. *Int J Radiat Oncol Biol Phys* 2004;59:488–494.

219. Nishijima W, Takooda S, Tokita N. Analyses of distant metastases in squamous cell carcinoma of the head and neck and lesions above the clavicle at autopsy. *Arch Otolaryngol Head Neck Surg* 1993;119:65.

220. Nordgren M, Abendstein H, Jannert M, et al. Health-related quality of life five years after diagnosis of laryngeal carcinoma. *Int J Radiat Oncol Biol Phys* 2003;56:1333–1343.

221. Nordgren M, Jannert M, Boysen M, et al. Health-related quality of life in patients with pharyngeal carcinoma: a five-year follow up. *Head Neck* 2006;28:339–349.

222. Nowak P, van Dieren E, van Sornsen de Koste J, et al. Treatment portals for elective radiotherapy of the neck: an inventory in The Netherlands. *Radiother Oncol* 1997;43:81–86.

223. Nowak PJ, Wijers OB, Lagerwaard FJ, et al. A three-demensional CT-based target definition for elective irradiation of the neck. *Int J Radiat Oncol Biol Phys* 1999;45:33–39.

224. Oreggia F, Stefani EDE, Deneo-Pelligrini H. Carcinoma of the tonsil: A retrospective analysis of prognostic factors. *Arch Otolaryngol* 1983;109:305–309.

225. O'Sullivan BWP, Grice B. Assesment of contralateral neck failure in carcinoma

treated with ipsilateral radiotherapy. *Clin Invest Med* 1997;20[4 Suppl]:S94(abstr 524) .

226. Parsons JT, Mendenhall WM, Stringer SP, et al. Squamous cell carcinoma of the oropharynx. Surgery, radiation therapy, or both. *Cancer* 2002;22:2967–2980.
227. Parsons JT, Million RR, Cassisi NJ. Carcinoma of the base of the tongue: Results of radical irradiation with surgery reserved for irradiation failure. *Laryngoscope* 1982;92:689.
228. Pasma K, Dirkx M, Kroonwijk M, et al. Dosimetric verification of intensity modulated beams produced with dynamic multileaf collimation using an electronic portal imaging device. *Med Phys.* 1999;26:2373–2378.
229. Peiffert D, Pernot M, Malissard L. Salvage irradiation by brachytherapy of velotonsillar squamous cell carcinoma in a previously irradiated field: results in 73 cases. *Int J Radiat Oncol Biol Phys* 1994;29:681–686.
230. Penagaricano J. Step-and-shoot IMRT vs. helical tomotherapy: in regard to van Vulpen et al. *Int J Radiat Oncol Biol Phys* 2005;62; 1535–1539. Int J Radiat Oncol Biol Phys. 2006;64:328.
231. Perez CA, Bradley J, Chao CK, et al. Functional imaging in treatment planning in radiation therapy: a review. *Rays* 2002;27:157–173.
232. Perez CA, Brady LW, Halperon EG, et al. *Principles and practice of radiation oncology*. Philadelphia: Lippincott Williams & Wilkins; 2004:1022–1070.
233. Perez CA, Carmichael T, Devineni VR. Carcinoma of the tonsillar fossa: a nonrandomized comparison of irradiation alone or combined with surgery: Long-term results. *Head Neck* 1991;13:282–290.
234. Perez CA, Patel MM, Chao KSC. Carcinoma of the tonsillar fossa: Prognostic factors and long-term therapy outcome. *Int J Radiat Oncol Biol Phys* 1998;42:1077–1084.
235. Pernot M, Hoffstetter S, Pfeiffert D, et al. Role of interstitial brachytherapy in oral and oropharyngeal carcinoma: reflection of a series of 1344 patients treated at the time of initial presentation. *Otolaryngol Head Neck Surg* 1996;115:519–526.
236. Pernot M, Malissard L, Taghian A. Velotonsillar squamous cell carcinoma: 277 cases treated by combined external irradiation and brachytherapy—results according to extension, localization and dose rate. *Int J Radiat Oncol Biol Phys* 1992;23:715–723.
237. Petruson K, Mercke C, Lundberg LM, et al. Longitudinal evaluation of patients with cancer in the oral tongue, tonsils, or base of tongue. Does interstitial radiation dose affect quality of life? *Brachytherapy* 2005;4:271–277.
238. Pignon JP, Bourhis JD. For the Meta-analysis of Chemotherapy on Head and Neck Cancer (MACH-NC) Collaborative Group. Chemotherapy added to locoregional treatment for head and neck squamous-cell carcinoma: three meta-analyses of updated individual data. *Lancet* 2000;355:949–955.
239. Ploquin N, Song W, Lau H, et al. Intensity modulated radiation therapy for oropharyngeal cancer: the sensitivity of plan objectives and constraints to set-up uncertainty. *Phys Med Biol.* 2005;50:3515–33.
240. Pol van dM, Levendag PC, Bree dR, et al. Radical radiotherapy compared with surgery for advanced squamous cell carcinoma of the base of tongue. *Brachytherapy* 2004;3:78–86.
241. Pommier P, Bolot G, Martel I. Salvage brachytherapy of posterior pharyngeal wall squamous cell carcinoma in a previously irradiated area. *Int J Radiat Oncol Biol Phys.* 1997;38:53–58.
242. Pradhan S, Rajpal RM, Kothary PM. Surgical management of postradiation residual recurrent cancer of the base of the tongue. *J. Surg Oncol* 1980;14:201–206.
243. Puri D, Chou W, Lee N. Intensity-modulated radiation therapy in head and neck cancers dosimetric advantages and update of clinical results. *Am J Clin Oncol* 2005;28:415–423.
244. Puthawala AA, Syed AMN, Eads DL. Limited external beam interstitial 192 Iridium irradiation in the treatment of carcinoma of the base of the tongue: a ten year experience. *Int J Radiat Oncol Biol Phys* 1988;14:839–848.
245. Puthawala AA, Syed AMN, Eads DL. Limited external irradiation and interstitial 192 iridium implant in the treatment of squamous cell carcinoma of the tonsillar region. *Int J Radiat Oncol Biol Phys* 1985;11;1595–1602.
246. Rabuzzi DD, Mickler AS, Clutter DJ, et al. Treatment results of combined high-dose preoperative radiotherapy and surgery for oropharyngeal cancer. *Laryngoscope*. 1982;92[9 Pt 1]:989–992.
247. Radiation Therapy Oncology Group (RTOG) study protocol H0022.Available at: www.rtog.org. Accessed
248. Raymond WM, William JW. Quality of life of patients with recurrent nasopharyngeal carcinoma treated with nasopharyngectomy using the maxillary swing approach. *Otolaryngol Head Neck Surg* 2006;132:309–316.
249. Regueiro CA, Milan I, de la TA. Influence of boost technique (external beam radiotherapy of brachytherapy) on the outcome of patients with carcinoma of the base of the tongue. *Acta Oncol* 1995;34:225–233.
250. Remmler D, Medina J, Byers RM. Treatment of choice for squamous carcinoma of the tonsillar fossa. *Head Neck Surg* 1985;7:206–211.
251. Reynaert N, Coghe M, De Smedt B, et al. The importance of accurate linear accelerator head modelling for IMRT Monte Carlo calculations. *Phys. Med. Biol.* 2005, 50, 831–846.
252. Reynaert N, Van Der Marck S, Schaart D, et al. Monte Carlo treatment planning—an introduction. Report 16 of the Netherlands Commission on Radiation Dosimetry, 2006. Available at: www. ncs-dos. org. Accessed
253. Ringash J, Bezjak A. A structured review of quality of life instruments for head and neck cancer patients. *Head Neck* 2001;23:201–213.
254. Robbins K. Integrating radiological criteria into the classification of cervical lymph node disease. *Arch Otolaryngol Head Neck Surg* 1999;125:285–287.
255. Robbins KT, Clayman G, Levine PA, et al. Neck dissection classification update: revisions proposed by the American Head and Neck Society and the American Academy of Otolaryngology—Head and Neck Surgery. *Arch Otolaryngol Head Neck Surg*. 2002;128:751–758.
256. Robbins KT, Medina JE, Wolfe GT, et al. Standardizing neck dissection terminology. Official report of the academy's committee for head and neck surgery and oncology. *Arch Otolaryngol Head Neck Surg* 1991;117:601–605.
257. Robbins KT, Samant S, Vieira F, et al. Presurgical cytoreduction of oral cancer using intra-arterial cisplatin and limited concomitant radiation therapy (Neo-Radplat). *Arch Otolaryngol Head Neck Surg* 2004;130:28–32.
258. Robertson ML, Gleich LL, Barrett WL. Base-of-tongue cancer: survival, function, and quality of life after external-beam irradiation and brachytherapy. *Laryngoscope* 2001;111:1362–1365.
259. Roesink JM, Moerland MA, Battermann JJ. Quantitative dose volume response analysis of changes in parotid gland function after radiotherapy in the head-and-neck region. *Int J Radiat Oncol Biol Phys* 2001;51:938–946.
260. Roesink JM, Schipper M, Busschers W. A comparison of mean parotid gland dose with measure of parotid gland function after radiotherapy for head-and-neck cancer: implications for future trials. *Int J Radiat Oncol Biol Phys* 2005;63:1006–1009.
261. Rosenthal DI, Kian AK. Altered radiation therapy fractionation, chemoradiation, and patient selection for the treatment of head and neck squamous carcinoma. *Semin Radiat Oncol* 2004;14:153–166.
262. Rouviere H. *Anatomy of the human lymphatic system*. Ann Arbor, MI: Edwards Brothers; 1938.
263. Roy S, Tibesar RJ, Daly K, et al. Role of planned neck dissection for advanced metastic disease in tongue base or tonsil squamous cell carcinoom treated with radiotherapy. *Head Neck* 2002;24:474–481.
264. Salama JK, Vokes EE, Chmura SJ, et al. Long-term outcome of concurrent chemotherapy and reirradiation for recurrent and second primary head-and-neck squamous cell carcinoma. *Int J Radiat Oncol Biol Phys* 2006;64:382–391.
265. Samant S, Kumar P, Wan J. Concomitant radiation therapy and targeted cisplatin chemotherapy for the treatment of advanced pyriform sinus carcinoma: disease control and preservation or organ function. *Head Neck* 1999;21:595–601.
266. Santvoort van J, Heijmen B. Dynamic multileaf collimation without 'tongue-and-groove' underdosage effects. *Phys Med Biol.* 1996;41:2091–105.
267. Sartar CI. Biological modifiers as potential radiosensitizers: targeting the epidermal growth factor receptor family. *Semin Oncol* 2000. 27:15–20.
268. Schuller DE, McGuirt WF, Krause CJ, et al. Increased survival with surgery alone vs. combined therapy. *Laryngoscope.* 1979;98:582–594.
269. Scrimger R, Stavrev P, Parliament M, et al. A phenomenological model describing flow reduction for parotid gland irradiation with intensity-modulated radiotherapy (IMRT): Evidence of significant recovery effect. *Int J Radiat Oncol Biol Phys* 2004;60:178–185.
270. Seco J, Adams E, Bidmead M, et al. IMRT treatments assessed with a Monte Carlo dose calculation engine. *Phys Med Biol.* 2005: 50, 817–830.
271. *SEER cancer statistics review, 1973—1992*. Bethesda, MD: US Dept of Health and Human Services, National Cancer Institute;1995. Publication No. 96–2789.
272. Seikaly H, Rieger J, Wolfaardt J. Functional outcomes after primary oropharyngeal cancer resection and reconstruction with the radial forearm free flap. *Laryngoscope* 2003;113:897–904.
273. Selek U, Garden AS, Morrison WH. Radiation therapy for early-stage carcinoma of the oropharynx. *Int J Radiat Oncol Biol Phys* 2004;59:743–751.
274. Senan S, Levendag PC. Brachytherapy for recurrent head and neck cancer. *Hematol Oncol Clin North Am* 1999;13:225–233.
275. Sessions DG, Lenox J, Spector GJ, et al. Analysis of treatment results for base of tongue cancer. *Laryngoscope* 2003;113:1252–1261
276. Shah J. Patterns of cervical lymph node metastases from squamous carcinomas of the upper aerodigestive tract. *Am J Surg* 1990;160:405–409.
277. Shah JP.Candela FC, Poddar AK. The patterns of cervical lymph node metastasis from squamous carcinoma of the oral cavity. *Cancer* 1990;66:109–113.
278. Shalev S. Treatment verification using digital imaging. In: Smith AR, ed. *Radiation therapy physics*. Berlin: Springer; 1995:155–173.
279. Sham JST, Choy D, Wei WI. Nasopharyngeal carcinoma: orderly neck node spread. *Int J Radiat Oncol Biol Phys* 1990;19:929–933.
280. Shiley SG, Hargunani CA, Skoner JM, et al. Swallowing function after chemoradiation for advanced stage oropharyngeal cancer. *Otolaryn Head Neck Surg* 2006; 134:455–459.
281. Skoner JM, Andersen PE, Cohen JI. Swallowing function and tracheotomy dependence after combined-modality treatment including free tissue transfer for advanced-stage oropharyngeal cancer. *Laryngoscope* 2003;113:1294–1298.
282. Sohn HG, Har-El G. Neck dissection prior to radiation therapy for squamous cell carcinoma of tongue base. *Am J Otolaryngol* 2002;23:138–141.
283. Som PM, Curtin HD, Mancuso AA. An imaging-based classification for the cervical nodes designed as an adjunct to recent clinically based nodal classifications. *Arch Otolaryngol Head Neck Surg* 1999;125:388–396.
284. Son YH, Kacinski BM. Therapeutic concepts of brachytherapy/megavoltage in sequence for pharyngeal wall cancers. Results of integrated dose therapy. *Cancer* 1987;59:1268–1273.
285. Spanos WJ Jr, Shukovsky LJ, Fletcher GH. Time, dose, and tumor volume relationships in irradiation of squamous cell carcinomas of the base of the tongue. *Cancer* 1976;37:2591.
286. Spiro RH, Kelly J, Vega AL. Squamous carcinoma of the posterior pharyngeal wall *Am J Surg*. 1990;160:420–423.
287. Spiro RH, Koss LG, Hajdu SI. Tumors of minor salivary gland origin. *Cancer* 1973;31:117–129.
288. Staar S. Intensified hyperfractionated accelerated radiotherapy limits the additional benefit of simultaneous chemotherapy -results of a multicentric randomized German trial in advanced head-and-neck cancer. *Int J Radiat Oncol Biol Phys* 2001;50:1161–1171.
289. Stroom J, de Boer J, Huizenga H, et al. Inclusion of geometrical uncertainties in radiotherapy treatment planning by means of coverage probability. *Int J Radiat Oncol Biol Phys* 1999;43:905–919.
290. Stroom J, Heijmen B. Geometrical uncertainties, radiotherapy planning margins, and the ICRU-62 report. *Radiother Oncol* 2002;64:75–83.
291. Su CK, Bhattacharaya J, Wang CC. Role of neck surgery in conjunction with radiation in regional control of node positive cancer of the oropharynx. *Am J Clin Oncol* 2002;25:109–116.
292. Suntharalingam M. The role of concurrent chemotherapy and radiation in the management of patients with squamous cell carcinomas of the head and neck. *Semin Oncol* 2003;30:37–45.
293. Takacsi-Nagy ZP, Oberna F. Interstitial high-dose-rate brachytherapy in the treatment of base of tongue carcinoma. *Strahlenther Onkol* 2004;180:768–775.
294. Talton BM, Elkon D, Kim J. Cancer of the posterior hypopharyngeal wall. *Int J Radiat Oncol Biol Phys* 1981;7:597–599.
295. Taylor SG IV, Murthy AK, Vannetzell JM. Randomized comparison of neoadjuvant cisplatin and fluorouracil infusion followed by radiation versus concomitant treatment in head and neck cancer. *J Clin Oncol* 1994;12:385–395.
296. Teichgraeber JF, McConnel FM. Treatment of posterior pharyngeal wall carcinoma. *Otolaryngol Head Neck Surg.* 1994;94:287–290.
297. Terhaard CHJ, Braam P, Roesink. Significant impovement of parotid flow of IMRT compared to conventional radiotherapy in oropharyngeal cancer. *Int J Radiat Oncol Biol Phys* 2005;63: S372.

298. Thorstad W, Chao K, Haughey B. Toxicity and compliance of subcutaneous amifostine in patients undergoing postoperative intensity-modulated radiation therapy for head and neck cancer. *Semin Oncol.* 2004;31[6 Suppl 18] 8–12.

299. Tiwari RM, Ardenne vA, Leemans CR. Advanced squamous cell carcinoma of the base of the tongue treated with surgery and post-operative radiotherapy. *Eur J Surg Oncol* 2000;26:556–560.

300. Tuyns AT, Esteve J, Raymond L. Cancer of the larynx/hypopharynx, tobacco and alcohol: IARC International case-control study of Turin and Varese (Italy), Zaragosa and Navarra (Spain), Geneva (Switzerland) and Calvados (France). *Int J Cancer* 1988;41:483–491.

301. Vallis MP, Cleeland J, Bradley PJ. Radiation therapy of squamous carcinoma of the tonsil: an analysis of prognostic factors and of treatment failures. *Br J Radiol* 1986;12:251–256.

302. Verdonck-de Leeuw IM, Keus RB, et al. Consequences of voice impairment in daily life for patients following radiotherapy for early glottic cancer: Voice quality, vocal function, and vocal performance. *Int Radiat Oncol Biol Phys* 1999;44:1071–1078.

303. Verdonck-de Leeuw IM, Mahieu HF. Vocal aging and the impact in daily life: a longitudinal study. *J Voice* 2004;18:193–202.

304. Vieira S, Dirkx M, Heijmen B, et al. SIFT: A Method to verify the IMRT fluence delivered during patient treatment using an electronic portal imaging device. *Int. J. Radiat. Oncol Biol Phys.* 2004;60:981–993.

305. Vieira S, Dirkx M, Pasma K, et al. Fast and accurate leaf verification for dynamic multileaf collimation using an electronic portal imaging device. *Med Phys.* 2002;29:2034–40.

306. Vieira S, Kaatee R, Dirkx M, et al. Two-dimensional measurement of photon beam attenuation by the treatment couch and immobilization devices using an electronic portal imaging device. *Med Phys.* 2003;30:2981–7.

307. Vikram B, Hilaris BS. A non-looping afterloading technique for interstitial implants of the base of the tongue. *Int J Radiat Oncol Biol Phys.* 1981;7:419–422.

308. Vikram B, Strong E, Shah J, et al. A non-looping afterloading technique for base of tongue implants: results in the first 20 patients. *Int J Radiat Oncol Biol Phys.* 1985;11:1853–1855.

309. Vokes EE. Induction chemotherapy followed by concomitant chemoradiotherapy for advanced head and neck cancer: impact on the natural history of the disease. *J Clin Oncol* 1995;13:876–883.

310. Vulpen M, van Field C, Raaijmakers C, et al. Comparing step-and-shoot IMRT with dynamic helical tomotherapy IMRT plans for head-and-neck cancer. *Int J Radiat Oncol Biol Phys.* 2005;62:1535–1539.

311. Wang CC, Montgomery W, Efird J. Local control of oropharyngeal carcinoma by irradiation alone. *Laryngoscope* 1995;102:529–533.

312. Wang CJ, Huang EY, Hsu HC, et al. The degree and time-course assessment of radiation-induced trismus occurring after radiotherapy for nasopharyngeal cancer. *Laryngoscope* 2005;115:1458–1460.

313. Wang MB, Kuber N, Kerner MM, et al. Tonsillar carcinoma: analysis of treatment results. *J Otolaryngol* 1998;27:263–269.

314. Ware JJ, Sherbourne CD. The MOS 36-item short-form health survey (SF—36): I. Conceptual framework and item selection. *Med Care* 1992;30:473–483.

315. Warkentin B, Stavrev P, Stavreva N, et al. A TCP-NTCP estimation module using DVHs and known radiobiological models and parameter sets. *J Appl Clin Med Phys* 2004;5:50–63.

316. Weichert KA, Aron B, Maltz R. Carcinoma of the tonsil: treatment by a planned combination of radiation and surgery. *Int J Radiat Oncol Biol Phys* 1976;1:505–508.

317. Wijers OB, Levendag PC, Braaksma MMJ. Patients with head and neck cancer cured by radiation therapy: a survey of the dry mouth syndrome in long-term survivors. *Head Neck* 2002;24:737–747.

318. Wijers OB, Levendag PC, Tan T, et al. A simplified CT-based definition of the lymphnode levels in the node negative neck. *Radiother Oncol* 1999;1:35–42.

319. Wingo PA, Tong T, Bolden S. Cancer statistics, 1996. *Ca Cancer J Clin* 1996;46:5–27.

320. Withers HR, Peters LJ, Taylor JMG. Late normal tissue sequelae from radiation therapy for carcinoma of the tonsil: patterns of fractionation study of radiobiology. *Int J Radiat Oncol Biol Phys* 1995;33:563–568.

321. Withers HR, Peters LJ, Taylor JMG. Local control of carcinoma of the tonsil by radiation therapy: an analysis of patterns of fractionation in nine institutions. *Int J Radiat Oncol Biol Phys* 1995;33:549–562.

322. Withers HR. Local control of carcinoma of the tonsil by radiation therapy: an analysis of patterns of fractionation in nine institutions. *Int J Radiat Oncol Biol Phys* 1995;33:549–562.

323. Wong CS, Ang KK, Fletcher GH, et al. Definitive radiotherapy for squamous cell carcinoma of the Tonsillar Fossa. *Int J Radiat Oncol Biol Phys* 1989;13:657–662.

324. Wu Q, Manning M, Schmidt-Ullrich R, et al. The potential for sparing of parotids and escalation of biologically effective dose with intensity-modulated radiation treatments of head and neck cancers: a treatment design study. *Int J Radiat Oncol Biol Phys.* 2000;46:195–205.

325. Wu Q, Mohan R, Morris M, et al. Simultaneous integrated boost intensity-modulated radiotherapy for locally advanced head-and-neck squamous cell carcinomas. I: dosimetric results. *Int J Radiat Oncol Biol Phys* 2003;56:573–585.

326. Yoshida K, Inoue T, Inoue T. Treatment results of radiotherapy with or without surgery for posterior pharyngeal wall cancer of oropharynx and hypopharynx: prognostic value of tumor extension. *Radiat Med* 2004;22:30–36.

327. Yu L, Vikram B, Chadha M. High dose rate brachytherapy in patients with cancer of the head and neck. *Endocur Hyperthermia Oncology* 1996;12:1–6.

328. Zijtveld van M, Dirkx M, De Boer J, et al. 3D dose reconstruction for clinical evaluation of IMRT pretreatment verification with an EPID. *Radiother Oncol.* 2007;82:201–207.

329. Zijtveld van M, Dirkx M, De Boer J. Dosimetric pretreatment verification of IMRT using an EPID; clinical experience. *Radiother Oncol.* 2006;81:168–175.

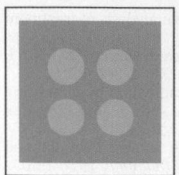

Chapter 43
Hypopharynx Cancer

Hiral K. Shah, Deepak Khuntia, Henry T. Hoffman, Paul M. Harari

There is a strong association between tobacco use and the development of hypopharynx cancer (13,59,68). Due to the rich lymphatic network in this anatomic region, patients commonly present with regional nodal metastases. Many hypopharynx cancer patients also carry significant medical comorbidities and social issues that present additional challenges to the successful delivery of aggressive cancer therapy. As for all complex tumors of the head and neck region, multidisciplinary evaluation and management is critical and should involve a head and neck surgeon, radiation oncologist, medical oncologist, nurse, nutritionist, speech/swallow therapist, and social worker. Although a selected cohort of early stage tumors may be amenable to organ preservation surgery, more radical surgery such as laryngopharyngectomy is often required for patients who undergo a primary operative approach for hypopharynx cancer. This ablative procedure can induce significant cosmetic and functional changes, and postsurgical rehabilitation efforts guided by knowledgeable professionals are very important to assist in patient adaptation. Increasingly, hypopharynx cancer patients are being considered for nonoperative treatment approaches using definitive radiation or chemoradiation as a means of obtaining tumor control with preservation of organ function. Regardless of the specific treatment approach, all patients require active rehabilitation therapy in an effort to maximize their ultimate speech and swallow function. Despite stepwise advances in the diagnosis and treatment of hypopharynx cancer, the overall outcome for these patients is relatively poor compared with other head and neck cancer sites. As with most tumors of the head and neck region, there is significant interest in combining molecular targeted therapies with traditional cytotoxic therapy in an effort to further improve outcome.

Anatomy

The hypopharynx, sometimes referred to as the laryngopharynx, is contiguous superiorly with the oropharynx and inferiorly with the cervical esophagus (Fig. 43.1). As general landmarks, the superior border of the hypopharynx is demarcated by the hyoid bone and the inferior border by the cricoid cartilage. With regard to cancer diagnosis and staging, there are three primary anatomic subsites within the hypopharynx: the bilateral pyriform sinuses, the postcricoid region, and the posterior pharyngeal wall.

The pyriform sinuses are essentially inverted pyramids with the medial, lateral, and anterior walls narrowing inferiorly to form the apices. Posteriorly, the pyriform sinuses are open and contiguous with the pharyngeal walls. Superiorly, the sinuses are surrounded by the thyrohyoid membrane through which passes the internal branch of the superior laryngeal nerve. Tumor involvement of the sensory branches of this nerve can result in referred otalgia. The postcricoid region is comprised of the mucosa overlying the cricoid cartilage, with the arytenoid and esophageal mucosa forming the superior and inferior borders, respectively. The posterior pharyngeal wall is predominantly comprised of squamous mucosa covering the middle and inferior pharyngeal constrictor muscles and is separated from the

prevertebral fascia by the retropharyngeal space. Typically, the mucosa lining the pharyngeal wall is <1 cm in thickness and provides a minimal barrier to direct tumor infiltration. The posterior pharyngeal wall is contiguous with the lateral wall of the pyriform sinus (Fig. 43.2A,B).

Sensory innervation of the hypopharynx is provided by the internal branch of the superior laryngeal nerve as well as fibers deriving from the glossopharyngeal nerve. The recurrent laryngeal nerve and the pharyngeal plexus provide the primary motor supply. The arterial supply of the hypopharynx is derived primarily from branches of the external carotid artery: superior thyroid arteries, ascending pharyngeal arteries, and lingual arteries.

There is a rich network of lymphatics within the hypopharynx that drain directly through the thyrohyoid membrane and into the jugulodigastric lymph nodes, most commonly involving the subdigastric node. Additionally, there may be direct drainage into the spinal accessory nodes. Tumors involving the posterior pharyngeal wall can also drain into the retropharyngeal nodes, including the most cephalad retropharyngeal nodes of Rouviere.

Epidemiology and Etiology

Hypopharynx cancers are relatively uncommon. Approximately 2,500 to 3,000 cases are diagnosed annually in the United States. The pyriform sinus is the most common subsite of origin comprising 65% to 75% of hypopharynx cases (15). Although it is sometimes difficult to definitively assign tumor origin to a single subsite, approximately 10% to 20% of hypopharynx tumors arise from the posterior pharyngeal wall and 5% to 15% originate from the postcricoid region (5). Due to the rich lymphatic drainage of the hypopharynx, at least 50% of patients will manifest clinically positive cervical lymph nodes at the time of diagnosis (43). Jugular chain nodes, levels II through IV, as well as retropharyngeal nodes, are all at high risk to harbor regional metastases in patients with hypopharynx cancer. In parallel to cancers of the nasopharynx, retropharyngeal nodes may be the first site of nodal spread. Postcricoid tumors may also spread directly to pre- and paratracheal nodal basins. Due to the high propensity for advanced primary disease as well as regional nodal involvement, the majority of hypopharynx cancer patients present with stage III and IV disease. In a retrospective study from Washington University, 87% of patients with cancers of the pyriform sinus and 82% of patients with posterior pharyngeal wall tumors presented with stage III or IV disease (65).

Over 90% of patients with hypopharynx cancer report past cigarette use (40). Alcohol appears to potentiate the carcinogenic effects of tobacco but in isolation is not clearly associated with an increased risk of developing hypopharynx cancer. The index hypopharynx cancer often occurs within a field of diseased mucosa characterized by high-grade dysplasia. This "field cancerization" reflects widespread mucosal exposure to carcinogens and is responsible for the high rate of synchronous and metachronous primary tumors identified in patients with

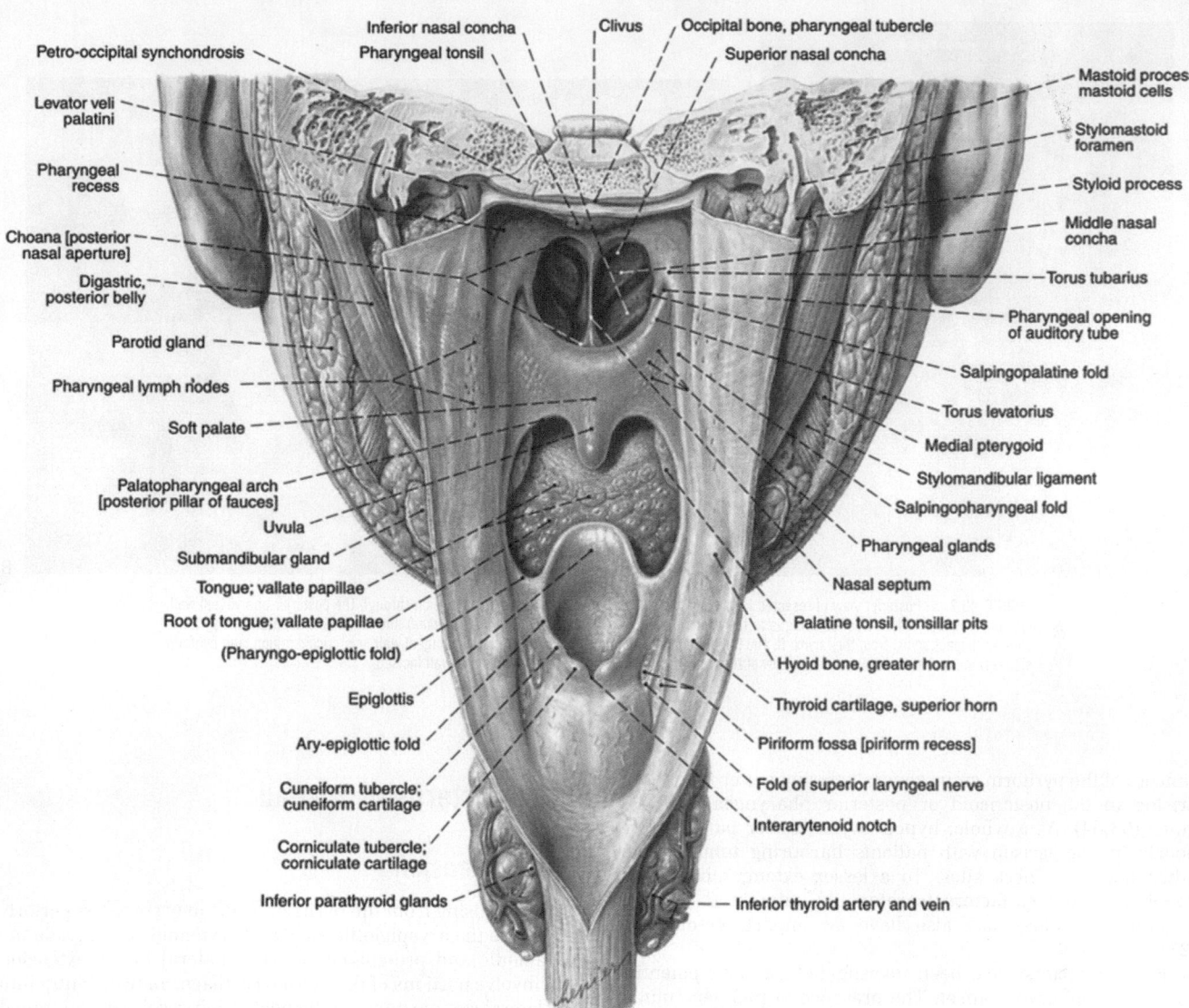

FIGURE 43.1. Posterior view of the hypopharynx shows the relationship of the pyriform sinus, pharyngeal wall, and postcricoid region within the head and neck. (From Sobotta J. *Atlas of human anatomy,* vol. I. Munich: Lippincott Williams & Wilkins, 2001, with permission.)

hypopharynx cancer. Successful counseling with particular emphasis on smoking cessation can enhance treatment tolerance and diminish the risk of developing subsequent cancers of the upper aerodigestive tract. Patients with occupational exposure to coal dust, steel dust, iron compounds, and fumes have also shown an increased risk for developing hypopharynx cancer (6,60). Overall, the incidence of hypopharynx cancer has shown some gradual decline in the United States. From 1975 to 2001 the incidence decreased by approximately 35%, perhaps as a result of smoking cessation efforts (21).

Human papilloma virus (HPV) infection is well established as a risk factor for the development of squamous-cell carcinoma of the gynecologic tract, particularly in the uterine cervix. The relationship between HPV and head and neck cancer is only recently becoming better appreciated, particularly for cancers of the nasopharynx and oropharynx. Studies have demonstrated that approximately 20% to 25% of patients with hypopharynx cancer test positive for HPV DNA (42,50). Currently, the clinical implications of the presence of HPV in hypopharynx cancer are yet to be defined.

There is a recognized increased risk of developing cancers of the postcricoid region for patients with Plummer Vinson syn-

drome, characterized by iron-deficiency anemia, hypopharyngeal webs, weight loss, and dysphagia (75). Favorable changes in the epidemiology of hypopharynx cancer have resulted from changes in nutrition. The addition of iron to flour has made Plummer Vinson syndrome quite rare in the upper midwestern United States and Scandinavian countries where it was formerly more common. An associated decrease in hypopharynx cancer involving the postcricoid region has followed.

Prognostic Factors

Several prognostic factors have been identified for patients with hypopharynx cancer. Age, particularly >70 years, has been identified as an unfavorable predictor of outcome (24). This may simply reflect the diminished likelihood of elderly patients to successfully tolerate the aggressive therapy approaches required for locoregionally advanced cancers of the head and neck. Women have been found to achieve somewhat improved outcomes compared to men, although this may in part be a manifestation of earlier stage disease at diagnosis (63,64). In addition, tumor location has an impact on outcome with

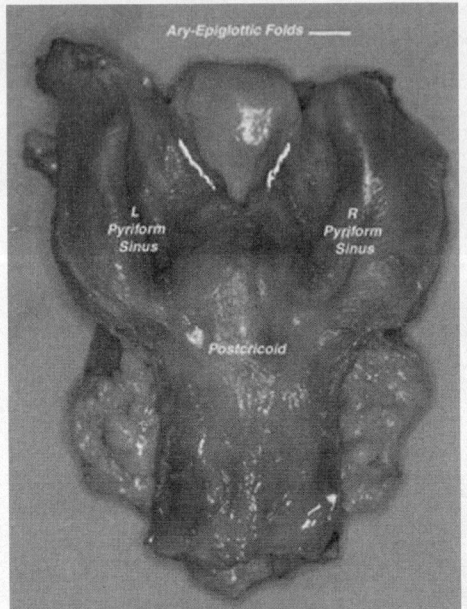
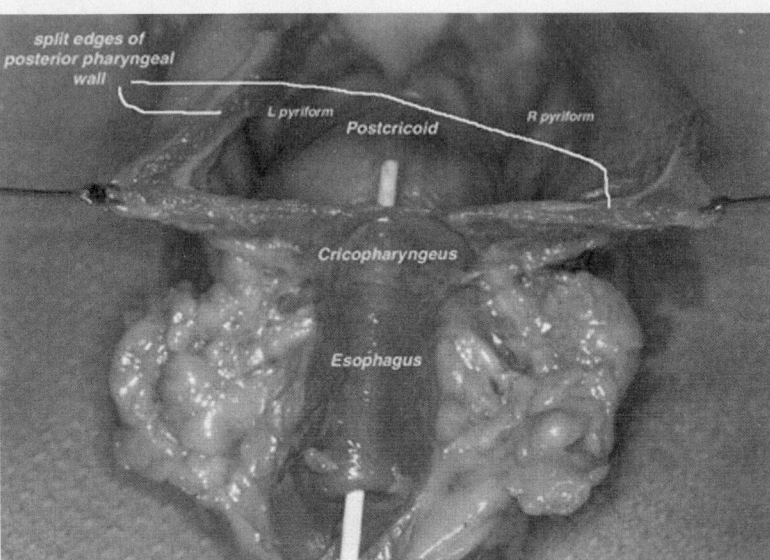

FIGURE 43.2. A: Posterior view of resected larynx and hypopharynx specimen afforded by incision through the posterior pharyngeal wall, cricopharyngeus, and cervical esophagus in the posterior midline. The aryepiglottic folds (*marked*) and arytenoids separate the pyriform sinuses (hypopharynx) from the larynx. **B:** The three primary anatomic subsites (posterior pharyngeal wall, postcricoid region, and pyriform sinuses) are revealed in this posterior view of the hypopharynx with the posterior pharyngeal wall incised.

cancers of the pyriform sinus generally faring better than those arising in the postcricoid or posterior pharyngeal wall regions (63,64). As a whole, hypopharynx cancer patients fare poorly in comparison with patients harboring tumors from other head and neck sites. To a lesser extent, tobacco, alcohol, and dietary factors (carotenoids, vitamin C, vitamin E, and flavonoids) may also have an impact on outcome (23).

Biologic factors have been investigated for their potential role in hypopharynx cancer. The presence of p53 gene mutations have been associated with bulkier tumors and younger patients along with higher expression of the epidermal growth factor receptor (EGFR). However, p53 has not shown correlation with multiple primary tumors, tumor grade, or DNA ploidy (15,28). Further, definitive data in hypopharynx cancer does not exist correlating a prognostic significance of EGFR expression with overall outcome (29).

:: Staging

The most commonly used system for staging hypopharynx cancer is the American Joint Committee on Cancer (AJCC) 2002 edition of their staging manual, which is based on a combination of clinical and radiographic data (Table 43.1) (30). The nodal and group staging is similar to other sites within the pharynx with the exception of nasopharynx. One must always exercise good clinical judgment when designing treatment recommendations based on AJCC staging. With specific regard to hypopharynx cancer, the AJCC staging system does not differentiate the specific tumor subsite or number of walls invaded by tumor that may have prognostic significance as well as management implications. Moreover, patient factors including age, comorbid medical conditions, and motivation for organ preservation are beyond the scope of the staging system, but nevertheless represent important factors for consideration with each individual patient.

:: Patterns of Spread

Local Extension

Cancers arising from the pyriform sinus may spread superiorly to involve the aryepiglottic folds and arytenoids and invade the paraglottic and pre-epiglottic space. Lateral tumor extension can involve portions of the thyroid cartilage, allowing entry into the lateral compartment of the neck. High-resolution computed tomography (CT) or magnetic resonance imaging (MRI) is often useful for optimal assessment regarding the extent of tumor invasion. For tumors arising from the medial wall, the most common site of involvement for pyriform sinus tumors, there is a likelihood of tumor involvement of intrinsic muscles of the

Table 43.1	AMERICAN JOINT COMMITTEE ON CANCER 2002 T STAGING FOR HYPOPHARYNX CANCER

T Stage

T1	Limited to 1 subsite of the hypopharynx and ≤2 cm in greatest dimension
T2	Tumor invades more than 1 subsite of the hypopharynx or an adjacent site, or measures >2 cm but ≤4 cm in greatest diameter without fixation of hemilarynx
T3	Tumor measures >4 cm in greatest dimension or with fixation of hemilarynx
T4a	Invades thyroid/cricoid cartilage, hyoid bone, thyroid gland, esophagus, or central compartment soft tissue, which includes prelaryngeal strap muscles and subcutaneous fat
T4b	Tumor invades prevertebral fascia, encases carotid artery, or involves mediastinal structures

From Frederick L, Greene DLP, Fleming ID, et al. *AJCC cancer staging manual.* New York: Springer, 2002, with permission.

larynx resulting in vocal cord fixation. Inferior tumor extension beyond the apex can involve the thyroid gland.

Cancers arising within the postcricoid region can extend circumferentially to involve the cricoid cartilage or anteriorly to involve the larynx with resultant vocal cord fixation. Tumor involvement of the recurrent laryngeal nerve can also precipitate vocal cord fixation. Primary postcricoid tumors are often quite extensive and can involve the pyriform sinus, trachea, or esophagus. As a result, these tumors generally carry a worse prognosis in comparison to tumors from other subsites of the hypopharynx (66). Nodal spread to the paratracheal nodes and inferior deep cervical nodes is not uncommon. Tumor arising from the posterior pharyngeal wall can extend to involve the oropharynx superiorly, the cervical esophagus inferiorly, and the prevertebral fascia and retropharyngeal space posteriorly.

Many cancers of the hypopharynx have a propensity for submucosal spread. It can therefore be difficult to accurately quantify the full microscopic extent of disease. This is particularly true for cancers of the posterior pharyngeal wall and postcricoid regions. Careful study through serial sectioning of surgical specimens has identified that 60% of hypopharynx cancers demonstrate subclinical spread with a range of 10 mm superiorly, 25 mm medially, 20 mm laterally, and 20 mm inferiorly (39). This extensive pattern of tumor infiltration can present considerable challenges in the effort to achieve clear surgical margins or full dosimetric coverage with radiotherapy.

Regional Disease

Lymphatics of the pyriform sinus can drain through the thyrohyoid membrane, across the pretracheal nodes, and into level II and III cervical nodes (Table 43.2). Tumors arising from the posterior pharyngeal wall can involve the retropharyngeal nodes (Rouviere's nodes) extending cephalad to the base of skull. In light of cross-draining lymphatics, there is a significant risk of bilateral cervical adenopathy associated with cancers arising in the hypopharynx (51) (Fig. 43.3).

Distant Metastases

The most common site for distant metastasis to develop in patients with cancer of the hypopharynx is the lung. Approximately one quarter of patients diagnosed with hypopharynx cancer either present with distant metastasis or develop them at

Table 43.2	INCIDENCE OF LYMPH NODE METASTASIS AT PRESENTATION BASED ON NODAL GROUP	
Nodal Group	**Ipsilateral (%)**	**Contralateral (%)**
I	1	0
II	72	9
III	55	3
IV	21	2
V	15	2
Supraclavicular	3	1
Paratracheal	8.3	—

some time during the course of their disease (48). For those patients not rendered free of locoregional disease following initial therapy, the incidence of distant metastases increases notably with the length of time following initial treatment (45).

Field Cancerization

Carcinogens can induce dysplastic changes throughout the mucosa of the upper aerodigestive tract, leading to an increased risk for field cancerization that enhances the likelihood of synchronous or metachronous secondary primary tumors. Approximately 7% of patients with hypopharynx cancer will manifest a secondary primary tumor at initial diagnosis and between 10% to 20% will develop a secondary primary tumor over time. In fact, this second tumor risk is a significant cause of mortality in patients who survive >2 years following initial treatment (38).

Clinical Presentation

In light of the nonspecific nature of early symptoms, the majority of patients with cancers of the hypopharynx present with advanced local and/or regional disease. Frequently, there is a delay between presentation and diagnosis as patients are often managed for presumed infectious or gastrointestinal etiology. The majority of symptoms are related to local tumor spread including dysphagia and odynophagia. There may be frank esophageal obstruction, invasion of constrictor muscles, prevertebral space invasion, or strap muscle invasion. Common

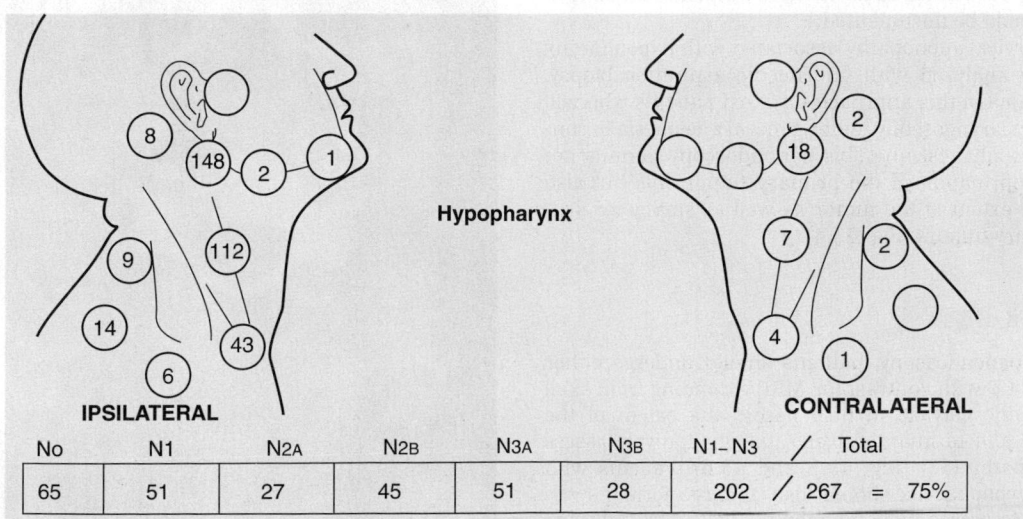

FIGURE 43.3. Nodal distribution patterns for a series of 267 patients with hypopharynx cancer as summarized by admission records at the M.D. Anderson Hospital (From Lindberg R. Distribution of cervical lymph node metastases from squamous cell carcinoma of the upper respiratory and digestive tracts. *Cancer* 1972;29:1446–1449, with permission.)

Clinical Radiation Oncology

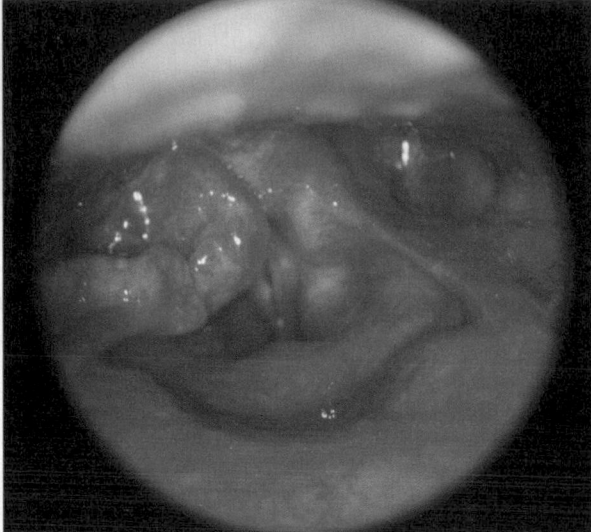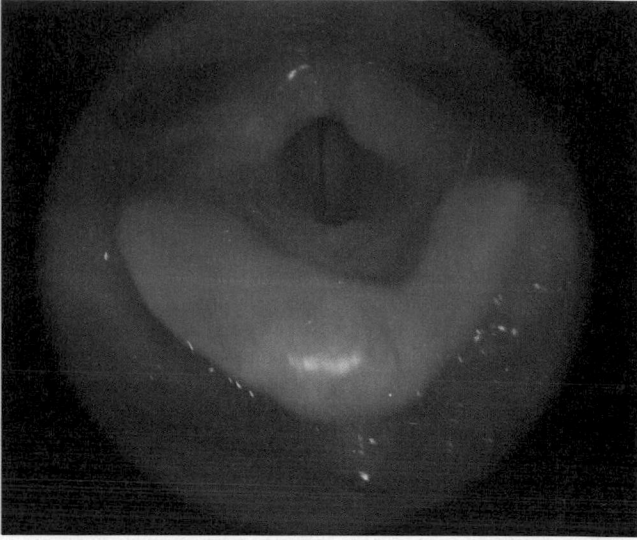

FIGURE 43.4. A: Outpatient clinic photograph taken through a rigid endoscope mounted with a 35-mm camera of a newly diagnosed exophytic T2 tumor arising from the right pyriform sinus with involvement of the adjacent aryepiglottic fold. There was no compromise of vocal cord mobility and clinical staging of the primary lesion was T2. **B:** Photographic examination 1 year following 70 Gy radiation (intensity-modulated radiation therapy) and concurrent cisplatin chemotherapy with compete tumor regression and excellent functional status of the laryngopharynx. Note mild to moderate mucosal edema of supraglottic structures following high-dose radiation.

presenting signs and symptoms include dysphagia, sore throat, hoarseness, weight loss >10 pounds, and neck mass. The majority of patients present with more than one of these signs and symptoms (70). Selected patients may first come to medical attention with complaints of unilateral ear pain (referred otalgia) due to tumor involvement of the nerve of Arnold, a branch of the superior laryngeal nerve.

A comprehensive work-up for patients with cancers of the hypopharynx should include a detailed history focusing on the duration of symptoms, amount of weight loss, the presence of otalgia, changes in voice quality, and degree of dysphagia. Factors such as previous history of an upper aerodigestive tract malignancy and smoking are important. A detailed physical examination should include direct and indirect visualization of the full laryngopharyngeal axis with particular attention to the size, location, and anatomic positioning of the primary tumor as well as the mobility status of the true vocal cords. Dentition and oral health should be assessed. If the patient presents with cervical adenopathy, the size, number, location, texture, and mobility of those nodes should be documented.

Although cervical adenopathy associated with hypopharynx cancer may be analyzed with fine needle aspiration biopsy, there is little value in this approach for most patients who will undergo a direct laryngoscopy under general anesthesia in conjunction with esophagoscopy. This panendoscopy permits not only biopsy confirmation of the primary tumor site, but also mapping of the extent of the tumor as well as survey for synchronous primary tumors (Fig. 43.4).

Staging Work-Up

In addition to panendoscopy, patients should undergo either high-resolution CT with contrast (or MRI) extending from skull base to below the clavicle to help assess the extent of the primary tumor and to quantitatively and qualitatively assess cervical adenopathy (53) (Fig. 43.5 and 43.6). Patients with cancer of the hypopharynx should also undergo formal swallow evaluation to assess their functional swallow capacity before the initiation of therapy. This analysis may be done as a "bedside" study of swallowing capacity, a fiberoptic endoscopic swallowing evaluation (FEES), or through the more definitive fluoroscopic barium swallow study. This modified barium swallow study is called a cookie swallow, videopharyngogram, or oropharyngeal motility study (OPMS). Either a chest x-ray or CT is recommended to assess the presence of pulmonary metastasis.

F-18-deoxyglucose or fluorodeoxyglucose/positron emission tomography ([18]FDG-PET) imaging is increasingly used to help assess the extent of the primary tumor and regional adenopathy as well as the presence of distant metastasis. FDG-PET is becoming an increasingly valuable adjunct to CT and/or MRI in the radiation treatment planning process, particularly for patients treated with conformal IMRT or tomotherapy techniques. Di Martino et al. (22) compared CT, PET, color-coded duplex sonography, palpation, and panendoscopy in assessment of

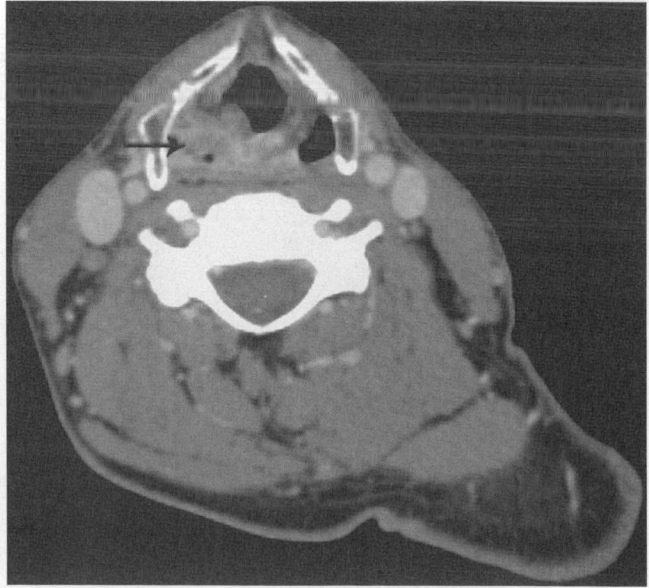

FIGURE 43.5. Axial computed tomography image from the same case as Figure 43.4 depicting the T2 hypopharynx tumor involving the right pyriform sinus.

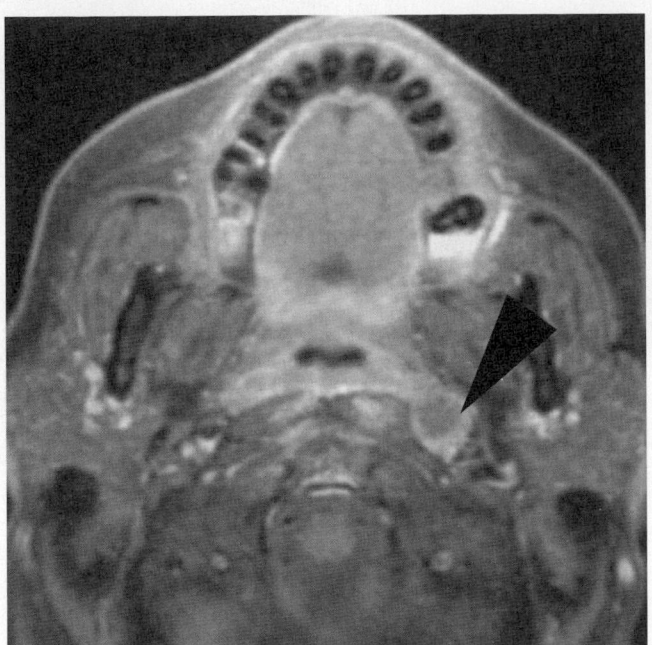

FIGURE 43.6. Axial gadolinium-enhanced T1-weighted MRI scan with fat-saturation depicting metastatic lateral retropharyngeal node with evidence of central necrosis and peripheral enhancement.

tumor and nodal status. The results of this study are summarized in Table 43.3 and support the promising sensitivity and specificity of PET scanning in head and neck cancers. Schwartz et al. (59) examined standardized uptake value (SUV) of primary and nodal metastasis in head and neck cancer patients and their relationship to clinical outcome. A primary tumor SUV >9.0 was associated with a significantly lower local recurrence-free survival and disease-free survival (DFS). There was no correlation between nodal SUV and clinical outcome.

Pathological Classification

Review of the National Cancer Data Base (NCDB) Benchmark Reports identified 3,519 cases of hypopharynx cancer reported from 1,542 hospitals during 2000 and 2001. Over 93% of the cases were reported as squamous-cell carcinoma with "other specified types" representing 6.9% of cases (53). On rare occa-

Table 43.3	COMPARISON OF VARIOUS MODALITIES FOR STAGING			
	Sensitivity (%)		Specificity (%)	
	T	N	T	N
Panendoscopy	95	—	85	—
PET	95	84	92	90
CDDS	74	84	75	96
CT	68	84	69	88
Palpation	—	63	—	96

CDDS, color-coded duplex sonography; CT, computed tomography; N, nodal stage; PET, positron emission tomography; T, tumor stage
From Di Martino E, Nowak B, Hassan HA, et al. Diagnosis and staging of head and neck cancer: a comparison of modern imaging modalities (positron emission tomography, computed tomography, color-coded duplex sonography) with panendoscopic and histopathologic findings. *Arch Otolaryngol Head Neck Surg* 2000;126:1457–1461, with permission.

sion, lymphoma, sarcoma, adenocarcinoma, or adenoid cystic carcinoma may present in the hypopharynx, but each histology makes up <0.5% of overall hypopharynx cancer diagnoses (21).

Pretreatment Evaluation

Many patients with hypopharynx cancer present with concurrent medical and social comorbidities that require consideration before initiating cancer-directed therapy. Commonly, there is a progressive history of dysphagia and odynophagia with associated weight loss. Whether these patients are treated with surgical or nonsurgical approaches, a gastrostomy tube may need to be considered as a temporary measure. It is important to optimize or at least stabilize the patient's nutritional status prior to initiating definitive therapy.

It is valuable for hypopharynx cancer patients to undergo evaluation by a speech and swallow therapist to evaluate the degree of dysfunction prior to therapy. Patients may be able to use adaptive techniques to improve the effectiveness and safety of their oral intake. Additionally, close follow-up with the same speech and swallow therapist is highly desirable during and after therapy to maximize the patient's long-term functional capabilities.

Since many hypopharynx patients have an active history of alcohol and tobacco use, it is important to counsel accordingly and encourage all patients to take advantage of methods and programs to facilitate smoking and alcohol cessation. All patients should undergo comprehensive dental evaluation and cleaning as well as basic education regarding oral hygiene. For patients treated with conventional radiation therapy techniques there is a significant likelihood of long-term xerostomia that can promote dental decay. If existing dentition is in poor condition, dental extractions should be considered prior to therapy, particularly for teeth that will reside within the high-dose radiation region. Typically 10 to 14 days are required following dental extractions to allow for healing prior to the initiation of radiation therapy. Custom fluoride carrier trays should be fabricated and discussed for long-term use in an effort to diminish the rate of dental decay for patients with chronic xerostomia.

Finally, many patients with hypopharynx cancer will have social issues including lack of family support, financial limitations, transportation issues, poor nutrition, and hygiene habits that may hamper their ability to successfully receive adequate care. Often, the involvement of a case manager or social worker is of central importance to assist patients who require support both during as well as following cancer therapy.

Management

T1–2 Tumors

Surgery

Contemporary indications for primary surgical management of patients with early cancers of the hypopharynx include those with a history of previous head and neck radiation, those in whom organ conservation approaches are deemed possible (a relatively small proportion of cases), and those who refuse radiation. Even for hypopharynx cancer patients who will receive nonoperative treatment approaches, it remains critical for the head and neck surgeon to remain actively involved. The role of the surgeon in these cases may include endoscopic biopsy with detailed assessment of tumor extent, methods to secure the airway (tracheotomy or laser debulking), and methods to ensure adequate nutrition (gastrostomy).

Patients with hypopharynx cancer also require careful evaluation regarding regional nodal metastases. For N0–1 patients treated with primary radiation or chemoradiation approaches, adjuvant neck dissection is generally unnecessary. However, for patients presenting with N2–3 neck disease, careful evaluation of tumor response in the neck is important to help gauge the potential value of adjuvant neck dissection following radiation or chemoradiation. Although an increasing number of reports suggest that detailed imaging of the neck 8 to 12 weeks postradiation with FDG-PET can serve as a valuable guide to help select those patients warranting adjuvant neck dissection, many institutions mandate adjuvant neck dissection for all patients presenting with N2–3 neck disease in an effort to maximize regional disease control. Both approaches are readily defendable at present (10,56,67,68,74). If neck dissection is performed, this provides an opportunity for the surgeon to reassess the primary tumor site under anesthesia with directed biopsy if suspicious for residual disease. If residual disease at the primary site is highly suspected or confirmed by biopsy several months following completion of radiation or chemoradiation, this will prompt consideration regarding the feasibility and advisability of salvage surgery options.

A selected cohort of T1 and T2 hypopharynx cancers may lend themselves to surgical excision. These favorable subsites include the upper pyriform sinus and the posterior pharyngeal wall. The standard supraglottic laryngectomy encompasses the aryepiglottic fold and may be extended to include part of the arytenoids, base of tongue, and upper pyriform sinus. Small cancers isolated to the posterior pharyngeal wall may be removed by endoscopic laser resection or removal using an open approach. Dysphagia requiring no food by mouth status is common from the open approach, especially if reconstruction of the posterior wall is effected with an adynamic and insensate free flap. Relative contraindications to organ conservation surgery for hypopharynx cancers include transglottic tumor extension, cartilage invasion, vocal fold paralysis, postcricoid invasion, deep pyriform sinus invasion, and extension beyond the larynx.

Innovations with free flap reconstruction have permitted retention of speech and swallowing and breathing functions of the larynx despite extensive resection by way of a hemilaryngopharyngectomy. The temporoparietal flap and radial forearm free flap coupled with rigid cartilaginous support have been employed to retain function in patients with hypopharynx cancers without extension to the postcricoid region or apex of the pyriform sinus (58,71).

Radiation

Curative radiation therapy (RT) is generally the preferred treatment option for patients with T1–2 hypopharynx tumors. This approach affords good potential for organ preservation without compromise in clinical outcome. A classical course of radiation therapy for hypopharynx cancer lasts 6 to 7 weeks, with treatment delivered 5 days per week. Conventional treatment involves a shrinking field technique that initiates with opposed lateral fields encompassing the primary tumor and upper neck lymphatics with a matched anterior field to complete treatment of the lower neck. One of the most common worldwide fractionation regimens involves the delivery of 2 Gy daily fractions to 70 Gy over 7 weeks. Altered fractionation techniques including hyperfractionation (e.g., 1.1 to 1.4 Gy twice daily) and accelerated fractionation (e.g., six fraction per week or concomitant boost regimens) have demonstrated improved locoregional control rates for head and neck cancer patients (31,54,61). A recent meta-analysis examined 15 trials that compared conventional fractionation to altered fractionation, either hyperfractionation or accelerated fractionation. The study demonstrated a small but statistically significant survival benefit of 3.4% at 5 years with altered fractionation. The benefit was higher with hyper-

fractionation compared to accelerated fractionation and was more pronounced for patients younger than age 50 (9). Due to the high likelihood of subclinical nodal metastases, even in the clinically N0 neck, patients traditionally receive comprehensive radiation to encompass nodal regions from skull base to clavicle. Due to the varying thickness of the head and neck, custom compensators or wedges should be used for the lateral fields to obtain a more homogeneous dose distribution. Shrinking field techniques to spare direct spinal cord dose after ~45 Gy, as well as final mucosal field reductions after 54 to 60 Gy are often appropriate with posterior neck boosting with electrons to complete the nodal dosing without excessive dose to the spinal cord.

Over the past 10 to 15 years, the use of three-dimensional CT-based planning has become routine in the management of head and neck cancer patients (Fig. 43.7). CT-based planning allows precise delineation of target volume and visualization of dose distributions (Fig. 43.8).

Early T-stage hypopharynx patients with N0–1 neck disease can be considered for treatment with radiation alone or concurrent radiation plus chemotherapy. In this setting, gross disease should receive 70 Gy and the contralateral neck (N0) should receive 50 to 54 Gy. With T1-N0 lesions, patients may achieve 5-year disease-specific survival (DSS) on the order of 90%, while T2-N0 lesions may achieve DSS of >70% (52). (Tables 43.4 and 43.5).

Patients with advanced N2–3 neck disease are often considered for postradiotherapy or postchemoradiotherapy neck dissection in an effort to maximize the likelihood of neck control (47). Several recent studies, including one from the University of Iowa, have assessed the value of a postradiation FDG-PET to help select those patients who might benefit most from subsequent neck dissection. For complete clinical responders, the Iowa study concluded that FDG-PET in this setting has a very high negative predictive value. The authors suggest that FDG-PET may be a valuable tool to help determine which patients should undergo adjuvant neck dissection versus observation following the completion of head and neck radiation or chemoradiotherapy (79).

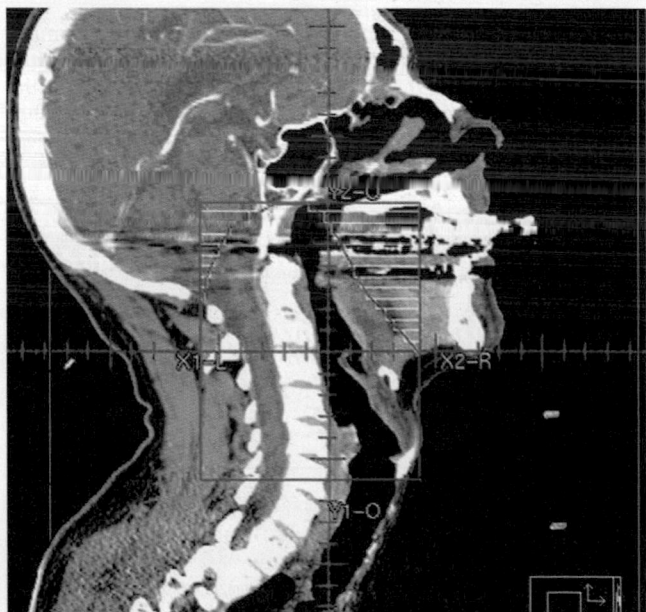

FIGURE 43.7. Digitally reconstructed radiograph depicting a classical lateral field designed to encompass the T2 pyriform sinus cancer from Figures 43.4 and 43.5 plus bilateral cervical lymphatics from skull base to cricoid, with a matching anterior low neck field to extend the lymphatic coverage to the level of the clavicle.

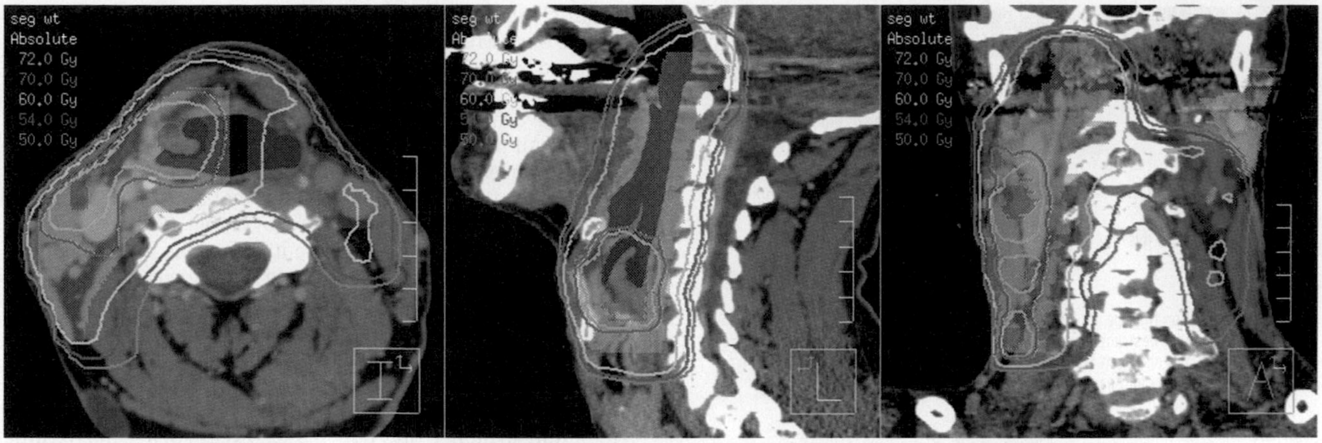

FIGURE 43.8. Transverse, sagittal and coronal treatment planning images depicting head and neck intensity-modulated radiation therapy isodose distributions for patient with a T2 N2b M0 right pyriform sinus cancer (same case as depicted in Fig. 43.4A). Prescriptions included 70 Gy to the gross tumor volume, 60 Gy to the high risk clinical target volume 1 and 54 Gy to the lower risk clinical target volume 2. The left parotid gland received a mean dose of 22 Gy.

Squamous-cell carcinomas of the head and neck are rapidly proliferating tumors. There has been significant interest over the past several decades in the use of intensified radiation fractionation schedules to counter rapid tumor cell repopulation as a means of improving outcome in head and neck cancer patients treated with radiation alone. The Radiation Therapy Oncology Group (RTOG 9003) altered fractionation in a randomized trial comparing conventional fractionation to hyperfractionation, split-course, and concomitant boost techniques and demonstrated a significant improvement in DFS for the hyperfractionation and concomitant boost arms (31) (Table 43.6). Hypopharynx patients were included within the study cohort for this randomized trial. These altered fractionation regimens were associated with higher incidence of grade 3 or worse acute mucosal toxicity but no significant difference in overall chronic toxicity at 2 years following completion of treatment.

In the past several years, there has been significant interest in the use of intensity-modulated radiation therapy (IMRT) in head and neck cancer as a means of diminishing normal tissue toxicities, particularly xerostomia resulting from irradiation of major salivary glands. Excellent candidates for IMRT include patients with unilateral T1–3 primary lesions with ≤N2b neck disease. In light of the high-dose gradients that can accompany highly conformal plans, a critical component of successful IMRT delivery is the use of an accurate and reproducible localization system. At several centers, the use of an optically guided localization system is used to enhance treatment precision for patients undergoing IMRT for head and neck cancer (41) (Fig. 43.9). The cephalad margin of the N0 contralateral neck may often be limited to the C1–2 interspace in an effort to further improve parotid gland sparing (24,25).

T3–4 Resectable

Surgery

Favorable T3 hypopharynx cancers that present in the upper aspect of the pyriform sinus and permit full extirpation by either an extended supraglottic laryngectomy or extended vertical partial laryngopharyngectomy with free flap reconstruction are possible but infrequent. Many T3 and T4 hypopharynx cancers that are treated surgically will require total laryngectomy with efforts to preserve a posterior strip of the hypopharynx spanning the oropharynx to the esophagus. This preserved posterior wall of the hypopharynx may be tubed and closed on itself in selected cases. In the past it was common practice to accept primary reconstruction of this segment as adequate for swallowing with closure over a nasogastric tube. More recently primary closure has been discouraged for cases with less than a 3 to 3.5 cm width of posterior pharyngeal wall mucosa to tube on itself. Most commonly superior swallowing results when the anterior and lateral walls of the remaining hypopharynx are reconstructed with either pedicled or free flap reconstruction.

For more bulky tumors of the hypopharynx, total laryngopharyngectomy is required and refers to removal of the larynx and the entire hypopharynx. This procedure creates a gap between the oropharynx and esophagus that can be reconstructed with a tubed fasciocutaneous flap such as the radial forearm free flap or lateral thigh flap, a free jejunum, or a tubed pedicled myocutaneous flap. The myocutaneous flaps are technically difficult to tube due to the bulk of the fat and muscle underlying the skin paddle.

Laryngopharyngectomy with esophagectomy may be performed if the hypopharynx cancer extends inferior to the

	GENERAL ANATOMIC LANDMARKS FOR FIELD DESIGN USING CONVENTIONAL HEAD AND NECK RADIOTHERAPY FOR HYPOPHARYNX CANCER	
Table 43.4	

Superior border	Include base of skull
Posterior border	Behind vertebral spinous processes (or further if required to cover metastatic cervical lymph nodes)
Inferior border	Lower aspect of cricoid cartilage unless extensive caudal tumor extension
Anterior border	Flash skin at level of thyroid cartilage

For T1 lesions, classical dose is 66 to 70 Gy in 2-Gy daily fractions. For T2–4 lesions consider altered fractionation regimens and/or concurrent cisplatin-based chemotherapy particularly for patients <70 years of age. Gross disease should generally receive 70 Gy with concurrent chemotherapy.

Table 43.5	GENERAL TREATMENT RECOMMENDATIONS BASED ON HYPOPHARYNX TUMOR STAGE
Stage I	Radiation alone or voice preservation surgery if feasible
Stage II	Radiation alone
Stage III and IV with functional laryngopharynx	Concurrent chemoradiation followed by selective neck dissection
Stage III and IV with dysfunctional laryngopharynx[a]	Laryngopharyngectomy with adjuvant RT or CRT

CRT, chemoradiation therapy; RT, radiation therapy
[a]Patients with bulky, destructive tumors that severely compromise the airway, destroy cartilage, bone, and deep soft tissue are often best served with immediate laryngopharyngectomy and postoperative radiation or chemoradiation.

cricopharyngeus to ensure the inferior margin. In this case, reconstruction with a gastric pull-up or colon interposition are options used to restore the conduit for food and saliva extending from the oropharynx to the stomach.

Postoperative Radiation Therapy

In light of the deeply infiltrative nature of advanced hypopharynx cancers that are treated with initial surgical resection, the vast majority of patients are recommended to undergo adjuvant radiation therapy in an effort to enhance locoregional control rates. Classical indications for postoperative radiation include T4 primary tumors, close or positive microscopic margins, cartilage/bony invasion, >1 metastatic lymph node, or the presence of extracapsular extension (ECE). Conventional therapy involves the use of shrinking field techniques, as described previously, to deliver 54 to 63 Gy to all areas at risk and a boost to 60 to 66 Gy to regions of ECE and/or positive margins. The entire cervical nodal chain from the skull base to the clavicle bilaterally should be included. IMRT techniques may be considered in an attempt to reduce radiation dose to normal tissue structures such as the contralateral parotid gland and thereby preserve better salivary function.

Recently, the role of concurrent chemotherapy along with postoperative radiation has been evaluated in prospective randomized trials by the RTOG and European Organization for Research and Treatment of Cancer (EORTC). Eligibility criteria in the RTOG trial included patients with two or more positive nodes, ECE, or microscopically positive margins. All patients received 60 Gy alone or with concurrent cisplatin 100 mg/m[2] every 3 weeks. This trial demonstrated an improvement in locoregional control and DFS for patients who received con-

current chemoradiotherapy. However, no significant benefit in absolute survival was confirmed (Table 43.7) (20). The EORTC conducted a similar trial that included patients with stage III (except T3 N0 larynx), stage IV, and patients with stage I or II with positive margins, lymphovascular invasion, and perineural invasion. All patients received 66 Gy alone or with cisplatin at 100 mg/m[2] every 3 weeks. This trial demonstrated a significant improvement in progression-free survival and overall survival with the addition of chemotherapy (6) (Table 43.8).

Although the studies above identify that the addition of cisplatin chemotherapy to postoperative radiation can improve tumor control outcome for specific categories of high-risk patients, it is clear that this modest benefit comes at the expense of additional toxicity. Careful clinical judgment regarding the selection of patients most likely to tolerate and thereby benefit from this approach is warranted. In the definitive treatment setting, there is mounting evidence that patients >70 years of age derive little to no benefit from the addition of systemic chemotherapy to radiation in head and neck cancer (9,55). This is quite likely to be true in the postoperative head and neck cancer treatment setting as well. The inadvertent introduction of treatment breaks during the adjuvant radiation course can easily compromise the potential benefits of the combined modality therapy in this setting.

There is considerable interest in the use of molecular targeted therapies in the treatment of head and neck cancer patients. The most mature clinical data set in head and neck cancer involves the use of EGFR inhibitors such as cetuximab (monoclonal antibody against the EGFR). An international phase III trial comparing high-dose radiation alone versus radiation plus cetuximab in advanced head and neck cancer patients confirmed a locoregional control improvement (10% at 3 years) and overall survival advantage (10% at 3 years) with the addition of cetuximab (7). A relatively small subset of patients with hypopharynx cancer were enrolled in this study of 424 patients, and this subset did not demonstrate a clear advantage with use of the EGFR inhibitor treatment. Ongoing trials to examine the potential value of adding cetuximab to concurrent chemoradiation approaches in advanced head and neck cancer are in progress in both the definitive and high-risk postoperative settings.

Definitive Radiation Therapy

There are several reasons why hypopharynx cancer patients who are technically resectable may not undergo primary surgery. These include age (e.g., patients >70 or 80 years old), the presence of significant medical comorbidities and/or patient unwillingness to accept total laryngectomy. Curative-intent radiation or chemoradiation is often pursued in these settings. Conventional radiation therapy commonly involves a shrinking three-field technique to deliver ~70 Gy in 2 Gy daily fractions to areas of gross disease and 50 to 60 Gy to areas of microscopic disease. If patients are scheduled to undergo postradiotherapy neck dissection, then gross nodal disease can be limited to 60 to 63 Gy. If patients are not candidates for postradiotherapy neck dissection, then gross nodal disease should be carried to 70 Gy. Altered fractionation regimens such as hyperfractionation or accelerated fractionation should be considered for patients being treated with radiation alone, as this approach has been demonstrated to improve the likelihood of locoregional tumor control (31).

In patients with adequate performance status, concurrent chemoradiation strategies using platinum-based chemotherapy should be considered. The most comprehensive meta-analysis to examine the benefit of chemotherapy in advanced head and neck cancer confirms a small but significant survival advantage for the use of chemotherapy, with the best gains observed with the use of concurrent platinum-based regimens (8%) (9,55).

Table 43.6	LOCAL REGIONAL CONTROL IN RADIATION THERAPY ONCOLOGY GROUP 9003			
	Arm 1[a] (%)	Arm 2[b] (%)	Arm 3[c] (%)	Arm 4[d] (%)
2-year local failure rate	43.7	37.8	43.0	36.9
2-year nodal failure rate	32.1	26.6	30.8	33.3

[a]Arm 1: Standard fractionation at 2 Gy/fraction to 70 Gy in 7 weeks.
[b]Arm 2: Hyperfractionation at 1.2 Gy/fraction b.i.d. to 81.6 Gy over 7 weeks.
[c]Arm 3: Accelerated fractionation with split at 1.6 Gy/fraction b.i.d. to 67.2 Gy over 6 weeks with a 2 week break at 38.4 Gy.
[d]Arm 4: Concomitant boost to 72 Gy over 6 weeks.
From Fu KK, Pajak TF, Trotti A, et al. A Radiation Therapy Oncology Group (RTOG) phase III randomized study to compare hyperfractionation and two variants of accelerated fractionation to standard fractionation radiotherapy for head and neck squamous cell carcinomas: first report of RTOG 9003 [see comment]. Int J Radiat Oncol Biol Phys 2000;48:7–16, with permission.

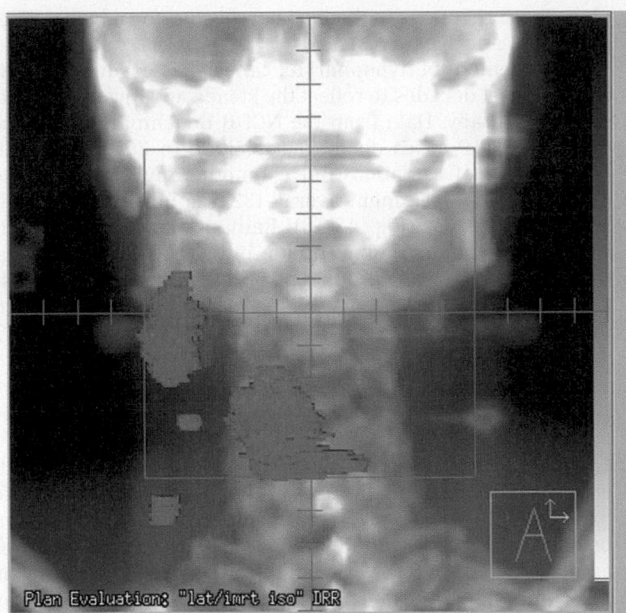
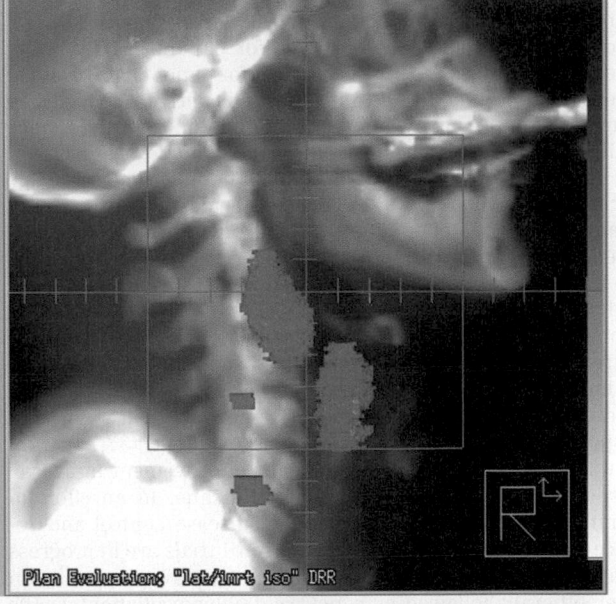
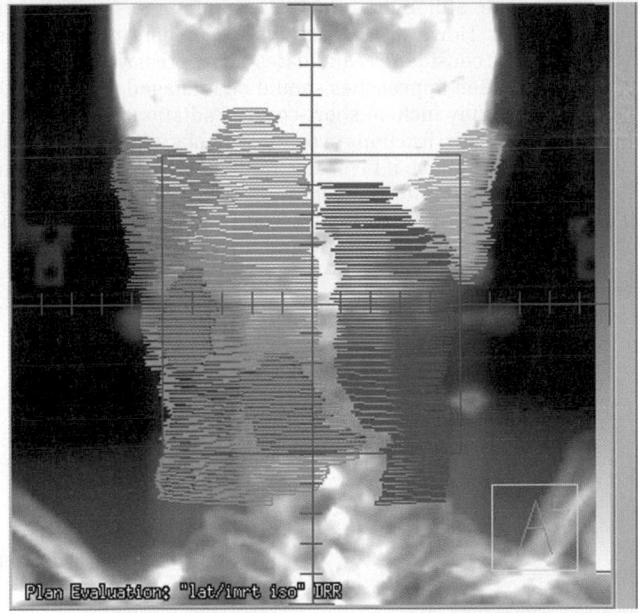
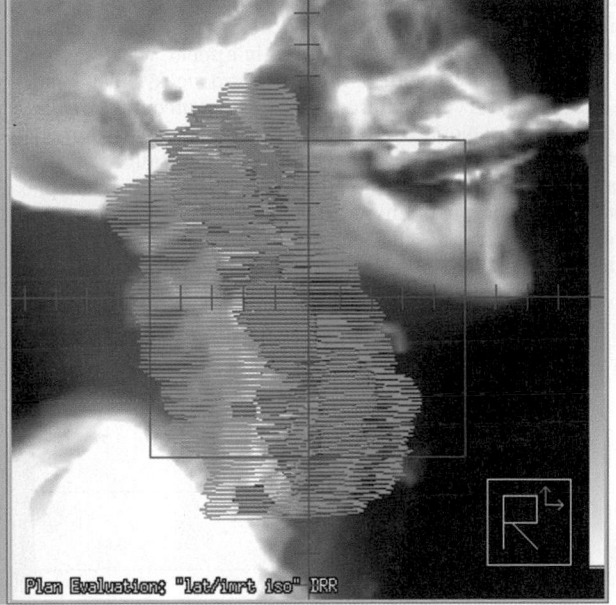

FIGURE 43.9. Beam's eye projections of intensity-modulated radiation therapy target contours for patient with T2 N2b M0 tumor of the right pyriform sinus (same case as depicted in Figs. 43.4, 43.5, and 43.9). **A,B:** Depict anterior and lateral projections highlighting the gross tumor volume (red , 70 Gy). **C,D:** Depict the same projections highlighting high-risk clinical target volume 1 (green, 60 Gy), low risk clinical target volume 2 (blue, 54 Gy), and bilateral parotid glands.

Table 43.7	RESULTS OF RADIATION THERAPY ONCOLOGY GROUP POSTOP CHEMORADIATION TRIAL		
	Arm 1[a] (%)	Arm 2[b] (%)	p
2-year locoregional control	72	82	0.003
2-year DM	23	20	NS

DM, distant metastasis; NS, nonsignificant
[a]Arm 1: 60 Gy in 6 weeks.
[b]Arm 2: 60 Gy in 6 weeks with concurrent cisplatin (100 mg/m^2) days 1, 22, and 43.
From Cooper JS, Pajak TF, Forasiere AA, et al. Postoperative concurrent radiotherapy and chemotherapy for high-risk squamous-cell carcinoma of the head and neck [see comment]. *N Engl J Med* 2004;350:1937–1944, with permission.

Table 43.8	RESULTS OF EUROPEAN ORGANISATION FOR RESEARCH AND TREATMENT OF CANCER POSTOP CHEMORADIATION TRIAL				
	Arm 1[a]		Arm 2[b]		
	Median	5 Year (%)	Median	5 Year (%)	p
PFS	23 months	36	55 months	47	0.04
OS	32 months	40	72 months	53	0.02

OS, overall survival; PFS, progression free survival
[a]Arm 1: Radiation therapy alone 66 Gy in 6.5 weeks.
[b]Arm 2: 66 Gy in 6.5 weeks with concurrent cisplatin (100 mg/m^2) days 1, 22, and 43.
From Bernier J, Domenge C, Ozsahin M, et al. Hypopharative irradiation with or without concomitant chemotherapy for locally advanced head and neck cancer [see comment]. *N Engl J Med* 2004;350:1945–1952, with permission.

However, this meta-analysis also confirms a steadily decreasing benefit for the use of chemotherapy with advancing patient age, such that no advantage is observed for patients >70 years of age. This same loss of statistical benefit for patients >70 years of age is also observed for the outcome gains derived from altered fractionation over conventional fractionation. Therefore, once daily radiation regimens (conventional technique or IMRT) may be quite reasonable for hypopharynx patients >70 years of age (or selected patients with modest performance status) rather than intensified fractionation regimens or the use of concurrent chemotherapy.

Recently, there has been renewed interest in the concept of induction chemotherapy approaches for patients with locoregionally advanced head and neck cancer, particularly with the introduction of taxane-containing regimens that offer promise to improve tumor response rates. Two randomized trials have been reported that compare induction 5-fluorouacil (5-FU) and cisplatin versus 5-FU, cisplatin, plus a taxane (37,73). Preliminary reports suggest a significant improvement in overall response rate with the addition of a taxane. In an effort to simultaneously enhance locoregional disease control and reduce distant metastases, several phase III trials are in progress that compare this sequential approach (triple agent induction chemotherapy followed by concurrent chemoradiation) versus concurrent chemoradiation (current standard of care) for patients with locoregionally advanced head and neck cancer (1). These aggressive approaches certainly appear worthy of controlled clinical investigation for head and neck subsites such as the hypopharynx, where the overall outcomes are poor and both locoregional control and distant metastases present a formidable challenge. Nevertheless, maturation of these trials is important before the ad hoc adoption of such complex, costly, and toxic treatment strategies. Careful assessment of tumor control, survival, and long-term functional outcome dovetailed with quality of life evaluation will be important to help place these regimens in the best perspective for advanced head and neck cancer patients.

Management of hypopharynx cancer has gradually evolved over the past decades to reflect the steady advancement of nonsurgical therapy. Data from the NCDB Benchmark reports addressing 3,519 cases diagnosed in 2000 to 2001 reveals the combination of radiation and chemotherapy to be the most common initial treatment overall (32.5%) for all stages of hypopharynx cancer (Fig. 43.10). Radiation as a single modality therapy was the most common initial treatment for stage I hypopharynx cancer (34%) followed by surgery alone (19.4%) as next most common (Fig. 43.11A). Chemoradiation was the most common treatment for stage II (34.4%), stage III (37%), and stage IV (35.7%) disease (Figs. 43.11B–D) (53).

Unresectable, Nonmetastatic Disease

The management of patients with unresectable locoregional disease without distant metastases is dependent on patient performance status. A patient with a good performance status may be offered definitive radiotherapy or concurrent chemotherapy as discussed above. In a randomized Intergroup trial of unresectable head and neck cancers, the addition of high-dose cisplatin to radiation was found to improve survival versus radiation alone, although at the expense of increased toxicity (2) (Table 43.9). However, patients with poor performance status who are not considered candidates for aggressive radiation or chemoradiation approaches should be managed with palliative intent. This may include short-course radiation regimens such as 4 to 5 Gy of five fractions over 1 to 2 weeks with a repeat of the same 3 weeks hence if favorable initial tolerance and response is achieved. Systemic chemotherapy alone can be considered, although for poor performance status patients, best supportive care with medical therapy and airway control may also be appropriate.

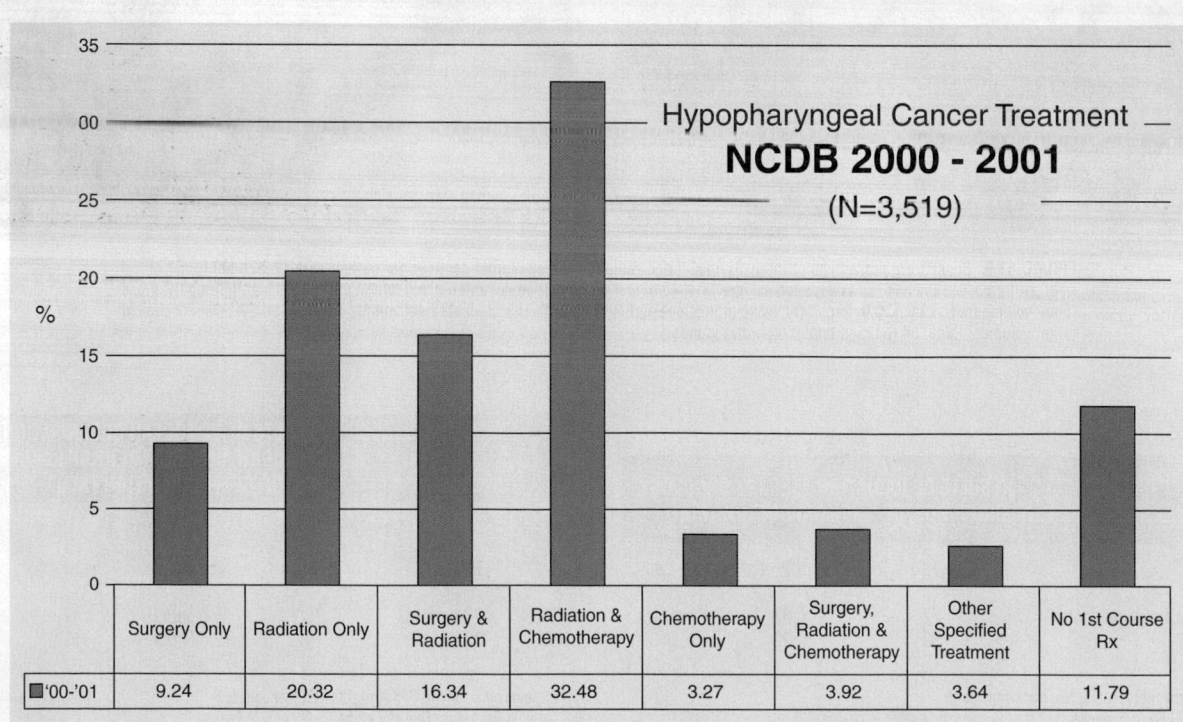

	Surgery Only	Radiation Only	Surgery & Radiation	Radiation & Chemotherapy	Chemotherapy Only	Surgery, Radiation & Chemotherapy	Other Specified Treatment	No 1st Course Rx
■ '00-'01	9.24	20.32	16.34	32.48	3.27	3.92	3.64	11.79

FIGURE 43.10. Among all cases reported from the National Cancer Data Base in the Benchmark Reports for 2000 and 2001, the majority (32.5%) received initial treatment using a combination of radiation and chemotherapy. (From National Cancer Data Base. *Commission on cancer.* American College of Surgeons. Benchmark Reports, v 3.0; November 6, 2005, with permission.)

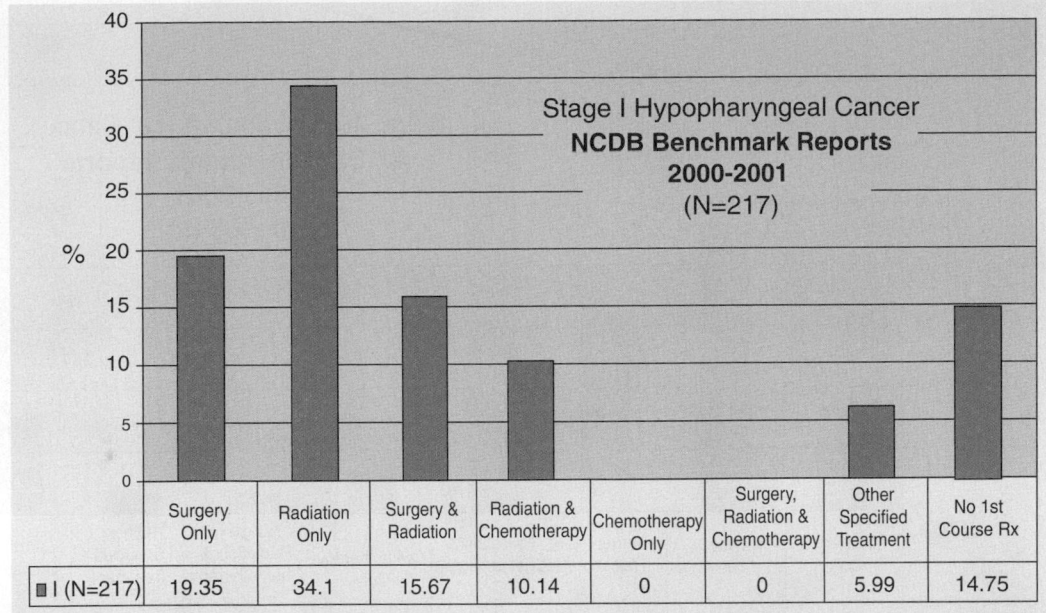

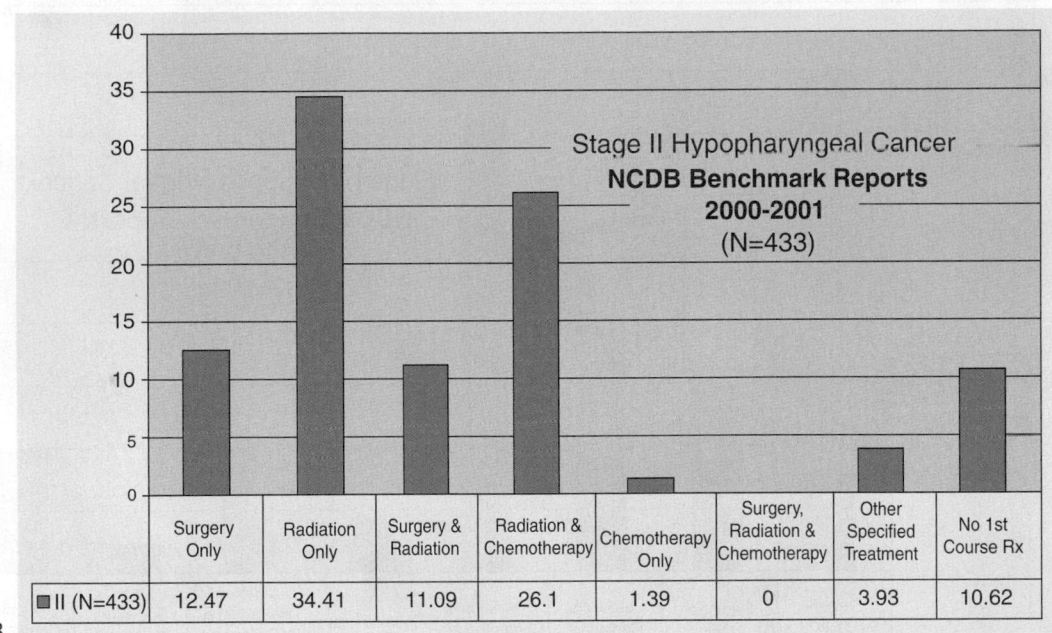

FIGURE 43.11. A: Breakdown of treatment approach according to stage revealed that the few stage I cancers (6.2% of all stages) were primarily treated with the single modality therapy of either radiation (34.1%) or surgery (19.4%). **B:** Radiation alone (34.1%) was the modality most commonly used as initial treatment for the 12.3% of hypopharynx cancers classified as stage II. Radiation combined with chemotherapy was used in 26.1% of stage II cases. (*continued*)

Metastatic Disease

As many as one quarter of hypopharynx cancer patients will develop metastatic disease at some point in their clinical course. In this setting, treatment is palliative and should be delivered to maximize or help maintain quality of life. If patients are having difficulty with local pain, bleeding, or swallowing, palliative short-course radiation therapy can be delivered as described above. Surgery may also provide a reasonable palliative option for selected patients who have incurable disease but significant symptoms related to their localized disease. If aspiration of secretions (despite no food by mouth status and enteral feedings) persists, laryngopharyngectomy may afford a reasonable option to discuss with the patient and family members. Similarly, complete stenosis of the pharynx or upper esophagus due to

tumor (or following treatment) may leave a patient with constant need for suctioning his or her own secretions. In selected patients, laryngopharyngectomy with gastric pull-up may be a reasonable palliative option. Finally, G-tube placement can be considered for patients who do not wish to pursue palliative radiation therapy or surgery. Many patients in this setting will benefit from narcotic analgesics for pain management.

Patients with adequate or good performance status should be considered for palliative chemotherapy. Several agents have shown response for recurrent and metastatic (head and neck) cancer including cisplatin, carboplatin, 5-FU, methotrexate, docetaxel, or combination regimens based on platinum or taxane and the more recent introduction of molecular targeted therapies including the EGFR inhibitors (17,19). A randomized trial has been reported comparing the efficacy of cisplatin

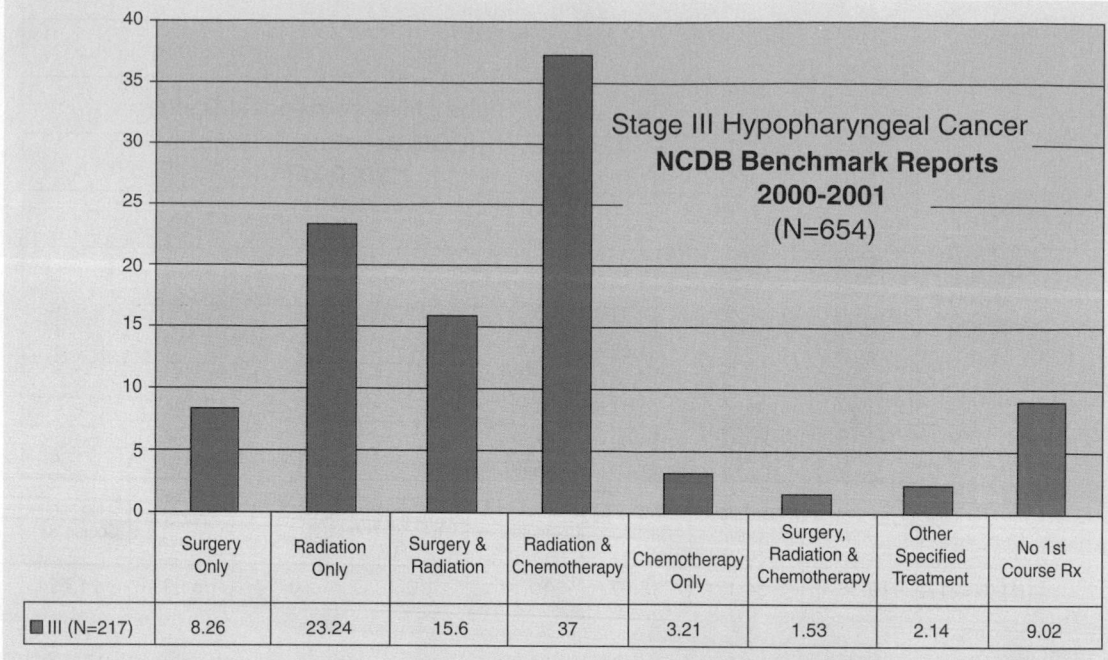

	Surgery Only	Radiation Only	Surgery & Radiation	Radiation & Chemotherapy	Chemotherapy Only	Surgery, Radiation & Chemotherapy	Other Specified Treatment	No 1st Course Rx
■ III (N=217)	8.26	23.24	15.6	37	3.21	1.53	2.14	9.02

C

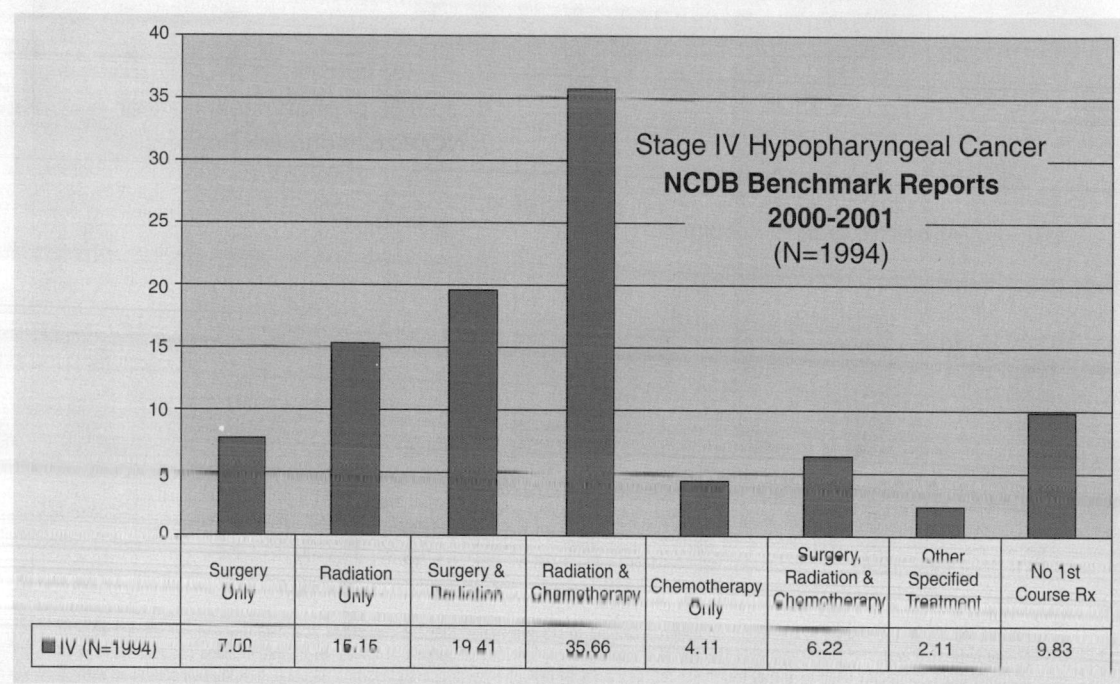

	Surgery Only	Radiation Only	Surgery & Radiation	Radiation & Chemotherapy	Chemotherapy Only	Surgery, Radiation & Chemotherapy	Other Specified Treatment	No 1st Course Rx
■ IV (N=1994)	7.50	15.15	19.41	35.66	4.11	6.22	2.11	9.83

D

FIGURE 43.11. (*Continued*) **C:** Stage III hypopharynx cancer was most commonly treated with radiation combined with chemotherapy (37%) or radiation alone (23.2%). **D:** Stage IV hypopharynx cancer was most commonly treated with either chemoradiation (35.7%) or surgery with postoperative radiation (19.4%). (From National Cancer Data Base. *Commission on cancer.* American College of Surgeons. Benchmark Reports, v 3.0; November 6, 2005, with permission.)

alone compared with two multiagent regimens: (a) cisplatin and 5-FU and (b) cisplatin, 5-FU, bleomycin, and vincristine. Although the combination regimens demonstrated higher tumor response rates, this did not translate into a significant difference in median survival between the three arms. The combination arms were more toxic (16). In the 1990s there was significant interest in incorporating taxanes into regimens for recurrent and metastatic head and neck cancer. A randomized trial comparing cisplatin and 5-FU to cisplatin and paclitaxel demonstrated similar response rates, median survival, and 1-year survival. The cisplatin and 5-FU arm was more toxic to administer (33). There has also been significant interest in incorporating targeted ther-

apies such as the EGFR inhibitors for head and neck cancer patients with metastatic or recurrent disease. These agents generally elicit modest response rates when given as single agents. For example, cetuximab, gefitinib, and erlotinib have generated response rates of 13%, 11%, and 4%, respectively as single agents in head and neck cancer (18,62,72). There is interest in combining traditional cytotoxic chemotherapy agents with targeted agents to improve overall outcomes. A trial comparing cisplatin alone or in combination with cetuximab demonstrated improved response rates with cetuximab, but no significant improvement in progression-free survival or overall survival (13).

Table 43.9	CONCURRENT CHEMORADIATION IN UNRESECTABLE HEAD AND NECK CANCER			
	Arm 1[a] (%)	Arm 2[b] (%)	Arm 3[c] (%)	p
Acute ≥ grade III toxicity	52	89	7	<0.001
3-year OS	23	37	27%	Arm A vs. B (p = 0.014) Arm A vs. C (p = NS)

OS, overall survival; RT, radiation therapy
[a]Arm 1: RT alone 70 Gy, 7 weeks.
[b]Arm 2: RT to 70 Gy in 7 weeks with concurrent cisplatin (100 mg/m^2) days 1, 22, and 43.
[c]Arm 3: 60 to 70 Gy split course RT with concurrent cisplatin (75 mg/m^2) day 1 and 5-FU (1,000 mg/m^2/d) as a 96-hour continuous infusion.
From Adelstein DJ, Li Y, Adams GL, et al. An intergroup phase III comparison of standard radiation therapy and two schedules of concurrent chemoradiotherapy in patients with unresectable squamous cell head and neck cancer. *J Clin Oncol* 2003;21:92–98, with permission.

Complications

Surgery

The complications from surgery generally fall within the confines of bleeding, infection, reaction to the anesthesia, and damage to structures around or in the field of surgery. The damage to the laryngopharynx that occurs in the course of removing those tissues involved by cancer necessarily interferes with key laryngeal functions: breathing, swallowing, and speaking.

If an effort is made to preserve laryngeal function, some compromise may be required. A long-term tracheotomy, no food by mouth status with the use of gastrostomy feedings, and/or significant dysphonia are not uncommon for patients with hypopharynx cancer treated with conservation laryngeal surgery. These same complications may attend the more comprehensive laryngopharyngectomy as well. Stenosis of the neopharynx, difficulty with alaryngeal speech, and stomal stenosis may compromise the same functions ordinarily ascribed to the larynx. For all open surgical approaches, the risk of a salivary fistula is greatest for those patients previously treated with radiation. Although salivary fistulas are rare with endoscopic approaches, they have occurred in cases requiring aggressive laser resection.

Radiation Therapy

During a course of head and neck radiation therapy, there are predictable side effects that are experienced by the majority of patients: mucositis, fatigue, loss of taste acuity, radiation dermatitis, and xerostomia. Typically patients will begin to experience mucositis during the 3rd week of radiotherapy. This initially manifests as mucosal blanching within the treatment field, but can progress to patchy or confluent mucositis. Initially patients can be treated with an over-the-counter pain reliever, but once patients develop grade II or III mucositis, they will commonly require narcotic analgesics for adequate pain control. The combination of dysphagia and mucositis can result in significant nutritional compromise, necessitating intravenous hydration and parenteral nutritional supplementation. Nausea associated with treatment can also further complicate the nutritional status. These acute toxicities can become particularly pronounced in the setting of intensified radiation fractionation schedules and/or combined chemoradiotherapy. Patients may require prophylactic antiemetics. In patients receiving concurrent radiotherapy and platinum-based chemotherapy, there is

clear potential for myelosuppression; therefore, blood counts should be monitored regularly. Signs or symptoms of infection should be addressed promptly. Finally, xerostomia can become problematic during the course of radiation. Ultimately, patients can be reassured that the majority of these side effects, with the exception of xerostomia, are temporary and will resolve several weeks to months following completion of therapy.

As noted, one of the acute side effects of radiotherapy that can become permanent is xerostomia. Chemical and physical modifiers of the radiation response have been utilized to reduce long-term xerostomia. The free-radical scavenger amifostine has the potential to reduce radiation effects on normal tissues if administered just prior to each radiation fraction. A randomized phase III trial demonstrated a reduction in the severity of the acute and chronic grade 2 or higher xerostomia in patients who received amifostine during RT (11). Dose-limiting toxicities commonly include hypotension and nausea. However, more recent reviews have called into question the ultimate value of amifostine in patients with advanced head and neck cancer, and currently there is no universal standard recommendation across treatment centers for the use of this radioprotector (40,76).

IMRT or tomotherapy techniques allow the clinician to physically modify the radiation dose distribution in an effort to spare critical normal tissues. This approach has been used increasingly for (head and neck) cancer patients to reduce radiation dose to the major salivary glands. A dosimetric analysis comparing radiation dose to the parotid gland and postradiation salivary function demonstrates that limiting mean dose to the parotid gland to <26 Gy is associated with improved postradiation salivary function (25).

In some cases, hypopharynx cancer patients who complete a course of radiation therapy will be noted to have persistent laryngeal edema on subsequent follow-up visits. Although in the early posttreatment phase (in fact up to 24 months), significant or newfound edema should raise suspicion regarding the possibility of persistent or recurrent disease, the majority of patients who receive high-dose radiation across major segments of the larynx and hypopharynx will manifest some degree of edema, mucosal congestion, and eventual fibrosis (see Fig. 43.4B). Generally, this collateral damage is a tolerable chronic toxicity with modest impact on patient quality of life. However, in approximately 10% to 15% of patients, this edema is severe enough to cause significant airway and swallow function compromise requiring tracheostomy.

Outcomes

There are several institutional reports of radiation therapy alone in the management of hypopharynx cancer. It is difficult to compare directly the results between surgically treated patients and radiation treated patients because there is often a selection bias whereby some patients are selected for surgery and others referred for radiotherapy. The University of Florida has systematically reported their results with radiation alone for patients with hypopharynx cancer (Tables 43.10–43.12) (3,27).

In an effort to examine the potential for organ preservation in patients with advanced cancers of the hypopharynx, the EORTC conducted a randomized trial for patients who would require total laryngectomy as a surgical approach. This trial randomly allocated patients to induction chemotherapy with cisplatin and 5-florouracil followed by definitive radiation versus primary surgical resection and postoperative radiation. With a median follow-up of 10 years, this trial demonstrated no significant difference in 5- or 10-year overall survival or progression-free survival. Of note, two thirds of living patients in the chemoradiotherapy arm were able to retain their larynx (43).

Table 43.10	LOCAL CONTROL FOR CARCINOMA OF THE POSTERIOR PHARYNGEAL WALL TREATED WITH RADIATION ALONE			
	Local Control after RT		Ultimate Local Control after Salvage	
Stage	2 Year (%)	5 Year (%)	2 Year (%)	5 Year (%)
T1	100	100	100	100
T2	79	74	86	81
T3	59	49	66	66
T4	36	36	36	36

RT, radiation therapy
From Amdur RJ, Mendenhall WM, Stringer SP, et al. Organ preservation with radiotherapy for T1-T2 carcinoma of the pyriform sinus. *Head Neck* 2001;23:353–362, with permission.

Table 43.12	CAUSE-SPECIFIC AND OVERALL SURVIVAL FOR CARCINOMA OF THE PYRIFORM SINUS TREATED WITH RADIATION ALONE	
AJCC Stage	5-Year Cause-Specific Survival (%)	5-Year Overall Survival (%)
I	—	57
II	96	61
III	62	41
IVa	49	29
IVb	33	25

AJCC, American Joint Committee on Cancer
From Amdur RJ, Mendenhall WM, Stringer SP, et al. Organ preservation with radiotherapy for T1-T2 carcinoma of the pyriform sinus. *Head Neck* 2001;23:353–362.

Long-Term Follow-Up

Regardless of whether patients undergo primary surgery or radiation therapy, there is value in close posttreatment surveillance by head and neck surgeon and radiation oncologist. During the first 6 months after treatment, patients should be followed every 4 to 6 weeks with clinical examination, including fiberoptic nasopharyngoscopy. Recommended guidelines include a follow-up visit every 1 to 3 months during the first year, every 2 to 4 months for the second year, every 4 to 6 months for years 3 through 5, and every 6 to 12 months thereafter. Additionally, if the patient received comprehensive head and neck radiation, the serum thyrotropin should be measured every 6 to 12 months. Imaging evaluation of the neck most commonly with CT or MRI scan are obtained at 3 to 6 month intervals during the first 2 years or as indicated based on clinical findings. Functional imaging with [18]FDG-PET can sometimes prove valuable to help differentiate posttreatment fibrosis from persistent or recurrent disease.

A study by Hermans et al. (36) examined findings on CT scan of the neck 3 to 4 months following completion of radiation therapy for patients with larynx or hypopharynx cancer to examine correlation with long-term outcome. The authors suggest that in patients achieving complete radiographic resolution of all pretreatment disease, the likelihood of subsequent local failure is very small. These patients might therefore undergo routine clinical examination with repeat imaging reserved for instances where the clinical examination becomes suspicious for recurrence. For patients who achieved <50% reduction in tumor volume or retained a mass ≥1 cm on the posttreatment imaging study, the likelihood of local failure was 100% and 30%, respectively. In these patients, repeat CT at 3 to 4 months, FDG PET, or biopsy is therefore recommended. Preliminary reports indicate that the results of the first post-RT FDG-PET scan may be a strong predictor of developing locoregional disease recurrence (78).

In the posttreatment setting of hypopharynx cancer patients, the involvement of an experienced head and neck radiologist is highly desirable for optimal interpretation of imaging results. Soft-tissue changes following ablative surgery and reconstruction or following high-dose radiation or chemoradiation with resultant edema and fibrosis can be very difficult to differentiate from tumor, particularly for the inexperienced reader.

Management of Recurrence

After completion of treatment, patients should be followed closely for signs of recurrent or persistent disease. If recurrence is suspected, this should generally be confirmed by biopsy. If biopsy is confirmatory, then the patient should undergo complete restaging to assess the extent of disease. In the setting of local or regional disease alone, patients treated with initial radiation or chemoradiation can be considered for surgical salvage therapy. Although salvage surgery following comprehensive head and neck radiation and chemotherapy presents several resection and reconstructive healing challenges for the surgeon, selected patients may still derive long-term benefit from this approach. Recurrent patients who initially received comprehensive head and neck radiation have traditionally not been considered good candidates for repeat high-dose radiation in light of normal tissue tolerances. However, with the advent of highly conformal radiation delivery techniques, selected patients may benefit from reirradiation approaches in conjunction with systemic chemotherapy (77). Many patients with recurrent disease, however, are not good candidates for aggressive surgery or radiation salvage therapy and are best served with systemic chemotherapy and/or best supportive care approaches.

In the setting of distant metastatic disease, further treatment will focus on palliative goals. If the patient is experiencing significant local symptoms in the setting of asymptomatic distant metastases, palliative surgery or radiation may still warrant

Table 43.11	CAUSE-SPECIFIC AND OVERALL SURVIVAL FOR CARCINOMA OF THE POSTERIOR PHARYNGEAL WALL TREATED WITH RADIATION ALONE (28)	
AJCC Stage	5-Year Overall Survival (%)	5-Year Cause-Specific Survival (%)
I	50	100
II	36	72
III	26	56
IVa	28	75
IVb	5	29

AJCC, American Joint Committee on Cancer
From Fein DA, Mendenhall WM, Parsons JT, et al. Pharyngeal wall carcinoma treated with radiotherapy: impact of treatment technique and fractionation. *Int J Radiat Oncol Biol Phys* 1993;26:751–757, with permission.

consideration. Most patients with distant metastatic disease and adequate performance status should be considered for systemic therapy and/or best supportive care options.

Quality of Life

Assessment of parameters including functional status, organ preservation, treatment cost, and patient-assessment of quality of life play an increasingly important role in the evaluation of overall treatment efficacy. For larynx and hypopharynx cancer patients, a focus of contemporary clinical investigation has been the study of treatments designed to preserve laryngeal function for patients traditionally treated with total laryngectomy. A frequently cited but somewhat controversial study by McNeil et al. (46) employed a questionnaire administered to healthy individuals and concluded that some might forgo total laryngectomy in favor of alternative therapy even if this choice diminished their ultimate chance for cure. A more recent report by El-Deiry et al. (26) evaluated long-term quality of life in a matched pair analysis comparing the surgical and nonsurgical treatment of patients with advanced head and neck cancer involving the oropharynx, hypopharynx, and larynx. Although patients in the surgery arm demonstrated worse speech outcomes than those treated with chemoradiation, this difference did not carry over to the overall quality of life score. These investigators concluded that, although it seems reasonable that organ preservation (nonsurgical) treatment will uniformly result in a higher quality of life, the complexities of human adjustment and multitude of potential treatment effects render this assumption invalid for many patients.

There have been relatively few prospective assessments of quality of life following treatment for head and neck cancer. In a subset of locally advanced patients requiring radical surgery such as total laryngectomy and partial pharyngectomy, the functional deficits are predictable. However, for patients undergoing "organ preservation" with radiation alone or in combination with chemotherapy, it can be difficult to assess the true extent and quality of organ preservation. Regardless of the primary treatment approach, these patients often require long-term speech, swallow, and dental rehabilitation. A study from Meyer et al. (49) retrospectively assessed speech intelligibility and quality of life in survivors of head and neck cancer. A total of 64 patients were enrolled; 31 underwent RT alone, five surgery alone, and 28 received both. All patients underwent comprehensive subjective and objective testing of speech function and quality of life. They found significant subjective and objective deficits in speech and quality of life even 5 years after completion of therapy. Terrell et al. (69) reported the results of a self-administered health survey of 570 patients at a Veteran's Administration hospital that demonstrated that the single most notable event having a negative impact on Quality of life was placement of a feeding tube. This was followed by medical comorbid conditions, presence of a tracheotomy tube, chemotherapy, and neck dissection.

A prospective study on quality of life utilizing the EORTC QLQ-C30 and QLQ-head and neck 35 questionnaires was conducted in Sweden on 357 patients. This study found that quality of life issues were significantly associated with the site of origin, with stage at diagnosis being the most important predictor. Additionally, patients with hypopharynx cancer exhibited the poorest quality of life (35). A study from the University of South Carolina compared swallow related quality of life after surgery or radiotherapy for head and neck cancer using a dysphagia risk factor survey, the M.D. Anderson Dysphagia Inventory (MDADI). They found significantly better scores on the emotional and functional components of the MDADI for patients undergoing chemoradiation compared to those undergoing surgery followed by radiation (34).

Conclusion

Patients with cancers of the hypopharynx commonly present with advanced disease associated with varying degrees of compromise in speech and/or swallow function. Many hypopharynx cancer patients also carry significant medical and social comorbidities. Typically, small T1–2 lesions can be managed with either primary radiation or surgery with similar clinical outcome. For intermediate stage disease that would require laryngopharyngectomy for the surgical approach, an increasingly preferred treatment option is combined chemoradiation that has demonstrated equivalence to immediate surgery in cancer survival, however, with improved organ preservation and functional outcome. For bulky hypopharynx tumors with significant airway compromise, laryngeal distortion, and cartilage destruction, it is generally best to proceed with definitive surgery with postoperative radiation or chemoradiation. Despite an aggressive approach in the overall management of hypopharynx cancer patients, ultimate cure rates remain quite poor. There are relatively few early stage patients, and for many advanced stage patients it is difficult to achieve long-term control. Even for those patients with excellent response to therapy, there exists a continuous risk for the development of second malignancies, particularly of the upper aerodigestive track with long-term follow-up. Posttreatment patients often require aggressive speech and swallow therapy to maximize their functional outcome. There is significant interest in the incorporation of molecular targeted therapies in combination with traditional cytotoxic therapy and radiation in an effort to improve outcomes.

Acknowledgments

We acknowledge the assistance of Lindell R. Gentry, M.D., Charles W. Hodge, M.D., and Wolfgang Tome, Ph.D. in image editing and collection and Gregory Allen, M.D., Ph.D. for reference editing.

References

1. Adelstein DJ, Leblanc M. Does induction chemotherapy have a role in the management of locoregionally advanced squamous cell head and neck cancer? *J Clin Oncol* 2006;24:2624–2628.
2. Adelstein DJ, Li Y, Adams GL, et al. An intergroup phase III comparison of standard radiation therapy and two schedules of concurrent chemoradiotherapy in patients with unresectable squamous cell head and neck cancer. *J Clin Oncol* 2003;21:92–98.
3. Amdur RJ, Mendenhall WM, Stringer SP, et al. Organ preservation with radiotherapy for T1-T2 carcinoma of the pyriform sinus. *Head Neck* 2001;23:353–362.
4. Barnes L, Johnson JT. Pathologic and clinical considerations in the evaluation of major head and neck specimens resected for cancer. Part I. *Pathol Ann* 1986;21:173–250.
5. Bernier J, Domenge C, Ozsahin M, et al. Postoperative irradiation with or without concomitant chemotherapy for locally advanced head and neck cancer [see comment]. *N Engl J Med* 2004;350:1945–1952.
6. Boffetta P, Richiardi L, Berrino F, et al. Occupation and larynx and hypopharynx cancer: an international case-control study in France, Italy, Spain, and Switzerland. *Cancer Causes Control* 2003;14:203–212.
7. Bonner JA, Harari PM, Giralt J, et al. Radiotherapy plus cetuximab for squamous-cell carcinoma of the head and neck. *N Engl J Med* 2006;354:567–578.
8. Bourhis J, Overgaard J, Audry H, et al. Hyperfractionated or accelerated radiotherapy in head and neck cancer: a meta-analysis. *Lancet* 2006;368:843–854.
9. Bourhis J, LeMaitre J, Pignon J, Ang K, et al. Impact of age on treatment effect in locally advanced head and neck cancer (HNC): two individual patient data meta-analyses. *J Clin Oncol* 2006;24:5501.
10. Boyd TS, Harari PM, Tannehill SP, et al. Planned postradiotherapy neck dissection in patients with advanced head and neck cancer. *Head Neck* 1998;20:132–137.
11. Brizel DM, Wasserman TH, Henke M, et al. Phase III randomized trial of amifostine as a radioprotector in head and neck cancer [see comment]. [Erratum appears in *J Clin Oncol* 2000;18(24):4110–4111.] *J Clin Oncol* 2000;18:3339–3345.
12. Brugere J, Guenel P, Leclerc A, et al. Differential effects of tobacco and alcohol in cancer of the larynx, pharynx, and mouth. *Cancer* 1986;57:391–395.
13. Burtness B, Goldwasser MA, Flood W, et al. Phase III randomized trial of cisplatin plus placebo compared with cisplatin plus cetuximab in metastatic/recurrent head and neck cancer: an Eastern Cooperative Oncology Group study. *J Clin Oncol* 2005;23:8646–8654.
14. Carpenter RJ 3rd, DeSanto LW. Cancer of the hypopharynx. *Surg Clin North Am* 1977;57:723–735.

15. Chang F, Syrjanen S, Syrjanen K. Implications of the p53 tumor-suppressor gene in clinical oncology. *J Clin Oncol* 1995;13:1009–1022.
16. Clavel M, Vermorken JB, Cognetti F, et al. Randomized comparison of cisplatin, methotrexate, bleomycin and vincristine (CABO) versus cisplatin and 5-fluorouracil (CF) versus cisplatin (C) in recurrent or metastatic squamous cell carcinoma of the head and neck. A phase III study of the EORTC Head and Neck Cancer Cooperative Group. *Ann Oncol* 1994;5:521–526.
17. Cohen EE. Role of epidermal growth factor receptor pathway-targeted therapy in patients with recurrent and/or metastatic squamous cell carcinoma of the head and neck. *J Clin Oncol* 2006;24:2659–2665.
18. Cohen EE, Rosen F, Stadler WM, et al. Phase II trial of ZD1839 in recurrent or metastatic squamous cell carcinoma of the head and neck. *J Clin Oncol* 2003;21:1980–1987.
19. Colevas AD. Chemotherapy options for patients with metastatic or recurrent squamous cell carcinoma of the head and neck. *J Clin Oncol* 2006;24:2644–2652.
20. Cooper JS, Pajak TF, Forastiere AA, et al. Postoperative concurrent radiotherapy and chemotherapy for high-risk squamous-cell carcinoma of the head and neck [see comment]. *N Engl J Med* 2004;350:1937–1944.
21. Davies L, Welch HG. Epidemiology of head and neck cancer in the United States. *Otolaryngol Head Neck Surg* 2006;135:451–457.
22. Di Martino E, Nowak B, Hassan HA, et al. Diagnosis and staging of head and neck cancer: a comparison of modern imaging modalities (positron emission tomography, computed tomography, color-coded duplex sonography) with panendoscopic and histopathologic findings. *Arch Otolaryngol Head Neck Surg* 2000;126:1457–1461.
23. Dikshit RP, Boffetta P, Bouchardy C, et al. Lifestyle habits as prognostic factors in survival of laryngeal and hypopharyngeal cancer: a multicentric European study. *Int J Cancer* 2005;117:992–995.
24. Eisbruch A, Ship JA, Dawson LA, et al. Salivary gland sparing and improved target irradiation by conformal and intensity modulated irradiation of head and neck cancer. *World J Surg* 2003;27:832–837.
25. Eisbruch A, Ten Haken RK, Kim HM, et al. Dose, volume, and function relationships in parotid salivary glands following conformal and intensity-modulated irradiation of head and neck cancer [see comment]. *Int J Radiat Oncol Biol Phys* 1999;45:577–587.
26. El-Deiry M, Funk GF, Nalwa S, et al. Long-term quality of life for surgical and nonsurgical treatment of head and neck cancer. *Arch Otolaryngol Head Neck Surg* 2005;131:879–885.
27. Fein DA, Mendenhall WM, Parsons JT, et al. Pharyngeal wall carcinoma treated with radiotherapy: impact of treatment technique and fractionation. *Int J Radiat Oncol Biol Phys* 1993;26:751–757.
28. Frank JL, Bur ME, Garb JL, et al. p53 tumor suppressor oncogene expression in squamous cell carcinoma of the hypopharynx. *Cancer* 1994;73:181–186.
29. Frank JL, Garb JL, Banson BB, et al. Epidermal growth factor receptor expression in squamous cell carcinoma of the hypopharynx. *Surg Oncol* 1993;2:161–167.
30. Frederick L, Greene DLP, Fleming ID, et al. *AJCC cancer staging manual.* New York: Springer, 2002.
31. Fu KK, Pajak TF, Trotti A, et al. A Radiation Therapy Oncology Group (RTOG) phase III randomized study to compare hyperfractionation and two variants of accelerated fractionation to standard fractionation radiotherapy for head and neck squamous cell carcinomas: first report of RTOG 9003. *Int J Radiat Oncol Biol Phys* 2000;48:7–16.
32. Gibson MK, Li Y, Murphy B, et al. Randomized phase III evaluation of cisplatin plus fluorouracil versus cisplatin plus paclitaxel in advanced head and neck cancer (E1395): an intergroup trial of the Eastern Cooperative Oncology Group. *J Clin Oncol* 2005;23:3562–3567.
33. Gillespie MB, Brodsky MB, Day TA, et al. Swallowing-related quality of life after head and neck cancer treatment. *Laryngoscope* 2004;114:1362–1367.
34. Hammerlid E, Bjordal K, Ahlner-Elmqvist M, et al. A prospective study of quality of life in head and neck cancer patients. Part I: at diagnosis. *Laryngoscope* 2001;111:669–680.
35. Hermans R, Pameijer FA, Mancuso AA, et al. Laryngeal or hypopharyngeal squamous cell carcinoma: can follow-up CT after definitive radiation therapy be used to detect local failure earlier than clinical examination alone? *Radiology* 2000;214:683–687.
36. Hitt R, Lopez-Pousa A, Martinez-Trufero J, et al. Phase III study comparing cisplatin plus fluorouracil to paclitaxel, cisplatin, and fluorouracil induction chemotherapy followed by chemoradiotherapy in locally advanced head and neck cancer. *J Clin Oncol* 2005;23:8636–8645.
37. Ho CM, Lam KH, Wei WI, et al. Squamous cell carcinoma of the hypopharynx—analysis of treatment results. *Head Neck* 1993;15:405–412.
38. Hoffman HT, Karnell LH, Shah JP, et al. Hypopharyngeal cancer patient care evaluation. *Laryngoscope* 1997;107:1005–1017.
39. Hong TS, Tome WA, Chappell RJ, et al. The impact of daily setup variations on head-and-neck intensity-modulated radiation therapy. *Int J Radiat Oncol Biol Phys* 2005;61:779–788.
40. Jellema AP, Slotman BJ, Muller MJ, et al. Radiotherapy alone, versus radiotherapy with amifostine 3 times weekly, versus radiotherapy with amifostine 5 times weekly: a prospective randomized study in squamous cell head and neck cancer. *Cancer* 2006;107:544–553.
41. Keane TJ. Carcinoma of the hypopharynx. *J Otolaryngol* 1982;11:227–231.
42. Klussmann JP, Weissenborn SJ, Wieland U, et al. Prevalence, distribution, and viral load of human papillomavirus 16 DNA in tonsillar carcinomas. *Cancer* 2001;92:2875–2884.
43. Lefebvre JL, Chevalier D, Luboinski B, et al. Larynx preservation in pyriform sinus cancer: preliminary results of a European Organization for Research and Treatment of Cancer phase III trial. EORTC Head and Neck Cancer Cooperative Group [see comment]. *J Natl Cancer Inst* 1996;88:890–899.
44. Lindberg R. Distribution of cervical lymph node metastases from squamous cell carcinoma of the upper respiratory and digestive tracts. *Cancer* 1972;29:1446–1449.
45. Marks JE, Kurnik B, Powers WE, et al. Carcinoma of the pyriform sinus. An analysis of treatment results and patterns of failure. *Cancer* 1978;41:1008–1015.
46. McNeil BJ, Weichselbaum R, Pauker SG. Speech and survival: tradeoffs between quality and quantity of life in laryngeal cancer. *N Engl J Med* 1981;305:982–987.
47. Mendenhall WM, Million RR, Cassisi NJ. Squamous cell carcinoma of the head and neck treated with radiation therapy: the role of neck dissection for clinically positive neck nodes. *Int J Radiat Oncol Biol Phys* 1986;12:733–740.
48. Merino OR, Lindberg RD, Fletcher GH. An analysis of distant metastases from squamous cell carcinoma of the upper respiratory and digestive tracts. *Cancer* 1977;40:145–151.
49. Meyer TK, Kuhn JC, Campbell BH, et al. Speech intelligibility and quality of life in head and neck cancer survivors. *Laryngoscope* 2004;114:1977–1981.
50. Mineta H, Ogino T, Amano HM, et al. Human papilloma virus (HPV) type 16 and 18 detected in head and neck squamous cell carcinoma. *Anticancer Res* 1998;18:4765–4768.
51. Mukherji SK, Armao D, Joshi VM. Cervical nodal metastases in squamous cell carcinoma of the head and neck: what to expect. *Head Neck* 2001;23:995–1005.
52. Nakamura K, Shioyama Y, Kawashima M, et al. Multi-institutional analysis of early squamous cell carcinoma of the hypopharynx treated with radical radiotherapy. *Int J Radiat Oncol Biol Phys* 2006;65:1045–1050.
53. NCDB [National Cancer Data Base]. *Commission on cancer.* American College of Surgeons. Benchmark Reports, v 3.0. Journal November 6, 2005.
54. Overgaard J, Hansen HS, Specht L, et al. Five compared with six fractions per week of conventional radiotherapy of squamous-cell carcinoma of head and neck: DAHANCA 6 and 7 randomised controlled trial. *Lancet* 2003;362:933–940.
55. Pignon JP, Bourhis J, Domenge C, et al. Chemotherapy added to locoregional treatment for head and neck squamous-cell carcinoma: three meta-analyses of updated individual data. MACH-NC Collaborative Group. Meta-analysis of chemotherapy on head and neck cancer [see comment]. *Lancet* 2000;355:949–955.
56. Robbins KT, Wong FS, Kumar P, et al. Efficacy of targeted chemoradiation and planned selective neck dissection to control bulky nodal disease in advanced head and neck cancer. *Arch Otolaryngol Head Neck Surg* 1999;125:670–675.
57. Schechter GL, Kalafsky JT. Cancer of the hypopharynx and cervical esophagus: management concepts. *Oncology (Huntingt)* 1988;2:17–24, 34–35.
58. Schwager K, Hoppe F, Hagen R, et al. Free-flap reconstruction for laryngeal preservation after partial laryngectomy in patients with extended tumors of the oropharynx and hypopharynx. *Eur Arch Otorhinolaryngology* 1999;256:280–282.
59. Schwartz DL, Rajendran J, Yueh B, et al. FDG-PET prediction of head and neck squamous cell cancer outcomes. *Arch Otolaryngol Head Neck Surg* 2004;130:1361–1367.
60. Shangina O, Brennan P, Szeszenia-Dabrowska N, et al. Occupational exposure and laryngeal and hypopharyngeal cancer risk in central and eastern Europe. *Am J Epidemiol* 2006;164:367–375.
61. Skladowski K, Maciejewski B, Golen M, et al. Continuous accelerated 7-days-a-week radiotherapy for head-and-neck cancer: long-term results of phase III clinical trial. *Int J Radiat Oncol Biol Phys* 2006;66:706–713.
62. Soulieres D, Senzer NN, Vokes EE, et al. Multicenter phase II study of erlotinib, an oral epidermal growth factor receptor tyrosine kinase inhibitor, in patients with recurrent or metastatic squamous cell cancer of the head and neck. *J Clin Oncol* 2004;22:77–85.
63. Spector JG, Sessions DG, Emami B, et al. Squamous cell carcinomas of the aryepiglottic fold: therapeutic results and long-term follow-up. *Laryngoscope* 1995;105:734–746.
64. Spector JG, Sessions DG, Emami B, et al. Squamous cell carcinoma of the pyriform sinus: a nonrandomized comparison of therapeutic modalities and long-term results. *Laryngoscope* 1995;105:397–406.
65. Spector JG, Sessions DG, Haughey BH, et al. Delayed regional metastases, distant metastases, and second primary malignancies in squamous cell carcinomas of the larynx and hypopharynx. *Laryngoscope* 2001;111:1079–1087.
66. Spitz MR. Epidemiology and risk factors for head and neck cancer. *Semin Oncol* 1994;21:281–288.
67. Stenson KM, Haraf DJ, Pelzer H, et al. The role of cervical lymphadenectomy after aggressive concomitant chemoradiotherapy: the feasibility of selective neck dissection. *Arch Otolaryngol Head Neck Surg* 2000;126:950–956.
68. Strasser MD, Gleich LL, Miller MA, et al. Management implications of evaluating the N2 and N3 neck after organ preservation therapy. *Laryngoscope* 1999;109:1776–1780.
69. Terrell JE, Ronis DL, Fowler KE, et al. Clinical predictors of quality of life in patients with head and neck cancer. *Arch Otolaryngol Head Neck Surg* 2004;130:401–408.
70. Thawley SE. *Comprehensive management of head and neck tumors.* Philadelphia: WB Saunders, 1999.
71. Urken ML, Blackwell K, Biller HF. Reconstruction of the laryngopharynx after hemicricoid/hemithyroid cartilage resection. Preliminary functional results. *Arch Otolaryngol Head Neck Surg* 1997;123:1213–1222.
72. Vermorken JB, Bourhis J, Trigo J, et al. Cetuximab in recurrent/metastatic (R&M) squamous cell carcinoma of the head and neck (SCCHN) refractory to first-line platinum-based therapies. *J Clin Oncol* 2005;23(No 16S):5505.
73. Vermorken JB, Remenar E, van Herpen C, et al. Standard cisplatin/infusional 5-flourouracil (PF) vs docetaxel (T) plus PF (TPF) as neoadjuvant chemotherapy for nonresectable locally advanced squamous cell carcinoma of the head and neck (LA-SCHHN): a phase III trial of the EORTC Head and Neck Cancer Group (EORTC 24971). *J Clin Oncol* 2004; (No 14S):5508.
74. Wang SJ, Wang MB, Yip H, et al. Combined radiotherapy with planned neck dissection for small head and neck cancers with advanced cervical metastases. *Laryngoscope* 2000;110:1794–1797.
75. Ward PH, Hanson DG. Reflux as an etiological factor of carcinoma of the laryngopharynx [see comment]. *Laryngoscope* 1988;98:1195–1199.
76. Wasserman TH, Brizel DM, Henke M, et al. Influence of intravenous amifostine on xerostomia, tumor control, and survival after radiotherapy for head-and-neck cancer: 2-year follow-up of a prospective, randomized, phase III trial. *Int J Radiat Oncol Biol Phys* 2005;63:985–990.
77. Wong SJ, Machtay M, Li Y. Locally recurrent, previously irradiated head and neck cancer: concurrent re-irradiation and chemotherapy, or chemotherapy alone? *J Clin Oncol* 2006;24:2653–2658.
78. Yao M, Graham MM, Smith RB, et al. Value of FDG PET in assessment of treatment response and surveillance in head-and-neck cancer patients after intensity modulated radiation treatment: a preliminary report. *Int J Radiat Oncol Biol Phys* 2004;60:1410–1418.
79. Yao M, Smith RB, Graham MM, et al. The role of FDG PET in management of neck metastasis from head-and-neck cancer after definitive radiation treatment. *Int J Radiat Oncol Biol Phys* 2005;63:991–999.

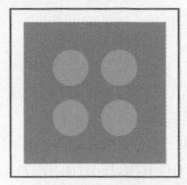

Chapter 44
Larynx

William M. Mendenhall, Russell W. Hinerman, Robert J. Amdur, Anthony A. Mancuso, Douglas B. Villaret, John W. Werning

Anatomy

The larynx is divided into the supraglottic, glottic, and subglottic regions. The supraglottic larynx consists of the epiglottis, the false vocal cords, the ventricles, and the aryepiglottic folds, including the arytenoids. The glottis includes the true vocal cords and the anterior commissure. The subglottis is located below the vocal cords (Figs. 44.1 and 44.2) (12).

The lateral line of demarcation between the glottis and supraglottic larynx is the apex of the ventricle. The demarcation between the glottis and subglottis is ill-defined, but the subglottis is considered to extend from a point 5 mm below the free margin of the vocal cord to the inferior border of the cricoid cartilage or 10 mm below the apex of the ventricle.

The vocal cords vary from 3 to 5 mm in thickness. Technically, the vocal cords terminate posteriorly with their attachment to the vocal process. The mucosa between the arytenoids is called the *posterior commissure*.

The shell of the larynx is formed by the hyoid bone, thyroid cartilage, and cricoid cartilage; the cricoid cartilage is the only complete ring. The more mobile interior framework is composed of the heart-shaped epiglottis and the arytenoid, corniculate, and cuneiform cartilages. The corniculate and cuneiform cartilages produce small, rounded bulges at the posterior end of each aryepiglottic fold.

The thyroid and the cricoid cartilages and a portion of the arytenoid cartilage are hyaline cartilage and may partially ossify with age, particularly in men. The epiglottis is elastic cartilage; ossification does not occur, and even focal calcification is rare (57).

The external laryngeal framework is linked together by the thyrohyoid, the cricothyroid, and the cricotracheal ligaments or membranes (Figs. 44.3 and 44.4) (12).

The epiglottis is joined superiorly to the hyoid bone by the hyoepiglottic ligament. The epiglottis is joined to the thyroid cartilage by the thyroepiglottic ligament at a point just below the thyroid notch and above the anterior commissure. The arrangement of the ligaments that connect the cricoid and arytenoid cartilages and form the vocal ligaments, which are part of the true vocal cords, is shown in Fig. 44.2B (12). The conus elasticus (cricovocal ligament) is the lower portion of the elastic membrane that connects the inferior framework. It connects the upper surface of the cricoid, the vocal process of the arytenoid, and the lower thyroid cartilage; its free border is thickened into the vocal ligament.

The vocal ligaments and muscles attach to the vocal process of the arytenoid posteriorly and the thyroid cartilage anteriorly. The intrinsic muscles of the larynx, which primarily control the movement of the cords, are presented in Figures 44.2 and 44.3 (12). The extrinsic muscles are concerned primarily with swallowing. The cricothyroid muscle produces tension and elongation of the vocal cords and is innervated by the superior laryngeal nerve (Fig. 44.4) (12).

The preepiglottic and paraglottic fat spaces are essentially one contiguous space lying between the external framework of the thyroid cartilage and hyoid bone and the inner framework of the epiglottis and intrinsic muscles. Lam and Wong (49) showed that there are thin membranous septa between the paraglottic and preepiglottic space that are capable of holding a tumor in check to a limited degree. The space is traversed by blood and lymphatic vessels and nerves. Because few capillary lymphatics arise in this area, invasion of the fat space should only be associated indirectly with lymph node metastases. The fat space is limited by the conus elasticus inferiorly, the thyroid ala, the thyrohyoid membrane, the hyoid bone anterolaterally, the hyoepiglottic ligament superiorly; and the fascia of the intrinsic muscles on the medial side. Posteriorly, it is adjacent to the anterior wall of the pyriform sinus.

The laryngeal surface of the epiglottis and the free margin of the vocal cords are squamous epithelium, and the remainder is usually pseudostratified ciliated columnar epithelium. Beneath the epithelium of the free edge of the vocal cord is the lamina propria, which can be divided into three layers. There is no true submucosal layer along the free margin of the vocal fold (40). The laryngeal arteries are branches of the superior and inferior thyroid arteries.

The intrinsic muscles of the larynx are innervated by the recurrent laryngeal nerve. The cricothyroid muscle, an intrinsic muscle responsible for tensing the vocal cords, is supplied by a branch of the superior laryngeal nerve; isolated damage to this nerve causes a bowing of the true vocal cord, which continues to be mobile, but the voice may become hoarse.

The supraglottic structures have a rich capillary lymphatic plexus; the trunks pass through the preepiglottic space and the thyrohyoid membrane and terminate mainly in the subdigastric lymph nodes; a few drain to the middle internal jugular chain lymph nodes.

There are essentially no capillary lymphatics of the true vocal cords; as a result, lymphatic spread from glottic cancer occurs only if tumor extends to supraglottic or subglottic areas.

The subglottic area has relatively few capillary lymphatics. The lymphatic trunks pass through the cricothyroid membrane to the pretracheal (Delphian) lymph nodes in the region of the thyroid isthmus. The subglottic area also drains posteriorly through the cricotracheal membrane, with some trunks going to the paratracheal lymph nodes and others continuing to the inferior jugular chain.

Epidemiology and Risk Factors

Cancer of the larynx represents about 2% of the total cancer risk and is the most common head and neck cancer (skin excluded). In 2003 in the United States, there were approximately 9500 new cases of cancer of the larynx (7100 men and 2400 women) and about 3800 deaths from laryngeal cancer (43). Based on 1973–1998 U.S. data, at diagnosis, about 51% of the cases remain localized, 29% have regional spread, and 15% have distant

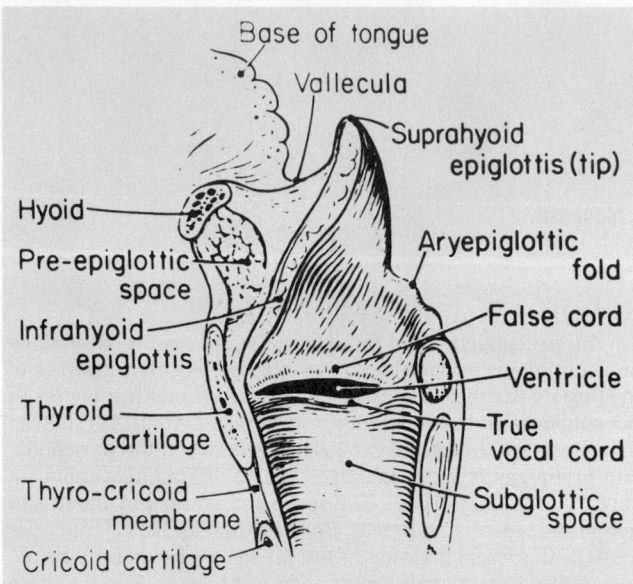

FIGURE 44.1. Diagrammatic sagittal section of the larynx. (Redrawn from Sabotta J. In: Clemente CD, ed. *Anatomy: A Regional Atlas of the Human Body.* Philadelphia: Lea & Febiger; 1975. Copyright 1975, Munich: Urban & Schwarzenberg.)

metastases (93). The ratio of glottic to supraglottic carcinoma is approximately 3:1.

Cancer of the larynx is strongly related to cigarette smoking. The risk of tobacco-related cancers of the upper alimentary and respiratory tracts declines among ex-smokers after 5 years and is said to approach the risk of nonsmokers after 10 years of abstention (120). The role of alcohol in provoking laryngeal cancer remains unclear (111). Some evidence exists that heavy marijuana smoking may be associated with laryngeal cancer in young patients.

Patterns of Spread

Local Spread

Although supraglottic and glottic lesions tend to remain confined to their original compartments, there is no anatomic barrier to growth from one area to the next. Glottic lesions tend to be slow-growing, but after they increase in size, they quickly extend to the supraglottic and subglottic areas. Supraglottic lesions do not often start near the vocal cords. Involvement of the cords on their external epithelial surface is a late phenomenon, but submucosal extension by way of the paraglottic space occurs earlier.

The fat space is an important avenue of submucosal tumor spread for infrahyoid epiglottis, false cord, and true vocal cord lesions. As the false cord and the true vocal cord lesions penetrate anteriorly and laterally, they quickly encounter the tough perichondrium of the thyroid cartilage and may eventually be shunted by the conus elasticus (lateral cricothyroid membrane) out of the larynx via the cricothyroid space. Thyroid cartilage invasion usually occurs in the ossified section of the cartilage, commonly in the region of the anterior commissure tendon or the junction of the anterior one-fourth and the posterior three-fourths of the thyroid lamina (5).

Fixation of the vocal cord from laryngeal cancer is usually caused by invasion or destruction of the vocal cord muscle, invasion of the cricoarytenoid muscle or joint, or, rarely, invasion of the recurrent laryngeal nerve. Perineural spread is uncommon in laryngeal malignancies.

Supraglottic Larynx

Suprahyoid Epiglottis

A lesion of the suprahyoid epiglottis may produce a huge exophytic mass with little tendency to destroy cartilage or spread

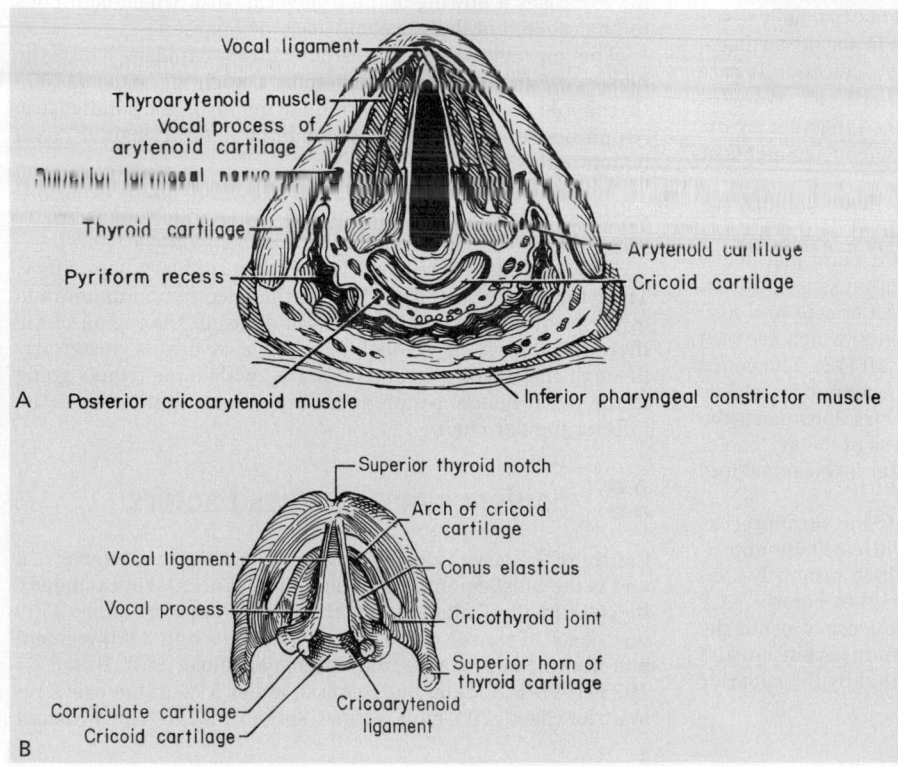

FIGURE 44.2. A: Cross-section of larynx at the level of the vocal cords. **B:** Framework of the larynx. (Redrawn from Sabotta J. In: Clemente CD, ed. *Anatomy: A Regional Atlas of the Human Body.* Philadelphia: Lea & Febiger; 1975. Copyright 1975, Munich: Urban & Schwarzenberg.)

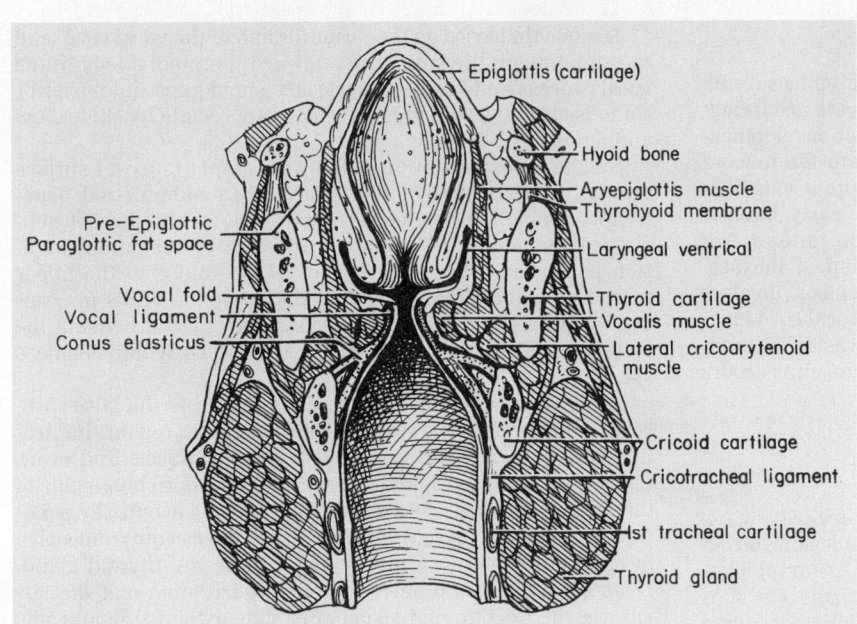

FIGURE 44.3. Diagram of the coronal view of the larynx. (Redrawn from Sabotta J. In: Clemente CD, ed. *Anatomy: A Regional Atlas of the Human Body.* Philadelphia: Lea & Febiger; 1975. Copyright 1975, Munich: Urban & Schwarzenberg.)

to adjacent structures. Other lesions may infiltrate the tip and destroy cartilage. The destructive lesions tend to invade the vallecula and preepiglottic space, the lateral pharyngeal walls, and the remainder of the supraglottic larynx.

Infrahyoid Epiglottis

Lesions of the infrahyoid epiglottis tend to produce irregular tumor nodules and simultaneously invade the porous epiglottic cartilage and thyroepiglottic ligament into the preepiglottic fat space and extend toward the vallecula and base of the tongue. The thick hyoepiglottic ligament is an effective tumor barrier. However, the tumor may present in the vallecula and base of tongue without involving the suprahyoid epiglottis.

Lesions of the infrahyoid epiglottis grow circumferentially to involve the false cords, aryepiglottic folds, medial wall of the pyriform sinus, and the pharyngoepiglottic fold. Invasion of the anterior commissure and cords and anterior subglottic extension usually occur only in advanced lesions. Infrahyoid epiglottic lesions that extend onto or below the vocal cords are at a high risk for thyroid cartilage invasion, even if the cords are mobile (91).

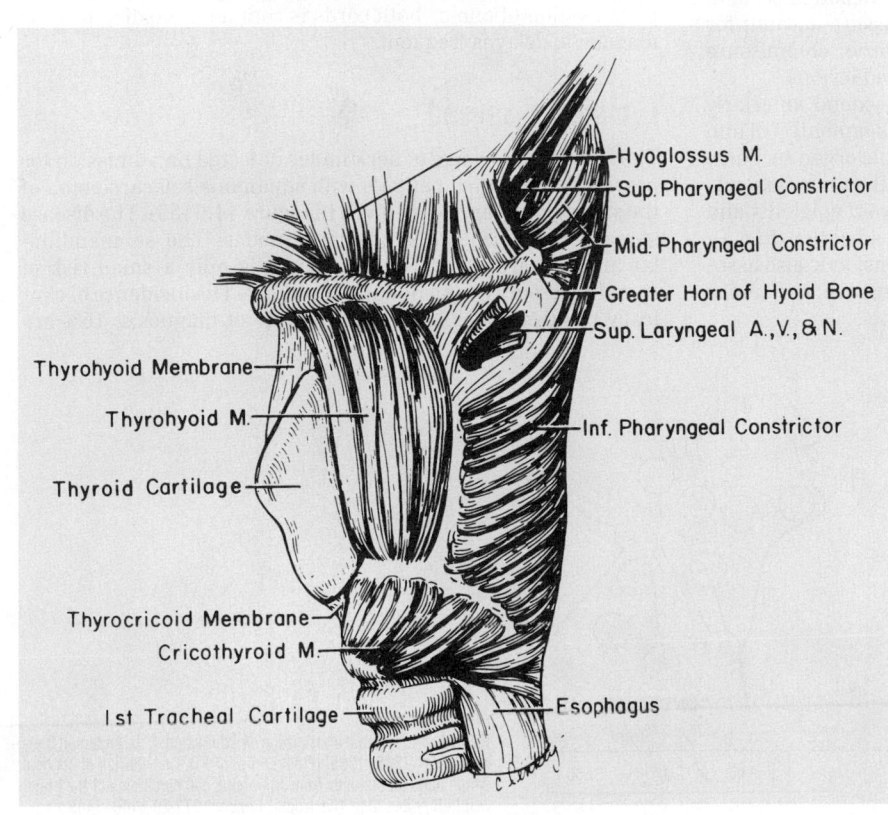

FIGURE 44.4. External view of the larynx. (Sabotta J. In: Clemente CD, ed: *Anatomy: A Regional Atlas of the Human Body.* Philadelphia: Lea & Febiger; 1975. Copyright 1975, Munich: Urban & Schwarzenberg.)

False Cord

Early false cord carcinomas, which are usually submucosal with little exophytic component, are difficult to delineate accurately. They involve the paraglottic fat space early in their development and may spread a considerable distance beneath the mucosa without producing physical signs. These carcinomas extend to the perichondrium of the thyroid cartilage quite early, but cartilage invasion is a late phenomenon. Extension to the lower portion of the infrahyoid epiglottis and invasion of the pre-epiglottic space are common. Submucosal extension involves the true vocal cord, which may appear normal. Vocal cord invasion is often associated with thyroid cartilage invasion. Submucosal extension to the medial wall of the pyriform sinus occurs early.

Aryepiglottic Fold/Arytenoid

Early lesions of the aryepiglottic fold/arytenoid are usually exophytic. It may be difficult to decide whether the lesion started on the medial wall of the pyriform sinus or on the aryepiglottic fold. As the lesions enlarge, they extend to adjacent sites and eventually cause fixation of the larynx, which is usually a result of involvement of the cricoarytenoid muscle or joint or, rarely, invasion of the recurrent laryngeal nerve. Computed tomography (CT) may distinguish the cause of fixation. Advanced lesions invade the thyroid, epiglottic, and cricoid cartilages and eventually invade the pyriform sinus and postcricoid area.

Glottic Larynx

Most lesions of the true vocal cord begin on the free margin and upper surface of the cord. When diagnosed, about two-thirds are confined to the cords, usually one cord. The anterior portion of the cord is the most common site. Anterior commissure involvement, which is common, is said to occur when no tumor-free cord can be seen anteriorly; if the lesion crosses to the opposite cord, anterior commissure invasion is certain. Small lesions isolated to the anterior commissure account for only 1% to 2% of cases. Extension to the posterior commissure area is uncommon, occurring only in advanced lesions.

Tumors at the anterior commissure may extend anteriorly via the anterior commissure tendon (Broyles' ligament) (10) into the thyroid cartilage. Kirchner (46), using whole organ sections, showed that such extension is unusual unless the tumor extends off the vocal cord onto the base of the infrahyoid epiglottis and suggested that the tendon serves as more of a barrier than an avenue of tumor spread. Early subglottic extension is also associated with involvement of the anterior commissure, and tumor may grow through the cricothyroid membrane.

Lesions that arise on the posterior half of the vocal cord tend to extend along the submucosa toward the medial side of the vocal process and invade the cricoarytenoid joint and posterior commissure; this spread is difficult to appreciate by clinical examination.

Subglottic extension may occur by simple mucosal surface growth, but it more commonly occurs by submucosal penetration beneath the conus elasticus. One centimeter of subglottic extension anteriorly or 4 to 5 mm of subglottic extension posteriorly brings the border of the tumor to the upper margin of the cricoid, exceeding the anatomic limits for conventional hemilaryngectomy. Lesions may spread beneath the epithelium along the length of the vocal cord within Reinke's space (84).

As vocal cord lesions enlarge, they extend to the false cord, vocal process of the arytenoid, and subglottic region. Infiltrative lesions invade the vocal ligament and muscle and eventually reach the paraglottic space and the perichondrium of the thyroid cartilage. Advanced glottic lesions eventually penetrate through the thyroid cartilage or via the cricothyroid space to enter the neck, where they may invade the thyroid gland. Lesions involving the anterior commissure often exit the larynx via the cricothyroid space after they extend subglottically (84).

A fixed cord that is associated with a lesion having less than 1 cm of subglottic extension and no false cord involvement does not ordinarily indicate invasion of the thyroid cartilage (46). If the false cord is also involved, cartilage invasion is likely.

Subglottic Larynx

Subglottic cancers are rare. Most involve the inferior surface of the vocal cords by the time they are diagnosed, so it is difficult to know whether the tumor started on the undersurface of the vocal cord or in the true subglottic larynx. Because early diagnosis is uncommon, most lesions are bilateral or circumferential at discovery. They involve the cricoid cartilages in the early stage because there is no intervening muscle layer. Partial or complete fixation of one or both cords is common; misdiagnosis or diagnostic delay is frequent.

Lymphatic Spread

The location and stage of neck nodes detected on admission for previously untreated patients with squamous cell carcinoma of the supraglottic larynx are given in Figure 44.5 (55). The disease spreads mainly to the subdigastric nodes. The submandibular area is rarely involved, and there is only a small risk of spinal accessory lymph node involvement. The incidence of clinically positive nodes is 55% at the time of diagnosis; 16% are

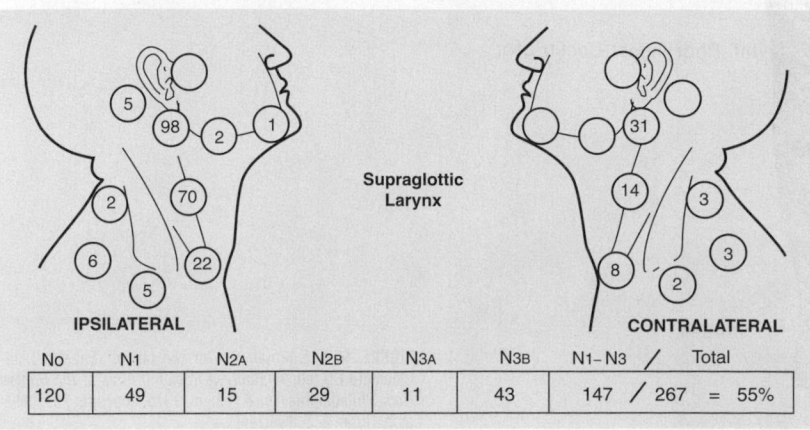

No	N1	N2A	N2B	N3A	N3B	N1–N3 /	Total
120	49	15	29	11	43	147 /	267 = 55%

FIGURE 44.5. Nodal distribution on admission, M.D. Anderson Cancer Center, 1948–1965. (From Lindberg RD. Distribution of cervical lymph node metastases from squamous cell carcinoma of the upper respiratory and digestive tracts. *Cancer* 1972;29:1446–1449.)

bilateral (55). Elective neck dissection shows pathologically positive nodes in 16% of cases; observation of initially node-negative necks eventually identifies the appearance of positive nodes in 33% of cases (18,81). Spread to the pyriform sinus, vallecula, and base of the tongue increases the risk of lymph node metastases. The risk of late-appearing contralateral lymph node metastasis is 37% if the ipsilateral neck is pathologically positive, but the risk is unrelated to whether the nodes in the ipsilateral neck were palpable before neck dissection.

In carcinoma of the vocal cord, the incidence of clinically positive lymph nodes at diagnosis approaches zero for T1 lesions and less than 2% for T2 lesions (66). The incidence of neck metastases increases to 20% to 30% for T3 and T4 lesions. Supraglottic spread is associated with metastasis to the jugulodigastric nodes. Anterior commissure and anterior subglottic invasion are associated with involvement of the midline pretracheal lymph node (Delphian node).

Lederman (52) reported a 10% incidence of positive lymph nodes in 73 patients with subglottic carcinoma.

Clinical Presentation

Carcinoma arising on the true vocal cords produces hoarseness at a very early stage. Sore throat, ear pain, pain localized to the thyroid cartilage, and airway obstruction are features of advanced lesions.

Hoarseness is not a prominent symptom of cancer of the supraglottic larynx until the lesion becomes quite extensive. Pain on swallowing, usually mild, is the most frequent initial symptom, often described as a sore throat. Some patients report a sensation of a "lump in the throat." Pain is referred to the ear by way of the vagus nerve and auricular nerve of Arnold. A mass in the neck may be the first sign of a supraglottic cancer. Late symptoms include weight loss, foul breath, dysphagia, and aspiration.

Diagnostic Work-Up

Physical Examination

Flexible fiberoptic endoscopes are now used routinely as a complement to the laryngeal mirror examination. The mirror often provides the best view of the posterior pharyngeal wall. The flexible fiberoptic laryngoscope is inserted through the nose and is useful in more difficult cases.

Determination of the mobility of the vocal cords frequently requires multiple examinations because the subtle distinctions between mobile, partially fixed, and fixed cords are often challenging, apparently changing from examination to examination. A cord that appeared mobile to the surgeon before direct laryngoscopy may exhibit impaired motion or even fixation after biopsy.

Ulceration of the infrahyoid epiglottis or fullness of the vallecula is an indirect sign of preepiglottic space invasion. Palpation of diffuse, firm fullness above the thyroid notch with widening of the space between the hyoid and the thyroid cartilages signifies invasion of the preepiglottic space. The preepiglottic fat space is a low-density area on the CT scan, and changes resulting from tumor invasion are easily seen.

Postcricoid extension may be suspected when the laryngeal click disappears on physical examination. Postcricoid tumor may cause the thyroid cartilage to protrude anteriorly, producing a fullness of the neck.

Invasion of the thyroid cartilage remains a difficult clinical diagnosis. Localized pain or tenderness to palpation or a small bulge over one ala of the thyroid cartilage is suggestive.

Radiographic Studies

CT scan with contrast enhancement is the method of choice for studying the larynx (Fig. 44.6) (72). The CT scan should be performed before biopsy so that abnormalities that may be caused by the biopsy are not confused with tumor. CT is preferred to magnetic resonance imaging (MRI) because the longer scanning time for MRI results in motion artifact (73). CT slices 1 to 2-mm thick are obtained at 1– to 2-mm intervals through the larynx and at 3-mm intervals for the remainder of the study. Thinner sections (1 to 2 mm through the larynx) facilitate high-quality multiplanar reformations. The gantry is angled so that the scan slices are parallel to the plane of the true vocal cords. It is also necessary to obtain a CT scan of the entire neck to detect positive, nonpalpable lymph nodes. Positive retropharyngeal nodes may be present at diagnosis in patients with laryngeal cancer who have advanced neck disease (59). Retropharyngeal adenopathy is often not apparent on physical examination but is usually appreciated on CT scan.

Contrast enhancement helps to outline the blood vessels and thyroid gland. Tumor is often enhanced, probably because of reactive inflammatory changes. In addition to CT, MRI may be obtained to define subtle exolaryngeal spread or early cartilage destruction. The value of MRI for detecting early cartilage destruction is open to speculation. Sagittal MRI may be useful in detecting early invasion of the base of the tongue.

Vocal Cord Carcinoma

Although the CT scan does not show minimal mucosal lesions and is generally not helpful for well-defined, easily visualized T1 or early T2 vocal cord carcinomas, it is almost always obtained. CT is excellent for determining subglottic extension and is often used in selected T1 and most T2 lesions for this reason alone. CT scanning is useful in the diagnosis of moderately advanced and advanced lesions; it is excellent for demonstrating extension outside the larynx into the soft tissues of the neck and has potential for determining thyroid or cricoid cartilage invasion, which tends to occur at the edges of the cartilage rather than on the face. Early cartilage involvement is difficult to detect with axial scans, but it may be demonstrated by coronal or sagittal scanning techniques. If the low-density plane of the paraglottic space is intact, cartilage is probably not invaded by tumor.

Archer et al. (6) correlated CT findings with the incidence of cartilage or bone invasion on whole-organ sections. For 12 of 14 patients with pathologic evidence of cartilage invasion, the average diameter of the tumor in two dimensions was more than 16 mm, and the lesion was located below the top of the arytenoid. Lesions in which the maximum diameter lay above the top of the arytenoid had a low incidence of cartilage invasion (6).

Supraglottic Carcinoma

The CT scan provides an excellent means for viewing the preepiglottic and paraglottic fat spaces. Soft tissue extension into the neck or base of the tongue can also be seen. The CT scan is also useful for determining extension to the subglottic areas (57).

Diagnostic procedures for laryngeal cancer at the University of Florida are summarized in Table 44.1 (65). A CT scan is usually performed for all patients; MRI is obtained in a small subset of patients with questionable findings on CT. Positron emission tomography is not routinely obtained. Direct laryngoscopy and biopsy with frozen section are usually performed with the patient under general anesthesia. The ventricles, subglottic area, apex of the pyriform sinus, and postcricoid area must be carefully examined because these areas are not consistently seen by

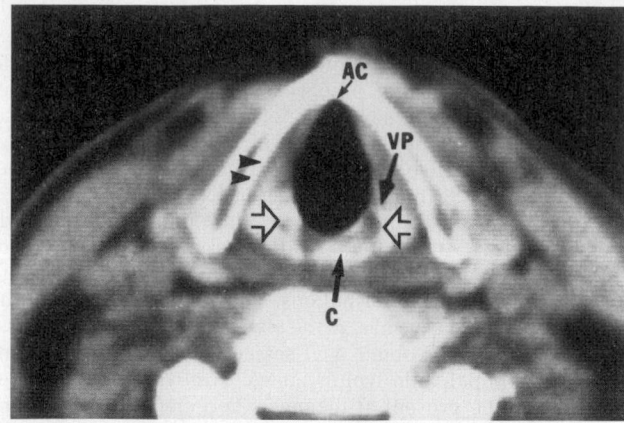

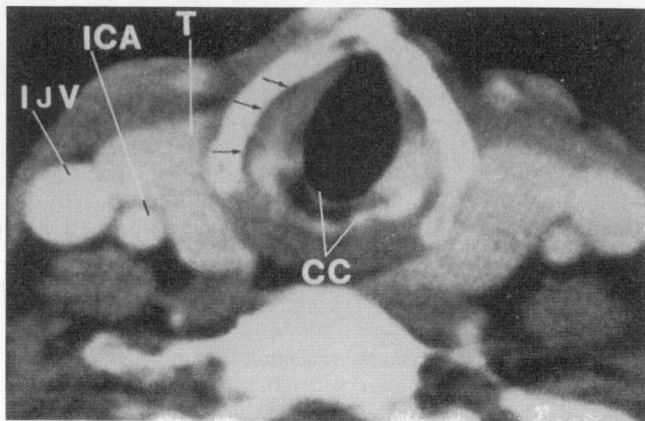

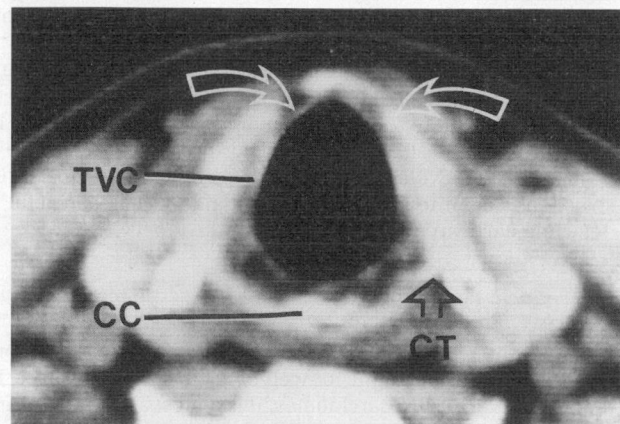

FIGURE 44.6. A: Normal computed tomography (CT) anatomy of the midplane of the true vocal cords. *Open arrows* indicate arytenoid cartilages. The top of the cricoid cartilage (C) is partially visualized at this level. The vocal process (VP) of the left arytenoid cartilage is demonstrated. A narrow, low-density plane is seen between the right true vocal cord and the thyroid lamina (*arrowheads*); this is the inferior part of the paraglottic fat space. Notice the complete lack of tissue at the anterior commissure (AC). *Any tissue density here should be considered abnormal.* **B:** Normal CT anatomy just below the midplane of the vocal cords. *Arrows* indicate low-density lower paraglottic fat space. The fibrofatty tissue in this space facilitates separation of the vocal cord and the adjacent thyroid lamina. If this clear space is maintained in the face of the thyroid lamina irregularity adjacent to the tumor, the lamina abnormality can be attributed to uneven calcification rather than tumor destruction. The posterior portion (lamina) of the cricoid cartilage (CC) is seen. The outer and inner cortex of the cartilage is calcified; an intervening marrow space has lower density. The vertical height of the lamina is 2 to 3 cm. There is incomplete calcification of the thyroid cartilage anteriorly. IJV, internal jugular vein; ICA, internal carotid artery; T, thyroid gland. **C:** Normal CT anatomy 5 mm below the free margin of the true vocal cord (TVC). The vocal cord appears thin because of abduction during scanning. There is incomplete bilateral paramedian calcification and thinning of the thyroid lamina (arrows). Notice the normal lack of tissue density between the airway and the anterior arch of the thyroid cartilage. CC, cricoid cartilage; CT, cricothyroid joint. (From Million RR, Cassisi NJ. Larynx. In Million RR, Cassisi NJ, eds. *Management of Head and Neck Cancer: A Multidisciplinary Approach.* Philadelphia: JB Lippincott; 1984:315–364.)

Table 44.1 DIAGNOSTIC WORK-UP FOR CARCINOMA OF THE LARYNX

General
  History
  Physical examination
  Indirect laryngoscopy
  Direct laryngoscopy
  Biopsies
Radiographic studies
  Chest x-ray films
  Computed tomography with contrast enhancement (before biopsy)
  Magnetic resonance imaging (selected cases)

From Mendenhall WM, Parsons JT, Mancuso AA, et al. In: Perez CA, Brady LW, eds. *Principles and Practice of Radiation Oncology,* 4th ed. Philadelphia: Lippincott-Raven: 1998.

indirect examinations. Fiberoptic telescopes (0 and 30 degrees) are introduced through the laryngoscope for inspection of these areas. A generous biopsy specimen is taken from the obvious lesion; additional biopsy specimens may be obtained from suspicious areas and from areas grossly involved. The mucosa of the margin of the cord may be stripped to provide adequate tissue if the lesion is distributed superficially along the cord and is not obviously a carcinoma.

Staging

The 2002 American Joint Committee on Cancer (AJCC) (3) staging system for laryngeal primary cancer is listed in Table 44.2. T2 glottic cancers are stratified into those with normal (T2A) and impaired (T2B) vocal cord mobility. For lesions arising in the supraglottis, the sites of origin include false cords, aryepiglottic folds, suprahyoid epiglottis, infrahyoid epiglottis, pharyngoepiglottic folds, and arytenoids. Only in the early T-stages can one identify the specific site of origin with certainty. As the lesion enlarges, the site of origin is an educated guess

Table 44.2 | STAGING OF LARYNGEAL CANCER

Supraglottis

T1	Tumor limited to one subsite of supraglottis with normal vocal cord mobility
T2	Tumor invades mucosa of more than one adjacent subsite of supraglottis or glottis or region outside the supraglottis (e.g., mucosa of base of tongue, vallecula, medial wall of pyriform sinus) without fixation of the larynx
T3	Tumor limited to larynx with vocal cord fixation and/or invades any of the following: Postcricoid area, preepiglottic tissues, paraglottic space, and/or minor thyroid erosion (e.g., inner cortex)
T4a	Tumor invades through the thyroid cartilage and/or invades beyond the larynx (e.g., trachea, soft tissues of neck including deep extrinsic muscles of the tongue, strap muscles, thyroid, or esophagus)
T4b	Tumor invades prevertebral space, encases carotid artery, or invades mediastinal structures

Glottis

T1	Tumor limited to vocal cord(s) (may involve anterior or posterior commissure) with normal mobility
T1a	Tumor limited to one vocal cord
T1b	Tumor involves both vocal cords
T2	Tumor extends to supraglottis and/or subglottis, and/or with impaired vocal cord mobility
T3	Tumor limited to the larynx with vocal cord fixation and/or invades paraglottic space, and/or minor thyroid cartilage erosion (e.g., inner cortex)
T4a	Tumor invades through the thyroid cartilage and/or invades tissues beyond the larynx (trachea, soft tissues of neck including deep extrinsic muscles of the tongue, strap muscles, thyroid, or esophagus)
T4b	Tumor invades prevertebral space, encases carotid artery, or invades mediastinal structures

Modified from American Joint Committee on Cancer. *Manual for Staging of Cancer*, 6th ed. New York: Springer-Verlag; 2002:47–57.

based on the location of the greatest bulk of tumor. The major difference between the 1998 and 2002 staging systems is that a glottic cancer that invades the paraglottic space is upstaged to T3 in the latter system, even with mobile vocal cords, resulting in significant stage migration. Additionally, T4 has been stratified into T4A and T4B, based on resectability.

Pathologic Classification

Nearly all malignant tumors of the larynx arise from the surface epithelium and therefore are squamous cell carcinoma or one of its variants.

Carcinoma *in situ* occurs frequently on the vocal cords. Differentiating among dysplasia, carcinoma *in situ*, squamous cell carcinoma with microinvasion, and true invasive carcinoma is a problem that the pathologist and the clinician frequently confront.

Most vocal cord carcinomas are well or moderately well differentiated. In a few cases, an apparent carcinoma and sarcoma occur together, but most of these are actually a spindle-cell carcinoma (i.e., squamous cell carcinoma with a spindle-cell stromal reaction).

Verrucous carcinoma occurs in 1% to 2% of patients with carcinoma of the vocal cord. The histologic diagnosis is difficult and must correlate with the gross appearance of the lesion.

Small cell neuroendocrine carcinoma is rarely diagnosed in the supraglottic larynx, but it should be recognized because of its biologic potential for rapid growth, early dissemination, and responsiveness to chemotherapy.

Minor salivary gland tumors arise from the mucous glands in the supraglottic and subglottic larynx, but they are rare (31).

Even rarer are chemodectoma, carcinoid, soft tissue sarcoma, malignant lymphoma, or plasmacytoma. Benign chondromas and osteochondromas are reported, but their malignant counterparts are rare.

Prognostic Factors

The extent of the primary lesion and neck disease are the major determinants of prognosis. The likelihood of local control is determined primarily by T-stage; there are conflicting data pertaining to a possible inverse relationship between N-stage

and local control. The likelihood of locoregional control is impacted primarily by the overall AJCC stage, which accounts for both T- and N-stages. AJCC stage and N-stage are the major determinants of cause-specific survival. Additionally, within each N-stage, patients with positive nodes in the low neck below the level of the thyroid notch tend to have a lower cause-specific survival rate compared with those with disease confined to the upper neck. In general, women tend to have a better prognosis than men.

Treatment Selection and Technique: Vocal Cord Carcinoma

Selection of Treatment Modality

In treating vocal cord carcinoma, the goal is cure with the best functional result and the least risk of a serious complication. Patients may be considered to be in an early group if the chance of cure with larynx preservation is high, they are in a moderately advanced group if the likelihood of local control is 60% to 70% but the chance of cure is still good, and they are in an advanced group if the chance of cure is moderate and the likelihood of laryngeal preservation is relatively low. The early group may be treated initially by radiation therapy or, in selected cases, by partial laryngectomy. The moderately advanced group may be treated with either irradiation with laryngectomy reserved for relapse or by total laryngectomy with or without adjuvant postoperative irradiation. The obvious advantage of the former strategy, which we use at the University of Florida, is that there is a fairly good chance that the larynx will be preserved. Although some patients may be rehabilitated with a tracheoesophageal puncture after laryngectomy, only about 20% of patients use this device long term and the majority use an electric larynx (62). The advanced group is treated with total laryngectomy and neck dissection with or without adjuvant radiation therapy or by radiation therapy and adjuvant chemotherapy (68). Data suggest that if patients whose tumors show a partial or complete response to two to three cycles of neoadjuvant chemotherapy are then given high-dose radiation therapy, the cure rates are comparable with those obtained with initial total laryngectomy (16). Another less expensive and less toxic method to select patients likely to be cured by radiation therapy alone is to calculate the primary tumor volume on pretreatment CT or MRI. Data indicate that primary tumor volume is inversely related to the probability of local control after irradiation (61,64). Recent data indicate that whereas induction chemotherapy probably does not improve the likelihood of locoregional control and survival, concomitant chemotherapy and irradiation results in an improved possibility of cure compared with irradiation alone (23,68,90). There is a subset of patients with high volume, unfavorable, advanced cancers who may be cured by chemoradiation but have a useless larynx and permanent tracheostomy and/or gastrostomy (61). These patients are best treated with a total laryngectomy, neck dissection, and postoperative irradiation.

Carcinoma *in Situ*

Lesions diagnosed as carcinoma *in situ* may sometimes be controlled by stripping the cord. However, it is difficult to exclude the possibility of microinvasion on these specimens. Recurrence is frequent, and the cord may become thickened and the voice hoarse with repeated stripping. Localized carcinoma *in situ* can also be excised using the CO_2 laser.

Early radiation therapy for carcinoma *in situ* often means a better chance of preserving a good voice, especially as many patients with this diagnosis eventually receive this treatment (28).

Many patients with a diagnosis of carcinoma *in situ* have obvious lesions that probably contain invasive carcinoma. We have often proceeded with radiation therapy rather than put the patient through a repeated biopsy procedure.

Early Vocal Cord Carcinoma

In most centers, irradiation is the initial treatment prescribed for T1 and T2 lesions, with surgery reserved for salvage after radiation therapy failure (60,71). Although hemilaryngectomy or cordectomy produces comparable cure rates for selected T1 and T2 vocal cord lesions, irradiation is generally preferred (71,79). Supracricoid laryngectomy, as reported by Laccourreye et al. (47) is a procedure designed to remove moderate-sized cancers involving the supraglottic and glottic larynx. The larynx may be removed with preservation of the cricoid and the arytenoid with its neurovascular innervation, the defect is closed by approximating the base of the tongue to the remaining larynx. The oncologic and functional results of this procedure in selected patients are reported to be excellent. Transoral laser excision also may provide high cure rates for select patients with small, well-defined lesions limited to the midthird of one true cord (58,103). A small subset of transoral laser surgeons, notably Professor Steiner, use this technique successfully in moderately advanced cancers (71). The major advantage of irradiation compared with partial laryngectomy is better quality of the voice. Partial laryngectomy finds its major use as salvage surgery in suitable cases after irradiation failure. Even if the patient has a local recurrence after salvage partial laryngectomy, there is a third chance with total laryngectomy, which may still be successful.

Verrucous lesions have the reputation of being unresponsive to radiation therapy and, in some instances, converting into invasive, often anaplastic, metastasizing lesions. Partial laryngectomy is recommended for early verrucous carcinoma of the glottis, but irradiation is recommended if the alternative is total laryngectomy. We have observed typical verrucous lesions that have disappeared with radiation therapy and not recurred. O'Sullivan et al. (80) also have made this observation. Additionally, a variety of tumors that recur after unsuccessful treatment (with surgery, radiation therapy, and/or chemotherapy) are more likely to exhibit more aggressive behavior.

Moderately Advanced Vocal Cord Cancer

Fixed-cord lesions (T3) may be subdivided into relatively favorable or unfavorable lesions. Patients with unfavorable lesions usually have extensive bilateral disease with a compromised airway and are considered to be in the advanced group. Patients with favorable T3 lesions have disease confined mostly to one side of the larynx, have a good airway, and are reliable for follow-up. Some degree of supraglottic and subglottic extension usually exists. The extent of disease and tumor volume, in particular, are related to the likelihood of control after radiation therapy (61).

The patient with a favorable lesion is advised of the alternatives of irradiation with surgical salvage or immediate total laryngectomy. Recent data suggest that the likelihood of locoregional control is better after some altered fractionation schedules compared with conventional once-daily radiation therapy (24,68). Follow-up examinations are recommended every 4 to 6 weeks for the first year, every 6 to 8 weeks for the second year, every 3 months for the third year, every 6 months for the fourth and fifth years, and annually thereafter. The patient must understand that total laryngectomy may be recommended purely on clinical grounds without biopsy-proven recurrence and that the risk of laryngeal osteochondronecrosis is about 5%.

Evaluation of cord mobility after 50.4 Gy or at the end of radiation therapy has not been helpful in predicting local control (64). Some patients in whom the vocal cord remained fixed have had local tumor control of the disease for 2 years or longer after radiation therapy.

The major difficulty in using irradiation for the more advanced lesions is distinguishing radiation edema from local recurrence during follow-up examinations (87). Progressive laryngeal edema, persistent throat pain, or fixation of a previously mobile vocal cord frequently signifies recurrent disease in the larynx, although a few patients with these findings remain disease-free with long-term follow-up.

Extended hemilaryngectomy has been used by a few surgeons in the treatment of well-lateralized fixed-cord lesions. A permanent tracheostomy is usually required because a portion of the cricoid is resected, but a useful voice may be retained (88).

Advanced Vocal Cord Carcinoma

Advanced lesions usually show extensive subglottic and supraglottic extension, bilateral glottic involvement, and invasion of the thyroid, cricoid, or arytenoid cartilage, or frequently all three (5,6). The airway is compromised, necessitating a tracheostomy at the time of direct laryngoscopy in approximately 30% of patients. Clinically positive lymph nodes are found in about 25% to 30% of patients.

The mainstay of treatment is total laryngectomy, with or without adjuvant radiation therapy. The most frequent sites of local failure after total laryngectomy are around the tracheal stoma, in the base of tongue, and in the neck lymph nodes or soft tissues of the neck. If the neck has clinically negative findings before surgery and if postoperative irradiation is planned, neck dissection may be withheld, and radiation therapy may be used to treat both sides of the neck. However, in practice, most surgeons prefer to perform elective bilateral selective (levels II-IV) neck dissections in conjunction with a total laryngectomy for T3N0 or T4N0 laryngeal cancer, even if postoperative irradiation is planned. If the lymph nodes are clinically positive, a therapeutic neck dissection is performed at the time of laryngectomy.

The indications for postoperative radiation therapy include close or positive margins, significant subglottic extension (1 cm or more), cartilage invasion, perineural invasion, endothelial-lined space invasion, extension of the primary tumor into the soft tissues of the neck, multiple positive neck nodes, extracapsular extension, and control of subclinical disease in the opposite neck (2,41). Preoperative irradiation is indicated for patients who have fixed neck nodes, have had an emergency tracheotomy through tumor, or have direct extension of tumor involving the skin.

Definitive irradiation is prescribed for the patient who refuses total laryngectomy or is medically unsuitable for major surgery.

As previously stated, there is evidence that two to three cycles of neoadjuvant chemotherapy followed by radiation therapy in patients obtaining at least a partial response may provide a moderate likelihood of larynx preservation without compromising cure (16). Recent data suggest that concomitant chemotherapy and irradiation is more efficacious than irradiation alone or induction chemotherapy followed by radiation therapy (23,90). The optimal combination of concomitant chemotherapy and irradiation is unclear (68).

A randomized intergroup trial (Radiation Therapy Oncology Group 91–11) compared three treatment arms: Arm A, three cycles of induction cisplatin and fluorouracil followed by irradiation in complete and partial responders; Arm B, radiation therapy and concomitant cisplatin (100 mg/m^2 on days 1, 22, and 43 of radiation therapy); and Arm C, once-daily irradiation (70 Gy in 35 fractions during 7 weeks) alone (23). Five hundred forty-seven patients were randomized and followed for a median of 3.8 years; 518 patients were evaluable. The rates of larynx preservation were: Arm A, 72%; Arm B, 84%; and Arm C, 67%. The rates of larynx presentation were significantly improved for Arm B; there was no significant difference between Arm A and Arm C. The 5-year survival rates were similar for the three treatment groups: Arm A, 55%; Arm B, 54%; and Arm C, 56%. The likelihood of developing distant metastases was lower for the two groups of patients that received adjuvant chemotherapy.

Surgical Treatment

Cordectomy is an excision of the vocal cord and may be performed by the transoral approach usually with a laser or externally by a thyrotomy. Its use is usually confined to small lesions of the middle third of the cord. After cordectomy, a pseudocord is formed, and the patient has a useful, if somewhat harsh, voice.

Vertical partial laryngectomy (i.e., hemilaryngectomy) allows removal of limited cord lesions with preservation of voice. One entire cord with as much as a third of the opposite cord with the adjacent thyroid cartilage is the maximum cordal involvement suitable for surgery in men; women have a smaller larynx, and usually only one vocal cord may be removed without compromising the airway. Partial fixation of one cord is not a contraindication to hemilaryngectomy, but only a few surgeons have attempted hemilaryngectomy for selected fixed-cord lesions. The maximum subglottic extension suitable for hemilaryngectomy is 8 to 9 mm anteriorly and 5 mm posteriorly; this limit is necessary to preserve the integrity of the cricoid. Tumor extension to the epiglottis, false cord, or both arytenoids is a contraindication to hemilaryngectomy.

Supracricoid partial laryngectomy is used for selected T2 and T3 glottic carcinomas and entails removal of both true and false cords as well as the entire thyroid cartilage. The cricoid is sutured to the epiglottis and hyoid (cricohyoidopexy).

Total laryngectomy with or without neck dissection is the operation of choice for advanced lesions and as a salvage procedure for radiation therapy failures in lesions that are not suited for conservation surgery. The entire larynx is removed, and the pharynx is reconstructed. A permanent tracheostomy

is required. Speech may be reconstituted with a prosthesis or with an electrolarynx. One hundred four (63%) of 166 patients entered into the surgery and postoperative irradiation arm of the Veterans Affairs Laryngeal Cancer Study Group randomized trial were evaluable for communication status at 2 years after treatment (38). Ninety-six patients had undergone a total laryngectomy and communicated as follows: Tracheoesophageal, 27 (28%); esophageal, 5 (5%); artificial larynx, 47 (50%); nonvocal, 7 (7%); and no data, 10 (10%) (38). One hundred seventy-three patients underwent total laryngectomy and postoperative radiotherapy at the University of Florida and 69 patients were evaluable for 5 years or longer (62). Voice rehabilitation was accomplished as follows: Tracheoesophageal, 19%; artificial larynx, 57%; esophageal, 3%; nonvocal, 14%; and no data, 7%.

Radiation Therapy Technique

Irradiation for T1 or T2 vocal cord cancer is delivered by small portals covering only the primary lesion. The cervical lymph node chain is not electively treated. For T1 lesions, radiation therapy portals extend from the thyroid notch superiorly to the inferior border of the cricoid and fall off anteriorly. The posterior border depends on the posterior extension of the tumor (73). For T2 tumors, the field is extended depending on the anatomic distribution of the tumor. The field size ranges from 4 × 4 cm to 5 × 5 cm (plus an additional 1 cm of "flash" anteriorly) and is occasionally 6 × 6 cm for a large T2 lesion. Portals larger than this increase the risk of edema without improving the cure rate.

A commonly used dose-fractionation schedule at many institutions is 66 Gy for T1 lesions and 70 Gy for T2 cancers given in 2-Gy fractions. Evidence suggests that increasing the dose per fraction may improve the likelihood of local control (4,19,36,37,45,69,97,119). Ample data suggest that 1.8 Gy once daily results in significantly lower local control rates compared with 2 Gy once daily (45). Yamakazi et al. (121) recently reported a prospective trial in which patients with T1N0 squamous cell carcinoma of the glottic larynx were randomized to definitive radiotherapy at 2 Gy per fraction or 2.25 Gy per fraction. The 5-year local control rates were 77% after 2 Gy per fraction and 92% after 2.25 Gy per fraction ($p = .004$); there was no difference in either acute or late toxicity. Patients with T1 or T2 vocal cord cancer who are treated with once-a-day fractionation at the University of Florida are irradiated with 2.25 Gy per fraction; the dose-fractionation schemes used are shown as follows: Tis–T2 A, 63 Gy in 28 fractions; and T2B, 65.25 Gy in 29 fractions.

At the University of Florida, patients are treated in the supine position; the field borders for a patient with a T1N0 cancer are depicted in Fig. 44.7 (73). The field is checked by the physician at the treatment machine according to palpable anatomic landmarks. This allows the treatment volume to be kept at a minimum and reduces the risk of geographic miss. A three-field technique, using 4-or 6-MV x-rays, is used to deliver approximately 95% of the dose through opposed lateral wedged fields weighted to the side of the lesion; the remaining dose is delivered by an anterior field shifted 0.5 cm toward the side of the lesion (Fig. 44.8) (73). The tumor dose is usually specified at the 95% normalized isodose line.

Irradiation of T3 and T4 lesions requires larger portals, which include the jugulodigastric and middle jugular lymph nodes (Fig. 44.9) (74,85). The inferior jugular lymph nodes are included in a separate low-neck portal. Patients treated at the University of Florida are irradiated in a continuous-course twice daily at 1.2 Gy per fraction to a total dose of 74.4 Gy. The portals are reduced after 45.6 Gy in 38 fractions; the reduced portals cover only the primary lesion.

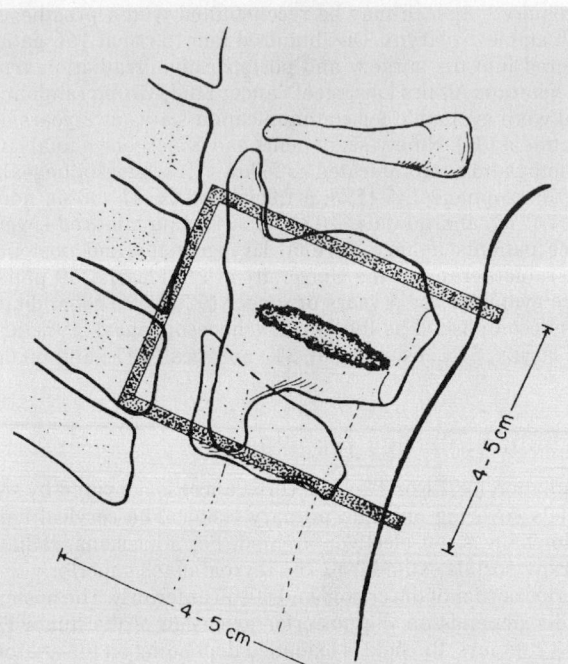

FIGURE 44.7. Treatment portal for early glottic carcinoma. The top border is adjusted according to the lesion. The middle of the thyroid notch is the landmark for very early lesions, and the top of the notch is the marker for larger lesions or those with minimal supraglottic extension. The posterior border is 1 cm posterior to the back edge of the thyroid cartilage if the lesion is confined to the anterior two thirds of the vocal cord; if the posterior one third of the vocal cord is involved, the posterior border is placed 1 to 1.5 cm behind the cartilage. The inferior border is placed at the bottom of the cricoid cartilage if there is no subglottic extension. (From Million RR, Cassisi NJ, Mancuso AA. Larynx. In: Million RR, Cassisi NJ, eds. *Management of head and neck cancer: A multidisciplinary approach,* 2nd ed. Philadelphia: JB Lippincott; 1994:431–497. Copyright 1988 by Elsevier Science, Inc.)

Intensity-modulated radiation therapy (IMRT) is employed if there is a clear advantage associated with this technique. Disadvantages associated with IMRT include increased dose inhomogeneity, increased total body dose, and increased labor and expense. The most common indications for IMRT for laryngeal cancers are the occasional patients with a node-positive T3–T4 cancer in which the retropharyngeal nodes are electively

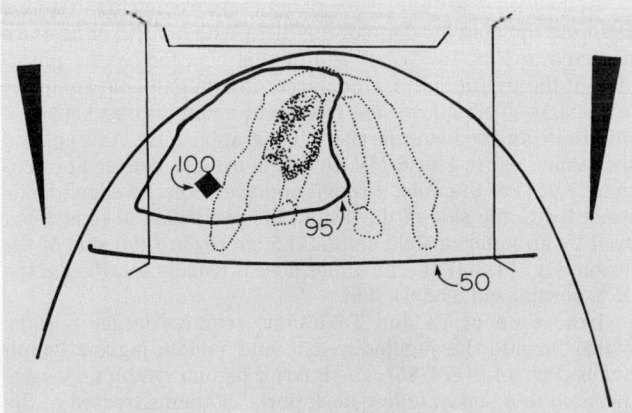

FIGURE 44.8. Normalized isodose distribution for three-field technique for treatment of a tumor involving the anterior two thirds of one true vocal cord. The dose is specified at the 95% isodose line. (From Million RR, Cassisi NJ, Mancuso AA. Larynx. In: Million RR, Cassisi NJ, eds. *Management of head and neck cancer: A multidisciplinary approach,* 2nd ed. Philadelphia: JB Lippincott; 1994:431–503.)

irradiated and the dose to the contralateral parotid gland reduced and/or a difficult low match between the lateral fields used to treat the primary site and upper neck and the anterior low neck field in a patient with a short neck and large shoulders. In the latter instance, IMRT could be used to encompass the entire target volume and avoid the problem of field junctioning entirely. IMRT is especially useful for patients with extensive subglottic invasion where achieving an adequate inferior margin with conventional lateral portals may not be possible.

Evidence from both retrospective and randomized trials points to improved therapeutic ratios with altered fractionation schedules (68). Given that irradiation is effective treatment for head and neck primary squamous cell carcinoma, it should not be surprising that higher doses of irradiation given more intensively would be more effective at providing tumor control. Because most observers have noted no increase in late toxicity with the various regimens, it generally is concluded that these schedules yield an improved therapeutic ratio. A recently updated Radiation Therapy Oncology Group 90–03 trial (24,109) reported on 1,073 patients who were randomly selected to receive one of four fractionation schedules:

a. Standard fractionation: 2 Gy per fraction, once a day, 5 days a week, to a total dose of 70 Gy in 35 fractions during 7 weeks;

b. Hyperfractionation: 1.2 Gy per fraction, twice daily ($\geq$6 hours apart), 5 days a week, to a total dose of 81.6 Gy in 68 fractions during 7 weeks;

c. Accelerated fractionation with split: 1.6 Gy per fraction, twice daily ($\geq$6 hours apart), 5 days a week, to a total dose of 67.2 Gy in 42 fractions during 6 weeks, including a 2-week rest after 38.4 Gy, or;

d. Accelerated fractionation with concomitant boost: 1.8 Gy per fraction, once a day, 5 days a week to a large field, plus 1.5 Gy per fraction once a day to a boost field given 6 or more hours after treatment of the large field for the last 12 treatments days, to a total dose of 72 Gy in 42 fractions during 6 weeks.

The 5-year locoregional failure rates were standard fractionation, 59%; hyperfractionation, 51%; accelerated split course, 58%; and concomitant boost, 52%. Both the hyperfractionation and concomitant boost schedules yielded locoregional control rates that were significantly better than standard fractionation. There was a trend toward improved overall survival with hyperfractionation, but no difference in cause-specific survival. Acute toxicity was increased with all three altered fractionation schedules; there was a modest increase in late effects with the concomitant boost schedule.

The treatment technique used for postoperative irradiation after total laryngectomy is depicted in Figure 44.10 (2). The treatment technique for preoperative irradiation is essentially the same as that used for irradiation alone. Alternatively, IMRT may be employed for the indications discussed previously.

Treatment of Recurrence

Most recurrences appear within 18 months, but late recurrences may appear after 5 years. The latter are likely second primary malignancies. The risk of metastatic disease in lymph nodes increases with local recurrence (63).

Recurrence after Radiation Therapy

With careful follow-up, recurrence is sometimes detected before the patient notices a return of hoarseness. There is often minimal lymphedema for 1 to 2 months after irradiation, which usually subsides or stabilizes. An increase in edema, particularly if associated with hoarseness or pain, suggests recurrence, even if there is no obvious tumor. Fixation of a previously mobile

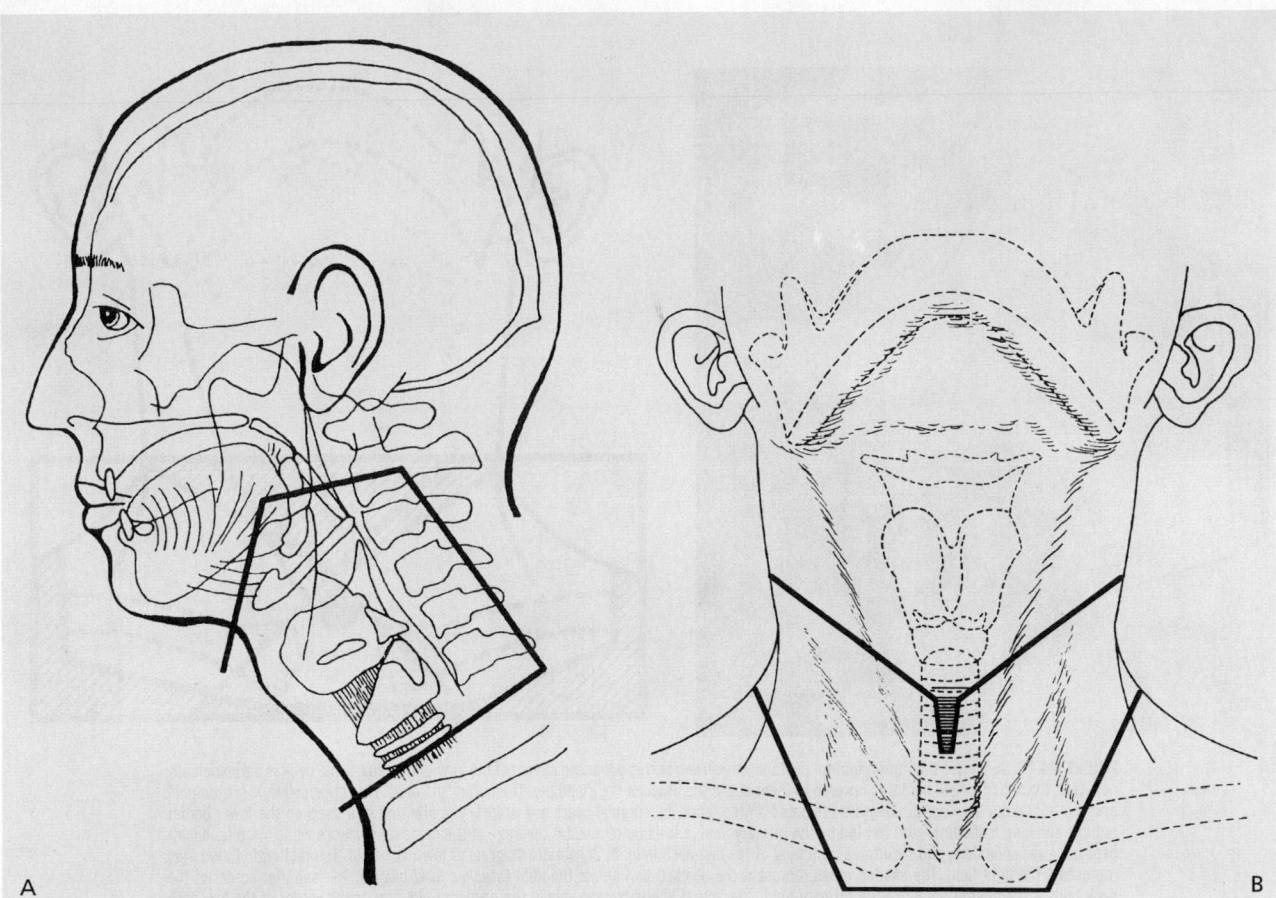

FIGURE 44.9. A: Radiation treatment technique for carcinoma of glottic larynx, stage T3-T4N0. The patient is treated supine, and the field is shaped with Lipowitz's metal. Anteriorly, the field is allowed to fall off. The entire pre-epiglottic space is included by encompassing the hyoid bone and epiglottis. The superior border (just above the angle of the mandible) includes the jugulodigastric lymph nodes. Posteriorly, a portion of the spinal cord must be included within the field to ensure adequate coverage of the midjugular lymph nodes; spinal accessory lymph nodes themselves are at little risk of involvement. The lower border is slanted to facilitate matching with the low neck field and to reduce the length of spinal cord in the high-dose field. The inferior border is placed at the bottom of the cricoid cartilage if the patient has no subglottic spread; in the presence of subglottic extension, the inferior border must be lowered according to the disease extent. **B:** Example of a low-neck portal for T3N0 glottic carcinoma. The main nodes al risk are the low jugular and lateral paratracheal. The Delphian node would be in the primary portal. A very narrow and short midline shield is used. ([A] Reprinted from Parsons JT, Mendenhall WM, Mancuso AA, et al. Twice-a-day radiotherapy for squamous cell carcinoma of the glottic larynx. *Head Neck* 1989;11:123–128, with permission. [B] Reprinted from Million RR, Cassisi NJ, Mancuso AA, et al. Management of the neck for squamous cell carcinoma. In: Million RR, Cassisi NJ, eds. *Management of head and neck cancer: A multidisciplinary approach,* 2 nd ed. Philadelphia: JB Lippincott; 1994:75–143, with permission.)

vocal cord usually implies local recurrence, but we have occasionally observed a patient who has experienced a fixed cord with an otherwise normal-appearing larynx and who has not shown evidence of recurrence.

It may be difficult to diagnose recurrence if the tumor is submucosal. Generous, deep biopsies are required. If recurrence is strongly suspected, laryngectomy may rarely be advised without biopsy-confirmed evidence of recurrence. Positron emission tomography may be useful to distinguish recurrent tumor from necrosis.

Radiation therapy failures may be salvaged by cordectomy, hemilaryngectomy, supracricoid partial laryngectomy, or total laryngectomy. Biller et al. (8) reported a 78% salvage rate by hemilaryngectomy for 18 selected patients in whom irradiation failed; total laryngectomy was eventually required in 2 patients. Only two patients died of cancer. These investigators offered guidelines for using hemilaryngectomy: Contralateral vocal cord is normal, arytenoid is not involved, subglottic extension does not exceed 5 mm, and vocal cord is not fixed. In our experience, 14 patients irradiated for T1 or T2 vocal cord cancers underwent a hemilaryngectomy after local recurrence and 8 were successfully salvaged (60).

Recurrence after Surgery

The rate of salvage by irradiation for recurrences or new tumors that appear after initial treatment by hemilaryngectomy is about 50%. Lee et al. (53) reported seven successes among 12 patients; one lesion was later controlled by total laryngectomy. Total laryngectomy can be used successfully to treat hemilaryngectomy failures not suitable for radiation therapy. Irradiation rarely cures patients with recurrence in the neck or stoma after total laryngectomy.

Treatment Selection and Technique: Supraglottic Larynx Carcinoma

Selection of Treatment Modality

Patients with supraglottic laryngeal carcinoma may be considered to be in an early or favorable group suitable for radiation therapy or conservation laryngectomy or an unfavorable group often requiring total laryngectomy.

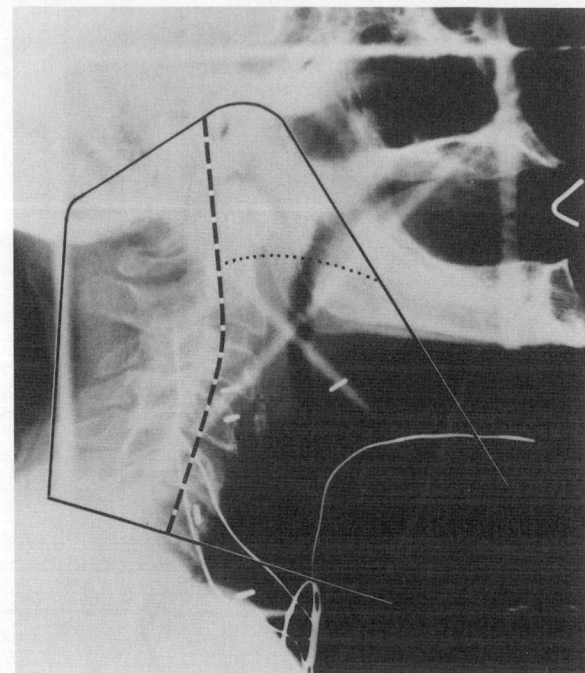
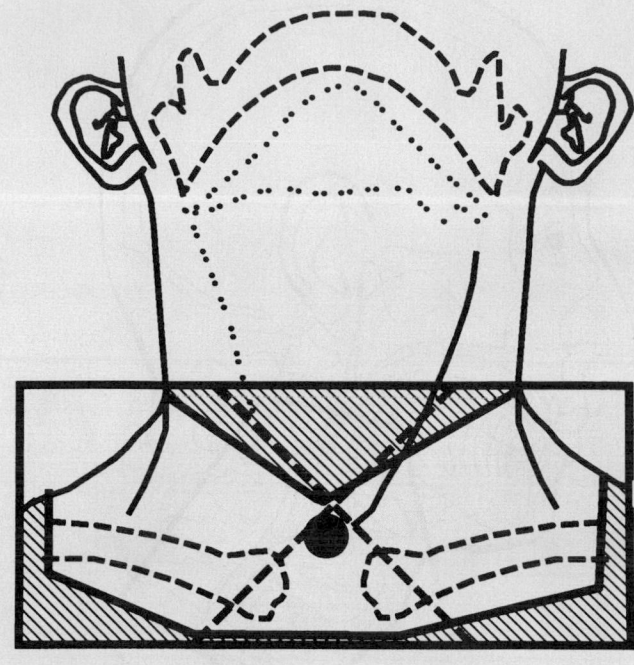

A

B

FIGURE 44.10. A: Typical simulation film for postoperative treatment of advanced cancer of the laryngopharynx. If the neck is pathologically negative, the superior field border is lowered to 2 cm above the angle of the mandible. The initial "off-cord" reduction (50 Gy) (*broken line*) and the final reduction (*dotted line*) are indicated. Wires mark the surgical scars and stoma. The slanting line used on the lower border reduces the length of spinal cord treated by the primary field, allows better caudal coverage of the mucosal surfaces while simultaneously bypassing the shoulders, and facilitates matching of the low-neck field. **B:** Schematic diagram of low-neck field. The rectangle (*solid line*) represents the light field. The shaded areas represent the blocked portions of the field (*stacked lead blocks*). The superior border of the neck field is the inferior border of the primary field. The actual line is treated only in the primary field. The upper border of the low-neck field assumes a V shape. In the midline of the patient, the apex of the V generally is at or close to the central axis (*broken lines*), so that the portal that treats the spinal cord is not divergent in its upper portion and diverges away from the primary fields in its lower portion. At the junction of the three fields, a short (2- to 3-cm) segment of spinal cord remains untreated by any of the three fields. (From Amdur RJ, Parsons JT, Mendenhall WM, et al. Postoperative irradiation for squamous cell carcinoma of the head and neck: An analysis of treatment results and complications. *Int J Radiat Oncol Biol Phys* 1989;16:25–36. Copyright 1989 by Elsevier Science, Inc.)

Early and Moderately Advanced Supraglottic Lesions

Treatment of the primary lesion for the early group is by external-beam irradiation or supraglottic laryngectomy, with or without adjuvant irradiation (39). Transoral laser excision is effective in experienced hands for small, selected lesions (103). Total laryngectomy is rarely indicated as the initial treatment for this group of patients and is reserved for treatment failures.

Radiation therapy and supraglottic laryngectomy are highly successful modes of therapy for early lesions (39). Approximately 50% of supraglottic laryngectomies performed at the University of Florida have been followed by postoperative irradiation because of neck disease and, less often, positive margins.

The decision to use radiation therapy or supraglottic laryngectomy depends on several factors including the anatomic extent of the tumor, medical condition of the patient, philosophy of the attending physician(s), and the inclination of the patient and family. Overall, about 80% of patients are treated initially by irradiation. Approximately half of the patients seen in our clinic whose lesions are technically suitable for a supraglottic laryngectomy are not suitable for medical reasons (e.g., inadequate pulmonary status or other major medical problems); these patients are treated with radiation therapy.

Analysis of local control by anatomic site within the supraglottic larynx shows no obvious differences in local control by irradiation for similarly staged lesions. Invasion of the pre-epiglottic space is not a contraindication to supraglottic laryn-

gectomy or irradiation. Primary tumor volume based on pretreatment CT is inversely related to local tumor control after radiation therapy (61). A large, bulky infiltrative lesion, especially one with extensive preepiglottic space invasion, is a common reason to select supraglottic laryngectomy.

The status of the neck often determines the selection of treatment of the primary lesion. Patients with clinically negative neck nodes have a high risk for occult neck disease and may be treated by radiation therapy or supraglottic laryngectomy and bilateral selective neck dissections, (levels II–IV).

If a patient has an early-stage primary lesion but advanced neck disease (N2b or N3), combined treatment is frequently necessary to control the neck disease (70). In these cases, the primary lesion is usually treated by irradiation alone, with surgery added to the treatment of the involved neck site(s). If the same patient were treated with supraglottic laryngectomy, neck dissection, and postoperative irradiation, the portals would unnecessarily cover the primary site and the neck. If the patient has early, resectable neck disease (N1 or N2a) and surgery is elected for the primary site, postoperative irradiation is added only because of unexpected findings (e.g., positive margins, multiple positive nodes, or extracapsular extension). We prefer to avoid routine high-dose preoperative or postoperative irradiation in conjunction with a supraglottic laryngectomy because the lymphedema of the remaining larynx may be considerable, although it eventually subsides. However, Lee et al. (54) from M.D. Anderson Cancer Center reported excellent results with combined supraglottic laryngectomy and postoperative irradiation for moderately advanced lesions.

Advanced Supraglottic Lesions

Although a subset of these patients may be suitable for a supraglottic or supracricoid laryngectomy, total laryngectomy is the main surgical option. Selected advanced lesions, especially those that are mainly exophytic, may be treated by radiation therapy and concomitant chemotherapy (90) with total laryngectomy reserved for irradiation failures.

For patients whose primary lesion is to be treated by a total or partial laryngectomy and who have resectable neck disease, surgery is the initial treatment, and postoperative irradiation is added if needed. If the neck disease is unresectable, preoperative radiation therapy is used. The indications for preoperative and postoperative irradiation have been previously outlined.

Surgical Treatment

Supraglottic Laryngectomy

Supraglottic laryngectomy is voice-sparing surgery that can be used successfully for selected lesions involving the epiglottis, a single arytenoid, the aryepiglottic fold, or the false vocal cord. Extension of the tumor to the true vocal cord, the anterior commissure, or both arytenoids; fixation of the vocal cord; or thyroid or cricoid cartilage invasion precludes supraglottic laryngectomy. The supraglottic laryngectomy may be extended to include the base of the tongue if one lingual artery is preserved.

All patients have difficulty swallowing with a tendency to aspirate immediately after surgery, but almost all learn to swallow again in a short time; motivation and the amount of tissue removed are key factors in learning to swallow again. Preoperatively, adequate pulmonary reserve is evaluated by blood gas determinations, function tests, chest roentgenography, and a work test involving walking the patient up two flights of stairs to determine tolerance to pulmonary stress. The voice quality is generally normal after supraglottic laryngectomy.

Supracricoid Laryngectomy

This procedure is an option for lesions extending from the supraglottis into one or both vocal cords. However, vocal cord fixation is a relative contraindication. At least one arytenoid must be preserved for successful decannulation and phonation. Extension to the cricoid and thyroid cartilage destruction also preclude its use. Phonation and respiratory function are reconstituted by approximating the cricoid to the hyoid (cricohyoidopexy).

Wide-Field Total Laryngectomy

Total laryngectomy is performed as previously described.

Radiation Therapy Technique

The primary lesion and both sides of the neck are treated with opposed lateral portals; wedges are used to compensate for the contour of the neck (Fig. 44.11) (73). The lower neck nodes are irradiated through a separate anterior portal. IMRT may be employed to spare one or both parotids and to avoid a low match line in the occasional patient with a short neck and large shoulders. We currently use the concomitant boost fractionation schedule when employing IMRT.

In the case of clinically positive nodes, an electron beam portal may be used to increase the dose to the posterior cervical nodes after the fields are reduced to avoid the spinal cord at 45 Gy. CT is obtained 4 weeks after completing radiotherapy, and a neck dissection is added if the residual cancer in the nodes is thought to exceed 5%; otherwise the patient is observed and a CT is repeated in 3 months (70).

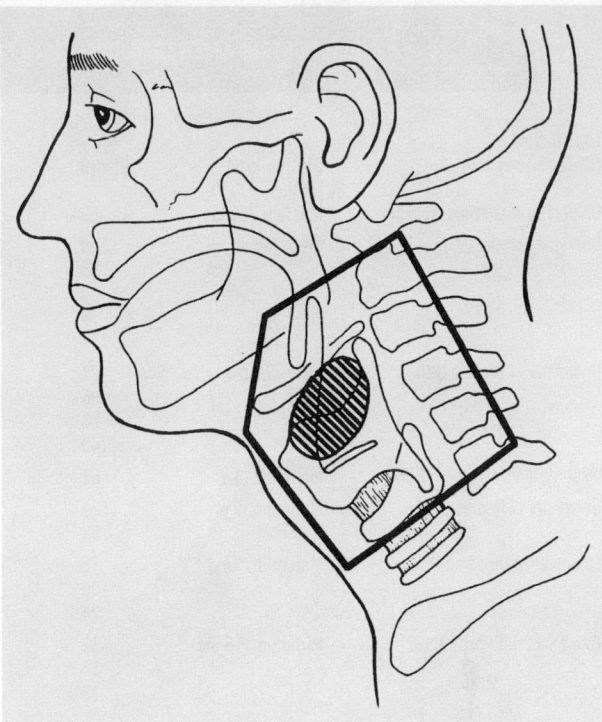

FIGURE 44.11. Example of the portal for a lesion of the lower epiglottis or false vocal cord and a neck with clinically negative findings. The subdigastric nodes are included but not the junctional nodes. Depending on the anatomy and tumor extent, the anterior border may fall off (i.e., "flash") or a small strip of skin may be shielded. (Reprinted from Million RR, Cassisi NJ, Mancuso AA, et al. Management of the neck for squamous cell carcinoma. In: Million RR, Cassisi NJ, eds. *Management of head and neck cancer: A multidisciplinary approach,* 2nd ed. Philadelphia; JB Lippincott; 1994:75–143, with permission.)

Patients experience a sore throat, loss of taste, and moderate dryness during irradiation. Edema of the arytenoids may occur and give a sensation of a lump in the throat. Tracheostomy is rarely necessary, even for bulky lesions.

Edema of the larynx may persist for several months to a year. Patients who continue to smoke heighten the side effects of dryness, dysphagia, and hoarseness.

Preoperative and Postoperative Treatment Technique

If total laryngectomy is required and the lesion is resectable, postoperative radiation therapy is preferred because there is no evidence that preoperative irradiation produces any better locoregional control or survival rates than surgery and postoperative radiation therapy. Irradiation is added for close or positive margins, invasion of soft tissues of the neck, significant subglottic extension (1 cm or more), thyroid cartilage invasion, multiple positive nodes, and extracapsular extension. The high-risk areas are usually the base of the tongue and the neck.

The dose for postoperative irradiation as a function of known residual disease is as follows: Negative margins, 60 Gy in 30 fractions; microscopically positive margins, 66 Gy in 33 fractions; and gross residual disease, 70 Gy in 35 fractions. All patients are treated with a continuous course, one fraction per day, 5 days per week. The lower neck is treated with doses to 50 Gy in 25 fractions at D_{max}. If there is subglottic extension, the dose to the stoma is boosted with electrons (usually 10 to 14 MeV) for an additional 10 Gy in five fractions. The treatment technique is shown in Fig. 44.10 (2). If postoperative irradiation is added after a supraglottic laryngectomy, the dose is lowered to 55.8 Gy

Table 44.3 LOCAL CONTROL AFTER TRANSORAL LASER EXCISION

Institution (Reference)	Follow-Up[a]	No. of Patients	Stage	Local Control (Interval) (%)	Local Control with Larynx Preservation (Interval) (%)	Ultimate Local Control (Interval) (%)
University of Göttingen (103)	Median, 78 mo	159	pTis-pT2	94 (NS)	99 (NS)	—
University of Kiel (95)	Mean, 40 mo	8	pTis	100 (NS)	—	—
		88	pT1a	92 (NS)	—	—
		10	pT1b	80 (NS)	—	—
		8	pT2	88 (NS)	—	—
		114	pTis-pT2	—	96 (NS)	—
University of Brescia (89)	Mean, 76 mo	21	pTis	81 (NS)	—	95[b] (5 y)
		96	pT1	82 (NS)	—	87[b] (5 y)
		23	pT2	74 (NS)	—	91[b] (5 y)
		140	pTis-pT2	80 (NS)	97 (NS)	—
Washington University (100)	Minimum, 3 y	61	T1	77 (NS)	90 (NS)	98 (NS)
University of Naples (76)	Minimum, 5 y	321	T1	82[b] (NS)	89[c] (NS)	—
		158	T2	60[b] (NS)	~ 67[c] (NS)	—
La Sapienza University (26)	Minimum, 3 y	12	Tis	100 (NS)	100 (NS)	—
		120	T1a	94 (NS)	100 (NS)	—
		24	T1b	91 (NS)	100 (NS)	—
Tata Memorial Hospital (92)	Minimum, 18 mo	52	T1a	90 (NS)	94 (NS)	—
		17	T1b	65 (NS)	88 (NS)	—
		13	T2	77 (NS)	92 (NS)	—

NS, not stated.
[a]Follow-up period for total number of patients.
[b]Ultimate local control with laser treatment alone.
[c]Locoregional control rate.
From Mendenhall WM, Werning JW, Hinerman RW, et al. Management of T1-T2 glottic carcinomas. *Cancer* 2004;100:1786–1792.

given in 1.8 Gy fractions. This dose produces acceptable rates of local control and laryngeal edema (94).

The treatment technique used for preoperative radiation therapy is essentially the same as that used for patients treated with irradiation alone, using doses of 50 to 60 Gy at 1.8 to 2 Gy per fraction. Thereafter, the dose is boosted to areas of unresectable disease (usually the neck) to total doses ranging from 66 to 70 Gy.

Treatment of Recurrence

Failures after supraglottic laryngectomy or radiation therapy can frequently be controlled by further treatment; therefore, recognition of recurrence should be vigorously pursued (39). Salvage of patients with recurrence after combined total laryngectomy and irradiation is uncommon. Stomal recurrences are occasionally controlled by radiation therapy or surgery.

Table 44.4 LOCAL CONTROL AFTER OPEN PARTIAL LARYNGECTOMY

Institution (Reference)	Follow-Up (y)	No. of Patients.	Stage	Local Control (Interval) (%)	Local Control with Larynx Preservation (Interval) (%)	Ultimate Local Control (Interval) (%)
Universitaire Timone (32)	NS	62	T1	100 (NS)	100 (NS)	—
		65	T2	92 (NS)	92 (NS)	—
Hôpital Saint Charles (13)	Minimum, 3	18	T1a	100 (NS)	—	—
		40	T1b	95 (NS)	—	—
		23	T2a	83 (NS)	—	—
Mayo Clinic (108)	Median, 6.6	159	Tis–T1	93 (5 y)	94 (NS)	100 (NS)
Hôpital Laënnec (48)	Minimum, 3	295	T1	89 (NS)	—	—
		90	T2a	74 (NS)	—	—
		31	T2b	68 (NS)	—	—
		416	T1–T2b	84 (NS)	—	97 (NS)
Washington University (100)	Minimum, 3	404	T1	92 (NS)	93 (NS)	99 (NS)
Washington University (101)	Minimum, 5	71	T2	93 (NS)	93 (NS)	99 (NS)

NS, not stated.
From Mendenhall WM, Werning JW, Hinerman RW, et al. Management of T1–T2 glottic carcinomas. *Cancer* 2004;100:1786–1792.

Table 44.5 LOCAL CONTROL AFTER RADIOTHERAPY

Institution (Reference)	Follow-Up[a] (y)	No. of Patients	Stage	Local Control (Interval) (%)	Local Control with Larynx Preservation (Interval) (%)	Ultimate Local Control (Interval) (%)
University of Florida (60)	Minimum, 2	230	T1a	94 (5 y)	98 (5 y)	
	Median, 9.9	61	T1b	93 (5 y)	95 (5 y)	98 (5 y)
		146	T2a	80 (5 y)	82 (5 y)	96 (5 y)
		82	T2b	72 (5 y)	76 (5 y)	96 (5 y)
Massachusetts General Hospital (114)	NS	665	T1	93 (5 y)	—	—
		145	T2a	77 (5 y)	—	—
		92	T2b	71 (5 y)	—	—
University of California (SF) (51)	Median, 9.7	315	T1	85 (5 y)	—	96[b] (5 y)
		83	T2	70 (5 y)	—	91[b] (5 y)
Princess Margaret Hospital (116)	Median, 6.8	403	T1a	91 (5 y)	—	—
		46	T1b	82 (5 y)	—	—
		286	T2	69 (5 y)	—	—
M.D. Anderson Hospital (29)	Median, 6.8	114	T2a	74 (5 y)	—	—
		116	T2b	70 (5 y)	—	—
		230	T2	72 (5 y)	—	91 (5 y)

NS, not stated; SF, San Francisco.
[a]Follow-up period for total number of patients.
[b]Local–regional control rates.
From Mendenhall WM, Werning JW, Hinerman RW, et al. Management of T1–T2 glottic carcinomas. *Cancer* 2004;100:1786–1792.

Table 44.6 SURVIVAL DATA

Institution (Reference)	Treatment	Follow-Up (y)	No. of Patients	Stage	Cause-Specific Survival (Interval) (%)	Absolute Survival (Interval) (%)
Washington University (100)	Laser	Minimum, 3	61	T1	95 (5 y)	84 (5 y)
University of Göttingen (103)	Laser	Median, 6.5	159	pTis–T2	100 (5 y)	87 (5 y)
University of Brescia (89)	Laser	Mean, 6.3	140	pTis–T2	98 (5 y)	93 (5 y)
Washington University (100)	OPL	Minimum, 3	404	T1	97 (5 y)	84 (5 y)
Mayo Clinic (108)	OPL	Median, 6.6	159	Tis-T1	—	84 (5 y)
Washington University (101)	OPL	Minimum, 5	71	T2	—	~ 92 (5 y)
University of Florida (60)	RT	Minimum, 2	230	T1a	98 (5 y)	82 (5 y)
		Median, 9.9	61	T1b	98 (5 y)	79 (5 y)
			146	T2a	95 (5 y)	77 (5 y)
			82	T2b	90 (5 y)	77 (5 y)
University of California (SF) (50)	RT	Median, 9.7	315	T1	96 (10 y)	65 (10 y)
			83	T2	91 (10 y)	63 (10 y)
Massachusetts General Hospital (114)	RT	NS	665	T1	98 (5 y)	—
			145	T2a	92 (5 y)	—
			92	T2b	84 (5 y)	—
M.D. Anderson Hospital (29)	RT	Median, 6.8	230	T2	92 (5 y)	73 (5 y)

OPL, open partial laryngectomy; RT, radiotherapy; SF, San Francisco; NS, not stated.
From Mendenhall WM, Werning JW, Hinerman RW, et al. Management of T1–T2 glottic carcinomas. *Cancer* 2004;100:1786–1792.

Table 44.7 STAGE T3 GLOTTIC CARCINOMA TREATED WITH IRRADIATION ALONE (NO CHEMOTHERAPY)

Investigator(s)	Institution	No. of Patients	Minimum Follow-Up (y)	Local Control (%)	Ultimate Control after Salvage Surgery (%)
Harwood et al. (34)	Princess Margaret (Toronto)	112	3	51	77
Wang (113)	Mass. General (Boston)	70	4	36	57
Fletcher et al. (21)	M.D. Anderson (Houston)	17	2	77	No data
Skolyszewski and Reinfuss (99)	15 European centers	91	3	50	No data
Stewart et al. (105)	Manchester (England)	67	10	57	67
Mills (75)	Capetown, South Africa	18	2	44	78
Mendenhall et al. (64)	U. Florida (Gainesville)	75	2	63	86

Modified from Parsons JT, Mendenhall WM, Mancuso AA, et al. Twice-a-day radiotherapy for T3 squamous cell carcinoma of the glottic larynx. *Head Neck* 1989;11:123–128.

Table 44.8	T3 GLOTTIC CARCINOMA TREATED AT THE UNIVERSITY OF FLORIDA, 1965–1988: 5-YEAR RESULTS	
Parameter	RT Alone (53 Patients) (%)	Surgery with or without Adjuvant RT (65 Patients) (%)
Locoregional control	62	75
Ultimate locoregional control	84	82
Absolute survival	55	45
Cause-specific survival	75	71

RT, radiotherapy.
Data from Mendenhall WM, Parsons JT, Stringer SP, et al. Stage T3 squamous cell carcinoma of the glottic larynx: A comparison of laryngectomy and irradiation. *Int J Radiat Oncol Biol Phys* 1992;23:725–732.

Table 44.10	PROPORTION OF PATIENTS SUITABLE FOR SUPRAGLOTTIC LARYNGECTOMY[a]	
Investigators	No. of Patients	No (%) with Supraglottic Laryngectomy
Ogura et al., 1975 (83)	263	177 (67)
Lutz et al., 1990 (56)	202	72 (36)
Lee et al., 1990 (54)	404	60 (15)
Weems et al., 1987 (118)	195	30 (15)
Gregor et al., 1996 (63)	89	26 (29)
Spriano et al., 1997 (102)	257	38 (14)

[a]Note: Some figures were estimated as closely as possible to fit table format if the information was not specifically stated in the cited reference.
From Hinerman RW, Mendenhall WM, Amdur RJ, et al. Carcinoma of the supraglottic larynx: Treatment results with radiotherapy alone or with planned neck dissection. *Head Neck* 2002;24:456–467.

Results of Treatment

Vocal Cord Cancer

The local control and survival rates after treatment of early-stage glottic carcinoma are depicted in Tables 44.3 through 44.6 (71). The local control and survival rates are similar for transoral laser excision, open partial laryngectomy, and radiotherapy. Larynx preservation rates are also comparable. Voice quality depends on the amount of tissue removed with partial laryngectomy and is probably similar for patients with limited lesions treated with laser to those undergoing radiotherapy and poorer for patients undergoing open partial laryngectomy (71).

Foote et al. (22) reported on 81 patients who underwent laryngectomy for T3 cancers at the Mayo Clinic between 1970 and 1981. Seventy-five patients underwent a total laryngectomy and 6 underwent a near-total laryngectomy; 53 patients received a neck dissection. No patient underwent adjuvant irradiation or chemotherapy. The 5-year rates of locoregional control, cause-specific survival, and absolute survival were 74%, 74%, and 54%, respectively. The results of definitive radiation therapy patients with T3 glottic carcinoma are depicted in Table 44.7 (85) and are similar to the surgical outcomes reported by Foote et al. (22).

The survival and control rates of patients with T3 fixed-cord lesions treated at the University of Florida are presented in Table 44.8 (67). There was no relationship between subsequent local control and whether the vocal cord remained fixed or became mobile during irradiation. The incidence of severe complications, including those after the initial treatment and any later

salvage procedures, was 15% after radiation therapy alone and 15% after surgery alone or combined with adjuvant irradiation. The vocal quality varied from fair to nearly normal.

The results of treatment of T4 vocal cord carcinoma in four surgical series and two radiotherapy series are summarized in Table 44.9 (35).

Parsons et al. (86) reviewed the literature and reported a local control rate of 62% in a series of 87 patients treated with irradiation alone for T4 glottic carcinoma.

Combined-Therapy Results

The proportion of patients suitable for a supraglottic laryngectomy is depicted in Table 44.10 (39). Depending on the referral patterns, a modest subset of patients is suitable for this operation. The extent of neck disease for patients treated with either surgery or radiotherapy is shown in Table 44.11 (39). In general, patients treated with supraglottic laryngectomy appropriately have earlier stage neck disease and would be anticipated to have a lower risk of distant failure and improved survival. The local control rates after transoral laser, radiotherapy, and supraglottic laryngectomy are summarized in Tables 44.12 through 44.14, respectively (39). In general, the local control rates after transoral laser excision are fairly good for patients with T1–T2 tumors and tend to deteriorate for those with more advanced disease. The local control rate are excellent for patients selected for supraglottic laryngectomy. However, the incidence of severe complications tends to be higher after supraglottic laryngectomy compared with radiotherapy and transoral laser excision (Table 44.15) (39).

Table 44.9	TREATMENT OF STAGE T4 GLOTTIC CARCINOMAS			
Investigator(s)	Tumor Stage	No. of Patients	Method of Treatment	Results (NED) (%)
Jesse (44)	T4N0-N+	48	Laryngectomy	54 at 4 y
Ogura et al. (82)	T4N0	11	Laryngectomy	45 at 3 y
Skolnick et al. (98)	T4N0	7	Laryngectomy	30 at 5 y
Vermund (110)	T4N0	31	Laryngectomy	35 at 5 y
Stewart and Jackson (106)	T4N0	13	Radiotherapy with surgery for salvage	38 at 5 y
Harwood et al. (35)	T4N0	56	Radiotherapy with surgery for salvage	49 at 5 y[a]

NED, no evidence of disease.
[a]Life-table method; uncorrected for deaths from intercurrent disease.
Modified from Harwood AR, Beal FA, Cummings BJ, et al. T4N0M0 glottic cancer: An analysis of dose-time-volume. *Int J Radiat Oncol Biol Phys* 1981;7:1507–1512.

Table 44.11 SUPRAGLOTTIC CARCINOMA: EXTENT OF NECK DISEASE VS. TREATMENT[a]

Investigator(s)	Treatment	No. of Patients	Extent of Neck Disease (%)
Bocca, 1991 (9)	SGL	537	94 N0–N1
Isaacs et al., 1998 (42)	SGL	39	74 N0–N1
Ogura et al., 1975 (83)	SGL	177	77 N0
Davis et al., 1991 (15)	Laser	14	93 N0
Zeitels et al., 1994 (122)	Laser	45	100 N0
Rudert et al., 1999 (96)	Laser	34	82 N0–N1
Ghossein et al., 1974 (30)	Radiation	203	53 N0
Hinerman et al., (39)	Radiation	274	54 N0

SGL = supraglottic laryngectomy.
[a]Note: Some figures were estimated as closely as possible to fit table format if the information was not specifically stated in the cited reference.
From Hinerman RW, Mendenhall WM, Amdur RJ, et al. Carcinoma of the supraglottic larynx: Treatment results with radiotherapy alone or with planned neck dissection. *Head Neck* 2002;24:456–467.

Table 44.12 SUPRAGLOTTIC LARYNX: LOCAL CONTROL AFTER TRANSORAL LASER EXCISION[a]

Investigator(s)	Staging	No. of Patients	Percent of Patients with T1 or T2 Tumors	Local Control (%) T1	T2	T3	T4
Davis et al., 1991 (15)	P	14 R	57	100	100	50	—
Steiner, 1993[b] (103)	P	81 R	72	—	76	77	100
Zeitels et al., 1994 (122)	ND	22	100	100	100	—	—
Zeitels et al., 1994 (122)	ND	23 R	65	100	92	63	—
Csanády et al., 1999 (14)	ND	23	100	70[c]		—	—
Rudert et al., 1999 (96)	P	34 R	50	100	75	78	38

P, pathologic staging; R, plus or minus radiotherapy; ND, type of staging not provided.
[a]Note: Some figures were estimated as closely as possible to fit table format if the information was not specifically stated in the cited reference.
[b]There were 51 glottic and 30 supraglottic carcinomas.
[c]Overall local control rates for T1 and T2.
From Hinerman RW, Mendenhall WM, Amdur RJ, et al. Carcinoma of the supraglottic larynx: Treatment results with radiotherapy alone or with planned neck dissection. *Head Neck* 2002;24:456–467.

Table 44.13 SUPRAGLOTTIC LARYNX: LOCAL CONTROL AFTER RADIOTHERAPY[a]

Investigators	Institution	No. of Patients	T1	T2	T3	T4
Fletcher and Hamberger, 1974 (20)	M.D. Anderson Hospital	173	88	79	62	47
Ghossein et al., 1974 (30)	Fondation Curie	203	94	73	46[b]	52
Wang and Montgomery, 1991 (115)	Massachusetts General Hospital	229 q.d.	73	60	54	26
		209 b.i.d.	89	89	71	91
Nakfoor et al., 1998 (77)	Massachusetts General Hospital	164	96	86	76	43
Sykes et al., 2000 (107)	Christie Hospital	331[b]	92[d]	81[d]	67[d]	73[d]
Hinerman et al., 2002 (39)	University of Florida[e]	274	100	86	62	62

q.d., once a day; b.i.d., twice a day.
[a]Note: Some figures were estimated as closely as possible to fit table format if the information was not specifically stated in the cited reference.
[b]All had cord fixation.
[c]All N0.
[d]After 17 were salvaged by total laryngectomies.
[e]By 1998 AJCC staging.
From Hinerman RW, Mendenhall WM, Amdur RJ, et al. Carcinoma of the supraglottic larynx: Treatment results with radiotherapy alone or with planned neck dissection. *Head Neck* 2002;24:456–467.

Clinical Radiation Oncology

Table 44.14   LOCAL CONTROL AFTER SUPRAGLOTTIC LARYNGECTOMY[a]

Investigator(s)	Institution	No. of Patients	Patients with T1 or T2 Tumors (%)	Local Control (%) T1	T2	T3	T4
Ogura et al., 1975 (83)	Washington University	177	78	—	94[b]		—
Bocca, 1991 (9)	Milan University						
Stage I		47	100	94	—	—	—
Stage II		252	100	—	82	—	—
Stage III		205	53	—	80[c]	—	—
Stage IV		33	70	—	67[d]	—	
Lee et al., 1990 (54)	M.D. Anderson Cancer Center	60	58	100	100	100	100
DeSanto, 1990 (17)	Mayo Clinic	70	100	100	100	—	—
Steiniger et al., 1997 (104)	Albany Medical College	29	83	—	97[a]	—	—
Spriano et al., 1997 (102)	Varese, Italy	54	100	96[e]	—	—	—
Burstein and Calcattera, 1985 (11)	University of California (LA)	40	58	100	85	94	100
Isaacs et al., 1998 (42)	University of Florida	33	76	100	78	71	100
Lutz et al., 1990 (56)	University of Pittsburgh	72	No data	—	99[f]	—	—

[a]Note: Some figures were estimated as closely as possible to fit table format if the information was not specifically stated in the cited reference.
[b]Overall local control rates for T1–T4.
[c]Overall local control rates for T1–T3.
[d]Overall local control rates for T2–T3.
[e]Overall local control rates for T1–T2.
[f]T stages were not specified.
From Hinerman RW, Mendenhall WM, Amdur RJ, et al. Carcinoma of the supraglottic larynx: Treatment results with radiotherapy alone or with planned neck dissection. *Head Neck* 2002;24:456–467.

Table 44.15   SUPRAGLOTTIC LARYNX: SEVERE COMPLICATIONS ACCORDING TO TREATMENT MODALITY[a]

Investigator(s)	Institution	No. (%) of Severe Complications
Radiotherapy		
Fletcher and Hamberger, 1974 (20)	M.D. Anderson Cancer Center	10/173 (6)
Ghossein et al., 1974 (30)	Fondation Curie	8/117 (7)
Nakfoor et al., 1998 (77)	Massachusetts General Hospital	12/169 (7)
Sykes et al., 2000 (107)	Christie Hospital	7/331 (2)
Hinerman et al. (39)	University of Florida	12/274 (4)
Supraglottic laryngectomy		
Lee et al., 1991 (54)	M.D. Anderson Cancer Center	9/63 (14)
Isaacs et al., 1998 (42)	University of Florida	14/34 (41)
Burstein and Calcaterra, 1985 (11)	University of California, Los Angeles	14/41 (34)
Steiniger et al., 1997 (104)	Albany Medical College	12/29 (41)
Spriano et al., 1997 (102)	Varese, Italy	13/54 (24)
Gall et al., 1977 (25)	Washington University	20/133 (15)
Weber et al., 1993 (117)	University of Pittsburgh	12/69 (17)
Beckhardt et al., 1994 (7)	University of Wisconsin	15/50 (30)
Transoral laser excision		
Rudert et al., 1999 (96)	University of Kiel, Germany	3/34 (9)
Zeitels et al., 1994 (122)	Massachusetts Eye and Ear Infirmary	2/45 (4)
Steiner, 1993[b] (103)	University of Gottingen, Germany	7/240 (3)
Davis et al., 1991 (15)	University of Utah, Salt Lake City	0/14 (0)
Csanády et al., 1999 (14)	Albert Szent Gyorgyi Medical University, Szeged, Hungary	0/23 (0)

[a]Note: Some figures were estimated as closely as possible to fit table format if the information was not specifically stated in the cited reference.
[b]Includes patients with glottic cancer.
From Hinerman RW, Mendenhall WM, Amdur RJ, et al. Carcinoma of the supraglottic larynx: Treatment results with radiotherapy alone or with planned neck dissection. *Head Neck* 2002;24:456–467.

Follow-Up Policy

Follow-up of patients with early lesions is planned for every 4 to 8 weeks for 2 years, every 3 months for the third year, and every 6 months for years 4 and 5, and then annually for life.

Follow-up of patients with vocal cord or supraglottic larynx lesions treated by radiation therapy or conservative surgery is almost more important than the treatment itself because early detection of recurrence usually results in salvage that may include cure with voice preservation.

If recurrence is suspected but the biopsy is negative, patients are reexamined at 2- to 4-week intervals until the matter is settled. The value of follow-up CT scans for detecting early local recurrence is investigational.

Wagenfeld et al. (112) studied 740 cases of glottic larynx cancer treated from 1965 to 1974 to determine the incidence of second respiratory tract malignancies. There was a minimum follow-up of 5 years. There were 48 second respiratory tract malignancies, although only 14 were expected. Twenty-five were in the lung, and 23 were scattered among other head and neck sites. Only 7 of the 23 second head and neck primary lesions resulted in death; these second lesions were frequently diagnosed in an early stage during routine follow-up for the glottic lesion.

Because the risk of a lethal lung primary lesion is nearly as great as that of dying of an early glottic carcinoma, it makes sense to obtain annual chest roentgenograms. Approximately 50% of patients who receive moderate-to-high dose radiotherapy to the entire thyroid gland will develop hypothyroidism within 5 years, so that thyroid functions are checked every 6 to 12 months and thyroid replacement is initiated if the thyroid-stimulating hormone level begins to rise (27).

Sequelae of Treatment

Surgical Sequelae

Neel et al. (78) reported a 26% incidence of nonfatal complications for cordectomy. Immediate postoperative complications included atelectasis and pneumonia, severe subcutaneous emphysema in the neck, bleeding from the tracheotomy site or larynx, wound complications, and airway obstruction requiring tracheotomy. Late complications included granulation tissue that had to be removed by direct laryngoscopy to exclude recurrences, extrusion of cartilage, laryngeal stenosis, and obstructing laryngeal web.

The postoperative complications and sequelae of hemilaryngectomy include chondritis, wound slough, inadequate glottic closure, and anterior commissure webs (25). The complications associated with supraglottic laryngectomy and total laryngectomy for supraglottic carcinomas include fistula (8%), carotid artery exposure or blowout (3% to 5%), infection or wound sloughing (3% to 7%), and fatal complications (3%) (25). The risk of complications increased if tumor margins were involved by tumor; there was no change in risk associated with age, sex, race, laryngeal site, stage of primary tumor, size of primary tumor, use of low-dose preoperative irradiation, or status of the positive nodes.

The incidence of complications after treatment of supraglottic carcinoma is depicted in Table 44.15 (39).

Radiation Therapy Sequelae

The acute reactions from the treatment of early vocal cord cancer using a tumor dose of 2.25 Gy per day to administer a total dose 63 Gy (^{60}Co, five fractions per week) are relatively mild. During the first 2 to 3 weeks, the voice may improve as the tumor regresses. The voice generally becomes hoarse again because of radiation-induced changes, even though the tumor continues to regress. A mild sore throat develops beginning at the end of the second week, but medication is usually not required. The voice begins to improve approximately 3 weeks after completion of treatment, usually reaching a plateau in 2 to 3 months. Patients with extensive lesions often recover a normal voice, although not as frequently as those with small tumors.

Edema of the larynx is the most common sequela after irradiation for glottic or supraglottic lesions. The rate of clearance of the edema is related to the irradiation dose, volume of tissue irradiated, addition of a neck dissection, continued use of alcohol and tobacco, and size and extent of the original lesion. Edema may be accentuated by a radical neck dissection and may require 6 to 12 months to subside.

Soft tissue necrosis leading to chondritis occurs in fewer than 1% of patients, usually in those who continue to smoke. Soft tissue and cartilage necroses mimic recurrence, with hoarseness, pain, and edema; a laryngectomy may be recommended as a last resort for fear of recurrent cancer, even though biopsy specimens show only necrosis.

Corticosteroids such as dexamethasone (Decadron) have been used to reduce radiation-induced edema after recurrence has been ruled out by biopsy. If ulceration and pain occur, administration of an antibiotic such as tetracycline may help. Of 519 patients with T1N0 or T2N0 vocal cord cancer treated at the University of Florida, 5 (1%) experienced severe complications (60), including total laryngectomy for a suspected local recurrence (1 patient), permanent tracheostomy for edema (3 patients), and a pharyngocutaneous fistula after a salvage total laryngectomy (1 patient).

In patients irradiated for supraglottic carcinoma, sore throat persists 3 to 4 weeks after completion of treatment. There is an associated dry mouth from irradiation of the salivary and parotid glands, a loss of taste, and a sensation of a lump in the throat. It is unusual for patients to require a tracheotomy before irradiation unless severe lymphedema develops at the time of direct laryngoscopy and biopsy. However, in patients who have recovered from the direct laryngoscopy and biopsy without obstruction, a tracheotomy has rarely been required during a fractionated course of radiation therapy.

Patients treated twice a day with 1.2 Gy fractions (continuous-course technique) to total doses of 74.4 to 76.8 Gy usually have more brisk acute reactions than those treated once a day with 2-Gy fractions. Approximately 20% treated with twice-a-day irradiation require temporary gastrostomy feeding tubes because they have difficulty in swallowing (1).

Examples of acute chondritis requiring discontinuation of treatment have not been seen, although most epiglottic lesions exhibit cartilage invasion.

The epiglottis, both suprahyoid and infrahyoid portions, remains thicker than normal for long periods of time, but this is not often associated with difficulty in swallowing, respiratory obstruction, or aspiration. The patient is cautioned to eat and drink slowly until the edema resolves. The false cord and arytenoids may develop some edema.

Lesions of the suprahyoid epiglottis frequently destroy the tip of the epiglottis, and it may require some time for the exposed cartilage to heal. Successful irradiation of infrahyoid epiglottis tumors is not associated with a high rate of necrosis, even though most of these lesions penetrate the porous epiglottic cartilage.

The incidence of severe late complications in 274 patients treated with radiation therapy alone or combined with neck dissection at the University of Florida was 4% (39).

Clinical Radiation Oncology

Acknowledgment

We thank the research support staff of the Department of Radiation Oncology, University of Florida, Gainesville, for their help with statistics, editing, and manuscript preparation

References

1. Al-Othman MOF, Amdur RJ, Morris CG, et al. Does feeding tube placement predict for long-term swallowing disability after radiotherapy for head and neck cancer? *Head Neck* 2003;25:741–747.
2. Amdur RJ, Parsons JT, Mendenhall WM, et al. Postoperative irradiation for squamous cell carcinoma of the head and neck: An analysis of treatment results and complications. *Int J Radiat Oncol Biol Phys* 1989;16:25–36.
3. American Joint Committee on Cancer. Larynx. *AJCC Cancer Staging Manual*, 6th ed. New York: Springer, 2002:47–57.
4. Amornmarn R, Prempree T, Jaiwatana J, et al. Radiation management of carcinoma of the tonsillar region. *Cancer* 1984;54:1293–1299.
5. Archer CR, Yeager VL, Herbold DR. Computed tomography vs. histology of laryngeal cancer: Their value in predicting laryngeal cartilage invasion. *Laryngoscope* 1983;93:140–147.
6. Archer CR, Yeager VL, Herbold DR. Improved diagnostic accuracy in laryngeal cancer using a new classification based on computed tomography. *Cancer* 1984;53:44–57.
7. Beckhardt RN, Murray JG, Ford CN, et al. Factors influencing functional outcome in supraglottic laryngectomy. *Head Neck* 1994;16:232–239.
8. Biller HF, Barnhill FR Jr, Ogura JH, et al. Hemilaryngectomy following radiation failure for carcinoma of the vocal cords. *Laryngoscope* 1970;80:249–253.
9. Bocca E, Sixteenth Daniel C, Baker, Jr. Memorial Lecture. Surgical management of supraglottic cancer and its lymph node metastases in a conservative perspective. *Ann Otol Rhinol Laryngol* 1991;100:261–267.
10. Broyles EN. The anterior commissure tendon. *Ann Otol Rhinol Laryngol* 1943;52:342–345.
11. Burstein FD, Calcaterra TC. Supraglottic laryngectomy: Series report and analysis of results. *Laryngoscope* 1985;95:833–836.
12. Clemente CD. *Anatomy: A regional atlas of the human body*. Philadelphia: Lea & Febiger; 1975.
13. Crampette L, Garrel R, Gardiner Q, et al. Modified subtotal laryngectomy with cricohyoidoepiglottopexy—Long term results in 81 patients. *Head Neck* 1999;21:95–103.
14. Csanády M, Iván L, Czigner J. Endoscopic CO$_2$ laser therapy of selected cases of supraglottic marginal tumors. *Eur Arch Otorhinolaryngol* 1999;256:392–394.
15. Davis RK, Kelly SM, Hayes J. Endoscopic CO$_2$ laser excisional biopsy of early supraglottic cancer. *Laryngoscope* 1991;101:680–683.
16. Department of Veterans Affairs Laryngeal Cancer Study Group. Induction chemotherapy plus radiation compared with surgery plus radiation in patients with advanced laryngeal cancer. *N Engl J Med* 1991;324:1685–1690.
17. DeSanto LW. Early supraglottic cancer. *Ann Otol Rhinol Laryngol* 1990;99:593–597.
18. Fletcher GH. Elective irradiation of subclinical disease in cancers of the head and neck. *Cancer* 1972;29:1450–1454.
19. Fletcher GH, Goepfert H. Larynx and pyriform sinus. In: Fletcher GH, ed. *Textbook of Radiotherapy*, 3rd ed. Philadelphia: Lea & Febiger; 1980:330–363.
20. Fletcher GH, Hamberger AD. Causes of failure in irradiation of squamous-cell carcinoma of the supraglottic larynx. *Radiology* 1974;111:697–700.
21. Fletcher GH, Lindberg RD, Jesse RH. Radiation therapy for cancer of the larynx and pyriform sinus. *Eye Ear Nose Throat Digest* 1969;31:58–67.
22. Foote RL, Olsen KD, Buskirk SJ, et al. Laryngectomy alone for T3 glottic cancer. *Head Neck* 1994;16:406–412.
23. Forastiere AA, Goepfert H, Maor M, et al. Concurrent chemotherapy and radiotherapy for organ preservation in advanced laryngeal cancer. *N Engl J Med* 2003;349:2091–2098.
24. Fu KK, Pajak TF, Trotti A, et al. A Radiation Therapy Oncology Group (RTOG) phase III randomized study to compare hyperfractionation and two variants of accelerated fractionation to standard fractionation radiotherapy for head and neck squamous cell carcinomas: First report of RTOG 9003. *Int J Radiat Oncol Biol Phys* 2000;48:7–16.
25. Gall AM, Sessions DG, Ogura JH. Complications following surgery for cancer of the larynx and hypopharynx. *Cancer* 1977;39:624–631.
26. Gallo A, de Vincentiis M, Manciocco V, et al. CO$_2$ laser cordectomy for early-stage glottic carcinoma: A long-term follow-up of 156 cases. *Laryngoscope* 2003;112:370–374.
27. Garcia-Serra A, Amdur RJ, Morris CG, et al. Thyroid function should be monitored following radiotherapy to the low neck. *Am J Clin Oncol* 2005;28:255–258.
28. Garcia-Serra A, Hinerman RW, Amdur RJ, et al. Radiotherapy for carcinoma in situ of the true vocal cords. *Head Neck* 2002;24:390–394.
29. Garden AS, Forster K, Wong PF, et al. Results of radiotherapy for T2N0 glottic carcinoma: Does the "2" stand for twice-daily treatment? *Int J Radiat Oncol Biol Phys* 2003;55:322–328.
30. Ghossein NA, Bataini JP, Ennuyer A, et al. Local control and site of failure in radically irradiated supraglottic laryngeal cancer. *Radiology* 1974;112:187–192.
31. Gindhart TD, Johnston WH, Chism SE, et al. Carcinoma of the larynx in childhood. *Cancer* 1980;46:1683–1687.
32. Giovanni A, Guelfucci B, Gras R, et al. Partial frontolateral laryngectomy with epiglottic reconstruction for management of early-stage glottic carcinoma. *Laryngoscope* 2001;111:663–668.
33. Gregor RT, Oei SS, Baris G, et al. Supraglottic laryngectomy with postoperative radiation versus primary radiation in the management of supraglottic laryngeal cancer. *Am J Otolaryngol* 1996;17:316–321.
34. Harwood AR, Beale FA, Cummings BJ, et al. T3 glottic cancer: An analysis of dose-time-volume factors. *Int J Radiat Oncol Biol Phys* 1980;6:675–680.
35. Harwood AR, Beale FA, Cummings BJ, et al. T4N0M0 glottic cancer: An analysis of dose-time-volume factors. *Int J Radiat Oncol Biol Phys* 1981;7:1507–1512.
36. Harwood AR, Beale FA, Cummings BJ, et al. T2 glottic cancer: An analysis of dose-time-volume factors. *Int J Radiat Oncol Biol Phys* 1981;7:1501–1505.
37. Harwood AR, Hawkins NV, Rider WD, et al. Radiotherapy of early glottic cancer. I. *Int J Radiat Oncol Biol Phys* 1979;5:473–476.
38. Hillman RE, Walsh MJ, Wolf GT, et al. Functional outcomes following treatment for advanced laryngeal cancer. Part I. Voice preservation in advanced laryngeal cancer. Part II. Laryngectomy rehabilitation: The state of the art in VA system. *Ann Otol Rhinol Laryngol* 1998;107:2–27.
39. Hinerman RW, Mendenhall WM, Amdur RJ, et al. Carcinoma of the supraglottic larynx: Treatment results with radiotherapy alone or with planned neck dissection. *Head Neck* 2002;24:456–467.
40. Hirano M. Structure and vibratory behavior of the vocal folds. In: Sawashima M, Cooper FS, eds. *Dynamic aspects of speech production: Current results, emerging problems, and new instrumentation*. Tokyo: University of Tokyo Press; 1977:13–27.
41. Huang DT, Johnson CR, Schmidt-Ullrich R, et al. Postoperative radiotherapy in head and neck carcinoma with extracapsular lymph node extension and/or positive resection margins: A comparative study. *Int J Radiat Oncol Biol Phys* 1992;23:737–742.
42. Isaacs JH.Jr, Slattery WH.III, Mendenhall WM, et al. Supraglottic laryngectomy. *Am J Otolaryngol* 1998;19:118–123.
43. Jemal A, Murray T, Samuels A, et al. Cancer statistics, 2003. *CA Cancer J Clin* 2003;53:5–26.
44. Jesse RH. The evaluation of treatment of patients with extensive squamous cancer of the vocal cords. *Laryngoscope* 1975;85:1424–1429.
45. Kim RY, Marks ME, Salter MM. Early-stage glottic cancer: Importance of dose fractionation in radiation therapy. *Radiology* 1992;182:273–275.
46. Kirchner JA. Staging as seen in serial sections. *Laryngoscope* 1975;85:1816–1821.
47. Laccourreye H, Laccourreye O, Weinstein G, et al. Supracricoid laryngectomy with cricohyoidoepiglottopexy: A partial laryngeal procedure for glottic carcinoma. *Ann Otol Rhinol Laryngol* 1990;99:421–426.
48. Laccourreye O, Weinstein G, Brasnu D, et al. A clinical trial of continuous cisplatin-fluorouracil induction chemotherapy and supracricoid partial laryngectomy for glottic carcinoma classified as T2. *Cancer* 1994;74:2781–2790.
49. Lam KH, Wong J. The preepiglottic and paraglottic spaces in relation to spread of carcinoma of the larynx. *Am J Otolaryngol* 1983;4:81–91.
50. Le Q-TX, Fu KK, Kroll S, et al. Influence of fraction size, total dose, and overall time on local control of T1–T2 glottic carcinoma. *Int J Radiat Oncol Biol Phys* 1997;39:115–126.
51. Le QT, Fu KK, Kroll S, et al. Influence of fraction size, total dose, and overall time on local control of T1–T2 glottic carcinoma. *Int J Radiat Oncol Biol Phys* 1997;39:115–126.
52. Lederman M. Place de la radiotherapie dans le traitment du cancer du larynx [The place of radiotherapy in the treatment of cancer of the larynx]. *Ann Radiol (Paris)* 1961;4:443–454.
53. Lee F, Perlmutter S, Ogura JH. Laryngeal radiation after hemilaryngectomy. *Laryngoscope* 1980;90:1534–1539.
54. Lee NK, Goepfert H, Wendt CD. Supraglottic laryngectomy for intermediate-stage cancer: U.T. M.D. Anderson Cancer Center experience with combined therapy. *Laryngoscope* 1990;100:831–836.
55. Lindberg RD. Distribution of cervical lymph node metastases from squamous cell carcinoma of the upper respiratory and digestive tracts. *Cancer* 1972;29:1446–1449.
56. Lutz CK, Johnson JT, Wagner RL, et al. Supraglottic carcinoma: Patterns of recurrence. *Ann Otol Rhinol Laryngol* 1990;99:12–17.
57. Mancuso AA, Hanafee WN. *Computed tomography and magnetic resonance imaging of the head and neck*, 2nd ed. Baltimore, MD: Williams & Wilkins; 1985.
58. McGuirt WF, Blalock D, Koufman JA, et al. Comparative voice results after laser resection or irradiation of T1 vocal cord carcinoma. *Arch Otolaryngol Head Neck Surg* 1994;120:951–955.
59. McLaughlin MP, Mendenhall WM, Mancuso AA, et al. Retropharyngeal adenopathy as a predictor of outcome in squamous cell carcinoma of the head and neck. *Head Neck* 1995;17:190–198.
60. Mendenhall WM, Amdur RJ, Morris CG, et al. T1-T2N0 squamous cell carcinoma of the glottic larynx treated with radiation therapy. *J Clin Oncol* 2001;19:4029–4036.
61. Mendenhall WM, Morris CG, Amdur RJ, et al. Parameters that predict local control following definitive radiotherapy for squamous cell carcinoma of the head and neck. *Head Neck* 2003;25:535–542.
62. Mendenhall WM, Morris CG, Stringer SP, et al. Voice rehabilitation after total laryngectomy and postoperative radiation therapy. *J Clin Oncol* 2002;20:2500–2505.
63. Mendenhall WM, Parsons JT, Brant TA, et al. Is elective neck treatment indicated for T2N0 squamous cell carcinoma of the glottic larynx? *Radiother Oncol* 1989;14:199–202.
64. Mendenhall WM, Parsons JT, Mancuso AA, et al, Cassisi NJ. Definitive radiotherapy for T3 squamous cell carcinoma of the glottic larynx. *J Clin Oncol* 1997;15:2394–2402.
65. Mendenhall WM, Parsons JT, Mancuso AA, et al. Larynx. In: Carlos A. Perez LWB, ed. *Principles and practice of radiation Oncology*, 3rd ed. Philadelphia: Lippincott-Raven; 1998:1069–1093.
66. Mendenhall WM, Parsons JT, Stringer SP, et al. T1-T2 vocal cord carcinoma: A basis for comparing the results of radiotherapy and surgery. *Head Neck Surg* 1988;10:373–377.
67. Mendenhall WM, Parsons JT, Stringer SP, et al. Stage T3 squamous cell carcinoma of the glottic larynx: A comparison of laryngectomy and irradiation. *Int J Radiat Oncol Biol Phys* 1992;23:725–732.
68. Mendenhall WM, Riggs CE, Amdur RJ, et al. Altered fractionation and/or adjuvant chemotherapy in definitive irradiation of squamous cell carcinoma of the head and neck. *Laryngoscope* 2003;113:546–551.
69. Mendenhall WM, Riggs CE, Cassisi NJ. Treatment of head and neck cancers. In: DeVita VT, Hellman S, Rosenberg SA, eds. *Cancer: Principles & practice of oncology*, 7th ed. Philadelphia: Lippincott Williams & Willkins; 2005:662–732.
70. Mendenhall WM, Villaret DB, Amdur RJ, et al. Planned neck dissection after

definitive radiotherapy for squamous cell carcinoma of the head and neck. *Head Neck* 2002;24:1012–1018.

71. Mendenhall WM, Werning JW, Hinerman RW, et al. Management of T1-T2 glottic carcinomas. *Cancer* 2004;100:1786–1792.

72. Million RR, Cassisi NJ. Larynx. In: Million RR, Cassisi NJ, eds. *Management of head and neck cancer: A multidisciplinary approach*, 1st ed. Philadelphia: JB Lippincott; 1984:315–364.

73. Million RR, Cassisi NJ, Mancuso AA. Larynx. In: Million RR, Cassisi NJ, eds. *Management of head and neck cancer: A multidisciplinary approach*, 2nd ed. Philadelphia: JB Lippincott; 1994:431–497.

74. Million RR, Cassisi NJ, Mancuso AA, et al. Management of the neck for squamous cell carcinoma. In: Million RR, Cassisi NJ, eds. *Management of head and neck cancer: A multidisciplinary approach*, 2nd ed. Philadelphia: JB Lippincott; 1994:75–142.

75. Mills EE. Early glottic carcinoma: Factors affecting radiation failure, results of treatment and sequelae. *Int J Radiat Oncol Biol Phys* 1979;5:811–817.

76. Motta G, Esposito E, Cassiano B, et al. T1-T2-T3 glottic tumors: Fifteen years experience with CO_2 laser. *Acta Otolaryngol Suppl* 1997;527:155–159.

77. Nakfoor BM, Spiro IJ, Wang CC, et al. Results of accelerated radiotherapy for supraglottic carcinoma: A Massachusetts General Hospital and Massachusetts Eye and Ear Infirmary experience. *Head Neck* 1998;20:379–384.

78. Neel HB, III, Devine KD, DeSanto LW. Laryngofissure and cordectomy for early cordal carcinoma: Outcome in 182 patients. *Otolaryngol Head Neck Surg* 1980;88:79–84.

79. O'Sullivan B, Mackillop W, Gilbert R, et al. Controversies in the management of laryngeal cancer: Results of an international survey of patterns of care. *Radiother Oncol* 1994;31:23–32.

80. O'Sullivan B, Warde P, Keane T, et al. Outcome following radiotherapy in verrucous carcinoma of the larynx. *Int J Radiat Oncol Biol Phys* 1995;32:611–617.

81. Ogura JH, Biller HF, Wette R. Elective neck dissection for pharyngeal and laryngeal cancers: An evaluation. *Ann Otol Rhinol Laryngol* 1971;80:646–651.

82. Ogura JH, Sessions DG, Ciralsky RH. Supraglottic carcinoma with extension to the arytenoid. *Laryngoscope* 1975;85:1327–1331.

83. Ogura JH, Sessions DG, Spector GJ. Conservation surgery for epidermoid carcinoma of the supraglottic larynx. *Laryngoscope* 1975;85:1808–1815.

84. Olofsson J, van Nostrand AWP. Growth and spread of laryngeal and hypopharyngeal carcinoma with reflections on the effect of preoperative irradiation: 139 cases studied by whole organ serial sectioning. *Acta Otolaryngol Suppl (Stockh)* 1973;308:1–84.

85. Parsons JT, Mendenhall WM, Mancuso AA, et al. Twice-a-day radiotherapy for T3 squamous cell carcinoma of the glottic larynx. *Head Neck* 1989;11:123–128.

86. Parsons JT, Mendenhall WM, Stringer SP, et al. T4 laryngeal carcinoma: Radiotherapy alone with surgery reserved for salvage. *Int J Radiat Oncol Biol Phys* 1998;40:549–552.

87. Parsons JT, Mendenhall WM, Stringer SP, et al. Salvage surgery following radiation failure in squamous cell carcinoma of the supraglottic larynx. *Int J Radiat Oncol Biol Phys* 1995;32:605–609.

88. Pearson BW, Woods RD, Hartman DE. Extended hemilaryngectomy for T3 glottic carcinoma with preservation of speech and swallowing. *Laryngoscope* 1980;90:1950–1961.

89. Peretti G, Nicolai P, Redaelli De Zinis LO, et al. Endoscopic CO_2 laser excision for Tis, T1, and T2 glottic carcinomas: Cure rate and prognostic factors. *Otolaryngol Head Neck Surg* 2000;123:124–131.

90. Pignon JP, Bourhis J, Domenge C, et al. MACH-NC (Meta-Analysis of Chemotherapy on Head and Neck Cancer) Collaborative Group. Chemotherapy added to locoregional treatment for head and neck squamous-cell carcinoma: Three meta-analyses of updated individual data. *Lancet* 2000;355:949–955.

91. Pillsbury HR, Kirchner JA. Clinical vs histopathologic staging in laryngeal cancer. *Arch Otolaryngol* 1979;105:157–159.

92. Pradhan SA, Pai PS, Neeli SI, et al. Transoral laser surgery for early glottic cancers. *Arch Otolaryngol Head Neck Surg* 2003;129:623–625.

93. Ries LAG, Eisner MP, Kosary CL, et al. SEER cancer statistics review, *1973–1998*. Bethesda, MD: National Cancer Institute; 2001.

94. Robbins KT, Davidson W, Peters LJ, et al. Conservation surgery for T2 and T3 carcinomas of the supraglottic larynx. *Arch Otolaryngol Head Neck Surg* 1988;114:421–426.

95. Rudert HH, Werner JA. Endoscopic resections of glottic and supraglottic carcinomas with the CO_2 laser. *Eur Arch Otorhinolaryngol* 1995;252:146–148.

96. Rudert HH, Werner JA, Höft S. Transoral carbon dioxide laser resection of supraglottic carcinoma. *Ann Otol Rhinol Laryngol* 1999;108:819–827.

97. Schwaibold F, Scariato A, Nunno M, et al. The effect of fraction size on control of early glottic cancer. *Int J Radiat Oncol Biol Phys* 1988;14:451–454.

98. Skolnik EM, Yee KF, Wheatley MA, et al. Carcinoma of the laryngeal glottis: Therapy and end results. *Laryngoscope* 1975;85:1453–1466.

99. Skolyszewski J, Reinfuss M. The results of radiotherapy of cancer of the larynx in six European countries. *Radiobiol Radiother (Berl)* 1981;22:32–43.

100. Spector JG, Sessions DG, Chao KS, et al. Stage I (T1 N0 M0) squamous cell carcinoma of the laryngeal glottis: Therapeutic results and voice preservation. *Head Neck* 1999;21:707–717.

101. Spector JG, Sessions DG, Chao KSC, et al. Management of stage II (T2N0M0) glottic carcinoma by radiotherapy and conservation surgery. *Head Neck* 1999;21:116–123.

102. Spriano G, Antognoni P, Piantanida R, et al. Conservative management of T1-T2N0 supraglottic cancer: A retrospective study. *Am J Otolaryngol* 1997;18:299–305.

103. Steiner W. Results of curative laser microsurgery of laryngeal carcinomas. *Am J Otolaryngol* 1993;14:116–121.

104. Steiniger JR, Parnes SM, Gardner GM. Morbidity of combined therapy for the treatment of supraglottic carcinoma: Supraglottic laryngectomy and radiotherapy. *Ann Otol Rhinol Laryngol* 1997;106:151–158.

105. Stewart JG, Brown JR, Palmer MK, et al. The management of glottic carcinoma by primary irradiation with surgery in reserve. *Laryngoscope* 1975;85:1477–1484.

106. Stewart JG, Jackson AW. The steepness of the dose response curve both for tumor cure and normal tissue injury. *Laryngoscope* 1975;85:1107–1111.

107. Sykes AJ, Slevin NJ, Gupta NK, et al. 331 cases of clinically node-negative supraglottic carcinoma of the larynx: A study of a modest size fixed field radiotherapy approach. *Int J Radiat Oncol Biol Phys* 2000;46:1109–1115.

108. Thomas JV, Olsen KD, Neel HB III, et al. Early glottic carcinoma treated with open laryngeal procedures. *Arch Otolaryngol Head Neck Surg* 1994;120:264–268.

109. Trotti A, Fu KK, Pajak TF, et al. Long term outcomes of RTOG 90-03: A comparison of hyperfractionation and two variants of accelerated fractionation to standard fractionation radiotherapy for head and neck squamous cell carcinoma. *Int J Radiat Oncol Biol Phys* 2005;63:S70–S71(abstr).

110. Vermund H. Role of radiotherapy in cancer of the larynx as related to the TNM system of staging. A review. *Cancer* 1970;25:485–504.

111. Vincent RG, Marchetta F. The relationship of the use of tobacco and alcohol to cancer of the oral cavity, pharynx or larynx. *Am J Surg* 1963;106:501–505.

112. Wagonfeld DJ, Harwood AR, Bryce DP, et al. Second primary respiratory tract malignancies in glottic carcinoma. *Cancer* 1980;46:1883–1886.

113. Wang CC. Radiation therapy of laryngeal tumors: Curative radiation therapy. In: Thawley SE, Panje WR, eds. *Comprehensive management of head and neck tumors*. Philadelphia: WB Saunders; 1987:906–919.

114. Wang CC. Carcinoma of the larynx. In: Wang CC, ed. *Radiation therapy for head and neck neoplasms*, 3rd ed. New York: Wiley-Liss, Inc; 1997:221–255.

115. Wang CC, Montgomery WM. Deciding on optimal management of supraglottic carcinoma. *Oncology* 1991;5:41–46.

116. Warde P, O'Sullivan B, Bristow RG, et al. T1–T2 glottic cancer managed by external beam radiotherapy: The influence of pretreatment hemoglobin on local control. *Int J Radiat Oncol Biol Phys* 1998;41:347–353.

117. Weber PC, Johnson JT, Myers EN. Impact of bilateral neck dissection on recovery following supraglottic laryngectomy. *Arch Otolaryngol Head Neck Surg* 1993;119:61–64.

118. Weems DH, Mendenhall WM, Parsons JT, et al. Squamous cell carcinoma of the supraglottic larynx treated with surgery and/or radiation therapy. *Int J Radiat Oncol Biol Phys* 1987;13:1483–1487.

119. Woodhouse RJ, Quivey JM, Fu KK, et al. Treatment of carcinoma of the vocal cord: A review of 20 years experience. *Laryngoscope* 1981;91:1155–1162.

120. Wynder EL. The epidemiology of cancers of the upper alimentary and upper respiratory tracts. *Laryngoscope* 1978;88:50–51.

121. Yamazaki H, Nishiyama K, Tanaka E, et al. Radiotherapy for early glottic carcinoma (T1N0M0): Results of prospective randomized study of radiation fraction size and overall treatment time. *Int J Radiat Oncol Biol Phys* 2006;64:77–82.

122. Zeitels SM, Koufman JA, Davis RK, et al. Endoscopic treatment of supraglottic and hypopharynx cancer. *Laryngoscope* 1994;104:71–78.

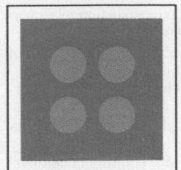

Chapter 45
Unusual Nonepithelial Tumors of the Head and Neck

Carlos A. Perez, Wade L. Thorstad

Glomus Tumors

Anatomy

Glomus bodies are found in the jugular bulb and along the tympanic (Jacobson) and auricular (Arnold) branch of the tenth nerve in the middle ear or in other anatomic sites (Fig. 45.1). Depending on the location, glomus tumors (chemodectoma or paraganglioma) can be classified as tympanic (middle ear), jugulare, or carotid vagal, or designated as originating from other locations, such as the larynx, adventitia of thoracic aorta, abdominal aorta, or surface of the lungs (56,152) (Fig. 45.2). These tissues are responsive to changes in oxygen and carbon dioxide tensions and pH.

Glomus tumors consist of large epithelioid (smooth muscle) cells with fine granular cytoplasm embedded in a rich capillary network and fibrous stroma with reticulin fibers, which derive from embryonic neural crest cells. Although histologically benign, they may extend along the lumen of the vein to regional lymph nodes, but rarely to distant sites.

Epidemiology

The mean age at diagnosis has been reported to be 44.7 years for carotid body tumors (196) and 52 years for glomus tympanicum (157). These tumors occur three or four times more frequently in women than in men, suggesting a possible estrogen influence (145,157,181). Glomus tumors may be familial; they also occur in multiple sites in 10% to 20% of patients (167,194).

Bilateral carotid glomus tumors were reported in six of 16 patients (38%) with a positive family history for these lesions but in only 17/206 patients (8%) without such a history (196). Multiple paragangliomas of the head and neck are rare (incidence of 10% of the total patients, but in familial cases it increases up to 35% to 50%) (167). In the head and neck region, the most common association is bilateral carotid body tumors or carotid body tumor associated with tympanic-jugular glomus.

Clinical Presentation

Glomus tumors may arise along the nerve roots. Glomus tumors of the middle ear may initially cause earache or discomfort. As they expand, eventually they produce pulsatile tinnitus, hearing loss, and, in later stages, cranial nerve paralysis resulting from invasion of the base of the skull in 10% to 15% of patients. Some patients endure ear symptoms for 3 to 5 years before seeking medical attention.

If the tumor invades the middle cranial fossa, symptoms may include temporoparietal headache, retro-orbital pain, proptosis, and paresis of cranial nerves V and VI. If the posterior fossa is involved, symptoms may include occipital headache, ataxia, and paresis of cranial nerves V to VII, IX, and XII; invasion of the jugular foramen causes paralysis of nerves IX to XI. Gaut et al. (95) described a case of a large intranasal glomus tumor that, at presentation, had eroded through the ethmoid roof to involve the floor of the anterior cranial fossa. The patient was treated with primary external-beam radiotherapy. To our knowledge,

this is the first report of an invasive glomus tumor of the head and neck.

Chemodectoma of the carotid body usually presents as a painless, slowly growing mass in the upper neck. Occasionally the mass may be pulsatile and may have an associated thrill or bruit. As it enlarges, the mass may extend into the parapharyngeal space and be visible on examination of the oropharynx. Very rarely these tumors may be malignant (171).

Metastases occur in 2% to 5% of cases (145,220).

Diagnostic Work-Up

Diagnostic evaluation for glomus tumors of the ear and base of skull is outlined in Table 45.1. In the majority of glomus tympanicum tumors, physical examination demonstrates a red, vascular middle ear mass, although occasionally it may be bluish or white (the latter resembling a cholesteatoma) (157). Audiography may demonstrate conductive hearing loss in the ear involved by tumor as noted in 33/49 patients evaluated by Larson et al. (157); four of 33 patients with conductive deficits also exhibited tympanic pulsations. Examination of the neck may occasionally demonstrate a mass in the neck that may be pulsatile or have a bruit or regional lymph node metastases.

Radiographic studies are invaluable in the diagnosis of these tumors. Plain mastoid radiographs never show the soft-tissue mass in the middle ear, although they frequently demonstrate clouding of the mastoid air cells, suggesting mastoiditis (157). High-resolution computed tomography (CT) with contrast has the highest degree of sensitivity and specificity to diagnose this tumor when located in the middle ear or jugular bulb; masses as small as 3 mm have been demonstrated in the middle ear. Tumor enhancement is similar to that of the temporalis muscle (157) (Fig. 45.3). In 46 patients with glomus tympanicum chemodectomas, there were no instances of local bony erosion; instead, the tumors engulfed the ossicular chain, bulged or protruded through the tympanic membrane, filled the middle ear, or extended into the eustachian tube orifice or aditus ad antrum. This pattern is in contrast to cholesteatomas, which typically destroy adjacent bony landmarks including the ossicles and progressively erode the petrous bones as they enlarge (157).

Magnification angiography is a sensitive and specific means of detecting glomus tympanicum tumors. This procedure should be performed after high-resolution thin-section CT scan (with contrast material), only when there is a question regarding the nature of the lesion or the location of the carotid canal. Findings include a hypervascular middle ear mass that first appears in the middle to late arterial phase, persists through the capillary phase, and quickly disappears in the venous phase without demonstrably early draining veins (162). Biopsy of an aberrant internal carotid artery can result in major neurologic sequelae or death.

Vogl et al. (275) reported on 40 patients with glomus tumors of the skull; diagnostic interpretations were correlated with histologic examination, digital subtraction angiography, CT, and clinical follow-up. Sixteen of 18 proven tumors were detected with spin-echo images alone. Although four high-flying jugular bulbs were misinterpreted as tumor because of similar signal

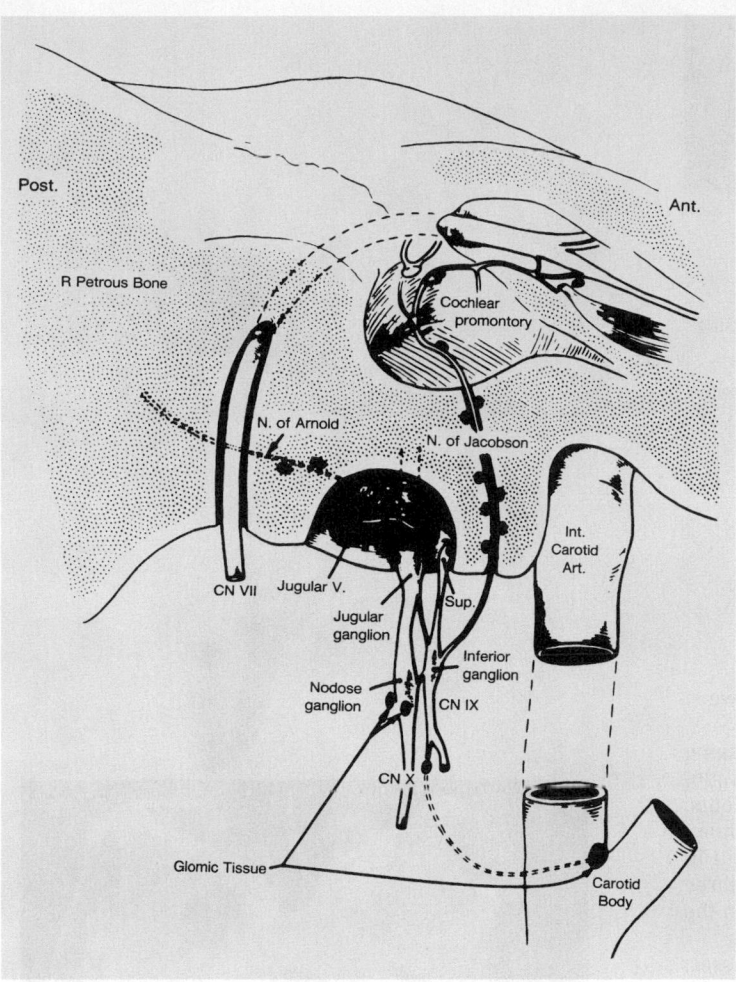

FIGURE 45.1. Anatomy of the region of the glomus jugulare. (From Hatfield PM, James AE, Schulz MN. Chemodectomas of the glomus jugulare. *Cancer* 1972;30:1165–1168, with permission.)

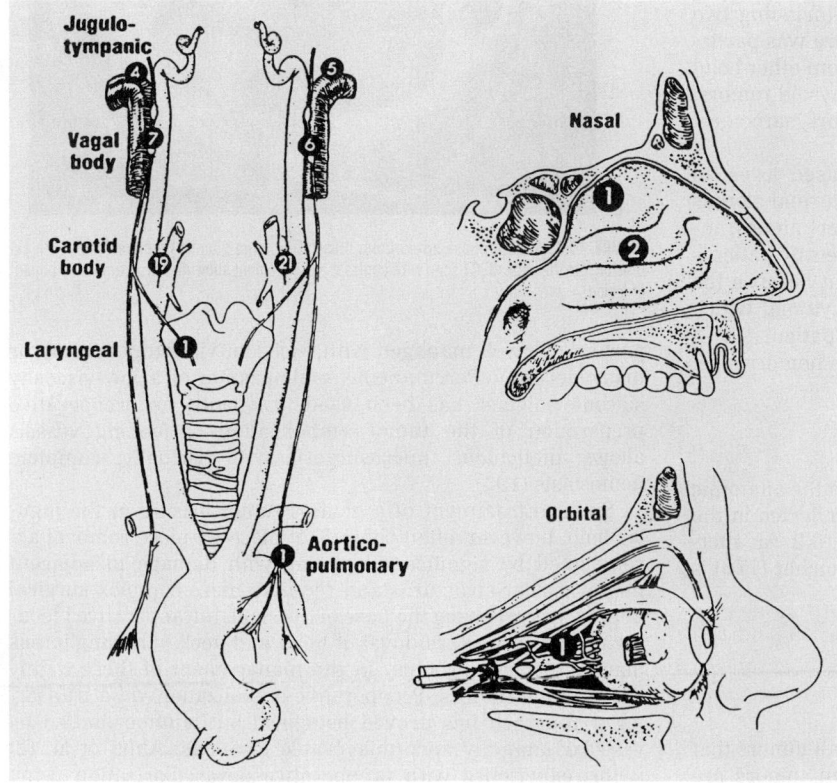

FIGURE 45.2. Distribution of paragangliomas of the head and neck region. Laterality was not specified in three patients with carotid body paragangliomas. The diagram does not include one left carotid body paraganglioma that was found incidentally at autopsy and a left vagal body paraganglioma that presented in a patient who had two other paragangliomas. (From Lack EE, Cubilla AL, Woodruff JM, et al. Paragangliomas of the head and neck region. *Cancer* 1977;39:3997–4009, with permission.)

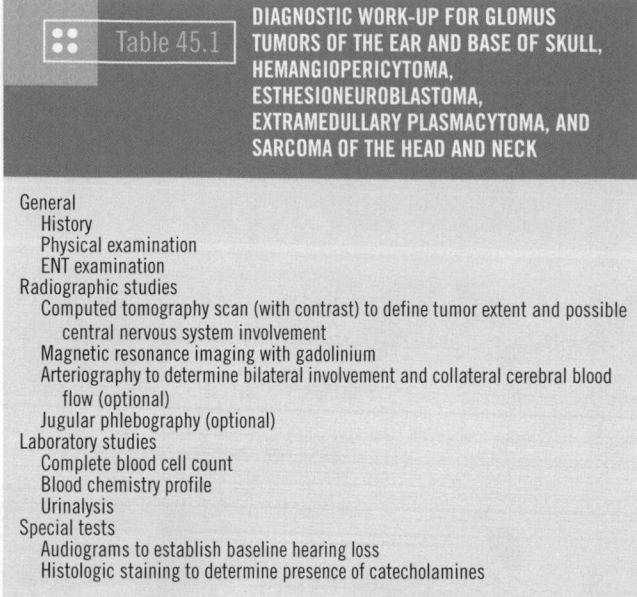

	DIAGNOSTIC WORK-UP FOR GLOMUS TUMORS OF THE EAR AND BASE OF SKULL, HEMANGIOPERICYTOMA, ESTHESIONEUROBLASTOMA, EXTRAMEDULLARY PLASMACYTOMA, AND SARCOMA OF THE HEAD AND NECK
Table 45.1	

General
  History
  Physical examination
  ENT examination
Radiographic studies
  Computed tomography scan (with contrast) to define tumor extent and possible
    central nervous system involvement
  Magnetic resonance imaging with gadolinium
  Arteriography to determine bilateral involvement and collateral cerebral blood
    flow (optional)
  Jugular phlebography (optional)
Laboratory studies
  Complete blood cell count
  Blood chemistry profile
  Urinalysis
Special tests
  Audiograms to establish baseline hearing loss
  Histologic staining to determine presence of catecholamines

intensity, combined evaluation allowed differentiation between tumor and sinusal blood flow in all cases.

Drape et al. (68) described magnetic resonance imaging (MRI) findings in 31 patients with a clinical suspicion of glomus tumor; gadoterate meglumine was injected in 19 patients. Twenty-seven of 28 pathologically confirmed glomus tumors were detected with MRI; a peripheral capsule was present in most tumors. The investigators were able to differentiate three subtypes of glomus tumors (vascular, solid, and myxoid) on the basis of relaxation times and enhancement characteristics.

Laird et al. (153) reported on 30 patients with neck masses; a bolus injection of ^{99m}Tc gluconate (20 mCi injected into the basilic vein) immediately followed by rapid injection of saline and scanning of the head and neck demonstrated glomus jugulare or carotid body tumors in seven patients, including two with clinically unsuspected tumors. The procedure was particularly useful in differentiating chemodectomas from other head and neck lesions such as thyroid tumors, parathyroid tumors, cystic hygromas, bronchogenic cysts, neural tumors, sarcomas, and lymph nodes.

Cytochemical techniques demonstrate increased levels of serotonin, epinephrine, and norepinephrine in normal glomus tissue of the carotid body. Histologic staining techniques, including chromatin and argentaffin reactions, identify patients with hormonally active tumors. This is important because the glomus tumor may coexist with a pheochromocytoma, which requires special preoperative preparation of the patient.

Biopsy of glomus tumors may result in severe hemorrhage.

Staging

The prognosis of these tumors is closely related to the anatomic location and the volume of the lesion, which is reflected in the Glasscock-Jackson classification shown in Table 45.2. An alternative classification proposed by McCabe and Fletcher (176) is presented in Table 45.3.

General Management

Surgery

Surgery is generally selected for treatment of small tumors that can be completely excised. Glomus tympanicum tumors are

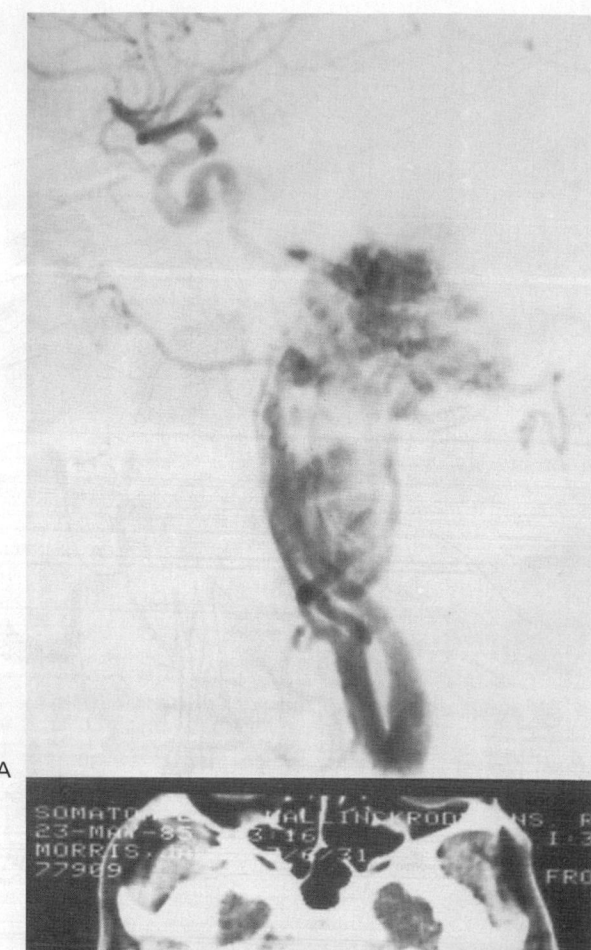

A

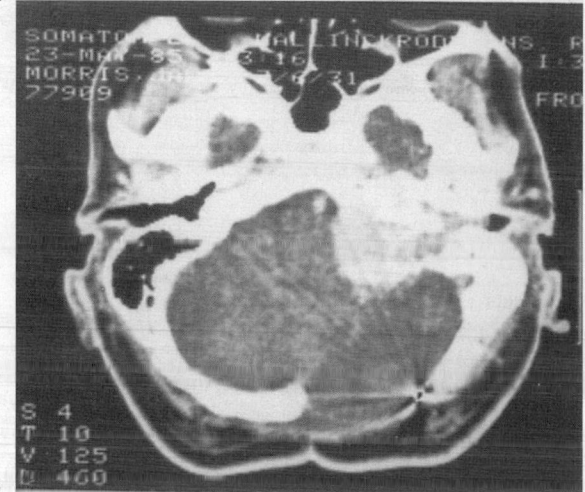

B

FIGURE 45.3. A: Late-phase arteriogram illustrating large glomus jugulare tumor with extension into the neck. **B:** CT scan with contrast enhancement showing intracranial component of lesion.

particularly well managed with excision, via tympanotomy or mastoidectomy. Percutaneous embolization of a low-viscosity silicone polymer has been used, frequently as preoperative preparation of the tumor embolization of feeding vessels allows meticulous microsurgery with virtually complete hemostasis (194).

Surgical treatment of a glomus tumor arising in the jugular bulb, however, often consists of piece-by-piece removal accompanied by significant bleeding with damage to adjacent neurovascular structures and requires more complex surgical approaches involving the base of the skull. Intraoperative bleeding during surgical removal of head and neck paragangliomas may be a major problem in the management of these highly vascularized tumors. Preoperative embolization via a transarterial approach has proved beneficial but is often limited by vascular anatomy and unfavorable locations. Abud et al. (2) report experience with preoperative devascularization using

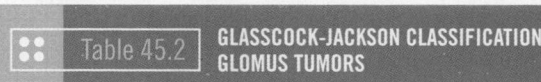

Table 45.2 | GLASSCOCK-JACKSON CLASSIFICATION OF GLOMUS TUMORS

Glomus tympanicum
I   Small mass limited to promontory
II Tumor completely filling middle ear space
III Tumor filling middle ear and extending into the mastoid
IV Tumor filling middle ear, extending into the mastoid or through tympanic membrane to fill the external auditory canal; may extend anterior to carotid

Glomus jugulare
I   Small tumor involving jugular bulb, middle ear, and mastoid
II Tumor extending under internal auditory canal; may have intracranial canal extension
III Tumor extending into petrous apex; may have intracranial canal extension
IV Tumor extending beyond petrous apex into clivus or infratemporal fossa; may have intracranial canal extension

From Jackson CG, Glasscock ME III, Harris PF. Glomus tumors: diagnosis, classification, and management of large lesions. *Arch Otolaryngol* 1982;108:401–406, with permission.

direct puncture and an intralesional injection of cyanoacrylate (acrylic glue) under fluoroscopic guidance in nine patients with head and neck paragangliomas. Angiograms showed that complete devascularization was achieved in all cervical glomus tumors, whereas subtotal devascularization was achieved in jugular paragangliomas, because the injection of acrylic glue was limited by the potential risk of reflux into normal brain via feeders from the internal carotid or vertebral artery. The tumors were surgically removed.

The local tumor control rate with surgery alone is only about 60%, and there is significant morbidity, particularly cranial nerve injury and bleeding.

In a retrospective review of all skull-base surgery cases treated at Baylor University 175 jugulotympanic glomus tumors and nine malignant cases (5.1%) were identified (171). The 5-year survival rate was 72%.

Radiation Therapy

Irradiation is frequently used in the treatment of glomus tumors, particularly for those in the tympanicum and jugulare bulb locations. Tumors with destruction of the petrous bone,

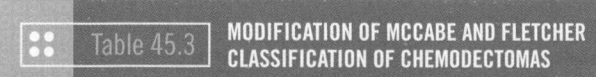

Table 45.3 | MODIFICATION OF MCCABE AND FLETCHER CLASSIFICATION OF CHEMODECTOMAS

Group I: Tympanic tumors
  Absence of bone destruction on x-rays of the mastoid bone and jugular fossa
  Absence of facial nerve weakness
  Intact eighth nerve with conductive deafness only
  Intact jugular foramen nerves (cranial nerves IX, X, and XI)

Group II: Tympanomastoid tumors
  X-ray evidence of bone destruction confined to the mastoid bone and not involving the petrous bone
  Normal or paretic seventh nerve
  Intact jugular foramen nerves
  No evidence of involvement of the superior bulb of the jugular vein on retrograde venogram

Group III: Petrosal and extrapetrosal tumors
  Destruction of the petrous bone, jugular fossa, and/or occipital bone on x-rays
  Positive findings on retrograde jugulography
  Evidence of destruction of the petrous or occipital bones on carotid arteriogram
  Jugular foramen syndrome (paresis of cranial nerves IX, X, or XI)
  Presence of metastasis

From Wang M-L, Hussey DH, Doornbos JF, et al. Chemodectoma of the temporal bone: a comparison of surgical and radiotherapeutic results. *Int J Radiat Oncol Biol Phys* 1988;14:643–648, with permission.

jugular fossa, or occipital bone or patients with jugular foramen syndrome are more reliably managed with irradiation (60,104,157,166,181,217,240). Some surgeons, such as Glasscock et al. (98) and Spector et al. (247), have questioned the effectiveness of radiation therapy in the treatment of chemodectomas because on histologic sections, obtained even many years after irradiation, it is possible to find chromophilic cells remaining in the tumor. However, there is also evidence of fibrosis and decreased vascularity (247). Suit and Gallager (256) demonstrated in a murine mammary carcinoma model that morphologically intact cells may have lost their reproductive ability after irradiation, which is the ultimate end point of cell killing. Furthermore, it is extremely unusual to observe clinical regrowth of a glomus tumor after irradiation, even if they do not regress completely.

Some reports describe successful combinations of surgery with either preoperative or postoperative irradiation (93,247), or preoperatively in an attempt to make an unresectable tumor operable, postoperatively when obvious tumor could not be resected.

Radiation Therapy Techniques

Radiation therapy techniques are determined by the location and extent of the tumor, which must be defined before treatment (53,185,249). Limited, usually bilateral, portals should be used for relatively localized glomus tumors, whether or not the treatment is combined with surgery (Fig. 45.4). Dickens et al. (63) used a three-field arrangement with a superior-inferior wedged and lateral open field, with a weighting of 1:1:0.33. Figure 45.5 shows superior-inferior 60-degree and 45-degree wedged filtered fields. Electrons (15 to 18 MeV) with a lateral portal or combined with cobalt-60 (^{60}Co) or 4- to 6-MV photons (20% to 25% of total tumor dose) render a good dose distribution (Fig. 45.6). In patients in whom tumor has spread into the posterior fossa, it may be necessary to use parallel opposed portals with 6- to 18-MV photons. Treatment is given at the rate of 1.8 to 2 Gy tumor dose per day with five treatments per week for a total tumor dose of 45 to 55 Gy in 5 weeks. Three-dimention (3D) conformal radiotherapy (RT) or image-guided radiation therapy (IMRT) are highly desirable techniques to treat these tumors, with excellent dose distributions (see Fig. 45.6). Table 45.4 summarizes the doses of irradiation recommended by several investigators and the probability of tumor control (185,249,280).

Leber et al. (158) reported on 13 patients with glomus tumors treated with radiosurgery because of recurrences after surgical removal in six patients. Histology was not available in seven patients, diagnosis was made from neuroradiological features only. Two patients had partial embolization before Gamma Knife (Elekta, Norcross, GA) treatment. Mean follow-up was 42 months (range, 14 to 72 months). Within the follow-up period there was no tumor progression and no clinical deterioration in any patient; 64% of the patients had an improvement of their symptoms, and in 36% the volume of the lesion decreased in size. There was no radiation-related morbidity.

Results of Therapy

The postirradiation change in tumor size is slow, with an increase in proliferative and perivascular fibrosis and minimal alterations in the chief epithelial cells (247). Histologic evaluation of tumor cell viability is not reliable (256). Despite the persistence of tumor both clinically and angiographically (166), amelioration of symptoms, absence of disease progression, and occasional return of cranial nerve function have been reported.

Seventeen patients were treated for glomus tympanicum tumors at Washington University (145). In five patients initial treatment consisted of irradiation alone, and all were

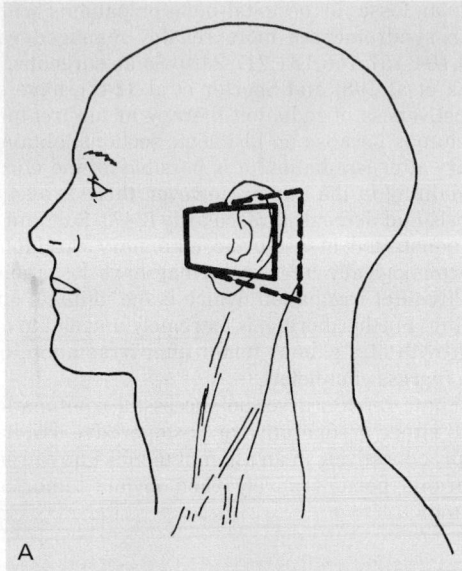

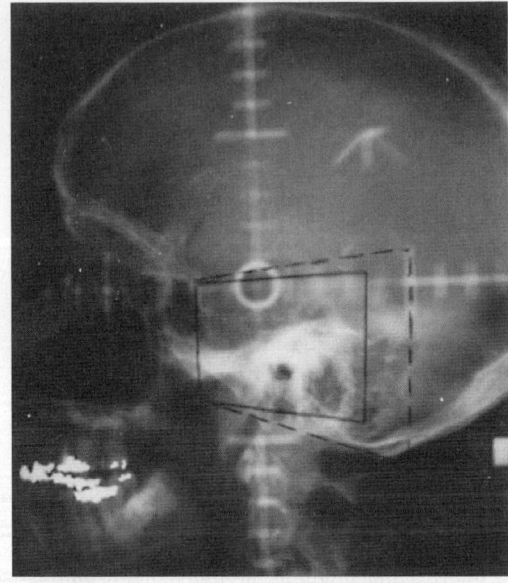

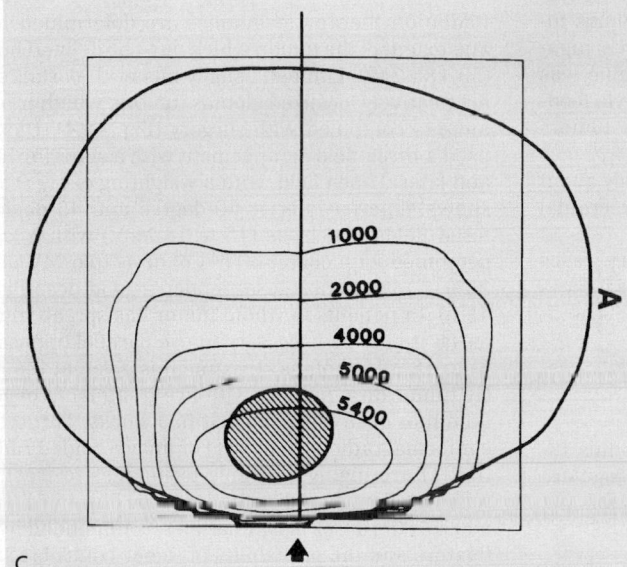

FIGURE 45.4 **A.** Portal used for relatively localized glomus tumor. **B.** Simulation film of patient with glomus tumor. **C.** Isodose distribution of a mixed-beam unilateral portal for a glomus tympanicum lesion (80% 16-MeV electrons, 20% 4-MV photons). (From Konefal JB, Pilepich MV, Spector GJ, et al. Radiation therapy in the treatment of chemodectomas. *Laryngoscope* 1987;97:1331–1335, with permission.)

tumorfree at last follow-up (4.5 years in one patient) or at death. Seven of eight patients irradiated for surgical recurrence were free of disease 4.5 to 19 years after irradiation. The remaining four patients were treated preoperatively or postoperatively; only one had recurrence and was salvaged surgically and tumorfree 10 years later. Of six patients with glomus jugulare lesions treated with irradiation, two with extensive lesions died of their disease, whereas the glomus tumor was controlled in four, including two patients with intracranial extension. Irradiation doses ranged from 46 to 52 Gy, with 86% to 100% tumor control with doses over 46 Gy and 50% (two of four) with doses below 46 Gy.

Of 19 patients treated with irradiation at the M.D. Anderson Cancer Center, five had only a biopsy without any surgical excision and 14 had partial excision (264). Ten patients had bony destruction; five of these had petrous pyramid and jugular foramen destruction, with accompanying multiple cranial nerve paralysis. Seventeen patients were treated with ^{60}Co anterior-posterior or superior-inferior wedged filtered fields, and two patients received electrons and photons (3:1) via a single

lateral field. Of 18 patients surviving a minimum of 5 years (13 surviving more than 10 years), all are alive and free of disease or have died of other causes.

Wang et al. (280) reported on 32 patients with tympanic chemodectomas; 13 treated with surgery alone, 15 with irradiation alone, and four with a combination of both modalities. The initial tumor control rate was 46% with surgery alone; ultimately 84% of patients were tumor-free after salvage with additional surgery. Although 78% survived 10 years, 31% developed complications. Of the patients treated with irradiation, 84% had initial local tumor control; 77% survived 10 years, and only 11% developed complications. The doses of irradiation used were slightly higher than those reported by others (mean 58.32 Gy). However, no improvement in tumor control was noted with higher doses. Complications occurred in two patients receiving 66 Gy.

In a compilation of several studies, Kim et al. (139) noted a 25% local failure rate in 83 patients treated with <40 Gy and 1.4% local failure in 142 patients receiving more than 40 Gy. Arthur (6) reported no recurrences in 24 patients treated with

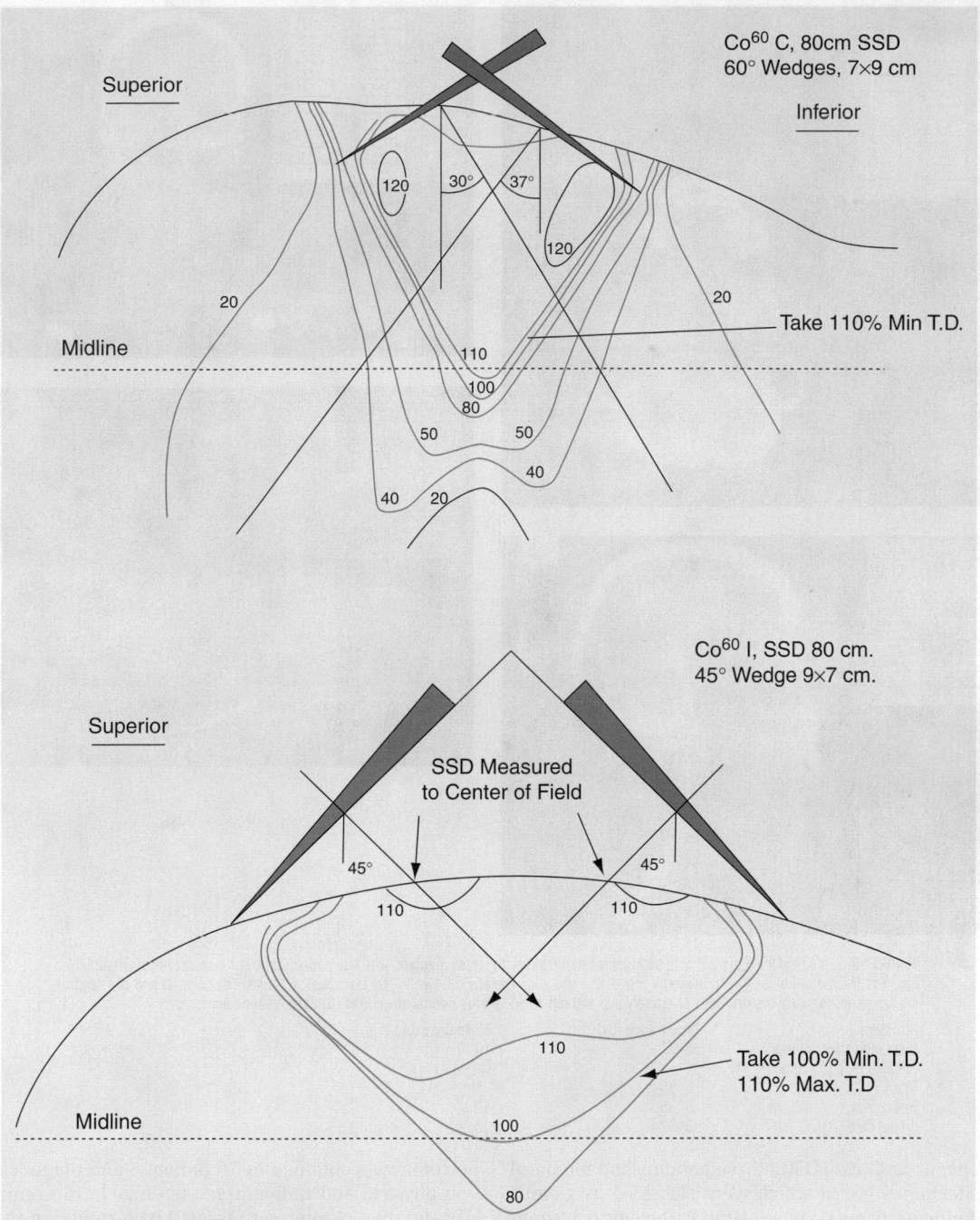

FIGURE 45.5. Isodose distributions using superior-inferior pairs of 60-degree **(A)** and 45-degree **(B)** converging wedge filtered ^{60}Co fields, demonstrating limited volume of irradiation. (From Tidwell TJ, Montague ED. Chemodectomas involving the temporal bone. *Radiology* 1975;116:147–149, with permission.)

doses of 45 to 50 Gy; only one failure was observed in a patient receiving 30 Gy in 15 fractions in 21 days. If the tolerances of the brain and brainstem to irradiation are considered, doses of 50 Gy (1.8- to 2-Gy fractions) are considered optimal for treatment of these lesions.

Powell et al. (216) reported on 84 patients with chemodectoma of the head and neck, 46 of which were in the glomus jugulare and tympanicum, treated with irradiation alone (45 to 50 Gy in 25 fractions). Local control of the lesion was 73% at 5 years. Thirty patients were treated with surgery after irradiation with no recurrences (median follow-up of 9 years). Four patients, treated with surgery alone, developed recurrences by 7 years. Four carotid body and glomus vagal tumors treated with irradiation were locally controlled at 1, 2, 8, and 11 years,

respectively. In 13 patients treated with surgery alone, the 15-year local control rate was 54%.

Mendenhall et al. (181) treated six chemodectomas of the carotid body and ganglion nodosum in four patients with doses of 40.8 to 48.5 Gy using ^{60}Co, 8-MV x-rays, or a combination of 8- and 17-MV x-rays. Lesions have remained stable in four patients 2 to 4.5 years after irradiation. Treatment results in a few patients with this type of tumor are summarized in Table 45.5.

Hinerman et al. (119) reported on 71 patients with 80 chemodectomas of the temporal bone, carotid bone, or glomus vagal treated with radiation therapy alone in 71 patients or subtotal resection and radiation therapy (eight tumors). Fourteen patients had undergone a previous treatment (surgery 11,

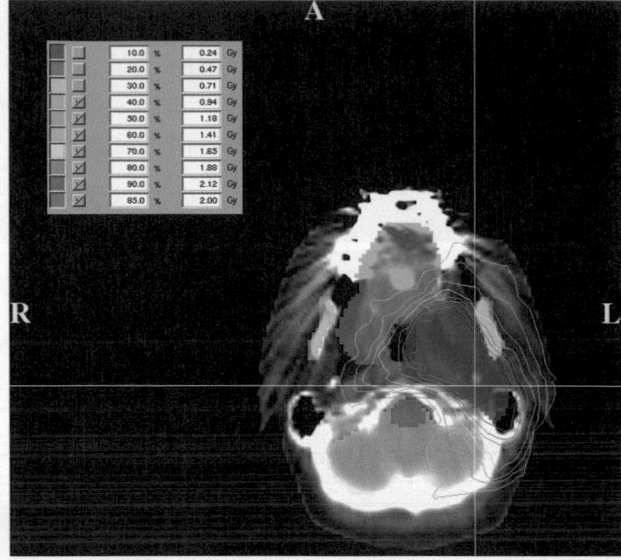

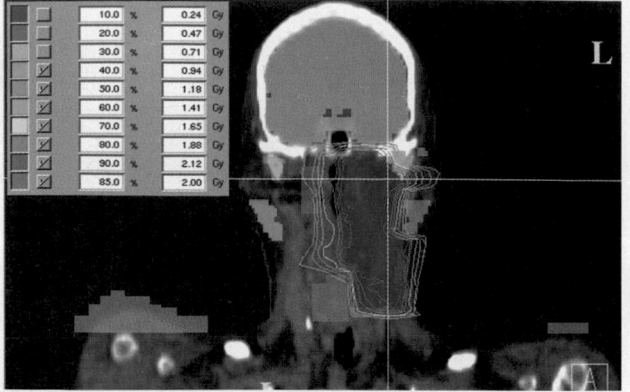

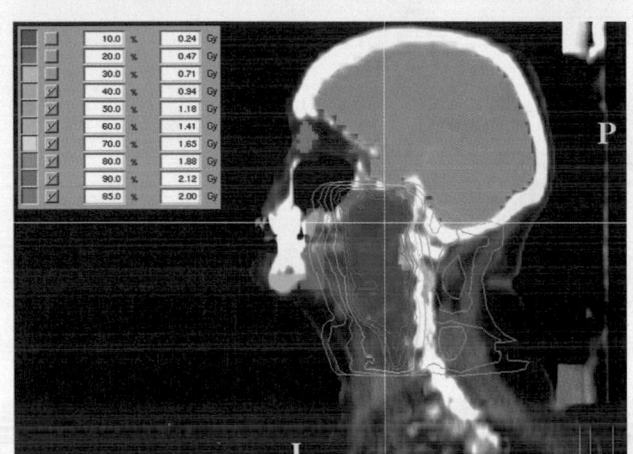

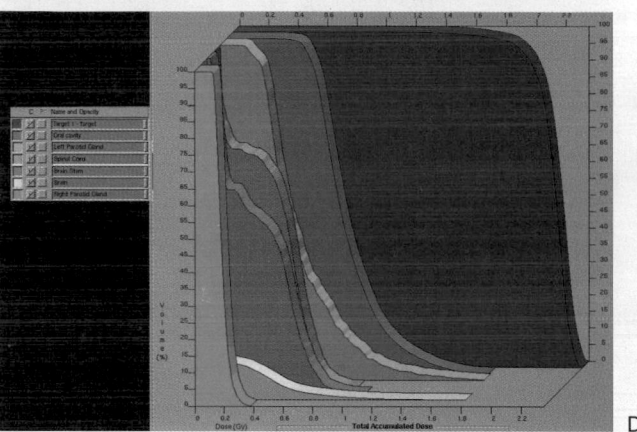

FIGURE 45.6. Female 59-years-old with an unusual malignant left glomus jugulare, who had a metastatic left upper cervical lymph node. She was treated definitively with intensity-modulated radiation therapy (66 Gy in 2-Gy fractions). **A:** Cross, **(B)** coronal, and **(C)** sagittal sections showing dose distributions at primary site and left neck, sparing normal structures **(D)** dose–volume histogram:

Structure	Dose Range (Gy)	Mean Dose (Gy)
Planning target volume (including left neck)	38–77	70
Brain	0–59	2
Brainstem	6–35	12
Spinal cord	0–32	13

irradiation one, or both two). Fifty-three patients had temporal bone chemodectomas, 46 of which were classified as glomus jugulare and nine as glomus tympanicum. Pathologic confirmation of chemodectomas was obtained in 21 patients and the diagnosis was made on physical or radiographic findings in the remaining 32 patients. Fifty patients were treated with radiation therapy alone and five with subtotal resection followed by postoperative radiation therapy for gross residual tumor. Median dose was 45 Gy with daily fractions of 1.5 to 2 Gy delivered with ^{60}Co, 6-MV, or 8-MV x-rays, or a combination of different beam energies. Twenty-eight patients were treated with ipsilateral wedge pair field arrangement, 18 with parallel-opposed fields; one patient was treated with stereotactic irradiation, and two were treated with three-dimensional conformal radiation therapy (3DCRT). Local control was obtained in 43 previously untreated lesions (93%) and in 11/12 (92%) previously chemodectomas. The results of treatment for temporal bone chemodectoma are summarized in Table 45.6.

Eighteen patients had 25 chemodectomas of carotid body and/or glomus vagal; 15 tumors originated in the carotid body and 10 in the glomus vagal. Pathologic confirmation of chemod-

ectoma was obtained in 10 patients, and diagnosis was based on physical and radiographic findings in the remaining eight. Twenty-two lesions were treated with radiation therapy alone, and two received postoperative radiation therapy after surgical resection for gross residual tumor with malignant changes and lymph node involvement. Patients with benign glomus tumors received 45 Gy in 25 fractions, in most instances, whereas patients with malignant carotid body tumors received 64.8 Gy to 70 Gy in 1.8 Gy fractions. Local tumor control was obtained in 14/15 carotid body and 10/10 glomus vagal (overall 96% tumor control) (274). The results of treatment for carotid body/glomus vagal are summarized in Table 45.7.

Complications were rare in patients treated with chemodectoma of the head and neck.

Hemangiopericytoma

Hemangiopericytomas are rare soft-tissue neoplasms that account for 3% to 5% of all soft-tissue sarcomas and 1% of all vascular tumors. Some 15% to 30% of all hemangiopericytomas

Clinical Radiation Oncology

Table 45.4 LOCAL CONTROL WITH RADIATION THERAPY FOR CHEMODECTOMA OF THE TEMPORAL BONE (GLOMUS TYMPANICUM AND JUGULARE)

Institution (Reference)	Local Control	Nominal Dosage Schedule
Princess Margaret Hospital (53)	42/45[a]	35 Gy/3 wk
Queen Elizabeth Hospital, Birmingham (6)	19/20[b]	45–50 Gy/4–5 wk
University of Washington (240)	10/13	8–65 Gy/4–7 wk
Rotterdamsch Radio-Therapeutisch Instituut, Netherlands (166)	19/19	40–60 Gy/4–6 wk
University of Minnesota (172)	13/14	30–60 Gy/3.5–7.5 wk
University of Virginia (104)	14/17	40–50 Gy/4–5 wk
University of Michigan	11/11	
Total	128/139 (92%)	

[a]Two patients listed as failures were salvaged with further treatments.
[b]One patient listed as a failure was salvaged with further radiation therapy.
Modified from Wang M-L, Hussey DH, Doornbos JF, et al. Chemodectoma of the temporal bone: a comparison of surgical and radiotherapeutic results. *Int J Radiat Oncol Biol Phys* 1987;14:643–648; and Springate SC, Weichselbaum RR. Radiation or surgery for chemodectoma of the temporal bone: a review of local control and complications. *Head Neck* 1990;12:303–307.

occur in the head and neck; of these, approximately 5% occur in the sinonasal area.

These tumors are believed to originate from the pericytes of Zimmerman extravascular cells morphologically resembling smooth muscle, found around the capillaries or from primitive mesenchymal cells. The function of the pericyte is uncertain but is believed to provide mechanical support for the capillaries having contractile function (254).

Epidemiology

Hemangiopericytomas is an unusual tumor; it represents approximately 1% of all vascular neoplasms; it occurs in both genders with equal frequency and is found primarily in adults. Only 45 cases of primary hemangiopericytomas of bone were described in the world literature in 1988.

In the head and neck, the most common sites are the nasal cavity and the paranasal sinuses, and usually, the orbital region, the parotid gland, and the neck (77,201,253).

Pathology

Hemangiopericytomas are composed of a proliferation of tightly packed pericytes around thin-walled endothelial-lined vascular channels ranging from capillary-sized vessels to large, gap-ing sinusoidal spaces (77). The tumor has a tendency to grow slowly and invade locally into adjacent structures. Although they are always well circumscribed and partially or completely surrounded by a pseudocapsule, benign tumors may be difficult to differentiate from malignant ones. However, prominent mitoses (greater than four per high-power field), foci of necrosis, and increased cellularity are suggestive of malignancy (77); the definitive sign is local recurrence or development of metastases. In general, tumors of the central nervous system, lower extremity, and mediastinum tend to be more malignant, with local recurrence occurring in up to 50% of cases (77). The final diagnosis of hemangiopericytomas is based on the histopathology and immunochemistry, and whether the tumor is benign or malignant is defined on the basis of the clinical history. Hemangiopericytomas located in the sinonasal area is generally benign.

Kowalski and Paulino (148) reviewed 12 cases of hemangiopericytomas. Proliferation index was assessed using an immunoperoxidase stain for MIB-1 (Ki-67). The mitotic index per 10 high power fields varied from 0 or 1 to 15. Proliferation indices using MIB-1 ranged from 2.6% to 52.5%. Clinical follow-up revealed three cases with recurrence all possessing proliferation indices of approximately 10%, indicating a more aggressive subset of hemangiopericytomas. Vuorinen et al. (278) found the proliferation index to be a poor predictor of prognosis.

Meningeal hemangiopericytomas almost always recur, despite seemingly complete removal due to infiltrative properties of hemangiopericytoma cells and not just higher proliferation potential. They often metastasize.

Clinical Presentation

Soft-tissue hemangiopericytoma is a firm, painless, slowly expanding mass that is often nodular and well localized. The skin overlying the mass does not have any discoloration or redness to indicate its vascular origin because the capillaries are emptied of the blood by compression of massive numbers of pericytes surrounding them (55,77).

In the head and neck, the tumor may constitute a polypoid, soft gray or red mass that grows slowly and may cause nasal obstruction. Epistaxis and nasal obstruction are common symptoms. The hemangiopericytomalike tumors of the nasal passages and paranasal sinuses differ slightly from those occurring elsewhere and probably represent a related but separate entity because they have little tendency toward recurrence or metastases regardless of the type of therapy.

Orbital hemangiopericytomas account for 3% of orbital malignancies and most frequently occur with painless proptosis (236). Hemangiopericytoma rarely originates in the lacrimal sac; it occurs in a younger age group than that of hemangiopericytoma of other locations. Charles et al. (42) reported on seven cases previously described and added one case.

Table 45.5 CHEMODECTOMAS OF THE CAROTID BODY AND GANGLION NODOSUM

Series (Reference)	No. of Patients	No. of Lesions	Dose (Gy)	Results[a]
Mitchell and Clyne (185)	6	6	37.5–55	5/6 controlled at 1.5–8 y
Lybeert et al. (166)	9	11	40–60[b]	9/9 controlled at 1.5–18 y
Mendenhall et al. (181)	4	6	40.8–48.5	4/4 controlled at 2–4.5 y

[a]Control is defined as regression or stabilization of local disease; no evidence of lymph node metastases.
[b]2 Gy per fraction.
Modified from Mendenhall WM, Million RR, Parsons JT, et al. Chemodectoma of the carotid body and ganglion nodosum treated with radiation therapy. *Int J Radiat Oncol Biol Phys* 1986;12:2175–2178.

::	Table 45.6	TEMPORAL BONE CHEMODECTOMAS: LOCAL CONTROL AFTER RADIATION THERAPY ALONE OR RADIATION THERAPY AND SURGERY		

Author (Reference)	No. of Patients	Percent Local Control	Follow-Up (y)
Larner et al. (156)	15	93 (RT alone)	Median, 16.2
Powell et al. (216)	46	90 (RT alone)	Median, 9
Wang et al. (280)	19	84 (RT ± surgery)	5–35
Konefal et al. (145)	23	83 (RT ± surgery)	Mean, 10.5
Pryzant et al. (217)	19	95 (RT ± surgery)	Mean, 11
Cole and Beiler (48)	30	97 (RT alone)	3–27
Boyle et al. (29)	9	100 (RT alone)	1–12
Schild et al. (232)	8	100 (RT ± surgery)	Median, 7.5
deJong et al. (60)	38	89 (RT ± surgery)	Median, 11.5
Hinerman et al. (119)	53	93 (RT ± surgery)	Mean, 15

RT, radiation therapy
From Hinerman RW, Mendenhall WM, Amdur RJ, et al. Definitive radiotherapy in the management of chemodectomas arising in the temporal bone, carotid body, and glomus vagale. *Head Neck* 2001;23:363–371, with permission.

Hemangiopericytoma may occur intracranially. When it arises in the brain, it is a solid mass attached to the meninges that grossly resembles a meningioma (128). These intracranial hemangiopericytomas carry a high risk of local failure (80%), as well as higher potential for dissemination. The mean time for local recurrence is 75 months (128).

The incidence of metastasis, which depends on the site of origin, can be 50% to 80%. Late metastases occurring 10 years after diagnosis are not uncommon.

On plain radiographs, hemangiopericytoma appears as a soft-tissue mass in the nasal cavity or other portions of the head and neck. A defect caused by pressure erosion of the surrounding bones may occur, and calcifications are rare. On arteriography, according to Yaghmai (293), hemangiopericytoma is the only vascular tumor that has some characteristic angiographic features that include radially arranged or spiderlike branching vessels around and inside the tumor and a long-standing, well-demarcated tumor stain. Intracranial tumors typically have arterial blood supply from both meningeal and cerebral connections, with one to three main feeders supplying many small corkscrewlike vessels (128). The most distinctive and constant feature of this tumor is its hypervascularity; this tissue characteristic also may be demonstrated with contrast-enhanced CT (201). Intracranially, the diffusely enhancing tumor may closely resemble a meningioma on CT. However, some CT signs may suggest hemangiopericytoma rather than meningioma: lack of calcification, scarce surrounding edema, and ringlike enhancement (198). Both CT and MRI scans are of special value in the delineation of the full extent of the tumor.

General Management

Complete surgical resection, if possible, combined with preoperative embolization of the tumor, is the treatment of choice. More extensive surgery is required in tumors that show features of malignancy. Many patients undergo surgical treatment after embolization of the feeding artery(ies).

For incompletely resected tumors, postoperative radiation therapy is used (184). The role of chemotherapy in this tumor is not well determined; a few reports have described partial tumor regression in some lesions treated with cytotoxic agents. Doxorubicin, alone or in combination-drug regimens, is the most effective agent for metastatic hemangiopericytoma, producing complete and partial remissions in 50% of cases (290). Other drugs prescribed when metastasis occurs are cyclophosphamide, dacarbazine, vincristine, and actinomycin-D (113).

Radiation Therapy Techniques

The role of radiation therapy alone in the management of hemangiopericytoma is controversial. The main role of irradiation is as an adjuvant after complete excision of the lesion or postoperatively for minimal residual disease (79,131,172,248). The tumor has been considered relatively radioresistant. Tumor doses of 60 to 65 Gy in 6 to 7 weeks are required to produce local tumor control in postoperative cases (128). Orbital hemangiopericytoma has been cured by surgery and postoperative irradiation to 65 Gy (236).

::	Table 45.7	CHEMODECTOMAS OF CAROTID BODY/GLOMUS VAGALE: RADIATION THERAPY ALONE OR RADIATION THERAPY AFTER SURGERY		

Author	No. of Patients	Local Control (%)	Follow-Up (y)
Valdagni and Amichetti (273)	7	100 (RT ± subtotal resection)	1–19
Verniers et al. (274)	22	100 (RT ± subtotal resection	Mean, 10
Powell et al. (216)	4	100 (RT alone)	Median, 9
Schild et al. (232)	2	100 (Subtotal resection + RT)	Median, 7.5
Cole and Beiler (48)	30[a]	97 (RT alone)	3–27
Hinerman et al. (119)	18	96 (RT ± resection)	Mean, 9

RT, radiation therapy
[a]Glomus jugulare and glomus vagale.
From Hinerman RW, Mendenhall WM, Amdur RJ, et al. Definitive radiotherapy in the management of chemodectomas arising in the temporal bone, carotid body, and glomus vagale. *Head Neck* 2001;23:363–371, with permission.

There appears to be a definite role for postoperative irradiation to the brain for primary hemangiopericytoma when radical surgery is performed because these tumors tend to recur after seemingly complete removal. Jha et al. (131) reported local tumor control in all patients treated with adjuvant external-beam irradiation postoperatively. Radiation therapy also has been used as a salvage procedure after local recurrence following initial surgery and/or chemotherapy.

The fields of irradiation should be wide, to encompass the tumor bed with a margin of at least 5 cm to safely avoid marginal recurrence. Portal arrangement and beam selection are similar to those used in treatment of malignant brain tumors or soft-tissue sarcomas.

Results of Therapy

Billings et al. (26) reported on 10 patients with hemangiopericytoma of the head and neck; seven tumors arose from soft-tissue sites and three from the mucosa. All patients underwent wide excision of the primary lesion with a local recurrence rate of 40%. Three patients developed metastatic lung disease 0 to 8 years after initial diagnosis. Each patient who developed metastatic disease had abundant mitoses on pathological review compared with rare or absent mitoses in the lesions that took a more benign course.

Patrice et al. (208) reported on 18 primary hemangioblastoma tumors (16 had no prior surgical resection and two were subtotally resected lesions) and 20 lesions treated after surgical failure with stereotactic irradiation (radiosurgery). Minimum tumor doses ranged from 12 to 20 Gy (median 15.5 Gy). With a median follow-up of 24.5 months (range 6 to 77 months), the 2-year actuarial survival was 88%, and the 3-year freedom from progression was 86%. Four of 22 patients died. Thirty-one of 36 evaluable tumors (86%) were controlled locally. None of the 18 primary tumors treated with definitive stereotactic irradiation failed. Of the 18 recurrent tumors, 13 (72%) were controlled. The median tumor volume of lesions that failed to be controlled was 7.85 cm^3 compared with 0.67 cm^3 for controlled lesions ($p = 0.0023$). There were no significant permanent complications attributable to the stereotactic irradiation.

Spitz et al. (248) published a report on 36 patients (older than 16 years) with hemangiopericytoma treated at the University of Texas M.D. Anderson Cancer Center. The median follow-up was 57 months. Twenty-eight patients (78%) underwent complete and potentially curative resection. Of the nine patients (32%) who had local recurrences, four (44%) had epidural tumors and three (33%) had retroperitoneal tumors, but none had extremity tumors. Ten patients had recurrences at distant sites. Of the 13 patients who experienced any form of disease recurrence, four had recurrences after a disease-free interval of more than 5 years. The 5-year actuarial survival rate for the entire group of 36 patients was 71%.

Carew et al. (36) reviewed the records of 12 patients with hemangiopericytomas of the head and neck. Five patients had lesions characterized as high or intermediate grade histologically, and seven had low-grade lesions. Nine patients were treated with curative intent; three presented either with pulmonary metastasis (two patients) or unresectable primary tumor (one patient) and were treated with radiation therapy and/or palliative doxorubicin-based chemotherapy. Patients treated with curative intent underwent a variety of surgical resections dictated by tumor location and size. Four patients received postoperative radiation therapy to a median dose of 60 Gy, for positive surgical margins (two patients), high-grade histology (one patient), or a recurrent lesion (one patient). The 5-year overall survival rate for patients treated surgically was 87.5%. A single mortality occurred in a patient with a recurrent high-grade lesion who failed at local, regional, and distant sites.

Payne et al. (209) described their experience in 12 patients with 15 intracranial hemangiopericytomas treated using gamma surgery. Clinical and radiographic follow-up of 3 to 56 months was available for 10 patients with 12 tumors. There was one tumor present at the time of initial gamma surgery in each patient. Two new tumors occurred in patients previously treated. Nine of the tumors decreased in volume and three remained stable. Four of the nine tumors that shrank later progressed at an average of 22 months after treatment. There were no complications and the quality of life following the procedure was maintained or improved in every case.

Chordomas

Anatomy

Chordomas are rare neoplasms of the axial skeleton that arise from the remnant of the primitive notochord (chorda dorsalis). About 50% arise in the sacrococcygeal area; 35% arise intracranially, where they typically involve the clivus, and the remaining 15% occur in the midline along the path of the notochord, primarily involving the cervical vertebrae (259).

Epidemiology

Chordomas are more common in patients in their 50s and 60s but can occur in all age groups. In children and young adults the prognosis and long-term survival appear to be better than in older patients (289). No risk factors have been identified. Male predominance is reported at a 2:1 to 3:1 ratio.

Natural History

Although slowly growing, chordomas are locally invasive, destroying bone and infiltrating soft tissues. Basisphenoidal chordomas tend to cause symptoms earlier and may be difficult to differentiate histologically from chondromas and chondrosarcomas and radiographically from craniopharyngiomas, pineal tumors, and hypophyseal and pontine gliomas. The lethality of these tumors rests on their critical location, aggressive local behavior, and extremely high local recurrence rate. The incidence of metastasis, which has been reported to be as high as 25%, is higher than previously believed and may be related to the long clinical history. The most common site of distant metastasis is the lungs, followed by liver and bone. Lymphatic spread is uncommon.

Pathology

Chordoma is a soft, lobulated tumor that may have areas of hemorrhage, cystic changes, or calcification. It is frequently encapsulated but may be nonencapsulated or pseudoencapsulated. Histologically, it is composed of cords or masses of large cells (physaliferous cells) with typical vacuoles and granules of glycogen in the cytoplasm and abundant intercellular mucoid material. Usually there are few mitotic cells. Heffelfinger et al. (114) postulated that a chondroid variant of chordoma may exist, being prevalent in the spheno-occipital area. Patients with this type of histologic variant have improved survival.

Aside from the previously mentioned histologic features, the prognostic factors that most influence the choice of treatment are location and local extent of tumor.

Clinical Presentation

Chordomas tend to originate from the clivus and chondrosarcomas from the temporal bone (141). Clinical symptoms vary with the location and extent of the tumor. In the head, extension may be intracranial or extracranial, into the sphenoid sinus, nasopharynx, clivus, and sellar and parasellar areas, with a resultant mass effect. In chordomas of the spheno-occipital region, the most common presenting symptom is headache. Other presentations include symptoms of pituitary insufficiency, nasal stuffiness, bitemporal hemianopsia, diplopia, and other cranial nerve deficits. Fuller and Bloom (88) reported on 13 patients with clivus chordoma, all of whom had multiple cranial nerve palsies. Facial pain was present in 11/13 patients.

Volpe et al. (277) reviewed the clinical features of 48 patients with chordoma and 49 patients with low-grade chondrosarcoma of the skull base. Twenty-five patients (52%) with chordoma and 24 patients (49%) with chondrosarcoma had ocular symptoms (diplopia or visual impairment) as the initial manifestation of the disease. Of the 59 patients (both groups) with diplopia, the diplopia was initially intermittent in 25 (42%). Headache and diplopia from abducens nerve palsy occurred in 22 patients (46%) with chordoma and 23 (47%) with chondrosarcoma.

Diagnostic Work-Up

The diagnostic work-up varies with the primary location of disease. Most patients have significant bony destruction, and some may have calcifications in the tumor; hence, plain films and, specifically, CT scans or MRI are very useful (67) (Table 45.8). In most cases, the soft-tissue component is much more extensive than initially appreciated, and a CT scan with contrast enhancement is required (Fig. 45.7A). CT and MRI are equivalent for demonstration of the presence and site of these tumors. MRI is inferior to CT in its ability to demonstrate bony destruction and intratumoral calcification (Fig. 45.7B) (197,258). MRI is superior to CT regarding the delineation of the exact extent of the tumor, which allows for better treatment planning (67). Because of availability and lower cost, CT appears to be the technique of choice for routine follow-up of previously treated patients (197).

Reliable signs of chordoma of the skull base are posterior extension to the pontine cistern; a lobulated, "honeycomb" appearance after gadolinium; the swollen appearance of the bone in the early stages; bone erosion on CT; and frequent extension to critical structures such as the circle of Willis, cavernous sinuses, and brainstem (67).

General Management

Because of their surgical inaccessibility and relative resistance to radiation therapy, clivus chordomas represent a formidable therapeutic challenge. The general management of the patient

is dictated by the anatomic location of the tumor and the direction and extent of spread. A surgical approach is recommended (when feasible), but complete surgical extirpation alone is unusual (230). Regression of preoperative symptoms without additional postoperative morbidity could be achieved by radical transoral tumor extirpation documented by MRI (234). Intracranial spread usually requires steroid coverage and therapy directed to correction of neurologic deficits that may be present. Because of the high incidence of local recurrence, combined surgical excision and irradiation is frequently used. No effective chemotherapeutic agent or combination of drugs has been identified.

Radiation Therapy Techniques

Irradiation techniques vary considerably, depending on the location of the tumor along the craniospinal axis. Basisphenoidal tumors usually are treated by a combination of parallel opposed lateral fields, anterior wedges, and photon and electron beam combinations, depending on the extent of the neoplasm. Precision radiation therapy planning, using CT and MRI, is required because high doses of external-beam radiation therapy are needed. Three-dimensional CRT or IMRT provide optimal dose distributions (Fig. 45.8).

The tumor usually surrounds the spinal cord and infiltrates vertebral bones. A combined technique using protons or electrons to boost the initial photon fields is generally applied. In the treatment of chordomas surrounding the spinal cord, IMRT can provide high-dose homogeneity and planning target volume (PTV) coverage. Frequent digital portal image-based setup control reduces random positioning errors for head and neck cancer patients immobilized with conventional thermoplastic masks. Gabriele et al. (90) treated a patient with incomplete resection of a vertebral chordoma surrounding C2-3 with a total dose of 58 Gy (International Commission of Radiation Units and Measurements point) in 2-Gy daily fractions. Beam arrangement consisted of seven 6 MV nonopposed coplanar IMRT fields using 120-leaf collimator in sliding window mode. To verify the daily setup, portal images at 0 degrees and 90 degrees were compared with the simulation images before treatment delivery (manual matching) and after treatment delivery (automatic anatomy matching). The mean dose to the PTV was 57.6 ± 2.1 Gy covering 95% of the PTV with the 95% isodose. The minimum dose to the PTV (D99) was 53.6 Gy in the overlapping area between the PTV and the spinal cord planning organ at risk volume (PRV). The maximum dose to the spinal cord was 42.2 Gy and to the spinal cord PRV (8 mm margin) 53.7 Gy. The mean dose to the parotid glands were 37.4 Gy (homolateral gland) and 19.5 Gy (contralateral gland). Average deviation in setup was -1.1 ± 2.5 mm (anterior-posterior), 2.4 ± 1.3 mm (latero-lateral), 0.7 ± 0.9 mm (craniocaudal) and -0.43 ± 1 degree (rotation).

Because of the slow proliferative nature of chordomas, high linear energy transfer may prove useful in their management, as it will be discussed later. Brachytherapy can be used for recurrent tumors of the base of skull or adjacent to the spine when a more aggressive surgical exposure is offered. Three of five chordomas were rendered stable when treated with iodine-94 (^{94}I) implants by Gutin et al. (105), performed with CT stereotactic technique. Kumar et al. (150) reported use of ^{94}I intraoperative interstitial implantation in two patients with recurrent chordomas. Disease was effectively controlled in both.

Results of Therapy

Photons

Although survival in some patients with chordoma may be long term, the salient feature of this unusual neoplasm is local

---

:: Table 45.8	**DIAGNOSTIC WORK-UP FOR CHORDOMA**

General
  History
  Physical examination
Radiologic studies
  Plain radiographs
  Computed tomography scan/magnetic resonance imaging
Laboratory studies
  Complete blood cell count
  Chemistry
  Urinalysis
Special studies
  Endocrinologic profile (clivus)
  Visual evaluations (clivus)

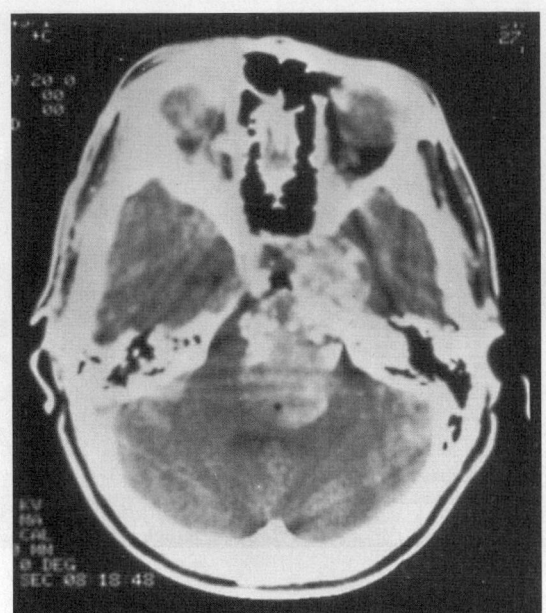
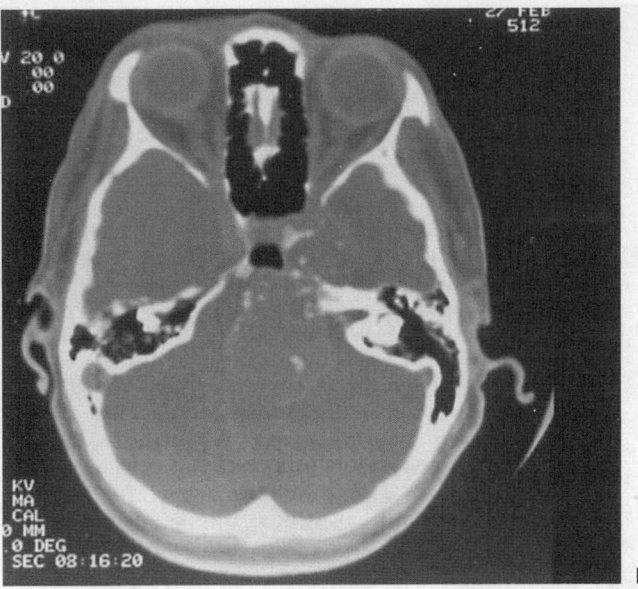

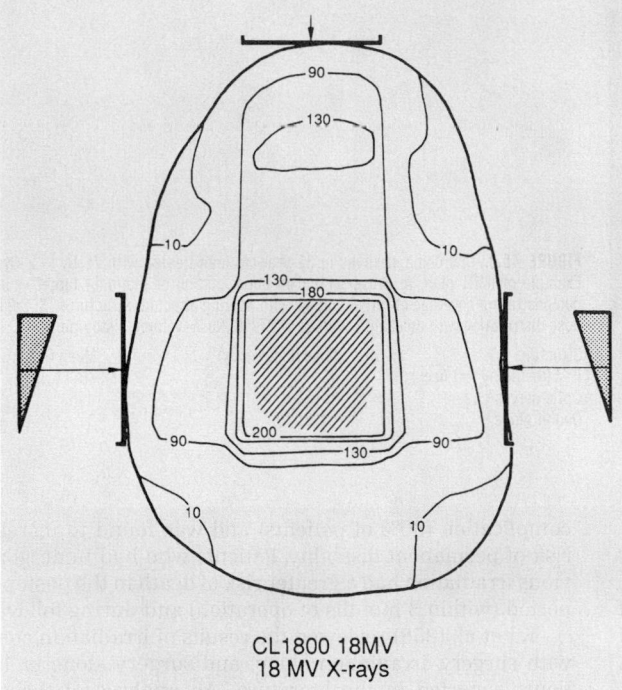

CL1800 18MV
18 MV X-rays

FIGURE 45.7. A: Contrast material-enhanced axial computed tomography scan demonstrates a large chordoma with extension into the posterior fossa and left parasellar region. **B:** Computed tomography scan photographed at bone windows shows the bony destruction and intratumoral calcifications. **C:** Treatment planning field arrangement for illustrated clivus chordoma using standard irradiation techniques with wedges on lateral points.

recurrence with eventual death. The course may be indolent, with multiple treatments for recurrences, but the overall 5-year diseasefree survival rate is <10% to 20%. At M.D. Anderson Cancer Center, of 19 patients treated definitively, three were alive and free of disease with relatively short follow-up of 3, 6, and 7.5 years, respectively. Fuller and Bloom (88), in 25 patients treated with external-beam irradiation, found 96% stabilization or reduction of pain; the overall actuarial survival rates were 44% and 17% at 5 and 10 years, respectively.

Catton et al. (37) analyzed the long-term results of treatment for patients with chordoma of the sacrum, base of skull, and mobile spine treated predominantly with postop-erative photon irradiation. In 20 base of skull chordomas, most of them irradiated with conventionally fractionated radiation to a median dose of 50 Gy in 25 fractions for 5 weeks (range 25 Gy to 50 Gy), median survival was 62 months (range 4 to 240 months) from diagnosis with no difference between clival and nonclival presentations. There was no survival advantage to patients receiving radiation doses >50 Gy (median 60 Gy) compared with lower doses <50 Gy (median 40 Gy). Hyperfractionation regimens did not influence the degree or duration of symptomatic response or progressionfree survival. Median survival after retreatment was 18 months.

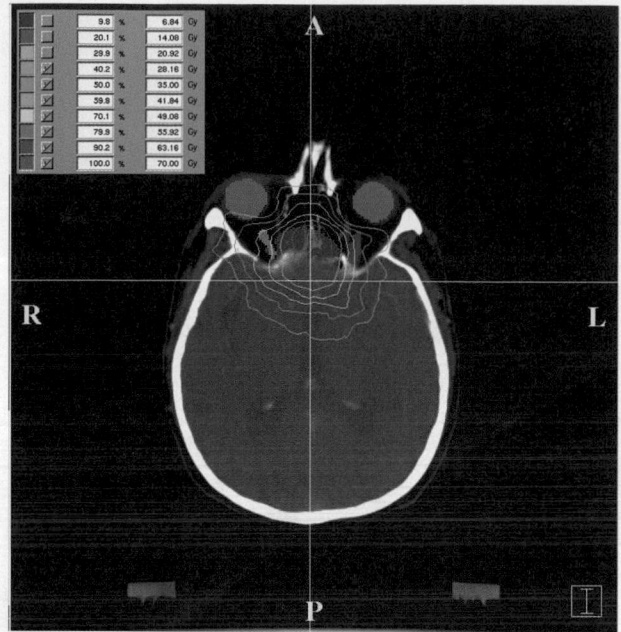

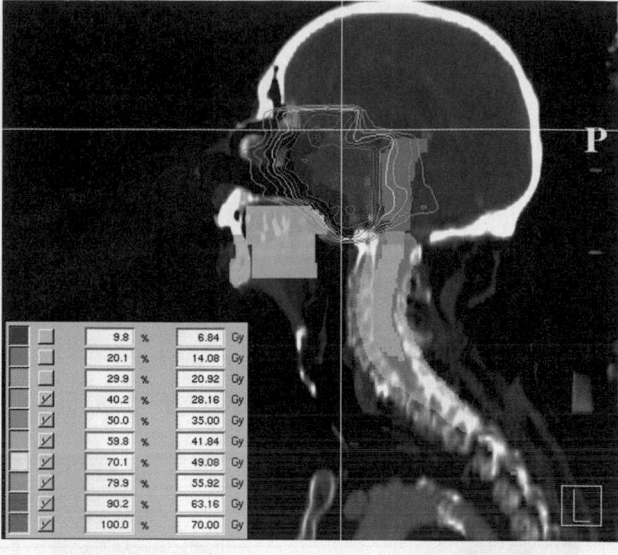

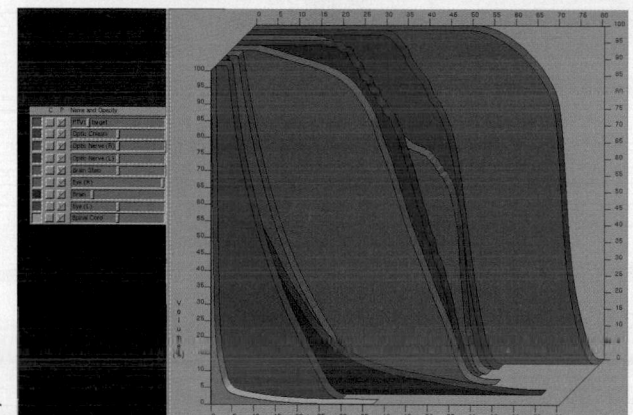

FIGURE 45.8. Chordoma of clivus in 81-year-old man treated with 70 Gy in 2-Gy fractions. Example of IMRT plan: **A:** Cross-section in upper portion of planning target volume (PTV), demonstrating coverage of target volume with sparing of ocular structures. **B:** Sagittal plane dose distribution with excellent coverage of PTV. **C:** Dose–volume histogram;

Structure	Dose Range (cGy)	Mean Dose (Gy)
PTV (including left neck)	60–75	70
Optic nerves/chasm	25–50	41
Ocular globe	3–30	12

Forsyth et al. (86) reported on 51 patients with intracranial chordomas (19 classified as chondroid) treated surgically (biopsy in 11 patients and subtotal removal or greater in 40); 39 patients received postoperative irradiation. At the time of the analysis, 17 patients were alive. The 5- and 10-year survival rates were 51% and 35%, respectively; 5-year survival was 36% for biopsy patients and 55% for those who had resection. Patients who underwent postoperative irradiation tended to have longer diseasefree survival times.

Gay et al. (96) analyzed the outcome of 46 patients with cranial base chordomas and 14 with chondrosarcomas treated with extensive surgical resection: 50% of them had been treated previously; 20% received postoperative irradiation. Nine patients with chordomas and two with chondrosarcomas died during the postoperative follow-up period. The 5-year recurrence-free survival rate for all patients was 76%. Chondrosarcomas had a better prognosis than chordomas (5-year recurrencefree survival rates of 90% and 65%, respectively) ($p = 0.09$). Patients who had undergone previous surgery had a greater risk of recurrence than did those who had not undergone previous surgery (5-year recurrencefree survival rates of 64% and 93%, respectively) ($p < 0.05$). Those with total or near-total resection had a better 5-year recurrencefree survival rate (84%) than did patients with partial or subtotal resection (64%) ($p < 0.05$). Postoperative leakage of cerebrospinal fluid was the most frequent complication (30% of patients) and was found to increase the risk of permanent disability. Patients who had undergone previous irradiation had a greater risk of death in the postoperative period (within 3 months of operation) and during follow-up.

Tai et al. (259) reviewed the results of irradiation combined with surgery, irradiation alone, and surgery alone in 159 patients reported in the literature. An analysis of the optimal biologically equivalent dose was performed using the linear-quadratic formula on 47 patients. With conventional photon irradiation no dose–response relationship was shown. Survival improved in patients undergoing surgery followed by irradiation.

Chetty et al. (45) reported on 18 chordomas, 61% of them occurred in the sphenoid region. Follow-up for 12 patients ranged from 3 to 170 months. Various combinations of surgery and radiation therapy were used. Mean survival was 73.4 months, with a survival rate of 50% (six of 12 patients).

Keisch et al. (138) reported on 21 patients with chordoma treated at our medical center: five had clival tumors, two had nasopharyngeal tumors, and one had a lumbar spine tumor. Nine patients were treated with surgery alone, eight had subtotal resection and postoperative irradiation, and four received irradiation alone after biopsy. The 5- and 10-year actuarial survival was significantly better in patients treated with surgery alone or surgery and irradiation than in those treated with radiation therapy alone (52%, 32%, and 0%, respectively) ($p =$ 0.02). Diseasefree survival of patients with base of skull tumors was not significantly different among the treatment groups.

Debus et al. (59) reported on 45 patients treated for chordoma or chondrosarcoma with postoperative fractionated 3D stereotactic radiation therapy. Median dose at isocenter was 66.6 Gy for chordomas and 64.9 Gy for chondrosarcomas. All chondrosarcomas achieved and maintained local tumor and recurrencefree status at 5-years follow-up. Local control rate of chordomas at 5 years was 50% and survival was 82%. Clinically significant late toxicity developed in only one patient.

Kondziolka et al. (144) assessed the use of radiosurgery in four patients with chordoma and two with chondrosarcoma (in five patients as adjuvant therapy for residual or recurrent tumors after surgical debulking; in one patient with a chordoma as primary treatment). No patient received fractionated external-beam irradiation. All tumors were <30 mm in diameter and were treated with 20 Gy to the tumor margin. During follow-up (mean 22 months; range 8 to 36 months), they found no progression of the treated tumor in any patient. Neurologic deficits before treatment improved in three patients; the other three patients remained in stable neurologic condition. Serial follow-up imaging studies demonstrated reduction in tumor size in two patients, and four patients had no tumor growth. One patient showed tumor progression outside the radiosurgical treatment volume.

Protons

The best results in the treatment of chordomas have been obtained with radical surgical procedures followed by high-dose proton irradiation. Berson et al. (22) described 45 patients with chordomas or chondrosarcomas at the base of the skull or cervical spine who were treated by subtotal resection and postoperative irradiation. Twenty-three patients were treated definitively by charged particles, 13 patients with photons and particles, and nine were treated for recurrent disease. Doses ranged from 36 to 80 Gy equivalent. There appeared to be significant benefit for patients with smaller tumor volumes (80% vs. 33% actuarial survival rate at 5 years). Patients treated for primary disease had a 78% actuarial local control rate at 2 years, whereas the rate for patients with recurrent disease was 33% (21).

Tatsuzaki and Urie (261) described the use of proton beam therapy at high doses for chordomas and chondrosarcomas of the base of the skull and cervical spine. Treatment delivered 74 cobalt gray equivalent (CGE) to the tumor while maintaining the central brainstem and central spinal cord at 48 CGE or less; and the surface of the brainstem, spinal cord, and optic structures at 60 CGE or less. Proton beam plans and 10-MV x-ray beam plans were developed with these assumptions and dose constraints. In all cases the proton beam plans delivered more dose to a larger percentage of the tumor volume, and the estimated tumor control probability was higher than with the x-ray plans. However, without precise positioning both the proton plans and the x-ray plans deteriorated, with a 12% to 25% decrease in estimated tumor control probability.

O'Connell et al. (193) reported on 62 patients with base of skull chordomas treated with proton beam irradiation (65 to 73.5 Gy equivalent); 29 patients (19 women and 10 men) experienced local failure, and 14 women (48%) and seven men (21%) died of disease. On histologic analysis, presence of more than 10% necrosis, prominent nucleoli, and tumor larger than 70 mm were significant predictors of short-term disease-specific survival. Chondroid chordoma and conventional chordomas had equivalent outcome.

Proton beam boosts have been recommended. Rich et al. (223) reported results in 48 patients with chordomas: 14 patients were treated with surgery and 17 with combination of partial surgical resection and irradiation, or irradiation alone after biopsy (15 patients) (Table 45.9). Various techniques were used to deliver doses of 45 to 80.4 Gy with photons alone or combined with 160-MeV protons, usually 2 Gy daily.

Fagundes et al. (80) updated the Massachusetts General Hospital experience with 204 patients treated for chordoma of the base of the skull or cervical spine. Sixty-three patients (31%) had treatment failures, which were local in 60 patients (29%) and the only site of failure in 49 patients. Two patients had regional lymph node relapse, and three developed surgical pathway recurrence. Thirteen patients relapsed in distant sites (especially lungs and bones). The 5-year actuarial survival rate after any relapse was 7%. There was no significant difference in survival for patients who had a local or distant failure. Two patients (1.4%) with local tumor control developed distant metastases in contrast with 10/60 patients (16%) who failed locally and distantly.

Terahara et al. (262) reported on 132 patients with skull base chordoma treated with combined photon and proton irradiation; in 115 patients dose-volume data and follow-up were available. The prescribed doses ranged from 66.6 CGE to 79.2 CGE (median of 68.9 CGE). The dose to the optic structures (optic nerves and chiasm), the brainstem surface, and the brainstem center was limited to 60, 64, and 53 CGE, respectively. Local failure developed in 42/115 patients, with the actuarial local tumor control rates at 5 and 10 years being 59% and 44% respectively. In a Cox multivariate analysis, the models equivalent

---

Table 45.9 PATIENT STATUS CORRELATED WITH TREATMENT AND RADIATION DOSE LEVEL IN CHORDOMA

Treatment					Cause of Failure				
Surgery	Irradiation	No. of Patients	NED	AWD	Local	Local + DM	DM	ID	Lost
Radical excision	None	8	4	0	2	0	0	1	1
Palliative excision	None	6	0	0	4	1	0	1	0
Partial excision	>60 Gy	5	4	0	0	1	0	0	0
	<60 Gy	12	0	3	6	2	0	0	1
Biopsy	>60 Gy	9	5	2	0	1	0	1	0
	<60 Gy	6	0	0	1	4	0	0	1
Total excision	Preoperative (50 Gy)	2	1	1	0	0	0	0	0
Totals		48	14	6	13	9	0	3	3

AWD, alive with disease; DM, distant metastasis; ID, intercurrent death; NED, no evidence of disease
From Rich TA, Schiller A, Suit HD, et al. Clinical and pathologic review of 48 cases of chordoma. *Cancer* 1985;56:182, with permission.

uniform dose (EUD) suggest that the probability of recurrence of skull-base chordomas depends on gender, target volume, and target dose inhomogeneity; EUD was shown to be a useful parameter to evaluate dose distribution for the target volume.

Hug et al. (123) analyzed treatment efficacy of fractionated proton radiation therapy administered for skull base 33 chordomas and 25 chondrosarcomas. Following various surgical procedures, residual tumor was present in 91% of patients; 59% demonstrated brainstem involvement. Target doses ranged from 64.8 to 79.2 (mean 70.7) CGE. The range of follow-up was 7 to 75 months (mean, 33 months). In 10 patients (17%) the treatment failed locally, resulting in local control rates of 92% (23/25 patients) for chondrosarcomas and 76% (25/33 patients) for chordomas. All tumors with volumes of 25 mL or less remained locally controlled compared with 56% of tumors larger than 25 mL ($p = 0.02$). Of patients without brainstem involvement 94% did not experience recurrence; whereas with brainstem involvement (and dose reduction because of brainstem tolerance constraints) the tumor control rate was 53% ($p = 0.04$). Actuarial 5-year survival rates were 100% for patients with chondrosarcoma and 79% for patients with chordoma. Grade 3 and 4 late toxicities were observed in four patients (7%) and were symptomatic in three (5%).

Benk et al. (18) described results in 18 children 4 to 18 years of age with base of skull or cervical spine chordomas who received fractionated high-dose postoperative irradiation using mixed-photon and 160-MeV proton beams. Median tumor dose was 69 CGE with a 1.8-CGE daily fraction. With a median follow-up of 72 months, the 5-year survival was 68%, and the 5-year diseasefree survival rate was 63%. Patients with cervical spine chordomas had a worse survival rate than did those with base of skull lesions ($p = 0.008$). The incidence of treatment-related morbidity was acceptable: two cases of growth hormone deficit corrected by hormone replacement, one temporal lobe necrosis, and one fibrosis of the temporalis muscle, improved by surgery.

A report on proton therapy for base of skull chordoma was published by the Royal College of Radiologists (228). They concluded that outcome after proton irradiation is superior to that reported for conventional photon irradiation. Radiation therapy schedules involving a mixed schedule of protons and photons have achieved an approximately 60% local tumor control rate at 5 years.

Sequelae of Treatment

In patients treated with high irradiation doses, as well as with charged particles, there is an increasing probability of sequelae including brain damage, spinal cord injury, bone or soft-tissue necrosis, and xerostomia. In a report by Berson et al. (22), three patients experienced unilateral visual loss, and four patients had radiation injury to the brainstem.

Santoni et al. (231) reported on the temporal lobe damage rate in 96 patients (75 primary and 21 recurrent tumors) treated with postoperative high-dose proton and photon irradiation for chordomas and chondrosarcomas of the base of the skull. All the patients were randomized to receive 66.6 or 72 CGE with conventional fractionation (1.8 CGE per day, five fractions a week) using opposed lateral fields for the photon component and a noncoplanar isocentric technique for the proton component. Of the 96 patients, 10 developed temporal lobe damage, (lateral in two and unilateral in eight). The cumulative temporal lobe damage incidence at 2 and 5 years was 7.6% and 13.2%, respectively. CT and MRI scans were evaluated for white matter changes; the MRI areas suggestive of temporal lobe damage in 10 patients were always separate from the tumor bed.

In patients receiving high-dose proton therapy for clivus tumors, Slater et al. (242) observed a 26% incidence of endocrine abnormalities at 3 years and 37% at 5 years, with hypothyroidism being the most frequent sequela. The dose to the pituitary in patients with abnormalities ranged from 63.1 to 67.7 Gy equivalent.

⠶ Lethal Midline Granuloma

Natural History and Pathology

Lethal midline granuloma (LMG) or midline malignant polymorphic reticulosis is a clinical entity characterized by progressive, unrelenting ulceration and necrosis of the midline facial tissues. LMG is associated with Epstein-Barr virus, which has at least two subtypes with different biologic properties that can be identified by their genomic configuration. The occurrence of the rare subtype 2 in LMG may relate to a covert immune defect (28). Considerable controversy exists regarding various disorders characterized by a necrotizing and granulomatous inflammation of the tissues of the upper respiratory tract and oral cavity. It is now clear that if infections and other known agents such as cocaine use, sarcoidosis, environmental toxins, and various neoplasms can be excluded, three clinicopathologic entities remain: Wegener's granulomatosis, LMG, and polymorphic reticulosis (PMR) (12). A review of the literature suggests that cases described as idiopathic midline destructive disease and PMR are a large evolutionary spectrum from almost benign to fatal malignant lymphoma (21).

Wegener's granulomatosis is an epithelioid necrotizing granulomatosis with vasculitis of small vessels. Systemic involvement of the kidneys and lungs is common.

PMR is an unusual disorder with distinctive clinical and pathologic features (177). Histologically, PMR is characterized by an atypical mixed lymphoid infiltration of the submucosa with extensive areas of necrosis, sometimes extending to bone or cartilage. The lesion consists of variable zones of small lymphocytes with scattered immunoblastic forms, abundant plasma cells with occasional eosinophilia, and histiocytosis (243). PMR has been considered a lymphoproliferative disorder; most, if not all, cases are peripheral T-cell lymphomas (163,283). Several authorities believe that PMR and systemic lymphomatoid granulomatosis are the same disease with the latter predominantly involving the lungs (94,163).

Idiopathic LMG describes a localized disorder not characterized by visceral lesions but by destruction of the midfacial area, which, if left untreated, is uniformly fatal. The histopathologic findings are nonspecific, with a relatively nondescript inflammatory reaction with acute and chronic inflammation and necrosis. Despite specific clinicopathologic features, the distinction between LMG and PMR is often difficult; although controversial, they may represent two phases of the same disease, with LMG remaining histologically benign or evolving into PMR. LMG occurs more frequently in men (94). Ages range from 21 to 64 years; almost half of the patients are in their 50s at presentation. Most patients have involvement of the nasal cavity (including destruction of the septum) and the paranasal sinuses (particularly maxillary antrum). The primary lesion may extend into the orbits, the oral cavity (palate, gingiva), and even the pharynx.

Characteristics of the three different diseases are outlined in Table 45.10.

Clinical Features and Diagnostic Work-Up

Clinical manifestations include progressive nasal discharge, obstruction, foul odor emanating from the nose, and, in later stages, pain in the nasal cavity, paranasal areas, and even in the orbits.

Examination discloses ulceration and necrosis in the nasal cavity, perforation or destruction of nasal septum and

Table 45.10	DIFFERENTIAL FEATURES OF THREE CLINICOPATHOLOGIC ENTITIES		
	Wegener's Granulomatosis	**Idiopathic Midline Granuloma**	**Polymorphic Reticulosis**
Disease features	Diffuse, inflammatory disease of upper airway, predominately sinuses and nose	Destructive extension to palate and facial soft tissues	Destructive lesion with destruction of bone and extension through soft tissues
Systemic involvement	Lungs, kidneys, small-vessel vasculitis may not have airway involvement	No	No
Associated with lymphoma	No	May remain benign or progress to lymphoma	Usually evolves to lymphoma
Histologic features	Necrotizing vasculitis with epithelioid granulomas, giant cells, and fibrinoid necrosis	Inflammatory reaction, nonspecific; granulomas and giant cells are infrequent	Characteristic atypical and polymorphic lymphoreticular cellular infiltrate; angiocentric growth patterns may simulate vasculitis, but fibrinoid necrosis is absent in vessel walls
Treatment	Chemotherapy	Radiation therapy	Chemotherapy; radiation therapy and chemotherapy

Modified from Bataskis JG. Wegener's granulomatosis and midline (non peeling) granuloma. *Head Neck Surg* 1979;1:213.

turbinates, and even ulceration of the nose. Edema of the face and eyelids may be noted, and the bridge of the nose may be sunken. Radiographic studies initially show soft-tissue swelling, mucosal thickening, and findings consistent with chronic sinusitis.

CT is invaluable in demonstrating the full extent of the tumor, including bone or cartilage destruction. In 13 patients presenting with LMG, CT proved essential for determining the extent of the disease, guiding biopsy, and planning radiation therapy (173). MRI was also helpful for the latter because it could distinguish fluid retained within the paranasal sinuses from solid masses and tumor from granulation tissue; it was of little value for detecting bone lysis. Eight patients proved to have T-cell lymphoma, two had Crohn's disease, in one the lesion was factitious, and two had granulomas without diagnostic histologic features.

General Management and Radiation Therapy Techniques

When treatment of these patients is planned, it is extremely important to exclude the diagnosis of Wegener's granulomatosis, a benign process that is commonly treated with antimicrobial agents, steroids, and systemic chemotherapy (94,190). Bona fide LMG does not respond to steroids; the treatment of choice is radiation therapy (64,89,237).

Target volume should encompass all areas of involvement, including adjacent areas at risk (i.e., for a lesion of the maxillary antrum it will include the antrum as well as all of the paranasal sinuses) with a 2- to 3-cm margin (106). Because marginal failures are a significant problem, wide margins are necessary for treatment of these patients (243).

Irradiation techniques are similar to those described for tumors of the paranasal sinuses, nasal cavity, or nasopharynx. Several investigators have described complete responses with doses of 30 to 50 Gy; most patients are treated with 35 to 45 Gy in 3 to 4.5 weeks (64,83,84,237). We recommend 45 to 50 Gy in 4.5 to 5.5 weeks in 1.8- to 2-Gy daily fractions.

Results of Therapy

Because of the rarity of this tumor, experience is limited. Fauci et al. (84) reported on 10 patients with extensive midline granuloma treated with irradiation. Three received 10 Gy, and all failed within 2 years (retreated with 40 to 46 Gy). The remaining seven patients received 40 to 50 Gy. Local control of disease

was 77%; two patients had local recurrences, one outside the initially irradiated volume.

The Mayo Clinic reports the most extensive experience in treatment of PMR or LMG with irradiation doses of 40 to 42 Gy (177). Of 20 patients irradiated for localized upper airway PMR, 13 were alive and well for an average of 9.5 years; two were alive and well with <1 year of follow-up; four were dead of other disease, and one was lost to follow-up.

In a study of 34 patients with PMR treated with primary radiation therapy except for one patient, Smalley et al. (243) found that a minimum dose of 42 Gy or a time-dose factor of 70 was necessary to achieve long-term local control. The most frequent failure site was within the original irradiation field. They believe that this problem should become much less significant with implementation of proper time-dose-fractionation schemes. Systemic failure occurred in 25% of their patients initially presenting with limited disease. The salvage of this subset of patients requires effective systemic chemotherapy. Also, Itami et al. (127) evaluated nine patients with locally confined nasal non-Hodgkin's lymphoma (NHL) treated with radiation therapy (all NHLs had T-lineage). Additionally, unique histological pictures of polymorphism, angiodestruction, and necrosis were seen in most cases, findings that are the histological features of PMR, which is the main cause of LMG. Although the disorder was considered to be locally limited at presentation, only three of the nine patients with nasal NHL could be induced into long-term remission with involved field radiotherapy (40 to 60 Gy) and distant extranodal spread was the primary cause of failure. Multimodality treatment using intensive chemotherapy and radiation therapy might improve the prognosis of these patients.

Fauci et al. (83) published a prospective study of 15 patients with systemic lymphomatoid granulomatosis. Of 13 patients treated with cyclophosphamide and prednisone, seven sustained complete remission (mean duration of remission, 5.2 ± 0.6 years). Two patients receiving only prednisone and six receiving cyclophosphamide and prednisone died. Six deaths were associated with biopsy-proven lymphoma; one was caused by a lymphomalike illness unproven by biopsy. The eighth death was caused by adenocarcinoma in a patient with lymphoma in remission. None of these patients received radiation therapy.

Chen et al. (43) reported their experience in 92 cases of LMG or centrofacial malignant lymphoma treated with radiation therapy. Twenty-five patients received combination chemotherapy, usually containing doxorubicin, cyclophosphamide, vincristine, and prednisone (CHOP) or other combinations, including CHOP or nitrogen mustard, vincristine, procarbazine, and prednisone (MOPP) in some patients. The nose was the most frequently involved site at initial presentation (85% of patients). Immunophenotyping in 36 patients showed T-cell lineage in 25 (69%) and B-cell in six (17%). The irradiation technique consisted of treating all involved and adjacent areas with doses of 30 to 75 Gy. Sixteen patients received neck irradiation (30 to 60 Gy). Daily fractions were 2 to 3 Gy in five weekly fractions. Actuarial survival rates were 59.5% at 5 years, 56.2% at 10 years, and 40.5% at 20 years. There was no significant difference in survival in patients receiving more or <50 Gy. A relapse in the midfacial region was noted in seven patients. Other relapse sites were lung and skin in three patients, para-aortic or inguinal lymph nodes in two patients, and brain in one. Survival of patients with recurrences was poor; 73% died within 8 months.

Hatta et al. (112) reviewed 18 patients (15 males and three females) with LMG (polymorphic reticulosis) (about 5.6% of patients with malignant head and neck tumors). Most of the 18 patients underwent both radiation therapy and chemotherapy (cyclophosphamide, vincristine, prednisone [COP], CHOP, methotrexate, leucovorin, doxorubicin, cyclophosphamide, vincristine, bleomycin, prednisone [MACOP-B]), but, since their disease had reached an advanced stage, three underwent radiation therapy only, three chemotherapy only, and one received no radical therapy. Of the 18 patients, 13 died of the disease; in six progress was confined to the local lesion. The 5-year cumulative survival rate was 15.7%. Fourteen autopsy studies revealed that tumor had invaded the liver (92.8%), lung (92.8%), and spleen (71.4%), and in all cases it was in leukemic patterns. Five cases were positive for ubiquitin carboxyl-terminal esterase L1 (ubiquitin thiolesterase) (UCHL-1) (CD45RO) and 10 cases were positive for lysozyme. All cases were positive for Ki-1 (CD30).

Sakata et al. (229) reported on 107 patients with stage I and II NHL of the head and neck treated with involved field radiation therapy for orbital, nasal, or paranasal lymphoma and extended field radiation for Waldeyer's ring or neck lymphoma (39 to 48 Gy). In the latter half of the study, adjuvant chemotherapy was administered. Of 107 patients, 95 achieved chemoradiation. Of the 12 patients who did not achieve chemoradiation, nine had nasal T-cell lymphoma (NTL) of the lethal midline granuloma (LMG-NTL) type. Only one patient who obtained chemoradiation relapsed in a previously irradiated area. LMG-NTL was the most significant prognostic factor on multivariate analysis ($p < 0.001$). Older patients also experienced a higher relative risk than patients of 60 years of age or less ($p = 0.0063$). Dose of adriamycin reached borderline significance ($p = 0.0600$). Radiotherapy is excellent for obtaining local control of head and neck NHL and LMG-NTL.

Chloroma

Natural History

Chloroma (granulocytic sarcoma, myeloblastoma) is a solid extramedullary tumor composed of early myeloid precursors usually associated with acute myelocytic leukemia (41); the most common sites of presentation are in the orbit and other craniofacial bones. The name chloroma (from the Greek *chloros*, meaning green) derives from the green color of affected tissues resulting from the presence of myeloperoxidase. Because not all deposits exhibit the characteristic green tint, the term "granulocytic sarcoma" seems more appropriate.

Granulocytic sarcomas were identified in 3% of 478 patients with acute chronic granulocytic leukemia; they can be seen with other myeloproliferative disorders, including polycythemia vera, hypereosinophilia, and myeloid metaplasia (189,190). In the absence of acute leukemia, granulocytic sarcoma is usu-

ally an ominous sign, suggesting imminent conversion to acute myelocytic leukemia or blast crisis (190). As survival rates for myelogenous leukemias improve, the number of patients who relapse with chloromas is increasing (189).

Children are affected more often than adults. Of 33 patients with orbital chloromas reported by Zimmerman and Font (294), 75% were in their first decade of life. Chloromas are found more frequently in children with the M4 and M5 acute myeloid leukemia subtypes of the French-American-British Cooperative Group Classification and are also associated with the 8:21 translocation. Chloromas may appear during bone marrow remission before an increase in blasts is detected in the bone marrow, so they may herald relapse (189,190).

Clinical Presentation and Diagnostic Work-Up

Intraorbital (retrobulbar) chloroma causes progressive exophthalmos or temporal swelling. Central nervous system involvement causes both local pressure phenomena and generalized elevation of intracranial pressure with headaches, nausea, and vomiting (188).

Intracerebral chloromas may manifest as the rare central nervous system (parenchymal) involvement of acute nonlymphocytic leukemia. Woo et al. (291) believe that intracerebral chloromas represent reactivation of sanctuary deposits of leukemic cells in the central nervous system originated from an initial hematogenous spread.

All patients require complete hematologic and neurologic testing as is true for any patient with suspected leukemia. Open biopsy remains the best diagnostic tool. Plain radiographic findings consist mainly of localized bone destruction with predominantly lytic lesions and associated soft-tissue masses in orbital and periorbital chloromas. Intracranial chloromas may exhibit intermediate or high attenuation in unenhanced CT scans, with intense, uniform enhancement after intravenous administration of contrast material. Confusion with meningioma, hematoma, solitary metastasis, and lymphoma may occur on CT scans (215,244).

Gallium-67 scintigraphy was used to detect unsuspected leukemic infiltrates (165), but is not used any longer. Currently positron emission tomography (PET) scanning may be more useful for this purpose and to assess tumor response to therapy.

Radiation Therapy Techniques

Chloromas are extremely radiosensitive; however, the optimal dose of irradiation has not been established. Response rates of leukemic infiltrates have been reported with doses as low as 4 Gy, yet the need for higher doses up to 30 Gy in certain locations of extramedullary leukemic infiltrates is well recognized (189,190). Although the literature is limited regarding the maximum dose needed for treatment of chloromas, it appears that 30 Gy is the maximum required for local control. In our limited experience, there appears to be a relationship between the size of the chloroma and the total dose of irradiation required for control. The target volume is the tumor mass and an adequate margin (2 to 3 cm). Irradiation techniques depend on the location of the infiltrate. For superficial lesions, electron beam is recommended. Orbital chloroma may constitute a radiation therapy emergency because visual loss is possible if the patient is not treated promptly.

Esthesioneuroblastoma

Esthesioneuroblastomas (ENB), first described by Berger and Luc (20), are rare tumors thought to arise in the olfactory receptors in the nasal mucosa or the cribriform plate of the ethmoid bone. The olfactory nerves perforate grooves in the ethmoid bone in the cribriform plate and continue into the subarachnoid spaces, accounting for the high incidence of intracranial extension (20,75).

Epidemiology

ENB constitutes 3% of all endonasal neoplasms. In the United States, according to the data from the Surveillance, Epidemiology, and the End Results Program, 84 cases of ENB were registered from 1978 to 1990 (72). About 945 cases have been reported in the world literature (31). The review authors' cases accounted for 198 and collaborative efforts accounted for 747 cases. Sex distribution was 53.6% male and 46.64% female. Kadish classification was applied to 563 cases; 103 (18.3%) class A, 182 (32.2%) class B, and 278 (49.4%) class C cases.

Herrold (117) induced olfactory neuroblastoma in the nasal cavity of hamsters by injection of dimethylnitrosamine and other nitroso derivatives. What role these agents may play in humans is unknown. No other risk factors have been identified. There appears to be a slight male predominance. The age incidence has a bimodal distribution, with peaks at 11 to 20 years and 40 to 60 years, the highest incidence at 51 to 60 years (75,143).

Natural History

Although others thought that EBN were of ectodermal origin, most observers believe the tumor to be of neuroectodermal origin in the olfactory epithelium (11,97). Most of these tumors occur high in the nasal cavity or in the lateral wall adjacent to the ethmoid. The tumor may spread to the opposite ethmoid bone, superiorly to the frontal sinus and anterior cranial fossa, posteriorly to the sphenoid sinus, nasopharynx, and base of skull, laterally to the orbits, forward to the frontonasal angle, or inferiorly to the nasal cavity and antrum (Fig. 45.9). Lymphatic spread may be to the subdigastric, posterior cervical, submaxillary, or preauricular nodes, as well as to the nodes of Rouviere.

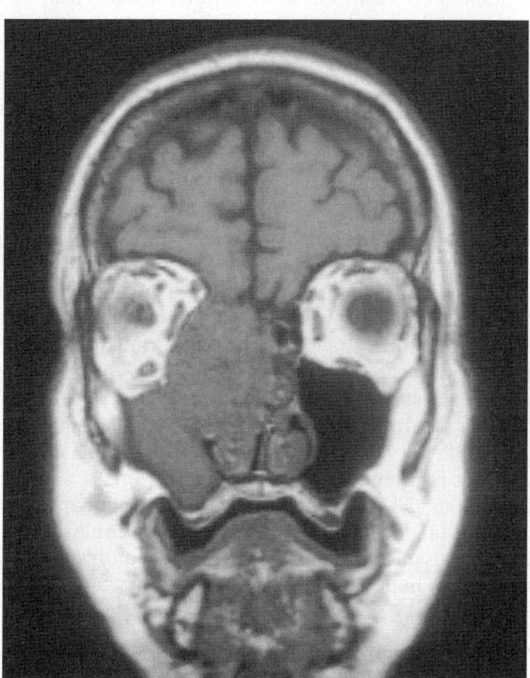

FIGURE 45.9. Coronal magnetic resonance imaging scan showing a large soft-tissue mass and bone destruction in the right ethmoidal maxillary sinuses and nasal cavity secondary to extensive (Kadish stage C) esthesioneuroblastoma.

The exact incidence of distant metastases is uncertain; it has been quoted to be as high as 50%, but this rate is influenced by the use of chemotherapy in high-risk patients.

Clinical Presentation

These tumors tend to be friable and bleed easily. The most common clinical symptoms are epistaxis and nasal blockage. Patients also may have local pain or headache, visual disturbances, rhinorrhea, tearing, proptosis, or swelling in the cheek (134). The symptoms may be associated with a mass in the neck.

Diagnostic Work-Up and Staging

Physical examination may show the inferior aspect of a polypoid friable mass in the nasal cavity. Ocular findings or a mass in the nasopharynx may be present. With early lesions, radiographs or CT or MRI may show only nonspecific opacification, soft-tissue swelling, and occasionally bone destruction (170,213,233). Octreotide is a somatostatin analog that, when coupled to a radioisotope, produces a scintigraphic image of neuroendocrine tumors (NET) expressing somatostatin type 2 (SSR 2) receptors. Octreotide scintigraphy (OS) may be useful in confirming the preoperative diagnosis of certain head and neck NET, such as paragangliomas, Merkel cell carcinomas, medullary thyroid carcinomas, and esthesioneuroblastomas. Bustillo et al. (34) carried out a retrospective study that compared the results of OS with the histopathologic diagnosis in 74 patients with head and neck NET. Of the 60 patients undergoing evaluation for suspected paraganglioma, OS was correctly positive in 36/37 patients with PG and correctly negative in 19/23 patients who did not exhibit PG (sensitivity of 97% and a specificity of 82%). There were 14 patients in the nonparaganglioma group. OS detected or diagnosed locoregional recurrences in two with esthesioneuroblastoma.

Table 45.1 outlines the suggested diagnostic work-up (214,253). MRI, especially with gadolinium contrast, may be used as a supplement or alternative to CT scanning (213). Kairemo et al. (135) described imaging findings in 17 olfactory neuroblastomas; CT provided the best information about the tumor and its local invasion into surrounding bone structures. MRI allowed an estimate of tumor spread into surrounding soft-tissue areas, such as the anterior cranial fossa and the retromaxillary space. Bone scintigraphy scan detected distant metastases.

In a review of 22 patients with a histologically proven olfactory neuroblastoma the tumors displayed a variety of imaging characteristics and aggressiveness (71). The expansile tendency of olfactory neuroblastoma is characterized by bowing of the sinus walls. The destructive aspect is manifested as tumor replacing the turbinates, septum, and sinus walls with extension into contiguous areas (Fig. 45.9 and 45.10). The density/signal and enhancement characteristics are nonspecific of olfactory neuroblastoma.

Although dopamine β-hydroxylase and catecholamines are produced by these tumors, their measurements or vanillylmandelic acid excretion levels have not proven clinically useful (71).

A staging system has been proposed by Kadish et al. (134) (Table 45.11).

Pathologic Features and Prognostic Factors

ENBs are polypoid, frequently reddish, soft, and vascular tumors with neuroblasts and neurocytes. Gerard-Marchant and Micheau (97) classified three histologic types. ENB contains epithelial components serving as a supporting stroma and have a nerve component that corresponds to the olfactory cells. Rosettes are the main feature, consisting of several rows of cells

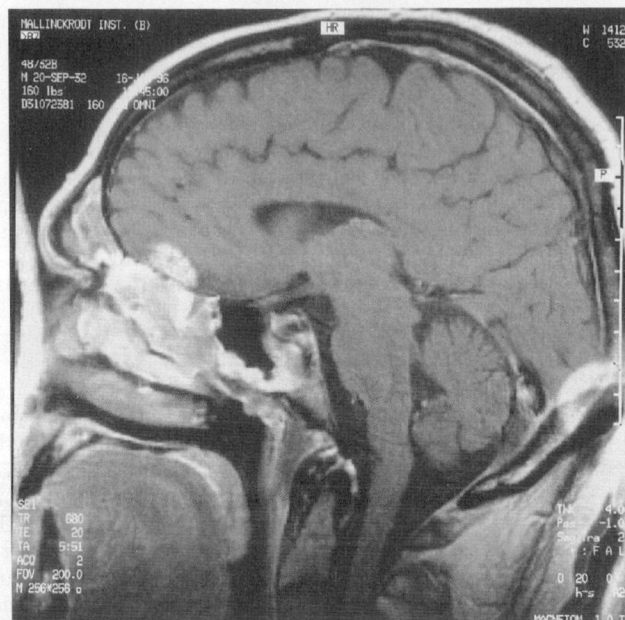
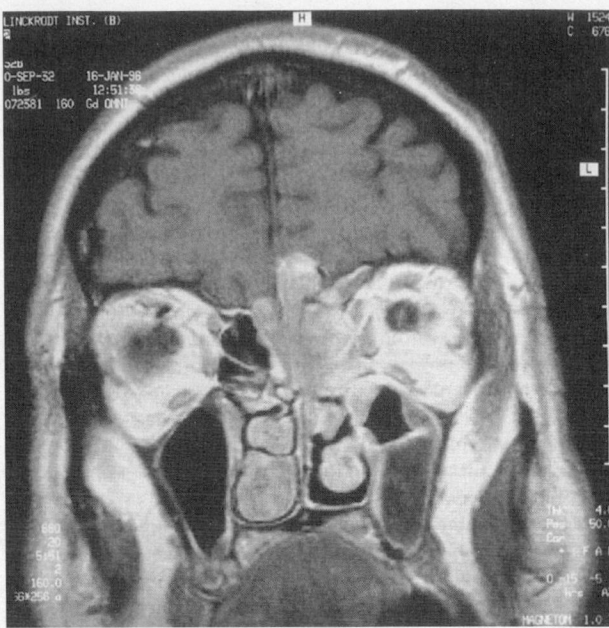

FIGURE 45.10. A,B: The sagittal and coronal views of a preoperative magnetic resonance imaging of a 56-year-old patient who was initially seen with a Kadish stage C tumor involving left nasal cavity and extending intracranially (*arrows*). (From Chao KSC, Kaplan C, Simpson JR, et al. Esthesioneuroblastoma: the impact of treatment modality. *Head Neck* 2001;23:749–757, with permission.)

arranged around the central area (11,252). ENBs may be confused with lymphoma or anaplastic carcinoma and have diffuse, regular distribution. ENBs contain many fibrils, which fill the central space of the rosette (called a pseudorosette). It has been suggested that the presence of chromaffin granules indicates a derivative from primitive neural crest cells. ENB must be distinguished from other poorly differentiated neoplasms including sinonasal undifferentiated carcinoma, which is derived from the Schneiderian epithelium. Sinonasal undifferentiated carcinoma lacks rosettes and intercellular fibrils (252).

Extension of the primary tumor based on the Kadish staging system (134) has been identified as the most important determinant of treatment outcome although this was not confirmed by Chao et al. (40). High-grade tumors had worse outcome in the reports from the Mayo Clinic and UCLA (85,91).

Argiris et al. (5) found in 16 patients with ENB, 11 of whom had Kadish stage B (50%) had brain involvement at presentation. Craniofacial resection was performed in 12 patients (81%); 14 received either preoperative or postoperative therapy (radiation therapy in 11 and chemotherapy in 4). The actuarial 5-year survival was 60%, diseasefree survival 33%, with a median follow-up of 4.3 years. The first site of failure was locoregional alone in 10/12 patients who progressed, and in six patients involved the brain or the meninges. Two patients were successfully salvaged.

Hyams (126) proposed a histologic grading system for ENB in which grade I tumors have an excellent prognosis and grade IV tumors are uniformly fatal. The Hyams grading system predated advanced craniofacial techniques, extensive use of immunohistochemistry, and the recognition of sinonasal undifferentiated carcinoma (SNUC) as a distinct entity. Miyamoto et al. (186) in a retrospective review of 12 patients with esthesioneuroblastoma and 14 with SNUC used the Kadish clinical stage and Hyams histopathologic system. Kadish staging was available for 26 patients (two patients with stage A tumors; seven with stage B, and 17 with stage C). Of the eight evaluable patients with Kadish stage A or B tumors, six remained disease free for more than 2 years compared with only 5/7 Kadish stage C tumors. Slides were available for Hyams grading in 21 patients (two patients with grade I tumors, four with grade II, four with grade III, and 11 with grade IV). Of the six patients with Hyams grade I or II tumors, four remained disease free for more than 2 years compared with only 4/15 patients with Hyams grade III or IV tumors. Three patients with Kadish stage C tumors (two with esthesioneuroblastoma, one with SNUC) and two patients with Hyams grade IV tumors (one with esthesioneuroblastoma and one with SNUC) survived for more than 5 years. They concluded that both the Hyams grading and the Kadish staging system can be used as independent predictors of outcome; patients with either advanced clinical stage or pathologic grade of ENB or SNUC have poor prognosis, but long-term survival is possible in these patients if aggressive treatment is used.

Papadaki et al. (204) analyzed 18 formalin-fixed paraffin-embedded olfactory neuroblastoma specimens (12 primary tumors and six recurrences or metastases) from 14 patients and concluded that p53 point mutation does not play an important role in the initial development of olfactory neuroblastoma; however, p53 wild-type hyperexpression may occur in subsets, show local aggressive behavior, and have a tendency for recurrence.

General Management

Surgery alone appears to be adequate treatment for small, low-grade tumors confined to the ethmoids in which negative surgical margins can be obtained (25). An ethmoidomaxillary

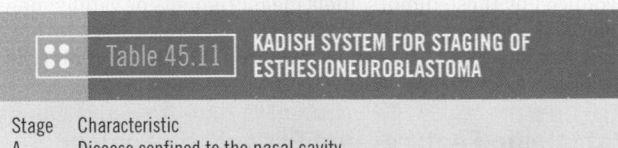

Table 45.11	KADISH SYSTEM FOR STAGING OF ESTHESIONEUROBLASTOMA

Stage	Characteristic
A	Disease confined to the nasal cavity
B	Disease confined to the nasal cavity and one or more paranasal sinuses
C	Disease extending beyond the nasal cavity or paranasal sinuses; includes involvement of the orbit, base of skull or intracranial cavity, cervical lymph nodes, or distant metastatic sites

From Kadish S, Goodman M, Wang CC. Olfactory neuroblastoma: a clinical analysis of 17 cases. *Cancer* 1976;37:1571–1576, with permission.

resection with or without orbital sparing is usually necessary. This procedure is combined with preoperative or postoperative irradiation (85,226). A complete resection with preservation of vital structures is achievable by using a craniofacial approach. The experience from the University of Virginia, however, has yielded no firm conclusions regarding whether craniofacial resection or more conservative surgery could be performed in early-stage disease (91).

Dias et al. (62) reported on 35 patients with ENB treated with gross tumor resection through a transfacial approach with postoperative RT in 11 patients, craniofacial resection (CFR) and postoperative RT in seven, exclusive RT in 14, CFR alone in one, and a combination of chemotherapy and RT in two. Radiation therapy median dose was 48 Gy. Analysis of survival showed that the Kadish classification best predicted disease-free survival ($p = 0.046$). The presence of regional and distant metastases adversely affected prognosis ($p <0.0001$ and $p = 0.01$, respectively). Craniofacial resection plus postoperative RT provided a better 5-year diseasefree survival rate (86%) compared with the other therapeutic options used ($p = 0.05$). The 5-year disease-specific survival rate was 64% and 43% for the low- and high-grade tumors, respectively ($p = 0.20$). Diseasefree survival was 46% and 24% at 5 and 10 years, respectively. Overall survival was 55% and 46% at 5 and 10 years of follow-up, respectively. Aggressive multimodality therapeutic strategies, particularly CFR and adjuvant RT, yielded the best treatment outcome.

Early lesions involving the ethmoids with little or no bony destruction or nerve invasion can be treated adequately by high-energy (photon or electron) radiation therapy with good cosmetic and functional results (20,85,143). Those with more extensive local disease benefit from surgery and adjuvant irradiation (20,40,214), although some have spoken against combined surgery and radiation therapy because of complications (13,256,302). Patients with locally advanced disease or high-grade tumors should receive aggressive treatment with combined modalities, such as surgery, radiation therapy, and chemotherapy.

Monroe et al. (187) described treatment results in 22 patients who received RT for ENB (equal numbers of males and females, median age of 54 years). The modified Kadish stage was A in one patient, B in four patients, C in 15 patients, and D in two patients. Treatment modalities included primary RT in six patients, preoperative RT in one patient, postoperative RT after craniofacial resection in 12 patients, and salvage RT in three patients treated for recurrence after surgery. Elective neck RT was performed in 11/20 patients (two patients had cervical metastases at presentation for RT). Rates of local tumor control, cause-specific survival, and absolute survival at 5 years were 59%, 54%, and 48%, respectively. The cause-specific survival rate at 5 years was lower after primary RT (17%) than after craniofacial resection and postoperative RT (56%). Cervical metastases occurred in 6/22 patients (27%). No neck recurrences occurred in 11 patients treated with elective neck RT compared with four neck recurrences in nine patients (44%) not receiving elective neck RT ($p = 0.02$). Their data and review of the current literature suggest a higher cervical failure rate than previously recognized; elective neck RT seems to correlate with improved nodal tumor control and should be considered in the treatment of esthesioneuroblastoma.

Rosenthal et al. (226) treated 72 adults with nonmetastatic, primary sinonasal neuroendocrine tumors (31 with ENB, 16 with SNUC, 18 with neuroendocrine carcinoma [NEC], and seven with small cell carcinoma [SmCC]). Patients with ENB usually were treated with surgery and/or radiotherapy; only 3/31 patients (9.7%) received radiation to regional lymphatics, and only 5/31 received chemotherapy. In contrast, patients with non-ENB histologies usually received chemotherapy (10/16 patients with SNUC, 12/18 patients with NEC, and 5/7 patients

with SmCC). With a median follow-up for surviving patients of 81.5 months, overall survival at 5 years was 93.1% for patients with ENB, 62.5% for SNUC, 64.2% for NEC, and 28.6% for SmCC ($p = 0.0029$). The local control tumor rate at 5 years also was superior for patients who had ENB (96.2%) compared with patients who had SNUC (78.6%), NEC (72.6%), or SmCC (66.7%) ($p = 0.04$). The regional failure (RF) rate at 5 years was 8.7% for patients with ENB, 15.6% for patients with SNUC, 12.9% for patients with NEC, and 44.4% for patients with SmCC. Additional late events increased the RF rate for patients with ENB to 31.9% at 10 years. The distant metastasis rate at 5 years was 0.0% for patients with ENB, 25.4% for patients with SNUC, 14.1% for patients with NEC, and 75.0% for patients with SmCC.

For advanced lesions, in which disseminated disease is likely, chemotherapy may improve tumor control and decrease the incidence of distant metastases. A combination of thiotepa, cyclophosphamide, doxorubicin, vincristine, nitrogen mustard, and actinomycin-D has been used (178). Wieden et al. (285) reported complete tumor regression and 2.7-year survival in a patient with extensive olfactory esthesioneuroblastoma treated with a combination of wide local excision, chemotherapy with cisplatin and 5-fluorouracil (5-FU), and irradiation (55.8 Gy).

A retrospective review of 10 patients with recurrent esthesioneuroblastoma treated with chemotherapy at the Mayo Clinic suggested that cisplatin-based chemotherapy is active in advanced, high-grade tumors (227). Survival from initial chemotherapy treatment was 44.5 months (range, 3 to 130 months) in patients with low-grade tumors and 26.5 months (range, 2 to 67 months) in patients with high-grade tumors.

Treatment, which could be classified in 898 reported cases, consisted of surgery alone in 24% (226 cases), radiation therapy alone in 18.4% (165 cases), combined surgery and radiation therapy in 43.2% (388 cases), chemotherapy in 13.2% (119 cases), and in 11 cases (1.2%) bone marrow transplant. In the reported cases follow-up could be evaluated in 477 cases, while in only 234 cases a 5-year follow-up was done; on these 20.5% had surgery only, 11.1% radiation therapy, and 68.4% combined surgery and radiation therapy. The best survival rates were obtained by combined therapy, 72.5% versus 62.5% with surgery alone and 53.8% with radiation therapy (31).

Elective Neck Treatment

Esthesioneuroblastoma has been shown to metastasize to the neck and remote sites. Although the sites of metastases are widely variable and often atypical, Olsen and DeSanto (196) reported cervical lymph nodes to be the most common site, developing in 10/21 patients (48%) in their series. Beitler et al. (16) found cervical lymph node metastases to be as common as local recurrence. In a literature review of 110 patients by Bailey and Barton (7), 24 patients (22%) had metastatic disease, with cervical lymph nodes being the most common site. Davis and Weissler (57) compiled a retrospective review of patients and found that the cumulative cervical metastasis rate reached 27% (55/207 patients). In general, because of the low incidence of cervical lymph node metastasis ($\leq$10%) in early-stage disease, elective irradiation of the neck or a dissection is not indicated (75). However, in patients with Kadish stage C disease, the cervical metastatic rate climbed to 44% (25/57 patients). As noted previously, Monroe et al. (187) observed cervical node metastasis in 6/22 patients (27%), incidence similar to that reported by other authors. In 11 patients they treated with elective neck RT no recurrences were noted, in contrast to 4/9 (44%) in patients not receiving elective neck RT. Thus, with advanced-stage disease, cervical nodes should be initially managed by irradiation, radical neck dissection, or a combination of both (57,75).

Clinical Radiation Oncology

Radiation Therapy Techniques

A combination of photons and electrons with anterior fields provides good coverage for limited ethmoidal disease when the tumor is confined anteriorly. Beam arrangement can be modified for disease extending into the orbit or maxillary sinus. Obturator or bolus may be needed postoperatively to compensate for tissue deficit. When intracranial or posterior extension is present or tumor has spread into the maxillary sinus, a pair of perpendicular (anteroposterior and lateral) portals with wedges or two lateral wedge fields in conjunction with an open anterior photon field will give good coverage of the treatment volume with the dose inhomogeneity around 10% to 20%. Incorporation of a vertex field eliminates the high inhomogeneous dose along the junction line of the conventional three-field technique. Treatment techniques are similar to those described for treatment of paranasal sinuses (see Chapter 39). The orbits can be spared or treated as the degree of extension dictates. Occasionally, an anterior electron beam field may be needed to supplement low-dose areas. When the electron beam is used over air cavities, some dosimetry problems result. Eye blocks must be positioned precisely to avoid undesirable side effects.

When combined therapy is used, preoperative doses of 45 Gy and postoperative doses of 50 to 60 Gy are indicated, depending on the status of the surgical margins. Doses of 65 to 70 Gy are delivered with irradiation alone in patients with inoperable tumors (137). Contrast-enhanced CT or MRI scans before initiation of treatment are crucial to demarcate extension of the tumor. Treatment planning with CT for determination of tumor extension is extremely important (239). Because of the proximity of esthesioneuroblastoma to the optic nerves, optic chasm, and the brainstem, the precision of treatment setup, target volume definition, and dose homogeneity dictate tumor control and the sequelae of treatment. Treatment techniques similar to those for paranasal sinuses may create "hot spots" along the optic tracks. High doses per fraction (exceeding 2 Gy) increase the possibility of late sequelae such as blindness and bone and brain necrosis (10,91).

Three-dimension CRT or IMRT provide alternatives to the conventional three-field technique frequently used to treat these tumors (Fig. 45.11). Special attention should be directed to reduce unnecessary irradiation to ocular structures. When occasionally a patient presents with cervical node metastasis IMRT is very helpful to optimally treat the primary tumor and the cervical lymphatics (Fig. 45.12)

Results of Therapy

Surgery and Irradiation

Radiation therapy is an important component in the management of esthesioneuroblastoma, but the optimal sequence when

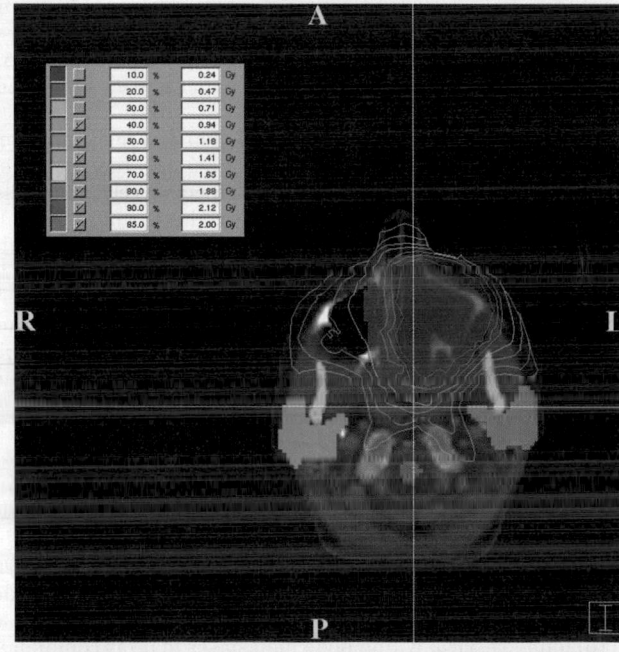

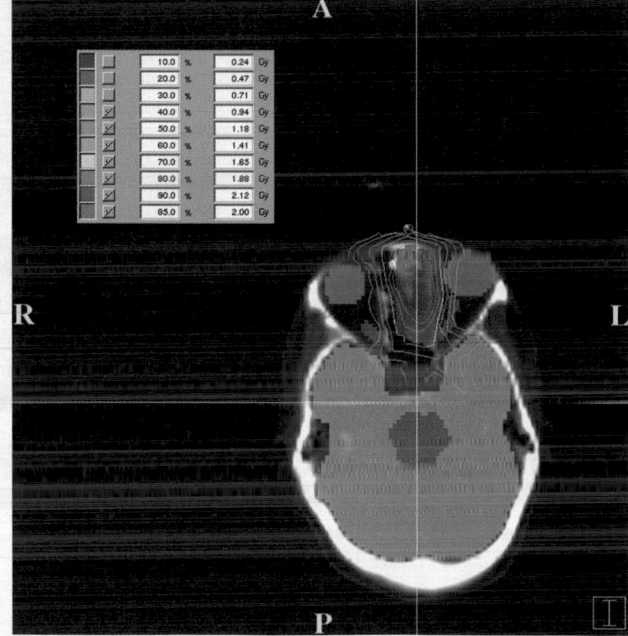

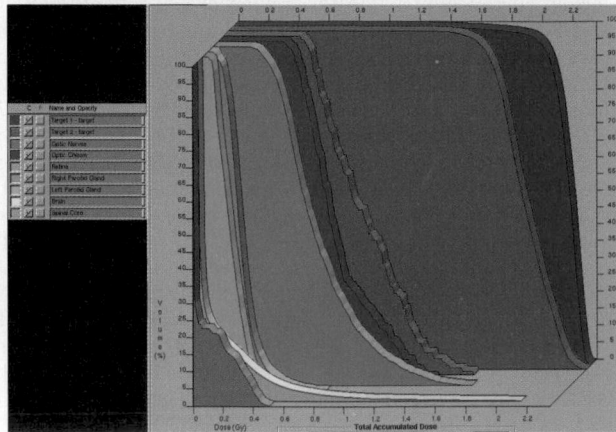

FIGURE 45.11. Esthesioneuroblastoma in a 35-year-old female, initially treated with a craniofacial surgical resection. Patient received postoperative intensity-modulated radiation therapy (2-Gy fractions). **A:** Cross-section illustrating coverage of ethmoidnasal and left maxillary antrum volume. **B:** Cross-section showing dose distribution in target volume with excellent sparing of ocular structures. **C:** Dose–volume histogram:

Structure	Dose Range (cGy)	Mean Dose (Gy)
Planning target volume 1	30–70	65
Planning target volume 2 (+ radiotherapy nasal??)	40–70	58
Optic chasm and nerves	13–42	24

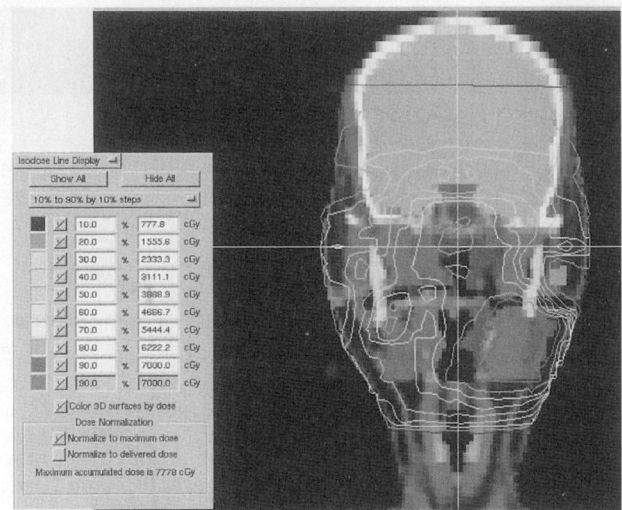

A

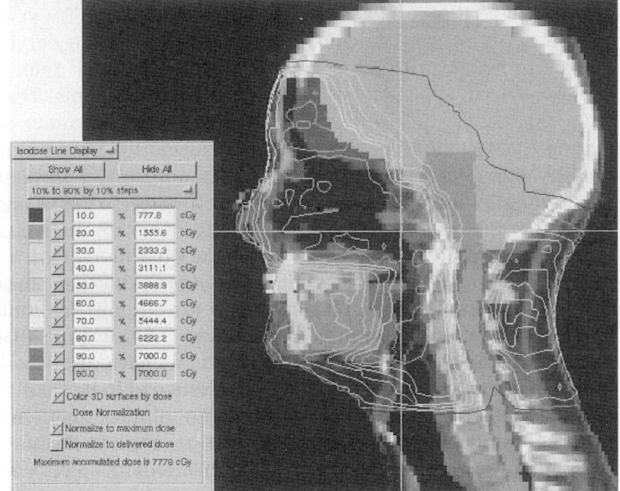

B

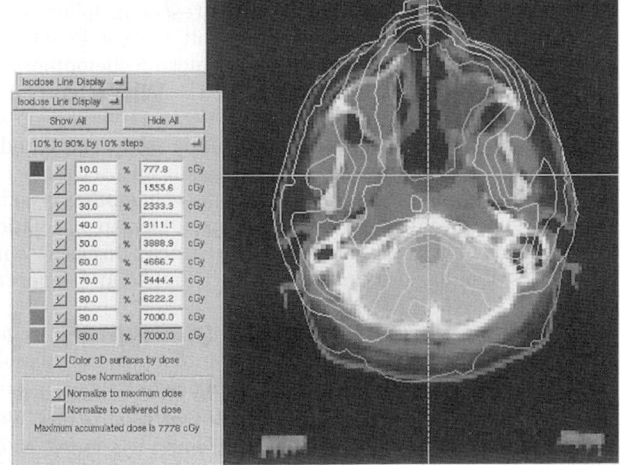

C

FIGURE 45.12. Patient with stage C esthesioneuroblastoma of ethmoid cells and nasal cavity who presented with a large left upper cervical lymph node metastasis. Intensity-modulated radiation therapy plans to deliver 70 Gy to primary tumor and cervical lymphadenopathy. **A:** Coronal, **(B)** sagittal, **(C)** cross-section dose distributions illustrate excellent coverage of all target volumes.

integrated with surgery is unknown. Dulguerov and Calcaterra (70) reported that 83% of patients who were treated with combined irradiation and surgery did not have recurrences. Eden et al. (72) reported no significant difference in survival whether preoperative or postoperative irradiation was given, but suggested improved local tumor control with preoperative irradiation. Technical factors may have contributed to a higher incidence of postoperative radiation therapy failures because three of five postoperative cases received <50 Gy; all three patients were treated with a single anterior field, which gives less homogeneous dose distribution throughout the treatment volume.

At M.D. Anderson Cancer Center, 11 patients were treated with combined surgery and irradiation in most instances. Four patients were alive and disease free at 2.5, 5, 8, and 12 years, respectively; two died of disease 4 and 5 years after treatment. One patient was lost to follow-up at 9 months with extensive disease and is presumed dead. Two patients died of complications but were free of disease.

Spaulding et al. (246) compared 30 patients treated in two time periods: 1969 to 1975 and 1976 to 1985. With the introduction of craniofacial resection, complex field megavoltage irradiation, and chemotherapy in stage C disease in 1976, the overall 2-year survival rate increased from 70% to 87%. For stage C disease, the survival rate increased from 50% to 88%.

Dzalitian et al. (71) described 19 cases of esthesioneuroblastoma, 18 of which were followed. Four patients with advanced disease received radiation therapy exclusively; three soon died of disease, and one patient died 5 years later, presumably of coronary occlusion. Combination radiation therapy and rhinotomy failed in five other patients, but three were salvaged surgically. Three of nine patients treated with surgery only were free of disease at 3 to 14 years. Five of six failures were salvaged with irradiation and surgery.

Foote et al. (85) updated the experience of the Mayo Clinic. Seventeen patients had disease confined to nasal cavity or paranasal sinuses (Kadish stage A and B), and 32 patients had more advanced disease. Treatment included gross total resection alone or combined with radiation therapy. The 5-year actuarial survival, diseasefree survival, and local tumor control rates were 69.1%, 54.8%, and 65.3%, respectively. Local tumor control was improved in patients who received postoperative irradiation (55.5 Gy) even after complete tumor resection.

Levine et al. (160) conducted a retrospective review of 35 patients; 6% of them presented with cervical metastasis, but ultimately 25.7% developed cervical metastases. Fourteen percent of the patients developed a local recurrence an average of 6 years after diagnosis, and in 37% ultimately at least one episode of metastatic disease occurred. The diseasefree survival was 80.4% at 8 years. Central nervous system complications occurred in 25.7% of patients, orbital complications in 22.9%, systemic posttreatment problems in 20%, and had chemotoxic sequelae in 18%. Eriksen et al. (78) carried out a retrospective review of 13 patients with esthesioneuroblastoma; according to the Kadish classification one patient had stage A disease, 5 patients stage B, and 7 patients stage C. The 5-year diseasefree survival was 51%. Forty-six percent of the patients experienced relapse, and despite intensive salvage therapy, median survival after recurrence was only 12 months.

Chao et al. (40) reported on 25 patients with esthesioneuroblastoma, ages ranging from 16 to 73 years (median, 37 years). The tumors were Kadish stage A in 3, stage B in 13, C in 8, and modified D in 1 (cervical nodal metastasis). Seventeen patients were treated with surgery and radiation therapy, six with irradiation alone, and two with surgery only. Eight patients received neoadjuvant chemotherapy. Median follow up was 8 years (range, 2 to 24 years). The 5-year actuarial overall survival, diseasefree survival, and local tumor control rates were 66.3%, 56.3%, and 73%, respectively. Kadish stage was not a significant prognosticator for local control or diseasefree

Table 45.12	RESULTS OF TREATMENT CORRELATED WITH MODALITY AND STAGE FOR ESTHESIONEUROBLASTOMA

	Stage A			Stage B			Stage C		
Modality[a]	Initial Treatment	For Recurrence	Total Control Rate(%)	Initial Treatment	For Recurrence	Total Control Rate(%)	Initial Treatment	For Recurrence	Total Control Rate(%)
Radiation therapy alone	2/5	5/5	70	4/7	3/4	64	1/5	1/1	33
Surgery alone	5/9	4/4	69	3/6	1/2	50	1/1	—	—
Radiation therapy and surgery	7/10	—	70	12/30	0/1	57	7/15	—	47

[a]All results reflect treatment of 78 patients, who were observed for 6 months to 32 years.
From Elkon D, Hightower SI, Lim ML, et al. Esthesioneuroblastoma. Cancer 1979;44:1087–1094, with permission.

survival. Five-year local tumor control was 87.4% for the combination of surgery and radiation therapy and 51.2% for irradiation alone. Two patients with Kadish stage A and B disease underwent surgical resection alone; both failed locally. In contrast, only 3/9 with Kadish stage A or B disease who received adjuvant radiation therapy had a local recurrence. With adjuvant radiation therapy, the surgical margin status did not influence local tumor control. Among the eight patients who received neoadjuvant chemotherapy, six patients showed no response, one had partial response, and one a complete response.

Simon et al. (241) reported on 13 patients with esthesioneuroblastoma or olfactory neuroblastoma; none of the patients had Kadish stage A disease, five had stage B, and eight had stage C. The majority of the patients were treated with a craniofacial resection or tumor removal through a rhinotomy approach. Two patients received neoadjuvant chemotherapy before surgical resection because of locally advanced tumor (cisplatin, ifosfamide, and etoposide). Twelve of the 13 patients received radiation therapy either initially or for salvage. Median dose of postoperative irradiation was 59.4 Gy; 1.8 Gy per day to fields encompassing the involved anatomy with a margin. The overall actuarial 5-year survival was 61% and 10-year 24%, and diseasefree survival rates were 56% and 42%, respectively.

Elkon et al. (75) compiled results for 97 patients treated with different modalities reported in the literature. Survival and tumor control in 78 patients, staged according to the Kadish system, are summarized in Table 45.12.

Chemotherapy and Irradiation

Wade et al. (279) reported that 8/13 patients (62%) had an objective response to cytotoxic agents (cyclophosphamide and vincristine). Eden et al. (72) described results in 16 patients with stage A or B disease and 24 with stage C disease treated with irradiation (median dose 50 Gy) and surgery for stage A and B disease, with the addition of chemotherapy (cyclophosphamide and vincristine) for stage C disease. Actuarial survival rates at 5 and 10 years were 78% and 71%, respectively. Locoregional failure developed in 15/40 patients; 68% of the failures were locoregional (including brain, neck, facial bone, and sinus). They had no recurrences at the primary tumor bed; all recurrences were either outside the irradiation field or at distant sites.

Preoperative neoadjuvant therapy may provide a valuable complement to radical craniofacial resection. Polin et al. (214) reviewed 34 patients with biopsy-proven esthesioneuroblastoma. In multivariate regression analysis, advanced age was predictive of decreased diseasefree survival ($p = 0.008$), whereas advanced Kadish stage was associated with a borderline higher rate of disease-related mortality ($p = 0.056$). Two thirds of the patients showed a significant reduction in tumor burden with adjuvant therapy. Patients with response to neoad-

juvant chemotherapy demonstrated a significantly lower rate of disease-related mortality ($p = 0.50$). The overall 5- and 10-year survival rates were 81% and 54.5%, respectively.

Forty patients were treated for esthesioneuroblastoma at Institut Gustave Roussy, France (97). Three had stage T1, seven T2, 15 T3, and 15 T4 lesions. At presentation the cervical metastatic rate was 18% and distant metastases were detected by bone marrow biopsy and bone scan in three patients. Treatment modalities included surgery alone in eight patients, radiation therapy alone in three patients, surgery plus radiation therapy in 11 patients, chemotherapy alone in two patients, chemotherapy plus radiation therapy in 10 patients, and chemotherapy plus surgery and radiation therapy in six patients. The 5-year survival rate was 51%. Multimodality treatment offered better survival (63% at 5 years) and diseasefree interval (54 months). Overall local, regional, and distant failure rates were 58%, 15%, and 40%, respectively. Distant metastases commonly occurred in bone (82%). Cervical metastasis was an unfavorable prognostic indicator (0% survival at 2 years).

Bhattacharyya et al. (24) reported on nine patients with esthesioneuroblastoma or neuroendocrine carcinoma of the paranasal sinuses treated with two cycles of cisplatin and etoposide followed by photon and stereotaxic proton radiation therapy totaling approximately 68 Gy to the primary site. Poor responders were treated with surgical resection followed by postoperative irradiation; in two cases, this was combined with two additional cycles of cisplatin and etoposide chemotherapy. Nine patients with a median Dilguerov T3 stage (range, T2 to T4) completed the treatment protocol, with mean follow-up after diagnosis of 20.5 months. Eight of nine patients exhibited a dramatic response to therapy, and resection was not required. One patient failed to respond to induction chemotherapy and received surgical therapy followed by postoperative radiation therapy. There have been no recurrences (mean diseasefree interval of 14 months). Complications were limited and generally transient.

In the University of Virginia series of five patients salvaged with high-dose chemotherapy and bone marrow transplantation, three were alive with no evidence of disease, whereas only 4/17 patients (24%) salvaged with surgery and chemotherapy or irradiation were alive with no evidence of disease. Although the indications for high-dose chemotherapy and bone marrow transplantation must be better defined, it is a promising alternative for patients with large tumors or those with recurrent tumor to whom no further local therapy (e.g., surgery or irradiation) can be safely given.

Sequelae of Treatment

In a few patients, depending on the dose of irradiation, long-term sequelae include bone necrosis, blindness, or painful eye reactions requiring enucleation (10,196,206).

Simon et al. (241), in 13 patients with olfactory esthesioneuroblastoma treated with surgery and radiation therapy, noted that visual impairment was the most common complication. One patients lost vision as a result of glaucoma and radiation retinopathy after receiving 67.34 Gy in 34 fractions. One patient treated with 61.76 Gy in 34 fractions developed a visual field defect and optic atrophy; she also had a nasal cutaneous fistula. One patient sustained intraoperative rupture of the ocular globe and subconjunctival hemorrhage.

Extramedullary Plasmacytomas

Solitary plasmacytomas are rare tumors of plasma cell origin making up 4% of all plasma cell tumors. Multiple myeloma occurs about 40 times more frequently than solitary plasmacytoma (142,200,288). Monoclonal extramedullary plasmacytoma (EMP) is a rare, low-grade lymphoma found predominantly in the head and neck region. Only since the introduction of immunophenotyping techniques two decades ago has it been possible to differentiate EMP from benign polyclonal plasma cell proliferation. Hotz et al. (122) reviewed the records of 24 patients with morphologically diagnosed EMP treated at their institution; only 14 patients had true monoclonal plasmacytoma. No EMP-related deaths occurred. Two patients had local recurrence, and two patients developed multiple myeloma. Diagnostic procedures exclude a benign polyclonal plasmacytoma, multiple myeloma, and solitary bone plasmacytoma. The slow natural progression of the disease and the rarity of secondary multiple myeloma favor nonmutilating local surgery whenever possible to avoid the long-term sequelae of radiation.

Epidemiology

The annual incidence of EMP is 0.04 cases per 100,000 population (178). They constitute only 0.5% of all upper respiratory tract malignancies. Male patients exceed female patients by a ratio of 4:1, and 75% of patients are 40 to 60 years of age (16,200,292).

In a detailed literature search of more than 400 publications between 1905 and 1997, EMP mainly occurred between the fourth and seventh decades of life (3). Seven hundred fourteen cases (82.2%) were found in the upper aerodigestive tract.

The most common sites in the head and neck are the nasopharynx, nasal cavity, paranasal sinuses, and tonsils.

Clinical Presentation and Diagnostic Work-Up

EMP of the head and neck area should be considered a separate entity because of its clinical behavior. The most common symptoms are nasal obstruction, local pain and swelling, and epistaxis.

Grossly, plasmacytomas tend to be sessile in the nasal cavity and paranasal sinuses and pedunculated in the nasopharynx and larynx. The masses are soft, pliable, and pale gray. The lesion may remain localized or may infiltrate and destroy the surrounding soft tissue and bone. The usual criteria for solitary plasmacytomas, either medullary or extramedullary, include a biopsy-proven plasma cell tumor with one or, at the most, two solitary foci, absence of Bence-Jones protein in the urine, bone marrow taken some distance from the primary site not involved by tumor (<10% of plasma cells), hemoglobin of 13 g/mL or more, and a normal serum protein level or serum electrophoresis at the time of the diagnosis. Basically, the diagnosis of solitary plasmacytoma is made by exclusion, that is, by eliminating the possibility of multiple myeloma (51). Diagnosis is based on histology along with special immunoperoxidase staining for immunoglobulin lambda and kappa light chains (281).

Dimopoulos et al. (65) noted that strict staging criteria, including normal MRI studies of the axial skeleton and the long bones and absence of monoclonal plasma cells detected by flow cytometry or PCR, are required for diagnosis of solitary plasmacytoma. Many patients enjoy prolonged diseasefree survival, but the incidence of systemic relapse is high. Careful microscopic and immunohistochemical studies are required for the correct diagnosis, because this disease can be confused with other malignancies, particularly lymphomas.

Six patients with primary EMP in the head and neck were examined with MRI (276); five lesions were oval and sharply demarcated without signs of infiltration, while the other lesion filled the parapharyngeal space bilaterally. On T2-weighted sequence, the lesions had moderate signal intensity. On plain T1-weighted sequences, the tumors were isointense or slightly hyperintense with respect to surrounding muscles; after administration of contrast medium, four lesions showed notable enhancement, with distinct central inhomogeneity.

Bone destruction is not a particularly bad prognostic sign, although some investigators report that it adversely affects prognosis (276). Bony invasion is common in the more malignant types (11).

Cervical lymph node metastasis from EMP varies with the site of the primary lesion and follows the same pattern of spread as squamous-cell carcinoma arising in a similar site. The reported incidence of lymph node metastasis ranges from 12% to 26% (142). The diagnostic work-up for EMP arising in the head and neck region is shown in Table 45.1.

The exact relationship between EMP and multiple myeloma is unclear; however, approximately 20% to 30% of EMP cases will convert to multiple myeloma (51,121,287).

General Management

Pedunculated EMP lesions may be treated by surgical excision because the chance of local recurrence is low. The treatment of choice for all other lesions is radiation therapy alone or combined with other modalities (109). In a review of 714 cases in the literature the following therapeutic strategies were used to treat patients with EMP of the upper aerodigestive tract: radiation therapy alone in 44.3%, combined therapy (surgery and irradiation) in 26.9%, and surgery alone in 21.9%. The median overall survival or recurrencefree survival was longer than 300 months for patients who underwent combined intervention (surgery and irradiation), for surgical intervention alone (median survival time, 156 months), and for radiation therapy alone (median survival time, 114 months). Overall, after treatment for EMP in the upper aerodigestive tract, 61.1% of all patients had no recurrence or conversion to systemic involvement (i.e., multiple myeloma); however, 22% had recurrence of EMP, and 16.1% had conversion to multiple myeloma.

Radiation Therapy Techniques

Irradiation techniques vary with the location of the primary tumor. The techniques are similar to those used for primary tumors in comparable locations (i.e., nasopharynx, tonsil, paranasal sinuses). Solitary plasmacytomas respond well to doses of 50 to 60 Gy in 2-Gy fractions. The local tumor control rate with radiation therapy alone is about 85%. Harwood et al. (109) summarized the literature but could not draw a dose–response curve from the data because of a lack of cases receiving low-dose radiation therapy. Nevertheless, there is a high risk of local recurrence with tumor doses below 30 Gy and a negligible risk for those treated at or above 40 Gy.

Wax et al. (281) reported on seven patients. Treatment consisted of radiation therapy in three cases, with doses ranging from 31.75 to 60 Gy. All patients have maintained local tumor control and had been followed for a minimum of 1.5 years, with an average of 3 years. One patient, treated with surgical excision, experienced a relapse at a distant site 6 years later.

The response to therapy of 32 patients with localized plasmacytoma were described by Shih et al. (238); 22 patients had solitary plasmacytoma of bone, and 10 had EMP. Median age for EMP was 63 years. Most EMPs occurred in the oronasopharynx (six cases) and paranasal sinuses (two cases). Seven patients with EMP received radiation therapy (47 to 65 Gy), and all achieved initial local tumor control. There was one local recurrence and multiple myeloma conversion in the EMP group. Local recurrence or dissemination was associated with the appearance of or an increase in M protein.

Holland et al. (121) reported on 14 cases of EMP, eight of which were in the head and neck. With doses of 46 to 62 Gy, the complete tumor response was 72%. No dose–response effect was observed.

Liebross et al. (162) described results in 22 patients with solitary EMP, in the head or neck in 19, usually in the nasal cavity or maxillary sinuses, bone destruction was found in 10/11 patients. Among all patients, serum myeloma protein was present in three patients (14%) and Bence Jones protein alone in two (9%). Radiation therapy was the sole treatment in 18/22 patients (median dose 50 Gy; range, 40 to 60 Gy); 5/7 patients with an EMP of oral cavity, oropharynx, nasopharynx, parotid, or larynx also received elective neck irradiation. Local tumor control was achieved in 21/22 patients (95%), and disease never recurred in regional nodes. Disappearance of myeloma protein occurred in 3/5 patients with an evaluable abnormality. Multiple myeloma developed in seven patients (32%), all within 5 years. The 5-year rate of freedom from progression to multiple myeloma was 56% and the median survival was 9.5 years. Chao et al. (40) reported on 16 patients with EMP and a median follow-up of 66 months. The head and neck region accounted for the majority of presentations (88%). A serum monoclonal paraprotein was found in three patients and bone erosion was identified in seven patients. All patients received local RT, although two patients also received elective nodal irradiation. The median RT dose was 45 Gy (range 40 to 50.4 Gy). Local tumor control was achieved in all patients (100%), however, regional recurrence outside the RT fields occurred in 2/16. Multiple myeloma (MM) developed in five patients (31%) all within 5 years. The 10-year myelomafree survival is 75% and 10-year overall survival is 54%.

Galieni et al. (92) reviewed 46 cases of EMP most frequently localized in the upper airways (37/46, 80%), with the mass being limited to a single site in all but seven patients in whom two contiguous sites were involved. The most frequent form of treatment was local radiation therapy. Thirty nine patients (85%) achieved complete remission, five (11%) a partial remission, and two (4%) did not respond to therapy. Local recurrence or recurrence at other sites occurred in 7.5% and 10%, respectively. Seven patients (15%) developed multiple myeloma. The 15-year survival rate was 78%.

Michalski et al. (182) described 10 patients with EMP treated with radiotherapy. One patient treated at relapse underwent surgical resection followed by postoperative RT. The disease was most frequently localized in the paranasal sinuses (50%). All nine patients who received definitive RT (40 to 50 Gy) achieved a complete response. Median follow-up period was 29 months. Four patients (40%) relapsed, three have died of their disease. Two patients with paranasal sinus disease subsequently relapsed with multiple myeloma at 10 months and 24 months, respectively. The relapse rate in neck nodes of 10% does not justify elective irradiation of the uninvolved neck.

Miller et al. (183) reported that tumor arose in the sinonasal/nasopharyngeal region in 11/20 patients (55%). The primary modality of treatment was radiation therapy (45 to 60 Gy). The mean follow-up was 60.2 months. In 15/20 cases, immunohistochemistry staining for immunoglobulin light chain production was conducted. One of the two cases (50%) classified as medullary plasmacytoma demonstrated conversion to multiple myeloma, whereas only 2/18 cases of EMP (11%) converted to multiple myeloma.

Ozsakin et al. (199) published a compilation of solitary plasmacytoma (42) in the head and neck. There were 258 patients with bone ($n = 206$) or extramedullary ($n = 52$) plasmacytomas without evidence of MM. Most ($n = 214$) of the patients received RT alone; 34 received chemotherapy and RT; and eight had surgery alone. The median radiation dose was 40 Gy. Median follow-up was 56 months (range 7 to 245 months). The median time for MM development was 21 moths (range 2 to 135 months), with a 5-year survival probability of 45% (Fig. 45.13A). The 5-year overall survival, diseasefree survival, and local control rates were 74%, 50%, and 86% respectively (Fig. 45.13B). On multivariate analyses, favorable factors were younger age and tumor size <4 cm for survival; age, extramedullary localization, and RT for diseasefree survival; and small tumor and RT for local control. Bone localization was the only predictor of MM development. No dose–response relationship was found for doses >30 Gy, even for larger tumors.

Tournier-Rangeard et al. (265), in a review of 17 patients with solitary EMP in the head and neck, noted a local tumor control of 100% for patients who received 45 Gy or greater dose to the CTV versus 50% with doses below 45 Gy ($p = 0.034$). Prognostic factor for 5-year disease-specific survival (81.6%) was local tumor control ($p = 0.058$). Prognostic factors for diseasefree survival (64.1%) were monoclonal immunoglobulin secretion ($p = 0.008$) and CTV dose >45 Gy ($p = 0.056$).

Table 45.13 summarizes the doses of irradiation and probability of tumor control reported by various investigators. Our limited experience confirms the efficacy of tumor doses of 45 to 50 Gy for local tumor control. In patients who had extensive disease, a higher dose (50 to 60 Gy) was used, as recommended by several investigators (51).

Nasopharyngeal Angiofibroma

Epidemiology

Juvenile nasopharyngeal angiofibroma (JNPA) is found more frequently in young pubertal boys (288); it has been shown to contain androgen receptors (4,81) and occasionally to regress with estrogen therapy. Hwang et al. (120) in 24 nasopharyngeal angiofibromas, detected androgen receptors in 18/24 (75%) cases, whereas only two (8.3%) were positive to progesterone. None of the 24 cases was positive for antibodies to estrogen.

JNPA comprises <0.05% of head and neck tumors (168). Patient age at presentation ranges from 9 to 30 years (52,272,288), with a median of 15 years. Females comprise <4% of the total cases (52). Some investigators have suggested chromosomal studies in affected women because this is mainly a male disease (39).

The tumor is believed to originate from the posterolateral wall of the nasal cavity where the sphenoidal process of the palatine bone meets the horizontal ala of the vomer and the roof of the pterygoid process (4) because it is always involved (39). Other investigators agree, because involution of tumor after irradiation usually occurs in this direction (235).

Clinical Presentation and Pathology

Symptoms usually occur 2 to 48 months before diagnosis (52). The most common complaints are nasal obstruction or epistaxis, followed by nasal voice or discharge, cheek swelling, proptosis, diplopia, hearing loss, and headaches (52). In a series by Witt et al. (288), 7/31 patients presented with anomalous sexual development.

Table 45.13	EXTRAMEDULLARY PLASMACYTOMA OF HEAD AND NECK TREATED BY RADIATION THERAPY					
Author	No. of Patients	No. of Males/ No. of Females	No. <50 yr of Age	Local Control	No. with Multiple Myeloma	Recommended Tumor Dose (Gy)[a]
Todd (312)	15	13/2	12	14/15	5	34.5–38 for 3 wk
Kotner and Wang (178)	16	10/6	12	12/16	4	40–50
Wiltshaw (339)	14	10/4	10	11/14	N/A	—
Woodruff et al. (344)	15	8/7	11	14/15	1	40–50
Bush et al. (42)	10	5/5	5	8/10	2	50–55
Harwood et al. (141)	22	18/4	16	18/22	4	35 for 3 wk
Kapadia et al. (167)	12	9/3	10	11/12	3	—
M.D. Anderson Hospital[b]	15	12/3	12	13/15	4	50
Total	119	85/34 (2.5:1)	88 (73.9%)	101/119 (84.9%)	23 (19.3%)	40–50

[a]10 Gy/wk unless otherwise stated.
[b]Updated, unpublished data of Corwin J.

Nasopharyngeal angiofibroma may initially extend into the nasal fossae and maxillary antrum and push the soft palate downward, then through the pterygopalatine fossa and superoanteriorly through the inferior orbital fissure or laterally through the pterygomaxillary fissure to the cheek and temporal regions (58).

Beham et al. (15) reported on 32 cases of nasopharyngeal angiofibroma. Most of the tumor vessels, which lacked elastic laminae, were characterized by vascular walls of irregular thickness and variable muscle content. In places endothelial cells were separated from the stroma by only a single attenuated layer of contractile cells, in some more fibrotic hyaline areas, the stromal cells displayed reactivity for smooth muscle actin. The irregularity of the vascular walls, together with the lack of elastic laminae and stromal fibers, explains the pronounced tendency for hemorrhage in these lesions.

Differential diagnosis includes fibrosarcoma, rhabdomyosarcoma, chronic sinusitis, arteriovenous malformation, lymphangioma, neurofibroma, pleomorphic adenoma, lymphoma, pyogenic granuloma, polyps, and hemangioma.

Diagnostic Work-Up

After the history and physical examination, CT scans with and without contrast should be obtained. The pattern of enhancement in this highly vascular tumor is diagnostic (164,192), and many investigators believe carotid angiograms are unnecessary (30) after CT diagnosis of the lesion, unless embolization, which is also controversial, is contemplated.

CT scans are especially helpful in regions involving thin bony structures (paranasal sinuses, orbits), where CT performs better than MRI. In the nasopharynx and parapharyngeal space MRI is superior to CT. Obtaining tumor volumetric data with spiral CT or MRI facilitates 3D treatment planning (102).

Seventy-two patients with JNPA were evaluated with CT and/or MRI (164). Origin of the tumor was in the pterygopalatine fossa at the aperture of the pterygoid (vidian) canal. The tumor extended posteriorly along the pterygoid canal with invasion of the cancellous bone of the pterygoid base and greater wing of the sphenoid in 60% of the patients. The inability to remove the tumor in toto was principally due to deep invasion of the sphenoid; 93% of recurrences occurred with this type of tumor extension.

If intracranial extension is noted and radiation therapy is contemplated, no further studies are indicated. If the lesion is extracranial and surgery is indicated, bilateral carotid angiograms will identify the feeding vessels and delineate the boundaries of the tumor (Fig. 45.13).

Biopsies are not indicated in all patients because of the potential for severe hemorrhage. It is important to perform a biopsy of the lesion when the clinical picture (sex, age, location, and behavior of the lesion) is not consistent with JNPA (250) because some lesions have proven to be sarcomas or chronic sinusitis (39). Two cases of fibrosarcoma have been reported in patients in their 40s (66).

Staging and Prognostic Factors

Two staging schemes have been proposed: (a) the system of Chandler et al. (39) (Table 45.14), and (b) a radiographic staging system by Sessions et al. (235). Stage Ia is limited to the nasopharynx and posterior nares; stage Ib extends to the paranasal sinuses; stages IIa, IIb, and IIc extend to other extracranial locations; and stage III is intracranial.

In a retrospective review of 44 cases of juvenile nasopharyngeal angiofibroma, invasion of the skull affected two thirds of the patients, and the rate of recurrence was 27.5% (116). Extensions to the intratemporal fossa, sphenoid sinus, base of pterygoids and clivus, the cavernous sinus (medial), foramen lacerum, and anterior fossa were correlated with more frequent recurrence. Long-term radiographic follow-up showed residual disease in nine asymptomatic patients: these remnants gradually involuted.

General Management

The decision of whether surgery or radiation therapy should be used depends in part on the initial extent of the disease. In patients with extracranial tumors (116,288), surgery is the treatment of choice and yields near-zero mortality or any long-term morbidity.

Tumor remnants in symptomfree patients should be kept under surveillance by repeated CT scanning, since involution may occur. Recurrent symptoms may be treated by radiation therapy rather than by extended surgery or combined procedures (39,61,116).

When there is intracranial tumor extension (seen in about 20% of patients) (130,288), the risk of surgically related death increases. In a literature review by Jones et al. (133), it was found to be 14% to 84%. Most of these patients are best treated with irradiation (54).

Some investigators recommend preoperative intraarterial tumor vessel embolization at the time of diagnostic bilateral carotid angiography, claiming a decrease in operative bleeding (154). Salvage with embolization of polyvinyl alcohol has been described (129). Others have reported anecdotal evidence of partial regression with the use of estrogens, believed to be

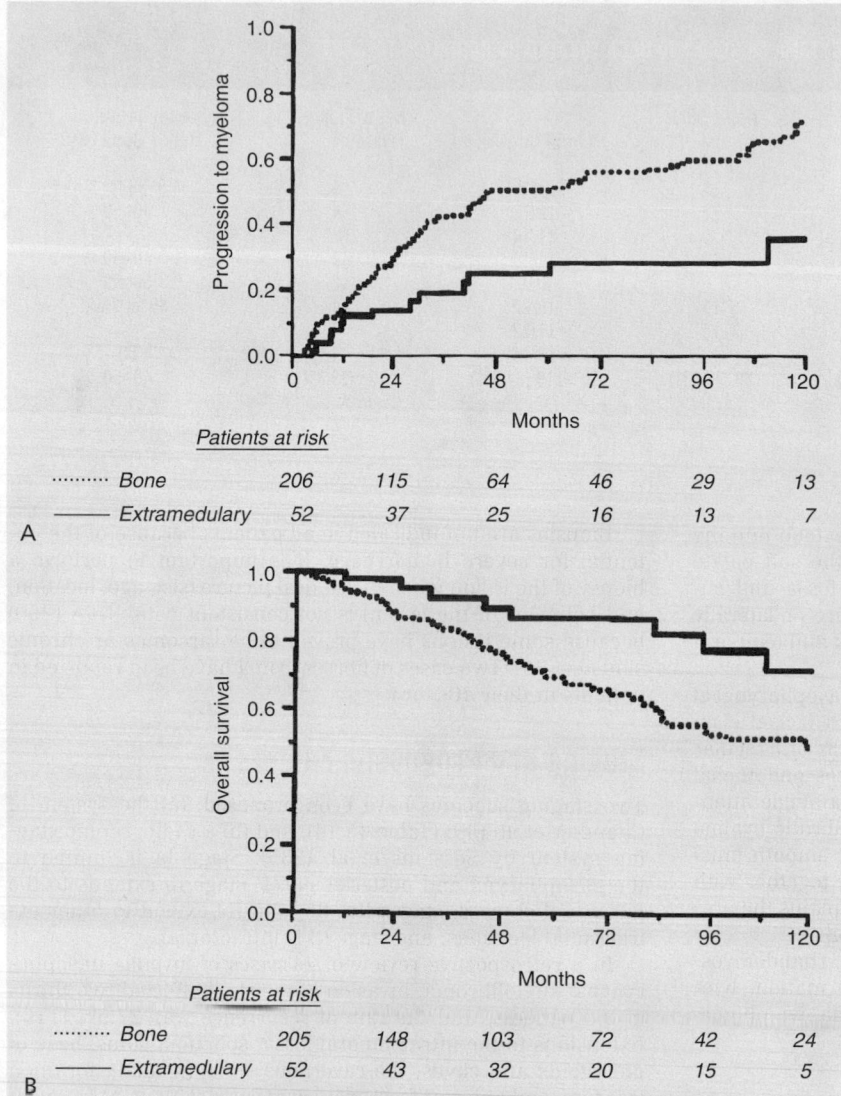

Patients at risk						
.... Bone	206	115	64	46	29	13
—— Extramedulary	52	37	25	16	13	7

Patients at risk						
.... Bone	205	148	103	72	42	24
—— Extramedulary	52	43	32	20	15	5

FIGURE 45.13. A: Probability of progression to multiple myeloma according to bone (*dotted line*) or extramedullary (*solid line*) solitary plasmacytoma ($p = 0.0009$). **B:** Overall survival correlated with bone (*dotted line*) or extramedullary (*solid line*) solitary plasmacytoma ($p = 0.04$). (From Özsakın M, Tsang RW, Poortmans P, et al. Outcomes and patterns of failure in solitary plasmacytoma: a multicenter rare cancer. Study of 258 patients. *Int J Rad Oncol Biol Phys* 2006;64:210–217, with permission.)

the result of feedback inhibition of the pituitary's production of gonadotropin-releasing hormone.

Although radiation therapy is equally effective in extracranial tumors, the low but existing risk of secondary malignancies should limit its use to the most advanced tumors only (10,154,284). In the experience of Cummings et al. (54) covering 20 years, only two radiation-related malignancies were noted (one skin, one thyroid).

	STAGING OF NASOPHARYNGEAL ANGIOFIBROMAS
Table 45.14	

Stage I	Confined to the nasopharynx
Stage II	Extension to nasal cavity and/or sphenoid sinus
Stage III	Extension to one or more: antrum, ethmoid, pterygomaxillary and infratemporal fossae, orbit, and/or cheek
Stage IV	Intracranial extension

From Chandler JR, Goulding R, Moskowitz L, et al. Nasopharyngeal angiofibromas: staging and management. *Ann Otol Rhinol Laryngol* 1984;93:322, with permission.

Radiation Therapy Techniques

Photon irradiation should be used for these patients, and fields must be individualized to cover the tumor completely with a margin (1 to 2 cm). Treatment portals are similar to those used in carcinoma of the nasopharynx (without irradiating the cervical lymph nodes) or carcinoma of the paranasal sinuses when these structures or the nasal cavity is involved. Opposing lateral portals are suitable in most patients, with larger fields and compensators used for tumors extending into the nose (Fig. 45.14). More extensive disease requires three-field or wedge-pair arrangements of 3DCRT or IMRT that can yield excellent dose distributions, particularly when there is nasopharyngeal or intracranial tumor extension. In all cases the eyes are protected as much as possible. The recommended tumor dose ranges from 30 Gy in 15 fractions in 3 weeks to 50 Gy in 24 to 28 fractions in 5 weeks (54). A conventional setup uses 6- to 18-MV photons to treat the lesion with parallel-opposed fields to 50 Gy (2-Gy fractions) (Fig. 45.15).

The advantages of IMRT for the treatment of extensive and/or recurrent JNPA has been described in three patients on whom the tumor affected the base of skull, pterygopalatine, and intratemporal fossae, posterior orbit, and nasopharynx (151).

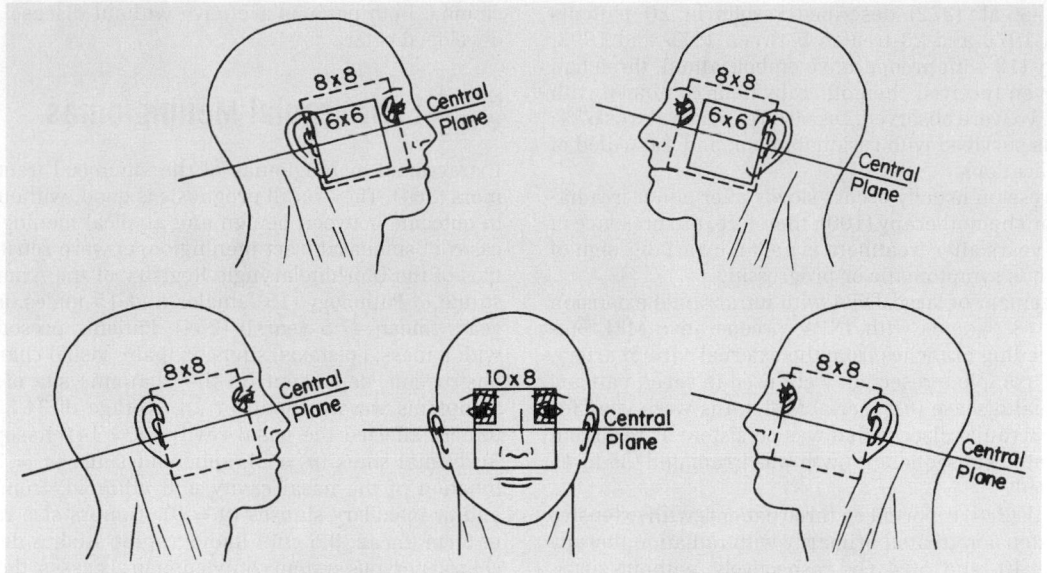

FIGURE 45.14. Diagrams of the most commonly used conventional field arrangements for treatment of nasopharynx angiofibroma: lateral opposed field pair and three-field technique. (From Cummings BJ, Blend R, Keane T. Primary radiation therapy for juvenile nasopharyngeal angiofibroma. *Laryngoscope* 1984;94:1599–1605, with permission.)

Tumor dose varied from 34 to 45 Gy. The tumor shrunk radiographically in all three cases, and there was no endoscopic evidence of disease in two cases at 15 months and 40 months. Late toxicity was limited to one episode of epistaxis and persistent rhinitis in one patient.

Results of Therapy

Jones et al. (133) reported the results of 40 patients with JNPA treated with surgery alone. With a mean follow-up of 17 months (6 to 36 months), the control rates according to the Sessions staging system were as follows: 100% (stages I and IIa), 83% (stage IIb), 80% (stage IIc), and 50% (stage III). All failures were controlled with irradiation ($n = 18$ patients), embolization ($n = 8$), or surgical resection ($n = 8$), and the other four were

observed only, demonstrating the extremely high salvage rate in this disease (126). These findings are consistent with other series reporting initial surgical control of 86% with an ultimate control rate of 96% (288).

In another report, 18 patients were treated with gross tumor excision; two cases with intracranial involvement required a combined neurosurgical-otolaryngologic approach (61). Recurrent intracranial disease was detected by MRI in three patients, who were treated with 35-, 36-, and 45-Gy external-beam irradiation. Extracranial tumor recurrences were re-excised in seven patients. All patients (followed up with serial MRI) are living without evidence of active disease.

Cummings et al. (54) treated 42 patients primarily with irradiation and 13 for postsurgical failures; all except six had biopsies. Nine had stage IV disease according to Chandler's staging system. Dose was 30 to 35 Gy in 14 to 16 fractions over a 3-week period. Follow-up ranged from 3 to 26 years. The control rate was 80% and was equivalent for all dose ranges. Local control was 89% and 74%, respectively, when three fields versus two fields were used. When the field size was more than 6 by 6 cm, the control rate was 83% versus 55% for smaller portals, indicating the importance of accurately determining the target volume, including any potential tumor extension. Of 11 recurrences, eight were controlled by a second course of irradiation and three by surgery. These tumors regress slowly, with 50% still present at 12 months. At 24 months, 23% of tumors were still present, and half of those recurred. Of the complete responders, only 1/33 had a recurrence. Robinson et al. (224) also found that objective responses after irradiation were noted within 6 months in 60% of patients and within 6 to 20 months in the other 40%. Symptoms, however, resolved in all patients within 6 months of treatment.

At the Mallinckrodt Institute of Radiology, Fields (written communication, 1989) reviewed our experience with 13 patients: 11 surgical failures and two primarily treated with irradiation. Intracranial extension was noted in 38% of patients. Follow-up ranged from 40 to 173 months. Doses ranged from 36 to 52 Gy, with a median of 48 Gy (1.8 to 2 Gy per fraction, 5 days a week). The control rate was 85%; patients failing irradiation were salvaged with embolization. Late morbidity was mostly xerostomia and dental decay.

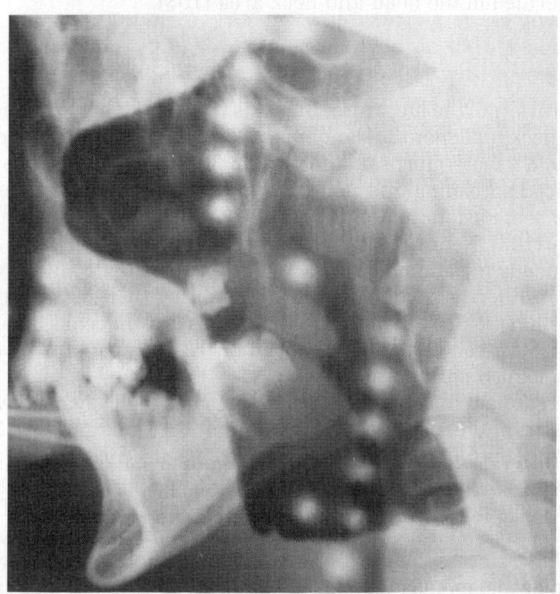

FIGURE 45.15. Example of conventional lateral portal used at the Mallinckrodt Institute of Radiology for nasopharyngeal angiofibroma.

Ungkanont et al. (272) described results in 20 patients treated before 1974 and 23 treated between 1975 and 1993: 31 had surgery (18 with preoperative embolization), three had irradiation, seven received chemotherapy (four combined with surgery), and two were observed. Disease-free survival was 67%; 28% of patients survived with residual tumor, and 4.6% died of surgical complications.

Tumor regression usually occurs slowly after either irradiation (54,172) or chemotherapy (100); therefore, the presence of tumor up to 2 years after treatment is not an invariable sign of failure unless it is symptomatic or progressing.

The management of large JNPA with intracranial extension is difficult. In 18 patients with JNPA, preoperative MRI, embolization of feeding branches from the external carotid artery, and attempted complete resection were used in seven patients with intracranial disease (61); serial MRI scans were used for follow-up. Intracranial disease that was persistent or recurrent and demonstrated subsequent growth was irradiated (35 to 45 Gy) or re-excised.

Wiatrak et al. (284) reported on three patients with extensive intracranial extension treated primarily with radiation therapy doses of 36.6, 40, and 50.4 Gy, respectively, without surgical tumor resection. Although there was no complete resolution of the tumors, significant improvement of symptoms was obtained without serious sequelae. Malignant degeneration in JNPA undergoing radiation therapy has been occasionally reported (16,54,224).

Goepfert et al. (100) reported on five patients with aggressive nasopharyngeal angiofibromas recurrent after extracranial resection and irradiation who were treated with chemotherapy. Doxorubicin (60 mg/m^2 intravenous [IV] push for 1 day) and dacarbazine (250 mg/m^2 IV drip for 5 days) were given, with courses being repeated every 3 to 4 weeks. In a second regimen, vincristine, dactinomycin, and cyclophosphamide were administered at usual doses. Excellent tumor regression was noted in all patients. Patients were disease free at 2, 3, 6, and 10 years.

Ochoa-Carrillo et al. (192) reported on 31 patients treated with surgery and/or radiation therapy. Surgery was the treatment chosen in patients with stage II and III disease, while radiation therapy was the treatment in stage IV, but it had low effectiveness, indicating the need to carefully investigate the value of craniofacial approaches in these tumors. Radiation therapy (30 to 55 Gy) was administered to 16 patients; seven with stage III persistent or recurrent tumor, and eight patients as initial treatment for stage IV disease. The disease-free interval of patients with stage III and IV disease was 80.3% and 19%, respectively, after 96 months of follow-up.

Tranbahuy et al. (267) reported on seven patients with juvenile angiofibroma who underwent direct tumoral embolization. This technique induced marked devascularization and necrosis of the tumor. No neurologic sequelae were encountered.

Sequelae of Therapy

Most investigators agree that surgical mortality increases with intracranial extension of the tumor. The most common radiation therapy sequelae include delayed growth secondary to hypopituitarism and decreased bone maturation (39). There are several well-documented cases of radiation-induced sarcomas in these patients (54,245) with doses ranging from 66 Gy to more than 90 Gy. Spagnolo et al. (245) reported on four patients treated with irradiation who later developed sarcoma. Chen and Bauer (44) reported the same findings in a patient receiving 66 Gy and followed up for 18 years. This patient was 48 years of age, so the original diagnosis of JNPA does not coincide clinically with typical JNPA. Cummings et al. (54) reported two neoplasms developing 13 and 14 years after irradiation; one was a basal cell carcinoma and one metastatic thyroid carcinoma. Both patients are alive without disease. Two patients developed cataracts.

Extracranial Meningiomas

Extracranial meningiomas of the sinonasal tract are rare tumors (264). The overall prognosis is good, without a difference in outcome between benign and atypical meningiomas. Thirty cases of sinonasal tract meningiomas were retrieved from the files of the Otorhinolaryngic Registry of the Armed Forces Institute of Pathology (15 females and 15 males, aged 13 to 88 years [mean 47.5 years]) (264). Patients presented clinically with a mass, epistaxis, sinusitis, pain, visual changes, or nasal obstruction, dependent on the anatomic site of involvement. Symptoms were present for an average of 31.3 months. The tumors affected the nasal cavity ($n = 14$), nasopharynx ($n = 3$), frontal sinus ($n = 2$), sphenoid sinus ($n = 2$), or a combination of the nasal cavity and ethmoid, frontal, sphenoid, and/or maxillary sinuses ($n = 9$). Tumors size ranged from 1 to 8 cm (mean, 3.5 cm). Radiographic studies demonstrated a central nervous system connection in six cases; the tumors often eroded the bones of the sinuses ($n = 18$) and involved the surrounding soft tissues, the orbit, and occasionally the base of the skull. Histologically, the tumors demonstrated features similar to intracranial meningiomas; the majority of the meningothelial type ($n = 23$), although there were three atypical meningiomas. Immunohistochemical studies confirmed the diagnosis with reactions for epithelial membrane antigen and vimentin (all tested). The differential diagnosis included paraganglioma, carcinoma, melanoma, psammomatoid ossifying fibroma, and angiofibroma.

Surgical excision was used in all patients. Three patients died with recurrent disease (mean, 1.2 years), one was alive with recurrent disease (25.6 years), and the remaining 24 patients were alive or had died of unrelated causes (mean, 13.9 years) at the time of last follow-up (two patients were lost to follow-up).

Nonlentiginous Melanoma

Malignant melanoma accounts for 11% of primary head and neck malignancies (8). Of all malignant melanomas, 20% to 35% are located in the head and neck area (108).

Cutaneous Melanoma

In a review of the literature, Batsakis (11) found that, of all head and neck malignant melanomas, 64% to 78% were cutaneous, 6% to 8% were mucosal, and 14% to 30% were ocular. The superficial spreading and nodular types of malignant melanoma have a metastatic potential of 10% to 30% and 50%, respectively (108). Neurotropic melanoma is an uncommon variant of cutaneous melanoma, with a higher propensity to invade peripheral nerves. A thorough evaluation with CT scans should determine if there is intracranial or base of the skull involvement; Beenken et al. (14) reported on 13 such patients, two of whom failed perineurally.

Treatment of cutaneous melanomas has typically been wide excision of the lesion with a minimum 3-cm margin (8). More recently, margins of at least 2 cm have been used in the head and neck area compared with wider margins for stage I melanomas, with equivalent success as noted by the local failure rate of 3% to 6% (155).

The Princess Margaret Hospital treated 16 patients with nodular melanomas with local excision and postoperative radiation therapy (50 Gy in 10 fractions over 2 weeks); 14 exhibited local tumor control, and six were alive and well 2 to 14 years after treatment. These results were comparable with those with wide local excision alone but with less morbidity and fewer cosmetic alterations. Later, at the same institution, Harwood and Cummings (108) treated five patients with definitive radiation therapy for superficial spreading melanoma of the head and neck area. All five lesions were locally controlled; one patient had a lymph node metastasis that was later controlled, and one died of distant metastases. They recommend treating these patients with 45 Gy in 10 fractions over 2 weeks to 50 Gy in 15 fractions in 3 weeks (107,111).

Harwood and Cummings (108) also reported results in 74 patients treated with three 8-Gy fractions given on days 0, 7, and 21 with shielding of the spinal cord, brain, and eye. Thirty patients were treated postoperatively after neck dissections if they had extracapsular extension, multiple nodal involvement, a node >3 cm, or residual disease. Tumor control in the neck was achieved in 26/30 patients (86.6%) with follow-up of 1 to 4 years. In four patients with microscopic residual disease at the primary site, this postoperative regimen controlled three of four lesions with follow-up of 1 to 3.5 years. The other 40 patients were treated either for gross (13 patients) or recurrent (27 patients) cutaneous melanoma. Complete response was observed in 15/40 lesions (37.5%) and partial response in 12. An update of Harwood's data (personal communication, 1989) showed a neck tumor control rate of 94% in 41 adjuvantly treated patients versus 57% in 48 patients with gross residual or recurrent tumors. He concluded that irradiation alone should be considered for treatment of superficial spreading melanomas when surgery is contraindicated or after a simple excision in all cases of nodular melanoma in which a wide excision may be contraindicated because of age, location, or medical condition. For nodal disease, patients with poor prognostic pathologic factors should receive postoperative irradiation. Recurrent or unresectable tumors also should be irradiated. He recommended high-dose fractions because the local control rate was 71% when the dose per fraction was >4 Gy and 25% with lower fractions (111).

Another approach to the treatment of recurrent or unresectable cutaneous melanomas is combined hyperthermia and high-fraction radiation therapy as reported by Emami et al. (76). The data support the use of high fractions for melanoma because Overgaard's complete response rate was 59% when fractions of more than 4 Gy were used and 33% for lower dose per fraction sizes. However, a randomized study by the Radiation Therapy Oncology Group comparing four fractions of 8 Gy given on days 0, 7, 14, and 21 and 20 fractions of 2.5 Gy in 5 weekly fractions showed no significant difference in tumor response (24.2% and 23.4% complete response and 35% partial response) (218).

Mucosal Melanomas

Primary mucosal melanomas of the head and neck area comprise 2% to 8% of the cases seen each year in the United States (13). They occur more commonly in countries such as Japan, where mucosal melanoma is found in 22% to 32% of patients with malignant melanoma (271). Most occur in the fifth to seventh decades of life; they are extremely rare in the first two decades (0.6% of mucosal melanomas) (91,269,270). The male-to-female ratio approaches 1:1 (269). A review by Batsakis et al. (13) of 204 mucosal melanomas showed 56.4% to be from the upper respiratory tract and 44% from the oral cavity and pharynx. Nasal cavity/paranasal tumors comprise <1% of malignant melanomas and 2% to 9% of head and neck melanomas (91,120). Pigmentation may precede the lesion in up to 28% of patients for more than 1 year (32). In the oral cavity, the most common location is the hard palate (up to 80%), followed in order of decreasing frequency by the upper gingiva and lower gingiva.

Diagnostic Work-Up

An excisional biopsy should be performed when feasible because some reports have suggested possible local or metastatic spread secondary to a punch or incisional biopsy (219), although this has not been noted in cutaneous melanomas (103). Batsakis et al. (13) found that one third of these lesions were amelanotic, and Hoki et al. (120) noted that 25% were amelanotic.

Metastatic melanoma to the mucosa of the head and neck area is less common (115). It can be differentiated from primary tumors by the presence of normal tissue between subepidermal tumor and the basal layer of melanocytes (13). In a review of the literature. The larynx, tongue, and tonsils are the most common locations for metastases (115).

Prognostic Factors

Batsakis et al. (13) found >0.5 mm invasion to be a poor prognostic factor. Trapp et al. (268) noted this to be true only in patients with more than 0.7 mm invasion. Lymph node involvement is not a prognostic factor. Mucosal melanomas fare worse than their cutaneous counterparts (137), suggesting a lack of immunologic competence (136,222).

Management and Results of Therapy

In a review of the Japanese literature, Umeda et al. (271) found a local tumor control rate for stage I and II disease of 58% (7/12) in surgically treated patients with oral melanomas and a minimum follow-up of 3 years. Similar rates of failure have been reported, even with radical en bloc excisions (20% to 42%). Because the main cause of treatment failure is distant metastases and because almost no patient has clinically evident nodal metastases at presentation, an elective neck node dissection is not recommended by some investigators (27). This subject is still controversial because 30% to 60% of patients may later develop nodal disease (23).

Ohya et al. (195) treated six patients with oral cavity melanomas with irradiation as a component of therapy (dose range 2,000 R to 8,900 R, five treated preoperatively, one postoperatively). All lesions were locally controlled with follow-up of 25 to 109 months; 3/7 patients were alive with 4 to 5 years of follow-up. Harwood and Cummings (108) treated 12 cases and added 12 cases from the literature for a total of 24 patients and 25 lesions. Local tumor control was achieved in 11/24 (9 to 54 months' follow-up). Six of seven tumors treated with 4-Gy fractions or larger were controlled, versus 5/18 treated with smaller fractions.

Postoperative radiation therapy was reported by Panje and Moran (203). Five patients were treated with ^{60}Co or 4-MV photons, 50 to 60 Gy, 1.5 to 2 Gy per fraction, over a period of 5 to 6 weeks. Only one patient showed local control; the other patients failed 6 to 12 months after irradiation.

Kingdom and Kaplan (140) described results in 13 patients with mucosal melanoma of the nasal cavity and paranasal sinuses treated with surgical resection. Eight had microscopically negative margins. Seven patients received postoperative irradiation (30 to 62 Gy). The neck was treated in three patients with doses of 30 to 50 Gy. The local tumor recurrence rate was 85% (11/13), with a mean interval from primary tumor treatment to recurrence of 16 months. Metastatic neck disease developed in two patients and distant metastases in four. Patients receiving postoperative irradiation had increased diseasefree interval and prolonged survival. Negative surgical margins were not predictive of a more favorable outcome. The investigators recommend resection of tumor with negative margins and postoperative irradiation for the treatment of all patients with mucosal malignant melanoma.

Patients with nasal cavity/paranasal mucosal melanoma have a median survival of 24 months. Five-year diseasefree survival rates of 25% have been reported (269). Patients with laryngeal melanoma had a 13% 5-year diseasefree survival rate (137). Because of the poor results obtained and because 37% of patients had associated adjacent pigmentation (222), some investigators recommend prophylactic excision of all melanocytic nevi. Because the results with irradiation are comparable with those of surgical series and because of the poor survival of these patients due to distant metastases and not locoregional failure, irradiation alone, with surgery for salvage, should be seriously considered as the primary treatment for mucosal melanomas of the head and neck (111).

Lentigo Maligna Melanoma

Natural History

Lentigo maligna (Hutchinson's melanotic freckle [124] or circumscribed precancerous melanosis of Dubreuilh) and its invasive counterpart, lentigo maligna melanoma (LMM), are well-recognized clinicopathologic entities (46). LMM comprises about 10% of all melanomas in the head and neck, occurs predominantly on the face and ears of elderly persons, and generally has a very long natural history, frequently reaching a large size before diagnosis. Approximately one third of lentigo maligna lesions, if left untreated, will eventually transform into invasive LMM.

Tannous et al. (260) hypothesized that lentigo maligna can be divided into two categories: one represents a pigmented lesion that is a precursor to melanoma, and the other melanoma in situ. Also, they hypothesized that in some patients there is a progression to malignant melanoma.

Clinical Presentation and Diagnostic Work-Up

These lesions appear as circumscribed and later as more diffuse areas of hyperpigmentation of the skin. They may develop some superficial nodularity and eventual ulceration as they become more invasive. In 10% of the latter patients, regional and distant metastases eventually develop. The 10% metastatic spread in LMM contrasts with the 25% metastatic tendency in nodular melanomas arising in superficial spreading melanomas and a 50% metastatic spread in nodular melanomas arising de novo.

The diagnostic work-up of these patients is similar to that of patients suspected of having malignant melanoma. Biopsies of the lesion are required to obtain histopathologic confirmation of the diagnosis. Careful physical examination must rule out any areas of extension or regional or distant spread.

General Management

The usual treatment of lentigo maligna and LMM has been surgery, with approximately 1- to 2-cm margin of normal skin (8).

Hill and Gramp (118) reported on 66 cases of lentigo malignant melanoma; 38% of which required two excisions or more to clear the tumor and 32% of cases showed evidence of invasive melanoma. Only one case has recurred thus far, and none have developed metastatic disease.

Because of the low incidence of regional lymph node metastases, elective lymph node dissection is not indicated. For larger lesions, wider surgical excision with skin grafting has been reported to give poor cosmetic results.

Cohen et al. (47) reported their experience with Mohs microsurgery, which was performed in 26 patients with lentigo maligna and 19 patients with lentigo maligna melanoma. After a median follow-up of 58 months (214.3 patient years), there was one recurrence, in a patient with five prior recurrences before Mohs micrographic surgery.

Kuflik and Gage (149) treated 30 patients with cryosurgery. Lesions ranged from 1.3 to 4.5 cm in diameter. Lesions recurred in two patients (recurrence rate of 6.6%) who were successfully retreated with cryosurgery. Eleven patients observed for more than 5 years showed no recurrences.

Radiation therapy with various techniques has been frequently used in the treatment of these patients, particularly those with larger lesions, because of minimal morbidity and generally excellent cosmetic results (Fig. 45.16).

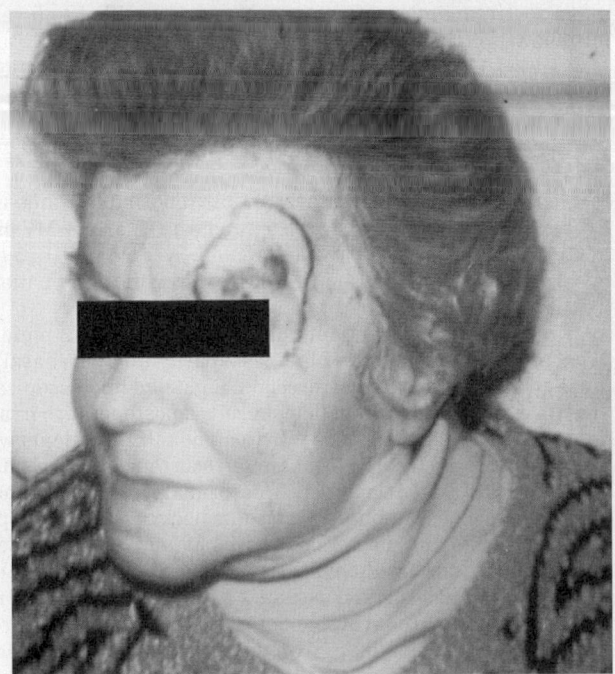
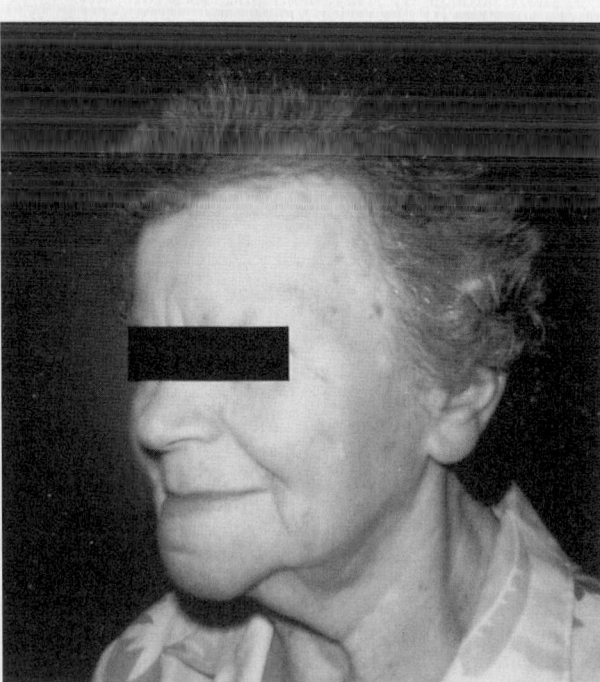

FIGURE 45.16. Lentigo maligna melanoma of face before **(A)** and 6 years after **(B)** 50 Gy in 25 fractions delivered with 9-MeV electrons and bolus.

Radiation Therapy Techniques

As in other skin lesions, the portals should be carefully designed to include the entire tumor with adequate margin (1 cm for lesions <2 cm and 2 cm for larger tumors). Because Miescher's irradiation technique used very superficial x-rays, with 50% depth dose being at approximately 1 mm, there is the possibility of local recurrence if dermal extension is unrecognized. Therefore, Harwood and Lawson (111) recommend using minimum x-ray energies of 100 keVp and preferably 140 to 175 keVp to treat these patients. Superficial x-rays (100 to 200 keVp) with adequate filtration or electrons (6 to 9 MeV) with appropriate thickness of bolus (about 1.5 cm) are adequate for most patients. Doses of 45 to 50 Gy in 15 to 25 fractions delivered over 3 to 5 weeks will control the disease in most patients. We recommend delivering 3 to 3.5 Gy, three times weekly, every other day, to a total of 50 Gy, depending on the size and thickness of the lesion. Elective irradiation of the regional lymphatics is not necessary.

Careful follow-up with clinical examinations and photographs of the lesion is essential to ascertain the continuing regression of the tumor.

In patients on whom surgical excision is performed, postoperative irradiation is recommended if positive margins are found (111). Doses are similar to those stated earlier.

Results of Therapy

Kopf et al. (146) reported six recurrences in 16 patients treated with 50 keV x-rays (500 cGy doses).

Harwood and Lawson (111) described 13 patients with lentigo maligna treated with radiation therapy: 11 had local tumor control, one had an edge recurrence salvaged by irradiation, and one had residual tumor (alive and well 11 years after treatment for the recurrence). One patient alive at 2 years refused further treatment. Of 19 patients irradiated for LMM, 17 had tumor control with radiation therapy alone for periods

ranging from 6 months to 6 years. One patient had a central recurrence that was salvaged by surgery (alive and well 5 years after treatment of recurrence). One patient died of intercurrent disease <3 months after irradiation. No patient has developed lymph node or distant metastases in either group.

Tsang et al. (269) described results in 54 patients treated with radiation therapy or surgery. Younger patients with smaller lesions were treated with surgical excision (18 patients) and achieved actuarial tumor control of 94% at 3 years. Older patients with larger lesions located in the head and neck area were treated by radiation therapy (36 patients), with an actuarial tumor control rate of 86% at 5 years. No patient developed metastatic melanoma. The late cosmetic appearance was acceptable in the majority of irradiated patients, with 11% showing poor cosmesis because of progressive skin pallor, atrophy, and telangiectasia in the treated area.

Sarcomas of the Head and Neck

Natural History

Sarcomas account for <1% of malignant neoplasms in the head and neck. The most frequent histological type is malignant fibrohistocytoma (29%), while the least common is liposarcoma (1%) (35). The histology is complex and requires immunochemical analysis including osteosarcoma, angiosarcoma, chondrosarcoma, hemangiosarcoma, leiomyosarcoma, liposarcoma, malignant fibrous sarcoma, rhabdomyosarcoma, malignant schwannoma, neurofibrosarcoma, and synovial sarcoma. Fibrosarcoma, angiosarcoma, leiomyosarcoma, and rhabdomyosarcoma are the most common types but this varies in published reports. Table 45.15 summarizes the distribution of various histologic types in 1,127 patients. Distribution of these sarcomas was 33% in the scalp or face, 26% in the orbit or paranasal sinuses, 14% arising from upper aerodigestive tract

Table 45.15   HISTOLOGIC DISTRIBUTION OF HEAD AND NECK SARCOMAS: REVIEW OF THE LITERATURE

Histology/Series	Weber et al. (282)	Tran et al. (226)	Greager et al. (101)	McKenna et al. (179)	Farhood et al. (82)	Eeles et al. (73)	Freedman et al. (87)	LeVay et al. (159)	Willers et al. (286)	Chao et al.[a]	Total (%)
Bone											
Osteosaroma	—	9	—	—	—	—	—	—	—	5	14 (1.2%)
Chrondosarcoma	—	16	—	—	—	—	—	—	—	—	16 (1.4%)
Fibrous											
Malignant fibrous histiocytoma	29	6	4	2	8	30	35	11	14	7	146 (13%)
Fibrosarcoma	20	20	12	2	51	8	38	6	5	5	167 (15%)
Muscle											
Leimyosarcoma	6	7	—	—	12	9	13	3	4	—	54 (4.9%)
Rhabdomyosarcoma	29	12	3	—	42	—	76	3	—	4	169 (15%)
Vaxular											
Angiosarcoma	24	26	3	2	17	3	25	5	11	4	120 (10%)
Hemangiopericytoma	—	3	3	2	10	—	23	2	—	—	43 (3.8%)
Fatty											
Liposarcoma	3	7	5	—	7	5	9	—	3	—	39 (3.6%)
Neural											
Malignant schwannoma	—	6	7	1	23[b]	16[b]	—	3	9	—	127 (11%)[b]
Neurofibrosarcoma	19	10	—	1			29	3	—	—	
Others											
Synovial sarcoma	4	2	3	2	6	7	—	2	4	—	30 (2.7%)
Low-grade tumor	11	13	9	—	—	4	46	5	6	—	94 (8.4%)
Miscellaneous	22	19	1	3	—	19	38	10	1	8	121 (10%)

[a]Unpublished data.
[b]Malignant schwannoma and neurofibrosarcoina combined.

including larynx, and 27% in the neck. Synovial sarcomas are rare soft-tissue malignancies in the head and neck region; they account for 3% to 5% of head and neck tumors. Histologic, immunohistochemical, and characteristic chromosomal translocation findings are necessary for diagnosis. The poor prognosis of this sarcoma justifies radical surgery with postoperative radiation.

Radiation-induced sarcoma of the head and neck is a rare long-term complication of treatment. The rarity of this tumor is reflected in the very few series reported in the English language medical literature (132,207). When they do occur, most appear at least 10 years following radiation therapy. There is a possibility of a postirradiation sarcoma whenever a suspicious lesion is seen, regardless of the amount of time that has passed since radiation therapy was administered. The original pathology should be re-examined to ensure that the original tumor was diagnosed correctly. Electron microscopy can be useful in differentiating sarcomatous-appearing epithelial lesions from true soft-tissue sarcomas.

The incidence of radiation-induced sarcomas of the head and neck is, however, likely to increase due to progressive aging of the population combined with improved survival in head and neck cancer patients. This problem can be extremely challenging and the overall outlook has been reported to be very bleak. Patel et al. (207) reviewed 69 cases reported in the English medical literature since 1966 and pooled this information with their experience in treatment of 10 patients. This group was compared for survival with 124 patients with a diagnosis of head and neck sarcoma registered on the Head and Neck Sarcoma database at the Royal Marsden Hospital. There was no site prediction for radiation-induced sarcoma of the head and neck, but malignant fibrous histiocytoma was the most common pathologic diagnosis. The period of latency between initial radiation therapy and diagnosis ranged from 9 to 45 years with a median of 17 years. Surgery was the mainstay of treatment, and follow-up ranged from 6 months to 15 years with a median of 48 months. The actuarial 5-year diseasefree survival rate in these patients was 60%.

Clinical Presentation and Diagnostic Work-Up

Clinical presentation varies with the primary site of disease.

Tumors arising from the aerodigestive tract usually present with nasal bleeding, a palpable mass in the neck, or difficulty in swallowing or breathing. Of tumors arising from the base of skull or the nerve sheath, cranial nerve deficit is the most common presentation. Diagnostic work-up follows that of soft-tissue sarcomas of other sites in the body. With early lesions, radiographs or CT may show only nonspecific opacification, soft-tissue swelling, and occasionally bone destruction. Table 45.1 outlines the suggested diagnostic work-up. MRI, especially with gadolinium contrast, may be used as a supplement or alternative to CT scanning (161). A CT scan of the chest is also mandatory for staging work-up.

The American Joint Committee on Cancer (AJCC) staging system for soft-tissue sarcomas is based on histologic grade, the tumor size and depth, and the presence of distant or nodal metastases. The staging system is the same as for sarcomas of the extremities, although specific staging for head and neck sarcomas is not standardized (49).

Prognostic Factors

Prognostic factors for predicting local recurrence or disease-free survival include anatomic site, treatment modality, tumor histology and grade, tumor size, extension of disease, and surgical margins (69,73,286).

A report from Royal Marsden Hospital showed anatomic location and treatment modality to be independent prognostic factors for local recurrence; tumors of the head had a better local recurrencefree survival than did those of the neck (73). Patients treated with a combination of surgery and radiation therapy had a better recurrencefree survival than did those treated with surgery or irradiation alone. The only significant independent prognostic factor for overall survival was the implementation of definitive surgery versus biopsy. In the above report, the prognostic impact of tumor stage and grade did not reach statistical significance. In contrast, Tran et al. (266) reported that 90% of patients with low-grade tumors were free of disease versus only 16% with high-grade lesions.

Bentz et al. (19) reviewed 111 head and neck sarcoma patients; median duration of follow-up was 51 months; the actuarial 5-year relapsefree disease-specific, and overall survivals were 55%, 52%, and 44% respectively. By multivariate analysis, size and grade significantly influenced all survivals, whereas margin status additionally influenced relapsefree survival.

In 352 patients treated at the Mayo Clinic for primary soft-tissue sarcoma of the head and neck, the 5-year overall survival for nonmetastasizing tumors such as dermatofibrosarcoma, protuberans, and desmoid tumors was 100%. Of the tumors with metastasizing potential that presented without lymph node metastasis or distant metastasis, the 5-year overall survival rate was 62.9% but decreased to 25% when lymph node or distant metastasis was detected at presentation (87).

In 109 soft-tissue sarcomas of all sites, a French study demonstrated that quality of the surgery was one of the most important variables for predicting local recurrences. Tumor size, surgical margins, presence of tumor necrosis, and adequacy of the excision correlated with metastasisfree survival (169).

In 57 patients with soft-tissue sarcomas of the head and neck treated at Massachusetts General Hospital, angiosarcoma had a considerably poorer prognosis than other histologies (257). In addition to tumor grade and size, direct tumor extension to neurovascular structures, bone, contiguous organs, and skin was associated with a higher incidence of distant metastasis. The actuarial 5-year freedom-from-distant-metastasis rates were 70% and 100% for tumors with or without direct extension, respectively.

General Management

Surgery is the preferred initial treatment modality for sarcomas (30). Unfortunately, it is often difficult to achieve complete resection of the tumor, and a high recurrence rate has been observed with surgery alone (82). Extracapsular enucleation of the tumor results in 90% local recurrence because of the presence of microscopic pseudopodia, which tend to grow through the pseudocapsule into the surrounding tissue and the presence of skipped lesions some distance from the main tumor mass. Pathologic analysis of the surgical bed often discloses microscopic extension of tumor. Farhood et al. (82), in a review of 176 cases of adult head and neck sarcomas, reported that the pathologic margins of surgical specimens obtained by wide local excision were positive in more than 50% of cases. This resulted in inferior overall survival for sarcomas of the head and neck when compared with extremity sarcomas (225). Wide local excision, with a 5-cm margin around the pseudocapsule in extremity sarcomas, is associated with better outcome, although approximately 20% will have local recurrence. The criteria for surgical resection are impractical for head and neck sarcomas because of anatomic limitations (49); wide local excision is rarely possible because the tumors extend beyond the confines of origin and in the proximity of vital neurovascular structures. Some retrospective studies have suggested improved local tumor control when combined surgery and external irradiation are used. In 130 patients with soft-tissue sarcomas of the head and neck treated with surgery alone at Royal Marsden Hospital, the overall 5-year survival was 50%; local tumor control was only 47%, and local recurrence was the cause of death in 63% of cases. Patients treated with combined-modality treatment (surgery and irradiation) had less extensive surgery, yet local recurrencefree survival was longer (73).

Radiation therapy, by external beam or brachytherapy, plays an important adjunctive role in the management, especially for tumors where en-bloc resection with negative margin is not possible (255,286). Chemotherapy regimens are available for soft-tissue neoplasms primarily designed to improve local tumor control (175). Survival is predicted on the incidence of local recurrence and risk of distant metastasis, both of which are influenced by tumor grade.

A systematic review of radiation therapy trials was performed by the Swedish Council of Technology Assessment in Health Care (SBU) (255). This synthesis of the literature on radiation therapy for soft-tissue sarcomas is based on data from five randomized trials. Moreover, data from six prospective studies, 25 retrospective studies, and three other articles were used. In total, 39 scientific articles were included, involving 4,579 patients. The results were compared with those of a similar overview from 1996 which included 3,344 patients. There was evidence that adjuvant radiotherapy improves local tumor control in combination with conservative surgery with negative, marginal, or minimal microscopic positive surgical margins. There are still insufficient data to establish that preoperative radiotherapy is favorable compared to postoperative radiotherapy in patients presenting primarily with large tumors. The preoperative setting results in more wound complications. There is no randomized study comparing external beam radiotherapy and brachytherapy. The data suggest that external beam radiotherapy and low–dose-rate brachytherapy result in comparable local control for high-grade tumors. Some patients with low-grade soft-tissue sarcomas benefit from external beam radiotherapy in terms of local control. Brachytherapy with a low dose rate for low-grade tumors seems to be of no benefit, but data are sparse. In two small studies investigating hyperfractionation schedules there was no indication of improvements compared to daily fractions of 2 Gy.

Mesenchymal chondrosarcoma of the sinonasal tract is a rare, malignant tumor of extraskeletal origin (141). Thirteen patients with sinonasal mesenchymal chondrosarcoma presented with nasal obstruction ($n = 8$), epistaxis ($n = 7$), or mass effect ($n = 4$), or a combination of these. The maxillary sinus was the most common site of involvement ($n = 9$), followed by the ethmoid sinuses ($n = 7$) and the nasal cavity ($n = 5$). All cases were managed by surgery with adjuvant radiation therapy ($n = 4$) and/or chemotherapy ($n = 3$). The overall mean survival was 12.1 years, although 5/6 patients who developed local recurrences died of disease (mean survival, 6.5 years). Six patients were alive and disease free (mean survival, 17.3 years), and two patients were lost to follow-up (141).

A multidisciplinary discussion before the initiation of treatment is required to formulate the best approach for radiation delivery, surgical technique, and mode of reconstruction.

Radiation Therapy Techniques

The general principles for radiation therapy of head and neck sarcomas are similar to those of soft-tissue sarcomas. Complete coverage of the surgical bed and scar with adequate margins (3 to 5 cm) is required (210). However, because of the proximity of critical and radiosensitive organs (eyes, spinal cord, brainstem), selecting optimal portal margins without seriously compromising the functioning of these organs is an art. Techniques similar to those used in epithelial tumors of the head and neck can be applied to sarcomas. In general, 55 to 60 Gy is needed for postoperative adjuvant irradiation, and an additional 10- to

15-Gy boost is recommended if the surgical margins are close (≤ 3 mm) or involved by tumor. Some institutions prefer preoperative irradiation of 45 to 50 Gy. Special attention should be directed to limiting the dose to critical structures. Use of a 3D treatment technique can be considered as demonstrated in Fig. 45.11.

Results of Therapy

Because of the propensity for sarcomas to invade the surrounding tissues, complete surgical clearance may be difficult (1). In a series from UCLA, attempted en-bloc resection left residual tumor at the surgical margins in 52/127 patients (266). The incidence of local recurrence was high (60%) with surgery alone.

In a retrospective report of 73 patients with sarcomas of the head and neck treated at Princess Margaret Hospital, the 5-year cause-specific survival was 62%, with a local recurrence rate of 41% and a distant metastasis rate of 31% (159). Extension to adjacent structures, high-grade tumor, and tumor >10 cm were associated with poor survival. Gross residual tumor after surgery was also associated with a high local recurrence rate (75%) despite the addition of radiation therapy. Patients with clear surgical margins or only microscopic involvement fared much more favorably and had a similar local tumor control rate (74% and 70%, respectively), provided adjuvant irradiation was given. Because of the difficulty in obtaining wide surgical margins, 68% of the patients died as a result of uncontrolled local disease. These data substantiate the importance of surgical margins as well as the contribution of adjuvant irradiation (159).

Colville et al. (49) reported on 41 male and 19 female patients treated with head and neck soft-tissue sarcomas, overall 5-year survival was 60%. Twenty-five patients had surgery alone, 20 surgery and pre- or postoperative radiation therapy and 15 received nonsurgical treatment. With mean follow-up of almost 4 years the 5-year local tumor control was 56% in the surgical and 40% in the nonsurgical group (more advanced and aggressive tumors). The 5-year survival was 70% and 40%, respectively.

Penel et al. (211) recorded their experience with 28 adult head and neck soft-tissue sarcomas. The median age was 45.7 years (range: 18 to 86). The male/female ratio was 15:13. The most common subtype was rhabdomyosarcoma (seven cases). Twenty-two patients presented with previous inadequate resection performed elsewhere before admission. Nineteen patients had surgery (complete resection in 13 cases). Associated treatments were neoadjuvant chemotherapy, adjuvant chemotherapy, and postoperative radiotherapy in 4, 3, and 10 cases, respectively. The 2-year overall survival rate was 56%.

Pandey et al. (202) reported on 22 cases of head and neck sarcomas (neck, lower jaw, tongue, cheek, scalp, and maxilla were the commonest sites affected). None of the patients had palpable neck nodes or distant metastasis at presentation. All the patients were treated with primary surgical resection, followed by adjuvant treatment in 14 cases (63.6%). After a median follow-up of 14.5 months, two patients died, six developed local recurrence, four developed metastatic disease, and another patient developed a second primary sarcoma. The overall 5-year survival was 80%, while the 5-year diseasefree survival rate was 24.1%.

Barker et al. (9) published a review of 44 patients diagnosed with nonmetastatic soft-tissue sarcoma in a head and neck. The most common tumor histologies included malignant fibrous histiocytoma (15 patients), angiosarcoma (nine patients), fibrosarcoma (six patients), and leiomyosarcoma (six patients). The median overall survival for all patients was 79 months. The actuarial 5-year local tumor control was 55% and was highly correlated with the extent of surgical excision: 25% for subtotal

			5-Year Actuarial Rates	
Author (Reference)	No. of Patients	Modalities	Local Control	Survival
Weber et al. (282)	188	S, R, C	—	Overall: 49.4% <5 cm
				Overall: 30.4% ≥5 cm
Greager et al. (101)	48	S, R, C	—	Disease free: 54%
Farhood et al. (82)	176	S, R, C	—	Overall: 55%
McKenna et al. (179)	16	S, R, C	75%	Disease free: 63%
Eeles et al. (73)	103[a]*	S, R, C	47%	Overall: 50%
LeVay et al. (159)	52	S, R, C	59%	Cause specific: 63%
Tran et al. (266)	164	S, R, C	41%	Overall: 66%
Willers et al. (286)	57	S, R, C	60%	Overall: 66%
Chao et al.[b]	33	S, R, C	49%	Disease free: 40%
Colville et al. (49)	60	S, R, C	50%	60%

Table 45.16   TREATMENT RESULTS OF ADULT SOFT-TISSUE SARCOMAS OF THE HEAD AND NECK

C, chemotherapy; R, radiation therapy; S, surgery
[a]Series based on adults and children, excluding angiosarcomas.
[b]Unpublished data.

resection/debulking, 65% for wide local excision, and 100% for radical excision. Local tumor control at 5 years was 60% for patients treated with both surgery and radiotherapy, 54% surgery alone, and 43% for radiation alone. Adjuvant radiation therapy significantly improved the local control rates (from 25% to 54%) for patients with close (<2 mm) or positive surgical margins. Of 14 patients with locoregional failure in whom salvage was attempted, nine (64%) were rendered disease free.

Rapidis et al. (221) reported on 25 patients with head and neck sarcomas with follow-up ranging from 8 to 144 months. Twenty-three patients were treated with surgery as the primary modality; 14 with surgery alone. Clear margins were obtained in all of them and local control was achieved in 12/13. The 5-year survival for the entire group was 40%. Reported results of treatment of soft-tissue sarcomas is summarized in Table 45.16.

Tumor Characteristics

Several series have shown that tumor grade and size dictate the outcome of patients with head and neck sarcomas such as leiomyosarcoma, rhabdomyosarcoma, and malignant fibrous sarcoma (50). Farhood et al. (82), in a review of 176 adult head and neck sarcomas, found that only 20% of the patients with high-grade tumors were alive 10 years after treatment, as opposed to 88% of patients with low-grade tumors. Greager et al. (101) noted mean survival of 98 months in patients with low-grade tumors smaller than 5 cm versus 15 months for those with high-grade lesions larger than 5 cm. Weber et al. (282) described a 45% 10-year survival rate for patients with tumors smaller than 5 cm versus 10% for those with tumors 5 cm or larger.

Many series have reported that chondrosarcoma is not a radiosensitive tumor, and radiation therapy has no role in it treatment. However, some reports have demonstrated the contribution of radiation therapy in this histology. Harwood et al. (110) reported that 6/12 patients with chondrosarcoma of the bone receiving irradiation alone were alive with no evidence of disease at periods ranging from 3 to 16 years. McNaney et al. (180) described a 65% survival rate at 2 years in 20 chondrosarcoma patients who received primary radiation therapy. Tumor grade was the most important prognostic factor.

Osteogenic sarcoma of the head and neck has a pattern of recurrence different from similar tumors elsewhere in the body. Head and neck osteosarcomas are usually high grade; they have a very high incidence of local recurrence but a lower risk of distant metastases. Several studies have used adjuvant irradiation and chemotherapy, which commonly results in improved locoregional tumor control and survival. Chambers and Mahoney (38) reported a 73% 5-year survival rate in patients with osteogenic sarcoma of the head and neck treated with high-dose preoperative irradiation followed by wide surgical excision. Similar observations were reported by Tran et al. (266).

Chemotherapy

Head and neck soft-tissue sarcomas frequently metastasize; 25% of patients in the UCLA study had distant metastases (266). The role of adjuvant chemotherapy to improve disease-free survival in sarcoma of the head and neck is controversial. The results were disappointing in a randomized trial conducted by the National Cancer Institute (99). Also, in a review of 11 randomized trials of adjuvant chemotherapy in nonextremity soft-tissue sarcomas, Elias and Antman (74) observed that none showed a statistically significant benefit in survival. Unlike with soft-tissue sarcomas of the extremities, in which distant metastasis is the most common cause of death, the majority of deaths in sarcomas of the head and neck are associated with local failure. Approximately half of the distant metastases were detected after local recurrence occurred (159). Chemotherapy did not appear to affect local tumor control (74).

McKenna et al. (179) reported on 16 adult patients with high-grade soft-tissue sarcomas of the head and neck treated with surgery, radiation therapy, and chemotherapy. With a median follow-up of 43 months, 12 patients (75%) achieved local tumor control, and 10 patients were disease free. In a series of 94 patients treated at UCLA (266), local control was achieved in 52% of those treated with surgery alone and 90% of those receiving adjuvant irradiation and/or chemotherapy.

For preoperative neoadjuvant chemotherapy, which supplements radiation therapy to downstage disease before surgery, satisfactory results are available only for sarcomas of extremities (212,227). The Institute Gustave-Roussy reported that two thirds of locally advanced lesions could be rendered operable after neoadjuvant chemotherapy and/or radiation therapy (227).

With the exception of rhabdomyosarcoma, postoperative adjuvant chemotherapy should be given only in a clinical trial setting.

References

1. Abbatucci J, Boulier N, deRanieri J, et al. Local control and survival in soft tissue sarcomas of the limbs, trunk walls, and head and neck: a study of 113 cases. *Int J Radiat Oncol Biol Phys* 1986;12:579–586.

2. Abud DG, Mounayer C, Benndorf G, et al. Intratumoral injection of cyanoacrylate glue in head and neck paragangliomas. *AJNR Am J Neuroradiol* 2004;29:1457–1462.
3. Alexiou C, Kau RJ, Dietzfelbinger H, et al. Extramedullary plasmacytoma: tumor occurrence and therapeutic concepts. *Cancer* 1999;85:2305–2314.
4. Antonelli AR, Cappiello J, Lorenzo DD, et al. Diagnosis, staging, and treatment of juvenile nasopharyngeal angiofibroma (JNA). *Laryngoscope* 1987;97:1319–1325.
5. Argiris A, Dutra J, Tseke P, et al. Esthesioneuroblastoma: the Northwestern University experience. *Laryngoscope* 2003;113:155–160.
6. Arthur K. Radiotherapy in chemodectoma of the glomus jugulare. *Clin Radiol* 1977;28:415–417.
7. Bailey B, Barton S. Olfactory neuroblastoma; management and prognosis. *Arch Otolaryngol Head Neck Surg* 1975;101:1–5.
8. Balch CM, Milton GW, Shaw HM, et al. Clinical management and treatment: results worldwide. In: Balch CM, Milton GW, eds. *Cutaneous melanoma*. Philadelphia: J.B. Lippincott, 1985;225.
9. Barker JL Jr, Paulino AC, Feeney S, et al. Locoregional treatment for adult soft tissue sarcomas of the head and neck: an institutional review. *Cancer J* 2003;9:49–57.
10. Baron SH. Brain radiation necrosis following treatment of an esthesioneuroblastoma (olfactory neurocytoma). *Laryngoscope* 1979;89:214–223.
11. Batsakis JG. In: *Tumors of the head and neck*, 2nd ed. Baltimore: Williams & Wilkins, 1979;474–475.
12. Batsakis JG. Wegener's granulomatosis and midline (non peeling) "granuloma." *Head Neck Surg* 1979;1:213–222.
13. Batsakis JG, Regezi JA, Solomon AR, et al. The pathology of head and neck tumors: mucosal melanomas. XIII. *Head Neck Surg* 1982;4:404–418.
14. Beenken S, Byers R, Smith JL, et al. Desmoplastic melanoma. *Arch Otolaryngol Head Neck Surg* 1989;115:374–379.
15. Beham A, Fletcher CD, Kainz J, et al. Nasopharyngeal angiofibroma: an immunohistochemical study of 32 cases. *Virchows Arch* 1993;423:2281–2285.
16. Beitler JJ, Fass DE, Brenner HA, et al. Esthesioneuroblastoma: is there a role for elective neck treatment? *Head Neck* 1991;13:321–326.
17. Benghiat A. Juvenile nasopharyngeal angiofibroma treated by radiotherapy. *J Laryngol Otol* 1986;100:351–356.
18. Benk V, Liebsch NJ, Munzenrider JE, et al. Base of skull and cervical spine chordomas in children treated by high-dose irradiation. *Int J Radiat Oncol Biol Phys* 1995;31:577–581.
19. Bentz BG, Singh B, Woodruff J, et al. Head and neck soft tissue sarcomas: a multivariate analysis of outcomes. *Ann Surg Oncol* 2004;11:619–628.
20. Berger L, Luc R. L'esthesioneuropitheliome olfacif. *Bull Cancer (Paris)* 1924;13:410–421.
21. Berrettini S, Segnini G, Bruschini P, et al. Lethal midline granuloma: a case of Ki-1 lymphoma. *Rev Laryngol Otol Rhinol (Bord)* 1993;114:37–42.
22. Berson AM, Castro JR, Petti P, et al. Charged particle irradiation of chordoma and chondrosarcoma of the base of skull and cervical spine: the Lawrence Berkeley Laboratory experience. *Int J Radiat Oncol Biol Phys* 1988;15:559–565.
23. Berthelsen A, Andersen AP, Jensen TS, et al. Melanomas of the mucosa in the oral cavity and the upper respiratory passages. *Cancer* 1984;54:907–912.
24. Bhattacharyya N, Thornton AF, Joseph MP, et al. Successful treatment of esthesioneuroblastoma and neuroendocrine carcinoma with combined chemotherapy and proton radiation. Results in 9 cases. *Arch Otolaryngol Head Neck Surg* 1997;123:34–40.
25. Biller HF, Lawson W, Sachdev V, et al. Esthesioneuroblastoma: surgical treatment without radiation. *Laryngoscope* 1990;100:1199–1201.
26. Billings KR, Fu YS, Calcaterra TC, et al. Hemangiopericytoma of the head and neck. *Am J Otolaryngol* 2000;21:238–243.
27. Blatchford SJ, Koopmann CF, Coulthard SW. Mucosal melanoma of the head and neck. *Laryngoscope* 1986;96:929–934.
28. Borisch B, Hennig I, Laeng RH, et al. Association of the subtype 2 of the Epstein-Barr virus with T-cell non-Hodgkin's lymphoma of the midline granuloma type. *Blood* 1993;82:858–864.
29. Boyle JO, Shimm DS, Coulthard SW. Radiation therapy for paragangliomas of the temporal bone. *Laryngoscope* 1990;100:896–901.
30. Bremer JW, Neel HB III, DeSanto LW, et al. Angiofibroma: treatment trends in 150 patients during 40 years. *Laryngoscope* 1986;96:1321–1329.
31. Broich G, Pagliari A, Ottaviani F. Esthesioneuroblastoma: a general review of the cases published since the discovery of the tumour in 1924. *Anticancer Res* 1997;17:2683–2706.
32. Buchner A, Hansen LS. Pigmented nevi of the oral mucosa: a clinicopathologic study of 36 new cases and review of 155 cases from the literature. II. Analysis of 191 cases. *Oral Surg* 1987;63:676–682.
33. Bush SE, Goffinet DR, Bagshaw MA. Extramedullary plasmacytoma of the head and neck. *Radiology* 1981;140:801–805.
34. Bustillo A, Telischi F, Weed D, et al. Octreotide scintigraphy in the head and neck. *Laryngoscope* 2004;114:434–440.
35. Cannizzaro MA, Cavallaro A, Veroux M, et al. A case of pleomorphic liposarcoma involving a parahypopharyngeal site. *Chirurgia Italiana* 2003;55:451–456.
36. Carew JF, Singh B, Kraus DH. Hemangiopericytoma of the head and neck. *Laryngoscope* 1999;109:1409–1411.
37. Catton C, O'Sullivan B, Bell R, et al. Chordoma: long-term follow-up after radical photon irradiation. *Radiother Oncol* 1996;41:67–72.
38. Chambers R, Mahoney W. Osteogenic sarcoma of the mandible. Current management. *Am J Surg* 1970;36:463–471.
39. Chandler JR, Goulding R, Moskowitz L, et al. Nasopharyngeal angiofibromas: staging and management. *Ann Otol Rhinol Laryngol* 1984;93:322–329.
40. Chao KSC, Kaplan C, Simpson JR, et al. Esthesioneuroblastoma: the impact of treatment modality. *Head Neck* 2001;23:749–757.
41. Chapman P, Johnson SAN. Mastoid chloroma relapse in acute myeloid leukemia. *J Laryngol Otol* 1980;94:1423–1427.
42. Charles NC, Palu RN, Jagirdar JS. Hemangiopericytoma of the lacrimal sac. *Arch Ophthalmol* 1998;116:1677–1680.
43. Chen HHW, Fong L, Su I-J, et al. Experience of radiotherapy in lethal midline granuloma with special emphasis on centrofacial T-cell lymphoma: a retrospective analysis covering a 34-year period. *Radiother Oncol* 1996;38:1–6.
44. Chen KTK, Bauer FW. Sarcomatous transformation of nasopharyngeal angiofibroma. *Cancer* 1982;49:369–371.
45. Chetty R, Levin CV, Kalan MR. Chordoma: a 20-year clinicopathologic review of the experience at Groote Schuur Hospital, Cape Town. *J Surg Oncol* 1991;46:261–264.
46. Clark WH, Miller MC. Lentigo maligna and lentigo malignant melanoma. *Am J Path* 1969;55:39–67.
47. Cohen LM, McCall MW, Zax RH. Mohs micrographic surgery for lentigo maligna and lentigo maligna melanoma: a follow-up study. *Dermatol Surg* 1998;24:673–677.
48. Cole JM, Beiler D. Long-term results of treatment for glomus jugulare and glomus vagale tumors with radiotherapy. *Laryngoscope* 1994;104:1461–1465.
49. Colville R, Charlton F, Kelly G, et al. Multidisciplinary management of head and neck sarcomas. *Head Neck* 2005;27:814–824.
50. Cormier JN, Pollock RE. Soft tissue sarcomas. *CA Cancer J Clin* 2004;54:94–109.
51. Corwin J, Lindberg RD. Solitary plasmacytoma of bone versus extramedullary plasmacytoma and their relationship to multiple myeloma. *Cancer* 1979;43:1007–1013.
52. Cummings BJ. The treatment of juvenile nasopharyngeal angiofibroma: the case for radiation therapy. *J Laryngol Otol* 1983;8[Suppl 1]:101–102.
53. Cummings BJ, Beale FA, Garrett PG, et al. The treatment of glomus tumors in the temporal bone by megavoltage radiation. *Cancer* 1984;53:2635–2640.
54. Cummings BJ, Blend R, Fitzpatrick P, et al. Primary radiation therapy for juvenile nasopharyngeal angiofibroma. *Laryngoscope* 1984;94:1599–1604.
55. Daugaard S, Hurltberg BM, Hou-Jenson K, et al. Clinical features of malignant haemangiopericytomas and haemangioendotheliosarcomas. *Acta Oncol* 1988;28A:209–213.
56. Davidson J, Gullane P. Glomus vagale tumors. *Otol Head Neck Surg* 1988;99:66–70.
57. Davis RE, Weissler MC. Esthesioneuroblastoma and neck metastasis. *Head Neck* 1992;14:447–482.
58. De SK, Das S, Dey D. Multiple extra-nasopharyngeal extensions of juvenile nasopharyngeal angiofibroma. *J Laryngol Otol* 1987;101:1083–1087.
59. Debus J, Schulz-Ertner D, Schad L, et al. Stereotactic fractionated radiotherapy for chordomas and chondrosarcomas of the skull base. *Int J Radiat Oncol Biol Phys* 2000;47:591–596.
60. deJong AL, Coker NJ, Jenkins HA, et al. Radiation therapy in the management of paragangliomas of the temporal bone. *Am J Otolaryngol* 1995;16:283–289.
61. Deschler DG, Kaplan MJ, Boles R. Treatment of large juvenile nasopharyngeal angiofibroma. *Otolaryngol Head Neck Surg* 1992;106:278–284.
62. Dias FL, Sa GM, Lima RA, et al. Patterns of failure and outcome in esthesioneuroblastoma. *Arch Otolaryngol Head Neck Surg* 2003;129:1186–1192.
63. Dickson RJ. Radiotherapy of lethal midline granuloma. *J Chron Dis* 1960;12:417–427.
64. Dickens WJ, Million RR, Cassisi NJ, et al. Chemodectomas arising in temporal bone structures. *Laryngoscope* 1982;92:188–191.
65. Dimopoulos MA, Kiamouris C, Moulopoulos LA. Solitary plasmacytoma of bone and extramedullary plasmacytoma. *Hematol Oncol Clin North Am* 1999;13:1249–1257.
66. Donald PJ. Sarcomatous degeneration in a nasopharyngeal angiofibroma. *Otolaryngol Head Neck Surg* 1979;87:42–46.
67. Doucet V, Peretti-Viton P, Figarella-Branger D, et al. MRI of intracranial chordomas. Extent of tumour and contrast enhancement: criteria for differential diagnosis. *Neuroradiology* 1997;39:571–576.
68. Drape JL, Idy-Peretti I, Goettmann S, et al. Sublingual glomus tumors: evaluation with MR imaging. *Radiology* 1995;195:507–515.
69. Dudhat SB, Mistry RC, Varughese T, et al. Prognostic factors in head and neck soft tissue sarcomas. *Cancer* 2000;54:868–872.
70. Dulguerov P, Calcaterra T. Esthesioneuroblastoma: the UCLA experience 1970–1990. *Laryngoscope* 1992;102:843–849.
71. Dzalitian M, Zuzko RD, Weiland LH, et al. Olfactory neuroblastoma. *Surg Clin North Am* 1977;57:751–762.
72. Eden BV, Debo RF, Larner JM, et al. Esthesioneuroblastoma. *Cancer* 1994;73:2556–2562.
73. Eeles R, Fisher C, Hern A, et al. Head and neck sarcomas: prognostic factors and implications for treatment. *Br J Cancer* 1993;68:201–207.
74. Elias A, Antman K. Adjuvant chemotherapy for soft tissue sarcoma: an approach in search of an effective regimen. *Semin Oncol* 1989;16:305–311.
75. Elkon D, Hightower SI, Lim ML, et al. Esthesioneuroblastoma. *Cancer* 1979;44:1087–1094.
76. Emami B, Perez CA, Konefal J, et al. Thermoradiotherapy of malignant melanoma. *Int J Hyperthermia* 1988;4:373–381.
77. Enzinger FM, Weiss SW. Hemangiopericytoma. In: Enzinger FM, Weiss SW, eds. *Soft tissue tumors*, 2nd ed. St. Louis, MO: C.V. Mosby, 1988;.
78. Eriksen JG, Bastholt L, Krogdahl AS, et al. Esthesioneuroblastoma: what is the optimal treatment? *Acta Oncol* 2000;39:231–235.
79. Espat NJ, Lewis JJ, Leung D, et al. Conventional hemangiopericytoma: modern analysis of outcome. *Cancer* 2002;95:1746–1751.
80. Fagundes MA, Hug EB, Liebsch NJ, et al. Radiation therapy for chordomas of the base of skull and cervical spine: patterns of failure and outcome after relapse. *Int J Radiat Oncol Biol Phys* 1995;33:579–584.
81. Farag MM, Ghanimah SE, Ragaie A, et al. Hormonal receptors in juvenile nasopharyngeal angiofibroma. *Laryngoscope* 1987;97:208–211.
82. Farhood A, Hajdu S, Shiu M, et al. Soft tissue sarcomas of the head and neck in adults. *Am J Surg* 1990;160:365–369.
83. Fauci AS, Hayes BF, Costa J, et al. Lymphomatoid granulomatosis: prospective clinical and therapeutic experience over 10 years. *N Engl J Med* 1982;306:68–74.
84. Fauci AS, Johnson RE, Wolff SM. Radiation therapy of midline granuloma. *Ann Intern Med* 1975;84:140–147.
85. Foote RL, Morita A, Ebersold MJ, et al. Esthesioneuroblastoma: the role of adjuvant radiation therapy. *Int J Radiat Oncol Biol Phys* 1993;27:835–842.
86. Forsyth PA, Cascino TL, Shaw EG, et al. Intracranial chordomas: a clinicopathological and prognostic study of 51 cases. *J Neurosurg* 1993;78:741–747.
87. Freedman A, Reiman H, Woods J. Soft-tissue sarcomas of the head and neck. *Am J Surg* 1989;158:367–372.
88. Fuller DB, Bloom JG. Radiotherapy for chordoma. *Int J Radiat Oncol Biol Phys* 1988;15:331–339.
89. Fuller PS, Haferman DR, Byrol RB, et al. Use of irradiation in lymphomatoid granulomatosis. *Chest* 1978;74:105–106.

90. Gabriele P, Macias V, Stasi M, et al. Feasibility of intensity-modulated radiation therapy in the treatment of advanced cervical chordoma. *Tumori* 2003;89:298–304.
91. Gadeberg CC, Hjelm-Hansen M, Sogaard H, et al. Malignant tumours of the paranasal sinuses and nasal cavity: a series of 180 patients. *Acta Radiol (Oncol)* 1984;23:181–187.
92. Galieni P, Cavo M, Pulsoni A, et al. Clinical outcome of extramedually plasmacytoma. *Haematologica* 2000;85:47–51.
93. Gardner G, Cocke EW, Robertson JT, et al. Glomus jugulare tumours: combined treatment. I. *J Otol Laryngol* 1981;95:437–454.
94. Gaulard P, Henni T, Marrolleau JP, et al. Lethal midline granuloma (polymorphic reticulosis) and lymphomatoid granulomatosis. *Cancer* 1988;62:705–710.
95. Gaut W, Jay AP, Robinson PA. Invasive glomus tumor of the nasal cavity. *Am J Otolaryngol* 2005;26:207–209.
96. Gay E, Sckhar LN, Rubinstein E, et al. Chordomas and chondrosarcomas of the cranial base: results and follow-up of 60 patients. *Neurosurgery* 1995;36:887–896.
97. Gerard-Marchant R, Michean C. Microscopic diagnosis of esthesioneuroblastomas: general review and report of five cases. *J Nat Cancer Inst* 1965;35:75–82.
98. Glasscock ME III, Jackson CG, Johnson GD, et al. Radiation therapy in chemodectoma treatment [Letter]. *Laryngoscope* 1988;98:465566.
99. Glenn J, Kinsella T, Glatstein E, et al. A randomized prospective trial of adjuvant chemotherapy in adults with soft tissue sarcomas of the head and neck, breast, and trunk. *Cancer* 1985;55:1206–1214.
100. Goepfert H, Cangir A, Lee YY. Chemotherapy for aggressive juvenile nasopharyngeal angiofibroma. *Arch Otolaryngol* 1985;111:285–289.
101. Greager J, Patel M, Briele H, et al. Soft tissue sarcomas of the adult head and neck. *Cancer* 1985;56:820–824.
102. Greese H, Nomayr A, Tomandl B, et al. 2D and 3D visualization of head and neck tumours from spiral-CT data. *Eur J Radiol* 2000;33:170–177.
103. Griffiths RW, Briggs JC. Biopsy procedures, primary wide excisional surgery and long-term prognosis in primary clinical stage I invasive cutaneous malignant melanoma. *Ann R Coll Surg Engl* 1985;67:75–78.
104. Grubb WV Jr, Lampe I. The role of radiation therapy in the treatment of chemodectomas of the glomus jugulare. *Laryngoscope* 1965;75:1861–1871.
105. Gutin PH, Leibel A, Hosobuchi Y, et al. Brachytherapy of recurrent tumors of the skull base and spine with iodine-125 sources. *Neurosurgery* 1987;20:938–945.
106. Halperin EC, Dosoretz MD, Goodman M, et al. Radiotherapy of polymorphic reticulosis. *Br J Radiol* 1982;55:645–649.
107. Harwood AR. Role of radiation therapy in the treatment of melanoma. In: Larson DL, Ballantyne AJ, Guillamondegui OM, eds. *Cancer in the neck: evaluation and treatment.* New York: Macmillan, 1986;243.
108. Harwood AR, Cummings BJ. Radiotherapy for mucosal melanomas. *Int J Radiat Oncol Biol Phys* 1982;8:1121–1126.
109. Harwood AR, Knowling MA, Bergsagel DE. Radiotherapy for extramedullary plasmacytoma of the head and neck. *Clin Radiol* 1981;32:31–36.
110. Harwood A, Kraybich I, Fornasier V. Radiotherapy of chondrosarcoma of bone. *Cancer* 1980;45:2769–2777.
111. Harwood AR, Lawson VG. Radiation therapy for melanomas of the head and neck. *Head Neck Surg* 1982;4:468–474.
112. Hatta C, Ishida M, Matsumoto T, et al. Cases of lethal midline granuloma (polymorphic reticulosis) at our department in a recent 10-year period. *J OtorhinoLaryngol Soc Jpn* 1993;96:879–885.
113. Heckmayr M, Gatzemeir U, Radenback D, et al. Pulmonary metastasizing hemangiopericytoma. *Am J Clin Oncol* 1988;11:636–642.
114. Heffelfinger MJ, Dahling DC, MacCarty CS, et al. Chordomas and cartilaginous tumors of the skull base cancer. *Cancer* 1973;32:410–420.
115. Henderson LT, Robbins KT, Weitzer S. Upper aerodigestive tract metastasis in disseminated melanoma. *Arch Otolaryngoal Head Neck Surg* 1986;112:659–663.
116. Herman P, Lot G, Chapot R, et al. Long-term follow-up of juvenile nasopharyngeal angiofibroma: analysis of recurrences. *Laryngoscope* 1999;109:140–147.
117. Herrold KM. Induction of olfactory neuroepithelial tumors in Syrian hamsters by dimethylnitrosamine. *Cancer* 1964;17:114–121.
118. Hill DC, Gramp AA. Surgical treatment of lentigo maligna and lentigo maligna melanoma. *Australas J Dermatol* 1999;40:25–30.
119. Hinerman RW, Mendenhall WM, Amdur RJ, et al. Definitive radiotherapy in the management of chemodectomas arising in the temporal bone, carotid body, and glomus vagale. *Head Neck* 2001;23:363–371.
120. Iloki K, Sambe S, Asakuru K, et al. Malignant melanoma in the maxillary sinus: a case successfully treated with radiotherapy. *Auris Nasus Larynx (Tokyo)* 1985;12:81–87.
121. Holland J, Trenkner DA, Wasserman TH, et al. Plasmacytoma: treatment results and conversion to myeloma. *Cancer* 1992;69:1513–1517.
122. Hotz MA, Schwaab G, Bosq J, et al. Extramedullary solitary plasmacytoma of the head and neck. A clinicopathological study. *Ann Otol Rhinol Laryngol* 1999;108:495–500.
123. Hug EB, Loredo LN, Slater JD, et al. Proton radiation therapy for chordomas and chondrosarcomas of the skull base. *J Neurosurg* 1999;91:432–439.
124. Hutchinson J. Notes on cancer and cancerous processes. *Arch Surg* 1890;2:218–224.
125. Hwang HC, Mills SE, Patterson K, et al. Expression of androgen receptors in nasopharyngeal angiofibroma: an immunohistochemical study of 24 cases. *Mod Pathol* 1998;11:1122–1126.
126. Hyams VJ. Tumors of the upper respiratory tract and ear. In: Hyams VJ, Batsakis JG, Michaels L, eds. *Atlas of tumor pathology*, 2nd ed. series, Fascicle 25. Washington, DC: Armed Forces Institute of Pathology, 1988;240–248.
127. Itami J, Itami M, Mikata A, et al. Non-Hodgkin's lymphoma confined to the nasal cavity: its relationship to the polymorphic reticulosis and results of radiation therapy. *Int J Radiat Oncol Biol Phys* 1991;20:797–802.
128. Jaaskelainen J, Servo A, Haltia M, et al. Intracranial hemangiopericytoma: radiology, surgery, radiotherapy and outcome in 21 patients. *Surg Neurol* 1985;23:227–236.
129. Jacobsson M, Petruson B, Svendsen P, et al. Juvenile nasopharyngeal angiofibroma: a report of eighteen cases. *Acta Otolaryngol* 1988;105:132–139.
130. Jafek BW, Krekorin EA, Kirsch WM, et al. Juvenile nasopharyngeal angiofibroma: the management of intracranial extension. *Head Neck Surg* 1979;2:119–128.
131. Jha N, McNeese M, Barkley HT, et al. Does radiotherapy have a role in hemangiopericytoma management? Report of 14 new cases and review of the literature. *Int J Radiat Oncol Biol Phys* 1987;13:1399–1402.
132. Johns MM, Concus AP, Beals TF, et al. Early-onset postirradiation sarcoma of the head and neck: report of three cases. *Ear Nose Throat J* 2002;81:402–406.
133. Jones GC, DeSanto LW, Bremer JW, et al. Juvenile angiofibromas. *Arch Otolarygol Head Neck Surg* 1986;112:1191–1193.
134. Kadish S, Goodman M, Wang CC. Olfactory neuroblastoma: a clinical analysis of 17 cases. *Cancer* 1976;37:1571–1576.
135. Kairemo KJ, Jekunen AP, Kestila MS, et al. Imaging of olfactory neuroblastoma–an analysis of 17 cases. *Auris Nasus Larynx* 1998;25:173–179.
136. Kanazawa T, Nishino H, Miyata M, et al. Haemangiopericytoma of infratemporal fossa. *J Laryngol Otol* 2001;115:77–79.
137. Kato T, Takematsu H, Tomita Y, et al. Malignant melanoma of mucous membranes. *Arch Dermatol* 1987;123:216–220.
138. Keisch ME, Garcia DM, Shibuya RB. Retrospective long-term follow-up analysis in 21 patients with chordomas of various sites treated at a single institution. *J Neurosurg* 1991;75:374–377.
139. Kim J-A, Elkon D, Lim M-L, et al. Optimum dose of radiotherapy for chemodectomas of the middle ear. *Int J Radiat Oncol Biol Phys* 1980;6:815–819.
140. Kingdom TT, Kaplan MJ. Mucosal melanoma of the nasal cavity and paranasal sinuses. *Head Neck* 1995;17:184–189.
141. Knott PD, Gannon FH, Thompson LD. Mesenchymal chondrosarcoma of the sinonasal tract; a clinicopathological study of 13 cases with a review of the literature. *Laryngoscope* 2003;113:783–790.
142. Knowling MA, Harwood AR, Bergsagel DE. Comparison of extramedullary plasmacytomas with solitary and multiple plasma cell tumors of bone. *J Clin Oncol* 1983;1:255–262.
143. Koka VN, Julieron M, Bourhis J, et al. Aesthesioneuroblastoma. *J Laryngol Otol* 1998;112:628–633.
144. Kondziolka D, Lunsford LD, Flickinger JC. The role of radiosurgery in the arrangement of chordoma and chondrosarcoma of the cranial base. *Neurosurgery* 1991;29:38–45.
145. Konefal JB, Pilepich MV, Spector GJH, et al. Radiation therapy in the treatment of chemodectomas. *Laryngoscope* 1987;97:1331–1335.
146. Kopf AW, Bart RS, Gladstein AH. Treatment of melanotic freckle with x-rays. *Arch Dermatol* 1976;112:801–807.
147. Koscielny S, Brauer B, Forster G. Hemangiopericytoma: a rare head and neck tumor. *Eur Arch Otorhinolaryngol* 2003;260:450–453.
148. Kowalski PJ, Paulino AF. Proliferation index as a prognostic marker in hemangiopericytoma of the head and neck. *Head Neck* 2001;23:492–496.
149. Kuflik EG, Gage AA. Cryosurgery for lentigo maligna. *J Am Acad Dermatol* 1994;31:75–78.
150. Kumar PP, Good RR, Skulkety ME, et al. Local control of clival and sacral chordoma after interstitial irradiation with iodine-125: new techniques for treatment of recurrent or unresectable chordomas. *Neurosurgery* 1988;22:479–483.
151. Kuppersmith RB, The BS, Donovan DT, et al. The use of intensity modulated radiotherapy for the treatment of extensive and recurrent juvenile angiofibroma. *Int J Pediatr Otorhinolaryngol* 2000;52:261–268.
152. Lack EE, Cubilla AL, Woodruff JM, et al. Paragangliomas of the head and neck region. *Cancer* 1977;39:3997–4009.
153. Laird JD, Ferguson WR, McIlrath EM, et al. Radionuclide angiography as the primary investigation in chemodectoma: concise communication. *J Nucl Med* 1983;24:475–483.
154. Lang DA, McKellar NJ, Lang W. Juvenile nasopharyngeal angiofibroma: the preferred treatment. *Scott Med J* 1983;28:64–66.
155. Lang NP, Stair JM, Degges RD, et al. Melanoma today does not require radical surgery. *Am J Surg* 1984;148:723–726.
156. Larner JM, Hahn SS, Spaulding CA, et al. Glomus jugulare tumors: long-term control by radiation therapy. *Cancer* 1992;69:1813–1817.
157. Larson TC III, Reese DF, Baker HL Jr, et al. Glomus tympanicum chemodectomas: radiographic and clinical characteristics. *Radiology* 1987;163:801–806.
158. Leber KA, Eustacchio S, Pendl G. Radiosurgery of glomus tumors: midterm results. *Stereotact Funct Neurosurg* 1999;72[Suppl 1]:53–59.
159. Levay J, O'Sullivan B, Catton C, et al. An assessment of prognostic factors in soft-tissue sarcoma of the head and neck. *Arch Otolaryngol Head Neck Surg* 1994;120:981–986.
160. Levine PA, Gallagher R, Cantrell RW. Esthesioneuroblastoma: reflections of a 21-year experience. *Laryngoscope* 1999;109:1539–1543.
161. Levine PA, Paling MR, Black WC, et al. MRI versus high resolution CT scanning: evaluation of the anterior skull base. *Otolaryngol Head Neck Surg* 1987;96:260–267.
162. Liebross RH, Ha CS, Cox JD, et al. Clinical course of solitary extramedullary plasmacytoma. *Radiother Oncol* 1999;52:245–249.
163. Lippman SM, Grogan TM, Spier EM, et al. Lethal midline granulomas with a novel T-cell phenotype as found in peripheral T-cell lymphoma. *Cancer* 1987;59:936–939.
164. Lloyd G, Howard D, Phelps P, et al. Juvenile angiofibroma: the lesions of 20 years of modern imaging. *J Laryngol Otol* 1999;113:127–134.
165. Luddy RE, Levy BE, Schwartz AD. 67Ga scintigraphy in granulocytic sarcoma. *Cancer* 1980;46:1357–1359.
166. Lybeert MLM, Van Andel JG, Eijkenboom WMH, et al. Radiotherapy of paragangliomas. *Clin Otolaryngol* 1984;9:105–109.
167. Magliulo G, Zardo F, Varacalli S, et al. Multiple paragangliomas of the head and neck. *Anal Otorrinolaringol Ibero Am* 2003;30:31–38.
168. Maharaj D, Fernandes CMC. Surgical experience with juvenile nasopharyngeal angiofibroma. *Ann Otolrhinollaryngol* 1989;98:269–272.
169. Mandard A, Petiot J, Marnay J, et al. Prognostic factors in soft tissue sarcomas: a multivariate analysis of 109 cases. *Cancer* 1989;63:1437–1451.
170. Manelfe C, Bonafe A, Fabre P, et al. Computed tomography in olfactory neuroblastoma. *J Comput Assist Tomogr* 1978;2:412–420.
171. Manolidis S, Shohet JA, Jackson CG, et al. Malignant glomus tumors. *Laryngoscope* 1999;109:30–34.
172. Mantravadi RVP. Radiation therapy for nonsquamous tumors of the head and neck. *Otolaryngol Clin North Am* 1986;19:741–754.
173. Marsot-Dupuch K, Cabane J, Raveau V, et al. Lethal midline granuloma: impact of imaging studies on the investigation and management of destructive mid facial disease in 13 patients. *Neuroradiology* 1992;34:155–161.

174. Maruyama Y. Radiotherapy of tympanojugular chemodectomas. *Radiology* 1972;105:659–663.
175. Mason M, Robinson M, Harmer C, et al. Intra-arterial adriamycin, conventionally fractionated radiotherapy and conservative surgery for soft tissue sarcomas. *Clin Oncol* 1992;4:32–35.
176. McCabe BF, Fletcher M. Selection of therapy of glomus jungulare tumors. *Arch Otolaryngol* 1969;89:156–159.
177. McDonald TJ, DeRemee RA, Harrison EG Jr, et al. The protean clinical features of polymorphic reticulosis (lethal midline granuloma). *Laryngoscope* 1976;86:936–945.
178. McElroy EA, Buckner JC, Lewis JE. Chemotherapy for advanced esthesioneuroblastoma: the Mayo Clinic experience. *Neurosurgery* 1998;42:1023–1027.
179. McKenna W, Barnes M, Kinsella T, et al. Combined modality treatment of adult soft tissue sarcomas of the head and neck. *Int J Radiat Oncol Biol Phys* 1987;13:1127–1133.
180. McNaney D, Lindberg R, Ayala A, et al. Fifteen year radiotherapy experience with chondrosarcoma of bone. *Int J Radiat Oncol Biol Phys* 1982;8:187–190.
181. Mendenhall WM, Million RR, Parsons JT, et al. Chemodectoma of the carotid body and ganglion nodosum treated with radiation therapy. *Int J Radiat Oncol Biol Phys* 1986;12:2175–2178.
182. Michalski VJ, Hall J, Henk JM et al. Definitive radiotherapy for extramedullary plasmacytomas of the head and neck. *Br J Radiol* 2003;76:738–741.
183. Miller FR, Lavertu P, Wanamaker JR, et al. Plasmacytomas of the head and neck. *Otolaryngol Head Neck Surg* 1998;119:614–618.
184. Mira JH, Chu FC, Fortner JC. The role of radiotherapy in the management of malignant hemangiopericytoma: report of 11 new cases and review of the literature. *Cancer* 1977;30:1254–1259.
185. Mitchell DC, Clyne CAC. Chemodectomas of the neck: the response to radiotherapy. *Br J Surg* 1985;72:903–905.
186. Miyamoto RC, Gleich LL, Biddinger PW, et al. Esthesioneuroblastoma and sinonasal undifferentiated carcinoma: impact of histological grading and clinical staging on survival and prognosis. *Laryngoscope* 2000;110:1262–1265.
187. Monroe AT, Hinerman RW, Amdur RJ, et al. Radiation therapy for esthesioneuroblastoma: rationale for elective neck irradiation. *Head Neck* 2003;25:529–534.
188. Muss HB, Maloney WC. Chloroma and other myeloblastic tumors. *Blood* 1973;42:721–728.
189. Neiman RS. The peripheral cell lymphomas come of age. *Mayo Clin Proc* 1986; 61:504–506.
190. Neiman RS, Barcos M, Berard C, et al. Granulocytic sarcoma: a clinicopathologic study of 61 biopsied cases. *Cancer* 1981;48:1426–1437.
191. Newman H, Rowe JF Jr, Phillips TL. Radiation therapy of the glomus jugulare tumor. *AJR Am J Roentgenol* 1973;118:663–669.
192. Ochoa-Carrillo FJ, Carrillo JF, Frias M. Staging and treatment of nasopharyngeal angiofibroma. *Eur Arch Otorhinolaryngol* 1997;254:200–204.
193. O'Connell JX, Renard LG, Liebsch NJ, et al. Base of skull chordoma: a correlative study of histologic and clinical features of 62 cases. *Cancer* 1994;74:2261–2267.
194. Ogura JH, Spector GJ, Gado M. Glomus jugulare and vagal. *Ann Otol Rhinol Laryngol* 1978;87:622–629.
195. Ohya T, Kudo K, Chen C-H, et al. Primary malignant melanomas of the oral mucosa. *Int J Oral Maxillofac Surg* 1987;16:496–499.
196. Olsen KD, DeSanto LW. Olfactory neuroblastoma: biologic and clinical behavior. *Arch Otolaryngol* 1983;109:797–802.
197. Oot RF, Melville GE, New PF, et al. The role of MR and CT in evaluating clival chordomas and chondrosarcomas. *AJR Am J Roentgenol* 1988;151:567–575.
198. Osborne DR, DuBois P, Drayer B, et al. Primary intracranial meningeal and spinal hemangiopericytomas: radiologic manifestations. *Am J Neuroradiol* 1981;2:69–74.
199. Ozsakin M, Tsang RW, Poortmans P, et al. Outcomes and patterns of failure in solitary plasmacytoma: a multicenter rare cancer network study of 258 patients. *Int J Rad Oncol* 2006;64(1):210.
200. Pahor AL. Extramedullary plasmacytoma of the head and neck, parotid, and submandibular salivary glands. *J Laryngol Otol* 1977;91:241–258.
201. Palacios E, Restrepo S, Mastrogiovanni L, et al. Sinonasal hemangiopericytomas: clinicopathologic and imaging findings. *Ear Nose Throat J* 2005;84(2):99–102.
202. Pandey M, Chandramohan K, Thomas C, et al. Soft tissue sarcoma of the head and neck region in adults. *Int J Oral Maxillofac Surg* 2003;32:43–48.
203. Panje WR, Moran WJ. Melanoma of the upper aerodigestive tract: a review of 21 cases. *Head Neck Surg* 1986;8:309–312.
204. Papadaki H, Kounelis S, Kapadia SB, et al. Relationship of p53 gene alterations with tumor progression and recurrence in olfactory neuroblastoma. *Am J Surg Pathol* 1996;20:715–721.
205. Parry DM, Li FP, Strong LC, et al. Carotid body tumors in humans: genetics and epidemiology. *J Natl Cancer Inst* 1982;68:573–578.
206. Parsons J, Bova F, Fitzgerald C, et al. Radiation retinopathy after external beam irradiation: analysis of time-dose factors. *Int J Radiat Oncol Biol Phys* 1994;30:765–773.
207. Patel SG, See AC, Williamson PA, et al. Radiation induced sarcoma of the head and neck. *Head Neck* 1999;21:346–354.
208. Patrice SJ, Sneed PK, Flickinger JC, et al. Radiosurgery for hemangioblastoma: results of a multi-institutional experience. *Int J Radiat Oncol Biol Phys* 1995;32[Suppl 1]:147(abstr).
209. Payne BR, Prasad D, Steiner M, et al. Gamma surgery for hemangiopericytomas. *Acta Neurochir (Wien)* 2000;142:527–536.
210. Pellitteri PK, Ferlito A, Bradley PJ, et al. Management of sarcomas of the head and neck in adults. *Oral Oncol* 2003;39:2–12.
211. Penel N, Van Haverbeke C, Lartigau E, et al. Head and neck soft tissue sarcomas of adult: prognostic value of surgery in multimodal therapeutic approach. *Oral Oncol* 2004;40:890–897.
212. Pezzi C, Pollock R, Evans H, et al. Preoperative chemotherapy for soft-tissue sarcomas of extremities. *Ann Surg* 1990;211:476–481.
213. Pickruth D, Heywang-Kobrunner SH, Speilmann RP. Computed tomography and magnetic resonance imaging features of olfactory neuroblastoma: an analysis of 22 cases. *Clin Otolaryngol* 1999;24:457–461.
214. Polin RS, Sheehan JP, Chenelle AG, et al. The role of preoperative adjuvant treatment in the management of esthesioneuroblastoma: the University of Virginia experience. *Neurosurgery* 1998;42:1029–1037.
215. Pomeranz SJ, Hawkins HH, Towbin R, et al. Granulocytic sarcoma (chloroma): CT manifestations. *Radiology* 1985;155:167–170.
216. Powell S, Peters N, Harmer C. Chemodectoma of the head and neck: results of treatment in 84 patients. *Int J Radiat Oncol Biol Phys* 1992;22:919–924.
217. Pryzant RM, Chou JL, Easley JD. Twenty year experience with radiation therapy for temporal bone chemodectomas. *Int J Radiat Oncol Biol Phys* 1989;17:1303–1307.
218. Radiation Therapy Oncology Group Protocol No. 8305. William T. Sause and Henry P. Plenk, Co-chairmen, 1988.
219. Rampen FH. Biopsy and survival of malignant melanoma. *J Am Acad Dermatol* 1985;12:385–388.
220. Rangawala AF, Sylvia LC, Becker SM. Soft tissue metastasis of a chemodectoma: a case report and review of the literature. *Cancer* 1978;42:2865–2869.
221. Rapidis AD, Gakiopoulou H, Stevrianos SD, et al. Sarcomas of the head and neck. Results from the treatment of 25 patients. *Eur J Surg Oncol* 2005;31:177–182.
222. Rapini RP, Golitz LE, Greer RO, et al. Primary malignant melanoma of the oral cavity: a review of 117 cases. *Cancer* 1985;55:1543–1551.
223. Rich TA, Schiller A, Suit HD, et al. Clinical and pathologic review of 48 cases of chordoma. *Cancer* 1985;56:182–187.
224. Robinson ACR, Khoury GG, Ash DV, et al. Evaluation of response following irradiation of juvenile angiofibromas. *Br J Radiol* 1989;62:245–247.
225. Robinson M, Barr L, Fisher C, et al. Treatment of extremity soft tissue sarcomas with surgery and radiotherapy. *Radiother Oncol* 1990;18:221–223.
226. Rosenthal DI, Barker JL, Jr, El-Naggar AK, et al. Sinonasal malignancies with neuroendocrine differentiation: patterns of failure according to histologic phenotype. *Cancer* 2004;101:2567–2573.
227. Rouesse J, Friedman S, Sevin D, et al. Preoperative induction chemotherapy in the treatment of locally advanced soft tissue sarcomas. *Cancer* 1987;80: 296–300.
228. Royal College of Radiologists Proton Therapy Working Party. Proton therapy for base of skull chordoma: a report for the Royal College of Radiologists. *Clin Oncol (R Coll Radiol)* 2000;12:75–79.
229. Sakata K, Hareyama M, Oouchi A, et al. Treatment of localized non-Hodgkin's lymphomas of the head and neck: focusing on cases of non-lethal midline granuloma. *Radiat Oncol Invest* 1998;6:161–169.
230. Saktor JP. Chordoma. *Int J Rad Oncol Bio Phys* 1981;7:913–915.
231. Santoni R, Liebsch N, Finkelstein DM, et al. Temporal lobe damage following surgery and high-dose photon and proton irradiation in 96 patients affected by chordomas and chondrosarcomas of the base of the skull. *Int J Radiat Oncol Biol Phys* 1998;41:59–68.
232. Schild SE, Foote RL, Buskirk SJ, et al. Results of radiotherapy for chemodectomas. *Mayo Clin Proc* 1992;67:537–540.
233. Schroth G, Gawehn J, Marquardt B, et al. MR imaging of esthesioneuroblastoma. *J Comput Assist Tomogr* 1986,10.316–319.
234. Seifer V, Laszig R. Transoral transpalatal neuroral of giant prenormosephalic clivus chordoma. *Acta Neurochir* 1991;112:141–146.
235. Sessions RB, Bryan RN, Naclerio RM, et al. Radiographic staging of juvenile angiofibroma. *Head Neck Surg* 1981;3:279–283.
236. Setzkorn RK, Lee DJ, Iliff NT, et al. Hemangiopericytoma of the orbit treated with conservative surgery and radiotherapy. *Arch Ophthalmol* 1987;105:1103–1105.
237. Shank BB, Kelley CD, Nisce LZ, et al. Radiation therapy in lymphomatoid granulomatosis. *Cancer* 1978;42:2572–2580.
238. Shih LY, Dunn P, Leung WM, et al. Localized plasmacytomas in Taiwan: comparison between extramedullary plasmacytoma and solitary plasmacytoma of bone. *Br J Cancer* 1995;71:128–133.
239. Sievers KW, Greess H, Baum U, et al. Paranasal sinuses and nasopharynx CT and MRI. *Eur J Radiol* 2000;33:185–202.
240. Simko TG, Griffin TW, Gerdes AJ, et al. The role of radiation therapy in the treatment of glomus jugulare tumors. *Cancer* 1978;42:104–106.
241. Simon JH, Zhen W, McCulloch TM, et al. Esthesioneuroblastoma: the University of Iowa experience 1978–1998. *Laryngoscope* 2001;111:488–493.
242. Slater JD, Austin-Seymour M, Munzenrider J, et al. Endocrine function following high dose proton therapy for tumors of the upper clivus. *Int J Radiat Oncol Biol Phys* 1988;15:607–611.
243. Smalley RS, Cupps RE, Anderson JA, et al. Polymorphic reticulosis limited to the upper aerodigestive tract: natural history and radiotherapeutic considerations. *Int J Radiat Oncol Biol Phys* 1988;15:599–605.
244. Sowers JJ, Moody PM, Naidich TP, et al. Radiographic features of granulocytic sarcoma (chloroma). *J Comput Assist Tomogr* 1979;3:226–233.
245. Spagnolo DV, Papadimitiou JM, Archer M. Postirradiation malignant fibrous histiocytoma arising in juvenile nasopharyngeal angiofibroma and producing alpha-1-antitrypsin. *Histopathology* 1984;8:339–352.
246. Spaulding CA, Kranyak MS, Constable WC, et al. Esthesioneuroblastoma: a comparison of two treatment eras. *Int J Radiat Oncol Biol Phys* 1988;15:581–590.
247. Spector GJ, Compagno J, Perez CA, et al. Glomus jugulare tumors: effects of radiotherapy. *Cancer* 1975;35:1316–1321.
248. Spitz FR, Bouvet M, Pisters PW, et al. Hemangiopericytoma: a 20-year single institution experience. *Ann Surg Oncol* 1998;5:350–355.
249. Springate SC, Weichselbaum RR. Radiation or surgery for chemodectoma of the temporal bone: a review of local control and complications. *Head Neck* 1990;12:303–307.
250. Standefer J, Holt GR, Brown WE Jr, et al. Combined intracranial and extracranial excision of nasopharyngeal angiofibroma. *Laryngoscope* 1983;93:772–779.
251. Stefiani S, Amarti A, Boulaadas M, et al. Synovial sarcoma of the head and neck: two cases report. *Rev Laryngol Otol Rhinol* 2005;126:53–56.
252. Stewart FM, Frierson HF, Levine PA, et al. Esthesioneuroblastoma. In: Williams CJ, Krikorian JG, Green MR, et al. eds. *Textbook of uncommon cancer*. New York: Wiley, 1988;63–65.
253. Stomeo F, Fois V, Cossu A, et al. Sinonasal haemangiopericytoma: a case report. *Eur Arch Otorhinolaryngol* 2004;261:555–557.
254. Stout AP. Hemangiopericytoma. Study of 25 new cases. *Cancer* 1949;2:1027–1054.
255. Strander H, Turesson I, Cavallin-Stahl E. A systematic overview of radiation therapy effects in soft tissue sarcomas. *Acta Oncol* 2003;42:516–531.
256. Suit HD, Gallager HS. Intact tumor cells in irradiated tissue. *Arch Pathol* 1964;78:648.
257. Suit HD, Mankin H, Wood W, et al. Treatment of the patient with stage M0 soft tissue sarcoma. *J Clin Oncol* 1988;6:854–862.
258. Sze G, Jichanco LS, Brant-Zawadski MN, et al. Chordomas: MR imaging. *Radiology* 1988;166:187–191.

259. Tai PT, Craighead P, Bagdon F. Optimization of radiotherapy for patients with cranial chordoma: a review of dose-response ratios for photon techniques. *Cancer* 1995;75:749–756.

260. Tannous ZS, Lerner LH, Duncan LM, et al. Progression to invasive melanoma from malignant melanoma in situ, lentigo maligna type. *Hum Pathol* 2000;31:705–708.

261. Tatsuzaki H, Urie MM. Importance of precise positioning for proton beam therapy in the base of skull and cervical spine. *Int J Radiat Oncol Biol Phys* 1991;21:757–765.

262. Terahara A, Niemierko A, Goitein M, et al. Analysis of the relationship between tumor dose inhomogeneity and local control in patients with skull base chordoma. *Int J Radiat Oncol Biol Phys* 1999;45:351–358.

263. Thompson LD, Gyure KA. Extracranial sinonasal tract meningiomas: a clinico-pathologic study of 30 cases with a review of the literature. *Am J Surg Pathol* 2000;34:640–650.

264. Tidwell TJ, Montague ED. Chemodectoma involving the temporal bone. *Radiology* 1975;116:147–149.

265. Tournier-Rangeard L, Lapeyre M, Graff-Caillaud P, et al. Radiotherapy for solitary extramedullary plasmacytoma in the head-and-neck region: a dose greater than 45 Gy to the target volume improves the local control. *Int J Radiat Oncol Biol Phys* 2006;64:1013–1017.

266. Tran L, Mark R, Meier R, et al. Sarcomas of the head and neck: prognostic factors and treatment strategies. *Cancer* 1992;70:169–177.

267. Tranbahuy P, Borsik M, Herman P, et al. Direct intratumoral embolization of juvenile angiofibroma. *Am J Otol* 1994;15:429–435.

268. Trapp TK, Fu YS, Calcaterra TC. Melanoma of the nasal and paranasal sinus mucosa. *Arch Otolaryngol Head Neck Surg* 1987;113:1086–1089.

269. Tsang RW, Liu IF, Wells W, et al. Lentigo maligna of the head and neck: results of treatment by radiotherapy. *Arch Dermatol* 1994;130:1008–1012.

270. Uehara T, Matsubara O, Kasuga T. Melanocytes in the nasal cavity and paranasal sinus. *Acta Pathol Jpn* 1987;37:1105–1114.

271. Umeda M, Mishima Y, Teranobu O, et al. Heterogeneity of primary malignant melanomas in oral mucosa: an analysis of 43 cases in Japan. *Pathology* 1988;20:234–241.

272. Ungkanont K, Byers RM, Weber RS, et al. Juvenile nasopharyngeal angiofibroma: an update of therapeutic management. *Head Neck* 1996;18:60–66.

273. Valdagni R, Amichetti M. Radiation therapy of carotid body tumors. *Am J Clin Oncol* 1990;13:45–48.

274. Verniers DA, Keus RB, Schouwenburg PF, et al. Radiation therapy, an important mode of treatment for head and neck chemodectomas. *Eur J Cancer* 1992;27:1028–1033.

275. Vogl TJ, Juergens M, Balzar JO, et al. Glomus tumors of the skull base: combined use of MR angiography and spin-echo imaging. *Radiology* 1994;192:1003–1010.

276. Vogl TJ, Steger W, Grevers G, et al. MR characteristics of primary extramedullary plasmacytoma in the head and neck. *AJNR Am J Neuroradiol* 1996;17:1349–1354.

277. Volpe NJ, Liebsch NJ, Munzenrider JE, et al. Neuro-ophthalmologic findings in chordoma and chondrosarcoma of the skull base. *Am J Ophthalmol* 1993;115:97–104.

278. Vuorinen V, Sallinen P, Haapsasalo H, et al. Outcome of 31 intracranial haemangiopericytomas: poor predictive value of cell proliferation indices. *Acta Neurochir (Wien)* 1996;138:1399–1408.

279. Wade PM Jr, Smith RE, Johns ME. Response of esthesioneuroblastoma to chemotherapy: report of five cases and review of the literature. *Cancer* 1984;53:1036–1041.

280. Wang M-L, Hussey DH, Doornbos JF, et al. Chemodectoma of the temporal bone: a comparison of surgical and radiotherapeutic results. *Int J Radiat Oncol Biol Phys* 1988;14:643–648.

281. Wax MK, Yun KJ, Omar RA. Extramedullary plasmacytomas of the head and neck. *Otolaryngol Head Neck Surg* 1993;109:877–885.

282. Weber R, Benjamin R, Peters L, et al. Soft tissue sarcomas of the head and neck in adolescents and adults. *Am J Surg* 1986;152:386–392.

283. Weis JW, Winter MW, Phyliky RL, et al. Peripheral T-cell lymphomas: histologic, immunohistologic and clinical classification. *Mayo Clin Proc* 1986;61:411–426.

284. Wiatrak BJ, Koopmann CF, Turrisi AT. Radiation therapy as an alternative to surgery in the management of intracranial juvenile nasopharyngeal angiofibroma. *Int J Pediatr Otorhinolaryngol* 1993;28:51–61.

285. Wieden PL, Yarington CT Jr, Richardson RG. Olfactory neuroblastoma: chemotherapy and radiotherapy for extensive disease. *Arch Otolaryngol* 1984;110:759–760.

286. Willers H, Hug E, Spiro I, et al. Adult soft tissue sarcomas of the head and neck treated by radiation and surgery or radiation alone: patterns of failure and prognostic factors. *Int J Radiat Oncol Biol Phys* 1995;33:585–593.

287. Wiltshaw E. The natural history of extramedullary plasmacytoma and its relation to solitary myeloma of bone and myelomatosis. *Medicine (Baltimore)* 1976;55:217–328.

288. Witt TR, Shah JP, Sternberg SS. Juvenile nasopharyngeal fibroma: a 30 year clinical review. *Am J Surg* 1983;46:521–525.

289. Wold LE, Laws ER. Cranial chordomas in children and young adults. *J Neurosurg* 1983;59:1043–1047.

290. Wong PP, Yagoda A. Chemotherapy of malignant hemangiopericytoma. *Cancer* 1978;41:1256–1260.

291. Woo E, Yue CP, Onann KE, et al. Intracerebral chloromas: report of a case and review of the literature. *Clin Neurol Neurosurg* 1986;88:135–139.

292. Woodruff RK, Whittle JM, Malpas JS. Solitary plasmacytoma. I. Extramedullary soft tissue plasmacytoma. *Cancer* 1979;43:2340–2343.

293. Yaghmai I. Angiographic manifestations of soft tissue and osseous hemangiopericytomas. *Radiology* 1978;126:652–659.

294. Zimmerman LCE, Font RL. Ophthalmologic manifestations of granulocytic sarcoma: a clinicopathologic study of 33 cases. *Am J Ophthalmol* 1975;80:975–990.

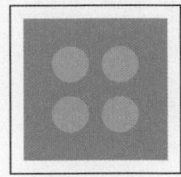

Chapter 46
Management of the Neck Including Unknown Primary Tumor

William M. Mendenhall, Robert J. Amdur, Russell W. Hinerman, Anthony A. Mancuso,
Douglas B. Villaret, John W. Werning

Anatomy

The incidence of lymph node metastases at the time of diagnosis is related to the relative density of the capillary lymphatic network (Table 46.1) (69). The nasopharynx and pyriform sinus have the most profuse capillary lymphatic networks, whereas the paranasal sinuses, middle ear, and true vocal cords have either sparse or no capillary lymphatics (101).

The location of the various lymph node groups in the head and neck is shown in Figure 46.1 (101). Under normal conditions, the right and left lymphatic networks do not shunt from one side to the other (33).

The *internal jugular chain* (IJC) lymph nodes lie adjacent to the internal jugular vein and extends from the skull base to the clavicle. The most superior group of lymph nodes in this chain lies near the base of the skull in the posterior aspect of the lateral pharyngeal space and is often referred to as the *parapharyngeal* or *junctional* lymph nodes. These lymph nodes lie deep to the sternocleidomastoid muscle, the posterior belly of the digastric muscle, and the tail of the parotid gland. The remaining IJC lymph nodes are artificially divided into the *subdigastric, middle jugular*, and *lower jugular* groups.

The *spinal accessory chain* lymph nodes (posterior cervical chain or posterior triangle lymph nodes) are distributed along the course of cranial nerve XI. The superior nodes of the spinal accessory chain blend with the upper IJC nodes.

The *supraclavicular* lymph nodes merge laterally with the spinal accessory chain lymph nodes and medially with the lower IJC lymph nodes.

There are three to six *submandibular* lymph nodes. They may be either preglandular or postglandular; there are no lymph nodes in the substance of the submandibular gland. The *submental* lymph nodes lie in the midline between the anterior bellies of the digastric muscles, anterior to the hyoid bone and external to the mylohyoid muscle.

The *lateral retropharyngeal* lymph nodes lie within the retropharyngeal space, which is bounded anteriorly by the pharyngeal constrictor muscles, superiorly by the skull base, and posteriorly by the prevertebral fascia. They are usually at the level of the C1 and C2 vertebral bodies but may be found as inferiorly as C3. The medial retropharyngeal nodes are small, inconstant intercalated nodes that are located near midline and empty into the lateral retropharyngeal lymph nodes.

The neck nodes are divided into levels as follows:

Level I, submental (IA) and submandibular (IB) nodes;
Level II, upper internal jugular nodes, from the skull base to the level of the hyoid bone;
Level III, middle internal jugular nodes, from the level of the hyoid bone to the omohyoid muscle;
Level IV, inferior internal jugular nodes, from the level of the omohyoid muscle to the clavicle;
Level V, spinal accessory lymph nodes; and
Level VI, anterior neck nodes, bounded by the hyoid bone, the sternum, and the common carotid arteries.

Included in level VI are the paratracheal, pretracheal, precricoid (Delphian), and tracheoesophageal groove nodes (106).

Natural History

The risk of lymph node metastases is influenced by the location of the primary tumor, histologic differentiation, size of the lesion, and the availability of capillary lymphatics (67). The estimated risk of subclinical disease in the clinically negative neck as a function of primary site and tumor (T) stage is shown in Table 46.2 (67). Recurrent lesions have a higher risk of lymphatic involvement than untreated lesions.

The relative incidence of clinically positive lymph nodes in the neck by anatomic site and T stage is shown in Table 46.3 (51). The most commonly involved lymph nodes in the head and neck are the subdigastric lymph nodes, followed by the midjugular lymph nodes. Lesions that are well lateralized almost always spread first to the ipsilateral neck nodes. Lesions on or near the midline, as well as lateralized base of tongue and nasopharyngeal lesions, may spread to both sides of the neck.

Theoretically, patients who have clinically positive lymph nodes on the ipsilateral side of the neck may be at risk for contralateral lymph node spread if the metastatic masses produce significant obstruction of the lymphatic trunks. In addition, patients who have undergone previous surgery on one side of the neck develop shunting of lymph across the submental region to the opposite side of the neck. When contralateral lymph node metastases occur, the subdigastric lymph nodes are most frequently involved, followed by the midjugular and lower jugular lymph node groups.

As tumor grows within a lymph node, the node becomes indurated and more rounded, and enlarges. Tumor eventually extends through the capsule of the lymph node and invades surrounding structures. Extension to the neurovascular bundle is common and may produce a mass that is considered fixed to palpation. The incidence of tumor involvement and the likelihood of capsular penetration as a function of lymph node size are shown in Table 46.4 (99).

The risk of lateral retropharyngeal lymph node involvement is related to primary site and neck stage (63); the medial retropharyngeal nodes are almost never the site of metastatic disease. The incidence of positive retropharyngeal nodes based on pretreatment computed tomography (CT) and, in selected cases, magnetic resonance imaging (MRI) is shown in Table 46.5 (63).

Diagnostic Work-Up

Physical Examination

The patient is examined in the sitting position, the examiner behind the patient with one hand on the occiput to flex the patient's head forward and the other hand on the side of the neck to be examined. To examine the IJC lymph nodes, which lie deep to

Table 46.1   INCIDENCE OF LYMPH NODE METASTASIS BY SITE OF PRIMARY DISEASE IN HEAD AND NECK SQUAMOUS CELL CARCINOMAS

Site	Nodes Positive at Presentation %	Nodes Negative Clinically, Positive Pathologically %	Nodes Initially Negative, Becoming Positive with No Neck Treatment %
Floor of mouth	30–59 (37,39,44)	40–50 (41,103)	20–35 (6,81)
Gingiva	18–52 (18,25,37,60)	19 (18)	17 (6,18)
Hard palate	13–24 (20,29,60)	ND	22 (6)
Buccal mucosa	9–31 (37,44)	ND	16 (6)
Oral tongue	34–65 (37,39,43,44)	25–54 (13,25,38,48,104)	38–52 (38,43,81,105)
Nasopharynx	86–90 (14,53,85)	ND	19–50[a] (42,86)
Anterior tonsillar pillar/ retromolar trigone	39–56 (8,45,52)	ND	10–15 (103)
Soft palate/uvula	37–56 (8,45,52)	ND	16–25 (52)
Tonsillar fossa	50–76 (14,39,45,47,53,85)	ND	22[b] (100)
Base of tongue	50–83 (45,85,88,93,103)	22 (88)	ND
Pharyngeal walls	50–71 (45,85,88,103)	66 (88)	ND
Supraglottic larynx	31–64 (39,74,103)	16–26 (88,96)	33 (33,96)
Hypopharynx	52–78 (25,83,88,103)	38 (88)	ND

ND, no data.
[a]T1N0 patients only.
[b]Patients received preoperative irradiation.
From Mendenhall WM, Million RR, Cassisi NJ. Elective neck irradiation in squamous-cell carcinoma of the head and neck. *Head Neck Surg* 1980;3:15–20, with permission.

the sternocleidomastoid muscle along the internal jugular vein, place the thumb and index finger around the sternocleidomastoid muscle in the form of a C and then gently proceed from the sternal notch to the angle of the mandible. Both sides of the neck should not be examined simultaneously. The submandibular and submental nodes may be evaluated by direct palpation of these areas as well as by a bimanual examination with the index finger placed in the floor of the mouth (84).

The following features of metastatic lymph nodes should be recorded: anatomic location, size, consistency, mobility, and

clinical impression as to whether the node is involved with cancer.

Radiographic Evaluation

CT, MRI, fluorodeoxyglucose positron emission tomography (FDG PET), and ultrasound may be used to evaluate cervical metastatic disease (58). At the University of Florida, CT remains the primary method of examination of most carcinomas arising in the upper aerodigestive tract and the regional lymphatic

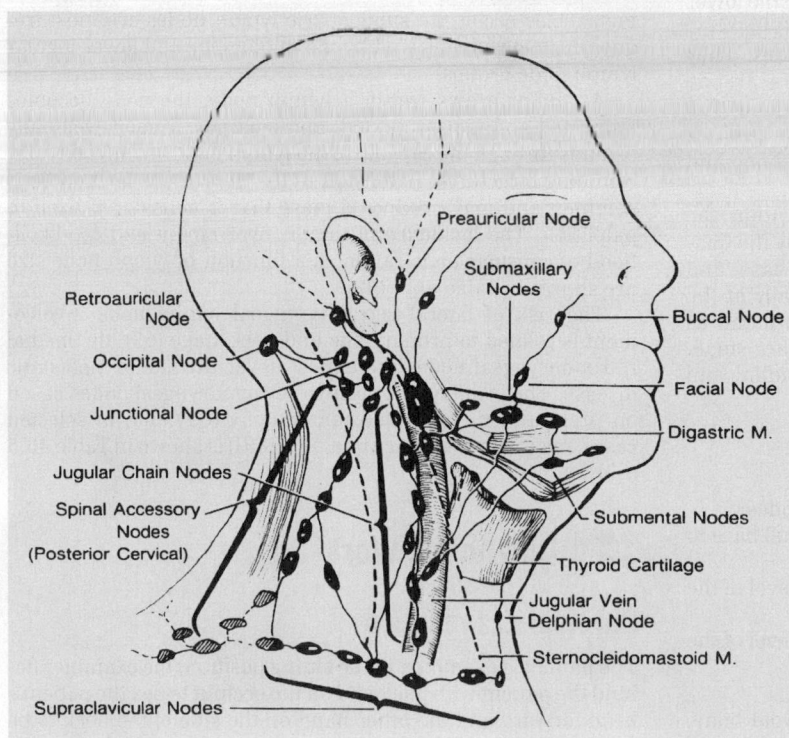

FIGURE 46.1. Arrangement of lymph nodes in the head and neck. (Redrawn from Rouviere H. *Anatomy of the human lymphatic system*. Tobias MJ, trans. Ann Arbor, MI: Edwards Brothers; 1938:27, with permission.)

| | Table 46.2 | DEFINITION OF RISK GROUPS | | |

Group	Estimated Risk of Subclinical Neck Disease %	Stage	Site
I Low risk	<20	T1	Floor of mouth, retromolar trigone, gingiva, hard palate, buccal mucosa
II Intermediate risk	20–30	T1	Oral tongue, soft palate, pharyngeal wall, supraglottic larynx, tonsil
		T2	Floor of mouth, oral tongue, retromolar trigone, gingiva, hard palate, buccal mucosa
III High risk	>30	T1–4	Nasopharynx, pyriform sinus, base of tongue
		T2–4	Soft palate, pharyngeal wall, supraglottic larynx, tonsil
		T3–4	Floor of mouth, oral tongue, retromolar trigone, gingiva, hard palate, buccal mucosa

From Mendenhall WM, Million RR. Elective neck irradiation for squamous cell carcinoma of the head and neck: analysis of time–dose factors and causes of failure. *Int J Radiat Oncol Biol Phys* 1986;12:741–746, with permission.

system. MRI is the primary study only in patients with nasopharyngeal malignancies. MRI also may be used in patients who are allergic to intravenous contrast medium. Ultrasound has been used mainly in Europe to evaluate the cervical nodes. FDG PET remains invalidated with regard to improving accuracy rates over those available with properly performed and interpreted CT.

Small metastases may be seen as lucent foci in normal-sized nodes. Such metastases have been identified and surgically confirmed in nodes as small as 6 to 8 mm; however, most subclinical disease in normal-sized nodes remains undetected on CT. FDG PET has a marginal capability to improve on CT in detecting the subclinical disease in small (less than 1 cm) nodes.

Lucent foci in normal-sized nodes must be differentiated from hilar fat or volume-averaging artifacts. As the metastasis grows, the node becomes more spherical than elliptical. Areas of necrosis are almost always present in nodal metastases larger than 2 cm. As the metastasis enlarges, the capsule of the node becomes hyperemic and is seen radiographically as a contrast-enhanced rim. When the capsule becomes indistinct and irregular along its outer margin, it is highly suggestive of early capsular penetration. Continued growth causes obliteration of the fat planes surrounding the nodes. Finally, no clear plane of normal tissue lies between the mass and the adjacent structures, at which point the clinician usually notes fixation (Fig. 46.2). Penetration of the prevertebral fascia and fixation to the scalene muscles are uncommon in untreated patients. Largely necrotic nodes may be negative on FDG PET examinations.

If a node shows evidence of capsular penetration and envelops more than 50% of the circumference of the carotid artery, clinical evidence of fixation to the artery is likely. Ultrasound and MRI may prove useful in evaluating tumor extension to the carotid, as suggested by CT. MRI tends to be better at excluding extension to the neurovascular bundle when it is suspected on CT, whereas ultrasound can help show invasion of the vessel wall, thus confirming focal extension to the artery.

Staging

The staging systems shown in Table 46.6 are those of the American Joint Committee on Cancer (AJCC). Because all University of Florida data presented in this chapter were analyzed using the 1983 AJCC staging system (4), both the 1983 and 2002 systems are outlined in Table 46.6. Stage N3C in the 1983 system is

rare and should alert the clinician to search for another primary lesion. The 2002 update of the AJCC staging system classifies bilateral or contralateral nodes not more than 6 cm in diameter as N2C; N3 is defined as a metastasis in a lymph node more than 6 cm in diameter. The AJCC nodal staging for nasopharyngeal carcinoma differs from other head and neck primary sites and will be discussed in the chapter devoted to that topic.

Surgery

Standard radical neck dissection involves removal of the superficial and deep cervical fascia with its lymph nodes in levels I to V in continuity with the sternocleidomastoid muscle, omohyoid muscle, internal and external jugular veins, spinal accessory nerve, and submandibular gland. Sacrifice of cranial nerve XI often, but not always, results in atrophy of the trapezius muscle, with resultant shoulder drop and discomfort.

Modified radical neck dissection removes the superficial and deep cervical fascia with its enclosed lymph nodes and leaves one or more of the nonlymphatic structures such as the sternocleidomastoid and digastric muscles, internal jugular vein, and spinal accessory nerve. Currently, almost all of the patients treated with neck dissection at our institution undergo this operation with at least preservation of cranial nerve XI. The advantages of the functional neck dissection are less cosmetic deformity and better function.

For a selective neck dissection, one or more of lymph node groups I to V are not removed. The advantage of the selective neck dissection is that it provides equivalent efficacy and less morbidity in appropriately selected cases. Supraomohyoid neck dissection removes the lymph nodes in levels I to III and is most commonly used for patients with small oral cavity cancers and a clinically negative neck. The lateral neck dissection entails removal of level II to IV nodes and is most often used in the treatment of laryngeal, oropharyngeal, and hypopharyngeal cancers. If significant metastatic adenopathy is encountered during a selective neck dissection, it should be converted to a radical or modified radical dissection.

An extended radical neck dissection implies removal of additional lymph node groups or nonlymphatic structures in addition to the structures removed in a radical neck dissection. Bilateral neck dissections may be performed simultaneously or separately (staged) in patients with bilateral neck disease, as long as one internal jugular vein can be preserved. At one time, simultaneous neck dissection appeared to be associated with a

Table 46.3 — CLINICALLY DETECTED NODAL METASTASES ON ADMISSION CORRELATED WITH T STAGE[a]

Primary Site	T Stage	N0 %	N1 %	N2–3 %
Oral tongue[b]	T1	86	10	4
	T2	70	19	11
	T3	52	16	31
	T4	24	10	66
Floor of mouth[b]	T1	89	9	2
	T2	71	18	10
	T3	56	20	24
	T4	46	10	43
Retromolar trigone/ anterior tonsillar pillar[c]	T1	88	2	9
	T2	62	18	20
	T3	46	21	33
	T4	32	18	50
Soft palate[c]	T1	92	0	8
	T2	64	12	24
	T3	35	26	39
	T4	33	11	56
Tonsillar fossa[c]	T1	30	41	30
	T2	32	14	54
	T3	30	18	52
	T4	10	13	76
Base of tongue[c]	T1	30	15	55
	T2	29	14	56
	T3	26	23	52
	T4	16	8	76
Oropharyngeal walls[c]	T1	75	0	25
	T2	70	10	20
	T3	33	22	44
	T4	24	24	52
Supraglottic larynx[d]	T1	61	10	29
	T2	58	16	26
	T3	16	25	40
	T4	26	18	41
Hypopharynx[e]	T1	37	21	42
	T2	30	20	49
	T3	21	26	54
	T4	26	15	58
Nasopharynx[f]	T1	8	11	82
	T2	16	12	72
	T3	12	9	80
	T4	17	6	78

[a]Data are those of 2,044 patients, M.D. Anderson Hospital, Houston, TX, 1948–1965
[b]T stage defined by Lindberg (51).
[c]T stage defined by Fletcher et al. (35).
[d]T stage defined by Fletcher et al. (36).
[e]T stage defined by MacComb et al. (55).
[f]T stage defined by Chen & Fletcher (19).
Modified from Lindberg RD. Distribution of cervical lymph node metastases from squamous cell carcinoma of the upper respiratory and digestive tracts. *Cancer* 1972;29:1446–1449, with permission.

Table 46.4 — RELATIONSHIP BETWEEN NODE SIZE, THE PRESENCE OF TUMOR IN THE NODE, AND CAPSULAR PENETRATION IN 519 NODES[a]

	Size of Node (cm)				
	1	2	3	4	≥5
Number of nodes	177	183	84	17	58
Percent positive	33	62	81	88	100
Percent positive with capsular penetration	14	26	49	71	76

[a]Data from the Institut Gustave-Roussy, Villejuif, France.
Modified from Richard JM, Sancho-Garnier H, Micheau C. Prognostic factors in cervical lymph node metastasis in upper respiratory and digestive tract carcinoma: study of 1713 cases during a 15-year period. *Laryngoscope* 1987;97:97–101, with permission.

	Table 46.5	**INCIDENCE OF POSITIVE RETROPHARYNGEAL NODES FOR VARIOUS PRIMARY SITES AND CLINICAL NECK STAGES (794 TUMORS)**		

	Clinical Neck Stage		
Primary Site	**N0 Neck No. %**	**N+ Neck^a No. %**	**Overall %**
Nasopharynx	2/5 (40)	12/14 (86)	74
Pharyngeal wall	6/37 (16)	12/56 (21)	19
Soft palate	1/21 (5)	6/32 (19)	13
Tonsillar region	2/56 (4)	14/120 (12)	9
Pyriform sinus or postcricoid area	0/55 (0)	7/81 (9)	5
Base of tongue	0/31 (0)	5/90 (6)	4
Supraglottic larynx	0/87 (0)	4/109 (4)	2

^{a}N +, neck nodes clinically involved (stages N1–3B).
From McLaughlin MP, Mendenhall WM, Mancuso AA, et al. Retropharyngeal adenopathy as a predictor of outcome in squamous cell carcinoma of the head and neck. *Head Neck* 1995;17:190–198, with permission.

higher incidence of complications and operative mortality compared with staged neck dissections (61,97). Our more recent experience suggests that this is no longer the case.

Complications of Neck Dissection

Complications of neck dissection include hematoma, seroma, lymphedema, wound infection, wound dehiscence, chyle fistula, damage to cranial nerves VII, X, XI, and XII, carotid exposure, and carotid rupture. The incidence of complications is higher when neck dissection is combined with resection of the primary lesion or when it follows a course of radiation therapy. The postoperative mortality rate for unilateral neck dissection after radiation therapy was 3% for patients treated between 1964 and 1982 (70).

The incidence of postoperative complications in a series of patients treated with radiation therapy to the primary lesion and neck followed by unilateral or bilateral neck dissection(s) is shown in Tables 46.7 (70) and 46.8 (102), respectively. Two of 10 patients undergoing a staged bilateral neck dissection experienced a moderately severe complication compared with 4 of 40 patients undergoing a simultaneous bilateral neck dissection. None of the 10 patients who underwent a staged bilateral neck dissection experienced a severe complication, compared

with 6 of 40 patients (15%) who underwent a simultaneous bilateral neck dissection (*p* = .24) (102).

Taylor et al. (108) analyzed the incidence of moderate (2+) and severe (3+) wound complications in a series of 205 patients who underwent a planned unilateral neck dissection after radiation therapy at the University of Florida. Radiation therapy was given once daily in 123 patients, twice daily in 80 patients, and with both techniques in the remaining 2 patients. The incidence of wound complications increased with total dose and dose per fraction (Fig. 46.3).

Radiation Therapy

Radiation therapy may be used in the treatment of cervical lymph node metastases as elective treatment when there are no palpable lymph nodes, as the only treatment for clinically positive lymph nodes (26), or as preoperative or postoperative treatment in combination with neck dissection for clinically positive lymph nodes (80).

The regional lymph nodes are considered in the treatment planning of the primary lesion. With clinically negative neck nodes, treatment planning depends on the estimated risk of subclinical disease in the nodes. With clinically positive lymph nodes, the plan is influenced by the number of lymph nodes, size, and location.

Elective Radiation Therapy of Cervical Lymph Nodes When the Primary Tumor Is Treated by Radiation Therapy

Factors that influence the decision to irradiate the neck electively are site and size of the primary lesion, histologic grade, difficulty in neck examination, relative morbidity for adding lymph node coverage, likelihood of the patient's returning for follow-up examinations, and suitability of the patient for a radical neck dissection if the tumor appears in the neck at a later date. Patients in whom the primary lesion is to be treated by radiation therapy, who have clinically negative nodes, and in whom the risk of subclinical disease is 20% or greater usually receive elective neck irradiation to a minimum dose equivalent to 45 to 50 Gy during 4.5 to 5 weeks (Table 46.2). Patients with lesions arising in the lip, nasal vestibule, nasal cavity, or paranasal sinuses have a low risk of subclinical neck disease, and the neck is not treated electively unless the lesion is recurrent, advanced, or poorly differentiated. Similarly, the risk of occult neck disease is essentially zero for T1 and 1.7% for T2

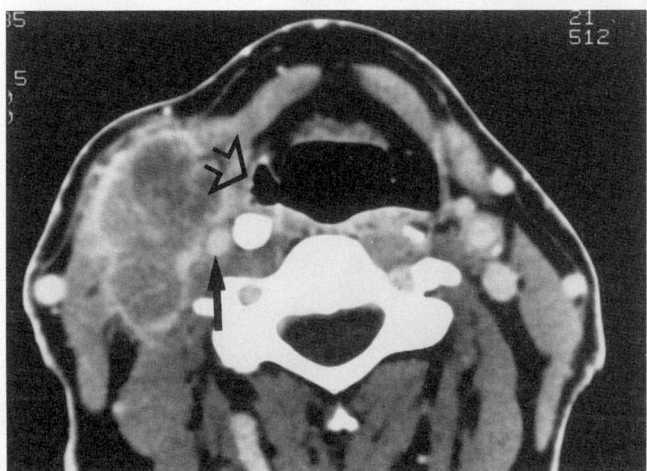

FIGURE 46.2. T1 squamous cell carcinoma of the lateral wall of the right pyriform sinus (*open arrow*) and a fixed N3B neck node that abuts but does not surround the carotid artery (*solid arrow*). (From Mendenhall WM, Parsons JT, Mancuso AA, et al. Head and neck: management of the neck. In: Perez CA, Brady LW, Halperin EC, et al., eds. *Principles and practice of radiation oncology.* Philadelphia: Lippincott Williams & Wilkins; 2004:1158–1178, with permission.)

Clinical Radiation Oncology

Table 46.6	1983 AND 2002 AMERICAN JOINT COMMITTEE ON CANCER STAGING FOR NECK LYMPH NODES
Stage	**Definition**
1983 Stage	
NX	Nodes cannot be assessed
N0	No clinically positive nodes
N1	Single clinically positive homolateral node ≤3 cm in diameter
N2	Single clinically positive homolateral node >3 cm but not >6 cm in diameter or multiple clinically positive homolateral nodes, none >6 cm in diameter
N2A	Single clinically positive homolateral node >3 cm but not >6 cm in diameter
N2B	Multiple clinically positive homolateral nodes, none >6 cm in diameter
N3A	Clinically positive homolateral node(s), one >6 cm in diameter
N3B	Bilateral clinically positive nodes (in this situation, each side of the neck should be staged separately (i.e., N3B, right; N2A, left; N1)
N3C	Contralateral clinically positive node(s) only
2002 Stage	
NX	Regional lymph nodes cannot be assessed
N0	No regional lymph node metastasis
N1	Metastasis in a single ipsilateral lymph node, ≤3 cm in greatest dimension
N2	Metastasis in a single ipsilateral lymph node, >3 cm but not >6 cm in greatest dimension, or in multiple ipsilateral lymph nodes, none >6 cm in greatest dimensions; or in bilateral or contralateral lymph nodes, none >6 cm in greatest dimension
N2A	Metastasis in single ipsilateral lymph node >3 cm but not >6 cm in greatest dimension
N2B	Metastasis in multiple ipsilateral lymph nodes, none >6 cm in greatest dimension
N2C	Metastasis in bilateral or contralateral lymph nodes, none >6 cm in greatest dimension
N3	Metastasis in a lymph node >6 cm in greatest dimension

From American Joint Committee on Cancer. *Manual for staging of cancer*, 2nd ed. Philadelphia: JB Lippincott; 1983:27; and American Joint Committee on Cancer. *Cancer staging manual*, 6th ed. New York: Springer-Verlag; 2002:25.

glottic carcinomas, and elective neck radiation therapy is not indicated (73,77).

The lateral treatment portals used to encompass cancers in the oropharynx, supraglottic larynx, and hypopharynx include the upper jugular and often the midjugular chain lymph nodes. Radiation portals used for primary lesions of the oral cavity, nasopharynx, glottis, nasal cavity, and paranasal sinuses must be enlarged to include the lymph nodes. The treatment portals for irradiation of the cervical lymph nodes must be designed in such a way as to minimize additional mucosal irradiation. A common error in irradiating oropharyngeal and nasopharyngeal cancers is to enlarge the lateral (primary) portals inferiorly to unnecessarily include all of the larynx in the lateral portals (Fig. 46.4) (76). Because the midneck is smaller in circumfer-ence than the upper neck, the total dose and dose per fraction are higher in the larynx than along the central axis of the beam, leading to "double trouble." Although a field junction through a positive node(s) may be avoided with intensity-modulated radiation therapy (IMRT), the larynx still receives a substantially higher dose compared with a separate anterior low neck portal with a midline laryngeal block junctioned at the thyroid notch (Figs. 46.5–44.7) (1). Treating an unnecessarily large field increases the acute and late effects of radiation therapy and, by increasing the risk of an unplanned split, reduces the probability of disease control (1,70).

Elective neck irradiation for early oral cavity lesions includes the submandibular and subdigastric lymph nodes. The midjugular and low jugular lymph nodes are treated as well

Table 46.7	POSTOPERATIVE COMPLICATIONS OF UNILATERAL NECK DISSECTION AFTER IRRADIATION TO THE PRIMARY LESION AND NECK (143 PATIENTS)

Complications	No. of Complications	No. of Second Operations to Repair Complication	Death
Salivary fistula	1	0	0
Wound breakdown	23	15	0
Bleeding	2	1	1
Pneumonia	2	0	1
Orocutaneous fistula	1	1	0
Lymphatic fistula	2	0	0
Pulmonary embolus	1	0	0
Cardiovascular problem	2	0	1
Sepsis	1	0	1
Total complications	35[a]	17	4[b]
Incidence	33/143 (23%)	17/143 (12%)	4/143 (3%)

[a]There were 35 complications in 33 patients.
[b]Deaths occurred 6, 7, 8, and 35 days after surgery.
From Mendenhall WM, Million RR, Cassisi NJ. Squamous cell carcinoma of the head and neck treated with radiation therapy: the role of neck dissection for clinically positive neck nodes. *Int J Radiat Oncol Biol Phys* 1986;12:733–740, with permission.

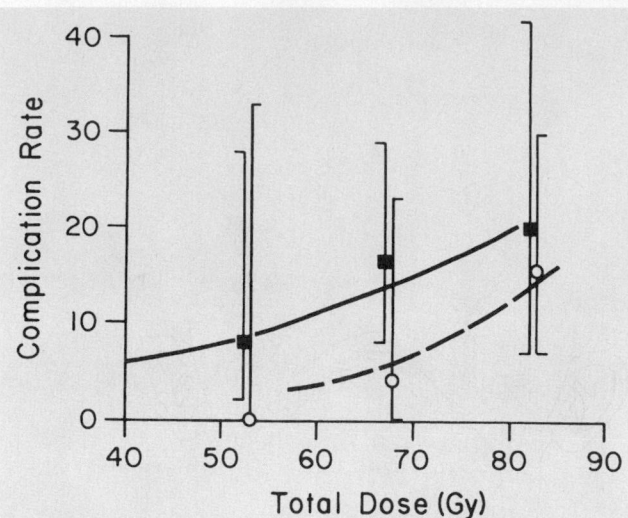

FIGURE 46.3. Complication rate (2+ or 3+) versus total dose. Separate analysis for once a day, (■ *solid curve*) and twice a day, (○ *dashed curve*). Data are plotted at the midpoints of the range 45 to 60 Gy, 60 to 70 Gy, and 75 to 90 Gy. Error bars denote 95% confidence intervals. The curves are the results of separate logistic regression analysis. (From Taylor JMG, Mendenhall WM, Parsons JT, et al. The influence of dose and time on wound complications following post-radiation neck dissection. *Int J Radiat Oncol Biol Phys* 1992;23:41–46, with permission.)

by using a narrow anterior field. For primary lesions located in the oropharynx, nasopharynx, supraglottic larynx, and hypopharynx, the lower neck nodes are also routinely included. The low neck is treated with a single anterior field (Fig. 46.8). A tapered midline larynx/trachea shield is added to protect the spinal cord, the larynx, and the pharynx. For primary lesions lying below the thyroid notch, a small midline tracheal block is placed in the low-neck field, primarily to avoid field overlap at the spinal cord. A 1-cm wide midline block made of Lipowitz's metal may be used to shield the trachea, esophagus, and spinal cord below the level of the cricoid.

Treatment of Clinically Positive Cervical Lymph Nodes When the Primary Tumor Is Treated by Radiation Therapy

The dose required to control a clinically positive lymph node that is included within the radiation portals depends on the size of the lymph node (26,107) and whether concomitant chemotherapy is administered. Relatively recent data suggest that advanced disease has a better chance of cure after altered fractionation and/or concomitant chemotherapy (79). Patients treated at our institution routinely receive hyperfractionation when using three-dimensional conformal radiotherapy and the concomitant boost technique when using IMRT, combined with weekly cisplatin 30 mg/m². Positive nodes receive approximately 70 to 74 Gy, regardless of size or rate of regression.

The decision to add a neck dissection after radiation therapy for multiple unilateral positive nodes or bilateral lymph node disease is individualized and is based on the diameter of the largest node, node fixation, and number of clinically positive nodes in the neck. If clinically positive lymph nodes disappear completely during radiation therapy, the likelihood of control by radiation therapy alone is improved, and a neck dissection may be withheld (10–12,56). Peters et al. (94) reported on 100 patients with node-positive squamous cell carcinoma of the oropharynx treated with concomitant boost radiotherapy between 1984 and 1993 at the M.D. Anderson Cancer Center (Houston, TX). Sixty-two patients had a complete response in

the neck and received no further therapy. Three patients (5%) subsequently developed an isolated recurrence in the neck and four patients (6%) developed a recurrence in the neck in conjunction with other sites of relapse. The 2-year neck disease control rates did not vary significantly with pretreatment nodal size: ≤3 cm, 87%, and >3 cm, 85%. The incidence of subcutaneous fibrosis was similar following irradiation alone compared with another group of patients who underwent a neck dissection in addition to radiation therapy. Johnson et al. (46) reported on 81 patients with node-positive stage III and IV squamous cell carcinoma of the head and neck treated with concomitant boost, accelerated hyperfractionated radiotherapy at the Medical College of Virginia (Richmond). Fifty-eight patients (72%) had a complete response in the neck and were followed; three patients (5%) subsequently developed an isolated recurrence in the neck and one additional patient developed recurrent cancer in the neck and in the primary site. The 3-year neck disease control rates were 94% for nodes ≤3 cm compared with 86% for those >3 cm.

Both of these series of patients received aggressive altered fractionated radiotherapy; it is unclear whether these data can be broadly extrapolated to patients with head and neck cancer from a variety of head and neck primary sites that are treated less aggressively. It is also unclear whether the addition of concomitant chemotherapy results in a lower likelihood of needing a neck dissection. Our policy at the University of Florida has changed to the extent that we now evaluate patients with clinically positive nodes with CT 4 weeks after irradiation and withhold neck dissection in the subset of patients with a complete response who are thought to have ≤5% risk of residual disease (50). Because the likelihood of successful salvage of a neck recurrence in an initially positive neck is 5% or less, we proceed with a neck dissection in borderline cases (15,54,68).

If a neck dissection is planned to follow radiation therapy in patients with clinically positive lymph nodes, the preoperative dose varies with the size and location of the lymph node, fixation, and response to radiation therapy. Preoperative doses of 50 Gy are sufficient for mobile lymph nodes 3 to 4 cm in size, but 60 Gy or more is recommended for 5- to 6-cm nodes and for fixed nodes. Lymph nodes measuring 7 to 8 cm are almost always fixed to adjacent structures and often require doses of 70 to 75 Gy for the surgeon to achieve a complete resection. If the lymph node lies behind the plane of the spinal cord, electrons may be used to boost the dose after the primary fields have been reduced off the spinal cord after 45 to 50 Gy (70).

Another technique commonly used for boosting the dose to the neck mass after spinal cord tolerance has been reached and the treatment to the primary lesion has been completed is opposed anterior and posterior fields with wedges. The final dose to the neck node (not to the entire neck) may be 70 to 80 Gy without exceeding the spinal cord tolerance (Fig. 46.9). The anterior and posterior wedge-pair technique is preferable to an appositional electron boost field because high-energy electron beams increase the skin and mucosal dose.

When the cervical lymph nodes are located superficially, sometimes within 1 cm from the skin or fixed to it, treatment with high-energy photon beams (≥6 MV) may underdose these nodes. Treatment should be initiated with ⁶⁰Co or 4-MV x-rays for the initial 45 to 50 Gy, after which a higher energy photon beam can be used to continue radiation therapy of the primary tumor if the neck nodes are clinically negative or if a neck dissection is planned to follow radiation therapy (Fig. 46.10). Parallel-opposed 6-MV x-ray beams may adequately treat the upper neck nodes included in the primary treatment fields; however, the supraclavicular nodes in the *en face* low-neck field may be underdosed with a 6-MV beam in very thin patients. Although electrons alone may be used to treat cervical nodes, it is preferable to combine them with photons because of the high surface dose with high-electron energies. Use of both

Clinical Radiation Oncology

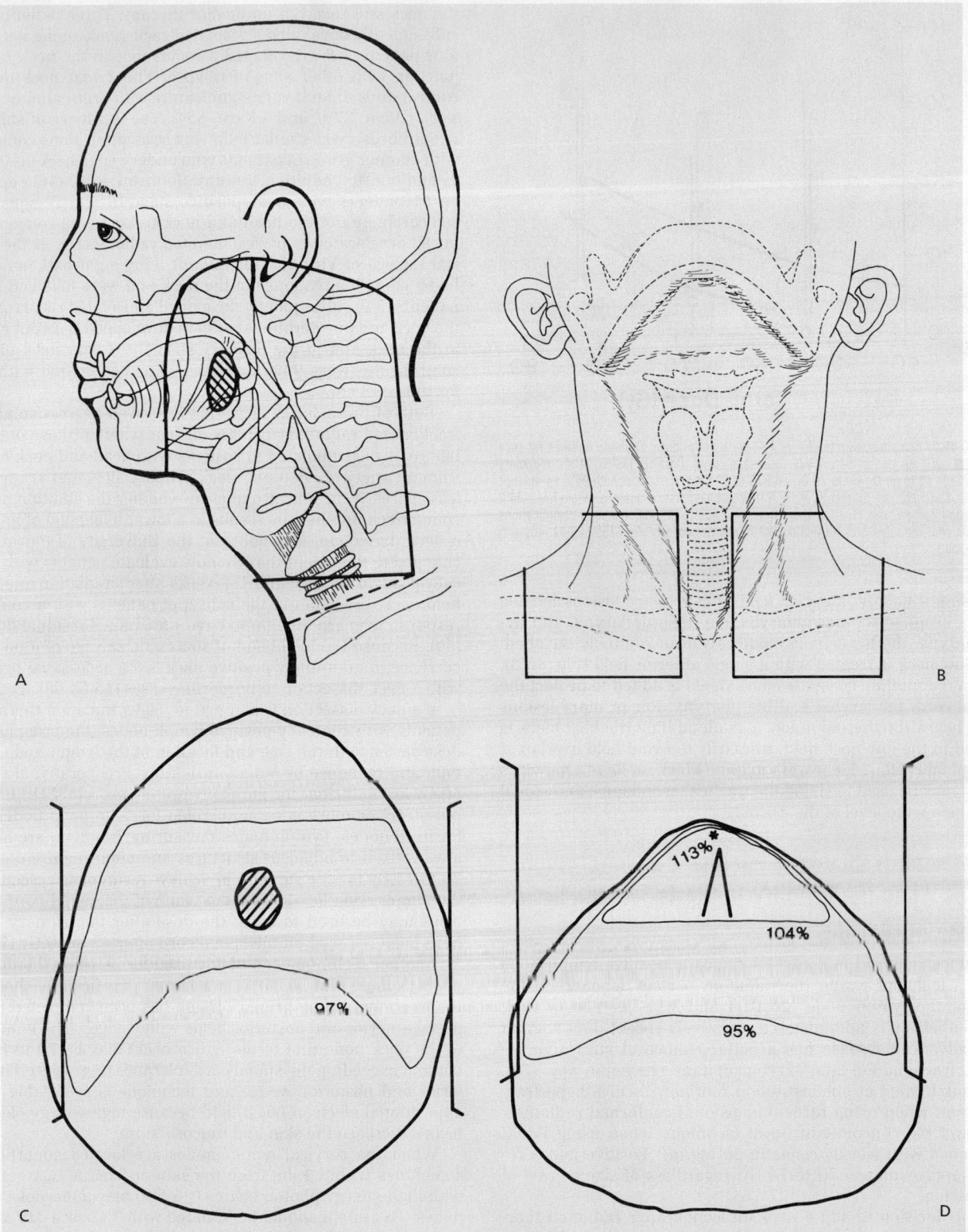

FIGURE 46.4. Carcinoma of the base of the tongue: large radiation portals. **A:** Parallel-opposed lateral portals include the primary lesion, larynx (*arrow*), hypopharynx, most of the cervical spinal cord, and the upper portion of the trachea and cervical esophagus. Treatment through this portal tangentially irradiates the skin of the anterior neck unnecessarily. If an anterior field is not used to irradiate the low neck, the inferior border of the lateral field may be placed near the clavicle (*dashed line*). **B:** Anterior low-neck portal. The wide midline tracheal block partially shields the low internal jugular lymph nodes, which are located adjacent to the trachea. The supraclavicular lymph nodes, which are less likely to be involved with tumor than the low jugular nodes, are adequately covered. **C:** Central axis dosimetry at the level of the base of tongue primary lesion. The contours were obtained from a RANDO phantom using parallel ^{60}Co fields weighted equally. The base of tongue tumor is outlined, and the tumor dose is specified at 97% of maximum dose. **D:** Off-axis contour through larynx. The minimum dose to the entire larynx is 104% of the maximum dose specified at the central axis, and *is maximum dose on this off-axis contour is 113%. If the base of tongue tumor dose is specified as 50 Gy at 2 Gy per fraction, the minimum larynx dose is 53.61 Gy at 2.14 Gy per fraction, and the maximum larynx dose is 58.25 Gy at 2.33 Gy per fraction. If the tumor dose is specified as 60 Gy at 2 Gy per fraction, the minimum larynx dose is 64.33 Gy at 2.14 Gy per fraction, and the maximum larynx dose is 69.9 Gy at 2.33 Gy per fraction. (From Mendenhall WM, Parsons JT, Million RR. Unnecessary irradiation of the normal larynx [editorial]. *Int J Radiat Oncol Biol Phys* 1990:18:1531–1533, with permission.)

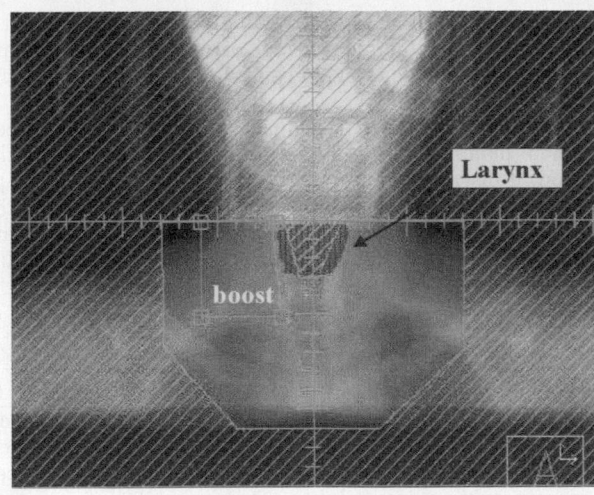
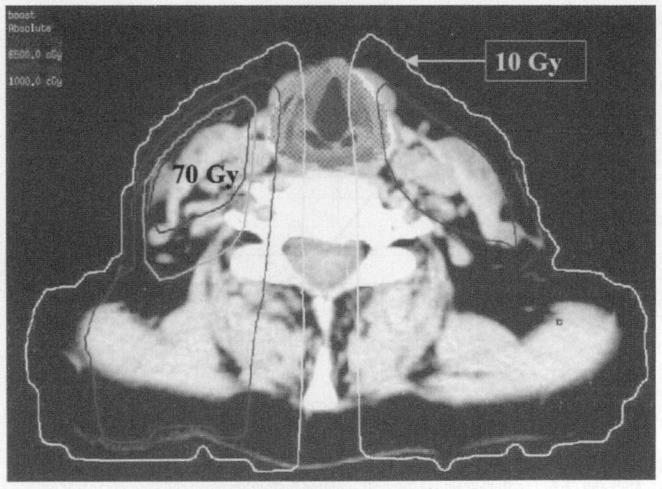

FIGURE 46.5. Laryngeal dose in a model patient with a stage T2N2b carcinoma of the tonsil with positive nodes on the right side at the level of the larynx. The primary site is irradiated with either intensity-modulated radiation therapy or lateral-opposed fields. The cervical lymphatics inferior to the primary site fields are treated with an anterior low-neck field. **A:** Digitally reconstructed radiograph of the low-neck fields. The larynx was contoured and appears as a red color-wash structure. The larynx is shielded with a narrow midline block that does not cover the entire width of the larynx (*arrow*). In this model patient, the entire low-neck field received 50 Gy, and then the field size was reduced to boost the positive nodes on the right of the larynx to 70 Gy. Irradiation was given with a 6-mV photon beam with source to axis distance of 100 cm. **B:** Axial dose distribution at the level of the true vocal cords showing that the dose to the central portion of the larynx is extremely low when the larynx is shielded in the anterior low-neck field. (From Amdur RJ, Li JG, Liu C, et al. Unnecessary laryngeal irradiation in the IMRT era. *Head Neck* 2004;26:257–264, with permission.)

20-MeV electrons and 17-MV x-rays is compared with treatment by 20-MeV electrons alone in a patient with a lateralized lesion of the oropharynx (Fig. 46.11) (16). The addition of the 17-MV x-rays to the 20-MeV electrons decreases the surface dose while still adequately irradiating the cervical nodes that are within the primary field. The addition of the x-ray beam also produces a dose distribution that is less affected by bone than that from the electron beam alone.

Large lymph nodes may not show much regression during the course of radiation therapy but often show significant regression from completion of treatment to the time that the patient returns for neck dissection, usually after 4 to 6 weeks. The mass frequently has a thick capsule that facilitates its removal at the time of neck dissection. It is preferable to add a neck dissection rather than treat with high-dose radiation therapy alone because the rate of disease control is higher, neck fibrosis

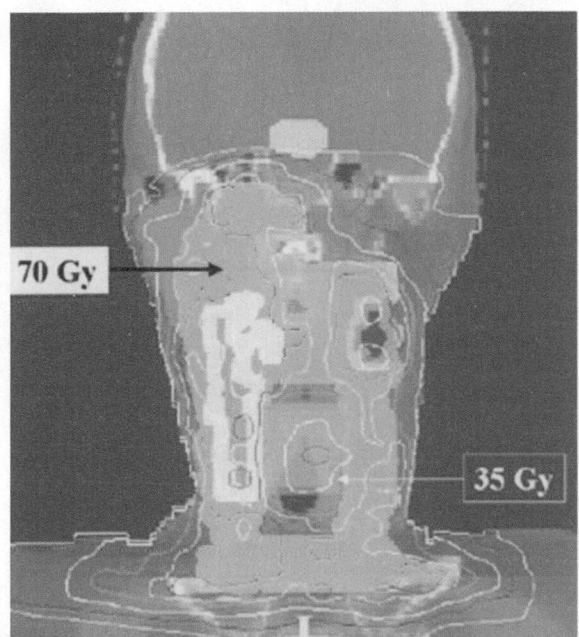
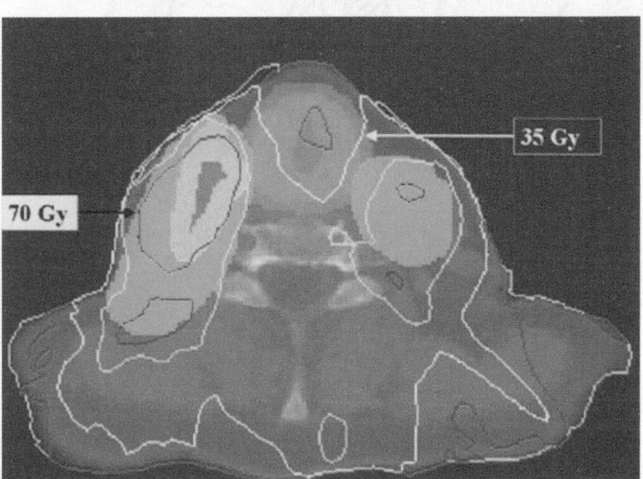

FIGURE 46.6. Dose distribution using IMRT as described in the text to treat the model patient with a stage T2N2b carcinoma of the tonsil with positive nodes on the right side at the level of the larynx. The plan was optimized to minimize the dose to the larynx while delivering 70 Gy to gross disease and 59.4 Gy to areas at risk for subclinical disease. **A:** Coronal projection near the middle of the larynx. **B:** Axial projection at the level of the true vocal cords. A comparison of Figs. 46.5B and 46.6B shows that sparing of the central portion of the larynx is shielded in an anterior low-neck field. (From Amdur RJ, Li JG, Liu C, et al. Unnecessary laryngeal irradiation in the IMRT era. *Head Neck* 2004;26:257–264, with permission.)

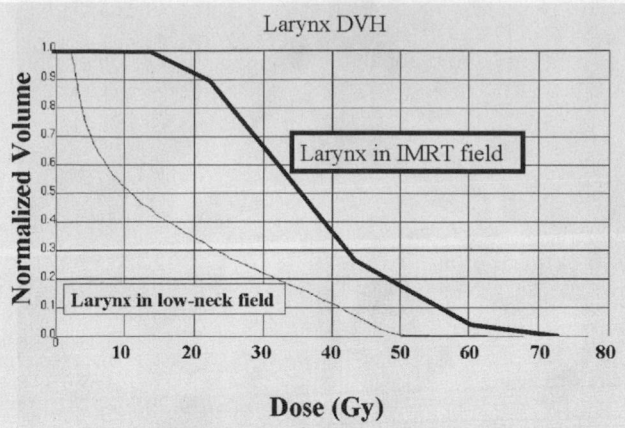

FIGURE 46.7. Dose-volume histogram (DVH) of the larynx for the model patient described in Figs. 46.5 and 46.6. The thicker line is the dose-volume histogram when the larynx is included in the intensity-modulated radiation therapy (IMRT) fields shown in Fig. 46.6. The thinner line is the dose-volume histogram when the larynx is shielded in the anterior low-neck field shown in Fig. 46.5. There is a major difference in the portion of the larynx that receives an extremely low dose. For example, when the larynx is included in the IMRT fields, the entire larynx receives more than 10 Gy, whereas when the larynx is shielded in the low-neck field, approximately 45% of the larynx receives less than 10 Gy. (From Amdur RJ, Li JG, Liu C, et al. Unnecessary laryngeal irradiation in the IMRT era. *Head Neck* 2004;26:257–264, with permission.)

is less pronounced, cranial nerve XII palsy due to entrapment is less frequent, and attempted salvage of a patient with neck failure after high-dose radiation therapy alone is seldom successful and often morbid.

Patients with bilateral neck disease require individualized treatment planning jointly by the radiation oncologist and the surgeon. If disease is minimal on one side, radiation therapy alone may be used to control the disease on that side of the neck, and a neck dissection may be used on the side with more disease. If major bilateral disease is present, bilateral neck dissection should follow radiation therapy.

Complications of Neck Irradiation

The complications of neck irradiation include subcutaneous fibrosis and lymphedema of the larynx and submentum. The latter complications may be minimized by sparing an anterior strip of skin when designing the parallel-opposed lateral portals used to encompass the primary lesion. The probability of complications is directly related to the radiation dose with little, if any, morbidity observed with the doses used for elective radiation therapy of the neck.

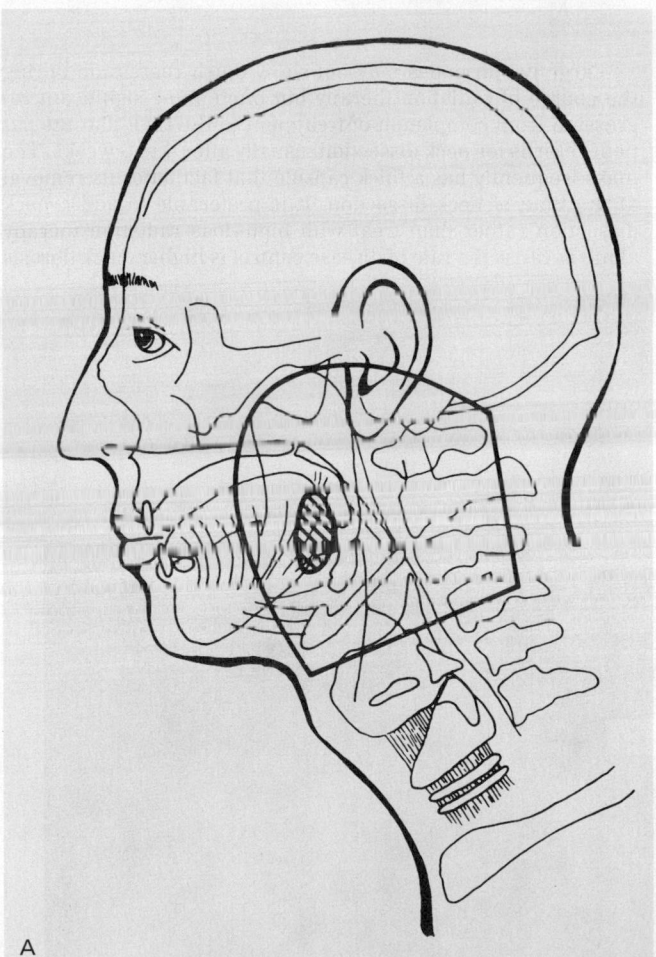

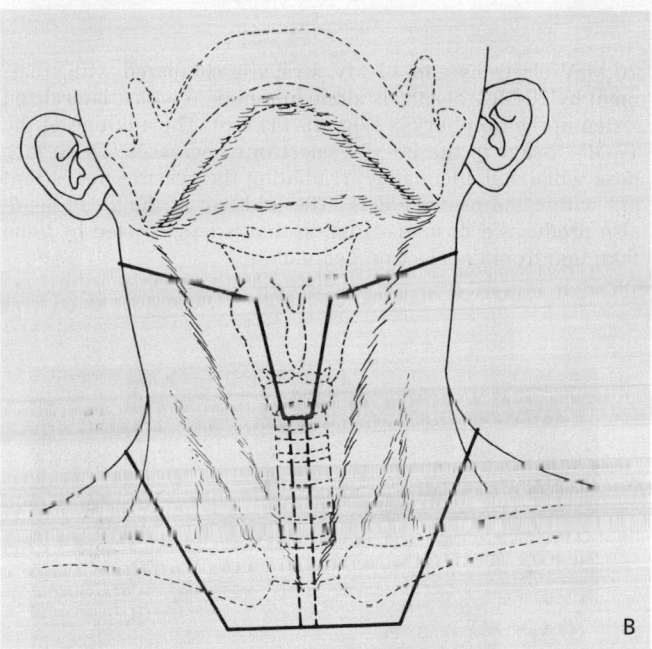

FIGURE 46.8. Lateral and anterior fields are used to irradiate a patient with a carcinoma limited to the base of tongue. **A:** Parallel-opposed fields include the primary lesion with a 2- to 3-cm inferior margin. The lower border of the field is placed at the thyroid notch and slants superiorly as the junction line proceeds posteriorly. This substantially reduces the amount of mucosal larynx, and spinal cord included in the primary treatment portals. **B:** *En face* low-neck portal with tapered midline larynx, and tapered midline larynx block. It is not necessary to treat the supraclavicular fossa unless clinically positive nodes are found in that particular hemineck. A 5-mm midline tracheal block may be placed in the low-neck portal *(dashed line)*. (From Mendenhall WM, Parsons JT, Million RR. Unnecessary irradiation of the normal larynx [editorial]. *Int J Radiat Oncol Biol Phys* 1990;18:1531–1533, with permission.)

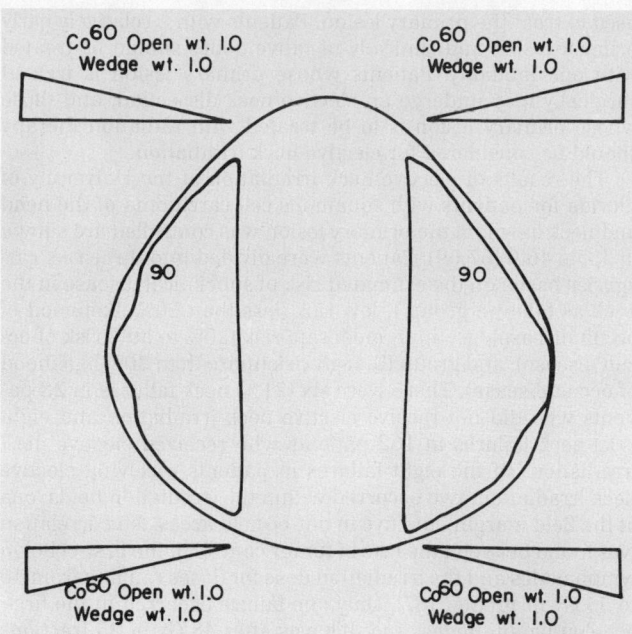

FIGURE 46.9. Dose distribution for anterior and posterior wedge ^{60}Co portals, with both fields weighted 1.0.

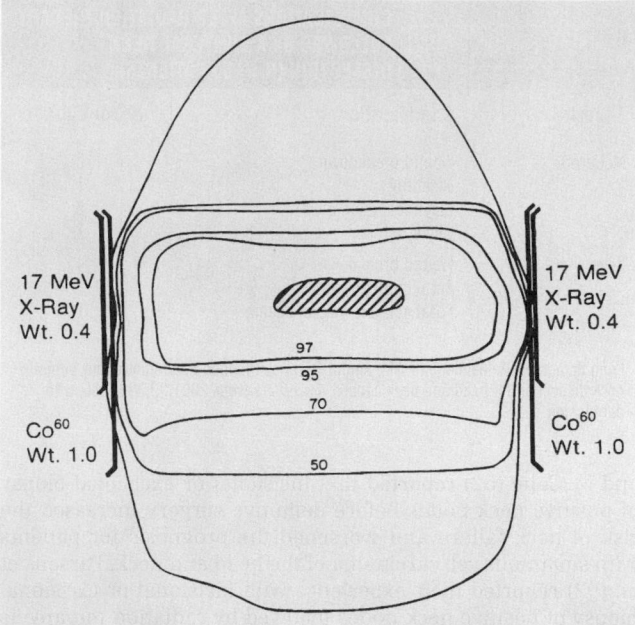

FIGURE 46.10. Dose distribution for parallel-opposed ^{60}Co portals, each weighted 1.0, with reduced 17-MV x-ray portals, each weighted 0.4.

Complications of neck treatment in patients who receive radiation therapy in conjunction with resection of the primary lesion and a neck dissection are essentially the same as those occurring after neck dissection. However, they occur with an increased incidence depending on the radiation dose and extent of surgery.

Treatment of the Neck after Incisional or Excisional Biopsy

Open biopsy of a clinically positive neck node before definitive treatment potentially spills tumor cells along tissue planes that may not be removed with a radical neck dissection. McGuirt

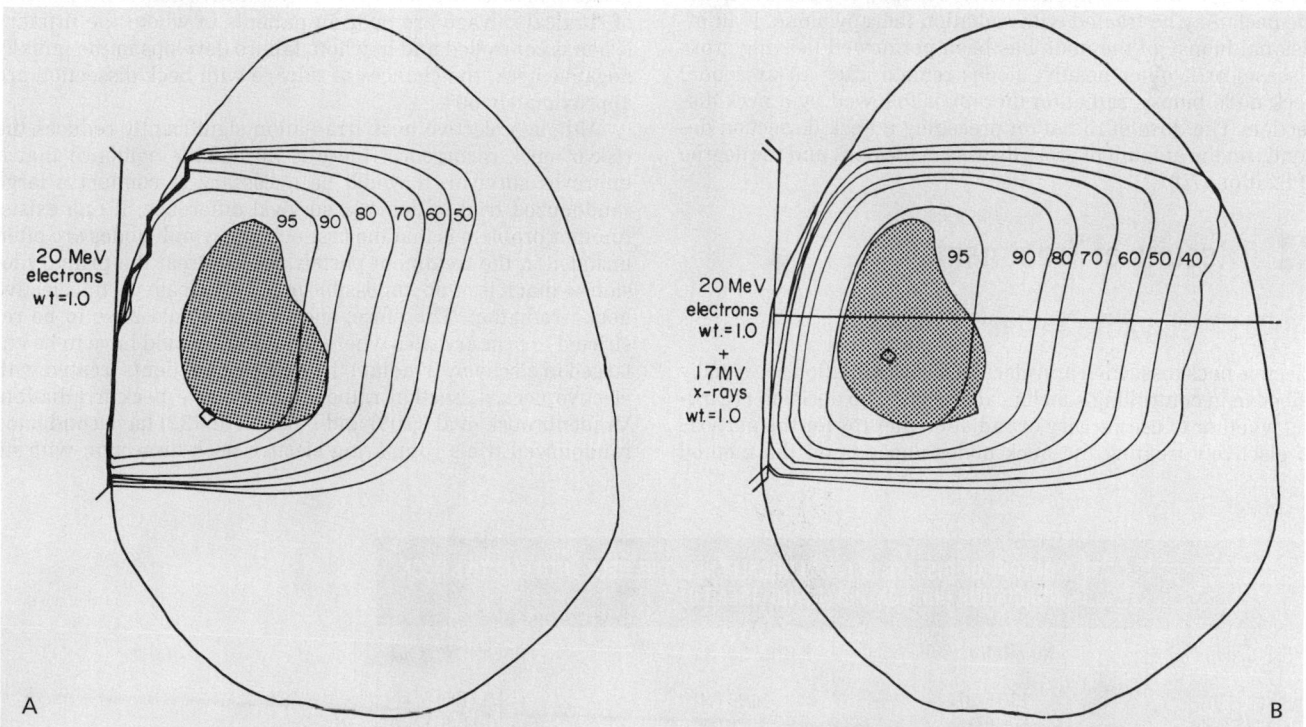

FIGURE 46.11. A: Dose distribution for 20-MeV electrons, field size, 8.5 × 8.5 cm; source-to-skin distance (SSD), 100 cm. **B:** Dose distribution for 20-MeV electrons, field size, 8.5 × 8.5 cm, and 17-MV x-rays, field size, 7 – 7 cm; SSD, 100 cm for both. The given doses are weighted 1 to 1. The addition of the 17-MV x-ray beam reduces the surface dose and gives a dose distribution that is affected less by bone. (From Bova FJ. Treatment planning for irradiation of head and neck cancer. In: Million RR, Cassisi NJ, eds. *Management of head and neck cancer: a multidisciplinary approach*, 2nd ed. Philadelphia: JB Lippincott; 1994: 1145–1146, with permission.)

Table 46.8	COMPLICATIONS AFTER RADIATION THERAPY FOLLOWED BY A BILATERAL NECK DISSECTION (N = 50 PATIENTS)	
Severity	Complication	No. of Patients
Moderate	Wound breakdown	2
	Bleeding	1
	Laryngeal edema	2
	Chyle fistula	1
Severe	Wound breakdown	4
	Fatal cardiac arrest	1
	Fatal acute laryngeal edema	1

From Somerset JD, Mendenhall WM, Amdur RJ, et al. Planned postradiotherapy bilateral neck dissection for head and neck cancer. *Am J Otolaryngol* 2001;22:383–386, with permission.

and McCabe (62) reported that incisional or excisional biopsy of positive neck nodes before definitive surgery increased the risk of neck failure and worsened the prognosis for patients with squamous cell carcinoma of the head and neck. Parsons et al. (92) reported their experience with incisional or excisional biopsy of positive neck nodes followed by radiation therapy as the initial step in the treatment of the patient; these data were updated by Mack et al. (57). After excisional biopsy of a single lymph node, radiation therapy alone to the primary lesion and to the neck resulted in a 95% rate of neck control (57). If residual disease remained in the neck after biopsy, radiation therapy followed by neck dissection was more successful than radiation therapy alone for controlling neck disease.

If the primary lesion is to be treated surgically, the patient's neck is also treated with preoperative radiation therapy to the primary lesion and neck, followed by resection. If the primary lesion is to be treated with radiation therapy, the patient is treated with radiation therapy. If there is no palpable disease remaining in the neck after excisional biopsy of a positive node, the neck may be treated with radiation therapy alone. If an incisional biopsy of the node has been performed (leaving gross disease) or if other positive nodes remain after an excisional neck node biopsy, radiation therapy is followed by a neck dissection. The dose of radiation preceding a neck dissection depends on the amount of gross disease in the neck and the degree of fixation (70).

Results of Treatment

Clinically Negative Nodes

Elective neck dissection and elective neck irradiation are equally effective in controlling subclinical disease. The decision regarding whether to use surgery or radiation therapy for the purpose of electively treating the neck nodes depends on the method used to treat the primary lesion. Patients with a relatively early primary lesion and clinically negative nodes should be treated with one modality. Patients whose primary lesion is treated surgically may undergo an elective neck dissection, and those whose primary lesion is to be treated with radiation therapy should be considered for elective neck irradiation.

The results of elective neck irradiation at the University of Florida for patients with squamous cell carcinoma of the head and neck in whom the primary lesion was controlled are shown in Table 46.9 (67,69). Patients were divided into three risk categories based on the estimated risk of subclinical disease in the neck as follows: group I, low risk (less than 20% likelihood of occult disease); group II, moderate risk (20% to 30% risk of occult disease); and group III, high risk (more than 30% likelihood of occult disease). There were six (21%) neck failures in 28 patients who did not receive elective neck irradiation and eight (5%) neck failures in 162 patients who received elective neck irradiation. Of the eight failures in patients receiving elective neck irradiation, two occurred within the irradiation fields, one at the field margin, and five in out-of-field areas. No correlation was found between the rate of tumor control in the first-echelon lymph nodes and the irradiation dose for doses ranging from 40 to 55 Gy or greater (67). Only one failure occurred in the first-echelon lymph nodes, and this was after 48 Gy in 25 fractions using continuous-course irradiation (67). The low neck, defined as that part of the neck located below the treatment portals used to treat the primary lesion, received either 50 Gy in 25 fractions or 40.5 Gy in 15 fractions, specified at D_{max} (0.5 cm depth). Both dose-fractionation protocols were equally effective in sterilizing subclinical disease in the low neck (75). Elective neck irradiation is equally efficacious for squamous cell carcinoma arising from various head and neck primary sites.

If the primary lesion recurs, there is a renewed risk of lymphatic spread to the neck even after elective neck irradiation has been administered because of the possibility of reseeding the neck lymphatics. In patients in whom primary failure occurs in addition to failure in the clinically negative nodes, the chances of surgical salvage are poor. In patients in whom the primary lesion is controlled and in whom failure develops in the initially negative neck, the chances of salvage with neck dissection are approximately 60%.

Although elective neck irradiation significantly reduces the risk of neck recurrence, there is no definite evidence that it improves survival. It would be necessary to conduct a large randomized trial to detect a survival difference, if one exists. Another problem is that the first-echelon lymph nodes are often included in the treatment portals used to treat the primary lesion so that it is often impossible to avoid at least partial elective neck irradiation. Therefore, such a trial would have to be restricted to primary sites where the portals would have to be enlarged to electively irradiate the neck or to patients treated with elective neck dissection rather than elective neck irradiation. Vandenbrouck et al. (109) and Fakih et al. (32) have conducted randomized trials comparing elective neck dissection with no

Table 46.9	CONTROL OF DISEASE IN THE CLINICALLY NEGATIVE NECK WITH ELECTIVE NECK IRRADIATION (NO. CONTROLLED/NO. TREATED)		
Risk Group (%)	No ENI No. (%)	Partial ENI No. (%)	Total ENI No. (%)
I (<20)	13/15 (87)	16/17 (94)	1/1 (100)
II (20–30)	6/9 (67)	34/38 (89)	10/11 (91)
III (>30)	3/4 (75)	32/33 (97)	61/62 (98)

ENI, elective neck irradiation.
From Mendenhall WM, Million RR. Elective neck irradiation for squamous cell carcinoma of the head and neck: analysis of time-dose factors and causes of failure. *Int J Radiat Oncol Biol Phys* 1986;12:741–746, with permission.

		NO						
Treatment	No Treatment	Partial Treatment	Complete Treatment	N1	N2A	N2B	N3A	N3B
Irradiation	—	15%	2%	15%	27%	27%	38%	34%
Surgery	55% (16/29)	35%	7%	11%	8%	23%	42%	41%
Combined	—	1/5	0/6	0%	0%	0%	23%	25%

Table 46.10   FAILURE OF INITIAL IPSILATERAL NECK TREATMENT: 596 PATIENTS WITH CARCINOMA OF THE TONSILLAR FOSSA, BASE OF TONGUE, SUPRAGLOTTIC LARYNX, OR HYPOPHARYNX[a]

[a]M.D. Anderson Cancer Center data; patients treated 1948–1967.
Modified from Barkley HT Jr, Fletcher GH, Jesse RH, et al. Management of cervical lymph node metastases in squamous cell carcinoma of the tonsillar fossa, base of tongue, supraglottic larynx, and hypopharynx. *Am J Surg* 1972;124:462–467, with permission.

elective neck treatment for patients with oral cavity carcinoma and oral tongue cancer, respectively. No survival advantage was noted for patients undergoing elective neck dissection in either study. However, because of the small number of patients in both trials, it is likely that even if a survival difference existed, it would have been missed.

Dearnaley et al. (24) reported a series of 148 patients treated with an interstitial implant, alone or combined with external-beam irradiation, for cancer of the tongue or floor of mouth. Of 131 patients with negative neck nodes at diagnosis, 59 (45%) received elective neck irradiation to a dose of 40 Gy or greater. A multivariate analysis showed that elective neck irradiation significantly improved survival and reduced the risk of dying of cancer. Piedbois et al. (95) reported a series of 233 patients with T1–2N0 carcinoma of the oral cavity treated with interstitial iridium brachytherapy: 123 patients received no elective neck treatment and 110 patients underwent an elective neck dissection. Patients who received an elective neck dissection tended to have more advanced primary lesions. Although the ultimate rates of neck control were similar, a multivariate analysis showed that elective neck dissection was significantly associated with improved survival.

Clinically Positive Nodes

The incidence of treatment failure in the neck by N stage and treatment category has been reported by the M.D. Anderson Cancer Center (Table 46.10) and the University of Florida (Table 46.11; Fig. 46.12) (9,78). In patients in whom the neck is

treated with combined modalities, radiation therapy precedes surgery when the primary site is to be treated with irradiation or when the node is fixed. Surgery precedes radiation therapy when the primary site is to be treated operatively and the nodes are resectable.

When the initial treatment is surgery, a neck dissection is sufficient treatment for patients with a single positive lymph node <3 cm unless there is extracapsular spread of disease. Radiation therapy may be added for control of subclinical disease in the contralateral side of the neck (Table 46.12) (9). The presence of multiple positive nodes in the surgical specimen is an indication for postoperative radiation therapy of the neck, especially when positive nodes are found at more that one level (2,49,99).

Olsen et al. (89) reported a series of 284 patients who underwent neck dissection at the Mayo Clinic for pathologic stage N1 and N2 squamous cell carcinoma of the head and neck; no patient received adjuvant therapy. Neck recurrence-free survival rates at 5 years were as follows: N1, 76%; N2, 60%; and overall, 69%. A multivariate analysis showed that four or more positive nodes (*p* = .005), invasion of lymphatic and/or vascular spaces (*p* = .003), invasion of soft tissue (*p* = .0008), and a desmoplastic stromal pattern (*p* = .0001) were significantly associated with an increased risk of recurrence in the neck (89).

The postoperative dose prescribed is usually 60 Gy in 30 fractions to 65 Gy in 35 fractions during 6 to 7 weeks for patients with negative margins; higher doses may be prescribed when residual disease is present in the neck (2,59,82). If radiation therapy is to be added after surgery, it is usually initiated within

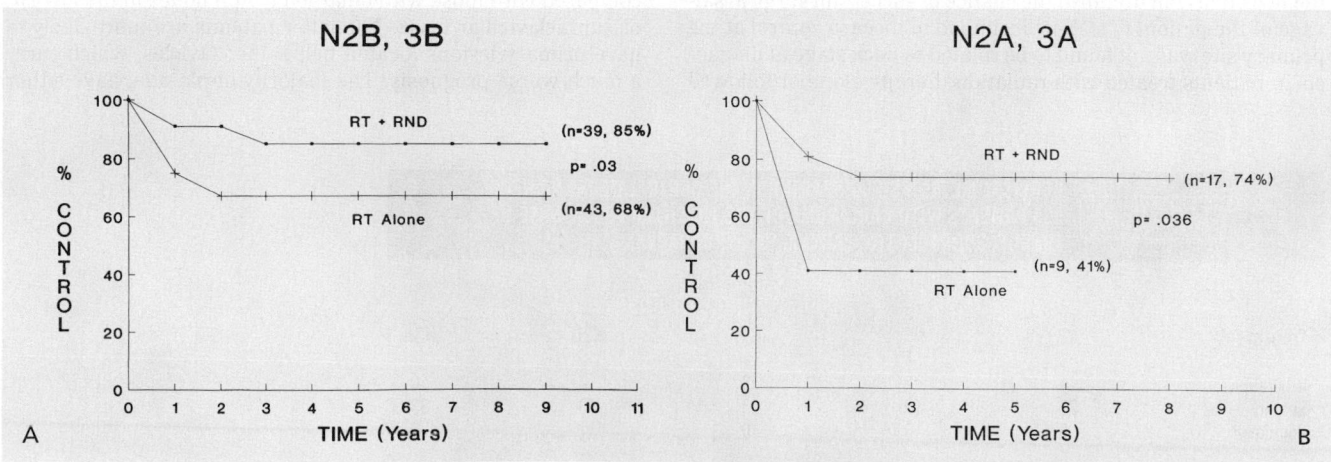

FIGURE 46.12. Rate of neck disease control (life table method [23]) for patients treated with twice-daily irradiation (RT) alone or combined with neck dissection (radiotherapy + RND) for clinically positive neck nodes. **A:** N2B, N3B. **B:** N2A, N3A. (From Parsons JT, Mendenhall WM, Cassisi NJ, et al. Neck dissection after twice-a-day radiotherapy: morbidity and recurrence rates. *Head Neck* 1989;11:400–404, with permission.)

Clinical Radiation Oncology

| Table 46.11 | FIVE-YEAR RATE OF NECK CONTROL BY 1983 AMERICAN JOINT COMMITTEE ON CANCER STAGE AND TREATMENT (459 PATIENTS; 593 HEMINECKS)[a] | | | | |

	Irradiation Alone		Irradiation + Neck Dissection		
Stage	No. Heminecks	Control (%)	No. Heminecks	Control (%)	Significance (p)
N1	215	86	38	93	.28
N2A	29	79	24	68	.60
N2B	138	70	80	91	<.01
N3A	29	33	40	69	<.01

[a]Excludes 67 heminecks on which incisional or excisional biopsy was done before treatment. University of Florida data; patients treated October 1964 to October 1985; analysis, December 1988 by Eric R. Ellis, MD.

4 to 6 weeks after the operation, although it has been reported that a delay to 10 weeks is not associated with an increased risk of neck failure (2).

The rate of control for neck nodes treated with radiation therapy alone as a function of node size, treatment scheme, and dose is shown in Table 46.13 (68). Radiation therapy alone is sufficient for patients with N1 (up to 2 cm) disease as long as the fraction size (2 Gy) and the total dose are sufficient (68). Radiation therapy followed by neck dissection has provided better rates of disease control than radiation therapy alone for patients with more advanced neck disease. The rate of neck disease control for patients treated with twice-daily irradiation, alone or followed by neck dissection, is depicted in Fig. 46.11 and shows a significant improvement in the control rates when neck dissection was added in selected cases (90,91). As shown in a multivariate analysis by Ellis et al. (27), the addition of neck dissection after radiation therapy is independently related to a significantly decreased risk of dying from cancer. At least 50 Gy should be given preoperatively to the lymph nodes, although doses vary according to the size and degree of fixation of the lymph node. For example, large, fixed lymph nodes require 70 to 75 Gy of preoperative irradiation (Table 46.14). The likelihood of disease control in each side of the neck treated with irradiation and neck dissection is decreased when the node is fixed before treatment or when residual tumor is found in the pathologic specimen (Tables 46.15 and 46.16) (70). No difference is seen in the rate of control as a function of the interval between radiation therapy and neck dissection when comparing patients who have surgery within 6 weeks with those who have neck dissection more than 6 weeks after radiation therapy (70). If a local recurrence occurs, prior combined treatment of the neck does not diminish the chance of successful surgical salvage of the patient (71). The likelihood of disease control at the primary site was not found to be related to neck stage at diagnosis in patients treated with radiation therapy alone or followed by neck dissection at the University of Florida (72); this finding is different from what others have reported (110).

Results after Incisional or Excisional Biopsy

Patients who have undergone an incisional or excisional biopsy of a metastatic lymph node before referral do not have an increased risk of neck failure or a decreased cure rate if radiation therapy is the next step in treatment (92). The likelihood of control and the cure rate are probably diminished if an operation without prior radiation therapy follows incisional or excisional biopsy of a metastatic neck node because of the risk that the biopsy procedure disseminated tumor cells into tissues not removed by neck dissection (61).

Ellis et al. (27,28) reported on 508 patients with 660 positive heminecks treated at the University of Florida with radiation therapy alone or followed by a planned neck dissection. Pretreatment node biopsy did not influence outcome when irradiation was the next step in treatment (Table 46.17) (27). The results of the forward stepwise log-rank tests of prognostic factors for predicting time to recurrence are shown in Table 46.18 (27).

Cervical Lymph Node Metastasis with Unknown Primary Tumor

In a small percentage of patients with enlarged cervical lymph nodes, the primary lesion cannot be found, even after extensive evaluation (7,31,64). Patients with enlarged lymph nodes in the upper neck have a good prognosis when treated aggressively, compared with those with enlarged lymph nodes in the low IJC or supraclavicular fossa. The latter patients are more likely to have primary lesions located below the clavicles, which carry a much worse prognosis. The majority of patients have either

| Table 46.12 | CERVICAL METASTASIS APPEARING IN THE CONTRALATERAL N0 NECK: 596 PATIENTS WITH CARCINOMA OF THE TONSILLAR FOSSA, BASE OF TONGUE, SUPRAGLOTTIC LARYNX, OR HYPOPHARYNX[a] | | | | |

	Stage (%)				
Treatment	N0	N1	N2A	N2B	N3A
Irradiation	4	2	9	7	0
Surgery	25	17	23	43	33
Combined	0	0	0	11	0

[a]M.D. Anderson Hospital data; patients treated 1948–1967.
Adapted from Barkley HT Jr, Fletcher GH, Jesse RH, et al. Management of cervical lymph node metastases in squamous cell carcinoma of the tonsillar fossa, base of tongue, supraglottic larynx, and hypopharynx. *Am J Surg* 1972;124:462–467, with permission.

Table 46.13 · LYMPH NODE DISEASE CONTROL BY RADIATION TREATMENT TECHNIQUE (NO. CONTROLLED/NO. TREATED)

Node Size (cm)	Continuous Course No. (%)	Split Course No. (%)	Excluded[a]	Total No. (%)
<1.0	5/5	2/2	1/1	8/8
1.0	29/35 (83)	19/23 (85)	3/4	51/62 (82)
1.5–2.0	43/49 (88)	20/24 (83)	5/9	68/82 (83)
2.5–3.0	14/19 (74)	10/18 (56)	0/3	24/40 (60)
3.5–6.0	14/20 (70)	10/17 (59)	0/1	24/38 (63)
≥7.0	0/2	0/5	0/1	0/8

Less than 50 Gy for nodes = 1.0 cm and <55 Gy for nodes = 1.5 cm.
Modified from Mendenhall WM, Million RR, Bova FJ. Analysis of time-dose factors in clinically positive neck nodes treated with irradiation alone in squamous cell carcinoma of the head and neck. *Int J Radiat Oncol Biol Phys* 1984;10:639–643, with permission.

Table 46.14 · CERVICAL LYMPH NODE DISEASE CONTROL WITH RADIATION THERAPY FOLLOWED BY NECK DISSECTION, WITH PRIMARY LESION TREATED INITIALLY BY RADIATION THERAPY (NO. CONTROLLED/NO. TREATED)[a]

Minimum Node Diameter (cm)	Minimum Node Dose (Gy) <50	50–50.99	60–69.99	≥70
<3	5/5	1/2	5/5	3/3
3–4	6/8	10/14	9/9	5/7
5–6	4/7	5/5	7/8	4/4
7–8	2/3	2/4	4/6	3/4
≥9	No data	1/1	2/4	0/1

[a]University of Florida data; patients treated 1964–1982; analysis 1984 by W. M. Mendenhall, MD. Ninety-one patients were treated with once-a-day fractionation, continuous, or split-course technique (100 heminecks).

Table 46.15 · CONTROL OF DISEASE IN THE NECK AS A FUNCTION OF NODE MOBILITY (109 PATIENTS; 121 HEMINECKS)

Size (cm)	Proportion of Fixed Nodes No. (%)	No. Heminecks Controlled/No. Treated Mobile or Tethered No. (%)	Fixed No. (%)
<3	1/23 (4)	19/22 (86)	1/1
3–4	4/44 (9)	33/40 (83)	2/4 (50)
5–6	9/27 (33)	17/18 (94)	6/9 (67)
7–8	10/21 (48)	8/11 (73)	5/10 (50)
≥9	3/6 (50)	2/3 (67)	1/3 (33)

From Mendenhall WM, Million RR, Cassisi NJ. Squamous cell carcinoma of the head and neck treated with radiation therapy: the role of neck dissection for clinically positive neck nodes. *Int J Radiat Oncol Biol Phys* 1986;12:733–740, with permission.

Table 46.16 · NECK DISEASE CONTROL AS A FUNCTION OF PATHOLOGIC FINDINGS IN THE NECK DISSECTION SPECIMEN (108 PATIENTS; 120 EVALUABLE HEMINECKS[a])

Size (cm)	Proportion with Positive Specimens No. (%)	No. Heminecks Controlled/No. Treated Negative Specimen No. (%)	Positive Specimen No. (%)
<3	10/23 (43)	13/13 (100)	7/10 (70)
3–4	22/43 (51)	20/21 (95)	14/22 (64)
5–6	10/27 (37)	17/17 (100)	6/10 (60)
7–8	12/21 (57)	8/9 (89)	5/12 (42)
≥9	4/6 (67)	2/2 (100)	1/4 (25)

[a]One patient was excluded because data were unavailable.
From Mendenhall WM, Million RR, Cassisi NJ. Squamous cell carcinoma of the head and neck treated with radiation therapy: the role of neck dissection for clinically positive neck nodes. *Int J Radiat Oncol Biol Phys* 1986;12:733–740, with permission.

Table 46.17 | **EFFECT OF NECK NODE BIOPSY ON 5-YEAR RATE OF NECK CONTROL (660 HEMINECKS)**

	No Neck Biopsy		Neck Biopsy		
Hemineck Stage	No. of Heminecks	Probability of Hemineck Control (%)	No. of Heminecks	Probability of Hemineck Control (%)	Significance of Difference Between Curves (p)
N1	253	87 ± 3	12	100	.22
N2A	53	73 ± 8	15	93 ± 6	.18
N2B	218	78 ± 3	23	72 ± 11	.86
N3A	69	54 ± 7	17	81 ± 10	.30

From Ellis ER, Mendenhall WM, Rao PV, et al. Incisional or excisional neck-node biopsy before definitive radiotherapy, alone or followed by neck dissection. *Head Neck* 1991;13:177–183, with permission.

Table 46.18 | **PROGNOSTIC FACTORS, IN ORDER OF THEIR IMPORTANCE, FOR PREDICTING THE TIME TO OCCURRENCE OF VARIOUS EVENTS**

Event	Rank Order	Factor	Level of Significance (p)
Recurrence in neck (n = 660 heminecks)	1	Increasing N stage	.0001
	2	Treatment of neck with RT alone	.0001
	3	Fixed nodes	.0001
	4	T stage[a]	.0350
Death with disease present (n = 508 patients)	1	Recurrence above clavicles	.0001
	2	Increasing N stage	.0003
	3	Fixed nodes	.0053
	4	Treatment of neck with RT alone	.0121
For occurrence of distant metastasis (n = 508 patients)	1	Recurrence above clavicles	.0001
	2	Increasing N stage	.0003
	3	Fixed nodes	.0704
	4	Nodes below thyroid notch	.1023

RT, radiation therapy.
[a]This factor is thought to be correlated with the censoring pattern.
From Ellis ER, Mendenhall WM, Rao PV, et al. Incisional or excisional neck-node biopsy before definitive radiotherapy, alone or followed by neck dissection. *Head Neck* 1991;13:177–183, with permission.

Table 46.19 | **DIAGNOSTIC WORK-UP FOR CERVICAL LYMPH NODE METASTASES: UNKNOWN PRIMARY TUMOR**

General
  History
  Physical examination
  Careful examination of the neck and supraclavicular regions
  Examination of oral cavity, pharynx, and larynx (indirect laryngectomy)
Radiographic studies
  Chest roentgenogram
  Computed tomography or magnetic resonance imaging scans of head and neck (special attention to nasopharynx, pharynx, and larynx)
Laboratory studies
  Complete blood cell count
  Blood chemistry profile
Direct laryngoscopy and directed biopsies
  Nasopharynx, both tonsils, base of tongue, both pyriform sinuses, and any suspicious or abnormal mucosal areas
  Fine-needle aspirate or core needle biopsy of the cervical node
  Tonsillectomy

Table 46.20	BIOPSY-PROVEN PRIMARY SITE VERSUS PHYSICAL AND RADIOGRAPHIC FINDINGS AND NUMBER OF PANENDOSCOPIES				
	No. of Patients with Biopsy-Proven Primary Site/No. of Patients Evaluated[b]				
		No. of Panendoscopies			
Patient Group[a]	1	2	3	Total Patients	
PEØ/RADØ	6/34 (18%)	0/7	1/1	7/42 (17%)	
PEØ/RAD⊕	19/34 (56%)	9/21 (43%)	1/1	29[c]/56 (52%)	
PE⊕/RADØ	4/6	1/3	No data	5/9 (56%)	
PE⊕/RAD⊕	11/16 (69%)	4/7	No data	15[d]/23 (65%)	
Total	40/90 (44%)	14/38 (37%)	2/2	56/130 (43%)	

Significance levels: 7/42 vs. 34/65, $p = .00023$; 7/42 vs. 15/23, $p = .00012$; 34/65 vs. 15/23, $p = .20413$.
[a]One of 29 patients had a positive FDG-SPECT scan and a negative CT of the head and neck; the remaining 28 patients had a positive CT and/or MR scan.
[b]Two of the 15 patients had a positive FDG-SPECT scan and a negative CT of the head and remaining 13 patients had a positive CT scan and/or MR scan.
Key: PE⊘ = no suggestive findings on physical examination; PE⊕ = suggestive of a primary site, but not definitely positive; RAD⊘ = no suggestive findings on radiographic findings; RAD⊕ = radiographic studies suggestive of primary site.
(Mendenhall WM, Mancuso AA, Parsons JT, et al. Diagnostic evaluation of squamous cell carcinoma metastatic to cervical lymph nodes from an unknown head and neck primary site. *Head Neck* 20(8):739–744, 1998).

squamous cell or poorly differentiated carcinoma. Those with adenocarcinoma almost always have a primary lesion below the clavicles, although if the nodes are located in the upper neck, one must exclude a salivary gland, thyroid, or parathyroid primary tumor. This section deals with patients presenting with squamous cell or poorly differentiated carcinoma in the upper or middle neck.

Patients should be evaluated with a thorough physical examination, including careful evaluation of the head and neck. A needle biopsy of the lymph node should be performed. After chest roentgenography, a CT or MRI of the head and neck is obtained to detect an unknown primary lesion arising from the mucosa of the head and neck. It is unclear whether FDG PET scans may identify primary lesions that would not otherwise be identifiable (87). The available data suggest that some patients will benefit from these studies. Direct laryngoscopy and examination under anesthesia are performed with directed biopsies of the nasopharynx, tonsils, base of the tongue, and pyriform sinuses, and of any abnormalities noted on CT or MRI or suspicious mucosal lesions noted at laryngoscopy. Patients with adequate lymphoid tissue in their tonsillar fossae should un-

dergo an ipsilateral tonsillectomy. The diagnostic evaluation for the patient with cervical metastasis from an unknown head and neck primary lesion is summarized in Table 46.19. The results of a diagnostic evaluation for an unknown primary site in 130 patients at the University of Florida are depicted in Table 46.20 (66). The primary site was discovered in more than 40% of patients and was most often located in the tonsillar fossa or base of tongue (Table 46.21).

Some patients may be cured with treatment directed only to the involved area of the neck (22); however, we usually irradiate the nasopharynx and oropharynx as well as both sides of the neck. The hypopharynx and larynx were irradiated as well until 1997 when we decided to eliminate them because they are rarely the site of the primary cancer and because irradiation of these sites significantly increases the morbidity of treatment. It is not necessary to irradiate the oral cavity unless the patient has submandibular adenopathy, in which case we either perform a neck dissection and observe the patient, or irradiate the oral cavity and oropharynx and not the nasopharynx. Patients are treated with parallel-opposed fields at 1.8 Gy per fraction to a midline dose of 64.8 Gy with reduction off the spinal cord at 45 Gy tumor dose (Fig. 46.13). An alternative is to use IMRT to spare the contralateral parotid gland in patients with ipsilateral neck nodes. The lower neck is treated through a separate *en face* anterior field.

Erkal et al. (31) reported on 126 patients treated with curative intent at the University of Florida between 1964 and 1997 with follow-up for at least 2 years. Radiation therapy was delivered to head and neck mucosal sites and both sides of the neck in 119 patients and to the neck alone in 7 patients. Twelve patients (10%) developed squamous cell carcinoma in a head and neck mucosal site at 0.5 to 10.9 years (median, 1.8 years) after treatment. The 5-year results were as follows: head and neck mucosal failure, 13%; neck node control, 78%; distant metastases, 14%; absolute survival, 47%; and cause-specific survival, 67%. Barker et al. (7) subsequently reported on 17 patients treated with the larynx-sparing technique previously described between 1997 and 2002 at our institution; none of these patients developed a head and neck mucosal squamous cell carcinoma after receiving radiation therapy.

Colletier et al. (21) reported on 136 patients treated with neck dissection followed by radiotherapy to head and neck mucosal sites and bilateral lymph nodes. Six percent of patients

Table 46.21	RESULTS OF DIAGNOSTIC EVALUATION OF 130 PATIENTS WITH SQUAMOUS CELL CARCINOMA FOR AN UNKNOWN HEAD AND NECK PRIMARY SITE—LOCATION OF THE PRIMARY LESION (58 LESIONS IN 56 PATIENTS)

Primary Site	No. of Patients (%)
Tonsillar fossa	25 (43)
Base of tongue	23 (39)
Pyriform sinus	5 (9)
Posterior pharyngeal wall	2 (3)
Lateral pharyngeal wall	1 (2)
Vallecula	1 (2)
Suprahyoid epiglottis	1 (2)

From Mendenhall WM, Mancuso AA, Parsons JT, et al. Diagnostic evaluation of squamous cell carcinoma metastatic to cervical lymph nodes from an unknown head and neck primary site. *Head Neck* 1998;20:739–744, with permission.

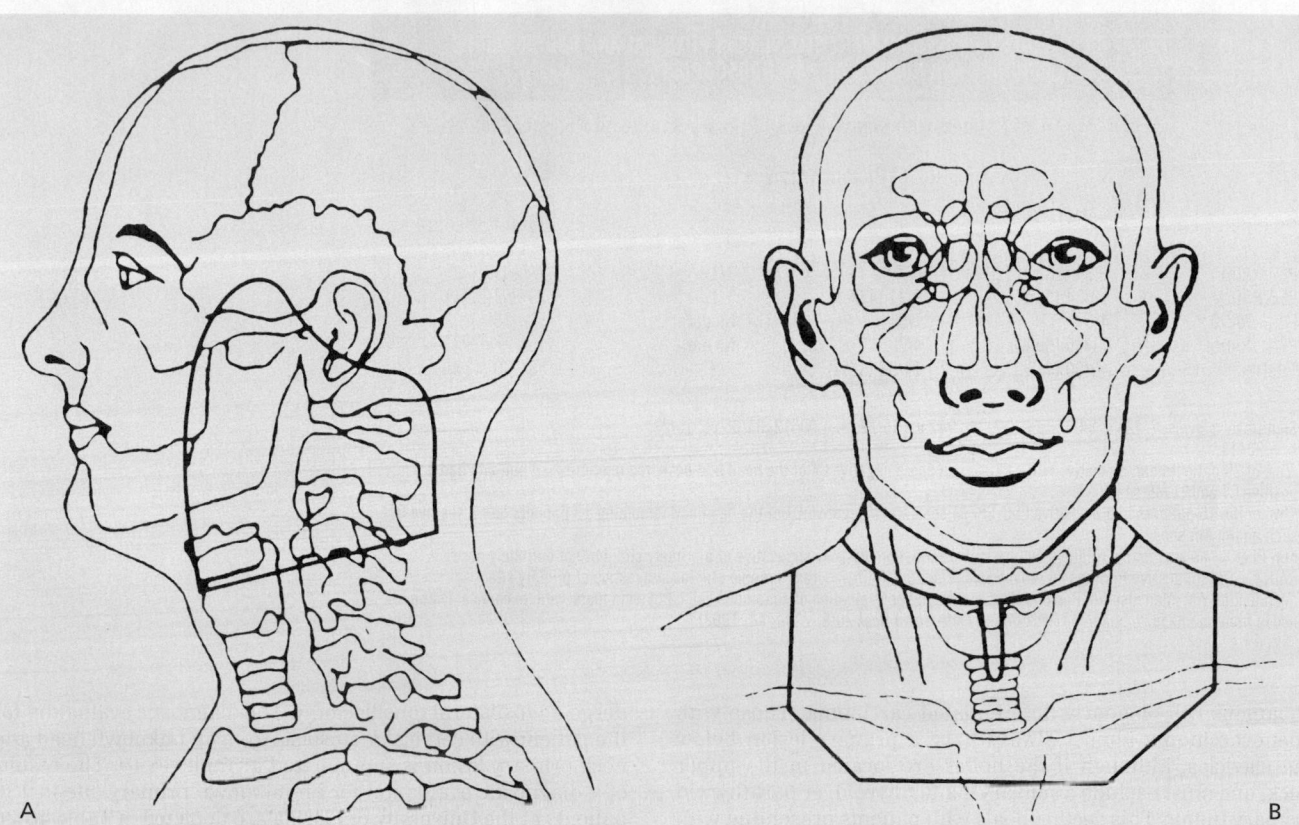

FIGURE 46.13. Radiation therapy portals used from 1997 to treat head and neck mucosal sites and upper cervical lymph nodes (**A**) and lower cervical and supraclavicular lymph nodes (**B**). The inferior border for lateral portals is placed at the superior anterior border of the thyroid cartilage, shielding the hypopharynx and larynx. (From Erkal HS, Mendenhall WM, Amdur RJ, et al. Squamous cell carcinomas metastatic to cervical lymph nodes from an unknown head-and-neck mucosal site treated with radiation therapy alone or in combination with neck dissection. *Int J Radiat Oncol Biol Phys* 2001;50:55–63, with permission.)

developed carcinomas in head and neck mucosal sites within radiotherapy portals, and 4% of patients developed carcinomas in head and neck mucosal sites outside radiotherapy portals. The absolute survival rate at 5 years was 60%. The authors recommended radiotherapy to head and neck mucosal sites.

Reddy and Marks (98) reported on 16 patients with radiotherapy to ipsilateral lymph nodes and 36 patients with radiotherapy to head and neck mucosal sites and bilateral lymph nodes. The authors concluded that radiotherapy reduced the rate of developing carcinomas in head and neck mucosal sites. For

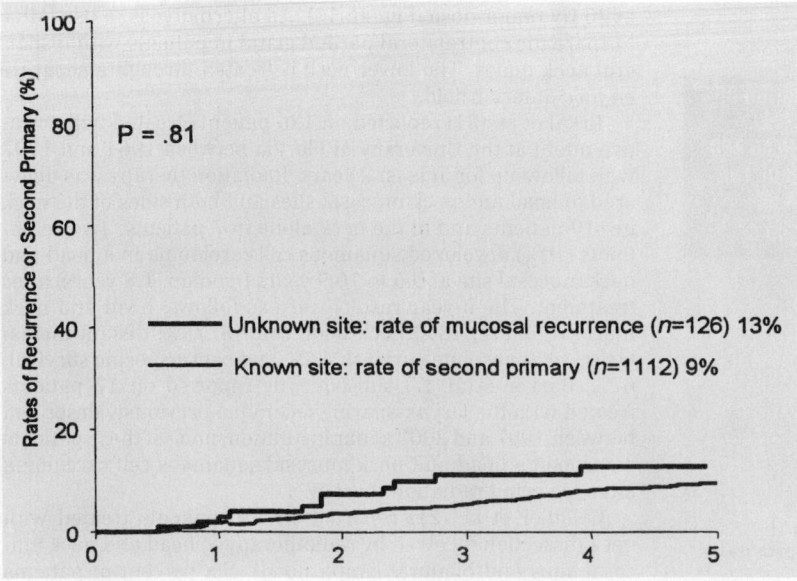

FIGURE 46.14. The rate of developing carcinomas in head and neck mucosal sites for patients treated for carcinomas with an unknown head and neck mucosal site compared with the rate of developing metachronous carcinomas in head and neck mucosal sites for patients treated for carcinomas with a known head and neck mucosal site. (From Erkal HS, Mendenhall WM, Amdur RJ, et al. Squamous cell carcinomas metastatic to cervical lymph nodes from an unknown head-and-neck mucosal site treated with radiation therapy alone or in combination with neck dissection. *Int J Radiat Oncol Biol Phys* 2001;50:55–63, with permission.)

patients with no radiotherapy to head and neck mucosal sites, the rate of developing carcinomas in head and neck mucosal sites was 46% and the absolute survival rate at 5 years was 47%. For patients treated with radiotherapy to head and neck mucosal sites, the rates were 8% and 53%, respectively. Grau et al. (40) reported on 273 patients treated with curative intent at five cancer centers in Denmark between 1975 and 1995 with surgery alone (23 patients), radiotherapy to the ipsilateral neck alone or combined with surgery (26 patients), and radiotherapy to the neck and head and neck mucosa alone or combined with surgery (224 patients). The ipsilateral oropharynx unintentionally received some irradiation in patients treated to the ipsilateral neck alone, depending on the treatment technique. The 5-year rates of freedom from failure in the head and neck mucosa were as follows: surgery alone, 45%; radiotherapy with or without surgery to the ipsilateral neck, 77%; and radiotherapy to the head and neck mucosa with or without surgery, 87%. The oropharynx, particularly the base of tongue, was the most common location of mucosal site failure.

The incidence of subsequent mucosal primary lesions was compared by Erkal et al. (31) for 1,112 patients with a known primary site (oropharynx, hypopharynx, and supraglottis) and a series of 126 patients treated for an unknown primary site at the University of Florida. The incidence of a subsequent mucosal head and neck cancer was similar for both groups, suggesting either that mucosal irradiation significantly reduced the risk of primary site failure or that patients with unknown primary sites have a much lower risk of a second primary head and neck cancer developing subsequently (Fig. 46.14) (31).

A subset of patients presenting with squamous cell carcinoma metastatic to the neck nodes from an unknown head and neck primary site are treated with palliative intent because of poor medical condition, extensive nodal involvement, and/or distant metastases at presentation. Treatment of the neck depends on the extent and location of the adenopathy. Forty of 166 patients (24%) were treated palliatively at the University of Florida between 1964 and 1997 (30). Treatment was delivered to the neck alone to a dose of 30 Gy in 10 fractions during 2 weeks or 20 Gy in two fractions with a 1-week interfraction interval. The nodal response rate was 65% and the symptomatic response rate was 57% at 1 year. The 1-year absolute and cause-specific survival rates were 25%.

The main complication of radiation therapy for patients treated for an unknown head and neck primary tumor is xerostomia. The complications of treatment of the neck, which have been discussed previously, depend on whether a neck dissection is added.

Acknowledgment

We thank the research support staff of the Department of Radiation Oncology, University of Florida, Gainesville, for their help with statistics, editing, and manuscript preparation.

References

1. Amdur RJ, Li JG, Liu C, et al. Unnecessary laryngeal irradiation in the IMRT era. *Head Neck* 2004;26:257–264.
2. Amdur RJ, Parsons JT, Mendenhall WM, et al. Postoperative irradiation for squamous cell carcinoma of the head and neck. an analysis of treatment results and complications. *Int J Radiat Oncol Biol Phys* 1989;16:25–36.
3. American Joint Committee on Cancer. *Manual for Staging of Cancer*, 2nd ed. Philadelphia: JB Lippincott;1983:27–39.
4. American Joint Committee on Cancer. *Manual for Staging of Cancer*, 2nd ed. Philadelphia: JB Lippincott;1983:37–42.
5. American Joint Committee on Cancer. Lip and oral cavity. In: Greene FL, Page DL, Fleming ID, et al, eds. *AJCC Cancer Staging Manual*, 6th ed. New York: Springer; 2002:23–32.
6. Ash CL. Oral cancer: a twenty-five year study. *Am J Roentgenol Radium Ther Nucl Med* 1962;87:417–430.
7. Barker CA, Morris CG, Mendenhall WM. Larynx-sparing radiotherapy for squamous cell carcinoma from an unknown head and neck primary site. *Am J Clin Oncol* 2005;28:445–448.
8. Barker JL, Fletcher GH. Time, dose and tumor volume relationships in megavoltage irradiation of squamous cell carcinomas of the retromolar trigone and anterior tonsillar pillar. *Int J Radiat Oncol Biol Phys* 1977;2:407–414.
9. Barkley HT Jr, Fletcher GH, Jesse RH, et al. Management of cervical lymph node metastases in squamous cell carcinoma of the tonsillar fossa, base of tongue, supraglottic larynx, and hypopharynx. *Am J Surg* 1972;124:462–467.
10. Bartelink H. Prognostic value of the regression rate of neck node metastases during radiotherapy. *Int J Radiat Oncol Biol Phys* 1983;9:993–996.
11. Bartelink H, Breur K, Hart G. Radiotherapy of lymph node metastases in patients with squamous cell carcinoma of the head and neck region. *Int J Radiat Oncol Biol Phys* 1982;8:983–989.
12. Bataini JP, Bernier J, Jaulerry C, et al. Impact of neck node radioresponsiveness of the regional control probability in patients with oropharynx and pharyngolarynx cancers managed by definitive radiotherapy. *Int J Radiat Oncol Biol Phys* 1987;13:817–824.
13. Beahrs OH, Devine KD, Henson SW Jr. Treatment of carcinoma of the tongue: end-results in 168 cases. *AMA Arch Surg* 1959;79:399–403.
14. Berger DS, Fletcher GH, Lindberg RD, et al. Elective irradiation of the neck lymphatics for squamous cell carcinomas of the nasopharynx and oropharynx. *Am J Roentgenol Radium Ther Nucl Med* 1971;111:66–72.
15. Bernier J, Bataini JP. Regional outcome in oropharyngeal and pharyngolaryngeal cancer treated with high dose per fraction radiotherapy. Analysis of neck disease response in 1646 cases. *Radiother Oncol* 1986;6:87–103.
16. Bova FJ. Treatment planning for irradiation of head and neck cancer. In: Million RR, Cassisi NJ, eds. *Management of head and neck cancer: a multidisciplinary approach*, 1st ed. Philadelphia: JB Lippincott;1984:209–230.
17. Bova FJ. Treatment planning for irradiation of head and neck cancer. In: Million RR, Cassisi NJ, eds. *Management of head and neck cancer: a multidisciplinary approach*, 2nd ed. Philadelphia: JB Lippincott;1994:291–309.
18. Cady B, Catlin D. Epidermoid carcinoma of the gum. A 20-year survey. *Cancer* 1969;23:551–569.
19. Chen KY, Fletcher GH. Malignant tumors of the nasopharynx. *Radiology* 1971;99:165–171.
20. Chung CK, Rahman SM, Lim ML, et al. Squamous cell carcinoma of the hard palate. *Int J Radiat Oncol Biol Phys* 1979;5:191–196.
21. Colletier PJ, Garden AS, Morrison WH, et al. Postoperative radiation for squamous cell carcinoma metastatic to cervical lymph nodes from an unknown primary site: outcomes and patterns of failure. *Head Neck* 1998;20:674–681.
22. Coster JR, Foote RL, Olsen KD, et al. Cervical nodal metastasis of squamous cell carcinoma of unknown origin: Indications for withholding radiation therapy. *Int J Radiat Oncol Biol Phys* 1992;23:743–749.
23. Cutler SJ, Ederer F. Maximum utilization of the life table method in analyzing survival. *J Chronic Dis* 1958;8:699–712.
24. Dearnaley DP, Dardoufas C, A'Hearn RP, et al. Interstitial irradiation for carcinoma of the tongue and floor of mouth: Royal Marsden Hospital experience 1970–1986. *Radiother Oncol* 1991;21:183–192.
25. Del Regato JA, Spjut HJ. *Ackerman and del Regato's cancer: diagnosis, treatment, and prognosis*, 5th ed. St. Louis, MO: CV Mosby; 1977:264–281, 341–345.
26. Dubray BM, Bataini JP, Bernier J, et al. Is reseeding from the primary a plausible cause of nodal failure? *Int J Radiat Oncol Biol Phys* 1993;25:9–15.
27. Ellis ER, Mendenhall WM, Rao PV, et al. Incision or excisional neck-node biopsy before definitive radiotherapy, alone or followed by neck dissection. *Head Neck* 1991;13:177–183.
28. Ellis ER, Mendenhall WM, Rao PV, et al. Does node location affect the incidence of distant metastases in head and neck squamous cell carcinoma? *Int J Radiat Oncol Biol Phys* 1989;17:293–297.
29. Eneroth CM, Hjertman L, Moberger G. Squamous cell carcinomas of the palate. *Acta Otolaryngol (Stockh)* 1972;73:418–427.
30. Erkal HS, Mendenhall WM, Amdur RJ, et al. Squamous cell carcinoma metastatic to cervical lymph nodes from an unknown head and neck mucosal site treated with radiation therapy with palliative intent. *Radiother Oncol* 2001;59:319–321.
31. Erkal HS, Mendenhall WM, Amdur RJ, et al. Squamous cell carcinomas metastatic to cervical lymph nodes from an unknown head-and-neck mucosal site treated with radiation therapy alone or in combination with neck dissection. *Int J Radiat Oncol Biol Phys* 2001;50:55–63.
32. Fakih AR, Rao RS, Borges AM, et al. Elective versus therapeutic neck dissection in early carcinoma of the oral tongue. *Am J Surg* 1989;158:309–313.
33. Fisch U. Lymphographische untersuchungen über das zervikale lymphsystem. *Fortschritte der Hals-Nasen-Ohren Heilkunde* 1966;14:53–162.
34. Fletcher GH. Elective irradiation of subclinical disease in cancers of the head and neck. *Cancer* 1972;29:1450–1454.
35. Fletcher GH, Jesse RH, Healey JE Jr, et al. Oropharynx. In: MacComb WS, Fletcher GH, eds. *Cancer of the head and neck*. Baltimore: Williams & Wilkins; 1967:179–212.
36. Fletcher GH, Jesse RH, Lindberg RD, et al. The place of radiotherapy in the management of the squamous cell carcinoma of the supraglottic larynx. *Am J Roentgenol Radium Ther Nucl Med* 1970;108:19–26.
37. Fletcher GH, MacComb WS, Braun EJ. Analysis of sites and causes of treatment failures in squamous cell carcinomas of the oral cavity. *Am J Roentgenol Radium Ther Nucl Med* 1960;83:405–411.
38. Frazell EL, Lucas JC Jr. Cancer of the tongue. Report of the management of 1554 patients. *Cancer* 1962;15:1085–1099.
39. Goffinet DR, Gilbert EH, Weiler SA, et al. Irradiation of clinically uninvolved cervical lymph nodes. *Can J Otolaryngol* 1975;4:927–933.
40. Grau C, Johansen LV, Jakobsen J, et al. Cervical lymph node metastases from unknown primary tumours: results from a national survey by the Danish Society for Head and Neck Oncology. *Radiother Oncol* 2000;55:121–129.
41. Hardingham M, Dalley VM, Shaw HJ. Cancer of the floor of the mouth: clinical features and results of treatment. *Clin Oncol* 1977;3:227–246.
42. Ho JH. An epidemiologic and clinical study of nasopharyngeal carcinoma. *Int J Radiat Oncol Biol Phys* 1978;4:183–198.
43. Horiuchi J, Adachi T. Some considerations on radiation therapy of tongue cancer. *Cancer* 1971;28:335–339.

44. Jesse RH, Barkley HT Jr, Lindberg RD, et al. Cancer of the oral cavity. Is elective neck dissection beneficial? *Am J Surg* 1970;120:505–508.

45. Jesse RH, Fletcher GH. Metastases in cervical lymph nodes from oropharyngeal carcinoma: treatment and results. *Am J Roentgenol Radium Ther Nucl Med* 1963;90:990–996.

46. Johnson CR, Silverman LN, Clay LB, et al. Radiotherapeutic management of bulky cervical lymphadenopathy in squamous cell carcinoma of the head and neck: is postradiotherapy neck dissection necessary? *Radiat Oncol Investig* 1998;6:52–57.

47. Kaplan R, Million RR, Cassisi NJ. Carcinoma of the tonsil: results of radical irradiation with surgery reserved for radiation failure. *Laryngoscope* 1977;87:600–607.

48. Kremen AJ. Results of surgical treatment of cancer of the tongue. *Surgery* 1956;39:49–53.

49. Lefebvre JL, Castelain B, De La Torre JC, et al. Lymph node invasion in hypopharynx and lateral epilarynx carcinoma: A prognostic factor. *Head Neck Surg* 1987;10:14–18.

50. Liauw SL, Mancuso AA, Amdur RJ. Postradiotherapy neck dissection for lymph node-positive head and neck cancer: the use of computed tomography to manage the neck. *J Clin Oncol* 2006;24:1421–1427.

51. Lindberg RD. Distribution of cervical lymph node metastases from squamous cell carcinoma of the upper respiratory and digestive tracts. *Cancer* 1972;29:1446–1449.

52. Lindberg RD, Barkley HT Jr, Jesse RH, et al. Evolution of the clinically negative neck in patients with squamous cell carcinoma of the faucial arch. *Am J Roentgenol Radium Ther Nucl Med* 1971;111:60–65.

53. Lindberg RD, Jesse RH. Treatment of cervical lymph node metastasis from primary lesions of the oropharynx, supraglottic larynx and hypopharynx. *Am J Roentgenol Radium Ther Nucl Med* 1968;102:132–137.

54. Mabanta SR, Mendenhall WM, Stringer SP, et al. Salvage treatment for neck recurrence after irradiation alone for head and neck squamous cell carcinoma with clinically positive neck nodes. *Head Neck* 1999;21:591–594.

55. MacComb WS, Healey JE Jr, McGraw JP, et al. Hypopharynx and cervical esophagus. In: MacComb WS, Fletcher GH, eds. *Cancer of the head and neck*. Baltimore: Williams & Wilkins Company; 1967:213–240.

56. Maciejewski B. Regression rate of metastatic neck lymph nodes after radiation treatment as a prognostic factor for local control. *Radiother Oncol* 1987;8:301–308.

57. Mack Y, Parsons JT, Mendenhall WM, et al. Squamous cell carcinoma of the head and neck: management after excisional biopsy of a solitary metastatic neck node. *Int J Radiat Oncol Biol Phys* 1993;25:619–622.

58. Mancuso AA, Hanafee WN. *Computed tomography and magnetic resonance imaging of the head and neck*, 2nd ed. Baltimore, MD: Williams & Wilkins; 1985.

59. Marcus RB Jr, Million RR, Cassisi NJ. Postoperative irradiation for squamous cell carcinomas of the head and neck: analysis of time-dose factors related to control above the clavicles. *Int J Radiat Oncol Biol Phys* 1979;5:1943–1949.

60. Martin CL, Craffey EJ. Cancer of the gums. *Am J Roentgenol Radium Ther Nucl Med* 1952;67:420–427.

61. McGuirt WF, McCabe BF. Significance of node biopsy before definitive treatment of cervical metastatic carcinoma. *Laryngoscope* 1978;88:594–597.

62. McGuirt WF, McCabe BF. Bilateral radical neck dissections. *Arch Otolaryngol* 1980;106:427–429.

63. McLaughlin MP, Mendenhall WM, Mancuso AA, et al. Retropharyngeal adenopathy as a predictor of outcome in squamous cell carcinoma of the head and neck. *Head Neck* 1995;17:190–198.

64. Mendenhall WM. Unknown primary squamous cell carcinoma of the head and neck. *Curr Cancer Ther Rev* 2005;1:167–174.

65. Mendenhall WM, Amdur RJ, Hinerman RW, et al. Head and Neck: management of the neck. In: Perez CA, Brady LW, Halperin EC, Schmidt-Ullrich RK, eds. *Principles and practice of radiation oncology*, 4th ed. Philadelphia: Lippincott Williams & Wilkins; 2004:1158–1178.

66. Mendenhall WM, Mancuso AA, Parsons JT, et al. Diagnostic evaluation of squamous cell carcinoma metastatic to cervical lymph nodes from an unknown head and neck primary site. *Head Neck* 1998;20:739–744.

67. Mendenhall WM, Million RR. Elective neck irradiation for squamous cell carcinoma of the head and neck: analysis of time-dose factors and causes of failure. *Int J Radiat Oncol Biol Phys* 1986;12:741–746.

68. Mendenhall WM, Million RR, Bova FJ. Analysis of time-dose factors in clinically positive neck nodes treated with irradiation alone in squamous cell carcinoma of the head and neck. *Int J Radiat Oncol Biol Phys* 1984;10:639–643.

69. Mendenhall WM, Million RR, Cassisi NJ. Elective neck irradiation in squamous-cell carcinoma of the head and neck. *Head Neck Surg* 1980;3:15–20.

70. Mendenhall WM, Million RR, Cassisi NJ. Squamous cell carcinoma of the head and neck treated with radiation therapy: the role of neck dissection for clinically positive neck nodes. *Int J Radiat Oncol Biol Phys* 1986;12:733–740.

71. Mendenhall WM, Parsons JT, Amdur RJ, et al. Squamous cell carcinoma of the head and neck treated with radiotherapy: does planned neck dissection reduce the change for successful surgical management of subsequent local recurrence? *Head Neck Surg* 1988;10:302–304.

72. Mendenhall WM, Parsons JT, Amdur RJ, et al. Squamous cell carcinoma of the head and neck treated with radiation therapy: the impact of neck stage on local control. *Int J Radiat Oncol Biol Phys* 1988;14:249–252.

73. Mendenhall WM, Parsons JT, Brant TA, et al. Is elective neck treatment indicated for T2N0 squamous cell carcinoma of the glottic larynx? *Radiother Oncol* 1989;14:199–202.

74. Mendenhall WM, Parsons JT, Mancuso AA, et al. Radiotherapy for squamous cell carcinoma of the supraglottic larynx: an alternative to surgery. *Head Neck* 1996;18:24–35.

75. Mendenhall WM, Parsons JT, Million RR. Elective lower neck irradiation: 5000 cGy/25 fractions versus 4050 cGy/15 fractions. *Int J Radiat Oncol Biol Phys* 1988;15:439–440.

76. Mendenhall WM, Parsons JT, Million RR. Unnecessary irradiation of the normal larynx [editorial]. *Int J Radiat Oncol Biol Phys* 1990;18:1531–1533.

77. Mendenhall WM, Parsons JT, Stringer SP, et al. T1-T2 vocal cord carcinoma: a basis for comparing the results of radiotherapy and surgery. *Head Neck Surg* 1988;10:373–377.

78. Mendenhall WM, Parsons JT, Stringer SP, et al. Squamous cell carcinoma of the head and neck treated with irradiation: management of the neck. *Semin Radiat Oncol* 1992;2:163–170.

79. Mendenhall WM, Riggs CE, Amdur RJ, et al. Altered fractionation and/or adjuvant chemotherapy in definitive irradiation of squamous cell carcinoma of the head and neck. *Laryngoscope* 2003;113:546–551.

80. Mendenhall WM, Villaret DB, Amdur RJ, et al. Planned neck dissection after definitive radiotherapy for squamous cell carcinoma of the head and neck. *Head Neck* 2002;24:1012–1018.

81. Million RR. Elective neck irradiation for TXN0 squamous carcinoma of the oral tongue and floor of mouth. *Cancer* 1974;34:149–155.

82. Million RR. Squamous cell carcinoma of the head and neck: combined therapy: surgery and postoperative irradiation [editorial]. *Int J Radiat Oncol Biol Phys* 1979;5:2161–2162.

83. Million RR, Cassisi NJ. Radical irradiation for carcinoma of the pyriform sinus. *Laryngoscope* 1981;91:439–450.

84. Million RR, Cassisi NJ, Mancuso AA, et al. Management of the neck for squamous cell carcinoma. In: Million RR, Cassisi NJ, eds. *Management of head and neck cancer: a multidisciplinary approach*, 2nd ed. Philadelphia: JB Lippincott;1994:75–142.

85. Million RR, Fletcher GH, Jesse RH. Evaluation of elective irradiation of the neck for squamous-cell carcinoma of the nasopharynx, tonsillar fossa, and base of tongue. *Radiology* 1963;80:975–988.

86. Moench HC, Phillips TL. Carcinoma of the nasopharynx. Review of 146 patients with emphasis on radiation dose and time factors. *Am J Surg* 1972;124:515–518.

87. Mukherji SK, Drane WE, Mancuso AA, et al. Occult primary tumors of the head and neck: detection with 2-[F-18] fluoro-2-deoxy-D-glucose SPECT. *Radiology* 1996;199:761–766.

88. Ogura JH, Biller HF, Wette R. Elective neck dissection for pharyngeal and laryngeal cancers: an evaluation. *Ann Otol Rhinol Laryngol* 1971;80:646–651.

89. Olsen KD, Caruso M, Foote RL, et al. Primary head and neck cancer. Histopathologic predictors of recurrence after neck dissection in patients with lymph node involvement. *Arch Otolaryngol Head Neck Surg* 1994;120:1370–1374.

90. Parsons JT, Mendenhall WM, Cassisi NJ, et al. Hyperfractionation for head and neck cancer. *Int J Radiat Oncol Biol Phys* 1988;14:649–658.

91. Parsons JT, Mendenhall WM, Cassisi NJ, et al. Neck dissection after twice-a-day radiotherapy: morbidity and recurrence rates. *Head Neck* 1989;11:400–404.

92. Parsons JT, Million RR, Cassisi NJ. The influence of excisional or incisional biopsy of metastatic neck nodes on the management of head and neck cancer. *Int J Radiat Oncol Biol Phys* 1985;11:1447–1454.

93. Parsons JT, Million RR, Cassisi NJ. Carcinoma of the base of the tongue: results of radical irradiation with surgery reserved for irradiation failure. *Laryngoscope* 1982;92:689–696.

94. Peters LJ, Weber RS, Morrison WH, et al. Neck surgery in patients with primary oropharyngeal cancer treated by radiotherapy. *Head Neck* 1996;18:552–559.

95. Piedbois P, Mazeron JJ, Haddad E, et al. Stage I-II squamous cell carcinoma of the oral cavity treated by iridium-192: is elective neck dissection indicated? *Radiother Oncol* 1991;21:100–106.

96. Putney FJ. Elective versus delayed neck dissection in cancer of the larynx. *Surg Gynecol Obstet* 1961;112:736–742.

97. Razack MS, Baffi R, Sako K. Bilateral radical neck dissection. *Cancer* 1981;47:197–199.

98. Reddy SP, Marks JE. Metastatic carcinoma in the cervical lymph nodes from an unknown primary site: results of bilateral neck plus mucosal irradiation vs. ipsilateral neck irradiation. *Int J Radiat Oncol Biol Phys* 1997;37:797–802.

99. Richard JM, Sancho-Garnier H, Micheau C, et al. Prognostic factors in cervical lymph node metastasis in upper respiratory and digestive tract carcinomas: study of 1,713 cases during a 15-year period. *Laryngoscope* 1987;97:97–101.

100. Rolander TL, Everts EC, Shumrick DA. Carcinoma of the tonsil: a planned combined therapy approach. *Laryngoscope* 1971;81:1199–1207.

101. Rouviére H. *Anatomy of the human lymphatic system*. Tobias MJ, trans. Ann Arbor, MI: Edwards Brothers; 1938:1–28, 77–78.

102. Somerset JD, Mendenhall WM, Amdur RJ, et al. Planned postradiotherapy bilateral neck dissection for head and neck cancer. *Am J Otolaryngol* 2001;22:383–386.

103. Southwick HW. Elective neck dissection for intraoral cancer. *JAMA* 1971;217:454–455.

104. Southwick HW, Slaughter DP, Trevino ET. Elective neck dissection for intraoral cancer. *AMA Arch Surg* 1960;80:905–909.

105. Spiro RH, Strong EW. Discontinuous partial glossectomy and radical neck dissection in selected patients with epidermoid carcinoma of the mobile tongue. *Am J Surg* 1973;126:544–546.

106. Stringer SP. Current concepts in surgical management of neck metastases from head and neck cancer. *Oncology* 1995;9:547–554.

107. Taylor JMG, Mendenhall WM, Lavey RS. Time-dose factors in positive neck nodes treated with irradiation only. *Radiother Oncol* 1991;22:167–173.

108. Taylor JMG, Mendenhall WM, Parsons JT. The influence of dose and time on wound complications following post-radiation neck dissection. *Int J Radiat Oncol Biol Phys* 1992;23:41–46.

109. Vandenbrouck C, Sancho-Garnier H, Chassagne D, et al. Elective versus therapeutic radical neck dissection in epidermoid carcinoma of the oral cavity. Results of a randomized clinical trial. *Cancer* 1980;46:386–390.

110. Wall TJ, Peters LJ, Brown BW, et al. Relationship between lymph nodal status and primary tumor control probability in tumors of the supraglottic larynx. *Int J Radiat Oncol Biol Phys* 1985;11:1895–1902.

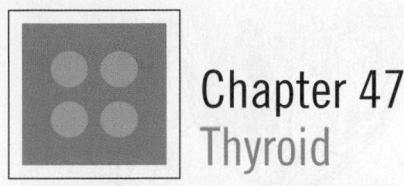

Chapter 47
Thyroid

Tamara E. Weiss, Perry W. Grigsby

Anatomy

The thyroid gland consists of right and left lobes, joined by an isthmus, which crosses the trachea at the second or third cartilaginous ring. A pyramidal lobe may extend superiorly from the isthmus or from one of the thyroid lobes (Fig. 47.1A). The thyroid gland has an average weight of 20 g. The parathyroid glands lie on the posterior surface of both thyroid lobes, and the recurrent laryngeal nerves are in a cleft between the trachea and esophagus, medial to the lateral aspect of both thyroid lobes.

The four major arteries supplying the thyroid are the paired superior thyroid arteries and the paired inferior thyroid arteries. A fifth artery arises from the aortic arch and enters the midline of the thyroid. A venous plexus forms under the fibrous capsule and contributes to confluences forming the superior and the middle thyroid veins; these veins enter the internal jugular veins. Occasionally, arising from the inferior poles are the inferior thyroid veins, which enter the innominate vein. Innervation of the gland is by the sympathetic and parasympathetic divisions of the autonomic nervous system.

Lymphatic drainage from the thyroid is in the superior, lateral, and inferior directions and generally follows the branches of the superior and inferior thyroid blood vessels (Fig. 47.1B). The superior lymphatic pathways drain the anterior and posterior portions of the thyroid lobes and the medial aspect of the gland adjacent to the isthmus. The collection trunks may cross anterior and superior to the isthmus and may communicate with the prelaryngeal nodes. A pyramidal lobe, if present, is included in the prelaryngeal collecting system. The collecting pathways from the prelaryngeal region and the anterior and medial aspects of the upper poles follow the blood vessels and continue to the superior subdigastric nodes of the internal jugular chain. The posterior portion of the upper lobes empties into collecting lymphatics that usually end in the superior and anterior internal jugular nodes. The lateral pathways follow the middle thyroid veins to the inferior and lateral nodes of the internal jugular chain; they chiefly drain the lateral lower half of each thyroid lobe. The inferior pathway drains the lower portion of the isthmus, the inferior poles, and the medial and posterior lower half of each thyroid lobe; they empty into the pretracheal and paratracheal lymph nodes.

Drainage pathways may lie adjacent to the thymus, and nodes in the area of the innominate veins may show metastatic disease from the lower poles and the inferior aspect of the isthmus. There appears to be free communication between the retropharyngeal and retroesophageal nodes and the recurrent laryngeal and paratracheal nodes. Anterior-superior mediastinal nodes are secondary nodes to the recurrent laryngeal and pretracheal nodal groups.

Epidemiology

Thyroid cancer comprises about 2% of all malignancies and accounts for less than 1% of all cancer deaths in the United States. According to the American Cancer Society, the number of new thyroid cancer cases for 2006 was estimated to be 30,180 (7,590 men and 22,590 women), with an estimated 1,500 deaths (630 men and 870 women) from the disease (7). Thyroid cancer is now the seventh most common cancer in women, with a 2% per year increase in incidence.

Radiation-Induced Thyroid Cancer

Thyroid gland exposure to ionizing radiation, particularly before puberty, is the only well-documented etiologic factor in thyroid cancer. One fourth of patients who receive between 0.02 Gy and several grays of external irradiation to the thyroid gland develop goiters; one fourth of these, or 7% of all individuals who receive external irradiation to the thyroid, develop cancer, usually papillary adenocarcinoma (51,122). In the past, external irradiation sometimes was used to treat children with conditions such as acne, fungus infections of the scalp, or an enlarged thymus gland, or to shrink enlarged tonsils or adenoids.

The Japanese population exposed to the atomic bomb in 1945 has been studied. The Hiroshima bomb contained a significant neutron component, but the Nagasaki bomb delivered almost pure γ-rays. Of a fixed population of 20,000 heavily and lightly exposed individuals systematically examined every second year since 1959, approximately 0.2% have developed thyroid cancer, mostly papillary adenocarcinoma. Women who were between 10 and 19 years old at the time of the bombings and were exposed to more than 0.5 Gy have a risk of thyroid cancer 8.8 times higher than that of women of similar age who were exposed to less than 0.01 Gy (103,120).

In 1954 Marshall Islanders were exposed to radioactive fallout from a nuclear test. Exposed persons and unexposed persons from nearby uncontaminated islands have been systematically studied annually. Thyroid gland irradiation was the result mainly of several short-lived, internally deposited radioiodine nuclides; external γ- and β-irradiation also contributed. By 1974, 34 of those exposed had developed thyroid lesions; 3 of the 34 lesions (1.3%) were cancers. The highest incidence of thyroid nodularity occurred in 19 persons who were irradiated before the age of 20 years. Their whole-body dose was estimated at 1.75 Gy and their thyroid dose at 12 Gy (140). The United States Department of Health and Human Services published a report of estimated exposures and thyroid doses received by the American people from ^{131}I in fallout following the Nevada atmospheric nuclear bomb tests. The tests were performed from 1952 through 1957. The report includes estimates of the thyroid dose by age, gender, and source and quantity of milk consumed, because milk was the source of most of the radioactive iodine exposure for most people. The report does not address the issue of the risk of thyroid cancer associated with thyroid doses from ^{131}I (106). The National Cancer Institute has developed a risk calculator to estimate the thyroid cancer risk from fallout from atomic bomb testing. The web address is http://ntsi131.nci.nih.gov.

Among irradiated U.S. populations, the highest incidence of thyroid cancer is in patients whose thyroid glands received external irradiation (e.g., treatment of tonsillitis). In two Chicago studies of patients with histories of tonsillitis treated with

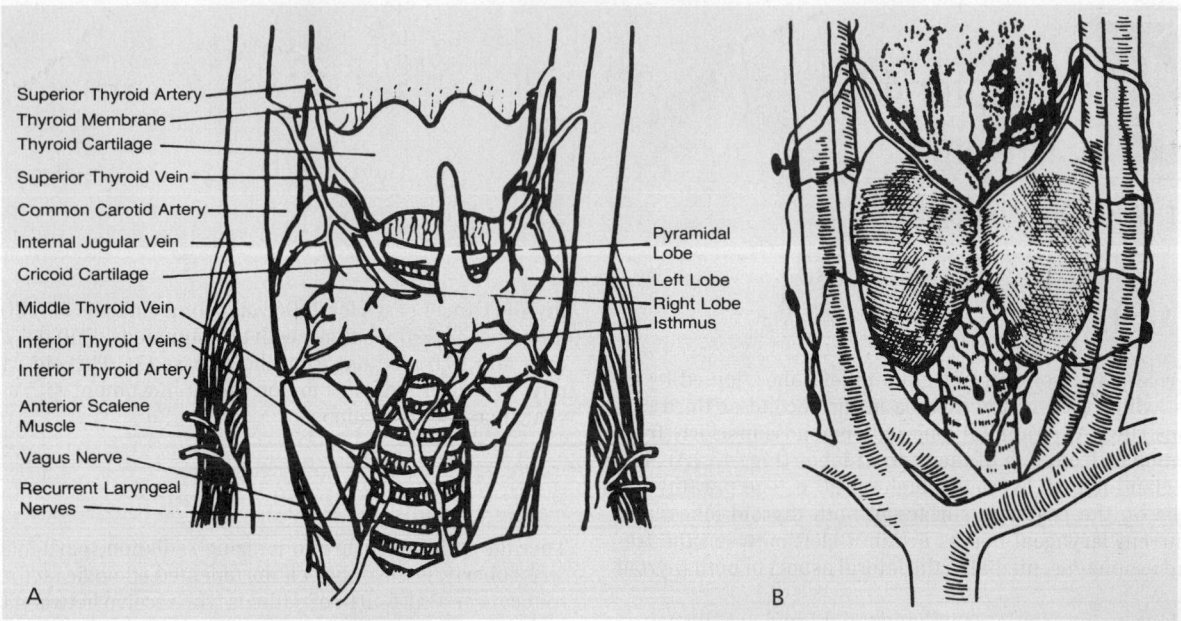

FIGURE 47.1. A: Anatomy of the thyroid. **B:** Lymphatic drainage of the thyroid. (From Mahomer HR, Caylor HD, Schlottnauer CF, et al. *Anat Rec* 1927:36:341, with permission.)

irradiation, 6% of those in one study and 7% in the other developed thyroid cancer (40). Thyroid cancer developed in 5% of a subgroup of Rochester patients in with nasopharyngeal lymphoid hyperplasia; the x-ray beam was directed at the tonsillar region. Other studies have shown that about 30% of patients with nodular disease in the thyroid after irradiation develop thyroid cancer. The prevalence of occult thyroid cancer found in two autopsy series of persons without radiation exposure was 5% and 22% (93).

According to Maxon et al. (96), external irradiation of the thyroid at doses greater than 2,000 rem is not clearly associated with thyroid cancer induction. With less than 2,000 rem of external irradiation, a linear no-threshold model suggests that children have absolute risks for thyroid cancer and for thyroid nodules of 4.2 and 12.3 cases per 10^6 persons per rem/year, respectively. Assuming that adults are half as sensitive as children to the induction of benign thyroid nodules by external irradiation, the risks of developing cancer or thyroid nodules for adults would be 4.2 and 8.2 cases per 10^6 persons per rem/year, respectively.

In April 1986, the Chernobyl nuclear reactor accident in the Soviet Union released substantial quantities of radioactive materials into the atmosphere and contaminated vast areas of Western and Eastern Europe. The radionuclides detected in the air included ^{131}I, ^{137}Cs, ^{99}Mo, and others. Iodine-131 is the easiest radionuclide to screen for in large populations of exposed persons. One study tested 58 individuals, 45 (78%) of whom had detectable quantities of radioiodine in the thyroid gland (23). The highest dose equivalent among adults was calculated as 5,180 mrem, which approximates that received from a diagnostic ^{131}I thyroid uptake test: 5 Ci of ^{131}I administered by mouth delivers between 6,500 to 9,000 mrem to an adult thyroid. Because of their smaller thyroid mass, children (younger than age 18 years) received higher radiation dose equivalents than did adults with similar uptake values. A 1-year-old child received a thyroid dose equivalent to 37,000 mrem for an uptake of 0.82 Ci; an adult thyroid gland concentrating this amount of ^{131}I would receive 471 mrem. Most of the test population, including two pregnant women, received negligible radiation dose equivalents to the thyroid.

In another study of the Chernobyl accident from Sweden, the time-activity curve for ^{131}I showed immediate uptake, with maximum uptake between 18 and 26 days after the accident (139). No measurable levels were observed after 93 days. This exposure may lead to a 0.1% increase in the incidence of thyroid cancer during a 25-year period.

Additional studies have shown a slight increase risk in the workers involved in the cleanup of Chernobyl who live in Estonia and Latvia (117). This was seen in those workers sent to Chernobyl in April and May 1986. This population is being screened for thyroid cancer and this may be contributing to this rise. Increased risk of thyroid cancer has also been shown in Belarus and Ukraine, with the higher rate in Belarus (68). A third study has shown that there is a significant increase in the number of thyroid cancer cases in children and adolescents living in Ukraine and Belarus at the time of the Chernobyl accident, with a 30% increase over baseline in Ukraine and 80% increase in Belarus (69).

Thyroid function abnormalities after neck irradiation for Hodgkin's disease have been reported (95). In one study among 50 disease-free patients 2 to 16 years after neck irradiation, 25 had abnormal thyroid studies: 8 were hypothyroid, 2 were hypothyroid and had abnormal scans, and 15 had abnormal scans. Of 15 patients with abnormal scans, 1 had elevated levels of thyroid-stimulating hormone (TSH) and another developed exophthalmos.

There have been isolated reports of thyroid cancer occurring years after ^{131}I therapy for hyperthyroidism. Many careful studies have concluded, however, that there is no correlation between the development of thyroid cancer and ^{131}I therapy for hyperthyroidism (65,137). No increase has been shown in infertility, spontaneous abortions, or congenital abnormalities among patients treated for hyperthyroidism with ^{131}I.

Clinical Manifestations and Diagnostic Work-Up

Early detection of thyroid cancer in the United States is hampered by the presence of approximately 300,000 benign nodules

Table 47.1 DIAGNOSTIC WORK-UP FOR THYROID TUMORS

Procedure	Finding	Significance
General		
History	External irradiation to head or neck between infancy and early adulthood	Known cause of thyroid cancer; also may result in benign lesions
	Family history of medullary thyroid cancer	Inherited in an autosomal dominant pattern
	Family or personal history of pheochromocytoma or hyperparathyroidism with or without mucosal neuromata	Suggestive of multiple endocrine neoplasia syndromes II or III with medullary thyroid cancer
	Diarrhea	Common in medullary thyroid cancer
Physical examination	Solitary thyroid nodule	Cancers more frequently found in solitary nodules
	Multiple nodules with a predominant or rapidly enlarging nodule	In multiple nodules containing cancer, neoplasm is usually in predominant nodule
	Thyroid fixation to adjacent structure	May indicate cancer
	Enlarged cervical lymph nodes in young person	May be only presenting symptom of occult thyroid cancer
	Goiter with unilateral vocal cord paralysis	Unusual except for anaplastic cancer
Special tests		
Fine-needle aspiration and biopsy	See text	See text
Catheterization	See text	See text
Imaging studies		
X-ray	Psammomatous calcifications	Suggests thyroid nodule is malignant
Ultrasound	Differentiates solid from cystic nodules	Solid nodules more often malignant
Computed tomography	Extent of primary tumor, metastases	Assists in treatment planning, assesses extent of tumor and response to therapy
Magnetic resonance imaging	See text	See text
Radionuclide procedures ^{99m}Tc or radioiodine imaging ^{201}Tl ^{125}I or ^{131}I-MIBG	Cold, warm, or hot nodule; single or multiple nodule	See text
Monoclonal antibodies		
Fluorescent imaging		
Laboratory studies		
Thyroglobulin	Postoperative value elevated	Indicates residual, recurrent, or metastatic differentiated thyroid cancer and correlates well with ^{131}I imaging detection of thyroid cancer
	Preoperative value elevated	Cannot distinguish between tumor and differentiated thyroid cancer
	Normal value	Supportive but not conclusive evidence of lack of disease
Calcitonin	Preoperative value elevated (basal or stimulated)	Indicates C-cell hyperplasia or medullary thyroid cancer (spontaneous or familial)
	Postoperative value (basal or stimulated)	Indicates residual, recurrent, or metastatic medullary thyroid cancer (spontaneous or familial)
	Normal level postoperatively after stimulation	Indicates lack of disease

among the U.S. population with clinically apparent goiters. No single historic factor, physical finding, or clinical laboratory test is pathognomonic for the detection of thyroid cancer, except for the serum calcitonin measurement used to detect medullary thyroid cancer. Rarely, benign or malignant tumors of the thyroid gland can lead to tracheal compression or invasion and cause acute tracheal obstruction or hemoptysis, requiring emergency total thyroidectomy. An outline of the diagnostic procedures for thyroid cancer is presented in Table 47.1. No differences in total serum levels of thyroxine (T_4) or triiodothyronine (T_3) separate benign and malignant disease.

A significant increase in the incidence of HLA-DR7 has been found among patients with non–radiation-associated thyroid cancer compared with normal controls. This finding was most noticeable with follicular and mixed papillary-follicular cancers. The frequency of HLA-DR7 was not increased in patients with radiation-associated thyroid cancer, but the interval from the date of irradiation to the onset of thyroid cancer was shorter in HLA-DR7–positive patients than in HLA-DR7–negative patients (138). The ret/PTC oncogene is an activated form of c-ret and may serve as a marker for the progression of papillary thyroid carcinoma. It appears to be unique in that its activation is re-stricted to papillary thyroid carcinoma. However, its activation appears to occur in only a minority of human papillary thyroid carcinomas (70).

Because medullary thyroid cancer often metastasizes to the anterior mediastinum, widening of that area on a radiograph in a patient with palpable thyroid abnormalities should result in the inclusion of medullary thyroid cancer in the differential diagnosis; however, this mediastinal finding also is seen with other types of thyroid cancers. In some patients, recognition of paraneoplastic syndromes associated with advanced medullary thyroid cancer can facilitate diagnosis. Approximately 20% to 30% of patients with proven medullary thyroid cancer, particularly those with metastatic disease, complain of persistent diarrhea (125). Prostaglandins, vasoactive intestinal polypeptide, and serotonin may be produced by the tumor singly or in combination and may be responsible for the diarrhea.

Serum calcitonin measurement, with or without the use of calcium or pentagastrin stimulation testing, is the key marker in detecting medullary thyroid cancer and its precursor C-cell hyperplasia and in managing postoperative patients, especially those with residual disease and metastases.

Imaging Studies

Standard Radiographs

The most common radiographic feature associated with thyroid nodules is intraglandular calcification, four types of which have been described: vascular, amorphous (usually large with irregular edges), plaquelike linear or curvilinear, and psammomatous (multiple, small, and discrete, suggesting a malignant tumor). Psammomatous calcifications are detectable radiographically in 50% of histologic specimens of papillary carcinoma, but clinical radiographs reveal them in only 10% of patients with papillary carcinoma.

Radionuclide Thyroid Imaging

Indications for thyroid imaging in suspected or proven thyroid cancer are anatomic and functional evaluation of a palpable thyroid nodule, detection of occult or minimal cancer in a high-risk patient, detection of primary tumor in a patient with known regional or distant thyroidal metastases, detection of regional or distant thyroid cancer metastases, and assessment of therapeutic effects. However, it must be stressed that the current preferred method for evaluating a solitary thyroid nodule is with ultrasound and subsequent fine-needle aspiration.

The four radiopharmaceuticals most commonly used for radionuclide imaging of the thyroid are ^{131}I, ^{125}I, ^{123}I, and ^{99m}Tc (Table 47.2). The use of ^{131}I for routine thyroid imaging is not indicated because it delivers a substantial radiation dose to the thyroid; ^{123}I and ^{99m}Tc provide better physical characteristics for imaging and deliver much lower radiation doses to the thyroid. Unlike ^{123}I and the other radioiodine imaging agents that are taken up and then organified by the thyroid, ^{99m}Tc is trapped by the thyroid but does not undergo organification. Iodine-131 is preferred in the postoperative management of differentiated thyroid cancer when searching for residual functioning thyroid gland tissue and functioning residual, recurrent, or metastatic thyroid tumor.

Several other radionuclide studies have been investigated in the evaluation of patients with thyroid carcinoma. These include ^{67}Ga imaging (61), [^{18}F]2-fluoro-2-deoxy D-glucose (FDG) (66), ^{201}Tl (16), ^{99m}Tc phosphates, and ^{99m}Tc-sulfur colloid liver imaging (58), [^{131}I]m-iodobenzylguanidine (35), radiolabeled monoclonal antibodies (84), and fluorescent thyroid scanning (110). FDG-PET (positron emission tomography) is advocated as the imaging modality of choice for patients with poorly differentiated thyroid cancer and those patients with an elevated thyroglobulin level and a negative total body ^{131}I scintigram.

A recent European multicenter study shows overall sensitivity of PET/computed tomography (CT) of 75% and specificity of 90%. This was evaluated further by evaluating patients with negative ^{131}I whole-body scans, showing PET to have 85% sensitivity and 90% specificity, compared with patients with positive ^{131}I whole-body scans, where PET has 65% sensitivity and 100% specificity. Thyroglobulin elevation >5 ng/mL also had improved sensitivity of 100% and specificity of 100% (33).

Another recent study showed improvement in PET scan quality in thyroid cancer patients when the patients were prepared with recombinant human TSH (rhTSH). Patients were imaged by PET scans if there was equivocal or positive thyroglobulin elevation and negative or equivocal ^{131}I whole-body scan and/or ultrasound/CT/magnetic resonance imaging (MRI). All patients underwent PET scan with TSH suppression, then TSH stimulation with rhTSH. The TSH-stimulated PET scans showed an increase in the number of lesions and lesions in more patients. All lesions were more intense. Several inflammatory lymph nodes did not significantly change under rhTSH stimulation (112).

Ultrasonography

Ultrasonography is a valuable tool for evaluating thyroid nodules because it differentiates solid from cystic nodules. Ideally, it is performed with a high-resolution, high-frequency (7.5- or 10-MHz) transducer. Ultrasound also may be useful in the postoperative evaluation of thyroid cancer patients (133,141). Ultrasound-guided biopsy can be an integral part of the evaluation for recurrent thyroid malignancy.

Computed Tomography and Magnetic Resonance Imaging

High-resolution CT provides an additional modality for thyroid cancer evaluation by defining the morphology of the thyroid gland and the anatomic extent of thyroid abnormalities in relation to the normal structures of the mediastinum and neck and by assisting in the radiologic detection of lung metastases and the assessment of therapy (Fig. 47.2) (132). As with cancers in other locations, CT is particularly valuable in the planning of external radiation therapy treatments. The tumor volume and the isodose distribution can be determined accurately (Fig. 47.2). CT with intravenous contrast inhibits uptake of radioiodine for scanning or treatment for 6 to 8 weeks because of the concentration of iodine in the intravenous contrast.

Because MRI may not be capable of differentiating benign from malignant tumors or determining functional status, it may have a limited role in the evaluation of patients with thyroid nodules or goiters (108). MRI does have three indications: assessment of substernal goiters, depiction of the overall extent of the thyroid mass and involvement of muscles, and identification of sites of thyroid cancer recurrence (4).

	Table 47.2	**RADIONUCLIDES USED FOR THYROID IMAGING**				
					Radiation Dose (mGy/MBq)	
Radionuclide	**Dose (MBq)**		**Principle Imaging Energy (keV)**	**Physical Half-Life**	**Total Body**	**Thyroid**
^{99m}Tc	185–370	IV	140	6.02 h	0.003–0.005	0.032–0.054
^{123}I	3.7–14.8	PO	159	13.2 h	0.005–0.011	2.973–5.405
^{123}I-MIBG	370	IV	159	13.2 h	0.005	0.595
^{125}I	1.85–3.7	PO	28, 35	60.7 d	0.004–0.011	10.81–21.62
^{131}I	1.11–1.85	PO	364	8.06 d	0.135–1.081	297.3–432.4
^{131}I-MIBG	18.5	IV	364	8.06 d	0.027	9.459
^{201}Tl	37–111	IV	68–80	73 h	0.016–0.081	0.116–0.251

IV, intravenous; PO, by mouth; MIBG, *m*-iodobenzylguanidine.

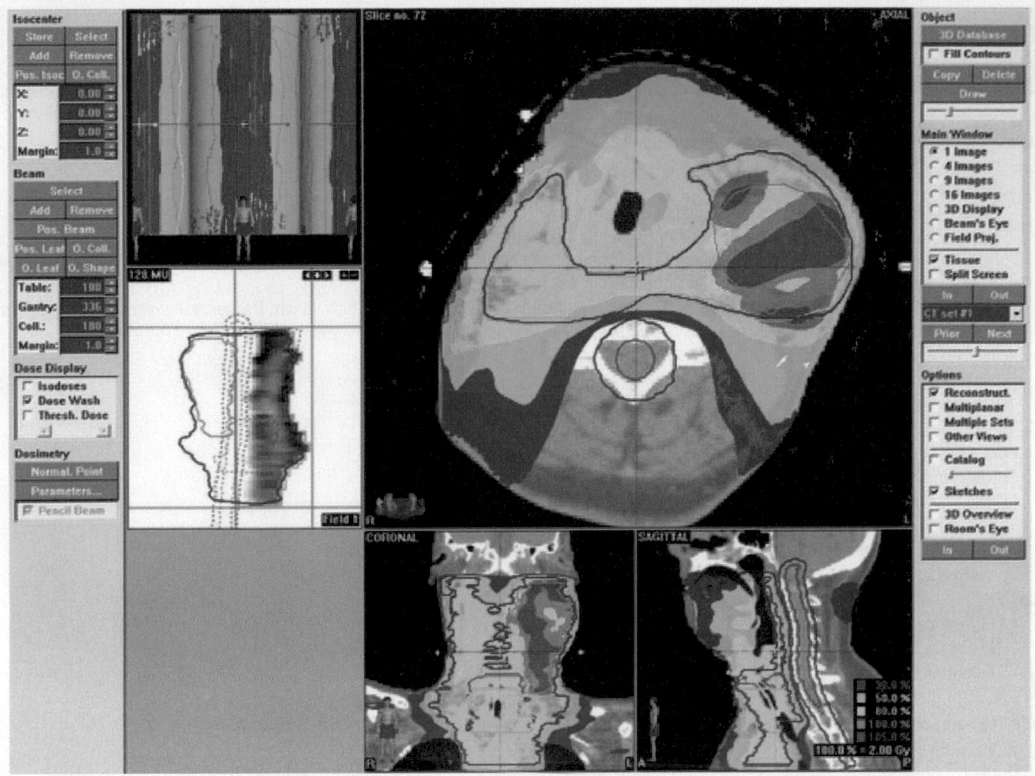

FIGURE 47.2. Intensity-modulated radiation therapy dose distribution to neck of patient with locally advanced thyroid cancer.

Fine-Needle Aspiration Biopsy

Fine-needle aspiration biopsy is a technique for obtaining follicular epithelial cells and minute tissue fragments for cytologic evaluation (48). The technique is used widely to differentiate benign from malignant nodules and has a reported accuracy as high as 95% (56). This technique has improved the presurgical evaluation of solitary nodules (44).

A cutting-needle biopsy using a Vim-Silverman or Tru-Cut needle may be performed to obtain larger tissue fragments for routine histologic examination. The technique should be used cautiously, if at all, for thoracic inlet nodules because large vessels at the inlet present a risk of acute airway obstruction from bleeding. Generally, cutting-needle biopsy is applied to nodules at least 2 cm in diameter, and preferably larger.

Staging

Because histologic diagnosis and patient age are important in determining the behavior and prognosis of thyroid cancer, these factors must be accounted for in the staging system. Staging of thyroid cancer is shown in Table 47.3. It is important to note that age is considered in the staging system and that all categories can be divided into *a* (solitary) and *b* (multifocal) types. Papillary or follicular lesions also are staged by patient age (less than 45 or older than 45 years old) (40). Pathologic staging of thyroid cancer tumors should be based on the *World Health Organization International Classification of Tumors* (156).

Pathologic Classification

Malignant thyroid neoplasms have been divided into four main types: papillary and mixed papillary-follicular, follicular,

medullary, and anaplastic. Rare tumors, comprising fewer than 5% of malignant tumors of the thyroid, include lymphoma, plasmacytoma, squamous cell and mucin-producing carcinoma, teratoma, sarcoma, carcinosarcoma, hemangioendothelioma, metastatic carcinoma to the thyroid, and thyroid cancer at unusual sites, including median aberrant thyroid, lateral aberrant thyroid, and struma ovarii (154).

Differentiated Thyroid Cancer

Differentiated thyroid cancer consists of papillary, mixed papillary-follicular, and follicular adenocarcinoma. These tumors arise from the thyroid follicular cells (i.e., endodermal origin) and can be treated with ^{131}I and thyroid-hormone suppression.

Papillary and Mixed Papillary-Follicular Cancers

Despite the differences in their histologic patterns, papillary and mixed papillary-follicular cancers are considered to represent a spectrum of neoplasms because they show biologic and clinicopathologic similarities. These neoplasms, representing the most common type of thyroid cancer, are usually slow-growing and indolent, with an excellent prognosis. They are multifocal in as many as 75% of patients, contain papillary structures, and may have a large follicular component, with psammoma bodies. These tumors are usually infiltrative and metastasize to regional lymph nodes through lymphatic channels; hematogenous metastases are uncommon.

Papillary cancer, including mixed papillary-follicular cancer, comprises 33% to 73% of malignant thyroid lesions. More than 90% of thyroid neoplasms found incidentally at autopsy are papillary cancers. This histologic type is the one most frequently encountered in thyroid glands previously exposed to irradiation (151). It is two to four times more common in females than in

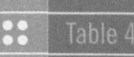

Table 47.3	DEFINITION OF TNM CATEGORIES AND STAGING IN CARCINOMA OF THE THYROID

Primary tumor (T)

NOTE: All categories may be subdivided: a, solitary tumor; b, multifocal tumor—measure the largest for classification.

TX	Primary tumor cannot be assessed
T0	No evidence of primary tumor
T1	Tumor ≤2 cm in greatest dimension limited to the thyroid
T2	Tumor <2 cm but not <4 cm in greatest dimension limited to the thyroid
T3	Tumor <4 cm in greatest dimension limited to the thyroid or any tumor with minimal extrathyroid or any tumor with minimal extrathyroid extension
T3	(e.g., extension to sternothyroid muscle or perithyroid soft tissues)
T4a	Tumor of any size extending beyond the thyroid capsule to invade subcutaneous soft tissues, larynx, trachea, esophagus, or recurrent laryngeal nerve
T4b	Tumor invades prevertebral fascia or encases carotid artery or mediastinal vessels.

All anaplastic carcinomas are considered T4 tumors.

T4a	Intrathyroidal anaplastic carcinoma—surgically resectable
T4b	Extrathyroidal anaplastic carcinoma—surgically unresectable

Regional lymph nodes (N)

Regional lymph nodes are the central compartment, lateral cervical, and upper mediastinal lymph nodes.

NX	Regional lymph nodes cannot be assessed
N0	No regional lymph-node metastasis
N1	Regional lymph-node metastasis
N1a	Metastasis to level VI (pretracheal, paratracheal, and prelaryngeal/Delphian lymph nodes)
N1b	Metastasis to unilateral, bilateral, or contralateral cervical or superior mediastinal lymph nodes

Distant metastasis (M)

MX	Presence of distant metastasis cannot be assessed
M0	No distant metastasis
M1	Distant metastasis

Stage grouping

Separate stage groupings are recommended for papillary or follicular, medullary, and anaplastic (undifferentiated) carcinoma

Papillary or follicular (under 45 years)

Stage I	Any T	Any N	M0
Stage II	Any T	Any N	M1

Papillary or follicular (45 years and older)

Stage I	T1	N0	M0
Stage II	T2	N0	M0
Stage III	T3	N0	M0
	T1	N1a	M0
	T2	N1a	M0
	T3	N1a	M0
Stage IVA	T4a	N0	M0
	T4a	N1a	M0
	T1	N1b	M0
	T2	N1b	M0
	T3	N1b	M0
	T4a	N1b	M0
Stage IVB	T4b	Any N	M0
Stage IVC	Any T	Any N	M1

Medullary carcinoma

Stage I	T1	N0	M0
Stage II	T2	N0	M0
Stage III	T3	N0	M0
	T1	N1a	M0
	T2	N1a	M0
	T3	N1a	M0
Stage IVA	T4a	N0	M0
	T4a	N1a	M0
	T1	N1b	M0
	T2	N1b	M0
	T3	N1b	M0
	T4a	N1b	M0
Stage IVB	T4b	Any N	M0
Stage IVC	Any T	Any N	M1

Anaplastic carcinoma

All anaplastic carcinomas are considered Stage IV

Stage IVA	T4a	Any N	M0
Stage IVB	T4b	Any N	M0
Stage IVC	Any T	Any N	M1

Histopathologic type

Papillary carcinoma (including follicular variant of papillary carcinoma)
Follicular carcinoma (including Hürthle cell carcinoma)
Medullary carcinoma
Undifferentiated (anaplastic) carcinoma

From Greene FL, Page DL, Fleming I, et al., eds. *AJCC cancer staging manual*, 6th ed. New York: Springer-Verlag; 2002, with permission.

males and occurs mostly in the third to fifth decades, although it can occur at any age. Papillary cancer accounts for 80% of thyroid cancers in the prepubertal age group. Tall-cell variant of papillary thyroid cancer and insular carcinoma recently have been described and appear to have a worse prognosis than typical papillary carcinoma of the thyroid (146).

Follicular Cancers

Follicular cancers are solitary, have a marked tendency to invade vascular channels, and metastasize hematogenously to distant sites. Lymph node metastases are uncommon. These cancers lack papillae, psammoma bodies, and ground-glass nuclei. They have the strongest propensity to concentrate ^{131}I.

Hürthle cell and primary clear cell carcinoma are classified as variants of follicular carcinoma. Follicular cancer comprises 14% to 33% of primary thyroid cancers and affects females two to three times as frequently as males. The average age at diagnosis is 50 to 58 years; this cancer occasionally is seen in children.

Medullary Thyroid Cancer

Medullary thyroid cancer is derived from parafollicular cells (C cells) that arise from the neuroectoderm and comprises 5% to 10% of all thyroid cancers. Approximately 80% of cases arise spontaneously, without apparent evidence of familial disease. The other 20% occur within familial multiple endocrine neoplasia syndromes (i.e., MEN IIa, IIb, or III) (119). Although medullary thyroid cancer itself does not concentrate ^{131}I, residual tumor in remaining thyroid gland tissue after surgery may be treatable with radioiodine because of iodine accumulation in follicular cells immediately adjacent to the medullary cancer cells; metastases may be treatable with ^{131}I-tagged monoclonal antibodies (62,126).

Anaplastic Cancer

Anaplastic thyroid cancer originates from the follicular cells of the thyroid; the disease features three histologic types: small cell, spindle cell, and giant cell. Tumors of this kind grow rapidly. Local invasion of structures (e.g., trachea) is followed by or concurrent with distant metastasis, and death usually occurs within 12 months of diagnosis.

Anaplastic cancer comprises about 5% of all malignant lesions of the thyroid. Patients range in age from 40 to 90 years, and women outnumber men 4 to 1. There is a history of goiter in 80% of these patients. It has been hypothesized that there is a transformation from a benign or low-grade malignant lesion to a highly malignant one.

Radiation-Induced Thyroid Cancer

The pathology of thyroid cancers in irradiated thyroids resembles that of spontaneous thyroid cancers; the well-differentiated papillary, follicular, and mixed papillary-follicular cancers predominate. The incidence of radiation-induced and spontaneous medullary and anaplastic thyroid cancers appears to be the same.

Although radiation-induced thyroid cancers have a well-differentiated appearance and respond well to treatment, they have a tendency to invade locally and to recur. Between one half and one third of patients have regional lymph node metastases when first operated (39). Distant metastases, usually to the lungs, exist in approximately 10% of patients at the time of initial surgery.

Prognostic Factors

Differentiated Thyroid Cancer

The most significant prognostic factors for papillary, mixed papillary-follicular, and follicular cancers are histologic pattern, patient age at diagnosis, and extent of local involvement.

Histology and Invasiveness

There are three types of papillary cancers. Occult sclerosing lesions, which comprise 12% to 28% of papillary cancers, are up to 1.5 cm in diameter, are confined to the thyroid, usually are not palpable, and are discovered incidentally during thyroid exploration after presentation with cervical lymph node metastases. Intrathyroidal lesions, which comprise 34% to 78% of papillary cancers, are apparent preoperatively, are larger than occult lesions, and are confined to the thyroid. Extrathyroidal lesions, which comprise 2% to 39% of papillary lesions, extend beyond the thyroid capsule to adjacent structures.

Young et al. (159) reviewed the effect of therapy in 214 patients with follicular thyroid cancer. Their study indicated that patients likely to die of this cancer have distant metastases at the time of initial presentation. If disease is confined to the neck at presentation, the overall prognosis is good, but it can be altered with the type of medical therapy. Both ^{131}I therapy and thyroid hormone therapy decreased the rate or recurrence.

Among those presenting with disease confined to the neck, the recurrence rate if thyroid nodules were less than 1.5 cm was 10%; with nodules larger than 1.5 cm, the recurrence rate was 8%. Neither lymph node involvement nor the extent of lymph node surgery affected recurrence rate. The recurrence rate was 7% if lymph nodes were involved but 11% if they were not. The duration of follow-up was not sufficient to allow conclusions about improved survival in patients with little or moderate invasion of the vasculature or thyroid nodule capsule (159). However, Rao et al. (119) found that poor prognostic factors for patients with pure follicular thyroid carcinoma were age greater than 40 years, tumor size greater than 5 cm, extrathyroidal extension, and distant metastasis. In a multivariate analysis of prognostic factors in 100 patients with follicular thyroid carcinoma, Brennan et al. (18) found that only age greater than 50 years, marked vascular invasion, and distant metastasis at the time of diagnosis were significant. Shaha et al. (129) also confirmed these results in a multivariate analysis of 228 patients with follicular thyroid carcinoma. They found high-risk factors to be age older than 45 years, Hürthle cell variety, extrathyroidal extension, tumor size exceeding 4 cm, and presence of distant metastasis.

Age

Mazzaferri et al. (98) reported that papillary cancer patients younger than 30 years of age had a higher recurrence rate than patients 30 years or older. Patients 40 years of age or older had a higher mortality rate than patients younger than 40 years.

In their study of differentiated thyroid cancer, Cady et al. (22) found that the overall recurrence risk was 10% and the death risk was 3% among women younger than 50 years of age; among patients with recurrent disease or metastases, only 30% died of disease. For women older than 50 years of age, the respective figures were 32%, 30%, and 89%.

Although it is uncommon, children and teenagers do develop thyroid carcinoma. Goepfert et al. (44) noted, in a study of patients younger than 20 years of age, that 85% of those with differentiated thyroid carcinoma had palpable cervical adenopathy, 11% had pulmonary metastasis, and, with a mean follow-up of 15.4 years, four had died as a result of their carcinoma. An

Clinical Radiation Oncology

update of the study of Goepfert et al. by Frankenthaler et al. (42) of 117 patients younger than 20 years of age with differentiated thyroid carcinoma indicated similar findings.

Lymph Node Involvement

In a Lahey Clinic series, survival was higher among patients with a greater number of involved lymph nodes in all histologically comparable groups (21). However, others have shown a poorer outcome for patients with positive lymph nodes.

In a recent analysis of the significance of lymph node metastasis at the time of initial diagnosis, Hughes et al. (66) performed a matched-pair analysis of patients with differentiated carcinoma of the thyroid. Their results demonstrate the problem of the significance (or lack of significance) of lymph node metastasis. There was no difference in overall survival between 100 patients with N1 disease and 100 patients with N0 disease. If age also was considered, then there was a significantly greater incidence of recurrence and a lower survival rate among those with N1 disease and age greater than 45 years (p =. 008). Among patients with N1 disease, patients younger than 45 years of age had better survival than those older than 45 years, but the difference was not statistically significant. One retrospective surgical series of 931 previously untreated patients with differentiated thyroid cancer found that female gender, multifocality, and regional lymph node involvement were favorable prognostic factors (128).

Medullary Thyroid Cancer

Medullary thyroid cancer has the potential for local and distant disease in some patients but may be benign in others. Dottorini et al. (36), in a study of 53 patients with medullary thyroid carcinoma, found stage of disease and postsurgical serum calcitonin level were the most significant and useful prognostic factors; survival did not correlate with immunohistochemical markers.

Anaplastic Thyroid Cancer

The prognostic factors for anaplastic thyroid cancer are a large, firm, bulky mass severely distorting the normal neck contour; frequent obstruction of the larynx, trachea, and esophagus by direct tumor extension; and poor response to any treatment modality. Although cervical lymph nodes usually are involved with tumor, they may be difficult to detect because of the extent of the primary tumor. Because the size of the tumor may make tracheostomy difficult or impossible, some degree of thyroidectomy may be required to establish an airway. Anaplastic cancer and other thyroid cancers can lead to obstruction of the superior vena cava. Most patients also may have metastases outside the neck at the time of diagnosis. It is not uncommon for patients to undergo complete resection of disease and to develop massive, locally recurrent disease 2 to 4 weeks postoperatively.

An analysis of prognostic factors in anaplastic thyroid cancers has recently been published, based on SEER data: 516 patients were identified, with registry entry between 1973 and 2000. Eight percent had intrathyroid tumors, 38% had extrathyroid tumors and/or lymph node involvement, and 43% had distant metastasis. Patient age <60 years with intrathyroidal disease were independent predictors of lower cause-specific mortality (74).

Thyroid Lymphoma

Junor et al. (72) reviewed 79 cases of primary non-Hodgkin's lymphoma of the thyroid, stages IE and IIE. In a univariate analysis, the presence of dysphagia, dyspnea, positive nodes, stage, and male gender all had a statistically significant detrimental influence on survival. Stage and dysphagia were the most influential individually, and a multivariate analysis indicated that the prognostic information in all of these features essentially was captured by just these two factors. A prognostic scoring index based on stage of disease and the presence of dysphagia was developed.

General Management

The treatment of spontaneous and radiation-induced thyroid cancers is the same. The treatment modalities include surgery, thyroid hormone therapy, ^{131}I therapy, external irradiation, and chemotherapy. The management of pediatric thyroid cancer has been described (63).

Postoperative external irradiation rarely is indicated for patients with microscopic or gross residual disease, as in the case of gross capsular invasion. External irradiation is indicated for patients with recurrence or extensive inoperable disease.

In follicular cancer (including Hürthle cell tumors) and mixed papillary-follicular cancer, the tumor and its metastatic sites usually take up ^{131}I after ablation of normal thyroid tissue. Indications for external irradiation include inoperable or recurrent disease, capsular infiltration, macroscopic or microscopic residual disease, failure after ^{131}I treatment, and critical metastases. If ^{131}I uptake is inadequate for therapeutic purposes after surgery for differentiated tumors, external irradiation is indicated if the tumor is inoperable, if there is gross residual disease in the operative field, if the connective tissue is invaded, or if there is extensive infiltration of the cervical lymph nodes (2).

Differentiated Thyroid Cancer

Surgery

The recommended initial therapy for differentiated thyroid cancer is near-total or total thyroidectomy. The exceptions are occult differentiated cancers and completely excised pure papillary cancers that are small and confined to one lobe. A near-total or total thyroidectomy may be necessary if additional management with ^{131}I is being considered.

Radical neck dissection has been abandoned in favor of the modified radical neck dissection for metastatic lymphadenopathy. Limited dissections of metastatic adenopathy in the cervical, jugular, paratracheal, and upper-mediastinal lymph nodes are performed with increasing frequency. Prophylactic node dissection is no longer used. A recent article by Shindo et al. (130) argues in favor of central compartment lymph node excision, showing a 29% incidence of central compartment lymph nodes in patients younger than 45 years and 39% in patients 45 or older. No cases of permanent vocal cord paralysis or permanent hypocalcemia were noted. There was a 1% incidence of transient vocal cord paresis, which resolved during 6 months. Knowledge of central lymph node status has management implications for the patients.

Mazzaferri et al. (98) showed that the extent of cervical lymph node surgery, ranging from radical neck to limited nodal dissection, did not affect recurrence or survival in patients with papillary thyroid cancer. Patients with metastatic cervical adenopathy had the same rate of recurrence regardless of the extent of surgery (98,159).

After total thyroidectomy for papillary cancer, the recurrence rate was 7.1% and the death rate was 0.3%; with subtotal thyroidectomy, the rates were 18.4% and 1.5%, respectively. If medical treatment only (i.e., ^{131}I and thyroid hormone suppression) was given after total thyroidectomy, the recurrence rate was 2.6% and the death rate was 0%. The use of thyroid hormone only also resulted in a 0% mortality rate, but the recurrence rate was 10%. Without ^{131}I or thyroid hormone therapy, the recurrence rate was 40% and the death rate 13.3% (98).

Young et al. (159), in a study of 214 patients with follicular thyroid carcinoma, found that the overall recurrence rate was not affected by positive cervical nodes or the extent of thyroid surgery. An increase in the recurrence rate was associated with extensive histologic invasion of the nodule capsule and thyroid. The postoperative recurrence rate was decreased by treatment with radioiodine and by thyroid hormone therapy. At 4 years, the recurrence rate was about 4% with thyroid hormone use only, 6% with ^{131}I and thyroid hormone together, and 22% without either treatment. But at 10 years, the recurrence rate was slightly greater than 10% with thyroid hormone only, 6% with both ^{131}I and thyroid hormone, and 33% without any medical therapy. The only deaths in their study attributable to thyroid cancer occurred in patients who presented with distant metastases (159).

The death rates for differentiated thyroid cancers have been evaluated by Beierwaltes (10). From 1935 to 1955, when less aggressive surgery was done and there was less use of ^{131}I, the death rate was 12.5% for papillary cancer and 11.7% for follicular cancer. Between 1957 and 1972, with more adequate surgery and more routine use of ^{131}I, the death rates for papillary and follicular cancer were 2.4% and 3.1%, respectively.

Hay et al. (61) developed a prognostic scoring system for surgical outcome in patients with papillary thyroid carcinoma. Their system (AGES) is based on patient *age*, tumor *grade*, *extent*, and *size*. This scoring system may aid the surgeon in determining whether ipsilateral lobectomy or bilateral lobar resection is the best surgical approach.

Iodine-131

Radioactive iodine is used to treat some papillary, mixed papillary-follicular, and follicular cancers. Hürthle cell cancer, a variant of follicular cancer, may respond to ^{131}I therapy. (See Appendix 47.1 for procedures for administration of [131]I.) Figure 47.3 is a flow diagram that offers a guide to the postoperative management and follow-up of patients with differentiated thyroid cancer; variations may occur at different medical centers. The Mallinckrodt Institute of Radiology guidelines for ablation are shown in Figure 47.4.

The indications for ^{131}I therapy in thyroid cancer are tumor greater than 1.0 to 1.5 cm, thyroid capsule invasion, vascular invasion, multifocal disease, soft-tissue invasion, postoperative residual disease in the neck, positive or close surgical margins, cervical or mediastinal nodal metastases, distant metastases, and recurrent disease. Iodine-131 delivers a high radiation dose to normal thyroid and thyroid cancer cells; one estimate is 0.1 Gy per microcurie of ^{131}I per gram of thyroid cancer tissue. Another estimate, considering a biologic half-life of 4 days for ^{131}I and a 0.1% uptake of the ^{131}I therapy dose per gram of tumor or tissue, is 150 Gy/mCi (9,64). However, the biologic half-life may be as short as 17 hours in postsurgical patients with thyroid carcinoma (80).

Thyroid tissue remaining in the thyroid bed after thyroidectomy may be ablated with [131]I. The ablation dose, administered after thyroidectomy, may vary from 30 to 100 mCi; more than one dose may be required, particularly with lower doses of [131]I. Reasons for thyroid ablation include the multifocality of differentiated tumors, the high frequency of contralateral lobe disease, and the possibility of transformation of a residual site of differentiated thyroid tumor to anaplastic cancer (73).

Thyroid ablation with ^{131}I given after near-total or total thyroidectomy prepares the patient for more definitive therapy by elevating TSH levels enough to expose cancerous tissue to TSH, thus facilitating ^{131}I uptake into metastases for localization and therapy and removing normal thyroid tissue to eliminate extraneous thyroglobulin sources. Thyroid ablation decreases the recurrence and mortality rates of differentiated thyroid cancer (67).

The question of appropriate doses of ^{131}I for the ablation of thyroid remnants remains controversial (9,10,12,33,82,118,131,147,153). Some investigators advocate the use of 30 mCi or less of ^{131}I in an attempt to decrease the potential morbidity and hospitalization associated with large radioiodine doses (5,9,33,82,118,130). However, with the Nuclear Regulatory Commission (NRC) rule changes of 1997, patients can be treated with large doses of ^{131}I on an outpatient basis. Studies indicate that the higher the initial dose of ^{131}I, the more successful the ablation and the less need for repeat administration of lower doses of [131]I (12,33,118). Beierwaltes (10) and Beierwaltes et al. (12) recommend a dose of not less than 100 mCi for residual ^{131}I uptake in the thyroid bed. They also suggest that an ablation dose of 100 to 149 mCi constitutes adjuvant therapy for occult metastases not detected by ^{131}I scanning (1 to 5 mCi), especially when pretreatment uptake of ^{131}I is low (<4%).

An area of development on the management of administration of ^{131}I for treatment of thyroid cancer patients is in the use of rhTSH. An international randomized trial has been performed using rhTSH for ablation of residual thyroid tissue using 3.7 GBq (100 mCi). Patients were randomized to treatment with the preparation regimen either of hypothyroidism or rhTSH. Dosimetry was performed to evaluate blood dose, remnant uptake, and area of uptake. The uptake values immediately posttreatment were comparable. Both groups had successful ablation of tissue by the criteria of no visible uptake or visible uptake with uptake percent of <0.1% on scans performed 8 months after ablation. Radioiodine kinetic studies showed the effective half-life in remnant tissue was shorter in the hypothyroid group, but the blood dose was lower in the euthyroid group (110). It has been approved in Europe for preparation of low-risk (T1 or T2 N0-1) patients since 2005 (29). Application for approval is pending in the United States.

Although no studies have confirmed whether low or high ablation doses are preferable, lower death and recurrence rates have been seen in patients in whom all traces of residual ^{131}I uptake are ablated (12,155). The use of 100 to 149 mCi of ^{131}I as an empiric ablation dose is attractive, given its apparent success in eliminating residual ^{131}I uptake after a single dose (12). Other investigators recommend that the amount of ^{131}I for adequate ablation should be determined by the individual patient's clearance of a tracer dose of radioiodine (8,9,67,94). If necessary, another dose of 75 to 100 mCi of ^{131}I may be administered 6 to 12 months after the initial dose.

Iodine-131 also may be used to treat recurrent differentiated thyroid carcinoma; postoperative residual disease in the neck or elsewhere; nodal metastases in cervical, mediastinal, hilar, or other sites; distant metastases in lungs, liver, bone, or other locations; and inoperable primary tumors (Fig. 47.5). The dose per treatment should be 150 to 250 mCi of ^{131}I, depending on the clinical situation. Individual doses less than 150 mCi are considered inadequate. The recommended maximum total dose (i.e., ablation and therapy) of ^{131}I is 800 to 1,000 mCi.

Iodine-131 therapy may be combined with external radiation therapy (142). The dose to metastases from ^{131}I may be calculated using single-photon emission computed tomography (SPECT) imaging. The SPECT dose estimates correlate with the clinical course of disease and may provide prognostic information (79).

In patients with unresectable or inoperable primary tumors, ^{131}I does not seem to affect the rate of tumor regression appreciably or to prolong survival. A combination of ^{131}I and external radiation therapy seems to offer the best results.

Beierwaltes et al. (11) established a threefold increase in survival time in patients whose metastases were eliminated by [131]I. Nemec et al. (107) showed that survival duration was

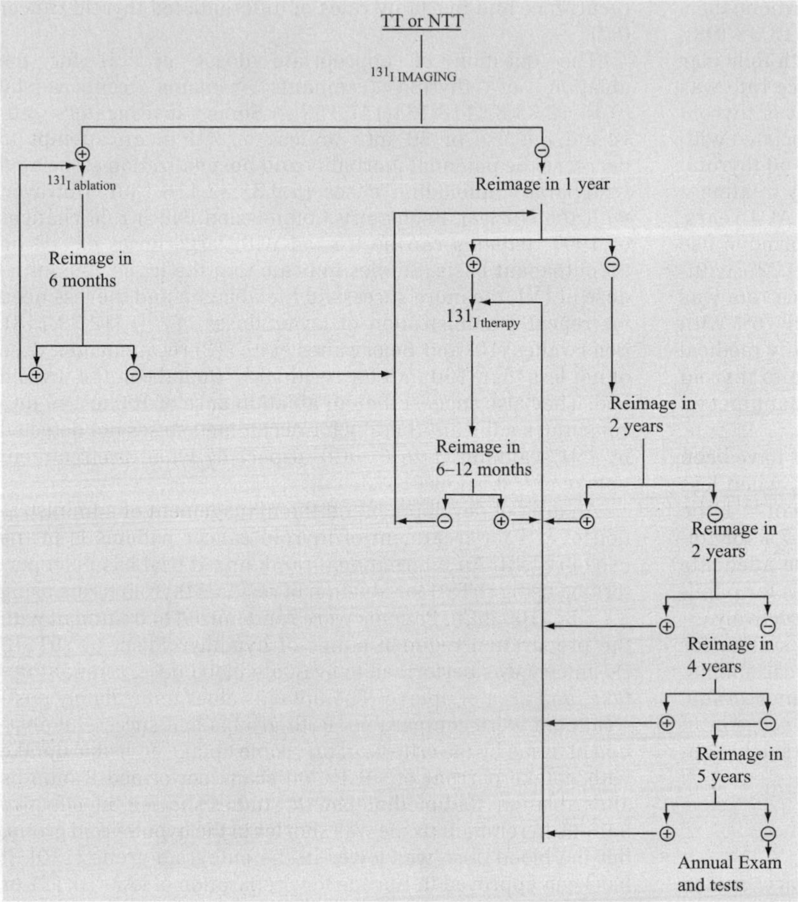

TT or NTT

^{131}I IMAGING

⊕

^{131}I ablation

Reimage in
6 months

⊕   ⊖

⊖

Reimage in 1 year

⊕   ⊖

^{131}I therapy

Reimage in
6–12 months

⊖   ⊕

Reimage in
2 years

Reimage in
2 years

⊕   ⊖

Reimage in
4 years

⊕   ⊖

Reimage in
5 years

⊕   ⊖

Annual Exam
and tests

FIGURE 47.3. Flow diagram for the postoperative management and follow-up of differentiated thyroid cancer.

significantly greater in patients treated with ^{131}I and that prognosis was adversely affected by bone metastases. In another study with ^{131}I, no patient with bone metastases was alive 10 years after treatment, and 11 (54%) of 20 patients with lung metastases were alive and free of disease 10 years after their initial therapy (19).

Total body imaging is done as early as 1 to 2 days or as late as 10 to 14 days after an ^{131}I ablation or therapy dose. No additional ^{131}I is given and no preparation of the patient is done. This imaging is performed because an ablative or therapeutic dose of ^{131}I may reveal additional lesions that were not detected with the lower scanning dose of ^{131}I used before ablation or therapy. Studies have confirmed this rationale (7,107).

External-Beam Radiation

External irradiation may be used after ^{131}I treatment if the cancer is nonfunctional (i.e., does not accumulate ^{131}I). This situation may occur in recurrent follicular cancers previously

treated with ^{131}I and may indicate that the cancer is becoming less differentiated and less functional. With gross residual disease, external irradiation may be given with up to 250 mCi of ^{131}I concurrently administered. Some researchers, however, caution that external irradiation should not precede ^{131}I therapy because it may jeopardize the success of the radioiodine treatment (14).

The external irradiation should encompass the thyroid bed and adjacent neck tissues. Treatment planning with CT is very helpful in ascertaining the depth and doses to the spinal cord.

Tubiana et al. (149) also advocated postoperative irradiation for patients with microscopic or macroscopic residual disease. Since 1956, their practice has been to deliver 50 Gy in 25 fractions in 5 weeks to the neck with a boost of 5 to 10 Gy to residual disease with ^{60}Co teletherapy. The spinal cord dose was limited to 42 Gy. They obtained a 5-year survival rate of 94% (62 of 66) for patients with complete surgery and 78% (76 of 97) for patients with incomplete surgery.

Farahati et al. (39) evaluated the role of adjuvant external irradiation in 238 patients with differentiated thyroid carcinoma. In their series, patients were treated with total thyroidectomy, postoperative radioiodine, and TSH-suppressive therapy with thyroid hormone. External irradiation was administered to 99 patients. Their analysis indicated that adjuvant external radiation therapy improves the rate of recurrence-free survival in patients older than 40 years with invasive papillary thyroid carcinoma and lymph node involvement.

A recent article from the University of Florida (100) reviewed a series of 42 patients treated with external-beam radiation therapy (EBRT) between 1962 and 2003. Most patients underwent surgery before EBRT. The volume covered included the thyroid bed, cervical lymph nodes, and upper mediastinum. Patients in the earlier years were treated with multifield

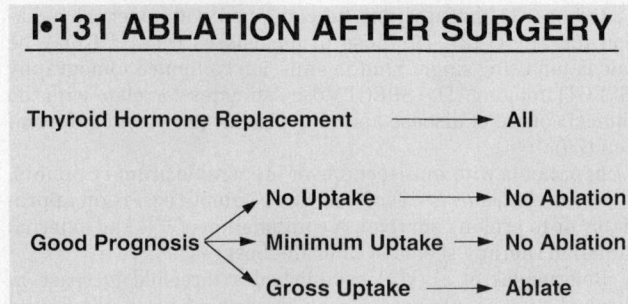

I•131 ABLATION AFTER SURGERY

Thyroid Hormone Replacement ──────► All

Good Prognosis
- No Uptake ──────► No Ablation
- Minimum Uptake ──► No Ablation
- Gross Uptake ──────► Ablate

FIGURE 47.4. The Mallinckrodt Institute of Radiology guidelines for thyroid ablation.

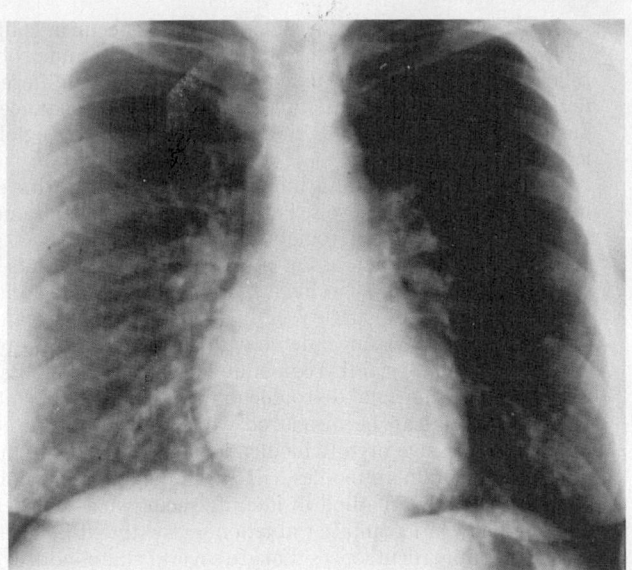
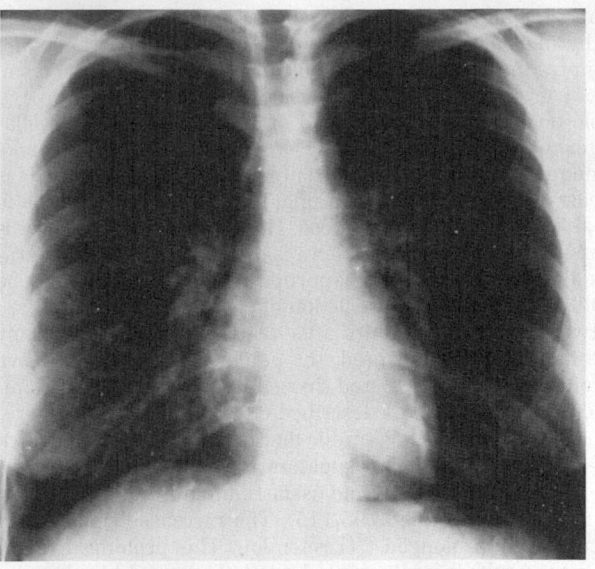

FIGURE 47.5. A: Posteroanterior chest radiograph of a patient with diffuse nodular bilateral pulmonary metastases from cancer of the thyroid. **B:** Posteroanterior radiograph of the same chest 1 year after administration of 150 mCi of [131]I. The pulmonary metastases have completely disappeared.

techniques and intensity-modulated radiation therapy (IMRT) from 2002. Median total doses were 64.9 Gy. 4 patients (9.5%) had locoregional recurrences. Patients with gross residual disease had 70% locoregional control versus 100% with microscopic disease. Cause-specific survival was 86% in those patients without metastasis, overall survival was 60%, 69% for patients with gross disease, compared with 90% with microscopic disease.

Another recent article showed decreased 10-year locoregional recurrence (8% with EBRT vs. 51% without EBRT) and 10-year progression-free survival (89% with vs. 39% without EBRT) in patients whose thyroid cancers invaded the trachea (74).

Inoperable, bulky disease should be approached with curative intent. Inoperable papillary thyroid carcinoma treated with local external irradiation has regressed markedly or disappeared, with patients surviving as long as 25 years. The treatment field should encompass the entire thyroid tumor, neck, and superior mediastinum (Fig. 47.6). A tumor dose of 65 to 70 Gy in 7 to 8 weeks in 1.8- to 2-Gy fractions is recommended.

Painful osseous metastases can be palliated by external radiation therapy, and prevention of pathologic fractures is a worthwhile goal. A medullary rod should be placed in long bones before external irradiation is administered if pathologic fracture is imminent or has occurred already. Brain, skeletal, hepatic, or subcutaneous metastases that press on vital structures should be treated with palliative external irradiation, ^{131}I therapy, or both. A dose of 45 Gy in 25 fractions in 5 weeks is adequate to achieve palliation. The patient's performance status and normal tissue tolerance must be considered in selecting the proper dose schedule.

Thyroid Hormone

Thyroid hormone-suppression therapy is effective in the management of differentiated thyroid cancer. All patients, regardless of the surgical procedure and between ^{131}I treatments, should be maintained on suppressive doses of long-acting thyroid medication, preferably L-thyroxine rather than desiccated thyroid, except for the patient who cannot tolerate L-thyroxine.

Because differentiated thyroid cancer grows under the stimulation of TSH, the goal of suppressive thyroid medication is to achieve a TSH level of 0.1 ng/mL. Periodic thyroid hormone measurements should be obtained to assess the degree of TSH suppression. Suppressive thyroid medication decreases the recurrence and mortality rates associated with differentiated thyroid cancer, particularly in patients with a large tumor burden, in whom the initial ^{131}I therapy may not be totally successful in eradicating all sites of thyroid cancer metastases and who might require subsequent ^{131}I treatment or other therapy.

Thyroid-Stimulating Hormone

Serum TSH has the greatest influence on ^{131}I uptake by normal thyroid cells and differentiated thyroid cancers; the latter are derived from follicular cells and have TSH receptors. The differentiated cancers respond to TSH in a fashion qualitatively similar to normal thyroid. In most, however, exposure to high concentrations of TSH is required to induce maximal uptake of [131]I (67). TSH levels may be elevated sufficiently within 2 weeks of total or near-total thyroidectomy.

Before ^{131}I is administered for whole-body imaging, initial ablation dose (if the patient was administered thyroid medication after surgery); repeat ablation dose; or ^{131}I therapy, thyroid hormone, or L-thyroxine must be discontinued for 2 to 4 weeks to allow the blood level of thyroid hormone to decrease and the TSH level to rise, enabling maximal stimulation of [131]I

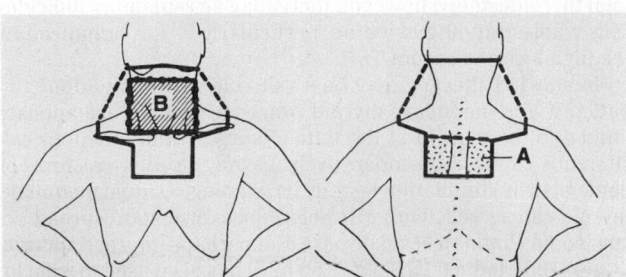

FIGURE 47.6. Diagrams of portals used in treatment of thyroid carcinoma. The A area *(right)* represents the posterior mediastinal portal used to increase the dose to these structures after the tolerance dose of the spinal cord has been reached with the large field (45 Gy). Additional irradiation also is delivered through an anteroposterior portal in the B area to the thyroid *(left).*

uptake. Cytomel can be used for 2 weeks prior to discontinuing all thyroid medication to help improve patient tolerance and minimize the potential period of symptomatic hypothyroidism. A TSH level of 30 IU/mL or greater is preferred before ^{131}I whole-body imaging, and a TSH of 50 IU/ml before ^{131}I ablation or therapy. Therapy usually can be instituted if ^{131}I uptake is adequate for imaging of thyroid metastases, as if the TSH is at least 30 IU/mL before scanning, it will be 50 by the time of the ablation or therapeutic dose. However, if the TSH level is greater than 50 IU/mL and there is no obvious ^{131}I uptake, radioiodine therapy may be inappropriate because there may be insufficient uptake for destruction of malignant tissues.

Twenty-four to 72 hours after an ^{131}I ablation or therapy dose has been administered, the patient is given suppressive thyroid medication. TSH and thyroid function levels are monitored and maintained as described elsewhere in this chapter.

Low-iodine diets and diuretic therapy to waste iodine, which are advocated by some investigators, may enhance ^{131}I radioiodine uptake by normal thyroid tissue remnants and thyroid cancer metastases (46,67,83,95,115). The increased uptake may be caused by prolonged ^{131}I retention. This prolonged retention also results in an increased whole-body and blood radiation dose; therefore, iodine depletion techniques should be used with caution.

Thyroglobulin

Thyroglobulin is produced by the thyroid gland only. Serum thyroglobulin levels are elevated in most patients with differentiated thyroid cancer before surgery, in most patients with follicular adenoma, and in some patients with other benign thyroid diseases. An elevated thyroglobulin level, therefore, cannot differentiate benign from malignant lesions preoperatively; very high levels of thyroglobulin suggest metastatic thyroid cancer (68). Athyrotic patients should not have circulating thyroglobulin.

The half-life of thyroglobulin is around 65 hours and takes nearly 1 month to clear the body after total thyroidectomy. Thyroglobulin antibodies are detected in about 20% of patients with thyroid cancer and interfere with the thyroglobulin assay, either underestimating or overestimating, based on the method of thyroglobulin determination. Thyroglobulin antibodies may resolve during 1 to 4 years after becoming athyreotic, but may not resolve at all. Increasing thyroglobulin antibodies can be a sign of residual or recurrent disease (155).

In patients with differentiated thyroid cancer after total thyroidectomy, the presence of serum thyroglobulin should indicate recurrent or residual thyroid neoplasm (67). Many studies have compared serum thyroglobulin levels and ^{131}I whole-body imaging for detecting recurrent disease (15,26,28,37,87,124). Thyroglobulin levels may be assessed whether or not the patient is receiving suppressive thyroid hormones. Nonsuppressed thyroglobulin values are not significantly greater than suppressed values in patients without residual disease. In patients with residual neoplasm, nonsuppressed values increase as the serum TSH level increases.

In 80% to 85% of patients, the thyroglobulin levels and ^{131}I imaging results agree, with abnormal ^{131}I scans seen in patients with elevated thyroglobulin levels; the reverse also holds. In 15% to 20% of cases, the results do not agree. Elevated thyroglobulin levels with normal ^{131}I scan results are believed to reflect greater sensitivity of the serum thyroglobulin for occult disease that is not detectable with imaging (3,13,15,87,127). However, Pineda et al. (113) have advocated the use of ^{131}I therapy for thyroid cancer patients with elevated thyroglobulin levels and negative diagnostic ^{131}I scans. They treated 17 patients with ^{131}I whose diagnostic scans were negative but whose serum thyroglobulin levels were elevated. In half of their patients, the serum thyroglobulin level normalized after treatment

with [131]I. Normal serum thyroglobulin levels occur in conjunction with an abnormal ^{131}I scan in 1.5% of patients and probably reflect some decrease in tumor function or tumor differentiation. However, Lubin et al. (90) demonstrated no instance of a positive whole-body scan with a negative serum thyroglobulin level in 58 patients.

Patients with bone and lung metastases tend to have the highest thyroglobulin levels. Patients with lymph node metastases have the lowest thyroglobulin levels (67,127).

Serum thyroglobulin assay is useful for most patients with differentiated cancer who have had a total thyroidectomy by surgery alone or by surgery with ^{131}I ablation. The value of thyroglobulin assays for patients with residual normal thyroid tissue is limited. Serial thyroglobulin levels should be obtained in all patients after total thyroidectomy to assist in their follow-up; these levels can be measured while the patient is receiving full suppressive thyroid medication. In patients who do not have thyroglobulin antibodies, rhTSH-stimulated thyroglobulin is a very sensitive method to identify recurrences early, once a whole-body ^{131}I scan after ablation or treatment is negative, and will identify recurrences that are several millimeters in size. This is becoming a very important tool in the long-term monitoring of patients with thyroid cancer.

Medullary and anaplastic cancers do not secrete thyroglobulin. Therefore, serum thyroglobulin levels cannot be used to monitor the clinical status of these patients (64).

Medullary Thyroid Cancer

Optimal management of medullary thyroid cancer involves early removal of the tumor, especially because localized medullary thyroid cancer has the capacity to metastasize early, whether or not the patient develops a virulent form of the disease. A schema for the evaluation and management of patients with medullary thyroid cancer is presented in Figure 47.7.

The surgical management and postoperative follow-up are similar for patients with spontaneous or familial medullary thyroid cancer. The operative procedure of choice is total thyroidectomy, especially because all patients with the hereditary form of medullary thyroid cancer have bilateral involvement of the thyroid. Even if tumor is seen only on microscopic examination (i.e., C-cell hyperplasia or microinvasive medullary thyroid cancer), the disease is usually multifocal. Because clinically occult medullary thyroid cancer that is grossly visible on cut section of the thyroid may have regional lymph node metastases, all lymph nodes in the central zone of the neck, from the hyoid bone to the sternal notch and laterally to the jugular veins, are resected. In patients with macroscopic lymph node involvement, a modified radical neck dissection is performed. More extensive local surgery has not been shown to be more efficacious.

The C cells in medullary thyroid cancer do not concentrate iodine and are not part of the thyroid follicular apparatus. After total thyroidectomy, however, there may be remaining follicular cells whose trapping of iodine, particularly ^{131}I, is enhanced by the high levels of serum TSH.

Iodine-131 therapy may be a valuable treatment adjunct in patients with medullary thyroid cancer whose disease appears limited to the thyroid at the time of surgery and in whom calcitonin is elevated postoperatively, basally, or after calcium- or pentagastrin-stimulation testing. Irradiating residual medullary thyroid cancer cells with ^{131}I before local or distant spread occurs could eliminate local disease and perhaps improve survival (32,62,126). Iodine-131 (e.g., 150 mCi) has been used to treat local residual medullary thyroid cancer after total thyroidectomy (62). The philosophy is that ^{131}I is taken up by the follicular cells and irradiates the adjacent C cells. This suggests that the C cells are radiosensitive (32,62). Iodine-131 therapy usually is not appropriate for the treatment of metastases to lymph nodes,

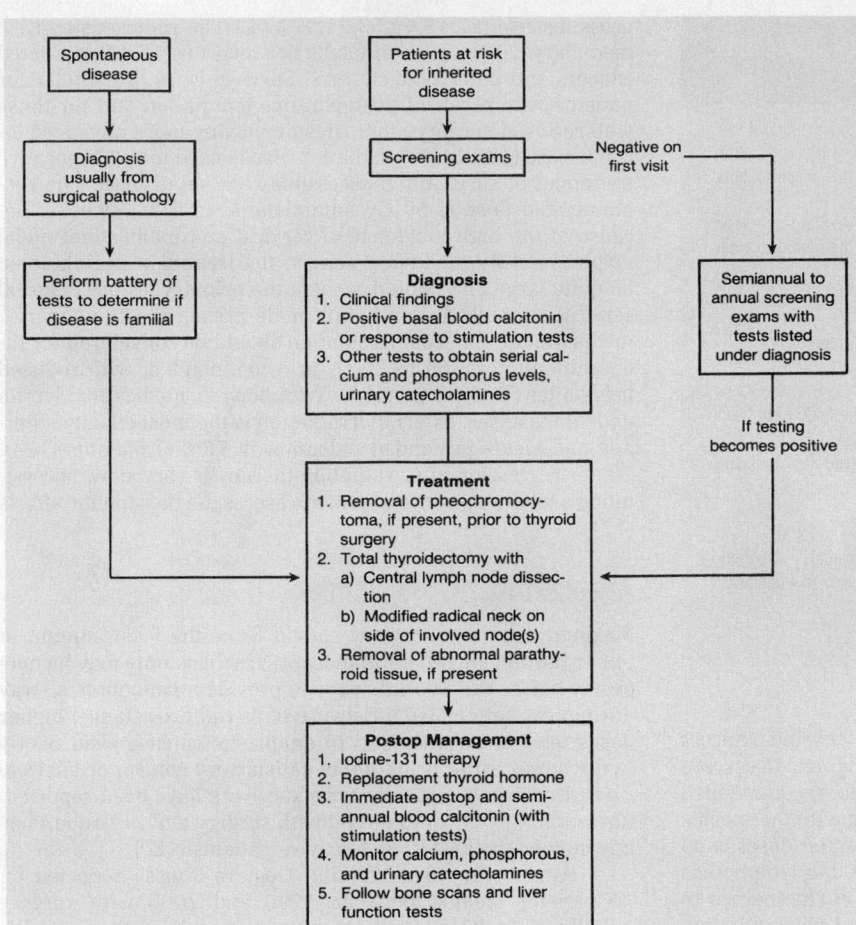

FIGURE 47.7. Schema for evaluation and management of sporadic and familial medullary thyroid cancer.

Clinical Radiation Oncology

bone, liver, lungs, or other sites because such metastases lack follicular cells and contain only C cells (101).

After total thyroidectomy, maintenance thyroid hormone therapy must be instituted. Because the C cells in medullary thyroid cancer are not under the control of TSH, there is no rationale for administering doses of thyroid hormone that are large enough to suppress TSH production, as is done for differentiated thyroid cancer.

Anaplastic Thyroid Cancer

Patients treated with combined surgery, irradiation, and chemotherapy appear to have the best results. Although the numbers were small, two factors seem significant in the group of survivors: they had a limited amount of disease, and all but one were treated with a combined therapeutic approach. The treatment of anaplastic cancer is discussed further in the next section.

Thyroid Lymphoma

Whereas excisional surgery and radiation therapy have resulted in a favorable outcome when non-Hodgkin's lymphoma is confined to the thyroid gland, controversy persists regarding the potential advantage of aggressive debulking over diagnostic biopsy alone when disease cannot be completely resected. In 62 patients who underwent primary surgery for non-Hodgkin's thyroid lymphoma, 50 patients had stage IE or IIE disease (116). Overall survival rates were 53% and 46% at 5 and 10 years, respectively; overall survival rates were 80% for stage IE confined to the thyroid, 58% for stage IE–extrathyroid, 50% for stage IIE, and 36% for stages IIIE and IVE, all at 5 years. Com-

plete remission was achieved in 88% of patients who underwent diagnostic biopsy plus adjuvant therapy alone, compared with 85% of patients in whom debulking plus adjuvant therapy was used. There was no difference in cause-specific survival between these two groups or between two subgroups who achieved complete remission. Relapse after complete remission occurred in 12 (26%) of 45 patients, only 2 of whom achieved long-term survival after salvage therapy. The role of surgery in non-Hodgkin's thyroid lymphoma is diminishing, and advances that further increase complete remission and relapse-free survival probably will not involve more aggressive surgical resections.

Matsuzuka et al. (93) described the clinical aspects of primary thyroid lymphoma. Treatment of thyroid lymphoma does not require resection of all lymphoma tissue or total thyroidectomy. The authors' successful treatment was radiation therapy combined with six courses of CHOP chemotherapy (cyclophosphamide, Adriamycin, vincristine, prednisolone). This mode of therapy improved the 8-year survival rate to almost 100%, regardless of the histologic type of malignancy.

Radiation Therapy Techniques

In contrast to ^{131}I, which is used for diagnosis and therapy for distant metastases of many thyroid cancers, external radiation therapy is effective for locoregional control of disease and in selected metastatic sites. External radiation therapy can be used alone or in combination with ^{131}I and is well tolerated. The indications for external irradiation in thyroid cancers are listed in Table 47.4.

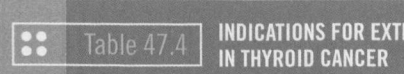

Table 47.4	**INDICATIONS FOR EXTERNAL IRRADIATION IN THYROID CANCER**

1. Primary therapy of thyroid cancer if unresectable locally, particularly if ^{131}I does not concentrate in tumor
2. Bulky tumor (e.g., mediastinal disease) large enough that it is uncontrollable by ^{131}I alone
3. Residual bulky tumor in the central neck, tracheal, and/or esophageal area or cervical nodal regions after thyroid surgery and removal of malignant cervical adenopathy that may not be controlled by ^{131}I alone
4. Skeletal metastases
   a. Concentration of ^{131}I small or absent
   b. Concern about a pathologic fracture, regardless of the degree of ^{131}I concentration
5. Brain metastases
6. Hepatic metastases if symptomatic or other treatment methods have been unsuccessfulg
7. Relief of pressure symptoms occurring in vital areas caused by soft-tissue masses
8. Superior vena cava syndrome
9. Continually recurring thyroid cancer regardless of ^{131}I accumulation
10. Recurrent or metastatic thyroid cancer occurring after maximal ^{131}I therapy
11. In sequence or conjunction with chemotherapy, particularly in anaplastic cancer
12. Preoperative therapy

Definitive external radiation therapy for thyroid cancers requires careful treatment planning because high doses are needed and serious injuries may occur. The recommended treatments can be found in the sections dealing with the specific tumor types. In general, carcinomas require higher doses of up to 60 to 70 Gy administered in about 7 weeks, but lymphomas need only about 30 to 36 Gy if combined with chemotherapy to 45 Gy in 4.5 to 5 weeks if patients are treated with radiation therapy alone.

IMRT is a developing technology that allows for improved coverage of the thyroid bed region, cervical and mediastinal lymph node regions at risk with sparing of critical normal tissues, for example, the spinal cord (109) (see Fig. 47.2)

A recent article from Memorial Sloan Kettering Cancer Center (123) reviewed a series of 20 patients treated between July 2001 and January 2004 with IMRT for nonanaplastic thyroid cancer. Doses used were 54 Gy to low-risk clinical target volume for microscopic disease (all regions of neck and superior mediastinum with negative pathology) and 59.4 to 63 Gy to high-risk clinical target volume (thyroid bed and areas of positive nodes). Areas of positive margins were treated to 63 to 66 Gy and areas of gross disease were treated to 63 to 70 Gy, with the dose later in the series 67.5 to 70 Gy. Planning target volume was expanded around the clinical target volume by 3 to 10 mm. Parotid gland dose was limited to 26 Gy, larynx to 70 Gy, and spinal cord to 45 Gy. With a median follow-up of 13 months (range, 1 to 28 months), two patients developed infield recurrence, both of whom had gross residual disease. One patient was treated to a total dose of 63 Gy, and the second was treated to 67.5 Gy at 2.25 Gy/fraction. Their 2-year progression-free survival rate was 85%. Six patients have died, four of metastatic disease. Acute side effects included acute mucositis and pharyngitis, skin toxicity, larynx toxicity, and L'Hermitte syndrome. Four patients required percutaneous gastrostomy (PEG) feeding tubes. Long-term side effects included pneumonitis, xerostomia, chronic dysphagia, and altered taste.

Medullary Thyroid Cancer

The effectiveness of external irradiation for medullary cancer is still controversial, but recent data indicate that it can be used in the curative treatment of patients with microscopic residual or gross disease (27,48,49,53,91,99,134). The radiosensitivity of medullary cancer probably falls between that of differentiated cancers and anaplastic cancers. Survival rates are similar for patients who received postoperative irradiation and for those who received surgery alone, despite having more advanced local disease (125,149). Irradiation also is used for postoperative treatment of surgically inaccessible residual disease. The recommended dose is 60 Gy administered in 6 to 7 weeks. Because of the high incidence of cervical and mediastinal nodal involvement by medullary cancer, the treatment portals must be quite large and should include the primary lesion, bilateral cervical supraclavicular lymph node areas, and the superior mediastinum. External irradiation should be considered for inoperable tumors; 65 to 70 Gy is recommended, with reduced fields after 55 to 60 Gy (135). With bony or mediastinal lymph node metastases, external irradiation is the most effective therapy and yields prolonged palliation in 75% of patients (124). Tumor regression after radiation therapy is very slow, necessitating a follow-up of many years to assess the therapeutic effects (124).

Anaplastic Thyroid Cancer

Maximal debulking surgery should leave the least amount of tumor burden for radiation therapy. Tracheostomy may be necessary before radiation therapy to provide an adequate airway during irradiation (107). Because of its radioresistance, higher doses tend to be delivered to anaplastic cancer; even 60 Gy in 6 weeks cannot bring about satisfactory control or survival rates. However, a few long-term survivors have been reported. Chemotherapy in combination with surgery and radiation therapy may be the best hope for these patients (120).

A recent study from Institut Gustave-Roussy reported on 30 patients treated between 1990 and 2000 with surgery initially, if feasible, chemotherapy with two cycles of Adriamycin/cisplatinum, followed by hyperfractionated radiotherapy, delivering 1.25 Gy twice daily to a total dose of 40 Gy, then four additional cycles of the same chemotherapy. If initially not feasible, surgery would be performed after completion of the chemo/radiotherapy if technically possible. Nineteen patients experienced complete local response at the end of this treatment regimen. Overall 1-year survival reported was 46%, and 3-year overall survival was 27%. Prognostic factors identified on multivariate analysis were tracheal extension (p =.03) and macroscopic complete resection (p =.04) (31).

Thyroid Lymphoma

Primary lymphoma of the thyroid gland is rare, comprising only 4% to 8% of all thyroid tumors and only 1.3% of all lymphomas. The predominant histologic type is diffuse histiocytic lymphoma; other types are poorly differentiated lymphocytic or mixed-cell lymphoma and Hodgkin's disease. As in other head and neck lymphomas, distant manifestation is common. Locally, the tumor may be quite bulky and may cause compression symptoms.

Treatment of thyroid lymphomas may involve the different modalities of surgery, radiation therapy, and chemotherapy. After a surgical procedure, postoperative radiation therapy of the neck and superior mediastinum to a minimum dose of 45 to 50 Gy should be adequate for local control of disease for most tumors. Among 91 cases of primary lymphomas of the thyroid treated between 1936 and 1996 at the Royal Marsden Hospital, the highest rates of local control and long-term survival were seen in patients who had complete surgical removal of gross tumor followed by radiation therapy (p <.005). This was in the earlier years. They were performing less extensive surgery in patients treated after 1990. Patients treated to doses of >40 Gy, when treated with radiation therapy alone as well as

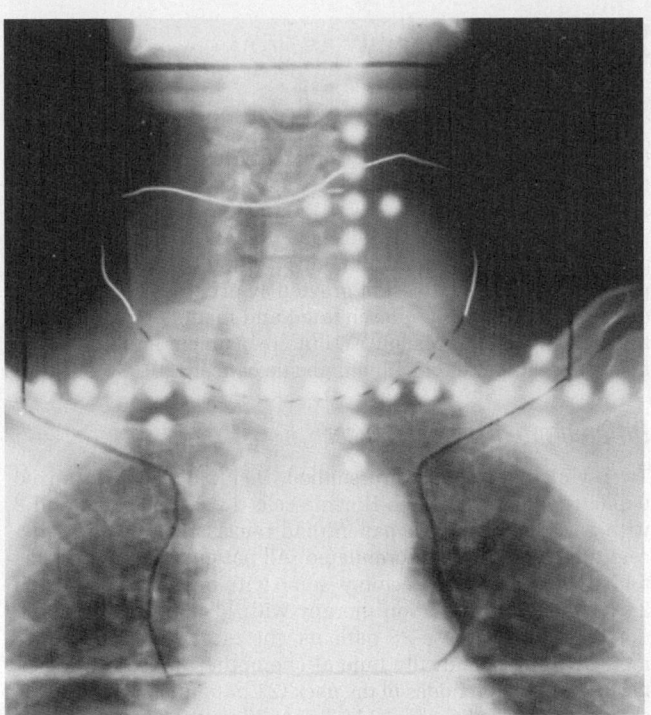

FIGURE 47.8. Anteroposterior simulation film of the initial large field, including the neck and mediastinum, in a patient with a large malignant lymphoma of the thyroid.

treatment with extended-field radiation therapy versus involved-field radiation therapy had improved local control. Survival was improved in the patients treated with extended-field radiation therapy when compared with involved-field radiation therapy (58). For tumors with adverse prognostic factors, such as large bulk, fixation, extracapsular extension, or retrosternal extension, Tupchong et al. (150) recommended the addition of chemotherapy because of the high risk of distant disease and local failure (Fig. 47.8).

Blair et al. (16) described their experience with 38 patients with primary thyroid lymphoma treated at the Mayo Clinic between 1965 and 1979. All patients were irradiated to approximately 40 Gy (range, 24 to 60 Gy) to the neck alone or to the neck and mediastinum. The 5-year disease-free survival rate was 59%. Patients with no gross residual disease at the beginning of radiation therapy had the least likelihood of recurrence. For stage IE and IIE primary thyroid lymphomas, they suggested that the radiation portal should include the neck, axillae, and mediastinum to a dose of 40 Gy.

Vigliotti et al. (154) treated a series of patients with stage IE and IIE thyroid lymphomas at the M.D. Anderson Cancer Center. Of 38 patients, 29 received radiation therapy: 15 alone and 14 in combination with chemotherapy. All patients received 40 Gy to the neck and upper mediastinum and 30 to 35 Gy to the lower mediastinum in 20 fractions during 4 weeks with cobalt teletherapy. The overall 5-year survival and disease-free survival rates were 72% and 64%, respectively. They concluded that radiation therapy alone was satisfactory for disease limited to the thyroid, with or without cervical adenopathy. However, they recommended combination chemotherapy for patients who had mediastinal tumor extensions.

A retrospective analysis of patients with primary malignant lymphoma of the thyroid was conducted by Logue et al. (89). A total of 32 patients with stage IE and 38 with stage IIE tumors were identified. A biopsy only was performed in 27 patients, lobectomy in 11 patients, subtotal thyroidectomy in 27 patients, and macroscopic thyroidectomy in 5 patients. All pa-

tients were treated with radiation therapy, but only two received chemotherapy. The overall relapse-free survival rate was 42%, with 60% for stage IE and 31% for stage IIE. Factors of prognostic significance for relapse and survival were stage, radiation therapy dose, stridor, retrosternal extension, and fixation.

Tsang et al. (147) retrospectively reviewed the records of patients treated at the Princess Margaret Hospital between 1978 and 1986. Of 39 patients with stage I or stage II disease, 18 were treated with radiation therapy alone, 3 with chemotherapy alone, and 18 with combined-modality therapy. Combined-modality therapy was used mainly in patients with large tumor bulk. The overall 5-year actuarial survival and cause-specific survival rates were 56% and 64%, respectively. The overall rate of relapse-free survival was 61% at 5 years. Among the 39 patients with stage I or stage II disease, 5-year actuarial survival, cause-specific survival, and relapse-free survival rates were 64%, 73%, and 66%, respectively. There were no significant differences in outcome between those treated with radiation therapy alone and those treated with combined-modality therapy (cause-specific survival, p = .25; relapse, p = .06). A univariate analysis showed that the only variable to reach statistical significance was tumor bulk. Age was marginally significant, but stage and histology were not statistically significant, possibly because of the fairly homogeneous distribution of patients in each of these variables. Patients with progression or relapse of lymphoma after initial treatment frequently died of disease. Isolated gastrointestinal relapses occurred in three cases, representing 27% of all relapses. Based on their findings that most patients with localized thyroid lymphoma require combined-modality therapy, the authors recommended radiation therapy alone only for a small, selected group of patients with stage I disease and small tumor bulk.

In an analysis of 211 patients with stage IE and IIE thyroid lymphoma treated at Yale, Doria et al. (35) concluded that the distant and overall relapse rates were significantly lower in patients receiving combined-modality therapy than in those receiving irradiation alone. Their analysis and review of the literature indicated that about 30% of patients with clinically localized disease will have distant relapse and that chemotherapy in addition to local irradiation can decrease the rates of distant and overall recurrence.

Sequelae of Therapy with Radioactive Iodine

Serious complications are rare after single doses of 200 mCi or less of ^{131}I (9,14,62). They are more common after larger single treatments or large cumulative doses. Van Nostrand et al. (152) reviewed the side effects of ^{131}I therapy for metastatic well-differentiated thyroid cancer after a mean follow-up of 15 months.

Early Sequelae

Early complications occur within 3 months of treatment. Acute illness (i.e., fatigue, headache, nausea, vomiting) may occur within 12 hours after administration of ^{131}I, but it occurs in fewer than 1% of patients.

Sialadenitis (i.e., swelling and pain in the salivary glands) occurs shortly after ^{131}I administration in about 5% to 10% of patients. It may last for a few days. This risk may be reduced by the use of lemon candy starting 48 hours after the administration of ^{131}-I, as shown in a recent article by Nagada et al. (104). This article showed a significant decrease in sialoadenitis, taste dysfunction, and xerostomia.

Edema of the neck after ^{131}I ablation of the thyroid has been reported (45). The clinical features of early neck edema after ^{131}I ablation are similar to those of angioneurotic edema. The neck edema responded well to corticosteroids.

Transient hyperthyroidism may occur after massive thyroid tissue destruction and subsequent release into circulation of large amounts of thyroid hormone. Thyroid storm is a potential complication in patients who are hyperthyroid from functioning metastatic disease (24,25,67,114,136). Pretreatment with antithyroid drugs, including β-adrenergic agents, can mediate the thyroid hormone storm after ^{131}I therapy (24). Patients with follicular thyroid cancer rarely may have hyperthyroidism produced by secretion of large amounts of thyroid hormone by the tumor.

Bone marrow suppression can be observed in almost all patients receiving ^{131}I therapy. Transient anemia, leukopenia, and thrombocytopenia have been reported (67). Permanent or severe marrow suppression has been reported with blood radiation doses greater than 2 Gy (86).

Transient vocal cord paralysis after ^{131}I ablation of residual thyroid gland after a near-total thyroidectomy has been reported (85). Pain, hemorrhage, and swelling in metastases after therapy presumably results from radiation-induced swelling and is analogous to radiation-associated thyroiditis (67). Sudden hemorrhage into functioning cerebral metastases and severe fatal cerebral edema in a patient with functioning cerebral metastases have been reported (67). Pretreatment with corticosteroids may avert serious complications of therapy, especially with brain metastases (64).

Long-Term Complications

Long-term complications are those that occur 3 months or longer after treatment. Radiation pneumonitis and pulmonary fibrosis have been associated with ^{131}I therapy, especially in the setting of diffuse-functioning lung metastases. To prevent radiation pneumonitis in this circumstance, a maximum of 80 mCi ^{131}I can be retained in the whole body 48 hours after treatment. Pneumonitis and pulmonary fibrosis may be managed with corticosteroids.

Permanent bone marrow suppression is rare. It occurs primarily in patients who received large cumulative doses of ^{131}I for bone metastases (67).

Leukemia as a complication of ^{131}I therapy is rare (<2%) (10,67). Patients who receive the largest amount of [131]I (>500 mCi total dose) in the shortest time interval appear to be the most susceptible to leukemia, especially if older than 50 years of age (67,158). Acute myelogenous leukemia is the most frequent type. Some authorities suggest waiting 1 year between ^{131}I therapies if the clinical situation is stable, but others suggest a 6- to 12-month interval (87).

Some authors have suggested that treatment with ^{131}I or external irradiation may be responsible for the occasional transformation of differentiated thyroid cancer to anaplastic cancer (67). However, Mazzaferri (97) and Mazzaferri et al. (98) found that more than half of the patients who developed anaplastic cancers had not received ^{131}I therapy. This finding suggests that the anaplastic transformation may relate more to the natural history of thyroid cancer (159).

Ovarian failure and azoospermia have been reported in patients after treatment with [131]I. In a series of patients previously treated with ^{131}I for thyroid cancer before the age of 20 years, there were no differences in infertility, miscarriage rate, prematurity, or congenital abnormalities compared with the general population (33,57,58). A recent review article suggests the testicular dose from 3.7 GBq (100 mCi) is 0.5 to 1.5 Gy per treatment, the dose that has been associated with azoospermia in animals (81).

Chemotherapy

Single-Agent Chemotherapy

Of 53 patients with thyroid cancer treated with doxorubicin (Adriamycin), about one-third achieved significant tumor regression and prolonged survival. Pulmonary metastasis was the most commonly responsive disease, followed by bone and regional metastatic disease in the neck. Another one third of the patients manifested arrest of previously progressive metastatic disease. Patients with differentiated and medullary cancer had the most significant responses, but doxorubicin had limited effectiveness in patients with anaplastic cancer (20).

Differentiated Thyroid Cancer

Twenty-eight patients were studied, including 10 with mixed papillary-follicular, 9 with Hürthle cell, 6 with follicular, and 2 with papillary cancer; 1 patient had unclassified primary thyroid tumor that was differentiated. All patients had undergone total or subtotal thyroidectomy (some with neck dissection) and 24 had received radiation therapy with ^{131}I, external irradiation, or both. In these 28 patients, the most common sites of metastatic disease at the time of chemotherapy were the soft tissues and lymph nodes of the neck (21 patients), the lungs, the skeleton, and the liver (1,3,11). Ten of 28 patients achieved partial remission of disease. The median duration of response and survival from initiation of chemotherapy was 8 and 17 months, respectively. Partial remissions occurred in four patients with mixed papillary-follicular cancer, in three with Hürthle cell cancer, in two with follicular cancer, and in the one patient with unclassified tumor. Median duration of survival for the 11 patients with no change in their disease was 12 months. Seven patients showed progressive disease despite doxorubicin chemotherapy; the median survival in these patients was only 6 months.

Medullary Thyroid Cancer

Seven patients (six men and one woman) with medullary thyroid cancer previously treated with thyroid surgery, neck dissection, ^{131}I, or external irradiation in various combinations were given doxorubicin. The median duration of disease before initiation of chemotherapy and the subsequent survival time were 36 and 19 months, respectively. Of the seven patients, three achieved a partial response of disease lasting 2, 21, and 39 months; another three patients showed no change for 4, 6, and 9 months. One patient died only 3 days after beginning chemotherapy and was considered an early death (20).

Anaplastic Thyroid Cancer

In 18 patients (median age, 68 years) with anaplastic cancer treated with doxorubicin, the median duration of disease from the time of diagnosis to chemotherapy was 4 months. Only 4 of the 18 patients showed any significant response to doxorubicin; 3 other patients had no change in their disease for brief periods (20). Median survival time was 2 months; six patients died within 3 weeks of beginning therapy, and two survived beyond 24 months from the initiation of therapy (28 and 38 months).

Multimodality Therapy

Anaplastic giant and spindle cell cancers are extremely malignant and seldom are controlled with radiation therapy alone. Chemotherapy has been advocated for this type of thyroid cancer (76–78). Tallroth et al. (143) reported the Swedish experience with anaplastic giant cell cancer at the Radiumhemmet. Of nine patients who received a three-drug program of bleomycin, cyclophosphamide, and 5-fluorouracil plus radiation therapy, only one patient (11%) survived (and lived 12 more years). Another group of 25 patients received three-drug chemotherapy and two-fractions-per-day radiation therapy. Three patients (12%) were free of disease, and the remaining 22 patients died of local disease and metastases. A third group of patients had preoperative and postoperative irradiation, three-drug chemotherapy, and surgery during remission, and the survival rate beyond 3 years was 12% (3 of 24 patients). The most recent protocol was that of weekly doxorubicin and radiation therapy; one of five patients remained alive longer than 10 months after treatment.

In 1987, Kim and Leeper (78) updated a report on a prospective protocol at Memorial Sloan-Kettering Cancer Center. Since 1979, 41 patients with locally advanced thyroid cancers were treated with a combination of low-dose doxorubicin and EBRT. Group 1 consisted of 22 patients with well-differentiated papillary, follicular, or mixed-type tumors. They received doxorubicin (10 mg/m^2) once a week before radiation therapy, which was given at a daily dose of 2 Gy, 5 days per week, to a total dose of 56 Gy. Group 2 had 19 patients with anaplastic giant and spindle cell cancers. They were given the same dose of doxorubicin but received their radiation twice a day, 3 days per week, at 1.6 Gy per fraction to a total dose of 57.6 Gy in 40 days. Local control rates at 2 years were 77% and 68%, respectively. Median survival was 4 years for group 1 and 1 year for group 2.

The use of debulking surgery in combination with hyperfractionated radiation therapy and low-dose doxorubicin has not been tested adequately in prospective, randomized studies. The literature continues to support this approach as the standard treatment regimen for these patients, however, and it may result in a 5-year survival rate of about 10% (88,144,145,153).

Patient Surveillance

Because the prognosis of patients with recurrent well-differentiated thyroid carcinoma is poor, it is assumed that the outcome for therapy of recurrent thyroid carcinoma will be better if the recurrence is detected early rather than late. Therefore, aggressive, long-term surveillance of these patients is necessary because recurrences may occur up to 40 years after the initial diagnosis of thyroid carcinoma.

Follow-up screening protocols for patients with differentiated thyroid carcinoma are not uniform and in general are constricted arbitrarily. Most studies have not addressed a specific long-term follow-up program; instead, they have assessed the efficacy of one or two tests in detecting persistent and recurrent disease. These tests include chest x-ray, bone scintigraphy, thallium-201 scintigraphy, ^{131}I scintigraphy, CT, MRI, ultrasonography, FDG-PET, and serum thyroglobulin determinations.

The current guidelines of the National Comprehensive Cancer Network (104) recommend long-term surveillance and maintenance with diagnostic whole-body ^{131}I scans and serum thyroglobulin measurements (in patients without serum antithyroglobulin antibodies) on a yearly basis until a negative scan is obtained, followed by annual thyroglobulin and antithyroglobulin antibodies. This recommendation is based on a study by Grigsby et al. (53), who found that the predictive value for relapse-free survival of one negative diagnostic ^{131}I study was 91% but that the predictive value for relapse-free survival of two negative diagnostic ^{131}I studies was 97% (p = .0197).

A major drawback in the performance of diagnostic ^{131}I scintigraphy is that patients must discontinue their thyroid hormone therapy for 2 to 4 weeks. Patients typically develop symptomatic hypothyroidism. The consequences of these periods of short-term hypothyroidism may include impaired work performance, personal safety, and difficult interpersonal relationships. To avoid the consequences of hypothyroidism and improve patient care, recombinant human thyrotropin (rTSH) has been developed for routine clinical use. Haugen et al. (60) have reported the results of a study of the comparison of rTSH and thyroid hormone withdrawal for the detection of thyroid remnants or cancer. The authors concluded that recombinant human TSH administration is a safe and effective means of stimulating radioiodine uptake and serum thyroglobulin levels in patients undergoing evaluation for thyroid cancer persistence and recurrence. The use of rTSH now has become standard in the evaluation and management of some patients with thyroid cancer.

Outpatient ^{131}I Therapy

The NRC promulgated new rules in 1997 that allow patients undergoing therapy with radiopharmaceuticals or permanent radioactive implants to be sent home immediately following their treatment. The new regulations most significantly affect the treatment of thyroid disease (primarily thyroid cancer) with ^{131}I. These changes present health care providers with the opportunity to improve patients' psychological well-being and quality of life, reduce health care costs, and reduce the potential for radiation exposure of the patient care staff.

The new rule is contained within Section 10, Code of Federal Regulations, Part 35 (10 CFR 35) "Medical Uses of Byproduct Material." The specific changes are noted in section 35.75 "Release of Individuals Containing Radiopharmaceuticals or Permanent Implants." Briefly stated, the new rule permits health care providers (licensees) to authorize the release from their control any individual who has received a radiopharmaceutical or permanent implant containing radioactive materials if the total effective dose equivalent (TEDE) to any other individual from exposure to the released individual is not likely to exceed 5 mSv (500 mrem). There are three additional requirements imposed by the new ruling:

1. It is required by 10 CFR 35.75 (b) that the licensee "provide the released individual with instructions, including written instructions, on actions recommended to maintain doses to other individual As Low As is Reasonably Achievable (ALARA) if the TEDE is likely to exceed 1 mSv (100 mrem)."
2. 10 CFR 35.75 (c) requires that the licensee "maintain a record of the basis for authorizing the release of an individual, for 3 years after the date of release, if the TEDE is calculated by
   1) using the retained activity rather than the activity administered,
   2) using an occupancy factor less than 0.25 at 1 m,
   3) using the biological or effective half-life, or
   (4) considering the shielding by tissue."
3. In 10 CFR 35.75 (d), the licensee is required to "maintain a record, for 3 years after the date of release, that instructions were provided to a breast-feeding woman if the radiation dose to the infant or child from continued breast-feeding could result in a TEDE exceeding 5 mSv (500 mrem)."

NRC Regulatory Guide 8.39 lists several common radionuclides and the activities and dose rates for authorizing patient release. Patients who receive ^{131}I may be released immediately if the administered activity is less than 33 mCi or if the exposure rate at 1 m is less than 7 mrem per hour. If both of these conditions are exceeded, then other immediate release criteria must be documented in accordance with 10 CFR 35.75 (a). If the administering physician chooses not to use the new-release criteria, patients still may be admitted to the hospital until the radionuclide has decayed and their body burden has been documented to be less than 33 mCi or their exposure rate at 1 m is less than 7 mrem per hour.

An alternative criterion for immediate release is based on a patient-specific calculation regarding the TEDE to the maximally exposed individual. This dose must be calculated to be less than 5 mSv (500 mrem). The NRC recommends that the patient-specific calculations be incorporated into a three-component model for radioactive iodine pharmacokinetics in patients with thyroid disease as set forth in Regulatory Guide 8.39. This three-component model makes several assumptions, including that the elimination of ^{131}I during the first 8 hours after administration is due to physical decay only; thereafter, the decay kinetics are regulated by the thyroidal component of elimination and physical decay. Additional assumptions are set forth by the NRC related to the occupancy factor for the maximally exposed individual and the uptake fractions and biologic half-lives of the extrathyroidal component and the thyroidal component.

The State University of New York at Stony Brook policy is to determine a 48-hour whole-body retention of ^{131}I or 24-hour uptake using [123]I. This measurement is made with a thyroid uptake detector. This whole-body retention percentage is a very conservative assumption of the long-lived thyroidal component. This retention percentage is inserted into the equation for the three-component model and the dose to infinity to the maximally exposed individual is determined. The maximum ^{131}I activity that can be administered to a patient who is to be released immediately then can be determined such that the dose to infinity to maximally exposed individuals is less than 5 mSv (500 mrem). This administered activity is determined easily from a graph of activities based on the whole-body retention percentage (Fig. 47.9). In practice, it is not uncommon to administer activities of 100 mCi to 250 mCi on an outpatient basis. Patients are admitted to the hospital for ^{131}I administration in the rare instance of medical necessity (i.e., hemodialysis, inability to comply with radiation precautions).

Although the NRC now allows for the administration of large amounts of ^{131}I on an outpatient basis, some physicians have been reluctant to adopt this policy. There is concern that the radiation exposure to household members of the patient will be excessive. Grigsby et al. (52) performed a study to measure the radiation exposure to household members from patients receiving outpatient ^{131}I therapy for thyroid carcinoma in accordance with the new NRC regulations. The study included 30 patients who received outpatient ^{131}I therapy following thyroidectomy for well-differentiated thyroid carcinoma. The study also included 65 household members and 17 household pets (dogs and cats). The main outcome measure of the study was to determine the radiation exposure to household members, pets, and four rooms in each home, as monitored with dosimeters for 10 days following ^{131}I administration. The patients received ^{131}I doses ranging from 76 to 150 mCi [131]I (mean, 116 mCi). The radiation dose to 65 household members ranged from 1 to 109 mrem (mean, 24 mrem). The dose to the 17 household pets ranged from 2 to 111 mrem (mean, 37 mrem). The mean dose to the four rooms ranged from 17 mrem (kitchen) to 58 mrem (bedroom). The authors concluded that ^{131}I doses to household members of patients receiving outpatient ^{131}I therapy were well below the limit (500 mrem) mandated by the new NRC regulations.

Appendix 47.1: Procedures for Administration of [131]I

Planning

Order ^{131}I at least 24 hours in advance. Schedule the patient for hospital admission.

Room Preparation

Cover the following with plastic bags: telephone receiver, telephone, food table, basin faucet handles, nurse call set, floor, toilet seat, and shower handles. Place radiation waste containers in the room for laundry and foods/paper.

Patient Preparation

Instruct the patient to wear foot coverings when ambulating. Instruct the patient to keep outside door closed and bathroom

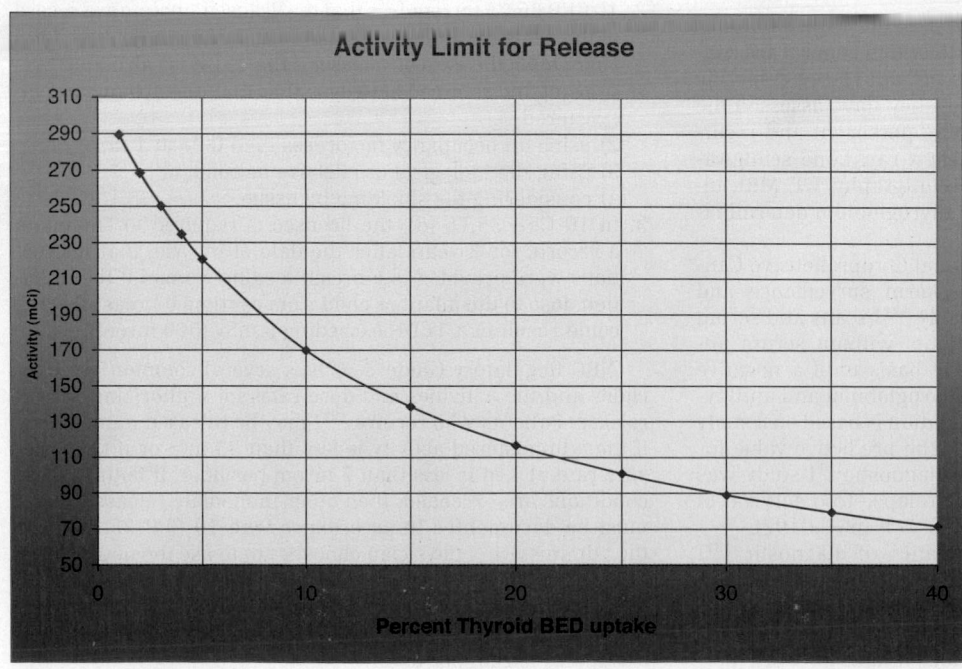

FIGURE 47.9. Graph showing relationship between percent uptake on thyroid carcinoma survey and maximal permissible dose for ^{131}I therapy on an outpatient basis.

door open at all times. Obtain vital signs and blood and urine samples (if needed) before ¹³¹I administration.

Administration

If administering liquid ¹³¹I, the patient must wear hospital gown with a "chuck" around neck and in lap. Personnel administering ¹³¹I should wear gown, gloves, and mask. Vial containing ¹³¹I should be vented in nuclear medicine hood to allow any volatile ¹³¹I to escape just before administration, if possible. During administration, the patient should sit on the side of the bed in front of the ¹³¹I, which is in a lead vial on a covered table. Open vial with T-bar, insert drinking straw, and put small amount of water in vial (along straw so it does not splash). Patient takes ¹³¹I through straw with additional water placed in lead vial to remove as much ¹³¹I as possible. Then the patient should swish and swallow several cups of water to rinse ¹³¹I from oral cavity. Do not remove straw from vial; bend it over and carefully place lead cap on to cover.

If administering ¹³¹I capsule, the patient is handed a container with the capsule and a moisture pack present within. The patient is instructed to verify his or her name is on the vial, then take the pill (not the moisture pack) and return the closed container to the physician.

Initial Survey

Within 15 minutes, measure the radiation exposure rate at 1 m from the midline of the patient's abdomen in both anteroposterior and lateral directions. Calculate the average. Patient may be released when same readings show less than 30 mCi of ¹³¹I or less than 7 mR/hour at 1 m, which is usually about 24 to 48 hours after 100 mCi was given, but is variable. An inventory or survey form with initial activity and exposure rate, nursing instructions, and decontamination form should be posted on the room door. Do not collect urine unless lead container is available and there is a specific reason to collect it.

Safety

At less than 30 mCi ¹³¹I (or exposure rate of 7 mr/hour at 1 m), discharge the patient.

Visiting is discouraged: limit to 0.5 hr/day per visitor; no pregnant women or children younger than 18 years should be allowed to visit. Visitors should sit in a designated chair across the room. If they come close to the patient, they should sit behind a lead shield. They should drink copious amounts of water to speed release of unused radioactivity, shower frequently, particularly before survey is performed so that ¹³¹I in clothing and on skin is not measured, and flush toilet several times after each use. Male patients should urinate seated. There should be no personal items except those to be disposed of at discharge. After discharge, patients should practice good personal hygiene for 1 to 2 days. Do not hold children closely for 2 to 3 days.

References

1. Abe Y, Ichikawa Y, Muraki T, et al. Thyrotropin (TSH) receptor and adenylate cyclase activity in human thyroid tumors: absence of high affinity receptor and loss of TJH responsiveness in undifferentiated thyroid carcinoma. *J Clin Endocrinol Metab* 1981;52:23–28.
2. Ampil FL. Postoperative external irradiation in thyroid carcinoma: a clinical experience of 20 treated patients and literature radiotherapy review. *J Surg Oncol* 1985;30:83–90.
3. Ashcraft MW, Van Herle AJ. The comparative value of serum thyroglobulin measurements and iodine 131 total body scans in the follow-up study of patients with treated differentiated thyroid cancer. *Am J Med* 1981;71:806–814.
4. Auffermann W, Clark OH, Thurnher S, et al. Recurrent thyroid carcinoma: characteristics on MR images. *Radiology* 1988;168:753–757.
5. Bal C, Padhy AK, Jana S, et al. Prospective randomized clinical trial to evaluate the optimal dose of 131I for remnant ablation in patients with differentiated thyroid carcinoma. *Cancer* 1996;77:2574–2580.
6. Balachandran S, Sayle BA. Value of thyroid carcinoma imaging after therapeutic doses of radioiodine. *Clin Nucl Med* 1981; 6:162–166.
7. Bandi P, Barber S, Boone M et al. Cancer Facts and Figures 2006. American Cancer Society. Available at: http://222.cancer.org/downloads/STT/CAFF2006pwsecured.pdf. Accessed March 1, 2006.
8. Becker DV, Hurley JR. Current status of radioiodine (I-131) treatment of hyperthyroidism. In: Freeman LH, Weissman HS, eds. *Nuclear medicine annual.* New York: Raven Press; 1982.
9. Becker DV, Hurley JR, Motazedi, et al. Ablation of postsurgical thyroid remnants in patients with differentiated thyroid cancer can be achieved with less whole body radiation. *J Nucl Med* 1982; 23:43(abstr).
10. Beierwaltes W. The treatment of thyroid carcinoma with radioactive iodine. *Semin Nucl Med* 1978;8:79–94.
11. Beierwaltes WH, Nishiyama RH, Thompson NW, et al. Survival time and "cure" in papillary and follicular thyroid carcinoma with distant metastases: statistics following University of Michigan therapy. *J Nucl Med* 1982;23:561–568.
12. Beierwaltes WH, Rabbani R, Dmuchowski, et al. An analysis of "ablation of thyroid remnants" with I-131 in 511 patients from 1947—1984: experience at the University of Michigan. *J Nucl Med* 1984;25:1287–1293.
13. Black EG, Cassoni A, Gimlette TM, et al. Serum thyroglobulin in thyroid cancer. *Lancet* 1981;2:443–445.
14. Blahd W. Nuclear medicine therapy of thyroid cancer. In: Thawley S, Panje W, Batsakis J, et al, eds. *Comprehensive management of head and neck tumors.* Philadelphia: WB Saunders; 1987.
15. Blahd WH, Drickman MV, Porter CW, et al. Serum thyroglobulin, a monitor of differentiated thyroid cancer in patients receiving thyroid hormone suppression therapy [concise communication]. *J Nucl Med* 1984;25:673.
16. Blair TJ, Evans RG, Buskirk GJ, et al. Radiotherapeutic management of primary thyroid lymphoma. *Int J Radiat Oncol Biol Phys* 1985;11:365.
17. Brendel AJ, Guyot M, Jeandot R, et al. Thallium-201 imaging in the follow-up of differentiated thyroid carcinoma. *J Nucl Med* 1988;29:1515–1520.
18. Brennan MD, Bergstralh EJ, van Heerden JA, et al. Follicular thyroid cancer treated at the Mayo Clinic, 1946 through 1970: Initial manifestations, pathologic findings, therapy, and outcome. *Mayo Clin Proc* 1991;66:11–22.
19. Brown AP, Greening WP, McCready VR, et al. Radioiodine treatment of metastatic thyroid carcinoma in the Royal Marsden Hospital experience. *Br J Radiol* 1984;57:323.
20. Burgess MA, Hill GS Jr. Chemotherapy in the management of thyroid cancer. In: Greenfield LD, ed. *Thyroid cancer.* Boca Raton, FL: CRC Press; 1978.
21. Cady B, Sedgwick CE, Meissner WA, et al. Changing clinical, pathologic, therapeutic and survival patterns in differentiated thyroid carcinoma. *Ann Surg* 1976; 184:541.
22. Cady B, Sedgwick CE, Meissner WA, et al. Risk factor analysis in differentiated thyroid cancer. *Cancer* 1979;43:810–820.
23. Castronovo FP.Jr. Iodine-131 thyroid burdens of European travelers returning to Boston after the Chernobyl accident [letter]. *N Engl J Med* 1986;315:1679.
24. Cerletty JM, Listwan WJ. Hyperthyroidism due to functioning metastatic thyroid carcinoma: precipitation of thyroid storm with therapeutic radioactive iodine. *JAMA* 1979;242:269.
25. Chapman CN, Sziklas JJ, Spencer RP, et al. Hyperthyroidism with metastatic follicular thyroid carcinoma. *J Nucl Med* 1984;25:466.
26. Charles MA. Comparison of serum thyroglobulin with iodine scans in thyroid cancer. *J Endocrinol Invest* 1982;5:267–271.
27. Chung CT, Sagerman RH, Ryoo MC. External irradiation for malignant thyroid tumors. *Radiology* 1980;136:753–756.
28. Colacchio TA, LoGerfo P, Calacchio DA, et al. Radioiodine total body scan versus serum thyroglobulin levels in follow-up of patients with thyroid cancer. *Surgery* 1982;91:42.
29. Cooper DS, Doherty GM, Haughn BR, et al. Management guidelines for patients with thyroid nodules and differentiated thyroid cancers. *Thyroid* 2006;16:1–33.
30. Cripa F, Alessi A, Geralli A et al. FDG PET in thyroid cancer. *Tumori* 2003;89:540–543,2003.
31. De Crevoisier R, BAudin E, Bachelot A et al. Combined treatment of anaplastic thyroid carcinoma with surgery, chemotherapy and hyperfractionated accelerated external radiotherapy. *Int J Radiat Oncol Biol Phys* 2004;60;1137–1143.
32. Deftos IJ, Stein MF. Radioiodine as an adjunct to the surgical treatment of medullary thyroid carcinoma. *J Clin Endocrinol Metab* 1980;50:967.
33. Degroot L, Reilly M. Comparison of 30- and 50-mCi doses of Iodine-131 for thyroid ablation. *Ann Intern Med* 1982;96:51–53.
34. Dobyns BM, Maloof K. The study and treatment of 199 cases of carcinoma of the thyroid with radioactive iodine. *J Clin Endocrinol* 1951;11:1323.
35. Doria R, Jekel J, Cooper DL. Thyroid lymphoma. *Cancer* 1994;73:200–206.
36. Dottorini ME, Assi A, Sironi M, et al. Multivariate analysis of patients with medullary thyroid carcinoma. *Cancer* 1996;77:1556–1565.
37. Echenique RL, Kasi L, Haynie TP, et al. Critical evaluation of serum thyroglobulin levels and I-131 scans in posttherapy patients with differentiated thyroid carcinoma [concise communication]. *J Nucl Med* 1982;23:235.
38. Endo K, Shiomi K, Kasagi K, et al. Imaging of medullary thyroid cancer with 131-I-MIBC. *Lancet* 1984;2:233.
39. Farahati J, Reiners C, Stuschke M, et al. Differentiated thyroid cancer. *Cancer* 1996;77:172–180.
40. Favus MJ, Schneider AB, Stachura ME, et al. Thyroid cancer occurring as a late consequence of head-and-neck irradiation. Evaluation of 1056 patients. *N Engl J Med* 1976;294:1019–1025.
41. Fleming ID, Cooper JS, Henson DE, et al. *AJCC cancer staging manual*, 5th ed. Philadelphia: Lippincott-Raven; 1997.
42. Frankenthaler RA, Sellin RV, Cangir A, et al. Lymph node metastasis from papillary-follicular thyroid carcinoma in young patients. *Am J Surg* 1990;160:341–343.
43. Gharib H, Goellner JR. Fine-needle aspiration biopsy of the thyroid: an appraisal. *Ann Intern Med* 1993;118:282–289.
44. Goepfert H, Dichtel WJ, Samaan NA. Thyroid cancer in children and teenagers. *Arch Otolaryngol* 1984;110:72–75.
45. Goolden AWG, Kam KC, Fitzpatrick ML, et al. Oedema of the neck after ablation of the thyroid with radioactive iodine. *Br J Radiol* 1986;59:583.
46. Goslings BM. Effect of a low iodine diet on I-131 therapy in follicular thyroid carcinomata. *J Endocrinol* 1975;64:30P(abstr).

47. Greenebaum E, Koss LG, Elequin F, et al. The diagnostic value of flow cytometric DNA measurements in follicular tumors of the thyroid gland. *Cancer* 1985;56:2011–2018.

48. Greenfield LD, George FW, III. The role of radiotherapy in the management of medullary thyroid cancer. *Int J Radiat Oncol Biol Phys* 1979;5[Suppl 1]:81.

49. Greenfield LD, Ucmakli A, George FW III, et al. The role of radiation therapy in the treatment of medullary thyroid cancer. *Contemp Surg* 1981;18:59.

50. Greene FL, Page DL, Fleming ID, et al., eds. *AJCC cancer staging manual*, 6th ed. New York: Springer-Verlag; 2002.

51. Greenspan FS. Radiation exposure and thyroid cancer. *JAMA* 1977;237:2089–2091.

52. Grigsby PG, Siegel BA, Baker S, et al. Radiation exposure from outpatient radioactive iodine (131I) therapy for thyroid carcinoma. *JAMA* 2000;283:2272–2274.

53. Grigsby PW, Baglan K, Siegel BA. Surveillance of patients to detect recurrent thyroid cancer. *Cancer* 1999;85:945–951.

54. Halnan KF. The non-surgical treatment of thyroid cancer. *Br J Surg* 1975;62:769.

55. Hamburger B, Gharib H, Melton LJ III, et al. Fine-needle aspiration biopsy of thyroid nodules. *Am J Med* 1982;73:381.

56. Handelsman DJ, Conway AJ, Donnelly PF, et al. Azoospermia after iodine-131 treatment for thyroid carcinoma. *Br Med J* 1980;281:1527.

57. Handelsman DJ, Turtle JR. Testicular damage after radioactive iodine (I-131) therapy for thyroid cancer. *Clin Endocrinol* 1983;18:465

58. Harrington KS, Michalaki VJ, Vini L et al. Management of non-Hodgkin's lymphoma of the thyroid lobe: the Royal Marsden experience. *Br J Radiol* 2005;78:405–410.

59. Hartshorne MF, Karl RD Jr, Cawthon MA, et al. Multiple imaging techniques demonstrate a medullary carcinoma of the thyroid. *Clin Nucl Med* 1983;8:628.

60. Haugen BR, Pacini F, Reiners C, et al. A comparison of recombinant human thyrotropin and thyroid hormone withdrawal for the detection of thyroid remnant or cancer. *J Clin Endocrinol Metab* 1999;84:3877–3885.

61. Hay I, Grant C, Taylor W, et al. Ipsilateral lobectomy versus bilateral lobar resection in papillary thyroid carcinoma: a retrospective analysis of surgical outcome using a novel prognostic scoring system. *Surgery* 1987;102:1088–1095.

62. Hellman DE, Kartchner M, van Antwerp JD, et al. Radioiodine in the treatment of medullary carcinoma of the thyroid. *J Clin Endocrinol Metab* 1979;48:451–455.

63. Herzog B. Thyroid gland diseases and tumors: surgical aspects. *Prog Pediatr Surg* 1983;16:15.

64. Higashi T, Ito K, Nishikawa Y, et al. Gallium-67 imaging in the evaluation of thyroid malignancy. *J Clin Nucl Med* 1988;13:792–799.

65. Holm LE, Dahlqvist I, Israelsson A, et al. Malignant thyroid tumors after iodine-131 therapy. *N Engl J Med* 1980;303:188–191.

66. Hughes CJ, Shaha AR, Shah JP, et al. Impact of lymph node metastasis in differentiated carcinoma of the thyroid: a matched-pair analysis. *Head Neck* 1996;18:127–132.

67. Hurley RJ, Becker DV. The use of radioiodine in the management of thyroid cancer. In: Freeman LM, Weissman HS, eds. *Nuclear medicine annual 1983*. New York: Raven Press; 1983.

68. Jacob P, Bogdanova TI, Buglova E et al. Thyroid cancer risk in areas of Ukraine and Belarus affected by the Chernobyl accident. *Radiat Res* 2006;165:1–8.

69. Jacob P, Bogdanova TI, Buglova E, et al. Thyroid cancer among Ukrainians and Belarusians who were children or adolescents at the time of the Chernobyl accident. *J Radiol Protect* 2006;26:51–67.

70. Jhiang SM, Mazzaferri EL. The ret/PTC oncogene in papillary thyroid carcinoma. *J Lab Clin Med* 1994;123:331–337.

71. Joensuu H, Ahonen A. Imaging and metastasis of thyroid carcinoma with fluorine-18 fluorodeoxyglucose. *J Nucl Med* 1987;28:910–914.

72. Junor EJ, Paul J, Reed NS. Primary non-Hodgkin's lymphoma of the thyroid. *Eur J Surg Oncol* 1992;18:313–321.

73. Kasai N, Sakamoto A. Malignant transformation of thyroid cancer: poorly differentiated cancer and anaplastic cancer transformation. *Gan No Rinsho* 1983;29:A7, 105–110.

74. Kebebew E, Greenspan FS, Clark OH, et al. Anaplastic thyroid carcinoma treatment outcomes and prognostic factors. *Cancer* 2005;103:1330–1335.

75. Keum KC, Suh YG, Koon WS, The role of postoperative external beam radiotherapy in the management of patients with papillary thyroid cancer invading the trachea. *Int J Radiat Oncol Biol Phys* 2006; in press.

76. Kim JH, Leeper RD. Combination Adriamycin and radiation therapy for locally advanced carcinoma of the thyroid gland. *Int J Radiat Oncol Biol Phys* 1983;9:565.

77. Kim JH, Leeper RD. Treatment of anaplastic giant and spindle cell carcinoma of the thyroid gland with combination Adriamycin and radiation therapy. *Cancer* 1983;52:954–957.

78. Kim JH, Leeper RD. Treatment of locally advanced thyroid carcinoma with combination doxorubicin and radiation therapy. *Cancer* 1987;60:2372–2375.

79. Koral KF, Alder RS, Carey JE, et al. Two-orthogonal-view method for quantification of rad dose to neck lesions in thyroid cancer therapy patients. *Med Phys* 1982;9:497–505.

80. Kovalic J, Grigsby P, Slessinger E. The relationship of clinical factors and radiation exposure rates from Iodine-131 treated thyroid carcinoma patients. *Med Dosim* 1990;15:209–215.

81. Krassas GE, Pontikides N. Male reproductive function in relation with thyroid alterations. *Best Pract Res Clin Endocrinol Metab* 2004;18:183–195.

82. Kuni CC, Klingensmith WC III. Failure of low doses of I-131 to ablate residual thyroid tissue following surgery for thyroid cancer. *Radiology* 1980;137:773–774.

83. Lakshmanan M, Schaffer A, Robbins J, et al. A simplified low iodine diet in I-131 scanning and therapy of thyroid cancer. *Clin Nucl Med* 1988;13:866–868.

84. Larson SM. Radiolabeled monoclonal anti-tumor antibodies in diagnosis and therapy. *J Nucl Med* 1985;26:538.

85. Lee TC, Harbert JC, Dejter SW, et al. Vocal cord paralysis following I-131 ablation of a postthyroidectomy remnant. *J Nucl Med* 1985;26:49–50.

86. Leeper RD, Simaoka K. Treatment of metastatic thyroid cancer. *Clin Endocrinol Metab* 1980;9:383.

87. Lemish I, Bennett F, Marten C, et al. A sensitive human thyroglobulin RIA to define clearly the presence or absence of functioning thyroid tissue. *J Nucl Med* 1984;25:49–55.

88. Levendag PC, DePorre PM, van Putten WL. Anaplastic carcinoma of the thyroid gland treated by radiation therapy. *Int J Radiat Oncol Biol Phys* 1993;26:125–128.

89. Logue JP, Hale RJ, Stewart AL, et al. Primary malignant lymphoma of the thyroid: A clinicopathological analysis. *Int J Radiat Oncol Biol Phys* 1992;22:929.

90. Lubin E, Mechlis-Frish S, Zatz S, et al. Serum thyroglobulin and Iodine-131 whole-body scan in the diagnosis and assessment of treatment for metastatic differentiated thyroid carcinoma. *J Nucl Med* 1994;35:257–262.

91. Lynn J, Gamvros OI, Taylor S. Medullary carcinoma of the thyroid. *World J Surg* 1981;5:27–32.

92. Martinez-Tello FJ, Martinez-Cabruja R, Fernandez-Martin J, et al. Occult carcinoma of the thyroid. *Cancer* 1993;71:4022–4029.

93. Matsuzuka F, Miyauchi A, Katayama S, et al. Clinical aspects of primary thyroid lymphoma: diagnosis and treatment based on our experience in 119 cases. *Thyroid* 1993;3:93–99.

94. Maxon HR, Englaro E, Thomas S, et al. Radioiodine-131 therapy for well-differentiated thyroid cancer—A quantitative radiation dosimetric approach: outcome and validation in 85 patients. *J Nucl Med* 1992;33:1132–1136.

95. Maxon HR, Thomas SR, Boehringer A, et al. Low iodine diet in I-131 ablation of thyroid remnant. *Clin Nucl Med* 1983;8:123.

96. Maxon HR, Thomas SR, Saenger EL, et al. Ionizing irradiation and the induction of clinically significant disease in the human thyroid gland. *Am J Med* 1977;63:967–978.

97. Mazzaferri E. Papillary thyroid carcinoma: a 10 year follow-up report of the impact of therapy in 576 patients. *Am J Med* 1981;70:511–518.

98. Mazzaferri E, Young R, Oertel J, et al. Papillary thyroid carcinoma: the impact of therapy in 576 patients. *Medicine* 1977;56:171–196.

99. McDay JB, Danoff BF. External beam radiotherapy in the management of locally invasive carcinoma of the thyroid. *Int J Radiat Oncol Biol Phys* 1978;4[Suppl 2]:226.

100. Meadows KM, Amdur RJ, Morris CG. External beam radiotherapy for differentiated thyroid cancer. *Am J Otolaryngol* 2006;74:24–28.

101. Michael BE, Forouhar FA, Spencer RP. Medullary thyroid carcinoma with radioiodide transport: Effects of iodine-131 therapy and lithium administration. *Clin Nucl Med* 1985;10:274.

102. Morgan GW, Freeman AP, McLean RG, et al. Late cardiac, thyroid, and pulmonary sequelae of mantle radiotherapy for Hodgkin's disease. *Int J Radiat Oncol Biol Phys* 1985;11:1925.

103. Morimoto J, Yoshimoto Y, Sato K, et al. Serum TSH, thyroglobulin, and thyroidal disorders in atomic bomb survivors exposed in youth: 30-year follow-up study. *J Nucl Med* 1987;28:1115.

104. Nagada K, Ishibashi T, Takei T et al. Does lemon candy decrease salivary gland damage after radioiodine therapy for thyroid cancer? *J Nucl Med* 2005;46: 261–266.

105. National Comprehensive Cancer Network thyroid carcinoma practice guidelines. 2005. Available at: www.nccn.org/professionals/physicians_gls/PDF/thyroid.pdf. Referenced December, 22, 2005.

106. National Institutes of Health. National Cancer Institute. *Estimated exposures and thyroid doses received by the American people from Iodine-131 in fallout following Nevada atmospheric nuclear bomb tests*. Bethesda, MD: U.S. Department of Health and Human Services, 1997.

107. Nemec J, Rohling S, Zamrazil V, et al. Comparison of the distribution of diagnostic and thyroablative I-131 in the evaluation of differentiated thyroid cancers. *J Nucl Med* 1979;20:92–97.

108. Noma S, Kanaoka M, Minami S, et al. Thyroid masses: MR imaging and pathological correlation. *Radiology* 1988;168:759–764.

109. Nutting CM, Convery C, Cosgrove VP, et al. Improvements in target coverage and reduced spinal cord irradiation using intensity modulated radiotherapy (IMRT) in patients with carcinoma of the thyroid gland. *Radiother Oncol* 2001;60: 173–180.

110. Pacini F, Ladenson PW, Schlumberger et al. Radioiodine ablation of thyroid remnants with recombinant human thyrotropin in differentiated thyroid carcinoma: results of an international randomized controlled study. *J Clin Endocrinol Metab* 2006;91:926–932.

111. Patton JA, Dandler MP, Partain CL. Prediction of benignancy of the solitary "cold" thyroid nodule by fluorescent scanning. *J Nucl Med* 1985;26:461.

112. Petrich T, Borner AR, Otto D, et al. Influence of rhTSH on [(18)F] fluorodeoxyglucose uptake by differentiated thyroid cancer. *Eur J Nucl Med Mol Imaging* 2002;29:641–647.

113. Pineda JD, Lee T, Ain K, et al. Iodine-131 therapy for thyroid cancer patients with elevated thyroglobulin and negative diagnostic scan. *J Clin Endocrinol Metab* 1995;80:1488 1492.

114. Pont A, Spratt D, Shinn JB. T3 toxicosis due to nonmetastatic follicular carcinoma for the thyroid. *West J Med* 1982;136:2455.

115. Powell MR, Blum AS. Maximizing radiation dose in radioiodine ablation of normal thyroid tissue and of thyroid cancer metastases. *Clin Nucl Med* 1984;9[Suppl1]:5.

116. Pyke CM, Grant CS, Habermann TM, et al. Non-Hodgkin's lymphoma of the thyroid: is more than biopsy necessary? *World J Surg* 1992;16:604–609.

117. Rahu M, Rahu K, Auvinen A et al. Cancer risk among Chernoble clean-up workers in Estonia and Latvia, 1986-1998. *Int J Cancer* e-publication 23 Jan 2006.

118. Ramacciotti C, Pretorius HT, Line BR, et al. Ablation of nonmalignant thyroid remnants with low doses of radioactive iodine [concise communication]. *J Nucl Med* 1982;23:483.

119. Rao RS, Parikh HK, Deshmane VH, et al. Prognostic factors in follicular carcinoma of the thyroid: a study of 198 cases. *Head Neck* 1996;18:118–126.

120. Razack MS, Sako K, Shimaoka K, et al. Radiation-associated thyroid carcinoma. *J Surg Oncol* 1980;14:287–291.

121. Rogers JD, Lindberg RD, Hill CS.Jr, et al. Spindle giant cell carcinoma of the thyroid: a different therapeutic approach. *Cancer* 1974;34:1328.

122. Rosenberg RD, Mettler FA.Jr, Moseley RD.Jr, et al. Thyroid radiation absorbed dose from diagnostic procedures in U.S population. *Radiology* 1985;156:183–185.

123. Rosenbluth BD, Serrano V, Happersett L et al. Intensity modulated radiation therapy for the treatment of nonanaplastic thyroid cancer. *Int J Radiat Oncol Biol Phys* 2005;63:1419–1426.

124. Roti E, Robuschi G, Emanuele R, et al. The value of serum thyroglobulin measurement as a marker of cancer recurrence in the follow-up for patients previously treated for differentiated thyroid tumor. *J Endocrinol Invest* 1982;5:43–46.

125. Rougier P, Parmentier C, Laplanche A, et al. Medullary thyroid carcinoma: prognostic factors and treatment. *Int J Radiat Oncol Biol Phys* 1983;9:161.

126. Saad MF, Guido JJ, Samaan NA. Radioactive iodine in the treatment of medullary carcinoma of the thyroid. *J Clin Endocrinol Metab* 1983;57:124.

127. Schatz H, Maser E, Teuber J, et al. The significance of serum thyroglobulin determination for monitoring of patients after thyroidectomy for differentiated thyroid carcinoma. *Verh Dtsch Ges Inn Med* 1981;87:587.

128. Shah JP, Loree TR, Dharker D, et al. Prognostic factors in differentiated carcinoma of the thyroid gland. *Am J Surg* 1992;164:658–661.
129. Shaha AR, Loree TR, Shah JP. Prognostic factors and risk group analysis in follicular carcinoma of the thyroid. *Surgery* 1995;118:1131–1136.
130. Shindo M, Wu J, Park E et al. The importance of central compartment elective lymph node excision in the staging and treatment of papillary thyroid cancer. *Arch Otolaryngol Head Neck Surg* in press.
131. Siddiqui AR, Edmondson J, Wellman HN, et al. Feasibility of low doses of I-131 for thyroid ablation in postsurgical patients with thyroid carcinoma. *Clin Nucl Med* 1986;6:158.
132. Silverman PM, Newman GE, Korobkin M, et al. Computed tomography in the evaluation of thyroid disease. *AJR Am J Roentgenol* 1984;141:897.
133. Simeone JF, Daniels GH, Hall DA, et al. Sonography in a follow-up of 100 patients with thyroid carcinoma. *AJR Am J Roentgenol* 1987;148:45–49.
134. Simpson W, Palmer J, Rosen I, et al. Management of medullary carcinoma of the thyroid. *Am J Surg* 1982;144:420.
135. Simpson W, Sutcliffe S, Gospodarowicz M. The thyroid. In: Moss W, Cox J, eds. *Radiation oncology: rationale, technique, results.* St. Louis: CV Mosby; 1989.
136. Smith R, Blum C, Benua RS, et al. Radioactive iodine treatment of metastatic thyroid carcinoma with clinical thyrotoxicosis. *Clin Nucl Med* 1985;10:874.
137. Spencer RP, Chapman CN, Rao H. Thyroid carcinoma after radioiodine therapy for hyperthyroidism: analysis based on age, latency, and administered dose of I-131. *Clin Nucl Med* 1983;8:216.
138. Sridama V, Hara Y, Fauchet R, et al. Association of differentiated thyroid carcinoma with HLA-DR7. *Cancer* 1985;56:1086.
139. Strand S-E, Erlandsson K, Löwenhielm P. Thyroid uptake of 131I and 133I from Chernobyl and the population of Southern Sweden. *J Nucl Med* 1988;29:1719.
140. Sutow WW, Conard RA, Thompson KH. Thyroid injury and effects on growth and development in the Marshallese children accidentally exposed to radioactive fallout. *CA Ca Bull* 1982;34:90.
141. Sutton RT, Reading CC, Charboneau JW. US-guided biopsy of neck masses and postoperative management of patients with thyroid cancer. *Radiology* 1988;168:769.
142. Syed AMN, Greenfield LD. The role of interstitial irradiation in the treatment of thyroid cancer. *Contemp Surg* 1980;17:36.
143. Tallroth E, Wallin G, Lundell G, et al. Multimodality treatment in anaplastic giant cell thyroid carcinoma. *Cancer* 1987;60:1428.
144. Tan RK, Finley RK, Driscoll D, et al. Anaplastic carcinoma of the thyroid: a 24-year experience. *Head Neck* 1995;17:41–48.
145. Tennvall J, Lundell G, Hallquist A, et al. Combined doxorubicin, hyperfractionated radiotherapy, and surgery in anaplastic thyroid carcinoma. *Cancer* 1994;74:1348–1354.
146. Terry JH, St John SA, Karkowski FJ, et al. Tall cell papillary thyroid cancer: incidence and prognosis. *Am J Surg* 1994;168:459–461.
147. Tsang RW, Gospodarowicz MK, Sutcliffe SB, et al. Non-Hodgkin's lymphoma of the thyroid gland: prognostic factors and treatment outcome. The Princess Margaret Hospital Lymphoma Group. *Int J Radiat Oncol Biol Phys* 1993;27:599–604.
148. Tubiana M. External radiotherapy and radioiodine in the treatment of thyroid cancer. *World J Surg* 1981;5:75.
149. Tubiana M, Haddad E, Schlumberger M, et al. External radiotherapy in thyroid cancers. *Cancer* 1985;55:2062–2071.
150. Tupchong L, Phil D, Hughes F, et al. Primary lymphoma of the thyroid: clinical features, prognostic factors, and results of treatment. *Int J Radiat Oncol Biol Phys* 1986;12:1813.
151. Turrin A, Pilotti S, Ricci SB. Characteristics of thyroid cancer following irradiation. *Int J Radiat Oncol Biol Phys* 1985;11:2149.
152. Van Nostrand D, Neutze J, Atkins F. Side effects of "rational dose" iodine-131 therapy for metastatic well differentiated thyroid carcinoma. *J Nucl Med* 1986;27:1519.
153. Venkatesh YSS, Ordonez NG, Schultz PN, et al. Anaplastic carcinoma of the thyroid. A clinicopathologic study of 121 cases. *Cancer* 1990;66:321–330.
154. Vigliotti A, Kong JS, Fuller LM, et al. Thyroid lymphomas stages IE and IIIE: comparative results for radiotherapy only, combination chemotherapy only, and multimodality treatment. *Int J Radiat Oncol Biol Phys* 1986;12:1807.
155. Waxman A, Ramanna L, Chapman N, et al. The significance of I-131 scan dose in patients with thyroid cancer: determination of ablation [concise communication]. *J Nucl Med* 1981;22:861.
156. Whitley RJ, Ain KB. Thyroglobulin: a specific serum marker for the management of thyroid cancer. *Clin Lab Med* 2004;24: 29–47.
157. World Health Organization. *International histological classification of tumors,* vols 1—25. Geneva: World Health Organization; 1957–1981.
158. Yoosufani Z, Slavin JD Jr, Hellman RM, et al. Preleukemia following large dose radioiodide therapy for metastatic thyroid carcinoma. *J Nucl Med* 1987;28:1348.
159. Young R, Mazzaferri E, Rahe A, et al. Pure follicular thyroid carcinoma: impact of therapy in 214 patients. *J Nucl Med* 1980;21:733–737.

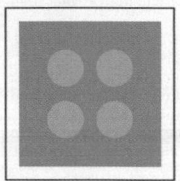

Chapter 48
Lung

Joe Y. Chang, Jeffrey D. Bradley, Ramaswamy Govindan, Ritsuko Komaki

Anatomy

In both lungs, the oblique fissure extends from the lung surface to the hilum and divides the upper and lower lobes. The right lung has three lobes as a result of a second fissure, the horizontal fissure. This fissure extends from the anterior margin into the oblique fissure and separates the middle lobe from the upper lobe (21). The left lung is composed of two lobes: an upper and lower lobe (21). The lingular portion of the left upper lobe corresponds to the middle lobe on the right. The lungs are coated by the visceral pleura, which extends into the fissures separating the lobes. The trachea enters the superior mediastinum and bifurcates approximately at the level of the fifth thoracic vertebra (77). The hila of the lungs contain the bronchi, pulmonary arteries, and veins; various branches from the pulmonary plexus; bronchial arteries and veins; and lymphatics (77).

The lung has a rich network of lymphatic vessels throughout its loose interstitial connective tissue, ultimately draining into the various lymph node stations, which may be divided into the following groups: intrapulmonary nodes (along the secondary bronchi), bronchopulmonary nodes (hilar nodes), mediastinal nodes, and supraclavicular or scalene nodes (14). Figure 48.1 shows regional nodal stations for lung cancer staging (4). The intrapulmonary lymph nodes may be related to segmental bronchi, or they may lie in the bifurcation of the branches of the pulmonary artery. The bronchopulmonary lymph nodes, situated either alongside the lower portions of the main bronchi (hilar lymph nodes) or at the bifurcations of the main bronchi into lobar bronchi (interlobar nodes) (20), comprise the hilar nodes, from a radiotherapeutic viewpoint. The mediastinal lymph nodes are divided in two groups: (a) superior, located above the bifurcation of the trachea (carina), including the upper paratracheal, pretracheal, retrotracheal, and lower paratracheal nodes (azygos nodes) and a group of nodes located in the aortic window; and (b) inferior, situated in the subcarinal region and inferior mediastinum, including the subcarinal, paraesophageal, and pulmonary ligament nodes.

The drainage for each pulmonary lobe is shown in Figure 48.2 (159). The lymph from the right upper lobe flows to the tracheobronchial lymph nodes. The lymph from the left upper lobe flows not only to the venous angle of the same side but also to the venous angle of the opposite superior mediastinum. The right and left lower lobe lymphatics drain into the subcarinal nodes and from there to the right superior mediastinum (the left lower lobe also may drain into the left superior mediastinum) and directly into the inferior mediastinal lymph nodes.

Epidemiology

Worldwide, lung cancer is the most common (1.35 million of 10.9 million new cases) and the deadliest (1.18 million of 6.7 million cancer-related deaths) form of cancer (171). The United States 2006 cancer statistics (93) showed that lung cancer is the second most common cancer for both men and women (92,700 or 13% of all cases, and 81,770 or 12% of all cases, respectively), but the number-one cancer killer in both sexes (90,330 men, 31% of all cancer-related deaths; and 72,1300 women, 26% of all cancer-related deaths). In fact, more people in the United States die of lung cancer than of the next three causes of cancer-related death—prostate cancer, breast cancer, and colorectal cancer—combined. Survival at 5 years measured by the Surveillance, Epidemiology, and End Results (SEER) program in the United States is 15%.

Between 1991 and 2002, the lung cancer incidence decreased 19.8% in men (1.8% reduction per year), but it increased 8% in women between 1990 and 1998 (1% increase per year) and subsequently decreased 2% between 1998 and 2002 (0.5% reduction per year). Lung cancer death rates for men have dropped by 19% during the past decade, whereas these rates continued to increase in women up to the year 2002 (93). This pattern of lung cancer is correlated with a change in the smoking pattern in men and women. Smoking is the primary risk factor in the development of lung cancer, accounting for 90% of cases in men and 70% in women (49,214). Lung carcinogenesis is known to occur from an accumulation of several genetic alterations, most commonly with p53 mutations and deletions on chromosomes 3p, 5q, 9p, 11p, and 17p. These alterations are more frequent in smokers than in nonsmokers (248). Patients with a history of lung cancer are at increased risk for a second lung cancer, at a rate of 1% to 2% per year. This rate increases for those survivors who continue to smoke (96). Industrial agents found in the environment, such as asbestos, coal tar fumes, nickel, chromium, arsenic, nickel, diesel exhaust,

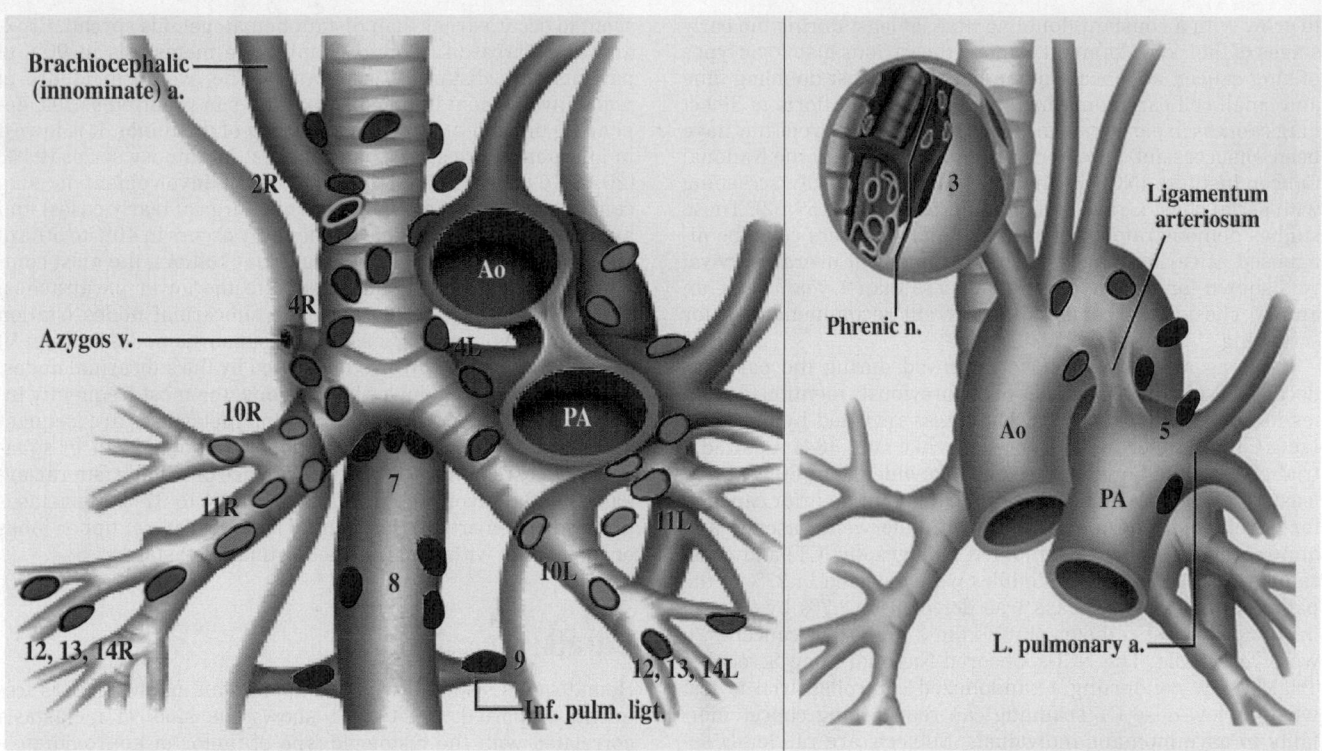

FIGURE 48.1. Regional nodal stations for lung cancer staging. N2 nodes include stations 1 to 9. N1 nodes include stations 10 to 14 Ao, aorta; PA, pulmonary aorta.

indoor radon, and radioactive materials, also have been related to the development of lung cancer. Adenocarcinoma surpassed squamous cell carcinoma as the most common subtype of lung cancer in both men and women in the mid-1980s. Adenocarcinoma has been more common in women since the 1950s and became the most common lung cancer diagnosis in men in 1990 (233). There are many theories that may explain a relative decrease in squamous and small cell carcinomas and the increase in adenocarcinomas. The introduction of filter cigarettes in the mid-1950s may have contributed by allowing smaller carcinogens to be deposited in the lung periphery. Filter use may have enticed smokers to take larger puffs and retain smoke longer to compensate for the lower nicotine yield. Smoking low-tar

filter cigarettes may increase the rate of adenocarcinoma because these cigarettes have a higher nitrate content, which has been shown to produce adenocarcinoma in laboratory animals (82,223,230).

:: | Natural History

It is often difficult to determine the site of origin of lung cancer. Garland et al. (66) studied 463 patients, 150 of whom had less advanced tumors that were suitable for determination of the site of origin: 58% of these tumors originated in the right lung and 42% in the left lung. Once established, tumors are likely

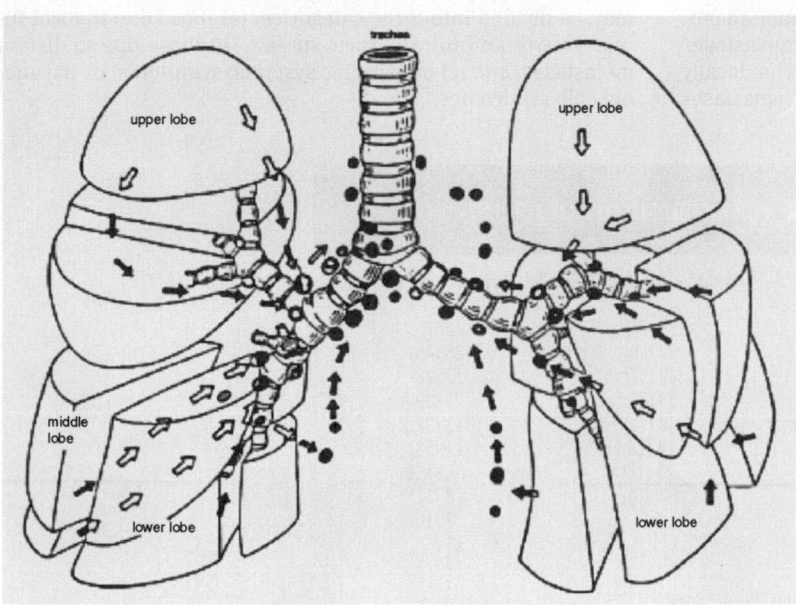

FIGURE 48.2. Primary lymphatic drainage for lung. (From Nagaishi C. *Functional anatomy and histology of the lung.* Baltimore: University Park Press; 1972, with permission.)

to grow with a constant doubling time, at least during the early stages of their development. Among the various histologic types of lung cancer, adenocarcinoma has the slowest doubling time and small cell carcinoma has the fastest (31). Efforts to detect lung cancers in earlier stages through screening programs have been unsuccessful. Screening programs funded by the National Cancer Institute (NCI) in the 1970s failed to justify screening with serial chest x-rays and sputum cytology (57,59,62). These studies demonstrated that although many cancers could be diagnosed at earlier stages, no improvement in overall survival was shown for screens at intervals less than 1 year. Thus, an annual chest x-ray remains the current recommendation for screening.

Imaging technologies have improved during the past two decades. With the deficiencies of the previously mentioned studies in mind, lung cancer screening was revisited by the Early Lung Cancer Detection Project, Henschke et al. (84) reported a trial of 1,000 patients at high risk (age older than 60 years, at least 10 pack-years of cigarette smoking, and no prior cancers) for development of lung cancer who underwent baseline and annual repeat low-dose computed tomography (CT) and chest radiography. Noncalcified nodules were detected in 27% of the patients. Malignant disease was detected in 2.7% by CT and in 0.7% by chest radiography. Of the 27 detected cancers, 26 were resectable. The NCI-sponsored National Lung Screening Trial is now conducting a randomized controlled trial to test whether low-dose CT scanning can reduce lung cancer mortality in asymptomatic individuals. Subjects are randomly collected to undergo screening with low-dose CT or chest x-ray. The National Lung Screening Trial will enroll 50,000 high-risk heavy smokers (and former heavy smokers who quit within 15 years before randomization), age 55 to 74 years. Participants will undergo an initial screening and two subsequent annual screenings and will be observed for a minimum of 4.5 years. Final analyses are expected in 2009 (72).

Patterns of Spread

The spread pattern of lung cancer may be divided into three pathways: local (intrathoracic), regional (lymphatic), and distant (hematogenous). Progression of lung cancer can be by any of these pathways in no particular order. A relation has been described between the incidence of local, regional, and distant spread and histologic type. Undifferentiated small cell carcinoma (oat cell cancer) has a higher incidence of distant metastasis than non–small cell cancers. Of the latter group, adenocarcinoma has shown higher potential for distant metastasis. Lung cancer may spread via hematogenous routes or locally within the lymphatics. In most cases, lymph node metastases seem to occur earlier than distant hematogenous spread. Croxatto and Barcat (41) found lymph node metastasis in 90% of patients with distant dissemination. The overall incidence of nodal involvement in lung cancer varies in reported series, depending on patient selection and stage of the tumor. It is lowest in lobectomy series (37%) and highest in autopsy series (94%) (20,87,164,168,186). Mediastinal nodal involvement in lung cancer also has been studied in both surgical (early cases) and autopsy series. Mediastinal adenopathy occurs in 40% to 50% of operative specimens (13). For right lung tumors, the most commonly involved mediastinal areas are the lower paratracheal nodes (station IV), followed by the subcarinal nodes (station VII). For left upper lobe lesions, the subaortic nodes (station V) are most commonly involved, followed by the subcarinal nodes. For lingular and left lower lobe lesions, the most frequently involved nodes are subcarinal (10). Skip metastases are frequent and occur more commonly in adenocarcinoma than in squamous cell carcinoma (129). The incidence of scalene (supraclavicular) nodal involvement ranges from 2% to 37%. Metastases to these nodes are predominantly from ipsilateral upper lobes or in patients with superior mediastinal metastases.

Extrathoracic Spread

Hematogenous spread with multiple organ involvement is frequently reported. Table 48.1 shows the sites of metastasis correlated with the histologic type of tumor in approximately 6,000 autopsy cases (131). Adrenal metastasis has been reported in 27.4% of patients with epidermoid carcinoma, in 35% to 40% of patients with small or large cell undifferentiated carcinoma, and in 42.9% of patients with adenocarcinoma (14). The abdominal lymph nodes were reported to be involved in more than 50% of patients with small cell undifferentiated carcinoma (81).

Clinical Presentation

Carcinoma of the lung is among the most insidious of all neoplasms. Some patients present with an asymptomatic lesion discovered incidentally on chest radiograph. However, the majority of lung cancers are discovered because of the development of a new or worsening clinical symptom or sign. Although no set of signs or symptoms is pathognomonic for lung cancer, they may be divided into three categories: (a) those due to local tumor growth and intrathoracic spread, (b) those due to distant metastases, and (c) nonspecific systemic symptoms, or paraneoplastic syndromes.

Table 48.1	SITE OF METASTASIS CORRELATED WITH HISTOLOGIC TYPE (AT AUTOPSY)			
Site of Metastasis	Squamous No. (%)	Small Cell No. (%)	Anaplastic No. (%)	Adenocarcinoma No. (%)
Lymph nodes	137 (52)	163 (83)	135 (74)	42 (73)
Liver	58 (21)	122 (62)	67 (36)	26 (45)
Adrenals	54 (19)	84 (42)	69 (37)	17 (28)
Bones	59 (21)	75 (37)	53 (28)	23 (39)
Brain	26 (15)	45 (40)	30 (22)	13 (37)
Kidney	39 (13)	28 (14.5)	24 (13.5)	11 (18)
Pancreas	9 (3.5)	46 (22)	25 (12)	3 (165)
Lung	31 (10)	13 (5)	15 (6)	8 (12)
Pleura	18 (5)	21 (9)	9 ( )	3 (165)
Total	255	191	179	56

From Line DH, Deeley TJ. The necropsy findings in carcinoma of the bronchus. *Br J Dis Chest* 1971;65:238–242, with permission.

Signs and Symptoms Related to Local Tumor Growth and Intrathoracic Spread

Signs and symptoms referable to the primary tumor vary depending on the location and size of the tumor. Centrally located tumors produce cough, a localized wheeze, hemoptysis, and symptoms and signs of airway obstruction and postobstructive pneumonitis such as dyspnea, fever, and productive cough. Peripheral tumors are more likely to be asymptomatic when they are small and confined within the lung; occasionally, cough and pleuritic chest pain may be evident.

Intrathoracic spread of lung cancer, either by direct extension or by lymphatic metastasis, is associated with a variety of sign and symptom complexes. Mediastinal invasion may be manifested as vague, poorly localized chest pain in association with other findings of nerve entrapment, vascular obstruction, and/or compression or invasion of the esophagus. One of the most common neurologic disorders arising from mediastinal involvement is hoarseness owing to entrapment of the recurrent laryngeal nerve. Because of its longer intrathoracic course, the left recurrent laryngeal nerve is more likely to be the source of hoarseness than the right recurrent laryngeal nerve. With recurrent laryngeal nerve paralysis, a patient may develop dysphagia for both solids and liquids, resulting in recurrent aspiration. Compression of the esophagus by the tumor also may lead to dysphagia. The formation of a tracheoesophageal or bronchoesophageal fistula, which occurs with a frequency of 0.16%, can be manifested by vigorous cough, especially on swallowing, and recurrent aspiration pneumonia. Involvement of the phrenic nerve is associated with hiccups early and leads later to paralysis and elevation of the hemidiaphragm with resulting dyspnea.

The principal vascular syndrome associated with the extension of lung cancer into the mediastinum is superior vena cava (SVC) syndrome, most commonly caused by invasion of the vein and extrinsic compression by the tumor but also by intraluminal thrombosis. Lung cancer accounts for 65% to 90% of all cases of SVC syndrome, and in approximately 85% of these cases the primary lung tumor is on the right, primarily in the right upper lobe or right mainstem bronchus. By cell type, small cell lung cancer (SCLC) predominates as the cause of SVC syndrome, followed by squamous cell carcinoma.

With apical tumors, the classic Pancoast's syndrome (lower brachial plexopathy, Horner's syndrome, and shoulder pain) may become manifest owing to local invasion of the lower brachial plexus (C8 and T1 nerve roots), satellite ganglion, and chest wall. The tumor may cause symptoms through involvement of the first or second rib or vertebrae and other nerve roots. The radiographic signs are those of an asymmetric apical cap or an apical mass. Most superior sulcus tumors are squamous cell carcinomas, although they may be adenocarcinomas or even SCLC, in 1% to 2% of cases, underscoring the importance of establishing a histologic diagnosis.

Approximately 15% of patients with lung cancer have pleural involvement at initial presentation, and 50% of patients with disseminated lung cancer develop pleural effusion during the course of their illness. A pleural effusion may be asymptomatic when small, but it is usually associated with dyspnea, cough, or chest pain. Pericardial involvement arises from direct extension of the tumor or as a result of retrograde spread through mediastinal and epicardial lymphatics. Lung cancer is the single most frequent source of pericardial metastases, accounting for 37% of reported cases.

Symptoms Due to Distant Metastasis

Approximately 60% of patients with SCLC and 30% to 40% of those with non–small cell lung cancer (NSCLC) present with stage IV metastatic disease. Although lung cancer can metastasize to virtually any organ site, the most common sites of hematogenous spread that are clinically apparent are the central nervous system (CNS), bones, liver, and adrenal glands. Many of these patients do not have symptoms that can be attributed to a specific distant site. Bone pain seems to be common. Symptoms related to liver involvement (right upper quadrant pain) are less common or nonspecific (nausea, weight loss, anemia). Involvement of the adrenal glands is often asymptomatic, and most adrenal metastases are discovered incidentally during staging evaluation or at autopsy. If symptomatic, it presents with unilateral pain in the ank, abdomen, or costovertebral angle. Much less commonly, signs or symptoms point to brain and CNS involvement. These can range from nonspecific headache or mental status change to focal or generalized seizures and localized weakness. Epidural and intramedullary spinal cord metastases may be the sole neurologic manifestations of lung cancer.

Nonspecific Systemic Symptoms and Paraneoplastic Syndromes

Systemic, nonspecific signs and symptoms are common in both SCLC and NSCLC. The 30% rate of anorexia is probably underreported. Weight loss, which is usually but not always accompanied by anorexia, occurs in approximately half of the patients, and generalized weakness occurs in one-third. Fever and anemia occur less frequently, in fewer than 20% of patients. Fever is generally not considered paraneoplastic in lung cancer patients; if present, it is usually associated with a documented infection (e.g., postobstructive pneumonia) or with liver metastases.

Paraneoplastic syndromes are condition associated with the cancer, which induce signs and symptoms away from the primary tumor or its metastasis. The major categories of paraneoplastic syndromes include endocrine, neurologic, cutaneous and musculoskeletal, and cardiovascular and hematological manifestations.

Diagnostic and Staging Work-Up

Determination of stage is important for therapeutic and prognostic implications. Careful initial diagnostic evaluation to define the location and to determine the extent of primary and metastatic tumor involvement is critical for the appropriate care of patients and radiotherapy target volume delineation. Staging procedures include history, physical examination, routine laboratory evaluations, chest x-ray, and chest CT scan with contrast. The CT scan should extend inferiorly to include upper abdomen and adrenal glands. In general, symptoms, physical signs, laboratory findings, or perceived risk of distant metastasis lead to an evaluation for distant metastatic disease. Additional tests such as bone scans and CT/magnetic resonance imaging (MRI) of the brain may be performed if initial assessments suggest metastases or for patients with stage II-III disease who are under consideration for aggressive local and combined modality treatments. Surgical staging of the mediastinum is considered standard if accurate evaluation of the nodal status is needed to determine therapy. The wider availability and use of fluorodeoxyglucose positron emission tomography (FDG-PET) for staging has modified this approach to staging mediastinal lymph nodes and distant metastases. The combination of CT scanning and PET scanning has greater sensitivity and specificity than CT scanning alone, and PET scan should be considered as a standard stage procedure. PET and CT imaging has changed the stage in 25% to 50% of cases in NSCLC compared with CT alone. If PET scan is performed, bone scan is not necessary.

Radiologic Examination

Chest x-ray remains the simplest method for identifying patients with lung cancer. It is still a preferred initial modality because of its availability, low cost, and low radiation dose. Lung lesions (usually >5 mm) and associated atelectasis, postobstructive pneumonitis, abscess, bronchiolitis, pleural reaction, rib erosion, pleural effusion, or bulky mediastinal lymphadenopathy may be identified on radiographs. CT scan remains the most effective noninvasive technique for evaluating suspected or known lung cancer and the mediastinum involvement. Unfortunately, the accuracy of CT scanning in identifying metastatic disease in mediastinal lymph nodes is highly variable, with sensitivity ranging from 51% to 95%. A lymph node size of 1 cm or more in the shortest diameter has been generally accepted as the criterion of abnormal nodal enlargement. However, approximately 8% to 15% of patients considered to have a negative CT scan for mediastinal nodal enlargement, with lymph nodes sized 1 cm or less, will ultimately be found to have mediastinal nodal involvement at the time of biopsy. Mediastinal lymph nodes that are more than 2 cm in diameter contain metastatic disease in more than 90% of cases. Lymph nodes that are 1.5 to 2 cm in size contain disease in more than 50% of cases, and nodes 1 to 1.5 cm in size harbor metastatic disease in 15% to 30% of cases. The negative predictive accuracy of CT scan is 85% to 92% for mediastinal lymph node metastases. Often, patients with lymph node involvement not found by CT scan but with metastases found at the time of thoracotomy can undergo complete resection, including removal of lymph nodes by complete mediastinal dissection. Survival rates are best for this group of patients with N2 disease compared with N2 disease identified by CT scan. FDG-PET scans detect new distant metastases that were not shown by CT or bone scan in about 30% of NSCLC patients and can help significantly with patient triage and significantly change the management of patients (135).

PET scanning can detect lesions >5 to 8 mm on the basis of an increased FDG uptake, and it has become a standard work up for NSCLC. If there is no evidence of distant metastatic disease on CT scan, FDG-PET scanning complements CT scan staging of the mediastinum and provides important information about distant metastases. The combination of CT scanning and PET scanning has greater sensitivity and specificity than CT scanning alone. Numerous nonrandomized studies of FDG-PET have evaluated mediastinal lymph nodes using surgery (i.e., mediastinoscopy and/or thoracotomy with mediastinal lymph node dissection) as the gold standard of comparison. A prospective trial studied the effect of FDG-PET on the staging of 102 patients with NSCLC and found that the sensitivity, specificity, negative predictive value, and positive predictive value of FDG-PET alone for the detection of mediastinal metastases were 91%, 86%, 95%, and 74%, respectively, as compared with CT scan alone, which had a sensitivity of 75% and a specificity of 66% (180). False-negative results from FDG-PET were seen in small tumors and when FDG-PET was unable to distinguish the primary lesion from contiguous lymphadenopathy. False-positive results were often caused by the presence of benign inflammatory disease such as abscesses and active granulomatous diseases, as well as by hypoxic conditions such as those that exist after radiotherapy. Treatment-induced hypermetabolic inammatory changes also may lead to difficulty in differentiating between treatment effects and those of the residual tumor. False-negative results have occurred primarily in tumors with low glucose metabolism (carcinoid and BAC) and in small tumors, owing to the limited spatial resolution of current PET scanners. For patients with clinically operable NSCLC, biopsy of mediastinal lymph nodes is recommended for nodes found on chest CT scan to be >1.0 cm in shortest transverse axis or found positive on FDG-PET scanning. Negative FDG-PET scanning does not preclude biopsy of radiographically enlarged mediastinal lymph nodes. Mediastinoscopy is necessary for the detection of cancer in mediastinal lymph nodes when the results of the CT scan and FDG-PET do not corroborate each other. In addition, FDG uptake on PET has been shown to have independent prognostic value in newly diagnosed NSCLC (198). The role of PET in measuring the biologic effects of anticancer therapy and in restaging after induction therapy awaits better standardization and large-scale experience (237). Integrated PET-CT provides more precise information on the exact location of focal abnormalities and improves the diagnostic accuracy of the staging of NSCLC (120).

Special Diagnostic Procedures

Sputum cytology remains a simple test with a positive predictive value that can approach 100%, but it has a sensitivity rate of only 10% to 15%. Fiberoptic bronchoscopy is an essential and standard technique for the evaluation of patients with pulmonary neoplasms; it remains the most important procedure for determining the endobronchial extent of disease, measuring tumor proximity to the carina and various bronchi and identifying unsuspected occult lesions that indicate multiplicity of disease. For lesions that are visible by endoscopy, an accurate histologic diagnosis can be achieved in more than 90% of cases. For central lesions, cytologic studies via washings and brushings, coupled with transbronchial fine-needle aspiration biopsy (TBFNA), heighten the diagnostic yield to greater than 95%. Peripheral lesions not visible endoscopically may be approached by cytologic studies of brushings and bronchioloalveolar lavage, which yield a diagnosis in 50% to 60% of patients. One of the most important applications of TBFNA is the evaluation of mediastinal lymphadenopathy, particularly for levels 2, 3, 4, 7, and 10. The true sensitivity and specificity of TBFNA seem to range from 14% to 50% and 96% to 100%, respectively. Thus, negative results require definitive operative confirmation, but the risk of a false-positive finding seems to be quite low (231). The advent of endoscopic sonography (bronchoscopic or esophageal) may improve the yield of TDNA to more than 80%.

CT-guided transthoracic percutaneous fine-needle aspiration biopsy can be used for poorly accessible sites in the lung, mediastinum, abdomen, and retroperitoneum. It has been shown to be more than 90% effective in establishing a final diagnosis with diagnostic accuracy rates greater than 97%, a false-positive rate of 1%, and a false negative rate ranging from 23% to 29%. Complications after transthoracic percutaneous fine-needle aspiration biopsy include pneumothorax (20% to 28%), with 5% to 7% requiring chest tube insertion; transient hemoptysis (2% to 4%); and, rarely, air embolism. Implantation of tumor cells along the needle tract has been reported in isolated cases but, again, is extremely rare (231).

Mediastinoscopy is the best method to evaluate the upper, middle peritracheal, and subcarinal lymph nodes. The accuracy of cervical mediastinoscopy ranges from 80% to 90%, and the false-negative rate ranges from 10% to 12%. The lymph node station most commonly missampled is the subcarinal region, which is difficult to access in some patients and challenging to biopsy completely in most patients. The subaortic and aortopulmonary window regions are inaccessible by standard cervical mediastinoscopy (208). "Anterior mediastinotomy" was originally described by McNeil and Chamberlain." It permits direct visual access to the anterior mediastinum through the second, third, or fourth anterior interspace. The procedure is used on the left side to evaluate disease in the subaortic and lateral aortic regions and the aortopulmonary window. Video-assisted thoracoscopy has enhanced the accuracy of diagnosis and staging of lung cancer and is very helpful for staging lung cancer in the presence of associated pleural disease and suspected mediastinal nodal spread. Video-assisted thoracoscopy has become a valuable adjunct to cervical mediastinoscopy and anterior mediastinotomy for evaluating the posterior mediastinum and the peritracheal, subazygous, hilar, and aortopulmonary window nodal regions.

Staging

The American Joint Committee on Cancer (AJCC) has adopted the TNM classification, originally proposed by Mountain et al. (151), which is based primarily on surgical findings. This staging system recently was revised (152,154) and is shown in Tables 48.2 and 48.3 and Fig. 48.3. This system was adopted by the AJCC and International Union Against Cancer in 1997. The stage serves as a guide for treatment modality and prognosis.

Pathologic Classification

The histologic classification of lung tumors was revised in 1999 and in 2004 (Table 48.4). The histologic types are based on analysis by light microscopy and with standard staining techniques. The four major types are squamous cell carcinoma, adenocarcinoma, large cell carcinoma (collectively known as NSCLC and reecting 90% of cases), and small cell undifferentiated carcinoma. The relative incidences of the various histologic types have changed gradually. In past decades, squamous cell carcinoma was the most common type, but in recent years it has

decreased in frequency and adenocarcinoma has increased to become the most common type (49%) in the United States. In some parts of the world, specifically Europe, squamous cell carcinoma is apparently still the most common type.

The majority of lung cancers are histologically heterogeneous. Lung neoplasms are generally classified by the

Table 48.3	STAGE GROUPING: TNM SUBSETS		
Stage	**TNM Subset**		
0	Carcinoma *in situ*		
IA	T1 N0 M0		
IB	T2 N0 M0		
IIA	T1 N1 M0		
IIB	T2 N1 M0	T3 N0 M0	
IIIA	T3 N1 M0	T1 N2 M0	
	T2 N2 M0	T3 N2 M0	
IIIB	T4 N0 M0	T4 N1 M0	T4 N2 M0
	T1 N3 M0	T2 N3 M0	T3 N3 M0
	T4 N3 M0		
IV	Any T, any N, any M		

From American Joint Committee on Cancer. *AJCC cancer staging manual*, 6th ed. New York: Spring-Verlag; 2002, with permission from Springer-Verlag.

Table 48.2	TNM DESCRIPTORS[a]
Primary tumor (T)	
TX	Primary tumor cannot be assessed, or tumor proven by the presence of malignant cells in sputum or bronchial washes but not visualized by imaging or bronchoscopy
T0	No evidence of primary tumor
Tis	Carcinoma *in situ*
T1	Tumor ≤3 cm in greatest dimension, surrounded by lung or visceral pleura, without bronchoscopic evidence of invasion more proximal than the lobar bronchus[a] (i.e., not in the main bronchus)
T2	Tumor with any of the following features of size or extent: <3 cm in greatest dimension; involves main bronchus, 2 cm or more distal to the carina; invades the visceral pleura; associated with atelectasis or obstructive pneumonitis that extends to the hilar region but does not involve the entire lung
T3	Tumor of any size that directly invades any of the following: chest wall (including superior sulcus tumors), diaphragm, mediastinal pleura, or parietal pericardium; or tumor in the main bronchus <2 cm distal to the carina, but without involvement of the carina; or associated atelectasis or obstructive pneumonitis of the entire lung
T4	Tumor of any size that invades any of the following: mediastinum, heart, great vessels, trachea, esophagus, vertebral body, or carina; or tumor with a malignant pleural or pericardial effusion,[b] or with satellite tumor nodule(s) within the ipsilateral primary tumor lobe of the lung
Regional lymph nodes (N)	
NX	Regional lymph nodes cannot be assessed
N0	No regional lymph node metastasis
N1	Metastasis to ipsilateral peribronchial and/or ipsilateral hilar lymph nodes, and intrapulmonary nodes involved by direct extension of the primary tumor
N2	Metastasis to ipsilateral mediastinal and/or subcarinal lymph node(s)
N3	Metastasis to contralateral mediastinal, contralateral hilar, ipsilateral or contralateral scalene, or supraclavicular lymph node(s)
Distant metastasis (M)	
MX	Presence of distant metastasis cannot be assessed
M0	No distant metastasis
M1	Distant metastasis[c]

[a]The uncommon superficial tumor of any size with its invasive component limited to the bronchial wall, which may extend proximal to the main bronchus, also is classified T1.
[b]Most pleural effusions associated with lung cancer are the result of tumor. However, there are a few patients in whom multiple cytopathologic examinations of pleural fluid are negative for tumor. In these cases, the fluid is nonbloody and is not an exudate. When these elements are clinical judgment dictate that the effusion is not related to the tumor, the effusion should be excluded as a staging element and the patient should be staged T1, T2, and T3. Pericardial effusion is classified according to the same rules.
[c]Separate metastatic tumor nodule(s) in the ipsilateral nonprimary tumor lobe(s) of the lung are also classified M1.
From American Joint Committee on Cancer. *AJCC cancer staging manual,* 6th ed. New York: Spring-Verlag; 2002, with permission from Springer-Verlag.

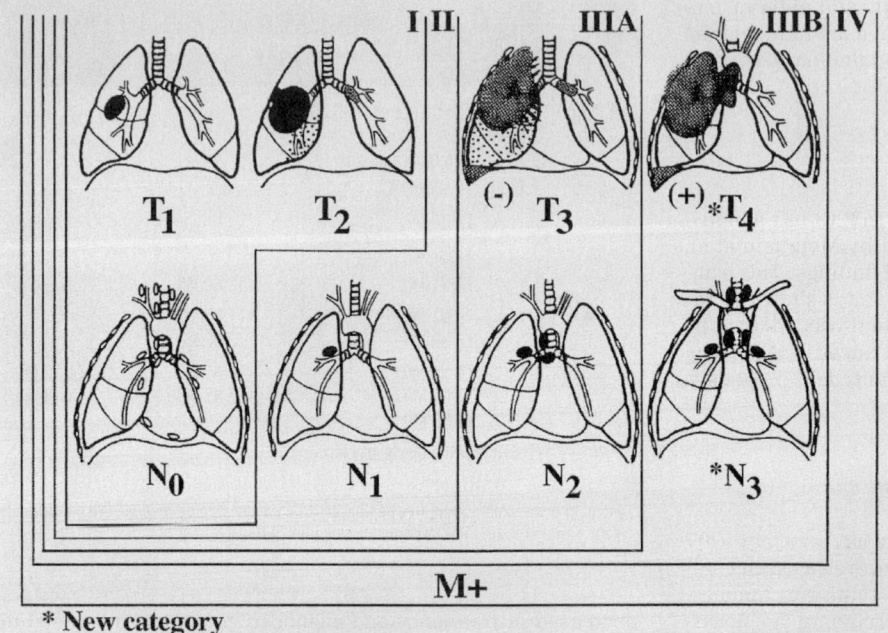

FIGURE 48.3. Anatomic stage grouping for non–small cell lung carcinoma.

best-differentiated region of the tumor and graded by its most poorly differentiated portion. For example, a tumor that shows characteristics of squamous differentiation by demonstrating the obvious presence of keratin pearl formation and intercellular bridges would be classified as a squamous cell carcinoma. If most of the cells of the remaining tumor did not show such features, the same tumor would be further labeled as a poorly differentiated squamous cell tumor.

Prognostic Factors

Prognostic factors for patients with lung cancer can be divided with regard to patient, tumor, and treatment-specific variables. Stanley (???) evaluated 77 prognostic factors in approximately 5,000 patients with inoperable carcinoma of the lung (V.A. Lung Group Protocols). The three most important prognostic factors affecting survival were patient-specific variables, including performance status (Karnofsky score), stage, and weight loss. It is generally believed that epidermoid carcinoma has the best prognosis, followed by adenocarcinoma and undifferentiated large cell carcinoma. However, the comparative prognosis of squamous cell versus adenocarcinoma of the lung remains controversial. Until recently, undifferentiated small cell carcinoma had the poorest prognosis, but prognosis has now improved because of more aggressive combined-modality treatments. The list of molecular prognostic markers continues to grow. Negative prognostic factors for NSCLC include mutations in the K-*ras* oncogene, deletion of tumor-suppressor genes (e.g., *p53*), *NCAM* (neural cell adhesion molecule) expression, elevated serum levels of neuron-specific enolase, overexpression of genes from the ErbB family including *ErbB-1* (epidermal growth factor receptor) and *ErbB-2* (Her2/*neu*), elevation of proliferative markers (Ki-67, cyclin D1, P16 loss, cyclin E, and cyclin B1), elevated angiogenesis markers (microvessel density, vascular endothelial growth factor receptors, and matrix metalloproteinases), and decreased apoptotic markers (apoptotic index, Fas cell surface receptors, and caspase-3). These factors have provided important clinical insights into the biology of lung cancer, and ongoing prospective studies using these biomarkers will have prognostic and therapeutic implications (28,202,236).

Table 48.4	WORLD HEALTH ORGANIZATION LUNG CANCER CLASSIFICATION

I. Epithelial tumors
  A. Benign
    1. Papillomas
    2. Adenoma
  B. Dysplasia/carcinoma *in situ*
  C. Malignant
    1. Squamous cell carcinoma
      a. Spindle cell variant
    2. Small cell carcinoma
      a. Oat cell carcinoma
      b. Intermediate cell type
      c. Combined oat cell carcinoma
    3. Adenocarcinoma
      a. Acinar
      b. Papillary
      c. Bronchioalveolar
      d. Solid carcinoma with mucin formation
    4. Large cell carcinoma
      a. Giant cell carcinoma
      b. Clear cell carcinoma
    5. Adenosquamous carcinoma
    6. Carcinoid tumor
    7. Bronchial gland carcinoma
    8. Others

II. Soft tissue tumors

III. Mesothelial tumors
  A. Benign
  B. Malignant

IV. Miscellaneous tumors
  A. Benign
  B. Malignant

V. Secondary tumors

VI. Unclassified tumors

VII. Tumorlike lesions

Adapted from Brambilla E, Travis WD, Colby TV, et al. The new World Health Organization classification of lung tumours. *Eur Respir J* 2001;18:1059–1068, with permission.

General Management

Non–Small Cell Lung Cancer

In patients with NSCLC, the most important prognostic factor is tumor stage. This factor largely determines treatment. Surgery is the standard mode of treatment of patients with stage I and II tumors and for selective patients with stage III tumors. Neoadjuvant or adjuvant therapy is recommended for many patients with stage II and III disease. Only about 20% of all patients presenting with lung cancer are suitable candidates for curative surgery. The use of combined-modality therapy including radiation and chemotherapy is recommended for locally advanced stage III disease. Patients with stage IV disease are treated with chemotherapy or palliative radiation therapy (RT) or with supportive therapy alone. Patients with histologically documented unresectable or inoperable stage I-III NSCLC are evaluated for definite radiotherapy with or without chemotherapy. If there are pressing symptomatic needs for palliation, such as significant obstruction of a major airway, severe hemoptysis, SVC obstruction, painful bony metastases in the weight-bearing areas, or symptomatic brain metastases, the initial treatment is radiotherapy with or without chemotherapy. If a patient has evidence of disseminated disease and there is no pressing need for radiotherapy, the approach includes consideration of systemic chemotherapy, or supportive therapy alone if the patient's general condition is not suitable for systemic chemotherapy.

Operable Tumors

Stage I and II Non-Small Cell Lung Cancer

The average 5-year survival rate for patients with stage I NSCLC is approximately 65% (range, 55% to 90.5%). Within this group, several factors seem to inuence survival: T status, tumor size independent of T status, and histology. The more favorable tumors are T1 squamous cell carcinoma and T1 BAC. Focal T1 N0 BAC has been reported to have a 5-year survival rate as high as 90.5% (45). Martini et al. (141) reported on 598 patients with stage I (N0) NSCLC who underwent dissection. There were 291 T1 and 307 T2 lesions. Mediastinal lymph node dissections were performed in 560 patients (94%). Overall survival rates of all patients with T1 N0 disease have been reported to be 82% at 5 years and 74% at 10 years, while those for patients with T2 N0 disease were 68% at 5 years and 60% at 10 years. In this series of 598 patients, the overall incidence of recurrence was 27% (local or regional, 7%; systemic, 20%). Second primary tumors developed in 206 patients (34%). Of these 206 tumors, 70 (34%) were second primary lung cancers, for an overall incidence of second primary lung cancers of 11.7% (70 of 598). This report concluded that (a) lymph node dissection is necessary to ensure accurate staging; (b) lesser resections such as wedge or segmental resection result in a high recurrence rate and reduced survival; and (c) second primary lung cancers are prevalent in long-term survivors.

The 1997 revision of the AJCC staging system for NSCLC reclassified these tumors as stage IA or IB, reflecting the better prognosis of patients with lesions less than 3 cm (155). The average 5-year survival rate for patients with stage II disease was 41.2% (range, 29% to 60%) (152,153).

The LCSG reported a randomized comparison of an anatomic lobectomy versus limited (wedge or segmental) resection for peripheral T1 pulmonary carcinomas (69). The locoregional recurrence rate for limited resection was three times greater than for lobectomy, 17% *versus* 6.4%. However, the report did not differentiate true local recurrences from regional nodal metastases. These recurrence rates are consistent with reports of nodal metastases in 17% and 37% of patients with

resected tumors measuring 1 to 2 cm and 2 to 3 cm, respectively (91). For this reason, an anatomic lobectomy is recommended in patients who are able to tolerate the procedure.

Postoperative adjuvant chemotherapy has been tested by several studies with promising results (182). Such an approach in selected patients (stage IB and above, see later section) may prolong survival with reasonable toxicity. This approach is becoming a standard of care in many cases of early-stage disease.

Stage III Non-Small Cell Lung Cancer

Approximately 25% to 40% of patients with NSCLC have stage III disease. Of these, approximately one-third present with potentially resectable disease, stage IIIA (T1–3 N2, T3 N1). The median survival duration for all patients with stage IIIA (clinical or surgical stage) disease treated with surgical resection is 12 months, and the 5-year survival rate is 9% to 15%. Within the stage IIIA subset, however, survival rates vary widely (152,153).

Patients with clinical (preoperative) N0 or N1 disease but pathologic (postresection) N2 disease survive longer than patients with clinical N2 disease, and 3- and 5-year survival rates of 47% and 34%, respectively, were reported for such patients (141). Pearson et al. (175) noted that patients with negative mediastinoscopic findings who were found to have N2 disease following resection had a 24% 5-year survival rate; the 5-year survival rate was only 9% for those who underwent resection after positive mediastinoscopy. Patients with "completely resected" pathologic N2 disease have a median 5-year survival rate approaching 22%. Approximately 33% of patients with stage IIIA disease (based on N2 nodal metastases) present with a single positive node, whereas the remainder present with multiple nodes involved at a single station or at multiple stations. Patients with multiple-station involvement have a significantly worse prognosis than patients with single-node involvement (142).

If patients are found to have N2 disease at diagnosis, combined-modality management is generally recommended. Participation in clinical trials is encouraged. Patients with stage IIIB disease are not considered candidates for surgical resection except for selective T4 tumors involving the carina and the SVC, aorta, or atrium or satellite lesions in the same lobe, limited vertebral involvement. However, special expertise is required and combined modality treatment is recommended.

Neoadjuvant (Induction) Treatment

Preoperative Irradiation

Despite the initial encouraging results of an institutional trial by Bloedorn et al. (18), two subsequent national collaborative studies failed to show any improvement in survival with the use of preoperative RT (212,240). However, many aspects of the study design and stratification in the latter two studies were criticized; all stages and histologies were included, and no appropriate stratification was performed. Treatment planning by simulators and modern megavoltage equipment were not used in either study. In a prospective randomized multi-institution trial of 478 patients with lung cancer, patients receiving preoperative irradiation (20 Gy in five fractions) followed by surgery were compared with patients receiving surgery alone. There was no difference in the 5-year survival rates among patients with stages I and II disease. However, the survival rates for stage III patients were 49.4% at 3 years and 29.2% at 5 years for the combined-therapy group compared with 28.1% and 15.8%, respectively, for the surgery-alone group (232).

Preoperative Chemotherapy

Patients with N0 disease usually have a very high cure rate and are not routinely candidates for neoadjuvant therapy. However,

Author/ Treatment	Patients	Responses (%)	Media Survival Time (mo)	3 Years (%)	5 Years (%)
TABLE 48.5 SURGERY ALONE VERSUS NEOADJUVANT CHEMOTHERAPY FOLLOWED BY SURGERY IN STAGE III NON–SMALL CELL LUNG CANCER					
Roth et al. (192)					
Surgery	32	—	14	19	15
CEP + S	28	35	21[a]	43	36
Rosell et al. (189)					
Surgery	30	—	10	5	0
MIP + S	30	60	22[a]	20	17

CEP, cyclophosphamide, etoposide, cisplatin; S, surgery; MIP, mitomycin, ifosfamide, cisplatin.
[a]$p < .05$.

patients with stage II (T1N1 and T2N1) disease, who have lower survival rates (25% to 50%) after surgical resection, and those with stage III disease, who have a very low survival rate, potentially could benefit from neoadjuvant therapy (88). Two randomized trials have been reported for patients with stage III cancers (Table 48.5).

At M.D. Anderson Cancer Center, 60 patients were randomized to undergo chemotherapy and surgery or surgery alone. Twenty-eight patients received three cycles of cyclophosphamide, etoposide, and cisplatin and then underwent surgery, and they were compared with 32 patients treated with surgery alone. The median survival durations were 64 months versus 11 months, favoring neoadjuvant chemotherapy. The 2-year survival rates were 56% in the neoadjuvant group and 15% in the surgery-only group ($p = .008$). In this study, the patients who had positive margins, multiple levels of positive lymph nodes, or extracapsular extension received postoperative radiotherapy (PORT) between 50 and 60 Gy, and only two patients developed local recurrences. Rosell et al. (189) from Barcelona randomized 60 patients treated with or without mitomycin C, ifosfamide, and cisplatin as neoadjuvant chemotherapy. Thirty patients received neoadjuvant chemotherapy followed by surgery, and the other half underwent surgery alone; the median survival duration was 26 months in the neoadjuvant group and 8 months in the surgery-only group. The 2-year survival rates were 29% among the patients who received neoadjuvant chemotherapy and 0% among the patients who received surgery alone, although both groups had PORT of 50 Gy in 5 weeks. The neoadjuvant chemotherapy group had an improved 2-year survival rate ($p = .001$).

Preoperative Chemoradiation

Almost all of the trials previously mentioned involved patients with stage IIIA disease. A similar approach also has been reported by Rusch et al. (194), who administered neoadjuvant treatment consisting of cisplatin plus VP-16 and concurrent irradiation, followed by surgery, to 51 patients with stage IIIB NSCLC (a subset of patients from a Southwest Oncology Group [SWOG] protocol). Thirty-two patients (63%) underwent resection of the primary tumor, with a 5.2% operative mortality rate. For all 51 patients, survival at 2 years was 39%. Most of the recurrences were distant. This study demonstrated the feasibility of such an approach in patients with more advanced stage IIIB disease. To study the issue of surgical resection after induction chemoradiation, the SWOG conducted a phase II trial of induction concurrent chemotherapy, cisplatin, and etoposide with thoracic RT (TRT) in 74 patients with biopsy-proven stage IIIA (N2) NSCLC. Study results suggested that this approach may

improve patient survival with reasonable toxicity. Median survival duration was 13 months, the 2-year survival rate was 37%, and the 3-year survival rate was 27%. Median survival duration of patients who had pathologic complete response of nodal disease was 30 months, while that of patients with residual nodal disease was 10 months ($p = .0005$). On the basis of the results from this study, the NCI had launched a phase III multicenter trial for patients with biopsy-proven N2 disease and potentially resectable NSCLC (NCI Protocol INT 139). Patients were stratified by performance status and T status and were randomized to receive induction chemoradiotherapy (45 Gy) followed by surgery or chemotherapy with definitive radiotherapy (61 Gy). All patients received an additional two courses of chemotherapy. Initial results, presented in 2003, showed better progression-free survival rate in the trimodality arm. Follow-up data, including survival data, were presented at the American Society for Clinical Oncology annual meeting in 2005 by Albain et al. (3). Study results confirmed significantly greater progression-free survival for trimodality arm. Survival curves were superimposed through year 2 and then separated. By year 5, an absolute survival benefit of 7% favored the surgery arm (odds ratio = 0.63 [0.36, 1.10]; $p = .10$). Subgroup analysis revealed better survival for patients who underwent a lobectomy ($p = .002$). However, trimodality therapy was not optimal when a pneumonectomy was required owing to the high mortality risk. Finally, N0 status at surgery significantly predicted a higher 5-year survival rate. The authors suggested that surgical resection after chemoradiation can be considered for fit patients when lobectomy is feasible.

The optimal regiment for induction treatment in N2 disease remains investigational. The Radiation Therapy Oncology Group (RTOG) is conducting a phase III study to compare induction chemotherapy versus induction chemoradiotherapy followed by surgical resection in pathologically proved N2 NSCLC.

Adjuvant Therapy

Postoperative Radiation Therapy

In general, postoperative RT is indicated in incomplete resections (close or positive margins) or positive mediastinal metastases (N2). Eradication of local cancer is a prerequisite for cure. As with any other tumor site, if surgical margins are close or positive, postoperative RT clearly is indicated for improvement of local tumor control. The definitions of positive, close, and clear surgical margins are rather arbitrary. Generally, if tumor cells are found at the surgical margins (usually inked), these are called *positive surgical margins*. If less than 0.5 cm of normal tissue is present adjacent to the tumor edge, the surgical margin usually is considered close; more than 1 cm of normal tissue is considered a clear surgical margin. Close or positive bronchial surgical resection margins can occur with peripherally located tumors, often attached to the chest wall, or with centrally located tumors. In these situations, a course of postoperative RT of 50 Gy for potential microscopic disease and 60 to 66 Gy for a positive margin in 2-Gy fractions usually is recommended. If, during thoracotomy, a complete and thorough resection of mediastinal nodes is performed and all nodes are negative, the course of postoperative RT for positive or close surgical margins can be directed to only a small volume related to the primary tumor. Lymph-bearing areas have not been treated prophylactically in this situation. Controversy exists regarding the role of postoperative adjuvant therapy for patients with resected N1 and N2 disease, with more data supporting adjuvant RT in N2 disease. The rationale for adjuvant RT stems for data-reporting patterns of failure following resection with 10% to 50% local regional failure and 20% to 40% distant failure. Numerous retrospective reports have been published on the potential benefits of postoperative adjuvant irradiation. Retrospective institutional reports suggest beneficial effects (37,105), but supporting data from controlled prospective randomized trials proving its efficacy are few and largely limited to improvement of local control.

PORT is currently contraindicated in patients with stage I completely resected disease on the basis of the PORT meta-analysis (183). Data for stage II and higher-stage disease neither support nor refute the use of PORT (because the hazard ratio error bars include 1.0), although it clearly improves regional control. The LCSG conducted a randomized study to evaluate postoperative radiotherapy in patients with complete resected stage II and IIIA squamous cell carcinoma of the lung (133). Only patients with hilar (N1) or mediastinal (N2) lymph node metastasis were included in the study. Patients on the adjuvant radiation arm were treated to 50 Gy in 5 weeks. No difference in overall survival was detected. However, patients receiving radiation had reduced local recurrence rates (3% vs. 41%), especially patients with N2 disease. There were four significant flaws in the design and conduct of this study: only squamous cell carcinoma was included; 11% of the patients of the irradiated patients had no regional-node metastasis and therefore would not have been advised to have postoperative irradiation; only 74% of the patients who were assigned to receive postoperative RT received within 5% of the total dose prescribed; and no quality assurance was performed to evaluate the treated irradiation volume.

The British Medical Research Council conducted a randomized trial for patients with completely resected T1–2 N1–2 M0 tumors (148). Patients randomized to the radiation arm received 40 Gy in 15 fractions, although 10% did not initiate such therapy. Results were reported by intention to treat. No survival advantage was seen for either group. However, adjuvant radiotherapy reduced local recurrences and the development of distant metastases, specifically bone metastases. On subgroup analysis, patients with N2 disease experienced fewer local recurrences, fewer distant metastases, and prolonged survival with the addition of radiotherapy. Patients with N1 disease did not benefit from RT.

The PORT meta-analysis (183) has been widely discussed because of the negative effect of RT on overall survival for all patients examined (stages I–III). Subgroup analysis identified that the decremental effect was statistically limited to patients with stage I disease and was nearly significant for stage II disease. There is a suggestion of benefit to PORT for patients with N2 disease that did not reach statistical significance. There are problems with the nine randomized trials that are included in this meta-analysis, including the inclusion of patients with stage I disease, four of the trials used hypofractionated treatment schedules, and seven of the trials used cobalt 60. These issues may have contributed significantly to the negative effect of RT on survival for the patients with stages I and II disease.

A recent publication from the SEER database included 7,465 patients with resected N0, N1, and N2 disease (116); 47% were treated with adjuvant RT. The median follow-up duration was 3.5 years. The use of PORT had no statistical impact on survival for the overall group. Subgroup analysis showed that PORT resulted in decreased survival for N0 (HR 1.176, confidence interval [CI] = 1.005–1.376) and N1 (HR 1.097, CI = 1.015–1.186) disease and a significant increase in survival for patients with N2 disease (HR 0.855, CI = 0.762–0.959).

Although these data from the PORT meta-analysis and SEER groups may not apply to modern radiotherapy techniques, they are further evidence that patients with resected N0 or N1 disease should not routinely receive radiotherapy. Megavoltage energies, conventional fraction sizes, and image-based treatment planning should be applied carefully to selected patients to minimize late complications.

Postoperative Chemotherapy

A meta-analysis in 1995 compared surgery alone with surgery followed by cisplatin-based chemotherapy. This study included eight trials and 1,394 patients and showed a 13% reduction in the risk of death, suggesting that adjuvant chemotherapy afforded an absolute benefit of 5% at 5 years ($p = .08$). This was not affected by patient sex, PS, age, or tumor histologic subtype (166). The International Adjuvant Lung Trial study included 1,867 patients who underwent randomization either to receive three or four cycles of adjuvant cisplatin-based chemotherapy or to undergo observation. The investigators concluded that cisplatin-based adjuvant chemotherapy prolonged survival among patients with completely resected NSCLC (8). During the American Society for Clinical Oncology 2004 annual meeting, two moderate-sized studies were reported to show a significant survival benefit of 15% at 5 years for the NCIC JBR10 study (241) and 12% at 4 years for the Cancer and Leukemia Group B (CALGB) 9633 study (225). In the ANITA trial, 8% survival benefit was observed in adjuvant chemotherapy arm (53). Furthermore, a Japanese meta-analysis of 2,003 patients randomized in six trials of uracil-tegafur showed a 5% benefit at 7 years (80), confirming the results of the Japanese Lung Cancer Research Group study (101). Supplementing surgery for NSCLC with chemotherapy (either adjuvant or neoadjuvant) is becoming the standard of care, and standardization, optimization, and individualization of this approach is expected in the near future (123).

Postoperative Adjuvant Chemoradiation

The role of adjuvant chemoradiotherapy remains controversial. Keller et al. (102) reported the results of this prospective randomized study designed to determine whether combination chemotherapy with cisplatin/etoposide and TRT was superior to TRT alone for patients with completely resected stage II or IIIa NSCLC. A total of four chemotherapy cycles was administered; the first two were given concomitantly with radiotherapy. Radiation was given in a daily fractionation sequence to a total dose of 50.4 Gy and was identical in the two treatment arms. The median follow-up was 44 months for 488 patients entered. Although the combined postoperative treatment was generally well tolerated, there was no decrease in the risk of intrathoracic recurrence for the experimental arm, nor was there evidence of a survival difference between the treatment arms. At this point, we conclude that there is no definitive evidence showing a meaningful clinical benefit for adjuvant concurrent chemotherapy and radiotherapy after resection of stage II or III NSCLC with negative margins.

The RTOG recently published the results of a phase II study using paclitaxel and carboplatin concurrently with adjuvant RT (25). Eighty-eight patients were accrued with stages II and IIIA disease and treated with 50.4 Gy in 28 fractions during 6 weeks during cycles 1 and 2 of chemotherapy. A boost of 10.8 Gy was given for patients with extracapsular extension or T3 lesions. Treatment compliance was good, with 93% completing RT and 86% completing chemotherapy. With a median follow up of 56.7 months, the median overall survival was 56.3 months with 1-, 2- and 3-year survival rates of 86%, 70%, and 61%, respectively. These phase II results compared favorably with the concurrent chemoRT arm of the previously described trial of Keller et al. (102), further supporting the need for a randomized trial testing sequential versus concurrent chemoRT for patients with resected N2 disease.

Summary

Recent studies have confirmed a survival benefit from adjuvant chemotherapy in NSCLC after surgical resection, and such a

Table 48.6 OUTCOME BY RADIATION THERAPY DOSE AND TREATMENT VOLUME FOR PATIENTS WITH STAGE I NON–SMALL CELL LUNG CANCER

Authors	No. Patients	Dose (Gy)	Local Field (%)	Grade 3–5 Toxicity	Intercurrent Death (%)	Overall Survival (%)		Cause-Specific Survival (%)	
						3 Yr	5 Yr	3 Yr	5 Yr
Dosoretz et al. (52)	152	76%, 60–69	Minority	0	11	—	10	—	—
Graham et al. (76)	103	Median, 60	20	1%	28	—	13	—	—
Haffty et al. (79)	43	59 continuous or 54 split	—	No obvious	—	36	21	—	—
Kaskowitz et al. (100)	53	Median, 63	<10	8%	27	19	6	33	13
Krol et al. (114)	108	60 or 65	100	0	34	31	15	42	31
Sandler et al. (197)	77	Median, 60	10	Minimal	16	17	14	22	17
Talton et al. (227)	77	60	0	0	—	21	17	—	—
Zhang et al. (247)	44	50%, 55–61; 50%, 69–70	0	1 myelitis	20	55	32	—	—
Sibley et al. (215)	141	Median, 64	27	1.5%	43	24	13	—	—

regimen has become standard treatment for resected stage IB to III NSCLC. Postoperation radiotherapy is indicated for patients with close or positive margins and/or resected N2 disease. If the resection margin is negative, and mediastinal nodes are positive, adjuvant chemotherapy should be given for two to four cycles followed by radiotherapy. If the resection margin is positive, postoperative radiotherapy should be given first, followed by adjuvant chemotherapy. The role of PORT in positive N1 disease remains controversial. Because of the potential long-term survival of the group of patients, chronic toxicity associated with PORT should be considered. For positive or close margins without N1 or N2 involvement, the target volume should be limited to the site of the positive margin only. The dose should be around 60 to 66 Gy. For gross positive margins (subtotal resection), patients should receive definitive therapy with concurrent chemoradiotherapy (see later discussion). For patients with N2 disease that has been surgically resected, the target volume should limited to the positive lymph node station plus or minus the ipsilateral hilum and subcarinal lymph node, depending on the location of primary cancer and whether full lymph node dissection was preformed during the surgery. The dose should be limited to about 50 Gy with standard fraction sizes.

Inoperable Non-Small Cell Lung Cancer

Definitive Radiation Therapy

Definitive Radiotherapy for Stage I/II
Patients who cannot undergo surgery because of their lung function, cardiac function, bleeding tendency, or other comorbid conditions, or patients who refuse surgery with stage I or II non–small cell carcinomas, should be considered for definitive RT. Results of retrospective studies are shown in Table 48.6. These studies suggest better results in patients with tumors smaller than 3 cm, in patients with excellent performance status, and in those given radiation doses of 60 Gy or more. Dosoretz et al. (50) reported that rates of distant metastasis were correlated to the size of the primary tumor. Incidences of metastasis in 3 years were 8% for cases with tumors smaller than 3 cm, 27% for tumors measuring 3 to 5 cm, and 50% for tumors larger than 5 cm. They reported that the local control rates at 3 years were 77% for 4-cm lesions and 48% for those larger than 4 cm.

As would be expected, the intercurrent death rates in this population are quite high (Table 48.6). Cause-specific survival is more descriptive of tumor control in the medically inoperable population but was poorly documented because of a lack of systematic image follow-up. In most previous studies, conventional fractionated radiotherapy (60 to 66 Gy in 1.8- or 2-Gy fractions) was used, with reported 5-year local control and overall survival

rates ranging from 30% to 50% and 10% to 30%, respectively (50,100). Several studies have reported a benefit from dose escalation, suggesting a dose-response relationship in both survival and local control in these patients (50,51,100,215). Because early-stage NSCLC is not inherently a systemic disease from diagnosis, and because local control is poor after conventional radiotherapy, research measures aimed at improving survival should put significant emphasis on improving local tumor obliteration.

Stereotactic Body Radiation Therapy. The development of three-dimensional conformal radiotherapy (3DCRT) and stereotactic body radiation therapy (SBRT) allows precise targeting and delivery of radiotherapy. SBRT for lung cancer uses elements of 3DCRT and also incorporates a variety of systems for taking cancer motion into consideration and decreasing setup uncertainty using image-guided radiotherapy techniques. These systems allow reduction of treatment volumes, facilitating hypofractionation with markedly increased daily doses and a significantly reduced overall treatment time. The combination of multiple beam angles to achieve sharp dose gradients, high-precision localization, and a high dose per fraction in extracranial locations is referred to as *SBRT*. This approach delivers a high biologic effective dose (BED) to the target while minimizing the normal tissue toxicities, which may translate into improved local control and survival.

Clinical Outcome and Biologically Effective Dose Consideration. Several studies have reported significantly improved local control and survival using SBRT in patients with stage I lung cancer. Onishi et al. (170) reported the delivery of 60 Gy to the planning target volume (PTV) in 10 fractions (6 Gy/fraction) in patients with stage I NSCLC. Six percent of the patients had local progression and 14% had distant or regional lymph node metastasis. Also, 9% experienced grade 2 or higher toxic effects. The 2-year overall survival rate was 58% in all patients and 83% in those with operable disease. Additionally, Nagata et al. (160) reported the delivery of 48 Gy to the isocenter in four fractions (12 Gy/fraction) during 5 to 13 days in patients with early-stage NSCLC. The local control rate was 98%, and the 5-year overall survival rate was 83% in patients with stage Ia disease and 72% in those with stage Ib disease. About 25% to 28% of the patients had regional lymph node metastasis. None of the patients had grade 3 or higher toxic effects. In a multi-institutional phase II study of patients with T1N0M0 NSCLC conducted by the Japan Clinical Oncology Group, researchers prescribed 48 Gy delivered in four fractions to the isocenter. In the United States, McGarry et al. (147) conducted a dose-escalation study using SBRT for stage I NSCLC. They prescribed delivery of radiation to the 80% isodose line and escalated the dose from 24 to 72 Gy (delivered in three fractions during 2 weeks). The local failure rate was 21%, and the regional and/or distant metastasis rate was about 30%. Most of the local failures occurred with doses less than 48 Gy. Grade 3 and higher toxic effects occurred with doses higher than 48 Gy. The dose regimen is considered too toxic for centrally located tumors and should be used only for peripheral lesions (2 cm away from the bronchus tree).

Currently, RTOG is conducting a phase II clinical study using 60 Gy in three fractions as described by McGarry et al. in patients with inoperable stage I and selective stage II peripheral located NSCLC. Recently, we reported our phase II study using SBRT in medically inoperable patients with stage I/II in both peripherally and centrally located NSCLC. When 70 Gy was delivered at 7 Gy/fraction to the gross target volume, the 1-, 2-, and 3-year local control rates were all 95% in all patients. The 1-, 2-, and 3-year overall survival rates were 100%, 91%, and 91%, respectively, in patients with stage I disease and 73%, 64%, and 64%, respectively, in those with stage II disease. Only 2.3% (1/43) of the patients had grade 3 pneumonitis (244).

The optimal regimen of dose and fractionation using SBRT remains unclear. Onishi et al. (169) retrospectively evaluated results from a Japanese multi-institutional SBRT study. Patients with stage I NSCLC (n = 245) were treated with hypofractionated high-dose SBRT in 13 institutions. A total dose of 18 to 75 Gy at the isocenter was administered in 1 to 22 fractions. The median calculated BED was 108 Gy (range, 57 to 180 Gy) and the median follow-up was 24 months. Pulmonary complications of grade >2 were observed in only six patients (2.4%). Local recurrence rate was 8.1% for BED ≥100 Gy compared with 26.4% for <100 Gy (*p* <.05). The 5-year overall survival rate of medically operable patients was 88.4% for BED ≥100 Gy compared with 69.4% for <100 Gy (*p* <.05). Their data showed that hypofractionated high-dose SBRT with BED <150 Gy was feasible and beneficial for curative treatment of patients with stage I NSCLC. For all treatment methods and schedules, local control and survival rates were better with BED ≥100 Gy compared with <100 Gy. Survival rates in medically operable, BED ≥100 Gy were comparable to those of surgery.

The BED, calculated using the linear quadratic equation BED = nd [1 + d/(α/β)] using an α/β of 10, was 96 Gy with delivery of 60 Gy in 10 fractions, 106 Gy with delivery of 48 Gy in 4 fractions, 119 Gy with delivery of 70 Gy in 10 fractions, and 180 Gy with delivery of 60 Gy in 3 fractions. When we consider optimal BED for SBRT, we need to keep in mind the potential long-term toxicity associated with SBRT, particularly for lesions close to critical structures such as tracheal, bronchus, vessels, nerves, esophagus, spinal cord, heart, and skin. Currently, the consensus is that BED must be >100 Gy and that the volume of critical structures receiving high BED (>80 Gy) should be minimized. Therefore, in general, only peripherally located disease should be treated with SBRT. For stage II disease, only selected disease such as chest wall involvement (T3N0M0) can be treated with SBRT. For patients with a central tumor location or N1 disease without further long-term toxicity data, a greater number of fractions and/or lower BED should be considered when using SBRT.

At M.D. Anderson Cancer Center, we reported our preliminary data using image-guided SBRT in early-stage NSCLC (32). Thirty-seven patients with pathologically confirmed stage I disease were treated with SBRT. All patients were staged with chest CT, PET, and brain MRI. Four-dimensional CT images were obtained in a General Electric simulator with the Varian RPM system. Internal gross target volume was delineated using maximal intensity projection that was created by combining the data

from the multiple four dimensional (4D) CT datasets at different breath phases (see later section for detail). Clinical target volume (CTV) was internal gross target volume plus an 8-mm margin, and a 3-mm setup uncertainty margin was added to form the PTV. Daily CT on-rail simulation was conducted during each fraction of radiotherapy. The prescribed dose was 50 Gy to PTV at a daily 12.5 Gy/fraction (daily SBRT for contiguous 4 days, BED = 112.5 Gy). Critical structures such as main bronchus, heart, and major vessels were excluded from the 40-Gy isodose line. Patients were followed every 3 months for 2 years with chest CT. PET scan was recommended 3 to 5 months after SBRT. Progression-free survival rate at the treated site in all cases was 100%, with a median follow up of 10 months. For stage Ia (T1N0M0) disease (n = 22), the complete response rate was 66.7% and the partial response was 28.8%. Stable disease was 4.5%. However, the complete response rate was 100% if PET was used for post-SBRT evaluation (n = 11). Mediastinal lymph node metastasis and distant metastasis developed in 4%. There was no grade II or above radiation pneumonitis in the patients with stage I disease, and no esophagitis was noted. Some patients (9.5%) developed grade II dermatitis at the treated site. All patients tolerated SBRT well without any symptoms during the SBRT. More patient study with long-term follow up is needed. Figure 48.4 shows a representative case with stage I NSCLC treated by SBRT that achieved complete clinical response.

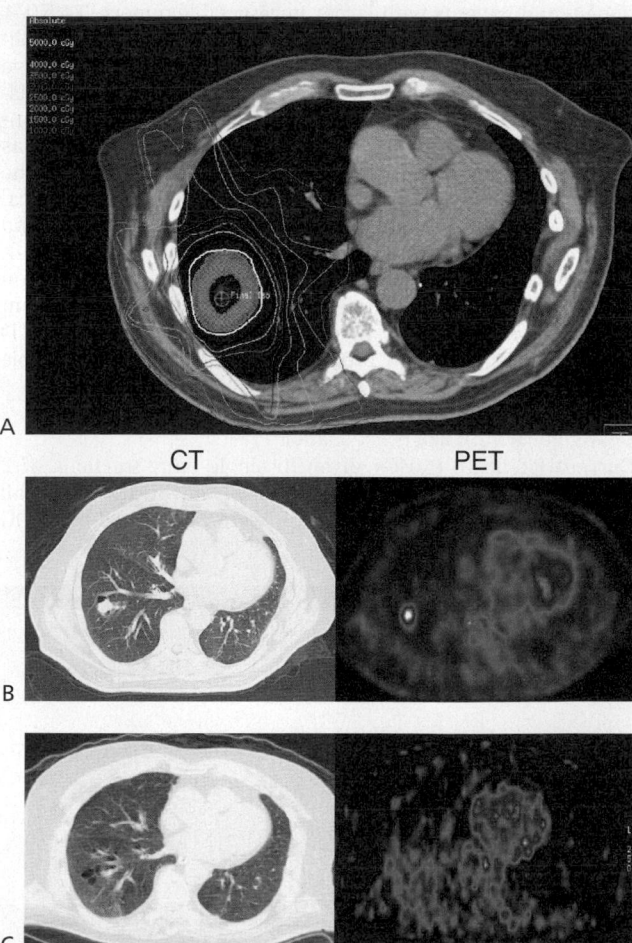

FIGURE 48.4. Stereotactic body radiation therapy (SBRT) in stage I non–small cell lung carcinoma (NSCLC). The patient was diagnosed as having T1N0M0 right lower lobe NSCLC and was treated with SBRT. **A:** Isodose distribution and target coverage with SBRT to a dose of 50 Gy in four fractions prescribed to planning target volume. **B:** Computed tomography (CT) and positron emission tomography (PET) before SBRT **C:** CT and PET 3 months after SBRT.

Phase II and phase III study to evaluate the role of SBRT in early-stage operable NSCLC is being considered by RTOG and the International Association for the Study of Lung Cancer.

Summary

Image-guided SBRT with delivery of BED >100 Gy is feasible and safe in the treatment of peripherally located inoperable stage I and selective II NSCLC. The 3- to 5-year local control and overall survival rates seem to be much better than those for conventional radiotherapy, and the toxicity is minimal. Particularly for stage Ia (T1N0M0) disease, SBRT achieved results comparable to those for surgical resection. SBRT is becoming the standard treatment for inoperable stage I NSCLC. To take tumor motion into consideration, image-guided SBRT is required and crucial. The optimal dose regimen remains unclear, but BED higher than 100 Gy seems to be needed. We need to balance the potential improvement of tumor control and treatment-related toxicities.

Definitive Radiotherapy in Stage III Non-Small Cell Lung Cancer

Definitive RT is indicated for approximately 40% of patients presenting with newly diagnosed NSCLC. This patient population consists of two groups: patients with localized lesions that are potentially resectable but are medically inoperable because of medical reasons (such as stage I/II disease as previously mentioned) and patients with larger unresectable tumors (T4 N0–1 or T1–4 N2–3). Most of the patients registered for RT have locoregionally advanced lung cancer (stage IIIA or IIIB). Definitive RT consists of a minimum dose of 60 to 75 Gy to the gross disease and 50 Gy to microscopic disease with standard fractionation (1.8 or 2 Gy/fraction). A minimal tumor dose of 60 Gy has been considered "standard" for the past 20 years. However, the optimal dose and regimen remain unclear. We know that local control with 60 Gy in stage III NSCLC is only about 30%, and a higher dose is required to improve local control and potential survival. However, toxicity associated with dose escalation limits the potential of dose escalation. 3DCRT and the recent development of intensity-modulated radiation therapy (IMRT) in lung cancer may allow further dose escalation with tolerable toxicity.

Conventional Dose and Fractionation

Current RT doses (60 Gy given in single daily fractions of 2 Gy) for patients with unresectable, locally advanced non–small cell carcinoma (stage IIIA and IIIB) were established by RTOG

73-01 (179). In this study, 375 patients with inoperable or unresectable stage III (T1N2, T2N2, T3N0, T3N1, T3N2) NSCLC (epidermoid, adenocarcinoma, or large cell undifferentiated carcinoma) were randomized to receive a dose of 40 Gy split-course or a 40-, 50-, or 60-Gy dose in continuous courses with daily doses of 2 Gy. At 2 to 3 years, survival was 15% to 20% for patients treated with 50 or 60 Gy compared with 10% for patients in the 40-Gy groups ($p = .10$). After 4 years, survival was comparable in all groups (4% to 6%). In patients treated with 40 Gy, the rates of intrathoracic failure were 44% and 52% compared with 33% to 45% in those treated with 50 or 60 Gy. The incidences of distant metastasis as detected by clinical or radiographic examination were 75% to 80% in all groups (177). In patients surviving 6 to 12 months, a statistically significant increased survival was noted when the intrathoracic tumor was controlled. Patients treated with 50 to 60 Gy and showing tumor control had a 3-year survival rate of 22% versus 10% if they had intrathoracic failure ($p = .05$). In patients treated with 40 Gy (split or continuous), the respective survival rates were 20% and 10% if the intrathoracic tumor was controlled ($p = 0.001$) (176).

Radiation Dose Escalation and Acceleration

From basic principles advocated by Fletcher (58), doses in the range of 80 to 100 Gy are required to sterilize the tumors frequently treated in bronchogenic carcinoma. There are two fundamental problems with the delivery of such doses in lung cancer: the high rate of distant metastases, the major contributor to tumor-related mortality, and the normal tissue toxicity of thoracic organs.

To improve survival rates for this population, some investigators set out to reduce local failures with intensified radiotherapy regimens. In 1983, the RTOG initiated a second dose-escalation trial in an effort to increase local control and survival. Hyperfractionation regimens (1.2 Gy twice daily) were used to decrease normal tissue toxicities (201). Five arms were tested: 60 Gy, 64.8 Gy, 69.6 Gy, 74.4 Gy, and 79 Gy. The best results were seen in a cohort of patients with good performance (Karnofsky performance score ≥ 70 and weight loss $\leq 50\%$) who received 69.6 Gy; the 1-year survival rate was 58% and the 3-year survival rate was 20%. In a later RTOG prospective phase III trial, hyperfractionated treatment to 69.6 Gy was compared with conventional irradiation (60 Gy) and chemoirradiation (see later discussion and Table 48.7).

Results for accelerated hyperfractionated radiotherapy schedules are given in Table 48.7. Saunders et al. (199) reported the results of a multicenter, European continuous, hyperfractionated, accelerated RT compared with standard

							Survival		
Regimen	Fractionation (Gy)	Fx/D	No. Fractions	Radiation Therapy Duration (d)	Total Dose (Gy)	1 Yr (%)	2 Yr (%)	Median	

Table 48.7　TRIAL OF ACCELERATED HYPERFRACTIONATED RADIATION THERAPY IN NON–SMALL CELL LUNG CANCER

Regimen	Fractionation (Gy)	Fx/D	No. Fractions	Radiation Therapy Duration (d)	Total Dose (Gy)	1 Yr (%)	2 Yr (%)	Median
Phase III randomized CHART Saunders et al. (199)	1.5	3	36	12	54	63	29	NA
RT alone	2	1	30	42	60	—	20	—
Phase II nonrandomized HART Mehta et al. (149)	1.5–1.8	3	36	15	57.6	57	NA	13 mo.

Fx/D, fraction per dose; CHART, continuous hyperfractionated accelerated radiation therapy; NA, not applicable; HART, hyperfractionated accelerated radiation therapy.

radiotherapy in NSCLC. Patients randomized to the experimental arm received 36 fractions of 1.5 Gy/fraction given as three fractions per day for 12 consecutive days, for a total dose of 54 Gy. The control arm received 2 Gy/fraction to 60 Gy during 6 weeks. Both 1- and 2-year survival rates were improved with the intensive radiotherapy course. There was no difference with respect to reported acute and late toxicities (13).

In a phase II hyperfractionated, accelerated RT trial sponsored by the Eastern Cooperative Oncology Group (ECOG 4593), 30 patients were treated with 1.5- to 1.8-Gy fractions three times per day during 16 days, for a total dose of 57.6 Gy (149). This protocol called for no treatments to be given on weekends. With a minimum follow-up of 19 months, the median survival was 13 months and the 1-year survival rate was 57%. This regimen is being compared with standard radiotherapy (60 Gy during 6 to 7 weeks) by ECOG in a phase III trial.

A trial from the Netherlands (207) intensified the radiation delivered using a concomitant-boost technique. Thirty-three patients with inoperable NSCLC were treated with 60 Gy in 20 fractions in 25 days. Fifteen patients received 40 Gy in 2-Gy fractions to the primary tumor and a part of the mediastinum, and 18 patients received the same dose to the primary tumor and the whole mediastinum. During each session, a simultaneous boost of 1 Gy was administered to the primary tumor. Moderate acute esophageal toxicity was observed in seven (22%) of 33 patients, and severe late toxicity was seen in one patient (3%). After a mean follow-up of 14 months, 17 patients (52%) had local tumor control, 13 patients (39%) developed a confirmed local recurrence within the treated area, and three patients (9%) had suspected tumor regrowth.

The RTOG recently completed a phase II dose-escalation study (RTOG 93–11) (23). Patients were treated with either radiation alone or radiation following neoadjuvant chemotherapy. Radiotherapy was planned with 3D conformal techniques with target volumes limited to the gross tumor volume (GTV) plus a margin. Because the study was designed to find the maximum tolerated radiation dose, the total volume of normal lung treated dictated the dose. Patients with smaller lung volumes irradiated were treated to higher doses according to the escalation schema. Total doses ranged between 70.9 and 90.3 Gy for the small-volume group and 70.9 to 77.4 Gy in the larger volume group. The daily fraction size was 2.15 Gy. RTOG 9311 showed that acute toxicity rates were acceptable for the dose up to 90.3 Gy (<15% grade 3 and above pneumonitis, and no esophagitis). However, late toxicities were more pronounced. Late radiation pneumonitis grade 3 and above occurred at a rate of 15% for patients with a V20 <25% treated to dose levels of 77.4 Gy or above with a fraction size of 2.15 Gy. For patients with a V20

of 25% to 37%, late pneumonitis grade 3 and above occurred at the rate of 15% for the doses of 70.9 Gy or above. The late grade 3 and above esophagitis occurred in <7% of the patients. The rate of late esophagitis was not directly correlated with doses but it may have been related to the volume of esophagus treated.

University of Michigan investigators performed a dose-escalation trial that included 106 patients with stages I-III NSCLC treated with 63 to 103 Gy in 2.1-Gy fractions using 3DCRT (113). Targets included only the primary tumor and any lymph nodes ≥1 cm. Eighty-one percent of the patients received no chemotherapy. The median survival was 19 months. Multivariate analysis revealed that weight loss ($p = .011$) and radiation dose ($p = .0006$) were significant predictors for overall survival. The 5-year overall survival rates were 4%, 22%, and 28% for patients receiving 63 to 69, 74 to 84, and 92 to 103 Gy, respectively. Radiation dose was the only significant predictor when multiple variables were included ($p = .015$). They concluded that higher dose radiation is associated with improved outcomes in patients treated within the range of 63 to 103 Gy.

Altered fractionation and/or dose escalation remain investigational for stage III NSCLC. For lung cancer, because of significant distant metastasis (>50%) and tumor motion during radiotherapy (>50% of tumors move >5 mm), chemotherapy and image-guided radiotherapy to take tumor motion into consideration play an important role in the management of NSCLC.

Definitive Chemoradiotherapy

Conventional radiotherapy alone resulted in a median survival of 10 months and a 5-year survival of 5%. To improve the outcome of treatment, chemotherapy was added to radiotherapy. Multiple phase III trials have demonstrated a survival advantage for the addition of chemotherapy to radiotherapy for NSCLC.

Chemotherapy and RT can be delivered sequentially or concurrently (Tables 48.8 and 48.9). The most well-known trial, reported by the CALGB (68), compared standard radiotherapy to 60 Gy to sequential cisplatin and vinblastine chemotherapy for two cycles followed by 60 Gy. Median and 5-year survivals were superior for the chemoradiation arm (13.8 months vs 9.7 months and 19% vs. 7%). These results led the RTOG to conduct a three-arm trial (RTOG 88–08) comparing standard radiotherapy, sequential chemoradiation (CALGB regimen), and 69.6-Gy hyperfractionated radiotherapy (200,201). Sequential chemotherapy was statistically superior to both standard radiation and hyperfractionation. Results for the hyperfractionated arm were not statistically different from those for

| **Table 48.8** | SEQUENTIAL CHEMOTHERAPY: RADIATION THERAPY FOR LOCALLY ADVANCED NON–SMALL CELL LUNG CANCER |

Authors	RT (Gy)	CT	Sequence	No. Patients	Median Survival (mo)	1 Yr	2 Yr	3 Yr	5 Yr
Dillman et al. (48)	60.0	—	—	77	9.7	40	13	11	7
	60.0	PV	CT→RT	79	13.8	55	26	23	19
Le Chevalier et al. (124)	65.0	—	—	177	10.0	41	14	4	—
	65.0	VCPC	CT→RT→CT	176	12.0	51	21	12	—
Sause et al. (201)	60.0	—	—	149	11.4	46	19	6	5
	60.0	PV	CT→ RT	151	13.2	60	32	15	8
	69.6	—	—	152	12	51	24	13	6

RT, radiation therapy; CT, chemotherapy; PV, cisplatin, vinblastine; MACC, methotrexate, doxorubicin, cyclophosphamide, lomustine; VCPC, vindesine, cyclophosphamide, cisplatin, lomustine.

Table 48.9 CONCURRENT (C) OR SEQUENTIAL (S) CHEMORADIOTHERAPY FOR STAGE III NON–SMALL CELL LUNG CARCINOMA							
		Median Survival (mo)		% Survival (yr)		% Esophagitis (Grade 3-4)	
Trial	No. of Patients	S	C	S	C	S	C
Furuse et al. (63)	314	13.3	16.5	8	16 (5)	4	23
Curran et al. (44)	400	14.6	17.1	12	21 (4)	5	26
Fournel et al. (60)	205	14.5	14.0	24	21 (4)	3	32

conventional radiation alone. Dillman et al. (48) later reported that a retrospective quality-control review identified 23% of cases in which portal films failed to completely encompass the tumor in the CALGB study. Two-dimensional radiotherapy was used for radiation treatment planning in all of these trials. Further efforts to improve local control and decrease distant metastasis led investigators to pursue additional strategies, including concurrent cisplatin-based chemotherapy with RT, combined chemotherapy and hyperfractionated RT, and new chemotherapeutic agents combined with RT.

Schaake-Koning et al. (203) compared radiotherapy alone with radiotherapy plus daily cisplatin or weekly cisplatin. There was no difference in distant failure rates between the groups with or without cisplatin. However, survival in the radiotherapy plus cisplatin group was 54%, 26%, and 16% at 1, 2 and 3 years, respectively, compared with 46%, 13%, and 2% in the radiotherapy-alone group ($p = .009$). Therefore, this study showed that a gain in local tumor control seems to have been translated into a gain in survival.

Furuse et al. (63) compared patients receiving two cycles of MVP (mitomycin, vindesine, and cisplatin) given every 28 days along with split-course RT (total dose of 56 Gy) with two cycles of MVP followed by continuous-course radiation (total dose of 56 Gy). The concurrent arm demonstrated an improved 5-year survival rate of 15.8%. A subsequent report demonstrated that the difference in survival was attributed to improved intrathoracic tumor control (64). Criticisms of this trial include the split-course radiotherapy used in the concurrent arm and the lower doses of radiotherapy used.

RTOG 9410 (44) conducted a three-arm randomized trial to analyze whether the concurrent delivery of cisplatin-based chemotherapy with TRT improves survival compared with the sequential delivery of these therapies for patients with locally advanced, unresected stage II-III NSCLC. The sequential arm included cisplatin (100 mg/m^2) and Vib (5 mg/m^2) with 60 Gy of radiotherapy. The concurrent arm used the same chemotherapy with 60 Gy of radiotherapy beginning on day 1 (CON-QD). The third arm employed concurrent cisplatin 50 mg/m^2 with oral etoposide 50 mg with 69.6 Gy in 1.2-Gy twice daily fractions beginning day 1 (CON-BID). For the 595 analyzable patients, the rates of acute grade 3 to 5 nonhematologic toxicity rates were higher with concurrent than sequential therapy, but late toxicity rates were similar (18% to 27%). With minimum and median potential follow-up times of 4.0 and 6.0 years, the median survival and 4-year survivals were 14.6 months and 12% (sequential arm), 17.0 months and 21% (CON-QD radiation therapy [RT]), and 15.2 months and 17% (CON-BID RT). The CON-QD RT arm had better survival than the sequential arm ($p = .046$). This report demonstrates the long-term survival benefit of the concurrent delivery of cisplatin-based chemotherapy with TRT as compared with the sequential delivery of these therapies. The locoregional failure rates were 50% (sequential arm), 43% (CON-QD), and 34% (CON-BID). The acute toxicities were higher in CON-BID with 68% grade 3 and above toxicities

compared with 48% in the CON-QD group. There was no significant difference in late toxicities and survival between these two groups. However, radiotherapy in field failure was improved in the CON-BID group. Higher toxicities in the CON-BID group may explain the lack of survival benefit. In RTOG 94-10, radiotherapy was based on two-dimensional planning, which is usually associated with higher toxicity.

A third trial comparing concurrent versus sequential chemoradiation, reported in 2001 and updated in 2005, also explored the use of consolidation chemotherapy (60). In this phase III trial from France, 205 patients were assigned to receive two cycles of cisplatin plus vinorelbine followed by 66 Gy of radiation versus cisplatin/etoposide and concurrent radiation to 66 Gy followed by two cycles of consolidation chemotherapy with cisplatin and vinorelbine. Local control rates were improved with the concurrent regimen (40% vs. 24%), and the median and 4-year survival times were numerically superior (but not statistically superior) for the concurrent arm (14.5 vs. 16.3 months and 14% vs. 21%). However, the incidence of grade 3 esophagitis was significantly higher in the concurrent arm (32% vs. 3%), and the toxic death rates were high on both arms (9.5% on the concurrent arm and 5.6% on the sequential arm).

These three phase III trials consistently demonstrated longer survival for the concurrent arms, and this difference was significant in two of the three trials. On the basis of these results, concurrent chemoradiation has become the standard of care since 2001. It is important to note that toxicity is significantly greater with concurrent chemotherapy.

In RTOG 9410, the locoregional failure after concurrent chemoradiotherapy was still around 34% to 43%. To improve the local control rate, three groups (RTOG, NCCTG, and the University of North Carolina) have separately performed radiation dose-escalation trials for this population and reported results supporting the safety of 74 Gy (22,206,220). Lee et al. (126) and Socinski et al. (220) conducted a phase I/II dose escalation clinical trial using high-dose 3DCRT (60 to 74 Gy) for inoperable stage IIIA/IIIB NSCLC with induction chemotherapy followed by concurrent chemoradiotherapy. They reported a 3-year survival rate of 36% and a 13% locoregional relapse rate as the only site of failure. For patients who finished radiotherapy, the 3-year survival rate was 45%. No grade 3 or above lung toxicities were reported; 8% of the patients developed grade 3/4 esophagitis. The same group is conducting higher dose escalation to up to 90 Gy (126,220). At 90 Gy, cases of bronchoesophageal fistula, bronchial stenosis, and fatal pulmonary hemoptysis were reported, although the incidence was still very low. One hundred twelve patients have been accrued, with a median follow-up of 4.9 years for surviving patients. The median survival was 24 months (range, 18 to 31 months). The 1-, 3-, and 5-year overall survival rates were 69% (60% to 77%), 36% (27% to 45%), and 24% (16% to 33%), respectively. The relatively longer follow-up of this population provides information about late complication risks. Late complications (defined as grade 3 or greater occurring >90 days after RT) occurred in

22% (25/112). Patients with complications seem to have longer survival than the overall group (p =.007). Late complications included bronchial stenosis (n = 3), fatal hemoptysis (n = 2), tracheoesophageal fistula (n = 1), esophageal stricture (n = 7), myocardial infarction (n = 5), pericardial disease (n = 4), and bone fracture (n = 6). Distant metastasis was still the major failure.

On the basis of promising local control and survival data with acceptable toxicity using 3DCRT to doses of 74 Gy with concurrent chemoradiotherapy, RTOG is planning to conduct a phase III study to compare a conventional dose of 60 Gy with 74-Gy radiotherapy using 3DCRT concurrently with weekly paclitaxel and carboplatin consolidative chemotherapy in patients with stage IIIA/B NSCLC.

Newer Chemoradiation Regimens

The most commonly used chemoradiation combination includes carboplatin and paclitaxel (Taxol). Selected phase II trials using paclitaxel, an inhibitor of normal microtubule function, and carboplatin have reported encouraging results (15,36,121). Paclitaxel has been shown to arrest cells in G2/M phase, the most radiosensitive phase of the cell cycle. The early response rates and survival rates appear promising in patients with unresectable stage III NSCLC. The reported grade 3 to 4 esophagitis and pneumonitis rates approach 26% to 46% and 17% to 22%, respectively, when chemotherapy is used concurrently with RT (36,121).

Other systemic therapies being tested in clinical trials include docetaxel (Taxotere), vinorelbine (Navelbine), gemcitabine (Gemzar), and irinotecan (Camptosar). In 2001, the CALGB (238) completed a three-arm randomized phase II study testing combinations of gemcitabine/cisplatin, paclitaxel/cisplatin, and vinorelbine/cisplatin with concurrent radiotherapy to 66 Gy (238). The results indicate the feasibility of administration of chemotherapy concurrently with these newer chemotherapeutic agents. Caution is advised when gemcitabine is delivered concurrently with radiation because of its enhanced radiosensitizing properties. Scalliet et al. (202) reported that three of eight patients had treatment-related deaths when a weekly dose of gemcitabine (1,000 mg/m^2) was used. The question of whether induction chemotherapy with two cycles of paclitaxel and carboplatin offers any survival advantage over the concurrent chemoradiation with weekly paclitaxel and carboplatin is being addressed in a closed but unreported CALGB study.

A novel concept of adding a possibly non–cross-resistant chemotherapy following the completion of concurrent chemoradiation was examined in a recent SWOG study. In this multi-institutional single-arm phase II study, 71 patients with unresectable stage IIIB NSCLC were treated with concurrent chemoradiation with cisplatin, etoposide, and TRT followed by three cycles of docetaxel (75 to 100 mg/m^2 given every 3 weeks) (122). The median survival was an impressive 27 months, and the projected 3-year survival was 47%. On the basis of this promising data, SWOG investigators now are conducting a phase III study comparing this regimen (cisplatin, etoposide, and radiation followed by three cycles of docetaxel) with an identical regimen followed by maintenance therapy with ZD 1839 (Iressa), a specific inhibitor of epidermal growth factor receptor (EGFR) tyrosine kinase.

The role of induction chemotherapy followed by concurrent chemoradiotherapy or concurrent chemoradiotherapy followed by consolidative chemotherapy remains investigational. Belani et al. (17) reported a multi-institutional randomized phase II study for locally advanced NSCLC. Patients were randomized to receive two cycles of induction paclitaxel (200 mg/m^2) and carboplatin (AUC = 6) followed by 63-Gy radiotherapy, two cycles of induction paclitaxel (200 mg/m^2)/carboplatin (AUC = 6) fol-

lowed by weekly paclitaxel (45 mg/m^2)/carboplatin (AUC = 2) with concurrent TRT 63.0 Gy (arm 2, induction/concurrent), or weekly paclitaxel (45 mg/m^2)/carboplatin (AUC = 2)/TRT (63.0 Gy) followed by two cycles of paclitaxel (200 mg/m^2)/carboplatin (AUC = 6; arm 3, concurrent/consolidation). The data showed that concurrent weekly paclitaxel, carboplatin, and TRT followed by consolidation chemotherapy seem to be associated with the best outcome, although this schedule was associated with greater toxicity.

Superior Sulcus Tumors of the Lung

Clinical Presentations

Superior sulcus tumors (SSTs) of the lung are uncommon lung cancers, accounting for only 3% of all lung cancer cases (111). SSTs may occur in three locations: anterior, where they invade major blood vessels such as the subclavian artery (Fig. 48.5A); middle, where they mainly invade the brachial plexus (particularly for SST located medially; Fig. 48.5B); and posterior, where they invade satellite ganglia or vertebral bodies with or without extension of the tumor into the foramen (Fig. 48.5C).

Symptoms and Signs Related to the Location of the Superior Sulcus Tumors

Pain from SSTs usually occurs in the shoulder and along the vertebral body or the scapula. One of important definitions of SST requires pain in the shoulder as it extremely rare that SST presents as a T2 lesion without pleural involvement. This pain is the result of the tumor localized at the apex of the lung and involving parietal pleura. Subsequently, the pain extends down the ulnar distribution of the ipsilateral arm to the elbow (which indicates involvement of T1) and eventually to the ulnar surface of the forearm and to the fourth and fifth fingers of the involved side of the hand (which indicates ulnar nerve involvement). If the C5-6 is involved by SST, the patient usually manifests atrophy of interdigital muscle (claw hand) because of dysfunction of the median nerve. If SST invades the C4-5, the patient manifests radial nerve involvement causing muscle atrophy of the ipsilateral palm. Once the sympathetic chain and the satellite ganglia are involved by the posteriorly located SST, patients usually develop Horner's syndrome manifesting ptosis, papillary miosis, and facial anhydrosis. The direct extension of the posterior SST into the first or second rib or vertebral bodies usually causes severe pain, and if the spinal canal or cord is involved, patients may be paralyzed. Patients usually do not show the pulmonary symptoms of hemoptysis, shortness of breath, and cough commonly associated with endobronchial lesions.

Diagnostic Images

MRI scans more accurately display the anatomy of SSTs than do CT scans (94% compared with 63%) (83). A sagittal section obtained by MRI can show extension of a SST to the posterior wall of the subclavian artery or involvement of the brachial plexus, vertebral body, or mediastinal lymph nodes. An axial CT scan cannot do this as easily because a CT scan is not as accurate as MRI in demonstrating invasion of the tumor into the foramen, spinal cord, or major blood vessels. Therefore, MRI is the better diagnostic method to demonstrate resectability of the SST. MRI of the brain is important for showing any micrometastasis; patients who have SST often present with brain metastases because of the location of the tumor and the fact that more of these patients have adenocarcinoma or large cell carcinoma of the lung, both of which are highly metastatic (108). When combined, MRI and CT can reveal extension of the SST into

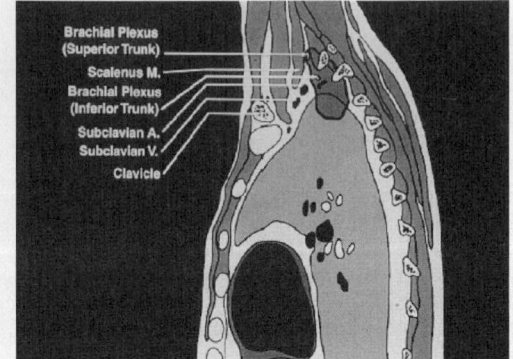

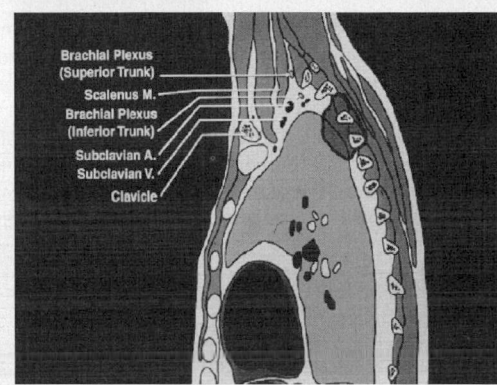

FIGURE 48.5. A: Anatomic relationship of an anteriorly located superior sulcus tumor to adjacent structures. **B:** Anatomic relationship of a medially located superior sulcus location to adjacent structures. **C:** Anatomic relationship of a posteriorly located superior sulcus location to adjacent structures. (From Komaki R, et al. *Semin Surg Oncol* 200;18:152–164, with permission).

the great vessels at the thoracic inlet, primarily the subclavian artery and vein; involvement of the trachea or esophagus; invasion into the brachial plexus; invasion of the chest wall; invasion into the vertebral bodies, foramen, and spinal cord; mediastinal lymph node involvement by metastasis or direct extension; and extrathoracic metastasis into the brain and upper abdomen. PET scan improves sensitivity and specificity, particularly for lymph node and distant metastasis as discussed in the diagnostic work-up.

Although the diagnosis of SST by diagnostic imaging is accurate in more than 95% of cases (173), cytologic or histologic confirmation of the definitive diagnosis is important because it might affect treatment. For example, one study found that 3% of SSTs were undifferentiated SCLCs, which can be treated as effectively with chemotherapy (97).

Mediastinoscopy

Staging is key to treatment strategy. Paulson (174) emphasized the importance of mediastinoscopy because his patients did very poorly if the mediastinal or hilar lymph nodes were involved: only three of 17 patients with hilar or mediastinal nodal involvement survived 1 year and none survived 2 years. In contrast, 44% of the patients with no nodal involvement survived 4 years or longer. Paulson also advocated scalene node biopsy for preoperative RT and subsequent surgery if the scalene nodes were palpable before initiation of treatment. Attar et al. (11) affirmed that adequate preoperative assessment is extremely important because those patients who had positive mediastinal lymph nodes died shortly after surgery. In his Toronto experience, Ginsberg (70) documented that stringent preoperative assessment of patients with SST ruled out surgery in 62 of 72 patients. As these reports illustrate, it is important to document the exact location of the SST as well as the extent of the disease because location will influence the resectability of the tumor and the radiation therapy dose arrangement.

Management

If resection is contraindicated, tumors can be treated with concurrent chemotherapy and RT. The contraindications for surgery include extensive invasion of the brachial plexus, subclavian artery, and vertebral bodies; mediastinal involvement (particularly perinodal), venous obstruction, and distant metastases (173).

Preoperative RT or Chemoradiotherapy and Surgical Resection

The combination of preoperative RT and subsequent surgical resection to treat SSTs first was reported by Shaw et al. (211) in 1961. Paulson (173–175) used this approach and updated it on several occasions. In brief, the SST, chest wall, and superior mediastinum were given 3,000 cGy per day in 10 fractions during 12 days. Three weeks after completion of RT, patients underwent *en bloc* resection of the tumor along with the involved chest wall including the entire first rib and posterior portion of the second and third ribs. The involved lung was resected by either lobectomy or segmental resection. The entire procedure was accompanied by dissection of the regional hilar and mediastinal lymph nodes. In a series reported by Paulson (174), 131 patients were administered preoperative RT to be followed by *en bloc* surgical resection. Of these, 78 patients (60%) completed preoperative RT followed by radical dissection. The operative mortality rate was 2.6%, and the overall survival rates were 31% at 5 years, 26% at 10 years, and 22% at 15 years. Three of 17 patients who had involvement of either the hilar or mediastinal lymph nodes survived 1 year, and none who had positive lymph nodes survived beyond 2 years. For the 61 patients who had no nodal involvement at the time of surgery, the 5-year survival was 44%, the 10-year survival was 33%, and the 15-year survival was 30%.

Ginsberg (70) reported on 72 patients with Pancoast's tumor: 50 of them had tumors deemed inoperable after screening, and only 10 patients underwent preoperative RT (3,000 cGy during 2 weeks) followed by resection. The 2-year survival of those 10 patients was 40%.

Martini (144) described the experience at the Memorial Sloan-Kettering Hospital during a 36-year period. Sixty-eight of 148 patients had surgery alone, and 48 patients had preoperative radiation followed by resection. Only 9% of the 68 patients who had surgery alone had completely resected tumors, compared with 23 patients who received preoperative radiation followed by complete resection. Martini (144) also claimed that, without CT or MRI, it was difficult to evaluate the resectability during that time. Martini also found that, if a tumor was not resectable at the time of surgery after preoperative RT, a combination of radon seed implants and external RT (40 Gy in 4 weeks) would provide better local tumor control and a survival rate comparable to that for external RT alone. The median survivals were 12 months and 6 months, respectively. Devine et al. (47) noted a 2-year survival of 29% and a 5-year survival of 14% in a series of patients who completed preoperative RT followed by surgery.

At M.D. Anderson Cancer Center (110), 143 patients with SSTs received single modality or combined treatment. Those patients with T3N0M0 tumors who had preoperative and postoperative RT, with or without chemotherapy, did extremely well and had a 5-year survival of 87%.

In a recently published phase II trial by SWOG (SWOG 9416) (195), patients with mediastinoscopy-negative T3–4 N0–1 NSCLC of the superior sulcus were treated with preoperative chemoradiation. The chemotherapy consisted of cisplatin and etoposide. The RT was delivered concurrently to a dose of 45 Gy. Ninety-two percent of patients had a complete resection following induction therapy; 65% of patients had a complete pathologic response or minimal microscopic residual disease. The 2-year overall survival rate was 55% for all patients and 70% for patients who had a complete resection.

Surgical Resection Followed by Postoperative RT with or without Chemotherapy

Martini and McCormack (143) reported on 170 patients with SST who were treated at Memorial Sloan-Kettering Cancer Center between 1938 and 1978. Among the 127 patients who underwent surgery, 20 patients had curative surgery after preoperative RT; their 5-year survival rate was 29%. The remaining 107 patients who underwent surgery received postoperative brachytherapy; their 5-year survival was 14%.

At M.D. Anderson Cancer Center, patients with stage T3-4N0-2M0 resectable SST undergo surgery followed by postoperative RT (1.2 Gy bid fractionation to a total dose of 60 Gy for negative margins and 64.8 GY for positive margins) and chemotherapy (oral VP-16 and cisplatin). At present, 33 patients are being treated on this protocol; the 2-year overall survival is 65%, and pain control has been excellent. In most cases of treatment failure, the patients had a distant metastasis (i.e., in the adrenal gland or lung) or a second malignancy in the lung.

In a group of patients reported by Dartevelle et al. (46), none of the patients received preoperative RT, 14% had surgery alone, and 86% had surgery followed by postoperative RT. The median follow-up was 2.5 years. The 2-year survival was 50%; the 5-year survival was 31%.

Patients who have not received preoperative RT but whose tumor margins are grossly positive need a definitive dose of RT (66 Gy without chemotherapy or 60 to 63 Gy with concurrent chemotherapy). Because most patients with SST present with adenocarcinoma or large cell carcinoma, prophylactic cranial irradiation needs to be considered early in the course of treatment.

Inoperable Superior Sulcus Tumors

Patients whose SSTs are considered to be medically inoperable or surgically unresectable should be considered candidates for curative or palliative RT with or without chemotherapy. Komaki et al. (111) reported on 36 patients with SST treated with external RT. All patients who survived beyond 2 years exhibited local control of the tumor. Between 1978 and 1983, an additional 32 patients with inoperable SST were studied. Relief of pain was achieved in 91% of all patients who presented with pain. Three-fourths of the patients with Horner's syndrome responded to the RT. The disease-free survival rates were 65% at 12 months, 38% at 24 months, 25% at 36 months, and 15% at 48 months. Again, no patient survived beyond 2 years if treatment failed locally. The patterns of failure showed that the brain was the most common site of distant metastasis after the completion of radiation (23 of 68 patients, 34%) (108).

Komaki et al. (111) reported on 85 patients with SST. The 60 patients who had medically or surgically inoperable SST and were treated by RT alone or RT with chemotherapy had a 2-year survival rate of 22%. In contrast, the 25 patients who had resectable tumors had a 2-year survival rate of 52%. In a more recent series, they reported on 77 patients who had unresectable or medically inoperable lesions; 45 patients received RT alone, and 32 had a combination of RT and chemotherapy. Those patients who received RT alone had an overall 5-year survival rate of 9% and a 5-year local tumor control of 51%. In contrast, patients who received combined RT (≥66 Gy given on a hyperfractionated regimen) and chemotherapy (oral VP-16 and cisplatin) had a 5-year survival rate of 36% and a 5-year local control rate of 63% (127). Patients who received sequential chemotherapy or concurrent chemotherapy with less than 66 Gy of radiation had a 5-year survival rate of only 7%. Twelve patients who received 66 Gy or more of radiation with either sequential or concurrent chemotherapy had a 5-year survival rate of 33% (110).

Summary

Because of the tumor location, which is associated with significant symptoms, patients with SST usually are diagnosed in the early stage of their disease without significant medistinal lymph node or distant metastasis, although the T stage could be advanced (T3, T4). Combined modality should be applied, and aggressive local treatment is recommended. Surgery plays an important role in the management. However, the procedure is challenging, and negative margins can be hard to achieve because of the surrounding critical structures. Either induction chemoradiotherapy or postoperative chemoradiotherapy should be considered. For patients who are not candidates for surgery resection, concurrent chemoradiotherapy is recommended and hyperfractionated radiotherapy should be considered to avoid long-term toxicity to the brachial plexus if high dose is planned, such as 69.6 Gy with 1.2 Gy/fraction given twice per day. 3DCRT or IMRT should be used. Because the tumor does not move significantly and critical structures need to be spared in this location, IMRT may play a better role than 3DCRT (Fig. 48.6).

Superior Vena Cava Syndrome

SVC syndrome is a medical emergency occasionally seen in patients with malignant neoplasia that requires immediate therapeutic action (204). Currently, 80% of cases of SVC syndrome result from bronchogenic carcinoma (7); malignant lymphoma accounts for 10% to 18% of the cases, and benign causes (e.g., goiter) account for 2% to 3%.

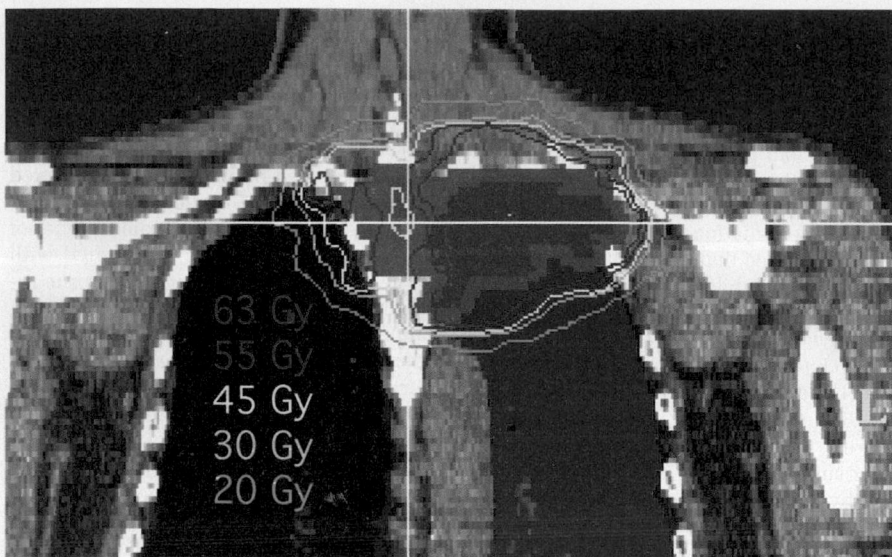

63 Gy
55 Gy
45 Gy
30 Gy
20 Gy

FIGURE 48.6. Intensity-modulated radiation therapy for inoperable superior sulcus tumor: 63 Gy to gross tumor volume (red) and 45 Gy to clinical target volume (orange).

This syndrome is produced by extrinsic compression of the SVC or intracaval thrombosis, which is seen in approximately 40% to 50% of patients with this syndrome. Work-up and establishment of diagnosis for patients with this syndrome depend on the severity of the symptoms. In patients with earlier symptoms and less severe respiratory distress, appropriate work-up including chest radiographs, CT scans, and bronchoscopy, and biopsy of tumor can be performed. However, in patients with full-blown SVC syndrome and severe respiratory distress, emergency therapy should be initiated and can be performed without tissue diagnosis.

Although it generally is believed that these patients have an extremely poor prognosis, approximately 10% to 20% survive longer than 2 years (7,216). Therefore, in the absence of distant metastasis, aggressive management and support are indicated. RT should be initiated as soon as possible. Patients initially should be given high dose fractions (3 to 4 Gy tumor dose) for 2 or 3 days, followed by additional daily doses of 1.8 to 2 Gy to complete the definitive course of RT (193). The recommended total tumor dose for patients with localized bronchogenic carcinoma is 60 to 70 Gy in 6 to 7 weeks. In patients with a diagnosis of small cell carcinoma presenting with SVC syndrome (see section Small Cell Lung Carcinoma), the mode of initial therapy is controversial; both RT and chemotherapy are effective.

Excellent symptomatic relief (disappearance of dyspnea, edema of the face, and distention of the neck and thoracic veins) has been observed in approximately 20% of patients with bronchogenic carcinoma. Good symptomatic improvement also has been noted in an additional 50% of patients with bronchogenic carcinoma. Only 15% of patients with bronchogenic carcinoma had minimal improvement, and 15% showed no significant response (216). Armstrong et al. (7) reported survival rates of 25% at 1 year and 10% at 3 years in 84 patients. Patients treated with initial high-dose RT followed by conventional therapy experienced faster and more durable symptomatic relief than patients treated with conventional fractionation at the initiation of the treatment (70% vs. 56%). Patients exhibiting symptomatic relief within 30 days had a significantly better survival rate than those who did not ($p = .002$). The addition of chemotherapy to irradiation at the initiation of treatment did not have any effect on the final outcome in two studies (7,128).

RT Techniques and Future Development

Three-Dimensional Conformal Radiation Therapy

With the advent of 3DCRT, traditional portals, target volumes, and beam arrangements have been questioned. Because of high local failure rates reported for NSCLC, one goal of 3DCRT is to increase the dose delivery to the gross tumor and/or minimize the dose to normal tissues. 3DCRT has several significant advantages: tumor and normal tissue delineation, image segmentation and display, accurate dose calculation, and the ability to manipulate beam geometry and weighting through the forward planning process. The importance of improved target delineation cannot be overemphasized. Once patients are immobilized and given a CT scan in the treatment position, the radiation oncologist can delineate the tumor and adjacent tissues in three dimensions, choose beam angles to maximize tumor coverage and/or minimize normal tissues treated, alter beam weighting, and perhaps alter couch angles for noncoplanar beam delivery. Conformal radiotherapy also enables the fusion of complementary imaging modalities, such as PET to aid in tumor delineation or single-photon emission computed tomography to choose beam angles. Purdy et al. (184) have provided an excellent overview of 3DCRT for purposes of reference.

The International Commission on Radiation Units Report No. 50 guidelines (90) for defining targets have been applied to the treatment of lung cancer. The GTV is the primary tumor and any grossly involved lymph nodes. The clinical tumor volume is the anatomically defined area thought to harbor micrometastasis (hilar or mediastinal lymph nodes or a margin around the grossly visible disease). The PTV accounts for physiologic organ motion during treatment and the inaccuracies of daily setup in fractionated therapy. In International Commission on Radiation Units Report 62, a new concept of the internal target volume (ITV) was proposed as representing the volume encompassing the clinical tumor volume and the internal margin to compensate for expected physiologic movements and variation in size, shape, and position of the clinical tumor volume during the radiotherapy. Details of target volume delineation will be discussed later.

Elective Nodal Irradiation

For many years, standard RT practice in the United States, with some recent exceptions (50,51,114,191,209), was to deliver 40 to 50 Gy to the electively irradiated regional-nodal areas (ipsilateral, contralateral, hilar, mediastinal, and occasionally supraclavicular areas) with an additional 20 Gy delivered to the primary tumor through reduced fields. This regimen was based on pathologic information regarding the high incidence of hilar and mediastinal node metastases in patients with bronchogenic carcinoma. Perez et al. (178), in an analysis of protocol compliance in 316 patients in the RTOG 73–01 trial, reported that in patients with radiographically negative lymph nodes, survival was higher in the group with no protocol variations who had adequate coverage of the hilar/mediastinal lymph nodes. However, the difference was not statistically significant ($p = .35$).

The rationale against elective nodal irradiation is the high local recurrence rates within the previously irradiated tumor volume and the high chance of distant metastasis: If gross disease cannot be controlled, why enlarge the irradiated volumes to include areas that might harbor microscopic disease? Three major factors have changed since RTOG 73-01 established standard irradiation doses and volumes: the use of chemotherapy, the advent of 3DCRT, and better staging and target delineation with PET. Emerging clinical data show that omitting prophylactic lymph node irradiation does not reduce the local control rate for patients receiving definitive radiotherapy, with isolated outside-field (field of radiotherapy) local recurrence rates less than 8%, particularly in patients with stage I disease and those who undergo PET scanning for staging (26,114,226). Dosoretz et al. (50) also observed no correlation of field size and treatment outcome; the lack of field size correlation was evident even when results were stratified according to tumor size.

Rosenzweig et al. (191) recently published results for a series of 171 patients treated definitively with 3DCRT to involved field volumes, without elective nodal irradiation. Only 6.4% of patients suffered elective nodal failures, including 1% ipsilateral supraclavicular, 3% contralateral supraclavicular, 4% ipsilateral inferior mediastinal, and 1% contralateral inferior mediastinal failure rates. Likewise, Senan et al. (209) reported similar low failure rates in untreated elective nodal areas in patients with stage III disease.

The explanation for these lower-than-expected elective nodal failure rates is twofold. First, incidental doses to the ipsilateral hilum, paratracheal, and subcarinal nodes approach 40 to 50 Gy when these regions are not intentionally irradiated (140). Second, lung cancer patients suffer from multiple causes of competing mortality, including their cancer and underlying comorbid illness. Patients may die of local failure, distant failure, or intercurrent illness without detection of elective nodal failures.

Staging of regional lymph nodes has been greatly enhanced with the help of PET. The addition of PET to clinical mediastinal staging with CT has improved the sensitivity and specificity to the range of 90% in comparison with CT alone. More accurate clinical staging with PET may allow the radiation oncologist to include involved hilar and mediastinal nodes that were not appreciated on the CT scan and reduce the probability of elective nodal failures. As the number of facilities with dedicated FDG-PET scanners increases, specifically combined PET/CT units, this technology will aid radiation oncologists in designing PTVs (26). Figure 48.7 illustrates PET/CT-based clinical stage compared with CT alone and its application in target delineation and treatment design using IMRT or 3DCRT.

Thus, in patients with NSCLC, it is important to deliver adequate doses of RT to involved nodal or mediastinal areas. Irradiation of other electively treated lymph nodes may not be necessary, particularly in patients staged with both CT and PET.

Target Volume Delineation

Gross Tumor Volume

GTV is defined as visible tumor by any imaging modality. The pulmonary extent of lung tumors should be delineated on pulmonary windows, and the mediastinal extent of tumors should be delineated using mediastinal windows. In general, a lymph node larger than 1 cm in shortest dimension on CT scan is considered to be positive because of higher than 15% involvement. The FDG-PET image is quite important for radiation treatment volume planning in stage III disease. Particularly, it can help to categorize suspect mediastinal/hilar lymph adenopathy and differentiate benign collapsed lung from tumor. Higher standard uptake values are predictive of metastatic disease and possible radiation resistance that may need to treat aggressively with stronger chemotherapy and higher radiation doses.

Clinical Target Volume

CTV is defined as the volume that contains gross and microscopic disease. In lung paranchymal disease, a radiographic–histopathologic study (71) demonstrated that GTV-to-CTV expansions of 6 mm for squamous cancers and 8 mm for adenocarcinomas are required to cover the gross tumor and microscopic disease with 95% accuracy. Expansions for other histologic types have not been determined, but a conservative approach would be to use 8 mm. An appropriate CTV for the mediastinum involvement has not been rigorously determined. We empirically use 8-mm expansions around involved nodes (either gross involvement or FDG-PET positivity). Obviously, these expansions should not necessarily be applied uniformly along all axes and should always be individualized based on the location of the primary tumor and involved lymph node. In the absence of radiographic proof of invasion, CTV of primary lesion should not extend into the chest wall or mediastinum. CTV expansions of lymph node disease should not extend into the major airways or lung.

Planning Target Volume

PTV is defined as CTV with a margin to account for daily setup error and target motion. Preliminary data at M.D. Anderson Cancer Center have shown that, when patients are immobilized with a Vac-Loc bag and T-bar, expansion along all axes of 7 mm accounts for 95% of the day-to-day set-up uncertainty. Setup uncertainty is likely both technique- and institution-dependent and should be measured individually for each technique.

Tumor motion consideration is critical for lung cancer radiotherapy. Our preliminary 4D CT study showed that more than 50% of the tumor moves more than 5 mm during the treatment and 13% moves more than 1 cm (possibly as high as 3 to 4 cm), particularly for the lesion close to the diaphragm. Tumor motion is best assessed individually for each patient. For patients with tumor motion of less than 5 mm, simple expansion for GTV margin is adequate. However, for the patients with significant tumor motion, particularly more than 1 cm, an individualized tumor motion margin should be considered. The treatment machine can be gated with respiration or the patient can use an assisted breath-hold technique or, possibly, an ITV-based approach can be used.

A commercially available system can be used to gate the linac (185). This technique uses an externally placed fiducial that is tracked as the patient breathes. The beam can be triggered at a chosen point in the respiratory cycle, typically end-expiration because this is the longest and most reproducible portion of the respiratory cycle. This requires that patients be able to breathe slowly in a regular pattern. Active breathing control and deep inspiration breath-hold are two techniques that have been pioneered to help patients hold their breaths at reproducible points

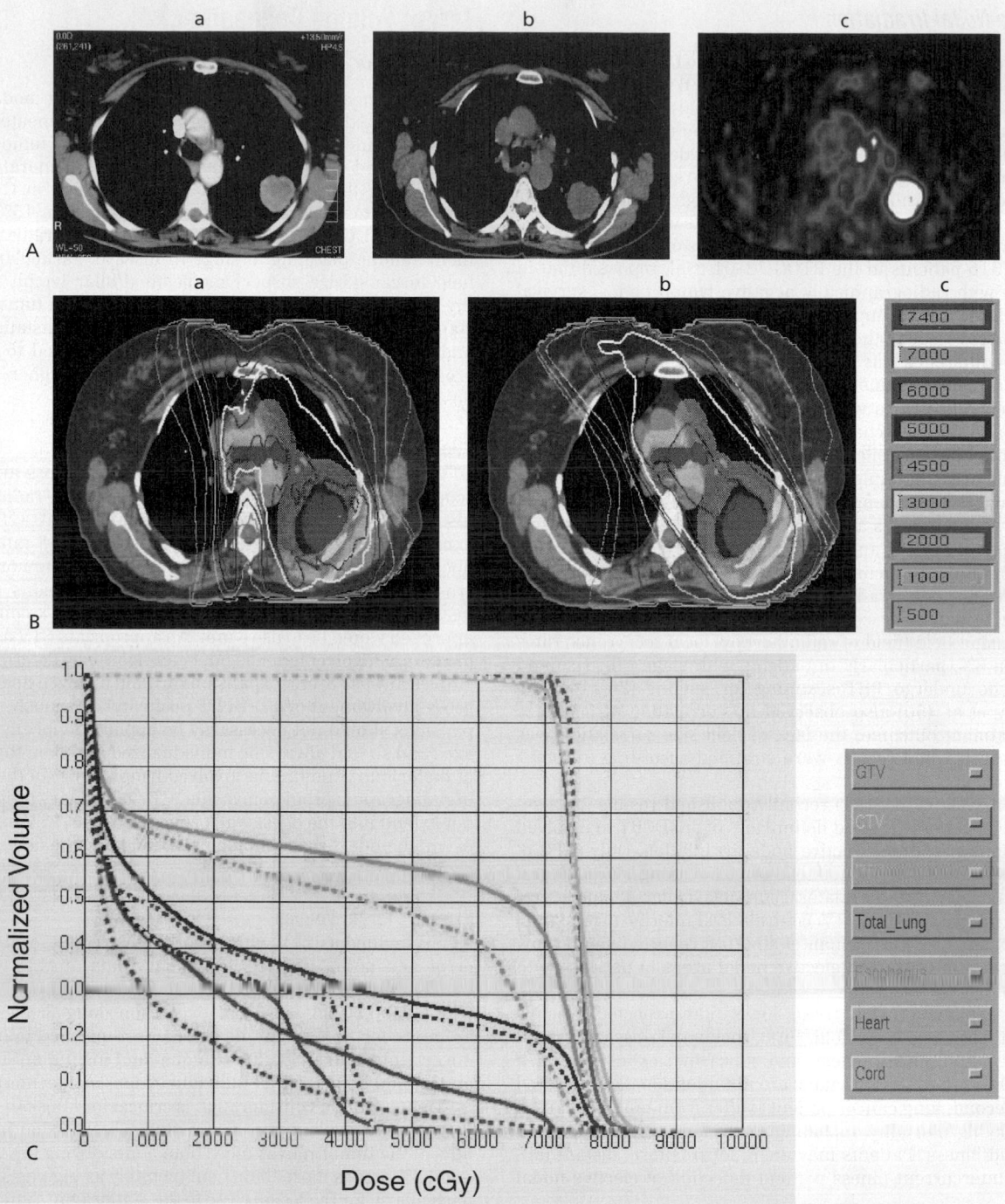

FIGURE 48.7. Positron emission tomography (PET) and computed tomograph (CT) based gross target volume delineation and radiotherapy planning using intensity-modulated radiation therapy (IMRT) or three-dimensional conformal radiation therapy (3DCRT). Transverse CT image demonstrates left upper love lesion with scattering small mediastinal lymph nodes (<1 cm; not large enough to be considered malignant). However, PET scan shows increased metabolic activity in both primary lesion and small mediastinal lymph nodes. Target volume is designed based on PET and CT image. Both 3DCRT and IMRT plans are conducted and compared. IMRT treatment planning improves spare of normal lung (V5, V10, V20), heart, and esophagus. **A:** Diagnostic image. **a:** CT with contrast; **b:** CT without contrast; **c:** PET. **B:** Isodose distribution of IMRT **(a)** and 3DCRT **(b)** treatment plans. **C:** Dose volume histogram comparison of 3DCRT and IMRT. *Solid line,* 3DCRT; *dashed line,* IMRT.

in the respiratory cycle (190,219). The radiation beam is then initiated. These two techniques limit patient respiratory excursion to fixed volumes. They limit diaphragm excursion to about 5 mm instead of 10 to 15 mm. These techniques require very cooperative patients who are able to hold their breath for at least 15 seconds.

Unfortunately, patients with poor pulmonary function (who would most benefit from reduction in irradiated lung volumes) are the patients least able to comply with breath-holding tech-

niques. Thus, it is not clear which is the best method to temporally immobilize lung tumors.

ITV is an expansion of CTV in which target motion is explicitly measured and taken into account as defined by International Commission on Radiation Units Report 62. Using new technologies such as multislice detectors and faster imaging reconstruction, it is now possible to image patients during real-time breathing and assess organ motion using 4D CT (162). To determine the ITV from the 4D CT images, the tumor volume

			Chemo/RT,
Organ	**RT Alone**	**Chemo/RT**	**Then Surgery**
Cord[a]	50 Gy	45 Gy	45 Gy
Lung[b]	MLD <20 Gy	MLD <20 Gy	MLD <20 Gy
	V20 <40%	V20 <35%	V20 <20%
		V10 <45%	V10 <40%
		V5 <65%	V40 <55%
Heart	V40 <50%	V40 <50%	V40 <50%
Esophagus	D_{max} <75 Gy	D_{max} <75 Gy	D_{max} <75 Gy
	V60 <50%	V55 <50%	V55 <50%
Kidney[c]	20 Gy (<50% of combined both kidneys or <75% of one side of kidney if another kidney is not functional)	Same as RT alone	Same as RT alone
Liver[d]	30 Gy (<40%)	Same as RT alone	Same as RT alone

Table 48.10 DOSE-VOLUME CONSTRAINTS FOR NORMAL TISSUES USING STANDARD FRACTIONATION TO TARGET VOLUME

Chemo, chemotherapy; RT, radiation therapy; MLD, mean lung dose

[a]We should take the treated volume size of spinal cord into consideration. The chance of spinal cord damage is increased as treated volume is increased. Physicians should consider off cord earlier if significant amount of spinal cord has received constraints dose. In general, spinal cord should not receive dose of <60 Gy even in very limited volume. Higher fraction size of radiation or higher daily dose will decrease the tolerance. If patient is treated with 3 Gy per fraction, the cord constrain should be around 40 Gy (based on biologic effective dose calculation).

[b]For patient receiving concurrent chemo/RT, V15 may also be an important parameter to be considered. V20 = effective lung volume (total lung volume – GTV) received ≥20 Gy.

[c]Consider kidney scan if large volume of one kidney will be treated to high dose.

outlined on the expiratory phase of the 4D images is registered on other phases of the images to create a union of target contours enclosing all possible positions of the target. The same principle can be applied to the images acquired with inspiration and expiration breath-holds. Attention should be paid to irregular breathing and variation in the breathing pattern over the course of the treatment, and the effects of such on the ITV margin.

Dose-Volume Constraint

It is extremely important not to exceed the maximum doses tolerated by sensitive and intrathoracic structures such as the lung, spinal cord, and heart. However, partial-volume normal tissue tolerances are not well understood. Special care should be exercised to restrict the radiation dose to the normal lung whenever possible. 3DCRT plan evaluation is more complex than two-dimensional isodose curve evaluation. Dose-volume histograms (DVHs) for all normal organs in the chest are evaluated for dose and volume of irradiation. DVH analysis still is being developed, but preliminary results indicate that it can predict the development of complications such as pneumonitis and lead to improved and more objective treatment planning (76,77,140–142). The common dose volume constraint used at M.D. Anderson is listed in Table 48.10 for reference. We discuss literature in the section Toxicity of Normal Tissue.

Intensity-Modulated Radiation Therapy

IMRT offers the benefit of dose escalation without causing greater toxic effects to surrounding normal tissue for patients with prostate or head and neck cancer (89). However, the application of IMRT to lung cancer has been delayed owing to general concern and the assumption that IMRT may deliver low

yet damaging doses to a larger volume of normal lung tissue. Moreover, the possible movement of a tumor because of respiration introduces another level of complexity to both the IMRT dosimetry and the technique used.

We investigated dosimetric improvement with respect to target dose, tumor conformity, and normal tissue-sparing, comparing IMRT with 3D CT for early and locally advanced NSCLC (132,158). We found that IMRT may be more suitable than 3D CT treatment planning for cases of advanced-stage disease with a larger GTV and thus a greater volume of normal lung involvement (Fig. 48.7). Using IMRT, the median absolute reduction in the percentage of lung volume irradiated above 10 and 20 Gy were 7% and 10%, respectively. This corresponded with decreases of more than 2 Gy in the mean total lung dose and 10% in the risk of radiation pneumonitis. The volumes of the heart and esophagus irradiated above 40 to 50 Gy and normal thoracic tissue irradiated above 10 to 40 Gy were reduced using the IMRT plans. In contradiction to common belief, the integral dose delivered to the patient was also reduced with IMRT in certain cases. There was a marginal increase in the spinal cord maximum dose and lung volume above 5 Gy in the IMRT plans in half of the cases, which could have been caused by the significant increase of monitor units and thus leakage dose in IMRT for the sliding window delivery technique used in these studies.

Although IMRT may be effective in reducing normal tissue toxicity and improving tumor coverage, its high-dose gradient and conformity require a high level of precision in dose delivery and tumor localization. In the meantime, the complexity introduced by tumor motion must be recognized when using IMRT. Unlike 3DCRT, IMRT treats only a portion of the target volume at a particular time. There is a great deal of concern as to whether target motion and collimator motion during IMRT delivery will have a significant interplay effect, thus degrading the planned dose distributions. For IMRT to be feasible and more effective in treating NSCLC, motion-reduction techniques should be explored further, such as breath-holding and tumor tracking. Our preliminary clinical data indicated that IMRT may reduce toxic effects in normal tissue in selected cases, particularly for tumor

Clinical Radiation Oncology

moves of less than 5 mm, and allow further dose escalation (245). We have recently developed IMRT guidelines for NSCLC using imaging-guided radiotherapy (33).

Guidelines for Lung Cancer IMRT Treatment

Patient Selection and Immobilization

Not every patient will benefit from IMRT treatment. On the basis of published data, patients with tumor located in the superior sulcus or close to the esophagus or spinal cord or patients with positive lymph nodes may benefit more from IMRT treatment. Earlier-stage, small mobile tumors may not be good candidates for IMRT treatment unless motion-mitigation techniques are involved. In addition, the conformal dose distribution and high-dose gradients in IMRT mandate improved patient immobilization.

Target Volume and Tumor Motion Considerations

IMRT for lung cancer requires a detailed understanding of chest radiographic anatomy, including both tumor volume and critical structures such as normal lung, esophagus, heart, and spinal cord. PET/CT is recommended for target delineation. On the basis of the available information, it is not necessary to treat uninvolved mediastinal lymph nodes or contralateral hilum or superior clavicular lymph nodes prophylactically. Only disease that can be seen with CT or PET needs to be included in the targeted volume. If a patient has mediastinal lymph node involvement, particularly for lower-lobe primary lung cancer, ipsilateral hilum and subcarinal lymph nodes may be treated. Organ motion during the treatment must be considered and addressed individually. Patients should be evaluated for regularity of breathing. responsiveness to feedback guidance, and breath-hold capability. On the basis of this evaluation, a treatment-delivery technique should be selected from free breathing, breath-hold, or other alternatives. 4D CT study is recommended for the treatment-planning purposes. At the least, tumor motion assessment should be conducted using fluoroscopy.

If the tumor moves <5 mm, the patient can be treated with free-breathing IMRT using ITV technique with an adequate margin. However, if significant tumor motion is anticipated, the patient should be treated with breath hold or other means of tumor tracking if such techniques can be used to freeze the tumor position at reproducible positions. Respiratory gated treatment may be considered, although it may have low duty cycle and residual tumor motion within the gating window. It is not clear at this time how accurately IMRT can deliver the dose to the target volume as planned when the tumor moves significantly and ITV technique is used. More 4D planning study for IMRT treatment is needed.

Tissue Heterogeneity Consideration

Because heterogeneity affects some beamlets more than others, resulting in a significant difference in dose distribution, heterogeneity correction should be applied for all IMRT lung cancer treatment plans.

Plan Evaluation and Quality Assurance

IMRT may cause cold spots or hot spots in unexpected locations that may not be reflected by the dose-volume distribution. Therefore, the isodose distribution on every image slide should be inspected. To reduce the potential increased low-dose (<10 Gy) delivery to the normal lung, fewer beams (five to seven beams) are recommended, in particular to reduce the beam delivery time and improve patient comfort. The physician should balance the concerns of dose inhomogeneity and lung tissue-sparing. Experienced IMRT planning and strict quality assurance for both mechanical and dosimetric accuracy for the treatment planning and delivery are mandatory.

Proton Radiotherapy in Non-Small Cell Lung Cancer

The proton is a charged particle that, compared with the photon, possesses a well-defined range of penetration determined by both the beam's energy and the density of the tissue through which it passes. As the proton beam penetrates the body, the particles slow down and deposit the dose sharply near the end of its range, a phenomenon known as the *Bragg peak*. By modulating the Bragg peak across the target volume, proton beams can deliver a full, localized, uniform dose of energy to the treatment site while sparing the surrounding normal tissues. The physics of the proton beam is ideal for treatments in which organ preservation is paramount, such as lung cancer. The preliminary clinical data from Shioyama et al. (213) and Bush et al. (29) using escalated/accelerated proton radiotherapy showed promising clinical results comparable to those of surgical resection in stage IA cases. Again, the accuracy of target delineation and tumor motion consideration are critical for both proton and photon treatment. Proton treatment is more sensitive to anatomic motion, position uncertainties, and tissue inhomogeneity (33).

In our preclinical study in M.D. Anderson Cancer Center, we found that proton radiotherapy significantly reduced dose to normal lungs, esophagus, spinal cord, and heart in both stage I and stage III NSCLC even with dose escalation (87.5 Gy for stage I and 74 Gy for stage III) compared with a standard dose of photon radiotherapy (66 Gy for stage I and 63 Gy for stage III) using either 3D or IMRT (34). We are conducting phase II clinical trials using imaging-guided dose escalated/accelerated proton radiotherapy for stage I (87.5 Gy with 2.5 Gy per fraction) and stage III (74 Gy with 2 Gy per fraction and concurrent chemotherapy) NSCLC.

Metastatic Non-Small Cell Lung Cancer

Rationale for Chemotherapy

Clearly, chemotherapy improves survival in patients with metastatic NSCLC (28). Cisplatin-based regimens have been shown to be superior to best supportive care (BSC) in improving outcome in patients with NSCLC (30,99). Four meta-analyses were conducted to determine whether chemotherapy is superior to BSC in advanced NSCLC (78,137,165,221). These studies reached a similar conclusion: administration of chemotherapy resulted in a modest but statistically significant prolongation in survival. Formal prospective analyses of quality-of-life (QOL) measures have revealed improvement in QOL measures for patients who received chemotherapy, whereas QOL measures declined for those on BSC (43,54). In addition, economic analyses favor chemotherapy over BSC by reducing hospitalization secondary to worsening of the disease.

Platinum-based chemotherapy, the recommended first-line chemotherapy, prolongs survival, improves symptom control, and yields superior QOL compared with BSC. This regimen has been shown to achieve overall response rate of 25% to 35%, time to progression of 4 to 6 months, median survival of 8 to 10 months, 1-year survival of 30% to 40% and 2-year survival of 10% to 15%. Patients with responsive or stable disease can continue to receive a total of four to six cycles of chemotherapy or until the disease progresses.

Effect of the "Newer Chemotherapeutic Agents" Introduced in the 1990s

Several new agents such as vinorelbine, paclitaxel, docetaxel, gemcitabine, and irinotecan became available in the 1990s. These new agents showed promising activity as single agents and in combination with a platinum compound in several phase II studies. In view of the promising response rates and acceptable toxicity profile, several of these agents have undergone extensive evaluation in the phase III setting.

Vinorelbine

Vinorelbine has been studied extensively in phase III settings. Vinorelbine as a single agent was compared with a combination of vindesine and cisplatin or vinorelbine and cisplatin in a randomized setting in patients with metastatic NSCLC (124,125). The median survival was 30 weeks for both the single-agent vinorelbine arm and the arm containing combination of vindesine and cisplatin. The combination of cisplatin and vinorelbine resulted in a median survival of 40 weeks. It was remarkable that, as a single agent, administration of vinorelbine had efficacy similar to that of a cisplatin-containing regimen but with substantially less toxicity. In a subsequent phase III study, the combination of cisplatin and vinorelbine was superior to therapy with cisplatin alone (243). In a third randomized study, cisplatin and vinorelbine were superior to a combination of 5-fluorouracil and leucovorin (30 compared with 22 weeks) (40). Vinorelbine as a single agent was found to be superior to BSC in elderly patients with metastatic NSCLC (229). This Elderly Lung Cancer Vinorelbine Italian Study reported not only an improvement in survival but also improvement in QOL parameters.

Paclitaxel

Several phase II studies reported encouraging response rates with the use of paclitaxel-containing chemotherapy regimens in patients with metastatic NSCLC (16,117,118). ECOG compared cisplatin and etoposide with cisplatin and paclitaxel (paclitaxel given during 24 hours of continuous infusion) and reported superior results with paclitaxel-based therapy (19). A European study reported similar survival results with cisplatin and paclitaxel compared with cisplatin and teniposide (median survival of 10 months), but the paclitaxel-containing arm was found to be less toxic (68). In a randomized study comparing cisplatin and etoposide with carboplatin and paclitaxel, there was no improvement in median survival, but the toxicities were much less with carboplatin and paclitaxel (16). In addition, the SWOG study reported a favorable toxicity profile with paclitaxel and carboplatin compared with cisplatin and vinorelbine (103). Once again, the median survival was identical in both arms in this study. With several phase II studies reporting encouraging activity and an acceptable toxicity profile, paclitaxel and carboplatin have become one of the commonly used chemotherapy regimens in patients with metastatic NSCLC.

Docetaxel

Several phase II studies have indicated reproducible activity for docetaxel in patients with metastatic NSCLC (28). In a phase III study presented in 2001, docetaxel and cisplatin and docetaxel and carboplatin were compared with a control arm of vinorelbine and cisplatin. The docetaxel and cisplatin combination was found to be marginally superior to vinorelbine and cisplatin (1-year survival rates: 47% compared with 42%, respectively; median survivals: 10.9 months compared with 10.0 months, respectively) (187).

Gemcitabine

Gemcitabine has been found to have promising activity in several phase II studies as a single agent or in combination with a wide variety of agents, including cisplatin, carboplatin, vinorelbine, paclitaxel, and docetaxel. In a randomized phase III study, the cisplatin and gemcitabine combination was found to be superior to the use of cisplatin alone (196). Two phase II studies have established the toxicity profile and the activity of gemcitabine and carboplatin (65).

Irinotecan

Irinotecan administered either weekly (100 mg/m²) or once every 3 weeks (350 mg/m²) is active as first-line therapy in patients with metastatic NSCLC, with response rates as high as 34% (119). Two phase III studies conducted in Japan have confirmed the activity of the irinotecan-based chemotherapy regimen in NSCLC. On the basis of these studies, the combination of irinotecan and cisplatin has become the standard of care in Japan for the treatment of metastatic NSCLC (209).

Nonplatinum Combinations in the Treatment of Metastatic NSCLC

There are no data to indicate that nonplatinum combinations are superior to platinum-based combination chemotherapy regimens in metastatic NSCLC. In a randomized phase III study comparing the combination of docetaxel and gemcitabine with docetaxel and cisplatin, there were no differences in survival (67).

Targeted Therapies or Biologic Agents

Several targeted therapies or biologic agents are undergoing extensive evaluation in patients with NSCLC. Some of these agents are administered orally and have a very favorable toxicity profile. If proven to be active, these agents alone or in combination with chemotherapy and/or radiotherapy potentially could have a significant impact in the outcome of patients with NSCLC.

Agents That Target EGFR or Receptor Tyrosine Kinases

Several new agents that target specific receptors or receptor tyrosine kinases now have become available for clinical research. The most promising among them is a class of compounds that target the EGFR or receptor tyrosine kinases. Agents that target EGFR tyrosine kinases have been studied recently in metastatic NSCLC. Randomized phase II/III studies have been completed recently with ZD 1839 (Iressa) and erlotinib (Tarceva). The preliminary data showed that erlotinib is associated with a trend toward improved progression-free and overall survival. In a phase II study of patients with relapsed NSCLC, OSI 774, another oral agent that targets EGFR tyrosine kinases, has been shown to produce a 1-year survival rate of approximately 40% with a very favorable toxicity profile (188). Cetuximab (C225), an antibody against RGFR, has been currently investigated for its role in concurrent chemoradiotherapy by RTOG.

Agents That Target Human Epidermal Growth Factor Receptor–2 (Her-2/Neu)

Initially, it was reported that nearly one third of patients with NSCLC had overexpression of Her-2/neu (205). It is becoming increasingly evident that the incidence of Her-2/neu overexpression is perhaps only around 10% in advanced NSCLC. The role of trastuzumab (Herceptin) as a single agent in patients with metastatic NSCLC currently is being studied by the CALGB group.

Agents That Inhibit Cyclooxygenase-2

It has been estimated that nearly 70% of NSCLC tumors express cyclooxygenase-2 (COX-2) (242). Inhibition of COX-2 has been known to promote apoptosis, to inhibit cell growth, and to be synergistic with chemotherapy (85,145,224). Several phase I/II studies are ongoing to assess the role of specific COX-2 inhibitors in combination with chemotherapy and radiotherapy in NSCLC.

Agents Targeting Vascular Endothelial Growth Factor

Bevacizumab (Avastin) is a recombinant monoclonal antibody that blocks vascular endothelial growth factor. On the basis of phase II/III clinical trials, the Eastern Cooperative Oncology Group (ECOG 4599) recommends bevacizumab in combination of paclitaxel and carboplatin as a new treatment for patients with stage IV nonsquamous NSCLC. As our knowledge of cancer biology evolves, molecular targets will continue to be an area of investigation. Other biologic targets under study include the vascular endothelial growth factor receptor and protein kinase c alpha.

▓▓ | Small Cell Lung Carcinoma

In the United States, approximately 40,000 persons received a diagnosis of SCLC during 2006, accounting for 20% to 25% of all lung cancer cases. Among those patients with SCLC, only one-fourth of them were expected to have limited disease in the thorax because the majority of those patients with SCLC already have disseminated disease in the thorax or extrathorax.

One important aspect of the management of SCLC is to distinguish the cytology or histology from that of NSCLC. Physical examination of patients with SCLC aims to identify prognostic indicators and clinical manifestations to distinguish them from patients with NSCLC. This is essential for determination of the type of treatment modality, aggressiveness of treatment, and other supportive management. When combined thoracic radiation therapy (TRT) and chemotherapy is given, conformal RT is used to reduce normal tissue toxicities such as esophagitis, pneumonitis, pericarditis, and myelitis. This is essential for these patients with limited-stage SCLC and good performance status who will need to tolerate acute toxicities during TRT/chemotherapy without break of TRT or modification of the dose of chemotherapy and/or TRT. Prophylactic cranial irradiation (PCI) has become a part of the standard management for patients with limited SCLC who have achieved complete response.

Pathology

The World Health Organization classification subdivides SCLC into three cell types (pure or classic, variant cell, and mixed), although there is no significant difference in outcome by subtype. Pure SCLC is more sensitive to chemotherapy and RT than is the variant cell type, although there is some controversy about whether the variant cell type significantly affects patient outcome. Aisner et al. (2) reviewed a series of 577 patients with limited SCLC treated by chemotherapy and RT on an ECOG protocol. There were 24 cases (4.4%) with the variant cell type. Complete response rates were 27% for patients with the variant cell type and 19% for patients with classic cell type ($p = .45$). The mixed-cell type should be treated as NSCLC rather than SCLC because its chemotherapeutic sensitivity and radiosensitivity are similar to those for NSCLC rather than SCLC.

Prognostic Factors

The most important prognostic factor for SCLC is stage (limited vs. extensive). Limited disease is confined to the hemithorax, although the presence of malignant pleural effusion will affect the outcome adversely. Patients who present with pleural effusion do worse than those without pleural effusion. However, the patients who have negative cytology of the pleural effusion do have better outcome than those with positive cytology. Extensive SCLC extends beyond the hemithorax, such as disease in both lungs, or extrathoracic extension often to the brain, leptomeninges, spinal cord, bone, bone marrow, adrenal gland, liver, pancreas, kidneys, small bowel, and pelvic contents. Patient factors influencing outcome are performance status and sex. Age is not a significant prognostic variable in patients with limited SCLC (218). However, patients older than 80 years will have limitations of the aggressive systemic treatment. Continuation of smoking will adversely affect the outcome. Other prognostic factors are elevated lactic dehydrogenase and alkaline phosphatase, low sodium, and possibly paraneoplastic syndromes, which include syndrome of inappropriate antidiuretic hormone, adrenocorticotropic hormone-producing syndrome, and Lambert-Eaton syndrome.

Staging Work-Up

The work-up to define SCLC is similar to that of NSCLC. The history and physical examination need to include any signs and symptoms related to paraneoplastic syndrome(s). It is also important for all patients to undergo MRI to rule out metastatic disease. Patients who achieve a complete response to the chemotherapy and radiotherapy are candidates for PCI. For patients with limited-stage disease, bone scan and bone marrow aspiration or biopsy are indicated if the lactic dehydrogenase is elevated, and thoracentesis is indicated if pleural effusion is present. Follow-up imaging studies and other work-up should be ordered as suggested by the Oncology Practice Guidelines of the National Comprehensive Cancer Network (161). PET scanning to evaluate the extent of lung cancer, including mediastinal nodal involvement, has become fairly accurate with the assistance of CT in NSCLC and may help in SCLC (180).

Treatment

Early-stage SCLC is diagnosed in fewer than 5% of SCLC patients. For patients with clinical stage I (T1-2, N0), complete resection with a lobectomy with mediastinal nodal dissection or sampling may be considered. However, mediastinoscopy should be performed to rule out occult nodal disease prior to resection. Postoperative chemotherapy should be considered even if surgical pathology shows no lymph node involvement. For patients with positive lymph node involvement after surgical resection, postoperative chemotherapy and radiotherapy should be considered. PCI should be considered in all cases.

Most patients with SCLC present with bulky and extensive lymph node involvement. Management of this group of SCLC has evolved from single chemotherapeutic agents in the 1940s and 1950s to multichemotherapeutic agents with TRT and PCI for limited SCLC in the 1990s (27). Feld et al. (56) reviewed eight series published between 1979 and 1987 and reported a rise in 2-year survival rates from a range of 10% to 15% to a range of 25% to 30%. Most, if not all, of the improvement in outcome was attributed to more effective combination chemotherapy regimens. Locoregional therapy alone, either surgery or RT, improved the short-term survival only slightly, primarily for a subset of patients with limited-stage disease with very rare 5-year survival. In a landmark trial conducted by the Medical Research Council in the 1960s, patients who were considered candidates for surgical resection by the standards of the time were randomized to thoracotomy with the intent of tumor removal or to definitive irradiation of the primary tumor and regional lymphatics (61). Radiation therapy resulted in slightly better mean survival duration (6.5 vs. 10 months; $p = .04$) with 1-, 2-, and 5-year survival rates of 22%, 10%, and 4%, respectively, compared with 21%, 4%, and 1% for the surgery arm. Of interest, the one 5-year survivor in the surgery arm was unable to receive surgery and was given RT. These studies led to the abandonment of surgery as a primary modality of treatment of SCLC with the possible exception of patients with solitary pulmonary nodules (86). A more recent approach is concurrent chemotherapy and TRT followed by aggressive systemic chemotherapy supported by granulocyte colony-stimulating factor, antibiotics, management of electrolytes, and erythropoetin-stimulating agent.

Combined Chemotherapy and Radiation Therapy

Although early development of distant metastasis is a critical problem, intrathoracic failure becomes more important once distant metastasis is controlled. Two meta-analyses, using different methods, confirmed the value of thoracic irradiation to decrease local recurrence and to improve survival. The study by Warde and Payne (239), based on results from 11 prospective randomized trials of chemotherapy with or without TRT, showed an absolute increase in overall survival of 5.4% at 2 years and in local control of 25% for patients with limited SCLC. Pignon et al. (181) collected data on 2,140 patients from 16 randomized trials comparing chemotherapy alone versus chemotherapy plus thoracic irradiation and found an improvement in absolute survival of 5.4% at 3 years. It is obvious that the effectiveness of both thoracic irradiation and systemic chemotherapy needs to be improved.

Concurrent TRT and Chemotherapy

The potential advantages from concurrent chemotherapy and RT are early use of both modalities, expectation and acceptance of greater toxicity, ability to plan RT more accurately, short overall treatment time (high-dose intensity), and possible sensitization of the tumor. The disadvantages are enhanced normal tissue toxicity (possible dose modification and/or possible treatment breaks) and an inability to assess response to either modality. In the 1970s, concurrent chemotherapy (cyclophosphamide, doxorubicin, and Oncovin) and TRT was tried at the National Cancer Institute (NCI), which successfully treated patients with limited SCLC, although the mortality rate from the treatment was 20% (98). Because of this high mortality, the use of concurrent TRT and doxorubicin was abandoned. Other strategies of concurrent RT and chemotherapy have been tried. McCracken et al. (146) reported results from a phase II trial of SWOG in which two courses of cisplatin, etoposide, and vincristine were given with concurrent RT using one fraction of 1.8 Gy per day, 5 days per week, to a total dose of 45 Gy. Additional chemotherapy with vincristine, methotrexate, and etoposide, alternating with doxorubicin and cyclophosphamide for 12 weeks, followed the concurrent therapy. They evaluated 154 patients; with a minimum period of observation of 3 years, the 2-year survival rate was 42% and the 4-year rate was 30%. Updated, this study showed a 5-year survival of 26% (92). Johnson et al. (94,95) and Turrisi et al. (234) reported a small series of patients treated with concurrent cisplatin and etoposide with accelerated fractionation: 1.5 Gy twice daily, 5 days per week, was given for 3 weeks for a total dose of 45 Gy. Two-year survival rates were 57% and 65% for the studies by Turrisi et al. (234) and Johnson et al. (95,98), respectively. Updated 4-year survival rates by Turrisi et al. (235) were 36%.

However, sequencing and timing of chemotherapy and TRT are still controversial. The National Cancer Institute of Canada clinical trial group (157) studied early versus late TRT in a randomized trial. Three hundred eight patients were randomized to receive early TRT, 40 Gy in 15 fractions during 3 weeks to the primary site with concurrent etoposide and cisplatin at week 3, or to receive late thoracic irradiation at week 15 with the same RT dose and concurrent chemotherapy. After completion of all chemotherapy and TRT, complete responders received PCI, 25 Gy in 10 fractions during 2 weeks. Although complete response rates did not significantly differ between the early and late TRT groups, progression-free survival ($p = .036$) and overall survival ($p = .008$) (Fig. 48.7) were significantly better in the early thoracic group. Patients in the late thoracic radiation group had significantly higher rates of brain metastases ($p = .006$). This study indicated that the early administration of TRT with concurrent chemotherapy improved survival, possibly by reducing the last clonogens in the primary.

The Japanese Clinical Oncology Group (JCOG) (73) reported a prospective randomized study for patients with limited SCLC treated by sequential or concurrent chemotherapy; 231 patients younger than 75 years of age with limited SCLC and good performance status were enrolled. Chemotherapy consisted of paclitaxel, 80 mg/m^2 on day 1 and etoposide, 100 mg/m^2 on days 1 through 3 every 3 weeks. Radiation therapy consisted of 45 Gy twice daily; the concurrent arm started chemotherapy and TRT on day 1 and the sequential arm started TRT after two cycles of chemotherapy. Chemotherapy was given for a total of four cycles. Their data showed significant improvement of survival with concurrent chemoradiotherapy compared with sequential chemotherapy and radiotherapy.

Fractionation

According to several phase II trials that have used thoracic irradiation twice daily with concurrent chemotherapy, median survivals ranged from 18 to 27 months and 2-year survivals ranged from 19% to 60%, with local control from 32% to 91% (95,234). Intergroup study 0096 (235) was conducted through ECOG and RTOG to investigate accelerated hyperfractionated RT versus daily fractionation of RT with concurrent cisplatin and etoposide for limited SCLC. The total dose for TRT was 45 Gy, with concurrent cisplatin and etoposide for four cycles. The cisplatin dose was 60 mg/m^2 day 1, and VP-16 was given intravenously 120 mg/m^2 on days 1, 3, and 5 and repeated every 21 days for four cycles. The daily fractionation group received 1.8 Gy per fraction per day with a total tumor dose of 45 Gy during 5 weeks compared with accelerated hyperfractionated RT (1.5 Gy twice daily fractionation with a 4- to 6-hour interfractional interval with a total tumor dose of 45 Gy in 30 fractions in 3 weeks). Those patients who achieved complete response were considered to receive prophylactic cranial radiation, 2.5 Gy × 10 fractions. Overall median survival for the entire group was 20 months, with a 2-year progression-free survival of 40%. Toxicities in the two arms were identical with the exception of acute grade 3 esophagitis, seen in 26% of the patients treated by twice daily and accelerated treatment and in 11% of the daily fraction group.

There has not been a significant difference in late toxicity of the esophagus. The treatment-related death rate was 2%. Overall concurrent chemotherapy and radiotherapy can be tolerated and efficacious, showing a 2-year survival of 40% by a large cooperative group, which is twice as good as a decade ago. Five-year survival has improved significantly by accelerated hyperfractionation (28%) compared with daily fractionation (21%) ($p = .043$) (235), which is a remarkable improvement of 5-year survival from a nationwide randomized study.

Dose of Thoracic Radiation

The radiation dose to the thorax is another controversial area (6,38). The National Cancer Institute of Canada reported an important study (39) to show dose response to the thorax. They found a clear dose response with increased thoracic progression-free survival by giving 37.5 Gy in 15 fractions in 3 weeks compared with 25 Gy in 10 fractions in 2 weeks as a consolidation after completion of cisplatin-etoposide and cyclophosphamide-doxorubicin-vincristine alternating or sequential chemotherapy. Arriagada et al. (9) at the Institute of Gustave-Roussy published a report of 173 patients with limited SCLC treated in two consecutive trials. The total dose of TRT increased from 45 Gy to 55 Gy, which was given by split courses interdigitating with chemotherapy. Their 3-year local control rates were 66%, 70%, and 70%, respectively, and 5-year survival rates were 16%, 16%, and 20%, respectively. There was a 10% rate of lethal toxicity without a significant difference depending on the dose. The authors concluded that there was no significant difference in local tumor control or survival with treatment between 45 Gy and 65 Gy when effective chemotherapy was given.

It is difficult to go to a higher dose by accelerated hyperfractionation without increasing acute esophagitis. On the basis of the Intergroup study results, Komaki et al. (112) developed a phase I study to increase TRT dose during boost treatment by reducing the treatment field for the second daily fraction. The dose was escalated from 50 to 64.8 Gy with concurrent oral etoposide and intravenous cisplatin. The result showed that the maximum tolerant dose was 61.2 Gy delivered in 5 weeks. A phase II RTOG study using this regimen has been closed, and the result will be available soon. A CALGB study also showed promising results with 36% 3-year survival with 70 Gy with 2 Gy per fraction of radiotherapy with concurrent chemotherapy. To this point, the optimal dose of radiotherapy in SCLC using modern 3DCRT with concurrent chemotherapy remains controversial. Off protocol, 45 Gy with 1.5 Gy per fraction given as a twice daily regimen is considered standard.

Volume of Thoracic Radiation

The volume of TRT to encompass prechemotherapy or postchemotherapy fields has been controversial. In the 1980s, there were significantly different survivals if the prechemotherapy volumes had not been encompassed. More recently, however, studies by Arriagada et al. (9), Kies et al. (104), and the Mayo Clinic (130) have not shown any significant difference in survival when patients received postchemotherapy volume encompassed by TRT compared with prechemotherapy volume irradiated. However, prechemotherapy CT scan should be reviewed to include the originally involved lymph node regions in the target volume. 3DCRT should be used to reduce normal tissue toxicity and still offer an adequate dose to the target volume.

Prophylactic Cranial Irradiation

The role of PCI has been controversial because of the lack of definitive input for improvement of overall survival and previously reported late neurotoxicities. However, the risk of brain metastasis from SCLC is correlated to the length of survival, and as more effective treatment extends life, a higher risk of brain metastasis has been observed (107). An autopsy series by Nugent et al. (167) found that 80% of patients who died 2 years after completion of treatment had metastases in the CNS, including the brain parenchyma, base of the skull, leptomeninges, or spinal cord. Better and less toxic treatment has been sought. Factors contributing to decreased late neurotoxicities include a lower total dose (24 to 30 Gy), smaller fraction size (2.0 to

2.5 Gy), timing of PCI, no concurrent chemotherapy, and less neurotoxic chemotherapy (106). Baseline and follow-up neuropsychologic tests showed that 83% (25/30) of patients with limited SCLC had evidence of cognitive dysfunction before PCI, and no significant differences were found from pretreatment tests after PCI. PCI has reduced brain recurrence significantly among the long-term survivors without obvious neurotoxicities, although the majority of studies have been done retrospectively (42,210).

Recently, the NCI in the United States (94) reported excellent results when 38 patients with limited SCLC were treated with etoposide and cisplatin with concurrent hyperfractionated RT, 1.5 Gy twice daily with a total dose of 45 Gy during 3 weeks. The 1-year actuarial survival was 83%, and the 2-year survival was 43%. The 5-year survival rate and median survival were 19% and 21.3 months, respectively. However, the CNS was the only site of initial relapse in 34% (13/38) of the patients. All 13 of these patients died of CNS metastasis. This study concluded that combined chemotherapy and RT for limited-stage SCLC resulted in a 2-year survival of 43%. However, the main cause of death among the patients was relapse of the original cancer, and isolated CNS metastasis caused more than 30% of the cancer deaths.

A meta-analysis reported in 1999 of seven prospectively randomized clinical trials found a disease-free and overall-survival advantage in those patients who underwent PCI compared with those not receiving PCI (12). Several problems with that report include the fact that four of the seven trials analyzed consisted of fewer than 100 total patients, which may undercut the validity of the statistical analyses. Also, approximately 14% of all 987 patients had extensive rather than limited disease. In addition, the dose fractionation of those patients who received PCI was not uniform. However, there was a trend in the reduction of brain relapses in the subset of PCI patients who were treated with at least 36 Gy of total radiation dose at the conventional 2-Gy fraction size. Finally, this meta-analysis made no attempt to determine the risk of long-term neurotoxicity in those receiving and not receiving PCI.

The optimal dose for PCI remains unclear. RTOG is conducting a phase II/III randomized study to compare different regimens of PCI, 25 Gy in 10 fractions, 36 Gy in 18 fractions, and 36 Gy in 24 fractions given as twice daily, in patients with limited-stage SCLC who achieve complete clinical response.

Summary

For limited-stage SCLC, concurrent chemoradiotherapy should be considered. Radiotherapy should be delivered to 45 Gy, given 1.5 Gy per fraction and twice daily, with concurrent cisplatin and etoposide chemotherapy. Patients should be encouraged to participate in research protocols using newer chemotherapy and/or dose escalation/escalation radiotherapy. PCI should be considered for complete clinical responders with a dose of 25 to 36 Gy.

Toxicity of Normal Tissue

Radiation-induced toxic effects in normal tissue are related to both dose and volume. In addition, the spatial arrangement of the functional subunits in the normal tissue is also critical. In the case of tissue in which the functional subunits are arranged in series, such as spinal cord, esophagus, tracheal, bronchus, vessels, and nerve, the integrity of each unit is important for organ function, and the elimination of any unit may result in significant toxicity. In this case, we should minimize the hot spots, particularly a very high dose, to these organs even for a small volume. In contrast, in tissues in which functional subunits are arranged in parallel, not serially, such as the lung, the integrity

Table 48.11	NORMAL TISSUE TOLERANCE OF THERAPEUTIC IRRADIATION: TRADITIONAL ESTIMATES

	TD$_{5/5}$ Volume[a]			
Organ	1/3	2/3	3/3	Selected End Point
Spinal cord	5,000	5,000	4,700	—
Lung	4,500	3,000	1,750	Pneumonitis
Heart	6,000	4,500	4,000	Pericarditis
Esophagus	6,000	5,800	5,500	Clinical stricture/perforation
Brachial plexus	6,200	6,100	6,000	Clinically apparent nerve damage
Thyroid	—	—	—	Not included

	TD$_{50}$ Volume			
Organ	1/3	2/3	3/3	Selected End Point
Spinal cord	7,000	7,000	—	—
Lung	6,500	4,000	2,450	Pneumonitis
Heart	7,000	5,500	5,000	Pericarditis
Esophagus	7,200	7,000	6,800	Clinical stricture/perforation
Brachial plexus	7,700	7,600	7,500	Clinically apparent nerve damage
Thyroid	—	—	—	Not included

[a]TD$_{5/5}$ and TD$_{50/5}$ represent the estimated dose for each organ volume or partial organ volume, resulting in a 1% to 5% risk and a 50% risk, respectively, at 5 years.
From Emami B, Lyman J, Brown A, et al. Tolerance of normal tissue to therapeutic irradiation. *Int J Radiat Oncol Biol Phys* 1991;21:109–122, with permission.

of each unit is less important; instead, the volume irradiated or spared plays a major role in complications in these tissues.

Emami et al. (55) published partial-volume irradiation parameters for various organs derived from an NCI-designated task force. Parameters were derived from a review of the literature and from clinical opinions of experienced radiation oncologists (Table 48.11). These data have served us for the last decade by defining partial organ tolerances. Toxicity end points are a 5% complication rate at 5 years (total dose [TD]$_{5/5}$) and a 50% complication rate at 5 years (TD$_{50/5}$) for different volumes irradiated. However, these toxicity parameters are incomplete and based on clinical data from two-dimensional radiotherapy alone without chemotherapy. The most important complications of radiotherapy in lung cancer are toxicity of the lung and esophagus. We discuss the current clinical data of these toxicities here, using 3DCRT with DVH analysis.

Lung Toxicity

Radiation-induced pneumonitis usually occurs after completion of radiotherapy, peaks at 2 months, and is stabilized or resolved around 6 to 12 months. It can be treated with corticosteroids such as prednisone 20 to 60 mg/day. Lung fibrosis occurs a few months after radiation and becomes chronic. Emerging clinical data based on 3DCRT in lung cancer have shown that mean lung dose (MLD), V5, V13, V20, and V30 are correlated with radiation lung injury. Graham recommended a cutpoint of V20 Gy at 40% with radiotherapy alone, at which 36% of patients developed grade 2 and above pneumonitis. He also reported that a total MLD of 20 Gy and above is associated with 24% grade 2 and above pneumonitis. Yorke et al. (246) reported that grade 3 and above pneumonitis correlated well with the MLD and V20. At MLD of 20 Gy, about 28% patients developed grade 3 and above pneumonitis. In addition, they reported strong correlations in the lower portion of the lungs and the ipsilateral lung. In a further analysis using a 3DCRT dose escalation study (from 70.2 to up to 90 Gy), they found a significant correlation between grade 3 and above pneumonitis and total, ipsilateral, and lower lung V5 to V40. When using a 20% rate of grade 3 and above

pneumonitis as a cut-off, V5, V10, and V20 of total lung were estimated to be around 58%, 48%, and 36%, respectively. Our data from M.D. Anderson supported these estimations. Currently, we recommend the use of MLD of 20 Gy and V5, V10, and V20 (GTV is excluded from lung volume calculation) of 65%, 45%, and 35%, respectively, as our cut-off threshold for lung cancer radiotherapy when concurrent chemotherapy is given (see Table 48.10). These cut-offs are based on current available information, and further modification may be needed when more mature data are available. More complicated calculations involve DVH reduction techniques, which reduce the DVH of an organ to a single effective uniform dose; effective lung dose (V$_{eff}$) (150); the NTCP calculation model (115,134); and the functional subunit model of Niemierko (163). These parameters have the disadvantages of a lack of clinical confirmation and technically difficult calculations.

Esophageal Toxicity

The radiotherapeutic management of thoracic malignancies often exposes the esophagus to high levels of ionizing radiation. After 2 to 3 weeks of conventionally fractionated radiotherapy, patients often complain of dysphagia and/or odynophagia that usually worsens toward the end of radiotherapy and peaks at the first week after completion of radiotherapy. This acute reaction to radiation can cause significant morbidity from dehydration and weight loss that can lead to treatment interruptions. The late reactions of the esophagus to radiation generally involve fibrosis of the organ that can lead to strictures. Patients may experience various degrees of dysphagia and may require endoscopic dilation. As with the acute reaction, rare cases may involve perforation or fistula formation.

The clinical and dosimetric predictors of acute and late esophagitis have become particularly important in the era of radiation dose escalation and concurrent chemoradiotherapy. Emami et al. (55) have reported that TD$_{5/5}$, TD$_{50/5}$ values in two-dimensional radiotherapy for stricture and perforation of the esophagus are 60 and 72 Gy in one-third of volume, respectively. Emerging clinical data based on 3DCRT indicated that, in general, the tolerance of the esophagus is around 60 Gy; however, the volume (particularly the length of circumference involvement) is very crucial. Singh et al. (217) reported that the threshold maximal esophageal point dose for grade 3-5 esophagitis was 58 Gy when concurrent chemoradiotherapy was given. The esophageal surface area receiving ≥55 Gy, the esophageal volume receiving ≥60 Gy (V60), and the use of concurrent chemotherapy were the most statistically significant predictive factors for acute esophagitis (24). For late toxicity, the length of the 100% of the circumference receiving ≥50 Gy (V50) percentage of surface area treated with ≥50 Gy, and maximal percentage of circumference ≥60 Gy are predictive for all grades of late toxicity (1,136). About 32% patients developed late esophageal toxicity if V50 >32% or the length of the 100% of the circumference >3.2 cm. Patients who received >80 Gy to any portion of the esophageal circumference have around a 50% chance for late toxicity. It should be noted that acute esophagitis (grade 2/3) is correlated significantly with V40 to V70 (35). In clinical practice, it is hard to avoid esophagitis totally when the target volume is close to the esophagus. Attention should be paid to minimize grade 3 and above toxicity. On the basis of available DVH data, to avoid severe acute and chronic toxicity, we suggest the thresholds of V55 <50% and maximal dose <75 Gy if concurrent chemotherapy is given (see Table 48.10).

Ongoing Investigations

The possible mechanisms to avoid or minimize lung and esophageal toxicity from RT can be broken down into improved radiation delivery, medical interventions to impede the inflammatory response of normal lung to irradiation, and the ability to predict inflammatory response based on genetic predisposition. IMRT has the potential to concentrate the prescribed radiation dose within the target volume and reduce the dose to surrounding normal structures; however, low-dose exposure (<5 Gy) to a larger volume of lung and tumor motion are the concerns, as previously discussed. Prospective clinical trials with IMRT and longer follow-up are needed. Also as previously discussed, proton radiotherapy may have a greater potential to spare more normal lung, particularly the low-dose region.

Attempts to modify the inflammatory response of irradiated lung are being investigated in various stages of clinical study. Tannehill et al. (228) showed that pretreatment with amifostine resulted in a lower incidence of esophagitis than would be expected with chemotherapy and radiation alone.

A phase III trial from Greece reported decreased rates of clinical pneumonitis, radiographic infiltrates, pulmonary fibrosis, and acute esophagitis in patients receiving amifostine (5). This phase III lung cancer trial was conducted comparing conventional radiation plus or minus amifostine given intravenously at 340 mg/m². The percentage of clinical grade 2 pneumonitis at 2 months was reduced from 49% to 16%. The percentage of x-ray evidence for pneumonitis grade 2 or more also was reduced, from 52% to 19% at 3 months following completion of therapy. The percentage of fibrosis at 6 months was reduced from 53% to 28%. This study showed a statistically significant reduction in esophagitis at weeks 3 to 6 of the RT. The percentages of complete and partial responses at 32 months were equal in the two treated arms.

Antonadou et al. (5) treated 68 patients in a small phase III randomized study with amifostine at 300 mg/m² in conjunction with radiation plus paclitaxel or carboplatin and/or radiation. Esophagitis and lung parenchymal toxicity were reduced by amifostine in all treatments with either paclitaxel and radiation or carboplatin and radiation.

Komaki et al. (109) at M.D. Anderson Cancer Center performed a phase III randomized study of chemoradiation with or without amifostine in patients with inoperable stage II and III NSCLC. Sixty patients were enrolled, of whom 53 could have

response evaluated. Patients received radiation at 1.2 Gy per fraction (two fractions per day for a total dose of 69.6 Gy), oral VP-16, and intravenous cisplatin. Patients received amifostine at 500 mg intravenously twice weekly within 1 hour before chemoradiation or the same chemoradiation without amifostine. Twenty-seven patients received amifostine, and 26 did not. Severe esophagitis was significantly lower in the amifostine group at 7% (2/27) than in the control group at 31% (8/26) ($p = .03$). Acute severe pneumonitis was lower in the amifostine group at 4% (1/27) than in the control group at 23% (6/26) ($p = .04$). Hypotension occurred in 70% of the amifostine patients, but only one patient discontinued treatment for this reason. Nausea and vomiting toxicity was not stated. Complete response in patients occurred in seven (26%) of the 27 patients who received amifostine compared with two (8%) of the 26 patients who did not ($p = .07$).

The RTOG conducted a phase III study of chemotherapy plus twice-daily radiation with or without amifostine in lung cancer (RTOG 98–01) (156), a total of 243 patients with stage II to IIIA/B NSCLC received induction paclitaxel and carboplatin followed by concurrent paclitaxel and carboplatin and hyperfractionated RT (69.6 Gy at 1.2 Gy twice daily). Patients were randomly assigned to amifostine 500 mg intravenously four times per week (any time between twice-daily radiotherapy) or no amifostine during chemoradiotherapy. In this study, amifostine did not significantly reduce grade 3 and above esophagitis in patients receiving hyperfractionated radiation and chemotherapy. However, patient self-assessments suggested an improvement of symptoms with amifostine. The issue of suboptimal timing of amifostine injection has been raised in this RTOG study. A multicenter study using subcutaneous injection of amifostine within 1 hour before radiotherapy is ongoing.

Clinically, there is a wide variation in the degree of acute pneumonitis and lung fibrosis in patients who have been treated similarly, suggesting a variation in lung radiosensitivity from person to person. One approach to increasing possibility of tumor control while maintaining an acceptable toxicity profile would be to identify sensitive patients before treatment. One possible approach to identifying sensitive patients will be to identify important cytokines or growth factors before or during therapy that correlate with the degree of pneumonitis or fibrosis. Prospective measurements of transforming growth factor-β indicate that this factor may be useful as a predictor of pulmonary fibrosis.

References

1. Ahn S, Kahn D, Zhou S, et al. Dosimetric and clinical predictors for radiation-induced esophageal injury. *Int J Radiat Oncol Biol Phys* 2005;61:335–347.
2. Aisner S, Finkelstein D, Ettinger D, et al. The clinical significance of variant-morphology small-cell carcinoma of the lung. *J Clin Oncol* 1990;8:402–408.
3. Albain K, Swann S, Rusch V, et al. Phase III study of concurrent chemotherapy and radiotherapy (CT/RT) vs CT/RT followed by surgical resection for stage IIIA (PN2) non-small cell lung cancer (NSCLC): outcomes update of North America Intergroup 0139 (RTOG 9309). *J Clin Oncol* 2005;23(165):7014.
4. American Joint Committee on Cancer. *AJCC cancer staging handbook*, Vol. 6th ed. Berlin: Springer-Verlag; 2002.
5. Antonadou D, Coliarakis N, Synodinou M, et al. Randomized phase III trial of radiation treatment +/- amifostine in patients with advanced-stage lung cancer. *Int J Radiat Oncol Biol Phys* 2001;51:915–922.
6. Ariyoshi Y, Fukuoka M, Furuse K, et al. Concurrent cisplatin-etoposide chemotherapy plus thoracic radiotherapy for limited-stage small cell lung cancer. Japanese Lung Cancer Chemotherapy Group in Japanese Clinical Oncology Group. *Jpn J Clin Oncol* 1994;24:275–281.
7. Armstrong B, Perez C, Simpson J, et al. Role of irradiation in the management of superior vena cava syndrome. *Int J Radiat Oncol Biol Phys* 1987;4:531–539.
8. Arriagada R, Bergman B, Dunant A, et al. Cisplatin-based adjuvant chemotherapy in patients with completely resected non-small-cell lung cancer. *N Engl J Med* 2004;350:351–360.
9. Arriagada R, Pellae-Cosset B, Ladron de Guevara J, et al. Alternating radiotherapy and chemotherapy schedules in limited small cell lung cancer: analysis of local chest recurrences. *Radiother Oncol* 1991;2:91–98.
10. Asamura H, Nakayama H, Kondo H, et al. Lobe-specific extent of systematic lymph node dissection for non-small cell lung carcinomas according to a retrospective study of metastasis and prognosis. *J Thorac Cardiovasc Surg* 1999;117:1102–1111.

11. Attar S, Miller J, Satterfield J, et al. Pancoast's tumor: irradiation or surgery? *Ann Thorac Surg* 1979;6:578–586.
12. Auperin A, Arriagada R, Pignon J, et al. Prophylactic cranial irradiation for patients with small-cell lung cancer in complete remission. *N Engl J Med* 1999;341:476–484.
13. Bailey A, Parmar M, Stephens R. Patient-reported short-term and long-term physical and psychologic symptoms: results of the continuous hyperfractionated accelerated [correction of accelerated] radiotherapy (CHART) randomized trial in non small-cell lung cancer. CHART Steering Committee. *J Clin Oncol* 1998;16:3082–3093.
14. Bearhs O, Henson D, Hutter R, et al. Manual for staging of cancer. In: Bearhs O, Henson D, Hutter R, et al., eds. 4th ed. Philadelphia: JB Lippincott; 1993.
15. Belani C, Aisner J, Day R. Weekly paclitaxel and carboplatin with simultaneous thoracic radiotherapy (TRT) for locally advanced non-small cell lung cancer (NSCLC): three year follow-up. *Proc Am Soc Clin Oncol of the American Society of Clinical Oncology* 1997;16:1608(abstr).
16. Belani C, Aisner J, Hiponia D, et al. Paclitaxel and carboplatin with and without filgrastim support in patients with metastatic non-small cell lung cancer. *Semin Oncol* 1995;22:7–12.
17. Belani C, Choy H, Bonomi P, et al. Combined chemoradiotherapy regimens of paclitaxel and carboplatin for locally advanced non-small-cell lung cancer: a randomized phase ii locally advanced multi-modality protocol. *J Clin Oncol* 2005;23:5883–5891.
18. Bloedern F, Cowley R, Cuccia C. Combined therapy: irradiation and surgery in the treatment of bronchogenic carcinoma. *Am J Radiol* 1961;85:175–181.
19. Bonomi P, Kim K, Kusler J, et al. Cisplatin/etoposide vs paclitaxel/cisplatin/G-CSF vs paclitaxel/cisplatin in non-small-cell lung cancer. *Oncology* 1997;11:9–10.
20. Borrie J. Primary carcinoma of the bronchus; prognosis following surgical resection; a clinico-pathological study of 200 patients. *Ann R Coll Surg Eng* 1952;10:165–186.
21. Boyden E. *Segmental anatomy of the lungs: a study of the patterns of the segmental bronchi and related pulmonary vessels.* Vol. New York: McGraw-Hill;1955.
22. Bradley J, Graham M, Suzanne S, et al. Phase I results of RTOG L-0117; a Phase I/II dose intensification study using 3DCRT and concurrent chemotherapy for patients with inoperable NSCLC. *Proc Am Soc Clin Oncol* 2005;23:16S(abstr).
23. Bradley J, Graham M, Winter K, et al. Toxicity and outcome results of RTOG 9311: a phase I-II dose-escalation study using three-dimensional conformal radiotherapy in patients with inoperable non-small-cell lung carcinoma. *Int J Radiat Oncol Biol Phys* 2005;61:318–328.
24. Bradley J, Leumwananonthachai N, Purdy J, et al. Gross tumor volume, critical prognostic factor in patients treated with three-dimensional conformal radiation therapy for non-small-cell lung carcinoma. *Int J Radiat Oncol Biol Phys* 2002;52:49–57.
25. Bradley J, Paulus R, Graham M, et al. Phase II trial of postoperative adjuvant paclitaxel/carboplatin and thoracic radiotherapy in resected stage ii and iiia non-small-cell lung cancer: promising long-term results of the Radiation Therapy Oncology Group—RTOG 9705. *J Clin Oncol* 2005;23:3480–3487.
26. Bradley J, Thorstad W, Mutic S, et al. Impact of FDG-PET on radiation therapy volume delineation in non-small-cell lung cancer. *Int J Radiat Oncol Biol Phys* 2004;59:78–86.
27. Bunn P, Ihde D. Small cell bronchogenic carcinoma: a review of therapeutic results. In: Livingston R, ed; 1981:169–208.
28. Bunn P, Kelly K. New chemotherapeutic agents prolong survival and improve quality of life in non-small cell lung cancer: a review of the literature and future directions. *Clin Cancer Res* 1998;4:1087–1100.
29. Bush D, Slater J, Shin B, et al. Hypofractionated proton beam radiotherapy for stage I lung cancer. *Chest* 2004;126:1198–1203.
30. Cellerino R, Tummarello D, Guidi F, et al. A randomized trial of alternating chemotherapy versus best supportive care in advanced non-small-cell lung cancer. *J Clin Oncol* 1991;9:1453–1461.
31. Chahinian A, Israel L. Rates and patterns of growth of lung cancer. In: Israel L, Chahinian A, eds. New York: Academic Press; 1976:63–79.
32. Chang J, Balter P, Liao Z, et al. Preliminary report of image-guided hypofractionated sterotactic body radiotherapy to treat patients with medically inoperable stage I or isolated peripheral lung recurrent non-small cell lung cancer. *Int J Radiat Oncol Biol Phys* 2006;66(3):5480.
33. Chang J, Liu H, Komaki R. Intensity modulated radiation therapy and proton radiotherapy for non-small cell lung cancer. *Curr Oncol Rep* 2005;7:255–259.
34. Chang J, Zhang X, Wang X, et al. Significant reduction of normal tissue dose by proton radiotherapy compared with three-dimensional conformal or intensity-modulated radiation therapy in Stage I or Stage III non-small-cell lung cancer. *Int J Radiat Oncol Biol Phys* 2006;65:1087–1096.
35. Chapet O, Kong F, Lee J, et al. Normal tissue complication probability modeling for acute esophagitis in patients treated with conformal radiation therapy for non-small cell lung cancer. *Radiother Oncol* 2005;77:176–181.
36. Choy H, Akerley W, Safran H, et al. Multiinstitutional phase II trial of paclitaxel, carboplatin, and concurrent radiation therapy for locally advanced non-small-cell lung cancer. *J Clin Oncol* 1998;16:3316–3322.
37. Chung C, Stryker J, O'Neill M, et al. Evaluation of adjuvant postoperative radiotherapy for lung cancer. *Int J Radiat Oncol Biol Phys* 1982;8:1877–1880.
38. Cox J. Dose-response in small cell carcinoma. *Int J Radiat Oncol Biol Phys* 1988;14:393–394.
39. Coy P, Hodson I, Payne D, et al. The effect of dose of thoracic irradiation on recurrence in patients with limited stage small cell lung cancer. Initial results of a Canadian Multicenter Randomized Trial. *Int J Radiat Oncol Biol Phys* 1988;14:219–226.
40. Crawford J, O'Rourke M, Schiller J, et al. Randomized trial of vinorelbine compared with fluorouracil plus leucovorin in patients with stage IV non-small-cell lung cancer. *J Clin Oncol* 1996;14:2774–2784.
41. Croxatto O, Barcat J. Lymph node metastasis in bronchogenic carcinoma. Study on its role in dissemination. *Johns Hopkins Med J* 1970;126:121–129.
42. Cull A, Gregor A, Hopwood P, et al. Neurological and cognitive impairment in long-term survivors of small cell lung cancer. *Eur J Cancer* 1994;30A:1067–1074.
43. Cullen M, Billingham L, Woodroffe C, et al. Mitomycin, ifosfamide, and cisplatin in unresectable non–small-cell lung cancer: Effects on survival and quality of life. *J Clin Oncol* 1999;17:3188–3194.
44. Curran W, Scott C, Langer C, et al. Long term benefit is observed in a phase III comparison of sequential vs concurrent chemo-radiation for patients with unresectable NSCLC:RTOG 9410. *Proc Am Soc Clin Oncol* 2003;61(abstr).
45. Daly R, Trastek V, Pairolero P, et al. Bronchoalveolar carcinoma: factors affecting survival. *Ann Thorac Surg* 1991;51:368–376.
46. Dartevelle P, Chapelier A, Macchiarini P, et al. Anterior transcervical-thoracic approach for radical resection of lung tumors invading the thoracic inlet. *J Thorac Cardiovasc Surg* 1993;105:1025–1034.
47. Devine J, Mendenhall W, Million R, et al. Carcinoma of the superior pulmonary sulcus treated with surgery and/or radiation therapy. *Cancer* 1986;5:941–943.
48. Dillman R, Seagren S, Propert K, et al. A randomized trial of induction chemotherapy plus high-dose radiation versus radiation alone in stage III non-small-cell lung cancer. *N Engl J Med* 1990;323:940–945.
49. Doll R, Peto R. The causes of cancer: quantitative estimates of avoidable risks of cancer in the United States today. *J Natl Cancer Inst* 1981;66:1191–1308.
50. Dosoretz D, Galmarini D, Rubenstein J, et al. Local control in medically inoperable lung cancer: an analysis of its importance in outcome and factors determining the probability of tumor eradication. *Int J Radiat Oncol Biol Phys* 1993;27:507–516.
51. Dosoretz D, Katin M, Blitzer P, et al. Medically inoperable lung carcinoma: the role of radiation therapy. *Semin Radiat Oncol* 1996;6:98–104.
52. Dosoretz D, Katin M, Blitzer P, et al. Radiation therapy in the management of medically inoperable carcinoma of the lung: results and implications for future treatment strategies. *Int J Radiat Oncol Biol Phys* 1992;24:3–9.
53. Douillard JY, Rosell R, Delena M, et al. Phase III adjuvant vinorelbine (N) and cisplatin (P) versus observation (OBS) in completely resected (stage I-III) non-small cell lung cancer (NSCLC) patients (pts): final results after 70-month median follow-up. *J Clin Oncol* 2005;23:16.
54. Ellis P, Smith I, Hardy J, et al. Symptom relief with MVP (mitomycin C, vinblastine and cisplatin) chemotherapy in advanced non-small-cell lung cancer. *Br J Cancer* 1995;71:366–370.
55. Emami B, Lyman J, Brown A, et al. Tolerance of normal tissue to therapeutic irradiation. *Int J Radiat Oncol Biol Phys* 1991;21:109–122.
56. Feld R, Ginsberg R, Payne D. Treatment of a small cell lung cancer. In: Roth J, Ruckdeschel J, Weisenburger T, eds. Philadelphia: WB Saunders; 1993:229–262.
57. Flehinger B, Melamed M, Zaman M, et al. Early lung cancer detection: results of the initial (prevalence) radiologic and cytologic screening in the Memorial Sloan-Kettering study. *Am Rev Respir Dis* 1984;130:555.
58. Fletcher G. Clinical dose response curves of human malignant epithelial tumours. *Br J Cancer* 1973;46:1–12.
59. Fontana R, Sanderson D, Taylor W, et al. Early lung cancer detection: results of the initial (prevalence) radiologic and cytologic screening in the Mayo Clinic study. *Am Rev Respir Dis* 1984;130:561.
60. Fournel P, Robinet G, Thomas P, et al. Randomized Phase III trial of sequential chemoradiotherapy compared with concurrent chemoradiotherapy in locally advanced non-small-cell lung cancer: Groupe Lyon-Saint-Etienne d'Oncologie Thoracique-Groupe Francais de Pneumo-Cancerologie NPC 95–01 Study. *J Clin Oncol* 2005;23:5910–5917.
61. Fox W, Scadding J. Treatment of oat-celled carcinoma of the bronchus. *Lancet* 1973;2:63–65.
62. Frost J, Ball W, Levin M, et al. Early lung cancer detection: results of the initial (prevalence) radiologic and cytologic screening in the Johns Hopkins study. *Am Rev Respir Dis* 1984;130:549.
63. Furuse K, Fukuoka M, Kawahara M, et al. Phase III study of concurrent versus sequential thoracic radiotherapy in combination with mitomycin, vindesine, and cisplatin in unresectable stage III non-small-cell lung cancer. *J Clin Oncol* 1999;17:2692–2699.
64. Furuse K, Hosoe S, Masuda T, et al. Impact of tumor control on survival in unresectable stage III non-small lung cancer (NSCLC) treated with concurrent thoracic radiotherapy (TRT) and chemotherapy (CT). *Proc Am Soc Clin Oncol* 2000;19:1893(abstr).
65. Gandara D, Edelman M, Lara P, et al. Gemcitabine in combination with new platinum compounds: an update. *Oncology* 1983;147:473–480.
66. Garland L, RL B, Coulson W, et al. The apparent sites of origin of carcinomas of the lung. *Radiology* 1962;78:1–11.
67. Georgoulias V, Papadakis E, Alexopoulos A, et al. Platinum-based and non-platinum-based chemotherapy in advanced non-small-cell lung cancer: a randomised multicentre trial. *Lancet* 2001;357:1478–1484.
68. Giaccone G, Postmus P, Splinter T, et al. Cisplatin/paclitaxel vs cisplatin/teniposide for advanced non-small-cell lung cancer. The EORTC lung cancer cooperative group. The European organization for research and treatment of cancer. *Oncology* 1997;11:11–14.
69. Ginsberg R, Rubinstein L. Randomized trial of lobectomy versus limited resection for T1 N0 non-small cell lung cancer. *Lung Cancer Study Group. Ann Thorac Surg* 1995;60:615–622.
70. Ginsberg R. Discussion of Attar S, Miller JE, Satterfield J. Pancoast's tumor: irradiation or surgery. *Ann Thorac Surg* 1979;28:578–586.
71. Giraud P, Antoine M, Larrouy A, et al. Evaluation of microscopic tumor extension in non-small-cell lung cancer for three-dimensional conformal radiotherapy planning. *Int J Radiat Oncol Biol Phys* 2000;48:1015–1024.
72. Gohagan J, Marcus P, Fagerstrom R, et al. Baseline findings of a randomized feasibility trial of lung cancer screening with spiral CT scan vs chest radiograph: the lung screening study of the national cancer institute. *Chest* 2004;126:114–121.
73. Goto K, Nishiwaki Y, Takasa M. Final results of a phase III study of concurrent versus sequential thoracic radiotherapy (TRT) in combination with cisplatin (P) and etopside (E) for limited-stage small-cell lung cancer (LD-SCLC): the Japan Clinical Oncology Group (JCOG) study. *Proc Am Soc Clin Oncol* 1999;18:468(abstr).
74. Graham M, Matthews J, Harms W, et al. Three-dimensional radiation treatment planning study for patients with carcinoma of the lung. *Int J Radiat Oncol Biol Phys* 1994;29:1105–1117.
75. Graham M, Purdy J, Emami B, et al. Clinical dose-volume histogram analysis for pneumonitis after 3D treatment for non-small cell lung cancer (NSCLC). *Int J Radiat Oncol Biol Phys* 1999;45:323–329.
76. Graham P, Gebski V, Stat M, et al. Radical radiotherapy for early nonsmall cell lung cancer. *Int J Radiat Oncol Biol Phys* 1995;31:261–266.
77. Gray H. *The anatomical basis of medicine and surgery*, 38th ed. New York: Churchill Livingston; 1995.
78. Grilli R, Oxman A, Julian J. Chemotherapy for advanced non-small-cell lung cancer: how much benefit is enough? *J Clin Oncol* 1993;11:1866–1872.

79. Haffty B, Goldberg N, Gerstley J, et al. Results of radical radiation therapy in clinical stage I, technically operable non-small cell lung cancer. *Int J Radiat Oncol Biol Phys* 1988;15:69–73.
80. Hamada C, Ohta M, Wada H, et al. Survival benefit of oral UFT for adjuvant chemotherapy after completely resected non-small lung cancer. *J Clin Oncol* 2004;22:7002.
81. Hansen H, Muggia F. Staging of inoperable patients with bronchogenic carcinoma with special reference to bone marrow examination and peritoneoscopy. *Cancer* 1972;30:1395–1401.
82. Hecht S, Hoffmann D. Tobacco-specific nitrosamines, an important group of carcinogens in tobacco and tobacco smoke. *Carcinogenesis* 1988;17:116–128.
83. Heelan R, Demas B, Caravelli J, et al. Superior sulcus tumors: CT and MR imaging. *Radiology* 1989;170:637–641.
84. Henschke C, Naidich D, Yankelevitz D, et al. Early lung cancer action project. *Cancer* 2001;92:153–159.
85. Hida T, Kozaki K, Muramatsu H, et al. Cyclooxygenase-2 inhibitor induces apoptosis and enhances cytotoxicity of various anticancer agents in non-small cell lung cancer cell lines. *Clin Cancer Res* 2000;6:2006–2011.
86. Higgins G, Shields T, Keehn R. The solitary pulmonary nodule. Ten-year follow-up of veterans administration-armed forces cooperative study. *Arch Surg* 1975;110:570–577.
87. Higginson J. Block dissection in pneumonectomy for carcinoma. *J Thorac Cardiovasc Surg* 1953;25:582–592.
88. Holmes E. Surgical adjuvant therapy of non-small cell lung cancer. *Chest* 1986;89:295–300.
89. Intensity Modulated Radiation Therapy Collaborative Working Group. Intensity-modulated radiotherapy: current status and issues of interest. *Int J Radiat Oncol Biol Phys* 2001;51:880–914.
90. International Commission on Radiation Units and Measurements. *Prescribing, recording, and reporting photon beam therapy*. Bethesda, MD: International Commission on Radiation Units and Measurements; 1993:50.
91. Ishida T, Yano T, Maeda K, et al. Strategy for lymphadenectomy in lung cancer three centimeters or less in diameter. *Ann Thorac Surg* 1990;50:708–713.
92. Janaki L, Rector D, Turrisi A. Patterns of failure and second malignancies from SWOG-8629: concurrent cisplatin, etoposide, vincristine, and once daily radiotherapy for the treatment of limited small cell lung cancer. *Proc Am Soc Clin Oncol* 1994;13:331(abstr).
93. Jemal A, Siegel R, Ward E, et al. Cancer statistics, 2006. *CA Cancer J Clin* 2006;56:106–130.
94. Johnson B, Bridges J, Sobczeck M, et al. Patients with limited-stage small-cell lung cancer treated with concurrent twice-daily chest radiotherapy and etoposide/cisplatin followed by cyclophosphamide, doxorubicin, and vincristine. *J Clin Oncol* 1996;14:806–813.
95. Johnson B, Salem C, Nesbitt J. Limited stage small cell lung cancer treated with concurrent hyperfractionated chest radiotherapy and etoside/cisplatin. *Lung Cancer* 1993;21–26.
96. Johnson B. Second lung cancers in patients after treatment for an initial lung cancer. *J Natl Cancer Inst* 1998;90:1335–1345.
97. Johnson D, Hainsworth J, Greco F. Pancoast's syndrome and small cell lung cancer. *Chest* 1982;82:602–606.
98. Johnson R, Brereton H, Kent C. Small-cell carcinoma of the lung: attempt to remedy causes of past therapeutic failure. *Lancet* 1976;2:289–291.
99. Kaasa S, Lund E, Thorud E, et al. Symptomatic treatment versus combination chemotherapy for patients with extensive non-small cell lung cancer. *Cancer* 1991;67:2443–2447.
100. Kaskowitz L, Graham M, Emami B, et al. Radiation therapy alone for stage I non-small cell lung cancer. *Int J Radiat Oncol Biol Phys* 1993;27:517–523.
101. Kato H, Ichinose Y, Ohta M, et al. A randomized trial of adjuvant chemotherapy with uracil-tegafur for adenocarcinoma of the lung. *N Engl J Med* 2004;350:1713–1721.
102. Keller S, Adak S, Wagner H, et al. A randomized trial of postoperative adjuvant therapy in patients with completely resected stage II or IIIa non-small-cell lung cancer. *N Engl J Med* 2000;343:1217–1222.
103. Kelly K, Crowley J, Bunn P, et al. Randomized phase III trial of paclitaxel plus carboplatin versus vinorelbine plus cisplatin in the treatment of patients with advanced non-small-cell lung cancer: a Southwest Oncology Group Trial. *J Clin Oncol* 2001;19:3210–3218.
104. Kies M, Mira J, Crowley J, et al. Multimodal therapy for limited small-cell lung cancer: a randomized study of induction combination chemotherapy with or without thoracic radiation in complete responders; and with wide-field versus reduced-field radiation in partial responders: a Southwest Oncology Group Study. *J Clin Oncol* 1987;5:592–600.
105. Kirsh M, Sloan H. Mediastinal metastases in bronchogenic carcinoma: influence of postoperative irradiation, cell type, and location. *Ann Thorac Surg* 1982;33:459–463.
106. Komaki R, Byhardt R, Anderson T, et al. What is the lowest effective biologic dose for prophylactic cranial irradiation. *Am J Clin Oncol* 1985;8:523.
107. Komaki R, Cox J, Whitson W. Risk of brain metastasis from small cell carcinoma of the lung related to length of survival and prophylactic irradiation. *Cancer Treat Rep* 1981;65:811.
108. Komaki R, Derus S, Perez-Tamayo C, et al. Risk of brain metastasis from small cell carcinoma of the lung related to length of survival and prophylactic irradiation. *Cancer* 1987;58:1649–1653.
109. Komaki R, Lee J, Kaplan B. Randomized phase II-III study of chemoradiation + amifostine in patients with inoperable stage II-III non-small cell lung cancer (NSCLC). *Proc Am Soc Clin Oncol* 2001;20:325(abstr).
110. Komaki R, Perkins P, Allen P, et al. Multidisciplinary approach for the management of superior sulcus tumors. *Proc Am Soc Clin Oncol* 1998;17:491(abstr).
111. Komaki R, Roh J, Cox J, et al. Superior sulcus tumors: results of irradiation of 36 patients. *Cancer* 1981;48:1563–1568.
112. Komaki R, Swann R, Ettinger D, et al. Phase I study of thoracic radiation dose escalation with concurrent chemotherapy for patients with limited small-cell lung cancer: report of Radiation Therapy Oncology Group (RTOG) protocol 97-12. *Int J Radiat Oncol Biol Phys* 2005;62:342–350.
113. Kong F, Ten Haken R, Schipper M, et al. High-dose radiation improved local tumor control and overall survival in patients with inoperable/unresectable non-small-cell lung cancer: long-term results of a radiation dose escalation study. *Int J Radiat Oncol Biol Phys* 2005;63:324–333.
114. Krol A, Aussems P, Noordijk E, et al. Local irradiation alone for peripheral Stage I lung cancer: could we omit the elective regional nodal irradiation? *Int J Radiat Oncol Biol Phys* 1996;34:297–302.
115. Kutcher G, Burman C, Brewster L, et al. Histogram reduction method for calculating complication probabilities for three-dimensional treatment planning evaluations. *Int J Radiat Oncol Biol Phys* 1991;21:137–146.
116. Lally B, Zelterman D, Colasanto J, et al. Postoperative radiotherapy for stage ii or iii non-small-cell lung cancer using the surveillance, epidemiology, and end results database. *J Clin Oncol* 2006;24:2998–3006.
117. Langer C, Leighton J, Comis R, et al. Paclitaxel and carboplatin in combination in the treatment of advanced non-small-cell lung cancer: a phase II toxicity, response, and survival analysis. *J Clin Oncol* 1995;13:1860–1870.
118. Langer C, Millenson M, O'Dwyer P, et al. Combination paclitaxel (1-hour) and carboplatin (AUC 7.5) in advanced non-small cell lung cancer: a phase II study by the Fox Chase Cancer Center Network. *Semin Oncol* 1996;23:35–41.
119. Langer C. Treatment of non-small-cell lung cancer in North America: the emerging role of irinotecan. *Oncology* 2001;15:13–18.
120. Lardinois D, Weder W, Hany T, et al. Staging of non-small-cell lung cancer with integrated positron-emission tomography and computed tomography. *N Engl J Med* 2003;348:2500–2507.
121. Lau D, Leigh B, Gandara D, et al. Twice-weekly paclitaxel and weekly carboplatin with concurrent thoracic radiation Followed by carboplatin/paclitaxel consolidation for stage III non-small-cell lung cancer: a California cancer consortium phase II trial. *J Clin Oncol* 2001;19:442–447.
122. Laurie G, Chansky J, Albain K, et al. Consolidation dcetaxel following concurrent chemoradiotherapy in pathologic stage IIIB non-small cell lung cancer (NSCLC) (SWOG9504): patterns of failure and updated survival. *Proc Am Soc Clin Oncol* 2001;1225(abstr).
123. Le Chevalier T, Arriagada R, Pignon J, et al. Should adjuvant chemotherapy become standard treatment in all patients with resected non-small-cell lung cancer. *Lancet Oncol* 2005;6:182–184.
124. Le Chevalier T, Brisgand D, Douillard J, et al. Randomized study of vinorelbine and cisplatin versus vindesine and cisplatin versus vinorelbine alone in advanced non-small-cell lung cancer: results of a European multicenter trial including 612 patients. *J Clin Oncol* 1994;12:360–367.
125. Le Chevalier T, Brisgand D, Soria JC, et al. Long term analysis of survival in the European randomized trial comparing vinorelbine/cisplatin to vindesine/cisplatin and vinorelbine alone in advanced non-small cell lung cancer. *Oncologist* 2001;6:8–11.
126. Lee C, Socinski M, Lin L, et al. High-dose 3D chemoradiotherapy trials in stage III non-small cell lung cancer (NSCLC) at the University of North Carolina: long-term follow up and late complications. *Proc Am Soc Clin Oncol* 2006;24:18S(abstr7145).
127. Lee JS, Komaki R, Fossella FV, et al. A pilot trial of hyperfractionated thoracic radiation therapy with concurrent cisplatin and oral etoposide for locally advanced inoperable non-small-cell lung cancer: a 5-year follow-up report. *Int J Radiat Oncol Biol Phys* 1998;42:479–486.
128. Levitt S, Jones TJ, Kilpatrick SJ, et al. Treatment of malignant superior vena caval obstruction. A randomized study. *Cancer* 1969;24:447–451.
129. Libshitz H, McKenna RJ, Mountain C. Patterns of mediastinal metastases in bronchogenic carcinoma. *Chest* 1986;90:229–232.
130. Liengswangwong V, Bonner JA, Shaw EG, et al. Limited-stage small-cell lung cancer: patterns of intrathoracic recurrence and the implications for thoracic radiotherapy. *J Clin Oncol* 1994;12:496–502.
131. Line D, Deeley T. The necropsy findings in carcinoma of the bronchus. *Br J Dis Chest* 1971;65:238–248.
132. Liu H, Wang X, Dong L, et al. Feasibility of sparing lung and other thoracic structures with intensity-modulated radiotherapy for non-small-cell lung cancer. *Int J Radiat Oncol Biol Phys* 2004;58:1268–1279.
133. Lung Cancer Study Group. Effects of postoperative mediastinal radiation on completely resected Stage II and Stage III epidermoid cancer of the lung. *N Engl J Med* 1986;315:1377–1381.
134. Lyman J, Wolbarst A. Optimization of radiation therapy. IV: a dose-volume histogram reduction algorithm. *Int J Radiat Oncol Biol Phys* 1989;17:433–436.
135. MacManus M, Hicks R, Matthews J, et al. High rate of detection of unsuspected distant metastases by PET in apparent stage III non-small-cell lung cancer: implications for radical radiation therapy. *Int J Radiat Oncol Biol Phys* 2001;50:287–293.
136. Maguire P, Sibley G, Zhou S, et al. Clinical and dosimetric predictors of radiation-induced esophageal toxicity. *Int J Radiat Oncol Biol Phys* 1999;45:97–103.
137. Marino P, Pampallona S, Preatoni A, et al. Chemotherapy vs supportive care in advanced non-small-cell lung cancer. Results of a meta-analysis of the literature. *Chest* 1994;106:861–865.
138. Martel M, Strawderman M, Hazuka M, et al. Volume and dose parameters for survival of non-small cell lung cancer patients. *Radiother Oncol* 1997;44:23–29.
139. Martel M, Ten Haken R, Hazuka M, et al. Dose-volume histogram and 3-D treatment planning evaluation of patients with pneumonitis. *Int J Radiat Oncol Biol Phys* 1994;28:575–581.
140. Martel MK, Sahijdak WM, Hayman JA, et al. Incidental dose to clinically negative nodes from conformal treatment fields for nonsmall cell lung cancer. *Int J Radiat Oncol Biol Phys* 1997;45:244.
141. Martini N, Bains MS, Burt ME, et al. Incidence of local recurrence and second primary tumors in resected stage I lung cancer. *J Thorac Cardiovasc Surg* 1995;109:120–129.
142. Martini N, Flehinger B, Zaman M, et al. Results of resection in non-oat cell carcinoma of the lung with mediastinal lymph node metastases. *Ann Surg* 1983;198:386–397.
143. Martini N, McCormack P. Therapy of stage III (nonmetastatic disease). *Semin Oncol* 1983;10:95–110.
144. Martini N. Discussion of Attar S, Miller JE, Satterfield J: Pancoast's tumor: irradiation or surgery? *Ann Surg* 1979;28:578–586.
145. Masferrer J, Leahy K, Koki A, et al. Antiangiogenic and antitumor activities of cyclooxygenase-2 inhibitors. *Cancer Res* 2000;60:1306–1311.
146. McCracken JD, Janaki LM, Crowley JJ, et al. Concurrent chemotherapy/radiotherapy for limited small-cell lung carcinoma: a Southwest Oncology Group Study. *J Clin Oncol* 1990;8:892–898.
147. McGarry R, Papiez L, Williams M, et al. Stereotactic body radiation therapy of early-stage non-small-cell lung carcinoma: phase I study. *Int J Radiat Oncol Biol Phys* 2005;63:1010–1015.

148. Medical Research Council Lung Cancer Working Party. The role of postoperative radiotherapy in non-small cell lung cancer: a multicentre randomised trial in patients with pathologically staged T1-T2, N1-N2, M0 disease. *Br J Cancer* 1996;74:632–639.
149. Mehta MP, Tannehill SP, Adak S, et al. Phase II trial of hyperfractionated accelerated radiation therapy for nonresectable non-small-cell lung cancer: results of Eastern Cooperative Oncology Group 4593. *J Clin Oncol* 1998;16:3518–3523.
150. Mohan R, Mageras G, Baldwin B, et al. Clinically relevant optimization of 3-D conformal treatments. *Med Phys* 1992;19:933–944.
151. Mountain C, Carr D, Anderson W. A system for the clinical staging of lung cancer. *Am J Roentgenol Radium Ther Nucl Med* 1974;120:130.
152. Mountain C, Dresler C. Regional lymph node classification for lung cancer staging. *Chest* 1997;111:1718–1723.
153. Mountain C. Prognostic implications of the International Staging System for Lung Cancer. *Semin Oncol* 1988;3:236–241.
154. Mountain C. The international system for staging lung cancer. *Semin Surg Oncol* 2000;18:106–115.
155. Mountain CF. Revisions in the International System for Staging Lung Cancer. *Chest* 1997;111:1710–1717.
156. Movsas B, Scott C, Langer C, et al. Randomized trial of amifostine in locally advanced non-small-cell lung cancer patients receiving chemotherapy and hyperfractionated radiation: Radiation Therapy Oncology Group Trial 98-01. *J Clin Oncol* 2005;23:2145–2154.
157. Murray N, Coy P, Pater JL, et al. Importance of timing for thoracic irradiation in the combined modality treatment of limited-stage small-cell lung cancer. The National Cancer Institute of Canada Clinical Trials Group. *J Clin Oncol* 1993;11:336–344.
158. Murshed H, Liu H, Liao Z, et al. Dose and volume reduction for normal lung using intensity-modulated radiotherapy for advanced-stage non-small-cell lung cancer. *Int J Radiat Oncol Biol Phys* 2004;58:1258–1267.
159. Nagaishi C. *Functional anatomy and histology of the lung*. Vol. Baltimore: University Park Press; 1972.
160. Nagata Y, Takayama K, Matsuo Y, et al. Clinical outcomes of a phase I/II study of 48 Gy of stereotactic body radiotherapy in 4 fractions for primary lung cancer using a stereotactic body frame. *Int J Radiat Oncol Biol Phys* 2005;63:1427–1431.
161. National Comprehensive Cancer Network. Oncology practice guideline. Small cell lung cancer. *Oncology* 1996;10:179–194.
162. Nehmeh S, Erdi Y, Pan T, et al. Four-dimensional (4D) PET/CT imaging of the thorax. *Med Phys* 2004;31:3179–3186.
163. Niemierko A. Reporting and analyzing dose distributions: a concept equivalent to uniform dose. *Med Phys* 1993;24:103–110.
164. Nohl-Oser H. An investigation of the anatomy of the lymphatic drainage of the lungs as shown by the lymphatic spread of bronchial carcinoma. *Ann R Coll Surg Eng* 1972;51:157–177.
165. Non-small cell lung cancer Collaborative Group. Chemotherapy in non-small cell lung cancer: a meta-analysis using updated data on individual patients from 52 randomized clinical trials. *BMJ* 1995;311:899–909.
166. Non-small Cell Lung Cancer Collaborative Group. Chemotherapy in non-small cell lung cancer: a meta-analysis using updated data on individual patients from 52 randomised clinical trials. *BMJ* 1995;311:899–909.
167. Nugent J, Bunn PJ, Matthews M, et al. CNS metastases in small cell bronchogenic carcinoma: increasing frequency and changing pattern with lengthening survival. *Cancer* 1979;44:1885–1893.
168. Ochsner A, Dixon J, DeBakey M. An analysis of 190 cases, 58 of which were successfully treated by pneumonectomy, with a review of the literature. *Clinics* 1945;3:1187.
169. Onishi H, Araki T, Shirato H, et al. Stereotactic hypofractionated high-dose irradiation for stage I non-small cell lung carcinoma clinical outcome in 245 subjects in a Japanese multiinstitutional study. *Cancer* 2004;101:1623–1631.
170. Onishi H, Kuriyama K, Komiyama T, et al. Clinical outcomes of stereotactic radiotherapy for stage I non-small cell lung cancer using a novel irradiation technique: patient self-controlled breath-hold and beam switching using a combination of linear accelerator and CT scanner. *Lung Cancer* 2004;45:45–55.
171. Parkin D, Bray F, Ferlay J, et al. Global cancer statistics, 2002. *CA Cancer J Clin* 2005;55:74–108.
172. Paulson D. Carcinomas in the superior pulmonary sulcus. *J Thorac Cardiovasc Surg* 1975;70:1095–1104.
173. Paulson D. Superior sulcus carcinomas. In: Sabiston DFS, eds. *Gibbons Surgery of the chest*. Philadelphia: WB Saunders; 1983:121–131.
174. Paulson D. Technical considerations of stage III disease: the "superior sulcus" lesion. In: Delarue NHE, eds. *International trends in general thoracic surgery*. Philadelphia: WB Saunders; 1985.
175. Pearson F, DeLarue N, Ilves R, et al. Significance of positive superior mediastinal nodes identified at mediastinoscopy in patients with resectable cancer of the lung. *J Thorac Cardiovasc Surg* 1982;83:1–11.
176. Perez C, Bauer M, Edelstein S, et al. Impact of tumor control on survival in carcinoma of the lung treated with irradiation. *Int J Radiat Oncol Biol Phys* 1986;12:539–547.
177. Perez C, Pajak T, Rubin P, et al. Long-term observations of the patterns of failure in patients with unresectable non-oat cell carcinoma of the lung treated with definitive radiotherapy. Report by the Radiation Therapy Oncology Group. *Cancer* 1987;59:1874–1881.
178. Perez C, Stanley K, Grundy G, et al. Impact of irradiation technique and tumor extent in tumor control and survival of patients with unresectable non-oat cell carcinoma of the lung: report by the Radiation Therapy Oncology Group. *Cancer* 1982;50:1091–1099.
179. Perez C, Stanley K, Rubin P, et al. A prospective randomized study of various irradiation doses and fractionation schedules in the treatment of inoperable non-oat-cell carcinoma of the lung. Preliminary report by the Radiation Therapy Oncology Group. *Cancer* 1980;45:2744–2753.
180. Pieterman R, van Putten J, Meuzelaar J, et al. Preoperative staging of non-small-cell lung cancer with positron-emission tomography. *N Engl J Med* 2000;343:254–261.
181. Pignon J, Arriagada R, Ihde D, et al. A meta-analysis of thoracic radiotherapy for small-cell lung cancer. *N Engl J Med* 1992;327:1818–1624.
182. Pisters K. Adjuvant chemotherapy for non-small-cell lung cancer—the smoke clears. *N Engl J Med* 2005;352:2640–2642.
183. Port Meta-analysis Trialists Group. Postoperative radiotherapy in nonsmall cell lung cancer: systematic review and meta-analysis of individual patient data from nine randomised clinical trials. *Lancet* 1998;352:257–263.
184. Purdy J, Perez C, Klein E, et al. *Three-dimensional conformal radiation therapy and intensity modulated radiation therapy: practical potential benefits and pitfalls*. Vol. New York: Lippincott, Williams & Wilkins; 2000.
185. Ramsey C, Scaperoth D, Arwood D, et al. Clinical efficacy of respiratory gated conformal radiation therapy. *Med Dosim* 1999;24:115–119.
186. Rienhoff W. The present status of the surgical treatment of carcinoma of the lung. *Ann Surg* 1947;125:541.
187. Rodriguez J, Plunzanska A, Gorbounova V, et al. A multicenter, randomized phase III study of doxetaxel + cisplatin (DC) and docetaxel + carboplatin (DCB) vs vinorelbine + cisplatin (VC) in chemotherapy-native patients with advanced metastatic non-small cell lung cancer. *Proc Am Soc Clin Oncol* 2001(abstr 1252).
188. Roman Perex Solar A, Huberman M, Karp D, et al. A phase II trial of the epidermal growth factor receptor (EGFR) tyrosine kinase inhibitor OSI-774, following platinum-based chemotherapy, in patients (pst) with advanced, EGFR-expressing, non-small cell lung cancer (NSCLC). *Proc Am Soc Clin Oncol* 2001(abstr 1235).
189. Rosell R, Gomez-Codina J, Camps C, et al. A randomized trial comparing preoperative chemotherapy plus surgery with surgery alone in patients with non-small-cell lung cancer. *N Engl J Med* 1994;330:153–158.
190. Rosenzweig K, Hanley J, Mah D, et al. The deep inspiration breath-hold technique in the treatment of inoperable non-small-cell lung cancer. *Int J Radiat Oncol Biol Phys* 2000;48:81–87.
191. Rosenzweig KE, Sim SE, Mychalczak B, et al. Elective nodal irradiation in the treatment of non-small-cell lung cancer with three-dimensional conformal radiation therapy. *Int J Radiat Oncol Biol Phys* 2001;50:681–685.
192. Roth J, Fossella F, Komaki R, et al. A randomized trial comparing perioperative chemotherapy and surgery with surgery alone in resectable stage IIIA non-small-cell lung cancer. *J Natl Cancer Inst* 1994;86:673–680.
193. Rubin P, Ciccio S. High daily dose for rapid decompression. In: Deeley T, ed. *Modern radiotherapy: carcinoma of the bronchus*. New York: Appleton-Century-Crofts; 1971:276–297.
194. Rusch V, Albain K, Crowley J, et al. Neoadjuvant therapy: a novel and effective treatment for stage IIIb non-small cell lung cancer. Southwest Oncology Group. *Ann Thorac Surg* 1994;58:290–295.
195. Rusch VW, Giroux DJ, Kraut MJ, et al. Induction chemoradiation and surgical resection for non-small cell lung carcinomas of the superior sulcus: Initial results of Southwest Oncology Group Trial 9416 (Intergroup Trial 0160). *J Thorac Cardiovasc Surg* 2001;121:472–483.
196. Sandler AB, Nemunaitis J, Denham C, et al. Phase III trial of gemcitabine plus cisplatin versus cisplatin alone in patients with locally advanced or metastatic non-small-cell lung cancer. *J Clin Oncol* 2000;18:122–130.
197. Sandler H, Curran W, Turrisi A 3rd. The influence of tumor size and pre-treatment staging on outcome following radiation therapy alone for stage I non-small cell lung cancer. *Int J Radiat Oncol Biol Phys* 1990;19:9–13.
198. Sasaki R, Komaki R, Macapinlac H, et al. [18F]Fluorodeoxyglucose uptake by positron emission tomography predicts outcome of non-small-cell lung cancer. *J Clin Oncol* 2005;23:1136–1143.
199. Saunders M, Dische S, Barrett A, et al. Continuous, hyperfractionated, accelerated radiotherapy (CHART) versus conventional radiotherapy in non-small cell lung cancer: mature data from the randomised multicentre trial. *Radiother Oncol* 1999;52:137–148.
200. Sause W, Kolesar P, Taylor SIV, et al. Final results of phase iii trial in regionally advanced unresectable non-small cell lung cancer: Radiation Therapy Oncology Group, Eastern Cooperative Oncology Group, and Southwest Oncology Group. *Chest* 2000;117:358–364.
201. Sause W, Scott C, Taylor S, et al. Radiation Therapy Oncology Group (RTOG) 88-08 and Eastern Cooperative Oncology Group (ECOG) 4588: preliminary results of a phase III trial in regionally advanced, unresectable non-small-cell lung cancer. *J Natl Cancer Inst* 1995;87:198–205.
202. Scalliet P, Goor C, Galdermans D. Gezmar (gemcitabine) with thoracic radiotherapy-a phase II pilot study in chemonaive patients with advance non-small-cell lung cancer (NSCLC). *Proc Am Soc Clin Oncol* 1998;17(abstr 499).
203. Schaake-Koning C, van den Bogaert W, Dalesio O F, J, et al. Effects of concomitant cisplatin and radiotherapy on inoperable non-small-cell lung cancer. *N Engl J Med* 1992;326:524–530.
204. Schechter M. The superior vena cava syndrome. *Am J Med* 1954;227:46–56.
205. Scheurle D, Jahanzeb M, Aronsohn R, et al. HER-2/neu expression in archival non-small cell lung carcinomas using FDA-approved Hercep test. *Anticancer Res* 2000;20:2091–2096.
206. Schild S, McGinnis WL, Graham D, et al. Results of a phase i trial of concurrent chemotherapy and escalating doses of radiation for unresectable non-small cell lung cancer. *Int J Radiat Oncol Biol Phys* 2005;63:S44(abstr 73).
207. Schuster-Uitterhoeve A, Hulshof M, Gonzalez G, et al. Feasibility of curative radiotherapy with a concomitant boost technique in 33 patients with non-small cell lung cancer (NSCLC). *Radiother Oncol* 1993;28:247–251.
208. Semik M, Netz B, Schmidt C, et al. Surgical exploration of the mediastinum: mediastinoscopy and intraoperative staging. *Lung Cancer* 2004;45:S55–S61.
209. Senan S, Burgers J, Samson M, et al. Can electivenodal irradiation be omitted in Stage III non-small cell lung cancer? An analysis of recurrences after sequential chemotherapy and "involved-field" radiotherapy to 70 Gy. *Int J Radiat Oncol Biol Phys* 2001;51:21.
210. Shaw E, Su J, Eagan R. Analysis of long-term survival and impact of prophylactic cranial irradiation in complete responders with small cell lung cancer: analysis of the Mayo Clinic and North Central Cancer Treatment Group data bases. *Proc Am Soc Clin Oncol* 1993;12(abstr 328).
211. Shaw R, Paulson D, Kee J. Treatment of the superior sulcus tumor by irradiation followed by resection. *Ann Surg* 1961;154:29–40.
212. Shields T. Pre-operative radiotherapy in the treatment of bronchial carcinoma. *Cancer* 1972;30:1388–1394.
213. Shioyama Y, Tokuuye K, Okumura T, et al. Clinical evaluation of proton radiotherapy for non-small-cell lung cancer. *Int J Radiat Oncol Biol Phys* 2003;56:7–13.
214. Shopland D. Tobacco use and its contribution to early cancer mortality with a special emphasis on cigarette smoking. *Environ Health Perspect* 1995;103:131–142.

215. Sibley G, Jamieson T, Marks L, et al. Radiotherapy alone for medically inoperable stage I non-small-cell lung cancer: the Duke experience. *Int J Radiat Oncol Biol Phys* 1998;40:149–154.

216. Simpson J, Perez C, Presant C. Superior vena cava syndrome. In: Yarbro J, Bornstein R, eds. *Oncologic emergencies.* New York: Grune & Stratton; 1980:43–72.

217. Singh AK, Lockett MA, Bradley JD. Predictors of radiation-induced esophageal toxicity in patients with non-small-cell lung cancer treated with three-dimensional conformal radiotherapy. *Int J Radiat Oncol Biol Phys* 2003;55:337–341.

218. Siu LL, Shepherd FA, Murray N, et al. Influence of age on the treatment of limited-stage small-cell lung cancer. *J Clin Oncol* 1996;14:821–828.

219. Sixel K, Aznar M, Ung Y. Deep inspiration breath hold to reduce irradiated heart volume in breast cancer patients. *Int J Radiat Oncol Biol Phys* 2001;49:199–204.

220. Socinski M, Rosenman J, Halle J, et al. Dose-escalating conformal thoracic radiation therapy with induction and concurrent carboplatin/paclitaxel in unresectable stage IIIA/B nonsmall cell lung carcinoma. *Cancer* 2001;92:1213–1223.

221. Souquet P, Chauvin F, Boissel J, et al. Polychemotherapy in advanced non small cell lung cancer: a meta-analysis. *Lancet* 1993;342:19–21.

222. Stanley K. Prognostic factors for survival in patients with inoperable lung cancer. *J Natl Cancer Inst* 1980;65:25–32.

223. Stellman S, Muscat J, Thompson T, et al. Risk of squamous cell carcinoma and adenocarcinoma of the lung in relation to lifetime filter cigarette smoking. *Cancer* 1997;80:382–388.

224. Stolina M, Sharma S, LIn Y. Specific inhibition of cyclooxygenase 2 restores antiumor reactivity by altering the balance of IL-10 and IL-12 synthesis. *J Immunol* 2000;164:361–370.

225. Strauss G, Herndon J, Maddaus M, et al. Randomized clinical trial of adjuvant chemotherapy with paclitaxel and carboplatin following resection in Stage IB non-small cell lung cancer (NSCLC): report of cancer and leukemia group B (CALGB) protocol 9633. *J Clin Oncol* 2004;22:7019.

226. Sulman E, Chang J, Liao Z, et al. Exclusion of elective nodal irradiation does not decrease local regional control of non-small cell lung cancer. *Int J Radiat Oncol Biol Phys* 2005;63:S226–S227.

227. Talton B, Constable W, Kersh C. Curative radiotherapy in non-small cell carcinoma of the lung. *Int J Radiat Oncol Biol Phys* 1990;19:15–21.

228. Tannehill SP, Mehta MP, Larson M, et al. Effect of amifostine on toxicities associated with sequential chemotherapy and radiation therapy for unresectable non-small-cell lung cancer: results of a phase II trial. *J Clin Oncol* 1997;15:2850–2857.

229. The Elderly Lung Cancer Vinorelbine Italian Study Group. Effects of vinorelbine on quality of life and survival of elderly patients with advanced non-small-cell lung cancer. *J Natl Cancer Inst* 1999;91:66–72.

230. Thun M, Lally C, Flannery J, et al. Cigarette smoking and changes in the histopathology of lung cancer. *J Natl Cancer Inst* 1997;89:1580–1586.

231. Toloza EM, Harpole L, Detterbeck F, et al. Invasive staging of non-small cell lung cancer: a review of the current evidence. *Chest* 2003;123:157S–166.

232. Trakhtenerg A, Kiseleva E, Pitskhelauri V. Preoperative radiotherapy in the combined treatment of lung cancer patients. *Neoplasma* 1988;35:459–465.

233. Trovo N, Minotel E, Fravelun G. Radiotherapy versus radiotherapy enhanced by cisplatin in stage III non-small cell lung cancer. *Int J Radiat Oncol Biol Phys* 1992;24:11–16.

234. Turrisi A, Glover D, Mason B. Long-term results of platinum, etoposide and twice daily thoracic radiotherapy for limited small cell lung cancer: results on 32 patients with 48 month minimum follow-up. *Proc Am Soc Clin Oncol* 1992;11 (abstr 292).

235. Turrisi AT, Kim K, Blum R, et al. Twice-daily compared with once-daily thoracic radiotherapy in limited small-cell lung cancer treated concurrently with cisplatin and etoposide. *N Engl J Med* 1999;340:265–271.

236. van Zandwijk N, Mooi W, Rodenhuis S. Prognostic factors in NSCLC: recent experiences. *Lung Cancer* 1995;12[Suppl]:S27–S233.

237. Vansteenkiste J, Fischer B, Dooms C, et al. Positron-emission tomography in prognostic and therapeutic assessment of lung cancer: systematic review. *Lancet Oncol* 2004;5:531–540.

238. Vokes E, Herndon J-I, Crawford J, et al. Randomized phase ii study of cisplatin with gemcitabine or paclitaxel or vinorelbine as induction chemotherapy followed by concomitant chemoradiotherapy for stage iiib non-small-cell lung cancer: Cancer and Leukemia Group B Study 9431. *J Clin Oncol* 2002;20:4191–4198.

239. Warde P, Payne D. Does thoracic irradiation improve survival and local control in limited-stage small-cell carcinoma of the lung? A meta-analysis. *J Clin Oncol* 1992;10:890–895.

240. Warren J. Pre-operative irradiation of cancer of the lung: final report of a therapeutic trial. *Cancer* 1975;36:914–925.

241. Winton T, Livingston R, Johnson D, et al. Vinorelbine plus cisplatin vs. observation in resected non-small-cell lung cancer. *N Engl J Med* 2005;352:2589–2597.

242. Wolff H, Saukkonen K, Anttila S, et al. Expression of cyclooxygenase-2 in human lung carcinoma. *Cancer Res* 1998;58:4997–5001.

243. Wozniak AJ, Crowley JJ, Balcerzak SP, et al. Randomized trial comparing cisplatin with cisplatin plus vinorelbine in the treatment of advanced non-small-cell lung cancer: a Southwest Oncology Group study. *J Clin Oncol* 1998;16:2459–2465.

244. Xia T, Li H, Sun Q, et al. Promising clinical outcome of stereotactic body radiation therapy for patients with inoperable Stage I/II non-small-cell lung cancer. *Int J Radiat Oncol Biol Phys* 2006;66:117–125.

245. Yom S, Liao Z, Liu H, et al. O-152 Analysis of acute toxicity results of intensity modulated radiationtherapy (IMRT) in the treatment of non-small cell lung cancer (NSCLC). *Lung Cancer* 2005;49:S52–S52.

246. Yorke E, Jackson A, Rosenzweig K, et al. Dose-volume factors contributing to the incidence of radiation pneumonitis in non-small-cell lung cancer patients treated with three-dimensional conformal radiation therapy. *Int J Radiat Oncol Biol Phys* 2002;54:329–339.

247. Zhang H, Yin W, Zhang L, et al. Curative radiotherapy of early operable non-small cell lung cancer. *Radiother Oncol* 1989;14:89–94.

248. Zienolddiny S, Ryberg D, Arab M, et al. Loss of heterozygosity is related to p53 mutations and smoking in lung cancer. *Br J Cancer* 2001;84:226–231.

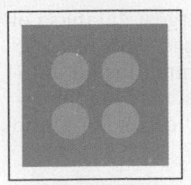

Chapter 49
Mediastinum and Trachea

Arthur Y. Hung, Tony Y. Eng, Todd J. Scarbrough, C. Dave Fuller, Charles R. Thomas, Jr.

Invasive thymomas and thymic carcinomas are relatively rare tumors, which together represent about 0.2% to 1.5% of all malignancies (56,459). Thymic carcinomas are rare and have been reported to account for only 0.06% of all thymic neoplasms. Arising from thymic, neurogenic, lymphatic, germinal, and mesenchymal tissues, these tumors are usually located in the anterior mediastinum but can be found in the posterior and middle mediastinum or neck. Lymphomas are the most common mediastinal tumor.

The anatomy of the mediastinum is trapezoidal in shape and is essentially the center of the thoracic cavity. It extends from the sternum anteriorly to the vertebral column posteriorly. The lungs and parietal pleurae are the lateral borders, the diaphragm is the floor, and the thoracic outlet of T1, its rib, and the manubrium form the roof (333). The mediastinum can be divided into three conceptual compartments as illustrated in Figure 49.1, but no anatomic barriers separate the compartments physically (51,138,437). The anterior mediastinum is the space anterior to the pericardium and great vessels and is occupied by the thymus, lymph nodes, and small vessels. The middle mediastinum is comprised of the heart, proximal great vessels, central airway structures, and lymph nodes. The posterior mediastinum is posterior to the heart and great vessels and contains the sympathetic chain ganglia, vagus nerve, thoracic duct, and esophagus. Table 49.1 lists the neoplastic masses that can occur and their typical compartment in the mediastinum.

Incidence of Primary Mediastinal Tumors

The frequency and prevalence of primary mediastinal tumors may be increasing (5,26,81,99). Adults generally develop thymic tumors and lymphomas, but germ cell tumors and carcinomas can also be found (99,496). Neurogenic tumors are usually seen in the pediatric population (26,164,165).

Thymomas

The thymus gland is an irregular lobulated lymphoepithelial organ in the anterior mediastinum. Embryologically, the thymus is derived from the endoderm of the lower portion of the third pharyngeal pouch and involutes during adulthood, gradually being replaced by adipose tissue. The blood supply is from the internal mammary arteries. The venous drainage is to the innominate and internal thoracic veins. The lymphatics drain into the lower cervical, internal mammary, and hilar nodes.

The vast majority of thymic tumors are thymomas, 90% of which are found in the anterosuperior mediastinum; other variants are found in the middle and posterior mediastinum or neck (329). Thymomas are epithelial tumors associated with an exuberant lymphoid component composed of immature cortical thymocytes. Although lymphomas, carcinoid tumors, and germ cell tumors may all arise within the thymus, only thymomas, thymic carcinomas, and thymolipomas arise from true thymic elements.

Epidemiology

Thymomas are exceedingly rare. The Surveillance, Epidemiology, and End Results (SEER) reported a thymoma incidence of 0.15 per 100,000 person-years (126). For patients with associated myasthenia gravis, the peak age is in the fourth decade, while in patients without myasthenia gravis, the peak age is in the seventh decade or later (271,293,334,352,364,388). According to the SEER data, thymoma incidence increased into the eighth decade of age and then decreased (126). The incidence was higher in males than females ($p = .007$) and was highest among Asians/Pacific Islanders (0.49 per 100,000 person-years).

Of anterior mediastinal masses, thymomas are the most common tumor comprising 30% (26,81,86,99,329,459). Of all mediastinal masses, thymomas represent 20% of the tumors in adults (154,270,437,496) and 15% in pediatric populations (329). Associations with Epstein-Barr virus, lymphoepitheliomas, radiation, and cytogenetic abnormalities have been suggested as possible precursors to disease (109,205,254,306,316, 457,497).

Natural History

Thymomas are generally characterized by an indolent growth pattern that can be locally invasive. In 30% to 40% of patients with a thymoma, myasthenia gravis is also present (256). The vast majority of thymomas are cytologically bland tumors and approximately half of them are noninvasive (31,35,37,89, 99,140,225,264,265,294,334,408,501). Roughly one-third are asymptomatic and found incidentally on a chest x-ray (264, 265,272). Of those with symptoms, 40% have symptoms relating to impingement by the intrathoracic mass ranging from cough, chest pain, dyspnea, hoarseness, super vena cava (SVC) obstruction, and even tumor hemorrhage (370). Another 30% of those with symptoms have systemic signs, and the remainder present with signs of myasthenia gravis.

Thymomas are associated with several parathymic syndromes, of which myasthenia gravis is the most common (400,431). The syndromes are autoimmune conditions such as benign cytopenia, hypogammaglobulinemia, and polymyositis and are reported to occur in 2% to 5% of patients (42,271,364, 400,431,502).

Myasthenia gravis is an autoimmune disease characterized by the presence of antibodies that react with nicotinic acetylcholine receptors in muscle and disrupt transmission at the neuromuscular junction (117). The cardinal features are weakness and fatigability of skeletal muscles, with the majority of patients exhibiting fatigue in ocular muscles first, including ptosis and diplopia. Generalized weakness develops in approximately 85% of patients. More severe cases involve the proximal limb girdle muscles, and in the worst cases it can even affect respiration (115,116,481). Myasthenia gravis occurs in approximately 45% of patients with thymomas with a range of 10% to 67% in series reporting over 100 patients (244,245,293,334,352,388). Conversely, only 10% to 15% of patients with myasthenia gravis have a thymoma (117,293,324). Roughly one fourth of patients with myasthenia gravis will have a normal thymus (59). Of the

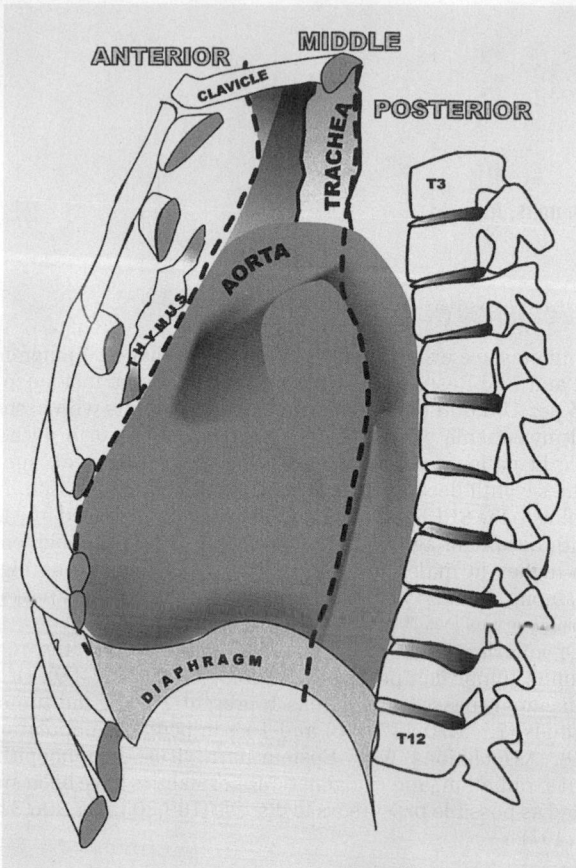

FIGURE 49.1. Anatomy of the mediastinum.

75% who have an abnormal thymus, only 15% to 20% will have a thymoma, while 60% will have thymic lymphoid hyperplasia (399). Thymectomy results in clinical improvement in most cases, even when the thymus is normal (49).

Other systemic symptoms may occur in 5% to 10% of patients with thymomas as part of a constellation of autoimmune disorders. Souadjian et al. (431) reviewed over 500 cases of thymoma and noted that 71% were associated with a systemic disease. These include erythroid and neutrophil hypoplasia, pancytopenia, Cushing's syndrome, DiGeorge syndrome, carcinoid syndrome, Lambert-Eaton syndrome, pernicious anemia, nephrotic syndrome, syndrome of inappropriate secretion of antidiuretic hormone, Whipple's disease, lupus erythematosus, pemphigus, myotonic dystrophy scleroderma, polymyositis, polyneuritis, myocarditis polyarthropathy, myotonic dystrophy, Sjogren's syndrome, Addison's disease, panhypopituitarism, sarcoidosis, hypogammaglobulinemia, ulcerative colitis, rheumatoid arthritis, Hashimoto's thyroiditis, hyperthyroidism, hyperparathyroidism, and thyroid carcinoma (61,82,302,329, 500). Other miscellaneous diseases include hypertrophic osteoarthropathy and chronic mucocutaneous candidiasis (302).

Additionally, some studies have reported an average of 15% higher than expected incidence of second primary malignancies in patients with thymomas over a normal population (42,282,305,431,479,502). In one study, the most notable excess risk for subsequent malignancy was for non-Hodgkin's lymphoma with digestive system and soft tissue sarcomas being elevated as well (126).

The vast majority of thymomas are indolent, but if the tumors spread, they most commonly implant regionally on the pleural surfaces and can cause pleural plaques, diaphragmatic masses,

and malignant pleural effusions (271). The largest database of thymomas reported lymphogenous metastasis in 1.8% of 1,093 patients, with 90% of those lymph nodes located in the anterior mediastinum (243). Rarely do thymomas spread hematogenously, but metastases have been reported to the liver, lung, and bone (211).

Diagnosis

Thymic tumors comprise 50% of all anterior mediastinal masses, the other 25% are lymphomas and various other tumors comprise the remainder (see Table 49.1) (99). The latter group often has characteristic radiographic findings (e.g., teratoma). Lymphomas often have other suggestive systemic symptoms or clinical findings, such as weight loss, fevers, and lymphadenopathy.

Biopsy can be performed via a fine-needle aspiration, bronchoscopy, mediastinoscopy, video-assisted thoracoscopy, or open biopsy. Often a clinical diagnosis is sufficient for a small thymoma in the setting of a patient with a parathymic syndrome. Traditionally biopsies were shunned because of concern of tumor spillage into the pleural space when the capsule was breached (323,424). No case of seeding of a needle tract or the biopsy site has been reported, and only three recurrences in thoracotomy scars have been reported (390,421). One series reported better survival in patients who underwent a preresection biopsy on multivariate analysis of 136 patients treated for thymomas ($p = .056$) (502). Many centers routinely obtain a biopsy for larger tumors (42,214,257,293,322,421,476).

The work-up begins with a careful evaluation for myasthenia gravis. Routine screening blood work for the common associated syndromes should be obtained along with a serum α-fetoprotein and β-hCG in men to rule out a germ cell tumor (423). Computed tomography (CT) imaging is the most valuable modality and commonly shows an anterior mediastinal mass (30,269,404,408). Magnetic resonance imaging (MRI) can provide more detail when needed and illustrates the musculoskeletal anatomy and aids in differentiating neurovascular structures of the mediastinum (58,255,460). The use of ^{18}F fluorodeoxyglucose positron emission tomography (FDG-PET) is under investigation and is confounded by the physiologic uptake of the thymus in children and young adults (130,250,278). Octreotide scanning has proven to be 100% accurate in a series of 17 patients (260).

Pathologic Classification

Thymomas have been extensively studied by pathologists because of the varied appearances and the frequent lack of classic malignant features. Many different classification systems have been proposed and used and are shown in Table 49.2. Indeed the terminology that has been used to describe thymomas has also been poorly defined. The major demarcation has been to describe thymomas as invasive versus noninvasive or alternately, "benign" versus malignant. However, recurrences and metastases after resection have been reported in all large series (105,293,388,403,477) regardless of stage or histologic subtype (7,8,28,34,42,271,293,304,321,334,352,373,388,403,477, 502). Even bland-appearing, noninvasive thymomas have the fundamental characteristics of a malignant tumor in the ability to recur and metastasize.

The most recent classification was proposed in 1999 and updated in 2004 by the World Health Organization (WHO) (398,466). However, a historical perspective of thymoma classification systems is necessary to interpret the literature. The earliest system proposed by Bernatz et al. (36) identified four categories based on predominant cell type: lymphocytic, epithelial, mixed, and spindle cell. But the predominant problem with this classification system, as with all systems, is the poor

Clinical Radiation Oncology

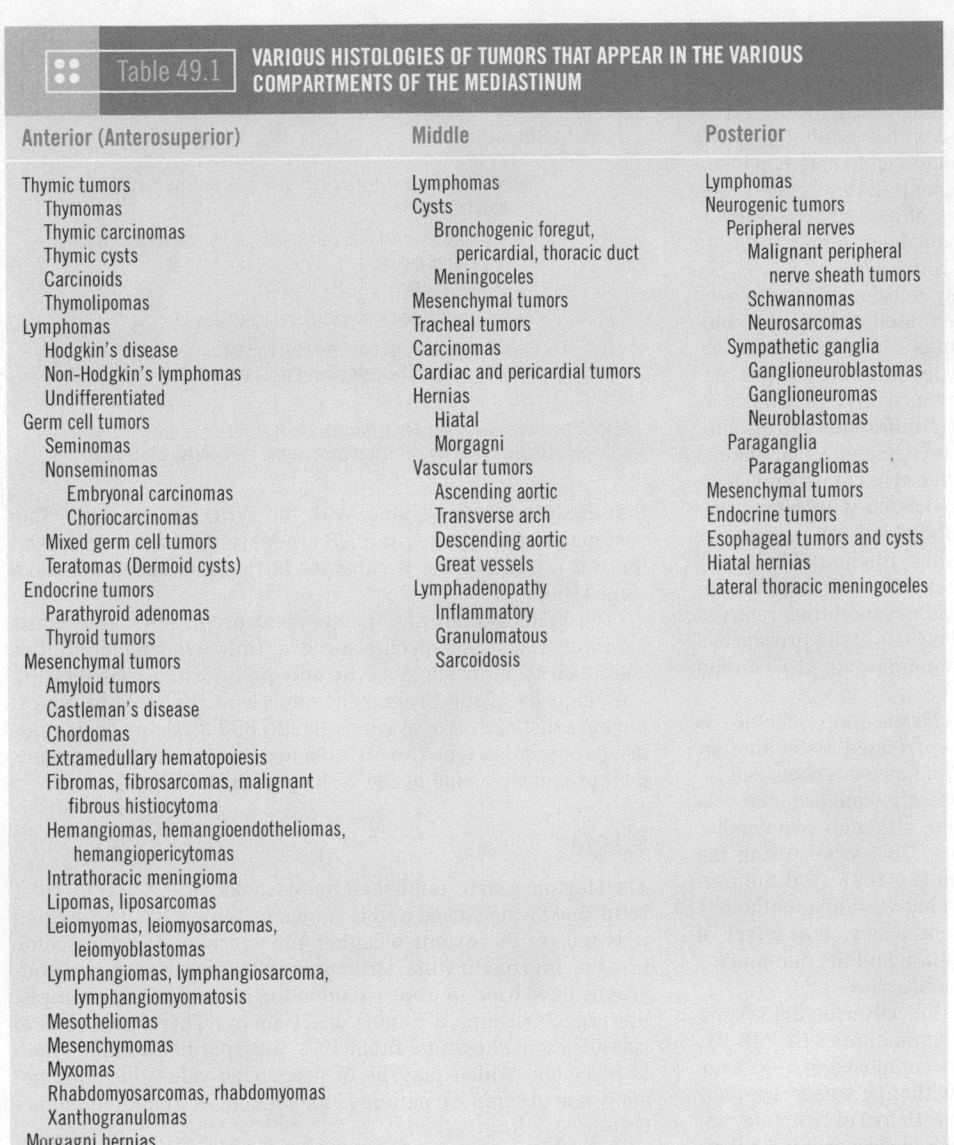

Table 49.1 VARIOUS HISTOLOGIES OF TUMORS THAT APPEAR IN THE VARIOUS COMPARTMENTS OF THE MEDIASTINUM

Anterior (Anterosuperior)	Middle	Posterior
Thymic tumors	Lymphomas	Lymphomas
Thymomas	Cysts	Neurogenic tumors
Thymic carcinomas	Bronchogenic foregut,	Peripheral nerves
Thymic cysts	pericardial, thoracic duct	Malignant peripheral
Carcinoids	Meningoceles	nerve sheath tumors
Thymolipomas	Mesenchymal tumors	Schwannomas
Lymphomas	Tracheal tumors	Neurosarcomas
Hodgkin's disease	Carcinomas	Sympathetic ganglia
Non-Hodgkin's lymphomas	Cardiac and pericardial tumors	Ganglioneuroblastomas
Undifferentiated	Hernias	Ganglioneuromas
Germ cell tumors	Hiatal	Neuroblastomas
Seminomas	Morgagni	Paraganglia
Nonseminomas	Vascular tumors	Paragangliomas
Embryonal carcinomas	Ascending aortic	Mesenchymal tumors
Choriocarcinomas	Transverse arch	Endocrine tumors
Mixed germ cell tumors	Descending aortic	Esophageal tumors and cysts
Teratomas (Dermoid cysts)	Great vessels	Hiatal hernias
Endocrine tumors	Lymphadenopathy	Lateral thoracic meningoceles
Parathyroid adenomas	Inflammatory	
Thyroid tumors	Granulomatous	
Mesenchymal tumors	Sarcoidosis	
Amyloid tumors		
Castleman's disease		
Chordomas		
Extramedullary hematopoiesis		
Fibromas, fibrosarcomas, malignant		
fibrous histiocytoma		
Hemangiomas, hemangioendotheliomas,		
hemangiopericytomas		
Intrathoracic meningioma		
Lipomas, liposarcomas		
Leiomyomas, leiomyosarcomas,		
leiomyoblastomas		
Lymphangiomas, lymphangiosarcoma,		
lymphangiomyomatosis		
Mesotheliomas		
Mesenchymomas		
Myxomas		
Rhabdomyosarcomas, rhabdomyomas		
Xanthogranulomas		
Morgagni hernias		

correlation with clinical prognosis. Verley and Hollmann (477) also identified four categories: spindle or oval, lymphocyte rich, differentiated epithelial cell rich, and undifferentiated epithelial. The first three types are cytologically bland, while the fourth category included pleomorphic tumors with a high number of mitoses and atypia that is also considered thymic carcinoma.

Unfortunately this categorization also had little correlation with prognosis.

Müller-Hermelink et al. (330) based their classification system on the fact that the thymus consists of different subsets of epithelial cells: cortical, medullary, mixed cortical and medullary, and well differentiated. Although this has been the

Table 49.2 THYMOMA CLASSIFICATION SYSTEMS (BY AUTHOR AND REFERENCE)

Bernatz et al. (37)	Müller-Hermelink et al. (330)	Suster and Moran (442)	Rosai and Sobin (398)
Spindle cell	Medullary	Thymoma, well differentiated	Type A
—	Mixed		Type AB
	Predominantly cortical		Type B1
Lymphocyte rich	Cortical		Type B2
Lymphoepithelial			
Epithelial rich	Well differentiated thymic carcinoma	Atypical thymoma	Type B3
—	High-grade thymic carcinoma	Thymic carcinoma	Type C

most widely used system, little association was found with the types of thymic epithelial cells from which these subtypes were thought to arise (248). Some studies were able to demonstrate associations such as cortical thymomas behaving more aggressively and being more often associated with myasthenia gravis (188,257,373,393,455,477), but the relationship between histologic types and prognosis was inconsistent (248,322,364,380). In multivariate analysis of large series of patients, the Müller-Hermelink classification system has not been found to be an independent predictor of survival (271,364,476).

Thymic carcinomas can be readily subclassified into well or poorly differentiated. Well-differentiated thymic carcinomas have features typical of thymomas but also contain areas of atypia and mitoses, but usually fewer than two per 10 high-power field (106). The incidence and prognosis of this group vary among studies. Poorly differentiated or, simply, thymic carcinomas are clearly recognized as a distinct group. The virtual absence of parathymic syndromes and clear-cut cellular atypia are consistently associated with poor prognosis. Thymic carcinomas can be subdivided into squamous cell, mucoepidermoid, basaloid, lymphoepitheliomalike, small cell/neuroendocrine, sarcomatoid, clear cell, and undifferentiated/anaplastic (444). Thymic carcinoid is sometimes referred to as a neuroendocrine thymic tumor because of the presence of neuroendocrine granules. Thymic carcinomas can also contain these granules.

A confounding problem of these classification schemes is that they could not be consistently correlated with another scheme (248). Additionally, when thymomas were classified independently by a panel of pathologists, the concordance was often as low as 35% within one system, although two smaller studies demonstrated a concordance of 78% when using the Müller-Hermelink classification system (79,101). Add the persistent problem of the poor correlation between histopathology of thymomas and their malignant potential as well as a lack of correlation with systemic syndromes (408), and the demand for a more consistent classification is obvious.

The WHO system is similar to the Müller-Hermelink system but recognizes six different types of thymic tumors (A, AB, B1, B2, B3, C) (436,466). Type A tumors are composed of neoplastic oval or spindle-shaped epithelial cells without atypia or lymphocytes. Type AB is similar to type A, but with foci of lymphocytes. Type B tumors consist of plump epithelioid cells and are subdivided into three subtypes as defined by an increasing proportion of epithelial cells and increasing atypia. Type B1 tumors resemble normal thymic cortex with areas similar to thymic medulla. Type B2 have scattered neoplastic epithelial cells with vesicular nuclei and distinct nucleoli among a heavy population of lymphocytes; perivascular spaces are prominent and a palisading effect of tumor cells along the perivascular spaces may be seen. Type B3 is composed of predominantly round or polygonal epithelial cells exhibiting mild atypia admixed with a minor component of lymphocytes; thus, this type resembles what others have described as well-differentiated thymic carcinoma. Thymic carcinomas are designated as type C tumors; these have clear-cut cytologic atypia and a cytoarchitecture resembling carcinoma distinctively unlike normal thymus tissue (106).

Since the WHO classification was proposed, the system has been evaluated. The concordance between different pathologists using the WHO system was 90% and 95% in two studies (69,369). But comparison of the WHO subtypes across studies demonstrated that the varying incidence of A and B subtypes was greater than could be ascribed to chance alone (106). The most clinically distinct subtypes are type B3, formerly known as well-differentiated thymic carcinomas, and type C, thymic carcinomas. There still exists marked variability in the clinical characteristics of patients with other WHO types. But there appears to be a good correlation with Masaoka stage in studies

that analyzed their patients with the WHO system (106). The vast majority of types A and AB are Masaoka stage I or II. And there is a trend of the B subtypes having increasing Masaoka stage (106).

The WHO system has independent prognostic value when focusing on disease-specific survival. Only two smaller studies continued to show stage as the only prognostic variable (106). The majority of the prognostic value is attributable to type C having a distinctly worse survival (226,353,391), but even studies that excluded type C were able to demonstrate the independent prognostic value of the WHO type (391,519).

Staging

The staging system published by Masaoka et al. (304) in 1981 is the most widely used and is shown in Table 49.3. The staging is based on the extent of either macroscopic or microscopic invasion into mediastinal structures at the time of surgery. Other groups have tried to improve upon the Masaoka. For example, the French Groupe d'Etudes des Tumeurs Thymiques (GETT) classification shown in Table 49.4, incorporates completeness of resection, which may be of prognostic value but does not allow one to compare patients independent of treatment factors (146).

Prognostic Factors

The two major prognostic factors that have consistently demonstrated prognostic value on multivariate analysis in large studies are invasiveness and completeness of resection (31,35,

Table 49.3		**MASAOKA STAGING SYSTEM FOR THYMOMAS**
Stage		**Description**
I		Macroscopically completely encapsulated, with no microscopic capsular invasion
II	a	Macroscopic invasion into surrounding mediastinal fatty tissue or mediastinal pleura
	b	Microscopic invasion into the capsule
III		Macroscopic invasion into surrounding organs
IV	a	Pleural or pericardial implants/dissemination
	b	Lymphogenous or hematogenous metastases

Adapted from Masaoka A, Monden Y, Nakahara K, et al. Follow-up study of thymomas with special reference to their clinical stages. *Cancer* 1981;48(10):2485–2492.

Table 49.4		**THYMOMA STAGING SYSTEM OF GETT**
Stage		**Description**
I	a	Encapsulated tumor, completely resected
	b	Macroscopically encapsulated tumor, completely resected Surgeon suspects mediastinal adhesions and potential capsular invasion
II		Invasive tumor, completely resected
III	a	Invasive tumor, subtotal resection
	b	Invasive tumor, biopsy only
IV	a	Distant pleural implants or supraclavicular metastasis
	b	Distant metastasis

GETT, Groupe d'Etudes des Tumeurs Thymiques
From Gamondes JP, Balawi A, Greenland T, et al. Seventeen years of surgical treatment of thymoma: factors influencing survival. *Eur J Cardiothorac Surg* 1991;5(2):124–131, with permission.

Table 49.5 | OVERALL SURVIVAL OF PATIENTS WITH THYMOMAS AT 5 AND 10 YEARS

Author (Reference)	Institution	Years of Inclusion	n	% R0	5-Year Survival				10-Year Survival			
					I	II	III	IV	I	II	III	IV
Kondo and Monden (244)	JACS	1990–1994	924	92	100	98	89	71	100	98	78	47
Regnard et al. (389)	CCML, Paris	1955–1993	307	85	89	87	68	66	80	78	47	30
Maggi et al. (293)	Torino	Pre-1991	241	88	89	71	72	59	87	60	64	40
Rena et al. (391)	Torino	1988–2000	175	84	100	100	100	100	100	100	85	—
Zhu et al. (517)	Fudan, Shanghai	1989–2002	175	89	100	96	78	57	—	—	—	—
Nakahara et al. (334)	Osaka	Pre-1988	141	80	100	92	88	47	100	84	77	47
Wilkins et al. (502)	Johns Hopkins	1957–1997	136	68	84	66	63	40	75	50	44	40
Rea et al. (384)	Padua	1970–2001	132	82	93	93	60	36	84	82	51	0
Blumberg et al. (42)	MSKCC	1949–1993	118	73	95	70	50	100	86	54	26	0
Quintanilla-Martinez et al. (380)	MGH	Pre-1994	116	94	100	100	70	70	100	100	60	0
Pan et al. (364)	Taipei	1961–1991	112	80	94	85	63	41	87	69	58	22
Elert et al. (124)	Wurzburg	1957–1988	102	—	83	90	46					

CCML, JACS, Japanese Association for Chest Surgery; MGH, Massachusetts General Hospital; MSKCC, Memorial Sloan-Kettering Cancer Center

37,42,56,87,100,105,265,271,304,351,352,364,388,472,476, 502). Stage has proven to be important in every large study (42,105,271,293,294,304,332,334,352,388,502). Overall survival at 15 years for stages I, II, III, and IV disease is reported to average 78%, 73%, 30%, and 8%, respectively and is shown in Table 49.5 (388). Disease-free survival rates at 10 years are on average 92%, 87%, 60%, and 35% for stages I, II, III, and IV, respectively, which is shown in Table 49.6 (87,105,352,380, 388).

The extent of resection is the other major prognostic factor consistently identified (42,150,388,458,495,502). Patients with an R0 resection have significantly improved survival over those with R1 or R2 resections (304,376). And while an R0 resection is almost always accomplished in stage I tumors, resectability rates decrease on average to 50% in stage III tumors (293,294,304,334). More recently, the WHO histology classification has also shown independent associations with prognosis. Table 49.7 summarizes the major studies reporting their analyses of stage, histology, and resection status as independent variables. Other potential prognostic factors are tumor size (>10 cm) and the presence of symptoms (42,271,373).

Older series reported that patients with the parathymic syndromes such as myasthenia gravis and other autoimmune diseases fared worse (42,87,501), but this has been contradicted by newer series (257,304,313,322,331,334,352,367, 373,388,472,502). Some studies have even reported signifi-

cantly better survival for patients with myasthenia gravis (293, 484,502). The explanation is likely due to earlier detection of thymomas (42,238,286,478). A recently reported study of 1,089 patients from Japan documented that myasthenia gravis was associated with 25% of the patients (245). Overall survival at 5 years was not significantly different for patients with stage III disease with myasthenia gravis versus without. For stage IV, 5-year overall survival was 85.1% for patients with myasthenia gravis versus 63.9% for patients without. An R0 resection was accomplished in a significantly higher proportion of patients with myasthenia gravis (60%) than those without (38%).

Age has been suggested as a prognostic factor. Patients younger than 30 to 40 have a better prognosis (87,271,476). Conversely, thymomas in children appear to have a more malignant course than those in adults (493). Fortunately, malignant thymomas in children are extremely rare (67).

General Management

Surgery

Surgical resection is the mainstay of treatment for thymomas. A complete en bloc surgical resection (R0) remains the treatment of choice for all thymomas regardless of invasiveness, except in rare advanced cases with extensive intrathoracic or extrathoracic metastasis. Fortunately, the vast majority (90% to 95%)

Table 49.6 | RECURRENCE RATES OF THYMOMAS

Author (Reference)	Study Years	Institution	n	% Receiving			5-Year Recurrence Rates			
				R0	Chemo	RT	I	II	III	IVa
Kondo and Monden (244)	1990–1994	JACS institutions	862	100	12	32	1	4	28	34
Regnard et al. (389)	1955–1993	ML, Paris	307	85	Few	Half	4	7	16	58
Maggi et al. (293)	Pre-1991	Torino	241	88	7	12	2	13	30	25
Wright et al. (507)	1972–2003	MGH	179	90	—	—	0	0	22	41
Rena et al. (391)	1988–2000	Torino	178	84	13	43	1.6	8.6	28	40
Zhu et al. (517)	1989–2002	Fudan, Shanghai	175	80	14	97	4	2.4	43	57
Cowen et al. (86)	1979–1990	FNCLCC	149	42	100	50	0	7	23	25
Wilkins and Castleman (501)	1957–1997	Johns Hopkins	136	68	7	37	8	10	24	0
Blumberg et al. (42)	1949–1993	MSKCC	118	73	32	58	4	21	47	80
Ruffini et al. (403)	1974–1993	Torino	114	100	—	25	5	10	30	33

FNCLCC, Federation Nationale des Centres de Lutte Contre le Cancer; JACS, Japanese Association for Chest Surgery; MGH, Massachusetts General Hospital; ML, Marie Lannelongue Hospital, Le Plessis-Robinson, France; MSKCC, Memorial Sloan-Kettering Cancer Center

Clinical Radiation Oncology

Table 49.7	RESULTS OF THE MULTIVARIATE ANALYSIS OF FACTORS PREDICTING THYMOMA-SPECIFIC SURVIVAL					
				Histology	Stage	R0
Author (Reference)	Institution	Years	n		*p*-Value	
Okamura et al. (354)	Osaka	1957–2000	273	0.05	0.0001	NS
Rieker et al. (394)	Heidelberg	1967–1998	218	<0.0024	<0.001	—
Wright et al. (507)	MGH	1972–2003	179	0.004	0.002	NS
Rena et al. (391)[a]	Torino	1988–2000	178	0.014	0.012	0.0001
Park et al. (369)[b]	Yonsei	1992–2002	150	0.019	<0.001	0.947
Rea et al. (384)[b]	Padua	1970–2001	132	0.0001	0.003	NS
Kondo et al. (246)[b]	Tokushima	1973–2001	100	NS	0.04	<0.05

MGH, Massachusetts General Hospital; NS, not statistically significant; R0, complete resection
[a]Type C excluded.
[b]Overall survival instead of disease-free survival.

of thymomas are localized (509). Operative mortality averages 2.5% (0.7% to 4.9%) (42,105,124,271,293,294,334,388). Resectability rates of stage I thymomas should approximate 100%. But for the higher stage thymomas, the resectability rates vary widely from 43% to 100% (average 85%) for stage II; from 0% to 89% (average 47%) for stage III; and from 0% to 78% (average 26%) for stage IV (105).

Because the completeness of resection is such an important prognostic factor, an aggressive surgical approach is justified to remove as much of the lesion as possible at the time of surgery. If a surgeon suspects residual microscopic disease may be present (an R1 operation), metallic clips should be placed to aid in delineating the radiation field. Whether subtotal resections are beneficial is controversial. Some authors have demonstrated better survival when a debulking operation was performed prior to adjuvant radiation therapy (87,244,293,304,321,334). Other investigators have reported no benefit over biopsy alone (42,87,146,293,326,334,388,476,484). Another large study found a significant difference in 5-year survival among patients undergoing subtotal versus biopsy only (64% vs. 36%), but little difference in 10-year survival, suggesting that the benefit may be only in intermediate-term survival (244). Because of the difficulties in controlling for residual disease after resections, selection bias, or other treatments, the data are unclear about whether subtotal resections are beneficial. It is very probable that a planned incomplete resection that leaves minimal residual disease will be advantageous, especially in the context of adjuvant radiation or chemotherapy.

Patients with stage I tumors have over 90% 5-year survival rates. Survival decreases slightly at 10 years (293,334,500). Local recurrences occur <5% of the time in this group. For stage II and III, surgery alone has recurrence rates in the range of 10% to 47%. Examining the causes of death in patients previously treated for a thymoma in series of more than 100 patients, 38% are related to thymoma (range 19% to 58%), 9% to postoperative causes (range 2% to 19%), 22% to myasthenia gravis (range 16% to 27%), 9% to other autoimmune diseases (range 2% to 19%), and 29% (range 8% to 47%) to unrelated causes (including other cancers) (87,271,293,294,321,334,352,380,388,477,502). Disease-free survival rates are shown in Table 49.6.

Recurrence

The overwhelming recurrence pattern for thymomas is locoregional. Eighty-one percent of recurrences are local, 9% distant, and 11% both (42,271,294,388,403,477). Most recurrences arise within 3 to 7 years (42,271,293,388,403,502). But recurrences may occur as late as 32 years after the initial resection (24,294,324,331,413). The treatment for recurrence is usually

surgical and adjuvant radiation (231,390,403). Most (50% to 75%) recurrences are operable, and of those that are operable, the reported rates of a successful R0 resection are 45% to 71% (42,105,390,403,471). For patients with a recurrence after a R0 resection, most studies show acceptable short- and long-term results (231,390), with 10-year actuarial survival in the range of 53% to 72% (105,355,390,403), while 10-year survival rates with an incomplete resection are reported to be 0% to 35% (105,355,388,390,403).

When recurrences are unresectable, radiation and chemotherapy have been used with modest results. The 5-year overall survival rates are reported to be 25% to 50% with poorer longer-term survival (42,105,153,293,403,471).

Radiation Therapy

Radiation therapy is often considered for the adjuvant setting in patients with resected stage II and III thymomas. Stage I thymomas have such a low recurrence rate after an R0 resection, so radiation is unlikely to improve upon the recurrence rate. The exact indications for radiation are controversial. Some authors recommend adjuvant radiation for all patients (321,334). Others recommend adjuvant radiation for stage II and III thymomas (87,116,244,388,500). And still others recommend radiation only in the circumstance of incomplete resection (172,298,299).

All of the data reporting on adjuvant radiation is retrospective and, because of the rarity of thymoma, spans many decades. Because stage and completeness of resection are the two most important prognostic factors, all the reported data on adjuvant radiation needs to be considered in the context of these factors. Among patients with stage II thymoma who have had a complete resection, several studies have reported a trend toward better control. The largest series reported no difference in recurrence rates (244), while one series reported worse results with adjuvant radiation (403). Haniuda et al. (173) identified that patients with fibrous adhesion to the mediastinal pleura without microscopic invasion benefited the most from postoperative therapy. The recurrence rates, with and without adhesion to the mediastinal pleura, were 36.4% versus 0%, respectively. And thus mediastinal pleura invasion may be another factor to consider.

For patients after an R0 resection for a stage III thymoma, many smaller series (<50 patients) have reported high control rates with adjuvant radiation. Urgesi et al. (472) reported no in-field recurrences in 33 patients but three recurrences out of the field, while other studies reported that the addition of radiation therapy did not appear to alter local or distant recurrences (42,172,244,298,299). Two studies combined their data for stage II and III patients with completely resected thymomas and demonstrated a nonsignificant trend toward a decreased rate of recurrence with adjuvant radiation (89,293).

Radiation has obviously been considered when a complete resection is not possible. For patients with thymomas who had a subtotal resection, two studies suggested a benefit to adjuvant radiation (89,293). Unfortunately both studies are small and, as always, subject to selection bias. Another study combining R0 and R1,2 resections of stage III thymomas demonstrated lower recurrence rates with adjuvant radiation in 44 patients. The actual recurrence rate with and without radiation was 40% versus 24%, respectively. The same author reported that adjuvant radiation appeared to lower the recurrence rate among stage IV patients with residual disease (89). Curran et al. (89) reported no mediastinal failures after radiation in 26 patients with incomplete resections for a stage III thymoma. In patients who did not receive radiation, the recurrence rate was 79% at 5 years. Other authors have concurred and reported very low rates of mediastinal failure for patients with gross residual disease who were treated with adjuvant radiation (76,472).

Radiation has been suggested for use in the neoadjuvant setting with the intent of reducing tumor burden and improving respectability, especially in the setting of gross invasion of critical structures (7,31,332,348,392,417,492,508). Response rates of up to 80% have been reported and describe a theoretical decrease in the potential for tumor seeding during surgery (87,89,293,348). The rates of R0 resections increased to 53% to 75% (7,392), which appears favorable when compared with the usual rates (~50%) of R0 resections of stage III thymomas (42,89,146,214,304,334,352,388). Ten-year survival does not appear to be better after preoperative radiation but the series are small (7,392,508).

In patients who are medically inoperable or for whom surgical resection is not possible, patients have been treated with radiation therapy alone with modest but acceptable results. Arakawa et al. (19) reported on 12 patients who presented with unresectable tumors and were treated with primary radiation therapy. Seven patients remained alive. Ciernik et al. (76) reported a 5-year survival of 87% in a small group of patients with stage III and IV disease who did not undergo resection. And Jackson and Ball (201) reported a 10-year survival of 44% for patients who received radiation following biopsies and/or incomplete resections. For patients with recurrences, Urgesi et al. (471) reported on the use of radiation alone in 21 patients with intrathoracic recurrences of thymoma. The 7-year survival of 70% was similar for those treated with radiation alone compared to those treated with surgery and adjuvant therapy. Although these results are informative, the use of preoperative and definitive radiation therapy without chemotherapy is no longer a primary consideration in the management of difficult thymomas.

In summary, the benefit from adjuvant radiation is unclear. Adjuvant radiation should be considered for any residual disease or incomplete resection regardless of stage. But for stage I patients, and many would argue also stage II, the recurrence rates are low enough that the benefit from radiation is marginal. For patients with stage III and IVa disease, the recurrence rates are high enough that the potential benefit from radiation cannot be dismissed, although the literature is not conclusive.

Chemotherapy

Thymomas have proven to be very sensitive to chemotherapy. A clinical response is seen in roughly two thirds of patients. Complete responses are seen about a third of the time (45,136,137,151,186,227,280–282,367,385). The duration of response ranges from 12 to 93 months. The ability of chemotherapy to impact long-term survival is more difficult to assess. In one retrospective analysis, chemotherapy reduced the rates of metastases to the lung, pleura, or other sites by half (17% vs. 38%; $p < .05$) among 90 patients. All patients had stage III or IV tumors and were treated with radiation and partial or no resection (87). Another study reported a nonsignificant trend toward better disease-free survival with the addition of chemotherapy (326).

The most promising use of chemotherapy is in the neoadjuvant setting. Analogous to the rationale for preoperative radiation, chemotherapy appears to be effective at rendering tumors more amenable to a complete resection. One study demonstrated that neoadjuvant chemotherapy is associated with improved survival in patients with stage III and IVa thymomas (286).

As with the literature on the effect of radiation, most of the series describing the use of chemotherapy are small and retrospective. The commonly employed drugs in combination chemotherapy are cisplatin, doxorubicin, and cyclophosphamide. One prospective intergroup study reported disappointing results with combined etoposide, ifosfamide, and cisplatin (281).

Besides cytotoxic agents, somatostatin analogs (i.e., octreotide) and high-dose corticosteroids have shown promise (362,363). One prospective study demonstrated a 47% response rate in 17 patients with resectable thymomas with two courses of glucocorticoid therapy before surgery (237). The pathophysiologic mechanism apparently exploits the ability of corticosteroids to induce apoptosis in CD4 plus CD8 plus double-positive immature thymocytes. Another prospective Eastern Cooperative Oncology Group study enrolled 42 patients with unresectable, advanced thymic malignancies in whom the octreotide scan was positive. Patients were treated with octreotide alone or with prednisone. Two patients had complete responses and 10 had partial responses, which led the investigators to conclude that octreotide alone had modest activity and prednisone improved the overall response rate (283). The most recent advances in targeted therapy are also being investigated and c-kit expression has been identified. The therapeutic implications of these observations remain to be determined.

Combined Modality Therapy

Some investigators have suggested that resectability and survival are improved with multimodality treatment by using chemotherapy preoperatively, surgery, and postoperative radiation and/or chemotherapy in patients with stage III or IV thymomas. Several institutions have conducted prospective accrual trials utilizing preoperative combination chemotherapy (227,289,385,476). The combinations all included cisplatin as well as some combination of cyclophosphamide, doxorubicin, vincristine, prednisone, and epirubicin. With these regimens, response rates were reported between 77% to 100% of the patients enrolled and are shown in Table 49.8. R0 resections were accomplished between 57% and 82% of the time. Pathological complete responses were seen in the range of 4% to 31% of the time. Overall survival at 5-years appears to be very favorable with these regimens ranging between 57% and 95% when considering the patients had unresectable stage III and IV thymomas (227,289,385,476). Also, all patients received postoperative radiation. These results appear superior to historical results for patients who underwent surgical resection alone. Multimodality therapy with preoperative combination chemotherapy with cisplatin, surgery, and postoperative radiation appears to deliver excellent results.

Reasonable results are also obtainable with combination chemotherapy and definitive radiation therapy. A prospective intergroup study reported 5-year survival of 52% for 26 patients who were treated with cisplatin, doxorubicin, and cyclophosphamide followed by radiation therapy for patients with unresectable thymomas. Median survival was 93 months.

| Table 49.8 | OUTCOMES AFTER COMBINED MODALITY THERAPY FOR THYMOMAS |

Author (Reference)	Institution	n	Preop Chemo	Adjuvant Therapy	% Response	% R0	% pCR	% 5-Year Survival
Lucchi et al. (286)	Pisa	36	cP, vp, epi	RT & Chemo	67	78	6	65 (est)
Venuta et al. (476)	Rome	25	cP, vp, epi	RT & Chemo	—	80	4	80
Kim et al. (227)	UT-MDACC	22	cyclo, doxo, cP, pred	RT & Chemo	77	82	18	95
Rea et al. (385)	Padua	16	cyclo, doxo, cP, vin	RT or Chemo	100	69	31	57
Yokoi et al. (513)	Tochigi	17	cyclo, doxo, pred	RT & Chemo	93	12	7	81

cP, cisplatin; cyclo, cyclophosphamide; doxo, doxorubicin; epi, epirubicin; pCR, pred, prednisone; RT, radiation therapy; UT-MDACC, vp, etoposide; vin, vincristine

Management of Myasthenia Gravis

Thymectomy has been an effective therapy for myasthenia gravis. The goals are to induce a remission or to reduce symptoms. Removal of normal-appearing thymuses improves symptoms in about half of patients with myasthenia gravis (46,127,203). Patients have higher acetylcholine receptor activity and titers of antistriated muscle antibodies are found in 80% to 90% of patients with myasthenia gravis (503). At centers with experience in the management of patients with myasthenia gravis preoperative and postoperatively, the mortality rate is essentially the same as that for general anesthesia (117).

Radiation therapy to the thymus has also been reported to be effective for the treatment of myasthenia gravis. Response rates and improvement of symptoms occurred in over 50% of patients after radiation (90,374,416). Radiation treatment alone for myasthenia gravis is really of historical interest, though, as surgical expertise and perioperative management of myasthenia gravis has improved.

Radiation Therapy Techniques

Radiation doses reported in the literature range from 30 to 60 Gy with standard fractionation (1.8 to 2.0 Gy). Postoperatively, the dose delivered is 45 to 50 Gy and higher for (+) margins or frank invasion. All radiation series are retrospective and subject to the same inherent limitations. One study did not identify a dose response (21), but two others did (311,326).

The treatment volume for a thymoma should encompass the entire thymus and any known sites of disease that are reasonable and safe to include. Nonregional pleural plaques would not be easily covered without compromising an inordinate volume of lung parenchyma. Because thymomas do not routinely spread through lymphatics, the draining nodal distributions do not need to be included (403). CT based planning is essential for targeting and accurate dosimetry of critical structures. As with all thoracic and mediastinal sites, the major critical structures include the spinal cord, lung parenchyma, pericardium, heart, and esophagus. The same guidelines used to treat lung cancer apply in minimizing dose to the noninvolved critical structures while accurately and reliably delivering treatment to a thoracic mass.

Thymic Carcinoma

Thymic carcinomas are less common than thymomas. Similar to thymomas, thymic carcinomas are thought to arise from thymic epithelium and commonly occur in the anterosuperior mediastinum. However, the clinical behavior of thymic carcinoma is different from thymoma. It is comparatively more aggressive with a higher propensity for capsular invasion. Patients frequently present with advanced disease and have a poorer 5-year survival than with thymomas (242,244,499).

Clinically, patients with thymic carcinoma may present initially with tussis, dyspnea, pleuritic chest pain, phrenic nerve palsy, or superior vena cava syndrome (63,212,242). Occasionally, associated paraneoplastic syndromes have also been observed (212,337,446). CT scans often demonstrate an irregular mass with necrotic, cystic, or calcified regions (63,379,419, 464). Approximately 80% of patients with thymic carcinoma may have radiographic evidence of invasion into adjacent structures in the mediastinum, and 40% may have evidence of mediastinal lymphadenopathy at presentation (112,212,253,262). Distant metastases to regional lymphatics, bone, liver, kidney, and lung are a common clinical feature (64,212,425,516). Bone scan, MRI, PET with ^{18}flourodeoxyglucose and ^{11}carbon labeled methionine (MET), and single-photon emission computer tomography (SPECT) have been utilized in both diagnosis and evaluation of therapeutic outcomes (4,213,250,406,410).

Thymic carcinomas are classified as type C thymic tumors by the WHO classification of human thymic epithelial neoplasms and are commonly staged utilizing the Masaoka clinical staging system for thymomas (93,304). As the histologic grade remains one of the most significant prognostic indicators, a revised histologic classification was proposed that broadly divides thymic carcinomas into high- and low-grade lesions (444). The majority of thymic carcinomas are undifferentiated high-grade lesions with anaplasia and marked cellular atypia, lacking the histologic features of a normal thymus (430); others may be adenocarcinomatous, sarcomatous, squamous, basaloid, mucoepidermoid, or lymphoepitheliallike histologically (63,345,445). Most variants of thymic carcinoma are highly lethal with frequent metastases to regional lymph nodes, bone, liver, and lung (379,443). Tumors in the low-grade histologic group are characterized by relatively favorable clinical courses and a low incidence of local recurrence and metastasis (176,347,395).

Owing to the paucity of experience, the ideal therapeutic regimen is unknown. Current management requires an aggressive multimodality approach, including primary surgical resection and the use of adjuvant cisplatin-based chemotherapy, often coupled with postoperative radiation therapy (156). Although incomplete resection does not necessarily preclude long-term survival if multimodality platinum-based therapy is used (182), complete resection is the cornerstone of treatment. Takeda et al. (452) observed a median survival of 57 months for patients with a complete resection versus 13 months for those without complete resection. Most studies employed adjuvant radiation therapy with a wide dose range of 40 to 70 Gy with standard fractionation scheme (1.8 to 2.0 Gy per fraction) (21,125,193,275,346,347,452). In a series of 26 patients treated with surgery and postoperative radiation without chemotherapy, Hsu et al. (193) observed a 77% 5-year overall survival rate. For patients with completely resected and subtotally resected tumor, the survival rates were 82% and 66%, respectively. The 5-year local control rate was 91% with a median radiation dose of 60 Gy.

In a cohort of 40 patients receiving either surgery and adjuvant radiation or definitive radiation therapy with or without chemotherapy, Ogawa et al. (347) noted 16 patients achieved complete resection, as well as an absence of local recurrence for patients with complete resection and adjuvant radiation with at least 50 Gy. Kondo and Monden (244) observed no survival benefit from the addition of adjuvant radiation to surgical resection in a retrospective multi-institutional study of 186 patients, although the authors stipulated that no definitive conclusions could be made regarding the role of adjuvant radiotherapy in thymic carcinoma due to retrospective nature of the study and subgroup sample size limitations. These studies seem to indicate that although local control is improved with radiation, a survival benefit remains to be demonstrated.

Thymic carcinoma is generally less responsive to chemotherapy than thymoma (62). The outcomes from chemotherapy alone are dismal. However, a significant beneficial effect has been seen in several studies with adjuvant cisplatin-based chemotherapy (241,335,380). Nakamura et al. (335) treated 10 patients with unresectable disease with platinum-based protocols with or without radiation therapy, and observed a median survival of 11 months. Yoh et al. (512) reported excellent preliminary results (42% response rate) with weekly chemotherapy of cisplatin, vincristine, doxorubicin, and etoposide for the treatment of advanced tumors. Other studies have showed favorable responses with various combinations of cisplatin, etoposide, ifosfamide, adriamycin, nedaplatin, doxorubicin, cyclophosphamide, and vincristine (232,241,280,281,287,335,512).

In a large multi-institutional study, the 5-year survival rates for patients with totally resected thymic carcinoma receiving chemotherapy, chemoradiation, radiotherapy alone, and no adjuvant treatment were 81.5%, 46.6%, 73.6%, and 72.2% respectively (244). Although few treatment recommendations may be made, for patients with resectable disease, complete surgical resection is the preferred initial therapeutic intervention (105,244,252,452,467). For unresectable lesions, neoadjuvant (preoperative) chemotherapy and/or thoracic radiotherapy appears reasonable. Ultimately, after complete resection, the most important prognostic factors are initial stage and tumor grade. Five-year survival rates for those patients with higher stage and grade neoplasms range between 15% to 20%, whereas patients with low-grade, localized disease may obtain 5-year survival rates of 80% to 90% (443,444).

Thymic Carcinoid

Thymic carcinoid tumors (neuroendocrine tumors) of the thymus are very rare, accounting for <5% of all neoplasms of the anterior mediastinum. They originate from the normal thymic Kulchitsky cells, which belong to the amine precursor uptake and decarboxylation (APUD) group (397). Thymic carcinoid tumors are often confused with thymomas due to their similar clinical appearance. Most patients with thymic carcinoid are men aged 30 to 50 years (male/female ratio: 3:1) (463). Approximately 50% are associated with endocrine disorders, such as multiple endocrine neoplasia (MEN −1), or secondary Cushing's syndrome (273,274,494). Patients may present with symptoms related to compression of normal structures (chest pain, dyspnea, cough, hoarseness, SVC syndrome) (102,397), or may be asymptomatic (274). Thymic carcinoids are best evaluated by CT or MRI in demonstrating local invasion of the surrounding structures (pericardium, great vessels, pleura, sternum) and intrathoracic/extrathoracic metastases. Most thymic carcinoids detected on radiographic studies are already advanced in stage, commonly metastasizing to regional lymph nodes. Metastases may be seen in 70% of patients within 8 years from initial diagnosis (22), which may explain their poor prognosis.

The Masaoka staging system for thymoma has been used to stage patients with thymic carcinoids (304,463). The WHO classifies thymic carcinoids as typical carcinoid, atypical carcinoid,

large cell neuroendocrine carcinoma, or small cell carcinoma (398,466), while the classification system proposed by Klemm and Moran (233) grades these tumors as well-differentiated (low grade), moderately differentiated (intermediate grade), or poorly differentiated (high grade). However, neither grading nor other histologic parameters have shown a consistent association with prognosis (463).

Complete surgical resection is the preferred method of treatment, although recurrence is common. Despite a lack of sufficient data, incomplete resections followed by adjuvant radiation and/or chemotherapy have shown some benefits without increased morbidity and mortality (22,120,274,483). Distant metastases to bone, liver, or skin occur in 30% to 40% of cases (498). Despite aggressive treatments, most patients do poorly; overall 5-year survival according to one report was 31%, with all 14 patients dead after 9 years (102). When associated with MEN1, thymic carcinoids tend to behave more malignantly. Most authors reported that all such patients eventually died of the disease (102,274,456). One study found that 5-year survival for cases without an associated endocrinopathy was about 70% and for those with an endocrinopathy, 35%.

Other Rare Tumors of the Thymus

Thymoliposarcoma was first described by Havlicek and Rosai (180) in 1984. This rare distinctive entity is considered the malignant counterpart of thymolipoma. Thymoliposarcoma occurs in adults, 36 to 77 years old, with a slight female predominance. Unlike its counterpart, no association with myasthenia gravis with thymoliposarcoma has been reported. It grows in an expansile manner with relatively low potential of distant metastasis in the absence of histologic dedifferentiation. Based on limited data in the literature, complete surgical resection or subtotal resection with adjuvant radiation therapy has been used for local control (180,192).

Malignant Mediastinal Germ Cell Tumors

Epidemiology

Primary extragonadal germ cell tumors comprise 2% to 5% of all germ cell tumors (169). Approximately two thirds of these tumors occur in the mediastinum (17,251,338). The mediastinum is the most common site of primary extragonadal germ cell tumors in young adults (490). However, germ cell tumors comprise ~10% of malignant mediastinal tumors and ~2% of mediastinal neoplasms (88,100). In a pooled analysis of 341 patients with mediastinal germ cell tumors treated over 20 years at 11 cancer centers, the median age of presentation was 33 for seminomatous tumors and 28 for nonseminomatous tumors (44).

Primary extragonadal germ cell tumors have a number of unexplained associations. Klinefelter's syndrome has been documented in patients with mediastinal germ cell tumors, but not in patients with testicular germ cell tumors (91,107,339,469). In one study, up to 20% of the patients with mediastinal germ cell tumors were found to have the karyotypic pattern of Klinefelter's syndrome, 47, XXY (6,343). A number of unusual malignant processes are associated with nonseminomatous germ cell tumors; associated hematologic malignancies include acute myeloid leukemia, acute nonlymphocytic leukemia, acute megakaryocytic leukemia, myelodysplastic syndrome, and malignant histiocytosis (66,170,340,341,343). In a pooled analysis of primary extragonadal germ cell tumors, 1/17 patients with primary mediastinal nonseminomatous germ cell tumors developed a fatal hematologic disorder after being diagnosed with the germ cell tumor (177).

Natural History

Primary extragonadal germ cell tumors arise along the midline of the body from the pineal gland, through the mediastinum and retroperitoneum, to the presacral areas. Although the origin of these primary extragonadal germ cell tumors remains controversial (60,139,167), they presumably arise from germ cells that migrate along the urogenital ridge during embryonic development (288,343). The embryologic urogenital ridge extends from C6 to L4 and after malignant transformation of displaced germ cells, explains the development of primary germ cell tumors outside the gonads.

Because primary gonadal germ cell tumors can spread to the retroperitoneum and mediastinum, although less commonly (338,343), a meticulous work-up must be performed to prevent overlooking an occult gonadal primary including a physical examination and testicular ultrasound. Despite the fact that primary mediastinal germ cell tumors have the same morphologic and histologic appearance as those of the testes, primary germ cell tumor of the mediastinum have a poorer prognosis and more aggressive behavior (11,149,217). Like germ cell tumor of the testes, they are divided into seminomatous and nonseminomatous tumors. Benign teratomas arise from germ cell elements, but they are not included in this discussion because they are nonmalignant and surgical resection is often curative.

Although primary mediastinal seminomatous germ cell tumors are radiation and chemo sensitive, the analogous nonseminomatous germ cell tumors have been categorized as poor risk disease in all staging systems (149). They are frequently invasive at the time of diagnosis, and approximately half will present with distant metastases of which lung is the most common site (44). Tumor markers can aid in diagnosis. The α-fetoprotein (AFP) is elevated in 75% of patients with a median of 2,500 ng/mL at diagnosis. The β-subunit of human chorionic gonadotropin (β-HCG) is elevated less than half of the time. And lactate dehydrogenase (LDH) is elevated in 50% of patients at presentation.

Clinical Presentation

As with most patients who have mediastinal tumors, local symptoms are usually caused by tumor compression or invasion of adjacent structures. Of patients with primary extragonadal germ cell tumor, 90% to 100% will have clinical symptoms (235). Dyspnea (25%), chest pain (23%), cough (17%), fever (13%), weight loss (11%), vena cava occlusion syndrome, and fatigue/weakness (6% each) are the most common symptoms (44,266,267). But many patients are asymptomatic and a mass is found incidentally on chest x-ray (303,358). A third of patients with seminomatous mediastinal germ cell tumors present with metastases. Of those with metastases, cervical lymph nodes are enlarged in 25%, but abdominal lymphadenopathy can also occur. For nonseminomatous germ cell tumors, distant metastases are much more common and the rates have been reported to be as high as 85% to 90% historically, but more recently appear in about 50% of patients at diagnosis (44,168,200,284,426).

Diagnostic Work-Up

Mediastinal germ cell tumors are usually readily detectable on chest x-rays with the majority of masses noted in the anterosuperior mediastinum. CT scans of the chest, abdomen, and pelvis are essential to evaluate the mass and screen for metastases and lymphadenopathy. As mentioned earlier, both a careful physical examination and testicular ultrasound should be performed to rule out an occult primary. Tumor markers, AFP, β-HCG, and

LDH levels can aid in diagnosis, evaluating treatment efficacy and monitoring for recurrence (53,99,121,204). Thus the determination of pretreatment and posttreatment baseline levels is essential.

The initial diagnosis of mediastinal germ cell tumors is usually achieved by a combination of CT, radiographs, sonograms, and tumor markers. In some instances, the tumor marker findings are sufficient to classify the lesion as an extragonadal nonseminomatous germ cell tumor without histologic confirmation, but histopathology is easily attainable through fine-needle aspiration with cytologic staining for tumor markers. False positive β-HCG levels have been reported (84,402).

Prognostic Factors

The most important prognostic factor for mediastinal extragonadal germ cell tumor is histologic type. Seminomas remain highly curable, while nonseminomatous histology, despite advances in therapy, is independently associated with poor progression-free and overall survival. The presence of metastases is also adversely associated with both progression-free and overall survival in both seminomatous and nonseminomatous histology. Elevation of β-HCG in nonseminomatous tumors is associated with inferior overall survival (44).

In a study of 104 patients with extragonadal mediastinal and retroperitoneal seminomas, the use of radiation therapy alone was associated with an inferior progression-free survival but not on multivariate analysis because only nine patients received radiation alone. Many factors were tested in this study and none were found to have significance on multivariate analysis including primary tumor size, the presence or location of metastatic disease, and the use of carboplatin instead of cisplatin (44).

General Management

Seminomatous Tumors

Seminomas are very sensitive to both radiation therapy and chemotherapy, and all patients with a seminomatous histology should be treated with curative intent, even in the setting of widely metastatic disease. The treatment has definitely evolved with the development of cisplatin-based chemotherapy regimens, and most patients should be initially treated with chemotherapy.

Historically, seminomatous tumors (and all mediastinal tumors) were treated surgically (152,343). Complete radical resection may be considered in selected patients if technically feasible and the patients do not want radiation or chemotherapy. Definitive radiation replaced surgical resection for patients with localized mediastinal seminomatous germ cell tumor with long-term survival rates of 60% to 80% despite having bulkier tumors referred for radiation alone (152,169,170,343). Radiation therapy had an initial advantage over chemotherapy by being more tolerable and less toxic, and patients were effectively salvaged with systemic chemotherapy following relapse (169).

Almost 30 years ago, Einhorn and Williams (122) at the University of Indiana first reported a 63% complete response rate with a median duration of 18 months in 19 patients with disseminated seminoma treated with cisplatin-based chemotherapy. In modern series, 92% of patients will achieve a favorable response to primary therapy, and a 5-year overall survival of >90% is standard (43).

Residual radiographic abnormalities after completing chemotherapy are not uncommon for patients with bulky mediastinal seminomas. The management of patients with residual radiographic abnormalities is still controversial. In 80% to 90% of patients, the residual masses represent dense fibrosis, and viable tumor is not detectable (327,343,378,415). Some have advocated surgical resection or biopsy of all postchemotherapy masses ≥ 3 cm (58,183,378,415). Still others have recommended close follow-up of these patients with early intervention if the mass enlarges on chest x-ray or CT scan, reserving resection, radiation, or salvage chemotherapy for progressive disease (170,171,343,415). The role of FDG-PET in predicting viable tumor is debatable and under investigation (33,148). Although seminomas are extremely sensitive to radiation therapy, radiation therapy delivered adjuvantly to postchemotherapy residual masses has not shown a significant benefit.

Radiation doses and treatment techniques for mediastinal seminomatous germ cell tumors have varied (29,55,77,135,195,470). Doses as low as 30 Gy to as high as 50 Gy have been recommended (29,88). Doses should be adjusted based on the size of the lesion, the history of chemotherapy exposure, and the clinical circumstances. The entire mediastinum should be encompassed with anteroposterior/posteroanterior fields with CT guidance. In the prechemotherapy era, marginal relapses occurred with smaller portals (470). Also in the historical context of the prechemotherapy era, the clinical target volume for definitive radiation alone often covered supraclavicular, cervical, and para-aortic lymph nodes (55,121,195,412). Extrapolating from prophylactic para-aortic node treatment in testicular seminomas, the contiguous lymphatic drainage sites for a mediastinal primary could be treated effectively with 20 Gy with minimal morbidity (209).

Mediastinal seminomatous germ cell tumors have been effectively treated with primary radiation therapy. Local tumor control of 89% to 100% and long-term survival of 50% to 80% has been reported in patients (25,55,88,343,470). Still, cisplatin-based combination chemotherapy is able to consistently provide >90% 5-year overall survival. But if chemotherapy is not an option, radiation is a viable alternative.

Nonseminomatous Germ Cell Tumors

The primary treatment for nonseminomatous germ cell tumor is intensive cisplatin-based combination chemotherapy, but surgical resection of all residual masses after first-line chemotherapy is recommended whenever technically possible, either as a one-stage or as a sequential procedure (178,220,342,506). Chemotherapy regimens include either cisplatin and etoposide or cisplatin, etoposide, and bleomycin. Patients typically respond favorably to treatment. And about one third of the time in testicular primaries, viable tumor is found at the time of resection of residual masses.

The role of radiation therapy has not been defined in nonseminomatous germ cell tumor. Radiation may have a role for unresectable residual masses given the high rate of persistent viable tumor and the poor rates of salvage therapy. Nonseminomatous germ cell tumors are also radiation sensitive but require higher doses than seminomatous tumors (224). Doses of 60 Gy or more may be necessary to achieve control.

For mediastinal nonseminomatous germ cell tumors, <5% of patients survived prior to the advent of cisplatin-based chemotherapy (121). With the use of cisplatin-based combination chemotherapy, long-term disease-free survival varies from 45% to 72% in more modern series incorporating postchemotherapy surgery (44,149,482). For patients who progress during or after initial chemotherapy, multiple salvage regimens have been used. Unfortunately, long-term survival for patients with relapsed mediastinal germ cell tumors is <10% (44,185,411). Thus surgical resection and even radiation therapy may play a role when no further effective chemotherapy is available.

▪▪ | Tracheal Carcinomas

Tracheal neoplasms are rare. Consequently, definitive statements regarding optimum management of these tumors is ham-

pered by the lack of any large prospective data set. The majority of informative data are derived from pooled population-based data sets or individual institutional series with a variety of treatment regimens. Several patterns emerge from a review of the retrospective data:

1. Surgical resection is the mainstay of therapy,
2. Local recurrence is a major pattern of failure, and
3. Adjuvant and definitive radiation appear effective.

Demographics

Primary tracheal malignancy is exceedingly uncommon, comprising approximately 0.1% to 0.4% of all diagnosed malignancies (191). Epidemiologic data from the SEER data set estimate an incidence of 0.2 per 100,000 persons in the United States; the true incidence of tracheal carcinomas is likely even lower (439). Traditionally, adenoid cystic carcinomas (formerly known as cylindromas) were considered the most common tracheal neoplasms, but recent reports suggest the most prevalent histology worldwide is squamous cell (60% to 90%) (272,301,511). Males are more often afflicted with tracheal cancers, with a SEER estimated incidence of 0.2 per 100,000, as compared to an incidence for females of 0.1 per 100,000 (439). Males are more commonly affected than females if the histology is of squamous origin (2 to 3:1), while the male to female ratio appears equivalent for adenoid cystic carcinomas (312). With squamous cell variants, the usual presenting age is the sixth decade of life; adenoid cystic carcinomas appear to present at a younger age. Other histologies include carcinoid, carcinosarcoma, granular cell tumor, hemangioma, neurogenic tumors, chondroma, and chondrosarcoma (15,16,20,47,48,54,72,98,104,110,113,128,129,143,194,199,207,210,229,230,240,247,276,285,292,295,296,310,320,328,336,365,375,383,407,422,428,432,434,462,474,477,485,488,510,518,520).

With >90% of patients in some series reporting tobacco use (487), it is likely associated with squamous cell carcinoma of the tracheas as it is with other squamous cell carcinomas of the upper aerodigestive tract (261).

Anatomy

The trachea is a fibrocartilaginous tube connecting the larynx superiorly and the mainstem bronchi inferiorly. The esophagus, thyroid, parathyroids, and trachea are derived from the same out-pouching of the embryonic foregut; the lungs arise from terminal tracheal buds. The blood supply of the trachea is as follows: inferior thyroidal arteries supply the superior trachea, while branches of the bronchial arteries supply the inferior portion. Arterial branches interdigitate between each cartilaginous ring (Fig. 49.2). The average adult trachea is 12 cm in length and 2 cm (females) to 2.3 cm (males) in diameter. In cross-section, the organ is "C" or "U" shaped. The upper border lies around the sixth or seventh cervical vertebra; the lower border around the fourth (full expiration) or sixth (full inspiration) thoracic vertebra. There are approximately two cartilaginous rings per centimeter. The posterior aspect of the trachea is membranous and is intimately associated with the esophagus.

Natural History

Tracheal carcinomas can present with a variety of symptoms: cough, dyspnea, dysphagia, and hemoptysis (3,518). Yang et al. (511) reported that cough (72% of patients) was the most frequently reported symptom, followed by dyspnea (66%), stridor (39%), hemoptysis (39%), and dysphonia (31%). For adenoid cystic carcinomas especially, asthma is a typical initial diagnosis, and these patients are often treated until their "refractory" chronic obstructive pulmonary disease is evaluated further

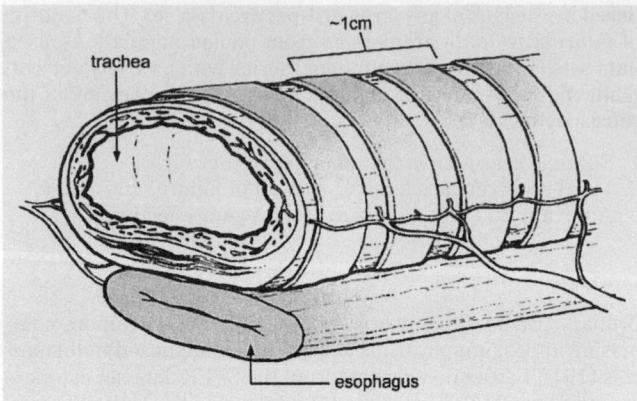

FIGURE 49.2. Representative schema of the trachea. Note the lateral longitudinal anastomotic artery running parallel to the organ and the intercartilaginous branches feeding each tracheal segment. The trachea resides in close proximity to the esophagus.

with bronchoscopy, typically after numerous "normal" chest radiographs (3,12,32,78,133,202,215,268,314,451,475,488). Hemoptysis appears more commonly in squamous cell carcinoma (461,511). Dysphagia is sometimes observed and has been noted as ominous (261). Recent data suggest that for patients with nonadenoid cystic/nonsquamous tracheal tumors, dyspnea at presentation was more frequent for benign tumors, while malignant tumors were associated with hemoptysis (143).

Adenoid cystic carcinomas are diagnosed with synchronous metastases in 40% to 50% of all cases (371). Despite this, survival is relatively prolonged, even in the face of distant metastases (114,142,159,239,461). In one series, median survival for these patients was 37 months (312), with median reported survival from time of diagnosis of approximately 5 years (487,511). When tumor spread occurs, it is almost always distant rather than to locoregional paratracheal lymph nodes. Local recurrence predominates, and recurrences 10 or more years after treatment are not uncommon (198,377,902).

In contrast to adenoid cystic carcinoma, squamous cell carcinoma demonstrates a more aggressive course. Reported median survival ranges from 6 to 12 months and depends on resectability (92,142,159,190,206,300,388,414,461). Local extension via paratracheal lymph nodes (approximately 30% at presentation) and distant metastases are frequent at presentation (158).

For other pathologic variants, the clinical course and natural history are difficult to accurately characterize, owing to paucity of reported data. Adenocarcinomas and sarcomas are thought to behave poorly (23,70,83,97,128,143,179,189,230, 259,317,357,396,405,418,429,473). Histologies such as granular cell tumor, carcinoid, lymphoma, leiomyoma, and small cell carcinoma have a variable prognosis yet seem to behave better than the squamous carcinomas, adenocarcinomas, or sarcomas (143).

Staging and Prognostic Factors

No universally accepted system for staging tracheal neoplasms has been adopted. A staging system proposed by Licht et al. (272) appears not to have predictable prognostic value. Past studies examining lymph node involvement found questionable, if any, significant adverse prognostic associations (158,388,511). However, more recent epidemiological data showed an association between nodal status and survival outcomes (38). Size and location of tumor seem to be important prognostically, likely relating to the extent of surgical resection necessary to remove the tumor and the fact that patients who have a carinal resection have higher postoperative mortal-

ity (12,38,162). More recently, Bhattacharyya (38) proposed a SEER-data validated staging system wherein stage I is defined as T1 N0 disease, stage II as T2 N0, stage III as T3 N0, and stage IV representing T4 N0 or any N1 disease. However, it remains to be seen whether this system will be implemented by clinicians or confirmed with clinical data sets.

General Management

Bronchoscopy is essential for diagnosis and preoperative surgical planning (3,85,157,309). In acute respiratory compromise, rigid bronchoscopy (see Fig. 49.2) may be indicated to allow "coring out" of the tracheal neoplasm (12,308,505). In a series by Mathisen and Grillo (307), of 56 patients with rigid bronchoscopy, symptomatic airway symptom improvement was observed in 90% of cases, with mild, easily controlled bleeding in 5%. Esophagoscopy is suggested in all patients to rule out esophageal invasion. A CT scan of the chest is indicated to aid in evaluation of tumor extension, resectability, involved lymph nodes, and pulmonary metastases (1–3,85,147,219,381,518).

Treatment Results

Resectability uniformly affords better mortality outcomes in reported series (157,159,160,388). And thus is the initial strategy for most tracheal primaries (2,92,144,157,158,184,258,291). Resection rates vary. For example, approximately 66% of tracheal primary cancers are resected at the Massachusetts General Hospital (157), yet registry data from the Netherlands demonstrate a resection rate of 12% (190). Just 10% of all patients treated in Denmark from 1978 to 1995 received a full resection (272). Contraindications to resection are surgeon dependent; Pearson et al. (371,372) recommends tracheal resection for select patients with adenoid cystic carcinoma with low-burden pulmonary metastases, yet many would consider a patient such as this unresectable (312).

The majority of patients receive median sternotomy and cervical collar excision, while extensive subglottic or high tracheal disease may require cervical exenteration with mediastinal tracheostomy (158,371,377). Margins may be compromised to ensure a functioning airway. Technical advances in surgical procedures, such as complete mobilization of the right hilar ligament, detachment/implantation of the left hilum, mobilization of the cervical trachea, carinal resection/reconstruction techniques, intrapericardial dissection techniques, have improved the ability to perform an R0 resection (160–162,241). Gaissert et al. (142,144) demonstrate resection rates improving from 68% to 82% and in-hospital mortality declining from 21% to 3% over a 40-year period.

After resection, postoperative radiation is usually recommended (142,144,157,159,308,309,487). Preoperative radiotherapy has also been attempted but less experience has been reported. Small retrospective series appear to show a benefit for adjuvant radiation. Chow et al. (74) showed that resection plus adjuvant radiation had a median survival of 61 months versus 16 months for those who received surgery alone. Regnard et al. (388) found that 31 patients who had a complete resection with adjuvant radiotherapy had a better 5-year survival than 27 patients without adjuvant radiation (74% vs. 53%; $p =$ NS). Additionally, postoperative radiation was also effective for incompletely resected patients (5-year survival, 45% vs. 0%; $p <$.05). The results of definitive therapy for tracheal tumors are presented in Table 49.9.

In unresectable tumors, radiation has been used alone. The best results have come from studies where doses >60 Gy have been given (132,206,297). Mornex et al. (325) report that the 5-year survival rate decreased from 12% for those receiving ≥ 56 Gy to 5% for those receiving lower doses. However, Chow et al. (74) caution against giving doses higher than 60 Gy, as

Table 49.9	RESULTS OF RESECTION WITH ADJUVANT IRRADIATION FOR PRIMARY TRACHEAL CARCINOMA		
Author (Reference)	**Histology**	**Treatment**	**Median Survival**
Grillo and Mathisen (159)	Squamous (n = 70)	Surgery ± RT[a]	34 mo
		RT	10 mo
	Adenoid cystic (n = 80)	Surgery ± RT[a]	118 mo
		RT	28 mo
Licht et al. (272)	—	Surgery alone (n = 6)	48% (5-y actuarial)
		RT alone (n = 35)	7%
		Laser/cautery ± RT (n = 24)	28%
		RT + chemo (n = 2)	0%
Chow et al. (74)	—	Surgery alone (n = 5)	16 mo
		RT alone (n = 12)	26 mo
		Surgery + RT (n = 5)	61 mo
Regnand et al. (388)	—	R0 + RT (n = 31)	74% (5-y actuarial)
		R0 (n = 27)	53% (p = NS)
		R1,2 + RT (n = 15)	47%
		R1,2 (n = 6)	0% (p <.05)
Maziak et al. (312)	Adenoid cystic (n = 35)	R0 ± RT (n = 14)[a]	9.8 y
		R1,2 + RT (n = 15)	7.5 y
		RT alone (n = 6)	6.2 y

R0, complete resection, R1,2, incomplete resection; RT, radiation therapy
[a]The minority received surgery alone.

three out of six patients with doses >60 Gy in his study had severe complications requiring surgical intervention (e.g., tracheoesophageal fistula, esophageal stricture, and severe tracheal crusting). Although none of the patients treated with <60 Gy (0/6) had late side effects, other authors have corroborated the concern of dose contributing to complications (155). Still, Chow et al. noted significantly better local control in patients who received >50 Gy in the adjuvant setting and >60 Gy in the definitive setting. In comparison, Fuwa et al. (141) reported reasonable results with implementing a novel endoluminal-centering catheter delivering a median dose for the group (external bean radiation therapy plus low-dose rate iridium-192) of 91 Gy, while reporting one treatment-related death 1 year

after therapy (113 Gy total dose). Harms et al. (175) report median doses of 60 Gy delivered with external bean radiation therapy and brachytherapy boosts of 15 to 18 Gy given with minimal Radiation Therapy Oncology Group grade 3 or 4 toxicity (8% of 25 patients). Data summarizing select radiotherapy-alone experiences in primary tracheal neoplasms are given in Table 49.10.

Combined chemoradiotherapy without resection has been attempted at some institutions, usually for nonsquamous histologies, with mixed results (461,480,487,515). Patients with squamous cell carcinoma have fared poorly, while those with small cell carcinoma or lymphoma have done better (236,272, 487,511).

Table 49.10	RETROSPECTIVE SERIES EXAMINING RADIOTHERAPY ALONE FOR PRIMARY TRACHEAL CARCINOMA			
Author (Reference)	**Histology**	**Treatment**	**Local Control**	**Survival**
Schraube et al. (414)	Squamous (n = 11)	46–60 Gy EBRT + 15–20 Gy HDR	6/11	31-mo median
Cheung (71)	Squamous (n = 20)	40–60 Gy	—	5-mo median
	Adenoid cystic (n = 4)	40–60 Gy		1-y median
Fields et al. (132)	Squamous (n = 17)	>60 Gy	5/6	25% 5 y (n = 18)
	Adenoid cystic (n = 1)	40–60 Gy	1/7	
		<40 Gy	0/4	
		>60 Gy	1/1	
Rostom and Morgan (401)	Squamous (n = 28)	60–70 Gy	16/24	11% (4-y actuarial)
	Adenoid cystic (n = 3)	<60 Gy	0/4	67% 4 y
		50–70 Gy		
Makarewick and Mross (297)		60 Gy EBRT + 6–12 Gy HDR (n = 8)	6/8	9.5-mo median (n = 23)
			1/3	
		40–60 Gy EBRT (n = 3)	0/12	
		<40 Gy (n = 12)		
Fuwa et al. (141)		EBRT + LDR (n = 4) (80–128 Gy)[a]	3/4	75% 3 y

EBRT external beam radiotherapy; HDR, high–dose rate brachytherapy; LDR, low–dose rate brachytherapy.
[a]One treatment related death in patient receiving 60 Gy RT + 53 Gy LDR iridium-192.

Radiation Techniques

No results have been reported that suggest patients would not benefit from adjuvant radiation therapy. For resected patients, 1 to 1.5 months of healing time should be allowed before beginning postoperative radiotherapy. Modern CT-based, three-dimentional conformal, or intensity-modlated radiation therapy (IMRT) treatment techniques should be used. In palliation or the setting of metastatic disease, aggressive treatment is warranted to prevent airway obstruction (325). External beam doses should be limited to 60 Gy. An intraluminal boost technique allows increasing dose (and hopefully control) with minimal added acute or late side effects (57,74,175,319,414,427).

Intraluminal brachytherapy is also useful in the palliative setting. Skowronek et al. (427) found, in a series of patients treated with 10 to 30 Gy in one to three fractions, that high-dose rate brachytherapy alone afforded prolonged survival and improved quality of life. In patients with locally extensive disease, the gravest complication is the development of a tracheoesophageal fistula after radiation, but this can also be impossible to avoid. For patients with emergent airway obstruction, rigid bronchoscopy should be performed instead of urgent radiotherapy.

The role of elective nodal irradiation for tracheal carcinoma is uncertain. As mentioned earlier, nodal status has not been found to be of prognostic significance; even cervical adenopathy was not associated with poorer outcome (511). Given the low proclivity of lymphatic spread for adenoid cystic carcinomas, elimination of elective nodal irradiation is certainly reasonable for this variant. Because local recurrence is the major factor influencing survival, nodal and regional failure patterns are not a main concern. Yet if mediastinal or cervical nodes are discovered at surgery or by CT, radiation to these regions is warranted.

Conclusion

Primary tracheal cancer is a rare neoplasm, and the majority of patients will present with squamous or adenoid cystic histologies. The optimal management for these tumors is a combined-modality approach incorporating surgical resection and postoperative radiation. For localized disease, the role of chemotherapy either alone or concurrent with radiation, is unknown.

▪▪ | Mediastinal Mesenchymal Tumors

Epidemiology

True mediastinal mesenchymal lesions (MMLs) are exceedingly rare tumors. Retrospective series document 2% to 8% of all mediastinal lesions as primary mesenchymal tumors; extrapolating these values estimates domestic incidence at approximately 0.1 to 0.2 per million (99,359–361). Approximately three quarters of mediastinal mesenchymal tumors are of lipomatous, lymphangitic, or vascular histology with the rest composed of unusual histologic variants (290). The age predilection is dependent on the specific histologic subtype (42,358–361,448).

Clinical Presentation and Work-Up

MMLs may arise in any of the three major component compartments of the mediastinum. Mesenchymal tumors that present in the pediatric population appear to be more malignant (39,448).

MMLs are able to achieve impressive sizes before detection, typically presenting with symptoms such as chest pain and dyspnea. At least one series suggests that symptomatic presentation is a harbinger of malignant character, with 80% of patients with malignant disease presenting as symptomatic versus 44% of patients with benign masses (99). Accurate histopathologic diagnosis is critical (448). Tissue can be obtained via mediastinoscopic biopsy, fine-needle aspiration, or endoscopy. The American Joint Committee on Cancer recommendations on staging for soft-tissue tumors can be applied.

Tumors of Adipose Tissue

Mediastinal lipomas are the most common mediastinal mesenchymal lesion; they comprise 1% to 5% of all lipomas (9,40,96,290). Lesions may be single or multiple in the mediastinum and may mimic cardiomegaly or pleural effusion on a chest x-ray. They are usually well circumscribed and encapsulated but can grow to 20 cm in size before detection (221,222). A gross total resection is almost always curative for these patients (163,165,344,453,491).

In contrast, liposarcomas consist of immature fat cells with malignant histology and behavior. Tumors often appear encapsulated and well circumscribed, even when invasion is present, thus the term pseudocapsule. A historical review noted that patients with well-circumscribed lesions had survivals ranging from 3 to 17 years, whereas patients with grossly invasive tumors died within 2 years (433). As with all sarcomas, prognosis depends on the grade of the lesion (52,234). Optimal treatment consists of surgical resection and adjuvant radiation therapy (514). Because well-differentiated tumors have little propensity for distant metastases, adjuvant radiation may be withheld after an R0 resection acknowledging the significant local recurrence rates of 20% to 30% (10,52,75,218,223,234).

Tumors of Lymph Tissue

Tumors arising from the vascular or lymphatic components of the mediastinum make up the bulk of the remaining MMLs (359–361). Lymphangiomas and hemangiomas are morphologically similar via light microscopy, and the presence of red blood cells or chyle within tumor lumen often serves as a primary diagnostic aid (491). Localized lymphangiomas are rare; more than 90% will have some degree of cervical extension (138). Lymphangiomatosis is usually seen in children and is characterized by synchronous widespread lymphangiomas. Mediastinal or pulmonary involvement carries a poor prognosis (11,50,66,96,120,449,450,454,486,491). Lymphangiosarcoma appears to be a malignant variant of lymphangiomas and should probably be treated as other soft-tissue sarcomas. Optimum treatment for lymphangiomas entails a full extirpation (350). The largest retrospective series of 25 patients with mediastinal and cervicomediastinal lymphangiomas reported excellent survival rates after surgical resection alone and that only one patient died of a complication from lymphangioma (368). Adjuvant radiation has little to offer and may actually be detrimental, with one report of postradiation transformation of a benign lymphangioma into a malignant lymphangiosarcoma (208,216,228). However, for symptomatic unresectable disease, radiation may be of benefit. Johnson et al. (208) described a young patient with surgically refractory chylothorax and lymphangioma who had prompt resolution after 20 Gy in 10 fractions of mediastinal irradiation. Another report demonstrated complete local control in three patients for large, unresectable lymphangiomas, which is concordant with other anecdotal reports for lymphangiomyomatosis (95,216).

Tumors of Vascular Tissue

MMLs with an endothelial origin include hemangiomas, hemangioendotheliomas, and hemangiopericytomas. Many of these tumors exhibit an indolent course, but hemangiopericytomas are notable for high rates of metastasis at presentation

(27,73,181,356). Hemangiomas may be capillary or cavernous. Cavernous hemangiomas (angiomyomas or hamartomatous) are distinguished from capillary hemangiomas by the presence of smooth muscle. Hemangiomas and hemangioendotheliomas are typically well circumscribed. Hemangioendotheliomas contain the hallmark cytoplasmic Weibel-Palade bodies (279,489).

Hemangiopericytomas arise from the capillary contractile pericytes of Zimmerman (73). Although most are indolent, recurrence and metastases have been observed many years after resection (187). Retrospective studies indicate high mitotic rates, and proliferative indices may portend malignant behavior (134,318). But long-term survival has still been reported with aggressive treatment of metastatic disease (118). Surgery remains the mainstay of therapy and is often curative (80). Because of their benign nature, hemangiomas or hemangioendotheliomas should not be treated with radiation (80). Radiation remains an option for incompletely resected hemangiopericytomas.

Miscellaneous Mediastinal Mesenchymal Lesions

A mélange of other MMLs have been occasionally encountered. These miscellaneous MMLs are primarily of musculoskeletal or connective tissue origin and are typically encountered in the posterior mediastinum (290). The routine treatment has been surgical excision and occasionally postoperative radiation therapy depending on the histology and clinical presentation (103,108,290,349,359–361,440,441).

Mediastinal Neurogenic Tumors

Epidemiology

Neurogenic tumors of the thorax arise in the posterior mediastinum from peripheral nerves, sympathetic ganglia, or mediastinal chemoreceptors. They account for about one third of all mediastinal neoplasms and are the most common cause of a posterior mediastinal mass (26,68,99,465). But they are extremely rare with an incidence of 0.5 per million in adults (99). Neuroblastoma is an aggressive variant of neurogenic tumors and is a disease of childhood. About 20% will occur in the mediastinum. Neuroblastoma is covered in the pediatric malignancy section of this book, Chapter XX. While neuroblastoma is more common in males and Caucasians, malignant neurogenic tumors have no gender predilection (18,277,386).

In adults, the majority of neurogenic tumors are benign schwannomas and neurofibromas in the setting of neurofibromatosis type 1 (NF-1) or von Recklinghausen's disease. Although schwannomas can reach a very large size before detection (491), resection can be completed for almost all patients and long-term local control ranges from 90% to 100% (13,277, 366,465).

Mediastinal paragangliomas have also been described. Paragangliomas are rare tumors that arise from extra-adrenal paraganglia and potentially are catecholamine secreting. Most tumors are benign, and surgical resection is usually curative, but more recent studies suggest that the risk of the tumor being malignant is >10% (94,123).

NF-1 is an autosomal dominant neurocutaneous disorder, with an estimated birth incidence of 1 in 2,500 (196). Individuals affected with NF-1 harbor an increased risk of developing both benign and malignant tumors. The most common tumor in individuals with NF-1 is the neurofibroma, a heterogeneous benign peripheral nerve sheath tumor (131,174). Neurofibromas can be discrete, focal cutaneous or subcutaneous growths, intraforaminal spinal tumors, or plexiform neurofibromas. Plexiform neurofibromas are composed of the same cell types as dermal neurofibromas but have an expanded extracellular matrix and a rich vascular supply (131). In one population study of 125 NF-1 patients, plexiform neurofibromas were clinically visible in 30% (197). Although malignant peripheral nerve sheath tumors (MPNSTs) develop in the general population, individuals with NF-1 have a significantly increased risk. Patients with NF-1 have almost a 10% lifetime risk of developing a MPNST (315,468). Because the majority of NF-1-associated MPNSTs arise within pre-existing plexiform neurofibromas, individuals with NF-1 and plexiform neurofibromas warrant increased surveillance.

In adults, the majority of malignant mediastinal neurogenic tumors are thus MPNSTs. In a recent retrospective review of one institution's experience, half of the patients had a MPNST with a trunk location (18). The authors did not differentiate between mediastinal and retroperitoneal locations, but this can be difficult given the lack of an anatomical barrier. Roughly a third of their patients had NF-1. The median age of presentation was 37 overall, but age 27 for patients with NF-1 and age 40 for patients without.

The other strong association for MPNSTs is prior radiation (41,111,435,504). In a series of patients treated at the Mayo Clinic over 20 years, almost 10% of their patients had a history of radiation exposure (504).

Natural History and General Management

The most common presentation is an asymptomatic mass on a routine chest x-ray (145,386). Symptoms of pain and nerve dysfunction can arise from compression when lesions are large or rapidly growing. MPNSTs are difficult to detect, metastasize rapidly, and thus carry a poor prognosis (119). Local invasion and bony destruction is often seen (263). Distant metastases can be seen in up to a third of patients at the time of presentation (435).

Management for patients with malignant mediastinal neurogenic tumors entails a multidisciplinary approach similar to the management of adult soft-tissue sarcomas. High-resolution CT imaging is essential, with an MRI to evaluate the neural and spinal anatomy if involvement is suspected (387). Surgical resection is the mainstay of therapy, and an R0 resection should be attempted but is often difficult in the mediastinum because of impingement on surrounding structures and the potential of a drastic neurologic deficit.

Consistent with the treatment of soft-tissue sarcomas, adjuvant radiation has been incorporated into the management of localized MPNSTs. The largest series published reports the results of 134 patients treated at the Mayo Clinic between 1975 and 1993 (504). Of those patients, only 25 had mediastinal tumors. An R0 operation was possible in 70%. In contrast, an earlier study noted only a 55% R0/R1 rate for mediastinal MPNSTs (249). A variety of radiation techniques were used in the Mayo series. About half of the patients received adjuvant radiation with a mean dose of 51 Gy postoperatively. Overall survival and local tumor control at 10 years was 42% and 50%, respectively, for the whole group of patients. The significant prognostic factors for overall survival on multivariate analysis were surgical margin status and history of radiation. For local control, surgical margin status, radiation dose, and the use of intraoperative radiation therapy or brachytherapy were significantly associated on multivariate analysis. Adjuvant radiation appears to have almost doubled local control rates from 40% to 73% at 3 years and 34% to 65% at 5 years ($p = .0004$). However, for survival, the result was suggestive but not significant with 5-year survival rates of 58% for those who received radiation compared with 43% for those who did not.

A more recent analysis also supports the use of radiation in the adjuvant setting for the treatment of MPNSTs (18). A review of 205 patients treated with localized MPNSTs of all body sites at the Istituto Nazionale per lo Studio e la Cura dei Tumori (Milan, Italy) over 25 years also reported a 43% disease-specific mortality rate at 10 years. Less than half of the patients received radiation therapy. The significant variables on multivariate analysis included tumor site, tumor size (>12 cm), surgical margin status, and the use of adjuvant radiation ($p = .016$). All the same factors except radiation, surprisingly, were significantly associated with local control on multivariate analysis. Patients who received radiation had fewer recurrences, but this was not statistically significant. About 30% of patients eventually developed distant metastases, of which the vast majority were pulmonary.

The delivery of radiation therapy for MPNSTs can be challenging. Because of the complicated issues in management, patients with these tumors should be treated at centers with extensive multidisciplinary experience in soft-tissue sarcomas. In the postoperative setting, the minimum dose for microscopic disease should be 60 Gy given over 30 fractions. Given the close proximity of the posterior mediastinum to the spinal cord, careful attention should be applied to immobilization and localization. A prone approach is likely more accurate and reliable by reducing the distance from the localization points to the treatment volume. On-board imaging with stereoscopic guidance can ensure daily accuracy. IMRT is often necessary to provide a concave dose distribution around the spinal cord. In the setting of gross residual disease, more dose may be beneficial but can be difficult or impossible to deliver given the normal tissue constraints.

For patients with unresectable disease, radiation can be delivered either alone or with agents that are typically used for soft-tissue sarcomas. Few agents have shown effectiveness for MPNST, and treatment regimens usually are with doxorubicin, ifosfamide, or a combination (409).

Significant progress has been made in recent years in elucidating the molecular genetics and biology of MPNST, especially in NF-1 patients. A variety of different genetic alterations have been reported in MPNSTs, but it is not clear whether any of these are causally related to tumorigenesis or malignant progression (166).

⠿ | Acknowledgment

The authors are grateful to Annelle Thomas for proofreading of the manuscript.

References

1. Aberle DR, Brown K, Young DA, et al. Imaging techniques in the evaluation of tracheobronchial neoplasms. *Chest* 1991;99(1):211–215.
2. Abudallo K, Romanoff H, Stern Z. Primary tumors of the thoracic trachea with special emphasis on surgical management. *Int Surg* 1976;61(6–7):347–349.
3. Adachi MM, Pamies RJ. Carcinoma of the trachea: a hidden tumor. *Hosp Pract (Off Ed)* 1993;28(7):81–84.
4. Adams S, Baum RP, Hertel A, et al. Metabolic (PET) and receptor (SPET) imaging of well- and less well-differentiated tumours: comparison with the expression of the Ki-67 antigen. *Nucl Med Commun* 1998;19(7):641–647.
5. Adkins RB Jr., Maples MD, Hainsworth JD. Primary malignant mediastinal tumors. *Ann Thorac Surg* 1984;38(6):648–659.
6. Aguirre D, Nieto K, Lazos M, et al. Extragonadal germ cell tumors are often associated with Klinefelter syndrome. *Hum Pathol* 2006;37(4):477–480.
7. Akaogi E, Ohara K, Mitsui K, et al. Preoperative radiotherapy and surgery for advanced thymoma with invasion to the great vessels. *J Surg Oncol* 1996;63(1):17–22.
8. Akwari OE, Payne WS, Onofrio BM, et al. Dumbbell neurogenic tumors of the mediastinum. Diagnosis and management. *Mayo Clin Proc* 1978;53(6):353–358.
9. Alden JF, Bjornson RB, Sterner ER, et al. Mediastinal lipoma. *Dis Chest* 1957;32(5):580–581.
10. Alho A, Eeg Larsen T. A case of multifocal liposarcoma? *Acta Orthop Scand* 1992;63(1):98–99.
11. Aliotta PJ, Castillo J, Englander LS, et al. Primary mediastinal germ cell tumors. Histologic patterns of treatment failures at autopsy. *Cancer* 1988;62(5):982–984.
12. Allen MS. Malignant tracheal tumors. *Mayo Clin Proc* 1993;68(7):680–684.
13. Almeida Netto MX, AW, Mediastinal tumors. *J Pneumol* 1984;10(1):15–24.
14. Alvarez OA, Kjellin I, Zuppan CW. Thoracic lymphangiomatosis in a child. *J Pediatr Hematol Oncol* 2004;26(2):136–141.
15. Amar YG, Nguyen LH, Manoukian JJ, et al. Granular cell tumor of the trachea in a child. *Int J Pediatr Otorhinolaryngol* 2002;62(1):75–80.
16. Amiraliev MA, Alekseev VI, Kolodiazhnyi AP, et al. [Carcinoid of the trachea simulating bronchial asthma (1 case)]. *Vopr Onkol* 1985;31(6):107–108.
17. Andac A, Mert B, Sevil B, et al. Adult primary extragonadal germ cell tumors: treatment results and long-term follow-up. *Med Pediatr Oncol* 2003;41(1):49–53.
18. Anghileri M, Miceli R, Fiore M, et al. Malignant peripheral nerve sheath tumors: prognostic factors and survival in a series of patients treated at a single institution. *Cancer* 2006;107(5):1065–1074.
19. Arakawa A, Yasunaga T, Saitoh Y, et al. Radiation therapy of invasive thymoma. *Int J Radiat Oncol Biol Phys* 1990;18(3):529–534.
20. Arevalo M, Ordi J, Renedo G, et al. Chondrosarcoma of the trachea. Report of a case. *Respiration* 1986;49(2):147–151.
21. Arriagada R, Bretel JJ, Caillaud JM, et al. Invasive carcinoma of the thymus. A multicenter retrospective review of 56 cases. *Eur J Cancer Clin Oncol* 1984;20(1):69–74.
22. Asbun HJ, Calabria RP, Calmes S, et al. Thymic carcinoid. *Am Surg* 1991;57(7):442–445.
23. Avilova OM, Vasilevskaia ZA. [Sarcoma of the trachea]. *Vrach Delo* 1974;5:34–36.
24. Awad WI, Symmans PJ, Dussek JE. Recurrence of stage I thymoma 32 years after total excision. *Ann Thorac Surg* 1998;66(6):2106–2108.
25. Aygun C, Slawson RG, Bajaj K, et al. Primary mediastinal seminoma. *Urology* 1984;23(2):109–117.
26. Azarow KS, Pearl RH, Zurcher R, et al. Primary mediastinal masses. A comparison of adult and pediatric populations. *J Thorac Cardiovasc Surg* 1993;106(1):67–72.
27. Backwinkel KD, Diddams JA. Hemangiopericytoma. Report of a case and comprehensive review of the literature. *Cancer* 1970;25(4):896–901.
28. Bader JL, Horowitz ME, Dewan R, et al. Intensive combined modality therapy of small round cell and undifferentiated sarcomas in children and young adults: local control and patterns of failure. *Radiother Oncol* 1989;16(3):189–201.
29. Bagshaw MA, McLaughlin WT, Earle JD. Definitive radiotherapy of primary mediastinal seminoma. *Am J Roentgenol Radium Ther Nucl Med* 1969;105(1):86–94.
30. Baron RL, Lee JK, Sagel SS, et al. Computed tomography of the abnormal thymus. *Radiology* 1982;142(1):127–134.
31. Batata MA, Martini N, Huvos AG, et al. Thymomas: clinicopathologic features, therapy, and prognosis. *Cancer* 1974;34(2):389–396.
32. Baydur A, Gottlieb LS. Adenoid cystic carcinoma (cylindroma) of the trachea masquerading as asthma. *JAMA* 1975;234(8):829–831.
33. Becherer A, De Santis M, Karanikas G, et al. FDG PET is superior to CT in the prediction of viable tumour in post-chemotherapy seminoma residuals. *Eur J Radiol* 2005;54(2):284–288.
34. Benjamin SP, McCormack LJ, Effler DB, et al. Primary tumors of the mediastinum. *Chest* 1972;62(3):297–303.
35. Bergh NP, Gatzinsky P, Larsson S, et al. Tumors of the thymus and thymic region: I. Clinicopathological studies on thymomas. *Ann Thorac Surg* 1978;25(2):91–98.
36. Bernatz PE, Harrison Eg, Clagett OT. Thymoma: a clinicopathologic study. *J West Soc Periodontol Periodontal Abstr* 1961;42:424–444.
37. Bernatz PE, Khonsari S, Harrison EG Jr., et al. Thymoma: factors influencing prognosis. *Surg Clin North Am* 1973;53(4):885–892.
38. Bhattacharyya N. Contemporary staging and prognosis for primary tracheal malignancies: a population-based analysis. *Otolaryngol Head Neck Surg* 2004;131(5):639–642.
39. Billmire DF. Germ cell, mesenchymal, and thymic tumors of the mediastinum. *Semin Pediatr Surg* 1999;8(2):85–91.
40. Blades B. Relative frequency and site of predilection of intrathoracic tumors. *Am J Surg* 1941;54:139–148.
41. Bloechle C, Peiper M, Schwarz R, et al. Post-irradiation soft tissue sarcoma. *Eur J Cancer* 1995;31A(1):31–34.
42. Blumberg D, Port JL, Weksler B, et al. Thymoma: a multivariate analysis of factors predicting survival. *Ann Thorac Surg* 1995;60(4):908–913, discussion 914.
43. Bokemeyer C, Droz JP, Horwich A, et al. Extragonadal seminoma: an international multicenter analysis of prognostic factors and long-term treatment outcome. *Cancer* 2001;91(7):1394–1401.
44. Bokemeyer C, Nichols CR, Droz JP, et al. Extragonadal germ cell tumors of the mediastinum and retroperitoneum: results from an international analysis. *J Clin Oncol* 2002;20(7):1864–1873.
45. Bonomi PD, Finkelstein D, Aisner S, et al. EST 2582 phase II trial of cisplatin in metastatic or recurrent thymoma. *Am J Clin Oncol* 1993;16(4):342–345.
46. Braitman H, Li W, Herrmann C Jr., et al. Surgery for thymic tumors. *Arch Surg* 1971;103(1):14–16.
47. Brewster DC, MacMillan IK, Edwards FR. Chondroma of the trachea: report of a case and review of the literature. *Ann Thorac Surg* 1975;19(5):576–584.
48. Briselli M, Mark GJ, Grillo HC. Tracheal carcinoids. *Cancer* 1978;42(6):2870–2879.
49. Buckingham JM, Howard FM Jr., Bernatz PE, et al. The value of thymectomy in myasthenia gravis: a computer-assisted matched study. *Ann Surg* 1976;184(4):453–458.
50. Bugaeva MI, Tararaev IA. [Lymphangiomatosis complicated by chylothorax]. *Sov Med* 1984;7:112–113.
51. Burkell CC, Cross JM, Kent HP, et al. Mass lesions of the mediastinum. *Curr Probl Surg* 1969;:2–57.
52. Burt M, Ihde JK, Hajdu SI, et al. Primary sarcomas of the mediastinum: results of therapy. *J Thorac Cardiovasc Surg* 1998;115(3):671–680.
53. Burt ME, Javadpour N. Germ-cell tumors in patients with apparently normal testes. *Cancer* 1981;47(7):1911–1915.
54. Burton DM, Heffner DK, Patow CA. Granular cell tumors of the trachea. *Laryngoscope* 1992;102(7):807–813.
55. Bush SE, Martinez A, Bagshaw MA. Primary mediastinal seminoma. *Cancer* 1981;48(8):1877–1882.
56. Cameron R, Loeher P, Thomas C. Neoplasms of the mediastinum. In: DeVita V, Hellman S, Rosenberg S, eds. *Cancer: principles and practice of oncology.* Philadelphia: Lippincott-Raven; 2000:1019–1036.
57. Carvalho Hde A, Figueiredo V, Pedreira WL Jr., et al. High dose-rate brachytherapy as a treatment option in primary tracheal tumors. *Clinics* 2005;60(4):299–304.
58. Casamassima F, Villari N, Fargnoli R, et al. Magnetic resonance imaging and high-resolution computed tomography in tumors of the lung and the mediastinum. *Radiother Oncol* 1988;11(1):21–29.

59. Castleman B. The pathology of the thymus gland in myasthenia gravis. *Ann N Y Acad Sci* 1966;135(1):496–505.
60. Chaganti RS, Rodriguez E, Mathew S. Origin of adult male mediastinal germ-cell tumours. *Lancet* 1994;343(8906):1130–1132.
61. Chahinian AP, Bhardwaj S, Meyer RJ, et al. Treatment of invasive or metastatic thymoma: report of eleven cases. *Cancer* 1981;47(7):1752–1761.
62. Chahinian AP. Chemotherapy of thymomas and thymic carcinomas. *Chest Surg Clin North Am* 2001;11(2):447–456.
63. Chalabreysse L, Etienne-Mastroianni B, Adeleine P, et al. Thymic carcinoma: a clinicopathological and immunohistological study of 19 cases. *Histopathology* 2004;44(4):367–374.
64. Chang HK, Wang CH, Liaw CC, et al. Prognosis of thymic carcinoma: analysis of 16 cases. *J Formos Med Assoc* 1992;91(8):764–769.
65. Chang JH, Newkirk J, Carlton G, et al. Generalized lymphangiomatosis with chylous ascites—treatment by peritoneo-venous shunting. *J Pediatr Surg* 1980; 15(6):748–750.
66. Chariot P, Monnet I, Gaulard P, et al. Systemic mastocytosis following mediastinal germ cell tumor: an association confirmed. *Hum Pathol* 1993;24(1):111–112.
67. Chatten J, Katz SM. Thymoma in a 12-year-old boy. *Cancer* 1976;37(2):953–957.
68. Chavez Espinosa JL, CFJ, Hoyer OH, Gomez Fernandez L. Endothoracic neurogenic neoplasm (analysis of 30 cases). *Rev Interam Radiol* 1980;5(2):49–54.
69. Chen G, Marx A, Wen-Hu C, et al. New WHO histologic classification predicts prognosis of thymic epithelial tumors: a clinicopathologic study of 200 thymoma cases from China. *Cancer* 2002;95(2):420–429.
70. Chen JS, Chang YL, Shu HS, et al. Surgical treatment of a primary tracheal angiosarcoma. *J Thorac Cardiovasc Surg* 2003;125(1):191–193.
71. Cheung AY. Radiotherapy for primary carcinoma of the trachea. *Radiother Oncol* 1989;14(4):279–285.
72. Chizh GI, Pichko RT. [Malignant carcinoid tumor of the trachea]. *Vestn Otorinolaringol* 1983(3):84–85.
73. Chnaris A, Barbetakis N, Efstathiou A, et al. Primary mediastinal hemangiopericytoma. *World J Surg Oncol* 2006;4:23.
74. Chow DC, Komaki R, Libshitz HI, et al. Treatment of primary neoplasms of the trachea. The role of radiation therapy. *Cancer* 1993;71(10):2946–2952.
75. Chung C, Lu CC, Chang SC, et al. Mediastinal liposarcoma with local recurrence: a case report. *Zhonghua Yi Xue Za Zhi (Taipei)* 1996;57(1):70–73.
76. Ciernik IF, Meier U, Lutolf UM. Prognostic factors and outcome of incompletely resected invasive thymoma following radiation therapy. *J Clin Oncol* 1994;12(7):1484–1490.
77. Clamon GH. Management of primary mediastinal seminoma. *Chest* 1983;83(2): 263–267.
78. Cleveland RH, Nice CM Jr., Ziskind J. Primary adenoid cystic carcinoma (cylindroma) of the trachea. *Radiology* 1977;122(3):597–600.
79. Close PM, Kirchner T, Uys CJ, et al. Reproducibility of a histogenetic classification of thymic epithelial tumours. *Histopathology* 1995;26(4):339–343.
80. Cohen AJ, Sbaschnig RJ, Hochholzer L, et al. Mediastinal hemangiomas. *Ann Thorac Surg* 1987;43(6):656–659.
81. Cohen AJ, Thompson L, Edwards FH, et al. Primary cysts and tumors of the mediastinum. *Ann Thorac Surg* 1991;51(3):378–384; discussion 385–386.
82. Cohen DJ, Ronnigen LD, Graeber GM, et al. Management of patients with malignant thymoma. *J Thorac Cardiovasc Surg* 1984;87(2):301–307.
83. Cohen SR, Landing BH, Isaacs H. Fibrous histiocytoma of the trachea. *Ann Otol Rhinol Laryngol Suppl* 1978;87(5 Pt 2)[Suppl 52]:2–4.
84. Cole LA, Rinne KM, Shahabi S, et al. False-positive hCG assay results leading to unnecessary surgery and chemotherapy and needless occurrences of diabetes and coma. *Clin Chem* 1999;45(2):313–314.
85. Compeau CG, Keshavjee S. Management of tracheal neoplasms. *Oncologist* 1996; 1(6):347–353.
86. Cowen D, Hannoun-Levi JM, Resbeut M, et al. Natural history and treatment of malignant thymoma. *Oncology (Williston Park)* 1998;12(7):1001–1005; discussion 1006.
87. Cowen D, Richaud P, Mornex F, et al. Thymoma: results of a multicentric retrospective series of 149 non-metastatic irradiated patients and review of the literature. FNCLCC trialists. Federation Nationale des Centres de Lutte Contre le Cancer. *Radiother Oncol* 1995;34(1):9–16.
88. Cox J. Primary malignant germinal tumors of the mediastinum: a study of 24 patients. *Cancer* 1975;36:1162.
89. Curran WJ Jr., Kornstein MJ, Brooks JJ, et al. Invasive thymoma: the role of mediastinal irradiation following complete or incomplete surgical resection. *J Clin Oncol* 1988;6(11):1722–1727.
90. Currier RD, Routh A, Hickman BT, et al. Thymus irradiation for myasthenia gravis. *Radiology* 1983;146(1):199–201.
91. Curry WA, McKay CE, Richardson RL, et al. Klinefelter's syndrome and mediastinal germ cell neoplasms. *J Urol* 1981;125(1):127–129.
92. D'Cunha J, Maddaus MA. Surgical treatment of tracheal and carinal tumors. *Chest Surg Clin North Am* 2003;13(1):95–110, vi.
93. Dadmanesh F, Sekihara T, Rosai J. Histologic typing of thymoma according to the new World Health Organization classification. *Chest Surg Clin North Am* 2001;11(2):407–420.
94. Dahia PL, Dahia PLM. Evolving concepts in pheochromocytoma and paraganglioma. *Curr Opin Oncol* 2006;18(1):1–8.
95. Dajee H, Woodhouse R. Lymphangiomatosis of the mediastinum with chylothorax and chylopericardium: role of radiation treatment. *J Thorac Cardiovasc Surg* 1994;108(3):594–595.
96. Daniel RA Jr., Diveley WL, Edwards WH, et al. Mediastinal tumors. *Ann Surg* 1960;151:783–795.
97. Daniels AC, Conner GH, Straus FH. Primary chondrosarcoma of the tracheobronchial tree. Report of a unique case and brief review. *Arch Pathol* 1967;84(6): 615–624.
98. Davies MJ, Hall DR, Ross BA. Rare tracheal tumours: two case reports of primary neurogenic tumours occurring in the trachea. *Respir Med* 1993;87(2): 145–146.
99. Davis RD Jr., Oldham HN Jr., Sabiston DC Jr. Primary cysts and neoplasms of the mediastinum: recent changes in clinical presentation, methods of diagnosis, management, and results. *Ann Thorac Surg* 1987;44(3):229–237.
100. Davis RD, Oldham HN, Sabiston DC The mediastinum. In: Sabiston DC, Spencer FC, eds. *Surgery of the chest*. Philadelphia: W.B. Saunders, 1995;.
101. Dawson A, Ibrahim NB, Gibbs AR. Observer variation in the histopathological classification of thymoma: correlation with prognosis. *J Clin Pathol* 1994;47(6): 519–523.
102. de Montpreville VT, Macchiarini P, Dulmet E. Thymic neuroendocrine carcinoma (carcinoid): a clinicopathologic study of fourteen cases. *J Thorac Cardiovasc Surg* 1996;111(1):134–141.
103. De Nictolis M, Goteri G, Campanati G, et al. Elastofibroma of the mediastinum. A previously undescribed benign tumor containing abnormal elastic fibers. *Am J Surg Pathol* 1995;19(3):364–367.
104. Desai DP, Maddalozzo J, Holinger LD. Granular cell tumor of the trachea. *Otolaryngol Head Neck Surg* 1999;120(4):595–598.
105. Detterbeck FC, Parsons AM. Thymic tumors. *Ann Thorac Surg* 2004;77(5):1860–1869.
106. Detterbeck FC. Clinical value of the WHO classification system of thymoma. *Ann Thorac Surg* 2006;81(6):2328–2334.
107. Dexeus FH, Logothetis CJ, Chong C, et al. Genetic abnormalities in men with germ cell tumors. *J Urol* 1988;140(1):80–84.
108. Dikshtein EA, Sadovnik EE. [Mesenchymoma of the mediastinum]. *Arkh Patol* 1985;47(12):59–61.
109. Dimery IW, Lee JS, Blick M, et al. Association of the Epstein-Barr virus with lymphoepithelioma of the thymus. *Cancer* 1988;61(12):2475–2480.
110. Dincer SI, Demir A, Kara HV, et al. Primary tracheal schwannoma: a case report. *Acta Chir Belg* 2006;106(2):254–256.
111. Dini M, Caldarella A, Lo Russo G, et al. [Malignant tumors of the peripheral nerve sheath (MPNST) after irradiation]. *Pathologica* 1997;89(4):441–445.
112. Do YS, Im JG, Lee BH, et al. CT findings in malignant tumors of thymic epithelium. *J Comput Assist Tomogr* 1995;19(2):192–197.
113. Dorfman J, Jamison BM, Morin JE. Primary tracheal schwannoma. *Ann Thorac Surg* 2000;69(1):280–281.
114. Douglas JG, Laramore GE, Austin-Seymour M, et al. Treatment of locally advanced adenoid cystic carcinoma of the head and neck with neutron radiotherapy. *Int J Radiat Oncol Biol Phys* 2000;46(3):551–557.
115. Drachman DB. Myasthenia gravis (first of two parts). *N Engl J Med* 1978;298(3): 136–142.
116. Drachman DB. Myasthenia gravis (second of two parts). *N Engl J Med* 1978;298(4): 186–193.
117. Drachman DB. Myasthenia gravis. *N Engl J Med* 1994;330(25):1797–1810.
118. Dube VE, Paulson JF. Metastatic hemangiopericytoma cured by radiotherapy. A case report. *J Bone Joint Surg Am* 1974;56(4):833–835.
119. Ducatman BS, Scheithauer BW, Piepgras DG, et al. Malignant peripheral nerve sheath tumors. A clinicopathologic study of 120 cases. *Cancer* 1986;57(10):2006–2021.
120. Economopoulos GC, Lewis JW Jr., Lee MW, et al. Carcinoid tumors of the thymus. *Ann Thorac Surg* 1990;50(1):58–61.
121. Economou JS, Trump DL, Holmes EC, et al. Management of primary germ cell tumors of the mediastinum. *J Thorac Cardiovasc Surg* 1982;83(5):643–649.
122. Einhorn LH, Williams SD. Chemotherapy of disseminated seminoma. *Cancer Clin Trials* 1980;3(4):307–313.
123. Elder EE, Elder G, Larsson C, et al. Pheochromocytoma and functional paraganglioma syndrome: no longer the 10% tumor. *J Surg Oncol* 2005;89(3):193–201.
124. Elert O, Buchwald J, Wolf K. Epithelial thymus tumors—therapy and prognosis. *Thorac Cardiovasc Surg* 1988;36(2):109–113.
125. Eng TY, Fuller CD, Jagirdar J, et al. Thymic carcinoma: state of the art review. *Int J Radiat Oncol Biol Phys* 2004;59(3):654–664.
126. Engels EA, Pfeiffer RM. Malignant thymoma in the United States: demographic patterns in incidence and associations with subsequent malignancies. *Int J Cancer* 2003;105(4):546–551.
127. Evoli A, Batocchi AP, Provenzano C, et al. Thymectomy in the treatment of myasthenia gravis: report of 247 patients. *J Neurol* 1988;235(5):272–276.
128. Fallahnejad M, Harrell D, Tucker J, et al. Chondrosarcoma of the trachea. Report of a case and five-year follow-up. *J Thorac Cardiovasc Surg* 1973;65(2): 210–213.
129. Farrell ML, Gluckman JL, Biddinger P. Tracheal chondrosarcoma: a case report. *Head Neck* 1998;20(6):568–572.
130. Ferdinand B, Gupta P, Kramer EL. Spectrum of thymic uptake at 18F-FDG PET. *Radiographics* 2004;24(6):1611–1616.
131. Ferner RE, Gutmann DH, Ferner RE, et al. International consensus statement on malignant peripheral nerve sheath tumors in neurofibromatosis. *Cancer Res* 2002;62(5):1573–1577.
132. Fields JN, Rigaud G, Emami BN. Primary tumors of the trachea. Results of radiation therapy. *Cancer* 1989;63(12):2429–2433.
133. Filatova NM. [Cancer of trachea presenting as bronchial asthma]. *Vrach Delo* 1977;5:58–59.
134. Finn WG, Goolsby CL, Rao MS. DNA flow cytometric analysis of hemangiopericytoma. *Am J Clin Pathol* 1994;101(2):181–185.
135. Fizazi K, Culine S, Droz JP, et al. Initial management of primary mediastinal seminoma: radiotherapy or cisplatin-based chemotherapy? *Eur J Cancer* 1998;34(3):347–352.
136. Fornasiero A, Daniele O, Ghiotto C, et al. Chemotherapy for invasive thymoma. A 13-year experience. *Cancer* 1991;68(1):30–33.
137. Fornasiero A, Daniele O, Ghiotto C, et al. Chemotherapy of invasive thymoma. *J Clin Oncol* 1990;8(8):1419–1423.
138. Fraser RS, PJ, Fraser RG, et al. The normal chest. In: Pare JAP, FG Fraser, eds. *Synopsis of diseases of the chest*. Philadelphia: W.B. Saunders,1994;1–116.
139. Friedman NB. The comparative morphogenesis of extragenital and gonadal teratoid tumors. *Cancer* 1951;4(2):265–276.
140. Fujimura S, Kondo T, Handa M, et al. Results of surgical treatment for thymoma based on 66 patients. *J Thorac Cardiovasc Surg* 1987;93(5):708–714.
141. Fuwa N, Ito Y, Matsumoto A, et al. The treatment results of 40 patients with localized endobronchial cancer with external beam irradiation and intraluminal irradiation using low dose rate (192)Ir thin wires with a new catheter. *Radiother Oncol* 2000;56(2):189–195.
142. Gaissert HA, Grillo HC, Shadmehr MB, et al. Long-term survival after resection of primary adenoid cystic and squamous cell carcinoma of the trachea and carina. *Ann Thorac Surg* 2004;78(6):1889–1896; discussion 1896–1897.
143. Gaissert HA, Grillo HC, Shadmehr MB, et al. Uncommon primary tracheal tumors. *Ann Thorac Surg* 2006;82(1):268–272; discussion 272–273.
144. Gaissert HA. Primary tracheal tumors. *Chest Surg Clin North Am* 2003;13(2):247–256.

145. Gale AW, Jelihovsky T, Grant AF, et al. Neurogenic tumors of the mediastinum. *Ann Thorac Surg* 1974;17(5):434–443.
146. Gamondes JP, Balawi A, Greenland T, et al. Seventeen years of surgical treatment of thymoma: factors influencing survival. *Eur J Cardiothorac Surg* 1991;5(3):124–131.
147. Gamsu G, Webb WR. Computed tomography of the trachea: normal and abnormal. *AJR Am J Roentgenol* 1982;139(2):321–326.
148. Ganjoo KN, Chan RJ, Sharma M, et al. Positron emission tomography scans in the evaluation of postchemotherapy residual masses in patients with seminoma. *J Clin Oncol* 1999;17(11):3457–3460.
149. Ganjoo KN, Rieger KM, Kesler KA, et al. Results of modern therapy for patients with mediastinal nonseminomatous germ cell tumors. *Cancer* 2000;88(5):1051–1056.
150. Gawrychowski J, RM, Gabriel A, et al. Thymoma—the usefulness of some prognostic factors for diagnosis and surgical treatment. *Eur J Surg Oncol* 2000;26:203–208.
151. Giaccone G, Ardizzoni A, Kirkpatrick A, et al. Cisplatin and etoposide combination chemotherapy for locally advanced or metastatic thymoma. A phase II study of the European Organization for Research and Treatment of Cancer Lung Cancer Cooperative Group. *J Clin Oncol* 1996;14(3):814–820.
152. Ginsberg RJ. Mediastinal germ cell tumors: the role of surgery. *Semin Thorac Cardiovasc Surg* 1992;4(1):51–54.
153. Goldel N, Boning L, Fredrik A, et al. Chemotherapy of invasive thymoma. A retrospective study of 22 cases. *Cancer* 1989;63(8):1493–1500.
154. Gonzales DG. The need for clinical studies in thymomas. *Radiother Oncol* 1991;21:75–76.
155. Green N, Kulber H, Landman M, et al. The experience with definitive irradiation of clinically limited squamous cell cancer of the trachea. *Int J Radiat Oncol Biol Phys* 1985;11(7):1401–1405.
156. Greene MA, Malias MA. Aggressive multimodality treatment of invasive thymic carcinoma. *J Thorac Cardiovasc Surg* 2003;125(2):434–436.
157. Grillo HC, Mathisen DJ, Wain JC Management of tumors of the trachea. *Oncology (Williston Park)* 1992;6(2):61–67; discussion 68, 70, 72.
158. Grillo HC, Mathisen DJ. Cervical exenteration. *Ann Thorac Surg* 1990;49(3):401–408; discussion 408–409.
159. Grillo HC, Mathisen DJ. Primary tracheal tumors: treatment and results. *Ann Thorac Surg* 1990;49(1):69–77.
160. Grillo HC. Management of tracheal tumors. *Am J Surg* 1982;143(6):697–700.
161. Grillo HC. New methods for the treatment of tracheal tumors. *Gp* 1965;32(6):78–85.
162. Grillo HC. Primary tracheal tumours. *Thorax* 1993;48(7):681–682.
163. Grosfeld JL, Skinner MA, Rescorla FJ, et al. Mediastinal tumors in children: experience with 196 cases. *Ann Surg Oncol* 1994;1(2):121–127.
164. Grosfeld JL, Weinberger M, Kilman JW, et al. Primary mediastinal neoplasms in infants and children. *Ann Thorac Surg* 1971;12(2):179–190.
165. Grosfeld JL. Primary tumors of the chest wall and mediastinum in children. *Semin Thorac Cardiovasc Surg* 1994;6(4):235–239.
166. Guha A, Lau N, Huvar I, et al. Ras-GTP levels are elevated in human NF1 peripheral nerve tumors. *Oncogene* 1996;12(3):507–513.
167. Hailemariam S, Engeler DS, Bannwart F, et al. Primary mediastinal germ cell tumor with intratubular germ cell neoplasia of the testis—further support for germ cell origin of these tumors: a case report. *Cancer* 1997;79(5):1031–1036.
168. Hainsworth JD, Einhorn LH, Williams SD, et al. Advanced extragonadal germ-cell tumors. Successful treatment with combination chemotherapy. *Ann Intern Med* 1982;97(1):7–11.
169. Hainsworth JD, Greco FA. Extragonadal germ cell tumors and unrecognized germ cell tumors. *Semin Oncol* 1992;19(2):119–127.
170. Hainsworth JD, Greco FA. Germ cell neoplasms and other malignancies of the mediastinum. *Cancer Treat Res* 2001;105:303–325.
171. Hainsworth JD, Hainsworth JD. Diagnosis, staging, and clinical characteristics of the patient with mediastinal germ cell carcinoma. *Chest Surg Clin North Am* 2002;12(4):665–672.
172. Haniuda M, Miyazawa M, Yoshida K, et al. Is postoperative radiotherapy for thymoma effective? *Ann Surg* 1996;224(2):219–224.
173. Haniuda M, Morimoto M, Nishimura H, et al. Adjuvant radiotherapy after complete resection of thymoma. *Ann Thorac Surg* 1992;54(2):311–315.
174. Harkin JC. Pathology of nerve sheath tumors. *Ann N Y Acad Sci* 1986;486:147–154.
175. Hemmer WD, Latz H, Becker et al., Treatment of primary tracheal carcinoma. The role of external and endoluminal radiotherapy. *Strahlenther Onkol* 2000. 176(1). p. 22–7.
176. Hartmann CA, Roth C, Minck C, et al. Thymic carcinoma. Report of five cases and review of the literature. *J Cancer Res Clin Oncol* 1990;116(1):69.
177. Hartmann JT, Nichols CR, Droz JP, et al. Hematologic disorders associated with primary mediastinal nonseminomatous germ cell tumors. *J Natl Cancer Inst* 2000;92(1):54–61.
178. Hartmann JT, Schmoll HJ, Kuczyk MA, et al. Postchemotherapy resections of residual masses from metastatic non-seminomatous testicular germ cell tumors. *Ann Oncol* 1997;8(6):531–538.
179. Harvey JC, Keen CW, Makowka L, et al. Adenocarcinoma of the trachea: palliative response to cobalt-60 irradiation. *Can J Surg* 1979;22(3):268–270.
180. Havlicek F, Rosai A. A sarcoma of thymic stroma with features of liposarcoma. *Am J Clin Pathol* 1984;82(2):217–224.
181. Hayashi A, Takamori S, Tayama K, et al. Primary hemangiopericytoma of the superior mediastinum: a case report. *Ann Thorac Cardiovasc Surg* 1998;4(5):283–285.
182. Hernandez-Ilizaliturri FJ, Tan D, Cipolla D, et al. Multimodality therapy for thymic carcinoma (TCA): results of a 30-year single-institution experience. *Am J Clin Oncol* 2004;27(1):68–72.
183. Herr HW, Sheinfeld J, Puc HS, et al. Surgery for a post-chemotherapy residual mass in seminoma. *J Urol* 1997;157(3):860–862.
184. Hetzel MR. Tracheal tumours: could treatment be better? *Clin Oncol (R Coll Radiol)* 1993;5(5):272–276.
185. Hidalgo M, Paz-Ares L, Rivera F, et al. Mediastinal non-seminomatous germ cell tumours (MNSGCT) treated with cisplatin-based combination chemotherapy. *Ann Oncol* 1997;8(6):555–559.
186. Highley M, Underhill CR, Parnis FX, et al. Treatment of invasive thymoma with single agent ifosfamide. *J Clin Oncol* 1999;17(9):2737–2744.
187. Hiraki A, Murakami T, Aoe K, et al. Recurrent superior mediastinal primary hemangiopericytoma 23 years after the complete initial excision: a case report. *Acta Med Okayama* 2006;60(3):197–200.
188. Ho FC, Fu KH, Lam SY, et al. Evaluation of a histogenetic classification for thymic epithelial tumours. *Histopathology* 1994;25(1):21–29.
189. Ho KL, Rassekh ZS. Rhabdomyosarcoma of the trachea: first reported case. *Hum Pathol* 1980;11[5 Suppl]:572–574.
190. Honings J, van Dijck JA, Verhagen AF, et al. Incidence and treatment of tracheal cancer: a nationwide study in the Netherlands. *Ann Surg Oncol* 2006;.
191. Houston HE, Payne WS, Harrison EG Jr., et al. Primary cancers of the trachea. *Arch Surg* 1969;99(2):132–140.
192. Howling SJ, Flint JD, Muller NL. Thymoliposarcoma: CT and pathologic findings. *Clin Radiol* 1999;54(5):341.
193. Hsu HC, Huang EY, Wang CJ, et al. Postoperative radiotherapy in thymic carcinoma: treatment results and prognostic factors. *Int J Radiat Oncol Biol Phys* 2002;52(3):801–805.
194. Hulka GF, Rothschild MA, Warner BW, et al. Carcinoid tumor of the trachea in a pediatric patient. *Otolaryngol Head Neck Surg* 1996;114(6):822–825.
195. Hurt RD, Bruckman JE, Farrow GM, et al. Primary anterior mediastinal seminoma. *Cancer* 1982;49(8):1658–1663.
196. Huson SM, Compston DA, Clark P, et al. A genetic study of von Recklinghausen neurofibromatosis in south east Wales. I. Prevalence, fitness, mutation rate, and effect of parental transmission on severity. *J Med Genet* 1989;26(11):704–711.
197. Huson SM, Harper PS, Compston DA. Von Recklinghausen neurofibromatosis. A clinical and population study in south-east Wales. *Brain* 1988;111(Pt 6):1355–1381.
198. Inoue H. [Long-term prognosis of adenoid cystic carcinoma of the trachea]. *Kyobu Geka* 1991;44(13):1121–1125.
199. Ipakchi R, Zager WH, de Baca ME, et al. Granular cell tumor of the trachea in pregnancy: a case report and review of literature. *Laryngoscope* 2004;114(1):143–147.
200. Israel A, Bosl GJ, Golbey RB, et al. The results of chemotherapy for extragonadal germ-cell tumors in the cisplatin era: the Memorial Sloan-Kettering Cancer Center experience (1975 to 1982). *J Clin Oncol* 1985;3(8):1073–1078.
201. Jackson MA, Ball DL. Post-operative radiotherapy in invasive thymoma. *Radiother Oncol* 1991;21(2):77.
202. Janower ML, Grillo HC, MacMillan AS Jr., et al. The radiological appearance of carcinoma of the trachea. *Radiology* 1970;96(1):39–43.
203. Jaretzki A 3rd, Wolff M. "Maximal" thymectomy for myasthenia gravis. Surgical anatomy and operative technique. *J Thorac Cardiovasc Surg* 1988;96(5):711–716.
204. Javadpour N The value of biologic markers in diagnosis and treatment of testicular cancer. *Semin Oncol* 1979;6(1):37–47.
205. Jensen MO, Antonenko D. Thyroid and thymic malignancy following childhood irradiation. *J Surg Oncol* 1992;50(3):206–208.
206. Jeremic B, Shibamoto Y, Acimovic L, et al. Radiotherapy for primary squamous cell carcinoma of the trachea. *Radiother Oncol* 1996;41(2):135–138.
207. Jobard P, Vandooren M, Baudouin J, et al. [Granular cell tumor of the trachea]. *Laval Med* 1966;37(5):602–604.
208. Johnson DW, Klazynski PT, Gordon WH, et al. Mediastinal lymphangioma and chylothorax: the role of radiotherapy. *Ann Thorac Surg* 1986;41(3):325–328.
209. Jones WG, Fossa SD, Mead GM, et al. Randomized trial of 30 versus 20 Gy in the adjuvant treatment of stage I testicular seminoma: a report on Medical Research Council Trial TE18, European Organisation for the Research and Treatment of Cancer Trial 30942 (ISRCTN18525328). *J Clin Oncol* 2005;23(6):1200–1208.
210. Jortay AM, Bisschop P. Chondroma of the trachea. *Acta Otorhinolaryngol Belg* 1998;52(3):247–251.
211. Jose B, Yu AT, Morgan TF, et al. Malignant thymoma with extrathoracic metastasis: a case report and review of literature. *J Surg Oncol* 1980;15(3):259–263.
212. Jung KJ, Lee KS, Han J, et al. Malignant thymic epithelial tumors: CT-pathologic correlation. *AJR Am J Roentgenol* 2001;176(2):433–439.
213. Kageyama M, Seto H, Shimizu M, et al. Thallium-201 single photon emission computed tomography in the evaluation of thymic carcinoma. *Radiat Med* 1994;12(5):237–239.
214. Kaiser LR, Martini N. Clinical management of thymomas: the Memorial Sloan-Kettering Cancer Center experience. In: Martini N, Vogt-Moykopf I, eds. *Thoracic surgery: frontiers and uncommon neoplasms*, Vol. 5. St. Louis: Mosby, 1989;176–183.
215. Kallenbach J, Song E, Zwi S. Haemoptysis with no radiological evidence of tumour—the value of early bronchoscopy. *S Afr Med J* 1981;59(16):556–558.
216. Kandil A, Rostom AY, Mourad WA, et al. Successful control of extensive thoracic lymphangiomatosis by irradiation. *Clin Oncol (R Coll Radiol)* 1997;9(6):407–411.
217. Kantoff P. Surgical and medical management of germ cell tumors of the chest. *Chest* 1993;103[4 Suppl]:331S–333S.
218. Kara M, Ozkan M, Dizbay Sak S, et al. Successful removal of a giant recurrent mediastinal liposarcoma involving both hemithoraces. *Eur J Cardiothorac Surg* 2001;20(3):647–649.
219. Karlan MS, Livingston PA, Baker DC Jr. Diagnosis of tracheal tumors. *Ann Otol Rhinol Laryngol* 1973;82(6):790–799.
220. Kay PH, Wells FC, Goldstraw P. A multidisciplinary approach to primary nonseminomatous germ cell tumors of the mediastinum. *Ann Thorac Surg* 1987;44(6):578–582.
221. Keeley JL, Gumbiner SH, Guzauskus AC, et al. Mediastinal lipoma; the successful removal of 1,700 gram mass; case report and review of recent literature of intrathoracic lipomas. *J Thorac Surg* 1953;25(3):316–323.
222. Keeley JL, Vana AJ. Lipomas of the mediastinum; 1940 to 1955. *Surg Gynecol Obstet* 1956;103(4):313–322.
223. Kendall SW, Williams EA, Hunt JB, et al. Recurrent primary liposarcoma of the pericardium: management by repeated resections. *Ann Thorac Surg* 1993;56(3):560–562.
224. Kersh CR, Eisert DR, Constable WC, et al. Primary malignant mediastinal germ-cell tumors and the contribution of radiotherapy: a southeastern multi-institutional study. *Am J Clin Oncol* 1987;10(4):302–306.
225. Kilman JW, Klassen KP. Thymoma. *Am J Surg* 1971;121(6):710–711.
226. Kim DJ, Yang WI, Choi SS, et al. Prognostic and clinical relevance of the World Health Organization schema for the classification of thymic epithelial tumors: a clinicopathologic study of 108 patients and literature review. *Chest* 2005;127(3):755–761.
227. Kim ES, Putnam JB, Komaki R, et al. Phase II study of a multidisciplinary

approach with induction chemotherapy, followed by surgical resection, radiation therapy, and consolidation chemotherapy for unresectable malignant thymomas: final report. *Lung Cancer* 2004;44(3):369–379.
228. King DF, Hirose FM, Gurevitch AW, et al. Lymphangiosarcoma following radiation therapy. *J Am Acad Dermatol* 1986;14(4):684.
229. Kintanar EB, Giordano TJ, Thompson NW, et al. Granular-cell tumor of trachea masquerading as Hurthle-cell neoplasm on fine-needle aspirate: a case report. *Diagn Cytopathol* 2000;22(6):379–382.
230. Kiriyama M, Masaoka A, Yamakawa Y, et al. Chondrosarcoma originating from the trachea. *Ann Thorac Surg* 1997;63(6):1772–1773.
231. Kirschner PA. Reoperation for thymoma: report of 23 cases. *Ann Thorac Surg* 1990;49(4):550.
232. Kitami A, Suzuki T, Suzuki S, et al. Effective treatment of thymic carcinoma with operation and combination chemotherapy against acute monocyte leukemia: case report and review of the literature. *Jpn J Clin Oncol* 1998;28(9):555–558.
233. Klemm KM, Moran CA. Primary neuroendocrine carcinomas of the thymus. *Semin Diagn Pathol* 1999;16(1):32–41.
234. Klimstra DS, Moran CA, Perino G, et al. Liposarcoma of the anterior mediastinum and thymus. A clinicopathologic study of 28 cases. *Am J Surg Pathol* 1995;19(7):782–791.
235. Knapp RH, Hurt RD, Payne WS, et al. Malignant germ cell tumors of the mediastinum. *J Thorac Cardiovasc Surg* 1985;89(1):82–89.
236. Kobayashi H, Nemoto Y, Namiki K, et al. Primary malignant lymphoma of the trachea and subglottic region. *Intern Med* 1992;31(5):655–658.
237. Kobayashi Y, Fujii Y, Yano M, et al. Preoperative steroid pulse therapy for invasive thymoma: clinical experience and mechanism of action. *Cancer* 2006;106(9):1901–1907.
238. Kohman LJ. Controversies in the management of malignant thymoma. *Chest* 1997;112[4 Suppl]:296S–300S.
239. Kohno N, Tateno H, Kawaida M, et al. Primary adenoid cystic carcinoma of the trachea: a case report of a twelve year survivor. *Keio J Med* 1995;44(1):30–32.
240. Koikkalainen K, Keskitalo E, Luosto R, et al. Carcinoid tumours and cylindromas of the tracheobronchial tree. *Ann Chir Gynaecol Fenn* 1974;63(4):332–341.
241. Koizumi T, Takabayashi Y, Yamagishi S, et al. Chemotherapy for advanced thymic carcinoma: clinical response to cisplatin, doxorubicin, vincristine, and cyclophosphamide (ADOC chemotherapy). *Am J Clin Oncol* 2002;25(3):266–268.
242. Kondo K, Monden Y. [Thymic carcinoma]. *Kyobu Geka* 2002;55[8 Suppl]:701–708.
243. Kondo K, Monden Y. Lymphogenous and hematogenous metastasis of thymic epithelial tumors. *Ann Thorac Surg* 2003;76(6):1859–1864; discussion 1864–1865.
244. Kondo K, Monden Y. Therapy for thymic epithelial tumors: a clinical study of 1,320 patients from Japan. *Ann Thorac Surg* 2003;76(3):878–884; discussion 884–885.
245. Kondo K, Monden Y. Thymoma and myasthenia gravis: a clinical study of 1,089 patients from Japan. *Ann Thorac Surg* 2005;79(1):219–224.
246. Kondo K, Yoshizawa K, Tsuyuguchi M, et al. WHO histologic classification is a prognostic indicator in thymoma. *Ann Thorac Surg* 2004;77(4):1183.
247. Kononov EP. [Carcinoid of the trachea]. *Zh Ushn Nos Gorl Bolezn* 1967;27(5):104.
248. Kornstein MJ, Curran WJ Jr., Turrisi AT 3rd, et al. Cortical versus medullary thymomas: a useful morphologic distinction? *Hum Pathol* 1988;19(11):1335–1339.
249. Kruger M, Uschinsky K, Engelmann C. [Surgical treatment of malignant thoracic schwannomas]. *Zentralbl Chir* 2001;126(3):223–228.
250. Kubota K, Yamada S, Kondo T, et al. PET imaging of primary mediastinal tumours. *Br J Cancer* 1996;73(7):882–886.
251. Kuhn MW, Weissbach L. Localization, incidence, diagnosis and treatment of extratesticular germ cell tumors. *Urol Int* 1985;40(3):166–172.
252. Kurup A, Loehrer PJ Sr. Thymoma and thymic carcinoma: therapeutic approaches. *Clin Lung Cancer* 2004;6(1):28–32.
253. Kushihashi T, Fujisawa H, Munechika H. Magnetic resonance imaging of thymic epithelial tumors. *Crit Rev Diagn Imaging* 1996;37(3):191–259.
254. Lam WW, Chan FL, Lau YL, et al. Paediatric thymoma: unusual occurrence in two siblings. *Pediatr Radiol* 1993;23(2):124–126.
255. Landwehr P, Schulte O, Lackner K. MR imaging of the chest: mediastinum and chest wall. *Eur Radiol* 1999;9(9):1737–1744.
256. Lara PN Jr. Malignant thymoma: current status and future directions. *Cancer Treat Rev* 2000;26(2):127–131.
257. Lardinois D, Rechsteiner R, Lang RH, et al. Prognostic relevance of Masaoka and Müller-Hermelink classification in patients with thymic tumors. *Ann Thorac Surg* 2000;69(5):1550–1555.
258. Larsson S, Cardillo G, Lepore V. Surgical management of tracheal tumours. *Scand J Thorac Cardiovasc Surg* 1987;21(2):97–103.
259. Larsson S, Lepore V, Cardillo G, et al. Primary tracheal rhabdomyosarcoma. Case report. *Scand J Thorac Cardiovasc Surg* 1989;23(3):293–295.
260. Lastoria S, Vergara E, Palmieri G, et al. In vivo detection of malignant thymic masses by indium-111-DTPA-D-Phe1-octreotide scintigraphy. *J Nucl Med* 1998;39(4):634–639.
261. Lee CH, Lin HC. Descriptive study of prognostic factors influencing survival of patients with primary tracheal tumors. *Changgeng Yi Xue Za Zhi* 1995;18(3):224–230.
262. Lee JD. CT findings in primary thymic carcinoma. *J Comput Assist Tomogr* 1991; 15:429–433.
263. Lee JY, Lee KS, Han J, et al. Spectrum of neurogenic tumors in the thorax: CT and pathologic findings. *J Comput Assist Tomogr* 1999;23(3):399–406.
264. Legg MA, Brady WJ. Pathology and clinical behavior of thymomas. a survey of 51 cases. *Cancer* 1965;18:1131–1144.
265. LeGolvan DP, Abell MR. Thymomas. *Cancer* 1977;39(5):2142–2157.
266. Lemarie E, Assouline PS, Diot P, et al. Primary mediastinal germ cell tumors. Results of a French retrospective study. *Chest* 1992;102(5):1477–1483.
267. Lemarie E, Lemarie E. [Malignant germinal tumours of the mediastinum: diagnosis and treatment]. *Rev Pneumol Clin* 2004;60(5 Pt 2):3S79–85.
268. Leonova LA, Mel'nikova VG. [Cancer of the trachea simulating bronchial asthma]. *Vrach Delo* 1972;4:107–108.
269. Levitt RG, Husband JE, Glazer HS. CT of primary germ-cell tumors of the mediastinum. *AJR Am J Roentgenol* 1984;142(1):73–78.
270. Lewis BD, Hurt RD, Payne WS, et al. Benign teratomas of the mediastinum. *J Thorac Cardiovasc Surg* 1983;86(5):727–731.
271. Lewis JE, Wick MR, Scheithauer BW, et al. Thymoma. A clinicopathologic review. *Cancer* 1987;60(11):2727–2743.
272. Licht PB, Friis S, Pettersson G. Tracheal cancer in Denmark: a nationwide study. *Eur J Cardiothorac Surg* 2001;19(3):339–345.
273. Lim LC, Tan MH, Eng C, et al. Thymic carcinoid in multiple endocrine neoplasia 1: genotype-phenotype correlation and prevention. *J Intern Med* 2006;259(4):428–432.
274. Lin FC, Lin CM, Hsieh CC, et al. Atypical thymic carcinoid and malignant somatostatinoma in type I multiple endocrine neoplasia syndrome: case report. *Am J Clin Oncol* 2003;26(3):270–272.
275. Lin JT, Wei-Shu W, Yen CC, et al. Stage IV thymic carcinoma: a study of 20 patients. *Am J Med Sci* 2005;330(4):172–175.
276. Littler ER. Asphyxia due to hemangioma in trachea. *J Thorac Cardiovasc Surg* 1963;45:552–558.
277. Liu HP, Yim AP, Wan J, et al. Thoracoscopic removal of intrathoracic neurogenic tumors: a combined Chinese experience. *Ann Surg* 2000;232(2):187–190.
278. Liu RS, Yeh SH, Huang MH, et al. Use of fluorine-18 fluorodeoxyglucose positron emission tomography in the detection of thymoma: a preliminary report. *Eur J Nucl Med* 1995;22(12):1402–1407.
279. Llombart-Bosch A, Peydro-Olaya A, Paris-Romeu F. Fine structure of a malignant hemangioendothelioma of the esophagus. *Virchows Arch* 1981;391(1):107–115.
280. Loehrer PJ Sr., Chen M, Kim K, et al. Cisplatin, doxorubicin, and cyclophosphamide plus thoracic radiation therapy for limited-stage unresectable thymoma: an intergroup trial. *J Clin Oncol* 1997;15(9):3093–3099.
281. Loehrer PJ Sr., Jiroutek M, Aisner S, et al. Combined etoposide, ifosfamide, and cisplatin in the treatment of patients with advanced thymoma and thymic carcinoma: an intergroup trial. *Cancer* 2001;91(11):2010–2015.
282. Loehrer PJ Sr., Kim K, Aisner SC, et al. Cisplatin plus doxorubicin plus cyclophosphamide in metastatic or recurrent thymoma: final results of an intergroup trial. The Eastern Cooperative Oncology Group, Southwest Oncology Group, and Southeastern Cancer Study Group. *J Clin Oncol* 1994;12(6):1164–1168.
283. Loehrer PJ Sr., Wang W, Johnson DH, et al. Octreotide alone or with prednisone in patients with advanced thymoma and thymic carcinoma: an Eastern Cooperative Oncology Group phase II trial. *J Clin Oncol* 2004;22(2):293–299.
284. Logothetis CJ, Samuels ML, Selig DE, et al. Chemotherapy of extragonadal germ cell tumors. *J Clin Oncol* 1985;3(3):316–325.
285. Low SY, Eng P, Thirugnanam A. Primary endotracheal neurogenic tumors. *Surg Endosc* 2004;18(2):348.
286. Lucchi M, Ambrogi MC, Duranti L, et al. Advanced stage thymomas and thymic carcinomas: results of multimodality treatments. *Ann Thorac Surg* 2005;79(6):1840–1844.
287. Lucchi M, Mussi A, Basolo F, et al. The multimodality treatment of thymic carcinoma. *Eur J Cardiothorac Surg* 2001;19(5):566–569.
288. Luna MA, Valenzuela-Tamariz J. Germ-cell tumors of the mediastinum, postmortem findings. *Am J Clin Pathol* 1976;65(4):450–454.
289. Macchiarini P, Chella A, Ducci F, et al. Neoadjuvant chemotherapy, surgery, and postoperative radiation therapy for invasive thymoma. *Cancer* 1991;68(4):706–713.
290. Macchiarini P, Ostertag H. Uncommon primary mediastinal tumours. *Lancet Oncol* 2004;5(2):107–118.
291. Macchiarini P. Primary tracheal tumours. *Lancet Oncol* 2006;7(1):83–91.
292. Madhumita K, Sreekumar KP, Malini H, et al. Tracheal haemangioma: case report. *J Laryngol Otol* 2004;118(8):655–658.
293. Maggi G, Casadio C, Cavallo A, et al. Thymoma: results of 241 operated cases. *Ann Thorac Surg* 1991;51(1):152–156.
294. Maggi G, Giaccone G, Donadio M, et al. Thymomas. A review of 169 cases, with particular reference to results of surgical treatment. *Cancer* 1986;58(3):765–776.
295. Maier HC. Hemangiomas of the subglottic region, trachea, and mediastinum in infancy and childhood. *Ann Thorac Surg* 1967;3(6):514–525.
296. Maish M, Vaporciyan AA. Chondrosarcoma arising in the trachea: a case report and review of the literature. *J Thorac Cardiovasc Surg* 2003;126(6):2077–2080.
297. Makarewicz R, Mross M. Radiation therapy alone in the treatment of tumours of the trachea. *Lung Cancer* 1998;20(3):169–174.
298. Mangi AA, Wain JC, Donahue DM, et al. Adjuvant radiation of stage III thymoma: is it necessary? *Ann Thorac Surg* 2005;79(6):1834–1839.
299. Mangi AA, Wright CD, Allan JS, et al. Adjuvant radiation therapy for stage II thymoma. *Ann Thorac Surg* 2002;74(4):1033–1037.
300. Manninen MP, Pukander JS, Flander MK, et al. Treatment of primary tracheal carcinoma in Finland in 1967–1985. *Acta Oncol* 1993;32(3):277–282.
301. Manninen MP. Symptoms and signs and their prognostic value in tracheal carcinoma. *Eur Arch Otorhinolaryngol* 1993;250(7):383–386.
302. Marchevsky AM, Kaneko M, Cohen BA. *Surgical pathology of the mediastinum. New York: Raven,* 1984;xi.
303. Martini N, Golbey RB, Hajdu SI, et al. Primary mediastinal germ cell tumors. *Cancer* 1974;33(3):763–769.
304. Masaoka A, Monden Y, Nakahara K, et al. Follow-up study of thymomas with special reference to their clinical stages. *Cancer* 1981;48(11):2485–2492.
305. Masaoka A, Yamakawa Y, Niwa H, et al. Thymectomy and malignancy. *Eur J Cardiothorac Surg* 1994;8(5):251–253.
306. Matani A, Dritsas C. Familial occurrence of thymoma. *Arch Pathol* 1973;95(2):90–91.
307. Mathisen DJ, Grillo HC. Endoscopic relief of malignant airway obstruction. *Ann Thorac Surg* 1989;48(4):469–473; discussion 473–475.
308. Mathisen DJ. Primary tracheal tumor management. *Surg Oncol Clin North Am* 1999;8(2):307.
309. Mathisen DJ. Tracheal tumors. *Chest Surg Clin North Am* 1996;6(4):875–898.
310. Matsuo T, Kinoshita S, Iwasaki K, et al. Chondrosarcoma of the trachea. A case report and literature review. *Acta Cytol* 1988;32(6):908–912.
311. Mayer R, Beham-Schmid C, Groell R, et al. Radiotherapy for invasive thymoma and thymic carcinoma. Clinicopathological review. *Strahlenther Onkol* 1999;175(6):271–278.
312. Maziak DE, Todd TR, Keshavjee SH, et al. Adenoid cystic carcinoma of the airway: thirty-two-year experience. *J Thorac Cardiovasc Surg* 1996;112(6):1522–1531; discussion 1531–1532.
313. McCart JA, Gaspar L, Inculet R, et al. Predictors of survival following surgical resection of thymoma. *J Surg Oncol* 1993;54(4):233–238.
314. McCarthy MJ, Rosado-de-Christenson ML. Tumors of the trachea. *J Thorac Imag* 1995;10(3):180–198.
315. McGaughran JM, Harris DI, Donnai D, et al. A clinical study of type 1 neurofibromatosis in north west England. *J Med Genet* 1999;36(3):197–203.

316. McGuire LJ, Huang DP, Teoh R, et al. Epstein-Barr virus genome in thymoma and thymic lymphoid hyperplasia. *Am J Pathol* 1988;131(3):385–390.
317. McKenzie GE, Rezek PR. Myosarcoma of trachea associated with Riedel struma. *AMA Arch Otolaryngol* 1953;57(1):22–39.
318. McMaster MJ, Soule EH, Ivins JC. Hemangiopericytoma. A clinicopathologic study and long-term follow-up of 60 patients. *Cancer* 1975;36(6):2232–2244.
319. Meyers BF, Mathisen DJ. Management of tracheal neoplasms. *Oncologist* 1997; 2(4):245–253.
320. Mikaelian DO, Cohn H, Israel H, et al. Granular cell tumor of the trachea. *Ann Otol Rhinol Laryngol* 1984;93(5 Pt 1):457–459.
321. Monden Y, Nakahara K, Iioka S, et al. Recurrence of thymoma: clinicopathological features, therapy, and prognosis. *Ann Thorac Surg* 1985;39(2):165–169.
322. Moore KH, McKenzie PR, Kennedy CW, et al. Thymoma: trends over time. *Ann Thorac Surg* 2001;72(1):203–207.
323. Moran CA, Travis WD, Rosado-de-Christenson M, et al. Thymomas presenting as pleural tumors. Report of eight cases. *Am J Surg Pathol* 1992;16(2):138–144.
324. Morgenthaler TI, Brown LR, Colby TV, et al. Thymoma. *Mayo Clin Proc* 1993; 68(11):1110–1123.
325. Mornex F, Coquard R, Danhier S, et al. Role of radiation therapy in the treatment of primary tracheal carcinoma. *Int J Radiat Oncol Biol Phys* 1998;41(2): 299–305.
326. Mornex F, Resbeut M, Richaud P, et al. Radiotherapy and chemotherapy for invasive thymomas: a multicentric retrospective review of 90 cases. The FNCLCC trialists. Federation Nationale des Centres de Lutte Contre le Cancer. *Int J Radiat Oncol Biol Phys* 1995;32(3):651–659.
327. Motzer R, Bosl G, Heelan R, et al. Residual mass: an indication for further therapy in patients with advanced seminoma following systemic chemotherapy. *J Clin Oncol* 1987;5(7):1064–1070.
328. Mulhollan TJ, Ro JY, el-Naggar AK, et al. Granular cell tumor of the biliary tree. *Am J Surg Pathol* 1992;16(2):204–206.
329. Mullen B, Richardson JD. Primary anterior mediastinal tumors in children and adults. *Ann Thorac Surg* 1986;42(3):338–345.
330. Müller-Hermelink HK, Marino M, Palestro G, et al. Immunohistological evidences of cortical and medullary differentiation in thymoma. *Virchows Arch* 1985;408(2–3):143–161.
331. Murakawa T, Nakajima J, Kohno T, et al. Results from surgical treatment for thymoma. 43 years of experience. *Jpn J Thorac Cardiovasc Surg* 2000;48(2):89–95.
332. Myojin M, Choi NC, Wright CD, et al. Stage III thymoma: pattern of failure after surgery and postoperative radiotherapy and its implication for future study. *Int J Radiat Oncol Biol Phys* 2000;46(4):927–933.
333. Nagaishi CUO, Nagasawa N. *Functional anatomy and histology of the lung*. Tokyo: Igaku Shoin, 1972.
334. Nakahara K, Ohno K, Hashimoto J, et al. Thymoma: results with complete resection and adjuvant postoperative irradiation in 141 consecutive patients. *J Thorac Cardiovasc Surg* 1988;95(6):1041–1047.
335. Nakamura Y, Kunitoh H, Kubota K, et al. Platinum-based chemotherapy with or without thoracic radiation therapy in patients with unresectable thymic carcinoma. *Jpn J Clin Oncol* 2000;30(9):385–388.
336. Nakano Y, Asakura K, Himi T, et al. Chondrosarcoma of larynx: a case successfully reconstructed after total cricoidectomy. *Auris Nasus Larynx* 1999;26(2):207–211.
337. Negron-Soto JM, Cascade PN. Squamous cell carcinoma of the thymus with paraneoplastic hypercalcemia. *Clin Imaging* 1995;19(2):122–124.
338. Nichols CR, Fox EP. Extragonadal and pediatric germ cell tumors. *Hematol Oncol Clin North Am* 1991;5(6):1189–1209.
339. Nichols CR, Heerema NA, Palmer C, et al. Klinefelter's syndrome associated with mediastinal germ cell neoplasms. *J Clin Oncol* 1987;5(8):1290–1294.
340. Nichols CR, Hoffman R, Einhorn LH, et al. Hematologic malignancies associated with primary mediastinal germ-cell tumors. *Ann Intern Med* 1985;102(5):603–609.
341. Nichols CR, Roth BJ, Heerema N, et al. Hematologic neoplasia associated with primary mediastinal germ-cell tumors. *N Engl J Med* 1990;322(20):1425–1429.
342. Nichols CR, Saxman S, Williams SD, et al. Primary mediastinal nonseminomatous germ cell tumors. A modern single institution experience. *Cancer* 1990;65(7): 1641–1646.
343. Nichols CR. Mediastinal germ cell tumors. *Semin Thorac Cardiovasc Surg* 1992; 4(1):45–50.
344. Nomimura T, Takahashi T, Kato Y, et al. [Mid mediastinal lipoma—a case report]. *Nippon Kyobu Geka Gakkai Zasshi* 1996;44(4):580–584.
345. Nonaka D, Klimstra D, Rosai J. Thymic mucoepidermoid carcinomas: a clinicopathologic study of 10 cases and review of the literature. *Am J Surg Pathol* 2004;28(11):1526–1531.
346. Nonaka T, Tamaki Y, Higuchi K, et al. The role of radiotherapy for thymic carcinoma. *Jpn J Clin Oncol* 2004;34(12):722–726.
347. Ogawa K, Toita T, Uno T, et al. Treatment and prognosis of thymic carcinoma: a retrospective analysis of 40 cases. *Cancer* 2002;94(12):3115–3119.
348. Ohara K, Okumura T, Sugahara S, et al. The role of preoperative radiotherapy for invasive thymoma. *Acta Oncol* 1990;29(4):425–429.
349. Okubo K, Kuwabara M, Ito K, et al. [A case of mediastinal fibrosarcoma]. *Nippon Kyobu Geka Gakkai Zasshi* 1995;43(2):221–225.
350. Okubo T, Okayasu T, Osaka Y, et al. [Surgical analysis of mediastinal lymphangioma—analysis of 7 cases]. *Nippon Kyobu Geka Gakkai Zasshi* 1992; 40(4):583–586.
351. Okumura M, Miyoshi S, Fujii Y, et al. Clinical and functional significance of WHO classification on human thymic epithelial neoplasms: a study of 146 consecutive tumors. *Am J Surg Pathol* 2001;25(1):103–110.
352. Okumura M, Miyoshi S, Takeuchi Y, et al. Results of surgical treatment of thymomas with special reference to the involved organs. *J Thorac Cardiovasc Surg* 1999;117(3):605–613.
353. Okumura M, Ohta M, Miyoshi S, et al. Oncological significance of WHO histological thymoma classification. A clinical study based on 286 patients. *Jpn J Thorac Cardiovasc Surg* 2002;50(5):189–194.
354. Okumura M, Ohta M, Tateyama H, et al. The World Health Organization histologic classification system reflects the oncologic behavior of thymoma: a clinical study of 273 patients. *Cancer* 2002;94(3):624–632.
355. Okumura M, Shiono H, Inoue M, et al. Outcome of surgical treatment for recurrent thymic epithelial tumors with reference to world health organization histologic classification system. *J Surg Oncol* 2007;95(1):40–44.
356. Osanai T, Kanazawa T, Nakamura K, et al. A case of primary cystic mediastinal hemangiopericytoma. *Arch Pathol Lab Med* 1994;118(5):575–577.
357. Outzen KE, Lunding J, Jakobsen J. Leiomyosarcoma of the trachea. *J Laryngol Otol* 1986;100(8):979–984.
358. Pachter MR, Lattes R. "Germinal" tumors of the mediastinum: a clinicopathologic study of adult teratomas, teratocarcinomas, choriocarcinomas and seminomas. *Dis Chest* 1964;45:301–310.
359. Pachter MR, Lattes R. Mesenchymal tumors of the mediastinum. I. Tumors of fibrous tissue, adipose tissue, smooth muscle, and striated muscle. *Cancer* 1963;16:74–94.
360. Pachter MR, Lattes R. Mesenchymal tumors of the mediastinum. II. Tumors of blood vascular origin. *Cancer* 1963;16:95–107.
361. Pachter MR, Lattes R. Mesenchymal tumors of the mediastinum. III. Tumors of lymph vascular origin. *Cancer* 1963;16:108–117.
362. Palmieri G, Lastoria S, Colao A, et al. Successful treatment of a patient with a thymoma and pure red-cell aplasia with octreotide and prednisone. *N Engl J Med* 1997;336(4):263–265.
363. Palmieri G, Montella L, Martignetti A, et al. Somatostatin analogs and prednisone in advanced refractory thymic tumors. *Cancer* 2002;94(5):1414–1420.
364. Pan CC, Wu HP, Yang CF, et al. The clinicopathological correlation of epithelial subtyping in thymoma: a study of 112 consecutive cases. *Hum Pathol* 1994;25(9):893–899.
365. Pant K, Bhagat R, Chawla R, et al. Primary carcinoid tumour of trachea. *Indian J Chest Dis Allied Sci* 1990;32(3):193–197.
366. Paris P. Mediastinal neural tumors, a report of 27 cases. *Diss Abstr Int [C]* 1991;52(3):418.
367. Park HS, Shin DM, Lee JS, et al. Thymoma. A retrospective study of 87 cases. *Cancer* 1994;73(10):2491–2498.
368. Park JG, Aubry MC, Godfrey JA, et al. Mediastinal lymphangioma: Mayo Clinic experience of 25 cases. *Mayo Clin Proc* 2006;81(9):1197–1203.
369. Park MS, Chung KY, Kim KD, et al. Prognosis of thymic epithelial tumors according to the new World Health Organization histologic classification. *Ann Thorac Surg* 2004;78(3):992–997; discussion 997–998.
370. Patterson GA. Thymomas. *Semin Thorac Cardiovasc Surg* 1992;4(1):39–44.
371. Pearson FG, Cooper JD. Experience with primary neoplasms of the trachea and carina. *Nippon Kyobu Geka Gakkai Zasshi* 1984;32(5):661–664.
372. Pearson FG, Thompson DW, Weissberg D, et al. Adenoid cystic carcinoma of the trachea. Experience with 16 patients managed by tracheal resection. *Ann Thorac Surg* 1974;18(1):16–29.
373. Pescarmona E, Rendina EA, Venuta F, et al. Analysis of prognostic factors and clinicopathological staging of thymoma. *Ann Thorac Surg* 1990;50(4):534–538.
374. Phillips TL, Buschke F. The role of radiation therapy in myasthenia gravis. *Calif Med* 1967;106(4):282–289.
375. Pogorzelski A, Zebrak J. [Tracheal hemangioma]. *Pediatr Pol* 1995;70(6):519–520.
376. Pollack A, Komaki R, Cox JD, et al. Thymoma: treatment and prognosis. *Int J Radiat Oncol Biol Phys* 1992;23(5):1037–1043.
377. Prommegger R, Salzer GM. Long-term results of surgery for adenoid cystic carcinoma of the trachea and bronchi. *Eur J Surg Oncol* 1998;24(5):440–444.
378. Puc HS, Heelan R, Mazumdar M, et al. Management of residual mass in advanced seminoma: results and recommendations from the Memorial Sloan-Kettering Cancer Center. *J Clin Oncol* 1996;14(2):454–460.
379. Quagliano PV. Thymic carcinoma: case reports and review. *J Thorac Imaging* 1996;11(1):66–74.
380. Quintanilla-Martinez L, Wilkins EW Jr., Choi N, et al. Thymoma. Histologic subclassification is an independent prognostic factor. *Cancer* 1994;74(2):606–617.
381. Rabkin I, Ovchinnikov VI, Tullo AL, et al. [Diagnosis of tumors of the trachea and main bronchi by computerized tomography]. *Vestn Rentgenol Radiol* 1993;3:5–9.
382. Ramsden D, Sheridan BF, Newton NC, et al. Adenoid cystic carcinoma of the head and neck: a report of 30 cases. *Aust N Z J Surg* 1973;43(2):102–108.
383. Raymond GS, Murray SK, Logan PM. Granular cell tumour of the trachea: case report. *Can Assoc Radiol J* 1997;48(1):48–50.
384. Rea F, Marulli G, Girardi R, et al. Long-term survival and prognostic factors in thymic epithelial tumours. *Eur J Cardiothorac Surg* 2004;26(2):412–418.
385. Rea F, Sartori F, Loy M, et al. Chemotherapy and operation for invasive thymoma. *J Thorac Cardiovasc Surg* 1993;106(3):543–549.
386. Reed JC, Hallet KK, Feigin DS. Neural tumors of the thorax: subject review from the AFIP. *Radiology* 1978;126(1):9–17.
387. Reeder LB. Neurogenic tumors of the mediastinum. *Semin Thorac Cardiovasc Surg* 2000;12(4):261–267.
388. Regnard JF, Fourquier P, Levasseur P. Results and prognostic factors in resections of primary tracheal tumors: a multicenter retrospective study. The French Society of Cardiovascular Surgery. *J Thorac Cardiovasc Surg* 1996;111(4):808–813; discussion 813–814.
389. Regnard JF, Magdeleinat P, Dromer C, et al. Prognostic factors and long-term results after thymoma resection: a series of 307 patients. *J Thorac Cardiovasc Surg* 1996;112(2):376–384.
390. Regnard JF, Zinzindohoue F, Magdeleinat P, et al. Results of re-resection for recurrent thymomas. *Ann Thorac Surg* 1997;64(6):1593–1598.
391. Rena O, Papalia E, Maggi G, et al. World Health Organization histologic classification: an independent prognostic factor in resected thymomas. *Lung Cancer* 2005;50(1):59–66.
392. Ribet M, Voisin C, Pruvot FR, et al. Lympho-epithelial thymomas. A retrospective study of 88 resections. *Eur J Cardiothorac Surg* 1988;2(4):261–264.
393. Ricci C, Rendina EA, Pescarmona EO, et al. Correlations between histological type, clinical behaviour, and prognosis in thymoma. *Thorax* 1989;44(6):455–460.
394. Rieker RJ, Hoegel J, Morresi-Hauf A, et al. Histologic classification of thymic epithelial tumors: comparison of established classification schemes. *Int J Cancer* 2002;98(6):900–906.
395. Ritter JH, Wick MR. Primary carcinomas of the thymus gland. *Semin Diagn Pathol* 1999;16(1):18–31.
396. Roncoroni AJ, Puy RJ, Goldman E, et al. Fibrosarcoma of the trachea with severe tracheal obstruction. *Thorax* 1973;28(6):777–781.
397. Rosai J, Higa E. Mediastinal endocrine neoplasm, of probable thymic origin, related to carcinoid tumor. Clinicopathologic study of 8 cases. *Cancer* 1972;29(4): 1061–1074.
398. Rosai J, Sobin LH. Histological typing of tumours of the thymus. In: Rosai J, Sobin L, eds. *WHO international histological classification of tumors*. Berlin, New York: Springer, 1999;9–14.

399. Rosenberg J. Neoplasms of the mediastinum. In: DeVita HS, VT Jr., Rosenberg SA, eds. *Cancer: principles and practice of oncology*. Philadelphia: Lippincott, 1989;706.
400. Rosenow EC 3rd, Hurley BT. Disorders of the thymus. A review. *Arch Intern Med* 1984;144(4):763–770.
401. Rostom AY, Morgan RL. Results of treating primary tumours of the trachea by irradiation. *Thorax* 1978;33(3):387–393.
402. Rotmensch S, Cole AL. False diagnosis and needless therapy of presumed malignant disease in women with false-positive human chorionic gonadotropin concentrations. *Lancet* 2000;355(9205):712–715.
403. Ruffini E, Mancuso M, Oliaro A, et al. Recurrence of thymoma: analysis of clinicopathologic features, treatment, and outcome. *J Thorac Cardiovasc Surg* 1997; 113(1):55–63.
404. Sagel SS, Aronberg DJ. Thoracic anatomy and mediastinum. In: Lee JKT, Sagel SS, Stanley RB, eds. *Computed body tomography*. New York: Raven Press, 1983;.
405. Saito H, Mizusawa A, Oketani N, et al. [Suspected leiomyosarcoma of the trachea]. *Nihon Kyobu Shikkan Gakkai Zasshi* 1997;35(4):420–425.
406. Sakai S, Murayama S, Soeda H, et al. Differential diagnosis between thymoma and non-thymoma by dynamic MR imaging. *Acta Radiol* 2002;43(3):262–268.
407. Salm R. Primary carcinoma of the trachea: a review. *Br J Dis Chest* 1964;58:61–72.
408. Salyer WR, Eggleston JC. Thymoma: a clinical and pathological study of 65 cases. *Cancer* 1976;37(1):229–249.
409. Santoro A, Tursz T, Mouridsen H, et al. Doxorubicin versus CYVADIC versus doxorubicin plus ifosfamide in first-line treatment of advanced soft tissue sarcomas: a randomized study of the European Organization for Research and Treatment of Cancer Soft Tissue and Bone Sarcoma Group. *J Clin Oncol* 1995;13(7):1537–1545.
410. Sasaki M, Kuwabara Y, Ichiya Y, et al. Differential diagnosis of thymic tumors using a combination of 11C-methionine PET and FDG PET. *J Nucl Med* 1999;40(10):1595–1601.
411. Saxman SB, Nichols CR, Einhorn LH. Salvage chemotherapy in patients with extragonadal nonseminomatous germ cell tumors: the Indiana University experience. *J Clin Oncol* 1994;12(7):1390–1393.
412. Schantz A, Sewall W, Castleman B. Mediastinal germinoma. A study of 21 cases with an excellent prognosis. *Cancer* 1972;30(5):1189–1194.
413. Schmidt R, Monig SP, Selzner M, et al. Surgical therapy of malignant thymoma. *J Cardiovasc Surg (Torino)* 1997;38(3):317–322.
414. Schraube P, Latz D, Wannenmacher M. Treatment of primary squamous cell carcinoma of the trachea: the role of radiation therapy. *Radiother Oncol* 1994; 33(3):254–258.
415. Schultz SM, Einhorn LH, Conces DJ Jr., et al. Management of postchemotherapy residual mass in patients with advanced seminoma: Indiana University experience. *J Clin Oncol* 1989;7(10):1497–1503.
416. Schulz MD, Schwab RS. Results of thymic (mediastinal) irradiation in patients with myasthenia gravis. *Ann N Y Acad Sci* 1971;183:303–307.
417. Sellors TH, Thackray AC, Thomson AD. Tumours of the thymus. A review of 88 operation cases. *Thorax* 1967;22(3):193–220.
418. Sennaroglu L, Sozeri B, Ataman M, et al. Malignant fibrous histiocytoma of the trachea. Case report. *Acta Otorhinolaryngol Belg* 1996;50(2):147–149.
419. Seto H, Kageyama M, Shimizu M, et al. Assessment of residual tumor viability in thymic carcinoma by sequential thallium-201 SPECT: comparison with CT and biopsy findings. *J Nucl Med* 1994;35(10):1659–1661.
420. Shahriari A, Odell JA. Cervical and thoracic components of multiorgan lymphangiomatosis managed surgically. *Ann Thorac Surg* 2001;71(2):694–696.
421. Shamji F, Pearson FG, Todd TR, et al. Results of surgical treatment for thymoma. *J Thorac Cardiovasc Surg* 1984;87(1):43–47.
422. Shi ML, Fan KH, Zhou CW, et al. [X-ray features of primary non-squamous cell carcinoma and other malignant neoplasms in the trachea and main bronchi—analysis of 23 cases]. *Zhonghua Zhong Liu Za Zhi* 1987;9(3):208–211.
423. Shields TW. Primary tumors and cysts of the mediastinum. In: Shields TW, ed. *General thoracic surgery*. Philadelphia: Lea & Febiger, 1983;927.
424. Shih DF, Wang JS, Tseng HH, et al. Primary pleural thymoma. *Arch Pathol Lab Med* 1997;121(1):79–82.
425. Shimosato Y, Kameya T, Nagai K, et al. Squamous cell carcinoma of the thymus. An analysis of eight cases. *Am J Surg Pathol* 1977;1(2):109–121.
426. Sickles EA, Belliveau RE, Wiernik PH. Primary mediastinal choriocarcinoma in the male. *Cancer* 1974;33(4):1196–1203.
427. Skowronek J, Piotrowski T, Mlynarczyk W, et al. Advanced tracheal carcinoma—a therapeutic significance of HDR brachytherapy in palliative treatment. *Neoplasma* 2004;51(4):313–318.
428. Slasky BS, Hardesty RL, Wilson S. Tracheal chondrosarcoma with an overview of other tumors of the trachea. *J Comput Tomogr* 1985;9(3):225–231.
429. Smirnov NM. [Sarcoma of the trachea]. *Zh Ushn Nos Gorl Bolezn* 1979(2):81–82.
430. Snover DC, Levine GD, Rosai J. Thymic carcinoma. Five distinctive histological variants. *Am J Surg Pathol* 1982;6(5):451–470.
431. Souadjian JV, Enriquez P, Silverstein MN, et al. The spectrum of diseases associated with thymoma. Coincidence or syndrome? *Arch Intern Med* 1974;134(2):374–379.
432. Spandow O, Lindholm CE. Granular cell tumour in a child's trachea—a diagnostic and therapeutic challenge. *Int J Pediatr Otorhinolaryngol* 1994;30(2):159–166.
433. Standerfer RJ, Armistead SH, Paneth M. Liposarcoma of the mediastinum: report of two cases and review of the literature. *Thorax* 1981;36(9):693–694.
434. Stieglitz F, Kitz R, Schafers HJ, et al. Granular cell tumor of the trachea in a child. *Ann Thorac Surg* 2005;79(2):e15–16.
435. Storm FK, Eilber FR, Mirra J, et al. Neurofibrosarcoma. *Cancer* 1980;45(1):126–129.
436. Strobel P, Marx A, Zettl A, et al. Thymoma and thymic carcinoma: an update of the WHO Classification 2004. *Surg Today* 2005;35(10):805–811.
437. Strollo DC, Rosado-de-Christenson ML, Jett JR. Primary mediastinal tumors: part II. Tumors of the middle and posterior mediastinum. *Chest* 1997;112(5):1344–1357.
438. Sumner TE, Volberg FM, Kiser PE, et al. Mediastinal cystic hygroma in children. *Pediatr Radiol* 1981;11(3):160–162.
439. Surveillance, Epidemiology, and End Results (SEER) Program SEER*Stat Database: Incidence—SEER 9 Regs Public-Use, Nov 2004 Sub (1973–2003), National Cancer Institute, DCCPS, Surveillance Research Program, Cancer Statistics Branch.
440. Suster S, Moran CA. Chordomas of the mediastinum: clinicopathologic, immunohistochemical, and ultrastructural study of six cases presenting as posterior mediastinal masses. *Hum Pathol* 1995;26(12):1354–1362.
441. Suster S, Moran CA. Malignant cartilaginous tumors of the mediastinum: clinicopathological study of six cases presenting as extraskeletal soft tissue masses. *Hum Pathol* 1997;28(5):588–594.
442. Suster S, Moran CA. Primary thymic epithelial neoplasms: spectrum of differentiation and histological features. *Semin Diagn Pathol* 1999;16(1):2.
443. Suster S, Moran CA. Thymic carcinoma: spectrum of differentiation and histologic types. *Pathology* 1998;30(2):111–122.
444. Suster S, Rosai J. Thymic carcinoma. A clinicopathologic study of 60 cases. *Cancer* 1991;67(4):1025–1032.
445. Suster S. Thymic carcinoma: update of current diagnostic criteria and histologic types. *Semin Diagn Pathol* 2005;22(3):198–212.
446. Suzuki K, Tanaka H, Shibusa T, et al. Parathyroid-hormone-related-protein-producing thymic carcinoma presenting as a giant extrathoracic mass. *Respiration* 1998;65(1):83–85.
447. Swain ME, Coblentz CL. Tracheal chondroma: CT appearance. *J Comput Assist Tomogr* 1988;12(6):1085–1086.
448. Swanson PE. Soft tissue neoplasma of the mediastinum. *Semin Diagn Pathol* 1991;8(1):14–34.
449. Swensen SJ, Hartman TE, Mayo JR, et al. Diffuse pulmonary lymphangiomatosis: CT findings. *J Comput Assist Tomogr* 1995;19(3):348–352.
450. Takahashi K, Takahashi H, Maeda K, et al. An adult case of lymphangiomatosis of the mediastinum, pulmonary interstitium and retroperitoneum complicated by chronic disseminated intravascular coagulation. *Eur Respir J* 1995;8(10):1799–1802.
451. Takami A, Okumura H, Maeda Y, et al. Primary tracheal lymphoma: case report and literature review. *Int J Hematol* 2005;82(4):338–342.
452. Takeda S, Sawabata N, Inoue M, et al. Thymic carcinoma. Clinical institutional experience with 15 patients. *Eur J Cardiothorac Surg* 2004;26(2):401–406.
453. Takeo S, Fukuyama S. Video-assisted thoracoscopic resection of a giant anterior mediastinal tumor (lipoma) using an original sternum-lifting technique. *Jpn J Thorac Cardiovasc Surg* 2005;53(10):565–568.
454. Tamay Z, Saribeyoglu E, Ones U, et al. Diffuse thoracic lymphangiomatosis with disseminated intravascular coagulation in a child. *J Pediatr Hematol Oncol* 2005;27(12):685–687.
455. Tan PH, Sng IT. Thymoma—a study of 60 cases in Singapore. *Histopathology* 1995;26(6):509–518.
456. Teh BT, Zedenius J, Kytola S, et al. Thymic carcinoids in multiple endocrine neoplasia type 1. *Ann Surg* 1998;228(1):99–105.
457. Teoh R, McGuire L, Wong K, et al. Increased incidence of thymoma in Chinese myasthenia gravis: possible relationship with Epstein-Barr virus. *Acta Neurol Scand* 1989;80(3):221–225.
458. Thomas CR Jr., Bonomi PD. Mediastinal tumors. *Curr Opin Oncol* 1991;3(2):335–343.
459. Thomas CR, Wright CD, Loehrer PJ. Thymoma: state of the art. *J Clin Oncol* 1999;17(7):2280–2289.
460. Thompson BH, Stabford W. MR Imaging of pulmonary and mediastinal malignancies. *MRI Clin North Am* 2000;8(4):729–739.
461. Thotathil ZS, Agarwal JP, Shrivastava SK, et al. Primary malignant tumors of the trachea—the Tata Memorial Hospital experience. *Med Princ Pract* 2004;13(2):69–73.
462. Tiedemann R. [Neurogenic tumors of the trachea]. *HNO* 1992;40(2):41–43.
463. Tiffet O, Nicholson AG, Ladas G, et al. A clinicopathologic study of 12 neuroendocrine tumors arising in the thymus. *Chest* 2003;124(1):141–146.
464. Tomiyama N, Johkoh T, Mihara N, et al. Using the World Health Organization classification of thymic epithelial neoplasms to describe CT findings. *AJR Am J Roentgenol* 2002;179(4):881–886.
465. Topcu S, Alper A, Gulhan E, et al. Neurogenic tumours of the mediastinum: a report of 60 cases. *Can Respir J* 2000;7(3):261–265.
466. Travis WD, World Health Organization, International Agency for Research on Cancer, et al. Pathology and genetics of tumours of the lung, pleura, thymus and heart. In: *World Health Organization classification of tumours*, Vol. 7. 2004, Lyon Oxford: IARC Press, 2004.
467. Tseng YL, Wang ST, Wu MH, et al. Thymic carcinoma: involvement of great vessels indicates poor prognosis. *Ann Thorac Surg* 2003;76(4):1041–1045.
468. Tucker T, Wolkenstein P, Revuz J, et al. Association between benign and malignant peripheral nerve sheath tumors in NF1. *Neurology* 2005;65(2):205–211.
469. Turner AR, MacDonald RN, Gilbert JA, et al. Mediastinal germ cell cancers in Klinefelter's syndrome. *Ann Intern Med* 1981;94(2):279.
470. Uematsu M, Kondo M, Dokiya T, et al. The role of radiotherapy in the treatment of primary mediastinal seminoma. *Radiother Oncol* 1992;24(4):226–230.
471. Urgesi A, Monetti U, Rossi G, et al. Aggressive treatment of intrathoracic recurrences of thymoma. *Radiother Oncol* 1992;24(4):221–225.
472. Urgesi A, Monetti U, Rossi G, et al. Role of radiation therapy in locally advanced thymoma. *Radiother Oncol* 1990;19(3):273–280.
473. Van Den Beukel JT, Wagenaar SJ, Vanderschueren R. Liposarcoma of the trachea. *Thorax* 1979;34(6):817–818.
474. van der Maten J, Blaauwgeers JL, Sutedja TG, et al. Granular cell tumors of the tracheobronchial tree. *J Thorac Cardiovasc Surg* 2003;126(3):740–743.
475. van Nostrand AW. Tracheal tumors—early diagnosis and treatment. *J Otolaryngol* 1977;6(1):74–84.
476. Venuta F, Rendina EA, Pescarmona EO, et al. Multimodality treatment of thymoma: a prospective study. *Ann Thorac Surg* 1997;64(6):1585–1591; discussion 1591–1592.
477. Verley JM, Hollmann KH. Thymoma. A comparative study of clinical stages, histologic features, and survival in 200 cases. *Cancer* 1985;55(5):1074–1086.
478. Verstandig AG, Epstein DM, Miller WT Jr., et al. Thymoma—report of 71 cases and a review. *Crit Rev Diagn Imaging* 1992;33(3):201–230.
479. Vessey MP, Doll R, Norman-Smith B, et al. Thymectomy and cancer: a further report. *Br J Cancer* 1979;39(2):193–195.
480. Videtic GM, Campbell C, Vincent MD. Primary chemoradiation as definitive treatment for unresectable cancer of the trachea. *Can Respir J* 2003;10(3): 143–144.
481. Vincent A, Palace J, Hilton-Jones D. Myasthenia gravis. *Lancet* 2001;357(9274): 2122–2128.
482. Walsh GL, Taylor GD, Nesbitt JC, et al. Intensive chemotherapy and radical

resections for primary nonseminomatous mediastinal germ cell tumors. *Ann Thorac Surg* 2000;69(2):337–343; discussion 343–344.

483. Wang DY, Chang DB, Kuo SH, et al. Carcinoid tumours of the thymus. *Thorax* 1994;49(4):357–360.

484. Wang LS, Huang MH, Lin TS, et al. Malignant thymoma. *Cancer* 1992;70(2):443–450.

485. Wang Y, Wang L, Zhang D. [Carcinoid of trachea and bronchus: a report of 20 cases]. *Zhonghua Zhong Liu Za Zhi* 2001;23(1):70–72.

486. Watts MA, Gibbons JA, Aaron BL. Mediastinal and osseous lymphangiomatosis: case report and review. *Ann Thorac Surg* 1982;34(3):324–328.

487. Webb BD, Walsh GL, Roberts DB, et al. Primary tracheal malignant neoplasms: the University of Texas M.D. Anderson Cancer Center experience. *J Am Coll Surg* 2006;202(2):237–246.

488. Weber AL, Grillo HC. Tracheal tumor: radiological, clinical and pathological evaluation. *Adv Otorhinolaryngol* 1978;24:170–176.

489. Weidner N. Atypical tumor of the mediastinum: epithelioid hemangioendothelioma containing metaplastic bone and osteoclastlike giant cells. *Ultrastruct Pathol* 1991;15(4–5):481–488.

490. Weiland K, Conley J. A primary germ cell tumor of the anterior mediastinum: a case report and discussion. *S D J Med* 2000;53(10):441–444.

491. Weiss SW, Goldblum JR, Enzinger FM. *Enzinger and Weiss's soft tissue tumors*, 4th ed. St. Louis: Mosby, 2001;xiv.

492. Weissberg D, Goldberg M, Pearson FG. Thymoma. *Ann Thorac Surg* 1973;16(2):141–147.

493. Welch KJ, Tapper D, Vawter GP. Surgical treatment of thymic cysts and neoplasms in children. *J Pediatr Surg* 1979;14(6):691–698.

494. Wen CC, Hsu YP, Sheu MH. Atypical carcinoid tumor of the thymus: a case report. *Chin J Radiol* 2003;28:317–321.

495. Whooley BP, Urschel JD, Antkowiak JG, et al. A 25-year thymoma treatment review. *J Exp Clin Cancer Res* 2000;19(1):3–5.

496. Whooley BP, Urschel JD, Antkowiak JG, et al. Primary tumors of the mediastinum. *J Surg Oncol* 1999;70(2):95–99.

497. Wick MR, Carney JA, Bernatz PE, et al. Primary mediastinal carcinoid tumors. *Am J Surg Pathol* 1982;6(3):195–205.

498. Wick MR, Rosai J. Neuroendocrine neoplasms of the mediastinum. *Semin Diagn Pathol* 1991;8(1):35–51.

499. Wick MR, Scheithauer BW, Weiland LH, et al. Primary thymic carcinomas. *Am J Surg Pathol* 1982;6(7):613–630.

500. Wilkens EW, Grillo HC, Scannell GEA. Role of staging in prognosis and management of thymoma. *Ann Thorac Surg* 1991;51:888–892.

501. Wilkins EW Jr., Castleman D. Thymoma: a continuing survey at the Massachusetts General Hospital. *Ann Thorac Surg* 1979;28(3):252–256.

502. Wilkins KB, Sheikh E, Green R, et al. Clinical and pathologic predictors of survival in patients with thymoma. *Ann Surg* 1999;230(4):562–572; discussion 572–574.

503. Williams CL, Hay JE, Huiatt TW, et al. Paraneoplastic IgG striational autoantibodies produced by clonal thymic B cells and in serum of patients with myasthenia gravis and thymoma react with titin. *Lab Invest* 1992;66(3):331–336.

504. Wong WW, Hirose T, Scheithauer BW, et al. Malignant peripheral nerve sheath tumor: analysis of treatment outcome. *Int J Radiat Oncol Biol Phys* 1998;42(2):351–360.

505. Wood DE. Management of malignant tracheobronchial obstruction. *Surg Clin North Am* 2002;82(3):621–642.

506. Wright CD, Kesler KA, Nichols CR, et al. Primary mediastinal nonseminomatous germ cell tumors. Results of a multimodality approach. *J Thorac Cardiovasc Surg* 1990;99(2):210–217.

507. Wright CD, Wain JC, Wong DR, et al. Predictors of recurrence in thymic tumors: importance of invasion, World Health Organization histology, and size. *J Thorac Cardiovasc Surg* 2005;130(5):1413–1421.

508. Yagi K, Hirata T, Fukuse T, et al. Surgical treatment for invasive thymoma, especially when the superior vena cava is invaded. *Ann Thorac Surg* 1996;61(2):521–524.

509. Yamakawa Y, Masaoka A, Hashimoto T, et al. A tentative tumor-node-metastasis classification of thymoma. *Cancer* 1991;68(9):1984–1987.

510. Yamamoto K, Alarcon JP, Armengod EB, et al. Tracheal carcinoid during pregnancy. *J Cardiovasc Surg (Torino)* 2004;45(5):525.

511. Yang KY, Chen YM, Huang MH, et al. Revisit of primary malignant neoplasms of the trachea: clinical characteristics and survival analysis. *Jpn J Clin Oncol* 1997;27(5):305–309.

512. Yoh K, Goto K, Ishii G, et al. Weekly chemotherapy with cisplatin, vincristine, doxorubicin, and etoposide is an effective treatment for advanced thymic carcinoma. *Cancer* 2003;98(5):926–931.

513. Yokoi K, Matsuguma H, Nakahara R, et al. Multidisciplinary treatment for advanced invasive thymoma with cisplatin, doxorubicin, and methylprednisolone. *Chest* 2005;128(4):145S-b–146.

514. Zagars GK, Goswitz MS, Pollack A. Liposarcoma: outcome and prognostic factors following conservation surgery and radiation therapy. *Int J Radiat Oncol Biol Phys* 1996;36(2):311–319.

515. Zhang HQ, Zhu ZJ, Peng DW, et al. [Primary tracheal carcinoma—report of 5 patients]. *Zhonghua Zhong Liu Za Zhi* 1988;10(1):45–47.

516. Zhang Z, Cui Y, Li B, et al. Thymic carcinoma (report of 14 cases) *Chin Med Sci J* 1997;12(4):252–255.

517. Zhu G, He S, Fu X, et al. Radiotherapy and prognostic factors for thymoma: a retrospective study of 175 patients. *Int J Radiat Oncol Biol Phys* 2004;60(4):1113–1119.

518. Zimmer W, DeLuca SA. Primary tracheal neoplasms: recognition, diagnosis and evaluation. *Am Fam Physician* 1992;45(6):2651–1657.

519. Zisis C, Rontogianni D, Tzavara C, et al. Prognostic factors in thymic epithelial tumors undergoing complete resection. *Ann Thorac Surg* 2005;80(3):1056–1062.

520. Zizmor J, Noyek AM, Lewis JS. Radiologic diagnosis of chondroma and chondrosarcoma of the larynx. *Arch Otolaryngol* 1975;101(4):232–234.

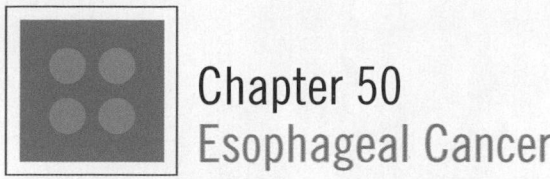

Chapter 50
Esophageal Cancer

Brian G. Czito, Albert S. Denittis, Christopher G. Willett

Less than 15% of patients diagnosed with esophageal cancer are cured, with half of the patients presenting with unresectable or metastatic disease. This chapter will review the natural history and treatment of esophageal cancer, including risk factors, staging, results of current therapeutic approaches, and future treatment strategies.

Anatomy

The esophagus is a thin-walled, hollow tube approximately 25 cm in length. It is lined with stratified keratinized squamous epithelium, extending from the cricopharyngeus muscle at the level of the cricoid cartilage superiorly to the gastroesophageal junction inferiorly. The lower third (5 to 10 cm) of the esophagus may contain glandular elements. Replacement of the stratified squamous epithelium with columnar epithelium is referred to as Barrett's esophagus, often occurring in the lower third. The Z-line refers to the endoscopically visible junction of the squamous and glandular epithelium. The four esophageal wall layers consist of an innermost epithelial layer, followed by an inner circular muscle layer, an outer longitudinal muscle layer, and an adventitia. No serosa is present, facilitating extra esophageal spread of disease.

The esophagus is frequently divided into cervical and thoracic components. The cervical esophagus begins at the cricopharyngeus muscle (approximately the C7 level or 15 cm from the incisors) and extends to the thoracic inlet (approximately T3 level or 18 cm from the incisors, at the level of the suprasternal notch). The thoracic esophagus extends from approximately the level of T3 to T10 or T11 (108). Endoscopically, the gastroesophageal (GE) junction is often defined as the point where the first gastric fold is encountered, although this may be a "theoretical" landmark. The location of the GE junction can be accurately defined histologically as the squamocolumnar junction.

Useful landmarks in reference to endoscopy include the carina (approximately 25 cm from the incisors) and the gastroesophageal junction (approximately 40 cm from the incisors). The American Joint Committee on Cancer (AJCC) has divided the esophagus into four regions: cervical, upper thoracic, midthoracic, and lower thoracic (8) (Fig. 50.1).

Siewert et al. (117) characterized cancer of the gastroesophageal junction according to the location of the tumor. If the tumor center is located >1 cm above the gastroesophageal junction (Z-line), the tumor is classified as a type I adenocarcinoma of the distal esophagus. If the tumor center is located within 1 cm cephalad to 2 cm caudad to the gastroesophageal junction, it is classified as type II. If the tumor center is located >2 cm below the gastroesophageal junction, the tumor is classified as type III. However, locally advanced/bulky tumors can make it difficult to accurately distinguish where tumors originated in relationship to the GE junction.

Lymphatic Drainage

The esophagus has an extensive, longitudinal interconnecting system of lymphatics. Lymphatic channels in the mucosa and submucosa communicate with the lymphatic channels in the muscle layers throughout. Lymph can travel the entire length of the esophagus before draining into lymph nodes (108), and thus the entire esophagus is at potential risk for lymphatic involvement. Up to 8 cm or more of "normal" tissue can exist between gross tumor and micrometastases "skip areas" secondary to this extensive lymphatic network (141). Additionally, as many as 71% of frozen tissue sections scored as margin-negative by conventional histopathology show involvement by lymphatic micrometastases with immunohistochemistry (62). Lymphatics of the esophagus drain into nodes that usually follow arteries, including the inferior thyroid artery, the bronchial and esophageal arteries, and the left gastric artery (celiac axis) (115) (Fig. 50.2).

Epidemiology and Risk Factors

Esophageal carcinoma is an uncommon malignancy, accounting for approximately 1% of all malignancy and 6% of all gastrointestinal malignancies. In 2004, there will be an estimated 15,560 new patients diagnosed with esophageal cancer in the United States and 13,940 deaths. Most cases occur in males, at a rate of 3.5:1 relative to female (67).

In the United States, there has been a dramatic rise in the incidence of adenocarcinoma of the esophagus, particularly in Caucasian males. In 1987, adenocarcinoma was reported to represent 34% and 12% of esophageal cancers in Caucasian men and women, versus 3% and 1% for African American men and women, respectively (20). Over the past 20 years, there has been an increase in the incidence of adenocarcinoma at a rate of 5% to 10% per year. This is a more rapid increase than any other cancer (20). As of 1998, esophageal adenocarcinoma accounted for almost 55% of all diagnosed cases in Caucasian men. African American men are more frequently diagnosed with squamous cell carcinoma (35,103) (Fig. 50.3).

The outcome for patients with esophageal carcinoma is bleak. In the 1990s, the 5-year survival rate for esophageal cancer was approximately 11%, with a median survival rate of approximately 9 months. Collectively, little difference in outcomes between histologic types has been observed (106).

Globally, the incidence of esophageal carcinoma varies widely. This malignancy is seen in high frequency in northern China, Iran, and Russia, near the Caspian Sea. Incidence rates can be as high as 100+ per 100,000 persons (70,85,109,145). Although the reasons for the geographic discrepancy are unknown, some reports have linked the arid climate and alkaline soil with these high-risk areas, as well as the ingestion of nitrosamines and inversely to the consumption of riboflavin, nicotinic acid, magnesium, and zinc (28,86). High-risk clusters have also been observed in South Africa, northern France, Hong Kong, and Brazil.

In North America and Western Europe, alcohol and tobacco use are the major risk factors for squamous cell carcinoma, accounting for 80% to 90% of cases (113). Reports have described the relative risk of esophageal cancer by the amount of alcohol

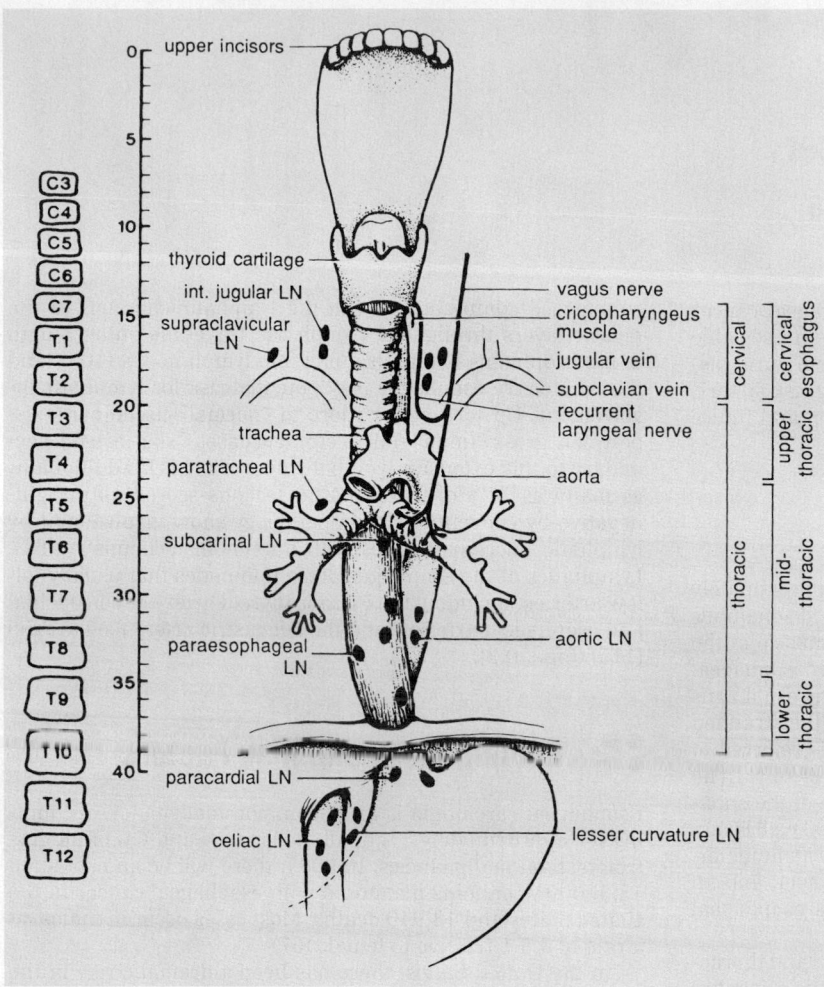

FIGURE 50.1. Anatomy of the esophagus. Note the lengths of the various segments of the esophagus from the upper central incisors and the two classification schemes for subdividing the esophagus. LN, lymph node

and tobacco consumed, including a relative risk of 155:1 when consuming >30 g per day of tobacco along with 121 g per day of alcohol (21).

In high-risk populations, diets of corn, wheat, millet, scant amounts of fruits, vegetables, and animal products are associated with increases in squamous cell carcinoma (136). Patients with Plummer-Vinson (Paterson-Kelly) syndrome, a condition

characterized by iron deficiency anemia and low riboflavin levels, are at an increased risk for oral cavity, hypopharyngeal, and esophageal cancer. Additionally, dietary intake of nitrosamines, nitrosamides, and N-nitroso compounds has been implicated in esophageal carcinoma. Examples of nitrate-rich foods include pickled vegetables, alcoholic beverages, cured meats, and fish (82,90).

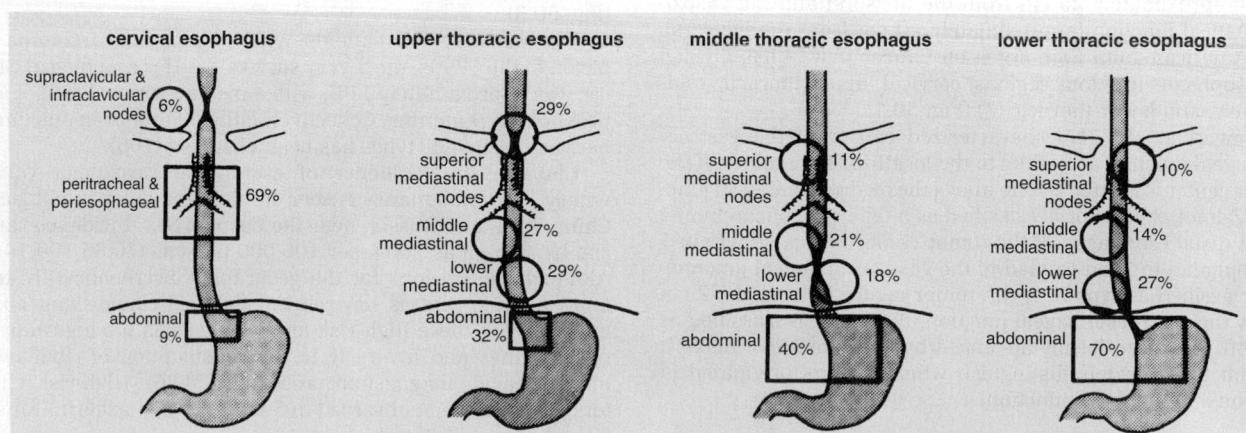

FIGURE 50.2. Positive lymph node distribution according to the location of the primary tumor. (Modified from Akiyama H, Tsurumaru M, Kawamura T, et al. Principles of surgical treatment for carcinoma of the esophagus: analysis of lymph node involvement. Circles represent potential sites of lymph node involvement while squares represent the dominant site of lymphatic spread. *Ann Surg* 1981;194:438; and Dormans E. Das Oesophaguscarcinoma: Ergebnisse der unter Mitarbeit von 39 pathologischen Instituten Deutschlands Durchgefuhrten Erhebung uber das Oesophaguscarcinomon [1925–1933]. *Z Krebforsch* 1939;49:86, with permission.)

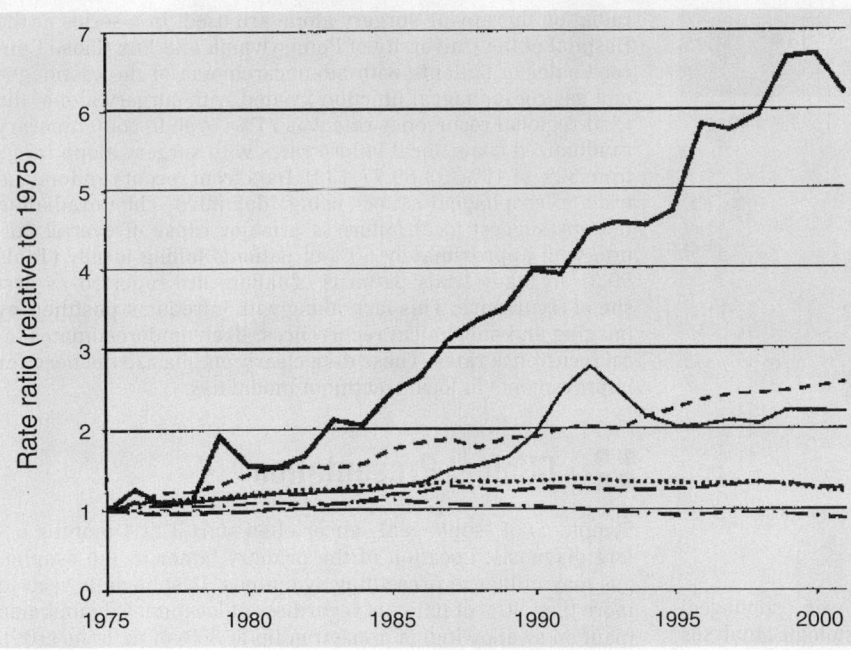

FIGURE 50.3. Relative change in incidence of esophageal adenocarcinoma and other malignancies (1975–2001). Data from the National Cancer Institute's Surveillance, Epidemiology, and End Results (SEER) program with age-adjustment using the 2000 U.S. standard population. Base line was the average incidence between 1973 and 1975. solid black line, esophageal adenocarcinoma; short dashed line, melanoma; line, prostate cancer; dashed line, breast cancer; dotted line, lung cancer; dashed and dotted line, colorectal cancer

Other risk factors associated with esophageal carcinoma include achalasia, caustic burns (especially lye corrosion), and tylosis. Achalasia of long duration (25 years) is associated with a 5% incidence of squamous cell carcinoma (10,61). Patients with tylosis (hyperkeratosis of the palms and soles and papilloma of the esophagus) have a reported 38% risk in developing esophageal cancer at a mean age of 45 years (57). Additionally, carcinoma of the esophagus occurs in 2% to 4% of patients with head and neck cancer.

Risk factors leading to the development of adenocarcinoma of the esophagus are not as well understood. Most esophageal adenocarcinomas tend to arise from the metaplastic columnar-lined epithelium known as Barrett's esophagus (122). Severe and long-standing gastroesophageal reflux disease (GERD) has clearly been shown to be a significant risk factor for Barrett's esophagus, which may lead to adenocarcinoma. It has been estimated that patients with long-standing severe reflux have a 44-fold risk of developing adenocarcinoma (74). In addition, smokers have a two- to threefold greater risk for developing esophageal adenocarcinoma versus nonsmokers (37,150). The relative risk of esophageal adenocarcinoma persists to three decades following smoking cessation, in contrast to a significant decline in similar patients with squamous cell carcinoma (58). Obesity has also been linked to a three- to fourfold risk of adenocarcinoma, possibly due to an increased risk of reflux (25). It has been estimated that a middle-aged patient with Barrett's esophagus has a 10% to 15% risk of developing esophageal adenocarcinoma during his or her lifetime (34).

Differences between tumor types as classified by Siewert include higher male to female ratios, increased incidence of hiatal hernia, GERD and Barrett's esophagus for type I tumors compared to types II and III, and more differentiated tumors observed in types I and II versus III (117).

Although many risk factors are associated with esophageal carcinoma, few studies have demonstrated a causal relationship leading to pathogenesis. Motesano et al. (94) reported possible genetic abnormalities involved in the genesis of esophageal cancer. In addition, possible differences in mechanisms of pathogenesis for squamous cell carcinoma and adenocarcinoma were described. Genetic abnormalities in squamous cell carcinoma include p53 mutations and multiple allelic losses at 3p and 9q, with amplification of cyclin D1 and epidermal growth factor receptor (EGFR). These mutations lead to cell hyperplasia, low-

and high-grade dysplasia, and ultimately, squamous cell carcinoma. In contrast, genetic abnormalities in adenocarcinoma include overexpression of p53, multiple allelic losses at 17p, 5q, and 13q, and amplification and overexpression of EGFR and human epidermal growth factor receptor 2 (HER-2). These abnormalities may be involved in the stepwise development of Barrett's esophagus, dysplasia, and, ultimately, adenocarcinoma. These differences suggest that squamous cell carcinoma and adenocarcinoma have different pathogeneses and therefore different etiologies. These mechanisms remain ill-defined.

Natural History and Patterns of Spread

Squamous cell carcinoma is characterized by extensive local growth and proclivity to lymph node metastases (55). Because the esophagus has no covering serosa, direct invasion of contiguous structures occurs early (100). Lesions in the upper esophagus can impinge on or invade the recurrent laryngeal nerves, carotid arteries, and trachea. If extraesophageal extension occurs in the mediastinum, tracheoesophageal or bronchoesophageal fistula may occur. Tumors in the lower third of the esophagus can invade the aorta or pericardium, resulting in mediastinitis, massive hemorrhage, or empyema (64).

For T1 lesions, the reported incidence of nodal spread is 14% to 21%; for T2 lesions, this rises to 38% to 60% (31,117). The location of involved lymph nodes is influenced by the origin of the primary tumor. Lymph node metastases are found in approximately 70% of patients at autopsy (5,19,39) (see Fig. 50.2). In patients with cervical lesions, lymph node metastases to the abdominal lymph nodes are rare. Distant hematogenous metastasis can occur at almost any site (9) (Table 50.1).

For lower esophageal and gastroesophageal junctional adenocarcinomas, approximately 70% of patients will have nodal metastases at presentation. This is influenced by tumoral depth of penetration, with nearly all T3-4 lesions exhibiting metastases in surgical series (Fig. 50.4). In patients with lower esophageal cancer, involvement of both mediastinal and abdominal lymph nodes is common (40) (Fig. 50.5). The incidence of abdominal nodal involvement increases as one proceeds distally in the esophagus to the gastroesophageal junction. For patients with tumors arising from the gastroesophageal junction, mediastinal involvement is less common. Nodal metastases

Table 50.1	DISTRIBUTION OF METASTASES BY ANATOMIC SITE	
Site	No. of Patients	Percentage
Lymph nodes	58	73
Lung	41	52
Liver	37	47
Adrenals	16	20
Diaphragm	15	19
Bronchus	13	17
Pleura	13	17
Stomach	12	15
Bone	11	14
Kidneys	10	13
Trachea	10	13
Pericardium	9	11
Pancreas	9	11

From Anderson LL, Lad TE. Autopsy findings in squamous-cell carcinoma of the esophagus. *Cancer* 1982;50:1587–1590, with permission.

above the level of the carina are rare in lower esophageal and junctional tumors (93). Additionally, histologic analyses of lower esophagus and gastroesophageal junction adenocarcinoma specimens suggest that many patients without nodal involvement on conventional histopathology actually have involvement when assessed by immunohistochemistry (116).

The primary direction for lymphatic flow for the lower esophagus is toward the abdomen. According to the classification by Siewert, nodal metastases are often seen in the mediastinum and abdomen for type I tumors, whereas type III tumors metastasize almost exclusively inferiorly, toward the celiac axis. Type II tumors are intermediate, preferentially spreading inferiorly and less frequently into the mediastinum. The primary value in the Siewert classification is to the guidance of appropriate type surgery (i.e., type I tumors are generally treated with esophagectomy and mediastinal lymph node resection, with types II and III approached through the abdomen) (117).

Patterns of Failure

Aisner et al. (4) and LePrise et al. (81) reviewed the patterns of failure in esophageal cancer after radical irradiation, radical surgery, or a combination of both (Table 50.2). These data suggest that high rates of local recurrence occur when either

radiation therapy or surgery alone are used. In a series at the Hospital of the University of Pennsylvania and Fox Chase Cancer Center of patients with adenocarcinoma of the esophagus and gastroesophageal junction treated with surgery alone, the local-regional recurrence rate was 77% (143). In contemporary randomized trials, local failure rates with surgery alone range from 32% to 45% (63,69,77,133). Data from recent randomized trials of esophageal cancer using "definitive" chemoradiation therapy suggest local failure is a major cause of overall failure, with approximately 50% of patients failing locally (Table 50.3). In many trials patterns of failure are reported as first site of recurrence. This fact, along with infrequent posttherapy imaging and subclinical recurrences, likely underestimates local recurrence rates. These data clearly emphasize the need for improvements in local treatment modalities.

Clinical Presentation

Symptoms of esophageal cancer often start 3 to 4 months before diagnosis. Location of the primary tumor in the esophagus may influence presenting symptoms. Dysphagia is seen in more than 90% of patients regardless of location. Odynophagia (pain on swallowing) is present in up to 50% of patients (109). Weight loss is common, with 40% to 70% of patients reporting a loss of >5% of total body weight. This extent of weight loss has been associated with a worse prognosis. Less frequent symptoms may include hoarseness, cough, and glossopharyngeal neuralgia (92).

Advanced lesions can produce signs and symptoms from tumor invasion into local structures. Hematemesis, hemoptysis, melena, dyspnea, and persistent cough secondary to tracheoesophageal or bronchoesophageal fistula may occur. Compression or invasion of the left recurrent laryngeal nerve or the phrenic nerves can cause dysphonia or hemidiaphragm paralysis. Superior vena cava syndrome and Horner's syndrome can also occur. Pleural effusion and exsanguination resulting from aortic communication may also be seen (109). Abdominal and back pain may occur with celiac axis nodal involvement with lower esophageal tumors.

Diagnostic Work-Up

After a thorough history and physical examination, all patients with suspected esophageal cancer should have a work-up similar to that outlined in Figure 50.6. Attention should be paid to cervical and supraclavicular lymph nodes. Basic blood counts

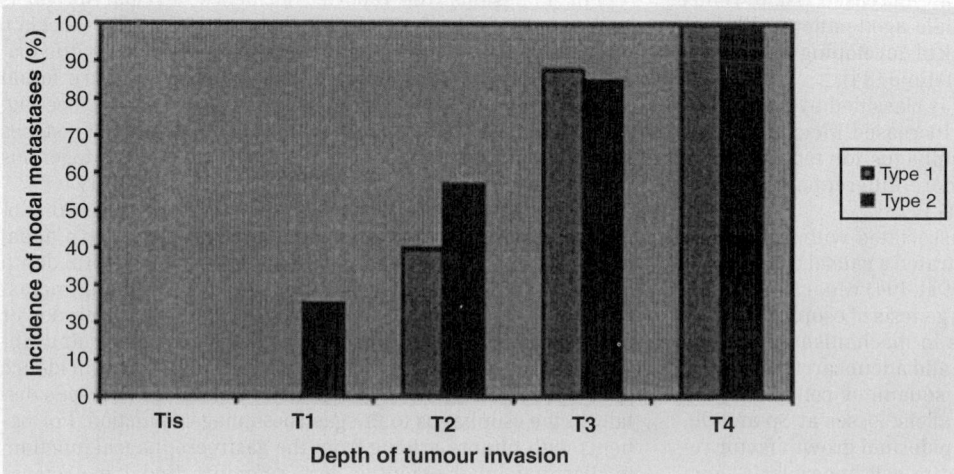

FIGURE 50.4. The incidence of nodal metastases related to depth of tumor invasion for adenocarcinoma.

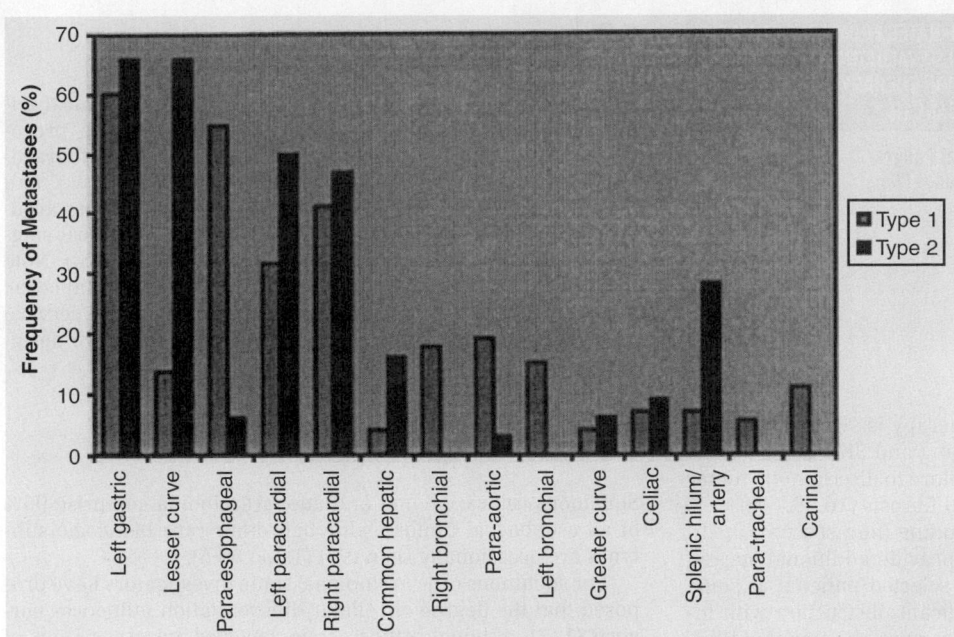

FIGURE 50.5. Distribution of nodal metastases by frequency of site involved for adenocarcinoma.

and a metabolic panel with liver function tests should be obtained.

Although the esophagogram may be used to define lesion extent, endoscopy is the best tool to diagnose and define such (129). During flexible endoscopy, biopsies and brushings should be taken of the primary site and suspicious areas harboring satellite lesions or submucosal spread. Additionally, accurate endoscopic measurement and characterization of tumor and gastroesophageal junction in relation to the incisors facilitates radiation treatment planning. Examination of the oral cavity, pharynx, larynx, and tracheobronchial tree may also be performed at the time of esophagoscopy in patients with squamous cell carcinomas given the high incidence of second tumors in the head and neck and upper airway (108). Additionally, bronchoscopy should be performed in patients with proximal malignancy to evaluate for the presence of tracheal or carinal

invasion, particularly for patients with tumors abutting these structures on computed tomography (CT). CT of the thorax and abdomen is critical to identify metastases to the liver, upper abdominal nodes, or adrenals. However, CT may not adequately assess periesophageal lymph node involvement or accurately define the true extent of the primary tumor (78,102). Conventional CT scan can accurately determine resectability in only 65% to 85% of cases. Furthermore, CT accurately predicts T stage in approximately 70% of cases and nodal involvement in only 50% to 70% of cases (53,71,105).

To assess periesophageal and celiac lymph node involvement and transmural extent of disease, endoscopic ultrasonography (EUS) should be performed. EUS provides accuracy rates of 85% to 90% for tumor invasion (T stage) and 75% to 80% for lymph node metastases, when matched to surgical pathology (68,73,107). However, the accuracy of endoscopic

Table 50.2 | PATTERNS OF FAILURE IN ESOPHAGEAL CANCER

Modality	No. of Patients	Recurrence (%)					
		Local	Marginal	Neck	Mediastinal	Local and Distant	Distant
Irradiation alone (30–80 Gy)	517	25–84	25	10–43	—	—	23–65
Radical surgery alone	266	21–50		44	33	—	17–65
							33 abdominal nodes
							17 liver 6 lung
Combined radiation therapy and surgery (primarily preoperative irradiation, 35–50 Gy usual dose)	2,078	22–87	53[a]	—	20[a]	—	7–43[b]
Radiation therapy and chemotherapy alone[c]	254	15–39	—	—	—	5–25	—
	—	—	—	—	—	—	6–25
Preoperative radiation therapy and chemotherapy[c]	150	2–36	—	—	—	5–38	16–29

[a]From one study.
[b]From two studies.
[c]Data from LePrise EA, Meunier BC, Etienne PL, et al. Sequential chemotherapy and radiotherapy for patients with squamous cell carcinoma of the esophagus. *Cancer* 1995;75:2.
Modified from Aisner J, Forastiere A, Aroney R. Patterns of recurrence for cancer of the lung and esophagus. In: Wittes RE, ed. *Cancer treatment symposia: proceedings of the Workshop on Patterns of Failure after Cancer Treatment,* vol 2. Washington, DC: U.S. Department of Health and Human Services, 1983:87, with permission.

Table 50.3	LOCAL FAILURE RATES FROM RANDOMIZED THERAPY TRIALS EVALUATING CHEMORADIATION THERAPY ALONE IN ESOPHAGEAL CANCER		
Study (Reference)	Dose (Gy)	Local Failure (crude) (%)	Local Failure (2-year) (%)
RTOG 85-01 (6)	50	45	47
INT 0123 (91)	50	55	52
INT 0123 (91)	64	50	56
German (123)	>60	51	58

ultrasound following neoadjuvant therapy is significantly less, ranging from 27% to 48% for T staging and 38% to 71% for N staging. This is possibly due to the failure to discriminate tumor from postradiation inflammation and fibrosis (16,75,149).

Surgical staging procedures, including thoracoscopy, mediastinoscopy, and laparoscopy, may provide additional staging information and are considered in selected patients at some institutions (66). Patients with significant obstruction with inability to maintain their weight may require placement of feeding jejunostomy. If surgery is planned, gastric tube placement is generally avoided given the stomach will ultimately serve as the "neoesophagus" following resection.

More recently, positron emission tomography (PET) has proven to be a valuable staging tool in esophageal cancer patients. The addition of PET to standard staging studies such as CT can improve the accuracy of detecting stage III and stage IV disease by 23% and 18%, respectively (17,46). Overall, it is estimated that PET will detect distant metastatic disease in approximately 20% of patients who are considered to have local regional disease only by CT. However, PET also appears to have a lower accuracy in detecting local nodal disease compared to CT alone or in combination with endoscopic ultrasound. Importantly, emerging data suggest that PET can be used to predict response to therapy, with "PET responders" experiencing significantly improved outcomes compared to "nonresponders." Additionally, PET has been used to predict therapeutic response to treatment early in the treatment course. This has led to investigation in early treatment response as measured by PET as a surrogate for therapeutic efficacy and clinical outcomes (142).

Staging Systems

Esophageal staging can be based on pathologic or clinical criteria. Pathologic staging is performed after invasive procedures including esophagectomy, mediastinotomy, or thoracotomy. Clinical staging is often employed with "definitive" and neoadjuvant chemoradiotherapy approaches and is less accurate. With the combination of CT, PET, and EUS, clinical staging closely correlates with pathologic stage (Table 50.4). Note the esophageal staging system is relatively unique in that celiac nodal metastases from a lower esophageal lesion and cervical nodal metastases from an upper esophageal lesion are designated M1a.

Pathologic Classification

Squamous cell carcinoma and adenocarcinoma comprise 95% of all esophageal tumors, although other rare histologic subtypes are occasionally seen (97) (Table 50.5).

For squamous cell carcinomas, some investigators have proposed that the degree of cellular differentiation influences survival (147), although others have reported no association of cellular differentiation to lymph node involvement or survival

Table 50.4	STAGING FOR CANCER OF THE ESOPHAGUS BY TUMOR, LYMPH NODE, AND METASTASIS		
Primary tumor (T)			
TX	Primary tumor cannot be assessed		
T0	No evidence of primary tumor		
Tis	Carcinoma *in situ*		
T1	Tumor invades lamina propria or submucosa		
T2	Tumor invades muscularis propria		
T3	Tumor invades adventitia		
T4	Tumor invades adjacent structures		
Regional lymph nodes (N)			
NX	Regional lymph nodes cannot be assessed		
N0	No regional lymph node metastasis		
N1	Regional lymph node metastasis		
Distant metastasis (M)			
MX	Presence of distant metastasis cannot be assessed		
M0	No distant metastasis		
M1	Distant metastasis		
Tumors of the lower thoracic esophagus			
M1a	Metastases in celiac lymph nodes		
M1b	Other distant metastases		
Tumors of the mid-thoracic esophagus			
M1a	Not applicable		
M1b	Nonregional lymph nodes and/or distant metastases		
Tumors of the upper thoracic esophagus			
M1a	Metastases in cervical nodes		
M1b	Other distant metastases		
Stage grouping			
Stage 0	Tis	N0	M0
Stage I	T1	N0	M0
Stage IIA	T2	N0	M0
	T3	N0	M0
Stage IIB	T1	N1	M0
	T2	N1	M0
Stage III	T3	N1	M0
	T4	Any N	M0
Stage IV	Any T	Any N	M1
Stage IVA	Any T	Any N	M1a
Stage IVB	Any T	Any N	M1b

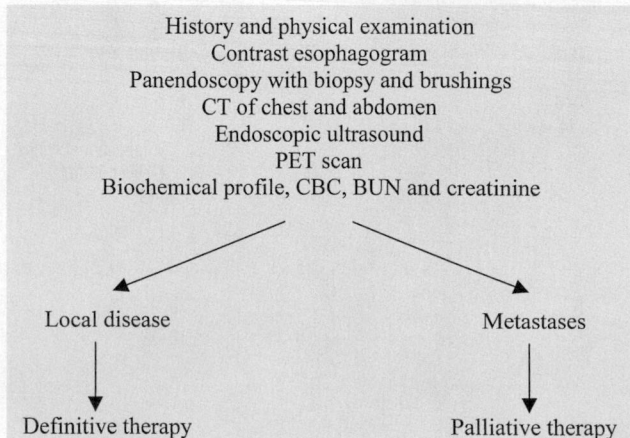

History and physical examination
Contrast esophagogram
Panendoscopy with biopsy and brushings
CT of chest and abdomen
Endoscopic ultrasound
PET scan
Biochemical profile, CBC, BUN and creatinine

Local disease → Definitive therapy

Metastases → Palliative therapy

FIGURE 50.6. Diagnostic work-up for esophageal cancer. BUN, blood urea nitrogen; CBC, completed blood cell count; CT, computed tomography; PET, positron emission tomography

Adapted from Fleming ID, Cooper JS, Henson DE, et al., eds. *American Joint Committee on Cancer: cancer staging manual*, 5th ed. New York: Spring-Verlag, 2002.

Table 50.5	PATHOLOGIC CLASSIFICATION OF MALIGNANT ESOPHAGEAL TUMORS

Epithelial tumors
Squamous cell carcinoma
  Well differentiated
  Moderately differentiated
  Poorly differentiated
Variants of squamous cell carcinoma
  Spindle cell carcinoma
  Pseudosarcoma and carcinosarcoma
  Verrucous carcinoma
  In situ carcinoma
Adenocarcinoma
  Adenoacanthoma
Adenoid cystic carcinoma (cylindroma)
Mucoepidermoid carcinoma
Adenosquamous carcinoma
Carcinoid
Small cell carcinoma

Nonepithelial tumors
Leiomyosarcoma
Malignant melanoma
Rhabdomyosarcoma
Myoblastoma
Choriocarcinoma
Lymphoma

From Rosenberg JC, Lichter AS, Leichman LP. Cancer of the esophagus. In: DeVita VT, Hellman S, Rosenberg SA, eds. *Cancer: principles and practice of oncology*, 3rd ed. Philadelphia: J.B. Lippincott, 1989;499, with permission.

(108). Pseudosarcoma is a variant of a poorly differentiated squamous cell carcinoma with spindle-shaped cells in the stroma resembling fibroblasts. Verrucous carcinoma is a well differentiated, papillary variant of squamous cell carcinoma (108). Squamous cell carcinoma *in situ* is rarely seen in the United States and should be distinguished from dysplasia (26,87,120).

Adenocarcinoma is now the predominant histologic type of esophageal cancer. Adenocarcinoma may arise from foci of ectopic gastric mucosa or intrinsic esophageal glands. However, it is believed the vast majority arises from Barrett's esophagus. If a focus of squamous cell metaplasia is found in an adenocarcinoma, the tumor may be referred to as an adenoacanthoma (129).

Adenoid cystic carcinomas are rare, with an incidence of 0.75%. Patients with this malignancy present around the sixth decade of life and have a median survival of only 9 months (44). Mucoepidermoid tumors (adenosquamous carcinomas) are more aggressive and carry a poor prognosis (131). The incidence of small-cell carcinoma is approximately 2%. Patients with these malignancies present in the sixth to eighth decades of life, and the lesion is usually located in the middle to lower esophagus in males (24,65). These are believed to originate in the argyrophilic cells in the esophagus and may produce paraneoplastic syndromes, such as antidiuretic hormone secretion and hypercalcemia (38). The clinical course of small-cell carcinoma is similar to that of small-cell carcinoma of the lung and may be responsive to chemotherapy and radiation therapy (65,131).

Nonepithelial tumors of the esophagus are rare. Among these, leiomyosarcomas are the most common. Twenty-five percent of patients with this tumor present with metastases (48,99,104). Histologically, these tumors have interlacing bundles of spindle-shaped cells. Less aggressive forms have fewer mitotic figures and less anaplasia. Prognosis has been reported to be more favorable than that of squamous cell carcinoma (131). In patients with Kaposi's sarcoma, gastrointestinal involvement of the esophagus can be seen (50).

Malignant melanoma is rare and can occur as a primary esophageal tumor or as a metastasis. These lesions are usually large and often covered by intact squamous mucosa with focal areas of ulceration. Spread is usually submucosal. Mean survival is approximately 7 months (83,121). Lymphoma comprises approximately 1% of esophageal malignancies. It is usually associated with direct extension from other organs, although primary esophageal lymphoma has been reported (98).

Prognostic Factors

Stage is the most important prognostic factor in estimating survival of esophageal cancer patients. Increasing depth of penetration (T stage), nodal involvement (N stage), and absence or presence of distant metastases (M stage) significantly influence outcome. Patients with distant metastases are very rarely curable. In addition to stage, other factors portend outcome. Tumor location in the esophagus has been reported to influence survival, with upper-third lesions experiencing improved outcomes versus lesions in the lower two-thirds (64,101). Tumor size may also impact outcome. One study reported a 2-year survival rate of 19.2% for patients with tumors <5 cm in size versus 1.9% for patients with tumors >9 cm (64). Increasing tumor size is also correlated with unresectability and higher rates of distant metastases. Histologic tumor type has also been reported as an independent prognostic factor in patients undergoing resection. Siewert et al. (118) analyzed over 1,000 patients undergoing resection and found a 5-year survival rate of 47% for patients with adenocarcinoma versus 37% with squamous cell carcinoma. Patients with early stage adenocarcinoma had a much lower incidence of nodal involvement versus their squamous cell carcinoma counter parts. However, other series have reported no survival differences by histology (6).

Women tend to fare better than men with regards to survival (64,101). Race may also be a factor; Hussey et al. (64) reported higher survival rates in Caucasians than African Americans. In contrast, a recent analysis of patients treated with radiation and chemotherapy showed no statistical survival difference between races (125). Age has also been found to be significant, with patients older than 65 years of age faring less well (101). Weight loss and low overall performance status also indicate poor prognosis (64). Deep ulceration of the tumor, sinus tract formation, and fistula formation are other poor prognostic factors (109). Lymphatic vessel invasion portends advanced stage and worse long-term survival (137).

The importance of obtaining uninvolved pathologic margins at resection is of significant importance with regards to long-term outcomes. An Intergroup study (discussed below) evaluating chemotherapy preceding and following esophagectomy showed outcomes were similar in patients undergoing R1 resection (positive microscopic margins), R2 resection (gross residual disease), or patients not undergoing resection at all. Only patients undergoing R0 resection (uninvolved margins) had a substantial chance of long-term disease-free survival (69). A patterns of care survey examined the outcomes of patients with adenocarcinoma and squamous cell carcinoma of the esophagus between 1996 and 1999. Patients were treated with radiation therapy across 59 institutions. On multivariate analysis, significant improvements in survival were seen in patients treated at centers with ≥500 new cancer patients per year, compared to centers seeing <500 (hazard ratio 1.32; $p = 0.03$) (126).

General Management

Treatment for esophageal carcinoma is characterized as curative or palliative. According to Pearson (101), only 20/100

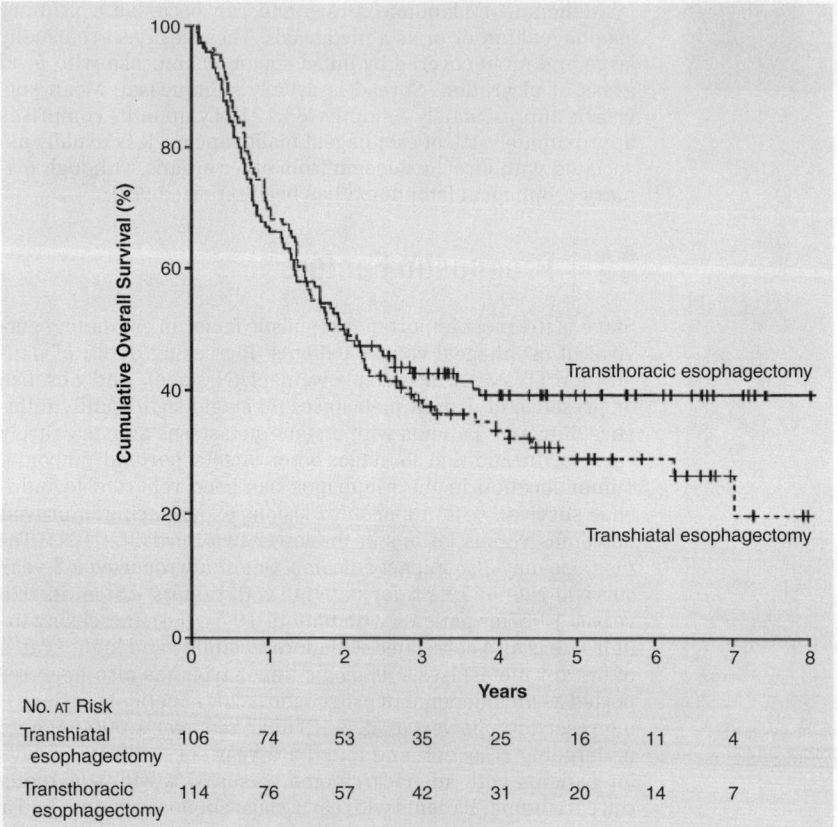

No. AT Risk

Transhiatal esophagectomy	106	74	53	35	25	16	11	4
Transthoracic esophagectomy	114	76	57	42	31	20	14	7

FIGURE 50.7. Overall survival among patients randomly assigned to transhiatal esophagectomy or transthoracic esophagectomy with extended en bloc lymphadenectomy. (Hulscher)

patients present with cancer of the esophagus that is truly localized to the esophagus, indicating that at the time of diagnosis, approximately 80/100 patients have locally advanced or distant disease.

Surgery with Curative Intent

Surgery of the thoracic esophagus requires a subtotal or total esophagectomy and is usually undertaken for lesions of the mid-III lower third of the thoracic esophagus and gastroesophageal junction. Patients with stage I to III and selected IVa tumors are often considered for potentially curative resection; however, aortic, tracheal, heart, or great vessel invasion may preclude resection. Esophagectomy may be accomplished by a number of techniques, including a transhiatal esophagectomy, right thoracotomy (Ivor-Lewis), left thoracotomy, or radical esophagectomy. Each technique has its advantages and disadvantages. Advantages of the transthoracic approach include better visualization with access and resection of the upper two thirds of the esophagus and mediastinal lymph nodes. Alternatively, the transhiatal approach has less morbidity than thoracotomy (including respiratory compromise) with easier access to anastomotic leaks (neck versus thorax). In any instance, achievement of negative margins at resection has been reported to be a significant prognostic factor and should be the goal of esophageal resection. In a study of 500 patients undergoing transthoracic resection, patients undergoing margin negative resection had a 5-year survival rate of 29% versus no 5-year survivors in patients with involved margins (43).

The Ivor-Lewis procedure is the classic approach to expose mid-esophageal lesions. A left thoracotomy procedure exposes lesions of the gastroesophageal junction. Transhiatal esophagectomy is performed without a thoracotomy and is useful in lower esophageal lesions, although direct visualization and dissection of varying mediastinal lymph nodes cannot be achieved. The optimal surgical approach is unknown. A ran-

domized trial comparing transhiatal versus transthoracic approaches in patients with adenocarcinoma showed no significant survival advantage to the later, although a possible trend was noted (5-year survival 29% vs. 39%; Fig. 50.7). However, perioperative mortality was also increased with the transthoracic approach (93).

Laparotomy can be performed before or concurrently with esophagectomy to rule out any disease below the diaphragm. Multiple reconstruction options are available following definitive surgery: esophagogastrostomy is the most widely used, using the stomach as a conduit to replace the esophagus. Patients with significant obstruction and inability to maintain their weight often require placement of feeding jejunostomy. If possible surgery is planned, gastric tube placement is generally avoided given the stomach will ultimately serve as the "neo-esophagus" following resection. Colon interposition, preferably with the left colon, can also be used, however, this approach is generally reserved for patients who have previously undergone gastric surgery or other procedures that have devascularized the stomach (108).

Squamous cell carcinoma of the cervical esophagus presents a difficult management situation. If surgery is performed, resection of portions of the pharynx, the entire larynx, thyroid gland, and the proximal esophagus is often required. Radical neck dissections are also carried out (109). Because of the significant morbidity and loss of organ function with surgery, chemoradiation alone has been frequently employed. The survival probability with definitive chemoradiotherapy is similar, without the major functional impairments, morbidity, and mortality associated with surgery (56).

Curative Combination Therapy

In the treatment of patients with esophageal cancer, an approach of radiation therapy with concurrent chemotherapy, with or without surgery, is frequently adopted. Multiagent chemotherapy with cisplatin and 5-fluorouracil (5-FU) is utilized most frequently. Taxanes, topoisomerase inhibitors, and antiepidermal growth factor receptor inhibitors with radiation therapy are under investigation.

Palliative Treatment

Palliative treatment is frequently used for the relief of symptoms of esophageal carcinoma, especially dysphagia (119). Surgical palliation involves resection and reconstruction, if possible, removing the bulk of the disease, potentially preventing abscess and fistula formation as well as bleeding. Substernal bypass with the colon or entire stomach has also been carried out (119). However, given the poor prognosis in patients with advanced disease and morbidity associated with resection, this approach is not commonly adopted and should be avoided in patients who can be managed with nonsurgical modalities.

Endoscopic dilatation is a reasonable alternative. When the lumen of the esophagus is dilated to 15 mm, dysphagia is often no longer experienced. Repeat dilatation is often required (109). Esophageal stenting with either conventional plastic stents or metallic self-expanding stents can also be used to maintain patency (112).

Palliative irradiation is frequently used to control the primary disease as well as distant metastases. Resolution of symptoms, especially pain and dysphagia, can be accomplished in up to 80% of patients (108). Palliative treatment regimens range from 30 Gy over 2 weeks (92) to 50 Gy over 5 weeks (108). Chemotherapy is also often used for palliation, either alone or in combination with radiation.

∷ | Radiation Therapy Techniques

Simulation

When patients are simulated, the radiation oncologist must know the extent of disease based on imaging (barium swallow, CT, PET) as well as endoscopy. During simulation, the patient is positioned, straightened, and immobilized on the simulation table. Arms are generally placed overhead. Palpable neck disease should be marked with a radio-opaque wire. Conventional simulation using fluoroscopy or CT-based simulation is appropriate. With either technique, the administration of oral contrast to delineate the esophagus is used. With conventional simulation (two-dimensional planning), frontal and lateral radiographs of the patient in the treatment position are obtained. For cervical and upper thoracic lesions, an immobilization mask may assist in an accurate reproducibility. Some authors recommend placing the patient in the prone position for treatment to displace the esophagus away from the spinal cord (120).

When three-dimensional (3D) conformal radiation therapy is used, the patient is placed on the CT simulator in the same treatment position, and a scan of the entire area of interest with margin is obtained. At minimum, 5-mm slices should be used, allowing accurate tumor characterization as well as improved quality of digitally reconstructed radiographs. Arterial phase IV contrast is generally used to delineate mediastinal and abdominal vascular nodal basins, including the celiac axis. The tumor and vital structures are then outlined on each slice on the treatment planning system, enabling a 3D treatment plan to be generated.

Treatment Planning

The fusion of CT-PET has been shown to prompt treatment modification of the gross tumor volume (GTV) and planning target volumes in a majority of patients, including lung volume considerations (148). A margin of 5 cm above and below the tumor is usually recommended to cover subclinical submucosal/nodal disease, as well as an approximate 2.5-cm radial margin. For disease located in the lower esophagus, the celiac axis and gastrohepatic ligament are often included based on patterns of spread data. The celiac axis is generally located at the level of T12 and can be identified on CT. Similarly, supraclavicular nodal basins are often included for upper esophageal lesions (109).

Because of the changing contour from the neck to the thoracic inlet, treatment of lesions in the upper third of the esophagus can present a difficult technical problem. Often, lesions in the upper cervical or postcricoid esophagus are treated from the laryngopharynx to the carina, depending on extent of disease. Supraclavicular and superior mediastinal nodes are irradiated electively. This can be achieved with lateral parallel opposed or oblique portals to the primary tumor and a single anterior field for the supraclavicular and superior mediastinal nodes (64). Another technique treats lesions in this region by means of a four-field box technique. A wax bolus is used to build up the lack of tissue above the shoulders, acting as a compensator. A high-energy beam (>15 MV) is used, and both sides of the neck are treated prophylactically. Other methods of treating lesions at the thoracic inlet include 140-degree arc rotations, anterior wedged pairs, and three- or four-field techniques using posterior oblique portals combined with a single anterior portal or anteroposterior-posteroanterior (AP) fields (64). More recently, intensity-modulated radiation therapy (IMRT)–based planning has facilitated the treatment of upper esophageal lesions (Fig. 50.8A,B). Strict normal tissue constraints, including normal lung and spinal cord, are important considerations using these techniques.

Lesions in the thoracic esophagus may be more simply approached. The inferior margin of the initial fields includes the gastroesophageal junction and, for lower or middle-third lesions, the celiac axis nodal basins as well as gastrohepatic ligament. Initial fields include anteroposterior-posteroanterior opposed portals and are treated to 30 to 36 Gy, after which oblique fields may be used, including an anterior field with posterior oblique pair (left and right posterior oblique) or opposed right anterior and left posterior oblique fields to 45 Gy, inclusive of the above nodal basins. Care should be taken to avoid as much of the heart as reasonably possible. Additionally, the kidney volume in the radiation field should be considered when treating the celiac axis in lower esophageal tumors. Reduced fields encompassing gross disease with an approximate 2-cm margin through oblique or lateral fields may then be used for an additional 5.4 Gy. Doses usually do not exceed 50 Gy (see below). Figures 50.9 and 50.10 show digitally reconstructed radiographs for a typical lower esophageal adenocarcinoma. Figure 50.11A,B illustrates dose distributions and a dose–volume histogram for a patient with lower esophageal adenocarcinoma using this approach.

In radiation therapy planning, normal tissue tolerance should always be considered. The spinal cord dose should generally be limited to 45 Gy using 1.8 Gy fractions. Efforts to minimize radiation to the heart, in particular the left ventricle in lower esophageal lesions, should be made. Adopting an "off heart" approach using oblique orientations (including right anterior and left posterior) may help facilitate this. Efforts to minimize dose to normal pulmonary tissues should be made, given there are emerging data suggesting volume of irradiated lung may correspond to postoperative complications and worsened pulmonary function (below). Frequently, the volume of irradiated lung can be minimized using a simple AP/PA approach. However, this often results in significant cardiac dose, particularly in lower esophagus and gastroesophageal junction tumors. Therefore, oblique orientations are used, resulting in increased volumes of normal lung being irradiated. When

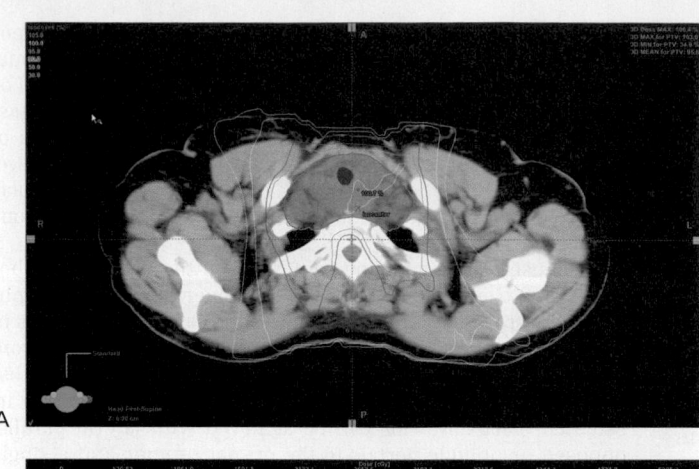

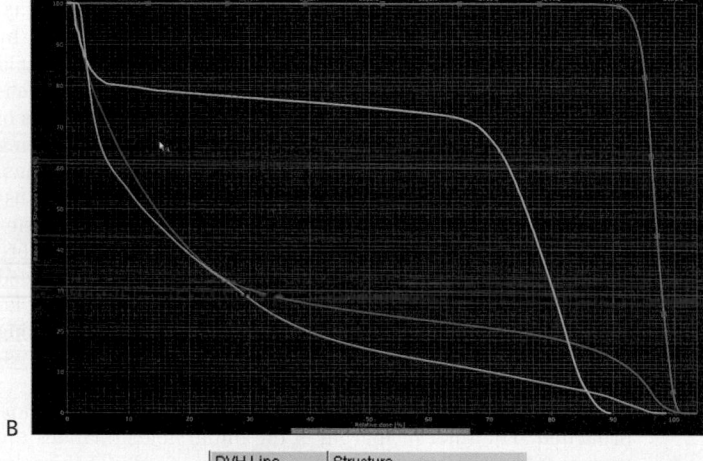

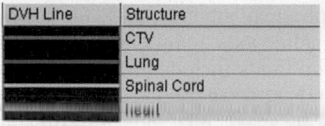

DVH Line	Structure
	CTV
	Lung
	Spinal Cord
	heart

FIGURE 50.8. A: Isodose curves of a patient with cervical esophageal lesion treated with an eight-field IMRT plan. **B:** Dose–volume histogram for patient treated to 50 to 40 cGy using an eight-field IMRT technique. CTV, clinical target volume. (Both photos courtesy of Zhiheng Wang, Ph.D.)

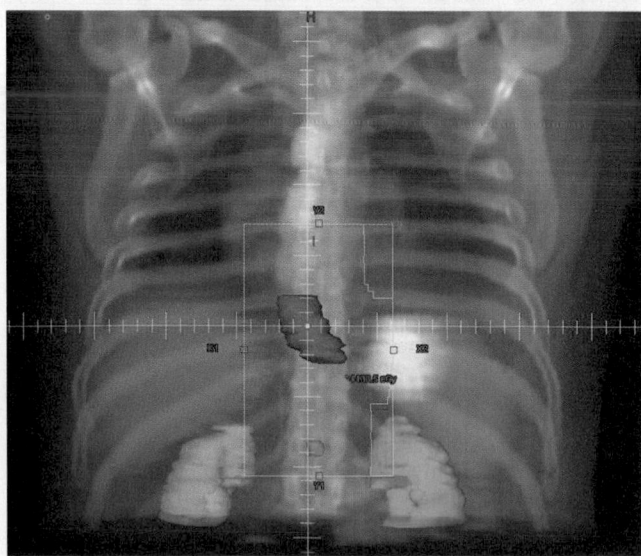

FIGURE 50.9. Digitally reconstructed radiograph for a typical lower esophageal lesion—AP view. gross tumor volume, red; celiac trunk, blue; right kidney, green; left kidney, blue (Courtesy of Rhonda May, CMD and Shiva Das, Ph.D.)

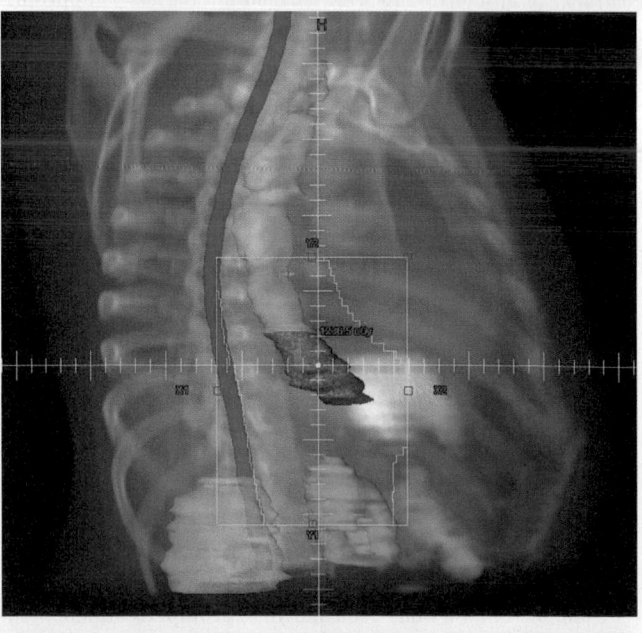

FIGURE 50.10. Right anterior oblique fields used to spare the left ventricle and spinal cord following initial AP/PA fields. (Courtesy of Rhonda May, CMD and Shiva Das, Ph.D.)

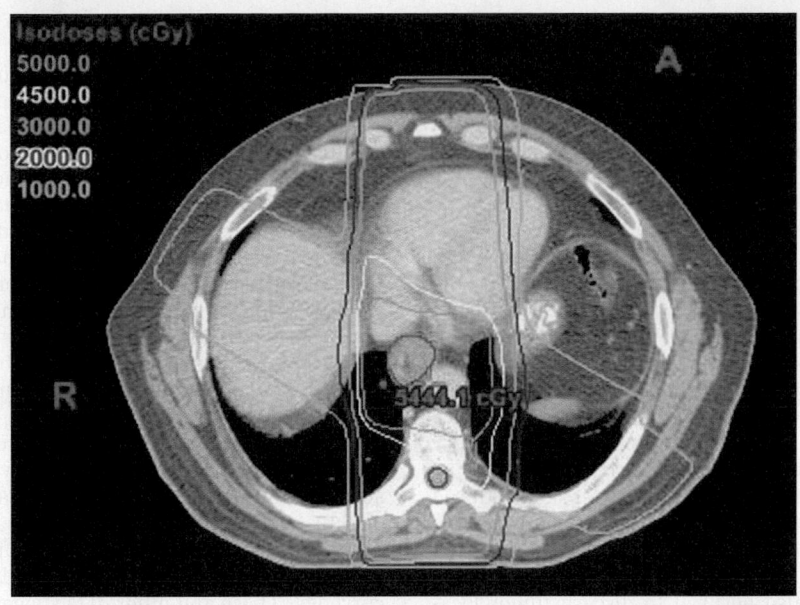

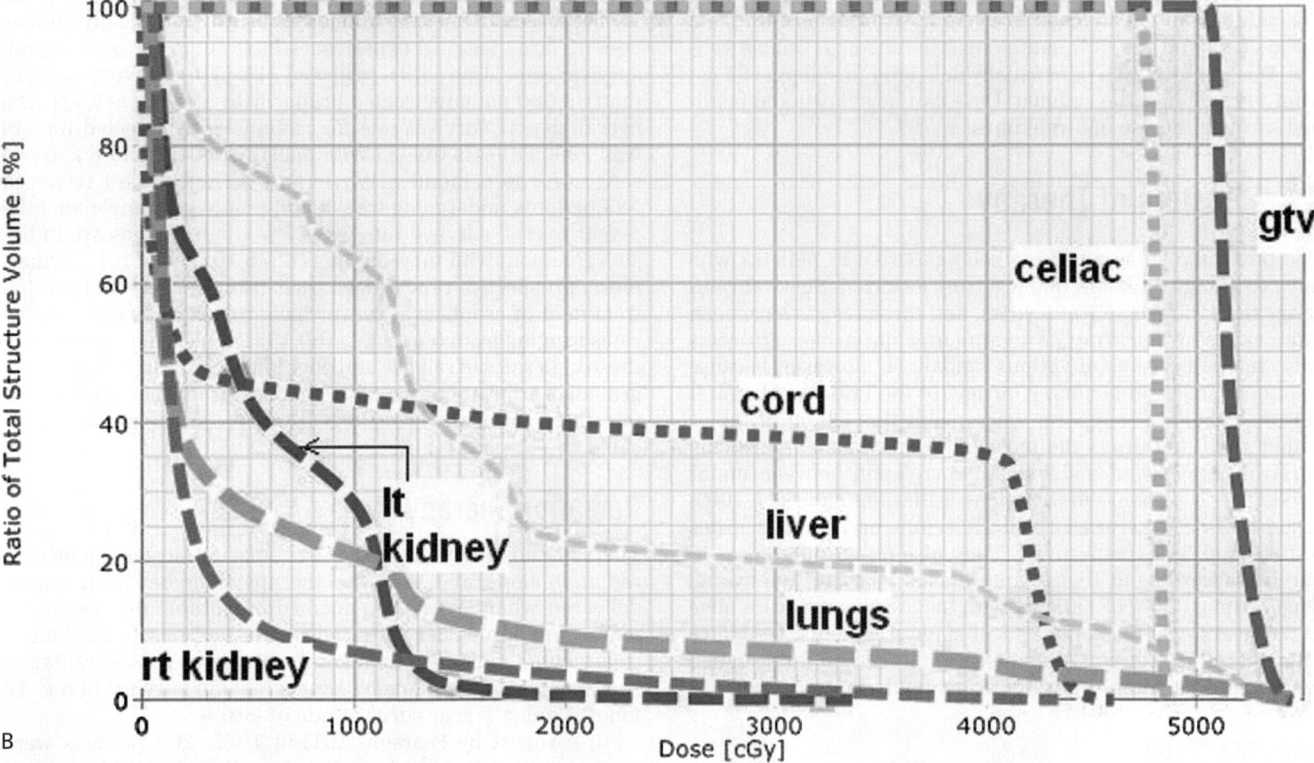

FIGURE 50.11. A: Dose distributions using computed tomography–generated dosimetry for a patient with an adenocarcinoma involving the lower esophagus. **B:** Dose–volume histogram for patient with a lower esophageal adenocarcinoma. (Both courtesy of Rhonda May, CMD and Shiva Das, Ph.D.)

given concurrent chemotherapy, dose to these fields should generally be limited to 13 to 15 Gy.

Doses of Radiation

Because local-regional failure is common after conventional chemoradiation, investigators have evaluated dose-escalation techniques. Minsky et al. (91) reported the results of Intergroup 0123, which randomized 236 patients with clinical stage T1-4, N0/1, M0 squamous cell or adenocarcinoma of the esophagus selected for nonsurgical therapy. Patients were randomized to receive 64.8 Gy versus 50.4 Gy, both with concurrent 5-FU and

cisplatin chemotherapy. Patients with cervical, mid-, or distal esophageal cancer were eligible with the exception of tumors within 2 cm of the gastroesophageal junction. Approximately 85% of patients had squamous cell histology. This study was closed after interim analysis showed no probability of superiority in the high-dose arm. No significant difference in median survival (13 vs. 18.1 months), 2-year survival (31% vs. 40%), or local-regional failure/persistence of disease (56% vs. 52%) was seen between the high-dose and standard-dose arms. Eleven treatment-related deaths occurred in the high-dose arm compared with two in the standard-dose arm, with 7/11 high-dose arm deaths occurring in patients who received 50.4 Gy or less.

The authors performed a separate survival analysis including only patients receiving the assigned radiation dose. Despite this, no survival advantage was noted in the high-dose arm. These authors concluded that higher radiation doses did not increase survival or local/regional control, and that the standard radiation dose for patients treated with concurrent 5-FU and cisplatin chemotherapy is 50.4 Gy.

Brachytherapy

In addition to external beam radiation therapy (EBRT), intracavitary therapy can be used with curative or palliative intent. The advantage of brachytherapy centers on exploitation of the inverse square law and quick dose falloff, thus sparing surrounding tissues from radiation while providing focal dose escalation. The radioactive source of choice is usually iridium-192 (^{192}Ir). High–dose-rate (HDR) techniques can deliver 100 to 400 Gy per hour, allowing treatment to be given in 5 to 10 minutes.

With brachytherapy, an afterloading catheter is introduced through the nose into the esophagus to the primary tumor site under fluoroscopic guidance. This is often performed with the patient on the simulation table. Contrast is used to define the tumor site. CT scan can also be used to discern tumor location. After localization films are taken and dosimetry generated, the catheter is then attached to a remote afterloader through a guide cable and the ^{192}Ir source inserted through remote control. Doses of 5 to 20 Gy are usually delivered to a depth of 1 cm from the center of the catheter. Dose can be shaped and modified through the use of dwell times.

Results of Therapy

The best survival results have been reported in patients who have esophageal tumors that are truly localized. Survival rates range from 25% to 35% at 5 years, and these results have been attained using an array of treatment approaches. Problems arise in comparisons of various modalities, however, because of patient selection factors. A review of the Princess Margaret Hospital data (15) supports the concept that extent of tumor rather than therapy is the most important factor influencing survival. They found a significant correlation between tumor (T) stage and response to treatment. T1 lesions showed a 100% response rate, whereas T2 and T3 lesions had response rates of 68% and 58%, respectively. They also found differences in survival according to T stage, metastasis (M) stage, and overall stage. Almost 20% of patients with stage I disease were alive at 3.5 years, whereas only 11% of stage II patients were alive after the same interval. All patients with stage III disease died within approximately 1.5 years following therapy.

Surgery Alone

Surgery remains the benchmark to which other modalities are compared. Surgery removes the tumor, a length of normal esophagus, and lymph nodes. Although multiple techniques exist in the resection of esophageal cancer, no clear "preferred" approach has emerged. Proponents of more extended resection (including transthoracic approaches) have advocated that such procedures result in a superior nodal clearance and therefore offer a more complete "oncologic" resection. As described previously, a trial from the Netherlands randomized 220 patients with esophageal adenocarcinoma to transhiatal esophagectomy alone or transthoracic esophagectomy with extended lymph node dissection. Patients undergoing transhiatal resection experienced significantly fewer pulmonary complications, chylous leaks, as well as significantly reduced ventilator dependence, intensive care unit, and hospital stays. At a median 4.7 year follow-up, no significant difference in local–regional re-

currence was seen between the two groups (32% transhiatal vs. 31% transthoracic). Furthermore, no significant differences were seen in median disease-free survival (1.4 years vs. 1.7 years; $p = 0.15$) or median overall survival (1.8 vs. 2.0 years; $p = 0.38$). However, there did appear to be a nonsignificant trend favoring the transthoracic approach in improved disease-free survival (5-year 27% vs 39%) and overall survival (5-year 29% vs. 39%) (see Fig. 50.7). The authors concluded that a transhiatal approach was associated with less morbidity relative to transthoracic surgery with no apparent survival advantage with either technique, although a trend toward improved survival with longer follow-up was seen (63). In summary, none of the surgical approaches to localized esophageal cancer has clearly been shown to be superior with regards to complications or outcomes, and no one standard surgical approach exists for esophageal cancer resection.

Following resection alone, local–regional relapse is a common mode of failure. Contemporary randomized trials with surgery-alone arms have reported local–regional failure rates of 32% to 45% (63,69,77,133). It should be remembered that patterns of failure reports often describe first site of failure only, potentially underreporting the true incidence of local–regional recurrence. These and other data suggest that even with modern surgical techniques, local–regional persistence of disease following resection remains a major problem. Additionally, studies pooling large surgical experiences have reported poor overall survival rates. One series reviewed 122 papers involving more than 83,000 patients treated primarily by surgery (41,42). The overall 5-year survival rate for patients with resected tumors was 12%. Patients treated with palliative intent had a survival range of 2 to 6 months. Whyte and Orringer (144) reviewed 583 patients undergoing transhiatal esophagectomy alone; the 5-year overall survival rate was 27%. Other studies are in basic agreement with these findings (2,76,101,114,119). Furthermore, prospective randomized trials using surgery alone in the treatment of esophageal cancer have reported 3-year survival rates ranging from 6% to 35% (69,133,139) (Table 50.6). Given these high rates of relapse and poor long-term survival, the integration of adjuvant or neoadjuvant chemoradiation approaches into the treatment of esophageal cancer is rational and indicated.

Radiation Therapy Alone

There are no randomized studies comparing surgery alone with radiation alone, and, radiation therapy alone has been usually delivered when lesions are deemed inoperable because of tumor extent or medical contraindications and/or when palliative treatment is indicated. In general, patients receiving radiation as a sole treatment modality have a median survival of 6 to 12 months and a 5-year survival rate of <10%.

In a report by Pearson (101) in 1977, 208 patients were treated with radiation alone. Patients received 50 Gy and had an unduplicated 5-year reported survival rate of 20%. An updated Edinburgh experience reported 2- and 5-year survival rates of 19% and 9%, respectively (95). A large review analyzing 49 series involving more than 8,400 patients treated primarily with radiation therapy found overall survival rates at 1, 2, and 5 years to be 18%, 8%, and 6%, respectively (42). Hancock and Glatstein (56) reviewed 9,511 patients and found only 5.8% were alive at 5 years. Okawa et al. (96) reported 5-year survival rates by stage. For patients with stage I disease, the 5-year survival rate was 20%; stage II, 10%; stage III, 3%; and stage IV, 0%. Overall, the 5-year survival rate was 9%. For cervical esophageal lesions treated with radiation alone, the cure rates are comparable with those in patients treated with surgery alone. Lederman (79) treated 263 patients with radiation therapy alone and reported 3- and 5-year survival rates of 11% and 7%, respectively. In more contemporary series, an

Table 50.6 | COMPARISON OF SURGERY ALONE ARMS IN RANDOMIZED STUDIES

Author (Reference)	Patients (Total)	Patients (Surgical)	Median Survival (Months)	2-Year Survival	3-Year Survival
Walsh et al. (139)	110	55	11	26	6
Urba et al. (133)	100	50	18	NA	15
Bosset et al. (23)	282	139	19	40	35
Kelsen et al. (69)	440	227	16	37	23
Medical Research Council (89)	802	402	13	34	NA

NA, not applicable

Intergroup randomized study (discussed below) comparing combined chemotherapy with 5-FU and cisplatin with radiotherapy (50 Gy) versus radiotherapy only (64 Gy) showed 3-year survival with radiotherapy alone was 0%. These and other data suggest that treatment with radiation therapy alone for esophageal cancer patients is palliative in the vast majority of patients (Table 50.7).

Preoperative Radiation Therapy

The use of preoperative radiation therapy has potential biologic and physical advantages, including increased resectability of tumors, increased tumor radioresponsiveness secondary to improved tumor oxygenation, a theoretical decreased likelihood of dissemination at the time of surgery, as well as avoidance of surgery in patients with rapidly progressive disease.

There are numerous nonrandomized studies reporting patient survival with preoperative radiation therapy. Hancock and Glatstein (56) reviewed 1,181 patients treated with preoperative irradiation. In their analysis, the overall 5-year survival rate was 6%, although in patients who completed preoperative therapy and esophageal resection, the 5-year survival rate was 14%. Marks et al. (88) treated 332 patients (101 resectable) with preoperative therapy and found 2- and 5-year survival rates of 23% and 14%, respectively.

There are at least five randomized studies comparing preoperative irradiation followed by surgery with surgery alone. These studies demonstrate no apparent clinical benefit to the use of preoperative radiation therapy alone (Table 50.8). Launois et al. (76) reported delivering 40 Gy over 8 to 12 days

with surgery 8 days later versus surgery alone. Resection rates were similar—70% and 58% for preoperative irradiation and for surgery alone, respectively. The 5-year survival rate after resection was 11.5% for those treated with surgery alone, compared with 9.5% for those treated with irradiation and surgery. The second randomized study, published by the European Organisation for Research and Treatment of Cancer (EORTC), used 33 Gy over 12 days (52). There was no significant difference in survival between those receiving preoperative irradiation and those receiving surgery alone. Arnott et al. (13) reported on 176 patients, 86 of whom were treated with esophagectomy alone versus 90 who were treated with preoperative radiation therapy. Preoperative radiation therapy was delivered with 4-MV photons using opposed fields, delivering 20 Gy at 2 Gy per fraction. Resectability and local failure were not reported. Patients receiving low-dose radiation therapy did not demonstrate a benefit in 5-year overall survival rates (17% vs. 9% for surgery and preoperative radiation, respectively; $p = 0.4$). Wang et al. (140) randomized 206 patients to surgery alone versus 40 Gy in 2-Gy fractions delivered preoperatively. No significant survival advantage was seen for patients receiving radiation therapy (35% vs. 30%; $p > 0.05$).

A recent meta-analysis from the Oeosophageal Cancer Collaborative Group updated data from five randomized trials of >1,100 patients comparing preoperative radiotherapy alone versus surgery alone. The majority of patients had squamous cell carcinoma. At a median follow-up of 9 years, the hazard ratio was 0.89, suggestive of an overall reduction in the risk of death of 11% and absolute survival benefit of 4% at 5 years with the use of preoperative radiotherapy. However, this was not statistically significant ($p = 0.06$). The authors concluded that there

Table 50.7 | RESULTS WITH EXTERNAL BEAM RADIATION THERAPY ALONE FOR ESOPHAGEAL CANCER

Author (Reference)	No. of Patients	Dose	2-Year Survival	5-Year Survival
Pearson (101)	288	50 Gy/4 wk (2.5 Gy/fr)	NR	17% (48/288)
Beatty et al. (15)	344	>40 Gy/<19 fr, >45 Gy/ <23 fr, >50 Gy/<3 mo	21%	0%
	176 curative[a]			
	168 palliative	Less than the curative doses	0%	0%
Schuchmann et al. (114)	127	>4,500 R	—	0%
		<4,500 R	—	0%
Newaishy et al. (95)	444 (all curative)	50–55 Gy/4 wk (2.5–2.75 Gy/fr)	—	9%
Okawa et al. (96)	288		NR	9%
DeRen (36)	678	60–69 Gy/6–8 wk, 5–10 Gy boost	11.4%	8%

fr, fraction; NR, not reported
[a]Thirty of the 176 radically treated patients had surgery plus irradiation.

| :: Table 50.8 | RANDOMIZED TRIALS OF PREOPERATIVE RADIATION THERAPY FOR ESOPHAGEAL CANCER |

Author (Reference)	Patients	Dose (Gy)	Fraction (Gy)	Local Failure		Survival (5-Year)	
				Surgery	RT + Surgery	Surgery	RT + Surgery
Launois et al. (76)	109	40	NA	NA	NA	12	10
Gignoux et al. (52)	229	33	3.3	67	46	8	10
Arnott et al. (13)[a]	176	20	2	NA	NA	17	9
Wang et al. (140)	160	40	2	NA	NA	30	35

NA, not applicable; RT, radiation therapy
[a]Both squamous and adenocarcinoma.

was no clear evidence that preoperative radiotherapy improves survival of patients with potentially resectable esophageal cancer (12).

In general, there were no differences in resectability rates, local failure, or survival in almost all reported individual studies. Interpretation of these varying studies is complicated by differences in radiation techniques, suboptimal radiation dose, and inadequate radiation volumes. Although preoperative radiation therapy alone may improve local control, there is no convincing data that it results in improved survival in esophageal cancer patients.

Postoperative Radiation Therapy

The main advantage to adjuvant versus neoadjuvant approaches is the knowledge of the pathological staging to appropriately select patients for therapy. Postoperative therapy may allow the radiation oncologist to treat areas at risk for recurrence while sparing otherwise normal radiosensitive structures, thereby decreasing toxicity. In addition, patients with pathologic T1N0 or metastatic disease may be spared treatment. Postoperative irradiation has historically been delivered to patients with esophageal cancer who have bulky tumors with gross residual disease or histologically proven microscopic residual disease. Potential disadvantages of postoperative radiation include limited tolerance of normal tissues following gastric pull-up or intestinal interposition and irradiation of a devascularized tumor bed.

Three randomized trails have assessed surgery alone versus surgery followed by postoperative radiation therapy. In a French trial, 221 patients with squamous cell carcinoma of the mid-lower esophagus undergoing esophagectomy were randomized to postoperative radiation therapy or no further treatment. Patients were stratified by extent of nodal involvement. Total dose was 45 to 55 Gy at 1.8 Gy per fraction, beginning within 3 months of surgery. Five-year survival in node negative patients was 38% versus 7% with involved nodes. No significant survival difference was seen in patients receiving postoperative radiation versus surgery alone. Rates of local regional recurrence were lower in patients receiving radiation therapy (85% vs. 70%; P = NS). However, in patients without nodal involvement, local–regional recurrence was significantly improved in patients receiving postoperative therapy (90% v. 65%; $p < 0.2$). The authors concluded that postoperative radiation therapy did not improve survival following resection for squamous cell carcinoma (127).

Investigators from the University of Hong Kong reported the results of 130 patients treated with postoperative radiation therapy versus surgery alone. Patients who underwent either curative or palliative resections were included in this trial. Radiation therapy was delivered to a total dose of 49 Gy (curative patients) or 52.5 Gy (palliative patients) using 3.5-Gy fractions. Most patients had squamous cell histology. Local recurrence was noted in 15% of patients receiving radiation and 31% of patients with surgery only ($p = 0.06$). In patients with squamous cell carcinoma, the local recurrence rate was 15% with radiation therapy versus 36% with surgery alone ($p = 0.02$). Median survival in patients was worse in patients receiving postoperative radiotherapy versus control patients (8.7 vs. 15.2 months; $p = 0.02$). A total of 10 patients undergoing surgery alone had tracheal bronchial recurrence resulting in death versus three patients receiving adjuvant radiation therapy ($p = 0.07$). The authors concluded that postoperative radiation therapy was associated with increased morbidity and death caused by irradiation injury as well as the early appearance of metastatic disease and a reduced overall survival, although patients receiving radiation therapy were less likely to have a tracheobronchial recurrence. The high rate of complications associated with radiation therapy in this study may possibly be related to the high dose per fraction and total dose delivered (47).

Lastly, a study conducted by Xiao et al. (146) randomized 549 patients to radical resection vs radical resection followed by radiation therapy. All patients had squamous cell carcinoma. The radiation dose delivered was 60 Gy in 6 weeks. Patients were classified into three groups: Group 1, no lymph node involvement; Group 2, one to two lymph nodes involved; Group 3, three or more lymph nodes involved. Results showed T stage, stage group, and the number of lymph nodes involved by tumor were highly predictive of survival. The 5-year survival for groups 1, 2, and 3 were 58.1%, 30.6%, and 14.4%, respectively. Local control and survival were improved in patients receiving postoperative irradiation. For patients with involved lymph nodes, 5-year survival for resection only patients versus patients receiving resection and radiation therapy were 17.6% and 34.1%, respectively ($p = 0.04$). In summary, postoperative radiation therapy may decrease local recurrence, particularly in the setting of involved margins, although the impact of this adjuvant treatment on overall survival remains less clear.

Postoperative Combined Chemoradiation

The role of adjuvant combined chemoradiation following resection of esophageal cancer has remained ill-defined. A large randomized Intergroup trial evaluating the role of adjuvant chemoradiation following surgery versus surgery alone for patients with adenocarcinoma of the stomach and GE junction was reported in 2001. In this study, a total of 556 patients with resected, margin-negative gastric or gastroesophageal junction adenocarcinoma were randomly assigned to surgery alone versus surgery with postoperative chemoradiotherapy. Treatment consisted of one cycle of 5-FU and leucovorin, followed by 45 Gy external beam irradiation concurrent with 5-FU, followed by two additional cycles of 5-FU and leucovorin. Approximately 20% of patients had lesions in the gastroesophageal junction. A significant survival advantage was seen in the adjuvantly treated group (median survival 27 months vs. 36 months; $p = 0.005$). On subset analysis, this benefit was detected in patients with gastroesophageal cancer (84). Therefore, in patients with stage Ib to IV, nonmetastatic GE junctional carcinoma, it is appropriate to advise adjuvant chemoradiotherapy in efforts to potentially improve upon local control and ultimate survival.

Preoperative Chemotherapy

Three large randomized trials have shown conflicting results with the use of neoadjuvant chemotherapy alone in the treatment of esophageal cancer. Kelsen et al. (69) reported the results of an Intergroup study randomizing 440 patients with squamous cell carcinoma and adenocarcinoma to receive either combined cisplatin or 5-FU chemotherapy for three cycles followed by resection, followed by a similar regimen of adjuvant chemotherapy, versus immediate resection with no chemotherapy. Results of this trial showed patients receiving neoadjuvant chemotherapy had a pathologic complete response rate of 2.5% at resection. There was no apparent survival advantage (3-year survival of 23% vs. 26%) in patients receiving chemotherapy. Additionally, rates of local failure (32% vs. 31%) and distant metastases development (41% vs. 50%) were not significantly different between the two groups. The authors concluded that neoadjuvant chemotherapy with cisplatin and 5-FU did not improve survival in patients with resectable esophageal cancer.

In contrast to the Intergroup study, a similar trial from the Medical Research Council (MRC) randomized 802 patients with squamous cell carcinoma or adenocarcinoma of the esophagus to either two cycles of combined cisplatin/5-FU chemotherapy versus surgery alone. Preoperative staging CT was not required, and radiation therapy was allowed in both treatment arms. Patients receiving neoadjuvant chemotherapy had a statistically improved 2-year survival (43% vs. 34%) (89). The reason for outcomes differences in these trials is not clear.

A recent large European study randomly assigned patients with resectable adenocarcinoma of the stomach, gastroesophageal junction, or lower esophagus to preoperative and postoperative chemotherapy with epirubicin, cisplatin, and 5-FU (ECF) versus surgery alone. Approximately one fourth of the patients had adenocarcinoma involving the lower esophagus or gastroesophageal junction. Patients receiving perioperative chemotherapy had a hazard ratio for death of 0.75, which was highly significant. Five-year survival in patients receiving chemotherapy was 36% versus 23% in patients undergoing surgery alone ($p = 0.009$). Subgroup analysis of patients with lower esophageal or gastroesophageal junction tumors showed benefit to the delivery of perioperative chemotherapy (33).

Urshel et al. (135) performed a meta-analysis of 11 randomized controlled trials including nearly 2,000 patients treated with neoadjuvant chemotherapy and surgery versus surgery alone in patients with resectable esophageal cancer. These authors did not demonstrate a survival benefit with the addition of neoadjuvant chemotherapy. In summary, the role of neoadjuvant chemotherapy alone in the setting of potentially resectable esophageal cancer remains controversial.

Preoperative Chemoradiation versus Surgery Alone

Walsh et al. (139) reported the first randomized study to evaluate the role of concurrent preoperative chemoradiation combined with surgery. One hundred ten patients with adenocarcinoma of the esophagus were randomized to receive cisplatin, 5-FU, and concurrent radiation therapy followed by surgery versus surgery alone. Combined modality patients received two courses of chemotherapy weeks 1 and 6. Patients were treated

using anteroposterior-posteroanterior fields (later changed to a three-field technique) to a total dose of 4,000 cGy in 15 fractions. Surgery was performed 4 to 6 weeks later, using five separate approaches. Median survival was 16 months with preoperative chemoradiation therapy compared to 11 months for the patients treated with surgery alone ($p = 0.01$). The 1-, 2-, and 3-year survival rates were 52%, 37%, and 32%, respectively, for patients who received multimodality therapy, and 44%, 26%, and 6%, respectively, for those patients assigned to surgery. These results were significant at 3 years ($p = 0.01$). The authors concluded neoadjuvant chemoradiation was superior to surgery alone in patients with resectable esophageal adenocarcinoma. This trial has been criticized for its poor surgery alone results, short follow-up, and lack of prerandomization CT staging.

Urba et al. (133) reported the results of 100 patients with nonmetastatic esophageal carcinoma (squamous and adenocarcinoma histology) randomized to receive preoperative chemoradiation followed by surgery versus transhiatal esophagectomy alone. Chemotherapy consisted of cisplatin, 5-FU, and vinblastine. Only 69% of the patients were able to receive the intended chemotherapy dose. Radiation was delivered at 1.5 Gy twice daily for 3 weeks to a total dose of 4,500 cGy. No elective nodal irradiation was performed. Surgery was performed on day 42. Tumors >5 cm, patient age >70 years, and squamous cell histology were associated with inferior survival. At median follow-up of 8 years, no significant difference in survival was seen between treatment arms, with a median survival of 17 months. However, 3-year survival rate was 16% in the surgery-alone arm versus 30% in the combined-modality arm ($p = 0.15$). A higher incidence of locoregional failure as first site of failure was seen in surgery-alone patients (42% vs. 19%;, $p = 0.02$). In patients experiencing pathologic complete response, a median survival of 50 months and a 3-year survival rate of 64% was seen, versus patients with residual tumor in the surgical specimen where median survival was 12 months with a 3-year survival rate of 19% ($p = 0.01$). The investigators stated that "Although this is not statistically significant, this suggests a possible trend to the benefit of multimodality therapy, but the sample size was too small to detect a more subtle survival difference," and that surgery should be continued as a standard of care.

Bosset et al. (23) reported an EORTC trial randomizing 282 patients with squamous cell carcinoma of the esophagus to either immediate surgical resection or preoperative therapy using concurrent cisplatin chemotherapy with radiation therapy. Patients were treated with split course radiotherapy with a 2-week interval, using 3.7 Gy per fraction to a total of 37 Gy. Postoperative mortality was significantly higher in patients receiving preoperative therapy (12% vs. 4%). Outcomes showed patients receiving neoadjuvant therapy experienced a significant improvement in disease-free survival, cancer-related mortality, margin-negative resection, and local control; however, no improvement in overall survival was seen versus patients undergoing surgery alone (median survival 18.6 months both groups). The authors concluded that neoadjuvant chemoradiation improved disease-free survival and local control in patients with squamous cell carcinoma of the esophagus, but had no impact on overall survival. The authors judged that the increase in postoperative mortality in the combined group "could be due to deleterious effects of the high-dose of radiation per fraction," among other factors, and believed that the dose of 3.7 Gy per fraction "probably had a detrimental effect." This trial has also been criticized for the split-course treatment approach as well as suboptimal chemotherapy.

Burmeister et al. (27) reported an Australian study randomizing 257 patients with adenocarcinoma and squamous cell carcinoma of the esophagus to surgery alone versus neoadjuvant therapy using concomitant 5-FU and cisplatin. Patient received 2.33 Gy per fraction to a total dose of 35 Gy. Patients undergoing

Table 50.9   RESULTS OF PREOPERATIVE COMBINED CHEMORADIATION VERSUS SURGERY ALONE—PHASE III TRIALS

Author (Reference)	Median Follow-Up (years)	Path	Regimen	No. of Patients	Path CR	3-Year Survival	Survival Difference
Urba et al. (133) (Mich)	8.2	SCC + adeno	5-FU-CDDP-Vinb/45 Gy S	50 50	28 —	CMT/S: 30% S alone: 16%	$p = 0.15$
Bosset et al. (23) (EORTC)	4.6	SCC	CDDP/37 Gy S	143 138	20 —	CMT/S: 33% S alone: 36%	NS
Walsh et al. (139) (Ire)	1.5	adeno	5-FU-CDDP/ 40 Gy S	58 55	22 —	CMT/S: 32% S alone: 6%	$p = 0.01$
Burmeister et al. (27) (Aus)	5.4	SCC+adeno	5-FU-CDDP/35 Gy S	128 128	16 —	CMT/S: 35% S alone: 31%	NS
Tepper et al. (128) (CALGB)	6.0	SCC+adeno	5-FU-CDDP/ 50 Gy S	30 26	40 —	CMT/S: 39% (5 y) S alone: 16% (5 y)	$p = 0.008$

adeno, adenocarcinoma; CDDP, cisplatin; CMT, combined modality therapy; 5-FU, 5-fluorouracil; S, surgery; SCC, squamous cell carcinoma; Vinb, vinblastine

neoadjuvant therapy had a 16% pathologic complete response rate at resection. Patients receiving neoadjuvant therapy were more likely to undergo curative resection and have negative lymph nodes on histologic examination. However, no significant improvement in median survival was seen (19 months vs. 22 months; hazard ratio 0.89; $p = 0.57$). On subset analysis, there appeared to be a trend toward improved survival in patients with squamous cell carcinoma undergoing neoadjuvant therapy versus surgery alone (progression-free survival hazard ratio 0.47; $p = 0.01$; overall survival hazard ratio 0.69; $p = 0.16$). The authors concluded that neoadjuvant chemoradiation as delivered in their study provided no obvious survival benefit in patients with esophageal cancer, although further study was warranted in patients with squamous cell carcinoma. Potential criticisms of this trial include delivery of a single chemotherapy cycle as well as delivery of lower radiation doses.

Preliminary trial results by the Cancer and Leukemia Group B (CALGB) described 56 patients (75% with adenocarcinoma) randomized to either surgery alone or neoadjuvant chemoradiation followed by surgical resection (128). Patients in the neoadjuvant therapy arm received cisplatin/5-FU based chemotherapy and 50.4 Gy of external beam radiation therapy at 1.8 Gy per fraction. This trial was closed prematurely due to poor accrual. In patients undergoing neoadjuvant therapy, pathologic complete response rate was 40%. A significant improvement in local control and survival was seen in patients receiving neoadjuvant combined-modality therapy (5-year survival 39% vs. 16%; $p = 0.008$). The authors concluded that neoadjuvant chemoradiation in patients with esophageal cancer significantly improves progression-free and overall survival (Table 50.9).

Because of the conflicting results in these studies, meta-analyses have been carried out. Fiorica et al. (45) analyzed six randomized controlled trials comparing neoadjuvant chemoradiation versus surgery. Some of these trials included suboptimal radiation techniques and sequential (versus concurrent) chemoradiation. The authors reported the odds ratio of death with neoadjuvant chemoradiation was significantly improved compared to surgery alone (0.53; $p = 0.03$). Additionally, patients undergoing neoadjuvant therapy experienced significant down-staging. The authors concluded chemoradiotherapy plus surgery significantly reduces mortality compared to surgery alone in patients with resectable disease. Urschel and Vasan (134) performed a meta-analysis of nine randomized controlled trials comparing neoadjuvant chemoradiation therapy with surgery versus surgery alone, comprising more than 1,100 patients. As above, multiple trials were deemed to have suboptimal radiation techniques and delivered sequential therapy. The 3-year survival odds ratio was 0.66, significantly

in favor of patients receiving neoadjuvant therapy. Additionally, when concurrent (as opposed to sequential) therapy alone was analyzed, an odds ratio of death of 0.45 was seen. These authors concluded that preoperative chemoradiation improves overall survival, margin negative resection rates, and local failure versus surgery alone. In summary, the available data suggest that neoadjuvant concurrent chemoradiation improves local control and modestly improves survival versus surgery alone in patients with resectable esophageal cancer.

Radiation Therapy Alone versus Chemoradiation

There are multiple randomized studies comparing radiation therapy alone with concurrent radiation and chemotherapy (6,11,110) as definitive therapy. However, many of these studies are handicapped by small patient numbers, substandard chemotherapy delivery, and the use of suboptimal radiotherapy techniques. This makes treatment results difficult to interpret. The landmark trial establishing the superiority of concurrent chemoradiation to radiation therapy alone was RTOG 8501. Herskovic et al. (59) reported results of this two-arm trial that treated 60 control patients with radiation alone to a total dose of 61 Gy versus 61 patients with 50 Gy of radiation therapy with concurrent chemotherapy. The chemotherapy protocol consisted of four planned courses of infusional 5-FU and cisplatin. Although less radiation was delivered in the concurrent-therapy arm, the results demonstrated a significant advantage of the combined-modality arm over the radiation-alone arm. The median survival in patients treated by radiation alone was 8.9 months compared with 12.5 months for those treated with combined therapy. The 2-year survival rate with the addition of chemotherapy improved from 10% to 38%, the incidence of local recurrence decreased from 24% to 16%, and the 2-year distant metastases rate decreased from 26% to 12%. Because of this highly significant survival difference, the randomization was stopped, and 69 additional patients were treated on the chemoradiation arm. Updated trial results from Al-Sarraf et al. (6) showed that at 5 years, survival rates were 30% and 0%, respectively, for chemoradiation and radiation therapy alone. Local recurrence rates were also decreased with the use of combined-modality therapy versus radiation alone (45% vs. 69%), and distant metastases were more frequent in the radiation-alone arm at 40% versus 12% for the combined-modality group. The incidence of acute toxicity, however, was higher for the combined-modality arm versus the radiation-alone arm (44% vs. 25%). Similarly, the incidence of life-threatening side effects, including hematologic toxicity and fistula formation, was increased from 3% to 20%. In conclusion, this study demonstrated a significant improvement in local control, median and overall survival, and distant metastases development with the addition of chemotherapy to radiation therapy, at the cost of increased side effects.

Comparison of outcomes data from "definitive" chemoradiation approaches suggests that survival with combined chemoradiation therapy is similar to that achieved by surgery alone. In previously discussed studies, median survivals of 14 to 20 months and 5-year survival rates of 20% to 30% were achieved with chemoradiation therapy alone; in comparison, with the MRC and Intergroup trials evaluating surgery alone, median survival rates were 13 to 16 months with 5-year survivals of approximately 20%. Additionally, local failure rates appear similar. For example, in the RTOG/Intergroup studies using chemoradiation therapy alone, local failure rates as a first site of failure range from 39% to 45%. In comparison, local failure rate for the Intergroup study evaluating surgery alone was 31%. However, this analysis was limited to patients undergoing R0 resection only (59% of patients) (69). This would undoubtedly be higher if considering all patients. Therefore, local failure and survival rates appear similar between "definitive" chemoradiation and surgical approaches.

Chemoradiation versus Chemoradiation Followed by Surgery

Two randomized trials have examined whether surgery is necessary following combined modality therapy. A report from French investigators randomized 445 patients with clinically resectable squamous cell or adenocarcinoma of the esophagus. All patients received concurrent 5-FU and cisplatin-based chemoradiation. Patients were allowed to be treated with one of two radiation regimens: 46 Gy over 4.5 weeks (continuous), or 30 Gy at 15 Gy per week (split course). Two hundred fifty-nine patients who had at least a partial response were then randomized to either surgery or additional combined modality therapy of 5-FU and cisplatin delivered concurrent with radiation (either an additional 20 Gy at 2 Gy per day or split course of 15 Gy). No significant difference in 2-year survival (34% vs. 40%; $p = 0.44$) or median survival (18 vs. 19 months) was seen between the groups. The death rate at 3 months following treatment was 9% in the surgery group versus 1% in the combined modality therapy alone group. Additionally, patients undergo-

ing surgery were found to have a worse quality of life. However, the rate of stent and dilatation requirement was higher in the nonsurgical arm. The results of this trial suggest that surgery following chemoradiation in responding patients does not further enhance survival (22).

In a study from Germany, 172 patients with potentially resectable squamous cell carcinoma of the esophagus received induction chemotherapy with 5-FU, leucovorin, etoposide, and cisplatin for three cycles, followed by concurrent etoposide and cisplatin with 40 Gy of external beam radiation therapy. Patients were then randomized to receive surgery versus continuing with combined chemoradiation (total radiation dose increased to 60 to 65 Gy, with or without brachytherapy). Local control was significantly improved in patients undergoing surgery (2-year local control 64% vs. 41%; $p < 0.05$). Despite this, no significant difference in survival was seen (median survival 16 vs. 15 months, 3-year survival 31% vs. 24%; $p = $ NS). The "severe" postoperative complication rate (including infection, leak) was 70%, and the hospital mortality rate was 11%. Overall treatment-related mortality was significantly higher in patients undergoing surgery (13% vs. 3.5%). In patients who did not respond to induction chemotherapy, 3-year survival was improved in patients undergoing surgery (18% vs. 9%). On regression analysis, only tumor response to induction chemotherapy was found to be a significant prognostic factor. An important caveat to this trial was that only approximately two thirds of patients in the surgery arm actually had surgery. The authors concluded that (a) surgery following combined modality therapy improves local control but had no impact on overall survival (Fig. 50.12A,B) and (b) nonresponders to induction chemotherapy may benefit from surgery, and it may be appropriate to individualize therapy based on response to induction treatment (123).

In a study describing national patterns of care from 1996 to 1999, practice standards for patients receiving radiation therapy for esophageal cancer were evaluated (126). The authors found that contemporarily treated patients had a decreased risk of death (hazard ratio 0.32) if treated with concurrent chemoradiotherapy followed by surgery compared with patients treated with chemoradiotherapy alone. In summary, although surgery following combined chemoradiation for esophageal cancer appears to improve local control of disease, its impact on ultimate survival remains controversial.

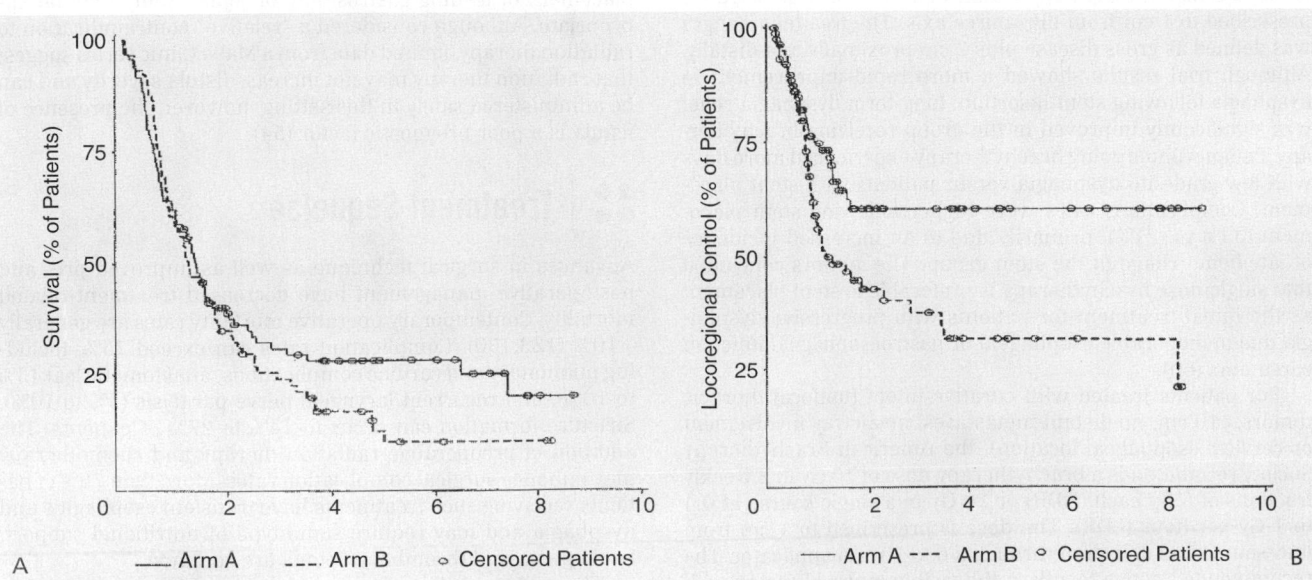

FIGURE 50.12. A: Overall survival-neoadjuvant therapy followed by surgery (arm A) versus chemoradiation alone (arm B). **B:** Local–regional control in patients undergoing neoadjuvant chemoradiation followed by surgery (arm A) versus "definitive" chemoradiation (arm B). (Stahl).

Brachytherapy

Gaspar et al. (49) reported the results of a prospective trial evaluating intraluminal brachytherapy in patients with nonoperable esophageal cancer. Patients initially received 50 Gy of external irradiation with concurrent chemotherapy, followed by a 2-week break and brachytherapy administration. Patients received either 15 Gy using HDR techniques over 3 consecutive weeks (5 Gy per fraction) or a single administration of 20 Gy using low-dose-rate (LDR) techniques. Dose was prescribed to 1 cm from the source axis. Treatments were accomplished by placement of a 10 to 12 French applicator inserted transnasally or transorally. The target length was defined as the pretreatment tumor length with 1-cm margin proximally and distally as determined by CT, barium swallow, and endoscopy. Both external irradiation and brachytherapy were given concurrently with 5-FU chemotherapy. Following the development of fistulas in six patients, the HDR dose was reduced to 10 Gy in two fractions, and the LDR arm was ultimately closed because of poor accrual. Results showed a median survival of 11 months in all patients. Local persistence/recurrence was observed in 63% of 49 eligible patients receiving HDR therapy. Six patients developed esophageal fistulas resulting in three deaths. These fistulas were deemed treatment related. The 1-year actuarial fistula development rate was 18%. The investigators conclude that esophageal brachytherapy, particularly in conjunction with chemotherapy, should be approached with caution (49). Review of other combined brachytherapy/EBRT series suggests fistula formation rates range from 0% to 12%, with a possible trend toward a higher incidence in patients receiving concurrent chemotherapy with brachytherapy. The incidence of brachytherapy-related mortality varies from 0% to 8%, with most series reporting rates at 4% or less (138).

Other studies have suggested that HDR brachytherapy is effective for palliation of dysphagia in up to 90% of patients (60). Danish investigators reported the results of a randomized trial of 209 patients with dysphagia due to inoperable esophageal or gastroesophageal junctional tumors. Patients were randomized to either endoscopic stent placement or single-dose HDR brachytherapy. Patient exclusion criteria included tumors >12 cm, tumors within 3 cm of the upper esophageal sphincter, deeply ulcerated tumors, tracheoesophageal fistula/tracheal involvement, presence of a pacemaker, and previous radiation treatment or stent placement. Brachytherapy was delivered through a flexible 1 cm applicator, delivering a dose of 12 Gy prescribed to 1 cm from the source axis. The treatment length was defined as gross disease plus 2 cm proximally and distally. Although trial results showed a more rapid improvement in dysphagia following stent insertion, long-term dysphagia relief was significantly improved in the group receiving brachytherapy. Patients undergoing brachytherapy experienced more days with low grade/no dysphagia versus patients with stent placement. Complications rates were higher following stent placement (33% vs. 21%), primarily due to an increased incidence of late hemorrhage in the stent group. The authors concluded that single-dose brachytherapy is preferable to stent placement as the initial treatment for patients with progressive dysphagia due to inoperable esophageal or gastroesophageal junction carcinoma (60).

For patients treated with curative intent (unifocal thoracic tumors <10 cm, no distant metastases, no airway involvement or cervical esophageal location), the American Brachytherapy Society recommends a brachytherapy dose of 10 Gy in 2 weekly fractions of 5 Gy each (HDR) or 20 Gy in a single course at 0.4 to 1 Gy per hour (LDR). The dose is prescribed to 1 cm from mid-source and delivered through a 6 to 10 mm applicator. The recommended active length is the visible mucosal tumor with a 1- to 2-cm proximal and distal margins (Fig. 50.13). Ideally, brachytherapy is started 2 to 3 weeks following completion of concurrent external irradiation/chemotherapy to allow mucositis resolution. Concurrent chemotherapy with brachytherapy is not recommended. In palliative cases, a similar approach is recommended, with delivery of 10 to 14 Gy in one or two fractions (HDR) or 20 to 25 Gy in a single course (LDR). In previously untreated patients with a short life expectancy (<3 months), a dose of 15 to 20 Gy in two to four fractions (HDR) or of 25 to 40 Gy (LDR) without external irradiation is recommended (Tables 50.10–50.12). In summary, the use of brachytherapy in the curative approach to esophageal cancer does not appear to significantly improve results achieved with combined external beam radiation therapy with chemotherapy alone.

Palliative Treatment

Although treatment advances have occurred in esophageal cancer over the past 20 years, the majority of patients diagnosed with this disease will die of their malignancy. Therefore, palliation remains an important goal. Dysphagia is a common presenting symptom and may significantly impair patient's quality of life. Radiation therapy has been used as an effective treatment for palliation. Many studies report a 60% to >80% rate of relief from dysphagia. Coia et al. (30) reported that nearly half of patients with baseline dysphagia experienced an improvement in swallowing within two weeks of treatment initiation. By the completion of the sixth week, over 80% experienced improvement. A median time to maximal improvement was approximately 1 month. Given the superior outcomes of patients receiving concurrent chemotherapy with radiation therapy in nonmetastatic disease, palliative chemoradiation is likely preferable to radiation alone for patients with advanced-stage esophageal carcinoma who have a good performance status. As described above, intraluminal brachytherapy has also been used for palliation of dysphagia. The previously described randomized trial from the Netherlands comparing intraluminal brachytherapy to stent placement showed that although patients undergoing stenting experienced a more rapid improvement in dysphagia, long-term palliation was significantly improved in patients treated with brachytherapy (60).

The palliative management of patients with tracheoesophageal fistula presents a clinical dilemma. Fistulization usually precludes surgery. These patients are often treated effectively with the placement of silicone-covered self-expanding metal stents, often obviating palliative surgery. Additionally, placement of feeding gastrostomy or jejunostomy may be appropriate. Although considered a "relative" contraindication to radiation therapy, limited data from a Mayo Clinic series suggest that radiation therapy may not increase fistula severity and can be administered safely in this setting; however, the presence of fistula is a poor prognostic factor (54).

░░ | Treatment Sequelae

Advances in surgical technique as well as improved pre- and postoperative management have decreased treatment-related mortality. Contemporary operative mortality rates are generally <10% (123,130). Complication rates can exceed 75%, including pulmonary and cardiac complications, anastomotic leak (5% to 10%), and recurrent laryngeal nerve paralysis (5% to 10%). Stricture formation can occur in 14% to 27% of patients. The addition of preoperative radiation therapy and chemotherapy may enhance surgical complication rates. More than 75% of patients receiving such treatments have transient esophagitis and dysphagia and may require some type of nutritional support. Leukopenia and thrombocytopenia are common.

The acute toxicities of radiation therapy include esophagitis, epidermitis, fatigue, and weight loss in most patients. Nausea and vomiting are common, particularly in patients with lower

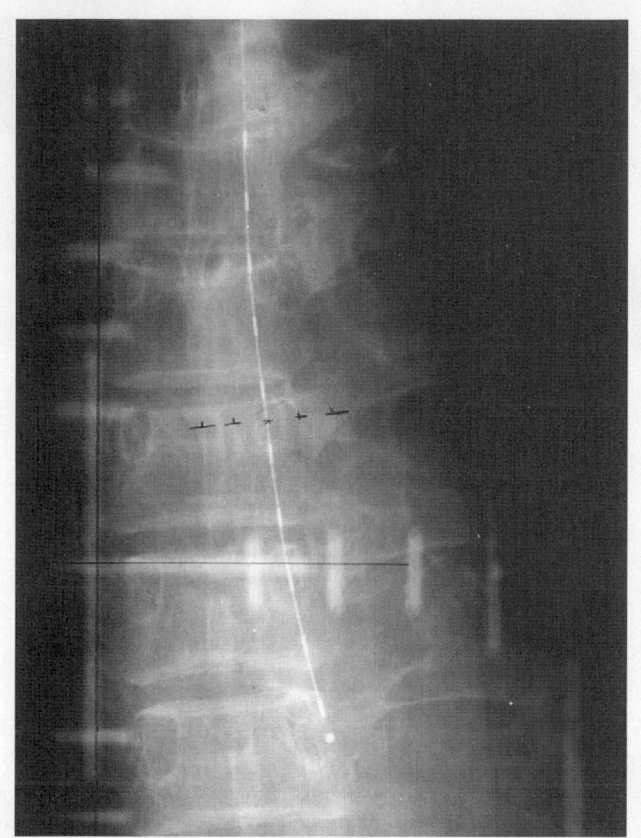

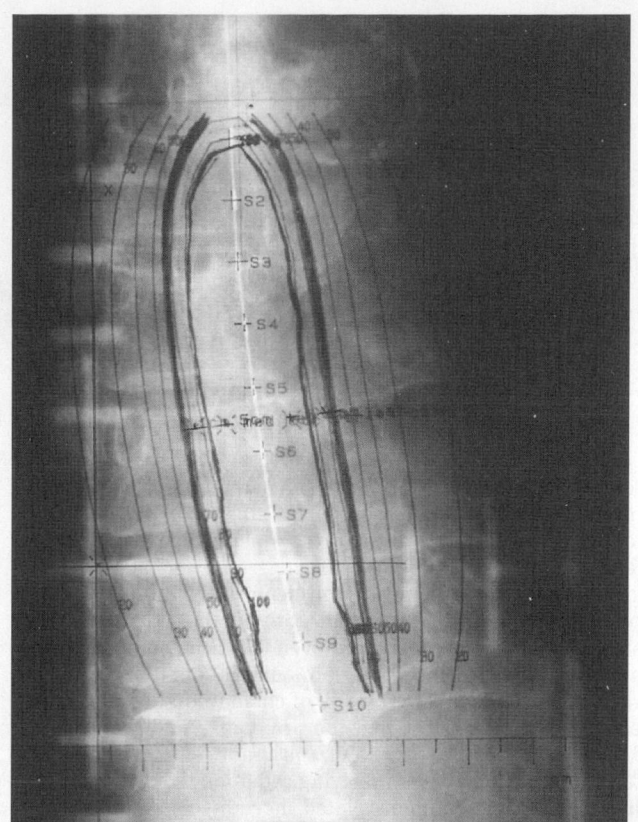

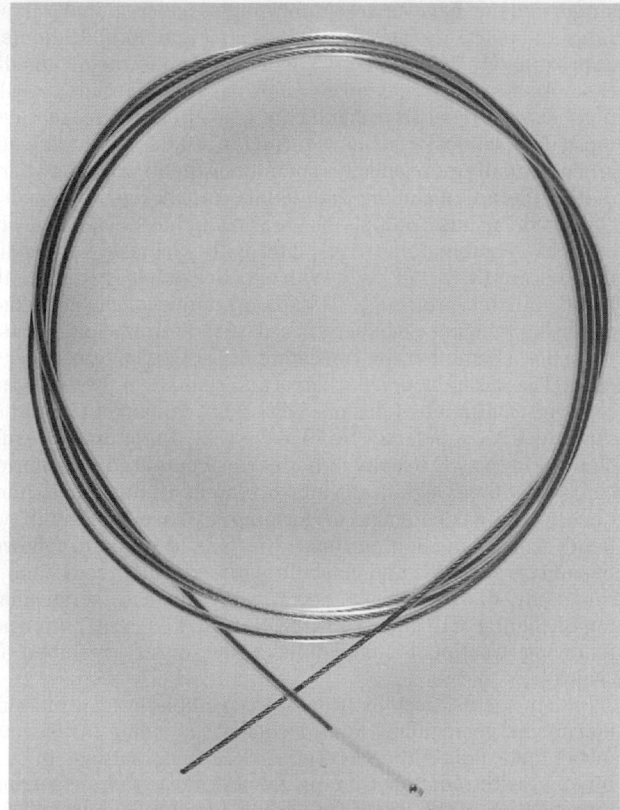

FIGURE 50.13. Iridium-192 (^{192}Ir) afterloading technique. **A:** Anterior dosimetry film for ^{192}Ir boost to mid-thoracic lesion. **B:** Anterior dose distribution for mid-thoracic lesion. **C:** ^{192}Ir afterloading catheter with closed end and guide wire in place. (Courtesy of the Department of Radiation Oncology, The Graduate Hospital, Philadelphia, with special thanks to Joan Pellak and Steve Yan.)

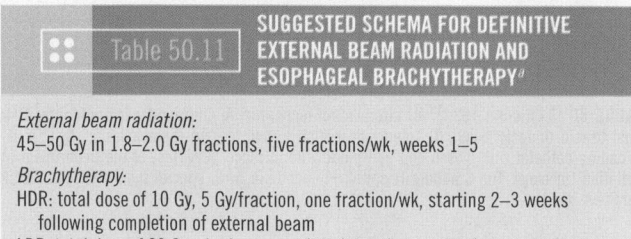

Table 50.10	SELECTION CRITERIA FOR BRACHYTHERAPY IN THE TREATMENT OF ESOPHAGEAL CANCER		
Good Candidates	**Poor Candidates**	**Contraindications**	
Primary tumor ≤10 cm length	Extra esophageal extension	Esophageal fistula	
Tumor confined to the esophageal wall	Tumor >10 cm in length	Cervical esophageal location	
Thoracic esophagus location	Regional lymphadenopathy	Stenosis which can not be bypassed	
No regional lymph node or systemic metastases	Tumor involving gastroesophageal junction or cardia		

esophageal and gastroesophageal junction tumors. Many symptoms resolve within 1 to 2 weeks of treatment completion. Pneumonitis has been seen, but is rare. A perforated esophagus is life threatening and may be characterized by substernal chest pain, a high pulse rate, fever, and hemorrhage (64). The addition of chemotherapy can significantly increase acute complications. Moderate to severe and even life-threatening toxicities have been reported in 50% to 66% of patients (29,59). In the previously discussed RTOG study of chemoradiation alone, patients treated with combined therapy had a higher incidence of acute grade 3 (44% vs. 25%) and grade 4 toxicity (20% vs. 3%) compared to patients receiving radiation therapy alone (6). Chemoradiation treatment-related mortality rates range from 0% to 3% (27,29,59,123,139).

The most common late effects following radiation therapy are stenosis and stricture formation. Stenosis can occur in more than 60% of patients. Stricture requiring dilatation has been reported to occur at least 15% to 20% of treated patients. Dysphagia may be relieved with two to three dilatations (29). Long-term results from the RTOG study showed that ≥late grade 3 toxicity was similar in the combined arm versus radiation-alone arm (29% vs. 23%). However, ≥grade 4 toxicity was higher in patients receiving combined modality therapy (10% vs. 2%) (32). Other complications include damage to organs within the radiation therapy volume, although this is uncommon. Recent studies have shown that significant declines in lung diffusion capacity and total lung capacity may occur in patients irradiated for esophageal cancer (51). In a report describing complications in patients receiving neoadjuvant combined modality therapy, 18% experienced pulmonary complications. These were significantly higher in patients where greater ≥40% of the lung volume received at least 10 Gy, and further increased in patients in whom ≥30% of the lung received at least 15 Gy (80). Chemotherapy may further increase the risk of late treatment-related toxicities.

Table 50.11	SUGGESTED SCHEMA FOR DEFINITIVE EXTERNAL BEAM RADIATION AND ESOPHAGEAL BRACHYTHERAPY[a]

External beam radiation:
45–50 Gy in 1.8–2.0 Gy fractions, five fractions/wk, weeks 1–5

Brachytherapy:
HDR: total dose of 10 Gy, 5 Gy/fraction, one fraction/wk, starting 2–3 weeks following completion of external beam
LDR: total dose of 20 Gy, single course, 0.4–1.0 Gy/h, starting 2–3 weeks from completion of external beam

HDR, high-dose rate; LDR, low-dose rate
[a]All doses specified 1 cm from mid-source or mid-dwell position.

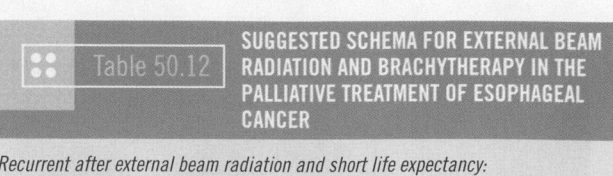

Table 50.12	SUGGESTED SCHEMA FOR EXTERNAL BEAM RADIATION AND BRACHYTHERAPY IN THE PALLIATIVE TREATMENT OF ESOPHAGEAL CANCER

Recurrent after external beam radiation and short life expectancy:
Brachytherapy:[a]
 HDR: total dose of 10–14 Gy, one or two fractions
 LDR: total dose of 20–40 Gy, one or two fractions, 0.4–1.0 Gy/h

No previous external beam radiation:
External beam radiation:
 30–40 Gy in 2–3 Gy fractions
Brachytherapy:[a]
 HDR: 10–14 Gy, one or two fractions
 LDR: total dose of 20–25 Gy, single course, 0.4–1.0 Gy/h

No previous external beam radiation, life expectancy >6 months:
External beam radiation:
 45–50 Gy in 1.8-2.0 Gy fractions, five fractions per week, weeks 1–5
Brachytherapy:[a]
 HDR: total dose of 10 Gy, 5 Gy/fraction, one fraction/week, starting 2–3 weeks following completion of external beam
 LDR: total dose of 20 Gy, single course, 0.4–1.0 Gy/h, starting 2–3 weeks following completion of external beam

HDR, high-dose rate; LDR, low-dose rate
[a]All doses specified 1 cm from mid-source or mid-dwell position.

Future Considerations

Although modest improvements in survival have been achieved by combining neoadjuvant chemoradiation therapy and surgery, patients treated with chemoradiation alone or with surgery alone have unacceptably high-local regional relapse rates and mortality rates (see Tables 50.3 and 50.6). Ultimately, approximately 75% of patients will succumb to metastatic disease. As described previously, efforts at radiation dose escalation have not resulted in significant gains in this disease. Given these data, clinical trials have turned to studies evaluating new and potentially more effective chemotherapeutic agents with radiation therapy, including traditional cytotoxic agents as well as "targeted" agents. Multiple phase II trials have evaluated preoperative combinations of cisplatin with paclitaxel with radiation therapy (3,10,111,130). With encouraging early results, the RTOG initiated protocol E-0113, a randomized phase II study assessing nonoperative therapies. The randomization included induction chemotherapy consisting of 5-FU, cisplatin, and paclitaxel versus induction paclitaxel and cisplatin only. Both arms received continuous-infusion 5-FU with concurrent radiation therapy 1.8 Gy per day to 50.4 Gy (72). Preliminary results showed increased toxicity in both arms compared to historical controls without significant improvements in outcomes. Additionally, the RTOG is also performing a phase II study (RTOG 0246) using induction paclitaxel, 5-FU, and cisplatin followed by concurrent 5-FU and cisplatin with external irradiation. In this study, there is no planned surgery. Instead, serial imaging including CT, endoscopy, EUS, and PET are performed following treatment completion, with surgery reserved for "salvage."

Other agents, such as irinotecan, oxaliplatin, capecitabine, epirubicin, gemcitabine, and docetaxel are being investigated in the metastatic setting as well as "curative" settings in combination with radiation therapy. Furthermore, there is ongoing investigation of the use of the vascular endothelial growth factor inhibitor bevacizumab as well as inhibitors of the epidermal growth factor receptors, including the antibody cetuximab and small molecule inhibitors gefitinib and erlotinib, in the treatment of esophageal cancer. All of these agents have radiosensitizing properties. The investigation of these agents with radiation therapy is the subject of future trials.

Summary

The prognosis for patients with carcinoma of the esophagus remains poor despite recent advances in combined-modality therapies. No firm recommendation can be made for managing locally advanced disease. The available data suggest that neoadjuvant chemoradiation may modestly improve outcomes in patients who are candidates for surgery. However, many patients are not able to tolerate surgery and combined chemoradiation may be more appropriate in selected patients, as definitive chemoradiation has resulted in survival rates comparable to surgery alone. Locoregional failure remains a significant pattern of relapse. For patients with stage IV disease, palliation with single-modality therapy or several modalities should be used and tailored to the patient's specific symptoms. Current unresolved issues include the following:

1. Is esophagectomy necessary after chemoradiation, and are there subsets of patients more likely to benefit from the addition of surgery than others?
2. Can introduction of newer chemotherapy/targeted agents in the neoadjuvant or definitive setting improve the results over "standard" chemoradiation with cisplatin and 5-FU?
3. Will new technologies such as 3D conformal therapy, PET-based planning, intensity-modulated radiation therapy, and image guided radiation therapy decrease complication rates and influence cure rates?
4. Will the identification of molecular prognostic markers allow "individualization" of treatments among patients?

References

1. Abdala E, Pisters P. Staging and preoperative evaluation of upper gastrointestinal malignancies *Sem Oncolo* 2004;31:513–529.
2. Adelstein DJ, Forman WB, Beavers B. Esophageal carcinoma. A six-year review of the Cleveland Veterans Administration Hospital experience. *Cancer* 1984;54:918–923.
3. Adelstein DJ, Rice T, Rybicki L, et al. Dose paclitaxel improve the chemoradiotherapy of locoregionally advanced esophageal cancer? A randomized comparison with fluorouracil-based therapy. *J Clin Oncol* 2000;18:2032.
4. Aisner J, Forastiere A, Aroney R. Patterns of recurrence for cancer of the lung and esophagus. *Cancer Treat Symp* 1983;2:87–105.
5. Akiyama H, Tsurumaru M, Kawamura T, et al. Principles of surgical treatment for carcinoma of the esophagus: analysis of lymph node involvement. *Ann Surg* 1981;194:438–446.
6. Al-Sarraf M, Martz K, Herskovic A, et al. Progress report of combined chemodiotherapy versus radiotherapy alone in patients with esophageal cancer: an Intergroup study. *J Clin Oncol* 1997;15:277–284.
7. American Cancer Society. *Cancer facts and figures—2005*. Atlanta: American Cancer Society, 2005.
8. American Joint Committee on Cancer. *Esophagus*, 6th ed. New York: Springer-Verlag, 2002.
9. Anderson LL, Lad TE. Autopsy findings in squamous-cell carcinoma of the esophagus. *Cancer* 1982;50:1587–1590.
10. Appleqvist P, Salmon M. Lye corrosion carcinoma of the esophagus. *Cancer* 1980;45:P2655.
11. Araujo C, Souhami L, Gil R, et al. A randomized trial comparing radiation therapy alone versus concomitant radiation therapy and chemotherapy in carcinoma of the thoracic esophagus. *Cancer* 1991;67:2258.
12. Arnott S, Duncan W, Gignoux M, et al. Preoperative radiotherapy for esophageal carcinoma: Oeosophageal Cancer Collaborative Group. *Cochran Data Base Cyst Rev* 2005;CD001799.
13. Arnott S, Duncan W, Kerr G, et al. Low dose preoperative radiotherapy for carcinoma of the oesophagus: results of a randomized trial. *Radiother Oncol* 1992;24:108–113.
14. Baquet C, Commisky P, Mack K, et al. Esophageal cancer epidemiology in blacks and whites: racial and gender disparities in incidence, mortality, survival rates and histology. *J Natl Med Assoc* 2005;97:1471–1478.
15. Beatty J, DeBoer G, Rider W. Carcinoma of the esophagus: pretreatment assessment, correlation of radiation treatment parameters with survival, and identification and management of radiation treatment failure. *Cancer* 1979;43:2254.
16. Beseth BD, Bedford R, Isacoff WH, et al. Endoscopic ultrasound does not accurately assess pathologic stage of esophageal cancer after neoadjuvant chemoradiotherapy. *Am Surg* 2000;66:827–831.
17. Blackstock AW, Farmer MR, Lovato J, et al. A prospective evaluation of the impact of 18-F-fluoro-deoxy-D-glucose positron emission tomography staging on survival for patients with locally advanced esophageal cancer. *Int J Radiat Oncol Biol Phys* 2006;64:455–460.
18. Blanke C, Chiappori A, Epstein B, et al. A phase II trial of neoadjuvant paclitaxel and cisplatin with radiotherapy followed by surgery and postoperative taxol with 5-FU and leucovorin in patients with locally advanced esophageal cancer. *Proc Am Soc Clin Oncol* 2000;19:248a.
19. Bloedorn F, Kasdorf H. *Radiotherapy in squamous cell carcinoma of the esophagus*, vol. 4. Chicago: Year Book Medical, 1971.
20. Blot WJ, McLaughlin J. The changing epidemiology of esophageal cancer. *Semin Oncol* 1999;26:2–8.
21. Blot WJ. Alcohol and cancer. *Cancer Res* 1992;52:2119.
22. Bedenne L, Michel P, Bouché O, et al. Chemoradiation followed by surgery compared with chemoradiation alone in squamous cancer of the esophagus: FFCD 9102. *J Clin Oncol* 2007;25(10):1155–1156.
23. Bosset J, Gignoux M, Triboulet J, et al. Chemoradiotherapy followed by surgery compared with surgery alone in squamous-cell cancer of the esophagus. *N Engl J Med* 1997;337:161–167.
24. Briggs J, Ibrahim N. Oat cell carcinoma of the oesophagus: a clinicopathologic study of 22 cases. *Histopathology* 1983;7:261.
25. Brown LM, Swanson CA, Gridley G, et al. Adenocarcinoma of the esophagus: role of obesity and diet. *J Natl Cancer Inst* 1995;87:104–109.
26. Burke E, Sturm J, Williamson D. The diagnosis of microscopic carcinoma of the esophagus. *Dig Dis* 1978;23:148.
27. Burmeister B, Smithers B, Gebski V, et al. Surgery alone versus chemoradiotherapy followed by surgery for respectable cancer of the oesophagus: a randomized controlled phase III trial. *Lancet* 2005;6:659–668.
28. Cheng K. The etiology of esophageal cancer in Chinese. *Semin Oncol* 1994;21:411–415.
29. Coia L, Engstrom P, Paul A, et al. Long-term results of infusional 5-FU, mitomycin-C, and radiation as primary management of esophageal carcinoma. *Int J Radiat Oncol Biol Phys* 1991;20:29–36.
30. Coia L, Soffen E, Schultheiss T, et al. Swallowing function in patients with esophageal cancer treated with concurrent radiation and chemotherapy. *Cancer* 1993;71:281.
31. Collard JM, Otte JB, Fiasse R, et al. Skeletonizing en bloc esophagectomy for cancer. *Ann Surg* 2001;234:25–32.
32. Cooper J, Guo M, Herskovic A, et al. Chemoradiotherapy of locally advanced esophageal cancer: long-term follow-up of a prospective randomized trial (RTOG 85-01). Radiation Therapy Oncology Group. *JAMA* 1999;281:1623–1627.
33. Cunningham D, Allum W, Stenning S, et al. Perioperative chemotherapy versus therapy alone for respectable gastroesophageal cancer. *N Engl J Med* 2006;355:11–20.
34. DeMeester TR. Clinical biology of the Barrett's metaplasia, dysplasia to carcinoma sequence. *Surg Oncol* 2001;10:91–102.
35. Denham JW, Burmeister BH, Lamb DS, et al. Factors influencing outcome following radio-chemotherapy for oesophageal cancer The Trans Tasman Radiation Oncology Group (TROG). *Radiother Oncol* 1996;40:31–43.
36. DeRen S. Ten-year follow up of esophageal cancer treated by radical radiation: anatomy of 869 patients. *Int J Radiat Oncol Biol Phys* 1989;16:32a.
37. Devesa S, Blot WJ, Fraumeni JF. Changing patterns in the incidence of esophageal and gastric carcinoma in the U.S. *Cancer* 1998;83:2049.
38. Doherty M, McIntyre M, Arnott S. Oat cell carcinoma of the esophagus: a report of six British patients with a review of the literature. *Int J Radiat Oncol Biol Phys* 1984;10:1477.
39. Dormans E. Das Oesophaguscarcinoma: Ergebnisse der unter Mitarbet von 29 Pathologischem Instituten Deutschlands Durchgefuhrten Erhebung uber das Oesophaguscarcinomon (1925–1933). *Z Krebforsch* 1939;49:86.
40. Dresner SM, Lamb PJ, Bennett MK, et al. The pattern of metastatic lymph node dissemination from adenocarcinoma of the esophagogastric junction. *Surgery* 2001;129:103–109.
41. Earlam R, Cuhna-Melo J. Oesophageal squamous cell carcinoma. II A critical review of radiotherapy. *Br J Surg* 1980;67:457–461.
42. Earlam R, Cuhna-Melo J. Oesophageal squamous cell carcinoma: I. A critical review of surgery. *Br J Surg* 1980;67:384.
43. Ellis F. Standard resection for cancer of the esophagus and cardia. *Surg Oncol Clin North Am* 1999;8:279–294.
44. Epstein J, Sears D, Tucker R. Carcinoma of the esophagus with adenoid cystic differentiation. *Cancer* 1984;53:1131.
45. Fiorica F, DiBona D, Schepis F, et al. Preoperative chemoradiotherapy for oesophageal cancer: a systematic review in meta-analysis. *Gut* 2004;53:925–930.
46. Flamen P, Lerut A, Van Cutsem E, et al. Utility of positron emission tomography for the staging of patients with potentially operable esophageal carcinoma. *J Clin Oncol* 2000;18:3202–3210.
47. Fok M, Sham JS, Choy D, et al. Postoperative radiotherapy for carcinoma of the esophagus: a prospective, randomized controlled study. *Surgery* 1993;113:138–147.
48. Gaede J, Postlethwait RW, Shelnurne J, et al. Leiomyosarcoma of the esophagus: report of two cases, one with associated squamous cell carcinoma. *J Thorac Cardiovasc Surg* 1978;75:740.
49. Gaspar L, Winter K, Kocha W, et al. A phase I/II study of external beam radiation, brachytherapy and concurrent chemotherapy for patients with localized carcinoma of the esophagus (Radiation Therapy Oncology Group Study 9207: final report). *Cancer* 2000;88:988–995.
50. Gelb A, Miller S. AIDS and gastroenterology. *Am J Gasterinterol* 1986;81:619.
51. Gergel T, Leichman L, Nava H, et al. Effective of concurrent radiation therapy and chemotherapy on pulmonary function in patients with esophageal cancer: dose-volume histogram analysis. *Cancer* 2002;8:451–460.
52. Gignoux M, Roussel A, Paillot B, et al. The value of preoperative radiotherapy in esophageal cancer: results of a study of the EORTC. *World J Surg* 1987;11:429–432.
53. Griffith JF, Chan AC, Chow LT, et al. Assessing chemotherapy response of squamous cell oesophageal carcinoma with spiral CT. *Br J Radiol* 1999;72:678–684.
54. Gschossman J, Bonner J, Foote R, et al. Malignant tracheal esophageal fistula in patients with esophageal cancer. *Cancer* 1993;72:1513–1521.
55. Halber MD, Daffner RH, Thompson WM. CT of the esophagus: I. Normal appearance. *AJR Am J Roentgenol* 1979;133:1047–1050.
56. Hancock S, Glatstein E. Radiation therapy of esophageal cancer. *Semin Oncol* 1984;11:144.
57. Harper P, Harper R, Howel-Evans A. Carcinoma of the esophagus with tylosis. *QJM* 1970;34:317.

Clinical Radiation Oncology

58. Heath E, Limburg P, Hawk E. Adenocarcinoma of the esophagus: risk factors and prevention. *Oncology* 2000;14:507–514, discussion 518–520, 522–523.
59. Herskovic A, Martz K, Al-Sarraf M, et al. Combined chemotherapy and radiotherapy compared with radiotherapy alone in patients with cancer of the esophagus. *N Engl J Med* 1992;326:1593.
60. Homs MY, Steyerberg EW, Eijkenboom WM, et al. Single-dose brachytherapy versus metal stent placement for the palliation of dysphagia from oesophageal cancer: multicentre randomised trial. *Lancet* 2004;364:1497–1504.
61. Hopkins R, Postlethwait R. Caustic burns and carcinoma of the esophagus. *Ann Surg* 1981;194:146.
62. Hosch S, Nikolas H, Stoecklein U, et al. Esophageal cancer: the mode of lymphatic tumor cell spread and its prognostic significance. *J Clin Oncol* 2001;19:1970–1975.
63. Hulscher JB, van Sandick JW, de Boer AG, et al. Extended transthoracic resection compared with limited transhiatal resection for adenocarcinoma of the esophagus. *N Engl J Med* 2002;347:1662–1669.
64. Hussey D, Barakley T, Bloedorn F. *Carcinoma of the esophagus*. 3rd ed. Philadelphia: Lea & Febiger, 1980.
65. Imai T, Sannohe Y, Okano H. Oat cell carcinoma (apudoma) of the esophagus. *Cancer* 1978;41:358.
66. Jaklitsch M, Harpole D, Healey E, et al. Current issues in the staging of esophageal cancer. *Semin Radiat Oncol* 1994;4:135.
67. Jemal A, Siegel R, Ward E, et al. Cancer statistics, 2007. *CA Cancer J Clin* 2007;57:43–46.
68. Kelly S, Harris KM, Berry E, et al. A systematic review of the staging performance of endoscopic ultrasound in gastro-oesophageal carcinoma. *Gut* 2001;49:534–539.
69. Kelsen D, Ginsberg R, Pagak T, et al. Chemotherapy followed by surgery compared with surgery alone for localized esophageal cancer. *N Engl J Med* 1998;339:1979–1985.
70. Kmet J, Mahboubi E. Esophageal cancer in the Caspian littoral of Iran: initial studies. *Science* 1972;175:846–853.
71. Kole AC, Plukker JT, Nieweg OE, et al. Positron emission tomography for staging of oesophageal and gastroesophageal malignancy. *Br J Cancer* 1998;78:521–527.
72. Komaki R, Winter K, Ajani A, et al. A randomized phase II study of two paclitaxel-based chemoradiotherapy regimens for patients with the non-operative esophageal carcinoma (RTOG 0113). *Int J Radiat Oncol Biol Phys* 2006;66[Suppl]: 579S–580S.
73. Konski A, Doss M, Milestone B, et al. The integration of 18-fluoro-deoxy-glucose positron emission tomography and endoscopic ultrasound in the treatment-planning process for esophageal carcinoma. *Int J Radiat Oncol Biol Phys* 2005;61:1123–1128.
74. Lagergren J, Bergstrom R, Lindgren A, et al. Symptomatic gastroesophageal reflux as a risk factor for esophageal adenocarcinoma. *N Engl J Med* 1999;340:825–831.
75. Laterza E, de Manzoni G, Guglielmi A, et al. Endoscopic ultrasonography in the staging of esophageal carcinoma after preoperative radiotherapy and chemotherapy. *Ann Thorac Surg* 1999;67:1466–1469.
76. Launois B, Delarue D, Campion J, et al. Preoperative radiotherapy for carcinoma of the esophagus. *Surg Gynecol Obstet* 1981;153:690.
77. Law S, Fok M, Wong J. Pattern of recurrence after oesophageal resection for cancer: clinical implications. *Br J Surg* 1996;83:107–111.
78. Lea JW, Prager RL, Bender HW Jr. The questionable role of computed tomography in preoperative staging of esophageal cancer. *Ann Thorac Surg* 1984;38:479–481.
79. Lederman M. Carcinoma of the oesophagus with special reference to the upper third: part I. Clinical considerations. *Br J Radiol* 1982;39:193.
80. Lee H, Vaporciyan A, Cox J, et al. Postoperative pulmonary complications after preoperative chemoradiation for esophageal carcinoma: correlation with pulmonary dose-volume histogram parameters. *Int J Radiat Oncol Biol Phys* 2003;57:1317–1322.
81. LePrise E, Meunier B, Etienne P, et al. Sequential chemotherapy and radiotherapy for patients with squamous cell carcinoma of the esophagus. *Cancer* 1995;75:2.
82. Lijinsky W. *Current concepts in the toxicology of nitrates, nitrites and nitrosamines*. Washington, DC: Hemisphere, 1979.
83. Ludwig M, Shaw R, Suto-Nagy G. Primary malignant melanoma of the esophagus. *Cancer* 1981;48:2528.
84. Macdonald J, Smalley S, Benedetti J, et al. Chemoradiotherapy after surgery compared with surgery wlone for adenocarcinoma of the stomach or gastroesophageal junction. *N Engl J Med* 2001;345:725–730.
85. Mahboubi M, Day N, Ghadrian P. *The negligible role of alcohol and tobacco in the etiology of esophageal cancer in Iran: a case-control study.* New York: Marcel Dekker, 1978.
86. Mahboubi M, Kmet J, Cook P. Esophageal cancer studies in the Caspian littoral of Iran: the Caspian Cancer Registry. *Br J Cancer* 1973;28:196.
87. Maimon H, Dreskin R, Coco A. Positive esophageal cytology without detectable neoplasm. *Gastrointest Endosc* 1974;20:156.
88. Marks R, Sorvas H, Wallace K, et al. Preoperative radiotherapy for carcinoma of the esophagus. *Cancer* 1976: 84.
89. Medical Research Council (MRC). Oesophageal Cancer Working Party. Surgical resection with or without preoperative chemotherapy in oesophageal cancer: a randomized controlled trial. *Lancet* 2002;359:1727–1733.
90. Miao C, Guo F, Zhang J. The relationship between fungi and nitrosamines and their precursors: II. The action of fungi isolated from grains in Linxian. *Med Ref* 1978;2:46.
91. Minsky B, Pajak T, Ginsberg R, et al. INT0123 (Radiation Therapy Oncology Group 94-05) phase III trial of combined-modality therapy for esophageal cancer high-dose versus standard dose radiation therapy. *J Clin Oncol* 2002;20:1167–1174.
92. Moertel C. *The esophagus*. 2nd ed. Philadelphia: Lea & Febiger, 1982.
93. Monig SP, Baldus SE, Zirbes TK, et al. Topographical distribution of lymph node metastasis in adenocarcinoma of the gastroesophageal junction. *Hepatogastroenterology* 2002;49:419–422.
94. Montesano R, Hollstein M, Hainaut P. Genetic alterations in esophageal cancer and their relevance to etiology and pathogenesis: a review. *Int J Cancer* 1996;69:225–235.
95. Newaishy G, Read G, Duncan W, et al. Results of radical radiotherapy of squamous cell carcinoma of the oesophagus. *Clin Radiol* 1982;33:347.
96. Okawa T, Kita M, Tanaka M, et al. Results of radiotherapy for inoperable locally advanced esophageal carcinoma. *Int J Radiat Oncol Biol Phys* 1989;17:49.
97. Oota K, Shin L. *Histological typing of gastric and oesophageal tumors*. Geneva: World Health Organization, 1977.
98. Orvidas L, McCaffrey T, Lewis F, et al. Lymphoma involving the esophagus [review]. *Ann Otol Rhinol Laryngol* 1994;102:843.
99. Partyka E, Sanowsksi R, Kozarek R. Endoscopic diagnosis of a giant esophageal leiomyosarcoma. *Am J Gasterinterol* 1981;75:135.
100. Pearson J, Leroux B. *Malignant tumors of the esophagus*. New York: Springer-Verlag, 1974.
101. Pearson J. The present status and future potential of radiotherapy in the management of esophageal cancer. *Cancer* 1977;39:882.
102. Picus D, Balfe DM, Koehler RE, et al. Computed tomography in the staging of esophageal carcinoma. *Radiology* 1983;146:433–438.
103. Pohl H, Welch HG. The role of overdiagnosis and reclassification in the marked increase of esophageal adenocarcinoma incidence. *J Natl Cancer Inst* 2005;97:142–146.
104. Postlethwait RW, Sealy W. *Surgery of the esophagus*. New York: Appleton-Century-Crofts, 1979.
105. Rankin SC, Taylor H, Cook GJ, et al. Computed tomography and positron emission tomography in the pre-operative staging of oesophageal carcinoma. *Clin Radiol* 1998;53:659–665.
106. Ries I, Kosary C, Hankey B, et al. *Cancer statistics review 1973–1974*. NIH publication No. 97-2789. Bethesda, MD: Department of Health and Human Services, 1997.
107. Rosch T. Endoscopic staging of esophageal cancer: a review of literature results. *Gastrointest Endosc Clin North Am* 1995;5:537.
108. Rosenberg J, Franklin R, Steiger Z. Squamous cell carcinoma of the thoracic esophagus: an interdisciplinary approach. *Curr Probl Cancer* 1981;5:6.
109. Rosenberg J, Lichter A, Leichman L. *Cancer of the esophagus*, 3rd ed. Philadelphia: J.B. Lippincott, 1989.
110. Roussell A, Jacob J, Haegele P, et al. Controlled clinical trial for the treatment of patients with inoperable esophageal carcinoma: a study of EORTC Gastrointestinal Tract Cancer Cooperative Group. *Rec Results Cancer Res* 1988: 110–121.
111. Safran H, Mitsumori M, Araki N, et al. Neoadjuvant paclitaxel, cisplatin, and radiation for esophageal carcinoma: a phase II study. *Proc Am Soc Clin Oncol* 1997;16:304a.
112. Schaer J, Katon R, Ivancev K, et al. Treatment of malignant esophageal obstruction with silicone-coated metallic self-expanding stents. *Gastrointest Endosc* 1992;38:7.
113. Schottenfeld D. Epidemiology of cancer of the esophagus. *Semin Oncol* 1984;11:92.
114. Schuchmann G, Heydorn W, Hall R, et al. Treatment of esophageal carcinoma: a retrospective review. *J Thorac Cardiovasc Surg* 1980;79:67.
115. Sharpiro A, Robillard G. The esophageal arteries. *Ann Surg* 1950;131:171.
116. Shurr P, Yekebas E, Kaifi J, et al. Lymphatic spread in micro involvement in adenocarcinoma of the esophagogastric junction. *J Surg Oncol* 2006;94:307–315.
117. Siewert JR, Marcus F, Werner M, et al. Adenocarcinoma of the esophagogastric junction: results of surgical therapy based on anatomical/topographic classification in 1,002 consecutive patients. *Ann Surg* 2000;232:353–361.
118. Siewert JR, Stein HJ, Feith M, et al. Histologic tumor type is an independent prognostic parameter in esophageal cancer: lessons from more than 1,000 consecutive resections at a single center in the Western world. *Ann Surg* 2001;234:360–367; discussion 368–369.
119. Skinner D. En bloc resection for neoplasms of the esophagus and cardia. *J Thorac Cardiovasc Surg* 1983;85:59.
120. Smoron G, O'Brien C, Sullivan C. Tumor localization and treatment technique for cancer of the esophagus. *Radiology* 1974;111:735.
121. Son Y. Primary mucosal malignant melanoma. Appraisal of role of radiation therapy. *Acta Radiol Oncol* 1980;19:177–181.
122. Spechler SJ. Barrett's esophagus. *Gastroenterologist* 1994;2:273–284.
123. Stahl M, Stuschke M, Lehmann N, et al. Chemoradiation with and without surgery in patients with locally advanced squamous cell carcinoma of the esophagus. *J Clin Oncol.*2005;23:2310–2317.
124. Stin H, Feith M, Siewert J. Cancer of the esophagogastric junction. *Surg Oncol* 2000;9:35–41.
125. Streeter O, Martz K, Gaspar L, et al. Does race influence survival for esophageal cancer patients treated on the radiation and chemotherapy arm of RTOG 85-01? *Int J Radiat Oncol Biol Phys* 1999;44:1047.
126. Suntharalingham M, Moughan J, Coia L, et al. Outcome results of the 1996–1999 patterns of care survey of the esophagus. *J Clin Oncol* 2005;23:2325.
127. Teniere P, Hay JM, Fingerhut A, et al. Postoperative radiation therapy does not increase survival after curative resection for squamous cell carcinoma of the middle and lower esophagus as shown by a multicenter controlled trial. French University Association for Surgical Research. *Surg Gynecol Obstet* 1991;173:123–130.
128. Tepper J, Krasna M, Niedzwiecki D, et al. Superiority of trimodality therapy to surgery alone in esophageal cancer: results of CALGB 9781. *J Clin Oncol 2006 ASCO Annual Meeting Proceedings, Part I* 2006;24:4012.
129. Thompson WM. Esophageal cancer. *Int J Radiat Oncol Biol Phys* 1983;9:1533–1565.
130. Tsuti S, Moriguchi S, Morita M, et al. Multivariate analysis of postoperative complications after esophageal resection. *Ann Thorac Surg* 1992;53:1052.
131. Turnbull A, Rosen P, Goodner J, et al. Primary malignant tumors of the esophagus other than typical epidermoid carcinoma. *Ann Thorac Surg* 1973;15:463.
132. Urba S, Orringer M, Iannettoni M, et al. A phase II trial of preoperative cisplatin, paclitaxel, and radiation therapy before trans-hiatal esophagectomy (THE) in patients with loco-regional esophageal cancer (CA). *Proc Am Soc Clin Oncol* 2000;19:248a.
133. Urba SG, Orringer MB, Turrisi A, et al. Randomized trial of preoperative chemoradiation versus surgery alone in patients with locoregional esophageal carcinoma. *J Clin Oncol* 2001;19:305–313.
134. Urschel J, Vasan H. A met-analysis of randomized controlled trials that compared neoadjuvant chemoradiation and surgery to surgery alone for resectable esophageal cancer. *Am J Surg* 2003;185:538–543.
135. Urshel J, Vasan H, Blewett C. A meta-analysis of randomized controlled trials that compared neoadjuvant chemotherapy and surgery to surgery alone for respectable esophageal cancer. *Am J Surg* 2002;183:274–279.
136. VanResenberg S. Epidemiologic and dietary evidence for a specific nutritional predisposition to esophageal cancer. *J Natl Cancer Inst* 1981;67:243.
137. von Rahden B, Stein HJ, Feith M, et al. Lymphatic vessel invasion as a prognostic factor in patients with primary resected adenocarcinoma of the esophagogastric junction. *J Clin Oncol* 2005;23:874–879.

138. Vuong T, Szego P, David M, et al. The safety and usefulness of high-dose-rate endoluminal brachytherapy as a boost in the treatment of patients with esophageal cancer with external beam radiation with or without chemotherapy. *Int J Radiat Oncol Biol Phys* 2005;63:758–764.

139. Walsh T, Noonan N, Hollywood D, et al. A comparison of multimodal therapy and surgery for esophageal adenocarcinoma. *N Engl J Med* 1996;335:462–467.

140. Wang M, Gu X, Huang G, et al. Randomized clinical trial on the combination of preoperative irradiation and surgery in the treatment of esophageal carcinoma: report on 206 patients. *Int J Radiat Oncol Biol Phys* 1989;16:325–327.

141. Watson W, Goodner J, Miller T, et al. Torek esophagectomy: the case against segmental resection for esophageal cancer. *J Thorac Surg* 1956;32:347.

142. Weber W, Ott K. Imaging of esophageal and gastric cancer. *Sem Oncolo* 2004;31:530–541.

143. Whittington R, Coia L, Haller D, et al. Adenocarcinoma of the esophagus and esophagogastric junction: the effects of single and combined modalities on the survival and patterns of failure following treatment. *Int J Radiat Oncol Biol Phys* 1990;19:593–603.

144. Whyte R, Orringer M. Surgery for carcinoma of the esophagus: the case for transhiatal esophagectomy. *Semin Radiat Oncol* 1994;4:146.

145. Wychulis A, Woolam G, Anderson H. Achalasia and carcinoma of the esophagus. *JAMA* 1971;215:1638.

146. Xiao Z, Yang Z, Miao Y, et al. Influence of number of metastatic lymph nodes on survival of curative resected thoracic esophageal cancer patients and value of radiotherapy: report of 549 cases. *Int J Radiat Oncol Biol Phys* 2005;62:82–90.

147. Yang C. Research on esophageal cancer in China: a review. *Cancer Res* 1980;40:2633.

148. Zabotto L, Touboul E, Lerouge D, et al. Impact of CT and 18F-deoxyglucose positron emission tomography image fusion for conformal radiotherapy in esophageal carcinoma. *Int J Radiat Oncol Biol Phys* 2005;63:340.

149. Zeccaro G, Rice T, Goldbloom J, et al. Endoscopic ultrasound can not determine suitability for esophagectomy after aggressive chemoradiotherapy for esophageal cancer. *Am J Gasterinterol* 1999;94:906–912.

150. Zhang Z, Kurtz R, Sun M. Adenocarcinoma of the esophagus and gastric cardia: medical conditions, tobacco, alcohol and socioeconomic factors. *Cancer Epidermiol Biomarkers Prev* 1996;5:761–768.

Clinical Radiation Oncology

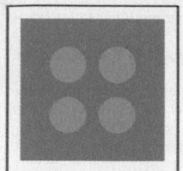

Chapter 51
Tumors of the Heart and Great Vessels

Rahul D. Tendulkar, Mark A. Chidel, Roger M. Macklis

Tumors of the Heart and Pericardium

Incidence and Epidemiology

Tumors of the heart and pericardium are reasonably rare and can arise as primary tumors or as secondary metastases from a known malignancy. Although involvement of the heart or pericardium is not uncommonly seen in the setting of malignancies such as Hodgkin's lymphoma, non-Hodgkin's lymphoma, lung cancer, and thymoma, the focus of this chapter is limited to tumors arising directly from the heart and pericardium.

The first described case of a cardiac tumor was by Albers in 1835 (17). Reynen (67) performed a compilation of autopsy series consisting of over 700,000 cases, finding 157 primary cardiac tumors. The overall incidence was 0.021%, with a range from 0% to 0.19%. Approximately 75% of primary tumors of the heart are benign, and about half of those are atrial myxomas arising from the interatrial septum (49,66,70). Lipomas, papillary fibroelastomas, and rhabdomyomas each account for approximately 10% of cases. Fibromas, hemangiomas, and teratomas are less common benign cardiac tumors (49). Cystic atrioventricular node tumors are extremely rare, but may lead to sudden death despite their small size (18). The Carney complex is an autosomal dominant syndrome comprised of cardiac myxoma, skin hyperpigmentation, and endocrinopathies, often associated with a mutation of the PRKAR1A gene (19,81). Variants include the LAMB (lentigines, atrial myxoma, mucocutaneous myxoma, and blue nevi) and NAME (nevi, atrial myxoma, myxoid neurofibroma, and ephelides) syndromes (18). Hamartomas, rhabdomyomas, and fibromas are diagnosed almost exclusively in children (56). Rhabdomyomas are the most common pediatric cardiac tumor and are associated with tuberous sclerosis.

Malignant primary tumors comprise the remaining 25%. It appears that malignant mesothelioma is the most common primary malignancy of the pericardium, although as of 1994, only 140 cases had been reported in the literature, and only a handful of case reports have been published since (3,4,37,39,58,74,75,79). Fibrosarcoma, angiosarcoma, and teratoma of the pericardium have also been documented (37,39). Primary malignancies of the myocardium comprise the bulk of the remaining cases, of which sarcomas account for the vast majority. Malignant fibrous histiocytoma, angiosarcoma, fibrosarcoma, and rhabdomyosarcoma are among the more common histologic types (48). Table 51.1 summarizes the relative frequency of specific subtypes of sarcoma that may be diagnosed. Lymphomas account for only about 2% of primary cardiac tumors, but the incidence appears to be increasing. Melanoma and carcinoma may also occur infrequently.

With advances in echocardiography, computed tomography (CT), and magnetic resonance imaging (MRI), the postmortem diagnosis of cardiac tumors is becoming less common. Surgical series seem to demonstrate an increase in the ratio of benign to malignant tumors, with malignant tumors accounting for only 10% of cases in a narrow range of 6% to 20% (13,20,25,52,53,56,59). This is likely the result of surgical management of benign myxoma, which accounts for over 80% of patients in some series, combined with changes in patient selection (13,20,53).

The majority of primary cardiac tumors arise in adults with a median age of 45 to 55 years (13,20,25,52,53,56,59). Among 533 cases in the database of the Armed Forces Institute of Pathology, McAllister and Fenoglio (49) noted that 83% of patients were adults. Infants (younger than 1 year of age) comprised 9% of the patients, and in this group, 96% of tumors were benign and only 4% were malignant. In a review of the data from the National Cancer Institute Surveillance, Epidemiology, and End Results (SEER) from 1973 to 1987, Mack (48) reported no sex predilection for the incidence of sarcoma of the mediastinum and heart.

Metastatic disease to the heart and pericardium occurs at a frequency much greater than that of primary tumors (2,26,34,38,40,44,68). In a review of more than 12,000 autopsies in Hong Kong, Lam et al. (40) noted that cardiac metastases were over 20 times more common than primary tumors. The majority of cases have involvement of the pericardium, whereas myocardial involvement is uncommon. In a review of autopsy series of patients with a known malignancy, Hanfling (34) noted the rate of reported cardiac involvement increased steadily from 1.5% in the late 1800s to 18.3% in 1960. Contemporary series indicate the rate of cardiac involvement is as high as 10% to 18% (34,38,44).

The sites of origin of cardiac metastases from solid tumors are summarized in Table 51.2. Lung cancer is the most common cause of cardiac metastases and accounts for nearly one half of cases. Upper gastrointestinal malignancies and breast cancer are also common causes of cardiac metastases, accounting for one fourth of cases. The remaining one fourth of cases arise from a wide variety of other malignancies. Melanoma is purported to have the highest propensity for metastatic spread to the heart and tends to involve the endocardium or myocardium (17). Cardiac metastases may also originate from lymphoma or leukemia. In 1960, Hanfling (34) reported that the proportion of cardiac metastases arising from these malignancies rivals that arising from solid tumors. Multiple medical advances in both chemotherapy and diagnosis have occurred since his report, and modern series consistently report that hematologic malignancies account for approximately 17% of cardiac metastases (2,26,38,40).

Anatomy

The heart is a hollow, conical organ with muscular walls. In the adult, it measures approximately 12 cm in length, 8 to 9 cm in width, and 6 cm in thickness. It is located in the inferior aspect of the middle mediastinum, with two-thirds lying to the left of midline and one-third to the right. The heart lies posterior to the sternum and rib cage, and anatomic landmarks on the chest wall may be used to approximate its position. The apex is located roughly 8 cm to the left of midline in the fifth intercostal space, and the base is at the level of the third costal cartilage. It rests on the diaphragm inferiorly. The heart receives its blood supply from the coronary arteries, which are located in the space between the myocardium and epicardium.

Table 51.1	DISTRIBUTION OF HISTOLOGIC SUBTYPES OF CARDIAC SARCOMA	
Subtype of Sarcoma	No. of Cases	Percentage of Cases
Angiosarcoma	105	28
Rhabdomyosarcoma	43	12
Undifferentiated/NOS	43	12
Fibrosarcoma	39	10
Malignant fibrous histiocytoma	33	9
Leiomyosarcoma	26	7
Liposarcoma	20	5
Other	64	17
Total	373	100

NOS, not otherwise specified.
Data compiled from references 13, 15, 48, 49, and 64.

The pericardial fat provides a smooth contour and is also located in this space. The heart has four chambers, two ventricles with thick muscular walls and two atria with thin muscular walls. Although the heart is not attached to surrounding organs, it is held in position by its association with the great vessels and the pericardium. The great vessels include the aorta, venae cava, pulmonary artery, and pulmonary veins, which arise from (or end in) the left ventricle, right atrium, right ventricle, and left atrium, respectively. The roots of the great vessels, along with the heart, are encompassed by the parietal pericardium. In combination with the epicardium, this fibrous layer provides a smooth cavity in which the heart can pump freely. Externally, the pericardium is adherent to, but separate from the mediastinal pleura, creating a potential space through which the phrenic nerve traverses (33).

Natural History

Pericardial Tumors

Primary malignant tumors of the pericardium are exceedingly rare and include mesothelioma, fibrosarcoma, angiosarcoma, and malignant teratoma (39). An American Medical Association survey of nearly 500,000 autopsies revealed a 0.0022% incidence of primary malignant pericardial neoplasms (74). Of 140 primary malignant pericardial mesotheliomas reported in the literature, only 28% of cases were diagnosed antemortem (37). Mesothelioma is the most common pericardial neoplasm and may either be confined to the pericardial sac at diagnosis or extend beyond it, involving the myocardium or mediastinal structures (3,37,79). Metastases have been documented by lymphatic and hematogenous routes to involve regional lymph nodes, lung, liver, brain, bone, and adrenal glands

Table 51.2	SITE OF ORIGIN FOR CARDIAC METASTASES	
Primary Tumor	No. of Patients	Percentage of Cases
Lung	271	47
Upper gastrointestinal[a]	107	19
Breast	42	7
Genitourinary–nonprostate	37	6
Melanoma	28	5
Other	93	16
Total	578	100

[a]Includes esophagus, stomach, small bowel, pancreas, and hepatobiliary primary tumors.
Data compiled from references 2, 26, 34, 38, 40, and 44.

(3,4,37,39,58,74,75,79). Despite the metastatic potential, pericardial tumors are more often fatal owing to local complications, such as restrictive pericarditis with resultant cardiac tamponade, arrhythmia due to myocardial invasion, or venae caval obstruction. Even if the tumor can be diagnosed antemortem, survival is poor. Typically, the onset of symptoms does not occur until the tumor is well advanced, and from that time the median survival is less than 6 months, with only a handful of patients surviving beyond 1 year (4,58,75). There are no clear risk factors for the development of pericardial mesothelioma. Although asbestos has been associated with pleural and peritoneal mesothelioma, no consistent relationship has been established in pericardial mesothelioma (3,37,79).

Tumors of the Myocardium

As noted previously, atrial myxomas are the most common benign tumors of the heart (13,20,25,52,53,56,59,72). Myxomas are diagnosed at a mean age of 45 to 55 years, but have been documented in infants and in octogenarians. Women appear to be affected twice as commonly as men. Typically, these tumors arise from the interatrial septum and grow into the adjacent chamber. The left atrium is the most common site of origin for myxoma, and this is six to seven times more common than myxoma of the right atrium. The tumor may also be located in the ventricles or the valves and can be bilateral. Benign myxomas tend to be slow growing and are minimally invasive and as such may have a long duration of symptoms before diagnosis. Although they are considered benign, the tumor can elicit dramatic symptoms from valvular insufficiency, congestive heart failure, and embolic phenomena. Surgical excision is the treatment of choice, with local recurrence rates ranging from 0% to 5.4%.

According to autopsy series, primary malignant tumors of the heart are approximately one-third as common as benign tumors. The median age at diagnosis is 30 to 40 years, slightly younger than that for benign tumors, and there is no sex predilection as seen in myxoma (48). In addition, there does not seem to be a predilection for site of the tumor in the heart, except for angiosarcomas, which tend to occur more frequently in the right atrium, and often present late with advanced disease and lung metastases (13,20,52,53,56). The duration of symptoms is on the order of months, and survival is poor. Even after attempts at curative resection, recurrences are common, and the median survival ranges from 6 to 18 months (13,15,20,25,52,53,56,59,64). The cause of death is most often complications of locally recurrent disease with invasion of adjacent chambers, valves, or pericardium. Tamponade, hemopericardium, and distant metastases are common (64). About 30% of primary cardiac sarcomas have distant metastases at the time of diagnosis (17). The incidence of hematogenous dissemination of a cardiac sarcoma may be explained by the high rate of blood flow through the heart.

Clinical Presentation

Tumors of the heart have been referred to as the "great imitators" of the cardiovascular system, and although there are no pathognomonic signs or symptoms, cardiac tumors can often be detected through careful attention to both cardiac and extracardiac manifestations of the disease (31,78). It is not surprising that tumors of the heart are often asymptomatic until they become more advanced (34). As the tumor enlarges, signs and symptoms result from disturbances of the normal heart function and are associated with the location of the tumor. The scope of clinical presentation is summarized in Table 51.3. Tumors involving the right heart may result in pulmonary emboli, pulmonary hypertension, tricuspid valve disease, or superior or inferior vena caval obstruction. Left-sided tumors can cause

Clinical Radiation Oncology

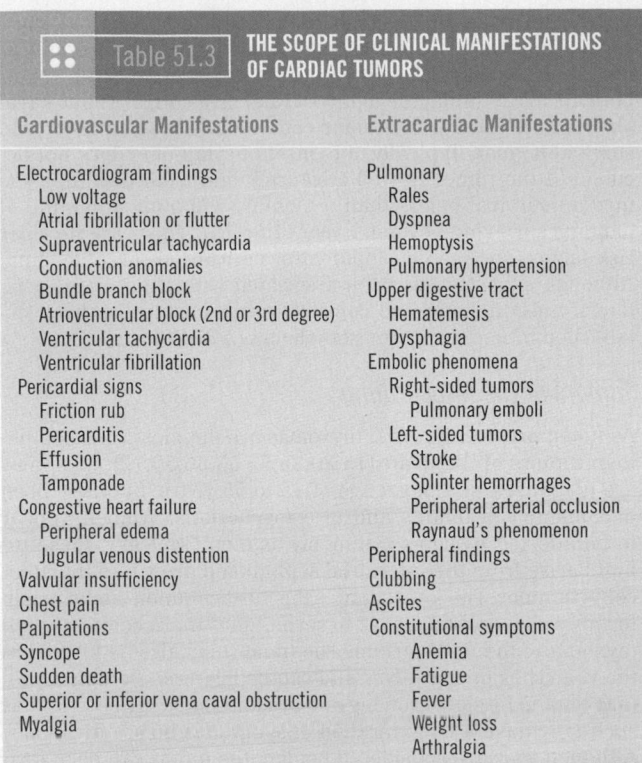

Table 51.3	THE SCOPE OF CLINICAL MANIFESTATIONS OF CARDIAC TUMORS	
Cardiovascular Manifestations	**Extracardiac Manifestations**	
Electrocardiogram findings	Pulmonary	
Low voltage	Rales	
Atrial fibrillation or flutter	Dyspnea	
Supraventricular tachycardia	Hemoptysis	
Conduction anomalies	Pulmonary hypertension	
Bundle branch block	Upper digestive tract	
Atrioventricular block (2nd or 3rd degree)	Hematemesis	
Ventricular tachycardia	Dysphagia	
Ventricular fibrillation	Embolic phenomena	
Pericardial signs	Right-sided tumors	
Friction rub	Pulmonary emboli	
Pericarditis	Left-sided tumors	
Effusion	Stroke	
Tamponade	Splinter hemorrhages	
Congestive heart failure	Peripheral arterial occlusion	
Peripheral edema	Raynaud's phenomenon	
Jugular venous distention	Peripheral findings	
Valvular insufficiency	Clubbing	
Chest pain	Ascites	
Palpitations	Constitutional symptoms	
Syncope	Anemia	
Sudden death	Fatigue	
Superior or inferior vena caval obstruction	Fever	
Myalgia	Weight loss	
	Arthralgia	

Table 51.4	DIAGNOSTIC EVALUATION FOR A SUSPECTED OR KNOWN CARDIAC TUMOR	
Required Studies	**Optional Studies**	
History	Cardiac catheterization, right- or left-sided	
Physical examination	Pressure and output measurements	
Blood work	Coronary angiography	
Complete blood count	Endomyocardial biopsy	
Liver function tests	Transesophageal echocardiography	
Renal profile	ECG-gated MRI	
Electrolytes	Radionuclide scintigraphy, including PET	
ECG	Pericardiocentesis	
Imaging	Staging for malignant tumors	
Chest radiography	CT of the abdomen, pelvis, and brain	
Transthoracic echocardiography	Bone scan	
Contrast-enhanced dynamic CT		

CT, computed tomography; ECG, electrocardiography; MRI, magnetic resonance imaging; PET, positron emission tomography

rapidly progressive congestive heart failure, which may be refractory to treatment. Mitral valve disease and thromboembolic phenomena may also result from tumors of the left heart. Arrhythmias are very common and are predominantly supraventricular tachycardia or nonspecific conduction anomalies (78). Specific presenting complaints are equally varied. Dyspnea is the most common presenting complaint and is noted in 5% to 60% of patients (2,15,42,61). Palpitations are frequently noted and may be positional. Syncope can also be positional; however, if the tumor protrudes into and obstructs a valve orifice, sudden death may result. Chest pain can be anginal, resulting from direct myocardial invasion or obstruction of the main coronary ostia. It can also be sharp, due to invasion of the pericardium, with resulting pericarditis. Constitutional symptoms also occur, with fever, malaise, anemia, and weight loss (2,15,34,42,61,78).

Physical examination may reveal tachycardia, murmur (which may be positional), pericardial rub, gallops, peripheral edema, jugular venous distention, rales, and stigmata of thromboembolic disease. Electrocardiography (ECG) most often reveals nonspecific ST- and T-wave changes, although low-voltage ECG, supraventricular tachycardia, bundle-branch block, or second-degree (type II) or third-degree atrioventricular node block may also be noted. Laboratory studies may reveal anemia, erythrocytosis, thrombocytosis, thrombocytopenia, leukocytosis, and elevated erythroid sedimentation rate (11,15,61,78).

Diagnostic Work-Up

Before the advent of echocardiography and angiography, 66% of tumors were diagnosed intraoperatively during exploration for suspected valvular disease. With current techniques, the diagnosis can be made reliably in the preoperative setting in almost 90% of cases (13). The diagnostic evaluation of patients with suspected cardiac tumors is presented in Table 51.4.

The physical examination and ECG findings were reviewed previously. The imaging techniques used in the diagnosis and evaluation of cardiac tumors include chest radiography, CT, MRI, echocardiography, radionuclide scintigraphy, and cardiac

catheterization. Although there is considerable overlap among these studies, each modality is unique and may offer advantages in evaluating the tumor. Chest radiography shows abnormalities in over 80% of patients. Unfortunately, abnormalities are usually nonspecific and therefore of limited usefulness. Findings include cardiomegaly, an abnormal cardiac contour, mediastinal widening, or evidence of congestive heart failure (1,14,78). Calcifications are present in up to 20% of cases, perhaps relating to the presence of valvular or pericardial disease (1,73). The finding of calcifications on imaging may also suggest the presence of a fibroma. In the setting of a malignant tumor, chest radiography may also reveal hilar nodal, pulmonary, or osseous metastatic disease.

Echocardiography, M-mode and two-dimensional, is the diagnostic procedure of choice among patients with suspected cardiac tumors. Either transthoracic (TTE) or transesophageal (TEE) techniques can be performed, yielding valuable information regarding size, shape, location, mobility, and areas of attachment (78). In a review of 533 primary cardiac tumors, Blondeau (13) found echocardiography provided a 98% diagnostic accuracy rate among the 437 patients for whom it was used. Bogren et al. (14) found that echocardiography detected abnormalities in 63 of 65 (97%) patients with primary cardiac tumors. With this high level of diagnostic yield, and because the use of TTE has no known side effects, it should be performed in all patients. TEE is a complementary procedure to TTE. It is clearly a more invasive procedure and is not required in all patients, although it may provide for better evaluation of right-sided tumors and of the left atrial appendage. In addition, it may be used for guidance during endomyocardial biopsy (28,47,55).

Cross-sectional imaging has also become indispensable in the evaluation of nonmyxomatous cardiac tumors. With the development of contrast-enhanced dynamic CT (Fig. 51.1), and ECG-gated MRI (Fig. 51.2), real-time imaging of the heart provides fine details of the tumor, with delineation of intraluminal, intramyocardial, and extracardiac extension (27,41,46,65,78). The findings may be used to prepare the surgical team, and if necessary can be used for planning purposes, should adjuvant therapy be required. Compared with chest radiographs, both CT and MRI are more sensitive in detecting metastatic disease. If these studies are positive, tissue diagnosis may be made without the need for endomyocardial biopsy or thoracotomy. If they have not been performed before surgery, CT of the brain, chest, and upper abdomen and a bone scan are recommended in the staging of malignant cardiac tumors.

Radionuclide imaging has been used in the evaluation of cardiac tumors. Gated cardiac blood pool scintigraphy has limited resolution, but may be able to detect tumors when other

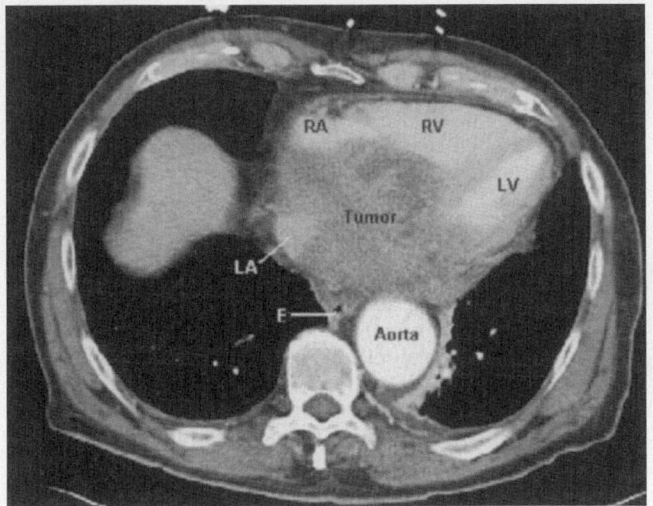

FIGURE 51.1. Computed tomography scan of a primary cardiac neoplasm arising from the left atrium. E, esophagus; LV, left ventricle; LA, left atrium; RA, right atrium; RV, right ventricle.

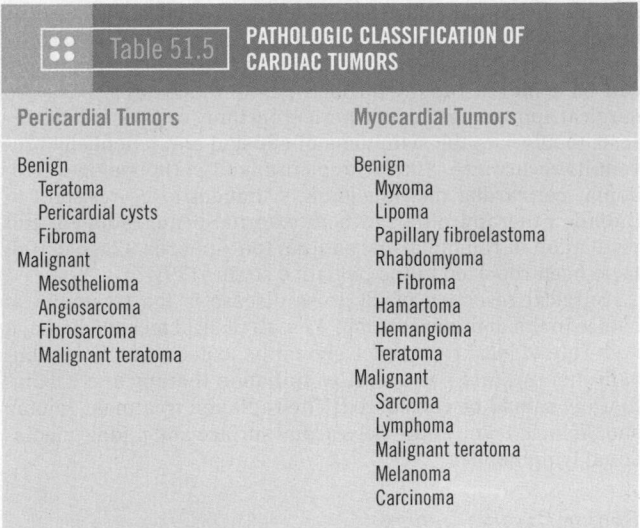

	PATHOLOGIC CLASSIFICATION OF CARDIAC TUMORS
Table 51.5	

Pericardial Tumors	Myocardial Tumors
Benign	Benign
Teratoma	Myxoma
Pericardial cysts	Lipoma
Fibroma	Papillary fibroelastoma
Malignant	Rhabdomyoma
Mesothelioma	Fibroma
Angiosarcoma	Hamartoma
Fibrosarcoma	Hemangioma
Malignant teratoma	Teratoma
	Malignant
	Sarcoma
	Lymphoma
	Malignant teratoma
	Melanoma
	Carcinoma

modalities have failed. Gallium 67 and thallium 201 scans may reveal intramyocardial invasion (14,78). Positron emission tomography (PET) is rapidly gaining favor in the staging of many cancers, and its usefulness in evaluating cardiac tumors is yet to be determined.

Cardiac catheterization was heavily utilized in the past, but its usefulness has diminished with the emergence of the noninvasive techniques noted previously. Catheterization may reveal wall structural or motion abnormalities, intracavitary filling defects, or evidence of neovascularization of the tumor (14,78). If a malignant tumor is suspected, endocardial biopsy may provide tissue for pathologic diagnosis. For patients who may undergo surgical resection of their tumor, catheterization is still recommended for the detection of coronary artery disease and pulmonary hypertension.

Staging System and Pathologic Classification

There is no accepted staging system available for cardiac tumors. With respect to pathologic classification, tumors of the heart and pericardium may be classified as primary, originating from the heart, or metastatic, originating from malignancies of other organs. Primary cardiac tumors can be further subclassified by the site of origin and by malignant potential (Table 51.5).

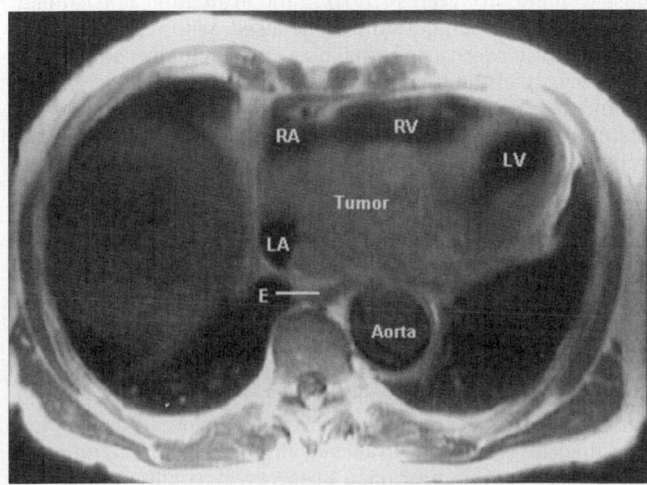

FIGURE 51.2. Magnetic resonance image of a primary cardiac neoplasm arising from the left atrium. E, esophagus; LV, left ventricle; LA, left atrium; RA, right atrium; RV, right ventricle.

Prognostic Factors

In general, the prognosis for patients with either primary or secondary malignant tumors of the heart is poor. The median survival of patients with malignant primary tumors is approximately 1 year, and both local and distant relapse is common. Blondeau (13) reported that angiosarcoma had a median survival of 2.14 years, compared with only 0.75 year for fibrosarcoma. Llombart-Cussac et al. (43), on the other hand, noted a worse survival for angiosarcomas due to their propensity to present late with advanced disease. Series from Burke et al. (15) and Putnam et al. (64) indicate that the histologic subtype does not appear to have prognostic value, although the microscopic finding of more than 10 mitoses per high-power field does portend a worse prognosis. Tazelaar et al. (77) also noted a worse outcome for tumors with high mitotic activity. Conversely, the ability to resect all gross tumor and a left atrial site of origin predict for longer survival (15,64). Although the duration of symptoms is typically short, some patients have a more protracted course, and outcome may be better in those with symptoms for more than 3 months before diagnosis (62). The use of adjuvant radiation therapy has been associated with longer survival (median, 22.7 months vs. 9.6 months) whereas adjuvant chemotherapy has provided mixed results (15,62). Given the retrospective nature of these studies, patient selection may be a source of bias. If a controlled, prospective study could be completed, it is unclear if it would confirm a survival improvement after adjuvant therapy.

The discovery and diagnosis of metastatic disease in the myocardium is rare in the antemortem setting, and hence prognostic factors have not been elucidated. Malignant pericardial effusion, on the other hand, is more easily diagnosed in life and can be appropriately palliated with pericardiocentesis, pericardotomy, or pericardial sclerosis. Among patients with metastases from a solid tumor, the median survival after the procedure is approximately 3 to 4 months, and appears to be improved with better performance status (6,23). The outcome among patients with lymphomatous involvement has not been documented.

Management of Cardiac Tumors

Primary Pericardial Tumors

Fewer than 150 primary pericardial malignant tumors have been reported in the literature to date, and less than one third of these were diagnosed during life (3,4,37,39,58,74,75,79).

Among those diagnosed before autopsy, locally advanced or metastatic disease is common, and palliative treatment may be the most appropriate option. Relief of pericardial tamponade can be achieved rapidly through pericardiocentesis. Palliative surgical approaches include pericardectomy or pericardial sclerosis to alleviate the symptoms of effusion and potentially prevent its recurrence. Similar to pleural and peritoneal mesothelioma, pericardial mesothelioma is thought to be resistant to radiation therapy, although both external-beam radiation and instillation of radiopharmaceuticals (phosphorus 32, gold 198) have been reported in the palliative setting (39,45).

Surgical resection of all gross disease is the treatment of choice in the definitive setting. As with pleural mesothelioma, a high rate of local recurrence should be expected without adjuvant therapy, and postoperative radiation therapy and chemotherapy should be considered. The radiation treatment volume should include the entire pericardial surface and middle mediastinal lymph nodes.

Benign Cardiac Tumors

The most common benign cardiac tumors are atrial myxomas in adults and rhabdomyomas in children. These are both treated surgically with low mortality rates and local control rates in excess of 95% (13,20,25,42,52,53,56,62). Endo et al. (25) reported an 86% 5-year overall survival rate after resection of atrial myxoma. Bogren et al. (14) found the 5-year survival rate was 87% for patients with myxoma and 76% for all patients treated for a benign cardiac tumor. Blondeau (13) reported 444 patients had resection of a myxoma with a 4% 30-day surgical mortality rate, a 1% late tumor- or treatment-related mortality rate, and only a 2% risk of local relapse. Given the high rate of cure, with an acceptable rate of morbidity, surgical resection without adjuvant chemotherapy or radiation is generally appropriate for benign primary cardiac neoplasms. Some rhabdomyomas may even regress spontaneously without the need for aggressive resection (57).

Malignant Primary Cardiac Neoplasms

Surgical resection is the primary treatment of choice for patients with primary malignant cardiac tumors. Unfortunately, local recurrence is often inevitable owing to the extent and invasiveness of the tumor. Even in the presence of a complete excision, local relapse is common and accounts for as much as one third of deaths. Sarcomas account for almost all primary malignant cardiac neoplasms, and the treatment principles should be similar to those for soft tissue sarcoma arising from other areas of the body. After complete or incomplete resection of the tumor, adjuvant radiation and chemotherapy may be used in an attempt to gain control of local and distant disease, respectively.

Anecdotal cases of orthotopic heart transplantation (OHT) for patients with malignant neoplasms of the heart have been described by Jamieson et al. (36) in the literature since the first reported case in 1981 (7,8,22,30,32,51,71,76,80). Although this technique should ideally achieve a complete tumor resection, the results have been mixed. There have been some case reports of long-term survivors, while many other patients have developed distant metastases and subsequent death within months of transplant. Some have attempted cardiac explantation, tumor removal, and autotransplantation (50). Although OHT has promise, theoretical dangers exist, including the potential protumor effect of immune suppression and the ability to tolerate adjuvant radiation therapy or chemotherapy.

Metastatic Tumors of the Heart and Pericardium

There is no known curative therapy for patients with metastatic disease to the heart. Palliative surgery has a role in both diagnosis and palliation for patients with malignant pericardial disease (6,23). Emergency pericardiocentesis or pericardotomy can alleviate cardiac tamponade and yield the diagnosis, and the instillation of a sclerosing agent, such as tetracycline, can often effectively prevent the reaccumulation of the pericardial effusion. Radiation may also be used to relieve symptoms of life-threatening outflow obstruction or pericardial disease.

Radiation Therapy Technique

For patients with a good performance status, radiation therapy is indicated for virtually all primary malignant cardiac tumors, either after resection or in the definitive setting for a tumor that is not resectable. For completely resected tumors with negative margins, doses of 45 to 50 Gy at 1.8 to 2 Gy per fraction appear reasonable. Should microscopic or gross residual disease remain, an additional 10- to 20-Gy boost should be considered to a smaller volume. The initial target should include all areas known to harbor tumor before surgery plus a generous margin of at least 2 cm. Among patients with pericardial mesothelioma, the entire pericardium should be included in the initial target volume. For tumors with a high propensity for nodal involvement (i.e., mesothelioma, angiosarcoma, rhabdomyosarcoma, carcinoma, or lymphoma), coverage of the middle and inferior mediastinal lymph nodes is also recommended. An anterior and posterior, parallel-opposed technique is adequate to cover the desired initial target volume. To limit the risk of radiation myelitis, preferential weighting to the anterior portal is recommended. If it is required, techniques such as opposed oblique fields or anterior wedged pair fields may be used for the boost target volume to obtain the desired dose to the target while limiting the dose to the spinal cord. One concern in using these techniques is the extent of normal tissue irradiation and the potential for severe toxicity, with respect not only to radiation-induced heart disease (RIHD), but to radiation pneumonitis and fibrosis. Some have reported the use of hyperfractionation to a dose of 70.5 Gy at 1.5 Gy per fraction with a radiosensitizer, iododeoxyuridine (54). More recently, the use of carbon-ion radiotherapy has been described for a case of cardiac angiosarcoma, using a dose of 64 Gy in 16 fractions over 4 weeks (5).

In the current era of CT planning, three-dimensional conformal techniques may provide a more homogeneous dose distribution and limit normal tissue irradiation. Intensity-modulated radiation therapy (IMRT) may also have a role in optimizing radiation to the heart. IMRT techniques allow for the selective intensification or reduction of dose to areas of specific concern. Both three-dimensional and IMRT planning systems utilize dose–volume histograms (DVH) in the evaluation of treatment plans. These techniques must be used with caution, however, because overly conformal plans may actually compromise the integrity of the treatment. Cardiac and respiratory motion should be considered during the planning process, and the planning target volume should be adequately expanded to account for this phenomenon. Motion can be evaluated using fluoroscopy or during the planning CT, if spiral CT technology is not used and if the images are obtained without respiratory gating. Representative isodose distributions for a three-dimensional conformal radiation therapy plan and the corresponding DVH data are shown in Figure 51.3.

The total dose able to be delivered is limited by cardiac and lung tolerance. Much of the available evidence on tolerance of the heart is based on patients previously treated for malignancies such as Hodgkin's lymphoma or breast cancer. In general, RIHD may be manifested as pericarditis, myocarditis, conduction defects, or coronary vascular disease (29,63). Damage to the pericardium is most often observed clinically. Risk factors for developing RIHD include total dose, dose per fraction, irradiated volume, radiation technique, age at exposure, and use

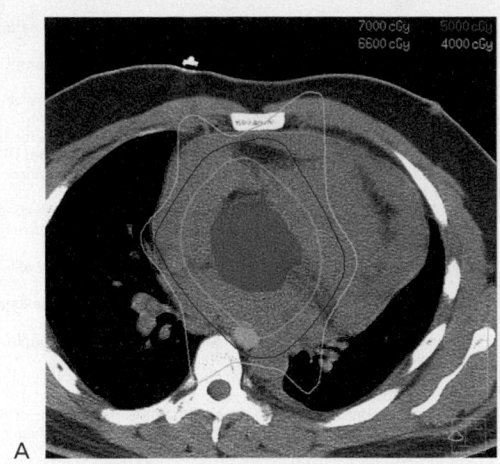 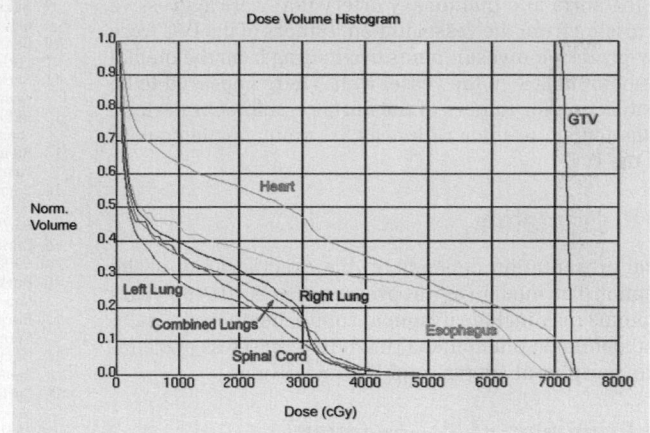

FIGURE 51.3. A sample three-dimensional (3D) conformal plan developed for a patient with an unresectable cardiac angiosarcoma **(A)**, and corresponding dose–volume histogram data for the 3D conformal plan **(B)**. GTV, gross tumor volume.

of concurrent or anthracycline-based chemotherapy. Emami et al. (24) estimated the TD5/5 for developing pericarditis to be 40 Gy for the whole heart, and 60 Gy for one third of the heart. However, current estimates of normal tissue tolerances tend to be conservative and may be underestimates (12,24).

Results of Therapy

In 1964 Sagerman et al. (69) published one of the earliest reports of adjuvant radiation for attempted cure. The patient was a 55-year-old with a primary cardiac fibromyxosarcoma. After incomplete resection, she underwent external-beam radiation therapy to a dose of 63 to 75 Gy to the primary site, with proper shielding of the spinal cord. As a result of the use of lateral fields, the left lung received 35 Gy to a large volume. The patient was treated with prophylactic steroids to prevent radiation pneumonitis and fibrosis. She died 8 months later with brain and lung metastases. Autopsy revealed complete sterilization of the primary tumor.

Despite the most aggressive treatment regimens, with surgical resection, postoperative radiation, and chemotherapy, the overall survival for patients with primary malignant cardiac tumors is poor. Operative mortality is relatively common at 8% to 9%, and is twice as high compared with that following resection of benign tumors. The median survival in most surgical series is in the range of 9 to 12 months (9,10,20,43,52,56,60,64), with outliers as low as 6 months (15,35,53) and as high as 18 months (13). Putnam et al. (64) reported a median survival of 11 months and a 2-year overall survival rate of only 14%. In this series, the authors also noted the importance of complete resection. For patients in whom complete resection was possible, the median survival was 24 months, compared with only 10 months for those with incomplete resection. Llombart-Cussac et al. (43) also noted improved survival with complete resection (22 months vs. 7 months). Burke et al. (15) reported significantly improved median survival of 12 months among patients who underwent adjuvant radiation, chemotherapy, or both, compared to 3 months in those who did not have adjuvant therapy. A group from Japan reported the first use of definitive carbon-ion radiotherapy in the treatment of a patient with cardiac angiosarcoma (5). After treatment, the tumor volume reduced by 86% and became negative on PET scan. After 18 months, the primary tumor remained controlled, but the patient had developed bilateral lung metastases 4 months after treatment.

The median survival for patients with metastatic disease to the heart is approximately 3 to 4 months, but long-term sur-

vival, as long as 3 years, has been documented and may be related to primary tumor histologic type and performance status (6,21,23). Pericardotomy or pericardial sclerosis appears to offer at least temporary control of tamponade and effusion in up to 90% of cases (6,23). Palliative treatment with radiation is well tolerated and is effective in controlling cardiac tamponade in approximately 60% of patients. Cham et al. (21) reported the results of radiotherapeutic palliation for 38 patients with secondary tumors of the heart and pericardium. Thirty-seven patients were noted to have pericardial involvement, nine also had invasion of the myocardium, and one had only endocardial involvement. The radiation dose was 25 to 30 Gy in 3 to 4 weeks for 32 patients. The dose was 15 to 20 Gy in 1.5 to 2 weeks for the remaining six patients, all of whom had lymphoreticular tumors. The overall response rate was 61%, with a median duration of response of 3 to 4 months. Lymphoreticular tumors had the best response rate (6 of 7 cases), followed by breast cancer (11 of 16 cases). Only 6 of the remaining 15 cases showed a response. Although the median survival among patients with metastases to the heart and pericardium is short, palliative efforts are not in vain because tamponade appears to be effectively controlled with the measures described here.

Treatment Sequelae

Late radiation-induced cardiac or pulmonary sequelae after the definitive treatment of cardiac tumors have not been well documented, probably as a result of the poor overall survival. The cardiotoxic effects of doxorubicin have been well documented, and there is evidence for increased risk when it is given in conjunction with radiation therapy (12); therefore, concurrent therapy should be avoided to the degree possible.

:: Tumors of the Great Vessels

The great vessels include the aorta, pulmonary artery, and the superior (SVC) and inferior vena cava (IVC). Tumors of these vessels are extremely rare. The literature consists mainly of case reports, and approximately 130 cases have been documented. As a whole, tumors of the great vessels are about as common as primary malignant pericardial mesothelioma. The only large series was conducted by Burke and Virmani (16). They evaluated 45 tumors on the files of the Armed Forces Institute of Pathology and found that all of the tumors were sarcomas, including intimal (undifferentiated) sarcoma, angiosarcoma, leiomyosarcoma, and synovial sarcoma. In contrast to the tumors of the aorta and pulmonary artery that were aggressive sarcomas arising from the vessel lumen, tumors of the IVC were mostly low-grade leiomyosarcomas originating from the medial layer of smooth muscle in the vessel wall. There appeared to be no sex predilection for tumors of the aorta or pulmonary artery, although the female-to-male ratio was 3:1 among patients with tumors of the IVC.

Clinical Presentation

The clinical presentation depends on the exact location of the primary tumor. The median age at presentation is 40 to 60 years (16). Symptoms may include dyspnea, cough, hemoptysis, pain, and thromboembolic phenomena, including pulseless extremities, stroke, peripheral edema, and SVC syndrome.

General Principles of Management

Resection of the tumor with graft reconstruction of the vessel is the treatment of choice. As with sarcomas of the heart, sarcoma of the great vessels should be treated with the same philosophy as used for treatment of soft tissue sarcoma. Postoperative radiation therapy should be considered for all patients, even those with low-grade tumors, because local recurrence would likely not be amenable to salvage surgical resection (15,16,53). The target volume varies depending on the site of the tumor, and normal tissue tolerances determine the maximally tolerated dose (24). Interstitial or endovascular brachytherapy may be useful to minimize radiation to normal tissues; however, the role of brachytherapy is yet to be defined. The role of chemotherapy also remains undefined.

Results of Therapy

Median survival depends on the location, resectability, and grade of the primary tumor. Burke and Virmani (16) reported the median survival was 5 months for aortic sarcoma, 23 months for sarcoma of the pulmonary artery, and 37 months for sarcoma of the IVC. Two patients with sarcoma of the SVC were alive and without disease 10 and 72 months posttreatment. Local relapse was documented in two patients, although metastatic disease occurred in 19 of 45 patients. The sites most commonly involved by metastases were the lung, liver, and bone. The peritoneum, adrenals, kidneys, skin, and lymph nodes were also noted.

⠿ | Acknowledgments

Dedicated to the memory of Adam Goldstein, M.D., University of Michigan Medical School, Class of 1995. The authors thank Nicole Pavelecky, Mary Jo Repasky, Twyla Willoughby, Ray Rodebaugh, and Thomas Carlson, M.D.

References

1. Abrams HL, Adams D, Grant HA. The radiology of tumors of the heart. *Radiol Clin North Am* 1971;9:299–326.
2. Adenle AD, Edwards JE. Clinical and pathologic features of metastatic neoplasms of the pericardium. *Chest* 1982;81:166–169.
3. Aggarwal P, Wali JP, Aggarwal J. Pericardial mesothelioma presenting as a mediastinal mass. *Singapore Med J* 1991;32:185–186.
4. Andersen JA, Hansen BF. Primary pericardial mesothelioma. *Dan Med Bull* 1974;21:195–200.
5. Aoka Y, Kamada T, Kawana M, et al. Primary cardiac angiosarcoma treated with carbon-ion radiotherapy. *Lancet Oncol* 2004;5:636–638.
6. Appelgvist P, Maamies T, Grohn P. Emergency pericardotomy as primary diagnostic and therapeutic procedure in malignant pericardial tamponade: Report of three cases and review of the literature. *J Surg Oncol* 1982;21:18.
7. Armitage JM, Kormos RL, Griffith BP, et al. Heart transplantation in patients with malignant disease. *J Heart Transplant* 1990;9:627–630.
8. Aufiero TX, Pae WE, Clemson BS, et al. Heart transplantation for tumor. *Ann Thorac Surg* 1993;56:1174–1176.
9. Bakaeen FG, Reardon MJ, Coselli JS, et al. Surgical outcome in 85 patients with primary cardiac tumors. *Am J Surg* 2003;186:641–647.
10. Bear PA, Moodie DS. Malignant primary cardiac tumors: The Cleveland Clinic experience, 1956 to 1986. *Chest* 1987;92:860–862.
11. Becker RC, Hobbs RE, Ratliff NB. Cardiac rhabdomyosarcoma: A case report and review of clinical and pathologic features. *Cleve Clin Q* 1984;51:83.
12. Billingham ME, Bristown MR, Glatstein E, et al. Adriamycin cardiotoxicity: Endomyocardial biopsy evidence of enhancement by radiation. *Am J Surg Pathol* 1977;1:17.
13. Blondeau P. Primary cardiac tumors: French studies of 533 cases. *Thorac Cardiovasc Surg* 1990;38:192–195(special issue).
14. Bogren HG, DeMaria AN, Mason DT. Imaging procedures in the detection of cardiac tumors, with emphasis on echocardiography: A review. *Cardiovasc Intervent Radiol* 1980;3:107–125.
15. Burke AP, Cowan D, Virmani R. Primary sarcomas of the heart. *Cancer* 1992;69:387–395.
16. Burke AP, Virmani R. Sarcomas of the great vessels: A clinicopathologic study. *Cancer* 1993;71:1761–1773.
17. Burke A, Virmani R. *Tumors of the heart and great vessels.* Washington, DC: Armed Forces Institute of Pathology, 1996.
18. Butany J, Nair V, Naseemuddin A, et al. Cardiac tumours: Diagnosis and management. *Lancet Oncol* 2005;6:219–228.
19. Carney JA, Hruska LS, Beauchamp GD, et al. Dominant inheritance of the complex of myxomas, spotty pigmentation, and endocrine overactivity. *Mayo Clin Proc* 1986;61:165–172.
20. Centofanti P, DiRosa E, Deorsola L, et al. Primary cardiac tumors: Early and late results of surgical management in 91 patients. *Ann Thorac Surg* 1999;68:1236–1241.
21. Cham WC, Freiman AH, Carstens PHB, et al. Radiation therapy of cardiac and pericardial metastases. *Radiology* 1975;114:701–704.
22. Crespo MG, Pulpon LA, Pradas G, et al. Heart transplantation for cardiac angiosarcoma: Should its indication be questioned? *J Heart Lung Transplant* 1993;12:527.
23. Davis S, Rambotti P, Grignani F. Intrapericardial tetracycline sclerosis in the treatment of malignant pericardial effusions: An analysis of thirty-three cases. *J Clin Oncol* 1984;2:631–636.
24. Emami B, Lyman J, Brown A, et al. Tolerance of normal tissue to therapeutic irradiation. *Int J Radiat Oncol Biol Phys* 1991;31:109–122.
25. Endo A, Ohtahara A, Kinugawa T, et al. Characteristics of 161 patients with cardiac tumors diagnosed during 1993 and 1994 in Japan. *Am J Cardiol* 1997;79:1708–1711.
26. Fabian JT, Rose AG. Tumours of the heart: A study of 89 cases. *S Afr Med J* 1982;61:71–77.
27. Freedberg RS, Kronzon I, Rumancik WM, et al. The contribution of magnetic resonance imaging to the evaluation of intracardiac tumors diagnosed by echocardiography. *Circulation* 1988;77:96–103.
28. Fye WB, Molina JE. Right atrial angiosarcoma: Echocardiographic diagnosis and surgical correlation. *Johns Hopkins Med J* 1980;147:111–116.
29. Gaya AM, Ashford RFU. Cardiac complications of radiation therapy. *Clinical Oncol* 2005;17:153–159.
30. Goldstein DJ, Oz MC, Rose EA, et al. Experience with heart transplantation for cardiac tumors. *J Heart Lung Transplant* 1995;14:382–386.
31. Goodwin JF. The spectrum of cardiac tumors. *Am J Cardiol* 1968;21:307–314.
32. Grandmougin D, Fayad G, Decoene C, et al. Total orthotopic heart transplantation for primary cardiac rhabdomyosarcoma: Factors influencing long-term survival. *Ann Thorac Surg* 2001;71:1438–1441.
33. Gray H, Goss CM, eds. *Anatomy of the human body,* 27th ed. Philadelphia: Lea & Febiger, 1959;579–582.
34. Hanfling SM. Metastatic cancer to the heart: Review of the literature and report of 127 cases. *Circulation* 1960;22:474–483.
35. Hermann MA, Shankerman RA, Edwards WD, et al. Primary cardiac angiosarcoma: A clinicopathologic study of six cases. *J Thorac Cardiovasc Surg* 1992;103:655–664.
36. Jamieson SW, Guadiani V, Reitz B, et al. Operative treatment of an unresectable tumor of the left ventricle. *J Thorac Cardiovasc Surg* 1981;81:797–799.
37. Kaul TK, Fields BL, Kahn DR. Primary malignant pericardial mesothelioma: A case report and review. *J Cardiovasc Surg* 1994;35:261–267.
38. Klatt EC, Heitz DR. Cardiac metastases. *Cancer* 1990;65:1456–1459.
39. Krasuski J, Frishman W. Malignant pericardial disease: Diagnosis and treatment. *Am Heart J* 1987;113:785.
40. Lam KY, Dickens P, Lam Chan AC. Tumors of the heart: A 20-year experience with a review of 12,485 consecutive autopsies. *Arch Pathol Lab Med* 1993;117:1027–1031.
41. Lipton MJ, Brundage BH, Higgins CB, et al. Clinical applications of dynamic computed tomography. *Prog Cardiovasc Dis* 1986;28:349–366.
42. Livi U, Bortolotti U, Milano A, et al. Cardiac myxomas: Results of 14 years' experience. *Thorac Cardiovasc Surg* 1984;32:143–147.
43. Llombart-Cussac A, Pivot X, Contesso G, et al. Adjuvant chemotherapy for primary cardiac sarcomas: The IGR experience. *Br J Cancer* 1998;78:1624–1628.
44. Lockwood WB, Broghamer WL. The changing prevalence of secondary cardiac neoplasms as related to cancer therapy. *Cancer* 1980;45:2659–2662.
45. Lokich JJ. The management of malignant pericardial effusions. *JAMA* 1973;224:1401–1404.
46. Lund JT, Ehman RL, Julsrud PR, et al. Cardiac masses: Assessment by MR imaging. *Am J Radiol* 1989;152:469–473.
47. Lynch M, Clements SD, Shanewise JS, et al. Right-sided cardiac tumors detected by transesophageal echocardiography and its usefulness in differentiating the benign from the malignant ones. *Am J Cardiol* 1997;79:781–784.
48. Mack TM. Sarcomas and other malignancies of the soft tissue, retroperitoneum, peritoneum, pleura, heart, mediastinum, and spleen. *Cancer* 1995;75:211–244.
49. McAllister HA, Fenoglio JJ. Tumors of the cardiovascular system. In: Hartman WH, Cowan WR, eds. *Atlas of tumor pathology.* 2nd ser, fascicle 15. Washington, DC: Armed Forces Institute of Pathology, 1978;1–3.
50. Mery GM, Reardon MJ, Haas J, et al. A combined modality approach to recurrent cardiac sarcoma resulting in a prolonged remission: A case report. *Chest* 2003;123:1766–1768.
51. Michler RE, Goldstein DJ. Treatment of cardiac tumors by orthotopic cardiac transplantation. *Semin Oncol* 1997;24:534–538.

52. Miralles A, Bracamonte L, Soncul H, et al. Cardiac tumors: Clinical experience and surgical results in 74 patients. *Ann Thorac Surg* 1991;52:886–895.

53. Molina JE, Edwards JE, Ward HB. Primary cardiac tumors: Experience at the University of Minnesota. *Thorac Cardiovasc Surg* 1990;38:183–191(special issue).

54. Movsas B. Primary cardiac sarcoma: A novel treatment approach. *Chest* 1998;114:648–652.

55. Mugge A, Daniel WG, Haverich A, et al. Diagnosis of noninfective cardiac mass lesions by two-dimensional echocardiography: Comparison of the transthoracic and transesophageal approaches. *Circulation* 1991;83:70–78.

56. Murphy MC, Sweeney MS, Putnam JB, et al. Surgical treatment of cardiac tumors: A 25-year experience. *Ann Thorac Surg* 1990;49:612–618.

57. Nir A, Tajik AJ, Freeman WK, et al. Tuberous sclerosis and cardiac rhabdomyoma. *Am J Cardiol* 1995;76:419–421.

58. Norman MG. Primary mesothelioma of the pericardium. *CMAJ* 1965;92:129–130.

59. Perchinsky MJ, Lichtenstein SV, Tyers GFO. Primary cardiac tumors: Forty years' experience with 71 patients. *Cancer* 1997;79:1809–1815.

60. Pessotto R, Silvestre G, Luciani GB, et al. Primary cardiac leiomyosarcoma: Seven-year survival with combined surgical and adjuvant therapy. *Int J Cardiol* 1997;60:91–94.

61. Peters MN, Hall RJ, Cooley DA, et al. The clinical syndrome of atrial myxoma. *JAMA* 1974;230:695–701.

62. Poole GV, Breyer RH, Holiday RH, et al. Tumors of the heart: Surgical considerations. *J Cardiovasc Surg* 1984;25:5.

63. Prosnitz RG, Chen YH, Marks LB. Cardiac toxicity following thoracic radiation. *Semin Oncol* 2005;32[2 Suppl 3]:S71–S80.

64. Putnam JB, Sweeney MS. Colon R, et al. Primary cardiac sarcomas. *Ann Thorac Surg* 1991;51:906–910.

65. Restrepo CS, Largoza A, Lemos DF, et al. CT and MR imaging findings of malignant cardiac tumors. *Curr Prob Diag Radiol* 2005;34:1–11.

66. Reynen K. Cardiac myxomas. *N Engl J Med* 1995;333:1610–1617.

67. Reynen K. Frequency of primary tumors of the heart. *Am J Cardiol* 1996;77:107.

68. Reynen K, Kockeritz U, Strasser RH. Metastases to the heart. *Ann Oncol* 2004;15:375–381.

69. Sagerman RH, Hurley E, Bagshaw MA. Successful sterilization of a primary cardiac sarcoma by supervoltage radiation therapy. *Am J Radiol* 1964;92:942–946.

70. Sarjeant JM, Butany J, Cusimano RJ. Cancer of the heart: Epidemiology and management of primary neoplasms and metastases. *Am J Cardiovasc Drugs* 2003;3:407–421.

71. Siebenmann R, Jenni R, Makek M, et al. Primary synovial sarcoma of the heart treated by heart transplantation. *J Cardiovasc Surg* 1990;99:567–568.

72. St. John Sutton MG, Mercier LA, Giuliani ER, et al. Atrial myxomas: A review of clinical experience in 40 patients. *Mayo Clin Proc* 1980;55:371–376.

73. Steiner RE. Radiologic aspects of cardiac tumors. *Am J Cardiol* 1968;21:344–355.

74. Strauss R, Merliss R. Primary tumor of the heart. *Arch Pathol* 1945;39:74–78.

75. Styman AL, MacAlpin RN. Primary pericardial mesothelioma: Report of two cases and review of the literature. *Am Heart J* 1971;8:760–769.

76. Talbot SM, Taub RN, Keohan ML, et al. Combined heart and lung transplantation for unresectable primary cardiac sarcoma. *J Thorac Cardiovasc Surg* 2002;124:1145–1148.

77. Tazelaar HD, Locke TJ, McGregor CG. Pathology of surgically excised primary cardiac neoplasms. *Mayo Clin Proc* 1992;67:957–965.

78. Thomas CR, Johnson GW Jr, Stoddard MF, et al. Primary malignant cardiac tumors: Update 1992. *Med Pediatr Oncol* 1992;20:519–531.

79. Thomason R, Schlegel W, Lucca M, et al. Primary malignant mesothelioma of the pericardium: Case report and literature review. *Texas Heart Inst J* 1994;21:170–174.

80. Uberfuhr P, Meiser B, Fuchs A, et al. Heart transplantation: An approach to treating primary cardiac sarcoma? *J Heart Lung Transplant* 2002;21:1135–1139.

81. Wilkes D, McDermott DA, Basson CT. Clinical phenotypes and molecular genetic mechanisms of Carney complex. *Lancet Oncol* 2005;6:501–508.

Clinical Radiation Oncology

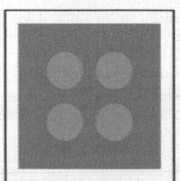

Chapter 52
Breast: Stage Tis

David E. Wazer, Douglas W. Arthur

Noninvasive carcinoma of the breast (stage Tis) includes Paget's disease of the nipple and two histopathologic entities that are distinct in both their clinical presentation and biologic potential: Lobular carcinoma *in situ* (LCIS) and ductal carcinoma *in situ* (DCIS). As a result of the increase in the use of mammography, these three histopathologic entities comprise a larger percentage of all breast cancer cases seen today. There remains considerable controversy regarding the optimal treatment approach and, as a consequence, treatment recommendations range from observation to breast conservation therapy to mastectomy. It is, therefore, important to understand the distinguishing pathologic appearances, biologic characteristics and natural history of these three noninvasive breast disease entities in order to appropriately formulate coherent treatment recommendations.

:: | Lobular Carcinoma *in Situ*

LCIS is characterized by multicentric breast involvement and consists of loose, discohesive epithelial cells that are large in size, variable in shape, and contain a normal cytoplasm to nucleus ratio (89). The extent of involvement of the lobular lumen ranges from simple filling to moderate-to-severe distention with extension into the adjacent extralobular ducts (124). As such, the lines of histologic delineation can become blurred between atypical ductal hyperplasia, LCIS, and, when ductal extension is seen, DCIS. This overlap of histologic morphology may complicate the interpretation of studies from different institutions (49,89,105,124).

LCIS has been reported to present with a multicentric distribution in up to 90% of mastectomy specimens, with bilateral involvement in 35% to 59% (89,105,124). LCIS cells are commonly estrogen-receptor positive, although overexpression of c-erbB-2 and p53 are uncommon (2,3,18,105). The loss of e-cadherin is often observed (2,64,129), and the absence of this adhesion molecule may explain the growth pattern seen with LCIS.

LCIS represents <15% of all noninvasive breast cancer (7,55,133). The majority of women are premenopausal at diagnosis, with an average age of 45 years (49,89,98). Risk factors for the development of LCIS correspond to those identified for invasive carcinoma (125). Because the male breast lacks lobular elements, this entity has not been described in men (49). As there are no clinical or mammographic indicators that are characteristic of LCIS, it is often detected as an incidental biopsy finding (89,105). In a minority of cases, LCIS can be detected with mammographic calcifications, but more commonly, calcifications are in adjacent tissue and are not histologically associated with LCIS (50,102,120). In excisional biopsy specimens, DCIS or invasive carcinoma are frequently identified even when LCIS is the sole histologic entity seen on core biopsy (24,47,74).

The presence of LCIS is considered a marker of increased risk for the subsequent development of invasive (usually ductal) carcinoma (7,49,55,98) that may be greatest for high-grade or more extensive lesions (86,89). This risk appears to be nearly equal for both breasts (22).

The question as to whether LCIS can serve as a direct precursor lesion to the subsequent development of invasive lobular carcinoma is unresolved. Some studies have suggested a clonal link of synchronously detected LCIS and invasive lobular carcinoma (60), whereas others have not (12). In an analysis of 182 patients with LCIS who were inadvertently enrolled on the National Surgical Adjuvant Breast and Project (NSABP) B-17 trial for DCIS and treated with lumpectomy only, there was a 14.4% in-breast tumor recurrence (IBTR) rate and a 7.8% contralateral breast tumor recurrence rate after a median follow-up of 12 years (44). Nine IBTR (5% of the total cohort) were invasive carcinoma and 17 (9% of the total cohort) were DCIS. Although the frequency of contralateral breast tumor recurrence rate was less than that of IBTR, the frequency of invasive contralateral breast tumor recurrence rate (5.6% of total cohort) was similar to invasive IBTR (5% of total cohort). Of note, all of the IBTR were documented to be at the site of the index lesion except for one, characterized as pure LCIS, that was found at a remote site.

Management for LCIS depends on whether it is associated with another malignancy (DCIS or invasive carcinoma) or if LCIS is the sole histologic diagnosis. Approximately 10% of early-stage breast cancers have an associated component of LCIS (1,81,103). The effect that the presence of LCIS has on the outcome of conservative management of early-stage breast cancer has only recently been evaluated. The most widely accepted treatment approach is to manage the breast according to the dominant malignant histology (DCIS or invasive carcinoma) and disregard the presence of LCIS. In such circumstances, it is not necessary to pursue additional surgery to obtain clear margins for LCIS (1,12,81,103).

If LCIS is the sole histologic diagnosis, treatment recommendations range from conservative to radical. When first described as an entity, the significance of LCIS was unknown and mastectomy was often performed (46). The high frequency of contralateral breast involvement was subsequently used to justify contralateral biopsy and even bilateral mastectomy (46,98). Observational studies after wide local excision alone have led to a better understanding of the natural history of this condition, and a more conservative approach is now commonly practiced (7,49,55). In patients with LCIS as the sole histologic diagnosis, the most widely accepted clinical practice is close observation with regular physical examination and mammographic surveillance (7,44,49,55,133). There is no role for radiotherapy in the management of LCIS. The fact that LCIS commonly involves both breasts makes treatment with unilateral mastectomy both inadequate and illogical. Bilateral prophylactic mastectomy is likely excessive in all but those patients believed to be at highest risk: Young age, diffuse high-grade lesion, and significant family history. A less radical prophylactic approach in high-risk patients is to consider the use of tamoxifen. Tamoxifen has demonstrated efficacy in the prevention of invasive carcinoma and, in the context of LCIS, has been shown to reduce risk by 56% (40,128).

Paget's Disease

The clinical presentation of crusting and eczematous changes of the nipple–areola complex were first described in 1856. However, it was not until 1874 that the association with an underlying breast cancer was reported by Sir James Paget (90). Paget's disease of the nipple is characterized by the presence of Paget's cells that are located throughout the epidermis (76). Paget's cells are large and have hyperchromatic, round-to-oval nuclei with abundant amphophilic-to-clear cytoplasm. Mitoses are commonly seen, and the cells can be found in clusters or individually in the basal layers. The fact that Paget's disease is associated with an underlying malignancy in more than 95% of cases has generated discussion regarding the origin of these malignant cells. The epidermotropic theory appears to be the prevailing opinion with the belief that the disease originates from the underlying *in situ* or invasive disease. This is supported by histologic evidence of intraepithelial extension, immunohistochemical studies, and evidence suggesting that the epidermal keratinocytes release a motility factor, heregulin-α, that results in the chemotaxis of Paget's cells that migrate to the overlying nipple epidermis (30,34).

Paget's disease is a rare entity representing <5% of all breast cancer cases (65,100) and is typically diagnosed in the fifth or sixth decade. Synchronous bilateral and male Paget's disease have been reported (30,57,77).

Patients with Paget's disease describe itching and burning of the nipple and areola. There is a slow progression toward a crusting eczematoid appearance that can extend to the periareolar skin. If neglected, bleeding, pain, and ulceration can occur (100,130). Alternatively, Paget's disease can be asymptomatic and present as a pathologic finding after incidental surgical removal of the nipple–areolar complex (63). The differential diagnosis includes superficial spreading melanoma, pagetoid squamous cell carcinoma *in situ*, and clear cells of Toker (68,76). A palpable mass is detected in approximately 50% of patients at diagnosis; in more than 90% of cases this will be an invasive carcinoma. In contrast, if no palpable mass is detected, 66% to

86% will have an underlying DCIS. These associated malignancies are usually located centrally, although they can occur elsewhere in the breast (21,30,100). Mammographic findings are frequent in the presence of a palpable mass, but normal mammograms are reported in as many as 50% of cases (61,100).

At presentation, clinical evaluation includes bilateral breast examination, mammography, and biopsy to confirm the diagnosis of Paget's disease and to fully evaluate the extent of the associated malignancy. The prognosis does not dependent on the diagnosis of Paget's disease, but rather on the associated malignancy. Therefore, local treatment as well as systemic and regional nodal disease risk management should be based on the associated disease.

Management of Paget's disease continues to evolve. Mastectomy was employed in the past but this has been increasingly supplanted by breast-conserving treatment (8,91,136). The infrequent occurrence of this disease entity, the range of disease presentations (nipple involvement with/without an underlying mass and association with invasive vs. noninvasive disease), and the variable extent of surgical resection has made the evaluation of treatment options difficult. Small series have described results with various forms of breast-conserving treatment including wide local surgical resection alone, radiotherapy alone, and wide excision followed by whole-breast radiotherapy. Conservative surgery alone for Paget's disease appears to be inadequate, with reported local recurrence rates of 25% to 40% (32,39,48,70,94,126). The use of radiotherapy alone has been reported as achieving an 85% local control rate in a small series of patients with Paget's disease of the nipple who presented without an associated palpable mass (121). However, this approach has not been widely adopted because of the undefined histologic type and extent of the underlying disease leading to uncertainty in field design and total radiation dose.

The combination of limited surgical resection and postoperative radiotherapy appears to be the most practical breast-conserving approach. Two studies have evaluated the combined use of surgery and radiotherapy in Paget's disease of the nipple. The European Organization for Research and Treatment of Cancer (EORTC) Study 10873 was a multi-institutional registry trial that reported a 5-year local recurrence rate of 5.2% (16). In this study, a complete excision with tumor-free margins of the nipple–areolar complex and underlying breast tissue was followed by whole-breast radiotherapy. The median follow-up was 6.4 years, and the majority of these patients were found to have an underlying DCIS without a palpable mass. A separate study consisted of a seven-institution collaborative review of 36 patients with Paget's disease without a palpable mass or mammographic density (78,93). Patient follow-up was a median of 9.4 years. The extent of surgical resection varied as patients underwent complete (69%) or partial (25%) excision of the nipple–areolar complex and underlying breast tissue, with 6% reported as biopsy only. The final margin status was documented as negative in 56%, positive in 6%, and unknown in 39%. All received whole-breast irradiation and most received an additional boost dose to the tumor bed. The actuarial rate of local failure as the only site of first recurrence was 9% at 5 years and 13% at both 10 and 15 years. Two additional patients recurred in the treated breast simultaneously with regional and distant metastasis at 69 and 122 months. Despite the differences in clinical, pathologic, and treatment factors, statistical evaluation did not identify any factors that significantly predicted for risk of local recurrence.

Current data suggest that a combined-modality approach that conserves the breast is an appropriate alternative to mastectomy in properly selected patients with underlying noninvasive or invasive carcinoma of limited extent. As with any breast-conserving approach, patients with multicentric disease extension should be excluded. Surgical resection should include the nipple–areolar complex with microscopically clear margins surrounding both the Paget's disease and the associated malignancy. Whole-breast radiotherapy is delivered with standard techniques. Management of regional nodes and the risk of systemic disease is dictated by the associated malignancy.

Ductal Carcinoma *in Situ*

Clinical Presentation and Epidemiology

DCIS is a neoplastic process that is confined to the ductal system of the breast and lacks histologic evidence of invasion. These cells neither disrupt the basement membrane nor involve the surrounding breast stroma. This entity lacks the ability to metastasize and is confined to the breast (20,26,88,99). Axillary-node involvement is rare (0% to 5%) and most likely is associated with an undetected focus of invasive carcinoma (112). Risk factors for the development of DCIS are the same as those identified for invasive carcinoma (125) including family history, reproductive events such as delayed age of first live birth and nulliparity, history of benign breast biopsy, and dietary factors such as alcohol consumption. Before the use of screening mammography, DCIS typically presented as a palpable mass or nipple discharge. An invasive component commonly was found, and pure DCIS rarely was encountered. The widespread use of mammography now routinely detects DCIS <1 cm in diameter and results in breast cancer-free survival rates that approach 100% (112).

With the increased use of mammography and as pathologists began to recognize DCIS as a pathologic entity, the incidence of DCIS has markedly increased (73,113,114). The incidence of DCIS in the United States rose from 4,800 cases in 1983 to now more than 50,000 cases annually, representing a 10-fold increase in only 20 years (19). Of the 215,990 new breast cancers diagnosed in 2004, 59,390 were noninvasive, of which 85% were DCIS (66). Of these, 90% are nonpalpable (34). Studies have shown that the rate of screen-detected DCIS increases with age despite the fact that it accounts for a progressively smaller proportion of the total breast cancers detected (33). The rate of DCIS detection has been reported to increase from 0.56 per 1,000 mammograms among women aged 40 to 49 years to 1.07 per 1,000 mammograms among women aged 70 to 84 years (33).

Mammography

Ninety-five percent of new cases of DCIS present with mammographic abnormalities, of which microcalcifications are most typical (123). Noncalcified mammographic abnormalities make up the remaining findings, with asymmetric densities identified in 10%, dominant masses in 8%, and abnormal galactograms (performed for evaluation of nipple discharge) in 6%. Linear and branching calcifications frequently are associated with high-grade DCIS and necrosis, whereas fine and granular calcifications are associated more commonly with low-grade DCIS (Fig. 52.1, A and B) (31,58,96,135).

Initial evaluation should include magnification views that allow for complete characterization of mammographic findings and determination of the need for biopsy. The extent of the lesion as determined mammographically may be used as a guide for excision; however, the size typically is underestimated by 1 to 2 cm when compared with pathologic measurements (58,104). Ultrasonography, digital mammography, and magnetic resonance imaging all have the potential to be helpful in the management of DCIS but have yet to be proven as an acceptable substitute for mammography in screening (106). In cases that present with nipple discharge and a negative mammogram, galactography may be helpful in determining the like-lihood of underlying DCIS versus papilloma (Fig. 52.1C) (92). Magnetic resonance imaging has the potential to refine clinical decision-making and surgical planning in select cases.

Pathology and Biology

The histologic diversity of DCIS can lead to difficulty in distinguishing it from other pathologic entities (88,99). The spectrum of DCIS extends from noncomedo, low-grade DCIS that can be similar in appearance to atypical ductal hyperplasia to comedo, high-grade DCIS. In addition, DCIS can extend into lobules, making it difficult to distinguish from LCIS (38). Traditionally, classification of DCIS has followed its architectural or morphologic appearance. The five subtypes of DCIS are comedo, solid, cribriform, micropapillary, and papillary (10,88,99) and it is common to encounter a mixture of subtypes within the same specimen (92). The characteristic features of each type are shown in Figure 52.2. Less common subtypes have been described and include apocrine, neuroendocrine, signet-cell cystic hypersecretory carcinoma, and clinging DCIS (71).

In 1997 a consensus conference committee was convened to reach an agreement on the pathologic classification of DCIS and the identification of specific features that may convey prognostic significance (26). Methods of processing and evaluating the pathologic specimen were also addressed. Rather than endorsing any specific classification system, the committee recommended and described features that should be documented for each case of DCIS, thus separating out important pathologic components and providing a comprehensive evaluation of the pathologic findings. These features include nuclear grade, presence of necrosis, polarization, and architectural pattern(s). The committee extended their recommendations to include margin status, lesion size, extent of microcalcifications, and correlation between specimen x-ray and mammographic findings. The DCIS Working Party of the EORTC arrived at similar conclusions and emphasized the importance of cytonuclear and architectural differentiation (97).

Three-dimensional examination and reconstruction techniques have resulted in a better understanding of the enormously complex structure of the mammary duct lobular system and the patterns by which DCIS can spread within the breast (51,84,85) (Fig. 52.3). Knowledge of the anatomy and distribution of DCIS within the mammary ductal tree can be useful in selecting patients for breast conservation and assuring maximal surgical clearance of the lesion while preserving an acceptable cosmetic result. For example, Ohtake et al. (84,85) studied the duct–lobular system with computer graphic reconstruction and found that the breast consists of 16 to 24 duct–lobular systems, each culminating in a corresponding collecting duct at the nipple. They also identified ductal anastomoses that established a connection between the various ductal–lobular units and provided a potential pathway for tumor extension and subsequent diffuse involvement (84,85). Their proposed model for the development of widespread intraductal tumor extension within the breast is seen in Figure 52.4.

Faverly et al. (37) have described DCIS growth pattern within the ductal tree and the implications for surgical excision. The growth patterns documented include unicentric (one area only), multicentric (two distinct areas separated by more than 4 cm), continuous (extension along ductal system without gaps), and discontinuous or multifocal (two or more areas separated by <4 cm). They found that in mammographically detected DCIS, a multicentric growth pattern was rare (less than 2%), with most cases showing an even distribution between discontinuous and continuous growth patterns. Of cases with a discontinuous growth pattern, 63% had foci separated by gaps that measured <5 mm, 83% had foci separated by <10 mm, and only 8% had foci separated by >10 mm. There was a correlation between differentiation and growth pattern such that 90% of poorly

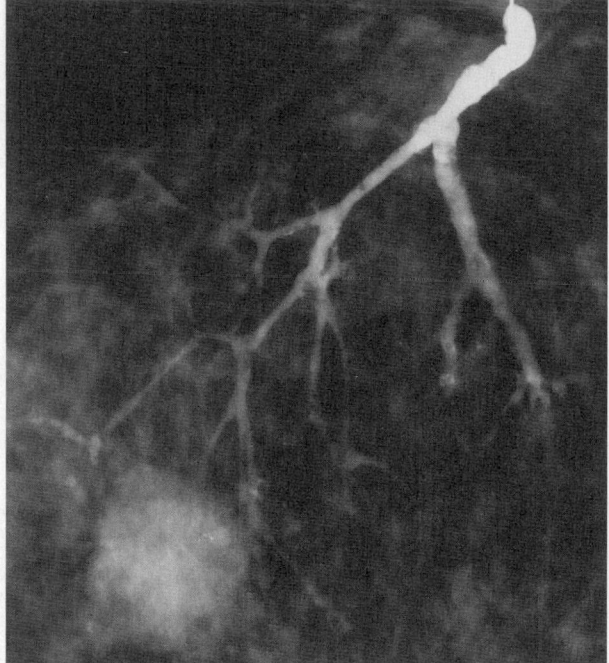

FIGURE 52.1. A: Linear and branching calcifications frequently associated with high-grade ductal carcinoma *in situ* (DCIS). **B:** Fine and granular calcifications commonly associated with low-grade DCIS. **C:** Galactogram with the multiple filling defects associated with DCIS.

differentiated DCIS showed a continuous growth pattern, whereas 70% of well-differentiated DCIS had a discontinuous growth pattern. Based on these findings, the authors concluded that a 1-cm margin of normal tissue around the lesion would lead to complete surgical clearance of histologically evident DCIS in 90% of cases.

DCIS is a precursor lesion to invasive ductal carcinoma and exists along an evolutionary continuum that starts with benign breast tissue and ends with an invasive breast carcinoma (4). This concept has been validated in several ways. For years, pathologists have recognized and documented confirmation of a histologic progression from benign breast cells to invasive breast cancer. The evolutionary concept is further supported by

the recognized association between the presence of DCIS and the subsequent increased risk of developing an invasive breast cancer (19,95,122). In some series, a 10-fold risk of developing an invasive lesion has been reported. Most importantly, the presence of shared identical genetic abnormalities between DCIS and synchronous invasive breast cancer demonstrates a clonal relationship of biologic progression (19,83,95,122). The biologic evolution from benign breast cells to invasive breast cancer occurs through highly diverse genetic mechanisms.

Genetic and molecular differences have been documented that differentiate DCIS from normal breast tissue. Genetic alterations have been evaluated with an analysis of loss of heterozygosity that has demonstrated gain or loss of multiple loci

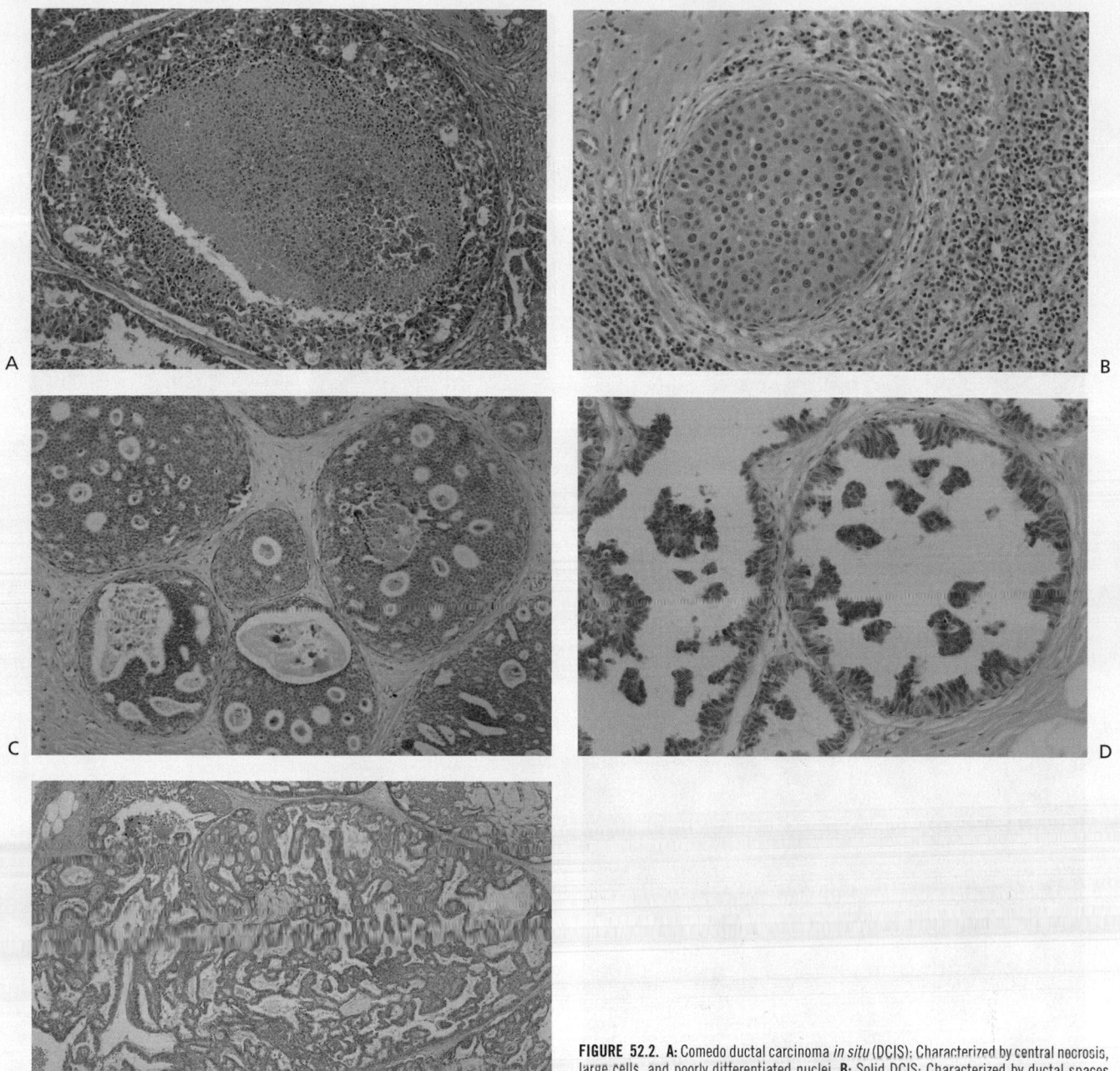

FIGURE 52.2. A: Comedo ductal carcinoma *in situ* (DCIS): Characterized by central necrosis, large cells, and poorly differentiated nuclei. **B:** Solid DCIS: Characterized by ductal spaces filled with neoplastic cells with limited necrosis. **C:** Cribriform DCIS: Characterized by micro-lumens and fenestrations. **D:** Micropapillary DCIS: Characterized by intraluminal projections with no fibrovascular core. **E:** Papillary DCIS: Characterized by intraluminal projections with a fibrovascular core.

(9,36,83,95,122). Loss of heterozygosity is not seen in normal breast tissue. The frequency of loss of heterozygosity correlates with histologic progression of breast tissue from benign to malignant. Loss of heterozygosity is seen in approximately 50% of atypical ductal hyperplasia. Among specimens harvested from cancerous breasts, 77% of noncomedo and 80% of comedo DCIS lesions share loss of heterozygosity with the synchronous invasive lesion in at least one locus (83).

Molecular markers have been studied in DCIS and are found to have a heterogeneous distribution of expression (19). The estrogen receptor is present in 70% of DCIS but the rate of expression is higher in low-grade lesions (90%) than in high-grade lesions (25%). This association with histologic grade is reversed for the rate of overexpression of HER2/neu proto-oncogene and the p53 tumor suppression gene. Approximately 50% of all DCIS lesions have overexpression of HER2/neu, and in 25% the p53

tumor suppressor gene is also detected. Both of these molecular markers are noted in <20% of low-grade lesions but are present in approximately two thirds of high-grade lesions.

Alterations in the surrounding breast parenchyma may also be seen with DCIS. High-grade DCIS, in particular, has been associated with the breakdown of the myoepithelial cell layer and basement membrane surrounding the ductal lumen (28), proliferation of fibroblasts, lymphocyte infiltration, and angiogenesis in the surrounding stromal tissues (52,53). Whether these stromal changes reflect important steps that facilitate primary tumor transformation or secondary alterations in response to ductal epithelium that is being transformed is unknown. Quantitative changes in the expression of genes related to cell motility, adhesion, and extracellular-matrix composition, all of which may be related to the acquisition of invasiveness, occur as DCIS evolves into invasive carcinoma (5).

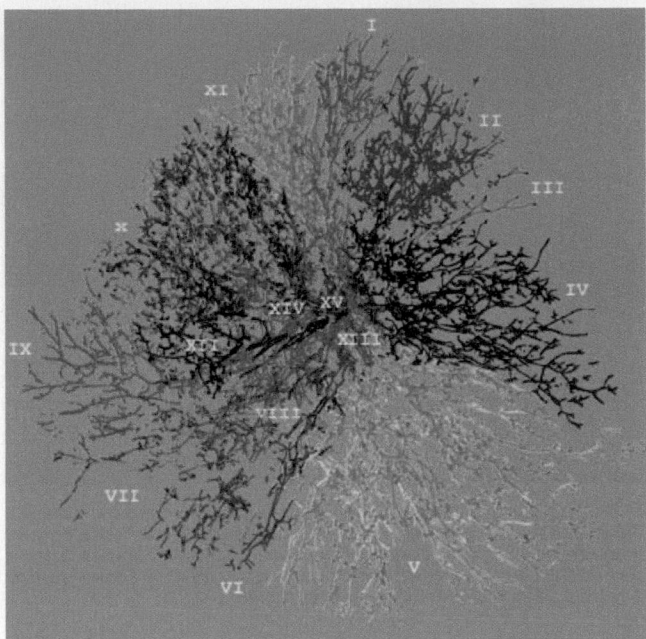

FIGURE 52.3. All ducts and their branches in an autopsy breast, viewed *en face*. Each Roman numeral refers to a different independent duct system. (From Going JJ, Moffat DF. Escaping from flatland: Clinical and biological aspects of human mammary duct anatomy in three dimensions. *J Pathol* 2004;203:538–544, with permission.)

Data suggest that DCIS represents a stage in the development of breast cancer in which most of the molecular changes that characterize invasive breast cancer are already present, although the lesion has not yet assumed a fully malignant phenotype. A final set of events, which probably includes gain of function by malignant cells and loss of function and integrity by surrounding normal tissues, is associated with the transition from a preinvasive DCIS lesion to invasive cancer. Most, if not all, clinically relevant features of breast cancer, such as hormone-receptor status, the level of oncogene expression, and histologic grade, are probably determined by the time DCIS has evolved (17,54,72,131).

An occult microinvasive tumor (one that does not exceed 0.1 cm in diameter) may be seen with some cases of DCIS. Such cases are classified as *microinvasive breast cancer* (115) and are generally treated according to the guidelines for invasive disease. Occult microinvasive tumors are most common in patients with DCIS lesions that are >2.5 cm in diameter (69), those presenting with palpable masses or nipple discharge, and those with high-grade DCIS or comedonecrosis (92, 107).

Natural History of DCIS

The overall incidence of DCIS in the general population is unclear. In an attempt to address this question, a small number of autopsy studies have been reported. One series examined 185 randomly selected breasts from 101 women in which a subgross sampling technique was used (6) and one or more foci of DCIS were found in 6% of cases. A review of seven autopsy series of women not known to have breast cancer during life showed a median prevalence of DCIS of 8.9% (range, 0% to 14.7%) (132). The fact that some autopsy series document a greater incidence of DCIS in asymptomatic women than most clinical series suggests either the possibility that DCIS is either underdiagnosed or that many cases are not clinically significant.

A primary consideration in the natural history of DCIS is the risk of progression to invasive carcinoma. The published evidence on the clinical course of untreated DCIS is sparse because it has been recognized as a distinct entity for only a relatively brief period, having been considered rare before the widespread use of mammography and having been treated most frequently by mastectomy. Those cases for which long-term follow-up data are available were grossly palpable DCIS, a form that may not be equivalent to the mammographic DCIS that is seen more commonly today. The few published long-term follow-up studies of DCIS after only biopsy document an overall incidence of subsequent invasive carcinoma of more than 36% (13,25,80,101). Most of these subsequent malignancies occur within 10 years, although as many as one-third may develop after 15 years (13,101).

Women with DCIS in one breast are at risk for a second tumor (either invasive or *in situ*) in the contralateral breast (56); the rate at which such tumors develop is similar to that among women with primary invasive breast cancer, approximately 0.5% to 1% per year.

DCIS is a part of the breast/ovarian cancer syndromes defined by BRCA1 and BRCA2, with mutation rates similar to those found for invasive breast cancer (23). These findings suggest that patients with DCIS with an appropriate personal or family history of breast and/or ovarian cancer should be screened and followed according to the same high-risk protocols as developed for invasive breast cancer.

Treatment Options for DCIS

Prognostic Factors and Their Interpretation

The goal of treatment with DCIS is prevention of local recurrence, with particular emphasis on the prevention of invasive breast cancer. Treatment decisions are largely based on information provided by mammography and, most especially, pathologic evaluation of the biopsy specimen. As such, in the consideration of treatment options it is important for the clinician to

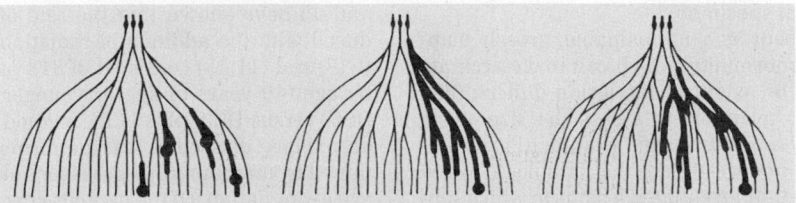

FIGURE 52.4. Models for the formation of widespread intraductal tumor extension over multiple mammary duct–lobular systems. *Narrow line*, normal mammary duct–lobular systems; *bold line*, intraductal tumor extension; *closed circle*, invasive tumor foci. **Left:** Multicentric development. **Middle:** Unicentric development with continuous intraductal tumor extension. **Right:** Unicentric development with continuous intraductal tumor extension through ductal anastomoses connecting adjacent duct–lobular systems. (From Ohtake T, Abe R, Kimijima I, et al. Intraductal extension of primary invasive breast carcinoma treated by breast—conservation surgery. *Cancer* 1995;76:32–45, with permission. Reprinted by permission of Wiley-Liss, Inc, a subsidiary of John Wiley & Sons, Inc.)

be aware of some of the technical limitations associated with the clinical and histopathologic assessment of DCIS.

Studies performed during the past two decades clearly have suggested that DCIS is not a single disease. Rather, this term encompasses a diverse group of lesions that differ with regard to their clinical presentation, mammographic features, extent and distribution within the breast, histologic characteristics, and biologic markers. Moreover, clinical follow-up studies have indicated that these lesions vary in their propensity to recur or progress to invasive breast cancer. As a consequence, a significant proportion of patients diagnosed with DCIS can be treated adequately with breast-conserving therapy (i.e., excision with or without radiation therapy). Which patients with DCIS can be treated safely with excision alone and which patients require radiation therapy after excision is a pressing clinical question. Attempts to resolve this issue have focused on the identification of risk factors for local recurrence after breast-conservation therapy for DCIS. With three exceptions (the prospectively randomized NSABP B-17, the EORTC 10853, and the United Kingdom Coordinating Committee on Cancer Research [UKCCCR] trials), all such studies have been retrospective in design. Nonetheless, a number of factors have been identified that may be important in defining local failure risk. These include symptomatic presentation (15,87,116), lesion size (108,116), histopathologic subtype (15), nuclear/cytologic grade (87,116,119), central necrosis (87,116,119), margin status (109,116,117), and patient age (15,42,117,127).

The relative importance of any histopathologic factor in predicting the probability of local recurrence and, in turn, selecting the appropriate therapeutic option for a given patient is unclear. This is partly the result of the inherent difficulty associated with the establishment of standardized and reproducible systems of pathologic classification, including such apparently straightforward assessments of grade, margin width, and lesion size.

Recent efforts to classify DCIS have been based primarily on the nuclear grade of the lesion and/or the presence or absence of necrosis. A number of studies have shown that there is an association between high nuclear grade and/or necrosis and the risk of local recurrence and progression to invasion (87,116,119). Although the criteria for histologic grading systems have been published, there are limited data regarding the ability of pathologists to apply them in a reproducible manner.

Several studies have shown that the status of the microscopic margins appears to be important in predicting the likelihood of recurrence in the breast for patients with both invasive breast cancer and DCIS treated with breast-conserving therapy (109,116,117). However, there are numerous technical problems in the evaluation of margins of breast-excision specimens. First, if a specimen is removed in more than one fragment, the margins cannot be evaluated. Second, there is no standardized method for sampling or reporting margins, and this process is subject to sampling error. Finally, it is often difficult to provide an accurate assessment of the margin width for patients who undergo a re-excision as the initial biopsy site can be eccentrically located in the surgical specimen.

Most DCIS lesions present as a nonpalpable, grossly inapparent mammographic abnormality, which can make accurate determination of the size or extent of the lesion difficult (Fig. 52.5). The two modalities available to assess the size of the lesion are mammography and pathologic examination. Mammography frequently will underestimate the pathologic extent of DCIS, particularly for well-differentiated lesions in which substantial areas of the tumor may not contain microcalcifications. Pathologic assessment of lesion size also can be difficult. Macroscopic examination of a specimen containing DCIS rarely reveals a grossly evident tumor that can be measured. Therefore, the assessment of the size of the lesion must be estimated from histologic sections.

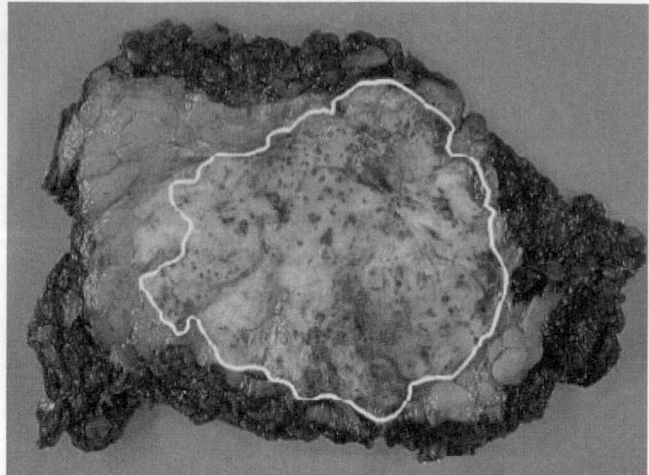

FIGURE 52.5. Extensive ductal carcinoma *in situ* (DCIS) in a mastectomy breast sectioned in the coronal plane. Every parenchymal structure (duct or lobule) within the marked perimeter is colonized by DCIS; outside that boundary there is none. (From Going JJ, Moffat DF. Escaping from flatland: Clinical and biological aspects of human mammary duct anatomy in three dimensions. *J Pathol* 2004;203:538–544, with permission.)

Mastectomy for DCIS

Mastectomy was the standard treatment of DCIS through the first four decades of its recognition as a distinct histopathologic entity. Mastectomy is a highly effective treatment for DCIS, with a locoregional control rate of 96% to 100% and cancer-specific mortality rates of 4% or less (111). No randomized study has compared mastectomy with breast-conservation treatment for DCIS. Therefore, the relative outcomes for mastectomy and breast-conservation treatment can be estimated only by reviewing nonrandomized, retrospective studies. Local treatment failure after mastectomy (111) may occur because of unrecognized invasive carcinoma that results in local recurrence or distant metastasis, or it may be the result of incomplete removal of breast tissue with the subsequent formation of a new primary tumor.

Data from some surgical trials (45) and large treatment registries (85) suggest that the rates of local or regional recurrence are significantly lower after mastectomy than after breast-conserving surgery, but there have been no significant differences in overall survival. Metastatic breast cancer can follow the recurrence of an invasive tumor or the development of cancer in the contralateral breast. However, death related to breast cancer within 10 years after the diagnosis of DCIS occurs in only 1% to 2% of all patients, irrespective of whether mastectomy or breast-conserving surgery was performed (35).

Breast Conservation for DCIS

Three prospective randomized studies of excision only versus excision plus breast irradiation for DCIS have been performed, and all have shown that the rate of local recurrence was reduced with the addition of radiation (Table 52.1). The NSABP B-17 trial (41,43) consisted of 818 patients who were stratified by age (49 years of age or younger vs. older than 49 years), DCIS versus DCIS plus LCIS, method of detection, and whether an axillary dissection was performed. Tumor size was determined by mammogram, gross pathologic measurement, or clinical examination. Of the patients enrolled, 83% had nonpalpable tumors. The 12-year rate of local recurrence was 15.7% with radiation and 31.7% without radiation (*p* <.000005) (Fig. 52.6). The average annual incidence rates of all ipsilateral breast tumor recurrences, ipsilateral noninvasive recurrences, and ipsilateral invasive recurrences were reduced with breast irradiation by 59%, 47%, and 71%, respectively. An analysis of clinical

Table 52.1	LUMPECTOMY VS. LUMPECTOMY AND WHOLE-BREAST RADIOTHERAPY: RANDOMIZED CLINICAL TRIALS FOR DUCTAL CARCINOMA *IN SITU* (DCIS)					
Trial Group	**No. of Patients**	**Follow-Up**	**Local Recurrence (cumulative %) DCIS + Invasive Carsinoma**			
			L	L+XRT	p value	
NSABP B-17	818	12-yr actuarial	31.7	15.7	<.000005	
EORTC 10853	1,010	10.2-yr median	25.0	15.0	<.0001	
UKCCCR	1,030	4.38-yr median	14.0	6.0	<.0001	

L, lumpectomy; L + XRT, lumpectomy and postoperative radiotherapy; NSABP, National Surgical Adjuvant Bowel and Breast Project; EORTC, European Organization for Research and Treatment of Cancer; UKCCCR, United Kingdom Coordinating Committee on Cancer Research.

variables showed that microcalcifications extending beyond a maximum dimension of >1 cm were associated with an elevated risk of breast recurrence. A central pathology review was performed, including a multivariate analysis of histopathologic variables (Table 52.2), that revealed only moderate/marked comedonecrosis as being significantly associated with local failure risk. Margin status (free vs. unknown/involved) was of borderline significance.

The EORTC 10853 trial (14,67) randomly allocated 1,010 patients with 5 cm or smaller DCIS and negative margins to excision versus excision plus breast irradiation. Lesions were nonpalpable in 79% of patients, and the mean maximal tumor diameter was approximately 2 cm. The 10-year rate of local recurrence was 15% for patients treated with radiation, as compared with 25% for patients treated without radiation (p <.0001). At a median follow-up of 10.2 years, radiation therapy resulted in risk reduction for both invasive and noninvasive breast relapse of 42%. As with the NSABP B-17 study, a central pathology review was performed (14,15). In a multivariate analysis (Table 52.3), factors associated with an increased risk of local recurrence were age 40 years or younger, clinically symptomatic presentation (nipple discharge or palpable mass), intermediate or poorly differentiated DCIS, solid and cribriform

histologic growth pattern, involved or uncertain margins, and treatment by local excision alone. The risk of invasive recurrence was not related to histologic type of DCIS, but the risk of distant metastasis was significantly higher in poorly differentiated DCIS compared with well-differentiated DCIS.

The EORTC 10853 trial did not allow the identification of an appropriate margin width for treatment with or without radiotherapy because the eligibility criteria did not require reporting of the margin status. Nonetheless, the central review of cases did provide some information regarding the relative importance of surgical margin as related to local failure risk. A recurrence rate of 24% at 4 years was observed in cases with close/involved margins after excision alone. Radiotherapy was not adequate to compensate for involved margins because even with the application of irradiation the recurrence rate was 20% in this group. These data and others (108,109,116,117) are strongly suggestive that obtaining a microscopic complete excision is essential for optimal local control in breast-conserving therapy for DCIS. Of further note, even in the group of DCIS cases for which margins could be considered optimal (i.e., those patients who underwent a surgical re-excision in which no residual DCIS was found), a 4-year local recurrence rate of 18% was observed when these patients were treated with surgery alone (15).

The UKCCCR DCIS Working group has also conducted a randomized trial investigating the role of adjuvant radiotherapy (59). With a 2 × 2 factorial protocol design, the aim of this study was to compare excision alone versus excision plus tamoxifen versus excision plus radiotherapy versus excision plus radiotherapy and tamoxifen. Tamoxifen was prescribed as 20 mg per day and radiotherapy was delivered through whole-breast tangential fields to a total dose of 50 Gy. Boost was not recommended. A total of 1,030 patients were enrolled. When reported with 4.38 year follow-up, the crude incidence of local recurrence was 14% of the patients who were treated with excision only and 6% when the excision was followed by radiotherapy. The addition of tamoxifen offered no benefit toward overall ipsilateral local control when administered in addition to radiotherapy; however, tamoxifen did appear to reduce the ipsilateral recurrence rate of DCIS (but not invasive carcinoma) in the absence of radiotherapy (59).

Subgroup analyses from randomized trials have demonstrated that the absolute benefits of radiotherapy are greater in women at increased risk for tumor recurrence, such as women with involved surgical margins (identified on retrospective pathologic review), younger women, and those with tumors that have high-grade or comedonecrotic features (14,15,41,43). However, radiotherapy lowers the incidence of recurrence among all subgroups, regardless of the baseline risk.

Patient age is an important prognostic variable for local recurrence after breast conservation for DCIS (15,42,117,127). In younger patients, DCIS more frequently contains adverse prognostic pathologic features and extends over a greater distance in the breast than in older patients (127). In series with

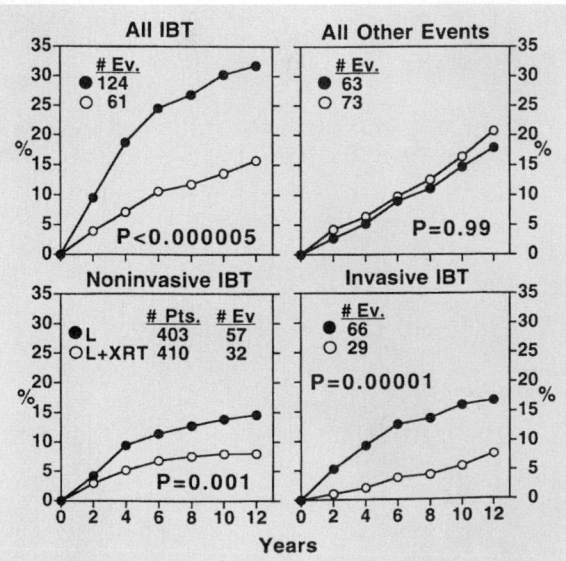

FIGURE 52.6. Cumulative incidence of all ipsilateral breast tumor (IBT) recurrences, noninvasive and invasive ipsilateral breast tumor recurrences, and of all other first events in women treated by lumpectomy (L) or lumpectomy and radiation therapy (L + XRT) in National Surgical Adjuvant Breast Project Protocol B-17. *P* values are comparisons of average annual rates of failure. # Ev, number of events; # Pts. Number of patients. (From Fisher B, Land S, Mamounas E, et al. Prevention of invasive breast cancer in women with ductal carcinoma in situ: An update of the National Surgical Adjuvant Breast and Bowel Project Experience. *Semin Oncol* 2001;28:400–418, with permission.)

Clinical Radiation Oncology

Table 52.2	ANNUALIZED RISK OF IPSILATERAL BREAST TUMOR RECURRENCE ACCORDING TO EXTENT OF COMEDONECROSIS AND MARGIN STATUS AS ADAPTED FROM NSABP B-17 (% RELAPSE PER PATIENT-YEAR)		
Histopathologic Variable	**Excision (%)**	**Excision Plus XRT (%)**	**_p_ Value**
Comedonecrosis			
Absent/slight	3.5	1.8	0.002
Moderate/marked	7.5	2.1	
Margin status			
Free	4.7	1.9	0.06
Uncertain/involved	7.2	2.5	

NSABP, National Surgical Adjuvant Breast and Bowel Project; XRT, external radiation therapy.

adequate follow-up, younger patients treated with lumpectomy and radiation therapy had a significantly higher rate of local recurrence than older patients, especially for invasive local recurrences (127). Some studies have suggested that careful attention to margin status and excising larger volumes of tissue can reduce this difference substantially (117,127). No available data show that younger patients have better long-term cancer-free survival rates if treated by mastectomy rather than lumpectomy and radiation therapy. Successful treatment of younger patients with DCIS with lumpectomy and radiation therapy requires careful attention to patient evaluation, selection, and surgical technique. When this is done, age at diagnosis should not be a contraindication to breast-conserving therapy.

A number of recent studies have attempted to identify and treat patients with highly selected favorable tumor characteristics with excision alone (i.e., without whole-breast irradiation)

and report 10-year local failure rates of 3% to 25% (109,111). A scoring system has been proposed (108) using histopathologic features including tumor size, grade, and margin width in an attempt to stratify patients according to local failure risk after excision plus or minus whole-breast irradiation. Each variable was assigned a score of 1 to 3, and the sum total defined the Van Nuys Prognostic Index. Although appealingly simple, this scheme (108) is drawn from the retrospective analysis of a patient cohort in which there exist a number of methodologic shortcomings and it has not been independently validated (29).

Wong et al. (134) performed a prospective study that attempted to identify patients with "low-risk" DCIS who can be spared whole-breast radiation therapy. This trial enrolled 158 patients with lesions that were mostly grade 1 or 2 and with a mammographic extent of ≤2.5 cm who were treated with wide excision, with final margins of ≥1 cm or a re-excision without

Table 52.3	CLINICAL AND HISTOLOGIC CHARACTERISTICS RELATED TO ANNUALIZED RISK OF LOCAL RECURRENCE AS ADAPTED FROM THE EORTC 10853 TRIAL (% RELAPSE PER PATIENT-YEAR)		
Characteristic	**Excision (%)**	**Excision Plus XRT (%)**	**_p_ Value**
Age (yr)			
>40	4.5	2.0	
≤40	11.3	5.8	0.001
Method of detection			
x-ray finding only	4.0	2.8	
Nipple discharge/palpable mass	6.8	5.0	0.015
Nuclear grade			
Low	3.3	1.0	
Intermediate	5.5	3.5	
High	7.0	4.5	0.001
Necrosis			
None	4.0	1.0	
Marked/moderate	5.0	4.0	0.018
Size (mm)			
<10	4.0	2.8	
10–20	8.8	1.3	
>20	17.8	2.3	0.2127
Margins			
Re-excision, no DCIS	4.5	1.8	
Free (>1 mm)	4.5	3.0	
Free (not specified)	3.5	3.0	
Close/involved (≤1 mm)	8.0	4.0	0.022
Architecture			
Clinging/micropapillary	2.0	0.8	
Cribriform	5.3	4.0	
Solid/comedo	7.0	3.8	0.001

EORTC, European Organization for Research and Treatment of Cancer; XRT, external radiation therapy; DCIS, ductal carcinoma _in situ_.

residual DCIS. Tamoxifen was not permitted. The median age was 51 years and the median follow-up was 40 months. The rate of ipsilateral local recurrence was 2.4% per patient-year, corresponding to a 5-year rate of 12%. Nine patients (69%) experienced recurrence of DCIS and four (31%) experienced recurrence with invasive carcinoma. These data provide prospective evidence that, despite margins of >1 cm, the local recurrence rate is substantial even in patients with small, grade 1 or 2 DCIS following treatment with wide excision alone.

Presently, the Radiation Therapy Oncology Group is conducting a prospective randomized trial to further assess the need for radiotherapy in low-risk DCIS. Following lumpectomy with ≥3 mm clear margins of resection, patients are stratified according to age (<50 vs. ≥50 years), tumor size (≤1 vs. >1 to 2.5 cm), margin status (negative re-excision vs. 3 to 9 vs. ≥10 mm), grade, and the use of tamoxifen (at the discretion of the managing physician). Following stratification, patients are randomized to whole-breast irradiation versus observation. The NSABP and Radiation Therapy Oncology Group have jointly launched a phase III accelerated partial-breast irradiation trial that randomly allocates patients between standard whole-breast irradiation following lumpectomy versus accelerated partial-breast irradiation to determine if in-breast control rates are comparable. As the in-breast failure patterns for DCIS suggest that treatment directed to the primary lesion plus a 2-cm margin should achieve local control rates that equate to whole-breast treatment approaches, patients with pure DCIS or DCIS and LCIS will be eligible for stratified randomization.

Follow-Up and Management of Recurrence

Ipsilateral tumor recurrences in patients with DCIS are usually detected on surveillance mammography, although one-quarter may be detected on the basis of changes on physical examination of the breast or chest wall (75,118). For this reason, patients should be scheduled for a baseline mammogram 6 to 12 months after initial therapy and at least annually thereafter. Distant breast cancer metastases in the absence of regional recurrence are unusual. Local recurrences after breast-conserving surgery and radiotherapy are generally treated with mastectomy. Selected patients with local recurrences who have not previously received radiotherapy may be candidates for local excision and radiotherapy. The clinical outcome of ipsilateral tumor recurrence is governed by the nature of the recurrence. Patients with recurrent DCIS have an excellent prognosis, with less than a 1% risk of further recurrence after salvage mastectomy. Patients with invasive recurrence after breast-conserving surgery for DCIS have a prognosis similar to those with early-stage breast cancer, with a 15% to 20% risk of metastatic recurrence at 8 years (118).

The Role of Tamoxifen for DCIS

The NSABP B-24 trial (42) compared excision plus radiotherapy to excision, radiotherapy, and tamoxifen. Patients who received tamoxifen had a decreased incidence of breast cancer events (invasive or noninvasive ipsilateral or contralateral breast cancer) compared with patients who did not receive tamoxifen (8.2% vs. 13.4% at 5 years, respectively; $p = .0009$), but no survival benefit was found. Tamoxifen therapy resulted in a 44% reduction in the risk of subsequent invasive tumor recurrence but had no significant effect on ipsilateral noninvasive breast recurrence (Table 52.4). Positive tumor margins were significantly associated with breast recurrence, and tamoxifen reduced ipsilateral breast failure by 22% with negative margins and 44% in cases with positive or unknown margins.

In contrast to the findings of the NSABP B-24 trial, the UKCCCR trial found that tamoxifen had no effect in reducing local recurrence rate when combined with whole-breast radiation therapy (Table 52.4). When used as single agent without radiation therapy after lumpectomy, tamoxifen had no effect on the incidence of invasive recurrence but did show a statistically significant reduction in the risk of DCIS recurrence (10% vs. 6%; $p = .03$) (59). As such, the role of tamoxifen for DCIS in the absence of whole-breast radiotherapy remains to be defined.

Because DCIS is a precursor to invasive breast cancer and shares many biologic features of invasive carcinoma, it is increasingly recognized as a target for preventive measures. In the largest trials of the prevention of primary breast cancer among women at high risk for breast cancer by virtue of age, family history, or prior benign breast disease, tamoxifen reduced the risk of DCIS by 50% to 70% (27,40).

A Decision Tree for DCIS

The management of DCIS requires the coordinated, multidisciplinary interaction of radiologists, surgeons, pathologists, and oncologists. Patients are first assessed to determine if they are candidates for breast-conserving surgery. Women with multicentric DCIS, as defined by the presence of two or more tumors in separate quadrants of the breast, and those with extensive or diffuse DCIS or suspicious-appearing microcalcifications throughout the breast are candidates for mastectomy, as are women in whom negative margins or acceptable cosmesis cannot be achieved with the use of breast-conserving surgery. Some women may prefer mastectomy to breast conservation in order to minimize the chance of ipsilateral recurrence or for other reasons. At present, there is no established role for the use of magnetic resonance imaging in screening patients for DCIS in determining whether breast-conserving surgery is an option.

Patients deemed to be appropriate candidates for breast conservation require complete surgical excision of the affected area. The extent of DCIS in the breast and the existing margin determine the likelihood of identifying residual disease on re-excision. Nearly half of patients with margins that are <1 mm have residual DCIS on re-excision (82). However, the optimal margin width for the management of DCIS is not known. At a minimum, there should be no tumor at the margin.

	No. of		Local Recurrence (cumulative %)		
Table 52.4	**TAMOXIFEN VS. NO TAMOXIFEN: RANDOMIZED CLINICAL TRIALS FOR DUCTAL CARCINOMA *IN SITU* (DCIS)**				
Trial Group	Patients	Follow-Up	DCIS + Invasive Carcinoma		
			−Tam	+Tam	*p* value
NSABP B-24	1,798	7-yr actuarial	11.1	7.7	.02
UKCCCR	1,576	4.38-yr median	15.0	13.0	.42

Tam, tamoxifen; NSABP, National Surgical Adjuvant Bowel and Breast Project; UKCCCR, United Kingdom Coordinating Committee on Cancer Research.

Clinical Radiation Oncology

Table 52.5　MANAGEMENT SCHEME FOR DUCTAL CARCINOMA *IN SITU* (DCIS)

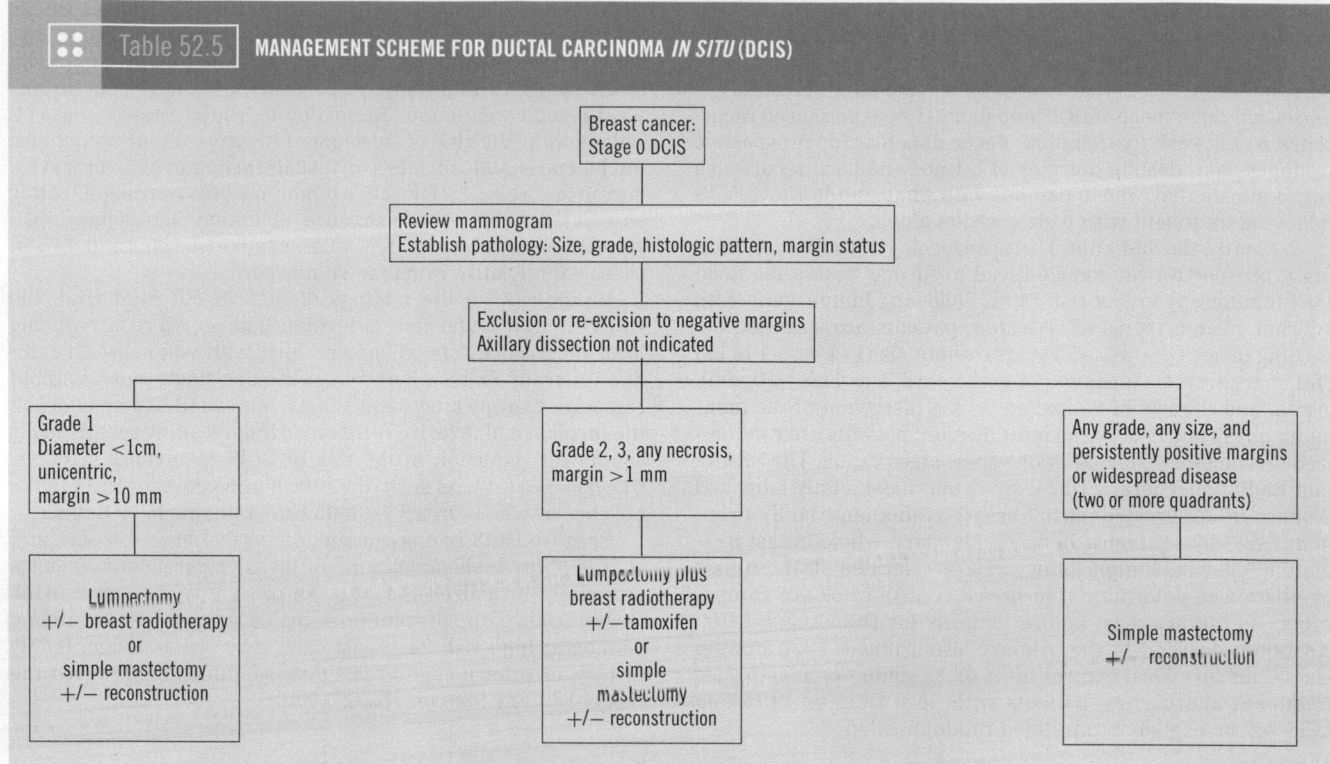

Neither dissection of axillary lymph nodes nor mapping of sentinel lymph nodes is routinely warranted in patients with DCIS because of the very low incidence of axillary metastases (110). Three to 13% of patients with DCIS, and a slightly greater percentage with DCIS and microinvasion, have isolated tumor cells in sentinel axillary lymph nodes (62). The prognostic significance of these cells is not clear. Clinical experience suggests that patients have a much better outcome than would be predicted by such rates of nodal metastases, and most instances represent micrometastases of unclear metastatic potential. However, sentinel lymph node mapping may be used in selected patients with a higher likelihood of occult invasive cancer—those with extensive, high-grade DCIS or palpable masses—and those undergoing mastectomy as sentinel node mapping cannot be performed afterward if invasive tumor is identified (79).

After breast-conserving surgery, radiotherapy is administered using tangential fields to the whole breast with a standard dose of 45 to 50 Gy delivered in daily fractions of 180 to 200 cGy. On the basis of extrapolation from data on the treatment of invasive breast cancer (11), a radiation boost to the tumor bed may be added to whole-breast treatment, particularly for women with close surgical margins, although the benefit of a boost in the management of DCIS is not established. There is no role for postmastectomy or nodal irradiation in the treatment of DCIS.

It is not yet possible to prospectively identify women who are at sufficiently low risk that radiotherapy may not be of some clinical advantage in preventing recurrences. After discussing the various options, patients may elect not to receive radiation treatment, but they must understand and accept the increased risk of recurrence that this choice probably entails.

In summary, despite considerable advances in our clinical knowledge base, the answer to the question "when should radiotherapy be used for DCIS?" remains complex and surrounded by considerable controversy. Two fundamental considerations must be emphasized:

1. A primary goal of breast-conserving therapy for DCIS is to achieve the best possible cosmetic outcome. Attempts to obtain wide surgical margins through deforming, large-volume breast excisions represent cosmetic failures and defeat the purpose of breast conservation.
2. Breast irradiation reduces the risk of subsequent invasive or noninvasive carcinoma in the treated breast and thus reduces the risk of the ultimate cosmetic failure: mastectomy

According to prospectively randomized trials of breast-conserving therapy for DCIS, radiotherapy reduces subsequent breast recurrence in all patient groups irrespective of prognostic risk factors. That is not to say, however, that radiotherapy must be used for all patients with DCIS. In all cases, a realistic and balanced discussion of the relative risks and benefits of treatment options should be presented to the patient. Reasonable estimates of breast recurrence during the ensuing decade with or without radiotherapy are available based on level I evidence from prospective clinical trials. A decision tree to assist in the selection of treatment options is presented in Table 52.5.

References

1. Abner AL, Connolly JL, Recht A, et al. The relationship between the presence and extent of lobular carcinoma *in situ* and the risk of local recurrence for patients with infiltrating carcinoma of the breast treated with conservative surgery and radiation therapy. *Cancer* 2000;88:1072–1077.
2. Acs G, Lawton TJ, Rebbeck TR, et al. Differential expression of e-cadherin in lobular and ductal neoplasms of the breast and its biologic and diagnostic implications. Anatomic Pathology. *Am J Clin Pathol* 2001;115:85–98.
3. Albonico G, Querzoli P, Ferretti S, et al. Biological profile of in situ breast cancer investigated by immunohistochemical technique. *Cancer Detect Prev* 1998;22:313–318.
4. Allred DC, Mohsin SK, Fuqua SAW. Histological and biological evolution of human premalignant breast disease. *Endocr Relat Cancer* 2001;8:47–61.
5. Allred DC, Wu Y, Tsimelzon A, et al. The progression of DCIS to IBC: A cDNA expression microarray study. *Breast Cancer Res Treat* 2002;76[Suppl1]:S81(abstr).
6. Alpers C, Wellings S. The prevalence of carcinoma *in situ* in normal and cancer associated breast. *Hum Pathol* 1985;16:796.
7. Andersen JA. Lobular carcinoma *in situ* of the breast—an approach to rational treatment. *Cancer* 1977;39:2597–2602.

8. Ashikari R, Park K, Huvos AG, et al. Paget's disease of the breast. *Cancer* 1970;26:680–685.
9. Aubele MM, Cummings MC, Mattis AE, et al. Accumulation of chromosomal imbalances from intraductal proliferative lesions to adjacent in situ and invasive ductal breast cancer. *Diagn Mol Pathol* 200;9:14–19.
10. Azzopardi JG. *Problems in breast pathology.* Philadelphia: WB Saunders; 1983.
11. Bartelink H, Horiot J-C, Poortmans P, et al. Recurrence rates after treatment of breast cancer with standard radiotherapy with or without additional radiation. *N Engl J Med* 2001;345:1378–1387.
12. Ben-David MA, Kleer CG, Paramagul C, et al. Is lobular carcinoma in situ as a component of breast carcinoma a risk factor for local failure after breast-conserving therapy?. *Cancer* 2006;106:28–34.
13. Betsill WL, Rosen PP, Lieberman PH, et al. Intraductal carcinoma: Long-term follow-up after treatment by biopsy alone. *JAMA* 1978;239:1863–1867.
14. Bijker N, Meijnen PH, Bogaerts J, et al. Radiotherapy in breast-conserving treatment for ductal carcinoma in situ (DCIS): Ten-year results of European organization for research and treatment of cancer (EORTC) randomized trial 10853. *J Clin Oncol* 2006;24:3381–3387.
15. Bijker N, Peterse JL, Duchateau L, et al. Risk factors for recurrence and metastasis after breast-conserving therapy for ductal carcinoma-in-situ: Analysis of European Organization for Research and Treatment of Cancer Trial 10853. *J Clin Oncol* 2001;19:2263–2271.
16. Bijker N, Rutgers EJT, Duchateau L, et al. Breast-conserving therapy for Paget disease of the nipple. *Cancer* 2001;91:472–477.
17. Buerger H, Otterbach F, Simon R, et al. Different genetic pathways in the evolution of invasive breast cancer are associated with distinct morphological subtypes. *J Pathol* 1999;189:521–526.
18. Bur ME, Zimarowski MJ, Schmitt SJ, et al. Estrogen receptor immunohistochemistry in carcinoma in situ of the breast. *Cancer* 1992;69:1174–1181.
19. Burstein HJ, Polyak K, Wong JS, et al. Ductal carcinoma in situ of the breast. *N Engl J Med* 2004;350:1430–1441.
20. Catzavelos C. Part III. The pathobiology of ductal carcinoma in situ. *Curr Probl Cancer* 2000;24:125–140.
21. Chaudary MA, Millis RR, Lane B, et al. Paget's disease of the nipple: A ten year review including clinical, pathological, and immunohistochemical findings. *Breast Cancer Res Treat* 1986;8:139–146.
22. Chuba PJ, Hamre MR, Yap J, et al. Bilateral risk for subsequent breast cancer after lobular carcinoma-in-situ: Analysis of surveillance, epidemiology, and end results data. *J Clin Oncol* 2005;23:5534–5541.
23. Claus EB, Petruzella S, Matloff E, et al. Prevalence of BRCA1 and BRCA2 mutations in women diagnosed with ductal carcinoma in situ. *JAMA* 2005;293:553–554.
24. Cohen MA. Cancer upgrades at excisional biopsy after diagnosis of atypical lobular hyperplasia or lobular carcinoma in situ core-needle biopsy: Some reasons why. *Radiology* 2004;231:617–621.
25. Collins LC, Tamimi RM, Baer HJ, et al. Outcome of patients with ductal carcinoma in situ untreated after diagnostic biopsy: Results from the Nurses' Health Study. *Cancer* 2005;103:1778–1784.
26. Consensus conference on the classification of ductal carcinoma in situ. *Cancer* 1997;80:1798–1802.
27. Cuzick J, Forbes J, Edwards R, et al. First results from the International Breast Cancer Intervention Study (IBIS-I): A randomised prevention trial. *Lancet* 2002;360:817–824.
28. Damiani S, Ludvikova M, Tomasic G, et al. Myoepithelial cells and basal lamina in poorly differentiated in situ duct carcinoma of the breast: An immunocytochemical study. *Virchows Arch* 1999;434:227–234.
29. de Mascarel I, Bonichon F, MacGrogan G, et al. Application of the Van Nuys prognostic index in a retrospective series of 367 ductal carcinomas in situ of the breast examined by serial macroscopic sectioning: Practical considerations. *Breast Cancer Res Treat* 2000;61:151–159.
30. Desai DC, Brennan EJ, Carp NZ. Paget's disease of the male breast. *Am Surg* 1996;62:1068–1072.
31. Dinkel H-P, Gassel AM, Tschammler A. Is the appearance of microcalcifications on mammography useful in predicting histological grade of malignancy in ductal cancer in situ?. *Br J Radiol* 2000;73:938–944.
32. Dixon AR, Galea RR. Pathogenesis and treatment of Paget's disease of the breast. *Cancer* 1981;48:835–829.
33. Ernster VL, Ballard-Barbash R, Barlow WE, et al. Detection of ductal carcinoma in situ in women undergoing screening mammography. *J Natl Cancer Inst* 2002;94:1546–1554.
34. Ernster VL, Barclay J, Kerlikowske K, et al. Incidence of and treatment for ductal carcinoma in situ of the breast. *JAMA* 1996;275:913–918.
35. Ernster VL, Barclay J, Kerlikowske K, et al. Mortality among women with ductal carcinoma in situ of the breast in the population-based Surveillance, Epidemiology, and End Results program. *Arch Intern Med* 2000;160:953–958.
36. Farabegoli F, Champeme MH, Bieche I, et al. Genetic pathways in the evolution of breast ductal carcinoma in situ. *J Pathol* 2002;196:280–286.
37. Faverly DRG, Burgers L, Bult P, et al. Three dimensional imaging of mammary ductal carcinoma in situ; clinical implications. *Semin Diagn Pathol* 1994;11:193–198.
38. Fechner RE. Epithelial alterations in the extralobular ducts of breasts with lobular carcinoma. *Arch Pathol* 1972;93:164–171.
39. Fischer B, Anderson S, Bryant J, et al. Twenty-year follow-up of a randomized trial comparing total mastectomy, lumpectomy, and lumpectomy plus irradiation for the treatment of invasive breast cancer. *N Engl J Med* 2002;347:1233–1241.
40. Fisher B, Costantino J, Wickerham DL, et al. Tamoxifen for prevention of breast cancer: Report of the national surgical adjuvant breast and bowel project P-1 study. *J Natl Cancer Inst* 1998;90:1371–1388.
41. Fisher B, Dignam J, Wolmark N, et al. Lumpectomy and radiation therapy for the treatment of intraductal breast cancer: Findings from National Surgical Adjuvant Breast and Bowel Project B-17. *J Clin Oncol* 1998;16:441–452.
42. Fisher B, Dignam J, Wolmark N, et al. Tamoxifen in treatment of intraductal breast cancer: National Surgical Adjuvant Breast and Bowel Project B-24 randomised controlled trial. *Lancet* 1999;353:1993–2000.
43. Fisher B, Land S, Mamounas E, et al. Prevention of invasive breast cancer in women with ductal carcinoma in situ: An update of the National Surgical Adjuvant Breast and Bowel Project Experience. *Semin Oncol* 2001;28:400–418.
44. Fisher ER, Land SR, Fisher B, et al. Pathologic findings from the National Surgical Adjuvant Breast and Bowel Project—twelve-year observations concerning lobular carcinoma in situ. *Cancer* 2004;100:238–244.
45. Fisher ER, Leeming R, Anderson S, et al. Conservative management of intraductal carcinoma (DCIS) of the breast. *J Surg Oncol* 1991;47:139–47.
46. Foote FW, Stewart FW. Lobular carcinoma in situ—a rare form of mammary cancer. *Am J Pathol* 1941;17:491–495.
47. Foster MC, Helvie MA, Gregory NE, et al. Lobular carcinoma in situ or atypical lobular hyperplasia at core-needle biopsy: Is excisional biopsy necessary? *Radiology* 2004;231:813–819.
48. Fourquet A, Campana F, Vielh P, et al. Paget's disease of the nipple without detectable breast tumor: Conservative management with radiation therapy. *Int J Radiat Oncol Biol Phys* 1987;13:1463–1465.
49. Frykberg ER, Bland KI. In situ breast carcinoma. *Adv Surg* 1993;26:29–72.
50. Georgian-Smith D, Lawton TJ. Calcifications of lobular carcinoma in situ of the breast: Radiologic-pathologic correlation. *Am J Roentgenol* 2001;176:1255–1259.
51. Going JJ, Moffat DF. Escaping from Flatland: Clinical and biological aspects of human mammary duct anatomy in three dimensions. *J Pathol* 2004;203:538–544.
52. Guidi AJ, Fischer L, Harris JR, et al. Microvessel density and distribution of ductal carcinoma in situ of the breast. *J Natl Cancer Inst* 1994;86:614–619.
53. Guidi AJ, Schnitt SJ, Fischer L, et al. Vascular permeability factor (vascular endothelial growth factor) expression and angiogenesis in patients with ductal carcinoma in situ of the breast. *Cancer* 1997;80:1945–1953.
54. Gupta SK, Douglas-Jones AG, Fenn N, et al. The clinical behavior of breast carcinoma is probably determined at the preinvasive stage (ductal carcinoma in situ). *Cancer* 1997;80:1740–1745.
55. Haagensen CD, Bodian C, Haagensen DE. *Lobular neoplasia (lobular carcinoma in situ). Breast carcinoma: Risk and detection.* Philadelphia: WB Saunders; 1981:238–292.
56. Habel LA, Moe RE, Daling JR, et al. Risk of contralateral breast cancer among women with carcinoma in situ of the breast. *Ann Surg* 1997;225:69–75.
57. Hayes R, Cummings B, Miller RAW, et al. Male Paget's disease of the breast. *J Cutan Med Surg* 2000;4:208–212.
58. Holland R, Hendriks J, Verbeek A, et al. Extent, distribution and mammographic/histological correlations of breast ductal carcinoma in situ. *Lancet* 1990;335:519–522.
59. Houghton J, George WD, Cuzick J, et al. Radiotherapy and tamoxifen in women with completely excised ductal carcinoma in situ of the breast in the UK, Australia, and New Zealand: Randomized controlled trial. *Lancet* 2003;362:95–102.
60. Hwang ES, Nyante SJ, Chen YY, et al. Clonality of lobular carcinoma in situ and synchronous invasive lobular carcinoma. *Cancer* 2004;100:2562–2572.
61. Ikeda DM, Helvie MA, Frank TS, et al. Paget disease of the nipple: Radiologic-pathologic correlation. *Radiology* 1993;189:89–94.
62. Intra M, Veronesi P, Mazzarol G, et al. Axillary sentinel lymph node biopsy in patients with pure ductal carcinoma in situ of the breast. *Arch Surg* 2003;138:309–313.
63. Inwang ER, Fentiman IS. Paget's disease of the nipple. *Br J Hosp Med* 1990;44:392–395.
64. Jacobs TW, Pliss N, Kouria G. Carcinomas in situ of the breast with indeterminate features. *Am J Surg Pathol* 2001;25:229–236.
65. Jamali FR, Ricci A, Deckers PJ. Paget's disease of the nipple-areola complex. *Surg Clin North Am* 1996;76:365–381.
66. Jemal A, Tiwari RC, Murray T, et al. Cancer statistics, 2004. *CA Cancer J Clin* 2004;54:8 29.
67. Julien JP, Bijker N, Fentiman IS, et al. Radiotherapy in breast-conserving treatment for ductal carcinoma in situ: First results of the EORTC randomised phase III trial 10853. EORTC Breast Cancer Cooperative Group and EORTC Radiotherapy Group. *Lancet* 2000;355:528–533.
68. Kohler S, Rouse RV, Smoller BR. The differential diagnosis of pagetoid cells in the epidermis. *Mod Pathol* 1998;11:79–92.
69. Lagios MD, Margolin FR, Westdahl PR, et al. Mammographically detected duct carcinoma in situ: Frequency of local recurrence following tylectomy and prognostic effect of nuclear grade on local recurrence. *Cancer* 1989;63:618–624.
70. Lagios MD, Westdahl PR, Marye RR, et al. Paget's disease of the nipple. *Cancer* 1984;54:545–551.
71. Lagios MD. Ductal carcinoma in situ: Controversies in diagnosis, biology, and treatment. *Breast J* 1995;1:68–78.
72. Lampejo OT, Barnes DM, Smith P, et al. Evaluation of infiltrating ductal carcinomas with a DCIS component: Correlation of the histologic type of the in situ component with grade of the infiltrating component. *Semin Diagn Pathol* 1994;11:215–222.
73. Lenhard RE Cancer statistics, a measure of progress. *CA Cancer J Clin* 1996;46:3–7.
74. Liberman L, Sama M, Susnik B, et al. Lobular carcinoma in situ at percutaneous breast biopsy: Surgical biopsy findings. *Am J Roentgenol* 1999;173:219–299.
75. Liberman L, Van Zee KJ, Dershaw DD, et al. Mammographic features of local recurrence in women who have undergone breast-conserving therapy for ductal carcinoma in situ. *Am J Roentgenol* 1997;168:489–493.
76. Lloyd J, Flanagan AM. Mammary and extramammary Paget's disease. *J Clin Pathol* 2000;53:742–749.
77. Markpoulos CH, Gogas H, Sampalis F, et al. Bilateral Paget's disease of the breast. *Eur J Gynaecol Oncol* 1997;18:495–496.
78. Marshall JK, Griffith KA, Haffty BG, et al. Conservative management of Paget disease of the breast with radiotherapy. *Cancer* 2003;97:2142–2149.
79. McMasters KM, Chao C, Wong SL, et al. Sentinel lymph node biopsy in patients with ductal carcinoma in situ: A proposal. *Cancer* 2002;95:15–20.
80. Millis RR, Thynne GSJ. In situ intraduct carcinoma of the breast: A long-term follow-up study. *Br J Surg* 1975;62:957–962.
81. Moran M, Haffty B. Lobular carcinoma in situ as a component of breast cancer: The long-term outcome in patients treated with breast-conservation therapy. *Int J Radiat Oncol Biol Phys* 1998;40:353–358.
82. Neuschatz AC, DiPetrillo T, Steinhoff M, et al. The value of breast lumpectomy margin assessment as a predictor of residual tumor burden in ductal carcinoma in situ of the breast. *Cancer* 2002;94:1917–1924.
83. O'Connell P, Pekkel V, Fuqua SA, et al. Analysis of loss of heterozygosity in 399 premalignant breast lesions at 15 genetic loci. *J Natl Cancer Inst* 1998;90:697–703.

84. Ohtake T, Abe R, Kimijima I, et al. Intraductal extension of primary invasive breast carcinoma treated by breast—conservation surgery. *Cancer* 1995;76:32–45.

85. Ohtake T, Kimijima I, Fukushima T, et al. Computer-assisted complete three-dimensional reconstruction of the mammary ductal/lobular systems. *Cancer* 2001;91:2263–2272.

86. Ottesen GL, Graversen HP, Blichert-Toft M, et al. Carcinoma in situ of the female breast. 10 year follow-up results of a prospective nationwide study. *Breast Cancer Res Treat* 2000;62:197–210.

87. Ottesen GL, Graversen HP, Blichert-Toft M, et al. Ductal carcinoma in situ of the female breast: Short-term results of a prospective nationwide study—The Danish Breast Cancer Cooperative Group. *Am J Surg Pathol* 1992;16:1183–1196.

88. Page DL, Anderson TJ. *Diagnostic histopathology of the breast.* Edinburgh: Churchill Livingstone; 1987.

89. Page DL, Kidd TE, Dupont WD, et al. Lobular neoplasia of the breast: Higher risk for subsequent invasive cancer predicted by more extensive disease. *Hum Pathol* 1991;22:1232–1239.

90. Paget J. On the disease of the mammary areola preceding cancer of the mammary gland. *St Bartholomew Hosp Rep* 1874;10:87–89.

91. Paone JF, Baker RR. Pathogenesis and treatment of Paget's disease of the breast. *Cancer* 1981;48:825–829.

92. Patchefsky AS, Schwartz GF, Finkelstein SD, et al. Heterogeneity of intraductal carcinoma of the breast. *Cancer* 1989;63:731–741.

93. Pierce LJ, Haffty BG, Solin LJ, et al. The conservative management of Paget's disease of the breast with radiotherapy. *Cancer* 1997;80:1065–1072.

94. Polgar C, Orosz Z, Kovacs T, et al. Breast-conserving therapy for Paget disease of the nipple. *Cancer* 2002;94:904–1905.

95. Radford DM, Phillips NHJ, Fair KL, et al. Allelic loss and the progression of breast cancer. *Cancer Res* 1995;55:5180–5183.

96. Recht A, Rutgers EJ, Fentiman IS, et al. The fourth EORTC DCIS consensus meeting (Chateau Marguette, Heemskerk, The Netherlands 23-24 January 1998)—conference report. *Eur J Cancer* 1998;34:1664–1669.

97. Recht A, van Dongen JA, Fentimen IS, et al. Third meeting of the DCIS Working Party of the EORTC (Fondazione Cini, Isola s. Giorgio, Venezia, 28 February 1994)—conference report. *Eur J Cancer* 1994;30A:1895–1901.

98. Rosen PP, Kosloff C, Lieberman PH, et al. Lobular carcinoma in situ of the breast. Detailed analysis of 99 patients with average follow-up of 24 years. *Am J Surg Pathol* 1978;2:225–251.

99. Rosen PP. *Rosen's breast pathology*, 1st ed. Philadelphia: Lippincott Raven; 1997:237–245.

100. Sakorafas GH, Blanchard K, Sarr MG, et al. Paget's disease of the breast. *Cancer Treat Rev* 2001;27:9–18.

101. Sanders ME, Schuyler PA, Dupont WD, et al. The natural history of low-grade ductal carcinoma in situ of the breast in women treated by biopsy only revealed over 30 years of long-term follow-up. *Cancer* 2005;103:2481–2484.

102. Sapino A, Frigerio A, Peterse JL, et al. Mammographically detected in situ lobular carcinomas of the breast. *Virchows Arch* 2000;436:421–430.

103. Sasson AR, Fowble B, Hanlon AL, et al. Lobular carcinoma in situ increases the risk of local recurrence in selected patients with stages I and II breast carcinoma treated with conservative surgery and radiation. *Cancer* 2001;91:1862–1869.

104. Satake H, Shimamoto K, Sawaki A, et al. Role of ultrasonography in the detection of intraductal spread of breast cancer: Correlation with pathologic findings, mammography and MR imaging. *Eur Radiol* 2000;10:1726–1732.

105. Schnitt SJ, Morrow M. Lobular carcinoma in situ: Current concepts and controversies. *Semin Diagn Pathol* 1999;16:209–223.

106. Schwartz GF, Solin LJ, Olivotto IA, et al. Consensus conference on the treatment of in situ ductal carcinoma of the breast, April 22–25, 1999. *Cancer* 2000;88:946–954.

107. Silver SA, Tavassoli FA. Mammary ductal carcinoma in situ with microinvasion. *Cancer* 1998;83:2300–2300.

108. Silverstein MJ, Lagios MD, Craig PH, et al. A prognostic index for ductal carcinoma in situ of the breast. *Cancer* 1996;77:2267–2274.

109. Silverstein MJ, Lagios MD, Groshen S, et al. The influence of margin width on local control of ductal carcinoma in situ of the breast. *N Engl J Med* 1999;340:1455–1461.

110. Silverstein MJ, Rosser RJ, Gierson ED, et al. Axillary lymph node dissection for intraductal breast carcinoma—is it indicated?. *Cancer* 1987;59:1819–1824.

111. Silverstein MJ, Van Nuys experience by treatment. In: Silverstein MJ, Lagios MD, Poller DN, et al., eds. *Ductal carcinoma in situ of the breast.* Philadelphia: Williams & Wilkins; 1997:443–447.

112. Silverstein MJ. Current management of noninvasive (in situ) breast cancer. *Adv Surg* 2000;34:17–41.

113. Simon MS, Lemanne D, Schwartz AG, et al. Recent trends in the incidence of in situ and invasive breast cancer in the Detroit Metropolitan area (1975–1988). *Cancer* 1993;71:769–774.

114. Simon MS, Schwartz AG, Martino S, et al. Trends in the diagnosis of in situ breast cancer in the Detroit Metropolitan area, 1973 to 1987. *Cancer* 1992;69:466–469.

115. Singletary SE, Allred C, Ashley P, et al. Revision of the American Joint Committee on Cancer staging system for breast cancer. *J Clin Oncol* 2002;20:3628–3636.

116. Sneige N, McNeese MD, Atkinson EN, et al. Ductal carcinoma in situ treated with lumpectomy and irradiation: Histopathological analysis of 49 specimens with emphasis on risk factors and long term results. *Hum Pathol* 1995;26:642–649.

117. Solin LJ, Fourquet A, Vicini FA, et al. Long-term outcome after breast-conservation treatment with radiation for mammographically detected ductal carcinoma in situ of the breast. *Cancer* 2005;103:1137–1146.

118. Solin LJ, Fourquet A, Vicini FA, et al. Salvage treatment for local recurrence after breast-conserving surgery and radiation as initial treatment for mammographically detected ductal carcinoma in situ of the breast. *Cancer* 2001;91:1090–1097.

119. Solin LJ, Yeh IT, Kurtz J, et al. Ductal carcinoma in situ (intraductal carcinoma) of the breast treated with breast-conserving surgery and definitive irradiation: Correlation of pathologic parameters with outcome of treatment. *Cancer* 1993;71:2532–2542.

120. Sonnenfeld MR, Frenna TH, Weidner N, et al. Lobular carcinoma in situ: Mammographic-pathologic correlation of results of needle-directed biopsy. *Radiology* 1991;181:363–367.

121. Stockdale AD, Brierly JD, White WF, et al. Radiotherapy for paget's disease of the nipple: A conservative alternative. *Lancet* 1989;2:664–666.

122. Stratton MR, Collins N, Lakhani SR, et al. Loss of heterozygosity in ductal carcinoma in situ of the breast. *J Pathol* 1995;175:195–201.

123. Tabar L, Gad A, Parsons WC, et al. Mammographic appearances of in situ carcinomas. In: Silverstein MJ, ed. *Ductal carcinoma in situ of the breast.* Baltimore: Williams & Wilkins; 1997:413–420.

124. Tavassoli FA. Lobular neoplasia. In: Tavassoli FA. *Pathology of the breast*, 2nd ed. New York: Elsevier; 1999:373–400.

125. Trentham-Dietz A, Newcomb PA, Storer BE, et al. Risk factors for carcinoma in situ of the breast. *Cancer Epidemiol Biomarkers Prev* 2000;9:697–703.

126. Veronesi U, Cascinelli N, Mariani L, et al. Twenty-year follow-up of randomized study comparing breast-conserving surgery with radical (Halstead) mastectomy for early breast cancer. *N Engl J Med* 2002;347:1227–1232.

127. Vicini FA, Recht A. Age at diagnosis and outcome for women with ductal carcinoma-in-situ of the breast: A critical review of the literature. *J Clin Oncol* 2002;20:2736–44.

128. Vogel VG, Costantino JP, Wickerham DL, et al. National Surgical Adjuvant Breast and Bowel Project Update: Prevention trials and endocrine therapy of ductal carcinoma in situ. *Clin CA Res* 2003;9:495s–501s.

129. Vos CB, Cleton-Jansen AM, Verx G, et al. E-cadherin inactivation in lobular carcinoma in situ of the breast: An early event in tumorigenesis. *Br J Cancer* 1997;76:1131–1133.

130. Ward KA, Burton JL, et al. Dermatological diseases of the breast in young women. *Clin Dermatol* 1997;15:45–52.

131. Warnberg F, Nordgren H, Bergkvist L, et al. Tumour markers in breast carcinoma correlate with grade rather than with invasiveness. *Br J Cancer* 2001;85:869–74.

132. Welch HG, Black WC. Using autopsy series to estimate the disease "reservoir" for ductal carcinoma in situ of the breast. How much more breast cancer can we find? *Ann Intern Med* 1997;127:1023–1028.

133. Wheeler JE, Enterline HT, Roseman JM, et al. Lobular carcinoma in situ of the breast—long term follow-up. *Cancer* 1974;34:554–563.

134. Wong JS, Kaelin CM, Troyan SL, et al. Prospective study of wide excision alone for ductal carcinoma in situ of the breast. *J Clin Oncol* 2006;24:1031–1036.

135. Wright B, Shumak R. Part II. Medical imaging of ductal carcinoma in situ. *Curr Probl Cancer* 2000;24:112–124.

136. Yim JH, Wick MR, Philpott GW, et al. Underlying pathology in mammary Paget's disease. *Ann Surg Oncol* 1997;4:287–292.

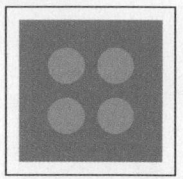

Chapter 53
Early Stage Breast Cancer

Bruce G. Haffty, Thomas A. Buchholz, Carlos A. Perez

Radiation therapy plays an essential and critical role in the management of breast cancer. In a general radiation oncology practice, breast cancer typically comprises approximately 25% of the total patient caseload. This chapter will provide an overview of general concepts in breast cancer and will then focus on management of early stage invasive disease. The conservative management of early stage disease by lumpectomy with or without radiation is a major focus of this chapter. Postmastectomy radiation, as well as advanced invasive disease and local–regional recurrence, will be covered in the advanced disease chapter that follows. Management of ductal carcinoma *in situ* and lobular carcinoma *in situ* are the focus of the previous chapter.

Anatomy

The female breast lies on the anterior chest wall superficial to the pectoralis major muscle (330). The breast can extend from the midline to near the midaxillary line and cranial-caudally from the second anterior rib to the sixth anterior rib. The upper-outer quadrant of the breast extends into the region of the low axilla and is frequently referred to as the axillary tail of Spence. This anatomical feature leads the upper-outer quadrant of the breast to contain a greater percentage of total breast tissue compared to the other quadrants, and, therefore, a greater percentage of breast cancers occur in this anatomical location.

The breast is made up of the mammary gland, fat, blood vessels, nerves, and lymphatics (330) (Fig. 53.1). The surface of the breast has deep attachments of fibrous septa, called *Cooper's ligament*, which run between the superficial fascia (attached to the skin) and the deep fascia (covering the pectoralis major and other muscles of the chest wall). Skin dimpling may be caused by tumors affecting these supporting structures. It is important to realize from a staging perspective that the chest wall includes the ribs, intercostal muscles, and serratus anterior muscle, but not the pectoral muscles.

The breast parenchyma is composed of lobules and ducts. The function of the lobules is to produce milk, and the function of the ducts is to transport lactation products to the nipple. The peripheral ducts converge into major lactiferous ducts, which then communicate with the nipple-areola complex. Most breast cancers develop at the interface between the ductal system and the lobules, a region called the terminal ductal lobular unit.

The breast parenchyma is intermixed with connective tissue, which has a rich vascular and lymphatic network. Mammary gland lymphatics begin in the interlobular or prelobular spaces, follow the ducts, and end in the subareolar network of lymphatics of the skin. The predominant lymphatic drainage of the breast is to axillary lymph nodes, which is commonly described in three levels, based on the relationship of the lymph node regions to the pectoralis minor muscle (Fig. 53.2). The level I axilla is caudal and lateral to the muscle, level II is beneath the muscle, and level III (also known as the infraclavicular region) is cranial and medial to the muscle. A standard axillary lymph node dissection resects the tissue and lymph nodes within levels I and II. It is very unusual to have involvement of level III of the axilla without disease in level I or II. The axillary

lymph nodes continue underneath the clavicle to become the supraclavicular lymph nodes, which can be involved in locally advanced breast cancers.

Lymphatics can also drain directly into the internal mammary lymph node chain (IMC), which are intrathoracic structures located in the parasternal space. Although these nodes are not usually visualized on computed tomography (CT), the anatomical region of the IMC can be determined by the internal mammary artery and vein, which are easily visualized by CT (Fig. 53.3), and usually lie 3 to 4 cm lateral to midline. When breast cancer involves the IMC, the majority of cases will have disease that is limited to lymph nodes in the first three interspaces. Regardless of the location within the breast, the axilla is the most common site of lymphatic involvement. However, breast cancers that develop in the medial, central, or lower breast more commonly drain to the IMC (in addition to the axilla) than those occurring in the lateral and upper quadrants.

The use of lymphoscintigraphy, by injecting technetium-99 radiocolloid into the peritumoral region, followed by scintillation scanning, is used now for sentinel lymph node imaging. This technique has helped to delineate primary lymphatic drainage patterns of breast cancer. In a study reported by Estourgie et al. (190) of 700 patients undergoing sentinel node mapping, the distribution of axillary and internal mammary drainage is summarized in Fig. 53.4. Even in inner-quadrant lesions, axillary drainage is more common than internal mammary drainage. However, internal mammary drainage was present in over 50% of lower inner-quadrant lesions.

Epidemiology

Breast cancer is the most frequently diagnosed cancer in women, and it is estimated that there will be 212,920 new cases of invasive breast cancer and 61,980 new cases of *in situ* breast cancers among women in the United States in 2006 (16,379). Primarily due to increased utilization of screening mammography, breast cancer incidence rates increased rapidly in the 1980s. It is estimated that 41,430 breast cancer deaths will occur in 2006, with breast cancer ranking second among cancer deaths in women (after lung cancer). In contrast to the significant number of breast cancer cases in women, it is expected that 1,720 cases of breast cancer will be diagnosed in men in 2006, with approximately 460 breast cancer deaths in men. Due to a combination of early detection, increased awareness, and improvements in therapy, death rates from breast cancer actually declined by approximately 2.3% per year from 1990 to 2002 (379). The decrease in breast cancer mortality is demonstrated in Fig. 53.5.

There is considerable geographic, ethnic, and racial variability in breast cancer incidence. Ethnicity and national origin rank highly as predictors of risk for breast cancer with up to a 10-fold variation throughout the world (461). Compared to other well-established risk factors such as age of menarche and menopause, age at first childbirth, and family history, geographic and ethnic variability is quite significant. It is likely that a complex interaction of multiple factors, including genetic,

1175

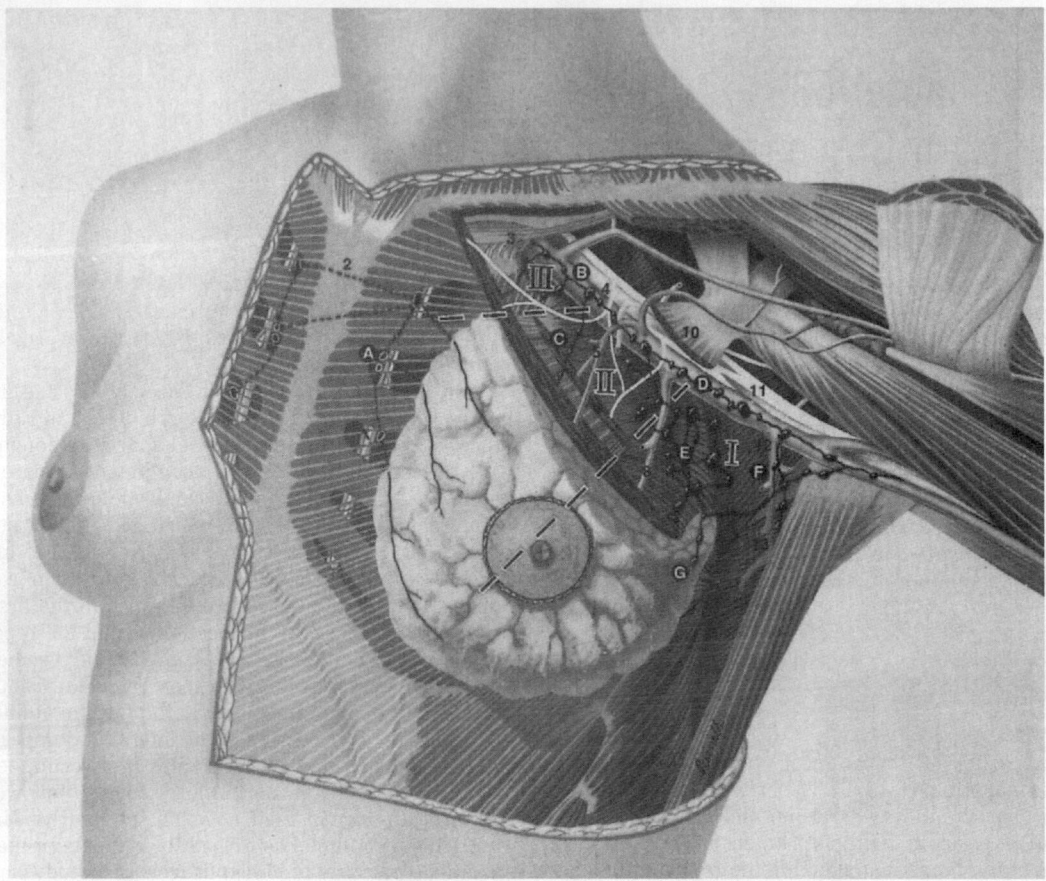

FIGURE 53.1. Anatomy of the breast and lymphatic drainage. (From Osborne MP. Breast development and anatomy. In: Harris JR, Hellman S, Henderson IC, et al., eds. *Breast diseases.* Philadelphia: J.B. Lippincott, 1987;1–14, with permission.)

environmental, and socioeconomic, contribute to the wide variability in age-adjusted incidence across populations.

The potential contribution of environmental factors and lifestyle is clearly demonstrated in the increasing incidence of breast cancers among Japanese American women and in trends of increasing incidence of breast cancer in Japan with recent changes in lifestyle. It is well recognized that the relatively low incidence of breast cancer in Asian immigrants to the United States has gradually increased as these immigrants have adapted to Western lifestyles (150). Rates of breast cancer over time in Japanese women in Los Angeles are now approaching the incidence in Caucasian women. In Japan, incidence rates have more than doubled from 1960 to 1990. This is likely a result of adaptation of Western lifestyles including fewer children, later marriage, increasing rates of obesity, and possibly dietary influences (112).

In the United States, the incidence of breast cancer in white women is higher than all other populations. Recent data from the National Cancer Institute's Surveillance, Epidemiology, and End Results (SEER) program report incidence rates of 141 cases per 100,000 white women, compared to 122 in African American, 97 in Asian Pacific Islander, 90 in Hispanics, and 58 in American/Alaskan Natives (379).

Although incidence is lower in African American women, the age of onset is younger and African American women are more likely to be diagnosed at a more advanced stage. Several studies have reported an earlier onset of breast cancer in African American compared to white women by approximately 10 years. Furthermore, several studies have reported, after correcting for stage, that African American women have more aggressive biology and a poorer overall prognosis (62,385).

Risk Factors

Table 53.1 summarizes the major risk factors associated with development of breast cancer. With the exception of female gender, increasing age is the most consistent and significant risk factor, with most populations demonstrating increasing incidence rates with age. Other risk factors include personal history and family history of breast cancer, nulliparity or late age at first childbirth, early menarche and late menopause, prior breast biopsy with hyperplasia or atypical hyperplasia, high breast tissue density, radiation exposure at a young age, alcohol consumption, and use of postmenopausal hormone therapy. Some of the national origin/ethnicity variability discussed above may be explained in part by differences in established risk factors, such as age of menarche, parity, and age at first childbirth. However, these factors explain only in part the variability observed in national origin, indicating that underlying genetic, environmental, and dietary factors are likely to contribute to the differences in the worldwide incidence of breast cancer (127). Breastfeeding, physical activity, and maintaining a healthy body weight have been demonstrated in various studies to be associated with a lower risk of breast cancer (127).

Age

The risk of breast cancer increases exponentially up to the age of menopause, at which time the rate of increase in the risk slows significantly. After the age of 80, the incidence of breast cancer begins to show a slight decline. For women in their late 30s, the annual increase in risk of developing breast cancer

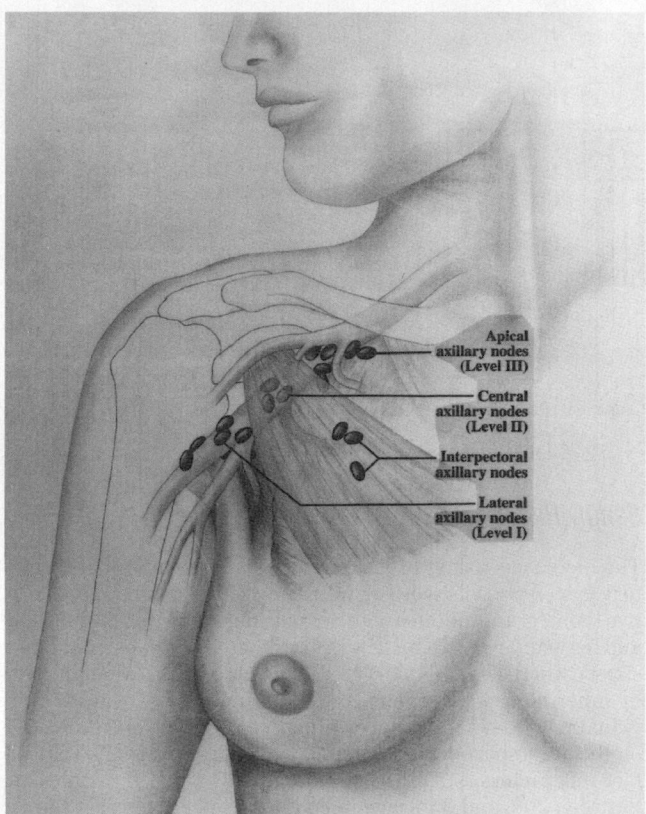

FIGURE 53.2. Location of the three levels of axillary lymph nodes. (Redrawn from Morrow M. Axillary node dissection: what role in managing BCa? *Contemp Oncol* 1994;8(4):16–27, copyright Medical Economics. Adapted from an illustration by John Daughterty, copyright 1994, with permission.)

is approximately 0.07% per year. This increases to 0.44% per year for women in their late 70s. Although these percentages may seem low, they represent only the risk for a given year; the lifetime risk is a summation of the annual breast cancer risks. Because younger women have a longer life expectancy than older women, younger women have a greater lifetime risk.

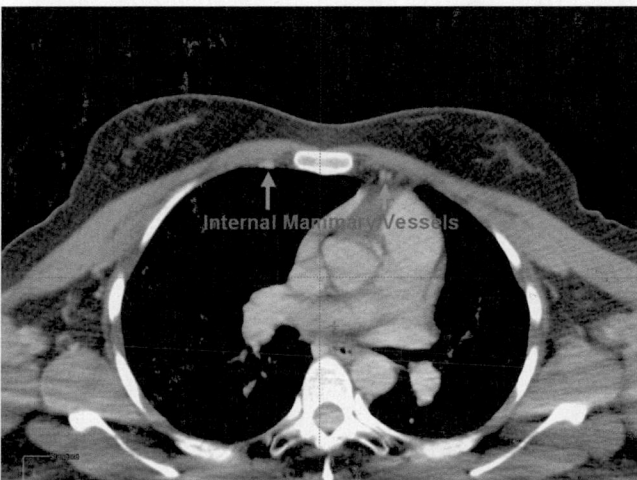

FIGURE 53.3. Treatment planning computed tomography scan of the chest demonstrating the location of the internal mammary vessels, which are typically located approximately 3 to 4 cm lateral to midline and approximately 3 cm deep to the surface. The internal mammary nodes are in close proximity to the vessels, with the most critical nodes being located in the first three intercostal spaces.

Only 0.43% of women develop breast cancer before the age of 40, whereas 4% of women develop breast cancer between the ages of 40 and 59 and 6.88% of women develop breast cancer between the ages of 60 and 79 (379).

Child Bearing/Parity/Breastfeeding

The protective effect of child bearing at younger ages on breast cancer risk is well established. In a worldwide case control study, MacMahon et al. (460,461) demonstrated a nearly linear relationship between relative risk of breast cancer and age at first birth, with women age 20 to 25 having nearly a 50% reduction in the relative risk of breast cancer compared to nulliparous women. Interestingly, for women whose first childbirth was over age 35, the risk appears greater than nulliparous women. Data on the effect of breastfeeding are not as strong as the data on age at first childbirth, but do suggest a protective effect. The Oxford Collaborative Group conducted an analysis of 47 studies evaluating breastfeeding and breast cancer risk and reported a decrease in relative risk of breast cancer by 4.3% for each 12 months of breastfeeding (69).

Ovarian Function

The relationship between ovarian function and breast cancer risk has long been recognized, with long menstrual history (early menarche and late menopause) contributing significantly to breast cancer risk. In experimental models and observational studies, removal of the ovaries reduces the risk of breast cancer (461). Women with surgically induced menopause have been shown to have significantly reduced risks of breast cancer compared to women whose menopause occurred naturally. In comparison with women whose menopause occurs between the ages of 45 and 54 (relative risk 1), women with early menopause before age 45 have a relative risk of breast cancer of 0.73 and women with late menopause at age >55 have a relative risk of 1.48. The data on early onset of menses and its association with breast cancer risk are also well established (461).

Exogenous Hormone

The risk of breast cancer associated with hormonal therapy has been controversial. A collaborative meta-analysis from 51 epidemiological studies of over 150,000 women did show an increased relative risk of 1.35 for current or recent users of hormonal replacement therapy (79). The authors reported that postmenopausal hormone replacement therapy increased the annual relative risk of developing breast cancer by 2.3% for each year of hormonal therapy. A recent randomized trial of postmenopausal hormone therapy from the Women's Health Initiative Study comparing estrogen and progestin with placebo was closed prematurely, demonstrating a 24% increase in breast cancer, coronary heart disease, stroke, and pulmonary emboli. This study of 46,000 women reported that the combined use of estrogen and progesterone increased the relative risk of breast cancer 8% compared with the risk in nonusers, whereas the use of estrogen alone increased the relative risk only 1% (636). Other studies have also demonstrated increased risks of breast cancer with long-term use of hormonal replacement therapy (657). However, short-term use of hormonal replacement, particularly in women with severe menopausal symptoms, has not been consistently associated with breast cancer risk. Although it is clear that there is an elevated risk of breast cancer with prolonged use of the combination of estrogen and progestin therapy, further studies are needed to assess the risks and benefits of different types of hormone replacement therapy for women who suffer severe menopausal symptoms. For women who have undergone hysterectomy, it seems that hormone replacement therapy with estrogen alone rather than estrogen and progesterone has

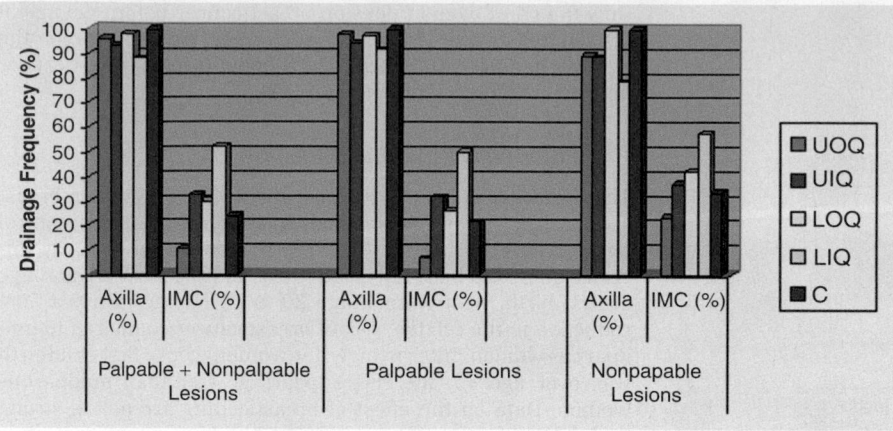

FIGURE 53.4. Distribution of lymphatic drainage of the breast to axillary and internal mammary chains according to the location within the breast. C, central; IMC, internal mammary chain; LIQ, lower inner quadrant; LOQ, lower outer quadrant; UIQ, upper inner quadrant; UOQ, upper outer quadrant; (Data extracted from study of 700 patients undergoing sentinel lymph node mapping by Estourgie SH, Nieweg OE, Olmos RA, et al. Lymphatic drainage patterns from the breast. *Ann Surg* 2004;239(2):232–237.)

a minimal effect on breast cancer risk. For women who have not undergone hysterectomy and who elect to be treated with hormone replacement therapy, combined estrogen and progesterone remains the standard for hormone replacement therapy to avoid the risk of endometrial cancer that is associated with unopposed estrogen replacement (657).

The use of oral contraceptives has not been consistently shown to increase the risk of breast cancer. There is some evidence that use of oral contraceptives for more than 4 years prior to first pregnancy increases the risk of breast cancer. Other studies, however, have not demonstrated increased risks of breast cancer, even with long-term exposures of >15 years (283,769).

Family History

The increased risk of breast cancer as a function of family history is well established. For women with a second-degree relative (aunt, grandmother) with breast cancer, the risk is about 1.5 and for women with a history in first-degree relatives (mother or sister), the risk is 1.7 to 2.5 (89). This may be explained in part by inheritance of a genetic condition that predisposes an individual to breast cancer development (e.g., mutations in BRCA1 or BRCA2); shared lifestyle; and inheritance of genes that affect risk factors, such as body habitus and age at menarche. Between 20% and 25% of women diagnosed with breast cancer have a positive family history of the disease, and approximately

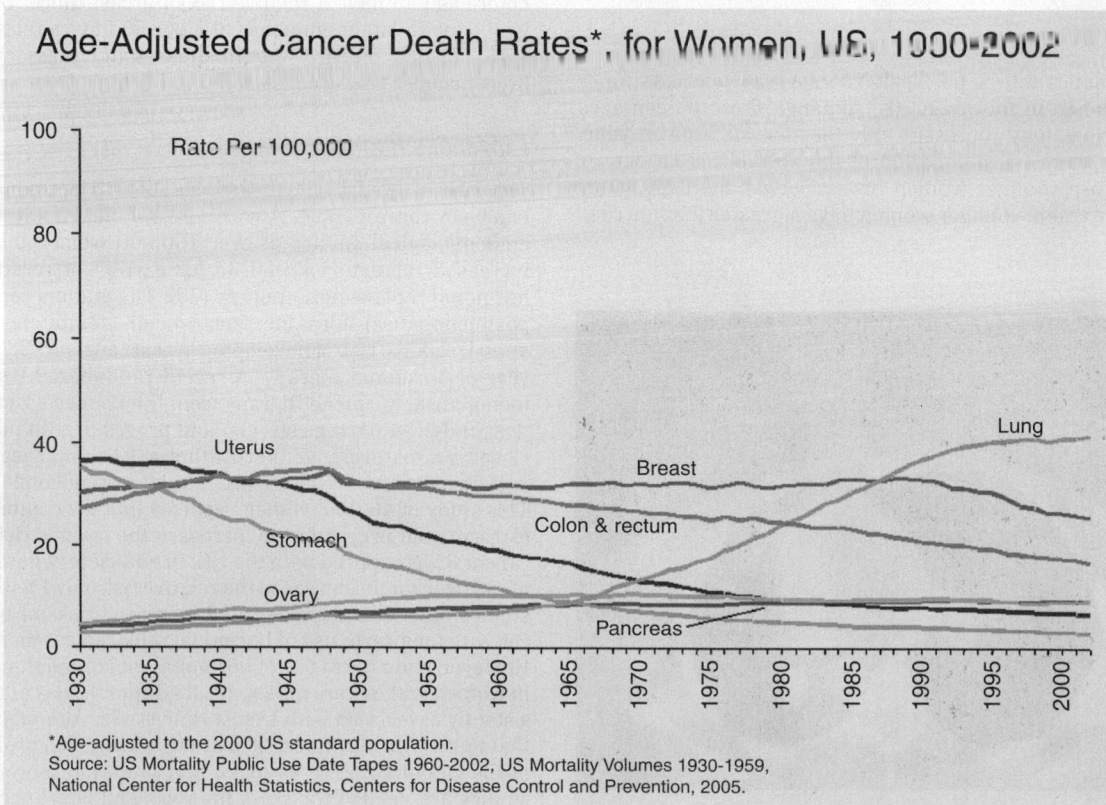

FIGURE 53.5. Age-adjusted cancer death rates for U.S. women, 1930–2002. Statistics show a recent decrease in breast cancer mortality, due to increase in screening detected malignancies and improvements in treatment. Age adjusted to the 2000 U.S. standard population. (From U.S. Mortality Public Use Data Tapes 1960–2002, U.S. Mortality Volumes 1930–1959, National Center for Health Statistics, Centers for Disease Control and Prevention, 2005.)

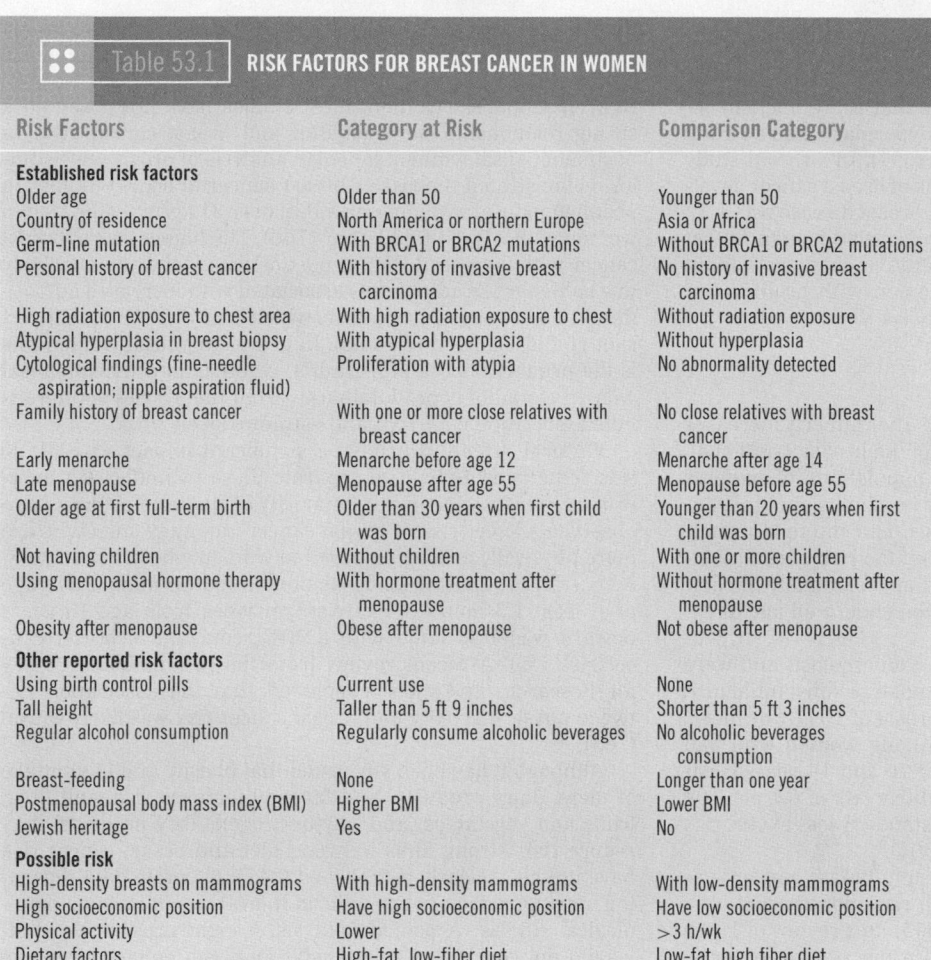

Risk Factors	Category at Risk	Comparison Category
Established risk factors		
Older age	Older than 50	Younger than 50
Country of residence	North America or northern Europe	Asia or Africa
Germ-line mutation	With BRCA1 or BRCA2 mutations	Without BRCA1 or BRCA2 mutations
Personal history of breast cancer	With history of invasive breast carcinoma	No history of invasive breast carcinoma
High radiation exposure to chest area	With high radiation exposure to chest	Without radiation exposure
Atypical hyperplasia in breast biopsy	With atypical hyperplasia	Without hyperplasia
Cytological findings (fine-needle aspiration; nipple aspiration fluid)	Proliferation with atypia	No abnormality detected
Family history of breast cancer	With one or more close relatives with breast cancer	No close relatives with breast cancer
Early menarche	Menarche before age 12	Menarche after age 14
Late menopause	Menopause after age 55	Menopause before age 55
Older age at first full-term birth	Older than 30 years when first child was born	Younger than 20 years when first child was born
Not having children	Without children	With one or more children
Using menopausal hormone therapy	With hormone treatment after menopause	Without hormone treatment after menopause
Obesity after menopause	Obese after menopause	Not obese after menopause
Other reported risk factors		
Using birth control pills	Current use	None
Tall height	Taller than 5 ft 9 inches	Shorter than 5 ft 3 inches
Regular alcohol consumption	Regularly consume alcoholic beverages	No alcoholic beverages consumption
Breast-feeding	None	Longer than one year
Postmenopausal body mass index (BMI)	Higher BMI	Lower BMI
Jewish heritage	Yes	No
Possible risk		
High-density breasts on mammograms	With high-density mammograms	With low-density mammograms
High socioeconomic position	Have high socioeconomic position	Have low socioeconomic position
Physical activity	Lower	>3 h/wk
Dietary factors	High-fat, low-fiber diet	Low-fat, high fiber diet

Table 53.1 RISK FACTORS FOR BREAST CANCER IN WOMEN

10% of women with breast cancer are from families who display an autosomal dominant pattern of breast cancer inheritance (625). The actual risk that family history conveys depends on the number of relatives affected and their age at diagnosis (having a first-degree relative with premenopausal breast cancer conveys a greater risk than does having a first-degree relative with postmenopausal cancer). Women with one first-degree relative affected by the disease have an increased relative risk of developing breast cancer two to three times that of women with no family history. Women with two or more first-degree relatives with a diagnosis of breast cancer have a still greater risk, four to six times that of women with no family history (89).

Women with a strong family history, particularly those with multiple first- and second-degree relatives, diagnosed with breast cancer in the premenopausal years are at risk for carrying mutations in the breast cancer susceptibility genes, BRCA1 or BRCA2. Although these mutations are present in <1% of the population and account for approximately 5% to 10% of all breast cancer cases, women carrying these mutations have a lifetime risk of developing breast cancer of up to 70% to 80% (625). Genetic counseling and/or testing should be considered in women at risk for carrying these mutations. Recently, the American Society of Clinical Oncology (ASCO) published guidelines for genetic testing (17). In the context of pre- and posttest counseling, ASCO recommends that "genetic testing be offered when:

1. The individual has personal or family history features suggestive of a genetic cancer susceptibility condition,
2. The test can be adequately interpreted, and

3. The results will aid in diagnosis or influence the medical or surgical management of the patient or family members at hereditary risk of cancer."

Personal History of Breast Cancer and History of "Benign" Breast Biopsy

Women with a prior history of breast cancer are at an elevated risk to develop a second contralateral breast cancer (811). Studies with long-term follow-up have demonstrated a risk of breast cancer in the contralateral breast of approximately 10% to 15%, depending on the patient population and length of follow-up (537). Patients treated for invasive breast cancer or ductal carcinoma *in situ* have similar risks of developing a contralateral breast cancer, which does not appear to be affected by the type of local therapy for the initial lesion. A recent analysis of ductal carcinoma *in situ* (DCIS) patients from the Connecticut Tumor Registry demonstrated a relative risk of developing contralateral breast cancer of 3.35 compared to women without a diagnosis of breast cancer (125). The risk of contralateral breast cancer as a function of prior radiation treatment is discussed in detail later.

Although women with a history of fibrocystic changes have been reported to have an elevated risk of breast cancer, recent evidence suggests that the majority of the elevated risk is due to the smaller proportion of women whose biopsy reveals atypical hyperplasia. Results from the Breast Cancer Detection Demonstration Project, which included over 280,000 women in 29 centers, demonstrated that women with atypical hyperplasia had 4.3 times the breast cancer risk of women without proliferative disease (95% confidence interval [CI], 1.7 to 11). In women with proliferative disease lacking atypical hyperplasia, the relative risk was 1.3 (95% CI, 0.77 to 2.2). In that study, the joint occurrence of family history and atypical hyperplasia had a strong synergistic effect on breast cancer risk (697). In a recent study by Hartmann et al. (336), the relative risk of breast cancer developing in women with biopsies of benign breast disease was 1.27 (1.15 to 1.41) for women with nonproliferative benign breast disease, 1.88 (1.66 to 2.12) for proliferative changes without atypia, and 4.24 (3.26 to 5.41) for women with proliferative changes with atypia.

Radiation Exposure

Exposure to ionizing radiation during or after puberty increases the risk for development of carcinoma of the breast. Land et al. (432,433) reviewed reports on three populations of patients exposed to ionizing radiation by atomic bombings, multiple fluoroscopic examinations for tuberculosis, and multiple examinations for mastitis. They concluded that the risk of radiation-induced cancer of the breast increased approximately linearly with increasing dose and was heavily dependent on age at exposure.

In a study of 31,710 women who had tuberculosis and were examined with repeated fluoroscopic studies, a substantial proportion (26.4%) received doses to the breast of 10 cGy or more; the breast cancer risk was greatest among women who had radiation exposure between the ages of 10 and 14 years (relative risk [RR], 4.5 per 1 cGy and an additive risk of 6.1 per 104 person-years per 1 cGy); there was substantially less excess risk with increasing age at first exposure (501).

A high risk of solid tumors, especially breast cancer, has been described in women treated with radiation therapy at a young age for Hodgkin's disease (135,355). In a review of 1,380 women treated at 15 institutions before the age of 16 years, breast cancer developed in 17 women, in seven after radiation therapy alone, and in 10 after irradiation and chemotherapy. Sixteen breast cancers appeared within or at the margin of the irradiation fields. The cumulative probability of breast cancer at 40 years of age was 35%. Women in this cohort of survivors had a risk of breast cancer 70 times higher than that of the general population (87).

In a recent study, relative risks of breast cancer were defined by radiation dose to the chest (0, 20 to <40 Gy, or ≥40 Gy). Estimates were from a case-controled study conducted within an international population-based cohort of 3,817 female survivors of Hodgkin's lymphoma diagnosed at age 30 years or younger. For a survivor who was treated at age 25 years with a chest radiation dose of at least 40 Gy without alkylating agents, estimated cumulative absolute risks of breast cancer by age 35, 45, and 55 years were 1.4% (95% CI, = 0.9 to 2.1), 11.1% (95% CI, 7.4 to 16.3), and 29.0% (95% CI, 20.2 to 40.1), respectively (750).

The risk of breast cancer associated with radiation exposure decreases sharply with increasing age at exposure, and even a small benefit to women of screening mammography would outweigh any possible risk of radiation-induced breast cancer (689). For women between 50 and 75 years of age, the benefit of annual screening mammography exceeds the radiation risk by a factor of almost 100, and for women aged 35 to 75 years the benefit of reduced mortality is projected to exceed the radiation risk by a factor of more than 75 (496).

Body Mass Index, Physical Activity, and Dietary Factors

The inherent complex interaction between body mass, physical activity, and diet complicates interpretation of epidemiologic studies correlating these factors with breast cancer risk.

Body mass index (BMI) has been clearly associated with breast cancer risk in a number of studies, but it appears to influence breast cancer risk predominantly in postmenopausal women. In premenopausal women, most studies have not observed a strong relationship between BMI and breast cancer risk. In postmenopausal women, a pooled analysis of prospective studies demonstrated the risk of breast cancer to be 30% higher in postmenopausal women with a BMI over 31 kg/m^2 compared to women with a BMI of 20 kg/m^2 (766). The higher risk of breast cancer with increased BMI in postmenopausal women is likely due to higher estradiol levels associated with increased adipose tissue and increased aromatase, which is involved in the conversion of androgens to estradiol. In postmenopausal women this is the primary source of estradiol, whereas in premenopausal women estradiol is predominantly from the ovaries so there is little association with BMI and estradiol levels.

Physical activity can have a significant impact on BMI, so it is sometimes difficult to separate these two effects in interpreting breast cancer risk. A majority of studies, however, have observed a lower risk of breast cancer among women who are more physically active compared to women who are sedentary. A recent case-control study demonstrated an annual average of at least 1.3 hours of exercise per week from age 10 years onward was associated with a 20% reduction in breast cancer risk (55). A recent review from the International Agency for Research on Cancer concluded that the association between physical activity and breast cancer risk was likely causal (763).

Although it has been suggested that obesity and high intake of meat, dairy products, and fat may increase risk, and fiber, fruits and vegetables, and phytoestrogens (soy products) may reduce risk, strong links between diet and breast cancer risk have not been clearly established (841). Accurate data regarding nutritional factors are difficult to evaluate in most epidemiological studies. A pooled analysis of eight prospective studies did not conclude a relationship between dietary fat intake and breast cancer risk. Similarly large prospective studies have failed to demonstrate an association between dietary fiber intake and breast cancer risk (363). Phytoestrogens found in soy products and many cereals, tea, and vegetables may reduce the effects of estrogen. Given the lower incidence of breast cancer in Asian countries with high soy intake, one might hypothesize a relationship between this dietary factor and breast cancer risk. Although animal studies suggest that high soy intake is protective, human studies have not been as conclusive.

Alcohol Consumption

In an analysis by the Oxford Group of 53 epidemiological studies, including 58,515 women with breast cancer and 95,067 women without breast cancer, women with daily consumption of four or more alcoholic drinks a day had a 50% higher breast cancer risk (319). The average consumption of alcohol reported was 6.0 g per day (about half a unit/drink of alcohol per day). Compared with women who reported drinking no alcohol, the relative risk of breast cancer was 1.32 (1.19 to 1.45; $p < .00001$) for an intake of 35 to 44 g per day of alcohol, and 1.46 (1.33 to 1.61; $p < .00001$) for ≥45 g per day of alcohol. The relative risk of breast cancer increased by 7.1% (95% CI, 5.5 to 8.7; $p < .00001$) for each additional drink of alcohol consumed on a daily basis.

Although the relationship between physical activity, BMI, and dietary factors may be difficult to separate, it is apparent that maintaining a sound, varied diet, limiting alcohol intake, avoiding obesity, and getting moderate physical activity are modifiable behaviors that can impact breast cancer risk (as well as other health-related issues) and they should be encouraged.

Mammographic Density

There is a large body of evidence suggesting a correlation between mammographic breast density and breast cancer risk (74,76,842). The risk of breast cancer associated with the highest category of density has been estimated to be two to six times greater than in the lowest category. Although the causal link between mammographic density remains poorly understood, breast density is in part attributable to genetic factors.

Byrne et al. (93) and Boyd et al. (75) noted that women with 75% or greater breast density parenchymal patterns on the mammogram had a fivefold greater risk of breast cancer. This parameter was independent of other prognostic factors, such as family history, age at first birth, or alcohol consumption.

Determining an Individual's Risk

It is important to consider the combination of risk factors when a generalized risk profile is determined. For example, combining age and family history indicates that a 40-year-old with two or more first-degree relatives with breast cancer has approximately the same annual risk of developing breast cancer as a 60-year-old with no risk factors (265). As mentioned earlier, despite this equivalence in annual risk, the 40-year-old used in this example has a much higher overall lifetime risk. Gail et al. (265) used these epidemiologic risk factors to derive a model for predicting an individual's annual and lifetime risks of breast cancer. In this model, an individual's annual risk of breast cancer is based on her present age, number of first-degree relatives with breast cancer, age at first birth, age at menarche, number of breast biopsies, and history of atypical ductal hyperplasia. The use of exogenous hormones is not considered in this model, and many of the other risk factors discussed above are not incorporated into this specific model.

Prevention and Genetic Screening

Approximately 10% of breast cancer patients have familial breast cancer, typically defined as breast cancer showing an autosomal dominant inheritance pattern (625). During the 1990s, germline mutations in three important tumor suppressor genes—p53, BRCA1, and BRCA2—were discovered in family members of individuals with familial breast cancer (100,354,462). All three genes have been shown unequivocally to predispose a woman to breast cancer.

Mutations in p53

Germline mutations in the p53 gene are very rare and result in *Li-Fraumeni syndrome,* named after two investigators who made significant contributions to the understanding of this condition (354). The p53 gene is one of the most important tumor suppressor genes and has been called the *guardian of the genome* because of its critical role in cellular pathways that recognize and direct a response to DNA injury. One consequence of a germline mutation in p53 is an increased risk for a variety of cancers, including childhood sarcomas, gynecologic tumors, and breast cancer. Breast cancer is the most common malignancy in patients with Li-Fraumeni syndrome; the lifetime risk is estimated to be 90% (354).

Mutations in BRCA1 and BRCA2

Studies of patients with familial breast cancer led to the discovery of BRCA1 in 1995 and BRCA2 in 1996. Similar to p53, both BRCA1 and BRCA2 are tumor suppressor genes that contribute to the stability of the genome by mediating the effects of the cel-

Table 53.2 PROBABILITY OF BRCA1 GERMLINE MUTATIONS IN VARIOUS CLINICAL SCENARIOS

Scenario	Probability (%)
Mother or father proven carrier	50
40-year-old with breast cancer and a first-degree relative with breast cancer	
Ashkenazic	20
Non-Ashkenazic	5
60-year-old with bilateral breast cancer and a first-degree relative with breast cancer	
Ashkenazic	20
Non-Ashkenazic	5
30-year-old with breast cancer and a first-degree relative with ovarian cancer	
Ashkenazic	50
Non-Ashkenazic	20

Data from Shattuck-Eidens D, Oliphant A, McClure M, et al. BRAC1 sequence analysis in women at high risk for susceptibility mutations. Risk factor analysis and implications for genetic testing. *JAMA* 1997;278:1242–1250.

lular response to DNA injury. Individuals with a germline mutation in BRCA1 have a lifetime risk of breast cancer of 65% to 85% (171,172). In addition, these individuals have an elevated lifetime risk of ovarian cancer, which may approach 50%. Other types of cancer that develop more frequently in BRCA1 carriers include colon cancer and prostate cancer. The lifetime risk of breast cancer for women with germline BRCA2 mutations mirrors that for women with BRCA1 mutations. BRCA2 mutation carriers are also at increased risk for ovarian cancer compared with the general population, but their risk is much less than the risk in women with BRCA1 mutations. BRCA2 is also associated with pancreatic cancer and male breast cancer. Genetic screening for germline mutations in BRCA1 and BRCA2 is now possible. Testing should be performed in centers equipped with genetic counseling programs designed to properly inform individuals of the social, economic, and legal consequences associated with genetic testing. Germline mutations in BRCA1 and BRCA2 are rare, occurring in fewer than 7% of patients with breast cancer. Thus, only a minority of breast cancer patients with a family history of the disease would be predicted to carry a mutation in one of these genes. Table 53.2 contains data concerning the probability of carrying a BRCA1 mutation based on an individual's age at cancer diagnosis, personal cancer history, and family cancer history and whether the individual is of Ashkenazic Jewish descent (677).

No definitive data exist on which to base screening recommendations for individuals with a proven germline mutation in a gene predisposing to the development of breast cancer. The American Society for Clinical Oncology (ASCO) has published a consensus statement recommending that these individuals undergo annual mammography and clinical and self-breast examination beginning at the age of 25 to 35 years (17). In addition, annual pelvic examinations with transvaginal sonography, color Doppler examinations of the ovaries, and measurement of serum CA-125 levels are recommended beginning at age 25 to 35 years. As will be discussed later, magnetic resonance imaging (MRI) has emerged as a promising screening tool for women at high risk for breast cancer.

Breast Cancer Prevention Strategies

Tamoxifen

Understanding of the role of estrogen and progesterone in breast cancer development has led to the development of pharmacologic strategies that could significantly decrease the incidence of breast cancer over the next two decades.

Several pharmaceuticals that affect the estrogenic pathways have been studied as chemopreventive agents, but the only agent for which mature data from clinical trials are available is tamoxifen (40,133,136,137,209,780). Interest in tamoxifen as a chemopreventive agent arose after a number of randomized trials designed to test the efficacy of hormonal therapy for invasive breast cancer reported that tamoxifen reduced the incidence of contralateral breast cancer. On the basis of these data, in 1992 the National Surgical Adjuvant Breast and Bowel Project (NSABP) began a randomized, placebo-controlled study (the P-1 trial) to test the efficacy of 5 years of tamoxifen use in the prevention of breast cancer (209). Between 1992 and 1997, 13,388 women with a 1.67% or greater predicted risk of developing breast cancer in 5 years were enrolled in this trial. Risk was assessed using a modification of the Gail model, which permitted enrollment of any woman older than 60 years of age and selected women younger than 60 years with additional risk factors that increased their annual risk to at least that of a 60-year-old. In addition, women with a history of lobular carcinoma *in situ* (LCIS) were included because their risk was believed to exceed the cutoff risk of 1.67%. Women were not allowed to use estrogen replacement therapy during their participation in the trial. The results of the P1 trial indicated that tamoxifen reduced the rates of invasive and noninvasive breast cancer by 49% and 50%, respectively. The benefit of tamoxifen was seen in all age groups (≤49 years, 50 to 59 years, ≥60 years). In addition, women with a history of atypical ductal hyperplasia had an 86% risk reduction, and women with a history of LCIS had a 56% risk reduction. Finally, the benefit was seen across all subgroups specified according to family history of breast cancer. Tamoxifen selectively reduced the incidence of estrogen receptor–positive tumors; estrogen receptor–negative tumors developed at an equal rate in the tamoxifen and placebo groups. No evidence was shown of a cardioprotective effect of tamoxifen in this trial, but the number of osteoporosis-related fractures was reduced in the tamoxifen-treated cohort. Tamoxifen increased the risk of developing stage I endometrial cancer (risk ratio of 2.53).

Although this study indicated that 5 years of tamoxifen use decreased the 5-year risk of developing breast cancer by about 50%, whether this result warrants the widespread use of tamoxifen for breast cancer prevention is controversial. In the NSABP report, 5 years of tamoxifen therapy in 6,576 women reduced the number of invasive or noninvasive breast cancer by 120 compared with the expected number. With the relatively short follow-up period of this important study, however, it was not possible to determine whether tamoxifen actually prevented this number of cases of breast cancer or rather simply delayed the onset of the disease.

More recently, a landmark study was published that compared tamoxifen to raloxifene as a preventative agent in postmenopausal women with breast cancer. Raloxifene, a drug that is primarily used in prevention of osteoporosis, had been shown in prior studies to decrease the incidence of breast cancers. The NSABP study of tamoxifen and raloxifene trial was a prospective, double-blind, randomized clinical trial (804). There were 19,747 postmenopausal women of mean age 58.5 years with increased 5-year breast cancer risk. Patients were randomized to oral tamoxifen (20 mg per day) or raloxifene (60 mg per day) for 5 years. There were 163 cases of invasive breast cancer in women assigned to tamoxifen and 168 in those assigned to raloxifene, which was not significantly different between the two arms. The main benefit of raloxifene was in toxicity. There were 36 cases of uterine cancer with tamoxifen and 23 with raloxifene. No differences were found for other invasive cancer sites, for ischemic heart disease events, or for stroke. Thromboembolic events also occurred less often in the raloxifene group. The number of osteoporotic fractures in the groups was similar, and there were fewer cataract surgeries in the group using raloxifene. There was no difference in the total number of deaths (101 for tamoxifen vs. 96 for raloxifene) or in causes of death. It appears from this study that raloxifene is as effective as tamoxifen in reducing the risk of invasive breast cancer and has a lower risk of thromboembolic events. Of note there were slightly more noninvasive cancers in the raloxifene group, but that was not statistically significant.

A comparison of the tamoxifen P1, P2, and other tamoxifen prevention trials is outlined in Table 50.9.

Prophylactic Surgery

An alternative strategy used to prevent breast cancer development is prophylactic surgical intervention. Hartmann et al. (335) analyzed outcomes in women with a family history of

Table 53.3	RESULTS OF CHEMO-PREVENTION TRIALS					
	Royal Marsden (tamoxifen vs. placebo) (587)	NSABP-P1 (tamoxifen vs. placebo) (209)	Italian (tamoxifen vs. placebo) (781)	IBIS-1 (tamoxifen vs. placebo) (136)	MORE (raloxifene vs. placebo) (133)	STAR (tamoxifen vs. raloxifene) (804)
Entry dates	1986–1996	1992–1997	1992–1997	1992–2001	1994–1999	1999–2005
Number randomized	2,494 (1,238 vs. 1,233)	6,681 vs. 6,707	2,700 vs. 2,708	3,573 vs. 3,566	2,557+2,572 vs. 2,576	9,726 vs. 9,745
Age (years)	30–70	≥35	35–70	35–70	66.5 (median)	≥35
Agent dose	Tamoxifen 20 mg	Tamoxifen 20 mg	Tamoxifen 20 mg	Tamoxifen 20 mg	Raloxifene 60 mg or 120 mg	Tamoxifen 20 mg, raloxifene 60 mg
Planned length (years) of treatment	5–8	5	5	5	4	5
Breast cancers						
Total	62 vs. 75	124 vs. 244	34 vs. 45	69 vs. 101	31/2 vs. 43	220 vs. 248
Invasive	54 vs. 64	89 vs. 175	28 vs. 40	64 vs. 85	22/2 vs. 39	163 vs. 168
Noninvasive	7 vs. 7	35 vs. 69	5 vs. 4	5 vs. 16	9/2 vs. 4	57 vs. 80
Unknown	1 vs. 4	—	1 vs. 1	—	—	—
Estrogen-recptor status (invasive only)						
Positive	31 vs. 44	41 vs. 130		44 vs. 63	10/2 vs. 31	115 vs. 109
Negative	17 vs. 10	38 vs. 31		19 vs. 19	9/2 vs. 4	44 vs. 51

IBIS, International Breast Cancer Intervention Study; MORE, Multiple Outcomes of Raloxifene Evaluation; NSABP, National Surgical Adjuvant Breast and Bowel Project; STAR, Study of Tamoxifen and Raloxifene.

breast cancer who underwent bilateral prophylactic mastectomy at the Mayo Clinic between 1960 and 1993. With a median follow-up time of 14 years, only four of the 639 treated patients developed breast cancer. According to the Gail model, 37.4 cases of breast cancer would have been expected to develop in this population, so the prophylactic surgery resulted in an 89.5% risk reduction ($p < .001$) (335).

As will be discussed later in the section on management of patients with BRCA1 and BRCA2 mutations, prophylactic oophorectomy in BRCA carriers also significantly reduces the risk of subsequent breast cancers in this population.

Breast cancer prevention strategies will continue to be a dynamic area of preclinical and clinical research in the near future.

Natural History and Origins

All forms of breast cancer are believed to develop as a consequence of unregulated cell growth and the development of phenotypic changes such as the ability to invade, recruit a new blood supply, and metastasize. These changes in phenotypes are secondary to the development of aberrations in genetic pathways. Some of these aberrations are inherited (germline mutations), whereas others develop during the life of a breast cell (somatic mutations). It is currently believed that most breast cancer is a consequence of a series of somatic mutations. As previously noted, only 20% to 25% of breast cancer patients have a history of breast cancer in a first-degree relative. However, it is possible that some women without a first-degree relative with breast cancer still inherit a genetic background that predisposes to breast cancer. These mutations may be insufficient to cause breast cancer unless accompanied by other mutations and, therefore, would be predicted to have a low penetrance. Historically, it has been much more difficult to discover low-penetrance mutations than to discover germline mutations that result in an autosomal dominant pattern of breast cancer development. However, with newer molecular techniques, such as deoxyribonucleic acid (DNA)–array assays, the identification of low-penetrance predisposing mutations may be more feasible.

Left untreated, breast cancer can have a variable clinical course. A classic paper by Bloom et al. (65) outlined the natural history of breast cancer patients seen between 1805 and 1933, not treated by surgery or irradiation, 250 of whom had a pathologic diagnosis of cancer. There were no patients with stage I disease, 2.4% with stage II, 23% with stage III, and 74% with stage IV. Survival in the untreated group was 3.6% compared to an overall survival of 34% in patients treated with radical or modified radical mastectomy with or without radiation.

Concepts regarding the natural history of breast cancer have undergone great evolution over the past 100 years, with a profound impact on the management of these patients. The Halsted (315) model was based on an orderly progression to the regional lymph nodes and from there to distant metastatic sites. Later, Keynes (399) and Crile et al. (130) suggested that breast cancer is a systemic disease, and that extensive surgery to achieve local tumor control was not as important as originally believed. This alternative hypothesis was fully demonstrated in both laboratory and clinical studies by Fisher (216), who advanced the concept that breast cancer, as a systemic process involving host–tumor interactions, would not show substantial effects on survival with variations in locoregional treatment. A third hypothesis put forward by Hellman (344) considers breast cancer as a heterogeneous disease with a spectrum extending from a tumor that remains localized throughout its course to one that disseminates systemically even when detected as a small lesion, suggesting that metastases are a function of tumor growth and progression factors.

The growth rate of a tumor in the breast is thought to be constant from the date of origin. Using estimates of doubling time, it would take an average of approximately 5 years for a tumor to reach palpable size, and those lesions with slower doubling time would have an even longer latent period (293).

The most common site of origin of breast cancer is the upper-outer quadrant (38.5%), followed by the central area (29%), the upper-inner quadrant (14.2%), the lower-outer quadrant (8.8%), and the lower-inner quadrant (5%) (293). These rates correlate with the amount of breast tissue in the various quadrants. Cancer is somewhat more common in the left than in the right breast and may appear in both breasts simultaneously (1% to 2%). As noted above, women with a history of breast cancer have a 10% to 15% risk of developing a new primary in the contralateral breast.

As the cancer grows, it travels along the ducts, eventually breaking through the basement membrane of the duct, invading adjacent lobules, ducts, fascial strands, and the mammary fat, spreading through the breast lymphatics and into the peripheral lymphatics. The tumor can grow through the wall of blood vessels, spread into the deep lymphatics of the dermis, and eventually produce edema of the skin (*peau d'orange*), which usually indicates that the superficial as well as the deep lymphatics are involved. Skin dimpling can be caused by involvement of *Cooper's ligament*. Ulceration and infiltration of overlying skin, which may develop late in the course of the disease, are usually preceded by fixation and localized redness of the skin over the tumor and are less frequently seen because of the current emphasis on screening and early diagnosis (293).

Axillary Spread

A common route of spread of breast carcinoma is first through the axillary lymph nodes, with the incidence increasing with larger tumors. Depending on mode of detection, tumor size, histology, and other clinical-pathological factors, between 10% and 40% of newly diagnosed stage T1 and T2 breast cancers have pathologic evidence of axillary nodal metastases. Voogd et al. (806) assessed 7,680 patients with documented invasive breast cancer; of 5,125 patients known to have clinically negative lymph nodes who underwent axillary dissection, 1,748 (34%) had positive lymph nodes at pathologic examination. Univariate analysis showed that lymph node metastases were associated with tumors larger than 1 cm ($p = .001$), moderate or poorly differentiated nuclear grade ($p = .005$), high fraction of cells in the growth phase (S phase) of the cell cycle ($p = .041$), presence of lymphatic vascular invasion ($p < .001$), and age younger than 60 years ($p = .01$).

Table 53.4 demonstrates the strong relationship between primary tumor size and axillary nodal involvement. Even patients with T1a and T1b disease have significant nodal involvement. Mustafa et al. (519) noted an overall frequency of axillary lymph node metastases in T1a and T1b lesions of 16%; integrating age, tumor size, and grade predicted the frequency of nodal metastases. Overall, patients with all three poor prognostic indicators had a 34% incidence of nodal involvement, and those with no poor prognostic factors had a 7% or less probability of nodal metastases. Gann et al. (271) reviewed 18,025 patients with a diagnosis of breast carcinoma from the American College of Surgeons database. On multivariate analysis, the following factors were independently associated with a greater likelihood of one or more positive lymph nodes: larger tumor size, young age, African American or Hispanic race, outer-half tumor location, poor or moderate differentiation, aneuploidy, and infiltrating ductal histologic type.

Although up to 30% to 40% of T1–2 clinically node-negative breast cancers may have pathologically involved lymph nodes, data from NSABP-04 suggest that less than half of clinically negative but pathologically positive axilla will experience a clinical

Table 53.4	INCIDENCE OF METASTATIC AXILLARY LYMPH NODES IN CARCINOMA OF BREAST CORRELATED WITH PRIMARY TUMOR SIZE				
	Tumor Size[a] (cm)				
Study (Reference)	≤0.5	0.6–1	1.0–2	2.1–3	3.1–5
Washington University[b]	3/55 (5%)	25/203 (12%)	59/294 (20%)	38/113 (34%)	9/31 (29%)
Tinnemans et al. (745)	1/13 (7.7%)	3/24 (12.5%)	13/44 (29.5%)	—	—
Silverstein et al. (682)	3/96 (3%)	27/156 (17%)	115/357 (32%)	145/330 (44%)[c]	—
Kambouris (389)	—	—	13/357 (32%)	15/25 (60%)	1/7 (14%)
Greco et al. (284)	—	40/306 (13%)	—	49/69 (71%)	
Fein et al. (198)	6/68 (9%)	7/48 (15%)	16/50 (32%)	—	—

[a]Number of patients with axillary metastasis/total number of patients with tumor size indicated.
[b]Unpublished data.
[c]T2 tumors (2–5 cm).

relapse in the axilla (212). In this study, operable breast cancer patients, who were primarily diagnosed with palpable breast tumors in the premammography era, were randomized to one of three arms: simple mastectomy without axillary dissection, simple mastectomy with axillary dissection, or simple mastectomy with comprehensive chest wall and regional nodal irradiation. In the arm undergoing axillary dissection, nodal positivity was approximately 40%. Nodal control was excellent (>97%) in this arm as well as in the arm treated with radiation. In the simple mastectomy arm, where no nodal treatment by radiation or dissection was administered, the axillary failure rate was approximately 20%. Assuming equal distribution among the arms, it is presumed the pathological involvement was approximately 40%, indicating that less than half of those with pathological involvement eventually failed clinically.

Nodal involvement has more recently been assessed by sentinel node techniques. Kamath et al. (388) analyzed 101 women with sentinel lymph node metastases on whom subsequent complete lymph node dissection was performed. Sentinel lymph node micrometastases (<2 mm) detected by cytokeratin staining were associated with a 7.6% (2/26) incidence of positive complete lymph node dissection, compared with a 25% (5/20) incidence when micrometastases were detected initially by routine hematoxylin-and-eosin (H&E) staining. Sentinel lymph node micrometastases, regardless of identification technique, conferred a risk of 15.2% (7/46) for nonsentinel lymph node involvement, which increased with larger tumors. Sentinel nodes are discussed in more detail later in the surgical management of breast cancer.

Internal Mammary Spread

Metastases to the internal mammary nodes (IMNs) are correlated with tumor size, are more frequent from medial half and central lesions, and occur more frequently when there is axillary node involvement (Table 53.5) (323). Veronesi et al. (777) found that, among women with tumors larger than 2 cm who were younger than 40 years of age and had positive axillary nodes, there was a 41% risk of having positive IMNs on IMN dissection; the corresponding risk for patients of that age with negative nodes was 16%. Sugg et al. (723) reviewed 286 patients with breast cancer who underwent IMN dissection. Positive IMNs were associated with primary tumor size (p <.0001) and the number of positive axillary nodes (p <.0001), but not with age or primary tumor location. Patients who had positive IMNs (25% of all patients) had a significantly worse overall 20-year disease-free survival rate than did patients with negative IMNs (p <.0001). Clinical failure of the internal mammary nodes is extremely rare, despite the evidence of pathological involvement from these studies. Most studies looking at nodal failure patterns report failure in the internal mammary region of <1% (242, 260, 299, 818, 808).

Supraclavicular Spread

Spread to supraclavicular lymph nodes usually allows involvement in the high axillary lymph nodes or IMNs depending on the location of the primary lesion. Chen et al. (110) reviewed 2,658 patients with invasive breast cancer who underwent surgery and adjuvant therapy. With a median follow-up period of 39 months, supraclavicular lymph node metastasis developed in 113 (4.3%). Young age (≤40 years), tumor size >3 cm, angiolymphatic invasion, negative estrogen receptor (ER) status, and DNA synthetic phase fraction >4% were significant for predicting supraclavicular metastasis on univariate analysis. Three predictive factors were significant after multivariate analysis: high histologic grade, more than four positive nodes, and axillary level II or III involved nodes. In patients

Table 53.5	INTERNAL MAMMARY NODE INVOLVEMENT RELATED TO LOCATION OF PRIMARY TUMOR AND TO AXILLARY NODE INVOLVEMENT				
	Location of Primary Tumor				
Axillary Involvement	Upper Inner Quadrant	Lower Inner Quadrant	Central	Upper Outer Quadrant	Lower Outer Quadrant
Axilla not involved[a]	20/143 (14%)	2/36 (6%)	5/76 (7%)	7/170 (4%)	2/40 (5%)
Axilla involved	47/105 (45%)	18/25 (72%)	65/140 (46%)	47/212 (22%)	10/53 (19%)
Total	67/248 (27%)	20/61 (33%)	70/216 (32%)	54/382 (14%)	12/93 (13%)

[a]Number of patients with internal mammary node involvement/total number of patients.
From Handley RS. Carcinoma of the breast. *Ann R Coll Surg Engl* 1975;57:59–66, with permission.

with axillary level I involved nodes and four or fewer positive nodes, the incidence of supraclavicular lymph node metastasis was 4.4%, but if axillary level III was involved, it increased to 15.1%.

Clinical failure in the supraclavicular fossa is relatively rare in patients with early stage breast cancer and is dependent on the degree of axillary involvement. For patients with no or minimal nodal involvement (<3 involved axillary nodes), supraclavicular failure is extremely rare. In an analysis of 691 patients with 0 to 3 nodes involved undergoing breast-conserving surgery and radiation therapy to tangential fields only without regional nodal irradiation, Galper et al. (269) reported failure in the supraclavicular fossa in 1.3% of patients.

Several studies have demonstrated that the failure rate in supraclavicular nodes, left untreated, may be as high as 20% in patients with advanced disease and/or more than four lymph nodes involved (207,219,220,722,797). In a cohort of 1,031 patients with operable breast cancer treated with mastectomy and level I or II node dissection plus adriamycin-based chemotherapy, but no radiation, Strom et al. (722) reported failure in the supraclavicular fossa was 8% at 10 years. Predictors of supraclavicular failure included four or more involved nodes and gross extranodal extension. In these subgroups, supraclavicular failure ranged from 14% to 19%. Radiation to the supraclavicular fossa in these higher-risk patients results in high local control rates, with isolated supraclavicular failures occurring in less that 1% of prophylactically treated nodes.

Systemic Spread

Using monoclonal antibodies to epithelial cytokeratins or tumor-associated cell membrane glycoproteins, carcinoma cells can be detected on cytologic bone marrow (or lymph node) preparations. Braun et al. (77) combined patient data from nine studies involving 4,703 patients with stage I, II, or III breast cancer. Micrometastasis was detected in 30.6% of the patients. With a median follow-up of 5.2 years, patients with bone marrow micrometastasis had larger tumors and tumors with a higher histologic grade and more often had lymph node metastases and hormone receptor-negative tumors, compared to those without bone marrow micrometastasis. The presence of micrometastasis was a significant prognostic factor for poorer overall survival (RR = 2.15; p <.001), breast cancer–specific survival (RR = 2.44; p <.001), disease-free survival (RR = 2.13), and distant-disease–free survival (RR = 2.33; p <.001 for all outcomes measures). In multivariate analysis, micrometastasis was an independent predictor of a poor outcome.

Local Control and Systemic Metastasis

Patients treated for breast cancer are at risk for local–regional failure as well as systemic metastasis. It is evident from the available literature that optimizing local control can impact systemic metastasis and survival, and similarly, systemic therapy has an impact on local control (124,300,358,803). Integration of systemic therapy with radiation will be discussed in detail later, but numerous studies have clearly demonstrated a significant improvement in local control with the use of radiation therapy and systemic therapy (both cytotoxic and hormonal) compared with radiation therapy without the use of systemic therapy (88,201,204,208,300,402). Appropriate integration of both local and systemic treatments through a multidisciplinary approach is thus essential to optimize outcome. Although there is some overlap, prognostic factors for local–regional control and systemic metastasis often differ.

For patients with early stage invasive breast cancer, even with appropriate systemic therapy, development of metastasis can vary from <5% in women with T1a disease and favorable histology, to over 40% for women with T2 tumors and pathologically involved lymph nodes. Similarly, local–regional failure rates can vary from <5% to over 40% depending on local treatment and prognostic factors for local failure (201,204,208, 246,302,768,778).

The impact of local control on systemic metastasis in breast cancer as well as other malignancies has been the subject of considerable debate and controversy. Although the benefits of local control with respect to cosmesis and quality of life are apparent, the independent effect of local control on systemic disease and survival has been questioned. Several studies have identified local control as an independent predictor of disease free and/or overall survival (111,202,241,302,307,778). Fisher et al. (202), in an analysis of patients treated in NSABP Protocol B-06, concluded that ipsilateral breast tumor recurrence was a harbinger, but not a cause, of distant metastases. Although mastectomy or breast irradiation after lumpectomy prevented expression of the marker (breast relapse), neither lowered the risk of distant metastases, which was determined by a host of prognostic factors.

More recent meta-analyses, however, have demonstrated a small but significant impact of local control on systemic metastasis and overall survival (124,803). A recent meta-analysis of randomized trials by Vinh-Hung et al. (803) comparing breast-conserving surgery without radiation to breast-conserving surgery with radiation confirms an approximate threefold reduction in local relapse with radiation therapy and an 8.6% improvement in mortality in the radiated cohorts.

One of the most convincing and authoritative studies related to this subject is the recent analysis of the Early Breast Cancer Trialists Collaborative Group (EBCTCG) (124). In this analysis over 42,000 women were enrolled in 78 randomized trials that compared 24 types of local treatment (radiotherapy vs. no radiotherapy, more vs. less surgery, or more surgery vs. radiotherapy). The EBCTCG attempted to relate the effect on local control to breast cancer mortality by grouping studies into whether the 5-year local relapse risk difference between the two comparisons of local therapy exceeded 10%. In those comparisons in which the difference in 5-year local recurrence risk was <10%, there was no impact on 15-year breast cancer mortality. However, there were 25,000 women enrolled in trials in whom the comparisons involved >10% differences in local control. In those studies, the difference in local recurrence risks at 5 years were 7% versus 26%, and the 15-year mortality risks were 44.6% versus 49.5% (p <.00001). The authors concluded that avoidance of a local recurrence in the conservatively managed breast or avoidance of a local–regional relapse after mastectomy had similar impact on breast cancer mortality. In the absence of any other cause of death, differences in local treatment that substantially affect local recurrence would avoid about one breast cancer death over 15 years for every four local relapses avoided. Figure 53.6 summarizes the results of this meta-analysis with respect to the impact of radiation on breast cancer mortality in both breast conservation and following mastectomy.

Another study, which supports the notion that local control influences survival, even in patients with known metastatic disease, is a report by Rapiti et al. (594). In 300 metastatic breast cancer patients recorded at the Geneva Cancer Registry between 1977 and 1996, they compared mortality risks from breast cancer between patients who had surgery of the primary breast tumor to those who had not and adjusted these risks for other prognostic factors. Women who had complete excision of the primary breast tumor with negative surgical margins had a 40% reduced risk of death due to breast cancer (hazard ratio [HR] = 0.6; 95% CI, 0.4 to 1.0; p = .049) compared with women who did not have surgery. The effect was most evident for women with bone metastasis only (HR, 0.2; 95% CI, 0.1 to 0.4; p = .001).

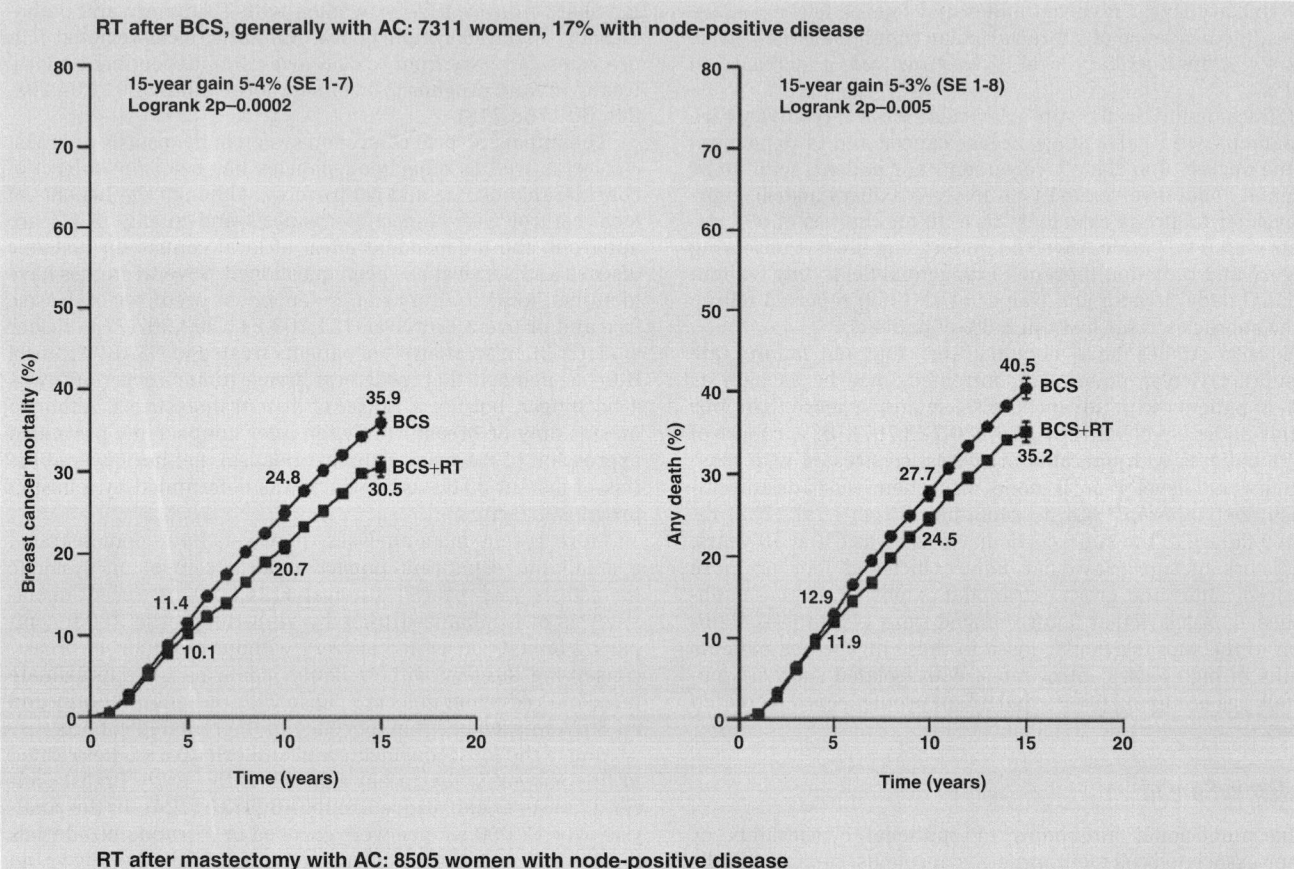

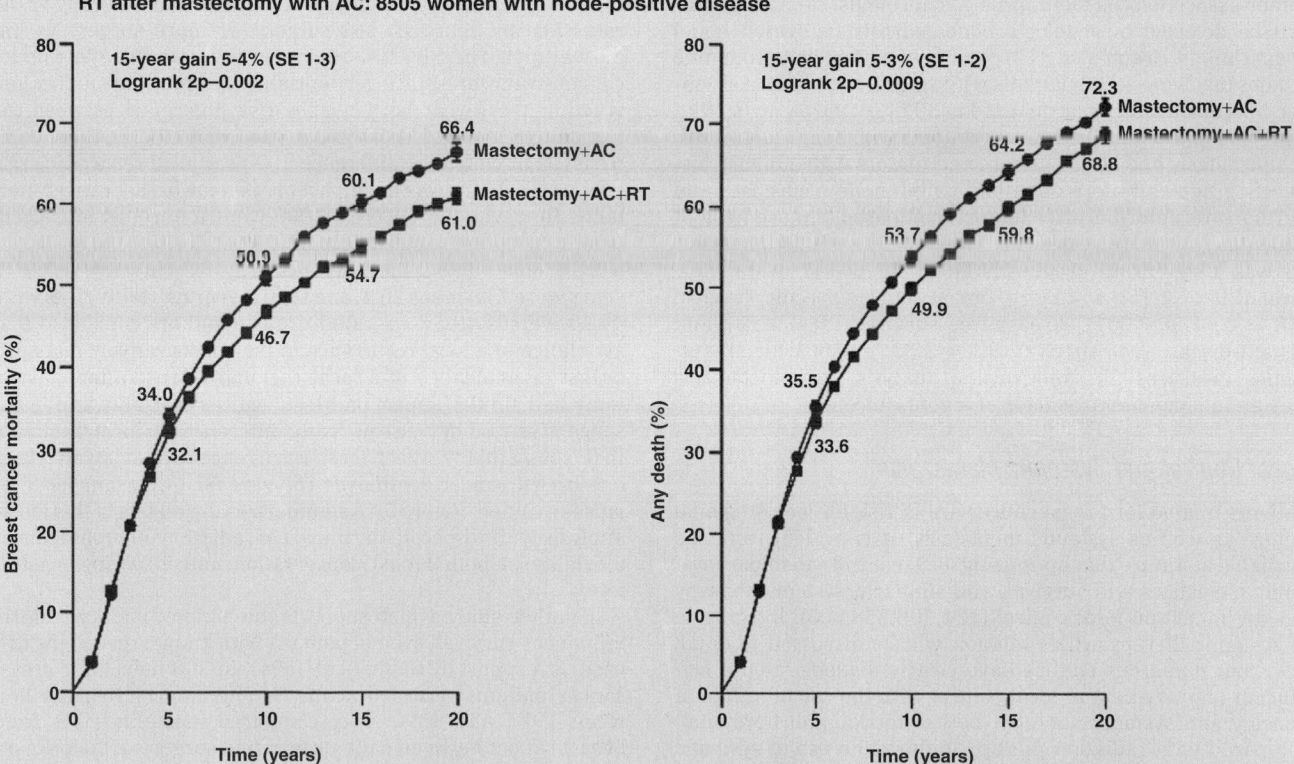

FIGURE 53.6. Effect of radiotherapy (RT) on breast cancer mortality and on all-cause mortality after breast-conserving surgery (BCS) or after mastectomy with axillary clearance (AC)—15- or 20-year probabilities. (From Clarke M, Collins R, Darby S, et al. Effects of radiotherapy and of differences in the extent of surgery for early breast cancer on local recurrence and 15-year survival: an overview of the randomised trials. *Lancet* 2005;366(0):2087–2106, with permission.)

Table 53.6	BREAST CANCER SCREENING GUIDELINES

Age Group	ACS (0)	ACR (0)	NCI (0)
20–39	BSE optional; CBE every 3 years.	Monthly BSE; CBE every 3 years.	No recommendation.
40–49	Annual mammography and CBE from 40 years.	Annual mammography and CBE from 40 years.	Mammography every 1–2 years.
>49	Annual mammography and CBE as long as a woman is in reasonably good health.	Annual mammography and monthly CBE as long as a woman is in reasonably good health.	Mammography every 1–2 years.
At increased risk	Consult with their doctors about the benefits and limitations of starting mammography screening earlier, having additional tests (i.e., breast ultrasound and MRI), or having more frequent examinations.	Consult with their physician about beginning mammography screening before age 40.	Seek expert medical advice about whether they should begin screening before age 40 and the frequency of screening.

ACR, American College of Radiology; ACS, American Cancer Society; BSE, breast self-examination; CBE, clinical breast examination; MRI, magnetic resonance imaging; NCI, National Cancer Institute.

Clinical Presentation

The majority of patients with T1 or T2 breast cancers present with a painless or slightly tender breast mass or have an abnormal screening mammogram. Patients with more advanced tumors may have breast tenderness, skin changes, bloody nipple discharge, or occasionally change in the shape and size of the breast. Rarely, patients may present with axillary lymphadenopathy or even distant metastasis. As noted previously, however, depending on tumor size, method of detection, and pathologic factors associated with the primary tumor, up to 30% to 40% of women with a clinically negative axilla may harbor subclinical pathologically involved axillary nodes.

The impact of delays in evaluation or treatment on the survival of patients with breast cancer is controversial. Richards et al. (615), in a review of 2,964 patients, found 942 (32%) who had symptoms for 12 or more weeks before their first hospital visit. Locally advanced or metastatic disease was detected in 32% of patients with delays compared with 10% of patients with intervals of <12 weeks between the onset of symptoms and hospital referral (*p* <.0001). Multivariate analysis showed that a longer duration of symptoms had a highly significant adverse influence on survival, but this was no longer evident when tumor size and stage were included in the model. Olivotto et al. (542) found that delays in diagnosis of 6 to 12 months led to an increased risk of larger tumor size and more lymph node metastases compared with patients diagnosed within 4 to 12 weeks of an abnormal screening mammogram result.

Screening in Breast Cancer

Mammography

Screening mammography has resulted in a shift in both the incidence and stage of patients presenting with breast cancer. In a simplified model described in Harris et al. (330), for every 1,000 screening mammograms, 80 women (8%) will be recalled for additional diagnostic imaging, 10 (1%) will require tissue diagnosis, and of those undergoing biopsy only three (0.3%) will have a malignancy.

There is a large body of evidence that early detection by mammography, followed by appropriate local, regional, and systemic treatment, is associated with reduced breast cancer mortality rates for women 50 years of age and older (181,183, 199,536,743). Although it remains an active area of debate, several authors (412,698) agree that screening mammography in women 40 to 49 years of age may reduce mortality from

breast cancer (183,185,200,411,412,697,698,731), and mammographic screening beginning at age 40 is encouraged in the majority of published guidelines (see Table 53.6). The reader is referred elsewhere for an extensive discussion of screening mammography studies (181,183,199). Selected series will be briefly discussed here and a summary of the classic screening mammography trials is summarized in Table 53.7. Collectively, these studies demonstrate a decrease in mortality and migration of patients from later stages of disease to earlier stages of disease with the use of screening mammography (21,181,183,199,411,413,697,698,728–730).

Sixteen-year results are available from the Health Insurance Plan study, which involved two systematically selected, randomly sampled groups of approximately 31,000 women aged 40 to 64 years who were offered screening examinations (675,676). Compared with the control group, which was observed and monitored, the mortality rate was reduced by approximately one-third in screened women 50 to 59 years of age. The survival difference between mammography-only and clinical examination-only cases appeared in years 7 to 10 after diagnosis. Although the greatest difference in mortality between screened and control group was detected in women 50 to 59 years of age when they entered the study, the differences are in favor of the study group at all ages.

Tabár et al. (728–730) demonstrated the benefit from mammography screening in two Swedish counties. In the group of women 20 to 69 years of age, there were 6,807 diagnosed with breast carcinoma over a 29-year period and 1,863 breast carcinoma deaths. The mortality rate from breast carcinoma diagnosed in women 40 to 69 years of age who were screened during the screening period (1988 to 1996) declined by 63% (RR, 0.37) compared with the breast carcinoma mortality rate during the period when no screening was available (1968 to 1977). The reduction in mortality rate observed during the service-screening period, adjusted for selection bias, was 48%. No significant change in breast carcinoma mortality rate was observed over the three periods in women who did not undergo screening.

In contrast to the above, a Canadian study revealed in women aged 50 to 59 years, the addition of annual mammography screening to physical examination had no effect on breast cancer mortality. Miller et al. (502) reported a study of 39,405 women (aged 50 to 59 years) randomly assigned to one of two study groups. By December 31, 1993, 622 invasive and 71 *in situ* breast cancers were observed in the mammography plus physical examination group, compared with 610 and 16, respectively, in the physical examination only group. At 13-year follow-up, the number of deaths from breast cancer was 107 in the mammography plus physical examination group and 105 in

Table 53.7	RANDOMIZED CONTROLLED TRIALS OF BREAST CANCER SCREENING

Trial and Years of Study (Reference)	Screening Protocol		Population				Relative Risk (95% Confidence Interval)
	Approach	Frequency	Age Group	Invited	Control	Follow-up (y)	
HIP (1963–1969) (675)	2V MM1 CBE	24 mo 4 rounds	40–49	14,432	14,701	18	0.77(0.53–1.11)
			50–64	16,568	16,299	18	0.80 (0.59–1.08)
Malmo (1976–1990) (21)	1 or 2 VMM	18–24 mo 5 rounds	45–49	13,528	12,242	12.7	0.64 (0.45–0.89)
			50–69	17,134	17,165	9	0.86 (0.64–1.16)
Kopparberg (1977–1985) (731)	1V MM	24 mo 4 rounds	40–49	9,650	5,009	20	0.76 (0.42–1.40)
			50–74	28,939	13,551	20	1.06 (0.65–1.76)
Ostergotland (1977–1985) (731)	1 V MM	24 mo 4 rounds	40–49	10,240	10,441	20	0.52 (0.39–0.70)
			50–74	28,229	26,830	20	0.81 (0.64–1.03)
Edinburgh (1979–1988) (10)	1 or 2 V MM CBE (initial)	24 mo 4 rounds	45–49	11,755	10,641	14	0.83 (0.54–1.27)
			50–64	11,245	12,359	10	0.85 (0.62–1.15)
CNBSS-1 (1980–1987) (503)	2 V MM CBE	12 mo 4–5 rounds	40–49	25,214	25,216	11–16	1.07 (0.75–1.52)
CNBSS-2 (1980–1987) (502)	2 V MM CBE	12 mo 4-5 rounds	50–59	19,711	19,694	13	1.02 (0.78–1.33)
Stockholm (1981–1985) (257)	1V MM	28 mo 2 rounds	40–49	14,185	7,985	11.4	1.01 (0.51–2.02)
			50–64	25,815	12,015	7	0.65 (0.4–1.08)
Gothenburg (61)	2 V MM	18 mo 5 rounds	39–49	11,724	14,217	12	0.56 (0.32–0.98)
			50–59	9,276	16,394	13	0.91 (0.61–1.36)

1 V MM, one-view mammography of each breast; 2 V MM, two-view mammography of each breast; CBE, clinical breast examination; CNBSS, Canadian Natural Breast Cancer Screening Studies; HIP, Health Insurance Plan.
Adapted from Smith, D'Orsi. In: Harris J, Lippman M, Morrow M, et al., eds. *Diseases of the breast.* Philadelphia: Lippincott Williams & Wilkins, 2004;Chapter 10.

the physical examination only group. The results of the Canadian study may be due to the unbalanced allocation of women with advanced cancers (large tumors, four or more positive nodes) to the screened group, the poor quality of the mammography in the trial, and an insufficient sample size (411,734).

Screening in Women Under Age 50

Although the majority of studies clearly support the impact of screening mammography on mortality in women over 50 years of age, data on screening younger women are more conflicting. Frisell and Lidbrink (257) presented updated data on breast cancer mortality for women younger than age 50 years from the Stockholm Mammographic Screening Trial. Approximately 40,000 women aged 40 to 64 years (14,842 aged 40 to 49 years) were randomized to a trial of breast cancer screening by single-view mammography alone; 20,000 women (7,103 aged 40 to 49) were randomized to a control group. In the 40- to 49-year age group, 24 and 12 breast cancer deaths were found in the study and control groups, respectively, after 11.4 years of follow-up. The RR of breast cancer death in screened versus nonscreened women was 1.08 (95% CI, 0.54 to 2.17).

A large trial was conducted in the United Kingdom involving 45,841 women aged 45 to 64 years who were offered annual screening by clinical examination and mammography; 63,636 were taught breast self-examination, and 127,117, for whom no extra services were provided, constituted a control population (759). After 16 years of follow-up, the breast cancer mortality rate was 27% lower in the two screening centers combined than in the four comparison centers. A 35% decrease in mortality rate was observed in mammographically screened women in all cohorts aged 45 to 64 years at entry. There was no evidence of less benefit in women aged 45 to 49 years at initial screening.

Several meta-analyses and overviews support the benefit of screening mammography in younger women. Kerlikowske et al. (397), in a meta-analysis of 13 selected studies, concluded that the overall RR for breast cancer mortality for women aged 50 to 74 years undergoing screening mammography com-

pared with those who did not was 0.74; in contrast, the RR in women aged 40 to 49 years was 0.93. Screening mammography significantly reduced breast cancer mortality rates in women 50 to 74 years of age, whereas there was no reduction in breast cancer mortality rates in women aged 40 to 49 years after 7 to 9 years of follow-up. Feig (195) reviewed the published literature and various issues concerning the potential benefit with mammographic screening of women 40 to 49 years of age. He concluded that with improved mammographic techniques, mortality could be reduced by 35% in women younger than 40 to 49 years of age with two-view annual mammographic screening. Wald et al. (810), in a meta-analysis of six randomized trials, observed a 15% reduction in mortality rate in women 40 to 49 years of age for whom a screening mammography was performed, compared with a reduction of 25% in women aged 50 to 74 years.

In the United States, screening mammography beginning at age 40 years is recommended for the general population (16). For some women at high risk for development of breast cancer, annual screening may be started at an earlier age. These women include those with a personal history of breast cancer, those who have had therapeutic radiation to the breast area especially for Hodgkin's lymphoma, BRCA-positive women, women with a family history of a first-degree relative with breast cancer at a young age, and women with a biopsy diagnosis of lobular carcinoma *in situ* or atypical ductal hyperplasia.

Screening mammography may impact the patterns of breast cancer management with increased use of breast-conservation treatment. Solin et al. (712) analyzed 206 newly diagnosed and treated breast cancers in 201 women from a health maintenance organization. Eligibility for conservation surgery and breast irradiation was significantly increased in women who had undergone mammographic screening compared with women who had not (88% and 60%, respectively) (p <.0001).

Despite some conflicting data in the large randomized trials and meta-analyses summarized above, there is general agreement that screening mammography can have a significant impact on stage of presentation of disease and breast cancer mortality. Given the incidence of breast cancer, promotion of screening for breast cancer is a major public health issue. The National Cancer Institute, American Cancer Society, and the American College of Radiology recommend a baseline mammogram at the age of 35 years (30 years in high-risk groups) (16,805). Repeat examinations should be carried out every 2 years beginning at 40 years of age. In women older than 50 years, mammograms should be performed annually. Risk factor information could be used to determine the optimal frequency of screening.

Digital versus Screen Film Mammography

There has been increased utilization of digital mammography for screening. This technology utilizes a special detector capable of transforming x-ray images into electronic digital image. Advantages include no film processing, faster image acquisition, and less call-backs due to the ability to manipulate the image digitally. Although the digital image resolution is significant, interpretation can be limited by the resolution of the monitor (690,691). In prospective direct comparisons of screen film to digital mammography, the sensitivity of digital and screen film techniques were not significantly different. Results of a large-scale American College of Radiology Imaging Network (ACRIN) trial of 49,000 women, which recently completed accrual, is awaited to further resolve this issue. Given the potential efficiencies and advantages of digital mammography, even with equivalent sensitivities many centers are moving in this direction.

Magnetic Resonance Imaging Screening

The role of MRI screening is rapidly evolving. Although MRI is unlikely to replace mammography for screening of the general population, its use in screening high-risk populations has recently been supported in several studies. In a prospective study by Lehman et al. (440), MRI detected otherwise occult contralateral breast cancers in 4% of women with a recent diagnosis of unilateral breast cancer. In 103 women with unilateral breast cancer, MRI detected four contralateral breast cancers, while mammography detected none. The increased yield was associated with 12% of women having an MRI recommended biopsy, resulting in a 33% positive predictive value.

For women at high risk for breast cancer due to strong family history and/or positive BRCA1–2 status, the standard screening techniques of breast self-examination, clinical breast examination, and mammography may be suboptimal. Nearly half of the cancers in this population are detected by physical examination between routine radiographic surveillance. In this population increased breast density and rapid proliferative rates likely contribute to the relative insensitivity of mammography. Although MRI has not yet been shown to impact on mortality, the sensitivity of MRI over mammography, clinical examination, and ultrasound in this high-risk population has been demonstrated in several studies (420,624,627,812,813). In a surveillance study, 236 women with BRCA1–2 mutations underwent one to three annual screenings with breast examination, mammography, MRI, and ultrasound. Of 22 cancers detected, 17 (77%) were detected by MRI, eight (36%) by mammography, seven (33%) by ultrasound, and two (9.1%) by breast examination. All four screening modalities combined had a sensitivity of 95%, which compared favorably to the 45% sensitivity for mammography and breast examination alone (812).

In a landmark study by Kriege et al. (420), 1,909 eligible women (cumulative lifetime risk of breast cancer of 15% or more) at high risk for familial breast cancer including 358 carriers of germ-line mutations) were screened with an annual MRI and mammography. Within a median follow-up period of 2.9 years, the screening program yielded 51 tumors. The sensitivity of clinical breast examination, mammography, and MRI for detecting invasive breast cancer was 17.9%, 33.3%, and 79.5%,

respectively, and the specificity was 98.1%, 95.0%, and 89.8%, respectively. The overall discriminating capacity of MRI was significantly better than that of mammography ($p < .05$). From this study, it appears that MRI is more sensitive than mammography in detecting tumors in women at high risk for familial breast cancer.

Ultrasound Screening

Although ultrasound is a useful tool as a supplement to mammography in the diagnosis of breast cancer, its use in routine screening of the general population has not been established (1,53,54,181). As with MRI, it is unlikely to replace mammography for screening the general population. However, it may have a role in screening high-risk populations. Currently, ACRIN has completed accrual of a prospective study evaluating ultrasound in screening high-risk women (1). The primary aim is to determine the diagnostic yield of malignancy using whole breast bilateral screening ultrasound combined with mammography versus mammography alone.

Screening by Physical Examination

Two studies have evaluated the effectiveness of screening by breast self-examination alone, the United Kingdom and the Canadian trials. Using Breast Cancer Registry data, Constanza and Foster (129,233) found fewer deaths from breast cancer (14% vs. 26%) and improved estimated 5-year survival rates (75% vs. 59%) among women who reported performing breast self-examination compared with those who did not. In the Breast Cancer Detection Demonstration Project, the estimated overall sensitivity of breast self-examination in detecting breast cancer was 26%, compared with 75% for the combination of clinical breast examination and mammography (668).

Baines et al. (37) reviewed the potential value of breast physical examination in 89,835 women participating in the Canadian National Breast Screening Study, 50% of whom did not have mammography and had only physical examinations performed by nurses. The authors concluded that physical examination of the breast by trained nurses was useful and cost-effective.

Clinical breast examination and self-examination may be complementary to mammography, perhaps detecting interval cancers in the 10% to 12% of cancers not visualized by mammography. Although it is evident that clinical screening is not as sensitive as mammography, the combination of clinical examination and mammography appears to yield optimal results in early detection.

Diagnosis and Work-Up

The work-up of a patient with a breast mass, including complete clinical and family history, is summarized in Table 53.8. The patient should be examined both sitting up and lying down (to confirm masses felt on the sitting-up examination and to detect lesions deeper in the breast or against the chest wall). Careful inspection of both breasts should be made, including size, form, and symmetry, changes in pigmentation, scaling or discharge from the nipple, and dilated veins or edema of the skin in a nonpregnant patient. The location, size, consistency, tenderness, and mobility of the palpable tumor should be recorded. It is useful to draw and photograph the projection of any suspect or palpable masses on the skin of the breast or nodal areas.

In addition to examination of the breast, careful evaluation of the axilla and supraclavicular node areas is mandatory. The number, consistency, tenderness, mobility or fixation, and size of lymph nodes should be noted. Clinically node-negative patients have pathologic involvement in 10% to 40% of cases (depending on primary tumor size), whereas no pathologic evidence of tumor is found in 25% to 30% of patients with clinically palpable axillary nodes.

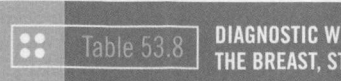

Table 53.8   DIAGNOSTIC WORK-UP FOR CARCINOMA OF THE BREAST, STAGES T1 AND T2

General
  History with emphasis on presenting symptoms, menstrual status, parity, family history of cancer, other risk factors
  Physical examination with emphasis on breast, axilla, supraclavicular area, abdomen

Special tests
  Biopsy (core biopsy directed by physical examination, ultrasound, or mammography as indicated, or needle localization)

Radiologic studies
  Before biopsy
  Mammography/ultrasonography
  Chest radiographs
  Magnetic resonance imaging of breast (selected cases)
  After positive biopsy
  Bone scan (when clinically indicated, for stage II or III disease or elevated serum alkaline phosphatase levels)
  Computed tomography of chest, abdomen and pelvis for stage II or III disease and/or abnormal liver function tests

Laboratory studies
  Complete blood cell count, blood chemistry
  Urinalysis

Other studies
  Hormone receptor status (ER, PR)
  HER2/neu status
  Consider genetic counseling/BRCA testing in selected cases

ER, estrogen receptor; PR, progesterone receptor

Examination of the abdomen for liver enlargement and evaluation for bony pain are also essential. Finally, a complete pelvic examination should be part of the overall evaluation of the patient, if not recently performed by the patient's other physicians.

Laboratory studies include a complete blood count and chemistry profile, including liver function tests (e.g., aspartate aminotransferase, alanine aminotransferase, lactate dehydrogenase, bilirubin).

Imaging in Breast Cancer Diagnosis and Work-up

Routine radiographic studies include chest radiography and bilateral mammograms. As clinically indicated, these may be supplemented by CT scanning, MRI, or positron emission tomography (PET) scans, bone scans, and plain radiographs of *symptomatic* bones, if clinically warranted.

Mammography

Mammography remains the most critical component of diagnostic imaging in breast cancer patients, and bilateral mammograms should be performed routinely in the work-up of the breast cancer patient. The Breast Imaging Reporting and Data Systems (BI-RADS) classification system, outlined in Table 53.9 has been widely adopted in classifying mammograms with respect to appropriate follow-up and/or intervention (546).

Kopans et al. (412) reviewed the advantages and disadvantages of diagnostic imaging techniques for evaluation of patients with breast cancer. Classically, breast carcinoma is seen as an ill-defined mass that may have spiculated margins (Fig. 53.7), although rarely cancers may also be seen with a knobby, lobulated, or even a smooth contour (ultrasonography may distinguish them from cystic masses). Architectural distortion of the breast tissue may be present. The appearance of linear, radiated, or spiculated changes around a central focus should always be considered suspect for carcinoma. The tumor may be hidden by dense parenchyma; review of previous mammogram compression views and sometimes ultrasonograms is very important in detecting subtle interval changes in the appearance of the breast (330).

Calcifications can be associated with either benign or malignant conditions of the breast. However, calcifications

Table 53.9   AMERICAN COLLEGE OF RADIOLOGY BREAST IMAGING REPORTING AND DATA SYSTEMS BI-RADS ASSESSMENT CATEGORIES—MAMMOGRAPHY

Complete Final Assessment Categories

Category 1 Negative	There is nothing to comment on. The breasts are symmetric and no masses, architectural disturbances, or suspect calcifications are present.
Category 2 Benign finding	This is also a negative mammogram, but the interpreter may wish to describe a finding. Involuting, calcified fibroadenomas, multiple secretory calcifications, fat-containing lesions such as oil cysts, lipomas, galactoceles, and mixed-density hamartomas all have characteristic appearances, and may be labeled with confidence. The interpreter might wish to describe intramammary lymph nodes, implants, and the like, while still concluding that there is no mammographic evidence of malignancy.
Category 3 Probably benign finding—short-interval follow-up suggested	A finding placed in this category should have a very high probability of being benign. It is not expected to change over the follow-up interval, but the radiologist would prefer to establish its stability. Data are becoming available that shed light on the efficacy of short-interval follow-up. At present, most approaches are intuitive. These will likely undergo future modification as more data accrue as to the validity of an approach, the interval required, and the type of findings that should be followed.
Category 4 Suspicious abnormality—biopsy should be considered	These are lesions that do not have the characteristic morphologies of breast cancer but have a definite probability of being malignant. The radiologist has sufficient concern to urge a biopsy. If possible, the relevant probabilities should be cited so that the patient and her physician can make the decision on the ultimate course of action.
Category 5 Highly suggestive of malignancy—appropriate action should be taken	These lesions have a high probability of being cancer.
Category 0 Need additional imaging evaluation	Finding for which additional imaging evaluation is needed. This is almost always used in a screening situation and should rarely be used after a full imaging workup. A recommendation for additional imaging evaluation includes the use of spot compression, magnification, special mammographic views, ultrasound, and so forth.

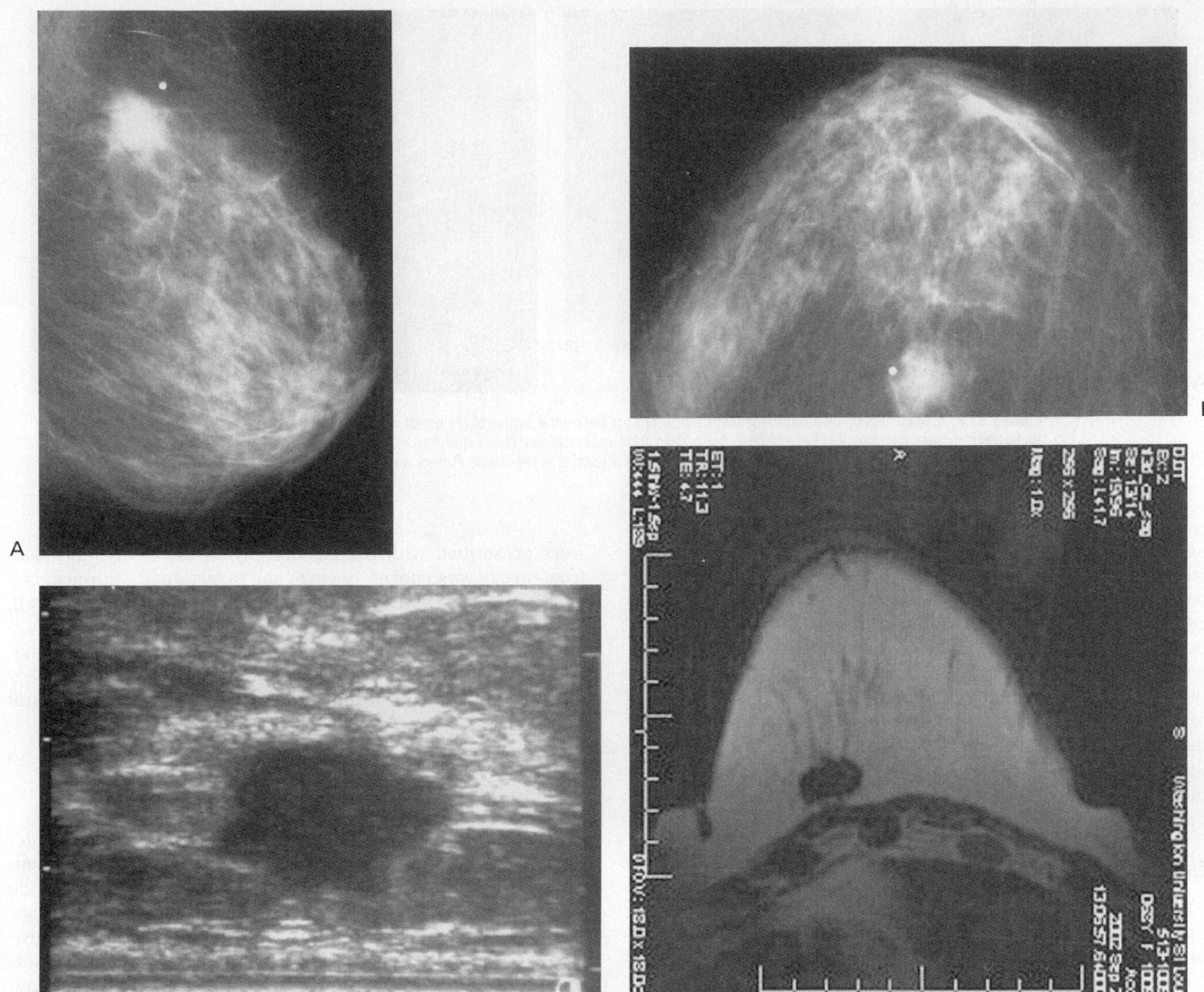

FIGURE 53.7. Medial-lateral (**A**) and cephalad-caudal (**B**) views of mammogram depicting a 1-cm mass with stellate margins deeply located in the upper quadrant of the left breast, histologically proven to be an invasive ductal carcinoma. **C:** Example of ultrasonogram of the breast showing a hypoechoic mass with "shadowing" deeper to the lesion, characteristic of invasive carcinoma. **D:** T1-weighted magnetic resonance image of the breast demonstrating a mass, that proved to be an invasive carcinoma.

associated with malignant tumors are typically 100 to 300 μm in size and are rodlike, tubular, branching, or punctate. Clusters of microcalcifications (more than five) are suggestive of intraductal disease, and in nonpalpable lesions needle localization aids in the diagnosis (Fig. 53.8). For patients undergoing biopsy of a suspicious mass or calcifications, about 30% will yield a diagnosis of malignancy (330). Solin et al. (712) noted that the use of mammographic needle localization breast biopsy increased from 3% in 1977 to 1978 to 26% in 1987 to 1988. The incidence of intraductal carcinoma referred for breast-conservation therapy increased from 6% to 13%.

The average sensitivity of mammography is approximately 90% (60% to 95%), and the specificity is 94% (50% to 98%). The positive predictive value is approximately 8% to 14% for screened patients, but is significantly higher for patients with symptoms or palpable masses (412). If microcalcifications were initially present, radiographs of the surgical specimen and postlumpectomy mammography are important to rule out residual disease for patients considering breast-conservation therapy (155). Lally et al. (431) reported on 114 patients with calcifications on mammography diagnosed with breast cancer. Of

these cases, 75 breasts at risk had no residual suspicious calcifications and proceeded to radiotherapy without further surgery or mammography. Thirty-six breasts at risk proceeded to radiation with either known suspicious calcifications or with nondocumented removal of calcifications after another excision. Of the 36 breasts, there were seven local failures and one regional failure. Of 34 breasts who underwent re-excision after detection of suspicious calcifications by preirradiation mammography, 20 (59%) were found to have residual disease. Patients with documented removal of suspicious calcifications were found to have better local control than patients without documented removal. In addition, the presence of calcifications on a preirradiation mammogram was associated with a high probability of detecting residual disease.

The radiation oncologist should be familiar with the difference between diagnostic and screening mammography, since a majority of conservatively treated breast cancer patients will have undergone diagnostic mammography prior to treatment, as well as in follow-up. Screening mammography refers to routine mammographic images in asymptomatic women and consists of two views: craniocaudal and mediolateral oblique of

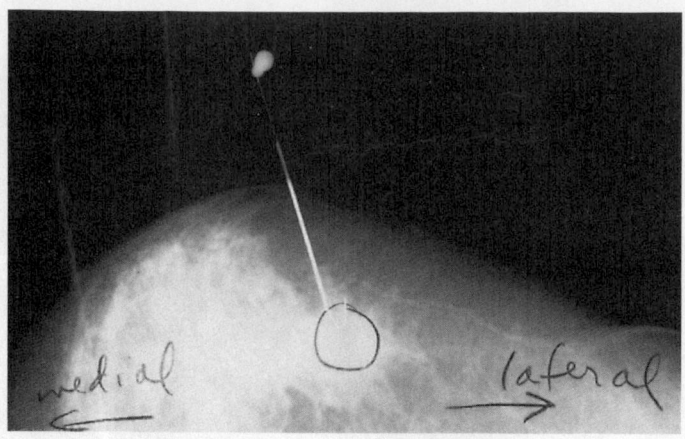
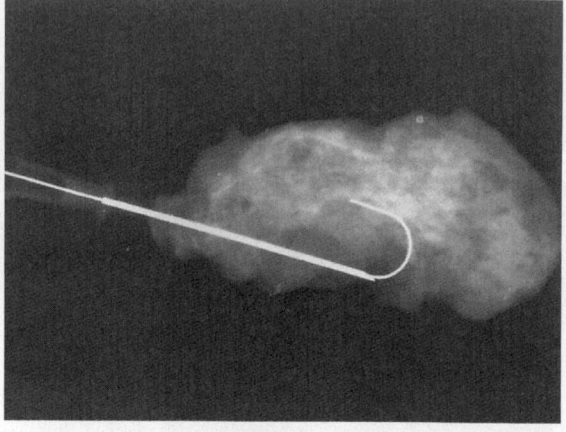

FIGURE 53.8. A: Mammogram demonstrating microcalcifications in the central portion of the breast with needle localization in place. **B:** Radiograph showing microcalcifications in the central portion of the wide excisional biopsy specimen. Pathologic diagnosis was intraductal carcinoma. Postlumpectomy mammogram showed no residual calcifications in the breast. Patient was treated with breast-conservation surgery and irradiation years ago and remains tumor free.

each breast. Diagnostic mammography is used to characterize abnormalities detected at screening or in women with palpable masses, employs additional magnification views, and is generally done with the radiologist present to determine the need for additional views and/or follow-up studies (330). Following breast conservation, most patients will undergo diagnostic mammograms, as additional images are often needed to rule out suspicious findings in the previously radiated breast. Some mammographers recommend reverting to screening studies after several years of stable mammography in the conservatively managed breast cancer patient.

Ultrasound

Ultrasound can be a useful tool to complement physical examination and mammography in the diagnosis and treatment of breast cancer. Its use as a screening tool is limited and is the focus of ongoing investigations, as previously noted. Ultrasonography has a reported sensitivity of 73% and specificity of 95% (696). It is very helpful in differentiating cysts from solid tumors (831), and its primary use is the identification and characterization of palpable and nonpalpable abnormalities of the breast detected by physical examination and/or mammography (330,696). In the evaluation of a palpable mass in 420 patients, if both mammography and ultrasound are negative, Soo et al. (715) reported the negative predictive value to be >99%. This was confirmed in a larger study of 3,516 patients from the Netherlands reported by Flobbe et al. (225).

In addition to complementing physical examination and mammography in diagnosis, ultrasound is often used as a guide for interventional procedures. Ultrasound-guided core biopsies are routinely performed in the diagnosis of breast cancer and have been shown to be more cost effective than stereotactic biopsy. Ultrasound can also be used for fine-needle aspiration biopsies, cyst aspirations, presurgical localizations, and evaluation of breast tissue surrounding implants in the evaluation of intracapsular and extracapsular rupture (330).

Ultrasound can also be used in the evaluation of the lumpectomy site for radiation treatment planning, localization of the boost, and evaluation of depth of the lumpectomy cavity for planning the radiation boost. In an analysis of 54 breasts undergoing boost planning for breast-conserving therapy, Ringash et al. (616) prospectively compared diagnostic ultrasound to the gold standard of surgical clips for localization of the lumpectomy site for electron boost irradiation. All patients had three to six surgical clips defining the excision cavity. Treatment fields

were prescribed with a 2-cm margin on the cavity, and electron energy was chosen to cover the target depth. Surgical clip position was assessed on orthogonal simulator films. Overall, 35/54 (65%) of localizations were adequate, 15/54 (28%) were marginal, and 4/54 (7%) were inadequate. They conclude that diagnostic ultrasound may be used to improve the accuracy of localization of the tumor bed when surgical clips are not present.

Magnetic Resonance Imaging

Although controversial for routine use, the use of MRI to supplement mammography in breast cancer diagnosis and treatment is rapidly increasing (see Fig. 53.7). In a review of MRI in the management of breast cancer, Hylton (365) summarized the potential for the current use of MRI: to complement mammography in screening; for differential diagnosis of questionable findings on physical examination, mammography, and ultrasound; and assessment of response in the neoadjuvant treatment of breast cancers.

In a recent retrospective study of MRI in the management of 441 women with breast cancer, Upponi and Warren (761) reported the indications for MRI studies were diagnostic in 176, monitoring chemotherapy in 126, and study of MRI screening for breast cancer in 139. MRI results were confusing or incorrect in 6% of the diagnostic group, 13% of the chemotherapy group, and 9% of the screening group. The authors report that MRI resulted in an increase in confidence or change in clinical plan in 46% of the diagnostic group, 72% of the chemotherapy group, and 80% of the screening group. In 44/283, MRI caused a beneficial change in the clinical plan based on conventional radiology.

Esserman et al. (188) reported that MRI successfully detected cancer in 55/58 cases. There were two false-positive and two false-negative results, including a nonsignificant enhancement of one lesion. The anatomic extent of disease was correctly identified in 98% of cases by MRI but in only 55% by mammography. The utility of MRI as an adjunct to mammography in problematic cases was investigated by Lee et al. (439). In 86 lesions with equivocal findings on mammography, positive findings were seen in 38 on MRI. Of these, 26 corresponded to areas of mammographic abnormalities. The remaining 12 sites were in areas where no abnormality had been suspected on mammography. Biopsies were performed on all 38 positive sites, and 10 (26%) were found to be malignant.

MRI has a clear role in the evaluation of patients who present with axillary metastasis with no evidence of a primary tumor in the breast by physical examination or mammography. In an analysis from Memorial Sloan-Kettering Cancer Center, Buchanan et al. (85) reported on 55 patients who presented with axillary adenopathy without evidence of distant disease. MRI revealed suspicious lesions in 76% (42/55). In 62% (26/42), the MRI finding proved to be the occult primary tumor, of whom 58% (15/26) were candidates for breast conservation. MRI did not identify the primary tumor in 25 women. Of these 25, 12 underwent mastectomy and cancer was found in 4/12. The authors concluded that breast MRI detects mammographically occult cancer in half of women with axillary metastases and is a valuable tool for patients with occult primary breast cancer.

The use of MRI in 207 women (212 breasts treated) undergoing breast-conserving therapy was reviewed in a study by Tillman et al. (743). All patients presented with clinical stage 0, I, or II disease. How breast MRI affected clinical management was assessed. The MRI findings affected the clinical management in 43 cases (20% of 212 breast cancers). Based on the pathology findings and the overall clinical course for each case, the breast MRI was judged to have had a strongly favorable effect on management in 18 cases (8%), a somewhat favorable effect in six cases (3%), an uncertain effect in five cases (2%), a somewhat unfavorable effect in 11 cases (5%), and a strongly unfavorable effect in three cases (1%). The effect of MRI was significantly greater when the MRI was performed before an excisional biopsy ($p = .0011$) or for larger tumors ($p = .0089$). The authors conclude that breast MRI appears to offer clinically useful information for determining optimal local treatment.

Computed Tomography

There is no established role for CT scans in routine staging of patients with early stage breast cancer. The need for iodine contrast material to differentiate benign from malignant conditions, high radiation dose, cost per study, and inability to detect small lesions precludes the use of CT for initial evaluation, except under special circumstances. Most patients with node-negative breast cancer do not need to undergo routine CT scans for staging, since the yield is exceeding low. A small percentage of women with very high-risk node-negative disease or with node-positive disease may be upstaged by routine CT scans and, although the yield is low, it is common practice to CT stage high-risk node-negative and node-positive breast cancer patients.

Many women undergoing breast-conserving surgery and radiation do have CT scans as part of radiation therapy treatment planning. Without the use of contrast and specific diagnostic imaging protocols, these scans should not be considered as part of a staging procedure. In a study of 153 extended CT scans performed as part of radiation treatment, however, Mehta and Goffinet (490) reported 11% revealed unexpected abnormalities, most of which were nonmalignant. Only 2/153 were found to have occult disease resulting in a change in stage.

Bone Scans

Routine bone scan at the time of initial treatment of stage I and II breast cancer is of limited value and should be reserved for patients with bone pain (741). In patients with stage I disease, the incidence of abnormalities on bone scan is approximately 2%, but a greater incidence of abnormalities is found in stages II (10%) and III (>20%) (91). In a group of 7,604 patients who had bone scan, of over 20,000 women operated on for breast cancer in Denmark, approximately 5% had abnormal study results (740). The incidence of abnormal scan results was greater in patients older than 60 years (8%) than in the younger group

(3%), most likely because of the many benign bone and joint disorders frequently seen in older women.

Koizumi et al. (406) reviewed records from 5,538 patients with breast cancer. The overall incidence of metastasis to bone was 2.13% (0% in patients with stage 0, 0.08% in stage I, 1.09% in stage II, 9.96% in stage III, and 34.04% in stage IV). Bone scans are more commonly recommended in patients with stage II larger tumors (>3 cm), aggressive histopathologic features, and in stage III or IV cancer.

Positron Emission Tomography Scanning

PET using ^{18}F-labeled fluorodeoxyglucose (FDG) scanning, although not a routine component of staging, is being used more frequently in breast cancer. Its application in patients on initial presentation with early stage disease has not been established. However, its potential role in patients with metastatic, advanced, and local–regional relapse of disease is rapidly evolving.

A study by Cachin et al. (95) evaluating PET in 47 women with metastatic breast cancer treated with high-dose chemotherapy reported that a complete response on PET was the most powerful predictor of survival.

In an analysis of PET scanning in 165 patients from British Columbia, Weiretal et al. (823) concluded that there are two clinical situations in which PET appears to be particularly valuable. The first is in the evaluation of patients who are suspected of having a tumor recurrence. The other is in identifying patients with multifocal or distant sites of malignancy who otherwise appear to have an isolated, potentially curable, local–regional recurrence.

Avril et al. (35) preoperatively evaluated 144 patients with masses suggestive of breast cancer with PET imaging. Of 185 breast tumors evaluated histologically, 132 were breast carcinomas and 53 were benign masses. Breast carcinomas were identified with an overall sensitivity of 64.4% for conventional image reading and 80.3% for sensitive image reading. Positive PET scans provided a high positive predictive value (96.6%) for breast cancer.

Schirrmeister et al. (658) also evaluated FDG PET scanning and compared it prospectively with standard staging procedures within 2 weeks before surgery in 117 women who had palpable breast tumors or lesions suggestive of cancer on mammography or ultrasonography. On biopsy, 89 patients were determined to have breast cancer and 28 benign tumors. For interpreting results as being breast cancer, FDG PET had a sensitivity of 93%, a specificity of 78%, an accuracy of 89%, a positive predictive value of 92%, and a negative predictive value of 96%. In detecting multifocal lesions, FDG PET was twice as sensitive (63%) as the combination of mammography and ultrasonography (32%). Distant metastases in three patients were missed with the standard staging procedures but detected with FDG PET. Because FDG PET had a false-negative rate of 20% for detection of lymph node metastases, this imaging method cannot replace histologic evaluation of axillary nodes.

Greco et al. (284) evaluated FDG PET for the preoperative detection of axillary metastases in 167 patients with T1–2 breast carcinomas who underwent axillary dissection following FDG PET. The overall sensitivity of lymph node staging with PET was 94.4% and the overall specificity was 86.3%; the overall accuracy was 89.8%. The PET scans had a positive predictive value of 84% and a negative predictive value of 95.3%.

Summary of Imaging for Breast Cancer

All women should undergo history and physical examination, with mammography and liver function tests. Ultrasound and/or MRI may be useful in selected cases to complement mammography. For women who have operable disease with normal liver function tests, surgical staging of the breast and node sampling is performed. For low-risk patients, no further staging is required. For women with more advanced disease and those being considered for neoadjuvant chemotherapy, preoperative staging would routinely include a bone scan, chest x-ray and CT, and/or abdominal ultrasound. PET scanning may be considered in selected cases.

Pathologic Studies

Histopathologic diagnosis may be obtained by fine-needle aspiration of cystic or solid masses or biopsies of solid masses; any fluid aspirated from the breast should be examined for malignant cells. Fine-needle aspiration of the breast is a simple, low-cost, accurate diagnostic technique that has been used for many years in Europe and is gaining increasing acceptance in the United States (831,847). A potential limitation of fine-needle aspiration is that it provides cytology and no tissue architecture. Therefore, while the presences of malignant cells can be detected, cytology from fine-needle aspiration cannot conclusively differentiate invasive from noninvasive disease. However, for lesions that are palpable or easily visualized on ultrasound, this method results in rapid and efficient diagnosis.

Stereotactic core needle biopsy is increasingly used to obtain a histologic diagnosis with high accuracy, particularly in small breast lesions (556). In 6,152 lesions sampled at multiple institutions, 817 (13.3%) showed infiltrating breast cancer, 167 (2.7%) showed intermediate or high-grade DCIS, and 213 (3.5%) showed atypical hyperplasia or low-grade DCIS. Complete agreement between the core biopsy and subsequent histologic sections was reached in 89.7% of lesions and partial agreement in 9.2%. Clinically significant complications occurred in only 6/3,765 cases (0.2%) for which follow-up was available.

Breast biopsy of any suspicious mass is mandatory. The biopsy usually can be done using local anesthesia; the patient should be informed of the nature of the lesion to allow for her greater participation in therapeutic decisions. There has been no evidence that delay in treatment up to 2 weeks after biopsy worsens prognosis (218).

In nonpalpable lesions, needle localization and radiographic techniques are necessary to identify the tissue to be removed. Failure to remove the mammographic abnormality has been reported in 0% to 8% of patients undergoing needle localization (434). The localizing wires should be left in place in the specimen and a radiograph obtained to ensure that the area of abnormality has been adequately excised. If the specimen radiograph does not document complete tumor removal, an immediate re-excision of the area at the tip of the wire should be carried out. However, specimen mammography may be of questionable benefit in the management or outcome of most patients undergoing image-guided, needle-localized breast biopsies. Bimston et al. (59) reviewed 164 patients who underwent 165 needle/dye-localized breast biopsies for suspect mammographic abnormalities. In only three (1.8%) did the patient clearly benefit from specimen mammography; in no patient was a malignant neoplasm missed.

If there is any question, particularly in patients with microcalcifications, a postbiopsy mammogram should be obtained to determine the completeness of tumor excision (330). The surgeon should prepare (orient) the specimen accordingly, and the margins of the resected breast tissue should be identified and inked before processing. The pathologist should be made aware of the nature of the lesion for appropriate processing of the specimen (664). Radiation oncologists should be familiar with the implications of the diagnostic procedures for carcinoma of the breast as active participants in a breast preservation therapeutic approach.

ER and progesterone receptor (PR) assays are routinely done in the United States in patients with breast cancer; these parameters are correlated with prognosis and tumor response to chemotherapeutic and hormonal agents (453,833). Immunohistochemical (IHC) techniques are commonly employed and correlate well with other hormonal receptor assays. Cellular assays measure the growth fraction (S-phase fraction [SPF]) of tumors, either by thymidine labeling index (TLI) or flow cytometry methods, and other tumor markers have prognostic implications, sometimes independent of tumor stage and hormone receptor status (498,499). HER-2/neu assay is being done routinely because overexpression is associated with poor prognosis, and these patients are currently being offered adjuvant therapy directed at HER2/neu. HER2/neu analysis by fluorescent *in situ* hybridization techniques has recently evolved as the standard for determining response to therapy directed at the HER2/neu oncogene (564,565).

Staging

Two staging systems are widely used for breast cancer: the American Joint Committee on Cancer (AJCC) (Table 53.10) (285) and the Union Internationale Contre le Cancer (UICC) (760) systems. Major changes were made for the sixth edition of the *AJCC Cancer Staging Manual,* the rationale of which was summarized in an article by Singletary et al. (688,689) include:

1. Micrometastases are distinguished from isolated tumor cells on the basis of size and histologic evidence of malignant activity.
2. Identifiers have been added to indicate the use of sentinel lymph node dissection and immunohistochemical or molecular analysis techniques.
3. Major classifications of lymph node status are designated according to the number of involved axillary lymph nodes as determined by routine hematoxylin-and-eosin (H&E) staining (preferred method) or by immunohistochemical staining.
4. The classification of metastasis to the infraclavicular lymph nodes has been added as N3. Metastasis to the supraclavicular lymph nodes has been reclassified as N3 rather than M1.
5. Metastasis to the IMNs, based on the method of detection and the presence or absence of axillary nodal involvement, has been reclassified. Microscopic involvement of the IMNs detected by sentinel lymph node dissection but not by imaging studies (excluding lymphoscintigraphy) or clinical examination is classified as N1. Macroscopic involvement of the IMNs detected by imaging studies (excluding lymphoscintigraphy) or by clinical examination is classified as N2 if it occurs in the absence of metastases to the axillary lymph nodes or as N3 if it occurs in the presence of metastases to the axillary lymph nodes.

The current AJCC staging for breast cancer does not include in the calculation of tumor size additional tumor found at the time of re-excision; this may result in understaging and undertreatment of patients with breast cancer (80). The Columbia staging system is important both historically and because it clearly identifies prognostic factors affecting operability (293). Figure 53.9 depicts the various clinical stages according to tumor and nodal characteristics.

Pathologic Classification

The World Health Organization (WHO) has classified proliferative conditions and tumors of the breast into the following categories: benign mammary dysplasias, benign or apparently benign tumors, carcinoma, sarcoma, carcinosarcoma, and unclassified tumors (654a). The AJCC has developed the alternative system shown in Table 53.11 (285).

Numerous detailed reports and monographs describe the pathologic features and clinical implications of carcinoma of the

Table 53.10 AMERICAN JOINT COMMITTEE ON CANCER STAGING OF BREAST CANCER

Primary Tumor (T)

Definitions for classifying the primary tumor (T) are the same for clinical and for pathologic classification. If the measurement is made by physical examination, the examiner will use the major headings (T1, T2, or T3). If other measurements, such as mammographic or pathologic measurements, are used, the subsets of T1 can be used. Tumors should be measured to the nearest 0.1-cm increment.

TX	Primary tumor cannot be assessed
T0	No evidence of primary tumor
Tis	Carcinoma *in situ*
Tis (DCIS)	Ductal carcinoma *in situ*
Tis (LCIS)	Lobular carcinoma *in situ*
Tis (Paget's)	Paget's disease of the nipple with no tumor

Note: Paget's disease associated with a tumor is classified according to the size of the tumor.

T1	Tumor 2 cm or less in greatest dimension
T1mic	Microinvasion 0.1 cm or less in greatest dimension
T1a	Tumor more than 0.1 cm but not more than 0.5 cm in greatest dimension
T1b	Tumor more than 0.5 cm but not more than 1 cm in greatest dimension
T1c	More than 1 cm but not more than 2 cm in greatest dimension
T2	Tumor more than 2 cm but not more than 5 cm in greatest dimension
T3	Tumor more than 5 cm in greatest dimension
T4	Tumor of any size with direct extension to chest wall[†] or skin, only as described below
T4a	Extension to chest wall, not including pectoralis muscle
T4b	Edema (including *peau d'orange*) or ulceration of the skin of the breast or satellite skin nodules confined to the same breast
T4c	Both (T4a and T4b)
T4d	Inflammatory carcinoma

Regional Lymph Nodes (N)

NX	Regional lymph nodes cannot be assessed (e.g., previously removed)
N0	No regional lymph node metastasis
N1	Metastasis to movable ipsilateral axillary lymph node(s)
N2	Metastasis to ipsilateral axillary lymph node(s) fixed or matted, or in clinically apparent[a] ipsilateral internal mammary nodes in the absence of clinically evident axillary lymph node metastasis
N2a	Metastasis in ipsilateral axillary lymph nodes fixed to one another (matted) or to other structures
N2b	Metastasis only in clinically apparent[a] ipsilateral internal mammary nodes and in the absence of clinically evident axillary lymph node metastasis
N3	Metastasis to ipsilateral mammary lymph node(s) with or without axillary lymph node involvement, or in clinically apparent[a] ipsilateral internal mammary lymph node(s) and in the presence of clinically evident axillary lymph node metastasis; or metastasis in ipsilateral supraclavicular lymph node(s) with or without axillary or internal mammary lymph node involvement
N3a	Metastasis in ipsilateral infraclavicular lymph node(s)
N3b	Metastasis in ipsilateral internal mammary lymph node(s) and axillary lymph node(s)
N3c	Metastasis in ipsilateral supraclavicular lymph node(s)

Pathologic Classification (pN)

pNX	Regional lymph nodes cannot be assessed (e.g., previously removed or not removed for pathologic study)
PN0	No regional lymph node metastasis histologically, no additional examination for isolated tumor cells (ITC)

Note: ITC are defined as single tumor cells or small cell clusters not greater than 0.2 mm, usually detected only by immunohistochemical (IHC) or molecular methods but which may be verified on hematoxylin and-eosin stains. ITCs do not usually show evidence of malignant activity (e.g., proliferation or stromal reaction).

pN0(i −)	No regional lymph node metastasis histologically, negative IHC
pN0(i+)	No regional lymph node metastasis histologically, positive IHC, no IHC cluster greater than 0.2 mm
pN0(mol −)	No regional lymph node metastasis histologically, negative molecular findings (reverse transcriptase polymerase chain reaction [RT-PCR])
pN0(mol+)	No regional lymph node metastasis histologically, positive molecular findings (RT-PCR)
pN1	Metastasis in 1 to 3 axillary lymph nodes, and/or in internal mammary nodes with microscopic disease detected by sentinel lymph node dissection but not clinically apparent[b]
pN1mi	Micrometastasis (greater than 0.2 mm, none larger than 2.0 cm)
pN1a	Metastasis in 1 to 3 axillary lymph nodes
pN1b	Metastasis in internal mammary nodes with microscopic disease detected by sentinel node dissection but not clinically apparent[c]
pN1c	Metastasis in 1 to 3 axillary lymph nodes and in internal mammary lymph nodes with microscopic disease detected by sentinel lymph node dissection but not clinically apparent[c]. (If associated with greater than 3 positive axillary lymph nodes, the internal mammary nodes are classified as Pn3b to reflect increased tumor burden.)
pN2	Metastasis in 4 to 9 axillary lymph nodes, or in clinically apparent[d] internal mammary lymph nodes in the absence of axillary lymph node metastasis
pN2a	Metastasis in 4 to 9 axillary lymph nodes (at least one tumor deposit greater than 2.0 mm)
pN2b	Metastasis in clinically apparent[b] internal mammary lymph nodes in the absence of axillary lymph node metastasis
pN3	Metastasis in 10 or more axillary lymph nodes, or in infraclavicular lymph nodes, or in clinically apparent[b] ipsilateral internal mammary lymph nodes in the presence of 1 or more positive axillary lymph nodes; or in more than 3 axillary lymph nodes with clinically negative microscopic metastasis in internal mammary lymph nodes or in ipsilateral supraclavicular lymph nodes
pN3a	Metastasis in 10 or more axillary lymph nodes (at least one tumor deposit greater than 2.0 mm), or metastasis to the infraclavicular lymph nodes
pN3b	Metastasis in clinically apparent[b] ipsilateral internal mammary lymph nodes in the presence of 1 or more positive axillary lymph nodes; or in more than 3 axillary lymph nodes and in internal mammary lymph nodes with microscopic disease detected by sentinel lymph node dissection but not clinically apparent[c]
pN3c	Metastasis in ipsilateral supraclavicular lymph nodes

Distant Metastasis (M)

MX	Distant metastasis cannot be assessed
M0	No distant metastasis
M1	Distant metastasis

[a]Clinically apparent is defined as detected by imaging studies (excluding lymphoscintigraphy) or by clinical examination or grossly visible pathologically.

[b]Clinically apparent is defined as detected by imaging studies (excluding lymphoscintigraphy) or by clinical examination.

[c]Not clinically apparent is defined as not detected by imaging studies (excluding lymphoscintigraphy) or by clinical examination.

From Greene FL, Page DL, Fleming ID, et al., eds. *AJCC cancer staging manual*, 6th ed. New York: Springer-Verlag, 2002:227–228, with permission.

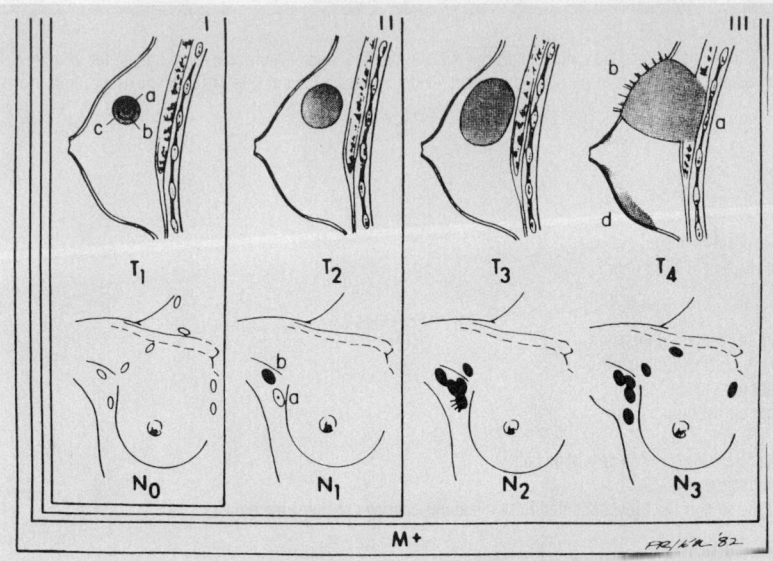

FIGURE 53.9. Clinical staging of carcinoma of the breast. Stages, in part, reflect curability by locoregional treatment modalities prognostically (surgery and radiation therapy). The equivalence of T and N categories are as follows: T2 = N1, T3 = N2, T4 = N3. The American Joint Committee on Cancer and Union Internationale Contre le Cancer classification systems use similar categories and stages. (From Langmuir VK, Poulter CA, Qazi R, et al. Breast cancer, In: Rubin P, ed. *Clinical oncology: a multidisciplinary approach for physicians and students*, 7th ed. Philadelphia: W.B. Saunders, 1993; with permission.)

breast, which are reviewed elsewhere (222,223,330,631,632). The radiation oncologist should be familiar with the histologic characteristics of breast cancer because many of them affect prognosis and may have important therapeutic implications. Brief descriptions of several types of carcinoma of the breast follow.

Microinvasive carcinoma is defined as "the extension of cancer cells beyond the basement membrane into the adjacent tissues with no focus more than 0.1 cm in greatest dimension." Lesions that fulfill this definition are staged as T1mic, a subset of T1 breast cancer. The AJCC staging manual further states that "when there are multiple foci of microinvasion, the size of only the largest focus is used to classify the microinvasion" and that the size of the individual foci should not be added together. Widely varying definitions of microinvasion have been used, and some differ substantially from that offered here (285).

Invasive (infiltrating) ductal carcinoma (IDC) is the most common type of breast cancer, comprising more than 50% of

all cases. It appears as solid cords or groups of ductal tumor cells varying in size and cytoplasmic content and degree of differentiation (846). Necrosis is rare, but lymphatic invasion may be present. An associated *in situ* component is frequently seen.

Tubular carcinoma is composed of tubular structures typically lined by a single layer of well-differentiated epithelium. The tubular cells simulate those of normal ducts or ductules, are arranged in multiglandular cribriform or adenocystic configurations, and are frequently associated with other *in situ* carcinomas of the breast (485). Tubular carcinomas have a nonaggressive growth pattern, with an excellent prognosis. A meta-analysis of 680 women showed an overall frequency of nodal metastasis of 13.8% (553). In view of the low incidence of axillary node metastases at presentation (7%) in low-risk tubular carcinoma of the breast (≤1 cm), some have advocated that axillary dissection may be omitted. In a retrospective review of 73 cases of tubular carcinoma, Sullivan et al. (725) reported treatment with conservative surgery (CS) plus radiation therapy in 67%, CS without radiation therapy in 18%, and mastectomy in 15%. The published literature of 529 conservatively treated tubular carcinomas was reviewed along with the 62 conservative cases from their series. No patients developed distant metastasis or died from disease. Local failure occurred in three (4%) of the cases. The literature review showed that adjuvant radiation therapy reduces local failure following CS for tubular carcinoma.

Medullary carcinoma is composed of cords and masses of large cells with reticular pleomorphic nuclei containing prominent nucleoli. There is a scant fibrous stroma, but lymphoid infiltrate is prominent. These tumors are microscopically and grossly well circumscribed. Prognosis, in general, is better than for other tumors. These tumors are more frequently seen in younger women and are commonly associated with patients with BRCA1 mutations (809).

Invasive lobular carcinoma (ILC) may be interspersed with LCIS; the cells appear singly or in small clusters in a targetoid or single-file pattern. Some scirrhous carcinomas probably are invasive lobular lesions; these tumors tend to be aggressive and multicentric and are prone to development of distant metastases. Du Toit et al. (168) reported five subtypes of lobular carcinomas in 171 cases and observed a 12-year actuarial survival rate of 100% for the tubulolobular subtype but of only 47% for the solid variant. Two other characteristics of invasive lobular carcinoma are that it is often "mammographically silent," meaning its detection or the full appreciation of extent of disease

Table 53.11	**AMERICAN JOINT COMMITTEE ON CANCER HISTOPATHOLOGIC CLASSIFICATION OF BREAST TUMORS**

In situ carcinomas
NOS
Intraductal (*in situ*)
Paget's disease and intraductal

Invasive carcinomas
NOS
Ductal
Inflammatory
Medullary, NOS
Medullary with lymphoid stroma
Mucinous
Papillary (predominantly micropapillary pattern)
Tubular
Lobular
Paget's disease
Undifferentiated
Squamous cell
Adenoid cystic
Secretory
Cribriform

NOS, not otherwise specified
From Greene FL, Page DL, Fleming ID, et al., eds. *AJCC cancer staging manual*, 6th ed. New York: Springer-Verlag, 2002, with permission.

is often not visualized mammographically, and they are much more commonly ER-positive than invasive ductal carcinoma. Infiltrating pleomorphic lobular carcinoma, an aggressive variant of ILC, was described in 38 cases; 29% of the specimens demonstrated signet ring cells (500).

Mucinous carcinoma, also called *mucoid* or *colloid carcinoma,* has been observed in older women with relatively long duration of symptoms (679). It is more likely to be devoid of a cellular reaction; necrosis and lymphatic invasion are very rare. It is slowly growing with a pushing border and has a low frequency of axillary lymph node metastasis. Survival is appreciably better than with IDC (531). Anan et al. (20) evaluated 76 patients with mucinous carcinoma (52 pure type and 24 mixed type). The incidence of lymphatic vessel invasion (4%) and nodal involvement (4%) were lower in pure mucinous carcinoma than in mixed carcinoma ($p <.05$). No nodal involvement occurred in patients with pure mucinous carcinoma <3 cm in diameter.

Adenocystic carcinoma is rarely found in the breast. Histologic features and clinical behavior are similar to its counterpart in the salivary gland and the upper respiratory tract (645). In 28 patients, only one had axillary node metastases; 22 were treated with mastectomy and six with local excision (with breast irradiation in five). With a median follow-up of 7 years, there were no local recurrences; the 5-year disease-free survival rate was 95% (27).

Invasive micropapillary carcinoma of the breast is characterized by growth of tumor cell clusters in prominent clear spaces resembling dilated angiolymphatic vessels. Nasser et al. (521) reported on 83 invasive micropapillary carcinomas; the mean tumor size was 4 cm, 22% invaded skin, 58% were poorly differentiated, and 71% were ER positive. Axillary node metastases were present in 77% of cases and were typically multiple (51% had three or more positive). Forty-six percent of the patients died from their disease (mean interval to death, 36 months). Skin involvement and nodal status were the only parameters predictive of poor survival ($p = .01$).

Metaplastic carcinoma is relatively rare. Park et al. (555) noted axillary lymph node metastasis in 6/15 patients (40%) in whom axillary node dissection was performed. A recent analysis by Beatty et al. (44) of the Swedish Cancer Institute identified 24 cases that were compared with typical breast cancer cases matched for age, date of diagnosis, stage, and ER/PR/HER2 status. The mean metaplastic primary tumor diameter was 2.5 cm. The histological/nuclear grade was high in 21/24 cases. ER and/or PR receptor status was negative in all cases. HER2 was negative in 10/11 cases tested. Epidermal growth factor receptor (EGFR) (HER1) was positive in 7/7 cases tested. Five-year survival was 83% (95% confidence interval, 66% to 100%). Comparison with matched typical breast cancer cases revealed no significant difference in multidisciplinary treatment patterns, recurrence, or survival. The increased expression of EGFR (HER1) provides an opportunity for targeted tumor therapy in these tumors.

In an analysis of the M.D. Anderson Cancer Center experience and the SEER database, Hennessey et al. (345) identified 100 patients with metaplastic sarcomatoid carcinoma and 213 patients in the SEER database with similar histology. They conclude that these are aggressive tumors with poor response to therapy and poor outcomes, also suggesting that studies evaluating novel targeted therapy are needed for these patients.

Spindle cell carcinoma of the breast, a variant of metaplastic carcinoma, includes a wide spectrum of lesions with mildly atypical features that may resemble fasciitis, fibromatosis, or myofibroblastic tumors. Unlike spindle cell carcinomas in general, they have no propensity for distant metastasis and should be termed *tumors* rather than *carcinomas*. Sneige et al. (705) studied 24 cases of fibromatosislike spindle cell breast carcinoma. Treatment consisted of local excision (seven cases) or modified radical mastectomy (13 cases), and was not specified

in four cases. In patients who underwent axillary nodal dissection, no lymph node metastases were found. Local recurrences developed in 2/6 patients who underwent local excision only.

Primary neuroendocrine small cell carcinoma is uncommon. Francois et al. (249) reported seven cases and Shin et al. (678) described nine cases. Immunohistochemical analysis showed consistent staining for cytokeratin markers but variable staining with neuroendocrine markers. The histologic type and prognosis are identical to those of lung cancer. It is important to distinguish these lesions from metastatic lung tumors or direct invasion of breast by Merkel cell carcinoma, lymphoma, or carcinoid tumor. It is reasonable to treat these patients with aggressive multiagent chemotherapy, excision of the primary tumor, and breast irradiation, although no data are available on the outcome of this approach.

Paget's disease describes involvement of the nipple by tumor. Most investigators agree that it represents extension of neoplasms from subjacent ducts in the nipple or metastases from an underlying carcinoma (811). The tumor seems to travel linearly down the ducts and may appear to be multicentric. There may be an associated subareolar tumor. Breast-conserving surgery followed by radiation is effective in this disease (58,476).

Cystosarcoma phyllodes is usually a benign lesion; in broad, fibrous beads that look "leaflike" are cystic clefts lined by a single layer of cells. These tumors are large; usually they are encapsulated, without invasion of the adjacent breast (293). The lesions frequently develop from pre-existing fibromas and have a long initial period of slow growth followed by a sudden, rapid increase in size. The grade (mitotic rate), surgical margins, and proliferative index have prognostic importance (184). In a report by Treves and Sunderland (752) of 77 patients, 18 lesions were classified as malignant, 18 as borderline, and 41 as benign. Distant metastases developed in nine patients with malignant tumors.

Primary mammary lymphomas are rare. In a study of 35 cases, including 16 primary lymphomas, diffuse large cell lymphoma was present in 10/16 primary and 14/18 secondary cases (26). Lymphoepithelial lesions in ducts and lobules and frequent vascular involvement were found in both primary and secondary cases. Immunohistochemistry studies of 13 tumors showed that 12 were B-cell in origin, and one a primary T-cell lymphoma. Survival was related to stage and histologic characteristics. Half of the patients with primary lymphoma had recurrent disease. Although some local recurrences were observed, recurrence in other extranodal sites predominated.

Sarcomas of the primary breast are occasionally seen. McGowan et al. (486) described 78 cases of primary breast sarcoma without metastatic disease (76 women, two men); 32 patients had malignant cystosarcoma phyllodes, and the others had stromal sarcomas (14 patients), angiosarcomas (eight patients), fibrosarcomas (seven patients), carcinosarcomas (five patients), liposarcomas (four patients), or other lesions (eight patients). The cause-specific survival rate was 48% the relapse-free rate was 42% and the local relapse-free rate was 75% at 10 years. No statistically significant difference in outcome was noted between those treated with conservation surgery and those undergoing mastectomy. Patients with negative margins had a significantly better local relapse-free rate than did those with positive margins (80% vs. 33%; $p = .009$).

Prognostic Factors for Survival and Metastasis

Carcinoma of the breast represents a wide spectrum of tumors with a variety of clinical, biological, and genetic characteristics resulting in a considerable variation in prognosis. It is important to understand, particularly from the radiation on-cologists' perspective, that prognostic factors for systemic re-lapses and prognostic factors for local relapse differ signifi-cantly. Furthermore, prognostic factors for local relapse after mastectomy differ substantially from prognostic factors for lo-cal relapse after lumpectomy and radiation (782). For example, tumor size and nodal status are clearly among the strongest pre-dictors of overall survival and metastasis and are also strong predictors of postmastectomy chest wall relapse when radia-tion is not used (330,604,830). However, these factors have not been consistently reported to be prognostic factors for breast relapse after cancer surgery. On the other hand, margin sta-tus is a strong predictor of relapse in the conservatively treated breast, but is not strongly correlated with distant metastasis (539,704,794). Young age is also a very strong predictor of lo-cal relapse after breast-conserving therapy, and although it has been shown to be predictive of systemic metastasis, the effect of young age on distant metastasis as an independent factor is clearly not as significant as it is for local relapse in the conser-vatively managed patient (850). Patients, as well as clinicians, often become confused regarding these issues, resulting in mis-conceptions regarding appropriate decision making and treat-ment. Below, prognostic factors for systemic relapse (i.e., distant metastasis, disease-free, and overall survival) are discussed. A more in-depth discussion of prognostic factors for local relapse following lumpectomy and radiation is included later in the section on selection factors for the conservative management of breast cancer. Prognostic factors related to postmastectomy chest wall recurrence for patients with early stage disease are discussed in Chapter 54.

There have been numerous studies correlating clinical and pathologic features of the primary tumor and/or nodal disease with prognosis. Over the past 20 years the rapid development and expansion of technology in molecular and genetic analysis has been accompanied by an exponential increase in studies evaluating molecular and genetic profiles of tumors as prog-nostic factors.

The College of American Pathologists presented a Consen-sus Statement in 1999 summarizing prognostic factors in breast cancer (223). Factors were category I if they were proven to be of prognostic importance and useful in clinical patient manage-ment. Category II factors had been extensively studied biologi-cally and clinically, but their importance remains to be validated in studies. Category III included all other factors not sufficiently studied to demonstrate their prognostic value.

Category I included tumor size, lymph node status, mi-crometastasis, histologic grade, mitotic count, and hormonal re-ceptor status. Category II included HER-2/neu expression, p53 mutations, lymphovascular invasion, and DNA ploidy. Category III included tumor angiogenesis, EGFR, transforming growth factor, Bcl-2, and cathepsin D overexpression.

More recently, based on advances in molecular techniques allowing for genetic profiling of tumors, additional molecular prognostic factors have been identified, which can further refine clinical decision making and are already being applied clinically. In this section, we will focus on the category I and category II factors and discuss more recently introduced promising prog-nostic factors that may influence distant metastasis and clinical management.

Tumor Size

The size of the primary tumor ranks among the strongest pre-dictors of distant metastasis, disease-free, and overall survival. Although tumor size correlates strongly with the presence and number of involved axillary lymph nodes, it is clearly an in-dependent prognostic factor. Among patients with documented node-negative disease, tumor size remains a strong and in-dependent predictor of disease-free and overall survival. In a

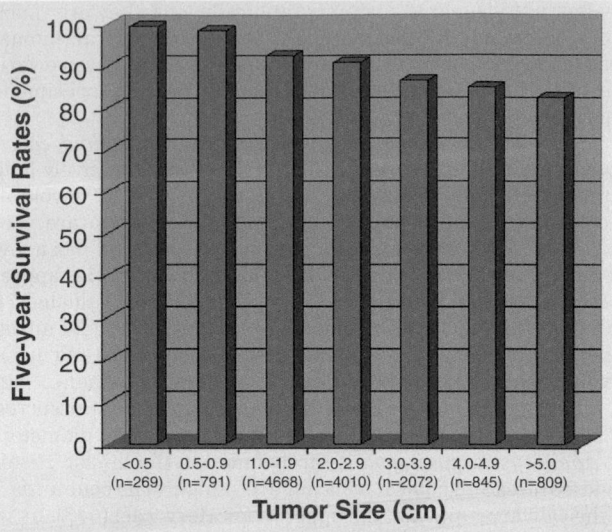

FIGURE 53.10. Five-year survival according to tumor size in node-negative breast cancers. (Data adapted from Carter CL, Allen C, Henson DE. Relation of tumor size, lymph node status and survival in 24,740 breast cancer cases. *Cancer* 1989;63:181–187.)

classic study with an over 20-year follow-up, Rosen et al. (632) reported a recurrence-free survival rate of 88% for tumors <1 cm, 72% for tumors 1.1 to 3 cm, and 59% for tumors 3.1 to 5 cm. In an analysis of 826 women with node-negative breast cancer treated by mastectomy at the University of Chicago with a median follow-up of 13.5 years, Quiet et al. (592) reported a 20-year disease-free survival of 79% for patients with tumors <2 cm, compared to 64% with tumors >2 cm. In multivariate analysis, the strongest predictor of outcome and time to relapse was pathologic tumor size. Survival as a function of primary tu-mor size in node-negative breast cancer patients is illustrated in Figure 53.10.

Axillary Nodal Status

Of all prognostic factors, nodal status continues to be the strongest predictor of disease-free and overall survival and is the primary factor that governs breast cancer staging (285) (Fig. 53.11). Although there is a direct relationship between the num-ber of axillary nodes involved and the risk of distant metastasis, the most commonly employed schema is to group patients into four prognostic categories (node negative, 1 to 3 involved nodes, 4 to 9 involved nodes, and >10 involved nodes). These nodal prognostic categories are employed in the N-staging of the cur-rent AJCC staging system. Although outcomes will continually improve as systemic therapies advance, data from previous NS-ABP trials treated primarily with local–regional therapy alone revealed 5-year survival rates of 82.8% for node negative, 73% for 1 to 3 positive nodes, 45.7% for 4 to 12 positive nodes, and 28.4% for >13 positive nodes (205,212,214,218).

Micrometastasis

The influence of microscopic disease in the lymph nodes has been the subject of several recent analyses due to the increased detection of micrometastasis in the era of sentinel lymph node biopsy. Most recent studies have demonstrated that by using a combination of blue dye and radiolabeled colloid techniques the sentinel node can be identified in >95% of cases (415,417,418). In experienced hands, false negative sentinel node rates are low (<10%), and prognosis of sentinel node-negative patients is similar to node-negative patients who have undergone a

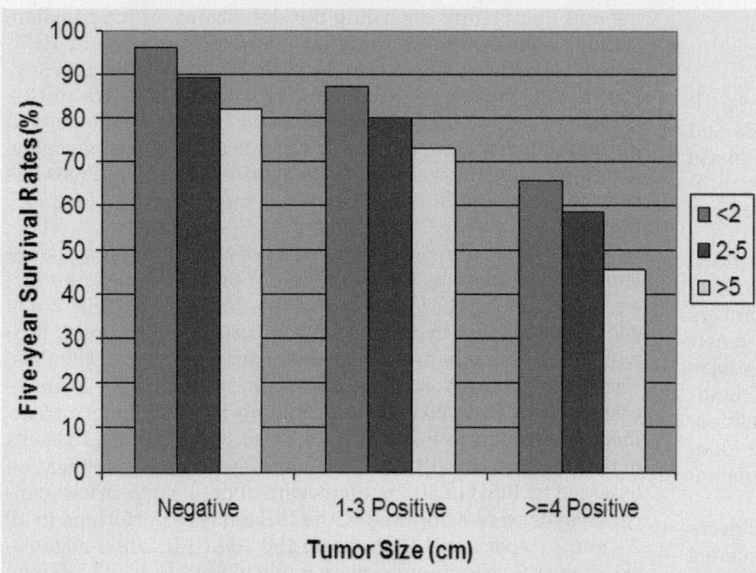

FIGURE 53.11. Five-year survival according to tumor size and nodal status. (Data adapted from Carter CL, Allen C, Henson DE. Relation of tumor size, lymph node status and survival in 24,740 breast cancer cases. *Cancer* 1989;63:181–187.)

complete axillary dissection. Although practice patterns are changing and the need for completion axillary dissection in sentinel node-positive patients has been challenged, the majority of sentinel node-positive patients go to complete axillary dissection where the prognosis will be governed by the number of axillary nodes involved.

Hansen et al. (326) evaluated the sentinel node in 696 women by H&E and IHC. With a median follow-up of 38 months the size of the sentinel node metastasis (<2 mm or >2 mm) was a significant prognostic factor. There was no difference in disease-free survival or overall survival, however between true node-negative and IHC only positive cases. Additional data from large databases will continue to emerge in the coming years to further refine the prognostic significance of micrometastasis and IHC only positive lymph node metastasis in breast cancer patients.

Tumor Type

The histologic subtype of invasive cancer has been shown to be of prognostic value in several studies. The tubular, mucinous, and medullary subtypes have been shown to have a more favorable prognosis, compared to invasive ductal (632,725,742,824). Invasive lobular tumors appear to have a prognosis similar to invasive ductal tumors (653). Poor prognostic categories include metaplastic, undifferentiated, and other rarer subtypes (221,330). In a classic analysis of 293 T2-N0 breast cancers with over 20-year follow-up treated by mastectomy, Rosen et al. (632) reported more favorable relapse rates in medullary, mucinous, tubular, and papillary subtypes, compared to invasive ductal and invasive lobular tumors.

Tumor Grade

Multiple tumor grading systems have been proposed in an effort to standardize and improve interobserver variability. The Scarff-Bloom-Richardson (66) classification system utilizes mitotic index, differentiation, and pleomorphism, each with scores of 1 to 3. Scores of 3 to 5 are well differentiated, 6 to 7 moderately differentiated, and 8 to 9 poorly differentiated. This system is commonly employed and has been shown to be of independent prognostic significance.

Elston and Ellis (185), of the Nottingham group, refined this methodology. The revised technique involves evaluation of three morphological features: the percentage of tubule formation, the

degree of nuclear pleomorphism, and an accurate mitotic count using a defined field area. A numerical scoring system is used and the overall grade is derived from a summation of individual scores for the three variables, and three grades of differentiation are used. Histological grade, assessed in 1,831 patients, shows a very strong correlation with prognosis; patients with grade I tumors have a significantly better survival than those with grade II and III tumors (*p* <.0001). If the protocol is followed, reproducible and consistent results regarding prognosis can be obtained.

Estrogen and Progesterone Hormonal Receptors in Tumor Cells

Several studies have indicated that patients with hormonal receptors have a significantly higher survival rate (487,488). Crowe et al. (132) studied 1,392 patients with carcinoma of the breast treated with modified radical mastectomy. ER-positive tumors (≥3 fmol/mg cytosol protein) were found in 1,063 patients (76.4%). Their 10-year overall survival rate of 65.9% was significantly better than the 56% rate in 329 patients with ER-negative tumors (*p* = .0001).

However, this correlation is not consistent with conflicting reports regarding the prognostic significance of hormonal receptor status (754). The apparent discrepancy in some of these reports may be explained by technical nuances. Esteban et al. (189) noted that quantitative immunohistochemistry of ERs provides results with better predictive value than the biochemically procured ones (261).

Tumors that express both ER and PR have the greatest benefit from hormonal therapy, but those containing only ER or PR still have significant responses. Two types of ERs, ER-α and ER-β, have now been identified. PR also exists in two forms, PR-A and PR-B (549). Patients with tumors negative for hormonal receptors have only a small probability of responding to hormonal therapy (549,833).

Lymphatic and Vascular Invasion

Lymphatic and vascular invasion (LVI) in the peritumoral region has been clearly demonstrated to be of independent prognostic significance in several studies (186,287,325,347,753). In the study by Rosen et al. (632), recurrence rate for LVI-positive stage I patients was 38% compared to 22% for LVI-negative patients.

Proliferative Indices/S-Phase/Thymidine Labeling Index

Various techniques for evaluating the proliferative rate of a tumor have been shown to correlate with distant metastasis and survival. The most common are the fraction of cells in S-phase (SPF), TLI, mitotic index, or antibodies directed against proliferative markers such as Ki-67 and PCNA (proliferating cell nuclear antigen).

Thymidine labeling represents the fraction of cells in the S-phase of the cell cycle and is based on the active incorporation of labeled thymidine into DNA; the TLI of primary breast cancers appears closely related to steroid receptor status and generally unrelated to pathologic stage. Retrospective analyses have shown that TLI is a prognostic indicator independent of tumor size, steroid receptors, and p53 and Bcl-2 protein expression. Together with patient age and tumor size, TLI is able to identify patients at different levels of risk for locoregional or distant metastases (13).

Wenger and Clark (825) concluded that despite different techniques and cutpoints, a higher SPF is in general associated with worse tumor grade, absence of steroid receptors, larger tumors, and positive axillary lymph nodes. Higher SPF is usually associated with worse disease-free and overall survival rates in both univariate and multivariate analyses.

Bryant et al. (84), in over 4,000 patients from NSABP Protocol B-14 who had ER-positive tumors and no axillary lymph node involvement, found a strong association between SPF and disease-free and overall survival rates.

DNA Ploidy Index

Most breast cancers exhibit a bimodal distribution of DNA values. DNA ploidy as measured by flow cytometry correlates with nuclear grade, with low-grade tumors being diploid and high-grade tumors being aneuploid (558). Ploidy was found to be associated with histologic type, tumor grade, and SPF values, but not with patient age, menopausal status, tumor size, axillary nodal status, ER status, or PR status (256). Diploid tumors tend to be ER positive, whereas aneuploid tumors are frequently ER-negative. Older patients are more likely to have hyperdiploid tumors (733). Diploid tumors tend to have a better prognosis than those with an aneuploid DNA distribution (180,387). Toikkanen et al. (746), in 351 patients monitored for a minimum of 22 years, observed a 25-year survival rate of 28% for patients with nondiploid tumors, in contrast to 48% for those with a diploid DNA pattern. In a European Organisation for Research and Treatment of Cancer (EORTC) trial evaluation of DNA, proliferative compartment was the most important predicting factor for overall survival and metastasis-free survival in 281 premenopausal, lymph node negative patients with invasive carcinoma of the breast (463).

Studies by Ewers et al. (192) and Fallenius et al. (194) also confirm the prognostic significance of DNA ploidy. Keyhani-Rofagha et al. (398) and Witzig et al. (834) reported no statistically significant prognostic significance of DNA ploidy.

HER-2/neu

The HER-2/neu proto-oncogene (also called c-erbB-2) located on chromosome 17 codes for a transmembrane glycoprotein, p185, which has tyrosine kinase activity and is homologous to the EGFR (692). It is amplified or overexpressed in up to 30% of in human breast carcinoma. Overexpression of the protein is associated with tumor aggressiveness and decreased disease-free survival in node-positive patients, with variable prognostic significance among node-negative patients. The conflicting reports regarding the prognostic significance of HER-2/neu may be related to interobserver variability in interpretation of stain-

ing and uncertainty regarding the significance of intermediate staining (564,565,692). Staining for overexpression of HER-2/neu is interpreted on a 0 to 3+ scale. The available data suggest that the majority of 0 to 1 staining is clearly negative and 3+ is clearly positive, while the classification of those patients with 2+ staining remains uncertain. Amplification of the oncogene identified using fluorescent *in situ* hybridization techniques has been found to be of more prognostic value (179,351,564,565, 692).

Variability in the prognostic value of HER-2/neu may be related to variability in interpretation of protein expression levels. Hoang et al. (351) compared the detection of HER-2/neu gene amplification by fluorescence *in situ* hybridization (FISH) with detection by immunohistochemistry using two antibodies. The low interobserver reproducibility in separating 2+ from 3+ cases necessitates further confirmation by FISH before treatment decisions are made. Birner et al. (60) correlated results of the Hercep test with HER-2/neu oncogene gene amplification assessed by FISH in 303 patients with node-positive breast cancer. Results were compared with FISH analysis performed in all 2+ and 3+ specimens (103 cases) and 104 HER-2/neu-negative specimens; 3+ carcinomas were found in 8.9% to 15.7% of specimens. FISH revealed that almost exclusively 3+ positive cases had HER-2/neu gene amplification. In univariate analysis, staining with the Hercep test revealed a worse prognosis in 3+ cases, which were significantly associated with lower ER levels and histologic grade III tumors.

More critical than its prognostic significance, however, is the predictive value of Herz/new status with respect to response to therapy and its value in identifying patients who may benefit from adjuvant targeted therapy directed at the protein (629). Several studies have demonstrated that HER-2/neu status may be predictive of response to hormonal therapy, resistance to alkylating agent–based chemotherapy, and response to taxanes (492,693).

Elledge et al. (179), in a study of 205 patients with ER-positive metastatic breast cancer who received tamoxifen as initial therapy, found that ER levels and Bcl-2 expression were significantly lower in patients who had HER-2–positive status. HER-2 status was not related to the response to tamoxifen, time to treatment failure, or survival rate.

p53 Gene

The p53 tumor suppressor gene encodes a nuclear phosphoprotein that is thought to be important to cell cycle regulation and DNA repair and that also may regulate induction of apoptosis by ionizing radiation (97,352). The p53 is most frequently mutated in sporadic breast cancer; alterations of this gene were identified in 43/192 tumors (22%) (97). Mutations of p53 were found more often in tumors of younger women ($p = .002$) and African American women ($p = .04$) and in tumors lacking ER ($p = .03$), PR ($p = .04$), or both ($p = .06$). In 843 cases of breast cancer, p53 mutations were not found in low-grade carcinomas (tubular, mucinous, papillary, and invasive cribriform types), but were observed in 4.2% of ILCs (6/140 cases), 15.5% of high-grade IDCs (99/640 cases), and 50% of pure medullary carcinomas (5/10 cases) (479). The overall survival rates were not significantly different in patients with mutant or wild-type p53 tumors. In another study of 156 patients with primary invasive breast cancer, overexpression of p53 protein emerged as a reliable and independent predictor for disease recurrence and reduced survival (255). Jansen et al. (377), in a study of 345 patients with breast cancer with a median follow-up of more than 10 years noted that Bcl-2 expression was not a prognostic factor, but p53 was an independent prognostic factor for overall survival ($p = .005$) and postrelapse survival ($p = .006$). However, p53 status was important only in the Bcl-2–positive subgroup.

The impact of p53 status on outcomes was reviewed by Thames et al. (739), who identified 301 studies on the influence of p53 overexpression, in which chemotherapy or radiotherapy was used alone or in combination with surgery. In an analysis of 45 studies meeting their selection criteria, they observed a nearly significant negative effect of p53 overexpression on outcome of treatment with cytotoxic drugs and radiation.

Urokinase-Type Plasminogen Activator and Plasminogen Activator Inhibitor Type

Urokinase-type plasminogen activator (UpA) and Plasminogen activator inhibitor-1 (PAI-1) have been shown in recent studies to have significant prognostic and predictive value (226,340). Node-negative patients with low UpA/PAI-1 have an excellent prognosis without systemic adjuvant therapy compared to patients whose tumors express high levels of UpA/PAI. Furthermore, the administration of chemotherapy was enhanced in those patients with high levels of UpA and PAI-1.

Genetic Profiling

Recent developments in DNA-microarray technologies allow for extensive profiling of tumors based on their gene expression signatures (340). Using this technology, investigators from the Netherlands Cancer Institute screened thousands of genes to develop a 70-gene prognostic signature, which in 295 women demonstrated a 10-year disease-free survival of 50.6% in 180 poor prognosis signature patients compared to 85.2% in 115 women with a favorable signature. In a recent validation study, the profiling outperformed classic prognostic criteria, but the magnitude of the prognostic value was not as strong (92,765,772).

An assay using gene profiling on paraffin-embedded specimens has been developed by Genomics Health Inc. (Redwood City, CA). The Oncotype DX assay is based on reverse transcriptase polymerase chain reaction assays to quantify expression of selected genes in paraffin-embedded tissues. A panel of 16 cancer-related genes and five reference genes were employed to compute a recurrence score (0 to 100), which is used to estimate odds of relapse over 10 years. Specimens from patients in NSABP trials with ER-positive tumors treated with tamoxifen alone were used to validate this scheme in which patients are categorized into low risk (<18 score), intermediate risk (18 to 30), or high risk (31 to 100). As shown in Fig. 53.12 the likelihood of distant metastasis is low in those patients with favorable scores treated with tamoxifen alone (552). These data can be used to determine which patients with ER-positive tumors and otherwise favorable factors may avoid chemotherapy, and aid the clinician and patient in clinical decision making.

Age

Although young age has consistently been shown to be a predictor of local relapse following breast-conserving surgery, there are conflicting data regarding its prognostic significance for distant metastasis and overall survival (105,116,147,245,379,782,850). The available data are confounded by the fact that younger women often present with palpable disease and have larger tumors with a higher percentage of positive nodes. Several studies, however, have shown that when corrected for stage, young age remains a significant prognostic factor for distant metastasis. In an analysis of 1,751 patients with nonmetastatic breast cancer, Vanlemmens et al. (773) demonstrated that younger women had a higher proportion of patients with ER-negative and high-grade tumors, and lower disease-free and breast cancer–specific survival. In multivariate analysis, young age at diagnosis was an independent poor prognostic factor. Kollias et al. (409), however, in an analysis of 2,879 patients age <70 with operable disease in the Nottingham database, demonstrated that the association of young age at diagnosis with a worse

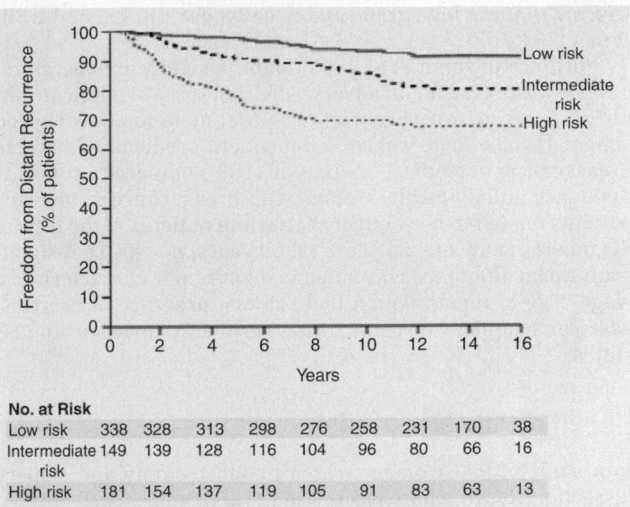

FIGURE 53.12. Outcome in patients with receptor-positive tumors treated with hormonal therapy broken down by recurrence score determined from gene profiling. (From Paik S, Shak S, Tang G, et al. A multigene assay to predict recurrence of tamoxifen-treated, node-negative breast cancer. *N Engl J Med* 2004;351:2817–2826, with permission.)

prognosis was explained by a higher proportion of poorly differentiated cancers in young women, and that young age itself had no influence on the prognosis of the individual. Although clearly not as valid as tumor size and nodal status, young age may be considered in combination with other prognostic factors in clinical decision making as a potential negative prognostic factor.

Race

African American women are commonly diagnosed with more advanced stages of breast cancer than white women (379). Simon and Severson (687), in a review of 10,502 women diagnosed with breast cancer (82% white and 18% African American), observed that African American women were more likely to present with regional or distant disease (45%) than white women (37%). White women had a better survival rate than African American women during the first 4 years after diagnosis (*p* <.0001), but there were no significant differences in survival by race in women who lived longer than 4 years (*p* = .64). Black women are more likely than whites to report that they have not had a mammogram within 3 years before diagnosis. However, history of mammographic screening accounted for <10% of the observed differences in stage at diagnosis (383).

In 75 black and 615 white women with stage I and II breast cancer treated with breast-conservation therapy and cyclophosphamide, methotrexate, 5-fluorouracil (CMF), with or without prednisone and tamoxifen, the 5-year actuarial local-only first failure rates were 5% for black women and 6% for white women (*p* = .53); regional-only failure 9% and 1%, respectively (*p* = .002); and regional recurrence as any component of first failure, 16% and 4%, respectively (*p* = .001) (572). The 5-year overall survival rate for the black patients was 82% versus 91% for the white patients (*p* = .01); the disease-free survival rates were 64% and 83%, respectively (*p* = .0002).

Eley et al. (176) reported on a study of 612 black and 518 white women aged 20 to 79 years with primary invasive breast cancer. After controlling for geographic site and age, the risk of dying was 2.2 times greater for blacks than whites. Adjustment for stage-reduced risk was from 2.2 to 1.7; further adjustment for sociodemographic variables had no effect. They concluded that approximately 75% of the racial difference in survival was explained by prognostic factors. Other studies have also indicated that black women more commonly develop breast cancers that are high grade and negative for ER, PR, and HER-2/neu (384,755).

Further, Newman et al. (523) found a significant overall recovery rate of 1.22 for an adverse effect of African American ethnicity on breast cancer mortality. Subset meta-analysis yielded similar results. Race was an independent predictor of a worse breast cancer outcome. Elmore et al. (182) compared a cohort of 100 black and 300 white women with breast cancer. The black patients tended to be younger than white patients at the time of diagnosis (mean age, 55 years vs. 60 years; $p = .001$). A significant racial difference was noted in eight tumor characteristics: stage, size of tumor, lymph node status, presence of necrosis, vascular/lymphatic invasion, DCIS, perineural invasion, and PR status.

Obesity/Body Mass Index

In a study of 923 women treated by mastectomy and axillary dissection, those who were obese (25% or more over optimal weight for height) at the time of primary breast cancer treatment 10 years after diagnosis were at significantly greater risk for recurrence (42%), compared with nonobese patients (32%; $p < .01$) (670). On multivariate analysis, obesity remained a statistically significant prognostic factor after controlling for tumor size, number of positive axillary lymph nodes, age at diagnosis, and adjuvant chemotherapy. Recurrent disease developed in 32% of obese patients compared with 19% of nonobese women.

Daling et al. (139), in a study of 1,177 women 45 years of age and younger who had invasive ductal breast carcinoma, found that women with breast carcinoma who were in the highest quartile of body mass index were 2.5 times more likely to die of their disease within 5 years of diagnosis compared with women in the lowest quartile of body mass index.

Smoking

High plasma levels of estrogens are associated with increased breast cancer risk. Manjer et al. (464), in an analysis of 792 women in a mammographic screening trial with a mean follow-up of 12.1 years, observed that 145 patients died of breast cancer. The RRs for smokers and exsmokers, compared with those who had never smoked, were 1.44 and 1.13, respectively. The association with smoking remained significant after adjustment for age, stage at diagnosis, and other potential confounders.

Pregnancy

Kroman et al. (421) investigated the prognostic effect of age at first birth and total parity in 10,703 women with primary breast cancer. After adjusting for age and stage of tumor, the number of full-term pregnancies had no prognostic value. However, women with primary childbirth between 20 and 29 years experienced a significantly reduced risk of death compared with women with primary childbirth before the age of 20 years (20 to 24 years, RR = 0.88; 25 to 29 years, RR = 0.80). Psyrri and Burtness (591) reviewed 117 articles and three abstracts referring to breast cancer in pregnancy. They concluded the prognosis of the pregnant breast cancer patient is similar to her stage-matched nonpregnant counterparts in most series. Management of breast cancer during and after pregnancy is discussed in detail later.

Although in the past it was thought that pregnancy after the diagnosis of breast cancer was associated with a worse prognosis, evidence suggests the contrary (357). Women with a history of breast cancer should be reassured that there is no strong evidence to suggest that subsequent pregnancy will increase the risk of recurrence.

Tumor Location

There is some evidence that medially located tumors have a poorer prognosis than laterally located tumors. An analysis of 45,880 patients from the SEER database by Gaffney et al. (260) demonstrated that the hazard ratio for inner quadrant location compared to outer quadrant was 1.27 for breast cancer specific survival and 1.11 for overall survival. Both were significant on multivariate analysis. Lohrisch et al. (454), in an analysis of 6,781 patients, also demonstrated a twofold risk of relapse and breast cancer death associated with high-risk medial breast tumors compared to lateral tumors. They postulate that this may be due to occult spread to internal mammary nodes. On the other hand, Janni et al. (376), in an analysis of 2,414 patients, concluded that there is no sufficient evidence to support any independent prognostic significance of tumor location in early breast cancer. However, medial tumor location may lead to the underestimation of axillary lymph node involvement.

Selected Other Prognostic Factors

A wide variety of other prognostic factors have been extensively evaluated. Although some of these have been promising in initial reports, these have not been applied in routine clinical decision-making. However, these markers may help to supplement information obtained with more established prognostic factors. Furthermore, with additional testing and validation, some of these markers may serve as targets for therapeutic interventions. Extensively evaluated and reported potentially useful prognostic factors include cathepsin D, vascular endothelial growth factor, epidermal growth factor, Bcl-2, carcinoembryonic antigen, prostate-specific antigen, E-cadheren, and others. The reader is referred elsewhere for an extensive review of molecular prognostic factors in breast cancer (634,635).

Serum Markers CA 15–3 and CA 27–29

CA 15–3 is a widely used tumor marker in carcinoma of the breast, but its role in the management of patients with early disease is controversial. O'Hanlon et al. (536) reported on 168 patients with stage I tumors; mean preoperative CA 15–3 levels at presentation were significantly elevated in these patients compared with others with benign disease. CA 15–3 levels were not elevated in patients with locoregional recurrences, but were significantly elevated in patients with bony metastases, and had a mean lead time of 6.3 months over bone scintigraphy. In 166 patients with stage II and III breast cancer, CA 27–29 had a high probability of predicting posttreatment recurrence, with a 5-month average lead time over chemical or imaging detection.

Management of Breast Cancer

Management of invasive breast cancer should be based on the clinical extent and pathologic characteristics of the tumor, in addition to the age of the patient (menopausal status), some biologic prognostic factors, and the preference and psychological profile of the individual patient, optimally in a multidisciplinary setting. Although surgical, medical, and radiation oncology remain the primary therapeutic disciplines in the management of breast cancer, the patient's management often is dependent on input from diagnostic radiology and pathology, the primary physician involved, and support services such as genetic counseling, social work, nursing, and others.

Chang et al. (106) analyzed the records of 75 women with 77 breast lesions examined in a multidisciplinary breast cancer center; the panel disagreed with treatment recommendations from the outside physicians in 32 cases (43%) and agreed in 41

(55%). For the 32 patients with a disagreement, the treatment recommendations were breast-conservation treatment instead of mastectomy (41%; $n = 14$) or re-excision (6%; $n = 2$), and further work-up instead of immediate definitive treatment in 10 (31%).

Patients with lesions smaller than 5 cm in diameter and some specific characteristics to be discussed later should be offered available options, with each modality thoroughly discussed. In some states, legislation has been enacted requiring treating physicians to comply with this practice.

Surgical Management of Breast Cancer

The surgical management of patients with early stage operable breast cancer addresses both the primary tumor and regional lymphatics (293,320,330). The primary tumor may be managed by mastectomy or lumpectomy, and the nodal regions may be surgically addressed by lymph node dissection or sentinel node biopsy. The radiation oncologist should be aware of the various surgical procedures, as it may influence the radiotherapeutic management. Procedures that remove the bulk of parenchymal breast tissue include the radical mastectomy, extended radical mastectomy, modified radical mastectomy, simple mastectomy (also referred to as total mastectomy), skin-sparing mastectomy, and nipple-sparing mastectomy. Partial mastectomy, lumpectomy, tylectomy, and quadrantectomy are collectively referred to as breast-conserving surgery.

Breast-conserving approaches, as well as the skin-sparing and nipple-sparing mastectomy, used in early stage breast cancers, are briefly discussed here as they are often used in early stage disease. Details of the mastectomy procedures are summarized in Chapter 54 (Table 54.3).

Skin-Sparing Mastectomy

Skin-sparing mastectomy is a standard mastectomy, with minimal skin sacrifice at the mastectomy site (330). This is often performed when immediate reconstruction is planned. This technique attempts to remove all breast tissue, but the preservation of skin provides cosmetic and reconstructive advantages. The procedure is oncologically sound and patients undergoing skin-sparing mastectomy do not require postmastectomy radiation unless they have risk factors that place them at higher risk (i.e., positive nodes, positive margins, large primary tumors), as discussed in Chapter 54.

Nipple-Sparing Mastectomy

The nipple-sparing mastectomy is distinct from the skin-sparing mastectomy in that the nipple and/or nipple areola complex are conserved. This procedure is more controversial and is not routinely employed in cancer patients. However, there have been recent studies employing this technique in combination with intraoperative electrons in patients with operable breast cancer (568).

Lumpectomy

Another treatment of breast cancer, initially described by Keynes in 1929 and 1937, combined breast-conserving surgery by wide local excision of the tumor followed by definitive irradiation to the intact breast (98,399,566,802). Various terms have been used to describe the surgical approach, including lumpectomy, wide local excision, breast-conserving surgery, tylectomy, tumorectomy, segmental mastectomy, partial mastectomy, and quadrantectomy. This approach, popular in Europe since 1950, has progressively gained acceptance in the United States since the early 1980s and is extensively discussed in this chapter. The NSABP recommends specific types of incisions depending

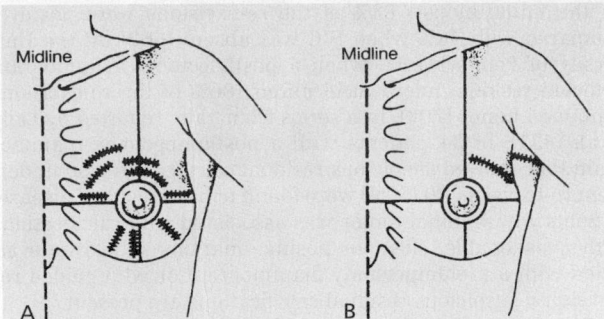

FIGURE 53.13. National Surgical Adjuvant Breast Project recommendations for the direction of incisions used for tumorectomy (**A**) and for axillary node dissection (**B**). (Courtesy of Bernard Fisher, M.D., Chairman, National Surgical Adjuvant Breast Project. From Bedwinek JM. Treatment of stage I and II adenocarcinoma of the breast by tumor excision and irradiation. *Int J Radiat Oncol Biol Phys* 1981;7:1553, with permission.)

on the location of the tumor (Fig. 53.13). The radiation oncologist may play an advisory role as in many cases the patient may be evaluated by both the surgeon and the radiation oncologist before the definitive operation.

The optimal extent of breast resection for treatment of T1–2 breast cancer has not been defined. Increasing the size of the resection may lower the risk of local recurrence but also has an adverse impact on the cosmetic outcome. Because cosmesis is a critical reason for performing tumor excision and irradiation instead of mastectomy, wide local excision with microscopically negative margins is preferable to segmental mastectomy or quadrantectomy. These last procedures are inferior cosmetically to a tylectomy and breast irradiation, usually with an electron beam or implant boost dose to the tumor bed.

Surgical removal of additional breast tissue surrounding the original excision site is indicated when margins are positive and there is a substantial probability that the tumor cell burden exceeds what can be controlled by the usual doses of radiation. The percentage of patients with residual tumor at the time of re-excision varies widely (32% to 62%), depending on the criteria used for taking a patient back to the operating room for more breast surgery. If the initial margins of resection are positive, 55% to 69% of re-excision specimens contain cancer cells, compared with 49% in cases with unknown margins (483,506,662,708). Sauter et al. (654) concluded that frozen-section analysis of re-excision lumpectomy margins is a safe and accurate technique that may eliminate the need for additional re-excision or higher-dose radiation boosts, resulting in better cosmesis. Tumor size alone is not usually considered an indication for re-excision in the absence of other factors.

Some authors have advocated re-excision of the primary site if the biopsy was performed at an outside hospital and margins of resection were unknown. Of one study of 210 patients having surgery at M.D. Anderson Cancer Center, 67 underwent re-excision after biopsies performed at other institutions, and invasive carcinoma was identified in 57% (506). An 8.2% incidence of breast recurrence (12/135 patients) was noted when the tumor excision was performed before referral to M.D. Anderson Cancer Center, but only 2% (4/210) when it was performed at that institution. At the Institut Gustave-Roussy, a breast recurrence rate of 10% was noted with outside excisions, compared with 5% in patients who had tumor excision at the Institut (122). Patients undergoing re-excision experienced a breast failure rate of only 3%.

Other factors that may have an impact on the rate of positive re-excisions include extensive intraductal carcinoma (EIC) and residual calcifications on a postlumpectomy preirradiation mammogram. At Harvard University, when EIC was detected on the initial biopsy, 88% of the re-excisions were positive, compared with 48% when EIC was absent (662). At the University of Pennsylvania, when a postlylectomy mammogram detected residual microcalcifications, 86% of the re-excisions contained tumor (708). In a series from Yale, reported by Lally et al. (431), of 34 patients with a postlumpectomy mammogram that showed suspicious residual calcification who underwent re-excision, 20 (59%) were found to have residual disease. Patients whose initial tumor was associated with calcifications with questionable, close, or positive margins should be evaluated with a prelumpectomy mammogram or with guided re-excision if suspicious residual calcifications are present.

Based on these findings, the authors recommend re-excision at the primary tumor site:

1. When the surgical procedure was less than a complete lumpectomy, such as an initial incisional biopsy or core biopsy,
2. When pathologic margins on the initial excisional biopsy are shown to be involved by tumor,
3. When there are residual suspicious microcalcifications on a postlumpectomy mammogram.

As will be discussed later, although re-excision for involved margins is indicated, selected patients with a focally involved margin may be treated with radiation therapy, without re-excision, following lumpectomy with acceptable local control rates.

In recent years, several reports have shown encouraging results with neoadjuvant chemotherapy, which allows breast-conserving surgery and irradiation to be used in a large proportion of patients with larger T2–3 tumors because they exhibit substantial regression (68,96). Neoadjuvant chemotherapy followed by breast conservation will be discussed in Chapter 54.

Choices between Mastectomy and Breast-Conserving Surgery in Early Stage Disease

For the majority of patients with early stage breast cancer, breast-conserving surgery (BCS) or mastectomy are both reasonable options, and patients are often conflicted regarding the choice. Patients should be reassured that provided they meet the criteria for breast-conserving surgery, all of the available medical evidence demonstrate equivalent long-term survival rates with both modalities.

A modified radical mastectomy may be preferable for some patients who wish to avoid radiation, for those in whom removal of clinical and radiographically apparent disease will result in a suboptimal cosmetic result, for those with diffusely positive margins that cannot be cleared with re-excision, and those with diffuse suspicious microcalcifications. Even patients who are ideally suited for breast-conserving therapy may have a personal preference for mastectomy, based on a number of factors.

Whelen et al. (828) reported on the decision-making process in 82 consecutive node-negative patients who were presented with a decision board of therapeutic choices (828). Overall, 95% of women chose lumpectomy and breast irradiation, and the reasons for choosing are summarized in Table 53.12. Kelemen et al. (395) evaluated the choice between breast-conserving surgery and modified radical mastectomy in 7,815 women with early stage breast cancer. There was a progressive increase from 16% to 47% in the use of breast-conserving therapy to treat tumors of all sizes over the 11 years of the study ($p < .0001$), and it was more frequently used for ≤ 2 cm tumors with an overall recovery rate of 2.46. Breast-conserving therapy was used at a slightly higher rate in medical centers than in community hospitals (31% vs. 28%; $p < .0001$); its use varied among geographic regions from a low of 24% in the southwestern United States to 36% in the Northeast and 40% in hospitals outside the continental United States ($p < .0001$). Local availability of radiation therapy did not influence choice of treatment.

In response to a questionnaire mailed to 2,405 oncologists from all three disciplines and 60 oncology nurses in the United States, Tannock and Belanger (733) noted that more than 60% thought that modified radical mastectomy and conservation surgery plus irradiation were equivalent options for patients with stage T1–2 carcinoma of the breast; 31% of the surgical oncologists favored the former and 35% of the radiation oncologists favored the latter approach. Medical oncologists were equally divided between the two procedures (14% and 18%, respectively).

In an analysis from Canada, Temple et al. (738) prospectively evaluated participants with a first diagnosis of localized unilateral breast cancer who were candidates for breast-conserving therapy or mastectomy. Of 157 patients between 1992 and 1995, 71.3% anticipated having BCS and 28.7% anticipated modified radical mastectomy. The patient, physician, and significant other were perceived to play a role in the decision process. The two top-ranked items perceived to have influenced treatment choice were the doctor's advice and possibility of complete cure. Most women (60%) participated in treatment choice to the degree that they preferred, but only 13.6% received their preferred amount of information. The type of planned surgery was predicted by the surgeon, contribution of the doctor as to choice of treatment, importance of breasts to sexuality, self-efficacy, and concerns about cancer recurrence from a multivariable

---

Table 53.12	**REASONS FOR CHOOSING BREAST IRRADIATION: MEAN IMPORTANCE**			
Reason	Consultation	Consultation and Checklist	Consultation and Decision Board	Overall
Reduces chance of local recurrence	4.50	5.00	4.75	4.77
Increases chance of surviving cancer	4.76	4.64	4.18	4.51
Prevents need for breast surgery in future	4.59	4.61	4.57	4.59
Prevents need for mastectomy	4.64	4.64	4.11	4.45
Doctor recommended irradiation	4.59	4.56	3.04[a]	4.02[b]
Side effects are acceptable	3.29	3.07	3.61	3.33[c]

[a] $p = .0006$ (three-way comparison).
[b] Doctor recommended irradiation versus other reasons ($p = .003$).
[c] Side effects are acceptable versus other reasons ($p = .0001$).
From Whelan TJ, Levine MN, Gafni A, et al. Breast irradiation postlumpectomy: development and evaluation of a decision instrument. *J Clin Oncol* 1995;13:847–853, with permission.

logistic regression model. The authors concluded that both patient and surgeon factors are important predictors of the type of planned surgery, but there is a gap between women's preferences and actual experiences with regard to information provided.

Some patients with early stage breast cancer will choose mastectomy to avoid the course of radiation, either due to the logistics of 6 weeks of therapy or due to fears of radiation therapy. It is likely over the next few years that more mature results and selection factors for treating women with accelerated partial breast irradiation will become available. For those women in whom the time commitment of treatment is an issue, this option may further impact the choice between mastectomy and BCS.

Patients selecting mastectomy should also be made aware that this procedure does not totally eliminate the need for radiation treatment. For patients with early stage operable breast cancer treated by modified radical mastectomy, postoperative irradiation of the chest wall and peripheral lymphatics may be indicated in selected patients with high-risk characteristics, positive nodes, and/or positive resection margins. Indications for postmastectomy radiation are discussed in Chapter 54.

Surgical Management of Axillary Lymph Nodes

An axillary node dissection or sentinel node biopsy is a standard component of the staging process for a majority of women with early stage invasive breast cancer (285,852). Although the role of complete axillary dissection is evolving, currently most patients with positive sentinel nodes will undergo completion axillary dissection. Clearly the procedure is most important for women in whom axillary nodal status will influence subsequent management with respect to adjuvant systemic therapy. The role of axillary dissection and sentinel node sampling, however, continues to evolve and is currently being evaluated in several trials. It is not uncommon for clinicians to avoid axillary staging if it is not going to influence management (306,605,680). This is relevant in elderly women with receptor-positive tumors who will receive hormonal therapy regardless of nodal status and are not felt to be candidates for cytotoxic chemotherapy. This issue also frequently arises in women of any age who undergo a sentinel node biopsy, which is positive, and have not undergone completion dissection. As will be discussed later, axillary radiation, as with axillary dissection, results in a high rate of regional control (306,605,680).

Axillary Node Dissection

The axillary contents are divided into three levels: level I represents tissue between the axillary vein and the latissimus dorsi muscle and the lateral border of the pectoralis minor muscle; level II is located between the lateral and medial borders of the pectoralis minor muscle; and level III is between the medial border of the pectoralis minor and Halsted's ligament (the apex of the axilla) (218,702,811) (see Figure 53.2). Thorough dissection of levels I and II has traditionally been the most common axillary surgical procedure in patients with clinically node-negative breast cancer. Complete axillary dissection, including level III, may be performed in patients with clinically positive lymph nodes. A higher incidence of breast and arm edema has been noted with level III axillary node dissection, and the benefit of dissecting the level III lymph nodes has not been demonstrated (595). Pigott et al. (584) reported on 146 patients treated with radical mastectomy (either modified or Halsted) for invasive ductal or lobular carcinoma of the breast. Eighty patients (55%) had histologically proven axillary lymph node metastases. If only the low (level I) axillary lymph nodes had been removed, 18 patients (25%) would have had metastases confined to levels II and III that would have gone undetected. However, only 1.4%

of patients showed positive level III lymph nodes if levels I and II were negative.

Approximately 20% to 40% of patients with carcinoma of the breast and clinically negative lymph nodes have pathologic evidence of lymph node metastases (140,211,214,330,811). Yet in patients with stage I or II breast cancer and clinically negative axillary lymph nodes, if an axillary dissection is not performed, axillary recurrence develops in only approximately 20% (212). In patients with clinically positive axilla, 20% to 30% have no histologic evidence of nodal metastatic disease (212).

Orr (548) performed a meta-analysis to examine possible survival benefits for axillary lymph node dissection in women with clinically negative axillae in six randomized, controlled trials comparing standard treatment (i.e., mastectomy and axillary lymph node dissection or segmentectomy and axillary lymph node dissection plus breast irradiation with standard treatment without axillary lymph node dissection). Approximately 3,000 patients were identified. All six trials demonstrated that prophylactic axillary lymph node dissection improved absolute survival rates anywhere from 4% to 16%. When the six trials were combined, the average survival benefit was 5.4%.

The necessity of axillary dissection has been questioned in selected patients with a low probability of nodal involvement. Silverstein et al. (680) reported positive axillary lymph nodes in only 3/96 (3%) patients with tumors 5 mm or less in diameter and in 27/156 (17%) patients with tumors 6 to 10 mm in diameter. They suggested eliminating axillary node dissection for T1a lesions but performing it routinely in patients with T1b and larger tumors. Iwasaki et al. (370), in a group of 823 patients with T1/N0/M0 invasive breast cancer, also identified a subgroup of patients who may have not needed to undergo axillary lymph node dissection. The incidence of axillary lymph node metastases in patients with clinical T1/N0/M0 invasive breast cancer was 25% (208/823). The frequency of nodal metastases correlated with tumor size: 1 cm or smaller, 17%; 1.5 cm or smaller, 25%; 2 cm or smaller, 29%. Mammography showed that patients with malignant calcification or speculation had a significantly higher rate of nodal metastases than those without these findings. Certain tumor types (medullary, mucinous, and tubular carcinoma) had lower positive rates for lymph node involvement. With regard to the histologic grade, lymph node positivity increased significantly with high-grade tumors.

In a randomized trial, evaluating the necessity of axillary dissection in older women, Martelli et al. (477) reported on 219 women, 65 to 80 years of age, with early breast cancer and clinically negative axillary nodes who were randomized to conservative breast surgery with or without axillary dissection. Tamoxifen was prescribed to all patients for 5 years. With a follow-up of 60 months, there were no significant differences in overall or breast cancer mortality or crude cumulative incidence of breast events between the two groups. Only two patients in the no axillary dissection arm (8 and 40 months after surgery) developed overt axillary involvement during follow-up. They conclude that older patients with T1-N0 breast cancer can be treated by conservative breast surgery and no axillary dissection without adversely affecting breast cancer mortality or overall survival.

Axillary recurrences after complete dissection range from 1% to 2%. DeBoer et al. (146) reported on 4,669 patients with invasive breast cancer who underwent axillary clearance. Fifty-nine patients (1.3%) experienced axillary recurrence with a median interval between initial treatment and diagnosis of axillary recurrence of 2.6 years. Surgery was part of the treatment of recurrence in 41/59 patients. Regional control of axillary recurrence was observed in 34 patients (58%). The 5-year actuarial survival rate for patients with axillary recurrence was 39%. Dewar et al. (160) reported on 558 patients with T1 and small T2 tumors treated with conservation therapy, including a lower axillary dissection in 374 patients (67%) and axillary clearance in 184 patients (33%). There was histologic evidence of axillary lymph node metastases in 36%. Only five patients relapsed in the axilla (at 5 years, 1.2%). Gerard et al. (274) also reported a 1.2% probability of axillary recurrence after axillary dissection without nodal irradiation in 195 patients with stage T1–2 tumors who were treated with conservation surgery and breast irradiation.

Sentinel Lymph Node Biopsies

In recent years there has been a substantial increase in the use of sentinel lymph node biopsies to stage patients with breast cancer. Patients are injected around the tumor with technetium-99 sulfur colloid and vital blue dye, and a hand-held gamma probe is used to identify areas of highest radioisotope uptake in the lymphatic system. The lymph nodes underlying this area (sentinel lymph nodes) are removed (120,417,465,466). The sentinel node procedure has been widely embraced as an acceptable standard for women with breast cancer. The procedure has a high degree of sensitivity and specificity (72,249,279,280, 288,368,416,471,515,532,619,699,786–788,852).

Although the current standard for patients with a positive sentinel node is to undergo completion axillary dissection, the necessity of this has been questioned and is the subject of ongoing clinical trials. As will be discussed later, for those patients undergoing breast-conserving therapy, radiation therapy results in a high possibility of regional nodal control, and may be considered in sentinel node-positive patients who do not undergo nodal dissection.

The Axillary Lymphatic Mapping Against Nodal Axillary Clearance (ALMANAC) trial is a multicenter randomized trial of 1,031 patients randomly assigned to sentinel node biopsy ($n = 515$) or standard axillary dissection ($n = 516$) (465). In this trial, Mansel et al. (465) reported the primary outcome measures, which were arm and shoulder morbidity and quality of life. Drain usage, length of hospital stay and resumption of normal activities after surgery were all highly significantly better in the sentinel lymph node group. In addition, patient-recorded quality of life and arm functioning scores were also significantly better, with no increase in anxiety levels in the sentinel node group. The authors conclude that sentinel node biopsy is the treatment of choice for patients who have early stage breast cancer and clinically negative nodes.

Veronesi et al. (786) also reported on a randomized trial of 516 patients with T1 tumors, randomized to either sentinel node biopsy or total axillary dissection. Axillary dissection was performed in the sentinel node group if the sentinel node contained metastases. In the axillary dissection group, the overall accuracy of the sentinel node status was 96.9%, the sensitivity 91.2%, and the specificity 100%. There was less pain and better arm mobility in the patients who underwent sentinel node biopsy only than in those who also underwent axillary dissection. There were 15 events associated with breast cancer in the axillary dissection group and 10 such events in the sentinel node group. Among the 167 patients who did not undergo axillary dissection, there were no cases of overt axillary metastasis during follow-up. A larger NSABP study addressing this issue has been completed but not yet reported.

Fifty percent of patients with sentinel lymph node metastases have no metastatic disease in nonsentinel lymph nodes on axillary lymph node dissection. Weiser et al. (823) assessed 1,000 patients undergoing sentinel lymph node biopsy; 231 (23%) had positive sentinel lymph nodes. Of these, 206 underwent completion axillary lymph node dissection. The likelihood of nonsentinel lymph node metastasis was inversely related to three clinicopathologic variables: tumor size 1 cm or smaller, absence of lymphovascular invasion, and sentinel lymph node micrometastases (≤ 2 mm). None of 24 patients with all three predictive factors had nonsentinel lymph node metastases, whereas 58% of patients with none of the factors had disease in the nonsentinel lymph nodes.

Weaver et al. (820) evaluated 443 patients with breast cancer. After sentinel node biopsies, a complete axillary lymph node dissection was performed. Original pathologic material was reviewed for 431 patients enrolled in this study and for 214 patients with node-negative disease. Metastases were detected in 16% of the sentinel lymph nodes and in 4% of the nonsentinel nodes (overall recovery, 4.3; $p < .001$). Occult metastases were detected in 4% of the sentinel lymph nodes and in 0.3% of the nonsentinel nodes. The probability of detecting metastases in nonsentinel nodes was more than 13 times greater in patients with positive sentinel lymph nodes than in patients with negative sentinel lymph nodes ($p < .001$).

The role of sentinel lymph node procedures in patients undergoing neoadjuvant chemotherapy is covered in Chapter 54.

Systemic Management of Breast Cancer

Systemic therapy is an essential component of both early stage node-negative breast cancer as well as advanced stage disease. Hormonal therapy, cytotoxic chemotherapy, and the more recently introduced biological therapies are routinely employed in the vast majority of patients with early stage breast cancer. For patients with all stages of breast cancer, systemic therapy has been shown to decrease the relative risk of relapse and mortality. However, there are subsets of patients with a very favorable prognosis and extremely low rate of relapse, in whom the risk reduction results in only a very small absolute benefit. At a recent consensus meeting at St. Galen, Switzerland, an expert panel proposed an algorithm for selection of systemic therapy in early stage breast cancer based on risk and responsiveness to endocrine therapy (280). The risk categories and selection of therapy are summarized in Tables 53.13 and 53.14.

The various systemic chemotherapy, hormonal therapy and biological therapy studies are summarized in detail in Chapter 51.

Radiation Therapy in the Management of Early Stage Invasive Breast Cancer

The radiation oncologist plays a critical role in the management of early stage breast cancer. As noted previously, the role of radiation therapy in postmastectomy radiation and in the neoadjuvant treatment of advanced breast cancers will be discussed in Chapter 54. The remainder of this chapter will primarily be focused on the role of radiation therapy in the conservative management of early stage invasive breast cancer.

Here we include an extensive discussion of the studies establishing breast-conserving surgery and radiation as the preferred standard of care for the majority of women with early stage invasive disease and studies evaluating the avoidance of radiation therapy in selected patients. Integration of radiation therapy with systemic therapy will be discussed, as will selection of patients for breast-conserving therapy. Risk factors for local relapse and controversies in the management of patients with special circumstances will be discussed. Technical issues in the delivery of radiation therapy for early stage breast cancer, including dosing and fractionation, matching techniques, and newer technical approaches will be presented. The rapidly evolving area of partial breast irradiation will also be discussed. Follow-up of the breast cancer patient and sequelae of treatment will be presented. Management of local relapse in the

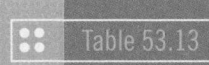

Table 53.13 — DEFINITION OF RISK CATEGORIES FOR PATIENTS WITH OPERATED BREAST CANCER

Risk category

Low risk[a]
Node negative AND *all* of the following features:
pT ≤2 cm, AND
Grade 1,[b] AND
Absence of peritumoral vascular invasion,[c] AND
HER2/neu gene neither overexpressed nor amplified,[d] AND
Age ≥35 years

Intermediate risk[e]
Node negative AND *at least one* of the following features:
pT >2 cm, OR
Grade 2-3,[b] OR
Presence of peritumoral vascular invasion,[c] OR
HER2/neu gene overexpressed or amplified,[d] OR
Age <35 years
Node positive (1–3 involved nodes) AND
HER2/neu gene neither overexpressed nor amplified[d]

High risk
Node positive (1–3 involved nodes) AND
HER2/neu gene overexpressed or amplified[d]
Node positive (4 or more involved nodes)

pT, pathological tumor size (i.e., size of the invasive component)
[a]Some panel members view pT1a and pT1b (i.e., pT <1 cm) tumors with node-negative disease as representing low risk even if higher grade and/or younger age.
[b]Histologic and/or nuclear grade.
[c]Peritumoral vascular invasion was considered controversial as a discriminatory feature of increased risk; its presence defined intermediate risk for node-negative disease, but did not influence risk category for node-positive disease.
[d]HER2/neu gene overexpression or amplification must be determined by quality-controlled assays using immunohistochemistry or fluorescence *in situ* hybridization analysis.
[e]Note that the intermediate-risk category includes both node-negative and node-positive 1–3 disease.
From Goldhirsch A, Glick JH, Gelber RD, et al. Meeting highlights: international expert consensus on the primary therapy of early breast cancer 2005. *Ann Oncol* 2005;16:1569–1583, with permission.

Table 53.14 — EXPERT CONSENSUS ON THE THERAPY OF BREAST CANCER

Risk Category[a]	Endocrine Responsive[b]	Endocrine Response Uncertain[b,c]	Endocrine Nonresponsive[b]
Low risk	ET	ET	Not applicable
	Nil[d]	Nil[d]	—
Intermediate risk	ET alone, or	CT → ET	CT
	CT → ET	(CT + ET)[e]	—
	(CT + ET)[e]	—	—
High risk	CT → ET	CT → ET	CT
	(CT + ET)[e]	(CT + ET)[e]	—

CT, chemotherapy; ET, endocrine therapy; Nil, no adjuvant systemic therapy
[a]See Table 53.13 for definitions of risk categories.
[b]Responsiveness to endocrine therapies is defined in the text.
[c]High levels of urokinase-type plasminogen activator (uPA) and its inhibitor, plasminogen activator inhibitor type 1 (PAI-1) as measured on tissue extracts using ELISA, are associated with increased uncertainty of endocrine responsiveness (Table 53.1).
[d]Indicates alternative treatment option in case of medical contraindications, preference of patient, or preference of physician.
[e]Clinical trial evidence suggests that chemotherapy and tamoxifen should be delivered sequentially, but no such data exist for aromatase inhibitors or ovarian function suppression/ablation. Hence, the option to deliver concurrent chemotherapy and some forms of endocrine therapy must be included. Specifically, concurrent GnRH analog given with chemotherapy for premenopausal women is acceptable (110,111).
From Goldhirsch, et al. Meeting highlights: international expert consensus on the primary therapy of early breast cancer 2005. *Ann Oncol* 2005;16(9):1569–1583.

conservatively treated breast and postmastectomy will be covered in Chapter 54. The role of radiation therapy in the management of DCIS and LCIS is also discussed in Chapter 54.

Breast-Conserving Therapy and Patient Selection

Breast-conserving surgery followed by radiation therapy to the intact breast is now clearly established as the most acceptable standard of care for the majority of women with early stage invasive breast cancer. In 1992, the *National Cancer Institute* published a monograph that stated that breast-conservation treatment is an appropriate method of primary therapy for most women with stage I or II breast cancer and is preferable because it provides survival equivalent to that of total mastectomy and axillary dissection while preserving the breast (790). Recommended techniques for breast-conservation treatment are wide local excision of the primary tumor, preferably with clear margins, axillary lymph node dissection, and breast irradiation (45 to 50 Gy), usually with a boost (10 to 20 Gy, depending on tumor size and status of the surgical margins). As will be discussed in detail under prognostic factors, although widely negative margins are desirable, patients with focally involved margins can be treated with radiation with excellent local control rates.

In addition to tumor control and survival, conservation of the breast with optimal cosmetic results is a crucial goal of this therapy, which is associated with improved psychoemotional adjustment of the patient to the diagnosis and treatment of carcinoma of the breast. It also enhances the acceptance by women of mammographic screening for early detection of this disease.

The widespread embracement of breast-conserving surgery followed by radiation therapy is based on numerous mature and well-documented studies, both prospectively designed randomized trials and large retrospective series of appropriately selected patients treated with breast conservation followed by radiation therapy.

It is important to select appropriate patients and tumors for breast-conservation therapy, with close consultation between the surgeon, medical oncologist, and the radiation oncologist and after thorough discussion of therapeutic alternatives with the patient. Risks and benefits of breast-conserving therapy compared to mastectomy should be discussed. Despite the clear evidence of equivalence, some patients will still prefer mastectomy, which remains an acceptable standard of care for all women with operable breast cancers. Although avoidance of radiation may be a primary rationale for some patients in choosing mastectomy, patients should realize that even with early stage operable disease postmastectomy radiation may be indicated based on the pathologic findings at mastectomy. It is likely that over the next several years, long-term results and selection factors for accelerated partial breast irradiation will become available and may further influence patient choices regarding breast-conserving surgery with more rapid radiation compared to mastectomy (31,310,795).

Ideally, patients electing breast-conserving surgery and radiation will have unicentric primary tumors that are less than 4 or 5 cm in diameter, as cosmesis is affected by the amount of tissue that must be removed in relation to the size of the breast (736). For patients in whom the size of the tumor, compared with the size of the breast, will result in an unacceptable cosmetic outcome, neoadjuvant chemotherapy followed by lumpectomy and radiation has been demonstrated to result in excellent breast-conservation rates (87,107,108). This will be discussed in detail in Chapter 54.

With careful attention to surgical margins, radiation technique, and the appropriate use of systemic therapy, local relapse rates in the majority of conservatively managed patients are low, and only a minority of patients with early stage invasive breast cancer are not suitable for breast-conserving therapy. There are several perceived relative "contraindications" to breast-conserving therapy, including patients with collagen vascular disease, germline mutations that predispose to breast cancer development, positive margins, more advanced disease, multicentric disease, those who are pregnant, and patients with prior radiation history. Although many of these factors require careful consideration and discussion between the treating physicians and the patient, as will be discussed in the section on special circumstances, selected patients faced with breast cancer in the setting of these controversial circumstances can be offered breast-conserving therapy with acceptable outcomes. Although some clinicians believe that patients at higher risk for development of local recurrence should not be treated with conservation surgery, there are relatively few absolute contraindications.

Perhaps with the exception of the patients with persistently positive diffuse margins and/or gross multicentric disease, where removal of clinically and radiographically apparent disease would result in an unacceptable cosmetic outcome, breast-conserving therapy followed by radiation can be offered to most women with early stage breast cancer, and may be offered to a high percentage of women with advanced cancers following neoadjuvant chemo- or hormonal therapy. The decision regarding breast-conserving therapy compared to mastectomy is often based on personal preference, as the available medical and scientific evidence suggests equivalent overall and disease-free survival in all subsets of patients.

Early Reports of Breast-Conserving Therapy

In 1937, Keynes (399) stated that "widespread operations based on the permeation theory of lymphatics and fascial planes have no real justification and the idea of conservative treatment of cancer of the breast may become less repugnant to us [surgeons]." He treated 325 patients with local removal of the breast tumor and radium implantation at the site of local incision as well as in the axilla. In 250 patients, the 5-year survival rate was 71% for group 1 (disease confined to the breast), 29% for group 2 (disease apparently confined to breast and axilla), and 23.6% for group 3 (advanced disease or inoperable cancer). At the time, the results were comparable with those achieved with radical mastectomy. Other early reports by Almiric et al. (14), Janjan et al. (375), Montague et al. (505), Peters (566), and Rissanen (620) paved the way for the development of randomized trials that have now clearly established breast-conserving surgery followed by radiation therapy as an accepted standard of care.

Randomized Studies Comparing Breast-Conserving Surgery Plus Radiation Therapy to Mastectomy

There have been numerous randomized trials that have clearly established breast-conserving surgery followed by radiation therapy as equivalent to mastectomy for appropriately selected patients with early stage breast cancer. Table 53.15 summarizes these randomized trials. In all of these trials, local tumor excision (tylectomy, lumpectomy), segmental mastectomy, or quadrantectomy combined with irradiation to the breast yielded survival and tumor control rates similar to those achieved with modified or classic radical mastectomy (201,203,446,767,768,778,789). Each of these randomized trials, as well as meta-analysis of the trials, clearly demonstrate equivalent mortality rates in conservatively treated patients compared with mastectomy (244,378,513).

The earliest prospective, randomized trial comparing breast conservation with radical mastectomy was conducted at Guy's Hospital in London. Three hundred and seventy women with stage I or II breast cancer were randomly assigned to receive either standard radical mastectomy or wide local excision plus irradiation (34). Although the rates of survival and distant metastasis were not significantly different for stage I disease, in stage II the recurrence rates in the breast and axilla were higher in the group treated with local excision and irradiation, and survival was significantly lower because of a higher rate of distant metastasis. Major weaknesses of this study were the low doses of irradiation used (35 to 38 Gy to the breast and 25 to 27 Gy to the axilla), probably patient selection, and surgical techniques.

Veronesi et al. (789) reported on 701 patients with tumors <2 cm in diameter and without palpable axillary nodes of whom 352 were randomly assigned to treatment with either quadrantectomy and axillary dissection plus irradiation (50 Gy in 5 weeks to the breast and 10 Gy boost) and 349 to radical (Halsted) mastectomy. Women with positive axillary lymph nodes also received 12 cycles of adjuvant chemotherapy with CMF. Actuarial 20-year overall and disease-free survival rates were comparable in the two groups (58%). The death rates from breast cancer were 26.1% and 24.3%, respectively. The incidence of local failure was 2.3% with mastectomy and 8.8% with quadrantectomy and irradiation. There was no difference in the incidence of contralateral breast cancer (10.2% and 8.7%, respectively) (778).

Fisher et al. (201,203) updated the results of the NSABP Protocol B-06 in 1,843 women with clinical stage I or II carcinoma of the breast <4 cm in diameter. Patients were randomly

	Institut Gustave-Roussy (1972–84) (650)	Milan (1973–80) (778)	NSABP B-06 (1976–84) (201)	NCI (1979–87) (586)	EORTC (1980–86) (767)	Danish (1983–89) (63)
No. of patients	179	701	1,219	237	874	904
Stage	1	1	1 and 2	1 and 2	1 and 2	1, 2, 3
Surgery	2-cm gross margin	Quadrantectomy	Lumpectomy	Gross excision	1-cm gross margin	Wide excision
Follow-up (y)	15	20	20	18	10	6
Overall survival						
CS+RT (%)	73	42	46	59	65	79
Mastectomy (%)	65	41	47	58	66	82
Local recurrence						
CS+RT (%)	9	9	14	22	20	3
Mastectomy (%)	14	2	10	6	12	4

Table 53.15 PROSPECTIVE RANDOMIZED TRIALS COMPARING CONSERVATIVE SURGERY AND RADIATION WITH MASTECTOMY FOR EARLY-STAGE BREAST CANCER

CT+RT, conservative therapy plus radiation therapy; EORTC, European Organization for Research tand Treatment of Cancer; NCI, National Cancer Institute; NSABP, National Surgical Adjuvant Breast and Bowel Project.

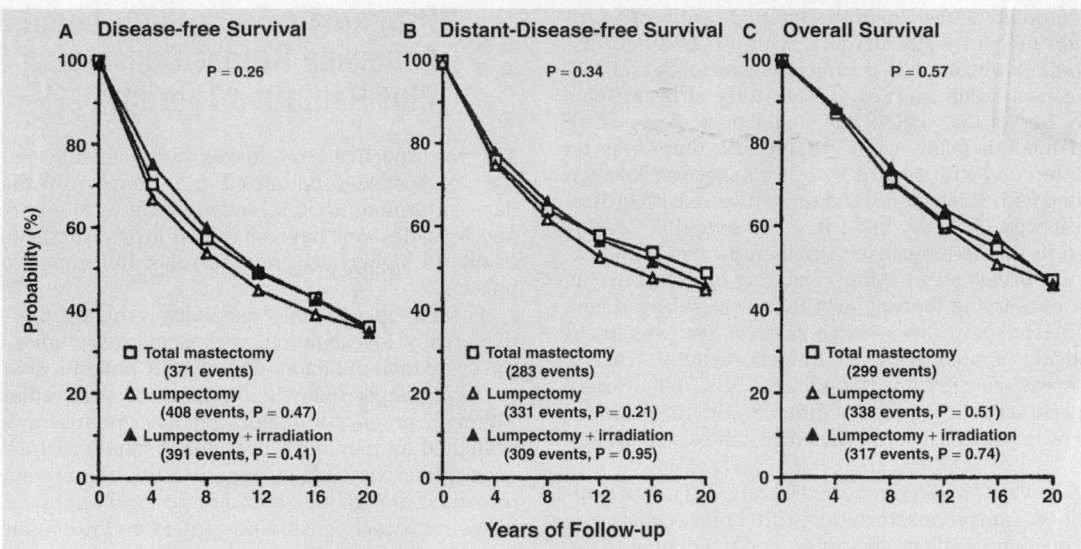

FIGURE 53.14. Life-table analysis showing disease-free survival among patients in the three cohorts who were treated by total mastectomy, lumpectomy, or lumpectomy and breast irradiation. The number of events includes those that occurred after the 20-year follow-up period. (From Fisher B, Anderson S, Bryant J, et al. Twenty-year follow-up of a randomized trial comparing total mastectomy, lumpectomy, and lumpectomy plus irradiation for the treatment of invasive breast cancer. *N Engl J Med* 2002;347(15):1233–1241, with permission.)

assigned to be treated with total mastectomy or lumpectomy (segmental mastectomy), with or without irradiation. Irradiated patients received 50 Gy to the breast through tangential fields irradiation and a boost to the operative site was not given. With 20-year follow-up, there was no significant difference in survival between patients treated with mastectomy, lumpectomy alone, or lumpectomy combined with irradiation (Fig. 53.14). For the patients treated with lumpectomy alone, the ipsilateral breast relapse rates were approximately 40% if the nodes were negative and 50% if they were positive. For patients treated with lumpectomy and irradiation, the corresponding rates were 10% for all patients and those with negative nodes and 5% for those with positive nodes, illustrating the interaction of irradiation and adjuvant chemotherapy in local tumor control. Cumulate incidence of ipsilateral breast tumor relapse in the lumpectomy alone compared to the lumpectomy and radiation arm is shown in Figure 53.15.

The Institut Gustave-Roussy conducted a prospective, randomized trial comparing mastectomy with local excision plus irradiation for women with cancers measuring 2 cm or less (649,650). The 15-year disease-free survival rate was 55% for the tumorectomy group and 45% for the mastectomy group (*p* = .23). The 15-year local recurrence rate was 9% in the conservation surgery and irradiation group and 14% in the mastectomy group.

The EORTC Breast Cancer Cooperative Group conducted a randomized trial of women with stage I or II breast cancer comparing modified radical mastectomy (420 patients) with breast-conservation therapy (448 patients) (767). The actuarial 8-year local tumor control rate was similar in both arms, 91% in the mastectomy group and 87% in the breast-conservation therapy group. There was one axillary recurrence in the mastectomy group and three in the conservation therapy group.

A Danish Cooperative Study carried out a similar randomized trial in 905 women (another 248 patients were treated with mastectomy or breast-conservation therapy according to preference without randomization) (64). High-risk patients (tumor >5 cm, invasion to skin or deep fascia, metastatic axillary lymph nodes) who were treated with breast-conservation therapy received radiation therapy to the regional lymph nodes. Those who were treated with mastectomy also received irradiation of the same target volume and all high-risk patients

received adjuvant CMF. At 6 years, the recurrence-free survival rate in 430 patients treated with breast-conservation therapy was 70%, compared with 66% in 429 patients treated with mastectomy. Overall survival rates were 79% and 82%, respectively. There were 12 breast relapses in the former group (3%) and 19 chest wall recurrences in the latter group (4%). In the breast-conservation therapy group, 31% of patients had excellent and 41% had satisfactory cosmesis.

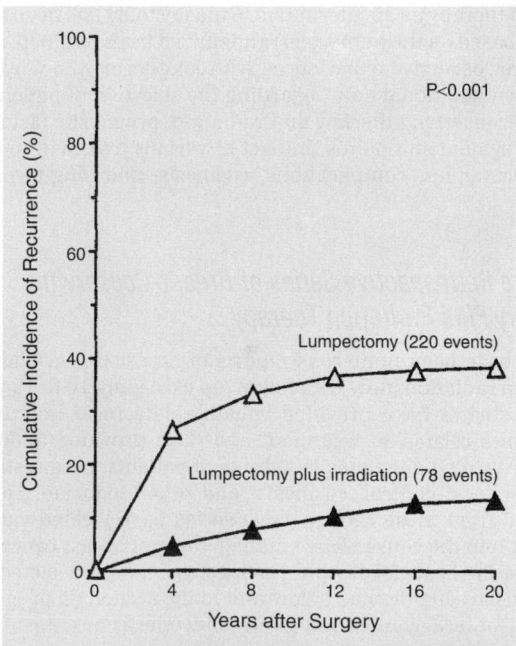

FIGURE 53.15. Cumulative incidence of ipsilateral breast recurrence after lumpectomy (*open diamonds*) or lumpectomy plus breast irradiation (*solid diamonds*) in 1,137 patients in the current-update cohort (cohort B) who had either negative or positive nodes and tumor-negative specimen margins. (From Fisher B, Anderson S, Bryant J, et al. Twenty-year follow-up of a randomized trial comparing total mastectomy, lumpectomy, and lumpectomy plus irradiation for the treatment of invasive breast cancer. *N Engl J Med* 2002;347(15):1233–1241, with permission.)

The U.S. National Cancer Institute reported results of a randomized study in which 122 patients with T1–2/N0/M0 disease were treated with modified radical mastectomy and 125 with breast-conservation therapy (45 to 50 Gy to breast plus 15- to 20-Gy boost) (371). Recently updated by Poggi et al. (586) with a median follow-up of 18.4 years, there was no detectable difference with regard to overall survival between patients treated with mastectomy and those treated with breast-conserving therapy (58% vs. 54%; $p = .67$ overall). Twenty-seven women in the breast-conserving therapy arm (22%) experienced an in-breast event. After censoring in-breast events in the breast-conserving therapy arm that were salvaged successfully by mastectomy, disease-free survival also was found to be statistically similar (67% in the mastectomy arm vs. 63% in the breast-conserving therapy arm; $p = .64$ overall). There was no statistically significant difference in the incidence of contralateral breast carcinoma between the two treatment groups.

Van Dongen et al. (767,768) reported on an EORTC trial comparing modified radical mastectomy with breast-conserving therapy (lumpectomy, axillary clearance, and irradiation to the breast, 50 Gy in 5 weeks and a 25-Gy boost with iridium implant) in 168 patients with stage I and 734 with stage II disease. Patients with microscopically incomplete excision of the tumor were included. Updated analysis from this trial with a median follow-up period of 13.4 years revealed locoregional recurrence rates were higher in the breast-conservation therapy group (10-year rate, 19.7%) than in the mastectomy group (10-year rate, 12.2%; $p = .0097$). The overall survival rate at 10 years was 66.1% for patients undergoing mastectomies and 65.2% for patients undergoing breast-conservation therapy ($p = .11$).

Additional Experiences with Breast-Conserving Surgery Plus Radiation Therapy

Although the acceptance of breast conservation therapy plus radiation therapy as an alternative to mastectomy has been established based on the numerous randomized trials outlined above, large retrospective experiences with long-term follow-up have provided additional data regarding the selection of patients for breast-conserving therapy and radiation, prognostic factors for local–regional end points, impact of various treatment policies and techniques, complications, cosmesis, and long-term outcomes.

Mature Retrospective Series of Breast-Conserving Surgery Plus Radiation Therapy

There have been numerous reports of breast-conserving therapy and radiation, now with follow-up exceeding 10 to 15 years. These studies have provided valuable data regarding technical issues related to treatment and have provided additional data regarding outcomes in subsets of patients, prognostic factors for local control, cosmesis, and other sequelae. Lessons learned from these retrospective series have yielded valuable insight into the conservative management of breast cancer and provide the basis for further prospective studies. Selected publications are highlighted below and in the section on prognostic factors for local control. Long-term outcome from some of these experiences are summarized in Table 53.16. Collectively these studies clearly show long-term outcomes that are consistent with the randomized trials noted above. Local failure rates will depend on follow-up, selection factors, and treatment as discussed later, but in general are expected to range between 0.5% and 1% per year.

Prognostic Factors for Local Relapse Following Breast-Conserving Surgery Plus Radiation Therapy

The retrospective experiences outlined above together with the prospective randomized trials have provided additional data confirming acceptable long-term local control, cosmesis, and toxicities and have identified prognostic factors that contribute to higher local relapse rates and impact on treatment policies.

Local relapse in the conservatively managed breast is an active area of investigation, with numerous studies dedicated to the evaluation of factors that identify patients at increased risk for local relapse following lumpectomy and radiation therapy. Although prognostic factors for local relapse are not as well evaluated as they have been for systemic relapse, there have been numerous studies demonstrating the prognostic value of molecular and genetic markers for local relapse. Local relapse following breast-conserving surgery and radiation can be governed by a complex array of host, primary tumor, and treatment factors, as demonstrated in Fig. 53.16.

Given the complex interaction of these factors, it is sometimes difficult to separate out the independent significance of any one factor. There have, however, been several factors that have been consistently reported in influencing local relapse in the conservatively managed breast cancer patient. Table 53.17 summarizes some of the more commonly reported prognostic factors for local relapse. The factors that most consistently have been reported to influence local relapse, namely, young age, margin status, and the use of systemic therapy, are discussed first, followed by other commonly evaluated prognostic factors.

Age

Young age has found consistently in numerous studies to be a risk factor for breast recurrence in conservation surgery and irradiation. Selected studies are summarized in Table 53.18.

Different investigators have used various age cutoffs, such as 40, 35, and 30 years. Kurtz et al. (427) reported a 19% incidence of local recurrence in 210 women younger than 40 years of age, compared with 9% in 1,172 older women. This observation correlated with EIC, high tumor grade, and a major mononuclear cell reaction. The Harvard Joint Center's inferior results in younger women also correlated with the presence of EIC (607). These findings have also been reported by other authors (121,151,771).

De la Rochefordiére et al. (147), in a study of 1,703 patients with stage I to III breast cancer, noted that younger patients had significantly lower survival rates and higher local and distant relapse rates than older patients. A log-linear function indicated a 4% decrease in recurrence for every year of age at diagnosis.

Fowble et al. (245), in 980 women with stage I and II breast cancer treated with breast-conservation therapy, reported that women younger than 35 years of age had a 53% 8-year relapse-free survival rate, compared with 67% for women 36 to 50 years and women older than 50 years of age (74%). Also, the incidence of breast recurrence was greater in the younger group (24%, 14%, and 12%, respectively; $p = .001$). Regional recurrence rates were 7%, 1%, and 1%, respectively ($p = .0002$).

One of the most significant and powerful studies correlating young age with local relapse was the large EORTC boost versus no boost trial (42). Overall in this study, young patient age was a

| | | Table 53.16 | CONSERVATION SURGERY AND IRRADIATION: NONRANDOMIZED STUDIES STAGE I AND II BREAST CANCER |

Study (Reference)	No. of Patients	Stage	Dose (Gy) Breast	Dose (Gy) Boost	Local Tumor Control (%)	Excellent or Good Cosmesis (%)	10-y Disease-Free Survival (%)
Amalric et al. (14)	1,440	I, II	60	15-20	80	90	74
Barr et al. (39)	411	I, II, III	48.4	20	88	NS	NS
Bartelink et al. (41)	585	T1,T2	50	25	98	NS	T1,92[a] T2,85
Calle et al. (99)	411	I, II	50	10	89	88	78
Clark et al. (119)	1,504	T1-2N0	40/3 wk	5-15	86	NS	70
Clarke et al. (122)	436	T1,T2	45	15	90	NS	—
Delouche et al. (151)	410	T1,T2	50–60	Yes	T1, 94 T2, 86	93	62.5
Dewar al. (159)	757	T0-2	45	15	92	—	69
Dubois et al. (169)	231	I	45	10–15	1,91	90	I-84
	161	II			84		II-75
Fagundes et al. (193)	425	T1,T2	50	10–15	92	77	74[b]
Fourquet et al. (236)	518	T1,T2	57–62	5–12	90	NS	NS
Fowble et al. (241)	697	I, II	50	10–15	91	93	I-79
							II-67
Gage et al. (262)	1,870	I, II	45–50	10–20	87	NS	NS
Haffty et al. (302)	433	I, II	48	10–20	92	NS	81
Kurtz et al. (423)	1,593	I, II	50–60	20	89	—	86
Leborgne et al. (438)	796	I, II	50	10–20	87[d]	NS	82[c]
Osborne et al. (550)	263	T1,T2	45	10	I, 85	—	I, 54
					11,81		II, 29
Pierquin et al. (581)	245	I, II	50	10–20	90	82	75[c]
Recht et al. (607)	366	I, II	50	10	II, 90	—	—
Sarrazin et al. (649)	179	T1smT2	45	15	II, 95	92	85[b]
Solin et al. (709)	217	T1	45–50	10–15	9592	9090	T1, 80[b]
	166	T2	45–50	10–15			T2, 69[b]
van Limbergen et al. (771)	235	T1,T2(3)	40–65	8–20	90	—	T1,75.4
							T2, 61.9
Vicini et al. (799)	1,396	I, II	50	10	92	87	NS
Vilcoq et al. (802)	314	T1,T2	50–55	10–20	90	—	84[b]

NS, not stated.
[a]6-y Disease-free survival.
[b]5-y Disease-free survival.
[c]15-y Disease-free survival.

significant predictor of local relapse. As shown in Figure 53.17 the use of a boost, as will be discussed later in management, was most effective in younger women. In a review of 3,602 women who underwent surgery (breast conservation 55% or mastectomy 45%) for early breast cancer and were rolled in EORTC

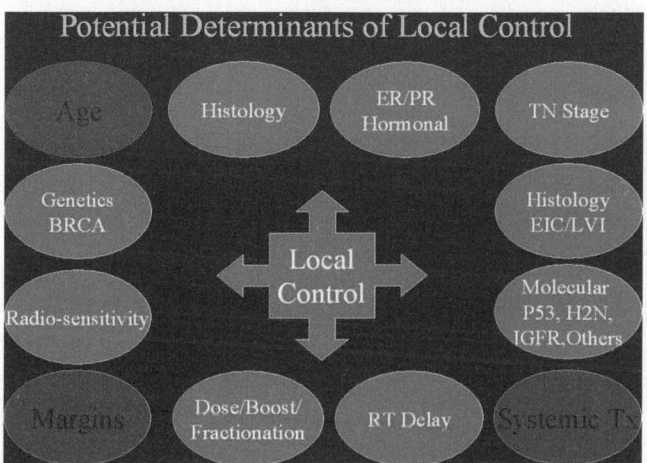

FIGURE 53.16. Schematic diagram of complex interaction of clinical and pathologic factors contributing to local control in the conservatively managed breast cancer patient. EIC/LVI, extensive intraductal carcinoma/lymphatic and vascular invasion; ER/PR, estrogen receptor/progesterone receptor; RT, radiotherapy; Tx, treatment.

studies, de Bock et al. (145) clearly demonstrated the impact of young age on local relapse. The results of multivariate analysis showed that younger age and breast conservation were risk factors for isolated locoregional recurrence (breast cancer under 35 years of age vs. over 50 years of age: hazard ratio 2.80 [95% CI, 1.41 to 5.60]; breast cancer age 35 to 50 years vs. over 50 years: hazard ratio 1.72 [95% CI, 1.17 to 2.54]; breast conservation: hazard ratio 1.82 [95% CI, 1.17 to 2.86]). After perioperative chemotherapy, less isolated locoregional recurrences were observed (hazard ratio: 0.63 [95% CI, 0.44 to 0.91]). It is concluded that young age and breast-conserving therapy are both independent predictors for isolated locoregional recurrence. The authors note that as an isolated locoregional recurrence is a potentially curable condition, women treated with breast conservation or diagnosed with breast cancer at a young age should be monitored closely to detect local recurrence at an early stage.

Numerous other studies, including studies by Chamber et al. (105), Nixon et al. (529), Kini et al. (404), Harrold et al. (334), Haas, et al. (294), and others have confirmed in univariate and multivariate analyses a significant correlation between younger age and local relapse rates. Although there is no apparent cut-off age where relapse rates significantly change, most of the studies have selected 35 or 40 years of age to demonstrate the differences. However, one study that compared the outcome of breast conservation in patients under 40 found that those under 35 had a higher risk of recurrence compared to those aged 36 to 40 (540).

Table 53.17   **SUMMARY OF RISK FACTORS FOR LOCAL RELAPSE**

Prognostic Factor	Effect	Strength of Data	Comment
Age	Young age increases local relapse	Multiple studies Upheld in multivariate analysis Few conflicting reports	Remains among the strongest factors
Margins	Positive margins increase local relapse	Multiple studies Upheld in multivariate analysis Few conflicting reports	Remains among the strongest factors Data on "close" margins are less consistent
Systemic therapy	Systemic therapy (chemo and hormonal) lowers risk of local relapse	Multiple studies support Some conflicting reports	May delay rather than counteract risk
Radiation dose	Higher doses decrease local relapse	Multiple studies support Confirmed in randomized trials (boost vs. no boost) Some conflicting data regarding doses above 50 Gy.	Interaction with margins and age Necessity of "boost" in women over 50 and with widely negative margins unclear
Extensive intraductal component	EIC positive tumors have higher rates of local relapse	Initial studies supportive Some confirmatory studies Some conflicting studies	Recent data suggest that negative margin status eliminates this as a risk factor
LCIS as a component	LCIS as a component increases risk of local relapse	Conflicting data with no clear consensus	Patients with LCIS are suitable candidates for BCS; debate remains regarding need for clear LCIS margins
Lobular histology	Lobular histology has higher local relapse rates	Conflicting data with no clear consensus	Should be treated similar to invasive ductal cancers
BRCA1-2	Higher late local relapses in BRCA1-2 patients	Several confirmatory studies Some conflicting data	Higher relapse rates related to late "new primaries"; this may be minimized by prophylactic hormonal manipulation
Tumor size	Larger tumors result in higher local relapses	Some confirmatory studies Several conflicting studies	Data is confounded by more frequent use of systemic therapy in larger tumors
Nodal status	Higher local relapse rates in node-positive patients	Several conflicting studies	As with tumor size, data are confounded by more frequent use of systemic therapy in node-positive patients
Receptor status	Higher local relapse rates in ER/PR negative patients	Some confirmatory studies Few conflicting studies No clear consensus	

EIC, extensive intraductal carcinoma; ER/PR, estrogen receptor/progesterone receptor; LCIS, lobular carcinoma *in situ*.

Margin Status

Positive margin status has been one of the most consistently reported factors associated with higher local relapse rates. Selected studies are summarized in Table 53.19. Due to the varying definitions of margin status and the complex interaction between margin status and use of systemic therapy, radiation dose, and patient age, there are conflicting conclusions regarding the influence of margin status on local relapse.

Definition of a negative margin is variable between institutions and in national studies. Although some consider no tumor cells seen on the inked margin, as defined by the NSABP, and others consider negative as margins of 1 or 2 mm beyond invasive cancer, of note, many of the studies evaluating margin

Table 53.18   **IPSILATERAL BREAST RECURRENCE RATES BY AGE**

Study (Reference)	Follow-Up (y)	≤35 Year		>35 Year	
		No. of Patients	Recurrence	No. of Patients	Recurrence
Clarke and Martinez (123)	5 (mean)	32	3 (9%)	424	21 (5%)
Fowble et al. (245)	8 (actuarial)	64	15 (24%)	916	119 (13%)
Haffty et al. (300)	8.2 (median)	34	5 (15%)	349	38 (11%)
Halverson et al. (316)	7 (actuarial)	37	3 (9%)	474	57 (12%)
Kini et al. (405)	10 (median)	—	24%	—	7%
Kurtz et al. (426)	11 (mean)	91	15 (16%)	1,291	129 (10%)
Matthews et al. (480)	≥2	72	11(15%)	306	15 (5%)
Nixon et al. (529)	8.3 (median)	107	15 (14%)	1,026	92 (9%)
Veronesi et al. (788)	6 (median)	95	9 (9%)	1,137	45 (4%)
Vicini et al. (799)	5 (actuarial)	65	14 (21%)	721	65 (9%)

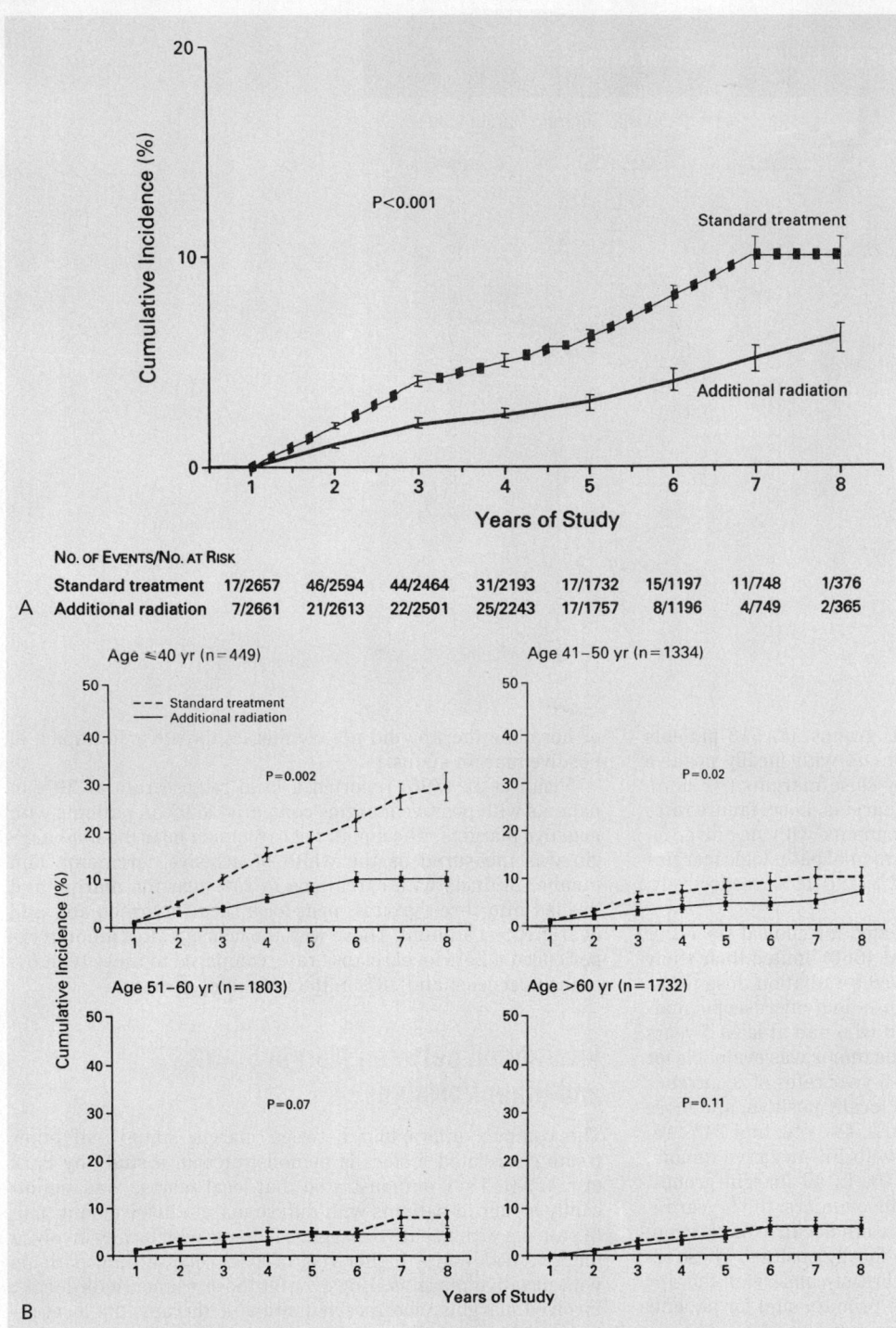

FIGURE 53.17. A: Cumulative incidence of recurrence of tumor in the ipsilateral breast after whole-breast irradiation at 50 Gy, with or without an additional dose to the tumor bed. **B:** Cumulative incidence of recurrence of tumor in the ipsilateral breast after whole-breast irradiation at 50 Gy, with or without an additional dose to the tumor bed, according to age. (From Bartelink H, Horiot J-C, Poortmans P, et al. Recurrence rates after treatment of breast cancer with standard radiotherapy with or without additional radiation. *N Engl J Med* 2001;345:1378–1387, with permission.)

status utilized pathological reports without a central rereview of the original pathology.

The degree of margin involvement (i.e., whether it is focally involved or more diffusely involved) also is a critical issue in determining the significance of margin involvement and how it should influence management. Although there are clearly conflicting reports, it is evident that obtaining a wide negative margin is desirable. However, a focally involved margin, particularly when re-excision is not technically feasible, as may be the case with a focally involved deep margin at the pectoralis facia, is not a contraindication to breast-conserving therapy.

Heimann et al. (343) analyzed 869 cases of stage I and II breast carcinoma in 852 women treated with breast-conserving

surgery and radiation therapy. The median follow-up was 43 months. Final microscopic margins were negative in 762 (88%), microscopically positive in 82 (9%), and unknown in 25 (3%) of the patients. In patients receiving boost radiation to the tumor bed, the local control rates at 5 years were 98% and 89%, respectively, for negative and positive margins (*p* <.01). When the margins of excision were microscopically positive, the tumor control rate was 91% if the total dose to the tumor bed was 60 Gy or greater compared with 76% for a dose of 60 Gy or less (*p* = .05).

Peterson et al. (567) evaluated the significance of final microscopic resection margin in 1,021 women with stage I or II invasive carcinoma of the breast treated with breast-conservation

Table 53.19	IPSILATERAL BREAST RECURRENCE RATES BY MARGINS			
		Recurrence Rates with Different Margin Status		
Study (Reference)	Follow-Up (y)	Positive (%)	Close (%)	Negative (%)
Anscher et al. (22)	5 actuarial	10	—	2
Bartelink et al. (41)	6 actuarial	7	—	2
Borger et al. (70)	5 actuarial	16	—	2
Clarke and Martinez (123)	5 mean	9	—	4
Dewar et al. (159)	10 actuarial	14	—	6
DiBiase et al. (162)	10 actuarial	33	—	12
Freedman et al. (250)	5 actuarial	12	14	7
Ghossein et al. (276)	7 median	10	—	12
Hartsell et al. (338)	3.4 median	11	—	2
Heimann et al. (343)	5 actuarial	11	—	2
Jobsen et al. (381)	10 actuarial	12	—	5
Park et al. (554)	8 crude rate	18	7	7
Peterson et al. (567)	8 actuarial	10	17	8
Pittinger et al. (585)	4.5 crude rate	25	2.9	3
Ryoo et al. (641)	3.5 median	—	13	8
Schnitt et al. (660)	6.2 median	13	4	2
Smitt et al. (704)	—	9	16	2
Solin et al. (713)	5 actuarial	2	11	7
Vicini et al. (796)	12 actuarial	30	18-24	9
Wazer et al. (818)	12 actuarial	17	9	5

therapy, who were divided into four groups: (a) 518 patients with negative margins, (b) 124 patients with focally positive margins, (c) 96 patients with focally close margins (≤2 mm), and (d) 283 patients with unknown margins. Local failure rates were not significantly different in patients with negative, focally positive, focally close, or unknown final pathologic margins of resection at 8 years (8%, 10%, 17%, and 16%, respectively; $p = .21$).

From a group of 607 patients treated for clinical stage I or II invasive breast cancer, Schnitt et al. (660) limited their study to 181 patients with IDC who received a radiation dose to the surgical site of 60 Gy or greater, whose final microscopic margins of resection were evaluable, and who had at least 5 years of follow-up. In 157 patients (87%), the tumor was evaluable for the presence or absence of EIC. The 5-year rates of recurrence among patients with negative, close, focally positive, and more than focally positive margins were 0%, 4%, 6%, and 21%, respectively. Among the 127 patients with EIC-negative tumors, the 5-year recurrence rate was <10% in all margin groups. Among the 30 patients with EIC-positive tumors, the 5-year recurrence rate was 0% when margins were negative or close but 50% when margins were more than focally positive. These results provide support for the use of breast-conserving therapy (including an irradiation boost to the primary site) for patients with EIC-positive tumors and negative margins.

In a similar analysis, Gage et al. (263) noted that patients with positive margins had a greater probability of breast relapse (21/131, 16%) than patients with negative margins (4/209, 2%). However, patients with focally positive margins had a failure rate of 9%. Patients with EIC and positive margins had the highest probability of breast relapse (8/19, 42%).

In an analysis of the Yale experience, Obedian and Haffty (539) reported a higher rate of local relapse among patients with positive margins. Patients were divided into four groups based on final pathologic margin status: negative ($n = 278$), close (within 2 mm, $n = 47$), positive ($n = 55$), or indeterminate ($n = 491$). Breast relapse-free survival at 10 years was 98% for patients with negative margins versus 98% for those with close margins versus 83% for those with positive margins versus 82% for those with indeterminate margins. Adjuvant chemotherapy

or hormone therapy did not counteract the adverse impact of positive margin status.

Vicini et al. (796) reported a local relapse rate of 30% in patients with positive margins compared to 9% in patients with negative margins. The amount of carcinoma near the final margin was measured as the width of invasive carcinoma and number of ducts with carcinoma in situ near the margin and divided into three groups: near-least, near-intermediate, and near-greatest amount. Those with the near-greatest amount experienced a 24% local relapse rate, compared to those with 6% in the near-least and 18% in the near-intermediate.

Interaction between Margin Status and Other Variables

The complex interaction between margin status and other treatment-related factors is demonstrated in a study by Park et al (554). They demonstrated that local relapse was significantly higher in patients with diffuse margin involvement than in patients with negative margins. Patients with focally involved margins also had a higher risk of local relapse than patients with negative margins. However, in those women with focally involved margins who received systemic therapy, the local relapse rate was similar to those with negative margins. Whether systemic therapy delays or negates the effect of a focally involved margin is a matter of debate, but clearly there are confounding factors that complicate interpretation of the available data.

Freedman et al. (250) studied 1,262 patients with clinical stage I or II breast cancer treated by breast-conserving surgery, axillary node dissection, and radiation therapy. The final margins were negative in 77%, positive in 12%, and close (≤2 mm) in 11%. The 5-year incidence of ipsilateral breast tumor recurrence was not significantly different between patients with negative (4%), positive (5%), or close (7%) margins. However, by 10 years, a significant difference in ipsilateral breast tumor recurrence became apparent (negative 7%, positive 12%, close 14%; $p = .04$). The 5-year cumulative ipsilateral breast tumor recurrence rate in patients with close or positive margins was 1% with adjuvant systemic therapy and 13% with no adjuvant therapy. However, by 10 years, the ipsilateral breast tumor recurrence rate was similar (18% vs. 14%) owing to more late failures in the patients who received adjuvant systemic therapy.

A study by Jobsen et al. (381) demonstrates some of the difficulties associated with interpretation of studies related to margin status and local relapse as it relates to other prognostic factors. In a study of 1,752 patients with known margin status and a median follow-up of 78 months, the 10-year local relapse rate was 5.6% and 12.2% for negative and positive margins, respectively. An interaction between age category and margin status was noted in relation to local relapse-free survival. The 5-year local relapse rate for women <40 years of age was 8.4% for negative margins and 36.9% for positive margins ($p = .005$). On the other hand the 5-year local relapse rate for women >40 years was 2.6% for negative and 2.2% for positive margins.

Although it is clear that margin status is a significant risk factor for local relapse, and negative margins are desirable, the available data suggest that patients with a focally involved margin are suitable candidates for breast-conserving therapy followed by radiation therapy to the intact breast.

Effect of Systemic Therapy on Local Control

The use of systemic therapy, in the form of adjuvant tamoxifen or adjuvant chemotherapy, has been clearly shown to impact local control in numerous retrospective and prospective randomized trials. Although it has been clearly demonstrated in randomized trials that chemotherapy and tamoxifen are not appropriate substitutes for radiation therapy, in patients who are treated with radiation therapy, the use of systemic therapy improves local control (88,201,204). As with the other critical prognostic factors, the degree to which systemic therapy influences local control is confounded by other factors.

In the NSABP B-06 trial, patients with lymph node–positive disease who were treated with radiation therapy and chemotherapy had an 8-year local recurrence rate of 5% compared with a local recurrence rate of 12% in lymph node–negative patients treated with surgery and radiation therapy alone (203). In the NSABP B-21 trial, tamoxifen similarly improved local control rates in patients with lymph node–negative breast tumors smaller than 1 cm. The crude rate of breast tumor recurrence was only 3% in women randomly assigned to undergo lumpectomy, radiation therapy, and tamoxifen compared with 7% in women treated with lumpectomy and radiation therapy alone (208). A retrospective analysis from the M.D. Anderson Cancer Center investigating the impact of systemic therapy on local control after breast-conservation therapy in patients with lymph node–negative breast cancer further confirmed these data (88). In this study, 277 patients treated with systemic therapy had improved 5-year (97.5% vs. 89.8%) and

10-year (95.6% vs. 85.2%) local control rates compared with 207 patients who received no systemic treatment. No statistically significant difference was evident in local control between patients treated with chemotherapy and those treated with tamoxifen alone ($p = .219$). In a Cox regression analysis, the use of systemic therapy was the most powerful clinical, pathologic, or treatment predictor of local control, producing a 3.3-fold reduction in the risk of local recurrence. Similar results have been reported in a series from Yale, where the risk of local relapse was lower among patients treated by breast-conserving surgery and radiation with adjuvant chemotherapy or adjuvant tamoxifen, compared to patients treated without adjuvant systemic therapy (308).

Table 53.20 summarizes several studies that have evaluated local control as a function of systemic therapy. It is evident that both hormonal therapy, as well as cytotoxic chemotherapy, influences local relapse rates.

Tumor Size

Although tumor size is clearly a strong predictor of systemic relapse and overall survival, its prognostic value in local relapse has not been consistently reported (Table 53.21). Differences are probably related to the treatment techniques used (e.g., completeness of tumor excision, use of irradiation boost) and the complex interaction of other prognostic factors as noted above.

Tumor Location

Location of the primary tumor within the breast is not known to be a contraindication to breast-conserving surgery, and any specific location is not associated with a higher local relapse rate. Haffty et al. (309), in a review of 1,014 patients with early breast cancer treated with breast-conservation therapy, identified 98 patients who had a central/subareolar tumor. Ten of 98 patients had the nipple–areola complex sacrificed at the time of surgery, whereas the remaining 88 patients had the entire area included in the boost cone-down field. The 10-year actuarial breast recurrence–free survival rate was 84%, the distant disease-free survival rate was 88%, and the overall survival rate was 79%, similar to patients with tumors in other locations. The nipple–areola complex could be preserved in most patients, and there were no significant complications. Thus, a subareolar breast cancer presentation was not a contraindication to breast-conserving therapy in early stage disease.

However, Gajdos et al. (267) reported on 95 women with tumors located within 2 cm of the border of the areola, considered to be subareolar carcinomas; 62 were treated with breast-conserving surgery and 33 with mastectomies. Radiation therapy was given to 87% of the breast-conserving surgery group and to 13% of the mastectomy group. The nipple–areola

---

Table 53.20 · IPSILATERAL BREAST RECURRENCE RATES BY SYSTEMIC TREATMENT (SysTx)

Study (Reference)	No. Patients	Follow-Up (y)	SysTx	With SysTx (%)	Without SysTx (%)	p
					Local Relapse	
NSABP-13 (213)	760	8	CTX	2.6	13	.001
NSABP-14 (210)	1400	10	Tam	3.4	10.3	.001
Buchholz et al. (88)	484	8	CTX+Tam	4.4	14.8	.004
Haffty et al. (300)	548	7	CTX+Tam	6	12	.02
Park et al. (positive margin) (554)	45	8	CTX	7	18	.05

CTX, chemotherapy; Tam, tamoxifen.

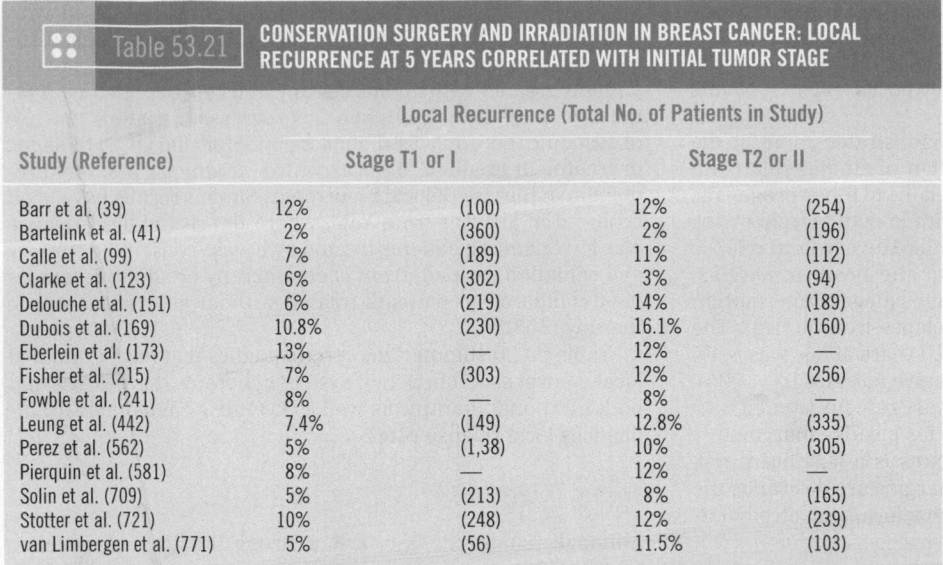

Table 53.21 CONSERVATION SURGERY AND IRRADIATION IN BREAST CANCER: LOCAL RECURRENCE AT 5 YEARS CORRELATED WITH INITIAL TUMOR STAGE

| Study (Reference) | Local Recurrence (Total No. of Patients in Study) | | | |
	Stage T1 or I		Stage T2 or II	
Barr et al. (39)	12%	(100)	12%	(254)
Bartelink et al. (41)	2%	(360)	2%	(196)
Calle et al. (99)	7%	(189)	11%	(112)
Clarke et al. (123)	6%	(302)	3%	(94)
Delouche et al. (151)	6%	(219)	14%	(189)
Dubois et al. (169)	10.8%	(230)	16.1%	(160)
Eberlein et al. (173)	13%	—	12%	—
Fisher et al. (215)	7%	(303)	12%	(256)
Fowble et al. (241)	8%	—	8%	—
Leung et al. (442)	7.4%	(149)	12.8%	(335)
Perez et al. (562)	5%	(1,38)	10%	(305)
Pierquin et al. (581)	8%	—	12%	—
Solin et al. (709)	5%	(213)	8%	(165)
Stotter et al. (721)	10%	(248)	12%	(239)
van Limbergen et al. (771)	5%	(56)	11.5%	(103)

complex was removed in 11 women in the breast-conserving group. On univariate analysis, variables significantly related to pathologic involvement of the nipple–areola complex were clinical involvement of the nipple–areola complex ($p = .001$), mammographic calcifications or Paget's disease ($p < .001$), pathologic tumor size ($p = .019$), and the presence of an EIC ($p = .098$). When radiation therapy was accounted for in multivariate analysis, the only variable significantly related to local recurrence in patients undergoing breast-conserving surgery was clinical involvement of the nipple–areola complex.

Extensive Intraductal Carcinoma

According to the Harvard definition of EIC, 25% or more of the primary tumor is intraductal carcinoma, and intraductal carcinoma is seen outside (adjacent to) the infiltrating tumor border (332). Fourquet et al. (236) reported a 30% incidence of EIC in 195 women younger than 45 years of age compared with 10.4% in 279 older women. EIC involving the primary tumor and adjacent tissues has been reported by some groups, particularly Harvard University and Marseilles, to be associated with a higher incidence of breast recurrences (331,425,427). In contrast, Clarke et al. (122), Fisher and Anderson (205), Fisher et al. (222), and van Limbergen et al. (771) found no significant impact on local tumor control with EIC. This difference may be related to the definition of EIC, adequacy of tumor excision, doses of irradiation delivered to the boost volume, as well as interactions with other factors. It has been reported by some that a somewhat higher breast relapse rate in EIC-positive patients was seen only in women younger than 40 years of age. Table 53.22 summarizes reports of breast relapse correlated with presence of EIC in selected studies.

Holland et al. (353) stated that an EIC component is associated with subsequent breast recurrence because of the presence of residual intraductal carcinoma in these patients. In a series of 214 women who underwent mastectomy, 71% of those with EIC had residual intraductal carcinoma, compared with 28% of those without that pathologic feature. In particular, 44% of the EIC-positive patients had prominent residual tumor compared with 3% of those who were EIC negative ($p < .00001$).

The impact of EIC on local relapse, however, appears to be minimized if negative margins are achieved. Although negative margins are desirable in all patients undergoing breast-conserving surgery, attention to margins in patients with EIC is particularly relevant, as a negative margin may decrease or eliminate the significance of EIC with respect to local failure.

Table 53.22 INCIDENCE OF BREAST RELAPSE CORRELATED WITH EXTENSIVE INTRADUCTAL CARCINOMA COMPONENT IN PRIMARY BREAST TUMOR ADJACENT BREAST

| Study (Reference) | Breast Recurrence at 5 Years (Total No. of Patients in Study) | | | |
	EIC Present		EIC Absent	
Bartelink et al. (41)	9%	(78)	2%	(203)
Boyages et al. (73)	24%	(165)	6%	(418)
Eberlein et al. (173)	27%	(165)	7%	(418)
Fisher et al. (222)	11%	(55)	9%	(366)
Fowble et al. (246)	22%	(22)	4%	(251)
Kurtz et al. (423)	18%	(105)	8%	(390)
Schnitt et al. (661)	15%	(132)	1%	(97)
Veronesi et al. (788)				
Quadrantectomy	10%	(21)	4%	(339)
Tumorectomy	30%	(37)	8%	(304)
Zafrani et al. (846)	11%	(62)	6%	(361)

EIC, extensive intraductal carcinoma

In a study from the Harvard group, Gage et al. (263) evaluated clinical stage I or II breast carcinoma treated with radiation therapy as part of breast-conserving therapy, of whom 343 had invasive ductal histology evaluable for an EIC, had inked margins that were evaluable for a review of their pathology slides, and received $\geq$60 Gy to the tumor bed. The 5-year rate of incidence of breast recurrences for patients with negative margins was 2%; for patients with positive margins, the rate was 16%. Among patients with negative margins, the 5-year rate of incidence of breast recurrences was 2% for all patients with close margins (negative $\leq$1 mm) and 3% for those with negative >1 mm margins. For patients with close margins, the rates were 2% and 0% for EIC-negative and EIC-positive tumors, respectively; the corresponding rates for patients with negative margins >1 mm were 1% and 14%. The 5-year rate of incidence of breast recurrences for patients with focally positive margins was 9% (9% for EIC-negative and 7% for EIC-positive patients). The 5-year crude rate of incidence of breast recurrences for patients with greater than focally positive margins was 28% (19% for EIC-negative and 42% for EIC-positive patients). The authors conclude that patients with negative margins of excision have a low rate of recurrence in the treated breast, whether the margin is >1 mm or $\leq$1 mm and whether the carcinoma is EIC negative or EIC positive. It appears from this study that although EIC may be a poor prognostic factor for local relapse, achievement of a negative margin eliminates EIC as a risk factor.

Histology

In general, studies that have evaluated local relapse in relation to histologic subtypes of breast cancer have not demonstrated higher relapse rates associated with specific histologic patterns. Weiss et al. (824) reported on 879 patients with stage I and II breast cancer treated with conservation surgery and irradiation. The patients were divided into seven groups based on histologic subtype: 368 patients with infiltrating and intraductal ductal carcinoma, 389 with IDC, 41 with ILC, 23 with combined infiltrating ductal and lobular carcinoma, 28 with medullary carcinoma, 12 with colloid carcinoma, and 18 with tubular carcinoma. There were no significant differences in 5-year actuarial overall survival, cause-specific survival, or relapse-free survival rates among the histologic categories. There was, however, a difference among the seven groups in distant metastasis only at first failure, with IDCs having the highest rate.

Thurman et al. (742), in an analysis of the Harvard series, identified 20 clinical stage I and II patients with mucinous carcinoma, 27 with medullary carcinoma, 28 with tubular carcinoma, and 1,055 with IDC. No significant difference was seen in the site of first failure between the four histologic types within the first 10 years after treatment. Local failure was significantly associated with age <50 years (p = .04), positive surgical margins (p = .007), lymphovascular invasion (p = .04), and presence of an extensive intraductal component (p <.001).

An analysis of medullary carcinomas treated conservatively was performed by the Yale group, who identified 46 cases of conservatively treated patients with medullary histology who were compared to 1,444 patients with infiltrating ductal carcinoma (809). The medullary cohort presented at a younger age with a higher percentage of patients in the 35 years or younger age group (26.1% vs. 6.6%; p <.00001). Twelve patients with medullary histology underwent genetic screening, and six patients were identified with deleterious mutations. This group showed greater association with BRCA1/2 mutations compared with screened patients in the control group (50.0% vs. 15.8%; p = .0035). The medullary cohort was also significantly associated with greater T stage and tumor size (37.0% vs. 17.2% T2; mean size 3.2 vs. 2.5 cm; p = .00097) as well as negative ER (84.9% vs. 37.6%; p <.00001) and PR (87.5% vs. 48.1%;

p = .00001) status. Breast relapse-free rates were not significantly different from the invasive ductal cancers (76.7% vs. 85.2%); however, 10-year distant relapse-free survival in the medullary cohort was significantly better than in the control group (94.9% vs. 77.5%; p = .028).

Tubular carcinomas treated with conservative surgery and radiation were reviewed by Sullivan et al. (725). They reviewed 62 of their own cases from Massachusetts General as well as 529 cases from the literature. They conclude that tubular carcinoma is associated with an excellent prognosis, but long-term follow-up is essential for detecting local failures. Adjuvant radiation therapy reduces the incidence of local failure following CS for tubular carcinoma. However, elderly women treated by CS may have a very low risk of local recurrence without adjuvant radiation therapy.

Infiltrating Lobular Carcinoma

A review of the literature strongly supports local tumor resection and breast irradiation as appropriate therapy for invasive lobular breast cancer, following the same guidelines used for invasive ductal tumors. Breast tumor control and survival after breast-conserving therapy are equivalent in patients with invasive ductal or lobular carcinoma. However, long-term follow-up is important because more lobular carcinoma local recurrences are late events.

Due to the presumed multicentric nature of lobular carcinomas, several groups have attempted to assess whether these subtypes are more prone to local failure with breast-conserving approaches. Schnitt et al. (663) compared the results of tumor excision and irradiation in 49 patients with stage I and II invasive lobular carcinomas and 561 patients with similar stages of invasive ductal carcinomas. The 5-year actuarial risk of local recurrence was similar for both groups (12% vs. 11%), and for IDC with or without an EIC, 23% and 5%, respectively.

Sastre-Garau et al. (653) evaluated 726 cases of ILC, 249 cases of mixed infiltrating ILC/IDC, and 10,061 cases of nonlobular infiltrating carcinoma (NLC). Follow-up was carried out on a subgroup of 5,846 cases. At diagnosis, ILC tumors were found to be larger than those with NLC, but lymph node involvement was lower in patients with ILC than in NLC. Multicentric lesions were not significantly more frequent in ILC than in NLC. The overall survival, locoregional control, disease-free interval, and metastatic spread rates were not different among the three groups. In 480 cases of ILC considered for conservation therapy, the local recurrence and overall survival rates were similar to those observed for IDC, but the pattern of metastatic dissemination was different.

Silverstein et al. (681) compared 161 patients with ILC and 1,138 patients with IDC. ILCs were larger, more difficult to diagnose clinically, and more difficult to excise completely. Nodal positivity for ILC was 32%, compared with 37% for IDC (p = .22). The 7-year disease-free survival rates were 74% for patients with ILC and 63% for those with IDC (p <.03). The 7-year cancer-specific survival rates were 83% and 77%, respectively (p <.04). The local breast failure rate was 5% in both the lobular and ductal carcinoma groups.

In an analysis of the University of Pennsylvania experience, Santiago et al. (646) compared 55 women with ILC to 1,093 women with IDC. There was no difference in the 10-year actuarial rates of overall survival (85% vs. 79%, respectively; p = .73), cause-specific survival (93% vs. 84%, respectively; p = .85), or freedom from distant metastases (81% vs. 80%, respectively; p = .76). The 10-year rates of local failure were 18% for patients with ILC and 12% for patients with IDC (p = .24), and the 10-year rates of contralateral breast carcinoma development for the two groups were 12% and 8%, respectively (p = .40).

Clinical Radiation Oncology

	Table 53.23	STUDIES EVALUATING LCIS AS A COMPONENT OF BREAST CANCER LOCAL RELAPSE IN BREAST-CONSERVING SURGERY

Study (Reference)	Patients and Controls		Follow-Up	Local Relapse		
	With LCIS	Without LCIS	(median in years)	With LCIS (%)	Without LCIS (%)	p
Moran and Haffty (508)	51	1,045	10.6	5	7	NS
Abner et al. (2)	119	1,062	13.4	13	12	NS
Ben-David et al. (48)	64	121	3.9	100	99.1	NS
Jolly et al. (382)	46	551	8.7	14	7	.04
Sasson et al. (652)	65	1,209	6.3	15	5	.001

LCIS, lobular carcinoma *in situ*; NS, not significant.

Lobular Carcinoma *In Situ* as a Component of Invasive Cancers

Several groups have evaluated whether patients with LCIS as a component of invasive cancer or DCIS was associated with higher local relapse rates. Conflicting results from these studies, as outlined in Table 53.23 preclude firm conclusions. Sasson et al. (652) noted that LCIS was present in 65 of 1,274 patients (5%) with stage I or II breast cancer. LCIS was more likely to be associated with an invasive lobular carcinoma (30/59 patients; 51%) than with IDC (26/1,125 patients; 2%). The 10-year cumulative incidence rate of ipsilateral breast tumor recurrence was 6% in women without LCIS compared with 29% in women with LCIS (*p* = .0003). In both groups, the majority of recurrences were invasive. The 10-year cumulative incidence rate of ipsilateral breast tumor recurrence in patients who received tamoxifen was 8% when LCIS was present compared with 6% when LCIS was absent (*p* = .46). In a series of 56 patients with an LCIS component, Jolly et al. (382) reported a higher risk of local relapse at 10 years (14%) compared to a rate of 7% in cases without an LCIS component. In multivariate analysis a component of LCIS was associated with a higher risk of local relapse.

However, studies from Yale, Harvard, and the University of Michigan failed to show a higher local relapse rate in patients with a component of LCIS. Abner et al. (2) reviewed 1,181 patients with stage I or II infiltrating ductal, infiltrating lobular, or infiltrating carcinoma with mixed features who had received at least 60 Gy to the tumor bed and had a minimum follow-up of 8 years. Of the 1,181 patients, 137 had detectable LCIS in or adjacent to the tumor. The 8-year local recurrence rate was not significantly increased for patients with LCIS overall or for the subgroup of patients with LCIS in or adjacent to the tumor. The risk of contralateral disease and of distant treatment failure also was unaffected by the presence or extent of LCIS (5% to 10% in all groups). Similar results were reported by Moran and Haffty (508) in an analysis of the Yale series where there was no statistically significant difference between patients with or without a component of LCIS in the 10-year overall survival (67% vs. 72%), distant disease-free survival (62% vs. 79%), or ipsilateral breast tumor recurrence-free survival (77% LCIS vs. 84% control). Ben-David et al. (48) reported the results on 64 cases treated at University of Michigan and also found no association between local failure and presence of LCIS. The presence of LCIS at the margins and the size and presence of multifocal LCIS did not alter the rate of local control.

Other Histologic Features

Clemente et al. (126), in 506 cases of infiltrating ductal carcinoma (T1–2/N0/M0), described peritumoral lymphatic infiltration in 6.9% of routinely evaluated specimens, whereas in a randomly selected group of 234 cases the frequency was 20%. Patients with peritumoral lymphatic infiltration had worse disease-free and total survival rates than those without this feature (*p* = .0001 for each), as well as more local recurrences (*p* = .0001) and a higher incidence of distant metastases (*p* = .0576).

Wong et al. (838), in a study of 234 patients with clinical T1/N0 breast cancer treated with breast-conservation surgery and radiation therapy, scored 180 patients as lymphatic vessel invasion negative and 54 as invasion positive (23 focal and 31 extensive). The local first failure rates were 14% and 22%, respectively. The percentages of regional distant failure (without local failure) were 12% and 21%, respectively. At 10 years, 60% of the lymphatic vessel invasion–negative patients remained free of any failure, compared with 50% of the lymphatic vessel invasion–positive patients.

Nodal Status

Although nodal status is the strongest predictor of distant metastasis and overall survival, most studies have not clearly demonstrated an effect of nodal status on local control in the conservatively managed breast cancer patient. This may be due to the fact that a majority of node-positive patients receive chemotherapy and/or hormonal therapy, which may counteract the effect of any minimal effect on local relapse. There are some data, however, that suggest an effect of nodal status on local relapse in conservatively managed patients. The Primary Therapy of Breast Cancer Study Group and others noted lower survival and a greater incidence of local recurrences in patients with positive axillary nodes after partial mastectomy (175,214,367,436,592). At the Institut Gustave-Roussy, among 336 patients, local recurrence was noted in 26% of those with and 6.5% of those without nodal involvement (649); the greater the number of nodes involved, the more likely the occurrence of local failure and the lower the survival rate (164,649). Increased incidence of breast relapse was also observed by van Limbergen et al. (771) in patients with N1b metastasis (8/42 patients, or 19%) and in those in whom three or more lymph nodes (4/14 patients, or 28.6%) compared with patients with N0 or N1a lymph nodes (14/187, 7.5%). However, more recent reports by several investigators noted lower survival rates but fewer breast relapses after breast-conservation therapy in patients with positive nodes. Again, this is likely a result of the interaction of irradiation to the breast with adjuvant chemotherapy. Since most node-positive patients receive chemotherapy, which is synergistic with radiation in lowering the local relapse rate, any potential adverse effect of positive nodes on local relapse may be lost.

Molecular Factors and Local Relapse

In comparison with an explosion of data regarding molecular markers as risk factors for overall survival and distant metastasis in breast cancer, there are relatively few data relating molecular markers to local relapse in the conservatively managed breast. There have been several studies, however, which demonstrate the potential application of molecular markers in predicting local–regional relapse in breast cancer patients (301,312,510). Particularly exciting is the potential to not only use these markers to identify patients at risk for relapse, but to consider the molecular markers as potential targets for therapeutic intervention and increasing radiation sensitivity. Several molecular markers have been shown in bench studies to be associated with radiation resistance, including p53, HER-2/neu, IGF-1R, and other markers associated with hypoxia (176,178,296,301,451,510,577,617,618,647,683,716, 758,848). Although there have been some consistent findings, to date there are many conflicting results and the numbers of events in any one series are not significant enough to base clinical decision making on. This is clearly an area that is ripe for further investigation, ideally with molecular studies linked to large clinical trials, to help to identify molecular markers predictive of local–regional outcomes and hopefully to identify potential targets for improving outcomes. Table 53.24 summarizes selected studies evaluating molecular markers for local–regional relapse in conservatively managed breast cancers.

Breast-Conserving Surgery without Radiation

Based on the mature data from the well-conducted randomized trials outlined above and on long-term follow-up from the several large retrospective series, it is apparent that breast-conserving surgery followed by radiation therapy is a safe and effective modality for the majority of women with early stage invasive breast cancer (330). Whether subsets of patients can be treated with breast-conserving surgery alone without irradiation has been the subject of considerable debate and several randomized trials. With the possible exception of selected elderly women, which will be discussed in a later section, subsets of patients in whom radiation therapy can be safely avoided have yet to be clearly identified. Collectively, the randomized studies to date consistently demonstrate approximately a threefold greater local relapse rate in the unirradiated cohorts (803). Although the majority of these trials did not demonstrate an impact on survival, recent pooled analysis of these randomized trials demonstrates a small, but statistically significant impact on mortality as a result of the omission of radiation.

Vinh-Hung et al. (803) conducted a pooled analysis of published randomized clinical trials that compared radiotherapy versus no radiotherapy after breast-conserving surgery. The outcomes studied were ipsilateral breast tumor recurrence and patient death from any cause. A search of the literature identified 15 trials with a pooled total of 9,422 patients available for analysis. The relative risk of ipsilateral breast tumor recurrence after breast-conserving surgery, comparing patients treated with no radiotherapy or radiotherapy, was 3.00 (95% CI, 2.65 to 3.40). Mortality data were available for 13 trials with a pooled total of 8,206 patients. The relative risk of mortality was 1.086 (95% CI, 1.003 to 1.175), corresponding to an estimated 8.6% (95% CI, 0.3 to 17.5) relative excess mortality if radiotherapy was omitted (Fig. 53.18A,B).

In an analysis from the Early Breast Cancer Trialists Collaborative Group, similar conclusions were reached evaluating various forms of local therapy (124). Within this meta-analysis were 7,300 women treated with breast-conserving surgery in

| Table 53.24 | MOLECULAR MARKERS IN THE LOCAL MANAGEMENT OF EARLY BREAST CANCER TREATED WITH BREAST-CONSERVING SURGERY PLUS RADIOTHERAPY |

Markers	Study (Reference)	Patient Population	Local Relapse
ER/PR	Silvestrini (684)	970 node negative	No correlation for either ER or PR
	Elkhuizen et al. (178)	195 case-control IBC	Higher frequency of PR-negative tumors in locally recurrent population (75% vs. 60%; *p* = .03)
	Vrieling et al. (807)	5,569 cases	Higher recurrence rate was observed in ER-negative or PR-negative tumors
	Grills et al. (286)	1,500 IBC	Regional nodal failure was associated with ER status on univariate analysis
	Choi et al. (114)	103 IBC	Neither ER nor PR correlated with local relapse rate; PR negativity was related with distant metastasis
	Pierce et al. (574)	867 IBC	Negative ER status was related to local failure
	Santiago et al. (647)	937 IBC	Negative PR status was related to local recurrence
HER2/neu	Haffty et al. (296)	20 case-control IBC	Higher expression of HER2/neu in patients experiencing local relapse (19% vs. 10%; *p* = .10)
	Pierce et al. (577)	137 IBC	HER2/neu correlated with extensive intraductal component but did not correlate to local relapse
	Kim et al. (401)	611 IBC	HER2/neu correlated with over all survival but not local relapse
	Choi et al. (114)	103 IBC	HER2/neu was not related with local or distant failure
	Harris et al. (329)	356 IBC	HER2/neu was not related to local failure
p53	Silvestrini et al. (686)	496 IBC	No correlation with p53 and local relapse
	Turner et al. (758)	94 IBC	p53 overexpression more common in locally recurrent group compared to locally controlled group (26% vs. 9%; *p* = .02)
	Elkhuizen et al. (178)	195 case-control IBC	p53 expression similar in locally recurrent and locally controlled group (21% vs. 23%; *p* = .61)
	Amornmarn et al. (19)	112 IBC	p53 expression associated with all local recurrence cases (only four local relapses in series)
	Choi et al. (114)	103 IBC	p53 was not related with local or distant failure
Proliferative markers	Choi et al. (114)	103 IBC	Ki-67 positivity was related with distant but not local failure
	Silvestrini et al. (685)	496 IBC	Thymidine-labeling index was not related with local failure
ATM mutation	Meyer et al. (497)	135 IBC	ATM gene alterations were not related to patient outcomes

ATM, ataxia telangiectasis mutations; ER, estrogen receptor; IBC, infiltrating breast cancer; PR, progesterone receptor

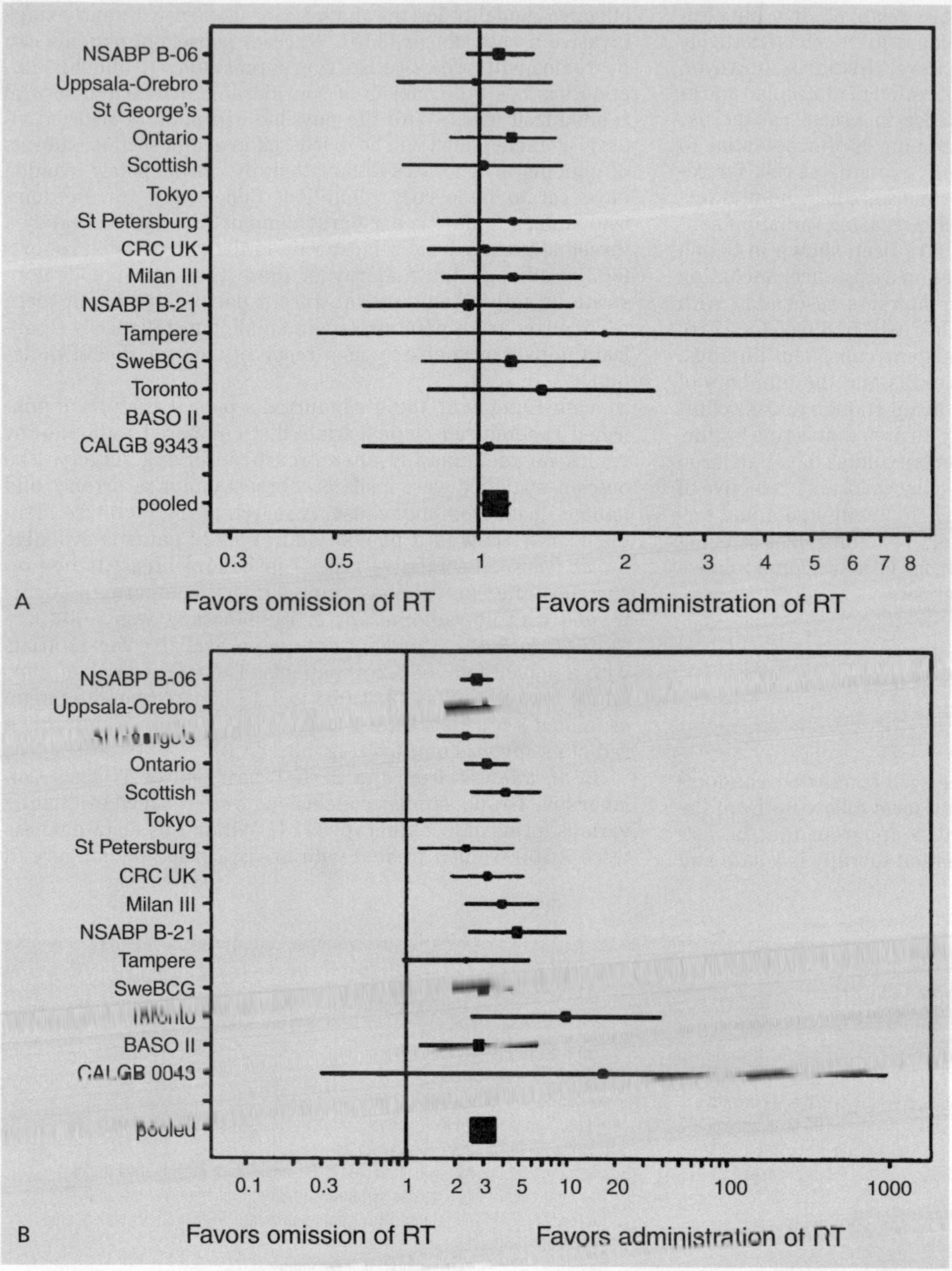

FIGURE 53.18 Meta-analysis of survival and local control in randomized trials comparing breast-conserving surgery with or without radiation. This meta-analysis demonstrated a three-fold reduction in local relapse and a small but significant increase in survival with the use of radiation therapy following lumpectomy. BASO, British Association of Surgical Oncology; CALGB, Cancer and Leukemia Group B; CRC, Clinical Research Council; NSABP, National Surgical Adjuvant Breast and Bowel Project; RT, radiotherapy; SweBCG, Swedish Breast Cancer Group (From Vinh-Hung V, Verschraegen C. Breast-conserving surgery with or without radiotherapy: pooled-analysis for risks of ipsilateral breast tumor recurrence and mortality. *J Natl Cancer Inst* 2004;96:115–121, with permission.)

trials randomizing patients to radiation therapy versus no radiation therapy. The majority included patients with axillary clearance of node-negative disease and generally were treated with radiation to the conserved breast alone. The reduction in local recurrence (mainly in the conserved breast) in patients treated with radiotherapy was highly significant ($p < .00001$) in every separate trial. As seen in Fig. 53.19, the recurrence rate ratio, comparing those allocated radiotherapy with those not, is about 0.3 in every trial, corresponding to a proportional reduction of 70%. Considering all 10 trials together, the 5-year risk of local recurrence is 7% among those allocated radiotherapy and 26% among those not, corresponding to an absolute reduction of 19% in this 5-year risk.

The proportional risk reduction for breast cancer mortality is much less than that for local recurrence, and none of the trial-specific breast cancer mortality results are clearly significant on their own. However, collectively there is a significant impact on breast cancer mortality (breast cancer death rate ratio 0.83,

SE 95% CI, 0.75 to 0.91; $p = .0002$), indicating a reduction of about one-sixth in the annual breast cancer mortality rate. The 15-year risk of death from breast cancer (in the hypothetical absence of other causes) is 30.5% among those allocated post-breast conserving surgery plus radiotherapy and 35.9% among those not (corresponding to an absolute reduction of 5.4%, SE 1.7).

Randomized Trials

Selected trials comparing breast-conserving surgery alone to breast-conserving surgery with radiation are summarized in Table 53.25.

The Uppsala-Orebro Breast Cancer Study Group reported on a trial in which women with stage I breast carcinoma were randomly assigned to be treated with either sector resection and axillary dissection plus 54 Gy breast irradiation (184 patients) or the same surgical procedure alone (197 patients) (447). The

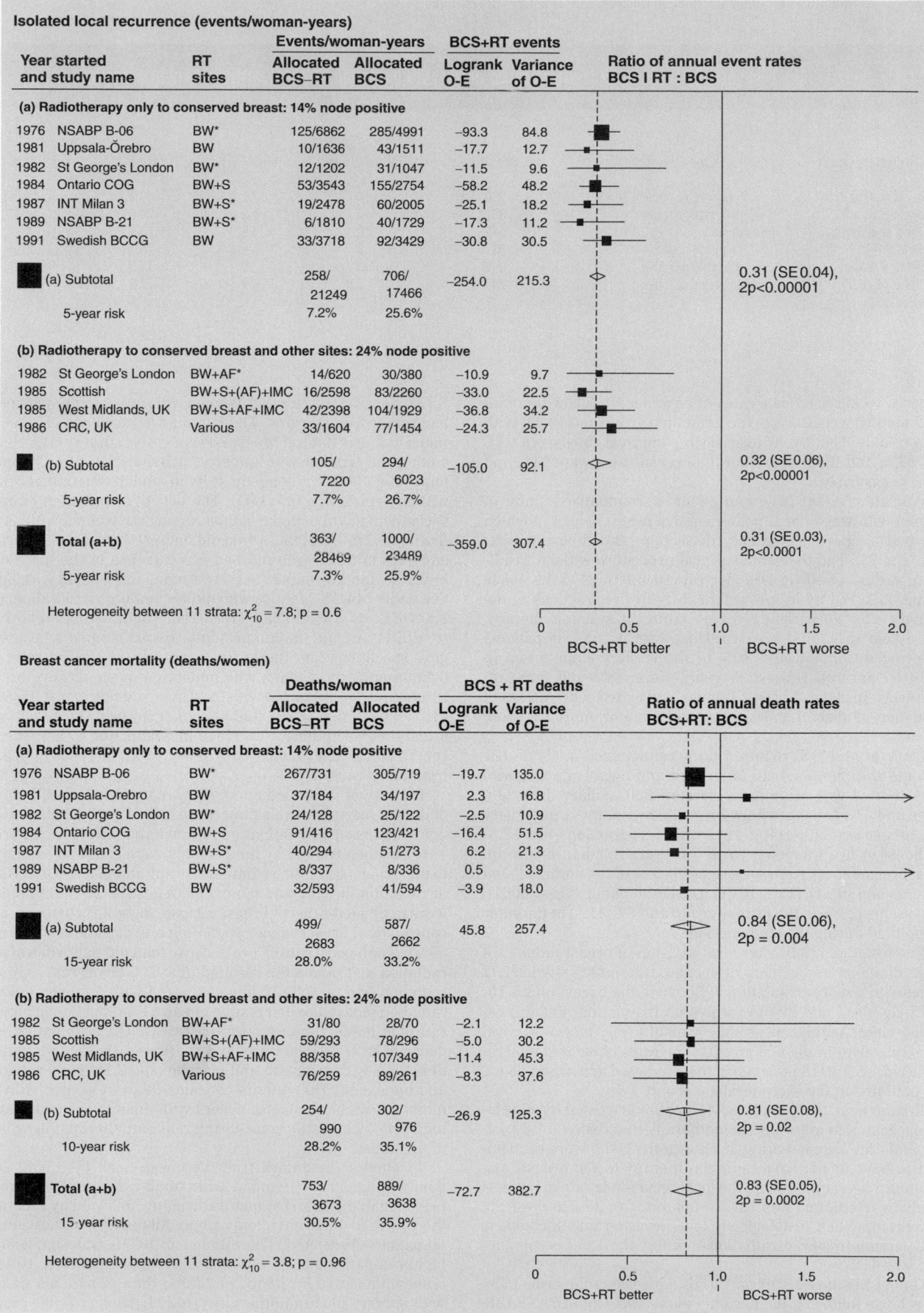

FIGURE 53.19. Meta-analysis of local control and survival from the Early Breast Cancer Trialists Collaborative Group (EBCTCG) demonstrating the impact of radiation therapy on both local control and survival in the management of breast cancer. AF, axillalfossa; BCS, breast-conserving surgery; BW, brcast/chest wall; IMC, internal mammary chain; O-E, observed-expected; RT, radiotherapy; SE, standard error. (From Clarke M, Collins R, Darby S, et al. Effects of radiotherapy and of differences in the extent of surgery for early breast cancer on local recurrence and 15-year survival: an overview of the randomised trials. *Lancet* 2005;366:2087–2106, with permission.)

Table 53.25	**RESULTS OF SELECTED RANDOMIZED TRIALS OF BREAST-CONSERVING SURGERY WITH OR WITHOUT RADIATION**					
					RT	
Study (Reference)	Criteria for Eligibility	No. of Patients	Follow-Up (y)	With (%)	Without (%)	p Value
Fisher et al. (201)	<4 cm node positive/negative	930	10	12.4	40.9	<.001
Liljegren et al. (447)	<2 cm node negative	381	10	8.5	24.0	.0001
Veronesi et al. (783)	<2.5 cm	579	10	5.8	23.5	<.001
Clark et al. (118)	<2 cm node negative	837	3	5.5	25.7	<.001
Fisher et al. (208)	<2 cm node negative	1,009	8	2.8	16.5	<.001
Winzer et al. (832)	<2 cm node negative	347	5.9	3.2	27.8	.001

actuarial local recurrence rates after a median follow-up of 63 to 65 months were 2.3% in the irradiated group and 18.4% with surgery only. The 5-year disease-free survival rates were 91% and 87%, and the 5-year overall survival rates were 91% and 90%, respectively.

Whelan et al. (826) reported on a randomized study of women with stage I or II node-negative breast cancer in which 403 had lumpectomy, axillary dissection, and breast irradiation, and 396 had the same surgical procedure without irradiation. A dose of 40 Gy was given in 16 fractions to the whole breast, followed by a boost of 12.5 Gy in five fractions to the primary site. No patient received adjuvant systemic therapy. The 5-year ipsilateral breast relapse rate was 8% in patients receiving irradiation and 30% in the surgery-alone group (p <.0001). Survival rates at 5 years were 88% and 86%, respectively. Ipsilateral breast relapse correlated with increased incidence of distant metastases and greater mortality from cancer.

Clark et al. (118) reported on a randomized study of 421 patients with tumors 4 cm or smaller and negative nodes who were treated with wide local excision and axillary dissection alone and 416 patients who were treated with the same surgery plus breast irradiation (40 Gy in 3 weeks 16 fractions, and 12.5-Gy boost in five fractions). With 7.6 years' median follow-up, breast recurrences were seen in 148 (35%) of the nonirradiated patients and in 147 (11%) of the irradiated patients (p <.0001); 99 patients (24%) in the former group and 87 (21%) in the latter group died during the study period.

Forrest et al. (232), after local excision of breast tumors <4 cm in diameter and axillary dissection, randomly assigned 291 patients to receive irradiation of 50 Gy to the breast plus a 10- to 15-Gy boost and 294 to receive no irradiation. Patients received either tamoxifen or six cycles of CMF. Overall survival was equivalent in the two groups. The rates of locoregional relapse were 6.1% (18 patients) in the irradiated group and 28.6% (84 patients) in the excision-alone group.

Renton et al. (613) analyzed 418 patients treated by wide local excision and adjuvant chemotherapy (tamoxifen if ER positive and CMF chemotherapy if ER negative) who were randomized to have or not have radiation therapy to the breast. At a minimum 5-year follow-up, the local recurrence rate in patients receiving irradiation was 13% compared with 35% in those not so treated. When histologically local excision was incomplete and patients received radiation therapy, the local recurrence rate was 17%.

One of the most significant trials addressing the issue of local relapse following lumpectomy alone was from the NSABP-06 (201). This trial included three arms, modified radical mastectomy, lumpectomy with radiation, and lumpectomy without radiation, and included both node-positive and node-negative patients. In this trial, breast irradiation decreased the likelihood of a recurrence in the ipsilateral breast in the group of 1,137 lumpectomy-treated women whose surgical specimens had tumor-free margins. The cumulative incidence of a recurrence in the ipsilateral breast 20 years after surgery was 14.3% among the women who underwent irradiation after lumpectomy and 39.2% among those who underwent lumpectomy without irradiation (p <.001), The benefit of radiation therapy was independent of nodal status. Among the women with negative nodes, 36.2% of those who did not receive radiation therapy and 17% of those who did had a recurrence in the ipsilateral breast within 20 years (p <.001). Among the women with positive nodes, 44.2% of those who did not undergo irradiation and 8.8% of those who did had a recurrence in the ipsilateral breast (p <.001). Among the lumpectomy-treated women whose surgical specimens had tumor-free margins, the hazard ratio for death among the women who underwent postoperative breast irradiation, as compared with those who did not, was 0.91 (95% CI, 0.77 to 1.06; p = .23). Radiation therapy was associated with a marginally significant decrease in deaths due to breast cancer. This decrease was partially offset by an increase in deaths from other causes.

Because of continued uncertainty regarding the need for radiation in more favorable tumors the NSABP continued to investigate this issue of elimination of irradiation. In the B-21 trial, 1,009 women treated by lumpectomy were randomly assigned to tamoxifen (n = 336), radiation therapy and placebo (n = 336), or radiation therapy and tamoxifen (n = 337) (204). End points were in divided rates of breast relapse, distant recurrence, and contralateral breast cancer. Radiation and placebo resulted in a 49% lower hazard rate of local relapse than did tamoxifen alone; radiation and tamoxifen resulted in a 63% lower rate than did radiation and placebo. When compared with tamoxifen alone, radiation plus tamoxifen resulted in an 81% reduction in hazard rate of in-breast tumor recurrence rate (IBTR). Cumulative incidence of local relapse through 8 years was 16.5% with tamoxifen, 9.3% with radiation and placebo, and 2.8% with radiation and tamoxifen. The authors concluded that in women with tumors ≤1 cm, local relapse occurs with enough frequency after lumpectomy to justify considering radiation therapy regardless of ER status.

In another landmark trial, Veronesi et al. (783,788) randomly assigned 567 women with small cancers of the breast (<2.5 cm in diameter) to quadrantectomy followed by radiation therapy or to quadrantectomy alone. All patients underwent total axillary dissection. The number of IBTRs was significantly higher in patients treated with surgery alone (59/273; 10-year crude cumulative incidence of 23.5%) than in patients treated with surgery plus radiotherapy (16/294; 10-year crude cumulative incidence of 5.8%). The difference in IBTR frequency between the two treatments was high in women up to 45 years of age, tending to decrease with increasing age up to no apparent difference in women older than 65 years. Overall survival curves for the two groups did not differ significantly (p = .326).

However, a limited survival advantage was evident after radiotherapy for node-positive women.

Other Nonrandomized Studies of Lumpectomy Alone

Lim et al. (449) recently updated a prospective single arm trial addressing omission of radiation for highly selected favorable patients from the Harvard group. Eighty-seven (of 90 planned) patients enrolled from 1986 until closure in 1992, when a predefined stopping boundary was crossed. Patients were required to have a unicentric, T1, pathologic node-negative invasive ductal, mucinous, or tubular carcinoma without an extensive intraductal component or lymphatic-vessel invasion. Surgery included local excision with margins of at least 1 cm or a negative re-excision. No radiation or systemic therapy was given. Nineteen patients (23%) had local recurrence as a first site of failure (average annual local recurrence: 3.5 per 100 patient-years of follow-up). The authors concluded that even in this highly selected cohort, a substantial risk of local recurrence occurred after breast-conserving surgery alone with margins of 1.0 cm or more.

McCready et al. (484) reported on a postmenopausal group of 244 patients with breast cancer treated with lumpectomy alone. With a median follow-up of 9.1 years, the overall breast relapse rate was 24% (59/244). On univariate analysis, smaller tumor size, negative nodes, positive ER status, and no lymphovascular or perineural invasion were associated with significantly lower relapse rates ($p < .05$). On multivariate analyses, lymphovascular or perineural invasion, age, and amount of DCIS were all significantly associated with greater risk of local relapse. The authors defined a low-risk subgroup (node-negative, younger than 65 years of age, no comedo, ER positive, no emboli) with a crude 10-year local recurrence rate of 9%.

Conservative Surgery Alone in Elderly Women

The available evidence clearly establishes lumpectomy followed by radiation as the standard of care for the majority of women with early stage invasive breast cancer. As noted in the numerous randomized trials reported above, lumpectomy alone results in a threefold increase in local relapse and compromised breast cancer related survival to a lesser degree (803). Given the lower reported local relapse rates in elderly women, however, the absolute benefit of radiation therapy following breast-conserving surgery may be less. The question of whether radiation can be eliminated following breast-conserving therapy has been addressed in both retrospective and more recently, carefully designed prospective randomized trials.

There is evidence from several retrospective and prospective series that elderly women may be spared radiation. Cooke et al. (128) identified 44 women treated with partial mastectomy, breast irradiation, and tamoxifen and compared them with 53 women treated in a similar fashion but without breast irradiation. At 39 months, the breast tumor recurrence rate was 5% with breast irradiation and 21% when irradiation was omitted. Of those not receiving irradiation, no breast relapses were seen in 22 patients older than 70 years of age at diagnosis, in contrast to eight breast recurrences in 31 patients younger than 70 years.

In the trial of quadrantectomy versus quadrantectomy plus radiation reported by Veronesi et al. (783), although there was a clear benefit in local control overall, the benefit was significant and apparent only in younger women; for patients over age 65 there was no significant benefit.

Gajdos et al. (266) noted that reported rates of local and distant recurrence for elderly patients were comparable with those for younger patients after both mastectomy and breast conservation. Ninety-eight of 920 patients older than 70 years of age were undertreated by conventional criteria. Undertreated elderly patients were significantly older (78 vs. 76 years; $p = .003$), were diagnosed with excisional biopsy more often (69% vs. 57%; $p = .069$), had fine-needle aspiration less frequently (22% vs. 38%; $p = .069$), and were more likely to have breast-conservation therapy (90% vs. 73%; $p = .004$). Local and distant disease-free survival rates for both groups were comparable. Tamoxifen treatment significantly reduced the chances for development of distant metastasis in node-negative elderly patients with invasive tumors ($p = .028$). Omission of chemotherapy had no impact on disease control in the elderly. Therefore, elderly women with favorable prognostic factors may be candidates for treatment with tumor resection and tamoxifen without irradiation or chemotherapy and with close follow-up.

Given the apparent biological differences in breast cancers in the elderly, as well as the logistical issues in daily radiation treatment, two recent randomized trials, published in the same issue of the *New England Journal of Medicine*, have addressed the issue of the need for radiation therapy in elderly women with early stage breast cancer (259,361). The first trial from the Cancer and Leukemia Group B (CALGB) and Radiation Therapy Oncology Group (RTOG) published by Hughes et al. (259), randomly assigned 636 women with clinical stage I, estrogen-receptor-positive breast carcinoma treated by lumpectomy to receive tamoxifen plus radiation therapy (317 women) or tamoxifen alone (319 women). The only significant difference between the two groups was in the rate of local or regional recurrence at 5 years (1% in the group given tamoxifen plus irradiation and 4% in the group given tamoxifen alone; $p < .001$). There were no significant differences between the two groups with regard to the rates of mastectomy for local recurrence, distant metastases, or 5-year rates of overall survival. The authors concluded that lumpectomy plus adjuvant therapy with tamoxifen alone is a reasonable choice for the treatment of women 70 years of age or older who have early, estrogen-receptor–positive breast cancer.

The second trial was a Canadian study published by Fyles et al. (259) of women 50 years of age or older who had T1–2 node-negative breast cancer. In this trial 769 women with early breast cancer with a tumor diameter of 5 cm or less were randomly assigned to receive breast irradiation plus tamoxifen (386 women) or tamoxifen alone (383 women). With a median follow-up of 5.6 years the rate of local relapse at 5 years was 7.7% in the tamoxifen group and 0.6% in the group given tamoxifen plus irradiation (hazard ratio, 8.3; 95% CI, 3.3 to 21.2; $p < .001$). The corresponding 5-year disease-free survival rates were 84% and 91%, respectively ($p = .004$). A subgroup analysis of 611 women with T1, receptor-positive tumors, similar to the CALGB cohorts, also indicated a benefit from radiotherapy with the 5-year rates of local relapse of 0.4% with tamoxifen plus radiotherapy and 5.9% with tamoxifen alone ($p < .001$). There was also a significant difference in the rate of axillary relapse at 5 years (2.5% in the tamoxifen group and 0.5% in the group given tamoxifen plus irradiation; $p = .049$), but there was no significant difference in the rates of distant relapse or overall survival. In both of these trials, women were not required to have surgical staging of the axilla, but did have clinically negative axilla in both; follow-up remains relatively short. Both studies show that even this favorable subgroup benefits from radiation with respect to local control, but the absolute benefit is small.

As a follow-up to the CALGB study, Smith et al. (700) conducted a detailed analysis of women over age 70 from the SEER-Medicare database. They identified 8,724 women aged 70 years or older treated with conservative surgery for small, lymph node-negative, estrogen-receptor–positive (or unknown receptor status) breast cancer. Using a proportional hazards model, they tested whether radiation therapy was associated with a lower risk of a combined outcome, defined as a second

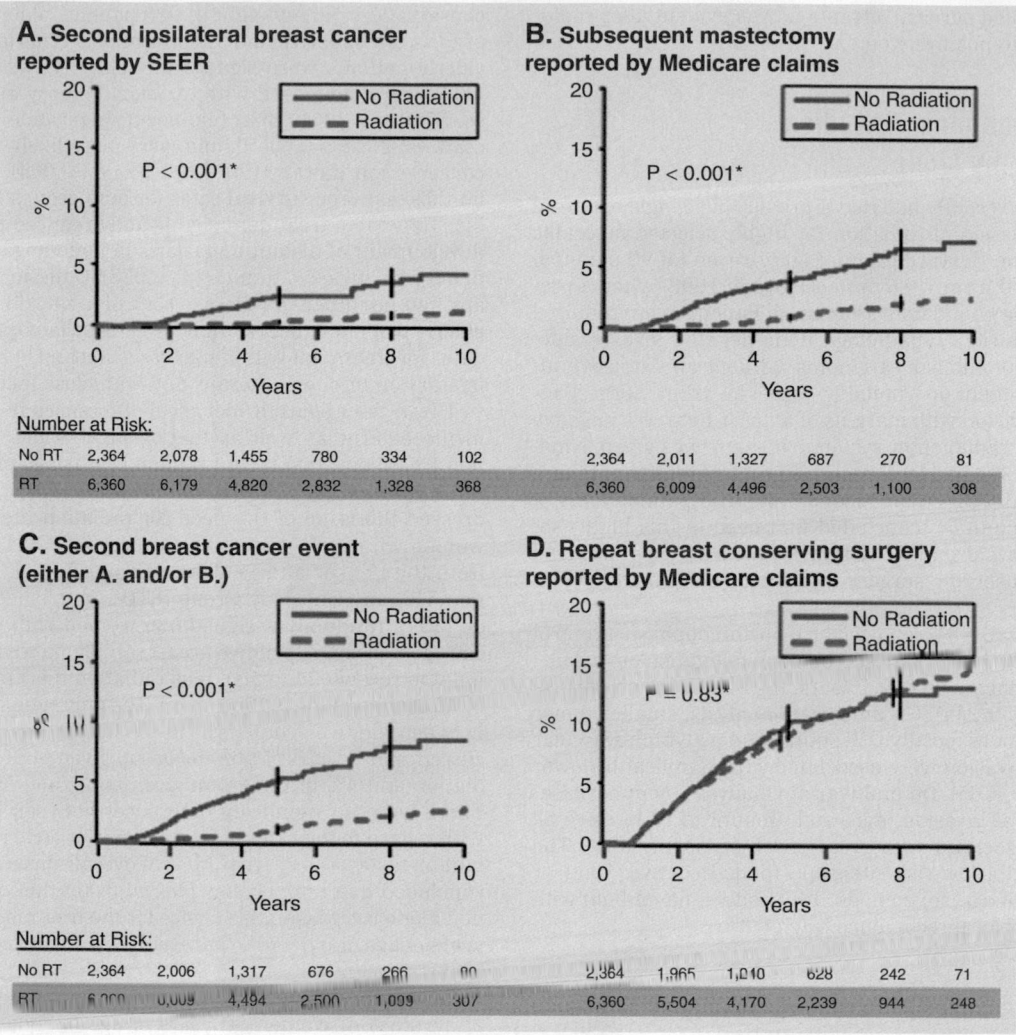

FIGURE 53.20. Association of radiation therapy with outcomes in elderly women. Patients were at risk for all outcomes beginning 9 months after diagnosis. **A:** Second ipsilateral breast cancer reported by Surveillance, Epidemiology, and End Results (SEER). This outcome was defined as a second ipsilateral, pathologically confirmed, invasive breast cancer. **B:** Subsequent mastectomy reported by Medicare claims. **C:** Second breast cancer event defined as a second ipsilateral, pathologically confirmed, invasive breast cancer reported by SEER data or as a subsequent mastectomy reported by Medicare claims. **D:** Repeat breast-conserving surgery as reported by Medicare claims. RT, radiation therapy. Error bars, 95% confidence intervals. *p values were calculated from a two-sided log-rank test. (From Smith BD, Gross CP, Smith GL, et al. Effectiveness of radiation therapy for older women with early breast cancer. *J Natl Cancer Inst* 2006;98:681–690, with permission.)

ipsilateral breast cancer reported by SEER and/or a subsequent mastectomy reported by Medicare claims. The results, summarized in Figure 53.20, were similar to those reported by the randomized studies above in that radiation therapy, compared with no radiation therapy, was associated with a lower risk of the combined outcome (hazard ratio 0.19; 95% CI, 0.14 to 0.28). Radiation therapy was associated with an absolute risk reduction of four events per 100 women at 5 years (from 5.1 events without radiation therapy to 1.1 with radiation therapy) and 5.7 events per 100 women at 8 years (from eight events without radiation therapy to 2.3 with radiation therapy) ($p < .001$).

Using a comorbidity analysis radiation therapy was most likely to benefit those aged 70 to 79 years without comorbidity (number needed to treat [NNT] to prevent one event = 21 to 22 patients) and was least likely to benefit those aged 80 years or older with moderate to severe comorbidity (NNT = 61 to 125 patients). The authors conclude that for older women with early breast cancer, radiation therapy was associated with a lower risk of a second ipsilateral breast cancer and subsequent mastectomy. Patients aged 70 to 79 years with minimal comorbidity were the most likely to benefit, and older patients with substantial comorbidity were least likely to benefit.

Collectively, these studies indicate that the benefit of radiation therapy for elderly women is significant in terms of local control, but this absolute benefit is relatively small and must be weighed against comorbidities and other competing risks. The two randomized trials and the SEER-MEDICARE analysis are summarized in Table 53.26. For women with favorable T1/N0 receptor–positive breast cancers, tamoxifen alone is a reasonable option that should be discussed. For patients with multiple comorbidities and shorter life expectancies, this option is often chosen. Our own preference in patients with low comorbidity and long life expectancy is to offer radiation, even in those over age 70 with estrogen-receptor–positive tumors.

Radiation Management of the Regional Lymphatics

Radiation therapy of the regional lymphatics remains one of the most variable aspects of breast-conserving therapy (104,374,605,648). The role of radiation therapy in management of the regional lymphatics is influenced by the risk of subclinical microscopic disease in regional nodal basins and

Table 53.26 FIVE-YEAR OUTCOME OF BREAST-CONSERVING SURGERY WITH OR WITHOUT RADIOTHERAPY IN ELDERLY WOMEN WITH BREAST CANCER

Study (Reference)	Age (y)	No. of Patients		Follow-Up	Ipsilateral Relapse			Axillary Relapse			Distant Relapse		
		CS	CS+RT		CS (%)	CS+RT (%)	p	CS (%)	CS+RT (%)	p	CS (%)	CS+RT (%)	p
Fyles et al. (259)	≥50	383	386	5.6 (median)	7.7	0.6	<.001	2.5	0.5	0.049	4.0	4.5	.69
Hughes et al. (361)	≥70	319	317	5.0 (median)	4.1	0.6	<.01	0.6	0	0.08	1.9	2.2	.77
Smith et al. (700)	≥70	2,364	6,360	>8	5.1	1.1	<.001	—	—	—	—	—	—

CS, conserving surgery; RT, radiation therapy.

patterns of failure. This risk is in part determined by disease characteristics and in part determined by the extent of surgical evaluation of the axilla, which has become increasingly relevant as a result of increased use of sentinel node and whether completion axillary dissections are performed for those patients with sentinel node-positive disease. Furthermore, clinicians differ significantly regarding their philosophy with respect to the treatment of subclinical microscopic disease, particularly as it relates to the internal mammary chain.

The issue of whether or not one treats the axilla in conservatively managed patients is further complicated by both uncertainty and misconceptions about the degree to which the axilla receives radiation from a standard tangential field. Although this will vary considerably, as will be discussed in the section on radiation techniques, tangential radiation ports will likely treat most level I nodes and a portion of level II nodes (659).

All of this uncertainty, debate, and controversy is well founded as there is little in the way of randomized data to establish a clear standard. Studies are under way randomizing high-risk node-negative and node-positive patients to treatment to the breast/chest wall only compared to the breast/chest wall and regional lymphatics. In the interim reliance on available

Table 53.27 TREATMENT POLICY FOR CONSERVATIVE MANAGEMENT OF EARLY STAGE INVASIVE BREAST CANCER

Treatment Volume	Indication	Fraction Size/Technique	Total Dose	Comment
Early Stage Invasive Breast Cancer				
Whole breast	Routinely following BCS	200 (prefer) or 180cGy/ tangents with wedges or dynamic wedges to optimize homogeneity	4,500–5,040 cGy	Consider omission of RT in elderly with stage I (estrogen receptor positive) and comorbidities
Boost	Routinely following whole breast	200 or 180 cGy (prefer 200)/ En face electrons	1,000–1,600 cGy to bring total dose to >6,000	May consider no boost for widely negative margins in women over 60
Accelerated whole breast	Patient convenience	266 cGy tangents with no nodal fields/no boost	4,250 cGy	
Accelerated partial breast	On protocol	3.4–3.8 Gy/ext beam conformal, interstitial, or MammoSite	3,400–3,850 cGy	
Treatment Policy for Regional Nodes				
Supraclav	• Clinical N2 or N3 disease • >4 +LN after axillary dissection • 1–3 +LN with high risk features • Node + sentinel lymph node with no dissection unless risk of additional axillary disease is very small • High risk[a] no dissection	180–200 (Prefer 200)/ AP or AP-PA	4,500–5,040 cGy	May omit with 1–3 positive nodes in select cases
Axilla	• N+ with extensive ECE • SN+ with no dissection • Inadequate axillary dissection • High risk[a] with no dissection	180–200/ AP—consider posterior axillary boost if suboptimal coverage with AP only	4,500–5,040 cGy	Axilla may be intentionally included with use of "high tangents"
Internal mammary	Individualized but consider for: • Positive axillary nodes with central and medial lesions • Stage III breast cancer • +SLN in the IM chain • +SLN in axilla with drainage to IM on lymphosintigraphy	180–200/ Partially wide tangents or separate IM electron/photon	4,500–5,040 [mb85]cGy	

AP/PA, anteroposterior/posteroanterior; BCS, breast-conserving surgery; ECE, extranodal tumor extension; IM, internal mammary; LN, lymph nodes; N+, node positive; SLN+, sentinal lymph node.
[a]High risk defined as estimated probability of nodal involvement >10% to 15%.

| Table 53.28 | AXILLARY RECURRENCE AFTER AXILLARY RADIATION IN CONSERVATIVELY MANAGED PATIENTS |

| Study (Reference) | No. of Patients | | | | Axillary Failure/No. of Failures (% Failure) | |
	N0	N1 (Clinical)	RT Dose (Gy)	Follow-Up (y)	N0	N1
Royal Marsden (550)	211	52	50/25	120 (min)	3 (1%)	15 (29%)
Institut Curie (94)	332	—	50/25	54 (ave)	7 (2%)	—
Santiago (36)	171	—	50/25	62 (med)	4 (2%)	—
Charlebourg (151)	281	—	50–70	60 (min)	4 (1%)	—
Henri Mondor (442)	446	47	69/33	120 (ave)	0 (0%)	3 (6%)
Groupe European (582)	1,040	181	45–70	>60 (med)	19 (2%)	7 (4%)
Tufts (817)	73	—	45/25	54	1 (1%)	—
JCRT (606)	335	35	44–55/22–30	73 (med)	3 (1%)	1 (3%)
Yale University (299)	590		46	>120	18 (2%)	—
JCRT (270)	292	126[a]	64–68	96	3 (1%)	3 (2%)

JCRT, Joint Center for Radiation Therapy; RT, radiation therapy.
[a]All the patients received limited axillary dissection; RT dose, radiotherapy dose to axilla, given as total dose in Gy/number of fractions.

retrospective data, calculated risks of subclinical disease, and patterns of failure form the basis for various treatment policies. Current treatment policies/guidelines at our institutions are outlined in Tables 53.27 and 53.28.

Although in the earlier years of breast-conservation therapy, node-negative as well as node-positive patients often received regional nodal treatment, most authors currently agree that it is not necessary to irradiate the regional lymphatics if the nodes are pathologically negative and an adequate axillary dissection has been performed (299,605,844). This general practice has now been extended to those patients with a negative sentinel node, since available studies have demonstrated a low rate of pathologically involved nodes after a negative sentinel node procedure performed by an experienced surgeon (277,415, 465).

However, noted previously, the clinically negative axilla harbors subclinical microscopic disease in up to 40% of patients

with early stage operable breast cancer (211), and both axillary dissection and axillary radiation result in high rates of regional nodal control (211,299,330,605,844).

Radiation Compared to Axillary Surgery

Sentinel node sampling, with or without full axillary dissection, is now the most common method of axillary management in women with early stage breast cancer. For patients in whom full axillary staging will not affect subsequent systemic management, who have not undergone any axillary staging procedure, or who have a positive sentinel node and did not undergo further axillary staging, axillary radiation has been shown to result in high rates of regional nodal control (299,330,605,612,844). Selected series demonstrating nodal control rates with radiation therapy in breast-conserving therapy are summarized in Table 53.28. Table 53.29 summarizes results of randomized

| Table 53.29 | AXILLARY FAILURE RATES IN PATIENTS IN RANDOMIZED TRIALS COMPARING AXILLARY TREATMENTS |

| Trials (Reference) | Study Design | No. of Patients | Follow-Up (month) | Positive LNs (%) | Axillary Failure Rates | | |
					AxD (%)	AxRT (%)	OBS (%)
NSABP B-04 (211)	M (AxD vs. AxRT vs. OBS)	1079	126 (ave)	40	1	3	19
Institut Curie (456)	CS (AxD vs. AxRT)	658	180 (med)	18	1	3	NA
Edinburgh (435)	M (AxD vs. AxRT)	275	72 (min)	30	1	14	NA
Guy's I (342)	M vs. CS (AxD vs. AxRT)	232	180 (min)	25	1	19	NA
Guy's II (342)	M vs. CS (AxD vs. AxRT)	258	120 (min)	31	1	13	NA
Manchester I (459)	M (AxRT vs. OBS)	714	60 (min)	NA	NA	19	37
Manchester II (614)	CS (AxRT vs. OBS)	708	65 (med)	NA	NA	10	23
International Breast Cancer Study Group (639)	M or CS (AxD vs. OBS)	454	79 (med)	14	0.4	NA	1.3
Italian Oncological Senology Group (784)	CS	435	63 (med)	NA	NA	0.5	1.5
Milan (477)	CS	219	60	23	1	NA	1.8

Positive LNs, incidence of pathologically involved lymph nodes in patients undergoing axillary lymph node dissection; AxD, axillary dissection; AxRT, axillary radiotherapy; CS, breast-conserving surgery; M, simple or radical mastectomy; OBS, observation; ave, average length of follow-up; min, minimum length of follow-up; med, median length of follow-up; NA, not applicable.

trials comparing axillary surgery to radiation and/or observation.

Retrospective Experiences

Haffty et al. (299) reported actuarial nodal control rates of 97% and 96% at 10 years for two groups of patients, 245 receiving irradiation alone without axillary dissection and 187 treated with irradiation to the supraclavicular lymph nodes and IMNs after axillary dissection. Minimal morbidity was associated with this treatment policy. Pejavar et al. (560) updated the Yale experience, demonstrating a 98% 5-year regional nodal control rate in 582 patients with invasive breast cancer treated by regional nodal irradiation without dissection compared to 98% 5-year nodal control rate in 1,440 patients treated by axillary dissection. Within this experience were 16 patients with positive sentinel nodes who did not undergo completion axillary dissection and were treated with radiation therapy. None of those sentinel node-positive patients recurred.

Galper et al. (270) estimated the efficacy of axillary radiation therapy after a positive sentinel node biopsy and evaluated the risk of regional nodal failure for patients with clinical stage I or II, clinically node-negative invasive breast cancer treated with either no dissection or a limited dissection (removal of five nodes or less) followed by axillary radiation therapy. Two hundred ninety-two patients had axillary radiation therapy instead of axillary dissection; 126 underwent axillary radiation therapy following limited node dissection. The median dose to the axilla was 46 Gy and to the supraclavicular fossa 45 Gy. Among patients found to have positive nodes on limited dissection, adjuvant chemotherapy and tamoxifen were administered to 81% and 7% of subjects, respectively. All patients had an 8-year follow-up. Six of the 418 patients (1.4%) had regional nodal failure within 8 years; four had simultaneous regional and distant recurrences; and two had isolated axillary failures. Three of the 292 patients (1%) with no axillary dissection, 0/84 patients with pathologically negative nodes, and 3/42 patients (7%) with pathologically involved nodes had regional node failure as a first site of failure.

A group of 511 patients with 519 stage I and II breast cancers treated with lumpectomy, with or without axillary dissection, and irradiation were reviewed by Halverson et al. (317). Management of the axilla consisted of irradiation after axillary dissection in 74, irradiation alone in 75, and observation in 21 patients; the extent of nodal irradiation was at the discretion of the attending radiation oncologist. Overall axillary recurrence was uncommon (1.2%) but was slightly more frequent after

irradiation alone (2.7%) than after surgery alone (0.3%; $p = .14$). There was no benefit for supplemental axillary irradiation after an axillary dissection yielding negative nodes or one to three positive nodes. Among the 21 patients in whom the axilla was not treated, axillary recurrence was not observed. Supraclavicular failures were rare in women with negative or one to three positive axillary lymph nodes (0.5%) and were not significantly affected by elective irradiation. IMN recurrence was seen in only one patient and was not influenced by elective internal mammary irradiation.

Randomized Studies

Randomized studies evaluating axillary treatment (dissection vs. observation vs. radiation) are summarized in Table 53.29. One of the largest and earliest comparisons of axillary surgery to radiation was the NSABP-04 study, in which operable clinically node-negative patients were randomly assigned to radical mastectomy, simple mastectomy, or simple mastectomy with radiation to the chest wall and regional lymphatics (212). The nodal relapse rate approached 20% in those assigned to simple mastectomy without radiation. The nodal control rate in the radical mastectomy arm and simple mastectomy plus radiation arm was comparable, with less than a 3% relapse rate in each of these arms.

A direct comparison of axillary treatment by dissection compared to radiation was recently reported by Louis-Sylvestre et al. (456), in which 658 patients with a breast carcinoma <3 cm in diameter and clinically uninvolved lymph nodes were randomly assigned to axillary dissection or axillary radiotherapy after breast-conserving surgery with radiation to the breast. Of the group undergoing dissection 21% of the patients in the axillary dissection group were node-positive. At 10 and 15 years, survival rates were identical in both groups (73.8% vs. 75.5% at 15 years). Recurrences in the axilla were less frequent in the axillary dissection group at 15 years (1% vs. 3%; $p = .04$) (Fig. 53.21). There was no difference in recurrence rates in the breast or supraclavicular region or distant metastases between the two groups.

Veronesi et al. (784) carried out a study in which women older than 45 years of age with breast cancer up to 1.2 cm were randomized, 214 of whom were treated with breast-conservation surgery and irradiation without axillary treatment and 221 with conservation surgery plus breast and axillary radiation therapy (50 Gy in 5 weeks). After a median follow-up of 63 months, overt axillary metastases were fewer than expected: three cases in the no axillary treatment group (1.5%) and one

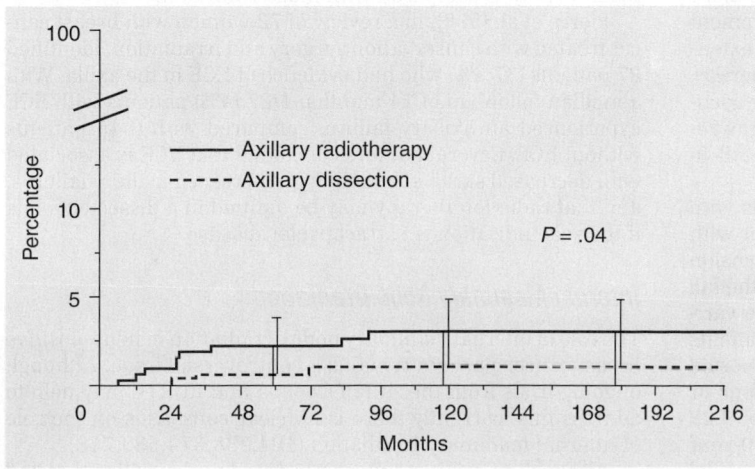

FIGURE 53.21. Associations between delay in postoperative radiotherapy (RT) and local recurrence rates (LRRs) in studies of the sequencing of adjuvant RT and chemotherapy for breast cancer. LRRs in patients who received delayed RT following initial chemotherapy are compared with the rates observed in those patients who received early RT by chemotherapy. Low-quality studies are indicated by an asterisk. CI, confidence interval; OR, (From Huang J, Barbera L, Brouwers M, et al. Does delay in starting treatment affect the outcomes of radiotherapy? A systematic review. *J Clin Oncol* 2003;21:555–563, with permission.)

in the radiation therapy group (0.5%). This study suggests that occult axillary metastases might never become clinically overt, and axillary dissection might be avoided in patients with small carcinomas and a clinically negative axilla. Axillary radiation therapy seems to protect the patients from axillary recurrence almost completely. It is possible that systemic therapy, the undamaged immunocompetent tissue in the axillary lymph nodes, and axillary irradiation may all be factors contributing to the low incidence of axillary failures in these patients. Also, in the patients receiving no axillary irradiation, it is highly likely that the level I lymph nodes were included in the standard tangential fields (605,659,839).

Irradiation of Lymphatics in Patients with Positive Axillary Lymph Nodes

Although there is a general consensus that radiation to the regional lymph nodes is not necessary in patients with pathologically node-negative disease, there is considerable variability in radiation to the regional lymphatics in patients with pathologically node-positive disease (242,269,299,489,605,612). Many radiation oncologists favor irradiation of the regional lymphatics in addition to the breast in node-positive women, while others favor no nodal irradiation, particularly in women with one to three positive nodes. Ongoing trials by the National Cancer Institute (NCI) of Canada and EORTC, which are randomizing high-risk node-negative and node-positive patients to treatment to the breast/chest wall alone or breast/chest wall and regional lymphatics, may help to resolve some of these issues.

Acknowledging the lack of definitive data and clear consensus, and allowing for flexibility depending on patient and physician preferences, the guidelines that the authors advocate are summarized in the lower section of Table 53.28. In general, the authors favor treatment of the supraclavicular fossa in patients with positive nodes. Treatment of the axilla and internal mammary will vary, with attention to the indications outlined in the table. Until results of the ongoing randomized trials of the NCI Canada (MA20) and EORTC are available, regional lymphatic irradiation will continue to be highly individualized based on physician and patient preferences.

Sarrazin et al. (650) carried out a randomized study comparing 88 patients treated with tumorectomy and irradiation and 91 patients treated with mastectomy. In a second randomization in the study, the patients with positive axillary lymph nodes in the first randomization were randomly assigned to receive or not receive nodal irradiation. There was no significant difference in overall survival between the two groups. Nevertheless, Yarnold (814) advised elective irradiation of the axilla and the supraclavicular fossa in selected patients, such as those with four or more metastatic axillary lymph nodes, involvement of the apex of the axilla, or gross extracapsular tumor extension, even if the patients are to receive adjuvant chemotherapy. These recommendations are supported by reports that document the benefit of postmastectomy irradiation in patients receiving chemotherapy, which are reviewed in more detail in Chapter 54.

Treatment of the axilla varies significantly in patients with positive nodes. For those patients with negative nodes, or with one to three positive nodes without extranodal tumor extension (ECE), there does not appear to be a benefit to targeting the full axilla (242,269,299,317,318,605). There is considerable variability regarding treatment of the full axilla, even in patients with multiple positive nodes. Mehta and Haffty (489) reported on the conservative management of 51 patients with four or more positive lymph nodes. With a median follow-up of 9.29 years, there were two nodal relapses, resulting in a 10-year nodal recurrence-free rate of 96%. Both patients with nodal relapses (one supraclavicular and one axillary/supraclavicular)

failed within the irradiated volume. Of the 40 patients treated to the supraclavicular fossa (omitting complete axillary radiation), none failed in the dissected axilla. It should be acknowledged, however, that the level I and a portion of level II nodes were likely included in the tangential breast irradiation field (659).

Fowble et al. (242) reported a 3% rate of isolated regional node recurrence (without simultaneous distant metastases) in 990 patients with clinical stage I or II breast cancer treated with breast-conserving surgery (with axillary sampling in 914) and irradiation. The most common site of regional failure was the axilla (17 patients), followed by the supraclavicular region (13 patients). Only the number of axillary lymph nodes removed at the time of initial axillary dissection was a significant prognostic factor for axillary recurrence.

Recht et al. (606) described a 2.3% incidence of regional nodal failure (38/1,624) in patients with stage I or II breast cancer treated with breast-conserving therapy (median follow-up, 77 months). In patients undergoing axillary dissection who were irradiated to the breast only, 9/420 (2.1%) with negative nodes and 1/47 (2.1%) with one to three positive nodes had an axillary failure. Supraclavicular failure occurred in eight patients with negative nodes (1.9%) and in none of those with positive nodes. In patients who did not have clinically suspect axillary lymph nodes and did not have axillary dissection but were treated with lymph node irradiation, the failure rate was 0.8% (3/355) in the axilla and 0.3% (1/364) in the supraclavicular area.

Extracapsular Extension

The risk of axillary recurrence after full dissection is low in patients with ECE, even without axillary lymph node irradiation. However, because these patients typically have more positive axillary lymph nodes than do patients without ECE, they are at risk for recurrence on that basis. Whether or not to treat the full axilla following dissection for patients with multiple positive nodes generally includes consideration of the extent of dissection, the degree of nodal involvement and extracapsular extension, and the degree to which the patient and physician are willing to accept some increased risk of lymphedema with full axillary radiation following dissection (330,605).

Hetelekidis et al. (347) evaluated 368 patients with T1–2 breast cancer and pathologically positive lymph nodes treated with breast-conserving therapy. The median number of sampled lymph nodes was 10. Twenty percent of the patients were treated with supraclavicular radiation therapy, and 64% received both axillary and supraclavicular radiation therapy (45 Gy). One hundred twenty-two patients (33%) had ECE. There was no significant correlation of either disease-free or overall survival or local–regional nodal, or distant failure rates in patients with ECE compared with those without it.

Pierce et al. (578), in a review of 72 women with breast cancer treated with conservation surgery and irradiation, identified 27 patients (37.5%) who had evidence of ECE in the axilla. With a median follow-up of 14 months, 1/27 (4%) patients with ECE experienced an axillary failure, compared with 0/45 patients without ECE. Several authors concluded that ECE is associated with decreased survival but not with increased axillary failures, and that radiation therapy may be omitted in a dissected axilla if the sole indication is extracapsular disease.

Internal Mammary Node Irradiation

The role of internal mammary nodal irradiation in node-positive breast cancer patients remains a controversial issue. Although ongoing trials from the NCI of Canada and EORTC may help to address this, currently there is no clear consensus on the role of internal mammary irradiation (104,238,374,538,718).

Although no trials conducted to date have specifically tested the effect of IMN irradiation, several surgical series comparing extended radical mastectomy and radical mastectomy, without adjuvant systemic therapy, have shown that extended radical mastectomy was associated with improved survival rates in patients with medial T1–2 tumors and positive axillary nodes (430,491). These surgical series and selected series evaluating internal mammary irradiation are summarized in Table 53.30.

The majority of randomized trials evaluating postoperative radiation therapy did include radiation to the internal mammary chain. However, it is difficult to distinguish whether the benefit derived from such treatment related specifically to radiation of the internal mammary chain, or to the breast/chest wall, supraclavicular and/or axillary treatment administered.

Freedman et al. (252) examined data regarding patterns of failure after elective IMN treatment. Although controversial, data from the prospective, randomized trials of IMN treatment do not seem to support elective dissection or irradiation. IMN irradiation did not contribute to survival, yet it raised the risk of cardiac toxic effects. Sentinel lymph node mapping provided an opportunity to examine the IMN chain in early breast cancer. It is possible that a biopsy of the "hot" nodes could be used to select patients who are most likely to benefit from additional regional therapy to these nodes.

Fowble et al. (238) compared the outcome in 1,383 women with stage I or II breast cancer who underwent wide excision, axillary node dissection with 10 or more nodes removed, and breast irradiation. A total of 114 women had radiation to the IMNs with deep tangents, and 1,269 did not. All axillary node–positive women received adjuvant chemotherapy or tamoxifen, or both. There were no significant differences in ipsilateral breast tumor recurrence, regional node recurrence, and initial or total distant metastases for the two groups. No IMN failures were observed among the 114 patients whose IMNs were treated, and only four IMN failures were found in the 1,269 other patients (two of whom had distant metastases). Similarly, 5- and 10-year actuarial overall and cause-specific survival rates were not significantly different.

In a series from Yale, Obedian and Haffty (538) found no difference in the 10-year disease-free survival rate after breast irradiation and excision, regardless of whether IMNs were irradiated. Of 984 patients with invasive breast cancer who were treated with conservative surgery and radiotherapy, patients were divided into two groups: those treated by intentionally targeting the internal mammary nodes ($n = 535$) and those treated without intentionally targeting the internal mammary nodes ($n = 411$). The decision not to use a separate internal mammary field was a result of a change in treatment policy over time and generally not based on number of nodes or tumor location. There were no significant differences between the groups with respect to age, ER/PR status, or use of adjuvant chemotherapy or hormone therapy. There were more patients with T2 tumors, positive nodes, medial lesions, indeterminate margins, and slightly longer follow-up in the group treated to the internal mammary chain. There were no significant differences between the groups with respect to overall survival or distant metastasis-free survival.

In a study by Stemmer et al. (718) of 100 node-positive patients scheduled to receive radiation to the internal mammary chain, 67 received the radiation and 33 did not due to technical difficulties. At a median follow-up of 77 months, disease-free survival was significantly prolonged in patients receiving internal mammary radiation compared to those without internal mammary radiation (73% vs. 52%; $p = .02$). A trend was seen for overall survival (78% vs. 64%; $p = .08$). Cox regression multivariate analysis found IMN radiotherapy to be significant both for disease-free and overall survival. There was no treatment-related mortality.

It is evident that data are conflicting and opinions regarding the role of internal mammary radiation remain unresolved. Until more definitive data become available, it is likely that patient and physician biases will dictate practice. The authors' approach is summarized in the lower portion of Table 53.28, acknowledging that uncertainties in the available data allow for substantial flexibility. The radiation oncologist, however, must be familiar with the various techniques to treat internal mammary nodes, which are summarized later in the section on techniques.

Sequencing Chemotherapy and Hormonal Therapy

Sequencing Chemoradiation in the Conservative Management of Breast Cancer

With the increasing use of systemic therapy in patients with early stage breast cancer, the integration of this treatment with surgery and radiation therapy has become an important clinical question. Initial retrospective series evaluating treatment sequencing suggest that a delay in the onset of radiation therapy to permit delivery of chemotherapy increased local recurrence rates (358,602,609,695). These data are summarized in a pooled analysis by Huang et al. (358). Ten retrospective studies involving 7,401 patients investigated the association between delay in initiating postoperative radiation therapy and local control in breast cancer (after lumpectomy in nine studies and lumpectomy or mastectomy in one study). Eight of these studies compared local control between patients who were treated more than 8 weeks after surgery and those treated within 8 weeks of surgery. The pooled random-effects odds ratio from the combined analysis was 1.62 (95% CI, 1.21 to 2.16), corresponding to an increase in the 5-year local recurrence rates (LRR) from 5.8% in those patients treated within 8 weeks to 9.1% in those patients treated between 9 and 16 weeks after surgery. In a separate analysis exploring the optimum sequencing of adjuvant radiation therapy and systemic chemotherapy after surgery for breast cancer from 11 retrospective series, the pooled random-effects odds ratio for these 11 studies was 2.28 (95% CI, 1.45 to 3.57), corresponding to an increase in the 5-year LRR from 6% in the radiation therapy–first group to 16.0% in the chemotherapy-first group (Fig. 53.21).

Most of these data are subject to criticism due to their retrospective nature, the fact that patients were treated in an earlier era with different surgical techniques, and lack of attention to margins and inclusion of heterogenous groups of patients with these caveats; there appears to be a trend toward higher local relapse rates with delays in radiation therapy, which appears to have been an appropriate concern with respect to integration of radiation therapy and chemotherapy in the conservatively managed patients.

Initial data regarding these concerns related to the delay in radiation while chemotherapy was being delivered led the Harvard group at Joint Center for Radiation Therapy (JCRT) to investigate the sequencing of radiation therapy and chemotherapy in a randomized prospective clinical trial (602,609). In this trial, women treated with breast-conserving surgery were randomly assigned to four cycles of doxorubicin-based combination chemotherapy, followed by radiation therapy or radiation therapy followed by four cycles of the same chemotherapy. In an update of this trial, Bellon et al. (46) reported no statistically significant treatment difference in the rates of freedom from any event, including breast cancer recurrence, contralateral breast cancer, second malignancy, or death (Fig. 53.22). The 10-year rate of any event was 46% for patients in the chemotherapy-first arm compared with 51% in the radiation-first arm. The 10-year rates of distant metastasis were 35% and 36% in the two arms, respectively; and the 10-year rates of death were 28% and 33%, respectively. For the 123 patients with negative margins, the crude local recurrence rates for

Table 53.30 — STUDIES EVALUATING IMPACT OF INTERNAL MAMMARY TREATMENT (SURGERY OR RADIATION) ON 10-YEAR SURVIVAL

Study (Reference)	Type of IMN Treatment	No. of Patients		Follow-Up (y)	Overall Survival			Distant Metastasis-Free Survival			Disease-Free Survival		
		With IMN Treatment	Without IMN Treatment		With IMN Treatment N (%)	Without IMN Treatment (%)	p value	Without IMN Treatment (%)	With IMN Treatment (%)	p value	Without IMN Treatment	With IMN Treatment	p value
Meier et al. (491)	Dissection	56	56	10	75	60.4	.130	—	—	—	—	—	—
Lacour et al. (430)	Dissection	750	703	10	56	53	.40	44	49	NS	—	—	—
Fowble et al. (238)	Radiation	114	1,259	6	80	81	.87	77	87	NS	82	87	.38
Obedian & Haffty (538)	Radiation	535	4.1	13	72	84	NS	—	—	—	—	—	—
Stemmer et al.[a] (718)	Radiation	67	33	6.4	78	64	.08	—	—	—	73	52	.02

IMN, internal mammary lymph nodes; NS, not significant.
[a]Survival data documented at the end point of follow-up.

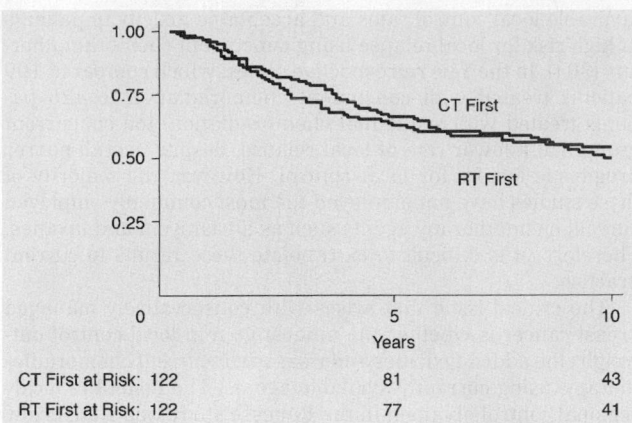

FIGURE 53.22. Event-free survival (including breast cancer recurrence, contralateral breast cancer, second malignancy, or death) by sequencing of chemotherapy (CT) and radiation therapy (RT) following breast-conserving therapy, from the Harvard randomized trial. (From Bellon JR, Come SE, Gelman RS, et al. Sequencing of chemotherapy and radiation therapy in early-stage breast cancer: updated results of a prospective randomized trial. *J Clin Oncol* 2005;23:1934–1940, with permission.)

chemotherapy-first and radiation-first patients were 6% and 13%, respectively. Corresponding rates of distant and regional recurrences were 18% and 26%, respectively. Among women with close margins ($n = 47$), crude local recurrence rates were 32% and 4%, respectively; distant/regional recurrences were 37% and 43%, respectively. In the group with positive margins ($n = 51$), local recurrences occurred in 23% of chemotherapy-first and 20% of radiation-first patients.

Although the JCRT study provided important data concerning treatment sequencing, this study predominantly focused on patients with lymph node positive disease. Investigators from the M.D. Anderson Cancer Center performed a retrospective analysis of sequencing of chemotherapy and radiation in 124 patients with lymph node–negative disease treated with breast-conservation surgery (86). In this series, 79% of the patients had negative margins. The 5-year actuarial rates of local control were 100% for the chemotherapy-first group (most commonly six cycles of doxorubicin-based chemotherapy) and 94% for the radiation-first group ($p = .351$). The 5-year recurrence-free sur-

vival rates for the chemotherapy-first and radiation-first groups were 92% and 77% ($p = .083$), respectively. These data again support an adjuvant-therapy schedule in which chemotherapy is delivered first. The median delays in radiation delivery were 6.7 months in the M.D. Anderson Cancer Center series and 16 weeks in the JCRT series.

More recently, with the addition of taxane-based chemotherapy to adriamycin-based regimens, concerns have arisen regarding the additional delays in initiating radiation therapy in conservatively managed patients. This was addressed in a recent study by Sartor et al. (651). In this randomized CALGB study evaluating doxorubicin with cyclophosphamide (AC) versus AC plus taxol (T), there were 345 conservatively managed patients. Although the sequencing was of radiation was not randomized, patients in the AC+T arm had radiation delayed by an additional 84 days (four 21 day cycles of taxol). Despite this added delay local–regional relapses were lower and the local–regional recurrence rates were lower in the AC+T compared to the AC alone arm (9.7% vs. 3.7%; $p = .04$). (The majority of patients in this randomized trial presumably had negative surgical margins.)

For the majority of patients undergoing breast-conserving surgery with negative margins, these data collectively indicate that administration of chemotherapy prior to radiation therapy does not result in excessive rates of local relapse, provided all modalities are given in a timely fashion without excessive delays. Whether patients with positive or close margins and/or other risk factors for local relapse would benefit from earlier administration of radiation remains an unresolved issue.

Concurrent Chemoradiation in Breast-Conserving Therapy

Although the concurrent use of chemoradiation therapy in conservatively managed breast cancer has fallen out of favor, there are data that suggest a high rate of local control in patients treated concurrently. These studies are summarized in Table 53.31. (The chemotherapy regimens used in these studies are no longer routinely employed because they are less effective.)

A recent randomized trial of concurrent versus sequential CMF chemotherapy was reported by Arcangeli et al. (25). A

Table 53.31 SELECTED STUDIES EVALUATION CONCURRENT CHEMORADIATION IN BREAST-CONSERVING SURGERY WITH RADIATION THERAPY

Study (Reference)	No. of Patients CON-CRT	No. of Patients Non-CON-CRT	Follow-Up (median)	Type of Chemo	Local Control CON-CRT	Local Control Non-CON-CRT	p	Toxicity with CON-CRT
Haffty et al. (305)	109	426	8.8 y	CMF (mainly)	92%	83%	<0.001	Cosmetic results, toxicities, and long-term complications acceptable
Bellon et al. (47)	112	—	7.8 y	CMF (prospective)	96%	—	—	—
Markiewicz et al. (473)	210	—	5.2 y for node-negative; 7.6 for node-positive	CF during radiation therapy flowed by further CMF	87% (10 y)	—	—	Cosmesis and complications acceptable
Rouesse et al. (638)	210	206	5.25 y	FNC for CON-CRT, FEC for sequential RT	97%	91%	0.01	Febrile neutropenia and grade 3–4 leukopenia significantly more frequent
Toledano et al. (747)	107	107	6.7 y	CNF	—	—	—	Increased incidence of grade 2 or greater late side effects.
Arcangeli et al. (25)	106	100	5.4 y	CMF	97%	96%	NS	Late toxicity and cosmesis not available yet

CF, oral cyclophosphamide/intravenous 5-fluorouracil; CMF, cyclophosphamide/methotrexate/5-fluofouracil; CNF, cyclophosphamide/mitoxantrone/5-fluorouracil; CON-CRT, concurrent chemotherapy; FEC, 5-fluorouracil/epirubicin/cyclophosphamide; FNC, 5-fluourouracil/mitoxantrone/cyclophosphamide; RT, radiation therapy.

total of 206 patients who had quadrantectomy and axillary dissection for breast cancer and were chosen to receive adjuvant CMF chemotherapy were randomized to concurrent or sequential radiotherapy. Radiotherapy was delivered only to the whole breast through tangential fields to a dose of 50 Gy in 20 fractions over 4 weeks, followed by an electron boost of 10 to 15 Gy in four to six fractions to the tumor bed. No differences in 5-year breast recurrence-free, metastasis-free, disease-free, and overall survival were observed in the two treatment groups. All patients completed the planned radiotherapy. No evidence of an increased risk of toxicity was observed between the two arms. No difference in radiotherapy and in the chemotherapy dose intensity was observed in the two groups. The authors concluded that in patients with negative surgical margins receiving adjuvant chemotherapy, radiotherapy can be delayed to up to 7 months. However, concurrent administration of CMF chemotherapy and radiotherapy was safe, and the authors suggest that such an approach might be reserved for patients at high risk of local recurrence.

Another randomized study of concurrent versus sequential radiation therapy was reported by Rouesse et al. (638). This study supports the concept that concurrent use of chemotherapy with radiation therapy improves local control in breast cancer. This trial compared concurrent chemoradiotherapy with FNC (5-fluourouracil 500 mg/m^2, mitoxantrone-12 mg/m^2, and cyclophosphamide 500 mg/m^2), to sequential FEC (5-fluorouracil 500 mg/m^2, epirubicin 60 mg/m^2, and cyclophosphamide 500 mg/m^2) followed by radiation in node-positive breast cancer in 650 women with operable breast cancer. All patients had node-positive disease and were randomized to sequential or concurrent chemoradiotherapy. Although there were no differences in disease-free or overall survival, local recurrences were significantly lower with concurrent therapy (3% vs. 7%). Of patients undergoing breast conservation, there were six local–regional relapses in the concurrent arm compared to 18 local–regional relapses in the sequential arm ($p = .01$). In multivariate Cox analysis, the sequential group had an increased risk of local–regional relapse compared to those in the concurrent group (RR 2.8, 95% CI, 1.1 to 7.2)

Toledano et al. (747) recently reported the results of the AR-COSEIN sequential versus concurrent adjuvant chemotherapy with radiation therapy after breast-conserving surgery. After breast-conserving surgery, patients were treated either with sequential treatment with chemotherapy first followed by radiation therapy (arm A) or chemotherapy administered concurrently with radiation therapy (arm B). In all patients, the chemotherapy regimen consisted of mitoxantrone (12 mg/m^2), 5-FU (500 mg/m^2), and cyclophosphamide (500 mg/m^2), six cycles (day 1 to day 21), Among the 214 evaluable patients, 107 were treated in each arm. Although local control was slightly superior in the concurrent arm, subcutaneous fibrosis, telangiectasia, skin pigmentation, and breast atrophy were significantly increased in arm B. No statistical difference was observed between the two arms of the study concerning grade 2 or greater pain, breast edema, or lymphedema.

Another randomized trial recently réported by Calais et al. (96), which is similar to the Rouesse study, compared concurrent radiotherapy with mitoxantrone, 5-FU, and cyclophosphamide to the same regimen followed by radiation therapy. Although toxicities were higher in the concurrent group, those patients with positive nodes had a significantly lower local relapse rate in the concurrent arm.

The concurrent use of chemotherapy and radiation following breast-conserving therapy has been reported in several nonrandomized studies. A prospective single arm study by Bellon et al. (47) also demonstrated favorable local control in a high-risk group of patients treated with concurrent CMF chemotherapy and reduced-dose radiation. Several other retrospective series, including one recently conducted from Yale, have demonstrated

favorable local control rates and acceptable toxicity in patients at high risk for local relapse using concurrent chemoradiotherapy (304). In the Yale retrospective series, which compared 109 patients treated with concurrent chemoradiation to 426 patients treated with sequential chemoradiation, the concurrent group had a lower rate of local relapse, despite overall poorer prognostic factors for local control. However, the majority of these studies have not employed the most commonly employed current chemotherapy agents such as adriamycin and taxanes. Therefore, it is difficult to extrapolate these results to current practice.

The critical issue that arises with conservatively managed breast cancer is whether the modest gain in local control outweighs the added toxicities and risks of concurrent chemoradiotherapy, using currently available agents. The benefit in local–regional control obtained in the Rouesse study was statistically significant, but it remains debatable whether the added toxicity of the concurrent program is worth the added risk. Potential issues with concurrent chemoradiation, as pointed out in a recent study by Burstein et al. (90), include high rates of radiation pneumonitis in patients treated with radiation given in combination with weekly paclitaxel. Although they observed more favorable results with less frequent dosing, this study highlights the importance of prospective evaluation of radiation in combination with newer chemotherapeutic agents. Furthermore, this study highlights the importance of the dosing and scheduling of the chemotherapy agents given in combination with radiation.

The challenge over the next few years will be to identify those patients who, when treated by the traditional approach of surgery followed by chemotherapy followed by radiation therapy, remain at elevated risk of local relapse. Also at risk may be subsets of patients treated with neoadjuvant chemotherapy followed by surgery followed by radiation. Those patients who, when treated by these traditional sequencing approaches, are at high risk of local relapse, are ideally suited for prospective evaluation of novel approaches using concurrent chemoradiation strategies. From such trials we can hopefully minimize local–regional relapse and optimize disease-free and overall survival, with acceptable treatment related morbidity.

Sequencing Tamoxifen and Radiation Therapy in Conservatively Managed Patients

The question of optimal scheduling of hormonal therapy and radiation has been raised due to theoretical concerns that tamoxifen may decrease the radiation sensitivity of tumors. In cell culture studies, tamoxifen causes arrest of breast cancer cells in culture in the relatively radioresistant G_0/G_1 phases of the cell cycle. Although there are conflicting data, suggesting both no effect and increased radiation sensitivity, clinicians and patients have been in a quandary regarding whether it is reasonable to begin tamoxifen during radiation. In addition, clinical studies have suggested increased pulmonary and breast fibrosis, possibly related to increased concentrations of transforming growth factor-β with the concurrent use of tamoxifen (52). In a retrospective case series, Wazer et al. (816) reported a trend for an adverse cosmetic outcome associated with breast fibrosis in patients treated with tamoxifen and breast irradiation given either concurrently or sequentially ($p = .06$), though this was not confirmed in other series (6,328,724).

Until recently, there were limited data concerning the effect of sequencing of tamoxifen on local relapse in the conservatively treated breast. A recent series of three separate retrospective series, however, performed independently but published simultaneously, reached similar conclusions that sequential or concurrent use of tamoxifen were both acceptable (6,328,575). These studies are summarized in Table 53.32. The largest study, by Ahn et al. (6) from the Yale group, compared 254 patients

Table 53.32 OUTCOMES OF CONCURRENT OR SEQUENTIAL TAMOXIFEN WITH RADIATION THERAPY IN EARLY STAGE BREAST CANCER

Study (Reference)	No. of Patients		Years of Follow-Up (median)	Total Local Relapse			Distant Metastasis			Secondary Malignancy			Complications
	CON-TAM	SEQ-TAM		CON-TAM (%)	SEQ-TAM (%)	p	CON-TAM (%)	SEQ-TAM (%)	p	CON-TAM (%)	SEQ-TAM (%)	p	
Ahn et al. (6)	254	241	10.0	5.9	7.5	.59	8.3	12.0	.16	17.3	15.8	.16	NA
Harris et al. (328)	174	104	8.6	4.0	4.8	.76	—	—	—	—	—	—	No significant difference between the two groups for arm edema, pneumonitis, and rib fracture
Pierce et al. (575)	202	107	10.3	15.8	14.0	.67	—	—	—	—	—	—	No significant differences between two groups for grade 3 or 4 toxicity; one grade 3 pulmonary toxicity observed in CON-TAM group

CON-TAM, concurrent tamoxifen; NA, not available; SEQ-TAM, sequential tamoxifen.

treated with concurrent tamoxifen and radiation therapy to 241 treated by radiation therapy followed by tamoxifen ($n = 241$). There were no significant differences in the risk of ipsilateral breast tumor recurrence, disease-free survival, or overall survival. The HR for ipsilateral breast tumor recurrence comparing sequential with concurrent tamoxifen and radiation therapy was 0.93 (95% CI, 0.42 to 2.05; $p = .86$). In this study, morbidity outcomes were not reported.

Another study, by Harris et al. (328), from the group at university of Pennsylvania compared 174 patients treated with concurrent tamoxifen and radiation therapy, with 104 patients treated with radiation therapy followed sequentially by tamoxifen. Similar to the Yale study, patients were accrued throughout a long period between 1980 and 1995, and again no significant differences in ipsilateral breast tumor recurrence, disease-free survival, or overall survival were observed between groups. The HR for ipsilateral breast tumor recurrence (sequential vs concurrent) was 1.23 (95% CI, 0.33 to 4.49; $p = .78$). In this study, breast edema and arm edema as well as cosmetic outcome and pneumonitis were analyzed, and no significant differences were observed.

The third study, by Pierce et al. (575), evaluated results from a randomized Southwest Oncology Group (SWOG) trial, in which patients were randomly assigned to cyclophosphamide, doxorubicin, and 5-fluorouracil (CAF), followed by tamoxifen; cyclophosphamide, methotrexate, and 5-fluorouracil (CMF); or CMF followed by tamoxifen. Although the sequencing of tamoxifen was not randomized, 202 patients received concurrent tamoxifen and radiation therapy and 107 received radiation therapy followed sequentially by tamoxifen. In this study, no differences were noted in the risk of ipsilateral breast tumor recurrence, disease-free survival, or survival between the radiation therapy followed sequentially by tamoxifen and the concurrent tamoxifen and radiation therapy groups. Patients who received concurrent tamoxifen and radiation therapy were more likely to receive radiation after chemotherapy, with less delay. The HR for risk of ipsilateral breast tumor recurrence (radiation therapy followed sequentially by tamoxifen vs. concurrent tamoxifen and radiation therapy) was 0.73 (95% CI, 0.26 to 2.04; $p = .54$).

Although these studies are limited by their retrospective design, they do offer some reassurance that the concurrent use of hormonal therapy with radiation therapy does not result in excessive rates of local relapse. A large randomized trial would be the appropriate next step in addressing this issue, but it is unclear whether this issue will be addressed by such a trial in the near future. Given the lack of more definitive data, it appears that either the concurrent or the sequential use of tamoxifen is acceptable in the conservatively managed breast cancer patient.

Breast-Conserving Therapy: Controversies and Special Circumstances

The available evidence from all of the retrospective and prospective trials above suggests that although there are clearly cohorts of patients who are at increased risk of local relapse, there are relatively few contraindications to breast-conserving therapy and there is little evidence that treatment of patients at higher risk for local relapse with breast-conserving therapy compromises overall survival. Careful attention to patient selection, surgical technique, and radiation technique, with the appropriate integration of systemic therapy, should minimize the probability of local relapse. There are several areas of controversy and special circumstances in the selection of patients for breast-conserving therapy that warrant specific discussion.

Breast-Conserving Surgery and Radiation in Familial Breast Cancer and Carriers of BRCA1-2 Mutations

There is considerable controversy and uncertainty regarding the role of breast-conserving surgery and radiation in carriers of BRCA1-2 mutations (11,312,623). It has been just over a decade since these two major breast cancer predisposition genes were identified. Genetic linkage studies from families at high risk for predisposing germline mutations have lead to the identification of the BRCA1-2 genes, and these two genes are thought to account for 5% to 10% of all breast cancers (100,171,172,228,229,625). Patients with either mutation have up to an 80% lifetime risk of developing breast cancer depending on variable penetrance of the gene. Inherited mutation of BRCA1 also confers a 20% to 40% lifetime risk of ovarian cancer. Typical patient characteristics of BRCA-associated breast cancer include young age at onset and bilateral involvement. The median age at breast cancer diagnosis is 40 for BRCA1 carriers and 45 for BRCA2 carriers (171,172,228,229,625). Tumor characteristics of BRCA1 carriers have been well described. Histopathologic features are often more aggressive, with high nuclear grade, aneuploidy, and high proliferation indices; tumors with a medullary component are more common. Estrogen and progesterone receptors are more likely to be negative when compared with BRCA2 or sporadic counterparts. Although there are some conflicting data, BRCA1-2 carriers with breast cancer appear to have equivalent survival when compared to age and stage-matched patients with sporadic disease (23,100,625,626,672).

The loci for BRCA1 and BRCA2 are chromosome 17q21 and chromosome 13q12-13, respectively (171,172,228,229,625). Both function as tumor suppressor genes and are involved in DNA double-strand break repair. The role of BRCA1-2 in DNA repair suggests the possibility of hypersensitivity to radiation, as well as the potential for radiation-induced complications including second tumors. DNA double-strand breaks caused by ionizing radiation in BRCA1-2 carriers could theoretically result in increased cell kill secondary to deficient repair mechanisms (516,520,530,625,677).

The risk of both contralateral primary breast cancer and ovarian cancer is substantially higher in patients with BRCA1-2 mutations than sporadic counterparts. An early publication by the Breast Cancer Linkage Consortium estimated a 64% risk of contralateral breast cancer by the age of 70 years in patients who have had BRCA1-associated breast cancer (100,588). The cumulative risk of ovarian cancer in these patients was 44% by age 70 years. Women with BRCA2 mutations have a risk of breast cancer similar to patients with BRCA1 mutations. There is a lesser risk of ovarian cancer, with a cumulative risk of <10% by age 70 years. These results have been interpreted with caution, as linkage studies are likely to overestimate the cancer risk associated with BRCA1-2 mutations. Several studies of known germline BRCA1-2 carriers have demonstrated a less pronounced increase in the rate of contralateral breast cancer compared with sporadic controls (100,588,625).

Early study of familiar breast cancer used positive family history as a surrogate for genetic predisposition. Many of the patients included likely did not harbor germline mutations of the BRCA1-2 genes. Seynaeve et al. (672), for the Dutch Cancer Society, investigated local recurrence after breast-conservation therapy in patients with ≥3 first-degree relatives with breast/ovarian cancer or BRCA1-2 families. Local recurrence rates were initially similar, but with longer follow-up there was a higher rate of recurrence in the hereditary group when compared with age-matched sporadic patients. Other studies of breast-conservation therapy in patients with a family history of breast cancer reported by Harrold et al. (334), Chabner

| Table 53.33 | RATE OF IPSILATERAL BREAST TUMOR RELAPSE IN BRCA MUTATION CARRIERS COMPARED TO SPORADIC CONTROLS |

Study (Reference)	No. of Patients Genetic	No. of Patients Sporadic	Follow-Up (y)	IBTR Sporadic (%)	IBTR Genetic (%)	p	Notes
Seyneave et al. (672)	87	174	10	16	30	.05	More recurrences elsewhere in cancers
Robson et al. (622)	28	277	10	6.9	22	.25	Only tested for founder mutations in Ashkenazic women
Robson et al. (626)	56	440	9.6	7	13	.68	As above
Haffty et al. (303)	23	135	12	21	46	.007	No oophorectomy or tamoxifen in BRCA group
Pierce et al. (576)	160	445	7.9	17	24	.19	HR for IBTR was significant in those carriers who did not undergo prophylactic oophorectomy

HR, hazard ratio; IBTR, in-breast tumor recurrence.

et al. (105), Haas et al. (294), and Freedman et al. (254) have not shown an increase in ipsilateral breast recurrence. Disparate results are expected, as family history is not the sole factor in genetic predisposition.

Turner et al. (757) published one of the first reports of ipsilateral breast tumor recurrence in patients with BRCA1-2 mutations in a pilot case-control study, which suggested a higher rate of late local relapses among BRCA1-2 mutation carriers. The majority of recurrences associated with a germline mutation occurred in a different quadrant of the breast and had distinct pathologic features. The longer time to recurrence, coupled with change in histology and tumor location, suggests that these events may be new primary cancers. Subsequent studies have confirmed these results, although there are conflicting reports. The risk of local and contralateral breast cancers as a function of BRCA1-2 status have been evaluated by numerous groups over the past 10 years (300,484,502,567,610–612,658,741). Selected studies are summarized in Table 53.33.

Robson et al. (622) studied breast-conservation therapy in Ashkenazic women with the BRCA gene founder mutations (BRCA1 185delAG, BRCA1 5382insC, and BRCA2 617delT). Archival tissue samples were retrieved from 305 women, and 28 BRCA gene founder mutations were detected. BRCA1-2 carriers had a nonsignificant trend toward increased ipsilateral breast cancer recurrence and decreased overall survival at 5 and 10 years. This trend may be related to the greater likelihood of young age and axillary lymph node involvement in women with BRCA founder mutations. On univariate analysis, age but not BRCA mutation status was associated with ipsilateral breast tumor recurrence. The significance of age was maintained on multivariate analysis, with a relative risk of 2.5. The risk of contralateral breast cancer at 5 and 10 years was 14.8% and 27%, respectively.

This series from Memorial Hospital was later combined with data from McGill University, yielding a total of 56 women with founder mutations (626). Again, BRCA1-2 carriers had an increased risk of contralateral breast cancer at a median follow-up of 9.7 years (27% vs. 8%; p <.001). Ipsilateral breast cancer recurrence for BRCA1-2 carriers was similar to noncarriers, and age <50 at diagnosis was the only significant predictor of metachronous ipsilateral disease (p = .002) (626). BRCA1 mutations were an independent predictor of breast cancer mortality on multivariate analysis, but only for women who did not receive chemotherapy. BRCA2 mutations had no impact on breast cancer–specific survival.

Haffty et al. (303) studied breast-conservation therapy in germline carriers with early onset breast cancer. One hundred and twenty-seven women diagnosed with breast cancer at age 42 years or younger agreed to undergo genetic testing, and 22 were found to have BRCA1-2 mutations. Adjuvant tamoxifen or oophorectomy were not used in any of the carriers of BRCA1-2 mutations. Patients in the genetic group were younger than sporadic patients, and this difference was significant on multivariate analysis. Treatment outcomes were compared with results from patients with sporadic disease. With a median follow-up of 12.7 years, the genetic group had a higher rate of ipsilateral (49% vs. 21%; p = .007) and contralateral breast events (42% vs. 9%; p = .001). Nine of the 11 ipsilateral breast recurrences were classified as second primary tumors, based on a difference in tumor location (n = 7) and/or histology (n = 8). The rate of ipsilateral and contralateral events was much higher than those reported in earlier series and may be attributable to both the young age of the patients at diagnosis and longer duration of follow-up. The proportion of relapse-free BRCA1-2 carriers was similar to noncarriers at 5 years, and then progressively declined with time (Fig. 53.23). It is promising that all of the second events in BRCA1-2 carriers were successfully salvaged and remained disease free. Steinmann et al. (717) confirmed the increased risk of developing ipsilateral second primaries in BRCA1-2 carriers and extended this concern to patients with bilateral breast cancer. Although the high rate of local relapses and contralateral events in these studies might be considered unacceptable, it is likely that the use of risk reduction strategies, such as tamoxifen and/or oophorectomy, would reduce these events to an acceptable level.

Although the data presented above present some apparent conflicting conclusions, a recent study by Pierce et al. (576) helped to resolve some of these issues. In a large collaborative study these authors evaluated a total of 160 BRCA1-2 mutation carriers with breast cancer matched to 445 controls with sporadic breast cancer (Fig. 53.24). Median follow-up was 7.9 years for mutation carriers and 6.7 years for controls. Although there was no significant difference in IBTR overall between carriers and controls (15-year estimates were 24% for carriers and 17% for controls, HR 1.37; p = .19), a subset analysis revealed higher rates of local relapse in those carriers who had not undergone prophylactic oophorectomy. Multivariate analyses for IBTR found BRCA1-2 mutation status to be an independent predictor of IBTR when carriers who had undergone oophorectomy were removed from analysis (HR 1.99; p = .04); the incidence of IBTR in carriers who had undergone oophorectomy was not significantly different from that in sporadic controls (p = .37). Contralateral breast cancers were significantly more frequent in carriers versus controls, with 10- and 15-year estimates of 26% and 39% for carriers and 3% and 7% for controls, respectively (HR 10.43; p <.0001). Tamoxifen use significantly reduced the risk of contralateral breast cancers in mutation carriers (HR 0.31; p = .05). Thus it appears that this study confirms the

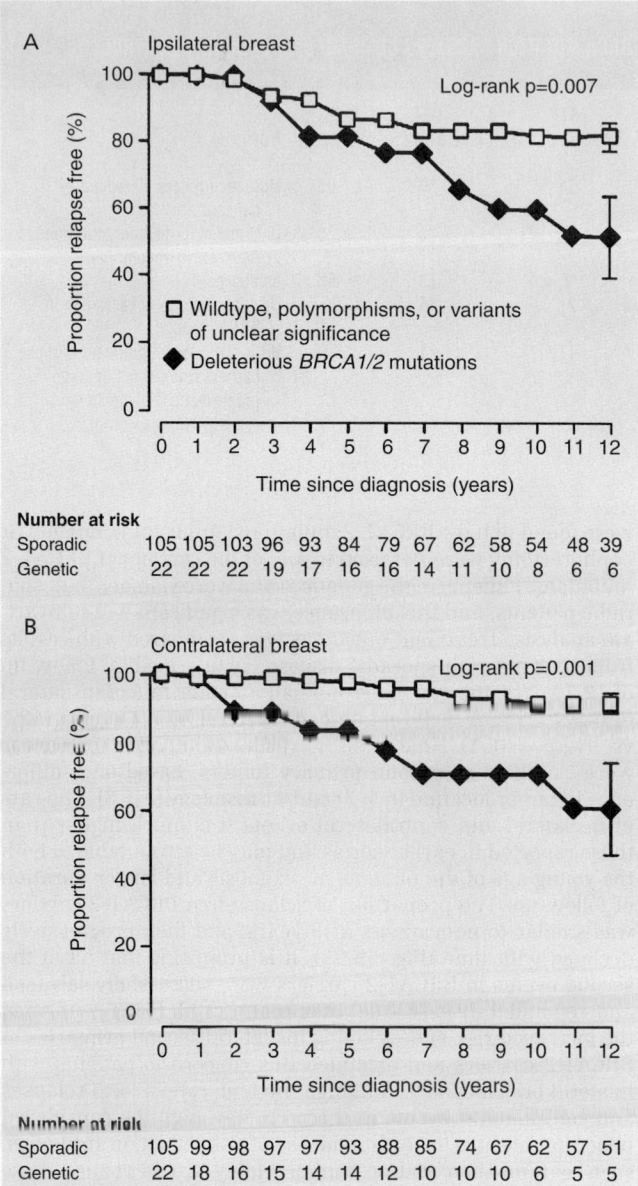

FIGURE 53.23. Risk of ipsilateral (**A**) and contralateral (**B**) breast tumor relapse as a function of BRCA1-2 mutation status in a cohort of conservatively managed breast cancer patients. (From Haffty BG, Harrold E, Khan AJ, et al. Outcome of conservatively managed early-onset breast cancer by BRCA1/2 status. *Lancet* 2002;359:1471–1477, with permission.)

findings of Haffty et al. that BRCA1-2 carriers have a high rate of both contralateral and ipsilateral breast events if they do not undergo specific measures to reduce the risk of subsequent breast cancers by undergoing oophorectomy and/or tamoxifen. Prophylactic mastectomy has been shown to significantly reduce the incidence of breast cancer in women with a family history of breast cancer and specifically women with BRCA1-2 mutations (335). This risk reduction strategy has complex emotional and psychological implications, and there are no data to suggest an improvement in survival when compared to close surveillance. Most preventative strategies have focused on primary prevention, but prophylactic strategies should also be considered at the time of breast cancer diagnosis. Oophorectomy and tamoxifen offer similar risk reduction for breast cancer patients with germline mutations. These agents have not been widely used in studies of conservatively managed breast cancer patients with

BRCA1-2 mutations. Their potential benefits must be weighed against the possible complications of premature menopause following oophorectomy and the side-effects of tamoxifen.

Women with BRCA1-2 mutations who underwent prophylactic oophorectomy to reduce the risk of ovarian cancer were found to have a decreased incidence of breast cancer. Rebbeck (600) studied the risk of breast cancer in 43 BRCA1 carriers with no history of breast or ovarian cancer who underwent prophylactic bilateral oophorectomy. When these patients were compared to BRCA1 controls who did not undergo oophorectomy, there was a significant reduction in breast cancer risk (HR 0.53). A follow-up report from Rebbeck et al. (598,599) for the Prevention and Observation of Surgical Endpoints (PROSE) study group identified 551 women with BRCA1-2 germline mutations and reported the incidence of ovarian and breast cancer in women who had undergone prophylactic oophorectomy and matched controls. Six women who underwent prophylactic oophorectomy were diagnosed with stage I ovarian cancer at the time of the procedure. With a median follow-up of 8 years, two women developed papillary serous peritoneal carcinoma after oophorectomy and 58 controls were diagnosed with ovarian cancer. After the exclusion of women who were diagnosed with cancer at surgery, oophorectomy reduced the risk of ovarian cancer by 96%. Oophorectomy also reduced the incidence of breast cancer in the subgroup of 241 women with no history of breast cancer or prophylactic mastectomy. Twenty-one (21.2%) of the 99 women who underwent prophylactic oophorectomy developed breast cancer versus 60/142 (42.3%) women in the control group (HR 0.47).

Kauff et al. (392) conducted a prospective study of the risk of gynecologic cancer and breast cancer in 170 BRCA1-2 carriers who chose to undergo surveillance or prophylactic oophorectomy. In the 98 women who chose prophylactic oophorectomy, three were later diagnosed with breast cancer and peritoneal cancer was diagnosed in one patient. The surveillance group of 72 patients yielded eight breast cancers, four ovarian cancers, and one peritoneal cancer. With a median follow-up of only 24 months, this prospective study supports an early reduction in breast and ovarian cancer risk with prophylactic oophorectomy.

In prospective trials, tamoxifen has been shown to reduce both the risk of breast cancer in high-risk women and the risk of contralateral breast cancer in patients with breast cancer (209,240). An analysis of the NSABP data from the P1 tamoxifen versus placebo P1 prevention trial identified 19 BRCA1-2 mutations in the 288 women who developed breast cancer (402). Five of the eight women with BRCA1 mutations had taken tamoxifen, versus 3/11 women with BRCA2 mutations. This represented a 62% reduction in breast cancer incidence for BRCA2 carriers, but no benefit for tamoxifen in BRCA1 carriers. The data set was small, however, with low power to detect a protective effect.

Narod et al. (520) studied tamoxifen and the risk of contralateral breast cancer in BRCA1-2 carriers. This collaborative effort compared women with bilateral breast cancer and women with unilateral breast cancer in a case-control study. Sixty-four (13%) BRCA1 mutation carriers used tamoxifen versus 39 (33%) BRCA2 carriers. This difference is expected as breast cancers associated with BRCA1 mutations are typically estrogen-receptor negative and BRCA2-associated breast cancers are commonly estrogen-receptor positive. Tamoxifen protected against contralateral breast cancer, with an odds ratio of 0.38 for BRCA1 carriers and 0.63 for BRCA2 carriers. The combined risk reduction for BRCA1 and BRCA2 carriers was 50%. The benefit of tamoxifen in BRCA1 carriers was possibly detected due to the larger sample size. This study also noted a reduction in contralateral breast cancer in patients who received oophorectomy. The odds ratio was 0.42, which is similar to the reduction in contralateral breast cancer noted with tamoxifen.

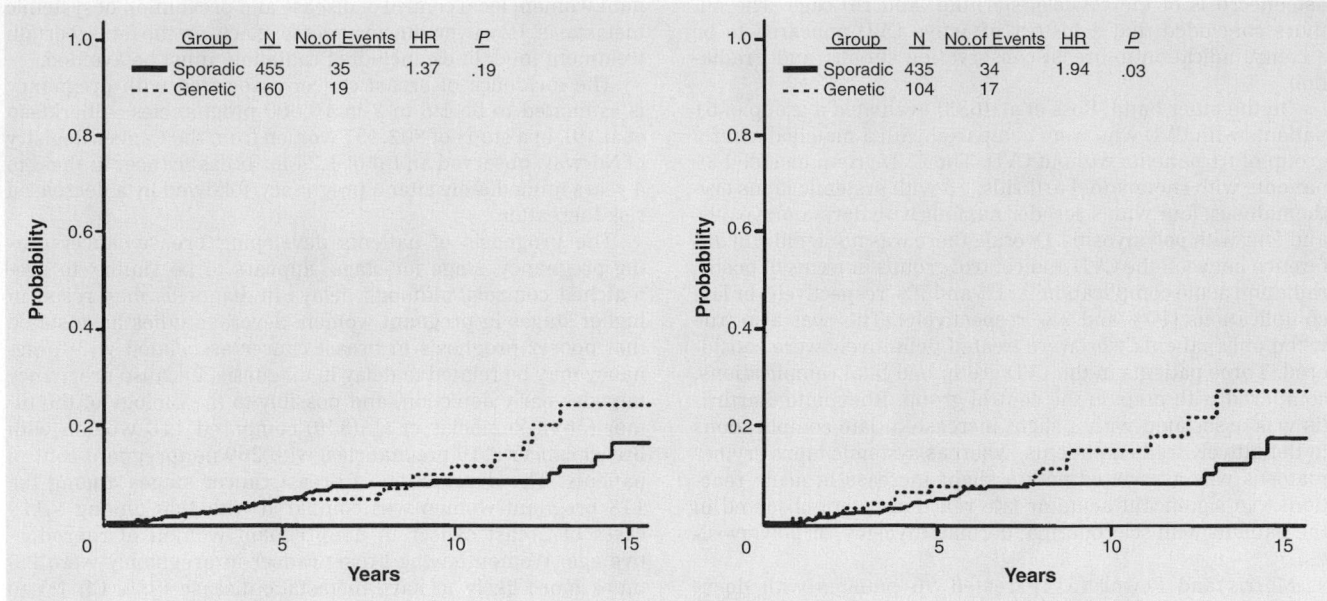

FIGURE 53.24. A: Risk of ipsilateral breast tumor relapse in BRCA carriers as a function of whether carriers had undergone prophylactic oophorectomy. **B:** In BRCA carriers who did not undergo oophorectomy, the risk of late local relapses was significantly greater than sporadic controls. (From Pierce LJ, Levin AM, Rebbeck TR, et al. Ten-year multi-institutional results of breast-conserving surgery and radiotherapy in BRCA1/2-associated stage I/II breast cancer. *J Clin Oncol* 2006;24:2437–2443, with permission.)

Although the conservative management of breast cancer in patients with BRCA1 and BRCA2 germline mutations warrants further study, the available evidence indicates that breast-conserving therapy followed by radiation therapy is an appropriate alternative to bilateral mastectomy in early stage breast cancer in these women. Theoretical concerns for radiation-induced complications have not been demonstrated (579). Although development of second primary tumors in the ipsilateral and contralateral breast remains a concern, prophylactic oophorectomy and tamoxifen appear to significantly reduce the probability of these secondary events (520,576,600,625). Prophylactic oophorectomy is even more critical in the risk-reduction strategy for the development of primary tumors of the ovary. For those women considering breast-conserving surgery and radiation therapy, strategies to reduce secondary events, including prophylactic oophorectomy as soon as child-bearing issues have been addressed and resolved, with or without tamoxifen or other hormonal agents as indicated, appears to be a

rational and viable option. Despite some evidence that tamoxifen reduces the risk of secondary breast cancers in patients who are carriers of BRCA1-2 mutations, the use of tamoxifen in BRCA1 breast cancer patients who are estrogen-receptor negative remains unresolved and controversial.

Collagen Vascular Disease

Increased acute and late effects of irradiation have been reported in patients with pre-existing collagen vascular disease (CVD). Selected studies addressing this issue are summarized in Table 53.34.

Fleck et al. (224) reported on five women in whom CVD developed 3 months to 10 years after radiation therapy and who had no complications. However, in three of four women with preexisting CVD severe complications developed, characterized by persistent moist desquamation, paresthesias in the ipsilateral arm, chest wall necrosis requiring surgical resection, and

Table 53.34   STUDIES EVALUATING COLLAGEN VASCULAR DISEASE IN BREAST-CONSERVING THERAPY

Study (Reference)	Total	CVD No. with Breast Cancer	Design	Findings
De Naeyer et al. (149)	3	1	Case report	Necrosis and progressive fibrosis
Fleck et al. (224)	9	4	Case report	Necrosis, brachial plexopathy, and severe moist desquamation
Robertson et al. (621)	2	2	Case report	Severe breast fibrosis, erythema, and pain
Chen et al. (109)	36	36	Case control	Late complication rates higher only in scleroderma
Morris et al. (514)	209	19	Retrospective	Increased radiation late effects appear in nonrheumatoid arthritis cases
Ross et al. (633)	61	?	Case control	No differences in acute/chronic complications
Phan et al. (571)	38	?	Case control	No difference was observed in the incidence of acute or late complications between the two groups.
Rakfal & Deutch (593)	6	4	Case report	No severe acute or late radiation complications

CVD, collagen vascular disease.

osteonecrosis of the clavicle, sternum, and rib cage. The authors concluded that a history of active CVD appeared to be a contraindication to breast-conservation surgery and irradiation.

On the other hand, Ross et al. (633) evaluated a group of 61 patients with CVD who were compared with a matched control group of 61 patients without CVD. The CVD group included 39 patients with rheumatoid arthritis, 13 with systemic lupus erythematosus, four with scleroderma, four with dermatomyositis, and four with polymyositis. Overall, there was no significant difference between the CVD and control groups in terms of postirradiation acute complications (11% and 7%, respectively) or late complications (10% and 7%, respectively). This was also true when only patients who were treated definitively were considered. Three patients in the CVD group had fatal complications, compared with none in the control group. Rheumatoid arthritis was associated with a slight increase in late complications in definitively treated patients, whereas systemic lupus erythematosus was associated with a slight increase in acute reactions. No significant acute or late reactions were observed in the patients with scleroderma, dermatomyositis, or polymyositis.

Morris and Powell (514) treated 96 patients with documented CVD with breast-conservation therapy (127 sites irradiated). Grade 3 or higher acute complications were seen in 15/127 (11.8%) sites, and the actuarial rate of significant late complications was 24% at 10 years. There was a single in-field sarcoma. Patients with rheumatoid arthritis had less severe late effects than those with other CVD (6% vs. 37% at 5 years; $p = .0001$).

In a study specifically evaluating conservatively treated breast cancer patients, Chen et al. (109) from the Yale group identified 36 patients with documented collagen vascular disease conservatively treated for early stage breast cancer between 1975 and 1998. All of these patients were treated with conventional radiation therapy to a median total dose of 64 Gy. Seventeen had rheumatoid arthritis, four had scleroderma, four had Raynaud's phenomenon, five had lupus erythematosus, two had Sjogren's disease, and four had polymyositis. Each of these patients was matched to two control patients without a history of CVD. Acute and late complications were assessed using a six-point scale from the toxicity criteria of the Radiation Therapy Oncology Group (RTOG) and the EORTC. No significant difference was detected between the collagen vascular disease and control groups with respect to acute complications (14% vs. 8%). With respect to late complications, a significant difference was observed (17% vs. 3%) between the two groups. However, when patients in the CVD group were analyzed by specific disease, this significance disappeared in all but the scleroderma group.

Collectively these data suggest that with the exception of patients with scleroderma, there does not appear to be a significantly greater late complication rate associated with CVD. Nevertheless, when patients with CVD are irradiated, it is prudent to limit the whole-breast dose to 45 Gy with 1.8-Gy fractions, use 6-MV photons, optimize homogeneity of dose distribution, avoid concurrent chemoirradiation, and discuss with patients the potential increased risks of radiation sequelae.

Pregnancy

Breast Cancer During Pregnancy

Breast cancer is the most common cancer diagnosed during pregnancy, and it represents a significant therapeutic challenge. Recently an expert international panel met and published general recommendations for breast cancer developing during pregnancy (455). The panel noted that the goal for the pregnant women with breast cancer is the same as that of the nonpreg-

nant women: local control of disease and prevention of systemic metastasis. However, due to adverse effects on the fetus, certain treatment modalities, including radiation, must be avoided.

The incidence of breast cancer associated with pregnancy is estimated to be 1.5 to 2 in 10,000 pregnancies. Alberktsen et al. (9), in a study of 802,457 women from the Cancer Registry of Norway, observed an RR of 1.24 for breast cancer in the 3 to 4 years immediately after a pregnancy, followed by a decreased risk thereafter.

The prognosis of patients developing breast cancer during pregnancy, stage for stage, appears to be similar to age-matched controls, although delays in diagnosis may result in higher stages in pregnant women. Several studies have stated that poorer prognosis in breast cancer associated with pregnancy may be related to delay in diagnosis, because pregnancy impedes early detection, and possibly to the biology of the tumor (569). Zemlickis et al. (849) compared 118 women with breast cancer (119 pregnancies) with 269 nonpregnant control patients. The distribution of breast cancer stages among the 118 pregnant women was compared with that among 5,115 cases of breast cancer in nonpregnant women of reproductive age. Women having breast cancer in pregnancy were 2.5 times more likely to have metastatic disease (95% CI, 1.1 to 5.3) and had a significantly lower chance of having stage I disease ($p = .015$). However, stage for stage survival of pregnant women did not differ from that of the control patients. A number of authors have commented on the high percentage of pregnant patients with lymph node involvement, compared with nonpregnant patients. Nugent and O'Connell (534) and others (5) have also suggested that the poorer outcome relates to the young age of the patient and not necessarily to the pregnancy (591).

In a review of the literature, Psyrri and Burtness (591) identified 117 articles and three abstracts related to breast cancer and pregnancy. Based on this extensive review, they conclude that delays in diagnosis may contribute to the higher proportion of patients with advanced stage at presentation, but the prognosis of the pregnant breast cancer patient is similar to her stage-matched nonpregnant counterparts in most series. As will be discussed below, selected chemotherapy agents can be administered during the second and third trimesters. Although therapeutic abortion is not necessary, women with high-risk disease may find this preferable. They also note that in women with known deleterious mutations in BRCA1-2, early pregnancy is not known to decrease subsequent breast cancer risk. In addition, the available evidence suggests that in women with a history of breast cancer, subsequent pregnancy does not increase the risk of recurrence.

In addition to requiring close coordination among multidisciplinary cancer caregivers, management of breast cancer during pregnancy also benefits from having obstetricians and pediatricians closely involved in therapeutic decision making. It is likely that as pregnancy in Western society is delayed to older ages the incidence of breast cancer developing during pregnancy will increase.

Breast cancers during pregnancy are almost universally diagnosed after an abnormal physical examination finding (591). There frequently may be a delay in diagnosis because breast mass is thought to represent obstructed milk ducts, and inflammatory changes of the breast may be misdiagnosed as cellulitis. For patients who present with a breast mass, a careful history and physical examination should be performed. The overall goal of managing breast cancer during pregnancy requires attention to both the mother and the fetus. Certain diagnostic and therapeutic interventions are known to be teratogenic and therefore are best avoided. Although theoretically a chest radiograph may be safely performed because the maximum dose to the fetus is <0.5 cGy, radiographic and scintigraphic imaging for staging should be minimized or deferred (147). Mammography is somewhat controversial, although the irradiation dose to the fetus is minimal (<0.5 mrem) (445). Ultrasound evaluations of the breast and lymph nodes can provide diagnostic information and serve as a method of guidance for core biopsy. Pathology of breast cancer during pregnancy is most frequently invasive ductal with high nuclear grade and lower rates of ER and PR positivity (591).

The management of the patient and the risks of certain interventions are also highly dependent on the week of gestation. In general, potentially harmful interventions carry the greatest risk during the period of organogenesis (first trimester) and are safest during the final trimester. For patients with operable disease, data suggest that surgery can be safely performed after the 12th week of pregnancy. The type of surgical procedure is dependent on the extent of disease and the trimester of the pregnancy (9,534,591,849). Few data exist concerning the safety and efficacy of sentinel lymph node biopsy. Although the blue dye used in sentinel lymph node surgery is not approved for use in pregnant patients, the estimated radiation dose to the fetus from the radiocolloid tracer is low. Except for radiation, treatment should not be altered or delayed because of pregnancy. Either a modified radical mastectomy or lumpectomy with axillary dissection is acceptable local treatment. Immediate breast reconstruction should not be performed.

Systemic chemotherapy with 5-fluorouracil, doxorubicin, cyclophosphamide (FAC) has been used in pregnancy. Investigators from M.D. Anderson reported a prospective series of 57 pregnant breast cancer patients who were treated on a single-arm, multidisciplinary, protocol with FAC in the adjuvant ($n = 32$) or neoadjuvant ($n = 25$) setting (313). Parents/guardians were surveyed by mail or telephone regarding outcomes of children exposed to chemotherapy *in utero*. All women who delivered had live births. One child had Down's syndrome and two had congenital anomalies (club foot; congenital bilateral ureteral reflux). The children are healthy and those in school are doing well, although two have special educational needs. They conclude that breast cancer can be treated with FAC chemotherapy during the second and third trimesters without significant short-term complications for the majority of children exposed to chemotherapy *in utero*. Longer follow-up of the children is needed to evaluate possible late side effects such as impaired cardiac function and fertility. Administration of chemotherapy in the first trimester is associated with a high risk of birth defects (17%, 24/139), in terms of probability of intrauterine growth retardation, prematurity, fetal malformation, or death this risk is less in the second and third trimesters (1.3%, 2/150) (163, 243).

As a general principle, hormonal therapy and radiation therapy should be avoided until after delivery. In one study, the estimated dose to the fetus from breast or chest wall radiation to a dose of 50 cGy is 2 cGy in the first trimester, 2.2 to 24.6 cGy during the second trimester, and 2.2 to 58.6 cGy during the third trimester. Dose to the fetus in the range 10 to 90 cGy during the first trimester have been associated with mental retardation (837).

When the patient chooses breast-conserving therapy, irradiation should be deferred until the fetus is delivered because 50 Gy delivered to the breast, even with external shielding, exposes the fetus to 0.1 to 0.15 Gy if it is small and contained in the true pelvis. During later gestation, when the fetus is larger and high in the abdomen, some fetal areas may receive as much as 2 Gy (837). In another study using a phantom (film dosimetry), doses to the pelvis ranged from 4.3 cGy with 4-MV x-rays to 15.8 cGy with cobalt-60 to the mid-pelvis (161).

Anatolak and Strom (24) determined fetal dose for a pregnant patient considering electron radiation therapy for a chest wall recurrence of breast cancer. Treatment was simulated using an anthropomorphic phantom. The measured dose to the unshielded fetus was 5.3 cGy, a level at which risk to the fetus is uncertain. Abdominal shielding, consisting of 6.6 cm of lead, was used to reduce the dose to the fetus to <1.5 cGy, a level considered to be of little risk. Using the lower (instead of upper) variable trimmer bars to define the field edge closest to the fetus resulted in an approximately 30% lower dose to the fetus.

Although there is some question whether there is any safe dose of irradiation to the fetus, Brent (81), in an extensive review of the literature, defined 0.05 Gy as a relatively safe upper limit of fetal exposure.

Pregnancy After Breast Cancer

Almost one-third of women of reproductive age in whom breast cancer later develops have had one or more pregnancies, and 70% of these pregnancies occur within 5 years of treatment (141). No data are available to suggest that subsequent pregnancy hastens or induces breast cancer recurrence. When matched by age and stage with nonpregnant patients, pregnant women with breast cancer do not have a worse outcome than nonpregnant patients with comparable stages. However, in patients receiving adjuvant chemotherapy, a minimum of 12 months between treatment and conception is advised. Breast-feeding is contraindicated in patients receiving chemotherapy because antineoplastic agents are excreted in the milk (534,569,591).

Sutton et al. (726) reviewed 227 women 35 years of age or younger at diagnosis who became pregnant after treatment with CAF adjuvant chemotherapy. Twenty-five patients had 33 pregnancies. The median interval between completion of chemotherapy and pregnancy was 12 months (range 0 to 87 months). Ten pregnancies were terminated, two ended in spontaneous abortion, two patients were still pregnant at the time of the report, and 19 produced normal full-term infants. The incidence of recurrence was 46% in patients without pregnancies, compared with 28% in those who had subsequent pregnancies. Similarly, 38% of patients without subsequent pregnancies were dead at the time of the report, compared with 12% of patients who became pregnant after chemotherapy treatment for breast cancer.

A population-based matched survival study assessed the risk of death for patients with breast cancer in relation to whether they delivered a live child subsequent to their cancer diagnosis (644). Among 2,548 women younger than 40 years of age diagnosed with carcinoma of the breast, 91 experienced subsequent deliveries (10 months or longer after the diagnosis), and 471 control patients were matched for stage, age, and year of breast cancer diagnosis. The control subjects had to survive at least the interval between the cancer diagnosis and the delivery of their matched counterparts. The control subjects had a 4.8-fold greater risk of death compared with those who delivered after the diagnosis of breast cancer. The authors' interpretation of this result was that there was a "healthy mother effect" (only women who felt healthy gave birth, and those who were affected by the disease did not). Nevertheless, six of eight deaths among the 91 patients who did give birth were related to breast cancer.

Dow et al. (166) evaluated treatment outcome and quality of life in 23 patients with subsequent pregnancies in a group of 1,624 patients treated with breast-conservation surgery and irradiation. This group was compared with 23 patients without subsequent pregnancies who were matched by age and stage at diagnosis and by time to pregnancy without recurrence. There were 32 pregnancies and 30 live births. Six of 23 (22%) women having children after breast cancer therapy had locally recurrent tumor, compared with 29% in the case-matched group. Contralateral breast cancer developed in one woman (4%) in

Clinical Radiation Oncology

the pregnancy group, compared with 11% in the case-matched group.

It may be helpful to suggest a waiting time (2 to 3 years) for the patient to regain health before attempting the physical stress of pregnancy and deferral of childbearing until after the period of greatest risk of recurrence of the tumor (141). The individual woman's prognosis, well-being, desire for children, support from spouse or significant other, and other sociodemographic factors must be carefully considered in this difficult decision-making process.

Lactation After Breast-Conservation Therapy

Successful breastfeeding, from the untreated as well as the treated breast, is possible after conservation surgery and irradiation. Higgins and Haffty (348) reviewed the records of 890 patients treated with radiation therapy for early stage (stage I or II) breast cancer. This series was recently updated by Moran et al. (509). Of over 3,000 patients treated from 1965 to 2003 a cohort of 21 premenopausal women who underwent breast-conserving therapy and subsequently sustained full-term pregnancies were identified. Lactation outcome parameters (breast swelling, ability to lactate, and volume of lactation in the treated and untreated breasts) were the main outcome measures. There were 28 pregnancies in 21 patients. One patient underwent bilateral breast treatment; therefore, a total of 22 breasts were irradiated. All patients interviewed reported little or no swelling of the treated breast during pregnancy. Of the patients studied, four (18.2%) elected pharmacological suppression of lactation. Of the remaining 18 breasts, lactation occurred in 10 (55.6%),

did not occur in seven (38.9%), and was unknown for one (5.5%). The volume was reported as significantly diminished in 80% of breasts treated. Lactation in the contralateral breast occurred in all patients who did not undergo pharmacological suppression. The authors confirm that successful lactation in the contralateral, untreated breast after breast-conserving therapy is expressed. In the treated breast, functional lactation is possible but is significantly diminished in the majority of patients. Tralins (749) reported results of a survey describing 53 women who became pregnant after conservation therapy and breast irradiation. Eighteen exhibited some lactation, and 13 (24.5%) were able to breastfeed from the involved breast. Pregnancy or lactation had no impact on prognosis; with a 5.4-year mean follow-up, the tumor-free survival rate was 82%.

Breast Irradiation in Patients Previously Irradiated for Hodgkin's Disease

There is an increased incidence of breast cancer in female patients who have previously undergone mantle irradiation for Hodgkin's disease. Numerous studies have demonstrated a significantly increased relative risk of breast cancer in women treated for Hodgkin's disease, with the risk significantly increasing with decreasing age of exposure. Table 53.35 summarizes the findings of several series.

Travis et al. (750) estimated that for a female Hodgkin's disease survivor who was treated at age 25 years with a chest radiation dose of at least 40 Gy without alkylating agents, cumulative absolute risks of breast cancer by age 35, 45, and 55

Table 53.35 | RISK OF SECONDARY BREAST CANCER DEVELOPMENT AFTER MANTLE RADIOTHERAPY FOR HODGKIN'S DISEASE

Study (Reference)	Population Total	Population Sex	Population Age (y)	Treatment	Average Follow-Up (y)	Interval to Breast Cancer Detection	Breast Cancer Cases Total	Breast Cancer Cases Age Range (y)	Relative Risk (95% CI)
Aisenberg et al. (8)	111	F		III + IV	18	8.5–25	14	23–49	—
			≤19						56 (23.3–107)
			20–29						7.0 (2.3–16.4)
			≥30						0.9 (0–5.3)
Chung et al. (115)	136	F	—	RT ± CT	14.8	6–22	11	30–63	AR = 55.1 cases/10,000 patient years
Carey et al. (101)	164	F	—	RT		11–17	4	37.3	5.45
Guibout et al. (290)	1,258	F	≥17	RT ± CT	16	16–28	4	30–34	7.01 (22–164)[a]
Huppe (355)	2,498	F/M	—	RT ± CT	—	—	25	—	4.1
Tinger et al. (744)	152	F	—	RT ± CT	>5	4–23	10	27–64	2.2
Bhatia et al. (57)	483	F	<16	RT ± CT	11.4	—	17	16–42	75.3
Mauch et al. (481)	349	F	3–69	RT ± CT	10.7	—	13	—	6.5 (3.5–11.2)
Salloum et al. (642)	144	F	—	RT ± CT	13.5	13.9–14	2	39–41	2 (0.6–7.4)
Hancock et al. (321)	885	F	—	RT ± CT	10	4.5–23	25	22–75	4.1 (2.6–5.9)
Prior and Pope (589)	777	F	—	RT ± CT	6.7	10–19	9	—	2.2
Tucker et al. (756)	1,507	F/M	—	RT ± CT	6.2	8	3	—	12 (2.3–35)
Kaldor et al. (386)	11,491	F	—	RT ± CT	1–20+	—	62	—	1.4
Travis et al. (751)	3,817	F	≤30	RT ± CT		7–30	105	27–57	3.2 (1.4–8.2)
Metayer et al. (495)	2,725	F	≤21	RT ± CT	10.5	—	52	—	4.9
Swerdlow et al. (727)	2,085	F	—	RT ± CT	1–15	—	19	—	14.4 (5.7–29.3)[b]
van Leeuwen et al. (770)	544	F	<40	RT ± CT	14.1	1–20+	27	—	5.2 (3.4–7.6)
Gervais-Fagnou et al. (275)	427	F	≤30	RT ± CT	12.3	9–25	15	30–52	10.6 (5.8–17)
Hudson et al. (360)	165	F	—	RT ± CT	15.1	3.6–24.9	6	—	33 (12–72)[a]
Wolden et al. (836)	207	F	<21	RT ± CT	13.1	8.5–27.9	16	—	26 (15–42)

AR, absolute risk; CI, confidence interval; CT, chemotherapy; F, female; M, male.
[a]Standardized incidence ratio.
[b]For patients treated at ages younger than 25 years.

years were 1.4% (95% CI, 0.9 to 2.1), 11.1% (95% CI, 7.4 to 16.3), and 29.0% (95% CI, 20.2 to 40.1), respectively.

Mastectomy has been recommended as the preferred treatment option in these women. Lumpectomy followed by breast irradiation has been considered by some to be contraindicated owing to the cumulative radiation dose to the breast. However, in selected patients using careful breast irradiation techniques that avoid significant overlap with the previous mantle port, anecdotal and retrospective reports in small numbers of patients suggest that it is possible to offer breast-conservation therapy. Therapeutic options and the potential increased risk of reirradiation sequelae should be thoroughly discussed with the patient. A second issue that should also be considered is the risk of the development of a new primary. Similar to patients with BRCA mutations, patients who have a history of breast cancer development after irradiation for Hodgkin's disease are at risk in the development of subsequent new primaries and may benefit from prevention strategies such as mastectomy.

Cutuli et al. (135) reported on a retrospective multicenter analysis in which 117 women and two men treated for Hodgkin's disease subsequently developed 133 breast cancers. Hodgkin's disease treatment was radiation therapy alone in 74 patients and combined modality with chemotherapy in 43 patients. Breast cancer occurred after a median interval of 16 years. Tumors were treated by mastectomy without ($n = 67$) or with ($n = 10$) irradiation. Forty-four tumors were treated with lumpectomy without ($n = 12$) or with ($n = 32$) radiation therapy. Another four received radiation therapy alone, and one had chemotherapy alone. Sixteen patients had isolated breast relapses, 39 had metastases, and 34 died. Young women treated for Hodgkin's disease should be carefully monitored in the long term by clinical examination, mammography, and ultrasonography. The authors suggested that a baseline mammography be performed 5 to 8 years after supradiaphragmatic irradiation (complete mantle or involved field) in patients treated before 30 years of age. Subsequently, mammography should be performed every 2 years or each year, depending on the characteristics of the breast tissue (e.g., density) and especially in the case of an association with other breast cancer risk factors.

Wolden et al. (835) described 71 cases of breast cancer in 65 survivors of Hodgkin's disease. Median age at diagnosis was 24.6 years for Hodgkin's disease and 42.6 years for breast cancer; the relative risk for invasive breast cancer after Hodgkin's disease was 4.7 compared with an age-matched cohort. Cancers were detected by self-examination in 63%, mammography in 30%, and by physical examination alone in 7%. The majority were of invasive ductal histology, and 27% had positive axillary nodes. The tumor was ER positive in 63% of the cases, and 25% of patients had an associated family history. The majority of tumors were smaller than 4 cm. Ninety-five percent of cases were managed by mastectomy because of prior irradiation, and two women underwent excisional biopsy with breast irradiation. One of these patients had tissue necrosis in the region of overlap with the prior mantle field. The incidence of bilateral breast cancer was 10%. The 10-year disease-specific survival rate for DCIS was 100%, stage I 88%, stage II 55%, stage III 60%, and stage IV 0%.

Recently Intra et al. (369) reported a novel approach with partial breast irradiation and intraoperative electrons. In a series of just three patients affected by breast cancer who had previously been treated with mantle radiation for Hodgkin's disease breast-conserving surgery and full-dose intraoperative radiotherapy with electrons were performed. A dose of 17 Gy (prescribed at 100% isodose) in one case and 21 Gy (at the 90% isodose) in two cases was delivered directly to the mammary gland without acute complications and with good cosmetic results.

One of the largest series using breast-conserving surgery with radiation therapy in patients previously treated for Hodgkin's disease is from Deutsch et al. (156). In this retrospective review, 12 women treated with radiotherapy with or without chemotherapy for Hodgkin's disease (11 patients) and non-Hodgkin's lymphoma (one patient) in whom breast cancer developed 10 to 29 years later were treated with lumpectomy and breast irradiation. Patients were treated with whole breast daily irradiation with a fractionation of 2 to 50 Gy with boost to the operative area. Six also received adjuvant chemotherapy for breast cancer. Breast irradiation was well tolerated without any unusual acute or chronic sequelae. They conclude that this may be an option for previously radiated Hodgkin's survivors who develop early stage breast cancer.

This controversial area will continue to evolve. Given the development of partial breast irradiation programs over the past several years, it is likely that data regarding reirradiation with partial breast programs will be reported (12,32). Clearly, however, Hodgkin's survivors and others who receive radiotherapy to breast at a young age are at high risk for developing breast cancers and should be carefully monitored. Women who develop breast cancer should be advised that mastectomy remains the treatment of choice. However, for patients highly motivated for breast preservation, anecdotal experiences using a variety of approaches have revealed acceptable toxicity and cosmesis.

Patients with More Than One Invasive Carcinoma (Multicentric Disease)

Multicentricity of breast cancer has been considered by some a contraindication to breast-conserving surgery, and suggested mastectomy as the preferred option (511). Conservation surgery and breast radiation therapy as an alternative to mastectomy is controversial in patients with two or more lesions in the same breast. Several studies have addressed this issue and it appears that the risk of relapse in the conservatively treated patient is slightly higher than if there is one lesion, but the risk may be acceptable in patients with two or perhaps three lesions provided these lesions are surgically excised with negative margins and there are no residual areas of suspicion on physical examination, mammogram, or imaging studies. Selected studies evaluating the conservative management of breast cancer in patients with multicentric disease are summarized in Table 53.36.

Kurtz et al. (424), in an analysis of 586 patients with unilateral stage I or II breast cancer treated with breast-conserving surgery and irradiation, found 61 patients who had two or more microscopic tumor nodules. After a median follow-up of 71 months, 15 patients (25%) had a recurrence in the treated breast, compared with 56 (11%) of 525 patients with single tumors ($p < .005$). Recurrence was noted more often in patients with multiple tumors diagnosed clinically or mammographically (8/22, 36%) than when multicentricity was apparent only on pathologic examination (7/39, 18%).

Wilson et al. (829) reviewed their experience in 1,060 patients treated with conservation surgery and breast irradiation of whom 13 (1.2%) presented with synchronous multicentric ipsilateral breast cancer. With a median follow-up of 71 months, 3/13 (23%) had an ipsilateral breast recurrence (72-month actuarial rate of 25%) compared with 12% in the single-lesion population. The use of conservation therapy in patients with more than one primary lesion should be considered with caution, and patients should be forewarned of the need for more extensive resections and the increased risk of breast relapse. Because resection of a larger volume of breast is required, cosmetic results may be compromised, and expectations may not be met. In such instances, a mastectomy may be the preferred approach.

Table 53.36 CONSERVATIVE SURGERY AND RADIATION IN THE TREATMENT OF MULTICENTRIC BREAST CANCER

Study (Reference)	Patients		Follow-Up (y)		Local Relapse Rate			Comment
	No. of SIBC	Controls	SIBC	Controls	SIBC (%)	Controls (%)	p Value	
Yale (829)	13	1,047	6	6	25	12	.403	Local recurrence rate in SIBC is greater than seen in patients with single lesions
JCRT (441)	10	707	5.3 (median)	6.3 (median)	40	11	.019	The presence of two or more primary tumors in the breast associated with a high likelihood of local recurrence
St Luke's (390)	36	19[a]	5	5	3	0	.54	No significant differences in the local or distant disease-free survival between the group treated with breast conservation and the group treated with mastectomy
Rush (339)	27	—	4.4 (median)	—	3.7	—	—	
France (424)	61	525	5.9 (median)	5.9 (median)	25	11	<.005	Macroscopically multiple breast cancers are at higher local failure risk, especially if multiplicity is clinically apparent, or if three or more gross nodules are seen on pathologic examination

SIBC, synchronous ipsilateral breast cancer.
[a]All are SIBC treated with mastectomy.

Conservation Surgery and Irradiation after Breast Augmentation

A growing number of breast cancers occur in women with prior augmentation mammoplasty. The stage of breast cancer at diagnosis in women who have undergone augmentation mammoplasty has been examined with conflicting results. In a retrospective review, Clark et al. (117) reported that 24% of 33 patients with augmented breasts and 42% of 1,735 patients with nonaugmented breasts had mammographically detected cancers (p = not significant). The incidence of DCIS in the two groups was similar (18% vs. 15%). Sizes of the mammographically detected tumors in the two groups were comparable. However, palpable tumors in the augmented group were significantly smaller than those in the nonaugmented group. Axillary lymph node involvement was detected in 19% of the augmented group and 41% of the nonaugmented group. Among those with mammographically detected tumors, there was no significant difference in axillary lymph node metastases between patients with augmented versus nonaugmented breasts (13% vs. 15%, respectively).

Patients with breast cancer with augmentations are currently being treated with conservation therapy, but no study has investigated the complications and cosmetic results of radiation therapy specifically in this group of women.

Breast-conservation therapy in 17 augmented patients with breast cancer was reported by Handel et al. (322), and 15 patients were available for follow-up. In 10 patients (67%), significant capsular contracture occurred in the irradiated breast an average of 12 weeks after completion of treatment. Four patients underwent revision surgery to correct symptoms arising from contracture. The authors concluded that irradiation of the breast for cancer in augmented women results in a high incidence of scar tissue contracture and poor cosmetic results.

In contrast, Guenther et al. (289) evaluated 20 women in whom breast cancer developed after augmentation mammoplasty (14 subcutaneous implants and 6 retromuscular implants). Patients were treated with wide local tumor excision

and level I and II axillary lymph node dissection. Irradiation was delivered to the breast (45 to 50 Gy), and a boost (14 to 21 Gy) was given to the tumor excision site with either photons, electrons, or iridium-192 (^{192}Ir) implant. With a median follow-up of 3.8 years (range, 6 months to 9.3 years), there were no local recurrences, although distant metastases developed in two patients. Seventeen patients (85%) had good or excellent cosmetic results.

Breast Conservation and Mammoplasty

Women with large, pendulous breasts have been documented to have poorer cosmetic outcomes when undergoing irradiation after breast-conservation surgery (thought to be caused by dose inhomogeneity) compared with women with small or medium-size breasts. Smith et al. (701) evaluated 10 women who had undergone bilateral reduction mammoplasty for breast malignancy followed by radiation therapy. A variety of reduction techniques were used to include the malignant lesions. Patients received 50 Gy in 25 fractions in 5 weeks after surgery. Radiation therapy was usually initiated within 4 weeks after surgery. With a follow-up of 37 months, no patients have had complications from the surgery or radiation therapy. No local recurrent malignancies have been detected. Cosmesis has been good to excellent in all patients.

Bilateral Carcinoma of the Breast

Among factors reported to be associated with an increased risk of bilateral breast carcinoma are younger age, family history of breast cancer, lobular carcinoma, multicentric disease, histologic differentiation of the primary tumor, parity, and positive PR status (350,356,444,526,610,667). The appearance may be synchronous (1% to 2%) or metachronous (5% to 8%). Synchronous breast carcinoma was defined as a contralateral cancer diagnosed within 1 year of initial diagnosis.

Patients with bilateral carcinoma have been treated with total or modified radical mastectomy. However, the available evidence clearly supports lumpectomy followed by breast irradiation as an acceptable alternative for appropriately selected women. Solin et al. (710) reported on 30 treated with breast-conservation therapy (11 with concurrent and 19 with metachronous carcinoma). A dose of 45 to 50 Gy was delivered to both breasts with tangential fields, in addition to a boost of 10 to 15 Gy with either iridium implant or electrons. The tangential fields were matched in the midline in 17 patients and overlapped by up to 3 cm in 10 patients. In the 60 treated breasts, the 5-year actuarial local failure rate was 6%. In 25 treated breasts with a minimum of 2 years of follow-up, 68% had excellent and 24% had good cosmetic results. The incidence of arm edema was 6%, similar to that reported in patients with unilateral disease.

Hungness et al. (362) reviewed their experience with 51 patients with bilateral synchronous breast cancer (2.1% of 2,382 treated for breast cancer during the same period). The first cancer was detected by palpation in 81% and by mammography in 14%. The corresponding figures for the contralateral cancer were 24% and 54%, respectively. The histologic type of cancer was identical in the two breasts in 29 patients (57%) and was different in 22 patients (43%). The overall 10-year survival rate was 66%.

Heron et al. (346) compared the outcomes in 1,315 patients (89.9%) with unilateral, 103 (7.1%) with metachronous, and 47 (3.0%) with synchronous breast carcinoma treated with either mastectomy or breast-conservation therapy. Patients with synchronous and metachronous bilateral carcinoma had a worse 8-year disease-free survival rate compared with patients with unilateral breast carcinoma, as well as increased risk of distant metastasis. In multivariate analysis, differences in local tumor control and overall survival were not statistically significant for patients who had bilateral or metachronous cancer compared with those who had unilateral disease.

Kollias et al. (408), in 3,210 women age 70 years or younger treated for primary operable breast cancer, identified 106 who had bilateral breast cancer; in 26 (0.8%) the disease was synchronous, and in 80 (24%) a contralateral breast cancer developed after treatment for an initial primary breast cancer. There was a significant difference in survival between women with unilateral breast cancer, synchronous bilateral breast cancers, and metachronous contralateral breast cancer, with survival rates at 16 years of 53.8%, 42.4%, and 60.1%, respectively ($p <.0001$), from the date of the diagnosis of the first primary tumor. There was no difference in survival between the three groups from the date of diagnosis of the second primary in cases of metachronous contralateral breast cancer ($p = .31$).

Ninety-five patients with bilateral carcinoma of the breast treated with mastectomy (60 patients), conservation of the breast (17 patients), or both (18 patients) were studied by Gustafsson et al. (291). Cumulative 5-year local tumor control rates were 94% for the 138 mastectomy patients and 90% for the 52 patients treated with breast-conservation therapy. Twenty-eight percent of the first carcinomas were stage I, compared with 43% of second carcinomas ($p <.05$), probably reflecting the close follow-up after initial treatment. The 5-year distant disease-free survival rate from treatment for the second carcinoma was 74%. The 5-year distant recurrence-free survival rate when second carcinomas were diagnosed within 5 years was 58%, compared with 95% for patients diagnosed more than 5 years after the first carcinoma.

De la Rouchefordiere et al. (148) reported on 149 patients with simultaneous bilateral breast cancer (diagnosed within 6 months). Of 298 tumors, 40% were T0 or T1, 45% T2, and 15% were T3 or T4. The majority (83%) were clinically node negative. Treatments were bilateral mastectomy in 43%, irradiation in 16%, and both in 41% of the patients. Fifty-one patients had bilateral breast-conserving therapy, and 24 were treated exclusively with irradiation. The 5-year disease-free survival rates were 70% to 86%, respectively, similar to those observed at the same institution in patients with unilateral tumors. Cosmesis was assessed in 48 patients and was acceptable in 37 (77%). The authors advised special attention should be paid to any possible overlap of the supraclavicular and internal mammary fields over the spinal cord; in one patient, spinal cord myelopathy developed at T6.

Freedman et al. (254) reviewed records of 116 patients with bilateral breast cancer and a breast cancer family history. The primary treatment was a breast-conserving procedure in 55 and a mastectomy in 61. Locoregional recurrences occurred in 4/46 cases treated with breast-conserving therapy, resulting in a 10-year actuarial locoregional tumor control rate of 83%. Of nine patients who did not receive radiation as a component of their breast-conserving therapy, locoregional recurrences developed in four (10-year locoregional control rate of 49%). The 10-year actuarial rates of locoregional control after mastectomy with and without radiation were 91% and 89%, respectively.

Fung et al. (258) reported on 55 women with stage 0, I, or II concurrent ($n = 12$) or sequential ($n = 43$) bilateral breast cancers treated with irradiation after breast-conserving surgery. The tangential fields were matched with no overlap in 40 patients (73%); there was overlap on skin of up to 4 cm in 14 patients (25%). For the 110 treated breast cancers, the 10-year actuarial local failure rate was 15%. Complications included breast edema (28%), arm edema (8%), pneumonitis (4%), cellulitis (3%), rib fracture (1%), and brachial plexopathy (1%). No patient had matchline fibrosis. For patients with a minimum of 3 years of relapse-free follow-up, the rate of excellent or good cosmetic outcome for 104 treated breasts was 85%.

Technical Issues in Radiation Management of Early Stage Disease

Treatment Position

Most patients are treated in the supine position, with the arm abducted (90 degrees or greater). Commercially available or custom made breast tilt boards with armrests that maintain the patient's daily position with the slope of the chest wall parallel to the table, often in combination with immobilization devices (e.g., alpha cradle, plastic molds), are typically used to reproduce daily positioning and minimize day-to-day set up errors (Fig. 53.25).

Other treatment positions have been used to improve the dosimetry in patients with large, pendulous breasts. A lateral decubitus position has been suggested by investigators at the Institut Curie, as shown in Figure 53.26 (131,235).

Irradiation in the prone position has been proposed by Merchant and McCormick (494), with reduction of dose in the high-dose region to 102% to 103% of the dose to the irradiated breast, as well as reduction of volume and dose to the underlying lung and heart and reduction of scattered dose to the contralateral breast. This technique is being increasingly employed and long-term follow-up data regarding outcomes and cosmesis are awaited. Patient positioning and a corresponding CT image are shown in Figures 53.27 and 53.28.

Treatment Volume

The entire breast and chest wall are included in the irradiated volume, as demonstrated in Figures 53.29 and 53.30. Radiopaque surgical clips placed at the margin of the tumor bed may assist in defining the target volume (707). The upper margin of the portals should be placed at the head of the clavicle to include the entire breast. The medial margin, if no internal mammary portal is used, should be at or 1 cm over the midline.

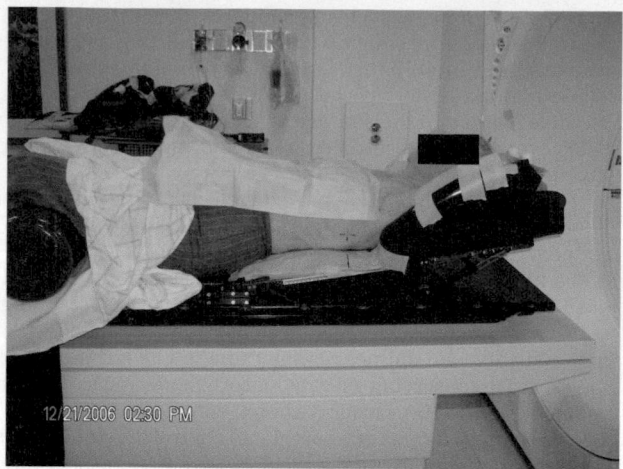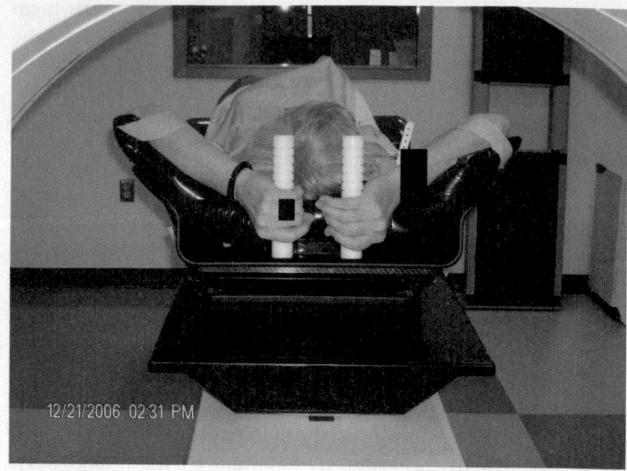

FIGURE 53.25. A,B: Patient immobilized for breast irradiation on a slant board with custom mold to minimize day-to-day positioning errors.

If an internal mammary field is used, the medial tangential portal is located at the lateral margin of the internal mammary field. (See discussion later on regional nodal irradiation.) The lateral-posterior margin should be placed 2 cm beyond all palpable breast tissue, which is usually near the mid-axillary line. The inferior margin is drawn 2 to 3 cm below the inframammary fold.

In patients treated with 6-MV or lower energy photons with wide tangential fields in whom separation is >22 cm there may be significant dose inhomogeneity in the breast; this may correlate with less satisfactory cosmetic results (507,736). This problem can be minimized by using higher energy photons (10 to 18

MV) to deliver all or a portion of the breast radiation (approximately 50%) as determined with treatment planning to maintain the inhomogeneity throughout the entire breast to 10% or less. If desired, the buildup of the beam may be modified with a "degrader." Bolus should be avoided in conservatively managed patients. A variety of immobilizing devices or molds may be constructed to support the breast in the treatment position (Fig. 53.31). A polyvinyl chloride, ring-shaped device, held by a strap, has been used around the breast to aid in positioning of patients with large, pendulous, or flaccid breasts. Skin reactions where material is in contact with the skin should be closely monitored (51).

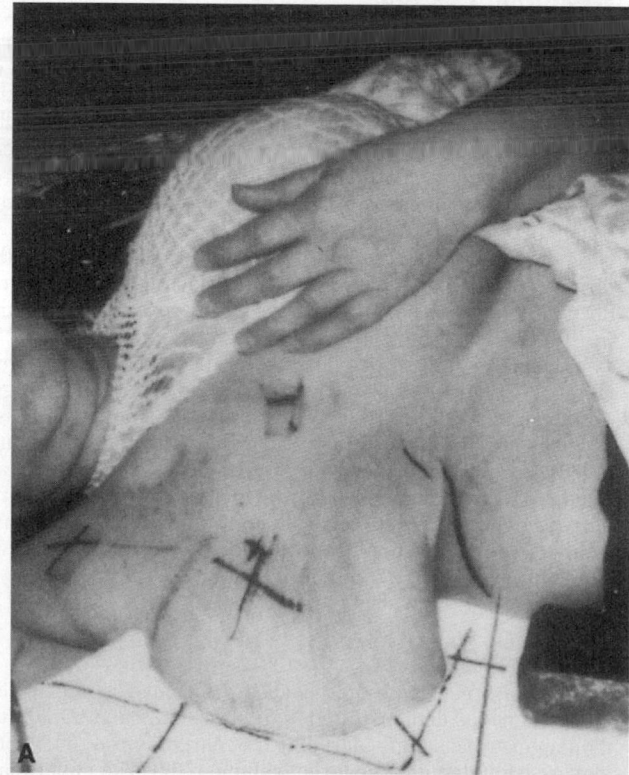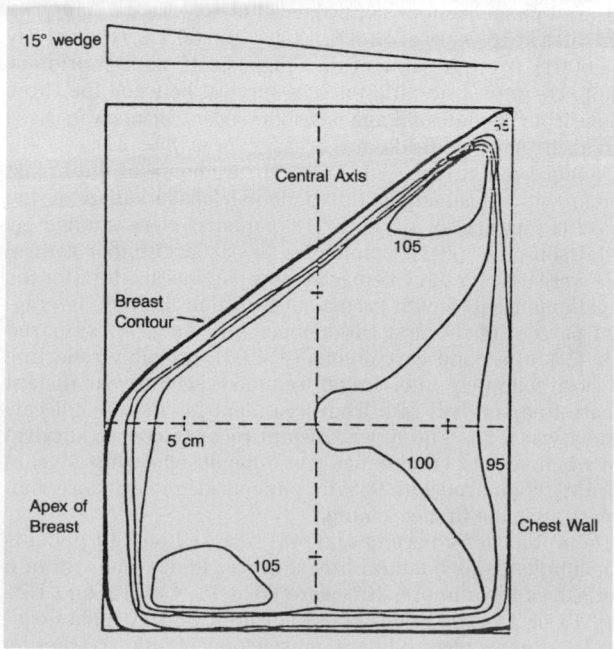

FIGURE 53.26. A: Patient with large, pendulous breast in lateral decubitus treatment position. **B:** Lateral decubitus isodose distribution with 15-degree wedge. (From Cross M, Elson HR, Aron BS. Breast-conservation radiation therapy technique for women with large breasts. *Int J Radiat Oncol Biol Phys* 1989;17:199, with permission.)

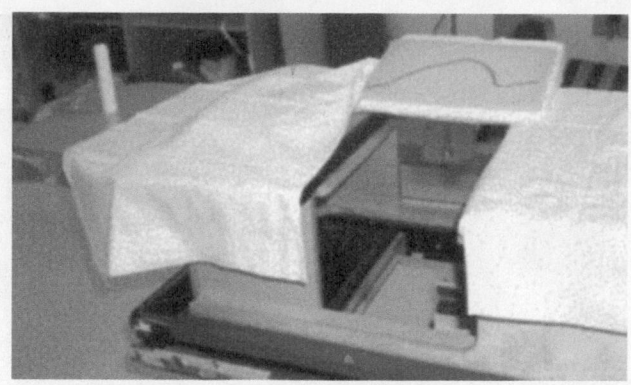
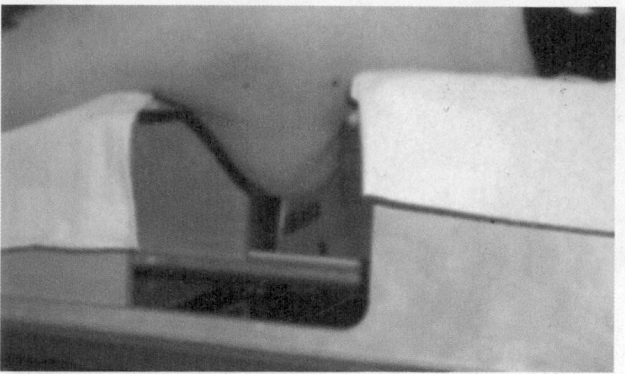

A | B

FIGURE 53.27. Prone breast board. **A:** Customized prone breast board with adjustable aperture and wedge for contralateral breast. **B:** Ipsilateral breast and anterior chest wall hang in dependent fashion away from thorax with ipsilateral arm placed above head. (From Goodman K, et al. Dosimetric analysis of a simplified intensity modulation technique for prone breast radiotherapy. *Int J Radiat Oncol Biol Phys* 2004;60(1):95–102, with permission.)

Alignment of the Tangential Beam with the Chest Wall Contour

The anterior chest wall slopes downward from the mid-chest to the neck. To make the posterior edge of the tangential beam follow this downward-sloping contour, the collimator of the tangential beam may be rotated, or the patient placed on a slant so that the slope of the chest wall is parallel to the table. An alternative is to make the deep posterior edge of the tangential beam follow the chest wall contour by means of a rotating beam splitter mounted on a tray without rotation of the collimator or using multileaf collimation. In this way, the superior edge of the tangential beam remains in the true vertical and matches perfectly the vertical inferior edge of the supraclavicular field if used.

Usually up to 2 to 3 cm of underlying lung is included in the tangential portals. The amount of lung included in the irradiated volume is greatly influenced by the portals used. Bornstein et al. (72) determined the amount of lung irradiated in 40 patients with breast cancer using CT scans for treatment planning in the treatment position. Parameters measured from simulator films included the perpendicular distance from the posterior tangential field edge to the posterior part of the anterior chest wall at the center of the field (central lung distance [CLD]), the maximum perpendicular distance from the posterior tangential field edge to the posterior part of the anterior chest wall (maximum lung distance [MLD]), and the length of lung as measured at the posterior tangential field edge on the simulator film (Fig. 53.32). The best predictor of the percentage of ipsilateral lung volume treated by the tangential fields was the CLD. A CLD of 1.5 cm predicted that approximately 6% of the ipsilateral lung would be included in the tangential field, a CLD of 2.5 cm, approximately 16%, and a CLD of 3.5 cm, approximately 26% of the ipsilateral lung (Fig. 53.33).

When the CLD is >3 cm, in treatment of the left breast, a significant volume of heart will also be irradiated. To avoid this, a medial tangential breast port (3 to 5 cm wide), somewhat similar to an internal mammary port, may be designed. The beam is angled 10 to 15 degrees laterally to conform to the angle of the medial breast port. The dose is prescribed to the posterior border of the chest wall as determined by CT scanning.

Special attention should be paid to minimizing the volume of heart irradiated. For the non–CT-based two-dimensional tangential technique in patients treated on the left side, the maximum dose to the heart and the percentage volume of heart included in the irradiated volume correlated with maximal heart

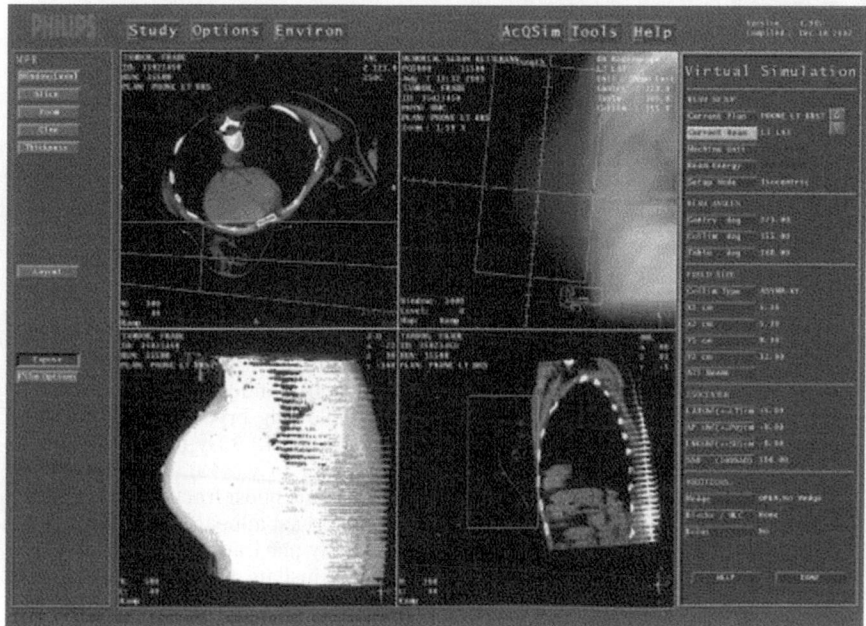

FIGURE 53.28. Computed tomography simulation images used to determine arrangement of tangent beams in prone breast irradiation. (From Goodman K, Hong L, Wagman R, et al. Dosimetric analysis of a simplified intensity modulation technique for prone breast radiotherapy. *Int J Radiat Oncol Biol Phys* 2004;60(1):95–102, with permission.)

Clinical Radiation Oncology

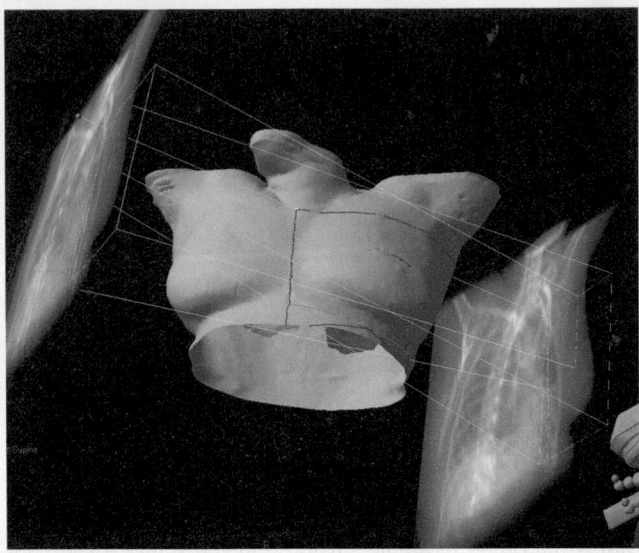

FIGURE 53.29. A tangential breast radiation field, demonstrating projection of tangential field on simulation film and patient surface.

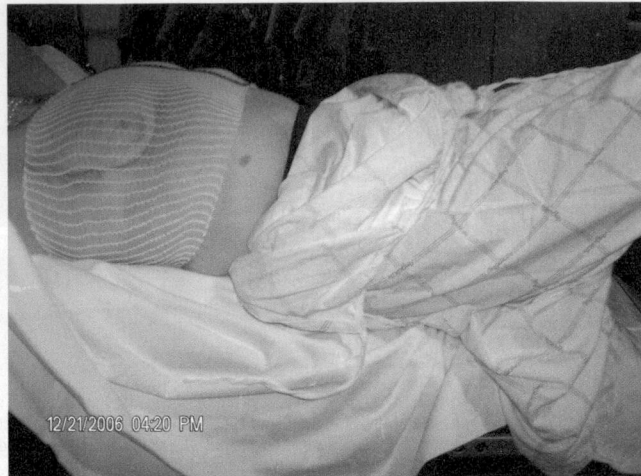

FIGURE 53.31. Immobilization material placed over breast tissue to help maintain day-to-day positioning of the breast.

distance (MHD) at different dose levels. Figure 53.34 plots the heart volume receiving 30 Gy versus MHD (solid dots) for 22 patients evaluated. The use of a medial breast port significantly decreased the volume of heart receiving high doses, whereas CT-based three-dimensional planning did not change the heart dose–volume histogram significantly from the non–CT-based tangential port technique. The medial breast port technique significantly decreased the mean percentage volume of heart receiving 20, 30, or 40 Gy compared with the tangential ports only. However, large MHD, heart located close to the chest wall, or thick chest wall are contraindications to using the medial breast technique if heart dose is a concern (410).

As will be discussed later in the section on cardiac sequelae, even small amounts of heart in the field can affect cardiac function. Marks et al. (475) have suggested the use of a cardiac block if the heart is in the tangential field, which can be supplemented by an electron field as shown in Figure 53.36. Use of short (10- to 15-second) treatments while the patient holds her breath is also feasible as a way of reducing cardiac radiation during left-sided breast cancer treatment (457).

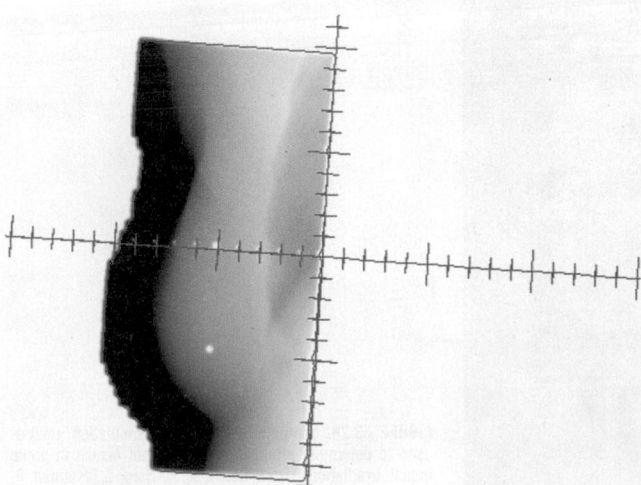

FIGURE 53.30. Examples of tangential port demonstrating breast tissue and approximately 2 cm of lung included in the field.

Doses of Radiation and Fractionation

Whole Breast Dose

With whole breast irradiation, tumor doses of approximately 45 to 50 Gy are delivered to the entire breast over 5 to 6 weeks (1.8- to 2-Gy tumor dose daily, five weekly fractions). Some authors have suggested daily fractions of 1.8 Gy for patients with large, pendulous breasts or when irradiation is combined with chemotherapy (47,473,601). Our preference is to use 2 Gy fractions to 50 Gy, since this is the scheme used in the vast majority of randomized trials using whole breast radiation therapy following conservative surgery.

Alternative fractionation schemes have been employed and have been shown to be acceptable. Whelan et al. (827), from the Ontario group, conducted a randomized trial comparing a shorter 16-fraction scheme over 22 days. Women with invasive breast cancer who were treated by lumpectomy and had pathologically clear resection margins and negative axillary lymph nodes were randomly assigned to receive whole breast irradiation of 42.5 Gy in 16 fractions over 22 days (short arm) or whole breast irradiation of 50 Gy in 25 fractions over 35 days (long arm). The primary outcome was local recurrence of invasive breast cancer in the treated breast and secondary outcomes was cosmetic result. There were 1,234 women randomly assigned to treatment, 622 to the short arm and 612 to the long arm. Five-year local recurrence-free survival was 97.2% in the short arm and 96.8% in the long arm. No difference in disease-free or overall survival rates was detected between study arms. The percentage of patients with an excellent or good global cosmetic outcome at 5 years were 76.8% and 77.4%, respectively. The authors concluded that the more convenient 22-day fractionation schedule appears to be an acceptable alternative to the 35-day schedule. It should be noted that no boost was employed in this trial.

In a randomized trial from the Royal Marsden, 719 patients with stage I or II breast cancer were randomly assigned to one of three fractionation schemes following breast-conserving therapy: 50 Gy in 25 fractions of 2 Gy; 42.9 Gy in 13 fractions of 3.3 Gy; or 39 Gy in 13 fractions of 3 Gy (843). Patients who received a boost all received the same boost fractionation scheme of 14 Gy in 2 Gy fractions. The breast appearance seemed to be superior in the 39 Gy in the 3 Gy per fraction arm. In a recent update of this trial, the risk of ipsilateral tumor relapse after 10 years was 12.1% (95% CI, 8.8 to 15.5) in the 50 Gy group, 14.8% (CI, 11.2 to 18.3) in the 39 Gy group, and 9.6% (CI, 6.7 to

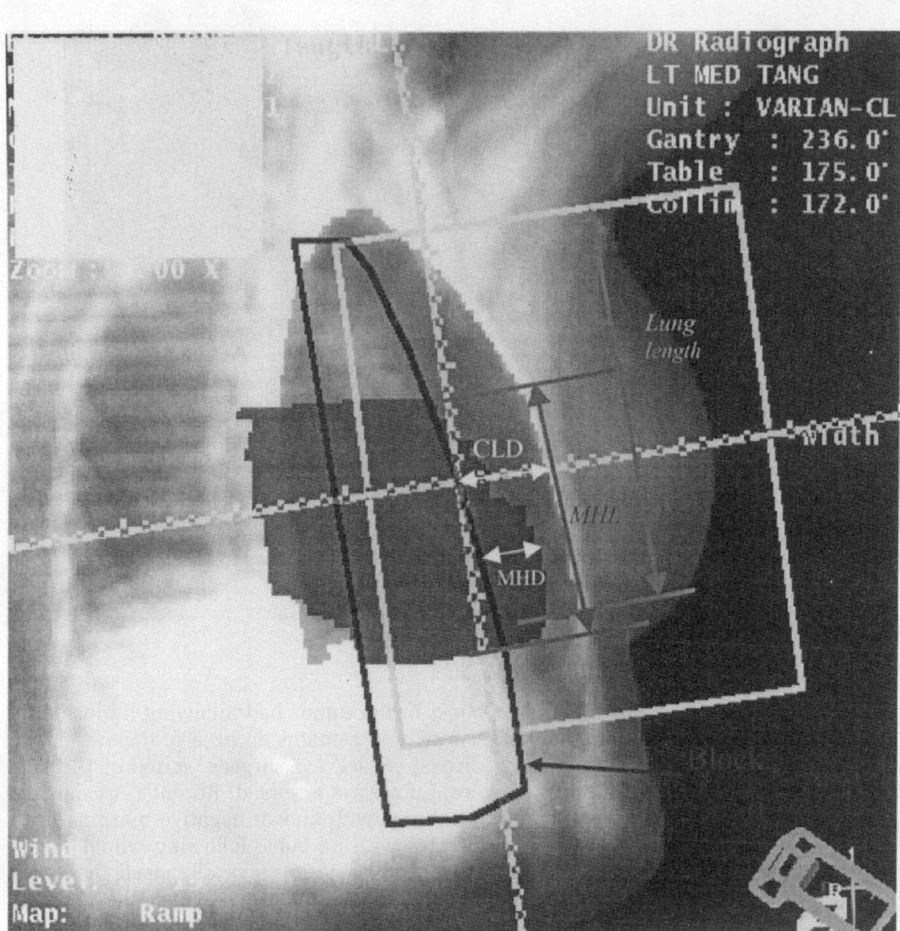

FIGURE 53.32. Measurement of the radiographic parameters using virtual simulator. The contoured heart is shown in black, the lung in gray. The central lung distance (CLD) is the lung distance in the projection of the tangential fields at the level of the central axis. Lung length is the vertical lung distance included in the radiation port. The maximal heart distance (MHD) is the width of heart in the tangent fields at its maximal level, whereas the maximal heart length (MHL) is the maximal length in tangential fields referring to the heart contour in a digitally reconstructed radiograph (DRR). (From Kong F-M, Klein EE, Bradley JD, et al. The impact of central lung distance, maximal heart distance, and radiation technique on the volumetric dose of the lung and heart for intact breast radiation. *Int J Radiat Oncol Biol Phys* 2002;54:963–971, with permission.)

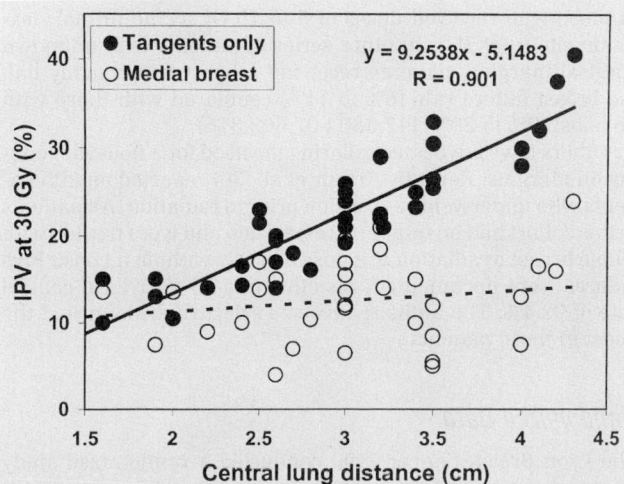

FIGURE 53.33. The relationship between percentage volume of ipsilateral lung and central lung distance using different techniques. Plan A (*solid dots*) is plotted as an example for tangential technique, whereas plan C (*clear dots*) is for the medial breast technique. The IPV 30 (percentage volume of ipsilateral lung at 30 Gy) increases linearly with increasing central lung distance (CLD) for the two-dimensional tangential technique, but appears independent of original CLD for the medial port technique. (From Kong F-M, Klein EE, Bradley JD, et al. The impact of central lung distance, maximal heart distance, and radiation technique on the volumetric dose of the lung and heart for intact breast radiation. *Int J Radiat Oncol Biol Phys* 2002;54:963–971, with permission.)

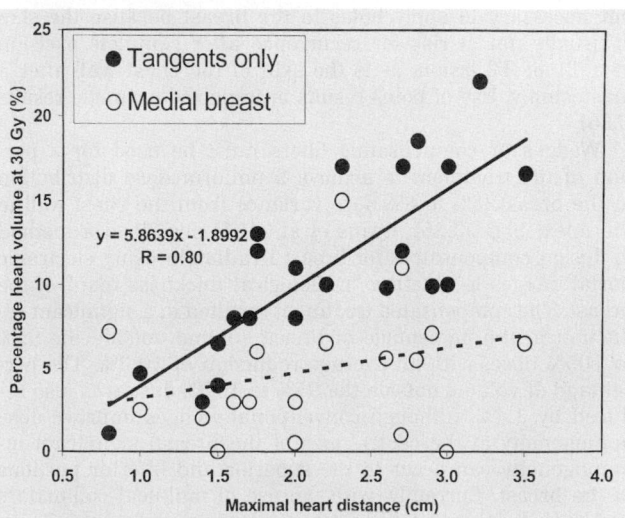

FIGURE 53.34. A plot of heart volume at 30 Gy versus maximal distance. Plans A (*solid dots*) and C (*clear dots*) for 30-Gy dose level are plotted for examples of tangential and medial breast technique, respectively. The PV30 of the heart (percentage volume of the heart at 30 Gy) increases almost linearly with increasing maximal heart distance (MHD) for two-dimensional technique, but seems to be independent of MDH for medial port technique. (From Kong F-M, Klein EE, Bradley JD, et al. The impact of central lung distance, maximal heart distance, and radiation technique on the volumetric dose of the lung and heart for intact breast radiation. *Int J Radiat Oncol Biol Phys* 2002;54:963–971, with permission.)

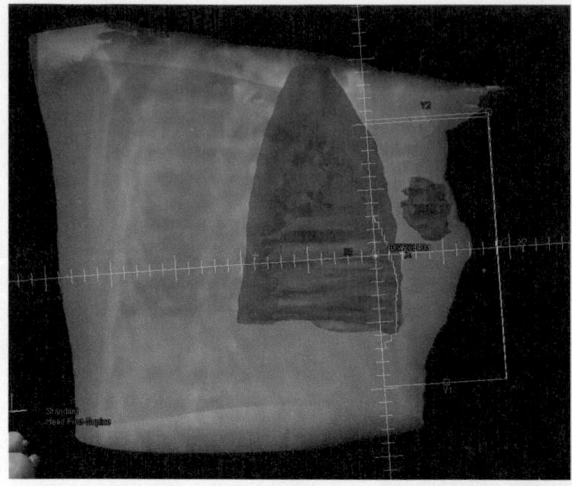
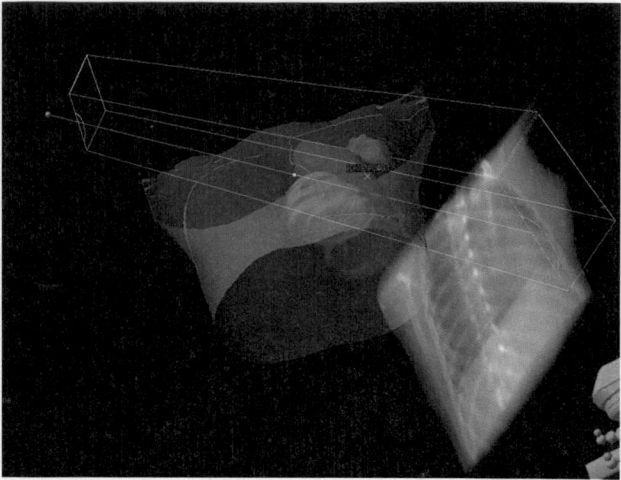

FIGURE 53.35. A: Left tangential breast field with heart block to shield left ventricle from radiation port. **B:** Projection of heart block on breast shields minimal amount of breast tissue. If necessary, a shadow electron field may be added to cover the portion of breast tissue shielded by heart block.

12.6) in the 42.9 Gy group (difference between 39 Gy and 42.9 Gy groups, χ^2 test; $p = .027$) (551).

A randomized trial from Hospital Necker in Paris compared 45 Gy in 25 fractions delivered in 5 weeks to 23 Gy delivered as 5 Gy on days 1 and 3 and 6.5 Gy on days 15 and 17. In patients treated by lumpectomy (56 in the conventional arm and 45 in the hypofractionation arm) the local–regional recurrence rate was similar (7% vs. 4%) (372).

Radiation Beams

X-ray energies of 4 to 6 MV are preferred to treat the breast. Photon energies >6 MV underdose superficial tissues beneath the skin surface, but higher-energy photons may be helpful in large breasts to decrease the integral breast dose. In these patients, the high-energy photon beam may be "degraded" to bring the maximum dose to more superficial tissues. It is not necessary to apply bolus to the breast because the skin is usually not at risk for recurrence after complete excision of a T1 or T2 lesion, as is the skin of the chest wall after a mastectomy. Use of bolus results in impaired cosmetic results (736).

Wedges or compensating filters must be used for a portion of the treatment to achieve a uniform dose distribution in the breast (5% to 8% dose variance from the chest wall to the apex; Fig. 53.36). Evans et al. (191) described a method to design compensators for breast irradiation using electronic portal images to obtain a "radiological thickness map" of the breast. The compensated treatment resulted in a significant reduction in the percentage of breast volume outside the 95% to 105% dose, with an average reduction of 10.2%. The percentage of volume outside the 95% to 107% dose was also reduced by 3.4%. Although conventional wedges improve dose homogeneity at the central axis of the breast, significant inhomogeneity can occur in the superior and inferior portions of the breast. Currently, with the use of multileaf collimators and more sophisticated treatment planning techniques, optimization of homogeneity throughout the breast can be achieved through the use of a variety of techniques. Dose homogeneity in a breast plan uncompensated (without wedges), with standard wedges, and with electronic dynamic wedge technique to improve homogeneity in the superior-inferior plane are outlined in Figure 53.37. These techniques are discussed in more detail later.

Boost to Tumor Site

The need for a boost to the tumor bed following lumpectomy and whole breast radiation remains an area of debate. In the earlier years of breast-conserving surgery, status of the surgical margins were not always assessed. Recent retrospective data suggest that patients with known negative margins have high local control rates with no boost following whole breast irradiation (30). Fisher et al. (206) have all raised the question of the need for a radiation dose boost at the excision site.

Most authors report that 65% to 80% of breast recurrences after conservation surgery and irradiation occur around the primary tumor site (99,111,222,241,298,333,423,607,702). These data provide a strong rationale for a tumor bed boost. Various series suggest that patients treated with higher doses have a greater probability of tumor control. Clark et al. (119) noted in 1,504 patients a greater incidence of failure at 10 years of 17% in those to whom no boost was delivered, compared with 11% in those who received doses of 5 to 15 Gy at the primary excision site ($p = .03$). In other series of patients with unknown surgical margins, patients receiving a boost had roughly half the breast failure rate (6% to 11%) compared with those with no boost (9% to 20%) (42,330,607,608,816).

Others have advocated tailoring the need for a boost depending on margins. Recently Arthur et al. (30) reported on 205 patients who underwent re-excision prior to radiation. All patients in this cohort had no tumor on re-excision and were treated with whole breast irradiation to a dose of 50 Gy without a boost. Five failures were documented, resulting in a 15-year local control rate of 92.4%. The authors advocate selective avoidance of the boost in these patients.

Randomized Data

The Lyon Breast Cancer Trial conducted a randomized study to assess the role of the boost in breast-conserving therapy in patients with stage I and II breast cancer (≤3 cm) who were treated with complete local tumor excision, axillary dissection, and 50 Gy to the breast in 20 fractions over 5 weeks, and randomly assigned to receive or not a boost of 10 Gy with electrons to the tumor bed (628). With a median follow-up of 3.3 years, at 5 years 10/521 women who received a boost (3.6%) and 20/503 (4.5%) who received no further treatment experienced a local breast relapse ($p = .044$).

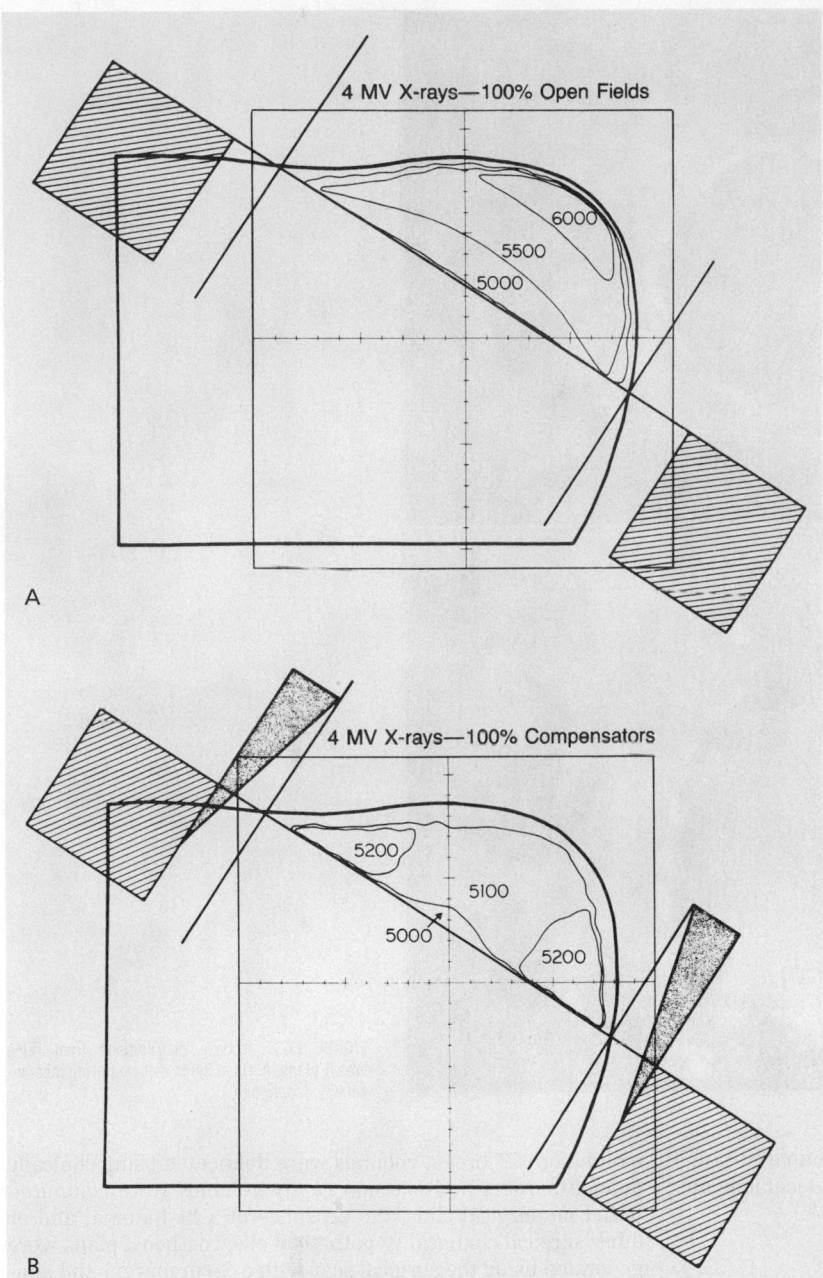

FIGURE 53.36. A: Isodose curves for 4-MV x-rays (source-axis distance, 80 cm) using tangential breast portals without compensators. Higher doses are delivered to the apex of the breast. **B:** Dose distribution using compensators for all treatments. **C:** Isodose curves using open fields for half of the treatment and compensators for the other half. **D:** Composite isodose curves for customized two-dimensional compensating filters, beam splitter for tangential fields, and internal mammary portal treated with 6-MV photons (16 Gy) and 12-MeV electrons (30 Gy).

Bartelink et al. (42) reported the results of the EORTC trial in which, after complete lumpectomy and axillary dissection, patients with stage I or II breast cancer received 50 Gy of radiation to the whole breast in 2-Gy fractions over a 5-week period and were randomly assigned to receive either no further local treatment (2,657 patients) or a boost of 16 Gy, usually given in eight fractions by electron beam (2,661 patients). With a median follow-up of 5.1 years, local recurrences were observed in 182/2,657 patients in the standard-treatment group and 109/2,661 patients in the additional-radiation group. The 5-year actuarial rates of local recurrence were 7.3% and 4.3%, respectively ($p < .001$, see Fig. 53.17A). Patients 40 years of age or younger benefited most; at 5 years, their rate of local recurrence was 19.5% with standard treatment and 10.2% with additional radiation (RR 0.46; 99% CI, 0.23 to 0.89; $p = .002$) (see Fig. 53.17B).

If a decision is made not to use a boost, careful assessment of lumpectomy margins is critical, as discussed in the following section.

Electron versus Interstitial Boosts

Before the widespread availability of electron beam therapy, interstitial brachytherapy or cone-down photon boost was popular. Experiences with interstitial boosts have been reported by several groups, using both high-dose-rate afterloading and low-dose-rate temporary implants (467,468,472,748,791,798). The reader is referred to these studies and the chapter on brachytherapy in this volume for a more extensive discussion of techniques related to interstitial tumor bed boosts. Currently, most institutions prefer electron beam boost because of its relative ease in setup, outpatient setting, lower cost, decreased time

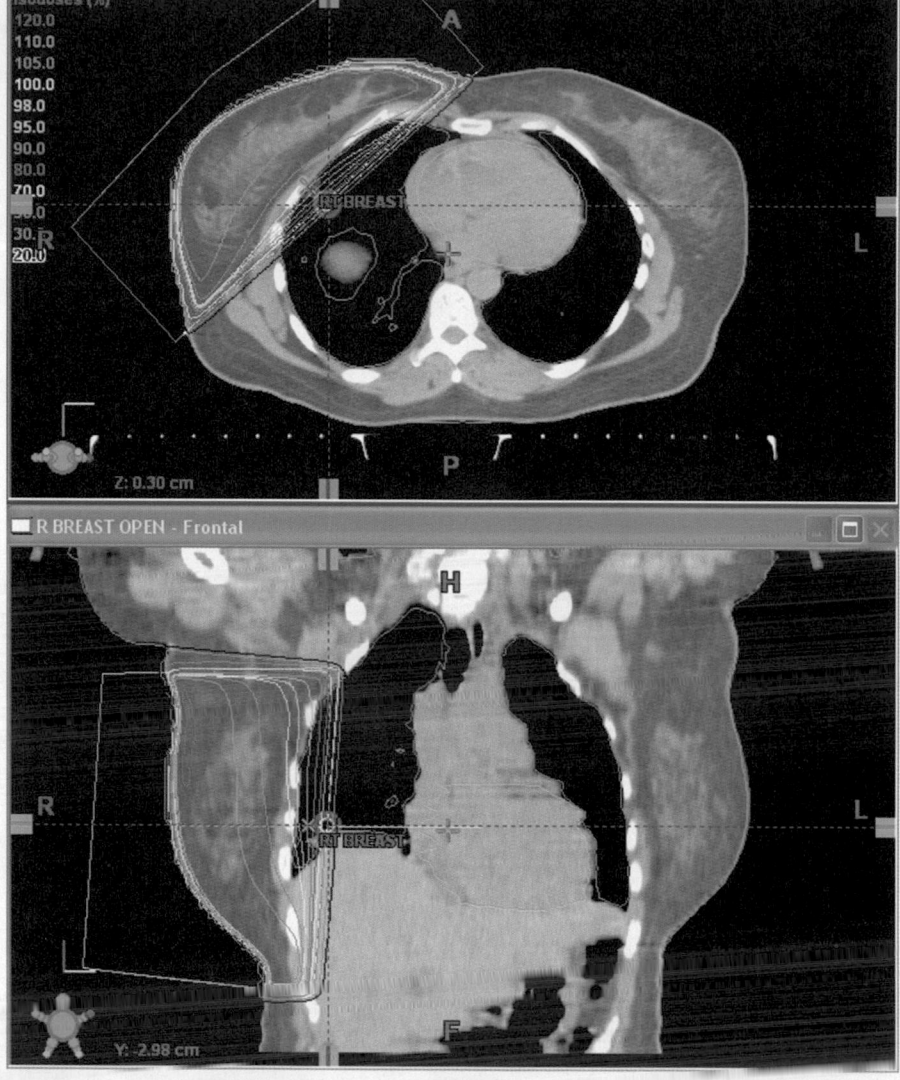

FIGURE 53.37. Isodose distributions from three breast plans. **A:** Open fields demonstrating inhomogeneity. (*continued*)

demands on the physician, and excellent results compared with ^{192}Ir implants. Cosmetic results with either boost technique at various institutions are summarized in Table 53.37.

Electron Boosts

The patient is positioned with the arm toward the head to flatten the breast contour, and may be rolled so that the tumor bed is parallel to the table and the accelerator head can point straight down onto the target volume. An electron energy is selected that covers the target volume depth (usual range is 9 to 16 MeV electrons), based on review of the physical examination, mammogram, ultrasound, CT, or other imaging used to ascertain the location and depth of the tumor or metallic surgical clips. The 90% prescription isodose line is limited to the chest wall to decrease dose to the lung. The clinical setup for electron boost involves marking the projection of the postlumpectomy volume on the skin and adding 2 to 3 cm in all directions.

Accurate target volume definition is critical with any boost technique. Methods vary from simple and unsophisticated (as described in the previous paragraph) to complex and expensive, such as ultrasound and CT definition of the target volume (541,703). The accuracy of using the scar to define the lumpectomy cavity has been questioned. In a study by Oh et al. (541) 30 women consecutively treated for 31 breast cancers had simulation CT scans performed before and after whole-breast

irradiation. CT breast volumes were delineated using clinically defined borders and excision cavity volumes were contoured based on surgical clips, the presence of a hematoma, and/or other surgical changes. Hypothetical electron boost plans were generated using the surgical scar with a 3-cm margin and analyzed for coverage. The volume reduction in the excision cavity was inversely correlated with time elapsed since surgery and body weight. The scar-guided hypothetical plans failed to cover the excision cavity adequately in 62% and 53.8% of cases using the pretreatment and postradiation CT, respectively.

Surgical clips are ideal for the localization of the tumor bed (197,703,707). The surgical clip method requires the cooperation of the surgical team. Despite the fact that it would theoretically take an infinite number of clips to define every extension of a typical tylectomy cavity, in practice six clips suffice (superficial, deep, medial, lateral, cephalad, and caudal). In a study reported by Denham et al. (152), surgical hemoclips were left *in situ* in 27 patients to demarcate the limits of the excision cavity. The position of these clips varied widely in relation to the patient's recollection of the position of the original lump, the surgical notes, and the surgical scar. Incomplete coverage of the excision cavity in the "coronal" (*en face*) plane using an electron field could have occurred in an estimated 10/24 (42%) cases had surgical clips not been left *in situ*. Depth of the surgical clips below the skin surface also varied markedly; in 19/26 (73%) cases, the clips were observed to be 3 cm or more below

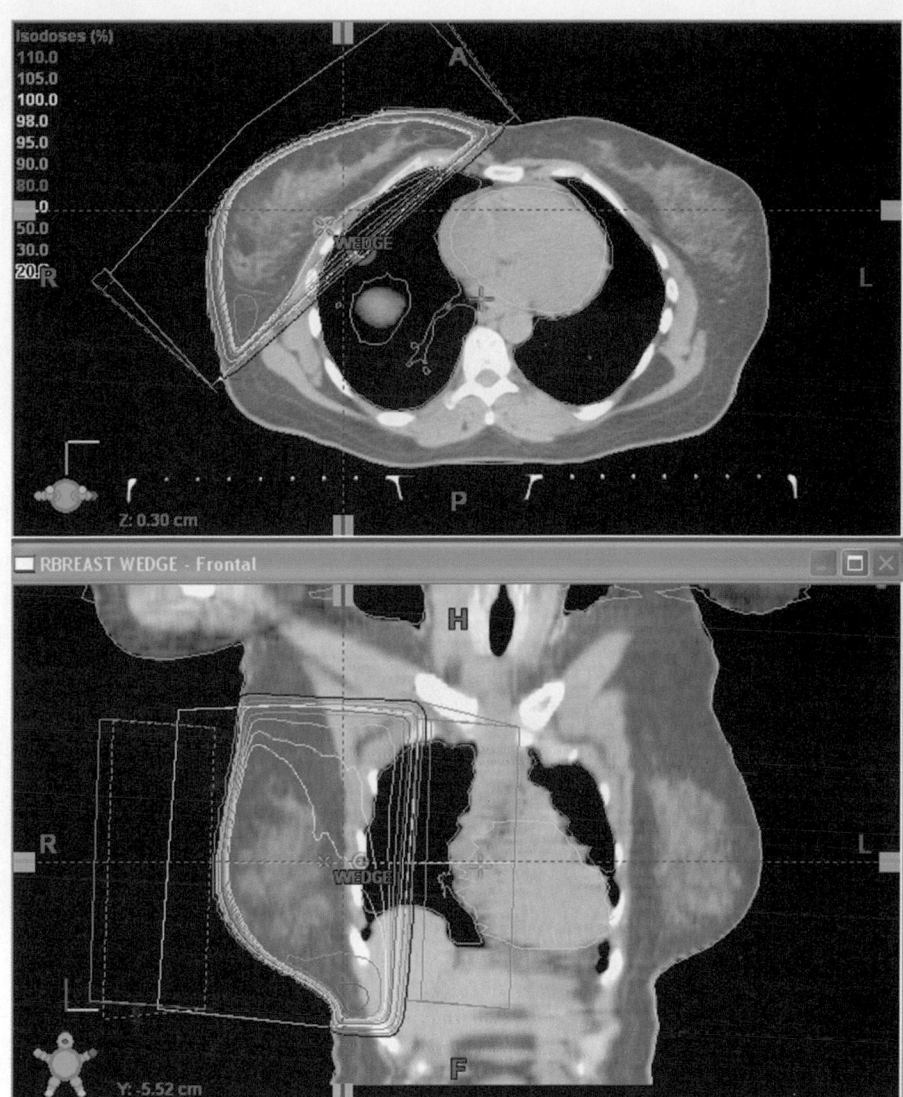

FIGURE 53.37. B: Standard wedges demonstrating improvement in central axis, but with a hot spot in the superior inferior plane. (*continued*)

the skin surface, whereas in only 5/26 (19.2%) cases were the clips found to be 2 cm or less deep to the surface. Had a 9-MeV electron beam been used to treat all of the patients, a major underdose of the excision cavity would have been likely in 21/26 evaluable cases (81%). Coverage would have improved to 11/26 (42%) had a 12-MeV beam been used.

In a British study, 50 patients treated with breast-conservation therapy had excision cavity boundaries marked by surgical clips (327). An electron beam boost field was initially planned to achieve a 2-cm margin. When evaluated by radiographs and the position of the surgical clips, the clinical field was found to be inadequate in 34 patients (68%). However, if 3-cm margins around this scar had been used, the median percentage of geographic misses would have been only 18.6%. Also, median distance from the center of the scar to the deepest clip was 3.8 cm, suggesting that electron beam energies of 12 MeV or higher can adequately cover most excision sites to volume. Nevertheless, in 10 patients the deepest clip was at 5 cm or greater depth.

Fein et al. (197) described a study of patients with stage I or II breast cancer treated with breast-conservation therapy; surgical clips were placed in the excision cavity in 556 patients, and no clips were placed in 808. After breast irradiation with tangential fields the primary tumor incision site was boosted with electron beam (14 to 20 Gy). The actuarial breast recurrence rates at 10 years were 11% in patients with clips and 5% in patients without clips ($p = .01$). Increased rates of breast recurrence were noted for patients with clips who had some of the following: no adjuvant treatment, unknown surgical margins, no re-excision, pathologic negative nodes, and outer location of primary tumor. The higher incidence of breast relapse may be related to a specific surgeon who had a breast recurrence rate of 21%, compared with 6% for the remainder of the surgeons ($p = .01$); the status of the margins was unknown in 48% of his patients, compared with 10% overall ($p = .001$). The authors concluded that failure to ink the surgical specimen and inadequate assessment of margins cannot be compensated by placement of surgical clips or treatment planning using CT to delineate the surgical bed. On the other hand, this study failed to show any benefit from use of surgical clips at the tumor excision margins to design the boost volume.

Ultrasonography can provide the depth of the biopsy cavity, as well as the other dimensions, for use in designing electron portal borders and selection of electron energy (616,703). Ultrasonography was used in 30 patients to measure breast thickness for determination of the most appropriate electron beam energy for the boost. In most patients, the depth was 4 cm or less, but in eight patients (32%), energy higher than 12 MeV should have been used to cover adequately the depth of the target volume (398).

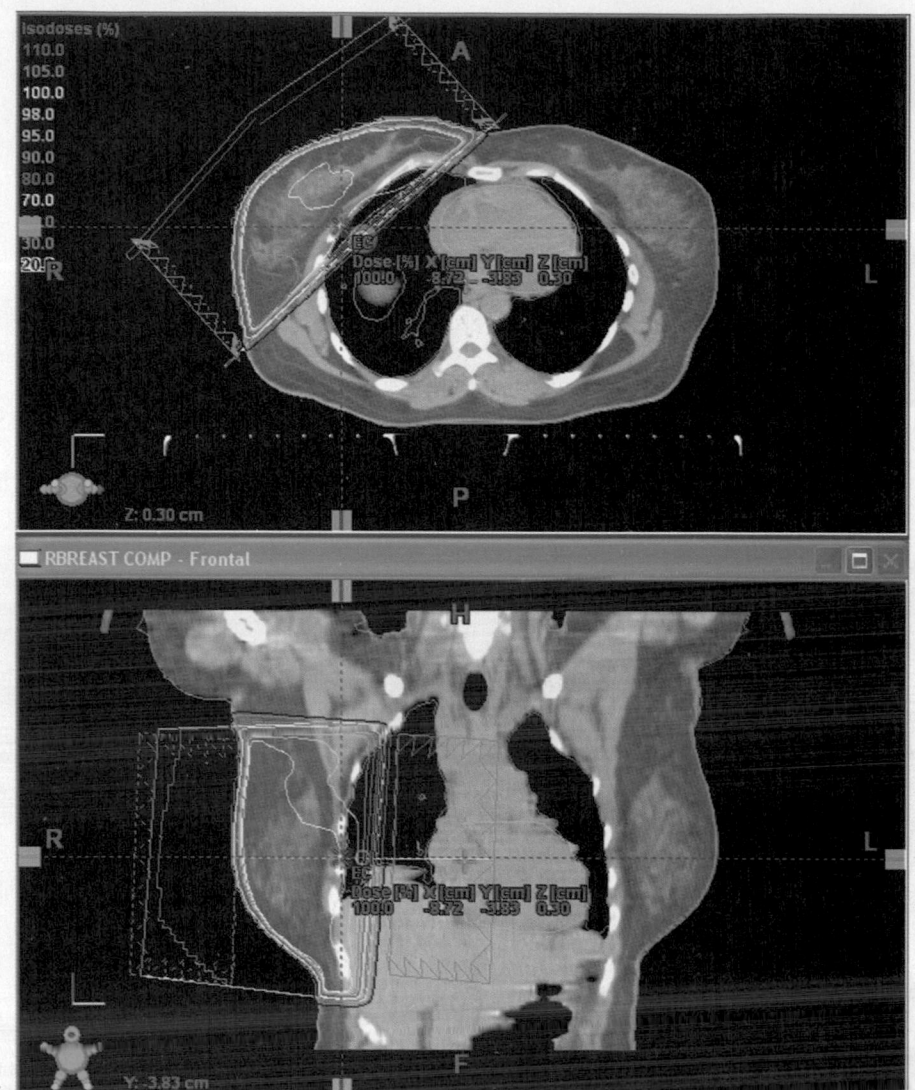

FIGURE 53.37. (*continued*) **C:** Dynamic wedge plan showing improved homogeneity in both the control axis as well as the superior-inferior plane.

CT-guided portal design should be done in the treatment position. This technique gives good definition of the depth of the chest wall, and has been shown to be similar to ultrasound in delineating the lumpectomy cavity (616,703). Delineation of the biopsy cavity becomes more difficult with increased interval from surgery. The combination of surgical clips with a treatment planning CT scan to define the lumpectomy site for electron boost is most ideal. In the absence of surgical clips, the CT scan evaluation of the biopsy cavity and/or postsurgical changes, in combination with clinical information including mammography findings, scar location, operative reports, and patient input, will provide accurate information regarding placement of the field and energy of the electron boost.

Irradiation of Regional Lymphatics

Radiation therapy to the breast/chest wall and regional lymphatics can be technically challenging and, as previously

Table 53.37			

EXCELLENT OR GOOD COSMETIC RESULTS WITH ELECTRON BEAM OR INTERSTITIAL BRACHYTHERAPY BOOST IN BREAST-CONSERVATION THERAPY

Study (Reference)	Electron Beam	Brachytherapy	Follow-Up
Fourquet et al. (234)	39/52 (75%)	48/68 (71 %)	3–7.3 y
Mansfield et al. (467)	357/376 (95%)	575/629 (91 %)	1 mo to 12 y
Olivotto et al. (543)	36/36 (100%)	298/497 (60%)	5 y
Perez et al. (563)	366/449 (81%)	97/129 (75%)	3–20 y
Ray & Fish (596)	97/107 (91%)	12/23 (52%)	6–120 mo
Touboul et al. (748)	104/126 (82%)	91/148 (61%)	29–139 mo
Vicini et al. (791)	(90%)	(88%)	59.3 mo (median)

discussed, remains one of the more variable and controversial aspects in management. A wide variety of available techniques, in combination with difficulties associated with matching fields, anatomic variability between patients, and lack of clear evidence regarding the superiority of any single approach, has resulted in a lack of consensus in regional nodal management.

Anatomic variation was highlighted in a study by Mansur et al. (469). They reported on 65 patients with breast cancer who had volumetric CT scanning in the treatment position. The IMNs and axillary lymph node regions were delineated according to a cross-sectional nodal atlas. The variable depths of IMNs at different intercostal spaces result in dose variations if the internal mammary port is treated with a single or inadequate electron beam energy. Axillary lymph nodes frequently overlapped the head of the humerus anteriorly when the arm was angled more than 90 degrees, but did not when the arm was angled 90 degrees or less. The larger the angle, the less the head of the humerus could be spared in the supraclavicular port.

Arthur et al. (29) evaluated treatment techniques for coverage of the intact breast and ipsilateral lymph node regions. Anatomic outlines were obtained from five randomly selected patients with CT scanning in treatment position (three with cancer of the left breast and two of the right). Three techniques used to treat ipsilateral breast and internal mammary and supraclavicular nodes (extended tangents, five-field, partially wide tangents) were configured and compared with a supraclavicular field matched to standard tangential fields. All of the treatment techniques covering IMNs included at least 10% more lung and heart volume than that covered by standard tangential fields. Because of increased chest wall thickness and depth of IMNs superiorly, complete coverage was not achieved with any technique if the IMN target extended superiorly into the medial supraclavicular field.

Goodman et al. (281) examined the relationship between tangential, anterior, and posterior radiation fields and regional lymph nodes, including level I to III axillary and supraclavicular lymph nodes in 55 patients who underwent CT scanning in the supine position. The mean depths of the level I to III axillary nodes were 4.6, 5.1, and 3.6 cm, respectively. The mean depth of the supraclavicular nodes was 3.9 cm. With the treatment using two tangential fields, level I axillary nodes appeared in the tangential portals in nine of nine patients, either alone or with other lymph node groups. In the three-field group, level I axillary nodes were in 16/16 tangential fields either alone or with level II nodes (eight patients). In eight patients, level III and the supraclavicular nodes were included in the anterior field, and in the other eight, levels II and III and the supraclavicular nodes were in the anterior field. There was considerable variation in the depth of supraclavicular and axillary lymph nodes in the fields in which these nodal groups appear and in the nodal group present in the posterior axillary boost field. To be certain that nodal groups to be treated are actually treated, as well as to minimize tissue irradiated, the authors recommended that before the placement of radiation fields the nodal groups be outlined on a CT scan. From a practical standpoint, whether this results in better tumor control than standard techniques has not been demonstrated.

Supraclavicular Lymph Nodes

The inferior border of the supraclavicular field is matched to the tangential field usually just below the clavicular head. The medial border is 1 cm across the midline, extending upward, following the medial border of the sternocleidomastoid muscle to the thyrocricoid groove. The lateral border is a vertical line at the level of the coracoid process, just medial to the humeral head. This field is angled approximately 10 to 15 degrees laterally to spare the cervical spine (Fig. 53.38). The typical width of the supraclavicular field is 7 to 9 cm. The supraclavicular field is

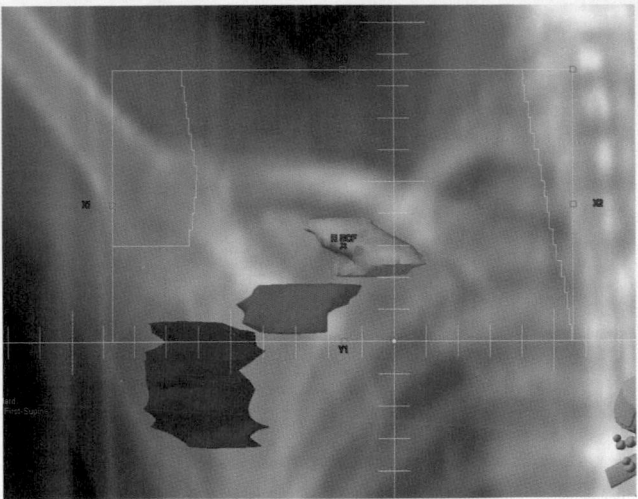

FIGURE 53.38. Supraclavicular and axillary field and field borders. Level I, II, and III nodes are demonstrated on the film. Note that level I nodes are included primarily in the tangential field in this case.

extended laterally to treat the full axilla, as clinically indicated. Figure 53.38 demonstrates a supraclavicular field with the supraclavicular, and level I, II, and III nodes are outlined. Level I as well as a portion of level II nodes will often be included in the tangential field; level III and supraclavicular nodes are covered in the supraclavicular field.

The total dose delivered to the supraclavicular field is 46 Gy-50 Gy at 1.8 to 2 Gy per day (calculated at a depth of 3 cm) in five fractions per week. Assessment of the depth of lymph nodes with ultrasound or CT scan treatment planning is useful to ensure adequate dose is delivered to the target. For patients in whom the target is deeper than 3 cm, higher energy photons or AP-PA treatment may be considered.

Axillary Lymph Nodes

When the axilla is treated in patients with positive nodes, or in patients with inadequate or undissected axillae, the supraclavicular field is extended laterally to cover at least two-thirds of the humeral head, as demonstrated in Figure 53.38. The dose to the midplane of the axilla from the supraclavicular field is calculated at a point approximately 2 cm inferior to the mid-portion of the clavicle. Depending on the dose distribution and patient's anatomy, a posterior axillary boost may be considered.

Posterior Axillary Boost

There is considerable debate regarding the necessity of a posterior axillary boost. Bentel et al. (50) questioned its necessity in a majority of patients. In 49 patients undergoing treatment-planning CT scanning in the treatment position, the maximum depth of the supraclavicular and axillary lymph nodes was measured on CT images and the relationship between the supraclavicular and axillary lymph node depth and patient diameter was determined. For an anterior field, the relative dose to the supraclavicular and axillary lymph nodes were calculated for a 6 MV photon beam. If an anterior 6-MV beam only is used to treat both supraclavicular and axillary lymph nodes, the dose to the axilla is within plus or minus 5% of the supraclavicular dose in 53% (26/49) patients and is 90% or more of the dose delivered to the supraclavicular nodes in 90% (44/49) of patients. The authors concluded that higher energy beams or anteroposterior/posteroanterior (AP/PA) supraclavicular axillary fields may

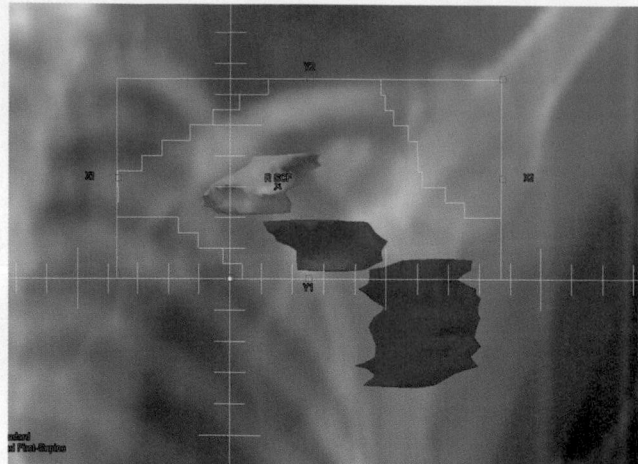

FIGURE 53.39. Posterior axillary field used to supplement the dose at midplane of the axilla. Note the small amount of lung included and the shielding of the humeral head (whenever possible).

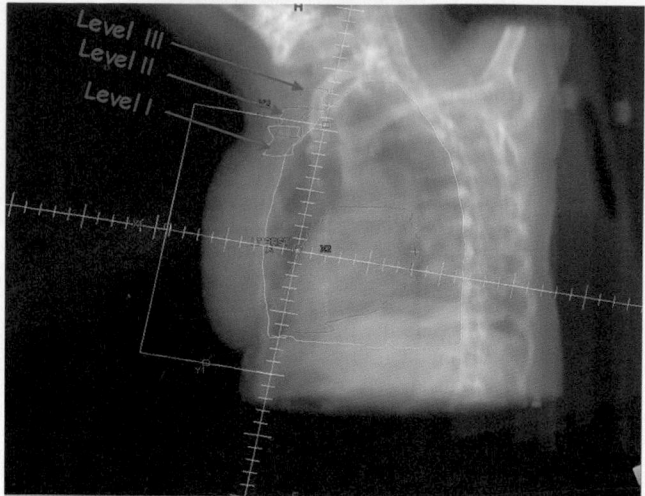

FIGURE 53.40. "High" tangential field shown coverage of level I and portion of level II nodes. With caudal edge of the field within 2 cm of the humeral head and leading edge approximately 2 cm from lung chest wall interface, the majority of nodes in level I and level II will be covered by this technique.

be reasonable when the axillary and supraclavicular nodes are deep.

The posterior axillary boost has been employed to supplement axillary dose. At the end of the treatments to the supraclavicular field, the dose to the midplane of the axilla may be supplemented by a posterior axillary field, as shown in Figure 53.39. Alternatively, the axilla should be contoured in CT-treatment planning as variation of the depth of the axilla from the AP skin surface varies from patient to patient and the supplement prescription point can be adjusted accordingly. If the dose is determined to be inadequate, a posterior boost may be employed. When a posterior axillary boost is used, the medial border of this field is drawn to allow 1.5 to 2 cm of lung to show on the portal film. If the inferior border is at the same level as the inferior border of the supraclavicular field, the lateral border just blocks falloff across the posterior axillary fold, the superior border splits the clavicle, and the superolateral border shields or splits the humeral head. Additional dose to the axilla midplane is usually administered to complete 46 to 50 Gy (2 Gy daily). When indicated, a boost of 10 to 15 Gy is delivered with reduced portals.

If the supraclavicular nodes are not felt to be at risk, a separate axillary field may not always be necessary to treat the axilla. In a study of 39 women with surgical clips in the axilla, Schlembach et al. (659) demonstrated that with tangential fields, placing the caudal border of the field within 2 cm of the humeral head and 2 cm deep to the chest wall-lung interface includes the majority of level I and level II lymph nodes (Fig. 53.40).

Internal Mammary Lymph Nodes

The benefit of irradiation of the IMNs is an unresolved issue because clinical failures at this site are very rare and the majority of patients at risk receive adjuvant therapy (252,538). However, the IMNs are difficult to treat because their exact location is often uncertain and the radiation fields that include them irradiate more normal tissue (49,573). Several techniques are used, the most common of which, a direct anterior field matched to tangential fields, was developed for postmastectomy radiation therapy and increases the volume of heart and lung tissue in the field. With this technique, the rising contour of the intact breast interferes with dosimetry, which may affect the traditional dose prescription point at depths of 4 to 5 cm and may prevent an easy match to the breast tangential fields. Including

the IMNs in the tangential fields (wide or deep tangents) may significantly increase the volume of irradiated lung and heart tissue and often includes a portion of the contralateral breast as well.

The medial border of the IMN field is the midline. The lateral border is usually 5 to 6 cm lateral to the midline. The superior border abuts the inferior border of the supraclavicular field and the inferior border is at the xiphoid or higher. If only the IMNs are to be treated, the superior border of the field is at the first intercostal space (superior border of the head of the clavicle). The field is set, as described previously, with an oblique incidence to match the medial tangential portal (Fig. 53.41).

The dose to the IMN field (45 to 50 Gy at 1.8 to 2 Gy per day) is calculated at a point 4 to 5 cm beneath the skin surface (depending on the thickness of anterior chest wall and ideally based on CT scan localization). Careful individualized planning and use of electrons of appropriate energy for all or a major portion of the IMN irradiation are necessary to minimize dose to the lung. To spare underlying lung, mediastinum, and spinal cord, electrons in the range of 12 to 16 MeV are preferred for a portion of the treatment, for example 14.4 to 16.2 Gy delivered with 4 to 6-MV photons and 30.6 to 32.4 Gy with electrons.

A solution that avoids matching of fields is the use of partially wide tangential fields to treat the internal mammary chain (671). Although IMNs can be imaged more clearly by radionuclide techniques, the nodes are typically located by identification of the internal mammary vessels, which can be seen on the CT simulator. The nodes in the first three intercostal spaces are thought to be most clinically significant. The medial border of the tangential field is moved 3 to 5 cm across the midline to cover the internal mammary nodes in the first three intercostal spaces. To minimize lung and cardiac exposure, a block is drawn in, as demonstrated in Figure 53.42, to block the inferior mediastinal nodes. The portal films should be inspected carefully to ensure that an excessive amount of lung or heart is not being irradiated. It is important to verify on the clinical setup that targeted breast tissue is not covered by the block.

Severin et al. (671) compared the partially wide tangent (PWT) technique of breast and internal mammary chain irradiation with photon/electron (P/E) and standard tangent (ST) techniques in terms of dose homogeneity within the breast and the dose to critical structures such as the heart and lung in 16 patients who underwent CT simulation for left-sided breast

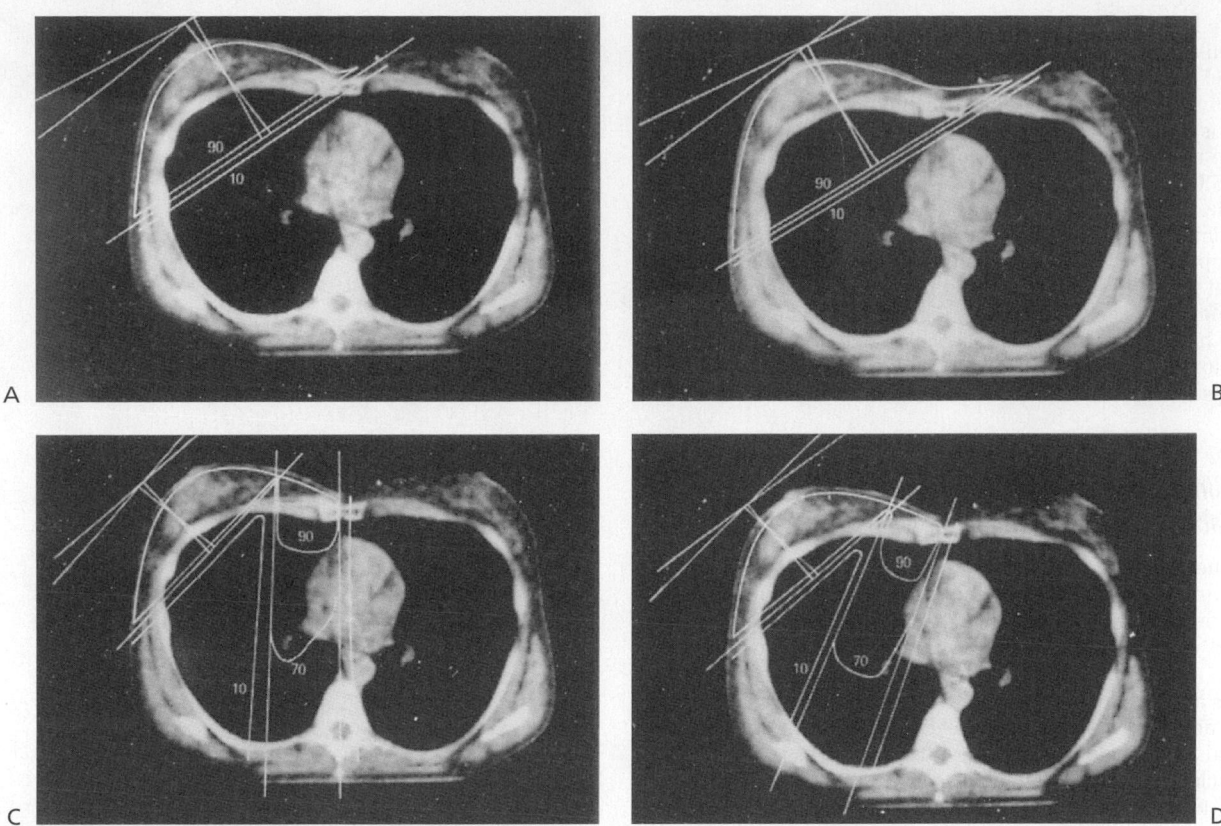

FIGURE 53.41. Irradiation of the breast: field configurations and isodose lines for 6-MV photons. **A:** "Standard tangents" technique. **B:** Deep tangents technique. **C:** *En face* internal mammary field (IMF) technique. **D:** Twenty-degree IMF technique. (From Roberson PL, Lichter AS, Bodner A, et al. Dose to lung in primary breast irradiation. *Int J Radiat Oncol Biol Phys* 1982;9:97–102, with permission.)

cancers. The mean dose to the left breast with the ST, P/E, and PWT techniques was 94.7%, 98.4%, and 96.5%, respectively ($p = .029$). The left lung received the lowest mean dose with the ST technique (13.9%) compared with PWT (22.8%) and P/E (24.3%). The internal mammary chain volume was most consistently treated with the PWT (mean dose 99%) versus P/E (86%)

and ST (38.4%) techniques, although this technique was associated with the greatest amount of contralateral breast (mean dose 5.8%) versus ST (3.2%) versus P/E (2.8%). The heart received the least dose with ST (mean dose 6.7%) versus PWT (10.3%) and P/E (19%). Pierce et al. (573), evaluating seven techniques of treating postmastectomy chest wall and lymphatics, also reported that the PWT technique was the most appropriate balance of target coverage and normal tissue sparing when irradiating the chest wall and internal mammary chain.

CT treatment planning is useful for irradiation of the IMN. Although the lymph nodes are most often not visible, the internal mammary vessels can be clearly seen and contoured on axial CT slices. This anatomic region can then be visualized in treatment field design and in dosimetry planning.

Matching the Tangential Fields with the Supraclavicular Field

A hot spot caused by divergence of the tangential beams into the supraclavicular field and of the supraclavicular beam into the tangential fields can exist just beneath the skin surface at the junction of the inferior border of the supraclavicular field and the superior border of the tangential fields (45). The sharp beam of a linear accelerator and the "horns" at the edge of this beam produce a marked increase in dose beneath the matchline if these divergences are not corrected. This increased dose may result in severe matchline fibrosis or even rib fracture.

There are numerous methods to adjust for divergence of the beams and minimize matchline fibrosis. The divergence of the tangential fields can be eliminated by angling the foot of the treatment couch away from the radiation source to direct the tangential beams inferiorly so that the superior edges of these

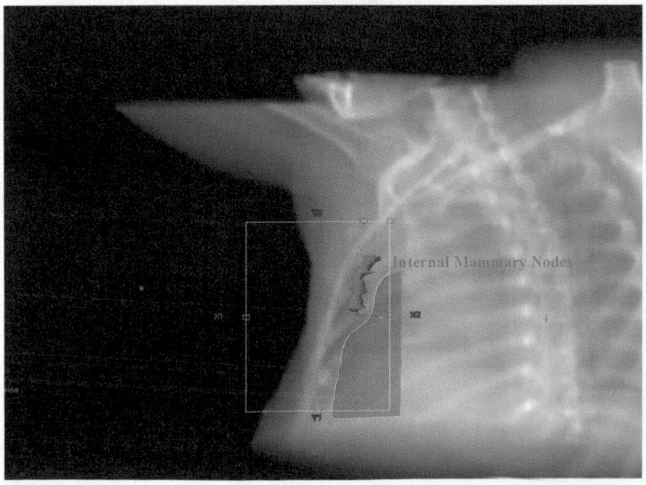

FIGURE 53.42. Partially wide tangential field covering internal mammary chain. The medial border of the tangential field is set 2 to 3 cm to the contralateral side to include the internal mammary chain. Below the fourth intercostals space, the field is blocked to minimize dose to the lung and/or heart. Projection of the field on the patient's surface demonstrates adequate coverage of the involved breast-chest wall with this technique. With this technique there may be a small amount of overlap onto the superior contralateral breast.

beams line up perfectly with the inferior border of the supra-clavicular field (Fig. 53.43). In addition, the collimator may be rotated to geometrically eliminate overlap at this junction. Al-ternatively, the "hanging block" technique, in which a vertical block is affixed to the superior portion of the collimator to block off the nonvertical portion of the tangential beam, can be used (Fig. 53.44).

The inferior divergence of the supraclavicular beam can be eliminated by blocking the inferior half of the beam. This can be accomplished with a beam splitter or with multileaf collimation so that the central, nondiverging portion of the beam becomes the inferior border of this field (Fig. 53.44B). The combination of the half-beam block supraclavicular field and the couch kick technique for the tangential field results in minimal overlap and has essentially eliminated the problem of matchline fibrosis.

The Single Isocenter Technique for Matching Supraclavicular and Tangential Fields

An alternative and attractive method for minimizing field matching problems between the supraclavicular and tangential fields is to use a technique that employs a single isocenter, placed at the junction of the supraclavicular and tangential fields, as demonstrated in Fig. 53.45. This single isocenter serves as the isocenter for both the supraclavicular/axillary ax-illary field and the tangential field, such that the nondivergent central axis single isocenter results in a perfect match of the supraclavicular and tangential fields (337). As demonstrated, when treating the supraclavicular field, the beam below the isocenter is completely blocked. The supraclavicular field is typ-ically angled 5% to 10% away from the spinal cord. Without moving the isocenter or patient, the tangential field is treated by closing the field above the isocenter and angling the beam to treat the tangential fields as demonstrated. Using this technique there is not an option for rotating the collimator. If the patient's anatomy and positioning is ideal, the tangential field is closed down to the central axis, an acceptable amount of lung is ex-posed (<3 cm), and no block may be required. In some cases the tangential field needs to be opened beyond the central axis and a block drawn to minimize lung exposure while maintain-ing coverage of the breast. Since much of the setup is performed on the CT simulator, it is critical when using this technique to clinically view the medial and lateral setups on the patient, to be sure that the entire breast is covered, the medial border is not extending to the contralateral breast, and the blocks are not covering any of the targeted breast tissue.

Matching the Tangential Fields with the Internal Mammary Field

When an internal mammary field is required, the match between it and the medial tangential field can be a problem if there is a significant amount of breast tissue beneath the matchline. In this situation, a cold spot can exist (Fig. 53.46). The effect may be negligible if the breast tissue beneath this matchline is thin (Fig. 53.46B), or it can be avoided including the internal mammary nodes in the tangential field as described above (Fig. 53.46C). Woudstra and van der Werf (840) described a technique using an oblique incidence of the internal mammary portal to match the orientation of the adjacent medial tangential portal; this results in a more homogeneous dose distribution at the junction of the two fields (Fig. 53.47). One potential advantage of the par-tially wide tangential field in the conservatively managed patient is that it avoids the problem of matching over breast tissue.

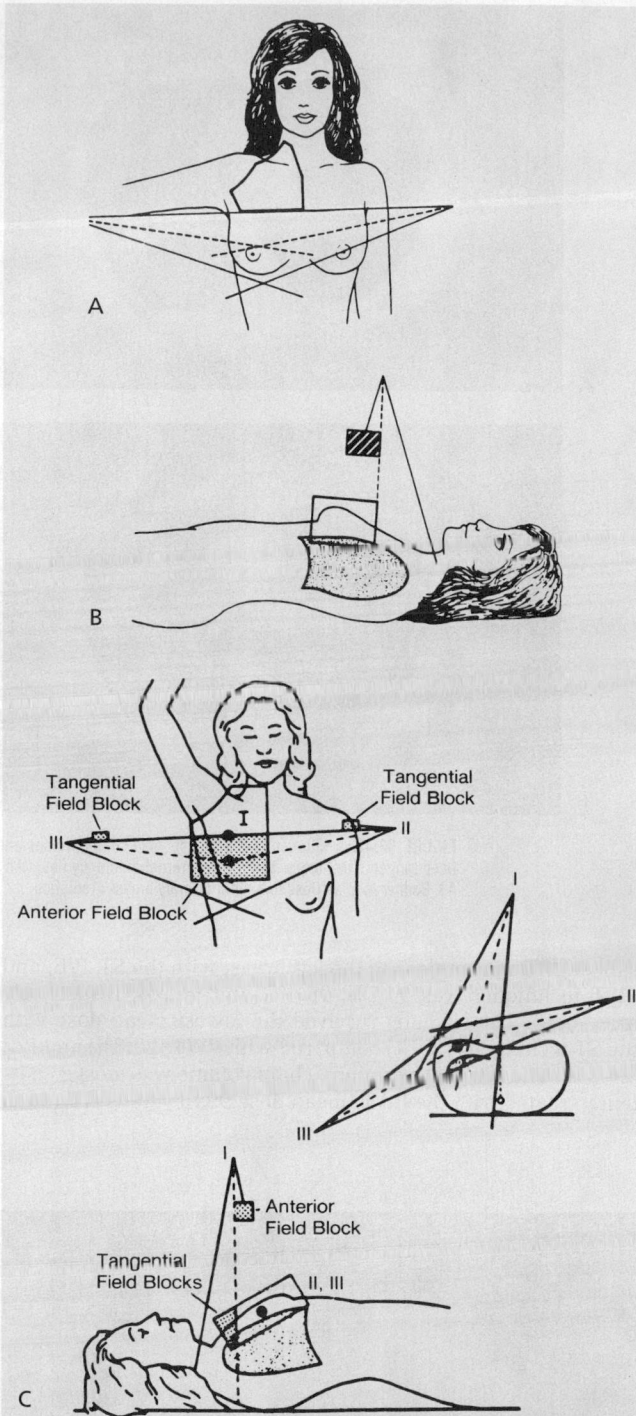

FIGURE 53.43. A: Inferior angulation of the tangential beams eliminates their divergence into the supraclavicular field. **B:** Splitting the supraclavicular beam eliminates its divergence down into the tangential field. (A and B from Bedwinek JM. Treatment of stage I and II ade-nocarcinoma of the breast by tumor excision and irradiation. *Int J Radiat Oncol Biol Phys* 1981;7:1553, with permission.) **C:** Three-field treatment beam geometry in irradiation of the intact breast and supraclavicular fields illustrated in coronal, cross-sectional, and sagittal projections. The supraclavicular and tangential field blocks are shaded. (C from Svensson GK, Chin LM, Siddon RL, et al. Breast treatment techniques at the Joint Center for Radiation Therapy. In: Harris JR, Hellman S, Silen W, eds. *Conservative management of breast can-cer: new surgical and radiotherapeutic techniques.* Philadelphia: J.B. Lippincott, 1983; with permission.)

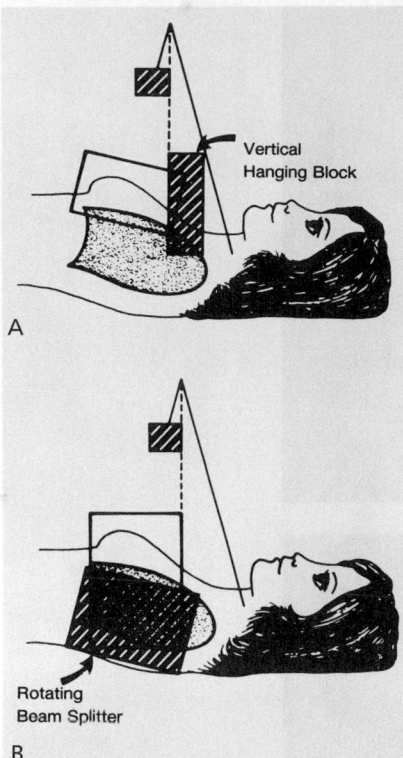

FIGURE 53.44. The superior edge of the tangential beams can be made perfectly vertical by means of the "hanging block" technique (**A**), or by avoiding collimator rotation with the use of a rotating beam splitter (**B**). (From Bedwinek JM. Treatment of stage I and II adenocarcinoma of the breast by tumor excision and irradiation. *Int J Radiat Oncol Biol Phys* 1981;7:1553, with permission.)

Irradiation Dose to the Contralateral Breast

Irradiation dose to the contralateral breast is of concern due to the potential long-term carcinogenic effect of scattered radiation. The data on risk of the contralateral breast are discussed extensively later. Although this risk appears to be minimal with modern techniques, the goal must be to expose all normal tissues not within the target volume to as low a dose as is reasonably achievable. Fraass et al. (247) measured the radiation dose to the contralateral breast in 16 women treated with 6-MV photon tangential fields and performed phantom measurements. For a typical treatment of 50 Gy, the contralateral breast received 0.5 to 2 Gy. Use of tangential fields only resulted in more dose delivered to the surface of the opposite breast, whereas use of the internal mammary field in addition to the tangential portals gave more dose deeper in the breast. Use of a 2.5-cm-thick lead shield over the contralateral breast during treatment with a medial tangential field reduced the dose to 35% of its original value. Similar shields used on the lateral tangential field had no protective effect. The authors recommended that wedges be used whenever possible on the lateral tangential fields rather than on the medial to decrease the dose to the contralateral breast.

A dosimetric study demonstrated that most of the scatter dose received by the opposite breast originates in the collimator and accessories of the accelerator, and it can be significantly decreased by increasing the distance between the source and the patient's skin (517). Therefore, an isocentric source-skin distance technique may be desirable. The use of half-field blocks (beam splitter) or, even better, independent jaws combined with tailored beam splitters or a multileaf collimator (MLC) following

the contour of the chest wall of the patient is very helpful in decreasing the dose to the contralateral breast.

Kelly et al. (396) reviewed the dose to the contralateral breast from breast irradiation with tangential fields using four different techniques. The highest dose was delivered with the use of cerrobend half-beam blocks (regardless of the proportion of wedge used). Remaining techniques gave similar dose ranges, with the lowest total dose produced by the asymmetric jaw with no medial wedge.

The clinical significance of this inadvertent radiation dose to the opposite breast is uncertain as various investigators have shown no increased risk of contralateral breast malignancy after treatment of the original breast by radiation therapy (206,525-537).

Three-Dimensional Conformal or Intensity-Modulated Radiation Therapy

Standard opposed tangential fields with appropriate use of wedges to optimize dose homogeneity remain the most commonly employed method for delivery of whole breast irradiation. A number of publications have explored the potential advantages of 3D conformal radiation therapy (3DCRT) or intensity-modulated radiation therapy (IMRT) to treat patients with breast cancer. Theoretically, 3DCRT involves a reduction in the volume of normal tissues receiving a high dose, with an increase in dose to the target volume that includes the tumor and a limited amount of normal tissue. IMRT potentially can further improve the dose distribution between the target and nontarget tissue, but may also increase the volume of tissue exposed to lower doses of radiation. As suggested in a recent review by Hall and Wuu (314), this may increase the risk of second malignancies, and one must carefully weigh the potential gains and limitations of advanced planning techniques.

Solin et al. (706) devised 38 three-dimensional treatment plans in two patients using multiple CT scan sections and compared various dose distributions. Breast inhomogeneity doses ranged from 5% to 10%. ^{60}Co produced greater inhomogeneities than 6-MV photons, with minimal improvement in tumor dose coverage. In contrast, 15-MV photons had significantly worse tumor coverage at shallow depths, although there was a slight reduction in hot spots. These authors were unable to identify any beam arrangement that improved dose distributions compared with standard tangential fields.

In a study of 26 patients irradiated to the intact breast with CT scanning-based three-dimensional treatment planning, Muren et al. (518) demonstrated a 50% reduction of the average excess cardiac mortality risk in left-side-treated patients using this technique. Their data showed, without consideration of patient or organ motion, that tangential breast irradiation with <1 cm of the heart and <2.5 cm of the lung in the treatment volume would lower the anticipated risk for cardiac mortality or pulmonary morbidity to <1%.

Cho et al. (113), in a comparison of various techniques in 12 patients with left-sided breast cancer, concluded that the lowest normal tissue complication probability values for heart and lungs were comparable between an oblique electron beam and the IMRT techniques compared with split-beam tangential fields. Fogliata et al. (227) also compared conventional photon beam, IMRT, and proton beam irradiation of the intact breast in five patients. Coverage of the planning target volume was comparable for the non-IMRT and IMRT techniques, but significantly less dose was delivered to the underlying lung with the proton beam technique.

Vicini et al. (800) reported on 281 patients treated with whole breast IMRT using multiple static MLC segments. Figure 53.48 shows a representative dose distribution. The median volume of breast receiving 105% of the prescribed dose

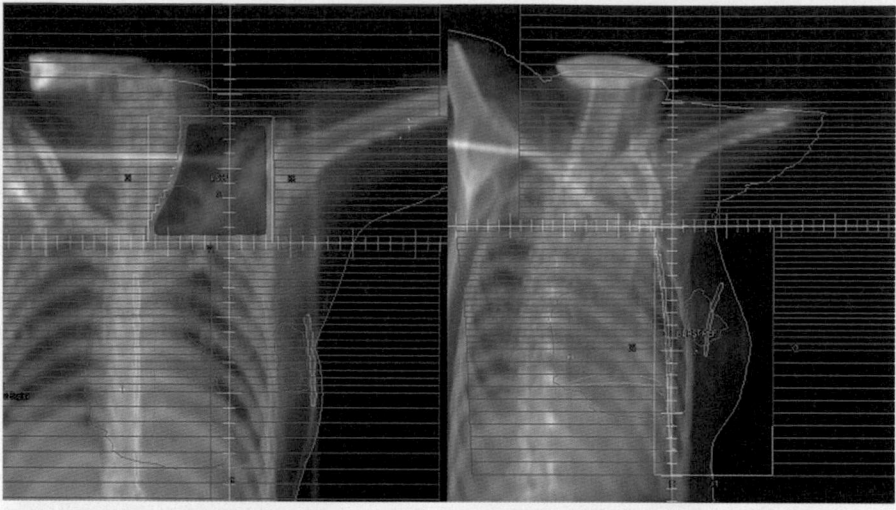

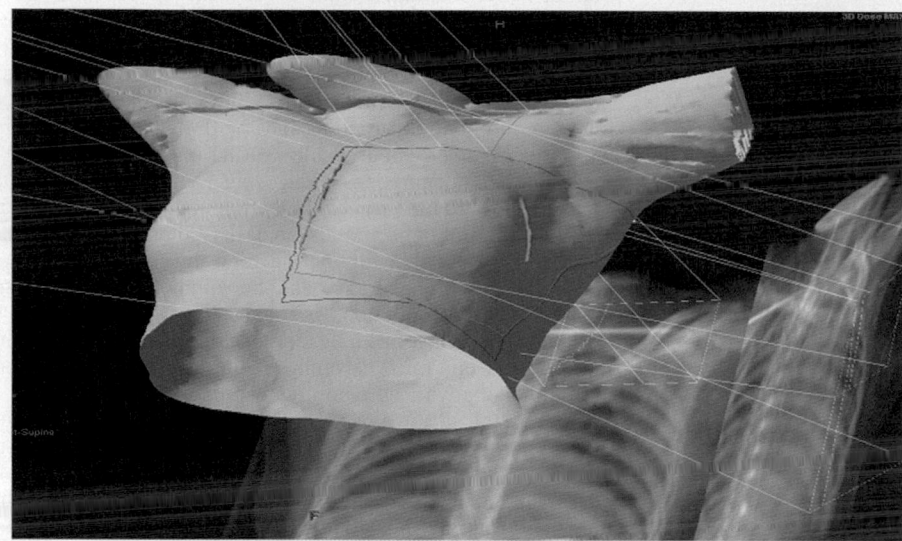

FIGURE 53.45. A: Mono-isocentric matching technique. Single isocenter is set at the match between the supraclavicular and tangential fields. The inferior portion of the beam is blocked for the supraclavicular treatment and the superior portion is blocked for the tangential field, with no movement of the isocenter, resulting in an ideal match. Blocks are drawn as indicated to shield lung and heart. The field should be viewed clinically to ensure that the blocks drawn to shield heart/lung to not block target tissue on the breast-chest wall. **B:** Projection of fields onto patient surface demonstrates perfect match of the supraclavicular and tangential fields.

was 11% (range 0% to 67.6%). The median breast volume receiving 110% of the prescribed dose was 0% (range 0% to 39%), and the median breast volume receiving 115% of the prescribed dose was also 0%. Only three (1%) experienced grade III toxicity. The cosmetic results at 12 months (95 patients analyzable) were rated as excellent/good in 94 patients (99%). No skin telangiec-

tasia, significant fibrosis, or persistent breast pain was noted. The authors concluded that the use of IMRT with a static MLC technique for tangential whole breast radiation therapy is an efficient method for achieving a uniform and standardized dose throughout the whole breast, and widespread implementation of this technology can be achieved with minimal imposition on

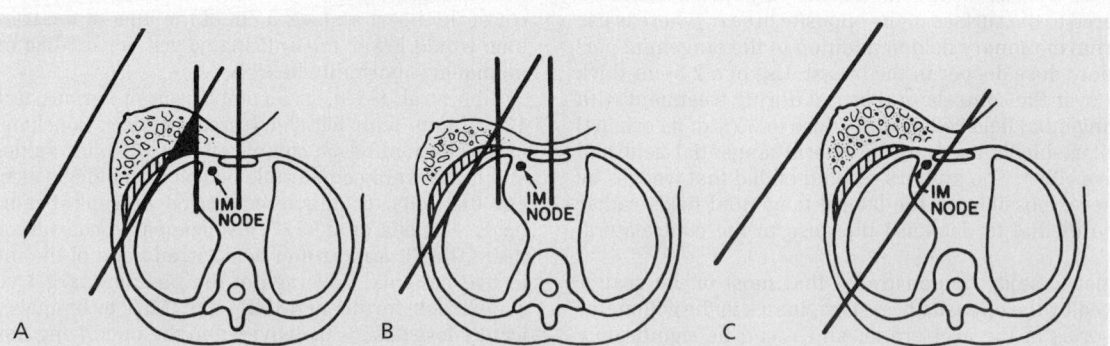

FIGURE 53.46. Diagrams showing several relationships between internal mammary and tangential fields. **A:** A significant cold region exists if the internal mammary (IM) tangential matchline overlies a large amount of breast tissue. **B:** The cold area may be negligible if the breast tissue beneath the matchline is thin. **C:** The lack of a separate IM field can result in irradiation of an excessive volume of lung, particularly in large-chested patients. (From Bedwinek JM. Treatment of stage I and II adenocarcinoma of the breast by tumor excision and irradiation. *Int J Radiat Oncol Biol Phys* 1981;7:1553, with permission.)

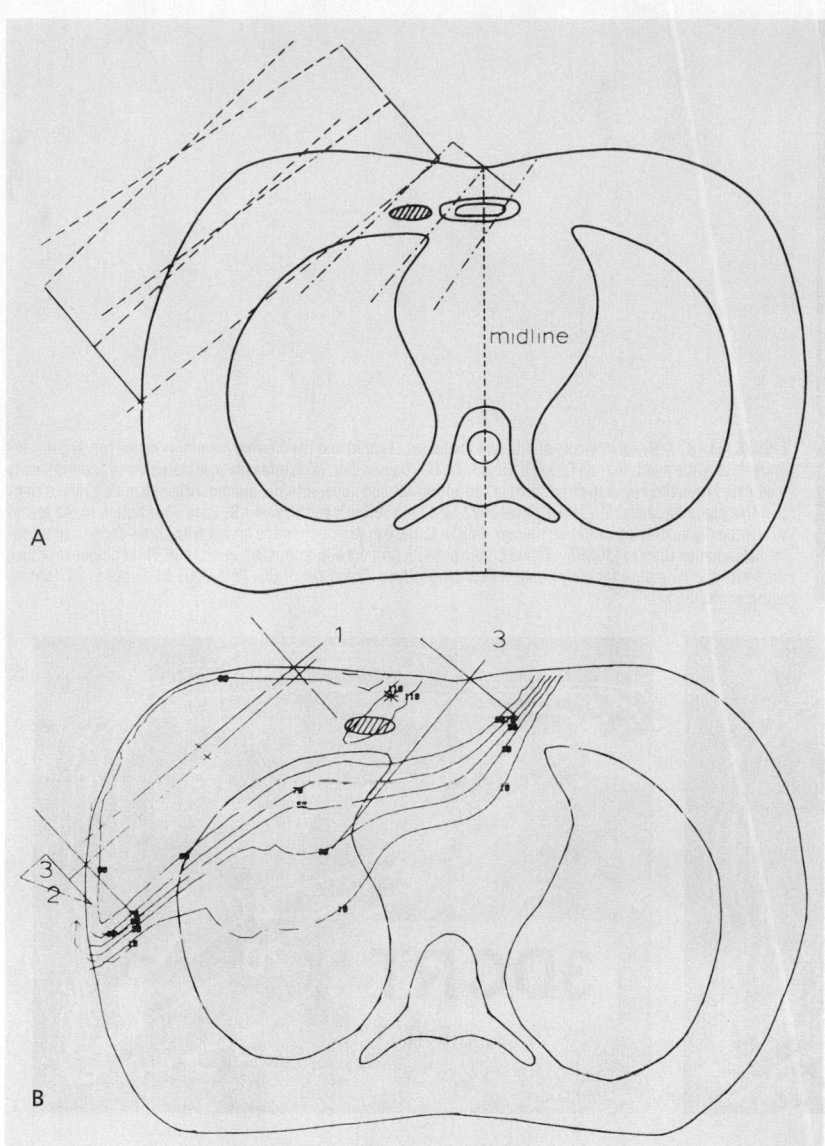

midline

A

B

FIGURE 53.47. A: An obliquely incident electron beam matched to the usual tangential beams. **B:** Isodose presentation of optimal matching of an obliquely incident electron beam to the tangential beams. The target volume is enclosed by the 90% isodose line (equals 40.5 Gy). Electron beam, 16 MeV; photon beam, 6 MV. (From Woudstra E, van der Werf H. Obliquely incident electron beams for irradiation of the internal mammary lymph nodes. *Radiother Oncol* 1987;10:209–215, with permission.)

clinic resources and time constraints. As demonstrated in Figure 53.48, optimized IMRT with 3DCRT were compared and a small reduction was reported in dose to the heart, lungs, and contralateral breast with IMRT.

In a recently reported trial of patients undergoing breast-conserving therapy, 358 patients undergoing whole breast irradiation were randomized to radiation to the breast with standard wedges or with IMRT. Those randomized to IMRT experienced significantly lower degrees of moist desquamation owing to the improved homogeneity with the IMRT techniques employed (583). Further follow-up and additional studies relating to the technical delivery of radiation therapy in early stage breast cancer will evolve rapidly in the next several years due to the rapid advances in technology.

It is important to recognize that the term *IMRT* has been used in various ways to describe breast cancer treatment. In some studies, IMRT is described as a method of three-dimensional dose compensation without a change in the gantry angles of predesigned tangential fields. In such instances, dose distribution has been improved, but the fields are not more conformal. Accordingly, low dose to other organs is not an issue. For others, IMRT attempts to improve conformality of the high-dose region by using multiple field angles that increase the volume of normal tissues that receive low radiation doses.

Accelerated Partial Breast Irradiation

The current standard of care for women with invasive breast cancer remains whole breast irradiation following breast-conserving surgery (522). With the notable exception of selected elderly women, omission of radiation therapy has now been proven in numerous randomized trials and meta-analysis to compromise local control, and to a lesser extent breast cancer-related mortality. For some women, the 6-week course of daily radiation with its associated time and travel issues is not feasible. In response to this, a wide variety of accelerated forms of treatment have been developed and proven safe and effective in short-term studies (32). These approaches include multicatheter interstitial implants placed around the excision cavity, single balloon catheter that can be afterloaded with a central radiation source (MammoSite, Cytyc Corporation, Marlborough, MA) which is placed into the excision cavity, external beam conformal partial breast irradiation, and

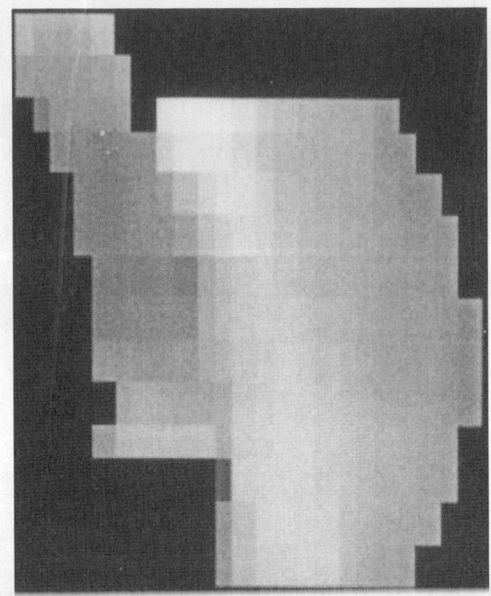

FIGURE 53.48. A: Beam intensity profile over the breast (*lighter*) and the internal mammary nodes (*darker*) to minimize dose to the heart. (A from Cho BCJ, Hurkmans CW, Damen EMF, et al. Intensity modulated versus non-intensity modulated radiotherapy in the treatment of the left breast and upper internal mammary lymph node chain: a comparative planning study. *Radiother Oncol* 2002;62:127–136, with permission.) **B:** Dose distribution to the breast with intensity modulated radiation therapy (IMRT). **C:** Dose distribution to the breast with three-dimensional conformal radiation therapy (3DCRT). (B and C from Keall PJ, Arnfield MR, Arthur DW, et al. An IMRT technique to reduce the heart and lung dose for early stage breast cancer. *Int J Radiat Oncol Biol Phys* 2001;51[Suppl 1]:247[abstr], with permission.)

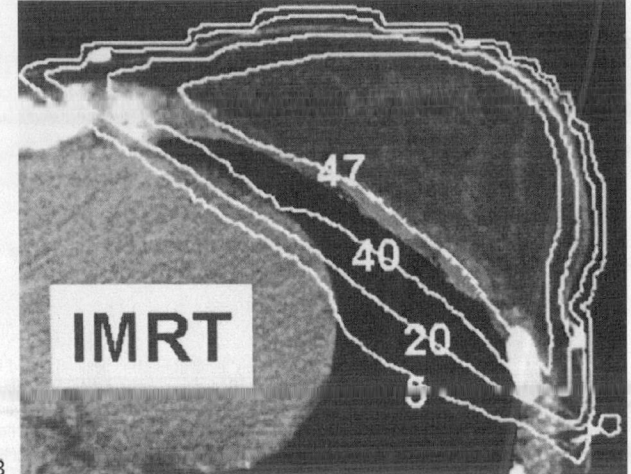

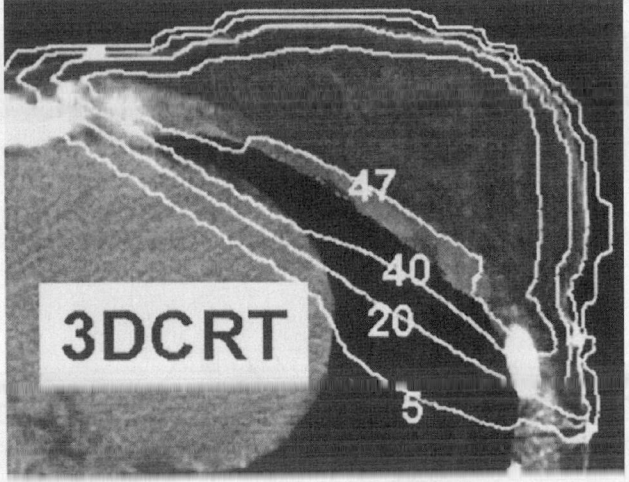

intraoperative single-dose irradiation. Although these techniques vary considerably, they share the common strategy of delivering the radiation to a smaller volume of breast tissue around the lumpectomy site, using fewer larger fractions delivered over a shorter time. The rationale behind this approach is that the majority of breast relapses occur at or near the lumpectomy site. Pathological studies from mastectomy specimens have demonstrated a lower probability of subclinical microscopic disease with increasing distance from the primary tumor (32,202,243,251,297,423,778,782,799). Although the early results clearly demonstrate the feasibility and acceptable toxicity of accelerated partial breast irradiation, this approach has not yet been demonstrated in a randomized trial to be equivalent to whole breast irradiation. There are several ongoing randomized trials that will attempt to answer the question of whether this approach is equivalent to whole breast irradiation for selected patients. The current NSABP-B39/RTOG-0413 is well under way with high enrollment (533). Although the mature results of this trial will not be available for several years, it should help to identify appropriate patients for this approach. Ongoing randomized trials investigating partial breast irradiation are summarized in Table 53.38. The NSABP-RTOG trial will randomize over 3,000 women with early stage breast cancer (including DCIS) to whole breast versus accelerated partial breast irradiation. This trial allows for any one

of three techniques of partial breast irradiation, namely, interstitial brachytherapy, MammoSite, or external beam conformal therapy (32). The techniques are selected based on the physician and/or patient preference prior to randomization. Fraction size is slightly higher for the external beam conformal (3.85 vs. 3.4 Gy), but all three employ twice daily radiation for a total of 10 treatments for a total dose of 38.5 or 34 Gy over 5 days. Each of the various techniques of partial breast irradiation is discussed below.

Multicatheter Interstitial Techniques

Experience is greatest with the multicatheter interstitial technique, as it was initially developed (and is still employed) as a boost technique following whole breast irradiation (428,793,819). As demonstrated in Figure 53.49, multiple catheters are generally positioned at 1- to 1.5-cm intervals, with the total number of catheters and planes employed dependent on the size, extent, and shape of the target. With refinements in image-guided techniques, this approach is generally quite adaptable to most cavities and locations within the breast. Due to its complexity, user dependence, and logistics, however, the use of this technique has been less widely embraced, compared to the MammoSite (described below) and external beam techniques.

Table 53.38	ONGOING RANDOMIZED TRIALS OF ACCELERATED PARTIAL BREAST IRRADIATION			
Institution/Trial	**Trial Design**	**No. of Cases**	**Control Arm**	**Experimental Arm**
NSABP B 39 RTOG 0413	Equivalence	3,000	50–50.4 Gy WB +/− 10–16 Gy boost	1. Interstitial Brachytx, **or** 2. MammoSite, **or** 3. 3D conformal EBRT
National Institute of Oncology Budapest, Hungary	Noninferiority	570	50 Gy WB	1. Interstitial Brachytx (5.2 Gy × 7) **or** 2. Electrons (50 Gy)
European Brachytherapy Breast Cancer GEC-ESTRO Working Group	Non inferiority, Nonirrelevant 3% difference	1,170	50–50.4 Gy WB + 10 Gy boost	Brachytherapy only 32.0 Gy 8 fractions HDR 30.3 Gy 7 fractions HDR 50 Gy PDR
European Institute of Oncology	Equivalence	824	50 Gy WB + 10 Gy boost	Intra-operative Single fraction EBRT 21 Gy × 1
University College of London	Equivalence	1,600	WB RT (per center) + boost	Intra-operative Single fraction EBRT 5 Gy × 1

EBRT, electron beam radiation therapy; HDR, high-dose radiation; PDR, pulsed dose rate; RT, radiation therapy; WB, whole breast.

Kuske et al. (429) recently reported the results of RTOG 95-17, a phase I and II study employing accelerated partial breast irradiation (APBI) using multiplane interstitial catheters in 99 women with early stage breast cancer. The inclusion criteria for this study included invasive nonlobular tumors ≤3 cm after lumpectomy with negative surgical margins and axillary dissection with zero to three positive axillary nodes without extracapsular extension. The patients were treated with either low-dose radiation (LDR) APBI (45 Gy in 3.5 to 5 days) or high-dose radiation (HDR) APBI (34 Gy in 10 twice-daily fractions within 5 days). Chemotherapy and/or tamoxifen were administered at the discretion of the treating physicians. Of the 99 women, 33 were treated with LDR and 66 with HDR APBI. Of the 66 patients treated with HDR APBI, two (3%) had grade 3 or 4 toxicity. Of the

33 patients treated with LDR, three (9%) had grade 3 or 4 toxicity during brachytherapy. No patient experienced late grade 4 toxicity; the rate of grade 3 toxicity was 18% for the LDR and 4% for the HDR groups.

Vicini et al. (794) reported on 133 cases of early stage breast cancer managed with lumpectomy and axillary lymph node dissection followed by interstitial implant alone (99 cases using LDR and 34 with HDR implant) to the tumor bed, matched to a control group treated with external beam from the same institution. The number of catheters per patient ranged from 11 to 18 (median 16). Tumor size ranged from 0.1 to 3 cm (median 1.1 cm), with margins of excision >2 mm. Patients treated with LDR implants received 50 Gy over 96 hours as an inpatient procedure and those treated with HDR implants received 32 Gy in

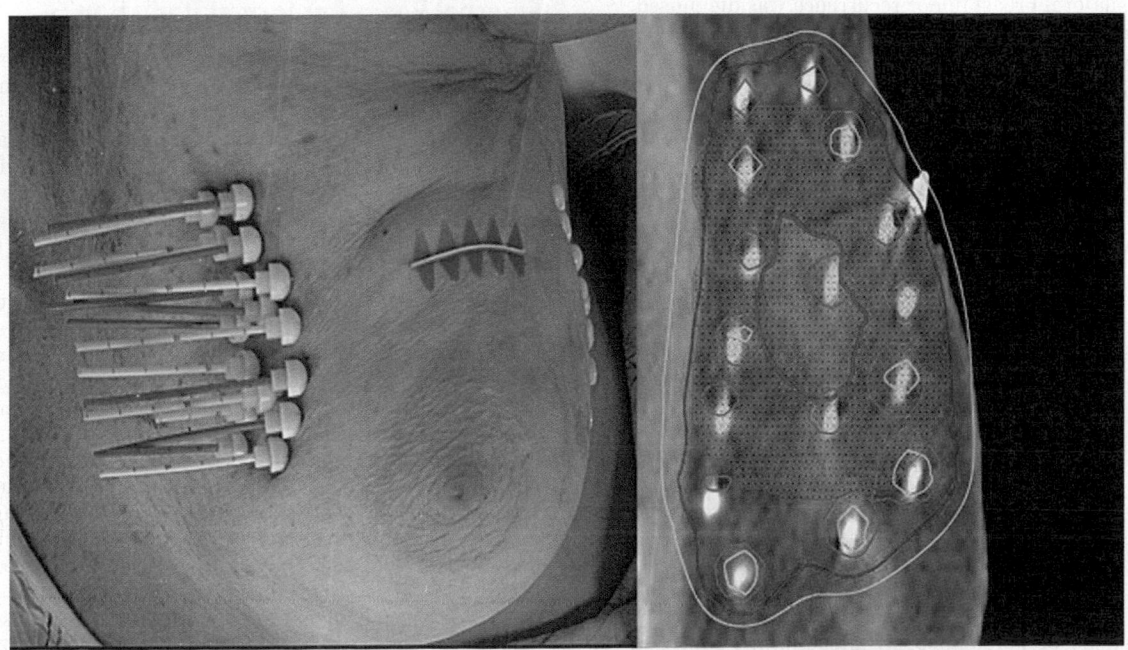

FIGURE 53.49. Partial breast irradiation demonstrating the multiplane interstitial implant technique. (From Arthur DW, Vicini FA. Accelerated partial breast irradiation as a part of breast-conservation therapy. *J Clin Oncol* 2005;23:1726–1735, with permission.)

eight fractions over 4 days (twice daily) as an outpatient procedure. The median follow-up for the external-beam radiation therapy group was 5.7 years versus 3.2 years for brachytherapy. No local or regional failures have been detected, and only one patient failed distantly in the HDR group. No significant adverse sequelae were noted, and cosmetic results were judged to be good or excellent in 98% of patients. No statistically significant differences were noted in the 5-year actuarial rates of ipsilateral breast (3% vs. 0%; $p = .17$) or locoregional failure (4% vs. 0%; $p = .37$) between patients treated with external-beam radiation therapy and those treated with brachytherapy alone.

Arthur et al. (31) used HDR brachytherapy (34 Gy in 10 fractions twice a day over 5 days) in 26 patients or LDR (45 Gy given at a dose rate of 45 to 50 cGy per hour) in 18 patients. After a median follow-up of 31 months (range 11 to 61 months), all patients remained locally controlled. Among patients receiving doxorubicin after brachytherapy, at a median follow-up of 12 months, recall reactions involving the skin overlying the implant site were observed in 42% of patients (6/14). On multivariate analysis, a recall reaction ($p = .0007$) and LDR brachytherapy ($p = .04$) were significant predictors of fibrosis and telangiectasis.

Wazer et al. (815) reported the results of APBI using HDR interstitial brachytherapy in a phase I and II single multi-institutional study in 33 women with early stage breast cancer. Eligible patients included those with T1, T2, N0, N1 ($\leq$3 nodes positive), and M0 tumors of nonlobular histologic features with negative surgical margins, no extracapsular lymph node extension, and a negative postexcision mammogram. High-activity ^{192}Ir was used to deliver 340 cGy per fraction, two fractions per day, for 5 consecutive days, to a total dose of 34 Gy to the target volume. The mean tumor size was 1.3 cm, and 55% of the patients had an extensive intraductal component. Three patients had positive axillary nodes. The RTOG late radiation morbidity scoring scheme was applied. Clinically evident fat necrosis occurred in eight patients at a median of 7.5 months after HDR brachytherapy completion. The only variables significantly associated with grade 3 or 4 toxicity were the number of source dwell positions and the volume of tissue encompassed by the prescription isodose shell. The global cosmetic scores after a minimum of 18 months' follow-up were zero cases with poor, four with fair, five with good, and 24 with excellent scores. One case of ipsilateral breast tumor recurrence was diagnosed.

Perera et al. (561) reported on 39 patients treated with HDR brachytherapy who were matched with patients treated with whole breast irradiation. All patients had a nonlobular history, and no patient had known positive margins. Breast radiation was 37.2 Gy (minimum dose to the lumpectomy site) in 10 fractions twice daily over 5 to 7 days in the brachytherapy group (group B). There were six ipsilateral breast recurrences in the brachytherapy group versus one in the control group, with a trend toward significance ($p = .059$). Four of the six recurrences in the brachytherapy group were outside the lumpectomy site. This study suggests that HDR brachytherapy alone to the lumpectomy site and without the routine use of systemic therapy is less effective than conventional whole breast radiation. A randomized clinical trial will shed more definitive light on this controversial subject.

MammoSite

MammoSite is an alternative method of delivering accelerated partial breast irradiation that has been widely embraced due to its simplicity and less dependence on user experience (32,33,394,795). The technique employs a single balloon catheter introduced into the lumpectomy site either at the time of lumpectomy or percutaneously after the procedure. In the current NSABP/RTOG clinical trial, patients cannot be randomized until after the lumpectomy procedure when final margins

and nodal status are known, and hence the device must be placed after the lumpectomy procedure. As shown in Figure 53.50, the catheter is located centrally within a distal balloon, which is inflated once the catheter is placed in the lumpectomy cavity. Adequacy of placement requires symmetry of the balloon, conformance of the balloon surface to the lumpectomy cavity, and a minimum distance between the surface of the balloon and skin of >5 mm (ideally >7 mm). Treatment is delivered via a high dose rate remote afterloading system to a circumferential 1 cm distance from the balloon surface. This technique is one of the three methods employed in the ongoing randomized trial, with a dose prescription of 3.4 Gy delivered at 1 cm twice daily to a total dose of 34 Gy over 5 days.

Although early experiences with this technique are promising, the results of the ongoing randomized trial will help to identify suitable patients. The most extensive experience with this technique has been reported by the American Society of Breast Surgeons MammoSite Registry Trial reported by Vicini et al. (795), which included 1,419 patients treated in 87 institutions. This was a nonrandomized single arm registration trial in which data were collected prospectively on clinical use of the MammoSite breast brachytherapy catheter for delivering breast irradiation. They reported on 1,237 patients (87% of enrolled patients) who received APBI (34 Gy prescribed to 1.0 cm in 10 fractions; 91% of the patients with invasive carcinoma (977/1,068 patients) had negative lymph node status, and 99% of all patients had negative margins. The median patient age was 65 years. Five hundred fifty-four catheters (45%) were placed with an open cavity at the time of lumpectomy, and 683 catheters (55%) were placed after lumpectomy. Skin spacing ranged from 2 to 75 mm (median 10 mm). In terms of cosmetic assessment, with relatively short follow-up, 95% of patients (1,030/1,084 patients) who had a cosmetic assessment had a good/excellent result at the last follow-up visit. At 12 months, cosmetic results were good/excellent in 92% of 248 evaluable patients. The median skin spacing ($\geq$7 mm vs. <7 mm) was associated significantly with a good/excellent cosmetic result (96.1% vs. 86.8%; $p = .0001$) overall and at 6 months ($p = .006$). One local recurrence (0.1%) was reported (new primary carcinoma). With short follow-up, this experience demonstrated acceptable toxicity and cosmesis.

External Beam Conformal Radiation

Although external beam conformal radiation has been developed only recently, it is the one that is most widely employed in the ongoing randomized trial (231,476,792). Recent data suggest that over 70% of patients in the randomized trial are opting for the three-dimensional conformal technique. Its widespread acceptance is likely due to the fact that it is totally noninvasive and delivers a homogenous dose distribution. Although the ongoing trial mandates supine position, Formenti (231) has advocated prone accelerated breast irradiation.

The technique, demonstrated in Figure 53.51, generally employs multiple conformal fields, although plans as simple as two opposing small conformal fields may be adequate. Challenges with this technique include daily positioning of the target, movement with breathing, and delivery of higher doses to surrounding normal breast tissue than with the brachytherapy. Nonetheless, this approach has been widely embraced and has been shown to be reproducible. In a phase I/II RTOG trial (study number 0319) of external beam conformal radiation, Vicini et al. (792) examined the use of three-dimensional conformal external beam radiation therapy to deliver accelerated partial breast irradiation. Reproducibility, as measured by technical feasibility, was the primary end point. This study was designed such that if fewer than five cases out of the first 42 patients evaluable were scored as unacceptable, the treatment would be considered reproducible. Patients received 38.5 Gy in 3.85

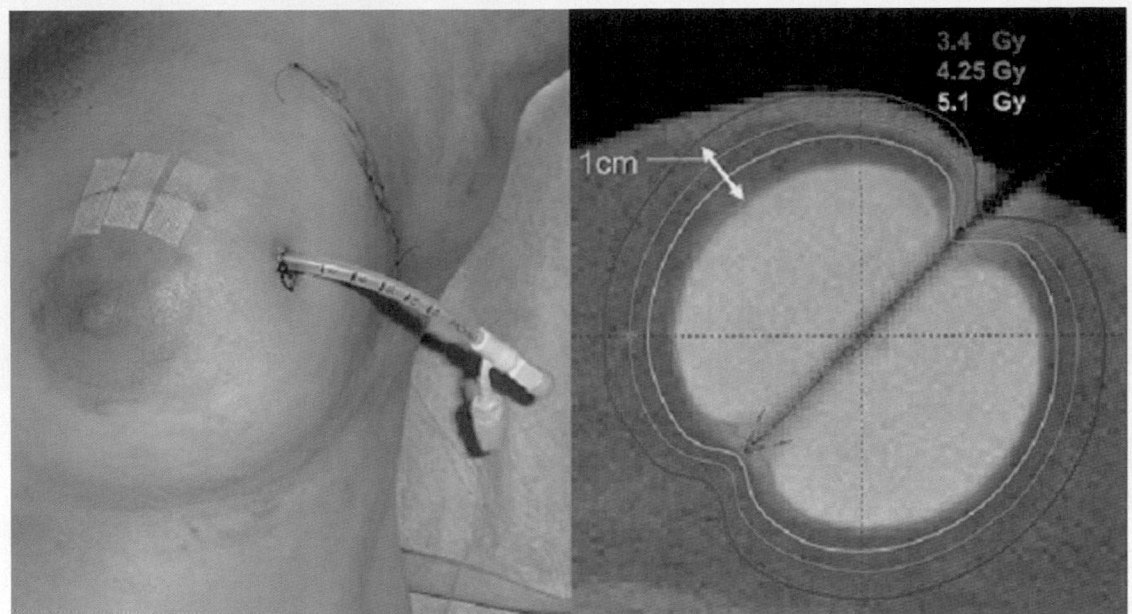

FIGURE 53.50. Partial breast irradiation demonstrating the MammoSite breast brachytherapy device. (From Arthur DW, Vicini FA. Accelerated partial breast irradiation as a part of breast-conservation therapy. *J Clin Oncol* 2005;23:1726–1735, with permission.)

Gy fractions delivered twice daily. The clinical target volume included the lumpectomy cavity plus a 10- to 15-mm margin bounded by 5 mm within the skin surface and the lung-chest wall interface. The planning target volume included the clinical target volume plus a 10-mm margin. A total of 58 patients were enrolled on this study over an 8 months period, five of whom were ineligible or did not receive protocol treatment. There were four cases with major variations and a total of 32 cases with minor variations in treatment plans. Based on this analysis the authors concluded that accelerated partial breast irradiation using three-dimensional conformal external beam radiation therapy was technically feasible and reproducible in

a multi-institutional trial using exceptionally strict dosimetric criteria.

Again, the ongoing randomized trial will help to further define acceptability and reproducibility of three-dimensional conformal external beam radiation as an option for women with early stage invasive breast cancer.

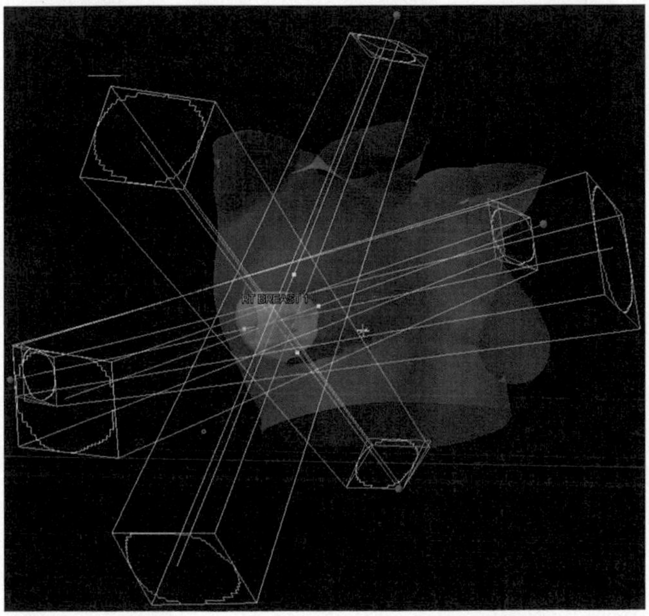

Intraoperative Accelerated Partial Breast Irradiation

Intraoperative accelerated partial breast irradiation has been most widely employed outside of the United States (544,779). The radiation is delivered in a single intraoperative dose to the lumpectomy site at the time of surgery, using intraoperative electrons or intraoperative photons. Vaidya et al. (762) describe a preliminary report using a 50 Kv spherical source to deliver a dose of 20 Gy at a depth of 1 cm, with acceptable toxicity.

Veronesi et al. (779) developed an intraoperative radiation therapy (IORT) technique for a breast quadrant after the removal of the primary carcinoma using a mobile linear accelerator with a robotic arm to deliver electron beams with energies from 3 to 9 MeV. The radiation is delivered directly to the mammary gland, and to spare the skin from radiation, the skin margins are stretched out of the radiation field (Fig. 53.52A,B). To protect the thoracic wall, an aluminum-lead disk is placed between the gland and the pectoralis muscle (Fig. 53.52C). Different dose levels were tested from 10 to 21 Gy without important side effects. They estimated that a single fraction of 21 Gy is equivalent to 60 Gy delivered in 30 fractions at 2 Gy per fraction. Seventeen patients received an IORT dose of 10 to 15 Gy as a boost to external radiation therapy, whereas 86 patients received 17, 19, or 21 Gy intraoperatively as their whole treatment. The follow-up time of the 101 patients ranged from 1 to 17 months (mean 8 months). The IORT treatment was very well accepted by all patients. The authors believe that single-dose IORT after breast resection for small mammary carcinomas may be an excellent alternative to the traditional postoperative radiation therapy. Based on these data the European Institute of Oncology has conducted a randomized trial, comparing this

FIGURE 53.51. Partial breast irradiation demonstrating the external beam conformal radiation technique.

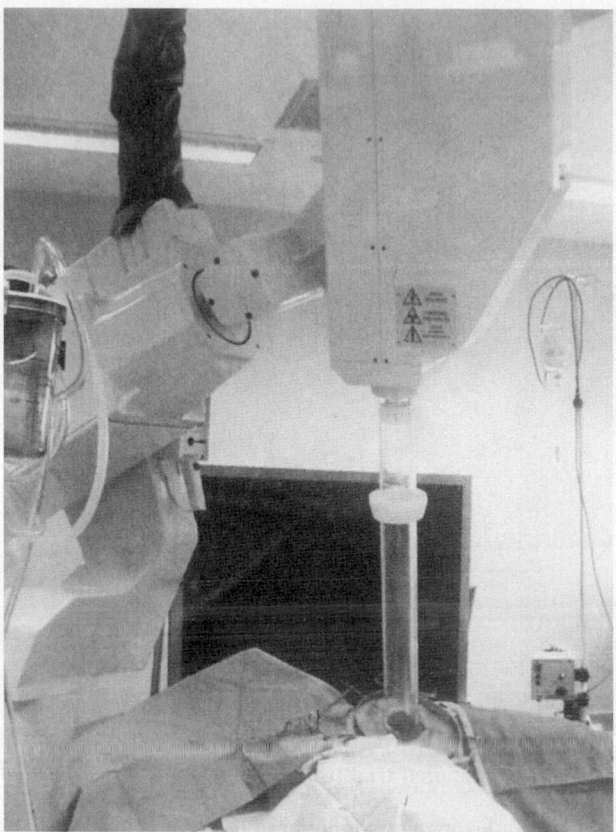

FIGURE 53.52. **A:** Linear electron beam accelerator in operating room during intraoperative radiation therapy. **B:** Proper placement of applicator in the breast. **C:** Before intraoperative radiation therapy delivery, an aluminum–lead disk (4 mm Al and 5 mm Pb thick) is placed between the deep face of residual breast and pectoralis muscle. (From Veronesi U, Oreechia R, Luini A, et al. A preliminary report on intraoperative radiotherapy (IORT) in limited-stage breast cancers that are conservatively treated. *Eur J Cancer* 2001;37: 2178–2183, with permission.)

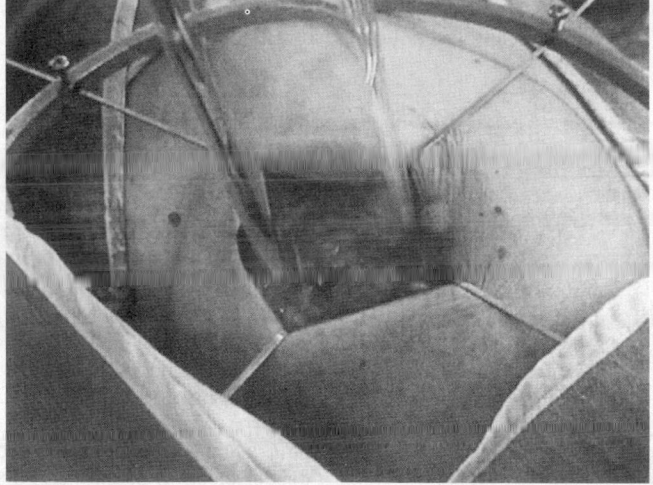

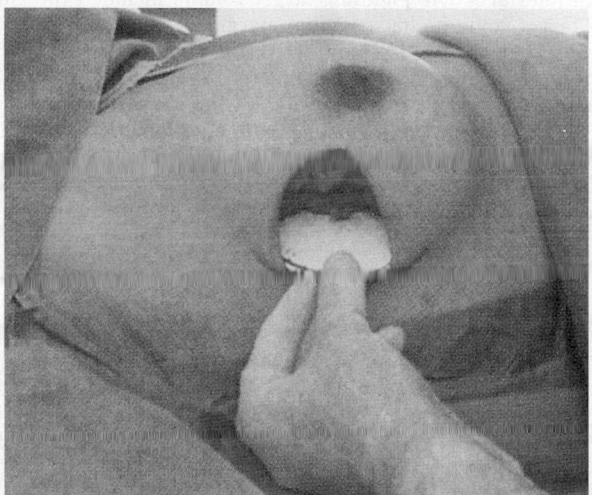

option to whole breast irradiation for selected patients, and results of this trial are eagerly awaited (544).

Cosmetic Outcomes and Sequelae

Cosmesis

Surgical, radiotherapeutic, chemotherapeutic, and host factors may influence cosmetic outcome (736). Surgical factors to be considered include extent of surgical resection, re-excision, orientation and length of the scar, closure or not of the tylectomy cavity, separate or continuous axilla-tylectomy scars, extent of the axillary dissection, and whether an ellipse of skin over the tumor was removed. Radiation therapy factors are doses to

the whole breast with tangential portals, homogeneity of dose throughout the breast (use of wedge or compensating filters), use of bolus, fractionation, overall duration of therapy including breaks, type and dose of boost, beam energy, and volume treated (whether peripheral lymphatic irradiation is administered). Chemotherapy issues include cytotoxic agents used, timing and sequence relative to radiation therapy, and doses and combinations of drugs. Host factors include size and shape of the breast, age, race, compliance with care and hygiene, concurrent medical illnesses (e.g., hypertension, diabetes, CVD), and intrinsic sensitivity to radiation.

Different methods have been used to evaluate breast cosmesis after breast-conservation therapy. Some are flawed because they do not establish strict guidelines or criteria for objectively judging cosmetic outcome. Pezner et al. (570) used scales and standard procedures for obtaining color slides to assess the cosmetic results of breast-conservation therapy, and other scales designed by various investigators were given to patients for comparison. The study demonstrated that observer-based consensus of cosmetic results is difficult to obtain with two commonly used scales, but by changing the scale gradations from four to two (zero to one vs. two to three satisfactory results), consensus exceeding 85% of observers can be obtained.

A commonly employed simple scale, developed by the Harvard group, employs a four-point scale: excellent, good, fair, and poor (630). At Washington University, questionnaires were completed by 458 patients and their radiation oncologists at regular 6-month intervals after treatment. Cosmetic outcome analysis of these patients was done for clinical and treatment-related factors (736). Approximately 80% of patients had excellent or good cosmesis (Fig. 53.53). Cosmetic results as a function of patient characteristics and radiation treatment factors are summarized in Tables 53.39 and 53.40. Clinical factors at presentation were analyzed by age, menopausal status, race, and tumor-related parameters of size, palpable status, and location. Patients older than 60 years of age had lower excellent cosmetic scores compared with patients 60 years of age or younger. Tumor size significantly influenced cosmetic outcome, most likely related to the volume of breast removed and perhaps boost dose. Cosmetic outcome by race indicated 40% of whites had an excellent cosmetic rating, compared with only 18% for African Americans. Thirty percent of African American patients received concurrent chemotherapy or hormonal therapy with irradiation, compared with 23% of white patients. Of African American patients, 14% were obese, 17% were hypertensive, 25% had both obesity and hypertension, and 4% had diabetes.

Poorer cosmetic outcomes in African American women have also been reported by Pierce et al. (572) and Tuomokuomo and Haffty (755). In the latter study, a detailed cosmetic analysis was performed on a subset of 20 African American patients and 20 white patients from the Yale database. The two groups were intentionally matched by age, follow-up, adjuvant therapy, and breast size and were asked to participate in a detailed cosmetic evaluation. With respect to overall cosmetic outcome and all specific cosmetic measures (edema, fibrosis, and pigmentation), African American patients fared more poorly than white patients. Overall cosmesis was good to excellent in 55% of African Americans, compared with 90% of whites.

Cosmesis may be affected by multiple breast and axillary surgical factors (736). The type of breast surgery is important, with patients undergoing excisional biopsy having the highest rate of excellent cosmesis (56%) compared with wide excision (35%) or quadrantectomy (13%; $p = .0001$). Scar orientation compliance with NSABP guidelines was a significant factor, with a 44% excellent cosmetic rating compared with 27% for patients with noncompliant scar orientations ($p = .0034$). Re-excision of the primary site also resulted in a lower rate of excellent cosmesis ($p = .0002$). Breast tissue resection of >100 cm^3 was associated with lower rates of excellent or good cosmesis, independent

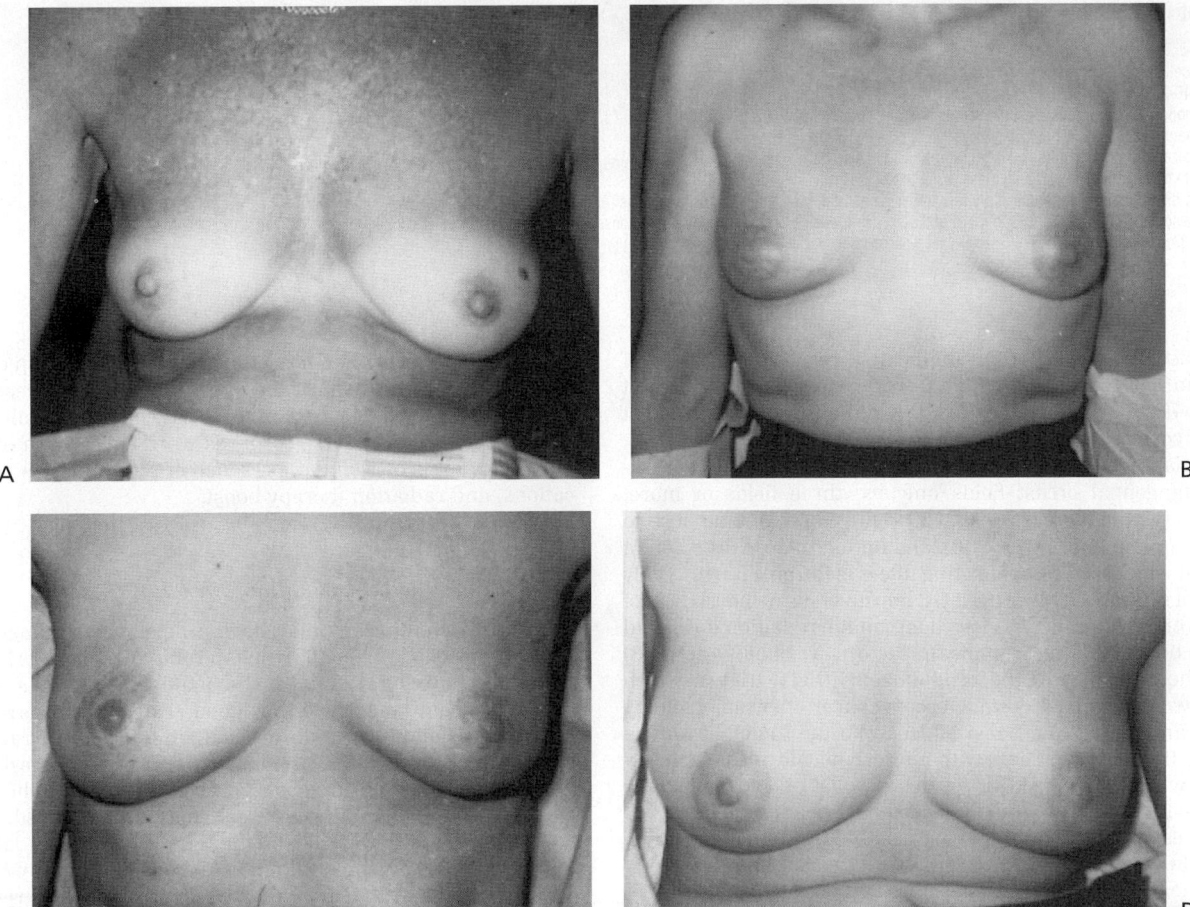

FIGURE 53.53. A–D: Photographs of patients showing excellent cosmetic results obtained with conservation surgery and irradiation for patients with T1 and T2 carcinomas of the breast. The patient in (C) has minimal telangiectasia in the area treated with a boost (upper region of left breast).

Table 53.39	COSMETIC RESULTS CORRELATED WITH PATIENT AND TUMOR CHARACTERISTICS

	No. of Patients	Cosmetic Score[a]			
		Excellent	Good	Fair	Poor
Age (y)					
$\leq$ 40	75	31 (41%)	33 (44%)	3 (4%)	8 (11%)
41–60	223	94 (42%)	92 (41%)	33 (15%)	4 (2%)
61–80	150	45 (30%)	71 (47%)	28 (19%)	6 (4%)
>80	10	3 (30%)	4 (40%)	3 (30%)	0
Menopausal status					
Premenopausal	141	63 (45%)	57 (40%)	11 (8%)	10 (7%)
Perimenopausal	31	15 (49%)	13 (42%)	3 (10%)	0
Postmenopausal l	280	94 (34%)	126 (45%)	52 (18%)	8 (3%)
Race					
White	406	164 (40%)	171 (42%)	56 (14%)	15 (4%)
Black	50	9 (18%)	27 (54%)	11 (22%)	3 (6%)
Tumor size (mm)					
<10	140	63 (45%)	58 (41%)	16 (11%)	3 (2%)
11–20	202	76 (38%)	90 (45%)	29 (14%)	7 (3%)
21–50	107	32 (30%)	47 (44%)	20 (19%)	8 (7%)
Palpable mass					
Yes	236	86 (36%)	107 (45%)	33 (14%)	10 (4%)
No	124	52 (42%)	60 (48%)	9 (7%)	3 (2%)
Primary location in breast					
Upper outer and axillary tail	238	93 (39%)	101 (42%)	36 (15%)	8 (3%)
Upper inner	72	30 (41%)	33 (45%)	6 (8%)	4 (5%)
Lower outer	55	22 (40%)	24 (44%)	7 (13%)	2 (3%)
Lower inner	38	12 (32%)	18 (47%)	8 (21%)	0
Central	59	16 (30%)	23 (43%)	10 (19%)	4 (7%)

[a]For excellent cosmetic score:
Age $\leq$40–60 y versus 61–>80 years, p = .001.
Premenopausal and perimenopausal versus postmenopausal, p = .02.
White versus black, p = .0034.
Tumor size <10–20 mm versus 21–50 mm, p = .05.
Palpable mass versus no palpable mass, p = .3976.
Primary site of upper outer and axillary tail, upper inner, and lower outer versus lower inner and central, p = .3407.
From Taylor ME, Perez CA, Halverson KJ, et al. Factors influencing cosmetic results after conservation therapy for breast cancer. *Int J Radiat Oncol Biol Phys* 1995;31:753–764, with permission.

of breast size (p = .0001). Similarly, a resected skin area of >20 cm² was correlated with a lower excellent cosmetic result (p = .045). Extent of axillary surgery did not significantly affect breast cosmesis.

Radiation factors affecting cosmesis included treatment volume (tangential breast fields only vs. three fields or more; p = .034), whole-breast dose >50 Gy (p = .024), total dose to the tumor site >65 Gy (p = .06), and optimum dose distribution created with use of compensating filters (see Table 53.40). Daily fraction size of 1.8 Gy versus 2 Gy, boost versus no boost, type of boost (brachytherapy vs. electrons), total irradiation dose, and use of bolus were not significant factors. Vrieling et al. (808) published a report of the randomized EORTC trial in which 5,318 women with early stage breast cancer after tumorectomy were randomized to a boost of 16 Gy to the tumor bed or no further treatment. Patients with microscopically incomplete excision were randomized to receive a boost of 10 Gy or 25 or 26 Gy with interstitial implant or external-beam radiation. Cosmetic results at 3 years were assessed in 731 women (364 with boost, 367 without boost) using digitizer measurements and displacement of the nipple cosmesis in the boost group was excellent in 33%, good in 38%, fair in 26%, and poor in 3%. In the no-boost group, the results were 42%, 44%, 13%, and 1%, respectively. The position of the nipple was the only moderately representative parameter of the overall cosmetic outcome.

Other measurements had no significant correlation with cosmesis. A global assessment of the appearance of the breast was thought to be a reliable method to assess cosmetic results. Factors associated with worse cosmesis were inferior tumor location, large excision volume, presence of postoperative complications, and radiation therapy boost.

Impact of Adjuvant Chemotherapy on Cosmesis

Adjuvant chemotherapy may have a deleterious influence on excellent to good cosmetic results (Table 53.41) (43,474,595, 630,736). In several studies, the main effect was a switch from "excellent" results to the "good" category. In particular, concomitant administration of chemotherapy and irradiation appears to have a more pronounced effect on cosmesis. The majority of studies using concurrent chemotherapy, however, employed agents that are no longer routinely employed.

Rose et al. (630) reported on the Harvard cosmesis data and found that 68% of women not receiving chemotherapy had an excellent result at 3 years, compared with 37% who received chemotherapy. Conversely, 9% of patients who did not receive chemotherapy were judged to have fair or poor cosmetic results, compared with 24% of those who received chemotherapy. These differences were mostly the result of an increase in breast

Table 53.40	COSMETIC RESULTS CORRELATED WITH RADIATION VOLUME, DOSE, AND BOOST TECHNIQUE					

	No. of Patients	Median Follow-Up (mo)	Cosmetic Score[a]			
			Excellent	Good	Fair	Poor
Type of radiation boost						
None	35	44	10 (29%)	13 (37%)	10 (28%)	2 (6%)
Electron	326	53	127 (39%)	147 (45%)	42 (13%)	10 (3%)
Implant	93	49	36 (39%)	40 (43%)	14 (15%)	3 (3%)
Daily fraction size without chemotherapy						
1.8 Gy	292	53	120 (41%)	126 (43%)	40 (14%)	6 (2%)
2.0 Gy	37	46	16 (43%)	14 (38%)	5 (14%)	2 (5%)
Daily fraction size with chemotherapy						
1.8 Gy	92	43	26 (28%)	47 (51%)	13 (14%)	6 (7%)
2.0 Gy	10	47	4 (40%)	2 (20%)	3 (30%)	1 (10%)
Treatment volume (field arrangements)						
Breast	302	48	125 (41%)	132 (44%)	39 (13%)	6 (2%)
Breast + supraclavicular nodes	29	67	6 (21%)	18 (62%)	4 (14%)	1 (3%)
Breast + supraclavicular + axillary nodes	74	53	23 (31%)	31 (42%)	14 (19%)	6 (8%)
Breast + internal mammary nodes (± supraclavicular and axillary nodes)	53	67	19 (36%)	19 (36%)	10 (19%)	5 (9%)
Radiation dose to the breast (Gy)						
45–47	267	40	106 (40%)	123 (46%)	33 (12%)	5 (2%)
47.01–50	101	59	43 (43%)	37 (37%)	18 (18%)	3 (3%)
50.01–52	75	78	21 (28%)	34 (45%)	15 (20%)	5 (7%)
51.01–62	5	76	0	1 (20%)	1 (20%)	3 (60%)
Total irradiation dose (breast and boost)						
≤ =55–65 Gy	384	50	149 (39%)	170 (44%)	53 (14%)	12 (3%)
≥ = 65.1 Gy	74	58	24 (32%)	30 (41%)	14 (19%)	6 (8%)

[a]For excellent cosmetic score:
No boost versus electron or implant, $p = .30$.
Daily fraction size of 1.8 versus 2 Gy without chemotherapy, $p = .9420$.
Daily fraction size of 1.8 versus 2 Gy with chemotherapy, $p = .4748$.
Breast versus breast and nodes, $p = .0340$.
Irradiation dose to breast of 45 to 50 Gy versus 50.01 to 62 Gy, $p = .0243$.
For excellent versus good cosmetic score regardless of total irradiation dose, $p = .06$.
From Taylor ME, Perez CA, Halverson KI, et al. Factors influencing cosmetic results after conservation therapy for breast cancer. *Int J Radiat Oncol Biol Phys* 1995;31:753-764, with permission.

retraction and, to a lesser extent, development of telangiectasia.

Taylor et al. (736) also reported impaired cosmetic outcome with concurrent administration of chemoradiation. Excellent cosmetic outcome was observed in 43% of patients receiving sequential chemotherapy, in 25% receiving concomitant chemoradiation, and in 41% receiving no adjuvant therapy ($p = .02$). The specific effect of methotrexate on cosmetic outcome was evaluated and the proportion of excellent cosmetic outcomes with methotrexate omitted was 41% versus 16% with methotrexate included. Good results were obtained in 23% versus 58%, fair results in 23% versus 26%, and poor results in 12% versus 0%, respectively ($p = .14$). Similarly, studies by Danoff et al. (142) and Markiewicz et al. (473,474) report no compromise of cosmesis in patients receiving concurrent chemoradiation if methotrexate was held during the radiation.

In a randomized trial of concurrent versus sequential radiation therapy, using 5-fluorouracil, cyclophosphamide, and mitoxantrone, Rouesse et al. (638) also reported comparable and

Table 53.41	IMPACT OF ADJUVANT CHEMOTHERAPY ON COSMESIS IN BREAST-CONSERVATION THERAPY		

		Good to Excellent Cosmesis (%)	
Institution (Reference)	Chemotherapy	Radiation Therapy without Chemotherapy	Radiation Therapy with Chemotherapy
Harvard University (43)	CMF, A	92	67
Palo Alto (595)	CMF	88	73
National Cancer Institute (142)	AC	80	70
University of Pennsylvania (473)	CMF ± P	89	81
Washington University (736)	CMF	81	78

A, doxorubicin; AC, doxorubicin, cyclophosphamide; CMF, cyclophosphamide, methotrexate, 5-fluorouracil; P, prednisone

acceptable cosmetic outcomes, whether patients were treated with sequential or concurrent chemotherapy.

Breast Cosmetic Surgery after Irradiation

Breast deformities after conservation therapy may represent difficult reconstructive problems (56). Correction of a locally damaged breast is a surgical challenge that can result in a fully restored breast if selection of the surgical procedure is properly carried out. In 37 patients who underwent correction of deformities after breast-conservation surgery, which included simple submuscular placement of traditional or expandable implants, breast reshaping, transposition of a latissimus dorsi muscle or musculocutaneous flap, transverse rectus abdominis muscle flap, and reverse abdominoplasty, aesthetic outcome was judged to be good or excellent in 78% of patients.

When *partial mastectomy*, a term that encompasses a diversity of excisional techniques, follows radiation therapy, breast defects characterized by parenchymal loss, nipple–areola complex distortion, and cutaneous abnormalities can occur. Slavin et al. (694) reported on eight patients who had reconstructive correction of an irradiated partial mastectomy deformity. Mammograms were obtained before and after the myocutaneous flap procedure. Six patients had reconstructions with latissimus dorsi flaps and two with rectus flaps. No patient underwent reconstruction sooner than 1 year after completion of radiation therapy for the entire group, a mean of 2.6 years elapsed from completion of radiation therapy to flap reconstruction of the breast. An aesthetic improvement of the partial mastectomy deformity was achieved in all eight patients. Complications consisted only of seroma formation in two patients after latissimus flap reconstruction. Mammographic evaluation revealed degeneration of the soft tissues of both types of flaps, a change that occurs as early as 6 months after operation and appears as a radiolucent area.

In a review of the M.D. Anderson Cancer Center experience, Kronowitz et al. (422) evaluated results of 69 patients who underwent repair of a partial mastectomy defect after radiation. They concluded that immediate repair of partial mastectomy defects with local tissues results in a lower risk of complications and better aesthetic outcomes than immediate repair of partial mastectomy defects with a latissimus dorsi flap.

Follow-Up of Patients Treated with Breast-Conservation Surgery and Irradiation

It is important to closely monitor patients treated with conservation surgery and irradiation because early detection of a local recurrence may allow for another wide local excision or a total mastectomy, without significantly compromising the overall survival of the patient (202,243,253,311,776,782,790). Although the optimal interval for follow-up mammography has not been determined, a postradiation bilateral diagnostic mammogram should be obtained within the first year following radiation therapy (154–156,821).

A careful history and physical examination are indicated every 3 to 6 months for 3 years and every 6 months for the following 2 years, and annually thereafter. In patients who underwent breast-conservation therapy, a diagnostic mammogram every 6 to 12 months for the first 2 years and yearly thereafter is sufficient unless the radiologist recommends more frequent examinations (154–156). Monthly breast self-examination should be emphasized for every patient, including demonstration of the examination in the upright and supine positions. At least yearly evaluation is mandatory even 10 years after therapy because of the possibility of late breast relapses and occasional distant metastases. According to the American Society of Clinical On-

cology's surveillance guidelines, intensive follow-up should be limited to high-risk patients with breast cancer, especially those who enter randomized clinical trials (18).

If there is strong evidence of suspect microcalcifications, masses, or architectural distortions of the breast after conservation surgery and irradiation, a biopsy should be obtained to rule out a recurrence. At times, these patients are difficult to evaluate. Posttreatment hematomas, fat necrosis, seromas, cysts, and scar tissue pose frequent dilemmas. Consultation with an experienced mammographer is essential.

Kollias et al. (407), in the United Kingdom, evaluated 5,102 contralateral screening mammograms performed biennially on 2,511 women aged 70 years and younger after treatment for primary operable breast cancer. Sixty-five metachronous contralateral breast cancers were identified: 21 (32%) at routine clinical examination, 24 (37%) at mammography, and 20 (31%) by patients between routine follow-up appointments. The prognostic features of metachronous cancers were better than or similar to those of the first cancer in 59/65 (91%) cases. Mammography may have contributed to the long-term survival of 16/26 women in whom the histologic characteristics of the first cancer predicted a good prognosis. The cancer detection rate with mammography for these women was 6.5 per 1,000 contralateral mammograms at a cost of 3,852 pounds sterling per cancer detected, suggesting that surveillance mammography of the contralateral breast is of value in women whose first cancer predicted a favorable prognosis.

Kramer et al. (419) assessed the efficacy of contrast-enhanced dynamic MRI compared with palpation, mammography, and ultrasonography in 33 patients after breast-conservation therapy. The sensitivities for the diagnosis of local recurrences were 51% for palpation, 67% for mammography, 85% for ultrasonography, and 91% for MRI. All multicentric local recurrences were diagnosed by MRI. Mammography did not diagnose 11 local recurrences in radiodense breast, and ultrasonography was able to diagnose eight of the 11, whereas MRI diagnosed 10 of the 11 recurrences. MRI may be useful as a complement to mammography and ultrasonography in the radiodense breast (194).

It is important to define the cost-benefit ratio of follow-up procedures. In a controlled trial in Italy, 655 women were randomly assigned to be monitored with an intensive surveillance program including physician visits, bone scan, liver ultrasonography, chest radiography, and laboratory tests after initial treatment for breast cancer (775). A control group of 665 women was monitored by their physicians with physical examination and only the clinically indicated tests. Both groups received a yearly mammogram. Compliance in both protocols was more than 80%. With a median follow-up of 71 months, there was no difference in overall survival between the two groups. There were 132 deaths (20%) in the intensive surveillance group and 122 deaths (18%) in the control group. Time to detection of recurrence and parameters related to quality of life were similar in both groups. Therefore, unnecessary tests are discouraged in the follow-up of patients treated for breast cancer.

Radiographic Findings after Breast-Conservation Therapy

Dershaw (155) summarized the most frequent mammographic findings: parenchymal distortion and fibrosis at the tumor excision site (secondary to surgical scar and irradiation), skin thickening, seen in 90% of patients, which may be diffuse or more prominent at the surgical excision site, and calcifications, due to fat necrosis, which are coarse and round and have radiolucent centers. Dershaw et al. (153) retrospectively reviewed the mammograms of 22 patients with local tumor recurrence that were usually associated with 10 or more calcifications

(17 patients, 77%). Recurrences commonly contained very suspect patterns of calcification, with linear forms in 15 cases (68%) and pleomorphic forms in 17 cases (77%). The distribution of calcifications was usually clustered (73%, 16/22) or segmental (18%, 4/22). Recurrences were characterized as obviously malignant in 77% of cases. The remainder were indeterminate, requiring biopsy. Therefore, women without worrisome mammographic patterns need not undergo breast biopsy. If the findings are stable, mammographic follow-up is sufficient. However, a change in number or characteristic pattern warrants a biopsy to rule out recurrent tumor. Mammographic findings were correlated with clinical observations in several studies (154,243,298,311,493,607,608,643,714). Figure 53.38 illustrates mammographically observed changes in a patient treated with breast-conservation therapy. Most changes are observed in the first 12 months after therapy, with stabilization achieved at 12 to 36 months after completion of therapy. Breast edema is mammographically present in virtually all patients at completion of therapy, with a steady high over 36 months and stabilization by 42 months (see Fig. 53.39).

Pretreatment and posttreatment mammograms were reviewed in 103 patients undergoing conservation therapy (78). The main posttreatment findings were a diffuse increase in parenchymal density with coarse stromal pattern, some parenchymal distortion, and thickening of the skin. Changes reached a peak at 9 months and slowly resolved over the next 2 years. At 31 to 33 months, 3/15 patients still had dense parenchyma, and six had skin thickening. Sixty-nine patients had fibroadenosis. Scar with retraction in the surgical area was observed on the mammograms of 71 patients. Fat necrosis was noted in two patients. During the 3-year follow-up, recurrent cancer was noted in two treated breasts, and contralateral breast cancer developed in three women.

Orel et al. (545) reported on 1,145 women with early breast cancer treated with lumpectomy and irradiation. One hundred two women with various mammographic and clinical findings later required biopsy at the treated site, and 58 had two sets of mammograms available for review (one within 3 months of the biopsy). Recurring cancer was documented in 38/58 (66%) patients. Thirteen (34%) of the recurrences were detected solely with mammography, and eight others were detected both mammographically and clinically. The positive predictive value for mammographic abnormalities was 72% (76% for soft tissue microcalcifications and 62% for other findings). Twenty-one recurrences (55%) were within the lumpectomy quadrant. Within the lumpectomy site, sensitivity was substantially better for physical examination (71%) than for mammography (43%). In the remaining breast outside the lumpectomy quadrant, mammography had a significantly higher sensitivity (71%) and positive predictive value (86%). The most common posttreatment findings reported by Orel et al. (545,547) and Stomper et al. (719) were calcifications alone (48%) or with a mass (29%), distortion of the breast parenchyma (20%), and inflammatory thickening of the breast skin.

Stomper et al. (719) reported on 50/1,600 patients with stage I or II invasive breast cancer treated with conservation surgery and irradiation on whom biopsies were performed within 4 months of a mammogram for suspected recurrence in the irradiated breast. The tumor was suspected based on mammography in only eight patients (35%), on physical examination in nine (39%), and on both in six (26%). The most common radiographic findings were calcifications with or without a mass. Histologic evidence of recurrent cancer was found in 23/45 (51%) biopsy specimens. Sixty-five percent of patients had recurrences at the primary site and 22% in other sites 13% were multifocal.

MRI is increasingly used in the evaluation of patients with equivocal mammographic findings. Viehweg et al. (801) followed 207 patients with breast cancer treated with breast-conservation therapy: 40 patients were examined 0 to 12 months and 167 patients later than 12 months after radiation therapy. Suspect or indeterminate findings were suggested by clinical examination or conventional imaging in 80 studies. In 127 women, MRI was performed in breast tissue that was difficult to assess owing to scarring or dense breast tissue. Recurrent carcinoma was confirmed in 27 patients by surgical biopsy. All 27 carcinomas, except for one with a slow signal increase, demonstrated early rise of signal intensity on dynamic T1-weighted, contrast-enhanced images. During the first year after therapy, the diagnostic accuracy was not improved by additional use of contrast-enhanced MRI because of strong and sometimes early and ill-circumscribed enhancement. Later than 12 months after therapy, enhancement decreased significantly and the false-positive calls could be reduced from 49 (conventional imaging) to 12 (conventional imaging plus MRI). A total of 12/26 recurrences and multifocality in 4/5 cases were diagnosed by MRI alone at this time.

Dao et al. (143) evaluated 35 women with breast carcinoma treated with conservation therapy who underwent posttreatment MRI. Nine patients had recurrent tumors, and 26 had a benign fibrotic mass confirmed at biopsy. In all cases, a localized hypointense area was present on plain spin-echo T1-weighted images. In all recurrent tumors, dynamic gadolinium-enhanced T1-weighted images demonstrated early increased signal intensity of the lesion within 3 minutes after bolus injection.

Drew et al. (167) also investigated MRI for screening for local recurrence after breast-conserving therapy. One hundred five patients were recruited for the study. Sixteen biopsies were performed and nine recurrences were confirmed histologically. The sensitivity for clinical examination, mammography, examination combined with mammography, and MRI alone for the detection of recurrent cancer were 89%, 67%, 100%, and 100%, respectively, and the specificity was 76%, 85%, 67%, and 93%. The authors concluded that combined clinical examination and mammography are as sensitive as MRI of the breast for the detection of locoregional recurrence, but MRI has greater specificity.

Sequelae of Irradiation in Breast Cancer

The most frequent complications associated with conservation surgery plus irradiation are arm or breast edema, breast fibrosis, painful mastitis or myositis, pneumonitis, and rib fracture. Apical pulmonary fibrosis is occasionally noted when the regional lymph nodes are irradiated (330,452,483,736,737,811).

Lymphedema/Breast Edema

Complications from axillary surgery, regardless of breast surgical procedure, have been reported by several authors. It should be emphasized that before the treatment of arm lymphedema after breast carcinoma it is mandatory to differentiate between treatment-associated complications and tumor recurrence in the regional lymphatics.

An extensive review of the literature related to arm edema following breast surgery was conducted by Erickson et al. (187). They found that arm edema is a common complication of breast cancer therapy that can result in substantial functional impairment and psychological morbidity. The risk of arm edema increases when axillary dissection and axillary radiation therapy are used. Preventive measures have not been well studied. Nonpharmacologic treatments, such as massage and exercise, have been shown to be effective therapies for lymphedema, but the effect of pharmacologic interventions remains uncertain. They conclude that as arm edema becomes more prevalent with the increasing survival of breast cancer patients, further research is needed to evaluate the efficacy of preventive strategies and therapeutic interventions (100).

Maunsell et al. (482) evaluated frequency of upper extremity problems from axillary surgery in 223 patients. At 3 months after surgery, 82% of patients reported at least one arm problem: swelling (24%), weakness (26%), some limitation in range of movement (32%), stiffness (40%), pain (55%), and numbness (58%). The frequency of these problems changed little 15 months later. Regardless of the type of mastectomy, women who underwent axillary dissection had more problems.

Clarke et al. (121) observed breast edema in approximately 20% of patients not undergoing axillary dissection, compared with 80% of those in whom this procedure was performed. The extent of the axillary dissection (medial or lateral to the tendon of the pectoralis minor) influences the incidence of breast or arm edema, with this complication being more frequent when more extensive axillary dissections are carried out (beyond level II—middle) (803). On the other hand, Dewar et al. (160) reported a greater incidence of upper limb sequelae in patients undergoing axillary surgery and irradiation (33.7%) or irradiation alone (26%) than in patients treated with axillary dissection only (7.2%). The most frequently noted complications were edema, impaired shoulder mobility, pain on movement, sensory or motor deficit, and pectoral muscle fibrosis.

Pain and discomfort after axillary lymph node dissection were significantly related to quality of life. Hack et al. (295), in 220 women with breast cancer who had undergone axillary lymph node dissection, noted that 73% had sensation of pain or discomfort, or the point of maximum arm-shoulder movement was different between the affected and nonaffected sides. Although more than half of the patients experienced pain-related discomfort and disability, patients in general reported a good quality of life and mental health. Younger women had significantly greater pain than older women. Patients with more than 13 lymph nodes dissected and patients receiving chemotherapy reported more pain.

Sentinel node sampling appears to be associated with a much lower degree of lymphedema (465). Sener et al. (669) reported that 9/303 patients (3%) who underwent only sentinel lymphadenectomy had lymphedema, compared with 20/117 patients (17%) who underwent sentinel lymphadenectomy combined with axillary dissection ($p < .0001$). Among 303 patients who underwent sentinel lymphadenectomy only, lymphedema developed in 8/155 patients (5%) who had tumors in the upper-outer quadrant and in 1/148 patients (0.7%) whose tumors were in other locations. The ALMANAC randomized trial also confirms lower morbidity and improved quality of life following sentinel node biopsy compared to axillary dissection (465).

Various treatment regimens have been used to treat lymphedema (512). The compression pump, along with skin care, exercise, and compression garments, is one. A second treatment is known as *complex decongestive physiotherapy* or *complex physical therapy*. Arm care, therapeutic exercises, manual lymph node drainage, and compression bandages or garments comprise this treatment regime. Decreases in lymphedema are noted if women are compliant with the prescribed treatment program.

Brorson et al. (83) reported on 20 patients with arm lymphedema after breast cancer treatment who underwent liposuction combined with controlled compression therapy or controlled compression therapy alone. Liposuction combined with controlled compression therapy reduced arm edema volume by (median) 115% (range 92% to 179%), whereas controlled compression therapy alone decreased arm edema volume by only 54% (range 7% to 81%; $p = .008$).

The incidence of breast or arm edema after conservation therapy varies and is related to performance and technique of axillary dissection (see Table 53.5), regardless of whether the axillary lymph nodes were irradiated and the dose of radiation delivered.

Skin/Breast Complications

A wide variety of symptoms may occur following radiation treatment to the conservatively treated breast. McCormick et al. (483) showed that breast swelling was the most frequently noted symptom (31% of patients), followed by muscle pain (on motion), incision site pain, and general breast discomfort (approximately 20%). Rib pain was noted by 13%. Forty-eight percent of patients reported more breast discomfort in the treated breast compared with the untreated breast during sexual activity (64 sexually active patients).

In addition to host factors such as such as collagen vascular disease and diabetes, underlying genetic factors may play a role in radiation complications. Iannuzzi et al. (366) evaluated 46 patients with early stage breast carcinoma who underwent limited surgery and breast irradiation. DNA was isolated from blood lymphocytes. Nine ataxia telangiectasis mutations (ATM) were identified in six patients (eight novel and one rare). The median follow-up was 3.2 years (range 1.3 to 19.3 years). All three patients (100%) who manifested grade 3 or 4 subcutaneous late sequelae possessed ATM mutations, whereas only 3/43 (7%) patients who did not have this form of severe toxicity harbored an ATM mutation ($p = .001$).

Skin effects after postlumpectomy radiation therapy may be affected more significantly by the increase in the dose of radiation per fraction than by the total dose. Gorodetsky et al. (282) studied 110 women with breast cancer who had been treated with lumpectomies and radiation therapy and normal controls using a viscoelasticity skin analyzer. With increasing age, the viscoelasticity of the skin decreased and anisotropy increased significantly. A small but significant increase in skin stiffness was noted with radiation therapy in the range of 45 to 50 Gy given in fractions of 1.8 Gy. A dose of 50 Gy given in fractions of 2.5 Gy produced a more pronounced effect.

Pseudosclerodermatosus panniculitis is an unusual variant of panniculitis seen as a complication of radiation therapy. Carrasco et al. (103) described four women in whom this unusual entity developed on the anterior chest and abdominal skin after they received radiation therapy for either breast carcinoma or painful bone metastases from breast carcinoma. Histopathologically, the epidermis and dermis of the involved area showed little or no evidence of radiodermatitis. The main findings were in subcutaneous tissue and consisted of thickened sclerotic septa composed of both thick and thin collagen bundles, and a lobular panniculitis characterized by lipophagic granulomas and scattered lymphocytes and plasma cells. This sequela should be distinguished from subcutaneous metastatic disease, cellulitis, or connective tissue diseases involving the subcutaneous fat.

Rayan et al. (597) reported on a randomized clinical trial of breast-conserving surgery and tamoxifen with or without radiation therapy in women 50 years of age and older treated for stage T1 or T2, node-negative breast cancer. A companion study to assess breast pain was carried out during the last 2 years of accrual to the trial, in which 86 patients participated. Forty-one received radiation therapy and tamoxifen and 45 tamoxifen alone. The median age was 70 years. Baseline pain and quality-of-life scores were similar for the two groups. At 3 months, patients receiving radiation therapy experienced more breast pain compared with those receiving tamoxifen alone, but this did not reach statistical significance. At 3 months, the pain scores for the radiation therapy and tamoxifen and tamoxifen groups were 2.39 and 1.83, respectively ($p = .47$). At 12 months, pain scores were lower and fairly similar in both groups, with a difference of 0.20 ($p = .71$).

Tamoxifen has been shown to induce secretion of tumor growth factor-β (TGF-β), which has been implicated in pathogenesis of radiation fibrosis. Li et al. (444a), in a study of 91 patients with T1 or T2 breast cancer, noted that TGF-β and the receptor-ligand complex appeared to be of clinical value in identifying patients at risk for development of postirradiation fibrosis of the breast. Wazer et al. (816) showed a trend toward decreased cosmesis in patients receiving tamoxifen. In a randomized study, pulmonary fibrosis developed in 15/24 (63%) women treated with 36.6 Gy in 12 fractions and tamoxifen, compared with 10/30 (33%) receiving irradiation alone. Also, 5/14 (36%) women treated with 40.9 Gy in 22 fractions and tamoxifen had lung fibrosis, compared with 2/16 (13%) 16 receiving irradiation alone (52). In contrast, Fowble et al. (237) observed no difference in cosmetic results or complications in 154 patients who received tamoxifen in combination with breast-conservation therapy compared with 337 patients who did not receive tamoxifen. The incidences of radiation pneumonitis were 0.2% and 0.3%, respectively. The sequence of tamoxifen, given concurrently or following radiation, has not been clearly shown to correlate with complications or cosmesis (6,328,724).

Markiewicz et al. (474) analyzed complications in 1,053 women with stage I or II breast cancer treated with breast-conserving therapy. Of this group, 206 received chemotherapy alone, 141 had hormonal therapy alone, 94 had both, and 612 received no adjuvant therapy. The incidence of grade 4 or 5 arm edema (≥ 2 cm difference in arm circumference) was 2% without chemotherapy and 8% with chemotherapy ($p = .00002$). However, the incidence of arm edema was not affected by sequencing or type of chemotherapy; it occurred in 10% and 7% of patients with sequential or concurrent treatment, respectively, and in 8% and 18% of patients treated with CMF or CAF, respectively. The incidence of clinical pneumonitis and rib fracture was not influenced by use of chemotherapy, sequencing of drugs, or use of hormonal therapy. The authors concluded that some chemotherapy could be given concurrently with radiation therapy to the breast without significant compromise of cosmetic results or sequelae of treatment.

Hyperbaric oxygen therapy has been shown to be effective in the treatment of some late radiation sequelae. Carl et al. (102) reported on 44 patients with persistent local symptoms after breast-conserving therapy. Hyperbaric oxygen therapy (100% oxygen at 240 kPa for 90-minute sessions) was administered to 32 patients for a median of 25 sessions (range 7 to 60 sessions). The remaining 12 patients declined hyperbaric treatment and acted as control subjects. The patients given hyperbaric oxygen therapy demonstrated a significant reduction in pain, edema, and erythema scores compared with untreated control subjects ($p < .001$). Seven of the 32 women who were treated with hyperbaric oxygen therapy were free of symptoms after treatment, whereas all 12 patients in the control group had persistent complaints. However, hyperbaric oxygen therapy did not have a significant effect on fibrosis and telangiectasia in the irradiated breast.

Brachial Plexopathy

Brachial plexus dysfunction is a possible complication of regional nodal radiation therapy. In a review of 1,624 patients, Pierce et al. (580) found that brachial plexus sequelae were observed in 1.8% of patients. They also found that the incidence of brachial plexopathy was significantly higher when the axillary dose was >50 Gy ($p = .004$). However, dose alone did not determine whether radiation damage would develop in a given patient. Treatment technique (two vs. three fields; $p = .0009$) and concomitant chemotherapy were also risk factors. Other investigators have found the incidence of this complication to be 1% or less (151,246). It is very important but difficult to distinguish between metastatic and radiation-induced brachial plexopathy.

Treatment for radiation brachial plexopathy consists of transdermal electrical nerve stimulation, dorsal column stimulators, neurolysis, and neurolysis with omentoplasty. Physical therapy, tricyclics, antiarrhythmics, anticonvulsives, nonsteroidal anti-inflammatory drugs, and steroids are helpful in therapy of both radiation-induced and metastatic brachial plexopathies (414).

Pritchard et al. (590) used hyperbaric oxygen in 34 volunteers with radiation-induced brachial plexopathy who were randomized to hyperbaric oxygen or a control group. The hyperbaric oxygen group breathed 100% oxygen for 100 minutes in a hyperbaric chamber (30 sessions over 6 weeks). The control group breathed a gas mixture equivalent to breathing 100% oxygen at surface pressure. Normalization of the warm sensory threshold was seen in two of the patients receiving hyperbaric oxygen therapy. Two cases with marked chronic arm lymphedema reported major improvement in arm volume. The authors concluded that there is no reliable evidence to support hyperbaric oxygen therapy to slow or reverse radiation-induced brachial plexopathy, although improvements in a warm sensory threshold suggest a therapeutic effect in long-standing arm lymphedema and justifies further investigation.

Pulmonary Sequelae

Symptomatic pneumonitis is infrequent. This clinical syndrome is noted one to several months after irradiation (393). Patients present with dry cough (88%), shortness of breath (35%), or fever (53%), and on radiographic studies a pulmonary infiltrate is observed in the irradiated volume (452). The risk for development of radiation pneumonitis may be related to the volume of lung irradiated (452,637).

The addition of regional nodal radiation therapy to breast irradiation significantly increases the incidence of symptomatic pneumonitis (1% without and 4% with regional node radiation therapy; $p < .001$). Combined axillary dissection and nodal irradiation results in a significantly higher incidence of arm edema compared with either alone (9.5% with axillary dissection, 6.1% with radiation therapy to the axilla and supraclavicular fossa, and 31% with combined modality therapy; $p < .001$) (637).

Lingos et al. (452) reported on radiation pneumonitis in a retrospective review of 1,624 patients treated with conservation surgery and irradiation. Overall, pneumonitis developed in 1% of patients. No patient had late or persisting pulmonary symptoms. The incidence of radiation pneumonitis was correlated with the combined use of chemotherapy and a supraclavicular field ($p = .0001$). Fourteen of 17 patients who had radiation pneumonitis also had IMNs treated. When patients treated with a three-field technique received chemotherapy concurrently with irradiation, the incidence of radiation pneumonitis was 8.8% (8/92), compared with 1.3% (3/236) for those who received sequential chemotherapy and irradiation to the breast only, and 0.5% (6/1,296) for those treated with irradiation to the breast only without chemotherapy ($p = .002$). In this study, the volume of lung irradiated did not correlate with the risk for development of radiation pneumonitis.

Taghian et al. (732), in 41 patients treated with radiation therapy and paclitaxel (21 concurrent, 20 sequential), also described a higher incidence of pneumonitis (14.6%) compared with control patients irradiated and not receiving chemotherapy (1.1%; $p < .0001$). Burstein et al. (90) also recently reported that the concurrent use of weekly paclitaxel with radiation result in high rates of pneumonitis. However, an analysis of patients treated with radiation as a component of a randomized trial in which 50% of the patients were treated with paclitaxel and 50% treated with a nontaxane regimen, found that the rates of pneumonitis were very low and not significantly different between the two arms (845).

The effect of tangential field technique on pulmonary function was reported by Lund et al. (458) in 25 patients treated with conservation surgery and irradiation. Dynamic and static lung

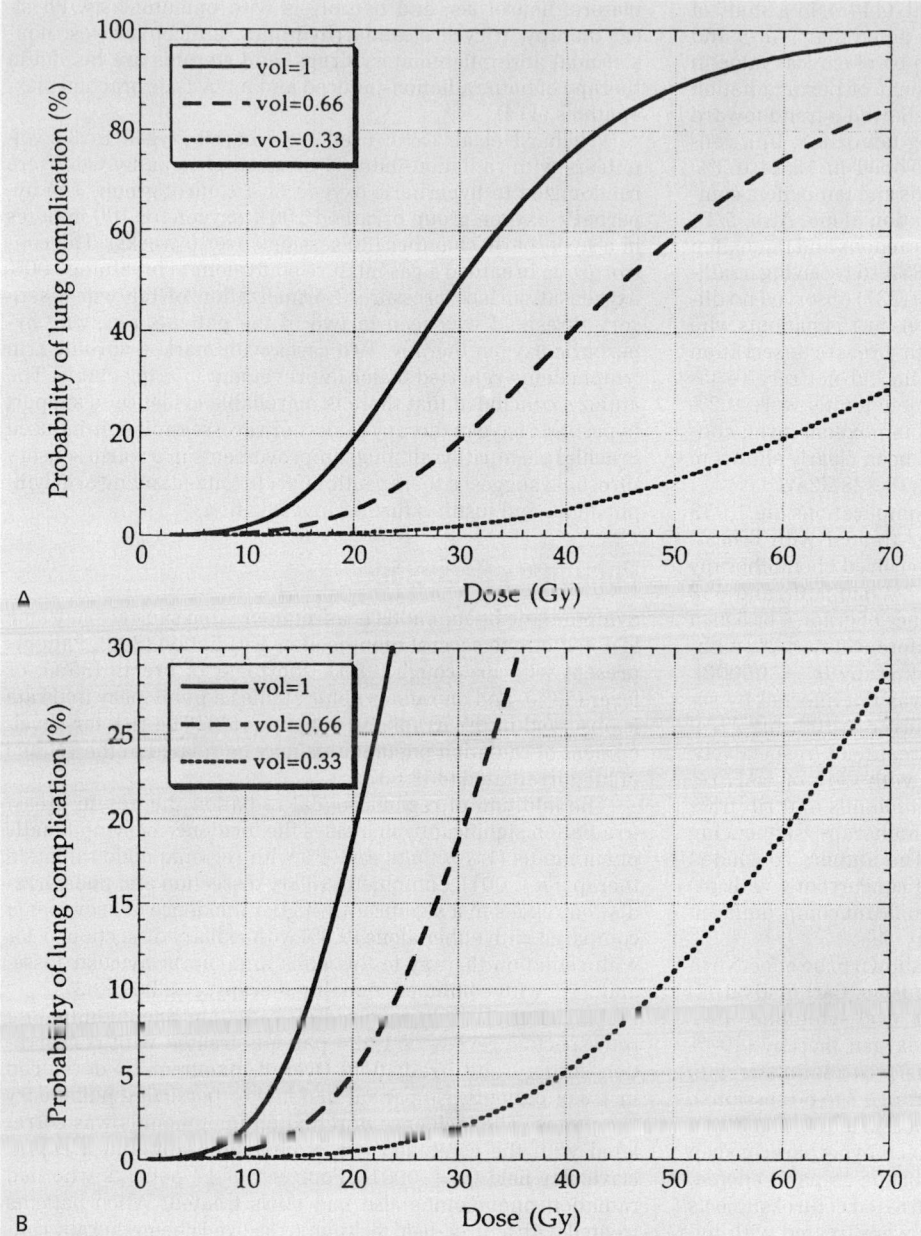

FIGURE 53.54. Probability of radiation pneumonitis versus dose. The relative lung volumes are 100%, 66%, and 33%. The curve parameters are $D_{50} = 30$ Gy, $\gamma = 1.01$, $s = 0.01$. The curves cover the probability range up to 100% **(A)**, and up to 30% (i.e., within the interval of the clinical data) **(B)**. (From Gagliardi G, Bjohle J, Lax I, et al. Radiation pneumonitis after breast cancer irradiation: analysis of the complication probability using the relative seriality model. *Int J Radiat Oncol Biol Phys* 2000;46:373–381, with permission.)

volumes, distribution of ventilation, and gas transfer were measured before irradiation and at varying intervals up to 1 year after completion of therapy. There was a small but statistically significant decrease in the forced vital capacity and forced expired volume in one second 3 months after irradiation ($p < .05$). These changes normalized within 1 year. The reduction in total lung capacity after 3 months almost achieved statistical significance ($p = .06$). These slight restrictive ventilatory changes are reversible and have no clinical importance.

Radiation pneumonitis was retrospectively assessed on the basis of clinical symptoms and radiologic findings using a serial organ model by Gagliardi et al (264). As demonstrated in Figure 53.54, a lung volume effect was relevant in the description of radiation pneumonitis. Lind et al. (450) measured pulmonary function 5 months after radiation therapy in 144 patients with node-positive stage II breast cancer. No deterioration of pulmonary function was detected among the patients who were treated with local radiation therapy. Patients undergoing locoregional radiation therapy showed a 5% mean reduction in

diffusion capacity ($p < .001$) and a 3% mean reduction in vital capacity ($p = .001$).

Cardiac Sequelae

The potential for excess cardiac morbidity associated with the use of radiation therapy in breast cancer has been extensively evaluated. It has been clearly demonstrated, based on data from randomized trials, overview, and meta-analysis, that when using older techniques, excess cardiac mortality from radiation offset some of the benefits that radiation therapy clearly produced with respect to breast cancer mortality (138,198,244). Although the evidence from more modern trials, using techniques that minimize exposure to the normal cardiac and pulmonary structures, have reduced cardiac toxicity, the radiation oncologist must be cognizant of the potential for adverse cardiac effects of incidental irradiation, particularly in the setting of left-sided breast cancers in patients receiving other cardiotoxic therapies, including adriamycin, epirubicin, and trastuzumab (673,674).

Earlier techniques of radiation therapy have clearly been implicated in excess cardiac mortality from large pools of randomized data. In an analysis of over 90,000 Swedish women, comparing left- to right-sided cancers, Darby et al. (144), from the Oxford group, reported excess ischemic heart disease mortality more than 10 years after initial treatment in the left sided cancer group (HR 1.13, 95% CI, 1.03 to 1.25; $p = .01$). The majority of cardiovascular deaths were from earlier studies using techniques that are no longer used. However, for patients treated after 1980, although the ratio was still 1.11, the confidence intervals were much larger (0.95 to 1.29), so the hazard remains uncertain for the more modern techniques.

Gyenes et al. (292) reported on the incidence of ischemic heart disease 15 to 20 years after adjuvant radiation therapy in 960 patients with breast cancer enrolled in the Stockholm Breast Cancer Trial. Of 37 long-term survivors, 20 received left-sided therapy and 17 received right-sided therapy or no therapy. Radiation therapy consisted of ^{60}Co tangential fields for preoperative treatment and electron beam portals, which included the IMNs, for postoperative therapy (45 to 50 Gy). Evaluation consisted of echocardiography (ECG), exercise stress tests with ^{99m}Tc myocardial perfusion scan, and careful history for cardiac risk factors. Results showed that 5/20 (25%) patients treated with left-sided radiation had defects on ^{99m}Tc scan, compared with none of 17 control patients ($p = .05$).

Paszat et al. (557) conducted a study of 25,570 cases of invasive female breast cancer that were linked to radiation therapy records from Ontario cancer centers. Postlumpectomy radiation therapy was administered to 1,555 patients on the left side and to 1,451 on the right side. Two percent of women with left-sided radiation therapy had a fatal myocardial infarction compared with 1% of women with right-sided radiation therapy ($p = .02$). Adjusting for age at diagnosis, the relative risk for fatal myocardial infarction with left-sided postlumpectomy radiation therapy was 2.10.

Rutqvist et al. (640) followed 684 patients with breast cancer treated with breast-conserving surgery and radiation therapy using tangential photon fields (48 to 52 Gy in 4.5 to 5.5 weeks). The median follow-up was 9 years. In 88% of patients, the target volume involved the breast only in the remaining patients, and regional nodes were irradiated. A control group included 4,996 patients with breast cancer who underwent mastectomies without postoperative radiation therapy. Twelve patients (1.8%) in the irradiated group had myocardial infarctions and five patients (0.7%) died as a result of myocardial infarctions. The relative risk for a myocardial infarction between the irradiated group and the control group was 0.6, and the relative risk for death was 0.4. The study presents no evidence that the risk for myocardial infarction is increased with radiation therapy after breast-conserving surgery no matter on which side the tumor was located. However, because the number of myocardial infarctions in the study was small, there is no way to rule out the possibility of cardiac problems in patients with left breast carcinomas.

Shapiro et al. (673) assessed the cardiac effects in 299 patients with breast cancer prospectively randomized to receive either five cycles or 10 cycles of cyclophosphamide and a doxorubicin intravenous bolus every 21 days. Of the 299 patients, 122 received radiation therapy. The risk of major cardiac events (congestive heart failure, acute myocardial infarction) was assessable in 276 patients, with a median follow-up of 6 years (range 0.5 to 19.4 years). The estimated risk of cardiac events per 100 patient-years was significantly higher for 10 cycles than for five cycles of chemotherapy (1.7 vs. 0.5; $p = .02$). The risk of cardiac events in the five-cycle patients, regardless of the cardiac radiation therapy dose-volume, did not differ significantly from rates of cardiac events predicted for a general female population. For patients receiving 10 cycles, the incidence of cardiac events was significantly increased (relative risk ratio 3.6; $p < .00003$) compared with the general population, particularly in groups that also received moderate- and high-dose-volume cardiac radiation therapy.

Cuzick et al. (138) updated cardiac toxicity data from eight randomized trials initiated before 1975 in which radiotherapy was the randomized option and surgery was the same for both treatment arms. An initial analysis of these trials demonstrated an increased all-cause mortality rate in 10-year survivors associated with radiation, but in the update this was no longer present. The initial increase mortality in the radiation arms was strongly influenced by the earliest trials, and more recent trials have found a nonsignificant net benefit in overall mortality associated with radiation therapy. However, an excess of cardiac deaths was apparent in both early and more recent trials ($p < .001$), but this was offset by a reduced number of deaths due to breast cancer, especially in more recent trials. Based on this, it is clearly prudent to use techniques that minimize cardiac dose.

Although clinical evidence of cardiac morbidity has decreased with modern techniques, care should be taken to exclude heart from the tangential radiation field. In an analysis of 114 patients, Marks et al. (475) assessed radiotherapy-induced left ventricular perfusion defects and whether these perfusion defects are related to changes in cardiac wall motion or alterations in ejection fraction. Patients were imaged 30 to 60 minutes after injection of technetium ^{99m} sestamibi or tetrofosmin. Postradiotherapy perfusion scans were compared with the preradiotherapy studies to assess for radiotherapy-induced perfusion defects as well as functional changes in wall motion and ejection fraction. The incidence of new perfusion defects 6, 12, 18, and 24 months after radiotherapy was 27%, 29%, 38%, and 42%, respectively. New defects occurred in approximately 10% to 20% and 50% to 60% of patients with <5%, and >5%, of their left ventricle included within the radiotherapy fields, respectively. The rates of wall motion abnormalities in patients with and without perfusion defects were 12% to 40% versus 0% to 9%. The authors note that radiation therapy causes volume-dependent perfusion defects in approximately 40% of patients within 2 years of radiotherapy, and that these perfusion defects are associated with corresponding wall-motion abnormalities. However, additional study is necessary to determine if these defects are associated with functional consequences.

Given these findings, the authors suggest the use of a heart block if needed to reduce or eliminate cardiac irradiation. CT-based three-dimensional treatment planning is used to design such cardiac blocks and select the optimal gantry angle to minimize the need for a heart block. There may be a small amount of breast tissue underdosed if the block overlies the medial inferior breast, but this tissue is typically <5%. In situations where the heart block may underdose the high-risk volume of the breast or chest wall, an "electron patch" can be used to treat the target tissue in the shadow of the heart block. A tangential field with a heart block is demonstrated in Figure 53.35.

Although it is clearly prudent to minimize exposure of the heart during radiation therapy, using modern techniques the available evidence does not suggest a higher incidence of cardiac mortality in left-sided radiation therapy.

Analysis of the randomized postmastectomy Danish trials, with over 10-year follow-up, showed no excess cardiac mortality with the use of postmastectomy radiation. Hojris et al. (352) reported the relative hazard of morbidity from ischemic heart disease among patients in the radiotherapy compared with the no-radiotherapy group was 0.86 (95% CI, 0.6 to 1.3), and that for death from ischemic heart disease the relative hazard was 0.84 (CI, 0.4 to 1.8). The hazard rate of morbidity from ischemic heart disease in the radiotherapy group compared with the no-radiotherapy group did not increase with time from treatment.

Patt et al. (559) analyzed data from the Surveillance, Epidemiology, and End Results–Medicare database for women who were diagnosed with nonmetastatic breast cancer from 1986 to 1993, had known disease laterality, underwent breast surgery, and received adjuvant radiotherapy. The study was comprised of 8,363 patients who had left-sided breast cancer and 7,907 who had right-sided breast cancer. With a mean follow-up of 9.5 years (range 0 to 15 years), there were no significant differences in patients with left- versus right-sided cancers for hospitalization for ischemic heart disease (9.9% vs. 9.7%), valvular heart disease (2.9% vs. 2.8%), conduction abnormalities (9.7% vs. 9.6%), or heart failure (9.7% vs. 9.7%). The adjusted hazard ratio for left- versus right-sided breast cancer was 1.05 (95% CI, 0.94 to 1.16) for ischemic heart disease, 1.07 (95% CI, 0.89 to 1.30) for valvular heart disease, 1.07 (95% CI, 0.96 to 1.19) for conduction abnormalities, and 1.05 (95% CI, 0.95 to 1.17) for heart failure.

Similar conclusions were reached by Nixon et al. (528), who reviewed 365 patients with 12-year follow-up who received irradiation to the left breast and 380 who received irradiation to the right breast as part of conservation therapy. Equivalent proportions from each group died of non–breast cancer causes (11%), including nine patients (2%) from each group who died from cardiac causes. Also, Vallis et al. (764), in a retrospective review of 2,128 women treated with lumpectomy and breast irradiation with a median follow-up of 10.2 years, noted that the incidence of myocardial infarction in the study cohort was comparable with that in an age-matched general population of women in Ontario.

Collectively, these data suggest no excess cardiac morbidity using tangential fields to treat left-sided breast cancers. However, it is prudent to minimize cardiac exposure in all patients, and particularly in those receiving left-sided radiation in combination with other potentially cardiotoxic drugs.

Risk of Stroke with Supraclavicular Radiation

For patients with node-positive disease undergoing supraclavicular radiation, there is a theoretical concern regarding the potential for development of accelerated carotid artery stenosis. In a recent study by Jagsi et al. (373) rates of stroke in 820 eligible early stage breast cancer patients treated with radiation therapy were compared with expected rates. Relationships between potential risk factors and actuarial rate of first stroke were analyzed. On multivariate analysis, only age ($p < .001$) and hypertension ($p = .003$) remained significant predictors of cardiovascular accident/transient ischemic attack. Age was the only significant predictor of cardiovascular accident alone ($p < .001$). This study found no significant association between supraclavicular radiotherapy and stroke after controlling for other factors. This study is in agreement with the findings of the Early Breast Cancer Trialists' Collaborative Group who reported the causes of non–breast cancer death in 32,800 patients treated in trials of surgery with and without radiotherapy. Although the incidence of heart disease was found to be significantly greater in those women who received radiotherapy, no significant excess mortality from radiotherapy was observed due to stroke.

Contralateral Breast Cancer and Irradiation

Although all patients with a diagnosis of breast cancer are at increased risk for developing contralateral breast cancer, the additional risk contributed by radiation treatment appears to be minimal, particularly when one uses modern techniques and maintains a dose to the contralateral breast that is as low as is reasonably achievable. Although this issue is often a concern raised by patients, the available data using modern radiation techniques do not suggest a significant increased risk of contralateral breast cancers in breast cancer patients who have been irradiated, in comparison to similar cohorts of breast cancer patients who have not undergone radiation (67,201, 330,525,537,811). Although there is some evidence suggesting a slight excess risk in women who are irradiated at a relatively young age (i.e., <45 years at diagnosis), the risk is extremely small and may be related to older techniques, and most experts would agree that the benefit of radiation far outweighs the risk (67). Nonetheless, it appears prudent to be aware of these potential risks and employ techniques that minimize scattered dose to the contralateral breast. As demonstrated in Table 53.42, the reported incidence of contralateral cancer in the majority of these studies of patients treated with conservative surgery and radiation do not appear to be elevated compared to those treated by mastectomy without radiation.

However, the EBCTCG overview analysis does suggest an elevated incidence of contralateral breast cancer in patients receiving radiation compared to those who did not receive radiation (124). This overview analysis of all randomized trials comparing radiation to surgery demonstrated an increased relative risk of contralateral breast cancers of 1.18 ($p = .002$). Although the excess risk appears to be driven primarily by older trials using antiquated techniques, these data do demonstrate the potential long-term effects of radiation-related secondary cancers and highlight the need to maintain dose to the contralateral breast as low as possible.

A report by Hankey et al. (324), involving 27,175 women treated for breast cancer between 1960 and 1975, disclosed an RR of 1.2 to 1.4 for development of cancer in the contralateral breast in irradiated patients compared with those who did not receive irradiation. The authors, however, concluded that the data did not indicate a pattern of relative risk consistent with an increased incidence of carcinoma in the opposite breast.

Boice et al. (67) evaluated the risk of second cancers associated with radiation therapy to the breast in 41,109 women with breast cancer who were registered in the Connecticut Tumor Registry between 1935 and 1982. They reviewed the records of 655 women in whom a second breast cancer developed 5 years or longer after initial treatment and compared the radiation exposure in these patients with the exposure in 1,189 matched control patients who did not have a second cancer. The average dose to the contralateral breast in women exposed to radiation was 2.82 Gy. The RR for development of a second breast cancer was 1.9 in the women who received radiation therapy, among patients who survived for 10 years or longer, the RR was 1.33. Women younger than 45 years of age had an RR of 1.59 for development of a second breast cancer, compared with 1.01 for older women. According to these authors, younger patients should be informed that, based on the results of this study, after 10 years the risk for development of a second cancer increases from 14% if they did not receive irradiation to 22% if they chose treatment involving irradiation.

On the other hand, Levitt and Mandell (443) estimated the dose delivered to the contralateral breast to be between 1 and 4 Gy. Assuming that 20,000 women undergo radiation therapy after conservation surgery, and using data on the risk for development of breast cancer after various doses of ionizing radiation, they concluded that fewer than one additional case of breast cancer would occur after 10 years. Storm et al. (720), in a case-controlled study of a registry-based cohort of patients with breast cancer in Denmark, also concluded there was little, if any, risk of radiation-induced breast cancer associated with exposure of adult breast tissue to low-dose irradiation.

Obedian et al. (537) compared 1,029 breast cancer patients treated with conservative surgery and radiation to a cohort of 1,387 breast cancer patients who underwent surgical treatment by mastectomy and who did not receive postoperative

Table 53.42	INCIDENCE OF CONTRALATERAL BREAST CANCER IN CARCINOMA OF THE BREAST TREATED WITH CONSERVATION SURGERY AND IRRADIATION OR MASTECTOMY	
Study (Reference)	**Conservation Therapy**	**Mastectomy**
Arriagada et al. (28)[a]	88 (14%)	91 (11%)
Broët et al. (82)	1,819 (3.8%)	1,815 (3.9%)
Clark et al. (119)	1,504 (3%)	—
Dewar et al. (159)	757 (6%)[b]	—
Hill-Keyser et al. (349)	1,801 (15.4%)[c]	—
Montague (506)	316 (1.9%)[d]	576 (5.2%)
Nielsen et al. (524)	—	No RT 1,545 (4%) RT 1,538 (5%)
Obedian et al. (537)	1,029 (10%)[e]	1,387 (10%)[e]
Recht et al. (607)	366 (9%)[f]	—
Rosen et al. (631)	—	RT, 76 (10.7%) No RT, 47 (9.4%)
Sarrazin et al. (650)	88 (9%)	91 (9%)
Veronesi et al. (778)	349 (5%)[g]	352 (5%)[g]

RT, radiation therapy
[a]Risk at 15 y (update of Sarrazin et al. data [650]).
[b]Actuarial relapse at 10 y.
[c]Actuarial risk at 20 y.
[d]Excludes simultaneous bilateral cancer.
[f]Actuarial risk at 5 y.
[e]Actuarial risk at 15 y.
[g]Actuarial risk at 12 y.

radiation during the same time period. The median follow-up was 14.6 years for the conservatively treated group and 16 years for the mastectomy group. The 15-year risk of any second malignancy was nearly identical for both cohorts (17.5% vs. 19%, respectively). The second breast malignancy rate at 15 years was 10% for both groups. In the subset of patients 45 years of age or younger at the time of treatment, the second breast and nonbreast malignancy rates at 15 years were 10% and 5% for patients undergoing breast-conserving therapy versus 7% and 4% for patients undergoing mastectomy (p = not statistically significant).

To address whether the radiation administered may influence the development of breast cancers on the contralateral side, Khan and Haffty (400) evaluated the location of contralateral breast cancers developing after radiation. There was not a preponderance of medial lesions developing in the contralateral group (where radiation dose would be higher), suggesting that there was no cause-effect relationship with respect to the prior radiation. In a study by Hill-Kayser et al. (349) the 20-year risk of contralateral breast cancer in 1,801 patients treated with breast-conserving surgery and radiation was 15.4%. They also demonstrated that the distribution of location of the contralateral tumors did not appear to be influenced by the prior irradiation.

In a recent update of the Danish randomized trials of postmastectomy radiation, Nielsen et al. (525) also do not report an excess risk of second malignancies in the contralateral breast in patients randomized to receive radiation. In this long-term follow-up performed among the 3,083 patients from the Danish Breast Cancer Cooperative Group 82B-C, randomized to postmastectomy radiation or not, there was no significance in the risk of contralateral breast cancers (6% radiotherapy vs. 5% no radiotherapy) between the two groups.

Incidence of Other Second Malignancies

The incidence of secondary malignancies, as with the issue of contralateral breast cancer, appears to be very low and it is evident that the appropriate use of radiation therapy far outweighs the risk of radiation-induced malignancy. Nonetheless, there is some evidence, with very long-term follow-up, of higher rates of secondary cancers. Although this may be more prevalent with older techniques, it is an important component of treatment planning to minimize dose to nontarget normal tissues. In addition to the excess risk of contralateral breast cancers discussed previously, the EBCTCG overview analysis did demonstrate an excess risk of secondary cancers of the lung, esophagus, leukemia, and sarcoma in all randomized trials of breast cancer that compared patients treated with and without radiation. The increased relative risk for each of these secondary malignancies as a function of radiation treatment for breast cancer was lung cancer, 1.61 (+/−0.18; p = .007); esophagus cancer, 2.06 (+/− 0.53; p = .05), leukemia, 1.71 (+/− 0.36; p = .03), and sarcoma, 2.34 (+/− 0.62; p = .03). The total relative risk for all secondary nonbreast malignancies was 1.20 (+/− 0.06; p = .001). Although the increased risk of secondary malignancies may be driven primarily by trials using older techniques, they highlight the importance of limiting dose to nontarget tissues.

Huang and Mackillop (359), in an analysis of 194,798 women from the SEER database who were diagnosed with invasive breast carcinoma (exclusive of those with distant metastasis) between 1973 and 1995, identified 54 women in a radiation therapy cohort and 81 women in a non-radiation therapy cohort in whom soft tissue sarcoma subsequently developed. In the radiation therapy cohort, the standardized incidence ratio was 26.2 for angiosarcoma and 2.5 for other sarcomas in the non-radiation therapy cohort, the standardized incidence ratios were 2.1 and 1.3 (95% CI, 1.0 to 1.7), respectively. The largest increase was observed in the chest wall breast. The elevated RR was significant even within 5 years of radiation therapy, but it reached a maximum between 5 to 10 years.

Karlsson et al. (391) quantified the risk of posttreatment sarcoma in 122,991 women with breast cancer in the Swedish Cancer Register. In this group 116 cases were found, giving a standardized incidence ratio of 1.9 per 10^4 women. The absolute risk was 1.3 per 10^4 person-years. There were 40 angiosarcomas and 76 sarcomas of other types. The sarcomas were located in the breast region or on the ipsilateral arm in 63% (67/106). In a case-control study, angiosarcoma correlated significantly with lymphedema of the arm (overall recovery, 0.5), but no correlation with previous irradiation was observed. However, for other histologic types of sarcomas, the risk increased linearly with the integral dose to 150 to 200 J and stabilized at higher energies. The risk was 2.4 for an energy of 50 J, approximately corresponding to the radiation of the breast after breast-conserving surgery.

More contemporary retrospective series have not reported an excess risk of secondary malignancies. However, interpretation of these series is limited by follow-up periods of <20 years, which may not be adequate. A study by Fowble et al. (239) that evaluated nonbreast malignancies, with approximately 9 years of follow-up, reported that the 10-year risk of second malignancy was 16% for all cancers, 7% for contralateral breast cancer, and 8% for all second non–breast cancer malignancies. Obedian et al. (537) also reported no increased risk of second nonbreast malignancies in patients treated with conservative surgery and radiation compared to a cohort treated with mastectomy without radiation during the same time interval. The 15-year risk of a second nonbreast malignancy was 11% for the radiation group and 10% for the mastectomy group.

Galper et al. (268) analyzed the risk for development of second nonbreast malignancies in 1,884 patients with clinical stage I or II breast cancer treated with excision and radiation therapy. By 8 years of follow-up 147 (8%) had a second nonbreast malignancy compared with the 127.7 expected from SEER. This corresponds to an absolute excess of 1% of the study population and a relative increase of 15% greater than expected from SEER ($p = .05$). Lung as a second nonbreast malignancy was observed in 33 women, 50% more than the 21.67 predicted by SEER ($p = .01$), although most of the lung malignancies occurred <5 years after treatment. Of seven sarcomas, three developed in the radiation field. Second nonbreast malignancies occurred in a substantial minority (8%) of patients treated with conservation surgery and radiation therapy. However, the absolute excess risk compared with the general population was very small (1%) and only evident after 5 years.

Ahsan and Neugut (7) reviewed SEER data in 220,806 women in whom breast cancer was diagnosed between January 1, 1973, and December 31, 1993. In women who had received radiation therapy for breast cancer, the RR for esophageal squamous cell carcinoma increased to 5.42 and the RR for esophageal adenocarcinoma increased to 4.22 10 years or more after radiation therapy. No increased risk was seen for either type of carcinoma among patients with breast cancer who did not receive radiation therapy.

The available evidence of the risk of lung cancer in patients undergoing radiation suggests that smoking and radiation may be synergistic in contributing to the risk of lung cancer. Ford et al. (230) analyzed smoking, radiation, and both exposures on lung carcinoma development in women who were treated previously for breast carcinoma in a case-control study of 280 female patients with a diagnosis of breast cancer prior to lung cancer. Smoking increased the odds of lung carcinoma in women without radiation (odds ratio 6.0; 95% CI, 3.6 to 10.1), but radiation did not increase lung carcinoma risk in nonsmoking women (overall recovery, 0.5; 95% CI, 0.3 to 1.1). The overall recovery rate for both radiation and smoking, compared with no radiation or smoking, was 9.0 (95% CI, 5.1 to 15.9). The authors conclude that smoking is a significant independent risk factor for lung carcinoma after breast carcinoma, but radiation alone was not. Smoking and radiation combined enhanced the effect of either alone.

Deutsch et al. (157), in a long-term analysis of the NSABP-04 and NSABP-06 trials, suggests an excess risk of lung cancers associated with the extent of radiation. The records of all patients who developed a recurrence in the lung or a new primary lung tumor were reviewed to determine the incidence and laterality of confirmed and probable primary lung carcinoma. For the NSABP-04 trial, which employed more comprehensive

radiation with larger lung volumes, there were a total of 23 subsequent confirmed and probable ipsilateral or contralateral primary lung carcinomas. In those patients who had received comprehensive postmastectomy radiotherapy, there was a statistically significant increase in the incidence of these new primary tumors ($p = .029$). With regard to the development of confirmed new primary ipsilateral lung carcinoma alone, the incidence was statistically significantly increased ($p = .013$) in those patients who had received radiotherapy as part of their treatment, and when confirmed and probable ipsilateral lung carcinomas were analyzed, there was a strong trend toward a statistically significant increase in those patients who had received radiotherapy ($p = .066$). For the NSABP B-06 trial (mean follow-up of 19 years), there was a total of 30 second primary lung carcinomas but no increase in either ipsilateral or contralateral primary tumors of the lung in those patients who had received radiotherapy. They conclude that extensive postmastectomy irradiation of the chest wall and regional lymphatic node areas, with consequent exposure of a greater volume of lung to higher doses as administered in the NSABP B-04 trial compared with postlumpectomy breast irradiation in the NSABP B-06 trial, was associated with an increased incidence of subsequent primary lung tumors, both ipsilateral and contralateral. Unfortunately, data regarding smoking were not available in this analysis.

Postirradiation Angiosarcoma of the Breast

Special attention should be paid to uncommon skin changes of the treated breast because clinical suspicion is the main clue to the diagnosis of postirradiation angiosarcoma. The primary therapy is simple mastectomy if wide tumor-free margins can be achieved. At this time, there is no clear indication for standard adjuvant chemotherapy or irradiation. Angiosarcomas arising in the field of radiation therapy are rare. Unlike other radiation-induced sarcomas, cutaneous angiosarcoma often occurs within a short time after irradiation. It is important to differentiate atypical vascular lesions from angiosarcoma, but currently there is no evidence that they represent a precursor to radiation-induced angiosarcoma. Deutsch and Rosenstein (158) reported an angiosarcoma arising in the breast more than 7 years after lumpectomy and breast irradiation. The initial appearance was very similar to late radiation dermatitis, and the true nature of the malignant lesion was not known for 23 months. Fineberg and Rosen (200) studied three patients with cutaneous angiosarcoma and four patients with atypical vascular lesions. All had breast-conserving surgery and axillary lymph node dissection, and six patients received conventional high energy postoperative doses of external beam radiation to the breast. Angiosarcoma was diagnosed 3.5, 3.7, and 5.25 years after radiation therapy. The three angiosarcomas were multifocal or diffuse and high grade, with solid cellular foci located mainly in the dermis. Two patients with angiosarcoma underwent mastectomy: one died 10 months after diagnosis with recurrent local angiosarcoma, and the other was alive and tumor free 2 months after diagnosis.

Feigenberg et al. (196) reported results of hyperfractionated radiation therapy in conjunction with surgery for angiosarcoma occurring after breast-conserving therapy in three patients. All three patients were treated initially with radical surgery for the angiosarcoma, but extensive recurrences were noted within 1 to 2 months of surgery. Because of the extremely rapid growth before and after surgery, hyperfractionated radiation therapy was used. Two of the patients underwent resection of the recurrence after radiation therapy, and neither specimen demonstrated any evidence of high-grade angiosarcoma. All three patients were alive without any recurrent disease 22, 38, and 39 months after treatment. For previously untreated angiosarcoma, the authors recommend hyperfractionated radiation therapy followed by surgery to enhance disease control, and in recurring tumors removing as much reirradiated tissue as possible.

Thirty-six cases of angiosarcoma after irradiation had been reported in the literature, and Edeiken et al. (174) presented two additional patients treated with breast-conserving treatment in whom angiosarcoma developed in the field of prior irradiation. Seven cases of angiosarcoma after radiation therapy for breast-conserving treatment of breast carcinoma had been reported, and the average time between the administration of radiation therapy and development of angiosarcoma was 8.6 years.

Marchal et al. (470) reported on nine breast angiosarcomas identified in a review of 18,115 patients who underwent breast-conserving treatment for carcinomas at 11 French cancer centers over a 20-year period ending in 1997. The estimated prevalence of angiosarcomas after breast-conserving therapy for carcinomas was 5/10,000, which is approximately the same as for primary angiosarcomas in healthy breasts. The patients had a mean age of 62.5 years when the primary breast cancer was treated and 69 years when the angiosarcoma was diagnosed. Most angiosarcomas were stage T1/N0/M0 and were treated with radical mastectomy; two patients underwent reirradiation, and two patients were given adjuvant chemotherapy. The time to the median survival after diagnosis of an angiosarcoma was 15.5 months. One patient was alive without progression of disease 32 months after a salvage mastectomy, and the rest had died.

In a series of 3,295 patients treated with conservative surgery and irradiation for breast cancer, Zucali et al. (851) observed three cases of soft tissue sarcoma in the irradiated breasts. It appears from these collective experiences that the risk of a second primary tumor in the irradiated breast is too low to justify modification of current policies of conservation therapy of breast cancer.

A rare complication after radical mastectomy is development of lymphangiosarcoma. It is associated with the development of lymphedema in the affected extremity and occurs in approximately 5/1,000 patients who have radical mastectomy and survive 5 years (478).

Cost-Benefit in Breast Cancer Treatment

Barlow et al. (38) compared the total medical care costs of breast-conservation therapy versus a mastectomy to 5 years after diagnosis in 1,675 women with early stage breast cancer, from a regional nonprofit health maintenance organization, who had initial diagnoses between 1990 and 1997 and were 35 years of age or older. These women were classified into four groups according to treatment: mastectomy only (group 1, $n = 183$), mastectomy plus adjuvant therapy (group 2, $n = 417$), breast-conservation therapy plus radiation therapy (group 3, $n = 405$), and breast-conservation therapy plus radiation therapy and adjuvant therapy (group 4, $n = 670$). At 6 months, the costs of the treatments differed significantly ($p < .001$). Breast-conservation therapy was more expensive than mastectomy. At 1 year, costs still differed significantly ($p < .001$) but were influenced more by the use of adjuvant therapy. By 5 years, the overall cost for breast-conservation therapy was lower than for a mastectomy, presumably due to costs of reconstruction and/or complications of mastectomy.

Warren et al. (814) linked data of women with breast cancer from the SEER cancer registries with their Medicare claims from 1990 through 1998. Initial care costs for the 6 months after diagnosis for women who underwent breast-conservation therapy and irradiation were approximately $450 per month higher than for women with modified radical mastectomy in the continuing-care phase, and costs for women undergoing breast-conserving surgery with radiation therapy were significantly less expensive than for modified radical mastectomy cases. The two groups had similar costs in the terminal-care phase. Long-term costs for women undergoing breast-conserving therapy with radiation therapy were not statistically different from those for women undergoing modified radical mastectomy.

Liljegren et al. (448) evaluated the cost-effectiveness of radiation therapy in a prospective, randomized trial of 381 women treated with sector resection plus axillary dissection with or without radiation therapy in stage I breast cancer. After a median follow-up of 5 years, 43 local recurrences, six of them in the radiation therapy group, had occurred ($p < .0001$). No differences in regional and distant metastases or survival rate were observed. Direct medical costs as well as indirect costs in terms of production lost during the treatment period and travel expenses were estimated from data in the medical records and the Swedish National Insurance Registry of each patient. Taking into account the cost of primary treatment, follow-up, cost of treatment of a local recurrence, travel expenses, and indirect costs (production lost), and excluding costs for treatment of regional and distant recurrence, the cost per avoided local recurrence at 5 years was $44,438. Adjustment of quality of life showed a cost for every gained quality-adjusted life-year to be approximately $210,526. These results stress the importance of identifying risk factors for local recurrence, a better understanding of the impact on quality of life of a local recurrence, and adding cost evaluations to clinical trials in early breast cancer.

Hayman et al. (341) performed a cost-utility analysis of electron beam boost using a Markov model. From a societal perspective, outcomes were measured in quality-adjusted life-years. On the basis of the Lyon trial, the electron beam boost was assumed to reduce local recurrences by approximately 2% at 10 years but to have no impact on survival. Direct medical, time, and travel costs were considered. The electron beam boost led to an additional cost of $2,008, an increase of 0.0065 quality-adjusted life-year, and an incremental cost-effectiveness ratio of over $300,000 quality-adjusted life-year. Even if patients do value a small cancer-risk reduction, the mean cost-effectiveness ratio remains high, at $70,859 quality-adjusted life-year, which is well above the commonly cited threshold for cost-effectiveness care ($50,000 quality-adjusted life-year). The electron beam boost is cost-effective only if patients place an unexpectedly high value on the small absolute reduction in local tumor recurrences achievable with it.

The development of accelerated partial breast irradiation, with its associated reduced number of treatments, has recently been evaluated with respect to its costs by Suh et al. (724). Treatment planning and delivery utilization data were modeled for eight different breast radiotherapy techniques:

1. Whole breast radiation: 60 Gy in 30 fractions;
2. Whole breast radiation: 50 Gy in 25 fractions;
3. Accelerated whole breast radiation: 42.5 Gy in 16 fractions;
4. Whole breast intensity-modulated radiotherapy (IMRT): 60 Gy in 30 fractions;
5. Accelerated partial breast irradiation, MammoSite: 34 Gy in 10 twice-daily fractions;
6. Accelerated partial breast HDR interstitial: 34 Gy in 10 twice-daily fractions;
7. Accelerated partial breast three-dimensional conformal radiotherapy (3DCRT): 38.5 Gy in 10 twice-daily fractions; or
8. Accelerated partial breast IMRT: 38.5 Gy in 10 twice-daily fractions.

Costs incurred by payer and patient (i.e., direct nonmedical costs; time and travel) were estimated and total societal costs were then calculated. The least expensive partial breast–based radiotherapy approaches were the external beam techniques (accelerated partial breast-3DCRT or IMRT). Any reduced cost to patients for the HDR brachytherapy-based accelerated partial breast regimens were overshadowed by substantial increases in cost to payers, resulting in higher total societal costs; the cost of HDR treatment delivery was primarily responsible for the increased direct medical cost. For the whole breast–based radiotherapy approaches, treating without a boost or with accelerated whole breast regimens reduced total costs. Overall, accelerated whole breast was the least costly of all the regimens, in terms of costs to society; accelerated partial breast approaches, in general, were favored over whole-breast techniques when only considering costs to patients.

Psychoemotional Aspects and Quality of Life in Patients with Breast Cancer

Approximately 25% to 35% of patients diagnosed with breast cancer have significant psychosocial distress manifested by anxiety or depression and some level of sexual dysfunction. These disruptive consequences of treatment remain bothersome for at least 2 years after initial therapy. Jensen (380), in a review of the literature studying psychosocial factors and their relation to breast cancer, revealed major methodological problems in evaluation of the data, including small sample size, retrospective design, lack of cross-referencing for other important factors, cross-referencing studies instead of longitudinal studies, and insufficient statistical analysis. Regarding psychosocial factors, some of the most valid studies indicate that the risk of getting breast cancer may be connected with difficulties in expressing feelings, especially ones of aggression coping strategy, the amount of stress, and the level of activity seem to be of possible influence on the prognosis. A possible connection between psycho and the immunologic system has been proposed, but there have been few data to support it.

The specific types, magnitude, and duration of emotional dysfunction of women undergoing breast-conservation therapy compared with those treated with mastectomy are highly variable, and although somewhat different, they require the attention and psychotherapeutic support of the treating physicians (655,656). Radical surgery produces more psychoemotional disruption in terms of feelings about body image, physical attractiveness, and sexuality, whereas lumpectomy and irradiation may interfere temporarily with the patient's lifestyle and may cause worries about cancer and the perceived adverse effects of irradiation. However, at present this assumption is not supported by research findings, but the fear of recurrence has been reported to be similar in women undergoing mastectomy or breast-conservation therapy.

A clinical decision analysis on the quality-adjusted life expectancy of patients with breast cancer, comparing a group treated with mastectomy and one treated with breast-conservation therapy, showed that breast-conservation therapy yields better quality-adjusted life expectancy than mastectomy. However, there are selected subgroups of patients who should preferably undergo mastectomy (774). Lasry and Margolese (437), in a comparison of psychological effects on some patients randomly assigned to NSABP Protocol B-06, noted that patients who underwent more radical surgery did not express less fear of cancer recurrence than those treated with lumpectomy. The expected tradeoff between breast conservation and increased fear of cancer recurrence did not occur.

Body image, as a component of self-concept, was compared by mailed questionnaires in 257 patients treated with mastectomy, mastectomy with delayed reconstruction, mastectomy with immediate reconstruction, or conservation therapy (504). When analysis of covariance with age was used, body image in the conservation therapy group was significantly more positive than in either the mastectomy group or the mastectomy with immediate reconstruction group. No differences in self-concept were evident among the four groups.

The advantage of breast-conservation therapy is psychological because preservation of the configuration of the body maintains the sensation of female identity and body image to a better extent than mastectomy (64). Breast-conservation therapy does not, however, reduce the high frequency of anxiety phenomena, mental instability, and depression. Psychosocial adjustment, body image, and sexual function were retrospectively assessed in 72 women who had partial and 147 women who had total mastectomy and immediate breast reconstruction (665,666). Questionnaires completed at a mean of 4 years after surgery (44% of questionnaires returned) showed that fewer than 20% of women reported good adjustment in the areas measured. There was no significant difference between the two groups with regard to body image, sexual attractiveness, or marital happiness. Of 184 women who answered the question, 109 (59%) believed that cancer had brought them closer to their partner, 44 (24%) saw no significant impact, and 31 (17%) believed that cancer had interfered with their relationships. There was no significant difference between the two surgery groups with regard to frequency of sexual expression, desire for sex, or actual sexual activity. Pleasure with breast caressing had decreased since cancer treatment for 44% of women with partial mastectomy and for 83% of those with mastectomy and breast reconstruction. With regard to satisfaction with appearance of the breast, there was no significant difference between the surgical groups.

Schain et al. (656) prospectively studied 142 women participating in clinical trials who were randomly assigned to undergo mastectomy or lumpectomy and radiation therapy. Baseline assessments were made before randomization and at 6, 12, and 24 months after treatment. At 6 months, patients receiving mastectomy reported significantly less control of events in their lives ($p = .003$) and more problems with sexual relations ($p = .021$) than did their conservatively treated counterparts. In addition, there were marked differences between patients receiving mastectomy and those undergoing lumpectomy and irradiation in the degree of distress over body image ($p = .059$ at 24 months). This study concluded that breast-conservation therapy protects a woman's perception of her body but does not, over time, contribute to more positive sexual adjustment.

Despite numerous studies of partial mastectomy and psychological morbidity in the first 24 months after surgery, little is known about the long-term psychosocial repercussions. Dorval et al (165) assessed the effect of the type of mastectomy on psychological adjustment in 124 breast carcinoma survivors, 47 of whom underwent partial mastectomy and 77 total mastectomy, 8 years after initial treatment. Interviews were also conducted 3 and 18 months after surgery. Psychological distress was assessed using the Psychiatric Symptom Index. No statistically significant differences between partial and total mastectomy were observed with respect to long-term quality of life. Among women younger than 50 years of age, partial mastectomy appeared to be protective against distress compared with total mastectomy ($p = .04$). In contrast, among women 50 years of age or older, partial mastectomy was associated with higher psychological distress.

With the increasing use of adjuvant chemotherapy in younger women with early stage breast cancer, the long-term impact on quality of life, effects of premature menopause, and changes in perceived sexual attractiveness must be given a high priority for research to improve posttreatment adjustment and satisfaction in these patients (272,273,666). Women who received chemotherapy were more likely to worry about breast cancer recurrence ($p = .001$), had sex less frequently ($p = .013$), tended to desire sex less frequently ($p = .032$), and had more vaginal dryness ($p < .001$) and dyspareunia ($p < .001$). Their ability to reach orgasm through intercourse tended to be reduced ($p = .043$), and their sexual satisfaction was significantly poorer ($p = .001$). The ability to have orgasm through noncoital caressing did not differ from that of other women. There was a significant correlation between the age of the patient and the frequency of sexual desire and activity.

In two large-scale clinical trials in Switzerland, adjuvant chemotherapy had a measurable effect on health-related quality of life, but this effect was transient and minor compared with the effect of patients' adjustment and coping after diagnosis and surgery (364).

Ganz et al. (272) conducted a survey of 864 breast cancer survivors. RAND Health Survey scores were as good or better than those of healthy, age-matched women, and the frequency of depression was similar to general population samples. Marital or partner adjustment was similar to that in normal healthy samples, and sexual functioning mirrored that of healthy, age-matched postmenopausal women. However, these breast cancer survivors reported higher rates of physical symptom (e.g., joint pains, headaches, and hot flashes) than healthy women. Sexual dysfunction occurred more frequently in women who had received chemotherapy (all ages), and in younger women who were no longer menstruating. In women 50 years of age and older, tamoxifen therapy was unrelated to sexual functioning. Clinicians should inquire about common symptoms to provide symptomatic management or counseling for these women.

Ganz et al. (273) also surveyed 1,096 women diagnosed with early stage breast cancer between 1 and 5 years earlier in two large metropolitan centers in the United States. Of the participants in the study, 356 had received tamoxifen alone, 180 chemotherapy alone, 395 chemotherapy and tamoxifen, and 265 received no adjuvant therapy. No significant differences in global quality of life or in depression scores were observed among the four treatment groups. The group receiving no adjuvant therapy had a physical functioning composite score that was at the mean for a normal population of healthy women, whereas those in the adjuvant treatment groups scored slightly lower. The mental health score was not significantly different among the four treatment groups and approximated scores from the normal population of healthy women. Overall, breast cancer survivors function at a high level, similar to healthy women without cancer. However, compared with survivors with no adjuvant therapy, those who received chemotherapy have significantly more sexual problems, and those treated with tamoxifen experience more vasomotor symptoms.

Nissen et al. (527) carried out a quality-of-life study in women 30 to 85 years of age with newly diagnosed breast carcinoma who underwent breast-conserving surgery ($n = 103$), mastectomy alone ($n = 55$), or mastectomy with reconstruction ($n = 40$). Quality of life was assessed after diagnosis (baseline) and at 1, 3, 6, 12, 18, and 24 months. Women who underwent mastectomy with reconstruction had greater mood disturbance ($p = .002$) and poorer well-being ($p = .002$) after baseline than women who had mastectomy alone, and these differences remained 18 months after surgery. The breast-conserving surgery and mastectomy-only groups did not differ significantly regarding well-being.

References

1. Aberle DR, Chiles C, Gatsonis C, et al. Imaging and cancer: research strategy of the American College of Radiology Imaging Network. *Radiology* 2005;235:741–751.
2. Abner AL, Connolly JL, Recht A, et al. The relation between the presence and extent of lobular carcinoma in situ and the risk of local recurrence for patients with infiltrating carcinoma of the breast treated with conservative surgery and radiation therapy. *Cancer* 2000;88:1072–1077.
3. Abner AL, Recht A, Eberlein T, et al. Prognosis following salvage mastectomy for recurrence in the breast after conservative surgery and radiation therapy for early-stage breast cancer. *J Clin Oncol* 1993;11:44–48.
4. Adair FE. Cancer of the breast. *Surg Clin North Am* 1953:313–327.
5. Adami HO, Malker B, Holmberg L, et al. The relation between survival and age at diagnosis in breast cancer. *N Engl J Med* 1986;315:559–563.
6. Ahn PH, Vu HT, Lannin D, et al. Sequence of radiotherapy with tamoxifen in conservatively managed breast cancer does not affect local relapse rates. *J Clin Oncol* 2005;23:17–23.
7. Ahsan H, Neugut AI. Radiation therapy for breast cancer and increased risk for esophageal carcinoma. *Ann Intern Med* 1998;128:114–117.
8. Aisenberg AC, Finkelstein DM, Doppke KP, et al. High risk of breast carcinoma after irradiation of young women with Hodgkin's disease. *Cancer* 1997;79:1203–1210.
9. Albrektsen G, Heuch I, Kvale G. The short-term and long-term effect of a pregnancy on breast cancer risk: a prospective study of 802,457 parous Norwegian women. *Br J Cancer* 1995;72:480–484.
10. Alexander FE, Anderson TJ, Brown HK, et al. 14 years of follow-up from the Edinburgh randomised trial of breast-cancer screening. *Lancet* 1999;353:1903–1908.
11. Alpert TE, Haffty BG. Conservative management of breast cancer in BRCA1/2 mutation carriers. *Clin Breast Cancer* 2004;5:37–42.
12. Alpert TE, Kuerer HM, Arthur DW, et al. Ipsilateral breast tumor recurrence after breast conservation therapy: outcomes of salvage mastectomy vs. salvage breast-conserving surgery and prognostic factors for salvage breast preservation. *Int J Radiat Oncol Biol Phys* 2005;63:845–851.
13. Amadori D, Silvestrini R. Prognostic and predictive value of thymidine labelling index in breast cancer. *Breast Cancer Res Treat* 1998;51:267–281.
14. Amalric R, Santamaria F, Robert F, et al. Radiation therapy with or without primary limited surgery for operable breast cancer: a 20-year experience at the Marseilles Cancer Institute. *Cancer* 1982;49:30–34.
15. Ambrosone CB, Freudenheim JL, Sinha R, et al. Breast cancer risk, meat consumption and N-acetyltransferase (NAT2) genetic polymorphisms. *Int J Cancer* 1998;75:825–830.
16. American Cancer Society. *Cancer facts and figures 2002*. Atlanta: American Cancer Society, 2002.
17. American Society of Clinical Oncology policy statement update: genetic testing for cancer susceptibility. *J Clin Oncol* 2003;21:2397–2406.
18. American Society of Clinical Oncology. Recommended breast cancer surveillance guidelines. *J Clin Oncol* 1997;15:2149–2156.
19. Amornmarn R, Bui MM, Prempree TB, et al. Molecular predictive factors for local recurrence and distant metastasis of breast cancer after lumpectomy with postoperative radiation therapy. *Ann Clin Lab Sci* 2000;30:33–40.
20. Anan K, Mitsuyama S, Tamae K, et al. Pathological features of mucinous carcinoma of the breast are favourable for breast-conserving therapy. *Eur J Surg Oncol* 2001;27:459–463.
21. Andersson I, Aspegren K, Janzon L, et al. Mammographic screening and mortality from breast cancer: the Malmo mammographic screening trial. *BMJ* 1988;297:943–948.
22. Anscher MS, Jones P, Prosnitz LR, et al. Local failure and margin status in early-stage breast carcinoma treated with conservation surgery and radiation therapy. *Ann Surg* 1993;218:22–28.
23. Ansquer Y, Gautier C, Fourquet A, et al. Survival in early-onset BRCA1 breast-cancer patients. Institut Curie Breast Cancer Group. *Lancet* 1998;352:541
24. Antolak JA, Strom EA. Fetal dose estimates for electron-beam treatment to the chest wall of a pregnant patient. *Med Phys* 1998;25:2388–2391.
25. Arcangeli G, Pinnaro P, Rambone R, et al. A phase III randomized study on the sequencing of radiotherapy and chemotherapy in the conservative management of early-stage breast cancer. *Int J Radiat Oncol Biol Phys* 2006;64:161–167.
26. Ariad S, Lewis D, Cohen R, et al. Breast lymphoma. A clinical and pathological review and 10-year treatment results. *S Afr Med J* 1995;85:85–89.
27. Arpino G, Clark GM, Mohsin S, et al. Adenoid cystic carcinoma of the breast: molecular markers, treatment, and clinical outcome. *Cancer* 2002;94:2119–2127.
28. Arriagada R, Le MG, Rochard F, et al. Conservative treatment versus mastectomy in early breast cancer: patterns of failure with 15 years of follow-up data. Institut Gustave-Roussy Breast Cancer Group. *J Clin Oncol* 1996;14:1558–1564.
29. Arthur DW, Arnfield MR, Warwicke LA, et al. Internal mammary node coverage: an investigation of presently accepted techniques. *Int J Radiat Oncol Biol Phys* 2000;48:139–146.
30. Arthur DW, Cuttino LW, Neuschatz AC, et al. Tumor bed boost omission after negative re-excision in breast-conservation treatment. *Ann Surg Oncol* 2006;13:794–801.
31. Arthur DW, Vicini FA, Kuske RR, et al. Accelerated partial breast irradiation: an updated report from the American Brachytherapy Society. *Brachytherapy* 2003;2:124–130.
32. Arthur DW, Vicini FA. Accelerated partial breast irradiation as a part of breast conservation therapy. *J Clin Oncol* 2005;23:1726–1735.
33. Arthur DW, Vicini FA. MammoSite RTS: the reporting of initial experiences and how to interpret. *Ann Surg Oncol* 2004;11:723–724.
34. Atkins H, Hayward JL, Klugman DJ, et al. Treatment of early breast cancer: a report after ten years of a clinical trial. *Br Med J* 1972;2:423–429.
35. Avril N, Rose CA, Schelling M, et al. Breast imaging with positron emission tomography and fluorine-18 fluorodeoxyglucose: use and limitations. *J Clin Oncol* 2000;18:3495–3502.
36. Baeza MR, Sole J, Leon A, et al. Conservative treatment of early breast cancer. *Int J Radiat Oncol Biol Phys* 1988;14:669–676.
37. Baines CJ, Miller AB, Bassett AA. Physical examination. Its role as a single screening modality in the Canadian National Breast Screening Study. *Cancer* 1989;63:1816–1822.
38. Barlow WE, Taplin SH, Yoshida CK, et al. Cost comparison of mastectomy versus breast-conserving therapy for early-stage breast cancer. *J Natl Cancer Inst* 2001;93:447–455.
39. Barr LC, Brunt AM, Goodman AG, et al. Uncontrolled local recurrence after treatment of breast cancer with breast conservation. *Cancer* 1989;64:1203–1207.
40. Barrett-Connor E, Mosca L, Collins P, et al. Effects of raloxifene on cardiovascular events and breast cancer in postmenopausal women. *N Engl J Med* 2006;355:125–137.
41. Bartelink H, Borger JH, van Dongen JA, et al. The impact of tumor size and histology on local control after breast-conserving therapy. *Radiother Oncol* 1988;11:297–303.
42. Bartelink H, Horiot JC, Poortmans P, et al. Recurrence rates after treatment of breast cancer with standard radiotherapy with or without additional radiation. *N Engl J Med* 2001;345:1378–1387.
43. Beadle GF, Come S, Henderson IC, et al. The effect of adjuvant chemotherapy on the cosmetic results after primary radiation treatment for early stage breast cancer. *Int J Radiat Oncol Biol Phys* 1984;10:2131–2137.
44. Beatty JD, Atwood M, Tickman R, et al. Metaplastic breast cancer: clinical significance. *Am J Surg* 2006;191:657–664.
45. Bedwinek JM, Brady L, Perez CA, et al. Irradiation as the primary management of

stage I and II adenocarcinoma of the breast: analysis of the RTOG breast registry. *Cancer Clin Trials* 1980;3:11–18.

46. Bellon JR, Come SE, Gelman RS, et al. Sequencing of chemotherapy and radiation therapy in early-stage breast cancer: updated results of a prospective randomized trial. *J Clin Oncol* 2005;23:1934–1940.

47. Bellon JR, Shulman LN, Come SE, et al. A prospective study of concurrent cyclophosphamide/methotrexate/5-fluorouracil and reduced-dose radiotherapy in patients with early-stage breast carcinoma. *Cancer* 2004;100:1358–1364.

48. Ben-David MA, Kleer CG, Paramagul C, et al. Is lobular carcinoma in situ as a component of breast carcinoma a risk factor for local failure after breast-conserving therapy? Results of a matched pair analysis. *Cancer* 2006;106:28–34.

49. Bentel G, Marks LB, Hardenbergh P, et al. Variability of the location of internal mammary vessels and glandular breast tissue in breast cancer patients undergoing routine CT-based treatment planning. *Int J Radiat Oncol Biol Phys* 1999;44:1017–1025.

50. Bentel GC, Marks LB, Hardenbergh PH, et al. Variability of the depth of supraclavicular and axillary lymph nodes in patients with breast cancer: is a posterior axillary boost field necessary? *Int J Radiat Oncol Biol Phys* 2000;47:755–758.

51. Bentel GC, Marks LB. A simple device to position large/flaccid breasts during tangential breast irradiation. *Int J Radiat Oncol Biol Phys* 1994;29:879–882.

52. Bentzen SM, Skoczylas JZ, Overgaard M, et al. Radiotherapy-related lung fibrosis enhanced by tamoxifen. *J Natl Cancer Inst* 1996;88:918–922.

53. Berg WA. Overview of breast imaging. *Semin Roentgenol* 2001;36:180–186.

54. Berg WA. Supplemental screening sonography in dense breasts. *Radiol Clin North Am* 2004;42:845–851, vi.

55. Bernstein L, Patel AV, Ursin G, et al. Lifetime recreational exercise activity and breast cancer risk among black women and white women. *J Natl Cancer Inst* 2005;97:1671–1679.

56. Berrino P, Campora E, Leone S, et al. Correction of type II breast deformities following conservative cancer surgery. *Plast Reconstr Surg* 1992;90:846–853.

57. Bhatia S, Robison LL, Oberlin O, et al. Breast cancer and other second neoplasms after childhood Hodgkin's disease. *N Engl J Med* 1996;334:745–751.

58. Bijker N, Rutgers EJ, Duchateau L, et al. Breast-conserving therapy for Paget disease of the nipple: a prospective European Organization for Research and Treatment of Cancer study of 61 patients. *Cancer* 2001;91:472–477.

59. Bimston DN, Bebb GG, Wagman LD. Is specimen mammography beneficial? *Arch Surg* 2000;135:1083–1086; discussion 1086–1089.

60. Birner P, Oberhuber G, Stani J, et al. Evaluation of the United States Food and Drug Administration-approved scoring and test system of HER 2 protein expression in breast cancer. *Clin Cancer Res* 2001;7:1669–1676.

61. Bjurstam N, Björneld L, Warwick J, et al. The Gothenburg Breast Screening Trial. *Cancer* 2003;97:2387–2396.

62. Blaszyk H, Vaughn CB, Hartmann A, et al. Novel pattern of p53 gene mutations in an American black cohort with high mortality from breast cancer. *Lancet* 1994;343:1195–1197.

63. Blichert-Toft M, Rose C, Andersen JA, et al. Danish randomized trial comparing breast conservation therapy with mastectomy: six years of life-table analysis. Danish Breast Cancer Cooperative Group. *J Natl Cancer Inst Monogr* 1992:19–25.

64. Blichert-Toft M. Breast-conserving therapy for mammary carcinoma: psychosocial aspects, indications and limitations. *Ann Med* 1992;24:445–451.

65. Bloom HJ, Richardson WW, Harries EJ. Natural history of untreated breast cancer (1805-1933). Comparison of untreated and treated cases according to histological grade of malignancy. *BMJ* 1962;5299:213–221.

66. Bloom HJ, Richardson WW. Histological grading and prognosis in breast cancer; a study of 1409 cases of which 359 have been followed for 15 years. *Br J Cancer* 1957;11:359–377.

67. Boice JD Jr., Harvey EB, Blettner M, et al. Cancer in the contralateral breast after radiotherapy for breast cancer. *N Engl J Med* 1992;326:781–785.

68. Bonadonna G, Veronesi U, Brambilla C, et al. Primary chemotherapy to avoid mastectomy in tumors with diameters of three centimeters or more. *J Natl Cancer Inst* 1990;82:1539–1545.

69. Bonadonna G, Veronesi U, Brambilla C, et al. Primary chemotherapy for resectable breast cancer. *Recent Results Cancer Res* 1993;127:113–117.

70. Borger J, Kemperman H, Hart A, et al. Risk factors in breast-conservation therapy. *J Clin Oncol* 1994;12:653–660.

71. Borgstein PJ, Pijpers R, Comans EF, et al. Sentinel lymph node biopsy in breast cancer: guidelines and pitfalls of lymphoscintigraphy and gamma probe detection. *J Am Coll Surg* 1998;186:275–283.

72. Bornstein BA, Cheng CW, Rhodes LM, et al. Can transmission measurements be used to predict the irradiated lung volume in the tangential fields in patients treated for breast cancer? *Int J Radiat Oncol Biol Phys* 1990;18:181–187.

73. Boyages J, Recht A, Connolly J, et al. Factors associated with local recurrence as a first site of failure following the conservative treatment of early breast cancer. *Recent Results Cancer Res* 1989;115:92–102.

74. Boyd NF, Dite GS, Stone J, et al. Heritability of mammographic density, a risk factor for breast cancer. *N Engl J Med* 2002;347:886–894.

75. Boyd NF, Lockwood GA, Byng JW, et al. Mammographic densities and breast cancer risk. *Cancer Epidemiol Biomarkers Prev* 1998;7:1133–1144.

76. Boyd NF, Stone J, Vogt KN, et al. Dietary fat and breast cancer risk revisited: a meta-analysis of the published literature. *Br J Cancer* 2003;89:1672–1685.

77. Braun S, Vogl FD, Naume B, et al. A pooled analysis of bone marrow micrometastasis in breast cancer. *N Engl J Med* 2005;353:793–802.

78. Braw M, Erlandsson I, Ewers SB, et al. Mammographic follow-up after breast conserving surgery and postoperative radiotherapy without boost irradiation for mammary carcinoma. *Acta Radiol* 1991;32:398–402.

79. Breast cancer and hormone replacement therapy: collaborative reanalysis of data from 51 epidemiological studies of 52,705 women with breast cancer and 108,411 women without breast cancer. Collaborative Group on Hormonal Factors in Breast Cancer. *Lancet* 1997;350:1047–1059.

80. Brenin DR, Morrow M. Accuracy of AJCC staging for breast cancer patients undergoing re-excision for positive margins. American Joint Committee on Cancer. *Ann Surg Oncol* 1998;5:719–723.

81. Brent RL. The effect of embryonic and fetal exposure to x-ray, microwaves, and ultrasound: counseling the pregnant and nonpregnant patient about these risks. *Semin Oncol* 1989;16:347–368.

82. Broët P, de la Rochefordiere A, Scholl SM, et al. Contralateral breast cancer: annual incidence and risk parameters. *J Clin Oncol* 1995;13:1578–1583.

83. Brorson H, Svensson H, Norrgren K, et al. Liposuction reduces arm lymphedema without significantly altering the already impaired lymph transport. *Lymphology* 1998;31:156–172.

84. Bryant J, Fisher B, Gunduz N, et al. S-phase fraction combined with other patient and tumor characteristics for the prognosis of node-negative, estrogen-receptor-positive breast cancer. *Breast Cancer Res Treat* 1998;51:239–253.

85. Buchanan CL, Morris EA, Dorn PL, et al. Utility of breast magnetic resonance imaging in patients with occult primary breast cancer. *Ann Surg Oncol* 2005;12:1045–1053.

86. Buchholz TA, Hunt KK, Amosson CM, et al. Sequencing of chemotherapy and radiation in lymph node-negative breast cancer. *Cancer J Sci Am* 1999;5:159–164.

87. Buchholz TA, Tu X, Ang KK, et al. Epidermal growth factor receptor expression correlates with poor survival in patients who have breast carcinoma treated with doxorubicin-based neoadjuvant chemotherapy. *Cancer* 2005;104:676–681.

88. Buchholz TA, Tucker SL, Erwin J, et al. Impact of systemic treatment on local control for patients with lymph node-negative breast cancer treated with breast-conservation therapy. *J Clin Oncol* 2001;19:2240–2246.

89. Burke W, Daly M, Garber J, et al. Recommendations for follow-up care of individuals with an inherited predisposition to cancer. II. BRCA1 and BRCA2. Cancer Genetics Studies Consortium. *JAMA* 1997;277:997–1003.

90. Burstein HJ, Bellon JR, Galper S, et al. Prospective evaluation of concurrent paclitaxel and radiation therapy after adjuvant doxorubicin and cyclophosphamide chemotherapy for stage II or III breast cancer. *Int J Radiat Oncol Biol Phys* 2006;64:496–504.

91. Butzelaar RM, van Dongen JA, van der Schoot JB, et al. Evaluation of routine preoperative bone scintigraphy in patients with breast cancer. *Eur J Cancer* 1977;13:19–21.

92. Buyse M, Loi S, van't Veer L, et al. Validation and clinical utility of a 70-gene prognostic signature for women with node-negative breast cancer. *J Natl Cancer Inst* 2006;98:1183–1192.

93. Byrne C, Schairer C, Wolfe J, et al. Mammographic features and breast cancer risk: effects with time, age, and menopause status. *J Natl Cancer Inst* 1995;87:1622–1629.

94. Cabanes PA, Salmon RJ, Vilcoq JR, et al. Value of axillary dissection in addition to lumpectomy and radiotherapy in early breast cancer. The Breast Carcinoma Collaborative Group of the Institut Curie. *Lancet* 1992;339:1245–1248.

95. Cachin F, Prince HM, Hogg A, et al. Powerful prognostic stratification by [18F]fluorodeoxyglucose positron emission tomography in patients with metastatic breast cancer treated with high-dose chemotherapy. *J Clin Oncol* 2006;24:3026–3031.

96. Calais G, Berger C, Descamps P, et al. Conservative treatment feasibility with induction chemotherapy, surgery, and radiotherapy for patients with breast carcinoma larger than 3 cm. *Cancer* 1994;74:1283–1288.

97. Caleffi M, Teague MW, Jensen RA, et al. p53 gene mutations and steroid receptor status in breast cancer. Clinicopathologic correlations and prognostic assessment. *Cancer* 1994;73:2147–2156.

98. Calle R, Pilleron JP, Schlienger P, et al. Conservative management of operable breast cancer: ten years experience at the Foundation Curie. *Cancer* 1978;42:2045–2053.

99. Calle R, Vilcoq JR, Zafrani B, et al. Local control and survival of breast cancer treated by limited surgery followed by irradiation. *Int J Radiat Oncol Biol Phys* 1986;12:873–878.

100. Cancer risks in BRCA2 mutation carriers. The Breast Cancer Linkage Consortium. *J Natl Cancer Inst* 1999;91:1310–1316.

101. Carey RW, Linggood RM, Wood W, et al. Breast cancer developing in four women cured of Hodgkin's disease. *Cancer* 1984;54:2234–2236.

102. Carl UM, Feldmeier JJ, Schmitt G, et al. Hyperbaric oxygen therapy for late sequelae in women receiving radiation after breast-conserving surgery. *Int J Radiat Oncol Biol Phys* 2001;49:1029–1031.

103. Carrasco L, Moreno C, Pastor MA, et al. Postirradiation pseudosclerodermatous panniculitis. *Am J Dermatopathol* 2001;23:283–287.

104. Ceilley E, Jagsi R, Goldberg S, et al. Radiotherapy for invasive breast cancer in North America and Europe: results of a survey. *Int J Radiat Oncol Biol Phys* 2005;61:365–373.

105. Chabner E, Nixon A, Gelman R, et al. Family history and treatment outcome in young women after breast-conserving surgery and radiation therapy for early-stage breast cancer. *J Clin Oncol* 1998;16:2045–2051.

106. Cheng JD, Maull JJ, Rohrbach DA, et al. The impact of a multidisciplinary breast cancer center on recommendations for patient management: the University of Pennsylvania experience. *Cancer* 2001;91:1231–1237.

107. Chen AM, Meric-Bernstam F, Hunt KK, et al. Breast conservation after neoadjuvant chemotherapy: the M.D. Anderson cancer center experience. *J Clin Oncol* 2004;22:2303–2312.

108. Chen AM, Meric-Bernstam F, Hunt KK, et al. Breast conservation after neoadjuvant chemotherapy. *Cancer* 2005;103:689–695.

109. Chen AM, Obedian E, Haffty BG. Breast-conserving therapy in the setting of collagen vascular disease. *Cancer J* 2001;7:480–491.

110. Chen SC, Chen MF, Hwang TL, et al. Prediction of supraclavicular lymph node metastasis in breast carcinoma. *Int J Radiat Oncol Biol Phys* 2002;52:614–619.

111. Cheng JC, Chen CM, Liu MC, et al. Locoregional failure of postmastectomy patients with 1-3 positive axillary lymph nodes without adjuvant radiotherapy. *Int J Radiat Oncol Biol Phys* 2002;52:980–988.

112. Chlebowski RT, Chen Z, Anderson GL, et al. Ethnicity and breast cancer: factors influencing differences in incidence and outcome. *J Natl Cancer Inst* 2005;97:439–448.

113. Cho BC, Hurkmans CW, Damen EM, et al. Intensity modulated versus non-intensity modulated radiotherapy in the treatment of the left breast and upper internal mammary lymph node chain: a comparative planning study. *Radiother Oncol* 2002;62:127–136.

114. Choi DH, Kim S, Rimm DL, et al. Immunohistochemical biomarkers in patients with early-onset breast carcinoma by tissue microarray. *Cancer J* 2005;11:404–411.

115. Chung CT, Bogart JA, Adams JF, et al. Increased risk of breast cancer in splenectomized patients undergoing radiation therapy for Hodgkin's disease. *Int J Radiat Oncol Biol Phys* 1997;37:405–409.

116. Chung M, Chang HR, Bland KI, et al. Younger women with breast carcinoma have a poorer prognosis than older women. *Cancer* 1996;77:97–103.

117. Clark CP 3rd, Peters GN, O'Brien KM. Cancer in the augmented breast. Diagnosis and prognosis. *Cancer* 1993;72:2170–2174.
118. Clark RM, Whelan T, Levine M, et al. Randomized clinical trial of breast irradiation following lumpectomy and axillary dissection for node-negative breast cancer: an update. Ontario Clinical Oncology Group. *J Natl Cancer Inst* 1996;88:1659–1664.
119. Clark RM, Wilkinson RH, Miceli PN, et al. Breast cancer. Experiences with conservation therapy. *Am J Clin Oncol* 1987;10:461–468.
120. Clarke D, Khonji NI, Mansel RE. Sentinel node biopsy in breast cancer: ALMANAC trial. *World J Surg* 2001;25:819–822.
121. Clarke D, Martinez A, Cox RS, et al. Breast edema following staging axillary node dissection in patients with breast carcinoma treated by radical radiotherapy. *Cancer* 1982;49:2295–2299.
122. Clarke DH, Le MG, Sarrazin D, et al. Analysis of local-regional relapses in patients with early breast cancers treated by excision and radiotherapy: experience of the Institut Gustave-Roussy. *Int J Radiat Oncol Biol Phys* 1985;11:137–145.
123. Clarke DH, Martinez AA. Identification of patients who are at high risk for locoregional breast cancer recurrence after conservative surgery and radiotherapy: a review article for surgeons, pathologists, and radiation and medical oncologists. *J Clin Oncol* 1992;10:474–483.
124. Clarke M, Collins R, Darby S, et al. Effects of radiotherapy and of differences in the extent of surgery for early breast cancer on local recurrence and 15-year survival: an overview of the randomised trials. *Lancet* 2005;366:2087-2106.
125. Claus EB, Stowe M, Carter D, et al. The risk of a contralateral breast cancer among women diagnosed with ductal and lobular breast carcinoma in situ: data from the Connecticut Tumor Registry. *Breast* 2003;12:451–456.
126. Clemente CG, Boracchi P, Andreola S, et al. Peritumoral lymphatic invasion in patients with node-negative mammary duct carcinoma. *Cancer* 1992;69:1396–1403.
127. Colditz GA. Epidemiology and prevention of breast cancer. *Cancer Epidemiol Biomarkers Prev* 2005;14:768–772.
128. Cooke AL, Perera F, Fisher B, et al. Tamoxifen with and without radiation after partial mastectomy in patients with involved nodes. *Int J Radiat Oncol Biol Phys* 1995;31:777–781.
129. Costanza MC, Foster RS Jr. Relationship between breast self-examination and death from breast cancer by age groups. *Cancer Detect Prev* 1984;7:103–108.
130. Crile G Jr., Cooperman A, Esselstyn CB Jr., et al. Results of partial mastectomy in 173 patients followed for from five to ten years. *Surg Gynecol Obstet* 1980;150:563–566.
131. Cross MA, Elson HR, Aron BS. Breast conservation radiation therapy technique for women with large breasts. *Int J Radiat Oncol Biol Phys* 1989;17:199–203.
132. Crowe JP Jr, Gordon NH, Hubay CA, et al. Estrogen receptor determination and long term survival of patients with carcinoma of the breast. *Surg Gynecol Obstet* 1991;173:273–278.
133. Cummings SR, Eckert S, Krueger KA, et al. The effect of raloxifene on risk of breast cancer in postmenopausal women: results from the MORE randomized trial. Multiple Outcomes of Raloxifene Evaluation. *JAMA* 1999;281:2189-2197.
134. Curtis RE, Boice JD Jr., Stovall M, et al. Risk of leukemia after chemotherapy and radiation treatment for breast cancer. *N Engl J Med* 1992;326:1745–1751.
135. Cutuli B, Borel C, Dhermain F, et al. Breast cancer occurred after treatment for Hodgkin's disease: analysis of 133 cases. *Radiother Oncol* 2001;59:247–255.
136. Cuzick J, Forbes J, Edwards R, et al. First results from the International Breast Cancer Intervention Study (IBIS-I): a randomised prevention trial. *Lancet* 2002;360:817–824.
137. Cuzick J, Powles T, Veronesi U, et al. Overview of the main outcomes in breast-cancer prevention trials. *Lancet* 2003;361:296–300.
138. Cuzick J, Stewart H, Peto R, et al. Overview of randomized trials of postoperative adjuvant radiotherapy in breast cancer. *Cancer Treat Rep* 1987;71:15–29.
139. Daling JR, Malone KE, Doody DR, et al. Relation of body mass index to tumor markers and survival among young women with invasive ductal breast carcinoma. *Cancer* 2001;92:720–729.
140. Danforth DN Jr, Findlay PA, McDonald HD, et al. Complete axillary lymph node dissection for stage I-II carcinoma of the breast. *J Clin Oncol* 1986;4:655–662.
141. Danforth DN Jr. How subsequent pregnancy affects outcome in women with a prior breast cancer. *Oncology (Williston Park)* 1991;5:23–30; discussion 30–21, 35.
142. Danoff BF, Goodman RL, Glick JH, et al. The effect of adjuvant chemotherapy on cosmesis and complications in patients with breast cancer treated by definitive irradiation. *Int J Radiat Oncol Biol Phys* 1983;9:1625–1630.
143. Dao TH, Rahmouni A, Campana F, et al. Tumor recurrence versus fibrosis in the irradiated breast: differentiation with dynamic gadolinium-enhanced MR imaging. *Radiology* 1993;187:751–755.
144. Darby SC, McGale P, Taylor CW, et al. Long-term mortality from heart disease and lung cancer after radiotherapy for early breast cancer: prospective cohort study of about 300,000 women in US SEER cancer registries. *Lancet Oncol* 2005;6:557–565.
145. de Bock GH, van der Hage JA, Putter H, et al. Isolated loco-regional recurrence of breast cancer is more common in young patients and following breast conserving therapy: long-term results of European Organisation for Research and Treatment of Cancer studies. *Eur J Cancer* 2006;42:351–356.
146. de Boer R, Hillen HF, Roumen RM, et al. Detection, treatment and outcome of axillary recurrence after axillary clearance for invasive breast cancer. *Br J Surg* 2001;88:118–122.
147. de la Rochefordiére A, Asselain B, Campana F, et al. Age as prognostic factor in premenopausal breast carcinoma. *Lancet* 1993;341:1039–1043.
148. de la Rochefordiére A, Asselain B, Scholl S, et al. Simultaneous bilateral breast carcinomas: a retrospective review of 149 cases. *Int J Radiat Oncol Biol Phys* 1994;30:35–41.
149. De Naeyer B, De Meerleer G, Braems S, et al. Collagen vascular diseases and radiation therapy: a critical review. *Int J Radiat Oncol Biol Phys* 1999;44:975–980.
150. Deapen D, Liu L, Perkins C, et al. Rapidly rising breast cancer incidence rates among Asian-American women. *Int J Cancer* 2002;99:747–750.
151. Delouche G, Bachelot F, Premont M, et al. Conservation treatment of early breast cancer: long term results and complications. *Int J Radiat Oncol Biol Phys* 1987;13:29–34.
152. Denham JW, Sillar RW, Clarke D. Boost dosage to the excision site following conservative surgery for breast cancer: it's easy to miss! *Clin Oncol (R Coll Radiol)* 1991;3:257–261.
153. Dershaw DD, Giess CS, McCormick B, et al. Patterns of mammographically detected calcifications after breast-conserving therapy associated with tumor recurrence. *Cancer* 1997;79:1355–1361.
154. Dershaw DD. Breast imaging and the conservative treatment of breast cancer. *Radiol Clin North Am* 2002;40:501–516.
155. Dershaw DD. Mammography in patients with breast cancer treated by breast conservation (lumpectomy with or without radiation). *AJR Am J Roentgenol* 1995;164:309–316.
156. Deutsch M, Gerszten K, Bloomer WD, et al. Lumpectomy and breast irradiation for breast cancer arising after previous radiotherapy for Hodgkin's disease or lymphoma. *Am J Clin Oncol* 2001;24:33–34.
157. Deutsch M, Land SR, Begovic M, et al. The incidence of lung carcinoma after surgery for breast carcinoma with and without postoperative radiotherapy. Results of National Surgical Adjuvant Breast and Bowel Project (NSABP) clinical trials B-04 and B-06. *Cancer* 2003;98:1362–1368.
158. Deutsch M, Rosenstein MM. Angiosarcoma of the breast mimicking radiation dermatitis arising after lumpectomy and breast irradiation: a case report. *Am J Clin Oncol* 1998;21:608–609.
159. Dewar JA, Arriagada R, Benhamou S, et al. Local relapse and contralateral tumor rates in patients with breast cancer treated with conservative surgery and radiotherapy (Institut Gustave Roussy 1970-1982). IGR Breast Cancer Group. *Cancer* 1995;76:2260–2265.
160. Dewar JA, Sarrazin D, Benhamou E, et al. Management of the axilla in conservatively treated breast cancer: 592 patients treated at Institut Gustave-Roussy. *Int J Radiat Oncol Biol Phys* 1987;13:475–481.
161. Diallo I, Lamon A, Shamsaldin A, et al. Estimation of the radiation dose delivered to any point outside the target volume per patient treated with external beam radiotherapy. *Radiother Oncol* 1996;38:269–271.
162. DiBiase SJ, Komarnicky LT, Heron DE, et al. Influence of radiation dose on positive surgical margins in women undergoing breast conservation therapy. *Int J Radiat Oncol Biol Phys* 2002;53:680–686.
163. Doll DC, Ringenberg QS, Yarbro JW. Antineoplastic agents and pregnancy. *Semin Oncol* 1989;16:337–346.
164. Donegan WL, Perez-Mesa CM, Watson FR. A biostatistical study of locally recurrent breast carcinoma. *Surg Gynecol Obstet* 1966;122:529–540.
165. Dorval M, Maunsell E, Deschenes L, et al. Type of mastectomy and quality of life for long term breast carcinoma survivors. *Cancer* 1998;83:2130–2138.
166. Dow KH, Harris JR, Roy C. Pregnancy after breast-conserving surgery and radiation therapy for breast cancer. *J Natl Cancer Inst Monogr* 1994:131–137.
167. Drew PJ, Kerin MJ, Turnbull LW, et al. Routine screening for local recurrence following breast-conserving therapy for cancer with dynamic contrast-enhanced magnetic resonance imaging of the breast. *Ann Surg Oncol* 1998;5:265–270.
168. du Toit RS, Locker AP, Ellis IO, et al. Invasive lobular carcinomas of the breast—the prognosis of histopathological subtypes. *Br J Cancer* 1989;60:605–609.
169. Dubois JB, Gary-Bobo J, Pourquier H, et al. Tumorectomy and radiotherapy in early breast cancer: a report on 392 patients. *Int J Radiat Oncol Biol Phys* 1988;15:1275–1282.
170. Dunst J, Steil B, Furch S, et al. Prognostic significance of local recurrence in breast cancer after postmastectomy radiotherapy. *Strahlenther Onkol* 2001;177:504–510.
171. Easton DF, Steele L, Fields P, et al. Cancer risks in two large breast cancer families linked to BRCA2 on chromosome 13q12-13. *Am J Hum Genet* 1997;61:120–128.
172. Easton DF. How many more breast cancer predisposition genes are there? *Breast Cancer Res* 1999;1:14–17.
173. Eberlein TJ, Connolly JL, Schnitt SJ, et al. Predictors of local recurrence following conservative breast surgery and radiation therapy. The influence of tumor size. *Arch Surg* 1990;125:771–775; discussion 775–777.
174. Edeiken S, Russo DP, Knecht J, et al. Angiosarcoma after tylectomy and radiation therapy for carcinoma of the breast. *Cancer* 1992;70:644–647.
175. Ege GN, Clark RM. Internal mammary lymphoscintigraphy in the conservative management of breast carcinoma: an update and recommendations for a new TNM staging. *Clin Radiol* 1985;36:469–472.
176. Eley JW, Hill HA, Chen VW, et al. Racial differences in survival from breast cancer. Results of the National Cancer Institute Black/White Cancer Survival Study. *JAMA* 1994;272:947–954.
177. Elkhuizen PH, Hermans J, Leer JW, et al. Isolated late local recurrences with high mitotic count and early local recurrences following breast-conserving therapy are associated with increased risk on distant metastasis. *Int J Radiat Oncol Biol Phys* 2001;50:387–396.
178. Elkhuizen PH, Voogd AC, van den Broek LC, et al. Risk factors for local recurrence after breast-conserving therapy for invasive carcinomas: a case-control study of histological factors and alterations in oncogene expression. *Int J Radiat Oncol Biol Phys* 1999;45:73–83.
179. Elledge RM, Green S, Ciocca D, et al. HER-2 expression and response to tamoxifen in estrogen receptor-positive breast cancer: a Southwest Oncology Group Study. *Clin Cancer Res* 1998;4:7–12.
180. Ellis CN, Frey ES, Burnette JJ, et al. The content of tumor DNA as an indicator of prognosis in patients with T1N0M0 and T2N0M0 carcinoma of the breast. *Surgery* 1989;106:133–138.
181. Elmore JG, Armstrong K, Lehman CD, et al. Screening for breast cancer. *JAMA* 2005;293:1245–1256.
182. Elmore JG, Moceri VM, Carter D, et al. Breast carcinoma tumor characteristics in black and white women. *Cancer* 1998;83:2509–2515.
183. Elmore JG, Reisch LM, Barton MB, et al. Efficacy of breast cancer screening in the community according to risk level. *J Natl Cancer Inst* 2005;97:1035–1043.
184. el-Naggar AK, Ro JY, McLemore D, et al. DNA content and proliferative activity of cystosarcoma phyllodes of the breast. Potential prognostic significance. *Am J Clin Pathol* 1990;93:480–485.
185. Elston CW, Ellis IO. Pathological prognostic factors in breast cancer. I. The value of histological grade in breast cancer: experience from a large study with long-term follow-up. *Histopathology* 1991;19:403–410.
186. Epstein AH, Connolly JL, Gelman R, et al. The predictors of distant relapse following conservative surgery and radiotherapy for early breast cancer are

similar to those following mastectomy. *Int J Radiat Oncol Biol Phys* 1989;17:755-760.

187. Erickson VS, Pearson ML, Ganz PA, et al. Arm edema in breast cancer patients. *J Natl Cancer Inst* 2001;93:96–111.

188. Esserman L, Hylton N, Yassa L, et al. Utility of magnetic resonance imaging in the management of breast cancer: evidence for improved preoperative staging. *J Clin Oncol* 1999;17:110–119.

189. Esteban JM, Felder B, Ahn C, et al. Prognostic relevance of carcinoembryonic antigen and estrogen receptor status in breast cancer patients. *Cancer* 1994;74:1575–1583.

190. Estourgie SH, Nieweg OE, Olmos RA, et al. Lymphatic drainage patterns from the breast. *Ann Surg* 2004;239:232–237.

191. Evans PM, Donovan EM, Fenton N, et al. Practical implementation of compensators in breast radiotherapy. *Radiother Oncol* 1998;49:255–265.

192. Ewers SB, Langstrom E, Baldetorp B, et al. Flow-cytometric DNA analysis in primary breast carcinomas and clinicopathological correlations. *Cytometry* 1984;5:408–419.

193. Fagundes MA, Fagundes HM, Brito CS, et al. Breast-conserving surgery and definitive radiation: a comparison between quadrantectomy and local excision with special focus on local-regional control and cosmesis. *Int J Radiat Oncol Biol Phys* 1993;27:553–560.

194. Fallenius AG, Franzen SA, Auer GU. Predictive value of nuclear DNA content in breast cancer in relation to clinical and morphologic factors. A retrospective study of 227 consecutive cases. *Cancer* 1988;62:521–530.

195. Feig SA. Estimation of currently attainable benefit from mammographic screening of women aged 40-49 years. *Cancer* 1995;75:2412–2419.

196. Feigenberg SJ, Mendenhall NP, Reith JD, et al. Angiosarcoma after breast-conserving therapy: experience with hyperfractionated radiotherapy. *Int J Radiat Oncol Biol Phys* 2002;52:620–626.

197. Fein DA, Fowble BL, Hanlon AL, et al. Does the placement of surgical clips within the excision cavity influence local control for patients treated with breast-conserving surgery and irradiation. *Int J Radiat Oncol Biol Phys* 1996;34:1009–1017.

198. Fein DA, Fowble BL, Hanlon AL, et al. Identification of women with T1-T2 breast cancer at low risk of positive axillary nodes. *J Surg Oncol* 1997;65:34–39.

199. Fenton JJ, Barton MB, Geiger AM, et al. Screening clinical breast examination: how often does it miss lethal breast cancer? *J Natl Cancer Inst Monogr* 2005;35:67–71.

200. Fineberg S, Rosen PP. Cutaneous angiosarcoma and atypical vascular lesions of the skin and breast after radiation therapy for breast carcinoma. *Am J Clin Pathol* 1994;102:757–763.

201. Fisher B, Anderson S, Bryant J, et al. Twenty-year follow-up of a randomized trial comparing total mastectomy, lumpectomy, and lumpectomy plus irradiation for the treatment of invasive breast cancer. *N Engl J Med* 2002;347:1233–1241.

202. Fisher B, Anderson S, Fisher ER, et al. Significance of ipsilateral breast tumour recurrence after lumpectomy. *Lancet* 1991;338:327–331.

203. Fisher B, Anderson S, Redmond CK, et al. Reanalysis and results after 12 years of follow-up in a randomized clinical trial comparing total mastectomy with lumpectomy with or without irradiation in the treatment of breast cancer. *N Engl J Med* 1995;333:1456–1461.

204. Fisher B, Anderson S, Tan-Chiu E, et al. Tamoxifen and chemotherapy for axillary node-negative, estrogen receptor-negative breast cancer: findings from National Surgical Adjuvant Breast and Bowel Project B-23. *J Clin Oncol* 2001;19:931–942.

205. Fisher B, Anderson S. Conservative surgery for the management of invasive and noninvasive carcinoma of the breast: NSABP trials. National Surgical Adjuvant Breast and Bowel Project. *World J Surg* 1994;18:63–69.

206. Fisher B, Bauer M, Margolese R, et al. Five-year results of a randomized clinical trial comparing total mastectomy and segmental mastectomy with or without radiation in the treatment of breast cancer. *N Engl J Med* 1985;312:665–673.

207. Fisher B, Bauer M, Wickerham DL, et al. Relation of number of positive axillary nodes to the prognosis of patients with primary breast cancer. An NSABP update. *Cancer* 1983;52:1551–1557.

208. Fisher B, Bryant J, Dignam JJ, et al. Tamoxifen, radiation therapy, or both for prevention of ipsilateral breast tumor recurrence after lumpectomy in women with invasive breast cancers of one centimeter or less. *J Clin Oncol* 2002;20:4141–4149.

209. Fisher B, Costantino JP, Wickerham DL, et al. Tamoxifen for prevention of breast cancer: report of the National Surgical Adjuvant Breast and Bowel Project P-1 Study. *J Natl Cancer Inst* 1998;90:1371–1388.

210. Fisher B, Dignam J, Wolmark N, et al. Tamoxifen and chemotherapy for lymph node-negative, estrogen receptor-positive breast cancer. *J Natl Cancer Inst* 1997;89:1673–1682.

211. Fisher B, Jeong JH, Anderson S, et al. Twenty-five-year follow-up of a randomized trial comparing radical mastectomy, total mastectomy, and total mastectomy followed by irradiation. *N Engl J Med* 2002;347:567–575.

212. Fisher B, Montague E, Redmond C, et al. Findings from NSABP Protocol No. B-04-comparison of radical mastectomy with alternative treatments for primary breast cancer. I. Radiation compliance and its relation to treatment outcome. *Cancer* 1980;46:1–13.

213. Fisher B, Redmond C, Dimitrov NV, et al. A randomized clinical trial evaluating sequential methotrexate and fluorouracil in the treatment of patients with node-negative breast cancer who have estrogen-receptor-negative tumors. *N Engl J Med* 1989;320:473–478.

214. Fisher B, Redmond C, Fisher ER. The contribution of recent NSABP clinical trials of primary breast cancer therapy to an understanding of tumor biology—an overview of findings. *Cancer* 1980;46:1009–1025.

215. Fisher B, Wickerham DL, Deutsch M, et al. Breast tumor recurrence following lumpectomy with and without breast irradiation: an overview of recent NSABP findings. *Semin Surg Oncol* 1992;8:153–160.

216. Fisher B. Laboratory and clinical research in breast cancer, a personal adventure. The David A Karnovsky Memorial Lecture. *Cancer Research* 1980;40:3863–3874.

218. Fisher B. *Some thoughts concerning the primary therapy of breast cancer*. Berlin: Springer-Verlag, 1976.

219. Fisher BJ, Perera FE, Cooke AL, et al. Extracapsular axillary node extension in patients receiving adjuvant systemic therapy: an indication for radiotherapy? *Int J Radiat Oncol Biol Phys* 1997;38:551–559.

220. Fisher BJ, Perera FE, Cooke AL, et al. Long-term follow-up of axillary node-positive breast cancer patients receiving adjuvant systemic therapy alone: patterns of recurrence. *Int J Radiat Oncol Biol Phys* 1997;38:541–550.

221. Fisher ER, Gregorio RM, Fisher B, et al. The pathology of invasive breast cancer. A syllabus derived from findings of the National Surgical Adjuvant Breast Project (protocol no. 4). *Cancer* 1975;36:1–85.

222. Fisher ER, Sass R, Fisher B, et al. Pathologic findings from the National Surgical Adjuvant Breast Project (protocol 6). II. Relation of local breast recurrence to multicentricity. *Cancer* 1986;57:1717–1724.

223. Fitzgibbons PL, Page DL, Weaver D, et al. Prognostic factors in breast cancer. College of American Pathologists Consensus Statement 1999. *Arch Pathol Lab Med* 2000;124:966–978.

224. Fleck R, McNeese MD, Ellerbroek NA, et al. Consequences of breast irradiation in patients with pre-existing collagen vascular diseases. *Int J Radiat Oncol Biol Phys* 1989;17:829–833.

225. Flobbe K, Bosch AM, Kessels AG, et al. The additional diagnostic value of ultrasonography in the diagnosis of breast cancer. *Arch Intern Med* 2003;163:1194–1199.

226. Foekens JA, Peters HA, Look MP, et al. The urokinase system of plasminogen activation and prognosis in 2780 breast cancer patients. *Cancer Res* 2000;60:636–643.

227. Fogliata A, Bolsi A, Cozzi L. Critical appraisal of treatment techniques based on conventional photon beams, intensity modulated photon beams and proton beams for therapy of intact breast. *Radiother Oncol* 2002;62:137–145.

228. Ford D, Easton DF, Peto J. Estimates of the gene frequency of BRCA1 and its contribution to breast and ovarian cancer incidence. *Am J Hum Genet* 1995;57:1457–1462.

229. Ford D, Easton DF, Stratton M, et al. Genetic heterogeneity and penetrance analysis of the BRCA1 and BRCA2 genes in breast cancer families. The Breast Cancer Linkage Consortium. *Am J Hum Genet* 1998;62:676–689.

230. Ford MB, Sigurdson AJ, Petrulis ES, et al. Effects of smoking and radiotherapy on lung carcinoma in breast carcinoma survivors. *Cancer* 2003;98:1457–1464.

231. Formenti SC. External-beam partial-breast irradiation. *Semin Radiat Oncol* 2005;15:92–99.

232. Forrest AP, Stewart HJ, Everington D, et al. Randomised controlled trial of conservation therapy for breast cancer: 6-year analysis of the Scottish trial. Scottish Cancer Trials Breast Group, *Lancet* 1996,348.708–713.

233. Foster RS Jr, Costanza MC. Breast self-examination practices and breast cancer survival. *Cancer* 1984;53:999–1005.

234. Fourquet A, Campana F, Mosseri V, et al. Iridium-192 versus cobalt-60 boost in 3-7 cm breast cancer treated by irradiation alone: final results of a randomized trial. *Radiother Oncol* 1995;34:114–120.

235. Fourquet A, Campana F, Rosenwald JC, et al. Breast irradiation in the lateral decubitus position: technique of the Institut Curie. *Radiother Oncol* 1991;22:261–265.

236. Fourquet A, Campana F, Zafrani B, et al. Prognostic factors of breast recurrence in the conservative management of early breast cancer: a 25-year follow-up. *Int J Radiat Oncol Biol Phys* 1989;17:719–725.

237. Fowble B, Fein DA, Hanlon AL, et al. The impact of tamoxifen on breast recurrence, cosmesis, complications, and survival in estrogen receptor-positive early-stage breast cancer. *Int J Radiat Oncol Biol Phys* 1996;35:669–677.

238. Fowble B, Hanlon A, Freedman G, et al. Internal mammary node irradiation neither decreases distant metastases nor improves survival in stage I and II breast cancer. *Int J Radiat Oncol Biol Phys* 2000;47:883–894.

239. Fowble B, Hanlon A, Freedman G, et al. Second cancers after conservative surgery and radiation for stages I-II breast cancer: identifying a subset of women at increased risk. *Int J Radiat Oncol Biol Phys* 2001;51:679–690.

240. Fowble B, Hanlon AL, Patchefsky A, et al. The presence of proliferative breast disease with atypia does not significantly influence outcome in early-stage invasive breast cancer treated with conservative surgery and radiation. *Int J Radiat Oncol Biol Phys* 1998;42:105–115.

241. Fowble B, Solin LJ, Schultz DJ, et al. Breast recurrence following conservative surgery and radiation: patterns of failure, prognosis, and pathologic findings from mastectomy specimens with implications for treatment. *Int J Radiat Oncol Biol Phys* 1990;19:833–842.

242. Fowble B, Solin LJ, Schultz DJ, et al. Frequency, sites of relapse, and outcome of regional node failures following conservative surgery and radiation for early breast cancer. *Int J Radiat Oncol Biol Phys* 1989;17:703–710.

243. Fowble B. Ipsilateral breast tumor recurrence following breast-conserving surgery for early-stage invasive cancer. *Acta Oncol* 1999;38[Suppl 13]:9–17.

244. Fowble B. Postmastectomy radiation in patients with one to three positive axillary nodes receiving adjuvant chemotherapy: an unresolved issue. *Semin Radiat Oncol* 1999;9:230–240.

245. Fowble BL, Schultz DJ, Overmoyer B, et al. The influence of young age on outcome in early stage breast cancer. *Int J Radiat Oncol Biol Phys* 1994;30:23–33.

246. Fowble BL, Solin LJ, Schultz DJ, et al. Ten year results of conservative surgery and irradiation for stage I and II breast cancer. *Int J Radiat Oncol Biol Phys* 1991;21:269–277.

247. Fraass BA, Roberson PL, Lichter AS. Dose to the contralateral breast due to primary breast irradiation. *Int J Radiat Oncol Biol Phys* 1985;11:485–497.

248. Fraile M, Rull M, Julian FJ, et al. Sentinel node biopsy as a practical alternative to axillary lymph node dissection in breast cancer patients: an approach to its validity. *Ann Oncol* 2000;11:701–705.

249. Francois A, Chatikhine VA, Chevallier B, et al. Neuroendocrine primary small cell carcinoma of the breast. Report of a case and review of the literature. *Am J Clin Oncol* 1995;18:133–138.

250. Freedman G, Fowble B, Hanlon A, et al. Patients with early stage invasive cancer with close or positive margins treated with conservative surgery and radiation have an increased risk of breast recurrence that is delayed by adjuvant systemic therapy. *Int J Radiat Oncol Biol Phys* 1999;44:1005–1015.

251. Freedman GM, Anderson PR, Hanlon AL, et al. Pattern of local recurrence after conservative surgery and whole-breast irradiation. *Int J Radiat Oncol Biol Phys* 2005;61:1328–1336.

252. Freedman GM, Fowble BL, Nicolaou N, et al. Should internal mammary lymph nodes in breast cancer be a target for the radiation oncologist? *Int J Radiat Oncol Biol Phys* 2000;46:805–814.

253. Freedman GM, Fowble BL. Local recurrence after mastectomy or

breast-conserving surgery and radiation. *Oncology (Williston Park)* 2000;14:1561–1581; discussion 1581–1562, 1582–1564.
254. Freedman LM, Buchholz TA, Thames HD, et al. Local-regional control in breast cancer patients with a possible genetic predisposition. *Int J Radiat Oncol Biol Phys* 2000;48:951–957.
255. Friedrichs K, Gluba S, Eidtmann H, et al. Overexpression of p53 and prognosis in breast cancer. *Cancer* 1993;72:3641–3647.
256. Frierson HF Jr. Ploidy analysis and S-phase fraction determination by flow cytometry of invasive adenocarcinomas of the breast. *Am J Surg Pathol* 1991;15:358–367.
257. Frisell J, Lidbrink E. The Stockholm Mammographic Screening Trial: risks and benefits in age group 40-49 years. *J Natl Cancer Inst Monogr* 1997:49–51.
258. Fung MC, Schultz DJ, Solin LJ. Early-stage bilateral breast cancer treated with breast-conserving surgery and definitive irradiation: the University of Pennsylvania experience. *Int J Radiat Oncol Biol Phys* 1997;38:959–967.
259. Fyles AW, McCready DR, Manchul LA, et al. Tamoxifen with or without breast irradiation in women 50 years of age or older with early breast cancer. *N Engl J Med* 2004;351:963–970.
260. Gaffney DK, Tsodikov A, Wiggins CL. Diminished survival in patients with inner versus outer quadrant breast cancers. *J Clin Oncol* 2003;21:467–472.
261. Gaffney EV, Halpin DP, Blakemore WS. Relationship between low estrogen receptor values and other prognostic factors in primary breast tumors. *Surgery* 1995;117:241–246.
262. Gage I, Recht A, Gelman R, et al. Long-term outcome following breast-conserving surgery and radiation therapy. *Int J Radiat Oncol Biol Phys* 1995;33:245–251.
263. Gage I, Schnitt SJ, Nixon AJ, et al. Pathologic margin involvement and the risk of recurrence in patients treated with breast-conserving therapy. *Cancer* 1996;78:1921–1928.
264. Gagliardi G, Bjohle J, Lax I, et al. Radiation pneumonitis after breast cancer irradiation: analysis of the complication probability using the relative seriality model. *Int J Radiat Oncol Biol Phys* 2000;46:373–381.
265. Gail MH, Brinton LA, Byar DP, et al. Projecting individualized probabilities of developing breast cancer for white females who are being examined annually. *J Natl Cancer Inst* 1989;81:1879–1886.
266. Gajdos C, Tartter PI, Bleiweiss IJ, et al. The consequence of undertreating breast cancer in the elderly. *J Am Coll Surg* 2001;192:698–707.
267. Gajdos C, Tartter PI, Bleiweiss IJ. Subareolar breast cancers. *Am J Surg* 2000;180:167–170.
268. Galper S, Gelman R, Recht A, et al. Second nonbreast malignancies after conservative surgery and radiation therapy for early-stage breast cancer. *Int J Radiat Oncol Biol Phys* 2002;52:406–414.
269. Galper S, Recht A, Silver B, et al. Factors associated with regional nodal failure in patients with early stage breast cancer with 0-3 positive axillary nodes following tangential irradiation alone. *Int J Radiat Oncol Biol Phys* 1999;45:1157–1166.
270. Galper S, Recht A, Silver B, et al. Is radiation alone adequate treatment to the axilla for patients with limited axillary surgery? Implications for treatment after a positive sentinel node biopsy. *Int J Radiat Oncol Biol Phys* 2000;48:125–132.
271. Gann PH, Colilla SA, Gapstur SM, et al. Factors associated with axillary lymph node metastasis from breast carcinoma: descriptive and predictive analyses. *Cancer* 1999;86:1511–1519.
272. Ganz PA, Rowland JH, Desmond K, et al. Life after breast cancer: understanding women's health-related quality of life and sexual functioning. *J Clin Oncol* 1998;16:501–514.
273. Ganz PA, Rowland JH, Meyerowitz BE, et al. Impact of different adjuvant therapy strategies on quality of life in breast cancer survivors. *Recent Results Cancer Res* 1998;152:396–411.
274. Gerard JP, Montbarbon JF, Chassard JL, et al. Conservative treatment of early carcinoma of the breast: significance of axillary dissection and iridium implant. *Radiother Oncol* 1985;3:17–22.
275. Gervais-Fagnou DD, Girouard C, Laperriere N, et al. Breast cancer in women following supradiaphragmatic irradiation for Hodgkin's disease. *Oncology* 1999;57:224–231.
276. Ghossein NA, Vilcoq J, Stacey P, et al. Is it necessary to irradiate the breast after conservative surgery for localized cancer? *Arch Surg* 1987;122:913–917.
277. Giuliano AE, Haigh PI, Brennan MB, et al. Prospective observational study of sentinel lymphadenectomy without further axillary dissection in patients with sentinel node-negative breast cancer. *J Clin Oncol* 2000;18:2553–2559.
278. Giuliano AE, Jones RC, Brennan M, et al. Sentinel lymphadenectomy in breast cancer. *J Clin Oncol* 1997;15:2345–2350.
279. Giuliano AE, Kirgan DM, Guenther JM, et al. Lymphatic mapping and sentinel lymphadenectomy for breast cancer. *Ann Surg* 1994;220:391–398; discussion 398–401.
280. Goldhirsch A, Glick JH, Gelber RD, et al. Meeting highlights: international expert consensus on the primary therapy of early breast cancer 2005. *Ann Oncol* 2005;16:1569–1583.
281. Goodman RL, Grann A, Saracco P, et al. The relationship between radiation fields and regional lymph nodes in carcinoma of the breast. *Int J Radiat Oncol Biol Phys* 2001;50:99–105.
282. Gorodetsky R, Lotan C, Piggot K, et al. Late effects of dose fractionation on the mechanical properties of breast skin following post-lumpectomy radiotherapy. *Int J Radiat Oncol Biol Phys* 1999;45:893–900.
283. Grabrick DM, Hartmann LC, Cerhan JR, et al. Risk of breast cancer with oral contraceptive use in women with a family history of breast cancer. *JAMA* 2000;284:1791–1798.
284. Greco M, Crippa F, Agresti R, et al. Axillary lymph node staging in breast cancer by 2-fluoro-2-deoxy-D-glucose-positron emission tomography: clinical evaluation and alternative management. *J Natl Cancer Inst* 2001;93:630–635.
285. Greene FL, Page DI, Fleming ID, et al., eds. *AJCC cancer staging manual*, 6th ed. New York: Springer-Verlag, 2002.
286. Grills IS, Kestin LL, Goldstein N, et al. Risk factors for regional nodal failure after breast-conserving therapy: regional nodal irradiation reduces rate of axillary failure in patients with four or more positive lymph nodes. *Int J Radiat Oncol Biol Phys* 2003;56:658–670.
287. Gruber G, Berclaz G, Altermatt HJ, et al. Can the addition of regional radiotherapy counterbalance important risk factors in breast cancer patients with extracapsular invasion of axillary lymph node metastases? *Strahlenther Onkol* 2003;179:661–666.
288. Guenther JM, Krishnamoorthy M, Tan LR. Sentinel lymphadenectomy for breast cancer in a community managed care setting. *Cancer J Sci Am* 1997;3:336–340.
289. Guenther JM, Tokita KM, Giuliano AE. Breast-conserving surgery and radiation after augmentation mammoplasty. *Cancer* 1994;73:2613–2618.
290. Guibout C, Adjadj E, Rubino C, et al. Malignant breast tumors after radiotherapy for a first cancer during childhood. *J Clin Oncol* 2005;23:197–204.
291. Gustafsson A, Tartter PI, Brower ST, et al. Prognosis of patients with bilateral carcinoma of the breast. *J Am Coll Surg* 1994;178:111–116.
292. Gyenes G, Fornander T, Carlens P, et al. Morbidity of ischemic heart disease in early breast cancer 15-20 years after adjuvant radiotherapy. *Int J Radiat Oncol Biol Phys* 1994;28:1235–1241.
293. Haagenson C. *Diseases of the breast*. Philadelphia: W.B. Saunders, 1986.
294. Haas JA, Schultz DJ, Peterson ME, et al. An analysis of age and family history on outcome after breast-conservation treatment: the University of Pennsylvania experience. *Cancer J Sci Am* 1998;4:308–315.
295. Hack TF, Cohen L, Katz J, et al. Physical and psychological morbidity after axillary lymph node dissection for breast cancer. *J Clin Oncol* 1999;17:143–149.
296. Haffty BG, Brown F, Carter D, et al. Evaluation of HER-2 neu oncoprotein expression as a prognostic indicator of local recurrence in conservatively treated breast cancer: a case-control study. *Int J Radiat Oncol Biol Phys* 1996;35:751–757.
297. Haffty BG, Carter D, Flynn SD, et al. Local recurrence versus new primary: clinical analysis of 82 breast relapses and potential applications for genetic fingerprinting. *Int J Radiat Oncol Biol Phys* 1993;27:575–583.
298. Haffty BG, Fischer D, Beinfield M, et al. Prognosis following local recurrence in the conservatively treated breast cancer patient. *Int J Radiat Oncol Biol Phys* 1991;21:293–298.
299. Haffty BG, Fischer D, Fischer JJ. Regional nodal irradiation in the conservative treatment of breast cancer. *Int J Radiat Oncol Biol Phys* 1990;19:859–865.
300. Haffty BG, Fischer D, Rose M, et al. Prognostic factors for local recurrence in the conservatively treated breast cancer patient: a cautious interpretation of the data. *J Clin Oncol* 1991;9:997–1003.
301. Haffty BG, Glazer PM. Molecular markers in clinical radiation oncology. *Oncogene* 2003;22:5915–5925.
302. Haffty BG, Goldberg NB, Fischer D, et al. Conservative surgery and radiation therapy in breast carcinoma: local recurrence and prognostic implications. *Int J Radiat Oncol Biol Phys* 1989;17:727–732.
303. Haffty BG, Harrold E, Khan AJ, et al. Outcome of conservatively managed early-onset breast cancer by BRCA1/2 status. *Lancet* 2002;359:1471–1477.
304. Haffty BG, Kim JH, Yang Q, et al. Concurrent chemo-radiation in the conservative management of breast cancer. *Int J Radiation Oncol Biol Phys* 2006;IN PRESS.
305. Haffty BG, Kim JH, Yang Q, et al. Concurrent chemo-radiation in the conservative management of breast cancer. *Int J Radiat Oncol Biol Phys* 2006;66:1306–1312.
306. Haffty BG, McKhann C, Beinfield M, et al. Breast conservation therapy without axillary dissection. A rational treatment strategy in selected patients. *Arch Surg* 1993;128:1315–1319; discussion 1319.
307. Haffty BG, Reiss M, Beinfield M, et al. Ipsilateral breast tumor recurrence as a predictor of distant disease: implications for systemic therapy at the time of local relapse. *J Clin Oncol* 1996;14:52–57.
308. Haffty BG, Wilmarth L, Wilson L, et al. Adjuvant systemic chemotherapy and hormonal therapy. Effect on local recurrence in the conservatively treated breast cancer patient. *Cancer* 1994;73:2543–2548.
309. Haffty BG, Wilson LD, Smith R, et al. Subareolar breast cancer: long-term results with conservative surgery and radiation therapy. *Int J Radiat Oncol Biol Phys* 1995;33:53–57.
310. Haffty BG. Accelerated partial breast irradiation: where do we go from here? *Breast J* 2005;11:303–305.
311. Haffty BG. Follow-up and salvage therapy for the conservatively treated breast cancer patient. *Semin Radiat Oncol* 1992;2:132–139.
312. Haffty BG. Molecular and genetic markers in the local-regional management of breast cancer. *Semin Radiat Oncol* 2002;12:329–340.
313. Hahn KM, Johnson PH, Gordon N, et al. Treatment of pregnant breast cancer patients and outcomes of children exposed to chemotherapy in utero. *Cancer* 2006;107:1219–1226.
314. Hall EJ, Wuu CS. Radiation-induced second cancers: the impact of 3D-CRT and IMRT. *Int J Radiat Oncol Biol Phys* 2003;56:83–88.
315. Halsted WS. The results of operations for the cure of cancer of the breast performed at Johns Hopkins Hospital from June 1889 to January 1894. *Johns Hopkins Hosp Bull* 1894;4:297.
316. Halverson KJ, Perez CA, Taylor ME, et al. Age as a prognostic factor for breast and regional nodal recurrence following breast conserving surgery and irradiation in stage I and II breast cancer. *Int J Radiat Oncol Biol Phys* 1993;27:1045–1050.
317. Halverson KJ, Taylor ME, Perez CA, et al. Management of the axilla in patients with breast cancers one centimeter or smaller. *Am J Clin Oncol* 1994;17:461–466.
318. Halverson KJ, Taylor ME, Perez CA, et al. Regional nodal management and patterns of failure following conservative surgery and radiation therapy for stage I and II breast cancer. *Int J Radiat Oncol Biol Phys* 1993;26:593–599.
319. Hamajima N, Hirose K, Tajima K, et al. Alcohol, tobacco and breast cancer—collaborative reanalysis of individual data from 53 epidemiological studies, including 58,515 women with breast cancer and 95,067 women without the disease. *Br J Cancer* 2002;87:1234–1245.
320. Hamilton T, Langlands AO, Prescott RJ. The treatment of operable cancer of the breast: A clinical trial in the south-east region of Scotland. *Br J Surg* 1974;61:758–761.
321. Hancock SL, Tucker MA, Hoppe RT. Breast cancer after treatment of Hodgkin's disease. *J Natl Cancer Inst* 1993;85:25–31.
322. Handel N, Lewinsky B, Silverstein MJ, et al. Conservation therapy for breast cancer following augmentation mammaplasty. *Plast Reconstr Surg* 1991;87:873–878.
323. Handley RS. Carcinoma of the breast. *Ann R Coll Surg Engl* 1975;57:59–66.
324. Hankey BF, Curtis RE, Naughton MD, et al. A retrospective cohort analysis of second breast cancer risk for primary breast cancer patients with an assessment of the effect of radiation therapy. *J Natl Cancer Inst* 1983;70:797–804.
325. Hanrahan EO, Valero V, Gonzalez-Angulo AM, et al. Prognosis and management of patients with node-negative invasive breast carcinoma that is 1 cm or smaller in size (stage 1; T1a,bN0M0): a review of the literature. *J Clin Oncol* 2006;24:2113–2122.

326. Hansen NM, Ye X, Grube BJ, et al. Manipulation of the primary breast tumor and the incidence of sentinel node metastases from invasive breast cancer. *Arch Surg* 2004;139:634–639; discussion 639–640.
327. Harrington KJ, Harrison M, Bayle P, et al. Surgical clips in planning the electron boost in breast cancer: a qualitative and quantitative evaluation. *Int J Radiat Oncol Biol Phys* 1996;34:579–584.
328. Harris EE, Christensen VJ, Hwang WT, et al. Impact of concurrent versus sequential tamoxifen with radiation therapy in early-stage breast cancer patients undergoing breast conservation treatment. *J Clin Oncol* 2005;23:11–16.
329. Harris EE, Hwang WT, Lee EA, et al. The impact of HER-2 status on local recurrence in women with stage I-II breast cancer treated with breast-conserving therapy. *Breast J* 2006;12:431–436.
330. Harris J, Lippman M, Morrow M, et al. *Diseases of the breast*. Philadelphia: Lippincott Williams & Wilkins, 2004.
331. Harris JR, Botnick L, Bloomer WD, et al. Primary radiation therapy for early breast cancer: the experience at the Joint Center for Radiation Therapy. *Int J Radiat Oncol Biol Phys* 1981;7:1549–1552.
332. Harris JR, Connolly JL, Schnitt SJ, et al. The use of pathologic features in selecting the extent of surgical resection necessary for breast cancer patients treated by primary radiation therapy. *Ann Surg* 1985;201:164–169.
333. Harris JR, Recht A, Amalric R, et al. Time course and prognosis of local recurrence following primary radiation therapy for early breast cancer. *J Clin Oncol* 1984;2:37–41.
334. Harrold EV, Turner BC, Matloff ET, et al. Local recurrence in the conservatively treated breast cancer patient: a correlation with age and family history. *Cancer J Sci Am* 1998;4:302–307.
335. Hartmann LC, Schaid DJ, Woods JE, et al. Efficacy of bilateral prophylactic mastectomy in women with a family history of breast cancer. *N Engl J Med* 1999;340:77–84.
336. Hartmann LC, Sellers TA, Frost MH, et al. Benign breast disease and the risk of breast cancer. *N Engl J Med* 2005;353:229–237.
337. Hartsell WF, Kelly CA, Schneider L, et al. A single isocenter three-field breast irradiation technique using an empiric simulation and asymmetric collimator. *Med Dosim* 1994;19:169–173.
338. Hartsell WF, Recine DC, Griem KL, et al. Delaying the initiation of intact breast irradiation for patients with lymph node positive breast cancer increases the risk of local recurrence. *Cancer* 1995;76:2497–2503.
339. Hartsell WF, Recine DC, Griem KL, et al. Should multicentric disease be an absolute contraindication to the use of breast-conserving therapy? *Int J Radiat Oncol Biol Phys* 1994;30:49–53.
340. Hayes DF. Prognostic and predictive factors revisited. *Breast* 2005;14:493–499.
341. Hayman JA, Hillner BE, Harris JR, et al. Cost-effectiveness of adding an electron-beam boost to tangential radiation therapy in patients with negative margins after conservative surgery for early-stage breast cancer. *J Clin Oncol* 2000;18:287–295.
342. Hayward J, Caleffi M. The significance of local control in the primary treatment of breast cancer. Lucy Wortham James clinical research award. *Arch Surg* 1987;122:1244–1247.
343. Heimann R, Powers C, Halpem HJ, et al. Breast preservation in stage I and II carcinoma of the breast. The University of Chicago experience. *Cancer* 1996;78:1722–1730.
344. Hellman S. Karnofsky Memorial Lecture. Natural history of small breast cancers. *J Clin Oncol* 1994;12:2229–2234.
345. Hennessy BT, Giordano S, Broglio K, et al. Biphasic metaplastic sarcomatoid carcinoma of the breast. *Ann Oncol* 2006;17:605–613.
346. Heron DE, Komarnicky LT, Hyslop T, et al. Bilateral breast carcinoma: risk factors and outcomes for patients with synchronous and metachronous disease. *Cancer* 2000;88:2739–2750.
347. Hetelekidis S, Schnitt SJ, Silver B, et al. The significance of extracapsular extension of axillary lymph node metastases in early-stage breast cancer. *Int J Radiat Oncol Biol Phys* 2000;46:31–34.
348. Higgins S, Haffty BG. Pregnancy and lactation after breast-conserving therapy for early stage breast cancer. *Cancer* 1994;73:2175–2180.
349. Hill-Kayser CE, Harris EE, Hwang WT, et al. Twenty-Year incidence and patterns of contralateral breast cancer after breast conservation treatment with radiation. *Int J Radiat Oncol Biol Phys* 2006.
350. Hislop TG, Elwood JM, Coldman AJ, et al. Second primary cancers of the breast: incidence and risk factors. *Br J Cancer* 1984;49:79–85.
351. Hoang MP, Sahin AA, Ordonez NG, et al. HER-2/neu gene amplification compared with HER-2/neu protein overexpression and interobserver reproducibility in invasive breast carcinoma. *Am J Clin Pathol* 2000;113:852–859.
352. Hojris I, Andersen J, Overgaard M, et al. Late treatment-related morbidity in breast cancer patients randomized to postmastectomy radiotherapy and systemic treatment versus systemic treatment alone. *Acta Oncol* 2000;39:355–372.
353. Holland R, Connolly JL, Gelman R, et al. The presence of an extensive intraductal component following a limited excision correlates with prominent residual disease in the remainder of the breast. *J Clin Oncol* 1990;8:113–118.
354. Hollstein M, Soussi T, Thomas G, et al. p53 gene alterations in human tumors: perspectives for cancer control. *Recent Results Cancer Res* 1997;143:369–389.
355. Hoppe RT. Hodgkin's disease: complications of therapy and excess mortality. *Ann Oncol* 1997;8[Suppl 1]:115–118.
356. Horn PL, Thompson WD. Risk of contralateral breast cancer. Associations with histologic, clinical, and therapeutic factors. *Cancer* 1988;62:412–424.
357. Hornstein E, Skornick Y, Rozin R. The management of breast carcinoma in pregnancy and lactation. *J Surg Oncol* 1982;21:179–182.
358. Huang J, Barbera L, Brouwers M, et al. Does delay in starting treatment affect the outcomes of radiotherapy? A systematic review. *J Clin Oncol* 2003;21:555–563.
359. Huang J, Mackillop WJ. Increased risk of soft tissue sarcoma after radiotherapy in women with breast carcinoma. *Cancer* 2001;92:172–180.
360. Hudson MM, Poquette CA, Lee J, et al. Increased mortality after successful treatment for Hodgkin's disease. *J Clin Oncol* 1998;16:3592–3600.
361. Hughes KS, Schnaper LA, Berry D, et al. Lumpectomy plus tamoxifen with or without irradiation in women 70 years of age or older with early breast cancer. *N Engl J Med* 2004;351:971–977.
362. Hungness ES, Safa M, Shaughnessy EA, et al. Bilateral synchronous breast cancer: mode of detection and comparison of histologic features between the 2 breasts. *Surgery* 2000;128:702–707.
363. Hunter DJ, Spiegelman D, Adami HO, et al. Non-dietary factors as risk factors for breast cancer, and as effect modifiers of the association of fat intake and risk of breast cancer. *Cancer Causes Control* 1997;8:49–56.
364. Hurny C, Bernhard J, Coates A. Quality of life assessment in the International Breast Cancer Study Group: past, present, and future. *Recent Results Cancer Res* 1998;152:390–395.
365. Hylton N. Magnetic resonance imaging of the breast: opportunities to improve breast cancer management. *J Clin Oncol* 2005;23:1678–1684.
366. Iannuzzi CM, Atencio DP, Green S, et al. ATM mutations in female breast cancer patients predict for an increase in radiation-induced late effects. *Int J Radiat Oncol Biol Phys* 2002;52:606–613.
367. Identification of breast cancer patients with high risk of early recurrence after radical mastectomy. II. Clinical and pathological correlations. A report of the Primary Therapy of Breast Cancer Study Group. *Cancer* 1978;42:2809–2826.
368. Ilum L, Bak M, Olsen KE, et al. Sentinel node localization in breast cancer patients using intradermal dye injection. *Acta Oncol* 2000;39:423–428.
369. Intra M, Leonardi MC, Gatti G, et al. Intraoperative radiotherapy during breast conserving surgery in patients previously treated with radiotherapy for Hodgkin's disease. *Tumori* 2004;90:13–16.
370. Iwasaki Y, Fukutomi T, Akashi-Tanaka S, et al. Axillary node metastasis from T1N0M0 breast cancer: possible avoidance of dissection in a subgroup. *Jpn J Clin Oncol* 1998;28:601–603.
371. Jacobson JA, Danforth DN, Cowan KH, et al. Ten-year results of a comparison of conservation with mastectomy in the treatment of stage I and II breast cancer. *N Engl J Med* 1995;332:907–90911.
372. Jacquillat C, Weil M, Baillet F, et al. Results of neoadjuvant chemotherapy and radiation therapy in the breast-conserving treatment of 250 patients with all stages of infiltrative breast cancer. *Cancer* 1990;66:119–129.
373. Jagsi R, Griffith KA, Koelling T, et al. Stroke rates and risk factors in patients treated with radiation therapy for early-stage breast cancer. *J Clin Oncol* 2006;24:2779–2785.
374. Jagsi R, Makris A, Goldberg S, et al. Intra-European differences in the radiotherapeutic management of breast cancer: a survey study. *Clin Oncol (R Coll Radiol)* 2006;18:369–375.
375. Janjan NA, Murray KJ, Conway P, et al. Prognosis for breast cancer surgery and radiation therapy compared with mastectomy alone. A retrospective analysis of 759 patients with stage I/II breast cancer. *Cancer* 1992;69:2842–2848.
376. Janni W, Rack B, Sommer H, et al. Intra-mammary tumor location does not influence prognosis but influences the prevalence of axillary lymph node metastases. *J Cancer Res Clin Oncol* 2003;129:503–510.
377. Janson RL, Joosten-Achjanie SR, Volovics A, et al. Relevance of the expression of bcl-2 in combination with p53 as a prognostic factor in breast cancer. *Anticancer Res* 1998;18:4455–4462.
378. Jatoi I, Proschan MA. Randomized trials of breast-conserving therapy versus mastectomy for primary breast cancer: a pooled analysis of updated results. *Am J Clin Oncol* 2005;28:289–294.
379. Jemal A, Siegel R, Ward E, et al. Cancer statistics, 2006. *CA Cancer J Clin* 2006;56:106–130.
380. Jensen AB. Psychosocial factors in breast cancer and their possible impact upon prognosis. *Cancer Treat Rev* 1991;18:191–210.
381. Jobsen JJ, van der Palen J, Ong F, et al. The value of a positive margin for invasive carcinoma in breast-conservative treatment in relation to local recurrence is limited to young women only. *Int J Radiat Oncol Biol Phys* 2003;57:724–731.
382. Jolly S, Kestin LL, Goldstein NS, et al. The impact of lobular carcinoma in situ in association with invasive breast cancer on the rate of local recurrence in patients with early-stage breast cancer treated with breast-conserving therapy. *Int J Radiat Oncol Biol Phys* 2006;66:365–371.
383. Jones BA, Kasl SV, Curnen MG, et al. Can mammography screening explain the race difference in stage at diagnosis of breast cancer? *Cancer* 1995;75:2103–2113.
384. Jones BA, Kasl SV, Howe CL, et al. African-American/White differences in breast carcinoma: p53 alterations and other tumor characteristics. *Cancer* 2004;101:1293–1301.
385. Joslyn SA, West MM. Racial differences in breast carcinoma survival. *Cancer* 2000;88:114–123.
386. Kaldor JM, Day NE, Band P, et al. Second malignancies following testicular cancer, ovarian cancer and Hodgkin's disease: an international collaborative study among cancer registries. *Int J Cancer* 1987;39:571–585.
387. Kallioniemi OP, Blanco G, Alavaikko M, et al. Tumour DNA ploidy as an independent prognostic factor in breast cancer. *Br J Cancer* 1987;56:637–642.
388. Kamath VJ, Giuliano R, Dauway EL, et al. Characteristics of the sentinel lymph node in breast cancer predict further involvement of higher-echelon nodes in the axilla: a study to evaluate the need for complete axillary lymph node dissection. *Arch Surg* 2001;136:688–692.
389. Kambouris AA. Axillary node metastases in relation to size and location of breast cancers: analysis of 147 patients. *Am Surg* 1996;62:519–524.
390. Kaplan J, Giron G, Tartter PI, et al. Breast conservation in patients with multiple ipsilateral synchronous cancers. *J Am Coll Surg* 2003;197:726–729.
391. Karlsson P, Holmberg E, Samuelsson A, et al. Soft tissue sarcoma after treatment for breast cancer—a Swedish population-based study. *Eur J Cancer* 1998;34:2068–2075.
392. Kauff ND, Satagopan JM, Robson ME, et al. Risk-reducing salpingo-oophorectomy in women with a BRCA1 or BRCA2 mutation. *N Engl J Med* 2002;346:1609–1615.
393. Kaufman J, Gunn W, Hartz AJ, et al. The pathophysiologic and roentgenologic effects of chest irradiation in breast carcinoma. *Int J Radiat Oncol Biol Phys* 1986;12:887–893.
394. Keisch M, Vicini F, Kuske RR, et al. Initial clinical experience with the MammoSite breast brachytherapy applicator in women with early-stage breast cancer treated with breast-conserving therapy. *Int J Radiat Oncol Biol Phys* 2003;55:289–293.
395. Kelemen JJ 3rd, Poulton T, Swartz MT, et al. Surgical treatment of early-stage breast cancer in the Department of Defense Healthcare System. *J Am Coll Surg* 2001;192:293–297.
396. Kelly CA, Wang XY, Chu JC, et al. Dose to contralateral breast: a comparison of four primary breast irradiation techniques. *Int J Radiat Oncol Biol Phys* 1996;34:727–732.
397. Kerlikowske K, Grady D, Rubin SM, et al. Efficacy of screening mammography. A meta-analysis. *JAMA* 1995;273:149–154.
398. Keyhani-Rofagha S, O'Toole RV, Farrar WB, et al. Is DNA ploidy an independent

prognostic indicator in infiltrative node-negative breast adenocarcinoma? *Cancer* 1990;65:1577–1582.
399. Keynes G. Carcinoma of the breast, the unorthodox view. *Proc Cardiff Med Soc* 1954;40.
400. Khan AJ, Haffty BG. The location of contralateral breast cancers after radiation therapy. *Breast J* 2001;7:331–336.
401. Kim S, Rimm D, Carter D, et al. BRCA status, molecular markers, and clinical variables in early, conservatively managed breast cancer. *Breast J* 2003;9:167–174.
402. King MC, Wieand S, Hale K, et al. Tamoxifen and breast cancer incidence among women with inherited mutations in BRCA1 and BRCA2: National Surgical Adjuvant Breast and Bowel Project (NSABP-P1) Breast Cancer Prevention Trial. *JAMA* 2001;286:2251–2256.
403. King RM, Welch JS, Martin JK Jr., et al. Carcinoma of the breast associated with pregnancy. *Surg Gynecol Obstet* 1985;160:228–232.
404. Kini VR, Vicini FA, Frazier R, et al. Mammographic, pathologic, and treatment-related factors associated with local recurrence in patients with early-stage breast cancer treated with breast conserving therapy. *Int J Radiat Oncol Biol Phys* 1999;43:341–346.
405. Kini VR, White JR, Horwitz EM, et al. Long-term results with breast-conserving therapy for patients with early stage breast carcinoma in a community hospital setting. *Cancer* 1998;82:127–133.
406. Koizumi M, Yoshimoto M, Kasumi F, et al. What do breast cancer patients benefit from staging bone scintigraphy? *Jpn J Clin Oncol* 2001;31:263–269.
407. Kollias J, Ellis IO, Elston CW, et al. Prognostic significance of synchronous and metachronous bilateral breast cancer. *World J Surg* 2001;25:1117–1124.
408. Kollias J, Evans AJ, Wilson AR, et al. Value of contralateral surveillance mammography for primary breast cancer follow-up. *World J Surg* 2000;24:983–987; discussion 988–989.
409. Kollias J, Murphy CA, Elston CW, et al. The prognosis of small primary breast cancers. *Eur J Cancer* 1999;35:908–912.
410. Kong FM, Klein EE, Bradley JD, et al. The impact of central lung distance, maximal heart distance, and radiation technique on the volumetric dose of the lung and heart for intact breast radiation. *Int J Radiat Oncol Biol Phys* 2002;54:963–971.
411. Kopans DB, Feig SA. The Canadian National Breast Screening Study: a critical review. *AJR Am J Roentgenol* 1993;161:755–760.
412. Kopans DB, Meyer JE, Sadowsky N. Breast imaging. *N Engl J Med* 1984;310:960–967.
413. Kopans DB. An overview of the breast cancer screening controversy. *J Natl Cancer Inst Monogr* 1997:1–3.
414. Kori SH. Diagnosis and management of brachial plexus lesions in cancer patients. *Oncology (Williston Park)* 1995;9:756–760; discussion 765.
415. Krag D, Harlow S, Julian T. Breast cancer and the NSABP-B32 sentinel node trial. *Breast Cancer* 2004;11:221–224; discussion 264–226.
416. Krag D, Weaver D, Ashikaga T, et al. The sentinel node in breast cancer—a multicenter validation study. *N Engl J Med* 1998;339:941–946.
417. Krag DN, Harlow S, Weaver D, et al. Radiolabeled sentinel node biopsy: collaborative trial with the National Cancer Institute. *World J Surg* 2001;25:823–828.
418. Krag DN, Julian TB, Harlow SP, et al. NSABP-32: Phase III, randomized trial comparing axillary resection with sentinel lymph node dissection: a description of the trial. *Ann Surg Oncol* 2004;11:208S–210S.
419. Kramer S, Schulz-Wendtland R, Hagedorn K, et al. Magnetic resonance imaging in the diagnosis of local recurrences in breast cancer. *Anticancer Res* 1998;18:2159–2161.
420. Kriege M, Brekelmans CT, Boetes C, et al. Efficacy of MRI and mammography for breast-cancer screening in women with a familial or genetic predisposition. *N Engl J Med* 2004;351:427–437.
421. Kroman N, Wohlfahrt J, Andersen KW, et al. Parity, age at first childbirth and the prognosis of primary breast cancer. *Br J Cancer* 1998;78:1529–1533.
422. Kronowitz SJ, Feledy JA, Hunt KK, et al. Determining the optimal approach to breast reconstruction after partial mastectomy. *Plast Reconstr Surg* 2006;117:1–11; discussion 12–14.
423. Kurtz JM, Amalric R, Brandone H, et al. Local recurrence after breast-conserving surgery and radiotherapy. Frequency, time course, and prognosis. *Cancer* 1989;63:1912–1917.
424. Kurtz JM, Jacquemier J, Amalric R, et al. Breast-conserving therapy for macroscopically multiple cancers. *Ann Surg* 1990;212:38–44.
425. Kurtz JM, Jacquemier J, Amalric R, et al. Risk factors for breast recurrence in premenopausal and postmenopausal patients with ductal cancers treated by conservation therapy. *Cancer* 1990;65:1867–1878.
426. Kurtz JM, Jacquemier J, Amalric R, et al. Why are local recurrences after breast-conserving therapy more frequent in younger patients? *J Clin Oncol* 1990;8:591–598.
427. Kurtz JM, Spitalier JM, Amalric R, et al. Mammary recurrences in women younger than forty. *Int J Radiat Oncol Biol Phys* 1988;15:271–276.
428. Kuske RR Jr. Breast brachytherapy. *Hematol Oncol Clin North Am* 1999;13:543-558, vi–vii.
429. Kuske RR, Winter K, Arthur DW, et al. Phase II trial of brachytherapy alone after lumpectomy for select breast cancer: toxicity analysis of RTOG 95-17. *Int J Radiat Oncol Biol Phys* 2006;65:45–51.
430. Lacour J, Bucalossi P, Cacers E, et al. Radical mastectomy versus radical mastectomy plus internal mammary dissection. Five-year results of an international cooperative study. *Cancer* 1976;37:206–214.
431. Lally BE, Haffty BG, Moran MS, et al. Management of suspicious or indeterminate calcifications and impact on local control. *Cancer* 2005;103:2236–2240.
432. Land CE, Boice JD Jr., Shore RE, et al. Breast cancer risk from low-dose exposures to ionizing radiation: results of parallel analysis of three exposed populations of women. *J Natl Cancer Inst* 1980;65:353–376.
433. Land CE. Studies of cancer and radiation dose among atomic bomb survivors. The example of breast cancer. *JAMA* 1995;274:402–407.
434. Landercasper J, Gundersen SB Jr., Gundersen AL, et al. Needle localization and biopsy of nonpalpable lesions of the breast. *Surg Gynecol Obstet* 1987;164:399–403.
435. Langlands AO, Prescott RJ, Hamilton T. A clinical trial in the management of operable cancer of the breast. *Br J Surg* 1980;67:170–174.
436. Lash TL, Silliman RA, Guadagnoli E, et al. The effect of less than definitive care on breast carcinoma recurrence and mortality. *Cancer* 2000;89:1739–1747.
437. Lasry JC, Margolese RG. Fear of recurrence, breast-conserving surgery, and the trade-off hypothesis. *Cancer* 1992;69:2111–2115.
438. Leborgne F, Leborgne JH, Ortega B, et al. Breast conservation treatment of early stage breast cancer: patterns of failure. *Int J Radiat Oncol Biol Phys* 1995;31:765–775.
439. Lee CH, Smith RC, Levine JA, et al. Clinical usefulness of MR imaging of the breast in the evaluation of the problematic mammogram. *AJR Am J Roentgenol* 1999;173:1323–1329.
440. Lehman CD, Blume JD, Thickman D, et al. Added cancer yield of MRI in screening the contralateral breast of women recently diagnosed with breast cancer: results from the International Breast Magnetic Resonance Consortium (IBMC) trial. *J Surg Oncol* 2005;92:9–15; discussion 15–16.
441. Leopold KA, Recht A, Schnitt SJ, et al. Results of conservative surgery and radiation therapy for multiple synchronous cancers of one breast. *Int J Radiat Oncol Biol Phys* 1989;16:11–16.
442. Leung S, Otmezguine Y, Calitchi E, et al. Locoregional recurrences following radical external beam irradiation and interstitial implantation for operable breast cancer—a twenty three year experience. *Radiother Oncol* 1986;5:1–10.
443. Levitt SH, Mandel J. Benefits versus risks in conservation surgery with irradiation for breast cancer. *Am J Med* 1984;77:93–100.
444. Lewis TR, Casey J, Buerk CA, et al. Incidence of lobular carcinoma in bilateral breast cancer. *Am J Surg* 1982;144:635–638.
444a. Li C, Wilson PB, Levine E, et al. TGF-beta levels in pre-treatment plasma identify breast cancer patients at risk of developing post-radiotherapy fibrosis. *Int J Cancer* 1999;84:155–159.
445. Liberman L, Giess CS, Dershaw DD, et al. Imaging of pregnancy-associated breast cancer. *Radiology* 1994;191:245–248.
446. Lichter AS, Fraass BA, Yanke B. Treatment techniques in the conservative management of breast cancer. *Semin Radiat Oncol* 1992;2:94–106.
447. Liljegren G, Holmberg L, Adami HO, et al. Sector resection with or without postoperative radiotherapy for stage I breast cancer: five-year results of a randomized trial. Uppsala-Orebro Breast Cancer Study Group. *J Natl Cancer Inst* 1994;86:717–722.
448. Liljegren G, Karlsson G, Bergh J, et al. The cost-effectiveness of routine postoperative radiotherapy after sector resection and axillary dissection for breast cancer stage I. Results from a randomized trial. *Ann Oncol* 1997;8:757–763.
449. Lim M, Bellon JR, Gelman R, et al. A prospective study of conservative surgery without radiation therapy in select patients with Stage I breast cancer. *Int J Radiat Oncol Biol Phys* 2006;65:1149–1154.
450. Lind PA, Rosfors S, Wennberg B, et al. Pulmonary function following adjuvant chemotherapy and radiotherapy for breast cancer and the issue of three-dimensional treatment planning. *Radiother Oncol* 1998;49:245–254.
451. Linderholm B, Tavelin B, Grankvist K, et al. Does vascular endothelial growth factor (VEGF) predict local relapse and survival in radiotherapy-treated node-negative breast cancer? *Br J Cancer* 1999;81:727–732.
452. Lingos TI, Recht A, Vicini F, et al. Radiation pneumonitis in breast cancer patients treated with conservative surgery and radiation therapy. *Int J Radiat Oncol Biol Phys* 1991;21:355–360.
453. Lippman ME, Allegra JC. Current concepts in cancer. Receptors in breast cancer. *N Engl J Med* 1978;299:930–933.
454. Lohrisch C, Jackson J, Jones A, et al. Relationship between tumor location and relapse in 6,781 women with early invasive breast cancer. *J Clin Oncol* 2000;18:2828–2835.
455. Loibl S, von Minckwitz G, Gwyn K, et al. Breast carcinoma during pregnancy. International recommendations from an expert meeting. *Cancer* 2006;106:237–246.
456. Louis-Sylvestre C, Clough K, Asselain B, et al. Axillary treatment in conservative management of operable breast cancer: dissection or radiotherapy? Results of a randomized study with 15 years of follow-up. *J Clin Oncol* 2004;22:97–101.
457. Lu HM, Cash E, Chen MH, et al. Reduction of cardiac volume in left-breast treatment fields by respiratory maneuvers: a CT study. *Int J Radiat Oncol Biol Phys* 2000;47:895–904.
458. Lund MB, Myhre KI, Melsom H, et al. The effect on pulmonary function of tangential field technique in radiotherapy for carcinoma of the breast. *Br J Radiol* 1991;64:520–523.
459. Lythgoe JP, Palmer MK. Manchester regional breast study—5 and 10 year results. *Br J Surg* 1982;69:693–696.
460. MacMahon B, Purde M, Cramer D, et al. Association of breast cancer risk with age at first and subsequent births: a study in the population of the Estonian Republic. *J Natl Cancer Inst* 1982;69:1035–1038.
461. MacMahon B. Epidemiology and the causes of breast cancer. *Int J Cancer* 2006;118:2373–2378.
462. Malkin D, Li FP, Strong LC, et al. Germ line p53 mutations in a familial syndrome of breast cancer, sarcomas, and other neoplasms. *Science* 1990;250:1233–1238.
463. Mandard AM, Denoux Y, Herlin P, et al. Prognostic value of DNA cytometry in 281 premenopausal patients with lymph node negative breast carcinoma randomized in a control trial: multivariate analysis with Ki-67 index, mitotic count, and microvessel density. *Cancer* 2000;89:1748–1757.
464. Manjer J, Berglund G, Bondesson L, et al. Breast cancer incidence in relation to smoking cessation. *Breast Cancer Res Treat* 2000;61:121–129.
465. Mansel RE, Fallowfield L, Kissin M, et al. Randomized multicenter trial of sentinel node biopsy versus standard axillary treatment in operable breast cancer: the ALMANAC Trial. *J Natl Cancer Inst* 2006;98:599–609.
466. Mansel RE, Goyal A, Newcombe RG. Internal mammary node drainage and its role in sentinel lymph node biopsy: the initial ALMANAC experience. *Clin Breast Cancer* 2004;5:279–284; discussion 285–276.
467. Mansfield CM, Komarnicky LT, Schwartz GF, et al. Perioperative implantation of iridium-192 as the boost technique for stage I and II breast cancer: results of a 10-year study of 655 patients. *Radiology* 1994;192:33–36.
468. Mansfield CM, Komarnicky LT, Schwartz GF, et al. Ten-year results in 1070 patients with stages I and II breast cancer treated by conservative surgery and radiation therapy. *Cancer* 1995;75:2328–2336.
469. Mansur DB, El Naqa I, Kong F, et al. Localization of internal mammary lymph nodes by CT simulation: implications for breast radiation therapy planning. *Radiother Oncol* 2004;73:355–357.
470. Marchal C, Weber B, de Lafontan B, et al. Nine breast angiosarcomas after conservative treatment for breast carcinoma: a survey from French comprehensive Cancer Centers. *Int J Radiat Oncol Biol Phys* 1999;44:113–119.

471. Mariani G, Villa G, Gipponi M, et al. Mapping sentinel lymph node in breast cancer by combined lymphoscintigraphy, blue-dye, and intraoperative gamma-probe. *Cancer Biother Radiopharm* 2000;15:245–252.
472. Mariani L, Salvadori B, Marubini E, et al. Ten year results of a randomised trial comparing two conservative treatment strategies for small size breast cancer. *Eur J Cancer* 1998;34:1156–1162.
473. Markiewicz DA, Fox KR, Schultz DJ, et al. Concurrent chemotherapy and radiation for breast conservation treatment of early-stage breast cancer. *Cancer J Sci Am* 1998;4:185–193.
474. Markiewicz DA, Schultz DJ, Haas JA, et al. The effects of sequence and type of chemotherapy and radiation therapy on cosmesis and complications after breast conservation therapy. *Int J Radiat Oncol Biol Phys* 1996;35:661–668.
475. Marks LB, Yu X, Prosnitz RG, et al. The incidence and functional consequences of RT-associated cardiac perfusion defects. *Int J Radiat Oncol Biol Phys* 2005;63:214–223.
476. Marshall JK, Griffith KA, Haffty BG, et al. Conservative management of Paget disease of the breast with radiotherapy: 10- and 15-year results. *Cancer* 2003;97:2142–2149.
477. Martelli G, Boracchi P, De Palo M, et al. A randomized trial comparing axillary dissection to no axillary dissection in older patients with T1N0 breast cancer: results after 5 years of follow-up. *Ann Surg* 2005;242:1–6; discussion 7–9.
478. Martin MB, Kon ND, Kawamoto EH, et al. Postmastectomy angiosarcoma. *Am Surg* 1984;50:541–545.
479. Martinazzi M, Crivelli F, Zampatti C, et al. Relationship between p53 expression and other prognostic factors in human breast carcinoma. An immunohistochemical study. *Am J Clin Pathol* 1993;100:213–217.
480. Matthews RH, McNeese MD, Montague ED, et al. Prognostic implications of age in breast cancer patients treated with tumorectomy and irradiation or with mastectomy. *Int J Radiat Oncol Biol Phys* 1988;14:659–663.
481. Mauch PM, Kalish LA, Marcus KC, et al. Second malignancies after treatment for laparotomy staged IA-IIIB Hodgkin's disease: long-term analysis of risk factors and outcome. *Blood* 1996;87:3625–3632.
482. Maunsell E, Brisson J, Deschenes L. Arm problems and psychological distress after surgery for breast cancer. *Can J Surg* 1993;36:315–320.
483. McCormick B, Yahalom J, Cox L, et al. The patients perception of her breast following radiation and limited surgery. *Int J Radiat Oncol Biol Phys* 1989;17:1299–1302.
484. McCready DR, Chapman JA, Hanna WM, et al. Factors associated with local breast cancer recurrence after lumpectomy alone: postmenopausal patients. *Ann Surg Oncol* 2000;7:562–567.
485. McDivitt RW, Stone KR, Craig RB, et al. A proposed classification of breast cancer based on kinetic information: derived from a comparison of risk factors in 168 primary operable breast cancers. *Cancer* 1986;57:269–276.
486. McGowan TS, Cummings BJ, O'Sullivan B, et al. An analysis of 78 breast sarcoma patients without distant metastases at presentation. *Int J Radiat Oncol Biol Phys* 2000;46:383–390.
487. McGuire WL, Clark GM. Prognostic factors and treatment decisions in axillary-node-negative breast cancer. *N Engl J Med* 1992;326:1756–1761.
488. McGuire WL, Tandon AK, Allred DC, et al. How to use prognostic factors in axillary node-negative breast cancer patients. *J Natl Cancer Inst* 1990;82:1006–1015.
489. Mehta K, Haffty BG. Long-term outcome in patients with four or more positive lymph nodes treated with conservative surgery and radiation therapy. *Int J Radiat Oncol Biol Phys* 1996;35:679–685.
490. Mehta VK, Goffinet DR. Unsuspected abnormalities noted on CT treatment planning scans obtained for breast and chest wall irradiation. *Int J Radiat Oncol Biol Phys* 2001;49:723–725.
491. Meier P, Ferguson DJ, Karrison T. A controlled trial of extended radical versus radical mastectomy. Ten-year results. *Cancer* 1989;63:188–195.
492. Menard S, Valagussa P, Pilotti S, et al. Response to cyclophosphamide, methotrexate, and fluorouracil in lymph node-positive breast cancer according to HER2 overexpression and other tumor biologic variables. *J Clin Oncol* 2001;19:329–335.
493. Mendelson EB. Evaluation of the postoperative breast. *Radiol Clin North Am* 1992;30:107–138.
494. Merchant TE, McCormick B. Prone position breast irradiation. *Int J Radiat Oncol Biol Phys* 1994;30:197–203.
495. Metayer C, Lynch CF, Clarke EA, et al. Second cancers among long-term survivors of Hodgkin's disease diagnosed in childhood and adolescence. *J Clin Oncol* 2000;18:2435–2443.
496. Mettler FA, Upton AC, Kelsey CA, et al. Benefits versus risks from mammography: a critical reassessment. *Cancer* 1996;77:903–909.
497. Meyer A, John E, Dork T, et al. Breast cancer in female carriers of ATM gene alterations: outcome of adjuvant radiotherapy. *Radiother Oncol* 2004;72:319–323.
498. Meyer JS, Friedman E, McCrate MM, et al. Prediction of early course of breast carcinoma by thymidine labeling. *Cancer* 1983;51:1879–1886.
499. Meyer JS, Province MA. S-phase fraction and nuclear size in long term prognosis of patients with breast cancer. *Cancer* 1994;74:2287–2299.
500. Middleton LP, Palacios DM, Bryant BR, et al. Pleomorphic lobular carcinoma: morphology, immunohistochemistry, and molecular analysis. *Am J Surg Pathol* 2000;24:1650–1656.
501. Miller AB, Howe GR, Sherman GJ, et al. Mortality from breast cancer after irradiation during fluoroscopic examinations in patients being treated for tuberculosis. *N Engl J Med* 1989;321:1285–1289.
502. Miller AB, To T, Baines CJ, et al. Canadian National Breast Screening Study-2: 13-year results of a randomized trial in women aged 50-59 years. *J Natl Cancer Inst* 2000;92:1490–1499.
503. Miller AB, To T, Baines CJ, et al. The Canadian National Breast Screening Study: update on breast cancer mortality. *J Natl Cancer Inst Monogr* 1997:37–41.
504. Mock V. Body image in women treated for breast cancer. *Nurs Res* 1993;42:153–157.
505. Montague ED, Paulus DD, Schell SR. Selection and follow-up of patients for conservation surgery and irradiation. *Front Radiat Ther Oncol* 1983;17:124–130.
506. Montague ED. Conservation surgery and radiation therapy in the treatment of operable breast cancer. *Cancer* 1984;53:700–704.
507. Moody AM, Mayles WP, Bliss JM, et al. The influence of breast size on late radiation effects and association with radiotherapy dose inhomogeneity. *Radiother Oncol* 1994;33:106–112.
508. Moran M, Haffty BG. Lobular carcinoma in situ as a component of breast cancer: the long-term outcome in patients treated with breast-conservation therapy. *Int J Radiat Oncol Biol Phys* 1998;40:353–358.
509. Moran MS, Colasanto JM, Haffty BG, et al. Effects of breast-conserving therapy on lactation after pregnancy. *Cancer J* 2005;11:399–403.
510. Moran MS, Haffty BG. Local-regional breast cancer recurrence: prognostic groups based on patterns of failure. *Breast J* 2002;8:81–87.
511. Morgenstern L, Kaufman PA, Friedman NB. The case against tylectomy for carcinoma of the breast. The factor of multicentricity. *Am J Surg* 1975;130: 251–258.
512. Morrell RM, Halyard MY, Schild SE, et al. Breast cancer-related lymphedema. *Mayo Clin Proc* 2005;80:1480–1484.
513. Morris AD, Morris RD, Wilson JF, et al. Breast-conserving therapy vs mastectomy in early-stage breast cancer: a meta-analysis of 10-year survival. *Cancer J Sci Am* 1997;3:6–12.
514. Morris MM, Powell SN. Irradiation in the setting of collagen vascular disease: acute and late complications. *J Clin Oncol* 1997;15:2728–2735.
515. Morrow M, Rademaker AW, Bethke KP, et al. Learning sentinel node biopsy: results of a prospective randomized trial of two techniques. *Surgery* 1999;126:714–720; discussion 720–722.
516. Moynahan ME, Pierce AJ, Jasin M. BRCA2 is required for homology-directed repair of chromosomal breaks. *Mol Cell* 2001;7:263–272.
517. Muller-Runkel R, Kalokhe UP. Scatter dose from tangential breast irradiation to the uninvolved breast. *Radiology* 1990;175:873–876.
518. Muren LP, Maurstad G, Hafslund R, et al. Cardiac and pulmonary doses and complication probabilities in standard and conformal tangential irradiation in conservative management of breast cancer. *Radiother Oncol* 2002;62:173–183.
519. Mustafa IA, Cole B, Wanebo HJ, et al. Prognostic analysis of survival in small breast cancers. *J Am Coll Surg* 1998;186:562–569.
520. Narod SA, Brunet JS, Ghadirian P, et al. Tamoxifen and risk of contralateral breast cancer in BRCA1 and BRCA2 mutation carriers: a case-control study. Hereditary Breast Cancer Clinical Study Group. *Lancet* 2000;356:1876–1881.
521. Nassar H, Wallis T, Andea A, et al. Clinicopathologic analysis of invasive micropapillary differentiation in breast carcinoma. *Mod Pathol* 2001;14:836–841.
522. National Institutes of Health consensus development conference statement: adjuvant therapy for breast cancer, November 1-3, 2000. *J Natl Cancer Inst Monogr* 2001;2001:5–15.
523. Newman LA, Mason J, Cote D, et al. African-American ethnicity, socioeconomic status, and breast cancer survival: a meta-analysis of 14 studies involving over 10,000 African-American and 40,000 White American patients with carcinoma of the breast. *Cancer* 2002;94:2844–2854.
524. Nielsen HM, Overgaard M, Grau C, et al. Loco-regional recurrence after mastectomy in high-risk breast cancer—risk and prognosis. An analysis of patients from the DBCG 82 b&c randomization trials. *Radiother Oncol* 2006;79:147–155.
525. Nielsen HM, Overgaard M, Grau C, et al. Study of failure pattern among high-risk breast cancer patients with or without postmastectomy radiotherapy in addition to adjuvant systemic therapy: long-term results from the Danish Breast Cancer Cooperative Group DBCG 82 b and c randomized studies. *J Clin Oncol* 2006;24:2268–2275.
526. Nielsen M, Christensen L, Andersen J. Contralateral cancerous breast lesions in women with clinical invasive breast carcinoma. *Cancer* 1986;57:897–903.
527. Nissen MJ, Swenson KK, Ritz LJ, et al. Quality of life after breast carcinoma surgery: a comparison of three surgical procedures. *Cancer* 2001;91:1238–1246.
528. Nixon AJ, Manola J, Gelman R, et al. No long-term increase in cardiac related mortality after breast-conserving surgery and radiation therapy using modern techniques. *J Clin Oncol* 1998;16:1374–1379
529. Nixon AJ, Neuberg D, Hayes DF, et al. Relationship of patient age to pathologic features of the tumor and prognosis for patients with stage I or II breast cancer. *J Clin Oncol* 1994;12:888–894.
530. Noguchi S, Kasugai T, Miki Y, et al. Clinicopathologic analysis of BRCA1- or BRCA2-associated hereditary breast carcinoma in Japanese women. *Cancer* 1999;85:2200–2205.
531. Norris HJ, Taylor HB. Prognosis of mucinous (gelatinous) carcinoma of the breast. *Cancer* 1965;18:879–885.
532. Nos C, Freneaux P, Louis-Sylvestre C, et al. Macroscopic quality control improves the reliability of blue dye-only sentinel lymph node biopsy in breast cancer. *Ann Surg Oncol* 2003;10:525–530.
533. NSABP-B39, RTOG-0413. (2005). *Vol. 2006.*
534. Nugent P, O'Connell TX. Breast cancer and pregnancy. *Arch Surg* 1985; 120:1221–1224.
535. O'Hanlon DM, Kerin MJ, Kent PJ, et al. A prospective evaluation of CA15-3 in stage I carcinoma of the breast. *J Am Coll Surg* 1995;180:210–212.
536. O'Malley MS, Fletcher SW. US Preventive Services Task Force. Screening for breast cancer with breast self-examination. A critical review. *JAMA* 1987;257:2196–2203.
537. Obedian E, Fischer DB, Haffty BG. Second malignancies after treatment of early-stage breast cancer: lumpectomy and radiation therapy versus mastectomy. *J Clin Oncol* 2000;18:2406–2412.
538. Obedian E, Haffty BG. Internal mammary nodal irradiation in conservatively-managed breast cancer patients: is there a benefit? *Int J Radiat Oncol Biol Phys* 1999;44:997–1003.
539. Obedian E, Haffty BG. Negative margin status improves local control in conservatively managed breast cancer patients. *Cancer J Sci Am* 2000;6:28–33.
540. Oh JL, Bonnen M, Outlaw ED, et al. The impact of young age on locoregional recurrence after doxorubicin-based breast conservation therapy in patients 40 years old or younger: How young is "young"? *Int J Radiat Oncol Biol Phys* 2006;65:1345–1352.
541. Oh KS, Kong FM, Griffith KA, et al. Planning the breast tumor bed boost: changes in the excision cavity volume and surgical scar location after breast-conserving surgery and whole-breast irradiation. *Int J Radiat Oncol Biol Phys* 2006;66(3):680–686.
542. Olivotto IA, Gomi A, Bancej C, et al. Influence of delay to diagnosis on prognostic indicators of screen-detected breast carcinoma. *Cancer* 2002;94:2143–2150.
543. Olivotto IA, Rose MA, Osteen RT, et al. Late cosmetic outcome after conservative surgery and radiotherapy:analysis of causes of cosmetic failure. *Int J Radiat Oncol Biol Phys* 1989;17:747–753.

544. Orecchia R, Veronesi U. Intraoperative electrons. *Semin Radiat Oncol* 2005; 15:76–83.
545. Orel SG, Fowble BL, Solin LJ, et al. Breast cancer recurrence after lumpectomy and radiation therapy for early-stage disease: prognostic significance of detection method. *Radiology* 1993;188:189–194.
546. Orel SG, Kay N, Reynolds C, et al. BI-RADS categorization as a predictor of malignancy. *Radiology* 1999;211:845–850.
547. Orel SG, Troupin RH, Patterson EA, et al. Breast cancer recurrence after lumpectomy and irradiation: role of mammography in detection. *Radiology* 1992;183:201–206.
548. Orr RK. The impact of prophylactic axillary node dissection on breast cancer survival—a Bayesian meta-analysis. *Ann Surg Oncol* 1999;6:109–116.
549. Osborne CK. Steroid hormone receptors in breast cancer management. *Breast Cancer Res Treat* 1998;51:227–238.
550. Osborne MP, Ormiston N, Harmer CL, et al. Breast conservation in the treatment of early breast cancer. A 20-year follow-up. *Cancer* 1984;53:349–355.
551. Owen JR, Ashton A, Bliss JM, et al. Effect of radiotherapy fraction size on tumour control in patients with early-stage breast cancer after local tumour excision: long-term results of a randomised trial. *Lancet Oncol* 2006;7:467–471.
552. Paik S, Shak S, Tang G, et al. A multigene assay to predict recurrence of tamoxifen-treated, node-negative breast cancer. *N Engl J Med* 2004;351:2817–2826.
553. Papadatos G, Rangan AM, Psarianos T, et al. Probability of axillary node involvement in patients with tubular carcinoma of the breast. *Br J Surg* 2001;88:860–864.
554. Park CC, Mitsumori M, Nixon A, et al. Outcome at 8 years after breast-conserving surgery and radiation therapy for invasive breast cancer: influence of margin status and systemic therapy on local recurrence. *J Clin Oncol* 2000;18:1668–1675.
555. Park JM, Han BK, Moon WK, et al. Metaplastic carcinoma of the breast: mammographic and sonographic findings. *J Clin Ultrasound* 2000;28:179–186.
556. Parker SH, Burbank F, Jackman RJ, et al. Percutaneous large-core breast biopsy: a multi-institutional study. *Radiology* 1994;193:359–364.
557. Paszat LF, Mackillop WJ, Groome PA, et al. Mortality from myocardial infarction following postlumpectomy radiotherapy for breast cancer: a population-based study in Ontario, Canada. *Int J Radiat Oncol Biol Phys* 1999;43:755–762.
558. Patek E, Johannisson E, Krauer F, et al. Microfluorometric grading of mammary tumors. A pilot study. *Anal Quant Cytol Histol* 1980;2:264–271.
559. Patt DA, Goodwin JS, Kuo YF, et al. Cardiac morbidity of adjuvant radiotherapy for breast cancer. *J Clin Oncol* 2005;23:7475–7482.
560. Pejavar S, Wilson LD, Haffty BG. Regional nodal recurrence in breast cancer patients treated with conservative surgery and radiation therapy (BCS+RT). *Int J Radiat Oncol Biol Phys* 1996.
560a. Penzer RD, Lorant JA, Terz J, et al. Wound-healing complications following biopsy of the irradiated breast. *Arch Surg* 1992;127:321–324.
561. Perera F, Yu E, Engel J, et al. Patterns of breast recurrence in a pilot study of brachytherapy confined to the lumpectomy site for early breast cancer with six years' minimum follow-up. *Int J Radiat Oncol Biol Phys* 2003;57:1239-1246.
562. Perez CA, Garcia DM, Kuske RR, et al. Organ preservation therapy in stage T1 and T2 carcinoma of the breast. *Front Radiat Ther Oncol* 1993;27:62–88.
563. Perez CA, Taylor ME, Halverson K, et al. Brachytherapy or electron beam boost in conservation therapy of carcinoma of the breast: a nonrandomized comparison. *Int J Radiat Oncol Biol Phys* 1996;34:995–1007.
564. Perez EA, Roche PC, Jenkins RB, et al. HER2 testing in patients with breast cancer: poor correlation between weak positivity by immunohistochemistry and gene amplification by fluorescence in situ hybridization. *Mayo Clin Proc* 2002;77:148–154.
565. Perez EA, Suman VJ, Davidson NE, et al. HER2 testing by local, central, and reference laboratories in specimens from the North Central Cancer Treatment Group N9831 intergroup adjuvant trial. *J Clin Oncol* 2006;24:3032–3038.
566. Peters MV. Wedge resection with or without radiation in early breast cancer. *Int J Radiat Oncol Biol Phys* 1977;2:1151–1156.
567. Peterson ME, Schultz DJ, Reynolds C, et al. Outcomes in breast cancer patients relative to margin status after treatment with breast-conserving surgery and radiation therapy: the University of Pennsylvania experience. *Int J Radiat Oncol Biol Phys* 1999;43:1029–1035.
568. Petit JY, Veronesi U, Orecchia R, et al. Nipple-sparing mastectomy in association with intra operative radiotherapy (ELIOT): a new type of mastectomy for breast cancer treatment. *Breast Cancer Res Treat* 2006;96:47–51.
569. Petrek JA. Breast cancer during pregnancy. *Cancer* 1994;74:518–527.
570. Pezner RD, Lipsett JA, Vora NL, et al. Limited usefulness of observer-based cosmesis scales employed to evaluate patients treated conservatively for breast cancer. *Int J Radiat Oncol Biol Phys* 1985;11:1117–1119.
571. Phan C, Mindrum M, Silverman C, et al. Matched-control retrospective study of the acute and late complications in patients with collagen vascular diseases treated with radiation therapy. *Cancer J* 2003;9:461–466.
572. Pierce L, Fowble B, Solin LJ, et al. Conservative surgery and radiation therapy in black women with early stage breast cancer. Patterns of failure and analysis of outcome. *Cancer* 1992;69:2831–2841.
573. Pierce LJ, Butler JB, Martel MK, et al. Postmastectomy radiotherapy of the chest wall: dosimetric comparison of common techniques. *Int J Radiat Oncol Biol Phys* 2002;52:1220–1230.
574. Pierce LJ, Griffith KA, Hayman JA, et al. Conservative surgery and radiotherapy for stage I/II breast cancer using lung density correction: 10-year and 15-year results. *Int J Radiat Oncol Biol Phys* 2005;61:1317–1327.
575. Pierce LJ, Hutchins LF, Green SR, et al. Sequencing of tamoxifen and radiotherapy after breast-conserving surgery in early-stage breast cancer. *J Clin Oncol* 2005;23:24–29.
576. Pierce LJ, Levin AM, Rebbeck TR, et al. Ten-year multi-institutional results of breast-conserving surgery and radiotherapy in BRCA1/2-associated stage I/II breast cancer. *J Clin Oncol* 2006;24:2437–2443.
577. Pierce LJ, Merino MJ, D'Angelo T, et al. Is c-erb B-2 a predictor for recurrent disease in early stage breast cancer? *Int J Radiat Oncol Biol Phys* 1994;28:395–403.
578. Pierce LJ, Oberman HA, Strawderman MH, et al. Microscopic extracapsular extension in the axilla: is this an indication for axillary radiotherapy? *Int J Radiat Oncol Biol Phys* 1995;33:253–259.
579. Pierce LJ, Strawderman M, Narod SA, et al. Effect of radiotherapy after breast-conserving treatment in women with breast cancer and germline BRCA1/2 mutations. *J Clin Oncol* 2000;18:3360–3369.
580. Pierce SM, Recht A, Lingos TI, et al. Long-term radiation complications following conservative surgery (CS) and radiation therapy (RT) in patients with early stage breast cancer. *Int J Radiat Oncol Biol Phys* 1992;23:915–923.
581. Pierquin B, Huart J, Raynal M, et al. Conservative treatment for breast cancer: long-term results (15 years). *Radiother Oncol* 1991;20:16–23.
582. Pierquin B, Mazeron JJ, Glaubiger D. Conservative treatment of breast cancer in Europe: report of the Groupe Europeen de Curietherapie. *Radiother Oncol* 1986;6:187–198.
583. Pignol J, Olivotto I, Rakovitch E, et al. *Proceedings of the ASTRO 48th Annual Meeting, Vol. 66, Number 3 Supplement 1*. Philadelphia: Elsevier, 2006.
584. Pigott J, Nichols R, Maddox WA, et al. Metastases to the upper levels of the axillary nodes in carcinoma of the breast and its implications for nodal sampling procedures. *Surg Gynecol Obstet* 1984;158:255–259.
585. Pittinger TP, Maronian NC, Poulter CA, et al. Importance of margin status in outcome of breast-conserving surgery for carcinoma. *Surgery* 1994;116:605–608; discussion 608–609.
586. Poggi MM, Danforth DN, Sciuto LC, et al. Eighteen-year results in the treatment of early breast carcinoma with mastectomy versus breast conservation therapy: the National Cancer Institute Randomized Trial. *Cancer* 2003;98:697–702.
587. Powles T, Eeles R, Ashley S, et al. Interim analysis of the incidence of breast cancer in the Royal Marsden Hospital tamoxifen randomised chemoprevention trial. *Lancet* 1998;352:98–101.
588. Prevalence and penetrance of BRCA1 and BRCA2 mutations in a population-based series of breast cancer cases. Anglian Breast Cancer Study Group. *Br J Cancer* 2000;83:1301–1308.
589. Prior P, Pope DJ. Hodgkin's disease: subsequent primary cancers in relation to treatment. *Br J Cancer* 1988;58:512–517.
590. Pritchard J, Anand P, Broome J, et al. Double-blind randomized phase II study of hyperbaric oxygen in patients with radiation-induced brachial plexopathy. *Radiother Oncol* 2001;58:279–286.
591. Psyrri A, Burtness B. Pregnancy-associated breast cancer. *Cancer J* 2005;11:83–95.
592. Quiet CA, Ferguson DJ, Weichselbaum RR, et al. Natural history of node-negative breast cancer: a study of 826 patients with long-term follow-up. *J Clin Oncol* 1995;13:1144–1151.
593. Rakfal SM, Deutsch M. Radiotherapy for malignancies associated with lupus: case reports of acute and late reactions. *Am J Clin Oncol* 1998;21:54–57.
594. Rapiti E, Verkooijen HM, Vlastos G, et al. Complete excision of primary breast tumor improves survival of patients with metastatic breast cancer at diagnosis. *J Clin Oncol* 2006;24:2743–2749.
595. Ray GR, Fish VJ, Marmor JB, et al. Impact of adjuvant chemotherapy on cosmesis and complications in stages I and II carcinoma of the breast treated by biopsy and radiation therapy. *Int J Radiat Oncol Biol Phys* 1984;10:837–841.
596. Ray GR, Fish VJ. Biopsy and definitive radiation therapy in stage I and II adenocarcinoma of the female breast: analysis of cosmesis and the role of electron beam supplementation. *Int J Radiat Oncol Biol Phys* 1983;9:813–818.
597. Rayan G, Dawson LA, Bezjak A, et al. Prospective comparison of breast pain in patients participating in a randomized trial of breast-conserving surgery and tamoxifen with or without radiotherapy. *Int J Radiat Oncol Biol Phys* 2003;55:154–161.
598. Rebbeck TR, Friebel T, Lynch HT, et al. Bilateral prophylactic mastectomy reduces breast cancer risk in BRCA1 and BRCA2 mutation carriers: the PROSE Study Group. *J Clin Oncol* 2004;22:1055–1062.
599. Rebbeck TR, Friebel T, Wagner T, et al. Effect of short-term hormone replacement therapy on breast cancer risk reduction after bilateral prophylactic oophorectomy in BRCA1 and BRCA2 mutation carriers: the PROSE Study Group. *J Clin Oncol* 2005;23:7804–7810.
600. Rebbeck TR. Prophylactic oophorectomy in BRCA1 and BRCA2 mutation carriers. *J Clin Oncol* 2000;18:100S–103S.
601. Recht A, Come SE, Gelman RS, et al. Integration of conservative surgery, radiotherapy, and chemotherapy for the treatment of early-stage, node-positive breast cancer: sequencing, timing, and outcome. *J Clin Oncol* 1991;9:1662–1667.
602. Recht A, Come SE, Henderson IC, et al. The sequencing of chemotherapy and radiation therapy after conservative surgery for early-stage breast cancer. *N Engl J Med* 1996;334:1356–1361.
603. Recht A, Connolly JL, Schnitt SJ, et al. The effect of young age on tumor recurrence in the treated breast after conservative surgery and radiotherapy. *Int J Radiat Oncol Biol Phys* 1988;14:3–10.
604. Recht A, Edge SB, Solin LJ, et al. Postmastectomy radiotherapy: clinical practice guidelines of the American Society of Clinical Oncology. *J Clin Oncol* 2001;19:1539–1569.
605. Recht A, Houlihan MJ. Axillary lymph nodes and breast cancer: a review. *Cancer* 1995;76:1491–1512.
606. Recht A, Pierce SM, Abner A, et al. Regional nodal failure after conservative surgery and radiotherapy for early-stage breast carcinoma. *J Clin Oncol* 1991;9:988–996.
607. Recht A, Silen W, Schnitt SJ, et al. Time-course of local recurrence following conservative surgery and radiotherapy for early stage breast cancer. *Int J Radiat Oncol Biol Phys* 1988;15:255–261.
608. Recht A, Silver B, Schnitt S, et al. Breast relapse following primary radiation therapy for early breast cancer. I. Classification, frequency and salvage. *Int J Radiat Oncol Biol Phys* 1985;11:1271–1276.
609. Recht A. Integration of systemic therapy and radiation therapy for patients with early-stage breast cancer treated with conservative surgery. *Clin Breast Cancer* 2003;4:104–113.
610. Recht A. Radiotherapy and surgery in early breast cancer. *N Engl J Med* 1996;334:989.
611. Recht A. Selection of patients with early stage invasive breast cancer for treatment with conservative surgery and radiation therapy. *Semin Oncol* 1996;23:19–30.
612. Recht A. Should irradiation replace dissection for patients with breast cancer with clinically negative axillary lymph nodes? *J Surg Oncol* 1999;72:184–192.
613. Renton SC, Gazet JC, Ford HT, et al. The importance of the resection margin in conservative surgery for breast cancer. *Eur J Surg Oncol* 1996;22:17–22.
614. Ribeiro GG, Magee B, Swindell R, et al. The Christie Hospital breast conservation trial: an update at 8 years from inception. *Clin Oncol (R Coll Radiol)* 1993;5:278–283.

615. Richards MA, Smith P, Ramirez AJ, et al. The influence on survival of delay in the presentation and treatment of symptomatic breast cancer. *Br J Cancer* 1999;79:858–864.

616. Ringash J, Whelan T, Elliott E, et al. Accuracy of ultrasound in localization of breast boost field. *Radiother Oncol* 2004;72:61–66.

617. Ringberg A, Anagnostaki L, Anderson H, et al. Cell biological factors in ductal carcinoma in situ (DCIS) of the breast-relationship to ipsilateral local recurrence and histopathological characteristics. *Eur J Cancer* 2001;37:1514–1522.

618. Ringberg A, Idvall I, Ferno M, et al. Ipsilateral local recurrence in relation to therapy and morphological characteristics in patients with ductal carcinoma in situ of the breast. *Eur J Surg Oncol* 2000;26:444–451.

619. Rink T, Heuser T, Fitz H, et al. Lymphoscintigraphic sentinel node imaging and gamma probe detection in breast cancer with Tc-99m nanocolloidal albumin: results of an optimized protocol. *Clin Nucl Med* 2001;26:293–298.

620. Rissanen PM. A comparison of conservative and radical surgery combined with radiotherapy in the treatment of stage I carcinoma of the breast. *Br J Radiol* 1969;42:423–426.

621. Robertson JM, Clarke DH, Pevzner MM, et al. Breast conservation therapy. Severe breast fibrosis after radiation therapy in patients with collagen vascular disease. *Cancer* 1991;68:502–508.

622. Robson M, Levin D, Federici M, et al. Breast conservation therapy for invasive breast cancer in Ashkenazi women with BRCA gene founder mutations. *J Natl Cancer Inst* 1999;91:2112–2117.

623. Robson M, Svahn T, McCormick B, et al. Appropriateness of breast-conserving treatment of breast carcinoma in women with germline mutations in BRCA1 or BRCA2: a clinic-based series. *Cancer* 2005;103:44–51.

624. Robson M. Breast cancer surveillance in women with hereditary risk due to BRCA1 or BRCA2 mutations. *Clin Breast Cancer* 2004;5:260–268; discussion 269–271.

625. Robson ME, Boyd J, Borgen PI, et al. Hereditary breast cancer. *Curr Probl Surg* 2001;38:387–480.

626. Robson ME, Chappuis PO, Satagopan J, et al. A combined analysis of outcome following breast cancer: differences in survival based on BRCA1/BRCA2 mutation status and administration of adjuvant treatment. *Breast Cancer Res* 2004;6:R8–R17.

627. Robson ME, Offit K. Breast MRI for women with hereditary cancer risk. *JAMA* 2004;292:1368–1370.

628. Romestaing P, Lehingue Y, Carrie C, et al. Role of a 10-Gy boost in the conservative treatment of early breast cancer: results of a randomized clinical trial in Lyon, France. *J Clin Oncol* 1997;15:963–968.

629. Romond EH, Perez EA, Bryant J, et al. Trastuzumab plus adjuvant chemotherapy for operable HER2-positive breast cancer. *N Engl J Med* 2005;353:1673–1684.

630. Rose MA, Olivotto I, Cady B, et al. Conservative surgery and radiation therapy for early breast cancer. Long-term cosmetic results. *Arch Surg* 1989;124:153–157.

631. Rosen PP, Groshen S, Kinne DW, et al. Contralateral breast carcinoma: an assessment of risk and prognosis in stage I (T1N0M0) and stage II (T1N1M0) patients with 20-year follow-up. *Surgery* 1989;106:904–910.

632. Rosen PR, Groshen S, Saigo PE, et al. A long-term follow-up study of survival in stage I (T1N0M0) and stage II (T1N1M0) breast carcinoma. *J Clin Oncol* 1989;7:355–366.

633. Ross JG, Hussey DH, Mayr NA, et al. Acute and late reactions to radiation therapy in patients with collagen vascular diseases. *Cancer* 1993;71:3744–3752.

634. Ross JS, Linette GP, Stec J, et al. Breast cancer biomarkers and molecular medicine. *Expert Rev Mol Diagn* 2003;3:573–585.

635. Ross JS, Linette GP, Stec J, et al. Breast cancer biomarkers and molecular medicine: part II. *Expert Rev Mol Diagn* 2004;4:169–188.

636. Rossouw JE, Anderson GL, Prentice RL, et al. Risks and benefits of estrogen plus progestin in healthy postmenopausal women: principal results From the Women's Health Initiative randomized controlled trial. *JAMA* 2002;288:321–333.

637. Rothwell RI, Kelly SA, Joslin CA. Radiation myelitis in patients treated for breast cancer. *Radiother Oncol* 1985;4:9–14.

638. Rouesse J, de la Lande B, Bertheault-Cvitkovic F, et al. A phase III randomized trial comparing adjuvant concomitant chemoradiotherapy versus standard adjuvant chemotherapy followed by radiotherapy in operable node-positive breast cancer: final results. *Int J Radiat Oncol Biol Phys* 2006;64:1072–1080.

639. Rudenstam CM, Zahrieh D, Forbes JF, et al. Randomized trial comparing axillary clearance versus no axillary clearance in older patients with breast cancer: first results of International Breast Cancer Study Group Trial 10-93. *J Clin Oncol* 2006;24:337–344.

640. Rutqvist LE, Liedberg A, Hammar N, et al. Myocardial infarction among women with early-stage breast cancer treated with conservative surgery and breast irradiation. *Int J Radiat Oncol Biol Phys* 1998;40:359–363.

641. Ryoo MC, Kagan AR, Wollin M, et al. Prognostic factors for recurrence and cosmesis in 393 patients after radiation therapy for early mammary carcinoma. *Radiology* 1989;172:555–559.

642. Salloum E, Doria R, Schubert W, et al. Second solid tumors in patients with Hodgkin's disease cured after radiation or chemotherapy plus adjuvant low-dose radiation. *J Clin Oncol* 1996;14:2435–2443.

643. Samuels JR, Haffty BG, Lee CH, et al. Breast conservation therapy in patients with mammographically undetected breast cancer. *Radiology* 1992;185:425–427.

644. Sankila R, Heinavaara S, Hakulinen T. Survival of breast cancer patients after subsequent term pregnancy: "healthy mother effect." *Am J Obstet Gynecol* 1994;170:818–823.

645. Santamaria G, Velasco M, Zanon G, et al. Adenoid cystic carcinoma of the breast: mammographic appearance and pathologic correlation. *AJR Am J Roentgenol* 1998;171:1679–1683.

646. Santiago RJ, Harris EE, Qin L, et al. Similar long-term results of breast-conservation treatment for stage I and II invasive lobular carcinoma compared with invasive ductal carcinoma of the breast: the University of Pennsylvania experience. *Cancer* 2005;103:2447–2454.

647. Santiago RJ, Wu L, Harris E, et al. Fifteen-year results of breast-conserving surgery and definitive irradiation for stage I and II breast carcinoma: the University of Pennsylvania experience. *Int J Radiat Oncol Biol Phys* 2004;58:233–240.

648. Sanuki-Fujimoto N. Benefits of axillary radiotherapy unclear in women with early stage breast cancer undergoing conservative breast surgery without axillary dissection. *Cancer Treat Rev* 2005;31:496–500.

649. Sarrazin D, Le M, Rouesse J, et al. Conservative treatment versus mastectomy in breast cancer tumors with macroscopic diameter of 20 millimeters or less. The experience of the Institut Gustave-Roussy. *Cancer* 1984;53:1209–1213.

650. Sarrazin D, Le MG, Arriagada R, et al. Ten-year results of a randomized trial comparing a conservative treatment to mastectomy in early breast cancer. *Radiother Oncol* 1989;14:177–184.

651. Sartor CI, Peterson BL, Woolf S, et al. Effect of addition of adjuvant paclitaxel on radiotherapy delivery and locoregional control of node-positive breast cancer: cancer and leukemia group B 9344. *J Clin Oncol* 2005;23:30–40.

652. Sasson AR, Fowble B, Hanlon AL, et al. Lobular carcinoma in situ increases the risk of local recurrence in selected patients with stages I and II breast carcinoma treated with conservative surgery and radiation. *Cancer* 2001;91:1862–1869.

653. Sastre-Garau X, Jouve M, Asselain B, et al. Infiltrating lobular carcinoma of the breast. Clinicopathologic analysis of 975 cases with reference to data on conservative therapy and metastatic patterns. *Cancer* 1996;77:113–120.

654. Sauter ER, Hoffman JP, Ottery FD, et al. Is frozen section analysis of reexcision lumpectomy margins worthwhile? Margin analysis in breast reexcisions. *Cancer* 1994;73:2607–2612.

654a. Scarff RW, Torloni H, et al. *Histological typing of breast tumors*. Geneva: World Health Organization, 1968.

655. Schain W, Edwards BK, Gorrell CR, et al. Psychosocial and physical outcomes of primary breast cancer therapy: mastectomy vs excisional biopsy and irradiation. *Breast Cancer Res Treat* 1983;3:377–382.

656. Schain WS, d'Angelo TM, Dunn ME, et al. Mastectomy versus conservative surgery and radiation therapy. Psychosocial consequences. *Cancer* 1994;73:1221–1228.

657. Schairer C, Lubin J, Troisi R, et al. Menopausal estrogen and estrogen-progestin replacement therapy and breast cancer risk. *JAMA* 2000;283:485–491.

658. Schirrmeister H, Kuhn T, Guhlmann A, et al. Fluorine-18 2-deoxy-2-fluoro-D-glucose PET in the preoperative staging of breast cancer: comparison with the standard staging procedures. *Eur J Nucl Med* 2001;28:351–358.

659. Schlembach PJ, Buchholz TA, Ross MI, et al. Relationship of sentinel and axillary level I-II lymph nodes to tangential fields used in breast irradiation. *Int J Radiat Oncol Biol Phys* 2001;51:671–678.

660. Schnitt SJ, Abner A, Gelman R, et al. The relationship between microscopic margins of resection and the risk of local recurrence in patients with breast cancer treated with breast-conserving surgery and radiation therapy. *Cancer* 1994;74:1746–1751.

661. Schnitt SJ, Connolly JL, Harris JR, et al. Pathologic predictors of early local recurrence in stage I and II breast cancer treated by primary radiation therapy. *Cancer* 1984;53:1049–1057.

662. Schnitt SJ, Connolly JL, Khettry U, et al. Pathologic findings on re-excision of the primary site in breast cancer patients considered for treatment by primary radiation therapy. *Cancer* 1987;59:675–681.

663. Schnitt SJ, Connolly JL, Recht A, et al. Influence of infiltrating lobular histology on local tumor control in breast cancer patients treated with conservative surgery and radiotherapy. *Cancer* 1989;64:448–454.

664. Schnitt SJ, Connolly JL. Processing and evaluation of breast excision specimens. A clinically oriented approach. *Am J Clin Pathol* 1992;98:125–137.

665. Schover LR, Yetman RJ, Tuason LJ, et al. Partial mastectomy and breast reconstruction. A comparison of their effects on psychosocial adjustment, body image, and sexuality. *Cancer* 1995;75:54–64.

666. Schover LR. Sexuality and body image in younger women with breast cancer. *J Natl Cancer Inst Monogr* 1994;177–182.

667. Sears HF, Janus C, McDermott A, et al. Bilateral breast carcinoma. prospective evaluation of factors assisting diagnosis. *J Surg Oncol* 1986;32:203–207.

668. Seidman H, Gelb SK, Silverberg E, et al. Survival experience in the Breast Cancer Detection Demonstration Project. *CA Cancer J Clin* 1987;37:258–290.

669. Sener SF, Winchester DJ, Martz CH, et al. Lymphedema after sentinel lymphadenectomy for breast carcinoma. *Cancer* 2001;92:748–752.

670. Senie RT, Rosen PP, Rhodes P, et al. Timing of breast carcinoma surgery during the menstrual cycle influences duration of disease-free survival. *Ann Intern Med* 1992;116:26–32.

671. Severin D, Connors S, Thompson H, et al. Breast radiotherapy with inclusion of internal mammary nodes: a comparison of techniques with three-dimensional planning. *Int J Radiat Oncol Biol Phys* 2003;55:633–644.

672. Seynaeve C, Verhoog LC, Van De Bosch LM, et al. Ipsilateral breast tumour recurrence in hereditary breast cancer following breast-conserving therapy. *Eur J Cancer* 2004;40:1150–1158.

673. Shapiro CL, Hardenbergh PH, Gelman R, et al. Cardiac effects of adjuvant doxorubicin and radiation therapy in breast cancer patients. *J Clin Oncol* 1998;16:3493–3501.

674. Shapiro CL, Recht A. Side effects of adjuvant treatment of breast cancer. *N Engl J Med* 2001;344:1997–2008.

675. Shapiro S, Venet W, Strax P, et al. Selection, follow-up, and analysis in the Health Insurance Plan Study: a randomized trial with breast cancer screening. *Natl Cancer Inst Monogr* 1985;67:65–74.

676. Shapiro S, Venet W, Strax P, et al. Ten- to fourteen-year effect of screening on breast cancer mortality. *J Natl Cancer Inst* 1982;69:349–355.

677. Shattuck-Eidens D, Oliphant A, McClure M, et al. BRCA1 sequence analysis in women at high risk for susceptibility mutations. Risk factor analysis and implications for genetic testing. *JAMA* 1997;278:1242–1250.

678. Shin SJ, DeLellis RA, Ying L, et al. Small cell carcinoma of the breast: a clinicopathologic and immunohistochemical study of nine patients. *Am J Surg Pathol* 2000;24:1231–1238.

679. Silverberg SG, Kay S, Chitale AR, et al. Colloid carcinoma of the breast. *Am J Clin Pathol* 1971;55:355–363.

680. Silverstein MJ, Gierson ED, Waisman JR, et al. Axillary lymph node dissection for T1a breast carcinoma. Is it indicated? *Cancer* 1994;73:664–667.

681. Silverstein MJ, Lewinsky BS, Waisman JR, et al. Infiltrating lobular carcinoma. Is it different from infiltrating duct carcinoma? *Cancer* 1994;73:1673–1677.

682. Silverstein MJ, Skinner KA, Lomis TJ. Predicting axillary nodal positivity in 2282 patients with breast carcinoma. *World J Surg* 2001;25:767–772.

683. Silvestrini R, Benini E, Veneroni S, et al. p53 and bcl-2 expression correlates with clinical outcome in a series of node-positive breast cancer patients. *J Clin Oncol* 1996;14:1604–1610.

684. Silvestrini R, Daidone MG, Luisi A, et al. Biologic and clinicopathologic factors as indicators of specific relapse types in node-negative breast cancer. *J Clin Oncol* 1995;13:697–704.

685. Silvestrini R, Daidone MG, Luisi A, et al. Cell proliferation in 3,800 node-negative

breast cancers: consistency over time of biological and clinical information provided by 3H-thymidine labelling index. *Int J Cancer* 1997;74:122–127.

686. Silvestrini R, Veneroni S, Benini E, et al. Expression of p53, glutathione S-transferase-pi, and Bcl-2 proteins and benefit from adjuvant radiotherapy in breast cancer. *J Natl Cancer Inst* 1997;89:639–645.
687. Simon MS, Severson RK. Racial differences in survival of female breast cancer in the Detroit metropolitan area. *Cancer* 1996;77:308–314.
688. Singletary SE, Allred C, Ashley P, et al. Staging system for breast cancer: revisions for the 6th edition of the *AJCC Cancer Staging Manual. Surg Clin North Am* 2003;83:803–819.
689. Singletary SE, Connolly JL. Breast cancer staging: working with the sixth edition of the *AJCC Cancer Staging Manual. CA Cancer J Clin* 2006;56:37–47; quiz 50–31.
690. Skaane P, Skjennald A, Young K, et al. Follow-up and final results of the Oslo I Study comparing screen-film mammography and full-field digital mammography with soft-copy reading. *Acta Radiol* 2005;46:679–689.
691. Skaane P, Skjennald A. Screen-film mammography versus full-field digital mammography with soft-copy reading: randomized trial in a population-based screening program—the Oslo II Study. *Radiology* 2004;232:197–204.
692. Slamon DJ, Clark GM, Wong SG, et al. Human breast cancer: correlation of relapse and survival with amplification of the HER-2/neu oncogene. *Science* 1987;235:177–182.
693. Slamon DJ, Romond EH, Perez EA. Advances in adjuvant therapy for breast cancer. *Clin Adv Hematol Oncol* 2006;4[Suppl 1]:4–9; discussion Suppl. 10; quiz 12 p following Suppl. 10.
694. Slavin SA, Love SM, Sadowsky NL. Reconstruction of the radiated partial mastectomy defect with autogenous tissues. *Plast Reconstr Surg* 1992;90:854–865; discussion 866–859.
695. Slotman BJ, Meyer OW, Njo KH, et al. Importance of timing of radiotherapy in breast conserving treatment for early stage breast cancer. *Radiother Oncol* 1994;30:206–212.
696. Smallwood JA, Guyer P, Dewbury K, et al. The accuracy of ultrasound in the diagnosis of breast disease. *Ann R Coll Surg Engl* 1986;68:19–22.
697. Smart CR, Byrne C, Smith RA, et al. Twenty-year follow-up of the breast cancers diagnosed during the Breast Cancer Detection Demonstration Project. *CA Cancer J Clin* 1997;47:134–149.
698. Smart CR, Hendrick RE, Rutledge JH 3rd, et al. Benefit of mammography screening in women ages 40 to 49 years. Current evidence from randomized controlled trials. *Cancer* 1995;75:1619–1626.
699. Smillie T, Hayashi A, Rusnak C, et al. Evaluation of feasibility and accuracy of sentinel node biopsy in early breast cancer. *Am J Surg* 2001;181:427–430.
700. Smith BD, Gross CP, Smith GL, et al. Effectiveness of radiation therapy for older women with early breast cancer. *J Natl Cancer Inst* 2006;98:681–690.
701. Smith ML, Evans GR, Gurlek A, et al. Reduction mammaplasty: its role in breast conservation surgery for early-stage breast cancer. *Ann Plast Surg* 1998;41:234–239.
702. Smith TE, Lee D, Turner BC, et al. True recurrence vs. new primary ipsilateral breast tumor relapse: an analysis of clinical and pathologic differences and their implications in natural history, prognoses, and therapeutic management. *Int J Radiat Oncol Biol Phys* 2000;48:1281–1289.
703. Smitt MC, Birdwell RL, Goffinet DR. Breast electron boost planning: comparison of CT and US. *Radiology* 2001;219:203–206.
704. Smitt MC, Nowels KW, Zdeblick MJ, et al. The importance of the lumpectomy surgical margin status in long-term results of breast conservation. *Cancer* 1995;76:259–267.
705. Sneige N, Yaziji H, Mandavilli SR, et al. Low-grade (fibromatosis-like) spindle cell carcinoma of the breast. *Am J Surg Pathol* 2001;25:1009–1016.
706. Solin LJ, Chu JC, Sontag MR, et al. Three-dimensional photon treatment planning of the intact breast. *Int J Radiat Oncol Biol Phys* 1991;21:193–203.
707. Solin LJ, Danoff BF, Schwartz GF, et al. A practical technique for the localization of the tumor volume in definitive irradiation of the breast. *Int J Radiat Oncol Biol Phys* 1985;11:1215–1220.
708. Solin LJ, Fowble B, Martz K, et al. Results of re-excisional biopsy of the primary tumor in preparation for definitive irradiation of patients with early stage breast cancer. *Int J Radiat Oncol Biol Phys* 1986;12:721–725.
709. Solin LJ, Fowble B, Martz KL, et al. Definitive irradiation for early stage breast cancer: the University of Pennsylvania experience. *Int J Radiat Oncol Biol Phys* 1988;14:235–242.
710. Solin LJ, Fowble BL, Schultz DJ, et al. Bilateral breast carcinoma treated with definitive irradiation. *Int J Radiat Oncol Biol Phys* 1989;17:263–271.
711. Solin LJ, Fowble BL, Schultz DJ, et al. The detection of local recurrence after definitive irradiation for early stage carcinoma of the breast. An analysis of the results of breast biopsies performed in previously irradiated breasts. *Cancer* 1990;65:2497–2502.
712. Solin LJ, Fowble BL, Schultz DJ, et al. The impact of mammography on the patterns of patients referred for definitive breast irradiation. *Cancer* 1990;65:1085–1089.
713. Solin LJ, Fowble BL, Schultz DJ, et al. The significance of the pathology margins of the tumor excision on the outcome of patients treated with definitive irradiation for early stage breast cancer. *Int J Radiat Oncol Biol Phys* 1991;21:279–287.
714. Solin LJ, Fowble BL, Troupin RH, et al. Biopsy results of new calcifications in the postirradiated breast. *Cancer* 1989;63:1956–1961.
715. Soo MS, Rosen EL, Baker JA, et al. Negative predictive value of sonography with mammography in patients with palpable breast lesions. *AJR Am J Roentgenol* 2001;177:1167–1170.
716. Stal O, Sullivan S, Wingren S, et al. c-erbB-2 expression and benefit from adjuvant chemotherapy and radiotherapy of breast cancer. *Eur J Cancer* 1995;31A:2185–2190.
717. Steinmann D, Bremer M, Rades D, et al. Mutations of the BRCA1 and BRCA2 genes in patients with bilateral breast cancer. *Br J Cancer* 2001;85:850–858.
718. Stemmer SM, Rizel S, Hardan I, et al. The role of irradiation of the internal mammary lymph nodes in high-risk stage II to IIIA breast cancer patients after high-dose chemotherapy: a prospective sequential nonrandomized study. *J Clin Oncol* 2003;21:2713–2718.
719. Stomper PC, Recht A, Berenberg AL, et al. Mammographic detection of recurrent cancer in the irradiated breast. *AJR Am J Roentgenol* 1987;148:39–43.
720. Storm HH, Andersson M, Boice JD, Jr., et al. Adjuvant radiotherapy and risk of contralateral breast cancer. *J Natl Cancer Inst* 1992;84:1245–1250.
721. Stotter AT, McNeese MD, Ames FC, et al. Predicting the rate and extent of locoregional failure after breast conservation therapy for early breast cancer. *Cancer* 1989;64:2217–2225.
722. Strom EA, Woodward WA, Katz A, et al. Clinical investigation: regional nodal failure patterns in breast cancer patients treated with mastectomy without radiotherapy. *Int J Radiat Oncol Biol Phys* 2005;63:1508–1513.
723. Sugg SL, Ferguson DJ, Posner MC, et al. Should internal mammary nodes be sampled in the sentinel lymph node era? *Ann Surg Oncol* 2000;7:188–192.
724. Suh WW, Pierce LJ, Vicini FA, et al. A cost comparison analysis of partial versus whole-breast irradiation after breast-conserving surgery for early-stage breast cancer. *Int J Radiat Oncol Biol Phys* 2005;62:790–796.
725. Sullivan T, Raad RA, Goldberg S, et al. Tubular carcinoma of the breast: a retrospective analysis and review of the literature. *Breast Cancer Res Treat* 2005;93:199–205.
726. Sutton R, Buzdar AU, Hortobagyi GN. Pregnancy and offspring after adjuvant chemotherapy in breast cancer patients. *Cancer* 1990;65:847–850.
727. Swerdlow AJ, Barber JA, Hudson GV, et al. Risk of second malignancy after Hodgkin's disease in a collaborative British cohort: the relation to age at treatment. *J Clin Oncol* 2000;18:498–509.
728. Tabár L, Duffy SW, Burhenne LW. New Swedish breast cancer detection results for women aged 40-49. *Cancer* 1993;72:1437–1448.
729. Tabár L, Duffy SW, Vitak B, et al. The natural history of breast carcinoma: what have we learned from screening? *Cancer* 1999;86:449–462.
730. Tabár L, Vitak B, Chen HH, et al. Beyond randomized controlled trials: organized mammographic screening substantially reduces breast carcinoma mortality. *Cancer* 2001;91:1724–1731.
731. Tabár L, Vitak B, Chen HH, et al. The Swedish two-county trial twenty years later. Updated mortality results and new insights from long-term follow-up. *Radiol Clin North Am* 2000;38:625–651.
732. Taghian AG, Assaad SI, Niemierko A, et al. Risk of pneumonitis in breast cancer patients treated with radiation therapy and combination chemotherapy with paclitaxel. *J Natl Cancer Inst* 2001;93:1806–1811.
733. Tannock IF, Belanger D. Use of a physician-directed questionnaire to define a consensus about management of breast cancer: implications for assessing costs and benefits of treatment. *J Natl Cancer Inst Monogr* 1992:137–142.
734. Tarone RE. The excess of patients with advanced breast cancer in young women screened with mammography in the Canadian National Breast Screening Study. *Cancer* 1995;75:997–1003.
735. Taylor IW, Musgrove EA, Friedlander ML, et al. The influence of age on the DNA ploidy levels of breast tumours. *Eur J Cancer Clin Oncol* 1983;19:623–628.
736. Taylor ME, Perez CA, Halverson KJ, et al. Factors influencing cosmetic results after conservation therapy for breast cancer. *Int J Radiat Oncol Biol Phys* 1995;31:753–764.
737. Taylor PJ, Cooper GG, Sarkar TK. Upper-limb arterial disease in women treated for breast cancer. *Br J Surg* 1995;82:1089–1091.
738. Temple WJ, Russell ML, Parsons LL, et al. Conservation surgery for breast cancer as the preferred choice: a prospective analysis. *J Clin Oncol* 2006;24:3367–3373.
739. Thames HD, Petersen C, Petersen S, et al. Immunohistochemically detected p53 mutations in epithelial tumors and results of treatment with chemotherapy and radiotherapy. A treatment-specific overview of the clinical data. *Strahlenther Onkol* 2002;178:411–421.
740. Thomsen HS, Lund JO, Munck O, et al. Experience with 7,604 bone scintigraphies at time of operation for breast cancer 1977-1987. *Dan Med Bull* 1989;36:481–483.
741. Thomsen HS, Lund JO, Munck O, et al. The value of pre-scheduled bone scintigraphies in breast cancer. *Acta Oncol* 1988;27:617–619.
742. Thurman SA, Schnitt SJ, Connolly JL, et al. Outcome after breast conserving therapy for patients with stage I or II mucinous, medullary, or tubular breast carcinoma. *Int J Radiat Oncol Biol Phys* 2004;59:152–159.
743. Tillman GF, Orel SG, Schnall MD, et al. Effect of breast magnetic resonance imaging on the clinical management of women with early-stage breast carcinoma. *J Clin Oncol* 2002;20:3413–3423.
744. Tinger A, Wasserman TH, Klein EE, et al. The incidence of breast cancer following mantle field radiation therapy as a function of dose and technique. *Int J Radiat Oncol Biol Phys* 1997;37:865–870.
745. Tinnemans JG, Wobbes T, Holland R, et al. Treatment and survival of female patients with nonpalpable breast carcinoma. *Ann Surg* 1989;209:249–253.
746. Toikkanen S, Joensuu H, Klemi P. The prognostic significance of nuclear DNA content in invasive breast cancer—a study with long-term follow-up. *Br J Cancer* 1989;60:693–700.
747. Toledano A, Garaud P, Serin D, et al. Concurrent administration of adjuvant chemotherapy and radiotherapy after breast-conservative surgery enhances late toxicities: long-term results of the ARCOSEIN multicenter randomized study. *Int J Radiat Oncol Biol Phys* 2006.
748. Touboul E, Belkacemi Y, Lefranc JP, et al. Early breast cancer: influence of type of boost (electrons vs iridium-192 implant) on local control and cosmesis after conservative surgery and radiation therapy. *Radiother Oncol* 1995;34:105–113.
749. Tralins AH. Lactation after conservative breast surgery combined with radiation therapy. *Am J Clin Oncol* 1995;18:40–43.
750. Travis LB, Hill D, Dores GM, et al. Cumulative absolute breast cancer risk for young women treated for Hodgkin lymphoma. *J Natl Cancer Inst* 2005;97:1428–1437.
751. Travis LB, Hill DA, Dores GM, et al. Breast cancer following radiotherapy and chemotherapy among young women with Hodgkin disease. *JAMA* 2003;290:465–475.
752. Treves N, Sunderland DA. Cystosarcoma phyllodes of the breast: a malignant and a benign tumor;a clinicopathological study of seventy-seven cases. *Cancer* 1951;4:1286–1332.
753. Truong PT, Yong CM, Abnousi F, et al. Lymphovascular invasion is associated with reduced locoregional control and survival in women with node-negative breast cancer treated with mastectomy and systemic therapy. *J Am Coll Surg* 2005;200:912–921.
754. Tsangaris TN, Knox SM, Cheek JH. Tumor hormone receptor status and recurrences in premenopausal patients with node-negative breast carcinoma. *Cancer* 1992;69:984–987.
755. Tuamokumo NL, Haffty BG. Clinical outcome and cosmesis in African-American patients treated with conservative surgery and radiation therapy. *Cancer J* 2003;9:313–320.

756. Tucker MA, Coleman CN, Cox RS, et al. Risk of second cancers after treatment for Hodgkin's disease. *N Engl J Med* 1988;318:76–81.

757. Turner BC, Glazer PM, Haffty BG. BRCA1/BRCA2 in breast-conserving therapy. *J Clin Oncol* 1999;17:3689.

758. Turner BC, Gumbs AA, Carbone CJ, et al. Mutant p53 protein overexpression in women with ipsilateral breast tumor recurrence following lumpectomy and radiation therapy. *Cancer* 2000;88:1091–1098.

759. UK Trial Group. 16-year mortality from breast cancer in the UK trial of early detection of breast cancer. *Lancet* 1999;353:1909–1914.

760. Union Internationale Contre le Cancer. *TNM atlas: illustrated guide to the classification of malignent tumours.* Berlin: Springer-Verlag, 1982.

761. Upponi SS, Warren RM. The diagnostic impact of contrast-enhanced MRI in management of breast disease. *Breast* 2006;15(6)322–324.

762. Vaidya JS, Baum M, Tobias JS, et al. The novel technique of delivering targeted intraoperative radiotherapy (Targit) for early breast cancer. *Eur J Surg Oncol* 2002;28:447–454.

763. Vainio H, Kaaks R, Bianchini F. Weight control and physical activity in cancer prevention: international evaluation of the evidence. *Eur J Cancer Prev* 2002;11[Suppl 2]:S94–S100.

764. Vallis KA, Pintilie M, Chong N, et al. Assessment of coronary heart disease morbidity and mortality after radiation therapy for early breast cancer. *J Clin Oncol* 2002;20:1036–1042.

765. van de Vijver MJ, He YD, van't Veer LJ, et al. A gene-expression signature as a predictor of survival in breast cancer. *N Engl J Med* 2002;347:1999–2009.

766. van den Brandt PA, Spiegelman D, Yaun SS, et al. Pooled analysis of prospective cohort studies on height, weight, and breast cancer risk. *Am J Epidemiol* 2000;152:514–527.

767. van Dongen JA, Bartelink H, Fentiman IS, et al. Randomized clinical trial to assess the value of breast-conserving therapy in stage I and II breast cancer, EORTC 10801 trial. *J Natl Cancer Inst Monogr* 1992:15–18.

768. van Dongen JA, Voogd AC, Fentiman IS, et al. Long-term results of a randomized trial comparing breast-conserving therapy with mastectomy: European Organization for Research and Treatment of Cancer 10801 trial. *J Natl Cancer Inst* 2000;92:1143–1150.

769. Van Hoften C, Burger H, Peeters PH, et al. Long-term oral contraceptive use increases breast cancer risk in women over 55 years of age: the DOM cohort. *Int J Cancer* 2000;87:591–594.

770. van Leeuwen FE, Klokman WJ, Veer MB, et al. Long-term risk of second malignancy in survivors of Hodgkin's disease treated during adolescence or young adulthood. *J Clin Oncol* 2000;18:487–497.

771. van Limbergen E, van den Bogaert W, van der Schueren E, et al. Tumor excision and radiotherapy as primary treatment of breast cancer. Analysis of patient and treatment parameters and local control. *Radiother Oncol* 1987;8:1–9.

772. van't Veer LJ, Paik S, Hayes DF. Gene expression profiling of breast cancer: a new tumor marker. *J Clin Oncol* 2005;23:1631–1635.

773. Vanlemmens L, Hebbar M, Peyrat JP, et al. Age as a prognostic factor in breast cancer. *Anticancer Res* 1998;18:1891–1896.

774. Verhoef LC, Stalpers LJ, Verbeek AL, et al. Breast-conserving treatment or mastectomy in early breast cancer: a clinical decision analysis with special reference to the risk of local recurrence. *Eur J Cancer* 1991;27:1132–1137.

775. Verhoog LC, Brekelmans CT, Seynaeve C, et al. Survival and tumour characteristics of breast-cancer patients with germline mutations of BRCA1. *Lancet* 1998;351:316–321.

776. Veronesi U, Banfi A, Salvadori B, et al. Breast conservation is the treatment of choice in small breast cancer: long term results of a randomized trial. *Eur J Cancer* 1990;26:668–670.

777. Veronesi U, Cascinelli N, Bufalino R, et al. Risk of internal mammary lymph node metastases and its relevance on prognosis of breast cancer patients. *Ann Surg* 1983;198:681–684.

778. Veronesi U, Cascinelli N, Mariani L, et al. Twenty-year follow-up of a randomized study comparing breast-conserving surgery with radical mastectomy for early breast cancer. *N Engl J Med* 2002;347:1227–1232.

779. Veronesi U, Gatti G, Luini A, et al. Full-dose intraoperative radiotherapy with electrons during breast-conserving surgery. *Arch Surg* 2003;138:1253–1256.

780. Veronesi U, Maisonneuve P, Rotmensz N, et al. Italian randomized trial among women with hysterectomy: tamoxifen and hormone-dependent breast cancer in high-risk women. *J Natl Cancer Inst* 2003;95:160–165.

781. Veronesi U, Maisonneuve P, Sacchini V, et al. Tamoxifen for breast cancer among hysterectomised women. *Lancet* 2002;359:1122–1124.

782. Veronesi U, Marubini E, Del Vecchio M, et al. Local recurrences and distant metastases after conservative breast cancer treatments: partly independent events. *J Natl Cancer Inst* 1995;87:19–27.

783. Veronesi U, Marubini E, Mariani L, et al. Radiotherapy after breast-conserving surgery in small breast carcinoma: long-term results of a randomized trial. *Ann Oncol* 2001;12:997–1003.

784. Veronesi U, Orecchia R, Zurrida S, et al. Avoiding axillary dissection in breast cancer surgery: a randomized trial to assess the role of axillary radiotherapy. *Ann Oncol* 2005;16:383–388.

785. Veronesi U, Paganelli G, Galimberti V, et al. Sentinel-node biopsy to avoid axillary dissection in breast cancer with clinically negative lymph-nodes. *Lancet* 1997;349:1864–1867.

786. Veronesi U, Paganelli G, Viale G, et al. A randomized comparison of sentinel-node biopsy with routine axillary dissection in breast cancer. *N Engl J Med* 2003;349:546–553.

787. Veronesi U, Paganelli G, Viale G, et al. Sentinel lymph node biopsy and axillary dissection in breast cancer: results in a large series. *J Natl Cancer Inst* 1999;91:368–373.

788. Veronesi U, Salvadori B, Luini A, et al. Conservative treatment of early breast cancer. Long-term results of 1232 cases treated with quadrantectomy, axillary dissection, and radiotherapy. *Ann Surg* 1990;211:250–259.

789. Veronesi U, Zucali R, Luini A. Local control and survival in early breast cancer: the Milan trial. *Int J Radiat Oncol Biol Phys* 1986;12:717–720.

790. Veronesi U. NIH consensus meeting on early breast cancer. *Eur J Cancer* 1990;26:843–844.

791. Vicini F, White J, Gustafson G, et al. The use of iodine-125 seeds as a substitute for iridium-192 seeds in temporary interstitial breast implants. *Int J Radiat Oncol Biol Phys* 1993;27:561–566.

792. Vicini F, Winter K, Straube W, et al. A phase I/II trial to evaluate three-dimensional conformal radiation therapy confined to the region of the lumpectomy cavity for stage I/II breast carcinoma: initial report of feasibility and reproducibility of Radiation Therapy Oncology Group (RTOG) Study 0319. *Int J Radiat Oncol Biol Phys* 2005;63:1531–1537.

793. Vicini FA, Arthur DW. Breast brachytherapy: North American experience. *Semin Radiat Oncol* 2005;15:108–115.

794. Vicini FA, Baglan KL, Kestin LL, et al. Accelerated treatment of breast cancer. *J Clin Oncol* 2001;19:1993–2001.

795. Vicini FA, Beitsch PD, Quiet CA, et al. First analysis of patient demographics, technical reproducibility, cosmesis, and early toxicity: results of the American Society of Breast Surgeons MammoSite breast brachytherapy trial. *Cancer* 2005;104:1138–1148.

796. Vicini FA, Goldstein NS, Pass H, et al. Use of pathologic factors to assist in establishing adequacy of excision before radiotherapy in patients treated with breast-conserving therapy. *Int J Radiat Oncol Biol Phys* 2004;60:86–94.

797. Vicini FA, Horwitz EM, Lacerna MD, et al. The role of regional nodal irradiation in the management of patients with early-stage breast cancer treated with breast-conserving therapy. *Int J Radiat Oncol Biol Phys* 1997;39:1069–1076.

798. Vicini FA, Kestin LL, Edmundson GK, et al. Dose-volume analysis for quality assurance of interstitial brachytherapy for breast cancer. *Int J Radiat Oncol Biol Phys* 1999;45:803–810.

799. Vicini FA, Recht A, Abner A, et al. Recurrence in the breast following conservative surgery and radiation therapy for early-stage breast cancer. *J Natl Cancer Inst Monogr* 1992:33–39.

800. Vicini FA, Sharpe M, Kestin L, et al. Optimizing breast cancer treatment efficacy with intensity-modulated radiotherapy. *Int J Radiat Oncol Biol Phys* 2002;54:1336–1344.

801. Viehweg P, Heinig A, Lampe D, et al. Retrospective analysis for evaluation of the value of contrast-enhanced MRI in patients treated with breast conservative therapy. *Magma* 1998;7:141–152.

802. Vilcoq JR, Calle R, Stacey P, et al. The outcome of treatment by tumorectomy and radiotherapy of patients with operable breast cancer. *Int J Radiat Oncol Biol Phys* 1981;7:1327–1332.

803. Vinh-Hung V, Verschraegen C. Breast-conserving surgery with or without radiotherapy: pooled-analysis for risks of ipsilateral breast tumor recurrence and mortality. *J Natl Cancer Inst* 2004;96:115–121.

804. Vogel VG, Costantino JP, Wickerham DL, et al. Effects of tamoxifen vs raloxifene on the risk of developing invasive breast cancer and other disease outcomes: the NSABP Study of Tamoxifen and Raloxifene (STAR) P-2 trial. *JAMA* 2006;295:2727–2741.

805. Volkers N. NCI replaces guidelines with statement of evidence. *J Natl Cancer Inst* 1994;86:14–15.

806. Voogd AC, Coebergh JW, Repelaer van Driel OJ, et al. The risk of nodal metastases in breast cancer patients with clinically negative lymph nodes: a population-based analysis. *Breast Cancer Res Treat* 2000;62:63–69.

807. Vrieling C, Collette L, Fourquet A, et al. Can patient-, treatment- and pathology-related characteristics explain the high local recurrence rate following breast-conserving therapy in young patients? *Eur J Cancer* 2003;39:932–944.

808. Vrieling C, Collette L, Fourquet A, et al. The influence of patient, tumor and treatment factors on the cosmetic results after breast-conserving therapy in the EORTC "boost vs. no boost" trial. EORTC Radiotherapy and Breast Cancer Cooperative Groups. *Radiother Oncol* 2000;55:219–232.

809. Vu-Nishino H, Tavassoli FA, Ahrens WA, et al. Clinicopathologic features and long-term outcome of patients with medullary breast carcinoma managed with breast-conserving therapy (BCT). *Int J Radiat Oncol Biol Phys* 2005;62:1040–1047.

810. Wald NJ, Hackshaw A. Chlamidine J. The efficacy and safety of periodic mammographic breast cancer screening: summary of report of the European Society of Mastology. *Clin Radiol* 1994;49:592–593.

811. Wallgren A, Bernier J, Gelber RD, et al. Timing of radiotherapy and chemotherapy following breast-conserving surgery for patients with node-positive breast cancer. International Breast Cancer Study Group. *Int J Radiat Oncol Biol Phys* 1996;35:649–659.

812. Warner E, Plewes DB, Hill KA, et al. Surveillance of BRCA1 and BRCA2 mutation carriers with magnetic resonance imaging, ultrasound, mammography, and clinical breast examination. *JAMA* 2004;292:1317–1325.

813. Warner E, Plewes DB, Shumak RS, et al. Comparison of breast magnetic resonance imaging, mammography, and ultrasound for surveillance of women at high risk for hereditary breast cancer. *J Clin Oncol* 2001;19:3524–3531.

814. Warren JL, Brown ML, Fay MP, et al. Costs of treatment for elderly women with early-stage breast cancer in fee-for-service settings. *J Clin Oncol* 2002;20:307–316.

815. Wazer DE, Berle L, Graham R, et al. Preliminary results of a phase I/II study of HDR brachytherapy alone for T1/T2 breast cancer. *Int J Radiat Oncol Biol Phys* 2002;53:889–897.

816. Wazer DE, DiPetrillo T, Schmidt-Ullrich R, et al. Factors influencing cosmetic outcome and complication risk after conservative surgery and radiotherapy for early-stage breast carcinoma. *J Clin Oncol* 1992;10:356–363.

817. Wazer DE, Erban JK, Robert NJ, et al. Breast conservation in elderly women for clinically negative axillary lymph nodes without axillary dissection. *Cancer* 1994;74:878–883.

818. Wazer DE, Jabro G, Ruthazer R, et al. Extent of margin positivity as a predictor for local recurrence after breast conserving irradiation. *Radiat Oncol Investig* 1999;7:111–117.

819. Wazer DE, Lowther D, Boyle T, et al. Clinically evident fat necrosis in women treated with high-dose-rate brachytherapy alone for early-stage breast cancer. *Int J Radiat Oncol Biol Phys* 2001;50:107–111.

820. Weaver DL, Krag DN, Ashikaga T, et al. Pathologic analysis of sentinel and nonsentinel lymph nodes in breast carcinoma: a multicenter study. *Cancer* 2000;88:1099–1107.

821. Weight SC, Windle R, Stotter AT. Optimizing surveillance mammography following breast conservation surgery. *Eur J Surg Oncol* 2002;28:11–13.

822. Weinstein SP, Orel SG, Heller R, et al. MR imaging of the breast in patients with invasive lobular carcinoma. *AJR Am J Roentgenol* 2001;176:399–406.

823. Weir L, Worsley D, Bernstein V. The value of FDG positron emission tomography in the management of patients with breast cancer. *Breast J* 2005;11(3):204–209.

824. Weiss MC, Fowble BL, Solin LJ, et al. Outcome of conservative therapy for

invasive breast cancer by histologic subtype. *Int J Radiat Oncol Biol Phys* 1992;23:941–947.

825. Wenger CR, Clark GM. S-phase fraction and breast cancer—a decade of experience. *Breast Cancer Res Treat* 1998;51:255–265.

826. Whelan T, Clark R, Roberts R, et al. Ipsilateral breast tumor recurrence postlumpectomy is predictive of subsequent mortality: results from a randomized trial. Investigators of the Ontario Clinical Oncology Group. *Int J Radiat Oncol Biol Phys* 1994;30:11–16.

827. Whelan T, MacKenzie R, Julian J, et al. Randomized trial of breast irradiation schedules after lumpectomy for women with lymph node-negative breast cancer. *J Natl Cancer Inst* 2002;94:1143–1150.

828. Whelan TJ, Levine MN, Gafni A, et al. Breast irradiation postlumpectomy: development and evaluation of a decision instrument. *J Clin Oncol* 1995;13:847–853.

829. Wilson LD, Beinfield M, McKhann CF, et al. Conservative surgery and radiation in the treatment of synchronous ipsilateral breast cancers. *Cancer* 1993;72:137–142.

830. Wilson LD, Haffty BG. National Residency Matching Program (NRMP) results for radiation oncology, 2004 update. *Int J Radiat Oncol Biol Phys* 2004;60:689–690.

831. Winchester D, Bernstein J, Paige M. *The early detection and diagnosis of breast cancer*. Atlanta: American Cancer Society, 1988;1–20.

832. Winzer KJ, Sauer R, Sauerbrei W, et al. Radiation therapy after breast-conserving surgery: first results of a randomised clinical trial in patients with low risk of recurrence. *Eur J Cancer* 2004;40:998–1005.

833. Wittliff JL. Steroid-hormone receptors in breast cancer. *Cancer* 1984;53:630–643.

834. Witzig TE, Ingle JN, Cha SS, et al. DNA ploidy and the percentage of cells in S-phase as prognostic factors for women with lymph node negative breast cancer. *Cancer* 1994;74:1752–1761.

835. Wolden SL, Hancock SL, Carlson RW, et al. Management of breast cancer after Hodgkin's disease. *J Clin Oncol* 2000;18:765–772.

836. Wolden SL, Lamborn KR, Cleary SF, et al. Second cancers following pediatric Hodgkin's disease. *J Clin Oncol* 1998;16:536–544.

837. Wolmark N, Dunn BK. The role of tamoxifen in breast cancer prevention: issues sparked by the NSABP Breast Cancer Prevention Trial (P-1). *Ann N Y Acad Sci* 2001;949:99–108.

838. Wong JS, O'Neill A, Recht A, et al. The relationship between lymphatic vessel invasion, tumor size, and pathologic nodal status: can we predict who can avoid a third field in the absence of axillary dissection? *Int J Radiat Oncol Biol Phys* 2000;48:133–137.

839. Wong JS, Recht A, Beard CJ, et al. Treatment outcome after tangential radiation therapy without axillary dissection in patients with early-stage breast cancer and clinically negative axillary nodes. *Int J Radiat Oncol Biol Phys* 1997;39:915–920.

840. Woudstra E, van der Werf H. Obliquely incident electron beams for irradiation of the internal mammary lymph nodes. *Radiother Oncol* 1987;10:209–215.

841. Wu AH, Pike MC, Stram DO. Meta-analysis: dietary fat intake, serum estrogen levels, and the risk of breast cancer. *J Natl Cancer Inst* 1999;91:529–534.

842. Yaffe M, Boyd N. Mammographic breast density and cancer risk: the radiological view. *Gynecol Endocrinol* 2005;21[Suppl 1]:6–11.

843. Yarnold J, Ashton A, Bliss J, et al. Fractionation sensitivity and dose response of late adverse effects in the breast after radiotherapy for early breast cancer: long-term results of a randomised trial. *Radiother Oncol* 2005;75:9–17.

844. Yarnold JR. Selective avoidance of lymphatic irradiation in the conservative management of breast cancer. *Radiother Oncol* 1984;2:79–92.

845. Yu TK, Whitman GJ, Thames HD, et al. Clinically relevant pneumonitis after sequential paclitaxel-based chemotherapy and radiotherapy in breast cancer patients. *J Natl Cancer Inst* 2004;96:1676–1681.

846. Zafrani B, Vielh P, Fourquet A, et al. Conservative treatment of early breast cancer: prognostic value of the ductal in situ component and other pathological variables on local control and survival. Long-term results. *Eur J Cancer Clin Oncol* 1989;25:1645–1650.

847. Zajdela A, Ghossein NA, Pilleron JP, et al. The value of aspiration cytology in the diagnosis of breast cancer: experience at the Foundation Curie. *Cancer* 1975;35:499–506.

848. Zellars RC, Hilsenbeck SG, Clark GM, et al. Prognostic value of p53 for local failure in mastectomy-treated breast cancer patients. *J Clin Oncol* 2000;18:1906–1913.

849. Zemlickis D, Lishner M, Degendorfer P, et al. Maternal and fetal outcome after breast cancer in pregnancy. *Am J Obstet Gynecol* 1992;166:781–787.

850. Zhou P, Gautam S, Recht A. Factors affecting outcome for young women with early stage invasive breast cancer treated with breast-conserving therapy. *Breast Cancer Res Treat* 2007;101(1):51–57.

851. Zucali R, Merson M, Placucci M, et al. Soft tissue sarcoma of the breast after conservative surgery and irradiation for early mammary cancer. *Radiother Oncol* 1994;30:271–273.

852. Zurrida S, Galimberti V, Orvieto E, et al. Radioguided sentinel node biopsy to avoid axillary dissection in breast cancer. *Ann Surg Oncol* 2000;7:28–31.

853. Zurrida S, Orecchia R, Galimberti V, et al. Axillary radiotherapy instead of axillary dissection: a randomized trial. Italian Oncological Senology Group. *Ann Surg Oncol* 2002;9:156–160.

Clinical Radiation Oncology

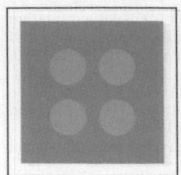

Chapter 54
Breast Cancer: Locally Advanced and Recurrent Disease, Postmastectomy Radiation, and Systemic Therapies

Thomas A. Buchholz, Bruce G. Haffty

Patients who present with locally advanced breast cancer are at risk for both distant and local-regional disease recurrence. Optimal treatment of locally advanced breast cancer requires a multidisciplinary approach that incorporates diagnostic imaging, chemotherapy, appropriate surgical intervention, radiation, and, if indicated, biological and hormonal therapies. The treatment outcome for an individual patient may depend on the degree to which this multidisciplinary approach is integrated and the expertise of the treatment team. This is especially important in the management of patients with locally advanced disease because the definition of optimal breast cancer treatment for such patients is constantly evolving and because such patients have the highest risk of disease recurrence without optimal treatment and require the most complex decision making.

The outcome for patients who have locally advanced breast cancer has improved dramatically over the past 30 years. Before the routine use of chemotherapy, most patients were treated with mastectomy, radiation, or a combination of the two; yet despite these approaches, most would develop distant metastases and die of the disease (50,64,65). The introduction of progressively more effective chemotherapy and hormone therapy regimens has significantly improved the prognosis. As additional improvements in systemic treatments further reduce the chance of dying from metastatic disease, the complete eradication of local-regional disease becomes increasingly more important.

This chapter focuses on the management of locally advanced breast cancer, with a particular focus on local regional control and radiation therapy. No consensus has been reached on the definition of "locally advanced breast cancer." Most commonly this term refers to stage III disease, meaning advanced primary or nodal disease without clinically evident systemic metastases. In addition to reviewing management strategies for stage III breast cancer, this chapter also reviews the role of postmastectomy radiation and systemic treatments for patients with all stages of invasive breast cancer. Management and outcome of locally recurrent breast cancer and selected unusual presentations of breast cancers are also discussed.

Epidemiology

Between 1980 and 1987, the incidence of breast cancer increased by approximately 4% each year, in part because of the increase in use of screening mammography, after which time breast cancer incidence has increase only 1% per year (10,20). Despite this increase in overall breast cancer incidence, the absolute numbers of cases diagnosed as locally advanced disease have remained relatively constant over time. For example, the proportion of tumors 3.0 cm or larger at diagnosis decreased 27% between 1980 and 1987, and in more recent years the percentage of tumors of this size has remained relatively stable (10,20). Two reasons have undoubtedly contributed to the decline in the percentage of cases of locally advanced disease at diagnosis. First, mammographic screening resulted in a larger proportion of patients being diagnosed with earlier disease stages. A second important contribution has been women's health initiatives and public education ef-

forts that have prompted women to seek medical care at the first sign of a breast mass. Finally, the medical community is better educated about appropriate standards for evaluating a breast mass.

Estimates of the percentage of breast cancers diagnosed as T3 disease or with lymph node involvement according to data from the Surveillance, Epidemiology, and End Results Program, as reported by the American Cancer Society, are shown in Table 54.1. Estimates indicate that 212,920 new cases of invasive breast cancer will be diagnosed in 2006, of which an estimated 12,775 new cases will have primary tumors over 5.0 cm and 63,876 new cases will have lymph node–positive disease at diagnosis (10,20).

Table 54.1 also includes data concerning the distribution of disease in whites and in African Americans (10,20). African American women with breast cancer more commonly present with advanced primary disease and lymph node–positive disease than do white women with breast cancer. This has been explained on the basis of both socioeconomic factors and biology. Specifically, African American women with breast cancer reportedly have less access to medical care and undergo screening mammography less often than do white women. African American women also more often have breast cancers that are of higher nuclear grade and more frequently have estrogen receptor (ER)-negative disease compared with white women (39,91).

In countries without mammography screening programs or poor access to health care, locally advanced breast cancer remains a more significant problem. In contrast to developed countries, the mortality rates from breast cancer have increased in these parts of the world, as shown in Figure 54.1 (106).

Inflammatory breast cancer is an important subcategory of locally advanced breast cancer that has a unique epidemiology, presentation, and biology. Inflammatory breast cancers are rare, accounting for only 2% of all breast cancers in the United States (90). Estimates indicate that approximately 4,000 cases of inflammatory breast cancer will be diagnosed in the United States in 2006. During the 1990s, the incidence of inflammatory breast cancer increased slightly. No known risk factors have been identified that are unique for the development of this form of breast cancer. However, the disease tends to occur in a younger population than does noninflammatory breast cancer. The proportion of African American women with breast cancer diagnosed with inflammatory breast cancer is higher than the proportion of white women with breast cancer. Lymph node involvement at the time of diagnosis is much more common in patients with inflammatory breast cancer than in those with noninflammatory breast cancer, and it is more common for patients with inflammatory breast cancer to have distant metastases at diagnosis (90).

Natural History

Natural History of Locally Advanced Disease

The outcome of patients who present with locally advanced breast cancer were once poor, but improvements in treatments

Table 54.1	ESTIMATES OF BREAST CANCER EXTENT OF DISEASE AT DIAGNOSIS FOR 2001–2002		
	All Races (%)	**White (%)**	**African American (%)**
Tumor ≤2.0 cm	66	67	53
Tumor 2.1–5.0 cm	28	27	37
Tumor >5.0 cm	6	6	10
Lymph node–negative	64	65	56
Lymph node–positive	30	29	35
Distant metastasis	6	6	9

Percentages calculated from the respective incidence values provided from Figures 3 and 4 of *Breast Cancer Facts and Figures 2005–2006*, published by the American Cancer Society.

have changed the prognosis considerably. Currently, many patients with locally advanced disease can be cured. As the disease grows within the breast, the tumor may infiltrate or invade the dermis or the chest wall. Skin retraction may occur because of tumor invasion of Cooper's ligaments, although this process can also be present in early stage disease. Tumor growth can also lead to infiltration or obstruction of the lymphatic drainage of the breast and breast skin, causing edema of the breast, known as peau d'orange. In addition, primary tumor growth increases the risk of spread through the lymphatics to involve regional lymph nodes and/or spread hematogenously to involve distant sites such as the liver, lung, bone, and brain.

Most advanced primary tumors are associated with axillary lymph node involvement at the time of diagnosis. The axillary lymph node region is divided into three levels, defined according to their relationship to the pectoralis minor muscle: Level I lymph nodes are inferolateral to the muscle, level II are beneath the muscle, and level III are superomedial to the pectoralis muscle (these lymph nodes are also called infraclavicular lymph nodes). Additional lymph nodes that may be involved in locally advanced breast cancer include Rotter's nodes, which are located between the pectoralis minor and pectoralis major muscles, and the supraclavicular and internal mammary lymph nodes. Figure 54.2 shows computed tomography (CT) scans from patients with locally advanced breast cancer presenting with involvement of the level II axilla (Fig. 54.2A), an infraclavicular lymph node (Fig. 54.2B), a Rotter's lymph node (Fig. 54.2C), and an internal mammary lymph node (Fig. 54.2D).

The clinical course of locally advanced breast cancer depends on several factors, including the specific disease characteristics at presentation, the biological features of the disease, and the treatment given. Without treatment, almost all locally advanced breast cancers eventually metastasize to visceral organs and become life threatening (64,65). Local disease progression can lead to ulceration of the breast skin, pain, bleeding, and infection. Progression of untreated regional lymphatic disease can cause pain, brachial plexopathy, arm edema, obstruction and thrombosis of the brachial vasculature, and skin ulceration.

Treatment advances have improved both survival times and survival rates for women with locally advanced breast cancer. Before the use of systemic treatment became routine, patients with advanced disease were treated with mastectomy, radiation therapy, or both and had 5-year survival rates of only 25% to 45% (50,64,65). Currently, 5-year survival rates approach 80% for patients with stage IIIA disease and 45% for patients with stage IIIB disease when treated with surgery, radiation therapy, and chemotherapy (74).

When assessing the survival of patients with stage III breast cancer, it is important to appreciate the heterogeneity of stage III disease. For example, an elderly woman with a neglected ER-positive, hormonally responsive, primary tumor that grew slowly but did not metastasize over a 1- to 2-year period will have a much more favorable prognosis compared to a young woman with an ER-negative T4 tumor that presented with a history of rapidly progressive disease.

Another important aspect to consider when evaluating the outcome of stage III breast cancer over time is the effect of stage migration. Improvements in diagnostic imaging increase the likelihood of detecting metastatic disease and thereby result in reclassifying some cases of stage III disease as stage IV. This reclassification artificially improves the outcome statistics for both stage III and stage IV disease. A similar effect was introduced by the 2003 change in the American Joint Commission of Cancer (AJCC) breast cancer staging system. That version of the staging system considers the number of positive lymph nodes in the pathological disease stage, but the previous version did not. Patients with four or more positive lymph nodes in the past would have been considered to have stage II disease but now are classified as having stage III disease. In an interesting study, authors compared the stage-specific long-term survival of a cohort of 1,350 patients with breast cancer staged according to the 1988 AJCC staging system or retrospectively restaged according to the 2003 AJCC system (150). Restaging led to most of the patients with four or more positive lymph nodes being moved from the stage II to the stage III category. These authors then compared the stage-specific survival of this same group of patients and found that the 10-year overall survival rates were significantly higher when the 2003 system was used, both for patients with stage II disease (76% [2003] vs. 65% [1988]; p <0.0001) and for those with stage IIIA disease (59% [2003] vs. 45% [1988]; p <0.0001) (150).

Natural History of Inflammatory Breast Cancer

Inflammatory breast cancer is a clinically defined subcategory of locally advanced breast cancer. The hallmarks of inflammatory breast cancer are rapid disease onset and the clinical findings of skin erythema, edema (peau d'orange), brawny breast induration, warmth, and asymmetric enlargement. Typically, extensive lymphovascular invasion by tumor emboli is present that involves the superficial dermal plexus of vessels in the papillary and high reticular dermis (63). It is critical to distinguish inflammatory breast cancers from locally advanced breast cancer with secondary lymphatic congestion. Neglected primary tumors can also lead to breast erythema, edema, warmth, and asymmetric enlargement, particularly when bulky axillary adenopathy impedes the normal lymphatic flow from the breast. However, the former has a history of rapid onset, while the latter tends to have a long interval between the first symptom and the presentation for medical treatment.

Despite the natural history of inflammatory breast cancer being one of rapid disease progression and early distant dissemination (9,63), in the United States, approximately 70% of patients with inflammatory breast cancer have evidence of localregional disease only at the time of diagnosis (146). Patients with inflammatory breast cancer typically have a worse clinical outcome than do other patients with T4 disease, suggesting that inflammatory breast cancer is a distinct biological entity (25). However, the prognosis for patients with inflammatory breast cancer has improved over time. Before the availability of combination chemotherapy, inflammatory breast cancer was almost uniformly fatal. Fewer than 5% of patients treated with surgery, radiation therapy, or both survived past 5 years, and the expected median survival time for such patients was <15 months (9). Local recurrence rates after surgery or radiation therapy were also high at approximately 50% (5,152). The introduction of doxorubicin-based chemotherapy improved outcomes (41,87). An evaluation of the outcome of patients

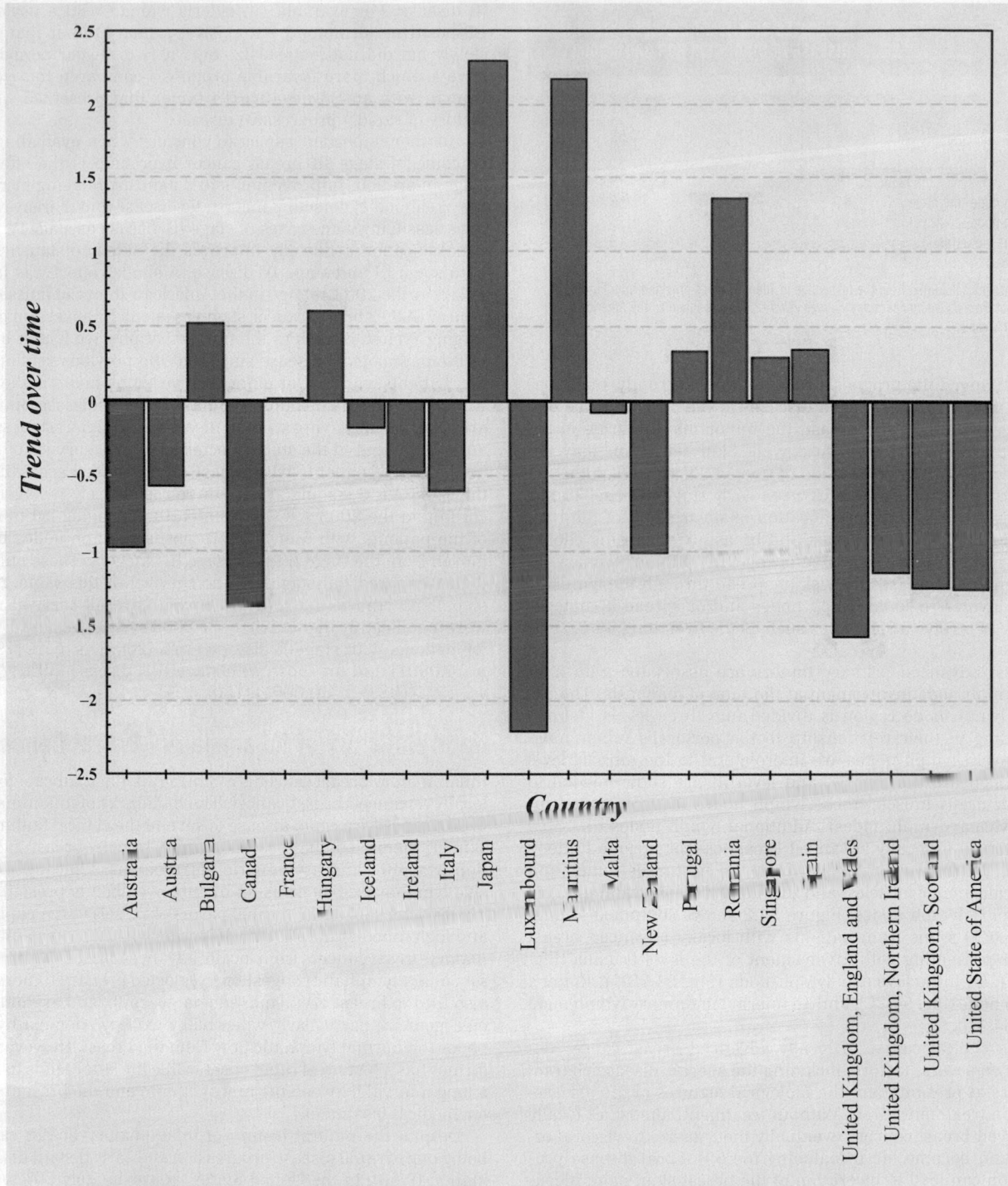

FIGURE 54.1. Breast cancer mortality trends between 1980–2000. As can be seen, the breast cancer mortality rates have decreased in Western countries such as the United States and the United Kingdom but have increased in other areas of the world. (From Trends in Worldwide Mortality Age-adjusted Rates, 2006.)

with inflammatory breast cancer registered in the Surveillance, Epidemiology, and End Results Program found that breast cancer–specific survival rates for patients with inflammatory breast cancer improved continuously throughout the 1990s (67). Currently, local control rates for patients treated with chemotherapy, mastectomy, and postmastectomy radiation now approach 70% to 80%, and 5-year survival rates are 30% to 40% (41,87).

Clinical Presentation of Locally Advanced Breast Cancer

Locally advanced breast cancer most commonly is diagnosed after a palpable mass is detected within the breast. Advanced disease can cause symptoms such as local or regional pain,

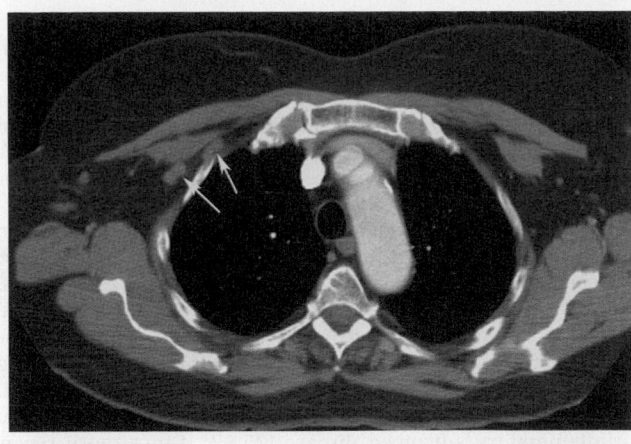
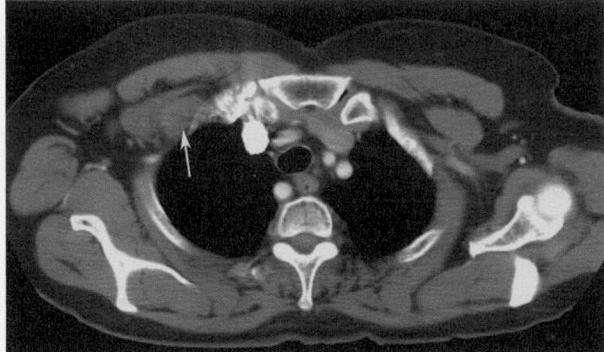
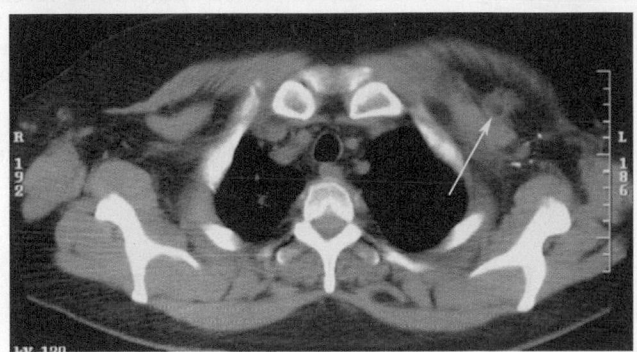
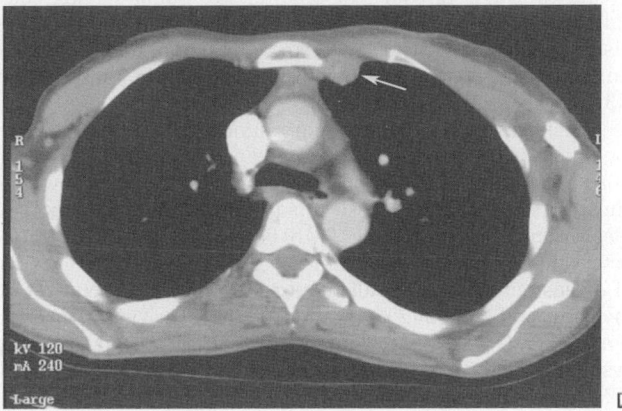

FIGURE 54.2. Computed tomography images of patients with lymph node involvement at the time of diagnosis. **A:** An image from a patient with involvement of axillary lymph nodes in the level II axilla. The white arrows show the involved lymph nodes, which are just beneath the pectoralis minor muscle. **B:** An involved level III axillary lymph node (*white arrow*) that extents superomedial to the pectoralis minor muscle. **C:** An involved Rotter's lymph node (white arrow), which is anterior to the pectoralis minor and beneath the pectoralis major muscle. **D:** An image from a patient with an involved internal mammary lymph node (*white arrow*).

bleeding, paresthesia, and paresis. As previously indicated, it is critically important to determine the onset of symptoms and the rate of disease progression to reach an accurate diagnosis as to whether an advanced breast cancer represents an inflammatory carcinoma.

Diagnostic Work-Up

For patients with locally advanced breast cancer, the workup should start with a careful history and physical examination. The breast examination should include notation of the breast symmetry as well as careful inspection for involvement or edema of the skin. Peau d'orange can sometimes be subtle and at times can be best detected through gentle compression of the dermis between two fingers, which can elicit an increased prominence of the hair follicles and skin thickening compared with the skin overlying the contralateral breast. This finding may be missed on a quick visual inspection. Other times, physical examination findings are more obvious. Figure 54.3 is a photograph of a patient with a neglected locally advanced breast cancer presenting with peau d'orange, inflammatory changes, breast retraction and involution, and effacement of the nipple-areola complex. Medical photographs are helpful to document the extent of visible abnormalities before treatment is begun and can be used to assess disease response to treatments.

The extent of palpable disease should also be measured and documented. Fixation of a breast mass to the pectoralis muscle or chest wall should be determined by assessing the mobility of the mass with the pectoralis muscle relaxed and contracted. Regional lymph nodes should be thoroughly evaluated by careful clinical examination with the patient in both supine and sitting positions. Clinical nodal evaluation may be supplemented with ultrasonographic imaging.

All cases of locally advanced disease require complete staging before initiation of therapy. Laboratory studies should include a complete blood cell count and serum chemistry profile with liver function tests. Radiographic studies should include a chest radiograph, a CT scan of the abdomen, a bone scan, and plain radiographs of symptomatic regions or areas of increased uptake on bone scans. Bone scans are recommended for all patients with locally advanced disease; up to 35% of patients with clinical stage III cancer can show abnormal bone scan results

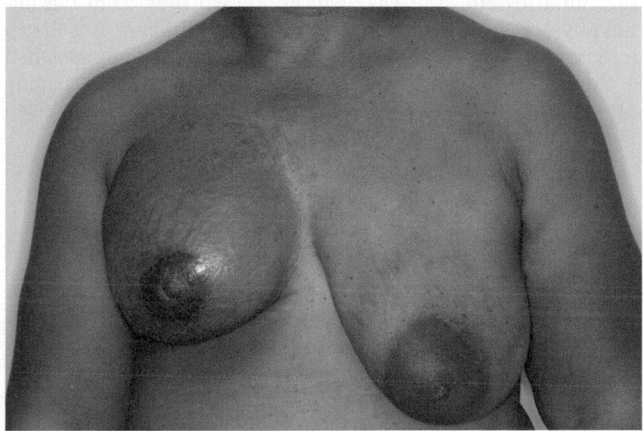

FIGURE 54.3. Photograph of a patient with a locally advanced noninflammatory right breast cancer at the time of diagnosis.

(3). If any neurologic symptoms suggestive of cerebral metastases are present, a contrast-enhanced CT scan or gadolinium-enhanced magnetic resonance imaging (MRI) scan of the brain should be obtained. Gadolinium-enhanced MRI is the preferred imaging technique if leptomeningeal carcinomatosis is suspected. The use of ^{18}F-fluorodeoxyglucose positron emission tomography (FDG-PET) for disease staging continues to be investigated, but to date this technique has not been shown to be any more useful clinically than conventional staging studies.

Staging of Locally Advanced Breast Cancer

A comprehensive discussion of disease staging systems for breast cancer is provided in Chapter 53. Some staging considerations are particularly relevant to patients with stage III disease. Stage III breast cancer can represent either T3 disease (tumors larger than 5.0 cm) with involved lymph nodes, N2 or N3 disease, or T4 disease (122).

Specific aspects of both primary tumor and nodal staging in locally advanced breast cancer warrant additional consideration. Specifically, T4 disease may represent invasion into the chest wall (T4a), tumors associated with breast edema or skin ulceration or satellite nodules (T4b) both invasion and T4b characteristics (T4c), or inflammatory breast cancer (T4d). Invasion of disease into the pectoralis major muscle without chest wall invasion and dimpling or fixation of the overlying skin does not qualify as T4 disease. Both clinical and pathological staging systems have been established for N2 and N3 disease. Clinical N2 disease signifies either involved axillary lymph nodes that are fixed to one another or to surrounding structures (N2a) or involved internal mammary lymph nodes without concurrent disease in the axilla (N2b), as determined by physical examination or imaging studies. Clinical N3 disease is disease that involves the infraclavicular region (N3a), both the axilla and internal mammary lymph nodes (N3b), or the supraclavicular region (N3c). Pathological N2 disease represents involvement of four to nine axillary lymph nodes with at least one focus measuring over 2.0 mm (N2a) or clinical involvement of internal mammary lymph nodes with pathologically negative axillary lymph nodes (N2b). Pathological N3 disease represents involvement of an infraclavicular lymph node or 10 or more involved lymph nodes with at least one focus measuring over 2.0 mm (N3a), clinical involvement of internal mammary lymph nodes with one to nine axillary lymph nodes involved, or pathological involvement of a sentinel internal mammary lymph node with four or more axillary lymph nodes involved (N3b), or a metastasis in the supraclavicular region (N3c) (122).

Currently, neoadjuvant chemotherapy is recommended for most patients with locally advanced breast cancer. Therefore, the initial extent of disease will be known only from the initial physical examination and radiographic findings. It is therefore imperative that disease in all patients be carefully assigned a clinical stage before any treatment is begun. These staging procedures may have clinical implications for treatments given later in the course of multimodality therapy.

Pathology and Biology of Locally Advanced Breast Cancer

The histopathology of locally advanced disease is relatively similar to that of early stage disease. Both infiltrating ductal carcinoma and lobular carcinoma can present as locally advanced disease. However, it is unusual for histologically "favorable" tumor types (e.g., tubular carcinoma, mucinous carcinoma, and medullary carcinoma) to present at advanced clinical stages unless the breast mass has been present for a long time.

The term *locally advanced breast cancer* encompasses a biological spectrum of diseases. Locally advanced disease that has developed between interval (annual) screening mammograms is most often ER-negative, with high nuclear grade and high proliferative index. In contrast, patients who present with extensive local-regional disease after years of medical neglect more often are found to have ER-positive disease with low nuclear grade and low proliferative index.

Inflammatory breast cancer also has biological characteristics that differ from those of noninflammatory breast cancer. Specifically, inflammatory cancer more often is of high histologic grade, shows high percentages of cells in S phase and aneuploidy, does not express the ER, and expresses high levels of p53 and epidermal growth factor (62,111). Interestingly, most investigators have found that HER2/neu overexpression is no more common in inflammatory breast cancer than in noninflammatory advanced disease (25,62). Other more recently discovered markers include the propensity of inflammatory tumors to overexpress RhoC GTPase and to lack the tumor suppressor gene WIPS3 (84,141). Finally, others have described that inflammatory breast cancers with loss of MUC-1 may be associated with poorer survival than tumors that express MUC-1. If these findings are confirmed and validated, markers such as these may prove to be useful for diagnosis and possibly as future therapeutic targets (84,141).

General Management and Treatment Results for Locally Advanced Breast Cancer

Locally advanced disease requires multimodality therapy aimed at eradicating all disease in the local-regional area and preventing distant disease recurrence. These goals are best achieved through the use of combined modality treatments that include chemotherapy, surgery, and radiation. In addition, ER-positive disease should be treated with hormonal therapy, and HER2/neu–positive disease should be treated with trastuzumab. Combined modality therapy has significantly improved the prognosis for patients with advanced breast cancer. As previously noted, the prognosis of patients with locally advanced disease treated in the era before chemotherapy was available was very poor, with 5-year survival rates of only 25% (50,64,65). In contrast, more recent single-institution studies have reported 5-year survival rates approaching 80% for patients with stage IIIA disease and 45% for patients with stage IIIB disease (74). National database studies also reflect improvements in survival over time. For example, a study evaluating the outcome of patients with lymph node–positive breast cancer demonstrated that 5-year survival rates were significantly better in the group treated in 1995 to 1999 than in the group treated in 1975 to 1979 (38) (Fig. 54.4). These survival statistics are likely to show continued improvement over time, because since 1999 several positive phase III clinical trials have shown that a new systemic treatment strategy may improve outcome among patients with lymph node–positive breast cancer. What is particularly exciting is that some of these advances represent incremental improvements in outcome over previous advances, so that when the benefits are added together the improvements over time become quite significant. As evidence of this improvement, an interesting study recently reported that between 1950 and 1980, the Food and Drug Administration approved fewer than five new systemic treatments for breast cancer during each decade; in contrast, six new agents were approved during the 1980s, and 12 new agents were approved during the 1990s (55). These new treatments are likely to continue to improve the prognosis for patients with advanced breast cancer during the decades to come, and the rate at which new agents for breast

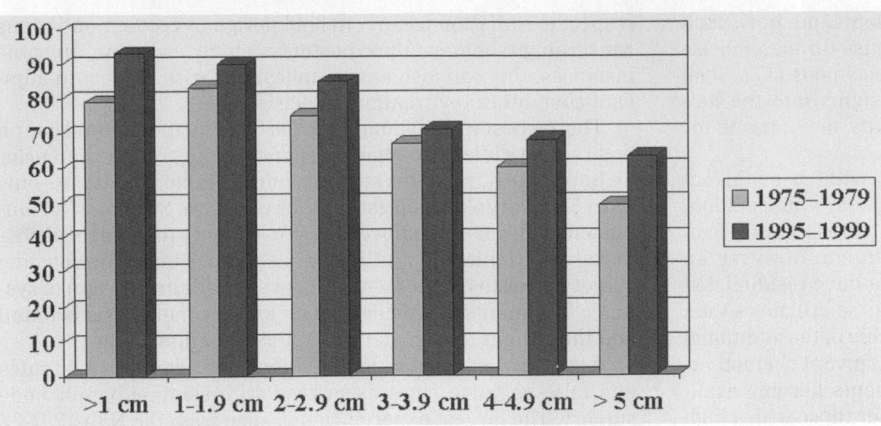

FIGURE 54.4. Five-year survival rates for patients with positive axillary lymph nodes according to tumor size and year of diagnosis. (Data from Elkin EB, Hudis C, Begg CB, et al. The effect of changes in tumor size on breast carcinoma survival in the U.S.: 1975–1999. *Cancer* 2005;104:1149–1157, with permission. Figure reprinted from Buchholz TA. Locally advanced breast cancer. In: *Handbook of radiation oncology.* Haffty BG, Wilson L, eds. 2006; Jones & Bartlett, Sudbury, MA, with permission.)

cancer treatment are introduced is expected to accelerate with identification of new therapeutic targets.

Overview of Treatment

Locally advanced breast cancer can present as either operable disease or inoperable disease. The current standard of treatment for all patients with inoperable breast cancer is to proceed with nooadjuvant chemotherapy as the initial therapy. Approximately 80% to 90% of patients with advanced breast cancer will show partial or complete clinical response to neoadjuvant chemotherapy (42,88), and most patients presenting with inoperable breast cancer become candidates for surgery after neoadjuvant treatment.

No criteria have been agreed on to distinguish inoperable from operable disease. In general, neoadjuvant chemotherapy is preferred if an initial surgical procedure is not likely to completely resect all gross disease with achievement of negative surgical margins. Most patients with T4 disease and all patients with inflammatory breast cancer should be given neoadjuvant chemotherapy to allow primary closure of the skin flaps of the mastectomy. For patients with operable stage IIIA disease surgery or neoadjuvant chemotherapy are equally good options. The advantages of each are highlighted below.

Neoadjuvant Chemotherapy: Advantages and Disadvantages

Neoadjuvant chemotherapy has become an increasingly popular treatment strategy for stage III breast cancer and selected cases of stage II breast cancer. The use of neoadjuvant chemotherapy has several potential advantages over the tra-

ditional sequence of surgery followed by adjuvant chemotherapy, but it also carries some disadvantages (Table 54.2). Several trials have clearly shown that neoadjuvant chemotherapy substantially reduces the size of the primary tumor and nodal metastases in more than 80% of cases. Accordingly, for patients with large primary tumors, the approach of using chemotherapy as the initial treatment has been shown to increase the probability that breast-conserving surgery can be performed (42,44,140,147). A second advantage of using chemotherapy first is that this sequence allows the response of the disease to a particular chemotherapy regimen to be assessed, which in turn could provide an opportunity to "cross over" to a different treatment regimen if disease in an individual patient shows little or no response to the first regimen. By doing so, a potentially effective second-line agent can be given rapidly, and the toxicity of an ineffective first regimen can be avoided.

Neoadjuvant chemotherapy has also been proven to be extremely valuable for clinical research. After several studies showed a strong correlation between the achievement of a pathological complete response (pCR; defined as no residual cancer being found in the postchemotherapy surgical specimen) and survival (42,88,147), investigators began using pCR rates as a short-term surrogate of the success of a chemotherapy regimen. Phase III randomized trials in which pCR rates were used as the primary end point have allowed the activity of two chemotherapy regimens to be compared with relatively small study populations and very short follow-up times relative to studies comparing two chemotherapy regimens used in an adjuvant setting. Neoadjuvant chemotherapy can also facilitate translational research to investigate the mechanisms of chemotherapy-induced cell death and chemotherapy resistance. For example, it has proven feasible to study changes

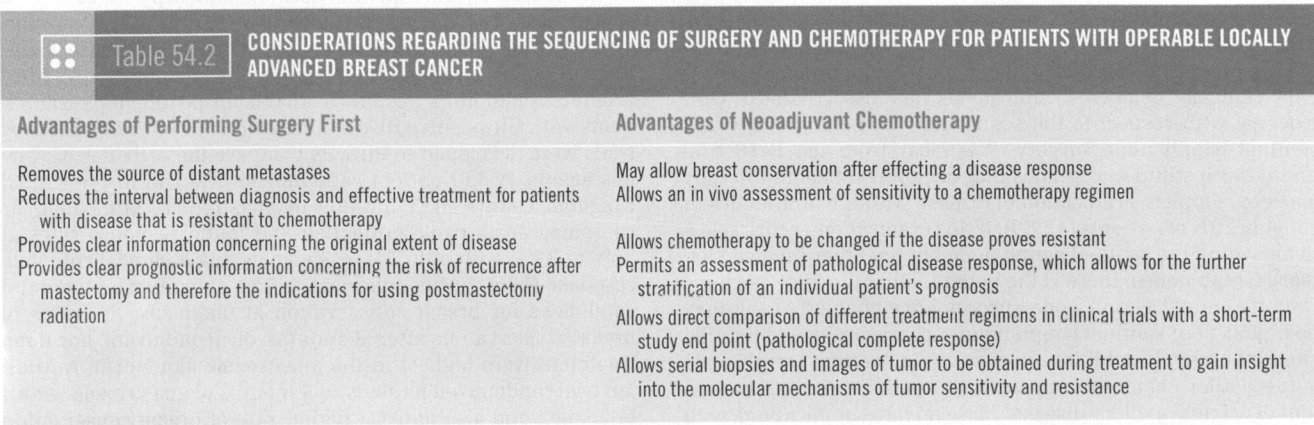

Table 54.2	**CONSIDERATIONS REGARDING THE SEQUENCING OF SURGERY AND CHEMOTHERAPY FOR PATIENTS WITH OPERABLE LOCALLY ADVANCED BREAST CANCER**

Advantages of Performing Surgery First	Advantages of Neoadjuvant Chemotherapy
Removes the source of distant metastases	May allow breast conservation after effecting a disease response
Reduces the interval between diagnosis and effective treatment for patients with disease that is resistant to chemotherapy	Allows an in vivo assessment of sensitivity to a chemotherapy regimen
Provides clear information concerning the original extent of disease	Allows chemotherapy to be changed if the disease proves resistant
Provides clear prognostic information concerning the risk of recurrence after mastectomy and therefore the indications for using postmastectomy radiation	Permits an assessment of pathological disease response, which allows for the further stratification of an individual patient's prognosis
	Allows direct comparison of different treatment regimens in clinical trials with a short-term study end point (pathological complete response)
	Allows serial biopsies and images of tumor to be obtained during treatment to gain insight into the molecular mechanisms of tumor sensitivity and resistance

in tumor genomes in response to treatment and how such changes correlate with chemotherapy response through the use of cDNA microarrays from serial biopsy specimens (17). Such studies are likely to provide significant insights into the heterogeneity of tumor response and to identify new targets for therapies.

Some have asserted that treatment with neoadjuvant chemotherapy also provides additional prognostic information. Clearly, the prognosis for patients with a pCR is better than the prognosis would have been before treatment. However, an equal percentage of patients will be found to have residual disease after chemotherapy, which confers a worse prognosis than originally anticipated. Therefore, the true value of the additional prognostic information from the use of neoadjuvant chemotherapy will come only when additional treatments become available that can positively influence prognosis for those with a high residual disease burden.

One theoretical advantage of neoadjuvant chemotherapy that has not been borne out in practice was the hope that earlier delivery of chemotherapy might improve survival for patients with locally advanced breast cancer. Clearly, most of the patients who present with advanced disease and subsequently die of that disease do so as a consequence of the progression of metastatic disease that was present at a microscopic level at the time of diagnosis. Therefore, the suggestion that initiating chemotherapy at diagnosis (when the micrometastatic tumor burden would be lowest) would improve outcome relative to delaying chemotherapy until after surgical resection was a rational one. This was further supported by preclinical animal studies showing that removal of the primary tumor could increase the growth rate of existing micrometastases and that treating animals with either chemotherapy or tamoxifen before resection of the primary tumor abrogated this adverse effect (43).

Two large randomized trials have been conducted to test the hypothesis that neoadjuvant chemotherapy could improve survival in patients with operable breast cancer. The first of these trials was the National Surgical Adjuvant Breast and Bowel Project (NSABP) B-18 study, in which 1,523 patients with operable breast cancer were randomly assigned to receive four cycles of doxorubicin and cyclophosphamide (AC) either before or after surgical treatment (12,147). After 9 years, the overall survival rates and disease-free survival rates were nearly identical between the two groups (p = 0.80 and p = 0.50, respectively). A second randomized prospective trial, conducted by the European Organization for Research and Treatment of Cancer (EORTC), confirmed these results and again found equivalent rates of survival and distant metastases between the neoadjuvant chemotherapy and adjuvant chemotherapy treatment groups (140). A recent meta-analysis of data from 3,946 patients treated in nine randomized trials comparing neoadjuvant with adjuvant chemotherapy in breast cancer found no statistical difference in the risk of death (risk ratio, 1.00), disease progression (risk ratio, 0.99), or distant disease recurrence (risk ratio, 0.94) (98).

The increasing use of neoadjuvant chemotherapy in patients with clinically negative lymph nodes has also created a controversy with respect to the sequencing of chemotherapy and sentinel lymph node surgery. It is clear from the B-18 trial and other institutional studies that neoadjuvant chemotherapy leads to complete eradication of disease within lymph nodes in roughly 20% of patients (42,89). If this eradication occurs selectively within the sentinel lymph node but not other involved axillary lymph nodes, there is the potential that the false-negative rate of sentinel lymph node surgery after chemotherapy may be higher than sentinel lymph node surgery performed prior to chemotherapy. In addition, performing a sentinel lymph node surgery after chemotherapy leads to an uncertainty of the extent of original axillary disease. This can have implications with

respect to radiation treatment field design or recommendations concerning whether to use postmastectomy radiation. In some instances, this can also have implications with respect to adjuvant chemotherapy treatment decisions.

There are some advantages to performing the sentinel lymph node surgery after neoadjuvant chemotherapy rather than prior to. Importantly, with this strategy, most commonly patients only have to undergo one surgery rather than two. Second, if a component of disease is removed prior to surgery, then the prognostic value of achieving a pCR is less certain. Finally, performing surgery prior to chemotherapy delays the administration of systemic treatments, particularly if an axillary metastasis is found and the patient then undergoes an axillary dissection.

A number of groups have studied the identification rates and false-negative rates associated with sentinel-lymph node surgery. The largest experience has been from the NSABP B-27 trial, which randomized 2,411 patients to one of three neoadjuvant chemotherapy regimens. A total of 428 of these patients had lymphatic mapping attempted. Successful identification of a sentinel lymph nodes was made in 85% and the false-negative rate was 11% (defined as the number of patients with positive nonsentinel lymph nodes with a negative sentinel lymph nodes divided by the total number of patients with positive axillary lymph nodes) (95).

A recent meta-analysis investigated 1,273 patients (21 published studies) treated with a sentinel lymph node biopsy with subsequent axillary dissection following neoadjuvant chemotherapy. These authors reported a pooled identification rate of 90% and false-negative rate of 12% (151). Since these outcomes are similar to those reported in multicenter studies in which sentinel lymph node surgery was performed prior to systemic therapy, delaying sentinel lymph node surgery until after chemotherapy appears acceptable.

Neoadjuvant Hormonal Therapy

There are fewer data concerning the long-term outcome of patients treated with hormone therapy prior to surgery. In part, this is because most patients treated with neoadjuvant systemic treatments for ER-positive breast cancers have the disease to an extent that necessitates both chemotherapy and hormonal treatments. However, interest in neoadjuvant hormonal therapy has increased after reports from studies that found patients with ER-positive disease to have a lower probability of achieving a pCR compared to those with ER-negative disease (120). For example, patients with lobular breast cancer, in who over 90% of tumors are ER-positive, have particularly low rates of pCR (33). In addition, some patients with ER-positive breast cancer that is locally advanced and/or lymph node–positive at presentation are not candidates for neoadjuvant chemotherapy due to comorbid medical conditions. For such patients, treatment with neoadjuvant hormonal therapy is a reasonable option (83).

Responses to neoadjuvant hormonal therapy occur over a slower period of time than those to neoadjuvant chemotherapy, and the rates of pCR with hormonal therapy are lower than those achievable with neoadjuvant chemotherapy. After aromatase inhibitors became available for postmenopausal patients with ER-positive disease, neoadjuvant hormone therapy trials were developed to directly compare the activities of various agents. A 330 patient randomized trial run in the United Kingdom compared 3 months of anastrozole, tamoxifen, or combined anastrozole/tamoxifen and found response rates of 36% to 39%, with only 1% to 3% achieving a clinical complete response (126). In the subgroup of 124 patients who were not candidates for breast conservation at diagnosis, the rates of breast conservation after 3 months of neoadjuvant hormone treatment were highest in the anastrozole alone arm. An Italian trial randomized patients to 3 months of anastrozole versus tamoxifen and also noted a higher rate of breast conservation after treatment with anastrozole alone versus tamoxifen alone. The overall response rates were similar to those in the United Kingdom study (21).

Breast Conservation Therapy after Neoadjuvant Chemotherapy

As noted, one of the potential benefits of neoadjuvant chemotherapy is that a large primary tumor will respond favorably to neoadjuvant chemotherapy, thereby rendering the disease amenable to a breast conservation surgical approach. One important consideration for performing breast-conserving surgery after neoadjuvant chemotherapy concerns the volume of surgical resection. This is less of a problem for patients with small initial primary tumors that shrink still further after neoadjuvant chemotherapy. However, for patients with T3 disease for whom initial breast-conserving surgery would be deforming, the volume of resection after neoadjuvant chemotherapy must be directed at the residual nidus rather than the original extent of disease. In some instances, neoadjuvant chemotherapy successfully shrinks large primary tumors to smaller residual niduses that can easily be resected in small volumes of tissue with good or excellent aesthetic outcomes. However, breast cancers can respond to neoadjuvant chemotherapy in a variety of ways, as shown in Figure 54.5. For tumors that shrink to a residual nidus, limited surgery would successfully resect the volume of residual disease, and the outcome, particularly for those with a pCR, would be expected to be excellent. However, in other cases, tumors respond favorably to neoadjuvant chemotherapy, but the residual disease is diffuse, multifocal, and scattered throughout the original tumor volume. In such cases, a small surgical resection carries the risk of leaving a residual disease burden within the breast. Careful selection of cases for breast conservation is therefore critical.

One of the first studies to provide findings regarding appropriate selection criteria for breast conservation after neoadjuvant chemotherapy examined 143 mastectomy specimens from patients given neoadjuvant chemotherapy to determine patterns of residual disease and their relationships to clinical factors. Only 23% of tumors had clinical and pathological features that would have predicted success with breast conservation. Important selection criteria included resolution of skin edema, favorable clinical response to neoadjuvant treatment, lack of multicentricity, and lack of extensive lymphovascular space invasion (123).

Since those findings were published, several groups have studied the clinical outcome of patients treated with breast conservation after neoadjuvant chemotherapy. In general, the outcome results have varied considerably across series, for several possible reasons. First, the selection criteria vary considerably across studies, and not surprisingly studies that include patients with positive surgical margins or inflammatory breast cancer tended to report higher rates of local recurrence (99,119). Similarly, some studies in which patients who achieved complete clinical resolution of disease could elect to forgo surgery showed higher recurrence rates (131). Other studies, however, predominantly from institutions with well-coordinated multidisciplinary teams and careful pathological analysis of the surgical specimen, have reported excellent outcomes (7,27).

Two of the most influential publications that addressed breast conservation after neoadjuvant chemotherapy were from the two largest randomized trials (NSABP B-18 and EORTC) comparing neoadjuvant chemotherapy with adjuvant chemotherapy for patients with stage II or stage III breast cancer. The conclusion in both studies was that neoadjuvant chemotherapy offered an advantage because breast conservation rates were higher in the neoadjuvant chemotherapy groups (42,140,147). However, it is important to recognize that approximately 60% of the patients enrolled in these studies were considered candidates for breast conservation at the time of diagnosis. Therefore, in the B-18 study, the improvement in breast conservation rates from 60% to 68% for patients treated with neoadjuvant chemotherapy essentially showed that 20% of initial mastectomy candidates (eight of 40 patients) could undergo breast conservation surgery instead after neoadjuvant chemotherapy. Not surprisingly, this increase was directly due to a higher percentage of patients with T3 disease being offered breast conservation after first responding to chemotherapy. Both studies reported that the overall breast recurrence risk in patients treated with neoadjuvant chemotherapy was not statistically different from that in patients treated with surgery first (42,140,147). However, in the B-18 study, the breast recurrence

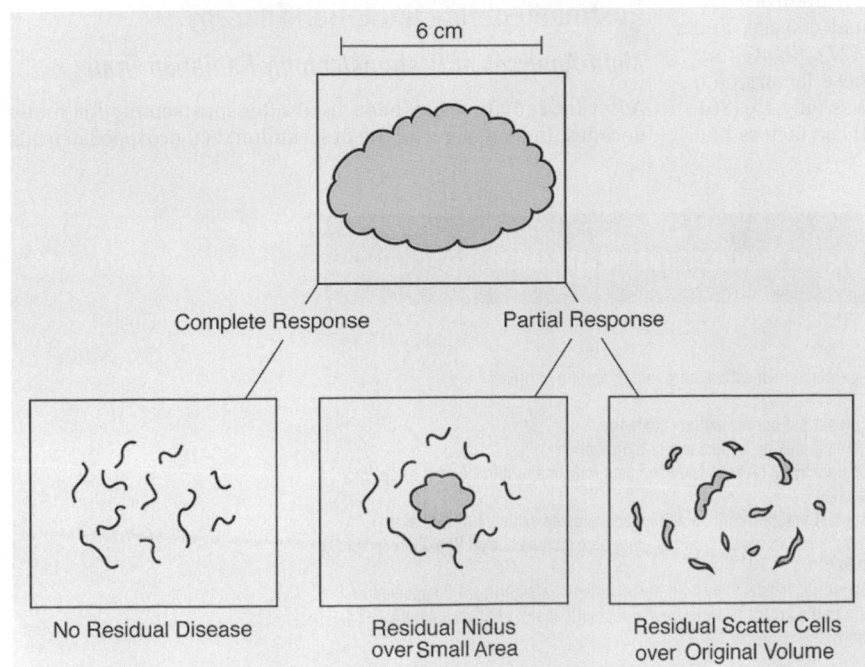

FIGURE 54.5. Three potential pathological outcomes of a primary tumor that responds to neoadjuvant chemotherapy. (From Buchholz TA, Hunt KK, Whitman GJ, et al. Neoadjuvant chemotherapy for breast carcinoma: Multidisciplinary considerations of benefits and risks. *Cancer* 2003;98:1150–1160, with permission).

rate in a subset of patients who initially would have required a mastectomy but were treated with breast conservation after a favorable response to neoadjuvant chemotherapy was twice that of the patients with smaller tumors who were treated with surgery first (15.7% vs. 7.6%, respectively) (147).

A meta-analysis of the nine randomized studies comparing neoadjuvant and adjuvant chemotherapy reported that the use of neoadjuvant chemotherapy was associated with an increase in the relative risk of local-regional recurrence relative to adjuvant chemotherapy (relative risk = 1.22, 95% confidence interval [CI] = 1.04 to 1.43) (98). This difference was largely influenced by the trials in which surgery was not performed and breast conservation after neoadjuvant chemotherapy was achieved with the use of radiation therapy alone (in those trials the relative risk was 1.53 and the 95% CI was 1.11 to 2.10) (98). These findings indicate that patients who achieve a complete clinical response would still benefit from a surgical procedure in addition to radiation.

Two of the largest studies showing acceptable outcomes for breast conservation after neoadjuvant chemotherapy have been from the Istituto Nazionale Tumori in Milan (7) and the University of Texas M.D. Anderson Cancer Center (27). The Milan experience consisted of 536 patients treated with neoadjuvant chemotherapy for a primary tumor 2.5 cm in diameter or larger. Eighty-five percent of these patients subsequently had breast-conserving surgery. However, it is important to note that the initial tumor size in more than half of these women was <4 cm, and thus these women may have been candidates for breast conservation at diagnosis. The 8-year rate of breast recurrence as a first site of failure in those treated with breast conservation was 6.8% (7). In the M.D. Anderson series, 340 carefully selected patients were treated with breast conservation therapy after showing a favorable response to chemotherapy (27). Patient selection criteria for the breast-conserving approach included having no residual T4 breast skin abnormalities, negative surgical margins, no multicentric disease, no residual malignant calcifications on postoperative mammogram, and the willingness and ability to undergo both surgery and radiation therapy. With these criteria, the outcome was favorable, with 5 and 10-year local recurrence rates of 5% and 10%, respectively, despite the fact that 72% of patients in the study had clinical stage IIB or III disease. Four factors were found to be independently associated with breast cancer recurrence and local-regional recurrence: Clinical N2 or N3 disease, lymphovascular space invasion, a multifocal pattern of residual disease, and residual disease larger than 2 cm in diameter (27). Eighty-four percent of patients had none or just one of these factors, and the recurrence rate at 10 years in this group was only 4% (26). In contrast, the 4% of patients with three of these factors had

a recurrence rate of 45%. Women with primary clinical T3 or T4 disease were at very low risk of recurrence if the tumor shrank to a solitary nidus or showed a pCR, but among patients with T3 or T4 tumors that broke up and left a multifocal pattern of residual disease the breast cancer recurrence rate was 20% (27). Research to determine whether MRI can predict which patients will have a multifocal pattern of residual disease is ongoing.

It is important to consider that patients with stage III breast cancer are at risk for local-regional recurrence even when mastectomy is performed. In addition, patients with advanced disease are at significant risk for distant metastases, which is an additional incentive to avoid removing the entire breast when breast-conserving surgery can be done with acceptably low recurrence rates. Recently, the investigators from M.D. Anderson Cancer Center applied the four prognostic criteria associated with breast recurrence in patients treated with neoadjuvant chemotherapy and breast conservation to a cohort of patients treated with neoadjuvant chemotherapy, mastectomy, and post-mastectomy radiation (78). These investigators found that for patients who had none or one of these factors, the results with either local-regional treatment approach were excellent and equivalent. Among patients with two factors, a nonsignificant trend was evident toward fewer local-regional recurrences with mastectomy, and for the small cohort of patients with three or four factors, mastectomy provided a statistically significant benefit.

Mastectomy

In the United States, mastectomy continues to be the most common local-regional treatment for breast cancer, particularly for patients with locally advanced disease. Several alternative mastectomy approaches are available for women with breast cancer (Table 54.3). A simple or total mastectomy resects the breast but not the axillary contents. For patients with clinical stage T1 or T2 N0 disease who are not interested in breast conservation, a total mastectomy with a sentinel lymph node dissection may be the treatment of choice. A modified radical mastectomy (removal of the breast plus a level I or II axillary dissection) remains the standard of care for patients with clinically positive lymph nodes or locally advanced disease.

Postmastectomy Radiation Therapy

Meta-Analyses of Postmastectomy Radiation Trials

Adjuvant radiation has been used after mastectomy for many decades. Indeed, some of the first randomized prospective trials

---

Table 54.3 — TYPES OF MASTECTOMIES USED AS TREATMENTS FOR BREAST CANCER

Surgical Therapies for Breast Cancer	Definition
Segmental mastectomy, lumpectomy, tylectomy	Removal of the primary tumor with a surrounding margin of breast tissue
Total or simple mastectomy	Removal of the breast but not the axillary contents
Modified radical mastectomy	Removal of the breast plus an axillary level I/II dissection
Radical mastectomy	Removal of the parenchyma breast tissue and pectoralis major muscle plus an axillary level I/II dissection
Extended radical mastectomy	Removal of the breast and pectoralis major muscle plus an axillary level I/II and internal mammary lymph node dissection, may also include a level III axillary lymph node dissection
Skin-sparing mastectomy	Total or modified radical mastectomy with preservation of a significant component of the native skin of the breast to optimize the aesthetic result of an immediate reconstruction

in medicine were done to investigate the efficacy of postmastectomy radiation. Despite this, significant controversy remains over the indications for its use. It is clear that mastectomy without radiation offers excellent local-regional control rates for most patients with noninvasive or stage I or IIA disease. In contrast, patients with stage III breast cancer (four or more positive lymph nodes or T3 or T4 primary tumors) have a clinically relevant risk of local-regional recurrence after mastectomy and thus would benefit from adjuvant radiation. What is less clear is whether radiation provides a survival advantage for patients with stage II breast cancer and one to three positive lymph nodes.

In 1987 Cuzik et al. (34) published the first meta-analysis of data from postmastectomy radiation therapy trials and reported that radiation use was associated with a poorer overall survival rate. In a subsequent analysis, the same group reported that postmastectomy radiation therapy decreased the breast cancer death rate but increased the nonbreast cancer death rate (35), which resulted in equivalent overall survival rates in the radiation and no-radiation groups. These analyses are mostly of historical interest because of the considerable heterogeneity in the surgical and radiation therapy treatments used in these trials as compared with modern-day treatment approaches. Moreover, these early trials often enrolled patients with early stage disease, who would not be predicted to derive any benefit from radiation therapy. Finally, the early studies of postmastectomy radiation predated the use of systemic therapy.

After the Cuzik meta-analyses, the Early Breast Cancer Trialists' Collaborative Group was formed and obtained the raw data from every randomized trial that investigated the role of radiation in breast cancer. Through the years, this group has published a series of meta-analyses that have provided important insights into the risks and benefits of postmastectomy radiation therapy (61). In the most recently published analysis based on data from 9,933 patients, postmastectomy radiation therapy reduced the 15-year isolated local-regional recurrence rates for patients with lymph node–positive disease from 29% to 8%. Importantly, this reduction led to a 5% decrease in the 15-year breast cancer mortality rate (60% vs. 55%) (60). For patients with lymph node–negative disease, a similar proportional reduction in local-regional recurrence was seen, but because the risk of recurrence was much lower, the reduction in the absolute local-regional recurrence risk was much smaller (8% for no-radiation vs. 3% radiation) (60). For these patients, this small improvement in local-regional recurrence was not associated with a difference in overall survival.

It is important to recognize the limitations of meta-analyses when considering the relevance of this large study to modern-day treatments for breast cancer. One problem with including trials dating back to the 1950s is that the radiation doses, fractionation patterns, treatment units, and field designs differ significantly from current standards. To minimize these confounding effects, Van de Steene et al. (139) conducted a similar meta-analysis but excluded trials that began before 1970, trials with small sample sizes, trials with relatively poor survival rates, and trials that used radiation fractionation schedules that are no longer in standard practice. When these studies were excluded, use of postmastectomy radiation therapy was associated with an even greater overall survival advantage. Moreover, adjuvant radiation probably can improve survival even further if the risk of dying from micrometastatic disease is minimized through the use of systemic therapy. To investigate this question, Whelan et al. (145) performed a meta-analysis of postmastectomy radiation trials that included systemic therapy for both treatment groups. In this analysis, the addition of radiation after mastectomy led to an even greater reduction in the risk of any recurrence (odds ratio, 0.69) and the risk of death (odds ratio, 0.83). Finally, a recent meta-analysis attempted to account for the quality of radiation delivery in these trials (54). In this study, the authors defined optimal dose as a between 40 to 60 Gy delivered in 2 Gy fractions and optimal treatment field arrangements as ones that included both the chest wall and the regional lymphatics. They then reanalyzed the data from the Early Breast Cancer Trialists' Collaborative Group according to the quality of radiation treatments and demonstrated that proportional reduction in local-regional recurrence was 80% for trials with optimal dose and treatment fields, compared to 70% and 64% for trials that were suboptimal with respect to dose or field arrangements, respectively. In addition, there was a statistically significant improvement in breast cancer mortality in the trials that used optimal radiation dose and treatment fields, but not in the other trials.

In summary, these meta-analyses have conclusively demonstrated that radiation has an important role in the management of locally advanced breast cancer. By reducing the risk of recurrence after mastectomy, radiation offers an incremental improvement in overall survival. Radiation seems to offer the greatest benefit when given using modern treatment techniques that minimize the risk of normal tissue injury and maximize the probability of tumor control and when given to patients who also receive systemic treatments.

Phase III Randomized Trials Investigating Postmastectomy Radiation

The most recent findings concerning the efficacy of postmastectomy radiation have come from 15- to 20-year outcome data from three randomized trials that investigated radiation therapy for patients with stage II or III breast cancer that also received systemic therapy. The largest of these studies was the Danish Breast Cancer Cooperative Group 82b trial, which randomly assigned 1,708 premenopausal women with stage II or III breast cancer to receive mastectomy followed by nine cycles of CMF (cyclophosphamide, methotrexate, and fluorouracil) chemotherapy or mastectomy, radiation therapy, and eight cycles of CMF chemotherapy (105). At the same time, this group also conducted the 82c trial, in which more than 1,300 postmenopausal women were randomly assigned to undergo mastectomy and 1 year of tamoxifen versus mastectomy, tamoxifen, and radiation therapy (106). Finally, a smaller trial, conducted in Vancouver, British Columbia, randomly assigned 318 premenopausal women with lymph node–positive disease to undergo mastectomy and CMF chemotherapy with or without postmastectomy radiation therapy (113). In all three of these studies, patients treated with radiation were at a lower long-term risk of isolated local-regional recurrence than were patients who did not undergo radiation therapy. Importantly, these improvements led to fewer patients developing metastatic disease and an improvement in overall survival (103,113). The results from these three trials are shown in Table 54.4.

Several important concepts can be ascertained from these studies. First, together these studies clearly demonstrate that by reducing local-regional recurrence, postmastectomy radiation therapy could improve overall survival. Second, these trials demonstrated that these patients had a clinically relevant risk of local-regional recurrence despite the use of either CMF chemotherapy or tamoxifen. These findings imply that the benefits of systemic treatments are predominantly to lower the competing risk of distant metastases, which makes the achievement of local-regional control more important.

One controversy that has arisen after the publication of these studies concerns the most appropriate indications for postmastectomy radiation. Specifically, these trials led to a debate as to whether postmastectomy radiation therapy is indicated for patients with stage II breast cancer with one to three positive lymph nodes. Most of the patients enrolled in the Danish and British Columbia trials had stage II disease with one to three

Table 54.4	LOCAL-REGIONAL RECURRENCE, RATES OF DISTANT METASTASIS, AND OVERALL SURVIVAL IN RANDOMIZED TRIALS COMPARING THE USE OF POSTMASTECTOMY RADIATION FOR PATIENTS TREATED WITH MASTECTOMY AND SYSTEMIC THERAPY

Trial (Reference)	Local-Regional Recurrence Rates (First Events Only)	Rates of Distant Metastasis	Survival Rates
Danish 82b (10 year) (105)			
Radiation	9%	Not provided	45%
No radiation	32%		54%
	$p < 0.0001$		$p < 0.0001$
Danish 82c (10 year) (106)			
Radiation	8%	Not provided	45%
No radiation	35%		36%
	$p < 0.0001$		$p = 0.03$
Danish 82b&c (18 year) (103)			
Radiation	14%	53%	Not provided
No radiation	49%	64%	
	$p < 0.0001$	$p < 0.0001$	
Vancouver, BC (20 year) (113)			
Radiation	13%	52%	47%
No radiation	39%	69%	37%
	$p < 0.0001$	$p = 0.004$	$p = 0.03$

positive lymph nodes (105,106,113). Accordingly, many have argued that these findings suggest all patients with lymph node–positive disease should receive radiation after mastectomy. The difficulty in interpreting these data, however, is that many patients in these trials did not undergo a formal level I or II axillary dissection. In the Danish studies, the median number of axillary lymph nodes resected was only seven (105), which is approximately 50% of the number reported from studies conducted in the United States. Also, 76% of the patients had fewer than 10 lymph nodes removed, and 15% had three or fewer lymph nodes removed (105). In the British Columbia trial, the median number of resected lymph nodes was 11 (112). Given the less extensive axillary surgery done in these studies, it is highly probable that some of the patients in these studies reported as having had one to three positive lymph nodes would have had four or more positive lymph nodes if a standard axillary dissection had been performed. Correspondingly, their risk of a chest wall or supraclavicular recurrence would be higher than that usually estimated for patients with one to three positive nodes. Moreover, failure to remove these additional involved axillary lymph nodes would predispose patients to axillary recurrence, which could be avoided by a more complete axillary dissection. Indeed, the most recent update of the Danish studies reported that 43% of all local-regional recurrences included recurrence in the axilla (103).

Another reason that the findings may not be transferable to other populations is that the local-regional recurrence risk for patients with one to three positive lymph nodes treated in these trials was much higher than for patients treated in the United States with standard modified radical mastectomy and systemic treatments. Specifically, the 18-year rate of isolated local-regional recurrence for the patients in the Danish studies treated with mastectomy and systemic treatment was 41% and the 18-year rate for the subgroup with one to three positive lymph nodes was 37% (103). In the British Columbia trial, the 20-year overall rate of local-regional recurrence was 39% (113), and findings concerning the risk in the subgroup with one to three positive lymph nodes were not provided. Furthermore, local-regional recurrences that developed concurrently with distant metastases or after distant metastases were not considered as local-regional events in either study. Therefore,

these rates probably underestimated the true percentage of patients who had persistent local-regional disease after mastectomy and systemic treatments.

Another cohort of patients in whom the use of postmastectomy radiation is controversial are those with pathological T3N0 disease. One reason for this controversy is that there are limited data regarding the risk of local-regional recurrence after mastectomy and systemic treatments in such patients. This lack of data is a consequence of the fact that the majority of breast cancers that are 5 cm or greater will have lymph node–positive disease, and that a large percentage of patients with clinical T3N0 disease are currently treated with neoadjuvant chemotherapy. Historically patients with pathological T3N0 disease who were treated with an initial mastectomy were recommended to receive postmastectomy radiation. However, two recent publications have indicated that the risk of local-regional recurrence is relatively low. Floyd et al. (46) published data concerning a multicenter study of 70 patients treated with mastectomy, systemic therapy, and no radiation for patients with pathological T3N0 disease and reported a 5-year local-regional recurrence of only 8%. Those who had LVSI had a 21% local-regional recurrence compared to a rate of only 4% for those without LVSI. Finally, of the patients who experienced a local-regional recurrence, 89% had the chest wall as their only site of recurrence. In addition, Taghian et al. (133) analyzed the outcome of 313 patients with pathological stage T3N0 disease who were treated with mastectomy, systemic treatments, and no radiation on NSABP clinical trials. The 10-year local-regional recurrences for this series were only 7%, with 24 of the 28 local-regional recurrences developing only on the chest wall.

Risks of Local-Regional Recurrence after Modified Radical Mastectomy and Systemic Treatment

The risks of recurrence in the Danish and British Columbia trials after mastectomy and chemotherapy were high relative to those reported from large series from the United States and from a European Cooperative Group. To help define the indications for radiation, several groups have recently conducted

	LOCAL-REGIONAL RECURRENCE RATES IN PATIENTS NOT TREATED WITH RADIATION AFTER MASTECTOMY IN RANDOMIZED CLINICAL TRIALS
Table 54.5	

Patterns-of-Failure Studies (Reference)	Number of Patients	Local-Regional Recurrence Rates at 10 Years (%)
ECOG (116)		
1–3 + LN	1,018	13
≥4 + LN	998	29
M.D. Anderson (82)		
1–3 +LN	466	12
≥4 + LN	419	27
NSABP (132)		
1–3 + LN	2,957	6–11
≥4 + LN	2,784	14–25
IBCSG (144)		
1–3 + LN	2,408	14–27
≥4 + LN	1,659	24–35

ECOG, Eastern Cooperative Oncology Group; IBCSG, International Breast Cancer Study Group; +LN, lymph-node positive.

	COFACTORS ASSOCIATED WITH A GREATER THAN 15% LOCAL-REGIONAL RECURRENCE AFTER MASTECTOMY AND CHEMOTHERAPY IN PATIENTS WITH ONE TO THREE POSITIVE LYMPH NODES
Table 54.6	

Study (Reference)	Number of Patients	Cofactors
Katz et al. (81,82)	466	Tumor size >4 cm Extracapsular extension >2 mm <10 lymph nodes removed 20% of lymph nodes involved Invasion of skin/nipple Invasion of pectoralis fascia Close or positive margins
Wallgren et al. (144)	2,408	Premenopausal, G2 or G3, LVSI Postmenopausal, G3 Postmenopausal, G2, T2 disease
Taghian et al. (132)	2,957	Age <50, T2 disease
Truong et al. (137)	821	Age <45 25% of lymph nodes involved ER-negative disease G3 disease Medial tumor location
Cheng et al. (28)	110	Age <40 Tumor size ≥3 cm Presence of LVSI No tamoxifen use

ER, estrogen receptor; LVSI, lymphovascular space invasion

studies to assess which patients are at risk for local-regional recurrence after treatment with a mastectomy that included a level I or II axillary dissection, systemic treatment, and no radiation. The results from the largest of these studies are summarized in Table 54.5 (82,116,132,144). In general, the findings suggest that the 10-year local-regional recurrence risk for patients with one to three positive lymph nodes was approximately 12% to 15%, which is nearly one-third of the local-regional recurrence rate in the no-radiation group of the British Columbia and Danish trials. The reasons for these lower risks are not clearly known but probably reflect differences in the surgical procedure performed. In addition, these studies reported outcomes at 10 years, whereas the randomized prospective studies reported outcome data at 18 and 20 years. In the Danish studies, the local-regional recurrence rate rose relatively consistently by 1% per year between the 10th and 25th follow-up years (103). Similarly, in the British Columbia randomized trial, approximately 20% of local-regional recurrences in the group that did not receive postmastectomy radiation developed after 10 years of follow-up (113).

Stage II breast cancer with one to three positive lymph nodes is also heterogeneous with respect to other prognostic factors that affect local-regional recurrence risk. Table 54.6 shows various cofactors that have been found to increase the risk of local-regional recurrence within this subgroup. Cheng et al. (28) analyzed 110 patients with a minimum follow-up of 25 months who were treated with modified radical mastectomy without radiation and had one to three positive axillary nodes (median number of nodes examined, 17) (28). Sixty-nine patients received adjuvant chemotherapy and 84 received adjuvant hormonal therapy with tamoxifen. These investigators defined four factors (age <40 years, tumor ≥3 cm, ER-negative disease, and lymphovascular invasion) that segregated the patients into a high-risk group (with three or four factors) and a low-risk group (with two or fewer factors). Tumor size was also found to be an important cofactor in work from M.D. Anderson, but those authors found a size of 4 cm to increase the risk. Finally, findings from the International Breast Cancer Study Group Trials I through VII found that premenopausal women with one to three positive lymph nodes had local-regional recurrence risks ranging from 19% to 27% if they had G2 or G3 disease with vascular invasion, but that risk was <15% if they had G1 disease with no

vascular invasion (144). Among postmenopausal women with one to three positive lymph nodes, those with G3 disease and tumors larger than 2 cm had a local-regional recurrence risk of 24% as compared with <15% for those with G1 or G2 disease with tumors smaller than 2 cm.

Margin status is another important corisk factor in this cohort. In an analysis of the 34 patients with close or positive margins whose primary tumor was smaller than 5 cm with zero to three positive axillary nodes and who received no postoperative radiation, Freedman et al. (51) reported a relatively high risk of local relapse, but only among younger women. Five chest wall recurrences appeared at a median interval of 26 months (range, seven to 127 months), resulting in an 8-year cumulative incidence of a chest wall recurrence of 18%. Patient age correlated with the cumulative incidence of chest wall recurrence at 8 years; the rate for women aged ≤50 years was 28% versus 0% for those older than 50 years (p = 0.04). Katz et al. (81) also found close or positive margins to be an independent risk factor for the development of local-regional recurrence after mastectomy, but in that series age did not affect this risk. The 10-year risk for the 29 patients with close or positive margins was 45%; the risk was 33% for those with pectoralis fascia invasion even when negative margins were achieved.

The presence of multicentric disease is strongly associated with other risk factors for local-regional recurrence, such as tumor size and nodal involvement. However, in patients with stage II disease with one to three positive lymph nodes, multicentric disease does not seem to elevate the risk of local-regional recurrence. Fowble et al. (49) reported that patients with multicentric disease without other strong risk factors for postmastectomy chest wall relapse had a 5-year actuarial risk of an isolated local-regional recurrence of 8%. By comparison, Katz et al. (81) found a 10-year recurrence risk of 37% for patients with multicentric disease, but limiting the analysis to only patients with one to three positive lymph nodes eliminated any association

Clinical Radiation Oncology

between multicentric or multifocal disease and local-regional recurrence.

Even if the risk of local-regional recurrence for most patients with one to three positive lymph nodes is relatively low after a modified radical mastectomy and chemotherapy, radiation could still provide a benefit. Indeed, Woodward et al. (149) found that the risk of local-regional recurrence after mastectomy and anthracycline-based chemotherapy was only 13% for patients with stage II disease and one to three positive lymph nodes. However, at the same institution, patients with similarly staged disease treated with postmastectomy radiation had a local-regional recurrence risk of only 3%. Whether this degree of benefit is clinically meaningful with respect to patient survival is unknown. A recent investigation of this question evaluated data from the Surveillance, Epidemiology and End Results Program concerning patients with T1 or T2 primary tumors treated with mastectomy. In that study, radiation use led to a 15% to 20% relative reduction in breast cancer mortality, but this reduction only became significant in a multivariate analysis of patients with seven or more positive lymph nodes (125). Because the treating physicians made the decisions concerning the use of radiation for the patients included in that database, unidentified biases could be present that affected these results. Indeed, other investigators, evaluating data from the same program on patients with T1 or T2 primary tumors with one to three positive lymph nodes, compared the outcome of those treated with breast-conserving surgery with radiation versus mastectomy without radiation (18). In that study, multivariate analyses showed that patients treated with breast conservation plus radiation had significantly improved survival compared with those treated with mastectomy without radiation. Again, unaccounted biases probably affected these results to some degree.

Both the American Society for Therapeutic Radiology and Oncology and the American Society of Clinical Oncology have published consensus statements recommending postmastectomy radiation therapy for women with four or more positive lymph nodes or advanced primary disease. Both statements included the recommendation that an additional trial be performed to further clarify the benefit of postmastectomy radiation therapy for women with stage II disease and one to three positive lymph nodes (71,114). Unfortunately, an Inter-Group trial designed to determine the benefits of postmastectomy radiation therapy for such patients closed owing to poor accrual. However, the SUPREMO (Selective Use of Postoperative Radiotherapy after Mastectomy) trial, recently opened in the United Kingdom and in the EORTC, may in the future provide answers to this question.

In summary, it is clear that postmastectomy radiation offers a significant benefit for patients in terms of a 20% to 40% risk of local-regional recurrence; therefore, it should be recommended for all such patients. It is reasonable to discuss the risks and benefits of radiation for patients with intermediate-risk disease, such as those with pathological stage II breast cancer. It is hoped that ongoing studies will further refine risk stratification within this subset by considering other cofactors such as margin status, lymphovascular space invasion, patient age, extent of axillary dissection, and presence of extracapsular disease.

Postmastectomy Radiation Therapy after Neoadjuvant Chemotherapy

In most cases, locally advanced breast cancer is currently treated with neoadjuvant chemotherapy as the initial therapeutic approach. As the use of neoadjuvant chemotherapy has become more common, new questions regarding the indications for postmastectomy radiation therapy have arisen. This is because historically the decision to administer radiation therapy

was made predominantly on the basis of the pathological extent of disease. However, neoadjuvant chemotherapy changes the extent of pathological disease in 80% to 90% of cases, and it is unclear whether and how the posttreatment pathological information should guide decisions regarding radiation treatment. What has been learned is that the correlations between pathological extent of disease and local-regional recurrence after mastectomy are different for patients treated with chemotherapy first compared with those treated with surgery first (16). Specifically, one study found that the local-regional recurrence rate associated with a particular pathological extent of disease after surgery was higher among patients treated with chemotherapy first than among patients treated with surgery first. This is not particularly surprising; in the neoadjuvant chemotherapy group, the pathologic examination represented residual disease after treatment, whereas in those treated with surgery first, the extent of disease represented untreated cancer. However, these findings imply that the risk of local-regional recurrence for patients given neoadjuvant chemotherapy is determined by both the pretreatment clinical stage and the extent of pathologically residual disease after chemotherapy.

Information on the efficacy of postmastectomy radiation therapy for patients treated with neoadjuvant chemotherapy is limited. One of the only published studies investigating this issue compared the outcomes of 579 patients who received neoadjuvant chemotherapy, mastectomy, and radiation therapy with those of 136 patients who were treated with neoadjuvant chemotherapy and mastectomy (79). Patients in this study had been treated in prospective trials, but radiation therapy was not a randomized variable in any of the trials, so significant imbalances in the prognostic factors were present between the two groups. Patients with worse disease characteristics were more often referred for and treated with radiation therapy, so the clinical disease stages were different in the two groups. Despite this, the local-regional recurrence rate was found to be significantly lower in the group treated with postmastectomy radiation therapy than in the group treated with neoadjuvant chemotherapy and mastectomy (10-year local-regional recurrence rates were 8% and 33%, respectively; p = 0.001). For patients with clinical stage III disease or extensive disease after chemotherapy, radiation led to significant improvements in local-regional recurrence, disease-specific survival, and overall survival rates. Multivariate analyses indicated that radiation was independently associated with a lower risk of local-regional recurrence (hazard ratio for not receiving radiation therapy –7.0; p <0.0001) and a lower risk of breast cancer death (hazard ratio for not receiving radiation therapy –2.03; p <0.0001) (79).

The same group of investigators has also shown that among patients with stage III disease who achieved a pCR, the local-regional recurrence rate for those treated with radiation therapy was 7% versus 33% for those who did not receive radiation therapy (p = 0.040). Radiation use in these patients was also associated with an improvement in survival. Finally, this group also tried to address which patients given neoadjuvant chemotherapy for clinical stage II breast cancer should receive radiation therapy. They examined 132 such patients who had not received radiation therapy and found that the small number of patients with clinical T3N0 disease and those with four or more positive lymph nodes had high rates of local-regional recurrence (53). However, the 42 patients with clinical stage II disease who had one to three positive lymph nodes after neoadjuvant chemotherapy had a relatively low rate of local-regional recurrence (5-year rate of 8%). It is hoped that data to better define the risk for such patients will be forthcoming from the patients treated with mastectomy in the NSABP B-18 trial.

These findings suggest that recommending postmastectomy radiation therapy is reasonable for all patients with clinical T3 or T4 tumors or clinical stage III disease regardless of their response to the chemotherapy regimen. In terms of clinical stage I or II breast cancer, postmastectomy radiation therapy should be recommended for patients with four or more positive lymph nodes after chemotherapy and for the unusual patient in whom the disease progresses and the primary tumor exceeds 5 cm in diameter. Clearly, however, additional studies are needed to quantify the local-regional recurrence risk for patients who present with T1 or T2 disease and have one to three positive lymph nodes after neoadjuvant chemotherapy.

Systemic Therapies

As previously indicated, systemic treatments play a critical role in the multidisciplinary management of both early stage and locally advanced breast cancer. There have been a number of recent advances in the systemic management of breast cancer and these improvements have contributed to the decreasing death rates recently noted for this disease.

Meta-Analyses

Similar to their meta-analyses of radiotherapy trials in breast cancer, the Early Breast Cancer Trialists' Collaborative Group has analyzed overviews of trials investigating chemotherapy and hormonal therapy for breast cancer. Their most recent meta-analysis was published in 2005, which evaluated data from almost 150,000 patients treated on 194 randomized trials that investigated chemotherapy or hormonal therapy (59). Only trials that began by 1995 were included, so no data were available concerning the efficacy of taxanes, aromatase inhibitors, or trastuzumab.

The use of chemotherapy was found to reduce the probability of recurrence and the risk of death for both patients with lymph node–positive disease and those with lymph node–negative disease (59). The proportional reduction in recurrence and breast cancer mortality achieved with chemotherapy was very similar for both groups. However, because patients with positive lymph nodes have a much greater risk of recurrence and death from disease, the absolute percentage who benefit from chemotherapy is greatest in this cohort. Use of multiagent chemotherapy resulted in an improved outcome compared to single-agent chemotherapy. In addition, there was a significant benefit in using anthracycline (FAC [fluorouracil, doxorubicin, and cyclophosphamide] or FEC [fluorouracil, epirubicin, and cyclophosphamide]) chemotherapy compared to CMF chemotherapy. Finally, the benefits of chemotherapy varied according to patient age, with patients less than 50 achieving a greater proportional reduction in the risk of recurrence (proportional reduction of 36%) than patients 50 to 69 years old (proportional reduction of 29%). The respective proportional reduction in the annual death rates for these cohorts was 38% and 20%. Using data from this analysis, Table 54.7 estimates the 5-year risk of recurrence and the absolute magnitude of benefit polychemotherapy by age and lymph node status (59).

Tamoxifen therapy also provides a significant benefit in reducing recurrence and improving survival for patients with ER-positive disease, with a 31% proportional reduction in the annual risk of breast cancer death rate (59). Tamoxifen provided a benefit for both younger and older patients with ER-positive or ER-unknown disease, but did not provide a benefit for patients with ER-negative disease. The data indicate that 5 years of tamoxifen therapy provided better outcomes compared to 1 to 2 years of treatment. For patients with ER-positive or ER-unknown lymph node–negative disease, tamoxifen treatment reduced the 5-year risk from 20.1% (no tamoxifen) to 11% (with tamoxifen). In the lymph node–positive cohort, the risks of recurrence were 40.8% versus 24.7%, respectively (59).

Table 54.7	BENEFITS OF POLYCHEMOTHERAPY VERSUS NO CHEMOTHERAPY IN REDUCING THE 5-YEAR RISK OF BREAST CANCER RECURRENCE	
Cohort	**Rates of Recurrence with and without Chemotherapy**	**Absolute Benefit (%)**
Age <50 LN–	17.5% vs. 27.4%	9.9
Age <50 LN+	40.6% vs. 55.2%	14.6
Age 50–69 LN–	14.3% vs. 19.6%	5.3
Age 50–69 LN+	36.7% vs. 42.6%	5.9

LN–, lymph node–negative; LN+, lymph node–positive
Data from Group EBCTC. Effects of chemotherapy and hormonal therapy for early breast cancer on recurrence and 15-year survival: An overview of the randomised trials. *Lancet* 2005;365:1687–1717, fig. 3.

This meta-analysis also found that the benefits of chemotherapy and tamoxifen therapy were additive for patients with ER-positive disease. The estimated cumulative reduction in the risk of mortality from combined anthracycline chemotherapy followed by tamoxifen in young women with ER-positive disease was estimated to be as high as 57% (59).

More Recent Advances: Chemotherapy

There have been important incremental advances beyond the standard of anthracycline chemotherapy in more recent years, most notably the introduction of taxanes. Three of the most important recent trials that have shown a benefit for adjuvant taxanes after anthracycline chemotherapy have been the CALGB 9344/Intergroup 0148 trial (73), the NSABP B-28 trial (96), and the BCIRG 001 trial (97). The design and results of these trials are given in Table 54.8. In aggregate, these trials have indicated that the addition of taxanes to anthracycline chemotherapy provides an additional reduction in the risk of recurrence in the adjuvant treatment of breast cancer.

These individual trial results have been confirmed in a meta-analysis of adjuvant taxane trials in breast cancer. This analysis revealed an improvement in both disease-free survival (absolute benefit estimated to be 3% to 5% for lymph node–positive patients at 5 years) and overall survival (absolute benefit estimated to be 2% to 3% for lymph node–positive patients at 5 years) (11).

Once taxanes became established as important component of adjuvant treatment of breast cancer, new trials began investigating the administration schedule of treatments. CALGB 9741/Intergroup trial randomized patients receiving AC (doxorubicin, cyclophosphamide) times four followed by paclitaxel times four or A times four, paclitaxel times four, C times four to a schedule that delivered the drugs every 3 weeks versus a "dose-dense" schedule of giving the chemotherapy with growth factor support every 2 weeks (30). The finding from this trial indicated that the dose-dense therapy further improved disease-free survival (4-years disease free survival rates were 82% [dose dense] vs. 75% [every 3-week administration]).

More Recent Advances: Hormonal Therapy

In addition to chemotherapy, hormonal therapy is indicated for all patients with ER- or PR-positive disease. Premenopausal

Table 54.8 | **REVIEW OF ADJUVANT TAXANE CHEMOTHERAPY TRIALS**

Trial (Reference)	Study Population	Randomization	Outcome
CALGB 9344 (73)	3,121 patients with lymph node–positive breast cancer	AC × 4 vs. AC × 4 followed by paclitaxel × 4	5-year DFS improved from 65% to 70%
NSABP B-28 (96)	3,060 patients with lymph node–positive breast cancer	AC × 4 vs. AC × 4 followed by paclitaxel × 4	5-year DFS improved from 72% to 76%
BCIRG 001 (97)	1,491 patients with lymph node–positive breast cancer	FAC × 6 vs. TAC × 6 (docetaxel/doxorubicin/cyclophosphamide)	5-year DFS improved from 68% to 75%

AC, doxorubicin, cyclophosphamide; DFS, disease-free survival; FAC, fluorouracil, doxorubicin, and cyclophosphamide; TAC, docetaxel, doxorubicin, cyclophosphamide

women who continue to have ovarian function after chemotherapy should receive tamoxifen as the preferred therapy. For postmenopausal women, the use of an aromatase inhibitor is equally appropriate. Aromatase inhibitors have proven to be a significant advance in hormonally responsive breast cancer. Unlike tamoxifen, which directly blocks the estrogen receptor on tumor cells, aromatase inhibitors provide beneficial effects by decreasing circulating estrogen by inhibiting the conversion of adrenal testosteronelike hormones into estrogen. Accordingly, aromatase inhibitors do not carry some of the same pro estrogenic effects that have been associated with tamoxifen, such as its potentially beneficial effects against osteoporosis and its potentially harmful effects of stimulating the endometrial lining.

After the safety and efficacy of aromatase inhibitors was established in postmenopausal women with ER-positive metastatic disease, these agents were studied in the adjuvant setting and also proved to be of clinical value. Table 54.9 reviews the results of three important recent adjuvant studies, in which the use of an aromatase inhibitor was found to be superior to the previously established standard of 5 years of tamoxifen therapy. Based on the results of these trials, there are a number of options for postmenopausal patients, including anastrozole for 5 years, letrozole for 5 years, initial tamoxifen for 2 to 3 years followed by exemestane, or tamoxifen for 5 years followed by 5 years of letrozole (31,58,75,134).

More Recent Advances: Trastuzumab

One of the most significant recent advances in breast cancer treatment has been the introduction of trastuzumab into the adjuvant treatment for patients with tumors that have gene amplification of the HER2/neu gene. In 2005, the initial results of a series of randomized prospective trials designed to evaluate whether the addition of trastuzumab increased the efficacy of adjuvant chemotherapy of patients with HER2/neu overexpression were published. The results of these studies were dramatic and indicated a significant incremental benefit for the use of trastuzumab over chemotherapy alone. Table 54.10 reviews the preliminary results of four of these studies (80,110,118,124). In the United States, the results of two similarly designed trials from the NSABP and the North Central Cancer Treatment Group were combined and indicated a 52% reduction in the relative risk of recurrence compared to anthracycline and taxane chemotherapy alone (118). In all trials, trastuzumab increased the risk for a decrease in cardiac ejection fraction, and it became more fully appreciated that patients who were treated with this agent require careful cardiac supervision. For most of these trials, patients who required radiation received trastuzumab concurrently during radiation treatments. To date, no increase in cardiac events or other serious sequelae have been reported as a consequence of the concurrent use of trastuzumab and radiation (109).

Table 54.9 | **REVIEW OF ADJUVANT AROMATASE INHIBITOR TRIALS**

Trial (Reference)	Study Population	Randomization	Outcome
ATAC (75)	9,356 postmenopausal patients	Arimidex × 5 years vs. tamoxifen × years vs. both	Arimidex reduced the relative risk of recurrence over tamoxifen by 23% (3.7% absolute reduction of the risk at 6 years), fewer contralateral breast cancers, fewer serious side effects
NCIC MA.17 (58)	5,187 postmenopausal patients	Letrozole vs. placebo × 5 years after 5 years of tamoxifen	Letrozole reduced the risk of distant recurrence and the risk of contralateral breast cancers, absolute benefit was 2.4% after 30 months median follow-up
Intergroup Exemestane Trial (31)	4,742 postmenopausal patients	2–3 years of tamoxifen then switching to exemestane vs. continuing tamoxifen × 5 years	Exemestane reduced the relative of recurrence over tamoxifen by 32% (4.7% absolute reduction of the risk at 3 years)
BIG 1-98 trial (134)	8,010 postmenopausal patients	Letrozole vs. letrozole + tamoxifen Tamoxifen vs. tamoxifen + letrozole	Comparing two letrozole first arms against two tamoxifen arms: 5-year recurrences were reduced by 19% and distant metastases reduced by 27% (2.6% absolute improvement in the 5-year disease free survival)

Trial (Reference)	Study Population	Randomization	Outcome
Table 54.10		**REVIEW OF TRIALS EVALUATING ADJUVANT TRASTUZUMAB WITH CHEMOTHERAPY FOR PATIENTS WITH HER2/NEU-POSITIVE BREAST CANCER**	
NSABP B-31 NCCTG N9831 (118)	3,351 patients with HER2/neu-positive disease, 94% had lymph node–positive disease	AC × 4 followed by paclitaxel × 4 with or with trastuzumab given concurrently with paclitaxel and as adjuvant therapy × 1 year	Trastuzumab reduced the relative risk of recurrence over chemotherapy alone by 52% (12% absolute reduction of the risk at 3 years), there was a 33% proportional reduction in the risk of death
HERA trial (110)	5,081 patients with HER2/neu-positive disease 68% had lymph node-positive disease	Minimum of 4 cycles of chemotherapy and then randomized to no trastuzumab vs. trastuzumab × 1 year vs. trastuzumab × 2 years	Trastuzumab × 1 year reduced the relative risk of recurrence over chemotherapy alone by 46% (8.4% absolute reduction of the risk at 3 years), there was insufficient follow-up to assess the trastuzumab × 2 years arm
FinHer Study (80)	232 patients with HER2/neu-positive, 84% had lymph node–positive disease	Docetaxel or vinorelbine × 3, FEC × 3 then randomized to no trastuzumab vs. trastuzumab × 9 weeks	Trastuzumab reduced the relative risk of recurrence or death over chemotherapy alone by 58% (11% absolute reduction of the risk at 3 years)
BCIRG 006 (124)	3,174 patients with HER2/neu-positive, 71% had lymph node–positive disease	AC × 4 + docetaxel × 4, with or with trastuzumab given concurrently with docetaxel and as adjuvant therapy × 1 year, third arm of docetaxel/carboplatinum/trastuzumab × 6 then as adjuvant therapy × 1 year	Trastuzumab reduced the relative risk of recurrence or death over chemotherapy alone by 39%

AC, doxorubicin, cyclophosphamide; FEC, fluorouracil, epirubicin, and cyclophosphamide.

Treatment Algorithms for Locally Advanced Breast Cancer

Figure 54.6 shows an algorithm for the management of patients with locally advanced operable cancer and patients who present with either operable or inoperable disease. Neoadjuvant chemotherapy is the preferred initial treatment for patients with inoperable disease and for selected patients with advanced but operable disease who are interested in being treated with breast conservation therapy. For such patients, neoadjuvant chemotherapy should consist of a regimen that contains either sequential or concurrent anthracyclines and taxanes. Some institutions elect to proceed with surgery after giving the anthracyclines but before giving the taxanes, whereas other institutions deliver all of the chemotherapy before surgery. A potential advantage of using all agents "up front" is that the chemotherapy course is not interrupted and therefore the treatment is given in the most dose-dense fashion.

After neoadjuvant chemotherapy, all patients should undergo surgical resection. Mastectomy remains the standard of care for most patients with locally advanced disease, but breast-conserving surgery can be considered for carefully selected patients. Axillary lymph node dissection should be performed for all patients with involved axillary lymph nodes at the time of presentation, regardless of the clinical response of axillary disease to neoadjuvant treatment. After surgery, adjuvant radiation to the breast, chest wall, and draining lymphatics should be offered to all patients with clinical stage III disease.

Some cases of advanced disease fail to respond to neoadjuvant chemotherapy, and such patients have a poor outcome. However, a small percentage of patients can achieve long-term

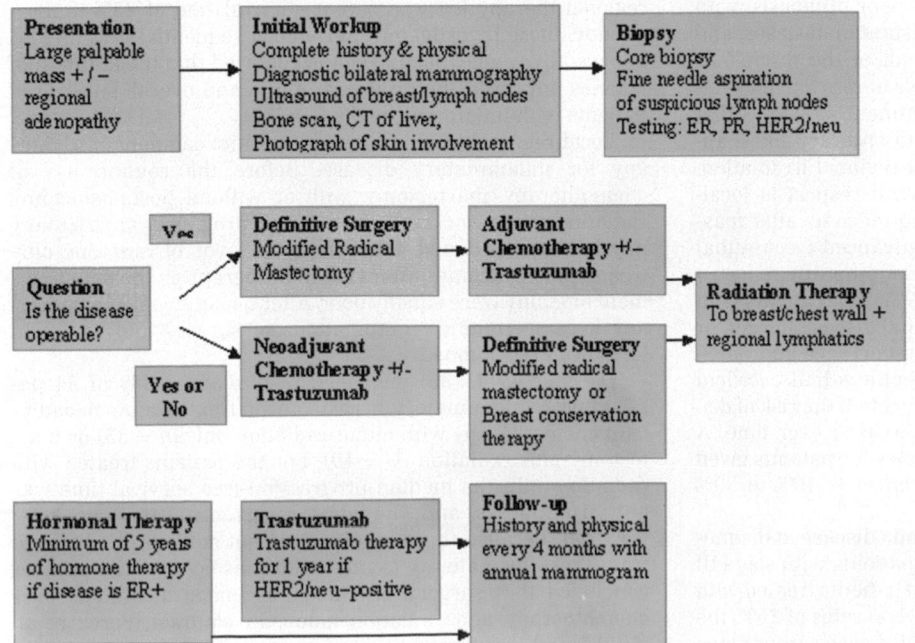

FIGURE 54.6. Flow diagram of work-up and treatment recommendations for patients who present with locally advanced breast cancer.

Clinical Radiation Oncology

survival with aggressive local-regional therapies. A study of 177 patients with advanced disease that was refractory to neoadjuvant chemotherapy reported a 10-year survival rate of 33% after aggressive local-regional treatments (14). Not surprisingly, those patients with ER-positive disease had the best outcome, in part because effective systemic therapies were still available to them.

For patients in whom the disease remains inoperable after neoadjuvant chemotherapy, preoperative or definitive radiation remains the treatment of choice. Surgeons and radiation oncologists need to carefully coordinate the care of such patients, and the future operability of the breast needs to be considered early in the treatment course because radiation-induced breast edema and erythema can mimic the clinical findings of advanced breast cancer. A study of 38 patients who underwent radiation therapy with or without mastectomy after the disease remained inoperable after neoadjuvant chemotherapy found that 46% were alive and 33% were free of distant disease at 5 years after treatment (77). Those patients who were able to undergo mastectomy after preoperative radiation had the best local-regional control. Preoperative radiation led to surgical complications in 9% of patients treated to <54 Gy but in 70% of the patients treated to doses of 54 Gy or more.

Some centers have piloted concurrent chemoradiation strategies as neoadjuvant approaches. In one recent study of the use of neoadjuvant paclitaxel followed by concurrent paclitaxel-radiation for patients with operable stage II or III breast cancer, 13 of the 38 patients (34%) experienced pCR and acceptably low treatment toxicity (24). Another group of investigators has also completed a phase I or II study of concurrent paclitaxel and radiation for 42 patients with locally advanced breast cancer and also found an excellent clinical response rate (91%) and a pCR rate of 16% (48). Again, acceptably low treatment toxicity was noted. However, because other investigators have found significant rates of pulmonary injury when paclitaxel and radiation were given concurrently to women with breast cancer, this approach is best taken within the context of a clinical research protocol.

Treatment Results for Locally Advanced Breast Cancer

As noted earlier in this chapter, stage III breast cancer historically has been associated with a very poor prognosis, with high rates of local-regional recurrence, distant metastases, and death. Currently, however, advances in all of the disciplines involved in breast cancer treatment have improved the outcome of such patients. With modern treatment strategies that include systemic therapy with taxanes and anthracyclines, appropriate surgical intervention, and local-regional irradiation, outcomes have significantly improved. With respect to local-regional control, a recent study evaluating outcome after mastectomy and radiation for patients with advanced disease that was initially treated with neoadjuvant chemotherapy reported a 10-year local-regional control rate of 89% (79). Patients with ER-negative disease and significant residual disease burden or skin invasion had rates of local-regional recurrence approaching 20%, whereas those without these features had excellent local-regional outcomes. As previously indicated, the risk of distant metastases has also significantly decreased over time. A reasonable estimate of 10-year survival rates for patients given modern treatments for stage III breast cancer is 40% to 50% (74).

Patients with supraclavicular lymph node disease at diagnosis have a poorer outcome than do other patients with stage III disease. However, because some studies of patients treated with chemotherapy have reported 10-year survival rates of 25%, the AJCC recently recategorized this stage of disease from stage

IV to stage IIIC (12). The local-regional management of such disease should be the same as for stage III disease. A recent study investigating the outcome of 70 patients with supraclavicular disease who were treated with neoadjuvant chemotherapy, surgery, and radiation reported a 5-year local-regional control rate of 77% and a 5-year overall survival rate of 47% (79). Patients in whom the supraclavicular disease showed a CR to neoadjuvant chemotherapy had better outcomes than did those with persistent disease after chemotherapy.

General Management and Treatment Results for Inflammatory Breast Cancer

Because inflammatory breast cancer is relatively uncommon, no data from randomized studies are available regarding the optimal therapeutic approach for this disease. In general, however, it is clear that management of inflammatory breast cancer requires carefully integrated care by a multidisciplinary team. Ideally, such patients should be evaluated in a multidisciplinary center by all specialists at the time of presentation to confirm the diagnosis of inflammatory disease, document the extent of disease (including photographs of areas of involved skin), and agree on a treatment plan. Inflammatory breast cancer is considered inoperable at presentation and should be treated initially with neoadjuvant chemotherapy (with consideration of trastuzumab if the tumor is HER2/neu-positive). Patients should be carefully monitored for response, and after achievement of the maximal clinical response, patients should be reevaluated for mastectomy. About 80% of patients with inflammatory breast cancer will achieve a clinical response and their disease will become operable (32). All patients should receive postmastectomy radiation therapy delivered to the chest wall and the draining lymphatics.

The optimal chemotherapy regimen for patients with inflammatory breast cancer includes both anthracyclines and taxanes. The introduction of anthracycline chemotherapy, when combined with local-regional treatments, provided the first evidence of treatment efficacy in this disease. Investigators at M.D. Anderson have conducted a series of single group prospective trials for patients with inflammatory breast cancer and found that neoadjuvant chemotherapy with FAC followed by local-regional therapy led to a 5-year survival rate of 25%. Subsequently, these investigators introduced sequential FAC or FEC followed by weekly paclitaxel and reported that the addition of taxanes improved the progression-free and overall survival of patients with inflammatory disease (32).

Local-regional treatment is an essential component of therapy for inflammatory disease. Before the routine use of chemotherapy, mastectomy, with or without postmastectomy radiation, was associated with a dismal prognosis, and so many physicians abandoned mastectomy in favor of radiation-only treatments. Outcomes after radiation therapy as the sole treatment modality were equally poor. After neoadjuvant chemotherapy became routine, combinations of surgery and radiation have been reevaluated.

De Boer et al. (36) published results of a study of 54 patients with inflammatory breast cancer treated after neoadjuvant chemotherapy with either radiation only (n = 35) or mastectomy plus radiation (n = 19). For the patients treated with radiation only, the median progression-free survival time was only 16 months and the local recurrence rate was 34%. However, because these results were not statistically different from those for patients treated with mastectomy, the authors concluded that surgery provided no clinical advantage over chemotherapy and radiation alone. In contrast, Perez et al. (108) found that the addition of mastectomy to local treatment significantly improved the outcome of inflammatory breast cancer treatment. Patients given neoadjuvant chemotherapy, mastectomy, and postmastectomy radiation had a local control rate of 79% and a 5-year disease-free survival of 40%. These data were also supported by Panades et al. (107), who evaluated 308 patients given chemotherapy as a component of their treatment and found that the 10-year local-recurrence-free survival rates were significantly better for patients who underwent mastectomy than for those who did not (about 60% vs. 34%, respectively; $p = 0.0001$), as were the 10-year breast cancer–specific survival rates (about 34% with mastectomy vs. 23% without; $p = 0.005$). A multivariate analysis that considered other potential prognostic factors found that the use of mastectomy remained a significant factor for improved local-recurrence-free survival ($p = 0.04$). Results from an M.D. Anderson study also confirmed these results, with multivariate analysis revealing that a complete or partial response to neoadjuvant chemotherapy, the use of radiotherapy, and the addition of mastectomy to the therapeutic regimen all significantly improved disease-specific survival (45).

More recent studies have focused on whether breast conservation can be safely performed for patients who achieved a CR to neoadjuvant chemotherapy (2,13,94,108). Some series have reported favorable control rates (2). However, Swain and Lippman (130) reported a local recurrence rate of 30%, despite their patients having achieved a clinical CR to neoadjuvant chemotherapy and multiple negative biopsies before irradiation. Low et al. (94) also reported a 40% local recurrence rate in 15 patients with inflammatory breast cancer treated with radiation therapy alone after a biopsy-proven CR. Finally, Brun et al. (13) reported a 54% local failure rate with attempts at breast conservation, and Chevallier et al. (29) reported a 61% local failure rate in patients treated with breast conservation after they had achieved a CR to neoadjuvant chemotherapy.

Radiation therapy also has an important role in the management of inflammatory breast cancer. After neoadjuvant chemotherapy and mastectomy, radiation use can be associated with local-regional control rates of over 80% (92). However, these results have been achieved with high-dose, aggressive treatments. Because inflammatory breast cancer has a rapid doubling time, investigators from M.D. Anderson investigated an accelerated hyperfractionated radiation delivery schedule in which 51 Gy is delivered to the chest wall, and draining lymphatic fields by giving 1.5 Gy twice a day. Subsequently, the chest wall is boosted to an additional 15 Gy, given in 10 fractions of 1.5 Gy twice daily. That approach was found to significantly improve local-regional disease control among patients treated to the 66-Gy total dose compared with a group treated only to 60 Gy on this schedule, with the respective 10-year local-regional control rates being 77% versus 58% ($p = 0.04$) (92). Statistically significant improvements were also seen in 5- and 10-year overall survival rates between these two groups ($p = 0.03$), and a trend toward improvement in 5- and 10-year disease-free survival rates was noted as well ($p = 0.06$). In a more recent update from these investigators in which the outcome of 192 patients treated with neoadjuvant chemotherapy, mastectomy, and postmastectomy radiation was evaluated, the authors reported a 5-year local-regional control rate of 84% (92). Factors associated with higher rates of local-regional control included partial response to chemotherapy, negative margins, three or fewer positive lymph nodes, and the use of taxane chemotherapy.

Clearly, great strides have been made over the past two decades in the management of inflammatory breast cancer, and patients whose disease is managed with trimodality therapy can have local-regional control rates exceeding 80% and 5-year survival rates of 40% or more. Improvements in systemic therapy will, it is hoped, further augment these results. For example, recent pilot results from the use of chemotherapy in combination with the EGFR–HER2/neu inhibitor lapatinib have shown favorable outcomes, and this strategy is currently being investigated in a larger phase II study.

General Management and Treatment Results for Locally or Regionally Recurrent Breast Cancer

The development of a local-regional recurrence after primary treatment of an invasive breast cancer, particularly for those treated with an initial mastectomy, often develops into a life-threatening condition. Accordingly, all patients should undergo disease restaging at the time of recurrence to rule out metastatic disease. All patients with local-regional recurrence should also have a biopsy for histopathological confirmation and for reevaluation of hormone receptor and HER2/neu status.

Local-regional recurrences are relatively uncommon, and patients with local-regional recurrences represent a heterogeneous group. Therefore, treatment strategies for must be tailored to individual cases.

Recurrence in the Breast after Breast Conservation Therapy

Mastectomy remains the standard salvage treatment for disease that recurs in the breast after breast-conserving treatment. Most such patients will have been previously treated with breast irradiation and therefore would not be candidates for a breast-conserving approach. However, some single institutional studies have investigated additional breast conserving surgery with or without radiation. Salvadori et al. (121) compared the outcome of 134 patients treated with mastectomy for a localized breast recurrence to 54 highly selected patients treated with a second breast conserving surgery alone. They found that a second breast recurrence was more common at 5 years in the re-excision group (19% vs. 4%). Komoike et al. (86) also reported a relatively high rate (30%) of a second breast relapse after local surgery only for recurrent disease. Experience with giving a second course of radiation therapy following local resection of a breast recurrence has also been limited, with most approaches being limited to a partial breast reirradiation strategy. Deutsch (37) treated 39 women with 50 Gy to the operative area using electrons after a repeat lumpectomy for an intact breast recurrence but reported a rate of second recurrence of 23%. Recht et al. (115) treated 17 ipsilateral breast tumor recurrence (IBTR) patients with pulse–dose-rate brachytherapy following repeat lumpectomy and noted a second breast recurrence in five patients. Finally, in the largest series to date, Hannoun-Levi et al. (69) treated 69 highly selected patients with interstitial brachytherapy after a second lumpectomy for an intact breast recurrence and after a median follow-up of 50 months reported that 11 (16%) developed a second recurrence. Grade 2 to 3 late complications developed in 0% to 32% of the patients depending on the radiation dose.

Patients with recurrence in the breast are also at risk of axillary metastases. Patients who initially underwent sentinel lymph node surgery should have an axillary lymph node dissection at the time of recurrence. The use of systemic therapy after breast recurrence needs to be decided on an individual basis according to the risk of metastatic disease, the previous systemic treatments used, and hormone receptor status.

Several investigators have investigated prognostic factors associated with outcome for patients with breast recurrence after treatment for an invasive breast cancer. Quite consistently through these studies is the finding that patients with a interval to development of recurrence of less than 2 years have a worse outcome than those who develop recurrent disease many years after treatment. In part, this may be explained by the hypothesis that early breast recurrences develop from repopulation of persistent microscopic disease, whereas some late breast recurrences represent a new primary tumor. Investigators from Yale University were among the first to provide insights into the prognostic importance of this distinction. These authors evaluated a series of 136 such patients and used clinical criteria to classify recurrences as either true recurrences or new primary tumors (127). New primary tumors were defined by one of the following: Location in the breast remote from the original tumor bed site, a change in histology, or a change from aneuploid to diploid status. Subsequently, investigators from M.D. Anderson undertook a similar analysis of 139 patients with in-breast recurrences. Both studies found that patients considered to have new primary tumors had significantly longer intervals between their initial primary tumor and the recurrence and had significantly lower rates of distant metastasis and death after the recurrence (76). These findings may be valuable in decisions regarding systemic treatments.

Reconstructive surgery can also be considered for patients treated with mastectomy, but the previous history of breast radiation may limit the success of implant-based procedures. Forman et al. (47) reported significant complications in six of the 10 patients in whom a tissue expander and implant was attempted after mastectomy in the setting of an ipsilateral breast recurrent treatment. Autologous tissue reconstruction may provide better outcomes. Moran et al. (100) reported on 11 patients who underwent free transverse rectus abdominis myocutaneous (TRAM) flaps with anastomosis to the thoracodorsal vessels in patients being treated for a breast recurrence. The complication rate was only 14%, and the aesthetic result was rated as excellent.

Local-Regional Recurrence after Mastectomy

Patients with recurrent disease after initial mastectomy have a worse prognosis than those with recurrent disease after initial breast conservation therapy. In the Canadian and the Danish prospective studies that evaluated postmastectomy radiation, patients who developed local-regional recurrence had very high rates of subsequently developing metastatic disease (102,103). In the Danish trial, the 5 year rate of distant metastatic disease development after an isolated local-regional recurrence was 73%, and the rate was no different for those in whom disease recurred after mastectomy only versus those with recurrent disease after mastectomy and radiation (102). Similarly, in the British Columbia trial, of the 39 patients who developed a local-regional recurrence, 37 eventually developed metastatic disease (113).

Several publications have provided insights into the factors of prognostic significance for patients with local-regional recurrence after mastectomy. One of the largest series was an analysis of the 535 patients who developed a postmastectomy recurrence after treatment in the Danish 82b and 82c randomized trials (102). In multivariate analyses, the investigators found the following factors to be associated with a poorer outcome: Large initial primary tumor and high number of positive lymph nodes, extracapsular extension, recurrence in the infraclavicular or supraclavicular regions, and a disease-free interval of <2 years. Other series have reported similar findings. In general, patients who present with chest wall recurrence, particularly those who have resectable disease and have not undergone radiation, have a greater probability of disease control and improved outcome. Investigators from M.D. Anderson found that initial nodal status, time to recurrence, and ability to use radiation to treat the recurrence were all independent predictors of outcome for patients with a chest wall recurrence (23). The 19 patients in whom these three factors were favorable had

a 5-year overall survival of 86% (median survival time, 141 months). The 5-year survival rate for the 89 patients who had one or two unfavorable features was 48% (median survival time, 54 months), and all 22 of the patients who had all three unfavorable factors died within 5 years of the recurrence (median survival, 16 months). Outcome for patients with T1 or T2 disease with one to three positive lymph nodes was just as poor after a local-regional recurrence as was the outcome for patients with four or more positive lymph nodes (22). In contrast, patients with initial lymph node–negative disease had a significantly better outcome.

Few data are available to quantify the benefits of systemic therapy for patients with local-regional recurrence. In one of the few series evaluating this issue, authors from British Columbia found in a nonrandomized study that use of chemotherapy at the time of recurrence reduced the probability of death from breast cancer, but this difference was not statistically significant compared with those who did not have chemotherapy at recurrence (p = 0.07). Finally, a randomized trial that investigated tamoxifen use versus no systemic therapy after salvage local therapy for patients with recurrent disease after mastectomy found an improvement in 5-year disease-free survival from 36% to 59% (p = 0.007) (8), supporting the use of systemic treatments in the management of patients with recurrent disease.

Investigators from M.D. Anderson conducted a series of four prospective single-group protocols evaluating systemic therapies for patients with either local-regional recurrence or metastatic disease that was converted to "no evidence of disease" after surgery, radiation, or both (70). The findings suggest that for patients with anthracycline-naive disease, the introduction of doxorubicin at the time of recurrence can lead to improved survival and more recently the use of docetaxel also seemed to lead to favorable outcomes for patients who had previously had anthracycline treatment. The 3-year disease-free survival rate for such patients was 58%.

The general management strategy for an isolated local-regional recurrence after mastectomy requires input from a multidisciplinary team. The initial evaluation should define the sites of disease involvement and determine whether the patient is able to undergo resection of all gross disease with negative surgical margins. Surgical therapy is recommended for patients with resectable disease, provided the patients can tolerate the surgery and the morbidity of the surgery is acceptable. After surgery, if the patients had not previously been given radiation therapy, they should receive comprehensive local-regional radiation. A study from Washington University found that patients who had radiation therapy to the chest wall and regional lymphatics had better outcomes than those in whom radiation fields were limited to the site of the recurrent disease (66). Finally, because patients with recurrent disease after mastectomy are at high risk of developing distant metastatic disease, those who have not been previously treated with anthracyclines or taxanes (or trastuzumab if the tumor is HER2/neu-positive) should strongly consider treatment with these agents (72). Patients with ER-positive disease should receive appropriate second-line endocrine therapy.

Patients presenting with bulky unresectable disease should be considered for neoadjuvant chemotherapy if active systemic agents are available. If the disease responds favorably, some of these patients may become candidates for surgical resection, which then can be consolidated with comprehensive radiation. The prognosis for those whose disease fails to respond is very poor, and radiation treatments alone are unlikely to render such patients free of disease. Nevertheless, aggressive local-regional radiation is often used to help stabilize the disease and to avoid the significant adverse consequences of uncontrolled growth of local-regional disease. The dose of radiation to be used depends on the presence or absence of gross disease and whether patients have previously undergone radiation therapy. For patients who have not had radiation therapy and do not have gross disease, we recommend comprehensive treatment to the chest wall and draining lymphatics to a dose of 50 to 54 Gy followed by a boost to the chest wall to 60 to 66 Gy. Hyperfractionated chest wall irradiation does not seem to provide any benefit over that of conventional therapy given once daily (4).

Regional Nodal Relapse

Patients with regional relapse have a less favorable prognosis than patients with intact breast or chest wall recurrences. In general, patients with isolated resectable disease in the low axilla should be treated with axillary dissection, comprehensive radiation to sites not previously treated including the chest wall, and systemic therapy. Most patients with recurrence in the supraclavicular fossa or internal mammary lymph nodes have unresectable disease. If active chemotherapy agents are available, it is reasonable to consider using neoadjuvant systemic treatment and consolidating with radiation at the point of maximal response. Woodward et al. (148) investigated the outcome of 140 patients with local-regional recurrence after mastectomy and doxorubicin chemotherapy and found that the 47 who had supraclavicular disease at the time of recurrence had a worse outcome than the remaining patients with recurrences in other sites (10-year disease-free survival of 5% vs. 39%, respectively; $p = 0.003$).

General Management and Treatment Results for Unusual Presentations of Breast Cancer

Axillary Metastases with Unknown Primary

The presentation of metastatic disease within axillary lymph nodes without an identifiable primary source is unusual, accounting for less than 1% of newly diagnosed breast cancer cases (85,142,143). Work-up for patients who present with axillary disease with an occult primary should initially be aimed at establishing the diagnosis and whether the disease represents a distant metastasis from a different site. Initial evaluation should include a history and physical examination (with particular attention to a skin examination to rule out an unsuspected truncal melanoma), routine serum studies, bilateral mammography, chest radiography, liver imaging, and bone scan. If no primary disease is detected with mammography, ultrasound and MRI scan of the breast is indicated. Cytological confirmation of disease within axillary lymph nodes can be obtained with ultrasound-guided fine needle aspiration. Tumor markers including ER, PR, and HER2/neu can and should be performed on the cytological specimens. Most individuals present with advanced nodal disease at presentation and are clinically staged as having T0N2–3 disease.

Modified radical mastectomy and postmastectomy radiation have been the historical local-regional treatments for patients with an occult breast primary and axillary metastases. Studies vary significantly with respect to the frequency with which a primary is found within the breast during pathological examination. In addition, most of these studies predate the use of MRI screening or other improvements in diagnostic imaging. In general, however, approximately two-thirds of the cases are found to have an invasive breast cancer found on pathological examination of a mastectomy specimen (85). Patients with inoperable nodal disease at presentation are treated with neoadjuvant chemotherapy prior to mastectomy. For such individuals, the probability of finding disease within the breast is likely even lower.

More recently, a number of investigators have investigated the safety of breast conservation therapy for patients with occult primary disease. An optimal treatment strategy for such patients can consist of neoadjuvant chemotherapy, reimaging of the breast to evaluate for calcifications resulting from tumor cell death, axillary dissection, and irradiation of the breast and draining lymphatics. Early attempts at breast conservation without breast irradiation resulted in high subsequent breast recurrence rates (6,40). More recent studies that incorporated breast irradiation have yielded better results. In one of the largest series, investigators from M.D. Anderson evaluated 45 patients treated over a 47-year period and compared the outcome of those treated with mastectomy ($n = 13$) to those treated with breast conservation ($n = 32$). These authors found equivalent rates of local-regional control, disease-free survival, and overall survival between the mastectomy and breast conservation cohorts. With a median follow-up of 7 years, only two of the 25 breast conservation patients who received breast irradiation developed a local recurrence (143).

Male Breast Cancer

Breast cancer developing in males is unusual. The American Cancer Society estimates that there will be 1,720 new cases of male breast cancer in the United States in 2006, which accounts for only 0.8% of the total new breast cancer cases. It was also estimated that 460 men will die of breast cancer during 2006 (10). The ratio of the number of deaths to new cases is 27% for males, compared to a ratio of 19% for females (10).

There are several known risk factors for male breast cancer. Similar to female breast cancer, breast cancer is more common in elderly men than young men. Some conditions that affect testosterone and estrogen levels can increase the risk of breast cancer in men. Examples of such conditions include a history of an undescended testicle, history of orchiectomy, and Klinefelter's syndrome (57). In addition, genetic conditions also can contribute and men with a family history of female breast cancer have an increased risk. More recently, germline mutations in the BRCA2 gene have been reported in 4% to 16% of men with breast cancer, and, unlike females, are more common than germline mutations in BRCA1 (52,104).

Males have a similar histopathological spectrum of breast cancers, with the exception of having lower rates of invasive lobular disease. In addition, male breast cancers more frequently are ER-positive (estimated rate of 90%) and HER2/neu-negative compared to female breast cancer (56). The presenting symptom for male breast cancer patients is typically a breast mass or axillary adenopathy. Most male breast cancer patients present with locally advanced disease. Diagnostic work-up is similar to that for female breast cancer and should include bilateral mammography. Treatment decisions are also similar to those used in women.

Mastectomy with or without postmastectomy radiation is the most common local-regional treatment approach. Investigators at M.D. Anderson reviewed 142 patients treated with mastectomy without radiation therapy and found that similar to female patients, margin status, number of positive nodes, and tumor size predicted for local-regional failure (16). Accordingly, decisions concerning postmastectomy radiation should be based on similar criteria used in the treatment of female breast cancer.

Similarly, systemic treatments are indicated for male breast cancer patients who have a clinically relevant risk of distant metastases. Data supporting the use of particular chemotherapy regimens are lacking given the rarity of the disease. In addition to chemotherapy, because most male breast cancers are hormonally responsive, tamoxifen is indicated for the majority of cases. Retrospective series have suggested that tamoxifen use can reduce the risk of recurrence and death (117). The role of aromatase inhibitors in males is currently under investigation.

Radiation Treatment Techniques after Mastectomy

Target Definitions

Traditionally, postmastectomy radiation therapy included treatment to the chest wall and draining lymphatics in the undissected axillary apex/supraclavicular fossa. It is clear from the pattern of failure studies from patients treated with mastectomy without radiation that the chest wall is the most common site of recurrent disease, accounting for two-thirds to three-quarters of all local-regional recurrences. It is also clear that patients with stage III disease (T3N1, T4, or pathological N2 or N3 disease) have a clinically relevant risk of recurrence in the axillary apex/supraclavicular fossa. A recent study of over 1,000 patients who did not receive radiation after treatment with mastectomy and chemotherapy found the 10-year risk of recurrence in the axillary apex/supraclavicular fossa to be 14% to 19% for patients with either four or more positive lymph nodes, 20% or greater positive lymph nodes, or extracapsular extension of disease that measured over 2 mm (129).

The benefit or radiation for treatment of the dissected level I or II axilla is less clear. In this same study, in which all patients had a standard axillary lymph node dissection (median number of lymph nodes recovered was 17), the 10-year risk of recurrence in this region was only 3%, and not predicted by the extent of axillary disease or extracapsular extension (129). In contrast, 13% of the patients treated in the no radiation arms of the Danish postmastectomy radiation trials and who developed a local-regional recurrence had the axilla as a component of their local-regional recurrence (103). The higher recurrence rate in the axilla likely was a consequence of a less extensive axillary level I or II dissection (median number of lymph nodes recovered was seven) in the Danish studies. These data together suggest that the decision to include the level I or II as a target for postmastectomy radiation in large part is determined by the completeness of the axillary dissection.

The treatment of the internal mammary lymph nodes for patients treated with postmastectomy radiation is controversial and the subject of ongoing phase III studies. The justification for including this region is based on previous experiences of dissecting the internal mammary chain, which found that up to 35% to 50% of patients with clinically advanced disease will have microscopic involvement of lymph nodes within this region (68,138). The randomized trials that have shown a survival advantage for postmastectomy radiation included the internal mammary lymph nodes within their treatment target volume (105,106,112). Finally, inclusion of the internal mammary lymph nodes provides a broader coverage of the chest wall, which may prove to be a secondary benefit in avoiding marginal misses.

When radiation is used after mastectomy for patients with stage II breast cancer, the appropriate target volumes are less clear. Patients with stage II breast cancer with one to three positive lymph nodes fail predominantly on the chest wall and have a much lower risk of recurrence in the axillary apex/supraclavicular fossa. In a site of failure analysis cited above, the risk of recurrence in the axilla/supraclavicular fossa for patients with one to three positive lymph nodes and no extracapsular extension was only 4% (129). For these reasons, some have advocated treatment of the chest wall only in such patients. However, the trials showing a survival advantage for the use of postmastectomy radiation included the axillary apex/supraclavicular fossa within the treatment fields.

CT simulation is very useful to more precisely delineate target volumes. For example, the internal mammary vessels within the first three intercostal interspaces, which are where lymph nodes at risk within this region are located, can be easily identified and contoured. Likewise, the depth of the level III axilla and supraclavicular fossa varies greatly according to individual anatomy and patient weight. Contouring the region helps to ensure that these targets fall within the desired isodose lines. A recent analysis that evaluated various dose prescriptions used for supraclavicular field treatments found that 6 MV photons prescribed to Dmax or a depth of 3 cm significantly underdosed contoured lymph node regions at risk in overweight and obese patients (defined according to patient body mass index) (93). Finally, for patients who require treatment to the low axilla, contouring the region at risk also helps to more precisely conform the dose distribution to the area in need of treatment.

Technique

Patients should be immobilized with their ipsilateral arm abducted (90 to 120 degrees) and externally rotated. In assessing arm position, it is important to have the soft tissues of the arm cranial to the junction of the tangent and supraclavicular fossa field. In addition, skin folds within the supraclavicular fossa should be avoided if possible. Patients are placed on a 10- to 15-degree angle board to flatten the slope of the chest wall in the region of the sternum. CT simulation is preferred in order to optimize target delineation as described above. Radio-opaque wires are placed on the mastectomy scar and the patient undergoes a treatment planning noncontrast CT scan. The border between the chest wall and the supraclavicular fields is typically placed at the bottom of the clavicular head. Appropriate isocenters and set-up points are determined and marked. Targeted areas of interest are then contoured on the CT slices.

Several techniques are available treat the chest wall and internal mammary lymph nodes. One of the more common methods is to use a 15- to 25-degree obliqued electron field to treat the medial chest wall and internal mammary lymph nodes. The lateral border of this field is then matched to a pair of photon tangent fields that treat the lateral chest wall and are created with matched nondivergent deep and cranial borders. A nondivergent cranial border is created through rotation of the couch, and a nondivergent deep border is achieved by over-rotating the gantry or a half-beam block. The collimators are rotated to match the chest wall slope, and any volume that extends into the supraclavicular field is blocked. An alternative technique that is particularly of benefit for patients with very little tissue between the lung and skin is to use three electron fields. The junction of such fields should be moved every week to minimize the consequences of the required gantry rotation necessary to make the fields apposition for the lateral chest wall. These fields are then matched to a supraclavicular/axillary apex field, which has been described in Chapter 53. For patients with advanced disease, the supraclavicular lateral field edge is often extended to give margin on the superior-lateral chest wall and to provide treatment of the anterior inter-pectoral Rotter's lymph nodes.

Figures 54.7, 54.8, and 54.9 show examples of matched electron, tangent fields; chest wall electron-only fields; and a supraclavicular/axillary apex field. All chest wall radiation fields should be designed to avoid irradiating the heart. The advantages of the field designs described above is that with the use of CT treatment planning, the beam arrangement, and selection of electron energies can be determined so that cardiac irradiation is avoided or minimized.

Dosimetry and Dose

Initial fields and target volumes should be treated to a total dose of 50 Gy in 25 fractions over 5 weeks. Three- to 5-mm bolus over the chest wall every other day or every day for 2 weeks (20 Gy total dose) and then as needed to ensure that a brisk radiation

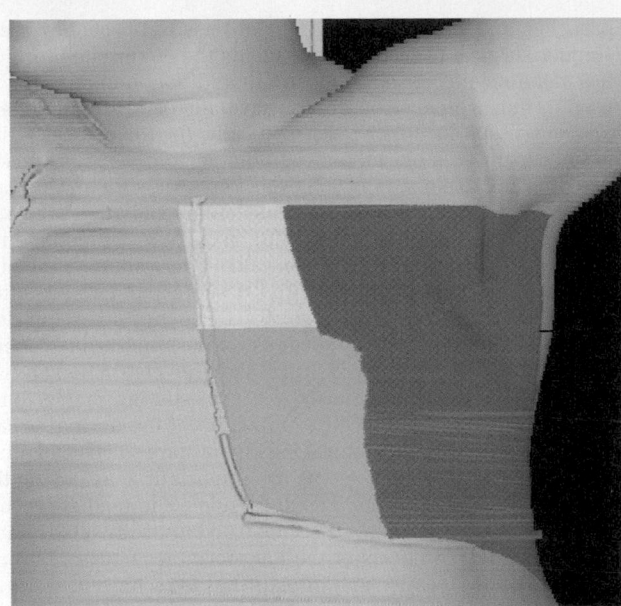

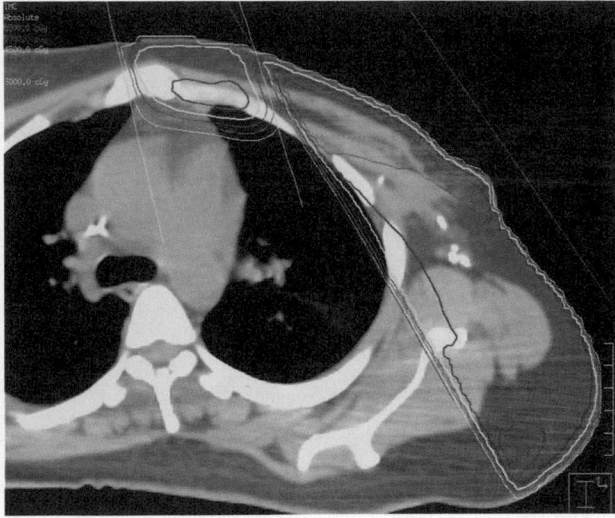

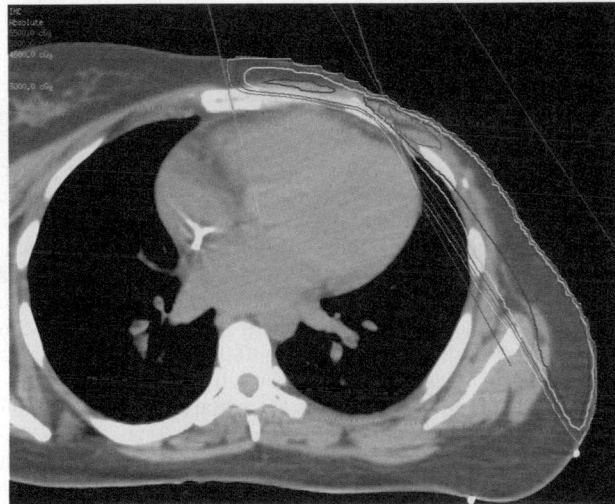

FIGURE 54.7. Images of radiation treatment fields to treat the chest wall and internal mammary lymph nodes. In this case, two medial electron fields were angled 15 degrees toward a matched pair of photon fields. The energy of the upper electron field is higher than the lower electron field in order to achieve coverage of the contoured internal mammary target while minimizing the dose to the heart. **A:** Shows a skin surface rendering of the fields. **B:** Shows an upper axial image. **C:** Shows a lower axial image in the region of the heart. (From Buchholz TA. Locally advanced breast cancer. In: *Handbook of radiation oncology.* Haffty BG, Wilson L, eds. 2006; Jones & Bartlett, Sudbury, M, with permission.)

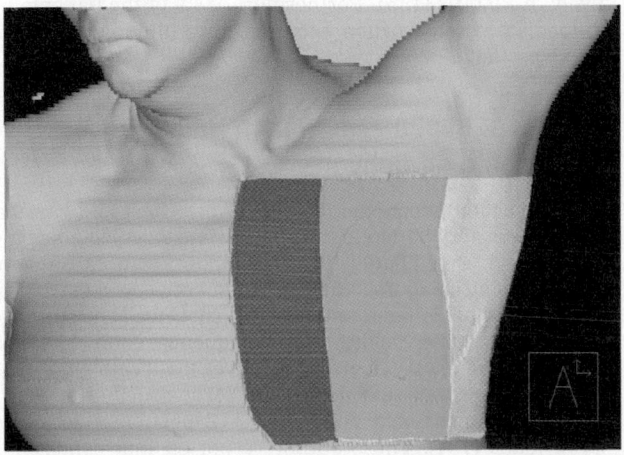

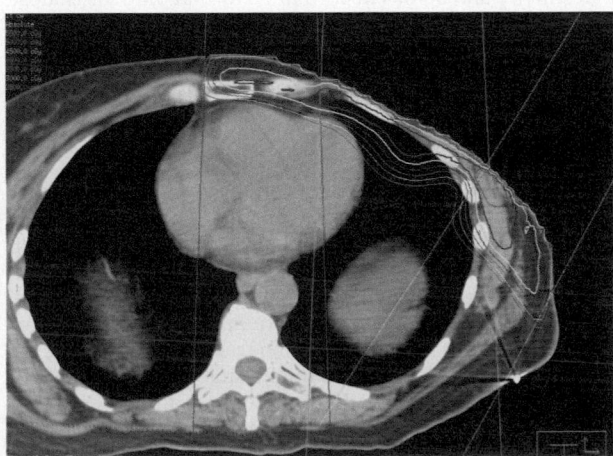

FIGURE 54.8. Images of radiation treatment fields using a match electron field technique to treat the chest wall and internal mammary lymph nodes. Three medial electron fields are matched on the skin. The junction between the middle and lateral fields are shifted weekly due to the differences in gantry angle. **A:** Shows a skin surface rendering of the fields. **B:** Shows an axial image of the fields.

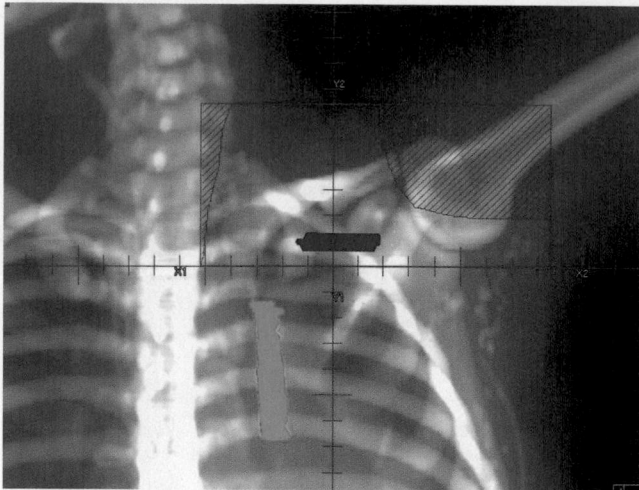

FIGURE 54.9. Image of a radiation treatment field used to treat the axillary apex/supraclavicular fossa. The level III region of the axillary and the upper internal mammary vessels have been contoured on axial CT images and reconstructed on this image. These contours are used to determine depth of dose prescription. (From Buchholz TA. Locally advanced breast cancer. In: *Handbook of radiation oncology*. Haffty BG, Wilson L, eds. 2006, Jones & Bartlett, Sudbury, MA, with permission.)

dermatitis develops. However, this dermatitis should not lead to a treatment interruption. There are no studies evaluating the optimal total dose, but in our institution we boost the chest wall with electron fields (5 to 10 cm beyond the mastectomy scar and covering the tumor bed location of the original primary) for an additional 10 Gy in five fractions over 1 week beyond the initial 50-Gy course. In addition, we boost all sites of unresected but initially involved adenopathy in the internal mammary, infraclavicular, and supraclavicular regions with a radiation boost. If ultrasonography has shown a resolution of disease in these areas down to 1 cm or less, we treat this region with an additional boost of 10 Gy. If more than 1 cm of disease persists, we increase the boost dose to 16 Gy.

Three-dimensional treatment planning systems allow for evaluation of dose distributions in multiple off-axis slices and calculations of dose using heterogeneity correction factors. Dose distributions can be modulated through standard wedge compensators or field-in-field techniques. Electron energies for the medial chest wall/internal mammary lymph node fields should ensure that the 90% isodose curve covers the contoured volume and avoids irradiation of the heart. In addition, the supraclavicular dosimetry should be checked to verify that the 90% isodose curve fully covers the undissected level III axilla.

Postmastectomy Radiation and Breast Reconstruction

Coordination of radiation and breast reconstruction is a commonly encountered issue for patients treated with mastectomy and requires clear communication between surgical oncologist, reconstructive/plastic surgeon, radiation oncologist, and the patient. There are many factors to consider regarding the issue of reconstruction and postmastectomy radiation, including ensuring the safety and efficacy of radiation treatments, ensuring the maximal quality of life for the patients, and achieving the optimal long-term aesthetic result from the procedure.

The two major classes of reconstruction are implant-based approaches and autologous tissue reconstruction. The two options for timing for the reconstruction are immediate (done at the time of mastectomy) or delayed (done after completion of radiation). There are advantages and disadvantages of both ap-

proaches and both timings. Implant-based approaches are a simpler surgical procedure that avoids the donor site morbidities of autologous tissue transfers. In addition, implants can be used in thin women who do not have adequate volume of autologous tissue in donor sites. Typically, for this procedure, a tissue expander is placed between the pectoralis major muscle and after full expansion is achieved, replaced with an implant. Most women treated with postmastectomy radiation who undergo implant-based reconstruction require an immediate reconstruction procedure. This is because after radiation the normal tissues are less compliant and tissue expanders are often unsuccessful and may cause rib fractures and other injuries. For women treated with autologous tissues, the reconstruction can be immediate or delayed. Immediate reconstruction has the benefit of being accompanied by a skin-sparing mastectomy, which preserves a significant component of the normal breast skins and preserves the natural inframammary sulcus and other skin envelopes. These elements are important to achieving the optimal cosmetic outcome. The downsides of immediate reconstruction relative to delayed reconstruction are twofold: Radiation has adverse effects of the long-term aesthetics of breast reconstructions, particularly implant-based reconstruction, and reconstruction has a negative effect on the design and delivery of radiation treatment fields.

Effects of Radiation on Reconstruction

The majority of patients who undergo an immediate reconstruction and require postmastectomy radiation will have an aesthetic change as a consequence of treatments. In general, implant-based reconstruction has high rates of late contraction, fibrosis, implant fixation, and a poor aesthetic outcome. Many of these changes begin 6 months after treatment and insidiously progress over time. Spear and Onyewu (128) reviewed the data on breast reconstruction with implants and found a 53% complication rate after radiation compared to a 10% rate in those who did not require radiation ($p < 0.001$). Other investigators have reported lower risks (1), although the length of follow-up and presentation of the data as an actuarial analysis are likely to have a significant effect of the findings.

Complications also develop for patients treated with an immediate autologous tissue reconstruction followed by radiation, although the effects, while common, may be less severe than implant-based approaches. Investigators from M.D. Anderson compared complications in patients treated with radiation and autologous tissue reconstruction. Those with an immediate reconstruction had a higher rate of complications compared to those with a delayed reconstruction (87.5% vs. 8.6%, respectively; $p < 0.001$) (135). Furthermore, 28% of the patients with immediate reconstruction required an additional flap to improve aesthetics.

Effects of Reconstruction on Radiation Treatment and Delivery

Reconstruction affects the contour of the chest and can make the delivery of radiation to the appropriate targeted areas more challenging. Overinflated tissue expanders can cause significantly sloping contours at field junction between chest wall and internal mammary fields and between chest wall and supraclavicular/axillary apex fields. As a consequence, compromises are sometimes necessary in order to deliver the treatment safely. A recent article evaluated the effects reconstruction had in radiation treatment field designs in 112 postmastectomy radiation plans (101). These authors reported that compromises in the field design were made in 52% of these cases because of the geometrical constraints caused by the reconstruction (33% were considered moderate compromises and 19% major compromises). In a matched control set treated with mastectomy without reconstruction, only 7% of cases had compromises in plans due to patient anatomy.

References

1. Anderson PR, Hanlon AL, Fowble BL, et al. Low complication rates are achievable after postmastectomy breast reconstruction and radiation therapy. *Int J Radiat Oncol Biol Phys* 2004;59:1080–1087.
2. Arthur DW, Schmidt-Ullrich RK, Friedman RB, et al. Accelerated superfractionated radiotherapy for inflammatory breast carcinoma: Complete response predicts outcome and allows for breast conservation. *Int J Radiat Oncol Biol Phys* 1999;44:289–296.
3. Baker RR, Holmes ER 3rd, Alderson PO, et al. An evaluation of bone scans as screening procedures for occult metastases in primary breast cancer. *Ann Surg* 1977;186:363–368.
4. Ballo MT, Strom EA, Prost H, et al. Local-regional control of recurrent breast carcinoma after mastectomy: Does hyperfractionated accelerated radiotherapy improve local control? *Int J Radiat Oncol Biol Phys* 1999;44:105–112.
5. Barker JL, Nelson AJ, Montague ED. Inflammatory carcinoma of the breast. *Radiology* 1976;121:173–176.
6. Bhatia SK, Saclarides TJ, Witt TR, et al. Hormone receptor studies in axillary metastases from occult breast cancers. *Cancer* 1987;59:1170–1172.
7. Bonadonna G, Valagussa P, Brambilla C, et al. Primary chemotherapy in operable breast cancer: Eight-year experience at the Milan Cancer Institute. *J Clin Oncol* 1998;16:93–100.
8. Borner M, Bacchi M, Goldhirsch A, et al. First isolated locoregional recurrence following mastectomy for breast cancer: Results of a phase III multicenter study comparing systemic treatment with observation after excision and radiation. Swiss Group for Clinical Cancer Research. *J Clin Oncol* 1994;12:2071–2077.
9. Bozzetti F, Saccozzi R, De Lena M, et al. Inflammatory cancer of the breast: Analysis of 114 cases. *J Surg Oncol* 1981;18:355–361.
10. *Breast Cancer Facts and Figures 2005–2006*. Atlanta, GA: American Cancer Society, 2006.
11. Bria E, Nistico C, Cuppone F, et al. Benefit of taxanes as adjuvant chemotherapy for early breast cancer: Pooled analysis of 15,500 patients. *Cancer* 2006;106:2337–2344.
12. Brito RA, Valero V, Buzdar AU, et al. Long-term results of combined-modality therapy for locally advanced breast cancer with ipsilateral supraclavicular metastases: The University of Texas M.D. Anderson Cancer Center experience. *J Clin Oncol* 2001;19:628–633.
13. Brun B, Otmezguine Y, Feuilhade F, et al. Treatment of inflammatory breast cancer with combination chemotherapy and mastectomy versus breast conservation. *Cancer* 1988;61:1096–1103.
14. Buchholz TA, Hill BS, Tucker SL, et al. Factors predictive of outcome in patients with breast cancer refractory to neoadjuvant chemotherapy. *Cancer J* 2001;7:413–420.
15. Buchholz TA, Hunt KK, Whitman GJ, et al. Neoadjuvant chemotherapy for breast carcinoma: Multidisciplinary considerations of benefits and risks. *Cancer* 2003;98:1150–1160.
16. Buchholz TA, Katz A, Strom EA, et al. Pathologic tumor size and lymph node status predict for different rates of locoregional recurrence after mastectomy for breast cancer patients treated with neoadjuvant versus adjuvant chemotherapy. *Int J Radiat Oncol Biol Phys* 2002;53:880–888.
17. Buchholz TA, Stivers DN, Stec J, et al. Global gene expression changes during neoadjuvant chemotherapy for human breast cancer. *Cancer J* 2002;8:461–468.
18. Buchholz TA, Woodward WA, Duan Z, et al. Radiation use and long-term survival in breast cancer patients with T1,T2 primary tumors and 1–3 positive axillary lymph nodes. *Int J Rad Oncol Biol Phys* 2006; in press.
19. Buchholz TA. Locally advanced breast cancer. In: Haffty BG, Wilson L, eds. *Handbook of radiation oncology*. 2006;S5.
20. *Cancer Facts and Figures 2006*. Atlanta, GA: American Cancer Society, 2006;19.
21. Cataliotti L, Buzdar AU, Noguchi S, et al. Comparison of anastrozole versus tamoxifen as preoperative therapy in postmenopausal women with hormone receptor-positive breast cancer: The Pre-Operative “Arimidex” Compared to Tamoxifen (PROACT) trial. *Cancer* 2006;106:2095–2103.
22. Chagpar A, Kuerer HM, Hunt KK, et al. Outcome of treatment for breast cancer patients with chest wall recurrence according to initial stage: Implications for postmastectomy radiation therapy. *Int J Radiat Oncol Biol Phys* 2003;57:128–135.
23. Chagpar A, Meric-Bernstam F, Hunt KK, et al. Chest wall recurrence after mastectomy does not always portend a dismal outcome. *Ann Surg Oncol* 2003;10:628–634.
24. Chakravarthy AB, Kelley MC, McLaren B, et al. Neoadjuvant concurrent paclitaxel and radiation in stage II/III breast cancer. *Clin Cancer Res* 2006;12:1570–1576.
25. Chang S, Parker S, Pham T, et al. Inflammatory breast carcinoma incidence and survival. The Surveillance Epidemiology and End Results (SEER) Program of the National Cancer Institute, 1975–1992. *Cancer* 1998;82:2366–2372.
26. Chen AM, Meric-Bernstam F, Hunt KK, et al. Breast conservation after neoadjuvant chemotherapy: A prognostic index for clinical decision-making. *Cancer* 2004;26.
27. Chen AM, Meric-Bernstam F, Hunt KK, et al. Breast-conserving therapy after neoadjuvant chemotherapy: The M.D. Anderson Cancer Center experience. *J Clin Oncol* 2004;22:2303–2312.
28. Cheng JC, Chen CM, Liu MC, et al. Locoregional failure of postmastectomy patients with 1–3 positive axillary lymph nodes without adjuvant radiotherapy. *Int J Radiat Oncol Biol Phys* 2002;52:980–988.
29. Chevallier B, Asselain B, Kunlin A, et al. Inflammatory breast cancer. Determination of prognostic factors by univariate and multivariate analysis. *Cancer* 1987;60:897–902.
30. Citron ML, Berry DA, Cirrincione C, et al. Randomized trial of dose-dense versus conventionally scheduled and sequential versus concurrent combination chemotherapy as postoperative adjuvant treatment of node-positive primary breast cancer: First report of Intergroup trial C9741/Cancer and Leukemia Group B trial 9741. *J Clin Oncol* 2003;21:1431–1439.
31. Coombes RC, Hall E, Gibson LJ, et al. Intergroup exemestane study. A randomized trial of exemestane after two to three years of tamoxifen therapy in postmenopausal women with primary breast cancer. *N Engl J Med* 2004;350:1081–1092.
32. Cristofanilli M, Gonzalez-Angulo A, Sneige N, et al. Invasive lobular carcinoma classic type: Response to primary chemotherapy and survival outcomes. *J Clin Oncol* 2005;23:41–48.
33. Cristofanilli M, Gonzalez-Angulo AM, Buzdar AU, et al. Paclitaxel improves the prognosis in estrogen receptor negative inflammatory breast cancer: The M.D. Anderson Cancer Center experience. *Clin Breast Cancer* 2004;4:415–419.
34. Cuzick J, Stewart H, Peto R, et al. Overview of randomized trials of postoperative adjuvant radiotherapy in breast cancer. *Cancer Treat Rep* 1987;71:15–29.
35. Cuzick J, Stewart H, Rutqvist L, et al. Cause-specific mortality in long-term survivors of breast cancer who participated in trials of radiotherapy. *J Clin Oncol* 1994;12:447–453.
36. De Boer RH, Allum WH, Ebbs SR, et al. Multimodality therapy in inflammatory breast cancer: Is there a place for surgery? *Ann Oncol* 2000;11:1147–1153.
37. Deutsch M. Repeat high-dose external beam irradiation for in-breast tumor recurrence after previous lumpectomy and whole breast irradiation. *Int J Radiat Oncol Biol Phys* 2002;53:687–691.
38. Elkin EB, Hudis C, Begg CB, et al. The effect of changes in tumor size on breast carcinoma survival in the U.S.: 1975–1999. *Cancer* 2005;104:1149–1157.
39. Elledge RM, Clark GH, Chamness GC, et al. Tumor biologic factors and breast cancer prognosis among white, Hispanic, and black women in the United States. *J Natl Cancer Inst* 1994;86:705–712.
40. Ellerbroek N, Holmes F, Singletary E, et al. Treatment of patients with isolated axillary nodal metastases from an occult primary carcinoma consistent with breast origin. *Cancer* 1990;66:1461–1467.
41. Fields JN, Perez CA, Kuske RR, et al. Inflammatory carcinoma of the breast: Treatment results on 107 patients. *Int J Radiat Oncol Biol Phys* 1989;17:249–255.
42. Fisher B, Brown A, Mamounas E, et al. Effect of preoperative chemotherapy on local-regional disease in women with operable breast cancer: Findings from National Surgical Adjuvant Breast and Bowel Project B-18. *J Clin Oncol* 1997;15:2483–2493.
43. Fisher B, Saffer E, Rudock C, et al. Effect of local or systemic treatment prior to primary tumor removal on the production and response to a serum growth-stimulating factor in mice. *Cancer Res* 1989;49:2002–2004.
44. Fisher ER, Wang J, Bryant J, et al. Pathobiology of preoperative chemotherapy: Findings from the National Surgical Adjuvant Breast and Bowel (NSABP) protocol B-18. *Cancer* 2002;95:681–695.
45. Fleming RY, Asmar L, Buzdar AU, et al. Effectiveness of mastectomy by response to induction chemotherapy for control in inflammatory breast carcinoma. *Ann Surg Oncol* 1997;4:452–461.
46. Floyd SR, Buchholz TA, Haffty BG, et al. Low local recurrence rate without postmastectomy radiation in node-negative breast cancer patients with tumors 5 CM and larger. *Int J Radiat Oncol Biol Phys* 2006;358–364.
47. Forman DL, Chiu J, Restifo RJ, et al. Breast reconstruction in previously irradiated patients using tissue expanders and implants: A potentially unfavorable result. *Ann Plast Surg* 1998;40:360–363; discussion 363–364.
48. Formenti SC, Volm M, Skinner KA, et al. Preoperative twice-weekly paclitaxel with concurrent radiation therapy followed by surgery and postoperative doxorubicin-based chemotherapy in locally advanced breast cancer: A phase I/II trial. *J Clin Oncol* 2003;21:864–870.
49. Fowble B, Yeh IT, Schultz DJ, et al. The role of mastectomy in patients with stage I–II breast cancer presenting with gross multifocal or multicentric disease or diffuse microcalcifications. *Int J Radiat Oncol Biol Phys* 1993;27:567–573.
50. Fracchia AA, Evans JF, Eisenberg BC. Stage III carcinoma of the breast—a detailed analysis. *Ann Surg* 1980;192:705.
51. Freedman GM, Fowble BL, Hanlon AL, et al. A close or positive margin after mastectomy is not an indication for chest wall irradiation except in women aged fifty or younger. *Int J Radiat Oncol Biol Phys* 1998;41:599–605.
52. Friedman LS, Gayther SA, Kurosaki T, et al. Mutation analysis of BRCA1 and BRCA2 in a male breast cancer population. *Am J Hum Genet* 1997;60:313–319.
53. Garg A, Strom EA, McNeese MD, et al. T3 disease at presentation or pathologic involvement of four or more lymph nodes predict for local-regional recurrence in stage II breast cancer treated with neoadjuvant chemotherapy and mastectomy without radiation. *Int J Rad Oncol Biol Phys* 2004;59:138–145.
54. Gebski V, Lagleva M, Keech A, et al. Survival effects of postmastectomy adjuvant radiation therapy using biologically equivalent doses: A clinical perspective. *J Natl Cancer Inst* 2006;98:26–38.
55. Giordano SH, Buzdar AU, Smith TL, et al. Is breast cancer survival improving? *Cancer* 2004;100:44–52.
56. Giordano SH, Cohen DS, Buzdar AU, et al. Breast carcinoma in men: A population-based study. *Cancer* 2004;101:51–57.
57. Giordano SH. A review of the diagnosis and management of male breast cancer. *Oncologist* 2005;10:471–479.
58. Goss PE, Ingle JN, Martino S, et al. A randomized trial of letrozole in postmenopausal women after five years of tamoxifen therapy for early-stage breast cancer. *N Engl J Med* 2003;349:1793–1802.
59. Group EBCTC. Effects of chemotherapy and hormonal therapy for early breast cancer on recurrence and 15-year survival: An overview of the randomised trials. *Lancet* 2005;365:1687–1717.
60. Group EBCTC. Effects of radiotherapy and of differences in the extent of surgery for early breast cancer on local recurrence and 15-year survival: An overview of the randomised trials. *Lancet* 2005;366:2087–2106.
61. Group EBCTC. Favourable and unfavourable effects on long-term survival of radiotherapy for early breast cancer: An overview of the randomised trials. *Lancet* 2000;355:1757–1770.
62. Guerin M, Gabillot M, Mathieu M, et al. Structure and expression c-erB-2 and EGFR receptor genes in inflammatory and non-inflammatory breast cancer: Prognostic significance. *Int J Cancer* 1989;43:201–208.
63. Haagensen C. *Diseases of the breast*, 2nd ed. Philadelphia: Saunders, 1971;576–584.
64. Haagensen CD, Cooley E. Radical mastectomy for mammary carcinoma. *Ann Surg* 1969;170:884.
65. Haagensen CD, Stout AP. Carcinoma of the breast: Criteria of inoperability. *Ann Surg* 1943;118:859–870.

66. Halverson KJ, Perez CA, Kuske RR, et al. Isolated local-regional recurrence of breast cancer following mastectomy: Radiotherapeutic management. *Int J Radiat Oncol Biol Phys* 1990;19:851–858.
67. Hance KW, Anderson WF, Devesa SS, et al. Trends in inflammatory breast carcinoma incidence and survival: The surveillance, epidemiology, and end results program at the National Cancer Institute. *J Natl Cancer Inst* 2005;97:966–975.
68. Handley RS. Carcinoma of the breast. *Ann R Coll Surg Engl* 1975;57:59–66.
69. Hannoun-Levi JM, Houvenaeghel G, Ellis S, et al. Partial breast irradiation as second conservative treatment for local breast cancer recurrence. *Int J Radiat Oncol Biol Phys* 2004;60:1385–1392.
70. Hanrahan EO, Broglio KR, Buzdar AU, et al. Combined-modality treatment for isolated recurrences of breast carcinoma: Update on 30 years of experience at the University of Texas M.D. Anderson Cancer Center and assessment of prognostic factors. *Cancer* 2005;104:1158–1171.
71. Harris JR, Halpin-Murphy P, McNeese M, et al. Consensus statement on postmastectomy radiation therapy. *Int J Rad Oncol Biol Phys* 1999;44:989–990.
72. Haylock BJ, Coppin CM, Jackson J, et al. Locoregional first recurrence after mastectomy: Prospective cohort studies with and without immediate chemotherapy. *Int J Radiat Oncol Biol Phys* 2000;46:355–362.
73. Henderson IC, Berry DA, Demetri GD, et al. Improved outcomes from adding sequential paclitaxel but not from escalating doxorubicin dose in an adjuvant chemotherapy regimen for patients with node-positive primary breast cancer. *J Clin Oncol* 2003;21:976–983.
74. Hortobagyi GN, Singletany EA, Buchholz TA. Locally advanced breast cancer. In: Singletary SE, Robb GL, GN H, eds. *Advanced therapy of breast disease*, 2nd ed. Hammilton, Ontario: B.C. Decker, Inc., 2004;498–508.
75. Howell A, Cuzick J, Baum M, et al. Results of the ATAC (Arimidex, tamoxifen, alone or in combination) trial after completion of 5 years' adjuvant treatment for breast cancer. *Lancet* 2005;365:60–62.
76. Huang E, Buchholz TA, Meric F, et al. Classifying local disease recurrences after breast conservation therapy based on location and histology: New primary tumors have more favorable outcomes than true local disease recurrences. *Cancer* 2002;95:2059–2067.
77. Huang E, McNeese MD, Strom EA, et al. Locoregional treatment outcomes for inoperable anthracycline-resistant breast cancer. *Int J Radiat Oncol Biol Phys* 2002;53:1225–1233.
78. Huang EH, Strom EA, Perkins GH, et al. Comparison of risk of local-regional recurrence after mastectomy or breast conservation therapy for patients treated with neoadjuvant chemotherapy and radiation stratified according to a prognostic index score. *Int J Radiat Oncol Biol Phys* 2006;352–357.
79. Huang EH, Tucker SL, Strom EA, et al. Postmastectomy radiation improves local-regional control and survival for selected patients with locally advanced breast cancer treated with neoadjuvant chemotherapy and mastectomy. *J Clin Oncol* 2004;22:4691–4699.
80. Joensuu H, Kellokumpu-Lehtinen PL, Bono P, et al. Adjuvant docetaxel or vinorelbine with or without trastuzumab for breast cancer. *N Engl J Med* 2006;354:809–820.
81. Katz A, Strom EA, Buchholz TA, et al. Loco-regional recurrence patterns following mastectomy and doxorubicin-based chemotherapy: Implications for postoperative irradiation. *J Clin Oncol* 2000;18:2817–2827.
82. Katz A, Strom EA, Buchholz TA, et al. The influence of pathologic tumor characteristics on locoregional recurrence rates following mastectomy. *Int J Rad Oncol Biol Phys* 2001;50:735–742.
83. Kaufmann M, Hortobagyi GN, Goldhirsch A, et al. Recommendations from an international expert panel on the use of neoadjuvant (primary) systemic treatment of operable breast cancer: An update. *J Clin Oncol* 2006;24:1940–1949.
84. Kleer CG, Zhang Y, Pan Q, et al. WISP3 and RhoC guanosine triphosphatase cooperate in the development of inflammatory breast cancer. *Breast Cancer Res* 2004;6:R110–R115.
85. Knapper WH. Management of occult breast cancer presenting as an axillary metastasis. *Semin Surg Oncol* 1991;7:311–313.
86. Komoike Y, Motomura K, Inaji H, et al. Repeat lumpectomy for patients with ipsilateral breast tumor recurrence after breast-conserving surgery. Preliminary results. *Oncology* 2003;64:1–6.
87. Krutchik AN, Buzdar AU, Blumenschein GR, et al. Combined chemoimmunotherapy and radiation therapy of inflammatory breast carcinoma. *J Surg Oncol* 1979;11:325–332.
88. Kuerer HM, Newman LA, Smith TL, et al. Clinical course of breast cancer patients with complete pathologic primary tumor and axillary lymph node response to doxorubicin-based neoadjuvant chemotherapy. *J Clin Oncol* 1999;17:460–469.
89. Kuerer HM, Sahin AA, Hunt KK, et al. Incidence and impact of documented eradication of breast cancer axillary lymph node metastases before surgery in patients treated with neoadjuvant chemotherapy. *Ann Surg* 1999;230:72–78.
90. Levine P, Steinhorn S, Ries L, et al. Inflammatory breast cancer. The experience of the Surveillance Epidemiology and End Results (SEER) program. *J Natl Cancer Inst* 1985;74:291–297.
91. Li CL, Malone KE, Daling JR. Differences in breast cancer hormone receptor status and histology by race and ethnicity among women 50 years of age and older. *Cancer Epidemiol Biomarkers Prev* 2002;11:601–607.
92. Liao Z, Strom EA, Buzdar AU, et al. Locoregional irradiation for inflammatory breast cancer: Effectiveness of dose escalation in decreasing recurrence. *Int J Radiat Oncol Biol Phys* 2000;47:1191–1200.
93. Liengsawangwong R, Yu T, Sun T, et al. Treatment optimization using Computed Tomography delineated targets should be used for supraclavicular radiation in breast cancer. *Int J Rad Oncol Biol Phys* 2006; in press.
94. Low JA, Berman AW, Steinberg SM, et al. Long-term follow-up for locally advanced and inflammatory breast cancer patients treated with multimodality therapy. *J Clin Oncol* 2004;22:4067–4074.
95. Mamounas EP, Brown A, Anderson S, et al. Sentinel node biopsy after neoadjuvant chemotherapy in breast cancer: Results from National Surgical Adjuvant Breast and Bowel Project Protocol B-27. *J Clin Oncol* 2005;23:2694–2702.
96. Mamounas EP, Bryant J, Lembersky BC, et al. Paclitaxel following doxorubicin/cyclophosphamide as adjuvant chemotherapy for node-positive breast cancer: Results from NSABP B-28. *Proc Annu Meet Am Soc Clin Oncol* 2003;22:(abstr 12).
97. Martin M, Peienkowski T, Mackey JR, et al. TAC improves disease free survival and overall survival over FAC in node positive early breast cancer patients, BCIRG 001: 55 months follow-up. *Breast Cancer Res Treat* 2003;82:A43(abstr).
98. Mauri D, Pavlidis N, Ioannidis JP. Neoadjuvant versus adjuvant systemic treatment in breast cancer: A meta-analysis. *J Natl Cancer Inst* 2005;97:188–194.
99. Mauriac L, MacGrogan G, Avril A, et al. Neoadjuvant chemotherapy for operable breast carcinoma larger than 3 cm: A unicentre randomized trial with a 124-month median follow-up. *Ann Oncol* 1999;10:47–52.
100. Moran SL, Serletti JM, Fox I. Immediate free TRAM reconstruction in lumpectomy and radiation failure patients. *Plast Reconstr Surg* 2000;106:1527–1531.
101. Motwani SB, Strom EA, Schechter NR, et al. The impact of immediate breast reconstruction on the technical delivery of postmastectomy radiotherapy. *Int J Radiat Oncol Biol Phys* 2006;76–82.
102. Nielsen HM, Overgaard M, Grau C, et al. Loco-regional recurrence after mastectomy in high-risk breast cancer—risk and prognosis. An analysis of patients from the DBCG 82 b&c randomization trials. *Radiother Oncol* 2006;79:147–155.
103. Nielsen HM, Overgaard M, Grau C, et al. Study of failure pattern among high-risk breast cancer patients with or without postmastectomy radiotherapy in addition to adjuvant systemic therapy: Long-term results from the Danish Breast Cancer Cooperative Group DBCG 82 b and c randomized studies. *J Clin Oncol* 2006;24:2268–2275.
104. Ottini L, Masala G, D'Amico C, et al. BRCA1 and BRCA2 mutation status and tumor characteristics in male breast cancer: A population-based study in Italy. *Cancer Res* 2003;63:342–347.
105. Overgaard M, Hansen PS, Overgaard J, et al. Postoperative radiotherapy in high-risk premenopausal women with breast cancer who receive adjuvant chemotherapy. *N Engl J Med* 1997;337:949–955.
106. Overgaard M, Jensen MB, Overgaard J, et al. Randomized trail evaluating postoperative radiotherapy in high risk postmenopausal breast cancer patients given adjuvant tamoxifen: Results from the DBCG 82c trial. *Lancet* 1999;353:1641–1648.
107. Panades M, Olivotto IA, Speers CH, et al. Evolving treatment strategies for inflammatory breast cancer: A population-based survival analysis. *J Clin Oncol* 2005;23:1941–1950.
108. Perez CA, Fields JN, Fracasso PM, et al. Management of locally advanced carcinoma of the breast. II. Inflammatory carcinoma. *Cancer* 1994;74:466–476.
109. Perez EA, Suman VJ, Davidson NE, et al. Effect of doxorubicin plus cyclophosphamide on left ventricular ejection fraction in patients with breast cancer in the North Central Cancer Treatment Group N9831 Intergroup Adjuvant Trial. *J Clin Oncol* 2004;22:3700–3704
110. Piccart-Gebhart MJ, Procter M, Leyland-Jones B, et al. Trastuzumab after adjuvant chemotherapy in HER2-positive breast cancer. *N Engl J Med* 2005;353:1659–1672.
111. Pro B, Cristofanilli M, Buzdar AU, et al. The evaluation of p53, HER-2/neu, and serial MDR protein expression as possible markers of chemoresistance and their use as prognostic markers in inflammatory breast cancer. *Proc Am Soc Clin Oncol* 1998;17:553a.
112. Ragaz J, Jackson SM, Le N, et al. Adjuvant radiotherapy and chemotherapy in node-positive premenopausal women with breast cancer. *N Engl J Med* 1997;337:956–962.
113. Ragaz J, Olivotto IA, Spinelli JJ, et al. Locoregional radiation therapy in patients with high-risk breast cancer receiving adjuvant chemotherapy: 20-year results of the British Columbia randomized trial. *J Natl Cancer Inst* 2005;97:116–126.
114. Recht A, Edge SB, Solin LJ, et al. Postmastectomy radiotherapy: Clinical practice guidelines of the American Society of Clinical Oncology. *J Clin Oncol* 2001;19:1539–1569.
115. Recht A, Gray R, Davidson NE, et al. Locoregional failure ten years after mastectomy and adjuvant chemotherapy with or without tamoxifen without irradiation: Experience of the Eastern Cooperative Oncology Group. *J Clin Oncol* 1999;17:1689–1700.
116. Resch A, Fellner C, Mock U, et al. Locally recurrent breast cancer: Pulse dose rate brachytherapy for repeat irradiation following lumpectomy—a second chance to preserve the breast. *Radiology* 2002;225:713–718.
117. Ribeiro G, Swindell R. Adjuvant tamoxifen for male breast cancer (MBC). *Br J Cancer* 1992;65:252–254.
118. Romond EH, Perez EA, Bryant J, et al. Trastuzumab plus adjuvant chemotherapy for operable HER2-positive breast cancer. *N Engl J Med* 2005;353:1673–1684.
119. Rouizer R, Extra JM, Carton M, et al. Primary chemotherapy for operable breast cancer: Incidence and prognostic significance of ipsilateral breast tumor recurrence after breast-conserving surgery. *J Clin Oncol* 2001;19:3828–3835.
120. Rouzier R, Pusztai L, Delaloge S, et al. Nomograms to predict pathologic complete response and metastasis-free survival after preoperative chemotherapy for breast cancer. *J Clin Oncol* 2005;23:8331–8339.
121. Salvadori B, Marubini E, Miceli R, et al. Reoperation for locally recurrent breast cancer in patients previously treated with conservative surgery. *Br J Surg* 1999;86:84–87.
122. Singletary SE, Greene FL. Revision of breast cancer staging: The 6th edition of the TNM Classification. *Semin Surg Oncol* 2003;21:53–59.
123. Singletary SE, McNeese MD, Hortobagyi GN. Feasibility of breast-conservation surgery after induction chemotherapy for locally advanced breast carcinoma. *Cancer* 1992;69:2849–2852.
124. Slamon D, Eiermann W, Robert N, et al. Phase III randomized trial comparing doxorubicin and cyclophosphamide followed by docetaxel (AC T) with doxorubicin and cyclophosphamide followed by docetaxel and trastuzumab (AC TH) with docetaxel, carboplatin and trastuzumab (TCH) in HER2 positive early breast cancer patients: BCIRG 006 study. *Breast Cancer Res Treat* 2005;94[Suppl 1]: (abstr 1).
125. Smith BD, Smith GL, Haffty BG, et al. Postmastectomy radiation and mortality in women with T1–2 node-positive breast cancer. *J Clin Oncol* 2005;23:1409–1419.
126. Smith IE, Dowsett M, Ebbs SR, et al. Neoadjuvant treatment of postmenopausal breast cancer with anastrozole, tamoxifen, or both in combination: The Immediate Preoperative Anastrozole, Tamoxifen, or Combined with Tamoxifen (IMPACT) multicenter double-blind randomized trial. *J Clin Oncol* 2005;23:5108–5116.
127. Smith TE, Lee D, Turner BC, et al. True recurrence vs. new primary ipsilateral breast tumor relapse: An analysis of clinical and pathologic differences and their implications in natural history, prognoses, and therapeutic management. *Int J Radiat Oncol Biol Phys* 2000;48:1281–1289.
128. Spear SL, Onyewu C. Staged breast reconstruction with saline-filled implants in the irradiated breast: Recent trends and therapeutic implications. *Plast Reconstr Surg* 2000;105:930–942.

129. Strom EA, Woodward WA, Katz A, et al. Clinical investigation: Regional nodal failure patterns in breast cancer patients treated with mastectomy without radiotherapy. *Int J Radiat Oncol Biol Phys* 2005;63:1508–1513.

130. Swain SM, Lippman ME. Treatment of patients with inflammatory breast cancer. *Important Adv Oncol* 1989;129–150.

131. Swain SM, Sorace RA, Bagley CS, et al. Neoadjuvant chemotherapy in the combined modality approach of locally advanced nonmetastatic breast cancer. *Cancer Res* 1987;47:3889–3894.

132. Taghian A, Jeong JH, Mamounas E, et al. Patterns of locoregional failure in patients with operable breast cancer treated by mastectomy and adjuvant chemotherapy with or without tamoxifen and without radiotherapy: Results from five National Surgical Adjuvant Breast and Bowel Project randomized clinical trials. *J Clin Oncol* 2004;22:4247–4254.

133. Taghian AG, Jeong JH, Mamounas EP, et al. Low locoregional recurrence rate among node-negative breast cancer patients with tumors 5 cm or larger treated by mastectomy, with or without adjuvant systemic therapy and without radiotherapy: Results from five National Surgical Adjuvant Breast and Bowel project randomized clinical trials. *J Clin Oncol* 2006;24:3927–3932.

134. Thurlimann B, Keshaviah A, Coates AS, et al. A comparison of letrozole and tamoxifen in postmenopausal women with early breast cancer. *N Engl J Med* 2005;353:2747–2757.

135. Tran NV, Chang DW, Gupta A, et al. Comparison of immediate and delayed free TRAM flap breast reconstruction in patients receiving postmastectomy radiation therapy. *Plast Reconstr Surg* 2001;108:78–82.

136. Trends in Worldwide Mortality Age-adjusted Rates; 2006;136.

137. Truong PT, Olivotto IA, Kader HA, et al. Selecting breast cancer patients with T1-T2 tumors and one to three positive axillary nodes at high postmastectomy locoregional recurrence risk for adjuvant radiotherapy. *Int J Radiat Oncol Biol Phys* 2005;61:1337–1347.

138. Urban JA, Marjani MA. Significance of internal mammary lymph node metastases in breast cancer. *Am J Roentgenol Radium Ther Nucl Med* 1971;111:130–136.

139. Van de Steene J, Soete G, Storme G. Adjuvant radiotherapy for breast cancer significantly improves overall survival: The missing link. *Radiother Oncol* 2000;55:263–272.

140. Van der Hage JA, Cornelis JH, van de Velde CJ, et al. Preoperative chemotherapy in primary operable breast cancer: Results from the European Organization for Research and Treatment of Cancer trial 10902. *J Clin Oncol* 2001;19:4224–4237.

141. Van Golen KL, Davies S, Wu ZF, et al. A novel putative low-affinity insulin-like growth factor-binding protein, LIBC (lost in inflammatory breast cancer), and RhoC GTPase correlate with the inflammatory breast cancer phenotype. *Clin Cancer Res* 1999;5:2511–2519.

142. Vezzoni P, Balestrazzi A, Bignami P, et al. Axillary lymph node metastases from occult carcinoma of the breast. *Tumori* 1979;65:87–91.

143. Vlastos G, Jean ME, Mirza AN, et al. Feasibility of breast preservation in the treatment of occult primary carcinoma presenting with axillary metastases. *Ann Surg Oncol* 2001;8:425–431.

144. Wallgren A, Bonetti M, Gelber RD, et al. Risk factors for locoregional recurrence among breast cancer patients: Results from International Breast Cancer Study Group Trials I through VII. *J Clin Oncol* 2003;21:1205–1213.

145. Whelan TJ, Julian J, Wright J, et al. Does locoregional radiation therapy improve survival in breast cancer? A meta-analysis. *J Clin Oncol* 2000;18:1220–1229.

146. Wingo PA, Jamison PM, Young JL, et al. Population-based statistics for women diagnosed with inflammatory breast cancer (United States). *Cancer Causes Control* 2004;15:321–328.

147. Wolmark N, Wang J, Mamounas E, et al. Preoperative chemotherapy in patients with operable breast cancer: Nine-year results from National Surgical Adjuvant Breast and Bowel Project B-18. *Cancer* 2001;30:96–102.

148. Woodward WA, Oh JL, Strom EA, et al. Maximizing curative potential for patients with isolated supraclavicular nodal recurrence after mastectomy and doxorubicin-base chemotherapy for breast cancer. *Proc Am Radium Soc* 2005;47 (abstr 67).

149. Woodward WA, Strom EA, Tucker SL, et al. Changes in the 2003 American Joint Committee on Cancer staging for breast cancer dramatically affect stage-specific survival. *J Clin Oncol* 2003;21:3244–3248.

150. Woodward WA, Strom EA, Tucker SL, et al. Locoregional recurrence after doxorubicin-based chemotherapy and postmastectomy radiation: Implications for patients with early stage disease and predictors for recurrence after radiation. *Int J Rad Oncol Biol Phys* 2003;57:336–344.

151. Xing Y, Foy M, Cox DD, et al. Meta-analysis of sentinel lymph node biopsy after preoperative chemotherapy in patients with breast cancer. *Br J Surg* 2006;93:539–546.

152. Zucali R, Uslenghi C, Kenda R, et al. Natural history and survival of inoperable breast cancer treated with radiotherapy and radiotherapy followed by radical mastectomy. *Cancer* 1976;37:1422–1431.

Clinical Radiation Oncology

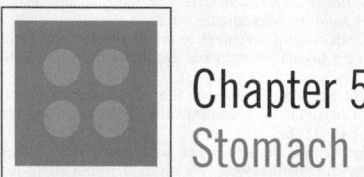

Chapter 55
Stomach

Christopher G. Willett, Leonard L. Gunderson

Anatomy

The stomach begins at the gastroesophageal (GE) junction, ends at the pylorus, and is apportioned into three parts. The cranial portion is the fundus (cardia). A plane passing through the incisura angularis on the lesser curvature divides the remainder of the stomach into the body and the pyloric portion (antrum). The anterior surface of the stomach is covered with peritoneum of the greater sac. At the left and cranially, it abuts the diaphragm. In view of the increasing incidence of gastric cancer at the GE junction, it is important to note that there is either no or variable visceral peritoneal covering at the most proximal portion of the GE junction (J;)). Positive radial margins at this site are often "true" positive margins, whereas many other positive margins in the stomach are free serosal margins unless the tumor is adherent to an adjacent organ or structure. The right portion of the anterior gastric surface is adjacent to the left lobe of the liver and the anterior abdominal wall. Posteriorly, the stomach is covered with peritoneum of the lesser sac or omental bursa. The stomach contacts many visceral structures; from superior to inferior, it is adjacent to the spleen, left adrenal gland, superior portion of the left kidney, ventral portion of the pancreas, and transverse colon. The hepatogastric ligament or lesser omentum is attached to the lesser curvature and contains the left gastric artery and the right gastric branch of the hepatic artery.

The stomach's vascular supply is derived from the celiac axis. The celiac artery usually has three branches: the left gastric artery, which supplies the upper right portion of the stomach; the common hepatic artery, which gives rise to the right gastric artery supplying the lower right portion of the stomach and the right gastroepiploic branch supplying the lower portion of the greater curvature; and the splenic artery, which gives rise to the left gastroepiploic supplying the upper portion of the greater curvature and the short gastric arteries supplying the fundus. Variations in this normal vascular supply are common. The celiac axis originates at or below the pedicle of T12 in approximately 75% of patients and at or above the pedicle of L1 in 25% of patients (74). The lymphatic drainage of the stomach follows the arterial supply. Although most lymphatics drain ultimately to the celiac nodal area, lymph-drainage sites can include the splenic hilum, supra-pancreatic nodal groups, porta hepatis, and gastroduodonal areas.

Epidemiology

Gastric cancer afflicted approximately 22,286 people in the United States in 2006 and resulted in about 11,430 deaths (56). During the past 60 years, there has been a significant decline in the incidence of gastric cancer in both sexes in Western countries. The causes of this decline are unknown (69,128). Although the overall decrease in gastric cancer incidence is encouraging, there has been a steady and rapid increase in the incidence of proximal and GE junction tumors over the past 20 years, especially in white males.

Risk factors implicated include high intake of smoked and salted foods, low intake of fruits and vegetables, low socioeconomic status, and decreased use of refrigeration (22,69). Pernicious anemia is associated with gastric cancer, with 5% to 10% of patients with pernicious anemia developing malignancies. Prior subtotal gastrectomy for benign lesions also carries a 2% to 5% risk of subsequent malignancies, with latency periods of 15 to 40 years (107). Villous adenomas are clearly premalignant; hyperplastic or hamartomatous polyps occur more frequently and are apparently benign. Gastric ulcers, per se, carry no increased risk, although previous distal gastrotomy for benign disease confers a 1.5- to threefold relative risk for development of gastric cancer, with a latency period of 15 to 20 years. The presence of *Helicobacter pylori* is associated with a three to six times greater risk of gastric cancer than if infection is absent. The increased association of *H. pylori* appears to be confined to those with distal gastric cancer and intestinal-type malignancy (46). Although this newly discovered association of *H. pylori* infection with gastric cancer may provide new insight into the pathogenesis of this tumor, only a small minority of infected people develop gastric carcinoma, and there are no known data regarding the screening of infected patients or the effect of treatment of infection on subsequent malignancy.

Patterns of Spread

Cancer of the stomach may extend directly into the omenta, pancreas, diaphragm, transverse colon or mesocolon, and

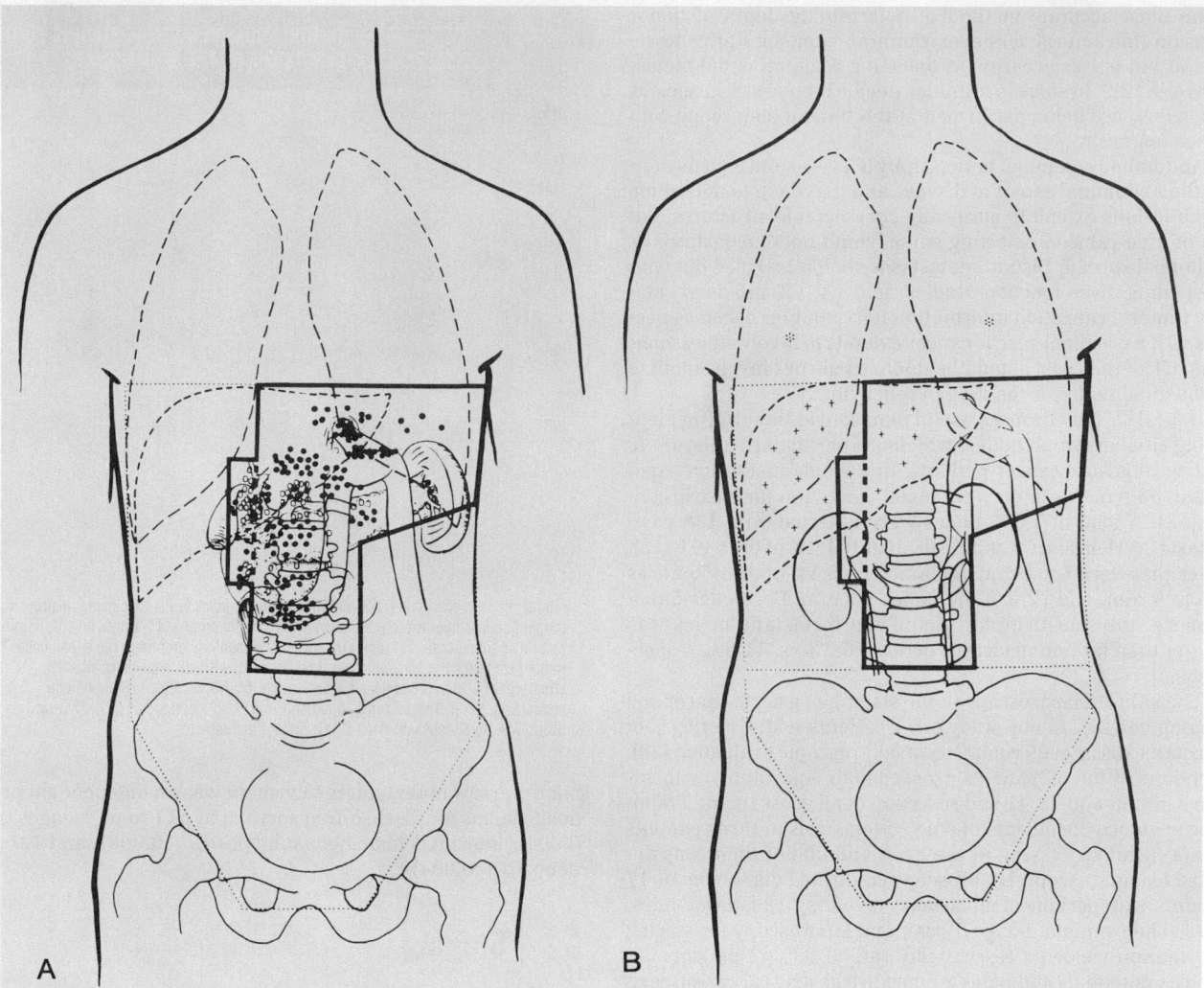

FIGURE 55.1. Patterns of failure in 82 evaluable patients in the University of Minnesota Reoperation series. **A:** Large bold circles indicate local failures in surrounding organs or tissues; large open circles indicate lymph node failures. **B:** Asterisk (*) indicates lung metastasis; plus (+) indicates liver metastasis. Superimposed irradiation portals encompass postsurgical gastric remnant, anastomoses, duodenal stump, gastric bed structures, and primary and secondary areas of lymph node drainage; broken lines represent upper and total abdomen fields. (From Gunderson LL, Sosin H. Adenocarcinoma of the stomach: areas of failure in a reoperation series [second or symptomatic looks]. Clinicopathologic correlation and implications for adjuvant therapy. *Int J Radiat Oncol Biol Phys* 1982;8:1, with permission.)

duodenum. Peritoneal contamination is possible after a lesion extends beyond the gastric wall to a free peritoneal (serosal) surface (101).

Microscopic or subclinical spread beyond the visible gross lesion occurs frequently because of the abundant lymphatic channels within the submucosal and subserosal layers of the gastric wall. The submucosal plexus is prominent in the esophagus and the subserosal plexus in the duodenum, allowing proximal and distal spread.

It is difficult to do a complete node dissection because of the numerous pathways of lymphatic drainage from the stomach (Fig. 55.1A). Initial drainage is to lymph nodes along the lesser and greater curvatures (i.e., gastric and gastroepiploic nodes) but also includes the celiac axis (i.e., porta hepatis, splenic suprapancreatic, and pancreaticoduodenal nodes), adjacent para-aortics, and distal paraesophageal system.

Gastric venous drainage is primarily to the liver by the portal system. Liver involvement is found in as many as 30% of patients at initial exploration, and it can occur as a result of both venous metastasis and direct extension (see Fig. 55.1B).

Clinical Presentation

The most common presenting symptoms are loss of appetite, abdominal discomfort, weight loss, weakness from anemia, nausea and vomiting, and tarry stools. Duration of symptoms is <3 months in almost 40% of patients and >1 year in 20%. Physical examination can reveal advanced disease, for which the presentation may be an abdominal mass (epigastric mass or liver), palpable left supraclavicular nodes, or a rectal shelf (peritoneal seeding).

Diagnostic Work-Up

Diagnosis usually is confirmed by upper gastrointestinal (GI) radiography and endoscopy. Double-contrast x-ray studies may reveal small lesions limited to the inner layers of the gastric wall. Endoscopy with direct vision, cytology, and biopsy yields the diagnosis in 90% or more of exophytic lesions, but infiltrative (linitis plastica), small (<3 cm), or cardia lesions are more difficult to diagnose endoscopically. Endoscopic ultrasonography is the most accurate method of determining depth of tumor invasion (intramural versus extramural extension) prior to resection but is less accurate in detecting regional nodal metastases (19,122). In some institutions needle biopsies of suspicious nodes now are being performed at the time of endoscopy with ultrasonography.

Abdominal computed tomography (CT) is useful in determining the abdominal extent of disease and may help to determine which lesions extend to surgically unresectable structures, but it is of little value in detecting small lymph node metastases or peritoneal spread. Distant metastases should be ruled out with chest films, liver function studies, and CT. CT provides valuable tumor localization information if irradiation becomes necessary. If a proximal gastric cancer extends to involve the esophagus, CT of the chest should be done to rule out involvement of mediastinal nodes or the lung parenchyma.

Helical CT may be more useful than conventional CT in identifying smaller lymph nodes, which are particularly relevant to staging of gastric cancer patients. In a single-institution experience, 58 patients underwent nodal dissection for gastric cancer (48). A total of 1,082 nodes were resected, and 138 were metastatic. Helical CT was able to identify 1.1% of the 649 lymph nodes that were 1 to 4 mm in diameter, 45.1% of the 355 nodes of 5 to 9 mm, and 72% of the nodes >9 mm. For nodes 5 mm or more, the sensitivity for identifying metastatic nodes was greater than for nonmetastatic nodes (75.2% vs. 41.8%, respectively).

The value of laparoscopy in the staging of gastric cancer still is being defined. In one study of 71 patients with CT criteria of resectable disease, 69 completed a laparoscopic evaluation (88). Forty-one of the 69 patients proceeded to laparotomy with curative intent, and 38/41 had resection of all gross tumor. Pathologic evidence documented hepatic metastasis in three patients with a negative CT scan of the liver, and one of them was detected by laparoscopy. Laparoscopy confirmed disease in 16/17 patients with peritoneal metastases (avoiding 12 laparotomies, 17%). The combination of CT scan and laparoscopy for staging information yielded a resectability rate of 93% in patients defined as potential candidates for curative gastric cancer surgery.

Treatment planning in gastric cancer patients would be improved by accurate preoperative classifications of key prognostic factors, especially depth of invasion (T category) and lymph node involvement (N category). A prospective study in 108 patients evaluated endogastric ultrasonography, CT, and intraoperative surgical assessment for T and N classification (154). Staging of the T category was correct with CT in 43% of the cases, with endoscopic ultrasonography in 86% of cases, and with intraoperative assessment in 56% of cases. Staging of N1 and N2 lymph nodes was correct with CT in 51% of the cases, with endoscopic ultrasound in 74%, and with intraoperative assessment in 54%. Advanced gastric tumors tended to be more accurately staged with CT; CT in general overstages the T category and understages the N category. Endoscopic ultrasound showed a high and similar accuracy for all the T categories, although it also tended to understage N categories. Finally, intraoperative assessment was equally accurate for all N categories, but tended to overstage early T stages and to understage N categories.

A report has analyzed prospectively the potential involvement of bone marrow at the time of radical surgery after obtaining material through aspiration and the use of monoclonal antibody CK-2 directed to component 18 of the intracellular cytokeratin (71). Among the 180 patients evaluated, 53% had a positive test for the presence of malignant cells in the bone marrow. The finding was correlated with pT ($p = 0.07$) and Borrmann's classification ($p = 0.02$) (13). The estimation of tumor cell contents in the bone marrow ($<3 \times 10^{(6)}$) was related significantly to overall and disease-free survival ($p = 0.04$ and $p <0.007$, respectively). The multivariate analyses detected that

	TUMOR, NODE, METASTASIS STAGING FOR
Table 55.1	**CARCINOMA OF THE STOMACH**

Stage	T[a]	N[a]	M[a]
0	Tis	0	0
IA	1	0	0
IB	1	1	0
	2	0	0
II	1	2	0
	2	1	0
	3	0	0
IIIA	2	2	0
	3	1	0
	4	0	0
IIIB	3	2	0
	4	1	0
IV	4	2	0
	1–3	3	0
	4	2–3	0
	Any	Any	0

[a]Tumor, node, metastasis (TNM) definitions are as follows: Tis, carcinoma in situ; intraepithelial tumor without invasion of the lamina propria; T1, tumor invades lamina propria or submucosa; T2, tumor invades the muscularis propria or the submucosa; T3, tumor penetrates the serosa (visceral peritoneum) without invasion of adjacent structures; T4, tumor invades adjacent structures; N0, no regional lymph node metastasis; N1, metastasis in 1–6 regional nodes; N2, metastasis in 7–15 regional nodes; M0, no distant metastasis; M1, distant metastasis.

bone marrow malignant involvement was an independent prognostic factor for disease-free survival in pT1 to pT2 stages ($p = 0.004$), intestinal histologic subtypes ($p <0.008$), and N0 patients ($p = 0.004$).

Staging

The current tumor, node, metastasis (TNM) system is depicted in Tables 55.1 and 55.2 (41). Portions of this system are compared with a modification of the Astler-Coller rectal system, which is suitable for all alimentary tract carcinomas (see Table 55.2) (57). The Astler-Coller system better describes the degree of extension beyond the wall (e.g., T3 includes any degree of extension beyond the serosa), but the TNM system better describes nodal involvement and the level of gastric invasion in lesions confined to the wall.

Pathology

Adenocarcinomas account for 90% to 95% of all gastric malignancies. Lymphomas, usually with an unfavorable histology, are the second most common malignancies. Rarely, leiomyosarcomas (2%), carcinoid tumors (1%), adenoacanthomas (1%), and squamous cell carcinomas (1%) occur.

The site of origin of gastric cancers within the stomach has changed in frequency in the United States over recent decades, and proximal lesions are being diagnosed and treated more frequently. Although the highest frequency is still in the antrum/distal stomach ($\sim 40\%$), the lowest frequency is now in the body rather than proximal portion of the stomach ($\sim 25\%$), with intermediate frequency in the proximal stomach and GE junction ($\sim 35\%$). Several investigators have reported an increased frequency of cardia lesions. Cardia lesions may have different epidemiologic factors, exhibit different tumor biology, and have an inferior prognosis from lesions in the other sites (64,73,90,96,151).

Table 55.2   STAGING SYSTEMS FOR GASTRIC CARCINOMA[a]

Staging System[b]		
Modified Astler-Coller	TNM	Characteristics
A	T1N0	Nodes negative; lesion limited to mucosa
B1	T2N0	Nodes negative; extension of lesion beyond mucosa but still within gastric wall
B2	T3N0	Nodes negative; extension beyond the entire wall (including serosa if present)
B3	T4N0	Node negative; beyond wall with adherence to or invasion of surrounding organs or structures
C1	Tis-2N1–3	Nodes positive; lesion limited to gastric wall
C2	T3N1–3	Nodes positive; extension of lesion through the entire wall (including serosa, if present)
C3	T4N1–3	Nodes positive; beyond wall with adherence to or invasion of surrounding organs or structures

[a]Also see Table 55.1.
[b]Comparison of tumor, node, metastasis (TNM) system (41) with a modification of the Astler-Coller rectal system by Gunderson and Sosin (59).

Gastric cancers sometimes are categorized according to Borrmann's five types. Type I tumors are polypoid or fungating; type II are ulcerating lesions surrounded by elevated borders; type III have ulceration with invasion of the gastric wall; type IV are diffusely infiltrating (linitis plastica); and type V are unclassifiable (13).

Prognostic Factors

The most important prognostic indicators reflect tumor extent. If hematogenous or transperitoneal spread is present, the outcome is uniformly fatal. Survival rates decrease with progressive tumor extension within or beyond the gastric wall (29,59,64,77). Lymph node involvement is important, as are the number and locations of nodes affected (31,64,77,100). Minimal node involvement adjacent to the primary lesion only moderately affects prognosis (29,93,100). The finding of either involved lymph nodes or complete wall penetration is usually not as ominous as the presence of both (Table 55.3) (29,57,77,100).

Flow cytometry is also prognostically valuable; aneuploidy is associated with unfavorable tumor location, lymph node metastasis, and primary tumor invasion (6,83,102). Unfavorable DNA flow cytometry correlates with a poor prognosis (6,85,104). The prognosis is worse for cardia lesions, and flow cytometry reveals a greater incidence of aneuploidy (102). The gross pathologic appearance of the primary lesion also reveals prognostic information, although it is not known whether this factor is independent of tumor stage. Patients with Borrmann type I and II tumors have relatively favorable 5-year survival rates, but patients with type IV (linitis plastica) fare poorly (4,5,93,142).

The molecular biology of gastric cancer reflects the heterogeneity of its causes and its histologic subtypes. Identification of the genetic and phenotypic variables existing among gastric cancers may lead to more directed therapeutic approaches and a more accurate prediction of clinical outcome. Changes that may affect the behavior of gastric tumor cells involve four major types of alterations. Loss of tumor suppressor gene function, especially inactivation of the p53 gene, certainly plays a critical role. The p53 gene is located on the short arm of chromosome 17 and plays a key role in tumor suppression and cell-cycle regulation (40). The p53 gene puts a brake on DNA replication and triggers programmed cell death in response to DNA damage (86). Loss of p53 function allows malignancy to develop, affects the effectiveness of chemotherapy and irradiation, and predisposes cells to genetic instability (75,106). The latter is particularly important because p53 mutations occur early (38).

A second major aberration affecting gastric epithelial cells is the impact of alterations in mismatch repair genes. Two such genes, hMSH3 and hMLH1, on chromosome 2 and 3, respectively, account for replication errors throughout the genome.

Table 55.3   EXTENT OF INITIAL DISEASE COMPARED WITH SURVIVAL RATES FOR CANCER OF THE STOMACH

Extent of Disease	5-Year Survival Rate (%)		≥5-Year Disease-Free Survival Rate (%)
	Dockerty (29)[a]	Kennedy (77)	Univ. of Minnesota Reoperation Series (59)
Negative Lymph Nodes			
Mucosa only	100	85	—
Beyond mucosa but within wall	61	52	—
Through wall	44	47	—
Positive Lymph Nodes			
Nodal extent	15	—	19
Regional only	—	17	—
Nonregional	—	6	—
Extent of Primary			
Within wall	—	—	40
Through wall	—	—	12

[a]Percentages are of those patients who left the hospital.

Mutations in these genes are implicated in cancer family syndromes and hereditary nonpolyposis colorectal cancer, a disease associated with an increased tendency for the development of gastric tumors (89). Mutations in these genes generate genetic instability and have the potential to lead to further alterations in oncogenes.

Two proto-oncogenes, C-met and K-sam, associate with scirrhous carcinoma of the stomach. The former encodes hepatocyte growth factor, which is a potent endogenous promoter of gastric epithelial cell growth (138). Its overexpression correlates with tumor progression and metastasis (137). The latter encodes a tyrosine kinase receptor family (137). In scirrhous carcinoma, c-met and k-sam amplification may occur independently. There is a tendency for k-sam to be activated in women younger than 40 years of age and c-met to be amplified in men older than 50 years of age (38,136).

Peptide receptors, including estrogen receptors and epidermal growth factor receptors, are associated with adverse prognoses (63,135). Epidermal growth factor receptors and epidermal growth factor levels correlate with higher rates of primary tumor infiltration, poorer histologic differentiation, and linitis plastica (152). The pathophysiologic relation between these peptide receptors and their association with poor prognoses is not understood.

Modern molecular biology observations confirm the heterogeneity of human gastric cancer. Genetic alterations detected and potentially associated with a worse prognosis include CD44 expression; telomerase reactivation; p53 gene inactivation; dysfunction of repair genes such as hMSH2 and hMLH1; overexpression of proto-oncogenes such as erb-B2, bcl-2, c-met, and k-sam; estrogenic receptor expression; and presence of viral genome (67). Gastric cancers with class II major histocompatibility complex antigen expression have a better prognosis, but the loss of expression is not an independent prognostic factor (135).

General Management

Surgical Management

Operative attempts are highly successful if disease is limited to the mucosa, but the incidence of such early lesions at diagnosis is <5% in most U.S. series. In Japan, the incidence of lesions initially confined to the mucosa or submucosa was only 3.8% in 1955 and 1956, but by 1966, as a result of screening procedures, this figure had increased to 34.5%, with corresponding survival rates of 90.9% (114).

Curative or palliative surgical resection is possible for 50% to 60% of patients at the time of initial disease presentation. However, only 25% to 40% are eligible for potentially curative resection.

No prospectively randomized trials have definitively established optimal surgical therapy (78). The preferred treatment for gastric carcinoma, especially for lesions arising in the body and antrum, is a radical subtotal resection. This operation removes approximately 80% of the stomach with the node-bearing tissue, the gastrohepatic and gastrocolic omenta, and the first portion of the duodenum. Larger or more proximal lesions require total gastrectomy. There appears to be no advantage to performing total gastrectomy if subtotal gastrectomy produces satisfactory margins (i.e., 5 cm) (33,118,128). Patients treated with total gastrectomy characteristically have 5-year survival rates of 10% to 15%, and those undergoing radical subtotal gastrectomy have 5-year survival rates of 25% to 45% (31,116,126). The inferior survivorship of patients undergoing total gastrectomy probably results from the larger tumors and unfavorable proximal lesions that prompt such a procedure. The value of splenectomy has not been addressed in prospec-

	POSITIVE MARGINS IN RESECTED
Table 55.4	**LONGITUDINAL GASTRIC SPECIMENS**

Study	No. of Margins Positive/No. Resected	Percentage
Whittington et al. (150)	34/106	32
Bleiberg et al. (10)	22/111	20
Regine and Mohiuddin (117)	31/120	26
Slot et al. (132)	16/58	28
Gez et al. (52)	7/22	32
Siewert et al. (129)	71/307	23
Gill et al. (54)	1/14	7
Allum et al. (2)	78/436	16
Total	260/1074	24

tive randomized trials, but retrospective Japanese data do not support a survival benefit (37,40).

The propensity for gastric carcinoma to spread via the submucosal lymphatics suggests that a 5.0-cm margin of normal tissue proximally and distally may be optimal. It may be necessary to include a portion of esophagus or duodenum to achieve adequate margins. Frozen-section pathologic evaluation of surgical margins has been advocated to confirm their adequacy (31). The importance of careful evaluation of longitudinal margins is emphasized in a number of series (Table 55.4) that have evaluated this issue and documented positive pathologic margins in approximately one quarter of "curatively" resected specimens (2,10,50,52,115,127,130,148). The approximate 25% positive longitudinal margin correlates almost precisely with the incidence of locoregional recurrence in the anastomosis or stump, as discussed in a later section of this chapter.

The issue of positive margins is also of importance with regard to radial or circumferential margins, which at present are not carefully evaluated. The incidence of radial margin positivity is not well reported in the literature (most of the series referenced in Table 55.4 addressed longitudinal margins alone). The increasing incidence of T3 and T4 GE tumors will result in an increasing incidence of microscopically positive radial margins. Because the particular tissue surrounding the GE junction and distal esophagus has no serosa, lesions that extend to the pathologic radial margin represent a true positive margin in a large percentage of cases.

The extent of lymph node dissection is controversial. Japanese researchers advocate complete lymph node removal to improve the rates of local control and survival. Several nonrandomized clinical trials suggested that extended lymphadenectomy may improve survival (23,32,84,110,111). Others (80) reported that increasingly radical lymphadenectomies failed to improve survival or reduce the risk of locoregional failure. Four prospective randomized trials of lymphadenectomies have been reported (11,12,17,18,25,26,119) and show no survival advantage with more extensive lymph node dissection. Morbidity and mortality rates have been significantly higher for patients undergoing more extensive nodal dissection. However, other important principles of lymph node dissection have been elucidated through these trials. The first is that, as more lymph node areas are dissected and as pathologic lymph node evaluation is more compulsive, considerable stage migration occurs. This stage migration produces an apparent improvement in stage-specific survival without improvement in survival in the group overall. In series with compulsive pathologic evaluation of these nodes (18), the likelihood of discovering lymph node metastasis increases markedly in both D1 dissections, which remove only the perigastric nodal areas, and D2 procedures, which also remove the celiac axis,

Table 55.5	PATTERNS OF FAILURE AFTER "CURATIVE" RESECTION OF GASTRIC CANCER		
	Incidence in Total Patient Group (%)		
Pattern of Failure	Clinical (85)	Univ. of Minnesota Reoperation[a]	Autopsy (51,60,68,133)
Locoregional[b]	38	67	80–93
Peritoneal seeding	28	41	30–43
Localized	—	19	—
Diffuse	—	22	—
Distant metastases	52	22	49

[a]107 patients at risk.
[b]Local or regional failure on basis of direct extension of tumor, lymphatic spread, or operative wound implant;one or more distant metastases on hematologic basis; abdominal involvement on basis of peritoneal seeding or peritoneal lymphatics.

splenic artery, and splenic hilar nodes. Finally, there is a small subset of patients who have limited metastasis in the celiac axis, superior pancreatic, or retroduodenal chains and may be cured by a D2 lymph node resection (30).

Endoscopic laser surgery has been applied successfully to patients with very early gastric cancer whose tumors were inoperable because of complicating medical illness. Small lesions that are pedunculated, noninvasive, and well differentiated have lymph node metastasis in <5% of cases and can be completely removed endoscopically in 75% of cases (47). Radiation therapy with chemotherapy may be considered as adjuvant therapy.

Noncurative gastrectomies may be indicated for lesions not resectable for cure. Some unresectable tumors may be debulked successfully, with sites of minimal residual disease marked judiciously with clips. This produces palliation and permits accurate delivery of postoperative radiation therapy.

Failure Patterns after Surgical Resection

Local regrowth failures in the tumor bed and regional lymph nodes and distant failures by hematogenous or peritoneal routes are common mechanisms of failure after "curative" resection in clinical, reoperative, and autopsy series (Tables 55.5 and 55.6) (57,60,68,109,133). For GE junction lesions, the liver and lungs are common sites of distant metastases. With gastric lesions that do not extend to the esophagus, the initial site of distant metastasis is usually the liver, and many failures could be prevented if an effective abdominal treatment could be combined with treatment to the tumor-node region. In the series of Landry et al. (85), 50/88 (57%) failing patients had disease progression within the abdomen only (97). Abdominal treatment also could address peritoneal seeding, which occurs in 23% to 43% of postgastrectomy patients (51,58,60,68,85,95,109,133).

Table 55.6	PATTERNS OF LOCOREGIONAL FAILURE AFTER RESECTION OF GASTRIC CANCER		
	Incidence(%)		
Failure Area	Clinical[a]	Reoperation[b]	Autopsy[c]
Gastric bed	21	54	52–68
Anastomosis or stumps	25	26	54–60
Abdominal or stab wound	—	5	—
Lymph node(s)	8	42	52

[a]130 patients at risk (95).
[b]107 patients at risk (57).
[c]92 patients at risk (133) and 28 patients at risk (51).

Locoregional failures occur commonly in organs and structures of the gastric bed and in lymph nodes (see Table 55.6). Failures in the anastomoses, gastric remnant, or duodenal stump also are frequent, as suggested by the incidence of positive longitudinal resection margins (see Table 55.4). As is true for most sites, clinical series underestimate the true incidence of locoregional failure when compared with reoperative or autopsy series (see Table 55.5). Progressive extension of the operative procedure to include routine splenectomy, omentectomy, and radical lymph node dissection neither improved survival nor decreased the incidence of locoregional failures in the University of Minnesota series (51,57). Subsequent failure in areas of initial node dissection occurred frequently, even with radical node dissections (57). The high rate of regional node relapse provides a partial explanation for the lack of survival benefit with a D2 (extended lymphadenectomy) versus D1 (limited lymphadenectomy) node dissection in the previously discussed phase III surgical trials.

Indications for Radiation Therapy

The results of the U.S. GI Intergroup Gastric Adjuvant Trial has changed the standard of care in the United States to the use of both chemotherapy and radiation therapy in the postoperative setting for patients with disease extension through the gastric wall and/or with nodes positive for tumor (91). Postoperative irradiation plus concurrent and maintenance 5FU (fluorouracil)–based chemotherapy is recommended for patients with stage IB, II, IIIA, IIIB, or IV with M0 gastric cancer (91). Quality control (QC) of irradiation field design was conducted during the cycle of chemotherapy given before the start of concurrent chemoirradiation (134). The up-front QC provided the mechanism to correct most of the major or minor deviations (35% incidence) in irradiation field design before the start of treatment and resulted in only a 6.5% final major deviation rate.

Radiation therapy, usually administered with concomitant 5FU-based chemotherapy, is indicated for locally confined gastric cancer that either is not technically resectable or occurs in medically inoperable patients. In this setting, therapy can be administered with curative or palliative intent, depending on the clinical situation. Those who undergo gastric resection with incomplete tumor resection or have truly positive margins of resection also are managed appropriately by combined-modality postoperative therapy.

Radiation Therapy Techniques

Idealized portals generated from patterns of failure data need to be modified on the basis of the individual patient's initial extent of disease (132,139). Based on the likely sites of locoregional

Table 55.7 GENERAL GUIDELINES OF IMPACT OF T AND N STAGE ON INCLUSION OF REMAINING STOMACH, TUMOR BED, AND NODAL SITES WITHIN IRRADIATION FIELDS			
TN Stage	Remaining Stomach[a]	Tumor Bed	Nodes
T1–T2 (not into subserosa) N0	N	N	N
T2N0 (into subserosa)[b]	Variable	Y	N
T3N0	Variable	Y	N
T4N0	Variable	Y	Variable
T1–2N+	Y	N	Y
T3–4N+	Y	Y	Y

[a]Inclusion of the remaining stomach is preferable in most patients if two thirds of one kidney can be excluded. This is dependent on the extent of surgical resection and uninvolved margins (in cm).
[b]Posterior wall T2N0 lesions, or those that extend beyond muscularis propria, especially tumors located in the proximal or distal stomach, are at risk for local relapse. In addition, patients with low-stage disease with close or positive surgical margins should be considered for treatment to the tumor bed.
(From Tepper JE, Gunderson LE. Radiation treatment parameters in the adjuvant postoperative therapy of gastric cancer. *Semin Radiat Oncol* 2002;12(2):187–195, with permission.)

failure (see Table 55.6), the gastric/tumor bed, anastomosis and gastric remnant, and regional lymphatics should be included in most patients (51,57,95,133). Major nodal chains at risk include the lesser and greater curvature; celiac axis; pancreaticoduodenal, splenic, suprapancreatic, and porta hepatis groups; and, in some, para-aortics to the level of mid-L3.

The relative risk of nodal metastases at a specific nodal location is dependent on both the site of origin of the primary tumor (139) and other factors including width and depth of invasion of the gastric wall. Tumors that originate in the proximal portion of the stomach and the GE junction have a higher propensity of spread to nodes in the mediastinum and pericardial region but a lower likelihood of involvement of nodes in the region of the gastric antrum, periduodenal area, and porta hepatis. Tumors that originate in the body of the stomach can spread to all nodal sites but have the highest likelihood of spreading to nodes along the greater and lesser curvature near the location of the primary tumor mass. Tumors that originate in the distal stomach, in the region of the gastric antrum, have a high likelihood of spread to the periduodenal, peripancreatic, and porta

hepatis nodes, whereas they have a lower likelihood of spread to the nodes near the cardia of the stomach, the periesophageal and mediastinal nodes, or to the splenic hilar nodes. Any tumor originating in the stomach has a high propensity of spread to nodes along the greater and lesser curvature, although they are most likely to spread to those sites in close anatomic proximity to the primary tumor mass.

Recently, guidelines for defining the clinical target volume for postoperative irradiation fields have been developed based on location and extent of the primary tumor (T stage) and location and extent of known nodal involvement (N stage) (141). Table 55.7 presents general guidelines on the impact of T and N stages on inclusion of the remaining stomach (gastric remnant), tumor bed, and nodal sites, whereas Tables 55.8 to 55.11 present treatment guidelines based on TN stage within each of the four primary sites (esophagogastric [EG] junction and proximal, mid, and distal stomach). In general, for patients with node-positive disease, there should be wide coverage of tumor bed, remaining stomach, resection margins, and nodal drainage regions. For node-negative disease, if there is a good surgical

Table 55.8 IMPACT OF SITE OF PRIMARY LESION AND TN STAGE ON IRRADIATION VOLUMES—ESOPHAGOGASTRIC JUNCTION (GENERAL GUIDELINES)				
Site of Primary and TN Stage	Remaining Stomach	Tumor Bed Volumes[a]	Nodal Volumes	Tolerance Organs or Structures
EG junction	If allows exclusion of two thirds right kidney	T-stage dependent	N-stage dependent	Heart, lung, spinal cord, kidneys, liver
T2N0 with invasion of subserosa	Variable dependent on surg-path findings[b]	Medial left hemidiaphragm; adjacent body of pancreas	None or perigastric, periesophageal[c]	
T3N0	Variable dependent on surg-path findings[b]	Medial left hemidiaphragm; adjacent body of pancreas	None or perigastric, periesophageal, mediastinal, celiac[c]	
T4N0	Preferable but dependent on surg-path findings[b]	As for T3N0 plus site(s) of adherence with 3–5 cm margin	Nodes related to site of adherence, ± perigastric, periesophageal, mediastinal, celiac	
T1–2N+	Preferable	Not indicated for T1, as above for T2 into subserosa	Periesophageal, mediastinal proximal perigastric, celiac	
T3–4N+	Preferable	As for T3, T4 N0	As for T1–2N+ and T4N0	

EG, esophagogastric; surg-path, surgical-pathologic.
[a]Use preoperative imaging (computed tomography [CT], barium swallow), surgical clips and postoperative imaging (CT, barium swallow).
[b]For tumors with wide (>5 cm) surgical margins confirmed pathologically, treatment of residual stomach is optional, especially if this would result in substantial increase in normal tissue morbidity.
[c]Optional node inclusion for T2–3 N0 lesions if adequate surgical node dissection (D2 dissection) and at least 10–15 nodes examined pathologically.
(From Tepper JE, Gunderson LE. Radiation treatment parameters in the adjuvant postoperative therapy of gastric cancer. *Semin Radiat Oncol* 2002;12(2):187–195, with permission.)

| Table 55.9 | **IMPACT OF SITE OF PRIMARY GASTRIC LESION AND TN STAGE ON IRRADIATION VOLUMES—CARDIA/PROXIMAL ONE-THIRD OF STOMACH (GENERAL GUIDELINES)** |

Site of Primary and TN Stage	Remaining Stomach	Tumor Bed Volumes[a]	Nodal Volumes	Tolerance Organ Structures
Cardia/proximal one-third of stomach	Preferred, but spare two-thirds of one kidney (usually right)	T-stage dependent	N-stage dependent	Kidneys, spinal cord, liver, heart, lung
T2N0 with invasion of subserosa	Variable dependent on surg-path findings[b]	Medial left hemidiaphragm, adjacent body of pancreas (± tail)	None or perigastric[c]	
T3N0	Variable dependent on surg-path findings[b]	Medial left hemidiaphragm, adjacent body of pancreas (± tail)	None or perigastric;optional: periesophageal, mediastinal, celiac[c]	
T4N0	Variable dependent on surg-path findings[b]	As for T3N0 plus site(s) of adherence with 3–5 cm margin	Nodes related to site of adherence, ± perigastric, periesophageal, mediastinal, celiac	
T1–2N+	Preferable	Not indicated for T1, as above for T2 into subserosa	Perigastric, celiac, splenic, suprapancreatic ± periesophageal, mediastinal, pancreaticoduodenal, porta hepatis[d]	
T3–4N+	Preferable	As for T3, T4N0	As for T1–2N+ and T4N0	

surg-path, surgical-pathologic

[a]Use preoperative imaging (computed tomography [CT], barium swallow), surgical clips, and postoperative imaging (CT, barium swallow).

[b]For tumors with wide (>5 cm) surgical margins confirmed pathologically, treatment of residual stomach is not necessary, especially if this would result in substantial increased normal tissue morbidity.

[c]Optional node inclusion for T2–3N0 lesions if adequate surgical node dissection (D2 dissection) and at least 10–15 nodes are examined pathologically.

[d]Pancreaticoduodenal and porta hepatis nodes are at low risk if nodal positivity is minimal (i.e., 1–2 positive nodes with 10–15 nodes examined), and this region does not need to be irradiated. Periesophageal and mediastinal nodes are at risk if there is esophageal extension.

(From Tepper JE, Gunderson LE. Radiation treatment parameters in the adjuvant postoperative therapy of gastric cancer. *Semin Radiat Oncol* 2002;12(2):187–195, with permission.)

resection with pathologic evaluation of at least 10 to 15 nodes, and there are wide surgical margins on the primary tumor (at least 5 cm), treatment of the nodal beds is optional. Treatment of the remaining stomach should depend on a balance of the likely normal tissue morbidity and the perceived risk of local relapse in the residual stomach.

Although parallel-opposed anteroposterior/posteroanterior (AP/PA) fields are a practical arrangement for tumor-bed and nodal irradiation, multifield techniques should be used if they can improve long-term tolerance of normal tissues. Tightly contoured AP/PA fields should be designed to spare as much normal tissue as possible (Figs. 55.2 and 55.3).

| Table 55.10 | **IMPACT OF SITE OF PRIMARY GASTRIC LESION AND TN STAGE ON IRRADIATION VOLUMES—BODY/MIDDLE ONE-THIRD OF STOMACH (GENERAL GUIDELINES)** |

Site of Primary and TN Stage	Remaining Stomach	Tumor Bed Volumes[a]	Nodal Volumes	Tolerance Organ Structures
Body/middle one-third of stomach	Yes—but spare two-thirds of one kidney	T-stage dependent	N-stage dependent—spare two-thirds of one kidney	Kidneys, spinal cord, liver
T2N0 with invasion of subserosa, especially post wall	Yes	Body of pancreas (± tail)	None or perigastric;optional: celiac, splenic, suprapancreatic, pancreaticoduodenal, porta hepatis[b]	
T3N0	Yes	Body of pancreas (± tail)	None or perigastric;optional: celiac, splenic, suprapancreatic, pancreaticoduodenal, porta hepatis[b]	
T4N0	Yes	As for T3N0 plus site(s) of adherence with 3–5 cm margin	Nodes related to site of adherence ± perigastric, celiac, splenic, suprapancreatic, pancreaticoduodenal, porta hepatis	
T1–2N+	Yes	Not indicated for T1;as for T2N0 with invasion of subserosa	Perigastric, celiac, splenic, suprapancreatic pancreaticoduodenal, porta hepatis	
T3–4N+	Yes	As for T3, T4N0	As for T1–2N+ and T4N0	

[a]Use preoperative imaging (computed tomography [CT], barium swallow), surgical clips, and postoperative imaging (CT, barium swallow).

[b]Optional node inclusion for T2–3N0 lesions if adequate surgical node dissection (D2 dissection) and at least 10–15 nodes examined pathologically.

(From Tepper JE, Gunderson LE. Radiation treatment parameters in the adjuvant postoperative therapy of gastric cancer. *Semin Radiat Oncol* 2002;12(2):187–195, with permission.)

:: Table 55.11	IMPACT OF SITE OF PRIMARY GASTRIC LESION AND TN STAGE ON IRRADIATION VOLUMES—ANTRUM/PYLORUS/DISTAL ONE-THIRD OF STOMACH (GENERAL GUIDELINES)			
Site of Primary and TN Stage	Remaining Stomach	Tumor Bed Volumes[a]	Tolerance Organ Nodal Volumes	Structures
Antrum/pylorus/distal one-third of stomach	Yes—but spare two-thirds of one kidney, usually left	T-stage dependent	N-stage dependent	Kidneys, liver, spinal cord
T2N0 with invasion of subserosa	Variable dependent on surg-path findings[b]	Head of pancreas, (± body), 1st and 2nd part of duodenum	None or perigastric;optional: pancreaticoduodenal, porta hepatis, celiac, suprapancreatic[c]	
T3N0	Variable dependent on surg-path findings[b]	Head of pancreas (± body), 1st and 2nd part of duodenum	None or perigastric;optional: pancreaticoduodenal, porta hepatis, celiac, suprapancreatic[c]	
T4N0	Preferable but dependent on surg-path findings[b]	As for T3N0 plus site(s) of adherence with 3–5 cm margin	Nodes related to site(s) of adherence ± perigastric, pancreaticoduodenal, porta hepatis, celiac, suprapancreatic	
T1–2N+	Preferable	Not indicated for T1;as for T2N0 with invasion of subserosa	Perigastric, pancreaticoduodenal, porta hepatis, celiac, suprapancreatic, optional—splenic hilum	
T3–4N+	Preferable	As for T3, T4N0	As for T1–2N+ and T4N0	

surg-path, surgical-pathologic
[a]Use preoperative imaging (computed tomography [CT], barium swallow), surgical clips, and postoperative imaging (CT, barium swallow).
[b]For tumors with wide (>5 cm) surgical margins confirmed pathologically, treatment of residual stomach is optional if this would result in substantial increased normal tissue morbidity.
[c]Optional node inclusion for T2–3N0 lesions if adequate surgical node dissection (D2 dissection) and at least 10–15 nodes examined pathologically.
(From Tepper JE, Gunderson LE. Radiation treatment parameters in the adjuvant postoperative therapy of gastric cancer. *Semin Radiat Oncol* 2002;12(2):187–195, with permission.)

More routine use of multiple field techniques should be considered when preoperative imaging exists to allow accurate reconstruction of target volumes. Single institution data suggest that multiple field arrangements may produce less toxicity (68). Although AP/PA fields can be weighted anteriorly to keep the spinal cord dose at acceptable levels using only parallel-opposed techniques, a four-field technique, if feasible, can spare spinal cord with improved dose homogeneity. Dependent on the posterior extent of the gastric fundus, either obliqued or more routine lateral portals can be used to deliver a 10- to 20-Gy

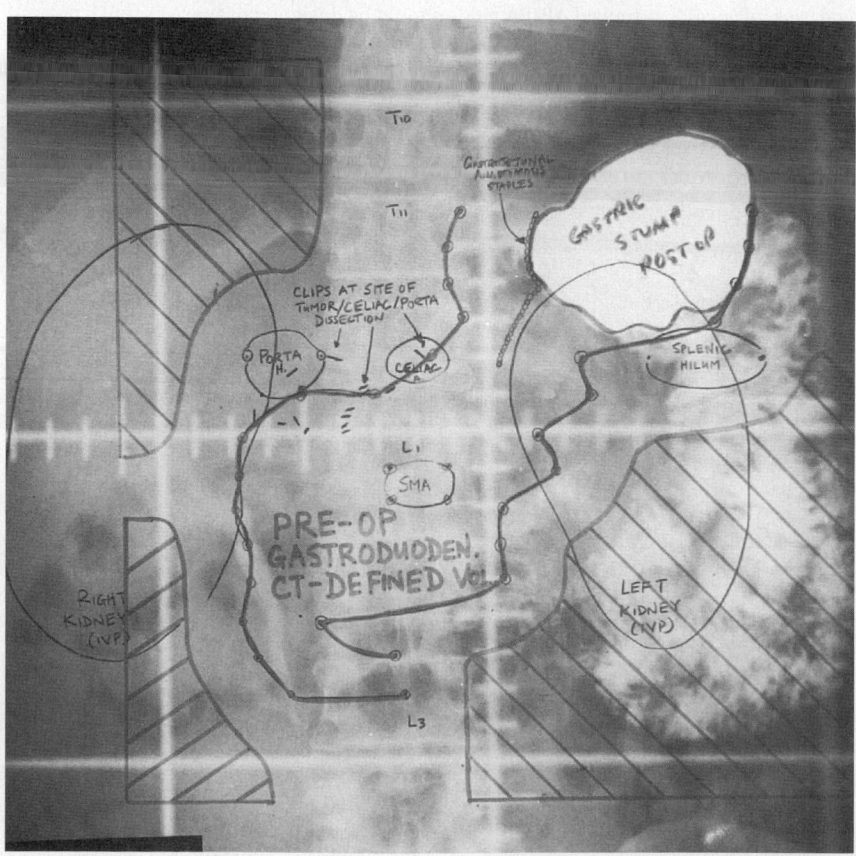

FIGURE 55.2. Simulation film for T3 antral tumor with two of five peritumoral lymph nodes metastatically involved (radical subtotal gastrectomy with D1 node dissection). Simulation film identifies areas at risk for recurrence, including preoperative gastric/tumor bed (defined by preoperative computed tomography [CT] scan), anastomotic sites and gastric stump (staple line seen on precontrast simulation films and marked on postintravenous pyelogram/postcontrast film), and regional lymphatics (celiac, porta hepatis, superior mesenteric artery, and splenic nodes identified on CT, and pancreaticoduodenal nodes lie in C-loop of duodenum identified by preoperative CT). The right kidney is spared for approximately three fourths of its volume, whereas the left kidney has about one third of its volume blocked. (From Smalley SS, Gunderson L, Tepper J, et al. Gastric surgical adjuvant radiotherapy consensus report: rationale and treatment implementation. *Int J Radiat Oncol Biol Phys* 2002;52:283–293, with permission.)

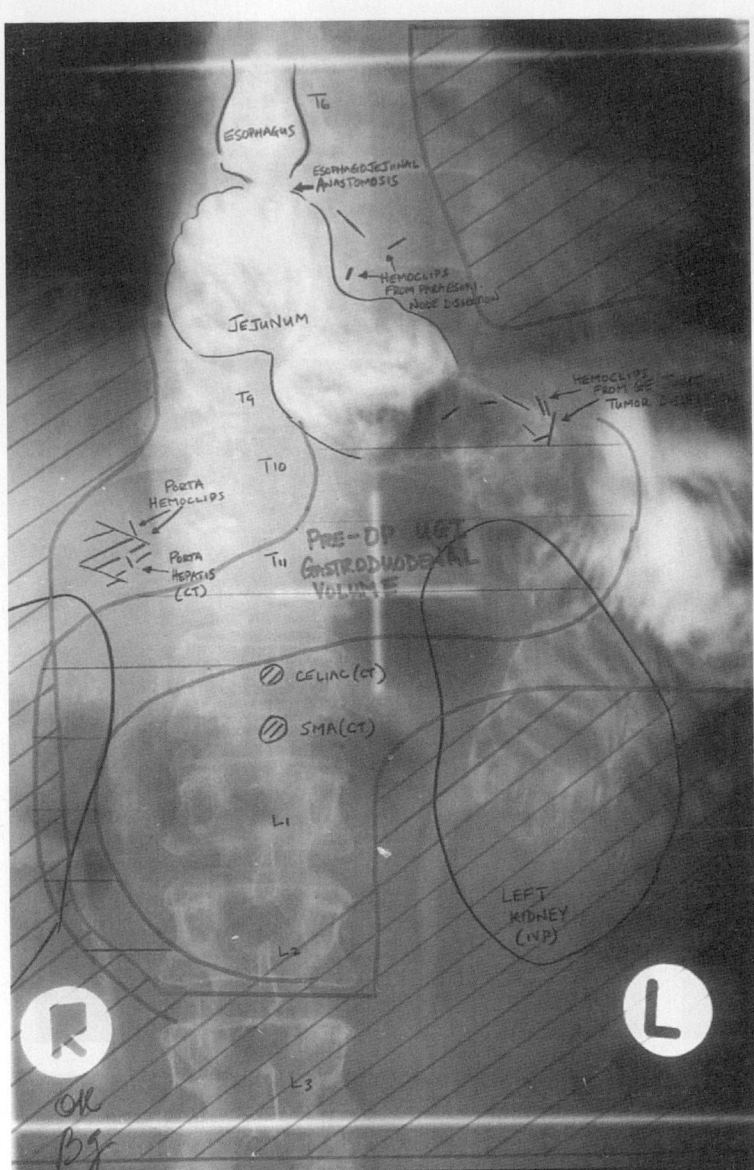

FIGURE 55.3. Simulation film for a T4 (diaphragm invasion) gastroesophageal junction tumor with four of 15 involved lymph nodes (total gastrectomy with modified R3 node dissection). Areas at risk for recurrence include preoperative gastric/tumor bed (defined by preoperative upper gastrointestinal radiographs and hemoclips placed at time of resection to mark tumor bed and diaphragm invasion), anastomotic sites and stump (anastomosis visualized at juncture of residual distal esophagus and jejunum), and regional lymphatics (including the celiac, porta hepatis, and pancreaticoduodenal areas as well as the distal paraesophageal nodes). (From Smalley SS, Gunderson L, Tepper J, et al. Gastric surgical adjuvant radiotherapy consensus report: rationale and treatment implementation. *Int J Radiat Oncol Biol Phys* 2002;52:283–293, with permission.)

component of irradiation to spare spinal cord or kidney. When lateral fields are used, liver and kidney tolerance limits the use of lateral fields to ≤20 Gy. With the wide availability of three-dimensional treatment-planning systems, it may be possible to target more accurately the high-risk volume and to use unconventional field arrangements to produce superior dose distributions. To accomplish this without marginal misses, it will be necessary to both carefully define and encompass the various target volumes because use of oblique or noncoplanar beams could exclude target volumes that would be included in AP/PA fields or nonoblique four-field techniques (AP/PA and laterals).

In the Massachusetts General Hospital and Mayo Clinic series, the average irradiation field measured 15 cm by 15 cm (58,66). With regimens using single daily fractions, the usual dose is 45 to 52 Gy delivered in 1.8- to 2.0-Gy fractions over 5 to 5.5 weeks, with a field reduction after 45 Gy. Reduced boost fields to small areas of residual disease and a small volume of stomach or small intestine sometimes can be cautiously carried to doses of 55 to 60 Gy with multifield techniques. In such instances, informed consent should include a discus-

sion of an increased risk of grade 3 to 4 gastrointestinal toxicity.

In most patients, a portion of both kidneys is within the treatment field, but at least two-thirds to three-fourths of one kidney should be excluded beyond a dose of 20 Gy. For proximal gastric lesions, 50% or more of the left kidney is commonly within the irradiation portal, and the right kidney must be appropriately spared. For distal lesions with narrow or positive duodenal margins, a similar amount of right kidney often is included, and every effort must be taken to spare enough left kidney to maintain function. Late renal sequelae have not been encountered with these techniques (58,115,149).

With proximal gastric lesions or lesions at the EG junction, a 3- to 5-cm margin of distal esophagus should be included; if the lesion extends through the entire gastric wall, a major portion of the left hemidiaphragm should be included (Fig. 55.4). In these circumstances, blocking can decrease the volume of irradiated heart. For unresectable lesions with moderate periesophageal extension, it may not be possible to exclude an adequate amount of heart with AP/PA fields, and the use of lateral fields for a portion of treatment may be indicated.

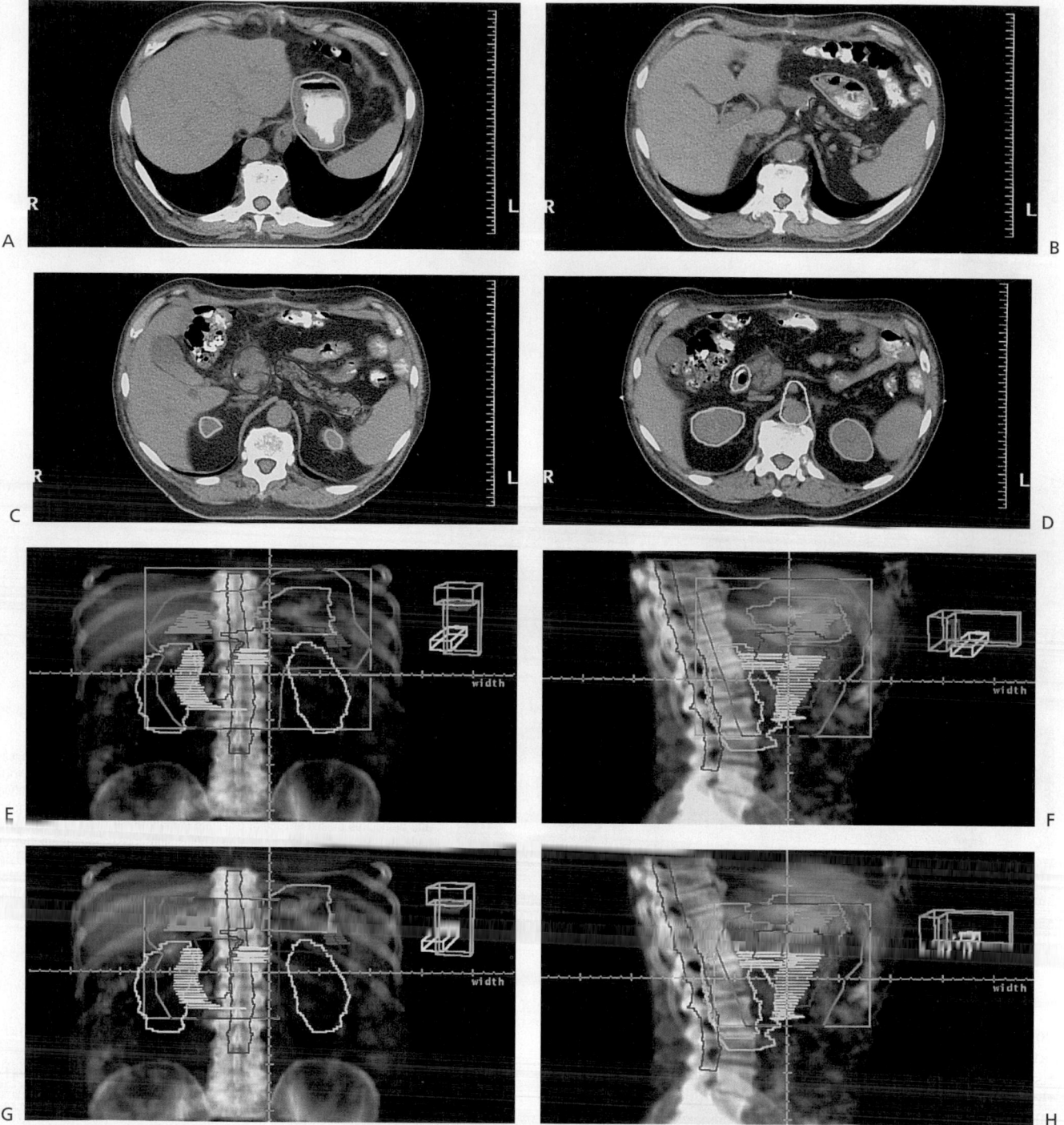

FIGURE 55.4. Optimized postoperative irradiation fields for patient with T3N1 antral primary (see Table 55.11). Structures of interest were delineated at time of computed tomography simulation (*A–D*), and irradiation fields were designed with the aid of digitally reconstructed radiographs (*E–H*). **A:** Gastric remnant (*teal*). **B:** Gastric remnant plus body/tail of pancreas (*dark blue*), splenic hilum (*salmon*), and porta hepatis (*medium blue*). that approximately 75% of the left kidney receives 20 Gy or less. **C:** Head of pancreas (*magenta*) and kidneys (*left, orange; right, light green*) are delineated in addition to body/tail of pancreas and splenic hilum. **D:** Celiac artery (*yellow*) and duodenum (*yellow–green*) are shown together with head of pancreas and kidneys. A four-field technique of AP (anteroposterior), PA (posteroanterior), and paired laterals was designed to include the gastric remnant (*teal*), tumor bed (head of pancreas [*magenta*], 1st and 2nd part of duodenum [*yellow–green cross hatched*]), pertinent nodal volumes (perigastric, pancreaticoduodenal, porta hepatic [*medium blue cross hatched*], celiac [*yellow cross hatched*], and suprapancreatic) and the optional nodal volume of splenic hilum (*salmon cross hatched*). **E:** Initial AP field (field margins as shown in medium blue exclude approximately two thirds of the left kidney while including about 50% of the right kidney). Exclusion of the optional splenic hilar nodes would have allowed additional, but minimal sparing of the left kidney in view of the adjacency of gastric antrum and splenic hilum. **F:** Initial right lateral field demonstrated exclusion of the spinal cord. **G:** Reduced AP field with exclusion of splenic hilar nodes and most of the gastric remnant. **H:** Reduced right lateral field. (*continued*)

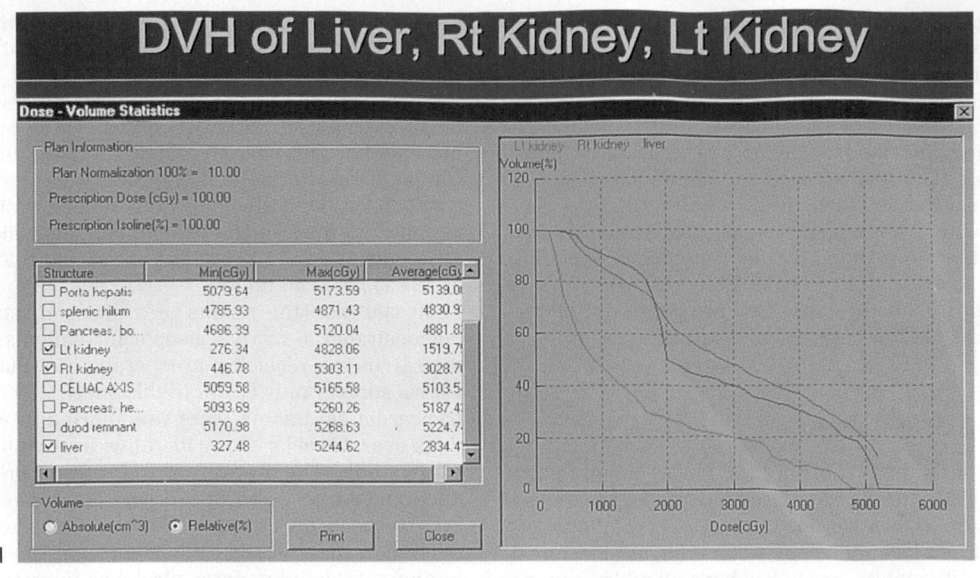

FIGURE 55.4. (*continued*) **I:** Dose-volume histogram (DVH) demonstrates that approximately 75% of the left kidney receives 20 Gy or less.

During therapy, patient tolerance, weight, and blood counts are checked at least weekly. If chemotherapy is used with irradiation, blood counts are obtained twice weekly.

Results of Therapy

Locally Advanced Unresectable or Subtotally Resected Gastric Cancer

For patients with locally advanced unresectable or subtotally resected gastric carcinoma, radiotherapeutic approaches with and without chemotherapy have been used because these tumors appear localized without clinically detectable metastases. Combined treatment with radiation therapy and chemotherapy appears to prolong survival but rarely results in long-term cure (98). Although only a modest effect on survival is seen, these studies have established, importantly, the foundation of contemporary combined modality therapy and have served as a stimulus to further clinical investigation in gastric cancer as well as other gastrointestinal disease sites. The results of these phase III studies have had a significant impact on clinical trial development in gastrointestinal malignancies (Table 55.12).

In 1969 Moertel et al. (98) reported the results of a prospective, controlled double-blind study of patients with locally advanced unresectable gastric cancer. In this study, 48 patients were randomized to 35 to 40 Gy of radiation therapy over 4 weeks with and without 5FU. Mean survival was 13 months in patients receiving radiation therapy and 5FU versus 5.9 months for the radiation therapy patients (p <0.01). These results demonstrated for the first time the clinical benefit of combining concurrent 5FU with radiation therapy and encouraged further investigation of combination therapy in gastric cancer and other gastrointestinal disease sites (esophageal, pancreatic, rectal, and anal carcinomas).

As a follow-up to this study, the Gastrointestinal Tumor Study Group examined the combination of 5FU/MeCCNU, or 1-(2-chloroethyl)-3-(4-methylcyclohexyl)-1 nitrosourea, and radiotherapy (50 Gy/split course/8 weeks) versus the same chemotherapy alone in locally advanced gastric cancer (49). Patients were eligible if the tumor involved regional lymph nodes or adjacent structures that could be completely resected en bloc. Of the 90 patients entered, 66 had a resection of the primary tumor. Of these, 23 had gross residual disease, 36 had microscopic residual, and seven had no documented residual disease. The study was closed prematurely because of an excess of early deaths in the combined chemotherapy–radiotherapy arm. The excessive early mortality of the combined-modality arm was attributed to early tumor progression and poor tolerance of the combined-modality regime. However, further follow-up beyond 3 years indicated continuing mortality among the chemotherapy-alone arm, whereas the combined chemoradiotherapy arm exhibited a plateau with 18% surviving 5 years.

Table 55.12	UNRESECTABLE OR RESIDUAL GASTRIC CANCER: TREATMENT RESULTS OF RANDOMIZED TRIALS				
Group or Institution	Treatment Arms	No. of Patients	EBRT Dose	Chemotherapy	Survival Results
Mayo Clinic (37)	EBRT + ChT vs. EBRT	48	35–40 Gy	5-FU	Increased survival for EBRT + 5FU with mean survival 13 months vs. 5.9 months and 3/25 (12%) vs. 0/23 5-year survival
GITSG (49)	EBRT + ChT vs. ChT	90	50 Gy split course	5FU + MeCCNU	Advantage in long-term survival with EBRT +ChT at 18% vs. 7% ($p < 0.05$)

ChT, chemotherapy; EBRT, external-beam radiation therapy; 5-Fu, 5-fluorouracil; GITSG, Gastrointestinal Tumor Study Group; MeCCNU, 1-(2-chloroethyl)-3- (4-methylcyclohexyl)-1 nitrosourea

Thus, despite an excess of early mortality, the combined-modality arm exhibited an overall superiority in 5-year survival. It is important to note that patients who had had their primary tumor resected experienced superior survival to those without resection. All of the survival benefit in patients receiving combined modality was in patients whose primary tumor had been resected. This trial showed that combined chemoradiation therapy is capable of rendering a substantial percentage of patients with microscopic residual gastric cancer free of disease. It furthermore supported the rationale of exploring chemoradiation adjuvant trials in completely resected patients at high risk of locoregional relapse because control of microscopic disease was able to cure a significant number of these patients.

Resectable Gastric Cancer

The recognition of the high rates of local and regional failure following surgery in patterns of failure analyses has served as the basis for clinical trials assessing the value of radiation therapy with and without chemotherapy as an adjuvant treatment (see Table 55.5). Although these studies have all addressed the important question of whether clinical outcome is enhanced by adjuvant radiation therapy, there has been marked variability in radiation dose and schedule, sequence with surgery (preoperatively, intraoperatively, or postoperatively), and the use of concurrent and maintenance chemotherapy (Table 55.13). These differences in study design may explain in part the conflicting results observed in phase III studies.

Two randomized phase III studies have studied the use of external beam radiation therapy (EBRT) with surgery (2,62,153). Although both studies used a similar radiation dose and schedule, sequence with surgery differed. In the British Stomach Cancer Group study, 436 patients were randomized to surgery alone; postoperative radiation therapy (45 to 50 Gy in 25 to 28 fractions); or cytotoxic chemotherapy with mitomycin, doxorubicin, and fluorouracil (FAM) (2,62). The 5-year survival for surgery alone was 20%, for surgery plus radiation therapy 12%, and for surgery plus chemotherapy 19%. In this study, no survival advantage was observed for patients who received postoperative EBRT, although there was an apparent improvement in local control, demonstrating that local disease could be affected by adjuvant radiation therapy. Locoregional failure was

documented in only 15/153 (10%) in the irradiation arm versus 39/145 (27%) in the surgery alone arm and 26/138 (19%) in the FAM group. Interpretation of the results is complicated by the inclusion of 171 patients undergoing resection with gross or microscopic residual carcinoma. These patients would not be candidates for current gastric surgical adjuvant trials in the United States. In addition, approximately one third of patients randomized to receive adjuvant treatment did not receive the assigned therapy. Of 153 patients randomized to the irradiation arm, only 104 (68%) received a dose of 40.5 Gy or more, and 36 (24%) received none.

In contrast, the results of a phase III study from Beijing demonstrated a survival benefit for patients with gastric cardia carcinoma receiving preoperative irradiation and surgery versus surgery only (153). In this study, 370 patients with gastric cardia carcinoma were randomized to 40 Gy in 20 fractions over 4 weeks of preoperative irradiation and surgery or surgery only. The 5-year survival rates of preoperative irradiation and surgery and the surgery alone group were 30% and 20%, respectively (10-year, 20% and 13%, respectively). These differences were statistically significant ($p = 0.009$). Further, local and regional nodal control was improved in patients undergoing preoperative irradiation and surgery (61%, 61%) versus surgery (48%, 45%) only. Morbidity and mortality rates were not increased in patients receiving preoperative irradiation and surgery.

An alternative approach to postoperative or preoperative irradiation is intraoperative radiation therapy (IORT) (61). The advantage of this technique is the ability to deliver a single large fraction (10 to 35 Gy) of radiation to the tumor or tumor bed while excluding or protecting surrounding normal tissue from the high-dose field. This approach permits high-dose irradiation with minimal normal tissue treatment. Two randomized trials have examined the efficacy of IORT in combination with surgery for patients with gastric carcinoma (1,129). Abe et al. (1) from Kyoto University performed a randomized trial for 211 patients with gastric cancer comparing surgery alone with surgery and intraoperative radiation (28 to 35 Gy). Patients were randomized based on hospital day of admission for surgery. For patients with tumor confined to the gastric wall, 5-year survival rates were similar for IORT and for resection alone. However, patients with Japanese stages II to IV disease who received IORT in conjunction with resection showed

			Survival		Local-Regional Relapse			
Series/Treatment Method	**Patients**	**Median (mos)**	**Long Term[a] (%)**	**P Value**	**N**	**%**	**P Value**	**Ref. No.**
1. Mayo Clinic (97)								96
a. Surgery alone	23	15	4	—	—	54	—	
b. Postop EBRT + 5FU	39	24	23	0.05	—	39	—	
2. British Stomach Group (62)								2,62
a. Surgery alone	145	—	20	—	39	27 (3 years)	—	
b. Postop ChT	138	—	19	—	26	19 (3 years)	—	
c. Postop EBRT	153	—	12	—	15	10 (3 years)	—	
3. China—Beijing (153)								151
a. Surgery alone	199	—	20	—	—	52	—	
b. Preop EBRT	171	—	30	0.009	—	39	<0.025	
4. Intergroup 0116 (91)						Disease-free survival (3 years)		90
a. Surgery alone	275	27	41	—		31	—	
b. Postop EBRT + ChT	281	36	50	0.005		48	<0.001	

Table 55.13 ADJUVANT IRRADIATION WITH AND WITHOUT CHEMOTHERAPY FOR RESECTED GASTRIC CANCER: TREATMENT RESULTS OF RANDOMIZED TRIALS

postop, postoperative; EBRT, external-beam radiation therapy; 5Fu, 5-fluorouracil; ChT, chemotherapy; preop, preoperative
[a]Long-term survival is 5-year data for Mayo Clinic and Beijing series, 3-year data for British and Intergroup 0116.

improved survival over patients who underwent resection without irradiation. Among patients with stage IV disease (who usually had local residual disease after maximal resection), there were no 5-year survivors who received surgery alone, but 15% of the patients who received IORT were alive at 5 years. The experience with IORT in gastric cancer at Kyoto University suggested that IORT may be beneficial in the treatment of locally advanced malignancies of the stomach.

To further evaluate this approach, Sindelar et al. (129) at the National Cancer Institute conducted a prospectively randomized-controlled trial comparing surgical resection and IORT with conventional therapy in gastric carcinoma. Patients in the experimental group underwent gastrectomy, and IORT was administered to their gastric bed (20 Gy). Patients in the control group underwent resection and postoperative EBRT to the upper abdomen (50 Gy in 25 fractions) for advanced-stage lesions extending beyond the gastric wall. Of the 100 patients screened for the study, 60 were randomized and underwent exploratory surgery. Nineteen patients were excluded intraoperatively because of unresectability or metastases, leaving 41 patients in the study. The median survival for patients with tumors of all stages was 25 months for the IORT group and 21 months for the control group (p = NS). Locoregional disease relapse occurred in seven of 16 (44%) IORT patients, and in 23/25 patients (92%) control patients (p <0.001). Complication rates were similar between IORT and control patients. Although IORT failed to afford a significant advantage over conventional therapy in overall survival, IORT did significantly improve control of locoregional disease. Based on these results, the use of IORT in gastric cancer remains investigational.

Because of the promising results in the early studies of combined-modality therapy for locally advanced unresectable or subtotally resected gastric cancer, investigators also have studied this combination in resectable gastric carcinoma. A small study from South Africa randomized 66 patients with resected gastric cancer (T1 to T3, N1 or N2, M0) to low-dose postoperative irradiation (20 Gy in eight fractions over 10 days) and 5FU or no further therapy (27). No difference in survival was observed between the patients undergoing surgery and adjuvant therapy and those undergoing surgery alone. Given the subtherapeutic doses of radiation used in this study, it is difficult to draw any conclusions as to the efficacy of adjuvant radiation therapy and 5FU.

In 1984 Moertel et al. (97) reported the results of a prospective randomized trial conducted at the Mayo Clinic with 62 patients with poor prognosis but completely resected gastric cancers who were randomized to either surgery alone or surgery followed by irradiation (37.5 Gy in 24 fractions over 4 to 5 weeks) with concurrent 5FU. A nonstratified, prerandomization scheme was used with a 2:3 ratio favoring treatment. Informed consent was requested of only the 39 patients randomized to treatment. Ten of the 39 refused further therapy and were observed. When analyzed by intent to treat, the adjuvant arm had statistically significant improvement in both relapse-free and overall survival (overall 5-year survival 23% vs. 4%; p <0.05). When patient outcome was compared with actual treatment received (29 adjuvant treatment, 33 surgery alone), 5-year survival still favored the adjuvant group (20% vs. 12%), but the differences were not statistically significant in view of the small patient numbers. The 10 patients who refused assignment to adjuvant treatment had more favorable prognostic findings than the other two groups of patients. When the two groups with equally poor prognostic factors were compared, the 5-year overall survival was 20% versus 4%, with an advantage to those receiving adjuvant treatment. When analyzed by treatment delivered, locoregional relapse was decreased with adjuvant treatments (54% incidence with surgery alone vs. 39% with irradiation and 5FU).

Because of these conflicting results, an Intergroup trial (INT 0116) was initiated to evaluate postoperative combined 5FU-based chemotherapy and irradiation to the gastric bed and regional nodes versus surgery only following resection of gastric cancer (91). Eligibility included patients with stages IB, II, IIIA, IIIB, and IV nonmetastatic adenocarcinoma of the stomach or GE junction. After an en bloc resection, 556 patients were randomized to either observation alone or postoperative combined-modality therapy consisting of 45 Gy in 25 fractions plus concurrent 5FU and leucovorin (4 days in week 1, 3 days in week 5) followed by two monthly 5-day cycles of 5FU and leucovorin. Nodal metastases were present in 85% of the cases. With 5 years of median follow-up, 3-year relapse-free survival was 48% for adjuvant treatment and 31% for observation (p = 0.001); 3-year overall survival was 50% for treatment and 41% for observation (p = 0.005). The median overall survival in the surgery-only group was 27 months, compared with 36 months in the chemoradiotherapy group; the hazard ratio for death was 1.35 (95% confidence interval, 1.09 to 1.66; p = 0.005). The hazard ratio for relapse in the surgery-only group as compared with the chemoradiotherapy group was 1.52 (95% confidence interval, 1.23 to 1.86; p <0.001). The median duration of relapse-free survival was 30 months in the chemoradiotherapy group and 19 months in the surgery-only group. Patterns of failure were based on the site of first relapse only and were categorized as local, regional, or distant. Local recurrence occurred in 29% of the patients who relapsed in the surgery-only group and 19% of those who relapsed in the chemoradiotherapy group. Regional relapse—typically abdominal carcinomatosis—was reported in 72% of those who relapsed in the surgery-only group and 65% of those who relapsed in the chemoradiotherapy group. Extra-abdominal distant metastases were diagnosed in 18% of those who relapsed in the surgery-only group and 33% of those who relapsed in the chemoradiotherapy group. Treatment was tolerable, with three (1%) toxic deaths. Grade 3 and 4 toxicity occurred in 41% and 32% of cases, respectively. The results of this large study demonstrate a clear survival advantage for the use of postoperative chemoradiation and strongly support the integration of postoperative chemoradiation into the routine care of patients with curatively resected high-risk carcinoma of the stomach and GE junction.

Since preoperative radiation therapy and chemotherapy have improved the surgical outcome in patients with rectal and esophageal cancer, this is a logical approach to explore in gastric cancer as well. Although no phase III trials have tested the value of preoperative radiation plus chemotherapy for patients with gastric cancer, two phase III trials for patients with esophagus cancer have included either lesions of the gastric cardia (143) or the esophagogastric junction (84). In both trials, the trimodality arm demonstrated an improvement in survival when compared with the control arm of surgery alone. The series by Walsh et al. (143) (adenocarcinoma of the esophagus or gastric cardia) demonstrated a median survival of 16 versus 11 months and 3-year survival of 32% versus 6% (p = 0.01), with the advantage to trimodality treatment. The U.S. GI Intergroup phase III trial (adenocarcinoma or squamous cell of esophagus or E-G junction), which closed prematurely due to low accrual, resulted in a median survival of 54 versus 21.6 months and 5-year survival of 39% versus 16% (p = 0.008), with an advantage to the trimodality arm.

Preoperative chemoradiation data for patients with gastric cancer is limited to phase II studies from single institutions and cooperative groups. M.D. Anderson Hospital has reported a study in which 33 patients completed a preoperative protocol that started with induction chemotherapy of 5FU, leucovorin, and cisplatin, followed by 45 Gy of radiation therapy in 25 fractions over 5 weeks. Infusional 5FU was administered concurrently with radiation therapy. In 28 patients (85%) of the patients, a gastrectomy was performed and D2 lymph node dissection was attempted. Pathological complete and partial response was found in 64% of all operated patients. These patients showed a significant longer median survival of 64 months in comparison with 13 months in patients with tumors not pathologically responding. In a study from the same institution, 41 patients with operable gastric cancer received two cycles of continuous 5FU, paclitaxel and cisplatin followed by 45 Gy of radiation therapy with concurrent 5FU and paclitaxel. An R0 resection was achieved in 78% of patients with pathological complete response of 25% and pathological partial response of 15%. Pathological response, R0 resection, and postoperative T and N stage were correlated with overall and disease-free survival. Recently, the Radiation Therapy Oncology Group reported the results of a phase II study of 49 patients undergoing induction 5FU, leucovorin, and cisplatin followed by concurrent radiation therapy and infusional 5FU and paclitaxel. Resection was attempted 5 to 6 weeks after radiation therapy and chemotherapy. The pathological complete response and R0 resection rates were 26% and 77%, respectively. At 1 year, more patients with tumors exhibiting a pathological complete response (89%) are living than patients with tumors who had a less favorable response (66%). Grade 4 toxicity occurred in 21% of patients. These data appear to support a study evaluating preoperative radiation therapy and chemotherapy versus postoperative radiation therapy and chemotherapy.

Palliative Radiation Therapy

Radiation therapy is capable of providing substantial palliation of local gastric cancer symptoms (16,34,44,61,81,94,99). It appears that 50% to 75% of patients can expect improvement of symptoms such as gastric outlet obstruction, pain from local tumor extension, and bleeding or biliary obstruction (81). The likelihood of benefit may increase with concomitant 5FU administration, with less tumor bulk, and if the patient's performance score is better before therapy (34,35,66,105). The median duration of palliation varies from 4 to 18 months in reports addressing this issue (34,35,92,105).

⠿ | Sequelae of Therapy

Anorexia, nausea, and fatigue are very common complaints during gastric radiation therapy, but our understanding of these problems is quite limited (14,28,42,131,144). Although visceral afferents may play some role in the acute emetogenic effects of radiation, other unknown factors, possibly chemical in nature and mediated by the chemoreceptor trigger zone, appear to be more important. Although selective serotonin (5-HT$_3$) antagonists effectively treat radiation-induced emesis, it is not clear

whether the mechanism of action is directed at the 5-HT$_3$ receptor alone or has an effect on inhibition of serotonin release (123). Other compounding factors may include the altered gastric motility and prolonged gastric emptying time observed in animal experiments as a response to irradiation (14,28,39,133).

Nutritional complications of treatment and myelosuppression, if concurrent chemotherapy is used during irradiation, can carry substantial morbidity and even occasional mortality from therapy. The Gastrointestinal Tumor Study Group reported a minimum 13% treatment-related mortality from nutritional problems or septic events on their concurrent chemoradiation arm (124), and almost 20% of the patients of Caudry et al. (21) were unable to complete therapy because of nutritional problems. However, others reported no severe or life-threatening nutritional compromise with aggressive chemoradiation (66,125,141). The toxic GI effects usually are managed with careful nutritional support and antiemetic therapy. It is our practice to proactively prescribe antiemetics at the initiation of therapy in patients undergoing aggressive upper abdominal irradiation.

Myelosuppression causing serious or, rarely, lethal toxicity also is reported in many of the combined-modality trials (61,66,125,141). If blood counts are monitored twice weekly during combined-modality therapy, serious problems with sepsis or bleeding should be uncommon (61,67,125).

Moderate doses of 16 to 36 Gy reduce secretion of pepsin and hydrochloric acid (20,55,122,133). For this reason, radiation therapy was once a common and successful therapy for peptic ulcer disease. Most of the gastric ulcers healed, but they recurred in approximately 40% of patients (20,55,133). Gastric-acid secretion decreased in almost all cases, with achlorhydria in 25% to 40% (47). The gastric-acid decrease usually persisted from 1 to 6 months, but 25% showed persistent decrease in acid production for 1 to 5 years or more.

Gastric late effects were categorized by the Walter Reed Group as dyspepsia, radiation gastritis, uncomplicated gastric ulcer, or gastric ulcer with perforation or obstruction (3,15,45). The associations between dose and these late effects are described in Table 55.14. These data suggest a 20% to 30% incidence of ulceration with doses of 45 to 59 Gy, with complications of these ulcers in 30% to 50% of the treated patients. Some caution is necessary in interpreting this experience because the Walter Reed cohort was treated with 200-keV photons or 1-MV photons using a larger skin distance, usually using only one field each day with daily fraction sizes of 3 Gy to mid line, which sometimes produced daily given doses of 4 to 6 Gy (15,45).

Most data suggest that gastric late effects are rare with doses of 40 to 52 Gy using conventional fractionation of 1.8 to 2.0 Gy. The relatively low risk of gastric late effects with

		Radiation Late Effects (%)[a]			
Dose (Gy)	# of Patients[b]	Dyspepsia	Gastritis	Ulcer	Complicated Ulcer[c]
<40	111	5	2	3	0
40–44.99	23	0	22	0	0
45–49.99	27	4	19	11	11
50–54.99	34	0	24	18	12
55–59.99	14	0	50	14	7
>60	8	0	0	13	38

⠿ Table 55.14 | **RADIATION DOSE COMPARED WITH LATE EFFECTS IN THE WALTER REED EXPERIENCE (3,15,45)**

[a]Results reported as number of patients with injury/total number of patients treated with this dose.
[b]Total number of patients treated at this dose.
[c]Ulcers complicated by obstruction or perforation.

doses <50 Gy is corroborated by many series using radiation therapy with or without chemotherapy for locally advanced gastric cancer (63,83,100,126,127,143). However, doses in the range of 50 to 55 Gy may produce variable gastric late effects, which in one series reached 9% (56). Doses of 60 Gy carried a 5% to 15% risk of gastric late effects (3,7,9,15,20,21,34,44,45, 47,55,56,60,63,72,74,105,112,120,121,142,143,149)(1274,).

The ability of histamine$_2$ (H$_2$) blockers and sucralfate to prevent the later development of radiation-induced gastric ulcerations is unproven. It may be reasonable to administer H$_2$ blockers prophylactically to patients receiving 45 Gy or more to any significant volume of the stomach or proximal duodenum.

Chemotherapy

Various combinations of active drugs have been reported to improve the response rate among patients with metastatic or locally unresectable gastric carcinoma (46). A combination of FAM has been associated with a 30% to 40% response rate and was the most widely prescribed regimen for patients with advanced disease in the 1980s (46). Despite an initial response rate of 64% when a combination of etoposide, doxorubicin, and cisplatin (EAP) was used by German investigators, in subsequent trials this regimen was considerably less effective and extremely toxic (76,87,113). A combination of fluorouracil, doxorubicin, and high-dose methotrexate (FAMTX) was associated with a significant improvement in the response rate, as compared with either EAP (76,150) or FAM (152). As a result of these studies, FAMTX became standard therapy for metastatic disease in the past decade.

In a British study of patients with unresectable or metastatic gastric and esophageal adenocarcinoma, 274 patients were randomized to either 5FU, doxorubicin, and methotrexate (FAMTX) or epirubicin, cisplatin, and continuous infusion 5FU (ECF) (145,146). ECF was associated with a superior response rate (45% vs. 21%; $p = 0.0002$), median survival (8.7 vs. 5.7 months; $p = 0.0006$ vs. 0.006) and 1-year survival (36% vs. 21%). Moreover, ECF was associated with a superior quality of life and less toxicity.

The ECF regimen has been explored in a perioperative approach as well. The Myoblast Autologous Grafting in Ischemic Cardiomyopathy (MAGIC) trial was initiated by the Medical Research Council (MRC) to address the question of perioperative chemotherapy (pre- and post-) in operable gastric cancer (24). In this study, 503 patients with adenocarcinoma of the stomach, lower esophagus, or gastroesophageal junction were randomly assigned to receive either three cycles of preoperative ECF chemotherapy followed by surgery and then another three cycles of postoperative ECF (250 patients) or surgery alone (253 patients). The resected tumors were significantly smaller and less advanced in the perioperative chemotherapy group. With a median follow-up of 4 years, 149 patients in the perioperative chemotherapy group and 170 in the surgery group had died. As compared with the surgery group, the perioperative chemotherapy group had statistically improved progression-free and overall survival rates.

In a separate phase II effort, 29 patients who had undergone a curative resection of esophagogastric adenocarcinoma received ECF for six cycles (18 weeks) postoperatively (8). The mean number of chemotherapy cycles delivered per patient was 5.2. Chemotherapy was well tolerated, with grade 3 or 4 toxicity as follows: leukopenia, 13.5%; nausea/vomiting, 10%; diarrhea, 3.5%; and thrombocytopenia, 3.5%. There were no treatment-related deaths. Overall, 3-year survival rate was 61.5%.

Following a curative resection of gastric adenocarcinoma, Neri et al. (104) randomized 103 patients with node-positive disease to postoperative epirubicin, leucovorin, and 5FU or observation. Three-year survival was 25% in the chemotherapy arm and 13% in the control arm. Median survival was 20.4 months for those patients who received chemotherapy compared with 13.6 months for those who did not receive postoperative therapy ($p < 0.01$). No long-term toxicity or cardiac toxicity was noted among patients treated with chemotherapy. Although postoperative epirubicin, 5FU, and leucovorin were associated with a significant improvement in survival, this study has been criticized for its small size.

Conclusions and Recommendations

Radiation therapy, usually administered with concomitant 5FU-based chemotherapy, is indicated for locally confined gastric cancer that either is not technically resectable or occurs in medically inoperable patients. In this setting, therapy can be administered with curative or palliative intent, depending on the clinical situation. Those who undergo gastric resection with incomplete tumor resection or have truly positive margins of resection are also appropriately managed by combined-modality therapy. Preferably, patients with locally advanced disease that is unresectable with negative margins would be identified preoperatively with endoscopic ultrasonography and CT staging. Preoperative chemoradiation then could precede an attempt at gross total resection, alone or in combination with IORT, and maintenance chemotherapy.

The results of the U.S. GI Intergroup Gastric Adjuvant Trial have changed the standard of care in the United States to the use of both chemotherapy and radiation therapy in the postoperative setting for patients with disease extension through the gastric wall and/or with nodes positive for tumor. Postoperative irradiation and concurrent and maintenance 5FU-based chemotherapy are recommended for patients with stage IB, II, IIIA, IIIB, or IV with M0 gastric cancer. Since extended node dissections were not commonly performed as a component of surgery in this trial, some have questioned whether postoperative chemoradiation would give added benefit following a D2 nodal resection. Although this is unlikely to be tested in a phase III trial, a recent South Korea analysis evaluated the potential role of postoperative chemoradiation in a series of 990 patients with D2 resection for gastric cancer who had high risk for relapse (80). Disease and patient characteristics and chemoradiation treatment factors paralleled the U.S. GI Intergroup phase III trial. Both recurrence free survival (RFS) and overall survival (OS) were improved in the 544 patients who received postoperative chemoradiation when compared with the 446 patients treated with surgery alone (5-year OS, 57 vs. 51%; $p = 0.02$; 5-year RFS 54.5 vs. 47.9%; $p = 0.016$).

Ongoing trials now are investigating new systemic agents with radiation therapy to establish efficacy compared with 5FU and leucovorin and to evaluate neoadjuvant approaches prior to resection. The current U.S. GI Intergroup postoperative adjuvant trial is testing 5FU infusion versus bolus 5FU leucovorin as the concurrent chemotherapy during radiation and ECF chemotherapy versus the 5FU leucovorin regimen as maintenance chemotherapy. On the basis of encouraging outcomes with phase II preoperative chemoradiation trials in patients with gastric cancer and phase III esophagus cancer trials, it would be appropriate to continue to evaluate this approach in patients with both potentially resectable as well as unresectable lesions.

The irradiation field design in the current phase III U.S. GI Intergroup trial is based on optimized field design related to both site of the primary lesion and TN stage of disease (139). With the wide availability of three-dimension conformal treatment planning systems, it may be possible to target more accurately the high-risk volume and to use unconventional field arrangements and/or IMRT to produce superior dose distributions. To accomplish this without marginal misses, however, it will be necessary to both carefully define and encompass the various target volumes (tumor bed, nodal sites at risk) since target volumes that would be included in AP/PA fields may be missed with other field arrangements (oblique, lateral, noncoplanar).

References

1. Abe M, Takahashi M, Ono K, et al. Japan gastric trials in intraoperative radiation therapy. *Int J Radiat Oncol Biol Phys* 1988;15:1431–1433.
2. Allum WH, Hallissey MT, Ward LC, et al. A controlled, prospective, randomized trial of adjuvant chemotherapy or radiotherapy in resectable gastric cancer: Interim report. *Br J Cancer* 1989;60:739.
3. Amory H, Brick I. Irradiation damage of the intestines following 1,000-KV roentgen therapy: Evaluation of tolerance dose. *Radiology* 1951;56:49.
4. Asakawa H, Otawa H, Yamada S, et al. Combination therapy of gastric carcinoma with radiation and chemotherapy. *Tohoku J Exp Med* 1982;137:445.
5. Asakawa H, Takeda T. High energy x-ray therapy of gastric carcinoma. *J Jpn Soc Cancer Ther* 1973;8:362.
6. Baba H, Korenaga D, Okamura T, et al. Prognostic significance of DNA content with special reference to age in gastric cancer. *Cancer* 1989;63:1768.
7. Ballon S, Berman M, Lagasse L, et al. Survival after extraperitoneal pelvic and para-aortic lymphadenectomy and radiation therapy in cervical carcinoma. *Obstet Gynecol* 1981;57:90.
8. Bamias A, Cunningham D, Nicolson V, et al. Adjuvant chemotherapy for esophagogastric cancer with epirubicin, cisplatin and infusional 5-fluorouracil (ECF): a Royal Marsden pilot study. *Br J Cancer* 1995;71:583–586.
9. Benetta G, Fraschini P, Labianca R, et al. The value of FAM polychemotherapy in advanced gastric cancer. *Proc Am Soc Clin Oncol* 1982;1:103.
10. Bleiberg H, Goffin JC, Dalesio O, et al. Adjuvant radiotherapy and chemotherapy in resectable gastric cancer: a randomized trial of the gastro-intestinal tract cancer cooperative group of the EORTC. *Eur J Surg Oncol* 1989;15:535.
11. Bonenkamp JJ, Sasako M, Van de Velde CJ, et al. Extended lymph node dissection for gastric cancer. *N Engl J Med* 1999;340:908–914.
12. Bonenkamp JJ, Songun I, Hermans J, et al. Randomized comparison of morbidity after D1 and D2 dissection for gastric cancer in 996 Dutch patients. *Lancet* 1995;345:745.
13. Borrmann R. Geschwulste des magens und duodenums. In: Henke F, Lanbarsch O, eds. *Handbuch der speziellen pathologischen anatomie and histologie*, vol 4. Berlin: Julius Springer, 1926;.
14. Brecher G, Cronkite E, Conard R, et al. Gastric lesions in experimental animals following single exposures to ionizing radiations. *Am J Pathol* 1958;34:105.
15. Brick I. Effects of million volt irradiation on the gastrointestinal tract. *Arch Intern Med* 1955;96:26.
16. Buffet C, Turner K. Letter to the editor. *Br J Surg* 1983;70:131.
17. Bunt AM, Hermans J, Smit VT, et al. Surgical/pathologic-stage migration confounds comparisons of gastric cancer survival rates between Japan and Western countries. *J Clin Oncol* 1995;13:19.
18. Bunt AM, Hogendoorn PC, van de Velde CJ, et al. Lymph node staging standards in gastric cancer. *J Clin Oncol* 1995;13:2309.
19. Caletti G, Ferrari A, Brocchi E, et al. Accuracy of endoscopic ultrasonography in the diagnosis and staging of gastric cancer and lymphoma. *Surgery* 1993;113:14.
20. Carpender J, Levin E, Clayman C, et al. Radiation in the therapy of peptic ulcer. *Am J Roentgenol* 1956;76:374.
21. Caudry M, Escarmant P, Maire JP, et al. Radiotherapy of gastric cancer with a three field combination: Feasibility, tolerance and survival. *Int J Radiat Oncol Biol Phys* 1987;13:1821.
22. Coggon D, Barker DJP, Cole RB, et al. Stomach cancer and food storage. *J Natl Cancer Inst* 1989;81:1178.
23. Csendes A. Invited commentary. *World J Surg* 1988;12:398.
24. Cunningham D, Allum WH, Stenning SP et al. Perioperative chemotherapy versus surgery alone for respectable gastroesophageal cancer. *New Engl J Med* 2006;355:11–20.
25. Cuschieri A, Weeden S, Fielding J, et al. Patient survival after D1 and D2 resections for gastric cancer: long-term results of the MRC randomized surgical trial. Surgical Cooperative Group. *Br J Cancer* 1999;79(9–10):1522.
26. Dent DM, Madden MV, Price SK. Randomized comparison of R1 and R2 gastrectomy for gastric carcinoma. *Br J Surg* 1988;75:110.
27. Dent DM, Werner ID, Novis B, et al. Prospective randomized trial of combined oncological therapy for gastric carcinoma. *Cancer* 1979;44:385–392.
28. Dickson H. Effect of x-irradiation on glucose absorption. *Am J Physiol* 1955;182:477.
29. Dockerty MB. Pathologic aspects of primary malignant neoplasms of the stomach. In: ReMine WH, Priestley JT, Berkson J, eds. *Cancer of the stomach*. Philadelphia: W.B. Saunders, 1964: 173.
30. Douglass HO, Clark JL, Barcewicz P, et al. Importance of the R_2 lymph node dissection in the surgical treatment of gastric cancer. *Proc Am Soc Clin Oncol* 1989;8:101.
31. Douglass HO, Nava HR. Gastric adenocarcinoma: Management of the primary disease. *Semin Oncol* 1985;12:32.
32. Dupont JB Jr, Lee JR, Burton GR, et al. Adenocarcinoma of the stomach: review of 1497 cases. *Cancer* 1978;41:941.
33. Emami B, Watring W, Tak W, et al. Para-aortic lymph node radiation in advanced cervical cancer. *Int J Radiat Oncol Biol Phys* 1980;6:1237.
34. Falkson G, Van Eden EB. A controlled clinical trial of fluorouracil plus imidazole carboxamide dimethyl triazeno plus vincristine plus bis-chloroethyl nitrosourea plus radiotherapy in stomach cancer. *Med Pediatr Oncol* 1976;2:111–117.
35. Falkson G. Halogenated pyrimidines as radiopotentiators in the treatment of stomach cancer. *Prog Biochem Pharmacol* 1965;1:695.
36. Fein R, Kelsen DP, Geller N, et al. Adenocarcinoma of the esophagus and gastroesophageal junction: prognostic factors and results of therapy. *Cancer* 1985;56:2512.
37. Fenoglio-Preiser CM, Noffsinger AE, Belli J, et al. Pathologic and phenotypic features of gastric cancer. *Semin Oncol* 1996;23:292–306.
38. Fenoglio-Preiser CM. The effect of oncogenes on biology and prognosis of surgically resected gastric cancer.
39. Fenton P, Dickson H. Changes in some gastrointestinal functions following x-irradiation. *Am J Physiol* 1954;177:528.
40. Finlay CA, Hinds PW, Levine AJ. The p53 proto-oncogene can act as a suppressor of transformation. *Cell* 1989;57:1083–1093.
41. Fleming ID, Cooper JS, Henson DE, et al. Stomach. In: *AJCC staging manual*, 5th ed. Philadelphia: J.B. Lippincott-Raven, 1997;71–76.
42. Fletcher G, Lindberg R, Caderao J, et al. Hyperbaric oxygen as a radiotherapeutic adjuvant in advanced cancer of the uterine cervix. *Cancer* 1977;39:617.
43. Fletcher G, Rutledge F. Extended field technique in the management of cancers of the uterine cervix. *Am J Roentgenol* 1972;114:116.
44. Freid JR, Goldberg H, Tenzel W, et al. Cobalt 60 beam therapy: three year's experience at Montefiore Hospital (New York). *Radiology* 1956;67:200.
45. Friedman M. Calculated risks of radiation injury of normal tissue in the treatment of cancer of the testis. *Proceedings of the Second National Cancer Conference*. Philadelphia: Lippincott-Raven Publishers, 1952;1:390.
46. Fuchs CS, Mayer RJ. Gastric carcinoma. *N Engl J Med* 1995;333:32.
47. Fukutomi H, Nakahara A. Endoscopic therapy of gastrointestinal cancer and its curability. *Gan To Kagaku Ryoho* 1988;4:1132.
48. Fukuya T, Honda H, Hayashi T, et al. Lymph node metastases: efficacy of the detection with helical CT in patients with gastric cancer. *Radiology* 1995;197:711.
49. Gastrointestinal Tumor Study Group. A comparison of combination chemotherapy and combined modality therapy for locally advanced gastric carcinoma. *Cancer* 1982;49:1771–1777.
50. Gez E, Sulkes A, Yablonsky-Peretz T, et al. Combined 5-fluorouracil (5-FU) and radiation therapy following resection of locally advanced gastric carcinoma. *J Surg Oncol* 1986;31:139.
51. Gilbertson VA. Results of treatment of stomach cancer: an appraisal of efforts for more extensive surgery and a report of 1938 cases. *Cancer* 1969;23:1305.
52. Gill PG, Jamieson GG, Denham J, et al. Treatment of adenocarcinoma of the cardia with synchronous chemotherapy and radiotherapy. *Br J Surg* 1990;77:1020.
53. Goldgraber M, Rubin C, Palmer W, et al. The early gastric response to irradiation: a serial biopsy study. *Gastroenterology* 1954;27:1.
54. Goldstein HM, Rogers LF, Fletcher GH, et al. Radiological manifestations of radiation induced injury to the normal upper gastrointestinal tract. *Radiology* 1975;117:135.
55. Goss CM. *Anatomy of the human body*. Philadelphia: Lea & Febiger, 1973.
56. Greenlee RT, Hill-Harmon MG, Murray T, et al. Cancer statistics 2006. *CA Cancer J Clin* 2006;56(2):106–130.
57. Gunderson LL. Gastric cancer—patterns of relapse after surgical resection. *Semin Radiat Oncol* 2002;12(2):150–161.
58. Gunderson LL, Hoskins B, Cohen AM, et al. Combined modality treatment of gastric cancer. *Int J Radiat Oncol Biol Phys* 1983;9:965.
59. Gunderson LL, Sosin H. Adenocarcinoma of the stomach: areas of failure in a reoperation series (second or symptomatic looks). Clinicopathologic correlation and implications for adjuvant therapy. *Int J Radiat Oncol Biol Phys* 1982;8:1.
60. Gunderson LL, Willett CG, Harrison LB, et al., eds. *Intraoperative irradiation: techniques and results*. Totowa, NJ: Humana Press, 1999.
61. Haas CD, Mansfield CM, Leichman LP, et al. Combined nonsimultaneous radiation therapy and chemotherapy with 5-FU, doxorubicin, and mitomycin for residual localized gastric adenocarcinoma: a Southwest Oncology Group pilot study. *Cancer Treat Rep* 1983;67:421.
62. Hallissey MT, Dunn JA, Ward LC, et al. The second British Stomach Cancer Group trial of adjuvant radiotherapy or chemotherapy in resectable gastric cancer: five year follow-up. *Lancet* 1994;343:1309–1312.
63. Harrison JD, Morris DL, Ellis IO, et al. The effect of tamoxifen and estrogen receptor status on survival in gastric carcinoma. *Cancer* 1989;64:1007.
64. Hartley LC, Evans E, Windsor CJ. Factors influencing prognosis in gastric cancer. *Aust NZ J Surg* 1987;57:5.
65. Henderson IWD, Lipowska B, Lougheed MN. Clinical evaluation of combined radiation and chemotherapy in gastrointestinal malignancies. *Am J Roentgenol Radium Ther Nucl Med* 1968;102:545.
66. Henning GT, Schild S, Stafford S. Results of irradiation or chemo-irradiation following resection of gastric cancer. *Int J Radiat Oncol Biol Phys* 2000;46:589–598.
67. Hilton DA, West KP. An evaluation of the prognostic significance of HLA-DR expression in gastric cancer. *Cancer* 1990;66:1154.
68. Horn RC. Carcinoma of the stomach: autopsy findings in untreated cases. *Gastroenterology* 1955;29:515.
69. Howson CP, Hiyama T, Wynder EL. The decline in gastric cancer: epidemiology of an unplanned triumph. *Epidemiol Rev* 1986;8:1.
70. Hughes R, Brewington K, Hanjani P, et al. Extended field irradiation for cervical cancer based on surgical staging. *Gynecol Oncol* 1980;9:153.
71. Janch KW, Heiss MM, Gruetzner V, et al. Prognostic significance of bone marrow micrometastases in patients with gastric cancer. *J Clin Oncol* 1996;14:1810–1817.
72. Jolles C, Freedman R, Hamberger A, et al. Complications of extended-field therapy for cervical carcinoma without prior surgery. *Int J Radiat Oncol Biol Phys* 1986;12:179.
73. Kalish RJ, Clancy PE, Orringer MB, et al. Clinical epidemiologic and morphologic comparison between adenocarcinomas arising in Barrett's esophageal mucosa and in the gastric cardia. *Gastroenterology* 1984;86:461.
74. Kao GD, Whittington R, Coia L. Anatomy of the celiac axis and superior mesenteric artery and its significance in radiation therapy. *Int J Radiat Oncol Biol Phys* 1992;25:131.
75. Kastan MB, Oyekwere O, Sidransky D, et al. Participation of p53 in the cell response to DNA damage. *Cancer Res* 1991;51:6304–6311.
76. Kelsen D, Atig O, Saltz L, et al. FAMTX versus etoposide, doxorubicin and cisplatin: a randomized trial in gastric cancer. *J Clin Oncol* 1992;10:541–548.
77. Kennedy BJ. TNM classification for stomach cancer. *Cancer* 1970;26:971.
78. Kern KA. Gastric cancer: a neoplastic enigma. *J Surg Oncol Suppl* 1989;1:34.
79. Kim GE, Shin HS, Seong JS, et al. The role of radiation treatment in management of extrahepatic biliary tract metastasis from gastric carcinoma. *Int J Radiat Oncol Biol Phys* 1994;28:711.
80. Kim S, Lim KH, Lee J, et al. An observational study suggesting clinical benefit for adjuvant postoperative chemoradiation in a population of over 500 cases after

gastric resection with D2 nodal dissection for adenocarcinoma of the stomach. *Int J Rad Onc Biol Phys* 2005;63:1279–1285.
81. Klaassen DJ, MacIntyre JM, Catton GE, et al. Treatment of locally unresectable cancer of the stomach and pancreas: a randomized comparison of 5-fluorouracil alone with radiation plus concurrent and maintenance 5-fluorouracil. An Eastern Cooperative Oncology Group study. *J Clin Oncol* 1985;3:373.
82. Kodama Y, Sugimachi K, Soejima K, et al. Evaluation of extensive lymph node dissection for carcinoma of the stomach. *World J Surg* 1981;5:241.
83. Korenaga D, Okamura T, Saito A, et al. DNA ploidy is closely linked to tumor invasion, lymph node metastasis, and prognosis in clinical gastric cancer. *Cancer* 1988;62:309.
84. Krasna M, Tepper JE, Niedzwiecki D, et al. Trimodality therapy is superior to surgery alone in esophageal cancer: results of CALGB 9871. 2006 Gastrointestinal Cancer Symposium, Abstract 4,p. 83.
85. Landry J, Tepper J, Wood W, et al. Analysis of survival and local control following surgery for gastric cancer. *Int J Radiat Oncol Biol Phys* 1990;191:1357.
86. Lane DP. Worrying about p53. *Curr Biol* 1989;2:581–583.
87. Lerner A, Gonin R, Steele G, et al. Etoposide, doxorubicin, and cisplatin chemotherapy for advanced gastric cancer: results of a phase II trial. *J Clin Oncol* 1992;10:536–540.
88. Loury AM, Mansfield PF, Leach SD, et al. Laparoscopic staging for gastric cancer. *Surgery* 1996;119:611–614.
89. Lynch HT, Smyrk TC, Watson P, et al. Genetics, natural history, tumor spectrum and pathology of hereditary non-polyposis colon cancer: an updated review. *Gastroenterology* 1993;104:1535–1549.
90. MacDonald JS, Cohn I, Gunderson LL. Carcinoma of the stomach. In: Hellman S, Rosenberg SA, eds. *Principles and practice of oncology*. Philadelphia: J.B. Lippincott, 1985;.
91. MacDonald JS, Smalley SR, Benedetti J, et al. Chemoradiotherapy after surgery compared with surgery alone for adenocarcinoma of the stomach or gastroesophageal junction. *N Engl J Med* 2001;345:725–730.
92. Mantell BS. Radiotherapy for dysphagia due to gastric carcinoma. *Br J Surg* 1982;69:69.
93. Maruta K, Shida H. Some factors which influence prognosis after surgery for advanced gastric cancer. *Ann Surg* 1968;167:313.
94. Maus JH, McCormick NA. Three years' clinical experience with rotation therapy with the theratron. *Am J Roentgenol* 1958;79:382.
95. McNeer G, Vandenberg H, Donn FY, et al. A critical evaluation of subtotal gastrectomy for the cure of cancer of the stomach. *Ann Surg* 1957;134:2.
96. Meyers WC, Damiano RJ, Postlethwait RW, et al. Adenocarcinoma of the stomach: changing patterns over the last 4 decades. *Ann Surg* 1987;205:1.
97. Moertel CG, Childs DS, O'Fallon JR, et al. Combined 5-fluorouracil and radiation therapy as a surgical adjuvant for poor prognosis gastric carcinoma. *J Clin Oncol* 1984;2:1249–1254
98. Moertel CG, Childs DS, Reitemeier RJ, et al. Combined 5 fluorouracil and supervoltage radiation therapy of locally unresectable gastrointestinal cancer. *Lancet* 1969;865:867.
99. Moertel CG, Rubin J, O'Connell MJ, et al. A phase II study of combined 5-fluorouracil, doxorubicin, and cisplatin in the treatment of advanced upper gastrointestinal adenocarcinomas. *J Clin Oncol* 1986;4:1053.
100. Nagatomo T, Amee I, Luffu S. Histologic criteria of serosal rupture and prognosis in gastric carcinoma. *Cancer* 1969;29:180.
101. Nakajima T, Harashima S, Hirata M, et al. Prognostic and therapeutic values of peritoneal cytology in gastric cancer. *Acta Cytol* 1978;22:225.
102. Nanus DM, Kelsen DP, Niedzwiecki D, et al. Flow cytometry as a predictive indicator in patients with operable gastric cancer. *J Clin Oncol* 1989;7:1105.
103. Nelson J, Boyce J, Macasaet M, et al. Incidence, significance, and follow-up of para-aortic lymph node metastases in late invasive carcinoma of the cervix. *Am J Obstet Gynecol* 1977;128:336.
104. Neri B, de Leonardis V, Romano S, et al. Adjuvant chemotherapy after gastric resection in node-positive cancer patients: a multicentre randomized study. *Br J Cancer* 1996;73:549–552.
105. Nordman E. Value of megavolt therapy in gastric carcinoma. *Bull Cancer (Paris)* 1976;63:217.
106. O'Connor PM, Jackman J, Jondle D, et al. Role of p53 tumor suppressor gene in cell cycle arrest and radiosensitivity of Burkitt's lymphoma cell lines. *Cancer Res* 1993;53:4776–4780.
107. Offerhaus GJA, Stadt J, Huibregtse K, et al. The mucosa of the gastric remnant harboring malignancy. *Cancer* 1989;64:698.
108. Okajima K. Surgical treatment of gastric cancer with specific reference to lymph node removal. *Acta Med Okayama* 1977;31:369.
109. Papachristou DN, Fortner JG. Local recurrence of gastric adenocarcinomas after gastrectomy. *J Surg Oncol* 1981;18:47.
110. Potish R, Adcock L, Jones T, et al. The morbidity and utility of peri-aortic radiotherapy in cervical carcinoma. *Gynecol Oncol* 1983;15:1.
111. Potish R, Twiggs L, Adcock L, et al. Para-aortic lymph node radiotherapy in cancer of the uterine corpus. *Obstet Gynecol* 1985;65:251.
112. Potish R, Twiggs L, Prem K, et al. The impact of extraperitoneal surgical staging on morbidity and tumor recurrence following radiotherapy for cervical carcinoma. *Am J Clin Oncol* 1984;7:245.
113. Preusser P, Wilke H, Achterrath W, et al. Phase II study of the combination of etoposide, doxorubicin, and cisplatin in advanced measurable gastric cancer. *J Clin Oncol* 1989;7:1310–1317.
114. Prolla J, Kobayashi S, Kirsner J. Gastric cancer: some recent improvements in diagnosis based upon the Japanese experience. *Arch Intern Med* 1969;124:238.
115. Regine WF, Mohiuddin M. Impact of adjuvant therapy on locally advanced adenocarcinoma of the stomach. *Int J Radiat Oncol Biol Phys* 1992;24:921.
116. ReMine WH, Priestley JT, Berkson J. *Cancer of the stomach*. Philadelphia: W.B. Saunders, 1964.
117. Robertson CS, Chung SC, Woods SD, et al. A prospective randomized trial comparing R1 subtotal gastrectomy with R3 total gastrectomy for antral cancer. *Am Surg* 1994;220:176.
118. Roswit B, Malsky SJ, Reid CB. Radiation tolerance of the gastrointestinal tract. In: Vaeth J, ed. *Frontiers of radiation therapy oncology*. Baltimore: University Park Press, 1972;160.
119. Rotman M, Moon S, John M, et al. Extended field para-aortic radiation in cervical carcinoma: the case for prophylactic treatment. *Int J Radiat Oncol Biol Phys* 1978;4:795.
120. Rubin P, Casarett G. *Clinical radiation pathology*. Philadelphia: W.B. Saunders, 1968;153.
121. Rubin S, Brookland R, Mikuta J, et al. Para-aortic nodal metastases in early cervical carcinoma: long-term survival following extended-field radiotherapy. *Gynecol Oncol* 1983;18:213.
122. Saito N, Takeshita K, Habu H, et al. The use of endoscopic ultrasound in determining the depth of cancer invasion in patients with gastric cancer. *Surg Endosc* 1991;5:14.
123. Scarantino CW, Ornitz RD, Hoffman LG, et al. On the mechanism of radiation-induced emesis: the role of serotonin. *Int J Radiat Oncol Biol Phys* 1994;30:825.
124. Schein PS, Novak J. A comparison of combination chemotherapy and combined modality therapy for locally advanced gastric carcinoma. *Cancer* 1982;49:1771.
125. Schein PS, Smith FP, Dritschillo A, et al. Phase I-II trial of combined modality FAM plus split-course radiation (FAM-RT-FAM) for locally advanced gastric and pancreatic cancer: a Mid-Atlantic Oncology Program study. *Proc Am Soc Clin Oncol* 1983;2:126.
126. Serlin O, Keehn RJ, Higgins GA, et al. Factors related to survival following resection for gastric carcinoma. *Cancer* 1977;40:1318.
127. Siewert JR, Lange J, Bottcher K, et al. Stomach cancer: the current situation from the surgical viewpoint. *Dtsch Med Wochenschr* 1987;112:622.
128. Silverberg E, Boring CC, Squires TS. Cancer statistics, 1990. *CA Cancer J Clin* 1990;40:9.
129. Sindelar WF, Kinsella TJ, Tepper JE, et al. Randomized trial of intraoperative radiotherapy in carcinoma of the stomach. *Amer J Surg* 1993;165:178–187.
130. Slot A, Meerwaldt JH, van Putten WLJ, et al. Adjuvant postoperative radiotherapy for gastric carcinoma with poor prognostic signs. *Radiother Oncol* 1989;16:269.
131. Smalley SR, Evans RG. Radiation morbidity to the gastrointestinal tract and liver. In: Plowman P, McElwain TJ, Meadows AT, eds. *The complications of cancer management*. London: Butterworth, 1989;.
132. Smalley SS, Gunderson L, Tepper J, et al. Gastric surgical adjuvant radiotherapy consensus report: rationale and treatment implementation. *Int J Radiat Oncol Biol Phys* 2002;52:283–293.
133. Stout AP. Pathology of carcinoma of the stomach. *Arch Surg* 1943;46:807.
134. Sugiyama K, Yonemura Y, Miyazaki I. Immunohistochemical study of epidermal growth factor and epidermal growth factor receptor in gastric carcinoma. *Cancer* 1989;63:1557.
135. Tahara E. Molecular mechanism of stomach carcinogenesis. *J Cancer Res Clin Oncol* 1993;119:265–272.
136. Tahara E, Semba S, Tahara H. Molecular biological observations in gastric cancer. *Semin Oncol* 1996;23:307–315.
137. Tahara E, Yokozaki H, Yasui W. Growth factors in gastric cancer. In: Nishi M, Tahara E, eds. *Gastric cancer*. Tokyo: Springer-Verlag, 1993;209–217.
138. Takahashi M, Ota S, Shimada T, et al. Hepatocyte growth factor is the most potent endogenous stimulant of rabbit gastric epithelial cell proliferation and migration in primary culture. *J Clin Invest* 1995;95:1994–2203.
139. Tepper JE, Gunderson LL. Radiation treatment parameters in the adjuvant postoperative therapy of gastric cancer. *Semin Radiat Oncol* 2002;12(2):187–195.
140. Tewfik H, Buchsbaum H, Latourette H, et al. Para-aortic lymph node irradiation in carcinoma of the cervix after exploratory laparotomy and biopsy-proven positive aortic nodes. *Int J Radiat Oncol Biol Phys* 1982;8:13.
141. Thirlwell MP, Keable HE, Kost K, et al. Combination of 5-fluorouracil (5-FU) plus semustine (MECCNU) with and without radiotherapy (RT) in advanced gastric and pancreatic carcinoma. *Proc Am Soc Clin Oncol* 1981;22:449.
142. Tsukiyama I, Akine Y, Kajiura Y, et al. Radiation therapy for advanced gastric cancer. *Int J Radiat Oncol Biol Phys* 1988;15:123.
143. Walsh TN, Noonau N, Hollywood D, et al. A comparison of multimodal therapy and surgery to esophageal adenocarcinoma. *N Engl J Med* 1996;335:462–467.
144. Wang S, Renzi A, Chinn H. Mechanism of emesis following x-irradiation. *Am J Physiol* 1958;193:335.
145. Waters JS, Norman, Cunningham D, et al. Long-term survival after epirubicin, cisplatin and fluorouracil for gastric cancer: results of a randomized trial. *Br J Cancer* 1999;80:269–272.
146. Webb A, Cunningham D, Scarffe JH, et al. Randomized trial comparing epirubicin, cisplatin, and fluorouracil versus fluorouracil, doxorubicin, and methotrexate in advanced esophagogastric cancer. *J Clin Oncol* 1997;15:261–267.
147. Welander C, Pierce V, Nori D, et al. Pretreatment laparotomy in carcinoma of the cervix. *Gynecol Oncol* 1981;12:336.
148. Whittington R, Coia LR, Haler DH, et al. Adenocarcinoma of the esophagus and esophago-gastric junction: The effects of single and combined modalities on the survival and patterns of failure following treatment. *Int J Radiat Oncol Biol Phys* 1990;19:593.
149. Willett CG, Tepper JE, Orlow E, et al. Renal complications secondary to radiation treatment of upper abdominal malignancies. *Int J Radiat Oncol Biol Phys* 1986;12:1601–1604.
150. Wils O, Klein H, Wagener D, et al. Sequential high-dose methotrexate and fluorouracil combined with doxorubicin: a step forward in the treatment of gastric cancer. *J Clin Oncol* 1991;9:827–831.
151. Yamada Y, Kato Y. Greater tendency for submucosal invasion in fundic area gastric carcinomas than those arising in the pyloric area. *Cancer* 1989;63:1757.
152. Yonemura Y, Ninimiya I, Ohoyama S, et al. Expression of e-erb B-2 oncoprotein in gastric carcinoma. Immunoreactivity for e-erb B-2 protein is an independent of poor short-term prognostic in patients with gastric carcinoma. *Cancer* 1991;62:2914.
153. Zhang ZX, Gu XZ, Yin WB, et al. Randomized clinical trial on the combination of preoperative irradiation and surgery in the treatment of adenocarcinoma of gastric cardia (AGC)—report on 370 patients. *Int J Radiat Oncol Biol Phys* 1998;42(5):929–934.
154. Ziegler K, Sanft C, Zimmer T, et al. Comparison of computed tomography, endosonography, and intraoperative assessment in TN staging of gastric carcinoma. *Gut* 1993;34:604–610.

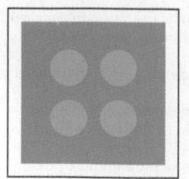

Chapter 56
Cancer of the Pancreas

Christopher G. Willett, Brian G. Czito, Johanna C. Bendell

Anatomy and Pathways of Spread

The pancreas lies in the retroperitoneal space of the upper abdomen at about the level of the first two lumbar vertebrae. It is divided into head (including the part called uncinate process), neck, body, and tail (Fig. 56.1). It has intimate contact with surrounding organs, including stomach, duodenum, jejunum, kidneys, and spleen as well as major vessels, which can be involved by direct tumor extension. Tumors in the head of the pancreas often invade or compress the common bile duct, causing jaundice and dilatation of the bile ducts and gallbladder.

The abundant pancreatic lymphatics have many connections with those of the duodenum. Regional drainage is to superior and inferior pancreaticoduodenal, porta hepatis, celiac, and superior mesenteric lymph nodes (2). With posterior tumor extension, para-aortic nodes are at risk. The main venous channels drain by the portal system to the liver. The lungs and pleura may also be involved because of posterior extension into tissues with venous drainage by the vena cava or its tributaries. Generalized peritoneal involvement is more common with carcinoma of the body and tail than with carcinoma of the head of the pancreas.

Epidemiology and Risk Factors

It is estimated that in 2006 there will have been 33,730 new cases of pancreatic cancer in the United States and 32,300 estimated deaths from the disease, making pancreatic cancer the fourth leading cause of cancer death in the United States (32). At present, surgery offers the only means of cure. Unfortunately, only 5% to 25% of patients present with tumors amenable to resection. Historically, patients undergoing resection of localized pancreatic carcinoma have a long-term survival of approximately 20% and a median survival of 13 to 20 months (23). Recent data suggest that the survival of patients who undergo resection of their pancreatic cancer may be improving, with contemporary 3-year survival rates around 30% (44). Patients who present with locally advanced and unresectable pancreatic cancer have a median survival of approximately 9 to 13 months, with rare long-term survival. The highest percentage (40% to 45%) of patients present with metastatic disease, which carries a shorter median survival of only 3 to 6 months (13).

Other pertinent epidemiological facts pancreatic cancer include: (a) age: incidence increases sharply after age 45 years; (b) female versus male (1.0 vs.1.3 incidence ratio); (c) race 14.8 per 100,000 (black males) versus 8.8 per 100,000 (general population). Risk factors of this malignancy include chronic pancreatitis, smoking, diabetes mellitus, and hereditary predisposition to pancreatic cancer or multiple cancers.

Clinical Presentation

Most patients with pancreatic cancer experience pain, weight loss, or jaundice. The initial presentation varies according to tumor location. Patients with tumors in the pancreatic body or tail usually present with pain and weight loss, while those in the head of the gland typically present with steatorrhea, weight loss, and jaundice. The recent onset of atypical diabetes mellitus, a history of recent but unexplained thrombophlebitis, or a previous attack of pancreatitis are often noted. Patients with pancreatic cancer rarely present with resectable disease because many of the presenting symptoms are nonspecific and are not investigated early or they result from local or systemic spread of disease. Positive physical findings, if any, are indicative of late-stage disease. These may include a palpable abdominal mass (i.e., pancreas, liver, or gallbladder due to biliary obstruction), supraclavicular nodes, or rectal shelf (i.e., peritoneal seeding).

Evaluation

In recent years, significant advances have been achieved in the imaging and staging of pancreatic cancer (94). Currently, the principal diagnostic tools are helical computed tomography (CT) scan, endoscopic ultrasound (EUS), and laparoscopy. These tools have facilitated the characterization of the primary tumor (resectable versus unresectable) as well as the identification of metastatic disease, so patients can be appropriately and reliably and triaged to operative and nonoperative therapies. With contemporary staging, the vast majority of patients with pancreatic cancer can be appropriately selected for surgery.

The most commonly used diagnostic and staging examination is an abdominal CT scan. Newer generation high-speed helical CT performed with contrast enhancement and thin section imaging allows high resolution, motion-free images of the pancreas and its surrounding structures to be obtained at varying phases of enhancement. Over 90% of patients deemed unresectable by CT are actually unresectable at operation. In addition, because tissue confirmation of malignancy is a necessary step prior to initiating therapy for patients with locally advanced tumors, CT can be utilized to facilitate fine-needle aspiration.

Advances in magnetic resonance imaging (MRI), including high resolution imaging, fast imaging, volume acquisitions, functional imaging, and MR cholangiopancreatograph have led to an improved ability of MRI to diagnose and stage pancreatic cancer (99).

Initial studies showed that positron emission tomography (PET) has a higher sensitivity, specificity, and accuracy than CT in diagnosing pancreatic carcinomas (42,70,80). PET is also more accurate than CT in identifying malignant pancreatic cystic lesions. New studies have compared PET-CT with PET in pancreatic cancers. Lemke et al. (42) studied 104 patients, with suspected pancreatic lesion. PET-CT software fusion had a higher sensitivity for malignancy detection than PET or CT alone (89% vs. 94% vs. 77%) but did not improve specificity (64%). All image modalities failed to stage lymph node involvement.

Another tool for staging and diagnosis is EUS. In this procedure, an endoscope with an ultrasound transducer at its tip is passed into the stomach and duodenum, where it provides high-resolution images of the pancreas and surrounding vessels and facilitates needle biopsies. Frequently, endoscopic ultrasound is

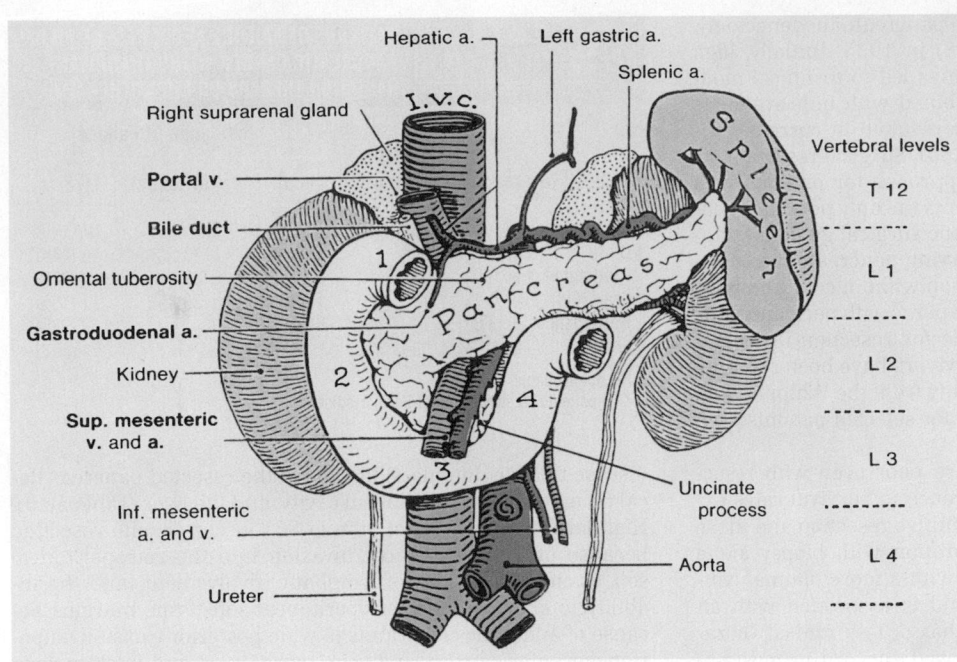

Hepatic a.   Left gastric a.

Splenic a.

Right suprarenal gland

I.V.C.

Portal v.

Bile duct

Omental tuberosity

Gastroduodenal a.

Kidney

Sup. mesenteric v. and a.

Inf. mesenteric a. and v.

Ureter

Spleen

Pancreas

Vertebral levels

T 12

L 1

L 2

L 3

Uncinate process

Aorta

L 4

FIGURE 56.1. Anatomy of the pancreas gland. a, artery; v, vein. Numbers 1–4 refer to portions of the duodenum. (From Moore KL. *Clinically oriented anatomy*, 2nd ed. Baltimore: Williams & Wilkins, 1985, with permission.)

performed in conjunction with endoscopic retrograde cholangiopancreatography (ERCP) (7). This combined diagnostic approach allows for staging, therapeutic stenting of the common bile duct when indicated, and retrieval of tumor cells by fine-needle aspiration without exposing the peritoneum to potential tumor seeding as may occur with CT-guided biopsies.

Because current imaging techniques cannot visualize small (1 to 2 mm) liver and peritoneal implants, staging laparoscopy has been used preoperatively to exclude intraperitoneal metastases. This technique can detect intraperitoneal metastases in up to 37% of patients with apparently locally advanced disease by CT (72). Patients with locally advanced disease with involved peritoneal washings or positive peritoneal biopsies have the same prognosis as those with metastatic disease. These patients are more appropriately treated with systemic therapies (16).

Staging

Staging has rarely been used in published series, and tumors are instead usually classified as resectable, unresectable, or metastatic. The current American Joint Committee on Cancer tumor, node, metastasis staging system is described in Table 56.1.

Pathologic Classification

Approximately 90% of pancreatic cancers are adenocarcinomas, and at least two-thirds are found in the head of the pancreas. Other cell types include islet cell tumors, cystadenomas, and cystadenocarcinomas; all have a much slower natural history than adenocarcinomas and are not considered in the section on treatment. The histopathology of lesions in the periampullary region of the head of the pancreas is of particular importance because different types of adenocarcinomas, originating from the pancreas, bile duct, ampullary region, or duodenum, carry very different prognoses (48).

Several molecular abnormalities have been implicated in contributing to the development of pancreatic cancer. At this time, four tumor suppressor genes have been implicated (p16,

p53, DPC4, and BRCA2), with incidences of 50% to 95% in all pancreatic tumors. Among oncogenes, K-ras activation is observed in 90% of these tumors. These molecular changes may become helpful in defining the precursor lesions with high likelihood of progressing into carcinomas and in characterizing pathologically ambiguous lesions. Screening may be another future application of these molecular markers (30).

General Management

Operative Considerations

More than 80% of patients present with advanced disease that is not amenable to curative resection (52,85), and 66% of patients are 65 years of age or older. The standard surgical treatment

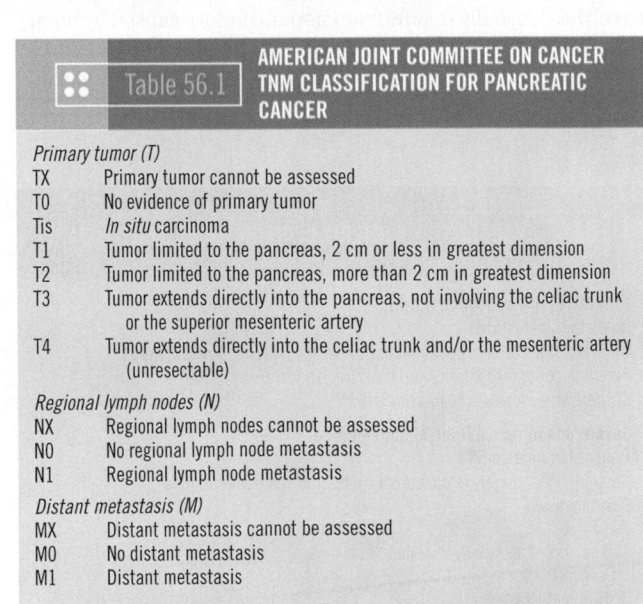

	AMERICAN JOINT COMMITTEE ON CANCER TNM CLASSIFICATION FOR PANCREATIC CANCER
Table 56.1	

Primary tumor (T)
TX	Primary tumor cannot be assessed
T0	No evidence of primary tumor
Tis	*In situ* carcinoma
T1	Tumor limited to the pancreas, 2 cm or less in greatest dimension
T2	Tumor limited to the pancreas, more than 2 cm in greatest dimension
T3	Tumor extends directly into the pancreas, not involving the celiac trunk or the superior mesenteric artery
T4	Tumor extends directly into the celiac trunk and/or the mesenteric artery (unresectable)

Regional lymph nodes (N)
NX	Regional lymph nodes cannot be assessed
N0	No regional lymph node metastasis
N1	Regional lymph node metastasis

Distant metastasis (M)
MX	Distant metastasis cannot be assessed
M0	No distant metastasis
M1	Distant metastasis

From American Joint Committee on Cancer. *AJCC cancer staging manual,* 6th ed. New York, Berlin, Hedelberg: Springer-Verlag, 2002;157–162, with permission.

for pancreatic cancer remains the pancreatoduodenectomy, first described by Whipple et al. (88) in 1935. Initially, high operative morbidity and mortality rates led to technical modifications of the operation that, combined with improvements in anesthesia and critical care, have resulted in current perioperative mortality rates of ≤2% (29,84). Surgical resection, as part of a multimodality treatment approach for patients with resectable pancreatic cancer, represents the only potentially curative treatment strategy (57,73). Some surgical guidelines appear well established. Pylorus-preserving pancreatoduodenectomy improves gastrointestinal function without compromising the oncologic management (39,78). Patients with peripancreatic lymph node involvement are suitable for resection (if technically possible) because long-term survivors have been reported (101). Because of the reduced morbidity from the Whipple et al. procedure, there is no age limitation for selected patients even at ages >80 years (45,75).

Although 5-year survival rates are poor even with resection (5% to 20%), a significant difference in survival rates exists between patients undergoing definitive resection and those receiving palliative bypass or exploration with biopsy alone (43). Although total pancreatectomy with a more optimal lymphadenectomy can be performed and is associated with an operative mortality rate similar to that of less radical "curative" procedures, this has not improved survival in most series. This question is affirmed in a prospective randomized trial whose preliminary results indicate that only 10% of patients with extensive retroperitoneal lymph nodes have these nodes involved as the only site (102). Finally, it is important to perform such surgical interventions at centers with high volumes and extensive experience (68,73,76). There are no universally accepted criteria for resectability other than absence of distant lymph node involvement and/or visceral, peritoneal, or extra-abdominal metastases. Some institutional differences are apparent for patients with locoregional disease and are based on different clinical experiences. Some generally accepted criteria that may be used to classify tumors into resectable, borderline resectable, and unresectable lesions are summarized in Table 56.2.

Areas of Failure and Cause of Death

For patients with locally unresectable tumors or metastatic disease, death usually results from hepatic failure caused by biliary obstruction by local tumor extension or hepatic replacement by metastases. For the 10% to 20% of patients undergoing a potentially curative pancreatoduodenectomy, three major sites of

Table 56.2	CRITERIA DEFINING RESECTABILITY STATUS

Resectable (head, body, and tail)
No distant metastases
Clear fat plane around celiac and superior mesenteric arteries (SMA)
Patent superior mesenteric vein (SMV)/portal vein
Borderline resectable (head and body)
Severe unilateral SMV/portal impingement
Tumor abutment on SMA
Gastroduodenal artery encasement up to origin at hepatic artery
Colon invasion
(Tail)
Adrenal, colon, or kidney invasion
Unresectable
Distant metastases
SMA or celiac encasement

From NCCN (National Comprehensive Cancer Network), version 2000, with permission.

Table 56.3	PATTERNS OF FAILURE AFTER RESECTION OF PANCREATIC CANCER WITHOUT ADJUVANT RADIATION THERAPY OR CHEMOTHERAPY

Author (Reference)	No. of Patients	Incidence of Failure		
		Local	Peritoneal	Liver
Tepper et al. (81)	26	13 (50%)	NA	NA
Griffin et al. (24)	36[a]	19 (53%)	11 (31%)	16 (44%)
Whittington et al. (90)	29	22 (85%)	6 (23%)	6 (23%)
Ozaki (60)	14	12 (86%)	5 (36%)	11 (79%)
Westerdahl et al. (87)	74	64 (86%)	NA	68 (92%)

NA, not available
[a]Ten patients received external-beam irradiation.

disease relapse dominate: the bed of the resected pancreas (local recurrence), the peritoneal cavity, and the liver (Table 56.3). High local failure rates of 50% to 86% occur despite resection because of frequent cancer invasion into the retroperitoneal soft tissues, high rates of lymphatic involvement, and the inability to achieve wide retroperitoneal soft-tissue margins because of anatomic constraints to wide posterior excision (superior mesenteric artery and vein, portal vein, and inferior vena cava). Careful pathologic examination of the posterior peripancreatic soft tissue margins indicates a high incidence (38%) of microscopic residual disease extending to these margins in patients undergoing resection (96). Therefore, tumor stage and grade and resection margin status are the best predictors of survival after surgery (1,96).

Radiation Therapy Techniques

Dose-Limiting Tissues

The dose-limiting organs for irradiation of upper-abdominal cancers are the small intestine, stomach, liver, kidneys, and spinal cord. Split-course regimens or precision multifield standard fraction techniques allow delivery of higher external-beam radiation doses than were previously accepted as tolerable, for example, split-course regimen of 60 Gy over 10 weeks (26) and precision irradiation techniques using 60 to 72 Gy over 7 to 9 weeks (90,93). Although precision techniques can spare the liver, kidney, and spinal cord, portions of the stomach and small bowel remain within the field. Because the long-term survival rate is low, the actual number of patients at long-term risk for small bowel or gastric complications is also small. Long-term complications may also be decreased because a much smaller volume of small bowel and stomach is included within the high-dose field. Three-dimensional conformal radiation therapy (3DCRT) and intensity-modulated radiation therapy (IMRT) currently are being investigated in patients with pancreatic cancer. Preliminary studies indicate that five to six conformal fields (28) or the 3D noncoplanar technique (9,17) can be designed to improve dose-volume characteristics over those of conventional four-field treatment designs, but the posterior wall of the stomach and the medial wall of the duodenum cannot usually be excluded from the high-dose volume.

Treatment Volumes and Doses

In patients undergoing surgery, clips should be placed to mark the extent of the lesion for later external irradiation. Used sparingly (e.g., a single small vascular clip placed in each location to mark superior, inferior, lateral, and medial margins), small clips produce only minimal interference on CT scans. Titanium clips

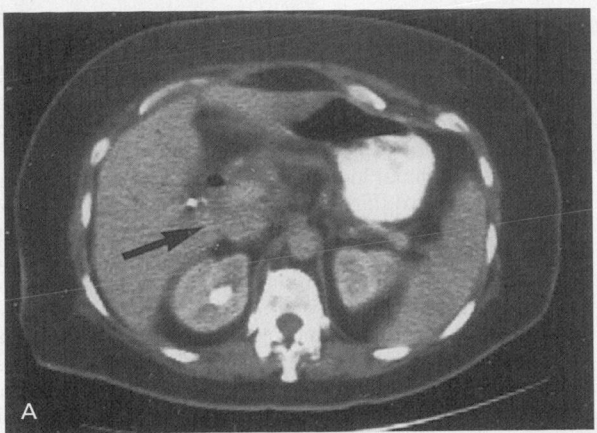

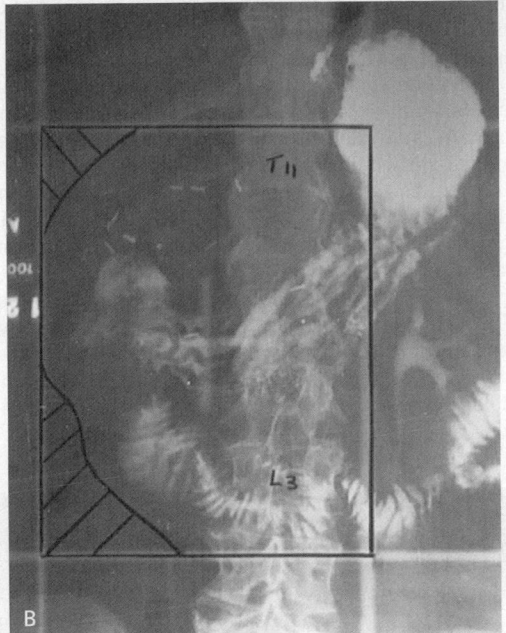

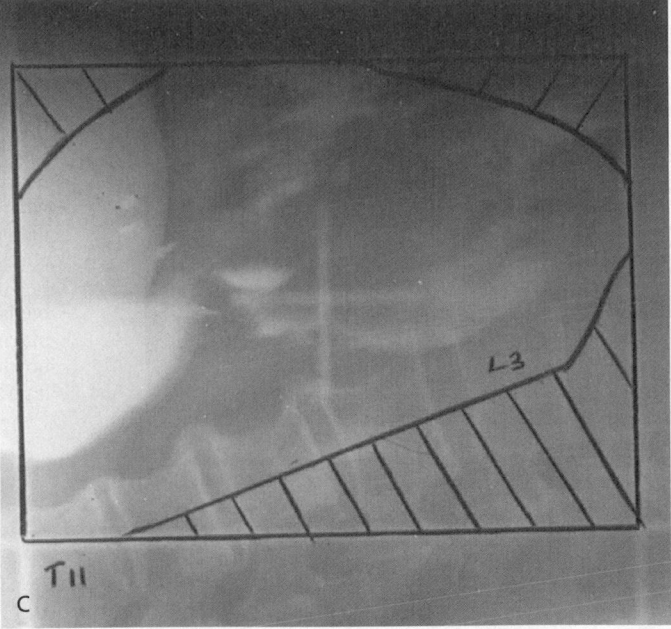

FIGURE 56.2. External beam four-field technique for pancreatic head lesion. **A:** The lesion on computed tomography scan. Note dilated pancreatic duct and relation of pancreas to duodenal loop and stomach. **B:** The anteroposterior/posteroanterior (AP/PA) field, which includes tumor with approximately 3-cm margin of the pancreas (body), the duodenal loop (plus approximately 50% of the right kidney), and the nodal area at risk. Most of the left kidney is shielded. **C:** The lateral field with an anterior margin 1.5 to 2.0 cm beyond gross disease and a posterior margin at least 1.5 cm behind front edge of vertebral body.

produce less CT interference but sometimes cannot be located on lateral simulation films because of their lesser density.

The patient should be supine during simulation and treatment. An initial set of anteroposterior (AP) and cross-table lateral films is obtained after injection of renal contrast medium to identify operative clips and renal position relative to the field center. Additional films can be obtained with contrast medium in the stomach and duodenal loop in unresected patients.

The intent of treatment is to use multiple field, fractionated, external-beam techniques with high-energy photons to deliver 45 to 50 Gy in 1.8-Gy fractions to tumor bed, unresected or residual tumor, and lymph node–bearing areas at risk. After 45 to 50.4 Gy, a boost field can be designed to include unresected or gross residual disease, as defined by CT scans and clips, while excluding most of the stomach and small bowel. With lesions in the head of the pancreas, major node groups include the pancreaticoduodenal, porta hepatis, celiac, and suprapancreatic nodes. The suprapancreatic node group is included with the body of the pancreas for a 3- to 5-cm margin beyond gross disease; however, more than two-thirds of the left kidney must be excluded from the anteroposterior/posteroanterior (AP/PA)

field because at least 50% of the right kidney is often in the field owing to duodenal inclusion. The entire duodenal loop with margin is included because pancreatic head lesions may invade the medial wall of the duodenum and place the entire circumference at risk, including the pancreaticoduodenal nodal basins (Fig. 56.2).

For head of pancreas lesions, the superior field extent is often at the middle or upper portion of the T11 vertebral body for adequate margins on the celiac vessels (T12, L1) and the inferior limit at the level L2–3 to include the superior mesenteric lymph nodes and third portion of the duodenum. The upper field extent is occasionally more superior with body lesions to obtain adequate margin on the primary lesion. With lateral fields, the anterior field margin is 1.5 to 2.0 cm beyond gross disease. The posterior margin is at least 1.5 cm behind the anterior portion of the vertebral body to allow adequate margins on para-aortic nodes, which are at risk with posterior tumor extension in head or body lesions. The lateral contribution usually is limited to 15 to 18 Gy because a moderate volume of kidney or liver may be in the irradiated volume (see Fig. 56.2); it is, therefore, important to reduce the weight of these beams accordingly because

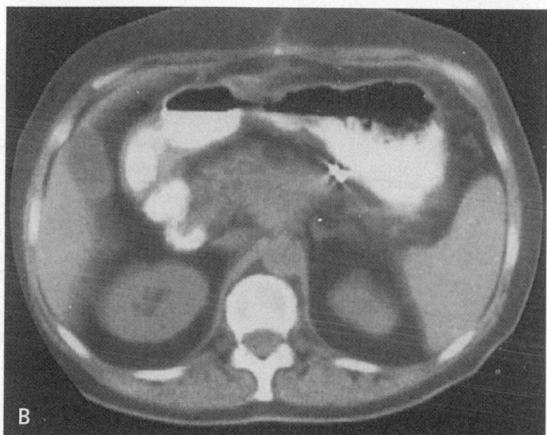

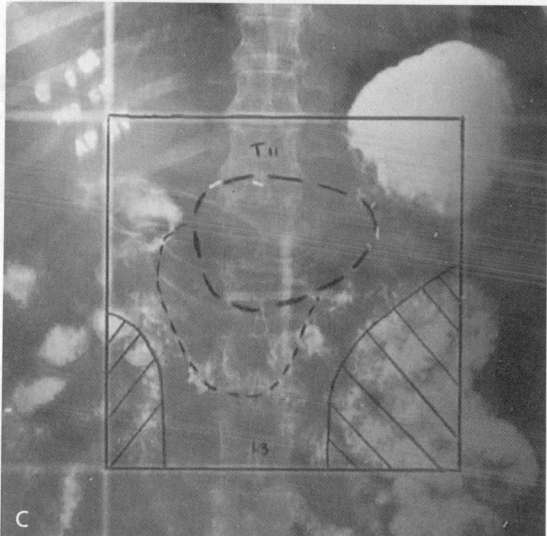

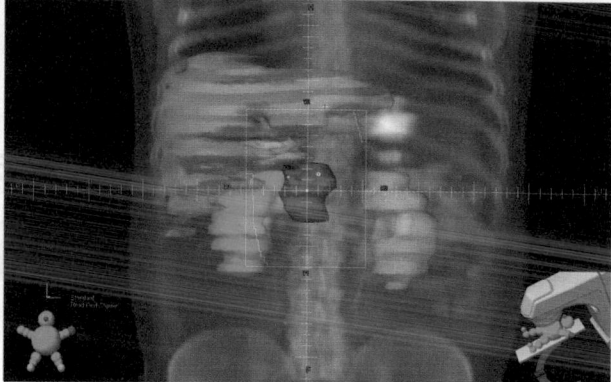

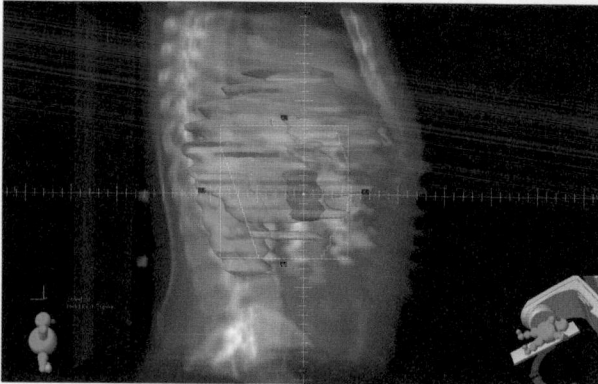

the risk of kidney damage is low if half of the volume is limited to 18 Gy or less (91).

With pancreatic body or tail lesions, at least 50% of the left kidney may need to be included to achieve adequate margins and to include node groups at risk (i.e., lateral suprapancreatic splenic artery and splenic hilum nodes). Because inclusion of the entire duodenal loop is not indicated with body or tail lesions, at least two thirds of the right kidney can be preserved, but with tailored blocks it is usually possible to cover pancreaticoduodenal and porta hepatis nodes adequately (Fig. 56.3).

CT-based treatment planning and 3DCRT techniques permit the construction of dose-volume histograms and the generation of treatment plans that optimize radiation dose delivery to tumor-bearing tissues and sparing of critical normal tissues. Normal tissue complication probabilities, according to classical clinical studies (12), can help accomplish this, although investigations are still under way (Fig. 56.4).

Further refinement of this approach is now being obtained by the use of IMRT. With this new technology, inverse treatment planning can be performed, permitting computer-based treatment optimization versus a standard "trial and error" planning approach. Second, a computer-controlled, nonuniform radiation treatment can be delivered to the target, permitting an even more precise and conformal dose pattern with further reductions in normal tissue irradiation. Evolution of these techniques will likely result in improved treatment tolerance and reduction of late morbidity. This is especially critical in this era of intensive chemoradiation protocols with their potential toxicity.

After resection, AP/PA and lateral fields are designed on the basis of preresection CT primary tumor volumes, operative clip placement, and postoperative CT nodal volumes (68). The only border that can be more restrictive is the anterior border on lateral fields because the primary tumor has been resected. This

FIGURE 56.3. External-beam four-field technique for body of pancreas lesion. **A:** Computed tomography (CT) scan showing right tumor extent of lesion marked with clips. **B:** CT scan of same patient showing left tumor extent marked with clips. The lesion extends posteriorly; note proximity of the tumor to the posterior wall of the stomach anteriorly. The normal glandular appearance of the head of the pancreas and its relation to the duodenum can be seen. **C:** The anteroposterior/posteroanterior (AP/PA) field showing lesion as reconstructed from CT and clips (*broken line*) and head of pancreas (*dotted line*). The field is extended to the left to get a 3- to 5-cm margin of uninvolved pancreas and additional nodal coverage (suprapancreatic with or without splenic). Although the pancreaticoduodenal and porta hepatis nodes are included, the entire duodenal loop does not need to be treated, and at least two thirds of the right kidney can be shielded. (From Gunderson LL, Margolis AR, Burhenne HJ, eds. *Alimentary tract radiology,* 3rd ed. St. Louis: C.V. Mosby, 1982, with permission.)

FIGURE 56.4. Three-dimensional conformal fields of patient with anteroposterior/posteroanterior arrangement **(A)** and right and left lateral arrangement **(B)** of patient with unrectable pancreatic cancer.

Table 56.4	**PROSPECTIVE, RANDOMIZED TRIALS FOR ADJUVANT THERAPY FOR PANCREATIC CANCER**			
Series (Reference)	**No. of Patients**	**Median Survival (months)**	**2-Year Survival (%)**	**5-Year Survival (%)**
GITSG (34)				
Treatment	21	21.0	43	19
Observation	22	10.9	18	5
Treatment (expanded cohort) (19)	30	18.0	46	NA
EORTC (37)				
Treatment	60	17.1	37	20
Observation	54	12.6	23	10
ESPAC-1 (54,55)				
Pooled data				
Chemotherapy	244	19.7	NA	NA
No chemotherapy	237	14.0	NA	NA
Chemoradiation	178	15.5	NA	NA
No chemoradiation	180	16.1	NA	NA
2 by 2 factorial				
Chemotherapy	147	20.1	40	21
No chemotherapy	142	15.5	30	8
Chemoradiation	145	15.9	29	10
No chemoradiation	144	17.9	41	20

EORTC, European Organisation for Research and Treatment of Cancer; ESPAC, European Study Group for Pancreatic Cancer; GITSG, Gastrointestinal Tumor Study Group; NA, not available

border is determined by vascular or nodal boundaries (porta hepatis, superior mesenteric, and celiac) as demonstrated on CT.

Radiation Therapy Results

Resectable Tumors: Adjuvant Therapy

After surgical resection of pancreatic cancer, local recurrence rates range from 50% to 86% and distant recurrence rate 40% to 90%, most commonly in the liver and/or peritoneum (24,60,81,87). For this reason, adjuvant radiation therapy, chemotherapy, and combined radiation and chemotherapy have been employed in an effort to improve patient outcomes (Table 56.4). Despite multiple trials, a definitive role for adjuvant therapy for resected pancreatic cancer has not been established.

Prospective Trials

The Gastrointestinal Tumor Study Group (GITSG) conducted the first prospective trial of adjuvant chemoradiotherapy for patients with resected pancreatic cancer and negative surgical margins. Patients were randomized to external beam radiation therapy (ERBT) to 40 Gy delivered in split-course fashion with concurrent 5-fluorouracil 500 mg/m^2 given as an intravenous bolus on the first three and last three days of radiation, followed by maintenance 5-FU for 2 years or until disease progression or to observation only (34). This trial was stopped early secondary to slow accrual (43 patients over 8 years), and a positive interim analysis showing that patients treated on the chemoradiotherapy arm experienced a survival benefit. Patients receiving chemoradiotherapy had a longer median survival (21 months vs. 11 months) and improved 2-year survival (43% vs. 19%). An additional 30 patients were later enrolled to receive adjuvant

chemoradiation. These additional patients confirmed the survival outcomes seen in the original trial with median survival of 18 months and a 2-year survival of 46% (19). The GITSG trial was criticized for many reasons: only 9% of patients received the planned 2-year maintenance chemotherapy, the radiation dose was low/split course, the number of patients was small, the accrual was slow, it had an unusually poor survival rate for the surgical control group, 25% of patients did not begin adjuvant therapy until over 10 weeks after resection, and 32% of the original treatment arm had violations of the scheduled radiation therapy. Nevertheless, this trial resulted in chemoradiation therapy being accepted as appropriate adjuvant therapy in the United States.

A second study sponsored by the European Organisation for Research and Treatment of Cancer (EORTC) sought to confirm the findings of the original GITSG study. In this trial, 218 patients with resected pancreas or other periampullary cancers were randomly assigned to receive 40 Gy of EBRT in a split-dose fashion with concurrent continuous infusional 5-FU or observation alone (37). This study showed no significant improvement ($p = .208$) in median survival (24 months vs. 19 months) or 2-year survival (51% vs. 41%). Interestingly, only 114 of the patients enrolled in the trial had pancreatic cancer, with the remaining patients having periampullary tumors. Subset analysis of the patients with primary pancreatic tumors showed a 2-year survival of 34% for treated patients versus 26% for the control group ($p = .099$). Limitations of this trial include no maintenance chemotherapy given in the treatment arm, patients with positive surgical margins were allowed on trial with no prospective assessment, the radiation dose was low, the number of patients was small, and the fact that 20% of patients assigned to treatment never received treatment.

The European Study Group for Pancreatic Cancer (ESPAC) then conducted the largest randomized trial evaluating adjuvant therapy for pancreatic cancer, ESPAC-1. Treating physicians were allowed to enroll their patients into one of three parallel randomized studies:

1. Chemoradiation versus no chemoradiation ($n = 69$), consisting of 20 Gy over 2 weeks with 5-FU 500 mg/m^2 on days 1 through 3, then repeated after a 2-week break;
2. Chemotherapy versus no chemotherapy ($n = 192$), consisting of bolus 5-FU (425 mg/m^2) and leucovorin (20 mg/m^2) given for 5 days every 28 days for 6 months; or
3. A 2 by 2 factorial design of 289 patients enrolled on chemoradiotherapy ($n = 73$), chemotherapy ($n = 75$), chemoradiotherapy with maintenance chemotherapy ($n = 72$), or observation ($n = 69$) (54,55).

The data from the treatment groups from all three parallel trials were then pooled for analysis. There was no survival difference between the 175 patients who received adjuvant chemoradiation and the 178 patients who did not receive therapy (median survival 15.5 months vs. 16.1 months; $p = .24$). There was, however, a survival benefit found for the patients who received adjuvant chemotherapy ($n = 238$) compared to those who did not ($n = 235$) (median survival 19.7 months vs. 14 months; $p = .0005$). On further follow-up, the 5-year survival rate for the patients who received chemotherapy was 21% versus 8% for those who did not.

Like its predecessors, the ESPAC-1 trial had many criticisms. These included:

1. Physicians were allowed to choose which of the three parallel trials to enroll patients on, creating potential bias.
2. Patients could receive "background" chemoradiation or chemotherapy as decided by their physician. Approximately one third of the patients enrolled on the chemotherapy versus no chemotherapy trial received "background" chemoradiation therapy or chemotherapy.

Table 56.5	SUMMARY RESULTS: PHASE III STUDIES OF POSTOPERATIVE RADIATION THERAPY AND CHEMOTHERAPY FOR PANCREATIC HEAD ADENOCARCINOMA SURVIVAL			
Study (Reference)	Median (Months)		3-Year Survival (%)	5-Year Survival (%)
GITSG[a] (34)				
5-FU/CRT ($n = 21$)	21		24	19
EORTC[b] (37)				
5-FU/CRT ($n = 60$)	17.1		30	20
RTOG 9704[c] (66)				
5-FU/CRT ($n = 221$)	16.9		21	—
Gem/CRT ($n = 221$)	20.6		32	—

CRT, chemoradiation therapy; EORTC, European Organisation for Research and Treatment of Cancer; 5-FU, 5-fluoroucil; Gem, gemcitabine; GITSG, Gastrointestinal Tumor Study Group; RTOG, Radiation Therapy Oncology Group
[a]Included patients with "negative" margins only.
[b]Included patients with T1–2 disease only and approximately 80% had negative margins.
[c]Included approximately 75% patients with T3–4 disease only and approximately 40% had negative margins.

3. The radiation was given in a split-dose fashion, with the treating physician judging the final treatment dose (40 Gy vs. 60 Gy).

4. In the chemoradiation versus no chemoradiation trial, no maintenance adjuvant chemotherapy was given, similar to the EORTC trial.

Although there was no benefit seen with adjuvant chemoradiation therapy, there was a benefit to adjuvant chemotherapy.

Building from the data showing potential benefit to adjuvant chemotherapy, investigators in Europe conducted a randomized phase III trial of adjuvant gemcitabine versus observation in patients with resected pancreatic cancer. Three hundred sixty-eight patients were enrolled to this trial and were randomized to gemcitabine 1,000 mg/m^2 intravenous days 1, 8, and 15 every 4 weeks for 6 months or observation (56). The primary end point was disease-free survival, and patients who were treated with gemcitabine had a statistically significantly longer disease-free survival (11.0 months vs 7.5 months) than those who had observation only. Overall survival data are awaiting maturity.

In the Radiation Therapy Oncology Group (RTOG) and Gastrointestinal Intergroup Trial 9704 phase III study, 538 patients with resected pancreatic cancer were randomized to either: (a) 3 weeks of continuous infusional 5-FU at 250 mg/m^2/day, followed by chemoradiation (50.4 Gy in 1.8 Gy daily fractions with continuous infusional 5-FU at 250 mg/m^2/day), then two 4-week courses of continuous infusional 5-FU at 250 mg/m^2/day beginning 3 to 5 weeks after completion of chemoradiation with 2 weeks' rest between courses, or (b) three weekly doses of gemcitabine at 1,000 mg/m^2/week followed by the same 5-FU–based chemoradiation as in the first arm, followed by 3 months of gemcitabine 1,000 mg/m^2 given weekly 3 out of every 4 weeks (66). Results showed a survival advantage in patients with resected pancreatic head carcinoma receiving maintenance gemcitabine versus maintenance 5-FU. The 3-year overall survival rate of 187 patients with resected pancreatic head carcinoma receiving maintenance gemcitabine with chemoradiation was 32%. In contrast, the 3-year overall survival rate of 194 patients receiving maintenance 5-FU with chemoradiation was 21%. Trial results of this study compared to other prospective studies are summarized in Table 56.5.

Single Institution Experiences

Reports of single-institution experiences with adjuvant therapy for resected pancreatic cancer have provided additional evidence to the benefit of adjuvant therapy. The largest of these series is from the Johns Hopkins Medical Institutions, where

investigators reported the results of a retrospective analysis of 174 patients were treated as follows:

1. EBRT (40 Gy to 45 Gy) with two 3-day courses of 5-FU at the beginning and end of radiation, followed by weekly bolus 5-FU (500 mg/m^2) for 4 months ($n = 99$),

2. EBRT (50.4 Gy to 57.6 Gy) to the pancreatic bed plus prophylactic hepatic irradiation (23.4 Gy to 27 Gy) given with infusional 5-FU (200 mg/m^2/day) plus leucovorin (5 mg/m^2/day) for 5 out of 7 days of the week for 4 months ($n = 21$), or

3. No therapy ($n = 53$) (100).

Patients who received adjuvant chemoradiation had a median survival of 20 months compared to 14 months for patients who were not treated. Two-year survival was 44% and 30%, respectively. There was no survival advantage to the more intensive adjuvant therapy. A follow-up report from this group of 616 patients with resected pancreatic cancer found adjuvant chemoradiation treatment as a strong predictor of outcome, with a hazard ratio of 0.5 (74).

Data with the highest seen survival after adjuvant therapy for pancreatic cancer come from a phase II trial done at Virginia Mason Clinic. Results from 43/53 enrolled patients on this study were reported in 2003. These patients were treated with EBRT to 50 Gy with concurrent chemotherapy with 5-FU 200 mg/m^2/day continuous infusion, cisplatin 70 mg/m^2 weekly, and interferon-α 3 million units subcutaneously every other day. After completion of chemoradiation, patients received 5-FU 200 mg/m^2/day continuous infusion on weeks 10 through 15 and 18 through 23 (61). The median survival, 2-year overall survival, and 5-year overall survival were 44 months, 58%, and 45%, respectively. With these encouraging data came significant toxicity, with 70% of patients experiencing grade 3 toxicities, and 42% of patients requiring hospitalization. The American College of Surgeons Oncology Group opened a larger, multicenter, phase II trial of 100 patients to further investigate this regimen, but this study closed secondary to poor accrual.

Neoadjuvant Therapy

Even after undergoing curative resection for pancreatic cancer, 80% to 85% of patients will recur. In addition, positive margins or nodal disease increases this rate of recurrence to 90% (8,96). The use of neoadjuvant chemoradiation offers another approach to improve on these figures for several reasons:

1. Approximately 25% of patients do not receive adjuvant therapy in a timely manner after surgery or do not receive it at all (74,77),

2. Given the high recurrence rates after surgical resection, pancreatic cancer is likely a systemic disease at the time of diagnosis in 80% to 85% of patients who appear to have resectable disease (14,86), and with neoadjuvant therapy, 20% to 40% of patients will be spared the morbidity of resection because their metastatic disease becomes clinically apparent (65),

3. Preoperative therapy could theoretically be less toxic and more effective as the chemotherapy and radiation would be given without the postsurgical issues of small bowel in the radiation field and decreased oxygenation and decreased drug delivery to the remaining tumor bed (89), and

4. Patients with local and unresectable lesions may be able to be downstaged to allow for surgical resection.

At M.D. Anderson Cancer Center, multiple trials of neoadjuvant 5-FU–based chemoradiation have been performed. The first trial treated 28 patients with 5-FU 300 mg/m^2/day continuous infusion with concurrent EBRT to 50.4 Gy over 5.5 weeks (15). Patients who underwent surgical resection also received intraoperative radiation therapy (IORT). Twenty-five percent of patients had evidence of metastatic disease on preoperative restaging. Fifteen percent had metastatic disease that was found on laparoscopy. For the patients who underwent surgery median survival was 18 months, and 41% had a pathologic partial response to therapy. However, 33% of patients treated on this study required hospitalization for gastrointestinal toxicity from therapy. For this reason, the next trials from this group focused on rapid fractionation EBRT. A prospective trial of 35 patients treated with EBRT to 30 Gy (3 Gy per fraction for 10 fractions) with concurrent 5-FU 300 mg/m^2/day continuous infusion found grade 3 nausea and vomiting in only 9% of patients with no grade 4 toxicities (63). Twenty-seven patients were taken to surgery and 20 patients underwent resection and IORT to 10 Gy to 15 Gy. Locoregional recurrence occurred in only 2/20 resected patients. Median survival for patients who underwent surgery was 25 months with a 3-year survival rate of 23%.

Phase I studies have attempted to build on the radiosensitization effects and the improved efficacy in advanced pancreatic cancer of gemcitabine in the neoadjuvant setting. Gemcitabine has also been studied in combination with other chemotherapy agents and EBRT in the neoadjuvant setting. A phase I study of 19 patients with pancreatic cancer evaluated the maximum tolerated dose (MTD) of cisplatin when given with gemcitabine at 1,000 mg/m^2 weekly with EBRT to 36 Gy given in 2.4 Gy fractions (53). Cisplatin was given on days 1 and 15 following gemcitabine. The MTD of cisplatin was 40 mg/m^2. Another trial from the M.D. Anderson Cancer Center evaluated a treatment schedule of gemcitabine 750 mg/m^2 and cisplatin 30 mg/m^2 given every 14 days for four treatments, followed by four weekly doses of gemcitabine at 400 mg/m^2 concurrent with 30 Gy of EBRT given as 3-Gy fractions over 2 weeks, beginning 2 days after the first dose of gemcitabine (97). Preliminary results of 37 patients showed 67% underwent resection, with 70% of the pathologic specimens showing necrosis of >50% of the tumor. This regimen, however, had significant toxicity, with 62% of patients requiring hospitalization (most due to biliary stent occlusion).

In radiobiologic models, paclitaxel may result in enhanced radiosensitization through:

1. Synchronization of tumor cells at G2/M, a relatively radiosensitive phase of cell cycle and
2. Tumor reoxygenation after apoptotic clearance of paclitaxel-damaged cells.

Pisters et al. (64) from M.D. Anderson Cancer Center have examined the use of paclitaxel as a radiation sensitizer in the neoadjuvant setting for pancreatic cancer. In this trial, 35 patients received paclitaxel 60 mg/m^2 weekly with concurrent EBRT to 30 Gy. Eighty percent underwent resection with 21% of pathology specimens showing >50% tumor necrosis. The 3-year survival for the patients who underwent preoperative therapy and resection was 28%. Hospitalization was required in 11% of patients for toxicity, primarily nausea and vomiting. These preliminary data show an increased toxicity without a significant improvement in histological response rate or survival.

Therapy for Locally Advanced Carcinoma

Patients with locally advanced carcinoma of the pancreas comprise a group of patients with an intermediate prognosis between resectable and metastatic patients. These patients have pancreatic tumors that are defined as surgically unresectable, but have no evidence of distant metastases. A tumor is considered to be unresectable if it has one of the following features:

1. Extensive peripancreatic lymph node involvement and/or distant metastases (typically to the liver or peritoneum),
2. Encasement or occlusion of the superior mesenteric vein (SMV) or SMV/portal vein confluence, or
3. Direct involvement of the superior mesenteric artery (SMA), inferior vena cava, aorta, or celiac axis.

However, recent advances in surgical technique may allow for resection of selected patients with tumors involving the SMV (41). Treatment with radiation and chemotherapy increases median survival for patients with locally advanced cancers to approximately 9 to 13 months, but rarely results in long-term survival. The therapeutic options of patients with locally advanced pancreatic cancer include EBRT with 5-FU chemotherapy, IORT, and more recently EBRT with novel chemotherapeutic and targeted agents. In evaluating the results of these various therapies, it is useful to remember that a median survival of 3 to 6 months has been reported for this subset of patients undergoing palliative gastric or biliary bypass only (25).

Prospective Trials

With the exception of one trial, conventional EBRT for locally advanced pancreatic cancer has been shown to improve survival when combined with 5-FU compared to EBRT alone or chemotherapy alone (Table 56.6). The Mayo Clinic undertook an early randomized trial in the 1960s in which 64 patients with locally unresectable, nonmetastatic pancreatic adenocarcinoma received 35 to 40 Gy of EBRT with concurrent 5-FU versus the same EBRT schedule plus placebo. A significant survival advantage was seen for patients receiving EBRT with 5-FU versus EBRT only (10.4 months vs. 6.3 months) (49).

GITSG followed with a similar study comparing EBRT alone to EBRT with concurrent and maintenance 5-FU. One hundred and ninety-four eligible patients with surgically confirmed unresectable and nonmetastatic pancreatic adenocarcinoma were randomized to receive 60 Gy of split course EBRT alone, 40 Gy of split course EBRT with two to three cycles of concurrent bolus 5-FU chemotherapy, or 60 Gy split course EBRT using a similar chemotherapy regimen. Patients in the latter groups received maintenance 5-FU after EBRT completion. The EBRT-alone arm was closed early as a result of an inferior survival rate. The 1-year survival rate in the two combined modality therapy arms was 38% and 36%, respectively, versus 11% in the EBRT-alone arm (50).

The second GITSG trial of this series randomized 157 eligible patients with unresectable disease to 60-Gy split course EBRT with concurrent and maintenance 5-FU from the previous trial or 40-Gy continuous course radiation with weekly concurrent doxorubicin chemotherapy, followed by maintenance

Table 56.6   PROSPECTIVE RANDOMIZED TRIALS FOR LOCALLY ADVANCED, UNRESECTABLE PANCREATIC CANCER

Series (Reference)	No. of Patients	Median Survival (Months)	Local Failure (%)	1-Year (%)	18-Month (%)
Mayo Clinic (49)					
EBRT (35–40 Gy/3–4 weeks) only	32	6.3	NS	6	6
EBRT (35–40 Gy/3–4 weeks) + 5-FU	32	10.4	NS	22	13
GITSG (18,50)					
EBRT (60 Gy/10 weeks) only	25	5.3	24	10	5
EBRT (40 Gy/6 weeks) + 5-FU	83	8.4	26	35	20
EBRT (60 Gy/10 weeks) + 5-FU	86	11.4	27	46	20
GITSG (21)					
EBRT (60 Gy/10 weeks) + 5-FU	73	8.5	58 (first site)	33	15
EBRT (40 Gy/4 weeks) + doxorubicin	70	7.6	51 (first site)	27	17
GITSG (20,22)					
EBRT (54 Gy/6 weeks) + 5-FU and SMF	22	9.7	45 (first site)	41	18
SMF only	21	7.4	48 (first site)	19	0
ECOG (36)					
FRRT (40 Gy/4 weeks) + 5-FU	47	8.3	32	26	11
5-FU only	44	8.2	32	32	21

EBRT, external beam radiation therapy; ECOG, Eastern Cooperative Oncology Group; 5-FU, 5-flurouracil; GITSG, Gastrointestinal Tumor Study Group; SMF, streptozocin, mitomycin-C, and 5-flurouracil.

doxorubicin and 5-FU. A significant increase in treatment-related toxicity was seen in the doxorubicin arm. However, no survival difference was observed between the two groups (median survival 37 vs. 33 weeks) (21). No clinical benefit was seen in substituting adriamycin for 5-FU.

A follow-up GITSG trial compared chemotherapy alone to chemoradiation, again in surgically confirmed unresectable tumors. Forty-three patients were randomized to receive combination streptozocin, mitomycin-C, and 5-FU (SMF) chemotherapy or 54 Gy of EBRT with two cycles of concurrent bolus 5-FU chemotherapy, followed by adjuvant SMF chemotherapy. The chemoradiation arm demonstrated a significant survival advantage over the chemotherapy alone arm (1-year survival 41% vs. 19%, respectively) (22).

In contrast to the results of the prior studies, the Eastern Cooperative Oncology Group (ECOG) reported no benefit to chemoradiation versus chemotherapy only. In this study, patients with unresectable, nonmetastatic pancreatic or gastric adenocarcinoma were randomized to receive either 5-FU chemotherapy alone or 40 Gy EBRT with concurrent bolus 5-FU during week 1. Patients with locally recurrent disease as well as patients undergoing surgery with residual disease were eligible for this trial. In the 91 analyzable pancreatic patients, no survival difference was observed between the two groups (median survival, 8.2 vs. 8.3 months) (36).

Continuous Infusional 5-Fluorouracil

The idea that continuous infusion 5-FU allows for increased cumulative drug dose to be given without a significant increase in toxicity and for a more protracted radiosensitization effect relative to bolus 5-FU has prompted its study in locally advanced pancreatic cancer. Trials of other gastrointestinal sites have shown an increased survival using continuous infusion 5-FU (58). Phase I and II trials have been performed in pancreatic cancer, showing that the use of infusional 5-FU is without excessive treatment-related toxicity and is effective (6,59,92). A phase I trial from ECOG found the MTD of continuous infusion 5-FU to be 250 mg/m^2/day with the dose-limiting toxicity being gastrointestinal. The progression-free survival at 1 year was 40% with a median survival of 11.9 months. The 2-year survival

rate for this trial was 18%. Although no randomized trials have been published, combined radiation therapy with infusional 5-FU is now commonly used, and combinations of chemotherapy with infusional 5-FU and radiation therapy for locally advanced pancreatic cancer are under investigation.

In addition, capecitabine, an oral 5-FU analog, in combination with radiation therapy for the treatment of pancreatic cancer has been reported (3). Dosing of capecitabine has been extrapolated from combined modality trials in rectal cancer to be about 1,600 mg/m^2/day divided twice a day during radiation treatment (83). No randomized trials have been reported with this combination. Of note, the combination of capecitabine and gemcitabine has been shown to be likely more efficacious than gemcitabine alone for patients with metastatic pancreatic cancer. There was a randomized trial of 533 patients with advanced pancreatic cancer who were treated with either single agent gemcitabine or gemcitabine plus capecitabine (10,27). The patients who received gemcitabine plus capecitabine had a statistically significant increase in response rate (14.2% vs. 7.1%; $p = .008$) and a statistically significant improvement in hazard ratio (HR) for overall survival (HR 0.80; 95% confidence interval [CI], 0.65 to 0.98). The confidence intervals for median survival for the two arms overlapped, however, with median survival in the gemcitabine plus capecitabine arm being 7.4 months (95% CI, 6.5 to 8.5) and in the gemcitabine arm 6 months (95% CI, 5.4 to 7.1 months). Further study of capecitabine in combination with radiation therapy is warranted.

In summary, with the exception of one study, conventional EBRT combined with 5-FU chemotherapy has been shown to offer a modest survival benefit for patients with locally advanced unresectable pancreatic cancer compared to radiation alone or chemotherapy alone. The median survival duration and 2-year survival rate for EBRT plus 5-FU are approximately 10 months and 12%, respectively. Because of these results, EBRT with 5-FU–based chemotherapy is a frequently employed therapy for these patients.

Increased EBRT Dosing

Because of the limited tolerance of normal tissue in the upper abdomen (liver, kidney, spinal cord, and bowel) to EBRT, total doses of only 45 to 54 Gy in 25 to 30 Gy fractions have usually been given. For an unresectable tumor, this dose of radiation is inadequate, as demonstrated by the high rates of local tumor progression and poor survival seen in both prospective and retrospective studies. For example, local progression occurred as first site of failure in 58% of patients treated to 60 Gy with concurrent 5-FU in the second GITSG trial (21). Similarly, the Mayo Clinic reported a local failure rate of 72% for 122 patients with unresectable pancreatic cancer treated with an EBRT dose of 40 to 60 Gy (69). An attempt has been made to evaluate whether an increased dose of radiation may improve outcomes. In a report from Thomas Jefferson University Hospital, 46 evaluable patients with unresectable disease by laparotomy were treated with 63 to 70 Gy EBRT with or without chemotherapy. Despite high-dose EBRT, the local failure rate was 78% (93).

Conversion of Locally Advanced Disease to Resectable

Because surgical resection of the primary tumor remains the only potentially curative treatment for pancreatic cancer, preoperative radiation has been studied to assess its ability to convert locally unresectable pancreatic cancer to resectable disease. In a study from New England Deaconess Hospital, 16 patients with locally advanced/unresectable pancreatic cancer were treated neoadjuvantly with 5-FU chemotherapy and 45 Gy of EBRT and infusional 5-FU. Of these 16 patients, only two (13%) were able to undergo resection (33). Similarly, investigators from Duke University reported that only 2/25 (8%) patients with locally advanced pancreatic cancer treated with 45 Gy of EBRT and 5-FU (with or without cisplatin or mitomycin-C) subsequently underwent complete resection with negative margins (89). A prospective study of 87 patients with locally advanced pancreatic cancer from Memorial Sloan-Kettering Cancer Center treated with combined modality therapy found three patients achieved a complete response. These patients were taken for resection and two were found to still have locally advanced disease and one was resected with negative margins only to recur and die 18 months later (35). These and other studies indicate that it is unlikely that currently utilized neoadjuvant chemoradiation can convert unresectable lesions to resectable ones and thereby increase the number of patients potentially cured with combined-modality therapy. It is important to remember that broadening the definition of a locally advanced pancreatic cancer will give the appearance of more optimistic results. If, however, one maintains a stringent CT-based definition of locally advanced pancreatic cancer that includes only arterial involvement (superior mesenteric artery or celiac axis invasion) or superior mesenteric or portal vein encasement or occlusion, successful down-staging to allow complete surgical resection will be an uncommon event with contemporary chemoradiation approaches.

Intraoperative Radiation Therapy

Because of the poor local control and results achieved with conventional EBRT and chemotherapy, specialized radiation therapy techniques that increase the radiation dose to the tumor volume have been used to improve local tumor control without significantly increasing normal tissue morbidity. These include iodine-125 implants and IORT as a dose escalation technique in combination with external beam irradiation and chemotherapy. A lower incidence of local failure in most series and improved median survival in some have been reported with these techniques when compared with conventional external beam irradiation, but it is uncertain whether this is due to superior treatment or case selection (69).

A recent study from investigators of the Massachusetts General Hospital reported the results of 150 patients treated with IORT and EBRT and chemotherapy (95). Although the study spanned nearly 25 years, it is relevant because it shows for the first time that long-term survival is possible for patients with unresectable pancreatic cancer. Although the 3- and 5-year survival rates (7%, 4%, respectively) are modest, they are not markedly different from the results reported in contemporary trials of resected pancreatic cancer patients (20%, 10%, respectively) or patients undergoing palliative pancreaticoduodenectomy (6.3%, 1.6%, respectively), especially when taking into account those patients with smaller tumors. For 25 patients treated with a small diameter applicator (5 or 6 cm), the 2- and 3-year actuarial survival rates were 27% and 17%, respectively. Furthermore, this study shows that postoperative and late treatment-related toxicity rates were acceptable. These study results support further study of selected patients with small, unresectable tumors into innovative protocols employing IORT.

Newer Chemotherapeutic Agents

Because of the high incidence of hepatic and peritoneal metastases and poor results with standard chemoradiotherapy, current and future research efforts include evaluation of EBRT with newer systemic agents including gemcitabine and paclitaxel. Interest in these agents is based on both their systemic cytotoxic effects and their radiosensitizing properties. Numerous investigators have pursued phase I and II studies combining EBRT with gemcitabine. Investigators from Wake Forest University and the University of North Carolina reported the results of a phase I trial of twice-weekly gemcitabine and 50.4 Gy of concurrent upper abdominal EBRT in 19 patients with unresectable/inoperable pancreatic adenocarcinoma. In this study, the maximum tolerated dose of gemcitabine was 40 mg/m^2. At this dose level, gemcitabine was well tolerated. Of eight patients with a minimum follow-up of 12 months, three remain alive, and one of these three has no evidence of disease progression (4). Following this trial the Cancer and Leukemia Group B (CALGB) began a phase II study of this regimen for locally advanced pancreatic cancer. Data from this trial show a median overall survival for 38 patients enrolled of 8.2 months (5). Using an alternate dosing scheme, McGinn et al. (47) investigated weekly full-dose gemcitabine combined with radiation therapy at escalating doses in a phase I trial of 37 patients with locally advanced or incompletely resected pancreatic cancer. These patients received two cycles of gemcitabine at 1,000 mg/m^2 on days 1, 8, and 15 of a 28-day cycle with concurrent EBRT during the first 3 weeks. An optimal dose of 36 Gy in 2.4 Gy fractions was determined and recommended for a phase II trial that has completed accrual (46).

Gemcitabine has also been studied in combination with 5-FU and radiation. ECOG performed a phase I trial of continuous infusion 5-FU at 200 mg/m^2, weekly gemcitabine at 50 to 100 mg/m^2, and 59.4 Gy of EBRT (79). The patients in this trial showed a significant amount of toxicity with five out of seven patients experiencing dose-limiting toxicities of gastric or duodenal ulcers, thrombocytopenia, or Stevens-Johnson syndrome. Because of these toxicities, the authors concluded that the combination of gemcitabine, 5-FU, and EBRT was not appropriate. However, the Massachusetts General Hospital, Dana Farber Cancer Center, and Brigham and Women's Hospital conducted a phase I or II study of continuous infusion 5-FU with weekly gemcitabine and concurrent 50.4 Gy of EBRT for locally advanced pancreatic cancer. In this study the MTD of weekly gemcitabine was 200 mg/m^2 when given with continuous infusion 5-FU at 200 mg/m^2 and concurrent EBRT. In this study, 32 patients were treated (13 at the MTD), and the severe toxicities were limited to one patient experiencing a grade 3 gastrointestinal bleed. The reason behind this is thought to be the lower dose of EBRT given, smaller treatment fields, and the continuous

Clinical Radiation Oncology

infusion 5-FU was given five days out of the week instead of seven (C. Fuchs, preliminary data). This dosage was used for investigation in a phase II multicenter trial through CALGB. Results from this trial are pending.

In a phase I trial at Brown University evaluating paclitaxel and 50 Gy of EBRT for patients with unresectable pancreatic and gastric cancers, the maximum tolerated dose of weekly paclitaxel with conventional irradiation was 50 mg/m^2 (71). The response rate was 31% among 13 evaluable pancreatic cancer patients. In the Brown University phase II study employing 50 Gy of EBRT with 50 mg/m^2/week of paclitaxel, 6/18 (33%) evaluable pancreatic cancer patients had a partial response; stable disease was observed in seven patients (39%); only one patient (6%) had local tumor progression after completion of treatment; and four (22%) have developed distant metastases. These data have led to an RTOG phase II study evaluating paclitaxel with EBRT for patients with unresectable pancreatic cancer (67). The median survival of 109 patients on this study was 11.2 months (95% CI, 10.1 to 12.3) with estimated 1- and 2-year survivals of 43% and 13%, respectively. External irradiation plus concurrent weekly paclitaxel was well tolerated when given with large-field radiotherapy. These data provided the basis for a RTOG trial using paclitaxel and irradiation combined with a second radiation sensitizer, gemcitabine, and a farnesyl transferase inhibitor.

Chemoradiation Effects on Quality of Life

Despite the potential survival benefits for patients with locally advanced pancreatic cancer receiving radiation therapy and chemotherapy, these gains are modest. With rare exception, all patients will ultimately succumb to their disease. In spite of this, significant palliative benefit can be achieved by chemoradiation. Pain, anorexia, fatigue, and clinical wasting are relatively common symptoms, which significantly impact the patient's quality of life. Although poorly documented in many studies, using the aforementioned techniques (including IORT), reports from larger series indicate complete pain relief can be obtained in as many as 50% to 80% of patients (82). Using EBRT alone with or without chemotherapy, approximately 35% to 65% of patients will experience pain resolution as well as some improvement in wasting and obstructive symptoms (11,21,26). Definite but less dramatic improvements in performance status and anorexic symptoms may be observed as well (11,26). Because of the high rate of mortality associated with this disease, quality of life should be one of the important end points in study design for these patients.

Targeted Therapies/Future Directions

As the biological basis of cancer is better understood, the use of cancer-specific targeted therapies is being increasingly investigated. There is preclinical evidence for either additive or synergistic effects for several of these approaches (such as antibodies against and vascular endothelial factor receptor [VEGF] and epidermal growth factor receptor [EGFR]) with both chemotherapy and radiation therapy, making these approaches especially promising. These targeted agents have been studied most extensively in the metastatic setting. Currently, the only targeted agent that has shown a statistically significant survival benefit in the metastatic setting compared to chemotherapy alone is erlotinib, an anti-EGFR tyrosine kinase inhibitor. However, the survival benefit is small, improving 1-year survival from 17% to 24% (51). The median progression-free survival and overall survival benefits for the gemcitabine plus erlotinib arm versus the gemcitabine plus placebo arm also showed a small benefit (3.75 vs. 3.55 months; $p = .003$ and 6.37 vs. 5.91 months; $p = .025$, respectively). A phase I study of erlotinib, gemcitabine, and radiation therapy for patients with locally advanced pan-

creatic cancer has found an MTD of erlotinib 100 mg daily, gemcitabine 40 mg/m^2 biweekly, and EBRT to 50.4 Gy (38). Of eight patients treated, seven have stable disease, and one patient was taken for R1 resection. Another phase I study has established an MTD for the combination of erlotinib, gemcitabine, paclitaxel, and radiation therapy for patients with locally advanced pancreatic cancer (31). Another EGFR inhibitor, cetuximab, has had promising phase II results in the metastatic setting. A phase II study of the EGFR-inhibiting antibody cetuximab plus gemcitabine enrolled 41 patients with advanced pancreatic cancer. In this study the response rate was 12%, with a median progression-free survival of 3.8 months and median overall survival of 7.1 months (98). A phase III randomized study of gemcitabine plus cetuximab versus placebo (Southwest Oncology Group S0205) has recently completed accrual, and results are eagerly awaited. Two small trials have reported preliminary results using cetuximab in combination with gemcitabine and radiation therapy for localized pancreatic cancer (40,62). These studies have found that cetuximab can be given at full dose with chemotherapy and radiation therapy without significantly increased toxicity. Efficacy results are pending.

Preclinical data have shown that inhibition of VEGF has radiosensitizing effects. The RTOG is currently undertaking a phase II study combining bevacizumab, an anti-VEGF antibody, with EBRT and capecitabine in the treatment of this group of patients. However, initially promising results in the metastatic setting have not shown benefit from the addition of an anti-VEGF antibody to chemotherapy. A phase II trial of the combination of gemcitabine and bevacizumab in 52 treated patients with advanced pancreatic cancer showed a response rate of 21%, a median progression-free survival of 5.4 months, and median overall survival of 8.8 months. The phase III randomized study of gemcitabine plus bevacizumab versus placebo (CALGB 80303), however, has finished accrual and was recently reported to show no benefit from the addition of bevacizumab to gemcitabine.

Summary

Pancreatic cancer remains one of the most formidable challenges in oncology. Newer imaging modalities have improved staging, thus facilitating treatment decisions. In the past 30 years, modest improvements in median survival have been attained for patients with locally advanced tumors treated by chemoradiation protocols. However, no significant impact on long-term survival has been accomplished. Local tumor control has been improved by the use of specialized radiation techniques, permitting safe dose escalation. Even with these techniques, it is not clear that a survival benefit is achieved given the proclivity of metastases in this malignancy. Trials are under way to test newer systemic agents that also act as potent radiosensitizers.

Despite the recognized limitations of current therapy, palliation can be achieved for a high percentage of patients by combined modality treatment. Quality of life should be considered a paramount end point in the care and protocol design of these patients. In patients with marginal or poor performance status, gemcitabine administration alone represents a reasonable alternative to combined modality therapy. Significant improvements in long-term survival will likely be achieved through ongoing attempts at exploitation of the basic biologic anomalies of this malignancy.

References

1. Allema JH, Reinders ME, van Gulik TM, et al. Prognostic factors for survival after pancreaticoduodenectomy for patients with carcinoma of the pancreatic head region. *Cancer* 1995;75(8):2069–2076.

2. American Joint Committee on Cancer. *AJCC cancer staging manual*, 6th ed. New York: Springer-Verlag, 2002.
3. Ben-Josef E, Shields AF, Vaishampayan U, et al. Intensity-modulated radiotherapy (IMRT) and concurrent capecitabine for pancreatic cancer. *Int J Radiat Oncol Biol Phys* 2004;59(2):454–459.
4. Blackstock AW, Bernard SA, Richards F, et al. Phase I trial of twice-weekly gemcitabine and concurrent radiation in patients with advanced pancreatic cancer. *J Clin Oncol* 1999;17(7):2208–2212.
5. Blackstock AW, Tepper JE, Niedwiecki D, et al. Cancer and leukemia group B (CALGB) 89805: phase II chemoradiation trial using gemcitabine in patients with locoregional adenocarcinoma of the pancreas. *Int J Gastrointest Cancer* 2003;34(2–3):107–116.
6. Boz G, De Paoli A, Innocente R, et al. Radiotherapy and continuous infusion 5-fluorouracil in patients with nonresectable pancreatic carcinoma. *Int J Radiat Oncol Biol Phys* 2001;51(3):736–740.
7. Brugge WR, Van Dam J. Pancreatic and biliary endoscopy. *N Engl J Med* 1999;341(24):1808–1816.
8. Cameron JL, Crist DW, Sitzmann JV, et al. Factors influencing survival after pancreaticoduodenectomy for pancreatic cancer. *Am J Surg* 1991;161(1):120–124; discussion 4–5.
9. Ceha HM, van Tienhoven G, Gouma DJ, et al. Feasibility and efficacy of high dose conformal radiotherapy for patients with locally advanced pancreatic carcinoma. *Cancer* 2000;89(11):2222–2229.
10. Cunningham D, Chau I, Stocken D, et al. GEM-CAP: phase III randomised comparison of gemcitabine with gemcitabine plus capecitabine in patients with advanced pancreatic cancer. In: *ECCO* 2005.
11. Dobelbower RR Jr., Borgelt BB, Strubler KA, et al. Precision radiotherapy for cancer of the pancreas: technique and results. *Int J Radiat Oncol Biol Phys* 1980;6(9):1127–1133.
12. Emami B, Lyman J, Brown A, et al. Tolerance of normal tissue to therapeutic irradiation. *Int J Radiat Oncol Biol Phys* 1991;21(1):109–122.
13. Evans D, Abbruzzese J, Willett C. *Cancer of the pancreas*, 6th ed. Philadelphia: Lippincott Williams & Wilkins, 2001.
14. Evans DB, Pisters PW, Lee JE, et al. Preoperative chemoradiation strategies for localized adenocarcinoma of the pancreas. *J Hepatobiliary Pancreat Surg* 1998;5(3):242–250.
15. Evans DB, Rich TA, Byrd DR, et al. Preoperative chemoradiation and pancreaticoduodenectomy for adenocarcinoma of the pancreas. *Arch Surg* 1992;127(11):1335–1339.
16. Fernandez-del Castillo C, Rattner DW, Warshaw AL. Further experience with laparoscopy and peritoneal cytology in the staging of pancreatic cancer. *Br J Surg* 1995;82(8):1127–1129.
17. Fine RM, Elshaikh MA, Pelley R, et al. Treatment outcome of 3D non-coplanar conformal radiotherapy and 5FU for resected pancreatic cancer (ASTRO 2001). *Int J Radiat Oncol Biol Phys* 2001;51:269.
18. Gastrointestinal Tumor Study Group. A multi-institutional comparative trial of radiation therapy alone and in combination with 5-fluorouracil for locally unresectable pancreatic carcinoma. *Ann Surg* 1979;189(2):205–208.
19. Gastrointestinal Tumor Study Group. Further evidence of effective adjuvant combined radiation and chemotherapy following curative resection of pancreatic cancer. *Cancer* 1987;59(12):2006–2010.
20. Gastrointestinal Tumor Study Group. Phase II studies of drug combinations in advanced pancreatic carcinoma: fluorouracil plus doxorubicin plus mitomycin C and two regimens of streptozotocin plus mitomycin C plus fluorouracil. *J Clin Oncol* 1986;4(12):1794–1798.
21. Gastrointestinal Tumor Study Group. Radiation therapy combined with adriamycin or 5-fluorouracil for the treatment of locally unresectable pancreatic carcinoma. *Cancer* 1985;56(11):2563–2568.
22. Gastrointestinal Tumor Study Group. Treatment of locally unresectable carcinoma of the pancreas: comparison of combined-modality therapy (chemotherapy plus radiotherapy) to chemotherapy alone. *J Natl Cancer Inst* 1988;80(10):751–755.
23. Geer RJ, Brennan MF. Prognostic indicators for survival after resection of pancreatic adenocarcinoma. *Am J Surg* 1993;165(1):68–73.
24. Griffin JF, Smalley SR, Jewell W, et al. Patterns of failure after curative resection of pancreatic carcinoma. *Cancer* 1990;66(1):56–61.
25. Gunderson LL, Haddock MG, Burch P, et al. Future role of radiotherapy as a component of treatment in biliopancreatic cancers. *Ann Oncol* 1999;10[Suppl 4]:291–295.
26. Haslam JB, Cavanaugh PJ, Stroup SL. Radiation therapy in the treatment of irresectable adenocarcinoma of the pancreas. *Cancer* 1973;32(6):1341–1345.
27. Herrmann R, Bodoky G, Ruhstaller T, et al. Gemcitabine (GEM) plus capecitabine (CAP) versus GEM alone in locally advanced or metastatic pancreatic cancer. Aspects of quality of life in a randomized phase III study of the Swiss Group for Clinical Cancer Research (SAKK) and the Central European Coo. *Eur J Cancer Suppl* 2005;3(2):203.
28. Higgins PD, Sohn JW, Fine RM, et al. Three-dimensional conformal pancreas treatment: comparison of four- to six-field techniques. *Int J Radiat Oncol Biol Phys* 1995;31(3):605–609.
29. Howard JM. Pancreatoduodenectomy: forty-one consecutive Whipple resections without an operative modality. *Ann Surg* 1968;168:629–640.
30. Hruban RH. 1999 update symposium. *J Am Coll Surg* 1998;187:429.
31. Iannitti D, Dipetrillo T, Barnett J, et al. Erlotinib and chemoradiation followed by maintenance erlotinib for locally advanced pancreatic cancer: a phase I study. *Am J Clin Oncol* 2005;28(6):570–575.
32. Jemal A, Siegel R, Ward E, et al. Cancer statistics, 2006. *CA Cancer J Clin* 2006;56(2):106–130.
33. Jessup JM, Steele G Jr., Mayer RJ, et al. Neoadjuvant therapy for unresectable pancreatic adenocarcinoma. *Arch Surg* 1993;128(5):559–564.
34. Kalser MH, Ellenberg SS. Pancreatic cancer. Adjuvant combined radiation and chemotherapy following curative resection. *Arch Surg* 1985;120(8):899–903.
35. Kim HJ, Czischke K, Brennan MF, et al. Does neoadjuvant chemoradiation downstage locally advanced pancreatic cancer? *J Gastrointest Surg* 2002;6(5):763–769.
36. Klaassen DJ, MacIntyre JM, Catton GE, et al. Treatment of locally unresectable cancer of the stomach and pancreas: a randomized comparison of 5-fluorouracil alone with radiation plus concurrent and maintenance 5-fluorouracil—an Eastern Cooperative Oncology Group study. *J Clin Oncol* 1985;3(3):373–378.
37. Klinkenbijl JH, Jeekel J, Sahmoud T, et al. Adjuvant radiotherapy and 5-fluorouracil after curative resection of cancer of the pancreas and periampullary region: phase III trial of the EORTC gastrointestinal tract cancer cooperative group. *Ann Surg* 1999;230(6):776–782; discussion 82–84.
38. Kortmansky J, O'Reilly E, Minsky B, et al. A phase I trial of erlotinib, gemcitabine, and radiation for patients with locally-advanced, unresectable pancreatic cancer. Paper presented at: ASCO Gastrointestinal Cancers Symposium, 2005. Abstract 133.
39. Kozuschek W, Reith HB, Waleczek H, et al. A comparison of long term results of the standard Whipple procedure and the pylorus preserving pancreatoduodenectomy. *J Am Coll Surg* 1994;178(5):443–453.
40. Krempien RC, Munter MW, Timke C, et al. Phase II study evaluating trimodal therapy with cetuximab intensity modulated radiotherapy (IMRT) and gemcitabine for patients with locally advanced pancreatic cancer (ISRCTN 56652283). *J Clin Oncol* 2006 ASCO Annual Meeting Proceedings Part I. Vol 24, no. 185, 2006, 4100.
41. Leach SD, Lee JE, Charnsangavej C, et al. Survival following pancreaticoduodenectomy with resection of the superior mesenteric-portal vein confluence for adenocarcinoma of the pancreatic head. *Br J Surg* 1998;85(5):611–617.
42. Lemke AJ, Niehues SM, Hosten N, et al. Retrospective digital image fusion of multidetector CT and 18F-FDG PET: clinical value in pancreatic lesions—a prospective study with 104 patients. *J Nucl Med* 2004;45(8):1279–1286.
43. Lillemoe KD. Current management of pancreatic carcinoma. *Ann Surg* 1995;221(2):133–148.
44. Lim JE, Chien MW, Earle CC. Prognostic factors following curative resection for pancreatic adenocarcinoma: a population-based, linked database analysis of 396 patients. *Ann Surg* 2003;237(1):74–85.
45. Magistrelli P, Masetti R, Coppola R, et al. Pancreatic resection for periampullary cancer in elderly patients. *Hepatogastroenterology* 1998;45(19):242–247.
46. McGinn CJ, Talamonti MS, Small W, et al. A phase II trial of full-dose gemcitabine with concurrent radiation therapy in patients with resectable or unresectable nonmetastatic pancreatic cancer. In: *GI ASCO*, 2004.
47. McGinn CJ, Zalupski MM, Shureiqi I, et al. Erlotinib plus gemcitabine compared with gemcitabine alone in patients with advanced pancreatic cancer: a phase III trial of the National Cancer Institute of Canada Trials Group. *J Clin Oncol* 2007;25:1960–1966.
48. Michelassi F, Erroi F, Dawson PJ, et al. Experience with 647 consecutive tumors of the duodenum, ampulla, head of the pancreas, and distal common bile duct. *Ann Surg* 1989;210(4):544–554; discussion 54–56.
49. Moertel CG, Childs DS Jr., Reitemeier RJ, et al. Combined 5-fluorouracil and supervoltage radiation therapy of locally unresectable gastrointestinal cancer. *Lancet* 1969;2(7626):865–867.
50. Moertel CG, Frytak S, Hahn RG, et al. Therapy of locally unresectable pancreatic carcinoma: a randomized comparison of high dose (6000 rads) radiation alone, moderate dose radiation (4000 rads + 5-fluorouracil), and high dose radiation + 5-fluorouracil: the Gastrointestinal Tumor Study Group. *Cancer* 1981;48(8):1705–1710.
51. Moore M, Goldstein D, Hamm J, et al. Erlotinib improves survival when added to gemcitabine in patients with advanced pancreatic cancer. A phase III trial of the National Cancer Institute of Canada Clinical Trials Group (NCIC-CTG). Paper presented at: ASCO Gastrointestinal Cancers Symposium, 2005.
52. Moosa AR. Surgical treatment of pancreatic cancer. *Am J Surg* 1986;152:503.
53. Muler JH, McGinn CJ, Normolle D, et al. Phase I trial using a time-to-event continual reassessment strategy for dose escalation of cisplatin combined with gemcitabine and radiation therapy in pancreatic cancer. *J Clin Oncol* 2004;22(2):238–243.
54. Neoptolemos JP, Dunn JA, Stocken DD, et al. Adjuvant chemoradiotherapy and chemotherapy in resectable pancreatic cancer: a randomised controlled trial. *Lancet* 2001;358(9293):1576–1585.
55. Neoptolemos JP, Stocken DD, Friess H, et al. A randomized trial of chemoradiotherapy and chemotherapy after resection of pancreatic cancer. *N Engl J Med* 2004;350(12):1200–1210.
56. Neuhaus P, Oettle H, Post S, et al. A randomised, prospective, multicenter, phase III trial of adjuvant chemotherapy with gemcitabine vs. observation in patients with resected pancreatic cancer. *JAMA*, 2007;297(3):267–277.
57. Niederhuber JE, Brennan MF, Menck HR. The National Cancer Data Base report on pancreatic cancer. *Cancer* 1995;76(9):1671–1677.
58. O'Connell MJ, Martenson JA, Wieand HS, et al. Improving adjuvant therapy for rectal cancer by combining protracted-infusion fluorouracil with radiation therapy after curative surgery. *N Engl J Med* 1994;331(8):502–507.
59. Osti MF, Costa AM, Bianciardi F, et al. Concomitant radiotherapy with protracted 5-fluorouracil infusion in locally advanced carcinoma of the pancreas: a phase II study. *Tumori* 2001;87(6):398–401.
60. Ozaki H. Improvement of pancreatic cancer treatment from the Japanese experience in the 1980s. *Int J Pancreatol* 1992;12(1):5–9.
61. Picozzi VJ, Kozarek RA, Traverso LW. Interferon-based adjuvant chemoradiation therapy after pancreaticoduodenectomy for pancreatic adenocarcinoma. *Am J Surg* 2003;185(5):476–480.
62. Pipas JM, Zaki B, Suriawinata AA, et al. Cetuximab, intensity-modulated radiotherapy (IMRT), and twice-weekly gemcitabine for pancreatic adenocarcinoma. In: *Proc Am Soc Clin Oncol*, 2006.
63. Pisters PW, Abbruzzese JL, Janjan NA, et al. Rapid-fractionation preoperative chemoradiation, pancreaticoduodenectomy, and intraoperative radiation therapy for resectable pancreatic adenocarcinoma. *J Clin Oncol* 1998;16(12):3843–3850.
64. Pisters PW, Wolff RA, Janjan NA, et al. Preoperative paclitaxel and concurrent rapid-fractionation radiation for resectable pancreatic adenocarcinoma: toxicities, histologic response rates, and event-free outcome. *J Clin Oncol* 2002;20(10):2537–2544.
65. Raut CP, Evans DB, Crane CH, et al. Neoadjuvant therapy for resectable pancreatic cancer. *Surg Oncol Clin North Am* 2004;13(4):639–661, ix.
66. Regine WF, Winter KW, Abrams R, et al. RTOG 9704 a phase III study of adjuvant pre and post chemoradiation (CRT) 5-FU vs. gemcitabine (G) for resected pancreatic adenocarcinoma. *J Clin Oncol* 2006 ASCO Annual Meetings Part I. Vol 24, No. 185, 2006, 14056.
67. Rich T, Harris J, Abrams R, et al. Phase II study of external irradiation and weekly paclitaxel for nonmetastatic, unresectable pancreatic cancer: RTOG-98-12. *Am J Clin Oncol* 2004;27(1):51–56.
68. Robinson EK, Lee JE, Lowy AM, et al. Reoperative pancreaticoduodenectomy for periampullary carcinoma. *Am J Surg* 1996;172(5):432–437; discussion 7–8.

69. Roldan GE, Gunderson LL, Nagorney DM, et al. External beam versus intraoperative and external beam irradiation for locally advanced pancreatic cancer. *Cancer* 1988;61(6):1110–1116.

70. Sachelarie I, Kerr K, Ghesani M, et al. Integrated PET-CT: evidence-based review of oncology indications. *Oncology (Williston Park)* 2005;19(4):481–490; discussion 90–92, 95–96.

71. Safran H, Akerman P, Cioffi W, et al. Paclitaxel and concurrent radiation therapy for locally advanced adenocarcinomas of the pancreas, stomach, and gastroesophageal junction. *Semin Radiat Oncol* 1999;9[2 Suppl 1]:53–57.

72. Shoup M, Winston C, Brennan MF, et al. Is there a role for staging laparoscopy in patients with locally advanced, unresectable pancreatic adenocarcinoma?. *J Gastrointest Surg* 2004;8(8):1068–1071.

73. Sohn TA, Lillemoe KD, Cameron JL, et al. Reexploration for periampullary carcinoma: resectability, perioperative results, pathology, and long-term outcome. *Ann Surg* 1999;229(3):393–400.

74. Sohn TA, Yeo CJ, Cameron JL, et al. Resected adenocarcinoma of the pancreas-616 patients: results, outcomes, and prognostic indicators. *J Gastrointest Surg* 2000;4(6):567–579.

75. Sohn TA, Yeo CJ, Cameron JL, et al. Should pancreaticoduodenectomy be performed in octogenarians?. *J Gastrointest Surg* 1998;2(3):207–216.

76. Sosa JA, Bowman HM, Gordon TA, et al. Importance of hospital volume in the overall management of pancreatic cancer. *Ann Surg* 1998;228(3):429–438.

77. Spitz FR, Abbruzzese JL, Lee JE, et al. Preoperative and postoperative chemoradiation strategies in patients treated with pancreaticoduodenectomy for adenocarcinoma of the pancreas. *J Clin Oncol* 1997;15(3):928–937.

78. Takao S, Aikou T, Shinchi H, et al. Comparison of relapse and long-term survival between pylorus-preserving and Whipple pancreaticoduodenectomy in periampullary cancer. *Am J Surg* 1998;176(5):467–470.

79. Talamonti MS, Catalano PJ, Vaughn DJ, et al. Eastern Cooperative Oncology Group phase I trial of protracted venous infusion fluorouracil plus weekly gemcitabine with concurrent radiation therapy in patients with locally advanced pancreas cancer: a regimen with unexpected early toxicity. *J Clin Oncol* 2000;18(19):3384–3389.

80. Tatsumi M, Cohode C, Mourtzikos K, et al. FDG-PET CT in evaluating patients with pancreatic cancer: Initial experience (abstract C24–417). Presented at: 89th Scientific Assembly and annual meeting of the Radiologic Society of North America, 2003.

81. Tepper J, Nardi G, Suitt H. Carcinoma of the pancreas: review of MGH experience from 1963 to 1973. Analysis of surgical failure and implications for radiation therapy. *Cancer* 1976;37(3):1519–1524.

82. Termuhlen PM, Evans DB, Willett CG. *IORT in pancreatic cancer*. Totowa, NJ: Humana Press, 1999.

83. Vaishampayan UN, Ben-Josef E, Philip PA, et al. A single-institution experience with concurrent capecitabine and radiation therapy in gastrointestinal malignancies. *Int J Radiat Oncol Biol Phys* 2002;53(3):675–679.

84. Warren KW, Braasch JW, Thum CW. Carcinoma of the pancreas. *Surg Clin North Am* 1968;48(3):601–618.

85. Warshaw AL, Fernandez-del Castillo C. Pancreatic carcinoma. *N Engl J Med* 1992;326(7):455–465.

86. Wayne JD, Abdalla EK, Wolff RA, et al. Localized adenocarcinoma of the pancreas: the rationale for preoperative chemoradiation. *Oncologist* 2002;7(1):34–45.

87. Westerdahl J, Andren-Sandberg A, Ihse I. Recurrence of exocrine pancreatic cancer—local or hepatic?. *Hepatogastroenterology* 1993;40(4):384–387.

88. Whipple AO, Parson WV, Mullin CR. Treatment of carcinoma of the ampulla of vater. *Ann Surg* 1935;102:763.

89. White RR, Tyler DS. Neoadjuvant therapy for pancreatic cancer: the Duke experience. *Surg Oncol Clin North Am* 2004;13(4):675–684, ix–x.

90. Whittington R, Bryer MP, Haller DG, et al. Adjuvant therapy of resected adenocarcinoma of the pancreas. *Int J Radiat Oncol Biol Phys* 1991;21(5):1137–1143.

91. Whittington R, Dobelbower RR, Mohiuddin M, et al. Radiotherapy of unresectable pancreatic carcinoma: a six year experience with 104 patients. *Int J Radiat Oncol Biol Phys* 1981;7(12):1639–1644.

92. Whittington R, Neuberg D, Tester WJ, et al. Protracted intravenous fluorouracil infusion with radiation therapy in the management of localized pancreaticobiliary carcinoma: a phase I Eastern Cooperative Oncology Group Trial. *J Clin Oncol* 1995;13(1):227–232.

93. Whittington R, Solin L, Mohiuddin M, et al. Multimodality therapy of localized unresectable pancreatic adenocarcinoma. *Cancer* 1984;54(9):1991–1998.

94. Willett CG, Czito BG, Bendell JC, et al. Locally advanced pancreatic cancer. *J Clin Oncol* 2005;23(20):4538–4544.

95. Willett CG, Del Castillo CF, Shih HA, et al. Long-term results of intraoperative electron beam irradiation (IOERT) for patients with unresectable pancreatic cancer. *Ann Surg* 2005;241(2):295–299.

96. Willett CG, Lewandrowski K, Warshaw AL, et al. Resection margins in carcinoma of the head of the pancreas. Implications for radiation therapy. *Ann Surg* 1993;217(2):144–148.

97. Wolff RA, Crane CH, Xiong HQ, et al. Preliminary analysis of preoperative systemic gemcitabine (GEM) and cisplatin (CIS) followed by GEM-based chemoradiation for resectable pancreatic adenocarcinoma. *J Clin Oncol*, 2004 ASCO Annual Meeting Proceedings Part I, Vol 22, 2004:156.

98. Xiong HQ, Rosenberg A, LoBugho A, et al. Cetuximab, a monoclonal antibody targeting the epidermal growth factor receptor, in combination with gemcitabine for advanced pancreatic cancer: a multicenter phase II trial. *J Clin Oncol* 2004;22(13):2610–2616.

99. Yeo C, Yeo T, Hruben R, et al. Cancer of the pancreas. In: DeVita V, Hellman S, Rosenberg S, eds., *Cancer: principles and practice of oncology*, 7th ed. Philadelphia: Lippincott Williams & Wilkins, 2007;957.

100. Yeo CJ, Abrams RA, Grochow LB, et al. Pancreaticoduodenectomy for pancreatic adenocarcinoma: postoperative adjuvant chemoradiation improves survival. A prospective, single-institution experience. *Ann Surg* 1997;225(5):621–633; discussion 33–36.

101. Yeo CJ, Cameron JL, Lillemoe KD, et al. Pancreaticoduodenectomy for cancer of the head of the pancreas. 201 patients. *Ann Surg* 1995;221(6):721–731; discussion 31–33.

102. Yeo CJ, Cameron JL, Sohn TA, et al. Pancreaticoduodenectomy with or without extended retroperitoneal lymphadenectomy for periampullary adenocarcinoma: comparison of morbidity and mortality and short-term outcome. *Ann Surg* 1999;229(5):613–622; discussion 22–24.

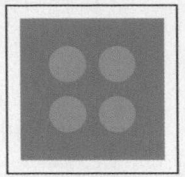

Chapter 57
Liver and Hepatobiliary Tract

Skye H. Cheng, Andrew T. Huang

⠿ | Liver Cancer

Primary liver cancer is one of the most common solid cancers (eighth overall and sixth in men) worldwide (164). The common histologies include hepatocellular carcinoma (HCC) cholangio-carcinoma, and rare neoplasms such as sarcoma and hepato-blastoma (23). The worldwide estimated deaths from liver cancer are more than 400,000 per year. Primary liver cancer is largely a problem of developing countries, in which 81% of the patients reside. There are high incidence rates in sub-Saharan Africa, eastern and southeastern Asia, and in Melanesia. Among the developed countries, the incidence is very low except in Japan, where 56% of the cases are due to infection with hepatitis C virus (151,164). The overall male and female sex ratio is ~2.6. The male predominance is more marked in the high-risk areas and less marked in the low-risk areas (151).

Patients developing liver cancer are usually asymptomatic other than those symptoms related to their chronic liver disease. Clinical symptoms are usually associated with advanced stage; the prognosis is dismal, with a 5-year survival 0% to 10%. Only one of five patients was amenable to curative resection in the past (119,209). With the implementation of screening programs with alpha-fetoprotein (AFP) and ultrasonography, improvement of surgical technique, and liver transplantation the resection rate can be increased to 30% to 50% (174,191).

Curability is associated with tumor stage, patient's performance, and liver function (190). The treatment options for early-stage disease include primary tumor resection, liver transplant, and local tumor ablation. There are no studies that compare these three treatments. In advanced-stage diseases, transcatheter arterial chemoembolization (TACE) is the only method proven to have survival benefit in a phase III study (121). Three-dimensional conformal radiotherapy (3DCRT) could be an adjunct treatment in highly selected patients whose large tumor is rendered nonviable after TACE (33,177).

⠿ | Hepatocellular Carcinoma

Topographic Anatomy

The liver is the largest solid organ of humans. Traditionally it is divided into left and right lobes separated by the falciform ligament. The surgeon needs to understand the spatial relationship of a tumor to the hepatic vascular system preoperatively to determine resectability. Fortunately, progress in imaging technique has made segmental division of the liver based on the anatomy of portal and hepatic veins feasible. The most common segmentation scheme proposed by Couinaud divides the liver parenchyma into right and left liver with four segments each (Fig. 57.1). The left part of the liver consists of caudate lobe (segment I), lateral segment (segments II and III), and medial segment (segment IV). The anatomic landmark between the medial segment and lateral segment is drawn between the gallbladder and inferior vena cava (the falciform ligament). The right part of the liver consists of anterior segments (segments V and VIII) and posterior segments (segments VI and VII). The anatomic landmark that separates the anterior from posterior segment is the right hepatic vein; the anatomic landmark that divides the anterior segment from the left medial segment is the middle hepatic vein. No good anatomic landmarks exist that further divide the anterior and posterior segments into superior and inferior subsegments (198).

Dynamic computerized tomography is very useful in distinctly defining segmental anatomy because the portal vein, hepatic vein, and inferior vena cava can be opacified at the same time (84,98).

Epidemiology

HCC is the most frequent primary cancer of the liver and ranks as the eighth most common cancer in the world. The age-standardized rate of incidence of liver cancer in 1990 worldwide was 14.7 per 100,000 men and 4.9 per 100,000 women. The male-to-female ratio was 3:1. High-risk regions are east and southeast Asia and sub-Saharan Africa (233). The highest incidence rate is seen in the male population of China, Taiwan, Korea, Thailand, Hong Kong, Singapore, Malaysia, Middle Africa, and Japan (27.6 to 35.8 per 100,000 populations) (209). In low-risk areas such as Australia, North America, and Europe, HCC occurs in only 1 to 3 per 100,000 people. However, the incidence of HCC has been rising in the United States, United Kingdom, and France during the past decade (44,48,58,200). The incidence of HCC approximately doubled between 1976 and 2000 in United States (127). The most likely reason for this rising incidence is the spread of hepatitis B and C virus infection (44,48,58,200).

Risk Factors

HCC is clearly associated with hepatitis B (HBV) and hepatitis C (HCV) viral infections and chronic liver disease. With persistent HBV infection, the risk of HCC increases by a factor of 100 (12). The risk of HCC is even much higher in patients who are HBeAg-positive compared with those who are HBeAg-negative (228). As is true for HBV, the relative risk of HCC among persons with chronic HCV infection and cirrhosis is also approximately 100 times the risk of uninfected persons (80). There also exists a synergistic interaction between the two viruses to cause HCC (29).

Other chronic liver-cell injury is also associated with the development of HCC. Chemical injury induced by ethanol, nitrites, hydrocarbons, solvents, organochlorine pesticides, primary metals, and polychlorinated biphenyls has been implicated (48,77). Ethanol is the most common culpable chemical agent and is thought to produce HCC through the development of liver cirrhosis or to play the role of a cocarcinogen. In a group of patients with HCV, there was a 1.5- to 2.5-fold greater risk of liver cirrhosis and HCC in the alcohol-drinking group compared with the alcohol-free group (96). Alcohol consumption is associated with accelerated progression of liver injury, higher frequency of liver cirrhosis, and higher incidence of HCC, and bears no relation to HCV replication (96,170).

Environmental toxins including aflatoxin, contaminated drinking water, and betel nut chewing may also be associated with the pathogenesis of HCC. Aflatoxins, well known

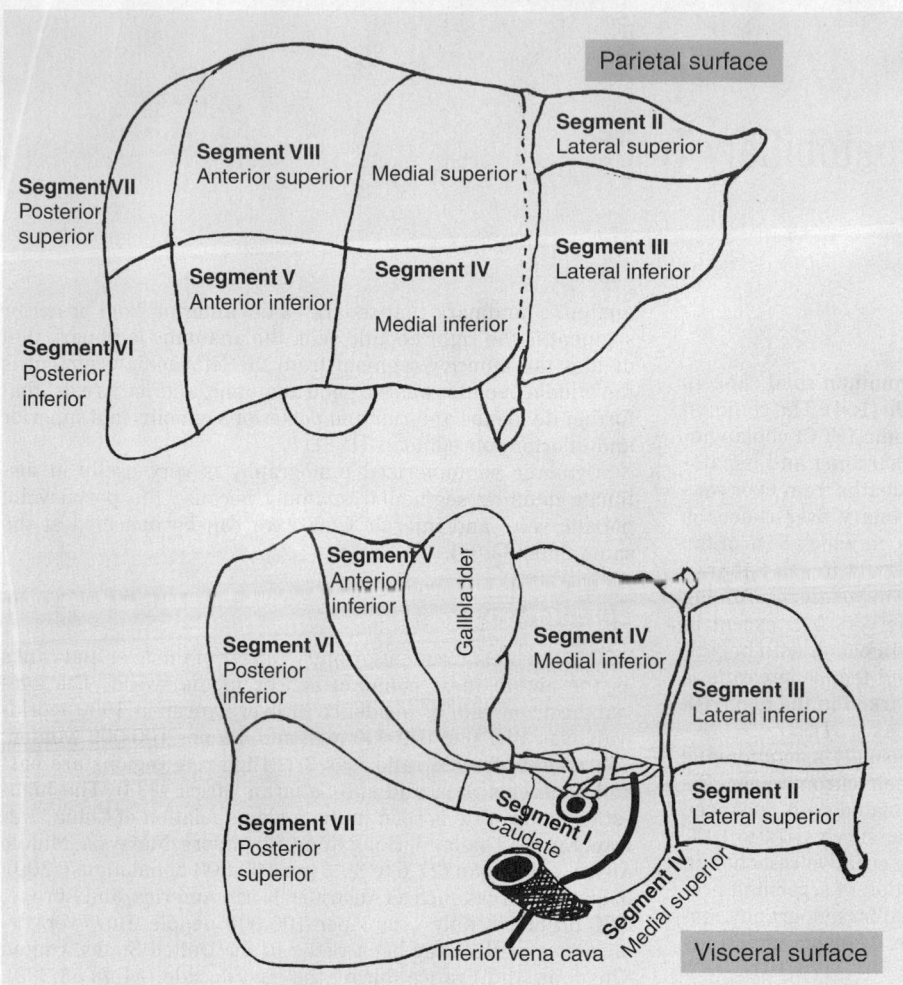

FIGURE 57.1. Segmentation schemes of the liver based on Couinaud's proposal.

hepatotoxic agents, are produced by the fungi, *Aspergillus flavus* and *Aspergillus parasiticus*. Aflatoxin could contaminate corn, soybeans, and peanuts. High rates of dietary aflatoxin intake have been associated with HCC (91,235). There is a synergistic interaction on HCC between chronic HBV infection and aflatoxin exposure (29). The risk of HCC increases dramatically when both factors are concurrently present.

Patients with hereditary liver disease, such as hemochromatosis, Wilson's disease, hereditary tyrosinemia, and type I glycogen storage disease, are at high risk of developing HCC (29,60). The common mechanism of developing HCC may be related to chronic injury and inflammation of the liver.

Prevention

The most effective ways of preventing HCC are to prevent HBV and HCV infection (195). A safe and effective vaccine for HBV has been available since 1982. A universal vaccination program for all newborns began in Taiwan in 1984; the incidence of HCC in children declined from 0.70 per 100,000 children between 1981 and 1986 to 0.36 between 1990 and 1994 (*p* <.01) (26). The development of a vaccine against HCV is more problematic because of the genetic heterogeneity of the virus. Strategies to prevent HCV infection and HCV-related HCC include blood screening, the use of disposable needles and syringes, the adoption of universal precaution for health care workers, and timely treatment of chronic HCV infection with interferon-alpha (13). Meta-analysis suggests that long-term interferon-alpha treatment may prevent the development of HCC in HCV-infected indi-

viduals. The preventive effect is more evident among sustained responders to interferon (13).

Surveillance

Surveillance for HCC has been widely applied; however, there is only one randomized controlled trial of surveillance versus no surveillance that has shown a survival benefit (238). The efficacy of surveillance is highly dependent on the incidence of HCC. Patients at high risk for developing HCC (i.e., annual rate of ≥1.5%) should be entered into surveillance programs (8,116). These patients include hepatitis B carriers who are (a) Asian men ≥40 years of age, (b) Asian women ≥50 years of age, (c) Africans ≥20 years of age, and (d) people with a family history of HCC. Patients with liver cirrhosis from any cause, such as hepatitis B and C, primary biliary disease, and hereditary hemochromatosis, are also candidates for surveillance (20).

Current recommendations for surveillance according to the American Association for the Study of Liver Diseases include (a) surveillance for HCC should be performed using ultrasonography, (b) AFP alone should not be used for screening unless ultrasound is not available, (c) Patients should be screened at 6- to 12-month intervals, and (d) the surveillance interval does not need to be shortened for patients at higher risk of HCC (20).

Clinical Presentation

HCC in the early stage is asymptomatic; it is generally detected by elevation of AFP and/or ultrasonography screening or is an incidental finding in search of other conditions such as chronic liver disease (236). Even in the advanced stage, some patients are still asymptomatic. Patients with symptoms usually suffer from chronic hepatitis and liver cirrhosis. Clinical symptoms include general fatigue, poor appetite, ascites, jaundice, upper gastrointestinal bleeding, splenomegaly, dilated abdominal veins, palmar erythema, gynecomastia, testicular atrophy, leg edema, and weight loss. Tumor-related symptoms include palpable mass in the upper abdomen (hepatomegaly), acute onset of pain (hemorrhage from tumor rupture) and dull pain in the right upper quadrant of abdomen, abdominal fullness, low-grade fever, obstructive jaundice, and splenomegaly (110). Very few individuals with HCC present initially with metastatic disease involving extrahepatic organs such as lungs, bone, adrenal glands, pancreas, and neck lymph nodes (211).

Diagnostic Work-Up

In a patient who is suspected of having HCC, the clinical history frequently includes a history of hepatitis, jaundice, blood transfusion, use of intravenous drugs, or exposure to aflatoxins. A family history of hepatitis or hemochromatosis is also an important indicator (234). Details concerning alcohol abuse and job descriptions related to industrial exposure to possible carcinogenic agents are also helpful.

The physical examination should include a search for signs of underlying liver disease such as jaundice, ascites, ankle edema, spider angioma on the anterior chest wall, palmar erythema, splenomegaly, increasing abdominal girth, and weight loss. Evaluation of the abdomen for liver size, existence of tumor masses, tenderness, and abdominal bruits should also be performed.

Blood tests should include serology for HBV and HCV, and AFP. If HBV or HCV serology is positive, quantitative HBV DNA or HCV RNA should be obtained (21). Evaluation of hepatic functional reserve includes prothrombin time, activated partial thromboplastin time, and serum albumin. Platelet, red cell, and white blood cell counts also should be obtained to look for simultaneous existence of portal hypertension and hypersplenism from liver cirrhosis. Fifteen-minute retention rate of indocyanine green (ICG) before treatment is very useful for determining resectability and/or the feasibility of radiation (33,76).

The diagnosis of HCC is often suspected in a patient with underlying liver disease such as cirrhosis or chronic viral hepatitis. In hepatitis or cirrhotic patients, any dominant solid nodule that is not clearly a hemangioma should be considered as HCC unless proven otherwise (68). Histologic diagnosis of HCC is recommended for patients who plan to have a nonsurgical therapy (197). Some investigators express their opinion that in patients having a nodule >2 cm in a cirrhotic liver with serum AFP >200 ng/mL and having the typical features of HCC on a dynamic imaging technique, biopsy is not necessarily warranted before surgery (14).

For surgical patients, there is a concern over the possibility of tumor seeding from biopsy or fine-needle aspiration (197). The reported magnitude of the risk ranges from 1.6% to 5% (54,87,97). In patients who have coagulopathy or significant ascites, biopsy or fine-needle aspiration may be contraindicated. At our institution, we routinely perform fine-needle aspirations including cellblocks under ultrasound guidance (55). Core biopsy of the mass is reserved for patients in whom we cannot make a definitive diagnosis by fine-needle aspirations with cellblocks. Coaxial cannula is used with fine-needle or core biopsies to reduce the chance of needle track seeding (124). In patients who have small hepatic nodules with diagnostic possibilities ranging from well-differentiated malignancy to benign disease, ultrasonographically guided needle-core biopsy should be considered (93).

Ultrasonography, computed tomography (CT), and magnetic resonance imaging (MRI) are the most common modalities used to evaluate tumors in the liver. Ultrasound examination of the liver is commonly used as a screening tool; small tumors are often hypoechoic. As the tumor grows, the echo pattern tends to become isoechoic or hyperechoic, and HCC can be difficult to distinguish from the surrounding liver (89). Nodules <1 cm should be followed with ultrasonography again at intervals of 3 to 6 months. Nodules between 1 and 2 cm in a cirrhotic liver should be investigated further with two dynamic studies, either a CT scan, contrast ultrasound, or MRI with contrast. Triphasic dynamic CT with unenhanced-, arterial-, portal venous-, and equilibrium-phase images is a useful tool to detect small HCC. The most sensitive phases during which to detect HCC nodules are the arterial and equilibrium phases (36,98).

Extrahepatic metastases are not common at presentation; they occur mainly in patients with T4 disease. The most common sites of metastasis are lung, abdominal lymph nodes, and bone (94). Routine metastatic surveys in patients with early-stage HCC are not recommended.

Staging

The prognosis in HCC patients is more complex because the underlying liver function also affects prognosis. Several factors have been identified as being important determinants of survival: the severity of underlying liver disease, the size and number of the tumor, vascular invasion, regional lymph node metastasis, and the presence of distant metastases. The most commonly used systems are the American Joint Committee on Cancer TNM staging system (Table 57.1) (72), Okuda staging systems (147), the Cancer of the Liver Italian Program (CLIP) scoring system (93), and the Barcelona-Clinic-Liver-Cancer staging system (89). In general, pathologic staging systems (such as TNM) predict prognosis better than do clinical systems, particularly when assessing the outcomes of resection. The Okuda and CLIP systems are more useful for predicting outcomes in patients with poor liver function who have advanced HCC.

Pathologic Classification

Histologic classification of malignant tumors of the liver includes HCC (conventional), HCC (fibrolamellar variant), cholangiocarcinoma (intrahepatic bile duct carcinoma), mixed hepatocellular cholangiocarcinoma, undifferentiated carcinoma, and hepatoblastoma. The fibrolamellar variant of HCC has a relatively better prognosis. It occurs more frequently in adolescents or young adults and has a more indolent clinical course than conventional HCC (163). Hepatoblastoma occurs most commonly in young children (median age, 13 to 16 months) and usually presents in an advanced stage (24,92).

General Management

HCC generally is a multicentric disease, especially when it is associated with HCV. The incidence of multicentric disease in HCV-related HCC (53.3%) is significantly higher ($p < .05$) than in the non-HCV-related HCC (7.7%) (75). The risk of multicentric occurrence increases with the progression of chronic liver disease and cirrhosis (107,167). Although multiple tumors occur less often in HBV-associated HCC than in HCV-associated HCC, the incidence of intrahepatic recurrence of HCC is significantly higher in patients with a sustained HBeAg-positive and high serum concentration of HBV DNA (105). Despite these observations, the mainstay of therapy is surgical resection. The majority of patients, however, are not eligible for surgery because of the extent of tumor involvement or underlying liver dysfunction. Several other treatment modalities

Table 57.1	**TNM CLASSIFICATION FOR HEPATOCELLULAR CARCINOMA AND INTRAHEPATIC BILE DUCT CANCER FROM THE AMERICAN JOINT COMMITTEE ON CANCER 2002 SYSTEM**		
Primary tumor (T)			
T0	No evidence of primary tumor		
T1	Solitary without vascular invasion		
T2	Solitary with vascular invasion, or multiple tumors none >5 cm		
T3	Multiple tumors >5 cm or tumor involving major branch of the portal or hepatic veins		
T4	Tumor with direct invasion of adjacent organs other than the gallbladder or with perforation of visceral peritoneum		
Regional lymph nodes (N)			
N0	No regional lymph node metastasis		
N1	Regional lymph node metastasis		
Distant metastasis (M)			
M0	No distant metastasis		
M1	Distant metastasis		
Stage Grouping			
Stage I	T1	N0	M0
Stage II	T2	N0	M0
Stage IIIA	T3	N0	M0
Stage IIIB	T4	N0	M0
Stage IIIC	Any T	N1	M0
Stage IV	Any T	Any N	M1

Modified from Greene F, Page D, Fleming I: *AJCC (American Joint Committee on Cancer) Cancer staging manual.* New York: Springer-Verlag; 2002:131.

are available, including liver transplantation, radiofrequency ablation (RFA), percutaneous ethanol or acetic acid ablation, TACE, cryoablation, radiation therapy, and systemic chemotherapy.

Surgical Resection

Surgical resection is a reliable method to obtain long-term disease control. The main limiting factor for resection is liver function. In virus-related HCC, the extent of surgical resection of hepatic tumor depends on the functional reserve of the remaining liver after surgery. Previously, the selection of patients for resection has been based on the Child-Pugh classification (Table 57.2), but this method is known to be inconsistent. Many Japanese and other Asian investigators rely on the ICG retention test (76). In Europe and the United States, selection of optimal candidates for resection is usually based on the assessment of the presence of portal hypertension, which is assessed clinically or by hepatic vein catheterization (19). Clinically significant portal hypertension is suspected when the platelet count is below 100,000/mm³) associated with significant splenomegaly. The goal of surgery is to remove gross tumor with a margin of 1 to 2 cm of normal liver.

Liver Transplantation

Many patients are inappropriate for definitive surgery because of underlying liver dysfunction. The increasing availability of liver transplantation has made this procedure an alternative to tumor resection for selected patients. Based on the Milan study and others, liver transplantation is an effective option for HCC patients (225). The selection criteria are solitary tumor 5 cm or up to three nodules with tumor size <3 cm. When these criteria are strictly applied, excellent overall 3- to 4-year actuarial (75% to 85%) and recurrence-free survival rates (83% to 92%) can be achieved (125,130,225). Risk factors of recurrence after transplantation include tumor size, number of tumors, vascular invasion, and persistence of HBV infection (15,130,162). A major disadvantage with orthotopic liver transplantation is the unpredictable, potentially long waiting time for donor organs (162).

Percutaneous Ablation

For patients with early-stage HCC who are not suitable for resection or transplantation, percutaneous ablation would be the treatment option (117,175). Destruction of tumor cells can be achieved by the injection of chemical substances (ethanol,

Table 57.2	**GRADING SYSTEM FOR CIRRHOSIS: THE CHILD-PUGH SCORE**				
Score	Bilirubin (mg/dL)	Albumin (g/dL)	Prothrombin Time (sec)	Hepatic Encephalopathy (grade)	Ascites
1	<2	>3.5	<4	None	None
2	2–3	2.8–3.5	4–6	1–2	Mild (detectable)
3	>3	<2.8	>6	3–4	Severe (tense)

Child class: A, 5 to 6; B, 7 to 9; C, >9.

Modified Child-Pugh classification of the severity of liver disease according to the degree of ascites, the plasma concentrations of bilirubin and albumin, the prothrombin time, and the degree of encephalopathy

acetic acid) or by modifying the temperature (radiofrequency, microwave, laser, cryotherapy). Ethanol injection is highly effective for small HCC. It achieves necrosis rate of 90% to 100% of the HCC <2 cm, but the necrosis rate could be reduced to 50% in HCC >3 cm (59,118,129).

RFA involves the local application of radiofrequency thermal energy to the lesion. RFA is a reasonable option for patients who do not meet resectability criteria for HCC, and yet are candidates for a liver-directed procedure based on the presence of liver-only disease. The best outcomes are in patients with a single tumor <4 cm in diameter. The efficacy in tumors >2 cm is better than with ethanol. Randomized control trials have shown that RFA provides better local disease control that could result in an improved survival (111,117,120,181).

Transcatheter Arterial Chemoembolization

Treatment combining intra-arterial embolization with lipiodol, an iodized oily contrast agent, and chemotherapy is believed to be most effective for unresectable tumors on the basis that HCC is a highly vascular tumor supplied mostly by the hepatic or adjoining arteries with a selectively higher drug localization aided by direct visualization during angiography (140,223). Despite two prospectively randomized studies failed to show significant survival benefit over conservative management in patients with unresectable HCC (1,159). Systematic review of randomized prospective studies in the more recent literature has shown TACE to have a positive impact on survival (121). For palliative purpose, TACE has been accepted as the standard treatment for patients with unresectable HCC, and it can be used selectively for tumors of different location and can be repeated if necessary (23,38).

Radiotherapy

HCC is a radiosensitive tumor (33). The major drawback of radiotherapy in treating HCC is the poor radiation tolerance of adjacent normal liver and the difficulty of tumor localization (49,62). Recent technological and conceptual developments in the field of radiation therapy, such as intensity-modulated radiation therapy, image-guided radiation therapy, and stereotactic body radiation therapy, have the potential to improve radiation treatments by conforming the delivered radiation dose distribution tightly to the tumor or target volume outline while sparing normal liver tissue from high-dose radiation (73,188). For patients with liver-confined disease treated with conformal radiotherapy with or without TACE, local control response rates ranged from 40% to 90%, and the median survival ranged from 10 to 25 months (78). Indications for conformal radiotherapy include large unresectable HCC, relieving portal vein thrombosis and obstructive jaundice, failure of prior TACE and as part of combined modality treatment with TACE, and percutaneous ab-

lation therapy (33,74,115,222). The combination of TACE and conformal radiotherapy in large unresectable HCC has not yet been defined in randomized trial.

Radiation Doses

The tumor response to radiotherapy and survival of patients with HCC are related to the dose delivered (45,74). Partial response was 18% to 23% in unresectable HCC treated with 21 Gy in seven fractions and increased to 48% with dose around 33 Gy (148,192). Seong et al. (179) irradiated 27 HCC patients who failed TACE and observed an objective response rate of 67% after a mean dose of 51.8 Gy $\pm$ 7.9 Gy. Dawson et al. (45) escalated radiation doses for unresectable hepatobiliary cancer and observed that patients who received radiation doses >70 Gy had better median survival (>16.4 months). It appears that the higher the radiation doses given, the higher the tumor response seen (Table 57.3).

Treatment Volumes

Although higher radiation doses have been shown to produce higher response, patients with HCC usually have liver cirrhosis, which forbids such doses. Published reports on 3DCRT with photon energy suggest that portions of the liver can be treated with acceptable complications. Lawrence et al. (109) have demonstrated the radiation doses of ~35 Gy can be tolerated for treatment of the whole liver, doses of ~42 Gy for 70% of the liver, ~52 Gy for 50% of the liver, and doses of ~70 Gy for 30% of the liver.

Lawrence et al. developed a normal tissue complication probability (NTCP) for intrahepatic malignancy. They designed a protocol in which each patient received the maximum possible dose while being subjected to a 10% risk of radiation-induced liver disease based on the NTCP model. The mean doses delivered according to this protocol were 56.6 $\pm$ 2.31Gy (range, 40.5 to 81 Gy). They observed a complication rate of 4.8% (95% confidence interval, 0% to 23.8%), a number that did not differ significantly from the predicted 8.8% calculated on the basis of the NTCP model (126). This model, however, was derived using patients with relatively normal liver function, and only 4 of 21 of their study population had HCC. The NTCP model for patients with impaired liver function requires further evaluation (32). Multivariate analyses demonstrated that the severity of hepatic cirrhosis was the only independent predictor for radiation-induced liver disease. For cirrhotic patients with Child-Pugh grade A, the hepatic radiation tolerance was mean dose to normal liver of 23 Gy (114).

ICG retention can be used to guide the treatment of HCC. In HCC patients with normal bilirubin and without ascites, if the ICG retention 15 minutes (ICG 15) is normal, the resection volume can be trisegmentectomy or bisegmentectomy; if ICG 15 is 10% to 19%, the resection volume can be left lobectomy or right monosegmentectomy; if ICG 15 is 20% to 29%, the

	RADIOTHERAPY WITH AND WITHOUT CHEMOTHERAPY FOR UNRESECTABLE HEPATOCELLULAR CARCINOMA
Table 57.3	

Series	Patient Number	Radiation Dose (Gy)	Chemotherapy	Response Rate (%)
Stillwagon et al. (192) (RTOG)	135	21, 3 q.d.	Concurrent ADR, 5-FU	22
Order et al. (148) (RTOG)	105	21, 3 q.d. + I^{131} 10–12 ×2 courses	Concurrent ADR and 5-FU	48
Seong et al. (179)	27	51.8 (mean), 1.8 q.d.	None	67
Dawson et al. (45)	25	58.5 (median), 1.5 b.i.d.	Concurrent HAI fluorodeoxyuridine	68

RTOG, Radiation Therapy Oncology Group; q.d., every day; ADR, doxorubicin; 5 FU, 5 fluorouracil; b.i.d., twice daily; HAI, hepatic arterial infusion.

Table 57.4	RADIATION TREATMENT GUIDELINES FOR HEPATOCELLULAR CARCINOMA

Nontumor Part of Liver	ICG (Gy)		
	≤10%	10.1%–20%	20.1%–30%
<1/3	40 (Gy)	No RT	No RT
1/3–1/2	50 (Gy)	40 (Gy)	No RT
>1/2	60 (Gy)	50 (Gy)	40 (Gy)

ICG, indocyanine green; RT, radiation therapy.
From Cheng SH, Lin YM, Chuang VP, et al. A pilot study of three-dimensional conformal radiotherapy in unresectable hepatocellular carcinoma. *J Gastroenterol Hepatol* 1999;14:1025–1033, with permission.

resection can be subsegmentectomy; if ICG 15 is 30% to 39%, the resection can be done to only limited area of the liver (95). Therefore, we propose a treatment guideline using ICG test for 3DCRT for patients with impaired liver function (Table 57.4). We advise no radiation treatment for patients with Child-Pugh class C liver cirrhosis or prolonged ICG retention unless only a very small portion of the liver is included in the radiation treatment fields (33).

Design of Treatment Field

The goal of conformal radiotherapy is to precisely target the tumor(s) and to reduce damage to the surrounding normal tissue. Respiratory organ motion probably is the largest intrafractional organ motion. Aruga et al. (9) studied organ motions involving the use of CT images obtained during both the static exhalation phase and static inhalation phase for upper abdomen irradiation. They found that the tumor shifted between the two respiratory phases. The variation ranged from 2.6 to 23.7 mm: from 0.4 to 5.9 mm in the lateral direction, 2.2 to 24.5 mm in the longitudinal direction, and 0.2 to 11.7 mm in the vertical direction. Breath-gating or breath-holding irradiation may help overcome the problem of respiratory movement during irradiation (144). In general, the radiation-field margin to the target in the lateral direction should be 6 to 9 mm, vertical direction 9 to 12 mm, superior direction 10 mm, and inferior direction 19 to 21 mm (11,183). Controlling, gating, or tracking respiratory motion or by the use of image-guided radiation therapy previously mentioned is currently under investigation (63).

Acute and Late Complications

The dose-limiting tissue injuries in radiation treatment for HCC include the liver, stomach, duodenum, bowels, and kidneys. Acute complications include general fatigue, transient elevation of liver function test, and nausea and vomiting (mainly for tumors in the left lobe of the liver), fever, and pancytopenia (33,179). Subacute and late complications include hepatic fail-

ure, radiation pneumonitis, and gastrointestinal bleeding (especially in tumor located in the inferior portion of the right lobe of the liver and radiation doses >50 Gy) (33,178). Hepatic failure can be avoided by an appropriate selection of patients and careful treatment planning.

Results of Combining TACE and Local Radiation Therapy

TACE alone rarely produces complete pathologic remission for HCC >5 cm, especially in the peripheral zone of the tumor (2,82). Additional therapy theoretically is required to eradicate the residual disease. The combination of TACE and conformal radiotherapy shows promising results in large HCC (Table 57.5). Guo and Yu (74) reported 107 patients with large unresectable HCC treated with TACE followed by external-beam irradiation. The greatest dimension of the tumors ranged from 5 to 18 cm. After a median follow-up interval of 24 months, the cumulative survival rates at 3 and 5 years were 28.4% and 15.8%, respectively, with a median survival of 18 months. Cheng et al. (33) reported 17 patients with unresectable HCC treated with TACE and conformal radiotherapy. The mean tumor size was 8.6 cm (range, 3.7 to 18 cm). The overall survival rate at 2 years was 58% and local progression-free tumor control was 83%. After 24 months of median follow-up, the median survival had not been reached, and 1 of 17 patients remained progression-free (Fig. 57.2). A retrospective analysis of 102 patients with unresectable HCC who were treated with or without local radiotherapy following TAE (without chemotherapy agents added during embolization) or percutaneous ethanol injection revealed that the 3-year survival rate of 44 patients in the radiation group was better than that of the no radiation group (81% vs. 55%) (230). Another study that combined TACE and local radiotherapy in 50 unresectable HCC patients reported a partial response rate of 66% and survival rates at 3 years of 43% (178). Wu et al. (221) reported 94 patients with HCC received 3DCRT combined with TACE. The response rate was 90.5% The overall survival rates at 1, 2, and 3 years were 93.6%, 53.8%, and 26.0%, respectively, with the median survival of 25 months. Although we do not know yet whether combined TACE and conformal radiotherapy is a superior treatment modality to TACE alone, the results of these studies suggest that in patients with large unresectable HCC, combined treatments could be a promising new treatment modality worthy of further investigation.

Chemotherapy

Systemic chemotherapy for HCC has limited value in clinical practice because only a small portion of patients obtain significant benefits at the price of remarkable toxicity (136). In general, cytotoxic therapy should be reserved for medically appropriate patients with adequate hepatic function, preferably administered within the context of a clinical trial. The side

Table 57.5	COMBINATION TACE AND LOCAL RADIOTHERAPY IN UNRESECTABLE HEPATOCELLULAR CARCINOMA

Series	Patient Number	Mean Tumor Size (cm)	Treatment	Overall Survival (3 yr) (%)	Median Survival (mo)
Guo and Yu (74)	107	10.2	TACE–RT	28	18
Cheng et al. (33)	17	8.6	TACE–RT–TACE	58 (2 yr)	>24
Yasuda et al. (230)	44	Range 3–8	TAE–RT	81	Not available
Seong et al. (178)	50	8.3	TACE–RT	43%	17
Wu et al. (221)	94	10.7	TACE–RT	26	25

TACE, transcatheter arterial chemoembolization; RT, radiation therapy.

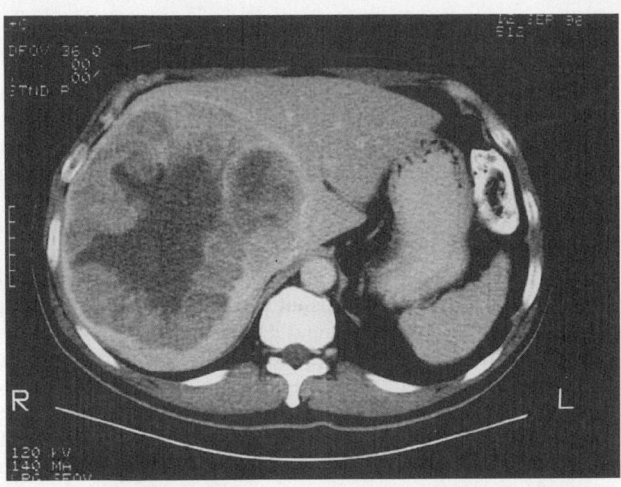

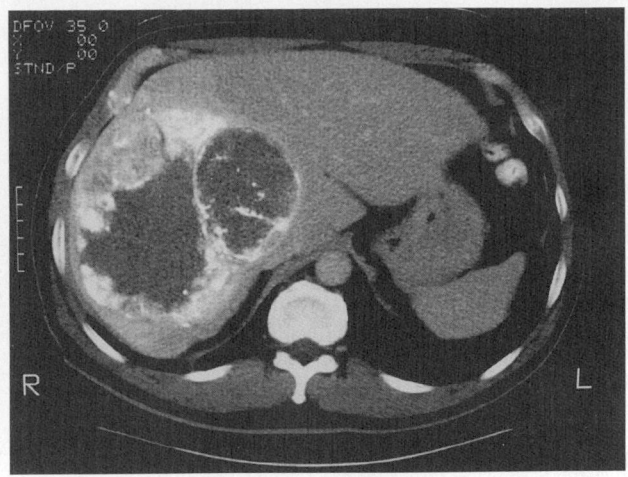

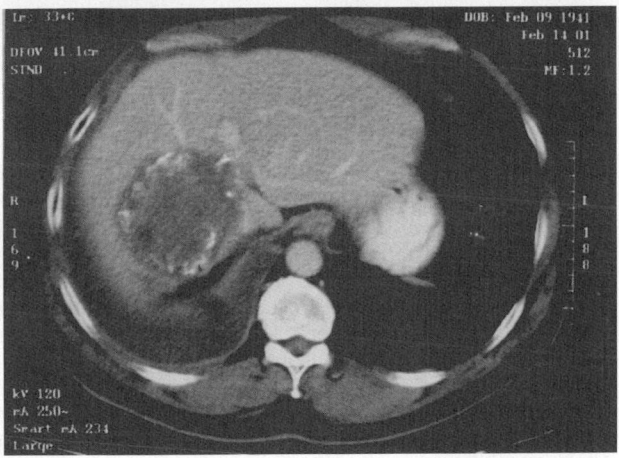

FIGURE 57.2. **A:** A 55-year-old man with hepatitis B virus infection developed a large hepatocellular carcinoma in right lobe of liver. The tumor measured 12 × 15 × 15 cm. Alpha-fetoprotein (AFP) was 901 ng/mL. **B:** After a first course of transcatheter arterial chemoembolization (TACE), his AFP dropped to 150 ng/mL. It rose to 440 ng/mL 3 months later. He had second TACE followed by three-dimensional conformal radiotherapy. This image was taken after the second TACE, revealing viable tumors in the peripheral zone of the main mass. **C:** Four years and 4 months after the first treatment, computed tomography revealed a nonenhancing tumor in the right lobe of the liver. His AFP remained <10 ng/mL after completion of radiotherapy.

effect profile of any chemotherapy regimen should be considered carefully in patients with advanced liver disease and a short life expectancy.

Several new drugs have been tested recently. One of the more promising of these drugs is gemcitabine. It has a low toxicity profile, but its antitumor activity in patients with advanced HCC is marginal: the response rate is 18% and the response duration is 35 weeks (229). Combination chemotherapy regimens have shown better responses. Leung et al. (112) reported on 50 patients treated with intravenous chemotherapy PIAF (cisplatin, doxorubicin, 5-fluorouracil [5-FU], and interferon-alpha). The partial response was 26% (13/50) and 4 patients achieved pathologic complete remission (112). Recent advances in molecular biology have uncovered the structures and/or functions of many cytokines thought to have a strong relationship with the mechanisms of the antitumor effect of biological therapies. Thalidomide, a sedative previously associated with severe fetal malformations, has limited value in the treatment of HCC (155,156). Molecular targeted therapy to the epidermal growth factor receptor and vascular endothelial growth factor has exhibited the potential to inhibit tumor growth of HCC (83,161,240).

Areas of Failure and Cause of Death

Survival of HCC after treatment depends on the clinical stage and liver function. Five-year survival in resectable HCC after partial hepatectomy is 50% to 73% in stage I patients, 30% to 56% in stage II patients, 10% to 29% in stage III patients, and ~10% in stage IV patients (50,168). The 5-year survival for patients with unresectable HCC is usually <10% (138). The major

cause of failure after resection is tumor recurrence within the liver; this observation still holds true for patients who undergo TACE alone. Extrahepatic metastases in advanced-stage HCC have become more common in recent years, related to improvements in the local treatment of intrahepatic disease (31,177).

Future Study

The overall treatment outcome in HCC is generally unsatisfactory. The main cause of failure is intrahepatic recurrence. Future efforts should be directed toward prevention of HBV and HCV infection through vaccination in hyperendemic regions, and perhaps through chemoprevention for individuals who are already infected and are persistent carriers. Other approaches include early diagnosis in high-risk populations and development of effective adjuvant treatments after resection.

Biliary Tract Cancer

Biliary tract cancers consist of cancer of the gallbladder, the bile ducts, and the ampulla of Vater. They are highly lethal because most are locally advanced at presentation. Gallbladder cancer is the most common cancer of the biliary tract and accounts for two thirds of these cancer patients, whereas bile duct cancer accounts for the remaining one-third (108). The term *cholangiocarcinoma* was used to describe cancers arising from the epithelial cells of the bile ducts, which include intrahepatic, perihilar, and distal extrahepatic biliary tree. At present, surgical excision of all detectable biliary tract cancers is associated with improvement in long-term survival. For unresectable tumors, the purpose of treatment is to palliate symptoms such as obstructive jaundice, biliary tract infection, pain, and ascites.

Cholangiocarcinoma

Topographic Anatomy

The bile ducts originate within the liver, with the left and right hepatic ducts joining to form the common hepatic duct. At the origin of the cystic duct, it becomes the common bile duct. The cystic duct drains bile from the gallbladder into the common bile duct. The gallbladder is adjacent to the undersurface of the liver.

There is a rich lymphatic network along the submucosa of bile ducts. The primary lymphatic drainage of the biliary tract is to the lymph nodes in the pericholedochal area, periportal region, hepatoduodenal ligament, common hepatic artery and pancreaticoduodenal groups (53,185,189).

Epidemiology and Risk Factors

Cholangiocarcinoma is a rare tumor in developed countries; there are approximately 5,000 cases per year in United States. However, it is one of the most common cancers in endemic areas of developing countries, as high as 87 per 100,000 people in northeast Thailand (25,215). Cholangiocarcinoma accounts for about 20% of the primary liver cancer in Western countries, and <10% in Asian nations that are endemic for HCC (28, 184).

A number of risk factors have been identified as important in the development of cholangiocarcinoma, most of which share a history of long-standing inflammation and chronic injury of the biliary epithelium (215). The major risk factor in Western countries is primary sclerosing cholangitis, which is closely associated with chronic inflammatory bowel disease, particularly ulcerative colitis (71). The risk of developing cholangiocarcinoma is higher in patients with primary sclerosing cholangitis, ulcerative colitis, and colonic neoplasm than in patients with primary sclerosing cholangitis and ulcerative colitis without colonic neoplasm (18). In Japan, patients with HCV infection have 1,000 times higher incidence than would be expected in the general population, and the accumulated rate of newly diagnosed cholangiocarcinoma is 1.6% at 5 years and 3.5% at 10 years (102). In Asia, chronic infections of the biliary tract and infestation by certain liver flukes, such as *Clonorchis sinensis* and *Opisthorchis viverinni* are associated with cholangiocarcinoma and hepatolithiasis (27). Hepatolithiasis itself is also a risk factor for cholangiocarcinoma; 5% to 10% of patients with intrahepatic stones develop this complication (34,106). Moreover, the combination of liver fluke infestation and nitrosamine exposure may explain the very high incidence of cholangiocarcinoma in northeast Thailand (152). Other risk factors, although rare, include congenital fibropolycystic disease of the biliary system such as choledochal cysts and Caroli's disease (cystic dilatation of intrahepatic bile ducts) (27).

The observed incidence and mortality of intrahepatic cholangiocarcinoma has increased in the past 3 decades in Japan, the United States, and the United Kingdom (127,151,153). In the United States, the age-adjusted mortality rate increased from 0.07 per 100,000 in 1973 to 0.69 per 100,000 in 1997, the estimated annual percent change of mortality was 9.44%. Better case ascertainment and diagnosis because of improved diagnostic imaging, use of image-guided biopsies, or increased use of endoscopic retrograde cholangiopancreatography (ERCP) cannot fully explain this observation (153,200).

Diagnosis

The most common presenting symptoms of biliary tract cancer are caused by obstruction of the bile duct and include painless jaundice, clay-colored stool, tea-colored urine, and pruritus. Other sign and symptoms include abdominal pain, fever, general malaise, abdominal distention, fullness, anorexia, and weight loss. The spectrum of cholangiocarcinoma can be classified into three broad groups: (a) intrahepatic, (b) perihilar, and (c) distal tumors. The age of onset is similar among the three groups and ranges from 60 to 65 years (142). Patients with extrahepatic tumor usually present with jaundice and tea-colored urine. Patients with intrahepatic tumors are less likely to be jaundiced and more likely to present with abdominal symptoms.

There are no reliable screening methods; early diagnosis is almost impossible even in patients with high-risk situations such as primary sclerosing cholangitis and hepatolithiasis (88). Some patients are diagnosed when screening blood work demonstrates elevation of alkaline phosphatase and γ glutamyl transferase. Ultrasonography and CT are the initial primary tools to evaluate biliary tract tumor (Table 57.6). Further tests include percutaneous transhepatic cholangiography, ERCP with brushing cytology, serum carbohydrate antigen 19-9 (CA 19–9) levels, radiologic imaging with dynamic CT scan, MRI, or both, and angiography.

A serum CA 19-9 value >100 U/mL has a sensitivity of ~75% and a specificity of ~80% (141). The optimal cut-off value for serum CA 19-9 that best discriminates between benign or malignant biliary tract diseases is influenced by the presence of cholangitis. Thus, in patients with symptoms of acute cholangitis, serum CA 19-9 concentrations should ideally be re-evaluated after recovery. The sensitivity of serum carcinoembryonic antigen (CEA) is low, helpful only in one third of patients (17). Biliary CEA levels increase significantly in patients with cholangiocarcinoma and also in patients with intrahepatic cholelithiasis (average, 50.3 to 57.4 ng/mL) compared with patients with benign strictures (average, 10.1 ng/mL) and patients with sclerosing cholangitis and choledochal cysts (average, 20.0 to 21.6 ng/mL) (141). Serum AFP may increase in some cases of cholangiocarcinoma, and this would suggest a diagnosis of mixed HCC and cholangiocarcinoma (139).

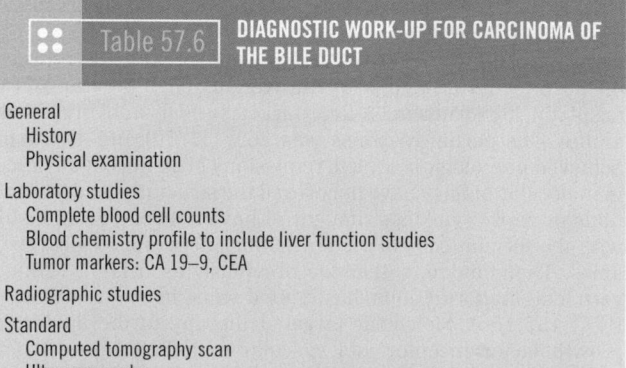

Table 57.6	DIAGNOSTIC WORK-UP FOR CARCINOMA OF THE BILE DUCT

General
  History
  Physical examination

Laboratory studies
  Complete blood cell counts
  Blood chemistry profile to include liver function studies
  Tumor markers: CA 19–9, CEA

Radiographic studies

Standard
  Computed tomography scan
  Ultrasonography
  Transhepatic cholangiography
  Endoscopic retrograde cholangiopancreatography

Optional
  Endoscopic ultrasound
  Magnetic resonance cholangiopancreatography
  Dynamic computed tomography scan
  Arteriography

Modified from Gunderson LL, Willett CG. Pancreas and hepatobiliary tract. In: Perez CA, Brady LW, eds. *Principles and practice of radiation oncology*, 3rd ed. New York: Lippincott-Raven Publishers;.

Cholangiocarcinoma is usually hypovascular or avascular at angiography. In dynamic CT, the majority of HCC demonstrate early enhancement followed by a continuous decrease in tumor attenuation over time. In contrast, tumor attenuation of cholangiocarcinoma increases during the delayed phase. CT frequently shows a hypodense hepatic lesion with peripheral enhancement and biliary dilatation (122,213). However, the extent of the exact proximal involvement along the bile duct tends to be underestimated by CT (201).

MRI also has been used to diagnose cholangiocarcinoma. Whether it offers any advantage in tumor delineation compared with CT is still being investigated (239). For hilar lesions (intrahepatic ductal dilatation with normal-caliber extrahepatic ducts), magnetic resonance cholangiopancreatography (MRCP) is emerging as the imaging technique of choice, and the use of invasive cholangiography, particularly ERCP, is diminishing (134). MRCP can provide information regarding not only the location, but also the cause of the obstruction. It provides the identification, characterization, and staging of the lesion, giving the clinician almost all the information necessary for the planning of adequate treatment (158).

Histologic diagnosis for cholangiocarcinoma is often achievable before surgical exploration with the use of brushing cytology at the time of ERCP or fine-needle aspiration from the tumor under CT or ultrasonographic guidance. Imaging-guided fine-needle percutaneous biopsy with cytology is a rapid and accurate diagnostic method in evaluating a wide range of hepatobiliary masses (43).

Pathology

Cholangiocarcinomas arise from the epithelium of the biliary tract; the majority of these cancers are adenocarcinomas. Rare histologies include squamous cell carcinoma, mucoepidermoid carcinoma, cystadenocarcinoma, and carcinoid tumor. Grossly, three subtypes of cholangiocarcinomas are identified: sclerosing, nodular, and papillary (25,219). Sclerosing tumors are characterized by an intense desmoplastic reaction. This type of tumor tends to invade the bile duct wall early, and as a result, is associated with low resectability and cure rates. Most cholangiocarcinomas are of this type (142). On the contrast, papillary histology has the most favorable prognosis (39). Microscopically, cholangiocarcinoma are classically well differentiated to undifferentiated. Cells tend to be cuboidal or low columnar and resemble biliary epithelium; mucin is always demonstrable in the cytoplasm. Bile duct obstruction can be associated with reactive hyperplasia of subepithelial mucous glands with or without cholangiocarcinoma (219). Cholangiocarcinomas frequently invade lymphatic, perineural, and periductal spaces, and portal tracts. Spreading along the lumen of large bile ducts can also be seen, especially in perihilar cholangiocarcinoma (101).

The differential diagnosis of cholangiocarcinoma from HCC can be further affirmed by positive reaction with CEA, CA 19-9, and immunohistochemistry with cytokeratin 19 (206). Mutations in the p53 tumor suppressor gene and K-ras proto-oncogene have been identified in cholangiocarcinoma (3,145,193). p53 overexpression and K-ras mutations are associated with a shortened survival (3).

Pathways of Tumor Spread

Bile duct cancers commonly spread by direct extension through the bile duct and the abundant lymphatic network in the submucosa. These tumors also commonly involve the surrounding structures by direct invasion. Lymph node metastasis in the porta hepatis and celiac axis are common. The lymph nodes in porta hepatis are more frequently involved with tumors in the intrahepatic duct and proximal extrahepatic bile duct and the pancreaticoduodenal nodes are more often involved with tumors in the distal bile duct (99,232).

The incidence of lymph node metastasis in intrahepatic cholangiocarcinoma ranges from 50% to 60% (207,227). Intrahepatic cholangiocarcinomas, irrespective of their intrahepatic location, mainly spread to the nodes in the hepatoduodenal ligament, then to the para-aortic nodes, retropancreatic nodes, or common hepatic artery node group. In addition, the left peripheral type or hilar type of cholangiocarcinoma tends to spread along the left gastric nodes through the lesser curvature (227). Lymph node metastasis in perihilar cholangiocarcinoma is common, which occurs in half of the patients, with the frequency of 43% in pericholedochal nodes, 31% in the periportal nodes, 27% in the common hepatic nodes, and 15% in the posterior pancreaticoduodenal nodes. The celiac and superior mesenteric nodes are rarely involved (99).

Lymph node metastasis in distal duct cancer is commonly observed near the duodenopancreatic regions. Yoshida et al. (232) examined 20 consecutive patients with distal bile duct cancer who underwent pancreaticoduodenectomy with extended lymph node dissection. Histologic evidence of lymph node metastasis was seen in 55% of the patients. The areas with frequent metastases were the posterior pancreaticoduodenal lymph nodes (35%), the nodes around the hepatoduodenal ligament (35%), and those around the common hepatic artery (30%). Para-aortic lymph node involvement occurred in 25% of patients and was significantly associated with pancreatic parenchymal invasion.

Staging

Cholangiocarcinoma in the intrahepatic bile ducts are staged similarly to HCC (Table 57.1). The American Joint Committee on Cancer TNM classifications for both hilar and distal cholangiocarcinoma were revised in 2002 (Table 57.7) (72). The current staging classification for cholangiocarcinoma does not predict overall survival or respectability (237). The most important prognostic factors for cholangiocarcinoma are resectability, regional lymph node metastasis, and distant metastasis.

General Management

Resection remains the primary treatment; 5-year survival rates after resection range from 10% to 40%, depending on the location of the primary tumor (142). Patients with unresectable cholangiocarcinoma generally have a very poor prognosis; chemotherapy and radiotherapy have been used but the results are disappointing (64).

Intrahepatic Cholangiocarcinoma

Intrahepatic cholangiocarcinoma accounts for 5% to 10% of all biliary tract cancers and constitutes 10% to 20% of primary liver malignancies. The resectability rate in all patients is only 30% to 50% (30,37). The outcomes after surgery for patients with lymph node metastasis are poor regardless of the sites of nodal metastasis; the 5-year survival rate in patients with lymph node metastasis was lower than that in patients without lymph node metastasis (0% vs. 51%; $p < .0001$) (227).

Factors that affect tumor recurrence include lymph node metastasis, presence of satellite nodules, positive resection margin, tumor size, and bilobar distribution (57,171,214,227). The patterns of failure after resection of intrahepatic cholangiocarcinoma are primarily in the liver (56%), regional lymph node (20%), and peritoneal seeding (24%) (226). The role of postoperative adjuvant radiotherapy with or without chemotherapy in the management of intrahepatic cholangiocarcinoma is controversial. The typical reports in the literature have small

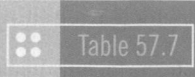

Table 57.7	AMERICAN JOINT COMMITTEE ON CANCER (AJCC) TNM CLASSIFICATION FOR BILIARY TRACT CANCER (GALLBLADDER, EXTRAHEPATIC BILE DUCT, AND AMPULLA OF VATER), 2002

Primary tumor (T)—Extrahepatic Bile Duct

Tx	Primary tumor cannot be assessed
T0	No evidence of primary tumor
Tis	Carcinoma *in situ*
T1	Tumor confined to the bile duct histologically
T2	Tumor invades beyond the wall of the bile duct
T3	Tumor invades the liver, gallbladder, pancreas, and/or unilateral branches of the portal vein (right or left) or hepatic artery (right or left)
T4	Tumor invades any of the following: main portal vein or its branches bilaterally, common hepatic artery, or other adjacent structures such as the colon, stomach, duodenum, or abdominal wall

Primary tumor (T)—Gallbladder

Tx, T0, Tis—Same as extrahepatic bile duct

T1	Tumor invades lamina propria or muscle layer
T1a	Tumor invades lamina propria
T1b	Tumor invades muscle layer
T2	Tumor invades perimuscular connective tissue; no extension beyond serosa or into liver
T3	Tumor perforates the serosa (visceral peritoneum) or directly invades into one adjacent organ, or both (≤2 cm into liver)
T4	Tumor extends >2 cm into liver and/or into two or more adjacent organs (stomach, duodenum, colon, pancreas, omentum, extrahepatic bile ducts)

Primary tumor (T)—Ampulla of Vater

Tx, T0, Tis	Same as extrahepatic bile duct
T1	Tumor limited to ampulla of Vater or sphincter Oddi
T2	Tumor invades duodenal wall
T3	Tumor invades <2 cm into the pancreas
T4	Tumor invades >2 cm into the pancreas and/or into other adjacent organs

Lymph node (N)—Gallbladder, bile duct, and Ampulla

Nx	Regional lymph node cannot be accessed
N0	No regional lymph node metastasis
N1	Regional lymph node metastasis[a]

Metastasis (M)

Mx	Distant metastasis cannot be accessed
M0	No distant metastasis
M1	Distant metastasis

AJCC stage groupings

Stage 0	Stage IIB
Tis, N0, M0	T1-T3, N1, M0
Stage IA	**Stage III**
T1, N0, M0	T4, any N, M0
Stage IB	**Stage IV**
T2, N0, M0	Any T, any N, M1
Stage IIA	
T3, N0, M0	

[a]Hilar, celiac, periduodenal, peripancreatic, and superior mesenteric nodes.
Modified from Greene F, Page D, Fleming I: *AJCC (American Joint Committee on Cancer) Cancer staging manual*. New York: Springer-Verlag; 2002:121.

numbers of patients, are retrospective, and have marked variations in radiation field and dose (231). A delineation of radiation fields based on patterns of failure analysis and lymph node spread of the disease will be necessary to rationally define the role of radiotherapy in any proposed phase III study. For unresectable cholangiocarcinoma, the purpose of treatment is palliative; however, some long-term survivals (a 4-year rate of 20%) have been observed in unresectable cholangiocarcinoma treated with conformal radiotherapy and intra-arterial infusion of fluorodeoxyuridine (172). Total hepatectomy with orthotopic liver transplantation also can be considered in this situation. However, early results of orthotopic liver transplantation have been disappointing, with rapid recurrence of disease (69). With highly selected patients and preoperative irradiation and chemotherapy, total hepatectomy with orthotopic liver transplantation performed in Mayo Clinic has been associated with prolonged disease-free and overall survival (47).

Perihilar Cholangiocarcinoma

Perihilar cholangiocarcinoma is the most common biliary tract carcinoma and accounts for 65% to 70% of tumors of the biliary tract (142). Perihilar tumors involving the bifurcation of the hepatic duct are also called *Klatskin tumors* (100). These tumors were further classified by Bismuth et al. (16) as tumors below the confluence of the left and right hepatic ducts (type I), tumors reaching the confluence (type II), tumors occluding the common hepatic duct and the right or the left hepatic duct (types IIIa and IIIb, respectively), and tumors that are multicentric or that involve the confluence and both the right and left hepatic ducts (type IV).

Only 25% to 79% of patients are amenable for surgical resection. Definitive surgery may involve combined bile duct and liver resection with caudate lobectomy (205). The 3-year survival rate was 55% for patients without involved nodes, 32% for patients with regional node metastasis, and 12% for patients with paraaortic node metastasis (99). In multivariate prognostic analysis, only lymph node metastases and curative resection have proven to be of independent prognostic significance (101).

The role of postoperative radiotherapy with or without chemotherapy in patients with completely resected cholangiocarcinoma remains unproven. A retrospective analysis from Johns Hopkins suggests that postoperative adjuvant radiation therapy does not improve survival (165). However, postoperative radiotherapy or chemoradiotherapy reduces the rate of local recurrence in patients with incomplete resection (196,204). In addition, many retrospective series and small phase II studies suggest superior outcomes for resected patients who receive external-beam radiation therapy with or without concomitant chemotherapy (66,133,216,220). For patients with microscopic residual disease after resection, a retrospective analysis from 63 patients with stage IV Klatskin tumor revealed that postoperative radiotherapy (with or without intraoperative radiotherapy) yielded significantly higher 5-year survival rates than in the resection alone group (33.9% vs. 13.5%) (204).

A retrospective study report from Mayo Clinic showed promising results in highly selected patients with unresectable hilar cholangiocarcinoma treated with preoperative radiotherapy and chemotherapy and orthotopic liver transplant (47). An update report from same group revealed that the 5-year survival in transplant patients was 80% and in resection-only patients it was 21% (169). Others also have reported similar promising results in these combined-modality treatments (79,194).

In general, patients with inoperable perihilar cholangiocarcinoma usually have obstructive jaundice and should be treated with endoscopic or percutaneous drainage and/or stent placement initially. External-beam radiotherapy alone rarely controls advanced disease. Combinations of external-beam radiotherapy, chemotherapy, and intraluminal brachytherapy may relieve pain and contribute to biliary decompression, and sometimes achieve long-term survival. The most active agents include 5-FU, gemcitabine, docetaxel, and oxaliplatin (4,217). The median survivals range from 17 to 21 months. In some cases, combined chemotherapy and radiotherapy could delay the progression of cholangiocarcinomas and await the chance for liver transplant (131,133).

Distal Bile Duct Carcinoma

Primary distal bile duct adenocarcinoma, which includes carcinoma of the ampulla of Vater, accounts for 25% to 30% of biliary tract carcinomas (142). Patients with distal duct carcinoma have the highest rate of curative resection as compared with proximal duct carcinoma. In an analysis of 171 patients who underwent surgical exploration at Mayo Clinic for extrahepatic cholangiocarcinoma from 1976 to 1985, the rate of curative resection (negative margins) by site of the primary tumor was 15% for proximal, 33% for midductal, and 56% for distal lesions (137). The prognosis of patients with distal duct carcinoma is also better than that of patients with proximal duct carcinoma (18).

The role of postoperative radiotherapy is uncertain. Investigators at Thomas Jefferson University found that postoperative radiotherapy did not improve survival in distal duct carcinoma after complete resection (6). However, studies of concurrent chemotherapy and radiotherapy show more promising results. Mehta et al. (128) from Stanford University treated 12 patients having unfavorable (mainly lymph node metastasis) ampullary carcinoma with concurrent radiotherapy and protracted venous infusion of 5-FU. Actuarial overall survival at 2 years was 89%, and median survival was 34 months. Another study conducted by the Eastern Cooperative Oncology Group revealed that unresectable pancreaticobiliary carcinoma treated with concomi-

tant radiotherapy and protracted intravenous infusion of 5-FU achieved a 2-year survival of 19% (220).

Radiation Therapy

Radiotherapy technique for intrahepatic cholangiocarcinoma is similar to treatment of HCC. The outcome of unresectable cholangiocarcinoma by radiotherapy alone is poor because of the poor tolerance of the surrounding organs. To enhance treatment effects, radiotherapy given with 5-FU–based chemotherapy is generally recommended (128,220). The dose-limiting surrounding organs include the liver, duodenum, stomach, and spinal cord.

Treatment Volumes

The extent of the tumor within the bile duct can be defined by percutaneous cholangiography, ERCP, and MRCP. However, the extraductal disease is difficult to define by any noninvasive procedure. Clip placement at the time of surgery is useful in delineating the extrahepatic portion of ductal lesions and in defining the primary tumor bed. With the incorporation of CT in radiation-treatment planning, and to reduce errors to a minimum, we advocate placing patients in treatment position when performing CT, using 1 to 3 mm per slice, and contrast medium to reconstruct the bile ducts and gross tumor volume (Fig. 57.3). The gross tumor volume (GTV) is defined as any visible tumor by CT and/or MRI. Clinical target volume (CTV) is defined as 1.5 cm margin to the GTV, especially along the bile duct and potential lymphatic drainage areas, which include nodes along the porta hepatis, pancreaticoduodenal system, and celiac axis (99,224,227,232). The planning target volume is defined by adding a margin of 0.5 to 1 cm to the CTV (133).

Radiation Doses

Initial setup of radiation fields is to include GTV and CTV; the radiation fields can be coplanar or noncoplanar. The planning target volume will be treated to 45 to 50 Gy in 1.8- to 2-Gy fractions given 5 days a week, using blocks if possible to exclude normal stomach, small intestine, kidney, and liver (133,210). Higher radiation doses are used only to treat the GTV with the application of 3DCRT (45). If boost-dose irradiation is feasible with brachytherapy techniques, the GTV is carried to 45 to 50 Gy with external techniques, and 20 to 30 Gy is delivered via an intraluminal the catheter (73). The most commonly employed brachytherapy technique for the biliary tract begins with the placement, by an invasive diagnostic radiologist, of a percutaneous drainage catheter through the area of tumor. The radiation oncologist then threads a catheter inside the drainage system catheter. When a low-dose-rate system is employed, a wire with Ir-192 is then placed at the desired location inside the catheter (5). If a remote high-dose-rate afterloading system is employed, then the appropriate dwell times and positions are selected and programmed. It is a matter of some debate as to where the brachytherapy prescription point should be placed. Some physicians select the tumor's peripheral edge, away from the catheter, as determined by CT or MRI. Other practitioners prefer a point 0.5 or 1 cm away from the catheter. It is important to be familiar with the valves used to direct bile flow in the drainage system lest, during the administration of brachytherapy, bile leaks onto the patient's skin and dressings. If the drainage system remains in place for a long period of time (i.e., a month), enteric bacterial colonization and biliary tract infection are common. The combination of external-beam irradiation and brachytherapy employed at Thomas Jefferson University resulted in 2-year and median survival rate increasing twofold when doses were brought up to >55 Gy (5). However, investigators at the University of Amsterdam reported no

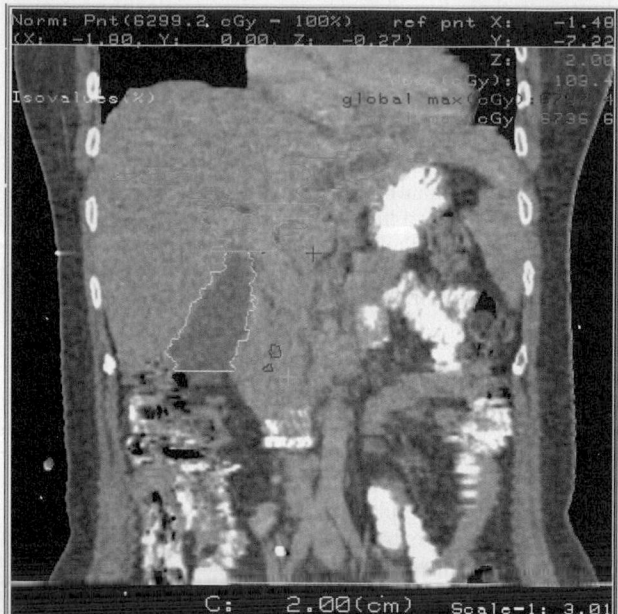

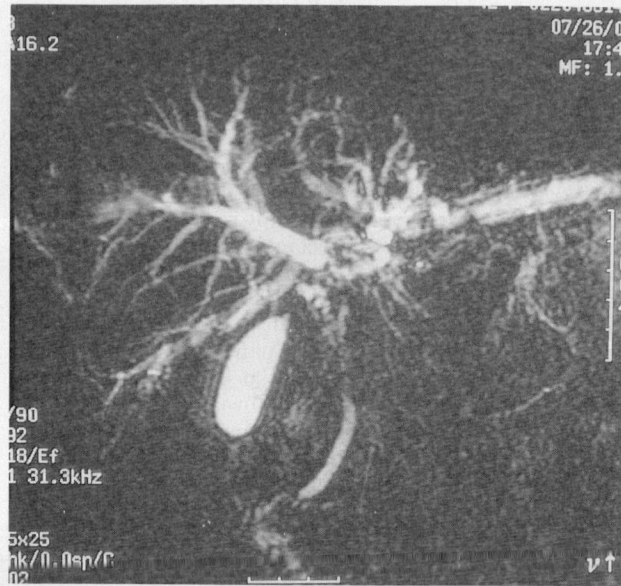

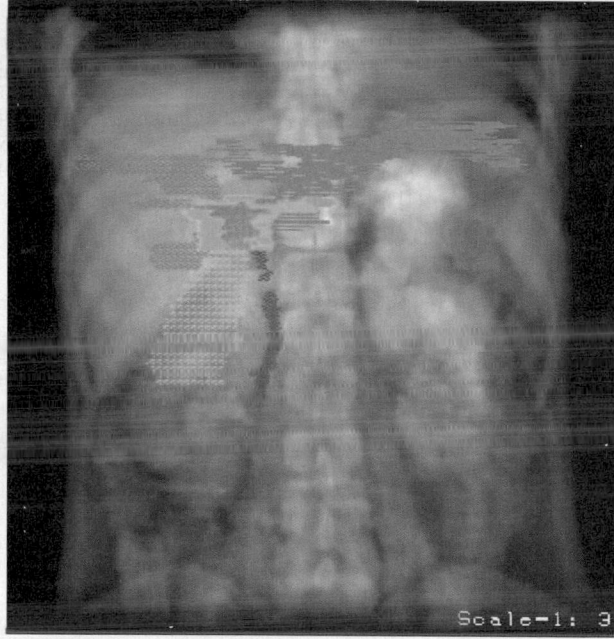

FIGURE 57.3. A: Computed tomography was performed in a 39-year-old woman who had cholangiocarcinoma of perihilar area. This film was reconstructed from a CT, which was obtained with 2 mm per slice. The tumor involved right and left hepatic duct (*green line*). **B:** Magnetic resonance cholangiopancreatography affirmed tumor extent. **C:** Digital reconstruction radiography revealed the gross tumor volume (green), and clinical target volume (purple).

improved survival at doses >55 Gy (70). The role of radiotherapy and its optimal dosage remains to be determined.

Acute and Late Complications

Acute complications of external-beam and intraluminal radiotherapy include nausea, vomiting, and transient elevation of transaminase. These effects are usually mild and tolerable (212).

Late complications are associated with radiation dose to surrounding organs. The most common complications are gastrointestinal bleeding, biliary bleeding, and duodenal stenosis (5,70,212). With external-beam doses of <55 Gy to the duodenum or stomach, the risk of severe gastrointestinal complications varies from 5% to 10%. At doses >55 Gy, one-third of patients develop severe problems.

Future Directions

There is a paucity of phase III studies for cholangiocarcinoma. We must rely on retrospective studies or prospective phase I-II trials. Further advances in treatment could potentially be made by: (a) defining when to use radiation and chemotherapy for high-risk patients after curative resection, (b) investigating the use of higher doses of conformal radiotherapy and chemotherapy in unresectable cholangiocarcinoma, and (c) identifying novel chemotherapeutic agents. Patients with unresectable cholangiocarcinoma should be offered clinical trials.

Adenocarcinoma of Gallbladder

Gallbladder carcinoma is not common; it is the fifth most common cancer of the gastrointestinal tract. The incidence indicates a large geographic variation and it accounts for approximately 5,000 new patients per year in the United States (10). Distinctly different from cholangiocarcinoma, the ratio of females to males is 2.5:1 (27). Cholelithiasis, anomalous junction of pancreaticobiliary ducts, and porcelain gallbladder are factors that predispose to gallbladder cancer (180). Cigarette smoking, alcohol consumption, and obesity may also increase the risk. Patients with polyps >10 mm in diameter may be at increased risk for gallbladder cancer (132,146). Chronic infection with *Salmonella typhi* and *Helicobacter bilis* is also associated with the risk of developing carcinoma of the gallbladder (56,123).

The most common clinical presentation is pain, followed by anorexia, nausea, or vomiting. Patients with early invasive gallbladder carcinoma are most often asymptomatic, or they have nonspecific symptoms that mimic or are due to cholelithiasis or cholecystitis. In general, gallbladder carcinoma is diagnosed late, which accounts for the poor prognosis (27). A French study of 724 patients revealed that only 4% of the patients had Tis lesions, 11% had T1 to T2 lesions, and 85% had T3 to T4 lesions (41). Five-year survival rates according to the National Cancer Data Base were Tis disease, 60%; T1N0, 39%; T2N0, 15%; and T3N0 or node-positive disease, 5% (51). However, improved outcomes have been noted in the last decade, and attributed to more aggressive surgery and the use of postoperative adjuvant therapy (143). Studies from Japan report a 5-year survival rate in stage I patients of 100%, stage II at 50% to 78%, stage III at 0% to 69%, and stage IV at 0% to 11% (182,203).

Lymphatic metastasis is initially to cystic and pericholedochal nodes and then to the pancreaticoduodenal system, with later potential spread to the rest of the celiac axis or the superior mesenteric or aortic nodes (182,208). The lymph node metastasis rate is associated with primary tumor stage: 0% to 2.5% in pT1a disease (involvement limited to the mucosa), 15% in T1b, disease, 62% in pT2 disease, and 81% in pT3/pT4 disease (182,187,218).

Surgery is the only potentially curative therapy, but only 10% to 30% of patients are eligible for resection (173). The standard surgical procedure is removal of the gallbladder, resection of various amounts of liver surrounding the gallbladder bed, resection of the extrahepatic bile duct, and dissection of the regional lymph nodes. Patients with jaundice should be considered for preoperative percutaneous transhepatic biliary drainage for relief of biliary obstruction. Overall, the curative resection rates for gallbladder carcinoma range from 10% to 30% in Western countries (113). The prognosis is related to the possibility of curative resection, primary tumor extension, and regional lymph node metastasis.

Patients with T1a disease often are cured after simple cholecystectomy and require no further adjuvant treatment (218). However, for patients with ≥T2 disease many reports support the benefit of radical resection; re-exploration is generally recommended (143,187,199). In more advanced disease, the role of adjuvant radiotherapy is uncertain. After "curative" resection, locoregional relapse in the tumor bed or regional nodes is common. Factors predicting recurrence are positive surgical margins, lymph node metastasis, and perineural invasion (35). Several retrospective analyses demonstrate that postoperative radiotherapy improved local control and survival (85,135,202). Benefits are also seen in patients who have microscopic residual tumors (202). Combination radiotherapy and chemotherapy with 5-FU also reveal similar benefits (46,61,104). However, there is lack of phase III studies. Whether combination treatment is better than single modality is still unknown.

Patients with stage III and IV disease are at high risk for distant metastasis. The most frequent sites of involvement are liver, peritoneum, and lung, with less frequent spread to ovaries, spleen, bones, and other organs (61,103). In general, patients who are locally unresectable should be referred for chemoradiotherapy. Median survival is improved in several retrospective studies (42,81). Systemic chemotherapy has had limited success in the treatment of advanced gallbladder carcinoma. Objective response rates range from 25% to 50%. Active agents include infusion 5-FU in combination regimens, leucovorin-modulated 5-FU, capecitabine, cisplatin, oxaliplatin, gemcitabine, and docetaxel. 5-FU and rIFN alpha-2b (65,149,154,157,160,186).

Other Rare Neoplasms

Primary sarcomas of the liver are extremely rare in adults and represent only 1% to 2% of primary liver cancers (40). Leiomyosarcoma is the most common histologic type, followed by malignant fibrous histiocytoma, epithelioid haemangioendothelioma, and angiosarcoma (166). Some patients with angiosarcoma have a history of occupational exposure to vinyl chloride monomer (86). Histologic grade of sarcoma is the only factor significantly associated with overall patient survival. Complete resection offers a chance of long-term survival (166).

Hemangioma is a benign lesion and generally is asymptomatic. For symptomatic hemangioma, the treatments of choice include steroids, interferon-alpha, arterial embolization, and surgery (90). If patients fail such treatments, radiotherapy may play a role. Long symptom-free survival times have been obtained with doses as low as 13 to 30 Gy during 2.5 to 4 weeks (150).

Hepatoblastoma is the most common malignant liver tumor of childhood. Children who have familial adenomatous polyposis are high risk to have hepatoblastoma. The risk of hepatoblastoma in these children is 700 to 7,500 times higher than in the general population (7,67). Surgery combined with chemotherapy has resulted in dramatic improvements in prognosis (52). With the combination of chemotherapy and surgery, 75% to 80% of patients may be cured (24). Preoperative chemotherapy often converts unresectable tumors to resectable and may facilitate surgery being performed with less blood loss and minimal technical complications (176).

⠓ Acknowledgment

The authors thank Ms. Yen-Chun Lin, Mr. Johns Chao-Ming Huang, and Dr. Chung Yih-Lin for their assistance in data collection, and Dr. Yu-Mong Lin for his invaluable comments on this chapter.

References

1. A comparison of lipiodol chemoembolization and conservative treatment for unresectable hepatocellular carcinoma. Groupe d'Etude et de Traitement du Carcinome Hepatocellulaire. *N Engl J Med* 1995;332:1256–1261.
2. Adachi E, Matsumata T, Nishizaki T, et al. Effects of preoperative transcatheter hepatic arterial chemoembolization for hepatocellular carcinoma. The relationship between postoperative course and tumor necrosis. *Cancer* 1993;72:3593–5598.
3. Ahrendt SA, Rashid A, Chow JT, et al. p53 overexpression and K-ras gene mutations in primary sclerosing cholangitis-associated biliary tract cancer. *J Hepatobiliary Pancreat Surg* 2000;7:426–431.
4. Alberts SR, Al-Khatib H, Mahoney MR, et al. Gemcitabine, 5-fluorouracil, and leucovorin in advanced biliary tract and gallbladder carcinoma: a North Central Cancer Treatment Group phase II trial. *Cancer* 2005;103:111–118.
5. Alden ME, Mohiuddin M: The impact of radiation dose in combined external beam and intraluminal Ir-192 brachytherapy for bile duct cancer. *Int J Radiat Oncol Biol Phys* 1994;28:945–951.
6. Alden ME, Waterman FM, Topham AK, et al. Cholangiocarcinoma: clinical significance of tumor location along the extrahepatic bile duct. *Radiology* 1995;197:511–516.
7. Aretz S, Koch A, Uhlhaas S, et al. Should children at risk for familial adenomatous polyposis be screened for hepatoblastoma and children with apparently sporadic hepatoblastoma be screened for APC germline mutations? *Pediatr Blood Cancer* 2006;47:811–818.
8. Arguedas MR, Chen VK, Eloubeidi MA, et al. Screening for hepatocellular carcinoma in patients with hepatitis C cirrhosis: a cost-utility analysis. *Am J Gastroenterol* 2003;98:679–690.
9. Aruga T, Itami J, Aruga M, et al. Target volume definition for upper abdominal irradiation using CT scans obtained during inhale and exhale phases. *Int J Radiat Oncol Biol Phys* 2000;48:465–469.

10. Baillie J: Tumors of the gallbladder and bile ducts. *J Clin Gastroenterol* 1999;29:14–21.
11. Balter JM, Lam KL, McGinn CJ, et al. Improvement of CT-based treatment-planning models of abdominal targets using static exhale imaging. *Int J Radiat Oncol Biol Phys* 1998;41:939–943.
12. Beasley RP, Hwang LY, Lin CC, et al. Hepatocellular carcinoma and hepatitis B virus. A prospective study of 22 707 men in Taiwan. *Lancet* 1981;2:1129–1133.
13. Benvegnu L, Alberti A: Risk factors and prevention of hepatocellular carcinoma in HCV infection. *Dig Dis Sci* 1996;41:49S–55S.
14. Bialecki ES, Ezenekwe AM, Brunt EM, et al. Comparison of liver biopsy and noninvasive methods for diagnosis of hepatocellular carcinoma. *Clin Gastroenterol Hepatol* 2006;4:361–368.
15. Bismuth H, Chiche L, Adam R, et al. Liver resection versus transplantation for hepatocellular carcinoma in cirrhotic patients. *Ann Surg* 1993;218:145–151.
16. Bismuth H, Nakache R, Diamond T: Management strategies in resection for hilar cholangiocarcinoma. *Ann Surg* 1992;215:31–38.
17. Bjornsson E, Kilander A, Olsson R: CA 19-9 and CEA are unreliable markers for cholangiocarcinoma in patients with primary sclerosing cholangitis. *Liver* 1999;19:501–508.
18. Bortolasi L, Burgart LJ, Tsiotos GG, et al. Adenocarcinoma of the distal bile duct. A clinicopathologic outcome analysis after curative resection. *Dig Surg* 2000;17:36–41.
19. Bruix J, Castells A, Bosch J, et al. Surgical resection of hepatocellular carcinoma in cirrhotic patients: prognostic value of preoperative portal pressure. *Gastroenterology* 1996;111:1018–1022.
20. Bruix J, Sherman M: Management of hepatocellular carcinoma. *Hepatology* 2005;42:1208–1236.
21. Buti M, Sanchez F, Cotrina M, et al. Quantitative hepatitis B virus DNA testing for the early prediction of the maintenance of response during lamivudine therapy in patients with chronic hepatitis B. *J Infect Dis* 2001;183:1277–1280.
22. Camma C, Giunta M, Andreone P, et al. Interferon and prevention of hepatocellular carcinoma in viral cirrhosis: an evidence-based approach. *J Hepatol* 2001;34:593–602.
23. Cance WG, Stewart AK, Menck HR: The National Cancer Data Base Report on treatment patterns for hepatocellular carcinomas: improved survival of surgically resected patients, 1985–1996. *Cancer* 2000;88:912–920.
24. Carceller A, Blanchard H, Champagne J, et al. Surgical resection and chemotherapy improve survival rate for patients with hepatoblastoma. *J Pediatr Surg* 2001;36:755–759.
25. Carriaga MT, Henson DE: Liver, gallbladder, extrahepatic bile ducts, and pancreas. *Cancer* 1995;75:171–190.
26. Chang MH, Chen CJ, Lai MS, et al. Universal hepatitis B vaccination in Taiwan and the incidence of hepatocellular carcinoma in children. Taiwan Childhood Hepatoma Study Group. *N Engl J Med* 1997;336:1855–1859.
27. Chao TC, Greager JA: Primary carcinoma of the gallbladder. *J Surg Oncol* 1991;46:215–221.
28. Chapman RW: Risk factors for biliary tract carcinogenesis. *Ann Oncol* 1999;10[Suppl 4]:308–311.
29. Chen CJ, Yu MW, Liaw YF: Epidemiological characteristics and risk factors of hepatocellular carcinoma. *J Gastroenterol Hepatol* 1997;12:S294–S308.
30. Chen MF, Jan YY, Jeng LB, et al. Intrahepatic cholangiocarcinoma in Taiwan. *J Hepatobiliary Pancreat Surg* 1999;6:136–141.
31. Cheng JC, Chuang VP, Cheng SH, et al. Local radiotherapy with or without transcatheter arterial chemoembolization for patients with unresectable hepatocellular carcinoma. *Int J Radiat Oncol Biol Phys* 2000;47:435–442.
32. Cheng JC, Wu JK, Huang CM, et al. Radiation-induced liver disease after three-dimensional conformal radiotherapy for patients with hepatocellular carcinoma: dosimetric analysis and implication. *Int J Radiat Oncol Biol Phys* 2002;54:156–162.
33. Cheng SH, Lin YM, Chuang VP, et al. A pilot study of three-dimensional conformal radiotherapy in unresectable hepatocellular carcinoma. *J Gastroenterol Hepatol* 1999;14:1025–1033.
34. Chijiiwa K, Ichimiya H, Kuroki S, et al. Late development of cholangiocarcinoma after the treatment of hepatolithiasis. *Surg Gynecol Obstet* 1993;177:279–282.
35. Chijiiwa K, Nakano K, Ueda J, et al. Surgical treatment of patients with T2 gallbladder carcinoma invading the subserosal layer. *J Am Coll Surg* 2001;192:600–607.
36. Cho JS, Kwag JG, Oh YR, et al. Detection and characterization of hepatocellular carcinoma: value of dynamic CT during the arterial dominant phase with uniphasic contrast medium injection. *J Comput Assist Tomogr* 1996;20:128–134.
37. Chu KM, Fan ST: Intrahepatic cholangiocarcinoma in Hong Kong. *J Hepatobiliary Pancreat Surg* 1999;6:149–153.
38. Chuang VP, Wallace S: Chemoembolization: transcatheter management of neoplasms. *Jama* 1981;245:1151–1152.
39. Chung C, Bautista N, O'Connell TX: Prognosis and treatment of bile duct carcinoma. *Am Surg* 1998;64:921–925.
40. Cioffi U, Quattrone P, De Simone M, et al. Primary multiple epithelioid leiomyosarcoma of the liver. *Hepatogastroenterology* 1996;43:1603–1605.
41. Cubertafond P, Mathonnet M, Gainant A, et al. Radical surgery for gallbladder cancer. Results of the French Surgical Association survey. *Hepatogastroenterology* 1999;46:1567–1571.
42. Czito BG, Hurwitz HI, Clough RW, et al. Adjuvant external-beam radiotherapy with concurrent chemotherapy after resection of primary gallbladder carcinoma: a 23-year experience. *Int J Radiat Oncol Biol Phys* 2005;62:1030–1034.
43. Dalton-Clarke HJ, Pearse E, Krause T, et al. Fine needle aspiration cytology and exfoliative biliary cytology in the diagnosis of hilar cholangiocarcinoma. *Eur J Surg Oncol* 1986;12:143–145.
44. Davila JA, Morgan RO, Shaib Y, et al. Hepatitis C infection and the increasing incidence of hepatocellular carcinoma: a population-based study. *Gastroenterology* 2004;127:1372–1380.
45. Dawson LA, McGinn CJ, Normolle D, et al. Escalated focal liver radiation and concurrent hepatic artery fluorodeoxyuridine for unresectable intrahepatic malignancies. *J Clin Oncol* 2000;18:2210–2218.
46. de Aretxabala X, Roa I, Burgos L, et al. Preoperative chemoradiotherapy in the treatment of gallbladder cancer. *Am Surg* 1999;65:241–246.
47. De Vreede I, Steers JL, Burch PA, et al. Prolonged disease-free survival after orthotopic liver transplantation plus adjuvant chemoirradiation for cholangiocarcinoma. *Liver Transpl* 2000;6:309–316.
48. Deuffic S, Poynard T, Buffat L, et al. Trends in primary liver cancer. *Lancet* 1998;351:214–215.
49. Dhir V, Swaroop VS, Mohandas KM, et al. Combination chemotherapy and radiation for palliation of hepatocellular carcinoma. *Am J Clin Oncol* 1992;15:304–307.
50. Dohmen K, Shirahama M, Onohara S, et al. Differences in survival based on the type of follow-up for the detection of hepatocellular carcinoma: an analysis of 547 patients. *Hepatol Res* 2000;18:110–121.
51. Donohue JH, Stewart AK, Menck HR: The National Cancer Data Base report on carcinoma of the gallbladder, 1989–1995. *Cancer* 1998;83:2618–2628.
52. Douglass EC: Hepatic malignancies in childhood and adolescence (hepatoblastoma, hepatocellular carcinoma, and embryonal sarcoma). *Cancer Treat Res* 1997;92:201–212.
53. Duda SH, Huppert PE, Schott U, et al. Percutaneous transhepatic intraductal biliary sonography for lymph node staging at 12.5 MHz in malignant bile duct obstruction: work in progress. *Cardiovasc Intervent Radiol* 1997;20:133–138.
54. Durand F, Regimbeau JM, Belghiti J, et al. Assessment of the benefits and risks of percutaneous biopsy before surgical resection of hepatocellular carcinoma. *J Hepatol* 2001;35:254–258.
55. Dusenbery D, Ferris JV, Thaete FL, et al. Percutaneous ultrasound-guided needle biopsy of hepatic mass lesions using a cytohistologic approach. Comparison of two needle types. *Am J Clin Pathol* 1995;104:583–587.
56. Dutta U, Garg PK, Kumar R, et al. Typhoid carriers among patients with gallstones are at increased risk for carcinoma of the gallbladder. *Am J Gastroenterol* 2000;95:784–787.
57. El Rassi ZE, Partensky C, Scoazec JY, et al. Peripheral cholangiocarcinoma: presentation, diagnosis, pathology and management. *Eur J Surg Oncol* 1999;25:375–380.
58. El Serag HB, Mason AC: Rising incidence of hepatocellular carcinoma in the United States. *N Engl J Med* 1999;340:745–750.
59. Ferrari FS, Stella A, Gambacorta D, et al. Treatment of large hepatocellular carcinoma: comparison between techniques and long term results. *Radiol Med (Torino)* 2004;108:356–371.
60. Fracanzani AL, Conte D, Fraquelli M, et al. Increased cancer risk in a cohort of 230 patients with hereditary hemochromatosis in comparison to matched control patients with non iron related chronic liver disease. *Hepatology* 2001;33:647–651.
61. Frezza EE, Mezghebe H: Gallbladder carcinoma: a 28 year experience. *Int Surg* 1997;82:295–300.
62. Friedman MA, Volberding PA, Cassidy MJ, et al. Therapy for hepatocellular cancer with intrahepatic arterial Adriamycin and 5-fluorouracil combined with whole-liver irradiation: a Northern California Oncology Group Study. *Cancer Treat Rep* 1979;63:1885–1888.
63. Fuss M, Salter BJ, Herman TS, et al. : External beam radiation therapy for hepatocellular carcinoma: potential of intensity-modulated and image-guided radiation therapy. *Gastroenterology* 2004;127:S206–S217.
64. Garner PD, Hall LD, Johnstone PA: Palliation of unresectable hilar cholangiocarcinoma. *J Surg Oncol* 2000;75:95–97.
65. Gebbia V, Majello E, Testa A, et al. Treatment of advanced adenocarcinomas of the exocrine pancreas and the gallbladder with 5-fluorouracil, high dose levofolinic acid and oral hydroxyurea on a weekly schedule. Results of a multicenter study of the Southern Italy Oncology Group (G.O.I.M.). *Cancer* 1996;78:1300–1307.
66. Gerhards MF, van Gulik TM, Gonzalez Gonzalez D, et al. Results of postoperative radiotherapy for resectable hilar cholangiocarcinoma. *World J Surg* 2003;27:173–179.
67. Giardiello FM, Offerhaus GJ, Krush AJ, et al. Risk of hepatoblastoma in familial adenomatous polyposis. *J Pediatr* 1991;119:766–768.
68. Gogel BM, Goldstein RM, Kuhn JA, et al. Diagnostic evaluation of hepatocellular carcinoma in a cirrhotic liver. *Oncology (Williston Park)* 2000;14:15–20.
69. Goldstein RM, Stone M, Tillery GW, et al. Is liver transplantation indicated for cholangiocarcinoma? *Am J Surg* 1993;166:768–772.
70. Gonzalez Gonzalez D, Gouma DJ, Rauws EA, et al. Role of radiotherapy, in particular intraluminal brachytherapy, in the treatment of proximal bile duct carcinoma. *Ann Oncol* 1999;10[Suppl 4]:215–220.
71. Gores GJ: Early detection and treatment of cholangiocarcinoma. *Liver Transpl* 2000;6:S30–S34.
72. Greene F, Page D, Fleming I: *American Joint Committee on Cancer: Cancer staging manual.* New York: Springer-Verlag; 2002:131.
73. Gunderson LL, Haddock MG, Foo ML, et al. Conformal irradiation for hepatobiliary malignancies. *Ann Oncol* 10[Suppl 4]:221–225.
74. Guo WJ, Yu EX: Evaluation of combined therapy with chemoembolization and irradiation for large hepatocellular carcinoma. *Br J Radiol* 2000;73:1091–1097.
75. Hanazaki K, Wakabayashi M, Sodeyama H, et al. Surgical outcome in cirrhotic patients with hepatitis C-related hepatocellular carcinoma. *Hepatogastroenterology* 2000;47:204–210.
76. Hashimoto M, Watanabe G: Hepatic parenchymal cell volume and the indocyanine green tolerance test. *J Surg Res* 2000;92:222–227.
77. Haverkos HW: Viruses, chemicals and co-carcinogenesis. *Oncogene* 2004;23:6492–6499.
78. Hawkins MA, Dawson LA: Radiation therapy for hepatocellular carcinoma: from palliation to cure. *Cancer* 2006;106:1653–1663.
79. Heimbach JK, Gores GJ, Haddock MG, et al. Liver transplantation for unresectable perihilar cholangiocarcinoma. *Semin Liver Dis* 2004;24:201–207.
80. Heintges T, Wands JR: Hepatitis C virus: epidemiology and transmission. *Hepatology* 1997;26:521–526.
81. Hejna M, Zielinski CC: Nonsurgical management of gallbladder cancer: cytotoxic treatment and radiotherapy. *Expert Rev Anticancer Ther* 2001;1:291–300.
82. Higuchi T, Kikuchi M, Okazaki M: Hepatocellular carcinoma after transcatheter hepatic arterial embolization. A histopathologic study of 84 resected cases. *Cancer* 1994;73:2259–2267.
83. Hopfner M, Sutter AP, Huether A, et al. Targeting the epidermal growth factor receptor by gefitinib for treatment of hepatocellular carcinoma. *J Hepatol* 2004;41:1008–1016.

84. Hori M, Murakami T, Kim T, et al. Sensitivity of double-phase helical CT during arterial portography for detection of hypervascular hepatocellular carcinoma. *J Comput Assist Tomogr* 1998;22:861–867.
85. Houry S, Haccart V, Huguier M, et al. Gallbladder cancer: role of radiation therapy. *Hepatogastroenterology* 1999;46:1578–1584.
86. Hozo I, Miric D, Bojic L, et al. Liver angiosarcoma and hemangiopericytoma after occupational exposure to vinyl chloride monomer. *Environ Health Perspect* 2000;108:793–795.
87. Huang GT, Sheu JC, Yang PM, et al. Ultrasound-guided cutting biopsy for the diagnosis of hepatocellular carcinoma—a study based on 420 patients. *J Hepatol* 1996;25:334–338.
88. Hultcrantz R, Olsson R, Danielsson A, et al. A 3-year prospective study on serum tumor markers used for detecting cholangiocarcinoma in patients with primary sclerosing cholangitis. *J Hepatol* 1999;30:669–673.
89. Ishiguchi T, Shimamoto K, Fukatsu H, et al. Radiologic diagnosis of hepatocellular carcinoma. *Semin Surg Oncol* 1996;12:164–169.
90. Iyer CP, Stanley P, Mahour GH: Hepatic hemangiomas in infants and children: a review of 30 cases. *Am Surg* 1996;62:356–360.
91. Jackson PE, Groopman JD: Aflatoxin and liver cancer. *Baillieres Best Pract Res Clin Gastroenterol* 1999;13:545–555.
92. Jung SE, Kim KH, Kim MY, et al. Clinical characteristics and prognosis of patients with hepatoblastoma. *World J Surg* 2001;25:126–130.
93. Kanematsu M, Hoshi H, Yamada T, et al. Small hepatic nodules in cirrhosis: ultrasonographic, CT, and MR imaging findings. *Abdom Imaging* 1999;24:47–55.
94. Katyal S, Oliver JH 3rd, Peterson MS, et al. Extrahepatic metastases of hepatocellular carcinoma. *Radiology* 2000;216:698–703.
95. Kawasaki S, Makuuchi M, Miyagawa S, et al. Results of hepatic resection for hepatocellular carcinoma. *World J Surg* 1995;19:31–34.
96. Khan KN, Yatsuhashi H: Effect of alcohol consumption on the progression of hepatitis C virus infection and risk of hepatocellular carcinoma in Japanese patients. *Alcohol Alcohol* 2000;35:286–295.
97. Kim SH, Lim HK, Lee WJ, et al. Needle-tract implantation in hepatocellular carcinoma: frequency and CT findings after biopsy with a 19.5-gauge automated biopsy gun. *Abdom Imaging* 2000;25:246–250.
98. Kim T, Murakami T, Takahashi S, et al. Optimal phases of dynamic CT for detecting hepatocellular carcinoma: evaluation of unenhanced and triple-phase images. *Abdom Imaging* 1999;24:473–480.
99. Kitagawa Y, Nagino M, Kamiya J, et al. Lymph node metastasis from hilar cholangiocarcinoma: audit of 110 patients who underwent regional and paraaortic node dissection. *Ann Surg* 2001;233:385–392.
100. Klatskin G: Adenocarcinoma of the hepatic duct at its bifurcation within the porta hepatis. An unusual tumor with distinctive clinical and pathological features. *Am J Med* 1965;38:241–256.
101. Klempnauer J, Ridder GJ, von Wasielewski R, et al. Resectional surgery of hilar cholangiocarcinoma: a multivariate analysis of prognostic factors. *J Clin Oncol* 1997;15:947–954.
102. Kobayashi M, Ikeda K, Saitoh S, et al. Incidence of primary cholangiocellular carcinoma of the liver in japanese patients with hepatitis C virus-related cirrhosis. *Cancer* 2000;88:2471–2477.
103. Kondo S, Nimura Y, Kamiya J, et al. Factors influencing postoperative hospital mortality and long-term survival after radical resection for stage IV gallbladder carcinoma. *World J Surg* 2003;27:272–277.
104. Kresl JJ, Schild SE, Henning GT, et al. Adjuvant external beam radiation therapy with concurrent chemotherapy in the management of gallbladder carcinoma. *Int J Radiat Oncol Biol Phys* 2002;52:167–175.
105. Kubo S, Hirohashi K, Tanaka H, et al. Virologic and biochemical changes and prognosis after liver resection for hepatitis B virus-related hepatocellular carcinoma. *Dig Surg* 2001;18:26–33.
106. Kubo S, Kinoshita H, Hirohashi K, et al. Hepatolithiasis associated with cholangiocarcinoma. *World J Surg* 1995;19:637–641.
107. Kubo S, Nishiguchi S, Hirohashi K, et al. Clinicopathological criteria for multicentricity of hepatocellular carcinoma and risk factors for such carcinogenesis. *Jpn J Cancer Res* 1998;89:419–426.
108. Landis SH, Murray T, Bolden S, et al. Cancer statistics, 1998. *CA Cancer J Clin* 1998;48:6–29.
109. Lawrence TS, Ten Haken RK, Kessler ML, et al. The use of 3-D dose volume analysis to predict radiation hepatitis. *Int J Radiat Oncol Biol Phys* 1992;23:781–788.
110. Lee CS, Sung JL, Hwang LY, et al. Surgical treatment of 109 patients with symptomatic and asymptomatic hepatocellular carcinoma. *Surgery* 1986;99:481–490.
111. Lencioni RA, Allgaier HP, Cioni D, et al. Small hepatocellular carcinoma in cirrhosis: randomized comparison of radio-frequency thermal ablation versus percutaneous ethanol injection. *Radiology* 2003;228:235–240.
112. Leung TW, Patt YZ, Lau WY, et al. Complete pathological remission is possible with systemic combination chemotherapy for inoperable hepatocellular carcinoma. *Clin Cancer Res* 1999;5:1676–1681.
113. Levin B: Gallbladder carcinoma. *Ann Oncol* 1999;10[Suppl 4]:129–130.
114. Liang SX, Zhu XD, Xu ZY, et al. Radiation-induced liver disease in three-dimensional conformal radiation therapy for primary liver carcinoma: the risk factors and hepatic radiation tolerance. *Int J Radiat Oncol Biol Phys* 2006;65:426–434.
115. Lin CS, Jen YM, Chiu SY, et al. Treatment of portal vein tumor thrombosis of hepatoma patients with either stereotactic radiotherapy or three-dimensional conformal radiotherapy. *Jpn J Clin Oncol* 2006;36:212–217.
116. Lin OS, Keeffe EB, Sanders GD, et al. Cost-effectiveness of screening for hepatocellular carcinoma in patients with cirrhosis due to chronic hepatitis C. *Aliment Pharmacol Ther* 2004;19:1159–1172.
117. Lin SM, Lin CJ, Lin CC, et al. Radiofrequency ablation improves prognosis compared with ethanol injection for hepatocellular carcinoma < or = 4 cm. *Gastroenterology* 2004;127:1714–1723.
118. Lin SM, Lin CJ, Lin CC, et al. Randomised controlled trial comparing percutaneous radiofrequency thermal ablation, percutaneous ethanol injection, and percutaneous acetic acid injection to treat hepatocellular carcinoma of 3 cm or less. *Gut* 2005;54:1151–1156.
119. Lin TY, Lee CS, Chen KM, et al. Role of surgery in the treatment of primary carcinoma of the liver: a 31-year experience. *Br J Surg* 1987;74:839–842.
120. Livraghi T, Lazzaroni S, Meloni F: Radiofrequency thermal ablation of hepatocellular carcinoma. *Eur J Ultrasound* 2001;13:159–166.
121. Llovet JM, Bruix J: Systematic review of randomized trials for unresectable hepatocellular carcinoma: chemoembolization improves survival. *Hepatology* 2003;37:429–442.
122. Loyer EM, Chin H, DuBrow RA, et al. Hepatocellular carcinoma and intrahepatic peripheral cholangiocarcinoma: enhancement patterns with quadruple phase helical CT—a comparative study. *Radiology* 1999;212:866–875.
123. Matsukura N, Yokomuro S, Yamada S, et al. Association between *Helicobacter bilis* in bile and biliary tract malignancies: *H. bilis* in bile from Japanese and Thai patients with benign and malignant diseases in the biliary tract. *Jpn J Cancer Res* 2002;93:842–847.
124. Maturen KE, Nghiem HV, Marrero JA, et al. Lack of tumor seeding of hepatocellular carcinoma after percutaneous needle biopsy using coaxial cutting needle technique. *AJR Am J Roentgenol* 2006;187:1184–1187.
125. Mazzaferro V, Regalia E, Doci R, et al. Liver transplantation for the treatment of small hepatocellular carcinomas in patients with cirrhosis. *N Engl J Med* 1996;334:693–699.
126. McGinn CJ, Ten Haken RK, Ensminger WD, et al. Treatment of intrahepatic cancers with radiation doses based on a normal tissue complication probability model. *J Clin Oncol* 1998;16:2246–2252.
127. McGlynn KA, Tarone RE, El-Serag HB: A comparison of trends in the incidence of hepatocellular carcinoma and intrahepatic cholangiocarcinoma in the United States. *Cancer Epidemiol Biomarkers Prev* 2006;15:1198–1203.
128. Mehta VK, Fisher GA, Ford JM, et al. Adjuvant chemoradiotherapy for "unfavorable" carcinoma of the ampulla of Vater: preliminary report. *Arch Surg* 2001;136:65–69.
129. Meloni F, Lazzaroni S, Livraghi T: Percutaneous ethanol injection: single session treatment. *Eur J Ultrasound* 2001;13:107–115.
130. Michel J, Suc B, Montpeyroux F, et al. Liver resection or transplantation for hepatocellular carcinoma? Retrospective analysis of 215 patients with cirrhosis. *J Hepatol* 1997;26:1274–1280.
131. Minsky BD, Kemeny N, Armstrong JG, et al. Extrahepatic biliary system cancer: an update of a combined modality approach. *Am J Clin Oncol* 1991;14:433–437.
132. Moerman CJ, Bueno-de-Mesquita HB: The epidemiology of gallbladder cancer: lifestyle related risk factors and limited surgical possibilities for prevention. *Hepatogastroenterology* 1999;46:1533–1539.
133. Morganti AG, Trodella L, Valentini V, et al. Combined modality treatment in unresectable extrahepatic biliary carcinoma. *Int J Radiat Oncol Biol Phys* 2000;46:913–919.
134. Motohara T, Semelka RC, Bader TR: MR cholangiopancreatography. *Radiol Clin North Am* 2003;41:89–96.
135. Nadler LH, McSherry CK: Carcinoma of the gallbladder: review of the literature and report on 56 cases at the Beth Israel Medical Center. *Mt Sinai J Med* 1992;59:47–52.
136. Nagahama H, Okada S, Okusaka T, et al. Predictive factors for tumor response to systemic chemotherapy in patients with hepatocellular carcinoma. *Jpn J Clin Oncol* 1997;27:321–324.
137. Nagorney DM, Donohue JH, Farnell MB, et al. Outcomes after curative resections of cholangiocarcinoma. *Arch Surg* 1993;128:871–879.
138. Nakamura H, Mitani T, Murakami T, et al. Five-year survival after transcatheter chemoembolization for hepatocellular carcinoma. *Cancer Chemother Pharmacol* 1994;33[Suppl]:S89–S92.
139. Nakamura S, Suzuki S, Sakaguchi T, et al. Surgical treatment of patients with mixed hepatocellular carcinoma and cholangiocarcinoma. *Cancer* 1996;78:1671–1676.
140. Nakao N, Kamino K, Miura K, et al. Transcatheter arterial embolization in hepatocellular carcinoma: a long-term follow-up. *Radiat Med* 1992;10:13–18.
141. Nakeeb A, Lipsett PA, Lillemoe KD, et al. Biliary carcinoembryonic antigen levels are a marker for cholangiocarcinoma. *Am J Surg* 1996;171:147–153.
142. Nakeeb A, Pitt HA, Sohn TA, et al. Cholangiocarcinoma. A spectrum of intrahepatic, perihilar, and distal tumors. *Ann Surg* 1996;224:463–475.
143. Nakeeb A, Tran KQ, Black MJ, et al. Improved survival in resected biliary malignancies. *Surgery* 2002;132:555–564.
144. Ohara K, Okumura T, Akisada M, et al. Irradiation synchronized with respiration gate. *Int J Radiat Oncol Biol Phys* 1989;17:853–857.
145. Ohashi K, Nakajima Y, Kanehiro H, et al. Ki-ras mutations and p53 protein expressions in intrahepatic cholangiocarcinomas: relation to gross tumor morphology. *Gastroenterology* 1995;109:1612–1617.
146. Okamoto M, Okamoto H, Kitahara F, et al. Ultrasonographic evidence of association of polyps and stones with gallbladder cancer. *Am J Gastroenterol* 1999;94:446–450.
147. Okuda K, Ohtsuki T, Obata H, et al. Natural history of hepatocellular carcinoma and prognosis in relation to treatment. Study of 850 patients. *Cancer* 1985;56:918–928.
148. Order SE, Stillwagon GB, Klein JL, et al. Iodine 131 antiferritin, a new treatment modality in hepatoma: a Radiation Therapy Oncology Group study. *J Clin Oncol* 1985;3:1573–1582.
149. Papakostas P, Kouroussis C, Androulakis N, et al. First-line chemotherapy with docetaxel for unresectable or metastatic carcinoma of the biliary tract. A multicentre phase II study. *Eur J Cancer* 2001;37:1833–1838.
150. Park WC, Rhillips R: The role of radiation therapy in the management of hemangiomas of the liver. *JAMA* 1970;212:1496–1498.
151. Parkin DM, Pisani P, Ferlay J: Estimates of the worldwide incidence of 25 major cancers in 1990. *Int J Cancer* 1999;80:827–841.
152. Parkin DM, Srivatanakul P, Khlat M, et al. Liver cancer in Thailand. I. A case-control study of cholangiocarcinoma. *Int J Cancer* 1991;48:323–328.
153. Patel T: Increasing incidence and mortality of primary intrahepatic cholangiocarcinoma in the United States. *Hepatology* 2001;33:1353–1357.
154. Patt YZ, Hassan MM, Aguayo A, et al. Oral capecitabine for the treatment of hepatocellular carcinoma, cholangiocarcinoma, and gallbladder carcinoma. *Cancer* 2004;101:578–586.
155. Patt YZ, Hassan MM, Lozano RD, et al. Durable clinical response of refractory hepatocellular carcinoma to orally administered thalidomide. *Am J Clin Oncol* 2000;23:319–321.
156. Patt YZ, Hassan MM, Lozano RD, et al. Thalidomide in the treatment of patients with hepatocellular carcinoma: a phase II trial. *Cancer* 2005;103:749–755.

157. Patt YZ, Jones DV Jr, Hoque A, et al. Phase II trial of intravenous flourouracil and subcutaneous interferon alfa-2b for biliary tract cancer. *J Clin Oncol* 1996;14:2311–2315.

158. Pavone P, Laghi A, Passariello R: MR cholangiopancreatography in malignant biliary obstruction. *Semin Ultrasound CT MR* 1999;20:317–323.

159. Pelletier G, Roche A, Ink O, et al. A randomized trial of hepatic arterial chemoembolization in patients with unresectable hepatocellular carcinoma. *J Hepatol* 1990;11:181–184.

160. Penz M, Kornek GV, Raderer M, et al. Phase II trial of two-weekly gemcitabine in patients with advanced biliary tract cancer. *Ann Oncol* 2001;12:183–186.

161. Philip PA, Mahoney MR, Allmer C, et al. Phase II study of Erlotinib (OSI-774) in patients with advanced hepatocellular cancer. *J Clin Oncol* 2005;23:6657–6663.

162. Philosophe B, Greig PD, Hemming AW, et al. Surgical management of hepatocellular carcinoma: resection or transplantation? *J Gastrointest Surg* 1998;2:21–27.

163. Pinna AD, Iwatsuki S, Lee RG, et al. Treatment of fibrolamellar hepatoma with subtotal hepatectomy or transplantation. *Hepatology* 1997;26:877–883.

164. Pisani P, Parkin DM, Bray F, et al. Estimates of the worldwide mortality from 25 cancers in 1990. *Int J Cancer* 1999;83:18–29.

165. Pitt HA, Nakeeb A, Abrams RA, et al. Perihilar cholangiocarcinoma. Postoperative radiotherapy does not improve survival. *Ann Surg* 1995;221:788–798.

166. Poggio JL, Nagorney DM, Nascimento AG, et al. Surgical treatment of adult primary hepatic sarcoma. *Br J Surg* 2000;87:1500–1505.

167. Poon RT, Fan ST, Ng IO, et al. Different risk factors and prognosis for early and late intrahepatic recurrence after resection of hepatocellular carcinoma. *Cancer* 2000;89:500–507.

168. Poon RT, Ng IO, Fan ST, et al. Clinicopathologic features of long-term survivors and disease-free survivors after resection of hepatocellular carcinoma: a study of a prospective cohort. *J Clin Oncol* 2001;19:3037–3044.

169. Rea DJ, Heimbach JK, Rosen CB, et al. Liver transplantation with neoadjuvant chemoradiation is more effective than resection for hilar cholangiocarcinoma. *Ann Surg* 2005;242:451–461.

170. Regev A, Jeffers LJ: Hepatitis C and alcohol. *Alcohol Clin Exp Res* 1999;23:1543–1551.

171. Roayaie S, Guarrera JV, Ye MQ, et al. Aggressive surgical treatment of intrahepatic cholangiocarcinoma: predictors of outcomes. *J Am Coll Surg* 1998;187:365–372.

172. Robertson JM, Lawrence TS, Andrews JC, et al. Long-term results of hepatic artery fluorodeoxyuridine and conformal radiation therapy for primary hepatobiliary cancers. *Int J Radiat Oncol Biol Phys* 1997;37:325–330.

173. Ruckert JC, Ruckert RI, Gellert K, et al. Surgery for carcinoma of the gallbladder. *Hepatogastroenterology* 1996;43:527–533.

174. Sasaki Y, Imaoka S, Nakano H, et al. Indications for hepatectomy for hepatocellular carcinoma: what stage of the disease is the best indication for surgery? *J Hepatobiliary Pancreat Surg* 1998;5:14–17.

175. Sato S, Shiratori Y, Imamura M, et al. Power Doppler signals after percutaneous ethanol injection therapy for hepatocellular carcinoma predict local recurrence of tumors: a prospective study using 199 consecutive patients. *J Hepatol* 2001;35:225–234.

176. Seo T, Ando H, Watanabe Y, et al. Treatment of hepatoblastoma: less extensive hepatectomy after effective preoperative chemotherapy with cisplatin and Adriamycin. *Surgery* 1998;123:407–414.

177. Seong J, Keum KC, Han KH, et al. Combined transcatheter arterial chemoembolization and local radiotherapy of unresectable hepatocellular carcinoma. *Int J Radiat Oncol Biol Phys* 1999;43:393–397.

178. Seong J, Park HC, Han KH, et al. Clinical results of 3-dimensional conformal radiotherapy combined with transarterial chemoembolization for hepatocellular carcinoma in the cirrhotic patients. *Hepatol Res* 2003;27:30–35.

179. Seong J, Park HC, Han KH, et al. Local radiotherapy for unresectable hepatocellular carcinoma patients who failed with transcatheter arterial chemoembolization. *Int J Radiat Oncol Biol Phys* 2000;47:1331–1335.

180. Sheth S, Bedford A, Chopra S: Primary gallbladder cancer: recognition of risk factors and the role of prophylactic cholecystectomy. *Am J Gastroenterol* 2000;95:1402–1410.

181. Shiina S, Teratani T, Obi S, et al. A randomized controlled trial of radiofrequency ablation with ethanol injection for small hepatocellular carcinoma. *Gastroenterology* 2005;129:122–130.

182. Shimada H, Endo I, Togo S, et al. The role of lymph node dissection in the treatment of gallbladder carcinoma. *Cancer* 1997;79:892–899.

183. Shimizu S, Shirato H, Xo B, et al. Three-dimensional movement of a liver tumor detected by high-speed magnetic resonance imaging. *Radiother Oncol* 1999;50:367–370.

184. Shin HR, Lee CU, Park HJ, et al. Hepatitis B and C virus, Clonorchis sinensis for the risk of liver cancer: a case-control study in Pusan, Korea. *Int J Epidemiol* 1996;25:933–940.

185. Shirabe K, Shimada M, Harimoto N, et al. Intrahepatic cholangiocarcinoma: its mode of spreading and therapeutic modalities. *Surgery* 2002;131:S159–S164.

186. Shirai Y, Ohtani T, Tsukada K, et al. Lymph node recurrence of gallbladder carcinoma successfully managed by systemic chemotherapy with 5-fluorouracil and mitomycin C: report of a 5-year survivor. *Eur J Surg Oncol* 1997;23:457–458.

187. Shirai Y, Yoshida K, Tsukada K, et al. Inapparent carcinoma of the gallbladder. An appraisal of a radical second operation after simple cholecystectomy. *Ann Surg* 1992;215:326–331.

188. Shirato H, Seppenwoolde Y, Kitamura K, et al. Intrafractional tumor motion: lung and liver. *Semin Radiat Oncol* 2004;14:10–18.

189. Silva MA, Tekin K, Aytekin F, et al. Surgery for hilar cholangiocarcinoma; a 10 year experience of a tertiary referral centre in the UK. *Eur J Surg Oncol* 2005;31:533–539.

190. Song TJ, Ip EW, Fong Y: Hepatocellular carcinoma: current surgical management. *Gastroenterology* 2004;127:S248–S260.

191. Sotiropoulos GC, Lang H, Frilling A, et al. Resectability of hepatocellular carcinoma: evaluation of 333 consecutive cases at a single hepatobiliary specialty center and systematic review of the literature. *Hepatogastroenterology* 2006;53:322–329.

192. Stillwagon GB, Order SE, Guse C, et al. 194 hepatocellular cancers treated by radiation and chemotherapy combinations: toxicity and response: a Radiation Therapy Oncology Group Study. *Int J Radiat Oncol Biol Phys* 1989;17:1223–1229.

193. Sturm PD, Baas IO, Clement MJ, et al. Alterations of the p53 tumor-suppressor gene and K-ras oncogene in perihilar cholangiocarcinomas from a high-incidence area. *Int J Cancer* 1998;78:695–698.

194. Sudan D, DeRoover A, Chinnakotla S, et al. Radiochemotherapy and transplantation allow long-term survival for nonresectable hilar cholangiocarcinoma. *Am J Transplant* 2002;2:774–779.

195. Sung JL: Prevention of hepatitis B and C virus infection for prevention of cirrhosis and hepatocellular carcinoma. *J Gastroenterol Hepatol* 1997;12:S370–S376.

196. Takada T, Amano H, Yasuda H, et al. Is postoperative adjuvant chemotherapy useful for gallbladder carcinoma? A phase III multicenter prospective randomized controlled trial in patients with resected pancreaticobiliary carcinoma. *Cancer* 2002;95:1685–1695.

197. Takamori R, Wong LL, Dang C, et al. Needle-tract implantation from hepatocellular cancer: is needle biopsy of the liver always necessary? *Liver Transpl* 2000;6:67–72.

198. Takayasu K, Okuda K: *Imaging in liver disease,* 1st ed. New York, Oxford University Press; 1997

199. Tashiro S, Konno T, Mochinaga M, et al. Treatment of carcinoma of the gallbladder in Japan. *Jpn J Surg* 1982;12:98–104.

200. Taylor-Robinson SD, Foster GR, Arora S, et al. Increase in primary liver cancer in the UK, 1979–94. *Lancet* 1997;350:1142–1143.

201. Tillich M, Mischinger HJ, Preisegger KH, et al. Multiphasic helical CT in diagnosis and staging of hilar cholangiocarcinoma. *AJR Am J Roentgenol* 1998;171:651–658.

202. Todoroki T, Kawamoto T, Otsuka M, et al. Benefits of combining radiotherapy with aggressive resection for stage IV gallbladder cancer. *Hepatogastroenterology* 1999;46:1585–1591.

203. Todoroki T, Kawamoto T, Takahashi H, et al. Treatment of gallbladder cancer by radical resection. *Br J Surg* 1999;86:622–627

204. Todoroki T, Ohara K, Kawamoto T, et al. Benefits of adjuvant radiotherapy after radical resection of locally advanced main hepatic duct carcinoma. *Int J Radiat Oncol Biol Phys* 2000;46:581–587.

205. Tsao JI, Nimura Y, Kamiya J, et al. Management of hilar cholangiocarcinoma: comparison of an American and a Japanese experience. *Ann Surg* 2000;232:166–174.

206. Tsuji M, Kashihara T, Terada N, et al. An immunohistochemical study of hepatic atypical adenomatous hyperplasia, hepatocellular carcinoma, and cholangiocarcinoma with alpha-fetoprotein, carcinoembryonic antigen, CA19-9, epithelial membrane antigen, and cytokeratins 18 and 19. *Pathol Int* 1999;49:310–317.

207. Tsuji T, Hiraoka T, Kanemitsu K, et al. Lymphatic spreading pattern of intrahepatic cholangiocarcinoma. *Surgery* 2001;129:401–407.

208. Tsukada K, Kurosaki I, Uchida K, et al. Lymph node spread from carcinoma of the gallbladder. *Cancer* 1997;80:661–667.

209. Tsuzuki T, Sugioka A, Ueda M, et al. Hepatic resection for hepatocellular carcinoma. *Surgery* 1990;107:511–520.

210. Urego M, Flickinger JC, Carr BI: Radiotherapy and multimodality management of cholangiocarcinoma. *Int J Radiat Oncol Biol Phys* 1999;44:121–126.

211. UyBarreta V, Mikesh C, Simmons B, et al. Atypical presentation of hepatocellular carcinoma. *South Med J* 2000;93:516–519.

212. Vallis KA, Benjamin IS, Munro AJ, et al. External beam and intraluminal radiotherapy for locally advanced bile duct cancer: role and tolerability. *Radiother Oncol* 1996;11:61–66.

213. Valls C, Guma A, Puig I, et al. Intrahepatic peripheral cholangiocarcinoma. CT evaluation. *Abdom Imaging* 2000;25.490–496.

214. Valverde A, Bonhomme N, Farges O, et al. Resection of intrahepatic cholangiocarcinoma: a Western experience. *J Hepatobiliary Pancreat Surg* 1999;6:122–127.

215. Vatanasapt V, Martin N, Sriplung H, et al. Cancer incidence in Thailand, 1988-1991. *Cancer Epidemiol Biomarkers Prev* 1995;4:475–483.

216. Verbeek PC, Van Leeuwen DJ, Van Der Heyde MN, et al. Does additive radiotherapy after hilar resection improve survival of cholangiocarcinoma? An analysis in sixty-four patients. *Ann Chir* 1991;45:350–354.

217. Verderame F, Russo A, Di Leo R, et al. Gemcitabine and oxaliplatin combination chemotherapy in advanced biliary tract cancers. *Ann Oncol* 2006;17:vii68–vii72.

218. Wakai T, Shirai Y, Yokoyama N, et al. Early gallbladder carcinoma does not warrant radical resection. *Br J Surg* 2001;88:675–678.

219. Weinbren K, Mutum SS: Pathological aspects of cholangiocarcinoma. *J Pathol* 1983;139:217–238.

220. Whittington R, Neuberg D, Tester WJ, et al. Protracted intravenous fluorouracil infusion with radiation therapy in the management of localized pancreaticobiliary carcinoma: a phase I Eastern Cooperative Oncology Group Trial. *J Clin Oncol* 1995;13:227–232.

221. Wu DH, Liu L, Chen LH: Therapeutic effects and prognostic factors in three-dimensional conformal radiotherapy combined with transcatheter arterial chemoembolization for hepatocellular carcinoma. *World J Gastroenterol* 2004;10:2184–2189.

222. Yamada K, Soejima T, Sugimoto K, et al. Pilot study of local radiotherapy for portal vein tumor thrombus in patients with unresectable hepatocellular carcinoma. *Jpn J Clin Oncol* 2001;31:147–152.

223. Yamada R, Kishi K, Sato M, et al. Transcatheter arterial chemoembolization (TACE) in the treatment of unresectable liver cancer. *World J Surg* 1995;19:795–800.

224. Yamaguchi K, Chijiiwa K, Saiki S, et al. Carcinoma of the extrahepatic bile duct: mode of spread and its prognostic implications. *Hepatogastroenterology* 1997;44:1256–1261.

225. Yamamoto J, Iwatsuki S, Kosuge T, et al. Should hepatomas be treated with hepatic resection or transplantation? *Cancer* 1999;86:1151–1158.

226. Yamamoto M, Takasaki K, Otsubo T, et al. Recurrence after surgical resection of intrahepatic cholangiocarcinoma. *J Hepatobiliary Pancreat Surg* 2001;8:154–157.

227. Yamamoto M, Takasaki K, Yoshikawa T: Lymph node metastasis in intrahepatic cholangiocarcinoma. *Jpn J Clin Oncol* 1999;29:147–150.

228. Yang HI, Lu SN, Liaw YF, et al. Hepatitis B e antigen and the risk of hepatocellular carcinoma. *N Engl J Med* 2002;347:168–174.

229. Yang TS, Lin YC, Chen JS, et al. Phase II study of gemcitabine in patients with advanced hepatocellular carcinoma. *Cancer* 2000;89:750–756.

230. Yasuda S, Ito H, Yoshikawa M, et al. Radiotherapy for large hepatocellular carcinoma combined with transcatheter arterial embolization and percutaneous ethanol injection therapy. *Int J Oncol* 1999;15:467–473.

231. Yeo CJ, Pitt HA, Cameron JL: Cholangiocarcinoma. *Surg Clin North Am* 1990;70: 1429–1447.

232. Yoshida T, Aramaki M, Bandoh T, et al. Para-aortic lymph node metastasis in carcinoma of the distal bile duct. *Hepatogastroenterology* 1998;45:2388–2391.

233. Yu MC, Yuan JM, Govindarajan S, et al. Epidemiology of hepatocellular carcinoma. *Can J Gastroenterol* 2000;14:703–709.

234. Yu MW, Chang HC, Liaw YF, et al. Familial risk of hepatocellular carcinoma among chronic hepatitis B carriers and their relatives. *J Natl Cancer Inst* 2000;92:1159–1164.

235. Yu SZ: Primary prevention of hepatocellular carcinoma. *J Gastroenterol Hepatol* 1995;10:674–682.

236. Yuen MF, Cheng CC, Lauder IJ, et al. Early detection of hepatocellular carcinoma increases the chance of treatment: Hong Kong experience. *Hepatology* 2000;31:330–335.

237. Zervos EE, Osborne D, Goldin SB, et al. Stage does not predict survival after resection of hilar cholangiocarcinomas promoting an aggressive operative approach. *Am J Surg* 2005;190:810–815.

238. Zhang BH, Yang BH, Tang ZY: Randomized controlled trial of screening for hepatocellular carcinoma. *J Cancer Res Clin Oncol* 2004;130:417–422.

239. Zhang Y, Uchida M, Abe T, et al. Intrahepatic peripheral cholangiocarcinoma: comparison of dynamic CT and dynamic MRI. *J Comput Assist Tomogr* 1999;23: 670–677.

240. Zhu AX, Blaszkowsky LS, Ryan DP, et al. Phase II study of gemcitabine and oxaliplatin in combination with bevacizumab in patients with advanced hepatocellular carcinoma. *J Clin Oncol* 2006;24:1898–1903.

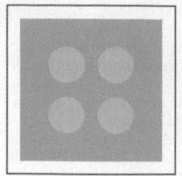

Chapter 58
Colon and Rectum

Mohammed Mohiuddin, Brian G. Czito, Christopher G. Willett

Anatomic Considerations and Patterns of Spread

The colorectum consists of the cecum, ascending colon, hepatic flexure, transverse colon, splenic flexure, descending colon, sigmoid colon, and rectum. Variability in the peritoneal investment, bowel mobility, and lymph node drainage of the colon and rectum presents unique therapeutic issues (77).

The posterior surfaces of the ascending and descending colon are often in direct contact with the retroperitoneum, while the anterior and lateral surfaces are draped with peritoneum (77). These posterior attachments can prevent significant mobility, increasing the difficulty of surgical resection. In contrast, the transverse colon is completely surrounded with peritoneum and supported on a long mesentery. As the sigmoid colon evolves distally into the rectum, the peritoneal coverage recedes. The rectum, approximately 12 to 15 cm in length, extends from the rectosigmoid junction to the puborectalis ring. The upper third of the rectum is draped with peritoneum anteriorly and on both sides. As the middle third of the rectum moves deeper into the pelvis, only the anterior surface is covered with peritoneum, which forms the posterior border of the rectouterine pouch or rectovesical space. The lowest third of the rectum is devoid of peritoneal covering and is in close proximity to adjacent structures including the bony pelvis (Fig. 58.1). Distal rectal tumors have no serosal barrier to invasion of adjacent structures and are more difficult to resect given the close confines of the deep pelvis (84).

Colonic nodal drainage consists of pericolic nodes and nodes in association with the vascular supply to the colon (i.e., mesenteric nodes). Because of the mobile and extensive nature of the colonic mesentery, complete regional lymph node coverage with radiotherapy (RT) is challenging but is usually well treated surgically. In contrast, the major regional groups for rectal nodal drainage can be covered within a reasonable RT field and include the perirectal, presacral, and internal iliac nodes (84).

Epidemiology, Molecular Cascade, Risk Factors, Hereditary Disease, and Clinical Presentation

Colorectal cancer remains a major worldwide health problem. In the United States alone, it is estimated that there will be 148,610 patients diagnosed with colon cancer and 55,170 deaths this year (83). World wide, approximately 1 million new cases per year are diagnosed, with 529,000 deaths (134). The median age is in the seventh decade; however, colorectal adenocarcinomas can occur any time in adulthood.

Although this malignancy may be linked to chemical carcinogens within the bowel lumen, it is not established whether these are ingested, the result of chemical activation of substances in the fecal stream, or a bacterial by-product (38,156). Environmental and dietary factors have been established as contributing to colorectal cancer. Factors shown to increase the risk of developing this disease include increasing age, male sex, family history of colorectal cancer, increasing height, increasing body mass index, processed meat intake, excessive alcohol intake, and low folate consumption. Of these risk factors, only increasing age, male sex, and excessive alcohol use have been found to be associated with rectal cancer (166). The value of consumption of fruits and vegetables in the prevention of colon and rectal cancer remains controversial, although recent studies have suggested that these associations may have been overstated (112). Contemporary prospective and randomized data do not support a high fiber diet in the prevention of colorectal cancer (66). Other studies have suggested that nonsteroidal anti-inflammatory drugs may serve in reducing colorectal cancer. The role of chemopreventive agents (carotenoids, aspirin, and other nonsteroidal anti-inflammatory drugs) in colorectal cancer is under active investigation.

A detailed discussion of the biologic and genetic pathways of development of colorectal cancer is beyond the scope of this chapter (38). In brief, it has been established that the development of colon cancer is a multifactorial process, involving changes in many genes including both proto-oncogenes and tumor suppressor genes. Colorectal cancers appear to arise through inactivation of the tumor suppressor genes adenomatous polyposis coli (APC) and P53 as well as mutations in the ras proto-oncogene.

Microsatellites are mutated short-repeat DNA sequences, usually consisting of one to five nucleotides (38). The majority of patients with hereditary nonpolyposis colorectal cancer (HNPCC) as well as a minority of sporadic colorectal cancers harbor microsatellite "instability." It has been shown that this instability occurs in patients with mutations in genes encoding enzymes that repair DNA replication errors. These defects in mismatch repair lead to high-frequency microsatellite instability. Studies have suggested that patients with tumors possessing a high frequency of microsatellite instability have a more favorable outcome and develop fewer metastases (60). Further elucidation of the genetic pathways in the development of colorectal cancer remains an active area of investigation and may ultimately impact therapy of this disease.

Colorectal cancer often produces minimal or no symptoms, emphasizing the need for screening programs in the general population. Many colorectal cancer symptoms are nonspecific, including changes in bowel habits, weakness, intermittent abdominal pain, nausea, and vomiting. The persistence of such symptoms as well as any evidence of iron deficiency anemia should be investigated.

The clinical presentation of colorectal cancer is determined largely by site of the tumor. Cancers of the right colon are often exophytic and commonly associated with iron deficiency anemia due to occult blood loss. During the past 20 years, the incidence of cancer of the right colon has increased and accounts for one third of large-bowel cancers. Many of these are diagnosed late. Cancers of the left colon and sigmoid colon are often deeply invasive, annular, and accompanied by obstruction and rectal bleeding. Rectal cancer frequently results in bleeding and alterations in bowel habits.

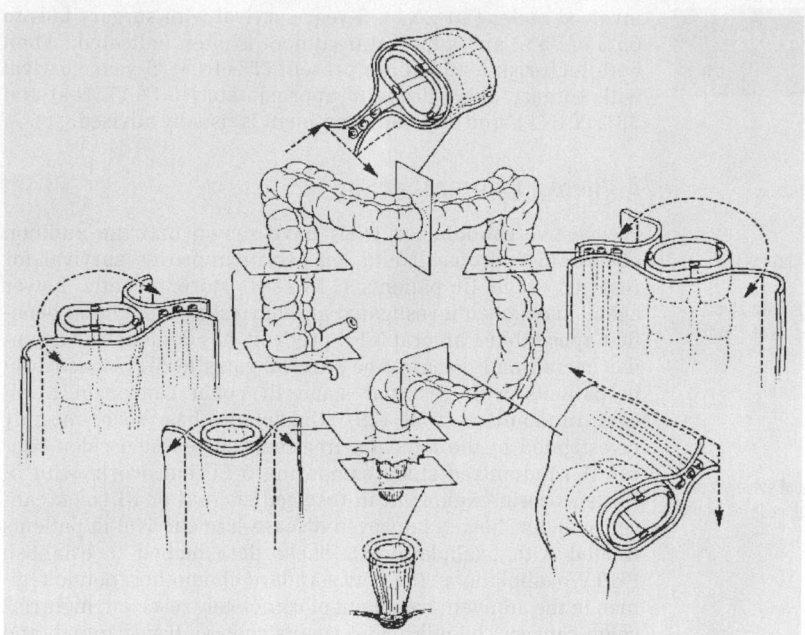

FIGURE 58.1. Idealized depiction of peritoneal relationships in the colon and rectum. The transverse and sigmoid colon are intraperitoneal, with a complete peritoneal covering (serosa) and mesentery. The ascending and descending colon are retroperitoneal, lack a true mesentery, and usually do not have a peritoneal covering posteriorly or laterally. The upper rectum begins above the peritoneal reflection and has peritoneum anteriorly and laterally. The lower half to two thirds of the rectum is below the peritoneal reflection (infraperitoneal). (From Gunderson LL, O'Connell MJ. The postoperative chemotherapy/irradiation adjuvant strategy. In: Cohen AF, Winawer SJ, Friedman MA, et al., eds. *Cancer of the colon, rectum, and anus.* New York: McGraw-Hill, 1995;631–645, with permission.)

Prevention and Early Detection

Neoplastic polyps, including tubular adenomas, villous adenomas, and tubulovillous adenomas, are precursors of colon cancers (38,179). Most colorectal cancers arise from pre-existing polyps. Patients with neoplastic polyps should be considered at high risk for large bowel cancer, and polypectomy may reduce this risk. With the availability of the flexible colonoscope and endoscopic polypectomy, polyps can be removed at a premalignant stage and patients followed closely.

Because the cumulative lifetime risk of developing colorectal cancer in the United States is about 6%, screening programs for the general population have been undertaken (153). The goal of screening is to detect preinvasive polyps or early invasive cancer. The presence of polyps increases the risk for cancer to approximately 15%. Data from programs in which proctoscopy is performed annually suggest that routinely scheduled polypectomy reduces the development of subsequent bowel cancer by 80% or more (156). The American Cancer Society has recommended screening should begin at age 50 in the average risk patient by either:

1. Annual fecal occult blood test and/or flexible sigmoidoscopy every 5 years,
2. Double contrast barium enema every 5 years, or
3. Colonoscopy every 10 years.

Intensive surveillance is recommended for patients at high risk (patients with adenomatous polyps, history of colorectal cancer, first-degree relative diagnosed with colorectal cancer or adenomas, inflammatory bowel disease, or high risk due to family history or genetic testing). Computed tomography (CT) colonography as well as genetic fecal testing are being studied as potential screening tools. Although screening methods can detect colorectal cancer at an early stage, <40% of patients are diagnosed with early disease, likely reflecting low rates of disease awareness as well as the infrequency of screening in eligible candidates (153).

Pathology and Pathways of Spread

Tumors of the colorectum arise in the mucosa and are virtually all (>90%) adenocarcinomas (38). Other histologic types include squamous cell carcinoma, carcinoid, leiomyosarcoma, and lymphoma. Most grading systems classify adenocarcinoma as well, either moderately or poorly differentiated.

Large bowel tumors invade from mucosa through the bowel wall and beyond, with involvement of lymphatic channels and lymph nodes. Hematogenous spread can occur, primarily to the lung and liver. There is little propensity for colon cancer to spread longitudinally within the bowel wall, in contrast to esophageal or gastric cancers.

Patient Evaluation/Staging

Pretreatment evaluation should include pathological confirmation of adenocarcinoma, colonoscopy to evaluate extent of tumor and rule out synchronous primaries (occurring in 3% to 5%), and baseline blood counts with liver function tests and carcinoembryonic antigen levels. Patients should undergo abdominal and pelvic CT scan as well as chest x-ray to evaluate extent of local regional disease as well as the presence or absence of distant metastases. Positron emission tomography (PET) scan, magnetic resonance imaging (MRI), and ultrasound may be useful in evaluating patients with oligometastatic disease who may be appropriate candidates for resection of metastatic disease with curative intent.

Prognostic factors influencing survival in colorectal cancer patients include depth of tumor invasion into and beyond the bowel wall, the number of involved regional lymph nodes, as well as the presence or absence of distant metastases. The tumor, node, metastasis (TNM) system of the American Joint Committee on Cancer can be used as a clinical (preoperative) or postoperative staging system (Tables 58.1 and 58.2).

Therapy of Colon Cancer

Surgery

Surgery is the primary treatment for patients with colonic tumors. Resection with curative intent is possible in approximately 75% of patients (156). Surgery of primary colon cancer is based on the anatomy and mechanisms by which this disease spreads. Adenocarcinomas of the colon may grow by direct extension into the lymphatics of the submucosa and bowel wall. To

▣ Table 58.1	COLORECTAL TUMOR, NODE, METASTASIS STAGING, 2002

Primary Tumor (T)

TX	Primary tumor cannot be assessed
T0	No evidence of primary tumor
Tis	Carcinoma in situ: Intraepithelial or invasion of lamina propria
T1	Tumor invades submucosa
T2	Tumor invades muscularis propria
T3	Tumor invades through the muscularis propria into the subserosa, or into non-peritonealized pericolic or perirectal tissues
T4	Tumor directly invades other organs or structures[a] and/or perforates visceral peritoneum (includes invasion of other segments of colon)

Regional Lymph Nodes (N)

NX	Regional lymph nodes cannot be assessed
N0	No regional lymph node metastasis
N1	Metastasis in one to three regional lymph nodes
N2	Metastasis in four or more regional lymph nodes (Tumor nodules in the pericolonic adipose tissue without evidence of residual lymph node are classified as a regional lymph node metastases)

Distant Metastasis (M)

MX	Distant metastasis cannot be assessed
M0	No distant metastasis
M1	Distant metastasis

[a]Direct invasion in T4 includes invasion of other segments of the colorectum by way of the serosa; for example, invasion of the sigmoid by a carcinoma of the cecum. Tumor that is adherent to other organs or structures, macroscopically, is classified as T4. However, if no tumor is present in the adhesion, microscopically, the classification should be pT3.
From Colon and rectum. In: *North American Joint Committee on Cancer staging manual*, 6th ed. New York: Springer, 2002, with permission.

avoid cutting across tumor in intramural lymphatics, sufficient lengths of bowel must be resected proximal and distal to the primary cancer. Colon cancer often extends through the serosa into mesenteric lymphatics that run along the blood vessels draining into the portal watershed at the root of the mesentery. Resection includes removal of the major lymphatic drainage system in the mesentery. Because anatomic resections designed to include named blood vessels also include the draining lymphatics, the boundaries for resecting large bowel cancer are relatively uniform. Right hemicolectomy, transverse colectomy, left hemicolectomy, and sigmoid resection are performed by adherence to surgical oncologic principles without major sacrifice of large bowel function.

Resection results in excellent cure rates for lesions limited to the bowel wall with negative nodes (average 5-year survival, 97% for T1N0; 85% to 90% for T2N0). With a single high-risk feature of extension beyond the colonic wall (T3–T4N0) or

▣ Table 58.2	AMERICAN JOINT COMMITTEE ON CANCER STAGE GROUPING

Stage	T	N	M	Dukes[a]	MAC[b]
0	Tis	N0	M0	—	—
I	T1	N0	M0	A	A
	T2	N0	M0	A	B1
IIA	T3	N0	M0	B	B2
IIB	T4	N0	M0	B	B3
IIIA	T1-T2	N1	M0	C	C1
IIIB	T3-T4	N1	M0	C	C2/C3
IIIC	Any T	N2	M0	C	C1/C2/C3
IV	Any T	Any N	M1	—	D

M, metastasis; N, node; T, tumor
[a]Dukes B is a composite of better (T3 N0 M0) and worse (T4 N0 M0) prognostic groups, as is Dukes C (Any TN1 M0 and Any T N2 M0).
[b]MAC is the modified Astler-Coller classification.

involved nodes (T0–2N+), 5-year survival with surgery falls to 65% to 75%, and adjuvant treatment is often indicated. When both high-risk features are present (T3–4N+), 5-year survival with surgery alone drops to approximately 50% (T3N+) and 35% (T4N+), and adjuvant treatment is usually advised.

Adjuvant Chemotherapy

Prospective randomized trials have shown that the addition of 5FU (5-fluorouacil) and leucovorin improves survival for resected stage III patients (118,130). More recently, newer agents have been investigated and have shown potential benefit. Capecitabine, an oral 5-FU prodrug, has demonstrated similar overall and disease free survival rates to 5-FU/leucovorin in patients with resected stage III colon cancer in a recent randomized trial (29). Oxaliplatin has been recently investigated in the adjuvant treatment of resected colon cancer. A randomized study comparing 5-FU/leucovorin with 5-FU/leucororin/oxaliplatin in resected stage II or III colon cancer patients showed improved disease-free survival in patients treated with oxaliplatin (8). These data helped to establish FU/LV/oxaliplatin as the new standard chemotherapeutic regimen in the adjuvant treatment of completely resected, high-risk colon cancer. The efficacy of agents such as bevacizumab and cetuximab as adjuvant therapy is being investigated.

Adjuvant Irradiation with or without Concurrent Chemotherapy

Because of the documented efficacy of adjuvant chemotherapy as well as the perception by many oncologists that colonic (as opposed to rectal) cancer is much more likely to relapse distantly than locally, there has been little evaluation of the efficacy of postoperative irradiation with chemotherapy. The potential indications for adjuvant radiation therapy in colon cancer are based on analyses of patterns of failure following resection (Table 58.3) (65,173). Advanced stage predicts for local failure in both colon and rectal cancers; however, local failure in colon cancer also depends on anatomic origin. The ascending and descending colon are considered "anatomically immobile," and their close proximity to the retroperitoneal tissues often limits wide surgical resection (Fig. 58.2). Limitations in achieving satisfactory circumferential margins increase the risk of residual disease and consequently local failure. In contrast, the mid-sigmoid and mid-transverse colon are relatively "mobile" with a wide mesentery, permitting the surgeon to obtain wide margins regardless of extent of disease invasion into the mesentery. Unless there is adjacent organ adherence/invasion by tumor, local failure at these sites is uncommon. Local failure rates for cecal, hepatic/splenic flexure, and proximal/distal sigmoid tumors are variable depending on the amount of mesentery present, tumor extension, and the adequacy of radial margins. When colon cancers adhere to or invade adjacent structures, local failure rates exceed 30% following surgery alone. In summary, local failure occurs in patients with colonic tumors where there are anatomic constraints on radial resection margins, including tumors adherent to or invading adjacent structures.

Until recently, data evaluating the use of adjuvant radiation therapy in high-risk colon cancer patients were limited to single-institution retrospective analyses (7,64,168,169). To summarize, these studies have suggested that operative bed failures in high-risk patients undergoing resection alone are at least 30%, and that the risk of local failure is reduced by the administration of adjuvant radiation therapy. These are discussed in detail below.

A report from the Massachusetts General Hospital (MGH) evaluated outcomes in high-risk patients undergoing resection followed by adjuvant radiation therapy and compared these

Table 58.3	FIVE-YEAR ACTUARIAL LOCAL CONTROL AND RELAPSE-FREE SURVIVAL AFTER SURGERY PLUS POSTOPERATIVE RADIOTHERAPY VS. SURGERY ALONE, ACCORDING TO STAGE—MASSACHUSETTS GENERAL HOSPITAL					
	Surgery Alone			**Surgery plus Postoperative Radiation**		
TNM Stage	**No. of Patients**	**LC (%)**	**RFS (%)**	**No. of Patients**	**LC (%)**	**RFS (%)**
T3N0	163	90	78	23	91	72
T4N0	83	69	63	54	93	79[a]
T3N+	100	64	48	55	70	47
T4N+	49	47	38	39	72	53[a]

LC, local control; RFS, relapse-free survival; TNM, tumor, node, metastasis
[a] <0.05.

to a similar cohort of patients treated over the same period undergoing surgery only. Irradiated patients included those with T4N0/N+, T3N+ disease (excluding mid-sigmoid and mid-transverse colon) and T3N0 patients with margins of <1 cm. A total of 171 patients received postoperative radiation, with 63 patients receiving concurrent chemotherapy, usually with bolus 5-FU (500 mg/m^2/d) for 3 consecutive days during the first and last weeks of radiation therapy. Radiation treatment was administered through parallel opposed or other multifield techniques to treat the tumor bed with an approximate 3- to 5-cm margin to a total dose of 45 Gy, followed by reduced fields to a total dose of 50.4 to 54 Gy. Draining nodes were included if thought to be at high risk for involvement. This cohort was compared to 395 patients with T3–4N0/N+ tumors undergoing surgery alone

during the same time period. Table 58.3 shows 5-year actuarial local control and relapse-free survival in the adjuvant group compared to patients undergoing surgery alone. Local control rates in T4N0 and T4N+ patients treated with radiation therapy were 93% and 72%, respectively versus 69% and 47%, respectively in patients undergoing surgery alone. Similarly, relapse-free survivals were 79% and 53%, respectively in T4N0/T4N+ patients undergoing adjuvant radiation, versus 63% and 38%, respectively undergoing surgery alone. No significant outcome differences were observed in patients with T3N0 and T3N+ lesions; however, there may be an element of selection bias in the radiation group given most patients were referred because of concerns of adequacy of local control following surgery alone. There was a trend toward improved local control in patients

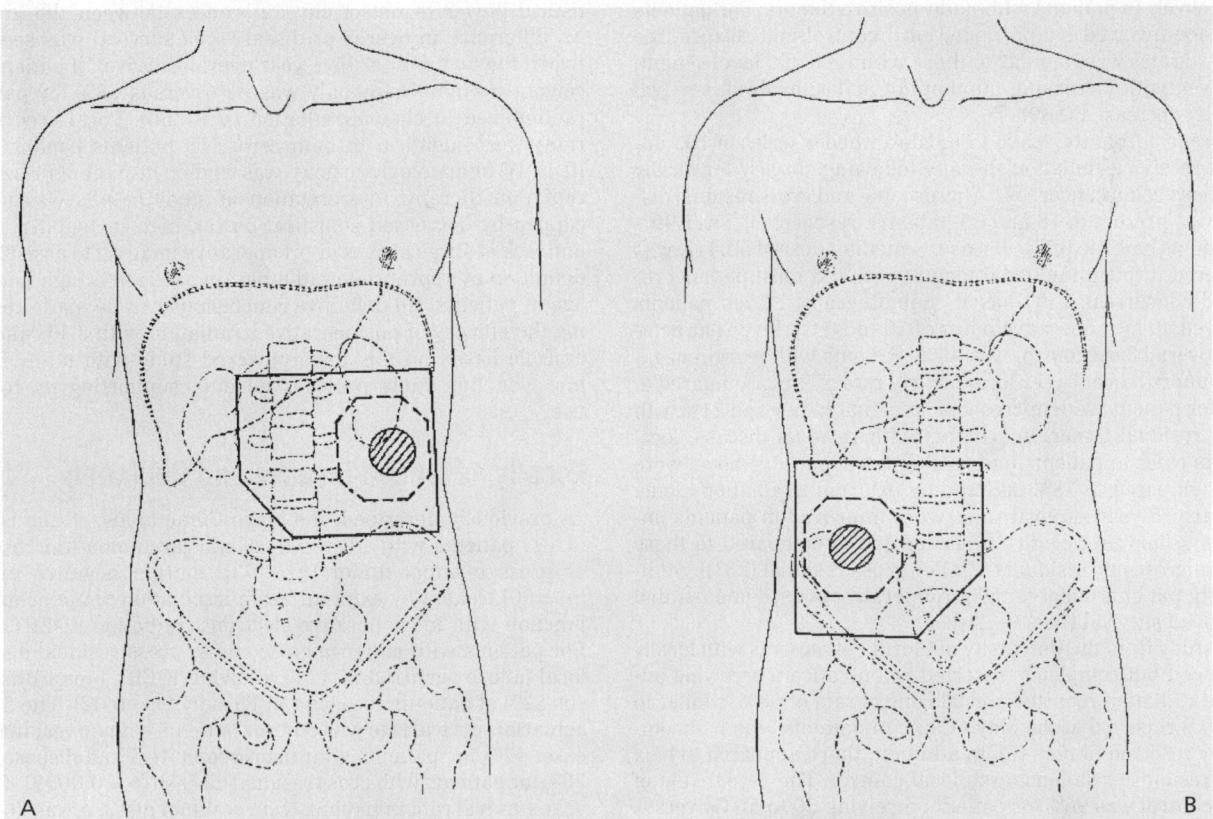

FIGURE 58.2. Idealized postoperative anteroposterior-posteroanterior irradiation fields of extrapelvic colon cancer (tumor bed and nodal regions). If treated preoperatively, lateral fields could be added based on imaging with computed tomography of the abdomen and colon radiograph. **A:** Para-aortic nodes are at risk, in addition to tumor bed, due to tumor adherence to posterior abdominal wall with descending colon cancer. **B:** External and common iliac nodes are at risk, in addition to tumor bed, from proximal ascending colon cancer. (From Gunderson LL, Martenson JA, Smalley SR, et al. Lower gastrointestinal cancer: Rationale, results, and techniques of treatment. *Front Radiat Ther Oncol* 1994;28:140–154, with permission.)

Table 58.4   FIVE-YEAR ACTUARIAL LOCAL CONTROL AND RELAPSE-FREE SURVIVAL OF ADJUVANTLY IRRADIATED PATIENTS BASED ON 5-FLUOROURACIL (5FU) ADMINISTRATION—MASSACHUSETTS GENERAL HOSPITAL

TNM Stage	Without 5FU			With 5FU		
	No. of Patients	LC (%)	RFS (%)	No. of Patients	LC (%)	RFS (%)
T3N0	16	87	69	7	100	80
T4N0	37	94	78	16	100	83
T3N+	41	69	48	14	70	43
T4N+	24	67	53	15	79	52

LC, local control; RFS, relapse-free survival; TNM, tumor, node, metastasis

receiving 5-FU (Table 58.4). The rate of acute enteritis in patients receiving irradiation and 5-FU was 16% versus 4% in patients undergoing irradiation only. This rate of enteritis is similar to data from studies of concurrent 5-FU and radiation therapy in rectal cancer. Late bowel complication rates were not increased by concomitant 5-FU administration. The conclusion was that patients with T4 tumors or tumors with abscess/fistula formation or margin positive resection may benefit from postoperative radiation. In an updated analysis from MGH, 152 patients with T4 tumors received adjuvant irradiation. On pathological examination, 42 patients had tumors with positive margins. For patients with negative margins the 10-year actuarial local control in T4N0 and T4N+ patients was 78% and 48%, respectively. In patients with node-negative tumors, the 10-year actuarial local control and relapse free survival rates were 87% and 58%, respectively, compared to 65% and 33%, respectively in patients with node-positive tumors. For patients with one involved lymph node, local control and relapse-free survival rates were similar to those without nodal involvement; however, with increasing numbers of nodes involved, survival steadily decreased (169).

A report from the Mayo Clinic described a series of 103 patients receiving radiation therapy following surgery for locally advanced colon cancer (64). Microscopic and gross residual disease was present in 18 and 35 patients, respectively. Over 90% of patients had T4N0/N+ disease. A median dose of 50.4 Gy was delivered through multifield techniques, and most patients received concurrent 5-FU–based chemotherapy. Eleven patients received an intraoperative boost of 10 to 20 Gy. Five-year actuarial overall local control was 40%. Patients with margin negative tumors had a 5-year local control rate of 90%, compared to 46% for patients with microscopic residual tumor and 21% with gross residual tumor. In patients with residual disease, local control rates in patients undergoing intraoperative boost were 89% compared to 18% undergoing external irradiation alone. Similarly, 5-year survival rates were improved in patients undergoing margin negative resection (66%) compared to those with microscopic residual (47%) or gross residual (23%). Additionally, patients undergoing intraoperative boost demonstrated improved survival (76% vs. 26%).

A study from the University of Florida of patients with locally advanced but completely resected colon cancers receiving adjuvant radiation reported a local control rate of 88%, similar to the 90% reported at the Mayo Clinic in patients who had completely resected tumors (7). In addition, there appeared to be a dose-response relationship to local control. The 5-year rate of local control was 96% for patients receiving 50 to 55 Gy versus 76% for patients receiving <50 Gy (p = 0.0095).

To assess whether the addition of radiation therapy to adjuvant chemotherapy would result in superior survival and local regional failure rates in resected, high-risk colon cancer patients, the U.S. Intergroup initiated a randomized prospective trial in 1992 (103). In this trial, patients with resected colon cancer were randomized to postoperative irradiation with 5-FU and levamisole or 5-FU and levamisole alone. Eligibility criteria included margin negative tumors with adherence to or invasion of surrounding structures (i.e., T4N0 or N+ disease, excluding peritoneal invasion) or tumors arising in the ascending or descending colon with metastatic regional nodes (T3N+). Patients were randomized to receive (a) weekly 5-FU combined with levamisole for 12 months' duration or (b) 5-FU and levamisole for 12 months with combined radiation therapy and chemotherapy beginning 1 month after the first 5-FU administration. The recommended total radiation dose was 45 Gy in 25 fractions over 5 weeks with an optional 5.4 Gy boost.

The initial trial accrual goal was 700 patients; however, the study was closed in 1996 due to poor accrual (222 patients; 189 evaluable). Therefore, total accrual was less than one third of the initial goals, and there was a decreased statistical power to detect any differences between the groups. No difference in overall or disease-free survival was seen between the two groups. Five-year overall survival of patients receiving chemotherapy only was 62% versus 58% for patients randomized to chemoirradiation (p >0.50). Local recurrence rates were identical in both arms (18 patients each). Grade III or IV hematologic toxicity was higher in patients receiving radiation therapy. Interpretation of study results was handicapped by decreased statistical power, high ineligibility rates, and lack of surgical clips or preoperative imaging to assist in the definition of appropriate radiotherapy fields in a high percentage of patients. No definitive conclusions can be made regarding the efficacy of postoperative irradiation with 5-FU and levamisole based on this underpowered study with many flaws; however, this study provides no data supporting its routine use.

Locally Advanced Disease and Palliation

As previously described, the Mayo Clinic analyzed the results of 103 patients with advanced colonic carcinoma (microscopic or gross residual tumor [n = 53]; margin negative tumors [n = 50] treated by external beam irradiation alone or in conjunction with intraoperative electron irradiation (IOERT) (64). For patients with either microscopic or gross residual disease, local failure occurred in 11% receiving IOERT plus EBRT versus 82% of patients receiving EBRT only (p = 0.02). The 5-year actuarial survival rate was 66% for patients with no residual disease, 47% for patients with microscopic residual disease, and 23% for patients with gross residual disease (p = 0.0009). The 5-year survival rate in patients with residual disease was 76% for patients receiving IOERT and 26% for patients receiving EBRT alone (p = 0.04).

For patients with metastatic disease, 5-FU–based chemotherapy is usually administered. Recent prospective randomized trials have shown that multiple agents improve survival in patients with metastatic colorectal cancer. Saltz et al.

(147) reported the results of a three-arm randomized trial comparing (a) irinotecan, 5-FU, and leucovorin (IFL) (b) 5-FU/leucovorin, or (c) irinotecan alone. Patients receiving IFL had an improved survival (median survival 14.8 months vs. 12.6 months; $p = 0.04$) and response rate (39% vs. 21%; $p < 0.001$) compared to 5-FU and leucovorin alone. The incidence of grade 3 or higher diarrhea was significantly higher with the three-drug regimen. Hurwitz et al. (80) reported a randomized trial comparing irinotecan, 5-FU, and leucovorin with or without bevacizumab, a monoclonal antibody directed against vascular endothelial growth factor (VEGF). Median survival was significantly improved in the bevacizumab arm (median survival 20.3 months vs. 15.6 months; $p < 0.001$). Additionally, response rates were improved in the bevacizumab containing arm (45% vs. 35%; $p = 0.004$). Cunningham et al. (37) randomized 329 patients with metastatic colorectal cancer refractory to irinotecan-based chemotherapy regimens to receive cetuximab (a monoclonal antibody directed against the epidermal growth factor [EGFR]) or cetuximab with irinotecan. Response rates in patients receiving combination therapy were significantly higher (23% vs. 11%; $p = 0.007$) as was median time to progression (4.1 vs. 1.5 months; $p < 0.001$). No difference in survival was observed. A study by Goldberg et al. (57) randomized 795 patients with previously untreated, metastatic colorectal cancer patients to receive (a) irinotecan, 5-FU, and leucovorin, (b) oxaliplatin, 5-FU, and leucovorin, or (c) irinotecan and oxaliplatin. Patients receiving oxaliplatin, 5-FU, and leucovorin had an improved median survival compared to those receiving irinotecan, 5-FU, and leucovorin or irinotecan and oxaliplatin (19.5 months vs. 15 months vs. 17.4 months; $p < 0.05$ for oxaliplatin containing regimens vs. irinotecan only regimen). Response rates in patients receiving 5-FU, leucovorin, and oxaliplatin were significantly higher than those receiving irinotecan, 5-FU, and leucovorin or irinotecan with oxaliplatin (45% vs. 31% vs. 35%; $p < 0.05$). Varying combinations of these drugs as well as other novel agents remain the focus of ongoing investigation in both the metastatic and nonmetastatic setting.

Palliative irradiation, sometimes in combination with 5-FU–based chemotherapy, is considered for patients with specific symptoms referable to metastatic disease—brain, bone, and other sites. The combination of radiation therapy and newer agents (capecitabine, irinotecan, oxaliplatin, bevacizumab, cetuximab) remains investigational.

Techniques of Irradiation

Treatment field design in colon cancer is based on patterns of failure data. As is true in the treatment of rectal carcinoma, great care must be taken in the design of postoperative treatment of adenocarcinoma of the colon. Field arrangement will vary depending on the site of the primary disease as well as areas judged to be at high risk for local recurrence (62). Patient positioning (supine, prone, decubitus) should be considered in planning. Small bowel is often a dose-limiting structure in this therapy, and it is often advantageous to position patients in the right or left decubitus position for at least a portion of their treatment, allowing displacement of the small bowel away from the treatment field. Immobilization devices may improve reproducibility. A small-bowel series defines small-bowel volume within the treatment field. It may be useful to compare films in both the decubitus and supine positions to determine the actual amount of small bowel displacement. CT-based planning may facilitate defining the tumor bed, determining beam orientation, as well as estimating the volume of small bowel included within the treatment fields. As in other abdominal malignancies, a portion of one kidney may be irradiated. Unilateral renal irradiation results in minimal long-term clinical sequelae,

assuming baseline function in the contralateral kidney is normal (174).

The total radiation dose used in the adjuvant treatment of colon carcinoma depends on the amount of suspected residual disease and tolerance constraints of surrounding normal tissue. Generally, an initial dose of 45 Gy in 25 fractions of 1.8 Gy per fraction is delivered through larger fields to the primary tumor and at-risk tissues. Reduced fields may be treated to 50 Gy if only a small portion of small bowel is included. For patient with T4 tumors, the general goal is to treat the tumor bed to a total dose of 54 to 60 Gy. Any treatment beyond 50 Gy mandates exclusion of all small bowel from the field. Spinal cord dose should be limited to 45 Gy. In addition, at least two thirds of one functional kidney should receive no more than 18 to 20 Gy and at least two thirds of the total liver volume should not receive more than 30 Gy. In a Mayo Clinic analysis, small bowel obstruction rates were lower when more than two treatment fields were used, and attempts should be made to implement multifield techniques, which may be aided by CT-based planning (150).

Generally, the primary tumor site should be covered with a 4- to 5-cm margin proximally and distally with 3- to 4-cm margin medially and laterally to cover areas of potential residual disease. The nodal basins in the mesentery beyond surgical margins are usually not treated as satisfactory margin clearance is obtained in these sites. An exception to this may be right colon tumors where both small bowel and right colon are supplied by ileocolic vessels, limiting the extent of resection. In some instances, treatment of the para-aortic nodes may be indicated, particularly with extensive retroperitoneal involvement by tumor. Treatment of proximal mesenteric nodes may be appropriate if nodes adjacent to the surgical or resection margin are involved. Figures 58.2 and 58.3 show idealized radiation fields for varying colonic sites including cecum, descending, as well as sigmoid cancer. In many situations, it may be appropriate to exclude treatment of para-aortic nodal basins, based on operative and pathological findings.

Conclusion

Subsets of patients with colon cancer have local recurrence rates similar to patients with rectal cancer if surgery only is undertaken. Because of encouraging pilot study results with postoperative irradiation with or without 5-FU for patients with resected high-risk colon cancers, and the positive results of 5-FU and levamisole in high-risk adjuvant colon cancer, an Intergroup randomized trial was undertaken, randomizing patients to 5-FU and levamisole or 5-FU and levamisole with tumor bed irradiation in patients at high risk for local recurrence following surgical resection. There was no benefit in survival in patients receiving adjuvant radiation therapy; however, interpretation of these results is handicapped by inadequate accrual and significant flaws that were previously discussed.

The value of adjuvant postoperative irradiation combined with systemic therapy for patients at high risk for local relapse is unlikely to ever be addressed in a definitive randomized trial. Treatment recommendations should be made on a case-by-case basis with existing data in the setting of an informed consent. Adjuvant tumor bed irradiation with concurrent 5-FU–based chemotherapy should be considered for patients with tumors (a) invading adjoining structures, (b) those complicated by perforation or fistula, and (c) where incomplete resection is performed.

The use of intraoperative irradiation as a supplement to EBRT in certain T4 tumors (i.e., those with uncertain margins) may also be appropriate. For patients with tumors adherent to or invading adjacent structures, the preferred treatment sequence would be preoperative EBRT plus 5-FU–based chemotherapy followed by resection with or without IOERT and

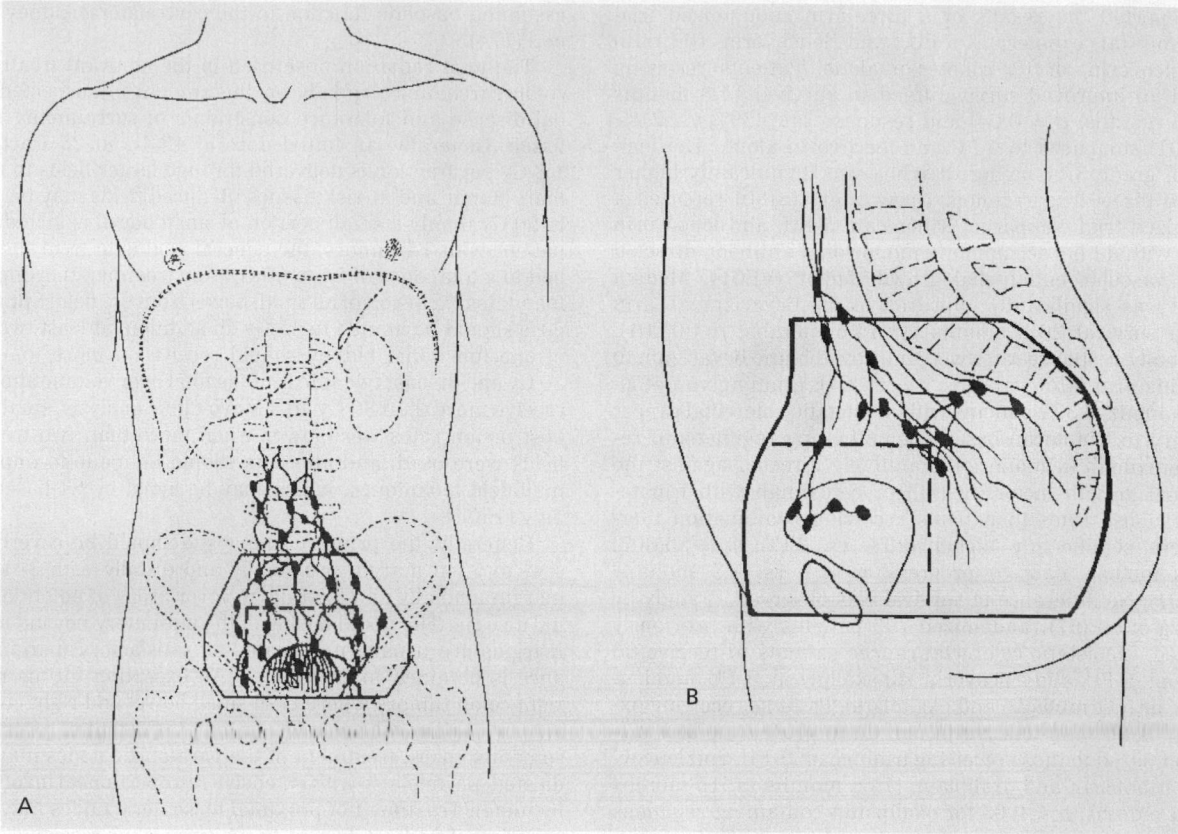

FIGURE 58.3. Idealized multiple-field preoperative or postoperative irradiation technique for a sigmoid colon cancer adherent to the bladder. Solid lines, large field; interrupted lines, boost field. **A:** Anteroposterior-posteroanterior. **B:** Paired laterals. (From Gunderson LL, Martenson JA, Smalley SR, et al. Lower gastrointestinal cancer: Rationale, results, and techniques of treatment. *Front Radiat Ther Oncol* 1994;28:140–154, with permission.)

postoperative systemic therapy, based on excellent results in preliminary IOERT reports from both U.S. and European institutions (146,150,171). A similar approach would be reasonable for patients with locally recurrent cancers or with regional nodal relapse (63,68,69,172).

Therapy of Rectal Cancer

Management of cancer of the rectum has undergone a dramatic change in the past decade. Until recently surgery had remained the primary treatment modality, but in spite of "curative" resections, a significant proportion of patients develop local recurrence of disease (20% to 50%) (136,142). Local tumor recurrence is highly correlated with both the depth of penetration of the tumor and the number of regional nodes involved by metastatic disease (41). Recent results of national cooperative group studies and several European randomized trials indicate that a multimodality treatment approach results in a significantly better outcome than surgery alone.

Defining the True Rectum and Impact of Tumor Location

Rectal cancer represents a spectrum of disease stages that needs careful definition to optimize multimodality treatment strategies, and defining the true rectum is of critical importance. Traditionally the rectum extends for 12 to 15 cm from the anal verge. The true surgical rectum begins at the anorectal ring, just proximal to the dentate line (47,102). This represents

the internal anal sphincteric muscle and is necessary for anal continence. It also represents the inferior limit for functional sphincter preservation surgery and defines the lymphatic watershed for rectal cancer spread. Tumors arising above the anorectal ring tend to metastasize along the distribution of the middle rectal vessels to the internal iliac lymph nodes as compared to tumors that may extend into the anal canal, which spread via nodes along the inferior rectal and external iliac pathways (5) (Fig. 58.4). Cancers that arise in the anal canal generally metastasize to the lungs rather than the liver, as is common with most true rectal cancers. The prognosis of patients worsens with more distal location of cancer, and these differences persist even with the addition of adjunctive therapy (96,160). The proximal and distal rectum have historically been defined by the level at which the peritoneum is reflected along the anterior surface of the rectum (usually at the level of S3) (91). This is a surgical observation and difficult to define in an intact patient. The middle valve of Hoston is a useful landmark that can often be identified endoscopically (usually about 6 cm from the anorectal ring), and can be used to differentiate proximal tumors from more distal lesions. All tumors that can be digitally palpated are generally considered distal cancers.

Prognostic Factors

Several prognostic factors, in addition to tumor location, have been shown to have a significant impact on tumor behavior (4). Tumor extent as defined by the American Joint Committee on Cancer (AJCC) staging clearly remains the dominant determinant of survival (155). Other patient factors such as

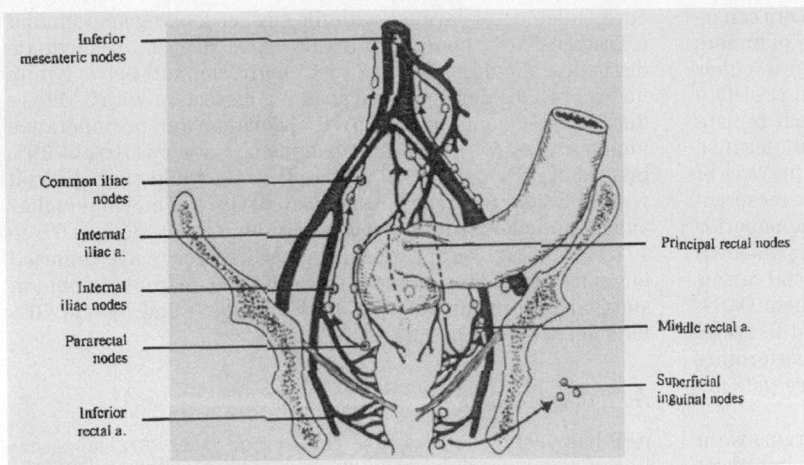

FIGURE 58.4. Lymphatics of the rectum.

age, gender, and ethnicity have little association with outcome but may affect choice of therapy (15,35,141). Histopathological grade is of borderline significance, however, and signet cell cancers have a particularly poor outcome (148). In some reports lymph-vascular invasion has been shown on univariate analysis to have a negative impact on survival (34,36). Circumferential tumors or those with total or near total obstruction (lumen <1 cm) respond very poorly, and tumors with deep central ulceration are associated with a high incidence of lymph node involvement (32,182). Tumor mobility remains a key factor in both choice and outcome of treatment (67,120). Mobile cancers have a much more favorable outcome as compared to tethered or fixed cancers. Some studies report that even among mobile cancers only 75% to 80% are completely resected with negative surgical margins (86). Surgery for fixed cancers has proven ineffective, and these tumors are often classified as unresectable. Tumor fixation, while harder to assess in the proximal rectum, is less often encountered without other adverse factors such as circumferential disease with obstruction or perforation (28). Tumor fixation is much more problematic in the distal rectum as the confines of the bony pelvis inhibits the surgeons ability to achieve adequate lateral/circumferential margins. Distal rectal cancers therefore require a more vigorous approach to adjuvant therapy than proximal cancers.

Imaging

Efforts to improve the clinical assessment of rectal cancers have been helped considerably with the evolution of new imaging modalities. Pelvic CT has been utilized extensively and is part of the routine work-up of patients. CT appears to be much more useful in identifying enlarged pelvic lymph nodes and metastasis outside the pelvis than the extent or stage of the primary tumor (48). Standard CT does not permit the visualization of the layers of the rectal wall, and, therefore, its utility in the assessment of small primary cancers is limited (82). The sensitivity of CT scan is reported as 50% to 80% accurate, with a 30% to 80% specificity (65% to 75% accurate for tumor staging and 55% to 65% accurate in mesorectal lymph node staging) (1). The ability of CT scans for detecting distant metastasis, including pelvic and para-aortic lymph nodes, is higher than for detecting perirectal nodal involvement (75% to 87% vs. 45%) (13,106). Any lymphadenopathy near the rectum seen on a CT scan should be considered abnormal.

Transrectal endoscopic ultrasound (EUS) techniques have been more helpful in efforts to clinically stage rectal cancers. EUS can be 80% to 95% accurate in tumor staging and 70% to 75% accurate in mesorectal lymph node staging (18,154). The transrectal ultrasound is very good at demonstrating layers of the rectal wall especially the mucosa, muscularis mucosa, submucosa, and muscularis propria (79,132). Its use is limited to lesions <14 cm from the anus and not applicable for the upper rectum or for stenosing tumors. EUS can also identify enlarged perirectal lymph nodes but is not effective outside of the perirectum (76). One area where EUS can be very useful is in determining extension of disease into the anal canal, which is an area that is poorly visualized on CT but of critical importance for planning sphincter preserving surgical procedures (61).

More recently, MRI techniques have been found to be of greater accuracy in defining the extent of rectal cancer extension and also determining the location and stage of tumor (21,25). Different approaches to MRI have been explored including the use of body coils, endorectal MRI and phased array techniques. Although MRI appears to have greater accuracy, it requires a significant learning curve but is becoming a greater part of the standard presurgical work-up for rectal cancer.

Body coil MRI, which first became available in the mid-1980s, has had an accuracy of 54% to 66% for T staging, but this has improved with the use of endorectal coil MRI with reported accuracy rates of 80% to 95% (16,90). A significant advantage of both endorectal coil and surface coil MRI is that it is less operator dependent and permits a larger field of view than EUS. It also allows assessment for proximal tumors and stenotic lesions where EUS is not an option. Another advantage of MRI is that it can detect involved lymph nodes on the basis of characteristics other than size. MRI can also be very helpful in determining the extent of lateral extension of disease, which is critical in predicting the adequacy of circumferential margins for surgical excision (17). Several studies using phased array MRI have reported accuracy rates of 80% to 97% in predicting lateral disease extent and have correlated the likelihood of tumor-free resection margin by visualizing tumor involvement of the mesorectal fascia (110).

All of these imaging techniques have advantages and limitations and should be considered complementary to a good physical examination. They are all less accurate in predicting response after neoadjuvant therapy with high rates of false positivity (51,161) and should be interpreted with caution in this setting.

Treatment

Surgery

Surgery remains the mainstay of curative treatment for carcinoma of the rectum. Surgical management depends on the stage and location of a tumor within the rectum. Early cancers can be managed with limited surgery; however, the majority of tumors tend to present as more advanced disease and require either a low anterior resection (LAR) or abdominoperineal resection (APR). The general principles of a surgical approach remain the removal of all gross and microscopic disease with negative proximal, distal, and circumferential margins. In the case of radical resection, this means removal of the adjacent mesorectal tissue containing the regional lymphatics and the superior hemorrhoidal artery pedicle. Several studies have now shown that the surgeon's experience with resection of colorectal cancer is an independent variable in the outcome of treatment (107). The Intergroup 0114 trial found that for stage II and III rectal cancers, APR rates were not only higher in hospitals performing low volume procedures (46% vs. 32%), but also more patients had positive resection margins (111).

Historically the distal and proximal resection margins were considered important determinants in outcome. A 5-cm distal margin of normal rectum was considered necessary for adequate surgical resection (20,58,139). However, several retrospective studies have shown that distal intramural spread of tumor is rare beyond 1.5 cm, and, therefore, a 2-cm distal margin is currently considered acceptable, except in lesions that are poorly differentiated or widely metastatic (137,163,175,180). The reduced requirement of 2-cm distal margin for adequate resection has lead to a significant increase in the likelihood of sphincter preservation procedures in this disease.

Radial Margin

The National Institute of Health Consensus Conference on Rectal Cancer indicated that the principal reason for local recurrence in resected rectal cancer appears to be related to the anatomic constraints in obtaining wide radial margins, even though the proximal and distal margins appear adequate (127). Quirke et al. (140), using whole mount specimens, found that 27% (14/52) of patients had spread to the lateral radial margin, even though the margins appeared negative with standard pathological assessment. Eighty-six percent of those with positive margins developed local regional recurrence of disease as compared to only 3% without lateral resection margin involvement. The mean surgical margin of resection has been shown to decrease with increasing stage of disease ranging from 14 mm for T1 cancers to 3 mm for T4 cancers, with a corresponding increase in local recurrence from 0% to 75% (128). A positive radial margin is an independent prognostic factor for local recurrence with a hazard ratio of 12:2, and for survival with a hazard ratio of 3:2 compared to patients with clear circumferential margins (2,70)

Total Mesorectal Excision

The high local recurrence of disease following standard APR or LAR (15% to 30%) has been thought by some to be due to blunt dissection that violates the planes of the mesorectal circumference (46). Lateral spread of disease has been shown to occur not only at the level of the tumor but distally within the mesorectum as well (31). Heald et al. (74) have recommended that en bloc removal of the tumor within the envelope of the endopelvic fascia is necessary to obtain adequate lateral clearance of disease and reduce the likelihood of local recurrence. Total mesorectal excision (TME), as they described, has now become the established standard for all radical rectal cancer resections and requires sharp dissection along the plane that separates the visceral from the parietal pelvic fascia with complete en bloc removal of the rectum so that all of the rectal mesentery remains within the envelope of the specimen (98). On gross pathology, a correct TME specimen will have a bilobed

encapsulated appearance with the surface looking smooth and unbroken like a lipoma. On pathological review, an adequate dissection should include 12 to 15 perirectal and pelvic lymph nodes (14,73). Careful nerve sparing dissection with TME reduces the incidence of retrograde ejaculation and postoperative impotence as compared to conventional surgery (10% to 29% instead of 25% to 75%) (71,104,158). TME, while more difficult with APR than LAR, may be associated with a somewhat higher anastomotic leak rate especially for low rectal lesions (15% to 17%) (86,87). Several series using TME surgery have reported low rates of local recurrence (4% to 7%) and an improvement in survival approaching 80% to 85% for stage II and 65% to 70% for stage III disease (9,22,45,72).

Abdominoperineal Resection

APR has been considered the gold standard for surgical resection of distal rectal cancer and requires removal of the primary tumor along with a complete proctectomy, leading to a permanent colostomy (85). Recent data suggest a decline in the rate of abdominoperineal resections being performed. APR is associated with a slightly higher morbidity and mortality than LAR and a worse quality of life related to changes in body image and depression due to the presence of a colostomy (59,177). There is also a higher risk of positive margins with APR as the mesorectum is very thin in the distal segment of the rectum and lateral margins are restricted by the close presence of the prostate in the male and vagina in females (105). The bony confines of the lower pelvis also restrict surgical access especially in males.

Low Anterior Resection

The availability of circular stapling devices has expanded the role of sphincter preservation surgical options in rectal cancers, and LARs are now being performed not just for cancers of the upper third of the rectum but also for middle and lower third cancers (95). Preserving adequate anorectal function becomes a bigger problem the more distal the level of anorectal anastomosis (183). Patients should have good anal sphincter continence prior to considering sphincter-preserving options. Patient age, pelvic anatomy, gender, and body habitus can affect suitability for sphincter preservation. A 2-cm distal margin of preserved normal rectum is considered optimal for preservation of good bowel function. In carefully selected patients a functional coloanal anastomosis can be achieved with significantly reduced margins for more distal cancers especially after neoadjuvant therapy. If LAR is planned following neoadjuvant radiation therapy, it is necessary to mobilize the splenic flexure to allow an unirradiated segment of the bowel to be used for an anastomosis. The latter can be performed with several techniques, either an end-to-end, side-to-end, or with a colonic J-pouch technique to maximize preservation of sphincter function (99,135). Several studies comparing results of LAR to APR have generally reported similar outcomes for local and distant recurrence rates and survival as long as all surgical margins are negative (88,124,176). The absence of a colostomy, while offering a better quality of life with LAR, can be compromised with bowel urgency and frequency or poor sphincter control (10).

Local Excision

Early rectal cancer may also be treated by local excision techniques, avoiding major surgery and a colostomy, but patients need to be carefully selected for these procedures. A transanal approach is usually associated with the least morbidity, but to be amenable for local excision, tumors generally need to be located <8 cm from the anal verge. An anal sphincter splitting approach can be used for tumors close to the anorectal junction, and occasionally a presacral Kraske approach can be used to access more proximal tumors. The adequacy of the resection needs to be full thickness into the fat, and it is important that the tumor be removed in one piece with at least a 1-cm margin without fragmentation so that careful assessment of margins can be performed. A primary closure of the defect of the rectum is then performed. The inability to sample perirectal and mesenteric lymph nodes can result in underestimation of the cancer stage. Lymph node metastases have been observed in 5% to 10% of T1 lesions and 20% to 35% of patients with T2 lesions (24). It is therefore necessary to restrict local excision to patients with low-risk tumors where the risk of recurrence is <10% (i.e., T1 or favorable T2 cancers). T1 lesions have excellent results with local excision alone, with 5-year control rates ranging from 82% to 97% and survival rates of 90% or better (53,126). The risk of perirectal nodal metastasis and high incidence of reported local failure rates for T2 cancers following local excision alone indicate the need for further adjuvant therapy (108).

Radiation Therapy Oncology Group (RTOG) Protocol 89-02 (145) examined the efficacy of local excision in a study of 65 patients with distal rectal cancers. Tumors had to have margins ≥3 mm, no LVI, no regional LN ≥2 cm by CT scan, and be grade 1 or 2 to be eligible for observation. T2 tumors with margins ≤3 mm received 59.4 to 65 Gy. Fourteen patients with T1 tumors were observed after surgery, whereas 13 patients with T1 tumors, 25 patients with T2 tumors, and 13 patients with T3 tumors received local excision with postoperative radiation of 50 to 65 Gy with 5-FU (1,000 mg for meter squared on days 1 to 3 and 29 to 31). None of the T1 tumors that had postoperative treatment had any relapse as compared to one distant metastasis and one local failure in the T1 observation arm. Five patients in the T2 group had relapses (two local, one distant, three both), and four patients in the T3 group suffered relapse (one distant, three both). Therefore, 20% of T2 and 23% of T3 tumors experienced local failure after local excision plus radiation chemotherapy. Therefore, while it is possible that highly selected T2 and limited T3 tumors may be treated with local excision and postoperative adjuvant therapy, the high locoregional failures makes this a nonstandard approach.

The Cancer and Leukemia Group B (CALGB) 8984 study provides some support for postoperative combined radiation and chemotherapy after local excision for T1 and T2 rectal cancers (157). Fifty-nine patients with T1 disease were treated with local excision alone, while 51 patients with T2 disease received adjuvant therapy consisting of T2 postoperative 54 Gy and 5-Fu (500 mg per meter squared on days of 1 to 3 and 29 to 31). T1 tumors had a 95% 4-year local control and 85% overall survival at 6 years as compared to T2 patients, who had a 85% local control and 70% overall survival. One out of two T1 local failures and four out five T2 local failures were salvaged by APR. Five T2 patients died with distant failure. Of note, 25% of the clinical T1 and T2 tumors were actually pathological T3. The 20% recurrence rate for T2 cancers in this trial and a 6-year disease-free survival rate of 71% is considerably inferior to the results of radical surgery with TME alone or neoadjuvant therapy followed by surgery. Therefore, although this study supports the use of adjuvant radiation and chemotherapy for adverse T1 and favorable T2 tumors, one should proceed with caution given the high local failure rate.

Based on the available data, local excision should be limited to tumors that are small (<4 cm), are clinically T1 or T2, well to moderately differentiated, and involve <40% of the circumference of the rectum. These tumors are usually mobile, polypoid, not ulcerated, and have favorable pathology including no lymphovascular or blood-vascular invasion (116).

Adjuvant Therapy

Postoperative

The problem of unacceptably high local recurrence after surgery has led to many studies exploring the potential benefit of postoperative adjuvant therapy (12,40). One of the advantages of postoperative radiation is the ability to selectively treat patients at high risk of local failure on the basis of pathologic stage. Disadvantages include a potentially hypoxic postsurgical bed, making radiation less effective and potentially higher complications due to increased small bowel in the radiation field, and a larger treatment volume, especially if the patient undergoes an APR and the perineal scar needs to be covered.

There have been several large trials of postoperative radiation with or without chemotherapy (3,94,138). In general, surgery alone has resulted in a 25% local failure rate and 40% to 50% overall survival for T3 or T4 or node-positive patients, while radiation with the addition of chemotherapy has yielded a lower local failure rate of 10% to 15% and higher overall survival rate of 50% to 60%.

The National Surgical Adjuvant Breast and Bowel Project (NSABP) R-01study randomized 555 patients into three arms after surgery: (a) observation, (b) postoperative chemotherapy of eight cycles of MOF (5FU, CCNU [semustine], and vincristine), and (c) postoperative radiation treatment alone of 46 to 47 Gy (49). Postoperative chemotherapy improved disease-free survival but not overall survival. The benefit of improved overall survival with MOF was restricted to men in subset analysis. Postoperative radiation treatment trended toward improved local control but not overall survival.

The NSABP R-02 study (182) enrolled 694 stage B and C patients and asked two questions in its study design: (a) Does the addition of radiation to chemotherapy improve outcome? and (b) Is MOF superior to 5-FU/LV in men? There were four treatment arms for males and two treatment arms for females. Five cycles of MOF were compared to six cycles of 5-FU/LV with or without radiation for the men. For women, 5-FU/LV was compared against additional radiation. The radiation dose was 50.4 Gy. At 5 years, the locoregional failure was 13% for the chemotherapy only arm as compared to 8% with the addition of radiation and chemotherapy. Additionally, 5-FU/LV showed better relapse-free survival and disease-free survival but not overall survival as compared to MOF. The conclusions of the two NSABP trials were that while postoperative radiation treatment did not appear to improve overall survival, there was an improvement in local control.

Two trials that did show an improvement in survival were the Gastrointestinal Tumor Study Group (GITSG) and North Central Cancer Treatment Group (NCCTG) studies. GITSG study was a four-arm trial of 227 patients with stage B2 and C rectal cancer who were randomized to either (a) surgery alone, (b) postoperative chemotherapy of bolus 5-FU (500 mg/m^2 in weeks 1 and 5 and methyl-CCNU (semustine given day 1), (c) postoperative radiation treatment of 40 to 48 Gy split course, or (d) postoperative chemotherapy and radiation therapy of 40 to 44 Gy plus bolus 5-FU (138). The severe acute toxicity was 61% in the combined modality treatment arm as compared to 31% with chemotherapy only and 18% with radiation only. In a 9-year update, postoperative chemotherapy and radiation therapy improved the overall survival to 54% versus 27% with observation after surgery. There was a prolonged time to recurrence and a decreased recurrence rate of 33% versus 55% with combined adjuvant treatment. Local failure rate was decreased to 10% versus 25% with surgery alone. Therefore, this trial concluded a significant overall survival advantage of nearly double for patients who had combined modality treatment after surgical resection.

The Mayo-NCCTG compared postoperative radiation therapy against postoperative radiation therapy and chemotherapy (94). Two hundred and four patients were included with T3 or T4 or node-positive tumors and all received one cycle of 5FU and semustine before randomization. The radiation dose was 45 to 50.4 Gy. The 5-year local regional failure was higher in the radiation only arm of 25% versus 15%, and the 5-year overall survival rate was 40% versus 55%. Combined postoperative chemotherapy and radiation therapy reduced recurrence by 34%, local recurrence by 46%, and distant metastases by 37%. Cancer deaths were reduced by 36%, and overall deaths were reduced by 29%.

Based on the results of these studies, the National Institute of Health Consensus Conference recommended that the combined use of radiation and chemotherapy is more effective than postoperative radiation alone, with a greater potential for improved survival, and is recommended. Several subsequent studies have attempted to delineate the kind of chemotherapy and delivery options in the combined modality treatment (129).

NCCTG 86-47-51 study compared chemotherapy regimens to be added to the postoperative radiation. Six hundred sixty stage II or III patients were randomized to systemic chemotherapy given (5-FU vs. 5-FU + semustine) and the method of delivery (bolus vs. continuous infusion 5-FU) (131). Nine weeks of chemotherapy were given followed by the experimental chemotherapy concurrently with 50.4 to 54 Gy radiation with additional chemotherapy thereafter. The bolus 5FU dose was 500 mg/m^2 on day 1 to 5 during weeks 1 and 5, whereas the continuous infusion 5-FU was 225 mg/m^2 per day. With a median follow-up of 46 months, there was a 27% improvement in relapse-free survival of 63% versus 53% in favor of continuous infusion 5-FU. The 4-year overall survival was 70% versus 60% in favor of continuous infusion. The time to relapse and the distant metastasis rate (31% vs. 40%) were also lower. There was no difference in local recurrence. Bolus 5-FU had a higher rate of leucopenia, while continuous infusion had more acute severe diarrhea. Semustine was of no additional benefit.

Intergroup 0114 study compared different chemotherapy regimens with radiation treatment for 1,695 patients (159). There were four arms of the study comparing (a) bolus 5-FU alone, (b) 5-FU and leucovorin, (c) 5FU plus levamisole, and (d) 5-FU and leucovorin plus levamisole. The levamisole was not given during the radiation treatment. The radiation treatment dose was 45 Gy with a 5.4- to 9-Gy boost to a total of 50.4 to 54 Gy. With a median follow-up of 7.4 years, there was no difference in overall survival or disease-free survival among the four groups. The three-drug regimen had a greater toxicity. Levamisole and leucovorin did not appear to add any benefit to the 5-FU.

Favorable T3N0

Several studies have shown that there may be a subset of tumors that might not need adjuvant therapy because of low risk of recurrence with surgery alone. Memorial Sloan-Kettering evaluated 95 patients with T3N0 rectal cancer treated by surgery alone (109). Seventy-nine patients underwent LAR and 16% underwent APR, both with sharp mesorectal excision. With 53.3-month follow-up, 6% had a local recurrence, 13% had distant metastases, and 3% had both local recurrence and distant metastases. Lymphovascular invasion was the only histological factor that was important for local recurrence. This study suggests that sharp mesorectal excision with LAR or APR for T3N0 rectal cancers results in low local recurrences of <10% without the use of adjuvant therapy.

In a retrospective review of 117 patients with T3N0 rectal cancer treated at MGH Willett et al. (170) reported that perirectal tumor invasion ≥2 mm, LVI, and poorly differentiated his-

tology were independent factors for increased risk of distant metastasis and worse relapse-free survival. Only depth of invasion was significant for local control. Of the 25 patients with favorable histological features (well differentiated/moderately differentiated, invading <2 mm into the perirectal fat, no LVI), the 10-year actuarial local control and relapse-free survival were 95% and 87%, respectively, as compared to 71% and 55% in the unfavorable group. Thus, a limited subset of patients with T3N0 rectal cancer may have an excellent outcome with surgery alone, but there are no randomized data to support the omission of adjuvant therapy for this group of patients at the present time.

Side Effects of Combined Chemoradiation

Although combined chemoradiation is the recommended approach for postoperative adjuvant therapy, it has to be kept in mind that the acute side effects can be considerably greater than postoperative radiation alone. In the NCCTG 79-47-51 study the incidence of nausea, vomiting, and diarrhea were significantly higher than with radiation alone (114). Patients also developed more stomatitis with mucosal ulceration and a slightly greater hematological toxicity as well (9% vs. 2%). Hydration is therefore critical in these patients as some patients may exhibit hypersensitivity to 5-FU with grade 4 diarrhea and an occasional death due to dehydration. Patients need to be supported with intravenous fluids and treatment interruption until the diarrhea is stabilized. Severe late toxicity was similar in both arms (7%). The incidence of diarrhea is greater with continuous infusion of 5-FU as compared to bolus 5-FU, and hand/foot syndrome is also more common in infusional therapy (97,114). In the Intergroup trials, 24% of patients receiving concurrent pelvic radiation and continuous infusion 5-FU experienced severe or life-threatening diarrhea (113). Chronic bowel injury was seen in 25% of the patients treated with postoperative radiation.

A key late side effect with postoperative radiation in patients undergoing low anterior resection is rectal urgency with frequent bowel movements, known as clustering. Patients can have six to 10 bowel movements in a short period of time, which can be quite distressing. There is also the likelihood of frequent nighttime bowel movements and occasional incontinence. These symptoms are related to the development in anastomotic strictures and fibrosis with lack of elasticity of the neo-rectum (93,101).

Treatment Technique for Postop Adjuvant Treatment

External-beam treatment portals for rectal carcinoma should always encompass the sites at greatest risk: The presacral space, the primary tumor site, and (for post-APR cases) the perineum. Other areas at risk include the internal iliac and distal common iliac nodes. The risk in the para-aortic region is sufficiently low, and the morbidity from treatment is sufficiently high to exclude this region from adjuvant rectal cancer radiation portals. The external iliac nodes should be covered for lesions extending to the dentate line.

In general, patients with rectal carcinoma should be treated in the prone position because this reduces the volume of small bowel within the pelvis (54). For patients with prior pelvic surgery, maneuvers to reduce volume of small bowel include treatment with a full bladder and the use of bowel-displacement techniques such as a belly board (foam board table with a cutout to allow the upper-abdominal contents to fall forward) or a foam board mound designed to push the full bladder posteriorly and cephalad (54). The use of shaped lateral fields reduces the dose to small bowel located in the anterior superior aspects of the pelvis.

If conventional (two-dimensional) treatment planning is used, a four-field (anteroposterior/posteroanterior [AP/PA]/right/left [R/L] lateral) or three-field (PA/R/L lateral) technique generally is used. The superior port edge is placed at the L4/L5 interspace—usually in the mid-L5 vertebral body. The distal port edge should be 5 cm below palpable tumor for patients receiving preoperative treatment. For postoperative cases the distal port edge is about 5 cm below the best estimate of the preoperative tumor bed and (if an APR has been performed) below the perineum. Anterior and posterior portals must have at least a 1.5-cm margin on the pelvic brim. There is an underappreciated incidence of lateral pelvic lymph node involvement that is not part of the routine resection of the rectum or the rectal mesentery.

Lateral treatment portals should encompass the entire sacrum posteriorly. A radiopaque marker should be placed at the posterior aspect of the anus to make certain that blocks in the posterior-inferior aspect of the portal do not impinge on targeted portions of anorectum. The anterior margin should be at least 4 cm anterior to the rectum, as determined by the rectal contrast placed at simulation. The use of intrarectal contrast during simulation ensures that the portals will be designed with the rectum at maximum distension. If the tumor has considerable extrarectal extension, then these guidelines should be modified to make certain that all macroscopic disease (determined by CT scan) is encompassed with about a 4-cm margin.

The usual dose given to pelvic portals is 4,500 cGy in 25 fractions of 180 cGy each. An additional boost is recommended for patients receiving postoperative radiation (164). Small bowel must be excluded from the boost volume after about 5,000 cGy. Typically, if small bowel cannot be excluded, the boost dose is 540 cGy. If it can be excluded, the usual boost dose is 900 cGy.

Recently, three-dimensional (3D) treatment planning has begun to be applied to rectal cancer (123). This is implemented best with careful attention to the concepts of clinical target volume (CTV) and planning target volumes (PTV). The initial CTV should include macroscopic disease with an approximately 2-cm margin in mesentery and within the course of the large bowel. In addition, the initial CTV should include rectal mesentery and nodal regions at risk.

Although there is no consensus on the optimum time for start of postoperative radiation, it is therefore recommended that treatment should begin 3 to 6 weeks after surgery.

Neoadjuvant Therapy

Considerable debate has evolved regarding the optimal approach to adjuvant therapy in rectal cancer. Although both pre- and postoperative adjuvant therapy can be effective, there has been a significant recent trend toward greater use of neoadjuvant treatment. Tumor down staging, improved resectability, and potential for expanded sphincter preservation options in the distal rectum also encourage the use of a neoadjuvant approach in the management of this disease. Historically several trials utilizing relatively moderate doses of preoperative radiation have been undertaken, with results consistently showing an improvement in local control but minimal or no improvement in overall survival (42,75,92). Recent studies from Europe have demonstrated that appropriate neoadjuvant preoperative radiation results in improvement of both local control and survival, and these results have had a significant impact on the current management of this disease (52,86).

The Swedish rectal preoperative radiation trial included 1,168 patients from 1987 to 1990 with resectable, Dukes A–C rectal cancer (133). Patients were randomized to 25 Gy in five fractions in 1 week followed by surgery 1 week later versus surgery alone. The surgery was rated as curative if margins were negative. With a median follow-up of 7 years there was a

significant reduction in local control in all three Dukes stages with preoperative radiation therapy as compared to surgery alone. The 5-year local recurrence with preoperative radiation treatment was 12% versus 27% for surgery alone. The local recurrence with preoperative radiation and curative surgery was 9% versus 23% with curative surgery alone. This study showed a 10% absolute overall survival advantage for preoperative radiation therapy of 58% versus 48% at 9 years ($p = 0.004$) and an advantage in cancer-specific survival among all patients of 74% in the preoperative arm versus 65% in the surgery only arm ($p = 0.002$).

One caveat of this study is that the surgery alone arm did not utilize TME, which may have resulted in an unacceptably high local failure rate of 27%. Late effects suggested more bowel movement frequency, incontinence, urgency, and soiling in the preoperative radiation treatment arm, although overall quality of life was rated good (19). This trial set the standard of care in many European centers, but the dose of 5 Gy times five fractions may induce significant acute and late toxicity, and the short interval between radiation and surgery may not have allowed sufficient time for tumor regression (downstaging) for improved sphincter preservation. Justification for a longer interval after preoperative radiation treatment before surgery was given by a French trial, Lyon 90–01, which delivered 39 Gy in 3 Gy per fraction without any chemotherapy preoperatively (50). Two hundred one patients were randomized after 6 to 8 weeks. The local control and overall survival after a median follow-up of 33 months were the same in both arms of the study. However, the pathological complete response was 7% versus 14% ($p = $ NSS) and the pathological down staging was 10% versus 26% ($p = 0.007$) in favor of the longer interval before surgery.

The TME experience by Heald et al. (74) suggested that TME alone is sufficient for achieving low local recurrence rates. A Dutch (CKVO 95–04) multicenter, phase III study of 1,861 patients was undertaken to evaluate the role of short course preoperative radiation with TME. Patients were randomized to TME alone versus 25 Gy in five fractions followed by TME surgery (86). No fixed tumors were included in the study, and half of the patients had T1 or T2 disease. The overall survival was the same in both arms of the study (82% at 2 years). However the local recurrence at 2 years was 8.2% in the TME-only arm as compared to 2.4% in the preoperative arm, highlighting the value of radiation treatment, even with TME. The sphincter preservation rate was the same in both arms, and there was no clear evidence of any downstaging effect. The perineal complication rate was slightly higher in the preoperative radiation arm of 26% versus 18% in the TME arm, while all other complications were equal. A more recent update indicates a higher incidence of sexual dysfunction and slower recovery of bowel function, more fecal incontinence, and generally poorer quality of life with short-course preoperative radiation.

Two meta-analyses of approximately 6,000 patients each were done to explore the benefit of preoperative radiation treatment. One analysis included 14 randomized controlled trials and reported that neoadjuvant radiation treatment was associated with significantly fewer local recurrences, improved specific survival, and an overall survival benefit (27). The second meta-analysis, provided by the Colorectal Cancer Collaborative Group, also reported on 14 randomized controlled trials (3). They noted a significant reduction in the risk of local recurrence and death from rectal cancer with preoperative radiotherapy.

Neoadjuvant Chemoradiation

The improvement in outcomes with combined chemoradiation and postoperative adjuvant therapy has led to similar recent approaches in the neoadjuvant therapy of this disease. In the

United States this has become widely accepted, but in other parts of the world several groups have undertaken studies to examine the potential benefit from neoadjuvant chemoradiation as compared to radiation alone.

Preoperative radiation therapy was compared with combined preoperative chemotherapy and radiation therapy in a French study (Fédération Francophone de la Canérologie Digestive), FFCD 9203 (56). Patients with resectable T3 and T4 tumors were randomized to 45 Gy of radiation alone versus radiation with concurrent bolus 5-FU (350 mg/m^2) plus leucovorin on days 1 to 5 during weeks 1 to 5. After surgery, four cycles of adjuvant chemotherapy were given. With a median follow-up of 69 months, there was an equivalent rate (51%) of sphincter-sparing surgery. Combined treatment led to improved pathological complete response rate of 11.4% versus 3.6% and an improved 5-year local failure rate of 8% versus 16.5%. There was, however, no difference in overall survival.

A similar study undertaken by the European Organization for Research and Treatment of Cancer (EORTC 22921) randomized patients to four arms, 45 Gy alone versus 45 Gy plus 5-FU leucovorin followed by surgery and patients further randomized to adjuvant therapy with 5-FU leucovorin (23). Results of the study indicate similar results to the French study with increased downstaging (14% versus 5.3%; $p = 0.0001$) with no difference in five-year survival (56% versus 54%). However, local control was significantly improved with the addition of chemotherapy. This information suggests that while there is less recurrence, there is no conclusive evidence that combined treatment offers a survival benefit compared to radiation alone. There was, however, a higher incidence of acute toxicity associated with combined chemoradiation.

In contrast to these studies, institutional experience from the United States does suggest significantly higher downstaging with the use of preoperative chemotherapy, and several institutional studies suggest an improvement in overall survival, and, therefore, notwithstanding the results from the randomized studies, most investigators currently utilize a combined modality approach to neoadjuvant therapy in this disease (149).

A study to determine whether a short course (5 Gy for five fractions) approach to neoadjuvant therapy is better than a protracted approach 50.4 Gy using 1.8 to 2 Gy fractions with concomitant bolus 5-FU and leucovorin given during weeks 1 and 5 was undertaken by the Polish rectal cancer group (26). Although a higher pathologic complete-response rate was seen with chemoradiation (16% vs. 1%), fewer positive radial margins (4% vs. 13%), and considerably reduced size of the tumor by approximately 1.9 cm no difference in the rate of sphincter preservation, local control or survival was seen.

There is considerable difference in the way chemotherapy has been administered in many of the trials undertaken and those that are ongoing. 5-FU has been used concurrent with radiation because of its well-established potentiating effect with radiation. However, several studies have used bolus 5-FU, while others have used leucovorin-modulated 5-FU during the first and last week of radiation. The results of the Intergroup study demonstrating a superiority of low-dose continuous infusion of 5-FU has been extrapolated to the neoadjuvant setting and appears to be the preferred approach to treatment (131). New drugs, including oxaliplatin, irinotecan, and oral fluoropyrimidines, have recently been shown to be effective in the treatment of metastatic colorectal cancer. These have now been incorporated into testing of new strategies with neoadjuvant therapy. Capecitabine is an oral fluoropyrimidine prodrug that is readily absorbed in the gastrointestinal tract and mimics the efficacy of continuous infusion 5-FU while avoiding the risk of side effects and complications due to a central line for CVI 5-FU (39). Capecitabine requires the presence of thymidine phosphorylase (TP) for conversion to the active form of 5-FU within the cells. TP is present in higher concentration in tumor cells, particularly

colorectal cancer than in normal tissues, and this potentially creates a therapeutic advantage for capecitabine as compared to intravenous 5-FU (151). Studies of capecitabine in combination with radiation have shown similar response rates to 5FU, and, therefore, this drug appears promising for trials in the neoadjuvant therapy (43,44,89). Capecitabine is generally given in two divided doses, 825 mg twice a day during the course of radiation treatment. Acute toxicity of diarrhea, stomatitis, nausea, and neutropenia are also somewhat less with capecitabine than with 5-FU/leucovorin, however, the incidence of hand/foot syndrome is higher with capecitabine (30).

Several newer options for neoadjuvant therapy include the addition of irinotecan or oxaliplatin to 5-FU and radiation (11,100,143,144). Early data from phase 1 and 2 trials suggest that an oxaliplatin dose of 60 mg/m^2 can be combined safely with continuous infusion 5-FU and standard radiation approaches with acceptable grade 3 toxicity and promising rates of pathological downstaging and with CR rates of 20% to 30%. Toxicity of irinotecan with a dose of 50 mg/m^2 once a week with continuous infusion 5-FU and radiation in the combined modality approach is somewhat higher but appears to be tolerable and also has yielded high response rates with complete responses of 25% to 30% (117). Ongoing phase III trials in the United States and Europe are evaluating capecitabine and oxaliplatin delivered neoadjuvantly with radiation therapy.

RTOG 00–12 is a randomized phase II study of neoadjuvant combined modality combined-modality radiation for distal rectal cancer. One-hundred and three patients with T3 or T4 distal rectal cancer (<9 cm from the dentate line) were randomized to continuous venous infusion 5-FU plus hyperfractionated radiation treatment of 55.2 to 60 Gy (1.2 Gy twice a day) versus continuous venous infusion 5-FU and irinotecan with conventional fractionation radiation of 50 to 54 Gy (1.8 Gy per fraction). The response rate between the two arms was similar with a pathological complete response rate of 28%, higher than in other studies (121).

Radiation dose is of critical importance in downstaging of cancer. The dose response of rectal cancer is steep in the dose range of 40 to 60 Gy. Several studies have shown the impact of radiation dose escalation on the rate of pathological complete response to neoadjuvant therapy (6,122). In a review of patients at Princess Margaret Hospital who received 40 Gy, 46 Gy, or 50 Gy in 2 Gy/fraction with continuous infusion 5-FU, the pathological complete response was 18%, 23%, and 33% respectively for the three dose levels (121). The two-year local relapse-free survival was 72%, 90%, 89% and disease-free survival 62%, 84%, and 78% for the 40 Gy, 46 Gy, and 50 Gy levels respectively (178). The overall survival was 72%, 94%, and 92% respectively. Doses of 46 Gy or 50 Gy were more effective than 40 Gy, but there was no difference between 46 or 50 Gy. Similar results have been reported from other studies as well.

Preoperative Versus Postoperative

Three phase III trials were conducted to compare preoperative versus postoperative chemoradiation treatment. The first trial was an RTOG 94-01/Intergroup 0417 trial that accrued 53 patients but closed early due to poor accrual. NSABP R-03 was scheduled to accrue 900 patients but also closed after accruing 267 patients (81). Patients with operable adenocarcinoma of the rectum were randomized (and stratified based on age and sex) to surgery followed by one cycle of 5-FU/LV and then concurrent bolus (weeks 1 and 5) 5-FU/LV with radiation treatment versus 5-FU/LV for 1 cycle then concurrent chemoradiation treatment followed by surgery. All patients received adjuvant 5-FU and leucovorin for four cycles. The study was underpowered, but the 1-year results showed a 10% sphincter preservation advantage in the preoperative arm (44% vs. 34%) with slightly higher grade 4 and 5 toxicity (34% vs. 23%) and diarrhea (24% vs. 12%) in this

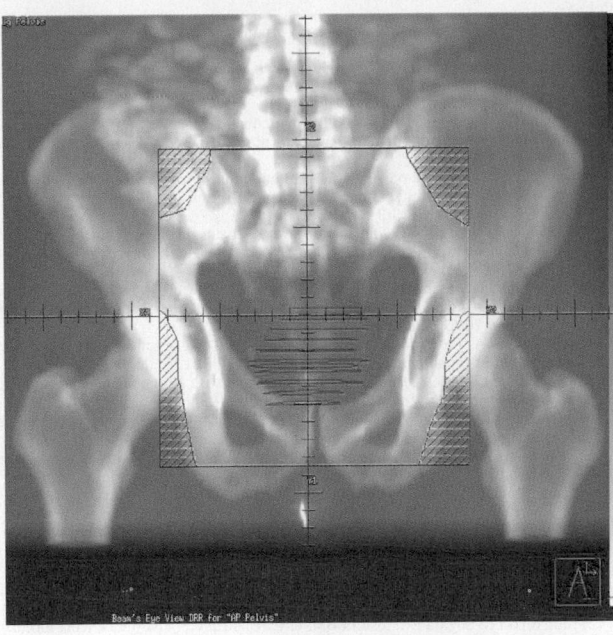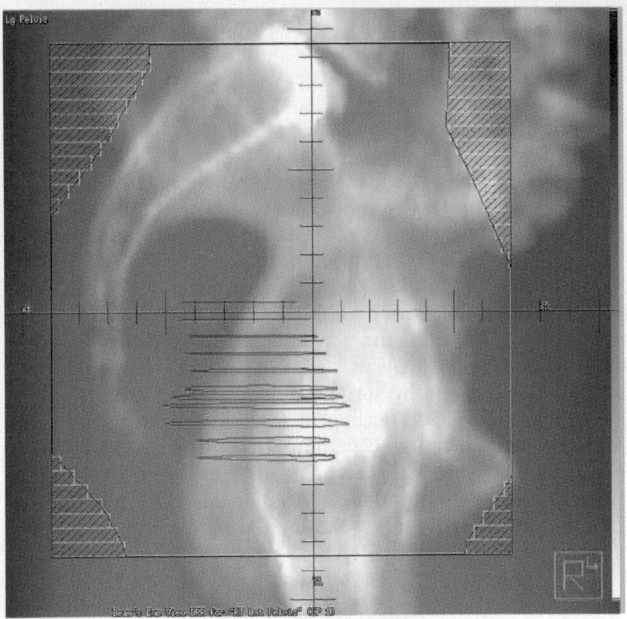

A   B

FIGURE 58.5. A: AP portal of patient with T4 rectal cancer. **B:** Lateral portal of a patient with T4 rectal cancer.

arm as well. The clinical complete response rate was 23%, and the pathological complete response rate was 10%. The disease-free survival at 1 year was 83% preop versus 78% postop (p = NSS).

The definitive phase III study in favor of preoperative radiation therapy was the CAO/ARO/AIO-94 study performed by the German Rectal Cancer group (149). Eight hundred twenty-three clinically staged T3 and T4 or node-positive rectal cancers were randomized to arm 1: Preoperative chemotherapy and radiation therapy followed by TME 6 weeks later, or arm 2: TME followed by postoperative chemotherapy and radiation therapy. The radiation therapy used was 50.4 Gy in 28 fractions with a 5.4 Gy as a small volume boost in the postoperative arm. The chemotherapy used was 5-FU given as 1 g/m^2 per day during the 1st and 5th weeks of radiotherapy as a 120-hour continuous infusion. Both arms received four additional cycles of 5-FU at 500 mg/m^2 per day for 5 days every 4 weeks. All surgeons were trained in the use of TME and were asked prior to treatment to evaluate the possibility of sphincter preservation. The 5-year results revealed a pelvic recurrence ratio of 6% versus 13% (p = 0.02) in favor of the preoperative arm. The distant recurrence rate was 36% versus 38% (p = NSS), disease-free survival was 68% versus 65% (p = NSS), and overall survival was 76% versus 74% (p = NSS) for preoperative radiation versus postoperative, respectively. There was significant tumor downstaging after preoperative combined modality treatment with an 8% pathological complete response rate. Nodal positivity was 25% in the preoperative versus 40% in the postoperative arm. The sphincter preservation rate in 188 patients with low-lying tumors (declared by the surgeon prior to randomization to require an APR) revealed that 39% versus 19% had a sphincter-preserving low anterior resection (p = 0.004) in the preoperative versus the postoperative arm. There were fewer acute (27% vs. 40%) and late toxicities (14% vs. 24%) in preoperative-treatment group. Thus, preoperative combined preoperative chemotherapy and radiation therapy resulted in significantly less local failures in the pelvis by half and also provided twice the sphincter preservation. Importantly, there was no difference in overall survival or disease-free survival between the two arms.

An example of radiation fields employed preoperatively are shown in Figure 58.5A,B. This patient received 45 Gy with four fields (AP/PA, right and left lateral) followed by field reductions to a dose of 50.4 to 54 Gy, as used with a patient with a T4 rectal cancer.

Locally Advanced Rectal Cancer

Clinical T4 tumors may not be resected completely due to tumor fixation. Preoperative radiation treatment is recommended to facilitate curative resections.

M.D. Anderson investigators demonstrated that preoperative chemotherapy and radiation therapy increased overall survival (80% vs. 60%), local control (95% vs. 66%), and the number of sphincter preserving procedures (35% vs. 7%) as compared to radiation alone (167). Memorial Sloan-Kettering Cancer Center reported a gross total resection rate of 97%, pathological complete response rate of 25%, 4-year local control of 70%, and 4-year overall survival of 67% when giving preoperative chemotherapy of 5-FU and leucovorin with 50.4 Gy of radiation followed by surgery (115). Preoperative radiation and chemotherapy resulted in improved resectability rates and possible improved local control and survival.

The IORT experience at MGH was reviewed by Nakfoor et al. (125). Preoperative continuous infusion 5-FU plus 50.4 to 54 Gy of radiation was given followed by a 4- to 6-week break and surgery. No intraoperative radiation was given if metastases were present at surgical exploration, if there were adequate margins >1 cm, or if there was less than T4 disease. Ten to 12.5 Gy were given for complete resection, 12.5 to 15 Gy for microscopic residual, and 17.5 to 20 Gy for gross residual disease. The 5-year local control was 90%, 65%, 55%, and the disease specific survival at 5 years was 65%, 45%, and 15%, for these three dose levels, respectively. The 5-year actuarial risk of complications was 15%, however. The risk of peripheral neuropathy was 20% for doses >15 Gy. IORT improves local control, especially with a gross total resection, but not survival for locally advanced rectal cancer.

Reirradiation

Recurrent rectal cancer is often approached the same way as T4 disease with an aggressive treatment plan of combined chemotherapy and radiation therapy followed by surgery and then adjuvant chemotherapy. At the time of surgery, IORT is considered. Approximately 10% of patients with T1 and T2N0 disease will fail locally after surgery, usually due to an inadequate lymph node dissection. The recurrences are found along the pelvic sidewall or in nonpelvic sidewall areas such as the uterus, prostate, or vagina. Because the pelvic sidewall is a difficult surgical resection, these recurrences face worse. The 5-year overall survival is approximately 20% (165). The local control is about 40% in patients with no prior radiation to 10% to 20% in patients who had prior radiation.

Forty-seven patients in an Italian retrospective study were treated with preoperative combined chemotherapy and radiation therapy (162). Patients who did not have prior radiation treatment received 45 Gy with continuous infusion 5-FU and mitomycin C followed by surgery and intraoperative radiation therapy of 10 to 15 Gy. Leucovorin and 5-FU were given for six to nine cycles adjuvantly. If patients had prior radiation treatment, they were given 23.4 Gy instead. The 5-year overall survival was 20% for all patients, 60% for resected tumors, 0% for unresected tumors, and 40% for patients treated by external beam, surgery, and IORT. The 5-year local control rate was 30% for all patients, 70% for completely resected tumors, 0% for unresectable tumors, and 80% for external beam, surgery, and IORT. Eighty-five percent had palliation of pain with a duration of 12 months.

Long-term results of reirradiation for patients with recurrent rectal carcinoma were reported by Mohiuddin et al. (119). One-hundred and three patients who developed locoregional recurrence after surgery with preoperative or postoperative radiation treatment (median dose 50.4 Gy) were reirradiated with concurrent 5FU continuous infusion. Patients were treated with opposed laterals or a three-field technique with a posterior field and two laterals to the presacral area and gross tumor volume with 2- to 4-cm margin. Patients received 30 Gy (1.2 Gy twice a day) or 30.6 Gy (1.8 Gy every day) followed by a boost of 6 to 20 Gy to gross tumor volume (2 cm margin). Forty-one patients were surgically explored after treatment, and 34 underwent resection, with six patients having sphincter sparing surgery. With immediate follow-up of 2 years, the 5-year overall survival rate was 19%. Patients who underwent resection had a higher survival rate with tolerable acute and late toxicity. Palliation of bleeding was achieved in 100% of patients.

References

1. Adalsteinsson B, Glimelius B, Graffman S, et al. Computed tomography in staging of rectal carcinoma. *Acta Radiol Diagn* 1985;26:45.
2. Adam IJ, Mohamdee MO, Martin IG, et al. Role of circumferential margin involvement in the local recurrence of rectal cancer. *Lancet* 1994;344:707.
3. Adjuvant radiotherapy for rectal cancer: A systematic overview of 8507 patients from 22 randomised trials. Colorectal Cancer Collaborative Group. *Lancet* 2001;358:1291.
4. AJCC (American Joint Committee on Cancer). In: Greene FL, Page DL, Fleming ID, et al., eds. *Cancer staging manual*, 6th ed. New York: Springer-Verlag, 2002;114.
5. Aldridge, MC, Phillips RKS, Hittinger R, Fry JS, et al. Influence of tumor site on presentation, management and subsequent outcome in large bowel cancer. *Br J Surg* 73:663–670.
6. Allal AS, Bieri S, Brundler MA. Preoperative hyperfractionated radiotherapy for locally advanced rectal cancers: A phase I-II trial. *Int J Radiat Oncol Biol Phys* 2002;54(4):1076–1081.
7. Amos EH, Mendenhall WM, McCarty PJ, et al. Postoperative radiotherapy for locally advanced colon cancer. *Ann Surg Oncol* 1996;3:431–436.
8. André T, Boni C, Mounedji-Boudiaf L, et al. Oxaliplatin, fluorouracil and leucovorin as adjuvant treatment for colon cancer. *N Engl J Med* 2004;350:2343–2351.
9. Arbman G, Nilsson E, Hallbook O, et al. Local recurrence following total mesorectal excision for rectal cancer. *Br J Surg* 1996;83:375.
10. Armendariz P, Ortiz H. Anterior resection: Do the patients perceive any clinical benefit? *Int J Colorectal Dis* 1996;11(4):191–195.
11. Aschele, C, Friso, ML, Pucciarelli, S, et al. A phase I-II study of weekly oxaliplatin, 5-fluorouracil continuous infusion and preoperative radiotherapy in locally advanced rectal cancer. *Ann Oncol* 2005;16:1140.
12. Balslev I, Pedersen M, Teglbjaerg PS, et al. Postoperative radiotherapy in Dukes' B and C carcinoma of the rectum and rectosigmoid. A randomized multicenter study. *Cancer* 1986;58:22.
13. Balthazar EJ, Megibow AJ, Hulnick D, et al. Carcinoma of the colon: Detection and preoperative staging by CT. *AJR Am J Roentgenol* 1988;150:301.
14. Baxter NN, Virnig DJ, Rothenberger DA, et al. Lymph node evaluation in colorectal cancer patients: A population-based study. *J Natl Cancer Inst* 2005;97:219.
15. Beahrs OH, Sanfelippo PM. Factors in prognosis of colon and rectal cancer. *Cancer* 1971;28:213.
16. Beets-Tan RG, Beets GL, Bortslap AC, et al. Preoperative assessment of local tumor extent in advanced rectal cancer: CT or high resolution MRI? *Abdom Imaging* 2000;25:533.
17. Beets-Tan RG, Beets GL, Vliegen RF, et al. Accuracy of magnetic resonance imaging in prediction of tumour-free resection margin in rectal cancer surgery. *Lancet* 2001;357:497.
18. Beynon J, Foy DM, Roe AM, et al. Endoluminal ultrasound in the assessment of local invasion in rectal cancer. *Br J Surg* 1986;73:474.
19. Birgisson. *JCO* 2005;23(34):8697–8705.
20. Black WA, Waugh JM. The intramural extension of carcinoma of the descending colon, sigmoid, and rectosigmoid: A pathologic study. *Surg Gynecol Obstet* 1948;87:457.
21. Blomqvist L, Machado M, Rubio C, et al. Rectal tumour staging: MR imaging using pelvic phased-array and endorectal coils vs endoscopic ultrasonography. *Eur Radiol* 2000;10:653.
22. Bolognese A, Cardi M, Muttillo IA, et al. Total mesorectal excision for surgical treatment of rectal cancer. *J Surg Oncol* 2000;74:21.
23. Bosset JF, Collette L, Calais G. Chemotherapy with preoperative radiotherapy in rectal cancer. *N Engl J Med* 2006;355:1114–1123.
24. Brodsky JT, Richard GK, Cohen AM, et al. Variables correlated with the risk of lymph node metastasis in early rectal cancer. *Cancer* 1992;69:322.
25. Brown G, Richards CJ, Bourne MW, et al. Morphologic predictors of lymph node status in rectal cancer with use of high-spatial-resolution MR imaging with histopathologic comparison. *Radiology* 2003;227:371.
26. Bujko K, Nowacki MP, Nasierowska-Gutt Mejer A, et al. Long-term results of a randomized trial comparing preoperative short course radiotherapy with preoperative conventionally fractionated chemoradiation for rectal cancer. *Br J Surg* 2006;93:1215–1223.
27. Camma C, Giunta M, Fiorica F, et al. Preoperative radiotherapy for resectable rectal cancer: A meta-analysis. *JAMA* 2000;284:1008.
28. Carraro PG, Segala M, Cesana BM, et al. Obstructing colonic cancer: Failure and survival patterns over a ten-year follow-up after one-stage curative surgery. *Dis Colon Rectum* 2001;44:243.
29. Cassidy J, Scheithauer W, McKendrick J, et al. Capecitabine (X) versus bolus 5-FU/LV as adjuvant therapy for colon cancer (the X-ACT study): Positive efficacy results of a phase III trial. *Proc Am Soc Clin Oncol (Post-Meeting Ed)* 2004;22(abstr 3509.
30. Cassidy J, Twelves C, Van Cutsem E, et al. First-line oral capecitabine therapy in metastatic colorectal cancer: A favorable safety profile compared with intravenous 5-fluorouracil/leucovorin. *Ann Oncol* 2002;13:566–572.
31. Cawthorn SJ, Parums DV, Gibbs NM, et al. Extent of mesorectal spread and involvement of lateral resection margin as prognostic factors after surgery for rectal cancer. *Lancet* 1990;335:1055.
32. Chapuis PH, Dent OF, Fisher R, et al. A multivariate analysis of clinical and pathological variables in prognosis after resection of large bowel cancer. *Br J Surg* 1985;72:698.
33. Colon and rectum. In: *North American Joint Committee on Cancer staging manual*, 6th ed. New York: Springer, 2002;113–124.
34. Compton CC, Fielding LP, Burgart LJ, et al. Prognostic factors in colorectal cancer: College of American Pathologists Consensus Statement 1999. *Arch Pathol Lab Med* 2000;124:979.
35. Copeland EM, Miller LD, Jones RS. Prognostic factors in carcinoma of the colon and rectum. *Am J Surg* 1968;116:875.
36. Crucitti F, Sofo L Doglietto GB, et al. Prognostic factors in colorectal cancer: Current status and new trends. *J Surg Oncol Suppl* 1991;2:76.
37. Cunningham D, Humblet Y, Siena S et al. Cetuximab monotherapy and cetuximab plus irinotecan in irinotecan-refractory metastatic colorectal cancer. *N Engl J Med* 2004;351:337–345.
38. Czito B, Willet C, Colon Cancer. In: Gundulon and Topper: Clinical Radiation Oncology, 2nd ed., Churchill Livingstone; p. 1101–1111; 2007.
39. Di Costanzo F, Sdrobolini A, Gasperoni S. Capecitabine, a new oral fluoropyrimidine for the treatment of colorectal cancer. *Crit Rev Oncol Hematol* 2000;35:101.
40. Douglass HO Jr, Moertel CG, Mayer RJ, et al. Survival after postoperative combination treatment of rectal cancer [letter]. *N Engl J Med* 1986;315:1294.
41. Dukes CE. The surgical pathology of rectal cancer. *Proc R Soc Med* 1943;37:131.
42. Duncan W. Adjuvant radiotherapy in rectal cancer: The MRC trials. *Br J Surg* 1985;72:S59–S62.
43. Dunst J, Reese T, Sutter T, et al. Phase I trial evaluating the concurrent combination of radiotherapy and capecitabine in rectal cancer. *J Clin Oncol* 2002;20:3983.
44. Dupuis O, Vie G, Lledo G, et al. Capecitabine chemoradiation in the preoperative treatment of patients with rectal adenocarcinoma: A phase II GERCOR trial. *Proc Am Soc Clin Oncol* 2004;22:254s(abstr).
45. Enker WE, Thaler HT, Cranor ML, et al. Total mesorectal excision in the operative treatment of carcinoma of the rectum. *J Am Coll Surg* 1995;181:335.
46. Enker WE. Operative consideration in rectal cancer – the pelvic dissection, cancer of the colon, rectum and anus. Ed. Cohen AM; 561–570.
47. Enker WE. Sphincter preserving options for rectal cancer. *Oncology* 10(11):1673–1689.
48. Farouk R, Nelson H, Radice E, et al. Accuracy of computed tomography in determining resectability for locally advanced primary or recurrent colorectal cancers. *Am J Surg* 1998;175:283.
49. Fisher B, Wolmark N, Rockette H, et al. Postoperative adjuvant chemotherapy or radiation therapy for rectal cancer: Results from NSABP protocol R-01. *J Natl Cancer Inst* 1988;80:21.
50. Francois Y, Nemoz CJ, Bauliex J, et al. Influence of the interval between preoperative radiation therapy and surgery on downstaging and on the rate of sphincter-sparing surgery for rectal cancer: The Lyon R90–01 randomized trial. *J Clin Oncol* 1999;17:2396–2402.
51. Freeny PC, Marks WM, Ryan JA, et al. Colorectal carcinoma evaluation with CT: Preoperative staging and detection of postoperative recurrence. *Radiology* 1986;158:347.
52. Frykholm GJ, Glimelius B, Pahlman L. Preoperative or postoperative irradiation in adenocarcinoma of the rectum: Final treatment results of a randomized trial and an evaluation of late secondary effects. *Dis Colon Rectum* 1993;36:564.
53. Gall FP, Hermanek P. Update of the German experience with local excision of rectal cancer. *Surg Oncol Clin North Am* 1992;1:99.

54. Gallagher M, Bereton I-ID, Rostock RA, et al. A prospective study of treatment techniques to minimize the volume of pelvic small bowel with reduction of acute and late effects associated with pelvic irradiation. *Int J Radiat Oncol Biol Phys* 1986;12:1565–1573.

55. Gerard A, Buyse M, Nordlinger B, et al. Preoperative radiotherapy as adjuvant treatment in rectal cancer. Final results of a randomized study of the European Organization for Research and Treatment of Cancer (EORTC). *Ann Surg* 1988;208:606.

56. Gerard J, Bonnetain F, Conroy T, et al. Preoperative (preop) radiotherapy (RT) + 5 FU/folinic acid (FA) in T3–4 rectal cancers: Results of the FFCD 9203 randomized trial. *J Clin Oncol* 2005;23:247S(abstr). Also available online at: www.asco.org/ac/1,1003,_12-002643-00_18-0034-00_19-0030989,00.asp (accessed June 9, 2005).

57. Goldberg RM, Sargent DJ, Morton RF, et al. A randomized controlled trial of fluorouracil plus leucovorin, irinotecan, and oxaliplatin combinations in patients with previously untreated metastatic colorectal cancer. *J Clin Oncol* 2004;22:23–30.

58. Grinnell RS. Distal intramural spread of carcinoma of the rectum and rectosigmoid. *Surg Gynecol Obstet* 1954;99:421.

59. Grumann MM, Noack EM, Hoffmann IA, et al. Comparison of quality of life in patients undergoing abdominoperineal extirpation or anterior resection for rectal cancer. *Ann Surg* 2001;233:149.

60. Gryfe R, Kim H, Hsieh E, et al. Tumor microsatellite instability and clinical outcome in young patients with colorectal cancer. *N Engl J Med* 2000;342:(2):6977.

61. Gualdi GF, Casciani E, Guadalaxara A, et al. Local staging of rectal cancer with transrectal ultrasound and endorectal magnetic resonance imaging: Comparison with histologic findings. *Dis Colon Rectum* 2000;43:338.

62. Gunderson LL, Martenson JA, Smalley SR, et al. Lower gastrointestinal cancer: Rationale, results and techniques of treatment. The lymphatic system and cancer. *Front Radiat Ther Oncol* 1994;28:140–154.

63. Gunderson LL, Nelson H, Martenson J, et al. Intraoperative electron and external beam irradiation with or without 5-FU and maximal surgical resection for previously unirradiated locally recurrent colorectal cancer. *Dis Colon Rectum* 1996;39:1380–1396.

64. Gunderson LL, Nelson H, Martenson J, et al. Locally advanced primary colorectal cancer. Intraoperative electron and external beam irradiation +/– 5-FU. *Int J Radiat Oncol Biol Phys* 1997;37:601–614.

65. Gunderson LL, Sosin H, Levitt S. Extrapelvic colon- areas of failure in a reoperation series: Implications for adjuvant therapy. *Int J Radiation Oncology Biol Phys* 1985;11:731–741.

66. Gustin DM, Brenner DE. Chemoprevention of colon cancer: Current status and future prospects. *Cancer Metastases Rev* 2002;21:323–348.

67. Habib NA, Peck MA, Sawyer CN, et al. Does fixity affect prognosis in the colorectal tumours? *Br J Surg* 1983;70:423–424.

68. Haddock MG, Gunderson LL, Nelson H, et al. Intraoperative irradiation for locally recurrent colorectal cancer in previously irradiated patients. *Int J Radiat Oncol Biol Phys* 2001;49:1267–1274.

69. Haddock MG, Nelson H, Donahue J, et al. IORT as a component of salvage therapy for colo-rectal cancer patients with advanced nodal metastases. *Int J Rad Oncol Biol Phys* 2003;56:966–973.

70. Hall NR, Finan PJ, al-Jaberi T, et al. Circumferential margin involvement after mesorectal excision of rectal cancer with curative intent. Predictor of survival but not local recurrence? *Dis Colon Rectum* 1998;41:979.

71. Havenga K, DeRuiter MC, Enker WE, et al. Anatomical basis of autonomic nerve-preserving total mesorectal excision for rectal cancer. *Br J Surg* 1996;83:384.

72. Havenga K, Enker WE, McDermott K, et al. Male and female sexual and urinary function after total mesorectal excision with autonomic nerve preservation for carcinoma of the rectum. *J Am Coll Surg* 1996;182:495.

73. Havenga K, Enker WE, Norstein J, et al. Improved survival and local control after total mesorectal excision or D3 lymphadenectomy in the treatment of primary rectal cancer: An international analysis of 1411 patients. *Eur J Surg Oncol* 1999;25:368.

74. Heald RJ, Husband EM, Ryall RD. The mesorectum in rectal cancer surgery—the clue to pelvic recurrence? *Br J Surg* 1982;69:613.

75. Higgins CA, Humphrey EW, Dwight RW, et al. Preoperative radiation and surgery for cancer of the rectum: Veterans Administration Surgical Oncology Group trial 11. *Cancer* 1986;58:352.

76. Hildebrandt U, Feifel G. Preoperative staging of rectal cancer by intrarectal ultrasound. *Dis Colon Rectum* 1985;28:42.

77. Horton J, Tepper J. In: Haffty B, Wilson L eds. *Colorectal cancer in handbook of radiation oncology*. Jones and Bartlett, 2006.

78. Horton KM, Abrams RA, Fishman EK. Spiral CT of colon cancer: Imaging features and role in management. *Radiographics* 2000;20:419.

79. Hulsmans FJH, Tio TL, Fockens P, et al. Assessment of tumor infiltration depth in rectal cancer with transrectal sonography: Caution is necessary. *Radiology* 1994;190:715.

80. Hurwitz H, Fehrenbacher L, Novotny W, et al. Bevacizumab plus irinotecan, fluorouracil, and leucovorin for metastatic colorectal cancer. *N Engl J Med* 2004;350:235–242.

81. Hyams DM, Mamounas EP, Petrelli N, et al. A clinical trial to evaluate the worth of preoperative multimodality therapy in patients with operable carcinoma of the rectum: A progress report of National Surgical Breast and Bowel Project Protocol R-03. *Dis Colon Rectum* 1997;40:131.

82. Isbister WH, al-Sanea O. The utility of pre-operative abdominal computerized tomography scanning in colorectal surgery. *J R Coll Surg Edinb* 1996;41:232.

83. Jemal A, Murray T, Ward E, et al. Cancer statistics, 2006. *CA Cancer J Clin* 2006;56:106–130.

84. Jessup JM, et al: Colon and rectum. In: Greene F, Page D, Fleming I, et al., eds. *AJCC cancer staging handbook*, 6th ed. New York: Springer-Verlag, 2002;137–138.

85. Jessup JM, Stewart AK, Menck HR. The National Cancer Data Base Report on patterns of care for adenocarcinoma of the rectum, 1985–1995. *Cancer* 1998;83:2408.

86. Kapiteijn E, Marijnen CA, Nagtegaal ID, et al. Preoperative radiotherapy combined with total mesorectal excision for resectable rectal cancer. *N Engl J Med* 2001;345:638.

87. Karanjia ND, Corder AP, Bearn P, et al. Leakage from stapled low anterior anastomosis after total mesorectal excision for carcinoma of the rectum. *Br J Surg* 1995;81:1224–1226.

88. Khalil es-SA, El Zohairy M, El-Shahawy M. Sphincter sparing procedures: Is it a standard for management of low rectal cancer. *J Egypt Natl Cancer Inst* 2004;16(4):210–215.

89. Kim JC, Kim TW, Kim JH, et al. Preoperative concurrent radiotherapy with capecitabine before total mesorectal excision in locally advanced rectal cancer. *Int J Radiat Oncol Biol Phys* 2005;63:346.

90. Kim NK, Kim MJ, Yun SH, et al. Comparative study of transrectal ultrasonography, pelvic computerized tomography, and magnetic resonance imaging in preoperative staging of rectal cancer. *Dis Colon Rectum* 1999;42:770.

91. Kirklin JW, Dockerty MB, Waugh JM. The role of the peritoneal reflection in the prognosis of carcinoma of the rectum and sigmoid colon. *Surg Gynecol Obstet* 1949;88:326–331.

92. Kligerman MM, Urdaneta N, Knowlton A, et al. Preoperative irradiation of rectosigmoid carcinoma including its regional lymph nodes. *Ani J Roentgenol Radium Ther Nucl Med* 1972;114:498–503.

93. Kollmorgen CF, Meagher AP, Wolff BG, et al. The long-term effect of adjuvant postoperative chemoradiotherapy for rectal carcinoma on bowel function. *Ann Surg* 1994;220:676.

94. Krook JE, Moertel CG, Gunderson LL, et al. Effective surgical adjuvant therapy for high-risk rectal carcinoma. *N Engl J Med* 1991;324:709.

95. Lavery IC, Lopez-Kostner F, Fazio VW, et al. Chances of cure are not compromised with sphincter-saving procedures for cancer of the lower third of the rectum. *Surgery* 1997;122:779.

96. Lingareddy V, Ahmad NR, Mohiuddin M. Palliative reirradiation for recurrent rectal cancer. *Int J Radiat Oncol Biol Phys* 1997;38:785.

97. Lokich JJ, Ahlgren JD, Gullo JJ, et al. A prospective randomized comparison of continuous infusion fluorouracil with a conventional bolus schedule in metastatic colorectal carcinoma: A mid-atlantic oncology program study. *J Clin Oncol* 1989;7425–432.

98. MacFarlane JK, Ryall RDH, Heald RJ. Mesorectal excision for rectal cancer. *Lancet* 1993;341:457.

99. Machado M, Nygren J, Goldman S, et al. Similar outcome after colonic pouch and side-to-end anastomosis in low anterior resection for rectal cancer: A prospective randomized trial. *Ann Surg* 2003;238:214.

100. Machiels JP, Duck L, Honhon B, et al. Phase II study of preoperative oxaliplatin, capecitabine and external beam radiotherapy in patients with rectal cancer: The RadIOxCape study. *Ann Oncol* 2005;16:1898.

101. Mak AC, Rich TA, Schultheiss TE, et al. Late complications of postoperative radiation therapy for cancer of the rectum and rectosigmoid. *Int J Radiat Oncol Biol Phys* 1994;28:597–603.

102. Marks GJ. The Enker article reviewed. *Oncology* 10(11):1690–1699.

103. Martenson JA, Willett CG, Sargent DJ, et al. A phase III study of adjuvant chemotherapy and radiation therapy compared with chemotherapy alone in the surgical adjuvant treatment of colon cancer: Results of Intergroup protocol 130. *J Clin Oncol* 2004;22(16):.

104. Masui H, Ike H, Yamaguchi S, et al. Male sexual function after autonomic nerve-preserving operation for rectal cancer. *Dis Colon Rectum* 1996;39:1140.

105. Matzel KE, Stadelmaier U, Muehldorfer S, et al. Continence after colorectal reconstruction following resection: Impact of level of anastomosis. *Int J Colorectal Dis* 1997;12:82.

106. McAndrew MR, Saba AK. Efficacy of routine preoperative computed tomography scans in colon cancer. *Am Surg* 1999;65:205.

107. McArdle CS, Hole D. Impact of variability among surgeons on postoperative morbidity and mortality and ultimate survival. *BMJ* 1991;302:1501.

108. Mellgren A, Sirivongs P, Rothenberger DA, et al. Is local excision adequate therapy for early rectal cancer? *Dis Colon Rectum* 2000;43:1064.

109. Merchant NB, Guillem JG, Paty PB, et al. T3N0 rectal cancer: Results following sharp mesorectal excision and no adjuvant therapy. *J Gastrointest Surg* 1999;3:642.

110. Meyenberger C, Huch Boni RA, Bertschinger P, et al. Endoscopic ultrasound and endorectal magnetic resonance imaging: A prospective, comparative study for preoperative staging and follow-up of rectal cancer. *Endoscopy* 1995;27:469.

111. Meyerhardt JA, Tepper JE, Niedzwiecki D, et al. Impact of hospital procedure volume on surgical operation and long-term outcomes in high-risk curatively resected rectal cancer: Findings from the intergroup 0114 study. *J Clin Oncol* 2004;22:166.

112. Michaels KB, Govannucci E, Joshipura KJ, et al. Prospective study of fruit and vegetable consumption and incidence of colon and rectal cancers. *J Natl Cancer Inst* 2000;92:1740–1752.

113. Miller AR, Martenson JA, Nelson H, et al. The incidence and clinical consequences of treatment-related bowel injury. *Int J Radiat Oncol Biol Phys* 1999;43:817.

114. Miller, RC, Sargent, DJ, Martenson, JA, et al. Acute diarrhea during adjuvant therapy for rectal cancer: A detailed analysis from a randomized intergroup trial. *Int J Radiat Oncol Biol Phys* 2002;54:409.

115. Minsky BD, Cohen AM, Keneny AJ, et al. Enhancement of radiation induced downstaging of rectal cancer by fluorouracil and high dose leucovorin chemotherapy. *J Clin Oncol* 1992;10:79–84.

116. Minsky BD, Rich T, Recht A, et al. Selection criteria for local excision with or without adjuvant radiation therapy for rectal cancer. *Cancer* 1989;63:1421.

117. Mitchell EP, Anné PR, Fry R, et al. Chemoradiation with CPT-11, 5-FU in neoadjuvant treatment of locally advanced or recurrent adenocarcinoma of the rectum: A phase I/II study update. *Proc Am Soc Clin Oncol* 2003;22:262(abstr 1052).

118. Moertel CG, Fleming TR, MacDonald JS, et al. Levamisole and fluorouracil for adjuvant therapy of resected colon carcinoma. *N Engl J Med* 1990;322:352–358.

119. Mohiuddin M, Marks G, Marks J. Long-term results of reirradiation for patients with recurrent rectal carcinoma. *Cancer* 2002;95:1144.

120. Mohiuddin M, Regine WF, Marks G. Prognostic significance of tumor fixation of rectal carcinoma: Implications for adjunctive radiation therapy. *Cancer* 1996;78(4):717–722.

121. Mohiuddin M, Winter K, Mitchell E, et al. Randomized phase II study of neoadjuvant combined-modality chemoradiation for distal rectal cancer: Radiation Therapy Oncology Group trial 0012. *J Clin Oncol* 2006;24:650.

122. Movas B, Hanlon AL, Lanciano R, et al. Phase I dose escalating trial of hyperfractionated pre-operative chemoradiation for locally advanced rectal cancer. *Int J Radiat Oncol Biol Phys* 1998;42(1):43–50.

123. Myerson Rh, Vaientini V, Birnbaum F, et al. A phase 1111 trial of three dimensionally planned concurrent boost radiotherapy and protracted venous infusion of SEC chemotherapy for locally advanced rectal carcinoma: Response to treatment. *Int J Radiat Ontol Biol Phys* 2001;50:1299–1308.

124. Nakagoe T, Ishikawa H, Sawai T, et al. Survival and recurrence after a sphincter-saving resection and abdominoperineal resection for adenocarcinoma of the rectum at or below the peritoneal reflection: A multivariate analysis. *Surg Today* 2004;34(1):32–39.
125. Nakfoor BM, Willett CG, Shellito PC, et al. The impact of 5-fluorouracil and intra-operative electron beam radiation therapy on the outcome of patients with locally advanced primary rectal and rectosigmoid cancer. *Ann Surg* 1998;228:194.
126. Nascimbeni R, Burgart LJ, Nivatvongs S, et al. Risk of lymph node metastasis in T1 carcinoma of the colon and rectum. *Dis Colon Rectum* 2002;45:200.
127. Nelson H, Petrelli N, Carlin A, et al. Guidelines 2000 for colon and rectal cancer surgery. *J Natl Cancer Inst* 2001;93:583.
128. Ng IOL, Luk IS, Yuen ST. Surgical lateral clearance margins in resected recta-carcinoma: A multivariate analysis of clinicopathologic features. *Cancer* 1993;71:191972–191976.
129. NIH consensus conference. *JAMA* 1990;264(11):1444–1450.
130. O'Connell MJ, Mailliard JA, Kahn MJ, et al. Controlled trial of 5-FU and low-dose leucovorin given for 6 months as postoperative adjuvant therapy for colon cancer. *J Clin Oncol* 1997;15:246–250.
131. O'Connell MJ, Martenson JA, Wieand HS, et al. Improving adjuvant therapy for rectal cancer by combining protracted-infusion 5-FU with radiation therapy after curative surgery. *N Engl J Med* 1994;331:502.
132. Orrom WJ, Wong WD, Rothenberger DA, et al. Endorectal ultrasound in the preoperative staging of rectal tumors: A learning experience. *Dis Colon Rectum* 1990;33:654.
133. Pahlman L, Glemelius B. Pre- or postoperative irradiation in rectal and rectosigmoid carcinoma. *Ann Surg* 1990;211:187–195.
134. Parkin D, Bray F, Ferlay J, et al. Global cancer statistics, 2003. *CA Cancer J Clin* 2005;55:74–108.
135. Paty PB, Enker WE, Cohen AM, et al. Long-term functional results of coloanal anastomosis for rectal cancer. *Am J Surg* 1994;167:90.
136. Pilipshen SJ, Heilwoil M, Quan SHQ, et al. Pattern of pelvic recurrence following definitive resections of rectal cancer. *Cancer* 1984;53:1354–1362.
137. Pollett WG, Nicholls RJ. The relationship between the extent of distal clearance and survival and local recurrence rates after curative anterior resection for carcinoma of the rectum. *Ann Surg* 1983;198:159.
138. Prolongation of the disease-free interval in surgically treated rectal carcinoma, Gastrointestinal Tumor Study Group. *N Engl J Med* 1985;312:1465.
139. Quer EA, Dahlin DC, Mayo CW. Retrograde intramural spread of carcinoma of the rectum and rectosigmoid, a microscopic study. *Surg Gynecol Obstet* 1953;96:24.
140. Quirke P, Durdey P, Dixon MF, et al. Local recurrence of rectal adenocarcinoma due to inadequate surgical resection. Histopathological study of lateral tumor spread and surgical excision. *Lancet* 1986;2:996.
141. Rankin FW, Broder AC. Factors influencing prognosis in carcinoma of the rectum. *Surg Gynecol Obstet* 1928;46:660–667.
142. Rich T, Gunderson LL, Lew R, et al. Patterns of recurrence of rectal cancer after potentially curative surgery. *Cancer* 1983;52:1317.
143. Rodel C, Grabenbauer GG, Papadopoulos T, et al. Phase I/II trial of capecitabine, oxaliplatin, and radiation for rectal cancer. *J Clin Oncol* 2003;21:3098.
144. Rosenthal D, Catalano P, Haller D, et al. ECOG 1297: A phase I study of preoperative radiation therapy (RT) with concurrent protracted continuous infusion 5-FU and dose escalating oxaliplatin followed by surgery, adjuvant 5-FU, and leucovorin for locally advanced (T3/4) rectal adenocarcinoma. *Proc Am Soc Clin Oncol* 2003;22:273(abstr 1094).
145. Russell AH, Harris J, Rosenberg PJ, et al. Anal sphincter conservation for patients with adenocarcinoma of the distal rectum: Long-term results of Radiation Therapy Oncology Group Protocol 89-02. *Int J Radiat Ontol Biol Phys* 2000;46:313–322.
146. Rutten H, Gosens M, Klaassenet R, et al. The treatment of locally recurrent rectal cancer with intraoperative electron beam radiotherapy (IOERRT). Presented at: Fourth International Symposium of the International Society of Intraoperative Radiation Therapy. March 17–19, 2005; Miami, FL.
147. Saltz LB, Cox JV, Blanke C, et al. Irinotecan plus fluorouracil and leucovorin for metastatic colorectal cancer. *N Engl J Med* 2000;343:905–914.
148. Sasaki O, Atkin WS, Sass JR. Mucinous carcinoma of the rectum. *Histopathology* 1987;11:259–272.
149. Sauer R, Becker H, Hohenberger W, et al. Preoperative versus postoperative chemoradiotherapy for rectal cancer. *N Engl J Med* 2004;351:1731–1740.
150. Schild SE, Gunderson LL, Haddock MW, et al. The treatment of locally advanced colon cancer. *Int J Radiat Oncol Biol Phys* 1997;37:51–58.
151. Schuller J, Cassidy J, Dumont E, et al. Preferential activation of capecitabine in tumor following oral administration to colorectal cancer patients. *Cancer Chemother Pharmacol* 2000;45:291.
152. Smalley SR, Benedetti J, Williamson S, et al. Intergroup 0144—phase III trial of 5-FU based chemotherapy regimens plus radiotherapy (XRT) in postoperative adjuvant rectal cancer. Bolus 5-FU vs prolonged venous infusion (PVI) before and after XRT + PVI vs bolus 5-FU + leucovorin + levamisole before and after XRT + bolus 5-FU + LV. *Proc Am Soc Clin Oncol* 2003;22:251A(abstr).
153. Smith R, Cokkinides V, Eyre H. American Cancer Society guidelines for the early detection of cancer, 2004. *CA Cancer J Clin* 2004;54:41–52.
154. Solomon MJ, McLeod RS. Endoluminal transrectal ultrasonography: Accuracy, reliability, and validity. *Dis Colon Rectum* 1993;36:200.
155. Spratt JS, Spjut HJ. Prevalence and prognosis of individual clinical and pathologic variables associated with colorectal carcinoma. *Cancer* 1967;20:18761985.
156. Steele G, Mayer R, Podolsky DK, et al. Cancer of the colon, rectum, and anus. In: *Cancer manual*, 9th ed. Boston: American Cancer Society, Massachusetts Division, 1996.
157. Steele GD Jr, Herndon SE, Bleday R, et al. Sphincter-sparing treatment for distal rectal adenocarcinoma. *Ann Surg Oncol* 1999;6:433–441.
158. Sugihara K, Moriya Y, Akasu T, et al. Pelvic autonomic nerve preservation for patients with rectal carcinoma. Oncologic and functional outcome. *Cancer* 1996;78:1871.
159. Tepper JE, O'Connell M, Petroni G, et al. Adjuvant postoperative fluorouracil-modulated chemotherapy combined with pelvic radiation therapy for rectal cancer. *J Clin Oncol* 1997;15:2030.
160. Third Report of the MRC Trial: Clinico-pathological features of prognostic significance in operable rectal cancer in 17 centres in the U.K. *Br J Surg* 1984;50:435–442.
161. Urban M, Rosen HR, Holbling N, et al. MR imaging for the preoperative planning of sphincter-saving surgery for tumors of the lower third of the rectum: Use of intravenous and endorectal contrast materials. *Radiology* 2000;214:503.
162. Valentini V, Morganti AG, et al. Preoperative hyperfractionated chemoradiation for locally recurrent rectal cancer in patients previously irradiated to the pelvis: A multicentric phase II study. *Int J Radiat Oncol Biol Phys* 64(4):1129–1139.
163. Vernava AM 3rd, Moran M, Rothenberger DA, et al. A prospective evaluation of distal margins in carcinoma of the rectum. *Surg Gynecol Obstet* 1992;175:333.
164. Vigliotti A, Rich TA, Romsdahl MM, et al. Postoperative adjuvant radiotherapy for adenocarcinoma of the rectum and rectosigmoid. *Int J Radiat Oncol Biol Phys* 1987;13:999–1006.
165. Wanebo HJ, Antoniuk P, Koness RJ, et al. Pelvic resection of recurrent rectal cancer: Technical considerations and outcomes. *Dis Colon Rectum* 1999;42:1438.
166. Wei EK, Govannucci E, Wu K. Comparison of risk factors for colon and rectal cancer. *Int J Cancer* 2004;108 (3):433–442.
167. Weinstein GD, Rich TA, Shumate CR, et al. Preoperative infusional chemoradiation and surgery with or without an electron beam intraoperative boost for advanced primary rectal cancer. *Int J Radiat Oncol Biol Phys* 1995;32(1):197–204.
168. Willett C, Fung C, Kaufman D, et al. Postoperative radiation therapy for high-risk colon carcinoma. *J Clin Oncol* 1993;11(6):1112–1117.
169. Willett C, Goldberg S, Shellito P, et al. Does postoperative radiation play a role in the adjuvant therapy of stage T4 colon cancer? *Cancer J Sci Am* 1999;5(4):242–247.
170. Willett CG, Badizadegan K, Ancukiewicz M, et al. Prognostic factors in stage T3N0 rectal cancer: Do all patients require postoperative pelvic irradiation and chemotherapy? *Dis Colon Rectum* 1999;42–167.
171. Willett CG, Shellito PC, Tepper JE, et al. Intraoperative electron beam radiation therapy for primary locally advanced rectal and rectosigmoid carcinoma. *J Clin Oncol* 1991;9:843–849.
172. Willett CG, Shellito PC, Tepper JE, et al. Intraoperative electron beam radiation therapy for recurrent locally advanced rectal and rectosigmoid carcinoma. *Cancer* 1991;67:1504–1508.
173. Willett CG, Tepper JE, Cohen AM, et al. Failure patterns following curative resection of colonic carcinoma. *Ann Surg* 1984;200:685–690.
174. Willett CG, Tepper JE, Orlow E, et al. Renal complications secondary to radiation treatment of upper abdominal malignancies. *Int J Radiat Oncol Biol Phys* 1986;12:1601–1604.
175. Williams NS, Dixon MF, Johnson D. Reappraisal of the 5 centimeter rule of distal excision for carcinoma of the rectum, a study of distal intramural spread and of patients' survival. *Br J Surg* 1983;70:150.
176. Williams NS, Durdey P, Johnston D. The outcome following sphincter-saving resection and abdominoperineal resection for low rectal cancer. *Br J Surg* 1985;72:595.
177. Williams NS, Johnston D. Survival and recurrence after sphincter saving resection and abdominoperineal resection for carcinoma of the middle third of the rectum. *Br J Surg* 1984;71:278.
178. Wiltshire KL, Ward IG, Swallow C, et al. Preoperative radiation with concurrent chemotherapy for resectable rectal cancer: Effect of dose escalation on pathologic complete response, local recurrence-free survival, disease-free survival, and overall survival. *Int J Radiat Oncol Biol Phys* 2006;64(3):709–716.
179. Winawer SJ, Zauber AG, Ho MH, et al. Prevention of colorectal cancer by colonoscopic polypectomy. *N Engl J Med* 1993;329:1977–1981.
180. Wolmark N, Fisher B. An analysis of survival and treatment failure following abdominoperineal and sphincter-saving resection in Dukes' B and C rectal carcinoma. A report of the NSABP clinical trials. National Surgical Adjuvant Breast and Bowel Project. *Ann Surg* 1986;204:480.
181. Wolmark N, Wieand HS, Hyams DM, et al. Randomized trial of postoperative adjuvant chemotherapy with or without radiotherapy for carcinoma of the rectum: National Surgical Adjuvant Breast and Bowel Project Protocol R-02. *J Natl Cancer Inst* 2000;92:388.
182. Wolmark N, Wieand HS, Rockette HE, et al. The prognostic significance of tumor location and bowel obstruction in Dukes B and C colorectal cancer. Findings from the NSABP clinical trials. *Ann Surg* 1983;198:743.
183. Zaheer S, Pemberton JH Farouk R, et al. Surgical treatment of adenocarcinoma of the rectum. *Ann Surg* 1998;227:800.

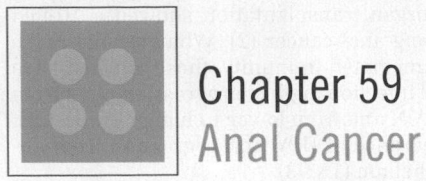

Chapter 59
Anal Cancer

Bernard J. Cummings, James D. Brierley

Anatomy

The anal canal is 3 to 4 cm in length, the posterior wall being longer than the anterior. The superior margin is determined clinically by the palpable upper border of the anal sphincter and puborectalis muscle of the anorectal ring. At this level, the rectal lumen narrows suddenly, and the anal canal passes inferiorly and posteriorly to its external opening, the anus. The distal end of the canal at the anal verge is the level at which the walls of the anal canal come into contact in their normal resting state; it approximates the palpable groove between the lower edge of the internal sphincter and the subcutaneous part of the external sphincter and the junction with true skin. The American Joint Committee on Cancer Clinical Staging (AJCC) (58) and the International Union Against Cancer (UICC) (112) recommend this definition of the anal canal, rather than a convention used by some centers under which carcinomas that are above or exactly astride the dentate line are classified as anal canal tumors and those lying mainly or entirely below that line are called anal margin tumors (Fig. 59.1). The terms *anal margin* and *perianal skin* are now generally used interchangeably. Perianal carcinomas are arbitrarily considered to be cancers arising from the skin within a 5-cm radius of the anal verge, although it has been suggested that this area might more logically be restricted to the puckered, pigmented skin surrounding the anus (130). Proposals for standardizing terminology and definitions of structures in the anal region have been presented (130).

Four different types of epithelium are found within the anal region (32). The perianal skin is similar to hair-bearing skin elsewhere. At the anal verge, the skin blends with a pale-colored zone, sometimes called the pecten, lined by modified squamous epithelium that lacks hair or glandular structures. This squamous zone merges just below the dentate or pectinate line, which marks the mucosal folds of the anal valves, with a transitional epithelium that incorporates features of rectal, urothelial, and squamous epithelium. The purplish red–colored transitional zone extends proximally for about 2 cm until pinker-appearing rectal glandular mucosa becomes dominant.

The major lymphatic pathways flow to three lymph node systems. The perianal skin, the anal verge, and the canal distal to the dentate line drain predominantly to the superficial inguinal nodes, with some communications to the femoral nodes and to the external iliac systems. Lymphatics from around and above the dentate line flow with those from the distal rectum to the internal pudendal, hypogastric, and obturator nodes of the internal iliac systems. The proximal canal drains to the perirectal and superior hemorrhoidal nodes of the inferior mesenteric system. There are numerous lymphatic connections between the various levels of the anal canal, and an intramural system links the lymphatics of the canal with those of the rectum.

The veins of the anal canal connect with both the systemic and the portal venous systems. Venous plexuses, which lie in and surround the mucosal and muscular structures of the anal wall, anastomose around the junction of the anal verge and distal canal. The veins draining the inferior parts of these plexuses communicate with the systemic venous system via the internal pudendal and internal veins, and those from the superior canal flow predominately to the inferior mesenteric vein and then to the portal system (50).

Anorectal continence is mediated by both cerebrospinal nerves and the autonomic system. The smooth muscle of the internal sphincter is supplied by parasympathetic fibers from the second, third, and fourth sacral segments as well as sympathetic fibers from the hypogastric plexus. The upper canal has selective sensitivity for intraluminal differences in pressure, and the autonomic nerves mediate both the inhibitor and facilitator reflexes of the internal sphincter. The striated muscle of the external sphincter is under voluntary control and innervated by the internal rectal nerve, a branch of the pudendal nerve arising from the second, third, and fourth sacral nerves. The internal rectal nerve also transmits pain, touch, and other sensations from the anal lining below the dentate line and from the perianal skin (50).

Pathologic Classification

The 2000 edition of the World Health Organization (WHO) classification of anal tumors describes intraepithelial and invasive neoplasms (35). The term *anal intraepithelial neoplasia* (AIN) is applied to precancerous changes in the epithelium of the anal canal and perianal skin. These epithelial changes have been reviewed elsewhere (1,134).

For invasive cancers, the term *squamous cell carcinoma* is applied to all the various subtypes, large-cell keratinizing and nonkeratinizing, and basaloid or cloacogenic, which were considered separate entities in the previous classification (35). Clinicians have for some years grouped these various subtypes as *epidermoid* cancers because of their similar natural history; the term "epidermoid" is not used in the WHO classification. About 85% to 90% of primary anal canal cancers are squamous cell type. The remaining 10% to 15% are predominantly adenocarcinomas, most of which arise from anal glands. Adenocarcinomas from the rectal-type mucosa in the upper canal are classified as primary rectal cancers. The WHO system retains as separate entities rare variants such as squamous cell carcinoma with mucous microcysts, small cell, and undifferentiated cancers.

Primary cancers of the perianal skin are similar to cancers of the skin in other sites. Most are squamous cell cancers, with occasional basal cell cancers and skin adnexal adenocarcinomas.

Epidemiology

Anal cancers are about one-tenth as common as cancers of the rectum. Cancers arise in the canal with three to four times the frequency of perianal cancers. In North America and Europe, anal canal cancers are more common in women than in men, although this difference is decreasing; perianal cancers occur with about equal frequency in both sexes. The annual incidence varies widely in different parts of the world, but has been increasing in North America and Europe over the past 40 years.

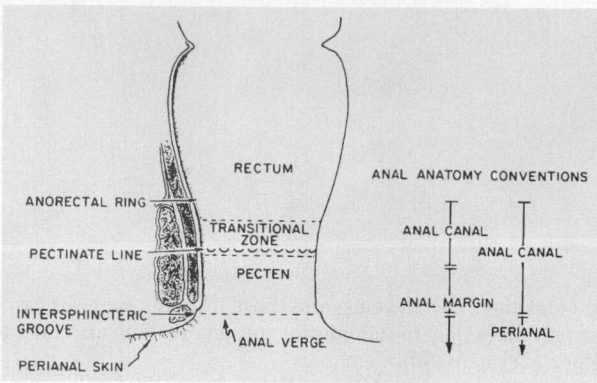

FIGURE 59.1. Anatomy of the anal region.

Although the annual incidence according to most cancer registries is just below 1 per 100,000, the annual age-adjusted rates in the U.S. Surveillance, Epidemiology, and End Results (SEER) registry for 1994 to 2000 had risen to 1.59 per 100,000 for males and 1.84 for females. The annual incidence of invasive and intraepithelial neoplasia almost doubled in both men and women between 1973 and 1979 and between 1994 and 2000 (68). The risk of anal cancer increases with age; the median age at diagnosis is from 60 to 65 years.

Risk Factors

The most significant risk factors so far identified are sexually transmissible viruses, immunosuppression, and tobacco smoking. The role of sexual practices and sexually transmissible agents has been investigated intensively. There are many similarities between anal cancer and uterine cervical cancer (134). Several specific types of human papilloma virus (HPV) are linked to cancer and precancerous lesions in the anogenital epithelium. These HPV types are readily transferred sexually. Subtypes of HPV with a high risk of association with cancer are type 16 in particular, and, to a lesser extent, types 18, 31, 33, 35, and others. These high-risk HPV types have been found in about 85% of anal squamous cancers in some series, more commonly in cancer of the canal than of the perianal skin (41). There is some geographic variation in the types of high-risk HPV found in anal cancer tissues (109). Case control studies suggest that a history of multiple sexual partners in homosexual or heterosexual relationships or of unprotected anal intercourse in males and in females (in the latter, before the age of 30) are predictive of an increased risk of AIN and invasive anal cancer (39). Compared to the overall annual incidence of anal cancer in white males in the United States of approximately 0.7 per 100,000, the estimated incidence in the male homosexual population, prior to the AIDS epidemic, ranged from about 12 to 37 per 100,000 (25).

Compromise of cell-mediated immunity reduces the ability to prevent or eliminate infection by viruses such as high-risk HPV. An increased risk of anal cancer is associated with at least two situations in which cell-mediated immunity is significantly altered: infection with human immune deficiency virus (HIV) and iatrogenic suppression of immunity in organ transplant patients. Interactions between HPV and HIV are complex. Although anal cancer has not been designated an AIDS-defining condition, data from the United States AIDS Cancer Registry linkage study showed that the rate of HPV-associated cancers and precursors was increased in HIV-infected persons for all anogenital sites compared with the general population. The relative risk for anal cancers was 6.8 in women and 37.9 in men (40). A national cohort study in Sweden of 5,931 patients

who had undergone organ transplantation showed a 10-fold excess risk of developing anal cancer (2). Whatever the cause of suppression of cell mediated immunity, those affected have increased rates of HPV infection, higher progression rates from normal epithelium to AIN and from lower to higher grade AIN, and lower rates of clearance of HPV and regression from abnormal to normal epithelium (18,93).

Because of the association between HIV and HPV infections and anal squamous cancer, it has been suggested that the increasing effectiveness of antiretroviral therapy may lead to longer survival of HIV-infected patients and an increased number with anal cancer (92). A review in 1999 of the effects of antiretroviral therapy showed a decrease in the incidence of Kaposi's sarcoma and lymphoma, but no significant reduction at that time in the incidence of less common malignancies such as anogenital cancers (63). The possible role of prophylactic and therapeutic vaccines against HPV in anal cancer has not been established (70).

Tobacco smoking is associated with up to a fourfold increase in risk in several case-control studies. Current smokers are at greater risk than past smokers (24,39).

Benign conditions such as fistulae, fissures, and hemorrhoids do not appear to predispose to cancer (43). Chronic anal inflammation due to inflammatory bowel disease has also been discounted as a risk factor. Using Danish health registers, a cohort study of 2,723 patients with Crohn's disease and 6,334 patients with ulcerative colitis who were followed for an average of 10 years found no significant increase in the incidence of anal cancer (42).

Natural History

Gervaz et al. (48) have proposed a molecular biological model of the pathogenesis of anal squamous carcinoma. There are some differences in the proposed pathways in immunocompetent and immunocompromised individuals. HPV infection is an initiating event in the majority of cases, but HPV DNA integration is necessary for the transition from low-grade to high-grade AIN and probably triggers the emergence of a monoclonal cell population. Loss of heterozygosity at 11q23 is the most consistent change found, and it appears to be independent of HIV status. In HIV-negative patients, progression toward invasive carcinoma appears to require, in addition, allele losses at chromosome regions harboring tumor suppressor genes such as 17p, 18q, and 5q. In HIV-positive patients, microsatellite instability, rather than chromosomal instability, may be a preferred pathway for progression toward invasive cancer.

Most squamous cell cancers of the anal region, especially the canal, are believed to be preceded by high-grade AIN (33). However, it has been estimated that no more than 1% of cases with AIN develop invasive cancer per year (74), a rate lower than that described for cervical intraepithelial neoplasia.

Anal dysplasia recurs frequently despite excision, laser ablation, or topical therapies, presumably because of persistence of the HPV infection with which it is associated (92,131). The natural history of AIN coexisting with anal cancers exposed to radiation, with or without chemotherapy, is unknown.

Squamous cancers of the anal canal spread most commonly by direct extension and lymphatic pathways. Hematogenous metastases are less common. Direct invasion from the anal mucosa into the sphincter muscles and perianal connective tissue spaces occurs early; in a series of 137 cases, cancers were confined to the mucosa and submucosa at diagnosis in only 12%, and to the sphincter muscles, without regional lymph node involvement, in only 34% (10). In about half the cases, anal cancers extend into the rectum and/or perianal skin. Invasion of the vaginal septum and vaginal mucosa is more common than invasion of the prostate gland, but anovaginal fistulas occur in fewer than 5% of women. Extensive tumors may infiltrate the pelvic walls.

Lymphatic invasion occurs relatively early. The overall risk of regional nodal involvement at diagnosis is about 25% (84). Pelvic lymph node metastases have been found in as many as 30% of patients treated by abdominoperineal resection (10,44,113). In an illustrative series, metastases were present in the superior hemorrhoidal nodes in 25% (15/61); in the external iliac, obturator, or hypogastric nodes in 30% (8/27); and in the inguinal nodes in 16% (12/74) of patients (113). Inguinal metastases are clinically detectable in up to approximately 20% of patients at initial diagnosis and are present subclinically in a further 10% to 20% (46,51,106,113). Nodal metastases were associated with 30% of cancers confined to the sphincter muscles and 60% of those that had extended through the sphincters or were more poorly differentiated (44). Lymphatic metastases increase in frequency with progressive enlargement of the primary cancer (44).

Extrapelvic metastases are identified at the time of first presentation in fewer than 10% of patients. They may occur via the portal or systemic venous systems or via lymphatics and are found most frequently in the liver and lungs.

Relapse after initial treatment is more common in the area of the primary tumor and the pelvic lymph nodes than in extrapelvic organs. Locoregional relapse rates of up to about 30% and extrapelvic failure rates up to about 20% are common (10,22,120,121). Overall 5-year survival rates are of the order of 55% to 65%.

Perianal cancers tend to grow locally and may extend into the anal canal. When the site of origin is in doubt, it is conventional to classify the cancer as arising in the anal canal. The ipsilateral inguinal nodes are the most common site of metastasis and are abnormal in from 5% to 20% of cases. Extrapelvic metastases are uncommon except in locally advanced cancer or those with nodal metastases. Overall 5-year cause-specific survival rates usually exceed 80%.

:: | Clinical Presentation

The symptoms of anal cancer are nonspecific, contributing to delay in presentation by the patient and in diagnosis by the physician of more than 6 months in a third of patients (31,116). Bleeding and anal discomfort are the most common symptoms and are reported by about half the patients (132). Less common complaints include awareness of an anal mass, pruritus, and anal discharge. Pain is uncommon but may be severe. In patients with tumors in the proximal canal there may be an alteration in bowel habits, but this is uncommon with distal cancers (132). Occasionally, asymptomatic tumors are found during physical examination or in the course of investigation of an inguinal node mass. Unsuspected microinvasive carcinoma is sometimes found in mucosa removed at hemorrhoidectomy (13).

Small carcinomas are often nodular or plaquelike, but larger tumors are more typically ulcerated and infiltrative. Coexisting benign conditions such as anogenital warts, hemorrhoids, and anal fissures may be present. Anal sphincter tone is usually preserved and may be increased by painful spasm. Gross fecal incontinence resulting from sphincter destruction occurs in fewer than 5% of patients, although some fecal soiling is common. Similarly, vaginal fistulas are uncommon. Rarely, extrapelvic metastases may be the only symptomatic feature or finding.

:: | Diagnostic Work-Up

The history and physical examination should stress features that delineate the extent of the primary tumor, including anal sphincter competence and possible extension to adjacent organs. A biopsy of the primary tumor is necessary to establish the diagnosis and the histologic type. General anesthesia may be needed to permit detailed pelvic and anorectal examination, which should include proctoscopy. Sigmoidoscopy and colonoscopy, although often performed, infrequently disclose colonic pathology (127). Physical examination should include detailed examination of the genital region, especially in patients who give a history of previous anogenital area dysplasia or cancer, genital warts, anal-receptive intercourse, or are HIV-positive.

Only the inguinal and low perirectal lymph nodes are accessible to clinical examination. Because lymph node enlargement may be caused by reactive hyperplasia in as many as half of those with palpable inguinal nodes, clinically suspicious nodes should be assessed histologically by needle biopsy or simple excision (132). Metastases in the internal iliac and superior hemorrhoidal node chains, about half of which are <0.5 cm in diameter (126), cannot be identified reliably by current techniques of lymphangiography, pelvic lymphoscintigraphy, computed tomography (CT), or magnetic resonance imaging (MRI). Recent advances in MRI with contrast agents such as ultrasmall superparamagnetic iron oxide (USPIO) may improve the identification of nodal metastases. The role of sentinel node biopsy, so far applied only to inguinal nodes, has not been established (20,26). Abdominal and pelvic CT or MRI are useful to identify liver metastases or enlarged node masses that may be accessible to image-guided aspiration biopsy, and to localize the kidneys when radiation therapy is to be used. A chest film is sufficient screening for pulmonary metastases. Skeletal studies are not indicated in the absence of focal symptoms. Transanorectal ultrasonography may help to identify the depth of tumor penetration into the anal wall and the presence of enlarged perirectal lymph nodes.

Examination of blood and serum should include full blood count, renal and liver function tests, and, if any risk factors are present, assessment of HIV antibody status.

:: | Staging

With the establishment of treatment strategies designed to preserve anorectal function, staging systems based on surgicopathologic parameters have been supplanted by clinical staging. The systems for anal canal and perianal cancers most commonly used are those proposed by the UICC (112) and the AJCC (58) (Tables 59.1 and 59.2). Most authors continue to report results by T (tumor) category or N (node) category rather than by composite TNM (tumor, node, metastasis) stages. Under the UICC/AJCC systems, the regional lymph nodes for anal canal cancer are the perirectal, internal iliac, and inguinal nodes. Spread to all other pelvic node groups, including the external iliac, common iliac, and sigmoid nodes, is classified as metastasis (M1). For perianal cancers, the regional nodes are the ipsilateral inguinal nodes.

:: | Prognostic Factors

Features related to the anatomic extent of disease generally provide the most prognostic value (21). The most adverse factor for survival is the presence of extrapelvic metastasis (55,115,117). When anal cancer is confined to the pelvis, the size of the primary tumor is the most useful predictor for local control and preservation of anorectal function and survival (22,52,107). Involvement of regional lymph nodes is an adverse factor for survival but not for control of the primary tumor (22,51).

Age and performance status have each been considered prognostic, but patient selection confounds interpretation, and

⠿ Table 59.1	**ANAL CANAL TNM CLASSIFICATION**

Primary Tumor (T)

TX	Primary tumor cannot be assessed
T0	No evidence of primary tumor
Tis	Carcinoma *in situ*
T1	Tumor 2 cm or less in greatest dimension
T2	Tumor more than 2 cm but not more than 5 cm in greatest dimension
T3	Tumor more than 5 cm in greatest dimension
T4	Tumor of any size invades adjacent organ(s) (e.g., vagina, urethra, bladder) (involvement of the sphincter muscle(s) *alone* is not classified as T4)

Regional Lymph Nodes (N)

NX	Regional lymph nodes cannot be assessed
N0	No regional lymph node metastasis
N1	Metastasis in perirectal lymph nodes(s)
N2	Metastasis in unilateral iliac and/or inguinal lymph node(s)
N3	Metastasis in perirectal and inguinal lymph nodes and/or bilateral internal iliac and/or inguinal lymph nodes

Distant Metastases (M)

MX	Distant metastasis cannot be assessed
M0	No distant metastasis
M1	Distant metastasis

Stage Grouping

Stage 0	Tis	N0	M0
Stage I	T1	N0	M0
Stage II	T2	N0	M0
	T3	N0	M0
Stage IIIA	T1	N1	M0
	T2	N1	M0
	T3	N1	M0
	T4	N0	M0
Stage IIIB	T4	N1	M0
	Any T	N2, N3	M0
Stage IV	Any T	Any N	M1

From Sobin LH, Wittekind C. *TNM classification of malignant tumours*, 6th ed. New York: Wiley-Liss, 2002.

⠿ Table 59.2	**PERIANAL SKIN TNM CLASSIFICATION**

Primary Tumor (T)

TX	Primary tumor (T)
T0	No evidence of primary tumor
Tis	Carcinoma *in situ*
T1	Tumor 2 cm or less in greatest dimension
T2	Tumor more than 2 cm but not more than 5 cm in greatest dimension
T3	Tumor more than 5 cm in greatest dimension
T4	Tumor invades deep extradermal structures (i.e., cartilage, skeletal muscle, or bone)

Regional Lymph Nodes (N)

NX	Regional lymph nodes cannot be assessed
N0	No regional lymph node metastasis
N1	Regional lymph node metastasis

Distant Metastasis (M)

MX	Distant metastasis cannot be assessed
M0	No distant metastasis
M1	Distant metastasis

Stage Grouping

Stage 0	Tis	N0	M0
Stage I	T1	N0	M0
Stage II	T2, T3	N0	M0
Stage III	T4	N0	M0
	Any T	N1	M0
Stage IV	Any T	Any N	M1

From Sobin LH, Wittekind C. *TNM classification of malignant tumours*, 6th ed. New York: Wiley-Liss, 2002.

the majority of elderly patients tolerate radical treatment (113,122). Women have a better prognosis in some series (6,52,84). Hemoglobin levels ≤10 g/L at presentation have been correlated with poor local control and survival rates (17). Serum markers such as carcinoembryonic antigen (CEA) and squamous cell carcinoma antigen (SCCA) have not proved consistent as aids to diagnosis or monitoring of treatment response. In HIV-positive patients high viral load, low lymphocyte CD4+ counts, and AIDS have been prognostic of poor local tumor control and survival, and, in some series, of impaired tolerance of radiation and chemotherapy (60,101).

Fenger (34) surveyed nearly 50 reports on cytogenetic, flow cytometric, immunohistochemical, and other factors and considered that these studies offered some insights on pathogenesis but did not help with selection of treatment or provide guidance on prognosis.

⠿ | Treatment of Anal Canal Cancer

Four randomized trials have established that the combination of radiation therapy, 5-fluorouracil, (5-FU), and mitomycin is the standard against which other treatments should be compared (3,6,36,121). Nonrandomized comparisons of radical resection with this radiation-chemotherapy combination (53,84), or with radiation therapy alone (22,95) have shown the ability of radiation-based regimens to produce survival rates at least equal to those of surgical series, while allowing preservation of anorectal function in the majority of patients.

⠿ | Combined-Modality Therapy

Primary Tumor

Interest in combined-modality therapy originated with the report in 1974 by Nigro et al. (88) of complete tumor regression in three patients treated by radiation therapy and concurrent 5-FU and mitomycin or porfiromycin before planned abdominoperineal resection. The effectiveness of this combination as a radical treatment, rather than as an adjuvant to surgery, has been demonstrated since in numerous nonrandomized studies and confirmed in randomized trials.

The randomized trials conducted by the United Kingdom Coordinating Committee for Cancer Research (UKCCCR) (121) and the European Organisation for Research on Treatment of Cancer (EORTC) (6) both showed significant improvement in control of the primary cancer and in colostomy-free survival in patients who received irradiation combined with chemotherapy. The larger UKCCCR trial also showed improved cause-specific survival. Although the overall survival rates of those who received radiation and chemotherapy were slightly better than those of the patients treated with radiation therapy alone, the advantage did not reach statistical significance in either trial (Table 59.3).

In the UKCCCR trial (121), 577 patients with all stages (UICC Staging System, 1987 edition, which is the same as the 2002 edition [112]) of squamous cell cancer of the anal canal or anal margin were randomly assigned to receive radiation alone or radiation combined with chemotherapy. Forty percent had primary cancers >5 cm in size (T3) or deeply invasive (T4), 20% were lymph node positive, and 2% had extrapelvic metastases. The radiation dose was 45 Gy in 20 to 25 fractions in 4 to 5 weeks. Those randomized to chemotherapy received 5-FU (1,000 mg/m^2/day for 4 days or 750 mg/m^2/day for 5 days) by continuous peripheral intravenous infusion in the first and final weeks of radiation treatment, plus mitomycin (12 mg/m^2)

	THREE-YEAR RESULTS OF RANDOMIZED TRIALS OF RADIATION ALONE (RT) VERSUS RADIATION, 5-FLUOROURACIL, AND MITOMYCIN C (RTCT) (PERCENTAGES)					
Table 59.3						
	UKCCCR (*n* = 577)			EORTC (*n* = 103)		
	RT	RTCT	*p* Value	RT	RTCT	*p* Value
Locoregional control	39	61	<.0001	55	65	0.02
Cause-specific survival	61	72	.02	NS	NS	NS
Overall survival	58	65	.25	65	70	0.17

EORTC, European Organisation for Research and Treatment of Cancer; NS, not stated; UKCCCR, UK Coordinating Committee for Cancer Research.
UKCCR figures from UKCCCR Anal Canal Cancer Trial Working Party. Epidermoid anal cancer: results from the UKCCCR randomized trial of radiotherapy alone versus radiotherapy, 5-fluorouracil and mitomycin C. *Lancet* 1996;348:1049–1054; EORTC figures from Bartelink H, Roelofsen F, Eschwege F, et al. Concomitant radiotherapy and chemotherapy is superior to radiotherapy alone in the treatment of locally advanced anal cancer: results of a phase III randomized trial of the European Organization for Research and Treatment of Cancer Radiotherapy and Gastrointestinal Cooperative Groups. *J Clin Oncol* 1997;15:2040–2049.

by bolus intravenous injection on day 1 of the first course of chemotherapy. The patients were reassessed clinically 6 weeks after treatment. If the primary tumor had not regressed by at least 50% (as occurred in 10% in each group), surgery was recommended; otherwise, the patients received an additional 15 Gy in six fractions by a perineal field or 25 Gy over 2 to 3 days by iridium-192 implant. Locoregional failure, defined as the presence of residual or recurrent cancer in the primary site or regional nodes, treatment-related morbidity requiring surgery, or inability to close a colostomy opened prior to treatment, was observed in 81/285 (28%) patients treated by radiation therapy and chemotherapy but in 147/283 (52%) patients who received irradiation only. Surgery that included colostomy was necessary for management of toxicity in 10 patients (3.5%) in each study group. There were six (2%) deaths due to treatment in the combined-modality arm and two (0.7%) in the irradiation-alone arm. Acute toxicity, other than hematologic, was considered comparable in each group. The mortality rate from anal cancer was significantly reduced in the combined-modality treated patients, but the overall survival rate was not improved.

In the EORTC study, 103 patients with advanced cancers of the anal canal were randomized in a trial of similar design (6). Eighty-five percent of those entered had category T3 or T4 cancers (112) and 51% had abnormal nodes. The radiation dose was 45 Gy in 25 fractions over 5 weeks. Chemotherapy included 5-FU (750 mg/m^2/day for 5 days) in weeks 1 and 5 of radiation, and a single dose of mitomycin (15 mg/m^2) by bolus intravenous injection on day 1 of the first course of 5-FU only. After 6 weeks, boost irradiation of 15 Gy (if complete clinical response to previous treatment had occurred) or 20 Gy (after partial response) was given by external-beam or interstitial irradiation. The probability of complete tumor regression was significantly improved after combined-modality treatment; the colostomy-free survival rate of the patients who received irradiation and chemotherapy was 58% at 3 years, compared with only 35% for those treated by irradiation alone. One of 51 patients who received combined modality treatment died of toxicity. Otherwise, acute and late toxicity rates did not differ markedly. The hazards to which patients with advanced anal cancer are subject are illustrated by the finding in this trial that the probability of surviving 3 years or more without relapse, major morbidity from treatment, or a colostomy was only about 30%.

The Radiation Therapy Oncology Group (RTOG) and Eastern Cooperative Oncology Group (ECOG) established in a randomized trial that the combination of mitomycin with 5-FU and radiation is more effective than 5-FU alone with radiation (36). In that study, 291 patients with cancers of the anal canal of any T and N category (RTOG staging system) who did not have evidence of extrapelvic metastases received 45 to 50.4 Gy in 25 to 28 fractions over 5 weeks plus two courses of 5-FU (1,000 mg/m^2/day by continuous peripheral intravenous infusion) over 4 days, with or without mitomycin (10 mg/m^2 by bolus intravenous injection) on the first day of each course of chemotherapy. Chemotherapy was administered in weeks 1 and 5 of radiation therapy. Approximately 40% had cancers larger than 5 cm or invading adjacent organs, and 17% had abnormal lymph nodes. Patients were required to undergo biopsy of the primary tumor site 6 weeks after irradiation and chemotherapy. Biopsies were positive in 15% of those who received 5-FU only and in 8% of those who received both mitomycin and 5-FU (*p* =.14). Patients with positive biopsies had the option of receiving an additional 9 Gy in five treatments concurrently with a 4-day infusion of 5-FU (1,000 mg/m^2/day) and a single injection of cisplatin (100 mg/m^2) if it was thought that anal function might still be salvaged. At 5 years, the rates of colostomy (11% vs. 22%; *p* =.02) significantly favored treatment with radiation, 5-FU, and mitomycin, although colostomy-free survival rates did not differ significantly. There was no significant difference in overall survival rates (67% vs. 65%), although the disease-free survival rate was improved by the three-agent combination (67% vs. 50%; *p* =.006). Acute hematologic toxicity was more common in the patients who received mitomycin, but the rates of other acute and late toxic effects were similar in each treatment group. Four of 146 (2.7%) patients who received both 5-FU and mitomycin suffered fatal toxicity as did 1/145 treated with radiation and 5-FU alone.

In a further trial by the RTOG (RTOG 9811), so far reported only in abstract (3), induction 5-FU and cisplatin followed by 5-FU and cisplatin concurrent with radiation failed to improve disease-free survival compared to 5-FU and mitomycin with radiation. This trial included a higher total radiation dose than the earlier RTOG randomized trial, based on analysis of non-randomized studies that suggested a dose-control relationship (17,103), and on pilot studies, which had demonstrated that a proportion of patients could tolerate uninterrupted radiation schedules of up to 59.4 Gy over 6.5 weeks with either concurrent mitomycin with 5-FU (66,67) or cisplatin with 5-FU (79). In RTOG 9811 (3), one study group received 59 Gy in 6.5 weeks (45 Gy in 1.8-Gy fractions), followed without interruption by 14 Gy in 2-Gy fractions), with concurrent 5-FU (1,000 mg/m^2/day) by continuous infusion on days 1 to 4 and 29 to 32 plus mitomycin 10 mg/m^2 intravenous bolus on days 1 and 29; the other group received 5-FU (1,000 mg/m^2/day) days 1 to 4, 29 to 32, 57 to 60, and 85 to 88 plus cisplatin (75 mg/m^2 bolus injection on days 1, 29, 57, and 85) with the same 59-Gy radiation schedule (start day 57). At the time of reporting, 598 patients were analyzable. Twenty-eight percent had primary cancers >5 cm in size, and 26% had clinically positive nodes. The preliminary results showed an actuarial 5-year disease-free rate of 56% for radiation, 5-FU, and mitomycin versus 48% for radiation, 5-FU, and cisplatin (*p* =.28), with overall survival rates of 69% for both arms. The 5-year colostomy rate was 10% for the mitomycin-containing arm and 20% for the cisplatin arm (*p* =.12). Acute grade 3 or 4 nonhematologic toxicity rates were 75% in each arm, but hematologic toxicity was higher in the mitomycin-containing arm (67% vs. 47%).

Several other randomized trials are in progress. The UKCCCR Anal Cancer Trial II incorporates a double randomization: the first compares 5-FU plus mitomycin with 5-FU plus cisplatin concurrently with radiation; the second compares two courses of adjuvant 5-FU plus cisplatin with no adjuvant therapy. The radiation dose is 50.4 Gy in 1.8-Gy fractions over 5.5 weeks without interruption.

The French Federation Francaise de Cancerolgie Digestive (FFCD 9804) trial also includes a double randomization: the first

Clinical Radiation Oncology

to two courses of neoadjuvant 5-FU and cisplatin and the second to different doses of boost irradiation. The base radiation dose is 45 Gy in 1.8-Gy fractions over 5 weeks with concurrent 5-FU and cisplatin in weeks 1 and 5. After a 2-week break, the patients receive either 15 Gy or 20 to 25 Gy, according to randomization and tumor response. Chemotherapy is not given during the boost radiation.

The EORTC 22011 trial compares single-dose mitomycin and weekly cisplatin given concurrently with radiation to mitomycin and prolonged continuous infusion 5-FU concurrently with radiation. The total radiation dose is 59.4 Gy, consisting of an initial 36 Gy in 1.8-Gy fractions over 4 weeks, followed after an interval of 2 weeks by a further 23.4 Gy in 2.5 weeks. Chemotherapy is given during both phases of radiation.

Results were not presented by T, N, or stage category in either of the randomized trials that compared radiation combined with chemotherapy to radiation alone (6,121). Five-year survival rates from nonrandomized series managed by 5-FU, mitomycin, and radiation are about 80% for cancers ≤2 cm in size (T1), 70% for tumors 2 to 5 cm (T2), 45% to 55% for larger or deeply invasive cancers (T3 or T4), and 65% to 75% overall. The corresponding local control rates (excluding salvage treatment) are about 90% to 100% (T1), 65% to 75% (T2), 40% to 55% (T3 or T4), and 60% overall (Table 59.4). Because of case mix and the preponderance of advanced cancers in many series, generally only about two-thirds of all patients treated retain anorectal function. No more than about 5% of patients overall have lost anorectal function because of treatment related complications.

Efforts to improve results have included increases in total radiation dose and shortening of overall treatment time (both discussed below), and exploration of combinations of radiation and chemotherapy other than 5-FU plus mitomycin. Bleomycin showed no apparent benefit in nonrandomized studies (38,49,90). Of greater, and continuing, interest has been the combination of radiation, 5-FU, and cisplatin, which has produced levels of tumor control comparable to those produced by radiation, 5-FU, and mitomycin (Table 59.5). This combination has proven effective against squamous cell cancers in other sites, and cisplatin may act as a radiation sensitizer, a property lacking in mitomycin as currently used in clinical practice. However, the first report from a randomized trial did not show any superiority for cisplatin and 5-FU over mitomycin and 5-FU (3).

Much remains to be learned about the mechanisms of interaction between radiation and chemotherapy in the treatment of cancer. The synergistic interactions of various combinations of radiation, 5-FU, mitomycin and cisplatin observed in some laboratory studies are difficult to evaluate clinically, and no trials designed to study such interactions have been performed. Also, there have not been formal comparisons of more prolonged, but less daily dose-intense infusions of 5-FU with the 96- to 120-hour infusions generally favored, nor of bolus injections with continuous infusions of 5-FU or cisplatin. In most series, the timing of delivery of chemotherapy each day relative to irradiation has not been tightly controlled, and the importance of scheduling is not known.

In order to try to confirm eradication of the cancer, random biopsies from the site of the primary tumor, and/or abnormal nodes, shortly after chemoradiation have been advocated by some but are not necessary. Elective biopsies at predetermined times do not appear to lead to better results than can be achieved by biopsies directed only to areas suspected clinically of harboring residual or recurrent cancer. A negative biopsy does not exclude the possibility of cancer regrowth (87,118). Residual masses at the site of the original anal cancer may take several months to resolve fully after chemoradiation or radiation therapy alone (22,107,118). Most authors now recommend biopsy only when persistent cancer is suspected clinically.

Treatment of local residual cancer or recurrence is planned according to the extent of disease, both locoregional and ex-

trapelvic, and the potential for preserving anorectal function. It may be possible to deliver further radiation and chemotherapy. If conservative treatment is not possible, surgery, usually abdominoperineal resection, should be considered. Although the similar overall survival rates in the trials of irradiation versus irradiation and chemotherapy are thought to reflect, in part, the ability of surgery to salvage some patients, the results of attempted salvage in many series are disappointing, with reports of high rates of unresectable cancer, further pelvic recurrence, and extrapelvic recurrences (4,59,89,102). This probably reflects the more adverse biologic characteristics of cancers not eradicated by radiation and chemotherapy. Results of attempted surgical salvage are worse in patients who present initially with locally advanced primary tumors or nodal metastases. Survival rates at 3 years after salvage surgery range from as low as 10% to better than 50%.

Lymph Node Metastases

Lymph node metastases can be eradicated by the same radiation and chemotherapy doses effective against the primary tumor. Data from patients managed by surgery show that, when patients are first diagnosed, pelvic nodes are present in about 30% and inguinal node metastases are detectable clinically in 15% to 20% (10,51,113). It is of interest that the reported incidence of clinically abnormal inguinal nodes in patients managed by radiation tends to be somewhat lower, in the range of 10% to 15% (46). Late failure in the inguinal nodes after surgery for the primary tumor, consistent with the presence of subclinical metastases at the time of original presentation, has been described in 15% to 25% (10,51,113). However, in one recent series in which the primary tumor was treated by radiation, without elective treatment of clinically normal inguinal nodes, late inguinal failure occurred in only 8% (46). Approaches to the management of inguinal node metastases vary from radical dissection to excision or needle biopsy of enlarged nodes followed by radiation therapy or radiation and chemotherapy (22,46,94). Local control of the involved inguinal nodal areas is very good, usually ≥80% (22,46,94). However, 5-year survival rates are usually 10% to 20% lower than in those who do not have demonstrable node metastases (22,46,120).

Prophylactic or therapeutic radical dissection of the inguinofemoral nodes is not necessary and carries a high risk of late morbidity (113). High-dose irradiation to the pelvis or groin areas after extensive nodal resections increases the risk of morbidity. Elective irradiation of clinically normal inguinal node areas, with or without chemotherapy, reduces the risk of late node failure in that area to <5% (22,94,120).

Control of subclinical pelvic node metastases by irradiation and chemotherapy can be inferred from the low failure rates reported in pelvic node sites. Although large pelvic node masses may respond completely to radiation and chemotherapy, control and cure rates in these patients are low, particularly if the metastatic nodes are attached to the pelvic walls.

Extrapelvic Metastases

Deaths from extrapelvic metastases alone are relatively infrequent. Extrapelvic metastases are identified in 10% to 20% of patients. In the UKCCCR trial group treated by radiation, 5-FU, and mitomycin, although 27% (21/77) of those dying from cancer had metastases only, this represented only 7% of that trial group (121). By comparison, 38 deaths (49% of cancer deaths) in that study arm were due to pelvic cancer only. The overall crude rate of metastasis in those who received radiation and chemotherapy was 10%, compared to 17% in those treated by radiation alone. In the EORTC trial, 17% of those treated by radiation and chemotherapy developed metastases, as did 21% of those treated by radiation only (6). These rates are similar

Table 59.4 SELECTED RESULTS OF CONCURRENT RADIATION, 5-FLUOROURACIL, AND MITOMYCIN C

Author (Reference)	Chemotherapy 5-FU[a]	Mitomycin-C	Radiation[b] (dose/fractions/time)	Primary Tumor Control		Serious Complications[c]	5-Year Survival
Leichman et al. (77)	1,000 mg/m² /24 h IVI D1-4 and D29-32	15 mg/m² D1 IVB	30 Gy/15/D1-21	31/34 (91%) (≤5 cm)	7/10 (70%) (>5 cm)	NS	80%, crude
Sischy et al. (111)	1,000 mg/m² /24 h IVI D2-5 and D28-31	10 mg/m² IVB D1	40.8 Gy/24/D1-35	22/26 (85%) (≤3 cm)	32/50 (64%) (≥3 cm)	2/79 (3%)	73%, 3-year actuarial
Cummings et al. (22)	1,000 mg/m² /24 h IVI D1-4 and D43-46	10 mg/m² IVB D1 and D43	48 Gy/24/D1-58 (split course)	15/17 (88%) (≤5 cm)	13/16 (81%) (>5 cm or T4)	1/33 (3%)	65%, actuarial
Cummings et al. (22)	1,000 mg/m² /24 h IVI D1-4 and D43-46	10 mg/m² IVB D1 and D43	50 Gy/20/D1-56 (split course)	10/10 (100%) (≤5 cm)	3/4 (75%) (>5 cm or T4)	5/14 (36%)	65%, actuarial
Schneider et al. (108)	1,000 mg/m² /24 h IVI D1-4 and D29-32	10 mg/m² IVB D1 and D29	50 Gy/25-28/D1-35 ± boost	21/22 (95%) (≤5 cm)	14/19 (74%) (>5 cm or T4)	3/41 (7%)	77%, actuarial
Tanum et al. (117,118)	1,000 mg/m² /24 h IVI D1-4	10-15 mg/m² IVB D1	50-54 Gy/25-27/D1-35	28/30 (93%) (≤5 cm)	42/56 (75%) (>5 cm or T4)	14/89 (16%)	72%, actuarial
Cummings et al. (22)	1,000 mg/m² /24 h IVI D1-4	10 mg/m² IVB D1	50 Gy/20/D1-28	3/3 (≤5 cm)	11/13 (85%) (>5 cm or T4)	10/16 (63%)	75%, actuarial
Doci et al. (27)	750 mg/m² /24 h IVI (120 h) D1-5/D43-47/D85-89	15 mg/m² IVB D1/D43/D85	54-60 Gy/30-33/D1-53 (split course)	28/38 (74%) (≤5 cm)	9/17 (53%) (>5 cm)	2/56 (4%)	81%, actuarial

IVB, intravenous bolus injection; IVI, continuous intravenous infusion; NS, not stated; T4, invading adjacent organs.

[a]All infusions were for 96 hr except where shown.

[b]All series used pelvic radiation fields tangential to perineum.

[c]Serious complications required surgery or were grade 3 or greater (RTOG scale).

Table 59.5 | **SELECTED RESULTS OF RADIATION, 5-FLUOROURACIL, AND CISPLATIN**

Author (Reference)	Chemotherapy 5-FU	Cisplatin	Radiation (dose/fractions/time)	Primary Tumor Complete Response	Survival
Concurrent					
Gerard et al. (45)	1,000 mg/m^2/24 h IVI (96 h) D1-4	25 mg/m^2 IVB D1-4	40 Gy/10/D1-17 plus boost D63-64	76/94/(81%)[a]	84% 5-year actuarial
Martenson et al. (79)	1,000 mg/m^2/24 h IVI (96 hr) D1-4, D43-46	75 mg/m^2 IVB D1, D43	59.4 Gy/33/D1-59 split at 36 Gy	13/19 (68%)	Maximum follow-up 33 mo
Doci et al. (28)	750 mg/m^2/24 h IVI (96 h) D1-4, D22-25, Some plus 3rd cycle	100 mg/m^2 IVB D1, D22 Some plus 3rd cycle	54 Gy/30/D1-42 Some plus boost	32/35 (91%) at 6 mo	Med. follow-up 37 mo
Hung et al. (62)	250 mg/m^2/24 h IVI (144 h) 6 d/wk D1-42	4 mg/m^2/24 h IVI (144 h) 6 d/wk D1-42	54 Gy/30/D1-42	76/92 (82%)[a]	91% 5-year actuarial
Induction Plus Concurrent					
Peiffert et al. (100)	800 mg/m^2/24 h IVI (96 h) D1-4, D29-32 D57-60, D85-88	80 mg/m^2 IVB D1, D29 D57, D85	45 Gy/25/D57-90 plus boost 20 Gy D134	25/29 (86%) at 2 mo	NS
Induction					
Brunet et al. (12)	1,000 mg/m^2/24 h IVI (120 h) D2-6, D22-25, D43-46	100 mg/m^2 IVB D1, D22, D43	45 Gy/25/D64-99 plus boost	17/19 (89%)	No cancer death, 10-40 mo
Alternating					
Roca et al. (104)	750 mg/m^2/24 h IVI (120 h) D2-7, D23-28	30 mg/m^2 IVB D1-2, D22-23	20 Gy/10/D8-21, D29-42, plus boost	14/17 (82%)	Med. follow-up 18 mo

IVB, intravenous bolus injection; IVI, continuous intravenous infusion; med, median; NS, not stated.
[a]Local control for at least 12 months; all other studies no report on long-term follow-up.

to those reported following management of the primary cancer and regional nodes by surgery or radiation therapy only. The median survival time after diagnosis of extrapelvic metastases ranges from 8 to 12 months (55,115). Anal cancer metastases have been relatively resistant so far to all chemotherapy, radiation treatment, or combined modality protocols. The most active combination is 5-FU and cisplatin, although complete or durable responses are uncommon. Many recently developed drugs and molecular targeted agents have not yet been evaluated.

The role of adjuvant systemic chemotherapy has not been established. Treatment with 5-FU and mitomycin for up to 1 year in patients found to have residual cancer at surgery after preoperative combined modality therapy did not reduce recurrence rates and produced considerable morbidity (82). The one or two courses of chemotherapy given concurrently with radiation improve locoregional control rates but are not sufficient to reduce the rates of systemic metastases significantly. Both induction (neoadjuvant) and adjuvant chemotherapy, principally with 5-FU and cisplatin, are currently being evaluated (3,12,64,81,100,114). The initial report of the first randomized trial of two courses of neoadjuvant 5-FU and cisplatin showed no benefit in disease-free or overall survival (3). The intent of the additional chemotherapy in these studies is principally to further improve locoregional control, but reduction of the rate of metastases is also sought.

Radiation Therapy

The use of radiation therapy alone, either brachytherapy or external beam, has been greatly reduced since the confirmation of improved outcome of combined modality therapy. Radiation alone is now recommended mainly to patients who are unable to undergo radiation plus chemotherapy, especially elderly pa-

tients (14), or for the treatment of smaller cancers up to about 3 to 4 cm in size. Selected results are shown in Table 59.6.

Surgery

Surgery is the principal treatment for anal intraepithelial neoplasia (110) but retains only a limited place in the initial management of primary invasive anal cancer. A few patients (<5% in most series) present with extensive tumors that have destroyed the competence of the anal sphincters or fistulized into the vagina. Eradication of cancer by irradiation with or without chemotherapy does not restore continence in such patients because the cancer is replaced by fibrous tissue rather than the specialized muscle of the anal sphincters. These patients may be managed by abdominoperineal resection with postoperative irradiation and chemotherapy, using drug schedules similar to those for primary treatment and radiation doses of about 45 Gy in 5 weeks. An alternative approach is to perform colostomy before irradiation and chemotherapy, followed by immediate or delayed resection. Severe stricturing of the canal may follow irradiation and chemotherapy in patients who have had a prior colostomy, making assessment of tumor control difficult. It is frequently not possible to close the colostomy later because of the stricture. However, patients with extensive or circumferential cancers who have not lost continence and in whom a colostomy can be avoided often respond well to irradiation and chemotherapy with long-term preservation of anorectal function. Surgery should be considered for any patient unable to tolerate radiation, with or without chemotherapy. Serious postradiation morbidity may require surgical management, but the frequency of such morbidity appears to be decreasing as radiation techniques improve.

Local excision, preserving anorectal function, is possible in some patients, although this approach is now usually restricted to small well-differentiated squamous cell cancers that have

Table 59.6 | **SELECTED RESULTS OF RADIATION THERAPY ALONE**

Author (Reference)	Radiation		Primary Tumor Control		Serious Complications— Colostomy	5-Year Survival
Newman et al. (86)	50 Gy/20/4 wk	8/9 (≤2 cm)	42/52 (81%) (≤5 cm)	13/20 (65%) (>5 cm or T4)	2	66%
Cummings et al. (23)	50 Gy/20/4 wk (some EB-I/I)	6/6 (≤2 cm)	19/29 (66%) (≤5 cm)	13/28 (46%) (>5 cm or T4)	6	61%
Martenson and Gunderson (78)	45-50 Gy/25-28/5-6 wk Plus boost to 55-67 Gy	9/9 (≤2 cm)	17/17 (100%) (≤5 cm)	—	2 temp.	94%, actuarial
Otim-Oyet et al. (91)	60-65 Gy/30-33/6-7 wk (some with boost)	2/2 (≤2 cm)	16/22 (73%) (≤4 cm)	8/17 (47%) (>4 cm)	1	56% cause-specific
Papillon and Montbarbon (95)	42 Gy/10/2.5 wk Plus I 20Gy at 8 wk	NS	29/39 (74%) (≤4 cm)	27/64 (42%) (>4 cm)	6	60%

EB, external beam; I, interstitial brachytherapy; NS, not stated; temp, temporary

not invaded the sphincter muscles and are located distal to the dentate line (56,57). This approach is based on the finding in surgical series that pararectal or superior hemorrhoidal system lymph node metastases were associated with <5% of well-differentiated squamous cell cancers <2 cm in size (10,44). Excision of small cancers, especially of the distal canal and anal verge, is more expedient and generally associated with less morbidity than radiation-based treatments.

Perianal Cancer

The most common histologic type of invasive cancer of the perianal skin is squamous cell carcinoma, usually keratinizing. Basal cell cancers and adenocarcinomas can also occur.

Wide local excision with a 1-cm margin is recommended for all histologic types, provided anal continence can be preserved (73). Radiation alone or in combination with chemotherapy is also effective (9,85), but may produce symptomatic long-term skin changes. Radiation-based protocols identical to those for anal canal cancer are preferred when anal continence would be impaired by surgery. In the UKCCCR trial, one in four patients had a cancer that arose in the perianal skin (anal margin). Results by site of cancer origin were not reported, but local control and cause-specific survival rates favored combined modality therapy (121).

The regional nodes for the perianal skin are the ipsilateral inguinal nodes. Perirectal and pelvic node metastases are uncommon unless the cancer involves the anal canal extensively. The risk of inguinal node metastases is about 10%, primarily with category T3 or T4 tumors or poorly differentiated cancers. Elective bilateral inguinal nodal irradiation may be considered for these tumors, with inclusion of the pelvic nodes if the anal canal is invaded. The management of abnormal inguinal nodes is similar to that for anal canal cancer.

The principles of management for the uncommon basal cell and adenocarcinomas of the perianal skin are similar to those for these histological types elsewhere on the skin.

Patients with HIV/AIDS

Patients with HIV infection, especially those with a history of anal-receptive intercourse, are at increased risk of anal squamous cell cancer. The median age at diagnosis is in the fourth decade, about 20 years earlier than in non-HIV infected patients. Anal cancers in several small series of HIV-infected patients have been treated by combined modality therapy or radiation alone (16,30,60,61,97,101). HIV-infected patients are at increased risk of toxicity, particularly in the perineal skin and anorectal mucosa, when treated with radiation with or without chemotherapy, although the mechanisms for this are not known (37). However, the more recent reports suggest that it is not necessary to electively modify standard protocols of radiation (with respect to dose, fractionation, or volume) and chemotherapy (either 5-FU and mitomycin, or 5-FU and cisplatin), but modifications should be based on the severity of side effects in each individual patient (16,60). Two factors may predict for heightened acute normal tissue toxicity and/or poor cancer control, namely, a CD4 count <200/μL at the start of treatment or the presence of AIDS (61,101), but these findings are not inevitably associated with poor tolerance. Concurrent antiretroviral therapy does not reliably reduce the severity or incidence of toxicity of radiation and chemotherapy (74). Complete primary cancer remission rates of about 70% or better are generally described, but it is difficult to obtain reliable data on long-term tumor control, particularly in patients with AIDS.

Adenocarcinomas

Most adenocarcinomas involving the anal canal arise from rectal-type mucosa that extends below the upper muscular boundary of the canal. They are generally treated similarly to those that arise in the rectum. The uncommon adenocarcinomas that develop from anal glands or in fistulae have also usually been managed by abdominoperineal resection. Five-year survival rates following surgery alone are commonly <50%, with local recurrence rates of about 25% (8,73,84,119). Any advantage from adjuvant radiation and chemotherapy is unknown, although, by analogy, protocols used for primary rectal cancers are sometimes applied. Other centers have treated these anal adenocarcinomas by the protocols developed for squamous cell cancers. Experience is limited, but anorectal function has been retained, and apparent cures have been reported following treatment with radiation alone or with radiation and chemotherapy (8,69).

Small Cell Carcinomas

Small cell carcinomas are rare cancers characterized by early metastases and have a poor prognosis (10). The primary tumor may be managed by surgery or radiation. Systemic chemotherapy similar to that used for small cell cancers that arise elsewhere may be combined with radiation for the primary tumor and used to treat metastases, but responses are generally limited.

Radiation Therapy Techniques

Anal Canal

The treatment volumes of interest are determined by the philosophy adopted with regard to which lymph node groups should be treated and whether the primary tumor and lymph nodes should be treated in continuity. Only well-differentiated squamous cell cancers ≤2 cm in size situated in the distal canal appear to have a risk of nodal metastases <5% (10,44). Treatment of larger cancers by interstitial brachytherapy alone resulted in failure in pelvic nodes above the treated volume in 16% (14/88) in one study (94). The finding in surgical series of histopathologically verified metastases in the pararectal and internal iliac nodes in up to 30% and in inguinal nodes in up to 20% has encouraged most centers to irradiate these node groups electively. As a result, planning target volumes may be extensive. There is some evidence that acute and late morbidity can be reduced by avoiding tangential irradiation to the sensitive skin of the perineum and external genitalia or, if techniques that require tangential irradiation are elected, by the use of daily fractions ≤2 Gy. The irregularities and curvatures of the perineum and lower pelvis make homogenous radiation distributions difficult to achieve. Measurements with *in vivo* thermoluminescent dosimeters found dose variations of as much as 10% from predicted levels in the region of the anocutaneous junction (129). Computerized dose planning systems may not provide accurate values at skin–air interfaces. Care must be taken as far as possible to avoid regions of excessive dose.

Whole Pelvis Techniques

Many radiation oncologists prefer to treat the primary tumor and the posterior pelvic and inguinal nodes in continuity. An anterior-posterior–opposed pair of fields is the most common arrangement. If the patient is prone, the anus can be visualized readily and bolus placed selectively over any perianal tumor extension. Alternatively, the patient may be treated supine to reduce some of the inhomogeneities produced by the natural curvatures of the pelvic soft tissues. The upper border of the field is placed at the lumbosacral junction if the intent is to include the common iliac, upper presacral, and rectosigmoid nodes in the treated volume. This border is commonly moved down during treatment to the lower end of the sacroiliac joints, thus encompassing only the perirectal, lower presacral, and internal iliac nodes (and, if the volume is sufficiently wide, the lower external iliac nodes), in order to lessen the risk of radiation enteritis (36) (Fig. 59.2). Some authors consider elective treatment of radiologically normal lymph nodes above the level of the lower border of the sacroiliac joints unnecessary (22,23,80). The inferior field border is placed 3-cm distal to the lowermost extension of the primary tumor, which should be indicated with a radio-opaque marker during simulation.

The position of the lateral borders depends on the philosophy adopted with respect to the desirability of treating a continuous homogenous volume or the preference to minimize irradiation of the femoral head and neck. Options include anterior and posterior fields of equal size encompassing the inguinal nodes; anterior and posterior fields of equal size, but restricted to include the medial borders of the pelvis only, the inguinal nodes being treated by anterior electron beams matched to the photon

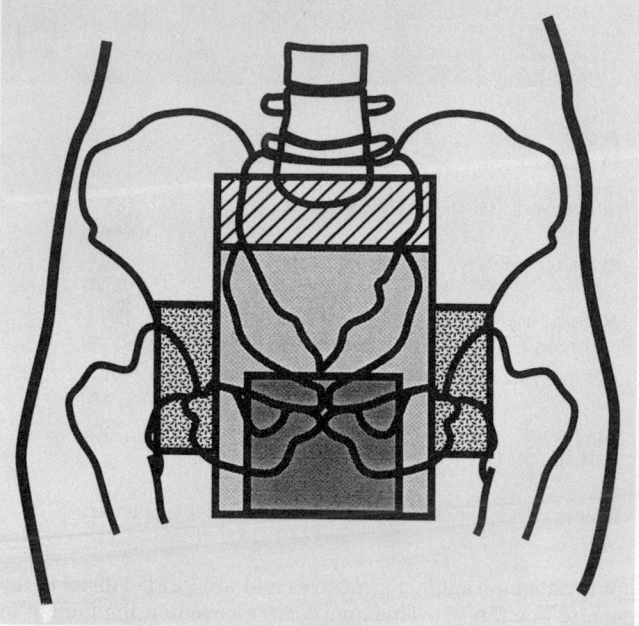

FIGURE 59.2. Example of radiation fields used to cover pelvis nodes and primary cancer. Upper border generally lowered from lumbosacral junction to lower border of sacroiliac joints part way through course. Fields are later reduced further to give higher dose to primary tumor. Separate anterior fields are applied to cover lateral inguinal nodes.

fields; and asymmetric photon fields, with a larger anterior field to cover the primary tumor, pelvic and inguinal nodes in continuity, and a posterior beam restricted to the primary tumor and pelvic nodes. In this latter arrangement, anterior electron beams are used to supplement the dose to the inguinal nodes to the desired level. The location and depth of the inguinal nodes should be obtained by axial imaging (75). When asymmetric and/or matched fields are used, there is potential for both over and under dosage (15). Considerable care is required in planning and in patient positioning.

Posterior Pelvis Techniques

If it is elected to irradiate the posterior pelvic tissues and inguinal nodes discontinuously for all or part of the prescription, or to treat the posterior pelvis only, the volume irradiated is reduced compared with that of whole-pelvis techniques. The anal canal and posterior pelvic nodes may be treated by multiple beam techniques. These are commonly three- or four-field techniques, such as a direct posterior or anterior-posterior/posterior-anterior (AP/PA) fields, and opposed lateral beams, analogous to those used for rectal cancer. Recently, multiple-field conformal techniques, including intensity-modulated radiation therapy (IMRT), have been described (15,83,125) (Fig. 59.3). Conformal techniques can reduce the mean dose to the perineum and external genitalia by about 30%. Although these techniques generally include beams tangential to the perineum, doses of at least 54 Gy in 1.8-Gy fractions can be delivered with only occasional need for treatment breaks due to skin or gastrointestinal toxicity (83,125). Early accounts of IMRT techniques have described the use of patient immobilization devices, but have not discussed the possible effects on dose distribution of internal organ motion.

Dose–Time Factors

All external-beam therapy is given by megavoltage equipment. The choice of beam energy should be based on the technique used and on the tissues to be included in the planning target volume and treated volume.

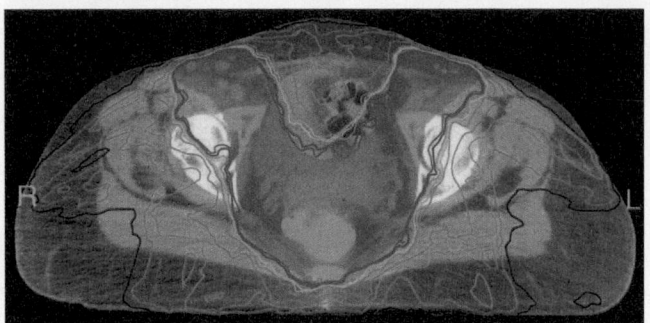

FIGURE 59.3. Transverse axial computed tomography of pelvis showing conformal intensity-modulated radiation therapy plan designed to include anorectum, posterior pelvic, internal iliac, and inguinal lymph nodes. (Image provided by Drs. R. Heimann and S. Johnson, University of Chicago.)

If external-beam irradiation is given without concurrent chemotherapy, it is usual, as in other cancers, to prescribe doses close to the tolerance of the normal tissues. There have been no studies to establish the optimum dose–time factors. A dose to the primary tumor of 60 to 65 Gy over 6 to 7 weeks, in 1.8- to 2-Gy fractions, is commonly prescribed. The primary tumor and regional nodes are encompassed to a dose of 40 to 45 Gy in 4 to 5 weeks, after which the volume is reduced. The smaller clinical target volume includes the primary tumor with a margin of 2 to 3 cm. This reduced volume may be treated as most appropriate by interstitial therapy, by external-beam therapy with a perineal field, or by multifield techniques (23,36,94). A dose of 15 to 20 Gy in 2 weeks is given to the reduced volume. If low–dose-rate interstitial radiation is used, a dose of 15 to 20 Gy at 0.5 cm from the plane of the implant over 24 hours (Paris system) is recommended (94). Proven or suspected metastases in the inguinal nodes and abnormal perirectal or pelvic nodes should be treated to the same total dose as the primary tumor.

Delivery of the final reduced volume treatment phase by brachytherapy is more common in Europe than in North America, where external beam treatment is favored. There are a number of reports of effective brachytherapy, including low–dose-rate (LDR) (96,99), pulsed–dose-rate (PDR) (47,105), and high–dose-rate (HDR) techniques (71,123). Brachytherapy has usually been given 2 to 8 weeks after external-beam therapy, although one schedule introduced HDR in the interval during split-course external beam therapy (71). There is no agreement on whether the treatment volume should include the full extent of the initial primary cancer (71,94,99,105) or only the tumor remaining at the time of implant (29). The brachytherapy dose depends on the composite dose of the total radiation prescription. Occasionally, significant toxicity has been encountered (98,105). Techniques to reduce the risk of serious toxicity by minimizing the volume irradiated (94,99), avoiding fully circumferential implants (94), and reducing the dose to the uninvolved anal circumference (29,47,94,105,123), have been described. The merits of adjuvants to brachytherapy such as intracavitary (76) or interstitial (72) hyperthermia or concurrent chemotherapy are unproven.

When radiation is given with concurrent 5-FU and mitomycin, or 5-FU and cisplatin, some modification of these dose–time guidelines is usual. The modifications are intended to reduce acute toxicity or are based on the successful outcomes of the lower dose radiation schedules initially introduced as surgical adjuvant therapy. Recent protocols, however, have sought to improve local control rates, particularly for larger tumors, by intensifying radiation or chemotherapy or both. Increases in total radiation doses and shortening of overall time of treatment by eliminating elective interruptions in radiation (split course therapy) have been advocated. When combined with 5-FU and mitomycin, radiation doses of as little as 30 Gy in 15 fractions

over 3 weeks have been shown to eradicate up to about 90% of cancers ≤3 cm in size. Higher doses, from 45 Gy in 25 fractions in 5 weeks to 54 Gy in 30 fractions in 6 weeks, sometimes supplemented by additional radiation after an interval of 6 to 8 weeks to a total of 60 to 65 Gy over a total time of about 12 weeks, have controlled from 65% to 75% of primary tumors >4 cm (see Table 59.4). Recent trials in North America have used 59 Gy in 32 fractions over 6.5 weeks (3,66,67,79); the effectiveness and tolerability of this schedule has not yet been reported in detail.

Short interruptions in external-beam treatment, generally of no more than 2 weeks but of up to 4 weeks in some series, were introduced into many combined modality protocols, either as elective breaks after about 3 weeks' treatment or as required by individual patients, to reduce the severity of acute anoproctitis and perineal dermatitis. Where further radiation was to be prescribed, based on the extent of clinical or histopathologic response to the first phase of treatment, longer intervals of 6 to 8 weeks were recommended to allow tumor regression. The possible adverse effects of split-course irradiation on the control of anal cancer have not been studied formally, but the limited data available on the potential tumor doubling time of anal cancer suggest that it is rapid, and of the order of 4 days (range 1 to 30 days; $n = 26$) (133), so some adverse effect may be expected from unnecessarily prolonged treatment. Overall treatment time was found to be more significant than the presence or absence of treatment interruptions in one study (54). In most studies that have considered treatment duration, better results have been achieved in patients who have had shorter treatment times (17,128). However, there are many potentially confounding factors in these nonrandomized comparisons, and the optimum treatment duration is not known. Several current studies seek to eliminate all interruptions or to reduce them to 2 weeks or less.

The rationale for escalating the total radiation dose is based on the observation in randomized and nonrandomized studies that the control rate of larger tumors was inferior to that of smaller cancers and analyses of nonrandomized studies that suggest a dose–control relationship (17,103). Review of 50 patients showed improved 5-year survival and local control rates following total radiation doses of 54 Gy or more (17). In another series of 34 patients with tumors >2 cm, local control rates were 38% (5/13) for those who received a total dose of <45 Gy, 69% (9/13) for 50 to 55 Gy, and 88% (7/8) for >60 Gy (103). The need to continue to review dose–time factors and techniques carefully is reflected by the finding of excessive acute and late toxicity when 5-FU and mitomycin were given concurrently with high-dose radiation, 50 Gy in 20 fractions of 2.5 Gy over 4 weeks, using anterior and posterior beams to 25 Gy followed by a three-field posterior pelvic technique for the remaining 25 Gy (22). In an RTOG phase II trial, 9/18 patients planned to receive an uninterrupted course of 59.4 Gy in 33 fractions over 6.5 weeks, with concurrent 5-FU and mitomycin, required a break in treatment of 2 weeks or more (66,67).

When clinically normal lymph nodes are irradiated electively, doses of about 36 Gy in 18 fractions in 3.5 weeks in combination with chemotherapy appear adequate (36), and doses as low as 24 Gy in 12 fractions in 2.5 weeks have been used successfully (22). Nodal metastases should be treated to the same dose as the primary cancer.

Perianal

If small (<4 cm) perianal cancers with low risk of regional node metastases are treated by radiation, a dose of 60 to 66 Gy in 2-Gy fractions over 6 weeks may be used. A direct perineal field is preferred as this minimizes the area of skin irradiated. Orthovoltage equipment may suffice, although electrons or low energy megavoltage photons (with bolus) are used more commonly. Care should be taken to flatten the perineum as much as possible to avoid areas of over or under dosage. Larger perianal cancers, or cancers invading the anal canal, are usually treated by the techniques and schedules of radiation and chemotherapy used for anal canal cancers. The upper border of the fields is usually placed at the lower end of the sacroiliac joints. The final phase of radiation may be given by direct perineal photon or electron therapy. Although brachytherapy may be used for the final phase, full treatment of perianal cancers by brachytherapy has been associated with high rates of necrosis in some series.

Sequelae of Therapy

Some nonrandomized series have described higher acute and late toxicity rates from combined modality therapy than those reported in the multicenter randomized trials. This probably results from use of different criteria for recording and reporting toxicity.

In programs that combined radiation therapy, 96-hour infusions of 5-FU and bolus injections of mitomycin, moderate leukopenia, thrombocytopenia, anoproctitis, and perineal dermatitis were recorded in about 30% of patients after doses of 25 to 30 Gy in 2.5 to 3 weeks (22,111). More profound proctitis and dermatitis occurred in up to 55% of those who received from 50 Gy in 4 to 5 weeks (22,118) to 59.4 Gy in 6.5 weeks (66). When cisplatin is substituted for mitomycin, marrow toxicity may be less, but at radiation doses of 59.4 Gy in 6.5 weeks, acute soft tissue toxicity rates are similar (3,79). All large studies of radiation, 5-FU, and mitomycin or cisplatin have reported an incidence (<2% overall) of mortality associated with acute toxicity, usually as a result of neutropenia with sepsis.

Serious late toxicity has not been reported after doses of 30 Gy in 3 weeks with 5-FU and mitomycin, but significant complications, often requiring surgery, have been recorded in about 5% to 15% of those receiving higher radiation doses. It is probable that those reports, many of which were retrospective, overlooked some treatment-related toxicity. For example, a large cohort study of 556 women aged 65 or over who developed anal cancer showed a higher risk of pelvic fracture, principally of the hip, in those who received radiation ($n = 399$) compared to those not irradiated ($n = 157$). The cumulative 5-year fracture rate was 14% versus 7.5% ($p < .01$) (7).

Less serious side effects are very common and may cause patients considerable discomfort (5,19,65,124). These include changes in anorectal function such as urgency and frequency of defecation, bleeding from anorectal telangiectasia, perineal dermatitis, dyspareunia, and impotence. These lower-grade side effects are usually managed medically with varying success. Systematic and prospective evaluation of the function of the anorectum and of other organs potentially affected by treatment has begun only recently, as have formal quality-of-life studies. There is often dissociation between a patient's account of anal and rectal function and continence and physiologic measurements of anorectal function, and the few studies in this area have been inconclusive (11,124). Prospective studies of pelvic organ function can be expected to assist the development of radiation treatment protocols by facilitating correlation of function with time–dose factors and radiation–chemotherapy interactions.

References

1. Abbasakoor F, Boulos PB. Anal intraepithelial neoplasia. *Br J Surg* 2005;92:277–290.
2. Adami J, Gabel H, Lindelof B, et al. Cancer risk following organ transplantation: a nation wide cohort study in Sweden. *Br J Cancer* 2003;89:1221–1227.
3. Ajani JA, Winter KA, Gunderson LL, et al. Intergroup RTOG 9811: a phase III randomized study of 5-fluorouracil, cisplatin and radiotherapy in carcinoma of the anal canal. Proceedings of the American Society of Clinical Oncology. *J Clin Oncol* 2006;24:1805(abstr).
4. Allal AS, Laurencet FM, Reymond MA, et al. Effectiveness of surgical salvage therapy for patients with locally uncontrolled anal carcinoma after sphincter-conserving surgery. *Cancer* 1999;86:405–409.
5. Allal AS, Sprangers MA, Laurencet F, et al. Assessment of long-term quality of life in patients with anal carcinomas treated by radiotherapy with or without chemotherapy. *Br J Cancer* 1999;80:1588–1594.
6. Bartelink H, Roelofsen F, Eschwege F, et al. Concomitant radiotherapy and chemotherapy is superior to radiotherapy alone in the treatment of locally advanced anal cancer: results of a phase III randomized trial of the European Organization for Research and Treatment of Cancer Radiotherapy and Gastrointestinal Cooperative Groups. *J Clin Oncol* 1997;15:2040–2049.
7. Baxter NN, Habermann EB, Tepper JE, et al. Risk of pelvic fractures in older women following pelvic irradiation. *JAMA* 2005;294:2587–2593.
8. Belkacemi Y, Berger C, Poortmans P, et al. Management of anal canal adenocarcinoma: a large retrospective study from the Rare Cancer Network. *Int J Radiat Oncol Biol Phys* 2003;56:1274–1283.
9. Bieri S, Allal AS, Kurtz JM. Sphincter-conserving treatment of carcinomas of the anal margin. *Acta Oncol* 2001;40:29–33.
10. Boman BM, Moertel CG, O'Connell M, et al. Carcinoma of the anal canal: a clinical and pathological study of 188 cases. *Cancer* 1984;54:114–125.
11. Broens P, Van Limbergen E, Penninckx F, et al. Clinical and manometric effects of combined external beam irradiation and brachytherapy for anal cancer. *Int J Colorectal Dis* 1998;13:68–72.
12. Brunet R, Becouarn Y, Pigneux J, et al. Cisplatin et fluorouracile en chimiothérapie neoadjuvante des carcinomas épidermoides du canal anal. *Lyon Chirurgical* 1990;87:77–79.
13. Cataldo PA, MacKeigan JM. The necessity of routine pathologic evaluation of hemorrhoidectomy specimens. *Surg Gynecol Obstet* 1992;174:302–304.
14. Chauveinc L, Buthaud X, Falxou MC, et al. Anal canal cancer treatment: practical limitations of routine prescription of concurrent chemotherapy and radiotherapy. *Br J Cancer* 2003;89:2057–2061.
15. Chen YJ, Liu A, Tsai PT, et al. Organ sparing by conformal avoidance intensity-modulated radiation therapy for anal cancer: dosimetric evaluation of coverage of pelvis and inguinal/femoral nodes. *Int J Radiat Oncol Biol Phys* 2005;63:274–281.
16. Cleator S, Fife K, Nelson M, et al. Treatment of HIV-associated invasive anal cancer with combined chemoradiation. *Eur J Cancer* 2000;36:754–758.
17. Constantinou EC, Daly W, Fung CY, et al. Time-dose considerations with treatment of anal cancer. *Int J Radiat Oncol Biol Phys* 1997;39:651–657.
18. Critchlow CW, Surawicz CM, Holmes KK, et al. Prospective study of high grade and intraepithelial neoplasia in a cohort of homosexual men: influence of HIV infection, immunosuppression and human papilloma virus infection. *AIDS* 1995;9:1255–1262.
19. Cummings BJ. Preservation of structure and function in epidermoid cancer of the anal canal. In: Rosenthal CJ, Rotman M, eds. *Infusion chemotherapy radiotherapy interactions: its biology and significance for organ salvage and prevention of second primary neoplasms.* Amsterdam: Elsevier Science Publishing Co., 1998;167–178.
20. Cummings BJ. Sentinel node biopsy for squamous cell carcinoma of the anus and anal margin. Discussion of Perera D et al. *Dis Colon Rectum* 2003;46:1030–1031.
21. Cummings BJ. Anal cancer. In: Gospodarowicz MK, O'Sullivan B, Sobin LH, eds. *Prognostic factors in cancer*, 3rd ed. Hoboken: John Wiley & Sons, 2006;139–142.
22. Cummings BJ, Keane TJ, O'Sullivan B, et al. Epidermoid anal cancer: treatment by radiation and 5-fluorouracil with and without mitomycin C. *Int J Radiat Oncol Biol Phys* 1991;21.1115–1125.
23. Cummings BJ, Keane TJ, Thomas GM, et al. Results and toxicity of the treatment of anal canal carcinoma by radiation therapy or radiation therapy and chemotherapy. *Cancer* 1984;54:2062–2068.
24. Daling JR, Sherman KJ, Hislop TG, et al. Cigarette smoking and the risk of anogenital cancer. *Am J Epidemiol* 1992;135:180–189.
25. Daling JR, Weiss NS, Klopfenstein LL, et al. Correlates of homosexual behavior and the incidence of anal cancer. *JAMA* 1982;247:1988–1990.
26. Damin DE, Rosito MA, Schwartsmann G. Sentinel lymph node in carcinoma of the anal canal: a review. *Eur J Surg Oncol* 2006;32:247–252.
27. Doci R, Zucali R, Bombelli L, et al. Combined chemoradiation therapy for anal cancer. *Ann Surg* 1992;215:150–156.
28. Doci R, Zucali R, La Monica G, et al. Primary chemoradiation therapy with fluorouracil and cisplatin for cancer of the anus: results in 35 consecutive patients. *J Clin Oncol* 1996;14:3121–3125.
29. Doniec JM, Schniewind B, Kovacs G, et al. Multimodal therapy of anal cancer aided by new endosonographic-guided brachytherapy. *Surg Endosc* 2006;20:673–678.
30. Edelman S, Johnstone PA. Combined modality therapy for HIV-infected patients with squamous cell carcinoma of the anus: outcomes and toxicities. *Int J Radiat Oncol Biol Phys* 2006;66:206–211.
31. Edwards AT, Morus LC, Goster ME, et al. Anal cancer: the case for earlier diagnosis. *J R Soc Med* 1991;84:395–397.
32. Fenger C. Histology of the anal canal. *Am J Surg Pathol* 1988;12:41–55.
33. Fenger C. Anal neoplasia and its precursors; facts and controversies. *Semin Diag Pathol* 1991;8:190–201.
34. Fenger C. Prognostic factors in anal carcinoma. *Pathology* 2002;34:573–578.
35. Fenger C, Frisch M, Marti MC, et al. Tumours of the anal canal. In: Hamilton SR, Aaltonen LA, eds. *Pathology and genetics of tumours of the digestive system.* Lyon: IARC Press, 2000;145–155.
36. Flam M, John M, Pajak TF, et al. The role of mitomycin C in combination with 5-fluorouracil and radiotherapy, and of salvage chemoradiation in the definitive nonsurgical treatment of epidermoid carcinoma of the anal canal: results of a phase III randomized Intergroup study. *J Clin Oncol* 1996;14:2527–2539.
37. Formenti SC, Chak L, Gill P, et al. Increased radiosensitivity of normal tissue fibroblasts in patients with acquired immunodeficiency syndrome (AIDS) and with Kaposi's sarcoma. *Int J Radiat Biol* 1995;68:411–412.
38. Friberg B, Svensson C, Goldman S, et al. The Swedish National Care Programme for anal carcinoma. Implementation and overall results. *Acta Oncol* 1998;37:25–32.

39. Frisch M. On the etiology of anal squamous carcinoma. *Dan Med Bull* 2002;49: 194–209.
40. Frisch M, Biggar RJ, Engels EA, et al. Association of cancer with AIDS-related immunosuppression in adults. *JAMA* 2001;285:1736–1745.
41. Frisch M, Fenger C, van den Brule AJ, et al. Variants of squamous cell carcinoma of the anal canal and perianal skin and their relation to human papilloma virus. *Cancer Res* 1999;59:753–757.
42. Frisch M, Johansen C. Anal carcinoma in inflammatory bowel disease. *Br J Cancer* 2000;83:89–90.
43. Frisch M, Olsen JH, Bautz A, et al. Benign anal lesions and the risk of anal cancer. *N Engl J Med* 1994;331:300–302.
44. Frost DB, Richards PC, Montague ED, et al. Epidermoid cancer of the anorectum. *Cancer* 1984;53:1285.
45. Gerard JP, Ayzac L, Hun D, et al. Treatment of anal canal carcinoma with high dose radiation therapy and concomitant fluorouracil-cisplatinum. Long term results in 95 patients. *Radiother Oncol* 1998;46:249–256.
46. Gerard JP, Chapet O, Samiei F, et al. Management of inguinal lymph node metastases in patients with carcinoma of the anal canal. Experience in a series of 270 patients treated in Lyon and review of the literature. *Cancer* 2001;92:77–84.
47. Gerard JP, Mauro F, Thomas L, et al. Treatment of squamous cell anal canal carcinoma with pulse dose rate brachytherapy. Feasibility study of a French Cooperative Group. *Radiother Oncol* 1999;51:129–131.
48. Gervaz P, Hirschel B, Morel P. Molecular biology of squamous cell carcinoma of the anus. *Br J Surg* 2006;93:531–538.
49. Glimelius B, Pahlman L. Radiation therapy of anal epidermoid carcinoma. *Int J Radiat Oncol Biol Phys* 1987;13:305–312.
50. Godlewski G, Prudhomme M. Embryology and anatomy of the anorectum. *Surg Clin North Am* 2000;80:319–343.
51. Golden GT, Horsley JS. Surgical management of epidermoid carcinoma of the anus. *Am J Surg* 1976;131:275–280.
52. Goldman S, Auer G, Erhardt K, et al. Prognostic significance of clinical stage, histologic grade, and nuclear DNA content in squamous cell carcinoma of the anus. *Dis Colon Rectum* 1987;30:444–448.
53. Goldman S, Glimelius B, Glas U, et al. Management of anal epidermoid carcinoma: an evaluation of treatment results in two population-based series. *Int J Colorectal Dis* 1989;4:234–243.
54. Graf R, Wust P, Hildebrandt B, et al. Impact of overall treatment time on local control of anal cancer treatment with radiochemotherapy. *Oncology* 2003;65: 14–22.
55. Greenall MJ, Quan SHQ, Decosse JJ. Epidermoid cancer of the anus. *Br J Surg* 1985;72[Suppl]:S97.
56. Greenall MJ, Quan SHQ, Stearns MW, et al. Epidermoid cancer of the anal margin. *Am J Surg* 1985;149:95–101.
57. Greenall MJ, Quan SHQ, Urmacher C, et al. Treatment of epidermoid carcinoma of the anal canal. *Surg Gynecol Obstet* 1985;161:509–517.
58. Greene FL, Page DL, Fleming D, et al. *AJCC cancer staging manual,* 6th ed. Philadelphia: Lippincott Raven, 2002.
59. Hill J, Slade A, Scholefield P, et al. Salvage abdominoperineal resection for anal carcinoma. *Int J Colorectal Dis* 1996;1:133–136.
60. Hoffman R, Welton ML, Klenche B, et al. The significance of pretreatment CD4 count on the outcome and treatment tolerance of HIV-positive patients with anal cancer. *Int J Radiat Oncol Biol Phys* 1999;44:127–131.
61. Holland JM, Swift PS. Tolerance of patients with human immunodeficiency virus and anal carcinoma to treatment with combined chemotherapy and radiation therapy. *Radiology* 1994;193:251–254.
62. Hung A, Crane C, Delclos M, et al. Cisplatin-based combined modality therapy for anal carcinoma: a wider therapeutic index. *Cancer* 2003;97:1195–1202.
63. International Collaboration on HIV and Cancer. Highly active antiretroviral therapy and incidence of cancer in human immunodeficiency virus-infected adults. *J Natl Cancer Inst* 2000;92:1823–1830.
64. James RD, David C, Neville D, et al. Chemoradiation and maintenance chemotherapy for patients with anal carcinoma: a phase II study of the UK Coordinating Committee for Cancer Research (UKCCCR) Anal Cancer Trial Working Party. *Proc Am Soc Clin Oncol* 2000;19:268a(abstr).
65. Jephcott CR, Pattiel C, Hay J. Quality of life after non-surgical treatment of anal carcinoma: a case control study of long-term survivors. *Clin Oncol* 2004;16:530–535.
66. John M, Pajak T, Flam M, et al. Dose acceleration in chemoradiation for anal cancer: Preliminary results of RTOG 9208. *Cancer J Sci Am* 1996;2:205–207.
67. John M, Pajak T, Krieg R, et al. Dose escalation without split-course chemoradiation for anal cancer: results of a Phase II RTOG study. Proceedings of the American Society of Therapeutic Radiology and Oncology. *Int J Radiat Oncol Biol Phys* 1997;39[Suppl 2]:203(abstr).
68. Johnson LG, Madeleine MM, Newcomer LM, et al. Anal cancer incidence and survival: the surveillance, epidemiology, and end results experience, 1973–2000. *Cancer* 2004;101:281–288.
69. Joon DL, Chao MW, Ngan SY, et al. Primary adenocarcinoma of the anus: a retrospective analysis. *Int J Radiat Oncol Biol Phys* 1999;45:1199–1205.
70. Kadish AS. Biology of anogenital neoplasia. In: Sparano JA, ed. *HIV and HTLV-1 associated malignancies*. Boston: Kluwer Academic Publishers, 2001; 267–286.
71. Kapp KS, Geyer E, Gebhart FH, et al. Experience with split-course external beam irradiation +/− chemotherapy and integrated Ir-192 high-dose-rate brachytherapy in the treatment of primary carcinomas of the anal canal. *Int J Radiat Oncol Biol Phys* 2001;49:997–1005.
72. Kapp KS, Kapp DS, Stuecklschweiger G, et al. Interstitial hyperthermia and high dose rate brachytherapy in the treatment of anal cancer: a phase I/II study. *Int J Radiat Oncol Biol Phys* 1993;28:189–199.
73. Klas JV, Rothenberger DA, Wong WD, et al. Malignant tumors of the anal canal. The spectrum of disease, treatment and outcomes. *Cancer* 1999;85:1686–1693.
74. Klencke BJ, Palefsky JM. Anal cancer: an HIV-associated cancer. *Hematol Oncol Clin North Am* 2003;17:859–872.
75. Koh WJ, Chiu M, Stelzer KJ, et al. Femoral vessel depth and the implications for groin node radiation. *Int J Radiat Oncol Biol Phys* 1993;27:969–974.
76. Kouloulias V, Plataniotis G, Kouvaris J, et al. Chemoradiotherapy combined with intracavity hyperthermia for anal cancer. *Am J Clin Oncol* 2005;28:91–99.
77. Leichman L, Nigro N, Vaitkevicius VK, et al. Cancer of the anal canal: model for preoperative adjuvant combined modality therapy. *Am J Med* 1985;78:211–215.
78. Martenson JA, Gunderson LL. External radiation therapy without chemotherapy in the management of anal cancer. *Cancer* 1993;71:1736–1740.
79. Martenson JA, Lipsitz SR, Wagner H, et al. Initial results of a phase II trial of radiation therapy, 5-fluorouracil and cisplatin for patients with anal cancer. *Int J Radiat Oncol Biol Phys* 1996;35:745–749.
80. Melcher AA, Sebag-Montefiore D. Concurrent chemoradiotherapy for squamous cell carcinoma of the anus using shrinking field radiotherapy technique without a boost. *Br J Cancer* 2003;88:1352–1357.
81. Meropol NJ, Niedzwiecki D, Shank B, et al. Combined modality therapy of poor risk anal canal carcinoma: a phase II study of the Cancer and Leukemia Group B (CALGB). *Proc Am Soc Clin Oncol* 1999;18:237a(abstr).
82. Michaelson RA, Magill GB, Quan SHQ, et al. Preoperative chemotherapy and radiation therapy in the management of anal epidermoid carcinoma. *Cancer* 1983;51:390–395.
83. Milano MT, Jani AB, Farry KJ, et al. Intensity-modulated radiation therapy (IMRT) in the treatment of anal cancer: toxicity and clinical outcome. *Int J Radiat Oncol Biol Phys* 2005;63:354–361.
84. Myerson RJ, Karnell LH, Menck HR. The National Cancer Data Base report on carcinoma of the anus. *Cancer* 1997;80:805–815.
85. Newlin HE, Zlotecki RA, Morris CG, et al. Squamous cell carcinoma of the anal margin. *J Surg Oncol* 2004;86:55–62.
86. Newman G, Calverley DC, Acker BD, et al. The management of carcinoma of the anal canal by external beam radiotherapy: experience in Vancouver 1971–1988. *Radiother Oncol* 1992;25:196–202.
87. Nigro ND. An evaluation of combined therapy for squamous cell cancer of the anal canal. *Dis Colon Rectum* 1984;27:763–766.
88. Nigro ND, Vaitkevicius VK, Considine B. Combined therapy for cancer of the anal canal: a preliminary report. *Dis Colon Rectum* 1974;17:354–356.
89. Nilsson PJ, Svensson C, Goldman S, et al. Salvage abdominoperineal resection in anal epidermoid cancer. *Br J Surg* 2002;89:1425–1429.
90. Nilsson PJ, Svensson C, Goldman S, et al. Epidermoid anal cancer: a review of a population-based series of 308 consecutive patients treated according to prospective protocols. *Int J Radiat Oncol Biol Phys* 2005;61:92–102.
91. Otim-Oyet D, Ford H, Fisher C, et al. Radical radiotherapy for carcinoma of the anal canal. *Clin Oncol* 1990;2:84–89.
92. Palefsky JM. Anal squamous intraepithelial lesions: relation to HIV and human papillomavirus infection. *J Acquir Immune Defic Syndr* 1999;21:542–548.
93. Palefsky JM, Holly EA, Hogeboom CJ, et al. Virologic, immunologic, and clinical parameters in the incidence and progression of anal squamous intraepithelial lesions in HIV-positive and HIV-negative homosexual men. *J Acquir Immune Def Synd* 1998;17:314–319.
94. Papillon J. *Rectal and anal cancers: conservative treatment by irradiation. an alternative to radical surgery*. Berlin: Springer-Verlag, 1982.
95. Papillon J, Montbarbon JF. Epidermoid carcinoma of the anal canal: a series of 276 cases. *Dis Colon Rectum* 1987;30:324–333.
96. Papillon J, Montbarbon JF, Gerard JP, et al. Interstitial curietherapy in the conservative treatment of anal and rectal cancers. *Int J Radiat Oncol Biol Phys* 1989;17:1161–1169.
97. Peddada AV, Smith DE, Rao AR, et al. Chemotherapy and low-dose radiotherapy in the treatment of HIV-infected patients with carcinoma of the anal canal. *Int J Radiat Oncol Biol Phys* 1997;37:1101–1105.
98. Peiffert D. Comment on pulsed dose rate (PDR) brachytherapy of anal carcinoma by Roed et al. (letter). *Radiother Oncol* 1997;44:296–297.
99. Peiffert D, Bey P, Pernot M, et al. Conservative treatment by irradiation of epidermoid cancers of the anal canal: prognostic factors of tumoral control and complications. *Int J Radiat Oncol Biol Phys* 1997;37:313–324.
100. Peiffert D, Giovanni M, Ducreux M, et al. High dose radiation therapy and neoadjuvant plus concomitant chemotherapy with 5 fluorouracil and cisplatin in patients with locally advanced squamous cell anal canal cancer: final results of a phase II study. *Ann Oncol* 2001;12:397–404.
101. Place RJ, Gregorcyk SG, Huber PJ, et al. Outcome analysis of HIV-positive patients with anal squamous cell carcinoma. *Dis Colon Rectum* 2001;44:506–512.
102. Renehan AG, Sanders MP, Schofield PF, et al. Patterns of local disease failure and outcome after salvage surgery in patients with anal cancer. *Br J Surg* 2005;92:605–614.
103. Rich TA, Ajani JA, Morrison WH, et al. Chemoradiation therapy for anal cancer: radiation plus continuous infusion of 5-fluorouracil with or without cisplatin. *Radiother Oncol* 1993;27:209–215.
104. Roca E, De Simone G, Barugel M, et al. A phase II study of alternating chemoradiotherapy including cisplatin in anal canal carcinoma. *Proc Am Soc Clin Oncol* 1990;9:128(abstr).
105. Roed H, Engelhonm SA, Svendsen LB, et al. Pulsed dose rate (PDR) brachytherapy of anal carcinoma. *Radiother Oncol* 1996;41:131–134.
106. Salmon RJ, Fenton J, Asselain B, et al. Treatment of epidermoid anal canal cancer. *Am J Surg* 1984;147:43–48.
107. Schlienger M, Touboul E, Mauban S, et al. Resultants du traitment de 286 cas de cancers epidermoides du canal dont 236 par irradiation a visée conservatrice. *Lyon Chirurgical* 1991;87:61–64.
108. Schneider IHF, Grabenbauer GG, Reck T, et al. Combined radiation and chemotherapy for epidermoid carcinoma of the anal canal. *Int J Colorectal Dis* 1992;7:192–196.
109. Scholefield JH, Kerr IB, Shepherd NA, et al. Human papillomavirus type 16 DNA in anal cancers from six different countries. *Gut* 1991;32:674–676.
110. Scholefield JH, Ogunbiji OA, Smith JH, et al. Treatment of anal intraepithelial neoplasia. *Br J Surg* 1994;81:1238–1240.
111. Sischy N, Doggett RL, Krall JM, et al. Definitive irradiation and chemotherapy for radiosensitization in management of anal carcinoma: interim report on Radiation Therapy Oncology Group Study No. 8314. *J Natl Cancer Inst* 1989;81:850–856.
112. Sobin LH, Wittekind C. *TNM classification of malignant tumours,* 6th ed. New York: Wiley-Liss, 2002.
113. Stearns MW, Urmacher C, Sternberg SS, et al. Cancer of the anal canal. *Curr Probl Cancer* 1980;4:1–44.
114. Svensson C, Goldman S, Friberg B, et al. Induction chemotherapy and radiotherapy in loco-regionally advanced epidermoid carcinoma of the anal canal. *Int J Radiat Oncol Biol Phys* 1998;41:863–867.
115. Tanum G. Treatment of relapsing anal carcinoma. *Acta Oncol* 1993;32:33–35.
116. Tanum G, Tveit K, Karlsen KO. Diagnosis of anal carcinoma—doctor's finger still the best? *Oncology* 1991;48:383–386.

117. Tanum G, Tveit K, Karlsen KO, et al. Chemotherapy and radiation therapy for anal carcinoma: survival and late morbidity. *Cancer* 1991;67:2462–2466.

118. Tanum G, Tveit K, Karlsen KO, et al. Chemoradiotherapy of anal carcinoma: tumour response and acute toxicity. *Oncology* 1993;50:14–17.

119. Tarazi R, Nelson RL. Anal adenocarcinoma: a comprehensive review. *Sem Surg Oncol* 1994;10:235–240.

120. Touboul E, Schlienger M, Buffat L, et al. Epidermoid carcinoma of the anal canal. *Cancer* 1994;73:1569–1579.

121. UKCCCR Anal Canal Cancer Trial Working Party. Epidermoid anal cancer: results from the UKCCCR randomized trial of radiotherapy alone versus radiotherapy, 5-fluorouracil and mitomycin C. *Lancet* 1996;348:1049–1054.

122. Valentini V, Morganti AG, Luzi S, et al. Is chemoradiation feasible in elderly patients? *Cancer* 1997;80:1387–1392.

123. Vordermark D, Flentje M, Sailer M, et al. Intracavitary after-loading boost in anal canal carcinoma. Results, function and quality of life. *Strahlenther Onkol* 2001;177:252–258.

124. Vordermark D, Sailer M, Flentje M, et al. Curative intent radiation therapy in anal carcinoma: quality of life and sphincter function. *Radiother Oncol* 1999;52:239–243.

125. Vuong T, Devic S, Belliveau P, et al. Contribution of conformal therapy in the treatment of anal canal carcinoma with combined chemotherapy and radiotherapy: results of a phase II study. *Int J Radiat Oncol Biol Phys* 2003;56:823–831.

126. Wade DS, Herrera L, Castillo NB, et al. Metastases to the lymph nodes in epidermoid carcinoma of the anal canal studied by a clearing technique. *Surg Gynecol Obstet* 1989;169:238–242.

127. Wasvary HJ, Barkel DC, Klein SN. Is total colonic evaluation for anal cancer necessary? *Am Surg* 2000;66:592–594.

128. Weber DC, Kurtz JM, Allal AS. The impact of gap duration on local control in anal canal carcinoma treated by split-course radiotherapy and concomitant chemotherapy. *Int J Radiat Oncol Biol Phys* 2001;50:675–680.

129. Weber DC, Nouet P, Kurtz JM, et al. Assessment of target dose delivery in anal cancer using in vivo thermoluminescent dosimetry. *Radiother Oncol* 2001;59:39–43.

130. Wendell-Smith CP. Anorectal nomenclature: fundamental terminology. *Dis Colon Rectum* 2000;43:1349–1358.

131. Williams AB, Darragh TM, Vranizan K, et al. Anal and cervical human papillomavirus infection and risk of anal and cervical epithelial abnormalities in human immunodeficiency virus-infected women. *Obstet Gynecol* 1994;83:205–211.

132. Wolfe HR, Bussey HJ. Squamous cell carcinoma of the anus. *Br J Surg* 1968;55:295–301.

133. Wong CS, Tsang RW, Cummings BJ, et al. Proliferation parameters in epidermoid carcinomas of the anal canal. *Radiother Oncol* 2000;56:349–353.

134. Zbar AP, Fenger C, Efron J, et al. The pathology and molecular biology of anal intraepithelial neoplasia: comparisons with cervical and vulvar intraepithelial carcinoma. *Int J Colorectal Dis* 2002;17:203–215.

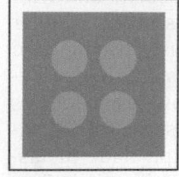

Chapter 60
Kidney, Renal Pelvis, and Ureter

Jeff M. Michalski

Anatomy

The kidneys are retroperitoneal structures located at the level between the 11th rib and the transverse process of the third lumbar vertebral body. Usually, the right kidney is slightly more inferior than the left with a position inferior to the right hepatic lobe. The renal axis runs parallel to the lateral margin of the psoas muscle. Each kidney is approximately 11 to 12 cm in length. The kidney is enveloped by a fibrous capsule and surrounded by perinephric fat, which is enveloped by Gerota's fascia. The organs adjacent to the right kidney include the liver superiorly, the duodenum and the vertebral bodies medially, and the transverse colon and small bowel anteriorly. On the left, the kidney abuts the spleen laterally; the stomach, pancreas, and vertebral bodies medially; and the small bowel and colon anteriorly. The kidneys are mobile organs that move vertically within the retroperitoneum on average 0.9 cm to 1.3 cm and as much as 4 cm during normal respiration (11,117, 137).

The caliceal collecting systems lie on the anteromedial surface of each kidney. The ureters course posteriorly and inferiorly, paralleling the lateral border of the psoas muscle until they curve anteriorly to join the bladder at the trigone.

The lymphatics of the kidney and renal pelvis drain along the renal vessels. The right kidney drains predominantly into the paracaval and interaortocaval lymph nodes, and the left kidney drains exclusively to the para-aortic lymph nodes (82). The lymphatic drainage of the ureter is segmented and diffuse and may involve any of the renal hilar, abdominal para-aortic, paracaval, common iliac, internal iliac, or external iliac lymph nodes.

Epidemiology and Risk Factors

The lesions discussed in this chapter are limited to adult renal cell carcinoma (e.g., hypernephroma, Grawitz's tumor) and transitional cell carcinoma of the collecting system and ureter.

Renal Cell Carcinoma

In 2006, the estimated number of new cases of kidney and other upper urinary tract cancers in the United States was 38,800, with more than 12,800 cancer deaths (60). These figures represent approximately 2% of all new cancers and cancer-related deaths. The average age at diagnosis is 55 to 60 years, and the tumors affect males more commonly than females, with a ratio of 1.5:1. A number of environmental (e.g., exposure to cadmium, thorium dioxide, petroleum products, and phenacetin-containing analgesics and tobacco use), occupational (e.g., leather tanners, shoe workers, asbestos workers), hormonal (e.g., diethylstilbestrol), cellular, and genetic factors have been associated with the development of renal cell carcinoma (71).

Long-term cigarette smoking is associated with an increased risk of developing renal cell carcinoma in men. High body weight and hypertension also are associated with a higher relative risk for development of these tumors (93).

The association of renal cell carcinoma and von Hippel–Lindau (VHL) disease has been long established (21). As many as 28% to 45% of people with VHL disease develop clear cell renal carcinoma (123). Chromosomal analysis of tumor cells from patients with familial renal cell carcinoma have revealed a proximal deletion in the short arm of chromosome 3 (65). These findings have led investigators to test sporadic cases of kidney cancer. Abnormalities of the short arm of chromosome 3 have been found in nonheritable renal cell carcinomas with high frequency (2). These findings suggest that these are not random alterations and that they may be involved in the origin of renal cell carcinoma. Several studies have shown that VHL mutation or VHL methylation with lack of expression of the gene account for 84% to 98% of sporadic cases of clear cell carcinoma of the kidney (12,70). The VHL gene product is a protein that in combination with ubiquitin ligase targets hypoxia-inducible factor (HIF) for proteolysis. The HIF-α subunit binds the VHL protein. In hypoxic conditions or in circumstances of defective VHL protein expression, HIF-α is not subject to proteolysis. The uninhibited HIF activity then leads to the overexpression of several hypoxia-inducible genes including vascular endothelial growth factor (VEGF) (58,140). Several studies of VEGF in renal cell carcinoma have shown nearly 100% expression of this protein or VEGF mRNA in tumor tissue (53,75,127,130). The papillary variant of renal cell carcinoma is not associated with VHL disease or its genetic variants.

Renal Pelvis and Ureter Cancer

Transitional cell carcinoma of the upper urinary tract accounts for 7% of all renal neoplasms and 5% of all urothelial malignancies (112). The incidence of bilateral upper urinary tract tumors is 1.5% to 2% for synchronous and 6% to 8% for asynchronous presentations (60). Renal pelvis tumor is found two to three times more commonly in men than in women, and the peak incidence is in the fifth and sixth decades of life. Upper urinary tract carcinoma is often a multifocal process; patients with cancer at one site in the upper urinary tract are at greater risk of developing transitional tumors elsewhere. About one-third of patients with upper urinary tract tumor develop bladder cancer (19).

Because the mucosal surfaces of the renal pelvis, ureter, and bladder have the same embryologic origin, many of the etiologic factors in renal pelvis and ureter tumors also apply to tumors of the urinary bladder. Urban residency, tobacco use, aminophenol exposure (e.g., benzidine, β-naphthylamine), renal stones, and analgesics (i.e., phenacetin abuse) have been associated with an increased risk for development of upper urinary tract tumors.

A chronic tubulointerstitial nephropathy endemic to the Balkan peninsula of Eastern Europe is associated with a high frequency of multifocal, slowly growing, superficial, papillary transitional cell cancer of the renal pelvis and ureter (107). The specific cause of this endemic nephropathy is unknown.

▪▪ | Natural History

Renal Cell Carcinoma

Primary renal cell tumors may spread by local infiltration through the renal capsule to involve the perinephric fat and Gerota's fascia. The tumor may grow directly along the venous channels to the renal vein or vena cava. Lymph node metastases occur with an incidence of 9% to 27% and most often involve the renal hilar, para-aortic, and paracaval lymph nodes (35,44). The renal vein is invaded by tumor in 21% of cases, and the inferior vena cava is invaded in as many as 4% of cases (141).

Of renal cell carcinomas, 7% are diagnosed incidentally at the time of radiologic evaluation for other diseases. Approximately 45% of patients with renal cell carcinoma have localized disease, 25% have regional disease, and about 30% have evidence of distant metastases at the time of diagnosis (44,119). Of patients with metastases, about 1% to 3% have solitary lesions (129). About half of the patients with renal cell carcinoma eventually develop metastatic disease (90).

Among patients presenting with metastatic renal cell carcinoma, the sites of distribution include lung (75%), soft tissue (36%), bone (20%), liver (18%), skin (8%), and central nervous system (8%) (80). Patients with metastatic disease at diagnosis have an extremely poor prognosis, with an expected survival of <5 years regardless of the site of metastasis (44,119).

Spontaneous regression of metastatic renal cell cancer after nephrectomy has been reported. In an extensive literature review, the incidence of regression of metastatic foci induced by nephrectomy was 0.8% (4/474 patients) (90). Patients who have local symptoms, such as hematuria, pain, hypertension, or other paraneoplastic syndromes, may benefit from a palliative nephrectomy. Cytoreductive surgery performed to prolong or increase the response of extrarenal disease in response to systemic therapy may be beneficial (6,34,88). Patients with a solitary metastatic lesion have a 5-year survival rate of 24% (compared with 4% for those with more than one metastatic focus), and they may benefit from aggressive therapy (38).

Renal Pelvis and Ureter Carcinoma

Upper urinary tract carcinoma is frequently a multifocal process. Patients with cancer at one site in the upper urinary tract are at significant risk for development of tumors elsewhere along the urothelium. The probability of multifocal occurrence is greatest in patients with large tumors and those with carcinoma *in situ*. Ureteral tumors tend to occur in the distal third of the ureter.

Transitional cell carcinoma of the upper urothelial tract may spread both by direct extension and by bloodborne and lymphatic metastases. Implantation of tumor cells in the bladder has been demonstrated, especially in previously traumatized areas. The incidence of lymph node metastasis is highly dependent on the grade of the primary tumor. Low-grade tumors have a very low metastatic propensity. In a series of 94 patients, none of 43 low-grade tumors had lymph node metastasis, compared with 3/22 tumors in patients with grade 3 or 4 tumors (26). Lymph node metastases were reported in 9/26 patients selected to receive postoperative radiation therapy (84).

▪▪ | Clinical Presentation

Renal Cell Carcinoma

Patients with renal cell carcinoma may present with an occult primary tumor or with signs and symptoms attributable to a local mass or systemic paraneoplastic syndromes. Gross hematuria, palpable flank mass, and pain describe a classic triad that occurs only in 5% to 10% of patients (121,122). Indeed, a finding of the classic triad often suggests advanced disease with a poor prognosis. The most frequent symptom associated with renal cell carcinoma is hematuria, either gross or microscopic. Renal cell carcinoma presenting as an incidental mass on a diagnostic imaging study ordered for other purposes accounts for 7% of all diagnoses and is associated with a very good prognosis (44,132).

A wide range of paraneoplastic syndromes has been associated with renal cell carcinoma. Parathyroidlike hormones, erythropoietin, renin, gonadotropins, placental lactogen, prolactin enteroglucagon, insulinlike hormones, adrenocorticotropic hormone, and prostaglandins have been identified in patients with renal cell carcinoma (29,126).

Renal Pelvis and Ureter Carcinoma

Gross or microscopic hematuria occurs in 70% to 95% of patients with renal pelvic or ureteral tumors (112). The other less common symptoms include pain (8% to 40%), bladder irritation (5% to 10%), or other constitutional symptoms (5%). About 10% to 20% of patients may present with a flank mass secondary to tumor or hydronephrosis.

▪▪ | Diagnostic Work-Up

Renal Cell Carcinoma

Renal masses are not uncommon, and most of them are benign. They frequently are diagnosed as an incidental finding during abdominal imaging for metastatic evaluation for an unrelated malignancy or other disease. An algorithm for the work-up of

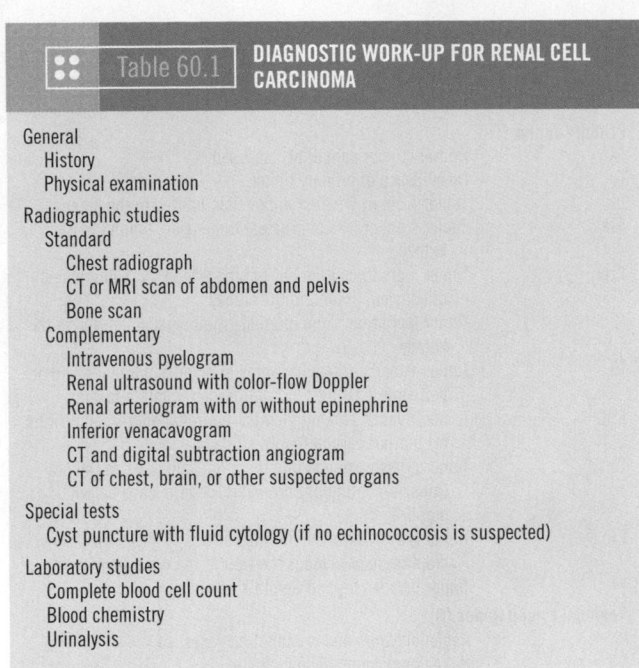

Table 60.1 DIAGNOSTIC WORK-UP FOR RENAL CELL CARCINOMA

General
    History
    Physical examination
Radiographic studies
    Standard
        Chest radiograph
        CT or MRI scan of abdomen and pelvis
        Bone scan
    Complementary
        Intravenous pyelogram
        Renal ultrasound with color-flow Doppler
        Renal arteriogram with or without epinephrine
        Inferior venacavogram
        CT and digital subtraction angiogram
        CT of chest, brain, or other suspected organs
Special tests
    Cyst puncture with fluid cytology (if no echinococcosis is suspected)
Laboratory studies
    Complete blood cell count
    Blood chemistry
    Urinalysis

CT, computed tomography; MRI, magnetic resonance imaging.

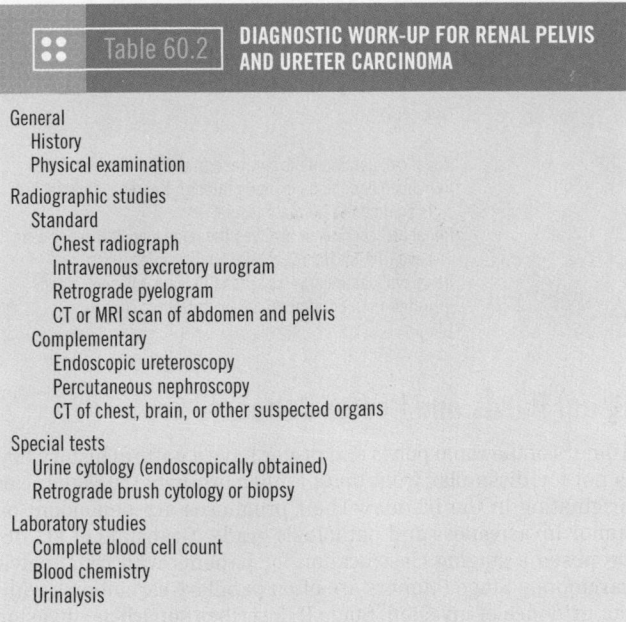

Table 60.2 DIAGNOSTIC WORK-UP FOR RENAL PELVIS AND URETER CARCINOMA

General
    History
    Physical examination
Radiographic studies
    Standard
        Chest radiograph
        Intravenous excretory urogram
        Retrograde pyelogram
        CT or MRI scan of abdomen and pelvis
    Complementary
        Endoscopic ureteroscopy
        Percutaneous nephroscopy
        CT of chest, brain, or other suspected organs
Special tests
    Urine cytology (endoscopically obtained)
    Retrograde brush cytology or biopsy
Laboratory studies
    Complete blood cell count
    Blood chemistry
    Urinalysis

CT, computed tomography; MRI, magnetic resonance imaging.

renal masses has been proposed (85). If computed tomography (CT) or ultrasound clearly identify the mass as a cyst, no further work-up is necessary. If a solid lesion is identified, then tumor removal by nephrectomy should be considered. In the case of small lesions, a follow-up CT scan to evaluate potential growth of the mass may raise the suspicion of malignancy. The diagnostic and staging work-up for renal cell carcinoma is given in Table 60.1. The diagnosis of renal cell carcinoma is established clinically and radiographically in most cases. Pathologic confirmation often is made at the time of curative nephrectomy. Once a radiographic diagnosis is made, a staging evaluation should be undertaken, which should include a complete history and physical examination, complete blood count, and liver and kidney function tests. A metastatic work-up should include a chest x-ray and CT or magnetic resonance imaging (MRI) scan of the abdomen and pelvis. Patients with symptoms suggestive of bony metastases and those with an elevated alkaline phosphatase level should undergo a bone scan. If metastatic lesions are detected, histologic confirmation should be made by biopsy of either the metastatic focus or the primary tumor. If renal vein or inferior vena cava invasion is suspected, ultrasound with color-flow Doppler may help define the extent of the tumor thrombus. Ultrasound is replacing the use of venacavography in the preoperative evaluation of patients with suspected venous invasion (85). Renal arteriography is sometimes helpful in planning surgery.

Renal Pelvis and Ureter Carcinoma

The diagnostic work-up for renal pelvis and ureter carcinoma is listed in Table 60.2. Intravenous urography frequently is used to evaluate patients with renal pelvis carcinoma. A filling defect in the renal pelvis or collecting system is the most common finding. Retrograde pyelography can be used to define the lower margin of a ureteral lesion, especially if there is significant proximal obstruction to flow of contrast from the renal pelvis. CT or MRI of the abdomen and pelvis before and after contrast administration gives useful information regarding the possible extension of tumor outside the collecting system (18). Urine cytology should be obtained endoscopically with a barbotage specimen. An ac-

curate cytologic diagnosis can be made in more than 80% of cases (27,55).

Staging

Renal Cell Carcinoma

In the United States, the staging system used most commonly by clinicians is the Robson modification of the Flocks and Kadesky system (Table 60.3) (35,114). Extension of tumor outside the renal capsule worsens the prognosis and thereby increases the stage of the patient's cancer. One drawback of this staging system is that patients with stage III cancers may have variable prognoses. Increasingly, the American Joint Committee on Cancer (AJCC) system is being utilized to stage patients with renal cell carcinoma (Table 60.4) (47). T1 and T2 cancers are completely within the renal parenchyma and have not invaded beyond the capsule. T3 tumors extend into major veins and invade the adrenal gland or perinephric tissues but do not extend beyond Gerota's fascia. T3a tumors invade the adrenal gland or perinephric tissues but do not extend beyond Gerota's fascia. Involvement of the renal vein or vena cava below the diaphragm defines T3b tumors, whereas T3c tumors involve gross tumor extending into the vena cava above the diaphragm. T4 tumors arise from the kidney and invade beyond Gerota's fascia. Regional lymph node metastases may involve spread to the renal hilar, paracaval, aortic, or retroperitoneal drainage sites. The node (N) stage classification depends on the size and number of lymph nodes involved. This staging system underwent significant modification in the 1997 edition. Tumors classified as T1 were changed from a limit of 2.5 cm to as large as 7 cm. Involvement of the renal vein in the absence of other extrarenal extension does not adversely affect survival. Patients with inferior vena cava (IVC) involvement above the diaphragm (T3c) have a worse survival rate than patients with tumors involving the renal vein or infradiaphragmatic IVC (T3b) (64). Patients with lymph node metastases (stage IIIB) have an inferior survival rate compared with patients whose tumor is confined to the renal vein or vena cava (stage IIIA) (121).

:: Table 60.3	ROBSON MODIFICATION OF THE FLOCKS AND KADESKY STAGING OF RENAL CELL CARCINOMA
Tumor Stage	**Description**
I	Renal cell carcinoma is confined to the kidneys
II	Renal cell carcinoma extends through the renal capsule but is confined to Gerota's fascia
III	Renal cell carcinoma involves the renal vein or inferior vena cava (IIIA) or the renal hilar lymph nodes (IIIB)
IV	Renal cell carcinoma has spread to local adjacent organs (other than adrenal gland) or to distant sites

Renal Pelvis and Ureter Cancer

Tumors of the renal pelvis and ureter have a natural history that is not too dissimilar from that of other urothelial malignancies originating in the bladder. Their prognoses are dependent on tumor invasiveness and pathologic grade. Grabstald et al. (46) proposed a staging classification for patients with renal pelvis carcinoma. Stage I tumors are often papillary carcinomas without evidence of invasion. Stage II describes superficial invasion limited to the lamina propria, and stage III tumors extend into the level of the muscularis. Stage IV describes cancers extending into adjacent structures or metastatic disease.

The 2002 AJCC staging classification for renal pelvis and ureter carcinoma is shown in Table 60.5 (47). Just as in the classification of Grabstald et al., the tumor (T) categories in the AJCC system depend on the extent of primary tumor invasion.

:: | Pathologic Classification

Renal Cell Carcinoma

The predominant histopathologic type of cancer that arises from the renal parenchyma is adenocarcinoma. Subtypes include clear cell carcinoma, which is the most predominant type, and granular cell carcinoma. A sarcomatoid variant represents 1% to 6% of renal cell carcinomas, and these tumors are associated with a significantly poorer prognosis (119).

Renal Pelvis and Ureter Carcinoma

More than 90% of malignant tumors arising from the renal pelvis and ureter are transitional cell carcinomas. Squamous cell carcinomas account for only 7% to 8%. Squamous cancers of the renal pelvis and ureter are often locally advanced and associated with a high local recurrence rate (7).

:: | Prognostic Factors

Renal Cell Carcinoma

The stage at initial presentation remains the most important prognostic factor for survival of patients with renal cell carcinoma. Survival statistics for patients with renal cell carcinoma have not changed much over the past 25 years. In 1969, Robson et al. (114) reported 5-year survival rates of 66% for stage I, 64% for stage II, 42% for stage III, and 11% for stage IV cancers. Table 60.6 lists survival by stage for patients treated primarily by radical nephrectomy over the past two decades.

The use of abdominal CT and ultrasound for nonmalignant medical illnesses has increased the frequency of diagnosis of incidental renal cell carcinomas. Patients who are discovered to have an incidental renal cell carcinoma have a 95% 5-year

:: Table 60.4	2002 AMERICAN JOINT COMMITTEE ON CANCER STAGING CLASSIFICATION FOR KIDNEY TUMORS

Primary Tumor (T)

TX	Primary tumor cannot be assessed
T0	No evidence of primary tumor
T1	Tumor 7 cm in greatest dimension, limited to the kidney
T1a	Tumor 4 cm or less in greatest dimension, limited to the kidney
T1b	Tumor more than 4 cm but not more than 7 cm in greatest dimension, limited to the kidney
T2	Tumor more than 7 cm in greatest dimension, limited to the kidney
T3	Tumor extends into major veins or invades adrenal gland or perinephric tissues but not beyond Gerota's fascia
T3a	Tumor invades adrenal gland or perirenal and/or renal sinus fat but not beyond Gerota's fascia
T3b	Tumor grossly extends into the renal vein or its segmental (muscle-containing) branches, or vena cava below diaphragm
T3c	Tumor grossly extends into the vena cava above the diaphragm or invades the wall of the vena cava
T4	Tumor invades beyond Gerota's fascia

Regional Lymph Nodes (N)[a]

NX	Regional lymph nodes cannot be assessed
N0	No regional lymph node metastasis
N1	Metastasis in a single regional lymph node
N2	Metastasis in more than one single lymph node
N3	Metastasis in a lymph node >5 cm in greatest dimension

Distant Metastasis (M)

MX	Presence of distant metastasis cannot be assessed
M0	No distant metastasis
M1	Distant metastasis

Stage Grouping

Stage I	T1	N0	M0
Stage II	T2	N0	M0
Stage III	T1	N1	M0
	T2	N1	M0
	T3	N0, N1	M0
	T3a	N0, N1	M0
	T3b	N0, N1	M0
	T3c	N0, N1	M0
Stage IV	T4	N0, N1	M0
	Any T	N2	M0
	Any T	Any N	M1

Histopathologic Grade

GX	Grade cannot be assessed
G1	Well differentiated
G2	Moderately well differentiated
G3–4	Poorly differentiated or undifferentiated

[a]Laterality does not affect the N classification.
Note: If a lymph node dissection is performed, then pathologic evaluation ordinarily would include at least eight nodes.
From Greene FL, Page DL, Fleming ID, et al. *AJCC cancer staging manual,* 6th ed. New York: Springer-Verlag, 2002, with permission.

survival rate, compared with 61% for patients who undergo abdominal imaging evaluation for genitourinary symptoms (132). The primary tumor size and clinical stages are significantly smaller and lower for patients who have no genitourinary symptoms compared with patients with symptoms (116).

The prognostic significance of renal vein or vena cava invasion has been the subject of considerable debate. A worse prognosis has been reported by some authors in patients with invasion of the renal vein or vena cava (77). The presence of vena cava involvement lowered the survival rate of patients with this finding, compared with patients presenting with distant metastases, in one series (44). Renal vein and IVC invasion was associated with an increased metastasis rate and inferior survival in a series reported by Ljungberg et al. (77). The opposite conclusion was made by Skinner et al. (121) in a review of

Table 60.5	2002 AMERICAN JOINT COMMITTEE ON CANCER STAGING CLASSIFICATION FOR RENAL PELVIS AND URETER TUMORS

Primary Tumor (T)

TX	Primary tumor cannot be assessed
T0	No evidence of primary tumor
Ta	Papillary noninvasive carcinoma
Tis	Carcinoma *in situ*
T1	Tumor invades subepithelial connective tissue
T2	Tumor invades muscularis
T3	(For renal pelvis only) Tumor invades beyond the muscularis into peripelvic fat or the renal parenchyma
T3	(For ureter only) Tumor invades beyond the muscularis into the periureteric fat
T4	Tumor invades adjacent organs or through the kidney into perinephric fat

Regional Lymph Nodes (N)[a]

NX	Regional lymph nodes cannot be assessed
N0	No regional lymph node metastasis
N1	Metastasis in a single lymph node, ≤ 2 cm in greatest dimension
N2	Metastasis in a single lymph node, >2 cm but ≤ 5 cm in greatest dimension, or multiple lymph nodes, ≤ 5 cm in greatest dimension
N3	Metastasis in a lymph node >5 cm in greatest dimension

Distant Metastasis (M)

MX	Distant metastasis cannot be assessed
M0	No distant metastasis
M1	Distant metastasis

Stage Grouping

Stage 0a	Ta	N0	M0
Stage 0is	Tis	N0	M0
Stage I	T1	N0	M0
Stage II	T2	N0	M0
Stage III	T3	N0	M0
Stage IV	T4	N0	M0
	Any T	N1, N2, N3	M0
	Any T	Any N	M1

Histopathologic Grade

GX	Grade cannot be assessed
G1	Well differentiated
G2	Moderately well differentiated
G3–4	Poorly differentiated or undifferentiated

[a]Laterality does not affect the N classification.
From Greene FL, Page DL, Fleming ID, et al. *AJCC cancer staging manual,* 6th ed. New York: Springer-Verlag, 2002, with permission.

309 cases treated by nephrectomy. As described previously, IVC invasion above the diaphragm (T3c) is associated with worse survival than renal vein invasion or IVC involvement below the diaphragm (T3b) (64). Renal vein or vena cava invasion often is associated with perinephric extension of the primary tumor. In patients with tumor involving only the renal vein or vena cava without perinephric invasion, the 5-year survival rate was 84%, comparable to that of patients with stage I cancers (45,128).

Lymph node metastases are associated with increased rates of local recurrence and distant metastasis (4,45,109,121). The overall risk of lymph node metastases is 20% (102,138). Pantuck et al. (102) retrospectively reviewed the treatment results of 900 patients and found that lymph node involvement was associated with larger, higher grade, and locally advanced tumors. Patients with lymph node metastases in radical nephrectomy specimens have a local failure rate of 21%, compared with only 4% in patients without lymph node metastases ($p = .0002$) (109). Patients with lymph node involvement and distant metastases have a worse 5-year survival rate than patients without nodal metastases (23% vs. 15%) (102). Bassil et al. (4) reported a 5-year survival rate of only 7% in patients with lymph node metastases; the extent of lymph node metastases did not influence outcome. Patients with distant metastases at initial presentation have a dismal prognosis, with an expected 5-year survival rate of 0% to 7% (4,128). A select group of patients with solitary metastases may have a 5-year survival rate of 25% to 35% (68,128).

Worsening pathologic grade is associated with poor 5-year disease-free survival (119,121). Fuhrman et al. (40) developed a four-tier grading system that is based on nuclear and nucleolar size, shape, and content. Tsui et al. (133) reported 5-year survival rates of 89%, 65%, and 46% for grades 1, 2, and 3 or 4, respectively. Papillary renal cell cancer has a 5-year survival rate that approaches 90% and metastasizes less frequently than clear cell renal carcinoma. The spindle cell or sarcomatoid variants of renal cell carcinoma are associated with a statistically significant inferior 5-year survival rate, compared with pure clear or clear and granular histologic variants (119,121). Nuclear morphology is a strong predictor of tumor stage and prognosis (40). High nuclear grade is associated with an increased incidence of advanced tumor stage, lymph node involvement, distant metastases, renal vein involvement, tumor size, and perirenal fat involvement. In a series of 190 patients reported by Bretheau et al. (13), the 5-year actuarial survival rates of patients with grade I, II, III, and IV tumors were 76%, 72%, 51%, and 35%, respectively. Sarcomatoid differentiation carries a significantly poorer prognosis than the clear cell or granular cell subtypes. Almost half of patients with sarcomatoid renal cell carcinoma have bone metastases at presentation.

Table 60.6	STAGE OF RENAL CELL CARCINOMA CORRELATED WITH SURVIVAL AFTER RADICAL NEPHRECTOMY

Author (Reference)	No. of Patients	5-Year Survival (%)			
		I	II	III	IV
Robson et al. (114)	88	66	64	42	11
Skinner et al. (121)	309	65	47	51	8
Waters and Richie (141)	130	51	59	12	0
McNichols et al. (87)	506	67	51	34	14
Selli et al. (119)	115	93	63	80	13
Golimbu et al. (45)	326	88	67	40	2
Dinney et al. (31)	314	73	68	51	20
Guinan et al. (48)	337	100	96	59	16
Javidan et al. (59)	381	95	88	59	10
Kinouchi et al. (66)	350	96	95	70	24
Tsui et al. (133)	643	91	74	67	32

The median survival time of patients with sarcomatoid renal cell cancer is only 6.6 months, compared with 19 months for other histologic types (118).

Nomograms and algorithms have been described to facilitate the determination of cancer-free survival in patients with renal cell carcinoma. Based on 601 patients treated at Memorial Sloan-Kettering Cancer Center with radical nephrectomy, Kattan et al. (63) used variables including patient symptoms (incidental, local, or systemic), histology (chromophobe, papillary, or conventional), tumor size, and pathologic stage to predict the risk of recurrence after surgery. Frank et al. (37) from the Mayo Clinic developed a predictive algorithm based on 1,801 patients treated with radical nephrectomy. This system combines stage, size, grade, and necrosis (SSIGN) to predict patient survival. Finally, Zisman et al. (147) from UCLA have developed an algorithm that utilizes AJCC TNM stage, Fuhrman's grade, and Eastern Cooperative Oncology Group (ECOG) performance status to divide patients into low-risk, intermediate-risk, and high-risk groups. This latter system has been validated using both single institutional series and a 4,202 patient data set from eight international centers (52,105,148).

Renal Pelvis and Ureter Carcinoma

The major prognostic factors in patients with renal pelvis or ureter carcinoma are initial stage and grade of the tumor. In a series of 127 patients, Corrado et al. (23) reported 5-year survival rates of 80%, 83%, 72%, 31%, and 16% for stage Ta, T1, T2, T3, and T4 tumors, respectively. Similar results have been described by Heney et al. (54), with 5-year survival rates ranging from 82% to 100% in patients with tumors confined to the mucosa versus 0% to 24% for tumors invading through the muscularis. Huben et al. (56) noted that patients with low-stage tumors had a median survival time of 91.1 months, compared with only 12.9 months in patients with higher stages (p = .004). In this series, a local recurrence rate of 25.9% was reported, with most occurring after simple nephrectomy or in patients with lymph node metastases. Charbit et al. (19) reported that 87% of patients with lymph node metastases died of their disease, compared with only 8% of patients without lymph node spread. In a series of 77 patients, Akdogan et al. (1) reported a worse disease-specific survival in patients with advanced stage disease.

High-grade tumors are associated with a higher incidence of metastasis and worse survival. Corrado et al. (23) reported 5-year survival rates of 83%, 75%, 52%, and 0% for grades 1 through 4, respectively. These results are comparable to those described by Heney et al. (54), who reported 100% survival for grade 1, 81% for grade 2, and 0% for grade 3. Local recurrence was identified in 3/24 patients with grade 3 tumors. No survival differences were seen for patients with papillary versus solid tumors. In the series of Charbit et al. (19), lymph node metastases were seen exclusively in patients with high-grade tumors. Of tumor-related deaths, 90% were in patients with high-grade tumors. Hall et al. (50) reported a retrospective series of 252 patients treated surgically for upper urinary tract transitional cell cancers. Significant factors for recurrence included high tumor grade and advanced clinical stage. By tumor stage, the 5-year disease-specific survivals were 100% for Ta or carcinoma *in situ*, 92% for T1, 73% for T2, and 41% for T3 cancers. Older patients and patients treated with parenchymal-sparing surgical procedures had higher rates of recurrence. In their series of 77 patients, Akdogan et al. (1) reported from a multivariate analysis that higher recurrence rates were associated with tumor location, higher grade, and advanced T stage. Tumors in the ureters were more likely to recur than tumors involving the renal pelvis. In a series of 86 patients, Park et al. (104) also reported a higher rate of recurrence in ureteral tumors, compared to those arising in the renal pelvis. A prior history

of bladder cancer has been reported to worsen the prognosis of patients with second urothelial cancers involving the upper tracts (1,92). From the Memorial Sloan-Kettering Cancer Center series of 129 patients, a multivariate analysis demonstrated that patients with advanced primary tumors and a prior history of bladder cancer were associated with worse disease-free survival (92).

Flow cytometry may aid in estimating long-term prognosis. In a multivariate analysis, Corrado et al. (23) demonstrated that, although stage and grade were the most important prognostic indices, DNA pattern (diploid vs. nondiploid) and the number of lesions (unifocal vs. multifocal) identified at initial diagnosis also determined prognosis. Patients with diploid tumors had a 79% survival rate, compared with only 46% in patients with nondiploid tumors (p = .0003). Recent data suggest that hypermethylation of the promoter region of patients with transitional cell cancers of the urothelium is associated with a worse prognosis. Tumors of the renal pelvis and ureters demonstrate hypermethylation in 94% of cases compared to 76% of similar appearing tumors in the bladder (p <.0001). Hypermethylation was also associated with higher tumor stage, tumor progression, and mortality (16).

General Management

Renal Cell Carcinoma

Surgery

The standard therapy for nonmetastatic renal cell carcinoma is radical nephrectomy. The results of patients treated primarily by radical nephrectomy are presented in Table 60.6. This operation is undertaken by a thoracoabdominal or transabdominal approach. Classically, a radical nephrectomy removes the malignant tumor along with the kidney, the adrenal gland, and the perinephric fat enclosed within Gerota's fascia. Regional lymph node dissection routinely is performed, although its benefit has not clearly been established. The European Organisation for Research and Treatment of Cancer (EORTC) has conducted a randomized trial of radical nephrectomy with or without an elective lymph node dissection. Preliminary results from that trial do not demonstrate an advantage to dissection of the lymph nodes (8). It is believed that elective removal of lymphatics that may contain microscopic disease is the only curative option for patients at risk (24). In a review of 900 patients undergoing nephrectomy for renal cell carcinoma, Pantuck et al. (102,103) reported that patients with lymph node metastases were three to four times more likely to have distant metastases. In patients with clinically negative nodes, there was no benefit to nodal dissection. In patients undergoing nephrectomy in the presence of known metastatic disease and clinically involved nodes, a lymph node dissection was associated with improved survival and appeared to improve response to immunotherapy.

Less aggressive operations than the classic radical nephrectomy may be considered in special circumstances. Improved preoperative assessment with CT can identify patients who have no significant risk of adrenal gland involvement (43). In 76% of cases, the adrenal gland can be spared at the time of surgery. Partial nephrectomy, or renal parenchyma-sparing surgery, has been used increasingly in patients who have early stage tumors or those with poor renal reserve or absence of a normal-functioning contralateral kidney. In a matched pair analysis of 164 patients undergoing nephron-sparing surgery at the Mayo Clinic, their disease-free survival rate was 79%, which compared favorably to 77% in patients undergoing radical nephrectomy (72). In 117 patients with renal tumors ≤4 cm undergoing partial nephrectomy at Memorial Sloan-Kettering Cancer Center, the 5-year freedom from recurrence was 98.6%

compared to 96.4% in a similar group of 173 patients undergoing radical nephrectomy. Compared to patients undergoing partial nephrectomy, those undergoing radical nephrectomy were at a higher risk of chronic renal insufficiency (86). There is some risk that sparing of the renal parenchyma may leave microscopic residual tumor or inadequately treat multifocal cancers (96,100,143). Partial nephrectomy has not been considered routine therapy for patients with a normal functioning contralateral kidney; however, this opinion has been challenged by some centers (73,81,83). Local recurrence rates of <10% and 5-year survival rates of 75% to 85% have been reported with a conservative surgical approach in patients selected for partial nephrectomy (108,122,131). Bilateral renal cell carcinoma occurs in 2% to 3% of patients. In these patients, renal parenchyma-sparing surgery is an attractive option because bilateral radical nephrectomy sentences the patient to a lifetime of renal dialysis or the need for a kidney transplant. Partial nephrectomy of the least-involved side, followed by either partial nephrectomy or radical nephrectomy of the remaining involved kidney, may retain enough functioning kidney to avoid dialysis or transplant. The second surgery may be performed after adequate recovery from the first operation (24).

Percutaneous ablative techniques such are radiofrequency ablation (149) or cryoablation (134,149) are gaining interest in the management of tumors <3 cm.

Radiation Therapy

Adenocarcinoma of the kidney is a variably radiosensitive neoplasm. *In vivo* experiments demonstrated a decrease in the rate of tumor transplantation in nude mice after pretreatment of human renal cell carcinoma cells with radiation therapy. These data support the existence of a theoretic benefit to preoperative irradiation in decreasing tumor shedding at the time of an operation (99). In another animal experiment, regression of renal cell carcinoma xenografts occurred in response to treatment with radioactive iodine–tagged monoclonal antibodies in mice, whereas those animals treated with untagged monoclonal antibodies demonstrated tumor growth (20). Still other *in vivo* data suggest that some renal cell cancer lines are resistant to conventionally fractionated radiation therapy schedules (94). Clinical experiences demonstrated very good subjective and objective response rates in patients receiving palliative irradiation for symptomatic metastases from renal cell carcinoma (30,36,51,57,98,144). Despite the favorable effect that irradiation has against this neoplasm in advanced disease, it has not convincingly improved the results of patients treated in an adjuvant setting for early stage disease.

There is some evidence that immunotherapy may enhance response to radiation therapy (94). In a murine model, the combination of pulmonary irradiation with vaccine therapy significantly reduced the rate of pulmonary metastases compared to pulmonary irradiation or vaccine therapy alone (95). In a clinical trial of 20 patients with metastatic renal cell carcinoma, Brinkmann et al. (14) reported that all patients experienced pain relief with three complete responses to a combination of radiation therapy and chemoimmunotherapy.

Historically, several retrospective series suggested a clinical benefit to adjuvant radiation therapy for renal cell carcinoma (35,113). Many of these series spanned several decades and predated modern staging, surgery, and radiation-therapy technologies. As with any retrospective series, these early reports can be appropriately criticized for inadequate balance between groups of patients treated in various ways over different periods. Some authors described theoretic benefits of preoperative radiation therapy, such as tumor shrinkage, increased resectability, and decreased tumor viability with fewer distant metastases because of lessened intraoperative seeding (115). Anecdotal reports of improved resectability were common and

warranted a study of preoperative radiation therapy in the context of a prospective clinical trial (35,113).

Two European studies were undertaken to test the efficacy of preoperative radiation therapy in renal cell cancer. A prospective randomized study of preoperative irradiation and nephrectomy versus nephrectomy alone was conducted in Rotterdam. No advantage was demonstrated in patients receiving radiation therapy with respect to overall survival or survival free of distant metastasis. In this trial, patients received a 30-Gy midplane dose to the involved kidney and regional lymph nodes, with 2-Gy daily fractions administered over a period of 3 weeks. Nephrectomy immediately followed completion of radiation therapy. Preoperative radiation therapy did appear to increase the rate of complete resectability in patients with locally advanced (T2, T3) tumors (135). This study was continued after the preliminary 1973 analysis. Later patients received 40-Gy preoperative radiation therapy. No benefit was demonstrated with preoperative irradiation, even at the higher radiation dose (136). In Sweden, a second prospective randomized clinical trial also was unable to demonstrate an advantage to patients receiving preoperative radiation therapy. In this trial, patients were randomly assigned to receive either 33-Gy preoperative irradiation in 15 fractions administered to the flank from a betatron unit before nephrectomy or nephrectomy alone. Patients receiving preoperative radiation therapy had a 5-year survival rate of 47%, compared with 63% for patients undergoing surgery alone (61).

Postoperative radiation therapy was reported to be beneficial in early retrospective studies (9,110). In a series reported by Rafla (110), patients receiving radiation therapy after nephrectomy had significantly better rates of survival and local control at 5 and 10 years than patients undergoing nephrectomy alone. No specific details regarding radiation therapy technique or dose were presented. The method by which patients were selected to receive or not receive radiation therapy was not described (p =.001). Other early series showed no advantage to postoperative radiation therapy (106).

Two prospective randomized studies testing the value of postoperative irradiation did not demonstrate an advantage to patients receiving radiation therapy after surgery. The first study from New Castle, United Kingdom, demonstrated an inferior survival for patients receiving radiation therapy compared with those treated with surgery alone (39). Local recurrence rates were not affected by the postoperative radiation therapy. No stratification of patients by tumor stage or grade was made. Four patients died of fatal hepatotoxicity after radiation therapy to a right-sided nephrectomy bed. Patients in this study received 55 Gy in 2.04-Gy daily fractions (71). A second randomized study conducted by the Copenhagen Renal Cancer Study Group compared patients with stage II or III renal cell cancer treated with nephrectomy alone with patients who received nephrectomy plus 50 Gy in 20 fractions to the kidney bed and regional ipsilateral and contralateral lymph nodes. No difference in relapse rate was found between the two study groups. There were significant complications involving the stomach, duodenum, and liver in 44% of patients receiving postoperative irradiation. In fact, 19% of deaths in the radiation therapy group were attributed to radiation-induced complications (69).

The four prospective randomized trials that have studied the effects of adjuvant radiation therapy seem to argue convincingly against its routine use in patients with renal cell carcinoma. There are some circumstances in which radiation therapy should be considered as part of the curative treatment for renal cell carcinoma. Radiation therapy has increased the resectability of locally advanced tumors in both prospective and retrospective series (113,136). Preoperative irradiation should be considered in patients with technically unresectable nonmetastatic tumors to convert them to resectable.

The lack of benefit from postoperative irradiation in the prospective clinical trials may be explained by poor patient selection and radiation-therapy technique. A retrospective review from Memorial Sloan-Kettering Cancer Center of 172 patients treated by radical nephrectomy demonstrated an overall local failure rate of only 5%. The majority of patients in this series had T1 or T2 tumors. Patients with lymph node metastases or positive margins had a significantly higher local failure rate of 21%, compared with 4% in patients without these bad prognostic features ($p = .002$) (109). This suggests that if a benefit from postoperative irradiation exists, it would be demonstrable only in patients with pathologic features that would increase their risk of local failure. Early stage tumors have an extremely good local control rate, and, therefore, radiation therapy would not be expected to play a beneficial role in patients with these tumors.

Kao et al. (62) reported that, in a retrospective series, 12 patients with high-risk, locally advanced tumors with perinephric invasion or surgically positive margins had a 100% local control rate if treated adjuvantly with postoperative irradiation. Patients received 41.4 to 63 Gy in 1.8- to 2-Gy fractions. The 5-year local failure rate was 30% in a comparable group of patients treated by surgery only during this same period ($p < .01$) (62). CT-based simulation and treatment planning in this series resulted in no serious late sequelae despite high radiation-therapy doses.

Another retrospective series demonstrated that 37 patients with T3 tumors had a statistically significant lower local failure rate (10%) when given postoperative irradiation, compared with 30 similar patients undergoing nephrectomy alone (37%) (124). Patients received a median dose of 46 Gy in 1.8- to 2-Gy fractions; CT-assisted treatment planning was used in most patients. Serious radiation-induced bowel sequelae occurred in only three patients (5%), each of whom was treated before routine use of CT-assisted treatment planning. This series has been updated and in 86 patients the risk of local recurrence was 16% and occurred exclusively in patients with T3b disease. These authors have now concluded that postoperative radiation therapy is not indicated for the patients with renal cell cancer (47). In a retrospective series of 186 patients with locally advanced renal cell carcinoma, 114 were administered postoperative radiation therapy (50-Gy median dose) (79). For the subgroup of patients with T3/N0 disease, radiation therapy reduced the rate of local recurrence from 15.8% to 8.8%. There was no impact on survival. No other subgroups benefited from the adjuvant radiation therapy.

These contemporary retrospective series have suggested a limited benefit to postoperative radiation therapy in patients selected because of a high risk of local recurrence (62,79,124). Based on this collection of both prospective and retrospective data, the following indications for radiation therapy should be considered: (a) unresectable nonmetastatic tumors and (b) incomplete resection with gross or microscopically positive margins. Although radiation therapy may decrease the local recurrence rate, an improvement in overall survival may not be demonstrated in this circumstance.

There are some data suggesting that high dose per fraction stereotactically delivered radiation therapy may have a role for patients with renal cell cancer. In a nude mice model of human renal cell cancer, Walsh et al. (139) demonstrated that radiation doses of 48 Gy delivered in three fractions resulted in a sustained decrease in tumor volume along with marked cytological changes. Beitler et al. (5) reported on nine patients who had refused surgery for the primary management of localized renal cell cancer and were subsequently treated with 40 Gy in five fractions using stereotactic body radiation therapy. With a median follow-up of 26.7 months, four of the nine patients had survived. One of the nine patients failed in the ipsilateral kidney, away from the initial radiation treatment volume, while

the other eight patients had durable local control. Wersall et al. (142) reported on eight patients treated with stereotactic radiation therapy to medically inoperable primary tumors using a radiation treatment schedule of 8 Gy in five fractions. Seven of the eight patients were locally controlled, and the median survival exceeded 58 months.

Systemic Therapy

Recent clinical trials of targeted molecular therapies have yielded encouraging results in patients with advanced renal cell cancer. Prior to these studies, conventional chemotherapy has demonstrated low response rates, typically with short durations (76,145). Other systemic therapies have been explored, including hormone therapy and immunotherapy. Based on encouraging animal models, progestational agents such as medroxyprogesterone acetate have been studied extensively in patients with renal cell carcinoma. Little objective benefit has been proven from the use of hormonal therapy (67). Immunologic therapies have yielded early encouraging results. Interferon-α has demonstrated activity in metastatic renal cell carcinoma, with objective response rates of 10% to 20% (76). Two randomized trials have demonstrated a survival advantage to interferon-α administered after radical nephrectomy in patients with metastatic disease (34,88). Therapy with interleukin-2 (IL-2), a lymphokine produced by activated T cells, resulted in complete response rates in 5% to 10% of selected patients with metastatic renal cell cancer, and another 10% to 15% demonstrated objective partial responses. These responses were generally of long duration (up to 2 years). IL-2 is the first biologic response modifier approved for clinical use in the United States (76). IL-2 therapy is not appropriate for all patients with metastatic renal cell carcinoma. Because of its cardiorespiratory, renal, gastrointestinal, and hematologic toxicities, patients being considered for its use must have good performance status. Because of its favorable effects on metastatic renal cell carcinoma in phase I and II clinical trials, IL-2 frequently is prescribed for this disease despite few data suggesting that it improves overall survival or is better than no therapy at all in unselected patients. The objective response rate in a series of phase II trials is 15%, with only 7% complete responses. The median response duration is 54 months. For the few patients who achieve a complete response, the duration of response exceeds 80 months (33).

The overexpression of VEGF associated with the mutation or silencing of the VHL gene provides a natural and attractive target for systemic therapy. The humanized anti-VEGF antibody, bevacizumab, has been investigated in a randomized phase II trial in patients with metastatic renal cell carcinoma. Patients receiving bevacizumab had a 4.8 month interval to progression compared to 2.5 months in patients receiving placebo (140). Tyrosine kinase inhibitors that target the VEGF pathway show promise in the management of advanced renal cell cancer. In a randomized phase II discontinuation trial, sorafenib, an oral inhibitor of both Raf kinase and the VEGF receptor, 50% of patients on the study drug showed no progression of disease compared to only 18% of patients who were receiving placebo ($p = .0077$) (111). The median time to progression for patients taking sorafenib was 24 weeks compared to 6 weeks in the control group ($p = .0087$). In a randomized phase III trial, sorafenib significantly prolonged progression-free survival (24 weeks) compared to placebo (12 weeks) ($p < .0001$) (32). Another tyrosine kinase inhibitor, sunitinib, targets both the VEGF and platelet-derived growth factor (PDGF) receptors. In a phase II trial, the oral administration of sunitinib yielded a 40% response rate with a median time to progression of 8.7 months (91). Both these tyrosine kinase inhibitors have favorable side-effect profiles and are generally well tolerated by patients. Similar to other anti-VEGF agents, these drugs can cause hypertension and may increase the risk of cardiovascular toxicities.

Clinical Radiation Oncology

Local Therapy for Metastatic and Recurrent Disease

For patients with metastatic renal cell carcinoma, palliative nephrectomy can relieve pain, hemorrhage, hypertension, or hypercalcemia induced by the primary tumor. Two prospective randomized trials have demonstrated that surgical removal of the primary tumor by radical nephrectomy improves response rates to systemic immunotherapy and improves survival. In an EORTC trial, 85 patients were randomized to receive five fractions of interferon-α either immediately or 4 to 6 weeks following radical nephrectomy. The time to progression was 5 months in the patients undergoing nephrectomy, compared to 3 months in the control patients ($p = .04$). Median duration of survival was 17 months in the surgical patients, compared to 7 months in the control patients ($p = .03$) (88). In a similar U.S. trial conducted by the Southwest Oncology Group, Flanigan et al. (34) randomized 241 patients to undergo radical nephrectomy followed by interferon α-2β or interferon α-2β alone. The median survival of the 120 patients undergoing nephrectomy was 11.1 months, compared to only 8.1 months in the 121 patients treated with immunotherapy alone ($p = .05$).

Resection of metastatic foci may be appropriate for patients who do not achieve adequate symptomatic relief from palliative radiation therapy. In some patients, resection of a solitary focus may allow for a prolonged disease-free interval, especially if the preceding disease-free interval was long and the patient has a good performance status (89,97).

Palliative radiation therapy is effective at relieving symptoms from metastatic renal cell cancer (36,51,74,98). A patient with a solitary bone metastasis may have a long survival time, and a sufficient radiation dose should be administered to allow durable pain relief. If surgery is used to remove a metastatic lesion, postoperative radiation therapy is indicated to prevent its recurrence. In a prospective phase II study using validated quality of life questionnaires, Lee et al. (74) from the Princess Margaret Hospital demonstrated that 83% of patients treated for pain had experienced significant pain relief with 30 Gy radiation delivered in 10 fractions. Palliation of neurologic symptoms from brain metastases, spinal-cord compression, or nerve invasion is not as successful as relief of pain from bone metastases (57,144).

Stereotactic radiosurgery has been successful at controlling and palliating metastatic sites from renal cell carcinoma (144). In 69 patients with brain metastases from renal cell cancer, Sheehan et al. (120) reported that in 63% of cases the lesions had decreased and in 33% they remained stable. In 48 patients with spinal metastases, Gerszten et al. (41) reported that 89% of patients experienced improvement in pain following single stereotactic treatments ranging in dose from 17.5 to 25 Gy. The volume of the spinal cord allowed to exceed 8 Gy was kept to <3 cm^3. In a series of 50 patients with metastatic renal cell carcinoma, Wersall et al. (142) reported that stereotactically delivered radiation to sites including the lung, liver, and adrenal resulted in complete regression in 30% of cases and either partial regression or stabilization of the lesions in 60%. Of 162 treated tumors, only three recurred. Dose and fractionation ranged from 8 Gy in four fractions, 10 Gy in four fractions, and 15 Gy in three fractions all delivered in 1 week.

Renal Pelvis and Ureter Carcinoma

Radical nephroureterectomy is an appropriate initial therapy for most patients with transitional cell carcinoma of the renal pelvis or ureter. This operation includes removal of the contents of Gerota's fascia, including the ipsilateral ureter with a cuff of bladder at its distal extent. Less radical surgeries have been plagued by high local or regional recurrence rates, sometimes approaching 30% (22). Hall et al. (50) reported an increased rate of recurrence when parenchymal sparing procedures were performed. Conservative surgical excision should be considered only in patients with low-grade, low-stage, solitary tumors in whom radical nephrectomy is not indicated because of poor kidney function or an absent contralateral kidney. In circumstances in which conservative resection is performed, postoperative radiation therapy should be considered. Conservative surgical options in selected cases include laparoscopic nephroureterectomy, nephrectomy and partial ureterectomy, endoscopic resection, and fulguration. The role of lymph node dissection in this disease is unclear. Patients who have the highest risk of lymph node metastases also have a high risk of systemic disease.

Few data support the routine use of adjuvant radiation therapy in transitional cell carcinoma of the renal pelvis or ureter. Radiation therapy may be beneficial in selected cases of high tumor stage (T3 or T4) and in patients with lymph node metastases. Retrospective data from Brookland and Richter (15) suggest a decreased local recurrence rate in patients treated with postoperative irradiation. Similar data were reported by Brady et al. (10) and Babaian et al. (3). Adjuvant irradiation in patients with high-stage transitional cell carcinoma of the renal pelvis and ureter has been associated with an increase in local control. Among 26 patients with stage T3 or T4/N0 or node-positive disease undergoing curative resections, 9/17 treated by surgery alone had local failure, compared with only one of nine who received adjuvant irradiation. In a multivariate analysis, the two factors associated with local failure were high tumor grade and lack of adjuvant radiation therapy (25). Clearly, for this uncommon tumor, the large patient numbers required to prove a benefit from adjuvant radiation therapy would require a cooperative group trial.

Patterns of recurrence were described in 252 patients undergoing surgery at the University of Texas Southwest Medical Center for transitional cell carcinoma of the upper urinary tract (50). Local recurrence occurred only 9% of the time, whereas new invasive urothelial tumors or distant metastases occurred in 69% and 22% of cases, respectively. Isolated local recurrences were rare. Another series from the Princess Margaret Hospital confirms the high rate of distant metastases. Although local failure occurred in 35% of patients with locally advanced disease, most patients also experienced distant metastases as well (17). Ozsahin et al. (101) conducted a retrospective review of 138 patients from the European Rare Cancer Network diagnosed with transitional cell cancer of the renal pelvis or ureters. After excluding 12 patients due to the presence of metastatic disease at presentation, all but three of the remaining patients underwent radical surgery ranging from nephrectomy to nephroureterectomy with or without lymph node dissection. A locoregional recurrence rate of 62% was reported following radical surgery alone. Radiation therapy was administered to 36% of the patients and generally covered the surgical bed without an attempt to cover the lymph nodes. Patients receiving radiation therapy were significantly more likely to have advanced, T4 disease ($p < .0001$) and tended to have higher-grade disease ($p = .06$). Although radiation therapy did not reduce the local recurrence rate compared to surgery alone, the authors admitted that selection bias and older radiation techniques may have prevented the detection of any benefit from adjuvant treatment.

The pathologic similarity of transitional cell carcinoma of the renal pelvis and ureter to bladder cancer has encouraged medical oncologists to use similar chemotherapeutic regimens in the management of upper-tract transitional cell carcinomas. The MVAC regimen developed at Memorial Sloan-Kettering Cancer Center combines methotrexate, vinblastine, doxorubicin, and cisplatin. Objective response rates of almost 70% have been reported in patients with metastatic transitional cell carcinoma of the bladder, ureter, and kidney (78,125). Palliative chemotherapy may be considered in patients with metastatic disease.

A series of 31 patients treated with adjuvant radiation therapy for nonmetastatic transitional cell cancer of the upper urinary tract was reported by Czito et al. (28). Nine patients also received chemotherapy consisting of methotrexate, cisplatin, and vinblastine prior to receiving radiation concurrent with cisplatin. The 5-year local–regional control rate was 67%. The 5-year overall and disease-specific survival appeared to be improved with the administration of concurrent chemotherapy. The overall survival for patients receiving concurrent chemotherapy and radiation therapy was 67% compared to 27% receiving postoperative radiation alone ($p = .01$). The disease-free survival for patients receiving concurrent chemotherapy and radiation therapy was 76% compared to 41% receiving postoperative radiation alone ($p = .06$).

Radiation Therapy Techniques

Renal Cell Carcinoma

Radiation therapy has been used in the management of patients with renal cell carcinoma in a number of circumstances including adjuvant therapy, either before or after definitive surgery, and as palliation for either local disease or distant metastases. In unresectable lesions, 40 to 50 Gy preoperative radiation therapy directed to the kidney tumor and regional lymphatics may improve resectability (136). Multiple-field techniques, similar to those described for postoperative radiation therapy, should be considered in patients receiving preoperative treatment.

CT-based treatment planning contributes to good local control with minimal morbidity. Careful definition of the target volume to encompass the nephrectomy bed, lymph node drainage sites, and surgical clips on the planning CT scan is important. Exclusive use of anterior-posterior field arrangements, particularly on the right side, is likely to result in irradiation of large volumes of bowel and liver beyond tolerance. Multiple-beam arrangements, including anterior, posterior, oblique, and lateral projections with beam's eye-view shaping and differential weighting of dose from each field, can optimize the radiation dose distribution to maximize target volume coverage while minimizing the dose to normal bowel or liver (Fig. 60.1). Total radiation doses of 45 to 50 Gy in 1.8- to 2-Gy daily fractions to the nephrectomy bed and regional lymph nodes with a boost to small volumes of microscopic or gross residual disease with an additional 10 to 15 Gy (total dose 50 to 60 Gy) are appropriate. Stein et al. (124) reported two scar recurrences and recommended that the incision site be included in the target volume. If the scar cannot be covered without increasing the amount of normal tissue irradiated, an additional electron beam field to treat the scar may be considered.

The high complication rates reported in the prospective trials of postoperative radiation therapy have taught radiation oncologists an important lesson regarding radiation therapy planning, patient selection, and the tolerance of the upper-abdominal viscera. Field projections and shaping should be selected to keep no more than 30% of the liver from receiving doses >36 to 40 Gy. The contralateral kidney dose should not exceed 20 Gy in 2 to 3 weeks. The spinal cord dose should be limited to 45 Gy in conventionally fractionated doses of 1.8 to 2 Gy per day. Intensity-modulated radiation therapy (IMRT) may be a reasonable consideration due the sensitivity of adjacent surrounding structures. If IMRT is considered, a plan to manage the

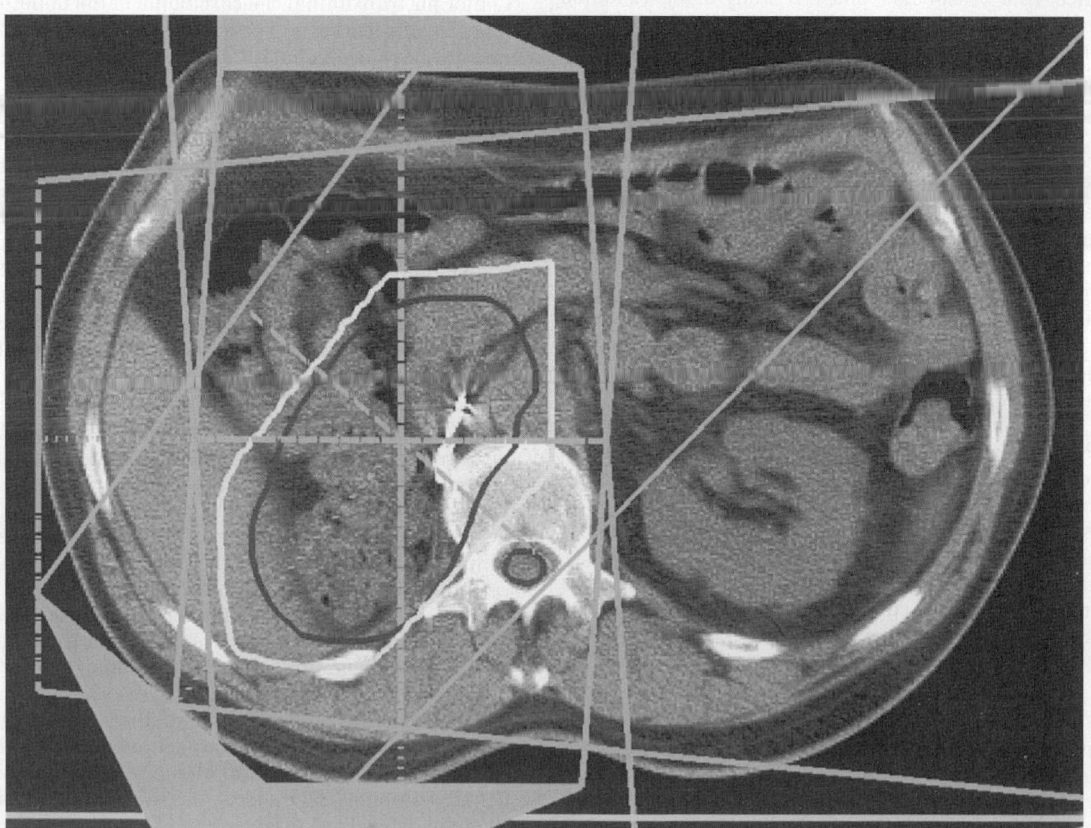

FIGURE 60.1. A computer tomography–based treatment plan using a combination of four fields (anterior, posterior, right lateral, and right posterior oblique) to cover the tumor bed (*dark oval*) with 54 Gy (isodose line displayed). This combination of fields and beam's-eye-view shaping allows sparing of the liver, bowel, and spinal cord.

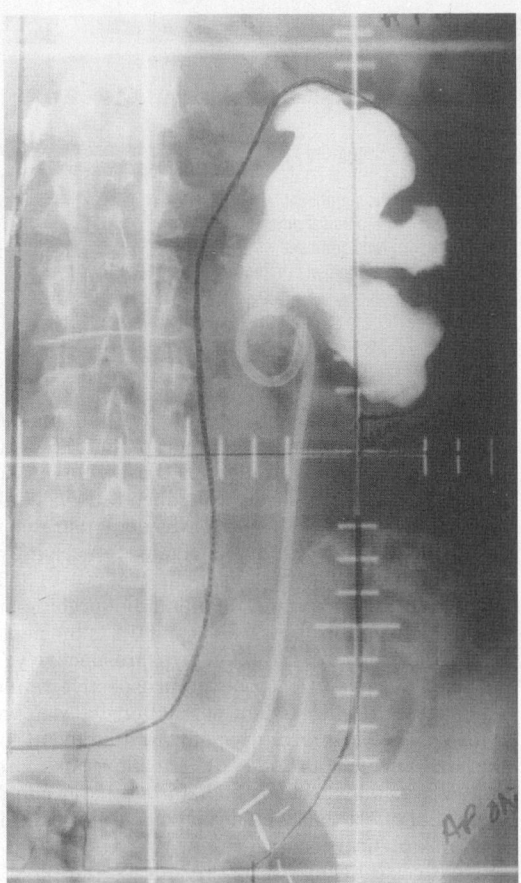 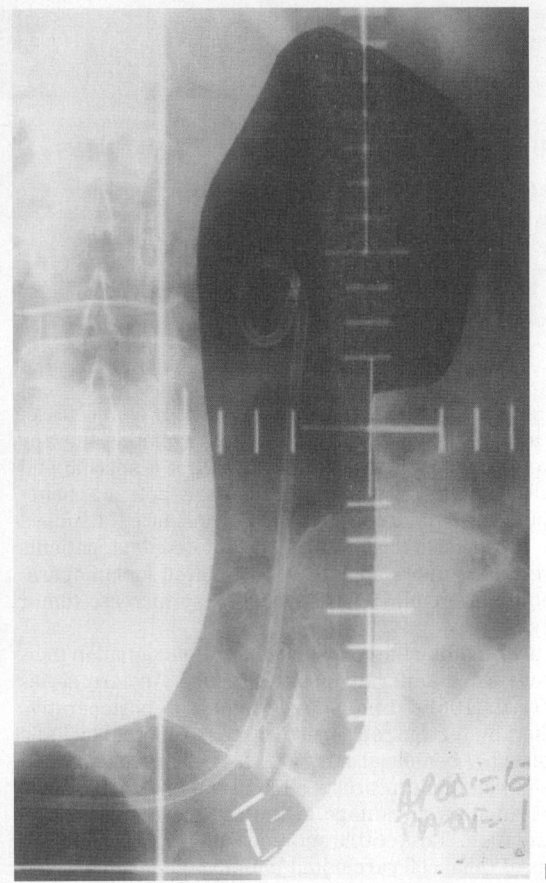

FIGURE 60.2. A: Final irradiation field for a patient with an unresectable transitional cell cancer of the renal pelvis and ureter. The contrast material outlines the renal pelvis and allows a block design to spare the renal parenchyma. The ureter is treated up to the insertion in the bladder. **B:** The "block check" film of the field designed in (A).

uncertainties in target localization such as gating or breathing control needs to be considered.

Because of the possibility of long survival even in the presence of distant metastases, aggressive treatment for palliation should be considered in patients who have limited metastatic disease with good performance status. Treatment fields should encompass metastatic foci with adequate (2- to 3-cm) margins. Radiation therapy doses of 35 to 40 Gy provide symptomatic relief in 64% to 84% of patients treated (36,51,98). Some series have reported higher symptomatic response rates with higher irradiation doses in renal cell carcinoma (98). A palliative dose of 45 to 50 Gy in 3 to 4.5 weeks may be considered.

Renal Pelvis and Ureter Carcinoma

Postoperative radiation therapy has been used in the management of renal pelvis and ureter cancers. For elective radiation therapy, the clinical target volume should include the renal fossa and the course of the ureter to the bladder wall at the ipsilateral trigone. The field encompassing these sites should be extended to cover the paracaval and para-aortic lymph nodes at risk of harboring metastatic disease (28). As in renal cell carcinoma, CT-based planning may facilitate dosimetric coverage of the regions at risk while minimizing dose to normal tissues. Radiation doses of 45 to 50 Gy at 1.8 to 2 Gy per day are appropriate to treat subclinical and microscopic disease. For more extensive disease (e.g., multiple positive nodes) or extensive positive margins, a boost of 5 to 10 Gy should be considered. For unresectable or gross residual disease, higher doses may be necessary. In this event, multiple-field arrangements includ-

ing oblique and lateral fields with field reductions are important to minimize toxicity to surrounding normal structures. CT-based simulation, three-dimensional treatment planning, and contrast-enhanced radiographs are helpful in defining the radiation therapy target volume (Fig. 60.2). Intensity modulated radiation therapy can be considered if organ motion is managed to avoid under dosing the planning target volume. Chemotherapy may allow a lower radiation dose for gross disease. Cozad et al. (25) reported on two patients with gross residual disease who achieved local tumor control with radiation doses of 45 and 50.4 Gy. One of these patients had a pathologically proven complete response at reoperation after receiving radiation therapy and concomitant MVAC.

Results of Therapy

Renal Cell Carcinoma

Adjuvant irradiation has made little impact in the modern management and outcome of most patients with renal cell carcinoma. The prospective randomized studies evaluating preoperative radiation therapy in the management of renal cell carcinoma show similar outcomes regardless of whether radiation therapy was administered. Table 60.7 summarizes the results of the prospective studies that have tested preoperative radiation therapy. Local tumor control, an important end point for evaluating the effectiveness of preoperative irradiation, was not reported in any of these prospective trials. The one benefit to preoperative radiation therapy that was suggested in the

| Table 60.7 | SURVIVAL AFTER NEPHRECTOMY OR PREOPERATIVE IRRADIATION AND NEPHRECTOMY FOR RENAL CELL CARCINOMA |

Author (Reference)	No. of Patients	Radiation Dose/ Fraction Size (Gy)	Treatment	5-Year Survival Rate (%)	Comments
van der Werf-Messing et al. (135,136)	85	—	N	50	No significant survival difference
	89	30–40/2	N + RT		
Juusela et al. (61)	50	—	N	63	No significant survival difference
	38	33/2.2	N + RT	47	

N, nephrectomy; RT, preoperative radiation therapy

Rotterdam study was an increase in the rate of complete resectability in patients with T3 tumors after radiation therapy (135). Because increased resectability was not a specific end point initially sought in this study design, this potential benefit of preoperative irradiation should be considered a subject for a future prospective trial. Lacking additional data, patients with unresectable tumors should be considered for preoperative radiation therapy of 45 Gy in an effort to increase tumor resectability.

Studies investigating the role of postoperative radiation therapy have not yielded uniformly positive results. An early series by Peeling et al. (106) did not show a benefit to postoperative radiation therapy. A large retrospective series reported by Rafla (110) suggested a beneficial effect of postoperative radiation therapy; however, modern prospective randomized trials have not demonstrated an advantage to the routine use of postoperative irradiation. Table 60.8 summarizes the results in selected series of renal cell carcinoma patients who were treated with postoperative radiation therapy. In the Rafla series, patients receiving radiation therapy had a 57% survival rate at 5 years, compared with 37% for patients treated by nephrectomy alone (110). He reported a local recurrence rate of 25% in patients undergoing nephrectomy versus 7% in patients undergoing nephrectomy followed by radiation therapy. In the prospective series reported by Fugitt et al. (39), patients receiving 55-Gy postoperative flank radiation therapy had 36% survival rate at 5 years, compared with 47% for those who did not receive radiation therapy. The local recurrence rate was only 7% in each group. Similarly, no advantage was demonstrated in the Copenhagen Renal Cancer Study (69). Patients receiving postoperative radiation therapy had a 5-year survival rate of 38%, which was inferior to the 63% rate of patients undergoing surgery alone. Local recurrence rates were 1% and 0% in the nephrectomy and nephrectomy-plus-irradiation arms, respectively. The low local recurrence rates in each of the prospective randomized studies suggest that the patient populations chosen were not likely to experience significant benefit from adjuvant local radiation therapy. Furthermore, the complication rates in each of these studies was unexpectedly high and probably compromised any beneficial effect that would have been identified in patients at high risk of local recurrence.

Two retrospective series readdress the possible beneficial effects of postoperative radiation therapy. The patients with renal cell carcinoma most likely to benefit from adjuvant radiation therapy are those with a significantly high risk of local failure. Patients with positive margins, regional lymph node metastases, or locally advanced tumors (T3 or T4) have a significantly higher risk of local failure than patients without these

| Table 60.8 | SURVIVAL AFTER NEPHRECTOMY OR NEPHRECTOMY AND POSTOPERATIVE RADIATION THERAPY FOR RENAL CELL CARCINOMA |

Author (Reference)	Stage	No. of Patients	Radiation Dose/Fraction Size (Gy)	Treatment	5-Year Survival Rate (%)	Local Recurrence (%)	RT-Related Mortality (%)	RT Complications (%)	Comments
Peeling et al. (106)	NS	96	—	N	52 (50/96)	NS	NS	NS	Retrospective study
		68	NS	N + RT	25 (17/63)	NS			
Rafla (110)	All	96	—	N	37 (35/94)	25	NS	NS	Retrospective study
		94	NS	N + RT	57 (46/81)	7			
Fugitt et al. (39)	NS	48	—	N	47 (17/35)	7	18	>20	Prospective randomized study
		52	55/2.04	N + RT	36 (14/39)	7			
Kjaer (68)	II, III	33	—	N	63[a]	1	19	44	Prospective randomized study
		32	55/2.5	N + RT	38[a]	0			
Stein et al. (124)	T2N0–T4N0	63	—	N	40	22	0	5	Retrospective study, CT-based planning
		56	46/1.8–2.0[b]	N + RT	50	9			
Kao et al. (62)	III–IV	12	—	N	62[c]	30	0	0	Retrospective study, CT-based planning
		12	45/1.8[c]	N + RT	75[c]	0			
Makarewicz et al. (79)	T3N0–T4N1	72	—	N	35.5	15.6	NS	NS	Retrospective study, significant LC benefit to T3N0 with RT
		114	50/1.8–2.0	N + RT	37.9				

CT, computed tomography; LC, local control; N, nephrectomy; NS, not stated; RT, radiation therapy
[a]Interpolated from graph; number at risk not known.
[b]Median dose.
[c]Disease-free survival.

findings (62,109,124). In a series reported by Stein et al. (124), the local recurrence rate for 30 patients with T3 tumors treated by nephrectomy alone was 37%, compared with only 10% in 37 patients treated with nephrectomy plus postoperative irradiation (p <.05). In a follow up to their original report, no benefit was seen to the elective administration of postoperative radiation therapy, even in the T3b patients whom they had originally described as having the highest risk of local recurrence (42). A local control advantage was suggested by Kao et al. (62). All 12 patients with capsular penetration, perinephric fat extension, or positive margins who received postoperative radiation therapy had local control with a 5-year disease-free survival rate of 75%, compared with a 30% local failure rate and a 62% disease-free survival rate in a comparable group of patients who received surgery alone (p <.01). In each of these series, patients at high risk of local failure were selected for adjuvant therapy, and radiation therapy was planned and delivered with the assistance of CT-based treatment planning.

Future studies should select patients who could potentially benefit from adjuvant radiation therapy. These include patients with high risk of local or regional failure, such as patients with positive margins or those with tumors involving the perinephric tissues. Patients with renal cell carcinoma confined to the kidney and/or renal vein have a low recurrence rate and a high survival rate after radical nephrectomy alone and should not be considered for adjuvant radiation therapy.

Renal Pelvis and Ureter Carcinoma

Tumors of the renal pelvis and ureter have a significantly high local recurrence rate after nephroureterectomy, particularly in patients with high-grade tumors or deep invasion (7). Data supporting the use of adjuvant radiation therapy in these cancers are sparse. An early report by Brookland and Richter (15) suggested a benefit for patients receiving adjuvant radiation therapy. Nine patients receiving postoperative irradiation (40 to 60 Gy [mean, 50 Gy] in 2-Gy fractions) had a lower local recurrence rate (11% vs. 46%) and a better survival rate (27% vs. 17%) than a group of 11 patients treated by surgery alone. This better outcome was seen despite the fact that the patients treated with radiation therapy had poorer prognostic features, such as high tumor grade, deep tumor invasion, or regional lymph node metastases. Babaian et al. (3) reported encouraging results for eight patients with deeply invasive ureter carcinoma treated with nephroureterectomy and postoperative radiation therapy. A local recurrence occurred in only one of eight patients after radiation therapy (40 to 60 Gy in 4 to 6 weeks). Cozad et al. (25) reported similar positive results in patients receiving adjuvant irradiation for renal pelvis and ureter cancer. Patients receiving postoperative radiation therapy had better local control and survival than patients treated with surgery alone. Five-year actuarial local control rates were 90% and 76%, respectively. Radiation therapy also provided substantial benefit to patients with unresectable tumors, allowing a median survival of 11 months, compared with only 4 months in patients managed without radiation therapy.

A report by Maulard-Durdux et al. (84) questioned the beneficial effects of adjuvant radiation therapy in transitional cell cancers of the upper urinary tract. Twenty-six patients received postoperative irradiation after radical surgery and were analyzed retrospectively. Radiation therapy (45 Gy) was administered to the local tumor site in eight patients, to the regional lymph nodes in three patients, and to both sites in 15 patients (58%). Because the survival rate in the irradiated patients was comparable to that seen in historical series of patients managed by surgery alone, the authors concluded that there was no advantage to adjuvant radiation therapy. However, local recurrences were seen in only one patient (4%) and nodal failure was seen in only four patients (15%). Two of the five local or regional failures occurred in sites that were not electively irradiated. The true infield failure rate was only 11.5% (3/26 patients). The distant failure rate was 54% in this series. A similar finding was reported by Ozsahin et al. (101) in a European multicenter retrospective analysis. In their series, 36% of the 138 patients received adjuvant postoperative radiation therapy, but there was no significant reduction in locoregional recurrences. Selection bias probably accounted for the lack of benefit as well as a high rate of distant metastases seen in the locally advanced-stage patients. The high rate of distant metastasis would warrant investigation of adjuvant systemic therapy in this situation. The low rate of infield irradiation failure suggests that there may indeed be an advantage to carefully planned postoperative local and regional lymph node irradiation. Hall et al. (49) have made a more compelling argument against routine use of postoperative radiation therapy. In 74 patients with stage III (n = 49) or stage IV (n = 25) transitional cell cancer of the upper urinary tract, there was no reduction in the rate of local recurrence with postoperative radiation therapy. In fact, the disease-free survival was worse in patients after receiving radiation therapy. Distant metastases were the most common site of failure. Isolated local recurrences were rare. In a series of 101 patients from Princess Margaret Hospital, postoperative radiation therapy was administered to 86 (17). Radiation treatment consisted of 36 Gy administered over 4 weeks—a relatively low dose. The rate of local failure in patients with T3–4/N0 or N+ disease was 35%, despite the radiation therapy. Distant metastases occurred in 53% of these same patients. Encouraging results have been reported by Czito et al. (28) when a combination of concurrent chemotherapy was administered to patients also receiving postoperative radiation therapy for locally advanced urothelial cancers of the upper urinary tracts. Collectively, these data argue that in the absence of effective systemic therapy, local radiation therapy is not likely to have a significant impact on cancer-free survival. Furthermore, low-dose radiation therapy, as administered in the Princess Margaret Hospital experience, is ineffective at preventing local tumor control. It is reasonable to consider adding systemic chemotherapy along with postoperative radiation therapy in patients who have locally advanced, positive surgical margins, or lymph node metastases.

:: | Sequelae of Radiation Therapy

The side effects and complications from radiation therapy for cancer of the kidney, renal pelvis, and ureters are similar to those expected from irradiation of the upper abdomen and pelvis. These side effects include nausea, vomiting, diarrhea, and abdominal cramping. Patients with right-sided tumors may have significant portions of the liver irradiated, and radiation-induced liver damage is possible. The Copenhagen Renal Cancer Study Group reported that 12/27 (44%) patients developed significant complications: three had biochemical changes indicating radiation hepatitis, three had duodenum and small-bowel stenosis, and six had duodenum and small-bowel bleeding (69). Surgery was performed on four of nine patients with bowel-related radiation therapy complications, and five patients died of treatment-related complications. The total radiation dose in this study was 50 Gy given in 2.5-Gy fractions per day—a fractionation schedule that may account for the high rate of complications. Fugitt et al. (39) also reported four cases of "liver" failure among 52 patients who received postoperative radiation therapy.

The complication rate after radiation therapy for tumors of the kidney and upper urinary tract is related to the total dose, fraction size, and technique of irradiation. CT-based simulation and three-dimensional treatment planning may decrease the risk of complications after elective radiation therapy in patients with upper urinary tract malignancies. In a series of 56 patients receiving 46 Gy postoperatively reported by Stein et al. (124), significant toxicity was seen in only three patients (5%). These three patients were treated before the routine use of CT-based treatment planning. In 12 patients receiving a median dose of 45 Gy reported by Kao et al. (62), no long-term treatment-related morbidity was identified.

References

1. Akdogan B, Dogan HS, Eskicorapci SY, et al. Prognostic significance of bladder tumor history and tumor location in upper tract transitional cell carcinoma. *J Urol* 2006;176:48–52.
2. Anglard P, Tory K, Brauch H, et al. Molecular analysis of genetic changes in the origin and development of renal cell carcinoma. *Cancer Res* 1991;51:1071–1077.
3. Babaian RJ, Johnson DE, Chan RC. Combination nephroureterectomy and postoperative radiotherapy for infiltrative ureteral carcinoma. *Int J Radiat Oncol Biol Phys* 1980;6:1229–1232.
4. Bassil B, Dosoretz DE, Prout GR Jr. Validation of the tumor, nodes and metastasis classification of renal cell carcinoma. *J Urol* 1985;134:450–454.
5. Beitler JJ, Makara D, Silverman P, et al. Definitive, high-dose-per-fraction, conformal, stereotactic external radiation for renal cell carcinoma. *Am J Clin Oncol* 2004;27:646–648.
6. Bennett RT, Lerner SE, Taub HC, et al. Cytoreductive surgery for stage IV renal cell carcinoma. *J Urol* 1995;154:32–34.
7. Blacher EJ, Johnson DE, Abdul-Karim FW, et al. Squamous cell carcinoma of renal pelvis. *Urology* 1985;25:124–126.
8. Blom JH, van Poppel H, Marechal JM, et al. Radical nephrectomy with and without lymph node dissection: preliminary results of the EORTC randomized phase III protocol 30881. EORTC Genitourinary Group. *Eur Urol* 1999;36:570–575.
9. Bloom HJ. Adjuvant therapy for adenocarcinoma of the kidney: present position and prospects. *Br J Urol* 1973;45:237–257.
10. Brady LW, Gislason GJ, Faust DS, et al. Radiation therapy. A valuable adjunct in the management of carcinoma of the ureter. *JAMA* 1968;206:2871–2874.
11. Brandner ED, Wu A, Chen H, et al. Abdominal organ motion measured using 4D CT. *Int J Radiat Oncol Biol Phys* 2006;65:554–560.
12. Brauch H, Weirich G, Brieger J, et al. VHL alterations in human clear cell renal cell carcinoma: association with advanced tumor stage and a novel hot spot mutation. *Cancer Res* 2000;60:1942–1948.
13. Bretheau D, Lechevallier E, de Fromont M, et al. Prognostic value of nuclear grade of renal cell carcinoma. *Cancer* 1995;76:2543–2549.
14. Brinkmann OA, Bruns F, Gosheger G, et al. Treatment of bone metastases and local recurrence from renal cell carcinoma with immunochemotherapy and radiation. *World J Urol* 2005;23:185–190.
15. Brookland RK, Richter MP. The postoperative irradiation of transitional cell carcinoma of the renal pelvis and ureter. *J Urol* 1985;133:952–955.
16. Catto JW, Azzouzi AR, Rehman I, et al. Promoter hypermethylation is associated with tumor location, stage, and subsequent progression in transitional cell carcinoma. *J Clin Oncol* 2005;23:2903–2910.
17. Catton CN, Warde P, Gospodarowica MK, et al. Transitional cell carcinoma of the renal pelvis and ureter; outcome and patterns of relapse in patients treated with postoperative radiation. *Urol Oncol* 1996;2:171–176.
18. Chahal R, Taylor K, Eardley I, et al. Patients at high risk for upper tract urothelial cancer: evaluation of hydronephrosis using high resolution magnetic resonance urography. *J Urol* 2005;174:478–482; quiz 801.
19. Charbit L, Gendreau MC, Mee S, et al. Tumors of the upper urinary tract: 10 years of experience. *J Urol* 1991;146:1243–1246.
20. Chiou RK, Vessella RL, Limas C, et al. Monoclonal antibody-targeted radiotherapy of renal cell carcinoma using a nude mouse model. *Cancer* 1988;61:1766–1775.
21. Christoferson LA, Gustafson MB, Petersen AG. Von Hippel-Lindau's disease. *JAMA* 1961;178:280–282.
22. Clayman RV, Lange PH, Fraley EE. Cancer of the upper urinary tract. In: Javadpour N, ed. *Principles and management of urologic cancer,* 2nd ed. Baltimore: Williams & Wilkins, 1983;
23. Corrado F, Ferri C, Mannini D, et al. Transitional cell carcinoma of the upper urinary tract: evaluation of prognostic factors by histopathology and flow cytometric analysis. *J Urol* 1991;146:1183–1186.
24. Couillard DR, deVere White RW. Surgery of renal cell carcinoma. *Urol Clin North Am* 1993;20:263–275.
25. Cozad SC, Smalley SR, Austenfeld M, et al. Adjuvant radiotherapy in high stage transitional cell carcinoma of the renal pelvis and ureter. *Int J Radiat Oncol Biol Phys* 1992;24:743–745.
26. Cozad SC, Smalley SR, Austenfeld M, et al. Transitional cell carcinoma of the renal pelvis or ureter: patterns of failure. *Urology* 1995;46:796–800.
27. Cullen TH, Popham RR, Voss HJ. Urine cytology and primary carcinoma of the renal pelvis and ureter. *Aust N Z J Surg* 1972;41:230–236.
28. Czito B, Zietman A, Kaufman D, et al. Adjuvant radiotherapy with and without concurrent chemotherapy for locally advanced transitional cell carcinoma of the renal pelvis and ureter. *J Urol* 2004;172:1271–1275.
29. Da Silva JL, Lacombe C, Bruneval P, et al. Tumor cells are the site of erythropoietin synthesis in human renal cancers associated with polycythemia. *Blood* 1990;75:577–582.
30. DiBiase SJ, Valicenti RK, Schultz D, et al. Palliative irradiation for focally symptomatic metastatic renal cell carcinoma: support for dose escalation based on a biological model. *J Urol* 1997;158:746–749.
31. Dinney CP, Awad SA, Gajewski JB, et al. Analysis of imaging modalities, staging systems, and prognostic indicators for renal cell carcinoma. *Urology* 1992;39:122–129.
32. Escudier B, Szczylik C, Eisen T, et al. Randomized phase III trial of the Raf kinase and VEGFR inhibitor sorafenib (BAY 43-9006) in patients with advanced renal cell carcinoma (RCC). 2005 ASCO Annual Meeting Proceedings. *J Clin Oncol* 2005;23:4510.
33. Fisher RI, Rosenberg SA, Fyfe G. Long-term survival update for high-dose recombinant interleukin-2 in patients with renal cell carcinoma. *Cancer J Sci Am* 2000;6:S55–S57.
34. Flanigan RC, Salmon SE, Blumenstein BA, et al. Nephrectomy followed by interferon alfa-2b compared with interferon alfa-2b alone for metastatic renal-cell cancer. *N Engl J Med* 2001;345:1655–1659.
35. Flocks RH, Kadesky MC. Malignant neoplasms of the kidney; an analysis of 353 patients followed five years or more. *J Urol* 1958;79:196–201.
36. Fossa SD, Kjolseth I, Lund G. Radiotherapy of metastases from renal cancer. *Eur Urol* 1982;8:340–342.
37. Frank I, Blute ML, Cheville JC, et al. An outcome prediction model for patients with clear cell renal cell carcinoma treated with radical nephrectomy based on tumor stage, size, grade and necrosis: the SSIGN score. *J Urol* 2002;168:2395–2400.
38. Frank W, Stuhldreher D, Saffrin R, et al. Stage IV renal cell carcinoma. *J Urol* 1994;152:1998–1999.
39. Fugitt RB, Wu GS, Martinelli LC. An evaluation of postoperative radiotherapy in hypernephroma treatment—a clinical trial. *Cancer* 1973;32:1332–1340.
40. Fuhrman SA, Lasky LC, Limas C. Prognostic significance of morphologic parameters in renal cell carcinoma. *Am J Surg Pathol* 1982;6:655–663.
41. Gerszten PC, Burton SA, Ozhasoglu C, et al. Stereotactic radiosurgery for spinal metastases from renal cell carcinoma. *J Neurosurg Spine* 2005;3:288–295.
42. Gez E, Libes M, Bar-Deroma R, et al. Postoperative irradiation in localized renal cell carcinoma: the Rambam Medical Center experience. *Tumori* 2002;88:500–502.
43. Gill IS, McClennan BL, Kerbl K, et al. Adrenal involvement from renal cell carcinoma: predictive value of computerized tomography. *J Urol* 1994;152:1082–1085.
44. Giuliani L, Giberti C, Martorana G, et al. Radical extensive surgery for renal cell carcinoma: long-term results and prognostic factors. *J Urol* 1990;143:468–473; discussion 473–474.
45. Golimbu M, Joshi P, Sperber A, et al. Renal cell carcinoma: survival and prognostic factors. *Urology* 1986;27:291–301.
46. Grabstald H, Whitmore WF, Melamed MR. Renal pelvic tumors. *JAMA* 1971;218:845–854.
47. Greene FL, Page DL, Flemming ID, et al. *AJCC cancer staging manual*. New York: Springer-Verlag, 2002.
48. Guinan P, Stuhldreher D, Frank W, et al. Report of 337 patients with renal cell carcinoma emphasizing 110 with stage IV disease and review of the literature. *J Surg Oncol* 1997;64:295–298.
49. Hall MC, Womack JS, Roehrborn CG, et al. Advanced transitional cell carcinoma of the upper urinary tract: patterns of failure, survival and impact of postoperative adjuvant radiotherapy. *J Urol* 1998;160:703–706.
50. Hall MC, Womack S, Sagalowsky AI, et al. Prognostic factors, recurrence, and survival in transitional cell carcinoma of the upper urinary tract: a 30-year experience in 252 patients. *Urology* 1998;52:594–601.
51. Halperin EC, Harisiadis L. The role of radiation therapy in the management of metastatic renal cell carcinoma. *Cancer* 1983;51:614–617.
52. Han KR, Bleumer I, Pantuck AJ, et al. Validation of an integrated staging system toward improved prognostication of patients with localized renal cell carcinoma in an international population. *J Urol* 2003;170:2221–2224.
53. Hemmerlein B, Kugler A, Ozisik R, et al. Vascular endothelial growth factor expression, angiogenesis, and necrosis in renal cell carcinomas. *Virchows Arch* 2001;439:645–652.
54. Heney NM, Nocks BN, Daly JJ, et al. Prognostic factors in carcinoma of the ureter. *J Urol* 1981;125:632–636.
55. Highman WJ. Transitional carcinoma of the upper urinary tract: a histological and cytopathological study. *J Clin Pathol* 1986;39:297–305.
56. Huben RP, Mounzer AM, Murphy GP. Tumor grade and stage as prognostic variables in upper tract urothelial tumors. *Cancer* 1988;62:2016–2020.
57. Huguenin PU, Kieser S, Glanzmann C, et al. Radiotherapy for metastatic carcinomas of the kidney or melanomas: an analysis using palliative end points. *Int J Radiat Oncol Biol Phys* 1998;41:401–405.
58. Iliopoulos O, Levy AP, Jiang C, et al. Negative regulation of hypoxia-inducible genes by the von Hippel-Lindau protein. *Proc Natl Acad Sci U S A* 1996;93:10595–10599.
59. Javidan J, Stricker HJ, Tamboli P, et al. Prognostic significance of the 1997 TNM classification of renal cell carcinoma. *J Urol* 1999;162:1277–1281.
60. Jemal A, Thomas A, Murray T, et al. Cancer statistics, 2006. *CA Cancer J Clin* 2006;56:106–130.
61. Juusela H, Malmio K, Alfthan O, et al. Preoperative irradiation in the treatment of renal adenocarcinoma. *Scand J Urol Nephrol* 1977;11:277–281.
62. Kao GD, Malkowicz SB, Whittington R, et al. Locally advanced renal cell carcinoma: low complication rate and efficacy of postnephrectomy radiation therapy planned with CT. *Radiology* 1994;193:725–730.
63. Kattan MW, Reuter V, Motzer RJ, et al. A postoperative prognostic nomogram for renal cell carcinoma. *J Urol* 2001;166:63–67.
64. Kim HL, Zisman A, Han KR, et al. Prognostic significance of venous thrombus in renal cell carcinoma. Are renal vein and inferior vena cava involvement different? *J Urol* 2004;171:588–591.
65. King CR, Schimke RN, Arthur T, et al. Proximal 3p deletion in renal cell carcinoma cells from a patient with von Hippel-Lindau disease. *Cancer Genet Cytogenet* 1987;27:345–348.
66. Kinouchi T, Saiki S, Meguro N, et al. Impact of tumor size on the clinical outcomes of patients with Robson state I renal cell carcinoma. *Cancer* 1999;85:689–695.
67. Kjaer M. The role of medroxyprogesterone acetate (MPA) in the treatment of renal adenocarcinoma. *Cancer Treat Rev* 1988;15:195–209.
68. Kjaer M. The treatment and prognosis of patients with renal adenocarcinoma with solitary metastasis. 10 year survival results. *Int J Radiat Oncol Biol Phys* 1987;13:619–621.
69. Kjaer M, Frederiksen PL, Engelholm SA. Postoperative radiotherapy in stage II and III renal adenocarcinoma. A randomized trial by the Copenhagen Renal Cancer Study Group. *Int J Radiat Oncol Biol Phys* 1987;13:665–672.
70. Kondo K, Yao M, Yoshida M, et al. Comprehensive mutational analysis of the VHL gene in sporadic renal cell carcinoma: relationship to clinicopathological parameters. *Genes Chromosomes Cancer* 2002;34:58–68.
71. Lai PP. Kidney, renal pelvis, and ureter. In: Perez CA, Brady LW, eds. *Principles and practice of radiation oncology*. Philadelphia: J.B. Lippincott, 1992;
72. Lau WK, Blute ML, Weaver AL, et al. Matched comparison of radical nephrectomy vs nephron-sparing surgery in patients with unilateral renal cell carcinoma and a normal contralateral kidney. *Mayo Clin Proc* 2000;75:1236–1242.
73. Lee CT, Katz J, Shi W, et al. Surgical management of renal tumors 4 cm or less in a contemporary cohort. *J Urol* 2000;163:730–736.

74. Lee J, Hodgson D, Chow E, et al. A phase II trial of palliative radiotherapy for metastatic renal cell carcinoma. *Cancer* 2005;104:1894–1900.
75. Lee JS, Kim HS, Jung JJ, et al. Expression of vascular endothelial growth factor in renal cell carcinoma and the relation to angiogenesis and p53 protein expression. *J Surg Oncol* 2001;77:55–60.
76. Linehan WM, Shipley WU, Parkinson DR. Cancer of the kidney and ureter. In: DeVita VT, Hellman S, Rosenberg SA, eds. *Cancer: principles and practice of oncology*, 4th ed. Philadelphia: J.B. Lippincott, 1993.
77. Ljungberg B, Stenling R, Osterdahl B, et al. Vein invasion in renal cell carcinoma: impact on metastatic behavior and survival. *J Urol* 1995;154:1681–1684.
78. Loehrer PJ Sr., Einhorn LH, Elson PJ, et al. A randomized comparison of cisplatin alone or in combination with methotrexate, vinblastine, and doxorubicin in patients with metastatic urothelial carcinoma: a cooperative group study. *J Clin Oncol* 1992;10:1066–1073.
79. Makarewicz R, Zarzycka M, Kulinska G, et al. The value of postoperative radiotherapy in advanced renal cell cancer. *Neoplasma* 1998;45:380–383.
80. Maldazys JD, deKernion JB. Prognostic factors in metastatic renal carcinoma. *J Urol* 1986;136:376–379.
81. Manikandan R, Srinivasan V, Rane A. Which is the real gold standard for small-volume renal tumors? Radical nephrectomy versus nephron-sparing surgery. *J Endourol* 2004;18:39–44.
82. Marshall FF, Powell KC. Lymphadenectomy for renal cell carcinoma: anatomical and therapeutic considerations. *J Urol* 1982;128:677–681.
83. Marshall FF, Taxy JB, Fishman EK, et al. The feasibility of surgical enucleation for renal cell carcinoma. *J Urol* 1986;135:231–234.
84. Maulard-Durdux C, Dufour B, Hennequin C, et al. Postoperative radiation therapy in 26 patients with invasive transitional cell carcinoma of the upper urinary tract: no impact on survival? *J Urol* 1996;155:115–117.
85. McClennan BL. Oncologic imaging. Staging and follow-up of renal and adrenal carcinoma. *Cancer* 1991;67:1199–1208.
86. McKiernan J, Simmons R, Katz J, et al. Natural history of chronic renal insufficiency after partial and radical nephrectomy. *Urology* 2002;59:816–820.
87. McNichols DW, Segura JW, DeWeerd JH. Renal cell carcinoma: long-term survival and late recurrence. *J Urol* 1981;126:17–23.
88. Mickisch GH, Garin A, van Poppel H, et al. Radical nephrectomy plus interferon-alfa-based immunotherapy compared with interferon alfa alone in metastatic renal-cell carcinoma: a randomised trial. *Lancet* 2001;358:966–970.
89. Middleton RG. Surgery for metastatic renal cell carcinoma. *J Urol* 1967;97:973–977.
90. Montie JE, Stewart BH, Straffon RA, et al. The role of adjunctive nephrectomy in patients with metastatic renal cell carcinoma. *J Urol* 1977;117:272–275.
91. Motzer RJ, Michaelson MD, Redman BG, et al. Activity of SU11248, a multitargeted inhibitor of vascular endothelial growth factor receptor and platelet-derived growth factor receptor, in patients with metastatic renal cell carcinoma. *J Clin Oncol* 2006;24:16–24.
92. Mullerad M, Russo P, Golijanin D, et al. Bladder cancer as a prognostic factor for upper tract transitional cell carcinoma. *J Urol* 2004;172:2177–2181.
93. Muscat JE, Hoffmann D, Wynder EL. The epidemiology of renal cell carcinoma. A second look. *Cancer* 1995;75:2552–2557.
94. Ning S, Trisler K, Wessels BW, et al. Radiobiologic studies of radioimmunotherapy and external beam radiotherapy in vitro and in vivo in human renal cell carcinoma xenografts. *Cancer* 1997;80:2519–2528.
95. Nishisaka N, Maini A, Kinoshita Y, et al. Immunotherapy for lung metastases of murine renal cell carcinoma: synergy between radiation and cytokine-producing tumor vaccines. *J Immunother* 1999;22:308–314.
96. Nissenkorn I, Bernheim J. Multicentricity in renal cell carcinoma. *J Urol* 1995;153:620–622.
97. O'Dea MJ, Zincke H, Utz DC, et al. The treatment of renal cell carcinoma with solitary metastasis. *J Urol* 1978;120:540–542.
98. Onufrey V, Mohiuddin M. Radiation therapy in the treatment of metastatic renal cell carcinoma. *Int J Radiat Oncol Biol Phys* 1985;11:2007–2009.
99. Otto U, Huland H, Baisch H, et al. Transplantation of human renal cell carcinoma into NMRI nu/nu mice. III. Effect of irradiation on tumor acceptance and tumor growth. *J Urol* 1985;134:170–174.
100. Oya M, Nakamura K, Baba S, et al. Intrarenal satellites of renal cell carcinoma: histopathologic manifestation and clinical implication. *Urology* 1995;46:161–164.
101. Ozsahin M, Zouhair A, Villa S, et al. Prognostic factors in urothelial renal pelvis and ureter tumours: a multicentre Rare Cancer Network study. *Eur J Cancer* 1999;35:738–743.
102. Pantuck AJ, Zisman A, Dorey F, et al. Renal cell carcinoma with retroperitoneal lymph nodes. Impact on survival and benefits of immunotherapy. *Cancer* 2003;97:2995–3002.
103. Pantuck AJ, Zisman A, Dorey F, et al. Renal cell carcinoma with retroperitoneal lymph nodes: role of lymph node dissection. *J Urol* 2003;169:2076–2083.
104. Park S, Hong B, Kim CS, et al. The impact of tumor location on prognosis of transitional cell carcinoma of the upper urinary tract. *J Urol* 2004;171:621–625.
105. Patard JJ, Kim HL, Lam JS, et al. Use of the University of California Los Angeles integrated staging system to predict survival in renal cell carcinoma: an international multicenter study. *J Clin Oncol* 2004;22:3316–3322.
106. Peeling WB, Mantell BS, Shepheard BG. Post-operative irradiation in the treatment of renal cell carcinoma. *Br J Urol* 1969;41:23–31.
107. Petkovic SD. Epidemiology and treatment of renal pelvic and ureteral tumors. *J Urol* 1975;114:858–865.
108. Provet J, Tessler A, Brown J, et al. Partial nephrectomy for renal cell carcinoma: indications, results and implications. *J Urol* 1991;145:472–476.
109. Rabinovitch RA, Zelefsky MJ, Gaynor JJ, et al. Patterns of failure following surgical resection of renal cell carcinoma: implications for adjuvant local and systemic therapy. *J Clin Oncol* 1994;12:206–212.
110. Rafla S. Renal cell carcinoma. Natural history and results of treatment. *Cancer* 1970;25:26–40.
111. Ratain MJ, Eisen T, Stadler WM, et al. Phase II placebo-controlled randomized discontinuation trial of sorafenib in patients with metastatic renal cell carcinoma. *J Clin Oncol* 2006;24:2505–2512.
112. Reitelman C, Sawczuk IS, Olsson CA, et al. Prognostic variables in patients with transitional cell carcinoma of the renal pelvis and proximal ureter. *J Urol* 1987;138:1144–1145.
113. Riches EW. The natural history of renal tumors. In: Riches EW, ed. *Tumors of the kidney and ureter*. Edinburgh: Williams & Wilkins, 1964:
114. Robson CJ, Churchill BM, Anderson W. The results of radical nephrectomy for renal cell carcinoma. *J Urol* 1969;101:297–301.
115. Rubin P, Keller B, Cox C, et al. Preoperative irradiation in renal cancer. Evaluation of radiation treatment plans. *Am J Roentgenol Radium Ther Nucl Med* 1975;123:114–121.
116. Russo P. The contemporary gold standard for T1 renal masses. *Am J Urol* 2004;2:214.
117. Schwartz LH, Richaud J, Buffat L, et al. Kidney mobility during respiration. *Radiother Oncol* 1994;32:84–86.
118. Sella A, Logothetis CJ, Ro JY, et al. Sarcomatoid renal cell carcinoma. A treatable entity. *Cancer* 1987;60:1313–1318.
119. Selli C, Hinshaw WM, Woodard BH, et al. Stratification of risk factors in renal cell carcinoma. *Cancer* 1983;52:899–903.
120. Sheehan JP, Sun MH, Kondziolka D, et al. Radiosurgery in patients with renal cell carcinoma metastasis to the brain: long-term outcomes and prognostic factors influencing survival and local tumor control. *J Neurosurg* 2003;98:342–349.
121. Skinner DG, Colvin RB, Vermillion CD, et al. Diagnosis and management of renal cell carcinoma. A clinical and pathologic study of 309 cases. *Cancer* 1971;28:1165–1177.
122. Smith RB, deKernion JB, Ehrlich RM, et al. Bilateral renal cell carcinoma and renal cell carcinoma in the solitary kidney. *J Urol* 1984;132:450–454.
123. Solomon D, Schwartz A. Renal pathology in von Hippel-Lindau disease. *Hum Pathol* 1988;19:1072–1079.
124. Stein M, Kuten A, Halpern J, et al. The value of postoperative irradiation in renal cell cancer. *Radiother Oncol* 1992;24:41–44.
125. Sternberg CN, Yagoda A, Scher HI, et al. Methotrexate, vinblastine, doxorubicin, and cisplatin for advanced transitional cell carcinoma of the urothelium. Efficacy and patterns of response and relapse. *Cancer* 1989;64:2448–2458.
126. Sufrin G, Mirand EA, Moore RH, et al. Hormones in renal cancer. *J Urol* 1977;117:433–438.
127. Takahashi A, Sasaki H, Kim SJ, et al. Markedly increased amounts of messenger RNAs for vascular endothelial growth factor and placenta growth factor in renal cell carcinoma associated with angiogenesis. *Cancer Res* 1994;54:4233–4237.
128. Thrasher JB, Paulson DF. Prognostic factors in renal cancer. *Urol Clin North Am* 1993;20:247–262.
129. Tolia BM, Whitmore WF Jr. Solitary metastasis from renal cell carcinoma. *J Urol* 1975;114:836–838.
130. Tomisawa M, Tokunaga T, Oshika Y, et al. Expression pattern of vascular endothelial growth factor isoform is closely correlated with tumour stage and vascularisation in renal cell carcinoma. *Eur J Cancer* 1999;35:133–137.
131. Topley M, Novick AC, Montie JE. Long-term results following partial nephrectomy for localized renal adenocarcinoma. *J Urol* 1984;131:1050–1052.
132. Tosaka A, Ohya K, Yamada K, et al. Incidence and properties of renal masses and asymptomatic renal cell carcinoma detected by abdominal ultrasonography. *J Urol* 1990;144:1097–1099.
133. Tsui KH, Shvarts O, Smith RB, et al. Prognostic indicators for renal cell carcinoma: a multivariate analysis of 643 patients using the revised 1997 TNM staging criteria. *J Urol* 2000;163:1090–1095; quiz 1295.
134. Uchida M, Imaide Y, Sugimoto K, et al. Percutaneous cryosurgery for renal tumours. *Br J Urol* 1995;75:132–136; discussion 136–137.
135. van der Werf-Messing B. Proceedings: carcinoma of the kidney. *Cancer* 1973; 32:1056–1061.
136. van der Werf-Messing B, van der Heul RO, Ledeboer RC. Renal cell carcinoma trial. *Strahlentherapie (Sonderb)* 1981;76:169–715.
137. van Sornsen de Koste JR, Senan S, Kleynen CE, et al. Renal mobility during uncoached quiet respiration: an analysis of 4DCT scans. *Int J Radiat Oncol Biol Phys* 2006;64:799–803.
138. Vasselli JR, Yang JC, Linehan WM, et al. Lack of retroperitoneal lymphadenopathy predicts survival of patients with metastatic renal cell carcinoma. *J Urol* 2001;166:68–72.
139. Walsh L, Stanfield JL, Cho LC, et al. Efficacy of ablative high-dose-per-fraction radiation for implanted human renal cell cancer in a nude mouse model. *Eur Urol* 2006;29:29.
140. Wang GL, Semenza GL. Purification and characterization of hypoxia-inducible factor 1. *J Biol Chem* 1995;270:1230–1237.
141. Waters WB, Richie JP. Aggressive surgical approach to renal cell carcinoma: review of 130 cases. *J Urol* 1979;122:306–309.
142. Wersall PJ, Blomgren H, Lax I, et al. Extracranial stereotactic radiotherapy for primary and metastatic renal cell carcinoma. *Radiother Oncol* 2005;77:88–95.
143. Whang M, O'Toole K, Bixon R, et al. The incidence of multifocal renal cell carcinoma in patients who are candidates for partial nephrectomy. *J Urol* 1995;154:968–970; discussion 970–971.
144. Wronski M, Maor MH, Davis BJ, et al. External radiation of brain metastases from renal carcinoma: a retrospective study of 119 patients from the M.D. Anderson Cancer Center. *Int J Radiat Oncol Biol Phys* 1997;37:753–759.
145. Yagoda A, Abi-Rached B, Petrylak D. Chemotherapy for advanced renal-cell carcinoma: 1983–1993. *Semin Oncol* 1995;22:42–60.
146. Yang JC, Haworth L, Sherry RM, et al. A randomized trial of bevacizumab, an anti-vascular endothelial growth factor antibody, for metastatic renal cancer. *N Engl J Med* 2003;349:427–434.
147. Zisman A, Pantuck AJ, Dorey F, et al. Improved prognostication of renal cell carcinoma using an integrated staging system. *J Clin Oncol* 2001;19:1649–1657.
148. Zisman A, Pantuck AJ, Wieder J, et al. Risk group assessment and clinical outcome algorithm to predict the natural history of patients with surgically resected renal cell carcinoma. *J Clin Oncol* 2002;20:4559–4566.
149. Zlotta AR, Wildschutz T, Raviv G, et al. Radiofrequency interstitial tumor ablation (RITA) is a possible new modality for treatment of renal cancer: ex vivo and in vivo experience. *J Endourol* 1997;11:251–258.

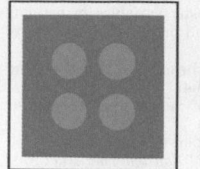

Chapter 61
Bladder

Zbigniew Petrovich, John P. Stein, Gabor Jozsef, Silvia C. Formenti

During the past 25 years there has been a steady decrease in the importance of definitive irradiation as a single modality therapy in the management of patients with carcinoma of the bladder. There has been a corresponding increase in the application of radical cystectomy and in the use of radiotherapy as a part of an organ-preservation multimodality therapeutic approach. This trend continues particularly in the United States and in the European Community. This chapter outlines the behavior of bladder cancer and presents evidence to support contemporary therapy of patients with this disease.

Anatomy of the Bladder

The bladder is a hollow, muscular organ that when empty lies within the pelvis, occupying the anterior portion of pelvic cavity just superior and posterior to the pubic bone. The bladder should be considered a true intra-abdominal organ that can project above the umbilicus when full. In infants, the true pelvis is shallow and the bladder neck is usually level with the upper border of the pubic symphysis. By puberty, the bladder has migrated to the confines of the deepened true pelvis.

The bladder is considered to have an apex, a superior surface, two inferolateral surfaces, a base or posterior surface, and a neck. The apex reaches a short distance cephalad above the pubic bone and ends as a fibrous cord which is a derivative of the urachus, a canal in the fetus connecting the bladder with the allantois. This fibrous cord extends from the apex of the bladder to the umbilicus between the peritoneum and the transversalis fascia. The superior surface is the only surface of the bladder that is covered by the peritoneum. This surface generally is associated with the uterus and ileum in women and with the ileum and sigmoid colon in men. The base of the bladder is posterior and is separated from the rectum by the vas deferens, seminal vesicles, and ureters in the male, and by the uterus and vagina in the female. The seminal vesicles form a V-shaped structure at the base of the bladder, with the vas deferens entering the middle of the so-called V. The ureters enter into the bladder slightly superior and lateral to the seminal vesicles, with the vas deferens coursing above and in a caudal direction to the ureters. The inferior and lateral surfaces of the bladder are in close relation with the pubic bone, the levator ani, and obturator internus muscles. The bladder is distinctly separate from the pubic bone by the retropubic space containing fat and fibroareolar tissue. The neck of the bladder is its most inferior portion adjacent to the prostate in men and the urethra in women. As the bladder distends with urine, the neck remains fixed in position, and the superior part will rise into the pelvic cavity. Anteroinferiorly and laterally, the bladder is cushioned from the pelvic sidewall by retropubic and perivesical fat and loose connective tissue. This perivesical space is called the space of Retzius.

The bladder mucosa is lined with transitional epithelium and appears smooth when the bladder is full; however, it contracts into numerous folds when it empties. The interureteral fold is a ridge at the bladder neck between the openings of the ureters into the bladder.

Epidemiology

Carcinoma of the bladder has been a well-recognized malignancy since the period of antiquity. In the United States bladder cancer is the second most common tumor of the genitourinary tract, and it is the second most common cause of death in genitourinary malignancy. In 1999 this tumor was diagnosed in 263,000 patients worldwide, representing 4% of all cancer (129). It is more common in males, with the incidence of 9.9 per 100,000, which makes it the eighth most important tumor in the world. The incidence in females is 2.3 per 100,000, which makes it 18th in incidence in the world. Bladder tumor is known for its wide geographic variation in the frequency of occurrence, with North America and North Africa being the highest and China the lowest. The estimated incidence and mortality of the common genitourinary malignancies in the United States in 2006 are shown respectively in Tables 61.1 and 61.2 (83). Carcinoma of the bladder in this country primarily affects males between 60 and 70 years of age, and its incidence is increasing.

In North Africa this tumor represents more than 30% of all cancers, is associated with bilharziasis, and it is primarily (more than 50%) squamous cell carcinoma (51). The associations of human papilloma virus and bacterial infections with bilharziasis are likely important factors in carcinogenesis of bladder cancer in this patient population. However, in North America and in the European Community a vast majority (more than 90%) of these tumors are transitional cell carcinomas (TCC), with adenocarcinoma and squamous cell carcinoma next in frequency (168). Small cell carcinoma and sarcoma are rarely diagnosed primary tumors of the bladder (100).

Carcinoma of the bladder has a well-documented history of environmental and industrial causative factors (153). Removal of these recognized industrial and environmental causative factors and an appropriate public health campaign are expected to reduce the incidence of bladder cancer from these causes. The strongest etiologic risk factor is the use of tobacco, which is responsible for about 50% of cases of bladder cancer in male patients in the United States (238).

Natural History

As many as 85% of patients diagnosed with TCC of the bladder have superficial low-grade tumors (Ta, T1), which are confined to the mucosa. Such lesions have a very high (70%) incidence of local recurrence, and 50% have disease progression following transurethral resection of the bladder (TURB) (15,136). The incidence of local recurrence is particularly high among patients with multiple lesions or those with high-grade superficial tumors (135). Of the 70% of patients who develop local recurrence, approximately one-third will have multiple recurrent lesions. Tumor progression to muscle-invasive disease at 5 years following the diagnosis has been reported in nearly 15% of these patients, whereas metastatic disease was seen in <5% and death from cancer was seen in nearly 9% of patients (89). In view of the propensity for tumor recurrence and progression

| Table 61.1 | **ESTIMATED INCIDENCE OF GENITOURINARY TUMORS IN THE UNITED STATES IN 2006** |

Tumor Site	Males	Females	Total
Prostate	234,460	—	234,460
Bladder	44,690	16,730	61,420
Kidney	24,650	14,240	38,890
Testis	8,250	—	8,250
Ureter	1,600	830	2,430
Total	313,650	31,800	345,450

From Jemal A, Siegel R, Ward E, et al. Cancer statistics, 2006. *Ca Cancer J Clin* 2006;56:106–130, with permission.

to a higher stage, patients with Ta, T1 disease require careful long-term follow-up.

A number of important risk factors for a progression to muscle-invasive disease have been identified. These factors include tumor grade, tumor size, the presence of solitary versus multiple lesions, history of prior recurrence(s), bladder neck involvement, and the presence of genetic risk factors (49,125,136). The recognition of these risk factors helps clinicians to target selected patients for more aggressive therapy at diagnosis.

Patients with Ta and T1 tumors, if followed for a long time, die as a result of bladder cancer in about 20% of cases, whereas an overwhelming (70%) majority are expected to die of other causes (132). Death from bladder cancer is twice as common in patients with T1 as opposed to Ta disease. An appropriate therapy in patients with Ta and T1 tumors is expected to modify the natural history of this disease.

Carcinoma *in situ* (Tis) presents another pathway to muscle-invasive disease. Tis may be associated with superficial papillary lesions or may arise *de novo,* which usually displays a more aggressive behavior leading to a greater probability of recurrence and muscle-invasive disease. A study of 31 Tis patients who received no specific therapy and were followed for a median of 64 months is of major interest (234). During the period of observation 52% of the study patients showed evidence of tumor progression to clinically significant muscle-invasive disease. The remaining 15 patients had a stable disease with 12 having subsequent tumor recurrence. This clearly demonstrated the importance of early and aggressive therapy in 90% of Tis patients.

Patients with muscle-invasive disease (T2, T3, and T4) tend to progress locally, with increasing tumor size and increasing depth of invasion leading to the involvement of extravesical structures and to metastatic disease, initially to the regional lymph nodes and subsequently to distant sites (230). The incidence of lymphadenopathy correlates well with the depth of tumor invasion in the bladder wall. Aggressive surgical therapy has shown to modify the natural history of this manifestation of bladder cancer (197). It is apparent that not all patients will

| Table 61.2 | **ESTIMATED MORTALITY IN GENITOURINARY MALIGNANCY IN THE UNITED STATES IN 2006** |

Site	Males	Females	Total
Prostate	27,350	—	27,350
Bladder	8,990	4,070	13,060
Kidney	8,230	4,710	12,840
Ureter	410	360	770
Testis	370	—	370

From Jemal A, Siegel R, Ward E, et al. Cancer statistics, 2006. *Ca Cancer J Clin* 2006;56:106–130, with permission.

follow this orderly tumor progression, with some showing early metastatic disease with relatively small primary tumors.

Diagnosis of metastatic disease in patients with carcinoma of the bladder is in an important and common event that tends to occur within the first 18 months of radical cystectomy. More than one-third of surgically treated patients develop distant metastasis, initially to the lung and bone and subsequently to multiple organs. The presence of distant metastasis is leading inevitably and rapidly to death (135,136). The risk factors for distant metastasis include depth of invasion (pT3b), direct tumor extension to the prostate, and pelvic lymphadenopathy (197).

Symptoms and Signs

Gross painless hematuria is the most common (75%) presenting sign of bladder cancer, with painless microscopic hematuria being less common. Nearly one in four patients present with irritative and obstructive symptoms and signs, which are frequently and incorrectly assumed to represent benign prostatic hyperplasia rather than bladder cancer. This factor results in delaying cystoscopy, thus compromising the patient's chance for early diagnosis and therapy. Nearly 20% of patients are asymptomatic or present with nonspecific symptoms or signs. Patients, particularly males who are past middle age, with even a single episode of painless hematuria need to be investigated for the presence of bladder cancer.

Diagnostic Work-Up

Patients should have detailed general and urologic history and physical examination followed by complete blood count and urinalysis. Cystoscopy with random biopsies or TURB if tumor has been identified also should be used. Cytology needs to be performed before and during cystoscopy. The role of cytology may be of major importance in making the initial diagnosis of transitional cell carcinoma as well as being a critical test in following patients after a definitive therapy. In case of positive biopsy for carcinoma, further and more directed work-up is required. Computed tomography (CT) of the pelvis and abdomen is essential because it provides an effective study to help with staging of known bladder cancer; evaluate the bladder, ureters, and kidneys; and assess for possible pelvic or periaortic lymphadenopathy. Major limitations of this imaging study include difficulty evaluating smaller bladder tumors; difficulty in making a diagnosis of a small extravesical tumor extension; problems evaluating areas of focal bladder wall edema, which may be a result of a recent biopsy; and particular difficulty evaluating the bladder following a definitive course of radiotherapy.

Magnetic resonance imaging (MRI) is an evolving imaging study in bladder cancer with similar limitations to those of CT. In a report on the value of MRI in staging of 143 patients with bladder cancer prior to EBRT, this imaging modality provided important data that helped to better define the true anatomic extent of the tumor and was an important predictor of prognosis (149).

Ultrasonography gained an important place in the staging of bladder cancer. The following ultrasound modes currently are used in the clinical practice: transabdominal, suprapubic, transrectal, and transurethral. Transrectal ultrasonography is not routinely used in patients with bladder cancer, whereas transurethral ultrasonography may help demonstrate the presence of transmural invasion. This technique is used infrequently in the United States and is much more popular in Scandinavia. Color Doppler study may help to differentiate between intravesical clot formation and bladder tumor. If distant metastasis is suspected, radiographs of the chest and bone scan are essential

| :: | Table 61.3 | STAGING OF PRIMARY BLADDER TUMORS (T-STAGE) |

T-Stage	Definition
Tx	Primary tumor cannot be assessed
T0	No evidence of primary tumor
Ta	Noninvasive papillary carcinoma
Tis	Carcinoma *in situ* (flat tumor)
T1	Tumor invades subepithelial connective tissue
T2	Tumor invades muscle
T2a	Tumor invades superficial muscle (inner half)
T2b	Tumor invades deep muscle (outer half)
T3	Tumor invades perivesical tissue
T3a	Microscopic invasion only
T3b	Macroscopic invasion (extravesical mass)
T4	Tumor invades prostate, uterus, vagina, pelvic wall, or abdominal wall
T4a	Tumor invades prostate, uterus, vagina
T4b	Tumor invades pelvic wall, abdominal wall

From American Joint Committee on Cancer. Urinary bladder. In: *AJCC cancer staging manual*, 5th ed. Philadelphia: Lippincott-Raven, 1997:241–243, with permission.

| :: | Table 61.5 | STAGE GROUPING |

Stage	T	N	M
0a	Ta	N0	M0
0is	Tis	N0	M0
I	T1	N0	M0
II	T2a	N0	M0
	T2b	N0	M0
III	T3a	N0	M0
	T3b	N0	M0
	T4a	N0	M0
IV	T4b	N0	M0
	Any T	N1	M0
	Any T	N2	M0
	Any T	N3	M0
	Any T	Any N	M1

American Joint Committee on Cancer. Urinary bladder. In: American Joint Committee on Cancer. *AJCC cancer staging manual*, 5th ed. Philadelphia: Lippincott-Raven, 1997:241 243.

diagnostic studies. Positron emission tomography is emerging as a very useful tool in staging of cancer of the bladder.

:: | Staging System

The TNM system recommended by the American Joint Committee on Cancer (3) currently is used for staging of bladder cancer. Tables 61.3, 61.4, and 61.5 define T (tumor), N (node), and M (metastasis) stages and stage grouping. Accurate clinical staging is imperative because it predicts a patient's prognosis and defines the optimal therapy (197). Pathologic staging is, as expected, more accurate in predicting tumor behavior than the clinical staging; however, both systems are of importance in the management of patients with bladder cancer.

In the near future it is expected that molecular genetics will help to better identify patients with more aggressive tumors, guiding clinicians in selecting appropriate therapy (36,136). Cytogenetic tests and molecular genetic studies such as DNA sequencing are already available to the clinic. The most promising and the most extensively used prognostic markers in bladder cancer are tumor suppressor genes such as p53 and retinoblastoma gene. It is anticipated that routine use of these new tests likely will make clinical and pathologic staging to a large extent obsolete.

| :: | Table 61.4 | STAGING SYSTEM FOR REGIONAL LYMPH NODES AND DISTANT METASTASIS |

N-Stage	Definition
Nx	Regional lymph nodes cannot be assessed
N0	No regional lymph node metastasis
N1	Metastasis in a single lymph node <2 cm in great dimension
N2	Metastasis in a single lymph node >2 cm but not >5 cm in greatest dimension; or multiple lymph nodes, none >5 cm in greatest dimension
N3	Metastasis in a lymph node >5 cm in greatest dimension
M-stage	
Mx	Distant metastasis cannot be assessed
M0	No distant metastasis
M1	Distant metastasis

From American Joint Committee on Cancer. Urinary bladder. In: *AJCC cancer staging manual*, 5th ed. Philadelphia: Lippincott-Raven, 1997:241–243, with permission.

:: | Pathology

In North America and Europe bladder cancer is represented by transitional cell carcinoma in more than 90% of cases. Squamous cell carcinoma represents approximately 5%, followed by adenocarcinoma. Other tumors such as small cell carcinoma, undifferentiated carcinoma, sarcoma, carcinosarcoma, and melanoma are very rare tumors of the bladder (6,101,102,168). Bladder tumors are histologically graded (G grade) as follows: GX, grade cannot be assessed; G1, well differentiated; G2, moderately differentiated; and G3 and G4, poorly differentiated or undifferentiated tumors (3). Tumor grade provides an important predictor of tumor behavior and helps in the selection of appropriate therapy.

:: | Treatment of Superficial Tumors

The most common presentation of bladder cancer is that of Ta and T1 tumor. TURB is the treatment of choice for these patients with superficial cancer. As it already has been discussed, tumor recurrence following TURB is found in 70% of patients, with 15% progressing to muscle-invasive disease (136). During the past 30 years multiple prospective randomized trials have been conducted in a search for optimal adjuvant intravesical therapy (91). Important risk factors have been identified, with 50% of patients assigned to a group with a low risk of recurrence, 30% to an intermediate group, and 20% to a high-risk group. This 20% of patients should be scheduled for a more aggressive therapy (91). A European Organisation for Research and Treatment of Cancer (EORTC) randomized trial compared treatment outcomes in 443 patients with superficial bladder cancer. The control group patients were treated with TURB alone, whereas the two treatment groups received 12 months of bladder instillations with doxorubicin or ethoglucid (90). The recurrence rate per year was 0.30 for the treatment groups and 0.68 for the TURB-alone group. Time to tumor recurrence was significantly longer in the intravesical chemotherapy patients, as compared to the control group (*p* <.001). It is of interest to note the incidence of tumor progression to muscle-invasive disease was similar (15%) for all three groups. Likewise, patient mortality rates were not affected by intravesical therapy. Similar benefits of intravesical chemotherapy in patients with Ta plus T1 transitional cell carcinoma were reported following meta-analysis of eight randomized trials (80). At 3 years following therapy, there was a 70% reduction in recurrence rate in patients receiving intravesical chemotherapy, as compared to those managed with TURB alone. The reported data on the use of intravesical Bacillus Calmette-Guerin (BCG) in this patient population with Ta plus T1 disease demonstrated a clear benefit of this form of intravesical immunotherapy (15,90).

Surgery

Management of High-Grade, Invasive Bladder Cancer

Although the majority of patients present with superficial bladder tumors, 20% to 40% will either present with or ultimately develop muscle invasive disease. Invasive bladder cancer is a lethal malignancy; if untreated over 85% of patients die of the disease within 2 years of diagnosis (144). Furthermore, a certain percentage of patients with high-grade bladder tumors without involvement of the lamina propria will recur/progress and/or fail intravesical management, and, too, may be best treated with an earlier cystectomy when survival outcomes are optimal (202).

The rationale for an aggressive treatment approach employing radical cystectomy for high-grade, invasive bladder cancer is based on several important observations. First, the best long-term survival rates, coupled with the lowest local recurrences, are seen following a definitive surgical approach removing the primary bladder tumor and regional lymph nodes (69,74,105,197,204). Second, the morbidity and mortality of radical cystectomy has substantially improved over the past several decades. Third, primary TCC of the bladder tends to be a tumor moderately sensitive to radiation therapy. Fourth, chemotherapy alone, or in combination with bladder-sparing protocols have not demonstrated equivalent long-term local control and survival rates compared to cystectomy (117). Fifth, radical cystectomy provides accurate pathologic staging of the primary bladder tumor (p stage) and regional lymph nodes, thus, selectively determining the need for adjuvant therapy based on precise pathologic evaluation. For the above mentioned reasons, radical cystectomy has become a standard and arguably the best form of definitive therapy for high-grade, invasive bladder cancer today.

The evolution and improvements in lower urinary tract reconstruction, particularly orthotopic diversion, has been a major component in enhancing the quality of life of patients requiring cystectomy. Currently, most men and women can safely undergo orthotopic lower urinary tract reconstruction to the native, intact urethra following cystectomy (200). Orthotopic reconstruction closely resembles the bladder in location and function, provides a continent means to store urine, and allows volitional voiding per urethra. The orthotopic neobladder eliminates the need for a cutaneous stoma, urostomy appliance, and the need for intermittent catheterization in most cases. These efforts have improved the quality of life of patients requiring removal of their bladder, and have also stimulated patients and physicians to consider radical cystectomy at an earlier more curable stage for high-grade, invasive bladder cancer (69).

A dedicated effort has been made to improve upon the surgical technique of radical cystectomy and to provide an acceptable form of urinary diversion, without compromise of a sound cancer operation (197,198,202). Certain technical issues regarding radical cystectomy and an appropriate lymph node dissection are critical to minimize local recurrence and positive surgical margins and to maximize cancer-specific survival. Attention to surgical detail is important in optimizing the successful functional outcomes of orthotopic diversion; maintaining the rhabdosphincter mechanism and urinary continence in these patients (198).

Radical cystectomy by definition implies the en bloc removal of the pelvic–iliac lymph nodes along with the pelvic organs anterior to the rectum: the bladder, urachus, prostate, seminal vesicles, and visceral peritoneum in men; the bladder, urachus, ovaries, fallopian tubes, uterus, cervix, vaginal cuff, and the anterior pelvic peritoneum in women. An appropriate lymphadenectomy is an important component of radical cystectomy and is related to the clinical outcomes of patients with high-grade, invasive bladder cancer. Evidence suggests that a more extended lymphadenectomy is beneficial in both lymph node–positive and lymph node–negative patients with bladder cancer (79,96,143,190,203). Although the exact limits of the lymphadenectomy for patients with bladder cancer undergoing cystectomy are currently debated, we have advocated an extended lymph node dissection with the boundaries to include: initiation at the level of the inferior mesenteric artery (superior limits of dissection), extending laterally over the inferior vena cava/aorta to the genitofemoral nerve (lateral limits of dissection), and distally to the lymph node of Cloquet medially (on Cooper's ligament) and the circumflex iliac vein laterally. This dissection includes bilaterally all obturator, hypogastric, presciatic, and presacral lymph nodes.

Radical cystectomy is an appropriate standard treatment for patients with high-grade, invasive bladder cancer. The clinical outcomes from the University of Southern California (USC) with this surgical approach and review of other contemporary cystectomy series are presented in Tables 61.6 and 61.7 (68,105,197). These results should provide a benchmark for outcomes to which other therapies can be compared.

Morbidity and Mortality of Radical Cystectomy and Lymphadenectomy

The early clinical results and outcomes with regard to the morbidity and mortality of radical cystectomy were disappointing. Lack of universal acceptance of this procedure was attributed to the considerable complication rate and the need for improvements in urinary diversion. Prior to 1970, the perioperative complication rate of radical cystectomy was approximately 35%, with a mortality rate of nearly 20%. However, with contemporary medical, surgical, and anesthetic techniques, along with better patient selection, the mortality and morbidity from radical cystectomy have dramatically decreased. We reported a 3% mortality rate in the USC series, which is similar to other contemporary reported studies of radical cystectomy (see Table 61.7) (68,105,118,197). Importantly, we found the administration of preoperative therapy (radiation and/or chemotherapy) and the form of urinary diversion performed (continent or incontinent) did not obviously increase the mortality rate of patients undergoing radical cystectomy (197).

The early complication rate following radical cystectomy should not be underestimated in this elderly group of patients. The median age of patients undergoing cystectomy in our series was 66 years. Of the 1,054 patients treated, 28% developed an early complication within the first 3 months of surgery (see Table 61.7.) (197). Early complications included all events related to the cystectomy, perioperative care, and urinary diversion. The administration of preoperative therapy (radiation and/or chemotherapy) and the form of urinary diversion did not significantly increase the early complication rate in these cystectomy patients. Most early complications following radical cystectomy are unrelated to the urinary diversion (85% diversion unrelated) and can be managed conservatively without the need for reoperation in approximately 90% of cases (193). In our

Table 61.6	CYSTECTOMY OUTCOMES IN SELECTED SINGLE INSTITUTION SERIES						Pathologic Subgroup		
Author (Reference)	Period (Years)	No. of Patients Male/Female	Median Age (years)	Median F/u (years)	Histology	% Op. Mort.	% OC	% EV	LN+
Stein et al. (197)	1971–1997	1054 (843/211)	66	10.2	TCC (94% high-grade)	3	56	20	24
Madersbacher et al. (105)	1985–2000	507 (400/-07)	66	3.75	TCC (95% high-grade)	7	43	33	24
Hautmann et al. (68)	1986–2003	788 (652/136)	66	2.9 yrs	TCC (82% high-grade)	5	63	19	18

EV, extravesical; LN, lymph node involved; OC, organ confined; Op., operative; TCC, transitional cell carcinoma.

Table 61.7	**THE MORBIDITY AND MORTALITY FOLLOWING RADICAL CYSTECTOMY AND EXTENDED LYMPHADENECTOMY IN 1,054 USC[a] PATIENTS STRATIFIED BY URINARY DIVERSION AND PREOPERATIVE THERAPY**			
Therapy	**Treatment**	**No. of Patients (%)**	**Perioperative Mortality[b] No. (%)**	**Early Complication[c] No. (%)**
Form of urinary diversion	Conduit[d]	278 (26)	8 (4)	83 (32)
	Continent[e]	776 (72)	19 (3)	209 (27)
Preoperative adjuvant therapy	None	884 (84)	26 (4)	247 (28)
	Radiotherapy (RT)	108 (10)	1 (2)	30 (32)
	Chemotherapy	49 (5)	0	12 (25)
	RT and chemotherapy	13 (2)	0	3 (23)
Total		1,054	27 (4)	292 (28)

[a]University of Southern California.
[b]Any death within 30 days of surgery or prior to discharge.
[c]Any complications within the first 4 months postoperative.
[d]Including ileal and colon conduits.
[e]Including continent cutaneous, orthotopic, and rectal reservoirs.
From Stein JP, Skinner DG, Montie JE. Radical cystectomy and pelvic lymphadenectomy in the treatment of infiltrative bladder cancer. In: Droller MJ, ed. *Bladder cancer: current diagnosis and treatment.* Totowa, NJ: Humana Press, 2001;267–304, with permission.

experience, the most common early diversion-unrelated complication is dehydration, while the most common early diversion-related complication following radical cystectomy is prolonged urinary leakage.

Although we observed that preoperative treatment with chemotherapy and/or radiation therapy does not increase the perioperative morbidity or morality, neoadjuvant treatment strategies have not been routinely employed in our patients prior to radical cystectomy for invasive bladder cancer. Preoperative radiation therapy is considered only in those patients with a history of a previous partial cystectomy or those who have experience extravesical tumor spill at the time of endoscopic management of the primary bladder tumor (182). Furthermore, although there has been a recent interest in the application of neoadjuvant chemotherapy in patients with muscle invasive bladder cancer (61), the routine administration of this is clearly a debatable issue (75). We continue to be advocates of postoperative adjuvant chemotherapy for high-risk patients based on accurate pathologic evaluation of the primary bladder tumor and regional lymph nodes (182,197).

Radical cystectomy may appropriately be performed in carefully selected elderly patients. We have evaluated the clinical outcomes of radical cystectomy in elderly patients (80 years of age or more) requiring therapy for bladder cancer (236). We found that in appropriately selected elderly individuals, the perioperative morbidity and mortality was similar to younger patients undergoing the same operation. These data are similar to other published reports (20,86). Collectively, this suggests that an aggressive surgical approach is a viable treatment strategy for properly selected elderly individuals who are in generally good health and require definitive management for bladder cancer. It is emphasized that physiologic age may be more important than chronologic age when determining appropriate candidacy for radical cystectomy. Proper patient selection, strict attention to perioperative details, along with a dedicated and meticulous team-oriented surgical approach, are critical components to minimize the morbidity and mortality of surgery and to ensure the best clinical outcomes in all patients following radical cystectomy.

Pathologic Stage and Subgroups

The pathologic stage of the primary bladder tumor and the presence of regional lymph node metastases are the most impor-

tant survival determinants in patients undergoing cystectomy for bladder cancer (68,105,197). These pathologic determinants may also be categorized into pathologic subgroups that provide risk stratification and direct the need for adjuvant therapy in the appropriately selected individual. Pathologic subgroups are defined as organ-confined, lymph node–negative tumors (P0, Pa, Pis, P1, P2a, P2b), nonorgan confined (extravesical) lymph node–negative tumors (P3, P4), and lymph node positive disease (N+); representing 56%, 20%, and 24% of patients respectively (68). The 5- and 10-year recurrence-free survival for the entire group of 1,054 patients in the USC series was 68% and 66%, respectively (Table 61.8). Most deaths occurred within the first 3 years following radical cystectomy and were attributed to bladder cancer recurrence. However, with longer follow-up (>3 years), most deaths in this elderly group of patients were primarily related to comorbid diseases unrelated to bladder cancer. This underscores the effective and durable outcomes of radical cystectomy.

Organ-Confined, Lymph Node–Negative Tumors

In the USC series, 56% of patients demonstrated pathologically organ-confined, lymph node–negative tumor (197). The outcomes in this pathologic subgroup were excellent (see Table 61.8) with the 5- and 10-year recurrence-free survival of 85% and 82%, respectively. No significant survival difference was observed when comparing superficially noninvasive (Pis, Pa), lamina propria invasive (P1), and muscle invasive (P2a, P2b) tumors as long as the tumor was confined to the bladder without evidence of lymph node involvement. Similar outcomes for patients with pathologic superficial bladder tumors following cystectomy have been previously reported (4,68,105). Collectively, these data support the treatment of patients with surgery when a tumor is confined to the bladder, without evidence of extravesical extension or lymph node metastasis. Treatment delays in patients with invasive bladder cancer should be avoided. Evidence suggests that prolonged delays may lead to more advanced pathologic stage and decreased survival in patients with muscle invasive bladder cancer (157). Furthermore, caution should be taken in delaying definitive therapy in patients with high risk, superficial bladder tumors, or those with superficial tumors that have not appropriately responded to conservative forms of therapy (202).

Clinical Radiation Oncology

Table 61.8   THE USC BLADDER CANCER STUDY OF RADICAL CYSTECTOMY. ESTIMATED PROBABILITY OF RF AND OS AT 5 AND 10 YEARS ACCORDING TO PATHOLOGIC STAGE

Pathologic Stage[a]	No. of Patients	Recurrence Free 5 Years prob s.e.	Recurrence Free 10 Years prob s.e.	Overall Survival 5 Years prob s.e.	Overall Survival 10 Years prob s.e.
Po, Pa, Pis N–[b]	208	0.89 +/– 0.02	0.85 +/– 0.03	0.85 +/– 0.03	0.67 +/– 0.04
N+[c]	5	0.60 +/– 0.22	0.60 +/– 0.22	0.40 +/– 0.22	0.40 +/– 0.22
No. of patients PoPaPis	213	0.88 +/– 0.02	0.85 +/– 0.03	0.84 +/– 0.03	0.67 +/– 0.04
P1 N–	194	0.83 +/– 0.03	0.78 +/– 0.04	0.76 +/– 0.03	0.52 +/– 0.04
N+	14	0.43 +/– 0.13	0.43 +/– 0.13	0.50 +/– 0.13	0.42 +/– 0.13
No. of patients P1	208	0.80 +/– 0.03	0.75 +/– 0.04	0.74 +/– 0.03	0.51 +/– 0.04
P2a N–	94	0.89 +/– 0.03	0.87 +/– 0.04	0.77 +/– 0.04	0.57 +/– 0.06
N+	21	0.50 +/– 0.11	0.50 +/– 0.11	0.52 +/– 0.11	0.52 +/– 0.11
No. of patients P2a	115	0.81 +/– 0.04	0.80 +/– 0.04	0.72 +/– 0.04	0.56 +/– 0.05
P2b N–	98	0.78 +/– 0.05	0.76 +/– 0.05	0.64 +/– 0.05	0.44 +/– 0.06
N+	35	0.41 +/– 0.09	0.37 +/– 0.09	0.40 +/– 0.08	0.26 +/– 0.08
No. of patients P2a	133	0.68 +/– 0.04	0.65 +/– 0.05	0.58 +/– 0.04	0.39 +/– 0.05
P3 N–	135	0.62 +/– 0.05	0.61 +/– 0.05	0.49 +/– 0.04	0.29 +/– 0.05
N+	113	0.29 +/– 0.05	0.29 +/– 0.05	0.24 +/– 0.04	0.12 +/– 0.04
No. of patients P3	248	0.47 +/– 0.04	0.46 +/– 0.04	0.38 +/– 0.03	0.22 +/– 0.03
P4a N–	79	0.50 +/– 0.06	0.45 +/– 0.07	0.44 +/– 0.06	0.23 +/– 0.06
N+	58	0.33 +/– 0.07	0.33 +/– 0.07	0.26 +/– 0.06	0.20 +/– 0.05
No. of patients P4a	137	0.44 +/– 0.05	0.41 +/– 0.05	0.33 +/– 0.04	0.22 +/– 0.04
Organ Confined[d] N–	594	0.85 +/– 0.02	0.82 +/– 0.02	0.78 +/– 0.02	0.56 +/– 0.02
N+	75	0.46 +/– 0.06	0.44 +/– 0.06	0.45 +/– 0.06	0.37 +/– 0.06
No. of patients	669	0.80 +/– 0.02	0.77 +/– 0.02	0.74 +/– 0.02	0.54 +/– 0.02
Extravesical[e] N–	214	0.58 +/– 0.04	0.55 +/– 0.04	0.47 +/– 0.04	0.27 +/– 0.04
N+	171	0.30 +/– 0.04	0.30 +/– 0.04	0.25 +/– 0.04	0.17 +/– 0.03
No. of patients	385	0.46 +/– 0.03	0.44 +/– 0.03	0.37 +/– 0.03	0.22 +/– 0.03
LN– patients	808	0.78 +/– 0.02	0.75 +/– 0.02	0.69 +/– 0.02	0.49 +/– 0.03
LN+ patients	246	0.35 +/– 0.03	0.34 +/– 0.03	0.31 +/– 0.03	0.23 +/– 0.03
Total	1,054	0.68 +/– 0.02	0.66 +/– 0.02	0.60 +/– 0.02	0.43 +/– 0.02

OS, overall survival; RF, recurrence-free, c. Overall survival; USC, University of Southern California
[a]AJCC staging of 1977 (American Joint Committee on Cancer. Urinary bladder. In: *AJCC cancer staging manual*, 5th ed. Philadelphia: Lippincott Raven, 1997:241–243).
[b]No lymph node involvement
[c]Lymph node metastasis
[d]Including Po, Pa, Pis, P1, P2a, P2b tumors.
[e]Including P3, P4 bladder tumors.
From Stein JP, Lieskovsky G, Cote R, et al. Radical cystectomy in the treatment of invasive bladder cancer: long-term results in 1,054 patients. *J Clin Oncol* 2001;19:666–675, with permission.

Extravesical, Lymph Node–Negative Tumors

Nonorgan confined (extravesical), lymph node–negative tumors were found in 20% of our patients undergoing cystectomy (see Table 61.8) (197). No obvious survival differences between extravesical P3 and P4 (node-negative) tumors were observed. The 5- and 10-year recurrence-free survival for this pathologic subgroup was 58% and 55%, respectively. Similar outcomes were reported by Madersbacher et al. (105) who demonstrated a 56% 5-year recurrence-free survival for the same pathologic subgroup. Patients with locally advanced tumors had higher recurrence rates and decreased survival compared to those with organ-confined, lymph node–negative tumors (145). The 1997 AJCC TNM Staging System stratifies extravesical tumor involvement (previously defined as pT3b) into microscopic (pT3a) and gross (pT3b) extravesical tumor extension (3). To determine the clinical significance of this new pathologic subgrouping, we evaluated the clinical outcomes in our group of patients following radical cystectomy with pathologic pT3 disease stratified by microscopic and gross extravesical tumor involvement (145). No significant difference was observed in the recurrence-free and overall survival in patients when evaluating for pT3a and pT3b extravesical extension. The incidence of lymph node involvement was similar (approximately 45%); however, the presence of lymph node involvement was associated with a higher risk of recurrence and worse survival compared to node-negative patients.

Lymph Node–Positive Disease

Despite an aggressive treatment philosophy and approach to bladder cancer, 24% of the USC patients demonstrated lymph node–positive disease at the time of cystectomy (see Table 61.6) (197). Furthermore, when one examines a large number of patients from eight contemporary series of radical cystectomy for TCC of the bladder, this incidence of 24% is nearly the same (Table 61.9). This underscores the metastatic capabilities of high-grade, invasive bladder cancer. Although patients with lymph node tumor involvement are a high-risk group of patients, nearly one third of these patients in our series were alive at 5 years. It is possible that the surgical approach employing an extended lymph node dissection provides some survival advantage in selected individuals with node-positive disease. The impact of adjuvant therapy in these patients, although difficult to critically assess and subject to selection bias, may also play a role in the outcomes of patients with lymph node–positive disease (105,197). In a separate analysis of lymph node–positive patients, we found that the administration of adjuvant chemotherapy was a significant and

Table 61.9 INCIDENCE OF LYMPH NODE METASTASIS FOLLOWING RADICAL CYSTECTOMY, CORRELATION TO PRIMARY TUMOR

Author (Reference)	Period (years)	No. of Patients	LN Met.[a] No. (%)	Bladder Tumor Stage[a] No. (%)				
				P0, Pis, Pa, P1	P2a	P2b	P3	P4
Poulsen et al. (142)	1990–1997	191	50 (26)	2 (4)	4 (18)	7 (25)	33 (51)	4 (43)
Vieweg et al. (223)	1980–1990	686	193 (28)	10 (10)	12 (9)	22 (23)	97 (42)	52 (41)
Leissner (95)	1999–2002	290	81 (28)	1 (3)	5 (13)	12 (22)	53 (43)	10 (50)
Stein et al. (197)	1971–1997	1,054	246 (24)	19 (5)	21 (18)	35 (27)	113 (44)	58 (42)
Vazina et al. (222)	1992–2002	176	43 (24)	1 (215)	10 (16)	—	20 (236)	12 (50)
Abdel-Latif et al. (1)	1997–1999	418	110 (26)	3 (215)	4 (7)	29 (25)	59 (48)	15 (65)
Madersbacher et al. (105)	1985–2000	507	124 (24)	2 (3)	26 (17)	—	64 (34)	32 (41)
Hautmann et al. (68)	1986–2003	788	142 (18)	2 (2)	31 (10)	—	73 (41)	36 (43)
Total		4,110	989 (24)					

LN Met., lymph node metastasis.
[a]AJCC Staging System of 1997 (American Joint Committee on Cancer. Urinary bladder. In: *AJCC cancer staging manual*, 5th ed. Philadelphia: Lippincott-Raven, 1997:241–243).

independent predictor for recurrence and overall survival in this group (190).

The prognosis in patients with lymph node–positive disease can be stratified by the number of lymph nodes involved (tumor burden), the stage of the primary tumor, and the presence of lymph node capsule perforation (114,197). In our cystectomy series, patients with less than five positive lymph nodes and those with lymph node–positive organ-confined bladder tumors had a significantly improved recurrence-free survival rate. Similar results with lymph node–positive tumors have been previously reported (96,223).

The number of lymph nodes involved with tumor and the extent of the lymph node dissection are both important variables for patients undergoing cystectomy for bladder cancer. We re-examined 246 patients with lymph node tumor involvement following radical cystectomy (190) to evaluate other prognostic factors in this high-risk group. This study simulated the concept of *lymph node density*, a prognostic factor that better stratifies lymph node–positive patients following radical cystectomy. Lymph node density is defined as the total number of positive lymph nodes divided by the total number of lymph nodes removed, which accounts for the extent of the lymph node dissection (number of lymph nodes removed) and the tumor burden (number of positive lymph nodes) following cystectomy for patients with lymph node–positive disease. Lymph node density therefore incorporates the concepts of tumor burden and the extent of lymphadenectomy. We found lymph node density to be a significant and independent prognostic variable in patients with lymph node metastases that may best stratify this high-risk group of patients (190). Future staging systems and the application of adjuvant therapy in clinical trials may consider applying these concepts to help better stratify this high-risk group of patients. Regardless, patients with any lymph node involvement remain at high risk for disease recurrence and should be considered for adjuvant treatment strategies.

Recurrence Following Radical Cystectomy

Recurrence following radical cystectomy for bladder cancer correlates well with the pathologic stage and subgroup (68,105,197). With long-term follow-up (median >10 years) recurrences in the USC series were classified as local (pelvic), distant, and urethral. Local recurrences were defined as those occurring within the soft tissue field of exenteration. Distant recurrences were defined as those occurring outside the pelvis, while urethral tumors were classified as a new primary tumor

occurring in the retained urethra. Overall, 30% of all patients in the USC series experienced a local or distant tumor recurrence (197). The median time to any recurrence was 12 months, with 86% of all patients developing their recurrences within the first 3 years of cystectomy. Of the 311 patients who developed a recurrence, the median time to distant recurrence was 12 months, while the median time to local recurrence was 18 months. Late tumor recurrences, defined as 5 years or more after surgery, do occur and underscore the need for lifelong follow-up.

Pelvic (Local) Recurrence

Radical cystectomy provides excellent local (pelvic) control of the disease. An overall local pelvic recurrence rate of 7% was observed in the USC series (197). Similar results have been reported by other investigators (Table 61.10) (68,105,197). Patients with organ confined, node-negative tumors demonstrated a 6% local recurrence rate, compared to a 13% incidence in those with nonorgan confined node-negative tumors. Patients at highest risk of a local recurrence (lymph node–positive disease) had a 13% local recurrence rate following cystectomy. The use of a high-dose short course of preoperative radiation therapy did not reduce the risk of pelvic recurrence (182). Nearly all patients suffering a pelvic recurrence following cystectomy will die of their disease, despite additional aggressive multimodal therapeutic efforts.

Metastatic (Distant) Recurrence

Recurrences following radical cystectomy are most commonly found at distant sites. Distant recurrence rates can also be stratified by pathologic subgroups. Patients with organ-confined, node-negative tumors demonstrated a 13% distant recurrence rate, which increased to 32% for those with extravesical lymph node–negative and 52% of patients with node-positive tumors (197). Patients at high risk for tumor recurrence should clearly be considered for adjuvant chemotherapy protocols. These results are similar to other large contemporary cystectomy series (see Table 61.9) (1).

Urethral Recurrence

Urethral tumor recurrence in patients with a history of bladder cancer following radical cystectomy represents a second manifestation of the multicentric defect of the primary transitional cell mucosa that led to the original bladder tumor. The term *urethral recurrence* is therefore somewhat misleading, suggesting a failure of definitive treatment of the bladder cancer. Rather,

Table 61.10 RECURRENCE-FREE SURVIVAL AND THE INCIDENCE OF RECURRENCE IN SELECTED STUDIES OF RADICAL CYSTECTOMY

Author/Series (Reference)	No. Patients	Median Follow-Up (mo.)	Recurrence-Free Survival (%)		Recurrence (%)	
			5 Year	10 Year	Local	Distant
Stein et al./USC (197)	1,054	122	68	66	7.3	22.2
Madersbacher et al./Bern (104)	507	45	62	50	7.9	35.3
Hautmann et al./Ulm (68)	788	53	65	59	9.3	17.8

most urethral tumors probably represent simply another occurrence of the transitional cell carcinoma in the remaining urothelium. As radical cystectomy has emerged as the most effective therapy for invasive bladder cancer, and as orthotopic diversion has increasingly been performed, the fate of the retained urethra has become an increasingly important oncologic issue.

The advent of orthotopic lower urinary tract reconstruction has provided a more natural voiding pattern in patients following radical cystectomy. Approximately 85% of all patients undergoing cystectomy for TCC of the bladder at USC receive an orthotopic neobladder substitute. From an oncologic perspective, only those with a positive surgical margin at the proximal urethra (distal to the apex of the prostate in men and just distal to the bladder neck in women) on intraoperative frozen section are absolutely excluded from orthotopic reconstruction. This enthusiasm to preserve the native urethra following radical cystectomy and allow for orthotopic reconstruction has rightfully increased concerns for a urethral recurrence in these patients.

Prior to the orthotopic era in women, urethral tumor recurrence was not an important oncologic issue because the entire urethra was removed at the time of cystectomy. With a better understanding of female pelvic anatomy and the inner vation of the rhabdosphincter and continence mechanism in women (23), along with the identification of various pathologic risk factors for urethral tumor involvement in these patients, orthotopic diversion has now become a commonly performed form of urinary diversion in women following cystectomy (195). Tumor involving the bladder neck is the most important risk factor for urethral tumor involvement in women (192,194). Although bladder neck involvement is a significant risk factor for urethral tumors, not all women with tumor involving the bladder neck will have urethral tumors. Approximately 50% of female patients with tumor at the bladder neck will have an uninvolved urethra free of tumor. In this situation, the patient may potentially be considered an appropriate candidate for orthotopic diversion. Furthermore, intraoperative frozen section analysis of the distal surgical margin is an accurate and reliable means to pathologically evaluate the proximal urethra (194). Utilizing this selection process, to date, we have not had a female urethral recurrence (195).

A growing population of male patients reconstructed to the urethra following cystectomy exists today. With longer follow-up, could this expose them to a greater risk for a urethral recurrence? The historical incidence of urethral recurrence in the retained urethra following cystectomy for bladder cancer ranges from 6% to 10% (47,48). Specific clinical and pathologic risk factors that have been identified to provided risk assessment for urethral recurrence include multifocal tumors, carcinoma *in situ*, tumor involvement of the prostate (particularly invasion of the prostatic stroma), and the form of urinary diversion (orthotopic or cutaneous) performed (47,66,98,191,204,207,213).

We evaluated our experience regarding a urethral recurrence in a large group of male patients undergoing radical cystectomy and urinary diversion for TCC of the bladder (191). In this study, we analyzed the clinical and pathological results of 768 consecutive male patients undergoing radical cystectomy with a median follow-up of 13 years. Of these 768 patients, 397 men (51%) underwent an orthotopic diversion (median follow-up 10 years) and 371 men (49%) underwent a cutaneous diversion (median follow-up 19 years). Overall, 45 patients (7%) developed a urethral recurrence. The median time to a urethral recurrence was 2 years (range 0.2 to 13.6 years). Of these 45 patients, 16 men (5%) had an orthotopic and 29 (9%) had a cutaneous form of urinary diversion (191).

In this cohort of male patients, multiple risk factors were analyzed with regards to urethral recurrence. In a multivariate analysis, two important variables were identified that significantly increased the risk of a urethral tumor recurrence following cystectomy including: (a) any prostate involvement and (b) the form of urinary diversion (191). The estimated 5-year probability of a urethral recurrence was 5% without prostate involvement, and increased to 12% and 18% with superficial (prostatic urethra and ducts) and invasive (stroma) prostate involvement, respectively. Patients undergoing an orthotopic diversion demonstrated a statistically significantly lower risk of urethral recurrence compared to those undergoing a cutaneous form of urinary diversion.

The follow-up and management of the urethra in male patients treated for high-grade invasive bladder cancer is of importance. The indications and timing of a prophylactic urethrectomy in those undergoing cystectomy and a cutaneous diversion is debatable. It may include urethrectomy at the time of cystectomy based on preoperative clinical parameters, based on the intraoperative frozen section analysis of the urethral margin, or a delayed urethrectomy based on final pathologic evaluation of the cystectomy specimen. These issues are best detailed with the patient preoperatively ensuring proper informed consent.

Our long-term experience provides some insight regarding the issues and management of the retained urethra in both men and women following cystectomy for bladder cancer. We believe that intraoperative frozen section analysis of the proximal urethra by an experienced pathologist is a reliable and accurate means to determine indications for orthotopic diversion in all patients. It has been our practice to perform an orthotopic neobladder in men and women whose intraoperative frozen section of the proximal urethra is free of tumor. This approach does not appear to increase the risk of a urethral recurrence in these patients (191,195). Male patients with known prostatic tumor involvement should not necessarily be excluded from an orthotopic substitute if the intraoperative biopsy is normal. Similarly, female patients with bladder neck involvement should not necessarily be excluded from an orthotopic neobladder if the intraoperative biopsy is also normal. All patients should be carefully counseled regarding the need for follow-up, the long-term risks of a urethral recurrence, and the possible need for urethrectomy following cystectomy.

The Importance of Surgical Technique

The dedication of the surgeon and technical commitment to a properly performed cystectomy and adequate lymphadenectomy is important to the success and optimal clinical outcomes for patients with high-grade bladder cancer. The importance of surgical technique is well illustrated in the role this may have played in a randomized multi-institutional cooperative group trial (62). In this prospective study, 270 underwent cystectomy with half of the patients receiving neoadjuvant chemotherapy. In a separate analysis of this trial, various surgical factors were subsequently analyzed (75). Of these 270 patients, 24 had no lymph node dissection, 98 had a limited dissection of the obturator lymph nodes only, and 146 patients had a so-called standard (not extended) pelvic lymph node dissection. The 5-year survival rates for these groups were 33%, 46%, and 60%, respectively. The median number of lymph nodes removed for the entire cohort was 10. Importantly, the survival rate for patients with <10 lymph nodes removed was significantly lower compared to patients with >10 lymph nodes removed; 44% versus 61%, respectively. In a multivariate analysis, the extent of the lymph node dissection, number of lymph nodes removed, and the number of cases performed by the individual surgeon were the most significant factors influencing survival in patients undergoing cystectomy for bladder cancer (75). It is emphasized that although this well-publicized study was not intended to analyze the surgical approach and/or technical differences in the treatment of bladder cancer, it is the surgical factors and not neoadjuvant chemotherapy that were most critical as predictors in the outcomes of these patients.

Summary of Surgical Therapy

The understanding that invasive bladder cancer is a lethal disease allowed the USC urologists to adopt an early and aggressive surgical approach. This included a radical cystectomy with a meticulous and extended bilateral pelvic iliac lymph node dissection. Radical cystectomy provides the best local pelvic control of the disease. In addition, this procedure provides accurate evaluation of the primary bladder tumor (p stage), along with the regional lymph nodes. Careful pathologic evaluation provides important prognostic information and allows for the application of adjuvant treatment strategies based on clear histopathologic determination, not clinical staging, which has been associated with significant errors in 30% to 50% of patients. This, coupled with the evolution and successful application of orthotopic lower urinary tract reconstruction in both men and women, has provided patients a more physiological and acceptable means to store and eliminate urine (118).

Current published data suggest that patients with extravesical tumor extension or with lymph node–positive disease are at increased risk for recurrence and should be considered for adjuvant chemotherapy protocols. Additionally, the application of molecular markers, based on pathologic staging and analysis, may also serve to identify patients at risk for tumor recurrence who may benefit from adjuvant therapy (196).

Radiotherapy

External Beam Radiotherapy

Definitive Radiotherapy

Because of the reported major progress in outcomes of radical cystectomy, development of orthotopic lower urinary tract reconstruction, and improved treatment results with the bladder preservation approach, since about 1985 radiotherapy alone has been used less frequently in the management of patients with bladder cancer. It became, however, an important part of a multimodality bladder conservation program, which also included TURB and chemotherapy. Radiotherapy alone applied with a curative intent was used extensively from the 1950s through the 1980s. It was inevitable that numerous studies attempted a comparison of treatment results obtained with radiotherapy versus those of radical cystectomy. Such comparisons were very difficult because each treatment modality was targeting a different patient population. Typically, patients selected for radical cystectomy had less advanced tumors at diagnosis, were younger, and were in a better general condition than patients selected for definitive irradiation (43,77). Additionally, patients were treated with radiotherapy based on clinical staging, whereas surgical patients frequently were staged pathologically. Nevertheless, multiple reports have been published demonstrating lower tumor control and survival rates in radiotherapy-treated patients (30,43,77).

In a report on 701 patients treated between 1977 and 1994 in western Sweden, the authors clearly stated that the 74 (10%) patients selected for definitive external beam radiation therapy (EBRT) (more than 60 Gy) were older and "unfit for surgery" (76). Yet, in their conclusion, they questioned the benefit of radiotherapy, which, as expected, showed results clearly inferior to those of surgery, with the 5-year survival for T2 and T3 tumors of only 15%. In another study of 534 patients, 263 (49%) were selected to receive preoperative radiotherapy followed by cystectomy, whereas 271 (51%) received definitive radiotherapy (43). The combined-therapy patients had better prognostic factors, including better T stage, than those treated with EBRT alone ($p < .001$). The 5-year survival rate for the 263 combined-therapy patients was 48%, whereas it was 22% for the 271 EBRT patients. In multivariate analysis the following parameters were found to be good prognostic factors predicting survival: clinical stage (T2 vs. T3 vs. T4; $p < .01$), age (<70 years vs. >70 years; $p < .01$), and hemoglobin level (>12 g/dL vs. 12 g/dL; $p < .01$).

A study of 384 patients reported in 1975 from Stanford University concluded that 30% to 40% of T3 patients are expected to be controlled with EBRT (57). Failure in the bladder with or without other organ involvement was noted in 217 (56%) patients. Severe bowel toxicity was recorded in 8% of patients, which included nine (4.7%) of those treated to the bladder only, and in 22 (11%) patients receiving pelvic irradiation with a final boost to the bladder.

Prognostic Factors

The well-recognized prognostic factors for overall and disease-free survival include tumor stage, tumor morphology, presence of intravesical versus extravesical tumor, completeness of TURB, presence of solitary versus multiple bladder tumors, presence of ureteric obstruction, presence of complete response (CR) after EBRT, and radiation dose (51,61,108,122,128,140,141,175). In a study of 342 patients, multiple bladder tumor ($p < .01$), presence of ureteric obstruction ($p < .001$), and higher T stage ($p = .044$) were good predictors of tumor recurrence in the bladder (108). Distant metastases were predicted well by higher T stage ($p = .03$) and presence of ureteric obstruction ($p = .003$). Some of the published reports showed the importance of hemoglobin level on tumor control and survival (59,146). The recognition of these important clinical prognostic factors is of major relevance in a more optimal selection of patients for definitive therapy.

In the past decade, major developments in molecular biology helped identify a new group of prognostic factors, which may better represent tumor behavior than the traditionally recognized parameters such as tumor stage or grade (127,180,196).

Multiple factors have been investigated, with the following showing greatest interest among oncologists interested in bladder cancer: expression of p53, p21, and retinoblastoma tumor suppressor genes, Ki67, and apoptotic index (21,36,42,65,93, 94,120,128,152,196). The factors obtained through immunohistochemical studies have obvious importance also in patients considered for radical cystectomy (42,74). The importance of these biologic factors in predicting prognosis, although promising, needs to be interpreted with caution until it is validated in prospective randomized trials.

Treatment Results

Early reports on treatment results obtained with EBRT in unselected patients, including those with T4 disease, demonstrated the incidence of local control exceeding 40% (8,38,57,58). A study from Western General Hospital, Edinburgh, conducted between 1971 and 1982, reported treatment results with definitive EBRT in 963 patients (38). Stage T1 was seen in 20%, T2 in 32%, T3 in 40%, and T4 in 8%. Treatment portals were limited to the bladder, and the most frequently used radiotherapy schedule was 55 Gy in 20 equal fractions. The overall 5- and 10-year survival rate for all patients was 30% and 18%, respectively. Survival correlated well with patient age ($p < .0001$), tumor grade, stage ($p < .0001$), tumor appearance (papillary, solid, or ulcerative; $p < .0001$), and the presence of CR at the end of radiotherapy ($p < .0001$). Complete tumor regression assessed cystoscopically was obtained in 46% of patients of whom 65% maintained CR. Local recurrence was diagnosed at 47% of patients at 5 years since EBRT and in 53% at 10 years. The incidence of distant metastasis correlated well ($p < .0001$) with tumor stage and tumor grade ($p < .0001$). At 10 years posttreatment 18% of T1 patients had metastatic disease; 28% of T2, 55% of T3, and 65% of T4 patients had metastatic disease. Severe late complications of radiotherapy were reported in 15% of patients, including 1% resulting in death. Another report from the United Kingdom on 704 patients demonstrated very similar treatment outcomes to that reported from Edinburgh, despite 37% of the study patients being treated having T4 disease (8). The same was true in early reports from the United States and Canada (57,58). It is important to point out that up to 70% of EBRT-treated patients lead a normal life with a well-functioning bladder (58). A study of 333 patients with T3 tumors treated with EBRT showed cystoscopically confirmed

CR in 41% (146). CR was influenced by the radiation dose and tumor grade, with grade 3 patients having the best incidence of CR (57%). CR was an important event because it influenced long-lasting tumor control and survival ($p < .0001$).

It is of interest to review contemporary reports on the use of EBRT in patients with bladder cancer. EBRT experience in a population-based study in Ontario, Canada, consisted of 1,372 (7%) patients who received radiotherapy out of 20,906 patients diagnosed with this disease within the period of the study (71). There has been a progressively smaller proportion of patients selected for EBRT, whereas a greater number was selected for surgery ($p = .001$). Patients receiving radiotherapy had a number of adverse prognostic factors as compared to those selected for surgical therapy. These factors included mean age (70 vs. 65 years; $p = .0001$) and the number of prior TURBs. No prior TURB was recorded in 12%, one TURB in 50%, two in 20%, and three or more in 17% of patients. Most patients received 60 Gy in 30 fractions, and 93% were treated with high-energy radiation beams. The 5-year overall survival was 28%, cystectomy-free survival was 25%, and cancer cause–specific survival was 41%. There was an important influence of age on survival. The 5 year survival of patients younger than 50 years of age was 50% as compared to 10% in those with older than age 80 years. This study's major conclusion was that radiotherapy alone has an important curative role in the management of patients with bladder cancer. In those with local recurrence a salvage cystectomy is a procedure of choice. Similar outcomes with EBRT were reported in other contemporary studies (30,44,59,71,83,122,140,166,175).

Interesting treatment results with EBRT in 120 T1 to T4 patients were reported from Royal Devon and Exeter Hospital in the United Kingdom (7). A total of 50 (42%) patients had T3 or T4 tumors. Patients received 50 Gy in 20 fractions, and the median follow-up was more than 6 years. The overall 5-year survival was 50%, with 67 (56%) patients developing a local recurrence. Of these 67 patients with local recurrence, 33 (49%) underwent a salvage cystectomy with subsequent median survival of 1 year.

A review of the world literature on treatment outcomes in EBRT-treated patients showed the following incidence of 5-year survival: T1, 35% to 71%; T2, 10% to 59%; T3, 10% to 38%; and T4, 0% to 16% (167). It is of importance to note that the addition of chemotherapy to EBRT has increased disease-free survival but has not improved the overall survival and failed

					Survival (%)	
Author (Reference)	N	Mean Age (Years)	Radiation Dose (Gy)	Tumor Stage	5 Year	10 Year
Duncan and Quilty (38)	963	66	55[a]	T1–T4	30	18
Blandy et al. (8)	704	68	55[a]	T1–T4	40	—
Goffinet et al. (57)	384	60	70	T1–T4	30	—
Goodman et al. (58)	470	66	50[a]	T2–T3	38	22
Quilty and Duncan (146)	333	67	55[a]	T3	26	15
Gospodarowicz et al. (59)	121	70	60	T2–T4b	32	—
Hayter et al. (71)	1,372	70	60	T2–T4	28	—
Jahnson et al. (83)	319	>70	64	T1–T4	28	8
Daehlin et al. (30)	90	71	64	T1–T4	29	14
Fossa et al. (43)	271	73	60	T2–T4	22	—
Bell et al. (7)	120	70	50[a]	T1–T4	50	—
Moonen et al. (122)	379	73	60	T2–T3	22	—
Total	5,526	70	60	T1–T4	31	15

Table 61.11   **TREATMENT RESULTS IN SELECTED STUDIES OF EXTERNAL BEAM RADIATION THERAPY**

EBRT, external beam radiation therapy.
[a]In 250 cGy daily fraction.

to reduce the incidence of distant metastasis (107,167). New treatment approaches with radiotherapy combined with hypoxic cell sensitizers and other promising agents need to be investigated in clinical trials (77,226). Treatment results in selected studies of 5,526 EBRT-treated patients are shown in Table 61.11.

As it has already been discussed, selection of patients for radiotherapy or for surgical treatment is not very well defined. It is of relevance to discuss factors influencing definitive therapy in patients with carcinoma of the bladder based on the published data from the Surveillance, Epidemiology, and End Results (SEER) program from 1992 to 1999, which involved a large number of patients from 11 geographic regions of the United States (88). In multivariate analysis the following factors were predicting selection for radical cystectomy: patient age, SEER site, and stage of disease, while patient race, age, sex, SEER site, and stage of disease were significant factors predicting the choice of radiotherapy. Stage of disease and the number of lymph nodes recovered at surgery were significant predictors of survival in radical cystectomy-treated patients. In radiotherapy-treated patients significant predictors of survival included age, sex, SEER site, and stage of disease. An additional important finding of this study was not offering definitive and potentially curative therapy to a substantial number of older patients, which could result in their long-term survival and a better quality of life. The reason for this selection process is not immediately apparent.

Pattern of Failure

Patients treated with EBRT have a high incidence of persistent tumor following the course of therapy as well as high incidence of local failure, which, in many studies, is about 50% (49,57,175). This incidence of failure depends on tumor stage and grade at diagnosis and, as expected, is higher than that reported in patients treated with radical cystectomy (197). However, the incidence of urethral recurrence at 3% in EBRT-treated patients is the same or lower than that reported in surgical series, which ranges from 0.7% to 18% (29). Distant metastasis represents the most common (up to 65%) site of failure in EBRT-treated and surgically treated patients (38,57). The incidence of metastatic disease is influenced by tumor stage and tumor grade ($p < .0001$) (37).

Treatment Schedules

The importance of radiation dose and treatment schedule was evaluated in a study of 379 patients with T2 and T3 tumors (121). Local recurrence in the bladder was noted in 137 (36%) patients, with the actuarial 5- and 10-year local control rate of 40% and 32%, respectively. In multivariate analysis, total radiation dose at 57.5 Gy was found to be an important factor predicting local control ($p = .004$). It is surprising that higher radiation doses in this study failed to increase the incidence of local control. Overall treatment time was only of borderline significance in obtaining local control ($p = .067$). This study contradicted earlier published data where overall treatment duration and total dose were important predictors of tumor control (104). A possible explanation for this difference is a relatively small (n = 77) number of patients in the second trial. Another retrospective study of 147 T2 and T3 patients demonstrated a lack of influence of overall treatment time on the incidence of local control and survival (33). It is apparent that the importance of total radiation dose and overall treatment duration on the incidence of local control needs to be determined in a prospective randomized trial. In the absence of such trials a recommended treatment schedule should consist of 60 to 66 Gy given at a 1.8- to 2-Gy daily fraction.

Altered Fractionation Schedules

The value of hyperfractionation schedules was investigated in a prospective randomized trial in patients with T2 to T4 tumors (125). The hyperfractionation schedule was 1 Gy given three times per day to a total dose of 84 Gy and it was compared with the conventional schedule of 2 Gy daily to a total of 64 Gy. Patients of both treatment groups completed their radiotherapy within 8 weeks, which included a 2-week rest period. Follow-up was at least 10 years. There was a 5- and 10-year survival and local-control benefit noted in patients receiving hyperfractionation regimen ($p = .003$). A 52% higher mortality rate was seen in the conventional schedule-treated patients than in those receiving multifraction per day radiotherapy. The incidence of late toxicity was not significantly different between patients of these two treatment groups.

A meta-analysis of two hyperfractionation randomized trials in patients with bladder cancer demonstrated decreased incidence of death ($p = .002$), increased probability of CR, and a better survival rate ($p = .001$) in patients treated with multifraction radiotherapy when compared with those receiving single daily fraction EBRT (210). The benefit of hyperfractionation in addition to bladder cancer also was seen in patients with head and neck or lung cancer. The greatest benefit, however, was seen in those with upper-respiratory and digestive-tract tumors.

The feasibility of accelerated fraction radiotherapy was tested in a study of 40 patients (123). A total dose of 66 Gy at 2 Gy daily given over a period of 6.5 weeks was selected as the standard treatment course. It subsequently was reduced to a 5- and then 4-week period. This required the use of two fractions a day to be given in the second part of the treatment course. A total of 15 (37%) patients had their treatment completed in 5 weeks, and 25 (63%) were done in 4 weeks. The 5-week patient group had no increased toxicity as compared to the conventional 2 Gy a day EBRT. However, of the 25 patients receiving the 4-week course, 16 (64%) had Radiation Therapy Oncology Group (RTOG) grade 3 toxicity, three (12%) had grade 4, and one (4%) patient had grade 5 toxicity. The 3-year actuarial incidence of grade 4 late bladder toxicity in this group of patients was 31%. The reported incidence of toxicity makes the 4-week course an unacceptable treatment schedule, whereas patients receiving the 5-week course had no toxicity higher than grade 3. The latter provides a possible alternative to the conventional radiotherapy schedule. Hypofractionation schedules are discussed in the next section of this chapter.

Salvage Cystectomy

The indications for salvage cystectomy include selected patients who have persistent disease following a full course of EBRT and those who present with recurrent disease at any time following irradiation. In one report on 704 patients treated with EBRT at the London Hospital between 1965 and 1974, 8% had salvage cystectomy (8). There was an unacceptably high mortality rate of 22% at 3 months with substantial other morbidity. In another study of 470 patients, surgical mortality was 11% (58). A total of 70 (15%) patients were selected for the salvage procedure for recurrent or persistent tumor following EBRT. The 5-year survival rate following cystectomy was 17%. In a more recent report on 32 salvage cystectomies the 5-year survival was about 50% (85). There was, however, a considerable late toxicity of this salvage therapy. Long-term need for salvage cystectomy was studied in 159 patients with T2 to T4 tumors (25). The incidence of salvage cystectomy was 24%, with a median time from EBRT of 12 months (range from 2 months to 10 years). The 5-year survival after the salvage procedure was 30%. Similar data were reported by other investigators (228).

It is of interest to note that salvage cystectomy in patients with radiotherapy failure also can be considered in association with a single-stage orthotopic lower urinary tract reconstruction. A USC study of 18 patients with local recurrence following EBRT of more than 60 Gy demonstrated safety and efficacy of this procedure (10). There was no mortality reported in this group of patients. The incidence of day continence was 67%, with night continence of 56%. It is apparent that salvage cystectomy should be considered in carefully selected patients with local recurrence following definitive pelvic irradiation.

Radiotherapy in Elderly Patients

Management of elderly patients who are diagnosed with muscle-invasive disease presents special problems. Frequently these patients have important coexisting medical conditions contraindicating the use of conventional bladder-sparing therapy or radical cystectomy. Radiotherapy alone consisting of a 6- to 7-week course of daily treatments may create a hardship on the patient and may need to be terminated prematurely. A no-treatment option is difficult to support because most patients are likely to experience distressing symptoms and signs of progressive disease such as pain, gross hematuria, frequency, and dysuria. In view of these problems with a major impact on patient quality of life, various hypofractionation treatment schedules have been investigated in a number of clinical trials. A complicating factor is a need for an appropriate (more than 55 Gy) total radiation dose, which was found in a study of 146 elderly patients to be an important predictor of response and survival (184).

A course of EBRT of up to 62.6 Gy in 30 fractions was given to 94 elderly (median age 78 years) patients (166). T1 to T2 tumors were present in 52 (53%) patients, and T3 to T4 were present in 42 (45%) patients. Median survival was 14 months, and the 5-year survival rate was 7%. Predictably, T stage and performance status were important factors predicting survival. A split course of radiotherapy may offer a good alternative course of treatment in this patient population (137).

A study of seven patients in poor general condition with locally advanced and severely symptomatic bladder cancer used a single fraction of 10 Gy given to the pelvis (19). All patients experienced rapid resolution of their symptoms, which included severe gross hematuria, pelvic pain, and ureteral obstruction. Median duration of response was 5 months, with a range of 2 to 8 months. It is of interest to note that four of these patients received three doses of 10 Gy at 3- to 4-week intervals. This treatment schedule should be used with caution in carefully selected patients in whom long-term survival is not expected. A study of 39 patients with locally advanced and symptomatic tumors used 30 Gy in 10 equal fractions given to the pelvis and showed a poor palliative response except for a reduction of gross hematuria (43,46). The conclusion of this study was that higher radiation doses are needed to obtain a better palliative effect in this patient population.

An interesting study in 65 elderly (median age 78 years) and frail patients was reported from Cardiff, United Kingdom (112). The stage distribution was 34 with T2 (52%), 24 with T3 (37%), and seven with T4a (11%). Nearly all (97%) had clinically N0 disease. The study was designed to obtain an optimal palliative benefit with minimal toxicity and minimal disruption to patient normal life. Two treatment schedules were used following TURB. The first schedule consisted of a total of 30 Gy given at weekly intervals of 6 Gy per fraction in 53 (82%) patients, and the second one was delivering 36 Gy also at 6 Gy per fraction in 12 (18%) patients. The highest (92%) incidence of palliation assessed at the 1-month follow-up was obtained in those with gross hematuria, whereas dysuria and frequency were relieved in only 24%. Complete relief of all symptoms was obtained in 51% of patients, with an additional 22% showing a substantial improvement for a median duration of 7 months. The median survival was 9 months (range 2 to 40 months). Acute gastrointestinal toxicity was common, with 12% of patients requiring hospitalization to treat this toxicity. Higher radiation dose did not increase treatment toxicity but also did not increase palliative effect or survival. The main criticism of this study is a denial of potentially curative radiotherapy to a subset of these patients. Similar outcomes with hypofractionation were obtained in a study of 70 (155) and another with 65 patients (86). A word of caution was introduced in a study of 123 patients managed with a hypofractionation schedule where 87% experienced treatment toxicity (76,160).

A prospective randomized trial was conducted in 500 patients to compare the outcome in two treatment groups. Group 1 received 35 Gy in 10 fractions and group 2 received 21 Gy in three fractions (37). There was no significant difference between the two treatment groups in important study end points, including palliative effect, toxicity, and survival. Despite the results of this study, which would favor a three-fraction treatment regimen, other investigators seriously questioned its benefits in elderly patients.

Preoperative Irradiation

Historically, the aims of preoperative radiotherapy included

1. Tumor size reduction in locally advanced, muscle-invasive disease, which would be expected to result in down staging and therefore make surgery easier,
2. Decrease in the incidence of local recurrence following radical cystectomy,
3. Decrease in the incidence of distant metastasis,
4. Improvement of survival, and
5. No increase in the incidence of surgical complications.

Important early work on preoperative irradiation was published by groups from M.D. Anderson Hospital and Memorial Sloan-Kettering Cancer Center (MSKCC) (111,230). Results of multiple clinical studies performed over the past 30 years showed no conclusive benefit of preoperative irradiation in reaching these defined goals. As a result, a routine use of preoperative irradiation remains controversial. The evidence for and against preoperative irradiation is presented.

Evidence Supporting Preoperative Radiotherapy

A study of 724 bladder cancer patients treated between 1954 and 1970 at M.D. Anderson Hospital in Houston included 125 (17%) patients who received planned preoperative irradiation (group I). Radiotherapy consisted of 50 Gy given in 25 equal fractions over a period of 5 weeks, and it was followed 6 weeks later by radical cystectomy (114). Treatment results in this group were compared with the 533 (74%) patients who received definitive radiotherapy alone (group II) and 61 (8%) of those who were treated with postoperative irradiation (group III). No information was provided as to the selection process used in the management of these patients. The 5- and 10-year survival was 23% and 20%, respectively, for group I, 16% and 8% for group II, and 40% and 14%, respectively, for group III patients (NS). The incidence of local failure was the lowest at 16% for group I, the highest at 45% for group II, and intermediate at 33% for group III. It is interesting that in 29% of the 125 group I patients no tumor was found in the bladder at radical cystectomy. A subsequent randomized trial compared treatment outcomes in the 35 patients receiving preoperative irradiation with 32 who received definitive radiotherapy only. The 5-year survival was 46% for the former and 16% for the latter group. The study conclusion was that there was a clear benefit of preoperative irradiation in patients with T3 tumors.

Results of a prospective randomized trial comparing preoperative radiotherapy (n = 98) with definitive pelvic irradiation (n = 91) in patients with deeply invasive bladder cancer were reported from Royal Marsden Hospital of London (9). Preoperative radiotherapy consisted of 40 Gy in 4 weeks, whereas definitive irradiation consisted of 60 Gy in 6 weeks. The 5-year survival in patients receiving the combined therapy was 38% versus 29% for those treated with radiotherapy alone (NS). This study demonstrated significant survival benefit of preoperative irradiation in patients younger than 60 years of age and males, with no benefit noted in older (>60 years of age) and female patients. It is of importance to note that tumor-stage reduction was obtained in 49% and no tumor was found in the resected specimen in 31% of patients receiving preoperative irradiation. The finding of no tumor in the cystectomy specimen in 31% of patients in this study was very similar to the 29% incidence of no residual tumor found in the M.D. Anderson report (114). Based on this study's outcomes the authors recommended a routine use of preoperative irradiation in younger (younger than 60 years of age) male patients with T3 bladder cancer, whereas older male and female patients with muscle-invasive disease should be considered for definitive irradiation with salvage cystectomy for tumor recurrence.

An important preoperative study comparing two sequentially given radiation schedules was reported by the group from MSKCC in New York (214). Group I (n = 119) received 40 Gy in 4 weeks with radical cystectomy performed more than 4 weeks later, and group II (n = 86) received 20 Gy in 5 days followed by immediate cystectomy. The 5-year disease-free survival was 43% for group I and 42% for group II patients with very similar incidence of pelvic recurrence in either group. Tumor recurrence was an important event because virtually all patients with recurrence were dead within 2 years of this diagnosis. The benefit of preoperative irradiation was most apparent among patients with deeply invasive or transmural tumors who showed twice as high 5-year survival rates than those treated for a similar disease with radical cystectomy alone.

A summary of the experience with preoperative irradiation in patients with bladder cancer at MSKCC presented four consecutive groups of patients treated in the same medical center (187,188). Group I (n = 137) patients were treated with radical cystectomy alone, group II (n = 119) received 40 Gy preoperative irradiation followed by cystectomy, group III (n = 86) received 20 Gy in 5 days followed by cystectomy, and group IV (n = 101) received the same treatment as group III between 1971 and 1974 (the most recently treated patients). The best survival was obtained in group IV patients, which was attributed to advances in surgery. The incidence of pelvic recurrence was the lowest in patients of the three groups who received preoperative irradiation. The incidence of distant metastases was similar for all patient groups, and it likely overshadowed the benefit of lower incidence of pelvic recurrence seen in those who received preoperative irradiation.

A strong support for the use of preoperative irradiation (50 Gy in 5 weeks) in patients with T3b bladder cancer was provided by a study reported from M.D. Anderson Cancer Center (22). The 5-year incidence of local control in the preoperative group (n = 92) was 91%, as compared to 72% for those treated with radical cystectomy alone (n = 43; p = .003). There was also a benefit of preoperative irradiation in terms of overall survival and disease-free survival and in freedom from distant metastasis (NS). In multivariate analysis, preoperative irradiation was an independent predictor of local control. The authors recommended a routine use of preoperative irradiation as an adjuvant therapy to surgery and chemotherapy in patients with T3b disease. In a related study from the same medical center the status of p53 was found to be an independent predictor of overall survival, disease-free survival, and freedom from distant metastasis (235). Preoperative irradiation was responsible

for down staging in 73% of the treated patients (139), whereas apoptosis index was predictive of down staging and had a positive relationship to response to radiotherapy (21). Important benefits of preoperative irradiation also were demonstrated in a study of 273 patients reported by Free University of Brussels (34).

Parsons and Million (131) examined published results of retrospective studies and six prospective randomized trials on the use of preoperative irradiation in patients with T3 bladder cancer. They compared the outcomes with those of similar patients treated with radical cystectomy alone. The authors disputed results of many published studies, which compared pathologic stage T3 patients treated with radical cystectomy with those clinically staged T3 and managed with preoperative irradiation followed by radical cystectomy. Such comparisons have inherent bias against the combined-treatment patients because they ignore the published data from several studies on the ability of preoperative irradiation to downstage the primary lesions in two thirds of the patients (range from 44% to 82%) or eliminate all tumor in the resected specimen in about one third of the treated patients (range from 14% to 43%). Based on a careful analysis of the published data the authors concluded that addition of preoperative irradiation to radical cystectomy improved clinical stage T3 patients' 5-year survival by 15% to 20% over that reported for patients treated with radical cystectomy alone. The recommended radiation dose for preoperative radiotherapy was 40 to 50 Gy given in 2-Gy daily increments and followed 4 to 6 weeks later by surgery. The authors felt that 20 Gy given over a period of 5 days was not a sufficient preoperative dose to downstage the primary lesion in an equal number of patients as seen in those receiving 40 to 50 Gy.

Evidence Against the Use of Preoperative Irradiation

In a study reported from USC conducted between 1979 and 1986, 97 high-grade muscle-invasive patients were treated with preoperative irradiation consisting of 16 Gy given in four equal fractions of 4 Gy each and followed by an immediate radical cystectomy (182). This group was compared with 248 patients of similar pathologic stage who underwent radical cystectomy between 1979 to 1986 and who received no adjuvant radiation or systemic chemotherapy. Notwithstanding the well-known limitations of nonrandomized comparisons, no difference in survival, the incidence of local control, or distant metastasis was noted between the two study groups. The treatment was well tolerated, and there was no increase in the incidence of complications following radical cystectomy. Based on this experience and because there was no apparent benefit noted, the routine use of preoperative irradiation at USC was discontinued.

A study on the use of preoperative irradiation in 121 patients with muscle-invasive or recurrent superficial cancer conducted at Umea University in Sweden used a 40 to 50 Gy dose given at 2-Gy daily increments (214). There was an unacceptably high incidence of treatment toxicity, which is difficult to explain based on the provided data of this study. It certainly is dissimilar to the other published reports on the treatment of patients with preoperative irradiation followed by radical cystectomy.

A prospective randomized trial of 154 T2 to T4a transitional cell carcinoma patients was conducted between 1983 and 1986 by the Danish Vesical Cancer Group (165). Patients randomized to preoperative irradiation (n = 66) received 40 Gy at 2-Gy daily fraction followed by radical cystectomy. This group was compared to similar patients who had received definitive radiotherapy (n = 88) consisting of 60 Gy. These patients included 27 with persistent tumor who subsequently were treated with salvage cystectomy. The treatment program was well tolerated by the study patients, with no additional toxicity of radical cystectomy attributed to preoperative irradiation. Survival of patients was better in the preoperative group; however, this difference did not reach statistical significance. Based on this study the authors felt that patients with muscle-invasive disease have two viable treatment options, with one allowing for the organ preservation with the use of definitive irradiation.

The role of preoperative irradiation in patients with muscle-invasive disease was examined and treatment outcomes were compared with those of radical cystectomy alone in a similar patient population using meta-analysis of the relevant published data of five randomized trials on this subject (81). There was no statistical difference observed in important treatment outcomes between the two studied groups of patients. The authors concluded that the "available clinical trial data do not support a role for routine use of preoperative radiation therapy in the treatment of muscle-invasive bladder cancer" (81). A similar conclusion was reached in a phase III study of 140 patients that compared surgery alone with surgery and preoperative irradiation (187).

Postoperative Radiotherapy

The main advantage of postoperative radiotherapy over the preoperative treatment is the availability of pathologic staging. This allows the administration of adjuvant irradiation only to those patients who have a high probability of tumor recurrence following radical cystectomy. No large clinical trials on the use of postoperative radiotherapy have been reported. It is of interest to review the RTOG phase II trial using a single fraction preoperative radiotherapy (5 Gy) followed by postoperative irradiation (45 Gy in 5 weeks) in pathologically determined high-risk patients (117). Of the study's 65 patients, 29 received preoperative and postoperative radiotherapy. The treatment program was very well tolerated, and there was no pelvic recurrence. The 3-year actuarial survival was 78%, and in the judgment of the study investigators it was better than the available alternative treatments. This therapeutic approach, however, was not followed in subsequent studies.

Treatment of Patients with Uncommon Bladder Tumors

Squamous cell carcinoma is an uncommon tumor in Europe and in North America. A retrospective study in 19 consecutive patients treated in Italy was reported in 2000 (168). None of the study patients had bilharziasis or spinal-cord injury. Involvement of the prostatic urethra was noted in nine (47%) patients, and the upper urinary tract was involved in an additional five (26%) patients. The majority (79%) of these patients were treated with radical cystectomy; one patient was treated with partial cystectomy, and the remaining three patients had TURB followed by EBRT. Neoadjuvant chemotherapy was given to four (21%) patients, and adjuvant chemotherapy was given to three (4%) patients. At a mean follow-up of 52 months, six (32%) patients were alive and free of disease. Pattern of failure was different from that of transitional cell carcinoma, with locoregional recurrence as a primary cause of death and relatively infrequent distant metastasis. A combination of radical surgery with adjuvant radiotherapy is a recommended treatment.

Two contemporary reports on the management of 19 patients with small cell carcinoma of the bladder were identified (6,101). Patients were treated with a combination of polychemotherapy and pelvic irradiation. Radiotherapy to the pelvis was given at 2 Gy per fraction to about 45 Gy to be followed by a 15-Gy dose to smaller fields. In the British Columbia Cancer Agency study of 14 patients, 10 were eligible for a chemoradiotherapy combination. The 2- and 5-year disease-free survival for these 10 patients was 70%. At the last follow-up 36% of patients were alive and free of tumor. However, all four patients treated with a palliative aim died of disease from 2 to 15 months of therapy. It is interesting that in surviving patients there was a 60% incidence of second primary lesions in the bladder within 3 years of therapy. Transitional cell carcinoma was the most common malignancy diagnosed in these patients.

Carcinosarcoma represents a heterogeneous group of very aggressive malignant lesions (102). The basic two variants are carcinosarcoma and sarcomatoid carcinoma. Most patients were treated with radical cystectomy or TURB with or without adjuvant radiotherapy and chemotherapy. Treatment outcomes were generally poor. Pathologic stage was the best predictor of survival, whereas histologic diagnosis was not a good predictor of outcome. Based on the limited published data on treatment results in patients with carcinosarcoma, it is difficult to recommend treatment policy. It appears that an aggressive multimodality treatment approach will produce an optimal outcome in selected patients with disease limited to the pelvis.

Particle Beams

Electron Beam

Electron beams have been used infrequently in the management of patients with bladder cancer, and at this time its application is of historical interest only. The authors do not recommend the use of electron beam for bladder cancer. On the other hand, intraoperative radiation therapy (IORT) is an important application for electron beam. A major problem relates to its cost because it requires a dedicated linear accelerator in the operating room or immediate access to the accelerator, with sterilizable beam-shaping devices. Radiation dose has to be given in a single fraction; therefore, the radiobiologic advantages of the expanded treatment time or the use of a conventional fractionation schedule is lost. In clinical trials IORT frequently was combined with EBRT. The intraoperative dose usually is delivered with a 4- to 9-MeV electron beam. The final choice of energy depends on the thickness of the target volume, and the typical radiation dose is 25 to 30 Gy (154). A recent review of IORT clearly demonstrated a high incidence of tumor control and a low incidence of severe toxicity in patients treated in contemporary clinical trials (173).

Of interest is a study reported in 2000 from France regarding 27 selected bladder cancer patients with muscle-invasive tumors (154). The treatment program consisted of TURB followed by 48-Gy EBRT given at 2 Gy per fraction with the 18-MV photon beam and cisplatin chemotherapy. This was followed with cystostomy and intraoperative 9-MeV EB delivering 15 Gy to the tumor site. The overall and salvage cystectomy 5-year survival was 53% and 48%, respectively. Of the 27 study patients, 10 (37%) developed distant metastasis and five (19%) had local recurrence. Treatment toxicity seems severe, with three patients developing mucosal necrosis and ureteral stenosis. The role of IORT for carcinoma of the bladder needs to be assessed in a prospective trial. Currently its use is not recommended outside of such studies.

Neutron Beam

It is of interest to review a prospective randomized trial comparing 4- to 8-MV photon beams versus a 15-MeV neutron beam in 108 patients with T2 and T3 tumors (138). The 1- and 5-year survival rates for both treatments groups were very similar, with greater toxicity being reported in those treated with neutron beam. Based on a lack of therapeutic gain, the use of a 15-MeV neutron beam with the treatment schedule reported in this study is not recommended in patients with carcinoma of the bladder.

Treatment Techniques

External Beam Radiotherapy

The use of high-energy photon beams (10 MV or more) is preferred in the treatment of patients with carcinoma of the bladder. The treatment volume initially includes the whole bladder, proximal urethra, and, in male patients, the prostate with the prostatic urethra and the regional lymphatics. The regional lymphatics adjacent to the bladder include hypogastric, external iliac, and obturator lymph nodes. Subsequently, patients receive radiotherapy to a smaller boost volume, which usually includes the bladder with about a 2-cm margin. A common definition of anatomic extent of the radiation portals is as follows:

1. The anterior–posterior fields extend laterally about 1.5 cm to the bony pelvis at its widest section with inferior corners excluded to protect the femoral heads.
2. The lateral fields extend anteriorly to about 1.5 to 2 cm from the most anterior aspect of the bladder as seen on an imaging study (CT). The posterior border lies about 2.5 cm posterior to the most posterior aspect of the bladder and falls within the rectum. Inferiorly, the tissue above the symphysis and the anal canal is blocked.
3. The inferior border is placed below the middle of the obturator foramen. The superior border is usually at the L5-S1 disc space.

There is, however, an ongoing debate whether the regional pelvic lymph nodes should be included in the radiation portals. The RTOG and some other investigators recommended the inclusion of the regional lymph nodes (177,211), while the recommendations of the Fourth International Consensus Meeting on Bladder Cancer are against this treatment policy (60,136). In the latter policy the bladder with a 2-cm margin is the recommended treatment volume. Digitally reconstructed radiographs of the induction radiation fields are shown in Figure 61.1A,B.

There is an additional controversy regarding the initial pelvic fields with regional lymph node inclusion with a full or empty bladder. The argument for the latter is that the overall irradiated volume is smaller. However, when treated with full bladder the distended organ is expected to push more of the small intestine and some part of the rectum out of the radiation field. The four-field box technique is used most frequently for the treatment of the initial large pelvic volume. It provides a relatively homogeneous dose distribution over the treated volume, while keeping the radiation dose outside this volume to about 50% of the intended tumor dose. Because much of the bladder is anterior to the coronal midplane, preferential weight can be given to the anterior field, relative to the posterior one. The preferential anterior weight and the shape of the external contour of the patient may cause a higher dose in the anterior part of the treatment volume, which easily can be reduced by applying appropriate wedges in the lateral fields. The treatment setup and the resulting dose distribution in the three principal planes are shown in Figure 61.2A–D.

The boost fields include either the whole bladder or only the involved part of the bladder with at least a 2-cm margin. These fields need to be set up and monitored with great care in view of the well-recognized bladder volume changes occurring during the treatment course (116). Although the most commonly used treatment technique is the four-field box with field sizes adjusted to the smaller boost volume, many other techniques can be employed, such as two lateral fields, three or four oblique fields, or rotational arc techniques. Treatment setup and dose distribution of the four-field box boost is shown in Figure 61.3A,B. As examples for other techniques, treatment setups and dose distributions of three oblique fields and bilateral arcs are shown in Figures 61.4A,B and 61.5A,B. The choice between these techniques depends on a number of factors such as the preference of the radiation oncologist, the tumor location, the target volume, and the dose delivered with the initial large pelvic portals to the dose-limiting structures such as femoral heads, rectum, and small intestines. There is a consensus, however, that when the desired treatment volume is the bladder only, the bladder should be treated empty. To decrease the overall irradiated volume, partial bladder boosts typically are treated with an empty bladder. However, consideration may be given to the treatment delivered with a full bladder if the target volume is relatively small and distending the bladder increases the distance between the target and the dose-limiting structures.

Because of the well-documented mobility of the bladder during the treatment, large enough margins have to be added to the intended target volume to accommodate its possible motion. Treating always with either an empty or full bladder can diminish, but not completely eliminate, the variation of the

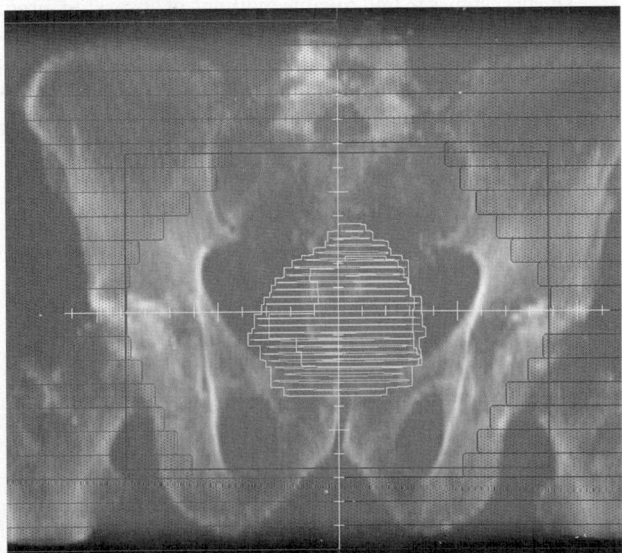
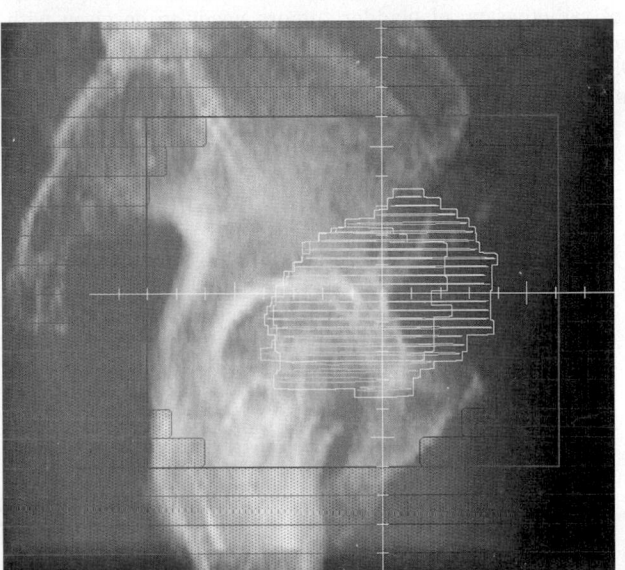

FIGURE 61.1. Digitally reconstructed radiographs of commonly used induction fields. **A:** Anterior–posterior portal. **B:** Right lateral portal.

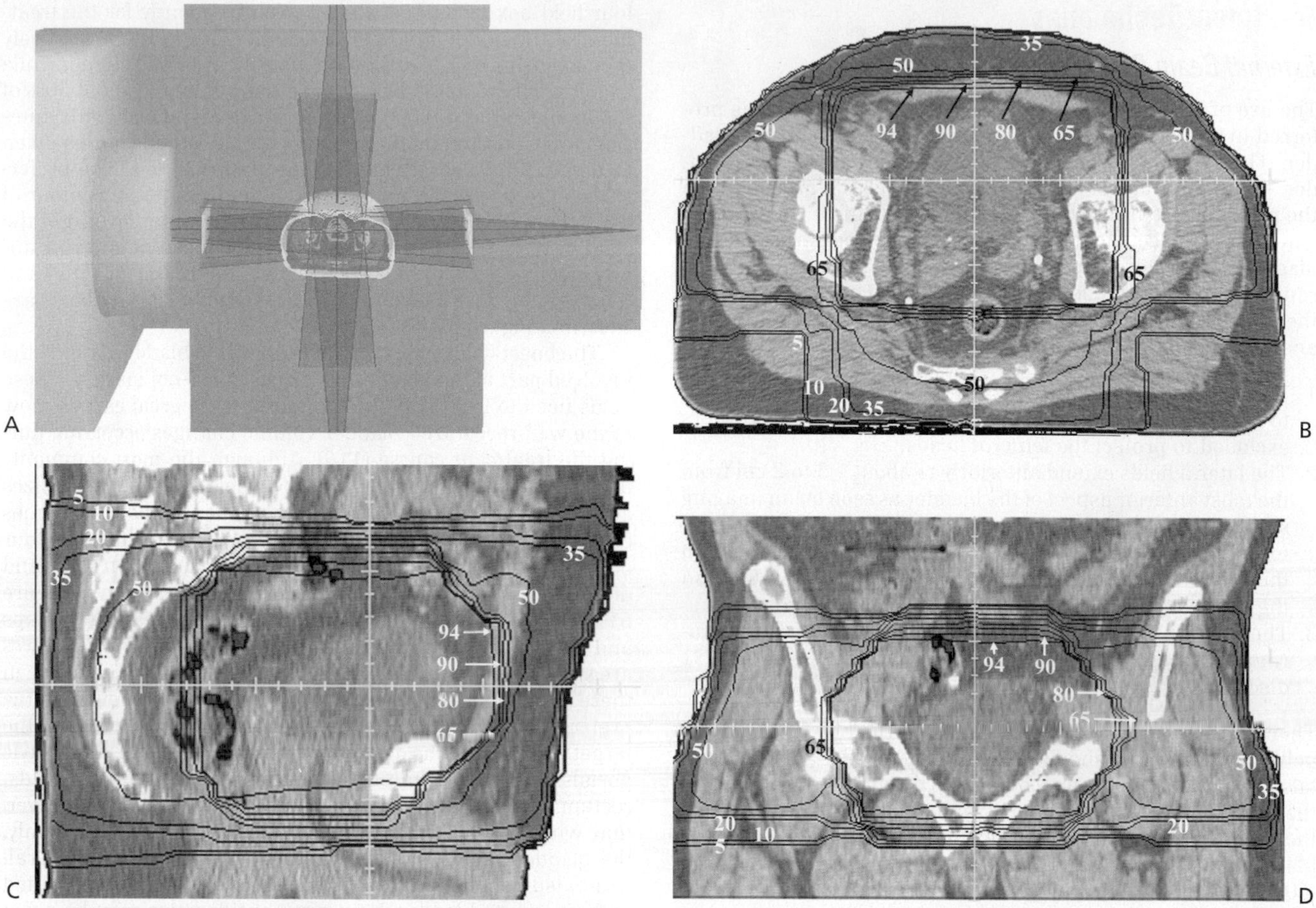

FIGURE 61.2. Field setup and radiation dose distribution of the initial pelvic fields. **A:** Four-field box technique. **B–D:** Dose distribution in the transverse, sagittal, and coronal planes.

location of the target volume. Neither can this variation be eliminated by using patient immobilization devices such as bean bags, thermoplastic sheets, or the like. The application of these devices still is recommended to increase the reproducibility of the patient setup and to limit the patient's movement during the treatment.

Due to the mobility of the bladder, strictly conformal (no margin) radiotherapy of bladder tumors needs to be given with great care to ensure targeting accuracy for every treatment (95,100). However, advanced localization techniques such as implanted markers and gating technology (the beam turns off if

a marker moves out of its permitted range) may make conformal therapy possible in the near future (171). Portal imaging systems are helpful in real-time monitoring of treatment accuracy (65). Given that the rapid development of techniques of conformal therapy inspired intensive research on new methods of external beam bladder irradiation, including conformal, intensity-modulated radiation therapy (IMRT), and adaptive techniques.

The first step is to find reliable methods of observing, predicting, and/or modeling the motion and deformation of the bladder. Easy access to CT (either conventional or onboard cone beam CT) makes repeat imaging feasible, thus the motion and

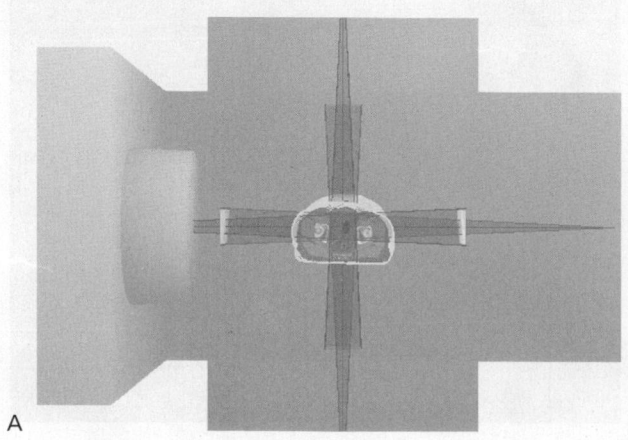

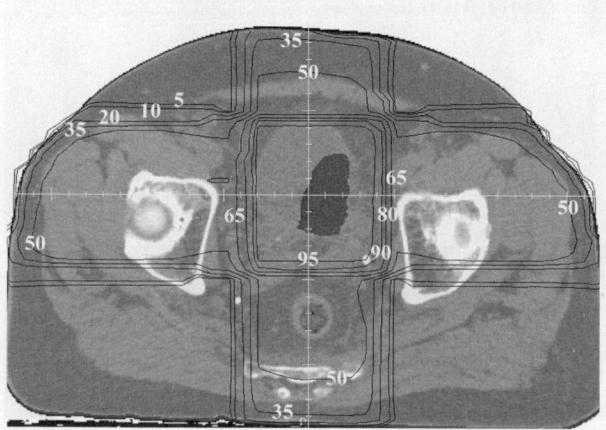

FIGURE 61.3. Fields setup and dose distribution in four-field boost. **A:** Four-field box setup. **B:** Dose distribution in the transverse plane.

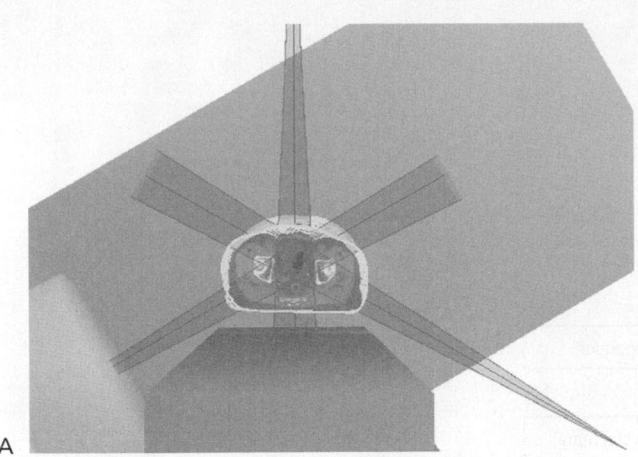
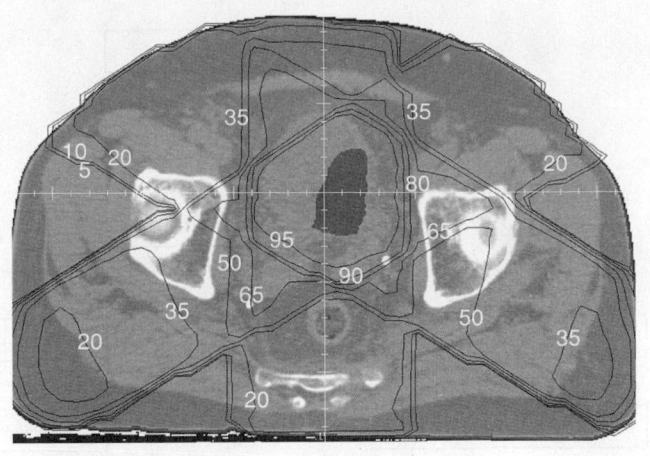

FIGURE 61.4. Portals setup and dose distribution of a three-field boost arrangement. **A:** Three-field setup. **B:** Dose distribution in the transverse plane.

deformation of the bladder can be observed. The repeat scans then can be used to:

1. Build an overall primary tumor volume (PTV), which will be treated during the entire session (113,124),
2. Modify the PTV as the treatment advances (image-guided radiation therapy [IGRT] and adaptive therapy) (142,147), or
3. Build mathematical models to predict the location and shape of the GTV and the adjacent organs (237).

At the present time appropriate margin selection and localization of the volume of the irradiated healthy tissues can be reduced, even with the conventional four-field technique. However, more conformal treatment techniques, like IMRT, tomotherapy, and so forth, can also be applied. Some relevant answers may be provided following completion in 2008 of an ongoing clinical trial (NCT00350688) at the Ottawa Hospital Regional Cancer Centre, Ontario, Canada, using helical tomotherapy IMRT in patients treated with a chemoradiation regimen.

The commonly accepted treatment schedule in patients with bladder cancer is 180 to 200 cGy per day to a total of 45 to 50 Gy to the whole pelvis, followed by a boost to a smaller volume to a combined total dose of 60 to 65 Gy.

Brachytherapy

Interstitial therapy in the United States is not a common part of management of patients with bladder cancer. However, brachytherapy commonly has been used for selected patients with bladder cancer in Europe and Japan. During the past 30 years, large clinical trials have been reported from Europe (119,132,156,189,216–218,232).

Contemporary brachytherapy for bladder cancer is limited almost exclusively to afterloaded interstitial therapy with iridium-192 (^{192}Ir) sources. The average photon energy of ^{192}Ir is 380 keV, which is lower than that of radium-226 (^{226}Ra) or cesium-137 (^{137}Cs) and, therefore, it better meets radiation safety requirements. The ^{192}Ir radiation still is penetrating enough to allow for an effective treatment at a 1- to 1.5-cm distance from a planar implant. ^{192}Ir has a half-life of 73.8 days, which necessitates source replacement every 3 to 4 months. The source(s) can be embedded in flexible wires to conform the implant to the contour of the bladder wall. Afterloading devices using ^{192}Ir sources, both in high– and low–dose-rate mode, are readily available, further increasing the flexibility of the treatment planning and ensuring the operator's safety (156,189,220,221).

A commonly accepted dimension of bladder tumors selected for brachytherapy is <5 cm. The tumor usually is treated with a single plane implant of three to five line sources: needles or catheters into which the radioactive sources will be loaded. The distance between line sources is about 1 cm. A single plane implant can be used to treat a 2- to 2.5-cm thick lesion; beyond that two-plane implants may become necessary. Needles or catheters used in brachytherapy are placed in the tumor during surgery. Flexible catheters of the afterloading technique can be removed without further surgery, whereas the removal of needles or tubes of the "classical" brachytherapy usually

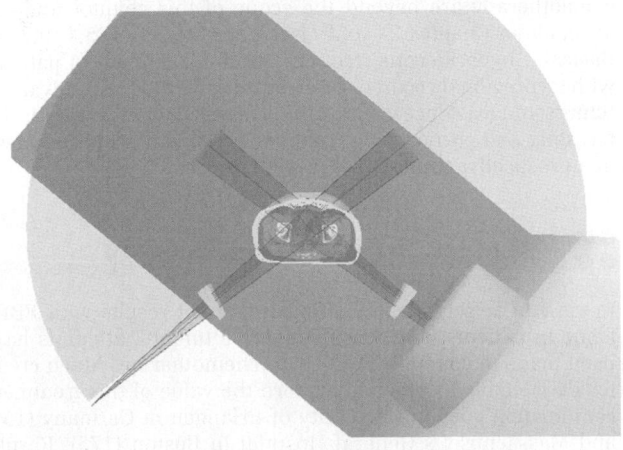
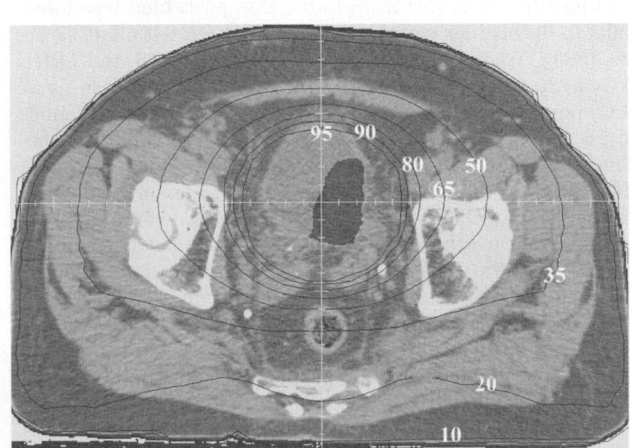

FIGURE 61.5. Field setup and dose distribution of a bilateral arc boost. **A:** Bilateral arc setup. **B:** Dose distribution in the transverse plane.

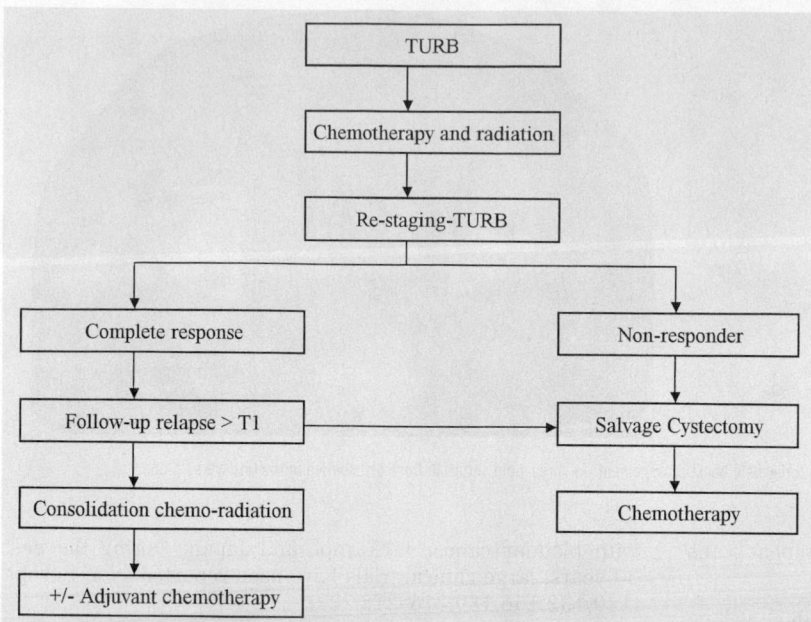

FIGURE 61.6. Schematic representation of the decision-making process in patients treated with a bladder-sparing approach.

require the reopening of the bladder. The use of contemporary treatment-planning process is recommended because it is expected to result in improved dose homogeneity and facilitate a better protection of the normal tissues (88,221).

Modern interstitial therapy in bladder cancer was introduced by Brigit Van Der Werf-Messing of Rotterdam, the Netherlands, initially with ^{226}Ra (216,217) and subsequently with ^{137}Cs (218,232). External beam radiotherapy was used successfully to reduce the incidence of scar recurrence and consisted of 10.5 Gy given in three fractions to the pelvis prior to the interstitial therapy. Excellent treatment outcomes were reported, with 5- and 10-year survival for T2 patients of 56% and 37%, respectively, and 39% and 19%, respectively, for those with T3 disease (216,217). A study of 98 poor-prognosis patients with T2 and T3 tumors was reported by Van Der Werf-Messing and Van Putten (218). The treatment protocol involved EBRT consisting of 40 Gy at 2.0 Gy per fraction followed by reduced dose ^{137}Cs implant. The 5-year survival in these poor-prognosis patients was 70%. Analysis of risk factors in extensive experience of the Rotterdam group identified the following parameters influencing prognosis: (a) tumor differentiation, (b) the number of prior TURB, (c) obstruction of ureter(s), (d) presence of vascular invasion; (e) T stage following preoperative EBRT, and (f) pathologic stage (232).

A more recent report from Rotterdam presented treatment results in 66 bladder cancer patients of whom 94% had T2 lesions (231). Treatment protocol consisted of TURB and EBRT (40 Gy in 20 equal fractions) followed by ^{192}Ir implant (30 Gy at 58 cGy per hour). A total of 42 (64%) patients had lymphadenectomy, whereas 16 (24%) had partial cystectomy. The 5-year incidence of freedom of local relapse and distant metastasis was 88% and 66%, respectively, with seven (11%) patients showing recurrence in the bladder and 16 (24%) having distant metastasis. The 5-year overall survival was 48%, whereas disease-free survival was 69%. The bladder preservation was obtained in 98% of the survivors. This treatment program was very well tolerated, with grade 3 RTOG toxicity seen in one (2%) patient. The authors strongly recommended the use of bladder preservation, as per their protocol, in properly selected patients with muscle-invasive disease.

A multicenter French study reported excellent treatment results in 205 patients of whom 177 (86%) were males. Of this group, 90% had transitional cell carcinoma with a mean tumor

size of 2.9 cm (155). Most of the study patients had pT1 (48%) or pT2 (32%) disease. The Rotterdam treatment protocol was followed with a short preoperative course of EBRT and ^{192}Ir implant. Partial cystectomy was performed in 118 (58%) patients. Tumor relapse in the bladder alone was seen in 25 (12%) patients, with an additional 12 (6%) patients who also had distant metastasis. A total of 21 (10%) patients developed distant metastasis. The 5-year survival by T stage was as follows: T1, 74%; T2, 63%; and T3, 47%. Bladder function was preserved in 96% of patients who survived. Acute treatment toxicity was noted in 26%, and late toxicity was seen in 14%, whereas three (1.5%) study patients died of surgical complications. Factors predictive of late toxicity included partial cystectomy, total dose of EBRT, and activity of the radioactive sources. Similar excellent treatment results with a low incidence of severe toxicity were recently reported from several centers in France and the Netherlands (32,119,132,215). It is apparent that brachytherapy in combination with EBRT represents an important modality in a conservative management of highly selected patients with carcinoma of the bladder.

Hyperthermia

Details on hyperthermia in combination with EBRT and/or chemotherapy are beyond the scope of this chapter and are available in Chapter 24 and elsewhere (24,111,135,149,219). Basically, hyperthermia may be a useful treatment in patients with locoregional recurrence or in those with locally advanced tumors and existence of contraindications to chemotherapy. Interesting and encouraging treatment results have been shown in a prospective randomized trial (219).

Bladder-Preservation Therapy

In view of largely disappointing treatment results with EBRT alone in patients with muscle-invasive tumors, attempts have been made to combine EBRT with chemotherapy. Much credit for early clinical studies to explore the value of this treatment combination goes to University of Erlangen in Germany (159) and Massachusetts General Hospital in Boston (175). Results of a phase I/II study conducted in the University of Erlangen

| Table 61.12 | TRIALS OF COMBINED MODALITY TREATMENT AND SELECTIVE ORGAN PRESERVATION |

Study/Author (Reference)	Combined Therapy Used	No. of Patients	5-Year Overall Survival (%)	5-Year Survival with Bladder Preservation (%)
RTOG 8512/Tester et al. (212)	EBRT + cisplatin	42	52	42
RTOG 8802/Tester et al. (211)	TURBT, MCV, EBRT + cisplatin	91	51	44 (4 y)
RTOG 8903/Shipley et al. (176)	TURBT, ± MCV, EBRT + cisplatin	123	49	38
Univ. Paris/Housset et al. (79)	TURBT, 5-FU, EBRT + cisplatin	120	63	NA
Erlangen-Germany/Rodel et al. (152)	TURBT, EBRT ± chemo (cisplatin, carboplatin, or cisplatin and 5-FU)	415 (RCT: cisplatin, 82; carboplatin, 61; 5-FU/cisplatin, 87)	50	42
MGH –Shipley 2003 (172)	TURBT, ± MCV, EBRT + cisplatin	190	54	45
RTOG 97-06/Hagan 2003 (63)	TURBT + accelerated EBRT + cisplatin and adjuvant MCV	52	61 (3-y projected)	48 (3-y projected)

EBRT, external beam radiotherapy; 5-FU, 5-fluorouracil; MCV, methotrexate, cisplatin, vinblastine; MGH, Massachusetts General Hospital; RTOG, Radiation Therapy Oncology Group; TURBT, transurethral resection of bladder tumor

in 67 patients with muscle-invasive carcinoma are of interest (159). Treatment protocol consisted of optimal TURB followed by 50.4 Gy EBRT given at 1.8 Gy daily with simultaneous cisplatin chemotherapy (25 mg/m^2 daily for 5 days during the first and last week of radiotherapy). CR assessed at 6 weeks of completion of therapy was obtained in 42 (75%) study patients and included 14 (88%) in T2, 27 (75%) in T3, and one (25%) in T4 lesions. Complete microscopically confirmed TURB was an important predictor of CR. The incidence of CR was better than that obtained in 62 similar patients treated in the same medical center with EBRT alone (p <.01). At 18 months posttreatment nine (18%) CR patients had a local recurrence. The 3-year survival for T1 was 73%; for T2 and T3 it was 68%, and for T4 patients it was 25%. The overall 3-year survival at 66% was not significantly different from that of matched control. The combined-therapy program was well tolerated without severe toxicity. Similar high incidence of CR in 70 T2 to T4 patients who were not candidates for radical cystectomy was reported by Shipley et al. (174) in 1987. From that point on combined-modality therapy has become a standard approach in patients seeking bladder-preservation therapy.

For the past two decades several phase II and III studies have evaluated combined modality treatments (Table 61.12). A variety of cytotoxic agents and combinations were used including MCV (methotrexate, cisplatin, vinblastine), cisplatin, 5-fluorouracil (5-Fu) with or without cisplatin and carboplatin (79). Newer agents such as paclitaxel and gemcitabine were also used as radiosensitizers (186). The reported CR in these trials ranged between 61% and 87%, with about one third of the patients undergoing cystectomy due to incomplete response. Moreover, in the past decade twice daily radiation therapy has evolved as the standard in the RTOG trials, originally inspired by a small trial from the University of Chicago (63,148). This approach was initially tested in a prospective, centrally randomized RTOG phase I or II trial of hyperfractionation as definitive radiation therapy for locally advanced squamous and transitional cell carcinoma of the bladder (27). The use of a combined twice daily radiotherapy with concurrent 5-FU and cisplatin was reported, and in more recent studies with concurrent paclitaxel and cisplatin (179,241). The radiation fields generally encompassed the pelvis to include the external and internal iliac lymph nodes in the PTV. A total dose of 40 to 45 Gy in 1.8 to 2 Gy per fraction was delivered to the PTV with an additional boost dose of 20 to 25 Gy to the primary tumor.

Chemoradiation delivered as initial, definitive treatment was originally reserved to patients unsuited for surgery (174). The results of a prospective multicenter study run by the National Bladder Cancer Group were published in 1987. Seventy patients with muscle invasive TCC, who were not candidates for cystectomy, were treated with EBRT and cisplatin. The overall CR rate was 70%, and it increased to 77% among the patients who completed the planned radiation treatment. Interestingly, the 4-year survival rate of patients achieving CR was significantly higher (57% vs. 11%; p <.01) than that of those who did not achieve CR.

The National Cancer Institute-Canada study, randomly assigned 99 patients with T2-4 bladder cancer to radiation (either definitive or neoadjuvant), with or without concurrent cisplatin. Chemoradiation improved local pelvic control (67% vs. 47%), but no difference was observed in the rate of distant relapse (26). Dunst et al. (39) published a single institution experience with 245 patients with invasive TCC treated with TURB and definitive radiation. One hundred and thirty-nine patients were treated with concurrent cisplatin or carboplatin. The single most important prognostic factor was the presence of residual disease after TURB. The extent of residual disease was classified R0 to R2 and correlated with the outcome. The patients without residual tumor (R0 at resection) had a 5-year survival of 80%, compared to 53% for those with R1 and 31% for those with R2. These differences were statistically significant (p <.01). Chemoradiation *per se* increased the rate of CR but had no impact on 5-year survival (52% vs. 50%), suggesting the presence of a subset of patients with tumors exquisitely sensitive to both the local and systemic effects of chemoradiation, as demonstrated by the coincidence of local response and a better 5-year survival rate.

A 15-year experience with chemoradiotherapy combination in 200 patients with carcinoma of the bladder was recently reported by a group from Ottawa Hospital, Canada (40). Chemotherapy consisted of three courses of intra-arterial cisplatin, while EBRT used 40 Gy to the pelvis with a 20 Gy boost to the bladder. CR was obtained in 166 (83%) of patients, while bladder preservation rate at a median follow-up of 34 months was 75%. Nearly the same excellent treatment results were reported in a study of 141 high-risk T1 patients by the group from University of Erlangen, Germany (227). The above results are very similar to those reported in multiple studies including those of RTOG and EORTC (35,151,172,176,178,212). The outcomes of contemporary organ-preservation trials resemble those reported by contemporary radical cystectomy studies. The obvious benefit of the conservatively treated patients is preservation of native bladder in a large majority of these patients.

The emerging evidence on the safety and feasibility of combined modality treatment led to the development of the current algorithm for bladder preservation (41). The algorithm reflects the main challenge of organ preservation (i.e., a clinical pathway that optimizes the chance to maintain a functional bladder while ensuring the same cancer-specific outcome of cystectomy). Key to the success of this approach is the correct selection of patients, with solitary TCC tumors, without extensive carcinoma *in situ*, and in general medical conditions compatible with platinum therapy. These candidates undergo TURB to achieve maximum removal of the tumor followed by an initial course of chemoradiation, an EBRT dose of approximately 40 Gy. Response to this first phase is assessed by biopsy at cystoscopy and urinary cytology. If both are negative for tumor (CR) a second course of chemoradiation follows (total dose of radiation is 64 to 65 Gy). If residual disease is documented, a cystectomy is recommended. Patients treated with bladder preservation are carefully followed by cystoscopy to ensure that early recurrences are promptly detected and salvaged by cystectomy.

Treatment Outcomes of Primary Cystectomy versus Organ Preservation

Comparing treatment outcomes from surgical series to those in studies that used a chemoradiotherapy combination with cystectomy for salvage is inappropriate because of inherent selection bias associated with treatment choice, as discussed earlier in this chapter. Conservative therapy is offered more often to older patients, patients with more advanced disease at diagnosis, or to those with serious comorbid conditions making surgery risky (16,158). Moreover, surgical assessment permits more accurate staging by histologically identifying disease, which is frequently clinically undetectable, thus inevitably underestimating the true extent of tumor in conservatively treated patients. Additionally, approximately 15% of patients are excluded at the time of cystectomy because of the identified extravesical tumor spread. Finally, because of the decrease in morbidity associated with modern radical cystectomy, more patients with earlier disease now are treated with surgery (197). This makes it difficult to compare outcomes achieved by current surgical series to those using irradiation in combination with chemotherapy, which typically treat patients with more advanced disease. As an example, a USC study published in 2001 demonstrated a 78% 5-year recurrence-free survival and 66% overall survival in patients treated with radical cystectomy (197). This series, however, also included patients with early disease, including 20% of those with noninvasive tumors. These results were superior to those reported from an earlier surgical series of 300 cystectomy patients from MSKCC, where the 5-year overall survival rate was 36% in patients with T2 to T4 disease (31). The most recent report from USC focused on the subset of pT2 tumors, demonstrating the clinical relevance of nodal involvement and its impact on survival (239).

Published data also from USC have shown that radical cystectomy is also feasible and well tolerated among elderly patients (236). Despite this major progress in the management of carcinoma of the bladder, approximately 40% to 50% of patients with muscle-invasive cancers are not cured by locoregional therapy and eventually die of metastatic bladder cancer. Additionally, even contemporary radical cystectomy for muscle-invasive cancer affects urinary and sexual function in both male and female patients, resulting in a significant impact on their quality of life.

Role of Systemic Therapy

In the metastatic disease setting, transitional cell carcinoma has demonstrated relative chemosensitivity. In contemporary phase II clinical trials, overall response rates are as high as 70% to 80%, with a 50% response rate maintained in phase III clinical trials (206). Importantly, a small but substantial minority of patients achieve a CR, with some long-term, durable responses observed. Currently, gemcitabine and cisplatin are the most widely used drugs as single agents, while the most commonly used platinum-based combination chemotherapy remains M-VAC (methotrexate, vinblastine, doxorubicin, and cisplatin) (18,52).

The high response rate to chemotherapy in the metastatic setting, albeit short lived, has led to the incorporation of chemotherapy in the definitive treatment of locally advanced bladder cancer either as preoperative treatment or in an "adjuvant" setting, as an adjunct to radical cystectomy or definitive radiotherapy. The rationale is to employ systemic therapy to aim at occult metastases present at the time of diagnosis of a muscle invasive tumor in hopes of preventing distant relapse.

Neoadjuvant Chemotherapy

Over the past two decades several studies have investigated the role of neoadjuvant chemotherapy with conflicting results. Phase I and II trials of neoadjuvant chemotherapy have reported overall response rates as high as 60% to 70%, out of which 30% were complete responses (205,224,233). In selected patients clinical down staging achieved by primary chemotherapy allowed operability (197). Six prospective randomized trials comparing single- (64,110) or multiple-agent (5,28,55,106) neoadjuvant chemotherapy with definitive local therapy have failed to demonstrate any significant survival advantage (109). Major limitations of these studies consist of the small number of patients and/or the choice of chemotherapy regimens that are currently considered suboptimal.

A large international prospective randomized trial of neoadjuvant chemotherapy prior to radical cystectomy or prior to EBRT demonstrated 32.5% pathologically proven CR but failed to demonstrate substantial benefit in survival, the results showing only a possible 5.5% difference in 3-year survival between the treatment groups (82). Several investigators attempted to find out whether, despite the negative results from the above-mentioned trials, a specific subset of patients could be identified that is likely to benefit from neoadjuvant chemotherapy. The Nordic Cooperative Bladder Cancer Study Group (107) randomized bladder cancer patients with clinical stage ranging from T1 G3 to T4a to receive two cycles of neoadjuvant cisplatin and doxorubicin versus no chemotherapy. Patients received a regimen of accelerated preoperative irradiation consisting of 20 Gy, at 4 Gy daily fractions for 5 consecutive days, followed by cystectomy. At subset analysis, a 12% survival benefit at 5 years was noted for those with T3 and T4 tumors (107). Similar outcome was noted in a study of 111 patients with T2 to T4 tumors treated with neoadjuvant M-VAC regimen at MSKCC (164). At a median follow-up of 5 years, patients with initial clinical extravesical extension who had experienced tumor down-staging by neoadjuvant chemotherapy had significantly better 5-year survival rates than those who had no down-staging (54% vs. 12%) (164).

The Nordic Cystectomy Trial II administered three preoperative cycles of cisplatin and methotrexate prior to cystectomy and compared the results to those of cystectomy alone (170). No preoperative radiation therapy was used in this study. Interestingly, despite a statistically significant pathological down staging (26.4% CR), no survival benefit was observed (5-year survival 53% vs. 46%; $p = $ NS). A similar study from M.D. Anderson Hospital compared three preoperative cycles of M-VAC chemotherapy followed by cystectomy, to cystectomy alone (62). The median survival was 77 months versus 44 months ($p = .06$) and the 5-year survival was 57% versus 43% ($p = .06$). Table 61.13 provides a summary of selected prospective randomized trials of neoadjuvant chemotherapy.

Table 61.13	PROSPECTIVE RANDOMIZED TRIALS COMPARING NEOADJUVANT CHEMOTHERAPY AND DEFINITIVE LOCAL TREATMENT ALONE			
Author (Reference)	Pts#	Standard Arm	Neoadjuvant Arm	Survival p-Value
Crawford et al. (28)	298	Cystectomy	M-VAC/cystectomy	NS
Wallace et al. (224)	296	Radiotherapy	CDDP/radiotherapy	NS
Pineiro et al. (107)	122	Cystectomy	CDDP/cystectomy	NS
Hall (64)	—	Cystectomy	CMV/cystectomy	NS
Bassi et al. (5)	206	Cystectomy	M-VAC/cystectomy	NS
Malmstrom et al. (106)	317	Cystectomy	MTX/CDDP/cystectomy	NS
Coppin et al. (26)	99	Preoperative radiotherapy/ cystectomy	Preoperative CDDP, and radiotherapy/cystectomy	NS
Sherif et al. (170)	317	Cystectomy	MTX/CDDP/cystectomy	NS
Grossman et al. (62)	317	Cystectomy	M-VAC/cystectomy	NS

CDDP, cisplatin; CMV cisplatin, methotrexate, and vinblastine; MTX, methotrexate; M-VAC, methotrexate, vinblastine, doxorubicin, and cisplatin

In 2004, the Advanced Bladder Cancer Overview Collaboration published a meta-analysis of 11 randomized clinical trials involving over 3,000 patients (2). Once the available published data were analyzed through the methodology of a meta-analysis, recipients of platinum-based combination chemotherapy were found to derive a significant benefit from systemic treatment, with overall survival increased from 45% to 50%. This effect was observed irrespective of the type of local treatment and did not vary between subgroups of patients. The hazard ratio (HR) tended to favor neoadjuvant multiagent chemotherapy (HR = 0.89, 95% confidence interval [CI] 0.81 to 0.98; $p = .022$), while there was no clear evidence supporting the use of single agent cisplatin. A recent phase III trial compared neoadjuvant chemotherapy plus cystectomy to cystectomy alone and reported a 5-year overall survival of 50% for the 307 patients assigned to the surgery alone arm (62).

Adjuvant Chemotherapy

Adjuvant chemotherapy, unlike its neoadjuvant counterpart, has the advantage of enabling a better patient selection based on the finding originated at surgical and pathological staging. The major disadvantages though, are the delay in systemic therapy and the inability to assess *in vivo* the individual response to chemotherapy. Five prospective randomized trials to test the benefit of adjuvant chemotherapy have been reported and are summarized in Table 61.14. Methodological flaws in these studies prevent a clear interpretation of the results: for instance, some of the chemotherapy agents used in these studies are no longer considered standard of care and sample sizes are gen-

erally inadequate to provide the statistical power to detect a significant difference in survival.

In 2006 the Advanced Bladder Cancer Meta-analysis Collaboration published a meta-analysis of six trials of adjuvant chemotherapy, after primary local treatment of bladder cancer (the five trials mentioned above and data from a study conducted by Otto et al. [129], published only as an abstract). The meta-analysis included 491 patients with stages T2 to T4a transitional cell carcinoma of the bladder. The overall HR for survival was 0.75 (95% CI, 0.6 to 0.96; $p = .019$), suggesting a 25% relative reduction in the risk of death for chemotherapy recipients compared to that of patients in the control arm. However, the impact of the trials that were stopped early because of toxicity removed a subset of patients actually not receiving the allocated treatment or not receiving salvage chemotherapy at recurrence, making it difficult to interpret results of the meta-analysis.

An EORTC Intergroup study (EORTC-30994) set to accrue 1,344 patients is currently being conducted. This important study may conclusively address the issue of adjuvant chemotherapy following cystectomy for TCC of the bladder. The trial will evaluate four cycles of adjuvant chemotherapy versus therapy at the time of relapse in high-risk patients with pT3 or pT4 or node positive disease. To facilitate accrual to the study the design allows for the individual investigators to select among three different chemotherapy regimens: standard-dose M-VAC, high-dose M-VAC, and gemcitabine/cisplatin combination. The results of this appropriately designed and sized randomized trial are needed before any definitive conclusions can be drawn on the value of adjuvant chemotherapy.

Table 61.14	RANDOMIZED TRIALS OF ADJUVANT CHEMOTHERAPY AFTER CYSTECTOMY			
Author (Reference)	N	Standard Arm	Adjuvant Arm	Results
Skinner et al. (181)	91	Cystectomy	Cystectomy + CAP	Benefit, but few patients received planned therapy.
Stockle et al. (208)	49	Cystectomy	Cystectomy + M-VAC	Benefit, but limited trial size, premature closure, and no therapy upon relapse.
Studer et al. (209)	80	Cystectomy	Cystectomy + CDDP	No benefit.
Freiha et al. (49)	55	Cystectomy	Cystectomy + CMV	Benefit limited to relapse-free survival.
Bono et al. (12)	83	Cystectomy	Cystectomy + CM	No benefit.

CAP, cisplatin, cyclophosphamide, and doxorubicin; CDDP, cisplatin; CM, cisplatin and methotrexate; CMV, cisplatin, methotrexate, and vinblastine; M-VAC, methotrexate, vinblastine, doxorubicin, and cisplatin

Treatment Toxicity and Its Impact on Quality of Life

Once a diagnosis of bladder cancer has been made, the patient's major concern is related to the loss of his/her bladder, resulting in a loss of the voiding function. Because bladder cancer is a common geriatric malignancy, concerns about loss of sexuality are also present but usually are less prominent than those reported by survivors of other genitourinary malignancies. Early stages of bladder cancer (T1-2) initially are managed by surgical removal of the tumor via TURB, followed by adjuvant topical treatment, usually with BCG or with intravesical chemotherapy (13,14). These treatments are generally well tolerated with toxicity limited to malaise and bone marrow suppression in <20% of patients (11). At a careful self-assessment, however, patients undergoing these treatments tend to report decreased sexual desire and painful intercourse (163).

The prognosis and management of muscle-invasive tumors are very different, and they are often more likely to affect patients' quality of life than the treatment of superficial tumors. When radiotherapy is the primary treatment modality, acute complications mainly consist of bladder irritability, resulting from mucositis with decreased bladder capacity, which is manifested by frequency, urge incontinence, and dysuria. The commonly used radiation-dose range from 60 to 65 Gy, at 180 to 200 cGy per day, may result in gastrointestinal toxicity such as diarrhea (usually mild) and anal irritation. These problems are almost never severe and occur toward the end of the treatment course. Late morbidity, conventionally defined as that occurring 3 months after completion of radiation treatment, is the result of interstitial fibrosis and contracture as well as obliterative endarteritis of the vessel perfusing the bladder. It manifests itself as painless hematuria; chronic frequency; and, in 5% to 11% of the cases, as contracted bladder (169,172,175,180). When bladder contracture occurs following radiotherapy, a careful differential diagnosis is required because 50% of the patients experiencing severe complications are found to have local tumor recurrence as the main cause for their symptoms.

An important quality of life study after TURB, chemotherapy, and radiation therapy for invasive bladder cancer was reported by a group from Massachusetts General Hospital (240). Seventy-one patients were treated with a trimodality strategy and remained disease free with intact bladders, underwent urodynamic studies, and completed a quality of life questionnaire. At a median follow-up of 6.3 years, 75% patients had normal bladder function by urodynamic studies. Reduced bladder compliance, as a late complication of radiation, was reported in 22%. Other bladder symptoms were relatively uncommon with continence problems reported in 19%, with 11% wearing pads (all women). Only one half of the patients reporting continence problems qualified them as distressful. Bowel symptoms occurred in 22% of the patients treated, but only 14% recorded any level of distress. The majority of men retained sexual function. In patients treated with EBRT as part of the organ-preservation approach, approximately 50% retained sexual potency (99,103), whereas 70% of women generally were able to conduct a normal sexual life.

Measures of quality of life after cystectomy were compared to those after radiotherapy in two European cross-sectional studies (17,72). Both of these studies reported urinary function results comparable to those cited by the Massachusetts General Hospital study (240). Bowel symptoms were more common in patients treated with radiation, but the differences were not statistically significant. As expected the self-reported adequate erectile function was significantly higher in irradiated patients than in patients undergoing cystectomy (38% compared to 8% to 13%).

In the past two decades, in patients with muscle-invasive bladder cancers managed with surgery, toxicity of radical cystectomy and its impact on quality of life has substantially improved, reflecting the major progress of urologic surgery (68,225). Nevertheless, radical cystectomy impacts many aspects of patient's life including urinary, sexual, and social functions. Furthermore, patients were found to undergo surgery and often were not psychologically prepared for this adjustment. An interesting study was conducted in Norway in 59 patients who completed a questionnaire before radical cystectomy regarding their quality of life expectation following surgery. Forty-nine relapse-free patients completed a comparable questionnaire after a median of 36 months following cystectomy (45). Most of the study patients reported the need for significant adjustments in their professional and social lives. This study could be biased by the fact that original assessment of quality of life was undertaken at the time of cancer diagnosis and discussion about cystectomy. This period for most individuals represents a very stressful time and it may not be representative of the true baseline patient's quality of life.

An important measure to help prevent or minimize the severity of some of the problems associated with radical cystectomy is to offer patients appropriate preoperative and postoperative counseling. Such an important service can only be optimally provided in major centers, which specialize in uro-oncology (68,183). Especially during the first few months following radical cystectomy, incontinence is the main concern for most patients. Although incontinence is a known side effect of surgery and patients are well informed about such a risk, it tends to have a profound impact on patients' self-esteem and has a major impact on the extent of patients' participation in social activities. Concerns about incontinence have been reported to become severe enough to induce withdrawal and depression (127).

It is apparent that the type of surgical procedure dramatically affects patients' quality of life (185). A prospective study conducted to evaluate quality of life in a cohort of patients who had undergone continent and incontinent urinary diversion was reported in 2000 (67). Predictably, continent reservoirs were associated with higher quality of life scores. Similarly, in a study of 192 bladder cancer patients operated on within the prior 5 years, the quality of life among recipients of continent urinary reservoirs with those receiving a wet urostomy was compared. Statistically significant superiority of continent reservoirs regarding all stoma-related items, patient global self-assessment of their quality of life (single item, $p <.005$), physical strength, mental capacity, leisure-time activities, and social competence were demonstrated ($p <.05$) (54).

Few studies have addressed the impact on quality of life of bladder-preservation therapy compared to that of radical cystectomy. A comparison was made through a self-administered questionnaire of 29 patients treated by a conservative approach, based on radiotherapy with or without chemotherapy, and 30 patients who had undergone cystectomy followed by urostomy (17). The two treatment groups reported important differences in quality of life adjustment. Quality of life following cystectomy, marked by the presence of stoma, was reduced by a lack of sexual activity and a worsened physical condition, but social and recreational life was little affected. Conversely, a low incidence of urinary symptoms and an acceptable sexual adjustment were found among the patients managed with the conservative therapy. In this group of patients the physical, psychologic, and sociorelational adjustments were also good. All subscale scores of quality of life were higher in the conservatively treated group as compared to the surgery-alone group. A statistically significant difference was noted in four of the six subscales tested (17). Some of the presented quality of life problems following radical cystectomy are not as relevant in contemporary practice with a wide and routine use of orthotopic diversions in male and female patients.

The late morbidity of cystectomy inevitably tends to affect patients' sexual life, with female patients in most cases being able to cope better than their male counterparts. As a consequence of radical cystectomy in the female patient, she is often left with a narrowed or foreshortened vagina, resulting in possible pain, numbness, or loss of sensation during sexual intercourse. To prevent scarring and foreshortening of the vagina, it is important to stress to the patient the necessity for regular daily use of vaginal dilators. The use of lubricants during sexual activity often is needed to compensate for the loss of natural vaginal lubrication. Loss of lubrication is multifactorial—it is caused by reduced blood flow in the reconstructed vagina and results from iatrogenic menopause because both ovaries were removed during surgery. A study of sexual function after cystectomy in women showed that five of the six women investigated reported either ceased or decreased sexual activity (126). In another study the main complaints included inhibited sexual desire, dyspareunia, and vaginal dryness (162).

As a consequence of radical cystectomy, male patients commonly face erectile dysfunction resulting from transection of the nerves responsible for erection and loss of ejaculation. Erectile dysfunction was reported by 91% of patients in a study on sexual function in men following a standard radical cystectomy (161). Approximately one half of these patients remained sexually active and were able to achieve orgasm. Probably because the orgasm was not accompanied by ejaculation, diminished intensity of the orgasm was reported in 53% of the patients in this study. The important contemporary modifications of radical cystectomy permitted 60% to 70% of patients to maintain their potency (108).

References

1. Abdel-Latif M, Abol-Enein H, El-Baz M, et al. Nodal involvement in bladder cancer cases treated with radical cystectomy: incidence and prognosis. *J Urol* 2004;172:85–89.
2. Advanced Bladder Cancer Overview Collaboration. Neoadjuvant chemotherapy for invasive bladder cancer. *Cochrane Database Syst Rev* 2004(1), CD005245.
3. American Joint Committee on Cancer. Urinary bladder. In: *AJCC cancer staging manual*, 5th ed. Philadelphia: Lippincott-Raven, 1997:241–243.
4. Amling CL, Thrasher JB, Frazier HA, et al. Radical cystectomy for stages Ta, Tis and T1 transitional cell carcinoma of the bladder. *J Urol* 1994;151: 31–35.
5. Bassi P, Pagano F, Pappagallo G, et al. Neo-adjuvant M-VAC of invasive bladder cancer. The G.U.O.N.E. multicenter phase III trial. *Eur Urol* 1998;33(1):142 (abstr 567).
6. Bastus R, Caballero JM, Gonzalez G, et al. Small cell carcinoma of the urinary bladder treated with chemotherapy and radiotherapy: results in five cases. *Eur Urol* 1999;35:323–326.
7. Bell CR, Lydon A, Kernick V, et al. Contemporary results of radical radiotherapy for bladder transitional cell carcinoma in a district general hospital with cancer-centre status. *BJU Int* 1999;83:613–618.
8. Blandy JP, England HR, Evans SJW, et al. T3 bladder cancer–the case for salvage cystectomy. *Br J Urol* 1980;52:506–510.
9. Bloom HJG, Hendry WF, Wallace DM, et al. Treatment of T3 bladder cancer: controlled trial of pre-operative radiotherapy and radical cystectomy versus radical radiotherapy. *Br J Urol* 1982;54:136–151.
10. Bochner BH, Figueroa AJ, Skinner EC, et al. Salvage radical cystoprostatectomy and orthotopic urinary diversion following radiation failure. *J Urol* 1998;160: 29–33.
11. Bohle A, Balck F, von Wietersheim J, et al. The quality of life during intravesical bacillus Calmette-Guerin therapy. *J Urol* 1996;155:1221–1226.
12. Bono AV, Benvenuti A, Gibba A, et al. Adjuvant chemotherapy in locally advanced bladder cancer. Final analysis of a controlled multicentre study. *Acta Urol Ital* 1997;11:5–8.
13. Bouffioux C, Denis L, Oosterlinck W, et al. Adjuvant chemotherapy of recurrent superficial transitional cell carcinoma: results of a European organization for research on treatment of cancer randomized trial comparing intravesical instillation of thiotepa, doxorubicin and cisplatin. The European Organization for Research on Treatment of Cancer Genitourinary Group. *J Urol* 1992;148:297–301.
14. Bouffioux C, Kurth K, Bono A, et al. Intravesical adjuvant chemotherapy for superficial transitional cell bladder carcinoma: results of 2 European Organization for Research and Treatment of Cancer randomized trials with mitomycin C and doxorubicin comparing early versus delayed instillations and short term versus long term treatment. The European Organization for Research on Treatment of Cancer Genitourinary Group. *J Urol* 1995;153:934–941.
15. Brake M, Loertzer H, Horsch R, et al. Long-term results of intravesical bacillus Calmette-Guerin therapy for stage T1 superficial bladder cancer. *Urology* 2000;55:673–678.
16. Brown AL Jr, Zietman AL, Shipley WU. An organ-preserving approach to muscle-invading transitional cell cancer of the bladder. *Hematol Oncol Clin North Am* 2001;15:345–358.
17. Caffo O, Fellin G, Graffer U, et al. Assessment of quality of life after cystectomy or conservative therapy for patients with infiltrating bladder carcinoma. A survey by a self-administered questionnaire. *Cancer* 1996;78:1089–1097.
18. Calabro F, Sternberg CN. State-of-the-art management of metastatic disease at initial presentation or recurrence. *World J Urol* 2006;24:543–556.
19. Chan RC, Bracken RB, Johnson DE. Single dose whole pelvis megavoltage irradiation for palliative control of hematuria or ureteral obstruction. *J Urol* 1979;122:750–751.
20. Chang SS, Alberts G, Cookson MS, et al. Radical cystectomy is safe in elderly patients at high risk. *J Urol* 2001;166:938–941.
21. Chyle V, Pollack A, Czerniak B, et al. Adoptosis and downstaging after preoperative radiotherapy for muscle-invasive bladder cancer. *Int J Radiat Oncol Biol Phys* 1996;35:281–287.
22. Cole CJ, Pollack A, Zagars GK, et al. Local control of muscle-invasive bladder cancer: preoperative radiotherapy and cystectomy versus cystectomy alone. *Int J Radiat Oncol Biol Phys* 1995;32:331–340.
23. Colleselli K, Stenzl A, Eder R, et al. The female urethral sphincter: a morphological and topographical study. *J Urol* 1998;160:49–50.
24. Colombo R, Lev A, Da Pozzo LF, et al. A new approach using local combined microwave hyperthermia and chemotherapy in superficial transitional bladder carcinoma treatment. *J Urol* 1995;153:959–963.
25. Cooke PW, Dunn JA, Latief T, et al. Long-term risk of salvage cystectomy after radiotherapy for muscle-invasive bladder cancer. *Eur Urol* 2000;38:279–286.
26. Coppin C, Gospodarowicz M, James K, et al. Improved local control of invasive bladder cancer by concurrent cisplatin and pre-operative or definitive radiation. *J Clin Oncol* 1996;14:2901–2907.
27. Cox JD, Guse C, Asbell S, et al. Tolerance of pelvic normal tissues to hyperfractionated radiation therapy: results of protocol 83-08 of the Radiation Therapy Oncology Group. *Int J Radiat Oncol Biol Phys* 1988;15:1331–1336.
28. Crawford ED, Natale RB, Burton H. Southwest Oncology Group Study (8710): trial of cystectomy alone versus neo-adjuvant M-VAC and cystectomy in patients with locally advanced bladder cancer (Intergroup trial 0080). *Prog Clin Biol Res* 1990;353:111–114.
29. Cresswell J, Roberts JT, Neal DE. Urethral recurrence after radical radiotherapy for bladder cancer. *J Urol* 2001;165:1135–1137.
30. Daehlin L, Haukaas S, Maartmann-Moe H, et al. Survival after radical treatment for transitional cell carcinoma of the bladder. *Eur J Surg Oncol* 1999;25: 66–70.
31. Dalbagni G, Genega E, Hashibe M, et al. Cystectomy for bladder cancer: a contemporary series. *J Urol* 2001;165:1111–1116.
32. De Crevoisier R, Ammor A, Court B, et al. Bladder-conserving surgery and interstitial brachytherapy for lymph node negative transitional cell carcinoma of the urinary bladder: results of a 28-year single institution experience. *Radiother Oncol* 2004;72:147–157.
33. De Neve W, Lybeert MLM, Goor C, et al. Radiotherapy for T2 and T3 carcinoma of the bladder: the influence of overall treatment time. *Radiother Oncol* 1995;36:183–188.
34. De Neve W, Lybeert MLM, Goor C, et al. T1 and T2 carcinoma of the urinary bladder: Long term results with external, preoperative, or interstitial radiotherapy. *Int J Radiat Oncol Biol Phys* 1992;23:299–304.
35. de Wit R. Overview of bladder cancer trials in the European Organization for Research and Treatment. *Cancer* 2003;97(8 Suppl):2120-2126.,
36. Del Muro XG, Condom E, Vigues F, et al. p53 and p21 expression levels predict organ preservation and survival in invasive bladder carcinoma treated with a combined-modality approach. *Cancer* 2004;100:1867–1859.
37. Duchesne GM, Bolger JJ, Griffiths GO, et al. A randomized trial of hypofractionated schedules of palliative radiotherapy in the management of bladder carcinoma: results of medical research council trial BA09. *Int J Radiat Oncol Biol Phys* 2000;47:379–388.
38. Duncan W, Quilty PM. The results of a series of 963 patients with transitional cell carcinoma of the urinary bladder primarily treated by radical megavoltage x-ray therapy. *Radiother Oncol* 1986;7:299–310.
39. Dunst J, Sauer R, Schrott KM, et al. Organ-sparing treatment of advanced bladder cancer: a 10-year experience. *Int J Radiat Oncol Biol Phys* 1994;30:261–268.
40. Eapen L, Stewart D, Collins J, et al. Effective bladder sparing therapy with intra-arterial cisplatin and radiotherapy for localized bladder cancer. *J Urol* 2004;172:1276–1280.
41. Efstathiou JA, Zietman AL, Kaufman DS, et al. Bladder-sparing approaches to invasive disease. *World J Urol* 2006;24(5):517–529.
42. Fleshner N, Kapusta L, Ezer D, et al. p53 nuclear accumulation is not associated with decreased disease-free survival in patients with node positive transitional cell carcinoma of the bladder. *J Urol* 2000;164:1177–1182.
43. Fossa SD, Aaronson N, Calais F, et al. Quality of life in patients with muscle-infiltrating bladder cancer and hormone-resistant prostatic cancer. *Eur Urol* 1989;16:335–339.
44. Fossa SD, Aass N, Ous S, et al. Survival after curative treatment of muscle-invasive bladder cancer. *Acta Oncol* 1996;35[Suppl 8]:59–65.
45. Fossa SD, Reitan JB, Ous S, et al. Life with an ileal conduit in cystectomized bladder cancer patients: expectations and experience. *Scand J Urol Nephrol* 1987;21:97–101.
46. Fossa SD. Pelvic palliation radiotherapy of advanced bladder cancer. *Int J Radiat Oncol Biol Phys* 1991;20:1379–1382.
47. Freeman JA, Esrig D, Stein JP, et al. Management of the patient with bladder cancer. Urethral recurrence. *Urol Clin North Am* 1994;21:645–651.
48. Freeman JA, Tarter TA, Esrig D, et al. Urethral recurrence in patients with orthotopic ileal neobladders. *J Urol* 1996;156:1615–1621.
49. Freiha F, Reese J, Torti FM. A randomized trial of radical cystectomy versus radical cystectomy plus cisplatin, vinblastine and methotrexate chemotherapy for muscle invasive bladder cancer. *J Urol* 1996;155:495–500.
50. Fujii Y, Fukui I, Kihara K, et al. Significance of bladder neck involvement of progression in superficial bladder cancer. *Eur Urol* 1998;33:464–468.
51. Fung CY, Shipley WU, Young RH, et al. Prognostic factors in invasive bladder carcinoma in a prospective trial of preoperative adjuvant chemotherapy and radiotherapy. *J Clin Oncol* 1991;9:1533–1542.
52. Gad El Mawla N, El Bolkany MN, Khaled HM. Bladder cancer in Africa: Update. *Semin Oncol* 2001;28:174–178.
53. Garcia JA, Dreicer R. Systemic chemotherapy for advanced bladder cancer: update and controversies. *J Clin Oncol* 2006;10(24):5545–5551.

54. Gerharz EW, Weingartner K, Dopatka T, et al. Quality of life after cystectomy and urinary diversion: results of a retrospective interdisciplinary study. *J Urol* 1997;158:778–785.
55. Ghersi D, Stewart LA, Parmar MKB, et al. Does neoadjuvant cisplatin-based chemotherapy improve the survival of patients with locally advanced bladder cancer: a meta-analysis of individual patient data from randomized clinical trials. *Br J Urol* 1995;75:206–213.
56. Gilsersleve J, Dearnaley DP, Evans PM, et al. A randomised trial of patients repositioning during radiotherapy using a megavoltage imaging system. *Radiother Oncol* 1994;31:161–168.
57. Goffinet DR, Schneider MJ, Glatstein EJ, et al. Bladder cancer: results of radiation therapy in 384 patients. *Radiology* 1975;117:149–153.
58. Goodman GB, Hislop G, Elwood JM, et al. Conservation of bladder function in patients with invasive bladder cancer treated by definitive irradiation and selective cystectomy. *Int J Radiat Oncol Biol Phys* 1981;7:569–573.
59. Gospodarowicz MK, Hawkins NV, Rawlings GA, et al. Radical radiotherapy for muscle invasive transitional cell carcinoma of the bladder: failure analysis. *J Urol* 1989;142:1448–1454.
60. Gospodarowicz MK, Quilty PM, Scalliet P, et al. The place of radiation therapy as definitive treatment of bladder cancer. *Int J Urol* 1995;2:41–48.
61. Greiner R, Skaleric C, Veraguth P. The prognostic significance of ureteral obstruction in carcinoma of the bladder. *Int J Radiat Oncol Biol Phys* 1977;2:1095–1100.
62. Grossman HB, Natale RB, Tangen CM, et al. Neoadjuvant chemotherapy plus cystectomy compared with cystectomy alone for locally advanced bladder cancer. *N Engl J Med* 2003;349:859–866.
63. Hagan MP, Winter KA, Kaufman DS, et al. RTOG 97-06: initial report of a phase I-II trial of selective bladder conservation using TURBT, twice-daily accelerated irradiation sensitized with cisplatin, and adjuvant MCV combination chemotherapy. *Int J Radiat Oncol Biol Phys* 2003;57:665–671.
64. Hall RR. Neoadjuvant CMV chemotherapy and cystectomy or radiotherapy in muscle invasive bladder cancer: first analysis of MRC/EORTC intercontinental trial. *Proc Am Soc Clin Oncol* 1996;15:244(abstr 612).
65. Harada S, Sato R, Nakamura R, et al. The correlation between spontaneous and radiation-induced apoptosis in T3B bladder cancer (histological grade G3), and the precedence between the two kinds of apoptosis for predicting clinical prognosis. *Int J Radiat Oncol Biol Phys* 2000;48:1059–1067.
66. Hardeman SW, Soloway MS. Urethral recurrence following radical cystectomy. *J Urol* 1990;144:666.
67. Hardt J, Filipas D, Hohenfellner R, et al. Quality of life in patients with bladder carcinoma after cystectomy: first results of a prospective study. *Qual Life Res* 2000;9:1–12.
68. Hart S, Skinner EC, Meyerowitz BE, et al. Quality of life after radical cystectomy for bladder cancer in patients with an ileal conduit, cutaneous or urethral kock pouch. *J Urol* 1999;162:77–81.
69. Hautmann RE, Gschwend JE, de Petriconi RC, et al. Cystectomy for transitional cell carcinoma of the bladder: results of a surgery-only series in the neobladder era. *J Urol* 2006;176:486–492.
70. Hautmann RE, Paiss T. Does the option of the ileal neobladder stimulate patient and physician decision towards earlier cystectomy? *J Urol* 1998;159:1845–1850.
71. Hayter CRR, Paszat LF, Groome PA, et al. A population-based study of the use and outcome of radical radiotherapy for invasive bladder cancer. *Int J Radiat Oncol Biol Phys* 1999;45:1239–1245.
72. Henningsohn L, Wijkstrom H, Dickman PW, et al. Distressful symptoms after radical radiotherapy for urinary bladder cancer. *Radiother Oncol* 2002;60:215–220.
73. Herr HW, Bochner BH, Dalbagni G, et al. Impact of the number of lymph nodes retrieved on outcome in patients with muscle invasive bladder cancer. *J Urol* 2002;167:1295–1298.
74. Herr HW, Bajorin DF, Scher HI, et al. Can p53 help select patients with invasive bladder cancer for bladder preservation? *J Urol* 1999;161:20–22.
75. Herr HW. Surgical factors in bladder cancer: more (nodes) + more (pathology) = less (mortality). *BJU Int* 2003;92:187–188.
76. Holmang S, Berghede G. Early complications and survival following short-term palliative radiotherapy in invasive bladder carcinoma. *J Urol* 1996;155:100–102.
77. Holmang S, Hedelin H, Borghede G, et al. Long-term follow-up of a bladder carcinoma cohort: questionable value of radical radiotherapy. *J Urol* 1997;157:1642–1646.
78. Hoskin PJ, Saunders MI, Dische S. Hypoxic radiosensitizers in radical radiotherapy for patients with bladder carcinoma. *Cancer* 1999;86:1322–1328.
79. Houssett M, Dufour E, Maulard-Durtux C, et al. Concomitant 5-fluorouracil-cisplatin and bifractionated split course radiation therapy for invasive bladder cancer. *Proc Am Soc Clin Oncol* 1997;16:319–325(abstr 1139).
80. Huncharek M, McGarry R, Kupelnick B. Impact of intravesical chemotherapy on recurrence rate of recurrent superficial transitional cell carcinoma of the bladder: results of a meta-analysis. *Anticancer Res* 2001;27:765–770.
81. Huncharek M, Muscat J, Geschwind JF. Planned preoperative radiation therapy in muscle invasive bladder cancer; results of a meta-analysis. *Anticancer Res* 1998;18:1931–1934.
82. International collaboration of trialists. Neoadjuvant cisplatin, methotrexate, and vinblastine chemotherapy for muscle-invasive bladder cancer: a randomised controlled trial. *Lancet* 1999;354:533–540.
83. Jahnson S, Pedersen J, Westman G. Bladder carcinoma—a 20-year review of radical irradiation therapy. *Radiother Oncol* 1991;22:111–117.
84. Jemal A, Siegel R, Ward E, et al. Cancer statistics, 2006. *Ca Cancer J Clin* 2006;56:106–130.
85. Johnson DE, Lamy S, Bracken JRB. Salvage cystectomy after radiation failure in patients with bladder carcinoma. *South Med J* 1977;70:1279–1281.
86. Jose CC, Price A, Norman A, et al. Hypofractionated radiotherapy for patients with carcinoma of the bladder. *Clin Oncol (R Coll Radiol)* 1999;11:330–333.
87. Koch MO, Smith JAJ. Influence of patient age and co-morbidity on outcome of a collaborative care pathway after radical prostatectomy and cystoprostatectomy. *J Urol* 1996;155:1681–1684.
88. Konety BR, Joslyn SA. Factors influencing aggressive therapy for bladder cancer: an analysis of data from the SEER program. *J Urol* 2003;170:1765–1771.
89. Kovacs G, Hebbinghaus D, Dennert P, et al. Conformal treatment planning for interstitial brachytherapy. *Strahlenther Onkol* 1996;172:469–474.
90. Kurth K, Tunn U, Ay R, et al. Adjuvant chemotherapy for superficial transitional cell bladder carcinoma: long-term results of a European organization for research and treatment of cancer randomized trial comparing doxorubicin, ethoglucid and transurethral resection alone. *J Urol* 1997;158:378–384.
91. Lam DL, Blumenstein BA, Crissman JD, et al. Maintenance bacillus Calmette-Guerin immunotherapy for recurrent TA, T1 and carcinoma in situ transitional cell carcinoma of the bladder: a randomized southwest oncology group study. *J Urol* 2000;163:1124–1129.
92. Lam DL, Van Meijden APM, Akaza H, et al. Intravesical chemo- and immunotherapy: how do we assess their effectiveness and what are their limitations and uses? Proceedings of the Fourth International Bladder Cancer Consensus Conference. *J Urol* 1995;2:23–25.
93. Lara PC, Perez S, Rey A, et al. Apoptosis in carcinoma of the bladder: relation with radiation treatment results. *Int J Radiat Oncol Biol Phys* 1999;43:1015–1019.
94. Lara PC, Rey A, Santana C, et al. The role of Ki67 proliferation assessment in predicting local control in bladder cancer patients treated by radical radiation therapy. *Radiother Oncol* 1998;49:163–167.
95. Larsen LE, Engelholm SA. The value of three-dimensional radiotherapy planning in advanced carcinoma of the urinary bladder based on computed tomography. *Acta Oncol* 1994;33:655–659.
96. Leissner J, Ghoneim MA, Abol-Enein H, et al. Extended radical lymphadenectomy in patients with urothelial bladder cancer: results of a prospective multicenter study. *J Urol* 2004;171:139–144.
97. Leissner J, Hohenfellner R, Thuroff JW, et al. Lymphadenectomy in patients with transitional cell carcinoma of the urinary bladder; significance for staging and prognosis. *BJU Int* 2000;85:817–823.
98. Levinson AK, Johnson DE, Wishnow KI. Indications for urethrectomy in an era of continent urinary diversion. *J Urol* 1990;144:73.
99. Little FA, Howard GC. Sexual function following radical radiotherapy for bladder cancer. *Radiother Oncol* 1998;48:87(abstr 344).
100. Logue JP, Sharrock CL, Cowan RA, et al. Clinical variability of target volume description in conformal radiotherapy planning. *Int J Radiat Oncol Biol Phys* 1998;41:929–931.
101. Lohrisch C, Murray N, Pickles T, et al. Small cell carcinoma of the bladder. *Cancer* 1999;86(11):2346–2352.
102. Lopez-Beltran A, Pacelli A, Rothenberg HJ, et al. Carcinosarcoma and sarcomatoid carcinoma of the bladder: clinicopathological study of 41 cases. *J Urol* 1998;159:1497–1503.
103. Lynch W, Jenkins B, Fowler C. The quality of life after radical radiotherapy for bladder cancer. *Br J Urol* 1992;70:519–521.
104. Maciejewski B, Majewski S. Dose fractionation and tumour repopulation in radiotherapy for bladder cancer. *Radiother Oncol* 1991;21:163–170.
105. Madersbacher S, Hochreiter W, Burkhard F, et al. Radical cystectomy for bladder cancer today—a homogenous series without neoadjuvant therapy. *J Clin Oncol* 2003;21:690–696.
106. Malmstrom PU, Rintala E, Wahlqvist R, et al. Five-year follow up of a prospective trial of radical cystectomy and neoadjuvant chemotherapy: Nordic Cystectomy Trial 1. *J Urol* 1996;155:1903–1906.
107. Malmstrom PU, Rintala E, Wahlqvist R, et al. Neoadjuvant cisplatin-methotrexate chemotherapy of invasive bladder cancer. Nordic Cystectomy Trial 2. *Eur Urol* 1999;35:60(abstr 238).
108. Mameghan H, Fisher R, Mameghan J, et al. Analysis of failure following definitive radiotherapy for invasive transitional cell carcinoma of the bladder. *Int J Radiat Oncol Biol Phys* 1995;31:247–254.
109. Marshall FF, Mostwin JL, Radebaugh LC, et al. [illegible] post[illegible] continence and potency. *J Urol* 1991;145:502–504.
110. Martinez-Pineiro JA, Gonzalez-Martin M, Arocena F, et al. Neoadjuvant cisplatin chemotherapy before radical cystectomy in invasive transitional cell carcinoma of the bladder: a prospective randomized phase III study. *J Urol* 1995;153:964–973
111. Matsui K, Takebayashi S, Watai K, et al. Combination radiotherapy of urinary bladder carcinoma with chemohyperthermia. *Int J Hyperthermia* 1991;7:19–20.
112. McLaren DB, Morrey D, Mason MD. Hypofractionated radiotherapy for muscle invasive bladder cancer in the elderly. *Radiother Oncol* 1997;43:171–174.
113. Meijer GJ, Rasch C, Remeijer P, et al. Three-dimensional analysis of delineation errors, setup errors, and organ motion during radiotherapy of bladder cancer. *Int J Radiat Oncol Biol Phys* 2003;55:1277–1287.
114. Miller LS. Bladder cancer. Superiority of preoperative irradiation and cystectomy in clinical stages B2 and C. *Cancer* 1977;39:973–980.
115. Mills RD, Turner WH, Fleischmann A, et al. Pelvic lymph node metastases from bladder cancer: outcome in 83 patients after radical cystectomy and pelvic lymphadenectomy. *J Urol* 2001;166:19–23.
116. Miralbell R, Nouet P, Rouzaud M, et al. Radiotherapy of bladder cancer: relevance of bladder volume changes in planning boost treatment. *Int J Radiat Oncol Biol Phys* 1998;41:741–746.
117. Mohiuddin M, Kramer S, Newall J, et al. Combined pre- and postoperative adjuvant radiotherapy for bladder cancer: results of RTOG/Jefferson study. *Cancer* 1981;47:2840–2843.
118. Montie JE. Against bladder sparing surgery. *J Urol* 1999;162:452–455.
119. Moonen L, Horenblas S, Van Der Voet JCM, et al. Bladder conservation in selected T1G3 and muscle-invasive T2-T3a bladder carcinoma using combination therapy of surgery and iridium-192 implantation. *Br J Urol* 1994;74:322–327.
120. Moonen L, Ong F, Gallee M, et al. Apoptosis, proliferation and p53, cyclin D1, and retinoblastoma gene expression in relation to radiation response in transitional cell carcinoma of the bladder. *Int J Radiat Oncol Biol Phys* 2001;49:1305–1310.
121. Moonen L, Van Der Voet H, de Nijis R, et al. Muscle-invasive bladder cancer treated with external beam radiation: influence of total dose, overall treatment time, and treatment interruption on local control. *Int J Radiat Oncol Biol Phys* 1998;42:525–530.
122. Moonen L, Van Der Voet H, de Nijis, R, et al. Muscle-invasive bladder cancer treated with external beam radiotherapy: pretreatment prognostic factors and the predictive value of cystoscopic re-evaluation during treatment. *Radiother Oncol* 1998;49:149–155.
123. Moonen L, Van Der Voet H, Horenblas S, et al. A feasibility study of accelerated fractionation in radiotherapy of carcinoma of the urinary bladder. *Int J Radiat Oncol Biol Phys* 1997;37:537–542.
124. Muren LP, Redpath AT, McLaren DB. Treatment margins and treatment fractionation in conformal radiotherapy of muscle-invading urinary bladder cancer. *Int J Radiat Oncol Biol Phys* 2004;71:65–71.
125. Naslund I, Nilsson B, Littbrand B. Hyperfractionated radiotherapy of bladder cancer. *Acta Oncol* 1994;33:397–402.

126. Nordstrom GM, Nyman CR. Male and female sexual function and activity following ileal conduit urinary diversion. *Br J Urol* 1992;70:33–39.

127. Ofman US. Preservation of function in genitourinary cancers: psychosexual and psychosocial issues. *Cancer Invest* 1995;13:125-131.

128. Osen I, Fossa SD, Majak B, et al. Prognostic factors in muscle-invasive bladder cancer treated with radiotherapy: an immunohistochemical study. *Br J Urol* 1998;81:862–869.

129. Otto T, Borgemann C, Krege S, et al. Adjuvant chemotherapy in locally advanced bladder cancer (PT3/PN1-2,M0): a phase III study. *Eur Urol* 2001;39[Suppl 5]: 147–151.

130. Parkin DM, Pisani P, Ferlay J. Global cancer statistics. *Ca Cancer J Clin* 1999;49:33–49.

131. Parsons JT, Million RR. Planned preoperative irradiation in the management of clinical stage B2-C (T3) bladder carcinoma. *Int J Radiat Oncol Biol Phys* 1988;14:797–810.

132. Pernot M, Hubert J, Guillemin F, et al. Combined surgery and brachytherapy in the treatment of some cancers of the bladder (partial cystectomy and interstitial iridium-192). *Radiother Oncol* 1996;38:115–120.

133. Petrovich Z, Baert L, Boyd SD, et al. Management of carcinoma of the bladder. *Am J Clin Oncol* 1998;21:217–222.

134. Petrovich Z, Baert L. Natural history of bladder carcinoma. In: Petrovich Z, Baert L, Brady LW, eds. *Carcinoma of the bladder. Innovations in management.* Berlin: Springer, 1997: 15–22.

135. Petrovich Z, Emami B, Kapp D, et al. Regional hyperthermia in patients with recurrent genitourinary cancer. *Am J Clin Oncol* 1991;14:472–477.

136. Petrovich Z, Jozsef G, Brady LW. Radiotherapy for carcinoma of the bladder. A review. *Am J Clin Oncol* 2001;24:1–9.

137. Phillips HA, Howard GCW. Split course radical radiotherapy for bladder cancer in the elderly: nonsense or common sense? A report of 76 patients. *Clin Oncol (R Coll Radiol)* 1996;8:35–38.

138. Pointon RS, Read G, Greene D. A randomised comparison of photons and 15 MeV neutrons for the treatment of carcinoma of the bladder. *Br J Radiol* 1985;58:219–224.

139. Pollack A, Zagars G, Cole CJ, et al. Significance of downstaging in muscle-invasive bladder cancer treated with preoperative radiotherapy. *Int J Radiat Oncol Biol Phys* 1997;37:41–49.

140. Pollack A, Zagars G. Radiotherapy for stage T3b transitional cell carcinoma of the bladder. *Semin Urol Oncol* 1996;14:86–95.

141. Pollack A, Zagars GK, Swanson DA. Muscle-invasive bladder cancer treated with external beam radiotherapy: Prognostic factors. *Int J Radiat Oncol Biol Phys* 1994;30:267–277.

142. Pos FJ, Hulshof M, Lebesque J, et al. Adaptive radiotherapy of for invasive bladder cancer: a feasibility study. *Int J Radiat Oncol Biol Phys* 2006;64:862–868.

143. Poulsen AL, Horn T, Steven K. Radical cystectomy: extending the limits of pelvic lymph node dissection improves survival for patients with bladder cancer confined to the bladder wall. *J Urol* 1998;160:2015–2020.

144. Prout G, Marshall VF. The prognosis with untreated bladder tumors. *Cancer* 1956;9:551–558.

145. Quek ML, Stein JP, Clark PE, et al. Microscopic and gross extravesical extension in pathologic staging of bladder cancer. *J Urol* 2004;171:640–645.

146. Quilty PM, Duncan W. Primary radical radiotherapy for T3 transitional cell cancer of the bladder an analysis of survival and control. *Int J Radiat Oncol Biol Phys* 1986;12:853–860.

147. Redpath AT, Muren LP. An optimization algorithm for determination of treatment margins around moving and deformable targets. *Radiother Oncol* 2005;77:194–201.

148. Richie JP, Weichselbaum R, Greenberger J, et al. Twice-a-day fractionation preoperative radiotherapy in patients with carcinoma of the bladder: preliminary report. *J Urol* 1981;125(2):179–181.

149. Rietbroek RC, Bakker PJM, Schilthuis MS, et al. Feasibility, toxicity, and preliminary results of weekly loco-regional hyperthermia and cisplatin in patients with previously irradiated recurrent cervical carcinoma or locally advanced bladder cancer. *Int J Radiat Oncol Biol Phys* 1996;34:887–893.

150. Robinson P, Collins CD, Ryder WDJ, et al. Relationship of MRI and clinical staging to outcome in invasive bladder cancer treated by radiotherapy. *Clin Radiol* 2000;55:301–306.

151. Rodel C, Grabenbauer GG, Kuhn R, et al. Combined-modality treatment and selective organ preservation in invasive bladder cancer: long-term results. *J Clin Oncol* 2002;20:3061–3069.

152. Rodel C, Grabenbauer GG, Rodel F, et al. Apoptosis, p53, BCL-2 and KI-67 in invasive bladder carcinoma: possible predictors for response to radiochemotherapy and successful bladder preservation. *Int J Radiat Oncol Biol Phys* 2000;46:1213–1221.

153. Ross RK, Paganini-Hill A, Henderson BE. Epidemiology of bladder cancer. In: Skinner DG, Lieskovsky G, eds. *Diagnosis and management of genitourinary cancer.* Philadelphia: W.B. Saunders, 1988: 23–31.

154. Rostom YA, Chapet O, Russo SM, et al. Intra-operative electron radiotherapy as a conservative treatment for infiltrating bladder cancer. *Eur J Cancer* 2000;36:1781–1787.

155. Rostom YA, Tahir S, Gershuny AR, et al. Once weekly irradiation for carcinoma of the bladder. *Int J Radiat Oncol Biol Phys* 1996;35:289–292.

156. Rozan R, Albuisson E, Donnarieix D, et al. Interstitial iridium-192 for bladder cancer (a multicentric survey: 205 patients). *Int J Radiat Oncol Biol Phys* 1992;24:469–477.

157. Sanchez-Ortiz RF, Huang WC, Mick R, et al. An interval longer than 12 weeks between the diagnosis of muscle invasion and cystectomy is associated with worse outcome in bladder carcinoma. *J Urol* 2003;169:110-115.

158. Sauer R, Birkenhake S, Kuhn R, et al. Efficacy of radiochemotherapy with platin derivatives compared to radiotherapy alone in organ-spring treatment of bladder cancer. *Int J Radiat Oncol Biol Phys* 1998;40:121–127.

159. Sauer R, Dunst J, Altendorf-Hofmann A, et al. Radiotherapy with and without cisplatin in bladder cancer. *Int J Radiat Oncol Biol Phys* 1990;19:687–691.

160. Scholten AN, Leer J-WH, Collins CD, et al. Hypofractionated radiotherapy for invasive bladder cancer. *Radiother Oncol* 1997;43:163–169.

161. Schover LR, Evans R, Von Eschenbach AC. Sexual rehabilitation and male radical cystectomy. *J Urol* 1986;136:1015–1017.

162. Schover LR, Von Eschenbach AC. Sexual function and female radical cystectomy: a case series. *J Urol* 1985;134:465–468.

163. Schover LR. Sexuality and fertility in urologic cancer patients. *Cancer* 1987;60:553–558.

164. Schultz PK, Herr HW, Zhang ZF, et al. Neoadjuvant chemotherapy for invasive bladder cancer: prognostic factors for survival of patients treated with M-VAC with 5-year follow-up. *J Clin Oncol* 1994;12:1394–1401.

165. Sell A, Jakobsen A, Nerstrom B, et al. Treatment of advanced bladder cancer category T2 T3 and T4a. *Scan J Urol Nephrol Suppl* 1991;138:193–201.

166. Sengelov L, Klintorp S, Havsteen H, et al. Treatment outcome following radiotherapy in elderly patients with bladder cancer. *Radiother Oncol* 1997;44:53–58.

167. Sengelov L, Von der Maase H. Radiotherapy in bladder cancer. *Radiother Oncol* 1999;52:1–14.

168. Serretta V, Pomara G, Piazza F, et al. Pure squamous cell carcinoma of the bladder in western countries. *Eur Urol* 2000;37:85–89.

169. Sheils RA, Nissenbaum MM, Mark SR, et al. Late radiation cystitis after treatment for carcinoma of the bladder. *S Afr Med J* 1986;70:727–728.

170. Sherif A, Rintala E, Mestad O, et al. Neoadjuvant cisplatin-methotrexate chemotherapy for invasive bladder cancer—Nordic Cystectomy Trial 2. *Scan J Urol Nephrol* 2002;36:419–425.

171. Shimizu S, Shirato H, Kitamura K, et al. Use of implanted marker and real time tracking of the marker for positioning of prostate and bladder cancers. *Int J Radiat Oncol Biol Phys* 2000;48:1591–1597.

172. Shipley WU, Kaufman DS, Tester WJ, et al. An overview of bladder cancer trials in the Radiation Therapy Oncology Group (RTOG). *Cancer* 2003;97[Suppl 8]:2115–2120.

173. Shipley WU, Kaufman SD, Prout GR Jr. Intraoperative radiation therapy in patients with bladder cancer. A review of techniques allowing improved tumor doses and providing high cure rates without loss of bladder function. *Cancer* 2006;60:1485–1488.

174. Shipley WU, Prout Jr GR, Einstein AB, et al. Treatment of invasive bladder cancer by cisplatin and radiation in patients unsuited for surgery. *JAMA* 1987;258:931–935.

175. Shipley WU, Rose M. Bladder cancer. The selection of patients for treatment by full-dose irradiation. *Cancer* 1985;55:2278–2284.

176. Shipley WU, Winter KA, Kaufman DS, et al. Phase III trial of neoadjuvant chemotherapy in patients with invasive bladder cancer treated with selective bladder preservation by combined radiation therapy and chemotherapy: initial results of radiation therapy oncology group 89–03. *J Clin Oncol* 1998;16:3576–3583.

177. Shipley WU, Zietman AL, Kaufman DS, et al. Bladder-conserving therapy for invasive bladder cancer using transurethral surgery, chemotherapy, and radiation therapy with patient selection by initial treatment response. In: Petrovich Z, Baert L, Brady LW, eds. *Carcinoma of the bladder.* Berlin: Springer, 1998: 197–204.

178. Shipley WU, Zietman AL, Kaufman DS, et al. Invasive bladder cancer: treatment strategies using transurethral surgery, chemotherapy and radiation therapy with selection for bladder conservation. *Int J Radiat Oncol Biol Phys* 1997;39:937–943.

179. Shipley WU, Zietman AL, Kaufman DS, et al. Selective bladder preservation by trimodality therapy for patients with muscularis propria-invasive bladder cancer and who are cystectomy candidates—the Massachusetts General Hospital and Radiation Therapy Oncology Group experiences. *Semin Radiat Oncol* 2005;15:36–41.

180. Shipley WU. Transitional research in bladder cancer. *Int J Radiat Oncol Biol Phys* 1996;35:411–412.

181. Skinner DG, Daniels JR, Russell CA, et al. The role of adjuvant chemotherapy following cystectomy for invasive bladder cancer: a prospective comparative trial. *J Urol* 1991;145:459–467.

182. Skinner DG, Lieskovsky G. Contemporary cystectomy with pelvic node dissection compared to preoperative radiation therapy plus cystectomy in management of invasive bladder cancer. *J Urol* 1984;131:1069–1072.

183. Skinner EC. Quality of life with reconstruction. *Semin Urol Oncol* 2001;19:56–58.

184. Smaaland R, Akslen LA, Tonder B, et al. Radical radiation treatment of invasive and locally advanced bladder carcinoma in elderly patients. *Br J Urol* 1991;67: 61–69.

185. Smith DB, Babaian FJ. Patient adjustment to an ileal conduit after radical cystectomy. *J Enterstom Ther* 1989;16:244–246.

186. Smith DC, Montie JE, Sandler HS, et al. A pilot trial of concurrent gemcitabine and radiotherapy as a bladder preserving strategy. *Proc Am Soc Clin Oncol* 2000;19:360(abstr 1419).

187. Smith JA Jr, Crawford ED, Paradelo JC, et al. Treatment of advanced bladder cancer with combined preoperative irradiation and radical cystectomy versus radical cystectomy alone: a phase III Intergroup study. *J Urol* 1997;157:805–808.

188. Smith JA Jr. Summary of preoperative irradiation and cystectomy for bladder cancer. *Semin Urol Oncol* 1997;15:86–93.

189. Soete G, Coen V, Verellen D, et al. A feasibility study of high dose rate brachytherapy in solitary urinary bladder cancer. *Int J Radiat Oncol Biol Phys* 1997;38:743–747.

190. Stein JP, Cai J, Groshen S, et al. Risk factors for patients with pelvic lymph node metastases following radical cystectomy with en bloc cystectomy: the concept of lymph node density. *J Urol* 2003;170:35–41.

191. Stein JP, Clark P, Miranda G, et al. Urethral tumor recurrence following cystectomy and urinary diversion: clinical and pathologic characteristics in 768 male patients. *J Urol* 2005;173:1163–1168.

192. Stein JP, Cote RJ, Freeman JA, et al. Indications for lower urinary tract reconstruction in women after cystectomy for bladder cancer: a pathological review of female cystectomy specimens. *J Urol* 1995;154:1329–1333.

193. Stein JP, Dunn MD, Quek ML, et al. The orthotopic T-pouch ileal neobladder: experience with 209 patients. *J Urol* 2004;172:584–587.

194. Stein JP, Esrig D, Freeman JA, et al. Prospective pathologic analysis of female cystectomy specimens: risk factors for orthotopic diversion in women. *Urology* 1998;51:951–955.

195. Stein JP, Ginsberg DA, Skinner DG. Indications and technique of the orthotopic neobladder in women. *Urol Clin North Am* 2002;29:725–734.

196. Stein JP, Grossfeld GD, Ginsberg DA, et al. Prognostic markers in bladder cancer: a contemporary review of the literature. *J Urol* 1998;160:645–659.

197. Stein JP, Lieskovsky G, Cote R, et al. Radical cystectomy in the treatment of invasive bladder cancer: long-term results in 1,054 patients. *J Clin Oncol* 2001;19: 666-675.

198. Stein JP, Quek MD, Skinner DG. Contemporary surgical techniques for continent urinary diversion: continence and potency preservation. In: *Atlas of the urologic clinics of North America,* 9th ed. Philadelphia: W.B. Saunders, 2001;147–173.

199. Stein JP, Skinner DG, Montie JE. Radical cystectomy and pelvic lymphadenectomy in the treatment of infiltrative bladder cancer. In: Droller MJ, ed. *Bladder cancer: current diagnosis and treatment.* Totowa, NJ: Humana Press, 2001;267–304.

200. Stein JP, Skinner DG. Orthotopic bladder replacement. In Walsh PC, Retik AB, Vaughan ED, et al., eds. *Campbell's urology*, 8th ed. Philadelphia: W.B. Saunders, 2002;3835–3864.

201. Stein JP, Skinner DG. Radical cystectomy in the female. In: *Atlas of urologic clinics of North America*, 5th ed. Philadelphia: W.B. Saunders, 1997;37–64.

202. Stein JP. Indications for early cystectomy. *Urology* 2003;62:591–595.

203. Stein JP. The role of lymphadenectomy in bladder cancer. *Am J Urol Rev* 2003;1:146–148.

204. Stenzl A, Bartsch G, Rogatsch H. The remnant urothelium after reconstructive bladder surgery. *Eur Urol* 2002;41:124–128.

205. Sternberg CN, Pansadoro V, Clabro F, et al. Neo-adjuvant chemotherapy and bladder preservation in locally advanced transitional cell carcinoma of the bladder. *Ann Oncol* 1999;10:1301–1305.

206. Sternberg CN. The treatment of advanced bladder cancer. *Ann Oncol* 1995;6:113–126.

207. Stockle M, Gokcebay E, Riedmiller H, et al. Urethral tumor recurrence after radical cystoprostatectomy: the case for primary cystoprostatectomy? *J Urol* 1990;143:41–46.

208. Stockle M, Meyenburg W, Wellek S, et al. Adjuvant polychemotherapy of nonorgan-confined bladder cancer after radical cystectomy revisited: long-term results of a controlled prospective study and further clinical experience. *J Urol* 1995;153:47–52.

209. Studer UE, Bacchi M, Biedermann C, et al. Adjuvant cisplatin chemotherapy following cystectomy for bladder cancer: results of a prospective randomized trial. *J Urol* 1994;152:81–84.

210. Stuschke M, Thames HD. Hyperfractionated radiotherapy of human tumors: overview of the randomized clinical trials. *Int J Radiat Oncol Biol Phys* 1997;37:259–267.

211. Tester W, Caplan R, Heaney J, et al. Neoadjuvant combined modality program with selective organ preservation for invasive bladder cancer: results of Radiation Therapy Oncology Group phase II trial 8802. *J Clin Oncol* 1996;14:119–126.

212. Tester W, Porter A, Asbell S, et al. Combined modality program with possible organ preservation for invasive bladder carcinoma: results of RTOG protocol 85-12. *Int J Radiat Oncol Biol Phys* 1993;25:783–790.

213. Tobisu K, Tanaka Y, Mizutani T, et al. Transitional cell carcinoma of the urethra in men following cystectomy for bladder cancer: multivariate analysis for risk factors. *J Urol* 1991;146:1551–1555.

214. Tomic R, Granfors T, Modig H. Morbidity after preoperative radiotherapy and cystectomy in patients with bladder cancer. *Scan J Urol* 1996;31:149–154.

215. Van Der Steen-Banasik EM, Visser AG, Reinders JG, et al. Saving bladders with brachytherapy: implantation technique and results. *Int J Radiat Oncol Biol Phys* 2002;53:622–629.

216. Van Der Werf-Messing BHP, Menon RS, Hop WCJ. Cancer of the urinary bladder category T2,T3 (NxM0) treated by interstitial radium implant: Second report. *Int J Radiat Oncol Biol Phys* 1983;9:481–485.

217. Van Der Werf-Messing BHP, Menon RS, Hop WCJ. Carcinoma of the urinary bladder category T3NxM0 treated by the combination of radium implant and external irradiation: second report. *Int J Radiat Oncol Biol Phys* 1983;9:177–180.

218. Van Der Werf-Messing BHP, Van Putten WLJ. Carcinoma of the urinary bladder category T2,3NxM0 treated by 40 Gy external irradiation followed by cesium[137] implant at reduced dose (50%), *Int J Radiat Oncol Biol Phys* 1989;10:1641–1651.

219. Van der Zee J, Gonzalez D, Van Rhoon GC, et al. Comparison of radiotherapy alone with radiotherapy plus hyperthermia in locally advanced pelvic tumours: a prospective, randomised, multicentre trial. Dutch Deep Hyperthermia Group. *Lancet* 2000;355:1119–1125.

220. Van Poppel H, Lievens Y, Van Limbergen E, et al. Brachytherapy with iridium 192 in bladder cancer. *Eur Urol* 2000;37:605–609.

221. Van't Riet A, te Loo JH, Mak ACA, et al. Evaluation of brachytherapy implants using the "natural" volume-dose histogram. *Radiother Oncol* 1993;26:82–84.

222. Vazina A, Dugi D, Shariat SF, et al. Stage specific lymph node metastasis mapping in radical cystectomy specimens. *J Urol* 2004;171:1830–1834.

223. Vieweg J, Gschwend JE, Herr HW, et al. Pelvic lymph node dissection can be curative in patients with node positive bladder cancer. *J Urol* 1999;161:449–454.

224. Wallace DMA, Raghavan D, Kelley K, et al. Neoadjuvant (pre-emptive) cisplatin therapy in invasive transitional cell carcinoma of the bladder. *Br J Urol* 1991;67:608–612.

225. Walsh PC, Mostwin JL. Radical prostatectomy and cystoprostatectomy with preservation of potency. Results using a new nerve-sparing technique. *Br J Urol* 1984;56:694–697.

226. Warde P, Gospodarowicz MK. New approaches in the use of radiation therapy in the treatment of infiltrative-cell cancer of the bladder. *World J Urol* 1997;15:125–133.

227. Weiss C, Woltze C, Engehausen DG, et al. Radiochemotherapy after transurethral resection for high-risk T1 bladder cancer: an alternative to intravesical therapy or early cystectomy?. *J Clin Oncol* 2006;24:2318–2324.

228. Whillis D, Howard GCW, Kerr GR, et al. Radical radiotherapy with salvage surgery for invasive bladder cancer: results following a reduction in radiation dose. *J R Coll Surg Edinb* 1992;37:42–45.

229. Whitmore WF Jr, Batata MA, Hilaria BS, et al. A comparative study of two preoperative radiation regimens with cystectomy for bladder cancer. *Cancer* 1977;40:1077–1086.

230. Wijkstrom H, Norming U, Lagerkvist M, et al. Evaluation of clinical staging before cystectomy in transitional cell bladder carcinoma: a long-term follow-up of 276 consecutive patients. *Br J Urol* 1998;81:686–691.

231. Wijnmaalen A, Helle PA, Koper PCM, et al. Muscle invasive bladder cancer treated by transurethral resection, followed by external beam radiation and interstitial iridium-192 *Int J Radiat Oncol Biol Phys* 1997;39:1043–1052.

232. Wijnmaalen A, Van Der Werf-Messing BHP. Factors influencing the prognosis in bladder cancer. *Int J Radiat Oncol Biol Phys* 1986;12:559–565.

233. Woehre H, Ous S, Klevmark B, et al. A bladder cancer multi-institutional experience with total cystectomy for muscle-invasive bladder cancer. *Cancer* 1993;72:3044–3051.

234. Wolf H, Melsen F, Pedersen SE. Natural history of carcinoma *in situ* of the urinary bladder. *Scand J Urol Nephrol* 1994;157:147–151.

235. Wu CS, Pollack A, Czerniak B, et al. Prognostic value of p53 in muscle-invasive bladder cancer treated with preoperative radiotherapy. *Urology* 1996;47:305–310.

236. X-23 Figueroa AJ, Stein JP, Dickinson M, et al. Radical cystectomy for elderly patients with bladder carcinoma: an updated experience with 404 patients. *Cancer* 1998;83:141–147.

237. Xiong L, Viswanathan A, Stewart AJ, et al. Deformable structure registration of bladder through surface mapping. *Med Phys* 206;33:1848–1856.

238. Yu MC, Ross RK. Epidemiology of bladder cancer. In: Petrovich Z, Baert L, Brady LW, eds. *Carcinoma of the bladder: innovations in management.* Berlin: Springer, 1987;1–13.

239. Yu RJ, Stein JP, Cai J, et al. Superficial (pT2a) and deep (pT2b) muscle invasion in pathological staging of bladder cancer following radical cystectomy. *J Urol* 2006;176:493–499.

240. Zietman AL, Sacco D, Skowronski U, et al. Organ conservation in invasive bladder cancer treated by trans-urethral resection, chemotherapy, and radiation: results of a urodynamic and quality of life study on long-term survivors. *J Urol* 2003;170:1772–1779.

241. Zietman AL, Shipley WU, Kaufman DS, et al. A phase I/II trial of transurethral surgery combined with concurrent cisplatin, 5 fluorouracil and twice daily radiation followed by selective bladder preservation in operable patients with muscle invading bladder cancer. *J Urol* 1998;160:1673–1677.

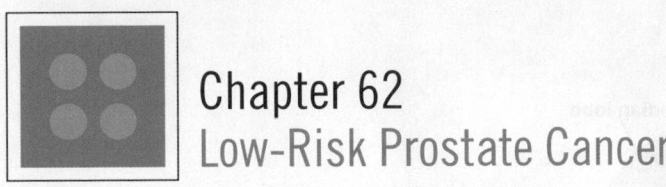

Chapter 62
Low-Risk Prostate Cancer

Michael J. Zelefsky, Richard K. Valicenti, Margie Hunt, Carlos A. Perez

Anatomy

Gross Anatomy and External Architecture

The prostate gland is an ovoid-shaped structure composed of fibrous, glandular, and muscular elements. It is located in the pelvis, adjacent to the rectum, bladder, dorsal and periprostatic venous complexes, pelvic sidewall musculature, the pelvic plexus, and cavernous nerves. Because of its shape, the prostate and the rectum curve away from each other as two convex surfaces. The prostate surrounds segments of the urethra before it passes through the genitourinary diaphragm (GUD) (Fig. 62.1). The male urethra is composed of five segments: the preprostatic urethra adjacent to the preprostatic sphincter; the prostatic urethra, which is from the verumontanum to the GUD; the membranous urethra as it courses through the GUD, which is surrounded by the external sphincter; the bulbar urethra in the penile bulb; and the penile urethra as it passes through the corpus spongiosum. The paired seminal vesicles are situated posterosuperiorly to the prostate gland and secrete seminal fluid into the bilateral ductus deferens as they become the ejaculatory ducts. These ducts transverse the prostate to join the urethra at the verumontanum (Fig. 62.1, right). At this point, the urethra changes it angulation by bending 30 to 40 degrees anteriorly.

The prostate is contained within a thin, fibrous adherent capsule that is structurally continuous with the stroma of the gland. The apex of the gland rests above the GUD. The GUD surrounds the membranous sphincter and may vary in length and thickness. The puboprostatic ligaments extend anteriorly from the surface of the gland to the pubic symphysis. The prostate is separated from the rectum posteriorly by Denonvilliers' fascia (retrovesical septum), which attaches above to the peritoneum and below to the GUD. It is this portion of the prostatic fascia that restricts posterior extension of prostatic carcinoma into the rectum. The lateral margins of the prostate are usually delineated against the levator ani muscles, forming the lateral prostatic sulci.

The anterior aspect of the prostate and the lateral pelvic floor are covered with the periprostatic fascia (Fig. 62.2). The endopelvic fascia lateral to the prostate gland contains neurovascular structures, including the venous plexus of Santorini, which is the primary drainage for the penis. This venous network, also referred to as the *dorsal vein complex,* covers the anterolateral surfaces of the prostate. The primary arterial blood supply to the prostate is via branches of the internal pudendal, inferior vesical, and middle hemorrhoidal arteries. The internal pudendal arteries also provide the blood flow to the penis. The nerves originate from the pelvic plexus, containing both sympathetic and parasympathetic fibers, and are distributed to the prostate, seminal vesicles, and the corpora cavernosa of the penis and urethra.

The prostatic apex is definable on diagnostic imaging and is important anatomically for radiation therapy treatment planning. Although the apex and the GUD, which surrounds the membranous sphincter, are easily visualized on coronal magnetic resonance imaging (MRI), it is important to recognize that the level of the GUD from the apex to the penile bulb may vary as Figure 62.3 indicates that the absence of an apical capsule contributes to the difficulty to discriminate the gland from the GUD during computed tomography (CT)-based treatment planning. Delineation of the neurovascular bundle is also limited on CT imaging.

Prostatic Zonal Anatomy

Zonal anatomy has essentially replaced lobar anatomy of the prostate. There are four zones of the prostate (Fig. 62.1): the peripheral zone (PZ), transition zone (TZ), central zone, and the anterior fibromuscular stroma zone. The central zone that surrounds the ejaculatory ducts has marked histologic differences from the PZ. It is the PZ, extending across the entire posterior surface of the gland, that is palpated on rectal examination and is the location of the most prostate cancers. The TZ is the location of benign prostatic hypertrophy. The anterior fibromuscular zone consists of an anterior band of fibromuscular tissue contiguous with bladder muscle and external sphincter. In young men, the PZ is the prominent zone, whereas the TZ becomes the dominant zone with age. It is important to note that there is no "median lobe" zone in this nomenclature, although such a "lobe" may be present in some prostate cancer patients and may have important implications for treatment planning and treatment selection. Histologically, the median lobe arises from the TZ or periurethral stroma, with varying proportions of fibrous, glandular, and muscle tissue.

Prostate Physiology

Histologically, the prostate consists of compound tubuloalveolar glands lined by two layers of cells. The glands are embedded in connective tissue comprising collagen and abundant smooth muscle that constitutes the prostatic stroma. This fibromuscular stroma functions both to control micturition by acting as a sphincter of the urethra and to express acidic prostatic secretions into the urethra by contracting during ejaculation.

The major function of the prostate is the production of seminal fluid that protects and nourishes the sperm after ejaculation. The prostate contributes approximately 30% to the seminal fluid, and the seminal vesicles, testicles, and bulbourethral glands provide the remaining 70%. Enzymes, including acid phosphatase and prostate-specific antigen (PSA), are secreted into the seminal fluid. PSA is a serine protease that is involved in the liquefaction of the seminal coagulum. Because PSA is produced primarily by benign and malignant prostatic epithelial cells and normally found at low concentrations in the serum, it is useful for prostate cancer screening and posttreatment monitoring of disease status.

The synthetic activity and growth of the prostate gland is regulated by androgens. The primary circulating androgen is testosterone. In the prostatic stroma, testosterone is converted to its active and more potent form, α-dihydrotestosterone, by 5-α-reductase. Secretory epithelial cells and stromal cells have intracellular androgen receptors. Dihydrotestosterone forms a complex with the dihydrotestosterone-binding domain of the

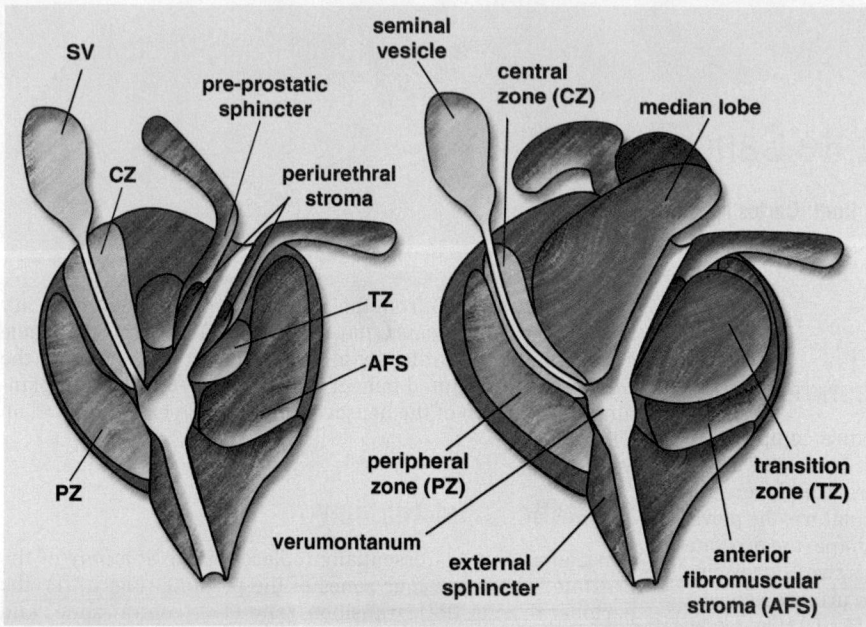

FIGURE 62.1. Zonal anatomy of the prostate. On the left, a young man with minimal transition zone (TZ) hypertrophy. Note that preprostatic sphincter and periejaculatory duct zone (central zone of McLean) are clearly defined. On the right, an older man with TZ hypertrophy, which effaces the preprostatic sphincter and compresses the periejaculatory duct zone. SV, seminal vesicle; CZ, central zone; AFS, anterior fibromuscular stroma; PZ, peripheral zone. (From McLaughlin PW, Troyer S, Berri S, et al. Functional anatomy of the prostate: implications for treatment planning. *Int J Radiat Oncol Biol Phys* 2005;63:479–491, with permission.)

androgen receptor, altering the structure of the DNA-binding domain such that it can reversibly bind DNA sequences known as *androgen response elements* in promoter or enhancer regions of androgen-regulated genes. The response includes stimulation of cell division, inhibition of apoptosis (programmed cell death), or cellular differentiation. In secretory epithelial cells, testosterone stimulation may result in the production and se-

cretion of prostatic fluid. These mechanisms are tightly regulated at many levels, from the hypothalamus secreting luteinizing hormone–releasing hormone to maintain testosterone levels in the blood, to the local regulation of 5-α-reductase in the prostate stroma. All of these factors acting at the same time determine the balance between cellular proliferation, cell death, and differentiation of a prostatic epithelial cell.

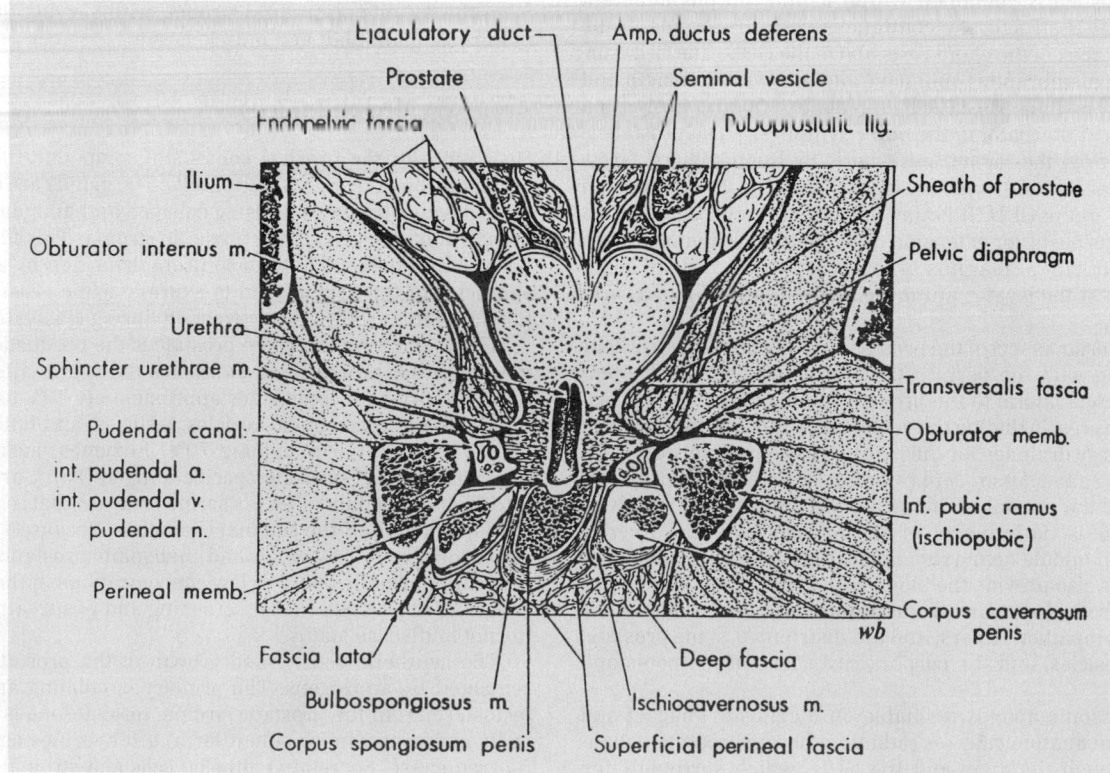

FIGURE 62.2. Frontal section of male pelvis at right angles to perineal membrane. (From Oelrich TM. The urethral sphincter muscle in the male. *Am J Anat* 1980;158:229–246, with permission.)

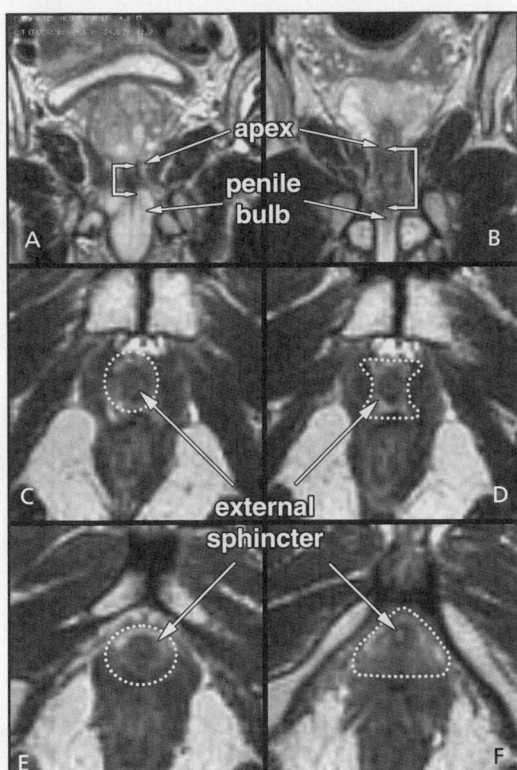

FIGURE 62.3. Variation in thickness of the genitourinary diagram (GUD) **(A,B)**. Levels of GUD from apex to penile bulb**(C–F)**. (From McLaughlin PW, Troyer S, Berri S, et al. Functional anatomy of the prostate: implications for treatment planning. *Int J Radiat Oncol Biol Phys* 2005;63:479–491, with permission.)

Epidemiology and Risk Factors

Clinical Incidence

Adenocarcinoma of the prostate is the most frequently diagnosed visceral cancer of men in the United States, accounting for 33% of nonskin cancers. The lifetime risk for American white and African American men is 18% and 21%, respectively. This corresponds with a lifetime risk of prostate-specific mortality of 3% and 5% (196,198). After large annual increases from 1988 to 1992, coinciding with the introduction of the PSA screening test, prostate cancer rates have leveled off since 1995 at approximately 140 per 100,000 men (Fig. 62.4). The overall incidence of the disease has more than doubled since 1985.

Perhaps because of widespread use of PSA screening and effective early treatment for localized disease, the age-adjusted death rates have begun to decrease. It was estimated that 234,500 new cases of prostate cancer would be diagnosed in 2006, but only approximately 27,400 patients would die of the disease. This compares with 189,000 new cases and 30,200 estimated deaths at the time of the last edition of this chapter in 2002. In 2007, carcinoma of the prostate may be surpassed by both colorectal cancer and lung cancer for causes of male cancer mortality.

Of the known or suspected risk factors for prostate cancer, the most important is age (Table 62.1). The median age at diagnosis is 68 years and the disease incidence escalates sharply with increasing age (11). The age-specific incidence for men younger than 65 years is only 51.7 per 100,000, but rises dramatically for men older than 65 years to 966.4 per 100,000 (293). According to autopsy data, 70% of men older than 80

years of age and 40% of men older than 50 years of age have pathologic evidence of cancer in the prostate (40).

Although the risk for development of histologic evidence of cancer in the prostate is fairly constant across countries and races, there is considerable variability in the incidence of clinically evident disease and mortality among different populations worldwide and in the United States (347).

The highest rates of prostate cancer are in Scandinavia, where it is the leading cause of male cancer death. The lowest recorded rates are in Asia. In the United States, incidence and mortality are higher among African Americans. A 30- to 50-fold difference in risk between African American men at the highest end of the spectrum and native Japanese at its lowest end has been reported. The mortality rates of prostate cancer in Japan have been dramatically increasing from 1960 to 2000, with differences between the United States, United Kingdom, France, and Italy decreasing (251). This increasing trend was noted for all age groups among Japanese males.

Risk Factors

Hormonal Influences

It is relatively well established that androgenic influences over time affect prostate carcinogenesis and disease progression (182). Generally, androgens are required for the development of prostate cancer, and it has been noted that men deficient in 2,5α–reductase are rarely diagnosed with benign prostatic hypertrophy or prostate cancer. In a study of 1,008 men, there was a positive correlation with plasma androstenedione levels and the development of prostate cancer (29). However, Gann et al. (132) found no clear association between individual hormone levels, including dihydrotestosterone, and the incidence of prostatic cancer. Yet, these investigators noted that high levels of testosterone in combination with low levels of the serum protein that binds testosterone, sex hormone–binding globulin, correlated with a higher risk of prostate cancer. Meikle et al. (263) observed a higher sex hormone–binding globulin level and a higher rate of testosterone synthesis in men with prostate cancer, compared with control subjects.

To date, the most conclusive evidence supporting the hormonal influence in the development of prostate cancer is from the Prostate Cancer Prevention Trial (407). This was the first large-scale, population-based trial testing the hypothesis that treatment with finasteride, which lowers intraprostatic dihydrotestosterone levels, prevents prostate cancer. In this trial, a total of 18,882 men, ≥55 years old, with normal digital rectal examination, and PSA level ≤3.0 ng/mL, were randomized to 7 years of finasteride (5 mg/day) or placebo. This study found that the prevalence of prostate cancer was reduced by 25% in men taking finasteride compared to placebo, with the prevalence of Gleason sum 7 to 10 tumors higher in the former group. It remains unclear whether this increase risk of high Gleason tumors is real or artifactual. Confirmations of these findings await the results of a second large-scale trial of another 5-α reductase inhibitor, dutasteride. This inhibitor affects both type 1 and type 2 forms of 5-α reductase, has antiandrogenic activity and promotes death in prostate cancer cell lines (231).

Dietary Influences

The development of prostate cancer may be attributed to both familial and environmental factors. Epidemiologic studies strongly suggest that a diet deficient in certain micronutrients is an important environmental risk factor. This has been supported through migration studies that indicate higher rates of prostate cancer in Asian men living in the United States compared with their counterparts in Japan or China (284,367). It

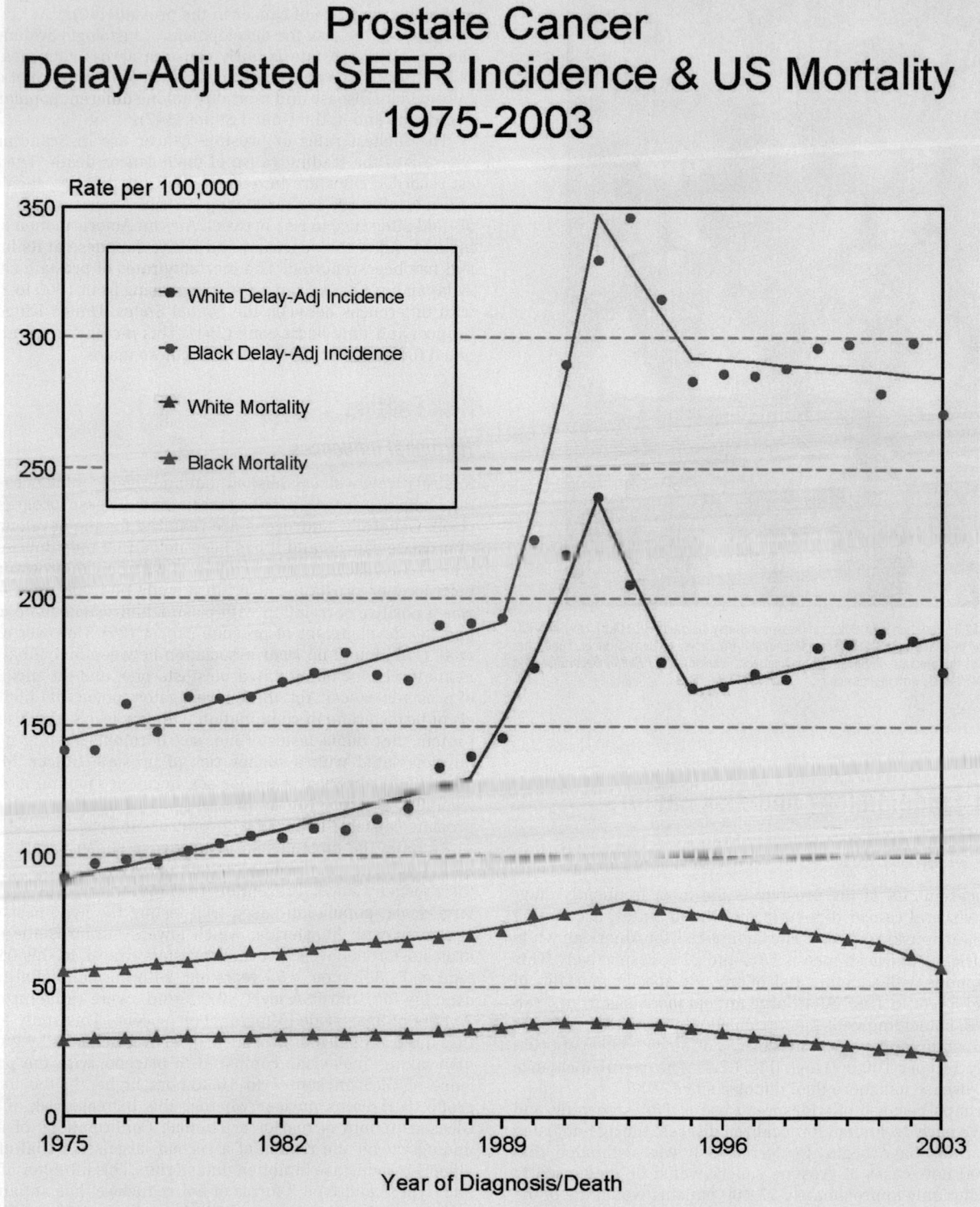

FIGURE 62.4. Surveillance, Epidemiology, and End Results (SEER) prostate cancer incidence and mortality rates, United States, 1975–2003. (SEER Cancer Statistics Review, 1975–2003. Available at: *http://seer.cancer.gov/cgi-bin/csr/1975_2003/, 2006.*)

has been postulated that nutritional factors play a role in stimulating the progression of microscopic disease. Salient features of the "Western diet" that differ from the traditional Asian diet are a high fat intake and low soy consumption. A Western diet has been associated with increased production of both androgens and estrogens, and a vegetarian diet with lower levels (176). There have been numerous case–control and cohort stud-

ies that have demonstrated an association between increased dietary fat intake and a higher risk of prostate cancer (122). Diets high in fat content may increase the relative risk of prostate cancer by a factor of 1.6 to 1.9 (207,365). In addition, several studies have shown that men with diets high in fiber and presumably lower in fat have a decreased risk of prostate cancer (275,370).

Clinical Radiation Oncology

| Table 62.1 | KNOWN OR SUSPECTED RISK FACTORS FOR PROSTATE CANCER |

Factor	Effect on Prostate Cancer Risk
Age	Increase
African American race	Increase
Geography	Scandinavia, high; Asia, low
Family history	Increase
Dietary fat	Increase
Agent Orange	May increase
Vasectomy	No effect
Benign prostatic conditions	No effect
Sexually transmitted diseases	No effect
Tobacco	Inconclusive data
Androgens	Inconclusive data

One prospective study (144) found that the type of fat intake was directly related to risk of prostate cancer. Red meat represented the food group with the strongest positive association with advanced cancer, with a relative risk of 2.64. Fat from dairy products (with the exception of butter) or fish was unrelated to risk. When analyzed by fatty acid type, only α-linolenic acid (an omega-3 fatty acid found in red meats and butter), not linoleic acid (omega-6 fatty acid found in fish oil), was implicated, with an increase in risk for prostate cancer of more than threefold. Conversely, a subsequent Canadian case-controlled study suggested that saturated fat consumption, not α-linolenic acid consumption, may play a role in prostate cancer progression (27). Finally, a Swedish study (163) of 406 men with prostate cancer and 1,208 without it (control subjects) demonstrated that body mass index and total amount of food consumed were independent risk factors.

Plant-based foods and their products, such as soy, tomatoes, cruciferous vegetables, and certain nutrients, are favorably associated with prostate cancer Frequently cited micronutrients that are related to prostate cancer development, progression, or mortality are summarized in Table 62.2. It is believed that these dietary factors contribute to antioxidant effects against DNA and cell damage.

Selenium is an essential trace nutrient that humans obtain through their diet of plants (related to soil composition, highest in Brazil nuts), animal products (highest in seafood), and present in nutritional supplements. There are experimental and epidemiologic data supporting the anticarcinogenic effects of selenium though apoptotic, angiogenic, or antioxidative pathways (69). Several large prospective studies have reported a 50% to 60% risk reduction in the development of prostate cancer in men with high levels of selenium as measured in their nails or plasma. Importantly, The Nutrition Prevention Trial identified a 50% reduction in prostate cancer risk in men blindly randomly assigned selenium supplements compared with placebo (112).

The beneficial effects of soy are attributed to isoflavones, one of several plant pigments found in soybeans. Isoflavones are a type of phytoestrogen, compounds that have weak estrogenic, antiestrogenic, and antioxidant effects that may all be protective against progression of prostate cancer in humans. These isoflavones, most significantly genistein and daidzein, have been shown to inhibit the growth of prostate cancer cell lines in nude mice (122). In particular, genistein has been shown to be a potent inhibitor of several steroid-metabolizing enzymes, such as aromatase, 5-α-reductase, and 17-β-hydroxysteroid dehydrogenase, as well as enzymes that are crucial to cellular proliferation, such as tyrosine kinase and topoisomerases I and II. Genistein is also an inhibitor of angiogenesis. It is estimated that Japanese men consume approximately 20 mg of isoflavones per day, whereas for Western men, the daily consumption is less than 1 mg/day. This is reflected in a mean plasma concentration of genistein of 180 ng/mL in Japanese men, compared with a level of <10 ng/mL for Western men (158).

Another protective nutrient is lycopene, prevalent in the Western diet, a carotenoid that is present in tomatoes, processed tomato products, and other fruits. It is one of the most potent antioxidants among dietary carotenoids. Although the antioxidant properties of lycopene are thought to be primarily responsible for its beneficial effects, other mechanisms may also be involved. In a review of 72 epidemiologic studies that investigated a link between cancer risk and consumption of tomato products, 57 linked tomato intake with a reduced risk; in 35 of those studies, the association was considered statistically significant (141). Two large, prospective studies reported a decrease in prostate cancer risk with higher tomato product consumption (139,279). Tomatoes were one of only four specific food items associated with significantly reduced prostate cancer risk in a prospective study of 14,000 Seventh-Day Adventist men (279). A prospective study (133) examined the relationship between the plasma concentration of several antioxidants and the risk for prostate cancer, using plasma samples obtained in the Physician's Health Study. Higher serum and tissue lycopene levels

| Table 62.2 | NUTRITIONAL RISK FACTORS FOR PROSTATE CANCER INCIDENCE, RECURRENCE, AND MORTALITY |

Food or Nutrient	Direction of Association with Prostate Cancer Risk	Direction of Association with Prostate Cancer Recurrence or Mortality	Overall Quality of Evidence
Selenium	Inverse		Strong
Tomato and lycopenes	Inverse	Inverse[a]	Good
Other carotenoids	Inverse	Inverse[a]	Good[a]
Vitamin E	Inverse (seen in smokers)	Inverse[a]	Good
Vitamin D	Inverse		Good
Calcium and dairy	Null to positive		Good
Red meat	Positive		Good
Fish/omega-3	Inverse	Inverse[a]	
Soy/isoflavones	Null to inverse	Null for PSA recurrence	Fair[a]
Tea/polyphenols	Null to inverse		Fair[a]
Zinc	Positive		Fair[a]
Heterocyclic amines	Positive		Fair[a]

[a]Limited data available.
Modified from Chan JM, Gann PH, Giovannucci, EL. Role of diet in prostate cancer development and progression. *J Clin Oncol* 2005;23:8152–8160.

were found to be inversely related to the incidence of prostate cancer development (134). In a recent meta-analysis of 21 studies, high intake of tomatoes was associated with a 10% to 20% risk reduction in prostate cancer, with lower risk due to cooked versus raw tomatoes (120).

Other micronutrients such as zinc and vitamins D and E have been studied and may have potential as chemopreventive agents (48,81,139,140,399). The data in support of these micronutrients are not as strong as the data in support of beneficial effects of selenium or lycopenes.

Familial Associations

Epidemiologic studies demonstrating familial clustering of prostate cancer were first reported in the 1960s (430). A large cohort study of the Utah Mormon population demonstrated a positive family history of prostate cancer in 6.6% of families of probands with prostate cancer and only 2.2% of families of probands without prostate cancer (430). A subsequent study using data from the Utah State Cancer Registry reported a familial relative risk of prostate cancer of 2.2 (55). Multiple studies have confirmed these findings, including a large case-control study from Johns Hopkins (384). Extensive cancer pedigrees were obtained from 691 prostate cancer cases and 640 spouse control subjects showing a twofold increased risk in men with a family history of prostate cancer in a single first-degree relative. There was a fivefold risk if there were two affected relatives, and the relative risk rose to 11 for three first-degree relatives with prostate cancer.

In a Canadian study (290), the frequency of prostate cancer detected in men who had a first-degree relative with a history of prostate cancer was 2.6 times greater than for men without such a history. Aprikian et al. (16), in a study of 2,968 patients, noted that prostate cancer was detected in 40% (1,300 patients) of men with a family history of prostate cancer, compared with 29% of 769 men without a family history (p <.0001). In a review of the epidemiology of prostate cancer, Giovannucci (139) reported that approximately 9% of cases may be attributed directly to a family history, although this may be as high as 43% among men younger than 55 years of age.

Despite the familial clustering of prostate cancer observed in these epidemiologic studies, causation cannot be inferred given the shared environmental factors among family members. Segregation analyses of cancer in multiple family members have been used to examine the role of genetic factors and inheritance patterns in prostate cancer. Segregation analysis is a statistical method used to determine the best-fitting model of inheritance for a particular disease in a study population. The largest segregation analysis of prostate cancer families suggested that the familial pattern was best explained by Mendelian inheritance of a rare, autosomal dominant gene in a subset of men with early-onset prostate cancer (57). The allele is highly penetrant, accounting for cancer by age 85 years in 88% of carriers compared with only 5% of noncarriers. Although this gene appears to be responsible for many of the early-onset cases, only 9% of all prostate cancers cases are in patients with this genetic predisposition, a percentage similar to that seen in both hereditary breast and colon cancers. Twin studies have also been used in the analysis of prostate cancer inheritance and have shown four to five times higher concordance rates for monozygotic twins (162).

Genetic and Molecular Influences

Researchers are now focusing on the molecular level to identify genetic alterations that may be involved in the multistep process of carcinogenesis. Progress in cytogenetic studies using polymerase chain reaction (PCR)–based polymorphism analysis has facilitated the identification of regions of the genome associated with various types of cancer. Linkage analysis is used to determine if there is an association between a particular genetic defect and clinical disease. There is ongoing investigation into the role of chromosomal deletions, oncogenes, and tumor suppressor genes in the initiation and progression of prostate cancer. Emerging data from analysis of DNA from high-risk families suggest that specific high-risk alleles exist for prostate cancer, as they do for other tumors. A major susceptibility locus for prostate cancer on the long arm of chromosome 1 (1q24-25) was identified through a genome-wide scan (372). The gene, *HPC1* (hereditary prostate cancer 1), has been linked to families with multiple members affected with an early average age at diagnosis (164). However, this association has not been identified in all studies. In addition to *HPC1*, six other loci have been studied (296). These six prostate cancer susceptibility genes with their alterations and phenotypic consequences are listed in Table 62.3.

Research delving into the molecular physiology of the prostate gland has also uncovered specific DNA sequences that may be related to the occurrence and progression of prostate cancer. It is well known that prostate cancer cells, like their normal counterparts, are usually sensitive to androgens, and their growth depends on androgen-stimulated cell division. Prostate cell growth is controlled by the interaction of circulating androgens, such as testosterone and dihydrotestosterone, with the androgen receptor. The androgen receptor gene contains a polymorphic CAG repeat sequence that encodes the portion of the receptor involved in DNA transcription. The length of the CAG repeat sequence was found to be inversely proportional to the activity of the androgen receptor; therefore, shorter CAG repeat sequences may be related to prostate cancer growth (68). Giovannucci et al. (145), in an analysis of the activity of the androgen receptor in men with prostate cancer, found that a shorter CAG repeat sequence in the androgen receptor gene predicts higher grade and more advanced stage of prostate cancer at diagnosis, as well as metastasis and mortality from the disease. Other studies found that the prevalence of short CAG repeats is higher among African Americans than whites (193), and that these sequences are longest among Chinese men (182). These findings may partly explain the higher risk for development of prostate cancer among African Americans and the lower risk in Asian countries.

In addition to these genetic alterations identified in prostate cancer, epigenetic changes such as abnormal DNA methylation have also been observed and may play a role in upregulation or loss of expression of genes (358). Millar et al. (278) have observed that abnormal methylation of specific sites throughout the genome of prostate cancer cells leads to loss of glutathione-S-transferase P1 (GSTP1) gene expression. The GSTP1 gene product is an enzyme that provides protection to mammalian cells against electrophilic metabolites of carcinogens and reactive oxygen species. Loss of GSTP1 may lead to a transition between proliferative inflammatory atrophy and prostatic intraepithelial neoplasia or prostate cancer (296).

Other Risk Factors

Chronic or recurrent inflammation may have a role in the development of prostate cancer, as has been recognized in many other human cancers. Although various microbial organisms have been identified to infect prostate tissue, the specific offending pathogen causing prostatitis has never been isolated. However, the specific cause may not be necessary as it is the host inflammatory response to an infection rather than the infectious agent itself that may lead to prostate cancer. In one large population-based study, prostate cancer risk was increased in men with a history of gonorrhea or syphilis (odds ratio, 1.6; 95% confidence interval, 1.2 to 2.1) (173). A criticism of such epidemiologic studies is the bias that men with symptomatic

Table 62.3 PROSTATE CANCER-SUSCEPTIBILITY GENES

Gene	Location	Alterations	Phenotypic Consequences
RNASEL	1q24-25	Base substitutions	Encodes endoribonuclease
ELAC2	17p11	Four-based deletion leading to premature protein truncation	
MSR1	8p22	Base insertion leading to premature termination	Unknown
		Base substitutions	Encodes subunits of class A macrophage-scavenger receptor
AR	Xq11-12	Polymorphic polyglutamine (CAG) and polyglycine (GGG) repeats	Encodes androgen receptor, and androgen dependent transcription factor
			Different polymorphic alleles may be associated with different transcription transactivation Activities
CYP17	10q24.3	Base substitution in transcriptional promoter	Encodes cytochrome P-450c17a, an enzyme that catalyzes key reactions in sex-steroid Biosynthesis
SRD5A2	2p23	Base substitutions	Encodes the predominant 5-α-reductase in the prostate, converts testosterone to dihydrotestosterone

Modified from Nelson WG, De Marzo AM, Isaacs WB. Prostate cancer. *N Engl J Med* 2003:349:366–381.

prostatitis compared with men without it are more likely to seek out care with urologists, have an increased serum PSA test, and have prostate biopsies (295).

Other risk factors for prostate cancer have been implicated, but have not been corroborated. Several reports have suggested an association between vasectomy and prostate cancer. In a prospective study of 10,055 vasectomized men and 37,800 non-vasectomized men, Giovannucci et al. (145) found an increased risk of 1.85 in the vasectomized men. In a retrospective study of 14,607 vasectomized or nonvasectomized men, the increased risk was 1.56 (142). A recent population-based case-control study of 923 new cases of prostate cancer among men aged 40 to 74 years from the New Zealand Cancer Registry showed no association between prostate cancer and vasectomy (87). Although there appears to be no definite etiologic relationship, it is possible that men undergoing vasectomy are more conscious of health care and more likely to be screened for prostate cancer (180). Circumcision has not been correlated with development of prostate cancer (349).

Armenian et al. (18), in a study of 296 patients with benign prostatic hyperplasia diagnosed either histologically or clinically and 299 age-matched control subjects observed from 7 to 27 years, found the incidence of prostatic cancer to be 3.7 times higher in the hyperplasia group than in the control group. This association was not observed by others (156).

Some studies correlated smoking with increased risk of prostate cancer (183), whereas another study did not find a significant correlation (125). In one analysis of 359 patients (104), a greater tumor-specific mortality rate among smokers than nonsmokers with stage A and D tumors was observed. No occupational factors have been confirmed as risks, but some evidence suggests that occupational exposure to cadmium and some aspects of farming may increase risks moderately, although these factors would account for only a small proportion of the total cases. Japanese men exposed to atomic bomb explosions in Hiroshima and Nagasaki have not had a significantly higher incidence of prostatic cancer (33).

Natural History

Local Growth Patterns

The studies of prostate morphology conducted by McNeal (261) showed that almost all prostatic carcinomas (>70%) develop in

the PZ of the prostate, whereas benign prostatic hyperplasia (>90%) arises from the TZ. In addition, examination of prostatectomy specimens revealed that small tumors tend to occur in the anteromedial gland, adjacent to the fibromuscular stroma, whereas larger, more advanced T stage tumors are often located in the posterior gland near the prostatic capsule (260,262).

Multifocality is characteristic of prostate cancer. On digital rectal examination (DRE), there may be one nodule or many, located unilaterally or bilaterally. Histologic and molecular studies of prostatectomy specimens of patients with prostate cancer have revealed that most contain a dominant or index tumor and one or more spatially separate, often heterogeneous tumors (47,52,155,330). Jewett (199) reported that multiple foci of disease were found throughout the prostate in 77% of prostatectomy specimens. Wise et al. (426) noted that only 17% of 486 patients treated by radical retropubic prostatectomy had one carcinoma detected by 3-mm step-section histologic examination. Of the 83% with multifocal disease, secondary cancers were mostly small; 58% were less than 0.5 cm³ in volume. Qian et al. (329), using fluorescence *in situ* hybridization to detect chromosomal abnormalities, found that an increasing incidence of chromosomal anomalies among specimens was positively correlated with progression from high-grade prostatic intraepithelial neoplasia to prostatic carcinoma. When lymph node involvement was present, there was usually evidence of one or more foci of the primary tumor sharing chromosomal anomalies with associated lymph node metastases, suggesting that just a single focus of carcinoma may give rise to metastases. This heterogeneity and multicentricity may account for the discrepancy between needle biopsy Gleason score and the grade determined from the dominant tumor in the prostatectomy specimen.

Tumors arising from the TZ tend to demonstrate a lower frequency of extracapsular extension and may harbor large volumes of disease with relatively high PSA levels but remain confined to the prostate. Despite a high PSA value (≥ 10 ng/mL), these tumors should be considered to have a favorable prognosis and managed accordingly. Noguchi et al. (299) described the histologic characteristics of 148 cases of TZ prostate cancer from radical prostatectomy (RP) specimens. Seventy percent were clinical stage T1c, with a preoperative serum PSA of 10 ng/mL or greater in almost two-thirds. Only 63% had a positive initial prostatic biopsy. On pathologic review, 80% had organ-confined disease and more than one third of cases had a cancer volume greater than 6 mL. When compared with 79

PZ cancers matched by volume, there were no differences in percentage Gleason grade 4/5, serum PSA, or prostate weight, although differences in clinical stage T1c to T2c and organ-confined cancer were highly significant. The actuarial 5-year PSA relapse–free survival rate was 71.5% among men with TZ cancer compared with 49.2% for those with PZ cancer.

PZ cancers tend to spread along the capsular surface of the gland, and may extend through the capsule of the gland, invade seminal vesicles and periprostatic tissues, and involve the bladder neck or the rectum. Clinical stage closely correlated with risk of extracapsular extension and disease progression (98,117,346). The incidence of microscopic tumor extension beyond the capsule of the gland (at the time of RP) in patients with clinically organ-confined disease ranges from 8% to 57% (63,414). Oesterling et al. (305), in an analysis of patients with stage T1c disease treated with RP, noted that 53% had pathologically organ-confined tumors, 35% had extracapsular extension, and 9% had seminal vesicle invasion. Of the last group, 66% had positive surgical margins, an incidence comparable with that for clinical stage T2 tumors. In a similar group of patients with T1c tumors, Epstein et al. (119) found that 34% had established extracapsular extension, 6% had seminal vesicle invasion, and 17% had positive surgical margins.

Pretreatment serum PSA is also predictive of extraprostatic extension and seminal vesicle invasion. The rate of organ-confined prostate cancer ranges from 53% to 67% for men with a PSA level between 4 and 10 ng/mL and from 31% to 56% for men with a PSA level between 10 and 20 ng/mL (209,010,017). D'Amico et al. (99), in a pathologic evaluation of 347 RP specimens, reported that none of 38 patients with PSA ≤4 ng/mL had seminal vesicle involvement, in contrast to 6% of 144 patients with PSA 4 to 10 ng/mL, 11% of 101 with PSA 10 to 20 ng/mL, 36% of 45 with PSA 20 to 40 ng/mL, and 42% of 19 with PSA >40 ng/mL. The incidence of positive surgical margins for these PSA subgroups was 11%, 20%, 33%, 56%, and 63%, respectively. The incidence of seminal vesicle involvement also is associated with the level of PSA, the Gleason score, and the clinical stage (100,387). Seminal vesicle involvement has been observed in from 10% of patients with A2 tumors to 30% of the patients with B2 lesions (60,416).

Roach (340) proposed a formula based on analysis of RP specimens to estimate the probability of extracapsular extension (ECE+) and seminal vesicle involvement (SV+):

$$ECE+ = 3/2\,PSA + (\text{Gleason score} - 3) \times 10$$
$$SV+ = PSA + (\text{Gleason score} - 6) \times 10$$

Regional Lymph Node Involvement

Tumor size and degree of differentiation affect the tendency of prostatic carcinoma to metastasize to regional lymphatics (127,319). With an increasing number of patients being diagnosed in earlier stages (as a result of screening PSA), there has been a decreased incidence of lymph node metastases in patients with clinical stage T1c and T2 tumors (307). In the low-risk prostate cancer patients, the risk of lymph node involvement is generally considered <10%.

Several groups (3,41,44,178,288,289,377) have developed models based on clinical or pathologic data that predict the risk of lymph node metastases. This information is important to decide whether a prostate cancer patient should be subjected to a staging lymphadenectomy (including laparoscopic technique) or considered for irradiation of the pelvic lymph nodes. Partin et al. (313) analyzed data from 703 patients and generated a nomogram for predicting nodal metastases based on three factors: clinical stage, preoperative PSA, and tumor biopsy grade. This model was validated in a larger multicenter study of 7,014 men and accurately predicted nodal metastases in 78% of patients (53). The negative predictive value was 99%. Bluestein

et al. (44) tested a model based on multivariate logistic regression analysis on 1,632 patients who underwent pelvic lymphadenectomy at the Mayo Clinic for staging of prostate cancer. Using this method, they determined that 29% of the patients with clinical stage T1a to T2c disease would have been spared pelvic lymphadenectomy with only a 3% rate of missed nodal metastases. Bishoff et al. (41) reported similar results demonstrating that 20% to 63% of patients with prostate cancer could be spared pelvic lymphadenectomy when accepting a 2% to 10% risk for missed nodal metastasis. These results suggest that many patients can be spared pelvic lymphadenectomy solely by analyzing preoperative PSA, Gleason grade, and clinical stage, without incurring an unacceptable risk for failing to identify regional metastasis (239).

Stock et al. (387), in a study of 99 patients who underwent laparoscopic lymph node dissection, correlated incidence of positive nodes with PSA, Gleason score, stage, and involvement of seminal vesicles. None of the patients with a Gleason score of 4 or lower, even those with PSA >20 ng/mL, had positive pelvic lymph nodes, and 8% in the group with Gleason scores of 5 or 6 and PSA levels of 4 to 10 ng/mL had positive nodes. However, the incidence of positive lymph nodes increased significantly (to 24%) in patients with PSA >20 ng/mL. These results are similar to those reported in patients treated with RP (44,313).

In an analysis of 2,144 patients treated at two institutions, Rees et al. (335) noted that only 30 (2.2%) of 1,390 patients with a negative DRE and either PSA of 5 ng/mL or less, Gleason score of 5 or less, or a combination of PSA <25 ng/mL and Gleason score of ≤7 had pelvic lymph node metastases.

Roach (340) suggested a formula based on pathologic findings in prostatectomy specimens to estimate the incidence of metastatic pelvic lymph nodes (Nodes+):

$$Nodes+ = 2/3\,PSA + (\text{Gleason score} - 6) \times 10$$

Prognosis is closely related to the presence of regional lymph node metastases; patients with positive pelvic lymph nodes have a significantly greater probability (>85% at 10 years) for development of distant metastasis than those with negative nodes (<20%) (135). However, a single nodal metastasis is not an unfavorable prognostic sign. In a study by Cheng et al. (73), 322 patients with positive lymph nodes after RP and bilateral pelvic lymphadenectomy were followed for a median of 6 years. Patients with prostate carcinoma who had multiple regional lymph node metastases had increased risk of death from disease, whereas patients with a single positive lymph node appeared to have a more favorable prognosis after RP and immediate adjuvant hormonal therapy. Prout et al. (327), in 92 patients with various stages of prostatic carcinoma, noted solitary lymph node metastasis in 11 (34%) of 32 patients with positive nodes. Bilateral pelvic lymph node involvement was present in 14 (58%) of 24 patients who had more than one metastatic lymph node. Only 2 (18%) of 11 patients with a single metastasis showed tumor progression, compared with 15 (76%) of 21 with multiple lymph node involvement. Golimbu et al. (150) noted a 10-year survival rate of 50% in patients with a single positive lymph node, compared with 20% for those with multiple lymph node involvement.

The prognostic significance of multiple involved lymph nodes should be considered with the extent of lymphadenectomy. Two recent studies have evaluated the anatomic extent of pelvic lymph node dissection on outcome (9,103). At Johns Hopkins University Hospital, two surgeons performed 4,000 radical prostatectomies with or without an extended lymph node dissection. The extended dissection removed more lymph nodes (mean 12 vs. 9; $p < .0001$) and detected more lymph node positive prostate cancer (3.2% vs 1.1%; $p < .0001$) than more limited procedure. If disease was found involving <15% of the extracted lymph nodes, extended lymph node dissection resulted in a more favorable 5-year PSA progression-free survival. Thus, in certain subgroups, an extended dissection may be beneficial. In another study, the number and percent of involved lymph nodes correlated with recurrence-free and overall survival (103). These results need additional validation in prospectively controlled studies.

Clinical Presentation and Diagnostic Work-Up

Screening Methods and Markers

Although DRE is still an essential element in screening and assigning clinical stage, only 25% to 50% of men with an abnormal DRE have cancer on biopsy. Moreover, because carcinoma of the prostate can be asymptomatic until attaining a significant size, if a patient presents with a palpable tumor, there is a significant risk that there already may be locally advanced or metastatic disease. With the advent of PSA screening, the diagnosis of prostate cancer may precede palpable disease on DRE and the symptoms of urinary obstruction or metastatic disease by many years. DRE is associated with 70% sensitivity and 50% specificity (59). In fact, 70% of cancers detected by PSA screening are confined to the prostate and 40% of cancers detected by PSA are not palpable (63). Nevertheless, the DRE should be used in combination with PSA screening because 25% of prostate cancers occur in men with normal PSA levels (22). The American Cancer Society, the American College of Radiology, and the American Urological Association recommend annual DRE and PSA screening test for men older than 50 years of age if their life expectancy is >10 years (22). For African American men or patients with a significant family history of prostate cancer, screening should be initiated at age 45 years (133).

PSA, initially identified and purified from prostatic tissue by Wang et al. (419) in 1979, is a protein with a molecular weight of 33,000. PSA is detected not only in prostatic tissue (normal tissue, benign hyperplasia, and malignant tumors) and in seminal fluid but in the sera of patients with prostatic cancer. It is localized in the cytoplasm of ductal epithelial cells and in secretory materials in ductal lamina (311). PSA has been detected with immunohistochemical techniques in pancreas and salivary glands and in women; therefore, it is not absolutely specific for prostatic epithelium (115). Although historically the normal value of PSA is 0.4 to 4 ng/mL for white males younger than 70 years old, it has been recently recommended that this upper limit of normal PSA level be adjusted to 2.6 ng/mL (328). Punglia et al. (328) carried out a logistic-regression analysis of 705 men who underwent a prostate biopsy in order to assess the probability of detecting prostate cancer in all the men studied in the cohort. They found that if biopsies were done only when the PSA value was >4.0 ng/mL, 82% of the cancers would have been missed. However, this recommendation should be taken with caution and is not ready for routine clinical practice because lowering the PSA threshold would potentially lead to overdiagnosis and overtreatment. In the absence of a randomized trial, it still remains unclear whether screening reduces mortality from prostate cancer.

Radioimmunoassays for prostatic acid phosphatase (PAP) have a sensitivity of approximately 10% and a specificity of about 90% for malignant tumors (59) and to a large extent have been superseded by PSA testing.

Stamey et al. (382) reported PSA and PAP measurements by radioimmunoassay in 2,200 serum samples from 699 patients, 378 of whom were known to have prostatic carcinoma. PSA was elevated in 122 of 127 patients with newly diagnosed prostatic carcinoma, whereas PAP was elevated in only 57 patients

with cancer and correlated less closely with tumor volume than did PSA. PSA was increased in 86% and PAP in 14% of the patients with benign prostatic hyperplasia. After RP for cancer, PSA routinely declines to undetectable levels, with an associated half-life of 2.2 days. PAP, if initially elevated, normalizes within 24 hours after surgery. Several authors concluded that PSA is more sensitive than PAP and DRE in the detection of prostatic carcinoma, and that PSA would be more useful in monitoring response and recurrence after therapy (187,360,382). A caveat is that both PSA and PAP may be elevated in benign prostatic hyperplasia. Hudson et al. (187) reported that only 3% of 168 men with benign prostatic hyperplasia had PSA levels >10 ng/mL, compared with 44% of 231 patients with prostatic carcinoma.

Several investigators (256,364,440) reported no significant impact of DRE on the plasma levels of PSA or PAP in patients with various prostatic abnormalities in whom blood samples were collected before, immediately after, and 30 minutes after rectal examination of the prostate. Others (83,232,310) have detected a significant increase in PSA after DRE. Ornstein et al. (310) noted an increase in both total and free PSA in 31% and 48% of men, respectively, at 1 hour after DRE. Matzkin et al. (254) found no significant change in PSA levels after inserting a urethral catheter and maintaining it for several days. Yet, significant PSA elevation has been demonstrated after prostatic massage, transrectal ultrasonography (TRUS), prostate biopsy, and transurethral resection of the prostate (TURP) (83,211,304,440). The kinetics of serum PSA elevation after DRE and needle biopsy were investigated in a Dutch study with few participants (46). Blood samples were taken at 1 minute, 30 minutes, 1, 3, 6, and 12 hours, and then every 24 hours until 5 days had elapsed. The peak levels were between 30 and 60 minutes after DRE and returned to baseline 24 to 72 hours after the examination. There was a threefold increase in PSA after needle biopsy, and only two of seven patients had returned to their baseline PSA at 5 days. Studies reporting the effect of ejaculation on PSA also have contradictory results. Some authors found no effect at all (174,385), whereas others have demonstrated that ejaculation increased PSA levels in 87% of 64 men evaluated with serial determinations (at 1, 6, 24, and 48 hours) (400). A return to baseline was observed in 92% of subjects by 24 hours and in 97% by 48 hours.

Nadler et al. (285) quantified causes of elevated PSA in 148 men with PSA >4 ng/mL (a finding suspect for cancer) and multiple negative biopsies. They were compared with 64 men who had a suspect DRE, multiple negative biopsies, and PSA of ≤4 ng/mL. Acute or chronic inflammation of the prostate was more prevalent in the high PSA group (63% vs. 27%; $p = .0001$). Patients with elevated PSA had significantly larger prostate volumes (median, 68 cm^3) than those without PSA elevation (median, 32.5 cm^3). Simultaneous regression analysis demonstrated that prostatic size accounted for 23%, inflammation for 7%, prostatic calculi for 3%, and nonisoechoic ultrasonographic lesions for 1% of the PSA serum variances.

The positive predictive value for PSA >4 ng/mL ranges from 31% to 54%. A greater yield is observed when elevated PSA is coupled with positive ultrasonographic and rectal examinations (111) (Table 62.4). The estimated rate of cancer detection by PSA screening ranges from 1.8% to 3.3%. The percentage of clinically localized tumors detected by PSA ranges from 81% to 97%. The percentage of pathologically localized tumors has ranged from 36% to 91%, and is significantly higher when serial PSA screening is done.

An important issue is the clinical significance of small tumors detected by PSA testing. Epstein et al. (118,119) identified subset of patients with potentially biologically insignificant tumors among men with clinical stage T1c disease who underwent RP. On multivariate analysis, the best model predicting insignificant tumor was PSA density <0.1 ng/mL per gram and no adverse pathologic findings on needle biopsy, or PSA density of 0.1 to

Table 62.4 | LIKELIHOOD OF DETECTING PROSTATE CANCER ON TRANSRECTAL BIOPSY FOR 2,054 MEN, AGED 40 TO 80 YEARS[a]

A. As a function of serum PSA level, independent of DRE result

PSA (ng/mL)	Age[b] (Yr)			
	<50	51–60	61–70	>71
<2.5	10	14	17	23
2.6–4.0	11	15	19	24
4.1–6.0	12	16	21	26
6.1–10.0	14	18	23	29
10.1–20.0	17	23	31	37
>20.0	40	49	60	69

B. As a function of patient age, serum PSA level, and DRE findings

PSA (ng/mL)	Age(Yr)							
	<50		51–60		61–70		71–80	
	DRE−	DRE+	DRE−	DRE+	DRE−	DRE+	DRE−	DRE+
<2.5	9	37	12	39	15	42	20	44
2.6–4.0	9	41	12	42	16	44	20	47
4.1–6.0	10	41	14	44	17	47	22	48
6.1–10.0	11	—	15	48	19	50	25	42
10.1–20.0	13	55	19	54	25	58	31	60
>20.0	22	82	45	74	43	81	59	84

PSA, prostate-specific antigen; DRE, digital rectal examination.
[a]Ninety-five percent confidence intervals are within 2% to 12% for all probabilities.
[b]Recorded at time of PSA collection.
From Potter SR, Horniger W, Tinzl M, et al. Age, prostate-specific antigen, and digital rectal examination as determinants of the probability of having prostate cancer. *Urology* 2001;57:1100–1104, with permission.

0.15 ng/mL per gram, with a low- to intermediate-grade cancer smaller than 3 mm found in only one needle biopsy core specimen. The positive predictive value of the model was 95%, with a negative predictive value of 66% (119). Dugan et al. (113) offered a definition of clinically insignificant cancer as a tumor that gives rise to no more than 20 cm³ of cancerous tissue in the prostate by the time of expected death and a Gleason score of <4 in patients 40 years old, 5 in 50- to 59-year-old patients, 6 in 60- to 69-year-old patients, and 7 in 70- to 79-year-old patients. Using these definitions, a review of 337 prostatectomy specimens showed that, for cancer volume doubling times of 2, 3, 4, and 6 years, clinically insignificant cancer was identified in 1 (0.3%), 13 (3.9%), 25 (7.4%), and 49 (14.5%) of specimens, respectively. Humphrey et al. (189) determined that in 11% to 30% of PSA-detected prostate cancers, the tumor volumes were <0.5 mL. Therefore, by these definitions, most men treated with RP (or radiation therapy) have clinically significant cancer.

The incidence of clinically unimportant cancers has been reported to be between 4% and 16% (119,154,306,404). Researchers at the Fred Hutchinson Cancer Center developed a computer model to estimate the rates of prostate cancer overdiagnosis because of PSA testing. Using the National Cancer Institute's Surveillance, Epidemiology, and End Results registry data as a comparison for their computer-generated incidence rates, they calculated overdiagnosis rates of 15% in whites and 37% in blacks. These men were predicted to have prostate cancer that would be detected only at autopsy (121). Conversely, an epidemiologic study randomizing men from Göteborg, Sweden, to PSA screening or a control group, demonstrated that screening did not lead to overdiagnosis of prostate cancer; rather, most cancers detected at PSA-guided screening would eventually develop into clinical, frequently fatal, disease (188).

Although PSA screening–detected cancers may be smaller, they may harbor aggressive disease. Investigators from the Netherlands studied 121 RP specimens from screened patients and found that screening-detected specimens were more likely to be pathologically organ-confined tumors and to have Gleason scores of <8 (177). However, 60% of screening-detected tumors contained areas with high-grade cancer (Gleason pattern 4 or 5) and 50% had a Gleason score of 7, suggesting that most of these tumors are clinically important. Preliminary results from a study of expectant management of patients with nonpalpable prostate cancer thought to have small-volume disease showed a 31% progression rate with a median follow-up of 23 months (58). Increased PSA density and decreased percentage free PSA correlated with progression of disease. Ninety-two percent of patients had curable disease at the time of their diagnosis of progression. These investigators conclude that observation with close follow-up may be a reasonable alternative for older men with a high likelihood of harboring small-volume prostate cancer.

Refinements of the PSA screening test have been introduced to increase the sensitivity and specificity of the test. It was anticipated that such approaches would be able to more readily find curable cancers in younger men and to avoid unnecessary biopsies of benign hypertrophic disease in older men. Unfortunately, none of these modifications listed in the following sections has proven reliable enough alone to base a treatment decision for the individual patient.

Prostate-Specific Antigen Density

PSA density relies on the fact that cancers produce less PSA per cell than nonmalignant prostatic tissues. It is calculated by dividing the serum PSA concentration by the volume of the prostate gland measured by TRUS. A higher PSA density is associated with malignancy.

Prostate-Specific Antigen Velocity

Another method is to obtain serial PSA measurements and calculate the rate of rise in PSA, or PSA velocity. A rate of rise of >0.75 ng/mL per year has been associated with a higher frequency of cancer. The Prostate Cancer Prevention Trial provides an opportunity to examine the risk of prostate cancer in men with a PSA value <4.0 ng/mL. In a recent secondary analysis, the investigators evaluate the significance of prediagnosis PSA velocity in assessing prostate cancer risk (406). They evaluated 20 different definitions of PSA velocity. PSA velocity did not contribute independent prognostic information. Only higher PSA level, abnormal DRE results, older age at biopsy, and African American race were predictive for high-grade disease (Gleason score ≥7). The value of prediagnosis PSA velocity has yet to be determined.

Free Prostate-Specific Antigen

Serum tests for the molecular forms of PSA (free versus complexed versus total) have been developed to discriminate between elevated PSA levels from benign prostatic hyperplasia versus cancer. This is based on the concept that PSA exists in serum in a complexed form bound to either α_1-antichymotrypsin or α_2-macroglobulin, two extracellular protease inhibitors. Bound to α_1-antichymotrypsin or α_2-macroglobulin, the enzyme is inactive but still detectable using conventional immunoassays. In a study of free PSA, complexed PSA, and total PSA (free + complexed), the complexed-to-total ratio was higher and free PSA lower in patients with prostate cancer relative to those with benign prostatic hyperplasia (247). Catalona et al. (64) reported on 113 patients with PSA levels between 4.1 and 10 ng/mL (63 with histologically confirmed benign prostatic hyperplasia, 30 with prostate cancer and enlarged gland, and 20 with cancer and a normal-sized gland). The median percentage of free PSA was 9.2% for men with cancer and a normal-sized gland, 15.9% for those with cancer and an enlarged gland, and 18.8% for those with benign prostatic hyperplasia (p <.001). Men with prostate cancer and either a normal or an enlarged gland had a significantly lower percentage of free PSA than men with benign prostatic hyperplasia only. At Washington University, a ratio of free to total PSA of ≤0.2 was most likely associated with prostate cancer, and with higher percentages with benign prostatic hypertrophy. A ratio of ≤0.15 was associated with a higher Gleason score and poorer prognosis (17).

Oesterling et al. (303) analyzed free, complexed, and total PSA in 422 healthy men aged 40 to 79 years. The respective recommended age-specific reference ranges (95th percentile) for the three forms were 0.5, 1, and 1 ng/mL for men aged 40 to 49 years; 0.7, 1.5, and 3 ng/mL for men aged 50 to 59 years; 1, 2, and 4 ng/mL for men aged 60 to 69 years; and 1.2, 3, and 5.5 ng/mL for men aged 70 to 79 years. Similar observations have been made by investigators at Johns Hopkins (62).

Reverse Transcriptase–Polymerase Chain Reaction Assay

Recent developments include using molecular biologic methods, particularly reverse transcriptase–PCR (RT-PCR), to measure markers by detecting low levels of messenger RNA (mRNA) for PSA and prostate-specific membrane antigen (PSMA) expressed by circulating metastatic prostate cancer cells (54,71,138,205,281). The assay is highly specific because the only cells expressing PSA in the peripheral blood are circulating prostate cancer cells. However, there is a wide range of sensitivities of detection of PSA-expressing cells in the peripheral blood reported in the literature (151).

Katz et al. (206), in 94 patients on whom RT-PCR assay for PSA mRNA was performed, reported an enhanced reaction in 26 (72%) of 36 patients who had extraprostatic tumor at the time of surgery. The test was negative in 51 (88%) of 58 patients with organ-confined disease. Six months after surgery, an increased PSA level was noted in 19% and 2% of the two groups, respectively. This bioassay may have significant staging value in patients who are candidates for RP.

Cama et al. (54) noted that, in contrast to the RT-PCR assay for PSA, the assay for PSMA did not correlate with pathologic stage of prostate cancer.

Oefelein et al. (301), using RT-PCR for PSA, identified positive cells in 20 (91%) of 22 operative field samples, and 4 (25%) of 16 had evidence of intraoperative hematogenous dissemination (p = .046). Their results suggest that tumor cell spillage and, less frequently, hematogenous dissemination may be associated with operative manipulation of the prostate during RP and may potentially represent the mechanism of failure after this treatment.

Israeli et al. (194), using the PCR assay, also reported circulating prostatic tumor cells in 2 (6.7%) of 30 men. However, prostate-specific membrane primer assay demonstrated tumor cells in 19 (63%) of 30 patients. All 16 negative control subjects had negative PSA and PSMA PCR results. Using PSA mRNA as a marker for prostatic epithelial cells, Seiden et al. (362) noted that 5 of 65 patients with clinically localized carcinoma of the prostate had PSA mRNA–detectable cells by transcription and PCR. On the other hand, 10 of 20 patients with hormone-refractory and progressive prostate cancer also demonstrated the same increased frequency of PSA mRNA–detectable cells.

Overall, most studies report a 0% PSA rate by RT-PCR in negative control cases, whereas the positive rate in the metastatic group ranges between 31% and 88% (281). However, 25% of men with localized prostate cancer who underwent RP and had specimen-confined disease had a positive PCR PSA assay (206). These men would be denied surgery if it was concluded that circulating prostate cancer cells are synonymous with incurable disease. A new approach is to use a combination of primers to improve the overall staging accuracy of RT-PCR. Preliminary work from the Cleveland Clinic suggests that combining RT-PCR for PSA and PSMA may improve the staging accuracy (152). Until the significance of a positive PCR assay is determined with long-term follow-up, RT-PCR remains experimental and should not change treatment recommendations.

Staging Work-Up

Patients with localized prostatic carcinoma are frequently asymptomatic; the diagnosis is often made with a screening PSA test. In the pre-PSA era, asymptomatic patients were diagnosed on the basis of palpating a hard nodule on DRE. Patients with locally advanced tumors have presented with bladder outlet obstructive symptoms such as urinary hesitancy, decreased force of the urinary stream, and postvoid dribbling as the tumor impinges on the membranous urethra. Chronic obstruction and bladder distention can lead to decreased compliance of the detrusor muscle that is manifested by symptoms of urinary frequency, urgency, and nocturia. Very early–stage disease (T1a or T1b) may occasionally be diagnosed at TURP for symptoms of bladder outlet obstruction caused by benign prostatic hyperplasia. With local invasion into the urethra or ejaculatory ducts, patients may experience hematuria or hematospermia. As the disease penetrates the capsule of the prostate, there may be invasion into the neurovascular bundles that course along the lateral aspects of the prostate, leading to erectile dysfunction. Disseminated disease frequently manifests as bone pain from distant osseous metastases.

A complete clinical history and a general physical examination including DRE are mandatory. The DRE is best performed with a well lubricated glove; the patient may be standing and bent over at the waist with his elbows resting comfortably on

Table 62.5	**DIAGNOSTIC WORK-UP FOR CARCINOMA OF THE PROSTATE**

Routine
    Clinical history and clinical examination
    Rectal examination

Laboratory
    Complete blood cell count, blood chemistry
    Serum PSA (total, free, percentage free)
    Plasma acid phosphatases (prostatic/total)

Radiographic imaging
    Magnetic resonance imaging with endorectal coil
    Radioisotope bone scan (PSA >20)
    Computed tomography of pelvis
    Chest radiograph (high risk for metastatic disease)
    Transrectal ultrasonography (for biopsy guidance)

Needle biopsy of prostate (transrectal, transperineal)
Staging lymph node dissection (high risk for lymph node metastases)

PSA, prostate-specific antigen.

a firm surface or in the lateral decubitus position on the examining table. The examiner should note the size of the gland, its overall consistency, and the presence of any firm areas. A typical neoplastic nodule of prostatic carcinoma is extremely firm, often not elevated above the surface of the gland, but surrounded by compressible prostatic tissue. The examiner should determine whether the lateral sulci are involved by tumor and also the degree of spread superiorly. In most patients the seminal vesicles cannot be palpated as discrete structures, and the finding of a firm area extending above the prostate suggests that the seminal vesicles are involved by malignancy. Only approximately 50% of prostatic nodules found on DRE are confirmed to be malignant on biopsy (199).

An abnormal DRE result, a consistently elevated PSA, or a combination of the two warrants a biopsy to establish a pathologic diagnosis. A TRUS-guided needle biopsy is the most common method for obtaining representative samples of the prostatic tissue. Six to 12 cores are taken, 3 to 6 from the right and 3 to 6 from the left. If clinically indicated by obstructive symptoms, a separate biopsy of the TZ is taken. The pathology report frequently includes the length of each core, and the length of each core that contains tumor.

Once the tissue diagnosis of prostate cancer is ascertained, the patient should undergo a staging work-up including laboratory data such as a baseline PSA, complete blood count, and testosterone level. The standard tests required in the evaluation of patients with prostatic carcinoma are listed in Table 62.5. Although a chest radiograph is recommended, a study of 236 patients undergoing RP showed abnormal findings in only 28 (11.9%), mostly related to cardiac or pulmonary problems or arterial hypertension; one primary lung cancer was found (332). According to the American College of Radiology appropriateness criteria, a chest radiograph should be performed as part of the initial staging only with suspected metastatic disease (342).

Imaging Studies

Diagnostic imaging studies have become an essential aspect of pretreatment evaluation and treatment selection. New techniques have allowed for more precise assessments of tumor location, volume, and extent, as well as biologic activity. As a result, clinical staging can be used more accurately as a prognostic factor for defining treatment options.

Transrectal Ultrasonography

The normal adult prostate imaged by TRUS appears as a symmetric, triangular, relatively homogeneous structure with an echogenic capsule. TRUS is used routinely for guidance during the transrectal biopsy and during prostate brachytherapy. However, only prostate cancers located in the peripheral zone can be reliably detected by ultrasonography. Attempts to characterize adenocarcinoma by pattern on TRUS have indicated that prostate cancers can have variable echogenicities. Rifkin et al. (338), in 443 men undergoing TRUS of the prostate, found 130 pathologically proven cancers and 313 cases of benign prostatic disease. Cancers were hyperechoic in 69% of the cases and had poorly defined margins, whereas benign lesions were hyperechoic in only 46% of the cases. The authors concluded that there are no specific characteristics on TRUS that reliably differentiate between benign prostatic disease and malignancy.

Chodak (75) and Chodak et al. (75), in a prospective, randomized study of TRUS in 216 men, reported a sensitivity of 86% but a specificity of only 41%; tumors smaller than 1 cm were the most difficult to detect. For staging purposes, Rifkin et al. (338) found a sensitivity of only 60% using TRUS to distinguish between T2 and T3 lesions.

Computed Tomography

The primary role of CT in prostate cancer is size determination of the prostate gland, radiation therapy treatment planning, and assessment of pelvic nodal metastases. Roach et al. (341) compared prostate volumes defined by MRI and CT and found a 32% increase in prostate volume when defined by noncontrast CT scan. Using image fusion, they identified four areas, including the posterior aspect, the posteroinferior apical aspect of the gland, the prostatic apex, and the neurovascular bundles, which tended to be areas of discrepancy between the two imaging modalities. Kagawa et al. (204), using CT-MRI fusion software for planning three-dimensional conformal radiation therapy (3DCRT), demonstrated that MRI was clearly superior to CT in defining the prostate apex, neurovascular bundles, and anterior rectal wall. The discrepancy in prostate location between the two imaging studies was also greatest at the apex and base of the gland.

CT lacks the soft tissue resolution needed to detect intraprostatic disease, capsular extension, or seminal vesical involvement. Moreover, for most patients with newly diagnosed prostate cancer, the incidence of positive lymph nodes is <5%; thus, there is little role for CT as a routine staging procedure (126,336). CT identification of pelvic adenopathy depends on lymph node enlargement, and the correlation between nodal size and metastatic involvement is poor (126,408,427).

Albertsen et al. (5) performed a population-based analysis to determine the positive yield of imaging studies performed on men with newly diagnosed prostate cancer. The positive yield of a CT scan was <12% for men with PSA 4 to 20 ng/mL. More than 10% of men with PSA >20 ng/mL and Gleason score 6 or greater were likely to have CT scans positive for extracapsular or metastatic disease. For combinations of high Gleason scores and PSA >50 ng/mL, the positive yield on CT scan was as high as 62%. Flanigan et al. (126) retrospectively studied 173 men who underwent preoperative CT scanning and found that none of the patients with a PSA <25 ng/mL had an abnormality by CT scan. Of 33 patients with PSA levels >25 ng/mL, 9 had nodal metastases, but only 3 (9%) of these 33 patients were correctly diagnosed by CT scanning. These authors concluded that routine preoperative CT scanning could not be justified in patients with a PSA <25 ng/mL. Although the histologic incidence of positive pelvic lymph nodes is substantial when PSA levels exceed 25 ng/mL, the sensitivity of CT for detecting positive nodes is only approximately 30% to 35% even at these levels (336).

Bone Scan

A close correlation exists between pretreatment PSA level and incidence of abnormal bone scan results (78,233). Given the low risk of osseous metastasis in patients with early-stage prostate cancer, the yield of a bone scan is low unless the PSA is >20 ng/mL or the patient complains of bone pain (78). In a retrospective analysis of 589 patients with untreated carcinoma of the prostate and PSA levels of ≤20 ng/mL, Rees et al. (336) reported that only 3 (1%) of 274 patients evaluated by bone scan and 3 (1%) of 262 patients evaluated by CT scan had evidence of metastatic disease. Only 1 of 108 patients with a PSA of ≤10 ng/mL had metastatic disease, and no patient with a Gleason score of ≤5 had an abnormal bone scan or CT scan result, or positive lymph nodes.

Huncharek and Muscat (190), in an analysis of 265 patients with localized carcinoma of the prostate, noted that no patients with PSA <4 ng/mL had a positive bone scan. In patients with PSA of 4.1 to 10 ng/mL and PSA of 10.1 to 20 ng/mL, 2.2% and 3.6%, respectively, had positive bone scans. In patients with PSA >20 ng/mL, 6.7% had a positive bone scan.

Albertsen et al. (5) analyzed prospective data from the Prostate Cancer Outcomes Study from 1995 and found that physicians ordered bone scans for approximately two thirds and CT for one third of all new patients. Less than 5% of the imaging studies yielded positive results. Only 1% of bone scans were positive for metastatic disease for men with PSA <10 ng/mL and Gleason score of ≤6. Only men with PSA >50 ng/mL and Gleason scores of 8 to 10 had positive yields on bone scan of >10%. The guidelines established by the American College of Radiology appropriateness criteria for pretreatment staging of clinically localized prostate cancer recommend that a radionuclide bone scan can be omitted from the work-up of low-risk patients, those with PSA of ≤10 ng/mL or Gleason score of 2 to 6.

From a clinical standpoint, a baseline bone scan may be helpful before treatment with radiation therapy, especially in elderly patients or those with a history of arthritis, to document degenerative changes that may later be interpreted as metastatic osseous disease. Bone scintigraphy in routine follow-up has no value because PSA is more sensitive in detecting recurrence, and treatment of asymptomatic bone metastases (except in cases of impending pathologic fracture) cannot be justified. Periodic PSA assessment is adequate for follow-up of these patients and bone scan should be limited to patients with rising PSA levels when clinically warranted (403).

Endorectal Magnetic Resonance Imaging

The major development in prostate imaging has come in the field of MRI. With the maturation of MRI technology, there have been significant improvements in MR technique and performance for imaging the prostate. Some of the recent advances include the use of the endorectal coil to improve spatial resolution, analytic image correction software to eliminate artifact, fast spin-echo imaging to reduce image acquisition time and provide higher signal-to-noise ratio, and the introduction of MR spectroscopy imaging (MRSI) to detect metabolic activity in the prostate (223). Moreover, increasing reader experience has greatly improved the accuracy of MRI staging for prostate cancer. Strict MRI criteria for the diagnosis of extracapsular extension have been elucidated. Nevertheless, there is still interobserver variability depending on the experience of the radiologist. One study has demonstrated that the specificity for diagnosis of extracapsular extension was 93% for senior readers and 94% for junior readers, whereas sensitivity was only 50% for senior readers and 14% for junior readers (438).

The appearance of the prostate and the information that can be gleaned for staging purposes depends on the MR technique used. On axial T1-weighted images, the prostate gland appears homogeneous and the zonal anatomy is not well appreciated (422). However, there is a much larger field of view, allowing for detection of locoregional adenopathy and suspected bony lesions (Fig. 62.5). Postbiopsy hemorrhage is evident on T1-weighted images as high T1 signal intensity (Fig. 62.5), which may be in the prostate, seminal vesicles, or both. This is an important observation because hemorrhage may mimic tumor on T2-weighted images, and because hemorrhage greatly limits the accuracy in the assessment of extracapsular extension (424).

The zonal anatomy of the prostate is clearly depicted on axial and coronal T2-weighted images. The vas deferens and seminal vesicals are also discernible on T2-weighted axial and coronal images, whereas the neurovascular bundles can be seen best on axial images (422) (Fig. 62.6). The penile root is better imaged on T2-weighted coronal sections, and is seen much more accurately than with CT. The peripheral zone is normally of high signal intensity, whereas tumor appears as low signal intensity. There are many other causes of low T2 signal intensity, including hemorrhage, prostatitis, hormone treatment, and radiation therapy. An area of low signal intensity can be attributed to hemorrhage if it causes high T1 signal intensity in the corresponding region. Low T2 signal intensity due to treatment (radiation or hormonal therapy) may be suspected when the signal change is diffuse and associated with a small, featureless prostate gland. Signs of extracapsular extension are a focal, irregular capsular bulge, asymmetry or invasion of the neurovascular bundles, and obliteration of the rectoprostatic angle (438).

Magnetic Resonance Spectroscopy Imaging

Spectroscopy is based on the principle that the electron cloud surrounding different chemical compounds shields the resonant atoms of interest to varying degrees depending on the specific atomic structure of the compound (439). This electron shielding causes the observed resonance frequency of the atoms to be slightly different and therefore identifiable. MRSI uses the pulse sequences from MRI, but instead of using the frequency information to provide spatial information, it is used to identify different chemical compounds. Because MRSI uses the same clinical MRI scanner, gradients, and radiofrequency coils as MRI, it can be added to an MRI examination and the metabolic data can then be overlaid directly on the corresponding anatomic images (223). This modality is particularly useful in the prostate because there are metabolic compounds that localize to regions of the prostate and can be used to distinguish between normal prostate cells and malignant cells. Human prostatic glandular cells produce large amounts of citrate during cellular metabolism that are secreted into the prostatic fluid, yielding concentrations 240 to 1,300 times greater than blood plasma concentrations. High levels of citrate are found in the glandular regions of the prostate such as the peripheral zone and lower levels in the transition and central zones. Choline is another metabolite found at intermediate levels in the normal prostate and seminal vesicles. On MRSI, regions of prostate cancer can be identified by differences in these two metabolite levels. A significant reduction in prostate citrate and a significant increase in prostate choline levels relative to the normal peripheral zone have been observed (223) (Fig. 62.7). These findings may correspond to a perturbation of cellular metabolism in malignant prostatic epithelial cells leading to less citrate production and secretion. The elevated levels of choline in prostate cancer may be attributed to the increased rate of cell proliferation, an increase in cell density in regions of cancer, and a change in the composition of the cell membrane leading to higher concentrations of choline-containing phospholipids (223). The result of MRSI is a metabolic map of the prostate corresponding

Clinical Radiation Oncology

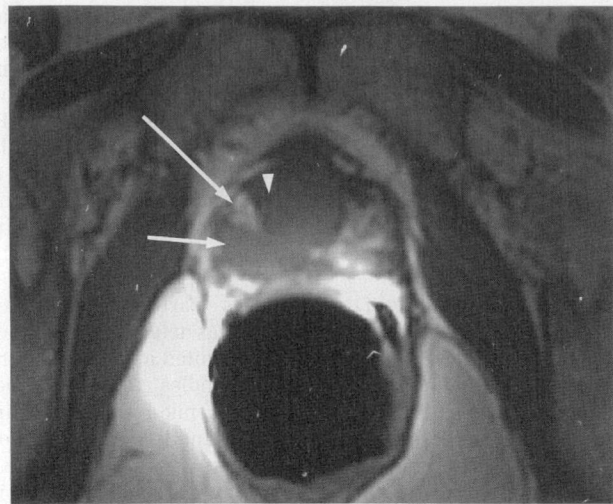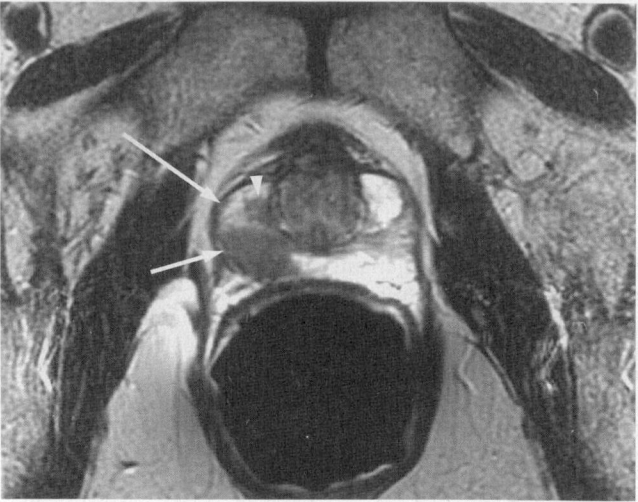

FIGURE 62.5. A: Normal T1-weighted axial magnetic resonance image. Age-related benign prostatic hyperplasia in the transition zone is evident (*long arrow*). The neurovascular bundles lie adjacent to the peripheral zone (*short arrow*). **B:** The T-2 weighted axial image of the same level of the gland demonstrates areas of low signal intensity adjacent to the postbiopsy hemorrhage that are suspect for tumor (*short arrows and arrowheads*). This is an example of the hemorrhagic exclusion sign. (Courtesy of Steven Eberhardt, MD.)

to normal and abnormal metabolic activity that can be used to pinpoint the location of prostatic tumors. This is exceptionally useful for accurate localization of prostate tumors and, in particular, when distinguishing between tumor and postbiopsy hemorrhage, which obscures MRI interpretations of prostate cancer. Moreover, there is great potential for the use of this technique for follow-up after treatment and in the development of more focused therapy.

The contribution of metabolic information gleaned from MRSI to MR anatomic imaging has improved the diagnostic accuracy of MRI both in localizing and staging prostate cancer (439). Investigators at the University of California, San Francisco (356) assessed the accuracy of combined MRSI and MRI for tumor detection and localization in 62 patients by comparing preoperative imaging results with histopathologic step-

section examination after prostatectomy. MRI tended to have a higher sensitivity and MRSI a higher specificity for detecting definite sites of cancer. The addition of MRSI significantly improved specificity over MRI alone. Compared with step-section pathology results, the specificity for tumor location with combined MRI and MRSI reached 91%. Combined MRI/MRSI allowed localization of cancer to a sextant of the prostate with a sensitivity of up to 95% compared with MRI alone, when either MRI or MRSI were positive. Moreover, a more recent study from

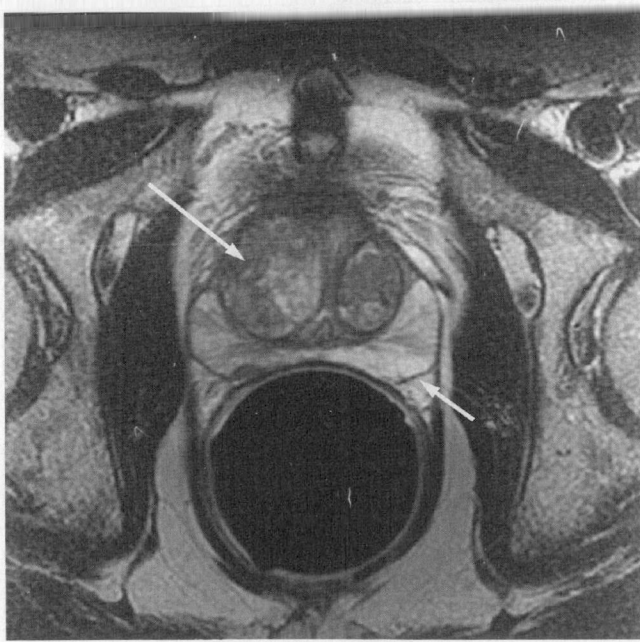

FIGURE 62.6. Normal T1-weighted axial magnetic resonance image. Age-related benign prostatic hyperplasia in the transition zone is evident (*long arrow*). The neurovascular bundles lie adjacent to the peripheral zone (*short arrow*). (Courtesy of Steven Eberhardt, MD.)

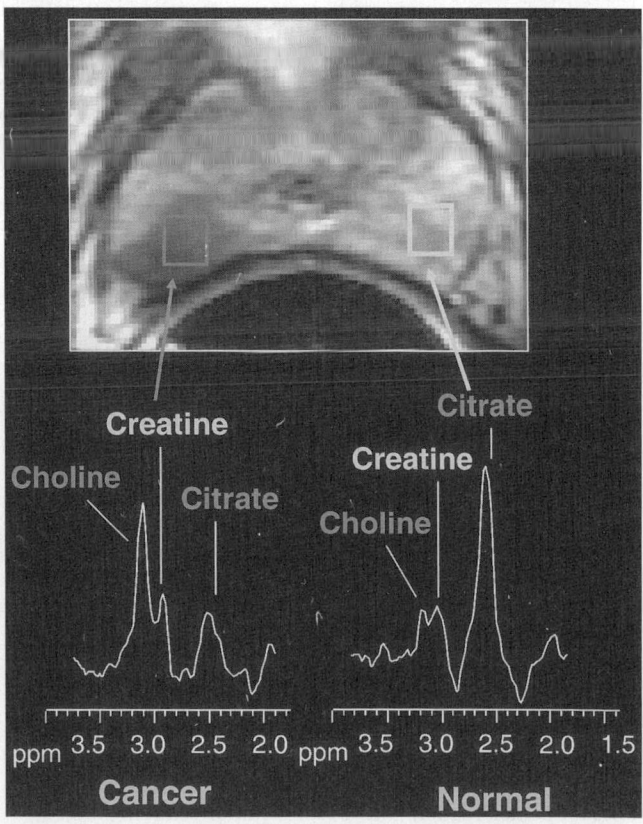

FIGURE 62.7. Three-dimensional ^{1}H magnetic resonance spectroscopic imaging. (Courtesy of Hedvig Hricak, MD.)

Chapter 62   Low-Risk Prostate Cancer   **1453**

University of California, San Francisco found MRI and MRSI are comparable with biopsy in accurately localizing intraprostatic cancer, and are more accurate than biopsy in the prostate apex (423).

In addition to improving prostate cancer localization, MRSI is complementary to MRI in staging and risk-stratifying patients with prostate cancer. Combined MRI/MRSI enhances the assessment of both extracapsular extension and seminal vesical invasion (438). Furthermore, the addition of MRSI to MRI improves the accuracy of less experienced MRI readers and reduces interobserver variability in the diagnosis of extracapsular extension (439). Emerging data suggest that metabolic information from MRSI may also be predictive of tumor aggressiveness. Preliminary MRI/MRSI studies have shown that citrate levels are lower in poorly differentiated prostate cancers, and choline levels may be elevated in more aggressive tumors with greater membrane phospholipid synthesis (224).

Risk Stratification Systems and Staging Classification

Based on tumor stage, pretreatment PSA, and biopsy Gleason score, PZ prostate cancer is generally grouped according to one of several risk stratification models (Table 62.6). These systems are useful to stratify disease-free survival, compare treatment results, and provide a means to appropriately recommend treatment options (100).

Traditionally clinical and pathologic staging systems were used alone to categorize outcome but now there are primarily used as component in risk-stratification systems. Nevertheless, it is critical to be familiar with the different updated staging systems in order to appropriately manage men with newly diagnosed prostate cancer. In 2003, the American Joint Committee on Cancer (AJCC) and International Union Against Cancer (UICC) updated the 1997 TNM classification system that replaced the older 1992 AJCC/UICC staging system and the Whitmore-Jewett system. The TNM staging system is based on separate designations for the primary tumor, regional nodes, and distant metastases. All information that is available before first definitive treatment may be used for clinical staging, including imaging studies. Advantages of the AJCC/UICC staging system include greater detail, allowing for more accurate patient risk assessment and stratification before treatment (11). In addition, this staging system better reflects the growing trend in early prostate cancer detection by PSA screening with the introduction in 1997 of a new category (T1c) for nonpalpable

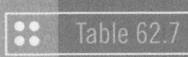

| Table 62.7 | **AMERICAN JOINT COMMITTEE TNM STAGING SYSTEM FOR PROSTATE CANCER (2003)** |

Primary tumor (T)
  TX Primary tumor cannot be assessed
  T0 No evidence of primary tumor
  T1 Clinically inapparent tumor neither palpable nor visible by imaging
  T1a Tumor incidental histologic finding in 5% or less of tissue resected
  T1b Tumor incidental histologic finding in more than 5% of tissue resected
  T1c Tumor identified by needle biopsy (e.g., because of elevated prostate-specific antigen)
  T2 Tumor confined within prostate
  T2a Tumor involves one lobe
  T2b Tumor involves more than half of a lobe but not both lobes
  T2c Tumor involves both lobes
  T3 Tumor extends through the prostate capsule
  T3a Extracapsular extension
  T3b Tumor invades seminal vesicle(s)
  T4 Tumor is fixed or invades adjacent structures other than seminal vesicles
  T4a Tumor invades bladder neck, external sphincter, or rectum
  T4b Tumor invades levator muscles or is fixed to pelvic wall, or both

Regional lymph nodes (N)
  NX Regional lymph nodes cannot be assessed
  N0 No regional node metastasis
  N1 Metastasis in single lymph node, ≤2 cm
  N2 Metastasis in a single node, >2 cm but not more than 5 cm
  N3 Metastasis in a node >5 cm

Distant metastasis (M)
  MX Presence of metastasis cannot be assessed
  M0 No distant metastasis
  M1 Distant metastasis
  M1a Nonregional lymph node(s)
  M1b Metastasis in bone(s)
  M1c Metastasis in other site(s)

cancers detected by biopsy because of an elevated PSA level. The 2003 staging system reestablishes the three divisions of T2 lesions that were used in the 1992 staging system. Tumor found in one or both lobes of the prostate by needle biopsy, but not palpable or visible by imaging, is classified as T1c. The 2003 AJCC/UICC staging system is summarized in Table 62.7.

Pathology

Adenocarcinoma, arising from peripheral acinar glands, is the most common tumor in the prostate. It is graded as well,

Table 62.6	**RISK GROUPING DEFINITIONS**		
Risk Group	Low	Intermediate	High
Seattle/MSKCC	PSA ≤10 ng/mL and GS 2-6 and stage T1-T2b	PSA >10 ng/mL or GS ≥7 or stage ≥T2c	Two or three of the intermediate risk factors
Mt. Sinai	PSA <10 ng/mL and GS 2-6 and stage T1-T2a	PSA 10.1-20 ng/mL or GS 7 or stage T2b	Two or three of the intermediate risks and/or PSA >20 ng/mL and/or GS 8-10 and/or stage ≥T2c
D'Amico	PSA <10 ng/mL and GS 2-6 and stage T1-T2a	PSA 10.1-20.0 ng/mL and/or GS 7 and/or stage T2b	PSA >20 ng/mL and/or GS 8-10 and/or stage ≥T2c

MSKCC, Memorial Sloan-Kettering Cancer Center; PSA, prostate-specific antigen; GS, Gleason score.
Modified from Sylvester JE, Blasko JC, Grimm, PD, et al. Ten-year biochemical relapse-free survival after external beam radiation and brachytherapy for localized prostate cancer: the Seattle experience. *Int J Radiat Oncol Biol Phys*. 2003;57:944–952.

Clinical Radiation Oncology

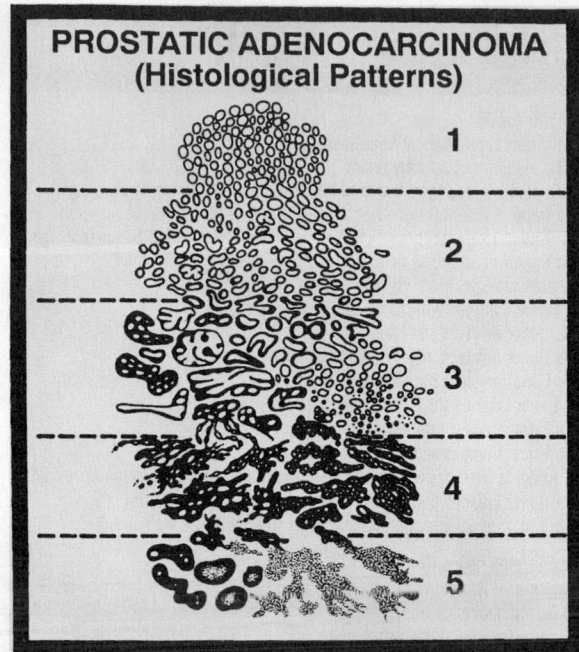

PROSTATIC ADENOCARCINOMA
(Histological Patterns)

1
2
3
4
5

FIGURE 62.8. Simplified drawing of histologic patterns, emphasizing degree of glandular differentiation and relation to stroma. All black in the drawing represents tumor tissue and glans with cytologic detail obscured except in right side of pattern 4, where tiny open structures are intended to suggest the "hypernephroid" pattern. (From Gleason DF, and the VA Cooperative Urological Research Group. Histologic grading and clinical staging of prostatic carcinoma. In: Tannenbaum M, ed. *Urologic pathology: the prostate.* Philadelphia: Lea & Febiger; 1977:171–198, with permission).

moderately, or poorly differentiated according to cellular characteristics such as nuclear content, number of nuclei, pleomorphism, gland formation, and invasion of the stroma (283).

Gleason (147,149) and Gleason and Mellinger (148) initially proposed a prognostic classification system based on the clinical stage and the degree of differentiation of primary and secondary morphologic patterns of the tumor, each graded from 1 to 5. Subsequently, only pathologic features were scored, resulting in the Gleason score that sums grades to yield nine discrete scores (range, 2 to 10; Fig. 62.8). The Gleason score is one of the strongest predictors of biologic behavior in prostate cancer, including invasiveness and metastatic potential; however, it is limited by its subjectiveness. There is significant interobserver and intraobserver variability reported using the Gleason grading system (80). In addition, the treatment with hormonal therapy agents can effect the pathologist's ability to accurately identify a Gleason score (14).

Moreover, grading errors may reflect sampling error because the needle biopsy samples a small fraction of the prostate gland and the grade of cancer obtained on needle biopsy may not always be representative of the actual histologic subtype or degree of differentiation of the tumor. Most studies demonstrate a tendency of pathologists to undergrade biopsy specimens. Johnstone et al. (202) noted that, compared with subsequent RP specimens, the incidence of correct grading of prostatic carcinoma from needle biopsies was 71%, with 23% undergrading and 6% overgrading. In a study from Memorial Sloan-Kettering Cancer Center (MSKCC), Gleason scores from 18-gauge needle biopsies were compared with radical retropubic prostatectomy specimens in 226 consecutive patients. The biopsy score was identical to the specimen score in 31% of cases, whereas 26% were discrepant by 2 or more Gleason scores. Overall, 54% of biopsies were undergraded and 15% were overgraded (85). University of Minnesota researchers found similar results from 466 patients (124). The biopsy grade was the same as that of the prostatectomy specimen in 54% of the patients, with up-

grading of the most common discordance in 75% of the well-differentiated tumors. When the biopsy grade was compared with the surgical pathologic stage, 49% of low-grade lesions and 82% of high-grade lesions in the biopsy had capsular penetration or locally advanced disease. A large, retrospective analysis (287) of the correlation between Gleason scores from biopsy and prostatectomy specimens and prediction of disease-free survival was carried out among 1,031 patients. Overall accuracy was 58.3%. When categorized by Gleason scores <7, 7, and >7, patients with tumors of Gleason score <7 on prostatectomy specimens had a significant survival advantage over those with Gleason scores <7 by biopsy, whereas disease-free survival was superior for patients with Gleason scores >7 by biopsy than those with Gleason scores >7 on prostatectomy specimens. The overall disease-free survival was similar among all patients with Gleason scores of 7. These data should be kept in mind when results of RP and irradiation are compared.

Predicting tumor extent and location using biopsy results was investigated by Humphrey et al. (189) in a correlative study of multiple parameters with pathologic features in 50 RP specimens. They noted that it was very difficult to predict tumor extent in the gland quadrants based on extent of tumor in the needle biopsy. There were 53 negative quadrant biopsies with carcinoma present in that quadrant in the RP specimen. Gregori et al. (157) evaluated the accuracy of sextant biopsies in predicting tumor location among 289 patients with clinically localized prostate cancer who underwent radical perineal prostatectomy. These investigators found that 33% of patients with a unilateral positive biopsy had cancer confined to one side of the gland, whereas 66% showed bilateral disease in the prostatectomy specimen.

The primary grade in the Gleason score provides additional prognostic information, particularly in Gleason score 7 prostate cancer. D'Amico et al. (96) studied pretreatment clinical and pathologic variables to predict time to postoperative PSA failure for patients with a PSA <10 ng/mL and T1c or T2a disease. They noted that 5-year PSA failure-free survival rates were not statistically different for patients with a biopsy Gleason score of 2 to 6 versus 3 + 4, but were significantly different for patients with a biopsy Gleason score of 2 to 6 versus 4 + 3 or 2 to 6 versus 8 to 10. Five-year biochemical control rates were 79%, 81%, 63%, and 10% for patients with biopsy Gleason scores of 2 to 6 (no grade 4 or 5), 3 + 4, 4 + 3, and 8 to 10, respectively. Makarov et al. (244) at Johns Hopkins evaluated 537 patients with Gleason score 7 tumors on biopsy to determine whether Gleason score 3 + 4 = 7 and 4 + 3 = 7 cancers behave differently regardless of the number of positive cores. Five variables (3 + 4 versus 4 + 3, number of positive cores, PSA, age, and DRE) were analyzed with respect to pathologic findings after RP. Postoperative Gleason score and pathologic stage significantly correlated with preoperative PSA and preoperative Gleason scores of 4 + 3 versus 3 + 4 on biopsy.

Stamey (380) and Stamey et al. (381,383) emphasized that, with regard to natural history of prostate cancer and prognosis, it is not just the Gleason score that is important, but how much of the tumor is present. In a study of histologic prognostic variables for PSA relapse among 372 men with prostate cancer followed for 3 years after retropubic prostatectomy, the most important variables predicting biochemical disease-free status for PZ cancers were percentage Gleason grade 4/5, cancer volume, serum PSA, and prostate weight (383). Percentage Gleason grade 4/5, cancer location in the PZ, cancer volume, and lymph node involvement had prognostic value in large-volume prostate cancer. These investigators also noted that TZ cancers have a better prognosis than PZ tumors because they are separated from the neurovascular bundles and the ejaculatory ducts by the compressed surgical capsule caused by expanding benign hyperplastic nodules (260). From the Stanford experience (298), cancer location in the PZ and percentage Gleason grade

4/5 were the most powerful predictors of biochemical failure in men whose cancer was ≥ 6 cm^3 and contained in the prostatic capsule. Preoperative serum PSA was not helpful in distinguishing biochemical failure rates in large-volume cancers regardless of whether they were organ confined.

D'Amico et al. (101,102) have shown that the percentage of positive prostate biopsies added clinically significant information regarding time to PSA failure among 960 men with PSA-detected or clinically palpable prostate cancer treated with RP. Investigators at the University of Michigan (297), in an analysis of preoperative factors, including clinical stage, PSA, biopsy Gleason score, greatest percentage of a biopsy core involved by cancer, number of biopsy cores containing cancer, and perineural invasion, found that only PSA, Gleason score, and greatest percentage of a biopsy core involved by cancer were highly predictive of PSA relapse-free survival on multivariate analysis. This additional prognostic information may identify patients who are candidates for adjuvant therapy after RP. In addition, with the use of radiation therapy, histologic features from prostatectomy specimens are not available to incorporate into prognostic models, and pretreatment risk stratification is important owing to the increasing use of nonsurgical treatment options.

Prostate core biopsy histologic features have been investigated for predicting extraprostatic extension and lymph node involvement. Researchers at the Mayo Clinic (361) compared biopsy specimen Gleason scores, percentage positive cores, and percentage surface area involved in all cores with pathologic stage determined from RP specimens. Multivariate analysis using these pathologic variables, in addition to patient age, clinical disease stage, and PSA, showed that the percentage of positive cores, initial serum PSA, and Gleason score of cancer in the needle biopsy were the only parameters that jointly predicted pathologic stage (T2 versus T3 disease). Narayan et al. (288) used the combination of preoperative PSA plus biopsy Gleason score in 932 patients who had undergone pelvic lymphadenectomy to predict risk of positive pelvic lymph nodes. Patients with biopsy Gleason scores ≤ 6 and preoperative PSA concentrations ≤ 10 ng/mL had <1% false-negative rate for pelvic lymph node metastases, suggesting that a staging pelvic lymphadenectomy is unnecessary.

Finally, the tumor histologic characteristics change with time and progression of disease. Cheng et al. (72) reported a trend toward histologic dedifferentiation when prostate carcinoma metastasized to regional lymph nodes. Among 242 patients treated with RP and pelvic lymphadenectomy at the Mayo Clinic, Gleason score in the lymph node metastases was higher than in the primary tumor in 45% of patients, lower in 12% of patients, and matched exactly in 43% of patients. The 5-year progression-free survival rate was significantly different between patients with histologic dedifferentiation and those without dedifferentiation.

Other Histologic Subtypes

Periurethral duct carcinoma is a separate clinicopathologic entity, usually consisting of a transitional cell type of carcinoma, although a mixture of glandular and transitional cells is also observed (30,213,255). Large anaplastic tumor cells cluster in the periurethral ducts and spread into the stroma. Frequent mitoses are seen (398). This tumor does not invade the perineural spaces as commonly as does adenocarcinoma of the prostate.

Reese et al. (337) reviewed 49 patients with *transitional cell carcinoma* of the prostate; 29 patients had stromal invasion and 20 had transitional cell carcinoma in the prostatic ducts only. Lymph node metastases were found in 14 (54%) of 26 patients with stromal invasion, compared with 4 (24%) of 17 with duct/acinar involvement. The 5-year survival rates were 80% for stromal node-negative, 45% for ductal node-negative, 55% for ductal node-positive, and 30% for stromal node-positive patients.

Ductal adenocarcinoma arises rarely from the major ducts. These tumors are usually papillary and on microscopic sections are composed of tall columnar cells with eosinophilic cytoplasm that may resemble endometrial carcinoma (56,277,397,443). Originally this lesion was thought to originate in the prostatic utricle, a müllerian remnant (265); however, most ductal adenocarcinomas are not derived from müllerian remnants and behave as acinar adenocarcinomas (155).

Most reports point to aggressive behavior, with invasion of the prostatic stroma and the bladder neck and metastases to the lymph nodes, bone, and lung. In most series, the majority of patients die of the tumors within 4 years (84,219). This tumor is moderately hormonally responsive and is sensitive to radiation therapy (84). The treatment of choice is RP (84,428). Kopelson et al. (213) reported a good prognosis in early stages; however, in stage C the 5-year survival rate was only 34.5%. They noted a 76% local tumor control rate and a 58% 5-year survival rate in patients treated with irradiation, in contrast to 14% local tumor control and 24% 5-year survival rates in patients not receiving this treatment. Brinker et al. (49) also observed a shortened average time to progression relative to a previous study group of men with acinar carcinoma among 58 patients treated with RP at Johns Hopkins.

Neuroendocrine tumors are a rare variant of a malignant tumor composed of small or carcinoidlike cells. Neuroendocrine cell substances found in these tumors include serotonin, neuron-specific enolase, chromogranin, calcitonin, and others. PAP and PSA are valuable to determine the prostatic origin of the tumor. Of 22 patients with stage T2 lesions, 4 died of the disease, and 3 of them had positive neuroendocrine cell findings. Of 20 patients with stage T3, 5 died of the disease, and all 5 had positive neuroendocrine cell features (82).

Mucinous carcinoma, not arising in major ducts or in the urethra, with positive histochemical stains for PAP, has been reported (116).

Sarcomatoid carcinoma is a rare tumor and is difficult to distinguish from a true sarcoma. There is coexistence of prostatic adenocarcinoma with sarcomatoid components that have spindle cells with large pleomorphic hyperchromatic nuclei. The pattern is that of a high-grade sarcoma in most patients, similar to the malignant fibrous histiocytoma of soft tissues. Mitotic figures range from 6 to 36 per 10 high-power fields. In 12 patients reported by Shannon et al. (366), tumor presentation was stage A or B in 4, C or D in 5, and unknown in 3 patients. Metastases data were available for 10 patients; the most common metastatic sites were bone (7 patients), lymph nodes (2 patients), lung (2 patients), liver (1 patient), and skin (1 patient). Immunostaining or electron microscopy demonstrated epithelial differentiation in the sarcomatoid areas in 6 of 11 patients on whom these studies were performed. All nine patients for whom follow-up data were available died of disease within 3 to 48 months after diagnosis. In three patients, sarcomatoid elements were part of the tumor at initial diagnosis; in the other nine, the sarcomatoid component was confirmed in subsequent evaluations after initial diagnosis (2 to 89 months). Four patients were treated with radiation therapy without beneficial result. These tumors are considered a very aggressive variant of prostatic adenocarcinoma.

Endometrioid tumors occasionally arise from the verumontanum. Endometrial glands and cells with numerous mitotic figures may be seen. These tumors may have an exophytic configuration in the prostatic urethra or infiltrate the adjacent tissues.

Adenoid cystic carcinoma is a rare tumor in the prostate (representing <0.1% of all tumors of this gland). The histologic appearance is similar to that of its salivary gland counterpart.

Other epithelial tumors, such as carcinoid or small cell carcinoma, have been reported in the prostate (24,137). The experience with these lesions is very limited, and in most patients behavior is highly aggressive and fatal (371). A review of the literature showed that in 130 patients reported with small cell carcinoma of the prostate, the 2-year survival rate was 3.6%, the 3-year rate was 1.8%, and 5-year rate was less than 1% (1). Squamous cell carcinoma originating primarily in the prostate is rare (153). Metastatic malignant tumors from other locations to the prostate are occasionally reported (153,201).

Sarcomas (leiomyosarcoma, rhabdomyosarcoma, or fibrosarcoma) constitute approximately 0.1% of all primary neoplasms of the prostate (398). Leiomyosarcoma is more common in middle-aged or older men, whereas rhabdomyosarcoma is found more frequently in younger patients. Several cases of malignant schwannoma have been described (359). These tumors tend to invade lymphatics and blood vessels, causing widespread regional lymphatic and distant metastases.

Carcinosarcoma of the prostate constitutes 0.1% of prostatic neoplasms. A mixture of adenocarcinoma invading the stroma and sarcomatous elements is seen histologically; smooth or striated muscle, fibroblasts, or other mesenchymal malignant cells may be identified.

Primary lymphoma of the prostate is rare, fewer than 100 cases having been reported. It accounted for only 0.1% of newly diagnosed lymphomas and only 0.09% of all prostatic neoplasias at M.D. Anderson Cancer Center (354).

General Management Trends in the United States

The optimal management of clinically localized prostate cancer remains controversial and is often a source of great frustration and anxiety for many patients who are compelled to make a decision regarding a treatment intervention for their disease. The practitioner must be aware that the natural history of this tumor is variable and influenced by multiple prognostic factors. All of the various forms of therapy for prostate cancer can affect quality of life and sexual function in varying degrees. In the process of counseling and discussing therapeutic options, it is important to present all available data regarding the variable natural history of this disease, prognostic significance of the diagnosis, potential therapeutic benefit of the various modalities, and immediate as well as late treatment-related sequelae. Life expectancy and quality of life considerations should be carefully discussed with the patient and spouse or significant other.

Based on the available data, when comparing patients with similar prognostic features, there are no significant differences in the biochemical and disease-free survival outcomes for patients with early stages of disease treated with RP, high-dose external-beam radiation therapy (EBRT), or interstitial implantation (97,220,457). In the absence of randomized trials demonstrating superiority of one treatment over another, there have been wide geographic variations in the preferred therapeutic intervention for early-stage prostate cancer currently practiced throughout the United States.

Observations from the CapSURE database (Cancer of the Prostate Strategic Urologic Research Endeavor), a registry of 10,000 men accrued from community-based urologic practices across the United States, has shed further light on practice patterns. Cooperberg et al. (86) reported an increasing trend for patients presenting at diagnosis with more favorable risk disease in 2001–2002 (47%) compared to 1989–1990 (31%). A lower percentage of high-risk patients (defined as PSA >20 ng/mL, Gleason 8-10 disease or T3-T4 disease) were noted on initial presentation (15% compared with 41%) for 2000–2001 and 1989–1990, respectively. Practice patterns have also changed in more recent years. The use of expectant management has decreased from 20% in 1993 to 8% in 2001. A slight decrease

in the use of prostatectomy and EBRT was reported with a significant increase in brachytherapy and primary androgen-deprivation therapy treatment interventions. Finally, there has been a steady increase in the use of neoadjuvant androgen-deprivation therapy in conjunction with planned radiotherapy. Comparing trends from 1989–1990 and 1999–2001, the use of neoadjuvant androgen deprivation has increased from 10% to 75% for those receiving EBRT, and 7% to 25% for those receiving brachytherapy.

Zelefsky et al. (444) reported significant changes of radiation therapy practice across the United States based on comparisons of the 1994 and 1999 surveys of the American College of Radiology Patterns of Care Survey. Overall, it was observed that, compared with the 1994 survey, there were significant changes in the practice and delivery of radiation therapy during the more recent survey period. Specifically, more patients, especially with favorable-risk disease, were treated with implantation compared with prior years. The implant-treated population was noted to be younger than the patients receiving EBRT. In the 1999 survey, higher doses of EBRT were more frequently delivered using 3DCRT techniques compared with what was reported in the 1994 survey. It was also noted that there was a substantial increase in recent years in the percentage of patients treated with androgen deprivation in conjunction with radiation therapy.

Several authors, including Adolfsson et al. (2) and Johansson et al. (200), have reported on patients, age 60 to more than 80 years, who, on histologic diagnosis of carcinoma of the prostate, were managed conservatively and observed without specific anticancer treatment until symptoms developed. Recently, a phase III randomized trial from the Scandinavian Prostate Cancer Group demonstrated the benefits of treatment intervention compared with an expectant management approach (39). In this study, 695 men were included with early stage T1 or T2 prostate cancer. The median follow-up was 8.2 years, the primary end point was death attributed to prostate cancer, and the secondary end point was overall survival. In the watchful waiting group, 8.9% died of disease compared with 4.6% in the RP group ($p = .02$). Men assigned to RP had a significantly lower incidence of distant metastases compared with those who underwent watchful waiting. However, the overall survival rates between the two groups were noted to be same.

In today's health environment in the United States, it is often not considered acceptable to delay definitive therapy for most patients with localized carcinoma of the prostate, except in selected elderly patients with low Gleason scores and low-volume disease based on the biopsy findings, as well as patients with significant medical comorbidities. Properly designed prospective clinical trials are critically needed to better define the efficacy and cost-effectiveness of various therapeutic approaches for localized carcinoma of the prostate.

Traditionally, the treatment options for patients with early-stage, clinically localized prostatic cancer (stages T1c or T2) have included RP, EBRT, or permanent interstitial implantation. Surgical techniques have significantly improved with the advent of the nerve-sparing operation popularized by Walsh (416), with a lower incidence of sexual impotence (approximately 30% to 60%, depending on the patient's age, tumor stage, and surgery extent) compared with classic RP (almost 100%), as well as improved methods available to reduce risks of posttreatment urinary incontinence. At the same time, the accuracy and safety of EBRT delivery have significantly improved with the emergence of 3DCRT and IMRT approaches. Permanent interstitial implantation using ultrasound-guided transperineal techniques and the recent developments of intraoperative conformal optimization for prostate brachytherapy have consistently improved the dose distributions for this treatment approach, leading to improved outcomes and decreased toxicities. For patients with intermediate-risk and selected unfavorable-risk features, in addition to high-dose EBRT alone, the combination of EBRT with permanent interstitial implantation or a high–dose-rate (HDR) brachytherapy boost represents appropriate treatment interventions in addition to RP.

Treatment Techniques

Radical Prostatectomy

RP, initially described by Young (436) in 1905 and popularized by Jewett (199), is a therapeutic option when the tumor is confined to the prostate; according to most urologists, it has no role in the management of gross extracapsular disease, seminal vesicle involvement, or in the presence of lymph node metastases. Two approaches for the classic RP are used: retropubic and perineal. The procedure consists of complete removal of the prostate and its surrounding capsule together with the seminal vesicles, the ampulla, and the vas deferens. The prostate is removed completely by excision of the urethra at the prostatomembranous junction, leaving no residual prostatic tissue at the apex. The retropubic approach is preferred by many urologic surgeons; this procedure also facilitates access for performing a bilateral pelvic lymph node dissection.

Walsh and Donker (417) described the anatomic basis for sexual impotence after RP and, based on that, reported on techniques to achieve a nerve-sparing approach. Through detailed anatomic studies, they demonstrated that the branches of the pelvic autonomic plexus that innervate the corpora cavernosa are located between the rectum and the urethra, along the lateral aspect of the prostate, and penetrate the urogenital diaphragm near or in the midmuscular wall of the urethra. Later they described the technique for radical retropubic prostatectomy with preservation of the neurovascular pedicle (416). They reported preservation of sexual function in 73% of 250 patients treated with this operation; the incidence of sexual impotence was correlated with the age of the patient at the time of surgery (418).

In the last 5 years there has been an increasing interest and practice of laparoscopic radical prostatectomy both in the United States and Europe. Advantages cited for the use of the laparoscopic procedure versus the open approach include improved visualization of the anatomy optical magnification, less blood loss, less postoperative pain, and more rapid resumption of normal activities (181) Preliminary functional and oncologic outcomes with this approach compare favorably to that achieved with open RP approaches. Robotic approaches are currently being used in some centers. The *Da Vinci* surgical system (Intuitive Surgical, Inc., Sunnyvale, CA) uses three multijoint robotic arms with one arm controlling the binocular endoscope and the other arms controlling small-wristed instruments. This system is controlled by the surgeon, who can be in a remote location from the patient, seated at an operative console. The stereoscopic view of the operative field provides the surgeon three-dimensional visualization with a 10-fold magnification. Fine and precise movements of the instruments can be achieved, and physiologic tremor can be eliminated. Whether such approaches would lead to significant improvements over surgical outcomes achieved with standard techniques is uncertain and will require prospective randomized studies.

Cryosurgery

Cryosurgery, in which tissues are coagulated by exposing them to very low temperatures with probes implanted through the perineum in the gland under ultrasonographic guidance, has been reintroduced in the treatment of prostate cancer after significant improvements in equipment design. In general, the procedure lasts on average for 2 to 3 hours and patients are discharged with a suprapubic tube or urethral catheter that remains in place for approximately 2 weeks.

Several reports have noted encouraging preliminary PSA relapse–free survival outcomes and posttreatment biopsy results after cryotherapy when used as the primary treatment for clinically localized prostate cancer (26,119,136). Yet there have also been reports documenting increased toxicity with cryotherapy, especially when used as a salvage intervention after a prior course of radiation therapy (194). Technical considerations and recent improvements in cryosurgical techniques have reduced the complications associated with the procedure. These improvements have included the use of multiple freeze–thaw cycles, urethral warming during the procedure, and the placement of thermocouples to maintain the temperatures to <40°C. More recently third-generation cryosurgery techniques have been used that use 17-gauge cryoprobes inserted via transrectal ultrasound guidance through a brachytherapylike template. Multiple mini-ice balls are created that coalesce and potentially provide more precision than standard cryotherapy techniques. Argon gas is used for freezing and helium gas for thawing. Early reports incorporating these enhancements have been promising, with associated decreased toxicity observed (168).

Radiation Therapy Techniques

Conventional External-Beam Radiation Therapy Techniques

Much of the current long-term radiation outcome data for the treatment of clinically localized prostate cancer are derived from patients treated in the 1970s. At that time, the treatment field size and portal configuration for radiation therapy were based on estimations of the anatomic boundaries of the prostate defined by plain-film radiography and by DRE. These techniques were suboptimal compared with the current ability to define the shape and location of the prostate with CT-assisted simulation and MRI. Furthermore, early conventional radiation therapy delivery methods limited the treatment volume to relatively small 6 × 6-cm to 8 × 8-cm fields using rotational arcs or a four-field box technique. Although usually sufficient for the treatment of small T1 and T2a tumors, reconstruction of such fields using CT imaging clearly demonstrated that even an 8 × 8-cm field size would be insufficient to encompass most prostates with locally advanced disease, especially when the seminal vesicles were at risk (401).

A variety of treatment techniques were used in the past, ranging from parallel-opposed anteroposterior portals with a perineal appositional field to lateral portals (box technique) or rotational fields to supplement the dose to the prostate (25,107,257). In general, four fields were used to treat the pelvis and prostate to an initial dose of 45 Gy, with a boost to 70 Gy or higher to the prostate only. For patients with node-positive disease, the initial fields were designed to cover the common iliac lymph nodes. The inferior margin of the pelvic fields was set 1.5 to 2 cm distal to the junction of the prostatic and membranous urethra (usually at or caudad to the bottom of the ischial tuberosities). The lateral margins were typically placed approximately 1 to 2 cm from the lateral bony pelvis (Fig. 62.9). The anterior margin of the lateral fields was placed 1.5 cm posterior to the projection of the anterior cortex of the pubic symphysis while posteriorly, the portals were designed to include the pelvic and presacral lymph nodes above the S3 segment, sparing the posterior rectal wall distal to this level. Some small bowel could usually be spared anteriorly, keeping in mind the anatomic location of the external iliac lymph nodes (Fig. 62.10).

Conformal and Intensity-Modulated Radiation Therapy Techniques

In the early to mid-1980s, three-dimensional (also known as conformal) treatment techniques became increasingly available. Although these techniques vary in some aspects, they

CARCINOMA OF PROSTATE - PORTALS

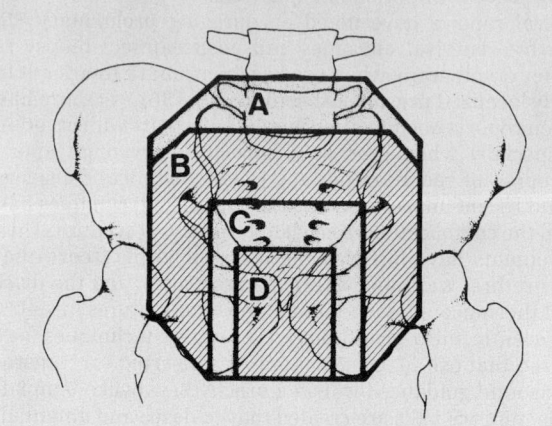

FIGURE 62.9. Diagrams of the pelvis showing volumes used to irradiate the prostate and pelvic lymph nodes. Lower margin is at or 1 cm below ischial tuberosities. At the Mallinckrodt Institute of Radiology, 15 × 15 cm portals at source-skin distance are used to stage A2 and B disease and for selected postoperative patients, whereas for stage C or D1 disease, 18–15 cm portals are used to cover all common iliac lymph nodes up to the bifurcation of the common iliac lymph nodes. Sizes of reduced fields are larger (up to 12 × 14 cm) when seminal vesicles or periprostatic tumors are irradiated compared with prostate boost only (up to 10 × 11 cm).

share certain common principles that offer significant advantages over conventional treatment techniques. CT-based images referenced to a reproducible patient position are used to localize the prostate and normal organs and to generate high-resolution 3D reconstructions of the patient. Treatment field directions are selected using beam's-eye-view techniques and the fields are shaped to conform to the patient's CT-defined target volume, thereby minimizing the volume of normal tissue irradiated. Conformal radiotherapy simulation, planning, and treatment incorporate various additional maneuvers to reduce treatment uncertainties and enhance setup reproducibility required during a protracted course of therapy.

IMRT is a relatively recent refinement of three-dimensional conformal techniques that uses treatment fields with highly irregular radiation intensity patterns to deliver exquisitely conformal radiation distributions. These intensity patterns are created using special "inverse" or "optimization" computer plan-

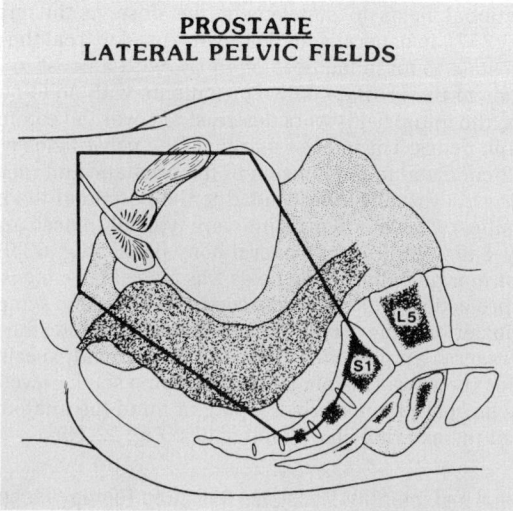

PROSTATE LATERAL PELVIC FIELDS

FIGURE 62.10. Lateral portal used in box technique to irradiate pelvic tissues and prostate. The anterior margin is 0.5 to 1 cm posterior to projected cortex of pubic symphysis. Presacral lymph nodes in included down to S3; inferiorly, the posterior wall of rectum is spared.

ning systems, the characteristics of which have been thoroughly summarized in several review articles (45,421). Rather than define each field shape and weight as is done in conventional treatment planning, planners of IMRT treatment specify the desired dose to the target and normal tissues using mathematical descriptions referred to as "constraints" or "objectives." Sophisticated optimization methods are then used to determine the intensity pattern for each treatment field that results in a dose distribution as close to the user-defined constraints as possible.

IMRT delivery is significantly more complex than conformal delivery as well. Delivery of an IMRT intensity pattern requires a computer-controlled beam-shaping apparatus on the linear accelerator known as a multileaf collimator (MLC). The MLC consists of many small individually moving leaves or fingers that can create arbitrary beam shapes. The MLC is used for IMRT delivery in either a static mode referred to as "step and shoot," which consists of multiple small, irregularly shaped fields delivered in sequence, or a dynamic mode (dynamic multileaf collimation) with the leaves moving during treatment to create the required irregular intensity patterns (379). Since its inception, IMRT has become a common and important method for treating prostate cancer and, through its ability to tightly conform the radiation to the shape of the target, has facilitated an escalation in dose at several institutions, including MSKCC.

In the following section, the 3DCRT and IMRT techniques used at MSKCC are highlighted with reference to similar techniques developed by others.

Immobilization, Simulation, and Computed Tomography Scanning

On the evening prior to simulation, patients undergo a standard bowel preparation. Immediately before the simulation procedure and CT scan the next day, the patient is asked to void his bladder. To visualize bowel in the vicinity of the prostate and seminal vesicles, a barium sulfate suspension is administered and the rectal lumen is visualized by inserting a rectal catheter.

The majority of the patients with prostate cancer at MSKCC are treated in a prone position, with the supine position reserved for those who are obese or have difficulty lying prone because of arthritis or other orthopaedic problems. Zelefsky et al. (454) compared treatment plans in both supine and prone positions and found the prone position was more suitable for the majority of the patients undergoing 3DCRT or IMRT treatment. For patients treated to doses ≥75.6 Gy, lower rectal wall doses and displacement of the bowel out of the treatment field were more often observed in the prone position. The prone position was also found to be technically reproducible and well tolerated by most patients. Others, however, have not observed the same superiority of the prone position (32,210,245,259,393). Stroom et al. (393) compared prostate and seminal vesicle movement in the supine and prone positions by evaluating serial CT scans in 15 supine and 15 prone patients. Although the overall variability in target position was slightly less for patients treated in the prone position, the systematic component of the organ motion was larger when patients were prone. Because the margin needed to compensate for systematic error is greater than that for random error, the authors concluded that the margins needed to account for organ motion were similar for the two positions. Malone et al. (245) observed more respiratory-induced prostate motion when patients were in the prone position. Fluoroscopic evaluation of the motion of implanted gold seeds was performed for patients in the supine and prone positions, with and without thermoplastic immobilization devices. Mean superior-inferior and anterior-posterior displacements of 2.9 ± 1.7 mm and 1.6 ± 1.1 mm, respectively, were observed for patients in the prone position with thermoplastic shells in place. Significant motion of ≥4 mm was observed in 23% of the patients. The authors suggested that this motion should be considered when designing treatment plans for patients in this position.

For immobilization, a thermoplastic mold is fabricated for simulation, CT scanning, and treatment to ensure that the patient is in the same treatment position during all procedures. The thermoplastic sheet is heated in warm water and molded to the patient's shape from the knees to midabdomen. Small sections of the mold are cut away to provide ports for marking and tattooing. The patient is scanned through an approximately 20 to 30 cm region around the prostate with a slice spacing and thickness of 3 mm. Before starting the CT planning study, several transverse images through the prostate and bladder are obtained to ensure that the rectal lumen is clearly visible, the bladder and rectum are not excessively filled, and the patient is properly positioned within the scan circle. Using the CT dataset, a "virtual simulation" is performed, using digitally reconstructed radiographs to localize the treatment area rather than conventional simulation films. The treatment isocenter is placed according to anatomic landmarks near the center of the prostate gland: midline, at the caudad aspect, and approximately 5 cm posterior to the symphysis pubis. The triangulation points for the isocenter are then tattooed, along with an additional alignment tattoo, along the sagittal line, approximately 10 cm superior to the isocenter. To ensure reproducible leg position, tattoos are placed on the back of the legs at the midshaft level, and the distance between the tattoos is recorded for future reference.

Target and Normal Tissue Contouring

The clinical target volume (CTV) is defined as the prostate and seminal vesicles. The planning target volume (PTV) is defined as the CTV with a margin to account for physical uncertainties including setup reproducibility, inter- and intrafractional organ motion. At MSKCC, a 1-cm margin is added to the CTV to form the PTV in all directions except posteriorly at the interface with the rectum, where the margin is reduced to 0.6 cm. Clinically, these margins were found to provide adequate target coverage based on a serial CT scan study evaluating organ motion during a course of 3DCRT (448). Normal tissues identified on each CT slice include the inner and outer walls of the rectum and bladder, the femoral heads, and the outer skin surface. Portions of the small bowel or sigmoid colon within 1 cm of the PTV are also contoured and taken into consideration, if necessary, during planning. In addition, the central 1-cm diameter portion of the prostate encompassing the prostatic urethra is defined for dosimetric consideration and evaluation during high-dose IMRT planning.

Accurate anatomic delineation of the prostate and, in particular, the prostatic apex, has been a topic of some controversy. Urethrography at the time of simulation as a method to accurately localize the apex has been advocated by some and extensively studied (7,88,280,351,353,394,425). Algan et al. (7) reviewed the location of the prostatic apex in 17 patients for whom MRI scan, retrograde urethrogram, and CT of the pelvis were obtained for 3D treatment planning. The location of the prostatic apex as determined by the urethrogram alone was, on average, 5.8 mm caudad to the location on the MRI, whereas the location of the prostatic apex as determined by CT/urethrogram was 3.1 mm caudad to that on MRI. If the prostatic apex is defined as 12 mm instead of 10 mm above the urethrogram tip (junction of membranous and prostatic urethra), the difference between the urethrogram and MRI locations of the prostatic apex is removed. Milosevic et al. (280) also found differences in the position of the prostatic apex between urethrogram, CT, and MR. In an evaluation of 20 patients, the authors found relatively poor correlation between MR and CT or MR and urethrogram in determining the height of the apex above the tuberosities. In response to concerns that the position of the prostate could be altered by the urethrogram itself, Mah et al. (243) performed sagittal MR scans immediately before and after urethrogram in 13 patients. No significant systematic motion of the prostate itself or the apex was observed, leading the authors to conclude that urethrography during simulation does not introduce localization error.

The contribution of MRI to improved accuracy and reproducibility of target localization in prostate cancer has also been well studied (106,333,341,413). Roach et al. (341) studied 10 patients with both MR and CT images of the prostate and noted that the prostate volume was 32% larger when defined by noncontrast CT than when determined by MRI. Areas of disagreement tended to occur in the posterior and posteroinferior-apical portions of the prostate, the apex (because of disagreement between urethrography and MRI), and the regions corresponding to the neurovascular bundle. Rasch et al. (333) also observed differences in CT- and MR-defined volumes. On average, the prostate and seminal vesicle volume defined on CT was 40% larger than that defined on MR. The CT-defined prostate was 8 mm larger at the base of the seminal vesicles and 6 mm larger at the prostatic apex. This difference was found to be significantly larger than interobserver variation.

Beam Selection and Planning

3DCRT Conformal Plans. The hallmark of 3D planning is the use of a multifield beam arrangement with field apertures designed using Bbeam's-eye-view projections that are conformal to the shape of the PTV, thereby shielding the normal tissues. At MSKCC, the standard 3D conformal beam arrangement consisted of six coplanar fields, including two lateral, two anterior and two oblique beams (237). Conformal apertures were drawn around the PTV adding a margin of approximately 5 to 6 mm in the axial directions to account for beam penumbra. This margin was sufficient dosimetrically in the axial plane because of the effect of the overlapping beams, whereas in the superior and inferior directions, a margin of 1 cm was typically necessary. For the beam shaping, multileaf collimation was used, which has effectively eliminated the handling of lead-cadmium alloy blocks. Several other beam arrangements have been proposed for 3DCRT, with the most common being the conformal four-field "box" (235,248,316,401).

Once the treatment fields and aperture shapes were defined, the dose distribution was calculated for a few representative planes, typically transverse, coronal, and sagittal planes through the isocenter. Dose-volume histograms were generated for the PTV, femoral heads, and rectal and bladder walls. If the bowel was located near the prostate and seminal vesicles, a dose calculation for the bowel was also done. For the MSKCC six-field plan, the two lateral beams typically delivered approximately half of the dose to the isocenter with the four oblique beams contributing the rest. The beam weights of the anterior oblique and posterior oblique beams were adjusted to obtain a uniform dose within the PTV and to place the hot spots away from the rectum. The plan was normalized so that the prescription isodose (100%) covered the PTV with a hot spot of 6% to 9% within the PTV. Although the portion of the rectal wall enclosed within the PTV was expected to receive the prescription dose, or slightly higher, the rectal wall volume receiving 75.6 Gy or more did not exceed 30%. Other normal tissue dose limits for these 3DCRT plans included limiting the maximum dose to the femurs to ≤68 Gy (90%), maximum dose to large bowel to ≤60 Gy (79%), and the maximum dose to small bowel to ≤50 Gy (66%).

Intensity-Modulated Radiation Therapy. Unlike 3DCRT treatment planning in which the planner defines the shape as well as the amount of radiation to be delivered from each treatment field, planners define dose "constraints" or "objectives" for the target and normal tissues, which describe the desired dose distribution in IMRT planning. These constraints typically consist of maximum or minimum dose limits on targets and dose and

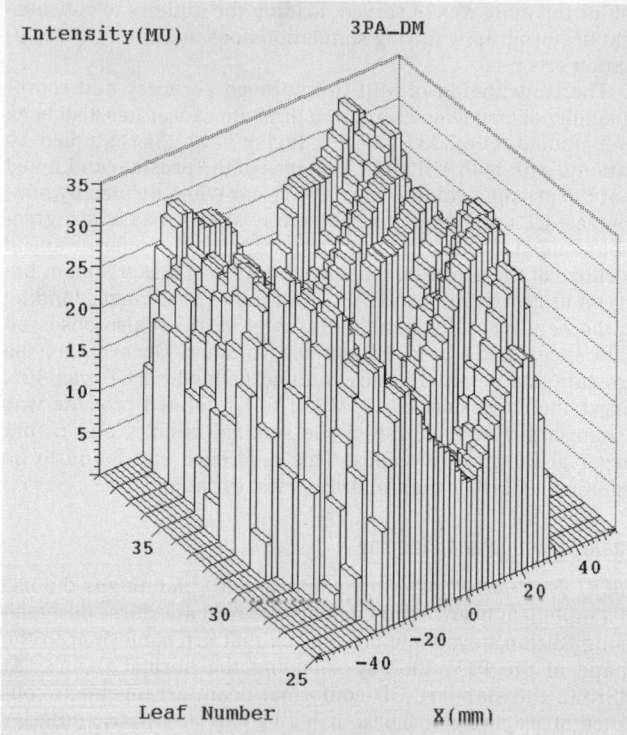

FIGURE 62.11. Radiation intensity pattern for a posterior intensity-modulated radiation therapy treatment field. Note the irregular shape of the intensity pattern and the relatively low intensity in the central section of the field, corresponding to the region overlying the rectum.

dose-volume limits on normal tissues. The planner specifies as many individual constraints for a specific target or normal tissue as desired, giving each its own weight or "penalty," reflective of its clinical importance. Using special computer software, these constraints drive a mathematical optimization of the radiation intensities of many small "beamlets" within each treatment field. The result of this optimization is a set of intensity patterns for the treatment fields and a dose distribution with characteristics as close as possible to the constraints entered by the planner. The MSKCC IMRT optimization algorithm was developed by Spirou and Chui (370) and relies on a conjugate gradient minimization to find the optimal intensity patterns and dose distribution. The IMRT intensity profiles are then converted to leaf motion using the algorithm of Spirou and Chui (379) for use during the dynamic MLC delivery. A typical intensity pattern for a posterior IMRT field for prostate treatment is shown in Figure 62.11.

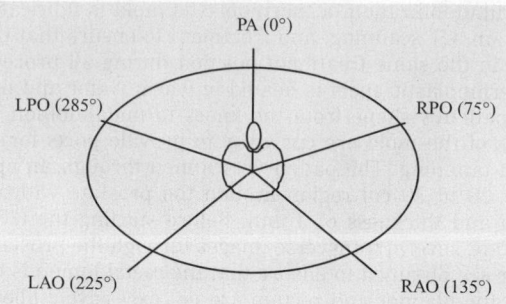

FIGURE 62.12. Schematic of the five-field beam arrangement used at Memorial Sloan-Kettering Cancer Center for intensity-modulated radiation therapy treatment of the prostate in the prone position. PA, posterior angle; RPO, right posterior oblique; RAO, right anterior oblique; LAO, left anterior oblique; LPO, left posterior oblique.

Because normal tissue shielding can be accomplished by modulating the beam intensity, IMRT beam directions are often somewhat nonintuitive and can differ significantly from those typically chosen for 3DCRT. Determination of appropriate target and normal tissue constraints can be tedious, and planners often repeat the optimization process multiple times, evaluating the dose distributions after each iteration and making small adjustments to the constraints before obtaining a final, acceptable plan. Most institutions performing IMRT planning set up templates that specify both the clinical goals of the dose distribution and initial target and normal tissue constraints for optimization. The MSKCC template for prostate IMRT planning to 81 Gy is shown in Table 62.8. Dose and dose-volume constraints for the PTV, PTV overlap with the rectum, and rectal and bladder walls are listed. It should be noted that constraint templates vary significantly between treatment planning systems; therefore, these constraints should be used only after a thorough evaluation on the user's system.

A variety of beam arrangements have been proposed for prostate IMRT treatment including multifield axial or noncoplanar arrangements in addition to intensity modulated arc therapy (51,326,437). At MSKCC, a standard arrangement of five 15-MV beams directed from the posterior, posterior oblique, and anterior oblique directions is used (Fig. 62.12). Primarily because of concern about increased risk of secondary cancers from higher neutron doses associated with IMRT treatment at high energies (165,166,215,216), some groups have proposed 6-MV IMRT techniques for the treatment of prostate cancer. As shown by Pirzkall et al. (318), however, a larger number of treatment fields may be necessary to achieve a dose distribution similar to that observed with 15-MV x-rays.

Table 62.8 OPTIMIZATION CONSTRAINT TEMPLATE AND PLANNING GOALS FOR MSKCC 81 GY AND IMRT PROSTATE TREATMENT

Structure	Optimization Constraints[a]			Treatment Plan Goals[b]	
	Max. Dose (Gy)/Penalty	Min. Dose (Gy)/Penalty	Volume (%)	Dose (Gy)	Volume (%)
PTV(excluding rectal overlap)	82.6/50	79.4 Gy/50	—	111% Max.	$V_{95} > 90$
PTV and rectum Overlap region	77.8/20	75.3 Gy/10	—	—	—
Rectal wall	77/20	—	—	75.6	30
Rectal wall	32.4/20	—	30	47	53
Bladder wall	79.4/35	—	—	—	—
Bladder wall	32.4/20	—	30	40	60

MSKCC, Memorial Sloan-Kettering Cancer Center; IMRT, intensity-modulated radiation therapy; Max., maximum; Min., minimum; PTV, planning target volume.
[a]Optimization constraints = initial target and normal tissue constraints entered into the IMRT optimization planning system.
[b]Treatment plan goals = dosimetric criteria used for evaluation and acceptance of an IMRT dose distribution.

The MSKCC clinical goals used to evaluate the IMRT dose distributions and dose-volume histograms for prostate patients are outlined in Table 62.8. These dosimetric guidelines defining acceptable target coverage, dose uniformity, and normal tissue doses have grown out of our 3DCRT and IMRT planning experience during the past 20 years and include several refinements resulting from retrospective outcome and toxicity analyses from our institution. Most notably, studies by Skwarchuk et al. (369) and Jackson et al. (196) retrospectively evaluating the rectal wall dose-volume histograms for patients treated to 70.2 and 75.6 Gy using 3DCRT techniques found that, on average, patients with late rectal bleeding had significantly higher rectal dose-volume histograms than patients who did not bleed. Both high- and intermediate-dose levels were found to be independently correlated with rectal bleeding. As a result of these studies, two rectal wall dose-volume histrogram limits were implemented and are routinely enforced at MSKCC when treating prostate cancer: no more than 30% of the rectal wall may receive more than 75.6 Gy and no more than 53% of the rectal wall can receive more than 47 Gy.

Typical dose distributions and dose-volume histograms for an 81 Gy IMRT plan are shown in Figures 62.13 and 62.14, respectively. The physician should carefully review the treatment plan and dose-volume histograms of the target and normal tissue structures to select the optimal treatment plan for the patient. Target coverage should be carefully assessed, as well the dose inhomogeneity and location of hot spots. In addition, careful attention should be given to determining if the treatment plan adequately meets acceptable dose constraints for the rectum, bladder, and bowel.

Standard Prescription Doses for 3DCRT and IMRT

Based on the results of a randomized trial from the M.D. Anderson Hospital (322), a radiation dose of 78 Gy (prescribed to the isocenter) would be appropriate for patients with PSA >10 ng/mL. Other institutions have demonstrated improved outcomes with higher radiation doses for all prognostic risk groups, including favorable-risk, early-stage disease. At MSKCC, 81 to 86 Gy are delivered to favorable-risk and intermediate/unfavorable-risk patients using IMRT. Daily fractions of 1.8 to 2 Gy, five fractions per week, are routinely used; however, others have reported encouraging results with a hypofractionated scheme delivering 70 Gy with fractions of 2.5 Gy (222,320). At MSKCC, the dose is prescribed to an isodose line that encompasses as much of the PTV as possible while still respecting the target and normal tissue goals listed in Table 62.8.

Typically, at least 90% to 95% of the PTV receives the prescription dose.

The usual dose delivered to the pelvic lymph nodes (when these lymph nodes are to be irradiated) is 45 Gy, with a subsequent boost to the prostate through reduced fields. 3DCRT and IMRT techniques have been used at MSKCC and elsewhere when pelvic lymph node irradiation is necessary, and observations indicate a significant reduction in bowel dose and improvement in the overall tolerance of therapy (21,66,300).

Treatment Delivery and Organ Motion Concerns

Movement of the prostate during treatment or between treatment fractions has long been a concern for prostate radiotherapy. A large number of studies investigating inter- and intrafractional motion of the prostate and seminal vesicles have been reported (4,15,23,28,34,77,93,105,186,210,227,263,294,345, 350,355,357,410,411,429,431,448). Most groups have measured prostate motion relative to bony landmarks through repeated imaging of implanted radio-opaque markers or serial CT studies. Although the reported magnitude of motion has varied, relatively little motion in the lateral direction and potentially significant movement in the anterior-posterior and superior-inferior directions has been consistently reported. Many studies have also observed a correlation between prostate and seminal vesicle motion and rectal or bladder filling.

Interfractional prostate motion was studied in approximately 50 patients by Crook et al. (93). Gold seeds implanted in the prostate were visualized on kilovolt radiographs taken at the simulation and approximately midway through treatment. Minimal prostate motion was observed in the lateral directions (0.1 to 0.5 cm) but inferior displacements of 0.5 and 1.0 cm or more were observed in 43% and 11% of their patients. Average displacement in the posterior direction was 0.72, 0.62, and 0.46 cm for seeds placed at the seminal vesicles, posterior aspect of the prostate, or apex of the gland, respectively; 60% of patients showed more than 0.5 cm posterior displacement of the prostate base, and 30% showed more than 1 cm.

Roeske et al. (345) evaluated 42 CT scans taken during the course of treatment on 10 patients. The standard deviations of the center of mass motion of the prostate were 0.7, 3.9, and 3.2 mm in the left-right, anterior-posterior, and superior-inferior directions, respectively. Corresponding data for center of mass motion of the seminal vesicles was 3.2, 7.3, and 4.1 mm. Motion of the prostate and seminal vesicles in the anteroposterior direction was strongly related to changes in rectal volume but only weakly related to bladder volume changes. For the prostate, a margin twice the patient group standard deviation

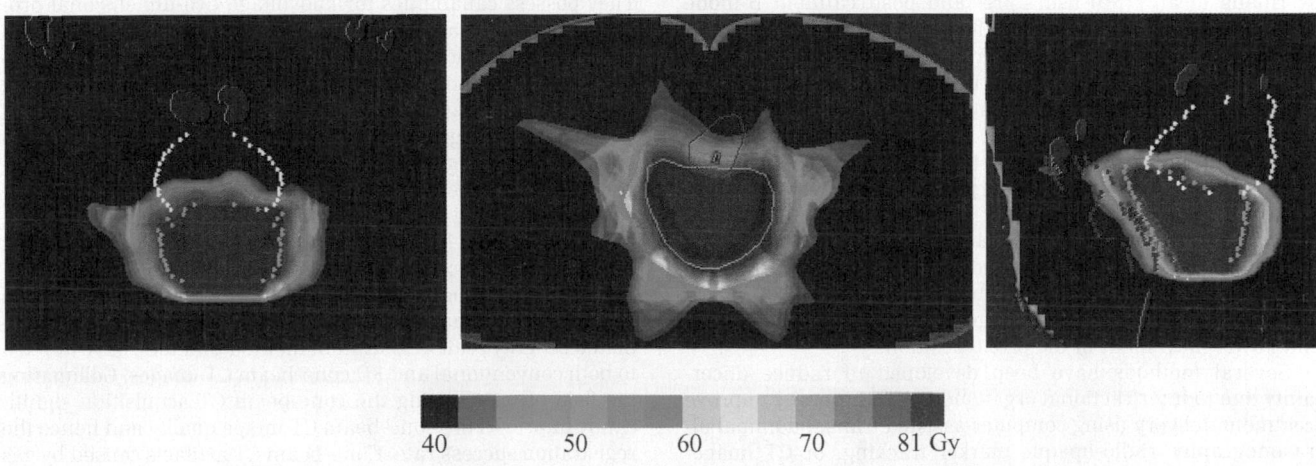

40   50   60   70   81 Gy

FIGURE 62.13. (Left to right): Axial, sagittal, and coronal color wash dose displays for an 81-Gy intensity-modulated radiation therapy prostate treatment. The structures outlined are the planning target volume (cyan), rectal (red), and bladder (yellow) walls.

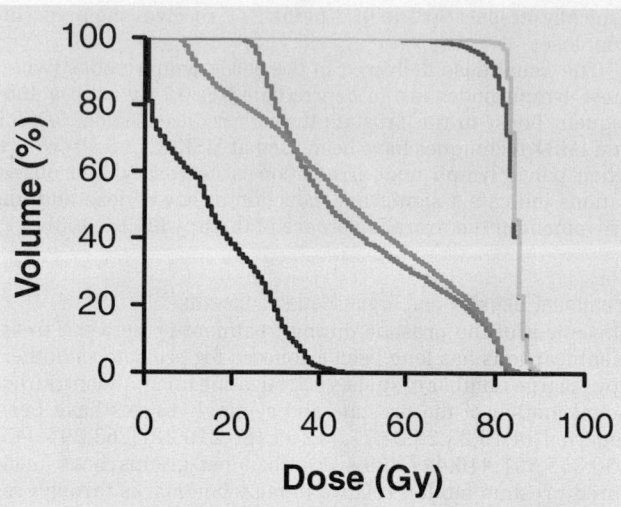

FIGURE 62.14. Typical dose-volume histogram for 81-Gy intensity-modulated radiation therapy prostate treatment. Dose-volume histograms are shown for the clinical target volume (yellow), planning target volume (orange), rectal wall (green), bladder wall (cyan), and femoral heads (purple).

(1.4 mm left-right, 7.8 mm anterior-posterior, and 6.4 mm superior-inferior) would have encompassed more than 95% of the center-of-mass motion.

Zelefsky and colleagues (448) obtained four serial CT studies for 50 patients (planning scan and three additional scans during the course of therapy). Prostate displacements in the anteroposterior and superoinferior directions were most frequently observed. The mean prostate motion in the anteroposterior, superoinferior, and left–right directions was 1.2, 0.5, and 0.6 mm, respectively. Anteroposterior movements were correlated with changes in rectal volume. Patients with large rectal volumes (>60 cm³) and large bladder volumes (>40 cm³) on the planning scan experienced a higher likelihood of having a 5-mm systematic displacement of the prostate and seminal vesicles, leading the authors to conclude that these patients may require more generous PTV margins to ensure adequate CTV coverage. However, among patients without large bladder and rectal volumes, a 1-cm margin around the CTV with a 6-mm margin at the prostate–rectal interface enclosed the posterior, anterior, superoinferior and left-right aspects of the CTV within the prescription dose level with a probability of 90%, 100%, 99% and 100%, respectively, indicating that the MSKCC margins provided adequate CTV coverage for most patients.

Intrafractional prostate motion was studied in 20 patients by Huang et al. (186) using pre- and posttreatment B-mode rectal ultrasound evaluations. Although the intrafractional motion was relatively insignificant in all directions, the predominant directions of motion were in the anterior and superior directions. Standard deviations of 0.4, 1.3, and 1.0 mm were observed in the lateral, anterior, and superior directions, respectively. A combination of real-time tumor tracking technology, fluoroscopy, and implanted gold markers were used by Kitamura et al. (210) to quantify intrafractional motion in 10 patients. Data were obtained with the patients in both supine and prone positions. The amplitude of the observed 3D motion was as much as 2.7 mm in the supine position and 24 mm in the prone position, indicating a great impact from respiration and bowel movement in the prone position.

Several methods have been developed to reduce uncertainty due to interfractional organ motion and thereby improve treatment delivery using computer-assisted transabdominal ultrasonography, radio-opaque marker tracking, or CT image-guidance. With the ultrasound system (BAT, Nomos Corporation, Sewickley, PA), patients are instructed to maintain a full bladder and are initially set up based on their tattoos in the supine position. The system is attached to the accelerator collimator and imports the coordinates of the isocenter as well as the target contours from the planning CT. Computer software facilitates 3D matching of the target contours with the prostate visualized on ultrasonography and determination of the necessary patient position modification. This system may not be reliable for patients who cannot maintain a full bladder and those with a large body habitus or other anatomic constraints because of anticipated poor image quality. It has also been noted that BAT measurements can be associated with a 2- to 3-mm error, which is sometimes in the range of the required shifts. Nevertheless, this system has been used by several investigators to verify the prostate position and results are consistent with improved accuracy of the daily treatment delivery (70,123,129,130,186,217,225,228,229,240,282,363). One such study, by Morr et al. (282), evaluated the BAT system on 23 patients undergoing IMRT treatment to the prostate. Once users of the system were sufficiently experienced, pretreatment ultrasound procedures could be performed in an average of about 5 minutes. Positional corrections averaged 2.6 ± 2.1 mm, 4.7 ± 2.7 mm, and 4.2 ± 2.8 mm in the lateral, anterior-posterior, and superior-inferior directions, respectively. The authors concluded that daily system use was feasible and resulted in clinically significant adjustments that would not have been possible using other conventional verification methods.

Recent technological advances have opened up the possibility of acquiring pre- or posttreatment megavoltage or kilovoltage CT images directly on the linear accelerator with the patient in the treatment position. One example of such a device, known as a tomotherapy unit (TomoTherapy Hi-ART, Madison, WI), consists of a 6-MV accelerator mounted within a CT-type gantry. Megavoltage CT images can be obtained prior to treatment, registered with the planning CT study, and the resulting positional corrections can then be applied prior to treatment. IMRT treatment is delivered through synchronized circular motion of the accelerator, couch translational motion, and multileaf collimation. Langen et al. (226) compared three methods of registering megavoltage CT images from a tomotherapy unit with the kilovoltage planning CT images and found that manual registration performed using implanted fiducial markers exhibited the least interobserver variability and agreed best with automatic registration computed from the center of mass of the three implanted fiducial markers.

Linac-based kilovoltage image guidance systems have recently become commercially available. These systems are comprised of a kilovoltage x-ray tube mounted 90 degrees from the accelerator head and a kilovotage imaging plate mounted 90 degrees from the standard megavoltage imaging device. They possess capabilities for kilovoltage two-dimensional projection imaging (radiographs), fluoroscopy, and 3D cone-beam CT, and are thus ideally suited for monitoring of inter- and intrafractional motion. Although little clinical experience using these kilovoltage gantry-mounted systems has been obtained to date, several groups have extensive experience monitoring and correcting for changes due to patient setup and organ motion with either two-dimensional electronic megavoltage portal imaging (EPID) or conventional CT systems (185,238, 250,373,374,432,434,435). As a result, several methods for fast prostate localization on CT images, appropriate for either off-line or on-line, image-guided radiotherapy have already been described. Smitsmans et al. (373,374) have developed an automated 3D gray scale registration method that they have applied to both conventional and 3D cone-beam CT images. Collimating the field of view during the cone-beam CT acquisition significantly improves the cone-beam CT image quality and hence the registration success rate. Cone-beam CT artifacts caused by gas pockets moving during the CT acquisition are the main cause of unsuccessful registration.

Hua et al. (185) have developed a semiautomatic method for localizing the prostate on pretreatment CT images based on manual identification of the posterior, anterior, left, and right extents of the prostate on the CT slices. The prostate displacement relative to the planning scan is then estimated through a simultaneous fitting of these "extents" to a finely spaced contour template from the planning scan. Identification of the prostatic extents on five pretreatment CT slices was found to be sufficient for reliable determination of the prostatic displacement. The approach of Yan et al. (435) has been to acquire an initial sequence of daily CT scans (typically 5 to 10 serial scans) from which the organ motion and patient setup inaccuracy can be reliably estimated. Based on these data, a confidence-limited PTV can be constructed that ensures, to within a defined statistical limit, that the CTV will receive a dose within a predefined tolerance. For example, the authors determined that a confidence-limited PTV constructed from daily CT scans obtained during the first week of 3DCRT treatment was sufficient to achieve a maximum dose reduction of $\leq 2\%$ in the CTV for at least 80% of the patients or a 4.5% reduction for 95% of the patients. IMRT treatment required 2 weeks of CT data to achieve the same level of dosimetric coverage. Referred to as adaptive radiotherapy, this off-line correction strategy is capable of excluding systematic error and compensating for random uncertainties. It requires serial scans, as previously outlined, and a single plan modification after the first or second week of therapy.

Brachytherapy For Early-Stage Disease: Treatment Techniques

Preplanned Transperineal Implantation Techniques

With the advent of transperineal CT and ultrasound-guided permanent prostatic implantation, the accuracy of isotope source placement has dramatically improved compared with older retropubic methods. The ultrasound-guided transperineal technique was initially described by Holm et al. (179) in 1983, and a large clinical experience was subsequently accumulated. This implantation technique evolved over the years into what is now known as the "Seattle Method," which uses a computer-generated preplanned approach. The technique can be described as follows: TRUS imaging is obtained before the planned procedure to assess the prostate volume. A computerized plan is generated from the transverse ultrasound images, producing isodose distributions and the ideal location of seeds within the gland to deliver the prescription dose to the prostate. Several days to weeks later, the implantation procedure is performed. Needles are then placed under ultrasonographic guidance through a perineal template according to the coordinates determined by the preplan. Radioactive seeds are individually deposited in the needle with the aid of an applicator or with preloaded seeds on a semirigid strand containing the preplanned number of seeds. In the latter case, this is accomplished by stabilizing the needle obturator that holds the seed column in a fixed position while the needle is withdrawn slowly, depositing a row or series of seeds within the gland. One of the inherent advantages of a stranded seed approach is the reduction of seed migration and embolization to the lung compared with the use of free seeds. While the embolization rate for stranded seeds is generally reported at <1%, the rate ranges from 5% to 72% in patients implanted with loose seeds. Among patients implanted with loose seeds, usually fewer than 2% of the implanted seeds are likely to migrate. There is no evidence of any adverse effect caused by seed embolization (308).

In general most brachytherapists use a modified peripheral loading technique for permanent interstitial implantation. This approach has been advocated by the Seattle group after observing a high rate of urethral complications during the early years of their experience with a homogenous loading pattern, which resulted in high urethral doses. Careful evaluation of the preplan with attention to dose-volume histogram analyses of both the target and normal tissues is essential to ensure that the dose to the urethra and rectum are within tolerance ranges and the prescription dose is being delivered to the prostate target. In a recent multi-institutional analysis there remains a great deal of variability within preplans as to acceptable target volume, seed strength, dose homogeneity, treatment margins, and extracapsular seed placement, although prostate brachytherapy prescription doses are uniform (272).

Intraoperative Planning Techniques for Prostate Brachytherapy

With the current availability of sophisticated treatment planning programs that can rapidly generate highly conformal dose distributions in the operating room, intraoperative planning for prostate brachytherapy has emerged as an attractive method for prostate brachytherapy. Intraoperative planning takes advantage of the opportunity of using real-time measurements of the prostate during the procedure while preplanning is often performed several weeks before implantation, frequently under different conditions than the actual operative procedure. Subtle changes in the position of the ultrasound probe as well as the distortion of the prostate associated with needle placement and subsequent edema can result in profound changes in the shape of the gland compared with the preplanned prostatic contour. Consequently, intraoperative adjustments of seed and needle placements are frequently required and the postplan CT-based dosimetry does not always correspond to the idealized preplan. Commercially available systems can track the placement of deposited seeds within the gland, which can provide feedback to the operator for the need to make adjustments to ensure target coverage and maintain constrained doses to the urethra and rectum. Yet, limitations still exist with such programs in their inability to reliably track and capture the exact coordinates of all of the deposited seeds on ultrasound because of difficulties with individual seed recognition using current ultrasound imaging techniques.

At MSKCC, an intraoperative conformal optimization and planning for ultrasound-based transperineal implant (TPI) that obviates the need for preplanning has been used (459). This technique involves a sophisticated optimization system that incorporates acceptable dose ranges allowed within the target as well as dose constraints for the rectal wall and urethra. An ultrasound probe is positioned in the rectum, and the prostate and normal anatomies are identified. Needles are inserted through the perineal template at the periphery of the prostate. The prostate is subsequently scanned from apex to base, and these 0.5-cm images are transferred to the treatment planning system using a PC-based video capture system. On the computer monitor, the prostate contours and the urethra are digitized on each axial image. Needle positions are identified on each image, and their coordinates are incorporated into a genetic algorithm optimization program. After the optimization program identifies the optimal seed-loading pattern and the dose calculations are completed, isodose displays are superimposed on each transverse ultrasound image and carefully evaluated. Dose-volume histograms for the target volume, rectum, and urethra are also carefully assessed. If portions of the target volume are found to be underdosed or higher urethral doses on selected images are observed, appropriate adjustments are made with the deletion of a seed or insertion of a new needle positions, and revised isodose distributions are immediately generated. The entire planning process from the contouring of images to the generation of the seed-loading pattern requires approximately 10 minutes. Seeds are then loaded with a standard applicator. Figure 62.15 shows a postimplantation CT image used for dosimetric evaluation.

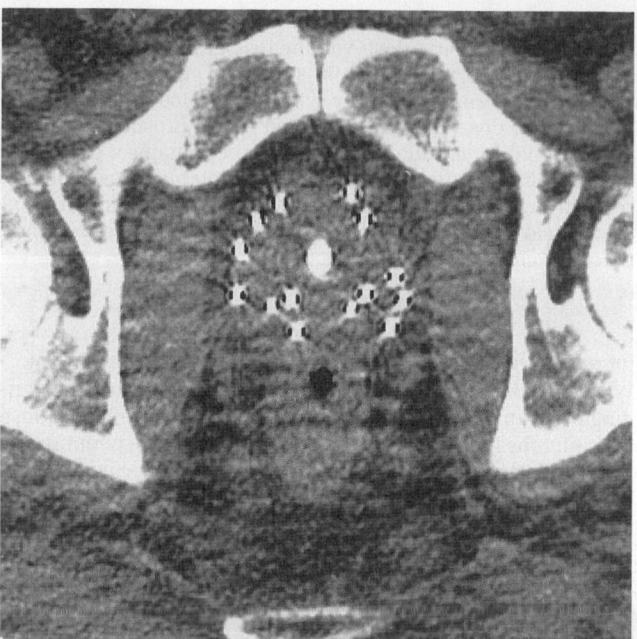

FIGURE 62.15. Postimplantation computed tomography scan after permanent transperineal ultrasound-guided seed implantation with urethral sparing.

Dose, Isotope, and Activity Considerations for Prostate Brachytherapy

In the retropubic implant era, 160 Gy was prescribed to a median peripheral dose, which assumed the prostate gland was in the configuration of a perfect ellipsoid. A reanalysis of the dosimetry of ^{125}I performed by Task Group 43 revealed that the actual dose delivered for a 160-Gy implant was approximately 10% lower (291). At present, the commonly used dose for interstitial implantation is 144 Gy prescribed to the isodose surface that completely encompasses the prostate as contoured from imaging studies. When ^{103}Pd became available, a lower prescription dose was recommended for this isotope (115 Gy). However, based on a consensus (National Institute of Standards and Technology 1999), the recommended prescription dose is approximately 10% higher or 125 Gy when ^{103}Pd is used (36).

There are clear physical differences between these two isotopes. The half-life of ^{125}I is 60 days, with a mean photon energy of 27 KeV and an initial dose rate of 7 cGy/hr. In contrast, the half-life of ^{103}Pd is 17 days, with a mean photon energy of 21 KeV and an initial dose rate of 19 cGy/hr. Dosimetric analyses of treatment plans performed with either isotope have not revealed significant differences between them (109). Most retrospective reports (67,266) have failed to demonstrate any benefit in terms of local tumor control or long-term complications for either isotope. A randomized trial has been conducted comparing ^{125}I with palladium-103 for the treatment of early-stage prostate cancer. To date, no difference in tumor control outcomes have been noted between the two arms of the study. Preliminary findings from this study have noted that patients treated with ^{103}Pd had more intense radiation prostatitis in the first month after implantation, but recovered from their radiation-related symptoms sooner than ^{125}I patients, consistent with palladium's shorter half-life (175).

Postimplantation Dosimetric Evaluation

Postimplantation dosimetric evaluation after prostate brachytherapy is recommended as the standard assessment of the quality of permanent interstitial implantation used for the treatment of prostate cancer (286). The adequacy of the target coverage with the intended prescription doses is evaluated with surrogate parameters such as volume of the prostate treated to 100% of the prescription dose (V_{100}) and the dose delivered to 90% of the prostate target (D_{90}). These parameters have been shown by several investigators to be associated with biochemical relapse and posttreatment biopsy outcomes (19,325,391). Equally important, other parameters of implant quality measure the dose exposure to the urethra and rectum. These measurements have been correlated with postimplantation urinary and rectal-related toxicities (167,270,375,460). Commercial software is routinely available to determine the coverage of the prostate and dose to critical normal tissue structures. Isodose curves and dose-volume histograms produce a detailed analysis of the radiation dose distribution relative to the prostate and surrounding normal tissues. Postimplantation evaluation is performed on the day of the procedure or 30 days after the procedure. The latter time point may be preferable when prostate edema is less significant after the implant and would less likely underestimate the prostate coverage with the prescription dose.

Bice et al. (38) examined multiple dosimetric parameters obtained from 50 prostate implants performed in 5 institutions using preplanning techniques. In that analysis, the average V_{100} (percentage volume of the prostate exposed to the prescription dose) for the respective five centers in ascending order was 77.5%, 84.3%, 87%, 88.4%, and 94.5%. Average maximal rectal doses calculated for each of the centers were 195, 263, 271, 292, and 354 Gy. No data were reported regarding urethral doses, although it was suggested that implants performed at centers that achieved higher percentages of target coverage with the prescription dose noted a concomitant increase in the central urethral dose (reflected in a greater percentage of the target volume receiving >150% of the prescription dose).

Zelefsky et al. (459) reported dosimetric outcome for intraoperative planning. The median V_{100}, V_{90}, and D_{90} (dose delivered to 90% of the prostate target) values for the intraoperative 3D technique were 96%, 98%, and 116%, respectively. In contrast, the V_{100}, V_{90}, and D_{90} values for a CT preplan and an ultrasound manual approach were 86%, 89%, and 88%, respectively, and 88%, 92%, and 94%, respectively (intraoperative optimization vs. other techniques; $p < .001$). A multivariate analysis determined that the intraoperative 3D technique (compared with other techniques) was an independent predictor of improved target coverage for each dosimetric parameter analyzed ($p < .001$). The maximum and average urethral doses were significantly lower with the intraoperative 3D technique compared with the other techniques, whereas a modest increase in the average rectal dose was also observed with the intraoperative 3D approach. Others have also demonstrated improved dosimetric outcomes with intraoperative planning techniques (209,253,274,388). A summary of published dosimetric outcomes after brachytherapy based on postimplantation CT-based dosimetric outcomes is shown in Table 62.9.

Investigators from the Joint Center for Radiation Therapy have reported the feasibility and early outcomes of TPI using intraoperative MRI instead of ultrasonography to guide seed placement (191,405). The CTV was defined as the peripheral zones identified on MRI; thus, seed placement was limited to the peripheral zones of the prostate, while the central and transitional zones were not implanted. Initial dosimetric analyses indicated that the median percentage of the CTV receiving the prescription dose was 94%. The median urethral D_{10} (dose to 10% of the urethral volume) was 210 Gy (range, 124 to 280 Gy) or 131% of the prescription dose.

Postimplantation evaluation is considered an important quality assurance procedure for prostate brachytherapy and provides important feedback to the brachytherapist concerning the quality of the implant performed and what corrections need

Table 62.9	POSTIMPLANT COMPUTED TOMOGRAPHY-BASED DOSIMETRIC PARAMETERS WITH PERMANENT PROSTATE BRACHYTHERAPY: TARGET COVERAGE AND NORMAL TISSUE DOSES					
Institution	V_{100}	D_{90} (Gy)	V_{150}	Rectal Dose	Urethral Dose
BC Cancer Agency	Loose, 90%	153	52.5%	V_{100} - 1.29 cm^3	NS
	Stranded, 91%	152	60%	V_{100} - 1.5 cm^2	
Mt. Sinai Medical Center (New York)	94%	175	56%	D_{30} - 46 Gy	D_{30} - 209
				D_{10} - 117 Gy	D_{10} - 220
Wheeling Medical Center (West Virginia)	95%	110%	55%	Mean, 78%	Mean, 120%
		167	68%	Maximum, 115%	Maximum, 141%
Memorial Sloan-Kettering Cancer Center	96%	173%	67%	Mean, 32%	Mean, 103%
				Maximum, 72%	Maximum, 129%

NS, Not stated.

to be made to optimize target coverage to reduce normal tissue dosing. Postimplantation dosimetric parameters also reflect the dose delivered to the prostate and may predict the likelihood of long-term tumor control outcomes. Stock et al. (386) reported that, among patients with low-risk disease who had an optimal dose based on retrospective postimplantation dosimetry evaluation (D_{90} >140 Gy; $n = 49$), the PSA relapse-free survival at 8 years was 94%, compared to 75% for those who received lower dose levels ($p = 0.02$).

Combination External-Beam Radiation Therapy and Brachytherapy

Although monotherapy approaches (EBRT alone or seed implantation alone) are appropriate treatment options for favorable-risk patients, combination of these treatment modalities is generally considered a more suitable treatment option patients with higher-risk disease. When a combined-modality approach is chosen for a patient, various treatment schemes have been used to integrate the brachytherapy with the EBRT. In general, 45 to 50 Gy of EBRT is delivered using conventional or conformal-based techniques to the prostate and periprostatic tissues. If a low–dose-rate boost is used, the brachytherapy prescription dose has been 90 Gy for ^{103}Pd implants and 110 Gy for ^{125}I implants. In the absence of clinical trials comparing HDR brachytherapy boosts versus low–dose-rate boosts, or the optimal sequence of therapy (brachytherapy boost preceding EBRT or vice versa), or the optimal isotope to be used for combined-modality therapy, there is no definitive evidence demonstrating the superiority of a particular treatment strategy over another.

A phase III trial, Radiation Therapy Oncology Group (RTOG) 0232, has recently been activated that compares permanent source brachytherapy as monotherapy to the combination of external-beam treatment followed by brachytherapy for patients with intermediate-risk prostate cancer. The primary end point of this study is survival outcome, and secondary end points include PSA relapse-free survival, distant metastases-free survival, and quality of life end points. Eligibility criteria for this study include clinical stage T1c-T2b, Gleason <7 with PSA 10 to 20 ng/mL or Gleason 7 with a PSA <10 ng/mL. The American Urological Association voiding symptom score should be ≤15 and prostate volume <60 g.

High-Dose-Rate Brachytherapy Techniques

HDR brachytherapy has been used as the brachytherapy component in combination with EBRT for the treatment of prostate cancer (208,214,249,252). In general, for this approach patients undergo transperineal placement of afterloading catheters in the prostate under ultrasonographic guidance. After CT-based treatment planning, several high-dose fractions,

ranging from 4 to 6 Gy each, are administered during an interval of 24 to 36 hours using ^{192}Ir. This treatment is followed by supplemental EBRT directed to the prostate and periprostatic tissues to a dose of 45 to 50.4 Gy using conventional fractionation. The Beaumont group has used fractionated outpatient HDR brachytherapy boosts interdigitated throughout the course of EBRT (208,249). Real-time intraoperative planning from the intraoperative ultrasonographic image was performed and each of three HDR boost treatments was delivered in the operating room under anesthesia. A dose-escalation study was implemented to increase gradually the dose per fraction delivered with the HDR boost from 5.5 Gy for three fractions to 10.5 Gy for three fractions. Improved outcomes with higher HDR boost doses were observed compared with outcomes achieved using lower dose levels. More recently, these investigators have used HDR brachytherapy as monotherapy without the addition of EBRT. The fractionation regimen was 38 Gy delivered in four fractions, two times daily during 2 days, and early tolerance and tumor control outcomes have been promising (159).

HDR brachytherapy offers several potential advantages over other techniques. Taking advantage of an afterloading approach, the radiation oncologist and physicist can more easily optimize the delivery of radiation therapy to the prostate and compensate for potential regions of underdosage ("cold spots") that may be present with permanent interstitial implantation. Further, this technique reduces radiation exposure to the radiation oncologist and others involved in the procedure compared with permanent interstitial implantation. Finally, HDR brachytherapy boosts may be radiobiologically more efficacious in terms of tumor cell kill for patients with increased tumor bulk or adverse prognostic features compared with low–dose-rate boosts such as ^{125}I or ^{103}Pd.

Results of Standard Treatment Interventions for Clinically Localized Prostate Cancer

Outcome with Radical Prostatectomy

Roehl et al. (344) have recently reported the outcome of 3,478 men who underwent RP for clinically localized prostate cancer at Washington University. In that report, the mean follow-up was 65 months. The overall biochemical recurrence rate at 10 years was 32% with a median time to failure of 28 months. The 10-year PSA relapse-free survival rates for patients with preoperative PSA levels <2.6, 2.6 to 4, 4.1 to 10, and >10 ng/mL were 91%, 78%, 74%, and 49%, respectively. Multivariate analysis revealed that predictors for PSA relapse-free survival outcomes included the preoperative PSA level, clinical tumor stage, Gleason sum, pathologic stage, and the treatment era. The 10-year cancer-specific and overall survival rates were 97% and

83%, respectively. The cancer-specific survival outcome was influenced by the pathologic stage ($p < .004$), Gleason sum ($p = 0.004$), and treatment era ($p = 0.04$). Of note, the 10-year biochemical relapse-free survival outcome was significantly different for those patients with pathologic Gleason 3 + 4 versus 4 + 3 (64% and 32%, respectively).

Han et al. (169) reported the long-term outcome of RP from the Johns Hopkins Hospital. In that report, 2,091 men underwent RP. In this series, 79% of patients had PSA levels <10 ng/mL and 62% of the patients had Gleason scores of ≤6. The mean follow-up was 6.3 years. The overall 10- and 15-year PSA relapse-free survival outcomes were 85% and 79%, respectively. The 10-year PSA control rates for patients with preoperative PSA values of 0 to 4, 4 to 10, 10.1 to 20, and >20 ng/mL were 91%, 79%, 57%, and 48%, respectively.

Bianco et al. (37) reported long-term outcome of RP in 1,746 patients treated at Baylor College of Medicine and MSKCC between 1983 and 2003 (206). The mean follow-up was 6 years. In this series, 76% and 70% of the patients had PSA ≤10 ng/mL and Gleason scores <7, respectively. Disease progression was defined as persistent elevation of the PSA >0.4 ng/mL before 1996 and 0.2 ng/mL afterwards, or the need for further therapeutic interventions. The incidence of positive surgical margins and organ-confined disease decreased with time; since 1995, 76% of patients had organ-confined disease with a 7% incidence of positive margins. The overall 10- and 15-year biochemical relapse-free survival outcomes were 77% and 75%, respectively. The 10-year PSA control rates for patients with preoperative PSA values of 0 to 4, 4 to 10, 10.1 to 20, and >20 ng/mL were 92%, 82%, 63% and 46%, respectively. The cancer-specific survival rates at 10 and 15 years were 95% and 89%, respectively. Among patients with positive surgical margins, the likelihood of disease-free progression at 10 years was 40% compared to 81%.

Amling et al. (13) from the Mayo Clinic reported the outcome of 2,782 patients with clinically localized prostate cancer treated between 1987 and 1993. They noted that among patients with pathologically confirmed T2,N0 disease, the 5- and 10-year PSA relapse-free survival rates were 82% and 68%, respectively. The highest risk of biochemical relapse was noted during the first 2 years after surgery, and only 6% of patients had a disease relapse after 5 years.

Outcome with Cryotherapy

A multi-institutional pooled analysis was performed that comprised 975 patients treated with cryosurgery in the management of their primary prostatic disease (242). The PSA relapse-free survival rates for patients with favorable, intermediate, and aggressive risk features were 75%, 71%, and 61%, respectively. The overall incidence of a positive biopsy after treatment was 8%. Bahn et al. (26) reported 7-year results for 590 patients who underwent primary cryotherapy for localized or locally advanced prostate cancer. The mean follow-up was 5.4 years. Using a cut-point of 0.5 ng/mL to define biochemical failure, the PSA relapse-free survival rates for low-, intermediate-, and high-risk patients were 61%, 68%, and 61%, respectively. Using a definition of three consecutive rising values from the nadir level (i.e., American Society for Therapeutic Radiology and Oncology [ASTRO] definition of biochemical failure [12]), the PSA relapse-free survival rates for low-, intermediate-, and high-risk patients were 92%, 89%, and 89%, respectively.

Outcome with Conventional External-Beam Radiation Therapy

The results of a large multi-institutional analysis comprising 4,839 patients with T1-T2 prostate cancer treated with EBRT

between 1986 and 1995 was reported by Kuban et al. (218). The median followup was 6.3 years. In this cohort, no patient received neoadjuvant androgen-deprivation therapy. Most of the patients included (70%) were treated with conventional EBRT and 30% were treated with 3DCRT planning techniques. Prescription doses ranged from 60 to 78 Gy. For the cohort of patients treated to dose levels <70 Gy, the median dose was 67 Gy; among those patients who received 70 Gy or more, the median dose in this cohort was 72 Gy. PSA failure was defined according to the ASTRO definition of three consecutive rising PSA values above the nadir value. The overall 8-year PSA control rates for patients with pretreatment PSA values of 0 to 4, 4 to 9.9, 10 to 20, and >20 to 30 ng/mL were 80%, 60%, 46% and 34%, respectively. The overall 8-year PSA control rates for patients with posttreatment nadir PSA values of 0 to 0.49, 0.5 to 0.99, 1 to 1.99, and ≥2.0 ng/mL were 93%, 88%, 86%, and 72%, respectively. Higher prescription dose levels of ≥72 Gy were associated with a significant decrease in PSA relapse rates, and these differences were most noted among patients with intermediate and higher risk disease. However, there was no apparent dose response for favorable-risk patients, yet the number of patients with favorable-risk features who received higher doses in this study was small.

The Role of Dose Escalation in Patients with Clinically Localized Disease

It has become clear that traditionally planned EBRT using conventional dose levels does not have the capacity to completely eradicate local prostatic disease in the majority of treated patients. Further, the results of conventional EBRT from the M.D. Anderson Hospital (461) demonstrate that even among patients with PSA <10 ng/mL, a continuous decline in the PSA relapse-free survival rate is observed with time, and no plateau is noted on these curves, especially among patients treated with lower radiation doses. With the increasing use of 3D conformal planning and availability of IMRT, prescription doses can be more reliably delivered to the prostate and lead to further improved outcomes. Single-institution studies have demonstrated excellent long-term biochemical outcomes for patients with intermediate and unfavorable risk disease. These studies led to the development of randomized trials that have now demonstrated improved PSA relapse-free survival outcomes, in particular for patients with intermediate risk and selected unfavorable risk disease.

Randomized Dose-Escalation Trials

Phase III randomized trials and several single-institution trials have confirmed the advantage of high-dose CRT for patients with localized prostate cancer. The results of the phase III trial from M.D. Anderson Hospital were reported by Pollack et al. (322). The study enrolled 301 patients with T1 to T3 prostate cancer, of whom 150 were treated to 70 Gy (conventional EBRT) and 151 were treated to 78 Gy (conventional EBRT followed by a 3D boost). The PSA relapse-free survival rates for the 78- and 70-Gy arms were 70% and 64%, respectively ($p = .03$). A significant advantage for dose escalation was detected among patients with pretreatment PSA levels >10 ng/mL. In this group, the PSA control rates for the 78- and 70-Gy arms were 62% and 43%, respectively ($p = .01$). However, among patients with PSA levels <10 ng/mL, no advantage for higher doses was observed. (Fig. 62.16).

Zietman et al. (461) reported the result of a randomized trial of 393 patients with T1-T2 prostate cancer with pretreatment PSA levels <15 ng/mL. Patients were randomized to receive conventional EBRT to a dose level of 70.2 Gy or 79.2 Gy. In both treatment arms, radiotherapy was delivered using a

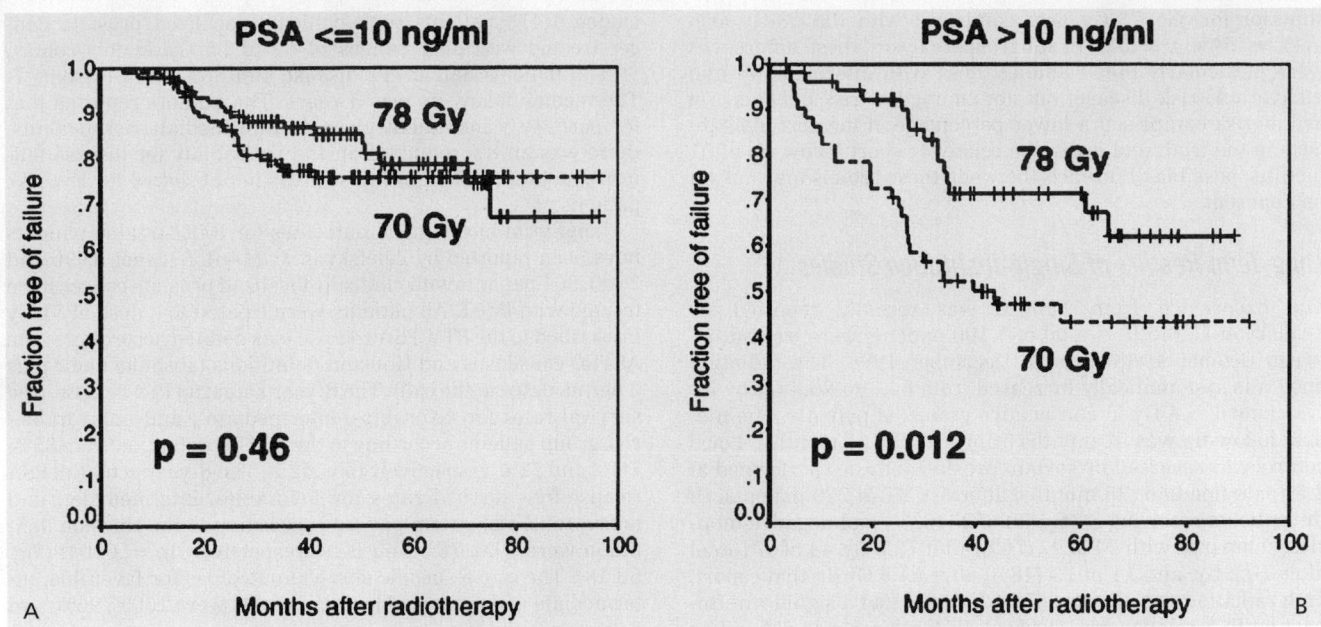

FIGURE 62.16. A,B: Actuarial prostate-specific antigen (PSA) relapse-free survival outcomes according to dose level. (From Pollack A, Zagars GK, Starkschall G, et al. Prostate cancer radiation dose response: results of the M.D. Anderson phase III randomized trial. *Int J Radiat Oncol Biol Phys* 2002;53:1097–1105, with permission).

combination of photon and proton beams. The median follow-up in this study was 5.5 years. The 5-year PSA relapse-free survival rates for the low- and high-dose arms was 61% and 80%, respectively, which represented a 49% risk reduction in biochemical failure. What was most noteworthy in this trial was that a clear advantage for higher dose was observed among the subset of patients with low-risk disease, which represented the majority of patients accrued to the trial (PSA <10 ng/mL, stage ≤T2a or Gleason score <6). In this subgroup of patients, a significant advantage for higher doses was observed, with an associated 51% risk reduction in biochemical relapse (80% vs. 60%

for higher versus lower doses; $p < .001$). A similar significant advantage for improved biochemical control was also observed when the subset of intermediate-risk patients were analyzed separately (81% vs. 63%; $p = .02$) (Fig. 62.17).

Recently, Peeters et al. (314) from the Netherlands Cancer Institute, reported the results of a randomized trial comparing 78 Gy of conventional photon radiotherapy to 68 Gy. Six hundred sixty-nine patients with T1-T4 disease were eligible and stratified by the use of neoadjuvant androgen-deprivation therapy, age, and treatment group. The median follow-up was 51 months. The 5-year PSA relapse-free survival outcome was

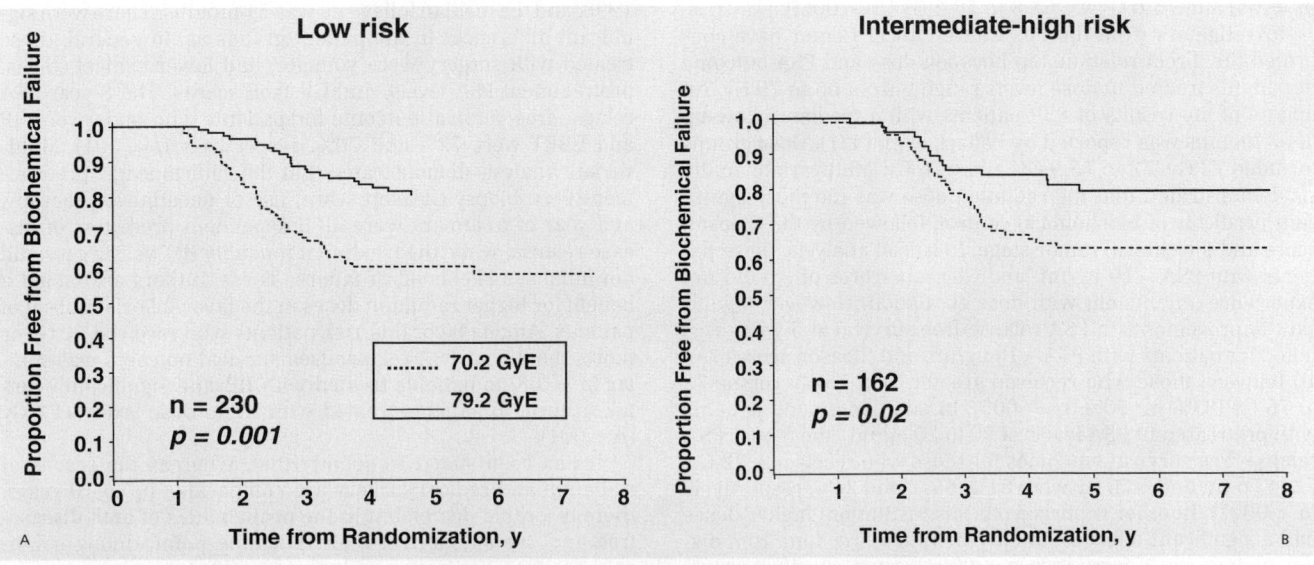

FIGURE 62.17. Freedom from biochemical failure (American Society for Therapeutic Radiology and Oncology [ASTRO] definition) following either conventional-dose (70.2 GyE [gray equivalents]) or high-dose (79.2 GyE) conformal radiation therapy analysis of these early cases is by risk subgroup. Low-risk patients have prostate-specific antigen level <10 ng/mL, stage ≤T2a tumors, and Gleason scores ≤6. (From Zietman AL, DeSilvio ML, Slater JD, et al. Comparison of conventional-dose vs high-dose conformal radiation therapy in clinically localized adenocarcinoma of the prostate: a randomized controlled trial. *JAMA* 2005;294:1233–1239, with permission).

superior for the 78-Gy arm compared with the 68-Gy arm (64% vs. 54%; $p = .02$). In subgroup analyses, these differences were particularly noted among those with intermediate- and unfavorable-risk disease, but not among low-risk patients. Yet as low-risk comprised a lower percentage of the accrued subjects in the trial, and given the relatively short follow-up of 51 months, possible differences between these groups may not yet be apparent.

Long-Term Results of Single-Institution Studies

The experience from MSKCC was recently reported by Zelefsky et al. (452). A total of 1,100 patients were treated between October 1988 through December 1998. The radiation dose was systematically increased from 64.8 to 86.4 Gy by increments of 5.4 Gy in consecutive groups of patients. The median follow-up was 52 months (range, 12 to 127 months). Local control was assessed by sextant prostate biopsies performed at 2.5 years (median, 35 months) after 3DCRT in 220 patients. Of the patients receiving 81 Gy, 30 of 33 (91%) had negative biopsies, compared with 74 of 97 (76%) after 75.6 Gy, 44 of 67 (66%) after 70.2 Gy, and 11 of 23 (48%) after 64.8 Gy. In that report, high radiation dose levels ($\geq$75.6 Gy) also had a significant impact on PSA relapse-free survival. PSA relapse was defined as three successive increases in the PSA value after a posttreatment nadir level was achieved. The date of failure was the midpoint in time between the last nonrising and the first-rising PSA value. For this analysis, patients were classified into prognostic groups according to pretreatment variables that independently affected the PSA outcome. Patients with stage T1 or T2 disease, pretreatment PSA $\leq$10 ng/mL, and Gleason score $\leq$6 were classified as a favorable-prognosis group. An increase in one of the variables classified the patient in the intermediate group, and an increase in two or more in the unfavorable-prognosis group. The 5-year actuarial PSA relapse-free survival rate for patients with favorable prognostic indicators who received 64.8 to 70.2 Gy was 80%, compared with 91% for those treated to $\geq$75.6 Gy ($p = .03$). For patients with an intermediate prognosis, the corresponding rates were, respectively, 47% and 70% ($n = .001$) and for the unfavorable prognosis group, 24% and 47% ($p = .04$). Furthermore, the 5-year PSA relapse-free survival rate for unfavorable-risk patients who received 81 Gy was 69%, compared with 19% for those treated to 75.6 Gy (81 Gy vs. 75.6 Gy [$p = .05$] and 75.6 Gy vs. 64.8 to 70.2 Gy [$p = .006$]).

Investigators from the Fox Chase Cancer Center have confirmed the direct relationship between dose and PSA outcome in patients treated to dose levels ranging from 66 to 79 Gy. An update of the results of 839 patients with a median follow-up of 63 months was reported by Pollack et al. (321). Dose groups included 72 Gy, 72 to 75.9 Gy, and $\geq$76 Gy. Multivariate analysis demonstrated that the radiation dose was the most significant predictor of biochemical control, followed by the Gleason score and the clinical tumor stage. In subset analysis, those patients with PSA <10 ng/mL and Gleason scores of $\leq$6 did not experience any benefit with dose escalation. However, significant improvements in PSA relapse-free survival at 5 years was noted for patients with PSA <10 ng/mL and Gleason scores 7 to 10 between those who received greater than 76 Gy versus 72 to 76 Gy (83% vs. 50%; $p = .005$). In addition among patients with pretreatment PSA levels of 10 to 20 ng/mL, the 5-year PSA relapse-free survival outcomes for those who received <72 Gy, 72 to 76 Gy, and >76 Gy were 81%, 65%, and 24%, respectively ($p < .0001$). In other reports from this institution, higher doses had a significant effect on the 5-year rate of freedom from distant metastasis (97% vs. 88%, $p = .0004$), cause-specific survival rate (99% vs. 94%, $p = .007$), and overall survival rate (88% vs. 79%, $p = .01$).

Symon et al. (396) reported the long-term outcome of high-dose 3DCRT from the University of Michigan. This report included 1,473 patients with clinically localized prostate cancer treated with dose ranges of 69 to 75 Gy. In this cohort, 90% of patients had T1-T2 disease and 88% had Gleason $\leq$7. The median follow-up was 3 years. The authors reported that for each 1-Gy increment given to intermediate-risk patients, there was an 8% reduction in the probability for disease failure. The benefit of higher doses was not observed for low-risk patients.

Long-term biochemical outcomes for IMRT-treated patients have been reported by Zelefsky et al. (446). Between 1996 and 2000, 561 patients with clinically localized prostate cancer were treated with IMRT. All patients were treated to a dose of 81 Gy prescribed to the PTV. PSA relapse was defined according to the ASTRO consensus and Houston definitions (absolute nadir plus 2 ng/mL dated at the call). The 8-year actuarial PSA relapse-free survival rates for favorable-, intermediate-, and unfavorable-risk group patients according to the ASTRO definition were 85%, 76%, and 72%, respectively ($p < .025$). The 8-year actuarial PSA relapse-free survival rates for favorable-, intermediate-, and unfavorable-risk group patients according to the Houston definition were 89%, 78% and 67%, respectively ($p = .0004$) (Fig. 62.18). The cause-specific survival outcomes for favorable, intermediate and unfavorable risk patients were 100%, 96%, and 84%, respectively.

Comparison of EBRT Outcomes with Surgery for Early-Stage Prostate Cancer

Because of a lack of randomized trials comparing the outcome of EBRT with surgery, retrospective nonrandomized comparisons have been made. A unique comparison was reported by Hanks et al. (170) of 104 patients who were pathologically staged as node-negative patients with early clinical stage disease. In this report, 104 patients with clinical stage A2 and B N0 disease underwent lymph node dissections and were treated in RTOG trial 77-06. The 10-year cause-specific mortality rate was 14%, with 87% of patients free of local recurrence, whereas the 10-year overall survival rate was similar to that for an age-matched control cohort generated by life tables (63% vs. 60%). Kupelian et al. (221) compared the 8-year outcomes of surgery and EBRT from the Cleveland Clinic. In this report, 1,054 patients were treated with surgery and 628 were treated with EBRT. Treatments (surgery or radiotherapy) were given between 1990 and 1998, and the median follow-up was 51 months. There were significant differences in the patient groups as, in general, those treated with surgery were younger, had lower clinical stages, pretreatment PSA levels, and Gleason scores. The 8-year PSA relapse-free survival outcome for patients who underwent RP and EBRT were 72% and 70%, respectively ($p = .01$). Multivariate analysis demonstrated that the clinical stage, pretreatment PSA, biopsy Gleason score, use of neoadjuvant therapy, and year of treatment were all independent predictors of disease relapse, while the treatment modality (RT vs. surgery) did not influence likelihood of failure. These authors also noted a benefit for higher radiation doses in the favorable-risk subset of patients. Among favorable-risk patients who received 72 Gy or more, the 8-year PSA relapse-free survival outcome was similar ($p = .08$) to patients treated with RP, and significantly better, in turn, to patients treated with RT to dose levels <72 Gy ($p < .001$).

It has been stated frequently that, whereas the results of radiation and radical surgery are comparable up to 10 years, there is a rapid decrement in the probabilities of both disease-free and overall survival after that time point among irradiated patients. Yet, such conclusions are likely erroneous owing to selection bias factors favoring a younger cohort with more favorable prognostic features who are more often chosen for surgery compared with radiation therapy. In addition, because of the lack of information in most radiation therapy series of

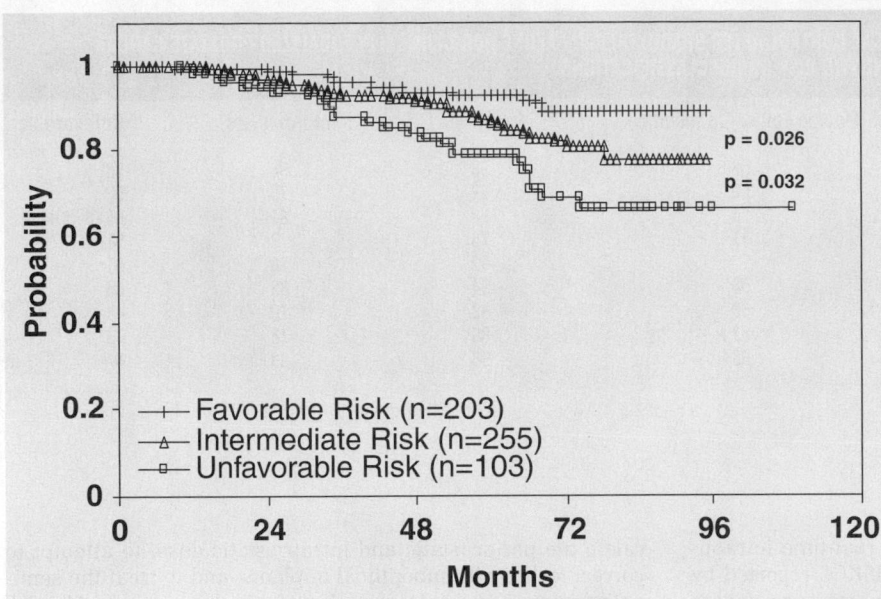

FIGURE 62.18. Actuarial prostate-specific antigen relapse-free survival outcomes for 81-Gy intensity-modulated radiation therapy, according to risk group. (From Zelefsky MJ, Chan H, Hunt M, et al. Long-term outcome of high dose intensity modulated radiation therapy for patients with clinically localized prostate cancer. *J Urol* 2006;176:1415–1419, with permission.)

Clinical Radiation Oncology

the pathologic status of the lymph nodes, patients with microscopic nodal disease will likely be included in radiation therapy reports, yet routinely excluded from surgical series.

Outcome with Brachytherapy

Similar to the predictors of biochemical outcome after EBRT for prostate cancer, PSA relapse-free survival after permanent seed implantation depends on several prognostic variables, including the pretreatment PSA, biopsy Gleason score, clinical stage, and the implant dose delivered to the target volume. In general, among patients with pretreatment PSA ≤ 10 ng/mL, TPI alone is associated with excellent biochemical outcome and appears comparable with other local interventions.

Grimm et al. (161) reported the outcome of 125 patients treated between 1988 and 1990 with ^{125}I permanent seed implantation and followed for a median of 81 months. For patients with low-risk disease (PSA <10, Gleason <7, and clinical stage $\leq$T2b) the 10-year PSA relapse-free survival outcome was 87%. Blasko et al. (42) reported the outcome of 230 patients treated with a median follow-up of 41 months with Pd-103. Most patients in this report had favorable risk features, whereas only approximately 30% and 20%, respectively, of the patients had Gleason scores >6 and PSA levels >10 ng/mL. The 7-year PSA relapse-free survival (with relapse defined as two consecutive rising PSA values) was 83%. Postimplantation biopsies were performed on 201 patients. The incidence of negative, indeterminate, and positive postimplant biopsies were 80%, 17%, and 3%, respectively.

Stone et al. (391) reported on 279 patients with T1-T2 prostate cancer treated with permanent ^{125}I prostate implantation. The median follow-up in that report was 6 years. The prescription dose was 160 Gy. The median postimplantation D_{90} was 164 Gy, with a range of 15 to 256 Gy. The 10 year PSA relapse-free survival outcomes for patients with low-risk disease was 91% compared to 63% for those with higher-risk disease (p <.001). Among patients whose postimplantation dosimetric evaluation revealed a D_{90} of >140 Gy ($n = 180$), the 10-year PSA relapse-free survival was 90% compared with 62% for patients with D_{90} doses <140 Gy ($n = 59$; p <.001). The D_{90} dose level (p <.0001) and the risk group ($p = .01$) were the only variables identified as highly predictive of PSA relapse-free survival outcome. Multivariate analysis identified the D_{90} dose levels >140 Gy (p <.0001) and low-risk group ($p = .01$) were

significant predictors for improved long-term biochemical outcome. In these patients, 185 (66%) underwent a postimplantation biopsy at a minimum of 2 years after treatment, of which 90% were negative. Among patients with low-risk disease, the incidence of a positive posttreatment biopsy was 4.5% compared with 15.5% for those with higher-risk disease ($p = .01$). Among patients who received a D_{90} dose of >140 Gy, the incidence of a positive posttreatment biopsy was 5% compared with 20.5% for those patients who received lower D_{90} dose levels ($p = .01$).

Potters et al. (325) reported on the outcome of 1,449 patients treated with brachytherapy, including patients treated with seed implantation alone or combined with EBRT. The median follow-up was 82 months. The 12-year PSA relapse-free survival according modified ASTRO definition for low-, intermediate-, and high-risk patients was 89%, 78%, and 63%, respectively ($p = .0001$). In these patients, the dose to 90% of the D_{90} correlated with biochemical tumor control outcomes. Multivariate analysis identified the following variables as independent predictors for improved long-term biochemical control: 90% of the D_{90} (p <.001), pretreatment PSA ($p = .001$), Gleason score ($p = .002$), percent positive cores ($p = .03$); while clinical stage, addition of hormones, and supplemental external radiotherapy did not impact on biochemical control.

Eleven institutions combined data on 2,693 patients treated with permanent interstitial brachytherapy monotherapy for T1-T2 prostate cancer (455). Of these patients, 1,831 (68%) were treated with ^{125}I (median dose, 144 Gy) and 862 (32%) were treated with Pd-103 (median dose, 108 Gy). The median follow-up was 63 months. The 8-year PSA relapse-free survival outcomes for favorable-, intermediate-, and unfavorable-risk patients were 82%, 70% and 48%, respectively (p <.001) according to the ASTRO consensus definition. Among patients in whom the dose to 90% of the prostate (D_{90}) was >130 Gy, the 8-year PSA relapse-free survival outcome was 90% compared with 73% for those with D_{90} dose levels $\leq$130 Gy (p <.001) The PSA nadir value at 3 years after implantation was associated with the long-term biochemical outcome. The 8-year PSA relapse-free survival outcomes were 92%, 86%, 79%, and 67%, respectively, for patients who achieved PSA nadir values of 0 to 0.49, 0.5 to 0.99, 1.0 to 1.99, and >2.0 ng/mL (p <.001). Among patients who were free of biochemical relapse at 8 years, the median nadir level was 0.1 ng/mL, and 90% of these patients achieved a nadir PSA level <0.6 ng/mL.

Table 62.10	FIVE-YEAR BIOCHEMICAL CONTROL AFTER BRACHYTHERAPY ALONE FOR CLINICALLY LOCALIZED PROSTATE CANCER ACCORDING TO PROGNOSTIC RISK GROUP CLASSIFICATIONS				
Study	Patients	Median Follow-Up (months)	Favorable	Intermediate	Unfavorable
Merrick (269)	688	58.6	98	98	88
Battermann (31)	351	50	89	75	57
Kollmeier (212)	243	75	88	81	65 (8-yr data)
Ash (19,20)	321 without HT	31	75	73	51
	346 with HT		92	76	51
Blasko (42)	403	58	94	82	65
Zelefsky (457)	269	63	82	70	48
Potters (323)	1449	82	89	78	63
Zelefsky (458)	367	63	96	89	N/A

HT, hormonal therapy; N/A, not applicable.

In an update of the 5-year outcome of real-time intraoperative planning for ^{125}I monotherapy at MSKCC reported by Zelefsky et al. (458), 367 patients with prostate cancer were treated with ^{125}I permanent interstitial implantation using a transrectal ultrasound-guided approach. Real-time intraoperative treatment planning, which incorporated inverse planning optimization, was used. The median follow-up time was 63 months. The median V_{100} and D_{90} values were 96% and 173 Gy, respectively. In 96% of cases, a D_{90} of >140 Gy was achieved. The median urethral and rectal doses were 100% and 33% of the prescription doses, respectively. The 5-year PSA relapse-free survival outcomes for favorable- and intermediate-risk patients according to the ASTRO definition were 96% and 89%, respectively. In these patients, no dosimetric parameter was identified that influenced the biochemical outcome. Table 62.10 summarizes the published biochemical outcomes after low-dose-rate interstitial seed implantation according to prognostic risk groups.

Outcome of Combination Brachytherapy and External Beam Radiation Therapy

Critz et al. (90) reported on 689 patients with early-stage prostate cancer treated with transperineal ultrasonography-guided implantation using ^{125}I followed 3 weeks later by the delivery of 45 Gy of conventional EBRT. The pretreatment PSA levels were ≤10 ng/mL and Gleason scores <7 in 73% and 76% of patients, respectively. No patients received neoadjuvant or adjuvant hormonal therapy. PSA relapse was defined as a PSA nadir level >0.2 ng/mL or a subsequent rising of PSA above this level. The median follow-up in that report was 4 years. The actuarial 5-year PSA relapse–free survival rates for patients with pretreatment PSA levels of 0 to 4 ng/mL (n = 50), >4 to 10 ng/mL (n = 451), >10 to 20 ng/mL (n = 144), and >20 ng/mL (n = 44) were 94%, 93%, 75%, and 69%, respectively.

Sylvester et al. (395) reported the Seattle Prostate Institute experience of 232 patients treated with combination of ^{125}I or [103]Pd brachytherapy in combination with EBRT. The mean follow-up in this group was 63 months. Projected 10-year biochemical relapse-free survival outcomes for patients defined according to the MS-KCC prognostic risk groupings were 85%, 77% and 45% for low-, intermediate-, and high-risk patient, respectively.

Combined-therapy regimens are often used for intermediate-risk and selected high-risk patients, yet its benefit over seed implantation alone is not established. There is a tendency to use combination therapy for various reasons in patients with higher-risk disease, including the potential to es-

calate the periprostatic and intraprostatic dose, to attempt to correct technically suboptimal implants, and to treat the seminal vesicles and/or pelvic lymph nodes in their entirety. Merrick et al. (273) have argued that excellent results can be achieved in such patients with brachytherapy alone without the need to use supplemental EBRT, especially if extraprostatic seed placement and careful implantation techniques are employed. Other retrospective reports have suggested poor biochemical outcomes when brachytherapy alone has been used for intermediate- and higher-risk patients. The role of combined therapy for intermediate-risk disease will likely be clarified with the results of RTOG 0232 trial. This phase III trial is currently randomizing patients with intermediate-risk disease to receive brachytherapy alone or with 45 Gy of EBRT. The study will accrue 1,520 patients with a primary end point of overall survival.

Outcome with High-Dose-Rate Brachytherapy

Galalae et al. (131) reported the combined results of three institutions' experience with high dose-rate brachytherapy combined with EBRT. In this report, 611 patients were treated and the median follow-up was 5 years. The 5-year PSA relapse-free survival outcomes were 96%, 88%, and 69% for favorable-, intermediate-, and unfavorable-risk patients, respectively. The use of short-course neoadjuvant androgen deprivation therapy did not impact on biochemical control or any other outcome parameter in this group of patients. Demanes et al. (108) reported on 209 patients treated with combined HDR brachytherapy and EBRT. With a median follow-up of 7 years, the 10-year biochemical control rates (ASTRO definition) were 90%, 87%, and 69%, for favorable-, intermediate-, and unfavorable-risk patients, respectively.

Yamada et al. (433) reported the experience from MS-KCC using HDR for selected intermediate- and high-risk patients. One hundred five consecutively treated between 1998 and 2004 were treated with HDR boost with [192]Ir (5.5 to 7.0 Gy) based on postimplant CT 3D treatment planning that used an in-house treatment plan optimization algorithm. The software used a genetic algorithm that was given dose constraints in a fashion similar to treatment planning tools developed at our institution for intensity-modulated prostate radiotherapy.

Dose constraints applied as parameters relative to the prescription dose included 100% target coverage, <120% maximum urethra dose, and rectal maximum dose ≤80% of the prescribed dose. 3DCRT (45 to 50.4 Gy) was also administered 3 weeks after the HDR procedure. With a median follow-up of 44 months, the 5-year PSA relapse-free survival outcomes for of low-, intermediate-, and high-risk patients were 100%, 98%, and 92%, respectively.

Acute and Late Treatment-Related Sequelae of Standard Treatment Interventions

Sequelae of Radical Prostatectomy

Complication rates after prostatectomy vary in the literature and recently have been shown to depend on the experience of the surgeon. Begg et al. (35) used the Medicare claim records from 11,522 patients who underwent prostatectomy between 1992 and 1996. Postoperative morbidity was found to be significantly reduced in hospitals that were considered to have high volume compared with lower volume ones (27% vs. 32%; $p = .03$) and among surgeons with a high-volume practice compared with lower volumes (26% vs. 32%; $p < .001$).

Immediate intraoperative/postoperative complications include pelvic pain and transient incontinence. Although intraoperative blood loss can range from 300 to 4,000 mL, meticulous surgical technique should reduce blood loss. The operative mortality rate has been reported to be 1% to 2%, but in experienced hands, the incidence is a fraction of 1%. The incidence of postoperative stress incontinence ranges from 5% to 57%.

Catalona et al. (61) reported on the complication rates in 1,870 patients who underwent RP. The authors reported a 2% incidence of a thromboembolic event and a 4% incidence of an anastomotic stricture. Recovery of urinary continence depended on the age of the patient. Among patients in their 50s, 60s, and 70s, the likelihood of persistent of urinary incontinence was 3%, 8%, and 13%, respectively. The incidence of impotence after bilateral and unilateral nerve-sparing surgery procedures was 53% and 32%, respectively. Bilateral nerve-sparing procedure was associated with improved potency preservation among patients who were younger than 70 years of age (71% vs. 48%; $p < .001$), whereas these differences were not significant in the older age group.

Bianco et al. (37) reported continence and potency outcomes in 1,472 patients who underwent surgery since 1991 and were operated on by a single surgeon. Among 1,288 patients who were continent prior to surgery, the actuarial likelihood of maintained continence was 91% at 12 months and 95% at 24 months. Of 785 patients with potency information available, the median time to erectile function recovery was 12 months, and the 2-year likelihood of potency preservation was 70%.

In a large review and comparison of two large series that reported on open prostatectomy and laparoscopic/robotic approaches (334), no significant differences were observed in perioperative and late complications. The incidence of major intraoperative complications, which included transfusions, was 6.6% versus 8.9% for open and laparoscopic techniques, respectively. The incidence of postoperative complications was 4.1% and 3.6% for open and laparoscopic approaches, respectively.

Sequelae of Cryotherapy

Many series have reported increased toxicity when cryotherapy has been used as salvage therapy after failed radiation therapy. However, toxicity is less often observed when cryotherapy is used in the primary management of disease. In a multi-institutional pooled analysis (242) comprising 975 patients treated with cryosurgery in the management of their primary prostatic disease, the incidence of impotence was 9%. Urinary incontinence was observed in 7.5%, and 13% required a TURP after therapy. Grade 4 urinary or rectal toxicity developed in 0.5%.

Sequelae of Conventional External-Beam Radiation Therapy

EBRT delivered with conventional techniques is fairly well tolerated, although grade 2 or higher acute rectal morbidity (discomfort, tenesmus, diarrhea) or urinary symptoms (frequency, nocturia, urgency, dysuria) requiring medication occur in approximately 60% of patients. Symptoms usually appear during the third week of treatment and resolve within days to weeks after treatment is completed. The incidence of late complications that develop ≥ 6 months after completion of treatment is significantly lower, whereas serious complications that require corrective surgical intervention are rare. An analysis of 1,020 patients treated in two large RTOG trials demonstrated an incidence of chronic urinary sequelae (i.e., cystitis, hematuria, urethral stricture, or bladder contracture) requiring hospitalization in 7.3% of cases, but the incidence of urinary toxicities requiring major surgical interventions was only 0.5% (230). More than half of chronic urinary complications were urethral strictures, occurring mostly in patients who had undergone a previous TURP. The incidence of chronic intestinal sequelae (chronic diarrhea, proctitis, rectal or anal stricture, rectal bleeding, or ulcer) requiring hospitalization for diagnosis and minor intervention was 3.3%, with 0.6% of patients experiencing bowel obstruction or perforation. Fatal complications were rare (0.2%).

Most complications attributed to radiation therapy are observed within the first 3 to 4 years after treatment, and the likelihood of complications developing after 5 years is low. The risk of complications is increased when radiation doses exceed 70 Gy. The risk of rectal toxicity has been correlated with the volume of the anterior rectal wall exposed to the higher doses of irradiation.

Sequelae of High-Dose Three-Dimensional Conformal Radiation Therapy Techniques

Michalski et al. (276) reported the toxicity outcomes of various risk groups enrolled in RTOG 9406, a phase I dose escalation study. The dose levels evaluated in this report included patients treated to the initial two dose levels of the study, 68.4 Gy and 73.8 Gy. The median follow-up times in these subgroups ranged from 2.2 to 3.4 years. The acute grade 2 bowel/rectal toxicity rates ranged from 16% to 25%. The crude incidence of late bowel/rectal toxicities ranged from 2% to 8%. With a median follow-up of 2.5 years, the crude late grade 2 and 3 gastrointestinal (GI) toxicities for those patients treated to 78 Gy (2-Gy fractions) was 22% and 2%, respectively.

Storey et al. (392) reported late rectal toxicity among patients treated on the phase III trial form the M.D. Anderson Hospital. The 5-year actuarial risks of late grade 2 rectal toxicity for the 70-Gy and 78-Gy dose level arms were 14% and 21%, respectively. In that report, the dose-volume histogram analyses of the patients treated to 78 Gy were analyzed to ascertain if there were any predictive patterns for late rectal toxicity. These investigators reported a significant correlation for the percentage of the rectum treated to 70 Gy or higher and the likelihood of late rectal toxicity. Patients with >25% of the rectal wall treated to 70 Gy or higher had a 37% risk of grade 2 rectal toxicity compared with 13% among patients who had <25% of the rectal wall exposed to these doses ($p = .05$).

Zelefsky et al. (447) reported the long-term tolerance of high-dose CRT at MSKCC. The 5-year actuarial rate of grade 2 rectal bleeding for patients receiving 64.8 to 70.2 Gy was 6%, compared with 17% for those treated to 75.6 Gy ($p < .001$). The 5-year actuarial rate of grade 3 or higher rectal toxicity was 1.2%, and no correlation between dose and the development of grade 3 complications was found within the range of 64.8 to 81 Gy. Multivariable analysis demonstrated the following variables as predictors of late rectal toxicity: prescription doses ≥75.6 Gy (p <.001), history of diabetes mellitus (p = .01), and the presence of acute GI symptoms during the course of treatment (p = .02). Predictors of late urinary symptoms included dose ≥75.6 Gy (p = .0008) and the presence of acute GI symptoms during the course of treatment (p <.001).

Peeters et al. (315) reported on the incidence of acute and late complications in a multicenter randomized trial comparing 68 Gy to 78 Gy 3DCRT. The median follow-up was 31 months. The 3-year incidence of grade 2 and higher GI and genitourinary (GU) toxicities for the 68-Gy dose arm was 23% and 28.5%, respectively. The 3-year incidence of grade 2 and higher GI and GU toxicities for the 78-Gy dose arm was 26.5% and 30%, respectively. The differences were not significant. However, the authors did note a significant increase in grade 3 rectal toxicity requiring laser cauterization for the higher dose arm. For patients treated to 78 Gy, the incidence of grade 3 rectal bleeding at 3 years was 10%, compared to 2% for those treated to 68 Gy. The following variables were found to be predictive of late GI toxicity: a history of abdominal surgery (p <0.001), and the presence of pretreatment GI symptoms (p = 0.001). The following variables were predictive of late GU toxicity: pretreatment urinary symptoms (p < 0.001), the use of neoadjuvant androgen deprivation therapy (p <.001), and prior transurethral resection of the prostate (p = .006).

In an attempt to improve further the conformality of the high-dose therapy plans and decrease the rate of grade 2 toxicity, an IMRT approach was introduced for the treatment of clinically localized disease. In this experience, IMRT had reduced the incidence of acute and late rectal effects compared with conventional 3DCRT, although acute and late urinary toxicities were not significantly different for the two methods (450–453). However, the combined rates of acute grade 1 and 2 rectal toxicities and the risk of late grade 2 rectal bleeding was significantly lower in the patients receiving IMRT (p = .05 and p =.0001, respectively). The 2-year actuarial rates of grade 2 rectal bleeding were 2% for IMRT and 10% for 3D-CRT (p <.001). In a recent update of 561 patients treated with IMRT to 81 Gy, the 8-year actuarial likelihood of developing grade 2 rectal bleeding was 1.6% (Fig. 62.19). Three patients (0.1%) experienced grade 3 rectal toxicity requiring either one or more transfusions or a laser cauterization procedure. No grade 4 rectal complications have been observed. The 8-year likelihood of developing late grade 2 and 3 (urethral strictures) urinary toxicities were 9% and 3%, respectively. Among patients who were potent prior to IMRT, 49% developed erectile dysfunction (446).

Urethral strictures have been observed in 1.5% of 1,100 patients treated with 3DCRT. Grade 3 hematuria requiring fulguration was observed in <0.5% of the patients. Among patients who previously underwent a TURP, a 4% incidence of stricture development after 3DCRT was observed (352). Other late urinary toxicities were not observed among patients with a prior history of a TURP. Lee et al. (236) observed a 2% incontinence rate among patients with a prior history of TURP who were treated with EBRT compared with a 0.2% rate in patients without a prior TURP. At the present time it does not appear that the use of IMRT has significantly reduced long-term urinary symptoms compared to conventional 3DCRT.

Potency Preservation with External-Beam Radiation Therapy

The rates of erectile dysfunction after EBRT have ranged from 6% to 84% (192). Investigators from the University of Chicago have reported potency rates after EBRT (246). With a median follow-up of 34 months, actuarial potency rates at 1, 20, 40, and 60 months were 96%, 75%, 59%, and 53%, respectively. Significant predictors of erectile dysfunction included pretreatment

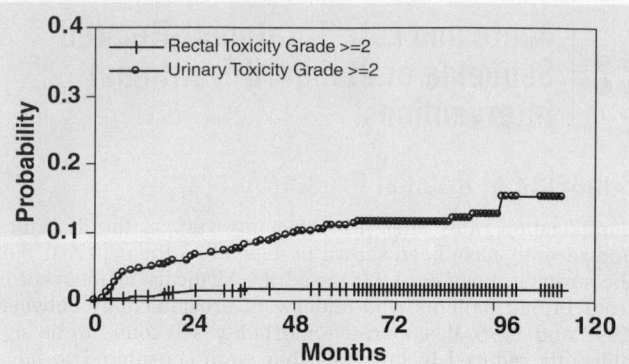

FIGURE 62.19. Actuarial likelihood of late grade 2 or greater rectal toxicities or late grade 2 or greater rectal toxicities. (From Zelefsky MJ, Chan H, Hunt M, et al. Long-term outcome of high dose intensity modulated radiation therapy for patients with clinically localized prostate cancer. *J Urol* 2006;176:1415–1419, with permission.)

potency status, diabetes, coronary artery disease, and androgen blockade. The reported rate of impotence with 3DCRT from MSKCC was 68% at 5 years, among patients treated to a dose ≥75.6 Gy (447). Aside from erectile dysfunction, other aspects of sexual dysfunction after radiotherapy include decreased volume of ejaculate, absence of ejaculate, decreased intensity of orgasm, and decreased libido. A summary of reported potency rates after treatment is shown in Table 62.11.

Significant limitations exist with the aforementioned reported potency preservation rates as the data are derived from retrospective analyses and information was often obtained without the use of validated questionnaires. Prospective studies suggest that when patients are assessed with validated tools, erectile dysfunction—defined as inability to achieve adequate erection sufficient for sexual intercourse—reaches 60% to 70%. What also complicates the interpretation of published incidence rates is the multifactorial nature of erectile dysfunction. The factors that impact erectile function include age, presence of medical comorbidities, antihypertensive medications, baseline erectile function, and the use of neoadjuvant and concurrent hormonal therapy.

Radiation-mediated impotence is likely multifactorial. However, it has been observed that 63% of patients evaluated for impotence after radiation therapy were diagnosed as having arteriogenic dysfunction, whereas 31% had cavernosal dysfunction. Only 3% were thought to have neurogenic impotence (449). Sildenafil administration results in significant improvement in erectile function (409,456). In one report, sildenafil improved erectile function in 74% of patients who underwent 3DCRT (median dose, 75.6 Gy), whereas 22% of patients had no response (456).

Low–Dose-Rate Brachytherapy: Acute and Late Toxicity

Urinary Toxicity

Acute urinary retention (AUR) is a known risk that can occur immediately after prostate brachytherapy, and the incidence varies in the literature. Crook et al. (91) studied 150 patients treated between 1999 and 2001 with prostate brachytherapy. In this group, 13% (n = 20) developed AUR. Of these 20 patients, 55% received prior androgen-deprivation therapy to decrease the size of the prostate prior to the procedure compared with 27% among patients who were not pretreated with androgen-deprivation therapy. A multivariate analysis revealed that larger prostate volumes and prior hormone therapy were each independent predictors of AUR.

| | Table 62.11 | INCIDENCE OF ERECTILE DYSFUNCTION AFTER RADIATION THERAPY FOR PROSTATE CANCER |

Study	Treatment	No. of Patients	Follow-Up (mo)	Erectile Dysfunction Incidence (%)
Mameghan et al. (245a)	ERT	42	55	45 at 2 yr
Roach et al. (340a)	ERT	60	21	38
Crook et al. (90a)	ERT	158	33	35
Mantz et al. (246a)	ERT	68	18	25 at 2 yr
Zelefsky et al. (447)	ERT	544	42	39
Pilepich et al. (317a)	ERT	230	54	72
Blasko et al. (41a)	BRT	469	38	≤70 yr of age: 15
				70 yr of age: 50
Stock et al. (386a)	BRT	65	18	21
Zelefsky et al. (456)	BRT	221	48	29
Merrick et al. (266a)	BRT	209	40	61 at 6 yr

ERT, external-beam radiation therapy; BRT, brachytherapy.
Adapted from Incrocci L, Slob AK, Levendag PC. Sexual (dys)function after radiotherapy for prostate cancer: a review. *Int J Radiat Oncol Biol Phys* 2002;52:681–693, with permission.

Terk et al. (402) noted a correlation of acute urinary retention (AUR) with baseline international prostate symptom score (IPSS) among 251 patients treated with prostate brachytherapy. The overall urinary retention rate was 5.5%. Among patients with preimplantation IPSS scores >20, 10 to 20, and <10, the rates of AUR after brachytherapy were 29%, 11%, and 2%, respectively. Merrick et al. (267) demonstrated an association between the volume of the TZ noted on MRI and the incidence of AUR. Among patients with MRI-defined TZ volumes of <50, 50 to 60, and >60 mL, the incidence of AUR was 0% (0/40), 33% (1/3), and 71% (5/7), respectively. In a subsequent analysis by investigators from the Princess Margaret Hospital (91), a multivariate analysis demonstrated that only the baseline urinary function and IPSS score were predictors of AUR, while TZ index was not significant predictor of this end point. These data, in combination with the lack of correlation of AUR with dose delivered to the urethra or prostate, suggest that the cause of AUR is most likely related trauma to the prostate gland.

In general, almost all patients after prostate brachytherapy develop acute urinary symptoms such as urinary frequency, urgency, and occasional urge incontinence. Depending on the isotope used, these symptoms often peak at 1 to 3 months after the procedure and subsequently gradually decline over the ensuing 3 to 6 months. Most patients significantly benefit with the use of an α-blocker, which ameliorates such symptoms in 60% to 70% of patients.

Grimm et al. (160) summarized the urinary acute and late symptoms of 310 patients who received ^{125}I or ^{103}Pd for localized disease. Approximately 90% of patients experienced grade 1–2 acute urinary symptoms, which included urinary frequency, urgency, and obstructive symptoms during the first 12 months after the procedure. Grade 3 acute toxicity was observed in 8% of patients, and 1.5% developed a grade 4 toxicity. Late grade 3 and 4 toxicities were observed in 7% and 1%, respectively. Urinary incontinence rates were as high as 48% among a small cohort of patients with a prior history of a TURP. Among those patients without a history of TURP and with modest gland volumes, the incidence of chronic urethritis and incontinence was found to be <3%.

Brown et al. (50) reported on 87 patients who underwent TPI, and urinary symptoms were carefully assessed after the procedure. Urinary effects such as frequency, nocturia, and dysuria generally developed 2 to 3 weeks postimplantation and peaked 3 to 4 months after the procedure. A gradual decline of the severity of symptoms was noted in approximately 75% of patients during the first 12 months. In this series, 41% of patients experienced acute grade 2–3 urinary morbidity, with 6% having grade 3 acute grade 3 urinary morbidity. After 12 months, 22% of patients experienced persistent urinary morbidity. Of this latter group, approximately 70% were characterized as having persistent grade 1 and 30% as having persistent grade 2–3 symptoms.

Several reports have demonstrated that acute urinary symptoms and late urinary morbidity after TPI correlate with the central target doses and the proximity of seed placement to the urethra. Stokes et al. (390) demonstrated a reduction in grade 2 symptoms (from 42% to 19%) when the central dose was reduced by placement of half-strength radioactive seeds in the periurethral area. Wallner et al. (415) have previously demonstrated a correlation of late urethral toxicity with the urethral dose from TPI. In that study the average maximal urethral dose among patients with late grade 2 and 3 urinary toxicities was 592 Gy, compared with 447 Gy for those who had minimal (grade 1) or no late urinary toxicity ($p = .03$). These dose levels, however, are unusual with modern treatment techniques. Zelefsky et al. (460) reported a reduced incidence of grade 2 acute urinary symptoms and more rapid resolution of symptoms with lower urethral doses achieved with an intraoperative real-time planning technique compared with a CT-based preplanned technique associated with higher urethral doses (Fig. 62.20). On the other hand, Allen et al. (10) have noted that prostate size, urethral dose, and isotope have no significant impact on late urinary morbidity, while continued smoking, the use of supplemental EBRT combined with brachytherapy, and the use of androgen-deprivation therapy were associated with an increased risk of late urinary morbidity.

Rectal Tolerance

Reports in the literature of grade 2 rectal toxicity after prostate brachytherapy range from 4% to 12%. The incidence of grade 3 or 4 rectal toxicity is unusual (<2%). Grade 2 symptoms manifest as rectal bleeding or increased mucous discharge. The onset of symptoms often peaks at 8 to 12 months and is self-limited in nature. Several reports have noted that rectal bleeding is associated with the rectal dose and its volume exposed to a particular dose. Snyder et al. (375) noted that the rectal volume in cubic centimeters exposed to the prescription dose of 160 Gy correlated with the incidence of grade 2 proctitis. For patients with 0.8 cc or less of rectal volume exposed to the prescription dose, no patient developed proctitis; from 0.8 to 1.8 cc approximately 8% of patients developed rectal bleeding. However, among patients with >1.8 cc of the rectal volume exposed to 160 Gy, almost 25% of patients developed rectal toxicity. Similarly, Han and Wallner (167) observed that the volume of the rectum receiving 100% of the prescription dose was 2.5 cc for those who

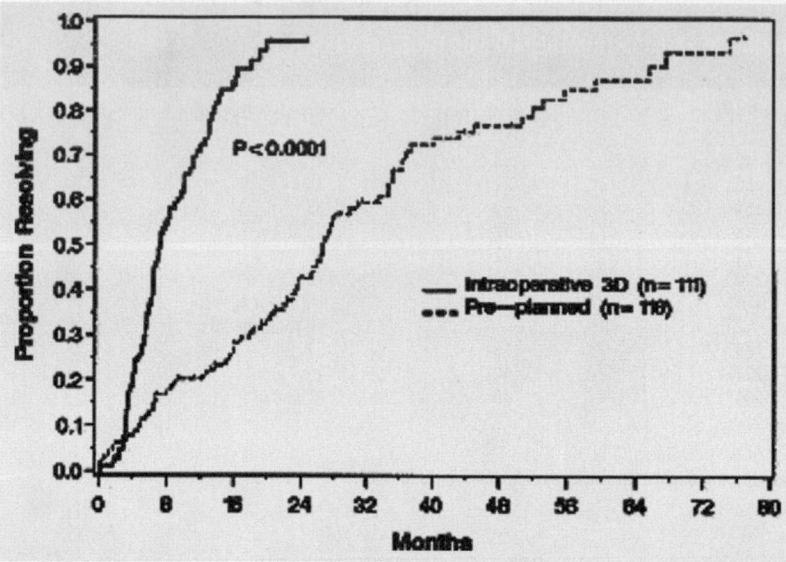

FIGURE 62.20. Time to resolution of urinary symptoms after brachytherapy using an intraoperative transrectal ultrasonography technique compared with a preplanned computed tomography-based transperineal technique. (From Zelefsky MJ, Yamada Y, Marion C, et al. Improved conformality and decreased toxicity with intraoperative computer-optimized transperineal ultrasound-guided prostate brachytherapy. *Int J Radiat Oncol Biol Phys* 2003;55:956–963, with permission.)

developed rectal bleeding and significantly lower (0.6 cc) for those who did not experience rectal bleeding ($p < .001$). Waterman and Dicker (420) also noted a correlation of rectal dose and the percentage of the rectal surface exposed to that dose and the incidence of rectal bleeding. In that report, tolerance dose (associated with a complication rate <5% of patients) for the rectum to low dose rate ^{125}I was 100, 150, and 200 Gy, respectively, to 30%, 20%, and 10% of the rectal surface.

Erectile Function

Erectile dysfunction after brachytherapy has been reported to occur from 20% to 80%. With longer follow-up observations, Zelefsky et al. (457) reported that, whereas the incidence of impotence at 2 years after implantation was 21%, the rate increased to 42% at 5 years after the procedure. Merrick et al. (271) observed a strong correlation with the dose to the penile bulb and proximal penis. Among patients whose dose to 50% of the penile bulb was <30%, the incidence of erectile dysfunction was 76%, compared to 31% for those with higher penile bulb doses. Similarly, among patients whose dose to 50% of the proximal penis and crura were <30%, the incidence of erectile dysfunction was 76%, compared to 31% for those who had higher penile bulb doses. These authors could not show a correlation with the dose delivered to the neurovascular bundle and long-term erectile dysfunction.

Excellent responses have been observed with sildenafil citrate in the treatment of posttreatment impotence after brachytherapy, with response rates up to 85% (268,331). In one study (325), the addition of neoadjuvant androgen deprivation had a significant impact on the potency preservation rate after prostate brachytherapy. Among patients treated with brachytherapy alone who developed impotence after implantation, 30 of 37 (81%) responded to sildenafil compared wit a response rate of 22 of 48 (46%) for patients who received neoadjuvant androgen-deprivation therapy in combination with brachytherapy ($p = .04$).

Sequelae of Combination EBRT and Low-Dose-Rate Brachytherapy

There is a paucity of information regarding the long-term tolerance of combined EBRT and brachytherapy for patients with localized prostate cancer. Critz et al. (89) reported grade ≥2 rec-

tal toxicities in 23% and grade ≥2 urinary toxicities in 20% of treated patients using this approach. The higher toxicity rates in this report may be attributed to their use of the retropubic open technique in some of these patients rather than a transperineal, ultrasound-guided technique. The tolerance profile for patients treated with combined EBRT and TPI at MSKCC was reported by Singh et al. (368). Four patients (6%) with acute urinary retention required Foley catheterization within 48 hours of the implant procedure. The catheter remained in place for median of 5 days. Twenty-three patients (42%) developed grade 2 urinary symptoms after completion of therapy requiring α-blocker medications. Three patients (4%) noted rare stress incontinence, and no patient described urge incontinence. Of the 65 patients treated, 45 (68%) reported at their last follow-up that their urinary symptoms had returned to their pretreatment level. Eight patients (13%) developed grade 2 rectal bleeding within 6 months from the completion of therapy. No grade 3 or 4 rectal toxicities were observed. Five patients (8%) reported increased frequency of bowel movements, which were managed with conservative measures. Forty-four of the patients (66%) were potent prior to the initiation of treatment. Of these, 17 (26%) developed erectile dysfunction.

Single-institution experiences have documented somewhat increased morbidity following combined treatment using conventional brachytherapy and EBRT techniques. The RTOG conducted a phase II study (RTOG P-0019) to assess the acute and late toxicity for patients with intermediate-risk, clinically localized prostate cancer (234). One hundred thirty-eight patients from 20 institutions were entered in this study. All patients were treated with EBRT (45 Gy/25 fractions) followed 2 to 6 weeks later by an interstitial implant using ^{125}I to deliver an additional 108 Gy. Thirty-five patients (27%) had preradiotherapy androgen deprivation. The median follow-up was 20 months. The most commonly reported acute toxicity was urinary frequency and dysuria. Acute Grade 3 toxicity was documented in 10/131 (7.6%) patients. No grade 4-5 acute toxicity has been observed. Late grade 3 toxicity has been observed in six men (five urinary, one bowel condition). The 18-month estimate of late grade 3 GU/GI toxicity is 3.3%. No late grade 4–5 toxicity has been observed. In the 61 men who reported no impotence at baseline and received no androgen deprivation, the 18-month rate of grade 2-3 impotence is 45.5% (95% confidence interval, 32.6–58.5%). These data suggest that, compared to brachytherapy alone, the acute and late morbidity observed in this multiinstitutional, cooperative group study is somewhat increased, which is consistent with previous reports from single institutions.

Morbidity of HDR Temporary Prostate Brachytherapy

The most common late GU morbidity is the development of urethral stricture. Most series have observed that urethral strictures are more common in men with a history of previous TURP. In most cases, the strictures can be managed with dilation in the office or in the outpatient surgical setting. Late GI morbidity can take the form of rectal bleeding, rectal ulcer, or (in rare cases) prostatorectal fistulae.

•• | Postirradiation Prostate-Specific •• | Antigen

A transient increase of PSA during radiation therapy, even as soon as the first fraction, has been reported in some patients (412,442). Because there is no prognostic significance to the PSA response during a course of radiation therapy, obtaining PSA levels during treatment is not necessary or recommended. Several investigators have carefully studied the PSA kinetics after a course of EBRT. According to the calculations of Ritter et al. (339), PSA half-life during radiation therapy ranges from 43 to 58.5 days, with an expected decline of 1.6% per day; Zagars et al. (442) reported a decline from 30 to 4.7 ng/mL at 3 months after irradiation.

PSA fluctuations are common in the follow-up period, and have been termed *PSA bounce*. Critz et al. (89) reported that 35% of patients after combined permanent interstitial implantation and EBRT experienced a transient rise in their PSA value after treatment. The median time from treatment to this bounce effect was 18 months, and 92% of the fluctuating levels were observed during the first 26 months after radiation therapy. These investigators reported fluctuations ranging from 0.11 to 15.8 ng/mL. Similar results have been reported by Cavanagh et al. (65) for patients treated with implantation alone or when combined with EBRT. Hanlon et al. (172) observed PSA bounce effect in approximately one third of patients treated with EBRT alone. In that series, the 5-year biochemical control rate for patients who experienced a PSA fluctuation was inferior to that in those patients who did not have a PSA bounce in their follow-up period (69% vs. 52%; $p = .02$). On the other hand, investigators from the M.D. Anderson Hospital (394) noted that of 964 patients treated with EBRT, only 12% experienced a PSA bounce, and that the 5-year PSA outcome was superior for those patients who experienced this PSA fluctuation compared with those who did not (82% vs. 58%; $p = .0001$).

Ciezki et al. (79) defined PSA bounce as an increased PSA level of at least 0.2 ng/mL greater than the nadir PSA with a subsequent PSA value declining back to the nadir level or lower. One hundred sixty-two patients were treated with a permanent ^{125}I implantation and followed for a minimum of 5 years. Using this definition of a PSA bounce, almost half of the patients (46%) experienced this phenomenon. The authors observed that the patients who experienced this fluctuation were more likely to be younger and less likely to develop a biochemical relapse. The authors also noted that PSA bounces generally occurred much sooner after treatment than a true PSA relapse. The median time to the first rise in PSA from the nadir was 15 months, compared with 30 months for an ASTRO-defined biochemical relapse or 22 months for a nadir +2 defined relapse. Other reports have defined PSA bounce in various ways and the literature needs to be interpreted for this reason with caution.

Although a low absolute PSA level or nadir value after radiation therapy has prognostic significance for improved disease-free survival, it is difficult to assign a specific PSA cut-point or nadir level as a definition of biochemical relapse. An ASTRO consensus panel has recommended a definition of biochemical relapse after EBRT as three consecutive rising PSA values from the nadir value. For clinical trials, this panel recommended that the date of failure should be considered the midpoint between the postirradiation nadir value and the first of three consecutive rises. It was also noted that although the nadir PSA level is considered a strong prognostic variable, no absolute level is considered a valid cut-point for reliably separating successful and unsuccessful outcomes. The recommendation was also made for PSA determinations at 3- to 4-month intervals during the first 2 years after treatments and every 6 months thereafter. The panel also recommended that a prostate rebiopsy is not necessary as a standard of care after a course of radiation therapy, and the absence of a rising PSA level after treatment is the most reliable indicator of tumor control (12). Recently, this definition of biochemical failure has been reassessed in another consensus panel (343). The panel recommended that the nadir + 2 definition (a rise by 2 ng/mL or more above the nadir PSA) be considered the standard definition for biochemical failure after EBRT with or without hormonal therapy. The panel also recommended that the date of failure be determined "at call" (not backdated). If the ASTRO consensus definition after EBRT were to be used, the reported date of biochemical control outcomes should be listed as 2 years short of the median follow-up.

Several studies have examined the significance of posttreatment PSA doubling time (PSADT). Following prostatectomy, in a single institutional experience, Pound et al. (324) noted that, for patients treated with RP, PSADT <10 months predicted the development of metastatic disease (3). Zelefsky et al. (445) reported on the impact of PSADT in a cohort of patients who developed biochemical relapse after EBRT. The PSADT for favorable-, intermediate-, and unfavorable-risk patients who developed a biochemical failure was 20.0, 13.2, and 8.2 months, respectively ($p < .001$). The 3-year incidence of DM for patients with PSADT of 0 to 3, 3 to 6, 6 to 12, and >12 months was 49%, 41%, 20%, and 7%, respectively ($p < .001$). Patients with PSADT of 0 to 3 and 3 to 6 months demonstrated a 7.0 and 6.6 increased hazard of developing distant metastases (DM) or death, respectively, compared with patients with a DT more than 12 months. Freedland et al. (128) noted that PSADT <9 months correlated with prostate cancer-specific mortality, but did not evaluate postprostatectomy PSADT as a surrogate for cause specific survival (CSS) (17). Using larger, multi-institutional databases, Albertsen et al. (5) and D'Amico et al. (94), noted that short PSADT correlated with an adverse effect on survival in patients treated with either prostatectomy or radiation therapy for prostate cancer. D'Amico et al. (94) assessed nonprospective data using Prentice's criteria and found that a PSADT <3 months was a surrogate end point for CSS.

Emerging data strongly correlate a rising PSA level with positive postirradiation prostate biopsies. Kabalin et al. (203), in an analysis of 27 patients, noted 100% positive biopsies in patients with abnormal PSA levels after irradiation. Dugan et al. (114) reported a significant correlation of negative postirradiation biopsies, depending on the PSA value (92% negative specimens with PSA <1 ng/mL, 50% with 1.1 to 2.5 ng/mL, and 29% with >2.5 ng/mL). The time from completion of radiation therapy has been shown to have an impact on the posttreatment biopsy outcome. Crook et al. (92) reported on 226 patients treated with conventional EBRT who underwent serial biopsies after treatment. At 13 months after radiation therapy, the incidence of a positive biopsy was 51%, but decreased to 30% for biopsies obtained at 30 months. Posttreatment biopsies require an experienced pathologist to interpret because of the significant radiation effect that takes place in the prostate that can easily be mistaken at times for residual disease. Immunohistochemical staining for high-molecular-weight keratin can often distinguish radiation atypia in benign glands from residual tumor.

:: | Acknowledgment

The authors are deeply indebted to Eve S. Ferdman for her editorial assistance.

References

1. Abbas F, Civantos F, Benedetto P, et al. Small cell carcinoma of the bladder and prostate. *Urology* 1995;46:617–630.
2. Adolfsson J, Steineck G, Whitmore WF Jr. Recent results of management of palpable clinical localized prostate cancer. *Cancer* 1993;72:310–322.
3. Alagiri M, Colton MD, Seidmon EJ, et al. The staging pelvic lymphadenectomy: implications as an adjunctive procedure for clinically localized prostate cancer. *Br J Urol* 1997;80:243–246.
4. Alasti H, Petric MP, Catton CN, et al. Portal imaging for evaluation of daily on-line set-up errors and off-line organ motion during conformal irradiation of carcinoma of the prostate. *Int J Radiat Oncol Biol Phys* 2001;49:869–884.
5. Albertsen PC, Hanley JA, Harlan LC, et al. The positive yield of imaging studies in the evaluation of men with newly diagnosed prostate cancer: a population based analysis. *J Urol* 2000;163:1138–1143.
6. Albertsen P, Hanley J, Penson D, et al. Validation of increasing prostate specific antigen as a predictor of prostate cancer death after treatment of localized prostate cancer with surgery or radiation. *J Urol* 2001;171:2221–2225.
7. Algan O, Hanks GE, Shaer AH. Localization of the prostatic apex for radiation treatment planning. *Int J Radiat Oncol Biol Phys* 1995;33:925–930.
8. Algan O, Hanks GE, Shaer AH. Localization of the prostatic apex for radiation treatment planning. *Int J Radiat Oncol Biol Phys* 1995;33:925–930.
9. Allaf ME, Palapattu GS, Trock BJ, et al. Anatomical extent of lymph node dissection: impact on men with clinically localized prostate cancer. *J Urol* 2004;172:1840–1844.
10. Allen ZA, Merrick GS, Butler WM, et al. Detailed urethral dosimetry in the evaluation of prostate brachytherapy-related urinary morbidity. *Int J Radiat Oncol Biol Phys* 2005;62:981–987.
11. American Joint Committee on Cancer. Prostate cancer. In: Greene FL, Page DR, Fleming ID, eds. *AJCC cancer staging manual*, 6th ed. New York: Springer-Verlag; 2003:309–316.
12. American Society for Therapeutic Radiology and Oncology. American Society for Therapeutic Radiology and Oncology consensus panel consensus statement: guidelines for PSA following radiation therapy. *Int J Radiat Oncol Biol Phys* 1997;37:1035–1041.
13. Amling CL, Blute ML, Bergstralh EJ, et al. Long-term hazard of progression after radical prostatectomy for clinically localized prostate cancer: continued risk of biochemical failure after 5 years. *J Urol* 2000;164:101–105.
14. Andriole G, Bostwick D, Civantos F, et al. The effects of 5alpha-reductase inhibitors on the natural history, detection and grading of prostate cancer: current state of knowledge. *J Urol* 2005;174:2098–1104.
15. Antolak JA, Rosen II, Childress CH, et al. Prostate target volume variations during a course of radiotherapy. *Int J Radiat Oncol Biol Phys* 1998;42:661–672.
16. Aprikian AG, Bazinet M, Plante M, et al. Family history and the risk of prostatic carcinoma in a high risk group of urological patients. *J Urol* 1995;161:101–106.
17. Arcangeli CG, Humphrey PA, Smith DS, et al. Percentage of free serum prostate-specific antigen as a predictor of pathologic features of prostate cancer in a screening population. *Urology* 1998;51:558–564.
18. Armenian HK, Lilienfeld AM, Diamond EL, et al. Relationship between benign prostatic hyperplasia and cancer of the prostate. *Lancet* 1974;2:115–117.
19. Ash D, Al-Qaisieh B, Bottomley D, et al. The correlation between D90 and outcome for I-125 seed implant monotherapy for localised prostate cancer. *Radiother Oncol* 2006;79:185–189.
20. Ash D, Al-Qaisieh B, Bottomley D, et al. The impact of hormone therapy on post-implant dosimetry and outcome following Iodine-125 implant monotherapy for localised prostate cancer. *Radiother Oncol* 2005;75:303–306.
21. Ashman JB, Zelefsky MJ, Hunt MS, et al. Whole pelvic radiotherapy for prostate cancer using 3D conformal and intensity-modulated radiotherapy. *Int J Radiat Oncol Biol Phys* 2005;63:765–771.
22. American Urological Association. AUA commentary: prostate-specific antigen best practice policy. *Oncology* 2000;14:267.
23. Aubry JF, Beaulieu L, Girouard LM, et al. Measurements of intrafraction motion and interfraction rotation of prostate by three-dimensional analysis of daily portal imaging with radiopaque markers. *Int J Radiat Oncol Biol Phys* 2004;60:30–39.
24. Azumi N, Shibuya H, Ishikura M. Primary prostatic carcinoid tumor with intracytoplasmic prostatic acid phosphatase and prostate-specific antigen. *Am J Surg Pathol* 1984;8:545–550.
25. Bagshaw MA, Cox RS, Ray GR. Status of radiation therapy of prostate cancer at Stanford University. *Monogr Natl Cancer Inst* 1988;7:47–60.
26. Bahn DK, Lee F, Badalament R, et al. Targeted cryoablation of the prostate: 7-year outcomes in the primary treatment of prostate cancer. *Urology* 2002;60:3–11.
27. Bairati I, Meyer F, Fradet Y. Dietary fat and advanced prostate cancer. *J Urol* 1998;159:1271–1275.
28. Balter JM, Sandler HM, Lam K, et al. Measurements of prostate movement over the course of routine radiotherapy using implanted markers. *Int J Radiat Oncol Biol Phys* 1995;31:113–118.
29. Barrett-Connor E, Garland C, McPhillips JB, et al. A prospective, population-based study of androstenedione, estrogens, and prostatic cancer. *Cancer Res* 1990;50:169–173.
30. Bates HR. Transitional cell carcinoma of the prostate. *J Urol* 1969;101:206–207.
31. Battermann JJ, Boon TA, Moerland MA. Results of permanent prostate brachytherapy, 13 years of experience at a single institution. *Radiother Oncol* 2004;71:23–28.
32. Bayley AJ, Catton CN, Haycocks T, et al. A randomized trial of supine vs. prone positioning in patients undergoing escalated dose conformal radiotherapy for prostate cancer. *Radiother Oncol* 2004;70:37–44.
33. Bean MA, Yatani R, Liu PI, et al. Prostatic carcinoma at autopsy in Hiroshima and Nagasaki, Japan. *Cancer* 1973;32:498–506.
34. Beard CJ, Kijewski P, Bussiére M, et al. Analysis of prostate and seminal vesicle motion: implications for treatment planning. *Int J Radiat Oncol Biol Phys* 1996;34:451–458.
35. Begg CB, Riedel ER, Bach PB, et al. Variations in morbidity after radical prostatectomy. *N Engl J Med* 2002;346:1138–1144.
36. Beyer D, Nath R, Butler W, et al. American Brachytherapy Society recommendations for clinical implementation of NIST-1999 standards for (103) palladium brachytherapy. *Int J Radiat Oncol Biol Phys* 2000;47:273–275.
37. Bianco FJ Jr, Scardino PT, Eastham JA. Radical prostatectomy: long-term cancer control and recovery of sexual and urinary function ("trifecta"). *Urology* 2005;66[Suppl]:83–94.
38. Bice WS Jr, Prestidge BR, Grimm PD, et al. Centralized multiinstitutional postimplant analysis for interstitial brachytherapy. *Int J Radiat Oncol Biol Phys* 1998;41:921–927.
39. Bill-Axelson A, Holmberg L, Ruutu M, et al. Radical prostatectomy versus watchful waiting in early prostate cancer. *N Engl J Med* 2005;352:1977–1984.
40. Billis A. Latent carcinoma and atypical lesions of prostate: an autopsy study. *Urology* 1986;28:324–329.
41. Bishoff JT, Reyes A, Thompson IM, et al. Pelvic lymphadenectomy can be omitted in selected patients with carcinoma of the prostate: development of a system of patient selection. *Urology* 1995;45:270–274.
41a. Blasko JC, Grimm PD, Ragde H. Brachytherapy and organ preservation in the management of carcinoma of the prostate. *Semin Radiat Oncol* 1993;3:240–249.
42. Blasko JC, Grimm PD, Sylvester JE, et al. Palladium 103 brachytherapy for prostate carcinoma. *Int J Radiat Oncol Biol Phys* 2000;46:839–850.
43. Blasko JC, Grimm PD, Sylvester JE, et al. The role of external beam radiotherapy with I-125/Pd-193 brachytherapy for prostate carcinoma. *Radiother Oncol* 2000;57:273–278.
44. Bluestein DL, Bostwick DG, Bergstralh EJ, et al. Eliminating the need for bilateral pelvic lymphadenectomy in select patients with prostate cancer. *J Urol* 1994;151:1315–1320.
45. Bortfeld T. Optimized planning using objectives and constraints. *Semin Radiat Oncol* 1999;9:20–34.
46. Bossens MM, Van Straalen JP, De Reijke TM, et al. Kinetics of prostate-specific antigen after manipulation of the prostate. *Eur J Cancer* 1995;31A:682–685.
47. Bostwick DG, Shan A, Qian J, et al. Independent origin of multiple foci of prostatic intraepithelial neoplasia: comparison with matched foci of prostate carcinoma. *Cancer* 1998;83:1995–2002.
48. Brawley OW, Parnes H. Prostate cancer prevention trials in the USA. *Eur J Cancer* 2000;36:1312–1315.
49. Brinker DA, Potter SR, Epstein JI. Ductal adenocarcinoma of the prostate diagnosed on needle biopsy: correlation with clinical and radical prostatectomy findings and progression. *Am J Surg Pathol* 1999;23:1471–1479.
50. Brown D, Colonias A, Miller R, et al. Urinary morbidity with a modified peripheral loading technique of transperineal ^{125}I prostate implantation. *Int J Radiat Oncol Biol Phys* 2000;47:53–360.
51. Burman C, Chui CS, Kutcher G, et al. Planning, delivery, and quality assurance of intensity-modulated radiotherapy using dynamic multileaf collimator: a strategy for large-scale implementation for the treatment of carcinoma of the prostate. *Int J Radiat Oncol Biol Phys* 1997;39:863–873.
52. Byar DP, Mostofi FK. Carcinoma of the prostate: prognostic evaluation of certain pathologic features in 208 radical prostatectomies. Examined by the step-section technique. *Cancer* 1972;30:5–13.
53. Caggianos I, Karakiewicz P, Eastham JA, et al. A preoperative nomogram identifying decreased risk of positive pelvic lymph nodes in patients with prostate cancer. *J Urol* 2003;170:1798–1803.
54. Cama C, Olsson CA, Raffo AJ, et al. Molecular staging of prostate cancer: II. A comparison of the applications of an enhanced reverse transcriptase polymerase chain reaction assay for prostate specific antigen versus prostate specific membrane antigen. *J Urol* 1995;153:1373–1378.
55. Cannon L, Bishop DT, Skolnick M. Genetic epidemiology of prostate cancer in the Utah Mormon genealogy. *Cancer Surv* 1982;1:47.
56. Carney JA, Kelalis PP. Endometrial carcinoma of the prostatic utricle. *Am J Clin Pathol* 1973;60:565–569.
57. Carter BS, Beaty TH, Steinberg GD, et al. Mendelian inheritance of familial prostate cancer. *Proc Natl Acad Sci U S A* 1992;89:3367–3371.
58. Carter HB, Walsh PC, Landis P, et al. Expectant management of nonpalpable prostate cancer with curative intent: preliminary results. *J Urol* 2002;167:1231–1234.
59. Catalona WJ. *Prostate cancer.* Orlando, FL: Grune & Stratton; 1984.
60. Catalona WJ, Bhis SW. Nerve-sparing radical prostatectomy: evaluation of results after 250 patients. *J Urol* 1990;143:538–544.
61. Catalona WJ, Carvalhal GF, Mager DE, et al. Potency, continence and complication rates in 1,870 consecutive radical retropubic prostatectomies. *J Urol* 1999;162:433–438.
62. Catalona WJ, Partin AW, Slawin KM, et al. Use of the percentage of free prostate-specific antigen to enhance differentiation of prostate cancer from benign prostatic disease: a prospective multicenter clinical trial. *JAMA* 1998;279:1542–1547.
63. Catalona WJ, Richie JP, Ahmann FR, et al. Comparison of digital rectal examination and serum prostate specific antigen in the early detection of prostate cancer: results of a multicenter clinical trial of 6,630 men. *J Urol* 1994;151:1283–1290.
64. Catalona WJ, Smith DS, Wolfert RL, et al. Evaluation of percentage of free serum prostate-specific antigen to improve specificity of prostate cancer screening. *JAMA* 1995;274:1214–1220.
65. Cavanagh W, Grimm PD, Sylvester JE, et al. Transient elevation of serum prostate-specific antigen following ^{125}I/^{103}Pd brachytherapy for localized prostate cancer. *Semin Urol Oncol* 2000;18:160–165.
66. Cavey ML, Bayouth JE, Colman M, et al. IMRT to escalate the dose to the prostate while treating the pelvic nodes. *Strahlenther Onkol* 2005;181:431–441.

67. Cha CM, Potters L, Ashley R, et al. Isotope selection for patients undergoing prostate brachytherapy. *Int J Radiat Oncol Biol Phys* 1999;45:391–395.

68. Chamberlain NL, Driver ED, Miesfeld RL. The length and location of CAG trinucleotide repeats in the androgen receptor N-terminal domain affect transactivation function. *Nucleic Acids Res* 1994;22:3181–3186.

69. Chan JM, Gann PH, Giovannucci EL, et al. Role of diet in prostate cancer development and progression. *J Clin Oncol* 2005;23:8152–8160.

70. Chandra A, Dong L, Huang E, et al. Experience of ultrasound-based daily prostate localization. *Int J Radiat Oncol Biol Phys* 2003;56:436–447.

71. Chang SS, Gaudin PB, Reuter VE, et al. Prostate-specific membrane antigen: much more than a prostate cancer marker. *Mol Urol* 1999;3:313–320.

72. Cheng L, Slezak J, Bergstralh EJ, et al. Dedifferentiation in the metastatic progression of prostate carcinoma. *Cancer* 1999;86:657–663.

73. Cheng L, Zincke H, Blute ML, et al. Risk of prostate carcinoma death in patients with lymph node metastasis. *Cancer* 2001;91:66–73.

74. Chodak GW. Additional therapy after prostatectomy: implications for patient counseling. *J Natl Cancer Inst* 1996;88:139–140.

75. Chodak GW, Wald V, Parmer E, et al. Comparison of digital examination and transrectal ultrasonography for the diagnosis of prostate cancer. *J Urol* 1986;135:951–954.

76. Chui CS, LoSasso T, Spirou S. Dose calculation for photon beams with intensity modulation generated by dynamic jaw or multileaf collimations. *Med Phys* 1994;21:1237–1244.

77. Chung PW, Haycocks T, Brown T, et al. On-line aSi portal imaging of implanted fiducial markers for the reduction of interfraction error during conformal radiotherapy of prostate carcinoma. *Int J Radiat Oncol Biol Phys* 2004;60:329–334.

78. Chybowski FM, Keller JJ, Bergstralh EJ, et al. Predicting radionuclide bone scan findings in patients with newly diagnosed, untreated prostate cancer: prostate specific antigen is superior to all other clinical parameters. *J Urol* 1991;145:313–318.

79. Ciezki J, Reddy CA, Garci J, et al. PSA kinetics after prostate brachytherapy: PSA bounce phenomenon and its implications for PSA doubling time. *Int J Radiat Oncol Biol Phys* 2006;64:512–517.

80. Cintra ML, Billis A. Histologic grading of prostatic adenocarcinoma: intraobserver reproducibility of the Mostofi, Gleason and Bocking grading systems. *Int Urol Nephrol* 1991;23:449–454.

81. Clark LC, Dalkin B, Krongrad A, et al. Decreased incidence of prostate cancer with selenium supplementation: results of a double-blind cancer prevention trial. *Br J Urol* 1998;81:730–734.

82. Cohen RS, Glezerson G, Hatlezee Z. Neuroendocrine cells: a new prognostic parameter in prostatic cancer. *Br J Urol* 1991;68:258–262.

83. Collins GN, Martin PJ, Wynn-Davies A, et al. The effect of digital rectal examination, flexible cystoscopy and prostatic biopsy on free and total prostate specific antigen, and the free-to-total prostate specific antigen ratio in clinical practice. *J Urol* 1997;57:1744–1747.

84. Colpaert C, Gentens P, Van Marck E. Ductal ("endometrioid") adenocarcinoma of the prostate. *Acta Urol Belg* 1998;66:29–32.

85. Cookson MS, Fleshner NE, Soloway SM, et al. Correlation between Gleason score of needle biopsy and radical prostatectomy specimen: accuracy and clinical implications. *J Urol* 1997;157:559–562.

86. Cooperberg MR, Broering JM, Litwin MS, et al. The contemporary management of prostate cancer in the United States: lessons from the cancer of the prostate strategic urologic research endeavor (CapSURE), a national disease registry. *J Urol* 2004;171:1393–1401.

87. Cox B, Sneyd MJ, Paul C, et al. Vasectomy and risk of prostate cancer. *JAMA* 2002;287:3110–3115.

88. Cox JA, Zagoria RJ, Raben M. Prostate cancer: comparison of retrograde urethrography and computed tomography in radiotherapy planning. *Int J Radiat Oncol Biol Phys* 1994;29:1119–1123.

89. Critz FA, Williams WH, Benton JB, et al. Prostate specific antigen bounce after radioactive seed implantation followed by external beam radiation for prostate cancer. *J Urol* 2000;163:1085–1089.

90. Critz FA, Williams WH, Levinson AK, et al. Simultaneous irradiation for prostate cancer: intermediate results with modern techniques. *J Urol* 2000;164:738–743.

90a. Crook J, Esche B, Futter N. Effect of pelvic radiotherapy for prostate cancer on bowel, bladder, and sexual function: the patient's perspective. *Urology* 1996;47:387–394.

91. Crook J, McLean M, Catton C, et al. Factors influencing risk of acute urinary retention after TRUS-guided permanent prostate seed implantation. *Int J Radiat Oncol Biol Phys* 2002;52:453–460.

92. Crook JM, Perry GA, Robertson S, et al. Routine prostate biopsies following radiotherapy for prostate cancer: results for 226 patients. *Urology* 1995;45:624–632.

93. Crook JM, Raymond Y, Salhani D, et al. Prostate motion during standard radiotherapy as assessed by fiducial markers. *Radiother Oncol* 1995;37:35–42.

94. D'Amico AV, Cote K, Loffredo M, et al. Determinants of prostate cancer specific survival following radiation therapy for patients with clinically localized prostate cancer. *J Clin Oncol* 2005;20:4567–4573.

95. D'Amico A, Moul J, Carroll P, et al. Surrogate end point for prostate cancer-specific mortality after radical prostatectomy or radiation therapy. *J Natl Cancer Inst* 2003;95:1376–1383.

96. D'Amico AV, Renshaw AA, Schultz D, et al. The impact of the biopsy Gleason score on PSA outcome for prostate cancer patients with PSA < or = 10 ng/mL and T1c,2a: implications for patient selection for prostate-only therapy. *Int J Radiat Oncol Biol Phys* 1999;45:847–851.

97. D'Amico AV, Whittington R, Kaplan I, et al. Equivalent biochemical failure-free survival after external beam radiation therapy or radical prostatectomy in patients with a pretreatment prostate specific antigen of 4 > 20 ng/mL. *Int J Radiat Oncol Biol Phys* 1997;37:1053–1058.

98. D'Amico AV, Whittington R, Malkowicz SB, et al. A multivariable analysis of clinical factors predicting for pathological features associated with local failure after radical prostatectomy for prostate cancer. *Int J Radiat Oncol Biol Phys* 1994;30:293–302.

99. D'Amico AV, Whittington R, Malkowicz SB, et al. A multivariate analysis of clinical and pathological factors that predict for prostate specific antigen failure after radical prostatectomy for prostate cancer. *J Urol* 1995;154:131–138.

100. D'Amico AV, Whittington R, Malkowicz SB, et al. Biochemical outcome after radical prostatectomy, external beam radiotherapy, or in interstitial radiation therapy for clinically localized prostate cancer. *JAMA* 1998;280:969–974.

101. D'Amico AV, Whittington R, Malkowicz SB, et al. Clinical utility of percent-positive prostate biopsies in predicting biochemical outcome after radical prostatectomy or external-beam radiation therapy for patients with clinically localized prostate cancer. *Mol Urol* 2000;4:171–175.

102. D'Amico AV, Whittington R, Malkowicz SB, et al. Clinical utility of the percentage of positive prostate biopsies in defining biochemical outcome after radical prostatectomy for patients with clinically localized prostate cancer. *J Clin Oncol* 2000;18:1164–1172.

103. Daneshmand S, Quek ML, Stein JP, et al. Prognosis of patients with lymph node positive prostate cancer following radical prostatectomy: long-term results. *J Urol* 2004;172:2252–2255.

104. Daniell HW. A worse prognosis for smokers with prostate cancer. *J Urol* 1995;154:153–157.

105. Dawson LA, Mah K, Franssen E, et al. Target position variability throughout prostate radiotherapy. *Int J Radiat Oncol Biol Phys* 1998;42:1155–1161.

106. Debois M, Oyen R, Maes F, et al. The contribution of magnetic resonance imaging to the three-dimensional treatment planning of localized prostate cancer. *Int J Radiat Oncol Biol Phys* 1999;45:857–865.

107. Del Regato JA, Trailings AH, Pittman DD. Twenty years follow-up of patients with inoperable cancer of the prostate (stage C) treated by radiotherapy: report of a National Cooperative Study. *Int J Radiat Oncol Biol Phys* 1993;26:197–201.

108. Demanes DJ, Rodriguez RR, Schour L, et al. High-dose-rate intensity-modulated brachytherapy with external beam radiotherapy for prostate cancer: California Endocurietherapy's 10–year results. *Int J Radiat Oncol Biol Phys* 2005;61:1306–1316.

109. Dicker AP, Lin CC, Leeper DB, et al. Isotope selection for permanent prostate implants? An evaluation of ^{103}Pd versus ^{125}I based on radiobiological effectiveness and dosimetry. *Semin Urol Oncol* 2000;18:152–159.

110. Donnelly BJ, Saliken JC, Ernst DS, et al. Prospective trial of cryosurgical ablation of the prostate: five-year results. *Urology* 2002;60:645–649.

111. Drachenberg DE, Brawer MK. Screening for prostate cancer. In: Vogelzang NJ, Shipley WU, et al., eds. *Comprehensive textbook of genitourinary oncology.* Philadelphia: Lippincott Williams & Wilkins; 2000:654–672.

112. Duffield-Lillico AJ, Dalkin BL, Reid ME, et al. Selenium supplementation, baseline plasma selenium status and incidence of prostate cancer: an analysis of the complete treatment period of the Nutritional Prevention of Cancer Trial. *BJU Int* 2003;91:608–612.

113. Dugan JA, Bostwick DG, Myers RP, et al. The definition and preoperative prediction of clinically insignificant prostate cancer. *JAMA* 1996;275:2888–2924.

114. Dugan TC, Shipley WU, Young RH, et al. Biopsy after external beam radiation therapy for adenocarcinoma of the prostate: correlation with original histological grade and current prostate specific antigen levels. *J Urol* 1991;146:1313–1316.

115. Elgamal A-ZA, Ectors NL, Sunardhi-Widyaputra S, et al. Detection of prostate specific antigen in pancreas and salivary glands: a potential impact on prostate cancer overestimation. *J Urol* 1996;156:464–468.

116. Epstein JI, Lieberman PH. Mucinous adenocarcinoma of the prostate gland. *Am J Surg Pathol* 1985;9:299–308.

117. Epstein JI, Pizov G, Walsh PC. Correlation of pathologic findings with progression after radical retropubic prostatectomy. *Cancer* 1993;71:3582–3593.

118. Epstein JI, Walsh PC, Brendler JB. Radical prostatectomy for impalpable prostate cancer: the Johns Hopkins experience with tumors found on transurethral resection (stage T1A and T1B) and on needle biopsy (stage T1C). *J Urol* 1994;152:1721–1729.

119. Epstein JI, Walsh PC, Carmichael M, et al. Pathologic and clinical findings to predict tumor extent of nonpalpable (stage T1c) prostate cancer. *JAMA* 1994;271:368–373.

120. Etminan M, Takkouche B, Caamano-Isorna F. The role of tomato products and lycopene in the prevention of prostate cancer: a meta-analysis of observational studies. *Cancer Epidemiol Biomarkers Prev* 2004;13:340–5.

121. Etzioni R, Penson DF, Legler JM, et al. Overdiagnosis due to prostate-specific antigen screening: lessons from U.S. prostate cancer incidence trends. *J Natl Cancer Inst* 2002;94:981–990.

122. Fair WR, Fleshner NE, Heston W. Cancer of the prostate: a nutritional disease? *Urology* 1997;50:840–848.

123. Falco T, Shenouda F, Kaufman C, et al. Ultrasound imaging for external-beam prostate treatment setup and dosimetric verification. *Med Dosim* 2002;27:271–273.

124. Fernandes ET, Sundaram CP, Long R, et al. Biopsy Gleason score: how does it correlate with the final pathological diagnosis in prostate cancer? *Br J Urol* 1997;79:615–617.

125. Fincham SM, Hill GB, Hanson J, et al. Epidemiology of prostatic cancer: a case-control study. *Prostate* 1990;17:189–206.

126. Flanigan RC, McKay TC, Olson M, et al. Limited efficacy of preoperative computed tomographic scanning for the evaluation of lymph node metastasis in patients before radical prostatectomy. *Urology* 1996;48:428–432.

127. Fowler JE, Whitmore WF. The incidence and extent of pelvic lymph node metastases in apparently localized prostatic cancer. *Cancer* 1981;47:1941–1945.

128. Freedland S, Humphreys E, Mangold L, et al. Risk of prostate cancer-specific mortality following biochemical recurrence after radical prostatectomy. *JAMA* 2005;294:433–439.

129. Fung AY, Enke CA, Ayyangar KM, et al. Prostate motion and isocenter adjustment from ultrasound-based localization during delivery of radiation therapy. *Int J Radiat Oncol Biol Phys* 2005;61:984–992.

130. Fuss M, Salter BJ, Cavanaugh SX, et al. Daily ultrasound-based image-guided targeting for radiotherapy of upper abdominal malignancies. *Int J Radiat Oncol Biol Phys* 2004;59:1245–1256.

131. Galalae RM, Martinez A, Mate T, et al. Long-term outcome by risk factors using conformal high-dose-rate brachytherapy (HDR-BT) boost with or without neoadjuvant androgen suppression for localized prostate cancer. *Int J Radiat Oncol Biol Phys* 2004;58:1048–1055.

132. Gann PH, Hennekens CH, Ma J, et al. Prospective study of sex hormone levels and risk of prostate cancer. *J Natl Cancer Inst* 1996;88:1118–1126.

133. Gann PH, Hennekens CH, Stampfer MJ. A prospective evaluation of plasma prostate-specific antigen for detection of prostate cancer. *JAMA* 1995;273:289–294.

134. Gann PH, Ma J, Giovannucci E, et al. Lower prostate cancer risk in men with

elevated plasma lycopene levels: results of a prospective analysis. *Cancer Res* 1999;59:1225–1230.

135. Gervasi LA, Mata J, Easley JD, et al. Prognostic significance of lymph node metastases in prostate cancer. *J Urol* 1989;142:332–336.

136. Ghafar MA, Johnson CW, De La Taille A, et al. Salvage cryotherapy using an argon based system for locally recurrent prostate cancer after radiation therapy: the Columbia experience. *J Urol* 2001;166:1333–1337.

137. Ghali VS, Garcia R. Prostatic adenocarcinoma with carcinoidal features producing adrenocorticotropic syndrome: immunohistochemical study and review of the literature. *Cancer* 1984;54:1043–1048.

138. Ghossein RA, Osman I, Bhattacharya S, et al. Detection of prostatic specific membrane antigen messenger RNA using immunobead reverse transcriptase polymerase chain reaction. *Diagn Mol Pathol* 1999;8:59–65.

139. Giovannucci E. Epidemiologic characteristics of prostate cancer. *Cancer* 1995;75:1766–1777.

140. Giovannucci E. Selenium and risk of prostate cancer. *Lancet* 1998;5:755–756.

141. Giovannucci E. Tomatoes, tomato-based products, lycopene, and cancer: review of the epidemiologic literature. *J Natl Cancer Inst* 1999;91:317–331.

142. Giovannucci E, Ascherio A, Rimm EB, et al. A prospective cohort study of vasectomy and prostate cancer in US men. *JAMA* 1993;269:873–877.

143. Giovannucci E, Ascherio A, Rimm EB, et al. Intake of carotenoids and retinol in relation to risk of prostate cancer. *J Natl Cancer Inst* 1995;87:1767–1776.

144. Giovannucci E, Rimm EB, Colditz GA, et al. A prospective study of dietary fat and risk of prostate cancer. *J Natl Cancer Inst* 1993;85:1538–1540.

145. Giovannucci E, Stampfer MJ, Krithivas K, et al. The CAG repeat within the androgen receptor gene and its relationship to prostate cancer. *Proc Natl Acad Sci U S A* 1997;94:3320–3323.

146. Giovannucci E, Tosteson TD, Speizer FE, et al. A retrospective cohort study of vasectomy and prostate cancer in US men. *JAMA* 1993;269:878–882.

147. Gleason DF. Histologic grade, clinical stage, and patient age in prostate cancer. *Monogr Natl Cancer Inst* 1988;7:15–18.

148. Gleason DF, Mellinger GT, VACURG, prediction of prognosis for prostatic adenocarcinoma by combined histological grading and clinical staging. *J Urol* 1974;111:58–64.

149. Gleason DF, Veterans Administration Cooperative Urological Research Group. Histologic grading and clinical staging of prostatic carcinoma. In: Tannenbaum M, ed. *Urologic pathology: the prostate.* Philadelphia: Lea & Febiger; 1977:171–198

150. Golimbu M, Provet J, Al-Askari S, et al. Radical prostatectomy for stage D1 prostatic cancer. *Urology* 1987;30:427–435.

151. Gomella LG, Raj GV, Moreno JG. Reverse transcriptase polymerase chain reaction for prostate specific antigen in the management of prostate cancer. *J Urol* 1997;158:326–337.

152. Grasso YZ, Gupta MK, Levin HS, et al. Combined nested RT-PCR assay for prostate-specific antigen and prostate-specific membrane antigen in prostate cancer patients: correlation with pathological stage. *Cancer Res* 1998;58:1456–1459.

153. Gray GF Jr, Marshall VF. Squamous carcinoma of the prostate. *J Urol* 1975;113:736–738.

154. Greene DR, Egawa S, Neerhut G, et al. The distribution of residual cancer in radical prostatectomy specimens in stage A prostate cancer. *J Urol* 1991;145:328–329.

155. Greene LF, Farrow GM, Ravitz JM, et al. Prostatic adenocarcinoma of ductal origin. *J Urol* 1979;121:303–305.

156. Greenwald PKV, Kirmss V, Polan AK, et al. Cancer of the prostate among men with benign prostatic hyperplasia. *J Natl Cancer Inst* 1974;53:335–340.

157. Gregori A, Vieweg J, Dahm P, et al. Comparison of ultrasound-guided biopsies and prostatectomy specimens: predictive accuracy of Gleason score and tumor after RP. *J Urol* 2001;66:66,TJ.

158. Griffiths K, Morton MS, Denis L. Certain aspects of molecular endocrinology that relate to the influence of dietary factors on the pathogenesis of prostate cancer. *Eur Urol* 1999;35:443–455.

159. Grills IS, Martinez AA, Hollander M, et al. High dose rate brachytherapy as prostate cancer monotherapy reduces toxicity compared to low dose rate palladium seeds. *J Urol* 2004;171:1098–1104.

160. Grimm PD, Blasko J, Ragde H, et al. Does brachytherapy have a role in the treatment of prostate cancer? *Hematol Oncol Clin North Am* 1996;10:653–673.

161. Grimm PD, Blasko J, Sylvester JE, et al. 10-year biochemical (prostate-specific antigen) control of prostate cancer with (125)I brachytherapy. *Int J Radiat Oncol Biol Phys* 2001;51:31–40.

162. Gronberg H, Damber L, Damber JE. Studies of genetic factors in prostate cancer in a twin population. *J Urol* 1994;152:1484–1487.

163. Gronberg H, Damber L, Damber JE. Total food consumption and body mass index in relation to prostate cancer risk: a case-control study in Sweden with prospectively collected exposure data. *J Urol* 1996;155:969–974.

164. Gronberg H, Isaacs SD, Smith JR, et al. Characteristics of prostate cancer in families potentially linked to the hereditary prostate cancer 1 (HPC1) locus. *JAMA* 1997;278:1251–1255.

165. Hall EJ. Intensity-modulated radiation therapy, protons, and the risk of second cancers. *Int J Radiat Oncol Biol Phys* 2006;65:1–7.

166. Hall EJ, Wuu CS. Radiation-induced second cancers: the impact of 3D-CRT and IMRT. *Int J Radiat Oncol Biol Phys* 2003;56:83–88.

167. Han BH, Wallner K. Dosimetric and radiographic correlates to prostate brachytherapy-related rectal complications. *Int J Cancer* 2001;96:372–378.

168. Han KR, Belldegrun AS. Third-generation cryosurgery for primary and recurrent prostate cancer. *BJU Int* 2004;93:14–18.

169. Han M, Partin AW, Zahurak M, et al. Biochemical (prostate specific antigen) recurrence probability following radical prostatectomy for clinically localized prostate cancer. *J Urol* 2003;169:517–523.

170. Hanks GE, Asbell S, Krall JM, et al. Outcome for lymph node dissection negative T-1b, T-2 (A-2, B) prostate cancer treated with external beam irradiation therapy in RTOG 77-06. *Int J Radiat Oncol Biol Phys* 1991;21:1099–1103.

171. Hanlon AL, Diratzouian H, Hanks GE. Posttreatment prostate-specific antigen nadir highly predictive of distant failure and death from prostate cancer. *Int J Radiat Oncol Biol Phys* 2002;53:297–303.

172. Hanlon AL, Pinover WH, Horwitz EM, et al. Patterns and fate of PSA bouncing following 3D-CRT. *Int J Radiat Oncol Biol Phys* 2001;50:845–849.

173. Hayes RB, Pottern LM, Strickler H, et al. Sexual behaviour, STDs and risks for prostate cancer. *Br J Cancer* 2000;82:718–725.

174. Heidenreich A, Vorreuther R, Neubauer S, et al. The influence of ejaculation on serum levels of prostate specific antigen. *J Urol* 1997;157:209–211.

175. Herstein A, Wallner K, Merrick G, et al. I-125 versus P-103 for low-risk prostate cancer: long-term morbidity outcomes from a prospective randomized multi-center controlled trial. *Cancer J* 2005;11:385–389.

176. Hill P, Wynder EL, Garbaczewski L, et al. Diet and urinary steroids in black and white North American men and black South African men. *Cancer Res* 1979;39:5101–5105.

177. Hoedemaeker RF, Rietbergen JB, Kranse R, et al. Histopathological prostate cancer characteristics at radical prostatectomy after population based screening. *J Urol* 2000;164:411–415.

178. Hoenig DM, Chi S, Porter C, et al. Risk of nodal metastases at laparoscopic pelvic lymphadenectomy using PSA, Gleason score, and clinical stage in men with localized prostate cancer. *J Endourol* 1997;11:263–265.

179. Holm H, Juul N, Pederson JF, et al. Transperineal iodine-125 seed implantation in prostatic cancer guided by transrectal ultrasonography. *J Urol* 1983;130:283–286.

180. Howards SS, Peterson HB. Vasectomy and prostate cancer, chance, bias, or a casual relationship? *JAMA* 1993;269:913–914.

181. Hoznek A, Samadi DB, Salomon L, et al. Laparoscopic radical prostatectomy: published series. *Curr Urol Rep* 2002;3:152–158.

182. Hsing AW, Gao YT, Wu G, et al. Polymorphic CAG and GGN repeat lengths in the androgen receptor gene and prostate cancer risk: a population-based case-control study in China. *Cancer Res* 2000;60:5111–5116.

183. Hsing AW, McLaughton JK, Schuman LM, et al. Diet, tobacco use, and fatal prostate cancer: results from the Lutheran Brotherhood cohort study. *Cancer Res* 1990;50:6836–6840.

184. Hsing AW, Reichardt JK, Stanczyk FZ. Hormones and prostate cancer: current perspectives and future directions. *Prostate* 2002;52:213–235.

185. Hua C, Lovelock DM, Mageras GS, et al. Development of a semi automatic alignment tool for accelerated localization of the prostate. *Int J Radiat Oncol Biol Phys* 2003;55:811–824.

186. Huang E, Dong L, Chandra A, et al. Intrafraction prostate motion during IMRT for prostate cancer. *Int J Radiat Oncol Biol Phys* 2002;53:261–268.

187. Hudson MA, Bahnson RR, Catalona WJ. Clinical use of prostate specific antigen in patients with prostate cancer. *J Urol* 1989;142:1011–1017.

188. Hugosson J, Aus G, Becker C, et al. Would prostate cancer detected by screening with prostate-specific antigen develop into clinical cancer if left undiagnosed? A comparison of two population-based studies in Sweden. *BJU Int* 2000;85:1078–1084.

189. Humphrey PA, Keetch DW, Smith DS, et al. Prospective characterisation of pathological features of prostatic carcinomas detected via serum prostate specific antigen based screening. *J Urol* 1996;155:816–820.

190. Huncharek M, Muscat J. Serum prostate-specific antigen as a predictor of radiographic staging studies in newly diagnosed prostate cancer. *Cancer Invest* 1995;13:31–35.

191. Hurwitz MD, Cormack R, Tempany CM, et al. Three dimensional real time magnetic resonance guided interstitial prostate brachytherapy optimizes radiation dose distribution resulting in a favorable acute side effect profile in patients with clinically localized prostate cancer. *Tech Urol* 2000;6:89–94.

192. Incrocci L, Slob AK, Levendag PC. Sexual (dys)function after radiotherapy for prostate cancer: a review. *Int J Radiat Oncol Biol Phys* 2002;52:681–693.

193. Irvine RA, Yu MC, Ross RK, et al. The CAG and GGC microsatellites of the androgen receptor gene are in linkage disequilibrium in men with prostate cancer. *Cancer Res* 1995;55:1937–1940.

194. Israeli RS, Miller WH Jr, Su SL, et al. Sensitive detection of prostatic hematogenous tumor cell dissemination using prostate specific antigen and prostate specific membrane-derived primers in the polymerase chain reaction. *J Urol* 1995;53:573–577.

195. Izawa JI, Ajam K, McGuire E, et al. Major surgery to manage definitively severe complications of salvage cryotherapy for prostate cancer. *J Urol* 2000;164:1978–1981.

196. Jackson A, Skwarchuk MW, Zelefsky MJ, et al. Late rectal bleeding after conformal radiotherapy of prostate cancer. II. Volume effects and dose-volume histograms. *Int J Radiat Oncol Biol Phys* 2001;49:685–698.

197. Jemal A, Siegel R, Ward E, et al. Cancer statistics, 2006. *CA Cancer J Clin* 2006;56:106–130.

198. Jemal A, Thomas T, Murray T, et al. Cancer statistics, 2002. *CA Cancer J Clin* 2002;52:23–47.

199. Jewett HJ. The present status of radical prostatectomy for stages A and B prostatic cancer. *Urol Clin North Am* 1975;2:105–124.

200. Johansson JE, Adami H-O, Andersson S-O, et al. High 10-year survival rate in patients with early, untreated prostatic cancer. *JAMA* 1992;267:2191–2196.

201. Johnson DE, Chalbaud R, Ayala AG. Secondary tumors of the prostate. *J Urol* 1974;112:507–508.

202. Johnstone PAS, Riffenburgh R, Saunders EL, et al. Grading inaccuracies in diagnostic biopsies revealing prostatic adenocarcinoma: implications for definitive radiation therapy. *Int J Radiat Oncol Biol Phys* 1995;32:479–482.

203. Kabalin JN, Hodge KK, McNeal JE, et al. Identification of residual cancer in the prostate following radiation therapy: role of transrectal ultrasound guided biopsy and prostate specific antigen. *J Urol* 1989;142:326–331.

204. Kagawa K, Lee WR, Schultheiss TE, et al. Initial clinical assessment of CT-MRI image fusion software in localization of the prostate for 3D conformal radiation therapy. *Int J Radiat Oncol Biol Phys* 1997;38:319–325.

205. Kantoff PW, Halabi S, Farmer DA, et al. Prognostic significance of reverse transcriptase polymerase chain reaction for prostate-specific antigen in men with hormone-refractory prostate cancer. *J Clin Oncol* 2001;19:3025–3028.

206. Katz AE, deVries DM, Begg MD, et al. Enhanced reverse transcriptase-polymerase chain reaction for prostate specific antigen as an indicator of true pathologic stage in patients with prostate cancer. *Cancer* 1995;75:1642–1648.

207. Kaul L, Hehmat MY, Kovi J, et al. The role of diet in prostate cancer. *Nutr Cancer* 1987;9:123–128.

208. Kestin LL, Martinez AA, Stromberg JS, et al. Matched-pair analysis of conformal high-dose rate brachytherapy boost versus external-beam radiation therapy alone for locally advanced prostate cancer. *J Clin Oncol* 2000;18:2869–2880.

209. Kini VR, Edmundson GK, Vicini FA, et al. Use of three-dimensional radiation

therapy planning tools and intraoperative ultrasound to evaluate high dose rate prostate brachytherapy implants. *Int J Radiat Oncol Biol Phys* 1999;43: 571–578.
210. Kitamura K, Shirato H, Seppenwoolde Y, et al. Three-dimensional intrafractional movement of prostate measured during real-time tumor-tracking radiotherapy in supine and prone treatment positions. *Int J Radiat Oncol Biol Phys* 2002;53:1117–1123.
211. Klomp ML, Hendrikx AJ, Keyzer J. The effect of transrectal ultrasonography (TRUS) including digital rectal examination (DRE) of the prostate on the level of prostate specific antigen (PSA). *Br J Urol* 1994;73:717–724.
212. Kollmeier MA, Stock RG, Stone N. Biochemical outcomes after prostate brachytherapy with 5-year minimal follow-up: importance of patient selection and implant quality. *Int J Radiat Oncol Biol Phys* 2003;57:645–653.
213. Kopelson G, Harisiadis L, Romas NA, et al. Periurethral prostatic duct carcinoma: clinical features and treatment results. *Cancer* 1978;42:2894–2902.
214. Kovacs G, Galalae R, Loch T, et al. Prostate preservation by combined external beam and HDR brachytherapy in nodal negative prostate cancer. *Strahlenther Onkol* 1999;175:87–88.
215. Kry SF, Salehpour M, Followill DS, et al. Out-of-field photon and neutron dose equivalents from step-and-shoot intensity-modulated radiation therapy. *Int J Radiat Oncol Biol Phys* 2005;62:1204–1216.
216. Kry SF, Salehpour M, Followill DS, et al. The calculated risk of fatal secondary malignancies from intensity-modulated radiation therapy. *Int J Radiat Oncol Biol Phys* 2005;62:1195–1203 [comment in 2005;64:1290–1291].
217. Kuban DA, Dong L, Cheung R, et al. Ultrasound-based localization. *Semin Radiat Oncol* 2005;15:180–191.
218. Kuban DA, Thames HD, Levy LB, et al. Long-term multi-institutional analysis of stage T1-T2 prostate cancer treated with radiotherapy in the PSA era. *Int J Radiat Oncol Biol Phys* 2003;57:915–928.
219. Kullu S, Ersev A, Simsek F, et al. Adenocarcinoma of the prostate with endometrioid features. *Int Urol Nephrol* 1991;23:577–580.
220. Kupelian P, Katcher J, Levin H, et al. External beam radiotherapy versus radical prostatectomy for clinical stage T1-T2 prostate cancer: therapeutic implications of stratification by pretreatment PSA levels and biopsy Gleason scores. *Cancer J Sci Am* 1997;37:78–87.
221. Kupelian PA, Potters L, Khuntia D, et al. Radical prostatectomy, external beam radiotherapy <72 Gy, external beam radiotherapy > or = 72 Gy, permanent seed implantation, or combined seeds/external beam radiotherapy for stage T1-T2 prostate cancer. *Int J Radiat Oncol Biol Phys* 2004;58:25–33.
222. Kupelian PA, Thakkar VV, Khuntia D, et al. Hypofractionated intensity-modulated radiotherapy (70 Gy and 2.5 Gy per fraction) for localized prostate cancer: long-term outcomes. *Int J Radiat Oncol Biol Phys* 2005;63:1463–1468.
223. Kurhanewicz, J, Vigneron DB, Males RG, et al. The prostate: MR imaging and spectroscopy. Present and future. *Radiol Clin North Am* 2000;38:115–138.
224. Kurhanewicz J, Vigneron DB, Nelson SJ. Three-dimensional magnetic resonance spectroscopic imaging of brain and prostate cancer. *Neoplasia* 2000;1: 166–189.
225. Langen KM, Pouliot J, Anezinos C, et al. Evaluation of ultrasound-based prostate localization for image-guided radiotherapy. *Int J Radiat Oncol Biol Phys* 2003;57:635–644.
226. Langen KM, Zhang Y, Andrews RD, et al. Initial experience with megavoltage (MV) CT guidance for daily prostate alignments. *Int J Radiat Oncol Biol Phys* 2005;62:1517–1524.
227. Lattanzi J, McNeeley S, Hanlon A, et al. Daily CT localization for correcting portal errors in the treatment of prostate cancer. *Int J Radiat Oncol Biol Phys* 1998;41:1079–1086.
228. Lattanzi J, McNeeley S, Hanlon A, et al. Ultrasound-based stereotactic guidance of precision conformal external beam radiotherapy in clinically localized prostate cancer. *Urology* 2000;55:73–78.
229. Lattanzi J, McNeeley S, Pinover W, et al. A comparison of daily CT localization to a daily ultrasound-based system in prostate cancer. *Int J Radiat Oncol Biol Phys* 1999;43:719–725 [comment in: 1999;43:705–706].
230. Lawton CA, Won M, Pilepich M, et al. Long-term treatment sequelae following external beam irradiation fro adenocarcinoma of the prostate: analysis of RTOG studies 7506 and 7706. *Int J Radiat Oncol Biol Phys* 1991;21:935–936.
231. Lazier CB, Thomas LN, Douglas RC, et al. Dutasteride, the dual 5alpha-reductase inhibitor, inhibits androgen action and promotes cell death in the LNCaP prostate cancer cell line. *Prostate* 2004;58:130–144.
232. Lechevallier E, Eghazarian C, Ortega JC, et al. Effect of digital rectal examination on serum complexed and free prostate-specific antigen and percentage of free prostate-specific antigen. *Urology* 1999;54:857–861.
233. Lee N, Fawaaz R, Olsson CA, et al. Which patients with newly diagnosed prostate cancer need a radionuclide bone scan? An analysis based on 631 patients. *Int J Radiat Oncol Biol Phys* 2000;48:1443–1446.
234. Lee WR, DeSilvio M, Lawton C, et al. A phase II study of external beam radiotherapy combined with permanent source brachytherapy for intermediate-risk, clinically localized adenocarcinoma of the prostate preliminary result of RTOG P-0019. *Int J Radiat Oncol Biol Phys* 2006;64:804–809.
235. Lee WR, Hanks GE, Hanlon AL, et al. Lateral shielding reduces rectal morbidity following high dose three-dimensional conformal radiation therapy for clinically localized prostate cancer: further evidence for a significant dose effect. *Int J Radiat Oncol Biol Phys* 1996;35:251–257 and comment in 1996;35:415–416.
236. Lee WR, Schultheiss TE, Hanlon AL, et al. Urinary incontinence following external-beam radiotherapy for clinically localized prostate cancer. *Urology* 1996;48:95–99.
237. Leibel SA, Kutcher GJ, Zelefsky MJ, et al. 3-D conformal radiotherapy for carcinoma of the prostate. Clinical experience at the Memorial Sloan-Kettering Cancer Center. *Front Radiat Ther Oncol* 1996;29:229–237.
238. Letourneau D, Martinez AA, Lockman D, et al. Assessment of residual error for online cone beam CT-guided treatment of prostate cancer patients. *Int J Radiat Oncol Biol Phys* 2006;62:1239–1246.
239. Link RE, Morton RA. Indications for pelvic lymphadenectomy in prostate cancer. *Urol Clin North Am* 2001;28:491–498.
240. Little DJ, Dong L, Levy LB, et al. Use of portal images and BAT ultrasonography to measure setup error and organ motion for prostate IMRT: implications for treatment margins. *Int J Radiat Oncol Biol Phys* 2003;56:1218–1224.
241. Locke J, Ellis W, Wallner K, et al. Risk factors for acute urinary retention requiring temporary intermittent catheterization after prostate brachytherapy: a prospective study. *Int J Radiat Oncol Biol Phys* 2002;52:712–719.
242. Long JP, Bahn D, Lee F, et al. Five-year retrospective, multi-institutional pooled analysis of cancer-related outcomes after cryosurgical ablation of the prostate. *Urology* 2001;57:518–523.
243. Mah D, Freedman G, Movsas G, et al. To move or not to move: measurements of prostate motion by urethrography using MRI. *Int J Radiat Oncol Biol Phys* 2001;50:847–951.
244. Makarov DV, Sanderson H, Partin AW, et al. Gleason score 7 prostate cancer on needle biopsy: is the prognostic difference in Gleason scores 4 + 3 and 3 + 4 independent of the number of involved cores? *J Urol* 2002;167:2440–2442.
245. Malone S, Crook JM, Kendal WS, et al. Respiratory-induced prostate motion: quantification and characterization. *Int J Radiat Oncol Biol Phys* 2000;48:105–109.
245a. Mameghan H, Fisher R, Watt WH, et al. Results of radiotherapy for localised prostatic carcinoma treated at the Prince of Wales Hospital, Sydney. *Med J Aust* 1991;154:317–326.
246. Mantz CA, Nautiyal J, Awan A, et al. Potency preservation following conformal radiotherapy for localized prostate cancer: impact of neoadjuvant androgen blockade, treatment technique, and patient-related factors. *Cancer J Sci Am* 1999;5:230–236.
246a. Mantz CA, Song P, Farhangi E, et al. Potency probability following conformal megavoltage radiotherapy using conventional doses for localized prostate cancer. *Int J Radiat Oncol Biol Phys* 1997;37:551–557.
247. Marley GM, Miller MC, et al. Free and complexed prostate-specific antigen serum ratios to predict probability of primary prostate cancer and benign prostatic hyperplasia. *Urology* 1996;48:16–22.
248. Marsh LH, Ten Haken RK, Sandler HM. A customized non-axial external beam technique for treatment of prostate carcinomas. *Med Dosim* 1992;17:123–127.
249. Martinez A. High dose rate brachytherapy for prostate cancer. In: Greco C, Zelefsky MJ, eds. *Radiotherapy for prostate cancer*. Amsterdam: Harwood Academic Publishers; 2000:279–286.
250. Martinez AA, Yan D, Lockman D, et al. Improvement in dose escalation using the process of adaptive radiotherapy combined with three-dimensional conformal or intensity-modulated beams for prostate cancer. *Int J Radiat Oncol Biol Phys* 2001;50:1226–1234.
251. Marugame T, Mizuno S. Comparison of prostate cancer mortality in five countries: France, Italy, Japan, UK and USA from the WHO mortality database (1960–2000). *Jpn J Clin Oncol* 2005;35:690–691.
252. Mate TP, Gottesman JE, Hatton J, et al. High dose-rate afterloading ^{192}iridium prostate brachytherapy: feasibility report. *Int J Radiat Oncol Biol Phys* 1998;41:525–533.
253. Matzkin H, Kaver I, Bramante-Schreiber L, et al. Comparison between two iodine-125 brachytherapy implant techniques: pre-planning and intra-operative by various dosimetry quality indicators. *Radiother Oncol* 2003;68:289–294.
254. Matzkin H, Laufer M, Chen J, et al. Effect of elective prolonged urethral catheterization on serum prostate-specific antigen concentration. *Urology* 1996;48:63–66.
255. Matzkin H, Soloway MS, Hardeman S. Transitional cell carcinoma of the prostate. *J Urol* 1991;146:1207–1212.
256. McAleer JK, Gerson LW, McMahon D, et al. Effect of digital rectal examination (and ejaculation) on serum prostate-specific antigen after twenty-four hours: a randomized, prospective study. *Urology* 1993;41:111–112.
257. McGowan DG. The value of extended field radiation therapy in carcinoma of the prostate. *Int J Radiat Oncol Biol Phys* 1981;7:1333–1339.
258. McLaughlin PW, Troyer S, Berri S, et al. Functional anatomy of the prostate: implications for treatment planning. *Int J Radiat Oncol Biol Phys* 2005;63:479–491.
259. McLaughlin PW, Wygoda A, Sahijdak W, et al. The effect of patient position ad treatment technique in conformal treatment of prostate cancer. *Int J Radiat Oncol Biol Phys* 1999;45:407–413.
260. McNeal JE. Cancer volume and site of origin of adenocarcinoma in the prostate: relationship to local and distant spread. *Hum Pathol* 1992;23:258–266.
261. McNeal JE. Origin and development of carcinoma of the prostate. *Cancer* 1969;23:24.
262. McNeal JE, Price HM, Redwine EA, et al. Stage A versus stage B adenocarcinoma of the prostate: morphological comparison and biological significance. *J Urol* 1988;139:61–65.
263. Melian E, Mageras GS, Fuks Z, et al. Variation in prostate position quantitation and implications for three-dimensional conformal treatment planning. *Int J Radiat Oncol Biol Phys* 1997;38:73–81.
264. Meikle AW, Smith JA, Stringham JD. Production, clearance, and metabolism of testosterone in men with prostatic cancer. *Prostate* 1987;10:25–31.
265. Melicow MM, Tannenbaum M. Endometrial carcinoma of uterus masculinus (prostatic utricle): report of six cases. *J Urol* 1971;106:892–902.
266. Merrick GS, Butler WM, Dorsey AT, et al. Potential role of various dosimetric quality indicators in prostate brachytherapy. *Int J Radiat Oncol Biol Phys* 1999;44:717–724.
266a. Merrick GS, Butler WM, Galbreath RW, et al. Erectile function after permanent prostate brachytherapy. *Int J Radiat Oncol Biol Phys* 2002;52:893–902.
267. Merrick GS, Butler WM, Galbreath RW, et al. Relationship between the transition zone index of the prostate gland and urinary morbidity after brachytherapy. *Urology* 2001;57:524–529.
268. Merrick GS, Butler WM, Wallner KE, et al. Erectile function after prostate brachytherapy. *Int J Radiat Oncol Biol Phys* 2005;62:437–447.
269. Merrick GS, Butler WM, Wallner KE, et al. Impact of supplemental external beam radiotherapy and/or androgen deprivation therapy on biochemical outcome after permanent prostate brachytherapy. *Int J Radiat Oncol Biol Phys* 2005;61: 32–43.
270. Merrick GS, Butler WM, Wallner KE, et al. The impact of radiation dose to the urethra on brachytherapy-related dysuria. *Brachytherapy* 2005;4:45–50.
271. Merrick GS, Butler WM, Wallner KE, et al. The importance of radiation doses to the penile bulb vs. crura in the development of postbrachytherapy erectile dysfunction. *Int J Radiat Oncol Biol Phys* 2002;54:1055–1062.
272. Merrick GS, Butler WM, Wallner KE, et al. Variability of prostate brachytherapy pre-implant dosimetry: a multi-institutional analysis. *Brachytherapy* 2005;4:241–251.
273. Merrick GS, Wallner KE, Butler WM, et al. Permanent prostate brachytherapy: is

supplemental external-beam radiation therapy necessary? *Oncology (Williston Park)* 2006;20:514–525.

274. Messing EM, Zhang JB, Rubens DJ, et al. Intraoperative optimized inverse planning for prostate brachytherapy: early experience. *Int J Radiat Oncol Biol Phys* 1999;44:801–808.

275. Mettlin C, Selenskas S, Natarajan N, et al. Beta-carotene and animal fats and their relationship to prostate cancer risk: a case-control study. *Cancer* 1989;64:605–612.

276. Michalski JM, Winter K, Purdy JA, et al. Toxicity after three-dimensional radiotherapy for prostate cancer on RTOG 9406 dose Level V. *Int J Radiat Oncol Biol Phys* 2005;62:706–713.

277. Millar DS, Ow KK, Paul CL, et al. Detailed methylation analysis of the glutathione S-transferase (GSTP1) gene in prostate cancer. *Oncogene* 1999;18:1313–1324.

278. Millar EK, Sharma NK, Lessells AM. Ductal (endometrioid) adenocarcinoma of the prostate: a clinicopathological study of 16 cases. *Histopathology* 1996;29:11–19.

279. Mills PK, Beeson WL, Phillips RL, et al. Cohort study of diet, lifestyle, and prostate cancer in Adventist men. *Cancer* 1989;64:598–604.

280. Milosevic M, Voruganti S, Blend R, et al. Magnetic resonance imaging (MRI) for localization of the prostatic apex: comparison to computed tomography (CT) and urethrography. *Radiother Oncol* 1998;47:277–284.

281. Moreno JG, Gomella LG. Circulating prostate cancer cells detected by reverse transcription-polymerase chain reaction (RT-PCR): what do they mean? *Cancer Control* 1998;5:507–512.

282. Morr J, DiPetrillo T, Tsai JS, et al. Implementation and utility of a daily ultrasound-based localization system with intensity-modulated radiotherapy for prostate cancer. *Int J Radiat Oncol Biol Phys* 2002;53:1124–1129.

283. Mostofi FK. Grading of prostatic carcinoma. *Cancer Chemother Rep* 1975;59:111–117.

284. Muir CS, Nectoux J, Straszewski J. The epidemiology of prostatic cancer: geographical distribution and time trends. *Acta Oncol* 1991;30:133–140.

285. Nadler RB, Humphrey PA, Smith DS, et al. Effect of inflammatory and benign prostatic hyperplasia on elevated serum prostate specific antigen levels. *J Urol* 1995;154:407–413.

286. Nag S, Bice W, DeWyngaert K, et al. The American Brachytherapy Society recommendations for permanent prostate brachytherapy postimplant dosimetric analysis. *Int J Radiat Oncol Biol Phys* 2000;46:221–230.

287. Narain V, Bianco FJ Jr, Grignon DJ, et al. How accurately does prostate biopsy Gleason score predict pathologic findings and disease free survival? *Prostate* 2001;49:185–190.

288. Narayan P, Fournier G, Gajendran V, et al. Utility of preoperative serum prostate-specific antigen concentration and biopsy Gleason score in predicting risk of pelvic lymph node metastases in prostate cancer. *Urology* 1994;44:519–524.

289. Narayan P, Gajendran V, Taylor SP, et al. The role of transrectal ultrasound-guided biopsy-based staging, preoperative serum prostate-specific antigen, and biopsy Gleason score in prediction of final pathologic diagnosis in prostate cancer. *Urology* 1995;46:205–212.

290. Narod SA, Dupont A, Cusan L, et al. The impact of family history on early detection of prostate cancer [letter]. *Nat Med* 1995;1:99–101.

291. Nath R, Anderson LL, Luxton G, et al. Dosimetry of interstitial brachytherapy sources: recommendations of the AAPM Radiation Committee Task Group No.43. *Med Phys* 1995;22:209–234.

292. National Cancer Institute sponsored study of classification of non-Hodgkin's lymphomas: summary and description of a working formulation for clinical usage. The Non-Hodgkin's Lymphoma Pathologic Classification Project. *Cancer* 1982;49:2112.

293. National Cancer Institute SEER cancer statistics review, 1973–1998. 2001. Available at: http://www.cdc.gov. Accessed

294. Nederveen AJ, Lagendijk H, van der Heide UA, et al. Comparison of megavolt age position verification for prostate irradiation based on bony anatomy and implanted fiducials. *Radiother Oncol* 2003;68:81–88.

295. Nelson WG, De Marzo AM, De Weese AM, et al. The role of inflammation in the pathogenesis of prostate cancer. *J Urol* 2004;172[5 Pt 2]:S6–12.

296. Nelson WG, De Marzo AM, Isaacs WB. Prostate cancer. *N Engl J Med* 2003;349:366–381.

297. Nelson CP, Rubin MA, Strawderman M, et al. Preoperative parameters for predicting early prostate cancer recurrence after radical prostatectomy. *Urology* 2002;59:740–745.

298. Noguchi M, Stamey TA, McNeal JE, et al. Preoperative serum prostate specific antigen does not reflect biochemical failure rates after radical prostatectomy in men with large volume cancers. *J Urol* 2000;164:1596–1600.

299. Noguchi M, Stamey TA, Neal JE, et al. An analysis of 148 consecutive transition zone cancers: clinical and histological characteristics. *J Urol* 2000;163:1751–1755.

300. Nutting CM, Convery DJ, Cosgrove VP, et al. Reduction of small and large bowel irradiation using an optimized intensity-modulated pelvic radiotherapy technique in patients with prostate cancer. *Int J Radiat Oncol Biol Phys* 2000;48:649–656.

301. Oefelein MG, Kaul K, Herz B, et al. Molecular detection of prostate epithelial cells from the surgical field and peripheral circulation during radical prostatectomy. *J Urol* 1996;155:238–242.

302. Oelrich TM. The urethral sphincter muscle in the male. *Am J Anat* 1980;158:229–246.

303. Oesterling JE, Jacobsen SJ, Klee GG, et al. Free, complexed and total serum prostate specific antigen: the establishment of appropriate reference ranges for their concentrations and ratios. *J Urol* 1995;154:1090–1095.

304. Oesterling JE, Rice DC, Glenski WJ, et al. Effect of cystoscopy, prostate biopsy and transurethral resection of prostate on serum prostate-specific antigen concentration. *Urology* 1993;42:276–282.

305. Oesterling JE, Suman VJ, Zincke H, et al. PSA-detected (clinical stage T1c or B1) prostate cancer. *Urol Clin North Am* 1994;20:293–302.

306. Ohori M, Wheeler TM, Dunn JK, et al. Pathological features and prognosis of prostate cancer detectable with current diagnostic tests. *J Urol* 1994;152:1714–1720.

307. Ohori M, Wheeler TM, Kattan MW, et al. Prognostic significance of positive margins in radical prostatectomy specimens. *J Urol* 1995;154:1818–1824.

308. Older RA, Synder B, Krupski TL, et al. Radioactive implant migration in patients treated for localized prostate cancer with interstitial brachytherapy. *J Urol* 2001;165:1590–1592.

309. Okotie OT, Aronson WJ, Wieder JA, et al. Predictors of metastatic disease in men with biochemical failure following radical prostatectomy. *J Urol* 2004;171:2260–2264.

310. Ornstein DK, Rao GS, Smith DS, et al. Effect of digital rectal examination and needle biopsy on serum total and percentage of free prostate specific antigen levels. *J Urol* 1997;157:195–198.

311. Papsidero LD, Kuriyama M, Wang MC, et al. Prostate antigen: a marker for human prostate epithelial cells. *J Natl Cancer Inst* 1981;66:37–42.

312. Partin AW, Kattan MW, Subong EN, et al. Combination of prostate-specific antigen, clinical stage, and Gleason score to predict pathological stage of localized prostate cancer: a multi-institutional update. *JAMA* 1997;277:1445–1451.

313. Partin AW, Yoo J, Carter HB, et al. The use of prostate specific antigen, clinical stage and Gleason score to predict pathological stage in men with localized prostate cancer. *J Urol* 1993;150:110–114.

314. Peeters ST, Heemsbergen WD, Koper PC, et al. Dose-response in radiotherapy for localized prostate cancer: results of the Dutch multicenter randomized phase III trial comparing 68 Gy of radiotherapy with 78 Gy. *J Clin Oncol* 2006;24:1990–1996.

315. Peeters ST, Heemsbergen WD, van Putten WL, et al. Acute and late complications after radiotherapy for prostate cancer: results of a multicenter randomized trial comparing 68 Gy to 78 Gy. *Int J Radiat Oncol Biol Phys* 2005;61:1019–1034.

316. Perez CA, Michalski J, Mansur D, et al. Three-dimensional conformal therapy versus standard radiation therapy in localized carcinoma of prostate: an update. *Clin Prostate Cancer* 2002;1:97–104.

317. Perrotti M, Pantuck A, Rabbani F, et al. Review of staging modalities in clinically localized prostate cancer. *Urology* 1999;54:208–214.

317a. Pilepich MV, Krall JM, al-Sarraf M, et al. Androgen deprivation with radiation therapy compared with radiation therapy alone for locally advanced prostatic carcinoma: a randomized comparative trial of the Radiation Therapy Oncology Group. *Urology* 1995;45:616–623.

318. Pirzkall A, Carol MP, Pickett B, et al. The effect of beam energy and number of fields on photon-based IMRT for deep-seated targets. *Int J Radiat Oncol Biol Phys* 2002;53:434–442.

319. Pisansky TM, Zincke H, Suman VJ, et al. Correlation of pretherapy prostate cancer characteristics with histologic findings from pelvic lymphadenectomy specimens. *Int J Radiat Oncol Biol Phys* 1996;34:33–39.

320. Pollack A, Hanlon AL, Horwitz EM, et al. Dosimetry and preliminary acute toxicity in the first 100 men treated for prostate cancer on a randomized hypofractionation dose escalation trial. *Int J Radiat Oncol Biol Phys* 2006;64:518–526.

321. Pollack A, Hanlon AL, Horwitz EM, et al. Prostate cancer radiotherapy dose response: an update of the Fox Chase experience. *J Urol* 2004;171:1132–1136.

322. Pollack A, Zagars GK, Starkschall G, et al. Prostate cancer radiation dose response: results of the M.D. Anderson phase III randomized trial. *Int J Radiat Oncol Biol Phys* 2002;53:1097–1105.

323. Potters L, Morgenstern C, Calugaru E, et al. 12-year outcomes following permanent prostate brachytherapy in patients with clinically localized prostate cancer. *J Urol* 2005;173:1562–1566.

324. Pound CR, Partin AW, Eisenberger MA, et al. Natural history of progression after PSA elevation following radical prostatectomy. *JAMA* 1999;281:1591–1597.

325. Potters L, Torre T, Fearn PA, et al. Potency after permanent prostate brachytherapy for localized prostate cancer. *Int J Radiat Oncol Biol Phys* 2001;50:1235–1242.

326. Price RA, Hanks GE, McNeeley SW, et al. Advantages of using noncoplanar vs. axial beam arrangements when treating prostate cancer with intensity-modulated radiation therapy and the step-and-shoot delivery method. *Int J Radiat Oncol Biol Phys* 2002;58:1256–1263.

327. Prout GR Jr, Heaney JA, Griffin P, et al. Nodal involvement as a prognostic indicator in patients with prostatic carcinoma. *J Urol* 1980;124:226–231.

328. Punglia RS, D'Amico AV, Catalona WJ, et al. Effect of verification bias on screening for prostate cancer by measurement of prostate-specific antigen. *N Engl J Med* 2003;349:335–342.

329. Qian J, Bostwick DG, Takahashi S, et al. Chromosomal anomalies in prostatic intraepithelial neoplasia and carcinoma detected by fluorescence in situ hybridization. *Cancer Res* 1995;55:5408–5414.

330. Qian J, Wollan P, Bostwick DG. The extent and multicentricity of high-grade prostatic intraepithelial neoplasia in clinically localized prostatic adenocarcinoma. *Hum Pathol* 1997;28:143–148.

331. Raina R, Agarwal A, Goyal KK, et al. Long-term potency after iodine-125 radiotherapy for prostate cancer and role of sildenafil citrate. *Urology* 2003;62:1103–1108.

332. Ranparia DJ, Hart L, Assimos DG. Utility of chest radiography and cystoscopy in the evaluation of patients with localized prostate cancer. *Urology* 1996;48:72–74.

333. Rasch C, Barillot I, Remeijer P, et al. Definition of the prostate in CT and MRI: a multi-observer study. *Int J Radiat Oncol Biol Phys* 1999;43:57–66.

334. Rassweiler J, Schulze M, Teber D, et al. Laparoscopic radical prostatectomy: functional and oncological outcomes. *Curr Opin Urol* 2004;14:75–82.

335. Rees MA, Campbell SC, Klein EA, et al. Validation of a model for predicting metastatic disease in the pelvic lymph nodes of patients with clinically localized prostate cancer. *J Urol* 1996;155:487(abstr).

336. Rees MA, McHugh TA, Door RP, et al. Assessment of the utility of bone scan, CT scan, and lymph node dissection in staging of patients with newly diagnosed prostate cancer. *J Urol* 1995;153:495 (abst.).

337. Reese JH, Freiha FS, Gelb AB, et al. Transitional cell carcinoma of the prostate in patients undergoing radical cystoprostatectomy. *J Urol* 1992;147:92–95.

338. Rifkin MD, Zerhouni EA, Gatsonis CA, et al. Comparison of magnetic resonance imaging and ultrasonography in staging early prostate cancer: results of a multi-institutional cooperative trial. *N Engl J Med* 1990;323:621–626.

339. Ritter MA, Messing EM, Shanahan TG, et al. Prostate-specific antigen as a predictor of radiotherapy response and patterns of failure in localized prostate cancer. *J Clin Oncol* 1992;10:1208–1217.

340. Roach M. Equations for predicting the pathologic stage of men with localized prostate cancer using the preoperative prostate specific antigen. *J Urol* 1993;150:1923–1924.

340a. Roach M 3rd, Chinn DM, Holland J, et al. A pilot survey of sexual function

and quality of life following 3D conformal radiotherapy for clinically localized prostate cancer. *Int J Radiat Oncol Biol Phys* 1996;35:869–874.
341. Roach M 3rd, Faillace-Akazawa P, Malfatti C, et al. Prostate volumes defined by magnetic resonance imaging and computerized tomographic scans for three-dimensional conformal radiotherapy. *Int J Radiat Oncol Biol Phys* 1996;35:1011–1018.
342. Roach M 3rd, Forman JD, Lee WR, et al. Staging evaluation for patients with adenocarcinoma of the prostate. American College of Radiology Appropriateness Criteria, ACR Web Site Edition, 2000. Available at: www.acr.org/departments/appropriateness_criteria/text.html. Accessed
343. Roach M 3rd, Hanks G, Thames H Jr, et al. Defining biochemical failure following radiotherapy with or without hormonal therapy in men with clinically localized prostate cancer: recommendations of the RTOG-ASTRO Phoenix Consensus Conference. *Int J Radiat Oncol Biol Phys* 2006;65:965–974.
344. Roehl KA, Han M, Ramos CG, et al. Cancer progression and survival rates following anatomical radical retropubic prostatectomy in 3,478 consecutive patients: long-term results. *J Urol* 2004;172:910–914.
345. Roeske JC, Forman JD, Mesina CF, et al. Evaluation of changes in the size and location of the prostate, seminal vesicles, bladder, and rectum during a course of external beam radiation therapy. *Int J Radiat Oncol Biol Phys* 1995;33:1321–1329.
346. Rosen MA, Goldstone L, Lapin S, et al. Frequency and location of extracapsular extension and positive surgical margins in radical prostatectomy specimens. *J Urol* 1992;148:331–337.
347. Ross RK, Coetzee GA, Reichardt J, et al. Does the racial-ethnic variation in prostate cancer risk have a hormonal basis? *Cancer* 1995;75:1778–1782.
348. Rosser CJ, Kuban DA, Levy LB, et al. Prostate specific antigen bounce phenomenon after external beam radiation for clinically localized prostate cancer. *J Urol* 2002;168:2001–2005.
349. Rotkin ID. Studies in the epidemiology of prostatic cancer: expanded sampling. *Cancer Treat Rep* 1977;61:173–179.
350. Rudat V, Schraube P, Oetzel D, et al. Combined error of patient positioning variability and prostate motion uncertainty in 3D conformal radiotherapy of localized prostate cancer. *Int J Radiat Oncol Biol Phys* 1996;35:1027–1034.
351. Sadeghi A, Kuisk H, Tran L, et al. Urethrography and ischial intertuberosity line in radiation therapy planning for prostate carcinoma. *Radiother Oncol* 1996;38:215–222.
352. Sandhu AS, Zelefsky MJ, Lee HJ, et al. Long-term urinary toxicity after 3-dimensionl conformal radiotherapy for prostate cancer in patients with prior history of transurethral resection. *Int J Radiat Oncol Biol Phys* 2000;48:643–647.
353. Sandler HM, Bree RL, McLaughlin PW, et al. Localization of the prostatic apex for radiation therapy using implanted markers. *Int J Radiat Oncol Biol Phys* 1993;27:915–919.
354. Sarris A, Dimopoulos M, Pugh W, et al. Primary lymphoma of the prostate: good outcome with doxorubicin-based combination chemotherapy. *J Urol* 1995;153:1852–1854.
355. Schallenkamp JM, Herman MG, Kruse JJ, et al. Prostate position relative to pelvic bony anatomy based on intraprostatic gold markers and electronic portal imaging. *Int J Radiat Oncol Biol Phys* 2005;63:800–811.
356. Scheidler J, Hricak H, Vigneron DB, et al. Prostate cancer: localization with three-dimensional proton MR spectroscopic imaging: clinicopathologic study. *Radiology* 1999;213:473–480.
357. Schild SE, Casale HE, Bellefontaine LP. Movements of the prostate due to rectal and bladder distension: implications for radiotherapy. *Med Dosim* 1993;18:13–15.
358. Schmutte C, Jones PA. Involvement of DNA methylation in human carcinogenesis. *Biol Chem* 1998;379:377–388.
359. Schuppler J. Malignant neurilemmoma of prostate gland. *J Urol* 1971;106:903–905.
360. Seamonds B, Yang N, Anderson K, et al. Evaluation of prostate-specific antigen and prostatic acid phosphatase as prostate cancer markers. *Urology* 1986;28:472–479.
361. Sebo TJ, Bock BJ, Cheville JC, et al. The percent of cores positive for cancer in prostate needle biopsy specimens is strongly predictive of tumor stage and volume at radical prostatectomy. *J Urol* 2000;163:174–178.
362. Seiden MV, Kantoff PW, Krithivas K, et al. Detection of circulating tumor cells in men with localized prostate cancer. *J Clin Oncol* 1994;12:2634–2639.
363. Serago CF, Chungbin SJ, Buskirk SJ, et al. Initial experience with ultrasound localization for positioning prostate cancer patients for external beam radiotherapy. *Int J Radiat Oncol Biol Phys* 2002;53:1130–1138.
364. Serel TA, Cetin M, Delibas N, et al. Effect of transrectal ultrasonography of the prostate on serum prostate-specific antigen levels and free/total prostate-specific antigen ratio. *Urol Int* 2000;64:24–26.
365. Severson RK, Grove JS, Nomura AM, et al, Body mass and prostatic cancer: a prospective study. *BMJ* 1988;297:713–715.
366. Shannon RL, Ro JY, Grignon DJ, et al. Sarcomatoid carcinoma of the prostate: a clinicopathologic study of 12 patients. *Cancer* 1992;69:2676–2682.
367. Shimizu H, Ross RK, Bernstein L, et al. Cancers of the prostate and breast among Japanese and white immigrants in Los Angeles County. *Cancer* 1991;63:963–966.
368. Singh A, Zelefsky MJ, Raben A, et al. Combined 3-dimensional conformal radiotherapy and transperineal Pd-103 permanent implantation for patients with intermediate and unfavorable risk prostate cancer. *Int J Cancer* 2000;90:275–280.
369. Skwarchuk MW, Jackson A, Zelefsky MJ, et al. Late rectal toxicity after conformal radiotherapy of prostate cancer (I): multivariate analysis and dose-response. *Int J Radiat Oncol Biol Phys* 2000;47:103–113.
370. Slattery ML, Schumacher MC, West DW, et al. Food consumption trends between adolescent and adult years and subsequent risk of prostate cancer. *Am J Clin Nutr* 1990;52:752–757.
371. Small EJ, Prins GS. Physiology and endocrinology of the prostate. In: Vogelzang NJ, Scardino PT, Shipley WU, et al., eds. *Comprehensive textbook of genitourinary oncology*. Baltimore: Williams & Wilkins; 1996:600–620.
372. Smith JR, Freije D, Carpten JD, et al. Major susceptibility locus for prostate cancer on chromosome 1 suggested by genome-wide search. *Science* 1996;274:1371–1374.
373. Smitsmans MH, de Bois J, Sonke JJ, et al. Automatic localization on cone-beam CT scans for high precision image-guided radiotherapy. *Int J Radiat Oncol Biol Phys* 2006;53:975–984.
374. Smitsmans MH, Wolthaus JW, Artigna X, et al. Automatic localization of the prostate for on-line or off-line image-guided radiotherapy. *Int J Radiat Oncol Biol Phys* 2004;60:623–635.
375. Snyder KM, Stock RG, Hong SM, et al. Defining the risk of developing grade 2 proctitis following 125I prostate brachytherapy using a rectal dose-volume histogram analysis. *Int J Radiat Oncol Biol Phys* 2001;50:335–341.
376. Spadinger I, Hilts M, Keyes M, et al. Prostate brachytherapy postimplant dosimetry: a comparison of suture-embedded and loose seed implants. *Brachytherapy* 2006;5:165–173.
377. Spevack L, Killion LT, West JC Jr, et al. Predicting the patient at low risk for lymph node metastasis with localized prostate cancer: an analysis of four statistical models. *Int J Radiat Oncol Biol Phys* 1996;34:543–547.
378. Spirou SV, Chui CS. A gradient inverse planning algorithm with dose-volume constraints. *Med Phys* 1998;25:321–33.
379. Spirou SV, Chui CS. Generation of arbitrary intensity profiles by dynamic jaws or multileaf collimators. *Med Phys* 1994;21:1031–1041.
380. Stamey TA. Some concerns about prostate cancer location, Gleason grade, and postradiation doubling times. *Int J Radiat Oncol Biol Phys* 1995;33:967–968.
381. Stamey TA, McNeal JE, Yemoto CM, et al. Biological determinants of cancer progression in men with prostate cancer. *JAMA* 1999;281:1395–1400.
382. Stamey TA, Yang N, Hay AR, et al. Prostate-specific antigen as a serum marker for adenocarcinoma of the prostate. *N Engl J Med* 1987;317:909–916.
383. Stamey TA, Yemoto CM, McNeal JE, et al. Prostate cancer is highly predictable: a prognostic equation based on all morphological variables in radical prostatectomy specimens. *J Urol* 2000;163:1155–1160.
384. Steinberg GD, Carter BS, Beaty TH, et al. Family history and the risk of prostate cancer. *Prostate* 1990;17:337–347.
385. Stenner J, Hoolthaus K, Mackenzie SH, et al. The effect of ejaculation on prostate-specific antigen in a prostate cancer-screening population. *Urology* 1998;51:455–459.
386. Stock RG, Stone NN, Dahlal M, et al. What is the optimal dose for 125I prostate implants? A dose-response analysis of biochemical control, post-treatment prostate biopsies, and long-term urinary symptoms. *Brachytherapy* 2002;1:83–89.
386a. Stock RG, Stone NN, DeWyngaert JK, et al. Prostate specific antigen findings and biopsy results following interactive ultrasound guided transperineal brachytherapy for early stage prostate carcinoma. *Cancer* 1996;77:2386–2392.
387. Stock RG, Stone NN, Ianuzzi C, et al. Seminal vesicle biopsy and laparoscopic pelvic lymph node dissection: implications for patient selection in the radiotherapeutic management of prostate cancer. *Int J Radiat Oncol Biol Phys* 1995;33:815–821.
388. Stock RG, Stone NN, Lo YC. Intraoperative dosimetric representation of the real-time ultrasound implant. *Tech Urol* 2000;6:95–98.
389. Stock RG, Stone NN, Lo YC, et al. Postimplant dosimetry for 125-I prostate implants: definitions and factors affecting outcome. *Int J Radiat Oncol Biol Phys* 2000;48:899–906.
390. Stokes SH, Real JD, Adams PW, et al. Transperineal ultrasound-guided radioactive seed implantation for organ confined carcinoma of the prostate. *Int J Radiat Oncol Biol Phys* 1997;37:337–341.
391. Stone NN, Stock RG, Unger P. Intermediate term biochemical-free progression and local control following 125Iodine brachytherapy for prostate cancer. *J Urol* 2005;173:803–807.
392. Storey MR, Pollack A, Zagars G, et al. Complications from radiotherapy dose escalation in prostate cancer: preliminary results of a randomized trial. *Int J Radiat Oncol Biol Phys* 2000;48:635–642.
393. Stroom JC, Koper PC, Kreovaar GA, et al. Internal organ motion in prostate cancer patients treated in prone and supine treatment position. *Radiother Oncol* 1999;51:237–248.
394. Sweeney PJ, Vijaykumar S, Sibley GS, et al. Comparison of CT-based treatment planning and retrograde urethrography in determining the prostatic apex at simulation. *Med Dosim* 1993;18:21–28.
395. Sylvester JE, Blasko JC, Grimm PD, et al. Ten-year biochemical relapse-free survival after external beam radiation and brachytherapy for localized prostate cancer: the Seattle experience. *Int J Radiat Oncol Biol Phys* 2003;57:944–952.
396. Symon Z, Griffith KA, McLaughlin PW, et al. Dose escalation for localized prostate cancer: substantial benefit observed with 3D conformal therapy. *Int J Radiat Oncol Biol Phys* 2003;57:384–390.
397. Tannenbaum M. Endometrial tumors and/or associated carcinomas of prostate. *Urology* 1975;6:372–375.
398. Tannenbaum M. Histology of the prostate gland. In: Tannenbaum M, ed. *Urologic pathology: the prostate*. Philadelphia: Lea & Febiger; 1977:312–315.
399. Tavani A, Gallus S, Franceschi S, et al. Calcium, dairy products, and the risk of prostate cancer. *Prostate* 2001;48:118–121.
400. Tchetgen M-B, Song JT, Strawderman M, et al. Ejaculation increases the serum prostate-specific antigen concentration. *Urology* 1996;47:511–516.
401. Ten Haken RK, Perez-Tamayo C, Tesse RJ, et al. Boost treatment of the prostate using shaped fixed fields. *Int J Radiat Oncol Biol Phys* 1989;16:193–200.
402. Terk MD, Stock RG, Stone NN. Identification of patients at increased risk for prolonged urinary retention following radioactive seed implantation of the prostate. *J Urol* 1998;160:1379–1382.
403. Terris MK, Klonecke AS, McDougall IR, et al. Utilization of bone scans in conjunction with prostate-specific antigen levels in the surveillance for recurrence of adenocarcinoma after radical prostatectomy. *J Nucl Med* 1991;32:1713–1717.
404. Terris MK, McNeal JE, Stamey TA. Detection of clinically significant prostate cancer by transrectal ultrasound-guided systematic biopsies. *J Urol* 1992;148:829–832.
405. Thomas MD, Cormack R, Tempany CM, et al. Identifying the predictors of acute urinary retention following magnetic resonance guided prostate brachytherapy. *Int J Radiat Oncol Biol Phys* 2000;47:905–908.
406. Thompson IM, Ankherst DP, Chi C, et al. Assessing prostate cancer risk: results from the Prostate Cancer Prevention Trial. *J Natl Cancer Inst* 2006;98:529–534.
407. Thompson IM, Goodman PJ, Tangen CM, et al. The influence of finasteride on the development of prostate cancer. *N Engl J Med* 2003;349:215–224.
408. Tiguert R, Gheiler EL, Tefilli MV, et al. Lymph node size does not correlate with the presence of prostate cancer metastasis. *Urology* 1999;53:367–371.
409. Valicenti RK, Choi E, Chen C, et al. Sildenafil citrate effectively reverses sexual

dysfunction induced by three-dimensional conformal radiation therapy. *Urology* 2001;57:769–773.

410. van Herk M, Bruce A, Kroes AP, et al. Quantification of organ motion during conformal radiotherapy of the prostate by three dimensional image registration. *Int J Radiat Oncol Biol Phys* 1995;33:1311–1320.

411. Vigneault E, Pouliot J, Laverdiere J, et al. Electronic portal imaging device detection of radiopaque markers for the evaluation of prostate position during megavoltage irradiation: a clinical study. *Int J Radiat Oncol Biol Phys* 1997;37:205–212.

412. Vijayakumar S, Quadri SF, Karison TG, et al. Localized prostate cancer: use of serial prostate-specific antigen measurements during radiation therapy. *Radiology* 1992;184:271–274.

413. Villeirs GM, Van Vaerenbergh K, Vakaet L, et al. Interobserver delineation variation using CT versus combined CT + MRI in intensity-modulated radiotherapy for prostate cancer. *Strahlenther Onkol* 2005;181:424–430.

414. Villers AA, McNeal JE, Freiha FS, et al. Development of prostatic carcinoma: morphometric and pathologic features of early stages. *Acta Oncol* 1991;30:145–151.

415. Wallner KE, Roy J, Harrison L, et al. Dosimetry guidelines to minimize urethral and rectal morbidity following transperineal I-125 prostate brachytherapy. *Int J Radiat Oncol Biol Phys* 1995;32:465–471.

416. Walsh PC. Radical retropubic prostatectomy with reduced morbidity: an anatomic approach. *Natl Cancer Inst Monogr* 1988;7:133–137.

417. Walsh PC, Donker PJ. Impotence following radical prostatectomy: insight into etiology and prevention. *J Urol* 1982;128:492–497.

418. Walsh PC, Lepor H, Eggleston JC. Radical prostatectomy with preservation of sexual function: anatomical and pathological considerations. *Prostate* 1983;4:432–485.

419. Wang MC, Valenzuela LA, Murphy GP, et al. Purification of a human prostatic specific antigen. *Invest Urol* 1979;17:159–163.

420. Waterman, FM, Dicker AP. Probability of late rectal morbidity in 125I prostate brachytherapy. *Int J Radiat Oncol Biol Phys* 2003;55:342–353.

421. Webb S. The physical basis of IMRT and inverse planning. *Br J Radiol* 2003;76:678–689.

422. Wefer AE, Hricak H. Imaging and staging of prostate cancer. In: Kantoff PW, D'Amico AV, eds. *Prostate cancer: principles and practice.* Philadelphia: Lippincott Williams & Wilkins; 2002:269–286.

423. Wefer AE, Hricak H, Vigneron DB, et al. Sextant localization of prostate cancer: comparison of sextant biopsy, magnetic resonance imaging and magnetic resonance spectroscopic imaging with step-section histology. *J Urol* 2000;164:400–404.

424. White S, Hricak H, Forstner R, et al. Prostate cancer: effect of postbiopsy hemorrhage on interpretation of MR images. *Radiology* 1995;195:385–390.

425. Wilder RB, Fone PD, Rademacher DE, et al. Localization of the prostatic apex for radiotherapy treatment planning using urethroscopy. *Int J Radiat Oncol Biol Phys* 1997;38:737–741.

426. Wise AM, Stamey TA, McNeal JE, et al. Morphologic and clinical significance of multifocal prostate cancers in radical prostatectomy specimens. *Urology* 2002;60:264–269.

427. Wolf JS Jr, Cher M, Dall'era M, et al. The use and accuracy of cross-sectional imaging and fine needle aspiration cytology for detection of pelvic lymph node metastases before radical prostatectomy. *Urology* 1995;153:993–999.

428. Wolfe JHN, Lloyd-Davis RW. The management of transitional cell carcinoma in the prostate. *Br J Urol* 1981;53:253–257.

429. Wong JR, Grimm L, Uematsu M, et al. Image-guided radiotherapy for prostate cancer by CT-linear accelerator combination: prostate movements and dosimetric considerations. *Int J Radiat Oncol Biol Phys* 2005;61:561–569.

430. Woolf CM. An investigation of familial aspects of carcinoma of the prostate. *Cancer* 1960;13:739.

431. Wu J, Haycocks T, Alasti H, et al. Positioning errors and prostate motion during conformal prostate radiotherapy using on-line isocentre set-up verification and implanted prostate markers. *Radiother Oncol* 2001;61:127–133.

432. Wu Q, Ivaldi G, Liang J, et al. Geometric and dosimetric evaluations of an online image-guided strategy for 3D-CRT of prostate cancer. *Int J Radiat Oncol Biol Phys* 2006;64:1596–1609.

433. Yamada Y, Bhatia S, Zaider M, et al. Favorable clinical outcomes of three-dimensional computer-optimized high-dose-rate prostate brachytherapy in the management of localized prostate cancer. *Brachytherapy* 2006;5:157–164.

434. Yan D, Lockman D, Brabbins D, et al. An off-line strategy for constructing a patient-specific planning target volume in adaptive treatment process for prostate cancer. *Int J Radiat Oncol Biol Phys* 2000;48:289–302.

435. Yan D, Wong J, Vicini F, et al. Adaptive modification of treatment planning to minimize the deleterious effects of treatment setup errors. *Int J Radiat Oncol Biol Phys* 1997;38:197–206.

436. Young HY. Early diagnosis and radical cure of carcinoma of the prostate: being a study of 40 cases and presentations of radical operation. *Bull Johns Hopkins Hosp* 1905;16:315–321.

437. Yu CX, Li XA, Ma L, et al. Clinical implementation of intensity-modulated arc therapy. *Int J Radiat Oncol Biol Phys* 2002;53:453–463.

438. Yu KK, Hricak H, Alagappan R, et al. Detection of extracapsular extension of prostate carcinoma with endorectal and phased-array coil MR imaging: multivariate feature analysis. *Radiology* 1997;202:697–702.

439. Yu KK, Scheidler J, Hricak H, et al. Prostate cancer: prediction of extracapsular extension by endorectal MR imaging and 3D 1 H-MR spectroscopic imaging. *Radiology* 1999;213:481–488.

440. Yuan JJ, Coplen DE, Petros JA, et al. Effects of rectal examination, prostatic massage, ultrasonography, and needle biopsy on serum prostate-specific antigen levels. *J Urol* 1992;147:810–814.

441. Zagars GK, Johnson DE, von Eschenbach AC, et al. Adjuvant estrogen following radiation therapy for stage C adenocarcinoma of the prostate: long-term results of a prospective randomized study. *Int J Radiat Oncol Biol Phys* 1988;14:1085–1091.

442. Zagars GK, Sherman NE, Babaian RJ. Prostatic-specific antigen and external beam radiation therapy in prostatic cancer. *Cancer* 1991;67:412–420.

443. Zaloudek C, Williams JW, Kempson RL. "Endometrial" adenocarcinoma of the prostate: a distinctive tumor of probably prostatic duct origin. *Cancer* 1976;37:2255–2262.

444. Zelefsky M, Moughan J, Owen J, et al. Changing trends in national practice for external beam radiotherapy for clinically localized prostate cancer: the 1999 Patterns of Care survey for prostate cancer. *Int J Radiat Oncol Biol Phys* 2004;59:1053–1061.

445. Zelefsky MJ, Ben-Porat L, Scher H, et al. Outcome predictors for the increasing PSA state after definitive external-beam radiotherapy for prostate cancer. *J Clin Oncol* 2005;23:826–831.

446. Zelefsky MJ, Chan H, Hunt M, et al. Long-term outcome of high dose intensity modulated radiation therapy for patients with clinically localized prostate cancer. *J Urol* 2006;176:1415–1419.

447. Zelefsky MJ, Cowen D, Fuks Z, et al. Long term tolerance of high dose three-dimensional radiotherapy in patients with localized prostate carcinoma. *Cancer* 1999;85:2460–2468.

448. Zelefsky MJ, Crean D, Mageras GS, et al. Quantification and predictors of prostate position variability in 50 patients evaluated with multiple CT scans during conformal radiotherapy. *Radiother Oncol* 1999;50:225–234.

449. Zelefsky MJ, Eid JF. Elucidating the etiology of erectile dysfunction after definitive therapy for prostatic cancer. *Int J Radiat Oncol Biol Phys* 1998;40:129–133.

450. Zelefsky MJ, Fuks Z, Happersett L, et al. Clinical experience with intensity modulated radiation therapy (IMRT) in prostate cancer. *Radiother Oncol* 2000;55:241–249.

451. Zelefsky MJ, Fuks Z, Hunt M, et al. High-dose intensity modulated radiation therapy for prostate cancer: early toxicity and biochemical outcome in 772 patients. *Int J Radiat Oncol Biol Phys* 2002;53:1111–1116.

452. Zelefsky MJ, Fuks Z, Hunt M, et al. High dose radiation delivered by intensity modulated conformal radiotherapy improves the outcome of localized prostate cancer. *J Urol* 2001;166:876–881.

453. Zelefsky MJ, Fuks Z, Leibel SA. Intensity-modulated radiation therapy for prostate cancer. *Semin Radiat Oncol* 2002;3:229–237.

454. Zelefsky MJ, Happersett L, Leibel S, et al. The effect of treatment positioning on normal tissue dose in patients with prostate cancer treated with three-dimensional conformal radiotherapy. *Int J Radiat Oncol Biol Phys* 1997;37:13–19.

455. Zelefsky MJ, Hollister DA, Levy LB, et al. Long-term multi-institutional analysis of stage T1-T2 prostate cancer treated with permanent brachytherapy. *Int J Radiat Oncol Biol Phys* 2005;63[Suppl 1]:S33.

456. Zelefsky MJ, McKee AB, Lee H, et al. Efficacy of oral sildenafil in patients with erectile dysfunction after radiotherapy for carcinoma of the prostate. *Urology* 1999;53:775–778.

457. Zelefsky MJ, Wallner KE, Ling CC, et al. Comparison of the 5-year outcome and morbidity of three dimensional conformal radiotherapy versus transperineal permanent iodine-125 implantation for early stage prostate cancer. *J Clin Oncol* 1999;17:517–522.

458. Zelefsky MJ, Yamada Y, Cohen G, et al. 5-year outcome of intraoperative conformal permanent I-125 interstitial implantation for patients with clinically localized prostate cancer. *Int J Radiat Oncol Biol Phys* 2007;67:65–70.

459. Zelefsky MJ, Yamada Y, Cohen G, et al. Postimplantation dosimetric analysis of permanent transperineal prostate implantation: improved dose distributions with an intraoperative computer-optimized conformal planning technique. *Int J Radiat Oncol Biol Phys* 2000;48:601–608.

460. Zelefsky MJ, Yamada Y, Marion C, et al. Improved conformality and decreased toxicity with intraoperative computer-optimized transperineal ultrasound-guided prostate brachytherapy. *Int J Radiat Oncol Biol Phys* 2003;5:956–963.

461. Zietman AL, DeSilvio ML, Slater JD, et al. Comparison of conventional-dose vs high-dose conformal radiation therapy in clinically localized adenocarcinoma of the prostate: a randomized controlled trial. *JAMA* 2005;294:1233–1239.

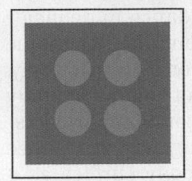

Chapter 63
Intermediate- and High-Risk Prostate Cancer

Hans T. Chung, Joycelyn L. Speight, Mack Roach, III

In 2005, an estimated 232,000 new cases of prostate cancer were diagnosed in the United States, representing about a third of all nondermatologic cancers (61). Prostate cancer was the second leading cause of cancer death in men, responsible for more than 30,000 deaths (61). Most of the patients destined to die from prostate cancer initially presented with unfavorable intermediate- or high-risk disease. This chapter focuses on the management of such patients. Since the last edition of this book, our understanding of prostate cancer has expanded substantially. With several prospective studies now demonstrating a survival advantage, hormonal therapy has become widely accepted as an integral part of treatment. Interest in adjuvant and salvage radiotherapy has been brought to the forefront with recently released prospective studies. With more mature data sets, our ability to prognosticate extends beyond merely biochemical control, but now includes prostate cancer-specific and overall mortality. Active cytotoxic agents have been identified in the metastatic setting, and as a result, their role in the adjuvant setting is the subject of intense scrutiny. Details on the management of low-risk prostate cancer and the background of prostate cancer in general can be found in Chapter 62.

Epidemiology

With increasing prostate-specific antigen (PSA) screening since the early 1990s, the clinical presentation of prostate cancer has changed dramatically, shifting from locally advanced or metastatic disease to clinically nonpalpable disease. Data from two national prostate cancer registries, the Cancer of the Prostate Strategic Urologic Research Endeavor (CaPSURE) and the Department of Defense Center for Prostate Disease Research (CPDR), highlight this stage migration (17,84). According to CaPSURE, the diagnosis of high-risk disease has seen a precipitous drop from 36.6% in 1989 to 1992 to 16.0% in 1999 to 2002 (17). Similarly, the proportion of patients presenting with a pretreatment PSA >20 ng/mL has dropped from 27.0% to 8.1% in the same time periods. Conversely, clinically nonpalpable disease (stage T1) has surged from 16.9% to 49.4%, respectively. Intermediate-risk disease has increased less dramatically from 33.8% to 37.2%, respectively. Data from CPDR mirror these findings. From 1988 to 1998, clinical stage T3 to T4 disease contracted from 19.2% to 4.4%, whereas T1c disease went from 0% to 47.8% (84).

Clinical Presentation

Patients with intermediate- or high-risk prostate cancer may present with locoregional symptoms, but this is not common. Lower urinary tract symptoms that may be seen include nocturia, urinary frequency, urgency, decreased flow, incomplete voiding, intermittent flow, or hesitancy. More bulky primary disease may present with difficulty in passing stool or even bloody stool. With increasing PSA and Gleason score, the risk of metastases increases. Metastatic spread is generally sequential, proceeding from the prostate to the pelvic lymph nodes then

bone. Thus patients with metastatic disease may present with renal failure, lymphedema of the lower extremities, and bone pain.

Prognostic Factors and Risk Classification Schemes

The traditional prognostic factors have been clinical T stage, presenting PSA, and Gleason score. To simplify treatment recommendations and prognostication, several risk classification schemes have been proposed by grouping patients with different clinical features, but similar biochemical outcome (28,136). The risk classification scheme proposed by D'Amico et al. (28) appears to be the most widely used and stratifies patients with clinically localized prostate cancer to three risk groups. Low-risk is defined as meeting all the criteria: T1c to T2a, PSA $\leq$10 ng/mL and Gleason score $\leq$6. Intermediate-risk is defined as T2b, PSA >10 but $\leq$20 ng/mL or Gleason score 7. High risk is any of the following: $\geq$T2c, PSA >20 ng/mL, or Gleason score 8 to 10. It has recently been validated using a study cohort of 7,316 men from two large cancer registries (CaPSURE and CPDR), and has also been found to predict for prostate cancer–specific mortality (PCSM) after radiotherapy (25).

Other pretreatment predictive factors have since been identified, including percentage of positive biopsy cores (PPC) and PSA velocity in radiotherapy and surgery-treated patients (27,29,66). D'Amico et al. (27) reported on the independent prognostic capabilities of PPC, calculated as the number of PPCs containing cancer divided by the total number of cores (27). In addition to PSA, Gleason score, and clinical T stage, PPC was also an independent predictor of PSA control. Interestingly, 76% of patients with intermediate-risk disease could be reclassified into either low- or high-risk disease. Specifically, those patients with <34% PPC had similar outcomes as low-risk patients (5-year PSA control 85% vs. 91%, respectively), whereas patients with more than 50% PPC had similar outcomes as high-risk patients (5-year PSA control 30% vs. 43%, respectively). The prognostic significance of PPC has also been reported to extend to PCSM in intermediate-risk patients (23). When stratified by $\leq$50% and >50% PPC, 7-year prostate cancer-specific survival was 100% versus 57% ($p = 0.004$), respectively. In patients treated with radical prostatectomy, high PPC is associated with adverse pathologic features like extracapsular extension, seminal vesicle invasion, positive surgical margins, lymphovascular invasion, perineural invasion, and pelvic lymph node involvement (41,44,78).

Pretreatment PSA velocity has recently been reported to be a significant independent predictor of PCSM (22,26). PSA velocity was calculated using linear regression modeling with at least two PSA measurements taken at least 6 months apart within 1 year prior to diagnosis. After adjusting for Gleason score and clinical T stage, a PSA velocity >2 ng/mL per year was a significant independent predictor of PSA recurrence ($p = 0.001$), PCSM ($p = 0.001$), and overall mortality ($p = 0.005$) (26). Moreover, it was associated with a 12-fold increase in the risk of PCSM when adjusted for other prognostic factors.

In summary, PSA velocity (>2 ng/mL per year) and PPC (>50%) have further refined our prognostic precision in addition to the traditional predictive factors (pretreatment PSA, Gleason score, clinical T stage). At the University of California–San Francisco (UCSF), the presence of either in intermediate-risk patients, as defined by the D'Amico classification, are considered as unfavorable intermediate- or high-risk disease. Single modality local therapy is likely not enough, but rather more aggressive treatment, such as hormonal therapy and pelvic irradiation, is indicated.

General Management

Radiation Therapy Techniques

For details on prostate only radiotherapy, please refer to Chapter 62. This section will focus on the implementation and toxicities of whole pelvic radiotherapy.

Whole Pelvic Irradiation

With conventional technique, pelvic irradiation is usually treated with a four-field box (Fig. 63.1). The target volume usually includes the prostate, seminal vesicles, obturator, and proximal internal and external iliac nodal regions. Occasionally common iliac, para-aortic, and even perirectal nodes are included in the initial target. The traditional field borders of the anteroposterior portals are as follows: Superior at the L5–S1 interspace, inferior at 2 cm distal to the membranous urethra (defined by the apex of the urethrogram peak), 1.5 to 2 cm lateral of the pelvic brim. Corner blocks are usually placed at all four corners to limit dose to the small bowel and femoral heads. In the lateral portals, the superior and inferior borders are placed at the same point as the anteroposterior portals; the anterior border is placed at the anterior most aspect of the pubic symphysis, and the posterior border is placed at the S2–S3 interspace. With CT planning, the prostate, seminal vesicles, rectum, small bowel, bladder, pelvic vessels, and penile bulb may be contoured to facilitate shielding of the rectum and small bowel.

The dosimetric advantages of intensity-modulated radiation therapy (IMRT) have led to its investigation in delivering pelvic radiotherapy. Compared to conventional technique, IMRT allows unprecedented sparing of nearby critical structures like the rectum, small bowel, bladder, and femoral heads (Figs. 63.2 and 63.3). Yet implementation of IMRT for pelvic radiotherapy has been somewhat hampered by the lack of guidance in delineating the nodal regions at risk. Whereas conventional technique involved simply placing field borders based on bony anatomy, IMRT requires the delineation of a nodal target volume. A study from Massachusetts General Hospital was recently reported using lymphotropic nanoparticle-enhanced magnetic resonance imaging (MRI) (115). As opposed to using bony surface as a landmark, the 69 identified lymph nodes from 18 patients more closely correlated with the vascular system. Ninety-five percent of the nodes were within 1.5 cm of a major vessel (internal and external iliac, common iliac, and aortocaval). There was no correlation between the size of the patient and the position of the nodes relative to vascular anatomic reference points such as the aortocaval and iliac bifurcations. In delineating a nodal target volume, the authors recommended a radial expansion of 2 cm (includes subclinical disease that is beyond the resolution of a computed tomography [CT] scan) around the iliac vessels at risk. These should include the distal 2.5 cm of the common iliacs from the iliac bifurcation, the proximal 9 cm of the external iliac vessels, and the proximal 8.5 cm of the internal iliac vessels.

In a study from UCSF, Wang et al. (129) compared the nodal target coverage by conventional field borders with IMRT. The nodes that were contoured included the obturator, internal/external iliac, common iliac, and presacral regions. In the conventional four-field plan, only 70.3% of the nodal target volume received the prescription dose of 45 Gy, whereas 96.2% was covered in the IMRT plan (*p* = 0.002). Even worse, conventional field placement led to 20.2% of the nodal target volume to receive <80% of the prescription dose. The rectal and bladder volume receiving 95% of the prescribed dose were significantly reduced with IMRT, with an absolute reduction of 23% and 80%, respectively.

Prostate Motion

With the shift to dose escalation and IMRT and its attendant high conformality around target structures, minimization of setup errors becomes critical. The previous technique of verification of the isocenter relied on obtaining weekly port films, which only allowed comparison of bony anatomy without any consideration of the prostate and did not account for prostate motion. Questions that have since emerged are:

1. How much does the prostate move on a daily basis (i.e., interfractional) and during each treatment (i.e., intrafractional)?

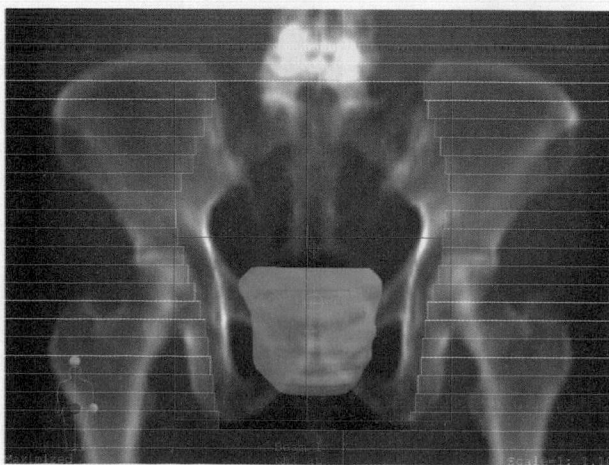
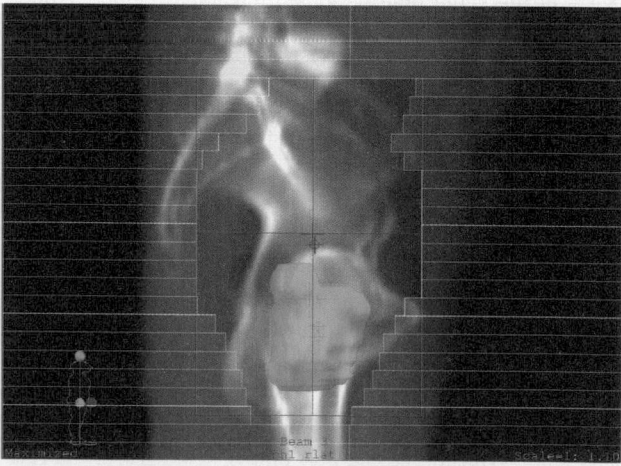

FIGURE 63.1. Typical field borders of whole pelvic radiotherapy based on bony anatomy. (Courtesy of Hans T. Chung, M.D., FRCPC, University of California–San Francisco.)

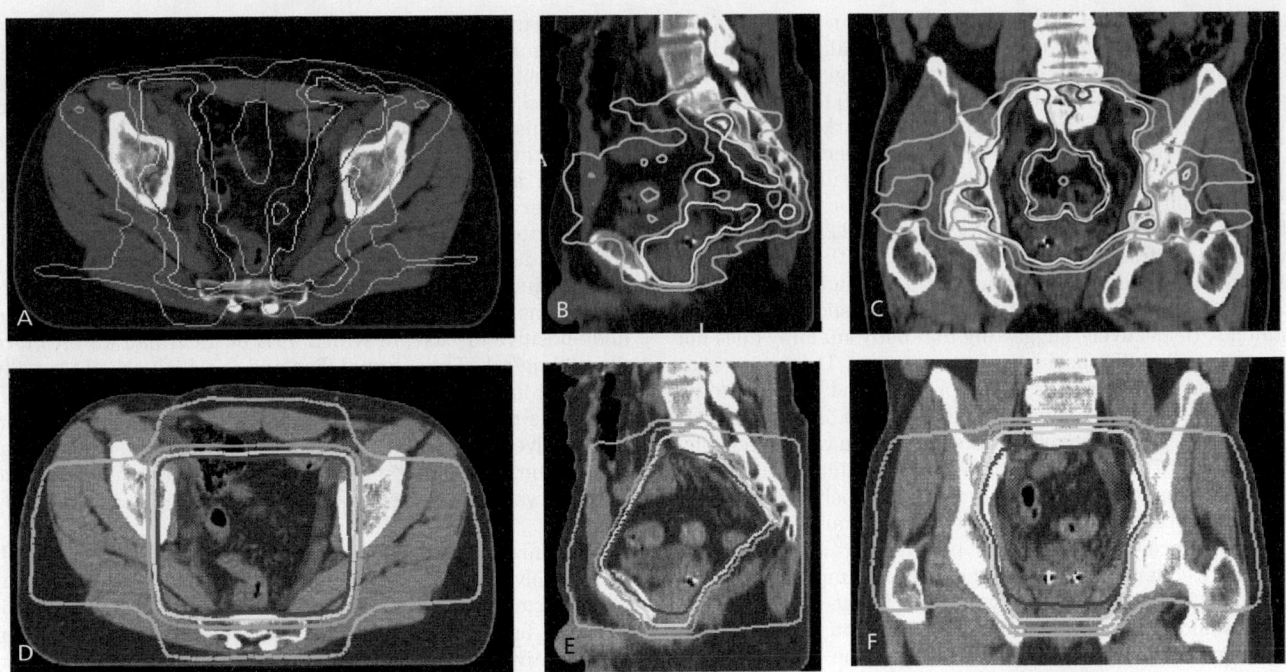

FIGURE 63.2. Comparison between IMRT and 3DCRT plans treating the pelvic nodes for the same patient. Isodose lines: Red—45 Gy; Yellow—42.75 Gy; Green—36 Gy; Blue—22.5 Gy. **A:** IMRT axial. **B:** IMRT sagittal. **C:** IMRT coronal. **D:** 3DCRT WP axial. **E:** 3DCRT WP sagittal. **F:** 3DCRT WP coronal. IMRT, intensity-modulated radiation therapy; 3DCRT, 3D conformal radiation therapy; WP, whole pelvic (Courtesy of Alice Wang-Chesebro, M.D., University of California–San Francisco.)

2. Is the positional relationship between the prostate and bony anatomy static (i.e., can bony anatomy be used as a surrogate of the prostate location)?

The use of fiducial gold seed markers and daily electronic portal imaging (EPI) with online correction is one such strategy. In a comprehensive study from the Mayo Clinic, the inter- and intrafractional motion of the prostate and pelvic bony anatomy in 20 prostate patients, each with three or four intraprostatic gold fiducial markers, and daily pretherapy and through-treatment EPI were reported (110). With more than 22,000 data points, Schallenkamp et al. (110) determined that the prostate moved as much as 9.1 mm (mean 2.5 mm) in the superior-inferior (SI), 16.3 mm (mean 3.7 mm) in

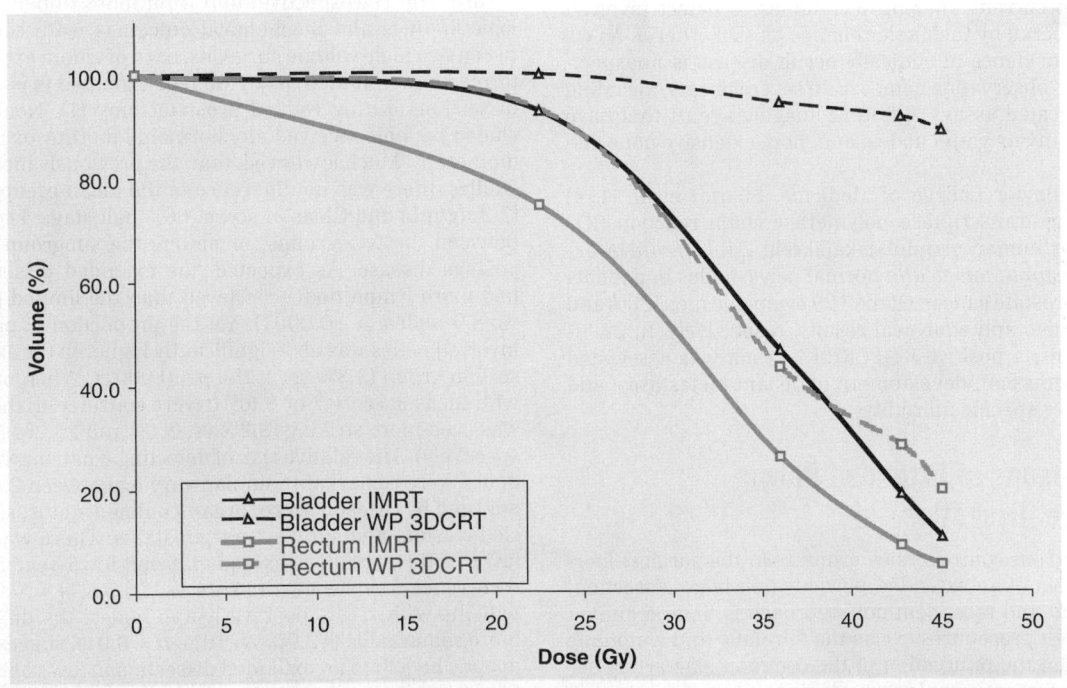

FIGURE 63.3. Comparison of dose volume histograms for rectum and bladder for whole-pelvic only phase using IMRT and 3DCRT plans. For both bladder and rectum, IMRT significantly reduced V45, V42.75, V36, and V22.5 ($p < 0.01$ for all comparisons) compared to 3DCRT plans. IMRT, intensity-modulated radiation therapy; 3DCRT, 3D conformal radiation therapy. (Courtesy of Alice Wang-Chesebro MD, University of California San Francisco.)

the anterior-posterior (AP), and 15.2 mm (mean 1.9 mm) in the right-left (RL) axes, prior to any efforts to localize the fields to the fiducial markers. In recommending a margin for setup and organ motion (i.e., clinical target volume [CTV] to planning target volumes [PTV] margin), without fiducial marker localization, SI, AP, and RL margins of 5.1, 7.3, 5 mm, respectively, were required to cover 95% of the CTV with the prescribed dose with a 95% probability. With a daily fiducial marker localization protocol, the margins can be reduced to 2.7, 2.9, and 2.8 mm, respectively. The interfractional three-dimentional (3D) displacements of the prostate and bony anatomy were 5.6 and 4.4 mm prior to localization and 2.8 and 4.4 mm after postlocalization adjustments, respectively, suggesting that bony anatomy does not accurately reflect the position of the prostate. The average intrafractional displacements of the prostate and bony anatomy were 0.1 and –0.5, 0.4 and 0.4, and 0.1 and 0.3 mm in the AP, SI, and RL axes, respectively. Marker migration was found to be minimal, with 79% within 1 mm and 96% within 1.5 mm. The latter results have been corroborated by Kupelian et al. (72), who demonstrated that the average absolute variation in intermarker distance was 1.01 ± 1.03 mm. Only 1% of the markers exhibited frequent movement, and it was found to be due to prostate deformation secondary to rectal filling.

If the nodal target volumes are assumed to correlate with bony anatomy, pelvic IMRT that is setup to the prostate gland by intraprostatic fiducial markers could lead to significant underdosing given the lack of correlation between the prostate and bony anatomy. In a preliminary analysis of patients treated at UCSF, Chen et al. (15) demonstrated that an isocenter shift of 5 or 10 mm in the superior direction could reduce nodal target coverage by 11% and 26%, respectively, with whole pelvic IMRT.

Biologic Rationale for Prophylactic Pelvic Irradiation

Incidence of Occult Lymph Node Involvement

The ability of current imaging techniques to detect involved nodes is hampered by their sole reliance on size criteria. As we will see, the incidence of clinically occult disease is unexpectedly high. This observation comes from several fronts, including more sophisticated assays, different imaging agents that have increased affinity to lymph nodes, and more extensive node dissection.

From the Baylor College of Medicine, Shariat et al. (114) studied reverse-transcriptase polymerase chain reaction (RT-PCR) assay for human glandular kallikrein 2 (hK2) mRNA expression in *histopathologically* normal pelvic nodes in patients with pT3N0 prostate cancer. Of the 199 evaluable men, 20% and 40% had positive and equivocal results, respectively. In multivariate analysis, a positive RT-PCR/hK2 result was associated with PSA progression, development of distant metastases, and prostate cancer-specific mortality.

Surgical Results of Extended Pelvic Lymph Node Dissection

One of the current controversies erupting in the surgical literature is the role of an extended pelvic lymph node dissection. The traditional and most common approach is to do a limited dissection. Both procedures excise the fibrofatty and lymphatic tissues between the bifurcation of the common iliac artery superiorly to the femoral canal inferiorly and to the pelvic sidewall laterally. The critical difference between the two procedures is that in the limited dissection, the posterior extent is carried to the obturator nerve, whereas in the extended dissection, it is extended to include the obturator vessels and internal iliac vein. A second important consideration, when reviewing surgical studies, is whether only hematoxylin and eosin (H&E) staining was performed, or more sensitive analyses were included, such as immunohistochemistry (IHC) or RT-PCR.

Bader et al. (7) conducted a prospective study of the anatomic extent of pelvic nodal involvement in a cohort of 365 men who underwent an extended lymph node dissection and radical prostatectomy. This study included men with clinically organ-confined disease on the basis of a CT scan and bone scan. The median number of nodes retrieved was 21. Despite using only H&E stains to evaluate the extracted nodes, 24% of patients had node-positive disease, of which 49% of them had a PSA more than 20 ng/mL. The internal iliac nodes, which are not usually dissected in a limited dissection, were involved in 58% of men with node-positive disease. Of note, 19% of node-positive men had involved nodes that were exclusively found in the internal iliac region, suggesting that the lymphatic drainage of prostate cancer is variable. The rate of problematic lymphocele was only 2%.

Heidenreich et al. (52) reported on the incidence of lymph node involvement between standard and extended pelvic lymphadenectomy in 203 patients. IHC staining was performed if the H&E findings were negative. There was no difference in preoperative PSA, clinical stage, Gleason score, or age between the two groups. The mean preoperative PSA was 15.9 ng/mL and the Gleason sum was 4.6 ± 2.3. There were more dissected nodes in the extended dissection group (28 vs. 11; $p <0.01$), at the expense of longer operative time (179 vs. 126 minutes; $p <0.03$). There were more than twice the number of patients with positive nodes (26% and 12%; $p <0.03$) in the extended dissection group, with 42% of all metastases lying outside the planes of a limited dissection. In patients deemed as high risk (Gleason score 7 to 10 and PSA ≥ 10.6 ng/mL) for lymph node metastasis, 60.9% of patients had histologically positive nodes. There was no difference in pelvic lymphocele or postoperative complications between the two groups. On that basis, Heidenreich et al. (52) have adopted a policy of performing an extended node dissection in high-risk patients.

In a large retrospective study from Johns Hopkins, the pathologic findings and biochemical outcomes were compared between two high-volume surgeons, each of whom exclusively performed either limited ($n = 1,865$) or extended ($n = 2,135$) node dissections during radical prostatectomy (1). None of the included patients received any hormonal therapy or adjuvant radiotherapy. Much lower risk than the previously mentioned two studies, there was no difference in the mean preoperative PSA (7.2 ng/mL) and Gleason score (66% had stage 4 to 6 disease) between the two groups, or among the subgroup with node-positive disease. As expected, the extended dissection group had more lymph nodes retrieved than the limited group (11.6 vs. 8.9 nodes; $p <0.0001$). Yet the proportion of patients with involved nodes was also significantly higher in the extended dissection group (3.3% vs. 1.2%; $p <0.0001$). When only patients with Gleason score 7 or 8 to 10 were considered, the difference was even more striking (8.2% vs. 2.4% and 23.2% vs. 8.9%, respectively). The relative risk of detecting a patient with involved nodes were remarkably similar, varying between 2.5 to 3 when adjusted by Gleason score, organ-confined status, seminal vesicle invasion, and surgical margin status. There was a trend in favor of the extended dissection group for 5-year biochemical recurrence-free survival (34.4% vs. 16.5%; $p = 0.07$). Among patients with <15% positive lymph nodes, the difference was more remarkable (42.9% vs. 10%; $p = 0.01$), suggesting a therapeutic benefit of an extended dissection in low volume disease. Clinically significant lymphoceles occurred in only 0.3% in the extended dissection group.

Using an intraoperative gamma probe and dynamic lymphoscintigraphy, Wawroschek et al. (130) found that about a third of sentinel lymph nodes were in areas outside of a limited node dissection, such as the presacral, hypogastric, and pararectal regions.

Novel Imaging Techniques

The role of lymphotropic superparamagnetic nanoparticles, given with MRI, has been recently reported (51). The nanoparticles are transported by lymphatic vessels, where they are filtered by lymph nodes. Lymph nodes that have been infiltrated by metastases will have distorted lymphatic flow, and thus will accumulate the nanoparticles. Of the histologically involved nodes, 71.4% did not meet the MRI size criteria for malignancy. The sensitivity (90.5% vs. 35.4%; p <0.001) and specificity (97.8% vs. 90.4%; p <0.001) of MRI with superparamagnetic nanoparticles was significantly better than conventional MRI. When only nodes that were between 5 to 10 mm in diameter on the short axis were considered, the sensitivity increased from 28.5% to 96.4% (p <0.001). It was also noted that there were nine cases where the involved node was seen in areas outside of the boundaries of a limited node dissection.

De Jong et al. (30) reported on C-choline positron emission tomography (PET) for preoperative nodal staging of prostate cancer. In contrast to (18)F-FDG PET, this radiolabeled agent does not suffer from radioactivity in the bladder, which can obscure nearby sites of metastases. The sensitivity, specificity, and accuracy were 80%, 96%, and 93%, respectively. In the 15 patients with histology-confirmed nodal disease, five patients had nodal disease in the common iliac region but otherwise had no involved nodes in the obturator region. In all five cases, (11)C-choline PET correctly detected them.

Implications for Radiotherapy

The surgical series suggests that an extended node dissection, not surprisingly, yields more dissected nodes. Perhaps more surprising is that more involved nodes are detected—despite negative preoperative imaging studies—suggesting that the harder one looks the more one finds. To further put this into perspective, these nodes are often found in areas (i.e., internal iliac and presacral nodes) that are traditionally not excavated by the more common limited node dissection, meaning that a significant proportion of higher-risk patients may have residual micrometastatic disease after surgery. The location of sentinel nodes have also been shown to be remarkably variable (130). Thus, some urologists have endorsed a more thorough node dissection in patients at higher risk of node involvement (6,52).

The second important concept to draw from the surgical studies is that taken together, these studies suggest that minimal lymph node involvement detected by an extended lymph node dissection does not necessarily lead to inevitable relapse. It is not difficult to surmise that patients with occult nodal disease who have been completely excised in an extended dissection would probably have a better outcome than the same patient with residual micrometastatic nodal disease after a limited dissection. Bader et al. (6,7) prospectively studied the outcomes of 92 patients with node-positive disease after radical prostatectomy and extended node dissection that was initially staged as clinically organ-confined prostate cancer. After 45 months, 39% of patients with only one positive node as compared to only 12% patients with two or more positive nodes were free of biochemical recurrence (p = 0.008). Although follow-up was short, prostate cancer-specific mortality was significantly different (8% vs. 33%, respectively; p = 0.004). In the prospective study of node-positive patients after radical prostatectomy by Messing et al. (79), in the observation arm, 18% had no evidence of disease at a median follow-up of 7.1 years. Of note, these patients had a limited node dissection (median number of nodes retrieved was 12). The main criticism of this argument

of improved outcomes with extended node dissection is that the effects of stage migration and lead time bias should not be discounted.

Collectively, these studies argue that an extended node dissection may yield a therapeutic benefit in the subgroup of patients with higher risk of nodal involvement yet have minimal nodal disease. This may in part be due to eradication of all tumor, but may also reflect the large individual variability of lymphatic drainage from the prostate gland (130). Can we extrapolate these results to pelvic radiotherapy? Is there a volume effect for pelvic radiotherapy as seen in the extent of lymph node dissection? The results from the Radiation Therapy Oncology Group (RTOG) 9413 would suggest so (96).

Although RTOG 9413 affirmed the role of whole-pelvic radiotherapy and neoadjuvant androgen suppression therapy (AST) in high-risk prostate cancer, there has been some lingering reluctance among radiation oncologists to deliver whole-pelvic radiotherapy, instead opting for "minipelvic" fields or omitting the pelvic field entirely (96). To reinforce this notion, secondary subgroup analysis of RTOG 9413 was recently presented, studying the volume-dependence of outcome (97). Because of the disparity in the time point at which the neoadjuvant and adjuvant AST arms became susceptible to relapse (i.e., end of both radiotherapy and AST), only patients (n = 649) who received neoadjuvant AST were included in this analysis. After stratifying by volume irradiated, the 7-year progression-free survival was 40%, 31%, and 27% in the groups that received whole-pelvic, minipelvic, and prostate-only radiotherapy (p = 0.02; Figure 63.4). There was no difference in acute grade ≥3 genitourinary or gastrointestinal toxicities among the three volumes. No difference was seen in the incidence of late grade ≥3 genitourinary toxicities between the whole-pelvic, minipelvic, and prostate-only radiotherapy groups at 48 months (3.0%, 2.4%, and 0%, respectively; p = 0.24). There was a small but significant increase in the incidence of late grade ≥3 gastrointestinal toxicities with larger fields at 48 months (4.3%, 1.2%, and 0%, respectively; p = 0.006). Of note, 3D conformal radiation therapy (3DCRT), let alone IMRT, was not routinely performed in this study. It is conceivable that with either modalities, late toxicities may be further decreased.

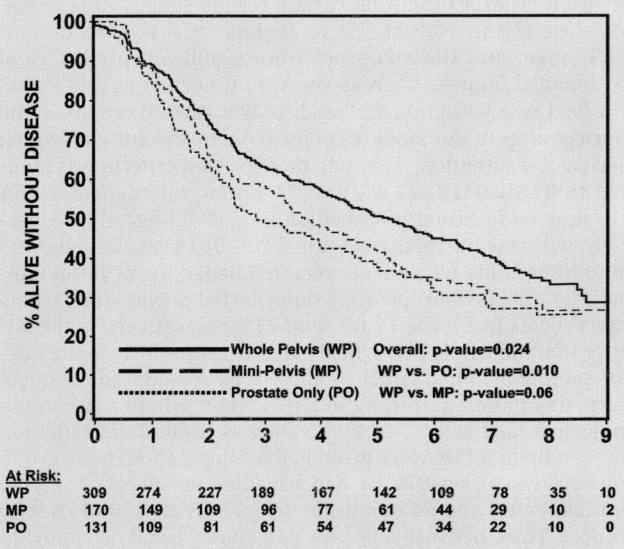

FIGURE 63.4. Progression-free survival of subgroup analysis of RTOG 9413 comparing whole-pelvic, minipelvic, and prostate-only radiotherapy. (From Roach M 3rd, DeSilvio M, Valicenti R, et al. Whole pelvic, "mini-pelvic" or prostate only external beam radiotherapy following neoadjuvant and concurrent hormonal therapy in patients treated on RTOG 9413. *Int J Radiat Oncol Biol Phys* 2006;66:647–653.)

The traditional pelvic radiotherapy volumes encompassed the obturator, external iliac nodes, and the distal portion of the common iliac nodes. Omitted are the internal iliac nodes. These borders reflect the regions excised by a limited node dissection and our concern for toxicities. Given the surgical data and our ability to deliver highly conformal radiotherapy (e.g., IMRT) that can minimize dose to nearby organs at risk (e.g., rectum, bowel, and bladder), perhaps we should consider expanding the target volume to include the internal iliac nodes. At UCSF, we recommend IMRT for pelvic irradiation. We routinely include the obturator, external and internal iliac, and distal portion of the common iliac nodes up to L5 to S1. As discussed earlier, investigators are currently studying the capabilities of IMRT in pelvic nodal treatment.

Radiation Oncology Trials

RTOG 9413 is a landmark trial that featured a two-by-two factorial randomization scheme to either prostate-only radiotherapy (PORT) or whole pelvic radiotherapy (WPRT) followed by a prostate boost, and either 4 months of neoadjuvant and concurrent hormones or 4 months of adjuvant hormones (96). Patients with an estimated nodal risk of >15% or T2c to T4 with a Gleason score of 6 or greater were eligible for the study. The 4-year progression-free survival was 54.2% and 47% in the combined WPRT arms and PORT arms ($p = 0.02$). When the four arms were analyzed separately, the neoadjuvant hormone and WPRT arm (59.6%) had a significantly better 4-year progression-free survival than the other three arms (44.3% to 49.8%; $p = 0.008$). Although there was no difference in acute (3% vs. 4%; $p = 0.39$) and late (2% vs. 2%; $p = 0.85$) grade 3 to 5 genitourinary (GU) morbidity, a trend toward increased acute (2% vs. 1%; $p = 0.06$) and late (1.7% vs. 0.6%; $p = 0.09$) grade 3 to 5 gastrointestinal (GI) morbidity was seen in the combined WPRT and prostate only arms, respectively.

One of the most common comments regarding RTOG 9413 is whether the beneficial finding of neoadjuvant hormones and WPRT still holds true in the dose-escalation era where doses of more than 80 Gy to the prostate alone can be given safely with IMRT. Retrospective data from Fox Chase Cancer Center were recently reported, investigating the effects of dose escalation, WPRT, and short-term hormones in the subgroup of patients who would otherwise be eligible for RTOG 9413 based on the inclusion criteria (58). Multivariate results suggest that radiation dose (70 to 72.9 vs. 73 to 76.9 vs. ≥77 Gy), PSA, clinical T stage, and Gleason score were significant predictors of biochemical failure, whereas short-term hormones and radiation field size were not. Although provocative, there are some shortcomings of this study, as pointed out by the authors, which merit closer attention. Although the inclusion criteria was identical to RTOG 9413, 42.4% and 31.4% of patients had a PSA <10 and 10 to 20 ng/mL (median PSA 10.95 ng/mL), respectively, whereas the median PSA in RTOG 9413 was 22.6 ng/mL. In addition, only 67 patients received neoadjuvant hormones. Radiation fields were prostate only, partial pelvic, and "whole pelvis" fields in 11.4%, 17.6%, and 71% respectively. In the latter group, the whole pelvic field extended superiorly to the inferior sacroiliac joints, which would not be considered adequate pelvic irradiation according to RTOG 9413, where a minimum unblocked field size of 16 by 16 cm was used. Total radiation doses of up to 82 Gy were given in the cohort, though the group that received at least 77 Gy had a median follow-up of only 30 months (vs. 62 and 54 months in the <73 Gy and 73 to 76.9 Gy groups). Thus, because only 16% patients received neoadjuvant hormonal therapy (NHT) and none received WPRT and the potential for selection bias (patients treated with NHT may have had worse disease than those not receiving NHT), these data do not make a compelling argument against WPRT and NHT acquired from a large phase III trial.

Vargas et al. (126) reported on the role of WPRT in a large cohort of patients treated at three institutions with external-beam radiotherapy and high–dose-rate brachytherapy. At the two German institutions, the policy was to give WPRT, whereas the American institution chose to irradiate the periprostatic area only (PORT). Of the 1,492 patients treated with this technique, 596 had an estimated nodal involvement of more than 15% based on the Roach formula, and they form the study cohort. Fifty-one percent received neoadjuvant/adjuvant hormones for ≤6 months, and 53.3% received WPRT. As opposed to the PORT group, the median PSA was higher (15.6 vs. 11.5 ng/mL), although both groups had a Gleason score of 7 and clinical T stage was slightly worse (T2b vs. T2a) in the WPRT group. Rather than show no difference, the 5-year actuarial PSA failure was significantly worse in the WPRT group (31.2% vs. 16.8%; $p <0.001$) as was clinical failure (17.6% vs. 7.9%; $p = 0.01$), suggesting an imbalance in predictors between the two groups. In multivariate analysis, Gleason score and clinical T stage were the only predictors of clinical failure, whereas PSA, use of hormones, WPRT and estimated risk of nodal involvement were not. Thus, the authors concluded that WPRT may not be beneficial in those with more than 15% risk of nodal involvement. Yet there are elements of the results and interpretation that are problematic. First, the authors chose to report only the median clinical T stage, PSA, and Gleason score (without p values) rather than provide a more detailed breakdown between the WPRT and PORT groups. Second, the findings of RTOG 9413 suggest a synergistic effect between neoadjuvant and concurrent hormones and WPRT. But it did not suggest that WPRT without hormones was beneficial. Rather than compare a subset of the study cohort that exclusively received WPRT and neoadjuvant hormones, this retrospective study included patients who did not receive hormones in their WPRT group. Finally, the multivariate analysis included WPRT and hormones as separate covariates.

Summary of University of California–San Francisco Recommendations

Whole Pelvic Radiotherapy

At UCSF, we recommend prophylactic whole pelvic IMRT to patients with an estimated nodal involvement of >15%, unfavorable intermediate- and high-risk prostate cancer. Our standard field arrangement are consistent with the fields recommended by Shih et al. (115) in their study on optimal delineation of nodal target volumes. The prostate boost is delivered with either IMRT, Iodine 125 (^{125}I) permanent seed or high–dose-rate (HDR) brachytherapy, although we prefer the latter approaches because of their ability to deliver maximal dose to the prostate. Brachytherapy is typically performed 1 to 2 weeks following pelvic radiotherapy. For T3 disease, we use an IMRT or HDR boost, which allows better coverage of extranodal disease.

Androgen Suppression Therapy

We give 2 months of neoadjuvant, then concurrent total androgen blockade using an luteinizing hormone-releasing hormone (LHRH) agonist and an antiandrogen. Two to 3 years of adjuvant hormones (only an LHRH agonist) is recommended for high-risk disease, but on occasion life-long androgen deprivation is used in patients with very high-risk disease (Table 63.1).

Volumes and Setup Variation

We routinely place three fiducial gold seed markers into the prostate under transrectal ultrasound guidance—two in the

	Low Risk	Favorable Intermediate Risk	Unfavorable Intermediate Risk	High Risk
TABLE 63.1 :: RECOMMENDATIONS OF PELVIC RADIOTHERAPY AND HORMONES				
Radiotherapy	PORT	PORT	WPRT	WPRT
Androgen suppression therapy	Not indicated	Neoadjuvant (2 months) Concurrent	Neoadjuvant (2 months) Concurrent ± Adjuvant	Neoadjuvant (2 months) Concurrent Adjuvant (24–36 months)

PORT, prostate-only radiotherapy; WPRT, whole-pelvic radiotherapy

Clinical Radiation Oncology

base and one in the apex. Each marker is approximately 1.1 mm in diameter and 3 mm in length. Using an amorphous silicon flat-panel detector, we perform daily electronic portal imaging (EPI) and make any necessary adjustments prior to each treatment. As such, we apply a 3-mm margin around the prostate gland and seminal vesicles in defining the PTV. At institutions without daily EPI to control for intra- and interfraction prostate motion, larger margins such as 0.5 to 1 cm should be considered.

Patients are instructed to empty their rectum with an enema prior to simulation. Patients are told to maintain a full bladder during simulation and treatment. A retrograde urethrogram is performed to assist in identifying the base of the prostate. Three-millimeter slice thickness is used for the CT simulation. The critical organs that are contoured include the penile bulb, small bowel, rectum, bladder, and femoral heads. The entire rectum is contoured from the anus to the rectosigmoid junction.

Intensity Modulated Radiotherapy Treatment Planning

For patients opting for definitive external-beam radiotherapy to the pelvis and prostate, we use a two-phase plan. The first phase delivers 25 to 30 fractions of 180 cGy per fraction (total 4,500 to 5,400 cGy) to the nodes, and 200 cGy per fraction (total 5,400 cGy) to the seminal vesicle and prostate PTV. The second phase is a cone-down boost to the prostate PTV alone with 10 to 11 fractions of 180 cGy per fraction. Therefore, the minimum total dose to the prostate (prescribed to the PTV) is 7,200 to 7,380 cGy. The usual isodose line that we prescribe to is 82% to 92%, meaning that the maximum dose in the prostate is as high as 120% of the prescribed dose (78 to 82 Gy). Both phases use a seven-field isocentric technique with 18-MV photons.

For pelvic radiotherapy followed by a brachytherapy boost, we deliver 25 fractions of 180 cGy per fraction to the nodes and prostate/seminal vesicle PTV (total dose 4,500 cGy). In postop patients opting for pelvic radiotherapy, we prescribe 25 fractions of 180 cGy to the nodes (total dose 4,500 cGy) and 200 cGy per fraction to the tumor bed PTV (total dose 5,000 cGy) then 9 fractions of 180 cGy per fraction to the prostate bed (total minimal PTV dose 6,620 cGy, maximum dose 7,800 cGy).

Toxicity of Pelvic Intensity Modulated Radiotherapy

In a study from Memorial Sloan-Kettering, the dosimetric outcomes of pelvic radiotherapy using two-dimensional (2D), 3DCRT, and IMRT were compared in 13 patients (4). The mean bowel dose was reduced by approximately 20% with 3DCRT and IMRT as compared to 2D planning ($p = 0.001$). Similarly, the bowel V45 was 41.7%, 22.6%, and 9.1% with 2D, 3DCRT, and IMRT. Rectal sparing was also evident with IMRT and 3DCRT.

The mean dose was 40.4, 37.3, and 27.3 Gy, respectively. The V25 was significantly better with IMRT (50.5%) as compared to 2D (91.7%) and 3DCRT (86.3%). Bladder V45 was significantly better with IMRT (87.2, 56.8, and 25.6%, respectively; $p <0.001$). Toxicity was minimal with no cases of acute grade 3 to 5 toxicities. Only one patient required medication for proctitis and none for diarrhea.

Jani et al. (60) retrospectively compared 15 patients who received pelvic IMRT versus 34 patients who received pelvic 3DCRT. The bladder (60.8% vs. 24.8%; $p = 0.04$) and rectal (65% vs. 25.1%; $p = 0.01$) V60 were significantly lower in the IMRT plans. The IMRT patients had significantly less acute GU but no difference in GI toxicities. Grade 3 (3% vs. 0%) and grade 2 GU (59% vs. 20%; $p <0.001$) toxicities were less with IMRT.

Dose Escalation

Perhaps the most polarized topic in prostate radiotherapy management is whether pelvic radiotherapy and/or hormonal therapy is needed in the setting of dose escalation. The crux of the argument for dose escalation in intermediate- and high-risk patients is that the relatively poor outcome observed in such patients may be due to inadequate doses of radiotherapy to the prostate itself, as suggested by postradiotherapy biopsy data, rather than occult metastatic disease. Therefore, some contend that dose escalation to the prostate obviates the need for pelvic radiation and/or hormonal therapy.

External-Beam Radiotherapy Alone

M.D. Anderson Cancer Center conducted a single-institution dose-escalation phase III trial comparing 70 with 78 Gy (93). The study included 301 patients with clinical stage T1 to T3 disease. The median PSA was 7.8 and Gleason score 8 to 10 was seen in 17% of patients. The prescription dose was specified to the isocenter. Radiotherapy was conventionally planned in the 70 Gy arm and in phase 1 of the 78 Gy arm; a conformal boost plan was used in the 78 Gy arm. No hormonal therapy was used. The 6-year PSA control was 70% versus 64% in favor of the 78 Gy arm ($p = 0.03$), but no survival difference was observed. Subgroup analyses suggested that the benefit of dose escalation is primarily in patients with a PSA >10 ng/mL (62% vs. 43%; $p = 0.012$), rather than when the PSA was 10 ng/mL or less ($p = 0.46$) or any Gleason score.

Proton Radiation Oncology Group (PROG) 9509 is a phase III trial of 393 men, comparing 19.8 GyE photon with 28.8 GyE proton boost to the prostate (138). All patients then received 50.4 Gy using photons to the prostate and seminal vesicles with 3DCRT. In the cohort, 32% and 8% had intermediate- and high-risk disease, respectively. Among the intermediate- and high-risk patients, high-dose therapy benefited only the intermediate-risk patients—5-year biochemical control was 81% versus 62.7% ($p = 0.02$). The lack of dose response seen in the high-risk group may have been due to the trial limiting the accrual to a PSA <15 ng/mL and T1b to T2b.

Zelefsky et al. (134) conducted a single-institution phase I and II study of dose escalation from 64.8 to 86.4 Gy to the prostate alone. Of note, these doses represented the minimum tumor dose, and radiotherapy was delivered by 3DCRT or IMRT. Of a total cohort of 1,100 patients, there were 405 and 416 patients with intermediate- and unfavorable (i.e., high-) risk disease, respectively. None of the patients received any adjuvant hormones. In the intermediate-risk group, doses of ≥75.6 Gy yielded significantly better PSA control rates than doses ≤70.2 Gy (p = 0.008). In the unfavorable risk group, 81 Gy improved 5-year biochemical control as compared to 75.6 Gy (67% vs. 43%; p = 0.05). Postradiation biopsies taken at 2.5 years seemed to support the contention that dose escalation was efficacious, even among intermediate- and unfavorable-risk patients. Whereas only 10% and 23% of patients who received 81 Gy and 75.6 Gy, respectively, had positive biopsies, 34% and 54% of patients who received 70.2 Gy and 64.8 Gy, respectively, had positive biopsies. For patients who received 75.6 Gy, the rates of positive biopsies increased as patients had less favorable disease—11%, 19%, and 30% in the favorable, intermediate, and unfavorable groups, respectively. It was observed that although doses of 81 Gy could be safely administered with 3DCRT, efforts to increase the dose further were not possible without IMRT. The overall grade 3 late rectal toxicity was 1%. In the cohort who received 75.6 Gy or greater using 3DCRT, grade 2 late rectal toxicity was 14%. Grade 3 urethral stricture or hematuria was seen in 1.5% of patients. The 5-year rate of grade 2 late urinary toxicity was 13%.

Updated results of a dose-escalation trial from Fox Chase Cancer Center were recently reported (92). All patients (n = 839) received conformal radiotherapy without hormones to total doses of 63 to 84 Gy, which was prescribed to the 95% isodose line. Fifty-three and 6% of patients had T2 and T3 disease and 29% and 14% had a PSA of 10 to 19.9 and ≥20 ng/mL, respectively. Multivariate analyses demonstrated that radiotherapy dose, PSA, Gleason score, and clinical T stage were significant predictors of biochemical failure. The group with a Gleason score of 7 to 10 and a PSA <10 ng/mL and the group with PSA 10 to 19.9 ng/mL (with any Gleason score) benefited from dose escalation. In the former group, 5-year biochemical failure was 70% versus 17% in the men who received <72 Gy and ≥76 Gy, respectively (p = 0.006). In the latter group, 5-year biochemical failure was 76%, 35%, and 21%, with <72 Gy, 72 to 75.9 Gy, and ≥76 Gy, respectively (p <0.0001). However, patients with a PSA <10 and a Gleason score of 2 to 6, or a PSA ≥20 Gy regardless of clinical T stage, did not benefit from increased dose.

A dose response has also been observed in patients with high-grade disease (Gleason score 8 to 10) (40,102). Roach et al. (102) reported that 83% of patients who received more than 71 Gy were free of progression compared to 0% with <71 Gy (p = 0.03). In a multi-institutional study of 180 patients with Gleason score 8 to 10 disease, 5-year PSA control was 88% and 65% in T1 and T2 disease with <70 and 70 to 75 Gy, respectively (p = 0.02). Five-year overall survival was 81%, 71%, and 59% after 75 to 80, 70 to 75, and <70 Gy, respectively (p = 0.04) (40).

To minimize follow-up and stage migration bias, Kupelian et al. (71) reported on the results of a multi-institutional retrospective study in 1,325 men treated between 1994 to 1995. Patients were stratified by radiation dose (<72 or ≥72 Gy); the median dose in both groups were 68.4 and 75.6 Gy, respectively. 3DCRT (vs. conventional) was used in 33% and 68%, respectively. No patients received hormonal therapy or pelvic irradiation. There were more advanced stage cancers (T2b to T2c, 32% vs. 42%) and higher median pretreatment PSA (8 vs. 9.2 ng/mL) in the high-dose group. In the cohort, 51% and 17% had intermediate-

and high-risk disease. In the intermediate-risk group, the 5-year biochemical disease-free survival was greater when at least 72 Gy was given (72% vs. 63%; p = 0.026). However, no dose response was seen in the low- and high-risk groups.

The biochemical outcomes of RTOG 9406, a phase I and II trial (n = 1,084) of sequential dose levels (68.4, 73.8, 79.2, 74, and 78 Gy) using 3DCRT, were recently reported (80). The third dose level (79.2 Gy) resulted in 5-year PSA control of 59%, 58%, and 47% in the low-, intermediate-, and high-risk groups (104). The acute and late toxicities of this dose level were acceptable, with no acute grade 3 to 5 and late grade 4 to 5 bladder or bowel toxicities. Late toxicities were absent or minimal (grade 1) in 81% of patients. Of 169 patients, only three patients had late grade 3 bladder toxicity (hemorrhagic cystitis). There was one case of late grade 3 bowel toxicity (hemorrhagic proctitis). These toxicity results were significantly less than historical data from RTOG 7506 and 7706. Based on these results among others, RTOG 0126, a phase III multi-institutional trial comparing 70.2 Gy with 79.2 Gy as a minimum PTV dose using 3DCRT or IMRT in intermediate-risk disease, is currently open for accrual.

External-Beam Radiotherapy with Brachytherapy Boost

According to the 1999 Patterns of Care Study of radiotherapy and brachytherapy, 46% of prostate cancer patients who received brachytherapy also received supplemental external-beam radiotherapy (XRT) (77). Rather than using XRT alone, where prostate doses are limited by nearby critical organs, many have combined the advantages of dose delivery by brachytherapy with the ability to irradiate a larger volume (e.g., periprostatic or whole pelvis) with XRT that would otherwise be beyond the reach of brachytherapy.

The Seattle Prostate Institute reported on the biochemical outcome of 232 consecutively treated patients with pelvic radiotherapy (45 Gy) followed by an ^{125}I (108 Gy) or palladium 103 (^{103}Pd) (100 Gy) brachytherapy boost (120). No hormones were given in this cohort. Patients received this combined treatment because of presumed higher risk disease on the basis of unfavorable risk factors, like high percentage of positive biopsy cores, perineural invasion, or bulky disease. Forty percent and 33% of patients had intermediate- and high-risk disease, respectively. Overall, the 10-year biochemical relapse-free survival was 70%. Ten-year biochemical control was 85%, 77%, and 45% in the low-, intermediate-, and high-risk groups.

From McMaster University, 104 patients with T2 and T3N0 disease and negative pelvic lymphadenectomy were randomly allocated to brachytherapy plus XRT or XRT alone (108). The XRT-only arm received 66 Gy to the isocenter, whereas the brachytherapy arm received 35 Gy using iridium 192 (^{192}Ir) seeds followed by XRT of 40 Gy (total dose 75 Gy). No adjuvant hormones were given. Intermediate- and high-risk disease constituted 40% and 60% of the cohort, respectively. All patients were conventionally planned using a four-field technique that encompassed the prostate and seminal vesicles with a 2 cm margin. After a median follow-up of 8.2 years, the 5-year biochemical failure rate was significantly less in the brachytherapy arm (29% vs. 61%; p = 0.002). The brachytherapy arm had improved biochemical control regardless of risk group. Of the 87% of patients who had a postirradiation prostate biopsy at 2 years, positive biopsies were significantly less in the brachytherapy arm (24% vs. 51%; p = 0.015). There was no difference in acute and late GI, GU, or sexual morbidity between the two arms.

The preliminary results of the first 165 intermediate-risk patients treated in a dose-reduction randomized trial were recently reported (128). Patients were randomized to either 20 or 44 Gy of preimplant supplemental XRT directed to the periprostatic region. All patients subsequently received ^{103}Pd brachytherapy (90 vs. 115 Gy, respectively). The median PSA was 7 and 6.7, respectively. The majority of patients had Gleason score 7 disease (83% and 75% in the 20 Gy and 44 Gy arms, respectively). Although the median follow-up was only 2.9 years, there was no difference in 3-year biochemical control between the 20 Gy and 44 Gy arms (83% vs. 88%, respectively; $p = 0.64$). With the short follow-up, it is difficult to draw conclusions from this study. It is also questionable how cytotoxic 20 Gy really is to presumed microscopic disease. Nonetheless, this study suggests that in patients with only one adverse feature (i.e., Gleason score 7), supplemental XRT to the periprostatic region may not be necessary.

In a preliminary report, Hsu et al. (55) demonstrated that high–dose-rate brachytherapy can be safely and efficaciously combined with WPRT and hormones. Among the 64 study patients, 44% had T3 disease, 23% had Gleason score 8 to 10 disease, and the mean estimated pelvic nodal risk was 25%. The 4-year disease-free survival rate was 92%, and there have been no prostate cancer deaths. There were two cases of perioperative hematuria, with one requiring a blood transfusion. One case of small bowel obstruction requiring resection was seen.

To see whether combined modality treatment could be implemented on a nationwide scale, RTOG P-0019, a phase II study of combined XRT with ^{125}I brachytherapy in intermediate-risk patients was initiated (75). The protocol mandated periprostatic XRT (45 Gy), followed by brachytherapy (108 Gy). There were no grade 4 or 5 acute and late toxicities. All grade 3 acute toxicities were urinary ($n = 10$), with urinary frequency ($n = 6$) the most common. There were six cases of grade 3 late toxicities, with five urinary and one proctitis. At 18-months, grade ≥ 2 erectile dysfunction was observed in 45.5%. Currently, there are two open RTOG studies of relevant interest. RTOG 0232 is a phase 2 trial comparing brachytherapy alone with combined brachytherapy and XRT in select intermediate-risk patients. RTOG 0321 is a phase 2 trial designed to estimate the rates of grade 3 late genitourinary and gastrointestinal toxicities with high–dose-rate brachytherapy and XRT in intermediate- and high-risk disease.

Despite the results of RTOG 9413, there has been ongoing controversy regarding whether pelvic radiotherapy or dose escalation is more important in terms of patient outcome. At UCSF, patients with unfavorable intermediate- or high-risk disease are offered combined AST and whole pelvic radiotherapy followed by a brachytherapy boost as a form of dose escalation or IMRT.

Androgen Suppression Therapy

AST has been increasingly used in combination with external-beam radiotherapy in the treatment of unfavorable intermediate- and high-risk adenocarcinoma of the prostate (12,13, 24,88–91). This practice is reflected in a recent CaPSURE report where the use of neoadjuvant hormones with radiotherapy increased from 9.8% to 74.6% in 1989 to 1992 and 1999 to 2001, respectively (16). Among high-risk patients, the use of neoadjuvant AST increased from 15.3% to 89.5% during the same periods, respectively (16).

Biologic Basis of Combining Androgen Suppression Therapy and Radiotherapy

Animal models have provided the basis for our understanding of the mechanism behind AST and radiotherapy. In the Shionogi *in vivo* tumor system, androgen-dependent tumors, designed to mimic prostate cancer, were implanted into SCID mice (139). The mice then received radiation and/or surgical orchiectomy at varying time sequences relative to each other. The results

showed that androgen ablation improved the tumor response to radiation and reflected a reduction in the radiotherapy dose needed to control 50% of tumors (TCD50). More provocative was the observation that the sequence of androgen ablation and radiotherapy was also relevant. When orchiectomy was performed prior to the delivery of radiotherapy, much lower doses of radiation were required to achieve a given level of tumor control than if performed after or during radiotherapy. Thus, increased overall cell kill appears to be one of the mechanisms responsible for the combined effects of androgen deprivation and radiotherapy.

More recently, Kaminski et al. (62) studied the effects of single-fraction radiotherapy and androgen ablation sequencing in the R33270G Dunning rat prostate tumor model on tumor volume growth kinetics. There were seven groups, including a sham group, radiotherapy (RT)-alone control groups, androgen deprivation alone group, and RT before, during, and after androgen deprivation. They found that the median posttreatment doubling time was significantly longer in the group that received radiotherapy after neoadjuvant androgen ablation compared to all the other treatment groups, including the radiotherapy with concurrent or adjuvant androgen deprivation groups. Therefore, the improved outcome after combined treatment may also be explained by diminished growth velocity in the surviving prostate cancer cells after treatment.

Clinical Trials Supporting Androgen Suppression Therapy and Radiotherapy

Thus far, there have been seven phase III randomized controlled trials and a meta-analysis published in the literature that compared radiotherapy alone with radiotherapy and AST. The trials can be broadly divided based on the era (e.g., pre-PSA) when they were conducted. With greater adoption of PSA screening, a dramatic stage migration was observed in the 1990s. The CaPSURE database demonstrated that high-risk disease decreased from 36.6% of patients diagnosed in 1989 to 1992 to 16.0% in 2000 to 2002 (17). In contrast, there has been a corresponding rise in low-risk disease from 29.5% to 46.8%, respectively (17). The pretreatment characteristics and outcome results of these seven trials are summarized in Tables 63.2 and 63.3, respectively.

High-Risk Prostate Cancer

As the first study to demonstrate a survival advantage with AST, the European Organization of Research and Treatment of Cancer (EORTC) 22863 study randomized 415 men with T1 and T2 and World Health Organization grade 3 disease, or T3 or T4 disease to either radiotherapy alone or 3 years of AST commenced on the first day of radiotherapy (13). Ninety-two percent of patients had T3 or T4 disease. All patients received WPRT and a prostate boost to a total dose of 70 Gy. Updated results demonstrated that after a median follow-up of 66 months, 5-year rates of biochemical control, disease-free survival, and overall survival were significantly in favor of the AST plus radiotherapy arm (12). AST reduced the risk of death by 49% and improved 5-year overall survival from 62% to 78% ($p < 0.0001$).

At around the same time, RTOG launched two companion trials—8531 and 8610—which were designed to target different subsets of high-risk patients. RTOG 8531 randomized 945 men with clinical stage T1 and T2N1, T3N0-1, or pT3 after radical prostatectomy to either radiotherapy or radiotherapy with indefinite AST beginning on the last day of radiotherapy (88). Like the EORTC trial, all patients received WPRT followed by a prostate boost to a total dose of 65 to 70 Gy. In the control arm, salvage AST was offered upon failure. In effect, this was a comparison between immediate versus delayed AST.

| :: Table 63.2 | SUMMARY OF PRETREATMENT CHARACTERISTICS OF RANDOMIZED CONTROLLED TRIALS OF RADIOTHERAPY ALONE VS. RADIOTHERAPY WITH ANDROGEN SUPPRESSION THERAPY | | | | | |

| | | | | Patient Characteristics | | |
Study (Reference)	Study Arms	No. of Patients	XRT Dose (Gy)	Clinical T Stage	Median PSA	Gleason Score
High Risk						
EORTC 22863 (12,13)	XRT alone	198	70	T3–T4 (92%)	≤10.1 (17%)	2–6 (28%)[a]
	XRT + AST	203			10–20 (16%)	7–10 (34%)
					20.1–40 (24%)	Unknown (38%)
					>40 (33%)	
					Unknown (7%)	
RTOG 8531 (88,91)	XRT alone	468	65–70	NR	24[b]	2–5 (13%)[a]
	XRT + AST	477				6–7 (49%)
						8–10 (29%)
						Unknown (9%)
RTOG 8610 (89,90)	XRT alone	230	65–70	T3–T4 (70%)	26.3[b]	2–6 (28%)[a]
	XRT + NHT, C-HT	226				7 (39%)
						8–10 (27%)
						Unknown (6%)
Quebec L-101 (74)	XRT alone	43	64			
	XRT + NHT	63		T2 (70%)	10.0	7–10 (27.4%)
	XRT + NHT, C-HT, AHT	55		T3 (30%)		
Granfors et al. (47)	XRT alone	46	65.05	T2 (65%)	NR	Grade 1 (12%)
	XRT + AST	45		T3–T4 (29%)		Grade 2 (70%)
						Grade 3 (18%)
Intermediate Risk						
BWH (24)	XRT alone	104	70.35	T1 (48%)	11	5–6 (27%)[a]
	XRT + NHT, C-HT, AHT	102		T2 (52%)		7 (58%)
						8–10 (15%)
TROG 96.01 (32)	XRT alone	270	66	T2 (60%)	15	2–6 (44%)
	NHT (3 months), CHT	265		T3–T4 (40%)		7 (38%)
	NHT (6 months), CHT	267				8–10 (17%)

AHT, adjuvant hormonal therapy; AST, androgen suppression therapy; BWH, Brigham and Women's Hospital; C-HT, concurrent hormonal therapy; CUOG, Canadian Urologic Oncology Group; EORTC, European Organization of Research and Treatment of Cancer; NHT, neoadjuvant hormonal therapy; NR, not recorded; PSA, prostate-specific antigen; RTOG, Radiation Therapy Oncology Group; TROG,Trans-Tasman Radiation Oncology Group; XRT, external-beam radiotherapy
[a]Gleason score distribution from central review.
[b]For RTOG 8531 and 8610, pretreatment PSA was available in only 44% and 28% of patients, respectively.

After a median follow-up of 5.6 years, the initial published report demonstrated that immediate AST improved biochemical control, but not overall survival in the entire cohort. Subgroup analyses identified a cluster of patients with centrally reviewed Gleason scores of 8 to 10 and not having undergone surgery who did have a survival advantage (66% vs. 55%; $p = 0.03$). The study has since been updated after a median follow-up of 7.6 years (91). At 10 years, the overall survival advantage seen with immediate AST now extends to the entire cohort (49% vs. 39%; $p = 0.002$), but was preferentially in the patients with a Gleason score of 7 to 10. Ten-year PCSM was significantly reduced in the immediate AST arm (16% vs. 22%; $p = 0.0052$).

RTOG 8610 randomized 456 patients with bulky T2 clinical stage T2-4N0-1 or a bulky primary tumor defined as >25 cm^2 prostate, to either radiotherapy alone or radiotherapy with 2 months of neoadjuvant and 2 months of concurrent AST (total 4 months) (89). The radiotherapy dose and technique was identical to RTOG 8531. Like RTOG 8531, the initial report (median follow-up 4.5 years) showed that AST improved 5-year progression-free survival but did not impact overall survival (89). With longer follow-up (median follow-up 6.7 years), the 8-year PCSM benefit from AST became more apparent (23% vs. 31%; $p = 0.05$), although there was no difference in overall survival (53% vs. 44%; $p = 0.10$) (90). On subgroup analysis of men with Gleason score 2 to 6 tumors, there was a significant overall survival benefit with AST at 8 years (70% vs. 52%; $p = 0.015$).

A meta-analysis of five consecutive RTOG phase III trials (including RTOG 8531 and 8610) provided further support for the combination of AST and radiotherapy (100). The meta-analysis

included 2,742 men treated between 1975 and 1992, and stratified them into four previously defined prognostic risk groups based on Gleason score, clinical T stage, and pelvic nodal involvement (99). PSA was not included in the risk groups because most of the studies were performed in the pre-PSA era. Whereas risk group 1 patients (i.e., low-risk) did not benefit from the addition of AST, risk groups 2 and 3 to 4 (i.e., intermediate- and high-risk, respectively) clearly benefited from the addition of short- and long-term AST, respectively, in terms of 8-year disease-specific survival and overall survival (100).

Conducted between 1991 and 1994, the Quebec L-101 study randomized 161 men with clinical stage T2 or T3 prostate cancer to one of three arms: Radiotherapy alone, 3 months of neoadjuvant AST plus radiotherapy, or 10 months of neoadjuvant, concurrent, adjuvant AST plus radiotherapy (73,74). The latter arm received 3-months of neoadjuvant AST, then continued for an additional 7 months during and after radiotherapy. Prostate-only radiotherapy to a dose of 6,400 cGy was used. The updated results had a median follow-up of 5 years and concluded that both arms containing AST had significantly improved 7-year PSA control rates better than the control arm (42% vs. 66% and 69%, respectively). There was no difference between the two experimental arms ($p = 0.6$). Granfors et al. (47) randomized 91 patients with T1 to T4, pN0-3 prostate cancer to radiotherapy alone or orchiectomy followed by radiotherapy. Patients were surgically staged with a pelvic lymphadenectomy. All patients received WPRT and a mean total prostate dose of 6,505 cGy. After a median follow-up of 9.3 years, clinical progression (61% vs. 31%; $p = 0.005$) and deaths from any

| Table 63.3 | SUMMARY OF OUTCOME RESULTS FROM RANDOMIZED CONTROLLED TRIALS OF RADIOTHERAPY ALONE VS. RADIOTHERAPY WITH ANDROGEN SUPPRESSION THERAPY |||||

Study (Reference)	Median Follow-Up (years)	Study Arms	5-Year Overall Survival	5-Year Cause-Specific Survival	5-Year Biochemical Control
High Risk					
EORTC 22863 (12,13)	5.5	XRT alone	62%	79%	45%
		XRT + AST	78%	94%	76%
			($p = 0.0002$)	($p = 0.0001$)	($p < 0.0001$)
RTOG 8531 (88,91)	7.6	XRT alone	71%	87%	21%
		XRT + AST	76%	91%	55%
			($p = 0.002$)	($p = 0.0052$)	($p < 0.0001$)
RTOG 8610 (89,90)	6.7	XRT alone	68%	80%	10%
		XRT + NHT	72%	85%	28%
			($p = 0.10$)	($p = 0.05$)	($p < 0.0001$)
Quebec L-101 (74)	5.0	XRT alone	NR	NR	58%
		XRT + NHT			76% ($p = 0.009$)
		XRT + NHT, C-HT, AHT			74% ($p = 0.003$)
Granfors et al. (47)	9.3	XRT alone	70%	75%	74%[a]
		XRT + AST	82%	85%	85%
			($p = 0.02$)	($p = 0.06$)	($p = 0.005$)
Intermediate Risk					
BWH (24)	4.5	XRT alone	78%	94%	55%
		XRT + NHT, C-HT, AHT	88%	100%	79%
			($p = 0.04$)	($p = 0.02$)	($p < 0.001$)
TROG 96.01 (32)	5.9	XRT alone	NR	91%	38%
		NHT (3 months), C-HT		92% ($p = 0.7$)	52% ($p - 0.002$)
		NHT (6 months), C-HT		94% ($p = 0.04$)	56% ($p < 0.0001$)

AHT, adjuvant hormonal therapy; AST, androgen suppression therapy; BWH, Brigham and Women's Hospital; C-HT, concurrent hormonal therapy; CUOG, Canadian Urologic Oncology Group; EORTC, European Organization of Research and Treatment of Cancer; NHT, neoadjuvant hormonal therapy; NR, not recorded; RTOG, Radiation Therapy Oncology Group; TROG, Trans-Tasman Radiation Oncology Group; XRT, external-beam radiotherapy
[a]Non-prostate-specific antigen progression-free survival.

cause (61% vs. 38%; $p = 0.02$) were significantly worse in the radiotherapy alone arm. However, in subgroup analyses, only patients with positive pelvic lymph nodes benefited from orchiectomy.

In summary, the studies consistently demonstrate that combining hormones with radiotherapy can confer a PSA control and survival advantage, and as such should be recommended in the high-risk group.

Intermediate-Risk Prostate Cancer

Two studies conducted in the PSA and 3DCRT era were recently published. As expected from the PSA stage migration, the participating patients in these trials are distinctly lower risk than the pioneering trials, and would be considered as intermediate-risk disease.

In a study from Brigham and Women's Hospital (BWH), 206 patients were randomly allocated to radiotherapy alone or 2 months each of total androgen blockade given before, during, and after radiotherapy for a total of 6 months (24). Low-risk patients were not eligible for this study. Whereas the pioneering studies were performed in an era when 3DCRT was still not widely available, this study exclusively utilized 3DCRT. Additionally, radiotherapy was confined to the prostate and seminal vesicles (i.e., WPRT was not performed). Nonetheless, after a median follow-up of only 4.52 years and a relatively small sample size, the AST arm had significantly improved 5-year PSA control (79% vs. 55%; $p < 0.001$), PCSM (0% vs. 6%; $p = 0.02$), and overall survival (88% vs. 78%; $p = 0.04$).

The Trans-Tasman Radiation Oncology Group (TROG) 96.01 study consisted of 802 men with locally advanced prostate cancer (32). A three-arm trial, patients were randomized to ra-

diotherapy alone, 3 months, or 6 months of neoadjuvant hormones with radiotherapy. The protocol prescription was 66 Gy to the prostate and seminal vesicles, without WPRT. Five-year PSA disease-free survival was significantly improved in the 3-month (52%; $p = 0.002$) and 6-month (56%; $p < 0.0001$) arms as compared to the control arm (38%). Although the 6-month arm (94%) showed significantly improved PCSM, the 3-month arm (92%) was not significantly different from the control arm (91%). Interestingly, 5-year distant failures were significantly less in the 6-month arm (13%) but not for the 3-month arm (22%) as compared to the control arm (19%).

Toxicities of Androgen Suppression

Having established that AST improves survival when combined with radiotherapy, enthusiasm has been somewhat tempered by the increasing recognition of AST's potentially serious complications (53,54). These include fatigue, weight gain, osteoporosis, depression, decreased cognitive function, erectile dysfunction, loss of libido, gynecomastia, anemia, decreased high-density lipoprotein, and hot flashes. In a recent study of 50,613 men with prostate cancer compiled from a linked database of Surveillance Epidemiology and End Results (SEER) and Medicare, the addition of AST significantly increased the risk of any fracture from 12.6% to 19.4%; fractures requiring hospitalization similarly increased from 2.37% to 5.19% (113). Recommendations on management of osteoporosis secondary to AST have since been published (33).

Furthermore, even after cessation of AST, testosterone levels may require a year or more before recovering to noncastrate levels. During this time, men are still exposed to the potential side effects of androgen deprivation. In a study by Pickles et al. (87), the overall median time for testosterone recovery to noncastrate levels after adjuvant AST and radiotherapy was 10 months. Testosterone recovery was dependent on the duration of the LHRH preparation, with 3- and 1-month preparations associated with a 16- and 8-month recovery time, respectively.

Sequencing of Androgen Suppression Therapy and Radiotherapy

Neoadjuvant therapy suggests delivery of the hormone prior to definitive radiation only. Yet the precise duration of androgen suppression is not so simple. One study found that the median time for testosterone recovery to noncastrate levels after cessation of AST was 10 months (87). In effect, these definitions are artificial since patients receiving neoadjuvant AST alone are in fact receiving concurrent and short-term adjuvant AST.

Optimal Timing of Androgen Suppression Therapy

RTOG 9413 randomized 1,323 men with an estimated risk of pelvic lymph node involvement exceeding 15% in a two-by-two factorial design: WPRT followed by prostate boost radiotherapy versus PORT, and 4 months of neoadjuvant and concurrent AST (commenced 2 months prior to starting radiotherapy) versus 4 months of adjuvant AST (96,101). Two thirds of the study patients had T2c to T4 disease and one third had a presenting PSA > 30 ng/mL. Seventy-three percent had a Gleason score of 7 to 10, and approximately one-quarter had an estimated pelvic nodal involvement >35%. After a median follow-up of 59.5 months, 4-year progression-free survival was significantly improved in the arm that received WPRT and neoadjuvant AST as compared to the other three arms (60% vs. 44% to 50%; $p = 0.008$); there was no significant difference between the other three arms (96). Because of the significant difference between the two WPRT arms, the conclusions were that the benefit was sequence dependent and that there was a favorable interaction between neoadjuvant AST and WPRT. Similarly, the lack of difference seen between the two PORT arms suggested that the benefit of AST was not sequence dependent when only the prostate was irradiated.

Duration of Androgen Suppression Therapy

Optimal Duration of Neoadjuvant Hormonal Therapy

To date, there are two published randomized trials evaluating the optimal duration of neoadjuvant AST. The Canadian Urologic Oncology Group (CUOG) study randomized 361 patients to either 3 or 8 months of neoadjuvant AST plus radiotherapy (20). The majority had intermediate- (43%) or high-risk (31%) disease. None received concurrent or adjuvant AST. There was no difference in 5-year overall survival or freedom from failure despite lower post-AST and postradiotherapy PSA nadir in the 8-month arm. Extracted 24 to 30 months after radiotherapy, rates of positive biopsies were also not significantly different (14% vs. 9%, respectively; $p = 0.34$). Testosterone recovery was in favor of the 3-month arm (95.5% vs. 88.7%; $p = 0.04$).

As previously discussed, TROG 96.01 is a three-arm study with a radiotherapy-alone control group (32). The other two arms were 3 and 6 months of neoadjuvant AST. An improvement in local control and biochemical disease-free survival was seen in both AST arms (52% to 56%) over the control arm (38%; $p < 0.005$), although the benefit seemed to be more pronounced in the 6-month arm. Prostate cancer–specific mortality was slightly less in the 6-month (6%) but not the 3-month arm (8%) as compared to the control arm (9%). Similar to the CUOG trial, there was no difference in biochemical control between the 3- and 6-month arms.

Recently completed accrual, RTOG 9910 compares 8 and 28 weeks of neoadjuvant total androgen blockade in intermediate-risk patients. With over 1,500 accrued patients, the results of this study will be eagerly anticipated. Until then, the available evidence suggests that neoadjuvant AST beyond 2 to 3 months is not beneficial.

Optimal Duration of Adjuvant Hormonal Therapy

As discussed, the Quebec L-101 trial randomized 161 intermediate-risk patients to either radiotherapy alone, 3-months of neoadjuvant AST and radiotherapy, or 10-months of neoadjuvant, concurrent, and adjuvant AST with radiotherapy (73,74). Although the two experimental arms had superior 7-year PSA control rates over the control arm, there was no difference between the two AST arms (69% vs. 66%; $p = 0.6$; see Table 63.4). In the subsequent confirmatory trial, Laverdiere's L-200 study, 296 intermediate-risk patients were randomized to either of the two experimental arms of L-101. After a median follow-up of 3.7 years, the 5-year biochemical control was identical in both arms at 70% (74).

Also previously discussed, in the meta-analysis of five consecutive RTOG randomized controlled prostate cancer trials (including RTOG 8531 and 8610), 2,742 men were stratified into four previously identified risk groups based on Gleason score, clinical T stage, and pelvic nodal involvement (99,100). Risk group 1 (i.e., "low risk") did not benefit from AST. However, risk group 2 (i.e., "intermediate risk") had significantly improved 8-year disease-specific survival from 83% to 98% ($p = 0.003$) with short-term AST. Risk groups 3 and 4 (i.e., "high risk") benefited from long-term AST; 8-year overall survival increased from 28% to 44%.

After RTOG 8610 demonstrated that short-term AST was beneficial, it served as the control arm in RTOG 9202, a phase III trial that sought to answer whether the addition of 24 months of adjuvant AST could improve outcome in high-risk patients (50). There were 1,514 men accrued to this trial, and whole-pelvic radiotherapy (44 to 50 Gy) and a prostate dose of 65 to 70 Gy was mandated. The median pretreatment PSA was 20.4 ng/mL, 55% had clinical T3 to T4 disease, and 23% had Gleason score 8 to 10 disease. After a median follow-up of 5.8 years, the long-term AST arm had superior 5-year PSA control (71.0% vs. 44.5%; $p < 0.0001$), prostate cancer-specific survival (94.6% vs. 91.2%; $p = 0.006$), but not overall survival. On subgroup analysis, long-term AST significantly improved overall survival and cause-specific survival in the patients with Gleason score 8 to 10, whereas no advantage was seen in Gleason score 2 to 7 disease.

Therefore, it appears that for intermediate-risk patients, short-term AST (3 to 4 months of neoadjuvant and concurrent) appears to be sufficient, whereas for high-risk patients, the addition of long-term (≥ 2 years) adjuvant AST appears to confer improved outcomes.

Radiation Volume and Hormonal Therapy Considerations

There have been 11 published phase III trials studying AST and radiotherapy. All five landmark trials—4 RTOG studies and EORTC 22863—mandated pelvic radiotherapy (12,50,90, 91,96). Among these studies, the pretreatment characteristics were remarkably similar—median PSA >20 ng/mL and 20% to 30% with a Gleason score of 8 to 10. Applying the Roach formula to calculate the estimated occult pelvic nodal involvement, this risk is probably at least 20% (101). In contrast, the two contemporary studies, BWH and TROG 96.01, did not use pelvic radiotherapy (24,32). Their pretreatment characteristics were strikingly different from the landmark trials—median PSA 11 to

Table 63.4		**SUMMARY OF OUTCOME RESULTS FROM RANDOMIZED CONTROLLED TRIALS STUDYING THE DURATION AND SEQUENCING OF ANDROGEN SUPPRESSION THERAPY**			
Study (Reference)	**Median Follow-Up (years)**	**Study Arms**	**5-Year Overall Survival**	**5-Year Cause-Specific Survival**	**5-Year Biochemical Control**
Duration of Neoadjuvant Trials					
CUOG (20)	3.7	NHT (3 months)	85%		61%
		NHT (8 months)	88% ($p = 0.13$)	NR	62% ($p = 0.88$)
TROG 96.01 (32)	5.9	XRT alone		91%	38%
		NHT (3 months), C-HT		92% ($p = 0.7$)	52% ($p = 0.002$)
		NHT (6 months), C-HT	NR	94% ($p = 0.04$)	56% ($p < 0.0001$)
Duration of Adjuvant Trials					
RTOG 9202 (50)	5.8	NHT (2 months), C-HT	78.5%	91.2%	44.5%
		NHT (2 months), C-HT, AHT (24 months)	80.0% ($p = 0.73$)	94.6% ($p = 0.006$)	72.0% ($p < 0.0001$)
Quebec L-101 (74)	5	XRT alone			58%
		XRT + NHT (3 months)	NR	NR	76% ($p = 0.009$)
		XRT + NHT, C-HT, AHT (10 months)			74% ($p = 0.003$)
Quebec L-200 (74)	3.7	NHT, C-HT (5 months)			70%
		NHT, C-HT, AHT (10 months)	NR	NR	70% ($p = 0.55$)[a]
Sequencing Trials					
RTOG 9413 (96)	5	WPRT + NHT (2 months), C-HT	89%	NR	69.7%
			84%		63.3%
		WPRT + AHT (4 months)	86%		57.2%
		PORT + NHT (2 months), C-HT	87%		63.5%
		PORT + AHT (4 months)	($p = 0.08$)[b]		($p = 0.048$)[b]

AHT, adjuvant hormonal therapy; C-HT, concurrent hormonal therapy; CUOG, Canadian Urologic Oncology Group; NR, not recorded; NHT, neoadjuvant hormonal therapy; PORT, prostate-only radiotherapy; RTOG, Radiation Therapy Oncology Group; TROG, Trans-Tasman Radiation Oncology Group; WPRT, whole pelvic radiotherapy; XRT, external-beam radiotherapy
[a] L-200 bNED rates are 4 years.
[b] RTOG 9413 outcome results are 4 years. bNED rates are actuarial, whereas OS rates are nonactuarial.

15, and 15% to 17% with Gleason score 8 to 10, respectively. The estimated pelvic nodal involvement is probably <15%. Thus, it appears that omitting pelvic radiotherapy in intermediate-risk patients will not deprive them of the benefits of AST.

Recommendations of Androgen Suppression Therapy

On the basis of 11 published phase III trials, there is currently level 1 evidence addressing the efficacy, duration, or timing of combining AST and radiotherapy. At UCSF, our practice regarding integrating pelvic radiotherapy and hormonal therapy are summarized in Table 63.1. However, it is important to consider that all 11 trials used doses <72 Gy that would be considered suboptimal by today's standard. Whether the benefit of AST remains in the current era of dose escalation is currently unclear and certainly merits study.

Definition of Prostate-Specific Antigen Relapse after Radiotherapy

Given the natural history of prostate cancer and the fact that PSA relapse precedes clinical failure by a number of years, most oncologists use PSA relapse, rightly or wrongly, as a surrogate measure of the success of treatment. In 1996, the American Society for Therapeutic Radiology and Oncology (ASTRO) developed a consensus definition of PSA relapse based on data sets of patients treated with external-beam radiotherapy alone (i.e.,

no hormones) (5). However, because of a lack of any other definitions, the ASTRO definition has been inappropriately applied to series using hormonal therapy as well. The ASTRO definition has also been criticized for follow-up bias, censoring artifact from backdating and poor correlation with clinical progression (124,127). To address these issues, RTOG-ASTRO cosponsored a conference in 2005 in Phoenix, Arizona, to develop a new definition, henceforth known as the *Phoenix definition* (98). PSA relapse is defined as a rise of 2 ng/mL or more above the absolute PSA nadir. This definition is only applicable to patients treated with external-beam radiotherapy with or without short-term hormonal therapy. The date of failure is taken at the time of meeting the definition and not backdated. Any salvage therapy initiated prior to meeting the criteria should also be declared as failure. With the Phoenix definition, sensitivity and specificity is 64% and 78%, respectively.

Chemotherapy and Prostate Cancer

Despite the advances made in the management of high-risk or locally advanced prostate cancer with the combination of androgen suppression therapy with radiotherapy, 5-year biochemical control remains at only 40% to 70% (50,96). In the RTOG 8610 AST and radiotherapy arm, the risk of distance metastases was 34% at 10 years (90). More alarming is a study that showed that the 10-year estimated rate of prostate cancer mortality was 24% in patients with high-risk disease (25). The poor outcome may be explained by the presence of micrometastases and androgen-independent clonogens. This has led researchers to investigate the use of cytotoxic chemotherapy in the locally advanced subgroup.

Chemotherapy for Hormone-Refractory Prostate Cancer

Mitoxantrone was one of the first agents to be shown in large phase III trials to exhibit activity toward hormone-refractory prostate cancer (HRPC) (11,63,122). Although none of the studies demonstrated a survival advantage, they nonetheless introduced the notion that a nonhormonal systemic agent may be active in prostate cancer. The first reported study was from National Cancer Institute of Canada (NCIC) where 161 men with symptomatic HRPC were randomized to either mitoxantrone and prednisone (M+P), or prednisone (P) alone (122). A reduction in pain was seen in the M+P arm as compared to the P arm (29% vs. 12%; $p = 0.01$). The median duration of palliation was longer in the M+P arm (43 vs. 18 weeks; $p < 0.0001$). Although there was no difference in survival, this may have been masked by the crossover of nonresponding patients in the P arm to mitoxantrone. Cancer and Leukemia Group B (CALGB) 9182 randomized 242 men with HRPC to mitoxantrone and hydrocortisone (M+H), or hydrocortisone alone, and similarly found that there was no difference in survival, although time to progressive disease was increased in the M+H arm (122). PSA decreased by more than 50% in 37.5% versus 21.5% ($p = 0.008$) in favor of the M+H arm. However, the improvement in quality of life was smaller than the NCIC study, which may be because more than a third of patients in the CALGB study had no or minimal pain and the poor quality of life survey response rate. In asymptomatic, progressive HRPC, Berry et al. (11) found that M+P improved time to progression as compared to P. PSA was reduced by more than 50% in 48% versus 24% of men ($p = 0.007$), respectively.

Another systemic agent that has been studied is estramustine, a radiosensitizer, estradiol conjugate and microtubule stabilizer (36,105). Its synergistic effect with other antimicrotubule agents, such as vinblastine, etoposide, paclitaxel, and docetaxel, has been studied in HRPC (56). A phase II study, CALGB 9780 evaluated estramustine, docetaxel, and prednisone in 46 men with progressive HRPC (110). Of the 24 patients who had measurable disease, three patients had a complete response and nine patients had a partial response. Although 56% of patients had grade 3 or 4 granulocytopenia, there were no cases of febrile neutropenia. Thromboembolic events occurred in 9% of patients. Other single-agent microtubule inhibitors have also been shown to exhibit activity against HRPC (81). Beer et al. (8) reported that weekly docetaxel reduced the PSA by at least 50% in 46% of patients, and improved pain in 48%. Similarly, Berry et al. (10) demonstrated that weekly docetaxel reduced PSA in 41% of patients by at least 50%.

It was not until two recent docetaxel-based studies where a survival advantage from a chemotherapeutic agent could finally be observed. TAX-327 was a three-arm trial of 1,006 men with HRPC (121). All patients received prednisone and were randomized to docetaxel given every 3 weeks, weekly docetaxel, or mitoxantrone (control arm). Although only 46% of patients in the docetaxel every 3 weeks arm completed the treatment, the median survival was significantly improved from 16.4 months in the control arm to 18.9 months. Furthermore, pain response rates, PSA, and quality of life scores were superior in the docetaxel every 3 weeks arm. A similar study was Southwest Oncology Group (SWOG) 9916, which randomized 674 men with progressive HRPC to either docetaxel every 3 weeks and estramustine (D+E) or mitoxantrone and prednisone (M+P) (85). The median survival (17.5 vs. 15.6 months; $p = 0.02$), progression-free survival (6.3 vs. 3.2 months; $p < 0.0001$), and PSA response (50% vs. 27%; $p < 0.0001$) were significantly better in the D+E

arm. In both studies, the docetaxel-based regimen had significantly higher rates of grade 3 to 4 toxicities.

Although the efficacy of chemotherapy is clear in HRPC, the optimal point at which to deliver chemotherapy remains unclear (83). For instance, it is not known whether chemotherapy is equally or more effective when given earlier in the disease spectrum, such as in the setting of a rising PSA after definitive treatment.

Chemotherapy in Locally Advanced Prostate Cancer

The encouraging activity of systemic agents in HRPC prompted researchers to evaluate those agents earlier in the disease spectrum where an androgen-independent agent is sorely needed. Although there have been no phase III trials, a number of phase I and II trials are beginning to emerge (45,82,83).

Febbo et al. (39) reported on a phase II study that tested 6 months of weekly docetaxel prior to surgery in 19 patients with high-risk localized prostate cancer. PSA levels decreased by at least 50% in 58% of the patients, with an average reduction of 64% after 6 months. Of note, testosterone levels remained stable, suggesting that the PSA decrease was androgen independent. Endorectal MRI showed that the prostate tumor volume had decreased by at least 25% and 50% in 68% and 21%, respectively, of patients. Only three patients had grade ≥ 3 toxicities. From the Cleveland Clinic, Dreicer et al. (34) performed a phase II study of 6 weeks of preop weekly docetaxel in 29 patients with locally advanced disease. As expected with the shorter course, PSA reduction was less dramatic; pre- and postchemotherapy PSA were 12 and 8.4 ng/mL, respectively ($p < 0.03$). Only 24% of patients had at least a 50% drop in PSA. In both studies, no pathologic complete responses were seen.

The combined effects of hormones and chemotherapy have also been studied. Konety et al. (69) reported that the median PSA nadir was only 0.17 ng/mL after 12 to 16 weeks of TEC (paclitaxel, estramustine phosphate, and carboplatin) prior to surgery. Pettaway et al. (86) reported that after 12 weeks of neoadjuvant ketoconazole and doxorubicin alternating with vinblastine and estramustine, 50% of the patients had an undetectable PSA yet no pathologic complete response was observed. CUOG-P01a is a Canadian multicenter, phase II study evaluating the pathologic effects of 6 months of neoadjuvant LHRH agonist and weekly docetaxel in 72 men with high-risk disease (46). Of the 64 patients who completed protocol therapy, two had a pathologic complete response and 10 had residual microfoci of cancer. The bottom line is that combining hormones and chemotherapy will result in 50% to 75% of patients achieving an undetectable PSA, although pathologic complete response is seldom seen.

Chemotherapy and Definitive Radiotherapy

Given the radiosensitizing properties of microtubule inhibitors, clinical studies looking at radiation and these agents are beginning to emerge. Khil et al. (67) evaluated the combination of radiotherapy and concurrent estramustine with ($n = 46$) or without ($n = 19$) vinblastine in 65 patients with locally advanced prostate cancer. Sixty patients completed concurrent chemoradiation. The remaining five patients had leukopenia ($n = 2$), superficial phlebitis ($n = 2$), and elevated liver enzymes ($n = 1$), but nonetheless completed the radiotherapy component. By 6 weeks, PSA levels were undetectable in 86% of patients. The 5-year biochemical control rates was 46% (PSA <1.5 ng/mL), but patients with initial PSA levels <50 ng/mL had considerably better outcome of 60% to 64%. There was one grade 3 leukopenia, one grade 3 small bowel toxicity, and one grade 4 radiation proctitis necessitating a diverting colostomy. Khil et al.

concluded that the primary benefit of this approach appeared to be in patients with a PSA of 20 to 50 ng/mL. Ben-Josef et al. (9) performed a pilot study with neoadjuvant estramustine and etoposide followed by concurrent estramustine and definitive 3DCRT radiotherapy in 16 patients with locally advanced disease. No treatment-related mortality was observed, but there was one case of deep vein thrombosis (DVT), one case of ischemic heart disease (IHD), and two cases of grade 3 leukopenia (but no neutropenic fever). Fourteen patients completed the protocol therapy. Of seven patients who had a prostate biopsy at 18 months after completing therapy, five had local control. Testosterone recovered at a median of 4.2 months after completing therapy in all patients.

Zelefsky et al. (135) reported on the outcomes of estramustine and vinblastine with more contemporary methods (3DCRT) and doses of radiotherapy (75.6 Gy). Twenty-three of 27 patients with locally advanced disease completed all three cycles, with the last cycle given concurrently with radiotherapy. The median PSA nadir was of an undetectable level, and the median time to PSA nadir was 6.1 months. The only chemotherapy-related grade 3 or greater toxicities were hematologic (two patients) and hepatotoxicity (two patients). At 2 years, the rate of late grade 2 GI toxicity was 20%; no late grade 3 or 4 GI toxicities were seen. The 2-year rates of late grade 2 and 3 GU toxicities were 25% and 12%, respectively. Because of empiric aspirin, no DVT or IHD were seen. Updated results (median follow-up 60 months) showed that the 5-year PSA control was 34%, with the median time to relapse of 12 months (103). Despite 22% of patients initially presenting with nodal disease, 78% remained metastasis-free. Testosterone levels recovered in 48% of patients.

In a phase I trial, Kumar et al. (70) reported that the maximally tolerated dose of weekly docetaxel given concurrently with 3DCRT in locally advanced disease was 20 mg/m^2 after grade 3 diarrhea was observed after 21.6 and 37.8 Gy in the 25 mg/m^2 dose level.

Such encouraging data have prompted the initiation of several phase III trials to determine the clinical role of chemotherapy in the high-risk setting. The preliminary results of RTOG 9902 were recently presented (106). All patients received 8 weeks of AST then radiotherapy (70.2 Gy) and long-term adjuvant AST. Patients were then randomized to with or without four cycles of adjuvant estramustine, VP-16, and paclitaxel. Warfarin was routinely given because of the risk of DVT associated with estramustine. Grade 4 or 5 toxicities were significantly higher in the chemotherapy arm (34 vs. 0 patients), and there were significantly more grade ≥3 GI, cardiovascular, and DVT toxicities in the chemotherapy arm. One-year actuarial rate of DVT was 8% despite intense anticoagulation. Study accrual was suspended and subsequently closed because of unacceptable risk of thromboembolic disease.

Future Directions

Recently open to accrual, RTOG 0521 is a phase III trial studying a different chemotherapy regimen than RTOG 9902. Notably, estramustine, thought to be associated with thromboembolic disease, was excluded. All patients will receive 2 months of neoadjuvant, concurrent and 24 months of adjuvant AST with radiotherapy. Patients are randomized to with or without six cycles of adjuvant docetaxel and prednisone. A second study open to accrual is from the Dana-Farber Cancer Institute and Sanofi-Aventis. Patients will be randomized to with or without docetaxel in combination with 6 months of AST and radiotherapy.

The past two decades were marked by advancement in the management of intermediate- and high-risk prostate cancer with hormonal therapy. As more active cytotoxic agents are identified and evaluated, the next decade may very well be her-

alded by the introduction of chemotherapy into our treatment schema. In summary, cytotoxic agents have been shown to improve survival in HRPC. Presently, it remains investigational in the adjuvant setting. Considering the poor prognosis of patients with locally advanced disease, its role in the management of such patients is the subject of intense research. The premise of this multimodality approach is that chemotherapy will address hormone-insensitive cancer cells, whereas hormonal therapy will address the hormone-sensitive cells.

Biochemical Failure after Radical Prostatectomy

After radical prostatectomy (RP), 10-year biochemical control rates are approximately 75% (49,57). Faced with similar issues as seen in radiotherapy, the definition of biochemical failure after RP is controversial (2,43). Generally, the most widely accepted definition of biochemical failure is a postoperative PSA that exceeds 0.2 ng/mL. Technically, the aim of radical prostatectomy is to remove the entire prostate gland and in turn, the postoperative PSA should be undetectable. However, the frequency of benign prostate tissue at the surgical margin is not uncommon, estimated to occur in 11% in one series (112). The difficulty in interpreting a rising PSA after surgery is determining whether it represents residual benign glands, isolated local recurrence, or distant metastases, as the management is vastly different. In the former, no further treatment is required, whereas potentially curative salvage therapy is available for locally recurrent disease, and palliative hormonal therapy with or without chemotherapy is indicated for distant recurrence. Distinguishing local from distant recurrence is made even more difficult by the fact that an initially rising PSA predates the development of clinically detectable metastatic disease by a number of years (94). Regardless of the initial post-RP PSA, it is imperative to establish a PSA trend before declaring biochemical recurrence. In a study by Amling et al. (2), 51% of men with an initial post-RP PSA of 0.20 to 0.29 did not have a subsequent rise in PSA. The inability of PSA to differentiate isolated local failure from distant failure after PSA relapse has led many investigators to study pretreatment and posttreatment predictive factors.

Predictive Factors after Biochemical Failure

Local versus Distant Recurrence

Positive surgical margins (PSM) and extracapsular extension (ECE) are associated with increased risk of PSA recurrence and presumed local recurrence (49,57). Rates of PSM have been reported to be 5% to 53%, with variations due to surgeon experience, surgical technique, preop PSA, clinical stage, and ECE (35,131). In a multicenter study of 5,831 men treated with radical prostatectomy from eight international institutions, the 5-year biochemical control rates were 83.8% and 53.1% for men with negative and PSM, respectively ($p = 0.0001$) (64).

Many investigators have reported on the merits of Gleason score, time to PSA relapse, postradiation PSA nadir, and PSA doubling time (PSA-DT) after PSA failure as a predictor of distant metastases versus local recurrence and PCSM (76,94,95,107,116,133,137). Pound et al. (94) reported that time to PSA recurrence ≤2 years after surgery, Gleason score of 8 to 10, and PSA-DT ≤10 months predicted for metastatic disease. Lee et al. (76) reported similar findings, with a PSA-DT of <12 months and an interval of <12 months from end of radiotherapy to PSA rise as significant independent predictors of distant failure. In a multi-institutional analysis of 4,839 patients treated with radiotherapy alone, PSA nadir and time to PSA nadir were significant independent predictors of biochemical and distant failure-free survival (95). Eight-year biochemical control was 75%, 52%, 41%, and 18% and distant failure-free survival was 97%, 96%, 91%, and 73% with a PSA nadir of 0 to 0.49, 0.5 to 0.99, 1 to 1.99, and $\geq$2 ng/mL, respectively (p <0.0001). A nomogram incorporating PSA-DT has been created to predict risk of distant metastases (116).

On the basis of these findings, D'Amico et al. (21) demonstrated that some of these prognostic factors could be used to predict for clinically insignificant postop PSA rises. A preop PSA <10 ng/mL, <T2a, Gleason score <7, and preop PSA velocity $\leq$0.5 ng/mL per year were associated with a postop PSA-DT $\geq$12 months or no PSA failure. Conversely, patients with a Gleason score of 7 to 10 and preop PSA velocity >2 ng/mL per year were associated with a postop PSA-DT <3 months. In the first scenario, the benign rise in PSA may represent residual benign prostate tissue, and thus salvage radiotherapy may not be required. In the latter scenario, more aggressive therapies such as hormonal therapy with chemotherapy should be offered on protocol. Although provocative, these results will need to be independently validated.

Prostate Cancer-Specific Mortality

Sandler et al. (107) observed that a PSA-DT of less than 12 months had significantly greater PCSM than when it was more than 12 months. A study from Johns Hopkins found similar results, with PSA-DT, Gleason score ($\leq$7 vs. 8 to 10), and disease-free interval ($\leq$3 vs. >3 years) independently associated with PCSM (42). Compiled from two multi-institutional databases with a cumulative cohort of 8,669 men treated with surgery or radiotherapy, CaPSURE and CPDR, Zhou et al. (137) showed that a PSA-DT of less than 3 months (p <0.0001) and Gleason score of 8 to 10 (p <0.0001) were significantly associated with PCSM.

Adjuvant Radiotherapy

The argument for adjuvant radiotherapy (ART) is that patients with positive surgical margins (PSM) and/or extracapsular extension (ECE) after radical prostatectomy are at an increased risk of local recurrence. Yet it is also known that having either ECE or PSM does not necessarily mean that local recurrence is inevitable. Epstein et al. (37) reported on 617 men with clinically confined disease treated with radical prostatectomy and found that despite ECE, the 10-year progression-free survival was 58.4% to 67.7% depending on the extent. By the same token, 10-year progression-free survival was 54.9% in men with PSM. Progression was independently predicted by Gleason score, PSM, and ECE.

How common are PSM and ECE seen? In a large series from Memorial Sloan-Kettering Cancer Center and Baylor College of Medicine, the outcome of 4,629 men with T1 to T3 prostate cancer were analyzed (35). Overall, PSM were seen in 20% of cases (range 0% to 48%). ECE was observed in 30.1% of cases. When only surgeons who had contributed more than 10 cases were considered, the rate of PSM ranged from 10% to 48%. Independent predictors of PSM were PSA, Gleason score, ECE, the surgeon, and surgical volume.

When one considers that data from CaPSURE show that 49% and 23% of intermediate- and high-risk patients had a radical prostatectomy from 1999 to 2001, the number of patients who potentially have PSM or ECE is by no means trivial (16). Yet only 8% of high-risk patients who were operated on received ART (18). The prevalence of understaging—deemed to be clinically organ-confined disease but later found to have pathologic stage T3 to T4 or node-positive disease—of prostate cancers was reported by Grossfeld et al. (48) to be 24%. Preop PSA, Gleason score, and percentage of positive biopsy cores were reported to be significant predictors of understaging.

Recently, the results of three large phase III trials, which evaluated the merits of adjuvant versus expectant management in postop patients with PSM and/or pT3 disease, were reported (14,119,132). EORTC 22911 consisted of 1,005 men with pT2-3N0 and at least one of the following risk factors: ECE, PSM, or seminal vesicle invasion (SVI). In the ART arm, radiation was commenced at a median of 90 days postop. ART consisted of 50 Gy in 25 fractions to a large volume that encompassed the surgical limits and subclinical disease, followed by 10 Gy boost given over five fractions to a reduced margin around the prostatic bed. The protocol salvage radiotherapy dose fractionation was 70 Gy in 35 fractions. The median preop (12.3 to 12.4 ng/mL) and postop PSA (0.2 ng/mL) were not significantly different between the two arms. The proportion of patients with risk factors in the delayed and adjuvant radiotherapy arms, respectively, are as follows: ECE (78.9% vs. 75.1%), SVI (25.4% vs. 25.5%), and PSM (63.0% vs. 62.2%). In the ART arm, 99.1% received at least the protocol dose of 60 Gy. Toxicity was surprisingly mild. Radiotherapy was interrupted due to toxicities in only 3.1%, with diarrhea responsible in eight of the 14 patients. In the ART arm, grade 3 diarrhea (5.3%) and urinary frequency (3.3%) were relatively low; the only grade 4 toxicity was urinary frequency (0.4%). There was no added risk of urinary incontinence with ART. The 5-year rates of grade 3 late toxicities was 2.6% (delayed arm) and 4.2% (ART arm; p = 0.0725). Five-year biochemical progression-free survival was significantly improved from 52.6% to 74.0% (p <0.0001) with ART, representing a 52% reduction in PSA relapse. Five-year locoregional failure was significantly lower in the ART arm (5.4% vs. 15.4%; p <0.0001). Of note, in the delayed arm, 163 (79%) of the 207 patients who relapsed were offered active treatment, of whom 69% (n = 113) received radiotherapy and 28% received hormonal therapy. Treatment in the delayed arm was initiated upon PSA relapse (61.3%) and locoregional progression (34.4%), and was commenced at a median time of 2.2 years. The limitations of this study were the use of conventional radiotherapy, suboptimal adjuvant dose, inclusion of patients with a potentially elevated postop PSA (10.7%), and variability in the management of relapsed patients in the delayed arm.

SWOG 8794 randomly assigned 473 node-negative patients initially treated with radical prostatectomy but found to have either PSM or pT3 (ECE and/or SVI) disease to ART or observation (119). Approximately half of patients had a detectable PSA following surgery. ART consisted of 60 to 64 Gy. The 5- and 10-year biochemical disease-free survival was significantly improved in the ART arm (61% vs. 38%, 47% vs. 23%, respectively). With a median follow-up of 9.7 years, there was a trend toward increased 10-year metastases-free survival (83% vs. 61%) and overall survival (74% vs. 63%) in favor of ART. Interestingly, in the subset of patients with SVI, ART conferred a benefit in biochemical disease-free survival (57% vs. 22%). In the observation arm, 32% of patients eventually received salvage radiotherapy. Hormonal therapy was initiated later (median 12.4 vs. 9.9 years) and less frequently (39% vs. 50%) in the ART arm.

From the German Cancer Society, ARO 96-02/AUO AP 09/95 randomized 385 patients from 22 centers with pT3 or PSM to either ART (60 Gy in 2 Gy fractions) or observation (132). Patients who were subsequently found to have a detectable postop PSA were categorized as progressive disease and given 66.6 Gy, regardless of the original randomization. 3DCRT was directed to the prostatic fossa and region of the seminal vesicles. Of the three phase III trials, this study had the shortest median follow-up of 40 months. Using intention-to-treat analysis of only patients who achieved an undetectable postop PSA, ART significantly improved progression-free survival (p <0.0001).

When analyzed according to the received treatment, 4-year progression-free survival was 81% versus 61% in favor of ART (p <0.0001). ART was very well tolerated, with only 3% reporting acute grade 3 bladder toxicity and none with grade 3 rectal toxicity (12% had grade 2 rectal toxicity). Late grade 2 and 3 rectal toxicity was seen in 3% and 0%, and bladder toxicity was observed in 5% and 2%, respectively. Of note, the compliance in the ART arm was surprisingly poor—21% did not proceed with radiotherapy.

The EORTC 22911, SWOG 8794, and ARO 96-02/AUO 09/95 provide consistent level 1 evidence that adjuvant radiotherapy is better than expectant management in terms of biochemical control, at an acceptable toxicity costs. It remains to be seen whether with longer follow-up this translates to an improvement in survival. Questions also remain whether the lessons learned from the definitive radiotherapy trials, such as pelvic radiotherapy, hormonal therapy, and dose escalation, have any role in the adjuvant setting. Furthermore, it is unclear whether a strategy of active surveillance with PSA tests and the early initiation of radiotherapy only when PSA has shown an upward trend can yield equivalent or better results. The advantage of such an approach is that perhaps the 50% of patients who do not relapse after surgery will be spared from radiotherapy. The disadvantage is that biochemical control may be compromised by waiting too long to intervene with definitive treatment, which could serve as a nidus for metastatic spread.

Adjuvant versus Salvage Radiotherapy

As discussed, the findings from EORTC 22911, SWOG 8794, and ARO 96-02/AUO 09/95 strongly advocate for the use of ART. Yet none of these trials address the concept of early salvage radiotherapy given when the PSA is still low. The attraction of this strategy is that only half of the patients with adverse pathologic features will relapse (37).

In a multi-institutional study, Stephenson et al. (118) reported on the outcomes and prognostic factors of 501 men who had salvage radiotherapy after a biochemical recurrence. Overall, 32% had a persistent detectable postop PSA. Seventeen percent of patients had preradiotherapy hormones (median duration of 3 months). The median radiation dose was 64.8 Gy, and 5% received pelvic irradiation. The median follow-up after surgery and radiotherapy were 81 and 45 months, respectively. In the entire cohort, the 4-year progression-free survival (PFS) was 45%, and 67% attained a PSA nadir of ≤0.1 ng/mL. Multivariate analyses demonstrated that Gleason score of 8 to 10, preradiotherapy PSA >2 ng/mL, negative margins, PSA-DT ≤10 months, and seminal vesicle invasion were associated with PSA progression. Supporting earlier intervention, preradiotherapy PSA of 0.6 ng/mL or less had significantly improved PFS than a PSA of 0.61 to 2 ng/mL (p = 0.006) and

more than 2 ng/mL (p <0.001). On subgroup analysis, 46 patients with no adverse prognostic factors had a 4-year PFS of 77%. Interestingly, the estimated outcome of subgroups of patients with seemingly adverse features yet had early salvage radiotherapy—preradiotherapy PSA ≤2 ng/mL—is not as futile as once thought. In the 77 patients with only PSA doubling time of ≤10 months as an adverse feature, the PFS was 64%. Similarly, in the group that had Gleason scores of 8 to 10 but a PSA-DT >10 months and positive surgical margins, the PFS was 81%. Patients who had delayed salvage radiotherapy (preradiotherapy PSA >2 ng/mL) had inferior PFS (12% to 22%).

Androgen Suppression Therapy and Postoperative Radiotherapy

Based on the established benefits of adding hormonal therapy to definitive radiotherapy, some investigators have extrapolated those results to the postoperative setting (19,31,38,65,68,117,123). The results are summarized in Table 63.5. All were retrospective studies, except for the subgroup analysis of RTOG 8531 by Corn et al. (19), with varying duration of hormonal therapy, median follow-up, and PSA failure definition.

In RTOG 8531, 141 postop patients with node-positive, ECE, and/or SVI were randomized to postoperative radiotherapy with immediate or delayed hormonal therapy (19). This subgroup received 60 to 65 Gy with optional nodal irradiation. Five-year freedom from biochemical relapse was 65% and 42% (p = 0.002) in favor of the adjuvant hormonal therapy arm. There was no difference in rates of distant metastases or overall survival. The addition of adjuvant hormonal therapy did not significantly change the toxicity profile.

In a systematic review, the complication-adjusted number needed to treat (NNT) method was used to evaluate the net benefit in terms of biochemical control in the context of hormone-related complications (59). The NNT method calculates the number of patients needed to receive hormonal therapy to improve biochemical control for one patient. The overall unadjusted NNT was 4.8. When adjusted for complications, the NNT varied from 4.8 to 5 depending on the assumptions made regarding toxicities of hormone. There was no significant difference when stratified by adjuvant or salvage radiotherapy. Jani et al. (59) noted that the magnitude of benefit was similar to the setting of hormonal and radiotherapy for an intact prostate.

Results are eagerly anticipated from RTOG 9601, which evaluated the role of hormonal therapy in adjuvant/salvage radiotherapy. Rather than an LHRH agonist, RTOG 9601 used 2 years of 150 mg daily of bicalutamide, a second-generation nonsteroidal antiandrogen. The eligibility criteria were as follows: pT3N0, pT2N0, and positive margins or biopsy-confirmed local

Table 63.5	SELECTED STUDIES COMPARING THE BIOCHEMICAL DISEASE-FREE SURVIVAL BETWEEN POSTOPERATIVE RADIOTHERAPY ALONE OR WITH HORMONAL THERAPY				
			Biochemical Disease-Free Survival	
Study (Reference)	Hormone Duration (months)	No. of Patients RT/RT+HT	RT Alone (%)	RT + HT (%)
Eulau et al. (38)	6	74/29	27	56
RTOG 8531 (19)	Indefinite	68/71	42	65
Song et al. (117)	4	31/30	39	39
de la Taille et al. (31)	4–6	18/34	32	61
Taylor et al. (123)	24	36/35	54	81
Katz et al. (65)	3	70/45	39	59
King et al. (68)	4	69/53	31	57

HT, hormonal therapy; RT, radiotherapy.

recurrence at time of rising PSA, and a study entry PSA ≥ 0.2 and ≤ 4 ng/mL (as persistent or relapse). The protocol mandates no pelvic irradiation and a total dose of 64.8 Gy given in 1.8 Gy fractions. In summary, the evidence to date—limited as it is—suggests that the inclusion of hormonal therapy to postoperative radiotherapy may be beneficial.

Postoperative Radiotherapy Dose Response

Currently, adjuvant radiotherapy doses of 60 to 64 Gy and salvage radiotherapy doses of 66 to 70 Gy appear to be the most commonly used. Valicenti et al. (125) reported on a dose-response effect in 86 patients with pT3N0 prostate cancer. None of the patients received hormonal therapy. Radiotherapy was given between 3 to 6 months after surgery in 90% of patients. The radiation dose ranged from 55 to 70.2 Gy (median dose 64.8 Gy). Among the 52 patients with an undetectable preradiotherapy PSA, 3-year PSA control was significantly better in patients who received 61.5 Gy or more than those who received a lower dose (91% vs. 57%; $p = 0.01$). In the 21 patients with a preradiotherapy PSA of 0.2 to 2 ng/mL, a dose response cut-off was seen with 64.8 Gy (79% vs. 33%; $p = 0.02$). These results were corroborated by Anscher et al. (3), who found that a salvage dose of more than 65 Gy was associated with improved disease-free survival.

University of California–San Francisco Recommendations of Postoperative Radiotherapy

All patients with adverse pathologic features (i.e., ECE, PSM, SVI) should be assessed by a radiation oncologist. Depending on the preop clinical features such as PSA kinetics, Gleason score, percentage of positive biopsy cores, and postop PSA nadir, a metastatic work-up may be warranted, if it has not been done already. In addition, we recommend a transrectal ultrasound of the tumor bed to assess and biopsy any residual prostate tissue. Patients with a postop PSA nadir <0.2 are offered adjuvant radiotherapy or active surveillance. In the latter option, patients return every 3 months for history and physical examination, digital rectal examination, and PSA measurement. If there is a clear rising trend in the PSA, salvage radiotherapy is offered.

Other important considerations are the patient's postop urinary function and estimated life expectancy. We tend to favor delaying radiotherapy in patients with significant urinary symptoms or incontinence secondary to the surgery, and patients with significant comorbidities such that the estimated life expectancy is less than 5 to 10 years.

We recommend patients to undergo implantation of two fiducial gold seed markers into the bladder neck and anastomotic site (111). For adjuvant patients, we prescribe 64 to 66 Gy, whereas for salvage patients, we use 70.2 Gy, both of which are in 1.8-Gy fractions. Whole pelvic radiotherapy to a dose of 45 Gy is considered depending on the extent of pelvic lymph node dissection, presence of seminal vesicle invasion, and the estimated nodal involvement. The same technique as described earlier in this chapter is used. With the results of RTOG 9601 pending, we tend to favor adding hormonal therapy.

References

1. Allaf ME, Palapattu GS, Trock BJ, et al. Anatomical extent of lymph node dissection: Impact on men with clinically localized prostate cancer. *J Urol* 2004;172:1840–1844.
2. Amling CL, Bergstralh EJ, Blute ML, et al. Defining prostate specific antigen progression after radical prostatectomy: What is the most appropriate cut point? *J Urol* 2001;165:1146–1151.
3. Anscher MS, Clough R, Dodge R. Radiotherapy for a rising prostate-specific antigen after radical prostatectomy: The first 10 years. *Int J Radiat Oncol Biol Phys* 2000;48:369–375.
4. Ashman JB, Zelefsky MJ, Hunt MS, et al. Whole pelvic radiotherapy for prostate cancer using 3D conformal and intensity-modulated radiotherapy. *Int J Radiat Oncol Biol Phys* 2005;63:765–771.
5. ASTRO Consensus statement: Guidelines for PSA following radiation therapy. American Society for Therapeutic Radiology and Oncology Consensus Panel [see comments]. *Int J Radiat Oncol Biol Phys* 1997;37:1035–1041.
6. Bader P, Burkhard FC, Markwalder R, et al. Disease progression and survival of patients with positive lymph nodes after radical prostatectomy. Is there a chance of cure? *J Urol* 2003;169:849–854.
7. Bader P, Burkhard FC, Markwalder R, et al. Is a limited lymph node dissection an adequate staging procedure for prostate cancer? *J Urol* 2002;168:514–518; discussion 518.
8. Beer TM, Pierce WC, Lowe BA, et al. Phase II study of weekly docetaxel in symptomatic androgen-independent prostate cancer. *Ann Oncol* 2001;12:1273–1279.
9. Ben-Josef E, Porter AT, Han S, et al. Neoadjuvant estramustine and etoposide followed by concurrent estramustine and definitive radiotherapy for locally advanced prostate cancer: Feasibility and preliminary results. *Int J Radiat Oncol Biol Phys* 2001;49:699–703.
10. Berry W, Dakhil S, Gregurich MA, et al. Phase II trial of single-agent weekly docetaxel in hormone-refractory, symptomatic, metastatic carcinoma of the prostate. *Semin Oncol* 2001;28:8–15.
11. Berry W, Dakhil S, Modiano M, et al. Phase III study of mitoxantrone plus low dose prednisone versus low dose prednisone alone in patients with asymptomatic hormone refractory prostate cancer. *J Urol* 2002;168:2439–2443.
12. Bolla M, Collette L, Blank L, et al. Long-term results with immediate androgen suppression and external irradiation in patients with locally advanced prostate cancer (an EORTC study): A phase III randomised trial. *Lancet* 2002;360:103–106.
13. Bolla M, Gonzalez D, Warde P, et al. Improved survival in patients with locally advanced prostate cancer treated with radiotherapy and goserelin [see comments]. *N Engl J Med* 1997;337:295–300.
14. Bolla M, van Poppel H, Collette L, et al. Postoperative radiotherapy after radical prostatectomy: A randomised controlled trial (EORTC trial 22911). *Lancet* 2005;366:572–578.
15. Chen H, Xia P, Verhey L, et al. Dosimetric consequences to the pelvic lymph nodes due to daily motion of the prostate. *Int J Radiat Oncol Biol Phys* 2004;60:S479.
16. Cooperberg MR, Grossfeld GD, Lubeck DP, et al. National practice patterns and time trends in androgen ablation for localized prostate cancer. *J Natl Cancer Inst* 2003;95:981–989.
17. Cooperberg MR, Lubeck DP, Mehta SS, et al. Time trends in clinical risk stratification for prostate cancer: Implications for outcomes (data from CaPSURE). *J Urol* 2003;170:S21–S25; discussion S26–S27.
18. Cooperberg MR, Moul JW, Carroll PR. The changing face of prostate cancer. *J Clin Oncol* 2005;23:8146–8151.
19. Corn BW, Winter K, Pilepich MV. Does androgen suppression enhance the efficacy of postoperative irradiation? A secondary analysis of RTOG 85-31. Radiation Therapy Oncology Group. *Urology* 1999;54:495–502.
20. Crook J, Ludgate C, Malone S, et al. Report of a multicenter Canadian phase III randomized trial of 3 months vs. 8 months neoadjuvant androgen deprivation before standard-dose radiotherapy for clinically localized prostate cancer. *Int J Radiat Oncol Biol Phys* 2001;60:15–23.
21. D'Amico AV, Chen M-H, Roehl KA, et al. Identifying patients at risk for significant versus clinically insignificant postoperative prostate-specific antigen failure. *J Clin Oncol* 2005;23:4975–4979.
22. D'Amico AV, Chen M-H, Roehl KA, et al. Preoperative PSA velocity and the risk of death from prostate cancer after radical prostatectomy. *N Engl J Med* 2004;351:125–135.
23. D'Amico AV, Keshaviah A, Manola J, et al. Clinical utility of the percentage of positive prostate biopsies in predicting prostate cancer-specific and overall survival after radiotherapy for patients with localized prostate cancer. *Int J Radiat Oncol Biol Phys* 2002;53:581–587.
24. D'Amico AV, Manola J, Loffredo M, et al. 6-month androgen suppression plus radiation therapy vs radiation therapy alone for patients with clinically localized prostate cancer: A randomized controlled trial. *JAMA* 2004;292:821–827.
25. D'Amico AV, Moul J, Carroll PR, et al. Cancer-specific mortality after surgery or radiation for patients with clinically localized prostate cancer managed during the prostate-specific antigen era. *J Clin Oncol* 2003;21:2163–2172.
26. D'Amico AV, Renshaw AA, Sussman B, et al. Pretreatment PSA velocity and risk of death from prostate cancer following external beam radiation therapy. *JAMA* 2005;294:440–447.
27. D'Amico AV, Schultz D, Silver B, et al. The clinical utility of the percent of positive prostate biopsies in predicting biochemical outcome following external-beam radiation therapy for patients with clinically localized prostate cancer. *Int J Radiat Oncol Biol Phys* 2001;49:679–684.
28. D'Amico AV, Whittington R, Malkowicz SB, et al. Biochemical outcome after radical prostatectomy, external beam radiation therapy, or interstitial radiation therapy for clinically localized prostate cancer [see comments]. *JAMA* 1998;280:969–974.
29. D'Amico AV, Whittington R, Malkowicz SB, et al. Clinical utility of the percentage of positive prostate biopsies in defining biochemical outcome after radical prostatectomy for patients with clinically localized prostate cancer [see comments]. *J Clin Oncol* 2000;18:1164–1172.
30. De Jong IJ, Pruim J, Elsinga PH, et al. Preoperative staging of pelvic lymph nodes in prostate cancer by 11C-choline PET. *J Nucl Med* 2003;44:331–335.
31. De la Taille A, Flam TA, Thiounn N, et al. Predictive factors of radiation therapy for patients with prostate specific antigen recurrence after radical prostatectomy. *BJU Int* 2002;90:887–892.
32. Denham JW, Steigler A, Lamb DS, et al. Short-term androgen deprivation and radiotherapy for locally advanced prostate cancer: Results from the Trans-Tasman Radiation Oncology Group 96.01 randomised controlled trial. *Lancet Oncol* 2005;6:841–850.
33. Diamond TH, Higano CS, Smith MR, et al. Osteoporosis in men with prostate carcinoma receiving androgen-deprivation therapy: Recommendations for diagnosis and therapies. *Cancer* 2004;100:892–899.
34. Dreicer R, Magi-Galluzzi C, Zhou M, et al. Phase II trial of neoadjuvant

docetaxel before radical prostatectomy for locally advanced prostate cancer. *Urology* 2004;63:1138–1142.
35. Eastham JA, Kattan MW, Riedel E, et al. Variations among individual surgeons in the rate of positive surgical margins in radical prostatectomy specimens. *J Urol* 2003;170:2292–2295.
36. Eklov S, Essand M, Carlsson J, et al. Radiation sensitization by estramustine studies on cultured human prostatic cancer cells. *Prostate* 1992;21:287–295.
37. Epstein JI, Partin AW, Sauvageot J, et al. Prediction of progression following radical prostatectomy. A multivariate analysis of 721 men with long-term follow-up. *Am J Surg Pathol* 1996;20:286–292.
38. Eulau SM, Tate DJ, Stamey TA, et al. Effect of combined transient androgen deprivation and irradiation following radical prostatectomy for prostatic cancer. *Int J Radiat Oncol Biol Phys* 1998;41:735–740.
39. Febbo PG, Richie JP, George DJ, et al. Neoadjuvant docetaxel before radical prostatectomy in patients with high-risk localized prostate cancer. *Clin Cancer Res* 2005;11:5233–5240.
40. Fiveash JB, Hanks G, Roach M, et al. 3D conformal radiation therapy (3DCRT) for high grade prostate cancer: A multi-institutional review. *Int J Radiat Oncol Biol Phys* 2000;47:335–342.
41. Freedland SJ, Csathy GS, Dorey F, et al. Percent prostate needle biopsy tissue with cancer is more predictive of biochemical failure or adverse pathology after radical prostatectomy than prostate specific antigen or Gleason score. *J Urol* 2002;167:516–520.
42. Freedland SJ, Humphreys EB, Mangold LA, et al. Risk of prostate cancer-specific mortality following biochemical recurrence after radical prostatectomy. *JAMA* 2005;294:433–439.
43. Freedland SJ, Sutter ME, Dorey F, et al. Defining the ideal cutpoint for determining PSA recurrence after radical prostatectomy. Prostate-specific antigen. *Urology* 2003;61:365–369.
44. Gancarczyk KJ, Wu H, McLeod DG, et al. Using the percentage of biopsy cores positive for cancer, pretreatment PSA, and highest biopsy Gleason sum to predict pathologic stage after radical prostatectomy: The Center for Prostate Disease Research nomograms. *Urology* 2003;61:589–595.
45. Gleave M, Kelly WK. High-risk localized prostate cancer: A case for early chemotherapy. *J Clin Oncol* 2005;23:8186–8191.
46. Gleave ME, Chi KN, Goldenberg L, et al. Multicentre phase II trial of combination neoadjuvant hormone therapy and weekly docetaxel prior to radical prostatectomy in high risk localized prostate cancer (CUOG-P01a). *J Clin Oncol (Meeting Abstracts)* 2004;22:4635.
47. Granfors T, Modig H, Damber JE, et al. Combined orchiectomy and external radiotherapy versus radiotherapy alone for nonmetastatic prostate cancer with or without pelvic lymph node involvement: A prospective randomized study. *J Urol* 1998;159:2030–2034.
48. Grossfeld GD, Chang JJ, Broering JM, et al. Under staging and under grading in a contemporary series of patients undergoing radical prostatectomy: Results from the Cancer of the Prostate Strategic Urologic Research Endeavor database. *J Urol* 2001;165:851–856.
49. Han M, Partin AW, Pound CR, et al. Long-term biochemical disease-free and cancer-specific survival following anatomic radical retropubic prostatectomy. The 15-year Johns Hopkins experience. *Urol Clin North Am* 2001;28:555–565.
50. Hanks GE, Pajak TF, Porter A, et al. Phase III trial of long-term adjuvant androgen deprivation after neoadjuvant hormonal cytoreduction and radiotherapy in locally advanced carcinoma of the prostate: The Radiation Therapy Oncology Group protocol 92-02. *J Clin Oncol* 2003;21:3972–3978.
51. Harisinghani MG, Barentsz J, Hahn PF, et al. Noninvasive detection of clinically occult lymph-node metastases in prostate cancer. *N Engl J Med* 2003;348:2491–2499.
52. Heidenreich A, Varga Z, Von Knobloch R. Extended pelvic lymphadenectomy in patients undergoing radical prostatectomy: High incidence of lymph node metastasis. *J Urol* 2002;167:1681–1686.
53. Hellerstedt BA, Pienta KJ. The current state of hormonal therapy for prostate cancer. *CA Cancer J Clin* 2002;52:154–179.
54. Higano CS. Side effects of androgen deprivation therapy: Monitoring and minimizing toxicity. *Urology* 2003;61:32–38.
55. Hsu IC, Cabrera AR, Weinberg V, et al. Combined modality treatment with high-dose-rate brachytherapy boost for locally advanced prostate cancer. *Brachytherapy* 2005;4:202–206.
56. Hudes G. Estramustine-based chemotherapy. *Semin Urol Oncol* 1997;15:13–19.
57. Hull GW, Rabbani F, Abbas F, et al. Cancer control with radical prostatectomy alone in 1,000 consecutive patients. *J Urol* 2002;167:528–534.
58. Jacob R, Hanlon AL, Horwitz EM, et al. Role of prostate dose escalation in patients with greater than 15% risk of pelvic lymph node involvement. *Int J Radiat Oncol Biol Phys* 2005;61:695–701.
59. Jani AB, Sokoloff M, Shalhav A, et al. Androgen ablation adjuvant to postprostatectomy radiotherapy: Complication-adjusted number needed to treat analysis. *Urology* 2004;64:976–981.
60. Jani AB, Su A, Milano MT. Intensity-modulated versus conventional pelvic radiotherapy for prostate cancer: Analysis of acute toxicity. *Urology* 2006;67:147–151.
61. Jemal A, Siegel R, Ward E, et al. Cancer statistics, 2006. *CA Cancer J Clin* 2006;56:106–130.
62. Kaminski JM, Hanlon AL, Joon DL, et al. Effect of sequencing of androgen deprivation and radiotherapy on prostate cancer growth. *Int J Radiat Oncol Biol Phys* 2003;57:24–28.
63. Kantoff PW, Halabi S, Conaway M, et al. Hydrocortisone with or without mitoxantrone in men with hormone-refractory prostate cancer: Results of the Cancer and Leukemia Group B 9182 Study. *J Clin Oncol* 1999;17:2506.
64. Karakiewicz PI, Eastham JA, Graefen M, et al. Prognostic impact of positive surgical margins in surgically treated prostate cancer: Multi-institutional assessment of 5831 patients. *Urology* 2005;66:1245–1250.
65. Katz MS, Zelefsky MJ, Venkatraman ES, et al. Predictors of biochemical outcome with salvage conformal radiotherapy after radical prostatectomy for prostate cancer. *J Clin Oncol* 2003;21:483–489.
66. Kestin LL, Goldstein NS, Vicini FA, et al. Percentage of positive biopsy cores as predictor of clinical outcome in prostate cancer treated with radiotherapy [comment]. *J Urol* 2002;168:1994–1999.
67. Khil MS, Kim JH, Bricker LJ, et al. Tumor control of locally advanced prostate cancer following combined estramustine, vinblastine, and radiation therapy. *Cancer J Sci Am* 1997;3:289–296.
68. King CR, Presti JC Jr. , Gill H, et al. Radiotherapy after radical prostatectomy: Does transient androgen suppression improve outcomes? *Int J Radiat Oncol Biol Phys* 2004;59:341–347.
69. Konety BR, Eastham JA, Reuter VE, et al. Feasibility of radical prostatectomy after neoadjuvant chemohormonal therapy for patients with high risk or locally advanced prostate cancer: Results of a phase I/II study. *J Urol* 2004;171:709–713.
70. Kumar P, Perrotti M, Weiss R, et al. Phase I trial of weekly docetaxel with concurrent three-dimensional conformal radiation therapy in the treatment of unfavorable localized adenocarcinoma of the prostate. *J Clin Oncol* 2004;22:1909–1915.
71. Kupelian P, Kuban D, Thames H, et al. Improved biochemical relapse-free survival with increased external radiation doses in patients with localized prostate cancer: The combined experience of nine institutions in patients treated in 1994 and 1995. *Int J Radiat Oncol Biol Phys* 2005;61:415–419.
72. Kupelian PA, Willoughby TR, Meeks SL, et al. Intraprostatic fiducials for localization of the prostate gland: Monitoring intermarker distances during radiation therapy to test for marker stability. *Int J Radiat Oncol Biol Phys* 2005;62:1291–1296.
73. Laverdiere J, Gomez JL, Cusan L, et al. Beneficial effect of combination hormonal therapy administered prior and following external beam radiation therapy in localized prostate cancer. *Int J Radiat Oncol Biol Phys* 1997;37:247–252.
74. Laverdiere J, Nabid A, De Bedoya LD, et al. The efficacy and sequencing of a short course of androgen suppression on freedom from biochemical failure when administered with radiation therapy for T2-T3 prostate cancer. *J Urol* 2004;171:1137–1140.
75. Lee WR, Desilvio M, Lawton C, et al. A phase II study of external beam radiotherapy combined with permanent source brachytherapy for intermediate-risk, clinically localized adenocarcinoma of the prostate: Preliminary results of RTOG P-0019. *Int J Radiat Oncol Biol Phys* 2006;64:804–809.
76. Lee WR, Hanks GE, Hanlon A. Increasing prostate-specific antigen profile following definitive radiation therapy for localized prostate cancer: Clinical observations. *J Clin Oncol* 1997;15:230–238.
77. Lee WR, Moughan J, Owen JB, et al. The 1999 patterns of care study of radiotherapy in localized prostate carcinoma: A comprehensive survey of prostate brachytherapy in the United States. *Cancer* 2003;98:1987–1994.
78. Lotan Y, Shariat SF, Khoddami SM, et al. The percent of biopsy cores positive for cancer is a predictor of advanced pathological stage and poor clinical outcomes in patients treated with radical prostatectomy. *J Urol* 2004;171:2209–2214.
79. Messing EM, Manola J, Sarosdy M, et al. Immediate hormonal therapy compared with observation after radical prostatectomy and pelvic lymphadenectomy in men with node-positive prostate cancer. *N Engl J Med* 1999;341:1781–1788.
80. Michalski JM, Winter KA, Roach M, et al. Clinical outcome of patients treated with 3D conformal radiation therapy 3D-CRT for prostate cancer on RTOG 9406. Presented at: Prostate Cancer Symposium. 2005; Orlando, FL.
81. Obasaju C, Hudes GR. Paclitaxel and docetaxel in prostate cancer. *Hematol Oncol Clin North Am* 2001;15:525–545.
82. Oh WK. An overview of chemotherapy trials in localized and recurrent nonmetastatic prostate cancer. *J Urol* 2004;172:S34–S37; discussion S37.
83. Oh WK. High-risk localized prostate cancer: Integrating chemotherapy. *Oncologist* 2005;10[Suppl 2]:18–22.
84. Paquette EL, Sun L, Paquette LR, et al. Improved prostate cancer-specific survival and other disease parameters: Impact of prostate-specific antigen testing. *Urology* 2002;60:756–759.
85. Petrylak DP, Tangen CM, Hussain MHA, et al. Docetaxel and estramustine compared with mitoxantrone and prednisone for advanced refractory prostate cancer. *N Engl J Med* 2004;351:1513–1520.
86. Pettaway CA, Pisters LL, Troncoso P, et al. Neoadjuvant chemotherapy and hormonal therapy followed by radical prostatectomy: Feasibility and preliminary results. *J Clin Oncol* 2000;18:1050–1057.
87. Pickles T, Agranovich A, Berthelet E, et al. Testosterone recovery following prolonged adjuvant androgen ablation for prostate carcinoma. *Cancer* 2002;94:362–367.
88. Pilepich MV, Caplan R, Byhardt RW, et al. Phase III trial of androgen suppression using goserelin in unfavorable-prognosis carcinoma of the prostate treated with definitive radiotherapy: Report of Radiation Therapy Oncology Group protocol 85-31. *J Clin Oncol* 1997;15:1013–1021.
89. Pilepich MV, Krall JM, al-Sarraf M, et al. Androgen deprivation with radiation therapy compared with radiation therapy alone for locally advanced prostatic carcinoma: A randomized comparative trial of the Radiation Therapy Oncology Group [see comments]. *Urology* 1995;45:616–623.
90. Pilepich MV, Winter K, John MJ, et al. Phase III radiation therapy oncology group (RTOG) trial 86-10 of androgen deprivation adjuvant to definitive radiotherapy in locally advanced carcinoma of the prostate. *Int J Radiat Oncol Biol Phys* 2001;50:1243–1252.
91. Pilepich MV, Winter K, Lawton CA, et al. Androgen suppression adjuvant to definitive radiotherapy in prostate carcinoma—long-term results of phase III RTOG 85-31. *Int J Radiat Oncol Biol Phys* 2005;61:1285–1290.
92. Pollack A, Hanlon AL, Horwitz EM, et al. Prostate cancer radiotherapy dose response: An update of the fox chase experience. *J Urol* 2004;171:1132–1136.
93. Pollack A, Zagars GK, Starkschall G, et al. Prostate cancer radiation dose response: Results of the M.D. Anderson phase III randomized trial. *Int J Radiat Oncol Biol Phys* 2002;53:1097–1105.
94. Pound CR, Partin AW, Eisenberger MA, et al. Natural history of progression after PSA elevation following radical prostatectomy. *JAMA* 1999;281:1591–1597.
95. Ray ME, Thames HD, Levy LB, et al. PSA nadir predicts biochemical and distant failures after external beam radiotherapy for prostate cancer: A multi-institutional analysis. *Int J Radiat Oncol Biol Phys* 2006;64:1140–1150.
96. Roach M 3rd, DeSilvio M, Lawton C, et al. Phase III trial comparing whole-pelvic versus prostate-only radiotherapy and neoadjuvant versus adjuvant combined androgen suppression: Radiation Therapy Oncology Group 9413. *J Clin Oncol* 2003;21:1904–1911.
97. Roach M 3rd, DeSilvio M, Valicenti R, et al. Whole pelvis, "mini-pelvis", or prostate-only external beam radiotherapy after neoadjuvant and concurrent hormonal therapy in patients treated in the Radiation Therapy Oncology Group 9413 trial. *Int J Radiat Oncol Biol Phys* 2006;66:647–653.
98. Roach M 3rd, Hanks G, Thames H Jr. , et al. Defining biochemical failure following radiotherapy with or without hormonal therapy in men with clinically localized prostate cancer: Recommendations of the RTOG-ASTRO Phoenix Consensus Conference. *Int J Radiat Oncol Biol Phys* 2006;65:965–974.

99. Roach M 3rd, Lu J, Pilepich MV, et al. Four prognostic groups predict long-term survival from prostate cancer following radiotherapy alone on Radiation Therapy Oncology Group clinical trials. *Int J Radiat Oncol Biol Phys* 2000;47:609–615.

100. Roach M 3rd, Lu J, Pilepich MV, et al. Predicting long-term survival, and the need for hormonal therapy: A meta-analysis of RTOG prostate cancer trials. *Int J Radiat Oncol Biol Phys* 2000;47:617–627.

101. Roach M 3rd, Marquez C, Yuo HS, et al. Predicting the risk of lymph node involvement using the pre-treatment prostate specific antigen and Gleason score in men with clinically localized prostate cancer. *Int J Radiat Oncol Biol Phys* 1994;28:33–37.

102. Roach M 3rd, Meehan S, Kroll S, et al. Radiotherapy for high grade clinically localized adenocarcinoma of the prostate. *J Urol* 1996;156:1719–1723.

103. Ryan CJ, Zelefsky MJ, Heller G, et al. Five-year outcomes after neoadjuvant chemotherapy and conformal radiotherapy in patients with high-risk localized prostate cancer. *Urology* 2004;64:90–94.

104. Ryu JK, Winter K, Michalski JM, et al. Interim report of toxicity from 3D conformal radiation therapy (3D-CRT) for prostate cancer on 3DOG/RTOG 9406, level III (79.2 Gy). *Int J Radiat Oncol Biol Phys* 2002;54:1036–1046.

105. Ryu S, Gabel M, Khil MS, et al. Estramustine: A novel radiation enhancer in human carcinoma cells. *Int J Radiat Oncol Biol Phys* 1994;30:99–104.

106. Sandler H, DeSilvio M, Pienta K, et al. Preliminary analysis of RTOG 9902: Increased toxicity observed with the use of adjuvant chemotherapy. Proceedings of the American Society Therapeutic Radiology and Oncology (ASTRO). *Int J Radiat Oncol Biol Phys* 2005;63:S123(abstr 203).

107. Sandler HM, Dunn RL, McLaughlin PW, et al. Overall survival after prostate-specific-antigen-detected recurrence following conformal radiation therapy. *Int J Radiat Oncol Biol Phys* 2000;48:629–633.

108. Sathya JR, Davis IR, Julian JA, et al. Randomized trial comparing iridium implant plus external-beam radiation therapy with external-beam radiation therapy alone in node-negative locally advanced cancer of the prostate. *J Clin Oncol* 2005;23:1192–1199.

109. Savarese DM, Halabi S, Hars V, et al. Phase II study of docetaxel, estramustine, and low-dose hydrocortisone in men with hormone-refractory prostate cancer: A final report of CALGB 9780. *J Clin Oncol* 2001;19:2509–2516.

110. Schallenkamp JM, Herman MG, Kruse JJ, et al. Prostate position relative to pelvic bony anatomy based on intraprostatic gold markers and electronic portal imaging. *Int J Radiat Oncol Biol Phys* 2005;63:800–811.

111. Schiffner DC, Gottschalk AR, Lometti M, et al. Daily electronic portal imaging of implanted gold seed fiducials in patients undergoing radiotherapy after radical prostatectomy. *Int J Radiat Oncol Biol Phys* 2007;67:610–619.

112. Shah R, Bassily N, Wei J, et al. Benign prostatic glands at surgical margins of radical prostatectomy specimens: Frequency and associated risk factors. *Urology* 2000;56:721–725.

113. Shahinian VB, Kuo YF, Freeman JL, et al. Risk of fracture after androgen deprivation for prostate cancer. *N Engl J Med* 2005;352:154–164.

114. Shariat SF, Kattan MW, Erdamar S, et al. Detection of clinically significant, occult prostate cancer metastases in lymph nodes using a splice variant-specific RT-PCR assay for human glandular kallikrein. *J Clin Oncol* 2003;21:1223–1231.

115. Shih HA, Harisinghani M, Zietman AL, et al. Mapping of nodal disease in locally advanced prostate cancer: Rethinking the clinical target volume for pelvic nodal irradiation based on vascular rather than bony anatomy. *Int J Radiat Oncol Biol Phys* 2005;63:1262–1269.

116. Slovin SF, Wilton AS, Heller G, et al. Time to detectable metastatic disease in patients with rising prostate-specific antigen values following surgery or radiation therapy. *Clin Cancer Res* 2005;11:8669–8673.

117. Song DY, Thompson TL, Ramakrishnan V, et al. Salvage radiotherapy for rising or persistent PSA after radical prostatectomy. *Urology* 2002;60:281–287.

118. Stephenson AJ, Shariat SF, Zelefsky MJ, et al. Salvage radiotherapy for recurrent prostate cancer after radical prostatectomy. *JAMA* 2004;291:1325–1332.

119. Swanson GP, Thompson IM, Tangen C. Phase III randomized study of adjuvant radiation therapy versus observation in patients with pathologic T3 prostate cancer (SWOG 8794). *Int J Radiat Oncol Biol Phys* 2005;63:S1.

120. Sylvester JE, Blasko JC, Grimm PD, et al. Ten-year biochemical relapse-free survival after external beam radiation and brachytherapy for localized prostate cancer: The Seattle experience. *Int J Radiat Oncol Biol Phys* 2003;57:944–952.

121. Tannock IF, de Wit R, Berry WR, et al. Docetaxel plus prednisone or mitoxantrone plus prednisone for advanced prostate cancer. *N Engl J Med* 2004;351:1502–1512.

122. Tannock IF, Osoba D, Stockler MR, et al. Chemotherapy with mitoxantrone plus prednisone or prednisone alone for symptomatic hormone-resistant prostate cancer: A Canadian randomized trial with palliative end points [see comments]. *J Clin Oncol* 1996;14:1756–1764.

123. Taylor N, Kelly JF, Kuban DA, et al. Adjuvant and salvage radiotherapy after radical prostatectomy for prostate cancer. *Int J Radiat Oncol Biol Phys* 2003;56:755–763.

124. Thames H, Kuban D, Levy L, et al. Comparison of alternative biochemical failure definitions based on clinical outcome in 4839 prostate cancer patients treated by external beam radiotherapy between 1986 and 1995. *Int J Radiat Oncol Biol Phys* 2003;57:929–943.

125. Valicenti RK, Gomella LG, Ismail M, et al. Effect of higher radiation dose on biochemical control after radical prostatectomy for PT3N0 prostate cancer. *Int J Radiat Oncol Biol Phys* 1998;42:501–506.

126. Vargas CE, Galalae R, Demanes J, et al. Lack of benefit of pelvic radiation in prostate cancer patients with a high risk of positive pelvic lymph nodes treated with high-dose radiation. *Int J Radiat Oncol Biol Phys* 2005;63:1474–1482.

127. Vicini FA, Kestin LL, Martinez AA. The importance of adequate follow-up in defining treatment success after external beam irradiation for prostate cancer [see comments]. *Int J Radiat Oncol Biol Phys* 1999;45:553–561.

128. Wallner K, Merrick G, True L, et al. 20 Gy versus 44 Gy supplemental beam radiation with Pd-103 prostate brachytherapy: Preliminary biochemical outcomes from a prospective randomized multi-center trial. *Radiother Oncol* 2005;75:307–310.

129. Wang-Chesebro A, Xia P, Coleman J, et al. Intensity-modulated radiotherapy improves lymph node coverage and dose to critical structures compared with three-dimensional conformal radiation therapy in clinically localized prostate cancer. *Int J Radiat Oncol Biol Phys* 2006;66:654–662.

130. Wawroschek F, Vogt H, Weckermann D, et al. Radioisotope guided pelvic lymph node dissection for prostate cancer. *J Urol* 2001;166:1715–1719.

131. Wieder JA, Soloway MS. Incidence, etiology, location, prevention and treatment of positive surgical margins after radical prostatectomy for prostate cancer. *J Urol* 1998;160:299–315.

132. Wiegel T, Bottke D, Willich N, et al. Phase III results of adjuvant radiotherapy (RT) versus "wait and see" (WS) in patients with pT3 prostate cancer following radical prostatectomy (RP) (ARO 96-02/AUO AP 09/95). *J Clin Oncol (Meeting Abstracts)* 2005;23:4513.

133. Zagars GK, Pollack A. Kinetics of serum prostate-specific antigen after external beam radiation for clinically localized prostate cancer. *Radiother Oncol* 1997;44:213–221.

134. Zelefsky MJ, Fuks Z, Hunt M, et al. High dose radiation delivered by intensity modulated conformal radiotherapy improves the outcome of localized prostate cancer. *J Urol* 2001;166:876–881.

135. Zelefsky MJ, Kelly WK, Scher HI, et al. Results of a phase II study using estramustine phosphate and vinblastine in combination with high-dose three-dimensional conformal radiotherapy for patients with locally advanced prostate cancer. *J Clin Oncol* 2000;18:1936–1941.

136. Zelefsky MJ, Leibel SA, Gaudin PB, et al. Dose escalation with three-dimensional conformal radiation therapy affects the outcome in prostate cancer. *Int J Radiat Oncol Biol Phys* 1998;41:491–500.

137. Zhou P, Chen M-H, McLeod D, et al. Predictors of prostate cancer-specific mortality after radical prostatectomy or radiation therapy. *J Clin Oncol* 2005;23:6992–6998.

138. Zietman AL, DeSilvio ML, Slater JD, et al. Comparison of conventional-dose vs high-dose conformal radiation therapy in clinically localized adenocarcinoma of the prostate: A randomized controlled trial. *JAMA* 2005;294:1233–1239.

139. Zietman AL, Prince EA, Nakfoor BM, et al. Androgen deprivation and radiation therapy: Sequencing studies using the Shionogi in vivo tumor system. *Int J Radiat Oncol Biol Phys* 1997;38:1067–1070.

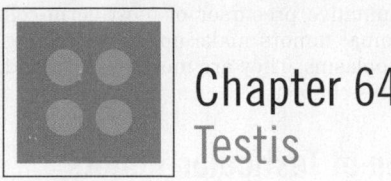

Chapter 64
Testis

Gerard C. Morton, Gillian M. Thomas

Anatomy

Knowledge of the lymphatic drainage of the testis is particularly important because surgical and radiotherapeutic management is predicated on knowledge of the probable site of lymphatic involvement in the infradiaphragmatic and subdiaphragmatic regions.

Four to eight collecting lymphatic trunks drain from the hilum of the testis and accompany the spermatic cord up to the internal inguinal ring along the course of the testicular veins. These lymphatic trunks continue cephalad with the vessels to drain into the retroperitoneal lymph glands between the levels of T11 and L4, but they are concentrated at the level of the L1 and L3 vertebrae. On the left the lymphatics drain primarily into the preaortic and para-aortic lymph nodes around the left renal hilum and thence to the interaortocaval nodes. On the right the first echelon of nodes are in the interaortocaval region, followed by the preaortic and para-aortic lymph nodes. Early lymphographic studies demonstrated rapid crossover from right to left as well as from left to right. Clinically, however, contralateral spread is mainly seen with right-sided tumors and rarely with left-sided tumors. In 15% to 20% of patients with testicular tumors, ipsilateral and contralateral nodes are involved (82).

Previous inguinal surgery may disrupt the lymphatic drainage and redirect it through the subcutaneous lymphatics of the anterior abdominal wall into the bilateral iliac nodes. The lymphatic drainage of the skin and subcutaneous tissues of the scrotum is into the inguinal and iliac nodes. From the retroperitoneal lumbar nodes, drainage occurs through the thoracic duct to lymph nodes in the mediastinum and supraclavicular fossae and occasionally to the axillary nodes.

Epidemiology

Testicular cancer is the most common malignancy among young men in North America and most western European countries. The median age at diagnosis is around 34 years, with almost 50% of incident cases between 20 and 34 years, and a further 20% between 35 and 44 years. Over 95% of testicular cancers are germ-cell tumors, either seminomas or nonseminomas. Nonseminomas have an age-specific incidence peak 10 years earlier than that of seminomas.

There is wide variation in incidence worldwide. The highest incidence has been reported in Denmark, Norway, and Switzerland and the lowest in eastern Europe and Asia. The incidence of testicular cancer has almost doubled in most Western countries over the past 25 years. Between 1973 and 2002, the incidence of testicular cancer in the United States increased from 3.6 per 100,000 to 6.8 per 100,000 in white males. No such trend was seen among black males in whom the incidence remained much lower at around 1 per 100,000 (87). It has been estimated that 8,250 new cases of testicular cancer will have been diagnosed in the United States in 2006, with 370 deaths (3). Despite the increased incidence, there has been a significant improvement in 5-year survival and reduction of mortality. The most dramatic reduction occurred in the 1970s when the mortality decreased from approximately 1 per 100,000 to 0.4 per 100,000 over a decade. Since then, there has been a continued more gradual decrease in mortality despite the increasing incidence. The 5-year survival rate in the United States has increased from 79% for those diagnosed in the mid-1970s to 96% for those diagnosed between 1995 and 2001.

Similar trends are also seen in most western European countries. In England and Wales, the age standardized incidence rate increased by 88% between 1971 and 1997, with a reduction in mortality rate of 71% in the same period (78). The incidence rate of testicular cancer has been increasing by 2.6% to 4.9% per year in northern Europe over the past three decades without evidence of attenuation in the trend (86). Both seminomas and nonseminomas demonstrate a similar temporal trend, although the proportion being diagnosed with seminomas has increased from 43% to 58% over the past two decades (79).

This temporal and geographic variation in incidence rates strongly suggests environmental etiological factors. The increasing incidence has paralleled decline in semen quality over the past several decades (51). It has been hypothesized that both testicular cancer and male subfertility may be caused by intrauterine exposure of the developing male embryo to factors that alter the hormonal balance (103). Although some studies have shown an increased testicular cancer risk in men born to mothers exposed to exogenous estrogens, other evidence supporting the "estrogen hypothesis" has been inconsistent (64).

Lower fertility and semen abnormality are associated with increased risk of testicular cancer (67). The association is similar for both seminomas and nonseminomas. In an analysis of over 32,000 men having sperm analysis at the sperm laboratory in Copenhagen, Denmark, men who had a low semen concentration, poor semen mobility, and high proportion of abnormal spermatozoa had a 9.3 relative risk of later being diagnosed with testicular cancer (49).

A history of undescended testicle has long been recognized as a risk factor (68). The odds ratio for the subsequent development of testicular cancer is around 4. The U.K. Testicular Cancer Study Group performed a case controlled study comparing 794 men with testicular cancer to age matched controls (23). The odds ratio associated with a history of undescended testis for all testicular cancer cases was 3.82. The odds ratio was 5.3 for seminoma and 3 for nonseminoma. The risk was highest for men over the age of 32 who had an odds ratio of 11.94 for pure seminoma and 5.1 for other histologies. This risk is further increased if the testis is intra-abdominal. If maldescent is unilateral, there is still an increased risk of developing a tumor in the contralateral normally descended testicle. Other factors that are associated with an increased risk of testicular cancer include having an inguinal hernia less than 15 years of age (odds ratio 3), a prior history of testis or groin injury, and any past history of sexually transmitted disease. Late puberty seems to have a protective effect.

There is no clear relationship between nutritional factors and exercise on testicular cancer risk. There is some evidence of a genetic component to the development of testis cancer. Fathers of sons with diagnosed cases have a twofold increased risk

Table 64.1	**RISK FACTORS FOR TESTICULAR CANCER**

Family history
History of cryptorchidism
Altered intrauterine hormonal environment
Low fertility
Abnormal sperm analysis
Immunosuppression

of themselves being diagnosed with a testicular cancer, while for brothers, the relative risk is over 12 (105). Certain chromosomal alterations, particularly loss of the short arm of chromosome 12, are commonly seen in germ-cell tumors.

There is an increased incidence of testicular cancer, both seminomas and nonseminomas in immunosuppressed patients (56). Testicular tumors represent the third most common AIDS-linked malignancy following Kaposi's sarcoma and non-Hodgkin's lymphoma, with a prevalence of 0.2% compared with 0.004% in the general male population. The interpretation of staging investigations for these patients can be difficult due to the frequency of AIDS-associated retroperitoneal lymphadenopathy, which can be mistaken for metastases. The overall cause-specific mortality rate is comparable to the mortality rate among testis cancer patients without immunosuppression.

In summary, germ-cell tumors are thought to arise in testes predisposed to the development of malignancy due to a combination of familial predisposition and intrauterine hormonal imbalance, later compounded by environmental factors and manifested by impaired spermatogenesis (Table 64.1).

Pathology

The vast majority (over 95%) of testicular neoplasms are germ-cell tumors. Germ-cell tumors are divided into seminomas and nonseminomas. Nonseminomas include embryonal carcinoma, yolk sac (endodermal sinus tumor), teratoma, choriocarcinoma, and mixed germ-cell tumors (Table 64.2). Intratubular germ-cell

Table 64.2	**CLASSIFICATION OF GERM-CELL TUMORS OF THE TESTIS**

Intratubular germ-cell neoplasia
Seminoma
    Classic type
    Spermatocytic type
Nonseminomatous germ-cell tumors
    Embryonal carcinoma
    Yolk sac (endodermal sinus) tumor
    Teratoma
        Mature
        Immature
        Teratoma with malignant transformation (with somatic carcinoma or
            sarcoma)
    Choriocarcinoma
    Mixed germ-cell tumors
Classification of Sex-Cord Stromal Tumors of the Testis
Leydig cell tumor
Sertoli cell tumor
Granulosa cell tumor
Fibroma-thecoma stromal tumor
Sex cord-stromal tumor with annular tubules
Gonadoblastoma
Sex cord-stromal tumor unclassified type

neoplasia (IGCN) is the putative precursor of most germ-cell neoplasms. Sex cord-stromal tumors make up the remaining 3% to 4% of testicular neoplasms. They are mostly benign and are beyond the scope of this chapter.

Classification of Testicular Tumors

Germ-Cell Tumors

Intratubular Germ-Cell Neoplasia

IGCN is thought to be the precursor lesion of most types of germ-cell tumors. Abnormal germ cells within the seminal tubules are commonly found adjacent to invasive seminal-cell tumors. Although initially termed carcinoma *in situ* (CIS), these cells are not of epithelial origin and are better termed intratubular germ-cell neoplasia or testicular intraepithelial neoplasia (TIN).

IGCN is found adjacent to testicular germ-cell tumors in over 95% of cases. It is also found in all clinical groups known to be at high risk for testicular cancer development: Cryptorchidism (2% to 4%), infertility (1%), ambiguous genitalia (25%), and contralateral testes of patients with testicular cancer (5%) (29).

ICGN is characterized by seminiferous tubules showing decreased spermatogenesis in which the normal constituents of the tubules are replaced by abnormal germ cells with the appearance of seminoma cells. These cells stain strongly for placental alkaline phosphatase (PLAP), whereas normal germ cells are negative.

IGCN has a 50% risk of developing into an invasive germ-cell tumor within 5 years. That risk probably approaches 100% by 8 years. There is strong evidence that IGCN is a precursor lesion of all types of germ-cell tumors except spermatocytic seminoma and infantile testicular tumors. It is hypothesized that the cells originate from primordial germ cells early during embryogenesis, possibly due to an excess of estrogens. They likely remain within the seminiferous tubules in a dormant stage until puberty when replication begins, possibly as a consequence of raised sex hormone levels. Transition to an invasive germ-cell tumor then occurs.

Seminoma

Classic Type

Seminoma is the most frequent germ-cell tumor, comprising over 50% of all germ-cell neoplasms. Serum level of human chorionic gonadotropin (HCG) is elevated in 15% to 30% of men at presentation, related to the presence of syncytiotrophoblastic cells. These may be identified in 7% of tumors on routine hematoxylin and eosin sections or by immunoperoxidase stains in 24%. Serum alpha-fetoprotein is not elevated in pure seminoma.

Grossly, seminoma is a soft tan-colored diffused multinodular mass. Focal necrosis is sometimes present. A prominent lymphocytic infiltrate is commonly seen within the fibrous stroma.

Anaplastic seminoma is no longer distinguished as a distinct entity. It was previously defined as a seminoma with a high mitotic count. It has since been found that the mitotic count is of no prognostic significance. Over 90% of seminomas will stain positive for a PLAP.

Spermatocytic Seminoma

Spermatocytic seminoma accounts for 2% of all testicular germ-cell tumors. It tends to occur in an older age group at a mean age of 54 years. It is important to differentiate spermatocytic seminoma from seminoma as the natural history and treatment is quite different. Spermatocytic seminoma is confined to the testes and is cured by orchidectomy. Only one case of metastatic spermatocytic seminoma has ever been reported (63). The cell of origin of spermatocytic seminoma is unknown. Unlike seminoma, it does not contain glycogen and stains negative for placental alkaline phosphatase. In fact, many authorities believe there is little to indicate that spermatocytic seminoma is of germ-cell origin.

Nonseminomatous Germ-Cell Tumors

Embryonal Carcinoma

Pure embryonal carcinoma makes up about 3% of all testicular germ-cell tumors and is a component of almost 50% of mixed germ-cell tumors. Over 80% of these tumors occur between the ages of 15 and 34 years.

Grossly, the tumor often exhibits a large area of hemorrhage and necrosis. Almost all embryonal carcinomas are PLAP positive and alpha-fetoprotein and HCG-positive cells are present in 33% and 21%, respectively.

Yolk Sac (Endodermal Sinus Tumor)

Pure yolk sac tumor makes up <2% of testicular tumors in adults but forms a component of 40% of mixed germ-cell tumors. It makes up 60% of germ-cell tumors in children. Eighty percent of pure yolk sac tumors occur in the first 2 years of life. It is associated with elevated serum levels of alpha-fetoprotein. Grossly, yolk sac tumors contain cystic spaces containing a gelatinous material. There is a variable amount of hemorrhage and necrosis. Microscopically, Schiller-Duval bodies are a characteristic feature.

Teratoma

Pure teratoma makes up 5% of all testicular germ-cell tumors. Teratomatous component may be seen in about 50% of mixed germ-cell tumors. In pure teratoma serum HCG and alpha-fetoprotein are normal. Mature teratoma consists of mature well-differentiated somatic tissues. Despite their benign appearance, metastases can occur. Immature teratoma contains immature elements in addition to varying amounts of well-differentiated tissue. Both mature and immature teratomas have a similar behavior. Teratoma with malignant transformation results from the development of a somatic carcinoma or sarcoma within the teratoma.

Choriocarcinoma

Pure choriocarcinoma is the rarest type of germ-cell tumor, accounting for less that 0.05% of lesions but present in about 4% of mixed germ-cell tumors. It is a highly aggressive neoplasm and often presents with metastatic disease, the primary lesion being occult. The serum HCG is elevated.

Mixed Germ-Cell Tumors

Mixed germ-cell tumors account for up to 50% of germ-cell tumors. Any of the above elements can be present in combination. Serum markers are elevated depending on the proportion of different elements present within.

Table 64.3   STAGE DISTRIBUTION OF SEMINOMA AT PRESENTATION AND EXPECTED RESULTS OF THERAPY

Stage	Stage Distribution (%)	Expected Survival (%)	No. of Patients Cured
I	85	99	84
II	11	95	10
III	4	80	3
Total	100		97

Natural History

Although the routes of dissemination are similar for seminomas and nonseminomatous tumors, the propensity for involvement of various sites at presentation differs. Pure seminoma has a much greater tendency to remain localized or involve only lymph nodes, while nonseminomatous germ-cell tumors of the testes more frequently spread by hematogenous routes. Pure seminoma is confined to the testis (stage I) in 85% of patients at presentation (Table 64.3). It spreads in an orderly fashion, initially to the drainage lymph nodes in the retroperitoneum (stage II). From the retroperitoneum, it spreads proximally to involve the next echelon of draining lymphatics in the mediastinum and supraclavicular fossae (stage IIIA disease). Only rarely and late does pure seminoma spread hematogenously to involve lung parenchyma (also stage IIIA), bone, liver, or brain (stage IIIC).

Clinical Presentation

A testicular tumor usually presents as a painless swelling in the scrotum, although pain, heaviness, and tenderness at presentation are not uncommon. Disease in the lymph nodes of the retroperitoneum may produce back pain or abdominal swelling. Widely disseminated parenchymal disease in lungs, liver, bone, or brain is rare but, if present, may produce systemic symptoms. Gynecomastia is a rare presentation of embryonal carcinoma and may be seen in association with the very uncommon sex cord-stromal tumors. Occasionally, patients present with metastatic germ-cell malignancies diagnosed by biopsy or elevated levels of serum tumor markers without evidence of a palpable mass in the testis. Occult primary disease in the testis is often detected by testicular ultrasound. If there is no evidence of a primary tumor in the testis, a diagnosis of an extratesticular germ-cell tumor, usually mediastinal, retroperitoneal, or pineal, may be made.

Diagnostic Work-Up

The tests necessary to evaluate patients with testicular cancer are listed in Table 64.4. A complete history should be taken, including information about previous inguinal or scrotal surgery, cryptorchidism, retractile testes, and orchiopexy. The physical examination should pay special attention to possible sites of lymph node metastases. Specifically, the abdomen should be examined to rule out the presence of large abdominal masses, and both supraclavicular regions should be palpated to rule out supraclavicular metastases. The contralateral testis should be examined clinically. The presence or absence of gynecomastia is an important observation.

If testicular tumor is suspected, testicular ultrasound should be performed. This usually demonstrates a solid mass within the testis, often with associated testicular microlithiasis (5). The

::	Table 64.4	**DIAGNOSTIC WORK-UP FOR TUMORS OF THE TESTIS**

General
History (document cryptorchidism and previous inguinal or scrotal surgery)
Physical examination
Laboratory Studies
Complete blood count
Biochemistry profile (including lactate dehydrogenase)
Serum assays
    α-fetoprotein (AFP)
    β-human chorionic gonadotropin
Surgery
Radical inguinal orchiectomy
Diagnostic Radiology
Chest x-ray films, posterior/anterior and lateral views
Computed tomography (CT) scan of abdomen and pelvis
CT scan of chest for nonseminomas and stage II seminomas
Ultrasound of contralateral testis
Special Studies
Semen analysis

appropriate surgical procedure to make the diagnosis and remove the primary tumor is a radical orchiectomy through an inguinal incision.

Laboratory Studies

A routine complete blood count and chemistry screen, including renal function tests, should be done. Pulmonary or renal function tests should be performed for patients who may receive bleomycin or combination chemotherapy.

Nonseminomatous germ-cell tumors of the testes are uniquely associated with reliable serum tumor markers: The β-subunit of human chorionic gonadotropin (β-HCG) and α-fetoprotein (AFP). One or both of these serum markers are elevated in 80% to 85% of patients with disseminated nonseminomatous disease. The metabolic half-life of AFP is approximately 5 days, and for β-HCG it is approximately 18 to 24 hours. Although β-HCG may be modestly elevated in 15% to 30% of patients with pure seminoma, usually any elevation of AFP connotes nonseminomatous disease. Serum tumor markers may be elevated in other circumstances or conditions, such as laboratory error, cross-reactivity with luteinizing hormone, marijuana use, hepatitis, or development of antibodies to the glycoproteins.

Serum PLAP is elevated in 50% of seminomas at presentation and has a serum half-life of 24 hours (34,50,52). For metastatic or recurrent disease it has a sensitivity of only 50% and a specificity of 90%, although lower in smokers. It therefore is of limited use in the evaluation and follow-up of patients.

If a testicular cancer is suspected, serum tumor markers should be assayed before and after orchiectomy, and interpretation of the levels of markers should take into account their metabolic half-lives. Serum tumor markers can document persistent or recurrent cancer after surgery or chemotherapy and may predict the responsiveness of nonseminomas to treatment. The level of β-HCG should decrease by 90% or more every 21 days with each successful treatment cycle of chemotherapy. A slow decline in β-HCG after treatment may imply suboptimal response to chemotherapy, permitting early implementation of salvage therapy before the development of overt resistance to chemotherapy develops. The decline of AFP is less predictable.

Semen analysis and banking of sperm should be considered for patients in whom treatment is likely to compromise fertility. With newer technologies it is possible to retrieve and bank sperm even with poorer quality sperm.

Radiographic Studies

Investigations should routinely include chest x-ray films for all patients and computed tomography (CT) of the thorax for any patient with nonseminomatous germ-cell tumors of the testis. CT scans of the abdomen and pelvis should be performed to evaluate the retroperitoneal nodal areas and assess the liver. CT of abdomen and pelvis relies on nodal size to assess the retroperitoneal nodes, with a sensitivity of 40% and a specificity of over 90% (12). There is considerable overlap between the size of normal and abnormal lymph nodes using a size limit of 10 mm to 20 mm (57). It therefore has limited ability to exclude the presence of disease, although enlarged lymph nodes in the appropriate clinical context (location, laterality, disease parameters) are very likely to be truly positive. Magnetic resonance imaging appears equivalent to CT in determining the size and location of retroperitoneal adenopathy.

Bipedal lymphangiography has a greater sensitivity than CT (71%) but a lower specificity (60%). It does not add to the diagnostic accuracy of a positive CT, but is able to demonstrate architectural abnormalities within normal-size lymph nodes (60).

Positron emission tomography (PET) has been shown to improve on the diagnostic accuracy of CT in early stage testicular cancer. It has a higher sensitivity (70%) and specificity (up to 100%) than CT (55). It is unable to detect lesions <5 mm in size or teratomas of any size (2) due to their very low metabolic activity. It also has an important role in evaluating residual retroperitoneal disease following chemotherapy, with a reported sensitivity and specificity in detecting viable tumor of 80% and 100%, respectively (8).

Baseline ultrasonography of the remaining testis should be performed. If the contralateral testis is atrophic and the patient under 30 years of age, there is a 30% risk of intratubular germ-cell neoplasia being present. Biopsy of the contralateral testis may be considered in this setting.

:: | Staging and Prognostic Factors

The Union Internationale Contre le Cancer (UICC) and the American Joint Committee on Cancer (AJCC) Staging and End-Results Reporting (1) classify patients by the features of the primary tumor (T), nodes (N), metastases (M), and level of serum (S) tumor marker (Table 64.5).

T stage is of prognostic value in early stage nonseminomas managed by orchidectomy alone—the relapse risk being around 20% for pT1 (stage IA) and 40% for pT2 (stage IB) with vascular invasion (83).

T stage is not useful in predicting risk of relapse in stage 1 seminomas, where tumor size and rete testis invasion are of independent prognostic value. In a pooled analysis of 638 patients with stage 1 managed by surveillance following orchiectomy, the relapse risk was 13% and 24% for tumors less than or greater than 4 cm, respectively (102).

The staging system classifies nodal disease by size (≤ 2 cm, 2 to 5 cm, and >5 cm in maximum dimension). The relapse risk for stage II seminoma after radiation therapy depends on the bulk of retroperitoneal disease. As can be seen from Table 64.6, the relapse risk is approximately 8% for stage IIA, 14% for stage IIB, and 28% for stage IIC. For patients with metastatic disease, differentiation is made between those with metastatic disease to nonregional nodes or lung (M1a) and those with nonpulmonary metastases (M1b). Serum tumor marker levels (S category) are based on the nadir value of AFP and HCG after orchidectomy. The serum level of LDH has prognostic value and is also included in staging.

The International Germ Cell Cancer Collaborative Group (IGCCCG) developed a widely accepted classification system for patients with metastatic germ-cell malignancies, which has

Clinical Radiation Oncology

Table 64.5 INTERNATIONAL UNION AGAINST CANCER AND AMERICAN JOINT COMMITTEE REPORTING SYSTEM

Primary Tumor (T) (Pathologic Classification)

pTx	Primary tumor cannot be assessed
pT0	No evidence of primary tumor (scar, etc.)
pTis	Intratubular, noninvasive
pT1	Tumor limited to testis and epididymis, no vascular/lymphatic invasion
pT2	Tumor limited to testis and epididymis, with vascular/lymphatic invasion or involvement of the tunica vaginalis
pT3	Tumor invades scrotum

Lymph Node (N)

N0	No regional node metastasis
N1	Metastasis in single or multiple nodes 2 cm or less in greatest dimension
N2	Metastasis in single or multiple nodes 2 to 5 cm greatest dimension
N3	Metastasis in lymph nodes >5 cm in maximum diameter

Distant Metastasis (M)

M0	No distant metastasis
M1a	Nonregional lymph node or pulmonary metastasis
M1b	Nonpulmonary visceral metastasis

Serum Tumor Markers (S)

Sx	Serum tumor markers not performed
S0	Serum tumor markers within normal limits
S1	LDH $<1.5 \times$ N and HCG $<5,000$ and AFP $<1,000$
S2	LDH 1.5–$10 \times$ N or HCG $5,000$–$50,000$ or AFP $1,000$–$10,000$
S3	LDH $>10 \times$ N or HCG $>50,000$ or AFP $>10,000$

Staging Groupings

IA	T1, N0, M0, S0
IB	T2-4, N0, M0, S0
IS	Any T, N0, M0, S1-3
IIA	Any T, N1, M0, S0/1
IIB	Any T, N2, M0, S0/1
IIC	Any T, N3, M0, S0/1
IIIA	Any T, Any N, M1a, S0/1
IIIB	Any T, Any N, M1a, S2
IIIC	Any T, Any N, M1b or S3

AFP, α-fetoprotein; HCG, human chorionic gonadotropin; LDH, lactate dehydrogenase

been incorporated into the TNM system (47) (Table 64.7). The prognostic classification is based on data collected on approximately 6,000 patients with metastatic germ-cell tumor from 10 countries during the platinum era. The classification was internally validated, as well as prospectively validated on a subsequent cohort of patients. The factors most strongly associated with a poor prognosis were mediastinal primary, nonpulmonary visceral metastases, or the presence of grossly elevated tumor markers (AFP $>10,000$ ng/mL, HCG $>50,000$ IU/L or lactate dehydrogenase [LDH] $>10 \times$ normal). Patients with nonseminomatous germ-cell tumors (NSGCT) were divided into three prognostic groups (good, intermediate, and poor prognosis) and seminomas into either good or intermediate prognostic groups (see Table 64.7). The good prognosis group comprises over 50%

Table 64.6 RELAPSE RATE FOLLOWING INFRADIAPHRAGMATIC PLUS OR MINUS MEDIASTINAL RADIOTHERAPY BY NODAL STAGE

	Stage IIA (≤ 2 cm)		Stage IIB (2–5 cm)		Stage IIC (>5 cm)	
Study (Reference)	N	Relapses	N	Relapses	N	Relapses
Chung et al. (19)	49	4	30	4	16	10
Classen et al. (22)	66	2	21	2	—	—
Zagars and Pollack (108)	6	0	38	5	25	3
Patterson et al. (74)	46	6	34	9	—	—
Bauman et al. (7)	29	2	10	1	4	2
Whipple et al. (106)	31	2	14	3	—	—
Vallis et al. (98)	26	1	22	2	5	2
Dosmann and Zagars (30)	55	7	13	4	—	—
Mason and Kearsley (62)	—	—	25[a]	1	24	6
Evensen et al. (33)	6	0	18	1	49	11
Total	314	24 (8%)	225	32 (14%)	123	34 (28%)

[a]Includes all tumors <5 cm.

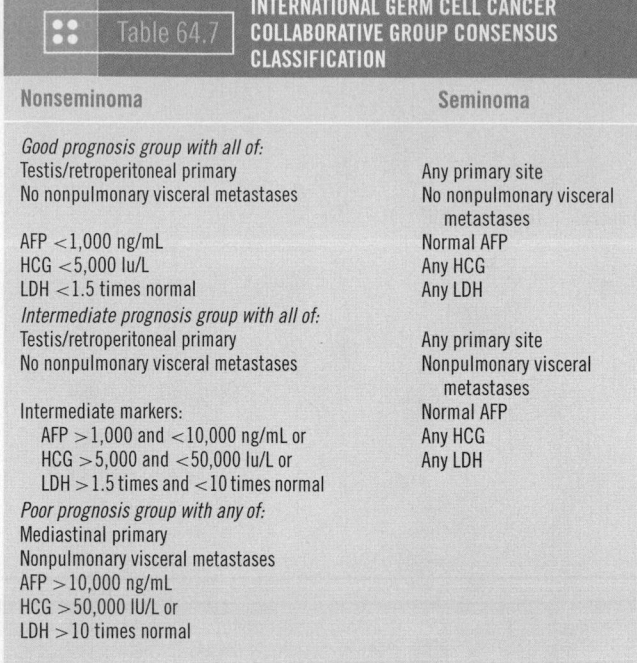

Table 64.7	INTERNATIONAL GERM CELL CANCER COLLABORATIVE GROUP CONSENSUS CLASSIFICATION	
Nonseminoma		**Seminoma**
Good prognosis group with all of:		
Testis/retroperitoneal primary		Any primary site
No nonpulmonary visceral metastases		No nonpulmonary visceral metastases
AFP <1,000 ng/mL		Normal AFP
HCG <5,000 Iu/L		Any HCG
LDH <1.5 times normal		Any LDH
Intermediate prognosis group with all of:		
Testis/retroperitoneal primary		Any primary site
No nonpulmonary visceral metastases		Nonpulmonary visceral metastases
Intermediate markers:		Normal AFP
AFP >1,000 and <10,000 ng/mL or		Any HCG
HCG >5,000 and <50,000 Iu/L or		Any LDH
LDH >1.5 times and <10 times normal		
Poor prognosis group with any of:		
Mediastinal primary		
Nonpulmonary visceral metastases		
AFP >10,000 ng/mL		
HCG >50,000 IU/L or		
LDH >10 times normal		

AFP, α-fetoprotein; HCG, human chorionic gonadotropin; LDH, lactate dehydrogenase

of all patients with metastatic NSGCTs and 90% of seminomas. It is associated with a 5-year survival rate of 91%. The intermediate prognosis group comprises over 25% of patients, and has a 5-year survival rate of 79%. The poor prognosis group comprises 15% to 20% of patients with NSGCT and has a 5-year survival rate of 48%.

The currently available staging systems allow a description of the anatomical extent of disease and have incorporated prognostic information from serum tumor markers to accurately reflect prognosis for metastatic disease.

General Management

The initial management of a suspected malignant germ-cell tumor of the testis consists of obtaining serum AFP and β-HCG measurements and then performing a radical (inguinal) orchiectomy with high ligation of the spermatic cord. Historically, it had been thought that scrotal violation (transscrotal orchiectomy, open testicular biopsy, or fine needle aspiration) compromised prognosis. Scrotal violation is associated with a slight increase in local recurrence rate compared with inguinal orchiectomy (2.9% vs. 0.4%, respectively), but is not associated with any difference in distant recurrence rates or overall survival (14). Orchiectomy is both diagnostic and therapeutic. Further management depends on pathologic diagnosis and the stage and extent of disease.

Seminoma

Adjuvant Radiotherapy

Patients with stage I seminoma have traditionally been managed with adjuvant radiotherapy to the retroperitoneal and ipsilateral pelvic nodes following orchiectomy. The subsequent relapse-free survival rate is around 97% (Table 64.8) and the disease-specific survival almost 100%. Although highly effective, adjuvant radiotherapy puts all patients at risk of long-term

treatment-related morbidity (particularly second cancer and infertility) and benefits only the 15% to 20% of patients harboring subclinical nodal disease. In order to reduce the overall morbidity of treatment, surveillance, reduced field radiotherapy, and adjuvant chemotherapy have evolved as alternative management strategies.

Surveillance

With the availability of highly effective radiation therapy and chemotherapy for salvage after relapse and with a low risk of occult retroperitoneal disease in well-staged patients, several investigators have examined a policy of postorchiectomy surveillance (Table 64.9).

With median reported follow-up of over 12 years in some series, data are now sufficiently mature to consider surveillance a standard option for patients with stage I seminoma following orchiectomy and is being widely adopted. In British Columbia, Canada, the proportion of patients managed by surveillance increased from 10% in 1992 to 33% in 2002 (97). A survey of U.S. and Canadian radiation oncologists reported that 78% offered surveillance as a management option (15), while a similar study in Australia and New Zealand reported a figure of 54% (46). Two-thirds of Canadian urologists reported offering surveillance as a management strategy, particularly where the perceived risk of relapse was low and the patient desired to preserve fertility (6).

Disease outcome with surveillance is detailed in Table 64.9. The seven reported series include 1,260 patients and all report very similar rates, timing, and patterns of recurrence. When managed by surveillance, about 20% of patients will relapse at a median time of around 14 months. In the series of 394 patients from Copenhagen, Denmark, median time to relapse was 13 months, with 87% occurring within the first 2 years and only 2% beyond 5 years (25). Choo et al. (16) reported very similar results from Toronto, with a median time to relapse of 13.6 months and only 2 of 88 patients relapsing after 5 years. In the Princess Margaret Hospital (PMH) series, the risk of relapse between 5 and 10 years was 4% (18). Given the small event rate in the individual reports, Warde et al. (102) have performed a pooled analysis from four series (PMH, Royal Marsden Hospital [RMH], Royal London Hospital, and the Danish Testicular Cancer Study Group). Individual patient data on 638 stage I seminoma patients managed by surveillance was obtained. With a median follow-up time of 7 years, the 5- and 10-year relapse-free rates were 82.3% and 78.7%, respectively. Most relapses (69%) occurred within the first 2 years of surgery, while 7% relapsed beyond 6 years. The 5-year cause-specific survival was 99.3%.

The predominant site of relapse is in the retroperitoneum (76% to 94%). Approximately 5% to 15% of patients relapse in the mediastinum or lungs, with inguinal relapse reported in 3% to 11%, usually only after previous scrotal interference. Following relapse, 74% to 82% of patients in the series were initially managed by radiation therapy, with a second relapse occurring in about 10% (6% to 16%). Second relapse almost always occurred at distant sites with a 90% to 95% rate of successfully salvage with chemotherapy.

Tumor size, presence of rete testis invasion, and patient age are most often associated with risk of relapse in the institutional series. In the pooled analysis, tumor size, the presence of rete testis invasion, and the presence of lymphovascular invasion were predictive of relapse on univariate analysis. On multivariate analysis, tumor size (hazard ratio = 2.0) and rete testis invasion (hazard ratio = 1.7) remained significant. The relapse-free rate decreased from 87.8% for tumors <4 cm without rete testis invasion to 68.5% for tumors >4 cm with rete testis invasion. Tyldesley et al. (97) also noted the importance of size >4 cm and rete testis invasion, reporting a 5-year relapse-free rate of

Table 64.8 PATTERNS OF RELAPSE AFTER ADJUVANT RADIATION THERAPY FOR STAGE I SEMINOMA

Author (Reference)	Number	Median Follow-Up (years)	Radiation Dose (Gy)	Fields	Number Relapsing	Para-Aortic/Renal Hilum	Pelvic/Inguinal	Distant	Cause-Specific Survival (%)
Fossa et al. (35)	365	9.1	36–40	DL	13 (4%)	1	7	6	99
Bauman et al. (7)	169	7.5	30	DL	5 (3%)	1	0	4	100
Fossa et al. (36)	236		30	DL	9 (4%)	0	0	9	100
	242	4.5	30	PA	9 (4%)	2	4	6	99.3
Melchior et al. (65)	87	7.7	36	DL	3 (3%)	0	0	3	100
	42	5.2	28	PA	1 (2%)	0	0	1	100
Logue et al. (59)	431	5.2	20	PA	15 (3%)	1	9	5	99
Santoni et al. (89)	487	10	30	DL ± Med; PA	21 (4%)	4	8	9	—
Classen et al. (21)	721	5.1	26	PA	26 (4%)	6	21	5	99.6
Garcia-Serra et al. (39)	57	15	25	DL ± Med	2 (4%)	0	0	2	96
Niazi et al. (70)	71	6.25	25	PA	1 (1%)	0	1	0	100
Bruns et al. (11)	80	7.1	20	Reduced PA	4 (5%)	1	3	0	100
	313		30	PA (88%)	10 (3%)	2	6	2	100
Jones et al. (50)	312	5.1	20	PA (89%)	11 (3%)	1	3	7	99.7
Oliver et al. (73)	904	4	20–30	PA (86%)	32 (4%)	3	10	19	99.9

DL, dog-leg; PA, para-aortic; Med, mediastinum

Table 64.9	SURVEILLANCE FOLLOWING ORCHIECTOMY FOR STAGE I SEMINOMA TESTIS					
Author (Reference)	Number	Median Follow-Up (months)	Relapse-Free Survival (%)	Proportion of Relapses Occurring in the Retroperitoneum (%)	Disease-Specific Survival (%)	Median Time to Relapse (months)
Horwich et al. (45)	103	62	82	94	100	15
von der Maase et al. (99)	261	48	80	94	99	14
Warde et al. (100)	201	73	85	91	99.5	17
Francis et al. (38)	120	55	82	94	100	4
Daugaard et al. (25)	394	60	83	87	100	13
Choo et al. (16)	88	145	80	76	100	14
Tyldesley et al. (97)	93	33	78	81	96	14

86%, 71%, and 50% in patients with no risk factor, one risk factor, or both risk factors, respectively. Choo et al. (16) also found a reduction in 10-year relapse-free rate from 86% to 52% in the presence of rete testis invasion.

Given the varying relapse risk with time and patterns of recurrence a reasonable surveillance policy involves four monthly assessments in the first 2 years, six monthly assessments in the third and fourth years, and annual assessments years 5 to 10. Assessment should include physical examination, CT scan of abdomen and pelvis, and chest x ray.

Surveillance is a slightly more costly approach to management than adjuvant nodal irradiation. Francis et al. (38) estimate that a policy of surveillance for 10 years was almost 39% more expensive than adjuvant radiotherapy in the United Kingdom. In Toronto, Canada, surveillance for 10 years was 43% more expensive than standard adjuvant treatment and follow-up (101). The main expense arose from the increased number of radiological investigations performed. With recommendations for less intense surveillance, this cost difference is likely less. Furthermore, it fails to take into account the longer-term cost of managing late radiation morbidities.

Surveillance should be contemplated and conducted only with a compliant patient and with an understanding that because of the risk of late relapse the patient should be monitored for at least 10 years. The survival rate of 99.5% from the large surveillance series indicates that this therapeutic option produces a result equivalent to that achieved with standard adjuvant retroperitoneal nodal irradiation and is a safe and effective alternative management, provided guidelines are followed.

Reduced Field Adjuvant Radiotherapy

About 60% of men undergoing "dog-leg" radiotherapy experience mild to moderate acute gastrointestinal toxicity, while under 5% experience moderate chronic toxicity (35). With longer follow-up there is also an increased risk of second malignancies within the target volume. As the predominant nodal drainage is to the para-aortic and renal hilar nodes, many investigators have questioned the need to include the pelvic nodes, and the use of para-aortic fields alone has been explored. A prospective multi-institution study from Germany reported a 99.6% disease-specific survival following para-aortic radiotherapy in 721 patients with stage I seminoma (21). With a median follow-up time of 61 months, the disease-free survival was 95.8%. No "in-field" recurrences occurred. On relapse, only 1.6% of patients had disease involving the ipsilateral pelvis and a further 0.6% experienced isolated pelvic nodal relapse. An ipsilateral pelvic relapse rate of around 2% has also been reported by other investigators following para-aortic radiotherapy alone (11,59,70). A clinical trial by the United Kingdom Medical Research Council randomized 478 men with stage I seminoma testis to either dog-leg or

para-aortic radiotherapy (36). The 3-year relapse-free survival was 96.6% and 96%, and overall survival 99.3% and 100%, following dog-leg and para-aortic fields, respectively. The pelvic relapse-free survival at 3 years was 100% in the dog-leg arm and 98.3% in the para-aortic arm. The omission of pelvic radiotherapy leads to a reduction in acute treatment toxicity (nausea, vomiting, myelosuppression) and a more rapid recovery of sperm count. Given a pelvic relapse rate of around 2%, it is considered reasonable by many not to treat the pelvic nodes and to treat the para-aortics alone. However, if the pelvic nodes are not treated, some ongoing surveillance of the pelvis with CT scanning will be required.

Adjuvant Chemotherapy

Adjuvant chemotherapy using single agent carboplatin has been proposed as a less toxic approach than radiotherapy for stage I seminoma. For men with advanced seminoma, carboplatin has significant efficacy with relatively low toxicity. Several series reported on the use of one or two cycles of carboplatin following orchiectomy (Table 64.10). Only one recurrence has been documented in a total of 235 reported stage I patients receiving two cycles of chemotherapy, while Dieckmann et al. (28) reported eight recurrences among 93 patients following a single course. Recurrences were all in the retroperitoneum and were readily salvaged with cisplatin-based chemotherapy. No deaths have been attributed to this approach, with a disease-specific survival of 100% in all the reported series. The Medical Research Council of the United Kingdom has performed a randomized comparison of single agent carboplatin and nodal irradiation in stage I seminoma (73). Almost 1,500 patients from 14 European countries were randomized to receive either adjuvant radiotherapy or one injection of carboplatin. Radiation was limited to para-aortic fields in 87%, the remainder also had inclusion of the ipsilateral pelvic nodes. With a median follow-up time of 4 years, the 3-year relapse-free survival rates were similar at 95.9% and 94.8% in the radiotherapy and carboplatin arms, respectively. In the adjuvant radiotherapy arm, the most common site of recurrence was either distant (57%) or in the pelvic nodes (31%). In the carboplatin arm, most of the relapses (74%) were in para-aortic nodes. Only one death from testicular cancer occurred in the radiotherapy group, with no cancer-related deaths in the chemotherapy group. Long-term toxicity (e.g., risk of leukemia) is unknown, but the regimen is well tolerated acutely with only mild myelotoxicity. Spermatogenesis recovers after carboplatin in a high proportion of cases (85).

Other authors have proposed a risk-adapted strategy, offering different management approaches based on individual risk of relapse. Aparicio et al. (4) performed a prospective study including 314 patients with stage I seminoma. Those with tumor size <4 cm and without rete testis invasion (100 patients) were managed by surveillance; "high-risk" patients with larger

Table 64.10	SINGLE AGENT CARBOPLATIN AS ADJUVANT TREATMENT FOLLOWING ORCHIDECTOMY FOR STAGE I SEMINOMA TESTIS			
Author (Reference)	N	Number of Cycles	Median Follow-Up (months)	Number of Relapses
Oliver et al. (72)	78	25 (1 cycle)	29	0
		53 (2 cycles)	54	1 (2%)
Krege et al. (54)	43	2	28	0
Dieckmann et al. (28)	125	93 (1 cycle)	48	8 (9%)
		32 (2 cycles)		0
Reiter et al. (84)	107	2	74	0
Oliver et al. (73)	573	1	48	27 (5%)
Aparicio et al. (4)	131[a]	2	34	7 (3.3%)

[a]All had high-risk stage I seminoma.

tumors and/or rete testis involvement (214 patients) received two courses of carboplatin. At a median follow-up of 34 months, relapse was observed in six patients on surveillance (6%) and in seven patients given carboplatin (3.3%). All relapsing patients were successfully managed by further chemotherapy, resulting in a 5-year survival rate of 100%.

It is clear that the survival of patients with stage I seminoma approaches 100% whatever treatment strategy is employed. The goal of management is to limit treatment morbidity without compromising chance of cure. For the compliant patient, surveillance is probably the option of choice. For patients not suitable for surveillance, adjuvant radiotherapy or adjuvant chemotherapy significantly reduces the risk of relapse. There are, however, limited data on the long-term efficacy or toxicity of adjuvant carboplatin. Furthermore, ongoing surveillance of the retroperitoneal nodes will still be required.

For patients with stage II seminoma, the recommended treatment depends on the bulk of retroperitoneal nodal disease. Radiotherapy of 25 to 35 Gy is the treatment of choice for patients with stage IIA or IIB seminoma (nodal disease up to 5 cm in maximal diameter). Irradiation of the para-aortic and ipsilateral pelvic nodes is a highly effective treatment strategy with a recurrence rate of <10% (see Table 64.6) and a disease-specific survival rate of 97% to 100%. The most common site of relapse following infradiaphragmatic radiotherapy is in the supraclavicular fossa or mediastinum, and as a result some authors recommend prophylactic supraclavicular irradiation (108). However, the proportion of patients destined to relapse exclusively in the supraclavicular fossa is small at <5%, and results with infradiaphragmatic irradiation alone with chemotherapy as salvage are excellent (19,22).

Disease control rates for stage IIA or IIB seminoma with single agent carboplatin appear inferior to that with radiotherapy. A phase II study by the German Testicular Cancer Study Group delivered three or four cycles of carboplatin to patients with stage IIA or stage IIB seminoma, respectively (53). The overall failure rate was 18%, with all relapses occurring in the retroperitoneum. Although carboplatin has been combined with radiotherapy in order to improve outcome (74), the reported relapse rate is within the range reported with radiotherapy alone.

Patients with stage IIC retroperitoneal disease (nodes >5 cm) are usually managed with systemic chemotherapy. Radiotherapy remains a treatment option, but the relapse rate of 30% is considered by many to be excessive. Chung et al. (19) report recurrence in 10 of 16 patients with stage IIC disease managed with radiotherapy compared to only one relapse in a similar group of 23 patients managed by chemotherapy. The choice of modality is also influenced by the size and location of the retroperitoneal nodal mass. If the mass is centrally located and does not overlie most of one kidney or significantly overlap the liver, primary radiation therapy remains an option. If the loca-

tion of the mass is such that the irradiation volume covers most of one kidney or significant volumes of the liver, then the potential morbidity of radiation therapy can be avoided by the use of primary cisplatin-containing combination chemotherapy (usually etoposide/cisplatin [EP] or bleomycin/etoposide/cisplatin [BEP]). For nodal disease >10 cm in diameter, the relapse rate is over 40% with radiotherapy, and these patients should be managed with systemic chemotherapy.

For the rare patient with stage III disease (i.e., supradiaphragmatic nodal disease or dissemination to parenchymal organs), or those with relapse following radiotherapy, the current standard therapy is three courses of BEP or four courses of EP chemotherapy. These patients are classified into either an intermediate prognosis or good prognosis group by the EGCCCG Consensus Classification, depending on the presence or absence of nonpulmonary visceral metastases, respectively (see Table 64.7). The 5-year survival is around 91% for good prognosis and 79% for intermediate prognosis patients. Despite initial favorable reports, single-agent carboplatin is not as effective as cisplatin-based combination treatment. In a pooled analysis of two randomized trials of 361 patients with metastatic seminoma, Bokemeyer et al. (9) reported an inferior progression-free (72% vs. 92%) and overall (89% vs. 94%) survival with carboplatin. Carboplatin monotherapy proved inferior to cisplatin-based combination therapy in all subgroups examined. The efficacy of carboplatin combinations (e.g., with ifosfamide or cyclophosphamide) has not been adequately tested.

For patients with stage II or III disease treated with primary chemotherapy, residual masses are present at 1 month in up to 80% of patients. Most of these then gradually regress over a period of several months. Management strategies involve the use of consolidative radiotherapy, surgical resection, or observation. In an effort to define the role of postchemotherapy radiotherapy, the Medical Research Council (MRC) Testicular Tumour Working Party conducted a retrospective review of patients with advanced seminoma managed by chemotherapy from 10 European centers (31). Of 302 patients identified, 174 (58%) had residual masses on completion of chemotherapy, with a subsequent 3-year progression-free survival of 85%. Approximately half of these patients underwent postchemotherapy radiotherapy, with selection based predominantly on institutional preference. Radiotherapy did not significantly influence the risk of progression, contributing an absolute increase in progression-free survival of only 2.3%. Instead, the most important prognostic factors for progression were the presence of prechemotherapy visceral metastases or raised LDH, or persistent visceral metastases postchemotherapy. At St. Bartholomew's Hospital, 43 of 107 patients (40%) with advanced seminoma had a residual mass postchemotherapy (81). Positive histology was found in three of 19 (15%) who underwent surgical exploration, while relapse at the site of the mass occurred in three others who were observed. Residual disease was only found in masses >3 cm in size. Of the 107 patients, 98 (92%) remained alive and free of recurrence. The largest report of surgical resection following chemotherapy comes from the Memorial Sloan-Kettering Cancer Centre (44). A total of 55 patients with advanced seminoma underwent resection or biopsy of residual mass within 4 weeks of chemotherapy. Of 27 with a mass >3 cm, eight (30%) had residual tumor. No viable tumor was found in any of the 28 patients with a residual mass <3 cm in maximal diameter.

From the above reports, it is clear that observation alone is adequate for a residual mass <3 cm in size. Two patterns of response to chemotherapy are evident on CT—the residual mass may be well defined with discrete, well-defined borders, or the mass may have indistinct borders merging into surrounding structures and resembling a fibrous plaque. The former are more amenable to surgical resection. Furthermore, if the tumor is well defined on CT, and measures more than 3 cm in greatest dimension, positive histology can be found in 50%. It is reasonable to resect these masses. If the mass is poorly defined, even if larger than 3 cm, the chance of finding positive histology is <10%. Resecting such a mass is hazardous, with risk of great vessel, ureteric, and small bowel injury. These should be observed. PET scan has been shown to have a high predictive value in the evaluation of postchemotherapy residual disease and can be further used to guide management.

Intratubular Germ-Cell Neoplasia

About 5% of men with testicular cancer will have intratubular germ-cell neoplasia in the contralateral testis. In 50% of cases, this will progress to invasive disease within 5 years. Surveillance is an option, but it is felt that eventually almost all cases will progress to invasive disease. Chemotherapy is not an effective treatment for IGCN. Cisplatin-based combination chemotherapy results in the temporary disappearance of IGCN from the contralateral testis, but it later recurs in a high proportion. The cumulative risk of recurrence is estimated at 21% and 42% at 5 and 10 years, respectively (17).

Radiotherapy is the treatment of choice for contralateral IGCN. Low-dose radiotherapy (16 to 20 Gy) is capable of eradicating IGCN while preserving most of the Leydig cell function. Ablation of germ cells in the remaining testis will result. However, almost all men with contralateral IGCN are already infertile (76). Several studies have shown the efficacy of radiotherapy in eliminating IGCN, and subsequent relapse is rare (20,75,91). Following radiotherapy, repeat biopsy shows a characteristic pattern of Sertoli-cell–only syndrome, with the disappearance of germ-cell elements. Some impairment of androgen production results, with clinical androgen deficiency in 20% to 25% of men following 18 to 20 Gy. Although it was suggested that doses as low as 14 Gy would be effective in eradicating IGCN with less impairment of testosterone production, recurrence and persistence of disease has been reported at these lower doses. Furthermore, serum testosterone declines at 3.6% per year following radiation in the 14 to 20 Gy range, with no dose dependency, leading most authors to recommend delivery of 18 to 20 Gy at 2 Gy per fraction.

Nonseminomatous Germ-Cell Tumors

A detailed discussion of the management of NSGCT is beyond the scope of this chapter. About half of all patients with NSGCT have clinical stage I disease at presentation. Options for management include surveillance, retroperitoneal node dissection, and adjuvant chemotherapy. All lead to a survival rate of close to 100%. Adjuvant radiotherapy has no role. Although capable

of preventing retroperitoneal relapse, the rate of distant relapse is the same as in patients offered surveillance (88). The relapse rate on surveillance is around 28% (range 13% to 37%) and the disease specific survival rate is 98% (range 95% to 100%) (92). The median time to relapse is 6 months, with almost all relapses occurring within 2 years. About 50% of relapses occur in the retroperitoneum and 25% in the lungs. Elevated tumor markers are found in over two thirds of relapsing patients, and there is 20% relapse rate with elevated markers only. Venous invasion, the presence of undifferentiated elements, and the absence of yolk sac elements independently predict for risk of relapse. The relapse risk increases from <5% to around 50% depending on the presence of these three risk factors.

Given the timing and pattern of relapse, it is recommended that a surveillance schedule should involve a physical examination, serum tumor marker levels, and chest x-ray every month in the 1st year, every 2 months in the 2nd year, every 3 months in the 3rd year, and every 6 months in the 4th and 5th years. CT scans of the abdomen and pelvis should be conducted every 1 month in the 1st year, every 4 months in the 2nd year, every 6 months in the 3rd year, and every 12 months in the 4th and 5th years (32).

Stage I NSGCT may alternatively be managed by retroperitoneal lymph node dissection (RPLND), resulting in an overall survival of 99%. Twenty percent to 30% of patients will be found to have pathologic stage II disease. Pathologic stage I disease has a reported relapse rate of about 11%, almost exclusively at distant sites, while pathologic stage II disease has a subsequent relapse rate of 20% to 30%, related to the extent of nodal involvement. This relapse rate can virtually be eliminated with the use of adjuvant chemotherapy, typically two cycles of BEP or EP. Modern surgical technique, specifically the use of modified nerve-sparing RPLND, has greatly reduced operative morbidity and has reduced the frequency of retrograde ejaculation to 5%.

Adjuvant chemotherapy with two cycles of BEP is an effective treatment strategy for patients with high-risk stage I disease. A large phase II MRC study concluded that two cycles of BEP reduced the relapse risk from an expected 50% to 2% (24). Substituting vincristine for etoposide (BOP) has similar efficacy with less alopecia, but results in unacceptable rates of neuropathy (93). Clinical stage I patients can therefore be managed by a policy of surveillance, RPLND, or adjuvant chemotherapy depending on patient preference, anticipated morbidity of treatment, and perceived risk of relapse.

Clinical stage IIA or IIB disease may be managed with either RPLND or primary chemotherapy (104). Between 11% and 25% of clinical stage II patients will be found to have pathologic stage I disease, with a subsequent relapse risk of around 10%. Subsequent surveillance is also appropriate for stage II disease with nodes <2 cm in diameter, where the relapse risk is around 25%. Relapse can be managed with salvage chemotherapy. For bulkier nodal disease, the risk of relapse is over 50% and immediate chemotherapy is often administered (53), which virtually eliminates risk of relapse, although surveillance is still an option. Either approach results in a survival of 98%.

If clinical stage II patients are managed with primary chemotherapy, typically three cycles of chemotherapy are used, resulting in a complete response in two-thirds, with a further third requiring a RPLND to remove a residual mass. Survival is similar whichever strategy is chosen. Following a primary RPLND, one third of patients relapse and require chemotherapy; following primary chemotherapy, one third of patients have a residual mass and require surgery.

Patients with stage IIC or III disease at presentation are managed with primary chemotherapy. One third of chemotherapy-treated patients have a radiographically apparent residual mass or masses after chemotherapy. In general, these should be excised. Although 30% to 50% will be found to have necrosis, 25%

to 40% are composed of teratoma and another 10% to 20% of undifferentiated carcinoma (71,80). Patients found to have necrosis or teratoma have a low risk of recurrence after surgical excision, but there is presumptive evidence that unresected teratoma may give rise to later relapse or progression. Patients with persistent carcinoma require additional chemotherapy but generally do well with this treatment.

Radiation therapy has no role in the management of patients with disseminated nonseminoma, with the exception of palliation or management of brain metastases in some patients. Newly diagnosed brain metastases, although rare, are still potentially curable. All require systemic chemotherapy. Resection should be considered of solitary metastases. On the other hand, if multiple metastases are present or if systemic therapy is urgently needed because of advanced systemic disease, it is certainly appropriate to proceed immediately with brain irradiation and systemic chemotherapy. Control of central nervous system disease is usually achieved; patients who do not attain durable complete remission usually fail systemically and not intracranially (10,93).

Radiation Therapy Techniques

For stage I disease, the clinical target volume (CTV) consists of the interaortocaval, preaortic, and para-aortic nodes. The left renal hilar nodes are included for left-sided tumors. The ipsilateral external iliac and common iliac nodes may also be included, particularly if there is concern about aberrant drainage. Inclusion of the inguinal scar, inguinal lymph nodes, or hemiscrotum is not warranted in the routine treatment of stage I disease. For stage II disease, a gross tumor volume (GTV) is identified from diagnostic imaging and the CTV also includes the ipsilateral pelvic nodes.

To cover the CTV with an appropriate margin, standard anatomical field borders have been used, classically the "dog-leg" or "hockey stick" technique. The superior border is placed between the T9 and T10 vertebral bodies, with the inferior border at the top of the obturator foramen. Some recommend using a lower superior border (T10/11 or T11/12 interspace) to reduce radiation dose to heart (11), and the inferior border may reasonably be raised to above the acetabulum to reduce the dose to testis. On the left, the lateral border is extended to include the left renal hilum, and customized shielding is positioned to reduce the amount of kidney irradiated. At the mid-L4 level the field is extended laterally to cover the ipsilateral external iliac nodes. Shielding is placed forming the "dog-leg" configuration (Fig. 64.1). Testicular shielding should be used if the patient wishes to preserve fertility (37). Traditional field placement based on bony anatomy provides adequate coverage of the nodal CTV for most patients. Individualized CT-based planning using large vessels as surrogates for nodal position may result in superior target dosimetry (61). Multileaf collimators now largely replace lead blocks to define the field shape.

If pelvic nodes are not being treated, the superior and lateral borders are largely as described above, although most use a lower superior border (e.g., T10/11). The inferior border is placed at the L5/S1 disc space (Fig. 64.2). Treatment is given using an anterior and posterior parallel opposed pair with 6 to 18 MV photons.

A wide range of dose and fractionation may be used. A dose of 25 Gy in 20 fractions is commonly used, although a similar dose at 2 Gy per fraction may be delivered over a shorter period of time. There is no benefit of treating to higher dose. The U.K. MRC and European Organization for Research and Treatment of Cancer (EORTC) have performed a randomized trial of 20 Gy in 10 fractions over 2 weeks and 30 Gy in 15 fractions over 3 weeks in 625 men with stage I seminoma (50). Almost 90% were treated with para-aortic fields. With a median follow-up of 61 months, 5-year relapse-free rates were similar at 97% and 96.4% in the 30 Gy and 20 Gy arms, respectively. Patients randomized to the 20 Gy arm had less early acute toxicity than those in the 30 Gy arm, although this difference

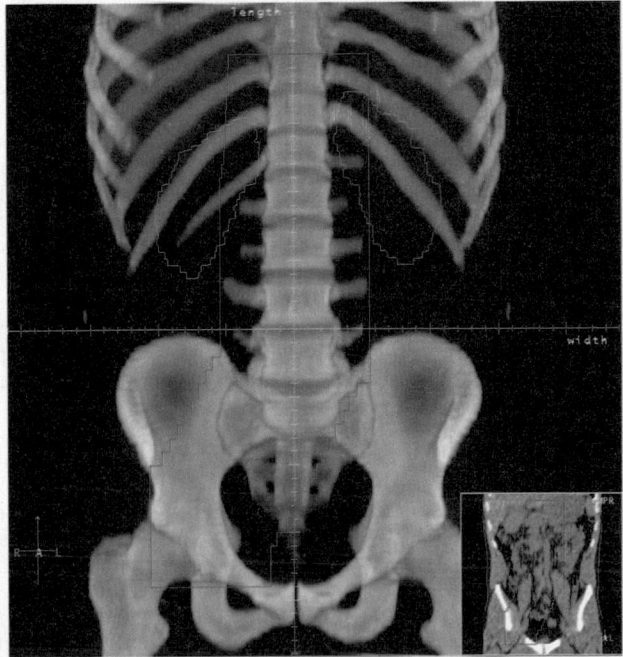
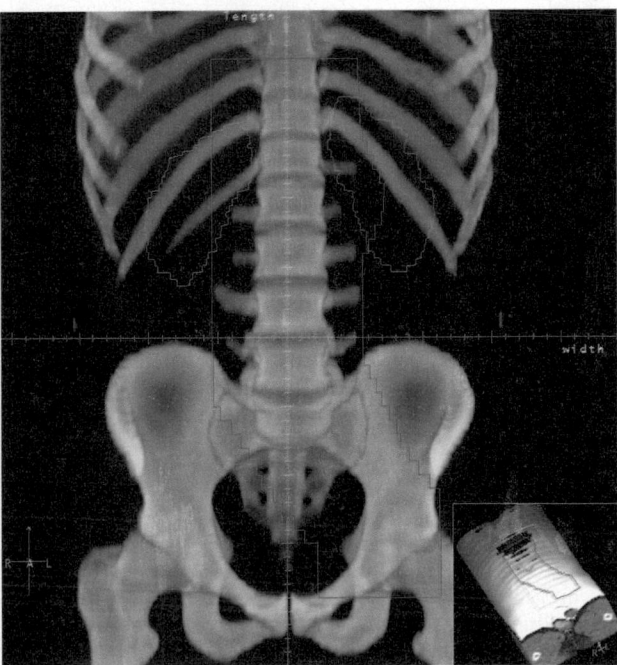

FIGURE 64.1. Classic dog-leg fields encompass the para-aortic and ipsilateral pelvic nodes. The superior border is at the T9/10 interspace, and the inferior border just above the obturator foramen (**A**). The lateral borders of the para-aortic field are at the tips of the lumbar transverse processes. For left sided tumors (**B**), the fields are often widened at the level of the renal hilum to include the hilar nodes. Acceptable modifications include reducing the superior border by one or two vertebral levels and raising the inferior border to above the acetabulum.

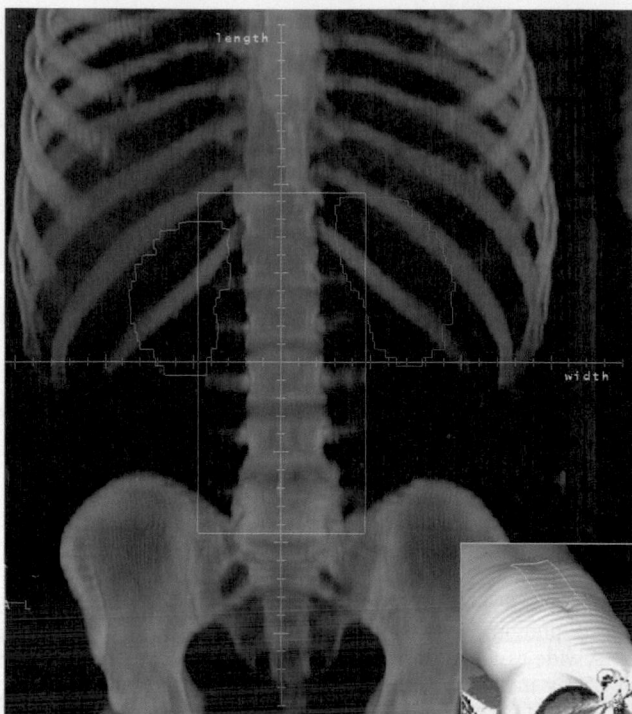

FIGURE 64.2. Para-aortic fields generally extend from the superior plate of T12 to the inferior border of L5. Laterally, the field edge is placed at the tips of the transverse processes, but may be expanded at the left renal hilum for left-sided tumors.

was no longer apparent at 12 weeks. Late toxicity has not been reported.

For stage IIA disease, standard dog-leg fields are used to treat the para-aortic and ipsilateral pelvic nodes. In a prospective study from Germany, a smaller treated volume was chosen: The superior border was set at the top of T11 and inferior border at the superior rim of the acetabulum (22). There appears to be little rationale for routine inclusion of the contralateral pelvic nodes, although the contralateral common iliac nodes may be included if there is concern about the risk of retrograde spread. For stage IIB disease (2 to 5 cm diameter), the field width should be appropriately widened to encompass the mass as visualized on CT with a margin of 2 cm (Fig. 64.3).

The optimal dose of radiation is unclear, with a range of acceptable dose and fractionations. Stage IIA disease is commonly treated to 25 Gy in 20 fractions, although other modern series recommend 26 to 30 Gy at 2 Gy per fraction. For stage IIB disease, the total radiation dose is usually increased to 35 Gy. The first 25 Gy is typically delivered to an initial volume, and a boost of 10 Gy in five fractions is given to a reduced field that encompasses the nodal mass with an adequate margin (see Figure 64.3C). Total doses between 26 Gy and 36 Gy at 2 Gy per fraction are also commonly used with excellent clinical outcome.

Stage IIC disease is treated by the same principles of radiation therapy as applied to stage IIB disease. In general, the abdominal fields are larger to encompass the known volume of disease. If a choice of primary radiation therapy has been made and the irradiation field of necessity encompasses most of one kidney, the field size should be reduced as the tumor shrinks. Initial shrinkage of large masses is often rapid, and abdominal CT scan repeated after the first 3 weeks of radiation therapy may allow significant reduction of the treatment volume while still encompassing the tumor mass. This allows at least two thirds of the kidney to be spared total doses higher than 18 Gy.

Results of Therapy

Seminoma

The outcome of treatment with currently available therapies depends on the stage and extent of disease at presentation. Table 64.3 shows the stage of disease at presentation and the expected survival for each group. The overall survival is around 97%.

For stage I disease, routine irradiation of the retroperitoneum and ipsilateral pelvic nodes results in 10-year relapse-free survival rates of 96% to 98% (see Table 64.8). Approximately 1% to 4% of patients relapse after infradiaphragmatic irradiation, usually within the first 3 years (58). The sites of relapse are usually evenly distributed between the mediastinum and distant sites. Occasional relapses occur as nonseminomatous germ-cell malignancies, even after careful review of the initial tumor, have shown a pure seminoma. Deaths from stage I seminoma are extremely rare. Most relapsing patients are salvaged with subsequent treatment, usually chemotherapy. Cause-specific survival rates in the large series are 99% to 100%.

The outcome for patients with stage II disease treated with infradiaphragmatic irradiation or infradiaphragmatic plus prophylactic mediastinal irradiation is shown in Table 64.6. Of 314 patients with nodes <2 cm in size, 24 (8%) developed a recurrence. Of 225 patients with nodal disease between 2 and 5 cm, recurrence occurred in 32 (14%). In the more contemporary prospective series reported by Classen et al., (22) disease-free survival was 95.3% for stage IIA and 88.9% for stage IIB despite the use of relatively small treatment fields. Relapse most commonly occurs in the mediastinum, supraclavicular nodes, and lungs. Cisplatin-based chemotherapy is able to salvage in excess of 80% of the relapses, leading to a 5-year cause specific survival rate of 96% to 100%.

Accumulated results of six series involving patients with masses >5 cm (stage IIC) suggest that the relapse rate after irradiation (usually including prophylactic mediastinal irradiation) is around 30% (see Table 64.6). Although the number of patients with stage IIC disease in any series is small, the overall survival rate appears to be over 90%. There is considerable variation in relapse rates reported between the different series. Mason and Kearsley (62) reported only two relapses in 12 patients with nodes between 5 and 10 cm, and four relapses in 12 patients with nodes >10 cm. The largest series of stage IIC patients comes from the Norwegian Radium Hospital (33). The relapse rate was 10% (two of 20) with nodes between 5 and 10 cm, and 31% (nine of 29) with nodes >10 cm. In the more recent report from the Princess Margaret Hospital, relapse occurred following infradiaphragmatic irradiation in eight of 14 patients with lymph nodes between 5 and 10 cm, and in both patients whose nodes were >10 cm. Only two of the 10 recurrences were solely "in-field." The majority of patients relapse at distant sites, such as in the neck or the mediastinum.

Because of the ability to salvage patients who relapse following radiotherapy with cisplatin-based combination chemotherapy, the survival results following primary radiotherapy or chemotherapy as initial therapy in patients with bulkier nodal disease are comparable. The potential toxicities of each approach must be evaluated for each patient, along with other factors influencing the choice of therapy.

For patients with stage IIC tumors >10 cm in diameter, relapse occurs in approximately 50% of the patients treated with initial radiation therapy, whether or not prophylactic mediastinal irradiation is given. Primary chemotherapy in patients with stage IIC disease has yielded a cumulative progression-free survival rate of over 90%. As discussed earlier, 30% to 50% of patients will have a residual mass detected on subsequent

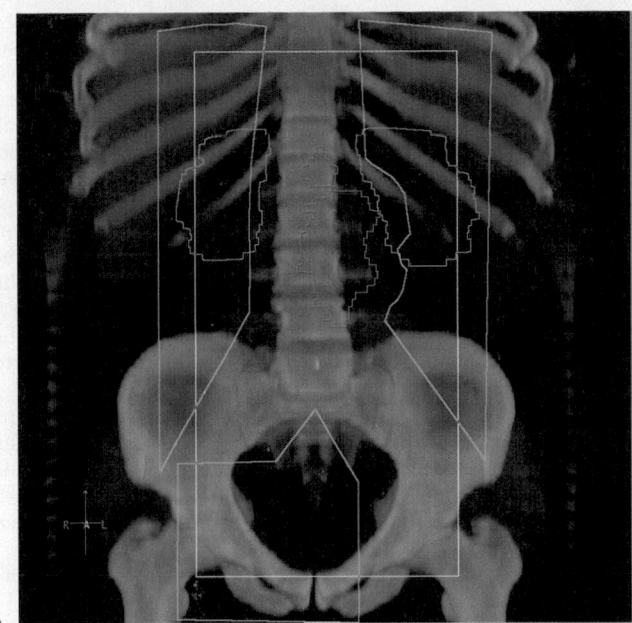

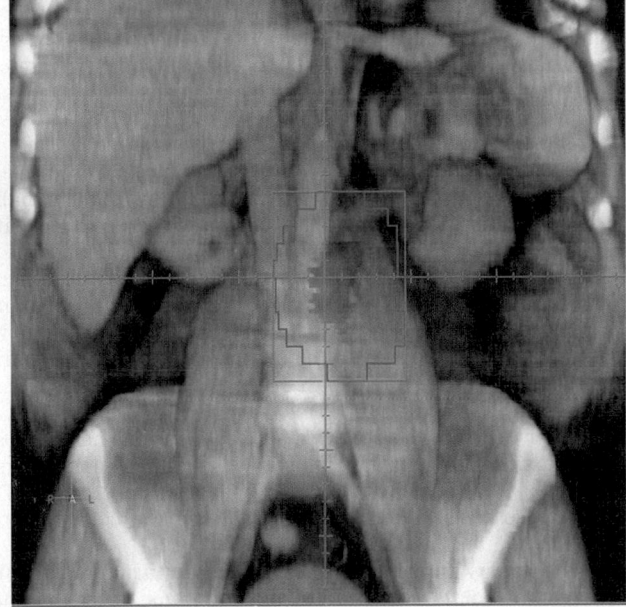

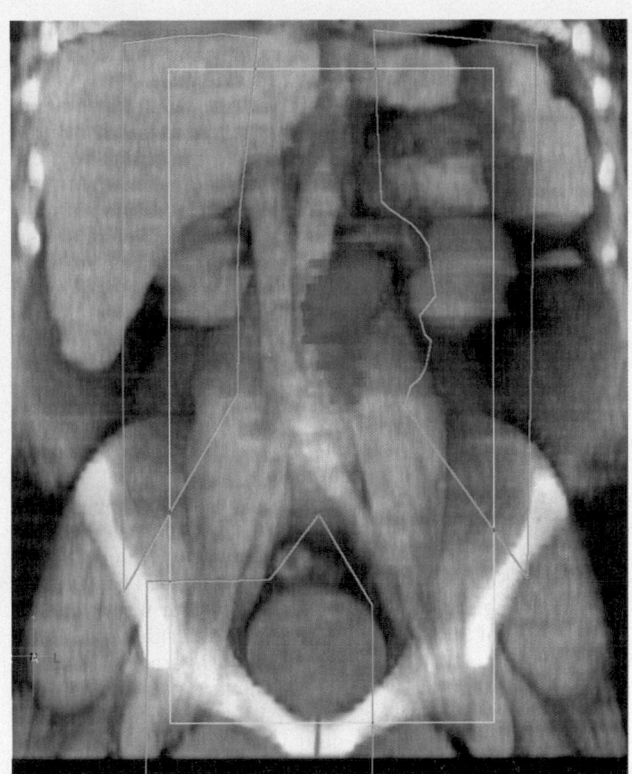

FIGURE 64.3. For stage IIb seminoma, the fields are widened to cover the gross nodal disease **(A,B)**. The inferior and lateral border on the contralateral side may be increased to include the contralateral common iliac nodes. Repeat CT scan **(C)** after 25 Gy demonstrates significant shrinkage of the mass, which then received a further 10 Gy in five fractions to the volume indicated.

CT imaging. The use of consolidation therapy after initial chemotherapy for bulky disease is gradually being abandoned. Surgery to remove residual masses is generally only considered for well-defined masses >3 cm or where the FDG-PET scan is positive. Due to the dense desmoplastic reaction induced by chemotherapy, surgery is usually technically difficult and often incomplete.

Cisplatin-based chemotherapy (BEP × 3 or EP × 4) is the standard treatment for patients with stage III seminoma, as well as for those with retroperitoneal masses >5 cm. Mencel et al. (66) reported that 93% of 142 patients with advanced seminoma achieved a favorable response to platinum-based chemotherapy, with an overall progression-free survival rate of 86%. Fifty-seven of 60 patients (95%) treated with four cycles of etoposide and platinum (EP) achieved a favorable response, and 55 (92%) remained progression free. Although it was expected that carboplatin would be a less toxic alternative to EP or BEP, subsequent randomized studies have shown it to be less effective.

A pooled analysis of 361 patients with metastatic seminoma included in two European clinical trials reported lower disease-free (72% vs. 92%) and overall survival (89% vs. 94%) for those randomized to the carboplatin arms.

Sequelae of Treatment

Radiation Therapy

The long-term sequelae of standard infradiaphragmatic irradiation for stage IA and IIA disease are related to the dose of radiation used (43). There appears to be no curative advantage for doses >25 Gy, but there is an increase in toxicity. In the MRC randomized trial comparing 30 Gy in 15 fractions delivered to either dog-leg or para-aortic fields, 33 of 478 patients (7%) were diagnosed with a peptic ulcer during follow-up. The occurrence rate was similar in both treatment arms. Very few patients report diarrhea as a long-term consequence, and the great majority of patients report a satisfactory quality of life, with a maintained body image and few side effects (13).

Approximately 50% of patients with testicular seminoma have some degree of impairment in spermatogenesis at the time of presentation. They have lower than average fertility both before and after diagnosis (77). Preirradiation impairment of spermatogenesis makes evaluation of the effects of irradiation on fertility difficult. It is unclear whether removal of the affected testis results in spontaneous amelioration of defects in spermatogenesis. Exposure of the remaining testis to therapeutic irradiation may further impair fertility, and the degree of impairment is dose dependent. Available data suggest that hormonal function and spermatogenesis may be compromised at dose levels as low as 0.5 Gy, and that cumulative doses above 2 Gy probably lead to permanent injury. Hahn et al. (42) reported the induction of aspermia in 10 of 14 patients who received over 65 cGy to the remaining testis. Aspermia was not detected at doses <50 cGy. Recovery of sperm in the semen occurred in the majority within 30 to 80 weeks of radiotherapy. A detailed assessment of fertility and sexual function was performed in the Southwest Oncology Group Study 8711 in a series of men following orchidectomy and radiotherapy for seminoma (41). Fourteen of 26 patients (54%) were subfertile at baseline, with a sperm count of <20,000 per mL. The average prescribed dose was 26 Gy in 1.6 Gy fractions, delivering a median dose of 79 cGy to the remaining testis. With a testicular dose below the median, the sperm count tended to drop to a nadir value around 6 months, with recovery of fertility by 12 months. With higher testicular dose, recovery of sperm count was further delayed. Jacobsen et al. (48) reported a 50% reduction in sperm count at 1 year in 21 men following dog-leg radiotherapy (median testis dose, 32 cGy). No change in sperm count was noted in 24 men treated with para-aortic fields (median testis dose 9cGy). Dog-leg radiotherapy also results in an elevation of serum follicle-stimulating hormone (FSH) levels, with no change in serum testosterone. FSH levels are highest within 6 months of radiotherapy and return to normal within 3 years. Use of para-aortic fields is not associated with significant alteration in endocrine profile. For men treated with dog leg fields, careful shielding of the remaining testis can reduce the dose received by the testis to between 1% and 2% of the prescription dose. With current radiation techniques, the great majority of men will return to baseline sperm concentrations and hormone levels with minimal impact on fertility.

It has been recognized for some time that patients are at increased risk of developing a second primary malignancy following treatment for testicular cancer. Travis et al. (96) investigated the occurrence of second malignancies among over 40,000 men who had undergone treatment for a testicular cancer between 1943 and 2001 from 14 population-based cancer registries in North America and Europe. The risk of developing a second solid tumor among 10-year survivors was almost twice that of the general population, with a relative risk (RR) of 1.9. The risk remained elevated for 35 years, with the highest RR for cancers of the stomach (RR = 4.0), pancreas (RR = 3.6), and bladder (RR = 2.7). There was also an increased risk of developing cancers of the lung, esophagus, colon, and pleura. An increased risk was found for both seminomas and nonseminomas and in patients treated with radiotherapy alone (RR = 2.0), chemotherapy alone (RR = 1.8), and both modalities (RR = 2.9). A case control study of leukemia risk in a cohort of 18,567 patients treated for testicular cancer between 1970 and 1993 has also been reported (95). Radiotherapy (mean dose 12.6 Gy to bone marrow) without chemotherapy was associated with a threefold elevated risk of leukemia. Risk increased with increasing dose of radiation to bone marrow, largely associated with the use of mediastinal irradiation. The cumulative dose of cisplatin was also predictive of excess leukemia risk, being

3.2 with the commonly administered dose. In absolute terms, it is estimated that 25 Gy to the retroperitoneum would result in nine excess cases of leukemia in 10,000 patients followed for 15 years. Commonly used doses of cisplatin might result in 16 excess cases. Although treatment factors are strongly implicated in the development of second primary malignancies following treatment, an excess risk of second cancers is seen even among testicular cancer patients who have just been observed. An increased rate of spontaneous chromosomal translocations is seen in lymphocytes of patients with early stage seminoma, compared to healthy controls (90). Following adjuvant radiotherapy, the translocation rate increases, before returning to preradiotherapy levels at around 30 months (69). It is hypothesized that this genomic instability may be a predisposing factor toward malignancy development.

Long-term survivors following radiotherapy for seminoma are also at increased risk of death from cardiac disease. Zagars et al. (107) have reported a cardiac standardized mortality ratio of 1.85 in patients followed out beyond 15 years. An excess risk was noted whether or not mediastinal radiotherapy was delivered.

Chemotherapy

Cisplatin-based chemotherapy is associated with alopecia and the potential for substantial nausea and vomiting. Modern antiemetics have improved gastrointestinal reactions. Serious short-term problems are myelosuppression, bleomycin-induced pulmonary fibrosis, and rarely, cisplatin nephrotoxicity. Myelosuppression and pulmonary fibrosis are fatal in 0.5% to 4% of treated patients.

A recently recognized effect of chemotherapy used in the treatment of germ-cell tumors is the risk of secondary malignancy. As discussed above, the cumulative dose of cisplatin strongly correlates with the risk of subsequent malignancy (95). Etoposide exposure increases the risk of leukemia. Morphologically, these leukemias are usually monocytic or myelomonocytic. Characteristic chromosomal translocations are frequently but not invariably present. The onset of leukemia is ordinarily closer to chemotherapy exposure than is the typical leukemia induced by alkylating agents.

Other late toxicities reported include high tone hearing loss, neurotoxicity, Raynaud's phenomenon, ischemic heart disease, hypertension, renal dysfunction, and pulmonary toxicity. Despite these observations, most patients have excellent overall health and functional status.

The fertility implications of chemotherapy are complex. BEP causes immediate azoospermia, but, with time, more than half of patients may recover normal or near-normal spermatogenesis (94). Permanent chemotherapy-related infertility is a rare event (27), and endocrine dysfunction only occurs with high cumulative doses of cisplatin (40).

References

1. *AJCC cancer staging manual*, 6th ed. New York: Springer-Verlag, 2006.
2. Albers P, Bender H, Yilmaz H, et al. Positron emission tomography in the clinical staging of patients with stage I and II testicular germ cell tumors. *Urology* 1999;53:808–811.
3. American Cancer Society. *Cancer facts and figures.* 2006.
4. Aparicio J, Germa JR, Garcia dM X, et al. Risk-adapted management for patients with clinical stage I seminoma: The Second Spanish Germ Cell Cancer Cooperative Group study. *J Clin Oncol* 2005;23:8717–8723.
5. Bach AM, Hann LE, Hadar O, et al. Testicular microlithiasis: What is its association with testicular cancer? *Radiology* 2001;220:70–75.
6. Bagnell S, Choo R, Klotz LH, et al. Practice patterns of Canadian urologists in the management of stage I testicular seminoma. *Can J Urol* 2004;11:2194–2199.
7. Bauman GS, Venkatesan VM, Ago CT, et al. Postoperative radiotherapy for stage I/II seminoma: Results for 212 patients. *Int J Radiat Oncol Biol Phys* 1998;42:313–317.
8. Becherer A, De Santis M, Karanikas G, et al. FDG PET is superior to CT in the prediction of viable tumour in post-chemotherapy seminoma residuals. *Eur J Radiol* 2005;54:284–288.

9. Bokemeyer C, Kollmannsberger C, Stenning S, et al. Metastatic seminoma treated with either single agent carboplatin or cisplatin-based combination chemotherapy: A pooled analysis of two randomised trials. *Br J Cancer* 2004;91:683–687.
10. Bokemeyer C, Nowak P, Haupt A, et al. Treatment of brain metastases in patients with testicular cancer. *J Clin Oncol* 1997;15:1449–1454.
11. Bruns F, Bremer M, Meyer A, et al. Adjuvant radiotherapy in stage I seminoma: Is there a role for further reduction of treatment volume? *Acta Oncol* 2005;44:142–148.
12. Bussar-Maatz R, Weissbach L. Retroperitoneal lymph node staging of testicular tumours. TNM Study Group. *Br J Urol* 1993;72:234–240.
13. Caffo O, Amichetti M, Tomio L, et al. Quality of life after radiotherapy for early-stage testicular seminoma. *Radiother Oncol* 2001;59:13–20.
14. Capelouto CC, Clark PE, Ransil BJ, et al. A review of scrotal violation in testicular cancer: Is adjuvant local therapy necessary? *J Urol* 1995;153:981–985.
15. Choo R, Sandler H, Warde P, et al. Survey of radiation oncologists: Practice patterns of the management of stage I seminoma of testis in Canada and a selected group in the United States. *Can J Urol* 2002;9:1479–1485.
16. Choo R, Thomas G, Woo T, et al. Long-term outcome of postorchiectomy surveillance for stage I testicular seminoma. *Int J Radiat Oncol Biol Phys* 2005;61:736–740.
17. Christensen TB, Daugaard G, Geertsen PF, et al. Effect of chemotherapy on carcinoma in situ of the testis. *Ann Oncol* 1998;9:657–660.
18. Chung P, Parker C, Panzarella T, et al. Surveillance in stage I testicular seminoma—risk of late relapse. *Can J Urol* 2002;9:1637–1640.
19. Chung PW, Gospodarowicz MK, Panzarella T, et al. Stage II testicular seminoma: Patterns of recurrence and outcome of treatment. *Eur Urol* 2004;45:754–759.
20. Classen J, Dieckmann K, Bamberg M, et al. Radiotherapy with 16 Gy may fail to eradicate testicular intraepithelial neoplasia: Preliminary communication of a dose-reduction trial of the German Testicular Cancer Study Group. *Br J Cancer* 2003;88:828–831.
21. Classen J, Schmidberger H, Meisner C, et al. Para-aortic irradiation for stage I testicular seminoma: Results of a prospective study in 675 patients. A trial of the German testicular cancer study group (GTCSG). *Br J Cancer* 2004;90:2305–2311.
22. Classen J, Schmidberger H, Meisner C, et al. Radiotherapy for stages IIA/B testicular seminoma: Final report of a prospective multicenter clinical trial. *J Clin Oncol* 2003;21:1101–1106.
23. Coupland CA, Chilvers CE, Davey G, et al. Risk factors for testicular germ cell tumours by histological tumour type. United Kingdom Testicular Cancer Study Group. *Br J Cancer* 1999;80:1859–1863.
24. Cullen MH, Stenning SP, Parkinson MC, et al. Short-course adjuvant chemotherapy in high-risk stage I nonseminomatous germ cell tumors of the testis: A Medical Research Council report. *J Clin Oncol* 1996;14:1106–1113.
25. Daugaard G, Petersen PM, Rorth M. Surveillance in stage I testicular cancer. *APMIS* 2003;111:76–83.
26. Dearnaley DP, Fossa SD, Kaye SB, et al. Adjuvant bleomycin, vincristine and cisplatin (BOP) for high-risk stage I non-seminomatous germ cell tumours: A prospective trial (MRC TE17). *Br J Cancer* 2005;92:2107–2113.
27. DeSantis M, Albrecht W, Holtl W, et al. Impact of cytotoxic treatment on long-term fertility in patients with germ-cell cancer. *Int J Cancer* 1999;83:864–865.
28. Dieckmann KP, Bruggeboes B, Pichlmeier U, et al. Adjuvant treatment of clinical stage I seminoma: Is a single course of carboplatin sufficient? *Urology* 2000;55:102–106.
29. Dieckmann KP, Skakkebaek NE. Carcinoma in situ of the testis: Review of biological and clinical features. *Int J Cancer* 1999;83:815–822.
30. Dosmann MA, Zagars GK. Post-orchiectomy radiotherapy for stages I and II testicular seminoma. *Int J Radiat Oncol Biol Phys* 1993;26:381–390.
31. Duchesne GM, Stenning SP, Aass N, et al. Radiotherapy after chemotherapy for metastatic seminoma—a diminishing role. MRC Testicular Tumour Working Party. *Eur J Cancer* 1997;33:829–835.
32. Ernst DS, Brasher P, Venner PM, et al. Compliance and outcome of patients with stage 1 non-seminomatous germ cell tumors (NSGCT) managed with surveillance programs in seven Canadian centres. *Can J Urol* 2005;12:2575–2580.
33. Evensen JF, Fossa SD, Kjellevold K, et al. Testicular seminoma: Analysis of treatment and failure for stage II disease. *Radiother Oncol* 1985;4:55–61.
34. Fatigante L, Ducci F, Campoccia S, et al. Long-term results in patients affected by testicular seminoma treated with radiotherapy: Risk of second malignancies. *Tumori* 2005;91:144–150.
35. Fossa SD, Aass N, Kaalhus O. Radiotherapy for testicular seminoma stage I: Treatment results and long-term post-irradiation morbidity in 365 patients. *Int J Radiat Oncol Biol Phys* 1989;16:383–388.
36. Fossa SD, Horwich A, Russell JM, et al. Optimal planning target volume for stage I testicular seminoma: A Medical Research Council randomized trial. Medical Research Council Testicular Tumor Working Group. *J Clin Oncol* 1999;17:1146.
37. Fraass BA, Kinsella TJ, Harrington FS, et al. Peripheral dose to the testes: The design and clinical use of a practical and effective gonadal shield. *Int J Radiat Oncol Biol Phys* 1985;11:609–615.
38. Francis R, Bower M, Brunstrom G, et al. Surveillance for stage I testicular germ cell tumours: Results and cost benefit analysis of management options. *Eur J Cancer* 2000;36:1925–1932.
39. Garcia-Serra AM, Zlotecki RA, Morris CG, et al. Long-term results of radiotherapy for early-stage testicular seminoma. *Am J Clin Oncol* 2005;28:119–124.
40. Gerl A, Muhlbayer D, Hansmann G, et al. The impact of chemotherapy on Leydig cell function in long term survivors of germ cell tumors. *Cancer* 2001;91:1297–1303.
41. Gordon W Jr., Siegmund K, Stanisic TH, et al. A study of reproductive function in patients with seminoma treated with radiotherapy and orchidectomy: (SWOG-8711). Southwest Oncology Group. *Int J Radiat Oncol Biol Phys* 1997;38:83–94.
42. Hahn EW, Feingold SM, Simpson L, et al. Recovery from aspermia induced by low-dose radiation in seminoma patients. *Cancer* 1982;50:337–340.
43. Hamilton C, Horwich A, Easton D, et al. Radiotherapy for stage I seminoma testis: Results of treatment and complications. *Radiother Oncol* 1986;6:115–120.
44. Herr HW, Sheinfeld J, Puc HS, et al. Surgery for a post-chemotherapy residual mass in seminoma. *J Urol* 1997;157:860–862.
45. Horwich A, Alsanjari N, A'Hern R, et al. Surveillance following orchidectomy for stage I testicular seminoma. *Br J Cancer* 1992;65:775–778.
46. Hruby G, Choo R, Jackson M, et al. Management preferences following radical inguinal orchidectomy for stage I testicular seminoma in Australasia. *Australas Radiol* 2002;46:280–284.
47. International Germ Cell Consensus Classification: A prognostic factor-based staging system for metastatic germ cell cancers. International Germ Cell Cancer Collaborative Group. *J.Clin.Oncol.* 1997;15:594–603.
48. Jacobsen KD, Olsen DR, Fossa K, et al. External beam abdominal radiotherapy in patients with seminoma stage I: Field type, testicular dose, and spermatogenesis. *Int J Radiat Oncol Biol Phys* 1997;38:95–102.
49. Jacobsen R, Bostofte E, Engholm G, et al. Risk of testicular cancer in men with abnormal semen characteristics: Cohort study. *BMJ* 2000;321:789–792.
50. Jones WG, Fossa SD, Mead GM, et al. Randomized trial of 30 versus 20 Gy in the adjuvant treatment of stage I testicular seminoma: A report on Medical Research Council Trial TE18, European Organisation for the Research and Treatment of Cancer Trial 30942 (ISRCTN18525328). *J Clin Oncol* 2005;23:1200–1208.
51. Jorgensen N, Asklund C, Carlsen E, et al. Coordinated European investigations of semen quality: Results from studies of Scandinavian young men is a matter of concern. *Int J Androl* 2006;29:54–61.
52. Koshida K, Uchibayashi T, Yamamoto H, et al. Significance of placental alkaline phosphatase (PLAP) in the monitoring of patients with seminoma. *Br J Urol* 1996;77:138–142.
53. Krege S, Boergermann C, Baschek R, et al. Single agent carboplatin for CS IIA/B testicular seminoma. A phase II study of the German Testicular Cancer Study Group (GTCSG). *Ann Oncol* 2006;17:276–280.
54. Krege S, Kalund G, Otto T, et al. Phase II study: Adjuvant single-agent carboplatin therapy for clinical stage I seminoma. *Eur Urol* 1997;31:405–407.
55. Lassen U, Daugaard G, Eigtved A, et al. Whole-body FDG-PET in patients with stage I non-seminomatous germ cell tumours. *Eur J Nucl Med Mol Imaging* 2003;30:396–402.
56. Leibovitch I, Baniel J, Rowland RG, et al. Malignant testicular neoplasms in immunosuppressed patients. *J Urol* 1996;155:1938–1942.
57. Leibovitch L, Foster RS, Kopecky KK, et al. Improved accuracy of computerized tomography based clinical staging in low stage nonseminomatous germ cell cancer using size criteria of retroperitoneal lymph nodes. *J Urol* 1995;154:1759–1763.
58. Livsey JE, Taylor B, Mobarek N, et al. Patterns of relapse following radiotherapy for stage I seminoma of the testis: Implications for follow-up. *Clin Oncol (R Coll Radiol)* 2001;13:296–300.
59. Logue JP, Harris MA, Livsey JE, et al. Short course para-aortic radiation for stage I seminoma of the testis. *Int J Radiat Oncol Biol Phys* 2003;57:1304–1309.
60. Marks LB, Shipley WU, Walker TG, et al. Role of lymphangiography in staging testicular seminoma. *Urology* 1991;38:264–266.
61. Martin JM, Joon DL, Ng N, et al. Towards individualised radiotherapy for stage I seminoma. *Radiother Oncol* 2005;76:251–256.
62. Mason BR, Kearsley JH. Radiotherapy for stage 2 testicular seminoma: The prognostic influence of tumor bulk. *J Clin Oncol* 1988;6:1856–1862.
63. Matoska J, Ondrus D, Hornak M. Metastatic spermatocytic seminoma. A case report with light microscopic, ultrastructural, and immunohistochemical findings. *Cancer* 1988;62:1197–1201.
64. McGlynn KA, Graubard BI, Nam JM, et al. Maternal hormone levels and risk of cryptorchism among populations at high and low risk of testicular germ cell tumors. *Cancer Epidemiol Biomarkers Prev* 2005;14:1732–1737.
65. Melchior D, Hammer P, Fimmers R, et al. Long term results and morbidity of paraaortic compared with paraaortic and iliac adjuvant radiation in clinical stage I seminoma. *Anticancer Res* 2001;21:2989–2993.
66. Mencel PJ, Motzer RJ, Mazumdar M, et al. Advanced seminoma: Treatment results, survival, and prognostic factors in 142 patients. *J Clin Oncol* 1994;12:120–126.
67. Moller H, Skakkebaek NE. Risk of testicular cancer in subfertile men: Case-control study. *BMJ* 1999;318:559–562.
68. Morrison AS. Cryptorchidism, hernia, and cancer of the testis. *J Natl Cancer Inst* 1976;56:731–733.
69. Muller I, Geinitz H, Braselmann H, et al. Time-course of radiation-induced chromosomal aberrations in tumor patients after radiotherapy. *Int J Radiat Oncol Biol Phys* 2005;63:1214–1220.
70. Niazi TM, Souhami L, Sultanem K, et al. Long-term results of para-aortic irradiation for patients with stage I seminoma of the testis. *Int J Radiat Oncol Biol Phys* 2005;61:741–744.
71. Nord C, Bjoro T, Ellingsen D, et al. Gonadal hormones in long-term survivors 10 years after treatment for unilateral testicular cancer. *Eur Urol* 2003;44:322–328.
72. Oliver RT, Edmonds PM, Ong JY, et al. Pilot studies of 2 and 1 course carboplatin as adjuvant for stage I seminoma: Should it be tested in a randomized trial against radiotherapy? *Int J Radiat Oncol Biol Phys* 1994;29:3–8.
73. Oliver RT, Mason MD, Mead GM, et al. Radiotherapy versus single-dose carboplatin in adjuvant treatment of stage I seminoma: A randomised trial. *Lancet* 2005;366:293–300.
74. Patterson H, Norman AR, Mitra SS, et al. Combination carboplatin and radiotherapy in the management of stage II testicular seminoma: Comparison with radiotherapy treatment alone. *Radiother Oncol* 2001;59:5–11.
75. Petersen PM, Giwercman A, Daugaard G, et al. Effect of graded testicular doses of radiotherapy in patients treated for carcinoma-in-situ in the testis. *J Clin Oncol* 2002;20:1537–1543.
76. Petersen PM, Giwercman A, Hansen SW, et al. Impaired testicular function in patients with carcinoma-in-situ of the testis. *J Clin Oncol* 1999;17:173–179.
77. Petersen PM, Skakkebaek NE, Vistisen K, et al. Semen quality and reproductive hormones before orchiectomy in men with testicular cancer. *J Clin Oncol* 1999;17:941–947.
78. Power DA, Brown RS, Brock CS, et al. Trends in testicular carcinoma in England and Wales, 1971–99. *BJU In.* 2001;87:361–365.
79. Powles TB, Bhardwa J, Shamash J, et al. The changing presentation of germ cell tumours of the testis between 1983 and 2002. *BJU Int* 2005;95:1197–1200.
80. Quek ML, Simma-Chiang V, Stein JP, et al. Postchemotherapy residual masses in advanced seminoma: Current management and outcomes. *Expert Rev Anticancer Ther* 2005;5:869–874.
81. Ravi R, Ong J, Oliver RT, et al. The management of residual masses after chemotherapy in metastatic seminoma. *BJU Int* 1999;83:649–653.
82. Ray B, Hajdu SI, Whitmore WF. Distribution of retroperitoneal lymph node metastases in testicular germinal tumors. *Cancer* 1974;33:340–348.
83. Read G, Stenning SP, Cullen MH, et al. Medical Research Council prospective study of surveillance for stage I testicular teratoma. Medical Research Council Testicular Tumors Working Party. *J Clin Oncol* 1992;10:1762–1768.

84. Reiter WJ, Brodowicz T, Alavi S, et al. Twelve-year experience with two courses of adjuvant single-agent carboplatin therapy for clinical stage I seminoma. *J Clin Oncol* 2001;19:101–104.

85. Reiter WJ, Kratzik C, Brodowicz T, et al. Sperm analysis and serum follicle-stimulating hormone levels before and after adjuvant single-agent carboplatin therapy for clinical stage I seminoma. *Urology* 1998;52:117–119.

86. Richiardi L, Bellocco R, Adami HO, et al. Testicular cancer incidence in eight northern European countries: Secular and recent trends. *Cancer Epidemiol Biomarkers Prev* 2004;13:2157–2166.

87. Ries LAG, Harkins D, Krapcho M, et al. *SEER cancer statistics review, 1975–2003*. Bethesda, MD: National Cancer Institute, 2006.

88. Rorth M, Jacobsen GK, von der MH, et al. Surveillance alone versus radiotherapy after orchiectomy for clinical stage I nonseminomatous testicular cancer. Danish Testicular Cancer Study Group. *J Clin Oncol* 1991;9:1543–1548.

89. Santoni R, Barbera F, Bertoni F, et al. Stage I seminoma of the testis: A bi-institutional retrospective analysis of patients treated with radiation therapy only. *BJU Int* 2003;92:47–52.

90. Schmidberger H, Virsik-Koepp P, Rave-Frank M, et al. Reciprocal translocations in patients with testicular seminoma before and after radiotherapy. *Int J Radiat Oncol Biol Phys* 2001;50:857–864.

91. Sedlmayer F, Holtl W, Kozak W, et al. Radiotherapy of testicular intraepithelial neoplasia (TIN): A novel treatment regimen for a rare disease. *Int J Radiat Oncol Biol Phys* 2001;50:909–913.

92. Sonneveld DJ, Koops HS, Sleijfer DT, et al. Surgery versus surveillance in stage I non-seminoma testicular cancer. *Semin Surg Oncol* 1999;17:230–239.

93. Spears WT, Morphis JG, Lester SG, et al. Brain metastases and testicular tumors: Long-term survival. *Int J Radiat Oncol Biol Phys* 1992;22:17–22.

94. Stephenson WT, Poirier SM, Rubin L, et al. Evaluation of reproductive capacity in germ cell tumor patients following treatment with cisplatin, etoposide, and bleomycin. *J Clin Oncol* 1995;13:2278–2280.

95. Travis LB, Andersson M, Gospodarowicz M, et al. Treatment-associated leukemia following testicular cancer. *J Natl Cancer Inst* 2000;92:1165–1171.

96. Travis LB, Fossa SD, Schonfeld SJ, et al. Second cancers among 40,576 testicular cancer patients: Focus on long-term survivors. *J Natl Cancer Inst* 2005;97:1354–1365.

97. Tyldesley S, Voduc D, McKenzie M, et al. Surveillance of stage I testicular seminoma: British Columbia Cancer Agency Experience 1992 to 2002. *Urology* 2006;67:594–598.

98. Vallis KA, Howard GC, Duncan W, et al. Radiotherapy for stages I and II testicular seminoma: Results and morbidity in 238 patients. *Br J Radiol* 1995;68:400–405.

99. Von der Maas, Specht L, Jacobsen GK, et al. Surveillance following orchidectomy for stage I seminoma of the testis. *Eur J Cancer* 1993;29A:1931–1934.

100. Warde P, Gospodarowicz MK, Banerjee D, et al. Prognostic factors for relapse in stage I testicular seminoma treated with surveillance. *J Urol* 1997;157:1705–1709.

101. Warde P, Gospodarowicz MK, Panzarella T, et al. Long term outcome and cost in the management of stage I testicular seminoma. *Can J Urol* 2000;7:967–972.

102. Warde P, Specht L, Horwich A, et al. Prognostic factors for relapse in stage I seminoma managed by surveillance: A pooled analysis. *J Clin Oncol* 2002;20:4448–4452.

103. Weir HK, Marrett LD, Kreiger N, et al. Pre-natal and peri-natal exposures and risk of testicular germ-cell cancer. *Int J Cancer* 2000;87:438–443.

104. Weissbach L, Bussar-Maatz R, Flechtner H, et al. RPLND or primary chemotherapy in clinical stage IIA/B nonseminomatous germ cell tumors? Results of a prospective multicenter trial including quality of life assessment. *Eur Urol* 2000;37:582–594.

105. Westergaard T, Olsen JH, Frisch M, et al. Cancer risk in fathers and brothers of testicular cancer patients in Denmark. A population-based study. *Int J Cancer* 1996;66:627–631.

106. Whipple GL, Sagerman RH, van Rooy EM. Long-term evaluation of postorchiectomy radiotherapy for stage II seminoma. *Am J Clin Oncol* 1997;20:196–201.

107. Zagars GK, Ballo MT, Lee AK, et al. Mortality after cure of testicular seminoma. *J Clin Oncol* 2004;22:640–647.

108. Zagars GK, Pollack A. Radiotherapy for stage II testicular seminoma. *Int J Radiat Oncol Biol Phys* 2001;51:643–649.

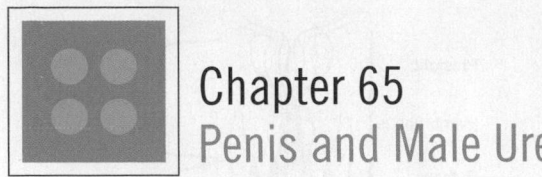

Chapter 65
Penis and Male Urethra

David B. Mansur, K.S. Clifford Chao

Anatomy

The basic structural components of the penis include two corpora cavernosa and the corpus spongiosum (Fig. 65.1A) (85). These are encased in a dense fascia (Buck's fascia), which is separated from the skin by a layer of loose connective tissue. Distally, the corpus spongiosum expands into the glans penis, which is covered by a skinfold known as the prepuce. The skin extends over and is firmly attached to the glans.

The male urethra is composed of a mucous membrane and the submucosa. It extends from the bladder neck to the external urethral meatus (Fig. 65.1B). The posterior urethra is subdivided into the membranous urethra, the portion passing through the urogenital diaphragm, and the prostatic urethra, which passes through the prostate. The anterior urethra passes through the corpus spongiosum and is subdivided into fossa navicularis (a widening within the glans); the penile urethra, which passes through the pendulous part of the penis; and the bulbous urethra, the dilated proximal portion of the anterior urethra. The prostatic urethra is covered by transitional epithelium only. The distal portion of the anterior urethra is covered by stratified squamous epithelium, which changes proximally to pseudostratified columnar epithelium. The columnar epithelium gradually changes into transitional epithelium in the membranous urethra.

The lymphatic channels of the prepuce and the skin of the shaft drain into the superficial inguinal nodes located above the fascia lata. The rich anastomotic network of the lymphatics within the penis and at the base of the penis means that for practical purposes lymphatic drainage may be considered bilateral. There is some disagreement as to whether the glans and the deep penile structures drain into the superficial or deep inguinal lymph nodes (those under the fascia lata). The so-called sentinel nodes located above and medial to the junction of the epigastric and saphenous veins have been identified as the primary drainage sites in carcinoma of the penis (Fig. 65.2) (13,68). Selective biopsy of this group of nodes is of obvious importance in assessment of tumor extent because if they are not involved by tumor, a complete nodal dissection may not be necessary. The reliability of this procedure has not been supported by some (95,96). Catalona (15) found that biopsy of the sentinel nodes showed false-negative results in 10% of Cabanas' patients who died of carcinoma (13).

The lymphatics of the fossa navicularis and the penile urethra follow the lymphatics of the penis to the superficial and deep inguinal lymph nodes. The lymphatics of the bulbomembranous and prostatic urethra may follow three routes. Some pass under the pubic symphysis to the external iliac nodes, some go to the obturator and internal iliac nodes, and others end in the presacral lymph nodes. The pelvic (iliac) lymph nodes rarely are involved in the absence of inguinal lymph-node involvement (19).

Epidemiology

Carcinoma of the penis is rare in the United States, where an estimated 1,100 new cases will be diagnosed each year (45).

The annual incidence is estimated to be one in 100,000 males, accounting for less than 1% of all cancers in men (19). There is increasing evidence that newborn circumcision has a preventive effect in the development of carcinoma of the penis (107). This tumor is extremely rare in circumcised Jewish men (19); circumcision performed early in life protects against carcinoma of the penis, but this is not true if the operation is done in adult life (108). The higher incidence in some areas of South America, Africa, and Asia seems to be related to the absence of the practice of neonatal circumcision. It has been shown that male circumcision is highly effective in preventing the development of penile carcinoma in Nigeria and Uganda (89,92). The high incidence of carcinoma of the penis in African-Americans has similarly been attributed to the lower percentage of African-Americans undergoing neonatal circumcision. Phimosis is common in men suffering from penile carcinoma. Smegma is carcinogenic in animals, yet the component of the smegma responsible for its carcinogenic effect has not been identified (19).

Boon and associates (10) observed an increased incidence of cervical carcinoma and penile carcinoma in Bali in a Hindu population in whom circumcision is rare and phimosis in adult males is high. They suggested that human papillomavirus (HPV) infection, estimated to be present in more than 75% of Balinese patients with genital carcinoma, may be a cofactor with impeded postcoital hygiene in genital carcinogenesis. In the Netherlands, where males usually are circumcised, the male is exclusively a vector of HPV but not a victim as in Bali. Martinez (77) in Puerto Rico and Graham and coworkers (43) in New York also noted a significantly higher incidence of carcinoma of the cervix in the wives of males with penile carcinoma. Other etiologic factors such as viruses (herpes simplex) and sexually transmitted disease (syphilis) have been implicated (30,113), but the evidence remains inconclusive (19).

Carcinoma of the male urethra is also rare. There are no recognized racial or geographic predisposing factors. Although the etiology remains unknown, there seems to be some correlation between the incidence of carcinoma of the urethra and chronic irritation (infection, sexually transmitted diseases, strictures). Significant past medical history of male patients with urethra cancer include sexually transmitted disease (24% to 37%), urethral stricture (35% to 54%), urethral trauma (7%), and urethral polyps (2%) (20,60). The part of the urethra covered by he transitional epithelium (prostatic and membranous urethra) may be susceptible to the same carcinogenic factors that affect the bladder and the upper urinary tract. Average age at presentation of these tumors is 58 to 60 years, although 10% occur in men younger than 40 years (19,20).

Natural History

Most carcinomas of the penis start within the preputial area, arising in the glans, coronal sulcus, or the prepuce itself. Lesions arising in the skin of the shaft are rare. In most patients, carcinoma of the penis is characterized by slow locoregional progression. The penis is handled and observed daily, yet there is often significant debate as to when patient recognition and

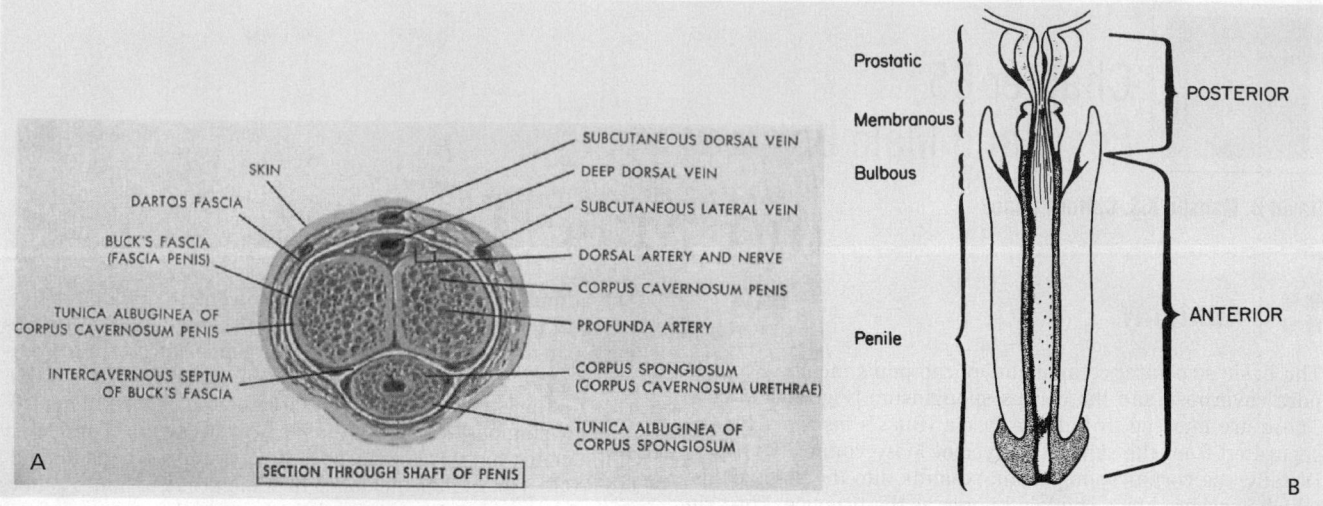

FIGURE 65.1. A: Cross section of penis shaft. (From Netter FH. *The CIBA collection of medical illustrations,* Volume 2. Reproductive system (85). Summit, NJ: CIBA Pharmaceutical, 1972, with permission.) **B:** Anatomic subdivisions of the male urethra.

medical diagnosis should have occurred. The patient may experience fear and embarrassment, which probably contributes to delayed diagnosis. Therefore expeditious diagnosis of all penile lesions should be the rule. Extensive primary lesions may involve the corpora cavernosa or even the abdominal wall. The inguinal lymph nodes are the most common site of metastatic spread. Pathologic evidence of nodal metastases is reported in about 35% of all patients and in approximately 50% of those with palpable lymph nodes (13,26,27,30) (Table 65.1).

Distant metastases are uncommon (about 10%), even in patients with advanced locoregional disease, and usually occur in patients with inguinal lymph-node involvement (54). These patients often die of septic complications, erosion of large vessels in the groin, or a combination of the two.

The natural history of carcinoma of the anterior urethra in the male is similar to that of carcinoma of the penis. Approximately 10% of tumors originate in the anterior urethra (20). Many tumors are low grade and progress slowly at primary and regional sites rather than spread to distal areas. Tumors of the penile urethra spread to the inguinal lymph nodes first, whereas those of the bulbomembranous and prostatic urethra metastasize first to the pelvic lymph nodes. Approximately one-third of men will present with either clinically or pathologically involved lymph nodes (20).

Urethral cancers tend to spread by direct extension to adjacent structures. Invasion into the vascular space of the corpus spongiosum in the periurethral tissues is common. Malignancies beginning in the bulbomembranous urethra often invade the deep structures of the perineum, including the urogenital diaphragm, prostate, and adjacent skin. In the majority of prostatic urethral tumors, the bulk of the prostate gland is invaded at the time of diagnosis. Hematogenous spread is uncommon except in advanced regional disease. Kaplan and colleagues (60) reported distant metastases in about 15% of patients; most had corpora cavernosa invasion at diagnosis.

Clinical Presentation

Carcinoma of the penis may present as either an infiltrative–ulcerative or an exophytic papillary lesion. Figure 65.3 demonstrates the localization of penile tumors in 259 patients from 14 cancer institutes in France. The glans and the prepuce were the predominant sites of the primary lesion, whereas tumors of the shaft were rare (104). Assessment of the primary lesion may be obscured by the presence of phimosis. Secondary infection and associated foul smell are quite common. Urethral obstruction is an unusual symptom of carcinoma of the penis. The most common presenting symptom is a mass, which occurs in more than two-thirds of patients. Ulceration is also common, occurring in approximately half of patients (27,112). In a collective series of 552 patients with penile carcinoma, the presenting symptoms were mass lesions (78%), pain or itching (12%), bleeding (7%), groin mass (7%), and urinary symptoms (4%)

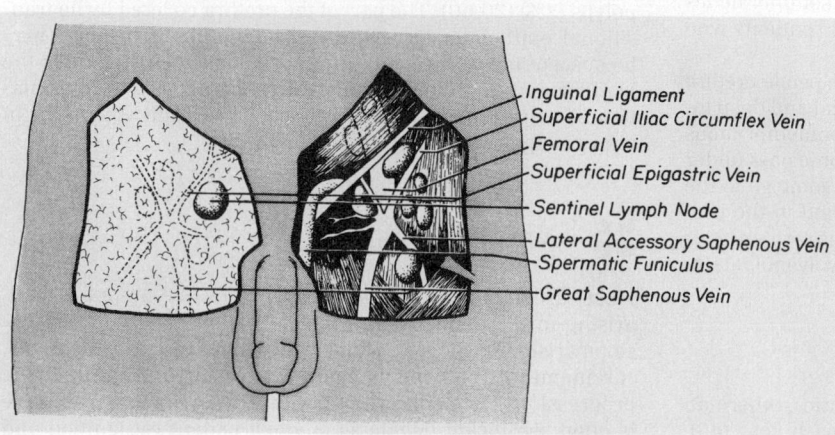

Inguinal Ligament
Superficial Iliac Circumflex Vein
Femoral Vein
Superficial Epigastric Vein
Sentinel Lymph Node
Lateral Accessory Saphenous Vein
Spermatic Funiculus
Great Saphenous Vein

FIGURE 65.2. Anatomic landmarks for inguinal lymph-node dissection. **Left:** Skin and immediately surrounding adipose tissue are removed to expose sentinel lymph node. Deep fatty stratum remains. Other lymph nodes and great saphenous vein and tributaries are indicated by dashed lines. **Right:** Sentinel lymph node and superficial and deep fascia are removed to expose other superficial and deep lymph nodes. (From Cabanas RM. An approach for the treatment of penile carcinoma. *Cancer* 1977;39:456–466, with permission.)

Table 65.1	PATHOLOGIC INCIDENCE OF METASTATIC LYMPH NODES IN PENILE CARCINOMA	
Investigator	Clinically Positive Nodes (%)	Total Patients (%)
Ekstrom and Edsmyr (30)	51	31
Jackson (54)	27	26
Derakhshani (27)	50	29
Barney (5)		50
Lenowitz and Graham (70)		35
Bassett (7)		33
Staubitz et al (113)		47
Jorstad (59)		37
Dean (24)		33
Fegen and Persky (33)	20	
deKernion et al (26)	62	
Gentil and Cavalcanti (37)	50	
Oota (90)	28	
Paymaster and Gangadharan (94)	50	

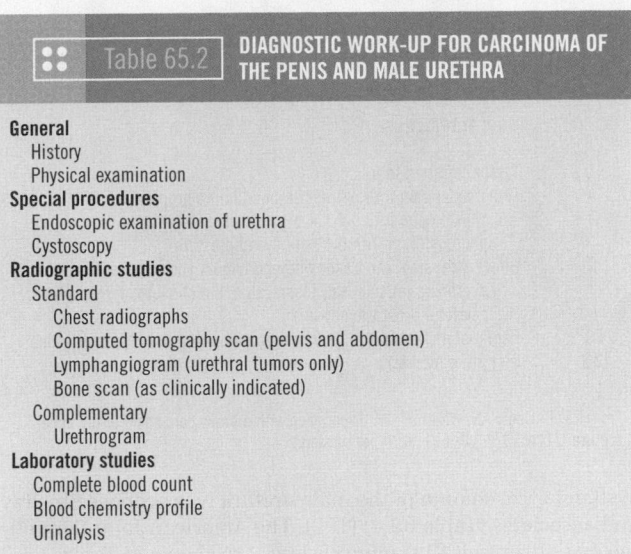

Table 65.2	DIAGNOSTIC WORK-UP FOR CARCINOMA OF THE PENIS AND MALE URETHRA

General
  History
  Physical examination
Special procedures
  Endoscopic examination of urethra
  Cystoscopy
Radiographic studies
  Standard
    Chest radiographs
    Computed tomography scan (pelvis and abdomen)
    Lymphangiogram (urethral tumors only)
    Bone scan (as clinically indicated)
  Complementary
    Urethrogram
Laboratory studies
  Complete blood count
  Blood chemistry profile
  Urinalysis

(48,51,84). Inguinal lymph nodes are palpable on presentation in 30% to 45% of patients (13,26,30,46,51,110); however, only half contain tumor (26,27). Enlargement of the lymph nodes often is related to inflammatory (infectious) processes. Administration of antibiotics over several weeks results in regression of inguinal lymph nodes in a substantial proportion of cases, and many have advocated this practice before the status of the regional lymph nodes is assessed definitively. Conversely, between 20% and 40% of patients with clinically negative inguinal lymph nodes have occult metastases (15,28,40,91,111).

Patients with urethral carcinoma most commonly present with obstructive symptoms (43%). Other presenting signs and symptoms include mass (28%), bleeding (20%), abscess (20%), and irritative symptoms (20%) (20). These symptoms often are attributed to urethritis or urethral stricture, which may precede

the development of urethral carcinoma and also may result in delay in diagnosis. The majority of urethral carcinomas occur in the bulbomembranous (posterior) region (61%), and tumors in this location have a worse prognosis compared to those arising in the anterior urethra (20).

Diagnostic Work-Up

Diagnostic studies required in the evaluation of patients with suspected or confirmed carcinoma of the penis and urethra are outlined in Table 65.2. Careful examination of the balanopreputial area may demonstrate small lesions. Urethroscopy and cystoscopy are essential. Inguinal lymph nodes should be evaluated thoroughly. Assessment of the regional lymphatics by lymphangiogram in carcinoma of the penis is of questionable value. The extensive inflammatory changes that are often present in the lymph nodes make interpretation of this procedure difficult. Computed tomography (CT) is useful in the identification of enlarged pelvic and periaortic lymph nodes in patients with involved inguinal lymph nodes.

In urethral carcinoma the inflammatory changes in the lymph nodes are less problematic, and lymphangiogram results are relatively reliable. CT scans of the pelvis and abdomen are useful in evaluating the pelvic and retroperitoneal lymphatics.

Staging

Among several staging systems proposed for classification of carcinoma of the penis, the one proposed by Jackson (54) is used most often (Table 65.3). The most commonly used staging

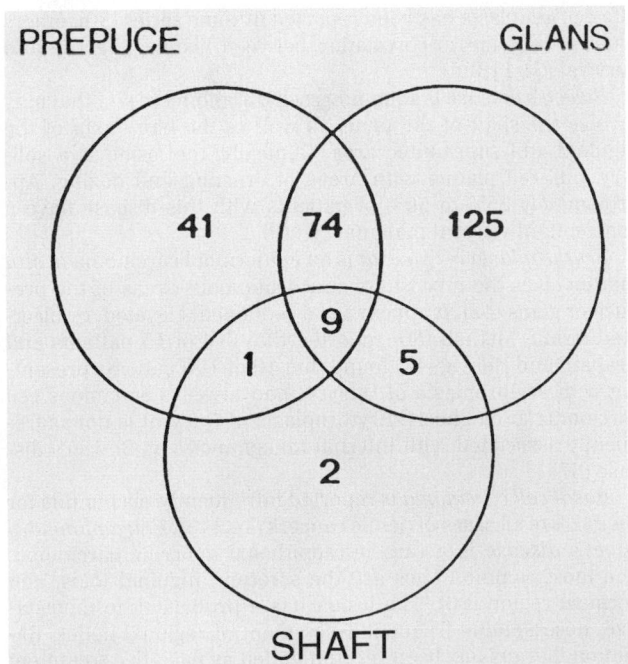

FIGURE 65.3. Localization of the primary tumor in 259 patients; each circle represents one anatomic compartment. Intersections indicate involvement of two or three compartments. Unknown: two. (From Rozan R, Albuisson E, Giraud B, et al. Interstitial brachytherapy for penile carcinoma: A multicentric survey (259 patients). *Radiother Oncol* 1995;36:83–93, with permission.)

Table 65.3	STAGING SYSTEM FOR CARCINOMA OF THE PENIS PROPOSED BY JACKSON
Stage	**Characteristics**
I	Tumor confined to glans and/or prepuce
II	Tumor extending onto shaft of penis
III	Tumor with malignant, but operable, inguinal lymph nodes
IV	Inoperable primary tumor extending off the shaft of the penis or inoperable groin nodes or distant metastases

(From Jackson SM. The treatment of carcinoma of the penis. *Br J Surg* 1966;53:33, with permission.)

Table 65.4	STAGING SYSTEM FOR MALE URETHRAL CARCINOMA PROPOSED BY RAY AND ASSOCIATES
Stage	**Characteristics**
0	Tumor confined to mucosa only
A	Tumor extension into but not beyond lamina propria
B	Tumor extension into but not beyond substance of corpus spongiosum or into but not beyond prostate
C	Direct extension into tissues beyond corpus spongiosum (corpora cavernosa, muscle, fat, fascia, skin, direct skeletal involvement) or beyond prostatic capsule
D1	Regional metastasis including inguinal and/or pelvic lymph nodes
D2	Distant metastasis

From Ray B, Canto AR, Whitmore WF. Experience with primary carcinoma of the male urethra. *J Urol* 1977;117:591, with permission.)

system for carcinoma of the male urethra was proposed by Ray and associates (Table 65.4) (102). The American Joint Committee on Cancer (AJCC) staging systems are shown in Tables 65.5 and 65.6 (34).

Pathologic Classification

Most malignant penile tumors are well-differentiated squamous cell carcinomas (4). Although an apparent adverse prognostic

Table 65.5	AMERICAN JOINT COMMITTEE ON CANCER STAGING SYSTEM FOR CARCINOMA OF THE PENIS

Primary tumor (T)

TX	Primary tumor cannot be assessed
T0	No evidence of primary tumor
Tis	Carcinoma *in situ*
Ta	Noninvasive verrucous carcinoma
T1	Tumor invades subepithelial connective tissue
T2	Tumor invades corpus spongiosum or cavernosum
T3	Tumor invades urethra or prostate
T4	Tumor invades other adjacent structures

Regional lymph nodes (N)

NX	Regional lymph nodes cannot be assessed
N0	No regional lymph-node metastasis
N1	Metastasis in a single superficial inguinal lymph node
N2	Metastasis in multiple or bilateral superficial inguinal lymph nodes
N3	Metastasis in deep inguinal or pelvic lymph node(s), unilateral or bilateral

Distant metastasis (M)

MX	Presence of distant metastasis cannot be assessed
M0	No distant metastasis
M1	Distant metastasis

Stage grouping

0	Tis	N0	
	Ta	N0	
I	T1	N0	
II	T1	N1	
	T2	N0	
	T2	N1	
III	T1	N2	
	T2	N2	
	T3	N0	
	T3	N1	
	T3	N2	
IV	T4	Any N	
	Any T	N3	
	Any T	Any N	M1

(From Fleming ID, Cooper JS, Henson DE, et al., eds. *Cancer staging manual*, edition 5. Philadelphia: JB Lippincott, 1997:217, with permission.)

Table 65.6	AMERICAN JOINT COMMITTEE ON CANCER STAGING SYSTEM OF CARCINOMA OF THE URETHRA

Primary tumor (T) (male and female)

TX	Primary tumor cannot be assessed
T0	No evidence of primary tumor
Ta	Noninvasive papillary, polypoid, or verrucous carcinoma
Tis	Carcinoma *in situ*
T1	Tumor invades subepithelial connective tissue
T2	Tumor invades corpus spongiosum or prostate or periurethral muscle
T3	Tumor invades corpus cavernosum or beyond prostatic capsule or the anterior vagina or bladder neck
T4	Tumor invades other adjacent organs

Regional lymph nodes (N)

NX	Regional lymph nodes cannot be assessed
N0	No regional lymph-node metastasis
N1	Metastasis in a single lymph node, ≤ 2 cm is greatest dimension
N2	Metastasis in a single lymph node, >2 cm in greatest dimension or metastases to multiple lymph nodes

Distant metastasis (M)

MX	Presence of distant metastasis cannot be assessed
M0	No distant metastasis
M1	Distant metastasis

Stage grouping

0a	Ta	N0	
0is	Tis	N0	
I	T1	N0	
II	T2	N0	
III	T1	N1	
	T2	N1	
	T3	N0	
	T3	N1	
IV	T4	N0	
	T4	N1	
	Any T	N2	
	Any T	Any N	M1

(From Fleming ID, Cooper JS, Henson DE, et al, eds. *Cancer staging manual*, edition 5. Philadelphia: JB Lippincott, 1997:217, with permission.)

effect of anaplasia has been reported in some series (30), others found no significant correlation between histologic grade and survival (51,113).

Bowen's disease is squamous cell carcinoma *in situ* that may involve the shaft of the penis as well as the hairy skin of the inguinal and suprapubic area. Clinically, the lesion is a solitary, dull-red plaque with areas of crusting and oozing. Approximately 25% to 50% of patients with this disease have a concomitant visceral malignancy (19).

Erythroplasia of Queyrat is an epidermoid carcinoma *in situ* that involves the mucosal or mucocutaneous areas of the prepuce or glans (42). It appears as a reddened, elevated, or ulcerated lesion. Mikhail (80) reported that five of 15 patients and Graham and Helwig (42) found that 10 of 100 patients presenting with erythroplasia of Queyrat had invasive squamous cell carcinoma at diagnosis. Erythroplasia of Queyrat is not as frequently associated with internal malignancies as Bowen's disease (87).

Basal cell carcinoma is reported infrequently, accounting for 1% to 2% of all cases of penile cancers (44,115). *Extramammary Paget's disease* is a rare intraepithelial apocrine carcinoma. The most common sites are the scrotum, inguinal folds, and perineal region (80). The lesion has a propensity to metastasize, necessitating frequent assessment of regional nodes. Radiation therapy has been recommended as palliative treatment (80).

Soft-tissue tumors are uncommon. Approximately half of the tumors are benign and may include angiomatous, neurogenous, myogenous, fibrous, and lymphoreticular tumors (25,74). Most soft-tissue tumors occur on the shaft.

PRIMARY MALIGNANCIES ASSOCIATED WITH SECONDARY CANCERS OF THE PENIS IN 219 PATIENTS Table 65.7	
Site of Primary Malignancy	Number of Patients
Genitourinary tract	
Bladder	65
Prostate	65
Kidney	23
Testis	10
Ureter	1
Gastrointestinal tract	
Rectum/sigmoid	34
Colon	1
Anus	1
Liver	1
Pancreas	1
Respiratory tract	
Lungs	8
Nasopharynx	1
Other	
Lymphosarcoma/reticulum cell sarcoma	4
Bone	2
Burkitt's lymphoma	1
Skin (malignant melanoma)	1

(From Powell BL, Craig JB, Muss HB. Secondary malignancies of the penis and epididymis: A case report and review of the literature. *J Clin Oncol* 1985;3:110–116, with permission.)

Primary lymphoma of the penis was reported in one patient with Peyronie's disease, without other evidence of lymphomatous involvement. Five cases of secondary involvement of the penis by lymphoma were reported in the literature (119).

Cancers *metastatic* to the penis are rare and usually represent late, advanced carcinomatosis. The most common neoplasms metastasizing to the penis are from the genitourinary organs, followed by the gastrointestinal and respiratory systems (Table 65.7). The predominant cell type is carcinoma, occurring in 202 of 219 cases (100). Sarcomas and tumors of unknown histologic type are rare. A palpable mass, swelling, nodule, or skin change frequently occurs. Priapism as an initial presenting feature or subsequent development occurs in 40% of patients (100).

The histologic subtypes in the Memorial Sloan-Kettering Cancer Center series of urethral cancers included squamous cell carcinoma (52%), transitional cell carcinoma (33%), epidermoid carcinoma (11%), adenocarcinoma (2%), and anaplastic carcinoma (2%) (20). Primary malignant melanoma arising from the urethra has been reported (39,88). The frequency of histologic type varies with site. More than 90% of carcinomas of the prostatic urethra are of transitional cell type. Adenocarcinomas occur only in the bulbomembranous urethra.

Prognostic Factors

The principal prognostic factors in carcinoma of the penis are extent of the primary lesion and status of the lymph nodes (112,118). The incidence of nodal involvement is related to the size, location, and grade of the primary lesion. Invasion of deep-seated structures (corpora cavernosa) carries a high risk of deep inguinal-node involvement.

Tumor-free regional nodes imply an excellent (80% to 90%) long-term survival or cure (26,110,118). Patients with involvement of the inguinal nodes fare considerably worse, and only 40% to 50% survive long term (26,73,110,118). Pelvic lymph-node involvement implies a still worse prognosis; less than 20% of these patients survive (13,26,51). Gerbaulet and Lambin (38) reported the results of 109 patients with carcinoma of the penis at Institut Gustave-Roussy. The actuarial survival rates of patients with negative nodes were 82% at 5 years and 59% at 10 years. For patients with positive nodes, the survival rates were 36% and 18%, respectively (Fig. 65.4). The number of positive lymph nodes also has been reported to have prognostic significance. Brkovic and coworkers reported a 5-year survival rate of 71% in patients with solitary inguinal lymph-node metastasis, compared to 33% in patients with multiple positive inguinal nodes (12).

Tumor differentiation was shown to be an important prognostic factor by Fraley and associates (35). None of nine patients with carcinoma *in situ,* one of 20 with well-differentiated lesions, five of 13 with moderately differentiated lesions, and three of four with poorly differentiated lesions died of their tumor. Other investigators have confirmed the prognostic significance of tumor grade (72,106,112,118).

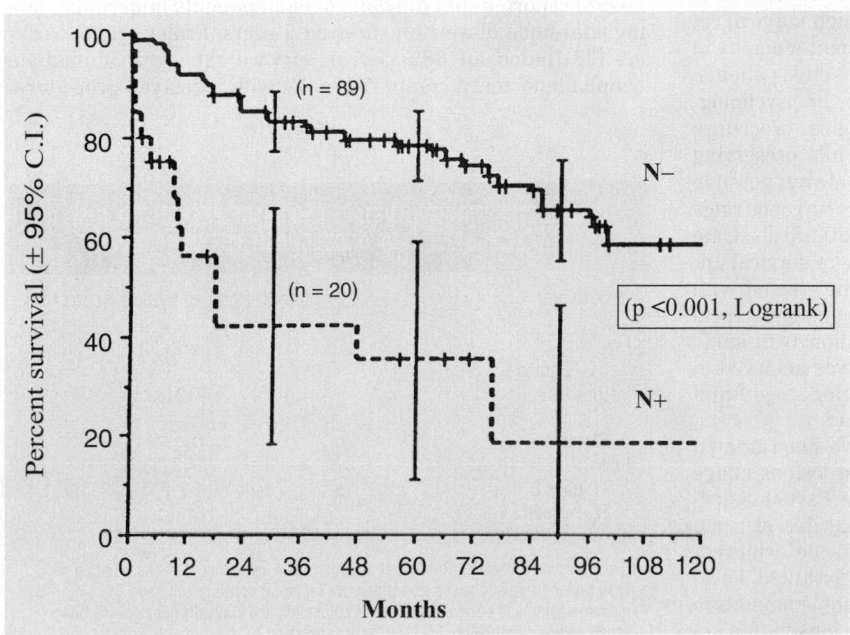

FIGURE 65.4. Actuarial survival of 109 patients treated at the Institut Gustave-Roussy. In patients with negative nodes, the actuarial survival is 82% at 5 years and 59% at 10 years. In patients with positive nodes, the survival is 36% and 18%, respectively. (From Gerbaulet A, Lambin P. Radiation therapy of cancer of the penis: Indications, advantages, and pitfalls. *Urol Clin North Am* 1992;19:325–332, with permission.)

Clinical Radiation Oncology

Carcinoma of the penis has been reported to have greater propensity to metastasize and have a poorer prognosis in patients younger than 50 years of age (35) and in patients older than 65 years of age (72). Soria and coworkers reported that younger age at presentation adversely affected disease-free survival but not overall survival (112). Conversely, Marcial and colleagues observed no difference in survival in relation to age (76).

The potential influence of HPV on prognosis was studied retrospectively in a cohort of patients treated surgically. HPV DNA was detected in paraffin-embedded specimens in 30% of patients. The presence of HPV had no prognostic significance with regard to lymph-node metastasis or overall survival (8). Overall prognosis in males with carcinoma of the urethra varies considerably with location of the primary lesion (20,41,63,65,67,75,82). Distal lesions generally have a prognosis similar to that of carcinoma of the penis. Lesions of the bulbomembranous urethra are usually quite extensive and are associated with a dismal prognosis. Dalbagni and colleagues reported a 5-year overall survival of 69% in patients with anterior tumors, compared to 26% in patients with posterior tumors (20). Other prognostic factors include lymph-node status and histology (superficial versus invasive) (20). Tumors of the prostatic urethra show prognostic features similar to those in bladder carcinoma. Superficial lesions have a good prognosis and may be managed with transurethral resection (67). Deeply invasive tumors have a greater tendency to develop inguinal/pelvic lymph-node and distant metastases.

General Management

Carcinoma of the Penis

Surgery

Treatment of patients with carcinoma of the penis generally is performed in two phases: initial management of the primary tumor and later treatment of the regional lymphatics. Surgical intervention at the primary site may range from local excision (including circumcision) or laser surgery (103) in a small group of highly selected patients (especially those with small lesions of the prepuce) to partial or total penectomy (1L,LT,TL). In very advanced proximal tumors, more aggressive resections such as total emasculation (penectomy, scrotectomy, orchiectomy) or cystoprostatectomy may be indicated (3). Although surgical resection is a highly effective and expedient treatment modality in most cases, it may not be acceptable to sexually active patients. Radical surgery, especially total penectomy, may be psychologically devastating to the patient. The ideal surgical procedure removes the disease with adequate margins while preserving sexual and urinary function, although this is not always possible because of the extent of disease. The high local recurrence rates described in some reports with limited surgery (50,53) illustrate the need for careful patient selection in choosing a surgical approach. Lesions confined to the prepuce may be treated with wide circumcision. Microsurgical techniques have shown local excision to be an acceptable and desirable option with small superficial lesions. A local control rate of 92% was achieved in 29 patients with a 5-year survival rate of 81% for stage I and 57% for stage II lesions (81).

Lesions on the glans penis traditionally have been treated by partial penectomy. Larger or more invasive lesions (stage III) can be treated by partial or total penectomy. Partial penectomy is the procedure of choice if surgical margins of 2 cm can be achieved. If an adequate margin cannot be achieved, total penectomy with perineal urethrotomy is warranted. Local (stump) recurrence is rare (19). It is possible for some patients to remain sexually active after partial penectomy. Jensen (55) re-

ported 45% of patients with 4 to 6 cm and 25% of patients with 2 to 4 cm of penile stump could perform sexual intercourse. D'Ancona and colleagues evaluated the quality of life in 14 patients treated with partial penectomy (22). Sexual function was reported to be normal or only slightly decreased in 64% of patients. Complete loss of sexual function was reported in 14% of patients.

Surgical Treatment of Inguinal Lymph Nodes

The clinical evaluation of inguinal lymph nodes in men with cancer of the penis is unreliable. Several series have shown the sensitivity of clinical staging of the nodes to be 40% to 60% and false-negative rates to be 10% to 20% (15,96). McDougal (79) reported the correlation between clinical findings and pathologic positivity of inguinal nodes in patients with penile carcinoma. For tumors with no invasion or superficial invasion, moderately or well differentiated, only 12% of clinically enlarged inguinal nodes were pathologically positive. However, 78% to 88% of invasive or poorly differentiated tumors metastasized to inguinal nodes regardless of clinical findings (79). In a prospective study involving 37 patients with clinically negative groins, Solsona and coworkers have demonstrated the predictive value of histologic grade and T stage in predicting the likelihood of occult-positive lymph nodes (111). Three groups were identified—low, intermediate, and high risk—with an incidence of occult-positive nodes of 0%, 33%, and 83%, respectively (Table 65.8). Given the unreliability of clinical assessment, a rationale exists to submit all patients to the staging and therapeutic benefits of radical inguinal lymph-node dissection. However, this procedure is associated with considerable morbidity. As many as one-half of patients will experience complications including wound necrosis or dehiscence, infection, lymphocele, erosion of femoral vessels, chronic lymphedema, thrombophlebitis, or pulmonary embolism (3,73). The morbidity of radical lymphadenectomy and the relative small percentage of patients with pathologic involvement of inguinal nodes has resulted in surveillance as initial management of regional lymph nodes in clinically negative patients at some centers. Of concern, however, are reports describing poor salvage rates after regional failure. McDougal reported a 5-year disease-free survival rate of 88% for patients with clinical stage II disease who underwent immediate lymphadenectomy, compared to 38% if delayed lymphadenectomy was performed (79). Johnson and Lo (58) reported that only one of eight patients undergoing late inguinal-node dissection survived 5 years. Fraley and coworkers (35) noted an 88% 5-year survival rate with immediate lymphadenectomy, compared to 8% with a delayed procedure.

Table 65.8	T STAGE AND GRADE PREDICT THE RISK OF OCCULT POSITIVE LYMPH NODES	
Risk Group	**Occult Positive Lymph Nodes (%)**
Low Tis, T1 grade 1	0/13 (0)
Intermediate T1 grade 2–3 T2 grade 1	4/12 (33.3)
High T2 grade 2 T2–3 grade 3	10/12 (83.3)

(From Solsona E, Iborra I, Rubio J, et al. Prospective validation of the association of local tumor stage and grade as a predictive factor for occult lymph node micrometastasis in patients with penile carcinoma and clinically negative inguinal lymph nodes. *J Urol* 2001;165:1506, with permission.)

Sentinel-node biopsy has been advocated as a less morbid means of evaluating inguinal nodes by some (13), but its reliability has been questioned by others (95,97). Catalona described a modified inguinal lymphadenectomy for patients with penile cancer and clinically negative groins (15,17). Long-term follow-up of nine patients reveals significantly less morbidity than the classic groin dissection designed by Daseler and associates (23). Extension of the nodal dissection into the pelvis to cover the iliac lymph nodes is justified in patients with evidence of inguinal involvement (positive biopsy of Cloquet's node). Approximately 20% of patients with pelvic lymph-node involvement can be salvaged by radical pelvic lymphadenectomy (13,117). As demonstrated in other anatomic sites such as the head and neck, uterine cervix, vagina, and vulva, patients with clinically negative lymph nodes who are at risk for microscopic nodal metastases (primary tumor beyond stage I or less than well-differentiated histology) can receive elective irradiation to the inguinal lymph nodes (50 Gy to 5 cm depth in 5 weeks) with a high probability of tumor control and low morbidity.

Radiation Therapy

The primary advantage of radiation therapy is preservation of the phallus. In the past, radiation therapy often used insufficient total dose and high dose per fraction along with poor technique resulting in underdosage or overdosage and a high incidence of injury to normal tissues. Although historically a wide variation of techniques, doses, and fractionation schemes have been used (1,30,32,54,83,86,99), improvement in the tumor control rate in some modern series using adequate total doses and small daily doses is noteworthy, resulting in a decreased incidence of treatment-related sequelae. Most patients who experience local failure after radiation therapy can be salvaged surgically. Several radiation modalities are used to deliver radiation to the penis, including megavoltage external-beam radiation therapy (EBRT), ^{192}Ir mold plesiotherapy, and interstitial implant using ^{192}Ir wires (49,78,98,99,103).

Inguinal lymph-node irradiation for clinically negative nodes is an integral component of successful radiotherapeutic management of this disease. Regional control has been achieved in 95% of cases. Without irradiation to the inguinal lymph nodes, as many as 20% of patients can be expected to develop positive nodes later (30,32). For palpable nodes, groin dissection may be necessary, accepting the likelihood of postoperative morbidity. Postoperative radiation therapy to the groin adds little to the morbidity but contributes significantly to locoregional tumor control. If the inguinal lymph nodes are treated, a CT scan helps define the depth and location of the inguinal lymph node, femoral artery, and veins, which is crucial, as indicated in Chapter 67.

Chemotherapy

The use of systemic chemotherapy either as an adjuvant or concomitantly with radiation therapy has not been fully investigated in patients with penile cancer. Chemoradiotherapy of squamous cell carcinoma of the anus (another HPV-related carcinoma) has been used with great success, resulting in high tumor control rates and organ preservation. Similar data in penile carcinoma are lacking, however. Modern multiagent chemotherapy regimens have overall response rates ranging from 15% to 55% in patients with advanced disease (Table 65.9). The agents most commonly used include platinum, methotrexate, and bleomycin. Additional clinical trials are needed to adequately define the role of chemotherapy in the management of cancer of the penis.

Carcinoma of the Male Urethra

Surgery or Radiation Therapy

The primary mode of therapy for carcinoma of the male urethra is surgical excision. Because of the rarity of this disease, comparison of the cure rates with radiation therapy or surgery is difficult. The principal advantage of irradiation is organ preservation. Noninvasive carcinoma of the proximal urethra can be treated with transurethral resection. In lesions of the distal urethra, results with either penectomy or radiation therapy are similar to those for carcinoma of the penis, and the 5-year survival rates are comparable (50% to 60%) (101). Involved regional lymph nodes are treated with lymphadenectomy.

Most patients, however, present with advanced invasive lesions, which are difficult to manage with either radical surgery or radiation therapy. The major problem is the high rate of local recurrence. In an attempt to improve the locoregional control rate, extended resections encompassing the inferior pubic rami, prostate, bladder, and perineum have been performed after preoperative radiation therapy. After a dose of 20 to 60 Gy, Klein and associates (65) performed an extended resection in seven patients with proximal urethral lesions. Locoregional failure was observed in two patients (29%).

Chemotherapy

Concomitant chemoradiotherapy has been investigated in only a few patients. However, these preliminary data are encouraging. Gheiler and colleagues reported their experience with multimodality treatment of 21 patients (10 women, 11 men) with urethral carcinoma at Wayne State (39). Treatment consisted of cisplatin and 5-fluorouracil (5-FU)–based chemotherapy for squamous cell carcinoma and concomitant external-beam irradiation. Patients with transitional cell carcinoma were treated with concomitant methotrexate, vinblastine, doxorubicin (Adriamycin), and cisplatin. Some patients underwent surgical resection following chemoradiation. With a median follow-up of 42 months, the overall disease-free survival rate was 62%. Of significance is the pathologic complete response rate of 87.5% in eight women undergoing resection following chemoradiation.

⠿ | Radiation Therapy Techniques

Carcinoma of the Penis

If indicated, circumcision must be performed before radiation therapy is initiated. The purpose of this procedure is to minimize radiation–therapy-associated morbidity: swelling, irritation of the skin, moist desquamation, and secondary infection. Although EBRT has become prevalent in the treatment of the primary lesion in carcinoma of the penis, plastic molds or interstitial implants still are used.

External-Beam Radiation Therapy

EBRT requires specially designed accessories (including bolus) necessary to achieve homogeneous dose distribution to the entire penis. Frequently, a plastic box with a central circular opening that can be fitted over the penis is used. The space between the skin and the box must be filled with tissue-equivalent material (Fig. 65.5). This box then can be treated with parallel-opposed megavoltage beams. An ingenious alternative to the box technique is the use of a water-filled container to envelop the penis while the patient is in a prone position (105).

Another more complex device consists of a Perspex tube attached to a baseplate resting on the skin (36). This is placed as

Table 65.9	MULTIAGENT CHEMOTHERAPY IN ADVANCED PENILE CARCINOMA					
	Agents	n	% Partial Response	% Complete Response	Median Survival (Months)	% Life-threatening Toxicity	% Fatal Toxicity
Hass et al (47)	Bleomycin Platinum Methotrexate	40	20	12.5	7	17	12.5
Corral et al (18)	Bleomycin Platinum Methotrexate	29	41	14	11.5	—	3.4
Kattan et al (61)	Varied (platinum based)	13	8	8	7.6	—	—

close as possible to the base of the penis, and a flexible tube is connected to a vacuum pump. The suction effect keeps the penis in a fixed position during treatment. Appropriate bolus is placed outside the tube. The patient also can be treated in the prone position, with the penis hanging through a small hole placed in the Perspex's cylinder. Fraction size in many of the reported series has been 2.5 to 3.5 Gy (total dose of 50 to 55 Gy), although a smaller daily fraction size (1.8 to 2.0 Gy) and a higher total dose are preferable. There is a well-established association between large fraction size and late tissue damage (Chapter 1). A total of 60 to 65 Gy, with the last 5 to 10 Gy delivered to a reduced portal, should result in a reduced incidence of late fibrosis.

Regional lymphatics may be treated with external-beam megavoltage irradiation. Both groins should be irradiated. The fields should include inguinal *and* pelvic (external iliac and hypogastric) lymph nodes (Fig. 65.6). The posterior pelvis may be partially spared by anterior loading of the beams (Chapter 67). Depending on the extent of the nodal disease and the proximity of the detectable tumor to the skin surface or the presence of skin invasion, application of a bolus to the inguinal area should be considered. If clinical and radiographic evaluation show no gross enlargement of the pelvic lymph nodes, the dose to these nodes may be limited to 50 Gy. In patients with palpable lymph nodes, doses of approximately 70 to 75 Gy over 7 to 8 weeks (1.8 to 2.0 Gy per day) with reducing fields (after 50 Gy) are advised. Alternatively, grossly involved nodes can be removed surgically either before or after inguinal radiation therapy.

Brachytherapy

A mold usually is built in the form of a box or cylinder with a central opening and channels for placement of radioactive sources (needles or wires) in the periphery of the device. The cylinder and sources should be long enough to prevent underdosage at the tip of the penis. A dose of 60 to 65 Gy at the surface and approximately 50 Gy at the center of the organ is delivered over 6 to 7 days. The mold can be applied either continuously, in which case an indwelling catheter should be in place, or intermittently. Intermittent application requires precise time-keeping. Alternatively, single- or double-plane implants can be used to deliver 60 to 70 Gy in 5 to 7 days (98). Salaverria and colleagues (106) point out that molds should be reserved for stage I and II tumors. We believe the same is true for interstitial implants. For additional technical details, see Chapter 18. In more extensive lesions involving the shaft of the penis, it is technically difficult to obtain an adequate margin with brachytherapy procedures, similar to the problem in performing a partial penectomy.

Carcinoma of the Male Urethra

Radiation therapy for carcinoma of the anterior (distal) urethra is similar to that for carcinoma of the penis; lesions of the bulbomembranous urethra can be treated with a set of parallel-opposed fields covering the groins and the pelvis, followed by perineal and inguinal boost. Lesions of the prostatic urethra can be treated with techniques and doses similar to those used for carcinoma of the prostate.

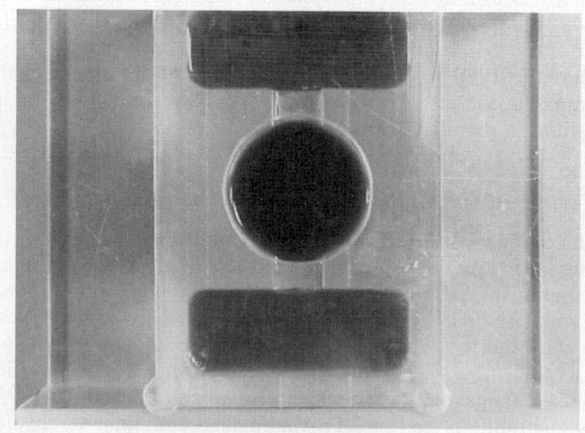
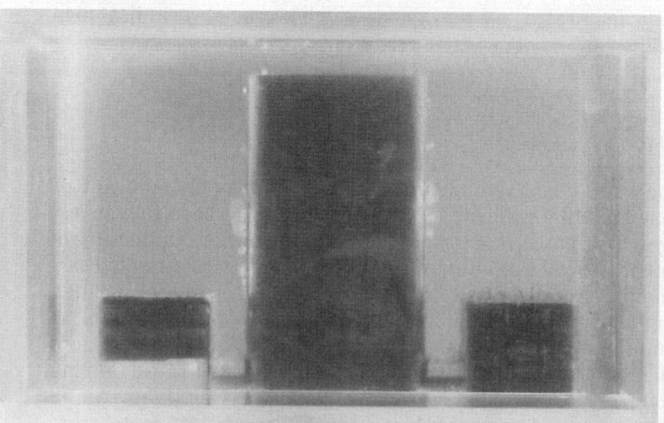

FIGURE 65.5. A: View from above of plastic box with central cylinder for external irradiation of the penis. Patient is treated in the prone position. The penis is placed in the central cylinder, and water is used to fill the surrounding volume in the box. Depth dose is calculated at the central point of box. **B:** Lateral view.

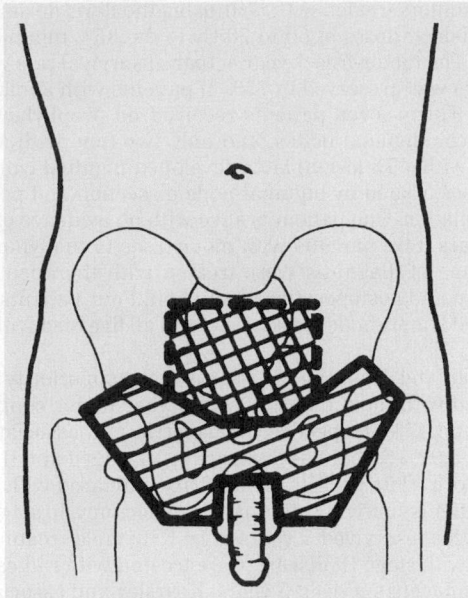

FIGURE 65.6. Portals encompassing inguinal and pelvic lymph nodes.

Results

Carcinoma of the Penis

At many institutions patients with carcinoma of the penis are treated surgically. A summary of selected modern surgical series is presented in Table 65.10. Ornellas and coworkers reported the results of 350 patients treated with surgery alone. Five-year disease-free survival was 62% for patients treated with immediate lymphadenectomy versus 8% in those treated with delayed lymphadenectomy. For all node-negative patients, 5-year disease-free survival was 87%, compared to 29% for node-positive patients (91). Boon (9) reported tumor control in 13 of 16 patients (81%) with carcinoma *in situ* or T1 and T2 tumors treated with wide local excision and lasers.

Radiation therapy has yielded comparable results at several institutions. Engelstad (32), Cade (14), Paterson and colleagues (93), Lederman (69), and Thurgar (116) reported 5-year survival rates ranging from 45% to 68% in groups of patients ranging from age 41 to 57 years treated with various irradiation techniques (mold, interstitial, external-beam). The ability of irradiation to control the tumor is closely associated with the stage of the disease.

The 20-year experience of the Institut Gustave-Rousy was reported by Soria and coworkers (112). One hundred and two patients with tumors less than 4 cm in diameter with less than 1-cm corpora cavernosa invasion were treated with a conservative approach consisting of limited surgery (biopsy, local excision, or therapeutic circumcision) and interstitial brachytherapy (65 to 70 Gy delivered over 5 to 7 days). Regional lymph nodes were not treated electively but were dissected in patients with clinically enlarged nodes. With a median follow-up of 111 months, the local tumor recurrence rate was 25%. A regional nodal recurrence developed in 21% of patients. Disease-free survival at 5 and 10 years was 56% and 42%, respectively. Overall survival at 5 and 10 years was 63% and 50%, respectively.

Grabstald and Keily (40) reported 90% local tumor control in 10 patients with stage I lesions treated with EBRT delivering 51 to 52 Gy over 6 weeks. Another series from M.D. Anderson Cancer Center demonstrated 80% local control and retention of the phallus in early-stage disease (48). Duncan and Jackson (29) also reported 90% local control for stage I lesions treated with a megavoltage treatment unit delivering 50 to 57 Gy over 3 weeks.

Irradiation of the involved regional lymph nodes in patients with carcinoma of the penis results in permanent control and cure in a substantial proportion of patients. In the classic series of Staubitz and associates (113), 13 patients with proven involvement of regional lymph nodes received radiation therapy to these nodes. Five of thirteen (38%) survived 5 years. Narayana and associates (84) reported two of 16 patients (12%) with histologically proven lymph-node metastases cured with radiation therapy. No data on radiation therapy are given for either series, precluding an assessment of the doses and fields.

Jackson (54) reported a 66% 5-year survival rate and 86% tumor control rate in 58 patients with stage I carcinoma of the penis treated with irradiation, compared with a 70% 5-year

Table 65.10	SURGICAL RESULTS IN PATIENTS WITH CARCINOMA OF THE PENIS				
			% Local Failure		
T Stage	**Author**	**n**	**Conserving Surgery**[a]	**Partial/Total Penile Amputation**	**% 5-Year Overall Survival**
T1	Brkovic et al (12)	22	56	0	77
	Horenblas et al (53)	—	10	—	—
	Lindegaard et al (72)	41	—	—	72
T2	Brkovic et al (12)	23	100	18	70
	Horenblas et al (53)	—	32	—	—
	Lindegaard et al (72)	26	—	—	55
T3/T4	Brkovic et al (12)	6	—	—	0
	Horenblas et al (53)	—	100	—	—
	Lindegaard et al (72)	6	—	—	10
T1–T4	Lindegaard et al (72)	63	35	5	—
	Derakhshani et al (27)	42	—	—	78
	Zouhair et al[b] (120)	16	—	25	—
	Lopes et al (73)	145			54

[a]Includes wide excision, laser ablation, radical circumcision.
[b]All patients treated with postoperative radiation therapy.

Clinical Radiation Oncology

survival rate and 81% tumor control rate in 27 surgically treated patients. In stage II, he observed six of 11 patients surviving 5 years and seven patients exhibiting tumor control in contrast to six surviving and eight showing tumor control in 12 surgically treated patients. In stage III, four of seven irradiated patients survived 5 years with tumor control, in contrast to two surviving and three with tumor control in seven treated with surgery only. Radium or cobalt molds produced the best sterilization of primary tumor; if irradiation had not controlled the primary lesion after 6 months, amputation of the penis was carried out, with a significant proportion of the patients salvaged. Two patients required amputation because of necrosis of the penis, and four developed severe phimosis, which was treated with meatotomy. Three of 37 patients (8%) initially treated surgically and 14 of 69 (20%) initially treated with irradiation developed inguinal lymph-node metastases. Overall, 8% of patients treated surgically and 10% of those irradiated died of inguinal lymph-node metastases and subsequent tumor spread.

Almgard and Edsmyr (1) reported tumor control in 12 of 17 patients treated with irradiation alone (superficial x-rays). Four patients underwent local radical excision for recurrence and survived from 10 to 30 years. In 17 additional patients local irradiation was followed by amputation of the penis, and 16 have been free of recurrence for 5 to 32 years. Marcial and associates (76) noted 5-year survival in four of six patients who received irradiation alone, in six of 11 who were given irradiation for frank persistence after limited surgery to the penis, and in six of eight to whom irradiation was administered postoperatively. Sixteen of 25 patients (64%) survived 5 years.

In a series of 145 patients reported by Knudsen and Brennhovd (66), 99 (68%) had recurrence, as did five of 14 patients (36%) treated by Johnson and colleagues (57) and 24 of 63 patients (38%) reported by Murrell and Williams (83). Haile and Delclos (49) reported tumor control and conservation of the penis in 16 of 20 patients (80%) treated with conservative radiation-therapy methods. Whereas irradiation alone or combined with a lymph-node dissection controlled lymph-node metastases smaller than 2 cm in four patients, radiation therapy was successful in controlling lymph-node metastases in only one of seven patients with N2 or N3 lymph nodes.

Sagerman and coworkers (105) reported tumor control in six of nine patients with stage I disease, two of three with stage II disease, and one of three with stage IV disease—all treated with irradiation alone. Two patients with stage I disease and one with stage II disease were surgically salvaged. Doses ranged from 45 Gy (15 fractions in 3 weeks) to 64 Gy (32 fractions in 6.5 weeks) with either orthovoltage x-rays or ^{60}Co and appropriate bolus. Good palliation was described in four of nine patients treated for inguinal lymph-node metastases to doses ranging from 20 (five fractions in 1 week) to 64 Gy. None of these patients survived more than 18 months.

Mazeron and associates (78) described tumor control in eight of nine patients with stage T1, 21 of 27 with T2, and 10 of 14

with T3 tumors treated with ^{192}Ir using the Paris dosimetry system, to deliver doses of 60 to 70 Gy to the 85% minimal tumor isodose. The tumor-free 5-year actuarial survival rate was 63%. The penis was preserved in 75% of patients with a follow-up of 8 years. Thirty-seven patients received no prophylactic treatment to the inguinal nodes, and only two (one with a T2 and another with a T3 lesion) later developed inguinal lymph-node metastases treated by inguinal-node dissection and postoperative irradiation. One patient is alive with no evidence of disease at 10 years. Five patients with metastases to the lymph nodes at the time of diagnosis were treated with therapeutic nodal dissection and postoperative irradiation. Four patients had uncontrolled lymph-node metastases, and all five died with distant disease.

Duncan and Jackson (29) discussed the superiority of EBRT compared with mold therapy, with 3-year tumor control rates of 90% and 47%, respectively. Salaverria and associates (106) reported a 92% 5-year survival rate in 13 stage I and II patients treated with ^{226}Ra or ^{192}Ir molds. This compared with 10 of 13 (77%) patients surviving after partial penectomy. In stage II, four of six patients survived 5 years after ^{192}Ir mold treatment. Ten patients with stage III disease were treated with radical amputation, and eight survived 5 years. Kearsley and associates (63) described a patient with locally advanced penile carcinoma and metastatic inguinal lymph nodes who was cured with irradiation alone—a remarkable achievement because most patients with stage IV die with locoregional and disseminated disease.

Tables 65.11 and 65.12 summarize tumor control rates achieved with EBRT alone or brachytherapy plus EBRT. Worth mentioning are the results of a multicenter report from France (104). With interstitial brachytherapy, no relationship was found between increasing dose and increasing local control with doses ranging from 60 to 65 Gy. Two variables have a significant impact on tumor recurrence: the maximum diameter of the tumor and deep infiltration of the disease.

Carcinoma of the Male Urethra

Historically, men with urethral carcinoma have been treated surgically. Dalbagni and associates have reported the outcome of 46 patients with carcinoma of the anterior and bulbar urethra treated at Memorial Sloan Kettering Cancer Center (20). The majority of patients were treated with definitive surgery. With a median follow-up of 125 months, the local control rate was 51%. The 5-year overall survival was 42%. Improved survival was seen in patients with anterior lesions (69%), compared to those with posterior lesions (26%).

Bracken and associates (11) described results in 11 patients with tumors at or anterior to the penoscrotal junction, eight of which were epidermoid carcinoma, two were transitional cell carcinoma, and one was melanoma. Three of four patients treated with total penectomy and perineal urethrostomy had tumor control. Partial penectomy controlled the local tumor in two

		Local Tumor Control		
Series	Modality	Stage I–II	Stage III–IV	Penis Preservation (%)
Duncan and Jackson (29)	Photon	16/20 (80%)		80
Haile and Delclos (49)	Photon	6/6 (100%)	2/2 (100%)	80
Kaushal and Harma (62)	^{60}Co	14/16 (88%)		93
Kelley et al (64)	Electron	10/10 (100%)		100
Pointon (99)	Photon	27/32 (84%)		
Sagerman et al (105)	Photon	9/12 (75%)	1/3 (33%)	

Table 65.11   RESULTS OF EXTERNAL-BEAM IRRADIATION FOR CARCINOMA OF THE PENIS

		Tumor Control		
Series	**Modality**	**Stage I–II**	**Stage III–IV**	**Penis Preservation (%)**
Almgard and Edsmyr (1)	ISI plus EBRT	14/16 (88%)[a]		
Chaudhary et al (16)	ISI	18/23 (78%)[a]		
Daly et al (21)	ISI	21/22 (95%)[a]		86%
El-Dimry et al (31)	Mold	17/23 (74%)[a]		
Gerbaulet and Lambin (38)	ISI	89/109 (82%)[a]		
Haile and Delclos (49)	Mold plus ISI	7/7 (100%)		
Jackson (54)	Mold	20/45 (44%)		44%
Knudson and Brennhovd (66)	Mold	46/145 (32%)[a]		
Mazeron et al (78)	ISI	29/36 (81%)[a]	10/14 (71%)	74%
Pierquin et al (98)	ISI	14/14 (100%)	12/31 (39%)	
Rozan et al (104)	ISI	162/184 (88%)[a]		78%
Rozan et al (104)	ISI plus EBRT	66/75 (88%)[a]		64%
Salaverria et al (106)	Mold	12/13 (92%)		77%
Soria et al (112)	ISI	26/102 (75%)[a]		53%
Suchaud et al (114) (56)	ISI	37/53 (70%)[a]		58%

Table 65.12 RESULTS OF BRACHYTHERAPY WITH OR WITHOUT EXTERNAL-BEAM RADIATION THERAPY FOR CARCINOMA OF THE PENIS

ISI, interstitial implant; EBRT, external-beam radiation therapy.
[a]All stages.

patients. The patient with melanoma had a local recurrence after operation. Two patients were treated with radiation therapy, and a third patient was treated with a combination of preoperative irradiation (45 Gy) and total penectomy. In all of these patients, tumor recurred locally. In four patients with inguinal lymph-node metastases, the regional disease was controlled by bilateral lymphadenectomy. All six patients in whom local and regional tumor was controlled remain alive and disease free at 1 to 20 years. In 16 patients, the urethral tumors arose posterior to the penoscrotal junction: 13 lesions were squamous cell carcinoma, two were transitional cell, and one was adenocarcinoma. Penectomy was performed in five patients, all of whom had tumor control and no evidence of recurrence 5 to 29 months after therapy. Two patients treated with local excision died of disease 14 and 18 months after surgery. Irradiation was used in three patients unsuccessfully, and all died of cancer 13 to 31 months after therapy.

Kaplan and colleagues (60) reported on 29 patients treated at Northwestern University and reviewed the literature. In their analysis, lesions of the distal urethra carried the best prognosis, and those in the bulbomembranous urethra had the worst. The results of 186 cases compiled by these authors are shown in Table 65.13. Five-year survival rates were 22% (16 of 71 patients) with tumors in the distal urethra, 10% (10 of 99 patients) with bulbomembranous urethra lesions, and 25% (four of 16 patients) with prostatic urethra tumors. Radiation therapy was used infrequently for these patients. Table 65.14 demonstrates equivalent local tumor control with either definitive radiation therapy or *en-bloc* resection.

The combination of radiation therapy and chemotherapy using 5-FU and mitomycin C has been reported for urethral carcinoma for organ preservation in locally advanced tumors. Reports by Baskin and Turzan (6), Johnson and colleagues (56), Licht and associates (71), and Shah and coworkers (109) support the efficacy of this combination for squamous cell carcinoma of the male and female urethra. Cleveland Clinic (71) reported results of patients with locally advanced squamous cell carcinoma of the urethra treated with concomitant chemoradiation including 5-FU ($1g/m^2$ intravenous infusion on days 1 to 4 and days 29 to 32) and mitomycin C ($50 mg/m^2$ bolus intravenous injection on day 1). EBRT (30 Gy in 15 fractions) to the pelvis and inguinal lymph nodes began on day 1. An additional 20-Gy tumor boost was given. Complete response was obtained in three patients, who remained disease-free after 43 months of follow-up. A patient with a T2N2M0 lesion treated with 30 Gy died of myocardial infarction several months after radiation therapy. Chemotherapy was well-tolerated and required no dose reduction or delay in treatment. One grade 3 acute toxicity (skin reaction) occurred that did not compromise the therapeutic plan. One patient developed urethral stricture that was managed successfully with urethral dilatation.

As previously described in this chapter, the largest chemoradiation experience for urethral carcinoma is the Wayne State experience (39). Concomitant 5-FU and cisplatin was used for squamous cell carcinoma, whereas concomitant methotrexate, vinblastine, Adriamycin (doxorubicin), and cisplatin (MVAC) was used for transitional cell carcinoma. A pathologic complete

Table 65.13 FIVE-YEAR SURVIVAL RATES IN 186 COLLECTED CASES OF MALE URETHRAL CARCINOMA CORRELATED WITH SITE

	No. of Patients	Five-Year Survival (%)
Distal urethra	71	22
Bulbomembranous urethra	99	10
Prostatic urethra	16	25

(Data from Kaplan GW, Bulkley GJ, Grayhack JT. Carcinoma of the male urethra. *J Urol* 1967;98:365–371, with permission.)

Table 65.14 LOCAL TUMOR CONTROL OF MALE URETHRAL CARCINOMA WITH RADIATION THERAPY OR EN-BLOC RESECTION

Modality	No. of Patients	No. Controlled
Radiation therapy		
Hopkins et al (52)	1	1
Kaplan et al (60)	11	9
Raghavaiah et al (101)	2	2
En-bloc resection		
Anderson and McAninch (2)	2	1
Klein et al (65)	7	5
Kaplan et al (60)	28	25

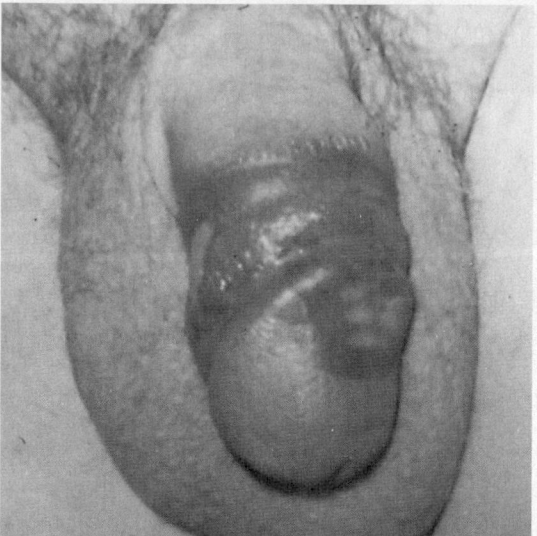 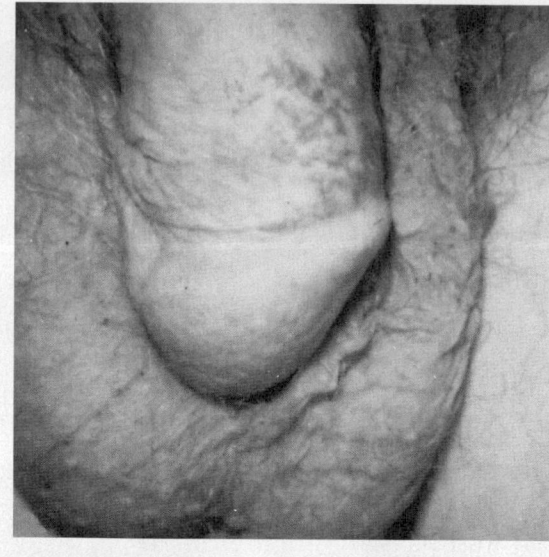

FIGURE 65.7. A: Squamous cell carcinoma of the balanopreputial region with extension into the glands (stage I). Patient was treated with 120 kVp x-rays, 0.3 mm Cu half-value layer, receiving 60-Gy skin dose in 5 weeks. **B:** Same patient 4 years later with no evidence of disease. Telangiectasis in present.

response was reported in 87.5% of women undergoing resection following chemoradiation. With a median follow-up of 42 months, the overall disease-free survival rate was 62%.

Sequelae of Treatment

Irradiation of the penis produces a brisk erythema, dry or moist desquamation, and swelling of the subcutaneous tissue of the shaft in virtually all patients. Although quite uncomfortable, these are reversible reactions that subside within a few weeks with conservative treatment. Telangiectasia is a common late consequence of radiation therapy and is usually asymptomatic (Fig. 65.7).

In the reported radiotherapy series, meatal–urethral strictures occur with a frequency of 0% to 40% (16,30,49,64,75,86). This incidence compares favorably with the incidence of urethral stricture following penectomy (27). Most strictures following radiation therapy are at the meatus.

Ulceration, necrosis of the glans, or necrosis of the skin of the shaft is a rare complication in modern series (16). Lymphedema of the legs has been reported following inguinal and pelvic radiation therapy, but the role of irradiation in the development of this complication remains controversial. Many patients with this symptom have active disease in the lymphatics that may be responsible for lymphatic blockage.

Of all male genitourinary cancers, penile cancer poses the greatest threat to sexual function and carries the most devastating psychologic impact as a result of penectomy. Despite recent advances in treatment, sexual function is not likely to be adequately preserved in some patients. These patients and their partners need information about the physical impairments after surgical intervention and should learn adjustment skills before undertaking treatment. Referral to a trained sexual consultant or therapist for help is indicated.

References

1. Almgard LE, Edsmyr F. Radiotherapy in treatment of patients with carcinoma of the penis. *Scand J Urol Nephrol* 1973;7:1–5.
2. Anderson K, McAninch J. Primary squamous carcinoma of the anterior urethra. *Urol* 1984;23:134–140.
3. Andriole GL, Miller DC, Colberg JW, et al. Surgical management of penile cancer. In: Vogelzang NJ, Scardino PT, Shipley WU, et al, eds. *Comprehensive textbook of genitourinary oncology*. Philadelphia: Lippincott Williams & Wilkins, 1999: 1057–1065.
4. Barnes RD, Sarembock LA, Abratt RP, et al. Carcinoma of the penis: The Groote Schuur Hospital experience. *J R Coll Surg Edinb* 1989;34:44–46.
5. Barney JD. Epithelioma of the penis: An analysis of 100 cases. *Ann Surg* 1907;46:890–914.
6. Baskin L, Turzan C. Carcinoma of the male urethra: Management of locally advanced disease with combined chemotherapy, radiotherapy, and penile-preserving surgery. *Urology* 1992;39:21.
7. Bassett JW. Carcinoma of the penis. *Cancer* 1952;5:530–538.
8. Bezerra ALR, Lopes A, Santiago GH, et al. Human papillomavirus as a prognostic factor in carcinoma of the penis. *Cancer* 2001;91:2315–2321.
9. Boon IA. Sapphire probe laser surgery for localized carcinoma of the penis. *Eur J Surg Oncol* 1988;14:193–195.
10. Boon ME, Susanti I, Tasche MJA, et al. Human papillomavirus (HPV)-associated male and female genital carcinomas in a Hindu population: The male as vector and victim. *Cancer* 1989;64:559–565.
11. Bracken RB, Henry R, Ordonez N. Primary carcinoma of the urethra. *South Med J* 1980;73:1003–1005.
12. Brkovic D, Kälble T, Dörsam J, et al. Surgical treatment of invasive penile cancer—the Heidelberg experience from 1968 to 1994. *Eur Urol* 1997;31:339–342.
13. Cabanas RM. An approach for the treatment of penile carcinoma. *Cancer* 1977; 39:456–466.
14. Cade S. *Malignant disease and its treatment by Radium*. Bristol: John Wright & Sons, 1940.
15. Catalona WJ. Modified inguinal lymphadenectomy for carcinoma of the penis with preservation of saphenous veins: Technique and preliminary results. *J Urol* 1988;140:306–310.
16. Chaudhary AJ, Ghosh S, Bhalavat RL, et al. Interstitial brachytherapy in carcinoma of the penis. *Strahlenther Onkol* 1999;175:17–20.
17. Colberg JW, Andriole GL, Catalona WJ. Long-term follow-up of men undergoing modified inguinal lymphadenectomy for carcinoma of the penis. *Br J Urol* 1997;79:54–57.
18. Corral DA, Sella A, Pettaway CA, et al. Combination chemotherapy for metastatic or locally advanced genitourinary squamous cell carcinoma: A phase II study of methotrexate, cisplatin and bleomycin. *J Urol* 1998;160:1770–1774.
19. Crawford ED, Dawkins CA. Cancer of the penis. In: Skinner DG, Lieskovsky G, eds. *Diagnosis and management of genitourinary cancer*. Philadelphia: W.B. Saunders, 1988: 549–563.
20. Dalbagni G, Zhang Z-F, Lacombe L, et al. Male urethra carcinoma: Analysis of treatment outcome. *Urol* 1999;53:1126–1132.
21. Daly N, Douchez J, Combes P. Treatment of carcinoma of the penis by iridium 192 wire implant. *Int J Radiat Oncol Biol Phys* 1982;8:1239–1243.
22. D'Ancona CAL, Botega NJ, De Moraes C, et al. Quality of life after partial penectomy for penile carcinoma. *Urol* 1997;50:593–596.
23. Daseler EH, Anson BH, Reimann AF. Radical excision of the inguinal and iliac lymph glands: A study based upon 450 anatomical dissections and upon supportive clinical observations. *Surg Gynecol Obstet* 1948;87:679–694.
24. Dean AL Jr. Epithelioma of the penis. *J Urol* 1935;33:252–283.
25. Dehner LP, Smith BH. Soft tissue tumors of the penis: A clinicopathologic study of 46 cases. *Cancer* 1970;25:1431–1447.
26. deKernion JB, Tynberg P, Persky L, et al. Carcinoma of the penis. *Cancer* 1970;32:1256–1262.
27. Derakhshani P, Neubauer S, Braun M, et al. Results and 10-year fol-low-up in patients with squamous cell carcinoma of the penis. *Urol Int* 1999;62:238–244.
28. Derrick FC Jr, Lynch KM Jr, Kretkowski RC, et al. Epidermoid carcinoma of the penis: Computer analysis of 87 cases. *J Urol* 1973;110:303–305.
29. Duncan W, Jackson SM. The treatment of early cancer of the penis with megavoltage x-rays. *Clin Radiol* 1972;23:246–248.
30. Ekstrom T, Edsmyr F. Cancer of the penis: A clinical study of 229 cases. *Acta Chir Scand* 1958;115:25–45.

31. El-Dimry M, Oliver R, Hope-Stone H, et al. Reappraisal of the role of radiotherapy and surgery in the management of carcinoma of the penis. *Br J Urol* 1984;56:724–728.
32. Engelstad RB. Treatment of cancer of the penis at the Norwegian Radium Hospital. *Radiology* 1948;60:801–806.
33. Fegen P, Persky L. Squamous cell carcinoma of the penis: Its treatment, with special reference to radical node dissection. *Arch Surg* 1969;99:117.
34. Fleming ID, Cooper JS, Henson DE, et al. *AJCC cancer staging manual*. Philadelphia: Lippincott-Raven, 1997.
35. Fraley EE, Zhang G, Sazama R, et al. Cancer of the penis: Prognosis and treatment plans. *Cancer* 1985;55:1618–1624.
36. Franzen L, Henriksson R, Karlsson N-O, et al. A technical device for irradiation in carcinoma of the penis [Letter]. *Acta Oncol* 1987;26:77–78.
37. Gentil F, Cavalcanti S. Total management of cancer of the penis. *Rev Inst Nac Cancer (Mexico)* 1964;15:321.
38. Gerbaulet A, Lambin P. Radiation therapy of cancer of the penis: Indications, advantages, and pitfalls. *Urol Clin North Am* 1992;19:325–332.
39. Gheiler EL, Tefilli MV, Tiguert R, et al. Management of primary urethral cancer. *Urol* 1998;52:487–493.
40. Grabstald H, Kelley CD. Radiation therapy of penile cancer: Six to ten-year follow-up. *Urology* 1980;15:575–576.
41. Grabstald H. Controversies concerning lymph node dissection for cancer of the penis. *Urol Clin North Am* 1980;7:793–799.
42. Graham JH, Helwig EB. Erythroplasia of Queyrat: A clinicopathologic and histochemical study. *Cancer* 1973;32:1396–1414.
43. Graham S, Priore R, Graham M, et al. Genital cancer in wives of penile cancer patients. *Cancer* 1979;44:1870–1874.
44. Greenbaum SS, Krull EA, Simmons EB. Basal cell carcinoma at the base of the penis: Case report. *Genitourin Med* 1989;64:128–129.
45. Greenlee RT. Cancer statistics, 2000: A benchmark for the new century. *CA Cancer J Clin* 2000;50:7–33.
46. Gursel EO, Georgountzos C, Uson AC. Penile cancer: Clinicopathologic study of 64 cases. *Urology* 1973;1:569–578.
47. Haas GP, Blumenstein BA, Gagliano RG, et al. Cisplatin, methotrexate and bleomycin for the treatment of carcinoma of the penis: A southwest oncology group study. *J Urol* 1999;161:1823–1825.
48. Haddad F. Letter to the editor. *J Urol* 1989;141:959.
49. Haile K, Delclos L. The place of radiation therapy in the treatment of carcinoma of the distal end of the penis. *Cancer* 1980;45:1980–1984.
50. Hanash K, Furlow W, Utz D. Carcinoma of the penis: A clinicopathologic study. *J Urol* 1970;104:291–297.
51. Hardner GJ, Bhanalaph T, Murphy GP, et al. Carcinoma of the penis: An analysis of therapy in 100 consecutive cases. *J Urol* 1972;108:428–430.
52. Hopkins S, Nag S, Soloway M. Primary carcinoma of the male urethra. *Urology* 1984;23:128–133.
53. Horenblas S, van Tinteren H, Delemarre JF, et al. Squamous cell carcinoma of the penis. II. Treatment of the primary tumor. *J Urol* 1992;147:1533–1538.
54. Jackson SM. The treatment of carcinoma of the penis. *Br J Surg* 1966;53:33–35.
55. Jensen M. Cancer of the penis in Denmark 1942 to 1962 (511 cases). *Dan Med Bull* 1977;24:66.
56. Johnson D, Kessler J, Ferrigni R, et al. Low dose combined chemotherapy/radiotherapy in the management of locally advanced urethral squamous cell carcinoma. *J Urol* 1989;141:615.
57. Johnson DE, Fuerst DE, Ayala AG. Carcinoma of the penis: Experience with 153 cases. *Urology* 1973;1:404–408.
58. Johnson DE, Lo RK. Management of regional lymph nodes in penile carcinoma. *Urology* 1984;24:308–311.
59. Jorstad LH. Carcinoma of the penis. *Am J Roentgenol* 1941;46:232–235.
60. Kaplan GW, Bulkley GJ, Grayhack JT. Carcinoma of the male urethra. *J Urol* 1967;98:365–371.
61. Kattan J, Culine S, Droz J-P, et al. Penile cancer chemotherapy: Twelve years' experience at Institut Gustave-Roussy. *Urol* 1993;42:559–562.
62. Kaushal V, Harma SC. Carcinoma of the penis. *Acta Oncol* 1987;26:413–417.
63. Kearsley JH, Roberts SJ, Bynaston B. Curative radiotherapy for stage IV carcinoma of the penis. *Med J Austral* 1986;145:474–475.
64. Kelley CD, Arthur K, Rogoff E, et al. Radiation therapy of penile cancer. *Urology* 1974;4:571–573.
65. Klein FA, Whitmore WF, Herr HW, et al. Inferior pubic rami resection with en bloc radical excision for invasive proximal urethral carcinoma. *Cancer* 1983;51:1238–1242.
66. Knudsen OA, Brennhovd IO. Radiotherapy in the treatment of the primary tumour in penile cancer. *Acta Chir Scand* 1967;113:69–71.
67. Konnak JW. Conservative management of low grade neoplasms of the male urethra: A preliminary report. *J Urol* 1980;123:175–177.
68. Kumar S, Ananthakrishnan N, Prema V. Predicting regional lymph node metastasis in carcinoma of the penis: a comparison between fine-needle aspiration cytology, sentinel lymph node biopsy and medial inguinal lymph node biopsy. *Br J Urol* 1998;81:453–457.
69. Lederman M. Radiotherapy of cancer of the penis. *Br J Urol* 1953;25:224–232.
70. Lenowitz H, Graham AP. Carcinoma of the penis. *J Urol* 1946;56:458–484.
71. Licht MR, Klein EA, Bukowski R, et al. Combination radiation and chemotherapy for the treatment of squamous cell carcinoma of the male and female urethra. *J Urol* 1995;153:1918–1920.
72. Lindegaard JC, Nielsen OS, Lundbeck FA, et al. A retrospective analysis of 82 cases of cancer of the penis. *Br J Urol* 1996;77:883–890.
73. Lopes A, Hidalgo GS, Kowalski LP, et al. Prognostic factors in carcinoma of the penis: Multivariate analysis of 145 patients treated with amputation and lymphadenectomy. *J Urol* 1996;156:1637–1642.
74. Malcaluso JN Jr, Sullivan JW, Tomberlin S. Glomus tumor of glans penis. *Urology* 1985;25:409–410.
75. Mandler JI, Pool TL. Primary carcinoma of the male urethra. *J Urol* 1966;96:67–72.
76. Marcial VA, Figueroa-Colon J, Marcial-Rojas RA, et al. Carcinoma of the penis. *Radiology* 1962;79:209–220.
77. Martinez I. Relationship of squamous cell carcinoma of the cervix uteri to squamous cell carcinoma of the penis. *Cancer* 1979;24:777–780.
78. Mazeron JJ, Langlois D, Lobo PA, et al. Interstitial radiation therapy for carcinoma of the penis using Iridium 192 wires: The Henri Mondor experience (1970–1979). *Int J Radiat Oncol Biol Phys* 1984;10:1891–1895.
79. McDougal WS, Kirchner FK, Jr., Edwards RH, et al. Treatment of carcinoma of the penis: The case for primary lymphadenectomy. *J Urol* 1986;136:38–41.
80. Mikhail GR. Cancers, precancers, and pseudocancer on the male genitalia: A review of clinical appearances, histopathology, and management. *J Dermatol Surg Oncol* 1980;6:1027–1035.
81. Mohs F, Snow S, Messing E, et al. Microscopically controlled surgery in the treatment of carcinoma of the penis. *J Urol* 1985;133:961.
82. Mullin EM, Anderson EE, Paulson DF. Carcinoma of the male urethra. *J Urol* 1974;112:610–613.
83. Murrell DS, Williams JL. Radiotherapy in the treatment of carcinoma of the penis. *Br J Urol* 1965;37:211–222.
84. Narayana AS, Olney LE, Loening SA, et al. Carcinoma of the penis: Analysis of 219 cases. *Cancer* 1982;49:2185–2191.
85. Netter FH. *The CIBA collection of medical illustrations, Vol. 2;* Reproductive System. Summit, NJ: CIBA Pharmaceutical, 1972.
86. Newaishy GA, Deeley TJ. Radiotherapy in the treatment of carcinoma of the penis. *Br J Radiol* 1968;41:519–521.
87. Nichols P. Pathology of cancer of penis. In: Skinner DG, Lieskovsky G, eds. *Diagnosis and management of genitourinary cancer*. Philadelphia: W.B. Saunders, 1988: 207–214.
88. Oliva E, Quinn TR, Amin MB, et al. Primary malignant melanoma of the urethra: a clinicopathologic analysis of 15 cases. *Am J Surg Pathol* 2000;24: 785–796.
89. Onuigbo WI. Carcinoma of skin of penis. *Br J Urol* 1985;57:465–466.
90. Oota K. Symposium de cancer del pene: Cancer of the penis in Japan. *Rev Inst Nac Cancer (Mexico)* 1964;15:289.
91. Ornellas AA, Seixas ALC, Marota A, et al. Surgical treatment of invasive squamous cell carcinoma of the penis: retrospective analysis of 350 cases. *J Urol* 1994;151:1244–1249.
92. Owor R. Carcinoma of the penis in Uganda. *IARC Sci Publ* 1984;63:493–497.
93. Paterson R, Tod MC, Russell MH. *The results of radium and x-ray therapy in malignant disease*. Edinburgh: Livingstone, 1950.
94. Paymaster JC, Gangadharan P. Carcinoma of the penis in India. *J Urol* 1967; 97:110.
95. Perinetti E, Crane DB, Catalona WJ. Unreliability of sentinel lymph node biopsy for staging penile carcinoma. *J Urol* 1980;124:734–735.
96. Persky L. Commentary: Problems and management of squamous cell carcinoma of the penis. In: Whitehead ED, Leiter E, eds. *Current operative urology*. Philadelphia: Harper & Row, 1984: 1180–1183.
97. Pettaway CA, Pisters LL, Dinney CP, et al. Sentinel lymph node dissection for penile carcinoma: the M.D. Anderson Cancer Center experience. *J Urol* 1995;154:1999–2003.
98. Pierquin B, Chassagne D, Chahbazian C, et al. *Brachytherapy*. St. Louis: Warren H. Green, 1978.
99. Pointon RCS. External beam therapy. *Proc R Soc Med* 1975;68:779–781.
100. Powell BL, Craig JB, Muss HB. Secondary malignancies of the penis and epididymis: A case report and review of the literature. *J Clin Oncol* 1985;3: 110–116.
101. Raghavaiah NV. Radiotherapy in the treatment of carcinoma of the male urethra. *Cancer* 1978;41:1313–1316.
102. Ray B, Canto AR, Whitmore WF. Experience with primary carcinoma of the male urethra. *J Urol* 1977;117:591–594.
103. Rosenberg SK. Carbon dioxide laser treatment of external genital lesions. *Urology* 1985;24:555.
104. Rozan R, Albuisson E, Giraud B, et al. Interstitial brachytherapy for penile carcinoma: A multicentric survey (259 patients). *Radiother Oncol* 1995;36: 83–93.
105. Sagerman RH, Yu WS, Chung CT, et al. External-beam irradiation of carcinoma of the penis. *Radiology* 1984;152:183–185.
106. Salaverria JC, Hope-Stone HF, Paris AMI, et al. Conservative treatment of carcinoma of the penis. *Br J Urol* 1979;51:32–37.
107. Schoen EJ, Oehrli M, Colby CJ, et al. The highly protective effect of newborn circumcision against invasive penile cancer. *Pediatrics* 2000;105:E36.
108. Schrek R, Lenowitz H. Etiologic facts in carcinoma of the penis. *Cancer Res* 1947;7:180–187.
109. Shah A, Kalra J, Silber L, et al. Squamous cell cancer of the female urethra: Successful treatment with chemoradiotherapy. *Urology* 1985;25:284.
110. Skinner DG, Leadbetter WF, Kelley SB. The surgical management of squamous cell carcinoma of the penis. *J Urol* 1972;107:273–277.
111. Solsona E, Iborra I, Rubio J, et al. Prospective validation of the association of local tumor stage and grade as a predictive factor for occult lymph node micrometastasis in patients with penile carcinoma and clinically negative inguinal lymph nodes. *J Urol* 2001;165:1506–1509.
112. Soria J-C, Fizazi K, Piron D, et al. Squamous cell carcinoma of the penis: Multivariate analysis of prognostic factors and natural history in a monocentric study with a conservative policy. *Ann Oncol* 1997;8:1089–1098.
113. Staubitz WJ, Lent MH, Oberkircher OJ. Carcinoma of the penis. *Cancer* 1955; 8:371–378.
114. Suchaud J, Kantor G, Richaud P. Curietherapie des cancers de la verge: Analyse d'une serie de 53 cas. *J Urol (Paris)* 1989;95:27–31.
115. Sulaiman MZ, Polazarz SV, Partington PE. Basal cell carcinoma of the penis: Case report. *Genitourin Med* 1989;64:128–129.
116. Thurgar CJL. *British practice in radiotherapy,* p. 194.London: Butterworth, 1955.
117. Vaeth JM, Green JP, Lowy RO. Radiation therapy of carcinoma of the penis. *AJR* 1970;108:130–135.
118. Villavicencio H, Rubio-Briones J, Regalado R, et al. Grade, local stage and growth pattern as prognostic factors in carcinoma of the penis. *Eur Urol* 1997;32:442–447.
119. Yu GSM, Nseyo UO, Carson JW. Primary penile lymphoma in a patient with Peyronie's disease. *J Urol* 1989;142:1076–1077.
120. Zouhair A, Coucke PA, Jeanneret W, et al. Radiation therapy alone or combined surgery and radiation therapy in squamous-cell carcinoma of the penis? *Eur J CA* 2001;37:198–203.

Clinical Radiation Oncology

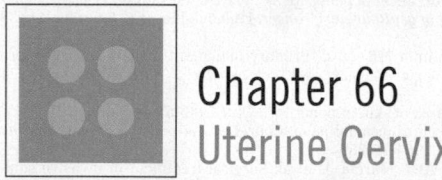

Chapter 66
Uterine Cervix

Carlos A. Perez, Brian D. Kavanagh

Anatomy

The uterus is a muscular hollow organ located in the midplane of the true pelvis, in an anteverted position, behind the bladder and in front of the rectum (Fig. 66.1), partially covered by peritoneum in its fundal portion and posteriorly; its anterior and lateral surfaces are related to the bladder and the broad ligaments, respectively. The corpus is separated from the cervix by a subtle constriction (the isthmus) and is divided into two regions: an upper or supravaginal portion above the ring containing the endocervical canal, and the vaginal portion, projecting in the vaginal vault.

The uterus is attached to the surrounding structures in the pelvis by two pairs of ligaments, the broad and the round ligaments (see Fig. 66.1). The broad ligament is a double layer of peritoneum extending from the lateral margin of the uterus to the lateral wall of the pelvis. It contains the fallopian tubes. The two layers of peritoneum forming the broad ligament enclose the *parametrium* as it reaches the uterus. Inferiorly, the broad ligament follows the plane of the pelvic floor and ends medially in the upper portion of the vagina (20).

The round ligament, a band of smooth muscle and connective tissue that contains small vessels and nerves, extends forward horizontally from its attachment in the anterolateral portion of the uterus to the lateral pelvic wall. The cord ascending from the lateral wall of the true pelvis crosses the pelvic brim and extends laterally to reach the abdominoinguinal ring, through which it leaves the abdomen to traverse the inguinal canal and terminates in the superficial fascia.

The uterosacral ligaments are paired supports for the lower uterus, extending from the uterus to the sacrum and running along the recto-uterine-peritoneal fields (20). The cardinal ligaments, also called *transverse cervical ligaments* (Mackenrodt's), are thickened connective tissue and fascia arising at the upper lateral margins of the cervix and inserting into the fascial covering of the pelvic diaphragm.

The uterus has a rich lymphatic network that drains principally into the paracervical lymph nodes; from there it goes to the external iliac (of which the obturator nodes are the innermost component) and the hypogastric lymph nodes. The pelvic lymphatics drain into the common iliac and the para-aortic lymph nodes. Lymphatics from the fundus pass laterally across the broad ligament continuous with those of the ovary, ascending along the ovarian vessels into the para-aortic lymph nodes. Some of the fundal lymphatics also drain into the external and internal common iliac lymph nodes (Fig. 66.2A).

The main artery supplying the uterus is the uterine artery, which originates from the anterior division of the hypogastric artery.

Because of the increasing use of intensity-modulated or image-guided radiation therapy (IMRT/IGRT) in the treatment of patients with gynecological malignancy, there is growing emphasis on imaging the pelvic anatomical structures, including lymph nodes for treatment planning (Fig 66.2B) (52). Finlay et al. (157) contoured pelvic blood vessels on computed tomography (CT) scans, as surrogates for lymph nodes in 45 patients and found this to be more accurate that bony landmarks for field delineation. Taylor et al. (601) used magnetic resonance imaging (MRI) to outline the pelvic lymph nodes in 20 patients and noted that with margins of 10 mm nodal coverage was 94% and with 15 mm 99%; with a modified 7-mm margin they ensured 99% nodal coverage with less volume of small bowel at risk.

Epidemiology

The American Cancer Society estimated that in 2007 there were 11,150 new cases of invasive carcinoma of the cervix in the United States and about 3,500 deaths, in addition to over 60,000 cases of carcinoma in situ (279). However, cervical cancer is highly prevalent in developing nations; it is estimated that close to 500,000 women worldwide develop this tumor and 233,000 die of the disease (262). Cervical cancer is more common in Latin America and less frequent in Jewish and European women and Fiji Islanders (250). Although some researchers have attributed the low frequency of cervical carcinoma in Jewish women to the circumcision of Jewish men (602), this low incidence has not been demonstrated in sexual partners of non-Jewish circumcised men. Lynch et al. (390) noted that although Ashkenazi women have an overall cancer risk comparable to other ethnic groups, it is still lower for carcinoma of the cervix, which occurs infrequently in Jewish women.

Carcinoma of the uterine cervix can be induced in experimental animals by application of hormonal or other chemical

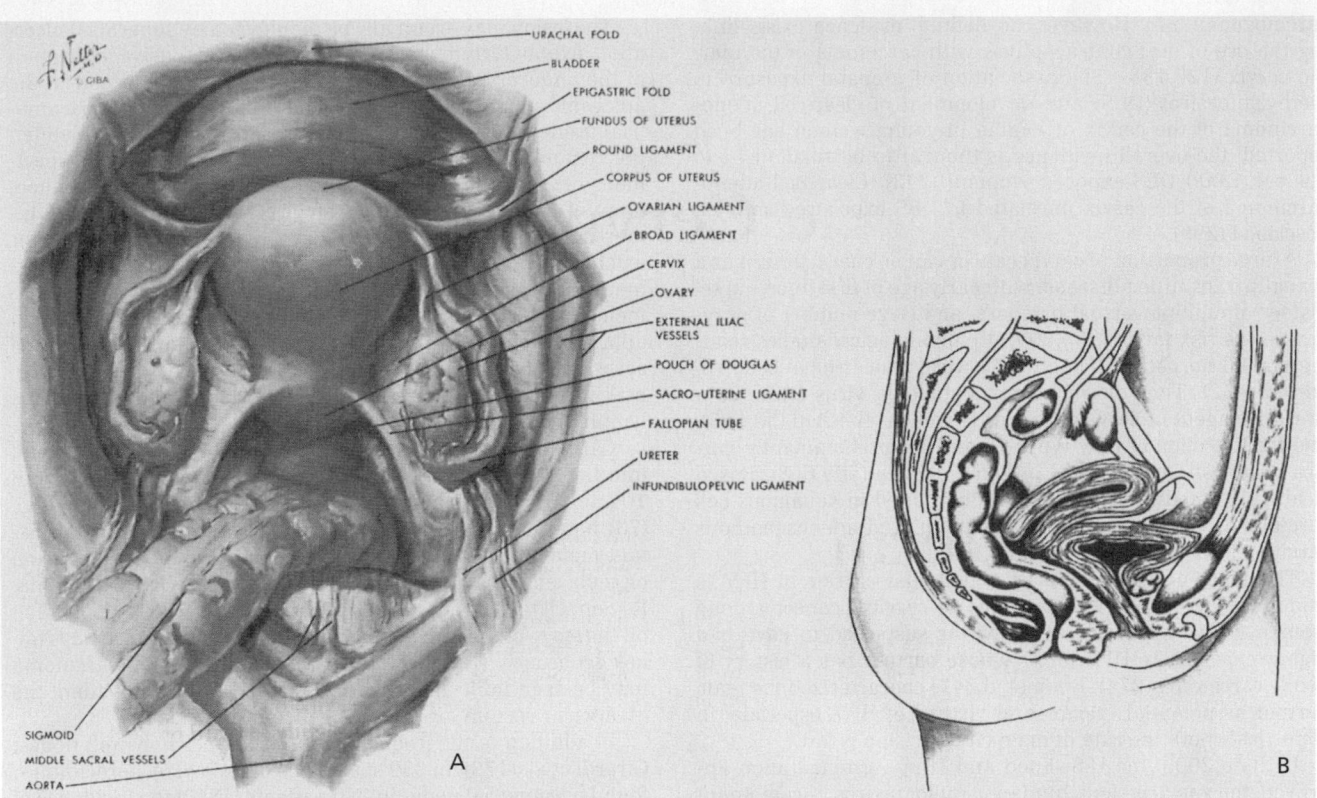

FIGURE 66.1. Anatomy of the pelvis observed from above **(A)** and on a sagittal view **(B)**, demonstrating the close relationship of the uterus to the bladder and the rectosigmoid. (A, © Copyright 1954, CIBA-GEIGY Corp. Reproduced from Netter F. *The CIBA collection of medical illustrations.* Summit, NJ: Ciba Pharmaceutical, 1972, with permission. All rights reserved.) (439)

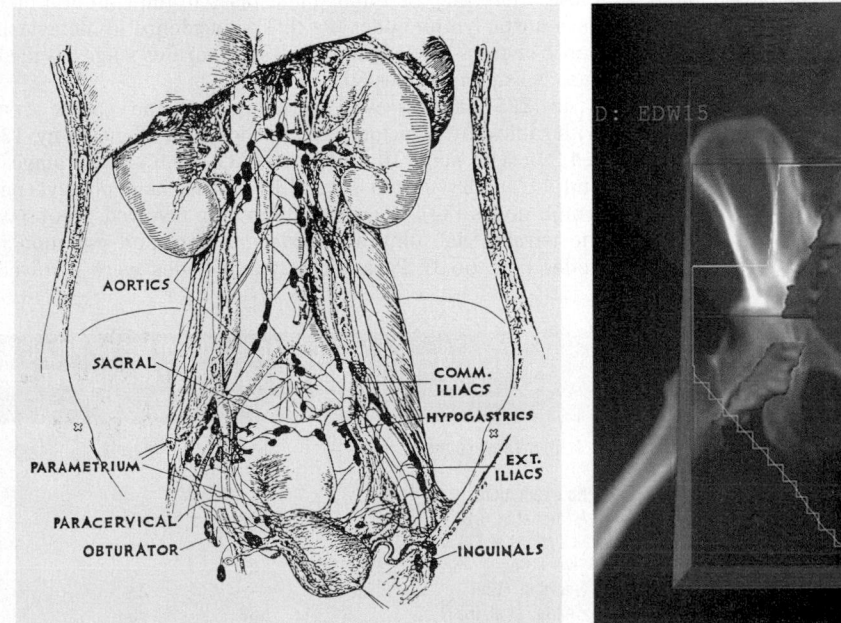

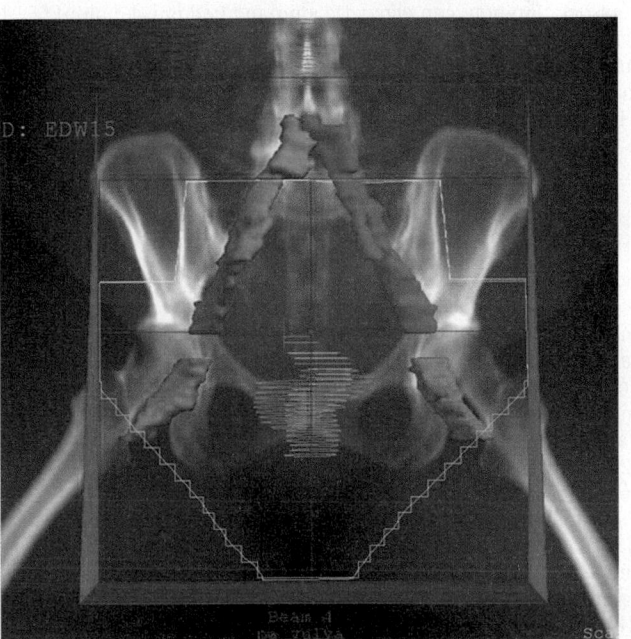

FIGURE 66.2. A: Lymph vessels and lymph nodes of the cervix and the body of the uterus. (From Henrikson E. The lymphatic spread of carcinoma of the cervix and of the body of the uterus: a study of 420 necropsies. *Am J Obstet Gynecol* 1949;58:924–942, with permission.). **B:** Three-dimensional reconstruction of location of pelvic and common iliac lymph nodes outlined on computed tomography scans in patient with carcinoma involving the distant vagina. Treatment portal is shown.

carcinogens (287). However, no definite evidence exists linking the use of oral contraceptives with carcinoma of the uterine cervix (127,188). The association of prenatal exposure to diethylstilbestrol (DES) and development of clear-cell adenocarcinoma of the cervix or vagina in young women has been reported; the overall incidence is thought to be small (0.14 to 1.4 per 1,000 DES-exposed women) (243). Clear cell adenocarcinoma of the cervix unrelated to DES exposure has been described (293).

A large proportion of cervix cancer can be characterized as a sexually transmitted disease, with early age of first intercourse, history of multiple sexual partners, and large number of pregnancies as risk factors (85,309). Epidemiological studies relating genital herpetic infection to cervical cancer have been reported (432). The role of human papilloma virus (HPV) as a causative agent of cervical cancer is well established (50,665), and the detection of HPV types 16 and 18, predominantly, carries prognostic importance in some studies (509,668). Bosch et al. (51) noted that HPV 16 predominated in squamous-cell carcinoma, whereas in adenocarcinoma and adenosquamous carcinoma HPV 18 predominated.

The male partner's role as a potential carrier of HPV is evidenced by the higher incidence of cervical cancer among women whose spouses are known or suspected to have had higher exposure to HPV (6) or whose partner has a history of penile carcinoma (274). Boon et al. (47) characterized the male partner as potential "vector and victim" of HPV, especially in countries where the rate of male circumcision is low.

In June 2006, the U.S. Food and Drug Administration approved the quadrivalent human papillomavirus recombinant vaccine for women 9 to 26 years for prevention of gynecological disease caused by HPV types 6, 11, 16, and 18. This is an exciting development and a landmark decision, heralded as a major advance in the prevention of cervical cancer that may have a worldwide impact on the incidence of this malignancy.

Other risk factors among HIV-positive women included racial/ethnic background (African American vs. white, relative risk [RR] = 1.64), current smoking (yes vs. no, RR = 1.55), and younger age (younger than 30 years vs. 40 years or older, RR = 1.75) (457).

An association between cigarette smoking and development of cervical cancer has been reported (32,187). A review of over 50 studies concluded that smoking was a cofactor for HPV infection and induction of cervical cancer (594). However, in the study by Agarwal et al. (6), cigarette smoking was not a risk factor.

Natural History and Patterns of Spread

Squamous-cell carcinoma of the uterine cervix usually originates at the squamous columnar junction (transformation zone) of the endocervical canal and the portio of the cervix. The lesion is frequently associated with severe cervical dysplasia and carcinoma in situ, usually progressing to invasive carcinoma over 10 to 20 years in the majority of patients (30,84).

The malignant process breaks through the basement membrane of the epithelium and invades the cervical stroma. Formerly, if the invasion was <3 mm, the lesion was classified as microinvasive or superficially invasive (84), a term not used in the International Federation of Gynecologists and Obstetricians (FIGO) staging, which classifies this tumor as Ia1. Invasion may progress, and in a modification of the FIGO staging schema (272), if a tumor is not grossly visible but has a depth of penetration of <5 mm and breadth of 7 mm or less, it is classified as stage IA2 invasive carcinoma; the incidence of metastatic pelvic lymph nodes is related to the depth of invasion, with an overall incidence of 3% to 8% (42,84).

The lesion may eventually be manifested by superficial ulceration, exophytic tumor in the ectocervix, or extensive infiltration of the endocervix. The tumor, if untreated, may spread to the adjacent vaginal fornices or to the paracervical and parametrial tissues (270), with eventual direct invasion of the bladder, the rectum, or both. Landoni et al. (352), in operative specimens of 230 radical hysterectomies with pelvic lymphadenectomy of patients with clinical stage IB and IIA, noted the tumor spreads endocervically equally in all directions; tumor extension into the vesicocervical ligament (anterior parametrium) was noted in 23% of cases, into the uterosacral ligaments (posterior parametrium) and the rectovaginal septum in approximately 15%, and into the parametria in 28% to 34% of cases. Paracervical extension was related to the depth of stromal invasion, tumor size, lymphatic invasion, and presence of lymph node metastasis.

Carcinoma of the uterine cervix has been found to extend into the lower uterine segment and the endometrial cavity in 10% to 30% of patients (470). Perez et al. (470) and Chao et al. (73) noted decreased survival and a greater incidence of distant metastases in patients with stromal endometrial invasion or replacement of normal endometrium by cervical carcinoma. Regional lymphatic or hematogenous spread occurs, depending on the stage of the tumor, but dissemination does not always follow an orderly sequence, and occasionally a small carcinoma may be seen infiltrating the pelvic lymph nodes, invading the bladder or rectum, or producing distant metastasis.

In addition to the frequently described pelvic lymph nodes, Girardi et al. (178), in 359 specimens of radical hysterectomies, found parametrial nodes in 280 patients (78%); the incidence of positive nodes was 11.4% in stage IB and 21.5% in stage IIB disease. With negative parametrial nodes, only 26% of patients had positive iliac lymph nodes, whereas 81% of patients with positive parametrial lymph nodes also had metastatic pelvic nodes. These data underscore the need to irradiate the parametrial tissues or carry out a complete bilateral pelvic lymphadenectomy in patients with invasive cervical carcinoma.

Carcinoma of the cervix may spread to the obturator lymph nodes (considered a medial group of the external iliac), to other external iliac nodes, and to the hypogastric lymph nodes. From these, there may be tumor metastases to the common iliac or para-aortic lymph nodes (242). The incidence of metastasis to pelvic or para-aortic lymph nodes for various stages of the disease is listed in Tables 66.1 and 66.2.

In 225 patients with carcinoma of the cervix treated with radical hysterectomy and pelvic lymphadenectomy, 13/91 (14.2%) with stage IB and IIA, 16/81 (19.8%) with stage IIB, and 11/40 (28%) with stage IIIB disease had positive pelvic lymph nodes (34). The most commonly involved groups were the parametrial, obturator, external iliac, and common iliac nodes (Fig. 66.3). Para-aortic lymph nodes were involved in

Table 66.1	PERCENTAGE OF INCIDENCE OF PELVIC NODE METASTASES IN CARCINOMA OF THE UTERINE CERVIX		
Author (Reference)	Stage I	Stage II	Stage III
No Irradiation			
Alvarez et al. (12)	12	—	—
Delgado et al. (117)	16	—	—
Piver & Chung (488)	27	—	—
Fine et al. (156)	—	23	37
Wharton et al. (651)	38	35	33
Postirradiation Lymphadenectomy			
Perez et al. (471)	7	—	—

Modified from Perez CA, DiSaia PJ, Knapp RC, et al. Gynecologic tumors. In: DeVita VT Jr, Hellman S, Rosenberg SA, eds. *Cancer: principles and practice of oncology*, 2nd ed. Philadelphia: JB Lippincott, 1985.

Table 66.2   METASTASES TO PARA-AORTIC LYMPH NODES IN CARCINOMA OF THE UTERINE CERVIX

Author (Reference)	Stage IB (%)	Stage IIA (%)	Stage IIB (%)	Stage IIIA (%)	Stage IIIB (%)	Stage IV (%)
Lagasse et al. (346)	8/143 (8)	4/22 (18)	19/58 (33)	0/3 (0)	19/61 (31)	1/4 (25)
Nelson et al. (437)	—	—	5/31 (16)	—	13/28 (46)	
Piver et al. (486)	—	—	6/46 (13)	—	18/49 (37)	4/7 (57)
Wharton et al. (651)	0/21 (0)	0/10 (0)	10/47 (21)	—	14/42 (33)	

Percentages are in parentheses.
Modified from Hoskins WJ, Perez CA, Young RC. Gynecologic tumors. In: DeVita VT Jr, Hellman S, Rosenberg SA, eds. *Cancer: principles and practice of oncology*, 3rd ed. Philadelphia: J.B. Lippincott, 1989.

3/91 (3.3%) patients with stage IB and IIA tumors 4 cm or less and in 5/38 patients (13.1%) with stage IIB and III disease.

Hematogenous dissemination through the venous plexus and the paracervical veins occurs less frequently but is relatively common with more advanced stages. In an analysis of 322 patients in whom distant metastases developed, the most frequently observed metastatic sites were the lung (21%), para-aortic lymph nodes (11%), abdominal cavity (8%), and supraclavicular lymph nodes (7%) (151). Bone metastases occurred in 16% of patients, most commonly to the lumbar and thoracic spine (Table 66.3). Spinal epidural compression from metastatic tumor, often involving lumbar segments, can occur rarely (15), and metastasis to the brain and the heart have been reported (372,394).

Clinical Presentation

Intraepithelial or early invasive carcinoma of the cervix can be detected before it becomes symptomatic by cytologic smears; Papanicolaou (Pap) smear, colposcopy and biopsies, and HPV testing have high specificity and sensitivity (94.5%)

Frequently, the first manifestation of abnormality is postcoital spotting, which may increase to metrorrhagia (intermenstrual bleeding) or more prominent menstrual bleeding (menorrhagia). Serosanguineous or yellowish, foul-smelling vaginal discharge may be noted in patients with advanced invasive carcinoma. If chronic bleeding occurs, the patient may complain of fatigue or other symptoms related to anemia.

Pain in the pelvis or hypogastrium may be caused by tumor necrosis or associated pelvic inflammatory disease. In patients with pain in the lumbosacral area, the possibility of para-aortic lymph node involvement with extension into the lumbosacral roots or hydronephrosis should be considered.

Urinary and rectal symptoms (hematuria, rectal bleeding) may appear in advanced stages as a consequence of invasion of the bladder or rectum by the neoplasm.

Diagnostic Work-Up

Every patient should be jointly evaluated by the radiation and gynecologic oncologists. After careful clinical history a general physical examination with attention to the supraclavicular (nodal) areas, abdomen, and liver, a careful pelvic examination should be carried out with as little discomfort to the patient as possible, without compromising the thoroughness of the evaluation (447). Pelvic examination should include inspection of external genitalia, vagina, and uterine cervix, rectal examination, and bimanual palpation of the pelvis. Pelvic examination under anesthesia is very important in the evaluation and clinical staging of these patients. Cystoscopy or rectosigmoidoscopy should be performed in all patients with stage IIB, III, and IVA disease or those with earlier stages who have a history of urinary or lower gastrointestinal tract disturbances. The diagnostic procedures for carcinoma of the cervix are presented in Table 66.4.

Screening

The American Cancer Society has recommended that asymptomatic women 20 years of age and older or sexually active younger than 20 years have annual Pap smears for 2 consecutive years and at least one every 3 years until the age of 65 years. The American College of Obstetricians and Gynecologists has strongly recommended that that Pap smears be obtained on an annual basis.

When obtaining the Pap smear, special attention should be directed to not using a lubricating agent (warm water on the speculum will suffice), to obtaining good "scrapings" from the cervix and vaginal posterior fornix (without blood), and to using a small brush to obtain an endocervical sample. The patient should be instructed not to cleanse with a douche before the examination, and specimens should be obtained for studies of

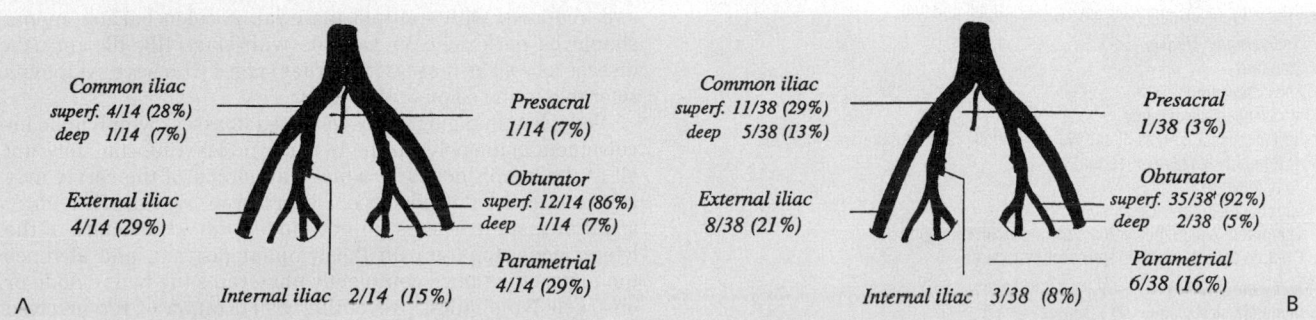

FIGURE 66.3.   A: Distribution of pelvic node metastases in 14 patients with stage IB to IIA cervical cancer, tumor size <4 cm, and **(B)** 38 patients with locally advanced cervical cancer treated with neoadjuvant chemotherapy. (From Benedetti-Panici P, Maneschi F, Scambia G, et al. Lymphatic spread of cervical cancer: an anatomical and pathological study based on 225 radical hysterectomies with systematic pelvic and aortic lymphadenectomy. *Gynecol Oncol* 1996;62:19–24, with permission.)

Table 66.3	**CARCINOMA OF THE UTERINE CERVIX (MALLINCKRODT INSTITUTE OF RADIOLOGY 1959–1986): ANATOMIC SITE OF FIRST METASTASIS**

Site	No. of Patients with Distant Metastases ($n = 322$)
Lung	69 (21%)
Para-aortic Nodes	37 (11%)
Abdominal cavity	26 (8%)
Supraclavicular nodes	21 (7%)
Spine	21 (7%)
Gastrointestinal tract	14 (4%)
Liver	13 (4%)
Inguinal nodes	10 (3%)
Miscellaneous	111 (35%)

From Fagundes H, Perez CA, Grigsby PW, et al. Distant metastases after irradiation alone in carcinoma of the uterine cervix. *Int J Radiat Oncol Biol Phys* 1992;24:197–204, with permission.

trichomonas. If the cytologic smear shows atypia or mild dysplasia (class II), the smear should be repeated no sooner than after 2 weeks, to allow representative cellular exfoliation.

Guidelines for reporting results of cervical and vaginal cytology were promulgated in 1988. The Bethesda system eliminated the classes of Pap cytology. The correlation between the cytologic diagnosis and subsequent histologic examination is over 90% (334). This system was modified in 1991 and in 2001 (565).

If the cytologic smear shows dysplasia or malignant cells, directed biopsies at colposcopy should be carried out immediately. Endocervical curettage must always be performed except in pregnant women. If the biopsy results are negative, the procedure should be repeated and, if necessary, a conization should be performed.

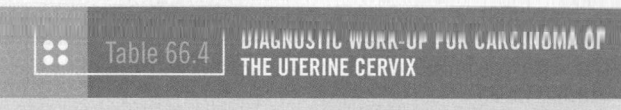

Table 66.4	**DIAGNOSTIC WORK-UP FOR CARCINOMA OF THE UTERINE CERVIX**

General
History
Physical examination, including bimanual pelvic and rectal examinations

Diagnostic procedures
Cytologic smears (Papanicolaou) if not bleeding
Colposcopy
Conization (subclinical tumor)
Punch biopsies (edge of gross tumor, four quadrants)
Dilatation and curettage
Cytoscopy, rectosigmoidoscopy (stages IIB, III, and IVA)

Radiographic studies
Standard
Chest radiography
Intravenous pyelography
Barium enema (stages III and IVA and earlier stages if there are symptoms referable to colon or rectum)
Complementary
Lymphangiography (optional)
Computed tomography or magnetic resonance imaging
Positron emission tomography scan (optional)

Laboratory studies
Complete blood count
Blood chemistry
Urinalysis

Conization/Loop Excision

Conization must be performed when no gross lesion of the cervix is noted and an endocervical tumor is suspected; the entire lesion cannot be seen with the colposcope; diagnosis of microinvasive carcinoma is made on biopsy; discrepancies are found between the cytologic and the histologic appearances of the lesion; or the patient is not reliable for continuous follow-up.

Conization involves a conical removal of a large portion of the ectocervix and endocervix. Cold biopsy specimens should always be obtained with a scalpel or other appropriate instrument. At least 50% of the endocervical canal should be removed without compromising the internal sphincter. Curettage of the remaining endocervical canal should be carried out.

Laser conization and loop diathermy excision have achieved some popularity in recent years. Loop excision or laser conization is frequently done in an office setting as an alternative to conization; loop excision is less expensive and more reliable than laser conization (505).

Biopsy

When a gross lesion of the cervix is present, multiple punch biopsies should be adequate to confirm the diagnosis of invasive carcinoma. Specimens should be obtained from any suspect area as well as in all four quadrants of the cervix and from any suspect areas in the vagina. It is important to obtain tissue from the periphery of the lesion with some adjoining normal tissue; biopsy specimens from central ulcerated or necrotic areas may not be adequate for diagnosis.

Dilatation and Curettage

Because possible upper extension of the tumor may modify the plan of therapy, fractional curettage of the endocervical canal and the endometrium is recommended at the time of initial evaluation, or during the first intracavitary radioisotope insertion if the patient is treated with radiation therapy.

Laboratory Studies

For invasive carcinoma, patients should have the following laboratory studies: complete peripheral blood evaluation, including hemogram, white blood cell count, differential and platelet count; blood chemistry profile, with particular attention to blood urea nitrogen, creatinine, and uric acid; liver function values; and urinalysis.

Imaging Studies

Traditionally, chest radiographs and intravenous pyelograms (IVP) were obtained in all patients for staging purposes. The IVP in many countries has been replaced by CT scan of the pelvis and abdomen with contrast material. A colon barium enema should be performed in patients with stage IIB, III, and IVA disease as well as those with earlier stages who have symptoms referable to the colon and rectum.

Pedal lymphangiography was used to assess lymph node involvement in the pelvic or para-aortic nodes. Unfortunately, not all of the lymph nodes to which carcinoma of the cervix may metastasize are opacified (i.e., obturator or hypogastric nodes), small metastatic lesions do not modify the architecture of the lymph node apparent on the lymphangiogram, and at times the metastatic tumor completely obliterates the lymph node or obstructs lymphatics, preventing visualization of the involved lymph nodes (478). Lagasse et al. (346) found the lymphangiogram to be unreliable as a basis for treatment decisions. This procedure has been replaced by CT scanning or MRI.

Table 66.5	COMPUTED TOMOGRAPHY SCAN IN THE EVALUATION OF PARA-AORTIC NODES				
Author (Reference)	No. of Cases	FIGO Stage	Sensitivity (%)	Specificity (%)	Accuracy (%)
Kilcheski et al. (314)	36	I–IV	—	80	—
Camilien et al. (67)	51	IB–IIA	67	100	100
Camilien et al. (67)	10	IIB–IV	67	100	90

FIGO, International Federation of Gynecologists and Obstetricians.
Modified from Camilien L, Gordon D, Fruchter RG, et al. Predictive value of computerized tomography in the presurgical evaluation of primary carcinoma of the cervix. *Gynecol Oncol* 1988;30:209–215, with permission.

If performed with intravenous (IV) contrast, CT scans substitute for IVP. The cervical tumor may be seen as an enlarged, irregular, hypoechoic cervix or as a mass with ill-defined margins. The overall accuracy of CT scanning in staging cervical cancer ranges from 63% to 88% (321). In the detection of lymph node abnormalities, the overall accuracy of conventional CT scanning is 77% to 85%, with a sensitivity of 44% and specificity of 93% (264).

Camilien et al. (67) reported on 61 patients with carcinoma of the cervix who had both preoperative CT scans and exploratory laparotomy; correlation of radiographic and surgical/pathologic findings showed that 75% of the enlarged pelvic lymph nodes on CT contained metastases and 97% of patients with negative nodes on CT scan were pathologically negative (specificity of 97%). However, histologically positive pelvic nodes were often missed on CT scan (sensitivity of 25%). The CT scan is more valuable in evaluation of the para-aortic lymph nodes (specificity of 100% and sensitivity of 67%; Table 66.5).

Shepherd et al. (554), in a retrospective study of CT scans in 56 patients with carcinoma of the cervix treated with irradiation, noted that tumor depth was correlated with lymph node involvement (p <0.01) and risk of death.

Heller et al. (239) reported a prospective evaluation of 320 patients with stage IIB to IVA carcinoma of the cervix entered into a Gynecologic Oncology Group (GOG) protocol in which preoperative CT scan, lymphangiography, and ultrasonography of the aortic area were performed. Para-aortic node dissection was done in patients with negative staging studies. Lymphangiography, CT scan, and ultrasonography had false-negative frequencies for pelvic lymph node evaluation of 14.2%, 25%, and 30%, respectively. The sensitivity was 79% for lymphangiography, 34% for CT scan, and 19% for ultrasonography and the specificity ratings were 73%, 96%, and 99%, respectively. Ultrasonography, therefore, is not reliable in preoperative detection of lymph node metastases, but it has limited value in evaluating extrauterine tumor involvement and may be used to detect uterine perforation, which can occur during intracavitary insertion (661).

MRI is being used more frequently for assessment of extracervical tumor extension (265), although it is somewhat more expensive. MRI is very useful in patients allergic to iodinated contrast material or impaired renal function. It is contraindicated in patients with pacemakers, cochlear implants, metallic prostheses, or large vascular clips. On T2-weighted images, a cervical cancer may be seen as a mass of intermediate signal intensity, usually of greater intensity than the fibrocervical stroma. On T1-weighted images, tumors are usually isointense with the normal cervix and may not be seen (24). Abnormal, irregular cervix margins, prominent parametrial strands, exocentric parametrial enlargement, and loss of parametrial fat planes on T1-weighted images or high signal in the parametria or cardinal/uterosacral ligaments on T2-weighted images are indicative of more extensive tumors (264,321,561). Parametrial tumor is easily identified on T2-weighted images from the low-intensity cervix and uterine ligaments.

Hawnaur et al. (236) compared pretreatment tumor staging and volume assessment by examination under anesthesia (EUA), transrectal ultrasonography (TRUS), and MRI in 60 patients with invasive carcinoma of the cervix. TRUS and MRI assigned the same tumor stage in only 30% of patients, and EUA and MRI agreed on tumor stage in an additional 27%. In cases of disagreement, the MRI staging correlated better with outcome than TRUS or EUA. Sixty-two percent of patients with enlarged lymph nodes on pretreatment MRI either died or had tumor recurrence or metastases. MRI was superior in assessing the full extent of bulky tumors and lymph node enlargement over both TRUS and EUA.

Hatano et al. (235) also evaluated MRI in 42 patients with advanced cervical cancer treated with external irradiation and high–dose-rate (HDR) brachytherapy. In biopsies performed immediately after radiation therapy (RT), no residual tumors were found in 36 patients (86%). The simultaneous MRI study demonstrated no high-signal intensity on T2-weighted images in 28 patients (75%). A high–signal-intensity area was observed in 14 patients, and this disappeared 3 months after RT in eight patients with a negative histologic study. The sensitivity, specificity, and accuracy of MRI tumor response studies at 3 months after radiation therapy were 100%. MRI studies performed at 30 Gy of external irradiation and 3 months after radiation therapy were predictive for local tumor control.

Postema et al. (494) compared MRI with pelvic examination (including under general anesthesia in selected patients) in 103 patients with invasive cervical carcinoma. The gold standard for comparing treatment decisions was based on surgicopathologic data available in 91 patients. MRI was better at identifying extracervical tumor spread, but it had more false-positive results. The pelvic examination led to correct treatment decisions in 89% of patients, with MRI not leading to an overall improvement in treatment decisions.

Also, in a study by Hansen et al. (230), clinical assessment was superior to low-field MRI in staging cervical cancer in 95 women on whom MRI examinations and clinical staging according to the FIGO recommendations were performed within 2 weeks after clinical diagnosis; the clinical staging correctly classified 57 patients (accuracy, 92%), compared with 52 patients with MRI using contrast enhancement (accuracy, 84%).

MRI dynamic enhancement during the first 2 weeks of radiation therapy may provide early prediction of tumor regression rate. In seven patients, tumor regression rates ranged from 2% to 15.2% per day and correlated positively with changes in both peak and mean tumor enhancement (p <0.01). A similar study was published by Gong et al. (181) and van de Bunt et al. (627). MRI also was found to be useful in providing accurate target volume definition in brachytherapy treatment planning (122).

Haider et al. (218) evaluated 56 patients with adenocarcinoma involving the cervix using MRI and noted that 42 (75%) had a visible mass. Findings were more prevalent in patients with primary adenocarcinoma of the endometrium, as characterized by a endometrial thickening (11 [73%] vs. 3 [13%]) endometrial cavity expansion by a mass (9 [60%] and 2 [9%] respectively) ($p = 0.003$).

Kodaira et al. (331) reviewed 84 patients with stage II cancer evaluated by MRI; all patients received intracavitary brachytherapy with (83) or without (1) external-beam radiation therapy (EBRT). The 5-year disease-free survival (DFS) of patients with maximal tumor size ($D_{max} \geq 50$ mm) was significantly lower (46.2%) than that for patients with $D_{max} < 50$ mm (88%; $p < 0.0001$).

Ebner et al. (136) reported that, in comparing MRI findings in 12 women with recurrent pelvic tumors and 10 with fibrotic mass (confirmed by laparotomy or biopsy in 21 patients), they were able to differentiate the two processes accurately in most instances. However, it is highly desirable to confirm abnormal or suspect lymph node radiographic findings with CT-guided fine-needle aspiration biopsies.

Corn et al. (96) evaluated endorectal coil MRI in 18 patients with cervical carcinoma (stages IB to IIIB); in seven patients, tumors were determined to be in a higher stage by endorectal coil MRI because of proximal vaginal involvement or the combination of proximal vaginal involvement and parametrial extension). Patients were treated with EBRT and low–dose rate (LDR) brachytherapy. Compared with those who had dark or intermediate signal, patients with bright signal characteristics tended to present with earlier stages, were less likely to have anemia, and more likely to have complete response to external irradiation.

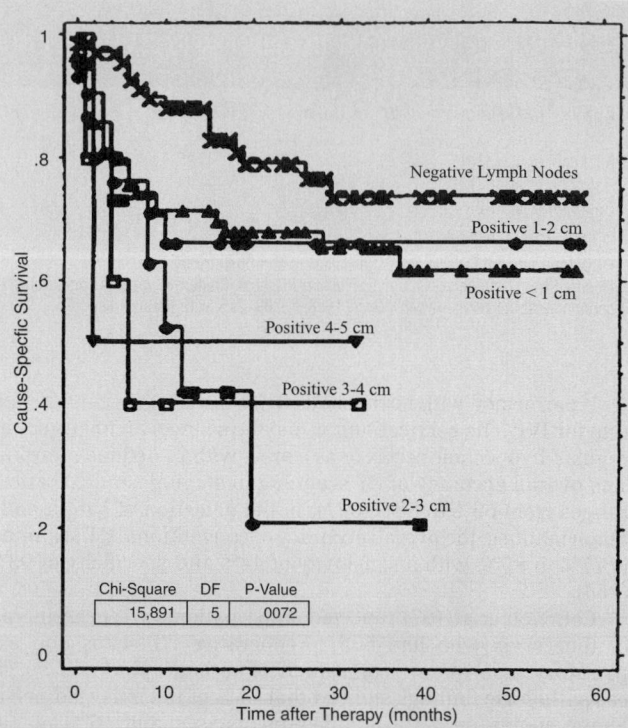

FIGURE 66.4. Cause specific survival in patients with carcinoma of the cervix correlated with pelvic lymph node status on posttreatment 2-[^{18}F]-fluoro-2-deoxy-D-glucose/positron emission tomography. (From Grigsby PW, Singh AK, Siegel BA, et al., Lymph node control in cervical cancer. *Int J Radiat Oncol Biol Phys* 2004;59:637–638, with permission.)

Positron Emission Tomography

Positron emission tomography (PET) scanning is increasingly used in the evaluation of patients with malignant neoplasia, including invasive cervical cancer, using 2-[^{18}F]-fluoro-2-deoxy-D-glucose (FDG). Rose et al. (521), in 32 patients with locally advanced carcinoma of the cervix, observed uptake in 91% of the primary tumors. Compared with surgical staging, PET scanning had a sensitivity of 75% and a specificity of 92% in detecting para-aortic metastasis.

Grigsby et al. (207) compared CT and FDG-PET scanning for lymph node staging in 101 patients with carcinoma of the cervix. CT demonstrated abnormally enlarged pelvic lymph nodes in 20 and para-aortic lymph nodes in seven patients, whereas PET demonstrated abnormal FDG uptake in pelvic lymph nodes in 67, in para-aortic lymph nodes in 21 and in supraclavicular lymph node in eight. The 2-year progression-free survival rate, based solely on para-aortic lymph node status, was 64% in CT-negative and PET-negative patients, 18% in CT-negative and PET-positive patients, and 14% in CT-positive and PET-positive patients ($p < 0.0001$). The most significant prognostic factor for progression-free survival was the presence of positive para-aortic lymph nodes on PET imaging ($p = 0.025$). The authors noted in 76 patients with no abnormal FDG uptake, 2-year survival was 86%, with persistent abnormal uptake 40% and no survivors in patients who developed new sites of abnormal uptake (206). In a follow-up study of 152 patients, the authors reported 5-year cause-specific survival (CSS) of 80% in 114 patients without abnormalities on posttherapy FDG-PET versus 32% in 20 with persistent uptake and no survivors in 18 with new sites of abnormal uptake (205). In another study on 208 patients, Grigsby et al. (208) noted a close correlation between doses of irradiation and number and size of positive lymph nodes with treatment failures and survival (Fig. 66.4).

Hope and Grigsby (257) performed FDG-PET scans in 58 patients with cervical carcinoma who had endometrial biopsy or dilatation and curettage; 36 (64%) had pathologic endometrial invasion (EI). Pelvic lymph node metastasis was more commonly detected in this group than in patients without EI (70% vs. 23%, respectively; $p < 0.001$) as were para-aortic node and supraclavicular node metastasis (30% vs. 0%, $p = 0.006$). Further, 2-year survival was 77% versus 50% and overall survival 92% versus 65%, respectively ($p = 0.047$).

Lin et al. (377) described the use of FDG-PET for brachytherapy treatment planning in 24 patients with cervical carcinoma, improving tumor coverage dose distribution, lowering dose to pelvic normal tissues, and improving outcome. Lin et al. (378), using FDG-PET in 32 patients with cervix carcinoma, observed a reduction in physiologic tumor volume of 50% occurring within 20 days from the initiation of radiation therapy.

Staging

The staging recommendations were last revised in 1995. Stage TIB includes all invasive tumors limited to the cervix larger than IA2. Stage TIB occult is no longer used. In 1995, FIGO modified the staging of stage IB lesions (confined to the cervix) into IB1, clinical lesions no >4 cm in size, and IB2, lesions >4 cm in size. There were no changes in the other stages, including the 1987 definitions of stages IA, IA1, and IA2 (553,621).

A parallel TNM staging system has been proposed by the American Joint Committee on Cancer (191). All histologic types should be included. When there is a disagreement regarding the staging, the earlier stage should be recorded (Table 66.6 and Fig. 66.5).

Kolstad (333) reviewed results of therapy in 643 patients with microinvasive carcinoma reclassified as stage IA1 or IA2.

Table 66.6   STAGING OF CARCINOMA OF THE UTERINE CERVIX

AJCC	FIGO	
Primary Tumor (T)		
TX		Primary tumor cannot be assessed
T0		No evidence of primary tumor
Tis		Carcinoma *in situ*
T1	I	Cervical carcinoma confined to uterus (extension to corpus should be disregarded)
T1a	IA	Preclinical invasive carcinoma, diagnosed by microscopy only
T1a1	IA1	Minimal microscopic stromal invasion
T1a2	IA2	Tumor with an invasive component 5 mm or less in depth taken from the base of the epithelium and 7 mm or less in horizontal spread
T1b	IB	Clinical lesions confined to the cervix or preclinical lesions greater than IA
	IB1	Clinical lesions no greater than 4 cm in size
	IB2	Clinical lesions greater than 4 cm in size
T2	II	Cervical carcinoma invades beyond uterus but not to the pelvic wall or to the lower third of vagina
T2a	IIA	Tumor without parametrial invasion
T2b	IIB	Tumor with parametrial invasion
T3	III	Cervical carcinoma extends to the pelvic wall and/or involves lower third of vagina and/or causes hydronephrosis or nonfunctioning kidney
T3a	IIIA	Tumor involves lower third of the vagina, with no extension to pelvic wall
T3b	IIIB	Tumor extends to pelvic wall and/or causes hydronephrosis or nonfunctioning kidney
T4[a]	IVA	Tumor invades mucosa of the bladder or rectum and/or extends beyond the true pelvis
Regional Lymph Nodes (N)		
Regional lymph nodes include paracervical, parametrial, hypogastric (obturator), common, internal and external iliac, presacral, and sacral.		
NX		Regional lymph nodes cannot be assessed
N0		No regional lymph node metastasis
N1		Regional lymph node metastasis
Distant Metastasis (M)		
MX		Presence of distant metastasis cannot be assessed
M0		No distant metastasis
M1	IVB	Distant metastasis

AJCC, American Joint Committee on Cancer; FIGO, International Federation of Gynecologists and Oncologists.
[a]Presence of bullous edema is not sufficient evidence to classify a tumor as T4.
Modified from Greene FL, Page DL, Flemming ID, et al. eds. *AJCC cancer staging manual*, 6th ed. New York: Springer, 2002;260, with permission.

Three of 232 patients with stage IA1 disease (1.3%) and 12/411 with stage IA2 (2.9%) had local recurrence in addition to four pelvic recurrences, confirming the validity of the staging modification.

The FIGO staging system is based on clinical evaluation (inspection, palpation, colposcopy); roentgenographic examination of the chest, kidneys, and skeleton and endocervical curettage and biopsies. Lymphangiograms, arteriograms, imaging findings, and laparoscopy or laparotomy findings should not be used for clinical staging.

Suspected invasion of the bladder or rectum should be confirmed by biopsy. Bullous edema of the bladder and swelling of the mucosa of the rectum are not accepted as definitive criteria for staging.

For a lesion to be classified as stage IIIB, the tumor should definitely extend to the lateral pelvic wall, although fixation is not required.

Patients with hydronephrosis or nonfunction of the kidney ascribed to extension of the tumor are classified as stage IIIB regardless of the pelvic findings. The currently used staging systems could be modified to accommodate some prognostic factors that have been reported, such as the significance of endometrial extension of cervical carcinoma, stromal invasion, and tumor volume in stage I and IIA carcinoma (barrel-shaped in the cervical or bulky tumor presentations), lymphatic/vascular permeation, and involvement of the lateral parametrium in stage IIB as opposed to the medial parametrium (478,489).

Surgical Staging

Some gynecologists have advocated the use of pretherapy laparotomy, particularly to evaluate the involvement of para-aortic lymph nodes. Recently, sentinel node biopsy in patients with cervical cancer has been used with encouraging results (120). The GOG prospectively evaluated 290 patients with carcinoma of the cervix (346); para-aortic node metastases were found in 19/58 (32.8%) patients with clinical stage IIB and 19/61 (31.1%) with stage IIIB disease.

A number of studies have compared the significance of para-aortic nodal metastases with other clinical and surgical findings with regard to progression-free survival and survival (578). In 626 patients treated on GOG randomized studies, the relative risk associated with positive para-aortic nodes was 11.0 for time to recurrence and 6.2 for survival time. In addition to the significant increase in risk of regional relapses, patients with para-aortic nodal metastasis are more likely to have extrapelvic failure (36).

Ketcham et al. (310) reported positive scalene fat pad biopsies in 7/36 (19%) patients with stage II, III, and IV carcinoma of the cervix and in 4/22 patients with postirradiation recurrences. However, this procedure is no longer routinely carried out at most institutions because of the low yield of positive specimens. Perez-Mesa and Spratt (479) found no supraclavicular node metastasis in 73 consecutive patients with various stages of cervical carcinoma. Manetta et al. (397) also did not detect scalene node metastasis in 24 patients with recurrent

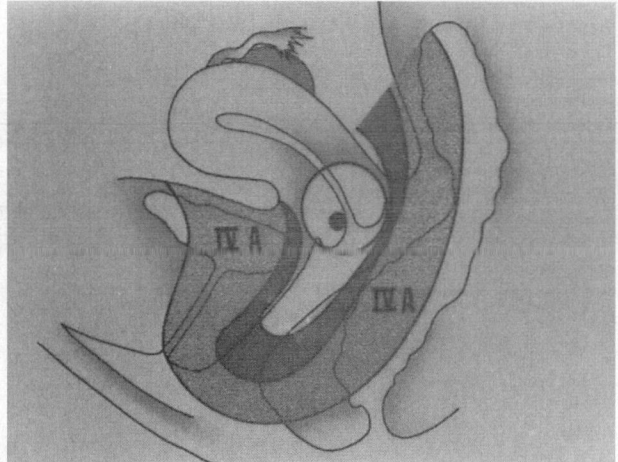

FIGURE 66.5. Diagrammatic representation of various anatomic stages of carcinoma of the uterine cervix, according to the Federation of Gynecologists and Obstetricians classification.

carcinoma of the cervix evaluated for exploration and possible pelvic exenteration.

Follow-Up

After treatment, patients should be regularly followed by both the radiation and the gynecologic oncologists. Careful history taking and a complete physical and pelvic/rectal examination usually is performed every month for the first 3 months after completion of irradiation, every 3 months for the remaining of the first year, every 4 months the second year, every 6 months during the third through fifth year, and yearly thereafter. The use of Pap smears for cervical and vaginal cytology as a follow-up study is controversial because of bizarre postirradiation cellular morphology that renders it difficult to distinguish postirradiation changes from residual or recurrent malignant cells (400,564). DNA analysis of postirradiation cytologic smears demonstrating atypia or dysplasia may provide ancillary information (109).

Rintala et al. (511) evaluated the reliability of cytologic analysis and atypia after radiation therapy in 89 patients treated for cervical carcinoma. A total of 697 Pap smears were taken; during the follow-up, 44 patients had recurrent disease, which was local in 17 (39%) cases. The rate of false-positive samples was only 3%. Radiation-induced atypia was detected in 28% of the Pap smears taken during the first 4 months after

radiation therapy, and its incidence decreased thereafter. In 1,000 patients treated with either surgery or radiation therapy at the M.D. Anderson Cancer Center for stage IB cervical cancer posttreatment, Pap smears did not detect a single asymptomatic recurrence among 133 patients with recurrent disease (41).

The presence of apparently viable tumor cells in the cytologic smear 3 months after irradiation should be evaluated with cervical biopsies, dilation and curettage, and careful examination under anesthesia, as indicated.

Complete blood counts and chemistry profile tests are obtained as clinically indicated. Chest radiography is commonly obtained on a yearly basis, usually for the first 5 years posttreatment, although its value to detect curable lung metastasis is not proven. If radiographs are consistently negative, obtaining them every other year thereafter may be sufficient.

Other imaging studies, such as CT, MRI, PET scanning, or bone scans, are obtained when clinically warranted. When persistent or recurrent tumor is suspected, biopsies should be obtained for histologic confirmation. If a biopsy is positive, immediate treatment should be instituted, as is discussed later.

Usually, hematometra after radiation therapy for cervical carcinoma is related to recurrent disease but occasionally may be related to estrogen replacement therapy, endometrial activity, and fibrosis and obliteration of the endocervix (634).

Pathologic Classification

Over 90% of tumors are squamous-cell carcinoma. Approximately 7% to 10% are classified as adenocarcinoma, and 1% to 2% are the clear-cell, mesonephric type.

Squamous-cell or epidermoid carcinoma is composed of cores and nests of epithelial cells arranged randomly; cells show central keratinization with cornified pearls and sometimes necrosis. Nonkeratinizing tumors may be seen. Electron microscopy may show desmosomes and tonofilaments. Squamous-cell carcinomas are divided into three types: large-cell keratinizing and nonkeratinizing and small cell type, and they are subdivided according to the degree of differentiation into well, moderately, or poorly differentiated.

Verrucous carcinoma is a variant of a very well-differentiated squamous-cell carcinoma that characteristically has a tendency to recur locally but not to metastasize (338). Mitotic activity is very low. It may be difficult to discriminate from a giant condyloma with cytologic atypia or from a well-differentiated invasive squamous carcinoma. Microscopically, verrucous carcinoma is exophytic, with an undulating, hyperkeratotic surface; the deep margin of a verrucous carcinoma is composed of large, bulbous masses that invade along a wide front in a "pushing" fashion.

Adenocarcinoma arises from the cylindrical mucosa of the endocervix or the mucus-secreting endocervical glands. Mucinous is the most common substage of adenocarcinoma. The endocervical adenocarcinoma may form mucosal glands lined by high columnar cells and produce tubular folds oriented in many directions. In another subtype, cells resemble those of the intestines; the epithelium tends to be pseudostratified and may contain goblet cells. The third variant is the signet-ring cell, which is rare and usually mixed with the endocervical or intestinal patterns.

Endometrioid carcinoma is the most common cell type of endocervical adenocarcinoma; the cells resemble those of the endometrium, and the presence of intracytoplasmic mucin in some cells may be seen in a substantial proportion of tumors. The World Health Organization recommends that endometrioid or endocervical types of adenocarcinoma be graded according to their architecture, based on the degree of gland formation (385).

Sometimes it is difficult to differentiate a primary endocervical adenocarcinoma from an endometrial tumor. Drescher et al. (126) described a higher incidence of involvement of the uterine corpus and the regional lymph nodes in 21 patients with adenocarcinoma compared with a similar number of patients with squamous-cell carcinoma. Chao et al. (71) and Contag et al. (93) described the use of microarray analysis for gene profiling (cDNA/RNA) to understand the molecular features of these tumors, which could aid in their classification. HPV has been identified in some subtypes of adenocarcinoma of the cervix (16).

A well-differentiated cervical adenocarcinoma has been improperly designated as *adenoma malignum* when it is truly a malignant tumor that invades adjacent tissues and may produce distant metastasis (559).

Adenosquamous carcinoma is relatively rare (2% to 5%) and consists of intermingled epithelial cell cores with squamous features and glandular structures. The squamous component is frequently nonkeratinizing. If the squamous component is benign metaplasia, the tumor is called *adenoacanthoma.*

Glassy cell carcinoma (1% to 2%) is considered a poorly differentiated adenosquamous tumor; it is rare and highly malignant. Survival is poor after surgery or irradiation. Ulbright and Gersell (622), in five cases of glassy cell carcinoma evaluated by light and electron microscopy, described both glandular and squamous differentiation. Littman et al. (379) reported only 4/13 patients, the majority with stage II disease, surviving 5 years (six had extrapelvic failures). Piura et al. (485) reported on five patients with cervical glassy cell carcinoma, three with stage IB1. All three patients were alive without disease 4, 12, and 18 months after diagnosis.

Adenoid cystic carcinoma is a rare variant of adenocarcinoma of the cervix (<1%) with an appearance similar to its counterparts in the salivary gland or the bronchial tree (184). The tumor is composed of nests and nodules of small carcinoma cells with a few characteristic cribriform patterns. Immunohistochemical findings for type IV collagen and laminin reveal intercellular cylinders composed of basement membrane material in the solid area without a cribriform pattern. They are locally aggressive and prone to metastasize (444).

Clear-cell carcinoma (mesonephric), not related to DES exposure, comprises approximately 2% of primary cervical adenocarcinomas and is thought to arise in mesonephric remnants (243). These tumors are submucosal, composed of clear and "hobnail" cells, and may grow in a tubular, glandular, papillary, or solid pattern. They appear at any age, with one-third occurring in women younger than 30 years of age. The clear cell is characterized by a voluminous cytoplasm filled with glycogen and the hobnail cell by single-cell apical projections into the neoplastic lumina. These tumors tend to be deeply positioned, with the bulk of the lesion on the stroma forming tubular structures, diffusely infiltrating the cervical stroma.

Clement et al. (89) described the clinicopathologic features in nine patients. Gross examination revealed polypoid or pedunculated masses that invaded the cervical wall in 50% of the hysterectomy specimens. On microscopic examination, five tumors contained basaloid carcinoma or squamous-cell carcinoma and four adenocarcinoma. In seven tumors, the sarcomatous component was homologous, usually resembling fibrosarcoma or endometrial stromal sarcoma, and two tumors contained heterologous sarcomatous elements. Cervical malignant müllerian mixed tumors, compared with their counterparts in the corpus, are more commonly confined at presentation and may have a better prognosis.

Small-cell carcinoma of the cervix, according to some authors, arises from endocervical argyrophilic cells or their precursors, multipotential neuroendocrine cells; however, some small-cell tumors do not contain morphologic evidence of neuroendocrine origin. Nuclear molding, absence of nucleoli, cell necrosis, and high mitotic activity are common. One-third to one-half stain positively for neuroendocrine markers such as chromogranin, serotonin, synaptophysin, or somatostatin. In the majority of patients, the cervical stroma is extensively infiltrated by single small round cells (2). Lymphatic and vascular invasion are significantly more common in small-cell carcinomas (noted in 58% of patients with stage IB disease; 40% of these patients had lymph node metastases at the time of radical surgery) (177). HPV 18 has been detected in the majority of these tumors (273).

Gersell et al. (177) described 15 patients with small-cell carcinoma; 13 showed cytokeratin on immunohistochemical studies, and at least one neuroendocrine marker was found in all 13 tumors (neuron-specific enolase, Leu-7, chromogranin, and synaptophysin). Invasion of vascular spaces was a prominent feature in seven tumors. Only three patients were alive 5, 11, and 78 months after treatment. In contrast, Van Nagell et al. (629), in an analysis of 25 patients, noted a 5-year survival rate of 54% for all stages of small-cell carcinoma, compared with 68% for matched large-cell nonkeratinizing squamous-cell and 74% for keratinizing squamous-cell carcinomas.

Basaloid carcinoma or adenoid-basal carcinoma, an extremely uncommon tumor, is characterized by nests or cords of small basaloid cells, prominent peripheral palisading of cells in the tumor nests, no significant stromal reaction or capillary space invasion, and an infiltrating growth pattern. Some authors have suggested a slow growth pattern with limited local invasiveness and low probability of lymph node metastases (107). Prognosis is excellent (358).

Primary sarcomas of the cervix have been occasionally described (e.g., leiomyosarcoma, rhabdomyosarcoma, stromal sarcoma, carcinosarcoma) (615).

Malignant lymphomas, primary or secondary in the cervix, have been sporadically reported. They behave, are classified, and should be treated as other lymphomas (148).

Metastasis of distant tumors to the uterine cervix are rare (about 4% of all tumors) and should be considered in the differential diagnosis. Metastasis from the breast, ovary, and kidney have been reported (53,464,557).

Prognostic Factors

Patient Factors

Age

According to some reports, age is not a prognostic factor in carcinoma of the cervix (116). Other authors have noted decreased survival in women younger than 35 or 40 years (108), who have a greater frequency of poorly differentiated tumors. In contrast, two European studies showed improved outcome for younger patients (407). This apparent contradiction may be explained by an analysis by Rutledge et al. (537), who showed an interaction between age and stage in the relative hazard plots for 250 patients younger than 35 years of age and matched control subjects. Mitchell et al. (413) evaluated 398 patients with stage I to III cervical carcinoma treated with radiation therapy. Patients were divided into nonelderly (35 to 69 years of age; $n = 338$) and elderly (≥ 70 years of age; $n = 60$) groups. Comorbid conditions in the elderly resulted in diminished ability to undergo intracavitary brachytherapy. Although the 5-year actuarial disease-free and CSS rates were comparable in the two groups, tumor recurrence and death from cervical cancer were more common beyond 5 years in the elderly group.

Race/Socioeconomic Status

Several authors have noted a correlation between racial or socioeconomic characteristics of patients and outcome of therapy (78,648). Mundt et al. (427) examined factors affecting outcome in 316 African American and 94 white patients undergoing RT for cervical cancer. With a median follow-up of 72.4 months, African Americans had a trend toward poorer 8-year cause-specific survival rates (47.9% vs. 60.6%; $p = 0.10$) compared with white patients. Factors correlating with poor outcome, present in the African American group, included lower hemoglobin (Hb) levels during RT ($p = 0.001$), lower median income ($p = 0.001$), and less frequent intracavitary brachytherapy ($p = 0.09$). Multivariate analysis demonstrated that race was not an independent prognostic factor after controlling for difference in patient, tumor, and treatment factors. Grigsby et al. (195), in 452 white and 124 African American women with stage II or III cancer of the cervix treated with RT alone, observed 5-year CSS rates for stage II of 66% and 61% ($p = 0.56$) and for stage III 38% and 47% ($p = 0.34$), respectively. Overall survival rates for stage II for the two racial groups were different (60% and 51%, respectively; $p = 0.02$) and may be related to non–cancer-related comorbidity factors.

Brooks et al. (56) evaluated 1,009 patients with invasive carcinoma of the cervix; 606 white, 354 African American, and 5% "other" races. African Americans were more likely to have Medicaid or to be uninsured (44% vs. 23%; $p = 0.001$) and were more likely to be admitted for an emergency or for a cancer-related complication ($p = 0.036$), to have comorbid illness ($p = 0.001$), to be admitted for a transfusion ($p = 0.01$), or to be treated with irradiation rather than surgery ($p = 0.001$). Racial differences existed in patterns of admission, type of therapy, and severity of illness.

Moreover, in an analysis of the 1994 Patterns of Care study of 471 cases of squamous-cell carcinoma treated in the United States and a randomly selected 215 additional cases from 17 institutions that admitted more than 40% minority patients, women who lived in low-income neighborhoods, who had only Medicaid coverage, or who were treated at large academic or minority-rich institutions tended to have a poorer initial performance status, higher-stage or bulky central tumor, and a lower pretreatment hemoglobin level (303).

General Medical Factors

Anemia and Tumor Hypoxia

Although stage, tumor volume, histologic type of the lesion, and vascular or lymphatic invasion are known to affect the prognosis of patients with cervical carcinoma, hemoglobin levels have also been the subject of extensive investigation in this regard.

Reviewing experimental data, Hirst (249) emphasized that in animal tumor models the opportunity to affect radiosensitivity by blood transfusion is transient. Blood transfusion is in general beneficial to the anemic patient with cancer, but it must be given as soon as possible before the first radiation dose to maximize its effects. Accounting for both the normal pulmonary and peripheral circulation and parallel flow through tumor tissue, Kavanagh et al. (308) calculated that decreasing hemoglobin–oxygen affinity should render a quantitatively greater decrease in radiobiologically hypoxic regions than what has been measured after the use of transfusions alone (586).

Using polarographic needle electrodes for direct tumor tissue oxygen measurements, investigators have reported worse outcomes for patients whose tumors have either a median partial pressure of oxygen (Po_2) level below 10 mm Hg (251) or a high percentage of Po_2 measurements below 5 mm Hg (330,518). Comparisons of intratumoral oxygen measurements before and after external-beam radiation therapy have usually indicated a trend toward improved oxygenation after radiation therapy (94,129), but the significance of posttreatment measurements is unclear (169). Hypoxic tumors are more likely to

recur locoregionally than well-oxygenated tumors regardless of whether surgery or radiation therapy is the primary local treatment (251).

Höckel et al. (251) reported higher 5-year disease-free survival rates in 21 patients in whom median oxygenation measured with polarographic needle electrodes was at least 10 mm Hg, in contrast to only 40% in 23 patients with a Po_2 <10 mm Hg.

Hypoxia-mediated genetic alterations such as inactivation or mutation of p53 are suspected to impart biologically aggressive traits (186).

Haensgen et al. (217), in 70 patients with stage IIB to IVA cervical cancer treated with EBRT and brachytherapy, analyzed biopsies for p53 transformed with a functionally inactive mutation (tp53) and DNA index measured by flow cytometry. *In vivo* oxygenation was measured with an Eppendorf probe, and patient hemoglobin levels were recorded. Patients with hemoglobin <11 g/dL had a 3-year survival rate of 27%, compared with 62% in those with hemoglobin ≥11 g/dL ($p = 0.006$). Of 70 tumors, 49 showed evidence of hypoxia (any reading of Po_2 <5 mm Hg) and a trend toward poorer survival compared with nonhypoxic tumors (48% vs. 70%; $p = 0.07$). Sixty of 70 tumors showed tp53 expression, which alone had no impact on survival (tp53 = 50% vs. wtp53 = 79%; $p = 0.11$). Hypoxic tumors had a significantly higher expression of tp53 ($p = 0.012$), whereas FIGO stage and anemia had no impact on p53 expression. Combining hypoxia and tp53 allowed stratification of subgroups with differing 3-year survival rates: tp53 ($n = 10$), 79%, and tp53 without hypoxia ($n = 44$), 47%. Flow cytometry demonstrated no effect of ploidy on survival. Advanced stage and pretreatment hemoglobin are independent prognostic factors in cervical carcinoma. Mutated or transformed tp53 was found more often in hypoxic tumors.

Notwithstanding the uncertain association between hypoxia and anemia, a randomized trial reported by Bush (64) 20 years ago remains an influential study; 132 patients with stage IIB to III cervical cancer were randomized to a control arm in which transfusions were given only if the hemoglobin level dropped below 10 g/dL, or an experimental arm in which transfusions were given to maintain the hemoglobin level at or above 12.5 g/dL. The results in the initial report suggested an improved outcome for patients in the experimental arm who received transfusions, but must understand the need to interpret the study results with caution in view of certain inherent biases in the analysis. As noted by Fyles et al. (168), there was not a statistically significant difference in outcome between treatment arms when compared by an intent-to-treat analysis. Second, the randomization was not stratified according to the potentially confounding influence of tumor size, and records of individual patients' tumor dimensions are not available. Finally, and perhaps most important, the thresholds for transfusion were based on anemia during therapy, not the initial hemoglobin. Although the subgroup analysis indicated a difference between patients in the control arm who received transfusion and patients in the experimental arm who received transfusion, only the least responsive patients in the control arm would likely continue to bleed during treatment and require a transfusion for a hemoglobin decrease below 10 g/dL, whereas the higher threshold for transfusion in the experimental group would have captured more patients already beginning to respond early in the course of treatment. Subsequently, Thomas (606) reviewed the Canadian experience and found that in 605 eligible patients with cervical cancer, 25% received blood transfusions, most frequently when Hb was below 100 g/L. On multivariate analysis baseline Hb was not a significant prognostic factor, but average weekly nadir during radiation therapy was significant (those with values higher than 120 g/L had lower incidence of local relapses and distant metastasis and better 5-year survival than patients with lower Hb levels).

Dunst et al. (130) studied 87 patients with squamous-cell cervical carcinoma treated with EBRT and HDR brachytherapy. Tumor oxygenation was measured with Eppendorf Po₂ before RT and at 19.8 Gy and angiogenesis was determined by microvessel density on biopsies. Pretreatment anemia had a significant impact on relapse rate (at 3 years, 6% in 20 patients with Hb >13 g/dL, 15% in 47 with Hb between 11 to 13 g/dL and 67% in 20 with Hb <11 g/dL). The 3-year overall survival was 79%, 64%, and 32%, respectively). Twenty-three tumors were poorly oxygenated (median Po₂ <15 mm Hg before RT and at 19.8 Gy) and 3-year survival was 38%, compared to 68% in patients with higher Po₂ ($p = 0.02$).

On the other hand, Eifel et al. (139), in a retrospective review of 2,997 patients with cervical cancer stage I or II treated with RT, found no impact of any Hb parameter on central, pelvic, or distant failures. Only tumor size and lymph node status were independent predictors of central recurrence ($p < 0.0001$) and tumor size, FIGO stage, lymph node status, and marginally transfusion during RT ($p = 0.04$) were correlated with disease-specific survival.

Munstedt et al. (426), in 183 patients who received adjuvant postradical surgery RT, noted that those with Hb <11 g/dL had lower recurrence-free and overall survival. Noteworthy, the difference was present mainly in a subgroup of women who had inadequate surgery.

The issue of whether blood transfusions to hemoglobin levels above 12 to 12.5 g/dL improve prognosis remains unsettled, but there are additional data to support that giving transfusions to maintain the average hemoglobin level during treatment at that level is beneficial. In a retrospective review of over 600 patients treated at seven different cancer centers in Canada, Grogan et al. (212) observed that the patients who maintained an average weekly hemoglobin level above 12 g/dL with or without transfusions had a significantly higher 5-year survival rate than patients with lower average weekly hemoglobin levels, regardless of the hemoglobin at presentation.

Many radiation oncologists routinely administer red blood cell transfusions (RBCT) to correct anemia before treatment with radiation therapy for cervical cancer, hoping at least for a generally favorable effect on the patient's sense of well-being and energy level if not also an impact on tumor radiosensitivity. Kapp et al. (297) reported on 204 patients who received red cell transfusion during RT when Hb level was <11 g/dL. Patients whose Hb was corrected (18.5%) had outcome similar to nontransfused patients. However, patient nonresponders to RBCT had decreased tumor control and survival.

Vaupel et al. (633), in a review of published data, concluded that maximum oxygenation of tumors is expected with Hb in the range of 12 to 14 g/dL for women and that higher Hb levels may not be better. This has implications for transfusions or administration of epoetin.

During the past decade, it has been established that recombinant human erythropoietin (EPO) provides an alternative means of sustaining or raising hemoglobin levels during radiation therapy. Typically, a dose of 200 U/kg per day 5 days per week would be expected to elevate hemoglobin by an average of 1 to 3 g/dL (133,356,637).

Dusenbery et al. (133), in 20 patients with carcinoma of the cervix with anemia, noted that EPO induced a prompt reticulocyte response (from 2.4% to 4.9%) by the beginning of radiation therapy. In the EPO group, the mean baseline hemoglobin level was 10.3 g/dL; by the second week it had increased to 12.2 g/dL, and by completion of radiation therapy, to 13.2 g/dL. Mean baseline hemoglobin level in concurrent control patients was 10.7 g/dL; at the completion of radiation therapy it was 10.4 g/dL.

Although it is clear that EPO can reduce the need for transfusions for anemic patients with cancer in a variety of settings, its effect on quality of life is less certain (547). Furthermore,

there is currently no proof that the use of EPO is in any way superior to transfusions with respect to impact on clinical outcome for patients receiving radiation therapy in particular, and transfusions are a less expensive option in most cases (305).

Other Medical Factors

Jenkin and Stryker (280) observed a higher incidence of pelvic recurrences and complications in patients with arterial hypertension (diastolic pressure >110 mm Hg).

Kapp and Lawrence (296) reported on 398 patients; patients with temperatures over 101°F had a higher incidence of distant metastases and a lower survival rate.

Tumor Factors

Tumor Volume

There is a close correlation between depth of stromal invasion, tumor size, and incidence of parametrial and pelvic node metastases and survival in patients with cervical cancer (12,117). In a study of women treated with radical hysterectomy, the 5-year disease-free survival rate was 90% in 181 patients stage IB1 (≤4 cm) and 72.8% in 48 patients with stage IB2 disease ($p = 0.02$) (155).

Toita et al. (614), in a review of 70 patients with stage IIB and IIIB carcinoma of the uterine cervix treated with RT alone, reported no significant correlation of 5-year DFS with size of the cervical tumor <60 mm (70% to 85%); however, in patients with tumor >60 mm, the 5-year DFS was 28.6%.

Piver and Chung (488) showed a greater incidence of lymphatic and distant metastasis and lower survival rates in patients with bulky and barrel-shaped stage IB and IIA tumors treated by radical hysterectomy (Table 66.7). Also, a higher incidence of pelvic recurrences and distant metastases and a decreased survival rate were reported by Fletcher (161), Eifel et al. (142), and Perez et al. (476) in patients with larger tumors treated with irradiation. In stages IB and IIA, higher radiation doses or combination with an extrafascial hysterectomy improved local tumor control (144,474).

Further, Leveque et al. (375), in patients with stage I to II adenocarcinoma of the cervix treated with RT alone or combined with radical surgery, noted that FIGO stage and pelvic node involvement were the most important parameters influencing overall survival. Silver et al. (558), in 93 patients with stage I adenocarcinoma of the cervix, described patient age and tumor grade as significant prognostic variables for survival ($p < 0.01$ and 0.01, respectively); tumor size was significant ($p < 0.01$) for survival and progression-free survival.

In contrast, Grigsby et al. (198), in patients with stage IB and IIA carcinoma of the cervix treated with preoperative irradiation and radical or conservative hysterectomy, observed no correlation of tumor volume with outcome. The 5-year pelvic failure rates for stage IB were 16% for tumors smaller than 3 cm and 9% for larger tumors ($p = 0.90$) and for stage IIA 22% for tumors both smaller or larger than 3 cm ($p = 0.75$).

Several retrospective studies have demonstrated decreased survival and a greater incidence of distant metastases in patients with endometrial extension of a primary cervical carcinoma (endometrial stromal invasion or replacement of the endometrium by tumor only) (470). Grimard et al. (211), on the other hand, confirmed those findings only in patients with stage IB tumors, but not in more advanced stages. Similar findings were noted by Noguchi et al. (445). Patients without uterine body invasion had a 5-year survival rate of 92.4% compared with 53.8% in patients with invasion.

| Table 66.7 | TREATMENT GUIDELINES FOR INVASIVE EPIDERMOID CARCINOMA OF CERVIX INCIDENTALLY FOUND AT SIMPLE (TOTAL) HYSTERECTOMY |

		External Irradiation (Gy)		LDR Intracavitary Ovoids Surface Dose (Gy)
Group	Tumor Extent	Whole Pelvis	Split Fields	
I	Microinvasion (≤3 mm invasion), margins clear	0	0	0–65
II	Fully invasive (>3 mm), margins clear	20	30	65
III	Microscopic residual (+ margins) or lymphatic permeation in groups I–II	30	20	70–75
IV	Gross residual "cut across tumor"	40	10–20	75–80
V	Recurrent tumor	40	10–20	80+ (interstitial therapy)

LDR, low–dose-rate.

Histology

Most reports have shown no significant correlation of survival or tumor behavior with the degree of differentiation of squamous-cell carcinoma or adenocarcinoma of the cervix (10,79,640).

Alfsen et al. (10) analyzed 417 adenocarcinomas and 88 other nonsquamous-cell carcinomas of the cervix; in patients with stage I, histological type, extension to the vagina or corpus uteri, tumor volume (>3,000 mm^3), infiltration depth (in thirds of the cervical wall), vascular invasion, lymph node metastases, treatment, and patient age were significant prognostic variables.

Although Reagan and Fu (507) demonstrated prognostic value of histologic differentiation in patients treated with irradiation, Crissman et al. (101) failed to observe a correlation between histologic parameters and patient survival.

Angiogenesis and Tumor Vascularity

Microvessel count is higher in patients with cervical neoplasia than in control patients and higher in patients who experience posttreatment recurrences. Obermair et al. (448), in 166 patients with stage IB cervical cancer, observed a 5-year survival rate of 89.7% in 102 patients whose tumors had a microvessel density of 20/field or less and 63% in 64 patients whose tumors had a microvessel density of >20/field (log rank p <0.0001). Similar findings were reported by Cooper et al. (95).

Loncaster et al. (383), in a retrospective study of 100 patients, found that vascular endothelial growth factor (VEGF) expression in tumor biopsies in advanced carcinoma of the cervix was associated with a poor prognosis.

Flow Cytometry Studies on DNA and Growth Fraction

Some authors have noted no significant difference in recurrence rates between patients with diploid or aneuploid tumors. Kristensen et al. (339), in a study 465 patients with invasive carcinoma of the uterine cervix on whom DNA index and S-phase fraction studies were performed, observed that neither ploidy level nor S-phase fraction had prognostic significance. On the contrary, Strang et al. (582) noted more relapses in tumors with an S-phase rate of 20% or greater.

Apoptosis and Radiation Response Markers

Wheeler et al. (652) evaluated levels of apoptosis as "predictors for tumor response" in 44 patients with stage IB adenocarcinoma of the cervix. Patients whose tumors had a baseline apoptosis level above the median value (2%) had better overall survival than those with lower than median levels ($p = 0.056$). Chung et al. (86), in pretreatment biopsy specimens of 48 patients with stage IIB squamous-cell carcinoma

of the uterine cervix treated with RT, found that those tumors with an apoptotic index above the median had better tumor control ($p = 0.0062$) and overall survival ($p = 0.0053$) than those whose tumors had a lower apoptotic index. Sheridan et al. (555), in a study of 39 patients with adenocarcinoma of the cervix, also noted that when the apoptotic index was quantified, the 5-year survival rates for women with tumors whose apoptotic index/mitotic index was greater or less than the median were 81% and 25%, respectively.

On the other hand, Paxton et al. (465) examined the percentage of apoptotic cells in 146 carcinomas of the cervix from patients scheduled to receive RT. The median apoptotic level was 0.73%. Patients were divided into two groups around the median. There was no statistically significant difference in outcome between the two groups.

Cerciello et al. (69), in 40 patients with stage IIA-IIIB cervix cancer treated with RT without chemotherapy, obtained biopsies before and after five fractions of RT. They observed significant changes in the cell cycle of cervical cancer, indicating intact G2/M checkpoint function, leading to the expectation that targeting compounds interfering with G2/M transition may enhance the effect of irradiation on cervix cancer.

Tsang et al. (619), in patients with carcinoma of the uterine cervix treated with irradiation, observed that the most significant factors for disease-free survival were large tumor size ($p = 0.01$), low hemoglobin ($p = 0.01$), labeling index (LI) flow cytometry (disease-free survival 67% for LI lower than 7%, 33% for LI of 7% or higher; $p = 0.03$), and potential doubling time ($T_{(pot)}$) (66% for $T_{(pot)}$ longer than 5 days, 35% for $T_{(pot)}$ of 5 days or less; $p = 0.04$). For small tumors (<6 cm in diameter), either a high LI (>7%) or a high apoptotic index (>1%) were associated with poorer disease-free survival.

West et al. (650) evaluated the intrinsic radiosensitivity of 145 tumor biopsies from patients with cervical carcinoma (in vitro survival fraction at 2 Gy using a clonogenic assay). Diploid tumors tended to be more radioresistant than aneuploid tumors ($p = 0.07$).

Bax, Bcl-2, c-erbB-2, p53

Bax protein serves as a positive regulator of apoptosis by forming heterodimers with bcl-2 protein, promoting cell survival; c-erbB-2 is a cell growth factor, and p53 a tumor suppressor gene. Ohno et al. (452) assessed the relation between apoptosis and the expression of Bax and Bcl-2 protein during RT for cervical carcinoma in 20 patients before and after administration of 9 Gy. The apoptotic cell index in tumor cells was 0.22% before irradiation and 1.20% after 9 Gy ($p = 0.0004$). The positive rate of Bax protein increased from 15% (in 3/20 patients) before irradiation to 60% (in 12/20 patients) after 9 Gy ($p = 0.0126$), suggesting that Bax protein is associated with apoptosis induced by fractionated radiation therapy. Wootipoom et al. (663), in 174 patients with cervical cancer, noted Bax, Bcl-2, and p53 expression in 68.4%, 25.9%, and 77.6% of the cases, respectively. Bax expression was associated with better survival, whereas Bcl-2 expression was associated with poor survival. Jain et al. (277) also found that neither Bcl-2 nor p53 expression were independent predictors of outcome in locally advanced cervical cancer.

Grace et al. (185), in a study of 105 patients with cervical cancer and 20 age-matched controls, noted a highly significant correlation between p53 and Bcl-2 expressions and HPV infection ($p = 0.00001$) and with various stages from dysplasia to invasive carcinoma.

Harima et al. (233), in 37 patients with stage IIIB cervical carcinoma treated with irradiation alone or combined with hyperthermia, noted that pelvic tumor control was associated with increased Bax expression: 10.5% (2/19) in the RT group versus 44.4% (8/18) in the thermoirradiation group ($p = 0.02$).

Mukherjee et al. (425) retrospectively analyzed 78 cases of stage II or IIB carcinoma of the cervix treated with RT followed by surgery 4 to 6 weeks later. On histologic examination of the surgical specimens, 40 cases (51%) showed a complete response to therapy. In the radioresistant cases, 15% (six cases) had positivity for Bcl-2 and p21 proteins, respectively, and 34% (13 cases) showed mutant p53 protein. None of the radiosensitive tumors were positive for these proteins. Seventy-five percent of the radiosensitive tumors (30 cases) were positive for the Bax antibody, whereas 81% of the radioresistant tumors (31 cases) were negative for Bax ($p < 0.01$). The presence of Bcl-2, p21, and p53 proteins could also be related to radioresistance of the tumors.

Altered expression of c-ercB-2 protein was shown to have prognostic significance in adenocarcinoma but not in squamous-cell carcinoma of the cervix (396).

The p53 gene controls entry into the S-phase of the cell cycle. Kainz et al. (292), in a study of 109 surgically treated patients, and Ebara et al. (135), in 46 patients with stage IIIB squamous-cell carcinoma of the cervix treated with RT alone, noted no significant difference in outcome, when correlated with p53 protein expression.

Cellular Oncogenes

Alterations in either the expression or function of cellular genes that control cell growth and differentiation have been investigated as prognostic markers in cervical cancer, but, as yet, the data based on small studies show no clear-cut useful marker.

The p27/Kip1 gene inhibits a variety of cyclin-dependent kinase complexes and regulates cell growth. Oka et al. (453) studied 202 biopsy specimens obtained from 77 patients with squamous-cell carcinoma of the cervix before and during RT for expression of p27 and p53 proteins. A high p27 LI before radiation therapy was associated significantly with good disease-free and metastasis-free survival rates. A high p53 LI before irradiation was associated with poor overall survival.

Both specific point mutations and amplification of *ras* genes have been noted, and overexpression of the ras gene p21 product is associated with a poor prognosis and increased frequency of lymph node involvement (237). Although loss of heterozygosity of the c-Ha-ras gene in squamous-cell carcinomas was not associated with advanced-stage disease, mutations were associated with a poor prognosis. In contrast, mutations of the Ki-ras gene have been detected in a small percentage of cervical adenocarcinomas, but have not been significantly associated with stage, grade, or survival (335,365).

The c-*myc* oncogene is amplified from three to 30 times in approximately 20% of squamous-cell carcinomas and is more frequent in high-stage compared with low-stage tumors. Overexpression of c-myc has been associated with a worse clinical outcome (275,512).

Gadd45 belongs to the class II family of DNA damage-inducible genes, and its role in DNA repair has been proved in many experimental models. Santucci et al. (543), in 14 patients with cervical cancer, found a correlation between the lack of gadd45 induction and a clinical response to irradiation (both local tumor control and disease-free survival) when a dose ranging from 18 to 25 Gy was delivered to the pelvis.

CD 34 is an antigen present in hemopoietic progenitor cells and is a sensitive marker for endothelial cells. In 62 patients with cervical cancer evaluated by Vieira et al. (636), CD 34 reactivity and higher microvessel density was associated with squamous-cell carcinoma.

CD 109 is a cell surface protein that was found to be expressed in cervical cancer more than in endometrial adenocarcinoma (669), which may have implications for development of new targeted therapy for cervical cancer.

Preoperative elevated CA 125 levels (cutoff value, 26 U/mL) were associated with depth of stromal invasion, lymphovascular invasion, and nodal metastasis in 116 patients with adenocarcinoma of the cervix. In patients with negative nodes, high CA 125 levels determined poor histopathological prognostic factors (618).

Carcinoembryonic Antigen

Tsai et al. (617) in 117 patients with adenocarcinoma of the cervix, 28 of whom had preoperative carcinoembryonic antigen (CEA) levels >5 ng/mL, noted a correlation with larger tumor size, deeper cervical invasion, and lymphovascular invasion ($p <0.001$). A Spanish study of 96 patients with invasive carcinoma of the cervix and seven with intraepithelial neoplasia showed elevated CEA levels in 33%, CA 19.9 in 32%, and CA 125 in 21.5% of patients (48). Specificity for each tumor maker was 98%. Increased CEA and CA 19.9 levels were found with more advanced stages of the disease and in patients with adenocarcinoma compared with squamous-cell carcinoma. At follow-up, all cases of progressive tumor or recurrence were detected by elevation of one of the three antigens. Specificity during follow-up was 92% for CEA and CA 125 and 92.6% for CA 19.9.

Cytokeratin Markers

In 80 patients with carcinoma of the cervix, expression of cytokeratin 10 and 13 and involucrin was found in 24%, 64%, and 53%, respectively (626). There was no difference in the expression of cytokeratin or involucrin between patients with positive or negative lymph nodes, although in the lymph node–positive group, survival was higher in patients lacking cytokeratin 13 expression ($p = 0.02$).

In another study of 272 patients with invasive carcinoma of the cervix with 1,053 samples, Bolli et al. (44) noted an elevation of squamous-cell carcinoma antigen (SCC-Ag) before treatment in 53% of 103 patients, increasing with advancing tumor stage at diagnosis. In 70 patients with recurrent tumor, 81% had elevated SCC-Ag. Ngan et al. (442) also identified elevation of serum SCC-Ag in 62% of 308 women with carcinoma of the cervix. Posttreatment SCC levels were raised in 69 patients (22.4%), and this was associated with a <5% 5-year survival rate, in contrast to 87% in women with normal SCC-Ag levels.

Hong et al. (254), in 401 patients with stage I to IV squamous-cell carcinoma of the cervix treated with RT, noted that the preirradiation SCC-Ag level strongly correlated with disease stage. A persistently elevated SCC-Ag level 3 months after RT was a stronger predictor for treatment failure than residual induration by pelvic examination, and it was associated with a higher incidence of distant metastasis.

Likewise, Micke et al. (409), in 141 patients with cervical cancer treated with RT, noted the pretherapy serum level of SCC-Ag was elevated in 72% (>2 ng/mL). Patients with a SCC below 7.2 U/mL had better tumor response than those with higher levels. After RT, 98% of patients in complete remission and 87% of those in partial remission had a serum level below the cutoff. In recurrent tumors, 82% of patients had a significant increase in serum levels before clinical manifestation of relapse (≤0.001). Hong et al. (256), in 1,031 patients with squamous-cell cervical cancer treated with RT with or without chemotherapy, noted that independent risk factors for local relapse were advanced stage and age <45 years; 5-year local relapse-free survival was higher (90%) if squamous-cell carcinomas antigen was less than two. This antigen may be a useful marker in the prognosis of patients with carcinoma of the uterine cervix.

Epstein-Barr, Transforming Growth Factor, β-Integrin, and Other Markers

Activity of Epstein-Barr virus antigen–specific killer T cells and shedding of Epstein-Barr virus were evaluated in 55 patients with carcinoma of the cervix (326). Activity was decreased in patients with cervical carcinoma compared with control patients; it became increasingly lower as the clinical stage of the disease advanced, and activity after treatment was clearly related to patient survival. These data may indicate an imbalance in local immunity against viral infection and impairment of T-cell immunity in patients with advanced cervical carcinoma.

In 79 patients undergoing radiation therapy for carcinoma of the cervix, pretreatment transforming growth factor-β_1 (TGF-β_1) levels were a significant prognostic factor for survival and local tumor control. There were weak significant correlations of TGF-β_1 levels with disease stage and the levels of circulating tumor markers (CA 125) (121). Hazelbag et al. (238) also assessed TGF-β_1 and plasminogen activator inhibitor (PAI-1) expression in 108 specimens of cervical carcinoma and noted that TGF was not associated with worse prognosis, whereas PAI-1 was.

Gruber et al. (213), in biopsies of 82 patients with cervical cancer, found that β_3-integrin was expressed in 50 (61%) and correlated it with higher incidence of locoregional recurrences and decreased survival.

Cyclooxigenases

Gaffney et al. (172), in 24 patients with carcinoma of the cervix treated with RT, observed that 5-year overall survival rates for tumors with low versus high COX-2 values were 75% and 35%, respectively ($p = 0.021$). COX-2 staining intensity was found to correlate positively with tumor size ($p = 0.022$).

Kim et al. (322) screened 84 patients with stage IIB squamous-cell and 21 with adenocarcinoma cervical cancer and found COX-2 expression more frequently in the adenocarcinoma group (57% vs. 24%; $p = 0.007$). The 5-year survival rate was 83% for COX-2 negative and 57% for COX-2 positive patients, regardless of histological subtype ($p = 0.001$). Pyo et al. (503) also showed that expression of COX-2 and coexpression of COX-2 and thymidine phosphorylase (TP) were correlated with high locoregional recurrence and lower survival. Moreover, Kang et al. (294), in 84 patients with cervix adenocarcinoma, observed a higher incidence of lymph node metastasis and decreased survival with elevated expression of COX-2

Hormonal Receptors

Suzuki et al. (590) investigated the expression of estrogen receptors and progesterone receptors (PgR) in biopsy specimens from cervical tumors before RT in 44 patients with cervical adenocarcinoma and 22 with adenosquamous-cell carcinomas treated. Staining for estrogen receptors or PgR was positive in 12 patients (19%). The estrogen receptor status did not correlate with the local tumor control, disease-free, or cause-specific survival. Disease-free survival rate of PgR-positive patients was signif-

icantly higher than that of PgR-negative patients ($p = 0.044$), but it was not statistically significant in relation to 5-year cause-specific survival or local tumor control.

HIV

In 120 patients with cervical cancer screened for HIV and treated with RT, Campbell et al. (68) observed a 4.2% positive HIV. These patients had more advanced tumors and duration of remission was shorter than in the HIV negative group. RT had no effect on the HIV titers. Women who are HIV positive or have acquired immunodeficiency syndrome associated with in situ or invasive carcinoma of the cervix are at a higher risk for tumor recurrence after treatment and death as a consequence of the malignant process (328,665).

General Management

Controversy continues between those who advocate radical surgery (58,380,478) and those who favor RT for the treatment of carcinoma of the uterine cervix. Russell et al. (534) noted that the of use of radiation as the sole therapy or as a component of the course of therapy has declined, coincident with a 32.3% increase in the use of hysterectomy alone and a 33.7% reduction in the use of radiation alone. A rise in the use of chemoradiation in patients with advanced stages was described by Eifel et al. (143) in a Patterns of Care record review (from 19% in 1996 to 63% in 1999). Moreover Barbera et al. (27) also reported a significant increase in the use of chemoradiation in Canada after the U.S. National Cancer Institute Bulletin on the subject (436).

The decline in use of irradiation may be related to earlier tumor detection in recent times because of greater awareness by physicians and patients, the widespread use of Pap smear screening, and the increased number of gynecologic oncologists, with a greater use of surgery in the treatment of patients with earlier cancer stages. Kapp and Giacca (295) offered new directions in radiation biology that potentially could have applications in the future treatment of patients with carcinoma of the cervix.

Patients should be treated with close collaboration between the gynecologic oncologist and the radiation oncologist, and an integrated team approach should be rigorously pursued. It is critical that the results of surgical series be reported based on the initial clinical staging, including all patients evaluated for that therapeutic modality, to make more meaningful comparisons with radiation therapy outcomes.

Carcinoma *In Situ*

Patients with carcinoma in situ, which may include those with severe dysplasia, are usually treated with a total abdominal hysterectomy with or without a small vaginal cuff. The decision to remove the ovaries depends on the age of the patient and status of the ovaries.

Occasionally, when the patient wishes to have more children, carcinoma in situ may be treated conservatively with a therapeutic conization (39), laser therapy, or cryotherapy (505). This approach should be judiciously selected when the extent of tumor allows it and the patient is reliable for continued follow-up (84). Conization microscopic margins are critical in decision making regarding a conservative approach or proceeding with a hysterectomy. A therapeutic hysterectomy can be performed 6 weeks after the conization.

Irradiation may be useful for the treatment of carcinoma in situ, particularly in patients with strong medical contraindications to surgery or when there is extension of the lesion to the vaginal wall or multifocal carcinoma in situ in both the cervix and the vagina (113,478).

In a group of 26 patients with carcinoma in situ treated at Washington University with intracavitary brachytherapy alone (approximately 5,000 mgh, 45 Gy to point A with LDR) with tandem and ovoids, no recurrences were recorded (201). Ogino et al. (449) used HDR brachytherapy in 14 patients with grade 3 cervical and six with grade 3 vaginal intraepithelial neoplasia (three with microinvasion) and six with recurrent cervical intraepithelial neoplasia after hysterectomy. Seventeen patients were treated with HDR brachytherapy alone, and three in combination with EBRT without surgery. The mean dose of HDR brachytherapy was 26.1 Gy (range, 20 to 30 Gy) prescribed at point A for intact uterus, or at 1 cm superior to the vaginal apex or 1 cm beyond vaginal mucosa for lesions of the vaginal stump. Fourteen patients were alive and six had died from intercurrent disease; none had recurrent disease. Rectal bleeding occurred in three patients and subsided spontaneously. Moderate and severe vaginal reactions were noted in two patients in whom the treatment included the entire vagina.

Stage IA

The definition of microinvasive (stage IA) carcinoma of the cervix lacks uniform diagnostic criteria; tumor volume in the stroma may be a more reliable criterion than depth of invasion to arrive at a definition of stage IA. Depth of invasion and tumor confluence have been identified as prognostic factors that should be taken into consideration in the planning of therapy (35). Conization is mandatory for more accurate diagnosis. According to Kolstad (333), lesions <1 mm in depth can be treated with conization, provided all margins are tumor free and continued careful follow-up is instituted. Raspagliesi et al. (506) used margins of 8 to 10 mm as guidelines for clearance in conization. Smaller margins or lymphovascular invasion in addition to depth of invasion were prognostic factors for recurrence.

Early invasive carcinoma of the cervix (stage IA2) is usually treated with a total abdominal or modified radical hysterectomy, but it can be treated with intracavitary radioactive sources alone (6,500 to 8,000 mgh, 60 to 75 Gy to point A, in two LDR insertions, respectively). With HDR brachytherapy the dose is approximately 36 to 45 Gy in 6 to 8 fractions, depending on tumor volume and depth of stromal invasion.

When the depth of penetration of the stroma by tumor is <3 mm, the incidence of lymph node metastasis is 1% or less, and a lymph node dissection or pelvic external irradiation is not warranted (201,478). With more extensive lesions, a Wertheim radical hysterectomy with pelvic lymphadenectomy is the preferred treatment. Tumor control with all treatment methods is over 95%, with patients eventually dying of intercurrent disease. Gadducci et al. (171) treated 30 patients with conization, 82 with total and 54 with radical hysterectomy; the recurrence rate was 10%, 4.9%, and 9.3%, respectively. None of 67 patients submitted to lymphadenectomy had positive pelvic nodes. In 98 patients with adenocarcinoma of the cervix none of 48 with depth of invasion (DOI) ≤5 mm had involved parametria or positive nodes, in contrast to 6/36 (16%) with DOI >5 mm (26).

Recently, in selected institutions, vaginal trachelectomy (removal of the cervix) and laparoscopic lymphadenectomy have been used to treat young patients with microinvasive carcinoma. The number of patients is small and follow-up is short, but preliminary results show a low incidence of recurrences (505).

Stages IB and IIA

The choice of definitive irradiation or radical surgery for stage IB and IIA carcinoma of the cervix remains controversial, and the preference for one procedure over the other depends on the institution, the gynecologic oncologist or radiation oncologist involved, the general condition of the patient, and characteristics of the lesion. An operation has been preferred by some in young

women to preserve the ovaries and the possibility of a more pliable vagina and better sexual activity after surgery. However, in some reports (18), ovarian function preservation has been observed in only 50% to 60% of surgically treated patients not receiving irradiation.

Another important alleged advantage of surgery is the opportunity to do a thorough pelvic and abdominal evaluation. However, surgical staging has not been shown to improve overall patient survival (437,651). Kupets et al. (343) assessed the value of debulking large nodes and concluded that the incremental overall benefit by stage was small. Exploratory laparotomy eliminates from the surgical group patients with more advanced disease. Delgado et al. (117) described a GOG study in which 1,125 patients were registered before surgery; 80 were ineligible after strict pathology review, an additional 129 patients were explored, but the hysterectomy was abandoned because of intraoperative complications in 49 patients or extent of disease beyond the uterus in 80 patients. Failure to account for these patients in other series overestimates the efficacy of radical surgery.

Few randomized trials have compared the results of radical hysterectomy with definitive RT. This subject is discussed further in the Results of Therapy section of this chapter.

Despite a slower regression after irradiation, reflecting cellular kinetics and a slow growth, no difference in tumor control or survival has been observed in adenocarcinomas compared with epidermoid carcinomas (200), although prognosis is related to tumor volume (141). Because of the predilection for endocervical involvement in adenocarcinoma, a combination of irradiation and conservative hysterectomy has been advocated by some authors (536), although results are comparable with those obtained with irradiation alone (200).

Bulky endocervical tumors and the so-called barrel-shaped cervix have a higher incidence of central recurrence, pelvic and para-aortic lymph node metastasis, and distant dissemination (160). Because of the inability of intracavitary sources to encompass the entire tumor in a high-dose volume, larger doses of external radiation to the whole pelvis or extrafascial hysterectomy, or both, have been advocated to improve therapeutic results (262). An extrafascial conservative hysterectomy has been recommended 6 weeks after completion of higher dose preoperative irradiation (20 Gy to the whole pelvis, additional 30 Gy to the parametria with midline shielding, and one intracavitary LDR insertion for 5,500 mgh, delivering approximately 50 Gy to point A, with a total dose to point A of 70 Gy). Higher doses of irradiation alone yield equivalent pelvic tumor control and survival rates (144,478). This subject is discussed further later in this chapter.

Stages IIB, III, and IVA

Patients with stage IIB and III tumors are treated with irradiation, usually combined with chemotherapy. Patients with stage IVA disease (bladder or rectal invasion) can be treated either with higher doses of external radiation to the whole pelvis, intracavitary insertions (total dose to point A with LDR brachytherapy about 90 Gy), and additional parametrial irradiation, or with pelvic exenteration (112), usually combined with chemotherapy. Niibe et al. (443), in analysis of 179 patients with stage IIIB adenocarcinoma, suggested that an optimal dose for these tumors was T-BED >10 or 100 Gy.

Numerous reports have been published on the concomitant use of irradiation and cytotoxic agents (hydroxyurea, cisplatin, and 5-fluorouracil [5FU], in some trials combined with mitomycin C) administered to obtain a radiosensitizing effect (83,98,459). Several publications show that chemotherapy combined with irradiation alone or after radical hysterectomy has value in the treatment of locally extensive squamous-cell carcinoma of the cervix, as it will be discussed in more detail later in this chapter.

Small-Cell Carcinoma of the Cervix

Small-cell carcinoma of the cervix, like its counterparts in the lung and other anatomic locations, has a high proliferation rate and marked propensity for regional lymph node and distant metastases. Miller et al. (410) demonstrated that all small-cell carcinomas of the cervix are aneuploid, compared with only 30% of large-cell nonkeratinizing squamous carcinomas. The incidence of lymphatic vascular space invasion is 80% to 90% (2), and lymph node metastases has been reported to be 40% to 67% (551). These patients must be evaluated in conjunction with a medical oncologist; the work-up should include bone marrow aspiration biopsy of the iliac crest and other tests to rule out metastatic spread. Furthermore, the basic therapy should include a combination of cytotoxic agents with pelvic EBRT and intracavitary brachytherapy to doses similar to those used in squamous-cell carcinoma, although some patients have been treated with radical surgery. As in carcinoma of the lung, it is probably more efficacious to administer two or three cycles of chemotherapy before the initiation of radiation therapy, if there is no acute bleeding. If bleeding is present, prompt institution of radiation therapy is necessary.

At Washington University, patients with small-cell carcinoma of the cervix are treated with the same irradiation techniques as outlined for other histologic varieties of cervical carcinoma in combination with multiagent chemotherapy. The most frequently prescribed drugs are cyclophosphamide (1,000 mg/m^2), doxorubicin (50 mg/m^2), and vincristine (1 mg/m^2) given every 3 or 4 weeks. Etoposide (VP-16) is being incorporated more frequently into some of the regimens (424). Depending on age and tolerance to therapy, the doses of radiation may be decreased by approximately 10%.

Hoskins et al. (261) used a multimodality regimen of four cycles of cisplatin and etoposide with concurrent locoregional RT in 11 women with small-cell carcinoma of the cervix. Prophylactic cranial irradiation was used in all patients except those with primary tumor progression. The 3-year overall and failure-free survival rates were 28%. Four patients were alive in first remission, the remaining seven died (two from toxicity, five from cancer). Toxicity of therapy was significant, with 70% experiencing severe neutropenia; 40% were admitted to the hospital for amount control.

Twelve patients with small-cell carcinoma of the cervix were treated with radical hysterectomy (five received postoperative RT for lymph node metastases and two for close margins). With a mean follow-up of 73 months, the disease-free survival rate was 36.4% compared with 71.6% for patients with non–small-cell carcinoma (551). Four of five patients who received postoperative irradiation died with pelvic recurrence and three also had disseminated metastases. However, only those with small lesions or those who received adjuvant irradiation were cured.

Delaloge et al. (114) reported only two of 10 patients with neuroendocrine small-cell carcinoma of the cervix surviving at 13 and 53 months after treatment, which included surgery, irradiation, and cisplatin/etoposide combination chemotherapy.

Boruta et al. (49) reviewed results in 11 of their own and 23 other patients with early stage neuroendocrine cervical carcinoma identified by a Medline search. Lymphovascular space invasion was present in 21/27 (78%) patients (seven unknown) and 15/29 (52%) had lymph node metastases. Fifteen patients were treated with platinum/etoposide (PE), seven with vincristine/doxorubicin/cyclophosphamide (VAC), two with alternating cycles of VAC and PE, and 10 with other chemotherapy regimens. Twenty women were treated with radiation therapy. The presence of lymph node metastases was a poor prognostic factor (p <0.001). PE and VAC chemotherapy was associated with increased survival (p <0.01).

Combination of Irradiation and Surgery

Preoperative Irradiation

At some institutions, the combination of preoperative irradiation and radical hysterectomy has been used in the treatment of patients with bulky stage IB and IIA tumors. Sometimes a LDR intracavitary insertion alone before surgery has been used (5,000 to 6,000 mgh). The rationale for use of an operation has been the alleged inability of irradiation to eradicate completely the metastatic tumor in the pelvic lymph nodes (478).

Postoperative Radiation Therapy after Radical Hysterectomy

Patients who have undergone radical hysterectomy with no preoperative radiation therapy at Washington University are considered for postoperative radiation therapy if they have high-risk prognostic factors, which include two or more positive pelvic lymph nodes, or patients with negative nodes who have microscopic positive or close (<3 mm) margins of resection, deep stromal invasion, or vascular/lymphatic permeation. These patients have intermediate risk of failure (117).

In a study of Alvarez et al. (12), high-risk and intermediate-risk patients had 56% survival, and low-risk patients a 92% survival. It is possible that negative-node patients with multiple intermediate risk factors may be at greater risk than patients with a single positive node (608). More than one-third of patients who have recurrences will present with extrapelvic disease (354). A randomized trial showed that postoperative pelvic irradiation alone (527) or combined with cisplatin and 5FU improve outcome in these patients (483).

In patients receiving postoperative irradiation, extreme care should be exercised in designing treatment techniques, including intracavitary insertions; because of the surgical extirpation of the uterus, the bladder and rectosigmoid may be closer to the radioactive sources than in the patient with an intact uterus. Furthermore, vascular supply may be affected by the surgical procedure, and adhesions can prevent immobilization of the small bowel loops that may be fixed in the pelvis.

Van den Berg et al. (628), in a project based on 47 lymphangiograms and 15 CT scans, asked radiation oncologists (n = 17) to define the clinical target volume (CTV) and planning target volume (PTV), and to delineate on simulation films the RT treatment portals to be used after a radical hysterectomy with lymph node dissection for stage IB or IIA cervical carcinoma with positive iliac lymph nodes. Large variations were observed in the portals used and in treatment techniques. From the digitized films, it appeared that in 50% of the cases the defined PTV was not covered adequately. Furthermore, 71% of the treatment plans would not cover the lateral borders of the reference PTV sufficiently. Thus, there is a need for a consensus in the design of standardized treatment volumes in these patients, particularly if IMRT will be used.

When metastatic pelvic lymph nodes are present, treatment has consisted of 50 Gy to the whole pelvis delivered with a four-field technique. Patients with positive common iliac or para-aortic node metastases should receive 50 Gy to the para-aortic region as well with extended fields. IMRT is particularly suited to treat these patients (150).

In patients not irradiated before surgery, for whom postoperative irradiation is indicated for deep stromal invasion in the cervix or close or positive surgical margins, an alternative is to deliver pelvic external irradiation (20 to 30 Gy to the whole pelvis and additional dose with a small midline block to complete 50 Gy to the parametria) in combination with an LDR intracavitary insertion for 65 Gy to the vaginal mucosa (approximately 1,800 mgh) or 30 to 36 Gy with HDR brachytherapy in five to six fractions, using colpostats or a cylinder (Fig. 66.6). At

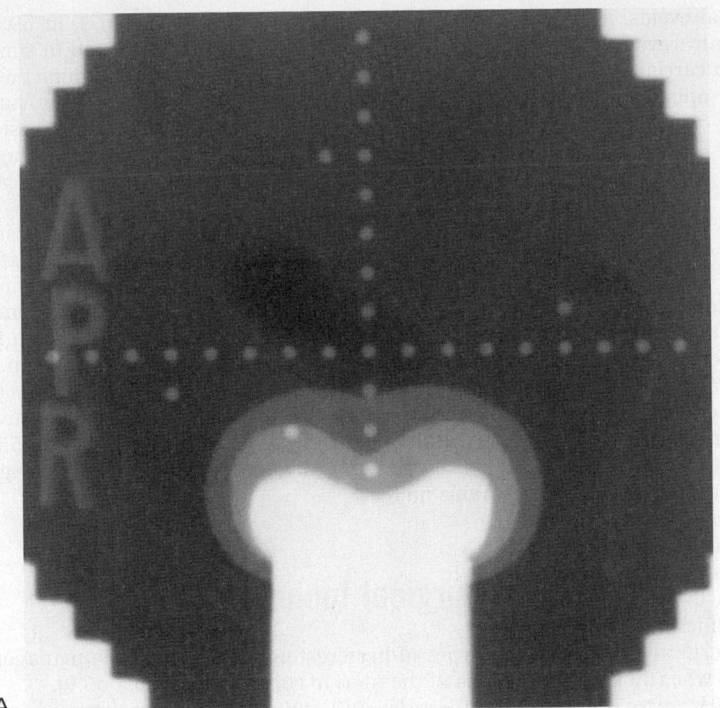

A

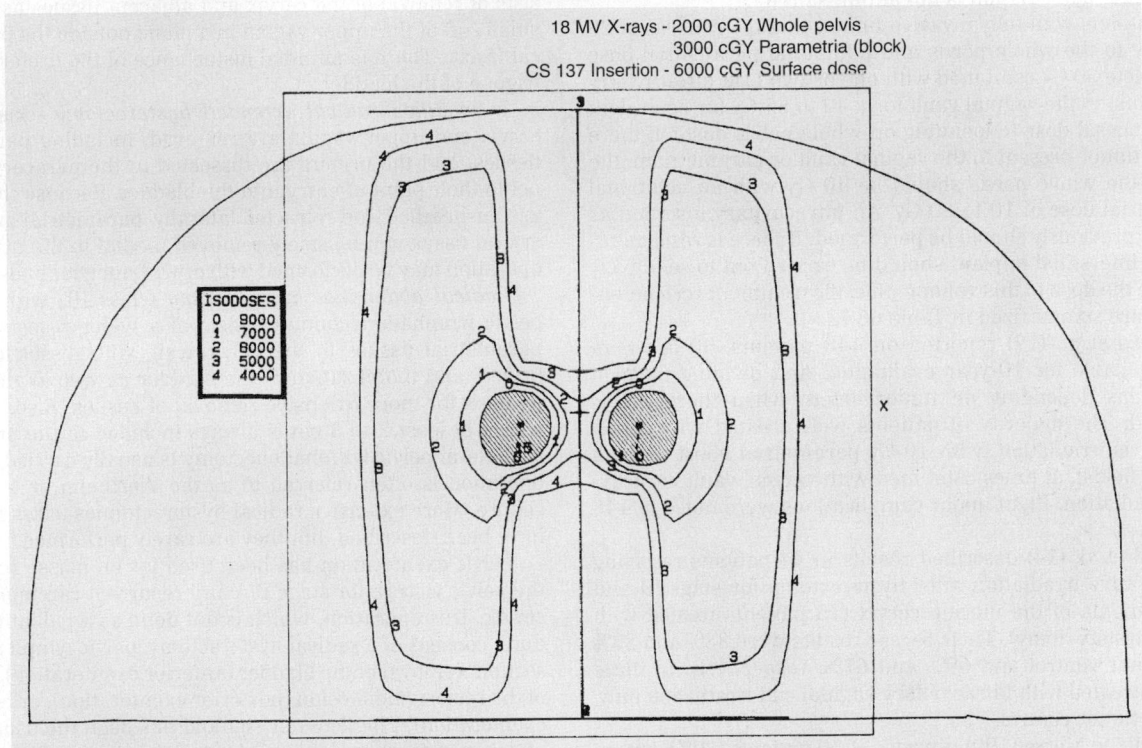

18 MV X-rays - 2000 cGY Whole pelvis
3000 cGY Parametria (block)
CS 137 Insertion - 6000 cGY Surface dose

ISODOSES	
0	9000
1	7000
2	6000
3	5000
4	4000

B

FIGURE 66.6. A: Anteroposterior localization film of the pelvis with a small midline wedge in a patient receiving postoperative irradiation after a radical hysterectomy. The wedge is designed to cover only the volume irradiated, with two ovoids inserted in the vaginal vault. **B:** Composite isodose curve through the midplane of the ovoids for patient receiving postoperative irradiation (20 Gy to the whole pelvis and 30 Gy to the parametria with small midline block and 60 Gy to the vaginal mucosa with brachytherapy insertion).

some institutions, external irradiation alone (50 Gy to the midplane of the pelvis) with a four field box technique has been used. Hong et al. (255) recommended, for node-negative patients with high risk factors, to irradiate only the low pelvis (median dose 50 Gy), which resulted in a reduction of grade 3 small bowel morbidity (3/149 = 2%) in comparison with patients treated to the whole pelvis (6/79 = 8%). Five-year disease-specific survival was 84% and 86%, respectively.

Because of the disruption of the anatomy due to parametrial and vaginal cuff resection, which would place potential foci of parametrial tumor at a distance from the vaginal ovoids, it has been recommended that postoperative vaginal intracavitary brachytherapy alone be used only for patients with carcinoma in situ (or with minimal invasive carcinoma, in our opinion) at the vaginal margin of resection (478).

Carcinoma of the Cervix Inadvertently Treated with a Simple Hysterectomy

Occasionally, a simple or total abdominal hysterectomy is performed, and invasive carcinoma of the cervix is incidentally found in the surgical specimen. In general, extrafascial abdominal hysterectomy is not curative because the paravaginal or paracervical soft tissues and vaginal cuff are not removed. Furthermore, it may be technically difficult to perform an adequate radical operation after previous simple hysterectomy (14). If only microinvasive carcinoma is found when a total or extrafascial hysterectomy with a wide cuff is performed, no additional therapy is necessary; for lesions with deeper stromal invasion, at most, one or two vaginal intracavitary insertion(s) to deliver a 65-Gy LDR mucosal dose (or 36 Gy at 0.5 cm in five or six fractions with HDR brachytherapy) to the vault is sufficient. If a less comprehensive resection was carried out, it is critical that these patients receive radiation therapy immediately when their postoperative status allows it, because the prognosis is worse if postoperative irradiation is not administered.

In patients with fully invasive tumor, therapy consists of 20 to 40 Gy to the whole pelvis and additional parametrial dose to complete 50 Gy combined with one or two LDR intracavitary insertion(s) to the vaginal vault for a 40 to 65 Gy (or equivalent HDR) mucosal dose (depending on whole pelvis dose). If there is gross tumor present in the vaginal vault or parametrium, the dose to the whole pelvis should be 40 Gy with an additional parametrial dose of 10 to 20 Gy. An intracavitary insertion as outlined previously should be performed. If there is residual tumor, an interstitial implant should be carried out to selectively increase the dose to this volume. Specific treatment recommendations are summarized in Table 66.7.

Andras et al. (19) reported on 148 patients, 90 of whom were available for 10-year evaluation, and dividing them in five groups depending on tumor extent when therapy was instituted. The majority of patients were treated with 50 Gy total-pelvis irradiation (with 10-Gy parametrial boost through reduced fields), at times combined with vaginal vault intracavitary irradiation. Eight major complications were noted in 148 patients.

Ampil et al. (14) described results in 44 patients receiving postoperative irradiation after hysterectomy for stage IB and IIA carcinoma of the uterine cervix (15 patients treated with radical hysterectomy). Their 5-year results were 88% and 83% local tumor control and 69% and 67%, respectively. In three patients treated with intracavitary vaginal cuff irradiation only, two had tumor control.

Green and Morse (190) reported 9/30 patients (30%) surviving 5 years after definitive radiation therapy for treatment of invasive cervical carcinoma after simple hysterectomy. The same authors noted that 14/32 patients retreated with another surgical procedure, usually a Wertheim hysterectomy, died within 5 years. They pointed out that the 5-year cure rate was 30% in patients treated within 1 year after the hysterectomy but was only 16% in those treated after 1 year. Thus, the time at which the patient is treated and the volume of tumor are important prognostic factors.

Crane and Schneider (99) described results in 18 patients treated with RT (with or without brachytherapy) for invasive carcinoma of the cervix discovered after simple hysterectomy. The 10-year actuarial local tumor control was 88%, and the overall survival rate 93%. Huerta et al. (267), in 59 patients with carcinoma of the cervix incidentally found in simple hysterectomy specimens (27 with gross residual tumor) who were treated with postoperative RT, reported a 3-year survival of 59%; factors affecting prognosis included gross residual tumor, time between hysterectomy and irradiation longer than 6 months, RT doses lower than 50 Gy, and histological tumor type.

Munstedt et al. (428) reported on 119 patients who received postoperative RT after radical hysterectomy and 80 after simple hysterectomy. There was a trend toward better survival in the radical hysterectomy group, but the authors concluded that postoperative RT is a good treatment in patients with invasive cervical cancer who undergo a simple hysterectomy. In another report of 105 patients with invasive cervical carcinoma found in inadequate surgery specimens treated with postoperative RT, 5-year pelvic tumor control was 72% and survival rate 55%. Late rectal toxicity was 19%, bladder 4.8%, and small bowel 14.3% (539) (Table 66.8).

Surgical Techniques

Several types of hysterectomy are used in the management of carcinoma of the uterine cervix (490) (Table 66.9).

Total (extrafascial) abdominal hysterectomy (class I) consists of removal of the cervix and adjacent tissues as well as a small cuff of the upper vagina in a plane outside the pubocervical fascia. There is minimal disturbance of the ureters and the trigone of the bladder.

In *modified radical extended hysterectomy* (class II), the cervix and upper vagina are removed, including paracervical tissues, and the ureters are dissected in the paracervical tunnel to their point of entry into the bladder. Because the ureters are unsheathed and retracted laterally, parametrial and paracervical tissue can be safely removed medial to the ureter. This operation may be performed with or without lymphadenectomy.

Radical abdominal hysterectomy (class III) with bilateral pelvic lymphadenectomy consists of a wider resection of the parametrial tissues to the pelvic wall, with dissection of the ureters and mobilization of the bladder as well as the rectum to allow for more extensive removal of tissues. Also, a vaginal cuff of at least 2 to 3 cm is always included in the procedure. A bilateral pelvic lymphadenectomy is usually carried out. This operation is often referred to as the Wertheim or Meigs procedure. More extensive radical hysterectomies (class IV and V) have been described, but they are rarely performed.

Pelvic exenteration has been used for en masse removal of the pelvic viscera for stage IVA and recurrent carcinoma of the cervix. This operation, which is not done as a palliative procedure, consists of a radical hysterectomy, pelvic lymph node dissection, removal of the bladder (anterior exenteration), removal of the rectosigmoid colon (posterior exenteration), or both (total exenteration). The ileum or sigmoid has been the usual means of achieving urinary diversion. Because some patients have a pelvic recurrence after radiation therapy, the transverse colon is used for the urinary conduit. Proof that there is no fixation to the pelvic wall and no extension of disease beyond the pelvis is mandatory. Metastases outside the pelvis, including those in para-aortic lymph nodes or any viscera, are absolute contraindications to the procedure. Bilateral ureteral obstruction secondary to tumor is also a relative contraindication (630). Patients with sacroiliac or hip pain or leg edema rarely benefit from this procedure and should be excluded on a clinical basis. In former years, pelvic exenteration was used in stage IVA carcinoma of the cervix with extension to the bladder. Modern radiation therapy has made this a rare indication for exenteration (337,412,625).

Table 66.8	RESULTS OF POSTOPERATIVE EXTERNAL IRRADIATION AFTER CONSERVATIVE HYSTERECTOMY IN EARLY STAGE CARCINOMA OF THE CERVIX[a]

			Survival		
Author (Reference)	No. of Patients	Local Control (%)	Percentage	Months	Severe Complications (%)[b]
Andras et al. (19)	80[c]	89	89	60	4
Ampil et al. (15)	27[c]	89	70	60	4
Saibishkumar et al. (539)	105	72	55	60	12

[a]Patients with postsurgery gross residual or recurrent disease before irradiation were excluded from the total number of cited cases.
[b]Remedial surgery was performed because of bowel or bladder damage in some patients in some series.
[c]All or some of the patients had additional vaginal cuff irradiation.
Modified from Ampil F, Datta R, Datta S. Elective postoperative external radiotherapy after hysterectomy in early-stage carcinoma of the cervix: is additional vaginal cuff irradiation necessary? *Cancer* 1987;60:280–288, with permission.

Pretreatment Laparotomy and Nodal Staging

Pretreatment extraperitoneal staging of patients with bulky or locally advanced cervical carcinoma may afford debulking of macroscopically positive lymph nodes without significantly increasing treatment-related morbidity and mortality. After extraperitoneal lymph node dissection, the use of high-energy photon beams and limiting the tumor dose to extended volumes in the para-aortic region to 50 Gy decreases the probability of complications (478). IMRT also enhances the sparing of adjacent abdominal normal tissues (150,493).

Cosin et al. (97) reviewed 266 patients with locally advanced cervical carcinoma who underwent extraperitoneal pelvic and para-aortic lymphadenectomy before RT. Patients were divided into four groups: group A had negative lymph nodes; B, resected, microscopic lymph node metastases; C, macroscopically positive lymph nodes that were resectable at the time of surgery; and D, unresectable lymph nodes. Lymph node metastases were detected in 50% of patients. All patients received EBRT and brachytherapy; patients with lymph node metastases received extended-field irradiation. Five- and 10-year disease-free survival rates were similar for all patients in groups B and C. All patients in group D recurred. There was a 10.5% incidence of severe radiation-related morbidity and a 1.1% incidence of treatment-related deaths.

Exploratory laparotomy and nodal staging to evaluate the presence of metastases to the pelvic or para-aortic nodes has had no demonstrated impact on survival (Table 66.10). A higher incidence of complications has been described when extensive transperitoneal para-aortic lymph node dissection is carried out (Table 66.11) and patients are later treated with definitive RT

(11.5% incidence of major complications with transperitoneal compared with 3.9% in the extraperitoneal lymphadenectomy group) ($p = 0.03$) (645).

Wharton et al. (651) reported on 120 patients with squamous carcinoma of the uterine cervix who had preirradiation celiotomy; 64 had metastasis to the lymph nodes (33% in the pelvis and 20% in the common iliac or para-aortic lymph nodes). There were 16 fatal complications, and 32 had major intestinal complications. Most patients with positive lymph nodes died with distant metastasis. Because of this negative experience, preirradiation laparotomy was discontinued at the M.D. Anderson Cancer Center, and the status of the lymph nodes was investigated with lymphangiography and verified when possible with percutaneous transabdominal needle biopsy.

Fine et al. (156) assessed severe radiation morbidity in 189 patients with carcinoma of the cervix who underwent pretherapy surgical staging by a retroperitoneal (67 patients) or transperitoneal (122 patients) approach; 79 patients had previously had a laparotomy. Patients subsequently received EBRT and brachytherapy with a median dose of 85 Gy to point A. In patients receiving para-aortic irradiation, a median of 45 Gy was administered. Of the 189 patients, 36 (34.9%) had radiation-induced complications requiring surgical repair or causing death; 47 received extended-field irradiation, and 13 (27.7%) had severe complications. The incidence of major treatment-related morbidity was similar (36.6%) in 15 patients who did not receive extended-field irradiation. There was a significant correlation between the incidence of complications and type of lymphadenectomy performed and whether the patient had a prior laparotomy (see Table 66.11). Patients who received <60 Gy to point A had significantly fewer complications (20%)

Table 66.9	TYPES OF ABDOMINAL HYSTERECTOMY

	Intrafascial	Extrafascial Type I	Modified Radical Type II	Radical Type III
Cervical Fascia	Partially removed	Completely removed	→→→→→	→→→→→
Vaginal cuff removal	None	Small rim removed	Proximal 1–2 cm removed	Upper third to half removed
Bladder	Partially mobilized	→→→→→	→→→→→	Mobilized
Rectum	Not mobilized	Rectovaginal septum partially mobilized	→→→→→	Mobilized
Ureters	Not mobilized	→→→→→	Unroofed in ureteral tunnel	Completely dissected to bladder entry
Cardinal ligaments	Resected medial to ureters	→→→→→	Resected at level of ureter	Resected at pelvic sidewall
Uterosacral ligaments	Resected at level of cervix	→→→→→	Partially resected	Resected at postpelvic insertion
Uterus	Removed	→→→→→	→→→→→	→→→→→
Cervix	Partially removed	Completely removed	→→→→→	→→→→→

[a]Type IV, extended radical hysterectomy (partial removal of bladder and/or ureter), in addition to type III.

Table 66.10	CARCINOMA OF THE UTERINE CERVIX: SURVIVAL AFTER STAGING LAPAROTOMY			
	Explored		Not Explored	
Stage	No. of Patients	Percentage Surviving	No. of Patients	Percentage Surviving
IIB	31	64.5	14	92.8
IIIA–IIIB	28	57.1	10	60.0

From Nelson JH, Macasaet MA, Lu T, et al. The incidence and significance of paraaortic lymph node metastases in late invasive carcinoma of the cervix. *Am J Obstet Gynecol* 1974;118:749–756, with permission.

than those receiving higher doses (44%). The 5-year survival was 42% for patients evaluated through a retroperitoneal and 36% for those evaluated through a transperitoneal approach.

Potish (497) pointed out that surgical staging provides prognostic data and can accurately lead to a relatively high cure rate for patients without nodal or peritoneal metastases. Potish et al. (496) noted that more than half of the patients with advanced cervical cancer with grossly positive pelvic nodes that were debulked survived, compared with none with unresectable lymph nodes, findings closely paralleling those of Inoue and Morita (269). The potential benefit of surgical debulking and irradiation will be small in patients with early or very advanced cervical carcinoma.

More recently, para-aortic node sampling has been performed through a laparoscopic approach; the procedure is well tolerated, recovery is prompt, and yield has been reported to be adequate (106,164).

Preservation of the Ovaries and Ovarian Function

In a survey of 124 patients who had undergone radical hysterectomy and lymphadenectomy with ovarian transposition, 68 responders were premenopausal at the time of surgery. Six of 30 women (30%) with ovarian preservation experienced early hormonal failure (five had one ovary and one patient had both preserved) (461). Combined-modality therapy may have a more pronounced effect on ovarian function than either irradiation or operation alone (159). Anderson et al. (18) noted that only 4/24 patients (17%) with ovarian transposition who received postoperative pelvic irradiation had continued ovarian function.

Feeney et al. (152) reported on 132 patients on whom lateral ovarian transposition was performed at the time of radical hysterectomy; 28 patients received postoperative pelvic irradiation. Fourteen of 28 patients (50%) who received pelvic irradiation had evidence of ovarian failure, in contrast to 3/104

patients (2.9%) on whom ovarian transposition was performed, without postoperative irradiation. Buekers et al. (59) also evaluated ovarian function in 102 patients with cervical cancer, 83 of whom underwent radical hysterectomy and 19 a staging laparotomy, all with ovarian preservation (80 included ovarian transposition); 26 patients received postoperative radiation therapy. After ovarian transposition without RT, 98% of patients retained ovarian function for a mean of 126 months, with menopause at a mean age of 45.8 years. When ovarian transposition and RT were added, 41% retained ovarian function for a mean of 43 months and experienced menopause at a mean age of 36.6 years.

Likewise, Morice et al. (421) reported on 107 patients treated for cervical cancer with radical hysterectomy and lymphadenectomy, 104 of whom (98%) had ovarian transposition to the paracolic gutters performed. Preservation of ovarian function was achieved in 100% for patients treated exclusively by surgery, 90% for those treated by postoperative vaginal brachytherapy, and 60% for patients treated by postoperative EBRT and vaginal brachytherapy.

Ovarian transposition or oophoropexy has been performed using laparoscopy, achieving continued hormonal function in 68% (8/11) and 50% (3/6) of the patients. Mean follow-up was 8.5 years, and mean radiation absorbed dose to the displaced ovaries was 26 Gy (363).

Stuckle et al. (580) performed laparoscopic lateral ovarian transposition during staging lymphadenectomy in 11 patients with carcinoma of the cervix treated with brachytherapy (11 cases), EBRT (nine cases), and chemotherapy (two cases). Ovarian preservation was achieved in 30% of the cases. Age was the most predictive factor for ovarian function preservation.

Radiation Therapy Techniques

Currently, the two main modalities of irradiation are external photon beam and brachytherapy. External irradiation is

Table 66.11	COMPLICATION RATE FOR PRETHERAPY SURGICAL STAGING			
	Transperitoneal (122/189; 64.6%)		Retroperitoneal (67/189; 35.4%)	
	Prior Laparotomy ($n = 52$), Group 1	No Prior Laparotomy ($n = 70$), Group 2	Prior Laparotomy ($n = 27$), Group 3	No Prior Laparotomy ($n = 40$), Group 4
Complications per Group	32 (61.5%)	25 (37.9%)	8 (29.6%)	1 (2.5%)
Percentage of total complications ($n = 66$)	48.5%	37.9%	12.1%	1.5%

From Fine BA, Hempling RE, Piver MS, et al. Severe radiation morbidity in carcinoma of the cervix: impact of pretherapy surgical staging and previous surgery. *Int J Radiat Oncol Biol Phys* 1995;31:717–723, with permission.

		CARCINOMA OF THE UTERINE CERVIX: WASHINGTON UNIVERSITY GUIDELINES FOR TREATMENT WITH IRRADIATION (LOW–DOSE-RATE BRACHYTHERAPY)					

Table 66.12

		External Irradiation (Gy)[a]		LDR Brachytherapy			
Tumor Stage	Tumor Extent	Whole Pelvis	Additional Parametrial Dose (Midline Shield)	Two Insertions (mgh)	Dose to Point A (Gy)[b]	Total Dose to Point A (Gy)	
IA		0	0	6,500–8,000	70	60–70	
IB (small)	Superficial ulceration; <2 cm in diameter or involving fewer than two quadrants	0	45	8,000	72	72	
IB (2–4 cm)	Four-quadrant involvement; no endocervical expansion	10	40	7,000	65–70	75–80	
IIA, IIB	Non–barrel-shaped type	20	30	8,000	65–70	85–90	
IB–IIA (bulky)[c] IIB, IIIA	Barrel-shaped cervix; parametrial extension	20	30	8,000	70	85–95	
IIIB	Parametrial involvement	20	40	8,000	70	85–95	
IIB, IIIB, IV	Poor pelvic anatomy; patients not readily treated with intracavitary insertions (barrel-shaped cervix not regressing; inability to locate external os)	40	20	6,500	50–55	90–95	

LDR, low–dose-rate.
Note: In patients older than 65 years of age or with history of previous pelvic inflammatory disease or pelvic surgery, reduce doses by 10%.
[a] 1.8 Gy/day, five weekly fractions, using 15 MV or higher photon beams, two portals treated daily.
[b] 0.6–0.8 Gy/h at point A.
[c] In stage IB and IIA, if complete regression is not obtained, perform extrafascial conservative hysterectomy (reduce brachytherapy dose to 6,000 mgh [55 Gy]).

used to treat the whole pelvis and the parametria including the common iliac and para-aortic lymph nodes, whereas central disease (cervix, vagina, and medial parametria) is primarily irradiated with intracavitary sources. The techniques described apply, with some individualization, to most patients with cervical carcinoma (Table 66.12).

External-Beam Irradiation

External-beam pelvic irradiation is delivered before intracavitary insertions in patients with

(a) Bulky cervical lesions or tumors beyond stage IIA to improve the geometry of the intracavitary application;
(b) Exophytic, easily bleeding tumors;
(c) Tumors with necrosis or infection; or
(d) Parametrial involvement.

Volume Treated

In treatment of invasive carcinoma of the uterine cervix, it is important to deliver adequate doses of irradiation not only to the primary tumor but to the pelvic lymph nodes to maximize tumor control (146,478). Greer et al. (193) reported on intraoperative retroperitoneal measurements carried out in 100 patients at the time of radical surgery. Both common iliac bifurcations were cephalad to the lumbosacral prominence in 87% of the patients. Therefore, the superior border of the pelvic portal should be at the L4-5 interspace to include all of the external iliac and hypogastric lymph nodes. This margin must be extended to the L3-4 interspace if common iliac nodal coverage is indicated. The width of the pelvis at the level of the obturator fossae averaged 12.3 cm, and the distance between the femoral arteries at the level of the inguinal rings averaged 14.6 cm. Posterior extension of the cardinal ligaments in their attachment to the pelvic side wall was consistently posterior to the rectum and extended to the sacral hollow. The uterosacral ligaments also extended posteriorly to the sacrum. These anatomic landmarks must be kept in mind in the correct design of lateral pelvic portals.

Greer et al. (194), based on anatomic and radiographic studies, used expanded pelvic radiation fields in 38 women with stage IIB and III cancers of the cervix. The median length and width of the anteroposterior–posteroanterior fields were 20 and 17.5 cm, respectively. Lateral fields had a median width of 16.5 cm and the posterior border encompassed the entire sacral silhouette.

Bonin et al. (45), in a review of 22 patients on whom detailed anatomic mapping of the anatomy of the pelvic lymph nodes was carried out by lymphangiography, concluded that if the criteria for adequacy of standard pelvic fields as defined by the GOG were applied (anteroposterior: 1.5-cm margin on the pelvic rim; lateral field anterior edge is a vertical line anterior to the pubic symphysis and posterior border), 10 patients (45%) would have had inadequate nodal coverage in the irradiation fields. The incompletely irradiated lymph nodes were in the lowest lateral external iliac group. However, if the irradiation portals are designed as we outline in this chapter and in previous publications, almost all of the pelvic lymph nodes would be within the irradiated volumes. With the advent of IMRT to treat gynecological tumors several authors have published guidelines emphasizing imaging methods to more accurately define target volumes, including lymph nodes (50,601).

For stage IB disease, conventional anteroposterior and posteroanterior portals 15 by 15 cm at the surface (approximately 16.5 cm at isocenter) are sufficient. For patients with stage IIA, IIB, III, and IVA carcinoma, somewhat larger portals (18 by 15 cm at surface, 20.5 by 16.5 cm at isocenter) are required to cover all of the common iliac nodes in addition to the cephalad half of the vagina (Fig. 66.7A). A 2-cm margin lateral to the bony pelvis is adequate. If there is no vaginal extension, the lower margin of the portal is at the inferior border of the obturator foramen.

When there is vaginal involvement, the entire length of this organ should be treated down to the introitus (Fig. 66.7B). It is very important to identify the distal extension of the tumor at the time of simulation by placing a radiopaque clip or bead on the vaginal wall or inserting a small rod with a radiopaque marker in the vagina (Fig. 66.8). Use of implanted cervical markers

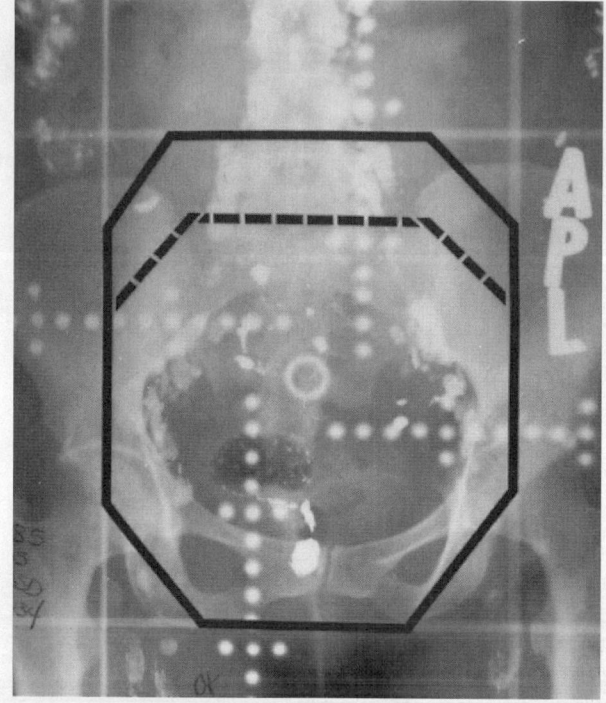

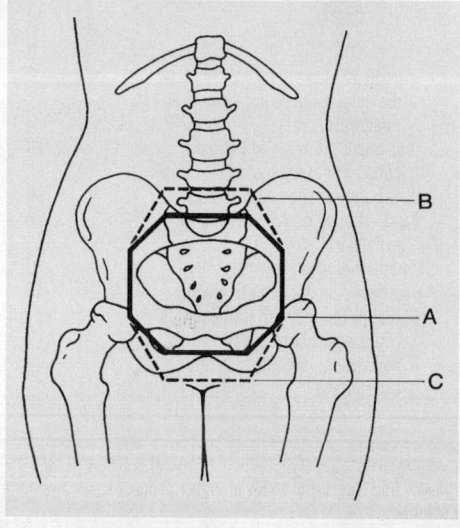

FIGURE 66.7. A: Anteroposterior simulation film of the pelvis illustrating portals used for external irradiation. The 15 by 15 cm portals at source-to-skin distance are used for stage IB (*broken line*), and 18 by 15 cm portals are used for more advanced disease (*solid line*). This allows better coverage of the common iliac lymph nodes. The distal margin is usually placed at the bottom of the obturator foramina. **B:** Diagram of pelvic portals used in external irradiation of carcinoma of uterine cervix. Standard portal for stage IB tumors is outlined (*solid line indicated as A*). When the common iliac nodes are to be covered, the upper margin is extended to the L4-5 space (*indicated in section B*). If there is vaginal tumor extension, the lower margin of the field is drawn at the introitus (*indicated in section C*).

to localize the vaginal apex or the cervix during simulation is more accurate than using a vaginal rod, according to Kim et al. (316); all patients showed a mean displacement of the cervical markers by the vaginal rod of 1.9 cm (range, 0.6 to 3.6 cm). The greatest displacement was cephalad (mean, 1.5 cm; range, 0.5 to 2.4 cm). Displacement was anterior in 5/8 patients, posterior in three patients, and lateral in four patients.

In patients with tumor involving the distal half of the vagina, the portals should be modified to cover the inguinal lymph nodes because of the increased probability of metastases (Fig. 66.9).

The lateral ports anterior margin is placed at the pubic symphysis; the posterior margin usually is designed to cover at least 50% of the rectum in stage IB tumors, and it should extend to the sacral hollow in patients with more advanced tumors (Fig. 66.10). The use of lateral fields allows a decrease in dose to the small bowel, but care must be taken to include all structures of interest (193,478,535).

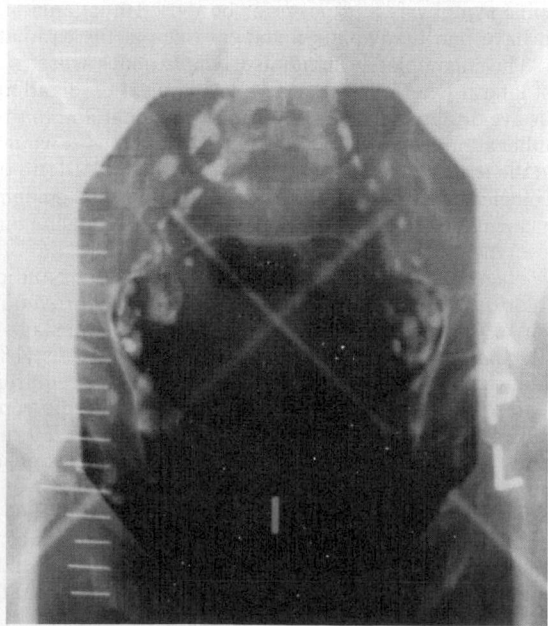

FIGURE 66.8. Anteroposterior simulation film of the pelvis showing a marker to indicate vaginal extension of tumor. The lymph nodes are opacified with contrast material.

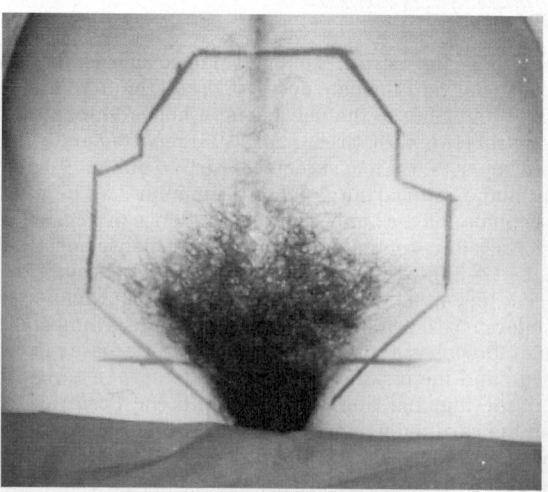

FIGURE 66.9. Lateral extension of pelvic portal to cover inguinal lymph nodes in a patient with tumor extension beyond the middle third of the vagina.

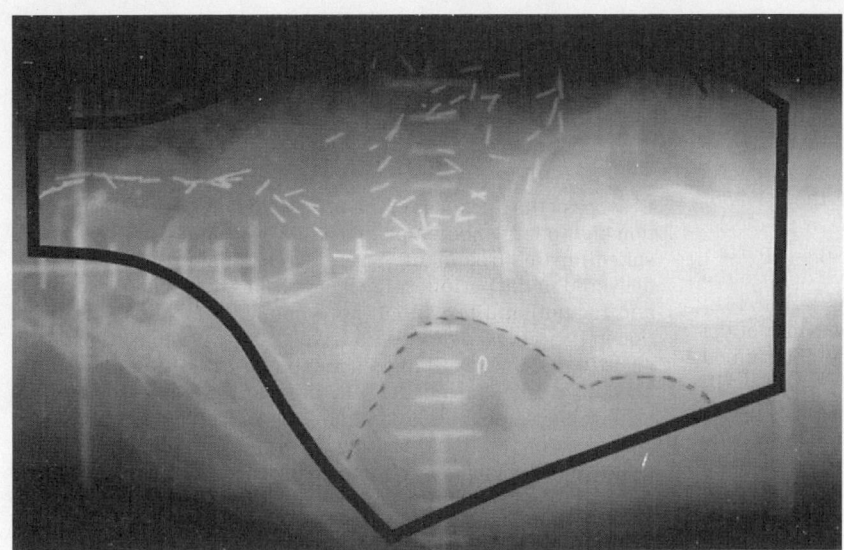

FIGURE 66.10. Lateral simulation film of the pelvis illustrating portals used for external irradiation. In this patient, treated after surgery, positions of pelvic lymph nodes are indicated with radiopaque surgical clips.

Zunino et al. (671) reviewed the appropriateness of radiation therapy box technique for cancer of the cervix in 35 sagittal MRIs and 10 lymphangiograms. An anatomic evaluation was conducted in cadavers to identify aortic bifurcation, lymph nodes, and uterus flexion. Dissection of female pelvises showed that the aortic bifurcation occurred at the inferior plate of L4 in 80% of the cadavers. The anatomic borders of the box technique used were the superior border of the anteroposterior–posteroanterior fields at the inferior edge of L4; inferior border at the inferior edge of the ischium; the lateral borders 2.5 cm outside of the bone pelvis rim; the anterior border of the lateral fields over the anterior edge of the pubic symphysis; and the posterior at the S2-3 interspace. In 50% of the patients with FIGO IB and in 67% with stage IIA disease, the posterior border of the lateral field was inadequate to encompass the PTV. In stage IIB, the posterior border was inadequate in eight patients (42%). In patients with stage IIB and IVA disease, the PTV was not encompassed. On the 35 sagittal MRIs, the placement of the posterior border of the lateral field was inadequate in 49% and the anterior border in 9% of the cases. The standard design of the lateral fields of the four-field technique based on anatomic bone references failed to encompass the PTV in a significant number of patients.

Further, Knocke et al. (329) used standard simulator planning, guided by bony landmarks for pelvic irradiation in 20 patients with primary cervical carcinoma, stages I to III, using four-field box technique. After defining the PTV with a three-dimensional (3D) planning system, the field configuration of the simulator planning was compared with a second one based on the defined PTV and evaluated regarding encompassment of the PTV by the treatment volume (International Commission on Radiation Units and Measurements [ICRU]). Planning by simulation resulted in one geographic miss, and in 10 more cases the coverage of the PTV by the treatment volume was inadequate. Three-dimensional treatment planning for pelvic irradiation of cervical carcinoma may reduce the treated volume, but further research must be done to determine whether the complication rate can be decreased as well.

Midline Shielding in Anteroposterior–Posteroanterior Portals

Depending on the institution and brachytherapy dose administered, midline shielding with rectangular or specially designed blocks are used for a portion of the external beam dose delivered with the anteroposterior–posteroanterior ports (478).

Wolfson et al. (658) compared the dose distribution in the pelvis with an individualized midline shield that conformed to the point A isodose line or a rectangular block in a retrospective review of 32 patients with invasive cervical carcinoma who underwent LDR brachytherapy. Patients were grouped as having a rectangular block (18 cases), customized block (five cases), or no block (nine cases). The point A isodose distribution from the implant was superimposed onto the whole pelvis simulation film. Approximately 72% of all cases (23/32) had tandem deviation up to 230 degrees, with a median of 50 degrees. This translated into a median percentage overdosage to point A right of 15% and left of 12.5%. Overall survival and incidence of chronic complications have not been affected by type of shielding (median follow-up of 17.7 months). Of 56 radiation facilities in the GOG surveyed concerning their use of a block, 34 (61%) responded; 88% (29/33) use a midline shield, most of them (76%) a rectangular central block that is not positioned with respect to possible tandem deviation.

Parametrial Boost

When parametrial tumor persists after 50 to 60 Gy is delivered to the parametria, an additional 10 Gy in five or six fractions may be delivered with reduced anteroposterior–posteroanterior portals (8 by 12 cm for unilateral and 12 by 12 cm portals for bilateral parametrial coverage). The central shield should be in place to protect the bladder and rectum.

Chao et al. (72) evaluated 343 patients with clinical stage IIIB cervical cancer treated with radiation therapy alone and identified 83 with clinical evidence of tumor in the uterosacral region. The average total dose, including external-beam and brachytherapy, to point A and the lateral pelvis was 80.3 to 86.5 Gy and 60.5 to 73.4 Gy, respectively. The external-beam dose to the lateral parametria was, on average, 10 Gy higher in patients with uterosacral involvement. The cumulative incidence of central/marginal failure at 5 years was significantly higher in the group of patients with uterosacral involvement (36%) compared with 21% for patients without involvement or unspecified involvement ($p = 0.002$). Lateral parametrial failure was similar for patients with and without uterosacral involvement (39% and 38% at 5 years, respectively; $p = 0.42$).

Para-Aortic Lymph Node Irradiation

If para-aortic node metastases are present or suspected, patients are treated with 45 to 50 Gy to the para-aortic area plus a 5 to 10 Gy boost to enlarged lymph nodes through reduced lateral or rotational portals. With conventional techniques, the para-aortic lymph nodes are irradiated either with an extended field that includes both the para-aortic nodes and the pelvis or through a separate portal (Fig. 66.11) (478,492). In this case, a "gap calculation" between the pelvic and para-aortic portals must be performed to avoid overlap and excessive dose to the small intestines. The upper margin of the field is at the T12-L1 interspace and the lower margin at L5-S1. The width of the para-aortic portals (in general, 8 to 10 cm) can be determined by CT scans, MRI, lymphangiography, FDG-PET scans, or IV pyelography outlining the ureters. The spinal cord dose (T12 to L2-3) should be kept below 45 Gy by interposing a 2-cm wide 5–half-value layer (HVL) shield on the posterior portal (usually after 40-Gy tumor dose) or using lateral ports and the kidneys below 1,800 cGy. A technique using four isocentric fields weighted 2:1 anteroposterior–posteroanterior over lateral portals and 1.8-Gy fractions was described by Russell et al. (532) to deliver high-dose therapy (56 to 61 Gy), with 7/14 patients alive and free of disease from 11 to 78 months. Kodaira et al. (332) evaluated a four-field para-aortic irradiation technique with 10-MV photons (mean, 50.4 Gy) in 97 patients with cervical cancer. The 5-year cause-specific survival rate was 32.2%. Grade 1 or 2 stomach and duodenum sequelae developed in 26.8%, grade 2 sequelae of small bowel in 3.1%, and grade 2 sequelae of bone in 3.1%.

Esthappan et al. (150) described a technique using CT and FDG-PET retroperitoneal to treat the para-aortic lymph nodes (50.4 and 59.4 Gy) with IMRT (Fig. 66.12). Acceptable dose distribution of the target volumes and sparing of the stomach, liver, and colon was achieved. Sparing of the spinal cord was dependent on the number and arrangements of the beams, as was the small bowel, sparing of which was limited because of overlap with the target volume. Adjusting number of beams and prescription parameters minimally improved kidney sparing.

Beam Energies

Because of the thickness of the pelvis, with conventional irradiation high-energy photon beams (10 MV or higher) are especially suited for this treatment. They decrease the dose of radiation delivered to the peripheral normal tissues (particularly bladder and rectum) and provide a more homogeneous dose distribution in the central pelvis. With lower-energy photons (Cobalt-60 or 4- to 6-MV x-rays), higher maximum doses must be given, and more complicated field arrangements should be used to achieve the same midplane tumor dose (three-field or four-field pelvic box or rotational techniques) while minimizing the dose to the bladder and rectum and to avoid subcutaneous fibrosis (Fig. 66.13) (253). Biggs and Russell (38) noted that the presence of a metallic prosthesis when using lateral fields or a box pelvic irradiation technique may result in a dose decrease of approximately 2% for 25-MV x-rays and average increases of 2% for 10-MV x-rays and 5% for ^{60}Co.

Allt (11) and Johns (285), in an update of a randomized study, reported better pelvic tumor control and survival and fewer complications in 65 patients with stage IIB and III cervical carcinoma treated with 22 MV photons compared with 61 treated with external irradiation with ^{60}Co, in addition to brachytherapy in both groups. In contrast, Holcomb et al. (253) compared outcome of 195 patients with stage IIB-IVA cervical carcinoma treated with ^{60}Co radiation therapy (group 1) and 53 treated with linear accelerators (group 2). There was no significant difference in overall survival, although there was a trend toward increasing pelvic recurrence in the ^{60}Co group (50.8%) compared with group 2 (35.8%; $p = 0.08$).

Hyperfractionated or Accelerated Hyperfractionated Radiation Therapy for Locally Advanced Cervix Cancer

MacLeod et al. (391) reported on a phase II trial of 61 patients with locally advanced cervical cancer treated with accelerated hyperfractionated radiation therapy (1.25 Gy administered twice daily at least 6 hours apart to a total pelvic dose of 57.5 Gy). A boost dose was administered with either LDR brachytherapy or EBRT to a smaller volume. Thirty patients had acute toxicity that required regular medication. One patient died of acute treatment-related toxicity. The overall 5-year survival was 27%, RFS was 36%, and actuarial local tumor control was 66%. There were eight severe late complications observed in seven patients, who required surgical intervention (actuarial rate of 27%). Five patients also required total hip replacement.

Viswanathan et al. (638) reported on 30 patients with stage II or III cervical cancer randomized to receive either hyperfractionation (15 patients) or conventional fractionation (15 patients). At 5 years, two patients in the hyperfractionation group and eight patients in the conventional treatment group had recurrent tumor ($p = 0.04$). Delayed bowel complications (grade 2 and 3) occurred in nine women in the hyperfractionation group and two patients in the conventional group ($p = 0.0006$).

The Radiation Therapy Oncology Group (RTOG 88-05) conducted a phase II trial of hyperfractionation (1.2 Gy to the whole pelvis twice daily at 4- to 6-hour intervals, 5 days per week) with brachytherapy in 81 patients with locally advanced carcinoma of the cervix. Total dose to the whole pelvis was 24 to 48 Gy, followed by one or two LDR intracavitary applications to deliver 85 Gy at point A and 65 Gy to the lateral pelvic nodes. Grigsby et al. (209) updated the results and noted that external

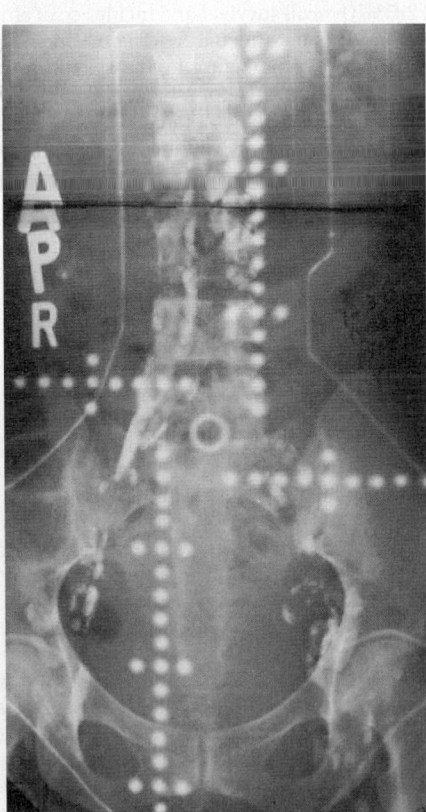

FIGURE 66.11. Simulation film of extended field for external irradiation of pelvic and para-aortic lymph nodes.

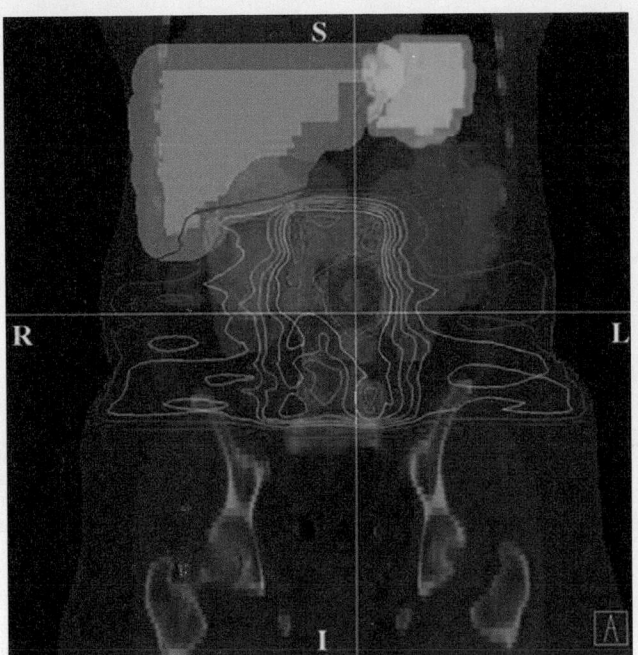
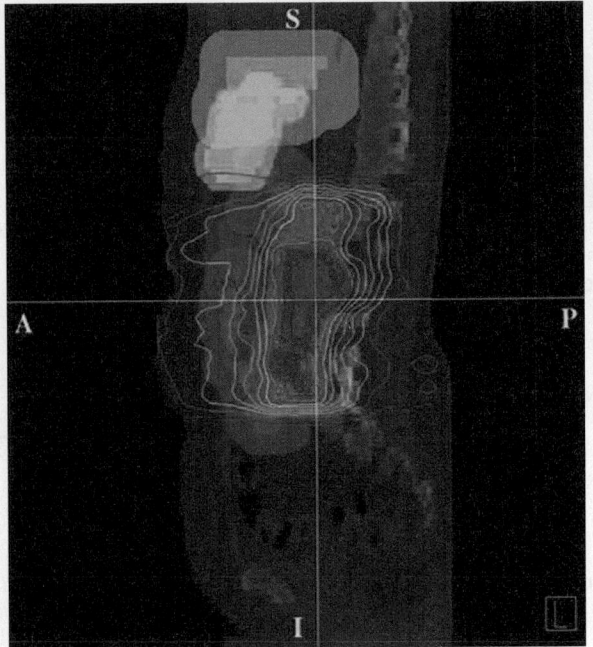
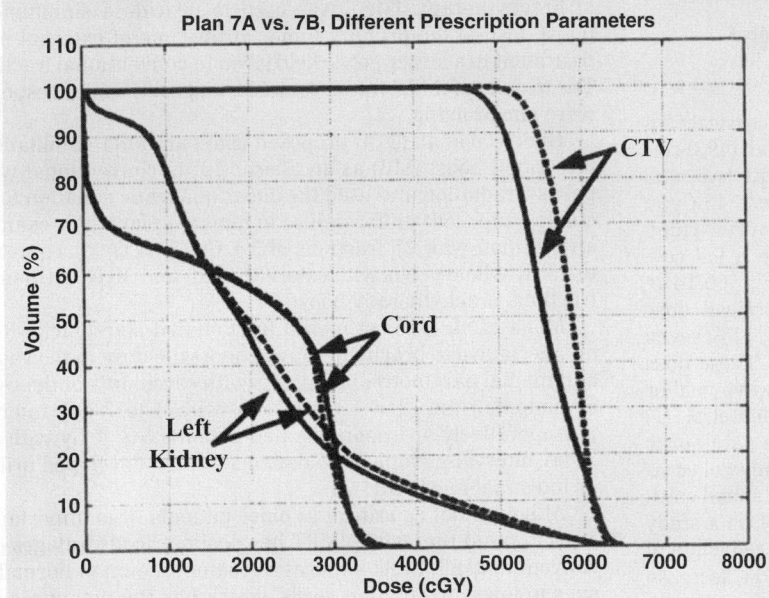

FIGURE 66.12. A,B: Example of treatment plan with intensity modulated radiation therapy for irradiation of para-aortic lymph nodes. **C:** Dose-volume histogram (DVH) illustrating sparing of left kidney and small intestine (*Plan 7A solid line; Plan 78B dashed line*). CTV, clinical target volume. (From Grigsby PW, Singh AK, Siegel BA, et al. Lymph node control in cervical cancer. *Int J Radiat Oncol Biol Phys* 2004;59:637–638, with permission.)

irradiation was completed in 71 (88%). The 5-year cumulative rates of grade 3 and 4 late effects for patients with stages IB2 or IIB tumors was 7% and at 8 years 10%, and with stage III or IVA disease, 12% at 5 years. The absolute survival was 48% at 8 years, and disease-free survival 33%, respectively. Comparison with historical control patients treated on other RTOG showed equivalent rates of pelvic tumor control, survival, and grade 3 and 4 toxicities at 3, 5, and 8 years, respectively.

Concomitant Boost

Kavanagh et al. (306) reported on 20 patients with FIGO stage III squamous-cell carcinoma of the cervix who were irradiated in a clinical trial involving a concomitant boost regimen. Patients re-

ceived 45 Gy to the pelvis in 25 fractions in 5 weeks. On Monday, Wednesday, and Friday of the last 3 weeks, an additional 1.6-Gy boost was given 6 hours after the whole pelvis treatment (14.4 Gy) through lateral fields encompassing the parametria and primary tumor, for a total tumor dose of 59.4 Gy. A single LDR brachytherapy procedure was performed within 1 week after the external-beam radiation therapy to raise the point A dose to 85 to 90 Gy in 42 days. Mean total treatment time was 46 days. Results were compared with patients treated with conventional radiation therapy during the same years. The 4-year actuarial tumor control rates were 78% in the concomitant boost and 70% in the conventional irradiation group (p = not significant). Only two patients receiving concomitant boost required a treatment break because of acute toxicity, but severe late

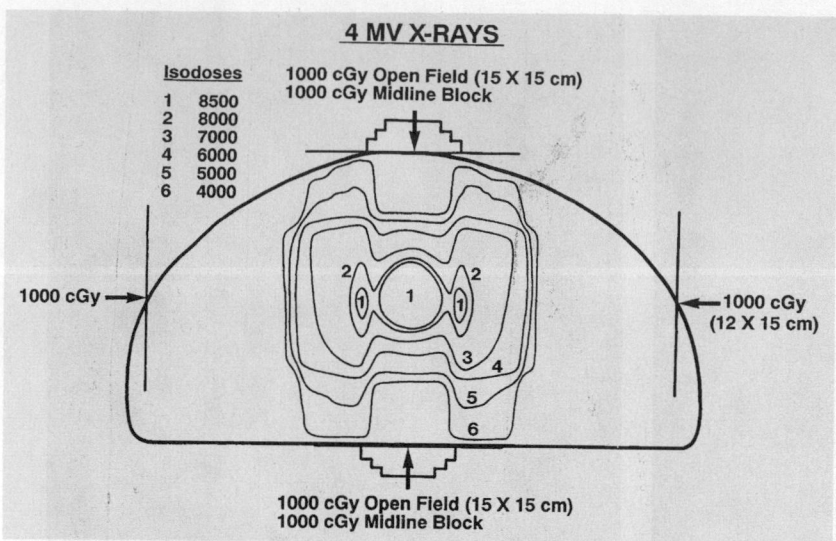

FIGURE 66.13. Example of isodose curves for "box" irradiation of the pelvis with low-energy photons. (From Perez CA, DiSaia PJ, Knapp RC, et al. Gynecologic tumors. In: DeVita V, Hellman S, Rosenberg SA, eds. *Cancer: principles and practice of oncology*, 2nd ed. Philadelphia: J.B. Lippincott, 1985; with permission.)

complications occurred in 8/20 patients. Further investigations into external-beam dose intensification should be conducted only with a more sophisticated technique than what was available during the time of the study to reduce toxicity.

Three-Dimensional or Intensity-Modulated Radiation Therapy

There is increasing experience with 3D or IMRT in cervical cancer, although results are preliminary. Portelance et al. (493) carried out IMRT as well as conventional planning with two- and four-field techniques in 10 patients. Prescription was 45 Gy in 25 fractions to the uterus and the pelvic and para-aortic lymph nodes. All IMRT plans were normalized to obtain a full coverage of the cervix with the 95% isodose curve (Fig. 66.14A). The volumes of small bowel receiving the prescribed dose (45 Gy) with IMRT technique were, with four fields, 11%; seven fields, 16%, and nine fields, 16.6% (Fig. 66.14B). These dose distributions were all significantly better than with two-field or four field conventional techniques (*p* <0.05.) Ahmed et al. (7) arrived at similar conclusions in five patients with para-aortic node metastasis, and they demonstrated the feasibility of escalating the dose to 60 Gy while sparing the kidneys, spinal cord, small bowel, and bone marrow. Heron et al. (245), in a study of 10 patients, showed that with IMRT there was a reduction of 52% in the small bowel volume receiving >30 Gy and a decrease of 66% for the rectum and 36% for the bladder, compared with 3D continuous radiation therapy (CRT). D'Souza et al. (105), in 10 patients, also noted a reduction of small bowel volume (33%) with IMRT compared with four-field pelvic RT; however, small volumes of bowel received 55 to 60 Gy with the IMRT plans. A patient prone position on a "belly board" was shown to reduce volume of small bowel irradiated (4).

Brixley et al. (55) and Lujan et al. (389) also used IMRT planning to spare the bone marrow of patients with gynecological tumors. Brixey et al. (55), in 36 patients, noted no significant difference in hematologic toxicity with IMRT or conventional RT alone; however, in patients receiving chemotherapy less grade 2 white blood cell toxicity was observed with IMRT (31.2% vs. 60%, respectively).

Uncertainties in the definition of target volumes when using 3D techniques have been identified (646). Bladder-filling control and accurate definition of margins for the PTV with image-guided position verification have been advocated to achieve a better application of IMRT (227). An example of dose distribution achieved with IMRT pelvic irradiation is illustrated in Fig. 66.15.

Early results with IMRT have been published. Kavanagh et al. (307) described the outcome of a small cohort of patients with stage IIB or IVA cervical cancer with medical illness or severe tumor-related anatomic distortion that limited delivery of brachytherapy. IMRT was used to provide a simultaneous boost dose to the primary tumor at the time of external-beam treatment to a larger pelvic field given in conventional fractions. The toxicity of IMRT was acceptable, and early tumor responses were encouraging.

Guerrero et al. (214) proposed using an IMRT simultaneous integrated boost (SIB) as an alternative to conventional whole pelvis irradiation and used the linear quadratic equation to calculate equivalent uniform dose in multiple plans. For example, an SIB plan with 25 fractions of 3.1 Gy (77.5 Gy) is equivalent to 45 Gy whole pelvis with external beam and 30 Gy HDR in five fractions brachytherapy boost.

Molla et al. (415) proposed fractionated stereotactic RT as an alternative to brachytherapy to boost the dose to the vaginal and medial parametria in patients with carcinoma of the cervix or endometrium (2 × 7 Gy to PTV with 1 to 7 day intervals postoperatively or in nonoperated patients 5 × 4 Gy with 2-to 3-day intervals). None of 16 patients treated developed urinary or intestinal morbidity.

Although not as critical in older patients, it is important to keep in mind that while IMRT has dosimetric advantages over conventional RT, IMRT exposes a greater amount of normal tissues to lower irradiation levels, which has the potential to increase the incidence of radiation-induced second cancers (224), a phenomenon already described with conventional RT techniques (43).

Brachytherapy

Several isotopes are available, although at present cesium-137 (^{137}Cs) is the most popular LDR source and iridium-192 (^{192}Ir) for HDR. Brachytherapy can be delivered with intracavitary techniques using a variety of applicators consisting of an intrauterine tandem and vaginal colpostats or, when necessary, vaginal cylinders, the majority of which are afterloading. Radiographs are always obtained using dummy sources, and the active sources can be inserted after the films have been reviewed and the position of the applicators judged to be satisfactory (Fig. 66.16). The vaginal packing is soaked in 40% iodinated contrast material to identify it on the radiographs.

Nag et al. (431) carried out a survey of brachytherapy practice for cervical cancer in the United States in 1995; of 521 responses, 206 (40%) did not perform any brachytherapy for

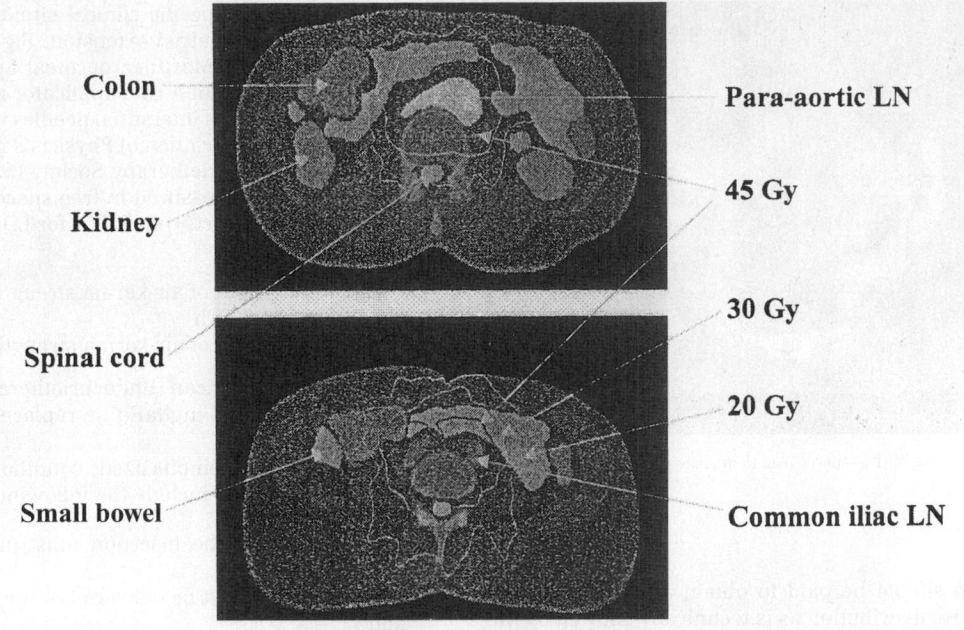

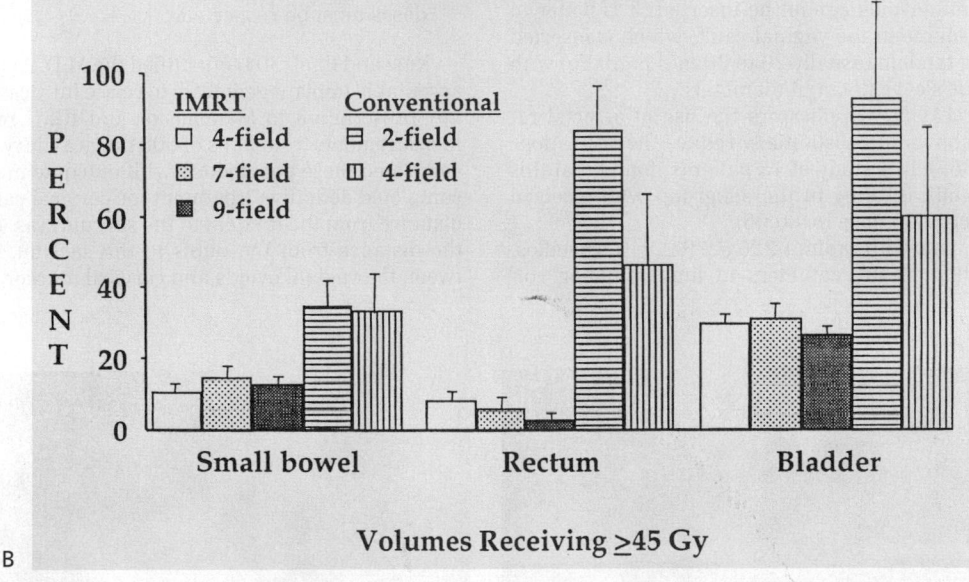

FIGURE 66.14. A: Axial views of intensity-modulated radiation therapy dose distribution. **B:** The functional volume of small bowel, rectum, and bladder receiving ≥45 Gy with IMRT or conventional techniques when 100% of the target volume (uterus) receives ≥95% of the prescription dose (45 Gy). (From Portelance L, Chao KSCC, Grigsby PW, et al. Intensity-modulated radiation therapy [(IMRT)] reduces small bowel and bladder doses in patients with cervical cancer receiving pelvic and para-aortic irradiation. *Int J Radiat Oncol Biol Phys* 2001;51:261–266, with permission.)

carcinoma of the cervix. For LDR treatments, the median pelvic EBRT dose was 45 to 50 Gy and the LDR brachytherapy dose was 42 and 45 Gy for early and advanced cancers, respectively. For HDR treatments, the median EBRT dose was 48 to 50 Gy and the median HDR dose was 29 and 30 Gy for early and advanced cancers, respectively. The median HDR dose per fraction was 6 Gy with a median of five fractions. Interstitial brachytherapy was used as a component of treatment in 6% of the patients by 21% of responders.

With regard to prescribing the doses, it is noteworthy that in 91 LDR applications with Fletcher-Suit applicators, Potish et al. (495) used linear least-squares regression to show that although there was a moderately good correlation between the milligram hours and dose to point A, it was markedly affected by the position of the colpostats and the tandem, making it difficult to formulate a simple conversion factor between the two systems.

Therefore, computer-generated dose distributions provide the best means of determining the doses to point A, point B, bladder, and rectum. ICRU Report 38 (271) defines the dose and volume specifications for reporting intracavitary therapy in gynecologic procedures.

Basic principles of the clinical application of brachytherapy and use of remote afterloading devices (LDR or HDR) are discussed in Chapters 19, 20, 21, and 22. In general, an intrauterine tandem with three or four sources [15 or 20-10-10-(10) mCi mgRaEq with LDR] is inserted in the uterus and two colpostats (2 cm in diameter, loaded with 20 mCi mgRaEq LDR sources) are placed in the vaginal vault and packed with iodoform gauze to deliver 0.6 to 0.8 Gy per hour to point A.

If the vaginal vault is narrow, it may be impossible to insert regular-sized colpostats, in which case miniovoids should be used (usually loaded with 10 mCi mgRaEq LDR sources).

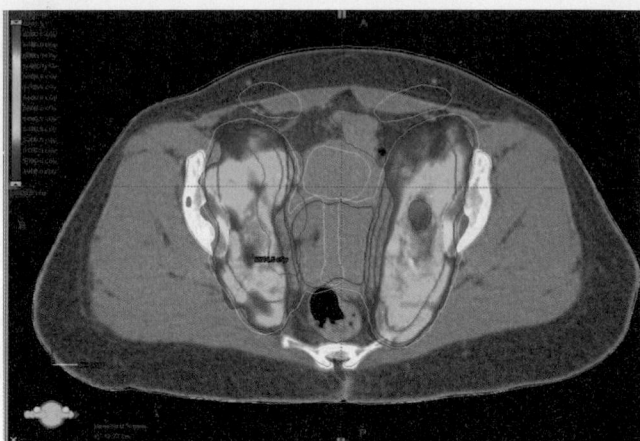

FIGURE 66.15. Illustration of IMRT treatment plan to irradiate pelvic lymph nodes, while sparing organs at risk.

Special attention should be paid to obtain as symmetric and homogeneous dose distribution as is technically allowed by the geometry of the cervix/vagina and the configuration of the tumor. When even miniovoids cannot be inserted, it is better to use a protruding source in the vaginal vault, which is inserted in the afterloading tandem (usually 20 to 30 mCi mgRaEq) with an overlying plastic sleeve (3 cm in diameter).

With HDR intracavitary applicators the use of a rectal retractor has been shown to substantially reduce the rectal dose (455). Lee et al. (368), in a study of 15 patients, found that this reduction was significant only in the subgroup who received >70% of the prescription dose (p <0.05).

Interstitial implants with radium-226 (^{226}Ra), ^{137}Cs needles, or ^{192}Ir afterloading plastic catheters to limited tumor vol-

umes are helpful in specific clinical situations (e.g., localized residual tumor, parametrial extension; Fig. 66.17). The use of Syed-Neblett and the Martinez perineal applicators has been discussed in Chapter 66. A ring applicator modified to allow simultaneous insertion of interstitial needles was described (325).

The American Association of Physicists in Medicine (13) and the American Endocurietherapy Society (656) recommend the air-kerma strength (measured in free space) to express source strength; the units are $cGy \cdot cm^2 \cdot h^{-1}$ for LDR and $cGy \cdot cm^2 \cdot s^{-1}$ for HDR sources:

1 Uh	= 1 unit of air-kerma strength for LDR sources
1 mgRaEq	= 8.23 Uh
1 Us	= 1 unit of air-kerma strength for HDR sources

Further, the American Endocurietherapy Society recommended that mgh and mgRaEq be replaced by the integrated reference air-kerma.

As Fletcher (160) emphasized, conditions for an adequate intracavitary insertion include the following:

(a) The geometry of the insertion must prevent underdosing around the cervix;
(b) Sufficient dose must be delivered to the paracervical areas; and
(c) Vaginal mucosal (and, we add, bladder and rectal) tolerance doses must be respected.

Katz and Eifel (304) quantified the M.D. Anderson criteria for acceptable implant geometry to relate intracavitary brachytherapy prescription to Manchester and ICRU reference doses in measurements from films of 808 intracavitary applications, and correlated these parameters with outcome in 396 patients who completed definitive treatment for cervical cancer. The median distance from the tandem to the sacrum was 4 cm, or one-third the distance from the pubis to the sacrum. The distance between the vaginal ovoids and cervical marker seeds was 7 mm,

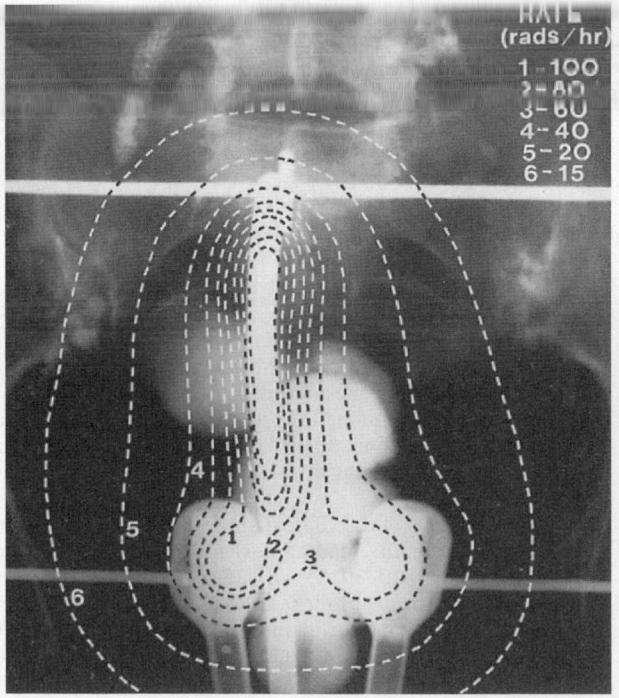
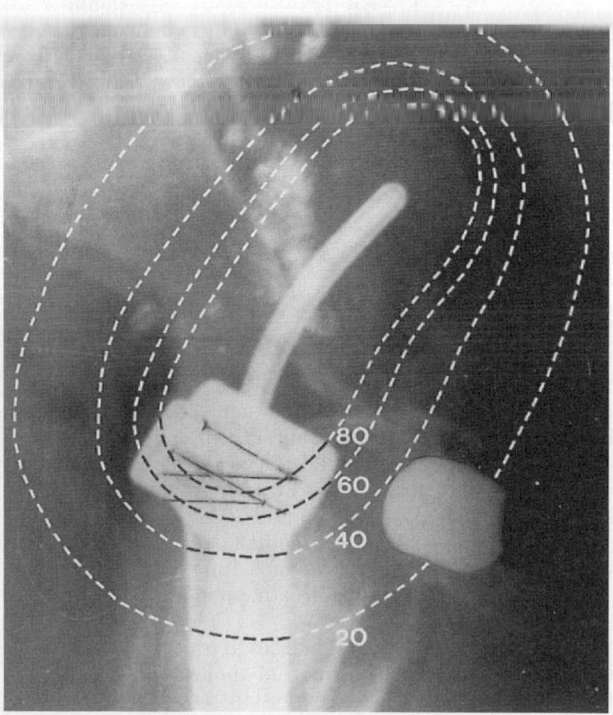

FIGURE 66.16. Anteroposterior **(A)** and lateral **(B)** radiographs of standard intracavitary insertion with afterloading Fletcher-Suit tandem and ovoids. Slight deviation of the tandem to the left is apparent. However, there is good symmetry between the tandem and ovoids. On the lateral projection, the tandem is crossing the ovoids near the center of the long axis. Radiopaque marker is present on the anterior lip of the cervix. A Foley balloon with Hypaque outlines the bladder neck.

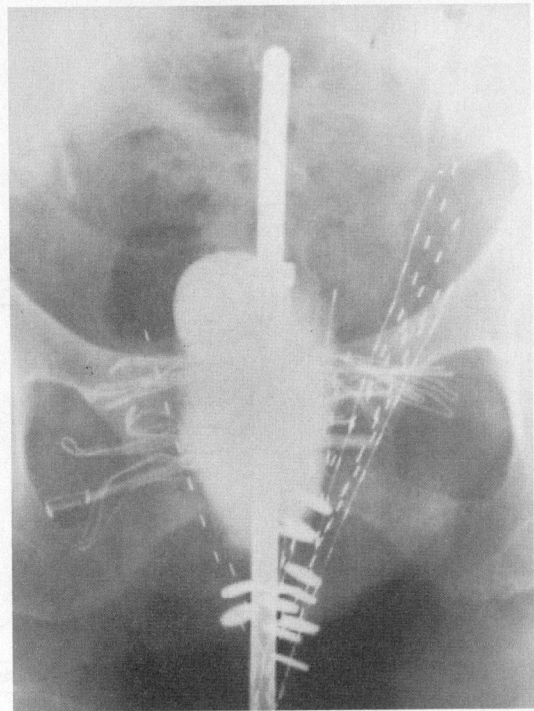
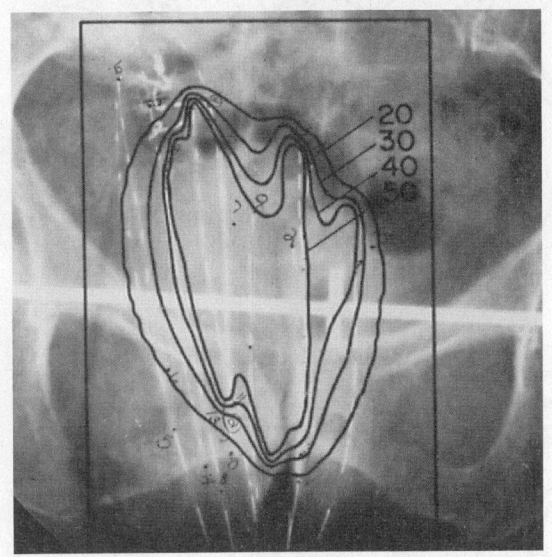

FIGURE 66.17. A: Example of left parametrial implant used to boost the dose in a patient in whom only an afterloading tandem was placed in combination with whole pelvis and parametrial irradiation for treatment of stage IIB carcinoma of the cervix. **B:** Example of afterloading iridium interstitial implant used to boost the dose in the right paravaginal and parametrial tissues in a patient with stage IIIB carcinoma of the cervix.

and the median distance between the tandem and the posterior edge of the ovoids was 50% of the ovoid length. In 92% of insertions, vaginal packing was posterior to or within 5 mm of a line that passed through the posterior edge of the ovoids, parallel to the tandem. The median doses to point A and rectal, bladder, and vaginal surface reference points were 87 Gy, 68 Gy, 70 Gy, and 125 Gy, respectively. The average ratios between the doses at bladder or rectal reference points and point A were somewhat greater when smaller vaginal applicators were used. There was no significant correlation between the doses to standard reference points and the rates of central recurrence or major complications.

Haie-Meder et al. (222) and Potter et al. (498) published explicit recommendations from the gynecological GEC ESTRO working group for dose prescription and specification of brachytherapy in cervix cancer based on volume parameters defined by 3D–image-based anatomy, physics, and radiobiology principles (Fig. 66.18). Specifications include dose to gross tumor volume (GTV), CTV, and pelvic organs at risk. The linear quadratic model is applied to both brachytherapy (BT) and external beam RT calculations. Lang et al. (353), in a multicenter study, confirmed the feasibility of these recommendations, with total doses to point A from both BT and EBRT, ranging from 85 to 91 Gy and to CTV within 69 to 73 cGy. Doses to organs at risk were comparable to those obtained with standard dosimetric methods, more accurately determined in dose–volume histograms.

Dose Rate Impact on Outcome

Haie-Meder et al. (220), in 204 patients with cervical cancer randomized to receive one of two preoperative LDR brachytherapy (0.4 or 0.8 Gy per hour), noted similar local tumor control (93%) and overall survival (85%) rates at 2 years with either dose rate. Grade 3 late complications were observed in 7% of patients treated with 0.4 Gy per hour and in 13% of patients

treated with 0.8 Gy per hour. There was one small bowel obstruction in the 0.4 Gy per hour group (1%) in contrast with five (5%) in the 0.8 Gy per hour group. Vesicovaginal fistulas were observed in 2% and 4%, respectively.

Fowler (162) analyzed results in 270 patients with carcinoma of the cervix treated with either 75 cGy per hour from manually loaded cesium or 150 cGy per hour by remote afterloading (440). There was an increase in grade 3 late complications from 4% to 22%, in spite of a reduction of 20% in dose, implying a rather large difference in biologic effect between the two systems. The effect of the increased dose rate was also described by Leborgne et al. (360). A Linear quadratic modeling was used to calculate biologically effective doses in the clinical protocols used. When the LDR was doubled, it was called medium dose rate (MDR). The maximum ratios calculated for the biologic effective doses of 16 Gy at MDR to 20 Gy at LDR were 1.06 to 1.15, assuming $\alpha/\beta = 4$ to 2 Gy, the latter being an unlikely extreme for rectal or urinary complications. The theoretically ideal dose reduction factors, calculated using the $t_{1/2}$ values derived from the clinical data, are in the range of 24% to 29% instead of 20%.

Rodrigus et al. (517) analyzed late complications in 143 patients with cervical cancer treated with two different brachytherapy schedules and external radiation. Seventy-seven patients had two intracavitary applications with a dose rate 0.54 Gy per hour and 66 patients with 1.07 Gy per hour. Because of the expected increase in complications with higher dose rate, the latter dose per application was reduced from 25 Gy to 20 Gy. Late intestinal and urinary complications were scored in 49/77 patients and in 46/68, respectively. Actuarial estimates at 5 years showed 42% and 54.1% late intestinal complications and 16.9% and 24.1% late urinary complications, respectively. Thus, despite the dose reduction, there was a clear dose rate effect on late morbidity. These studies emphasize the importance of dose rate of brachytherapy in carcinoma of the cervix.

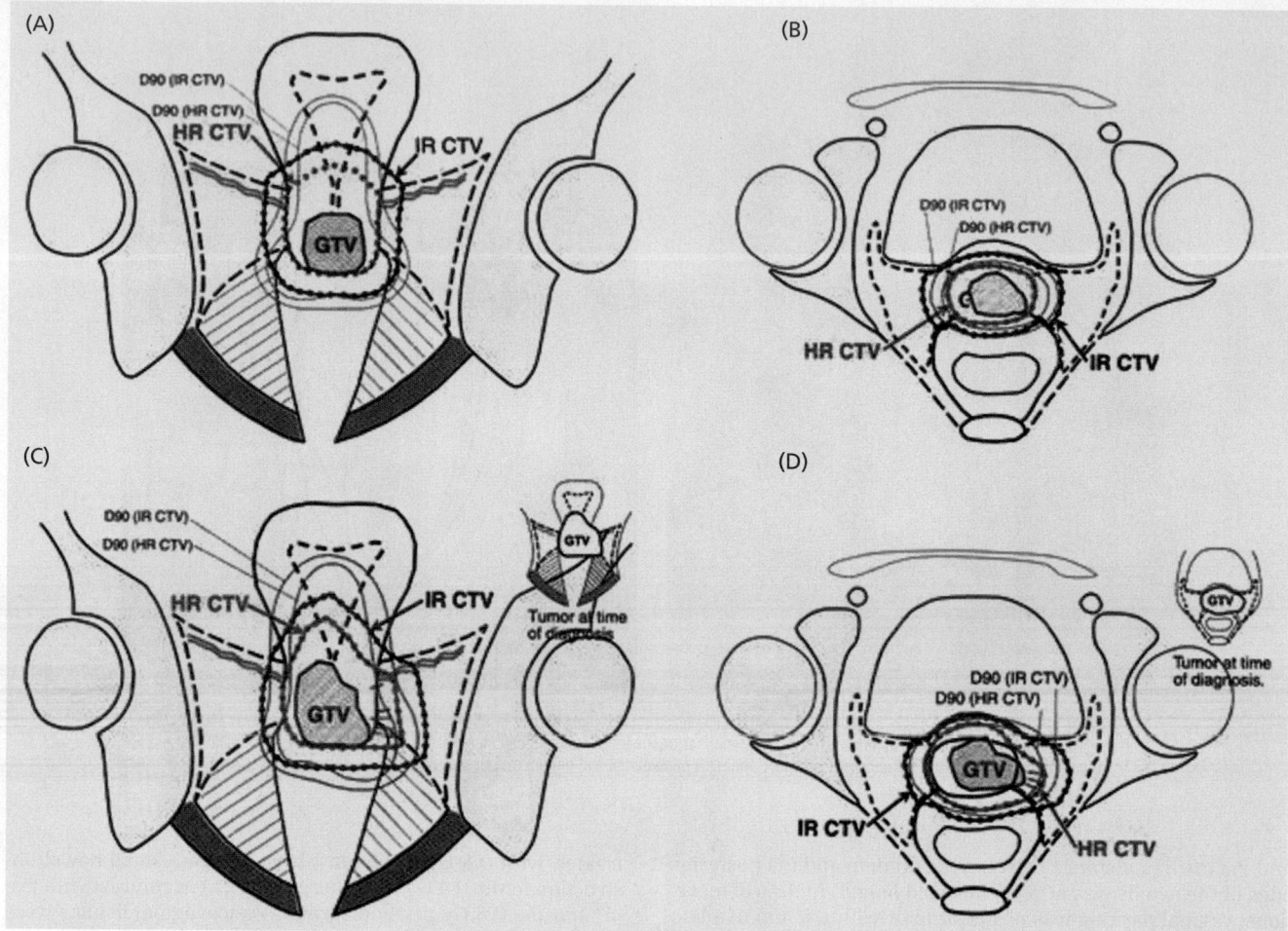

FIGURE 66.18. Diagrammatic representation of GTV and CTV for three-dimensional treatment planning in carcinoma of uterine cervix. Coronal **(A,C)** and transverse **(B,D)** sections for limited (A,B) and advanced (C,D) disease (*gray zones in left parametrium*). CTV, clinical target volume; GTV, gross tumor volume. (From Potter R, Haie-Meder C, Limbergen EV, et al. Recommendations from gynaecological (GYN) GEC ESTRO working group (II): Concepts and terms in 3D image based treatment planning in cervix brachytherapy–3D dose volume parameters and aspects of 3D image based anatomy, radiation physics, radiobiology. *Radiother Oncol* 2006;78:67–77, with permission.)

Low–Dose-Rate Brachytherapy

Intracavitary brachytherapy, with its rapid dose fall-off as a function of distance, yields a high dose to the uterus and paracervical tissues, but it is inadequate to treat the pelvic lymph nodes, and external irradiation is necessary to supplement the parametrial dose.

Rotmensch et al. (530) compared the outcome in 140 patients with early stage cervical cancer undergoing whole pelvis radiation therapy with one versus two LDR intracavitary brachytherapy applications. The two groups had similar 5-year local tumor control ($p = 0.83$), disease-free ($p = 0.23$), and cause-specific ($p = 0.29$) survival. Late complications were similar in the two groups. These results support the use of a single LDR application in patients with early stage disease undergoing definitive radiation therapy when 45-Gy external-beam pelvic irradiation is administered.

Perez et al. (474), in a retrospective analysis, noted that in patients with cervical cancer treated with radiation therapy alone for stage IB tumors <2 cm in diameter, the pelvic failure rate was under 10% with LDR doses of 70 to 80 Gy to point A, whereas for larger lesions, even doses of 85 to 90 Gy resulted in 25% to 37% pelvic failure rates. In stage IIB with LDR doses of 70 Gy to point A, the pelvic failure rate was approximately 50% compared with 20% in nonbulky and 30% in bulky tumors with doses >80 Gy. In stage III unilateral lesions, the pelvic fail-

ure rate was approximately 50% with 70 Gy or less to point A versus 35% with higher doses, and in bilateral or bulky tumors it was 60% with doses <70 Gy and 50% with higher doses.

Careful assessment of the quality of brachytherapy and dose distributions is critical. Suyama et al. (589) analyzed the minimal radiation dose to the peripheral area of the cervix in relation to local tumor failure using CT images taken at the time of intracavitary brachytherapy in 80 patients with carcinoma of the cervix. After CT scanning, isodose curves were superimposed on the CT images. Histograms of both the minimum percentage peripheral dose and the dose to the cervical area showed significant correlation in the local tumor control and local failure groups ($p < 0.001$).

Biology of High–Dose-Rate Brachytherapy for Cervical Carcinoma

To achieve tumor control using HDR equivalent to that with LDR brachytherapy, attention to the dose/fractionation schedule and to normal tissue doses is mandatory (165,223,455). In general, the α/β values for tumor and early responding tissues is approximately 10 (Gy_{10}), and for late-responding tissues 3 to 5 (Gy_{3-5}) (480). The values derived are not actual doses but biologically effective ones that take into consideration dose rate and impact of fraction size.

	HDR		LDR		
Stage	**Fractions**	**Dose Per Fraction (Gy)**	**Treatment Time (h)**	**Dose Rate (Gy/h)**	**Ratio of Total Doses (HDR/LDR)**
I	5.3 ± 0.40	7.6 ± 0.40	75.4 ± 7.3	0.87 ± 0.14	0.60 ± 0.13
II	4.7 ± 0.30	7.4 ± 0.30	80.2 ± 7.0	0.80 ± 0.11	0.54 ± 0.10
III	4.6 ± 0.40	7.4 ± 0.40	77.3 ± 8.9	0.87 ± 0.14	0.50 ± 0.11
IV	4.7 ± 0.70	7.5 ± 0.60	79.6 ± 18.5	0.89 ± 0.27	0.50 ± 0.21
All	4.82 ± 0.21	7.45 ± 0.20	78.1 ± 4.4	0.85 ± 0.07	0.54 ± 0.06

Table 66.13 — MEAN VALUES OF THE NUMBER OF FRACTIONS AND DOSE/FRACTION TO POINT A (FOR HIGH-DOSE RATE) AND TREATMENT TIME AND DOSE RATE (FOR LOW-DOSE RATE) WITH STANDARD ERRORS AND THE RATIO OF TOTAL DOSES

HDR, high–dose-rate; LDR, low–dose-rate.
From Orton CG, Seyedsadr M, Somany A. Comparison of high- and low-dose rate remote afterloading for cervix cancer and the importance of fractionation. *Int J Radiat Oncol Biol Phys* 1991;21:1425–1434, with permission.

Orton et al. (455) suggested an LDR-to-HDR reduction factor of 0.54 to 0.6 (Table 66.13). Patel et al. (463) calculated a similar correction factor of 0.58. These conversion factors are valid when three to five HDR fractions are used, but with a higher number of fractions (six to eight), the conversion factor is closer to 0.75.

Figure 66.19 illustrates late normal tissue effect, which is proportional to log cell kill, and the relationship to the number of HDR treatment fractions (163). Each full curve is calculated assuming the same log cell kill. Late damage rises sharply as the number of HDR fractions is decreased. When these curves are above the dashed lines that represent the maximum late effect of 70 Gy of LDR brachytherapy given at 0.5 Gy per hour, the risk of late complications increases. Displacing the bladder and rectum away from the HDR sources for the short duration of therapy may offset the radiobiologic disadvantage of using a few brachytherapy fractions (455).

Clinical Experience

There is increasing use of HDR sources in brachytherapy of carcinoma of the cervix; basic principles of brachytherapy are similar to those of LDR (642). At Washington University, patients are treated with HDR brachytherapy with a tandem or a vaginal cylinder, which is placed in the patient before each treatment with sedation and without anesthesia. An indwelling bladder catheter is used during the procedure, and gentle packing of the vagina with iodoform gauze helps to maintain the applicators in place. Their position is verified with anteroposterior and lateral pelvic radiographs taken before the actual HDR treatment in each application. The usual dose per fraction prescribed at 0.5-cm depth is 3 to 6 Gy, and three to six fractions are given once or twice weekly.

No randomized trials in the United States have compared HDR and LDR brachytherapy for cervical cancer, although some have been carried out in other countries (as described later). Each center has developed unique HDR treatment schedules, dose specification systems, and time–dose fractionation protocols that reflect their understanding of radiobiologic issues and their patient population base (5,247,520).

Roman et al. (520) do not use central blocking for any stage; at institutions that use a central block, a 5-HVL block is most commonly used. Wayne State University uses a step-wedge central shielding method (5). Most HDR insertions are performed weekly and are interdigitated by giving four fractions of EBRT per week with one HDR treatment per week (Fig. 66.20).

Treatment schedules integrating external-beam irradiation and brachytherapy were initially designed with regard to the disease stage and volume by Arai et al. (21). The number of HDR fractions used to treat cervical cancer varies among centers from as few as two to more than 10. The optimal time–dose–fractionation scheme and the technique for remote-control

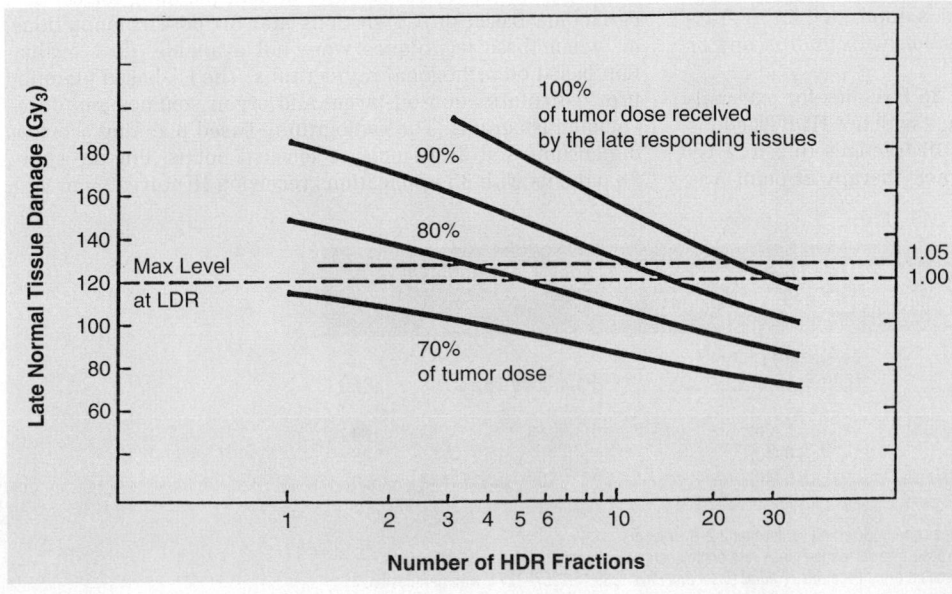

FIGURE 66.19. Relationship between number of high–dose-rate (HDR) fractions and late normal tissue effects. *Solid lines* show the increase in normal tissue late effects as the number of HDR fractions used to treat cervical cancer decreases. *Dotted lines* indicate the maximum level of late damage calculated for conventional low–dose-rate brachytherapy of 70 Gy at 0.5 Gy per hour for 140 hours, and an arbitrary level 5% above this. The intersection of the solid lines with the dotted lines indicates the number of HDR fractions needed to give equal late normal tissue effects. In this model, the dose to late-responding tissues should be kept at 83% of the tumor dose when treating with four to six HDR fractions. (Modified from Fowler JF. The radiobiology of brachytherapy. In: Martinez AA, Orton CG, Mould RF, eds. *Brachytherapy HDR and LDR.* Leersum, the Netherlands: Nucletron International BV, 1990;121–137, with permission.)

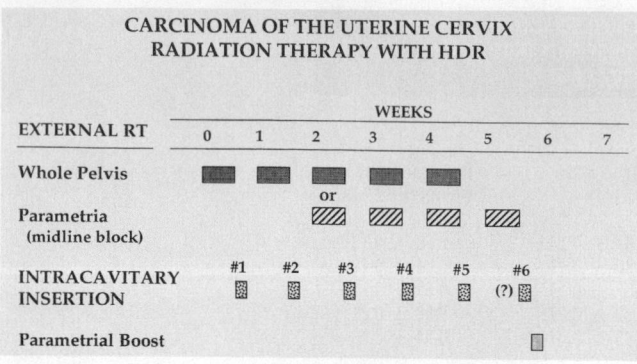

FIGURE 66.20. Schema of schedule for external radiation therapy and high–dose-rate brachytherapy in treatment of carcinoma of the uterine cervix at Washington University Medical Center.

afterloading intracavitary brachytherapy for cervical cancer have yet to be established through systematic clinical trials (429).

El-Baradie et al. (149) published a prospective study in which 45 patients with carcinoma of the uterine cervix were randomly allocated to either HDR or MDR. The external-beam radiation dose was the same in the two groups. The point A dose rate correction factor from LDR to HDR was 0.53, and from LDR to MDR 0.6. The 3-year survival and locoregional tumor control rates for both modalities were equivalent (62% and 67% for HDR and 68% and 74% for MDR). The rectal and bladder complication rates were the same in both groups (29% at 3 years). Tanaka et al. (596) also compared HDR and MDR brachytherapy in 150 and 56 patients, respectively. The survival was equivalent in the two groups; grade 2 or greater late toxicity tended to be higher in the HDR group (14% vs. 6%, respectively)

Orton et al. (455) noted that dose per fraction of HDR brachytherapy significantly influenced toxicity: Morbidity rates were highly significantly lower for point A doses/fractions of 7 Gy or less for both severe (1.28% vs. 3.44%; *p* <0.0001) and moderate plus severe injuries (7.56% vs. 19.51%; *p* <0.001). The effect of dose/fractionation on cure rates was equivocal.

Wayne State University uses a highly fractionated brachytherapy course with eight to 12 HDR fractions (5), which was chosen to keep the rectal dose for each HDR fraction to 2 to 2.5 Gy. The intracavitary technique uses an intrauterine stent so that applicators can be placed quickly without cervical dilatation and using little or no sedation. Treatment planning is performed on the initial insertion and is duplicated for all fractions by verifying the applicator position with fluoroscopy or radiographs.

Petereit et al. (482) uses 45 Gy in 25 fractions for external-beam irradiation to the pelvis combined with five HDR fractions (5.5 to 6 Gy per fraction) or four HDR fractions (6.5 to 7 Gy per fraction). The equivalent LDR brachytherapy at point A is

80 Gy with 67 Gy delivered to the bladder or the rectum, assuming these tissues receive 70% of the prescribed point A dose. For advanced stages, such as IIB or IIIB, the intracavitary dose may be increased to 7.5 Gy per fraction, to give an LDR equivalent dose of 85 to 90 Gy to point A. Petereit and Pearcey (480), based on their preliminary results and published reports in the literature, recommend the doses and fractionation schedules summarized in Tables 66.14 and 66.15.

Kuipers et al. (340) described a method to improve target coverage and locoregional tumor control with HDR tandem and ovoid applications, whereby HDR endocavitary and interstitial brachytherapy are applied in the same session for tumors with a lateral expansion of 25 mm or more from the axis of the cervical canal. Seventy-six combined applications were given to 41 patients. With a follow-up average of 23 months, in stage IIB tumors, 3-year DFS was 75%. No severe early or persistent late complications were observed.

Dose Specifications for High–Dose-Rate Brachytherapy

Dose specification reporting systems for HDR brachytherapy vary by institution. However, many combine the Tod and Meredith point A as a paracervical dose with ICRU Report 38 on bladder and rectal points (271). *In vivo* bladder and rectal dosimetry is performed during the HDR procedure by Roman et al. (520). Other centers obtain normal tissue doses from points located on dosimetry films and dose distribution curves.

Treatment planning for HDR brachytherapy can be accomplished by a variety of techniques, ranging from use of an atlas of applications and source loadings, to planning of only the initial insertion followed by replicating the insertion for subsequent treatments, to customized optimization of source loading for each HDR insertion (21). Himmelmann et al. (247) described individualized computer treatment planning and a reconstruction system used to achieve individual dosimetry. Computerized optimization of source position and the dwell time for each position is a potential advantage of HDR brachytherapy that can provide customized treatment planning on a case-by-case basis. However, customized optimization is not commonly performed because it increases the time needed for planning and requires experience on the part of the physics and dosimetry staff (605).

Three-Dimensional Brachytherapy Treatment Planning

Fellner et al. (153) compared treatment planning for cervical carcinoma based on CT sections and 3D dose computations, or, when these techniques were not available, dose evaluation based on orthogonal radiographs. The CT-based planning provides information on target and organ volumes and dose–volume histograms. The radiography-based planning provides dimensions and doses only at selected points. For the study, 28 patients with 35 applications receiving HDR treatment with

		CURRENT HIGH–DOSE-RATE FRACTIONATION SCHEDULES USED AT THE UNIVERSITY OF WISCONSIN FOR TREATING CERVICAL CANCER		
Table 66.14				
Stage	Whole Pelvis	Five HDR Fractions (LDR Equivalent)	Point A Gy 10	LQED
Stage I/II nonbulky	45 Gy	5.5 (35)	96	80
Stage I/II bulky	45 Gy	6.0 (40)	102	85
Stage IIIB	50.4 Gy	6.0 (40)	109	90

HDR, high–dose-rate; LDR, low–dose-rate; LQED, linear-quadratic effective dose for a 2-Gy fraction.
From Petereit DG, Sarkaria JN, Potter DM, et al. High-dose-rate versus low-dose-rate brachytherapy in the treatment of cervical cancer: analysis of tumor recurrence—the University of Wisconsin experience. *Int J Radiat Oncol Biol Phys* 1999;45:1267–1274, with permission.

Table 66.15		EQUIVALENT HIGH–DOSE-RATE FRACTIONATION SCHEDULES FOR CERVICAL CANCER		
Whole Pelvis	**Three HDR Fractions (LDR Equivalent)**	**Four HDR Fractions (LDR Equivalent)**	**Point A Gy 10**	**LQED**
45/25/1.8	8.0 Gy (35 Gy)	6.5 (35 Gy)	96	80
45/25/1.8	8.8 Gy (40 Gy)	7.2 (40 Gy)	102	85

HDR, high–dose-rate; LDR, low–dose-rate; LQED, linear-quadratic effective dose for a 2-Gy fraction.
From Petereit DG, Sarkaria JN, Potter DM, et al. High-dose-rate versus low-dose-rate brachytherapy in the treatment of cervical cancer: analysis of tumor recurrence—the University of Wisconsin experience. *Int J Radiat Oncol Biol Phys* 1999;45:1267–1274, with permission.

^{192}Ir were investigated. For a dose prescription of 7 Gy at point A, 83% (44 cm^3) of the CTV received at least 7 Gy.

Eich et al. (137), in 11 applications of HDR brachytherapy for cervical carcinoma, calculated doses to ICRU bulletin points on orthogonal radiographs, and the doses at rectum reference points were compared with *in vivo* measurements. The *in vivo* measurements were 1.5 Gy below the doses determined for the ICRU rectum reference point (4.05 ± 0.68 Gy vs. 6.11 ± 1.63 Gy). The advantages of *in vivo* dosimetry are easy practicability and the possibility to determine rectal dose during radiation. The advantages of computer-aided planning at ICRU reference points are that calculations are available before radiation and they can be taken into account for treatment planning.

Gebara et al. (175) estimated the external, internal, and common iliac dose rates using 3D CT-based dose calculations in tandem and ovoid brachytherapy in 30 patients with carcinoma of the uterine cervix treated with LDR brachytherapy using a CT-compatible Fletcher-Suit-Delclos device. Thirty-six implants were performed, and the authors concluded that the point B dose is similar to the maximum common iliac nodal dose.

DeWitt et al. (119), in 15 patients with cervical cancer, defined target and organs at risk for planning of HDR brachytherapy and established guidelines for volume and dose constraint parameters using image-guided inverse treatment planning. Pelloski et al. (468) compared CT-based volumetric calculations and ICRU reference point radiation doses in 60 patients with cervix cancer treated with LDR brachytherapy. Of 118 insertions performed, 93 were evaluated and the minimal dose delivered to the 2 or 3 cm of bladder or rectum (DBV2 and DRV2, respectively) were determined on dose–volume histogram (DVH). They concluded that the ICRU dose was a reasonable surrogate for the DRV2 but not for the DBV2. Furthermore, these calculations may not be applicable to other treatment guidelines or intracavitary applicators.

Dose Fractionation in High–Dose-Rate Brachytherapy

The relationship between dose and fractionation for HDR and LDR intracavitary irradiation of stage I and II carcinoma of the cervix was examined by Arai et al. (22). The dose rate at point A was 2 to 3 Gy per minute (120 to 180 Gy per hour) for HDR and 0.6 to 0.9 Gy per hour for LDR irradiation. Concurrent EBRT was given to the whole pelvis (23 to 30 Gy) followed by 25 to 30 Gy with central shielding, along with brachytherapy. They concluded that the optimal dose fractionation schedules for HDR brachytherapy were 28 ± 3 Gy in four to five fractions, 34 ± 4 Gy in eight to 10 fractions, or 40 ± 5 Gy in 12 to 14 fractions at point A.

The importance of adopting biologically based equivalent doses when switching from LDR to HDR brachytherapy is exemplified in a report by Newman (440) on 115 patients treated with external irradiation (40 to 50 Gy) and manual afterloading cesium sources delivering 60 Gy to point A with a dose rate of 0.75 Gy per hour, or a Selectron device with 40-mCi sources, which delivered from 0.75 to 1 Gy per hour to point A. Because

of the increased dose rate, the total intracavitary dose was reduced by 20%. Grade 3 genitourinary and gastrointestinal complications were observed in three of 87 patients (3.4%) treated with LDR, in contrast to 30/132 patients (22.7%) treated with the Selectron HDR sources. No significant differences in local tumor control and survival were found.

Chatani et al. (74) described a study in which 165 patients with carcinoma of the cervix were randomized to a HDR brachytherapy point A dose of 6 Gy (group A) or 7.5 Gy (group B) per fraction, both combined with external irradiation. The 5-year local failure rate was 16% in both groups, and distant failure rates were 23% and 29%, respectively ($p = 0.2955$). Moderate to severe complications requiring treatment were comparable (six patients, 7%) in the two groups.

Hama et al. (225) compared the effectiveness and safety of once versus twice-weekly HDR brachytherapy for cervical cancer in 124 patients treated with EBRT (50 Gy); 74 patients (group A) were treated with one HDR brachytherapy insertion weekly (three fractions of 7 Gy each to point A), and 50 patients (group B) were treated twice weekly (six fractions of 4.5 Gy each to point A). Overall survival rates were 65.2% and 65.3%, respectively ($p = 0.96$). Local recurrence-free survival rates were 69% for group A and 90% for group B ($p < 0.001$). The rate of grade 2 (moderate) and grade 3 (severe) complications was significantly lower for group B (6%) versus 32% in group A ($p < 0.001$).

Mayer et al. (405) compared HDR BT in two schedules to treat 210 patients with cervix cancer, one sequential (SRT) consisting of four fractions of 8 Gy followed by EBRT or continuous (CRT), consisting of five fractions of 6 Gy one session per week integrated with EBRT (four fraction per week). Total dose to point A was 68 to 70 Gy. Progression-free survival was 71% with CRT versus 56% with SRT ($p = 1.0$). Late bladder and rectal morbidity were 13% in the CRT and 25% in the SRT groups ($p = 0.037$), related to the higher dose per fraction (8 Gy).

Nam and Ahn (435) also compared, in a randomized study of 46 patients, two schedules of HDR BT (10 fractions of 3 Gy or five fractions of 5 Gy) followed by a small BT boost to residual tumor, in combination with EBRT (30.6 Gy to whole pelvis and 14.4 Gy to parametria with midline block). Three-year pelvic tumor control was 90% in both groups and disease-specific survival (DSS) 90.5% and 84.9% ($p = 0.64$), respectively. Late grade 2 or greater bladder or rectal morbidity was 23.8% and 9.1% ($p = 0.24$).

Liu et al. (381), based on the linear-quadratic model, developed isoeffect tables to convert traditional LDR doses and number of fractions to point A to HDR brachytherapy; depending on dose rate, different dose values can be calculated for various fractionation schedules. They predicted that, using therapeutic gain ratio, similar results would be obtained with either brachytherapy modality with two to four fractions of LDR and four to seven fractions of HDR.

The optimal time–dose–fractionation scheme for HDR brachytherapy for cervical cancer has yet to be established. The American Brachytherapy Society published recommendations for HDR brachytherapy for carcinoma of the cervix (429). Each institution should follow a consistent treatment policy, including complete documentation of treatment parameters and correlation with clinical outcome (pelvic tumor control, survival, and complications). The goals are to treat point A to at least a total LDR equivalent of 80 to 85 Gy for early stage disease and 85 to 90 Gy for advanced-stage disease. The pelvic sidewall dose recommendations are 50 to 55 Gy for early lesions and 55 to 65 Gy for advanced ones. As with LDR BT, every attempt should be made to keep the bladder and rectal doses below 80 Gy and 75 Gy LDR-equivalent doses, respectively. Interstitial brachytherapy should be considered when the tumor cannot be optimally encompassed by intracavitary brachytherapy. Some suggested dose and fractionation schemes for combining the external-beam radiation therapy with HDR brachytherapy for each stage of disease were presented, although they have not been thoroughly tested. It was emphasized that the responsibility for the medical decisions ultimately rests with the treating radiation oncologist.

Petereit and Pearcy (480), in a review of 24 HDR dose fractionation schedules published in the past three decades, found no dose relationship for either tumor control or late morbidity. They recommend that in the future all HDR publications for treatment of cervical cancer provide accurate and detailed fractionation and total-dose information. For additional discussion, see Chapters 21 and 22.

Results with Pulse–Dose Rate Brachytherapy

Rogers et al. (519) treated 52 patients with cervical carcinoma, 31 of which had staging laparotomy before radiation therapy. Brachytherapy was interstitial in 18 patients and intracavitary in 28. The median EBRT pelvis dose was 45 Gy in 25 fractions. Median total doses were 75.8 Gy to the implant volume with interstitial and 84.1 Gy to the A points with intracavitary at a median dose rate of 0.55 Gy per pulse per hour. Six patients had laparotomy-documented para-aortic node involvement and received EBRT to this site (45 Gy in 25 fractions). Thirty patients received concomitant weekly cisplatin chemotherapy (40 mg/m²). With a median follow-up of 25 months, the actuarial 4-year disease-free survival rates were 66% for the entire group (100% for stage IB, 69% for stage II, 68% for stage III/IVA, and 43% in patients treated for recurrences after surgery). Grade 4 complications occurred in two patients (4.3%). One patient (2.2%) had a grade 3 complication (frequent hematuria), and five (10.9%) had grade 2 complications.

Doses of Radiation

Stage IA (microinvasive) tumors are treated with intracavitary therapy only (LDR 60 Gy in one insertion or 75 to 80 Gy in two insertions to point A, or HDR 35 to 42 Gy in five to six insertions of 7 Gy to point A, one or two fractions per week).

The optimal dose for invasive carcinoma of the cervix is delivered with a combination of EBRT whole pelvis, intracavitary, and, at times, interstitial therapy. Some institutions such as ours use lower doses of whole pelvis external irradiation (10 Gy for stage IB and 20 Gy for stages IIA, IIB, and III) in addition to parametrial doses to complete 50 Gy in stage IB and IIA or 60 Gy to the involved parametrial tissues for more advanced stages. At Washington University, step-wedges designed in accordance with the isodose curves of the intracavitary applications are used to block the midline (Fig. 66.21). The LDR intracavitary insertions, usually two, deliver 7,000 to 7,500 mgh (65 to 70 Gy to point A) in stage IB tumors and 7,500 to 8,000 mgh (68 to 70 Gy to point A) for stage IIA, IIB, and III tumors. This technique affords a high central dose to the cervix, paracervical tissues, and parametria as well as a moderate homogeneous dose to the external iliac lymph nodes without exceeding the bladder and rectal tolerance doses (Fig. 66.22A).

Other institutions prefer higher doses of whole pelvis external irradiation (usually 40 to 45 Gy) with additional parametrial dose (with a midline 5-HVL rectangular block) to complete 50 Gy in patients with stage IB and IIA tumors and 55 to 60 Gy in patients with stage IIB, III, or IVA tumors. This is usually combined with one or two LDR intracavitary insertions for approximately 4,000 to 5,000 mgh (36 to 50 Gy to point A) to deliver a total dose of 85 to 95 Gy to point A, depending on the tumor volume and stage and age of the patient (Fig. 66.22B). We tend to reduce the total doses by 10% in women older than 70 years.

When 20 Gy is administered to the whole pelvis, for HDR brachytherapy the usual schedule is six fractions of 7 Gy or seven fractions of 6 Gy to point A. If 40 to 45 Gy is given to the whole pelvis, usually four fractions of 6 to 7 Gy to point A are administered.

Results of Therapy

When therapeutic results in invasive carcinoma of the cervix are evaluated, a direct comparison of surgically treated or irradiated patients is fraught with many uncertainties, including patient selection, reporting of surgical cases using staging determined by laparotomy findings, and different treatment techniques (670).

The impact of patient selection in results of surgical series was illustrated by Whitney and Stehman (654), who evaluated the frequency with which intended radical hysterectomy for cervical cancer is abandoned and the outcomes for those selected patients. In 1,127 patients with stage IB carcinoma of the cervix entered on GOG Protocol 49, 98 women (8.7%) were found at surgery to have extrauterine disease, and the proposed radical operation was abandoned. Subgroups of patients with extrapelvic disease (30) and pelvic extension (26), including grossly positive pelvis nodes (12), other pelvic implants (8), and gross serosal extension (2), were identified. Sixty-three (93%) patients subsequently underwent pelvic radiation therapy and brachytherapy. Para-aortic fields were added for eight patients who were found to have positive para-aortic nodes. The disease-free survival was shorter for patients whose radical procedure was abandoned than for those patients who underwent radical hysterectomy.

Stage IA

In 47 patients with microinvasive carcinoma treated at Washington University, 20 with intracavitary therapy only and 27 patients with combined external irradiation and intracavitary brachytherapy, only one patient had a pelvic recurrence and distant metastases 10 years later; the 5-year disease-free survival rate was 96% (201).

Webb et al. (644) analyzed lymph node status and survival rates of women with microinvasive cervical adenocarcinoma (FIGO stages IA1 and IA2) from the SEER database between 1988 and 1997. Among reported cases, 131 had stage IA1 and 170 had IA2 disease. Simple hysterectomy was done in 54 women with IA1 and 64 with IA2 disease and radical hysterectomy in 50 and 83 women, respectively. Only 1/140 women who had lymphadenectomy had a single positive lymph node. There were four tumor-related deaths (one with IA1 and three with IA2 disease). The survival rate was 98.7%.

Stages IB and IIA

The important contribution of external-beam irradiation to improve pelvic tumor control in larger lesions has been documented. Hamberger et al. (226), in 151 patients with stage IA or IB lesions <1 cm in diameter treated with intracavitary therapy

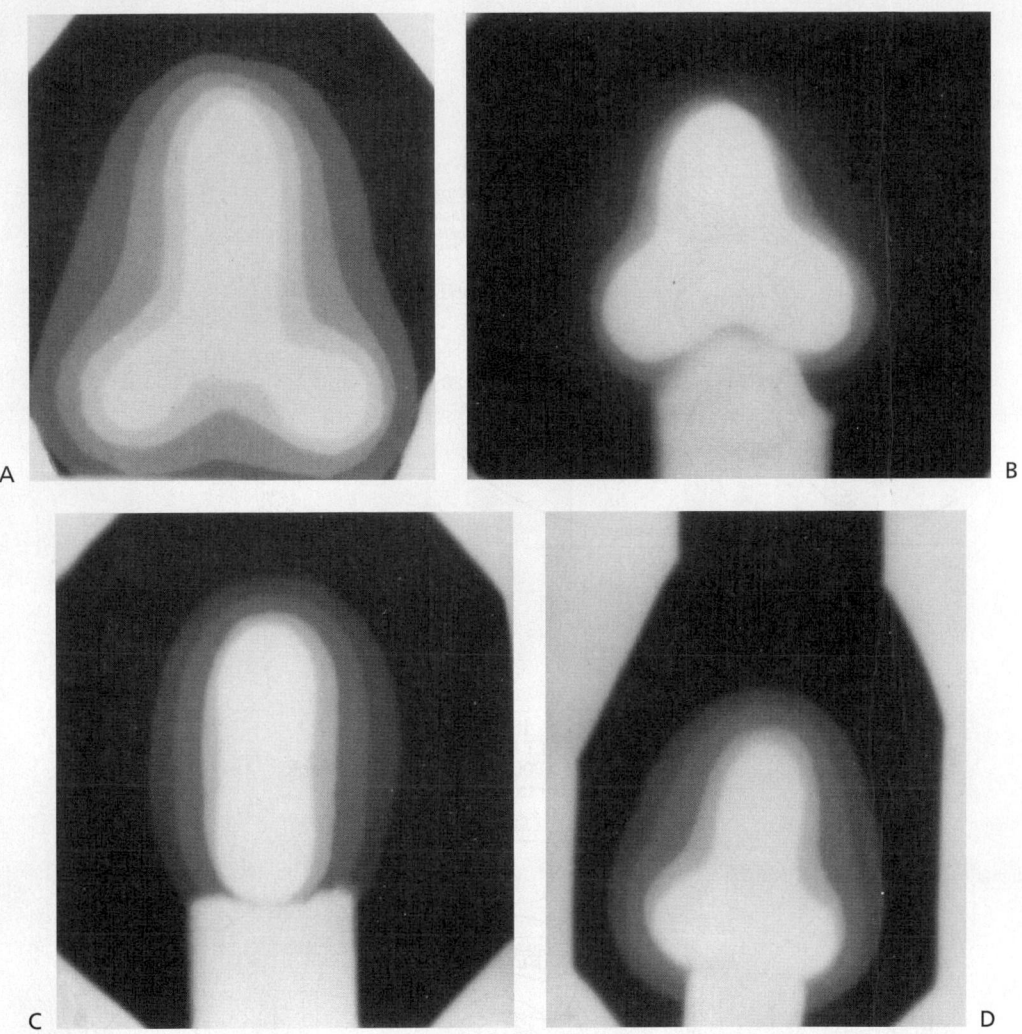

FIGURE 66.21. A–C: Examples of different step wedges used to shield the midline during external irradiation for carcinoma of uterine cervix. Wedges are designed according to the dose distribution obtained with brachytherapy sources. **D:** Localization film illustrating use of the midline wedge in a patient irradiated through extended fields. (A and B from Perez CA, DiSaia PJ, Knapp RC, et al. Gynecologic tumors. In: DeVita V, Hellman S, Rosenberg SA, eds. *Cancer: principles and practice of oncology,* 2nd ed. Philadelphia: J.B. Lippincott, 1985; with permission.

alone to high doses (8,640, 9,340, and 13,680 mgh), noted no failures in 41 patients with stage IA disease, and only 4/93 patients (4%) with stage IB, small-volume disease. However, 3/17 patients (18%) with more extensive stage IB lesions, treated with intracavitary therapy only, had regional failures. Only 3/151 patients (0.2%) had grade 3 complications.

Volterrani and Lombardi (639) reported 5-year survival of 82.6% in 23 patients with occult stage IB carcinoma of the cervix treated with intracavitary ^{226}Ra only (7,500 mgh) in contrast to only 64.8% in larger stage IB tumors and 50% in stage II. Unfortunately, the authors did not report the exact location of the failures. It is obvious that intracavitary therapy alone is grossly inadequate to irradiate larger primary tumors, including stage IB1.

With EBRT and BT, the usual 5-year survival rate for stage IB is 86% to 92%, and for stage IIA, approximately 75%. The overall pelvic failure rate in stage IB is approximately 5% to 8%, and in stage IIA, 15% to 20% (in half of the patients combined with distant metastases). Either surgery or adequate irradiation is equally effective in the treatment of stage IB and IIA carcinoma of the cervix; numerous noncontrolled studies support the merits of either modality with no significant difference in survival or pelvic tumor control (Tables 66.16 and Fig. 66.23). Saibishkumar et al. (541) published a retrospective review of

1,069 patients with cervical cancer treated with EBRT and BT to median point A dose of 81 Gy; 5-year overall pelvic tumor control was 63.9%, DFS 49.4%, and overall survival 51.8%. Late toxicity was observed in 1% to 2% of the patients.

Randomized Studies

A few randomized studies of radical operation and irradiation have been published; outcome with the two modalities is comparable. Newton (441) and Roddick and Greenlaw (516) reported, in prospectively randomized studies, equivalent survival and pelvic recurrence rates in patients with stage IB and IIA carcinoma of the uterine cervix treated with a radical hysterectomy or irradiation alone.

Landoni et al. (352) published results of a prospective, randomized trial of radiation therapy versus surgery; 469 women with stage IB and IIA cervical carcinoma were referred for treatment and 343 were randomized (172 to surgery and 171 to radiation therapy). Postoperative irradiation was delivered after surgery for women with surgical stage pT2b or greater, <3 mm of safe cervical stroma, and cut-through margins or positive pelvic nodes. Scheduled treatment was delivered to 169 and 158 women, respectively; 62/114 women with cervical diameters of <4 cm and 46/55 with >4 cm received radiation

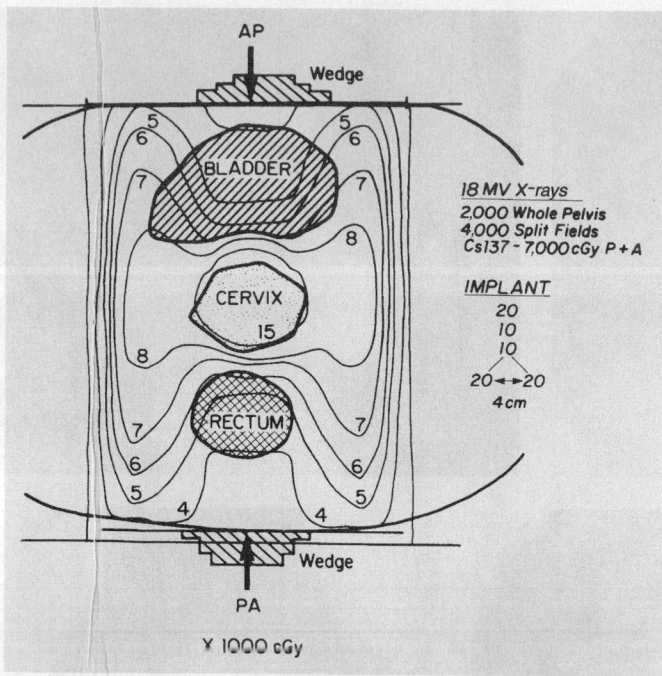

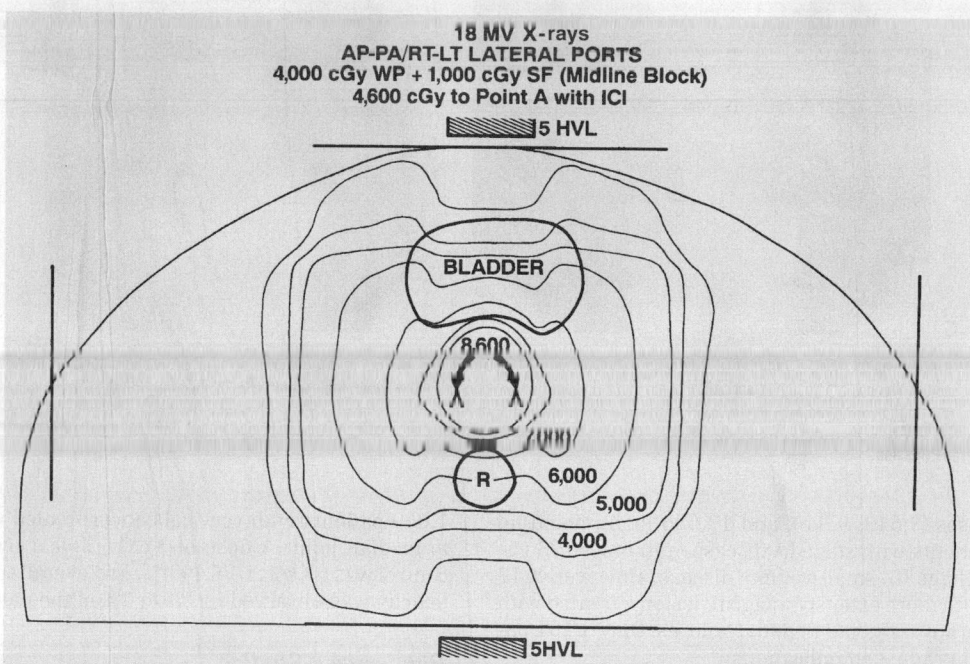

FIGURE 66.22. A: Composite isodose curves through point A for patient with carcinoma of uterine cervix treated with external irradiation and two intracavitary insertions. Doses and source arrangement are shown. High doses can be delivered to cervix and parametrial tissues with relative sparing of the bladder and rectum. **B:** Composite isodose curves through point A using 40-Gy whole pelvis dose and reduced brachytherapy dose (45 Gy to point A).

therapy. After a median follow-up of 87 months (range, 57 to 120 months), 5-year overall and disease-free survival rates were nearly identical in the surgery and radiation therapy groups (83% and 74%, respectively); recurrent disease developed in 86 women: 42 (25%) in the surgery group and 44 (26%) in the radiation therapy group (Fig. 66.24). Forty-eight patients (28%) in the surgery group had severe morbidity compared with 19 (12%) in the radiation therapy group ($p = 0.0004$; Table 66.17). The combination of surgery and radiation therapy had the worst morbidity, especially urologic complications.

Nonrandomized Studies

Kielbinska et al. (313), in a long-term study of 792 women treated with irradiation and 789 women treated with hysterectomy and irradiation for stage I cervical carcinoma, found no difference in survival, general health, incidence of recurrent carcinoma, or appearance of second primary malignancies.

Piver et al. (489) treated 103 women with stage IB cervical carcinoma with either radical hysterectomy and pelvic lymphadenectomy (if tumor <3 cm in greatest diameter) or

				FIVE-YEAR SURVIVAL OF PATIENTS WITH STAGES I AND II CARCINOMA OF THE UTERINE CERVIX TREATED WITH RADIATION THERAPY

Table 66.16 FIVE-YEAR SURVIVAL OF PATIENTS WITH STAGES I AND II CARCINOMA OF THE UTERINE CERVIX TREATED WITH RADIATION THERAPY

Study	Stage	No. of Patients	Survivors[a]	Percentage Survival
Fletcher (161)	IB	549	Actuarial	91.5
	IB and IIA	973	—	83.5
	IB and IIA	1,576	1,244	78.9
Perez et al. (471)	IB	312	Actuarial	87.0
	IIA	98	Actuarial	73.0
	I	—	—	83.5
	I and II	—	—	75.6
Rosseau et al. (525)	I	280	Absolute	83.0
	II	533	—	51.0

[a]Patients dead of intercurrent disease were included with survivors when data were available.
Modified from Hoskins WJ, Ford JH Jr, Lutz MH, et al. Radical hysterectomy and pelvic lymphadenectomy for the management of early invasive cancer of the cervix. *Gynecol Oncol* 1976;4:278–290, with permission.

irradiation (tumor >3 cm or medically inoperable). The 5-year disease-free survival rate was 92.3% for the surgical group and 91.1% for the radiation therapy group. Equivalent overall 5-year survival rates were noted.

In stage IB and IIA disease after a hysterectomy and lymphadenectomy (even combined with irradiation), patients with metastatic lymph nodes have survival rates that are approximately 50% of those of patients with negative nodes (284).

Einhorn et al. (147), in a nonrandomized study, observed a 100% 5-year survival rate in 49 patients with stage IB disease receiving combined therapy in comparison with 81% in 64 patients treated with irradiation alone. No difference was observed in 25 patients with stage IIA tumor treated with combined therapy and 40 patients treated with irradiation alone (5-year survival rate, 75%).

Perez et al. (471) reported on a prospectively randomized study of 118 patients with stage IB or IIA carcinoma of the uterine cervix in which patients were treated with RT alone or irradiation and surgery (20 Gy to the whole pelvis, one intracavitary insertion for 5,000 to 6,000 mgh, followed by a radical hysterectomy with pelvic lymphadenectomy 2 to 6 weeks later). In stage IB, the 5-year tumor-free survival was 80% and 82% ($p = 0.23$), respectively, and in stage IIA, 56% and 79%, respectively ($p = 0.13$). The incidence of grade 2 or 3 complications radiation alone was 13.8% and with preoperative irradiation and surgery 11%. Subsequently, Perez et al. (472) described results in 415 patients with stage IB or limited stage IIB treated with preoperative or postoperative irradiation and surgery. The 10-year cause-specific survival rate for patients with stage IB

nonbulky tumors treated with irradiation alone or irradiation combined with surgery was 84% with either modality. With bulky tumors (>5 cm), the 10-year rates were 61% and 68%, respectively ($p = 0.5$). For patients with stage IIA nonbulky tumors, the 10-year cause-specific survival rates were 66% and 71%, respectively, and with bulky tumors, 69% and 44%, respectively ($p = 0.05$). In patients with stage IIB nonbulky tumors treated with irradiation alone or combined with surgery, the 10-year cause-specific survival rates were 72% and 65%, respectively.

Stages IB and IIA (Bulky)

Mendenhall et al. (408) compared 75 patients in each group treated with irradiation alone or combined with surgery for bulky tumors and reported local tumor control of 74% and 76%, and absolute 54% and 52%. The authors currently reserve combining irradiation with an extrafascial hysterectomy for patients who have <25% tumor regression at the time of the first intracavitary application, who are medically operable, and in whom it is thought adequate surgical margins may be obtained.

Thoms et al. (611) reported on 363 patients with bulky endocervical carcinoma treated with curative intent (246 with irradiation alone and 117 with irradiation and surgery); 10-year survival was 45% and 64%, respectively. In a subset of 48 patients with similar tumors treated with irradiation alone and 45 with irradiation and surgery, the 10-year survival rates were comparable, and the pelvic tumor control rates were 90% and 87%, respectively.

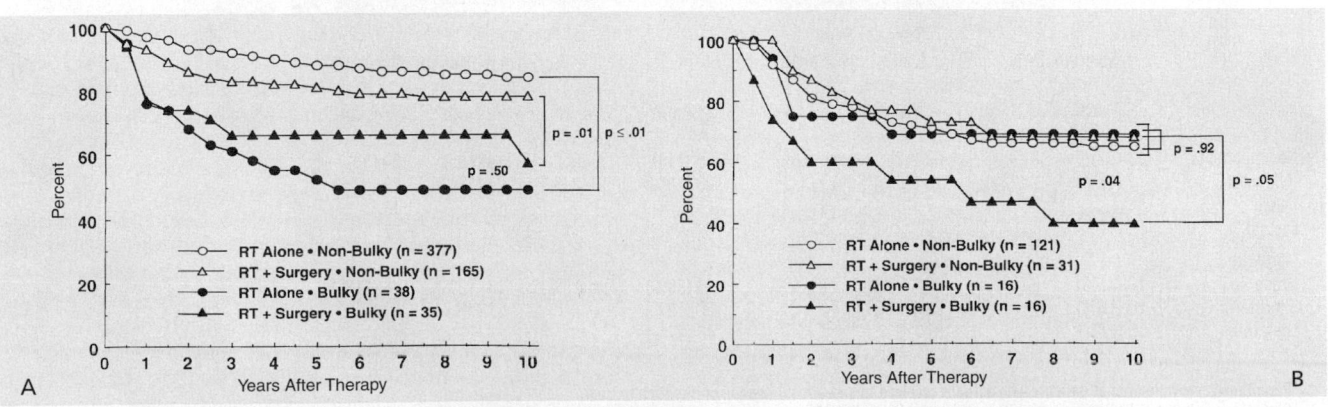

FIGURE 66.23. Disease-free survival of patients with stage IB **(A)** and IIA **(B)** carcinoma of uterine cervix treated with irradiation alone or combined with surgery. (Mallinckrodt Institute of Radiology, 1959–1989.) RT, radiation therapy.

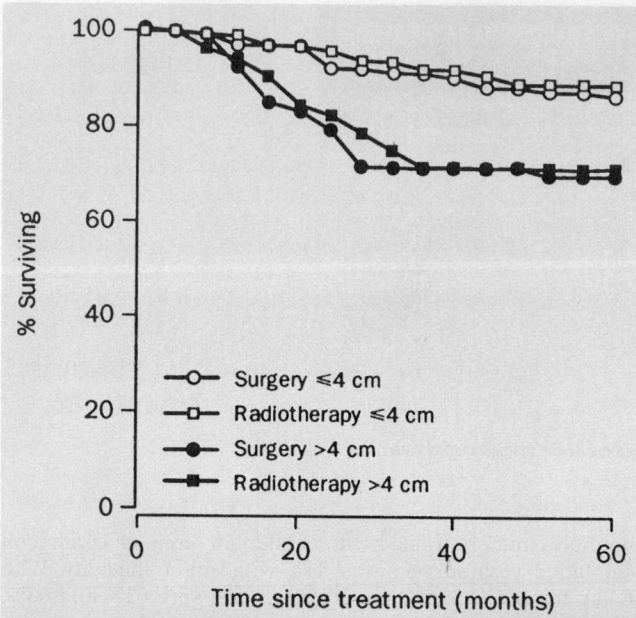

FIGURE 66.24. Overall actuarial survival of patients with carcinoma of the cervix randomized to treatment with radical surgery or radiation therapy, according to treatment group and cervical diameter. (From Landoni F, Maneo A, Colombo A, et al. Randomised study of radical surgery versus radiotherapy for stage IB-IIA cervical cancer. *Lancet* 1997;350:535–540, with permission.)

Eifel et al. (144) evaluated 1,526 patients, of whom 371 had tumors 6 cm or greater. There were biases in treatment selection, but a statistically significantly higher 10-year survival rate was noted in patients treated with irradiation and surgery (64% vs. 45%). Tumor diameter was highly significant as a prognostic factor, and they concluded that only patients with lesions >8 cm in diameter benefited from adjuvant hysterectomy. In the same study, 98 patients with stage IB and IIB bulky endocervical carcinomas (≥6 cm in diameter) were treated with RT alone. Twenty-four patients received <6,000 mgh of intracavitary treatment, and 73 received higher doses. Despite having somewhat more favorable tumors, patients who received <6,000 mgh had a higher rate of pelvic recurrence at 5 years (33%) than

those who received higher doses (16%; $p = 0.03$). Actuarial 5-year survival rates were 44% and 60% for low- and high-dose groups, respectively ($p = 0.14$).

Kim et al. (318) assessed the prognostic factors for pelvic tumor control in 40 patients with FIGO stage IB or IIA carcinoma, and 25 patients with stage IIB carcinoma classified as barrel-shaped (i.e., at least 5 cm in diameter) treated with curative intent. Seventy-two percent were treated with RT alone and 28% with RT and extrafascial hysterectomy. The extent of tumor regression after external-beam radiation therapy correlated with the likelihood of local tumor control ($p = 0.02$). For patients treated with radiation therapy alone, increased brachytherapy dose was associated with better local tumor control. The 10-year overall and cause-specific survival rates were 53% and 68%, respectively, and did not differ significantly between treatment groups.

Paley et al. (458) reported on 57 patients with barrel-shaped (mean diameter, 5 to 9 cm) cervical carcinoma treated with preoperative EBRT and BT (mean dose to point A, 79.6 Gy) followed by extrafascial hysterectomy 6 to 8 weeks later. Residual disease was present in 35 (61%) of the hysterectomy specimens; tumor sterilization correlated significantly with the mean dose to point A ($p = 0.016$). Ninety-five percent of the patients with negative specimens remained clinically free of disease at their last follow-up versus 31% of those with residual disease ($p < 0.001$).

The GOG and RTOG conducted a randomized phase III clinical trial in which 282 patients with carcinoma of the cervix measuring 4 cm or greater (exophytic or barrel-shaped) were treated with either external-beam and intracavitary irradiation or a slightly lower dose of intracavitary irradiation and the same pelvic EBRT followed by an extrafascial hysterectomy (311). The survival rates were 61.4% for irradiation alone and 64.4% for the combined irradiation and surgery group. The incidence of recurrences was 43.3% in the irradiation group compared to 34.5% with combined therapy ($p = 0.081$). The incidence of local recurrences was 25.8% 14.4%, respectively. The incidence of grade 3 and 4 sequelae of therapy was 10.5% and 9.8%, respectively. Thus, the addition of hysterectomy to standard irradiation did not significantly affect survival, although there was a small reduction in the local recurrence rate.

When combined therapy is used, the dose of irradiation delivered to the lymph nodes, the time of the operation, and the pathologic examination of the specimens are critical in

	Surgery						Radiation Therapy Alone		
	Surgery Only		Surgery Plus Radiation Therapy		Total				
	≤4 cm	>4 cm	≤4 cm	>4 cm	≤4 cm	>4 cm	≤4 cm	>4 cm
No. of patients[a]	53 (52)	9 (9)	62 (62)	46 (46)	115 (114)	55 (55)	114 (105)	54 (53)
Relapses	7 (13%)	2 (22%)	15 (26%)	17 (37%)	23 (20%)	19 (34%)	21 (18%)	23 (42%)
Pelvic	4	2	7	9	11	11	12	16
Distant	3	—	9	8	12	8	9	7
Morbidity								
Grade 2–3[b]	16 (31%)	3 (33%)	18 (29%)	11 (24%)	34 (30%)	14 (25%)	13 (12%)	6 (11%)
Short term	10 (16%)		22 (20%)		32 (19%)		11 (7%)	—
Long term	15 (24%)		31 (29%)		46 (27%)		25 (16%)	—

Table 66.17 RANDOMIZED TRIAL OF RADICAL SURGERY OR IRRADIATION IN STAGE I–II CERVICAL CANCER: RELAPSES AND MORBIDITY

[a]Parentheses show number of patients who actually received this treatment instead of intention to treat.
[b]Percentage calculated for number of patients who actually received treatment.
From Landoni F, Maneo A, Colombo A, et al. Randomised study of radical surgery versus radiotherapy for stage IB–IIA cervical cancer. *Lancet* 1997;350:535–540, with permission.

Table 66.18	STAGE IB CERVICAL CARCINOMA: 5-YEAR ESTIMATED DISEASE-FREE SURVIVAL CORRELATED WITH TREATMENT REGIMEN					
	Radical Hysterectomy and Pelvic Lymphadenectomy			External Pelvic Plus Intracavitary Irradiation		
Lesion Size (cm)	No. of Patients	Recurrence	Estimated 5-Year DFS	No. of Patients	Recurrence	Estimated 5-Year DFS
<1	18	0	100.0%	14	1 (7.1%)	92.3%
1–3	34	4 (11.8%)	87.5%	20	3 (15.0%)	94.4%
>3	3	0	100.0%	14	2 (14.3%)	84.6%
Total	55	4 (7.3%)	92.3%	48	6 (12.5%)	91.1%

DFS, disease-free survival.
Modified from Piver MS, Marchetti DL, Patton T, et al. Radical hysterectomy and pelvic lymphadenectomy versus radiation therapy for small (≤3 cm) stage IB cervical carcinoma. *Am J Clin Oncol* 1988;11:21–24, with permission.

determining the presence of postirradiation residual tumor (Table 66.18).

Perez et al. (470) noted that in patients with primary carcinoma of the uterine cervix who had endometrial stromal invasion or tumor only in the curettings, the addition of a hysterectomy did not improve the survival rate because most of the patients failed at distant sites.

Stages IIB, III, and IVA

Most patients with stage IIB tumors are treated with irradiation alone, and the 5-year survival rate is 60% to 65%. The pelvic failure rate ranges from 18% to 39%. In an analysis of the Patterns of Care Study in 157 patients who had stage IIB disease, Coia et al. (90) reported a better 4-year survival rate (67% and 54%) and in-field tumor control rate (78% and 68%) in patients with unilateral versus bilateral parametrial involvement, respectively. Similarly, in a review of 1,178 patients with stage IIB disease treated at Washington University, the 5-year survival rates were 70% with medial parametrial and 58% with lateral parametrial involvement ($p = 0.004$) (533). Kim et al. (320), in patients with stage IIB, found a correlation of point A dose and incidence of pelvic failures (Fig. 66.25). Before 1965, a pelvic lymphadenectomy was carried out at M.D. Anderson

Hospital after a full course of radiation therapy, but this procedure did not improve survival over irradiation alone and the complication rate was somewhat higher (161).

In stage IIIB carcinoma, the 5-year survival rates range from 25% to 48%, and pelvic failure rates range from 38% to 50% (161,417). Hanks et al. (228), reporting on the Patterns of Care Study, noted a 28% probability of 5-year survival in patients with stage III carcinoma of the cervix treated in a large number of facilities in the United States versus 60% survival in selected large centers (extended survey). Later, Komaki et al. (334) reported a significant increase in local pelvic tumor control (69%) in patients with stage III carcinoma of the cervix treated in 1983, compared with 37% and 49% in earlier periods ($p = 0.03$). The 5-year survival rate increased from 25% to 47% ($p = 0.02$). The improvement in pelvic tumor control may be associated with higher external beam doses, but more likely is related to the substantial increase in the percentage of patients receiving brachytherapy (96%) and more careful dosimetry and dose calculations for intracavitary therapy. They noted a decrease in major complications from 15% in the 1973 and 13% in the 1978 Patterns of Care Surveys to 7% in 1983. Montana et al. (418) reported that calculation of doses to the bladder and rectum were performed in 80% and 76% of patients, respectively, in the 1983 survey, which may also have resulted in decreased toxicity.

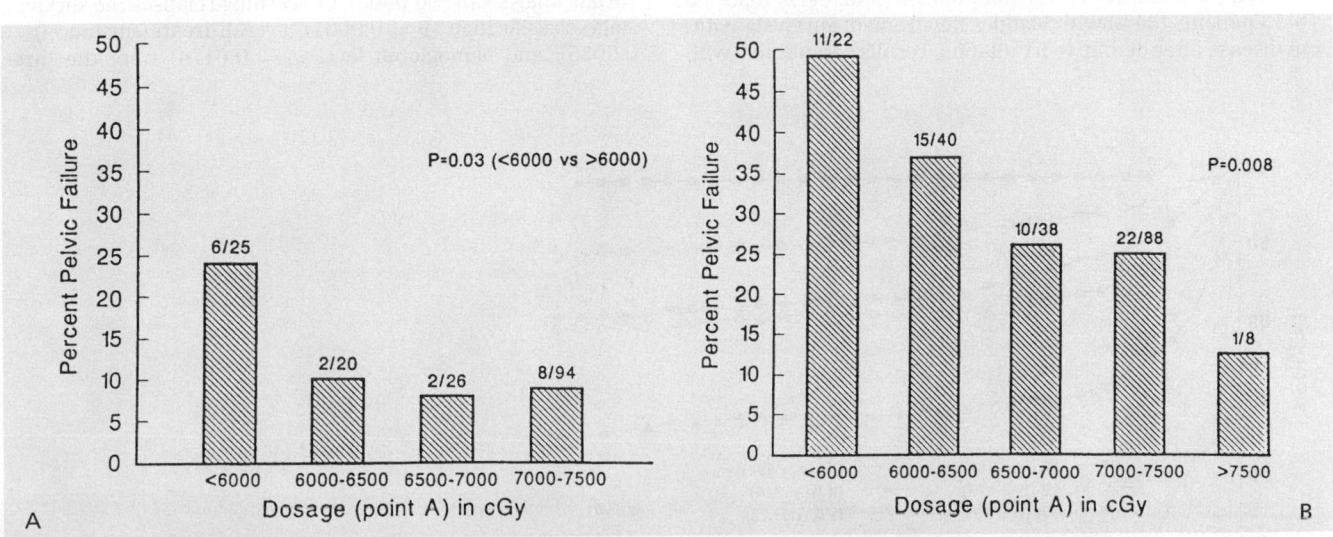

FIGURE 66.25. Relationships between pelvic failure and point A dose in stage IB **(A)** and stage IIB **(B)** cancer of the cervix. (From Kim RY, Trotti A, Wu C-J, et al. Radiation alone in the treatment of cancer of the uterine cervix: analysis of pelvic failure and dose response relationship. *Int J Radiat Oncol Biol Phys* 1989;17:973–978, with permission.)

Arthur et al. (23), in 89 patients with stage IIIB carcinoma of the cervix treated with external irradiation and brachytherapy, observed a locoregional tumor control rate of 22.5% and a disease-free survival rate of 15% in 16 patients treated with 78 Gy or lower doses to point A, in comparison with 53% and 47%, respectively, in 24 patients receiving higher doses.

Horiot et al. (259) reported the results of a French cooperative study of 1,383 patients with invasive carcinoma of the uterus treated with irradiation alone following the M.D. Anderson Hospital treatment guidelines. Survival and locoregional tumor control were similar in both groups, except in stage III, in which the pelvic and central failure rates were lower in the French patients, probably because of different tumor volumes or socioeconomic factors. Major urinary complications were noted in 2% of the patients and grade 3 bowel complications in 3% of the patients with stage I and IIA disease, and bowel complications in 7% of patients with IIB and III disease. Barillot et al. (28) updated the results in 642 patients; the analysis was divided into three periods: 1970 to 1978 (use of standard prescriptions), 1979 to 1984 (implementation of individual adjustments), and 1985 to 1994 (systematic individual adjustments). There was a significant reduction of the external radiation dose (above 40 Gy in 47% of patients before 1979 vs. 36% after 1984), use of parametrial boost (55% vs. 39%), of use of vaginal cylinder (28% vs. 11.5%), and of combined intracavitary and external irradiation volume (842 cm^3 vs. 503 cm^3 on average). The 5-year actuarial toxicity rates were grade 2, 23.5%; grade 3, 10%; and grade 4, 3%. The three main predictive factors for rectal and bladder sequelae were increased external radiation dose, higher dose rate at reference points, and whole-vagina brachytherapy. The disease-free survival rates observed with irradiation alone at Washington University Medical Center are shown in Figure 66.26.

Marcial et al. (399) described results of a randomized trial in 301 patients with stage IIB, III, and IVA carcinoma of the uterine cervix treated with split-course irradiation (10 fractions of 2.5 Gy, five weekly doses up to 25 Gy, followed by a rest period of 2 weeks, and an additional 25 Gy delivered in the same manner) or continuous irradiation (30 fractions of 1.7 Gy daily, five times per week, total dose 51 Gy) combined with LDR brachytherapy for 30 Gy to point A. There was no significant difference in tumor control, acute or late complications, or survival in the two groups.

In patients with stage IVA disease, the 5-year survival rates range from 18% (333) to 34%, and pelvic failures from 60% to 80% after definitive irradiation. Million et al. (412) reported 18/53 patients (34%) with bladder involvement surviving without disease after definitive irradiation, results comparable with those obtained with exenteration. Upadhyay et al. (625) noted 43% local tumor control and 18% 5-year survival rates in 44 patients with stage IVA carcinoma of the cervix treated with definitive radiation therapy.

Kramer et al. (337) reported on 48 patients with stage IVA carcinoma of the cervix treated with definitive RT. Patients with minimal parametrial involvement had a 5-year survival rate of 46% compared with only 5% for those with extensive parametrial tumor. The major complication rate was 22%, consisting mostly of vesicovaginal fistula in five patients.

Crozier et al. (102) described equivalent 5-year survival rates after salvage pelvic exenteration (37% in 35 patients with adenocarcinoma and 39% in 70 patients with squamous-cell carcinoma). In the adenocarcinoma group, 14/22 patients, and in the squamous cell-carcinoma group, 14/30 patients had distant metastases after pelvic exenteration.

Treatment of Elderly Patients

Oguchi et al. (451) reported on 23 patients 90 years of age or older treated with cervix carcinoma. Definitive radiation therapy was completed in 13 of the patients, and local tumor control at 6 months was attained in nine patients. Palliative RT was completed in 7/11, and palliation was observed in nine patients (81%). Seven patients were alive for 15 to 67 months. Fourteen patients died because of intercurrent disease or senility associated with active cancer, and two because of senility without evidence of cancer. The 2-year overall and relapse-free survival rates were 30% and 21%, respectively.

Multivariate Analysis

Fyles et al. (170), in 965 patients with invasive carcinoma of the cervix, identified FIGO stage as the most significant prognostic factor, followed by dose of irradiation to point A and overall time of radiation therapy. The 10-year survival rate was 62% in 743 patients receiving doses to point A of 85 Gy or higher, in contrast to 53% for 222 patients receiving lower doses. Patients with higher hemoglobin levels not receiving a transfusion (595) had a 10-year survival rate of 60% in contrast to 42% in 353 patients who were given transfusions for lower hemoglobin levels.

Chatani et al. (75), in 216 patients with stage IIB, III cervical carcinoma treated with a combination of external-beam and HDR brachytherapy, noted that overall treatment time was the most highly significant factor for local tumor control in multivariate analysis ($p = 0.0005$). Concerning relapse-free survival, stage classification ($p = 0.0001$), overall treatment time ($p = 0.0035$), and hemoglobin level ($p = 0.0174$) were the three

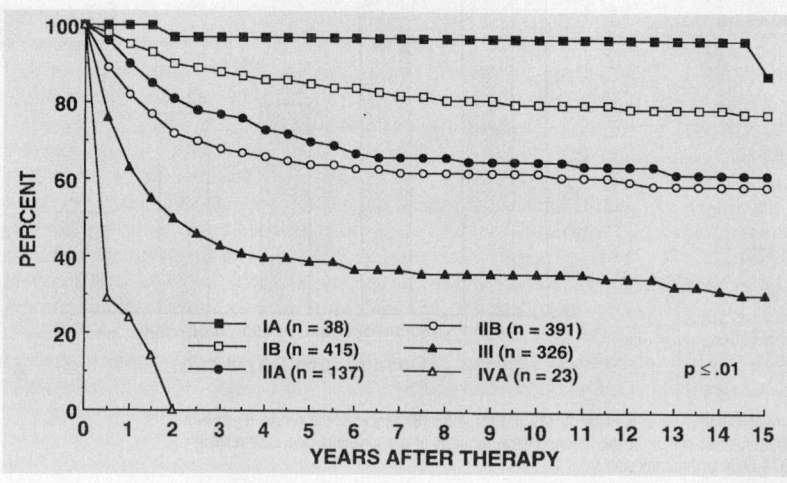

FIGURE 66.26. Disease-free survival for 1,330 patients with carcinoma of the cervix treated with irradiation alone at the Mallinckrodt Institute of Radiology (1959–1989).

most important prognostic factors; there was no relationship between treatment time and late complications.

Kapp et al. (299), in a study of 181 patients with FIGO stages IB to IV carcinoma of the cervix, documented that prognostic factors for patients treated with HDR are similar to those in previous series with LDR brachytherapy. In multivariate analysis, tumor size was the most powerful for pelvic tumor control and incidence of distant metastasis.

Interstitial Implants

Interstitial brachytherapy, discussed in detail in Chapter 20, has been used in the treatment of patients with cervical cancer (591). Because of the inability to insert an intracavitary tandem interstitial needle, implants were used at Washington University in 30 patients with stage IIB and in 37 with stage III carcinoma to deliver interstitial irradiation in the parametrium to supplement the dose delivered by external-beam and intracavitary brachytherapy. Despite the fact that the patients treated with interstitial implant were in a high-risk group, local tumor control was comparable with that of patients treated with standard techniques (474).

Pierquin et al. (484) described locoregional recurrences in 6% of 53 patients with T1, 11% in 47 with T2, and 42% of 19 patients with T3 primary tumors of the uterine cervix treated with a combination of external-beam irradiation and the Creteil method for interstitial implantation of ^{192}Ir sources in a plastic cervical-vaginal moulage and a uterine tandem.

Prempree (502) reported a 96% local tumor control rate and 61% 5-year disease-free survival rate in 23 patients with stage IIIB carcinoma of the cervix treated with a combination of external irradiation and intracavitary and interstitial implants to the parametrium. Overall, major complications were noted in 8% of the patients.

Martinez et al. (402), using the Martinez Universal Perineal Interstitial (MUPIT) applicator, treated 37 patients with advanced or recurrent carcinoma of the cervix and 26 with vaginal-urethral tumors. Doses of approximately 35 Gy were given, in addition to external irradiation (36 Gy to the whole pelvis and 14 Gy to the pelvic sidewall). They reported six local failures in the patients with cervical lesions and five in the group with vaginal-urethral tumors. The overall complication rate was 5.1%.

Nag et al. (430) reported on 31 patients with carcinoma of the cervix and eight with carcinoma of the vagina treated with external-beam radiation therapy and fluoroscopically guided interstitial brachytherapy. With a median follow-up of 36 months, 16 patients (51%) with cervical and five patients (62.5%) with vaginal carcinomas had local tumor control. The 5-year actuarial survival rates were 34% and 38% for cervical and vaginal cancers, respectively. Only one patient experienced grade 3 complications (2.5%).

Recio et al. (508) used laparoscopy at the time of interstitial brachytherapy in six patients with FIGO stages IIB to IVA cervical carcinoma, after completion of whole pelvis radiation; a total of 98 needles were inserted to deliver a median interstitial brachytherapy dose of 20 Gy. Eleven perforations in the pelvic peritoneum or bladder were identified during surgery in five of the six patients, leading to immediate repositioning of needles. No acute or short-term morbidity related to the procedure was noted.

Californium-252 or Neutrons

Maruyama and Muir (404) reported on 41 patients with stage IB cervix cancer treated with 40 to 50 Gy to the whole pelvis followed by a 5- to 15-Gy boost to the lateral pelvic wall and a single ^{252}Cf-neutron brachytherapy insertion in approximately 8 hours. Nearly total tumor clearance was achieved in over 90%

of the patients; tumor regression was more rapid in the ^{252}Cf group than in similar patients treated with ^{137}Cs and the same external-beam irradiation dose.

Maor et al. (398) published results in 156 patients with locally advanced cervical carcinoma treated at five institutions and randomized to receive external photons only to the pelvis (50 Gy in 25 fractions in 5 weeks) or mixed-beam external irradiation (three fractions a week of photons) to a total relative biologic effectiveness adjusted dose of 50 Gy over 5 weeks. All patients were scheduled to receive LDR intracavitary brachytherapy. Of 146 evaluable patients, 80 were treated with mixed-beam irradiation and 66 with photons. Only 50% of the patients in the mixed-beam group and 75% in the photon group underwent brachytherapy. The local tumor control at 2 years was 45% in the mixed-beam group and 52% in the photon group. Severe complications occurred in 19% of the mixed-beam and 11% of the photon-beam patients ($p < 0.13$). It was thought that the inferior outcome with neutrons may have resulted from the use of horizontal beams of varying energy and penetration.

Heavy Ions

Kato et al. (302) reported on 44 patients with locally advanced cervical cancer treated with carbon ion radiation therapy. Total whole pelvis dose was 52.8 to 72 Gy equivalent (GyE) in 16 fractions of 2.2 to 3 GyE and eight fractions local boost or 68 to 72.8 GyE (44.8 GyE and additional 24 or 28 GyE boost). The 5-year local tumor control was 45% and 79%, respectively. Eight patients developed major intestinal complications, which were surgically salvaged; they were associated with doses >60 GyE.

External-Beam Irradiation Alone

Occasionally, brachytherapy procedures cannot be performed because of medical reasons or unusual anatomic configuration of the pelvis or the tumor (i.e., extensive lesion, inability to identify the cervical canal). These patients may be treated with higher doses of external-beam irradiation alone, although treatment results are less than optimal.

Coia et al. (90), in an analysis of 565 patients with various stages of cervical carcinoma treated in the Patterns of Care Study, reported better survival (67%) and pelvic tumor control (78%) when patients were treated with external irradiation and brachytherapy compared with patients who had no intracavitary brachytherapy applications (36% 4-year survival and 47% in-field failure rates). Patients treated with two intracavitary applications had a higher 4-year survival rate (73%) and in-field tumor control rate (83%) than those receiving only one application (60% 4-year survival rate and 71% in-field tumor control rate).

Hanks et al. (228) and Montana et al. (417) reported a higher incidence of central pelvic recurrences in patients with stage III cervical carcinoma treated with external-beam therapy alone than in patients receiving brachytherapy in addition to external-beam irradiation (Table 66.19). The incidence of major complications was similar in both groups of patients.

Akine et al. (9) treated 104 patients with carcinoma of the uterine cervix with external irradiation alone (anteroposterior–posteroanterior or four-field box techniques) because of inability to perform intracavitary brachytherapy. Average doses delivered were 50 Gy to the whole pelvis, followed by additional doses with reduced portals to deliver a total of 60.8 Gy in 6 weeks, 72.3 Gy in 7.5 weeks, or 80.5 Gy in 8 weeks, with a daily dose of 1.9 or 2 Gy. The local tumor control rate was 27% for stage II, 19% for stage III, and 15% for stage IVA disease. The 5-year survival rates were 36%, 17%, and 5%, respectively. Four patients had major complications (usually proctitis) that required surgical treatment, and one patient died of rectal bleeding. Eight of 23 patients treated with conformal therapy

Table 66.19	CARCINOMA OF THE UTERINE CERVIX: INCIDENCE OF CENTRAL/PELVIC RECURRENCES CORRELATED WITH METHOD OF THERAPY			
		Incidence of Pelvic Failures		
Author (Reference)	Stage	External-Beam Only	External-Beam and Intracavitary	p Value
Hanks et al. (228)	III	33/38 (86%)	55/109 (50%)	0.0002
Montana et al. (417)	III	14/35 (40%)	12/37 (32%)	0.6725
Coia et al. (90)	I,II,III	(53%)	(22%)	<0.0100
Longsdon & Eifel[a] (382)	IIIB	641 (45%)	266 (24%)	<0.0001

[a]Five-year disease-free survival.
Modified from Stehman FR, Perez CA, Kurman RJ, et al. Uterine cervix. In: Hoskins WJ, Perez CA, Young RC, eds. *Principles and practice of gynecologic oncology,* 3rd ed. Philadelphia: Lippincott Williams & Wilkins, 2000:841–918.

had control of the tumor and survived 5 years without major complications.

Saibishkumar et al (540) treated 146 patients with cervix cancer with EBRT alone (60 to 66 Gy), because of unsuitability for brachytherapy; 5-year pelvic tumor control was 21.9% and DFS 11.6%.

Impact of Tumor Size on Outcome

Perez et al. (474), in an update of a previous report (476), reviewed 1,499 patients (stages IA to IVA) treated with definitive irradiation (combination of external-beam irradiation plus two intracavitary insertions to deliver doses of 70 to 90 Gy to point A). There was a close correlation between tumor size and extent with pelvic tumor control, incidence of distant metastasis, and disease-free survival in all stages. Eifel et al. (140), in a review of 1,526 patients with stage IB squamous-cell carcinoma of the uterine cervix treated with radiation therapy alone, noted pelvic tumor control in 97% of tumors <5 cm and in 84% of tumors 5 to 7 cm.

Impact of Prolongation of Treatment Time on Outcome

Several studies have described lower pelvic tumor control and survival rates in invasive carcinoma of the uterine cervix when the overall time in a course of irradiation is prolonged (115,167,179,350). Fyles et al. (167) reported approximately 1% loss of tumor control per day of prolongation of treatment time beyond 30 days in 830 patients with cervical carcinoma treated with irradiation alone. Lanciano et al. (350), in an analysis of 837 patients with squamous-cell carcinoma of the cervix from the Patterns of Care Study who were treated with irradiation and received doses of 66 Gy or greater, also described a 4-year actuarial in-field recurrence increase from 6% to 20% when total treatment time increased from 6 weeks or less to 10 weeks (p = 0.0001); this translated into significantly decreased survival.

Girinsky et al. (179), in 386 patients with stage IIB or III carcinoma of the cervix, also observed that the 10-year local recurrence–free survival rate decreased when overall treatment time exceeded 52 days. A 1.1% loss of pelvic tumor control per day was also observed in their regression analysis.

Perez et al. (473), in 1,330 patients treated with definitive irradiation, noted a major impact of prolongation of treatment time on pelvic tumor control in stages IB, IIA, and IIB (Fig. 66.27A,B). In stage III, although the rate of pelvic failure was higher with prolongation of treatment time, the difference was not statistically significant. There was also a strong correlation between overall treatment time and survival (Fig. 66.28A,B).

Regression analysis confirmed previous reports that prolongation of overall treatment time resulted in an increased failure rate of 0.59% per day in stage IB and IIA and 0.86% per day in stage IIB disease. Performance of all intracavitary insertions within 4.5 weeks from initiation of irradiation yielded lower pelvic failure rates (8.8% vs. 18% in stage IIB tumors; p ≤0.01).

In patients treated with radiation therapy, overall treatment time should be as short as possible, and any planned or unplanned interruptions or delays should be avoided. Timely integration of external-beam and intracavitary irradiation in patients with carcinoma of the uterine cervix is an important factor in improving pelvic tumor control.

Metastases to Para-Aortic Lymph Nodes

Para-aortic lymph node metastases are frequently combined with distant dissemination but are clinically apparent in only 10% to 20% of patients who have recurrences.

Nelson et al. (437) reported on 104 patients with stage II and III cervical carcinoma who had exploratory laparotomy and para-aortic lymph node biopsies; 12.5% of patients with stage IIA disease, 14.9% with stage IIB, and 38.4% with stage III disease had para-aortic lymph node metastases. They were treated with 60 Gy to the para-aortic region. Within 4 years, 50% of these patients had distant metastases and only one out of 13 was alive. There was no significant increase in complications in the patients receiving para-aortic irradiation (39% and 32%). They concluded that the main goal of exploratory laparotomy and para-aortic lymph node biopsy is to define the extent of disease.

Lovecchio et al. (388) noted a 50% 5-year survival rate in 36 patients with stage IB and IIA cervical carcinoma who had histologically confirmed para-aortic lymph node metastases treated with RT (including 45 Gy to the para-aortic lymph nodes). Fourteen of 31 evaluable patients had pelvic recurrences (12 combined with distant metastases). Unfortunately, the authors did not specify how many patients had para-aortic recurrences, although they reported four abdominal failures.

Stryker and Mortel (585) determined survival after extended-field treatment of para-aortic lymph node metastasis plus brachytherapy or pelvic boost in 35 patients; 5-year survival was 41.7% for 12 patients with microscopic para-aortic lymph node metastasis and 26.1% for 23 with grossly enlarged lymph nodes. Three patients (8.6%) had grade 4 morbidity.

Grigsby et al. (199) reviewed 43 patients with cervical cancer and biopsy-proven positive para-aortic lymph nodes treated with external irradiation to the pelvis and para-aortic regions (45 to 50 Gy) combined with brachytherapy. The 5-year overall survival rate was 32%, and the cause-specific survival rate was 49%. Tumor recurrence occurred in 20 patients (three in the pelvis, nine in pelvis and distant metastasis, and eight

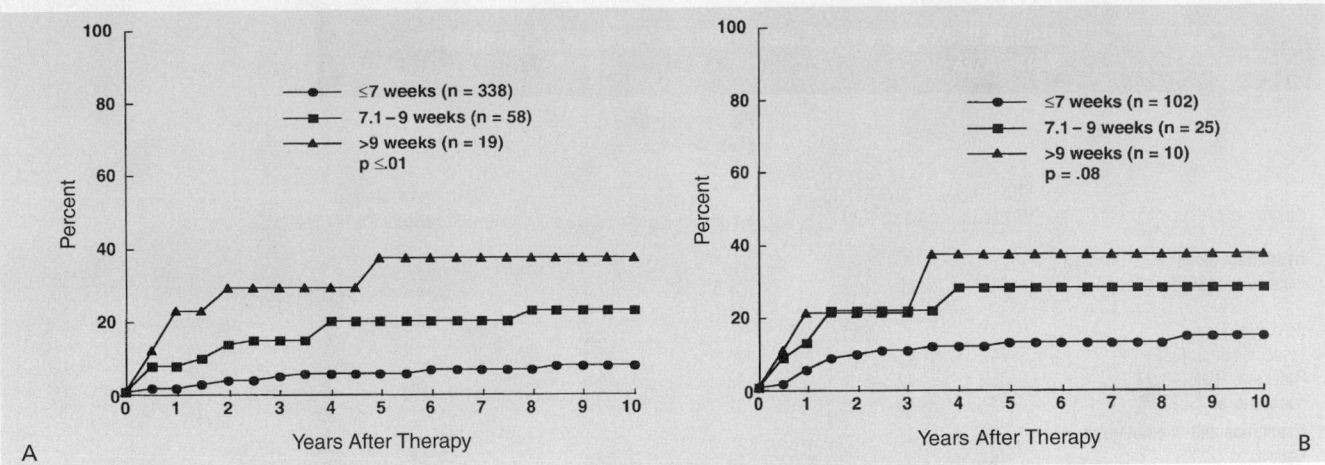

FIGURE 66.27. Pelvic failure rate correlated with length of treatment in stage IB **(A)** and IIA **(B)** carcinoma of the uterine cervix. (From Perez CA, Grigsby PW, Castro-Vita H, et al. Carcinoma of the uterine cervix: I. Impact of prolongation of treatment time and timing of brachytherapy on outcome of radiation therapy. *Int J Radiat Oncol Biol Phys* 1995;32:1275–1288, with permission.)

distant metastasis only). Severe grade 3 complications occurred in two patients (one had an enterovaginal fistula and the other radiation myelitis).

Hacker et al. (216), in 437 patients with invasive cervical carcinoma, 222 treated with radical hysterectomy and lymphadenectomy, identified 34 in whom resection of bulky pelvic or para-aortic lymph nodes was carried out without a complete lymphadenectomy. Thirty-three patients received pelvic external irradiation, and 28 combined pelvic and para-aortic extended-field irradiation (50.4 Gy in 1.8-Gy fractions using a four-field technique). Four cycles of cisplatin were administered to 23 patients. The 5-year survival was 80% in patients with pelvic and common iliac nodes and 48% in those with positive para-aortic lymph nodes. Serious long-term morbidity occurred in six patients (18%). Radiation enteritis was observed in five patients, leading to small bowel obstruction necessitating resection.

Grigsby et al. (196) evaluated twice-daily external irradiation to the pelvis and para-aortic nodes (1.2 Gy at 4- to 6-hour intervals, 5 days per week) combined with brachytherapy and concurrent chemotherapy in 29 patients with carcinoma of the cervix and positive para-aortic lymph nodes. EBRT doses were 24 to 48 Gy to the whole pelvis, 12 to 36 Gy parametrial boost,

and 48 Gy to the para-aortics with additional boost to a total dose of 54 to 58 Gy to known metastatic para-aortic sites. One or two LDR brachytherapy applications were performed to deliver a total dose of 85 Gy to point A. Cisplatin (75 mg/m^2, days 1 and 22) and 5FU (1,000 mg/m^2 per 24 hours for 4 days; days 1 and 22) were given for two or three cycles. Hyperfractionated external radiation therapy was completed in 86% (25/29). Radiation therapy toxicity was grade 2 in 34%, grade 3 in 21%, and grade 4 in 28%. An unacceptably high rate (31%, 9/29) of grade 4 nonhematologic toxicity was recorded. With a median follow-up of 18.9 months, at 2 years the overall survival rate was 47%, and the probability of locoregional failure was 49%.

Malfetano et al. (395) treated 67 patients with carcinoma of the cervix (44 with stage IIB and 23 with stage III disease) with cisplatin (1 mg/kg up to 60 mg weekly) and extended-field radiation therapy, including the para-aortic nodes, and brachytherapy; 75% were alive without evidence of disease with a mean follow-up of 47.5 months.

Chou et al. (82) treated 19 patients with isolated para-aortic lymph node metastasis from cervix cancer, 14 of them with chemoradiation, four with chemotherapy, and one with irradiation alone. Seven of the 14 patients receiving chemoradiation survived.

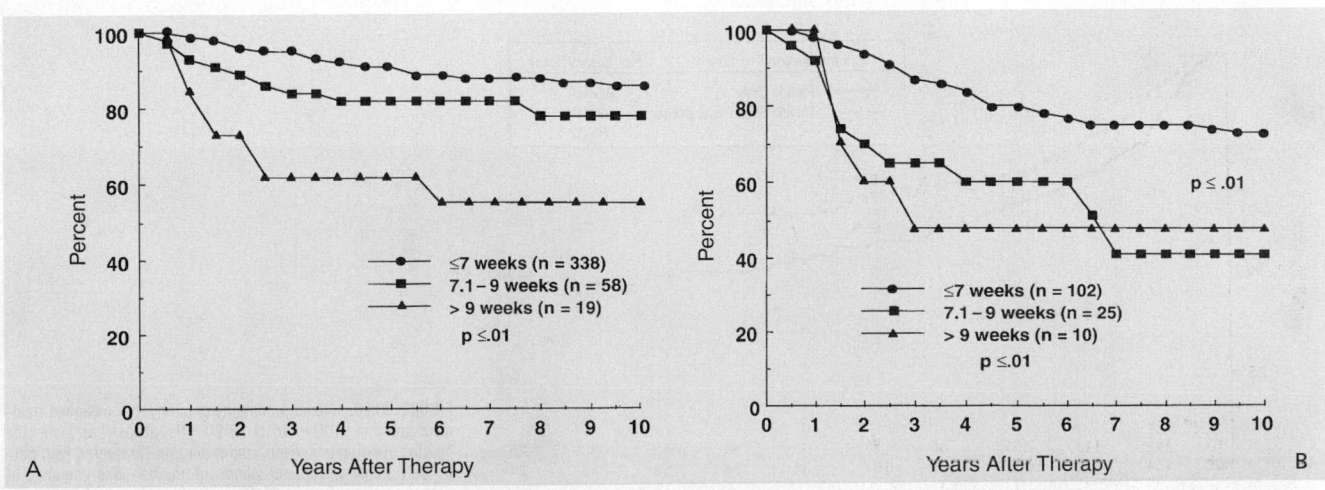

FIGURE 66.28. Cause-specific survival correlated with overall treatment time in stage IB **(A)** and IIA **(B)** carcinoma of the uterine cervix. (From Perez CA, Grigsby PW, Castro-Vita H, et al. Carcinoma of the uterine cervix: I. Impact of prolongation of treatment time and timing of brachytherapy on outcome of radiation therapy. *Int J Radiat Oncol Biol Phys* 1995;32:1275–1288, with permission.)

Table 66.20	RESULTS OF EXTENDED-FIELD IRRADIATION FOR PARA-AORTIC LYMPH NODE METASTASES				
Author (Reference)	No. of Patients	Para-Aortic Dose (Gy)	Percentage Disease-Free Survival		Incidence of Severe Complications (%)
			2–3 Years	5 Years	
Irradiation Alone					
Piver et al. (486) (two cohorts)	21	60	9.6	61.9	—
	10	44–50	43	10.0	—
Potish (497)	81	43.5–50.75	40	2.4	—
Lovecchio et al. (388)	36	45	70	50.0	—
Podczaski et al. (492)	35	42.5–51	38	29.0	9
Kodaira et al. (332)	97	50–70	32	—	—
Irradiation and Chemotherapy					
Chou et al. (82)	26	50	19	51.0	20
Kim et al. (319)	12	—	50	—	—
Singh et al. (560)	14	—	—	—	—
Varia et al. (631)	95	45	39[d]	14.0	—
Grigsby et al. (196)	29	48 (b.i.d.)	49	49.0	—
Malfetano et al. (395)	13	45	62	0	—
Podczaski et al. (492)[a]	33	42–51	37	31.0	9

[a]Only six patients treated with chemotherapy.
Modified from Goodman HM, Bowling MC, Nelson JH Jr. Cervical malignancies. In: Knapp RC, Berkowitz RS, eds. *Gynecologic oncology.* New York: Macmillan, 1986;225–273, with permission.

Goodman et al. (183) compiled survival statistics on patients with para-aortic lymph node metastasis and found an average 5-year survival rate of approximately 40% (Table 66.20).

Elective Para-Aortic Lymph Node Irradiation

Rotman et al. (527) for the RTOG (527) updated results of a randomized study of 337 patients with stage IIB carcinoma of the uterine cervix with no clinical or radiographic evidence of para-aortic lymphadenopathy who, in addition to standard pelvic irradiation, were randomized to electively receive or not 45 Gy to the para-aortic region (1.6- to 1,8-Gy fractions). The 10-year survival rate was 55% for patients receiving elective para-aortic irradiation and 44% for those treated to the pelvis only (p = 0.02; Fig. 66.29). The locoregional tumor control rate was similar (69% in the para-aortic node–irradiated group and 65% for

the pelvis-irradiated group). The 10-year grade 4 or 5 (major) complication rate was 8% in the group receiving para-aortic irradiation compared with 4% in patients treated with pelvic irradiation alone (p = 0.06).

A similar randomized study was reported by Haie et al. (219) and the European Organization for Research and Treatment of Cancer (EORTC) on 441 patients with cervical carcinoma, including stage III, who had no evidence of para-aortic lymph node involvement. In the study group, the para-aortic area either received or did not receive 45 Gy with external-beam irradiation. No statistically significant difference was found between the two treatment arms with regard to local tumor control, distant metastases, or survival. However, the incidence of para-aortic and distant metastases without pelvic failure was significantly higher in patients receiving pelvic irradiation alone. The incidence of small bowel injury was 0.9% in the pelvic irradiation and 2.3% in the pelvic and para-aortic

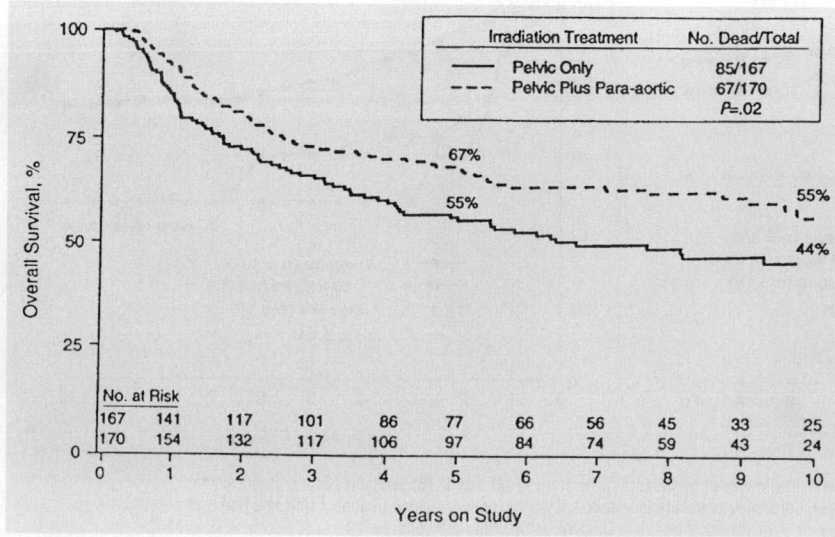

FIGURE 66.29. Overall probability of survival by assigned treatment group in RTOG Protocol 79-20. "No. at Risk" indicates the number of patients in each irradiation arm (presented with data for pelvic only on top) for whom information was complete at each year. (From Rotman M, Pajak TF, Choi K, et al. Prophylactic extended-field irradiation of para-aortic lymph nodes in stages IIB and bulky IB and IIA cervical carcinomas: ten-year treatment results of RTOG 79-20. *JAMA* 1996;274:387–393, with permission.)

Table 66.21	CARCINOMA OF THE UTERINE CERVIX: 5-YEAR DISEASE-FREE SURVIVAL RATES (MALLINCKRODT INSTITUTE OF RADIOLOGY, 1959–1982)					
	Irradiation Only			**Irradiation and Surgery**		
Stage	**Epidermoid (%)**	**Adenocarcinoma (%)**	***p* Value**	**Epidermoid (%)**	**Adenocarcinoma (%)**	***p* Value**
IA	29/29 (100)	2/2 (100)	—	8/8 (100)	2/2 (100)	—
IB	265/302 (87.7)	32/38 (84.2)	0.57	81/102 (79.4)	14/16 (87.5)	0.80
IIA	73/103 (70.9)	5/9 (55.6)	0.39	22/32 (68.8)	1/3 (33.3)	0.26
IIB	165/249 (66.3)	10/18 (55.6)	0.43	32/47 (68.1)	—	—
III	83/226 (36.7)	3/12 (25)	0.007	13/22 (59.1)	—	—

Modified from Grigsby PW, Perez CA, Kuske RR, et al. Adenocarcinoma of the uterine cervix: lack of evidence for a poor prognosis. *Radiother Oncol* 1988;12:289–296, with permission.

irradiation groups. A severe complication rate of 9% was observed in patients receiving para-aortic irradiation compared with 4.8% in those treated to the pelvis only.

Sood et al. (571) treated 54 patients with cervix cancer using extended fields (45 Gy) and HDR BT; 44 received concurrent cisplatin (20 mg/m2 per day for 5 days during the first and fourth week and once after the second HDR insertion). During a median follow-up of 28 months, six patients had died. The 3-year local tumor control was a 100% and 85%, respectively. Late toxicity was 10% and 6%, respectively.

Adenocarcinoma of the Cervix

Several authors have reported similar survival rates for equivalent stages of adenocarcinoma or squamous-cell carcinoma; clinical stage, volume of disease, and dose of irradiation were the most important prognostic factors (200,315). Grigsby et al. (200) found no difference in 5-year DFS in patients with adenocarcinoma of the cervix compared with squamous-cell treated with RT alone or combined with surgery (Table 66.21).

Similar observations were reported by Eifel et al. (138) in 229 patients with stage IB adenocarcinoma of the cervix. The 5-year survival rates were 72% versus 81% for squamous-cell carcinoma. The incidence of pelvic recurrence was similar (17% for adenocarcinoma and 13% for squamous-cell carcinoma). However, distant metastases were more frequent in patients with adenocarcinoma (37% vs. 21%; *p* <0.01). The survival rate in 165 patients who underwent adjuvant hysterectomy (78%) was not significantly different from that of patients who did not have a surgical procedure (71%). Later Eifel et al. (141) studied 334 patients with adenocarcinoma of the cervix. The 5-year relapse-free survival and locoregional control rates were 88% and 94%, respectively, in 91 patients with a normal-sized cervix, 64% and 82%, respectively, in 102 patients with lesions 3 to 5.9 cm in diameter, but only 45% and 81% in 22 patients with tumors >6 cm in diameter.

Fifty-eight patients with adenocarcinoma of the cervix treated with LDR or HDR brachytherapy and external pelvic irradiation were studied by Nakano et al. (433). The 10-year survival rates for stages I, II, III, and IV were 85.7%, 60%, 27.6%, and 9.1%, respectively. The local tumor control rate with HDR treatment was 45.5%, significantly lower than with LDR (85.7%) or mixed–dose-rate treatments (72.7%).

Kilgore et al. (315), in a study of 162 patients with adenocarcinoma compared with matched patients with squamous-cell carcinoma, found that clinical stage and lesion size were the most important prognostic factors. In patients with stage I tumors, no significant difference in survival was found when they were treated with radical surgery, irradiation alone, or irradiation combined with hysterectomy.

In contrast, Kjorstad et al. (327) reported a worse 5-year survival rate in 102 patients with adenocarcinoma (51%) compared with that of 1,900 patients with squamous-cell or other differentiated carcinomas (68%).

Comparison of Low–Dose-Rate and High–Dose-Rate Brachytherapy Results

Randomized Studies

A few randomized studies have been published comparing HDR and LDR brachytherapy for carcinoma of the cervix (215). A report by Shigematsu et al. (556), in patients with stage IIB or III disease treated with the HDR technique, showed higher 1-year local control (90%) with HDR versus 77% with LDR. The 5-year survival rate was 55% for both groups. Another trial including patients with stage IB, IIA, IIB, and III disease by Gupta et al. (215) showed similar local tumor control rates for both HDR and LDR (80% and 85%, respectively). However, the stage distributions in each group and the survival and complication rates were not described.

Teshima et al. (603) reported on a prospective, randomized study of 430 patients with carcinoma of the uterine cervix treated with either LDR (171 patients) or HDR (259 patients) brachytherapy combined with external irradiation. Cause-specific and overall survival rates were comparable for each clinical stage with either modality, except for stage I overall survival (Fig. 66.30). The conversion factor of total intracavitary dose from LDR to HDR was 0.5 to 0.53. With HDR, four fractions usually were delivered, and with LDR two fractions. The incidence of pelvic failures was comparable in both groups. The incidence of grade 2 and 3 morbidity was somewhat higher in the HDR group (approximately 10%) than in the LDR group (4%; *p* = 0.002).

Patel et al. (463) published a randomized trial of 482 patients with invasive squamous-cell carcinoma of the cervix. The overall local tumor control rate with LDR brachytherapy was 79.7% compared with 75.8% with HDR. The 5-year survival rates were 73% with LDR and 78% with HDR in stage I, 62% and 64%, respectively, in stage II, and 50% and 43% in stage III. The only statistically significant difference was the incidence of overall rectal complications, which was 19.9% for LDR compared with 6.4% for HDR. However, the incidences of more severe grade 3 and 4 complications were not significantly different (2.5% and 0.4%, respectively). Bladder morbidity was similar in both groups. Hareyama et al. (231) conducted a randomized study in 132 patients with stage II or IIIB cervical carcinoma treated with LDR or HDR BT and identical pelvic EBRT. The conversion factor from LDR to HDR was 0.588. The 5-year DSS with HDR for stage II and IIIB was 69% and 51%, respectively, and with LDR 87% and 60%, respectively. Pelvic tumor control was 89% and 73% and 100% and 70%, respectively, and grade 3 or

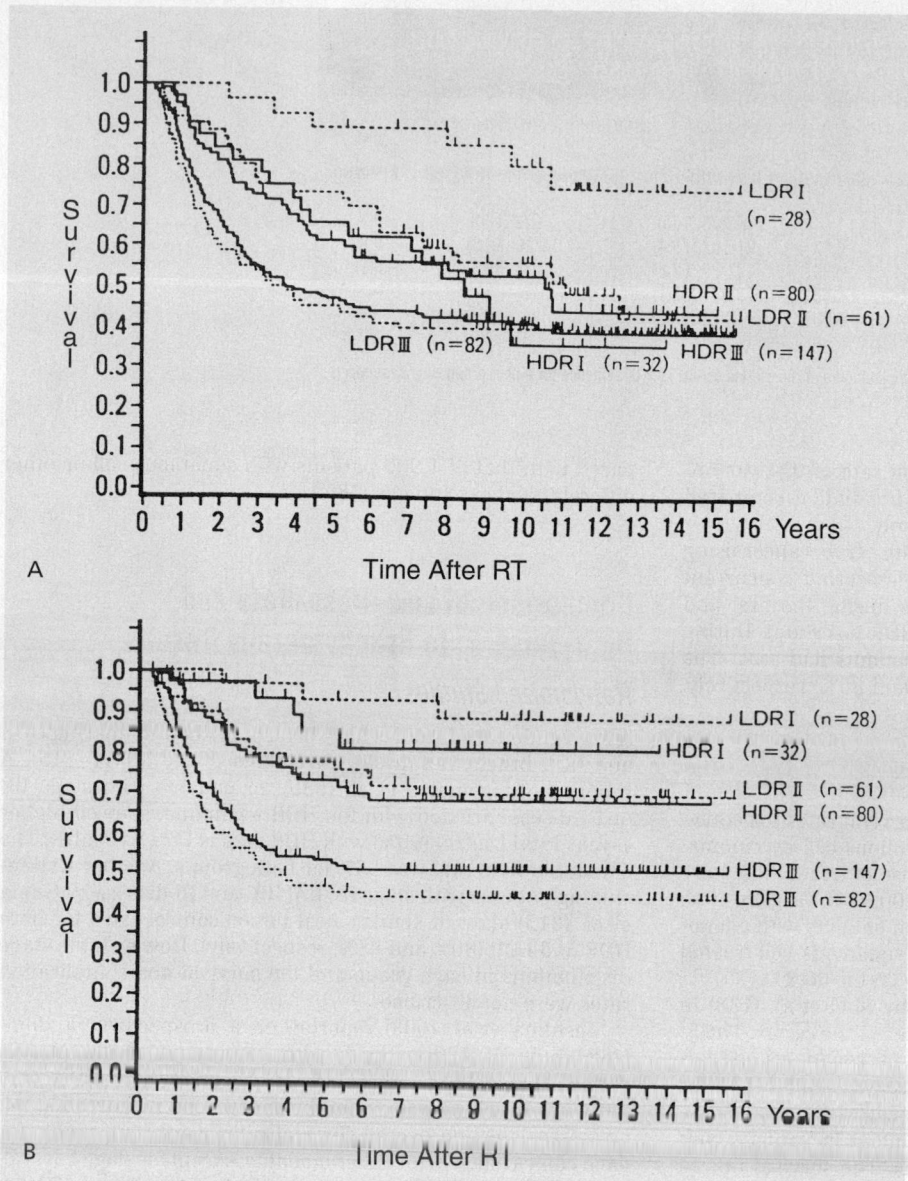

FIGURE 66.30. Actuarial survival rates **(A)** and actuarial cause-specific survival rates **(B)** of patients with carcinoma of the uterine cervix treated with LDR or HDR brachytherapy, correlated with stage and treatment group (January 1975 to August 1983). HDR, high-dose radiation, LDR, low dose radiation, RT, radiation therapy. (From Ieshima I, Inoue I, Ikeda H, et al. High dose rate and low-dose rate intracavitary therapy for carcinoma of the uterine cervix: final results of Osaka University Hospital. *Cancer* 1993;72:2409–2414, with permission.)

greater morbidity was 10% and 13%, respectively (differences were not statistically significant).

Lertsanguansinchai et al. (373) randomized 237 patients with cervical cancer to be treated with LDR (109 patients) or HDR (112 patients) brachytherapy and EBRT. Median follow-up was 40 and 37 months, respectively. Three-year pelvic tumor control was 89% and 86.4% and relapse-free survival 69% in both groups. Grade 3 or 4 morbidity was noted in 2.8% of LDR and 7.1% of the HDR patients ($p = 0.23$).

Nonrandomized Studies

Many nonrandomized studies compared the results of HDR with those of historic or concurrent control patients receiving LDR at the same institution (21,87,165,180,247,289). Most studies used point A as a reference point, although the definition of point A may have differed from center to center.

HDR dose per fraction at point A was 3 to 10 Gy; the number of fractions ranged from two to 13, and the number of fractions per week varied from one to three. Most centers used a schedule of 6 to 7 Gy per fraction per week for four to six fractions.

Table 66.22 illustrates the 5-year survival rates of patients who received HDR or LDR brachytherapy combined with external-beam irradiation for carcinoma of the cervix. Stage for stage, 5-year survival rates of patients treated with the HDR technique are comparable with those of historic or concurrent nonrandomized patients treated with LDR.

In an analysis of 198 patients treated with LDR brachytherapy at the University of Wisconsin, the 3-year survival rate was 66% versus 77% for 40 patients treated with HDR brachytherapy (545). Pelvic tumor control rate were 80% and 77%, respectively. The incidences of complications requiring hospitalization or surgery were 10% (20/198) and 2.5% (1/40), respectively.

Petereit et al. (482) updated the University of Wisconsin experience with 191 patients receiving LDR brachytherapy and 173 receiving HDR brachytherapy with equivalent external-beam radiation therapy techniques. The results are summarized in Tables 66.23 and 66.24. Pelvic tumor control and survival rates were comparable with the two techniques, except in stage III; in this subgroup, outcome was better with LDR brachytherapy, but this may be related to a lower HDR equivalent dose administered.

Table 66.22 HIGH–DOSE-RATE VERSUS LOW–DOSE-RATE BRACHYTHERAPY FOR CARCINOMA OF THE CERVIX: SURVIVAL

Author (Reference)	Stage	No. of Patients, HDR/LDR	HDR	LDR
Glaser (180)	I–III	493/288	59[a]	33[a] ($p = 0.001$)
Cikaric (87)	II	85/66	54	70
	III	52/120	37	43
Akine et al. (9)	IIB	20/83	67	56
	IIIB	37/212	54	38
Hareyama et al. (231)	I–II	61/61	69/51	87/60
Hsu et al. (266)	I–II	92/259	68	74
Ferrigno et al. (154)	I–III	118/190	55	69
Kuipers (339a)	I	21/32	76	80
	II	54/71	74	68
	III	36/42	36	48
Lertsanguansinchai et al. (373)	I–III	112/109	69	69
Shigematsu et al. (556)	IIB and III	143/106	55	55
Teshima et al. (603)	I–III	227/171	85/60	90/60
Arai et al. (21)	I	86/31	83	87
	II	173/125	71	75
	III	212/253	51	49
	IV	46/80	24	16

(5-Year Survival %)

HDR, high-dose-rate; LDR, low-dose-rate.
[a]Relapse-free survival.
Modified from Fu KK, Philips TL. High-dose rate versus low-dose rate intracavitary brachytherapy for carcinoma of the cervix. *Int J Radiat Oncol Biol Phys* 1990;19:791–796, with permission.

Le Pechoux et al. (359) treated 130 patients with cervical cancer with HDR brachytherapy (for stage I, 30 Gy in six weekly sessions) in combination with EBRT (50-Gy mean dose with midline shielding). Patients with more advanced disease received four sessions of biweekly brachytherapy for a total dose of 18 to 24 Gy and external irradiation (20 to 30 Gy to the whole pelvis, 50 to 66 Gy to parametria with midline shielding). The 5-year survival rates were 82% for patients with stage IIB and 47% with stage IIIB disease. There were four rectovaginal or vesicovaginal fistulas and one case of proctitis requiring colostomy. Survival, local tumor control, and morbidity were equivalent in 76 patients treated with 6 Gy once a week and in 54 patients receiving twice-weekly brachytherapy of 5 Gy per session.

Hsu et al. (266) treated 92 patients with cancer of the cervix with HDR brachytherapy, six fractions of 7 Gy per fraction (42 Gy) at point A (HDR-6); 57 received four fractions of 8 Gy per fraction (32 Gy) at point A (HDR-4). A twice-daily program was used for all patients receiving HDR in two split courses.

A historic control group of 259 patients was treated with LDR brachytherapy (40 Gy in two split courses). All patients received whole pelvis external irradiation of 36 to 45 Gy (mostly 40 Gy) before brachytherapy. Five-year local tumor control rates were equivalent in the three groups (82%, 85.5% for HDR, and 89.5% for LDR). Five-year survival rates were also comparable (67.7%, 77.9%, and 74.1%, respectively). However, late complications were lower in the HDR-4 group, which received treatment more biologically equivalent to the LDR regimen, than in patients in the HDR-6 group (11% vs. 25.6%).

Selke et al. (548) published results in 187 patients with primary carcinoma of the cervix treated with whole pelvis irradiation (46 Gy) and HDR brachytherapy with a dose rate to point A of 1.6 Gy per minute, decreasing to approximately 0.8 Gy per minute at the end of the 5-year study. Three HDR fractions (8 to 10 Gy to point A per fraction) were concurrently administered with the last 2 to 3 weeks of external irradiation. The 5-year actuarial survival rates were 72% for stage IB, 65% for

Table 66.23 UNIVERSITY OF WISCONSIN UPDATE: 3-YEAR SURVIVAL AND RELAPSE-FREE SURVIVAL RATES COMPARING HIGH–DOSE-RATE AND LOW–DOSE-RATE BRACHYTHERAPY FOR CERVICAL CANCER

	Survival[a]		Relapse-Free Survival[a]	
	HDR	LDR	HDR	LDR
Overall	62% (173)	67% (191)	63% (173)	70% (191)
Stage IB	86% (59)	82% (76)	85% (59)	81% (76)
Stage II	65% (64)	58% (65)	69% (64)	61% (65)
Stage IIIB	33% (50)	58% (50)	30% (50)	63% (50)

HDR, high-dose-rate; LDR, low-dose-rate.
[a]Number of patients is in parentheses.
From Petereit DG. Refresher course no. 103: high-dose rate brachytherapy for carcinoma of the cervix. Presented at the 40th Annual Meeting of the American Society for Therapeutic Radiology and Oncology, Phoenix, Arizona, October 1998, with permission.

Table 66.24	UNIVERSITY OF WISCONSIN UPDATE: 3-YEAR PELVIC TUMOR CONTROL AND DISTANT METASTASES RATES COMPARING HIGH–DOSE-RATE AND LOW–DOSE-RATE BRACHYTHERAPY FOR CERVICAL CANCER			
	Pelvic Tumor Control[a]		**Distant Metastases**[a]	
	HDR	**LDR**	**HDR**	**LDR**
Overall	71% (173)	82% (191)	20% (173)	15% (191)
Stage IB	85% (59)	91% (76)	8% (59)	7% (76)
Stage II	80% (64)	78% (65)	17% (64)	25% (65)
Stage IIIB	44% (50)	75% (50)	35% (50)	17% (50)

HDR, high–dose-rate; LDR, low–dose-rate.
[a]Number of patients is in parentheses.
From Petereit DG. Refresher course no. 103: high dose rate brachytherapy for carcinoma of the cervix. Presented at the 40th Annual Meeting of the American Society for Therapeutic Radiology and Oncology, Phoenix, Arizona, October 1998, with permission.

IIA, 66% for IIB, 66% for IIIA, and 45% for stage IIIB. With a median follow-up of 54 months, 23 patients had 25 complications; 13 (7.6%) were grade 3 or 4. Rectal complications were significantly higher in patients who received a total rectal dose higher than 54 Gy ($p = 0.045$).

Choi et al. (81) treated 136 patients with carcinoma of the cervix with external-beam whole pelvis irradiation (46 Gy in 23 fractions) and three weekly applications of HDR brachytherapy of 7 or 8 Gy per fraction to point A. The actuarial 5-year survival was 85% in stage IB, 64% in stage IIA, 70% in stage IIB, and 53% in stage IIIB. Grade 3 or higher complications occurred 3% to 7% of the patients. The most significant determinants of severe rectal complications were the addition of a lower vaginal tandem ($p < 0.01$), uterine tandem length longer than 5 cm, a total biologically effective dose to the rectum of more than 120 Gy, or stage III disease.

Kagei et al. (290) reported on 217 patients with carcinoma of the cervix (71 patients with stage II and 146 with stage III disease) who received whole pelvis EBRT (40 Gy in 20 fractions or 39.6 Gy in 22 fractions) and an additional 10 Gy in five fractions to the parametria followed by HDR brachytherapy. Cause-specific 5-year survival rates were 77% for stage II and 50% for stage III. Pelvic failure rates were 19% and 36% respectively. The rates of severe (grade 4) late complications were 2% for the rectum, 1% for the small intestine or sigmoid colon, and 1% for the bladder.

Takeshi et al. (595) treated 265 patients with stage III cervical carcinoma with external-beam radiation therapy (50.3 Gy) and intracavitary HDR brachytherapy (19.8 Gy). The 5-year overall survival, relapse-free survival, and locoregional event–free rates were 50.7%, 57.1%, and 71.2%, respectively. The 5-year incidence of major complications was 2.6% for bladder and 8.3% for rectum. The radiation dose in the subgroup with rectal complications was significantly greater than that in the subgroup without complications.

Wang et al. (641) reported treatment results in 173 patients with cervical carcinoma treated with HDR brachytherapy, whole pelvis irradiation (40 to 44 Gy in 20 to 22 fractions) followed by pelvic wall boost (6 to 14 Gy in three to seven fractions with central shielding). HDR brachytherapy delivered 7.2 Gy to point A in each of three applications, 1 to 2 weeks apart. Five-year pelvic tumor control rates were 94%, 87%, and 72% for stages IIA, IIB to IIIA, and IIIB to IVA, respectively. Five-year actuarial survival rates were 79%, 59%, and 41%, respectively. Sixty-six (38%) had rectal complications and 19 (11%) bladder complications. The 5-year actuarial rectal complication rates were 15%, 4%, and 3% for grades 2, 3, and 4, respectively.

Potter et al. (499) reported results in 148 patients treated with HDR brachytherapy and EBRT (48.6 to 50 Gy). Small tumors were treated with five to six fractions of 7 Gy at point A (25 Gy in the brachytherapy volume), which is isoeffective to 76 to 86 Gy at point A. Large tumors received three to four fractions of

7 Gy after 50 Gy of EBRT, which is isoeffective to 82 to 92 Gy at point A. Three-dimensional treatment planning for brachytherapy was based on conventional x-rays, and in 181/189 patients on CT scan. The mean brachytherapy dose was 16.2 Gy at the ICRU rectum reference point and 14.4 Gy at the ICRU bladder point. Taking into account the dose for EBRT, the mean isoeffective dose at the ICRU rectum reference point was 69.9 Gy. After a mean follow-up of 34 months, the actuarial late complication rate for grades 3 and 4 was 2.9% for bladder, 4% for bowel, 6.1% for rectum, and 30.6% for the vagina (shortening and obliteration).

Lorvidhaya et al. (386) reported the results in 1,992 patients with carcinoma of the cervix treated by external irradiation and HDR brachytherapy. There were 211 with stage IB, 225 with stage IIA, 902 with stage IIB, 14 with stage IIIA, 675 with stage IIIB, 16 with stage IVA, and 16 (0.8%) with stage IVB. With a median follow-up of 96 months, the actuarial 5-year disease-free survival rates were 70%, 59.4%, 46.1%, 32.3%, 7.8%, and 23,1%, respectively. The late complication rates (RTOG) for bowel and bladder combined were 7% for grade 3 and 1.9% for grade 4 complications.

Leborgne et al. (362) described a 4-year pelvic control rate of 93%, and a disease-free survival rate of 80% for 59 patients with stage IB to IIA disease treated with 18 Gy whole pelvis and 22 Gy to the parametria combined with six HDR fractions (14 Gy per hour to point A) of 7 Gy to point A, two in each treatment day with 6-hour intervals. The corresponding parameters for 29 patients with stage IIB disease were 79%, 75%, and 75%. The actuarial 4-year late grade 2 and 3 complication rate was 4.7%.

Ferrigno et al. (154) carried out a retrospective study of 190 patients treated with LDR and 118 with HDR brachytherapy in combination with pelvic EBRT for cervical cancer. For stage I or II patients, there was no difference in outcome; however, in the stage III group local tumor control was 58% with LDR and 50% with HDR ($p = 0.19$) and DFS was 49% versus 37% ($p = 0.03$). At 5 years, rectal sequelae were 16% versus 8% ($p = 0.03$), bladder 6% and 3% ($p = 0.13$), and small bowel 4.6% and 8.9% ($p = 0.17$).

Nakano et al. (434), in 1,148 patients with squamous-cell cervical cancer treated with external RT and HDR brachytherapy with 22 years median follow-up, the 10-year pelvic tumor control was 93% for stage IB, 82% for stage II, and 75% for stage III. Cause-specific survival was 89%, 74%, and 59%, respectively. Major sequelae were 4.4% in the rectosigmoid, 0.9% in the bladder, and 3.3% in the small intestine.

Kapp et al. (298) analyzed 720 ^{192}Ir HDR applications in 331 patients with gynecologic tumors to evaluate the dose to normal tissues. The ratio of bladder-base dose to bladder-neck dose was 1.5 for intracervical and 1.46 for intravaginal applications. CT-assisted dosimetry showed that the maximum doses to bladder and rectum were generally higher than those obtained from orthogonal films, with an average ratio of 1.44 for the bladder neck, 2.42 for the bladder base, and 1.37 for the rectum. If conventional methods are used for dosimetry, the authors recommended that doses to the bladder base should be routinely calculated because single-point measurements at the bladder neck seriously underestimate the dose to the bladder. Also, the rectal dose should be determined at several points over the length of the implant because of the wide range of anatomic variations.

Wright et al. (664) developed a questionnaire to elicit patient preference for two brachytherapy methods (one LDR or three HDR fractions and two HDR or five HDR fractions, assuming both methods to be isoeffective). The questionnaire was completed by 90 female staff members at their center, 18 previously treated patients, and 20 newly diagnosed patients. When both methods were assumed to be isoeffective, only 34% of the 38 patients preferred three HDR fractions to one LDR fraction. However, when HDR was assumed to be 2% more curative or 6% less toxic, 50% said they would prefer the HDR therapy. Both preference and strength of preference for LDR were significantly associated with a greater traveling distance for treatments.

Studies on resource utilization, such as published by Bastin et al. (31), and cost-effectiveness comparing LDR and HDR treatment should be carried out. These considerations have more relevance as we continue to debate the cost–benefit issues of HDR brachytherapy and health care costs.

Irradiation after Radical Hysterectomy

Only one randomized study has shown improved survival with postoperative pelvic irradiation (46 to 50.4 Gy in 23 to 28 fractions) after radical surgery in the presence of positive pelvic nodes or node-negative high-risk factors in women with stage IB cervical cancer treated by radical hysterectomy and pelvic lymphadenectomy. There were 277 eligible patients with at least two of the following risk factors: greater than one-third stromal invasion, capillary lymphatic space involvement, and large clinical tumor diameter; 137 patients randomized to pelvic radiation therapy and 140 to no further treatment. The results were updated by Rotman et al. (528); 24 (17%) patients in the irradiation group and 43 (30.7%) in the no further treatment group had cancer recurrences. In the radiation therapy group 27 patients died of cancer, and in the no further treatment group 40 died from cancer. There was a statistically significant reduction in risk of recurrence in the irradiation group, with recurrence-free rates at 2 years of 88% versus 79% for the irradiation and no further treatment groups, respectively. Over-

all survival difference did not reach statistical difference ($p = 0.074$) (Fig. 66.31). Severe or life-threatening (GOG grade 3 or 4) adverse effects occurred in nine patients (6.6%) in the radiation therapy group and three (2.1%) in the observation group.

Sundfør et al. (588) conducted a randomized study in which 122 patients with stage IIA and 20 with stage IIB cervix cancer were treated with intracavitary radium followed by either radical pelvic surgery including lymphadenectomy (group A, 72 patients) or EBRT (40 Gy) to the pelvis (group B, 70 patients). Postoperative RT (40 to 50 Gy) was given to patients in group A found to have node metastasis at operation. Fourteen patients in group A and 23 in group B died of recurrent cancer. The 10-year survival was 84% and 69%, respectively.

Treatment techniques may have an effect on outcome. Yamazaki et al. (667) compared 34 patients with cervical cancer treated with irregularly shaped four-field whole pelvis radiation therapy using CT simulation and 40 patients receiving whole pelvis EBRT with parallel-opposed fields in a nonrandomized study of postoperative radiation therapy consisting of 50 Gy in 25 fractions in 6 weeks. With a mean follow-up of 60 months, the actuarial 5-year pelvic tumor control was 94% with the two-field technique and 100% for the irregularly shaped four-field technique. The incidence of grade 2 or 3 bowel complications in the irregularly shaped technique group (2.9%, 1/34) was significantly lower than that in the two-field technique group (17.5%, 7/40; $p < 0.05$).

Burnett et al. (62) described a prosthetic silicone plastic device that is filled with saline and Renografin for x-ray visualization (capacity between 750 and 1,500 mL) to conform to the pelvis and exclude the small bowel from the irradiated volume. The device remains in place throughout the radiation therapy course and is removed through a small incision after draining the contents of the prosthesis. Seven devices had been placed to date of the report. In the postoperative period, there was one pulmonary embolism. All seven patients completed planned radiation therapy. The devices have been removed with no adhesions to the prosthesis.

Many nonrandomized reports on postoperative pelvic irradiation have been published (376,510); some are highlighted here.

Snijders-Keilholtz et al. (563) described results in 233 women who underwent radical hysterectomy for stage I or IIA cervical carcinoma; 156 were treated with surgery alone, and 77 received adjuvant radiation therapy for tumor-related high-risk prognostic factors. The most important prognostic factor for survival and disease-free survival was pelvic lymph node positivity; additional factors were depth of invasion and positive

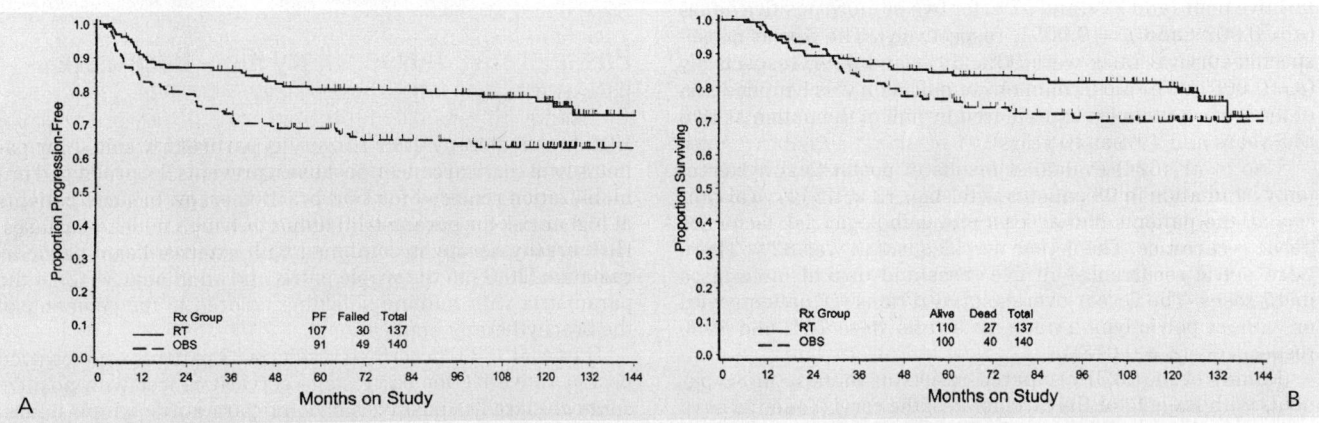

FIGURE 66.31. A: Recurrence-free survival and **(B)** overall survival of patients with stage IB carcinoma of the cervix, correlated with treatment method. (From Rotman M, Sedlis A, Piedmonte MR. A phase III randomized trial of postoperative pelvic irradiation in patients with stage IB cervical carcinoma with poor prognostic features: follow up of a Gynecologic Oncology Group study. *Int J Radiat Oncol Biol Phys* 2006;65:169–176, with permission.)

surgical margins. Twelve patients recurred after surgery alone, all in the pelvis (100%). Of the 23 recurrences after surgery and adjuvant radiation therapy, 13 were in the pelvis (56%; $p = 0.003$). Ten patients with poor prognostic factors and negative nodes received adjuvant radiation therapy, and none of these patients recurred. The incidence of severe gastrointestinal radiation-related side effects was 2%. The incidence of lymphedema of the leg was 11%, which was similar to that in the surgery-alone group.

Garipagaoglu et al. (173) investigated prognostic factors in 100 patients with stage IB or IIA cervical carcinoma treated with radical hysterectomy and postoperative irradiation. The 5-year overall survival, disease-free survival, and pelvic tumor control rates were 83.6%, 82.8%, and 91.8%, respectively. Pelvic lymph node metastasis ($p = 0.008$), interval between surgery and irradiation ($p = 0.001$), overall radiation therapy time ($p = 0.007$), and tumor size ($p = 0.028$) were significant factors for pelvic tumor control as well as for overall survival.

Kahousen et al. (291) reported on a GOG prospectively randomized, multicenter trial in which patients with stage IB or IIB cervical cancer treated with radical hysterectomy who had pelvic lymph node metastases or vascular invasion randomly received adjuvant chemotherapy (400 mg/m^2 carboplatin, and 30 mg bleomycin), or external pelvic radiation therapy, or no further treatment. After a median follow-up of 4.1 years (range, 2 to 7 years), there were no statistically significant differences ($p = 0.9539$) in disease-free survival rates among the three treatment arms, suggesting that adjuvant chemotherapy or radiation does not improve survival or recurrence rates in high-risk patients with cervical cancer after radical hysterectomy.

Gonzales et al. (182) reported that in 89 patients with stage IB or IIA cervical cancer with positive lymph nodes receiving postoperative irradiation, the 5- and 10-year survival rates were 60% and 51%, respectively. By comparison, 43 patients with negative lymph nodes had a survival rate of 85%. In the surviving patients, there were four gastrointestinal and seven genitourinary severe complications requiring surgical correction. In four patients, asymptomatic stenosis of the ureters was detected by IV pyelography performed routinely every year.

Russell et al. (?). In 66 patients receiving external irradiation for pelvic node metastasis after radical hysterectomy, observed a 65% 5-year survival rate. In contrast, in 15 patients who refused postoperative irradiation, only three (20%) survived 5 years.

Chatani et al. (76) reported on 128 patients with stage T1B to T2B carcinoma of the cervix who underwent radical hysterectomy with bilateral pelvic lymphadenectomy and postoperative EBRT. The 5-year local and distant failure rates were, respectively, 2% and 12% for negative nodes, 23% and 25% for one positive node, and 32% and 57%, for two or more positive nodes ($p = 0.0029$ and $p = 0.0051$, respectively). The 5-year cause-specific survival rates were 90%, 59%, and 42%, respectively ($p = 0.0001$). The most common complication was lymphedema of the lower extremity, experienced by half of the patients (42% at 5 years and 49% at 10 years).

Uno et al. (624) evaluated results of postradical hysterectomy irradiation in 98 patients with stage IB to IIB cervical cancer; all the patients had at least one pathologic risk factor for pelvic recurrence. The 5-year overall survival was 82%. There were pelvic recurrences in five cases and distant metastases in 15 cases. The 5-year overall survival rates for patients with or without pelvic lymph node metastasis were 76% and 89%, respectively ($p = 0.018$).

Kinney et al. (323) compared results of therapy in 82 patients with stage IB or IIA carcinoma of the cervix found to have pelvic lymph node metastases at Wertheim hysterectomy and bilateral lymphadenectomy without additional adjuvant therapy with 103 similar patients who received 50 Gy to the pelvis after surgery. The 5-year survival rate was 72% for the surgery-only patients and 64% for the group receiving adjuvant irradia-

tion. The incidences of pelvic recurrences were 67% and 27%, respectively. The lack of impact on overall survival in the irradiated patients is most likely related to a higher incidence of distant metastases, which may be a reflection of higher short-term survival and high-risk patient selection. Kinney et al. (324), in 117 patients treated with radical hysterectomy and pelvic lymphadenectomy, noted histologically proven nodal metastatic disease in 51 patients (44%; squamous cell in 35 and nonsquamous in 16). Nodal involvement was bilateral in 24 patients (47%). Para-aortic lymph node dissection was performed in 14 patients, and five had tumor involvement. Postoperative pelvic irradiation was administered to 29/51 patients (51.2 Gy, two fractions). Extended fields to the para-aortic area were used in six patients. The 5-year survival rates were 33% for the group receiving irradiation and 50% for the not irradiated group. Only one patient treated with postoperative irradiation had a pelvic failure, in contrast to seven patients not irradiated.

Inoue and Morita (269) described results in 72 patients treated with extended-field irradiation after radical surgery for nodal metastases from cervical cancer stage IB (37 patients), IIA (six patients), and IIB (29 patients). The median dose to para-aortic lymph nodes was 43.5 Gy and to the pelvis 45 Gy. The 5-year disease-free survival rates were 72% in 61 patients with squamous-cell carcinoma and 27% in 11 patients with nonsquamous-cell carcinoma. The 10-year disease-free survival rates were 88% for 22 patients with one positive node, 67% for 15 with two or three positive nodes, 64% for 16 with four to 17 positive nodes, and 20% for 10 patients with unresectable lymph nodes. Nineteen severe complications occurred in 17 patients; five were attributed to surgery, five to irradiation, and nine to both modalities. Four patients (5%) died of severe complications. Another six patients (8%) underwent major abdominal surgery for rectovaginal and ureterovaginal fistulas.

Mitsuhashi et al. (414) described an analysis of 108 patients with carcinoma of the cervix treated with postoperative EBRT to the pelvis followed by intravaginal cone boost with electron beam to the vaginal cuff. The 5-year cause-specific survival rates were 89% for 89 patients undergoing elective radiation therapy and 56% for 19 patients undergoing salvage irradiation ($p < 0.001$). Recurrent tumors at the vaginal cuff were observed in only two patients in the elective irradiation group. Vesicovaginal fistula developed in four patients; only one patient had grade 3 rectal complications.

It appears that a modest gain in survival may be observed in patients with pelvic lymph node metastasis from carcinoma of the uterine cervix who receive irradiation after various types of surgery (182,526). More recently, studies involving a comparison of radiation versus radiation with chemotherapy have addressed this issue and are discussed later.

Postoperative Intracavitary High–Dose-Rate Brachytherapy

HDR brachytherapy after surgery is particularly suited for patients with cervical cancer because it prevents the prolonged immobilization required for LDR brachytherapy. In some patients at higher risk for parametrial tumor or lymph node metastases, HDR brachytherapy is combined with external-beam pelvic irradiation (20 Gy to the whole pelvis and additional 30 Gy to the parametria with midline shielding tailored to the geometry of the brachytherapy applications).

Hart et al. (234) described results in 83 patients who received postoperative RT for early stage cervical cancer with positive surgical margins, positive pelvic or para-aortic lymph nodes, lymphovascular space invasion, or deep stromal invasion, or for disease discovered incidentally at simple hysterectomy. Twenty-eight patients were treated with LDR brachytherapy with or without EBRT and 55 with EBRT to the pelvis and HDR intracavitary. Of these 83 patients, 66 were evaluable (20 LDR and

46 HDR patients). Mean follow-up time was 101 months for the LDR group and 42 for the HDR group. The 5-year disease-free survival rate was 89% and 72%, local tumor control was 90% (18/20) and 89% (41/46), respectively. Three of 20 (15%) patients receiving LDR and 4/46 (9%) receiving HDR experienced grade 2 or 3 late treatment-related complications. No patient in either group had grade 4 or 5 complications.

Busch et al. (63) studied the outcome of 68 patients with cervical carcinoma—48 treated with radical hysterectomy and, because of risk factors, with postoperative RT (group 1), and 20 patients (group 2) pretreated with standard hysterectomy—admitted to the hospital for postoperative radiation therapy of the whole pelvis. Postoperative pelvic RT consisted of 39.6 Gy (box technique) and 6-Gy external-beam therapy to the pelvic lymph nodes, sparing the midline plus two HDR applications (7.5 Gy each), and survival, locoregional tumor control, and metastatic disease rates were nearly identical in both groups. Patients with positive lymph nodes had a worse prognosis (75% 3-year survival rate).

Atkovar et al. (25) described results in 126 patients treated with postoperative irradiation (median of 50 Gy in 5 weeks); 37 received vaginal cuff HDR brachytherapy (three fractions of 8 to 10 Gy at 5 mm, weekly). Overall and disease-free survival and locoregional tumor control rates were 71%, 69.9%, and 78.1%, respectively. Grade 2 and 3 complications developed in 5.5% of patients. Survival was the same in 67 patients treated with total abdominal hysterectomy and bilateral salpingo-oophorectomy and in 59 patients treated with radical hysterectomy and pelvic lymphadenectomy.

Sequelae of Treatment

Irradiation Alone

Acute Sequelae

Descriptions of sequelae vary among institutions because toxicity grading scales are not uniform and the scoring system for complications is not clearly stated in all reports. Dusenbery et al. (132) reported 21 (6.4%) life-threatening complications in 327/462 patient implants. Lanciano et al. (348), in 95 tandem and ovoid insertions for cervical cancer in 91 patients and for endometrial cancer in four, observed two uterine perforations and a vaginal laceration in two patients. Twenty-four percent of implants in 16 patients were associated with temperatures higher than 100.5°F. Five implants (5%) were removed because of presumed sepsis, pulmonary disease, arterial hypotension, change in mental status, and myocardial infarction.

Jhingran and Eifel (282), in 4,043 patients with carcinoma of the cervix who had undergone 7,662 intracavitary procedures, observed 11 (0.3%) documented or suspected thromboembolism, resulting in four deaths; the incidence of postimplant thromboembolism did not decrease significantly with the routine use of minidose heparin prophylaxis. Other life-threatening perioperative complications included myocardial infarction (one death in five patients), cerebrovascular accident (two patients), congestive heart failure (three patients), and halothane liver toxicity (two deaths). Intraoperative complications included uterine perforation (2.8%) and vaginal laceration (0.3%), which occurred more frequently in patients 60 years of age or older ($p < 0.01$).

Wollschlaeger et al. (659) reported morbidity during hospitalization in 128 patients with cervical carcinoma undergoing 110 LDR intracavitary brachytherapy insertions. Forty-two implants (24.7%) were associated with acute problems; the most common were fever/infection (14.1%) or gastrointestinal problems (5.9%).

Acute gastrointestinal side effects of pelvic irradiation include diarrhea, abdominal cramping, rectal discomfort, and oc-

casionally rectal bleeding, which may be caused by transient enteroproctitis. Patients with hemorrhoids may experience discomfort earlier than other patients. Diarrhea and abdominal cramping can be controlled with the oral administration of diphenoxylate hydrochloride, with loperamide, atropine sulfate, or opium preparations or emollients such as kaolin and pectin. Proctitis and rectal discomfort can be alleviated by small enemas with hydrocortisone and anti-inflammatory suppositories containing bismuth, benzyl benzoate, zinc oxide, or Peruvian balsam. Some suppositories contain cortisone. Small enemas with cod liver oil are also effective. A low-residue diet with no grease or spices and increased fiber in the stool (psyllium, polycarbophil) usually help to decrease gastrointestinal symptoms.

Genitourinary symptoms, secondary to cystourethritis, are dysuria, frequency, and nocturia. The urine is usually clear, although there may be microscopic or even gross hematuria. Methenamine mandelate and antispasmodics such as phenazopyridine hydrochloride or a smooth muscle antispasmodic such as flavoxate hydrochloride, hyoscyamine sulfate, oxybutynin chloride, or tolterodine tartrate can relieve symptoms. Fluid intake should be at least 2,000 to 2,500 mL daily. Urinary tract infections may occur; diagnosis should be established with appropriate urine culture studies, including sensitivity to sulfonamides and antibiotics. Therapy should be promptly instituted.

Erythema and dry or moist desquamation may develop in the perineum or intergluteal fold. Proper skin hygiene and topical application of petroleum jelly, petrolatum, or lanolin should relieve these symptoms. U.S.P. zinc oxide ointment and intensive skin care may be needed for severe cases.

Management of acute radiation vaginitis includes douching every day or at least three times weekly with a mixture of 1:5 hydrogen peroxide and water. Douching should be continued on a weekly basis until the mucositis has resolved or for 2 or 3 months as necessary. Superficial ulceration of the vagina responds to topical (intravaginal) estrogen creams, which stimulate epithelial regeneration within 3 months after irradiation. Use of vaginal dilators several times daily, started during the course of treatment, prevents vaginal stenosis. Psychoeducational intervention and motivation improve the compliance in use of dilators (278). More severe necrosis may require debridement on a weekly basis until healing takes place. Judicious use of biopsies is recommended to rule out persistent or recurrent cancer.

Late Sequelae

The incidence of major late sequelae of radiation therapy for stage I and IIA carcinoma of the cervix ranges from 3% to 5%, and for stage IIB and III, between 10% and 15%. The most frequent major sequelae for the various stages are listed in Tables 66.25 and 66.26. Injury to the gastrointestinal tract usually appears within the first 2 years after radiation therapy, whereas complications of the urinary tract are seen more frequently 3 to 5 years after treatment (327,469). Pedersen et al. (467), in a review of morbidity of radiation therapy in 442 patients with cervical cancer stages IIB, III, and IVA, recommended that actuarial estimates rather than frequency of sequelae be reported to avoid underestimation of risks of late morbidity after radiation therapy in long-term survivors. In fact, Eifel et al. (140), in 1,784 patients with stage IB carcinoma of the cervix, noted that the greatest risk of sequelae is in the first 3 years after therapy. The risk of rectal complications declined after the first 2 years of follow-up to 0.6% per year, whereas the risk of major urinary tract complications for survivors continued at 0.3% per year, with a 20-year actuarial risk of major complications of 14.4%.

Montana et al. (417), Perez et al. (475), and Pourquier et al. (500) noted a greater incidence of complications with higher doses of irradiation. Perez et al. (469) and Pourquier et al. (500)

Table 66.25 CARCINOMA OF THE UTERINE CERVIX: GRADE 2 SEQUELAE (WASHINGTON UNIVERSITY, 1959–1989)

	Stage				
	IB	IIA	IIB	III	IVA
Total no. of patients treated	415	137	391	326	23
Number of complications	51 (12%)	14 (10%)	65 (17%)	38 (12%)	3 (13%)
Rectum–rectosigmoid					
Rectal stricture	—	1	2	1	1
Proctitis	8	1	13	6	—
Rectal ulcer	1	—	—	2	1
Diverticulitis	—	—	1	—	—
Small bowel obstruction	2	—	3	4	—
Malabsorption	3	—	1	1	—
Urinary					
Chronic cystitis	—	2	12	4	—
Bladder ulcer	3	1	2	1	—
Incontinence	1	—	1	—	—
Urethral stricture	2	—	1	—	—
Extensive cystocele	—	—	—	3	—
Other					
Vaginal stenosis	21	4	7	6	1
Vault necrosis	8	2	2	5	—
Postoperative pelvic abscess	1	—	1	2	—
Lymphocyst	—	—	2	2	—
Pulmonary embolus	—	—	1	—	—
Subcutaneous fibrosis	1	—	—	—	—
Leg edema	—	—	7	3	—
Hemorrhage	—	—	1	—	—
Thrombosis of pelvic blood vessels	—	1	—	—	—
Arteriosclerosis	1	—	8	2	—
Thrombophlebitis	—	—	1	—	—
Pelvic fibrosis	—	1	—	—	—
Acute pelvic cellulitis	—	1	—	—	—
Neuritis	—	—	—	1	—

reported that with doses below 75 to 80 Gy delivered to limited volumes, grade 2 and 3 complications in the urinary tract and rectosigmoid were approximately 5%. However, the incidence increased to over 10% with higher doses of irradiation to these organs (Fig. 66.32). Doses higher than 80 Gy were also correlated with a greater incidence of small bowel injury (Fig. 66.33). The same analysis showed that patients who experienced sequelae of therapy had slightly better survival rates than patients without any complications. This was related to improved tumor control with higher doses of irradiation (469).

Perez et al. (475) quantitated the impact of total doses of irradiation, dose rate, and ratio of doses to bladder or rectum and point A on sequelae in 1,456 patients treated for cervical cancer with external-beam irradiation plus two LDR intracavitary insertions to deliver 70 to 90 Gy to point A. Median follow-up was 11 years. In stage IB, the frequency of grade 2 morbidity was 9%, and grade 3, 5%; in stages IIA, IIB, III, and IVA, the frequency of grade 2 morbidity was 10% to 12%, and of grade 3, 10%. The most frequent grade 2 urinary/rectal sequelae were cystitis and proctitis (0.7% to 3%). The most common grade 3 sequelae were vesicovaginal fistula (0.6% to 2% in patients with stage I to III tumors), rectovaginal fistula (0.8% to 3%), and intestinal obstruction (0.8% to 4%). In the bladder, doses below 80 Gy correlated with a <3% incidence of morbidity and 5% with higher doses ($p = 0.31$). In the rectosigmoid, the incidence of significant morbidity was <4% with doses below 75 Gy and increased to 9% with higher doses. For the small intestine, the incidence of morbidity was <1% with 50 Gy or less, 2% with 50 to 60 Gy, and 5% with higher doses to the lateral pelvic wall ($p = 0.04$). Multivariate analysis showed that dose to the rectal point was the only factor influencing rectosigmoid sequelae, and dose to the bladder point affected bladder morbidity (Table 66.25).

In a review of the Patterns of Care Study, Lanciano et al. (349) observed a 5-year actuarial rate of 14% for major late complications in 1,558 patients treated with irradiation for invasive carcinoma of the cervix. Women younger than 40 years of age or with a history of prior surgery or laparotomy for staging had a greater incidence of significant morbidity (15% to 18% vs. 8% to 9%). Also, EBRT dose per fraction >2 Gy, paracentral doses of 85 Gy or greater, and lateral parametrial doses higher than 60 Gy were independently associated with a higher complication rate.

Lee et al. (369), using 3 Gy fractions with EBRT, calculated the rectal point dose in the anterior wall at the level of the cervical os and noted that total higher BED (142.7 Gy) were associated with rectal sequelae compared with BED <131 Gy.

Mitchell et al. (413) evaluated 398 patients with stage I to III cervical carcinoma treated with radiation therapy. Patients were divided into nonelderly (35 to 69 years of age; $n = 338$) and elderly (≥ 70 years of age; $n = 60$) groups. The frequency and severity of acute and chronic sequelae were equivalent in both groups.

When late radiation proctitis occurs, initial treatment is the same as for acute proctitis. If the symptoms and rectal bleeding persist, laser treatment of rectal telangiectasis or ulcers is frequently beneficial. Roche et al. (515) treated six patients with hemorrhagic radiation-induced proctitis using outpatient intrarectal application of formaldehyde 4%. In four cases the bleeding ceased after the first formaldehyde application; two patients continued to bleed, but another application 3 weeks later definitively controlled the hemorrhage. There were no complications, such as burns or late stenosis of the deep layers of the rectum, and this technique was well tolerated. Rubinstein et al. (531) and Seow-Choen et al. (550) also reported

| Table 66.26 | CARCINOMA OF THE UTERINE CERVIX: GRADE 3 SEQUELAE (WASHINGTON UNIVERSITY, 1959–1989) |

	IB	IIA	IIB	III	IVA
Total no. of patients treated	415	137	391	326	23
Number of complications	26 (6%)	23 (17%)	57 (15%)	45 (14%)	2 (9%)
Rectum–Rectosigmoid					
Rectovaginal fistula	4	2	8	12	1
Rectouterine fistula	1	—	—	—	—
Colovaginal fistula	—	—	1	—	—
Rectal stricture	3	4	4	2	—
Proctitis	2	2	6	2	—
Rectal ulcer	—	—	1	—	—
Sigmoid perforation	1	—	3	1	—
Small Bowel					
Small bowel obstruction	3	5	12	8	—
Small bowel perforation	—	—	2	1	—
Enterocolic fistula	1	—	—	—	—
Enterocutaneous fistula	—	1	—	1	—
Enterovaginal fistula	—	—	1	—	—
Enteritis/cachexia	—	—	—	1	—
Urinary					
Vesicovaginal fistula	3	2	6	9	2
Ureterovaginal fistula	—	—	—	1	—
Cystitis	2	—	—	—	—
Bladder ulcer	—	—	—	1	—
Ureteral stricture	5	5	9	4	—
Other					
Postoperative pelvic abscess	—	—	1	1	—
Pulmonary embolus	—	—	1	—	—
Hemorrhage	—	—	1	2	—
Pelvic infection	1	—	—	—	—
Neuritis	—	1	1	—	—

treatment of radiation proctitis with a similar technique. Patients are sedated, a local anesthetic block is administered, and a sponge moistened with 4% formalin is applied for 4 minutes to each bleeding area of the rectum. Care is taken to protect the perianal skin from any caustic effects of the formalin.

Occasionally, a colostomy is necessary if conservation management fails. The importance of performing colonoscopy in patients with rectal bleeding, to exclude other lesions in the colon, including polyps or cancer, is emphasized.

Anal incontinence is occasionally observed. This sequela must be assessed in light of a report by Nelson et al. (438), who in a survey of 6,959 nonirradiated patients identified 153 (2.2%) who reported anal incontinence, without specific etiology. Thirty percent of incontinent subjects were older than 65 years of age, and 63% were women. Of those with anal incontinence, 36% were incontinent to solid feces, 54% to liquid feces, and 60% to gas.

Kim et al. (317) investigated the effects of radiation on anorectal function using manometry in 24 patients with carcinoma of the uterine cervix who had late radiation proctitis. These data were compared with those from 24 age-matched nonirradiated female volunteers. Regardless of the severity of proctitis symptoms, 75% of irradiated patients exhibited abnormal manometric parameters for sensory or motor functions. Radiation damage to nerves and to the external sphincter muscle were considered to be an important cause of motor dysfunction.

Quilty (504) noted a greater incidence of pelvic complications in patients treated with higher doses to the whole pelvis (40 to 50 Gy). The author commented that the intracavitary radium dose was not correlated with severe complications. Similar observations were made by Stryker et al. (584) in 132 patients, who recorded a 9% incidence of fistulas and a 14% incidence of

grade 2 and 3 complications after delivery of 50 Gy or higher to the whole pelvis (1.8-Gy daily dose) combined with intracavitary insertion. They recommended that the whole pelvis dose should not exceed 40 to 45 Gy when doses of approximately 40 Gy are delivered to point A with LDR intracavitary insertions.

Kuske et al. (344), comparing results of therapy in 99 patients with carcinoma of the cervix on whom minicolpostats were used, noted a 15% higher incidence of grade 2 and 3 complications, which was higher than the 8% incidence noted in a similar group of patients treated with regular colpostats during the same period ($p = 0.08$).

Perez et al. (469) reported that the incidence and type of complications with interstitial therapy at Washington University were approximately the same as in patients treated with intracavitary technique only. On the contrary, Kashibhatla et al. (300) noted 6% small bowel obstruction in 36 women with gynecological cancer treated with EBRT and interstitial brachytherapy, which was aggravated by previous abdominopelvic surgery. The 3-year risk of rectovaginal fistula was 18%, and it was significantly higher in patients who received total doses >76 Gy (100% vs. 7%; $p = 0.009$).

Irradiation of the para-aortic lymph nodes has been reported to cause increased morbidity, particularly if it is done after transperitoneal staging para-aortic lymphadenectomy. In a randomized study reported by Rotman et al. (527), a somewhat higher incidence of grade 2 and 3 complications was reported in 170 patients (10 complications) given 45 Gy to the para-aortic area in addition to standard pelvic irradiation, compared with five complications in 167 patients treated by pelvic irradiation only. The incidence of fatal (grade 5) complications was four and one, respectively. In a similar randomized

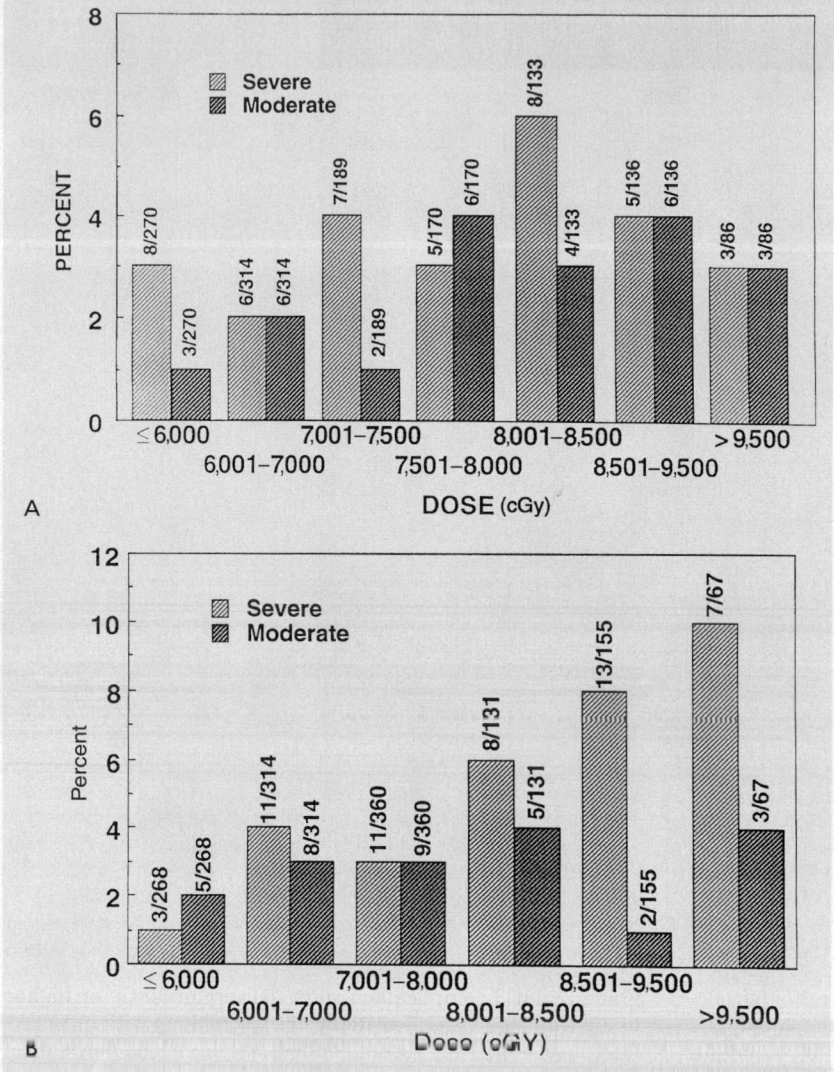

A

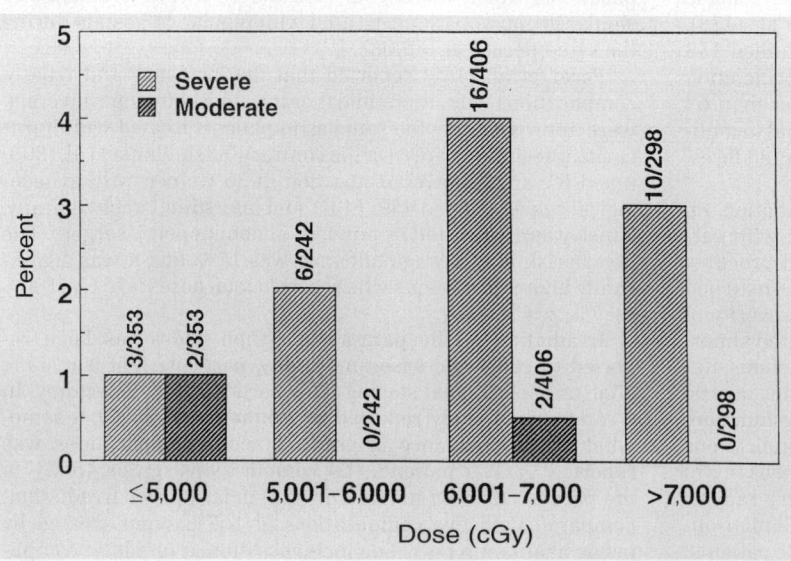

B

FIGURE 66.32. Incidence of moderate or severe genitourinary (**A**) or rectosigmoid (**B**) complications in patients with carcinoma of uterine cervix (all stages) treated with irradiation alone (external and brachytherapy). A greater frequency of complications is noted with maximum doses over 75 to 80 Gy to the bladder or rectum.

FIGURE 66.33. Incidence of moderate or severe complications in small intestine correlated with doses of irradiation.

study by Haie et al. and the EORTC (219), the incidence of grade 3 small bowel injury was 2.3% in the para-aortic irradiation group and 0.9% in the pelvic irradiation–only group. The overall incidences of severe complications were 9% and 4.8%, respectively.

Although it is common knowledge in the radiation oncology community, only a few sketchy reports have been published on the possible intolerance to pelvic irradiation in patients with inflammatory bowel disease (134,252). Willett et al. (655) reported on 28 patients with inflammatory bowel disease (10 with Crohn's disease, 18 with ulcerative colitis) who underwent external-beam abdominal or pelvic irradiation. Patients were treated either by specialized techniques (16 patients) to minimize small and large bowel irradiation or by conventional approaches (12 patients). The overall incidence of severe toxicity was 46% (13/28 patients), and six (21%) experienced severe acute toxicity necessitating cessation of radiation therapy. Late toxicity requiring hospitalization or surgical intervention was observed in 8/28 patients (29%). For patients treated with conventional approaches, the 5-year actuarial rate of late toxicity was 73% versus 23% for patients treated by specialized techniques ($p = 0.02$). In patients with inflammatory bowel disease undergoing abdominal or pelvic irradiation, judicious use of this modality must be observed.

On the contrary, Song et al. (567), in a review of 24 patients with a history of inflammatory bowel disease who received RT (median dose of 45 Gy in 1.8 to 3 Gy fractions) to fields encompassing some portion of the gastrointestinal tract, noted that five patients (21%) experienced acute intestinal toxicity of grade 3 or greater and two (8%) had grade 3 or greater late intestinal toxicity. Fifteen patients also received concurrent chemotherapy. The authors believed that the gastrointestinal toxicity in these patients was more modest than generally perceived. Also, Tiersten and Saltz (612) noted that five patients with inflammatory bowel disease and gastrointestinal malignancy completed planned radiation therapy (30 to 54 Gy), usually with concurrent 5FU, without difficulty.

Salama et al. (542) reported preliminary observations on acute toxicity with extended field IMRT in 13 patients with gynecological cancer. With median follow-up of 11 months, two patients treated with chemoradiation experienced grade 3 or higher morbidity and one (with history of previous surgeries) developed small bowel obstruction.

Levenback et al. (374) identified 116/1,784 patients (6.5%) with stage IB carcinoma of the cervix treated with irradiation in whom hemorrhagic cystitis developed, 23% grade 2 (repeated minor bleeding), and 18% grade 3 (hospitalization required for medical management). The median interval to onset of hematuria was 35.5 months. The risk of severe hematuria requiring surgical intervention was 1.4% at 10 years and 2.3% at 20 years. Minor episodes of hematuria are managed by antibiotic therapy. Cystoscopic, laser, or cautery treatment of bleeding points is indicated. Clot evacuation and continuous bladder irrigation are important elements in the acute management of patients with heavy bleeding. Occasionally, a urinary diversion is required for intractable severe hematuria.

In 13 patients with hemorrhagic cystitis treated with hyperbaric oxygen, all but one experienced durable cessation of hematuria (647). Lee et al. (364) also noted that, in 16/20 patients (80%) with hemorrhagic radiation cystitis, significant improvement was observed after treatment with hyperbaric oxygen at 2.5 atm (44 sessions).

Ureteral stricture at 20 years was observed in 2.5% of 1,784 patients with stage IB carcinoma of the cervix treated with irradiation (274 followed for up to 20 years or longer) (406). The most common presenting symptoms were flank pain and urinary tract infection. In five patients, ureteral stricture was complicated by a vesicovaginal fistula. Seven of 43 patients who had no evidence of cancer and hydroureter or hydronephrosis

died of radiation complications. Treatment of ureteral stenosis may consist of stenting or resection of the fibrotic segment and reimplantation of the ureter either with a ureteroneocystostomy or ureteroileocystostomy. In approximately half of the patients, diversion of urinary stream and ileal conduits are necessary. Occasionally, a nephrectomy is performed for removal of a nonfunctional kidney. Buglione et al. (60) reported a 10% incidence of late urinary morbidity and 1% ureteral fibrosis grade III or IV in 191 patients. They postulated the role of TGF-β_1 factor in the activation of fibroblasts and remodeling of extracellular matrix, which may be important in the induction of these sequelae.

Patients with gynecologic malignancies, including those receiving radiation therapy, are prone to development of urinary tract infections. Prasad et al. (501) collected 216 urine samples from 36 patients receiving pelvic irradiation, 12 of whom had urinary tract infection. The most common organisms isolated were *Escherichia coli*, followed by *Enterococcus* species. Appropriate urine bacterial studies and cultures are indicated in patients suspected of having superimposed urinary tract infection during the course of radiation therapy.

Parkin et al. (462) reported a 26% incidence of severe urinary symptoms (urgency, incontinence, and frequency) in patients treated with irradiation alone for cervical carcinoma. They carried out urodynamic studies in 42 women and compared them with 28 women having urodynamic evaluations before and after treatment. There was no difference in the mean maximum flow rate or mean *residual* volume in the two groups. However, mean volume of full bladder sensation was significantly lower in the postirradiation group than in the pretreatment group, as was the mean maximum cystometric capacity. This same dysfunction may be noted in approximately 10% of the general female population, and the incidence increases in older women (478).

Ureteroarterial fistula is a rare occurrence, and it is associated with a high mortality rate. When profuse urinary tract bleeding occurs in patients previously diagnosed with a gynecologic malignancy and treated with radiation therapy and extensive surgery, ureteroarterial fistula should be considered in the differential diagnoses (118).

Although extremely rare, lumbosacral plexopathy has been occasionally reported in patients treated for pelvic tumors with doses of 60 to 67.5 Gy. At Washington University, this syndrome was observed in four of 2,410 patients with cervical or endometrial carcinoma receiving 45 Gy to the para-aortic lymph nodes (without spinal cord shielding) or external pelvic irradiation (60 Gy to the parametria) and brachytherapy, with the lumbosacral plexus receiving total doses of 70 to 79 Gy (176). Lower extremity paralysis secondary to lumbosacral plexopathy was reported in one patient after standard radiation therapy for cervical cancer (3).

Patients previously reported as having radiation myelopathy to the lumbar spine may have suffered a lumbar and sacral nerve plexopathy instead of or in addition to the spinal cord injury. The differential diagnosis of plexopathy with recurrent tumors is sometimes difficult. In a comparison of 20 patients with lumbosacral plexopathy after irradiation and 30 patients with plexus damage from pelvic malignancy, Thomas et al. (610) noted that indolent leg weakness occurred early in radiation-induced plexopathy (pain occurred initially in 10% of patients, although ultimately it was present in 50%), whereas pain was most frequently associated with tumor plexopathy. Muscular weakness, numbness, and paresthesia are common in both groups. Electromyography showed abnormal myokymic discharges in 57% of patients, whereas this finding was very unusual in tumor-induced plexopathy. CT is extremely helpful in the detection of pelvic masses or bone destruction caused by tumor. The authors also reported extensive retroperitoneal fibrosis of the lumbosacral plexus in two patients and femoral nerve fibrosis with plexopathy in one patient. Although cystometrograms have demonstrated bladder atonicity in some cases, several authors have failed to observe bladder or rectal sphincter disturbances. Unfortunately, as in radiation myelopathy, the neurologic deficit is irreversible, and no effective therapy other supportive care has been found.

Other types of less severe, but still clinically significant sequelae have been described. Bruner et al. (57), in 90 patients treated with intracavitary irradiation for either carcinoma of the cervix (42 patients) or endometrial carcinoma (48 patients), 78 of whom also received external pelvic irradiation (44.5-Gy mean dose), noted that vaginal length decreased in most patients (at 24 months, in endometrial carcinoma from 8.8 cm to 7.8 cm, and in cervical carcinoma from 7.6 cm to 6.2 cm). Pretreatment sexual activity was reported by 31% of women in comparison with 43% after treatment. However, 22% of women reported a decrease in sexual frequency, and 37% a decrease in sexual satisfaction. This was correlated with increased dyspareunia, which was noted in 31% of women treated for carcinoma of the cervix and 44% of those treated for endometrial carcinoma. Grigsby et al. (204) described complex problems with sexual adjustment in women with gynecologic tumors treated with radiation therapy, with decreased frequency of sexual intercourse, desire, orgasm, and enjoyment of intercourse in 16% to 47% of patients.

Regular vaginal dilation is widely recommended to maintain vaginal health and sexual functioning; however, the compliance rate with this recommendation is not consistent. In a study to test the effectiveness of an "information-motivation-behavior skills" model, 32 women compliance was significantly improved (278,514). There was no evidence that the experimental intervention improved global sexual health. Jensen et al. (281) described persistent sexual dysfunction throughout 2 years after RT in 118 women; 85% had low or no sexual interest, 35% lack of vaginal lubrication, and 55% mild to severe dyspareunia. However, 63% of the sexually active patients before RT remained active, although with decreased frequency.

Grigsby et al. (203), in 1,313 patients with gynecologic tumors treated with radiation therapy, identified 207 who received pelvic irradiation to the inguinal areas, including the hips. Femoral neck fractures developed in 10 patients (4.8%); four were bilateral. The cumulative actuarial incidence of fracture was 11% at 5 years and 15% at 10 years. Most of the fractures occurred in patients receiving 45 to 63 Gy, and although radiation dose could not be correlated with the occurrence of fracture, no fractures were noted in patients receiving <42 Gy. Cigarette smoking and osteoporosis were significant prognostic factors for increased risk of fracture.

Blomlie et al. (40) described radiation-induced insufficiency fractures of the pelvis on MRI (characterized by edema on T1-weighted images) in 16/18 women (nine premenopausal and nine postmenopausal) with advanced cervical carcinoma. During the study, the fractures associated with edema subsided without treatment in 41/52 (79%) lesions in 15/16 (94%) patients. Moreno et al. (420) also described eight patients with pelvic cancer who developed insufficiency fractures after pelvic irradiation. The bone and CT scan showed abnormalities in the sacroiliac joint in all cases, and in the pubis in three cases.

In five patients, the initial diagnosis was bone metastases, which was incorrect. Treatment, consisting of nonsteroidal anti-inflammatory drugs and rest, led to symptomatic relief in all cases. These data should be evaluated in light of a report by Cummings et al. (103) of 9,516 women, 192 of whom sustained hip fractures not due to motor vehicle accidents. The incidence of hip fracture ranged from 1.1 per 1,000 woman-years when no risk factors were present to 27 per 1,000 woman-years in women with risk factors and low bone density.

Bye et al. (65) assessed health-related quality of life (HRQOL) 3 to 4 years after pelvic radiation therapy for carcinoma of the endometrium and cervix in 94 survivors, 79 (84%) of whom answered a survey. The treated women scored lower than the general population on role functioning (81.5 vs. 90.6; $p < 0.01$) and higher on diarrhea (23.8 vs. 9.5; $p < 0.01$). Compared with pretreatment conditions, an increase in cases with pain in the lower back, hips, and thighs was seen and was associated with deterioration in HRQOL.

Sequelae of High-Dose-Rate Brachytherapy

Petereit et al. (481) reported 16 acute events (9.5%) in 169 patients treated with HDR brachytherapy (128 with cervical cancer, also receiving external irradiation, and 41 medically inoperable endometrial carcinomas). The overall 30-day morbidity rate for the patients with cervical cancer was 5.5%, and the 30-day mortality rate was 1.6% (two patients, one died of pulmonary edema 12 days after first HDR insertion and the other had enteritis and died in a nursing home).

The complication rates for HDR and LDR techniques are usually equivalent (165,455). Petereit et al. (482) observed equivalent morbidity with LDR or HDR brachytherapy (Table 66.27). However, in the series by Cikaric (87), the rectal complication rate was significantly higher in the LDR group. Bladder complication rates reported, in general, are lower than rectal complication rates; again, except for the series by Cikaric (87) showing a higher complication rate with the LDR technique, there were no significant differences with the two techniques.

Ogino et al. (450), in 253 patients with invasive carcinoma of the cervix treated with HDR brachytherapy, noted that grade 4 rectal complications were not observed in patients with a time–dose factor below 130 or biologic equivalent dose lower than 147, assuming an α/β ratio of 3 Gy for late reactions.

Spontaneous intraperitoneal rupture of the urinary bladder, an extremely rare event, was reported by Fujikawa et al. (166) after radiation therapy for cervical cancer in 6/148 patients treated with HDR intracavitary brachytherapy combined with EBRT. All six patients underwent laparotomy and repair of the perforation; however, rerupture of the bladder occurred in three of these patients.

Clark et al. (88) reported on 43 patients treated with pelvic EBRT (46 Gy) and three HDR intracavitary treatments given weekly combined with concomitant chemotherapy (cisplatin, 30 mg/m² weekly) for advanced carcinoma of the cervix. At 40 months after treatment, 9/13 patients who received a dose to the rectal reference point greater than the prescribed point A

	Overall (%)	Genitourinary (%)	Rectum (%)	Small Bowel (%)
Table 66.27 UNIVERSITY OF WISCONSIN UPDATE: ACTUARIAL COMPLICATION RATE (GRADE 3 OR HIGHER) CORRELATED WITH ORGAN SITE AT 3 YEARS				
Low-dose rate	12	2.6	5.6	5.4
High-dose-rate	15	3.0	4.6	9.5

From Petereit DG. Refresher course no. 103: high dose rate brachytherapy for carcinoma of the cervix. Presented at the 40th Annual Meeting of the American Society for Therapeutic Radiology and Oncology, Phoenix, Arizona, October 1998, with permission.

dose had a 46% actuarial rate of serious (grade 3 and 4) rectal complications, compared with 14% in the remainder. A strong dose response was observed with a threshold for complications at a brachytherapy dose of 8 Gy per fraction.

Surgery

With improved anesthesia, surgical techniques, and antibiotic therapy, the mortality rate for radical hysterectomy with pelvic lymphadenectomy has decreased to 1% or less. The most frequent sequela after radical hysterectomy is urinary dysfunction, as a result of partial denervation of the detrusor muscle. Patients may have various degrees of loss of bladder sensation, inability to initiate voiding, residual urine retention, and incontinence.

Magrina et al. (392), in 375 patients treated with a modified radical hysterectomy for various gynecologic disorders, observed some form of postoperative (within 42 days of surgery) complications in 89 patients (24%). Patients who had a pelvic lymphadenectomy experienced a greater incidence of lower extremity lymphedema than those who did not undergo this procedure. Preoperative or postoperative pelvic irradiation was a significant predisposing factor for urinary tract infection, lymphedema, and bowel obstruction in these patients compared with those who did not receive pelvic irradiation.

Some loss of defecatory urge associated with chronic rectal dysfunction was observed by Barnes et al. (29) after radical hysterectomy. Manometric studies suggest a disruption of the spinal arcs controlling defecation.

Other complications include ureterovaginal fistula (the incidence of which has decreased to <3%), hemorrhage, infection, bowel obstruction, stricture and fibrosis of the intestine or rectosigmoid colon, and bladder and rectovaginal fistulas. Postsurgical complications are usually more amenable to correction than are late complications after irradiation.

Combined Irradiation and Surgery

When irradiation is combined with surgery, the complication rate tends to be somewhat higher, particularly because of injury to the ureter or the bladder (ureteral stricture or ureterovaginal or vesicovaginal fistula) (140). The dose of irradiation, technique, and the type of surgical procedure performed are important in determining the morbidity of combined therapy. Jacobs et al. (276), in 102 patients with invasive cervical carcinoma treated with low-dose preoperative irradiation and a radical hysterectomy with lymphadenectomy or high-dose preoperative irradiation and a conservative extrafascial hysterectomy, noted a major complication rate of 5%.

As discussed previously, a significant number of complications are associated with pretherapy staging laparotomy, particularly if irradiation (over 55 Gy) is given to metastatic para-aortic lymph nodes. The incidence of complications is between 5% and 20%, depending on the extent of the para-aortic lymph node dissection, use of transperitoneal or retroperitoneal approach for the operation, and dose of irradiation given (651).

Postoperative Irradiation

When postoperative radiation therapy is given to selected patients, further complications of the additional therapy are expected because of intestinal adhesions to denuded surfaces in the pelvis. Enteric complications, such as obstruction, fistula, or dysfunction, were observed in 24% of patients reported by Fiorica et al. (158). Other investigators, however, have reported no increase in the incidence of severe complications in patients treated with postoperative irradiation (355,563).

Montz et al. (419) evaluated bowel obstruction in 98 patients undergoing radical hysterectomy for a nonadnexal gynecologic malignancy. The incidence of small bowel obstruction was significantly higher ($p <0.05$) in patients who received concomitant radiation therapy (20%). None of these patients had recurrent disease at the time of small bowel obstruction. Findings at surgery consisted of minimal incisional adhesions but extensive matted small bowel adherent to the pelvic operative sites.

After combined treatment, some degree of lymphedema is frequently observed (30% to 40%).

Hormonal Replacement after Treatment of Cervical Cancer

After pelvic irradiation or bilateral salpingo-oophorectomy, usually carried out with a radical hysterectomy in patients treated for carcinoma of the uterine cervix, symptoms of menopause may occur. They can be treated with replacement hormones, although some gynecologists have expressed reservations. During the past 25 years, hormonal replacement therapy has been shown to reduce the risk of cardiovascular diseases, osteoporotic fractures, and colon carcinoma. On the other hand, there is a significant increase of the risk in breast cancer with prolonged use longer than 5 years.

Burger et al. (61) concluded that squamous-cell cancers of the cervix, vulva, and vagina are unlikely to be influenced by hormonal replacement therapy. In a study of women with ovarian cancer, 50 years of age or younger, estrogen replacement therapy did not have a negative influence on disease-free survival. Long-term hormonal replacement therapy in women treated for a gynecologic cancer must be based on the medical history of and discussion of risk with the individual patient (and her family when warranted). Usually, 0.625 to 1.25 mg of coagulated estrogen daily is sufficient (491,538,619).

⸭ | Palliative Irradiation

Frequently, the radiation oncologist is faced with the challenge of treating a patient with stage IVB or recurrent carcinoma who requires palliation of pelvic pain or bleeding. If vaginal bleeding is the main concern, a single LDR intracavitary insertion with tandem and colpostats for approximately 6,000 mgh (55 Gy to point A) suffices. If irradiation was delivered previously, lower intracavitary doses should be prescribed (4,000 to 5,000 mgh). Grigsby et al. (202) used two fractions of HDR brachytherapy with a ring applicator (once weekly) with control of bleeding in 14/15 patients.

Several high-dose fractionation schedules with external-beam radiation have been used. Spanos et al. (576) reported on a phase II study of daily multifractionated split-course irradiation in 142 patients with recurrent or metastatic disease in the pelvis. Irradiation consisted of 3.7 Gy per fraction given twice daily for 2 consecutive days, repeated at 3- to 6-week intervals for a total of three courses, aiming to a total tumor dose of 44.4 Gy. Occasionally, this regimen was combined with an LDR intracavitary insertion (4,500 mgh), blocking the midline for the last 14.4-Gy external dose. Twenty-seven patients survived more than 1 year. There were only two recorded cases of grade 3 toxicity (lower gastrointestinal tract). This study was expanded to a phase III protocol randomizing 136 patients between a short (2-week) or a longer (4-week) rest period between the split courses of irradiation (577). There was a trend toward increased acute toxicity in patients with shorter rest periods (5/58 vs. 0/68; $p = 0.07$). Late toxicity was not significantly different in the two groups. Pelvic tumor response was comparable in both groups (34% vs. 26%). Spanos et al. (575) reported a 6% complication rate in 290 patients treated in RTOG Protocol 85-02. No patient receiving <30 Gy experienced late toxicity. There was no significant difference in the incidence of complications for patients with a 2- or 4-week rest ($p = 0.47$).

Treatment of Recurrent Carcinoma of the Cervix

After Definitive Irradiation

Reirradiation of previously irradiated patients must be undertaken with extreme caution. It is very important to analyze the techniques used in the initial treatment (beam energy, volume, doses delivered with external or intracavitary irradiation). Also, the period of time between the two treatments must be taken into consideration because it is postulated that some repair of the initial damage may take place in the interval. However, it is foolhardy to assume that previously irradiated tissues will have the same tolerance as newly irradiated tissues. In general, external irradiation for recurrent tumor is given to limited volumes (40 to 45 Gy, 1.8-Gy tumor dose per fraction, preferentially using lateral portals). Occasionally, intracavitary or interstitial irradiation can be used to treat relatively circumscribed recurrences.

Sommers et al. (566) described the results of retreatment in 376 patients with recurrent carcinoma of the uterine cervix. Ninety-one patients received irradiation, mostly external (86.8%), occasionally combined with brachytherapy (7.7%) to control bleeding of central recurrences; brachytherapy alone was administered in 5.5% of patients. The usual dose for recurrent pelvic masses was 40 to 45 Gy and for para-aortic lymph node metastases 45 to 50 Gy in 5 weeks. Other metastatic sites were treated with 35 to 40 Gy in 3 to 4 weeks. Pelvic exenteration was attempted in 23 patients, only 10 of whom were deemed to be operable (43.5%), but it was completed in only seven. The probability of 5-year survival after treatment for recurrence was 30% with combined surgery and external irradiation, 12% with surgery alone, and 4% with external irradiation alone. The 5-year survival rate for 10 patients who underwent pelvic exenteration was 16%. Only 1% of the untreated patients survived 5 years. Six of 140 patients (4.3%) experienced grade 2 or 3 complications.

Selected patients with limited pelvic recurrences not fixed to the pelvic wall and without evidence of extrapelvic metastases can be potentially salvaged by radical hysterectomy or pelvic exenteration. Coleman et al. (91) described results in 50 patients who underwent radical hysterectomy for persistent (18 patients) or recurrent (32 patients) cervical cancer after primary radiation therapy. Lymph node metastases were identified in 5/39 patients (13%) in whom the lymph nodes were evaluated. The 5- and 10-year survival rates were 72% and 60%, respectively.

In 65 patients on whom pelvic exenteration was carried out at Memorial Sloan-Kettering Cancer Center, the 5-year survival rate was 23%. The operative mortality rate was 9.2% (357). The authors pointed out that the significant mortality and morbidity associated with this procedure preclude its use as palliative therapy.

Urinary diversion, either by nephrostomy or ileal bladder, may be of palliative value in patients with either recurrent carcinoma in the pelvis or complications. It must be kept in mind that diversion may prolong life but runs the risk of denying a terminally ill patient with cancer the oblivion and insensibility of uremia.

Kastritis et al. (301) treated 200 patients with stage IV or recurrent cervix cancer with platinum-based chemotherapy; response rate was 43.5% in 142 with squamous-cell and 53.5% in 58 with nonsquamous tumors ($p = 0.79$). Median survival was 11.57 and 19 months, respectively. Tinker et al. (613) treated 25 women for recurrent cervical cancer with carboplatin-paclitaxel and noted a 20% cure rate and 20% progression rate, with median survival of 21 months. Brewer et al. (54), in 32 women all of whom had previous chemotherapy and 29 previous RT, used cisplatin and gemcitabine, with a progression rate of 22% and median time to progression 3.5 months.

Para-Aortic Lymph Node Recurrences

Isolated recurrences in the para-aortic nodes after pelvic irradiation have been described in about 3% of patients and some may be salvaged with aggressive therapy. The advent of IMRT and IGRT makes treatment easier, with less morbidity.

Kim et al. (319) treated 12 patients with isolated para-aortic lymph node metastasis with hyperfractionated RT (60 Gy in 1.2 Gy fractions twice a day) and concurrent cisplatin-paclitaxel. Fields extended from superior plate of T12 to lower plate of L5. Three-year survival was 19%. Grade 3 or 4 hematologic toxicity developed in two patients. Singh et al. (560) detected 14 isolated para-aortic lymph node metastases in 816 patients previously treated with RT, who subsequently received RT to the para-aortic lymph node combined with concurrent chemotherapy. Seven patients survived 5 years.

Jhingran et al. (283), in a review of 1,955 patients treated with RT for cervix cancer, identified 120 with recurrent tumor above the pelvic fields. Initially, 10 had common iliac and five para-aortic node involvement. In 104 patients, recurrences were immediately adjacent to the upper borders of the RT fields. In 15 patients treated with curative intent for the para-aortic lymph node recurrence, 5 year survival was 25%.

After Previous Surgery

It is substantially easier to treat surgical recurrences with irradiation, which can salvage approximately 50% of patients with localized pelvic recurrences after surgery alone. A combination of whole pelvis external irradiation (20 to 40 Gy), depending on the volume of tumor, and additional parametrial dose with midline shielding for a total of 50 to 60 Gy are needed. In addition, one or two LDR intracavitary insertions (or equivalent HDR) that may cover either the vaginal vault or the entire vagina, depending on tumor volume, should be delivered. The total mucosal dose from the external and LDR intracavitary therapy can approach 140 Gy to the upper vagina and 95 Gy to the distal vagina without a high risk (240). It is extremely useful to combine these techniques with interstitial irradiation to boost the dose to residual. Doses of 20 to 35 Gy are administered with single, double-plane, or volume implants, depending on the extent of the tumor.

Larson et al. (354) observed 27 recurrences (11%) in 249 patients treated with radical hysterectomy and pelvic lymphadenectomy for stage IB carcinoma of the cervix; 17 (63%) had tumor recurrence in the pelvis or vulva; the other 10 patients had recurrences outside the pelvis. Eight of 15 patients (53%) treated with irradiation for an isolated recurrence in the pelvis or vulva were tumor free between 10 and 126 months after treatment of the recurrence (median, 48 months).

Ijaz et al. (268) reported on 50 patients treated with RT for an isolated pelvic recurrence of cervical carcinoma after radical hysterectomy; seven patients were treated with palliative intent using hypofractionated RT. The remaining 43 patients were treated with curative intent, 33 with RT only and 10 with cisplatin-based chemoirradiation. The overall 5-year survival rate was 33% for all 50 patients, 39% for the 43 patients treated with curative intent, and 25% for patients with isolated sidewall recurrences treated with curative intent. Three patients experienced late treatment complications.

Hille et al. (246) described results in 17 patients with recurrent cervix cancer (nine had a complete microscopically incomplete resection) treated with EBRT and BT to 50 to 65 Gy. The 5-year pelvic tumor control was 48% and RFS 24%.

Intraoperative Irradiation

Intraoperative radiation therapy (IORT) has been used for treatment of not only locally advanced but recurrent carcinoma of the cervix, with 3-year survival rates of 8% to 21% as reported by Mahé et al. (393) and Garton et al. (174), and a 5-year survival rate of 33% in 14 patients described by Kinney et al. (324). Patient selection may have had an impact on the different results. Abe and Shibamoto (1) noted that central recurrences, particularly in nonirradiated patients, and resection of the gross recurrent tumor in irradiated patients improve the benefit from IORT. Significant toxicity included peripheral nerve injury and ureteral stenosis (with doses higher than 15 to 20 Gy).

IORT was used in 70 patients with pelvic recurrences in a European cooperative study (393). Complete tumor resection was carried out in 30 patients, partial in 37, and unspecified in 3. Sixty-five patients had electron beam therapy (12 to 25 MeV), with mean doses of 18 Gy (10 to 25 Gy) after gross complete resection and 19 Gy (10 to 30 Gy) after partial resection. The 3-year overall survival rate was 8%. Grade 2 or 3 toxicity was observed in 19/70 patients (27%), with 10 complications being related to IORT.

Martinez-Monge et al. (403) reported a study of IORT in 26 patients with recurrent gynecologic tumors, some relapsing after full-dose radiation therapy (group 1) or recurrent disease after surgery (group 2). Cervical carcinoma was the initial tumor site of involvement in 18 patients. Treatment consisted of maximal surgical resection and IORT (10 to 25 Gy) to high-risk areas. Patients not previously irradiated also received external-beam irradiation (with or without chemotherapy) before or after surgery. There was one IORT-related incidence of motor neuropathy. The local tumor control rates were 33% and 77%; the 4-year actuarial survival for group 1 was 7% and the 6-year actuarial survival rate for group 2 was 33%.

Chemotherapy

Chemotherapy is being more extensively used in bulky and advanced cervical cancer; some cytotoxic agents have shown encouraging efficacy in patients with advanced and recurrent cervical carcinoma (662). Noteworthy, in a study of 41 patients who had weekly biopsies while receiving RT and chemotherapy for cervix cancer, increased tumor cell proliferation and accelerated repopulation was observed within 2 weeks from the initiation of therapy. Patients with a sustained yield and high S-phase fraction for two or more weeks were at increased risk for tumor progression (131).

Green et al. (189), in a search of medical databases for randomized trials of cervical cancer that compared RT with or without concurrent chemotherapy, identified 19 trials comprising 4,580 randomized patients, and they were the subjects of the meta-analysis. Concomitant chemotherapy and radiation improved tumor control and overall survival (RR 0.71; p <0.0001) and progression-free survival (RR 0.61; p <0.0001). The benefit was maximal in early stage (I and II) disease. The absolute survival benefit was 12%. Patients receiving chemoirradiation had a higher incidence of grade 3 or 4 hematologic and gastrointestinal toxicities.

Cisplatin is one of the most active cytotoxic agents in squamous-cell carcinoma of the uterine cervix (529). When cisplatin and irradiation are used concomitantly, substantial enhancement of cell killing is observe. Coughlin and Richmond (98) and Douple (125) suggested two mechanisms for radiation enhancement by platinum: (a) in hypoxic or oxygenated cells, free radicals with altered binding of platinum to DNA are formed at the time of irradiation; and (b) interaction inhibits repair of sublethal damage.

Cisplatin has been combined with other cytotoxic agents. Long et al. (384) conducted a randomized study comparing methotrexate, vinblastine, doxorubicin, and cisplatin (MVAC) or cisplatin/topotecan or cisplatin alone in patients with advanced cervical cancer. The MVAC arm was closed after four deaths in 63 patients occurred. In 294 patients assigned to the other arms response rate was 27% for cisplatin/topotecan and 13% for cisplatin alone, with median survival of 9.4 and 6.5 months, respectively. Other trials with cisplatin will be discussed later in this chapter.

Paclitaxel, a natural product found initially in the bark of the western yew tree, produces depolymerization and irreversible bundling of tubulin in the cell. It has been shown to have a radiosensitizing effect. Rose et al. (522) reported on a phase II study of 44 patients in which the starting dose was paclitaxel (135 mg/m^2, maximum 170 mg/m^2) infused over 24 hours, followed by cisplatin (75 mg/m^2) every 21 days. Forty patients (90.9%) had received prior radiation therapy. A median of six courses of chemotherapy was given. Of the 41 assessable patients, five (12.2%) had a complete response and 14 (34.1%) had a partial response.

Vinorelbine is a semisynthetic derivative of vinblastine. In a phase II trial in patients with prior irradiation, an 18% response rate was observed (464). A second phase II trial used the drug as neoadjuvant chemotherapy; in 42 patients, two complete and 17 partial responses (45%) were observed (345,422).

Irinotecan and topotecan are camptothecin derivatives whose cytotoxic mechanism is thought to target topoisomerase I (623). An international phase II trial reported a similar 21% response rate in patients predominantly with prior irradiation (one complete and eight partial responses among 42 patients) (635).

Gemcitabine, a nucleoside analog, showed a 4.5% partial response and 36% stable disease in 22 patients (546). In combination with cisplatin, it was evaluated in 32 women with previously treated cervix cancer (initial dose 800 mg/m^2 days 1 and 8 then every 28 days); there were seven (22%) partial responses and 12 stable disease responses (54).

Nonrandomized Studies of Chemotherapy and Irradiation

Numerous preliminary reports have been published on results of neoadjuvant/concomitant use of cisplatin and 5-fluorouracil (5-FU), with or without mitomycin C, combined with irradiation to treat patients with locally advanced or recurrent carcinoma of the cervix (46).

Trials with Cisplatin, 5-Fluorouracil, or Both

Perez and Grigsby (477) reported on 58 patients with locally advanced carcinoma of the cervix treated with concurrent 5-FU/cisplatin and irradiation, and compared the results with 257 patients with similar stages treated with irradiation alone during the same period. Pelvic tumor control, disease-free, and cause-specific survival were comparable. The incidence of rectal and bladder fistula was 7% in the chemoirradiation group and 4% with irradiation alone (p = 0.61).

Park et al. (459) described results in 113 patients with high-risk invasive cervical carcinoma treated with cisplatin and 5-FU. For adenocarcinoma, doxorubicin (45 mg/m^2 IV) was added. The patients subsequently received radiation therapy (not described in the publication). Compared with 77 patients treated with RT alone, in stage I or II tumors >4 cm, the 5-year survival rate was 78.3% with chemoirradiation and 48% with RT alone (p <0.01) and in stages III and IV 69.1% and 57.4%, respectively. Toxicity with combined chemoirradiation was not significantly enhanced compared with irradiation alone.

Sardi et al. (544) reported results of three courses of cisplatin, vincristine, and bleomycin (days 1 to 3) at 10-day intervals combined with RT in 205 unselected patients with stage IB cervix cancer (tumors >2 cm) who were divided at random into two groups treated with surgery and RT or neoadjucvant chemotherapy, surgery, and irradiation. After 67 months, no difference in survival was seen in patients with tumors 2 to 4 cm in both groups (77% for control patients vs. 82% with neoadjuvant chemotherapy), but statistically significant differences were seen in bulky tumors (>4 cm), 61% versus 80% in favor of neoadjuvant chemotherapy.

Souhami et al. (574) treated 50 patients with bulky, locally advanced carcinoma of the cervix with a combination of weekly cisplatin (30 mg/m^2) concurrent with RT. At 44 months, the actuarial survival rate was 65%, the total pelvic failure rate was 26%, and the distant metastasis rate was 24%. The incidence of late gastrointestinal toxicity was high, with 10 rectal ulcers (four colostomies required for severe bleeding), two rectovaginal fistulas, and two small bowel obstructions.

Park et al. (460) treated patients with stage I and II carcinoma of the cervix larger than 4 cm with RT alone, concurrent or sequential chemoradiation with cisplatin and 5-FU. The 30-month survival rates were 100% with concurrent chemoirradiation, 89.5% with sequential treatment, and 79.5% with irradiation alone ($p <0.05$).

Varia et al. (631) reported on GOG Protocol 125 that 87 patients with biopsy-confirmed para-aortic lymph nodes from cervical cancer were treated with extended-field irradiation (45 Gy in 1.5-Gy fractions) and higher doses to the pelvis (approximately 80 Gy to point A) in combination with 5-FU and cisplatin. The 3-year progression-free survival rate was 33%, and the overall survival rate was 39%. Grade 3 and 4 hematologic toxicity was noted in 13 patients (15%), chronic proctitis in three (3.5%), and four patients (4.6%) required surgery for rectal complications.

Lee et al. (366) treated 40 women with cervix cancer using 50 Gy EBRT and brachytherapy; in 25 three concurrent cycles of cisplatin/5-FU and in 15 six cycles of consolidation chemotherapy were given. There was no difference in 2-year survival between the two groups (98% to 100%). Grade 2 or greater hematologic toxicity was more frequent in the consolidation patients.

Grigsby et al. (199), in a prospective study of 65 patients with cervical cancer and node-negative on FDG-PET treated with RT alone (15 patients) or combined with concurrent weekly cisplatin (50 patients), noted a 5-year cause-specific survival of 78% and 74%, respectively. Severe complications included one RV fistula and one rectal stricture in the concurrent chemotherapy/RT group and one chemotherapy-related death.

Trials with Mitomycin C or Tirapazamine

Mitomycin C acts as an alkylating agent and inhibits DNA and RNA synthesis. Activation of mitomycin C is increased in hypoxic conditions, and thus it acts as a hypoxic radiosensitizer. Interstitial pneumonitis and pulmonary fibrosis are usually related to the dose of drug. Use of IV dexamethasone before administration of the drug may prevent pulmonary toxicity.

Christie et al. (83) described results in three groups of patients with stage IIB and III carcinoma of the cervix treated with pelvic irradiation and an intracavitary insertion combined with chemotherapy. Group A (64 patients) received 5-FU infusion during the first and last weeks of irradiation combined with mitomycin C (10 mg/m^2 IV). Group B (29 patients) received 5-FU without mitomycin C, and group C (84 patients) received irradiation alone. With median follow-up of 7.2 years, the 5-year survival rates were 56%, 32%, and 36%, and the local tumor control 73%, 53%, and 50%, respectively. Toxicity was greater

in group A (36% grade 3 and 4) compared with the 5-FU and irradiation group (14%) and the irradiation-alone group (20%).

Roberts et al. (513) reported on a trial in which 160 patients with locally advanced cervical cancer were randomized to receive RT alone (82 patients) or RT with concomitant mitomycin C (78 patients). The 4-year actuarial survival was 72% and 56%, respectively ($p = 0.13$), and the local recurrence-free survival rate was 78% and 63%, respectively ($p = 0.11$). There were no treatment-related deaths. No excess in nonhematologic toxicity has been observed with combined mitomycin C and irradiation.

Tirapazamine, a radiation sensitizer, with selective cytotoxic effect on hypoxic cells, was combined with cisplatin in 56 patients with recurrent or metastatic cancer. After six cycles given every 21 days, four complete and 13 partial responses were noted. Overall 6-month survival was 56%. Better response was seen in patients who had not received radiosensitizing chemotherapy previously (562).

Besides the usual hematologic and pelvic toxicity described in many of these studies with chemoradiation, Wun et al. (666), in a retrospective analysis of 75 patients with gynecological cancer who received erythropoietin and chemotherapy/RT, noted that 17 had upper or lower extremity thrombosis, in contrast to 2/72 who did not receive erythropoietin. Noteworthy, Anders et al. (17), in a review of the literature, reported 6/128 patients (4.7%) treated with chemptherapy/RT without erythropoietin developed grade 4 or 5 thrombosis toxicity.

Intra-Arterial Chemotherapy

Intra-arterial infusion of chemotherapeutic agents in cervical carcinoma was used for some years based on the distinct arterial supply to the tumor-bearing area. Unfortunately, the responses have been uncommon and short, and the toxicity and complication rates have been significant (423).

Onishi et al. (454) evaluated intra-arterial cisplatin through catheters inserted into both internal iliac arteries in cervix carcinoma. Patients were randomized into a concurrent intra-arterial infusion of platinum with RT (18 patients) or RT alone (15 patients). Five-year overall survival rates were 44.4% and 50%, respectively. In the group receiving intra-arterial infusion, grade 3 or 4 late bowel complications were seen in 44% and grade 3 or 4 myelosuppression in 33%, significantly more than in the RT group.

Randomized Studies of Chemotherapy and Irradiation

Hydroxyurea

The GOG carried out a trial of irradiation with either concomitant hydroxyurea (HOU) or a placebo in patients with stage IIIB or IVA cervix cancer (263). The study was criticized because patients were not surgically staged, half of the 190 patients were not evaluable, and radiation doses were low (478). Piver et al. (487) published an update of a study of 130 patients (13 with para-aortic lymph node metastasis), 75 of whom were surgically staged. Of 66 patients who underwent surgical staging, 33 received hydroxyurea and 33 a placebo in combination with irradiation. Of the patients who did not have surgical staging, 27 received hydroxyurea and 37 received placebo. The 2-year survival was higher in the HOU group.

In another larger randomized trial by the GOG reported by Stehman et al. (579), 296 surgically staged patients with stage IIB to IVA disease and negative para-aortic nodes were randomized to irradiation plus either hydroxyurea (139 patients) or misonidazole (157 patients). Survival was not statistically different between the regimens, with 33.8% deaths in the hydroxyurea and 38.9% deaths in the misonidazole groups

($p = 0.25$). Failure limited to the pelvis occurred in 18% of patients in the hydroxyurea group and 23.6% in the misonidazole group.

Noteworthy, in a randomized RTOG trial of patients with stage III disease, Leibel et al. (371) and Overgaard et al. (456) reported lower survival in patients receiving misonidazole than in the patients treated with irradiation alone.

Symonds et al. (592), in a review of seven randomized trials, found no evidence to support the use of HOU with RT in cervix cancer.

Cisplatin

Tattersall et al. (600) published a report of 71 patients with stage IB and IIA carcinoma of the cervix treated by radical hysterectomy who had metastatic pelvic lymph nodes and were entered into a randomized trial comparing pelvic RT alone or combined with three cycles of cisplatin (50 mg/m^2), vinblastine (4 mg/m^2), and bleomycin (15 mg), followed by the same pelvic irradiation. There was no difference in survival in the two groups.

Later, Tattersall et al. (598) reported on a randomized trial of 260 patients with stage IIB to IVA cervical cancer, 131 treated with pelvic irradiation (45 to 55 Gy followed by 30 to 35 Gy LDR brachytherapy), and 129 receiving chemotherapy (cisplatin and epirubicin at 3-week intervals for three cycles) followed by similar pelvic irradiation. Patients who received chemotherapy had a significantly higher pelvic failure rate (29% vs. 19%; $p < 0.003$) and inferior 3-year disease-free survival (40% vs. 50%) compared with those treated with RT alone ($p = 0.02$).

Souhami et al. (573) randomized 107 patients with stage IIIB carcinoma of the cervix to treatment with irradiation alone or combined with bleomycin, vincristine, mitomycin, and cisplatin (BOMP). The overall 5-year survival rate for the neoadjuvant-treated patients was 23% in contrast to 39% for those treated with irradiation alone ($p = 0.02$). Locoregional and distant failure rates were similar in both groups.

Chiara et al. (80) described a randomized study of patients with advanced carcinoma of the cervix (stages IIB and III) in which 46 patients were treated with irradiation alone or in combination with cisplatin. The actuarial 3-year progression-free survival rates were 72.4% and 59.3%, respectively.

Kumar et al. (342) reported a randomized trial in which 94 patients with carcinoma of the cervix were treated with chemotherapy (two cycles of bleomycin, ifosfamide-mesna, and cisplatin) followed by RT, and 90 patients were treated with irradiation alone. In the chemotherapy/RT group, 32-month survival was 63% for stage IIB and 50% for III and in the RT group, 59% for IIB and 27% for IIIB tumors (differences not statistically significant). There was no difference in radiation-induced toxicity between the two groups.

In a Swedish study (587), 47 patients with carcinoma of the cervix were randomized to be treated with irradiation alone (64.8 Gy, 1.8-Gy fractions) and 47 with a combination of three cycles of cisplatin and 5 days of 5-FU administered every third week, followed by the same pelvic irradiation. The 5-year disease-free survival rates were 70% with chemoirradiation and 57% with irradiation alone ($p = 0.07$). The incidences of pelvic recurrence were 60% and 47%, respectively, and for distant metastasis, 19% and 35%, respectively. Two patients in the chemoirradiation and one in the irradiation-alone group died as a consequence of therapy.

Tseng et al. (620) published results of a study in which patients with advanced carcinoma of the cervix were randomly assigned to either RT alone (60) or concurrent chemotherapy (cisplatin, vincristine, and bleomycin every 3 weeks for a total of four courses) and RT (62). After a median follow-up of 46.8 months, the disease-free survival and actuarial survival rates were 51.7% and 61.7% in the concurrent group and 53.2% and 64.5% in the RT group, respectively ($p = 0.27$). Treatment-

related toxicity was higher with the combination therapy compared with irradiation alone (36.7% vs. 17.7%; $p = 0.02$).

Randomized Studies in the United States

Results from several cooperative oncology groups demonstrated that cisplatin-based chemotherapy, when given concurrently with RT, prolongs survival in women with locally advanced cervical cancers, as well as in women with stage I to IIA disease who have metastatic disease in the pelvic lymph nodes, positive parametrial disease, or positive surgical margins at the time of primary surgery. However, Curtin et al. (104) completed a phase III trial in which 89 patients with high-risk stage IB or IIA undergoing radical hysterectomy and pelvic node dissection were randomized to be treated with postoperative cisplatin/bleomycin alone (44 patients) or combined with pelvic RT (45 patients). There were nine and 10 recurrences, respectively, and survival was equivalent.

The details of five other published studies were summarized by Lehman and Thomas (370) (Table 66.28) and discussed in detail.

The GOG conducted randomized Protocol 85 in which patients with carcinoma of the cervix, a clinical stage of IIB to IVA, and negative para-aortic nodes were treated with external pelvic irradiation (51 Gy) combined with 30 Gy to point A with LDR brachytherapy (653); 177 patients received 5-FU (IV infusion, 1 g/m^2 for 4 days) and cisplatin (50 mg/m^2 IV) on days 1, 29, and 30 to 33, and 191 patients received hydroxyurea (80 mg/kg orally twice weekly). With a median follow-up for survivors of 8.7 years, the 5-year survival rate in the cisplatin/5-FU arm was 60%, compared with 47% for women in the hydroxyurea arm.

After completion of GOG 85, the group opened GOG 120 for the same patient population (654), which was a three-arm randomized trial comparing irradiation plus hydroxyurea versus irradiation plus weekly cisplatin versus irradiation plus hydroxyurea, cisplatin, and 5-FU. In 526 evaluable patients with a median follow-up for survivors of 35 months, the 4-year survival rate for women in both the weekly cisplatin and irradiation arm and the irradiation, 5-FU, cisplatin arm was 69%, compared with 37% the hydroxyurea and irradiation arm ($p < 0.001$) Overall survival was also significantly better in the two patient groups receiving cisplatin. Hematologic toxicity was greater in the group treated with the three drugs compared with cisplatin or hydroxyurea alone.

The RTOG conducted a randomized study of 388 patients with stage IB to IIA larger than 5 cm, proven positive pelvic lymph nodes, or stage IIB to IVA carcinoma of the cervix in which patients were treated with either pelvic and para-aortic irradiation (best arm of RTOG Protocol 79-20) or pelvic irradiation and three cycles of concomitant chemotherapy with cisplatin (75 mg/m^2) and 4-day infusion of 5-FU (1,000 mg/m^2/per day) (466). Results were updated by Eifel et al. (145). With a median follow-up of 6.6 years for 228 survivors, the 8-year overall survival rate for women on the irradiation and cisplatin/5-FU arm was 67% versus 41% in the irradiation-only arm ($p < 0.0001$; Fig. 66.34). Disease-free survival rates were 66% and 36%, respectively. There were no significant differences in late complications in the treatment groups.

Southwest Oncology Group 8797 was a study for women with FIGO stage IA2, IB, or IIA carcinoma of the cervix with metastatic disease in the pelvic lymph nodes, positive parametrial involvement, or positive surgical margins at the time of primary radical hysterectomy with total pelvic lymphadenectomy. Patients had confirmed negative para-aortic lymph nodes; if the para-aortic lymph nodes were not sampled, the patients had confirmed negative common iliac lymph nodes. One hundred twenty-seven patients were randomized to be treated with pelvic EBRT with 5-FU infusion and cisplatin, and 116 were

| | Table 66.28 | DETAILS OF THE TREATMENT PROTOCOLS OF THE FIVE RANDOMIZED TRIALS THAT FORMED THE BASIS OF THE NATIONAL CANCER INSTITUTE ANNOUNCEMENT |

Author (Reference)	No. of Patients	Tumor Stage	Surgical Staging	Control Arm	Investigational Arm
Keys et al. (312)	369	Bulky IB (≥4 cm)	Completion hysterectomy	XRT	XRT + cisplatin (40 mg/m² IV weekly × 6 wk)
Whitney et al. (653)	368	IIB, III, IVA	Yes	XRT + hydroxyurea (80 mg/kg PO 2×/wk)	XRT + cisplatin (50 mg/m² IV days 1, 28) + 5-FU infusion (1 g/m²/day, days 2–5, 30–33)
Rose et al. (523)	526	IIB, III, IVA	Yes	XRT + hydroxyurea (3 g/m² PO 2×/wk)	XRT + cisplatin (40 mg/m² weekly × 6 wk) versus XRT + cisplatin (50 mg/m² IV days 1, 29) + 5-FU infusion (1 g/m²/day, days 1–4, 29–33) + hydroxyurea PO (2 g/m² 2×/wk × 6 wk)
Eifel et al. (145)	386	IIB, III, IVA, IB, IIA + tumor ≥5 cm or positive pelvic nodes	Yes	XRT (pelvic + para-aortic)	XRT + cisplatin (75 mg/m² IV day 1) + 5-FU infusion (1 g/m²/day, days 1–5 × 3 q3 wk)
Peters et al. (483)	243	IA2, IB, IIA (pathologic stage) + positive pelvis nodes and/or positive margins and/or microscopic involvement of parametria	Yes	XRT	XRT + cisplatin (70 mg/m² IV) + 5-FU infusion (1 g/m² days 1–5 × 4 q3 wk)

5-FU, 5-fluorouracil; XRT, pelvic external radiation therapy.
From Lehman M, Thomas G. Is concurrent chemotherapy and radiotherapy the new standard of care for locally advanced cervical cancer? *Int J Gynecol Oncol* 2001;11:87–99, with permission.

treated with irradiation alone. The 3-year survival for women on the adjuvant cisplatin/5-FU and RT arm was 87% compared with 77% for women on the pelvic irradiation arm (Fig. 66.35) (483). The difference is statistically significant.

In GOG 123, 183 women with bulky (≥4 cm) stage IB carcinoma of the cervix with negative pelvic and para-aortic nodes radiographically or surgically determined were randomized to be treated with pelvic EBRT and brachytherapy, followed by extrafascial hysterectomy, and 186 received EBRT and brachytherapy with weekly cisplatin (40 mg/m², total dose not to exceed 70 mg per week) followed by extrafascial hysterectomy (312). With a median follow-up for survivors of 35.7 months. The progression-free survival rate for women treated with irradiation and cisplatin was 79% compared with 63% for those treated with RT alone (*p* <0.001). The overall 3-year survival rates were 83% and 74%, respectively (*p* = 0.0008).

The results of these five randomized trials were summarized by Rose and Eifel (524) (Table 66.29).

Haie-Meder et al. (221), in a review of these trials, concluded that the published results have led to a modification in the standard of treatment in these poor-prognosis cervix cancers. Five of the randomized trials evidenced the superiority of cisplatin-based chemotherapy, but the optimal chemotherapeutic regimens remain to be defined.

In GOG Protocol 165, patients with stages IIB to IVA cervical cancer received either radiation therapy and concurrent weekly cisplatin (40 mg/m²) or radiation therapy and a protracted venous infusion (PVI) of 5-FU. Lanciano et al. (347) reported that the study was prematurely closed after an interim analysis showed a failure rate 35% higher and would not result in improved DFS with PVI 5-FU/RT compared with weekly cisplatin.

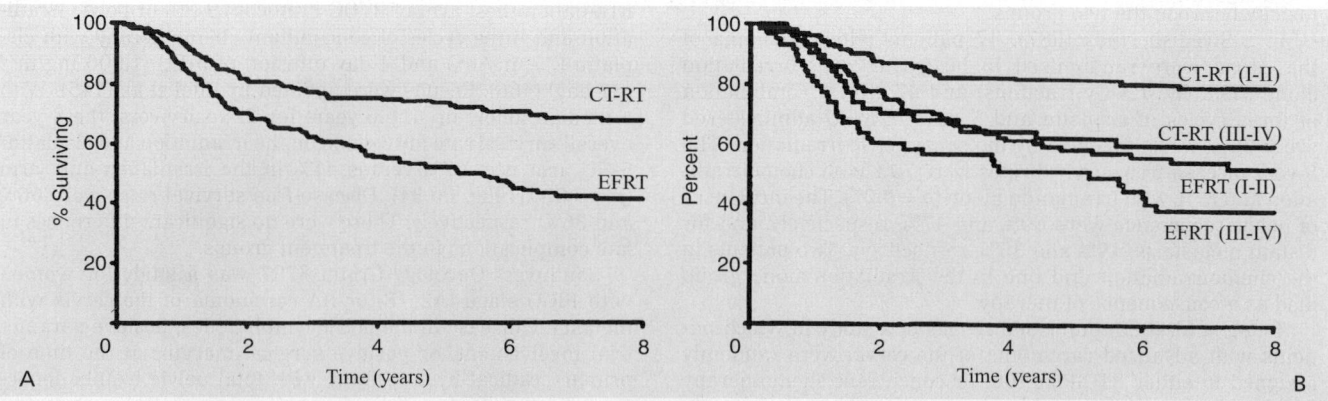

FIGURE 66.34. A,B: Overall survival rates of patients randomized to receive concurrent chemotherapy and pelvic radiation (CT-RT) or extended-field radiation therapy (EFRT; *p* = 0.004). **B:** Subgroups stratified by International Federation of Gynecology and Obstetrics stage. Numbers in parentheses indicate the number of patients at risk for recurrence at 3 or 5 years. (From Eifel PJ, Winter K, Morris M, et al. Pelvic irradiation with concurrent chemotherapy versus pelvic and para-aortic irradiation for high risk cervical cancer: an update of radiation therapy oncology group trial (RTOG 90-01). *J Clin Oncol* 2004;22:872–880, with permission.)

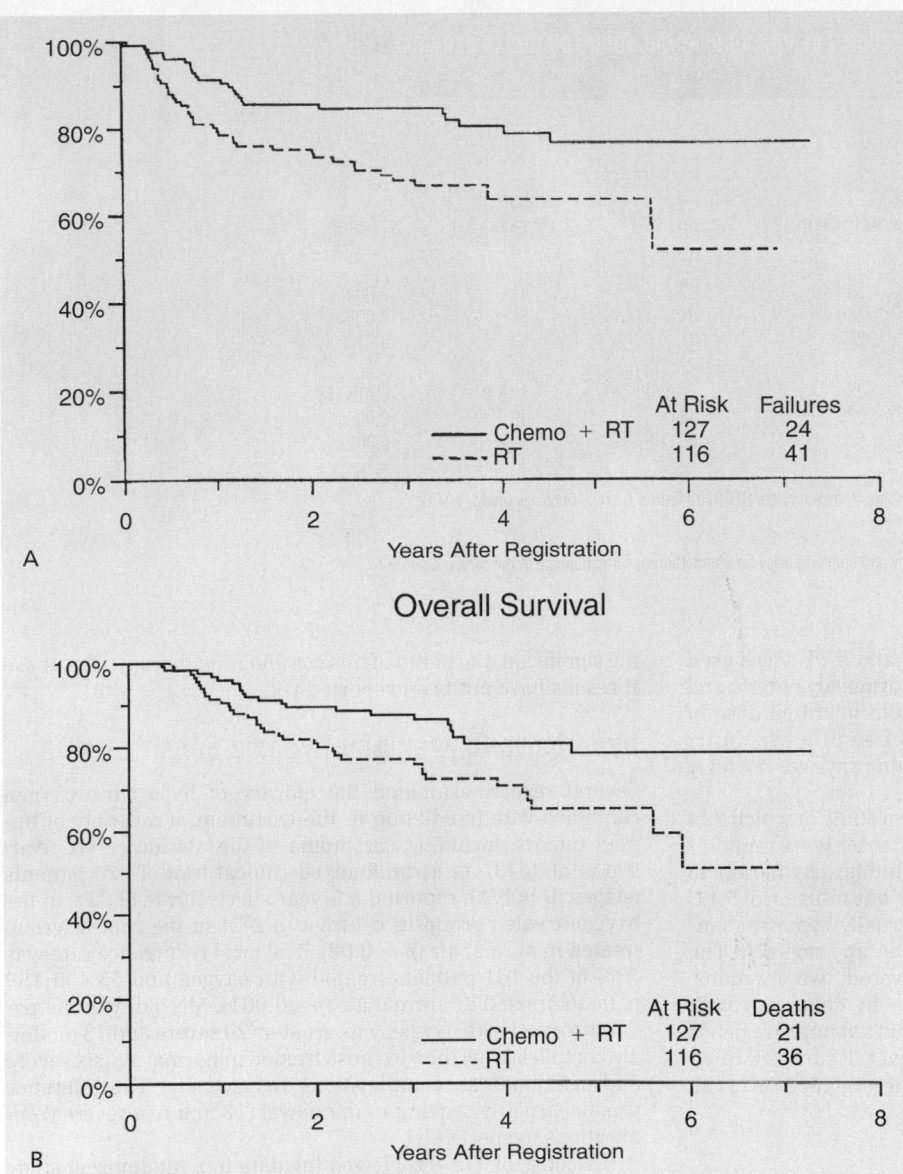

FIGURE 66.35. Progression-free **(A)** and overall **(B)** survival for 127 patients randomized to receive chemotherapy plus radiation therapy (Chemo+RT) and for 116 patients randomized to receive radiation therapy (RT) alone. (From Peters WA III, Liu PY, Barrett RJ, et al. Concurrent chemotherapy and pelvic radiation therapy compared with pelvic radiation therapy alone as adjuvant therapy after radical surgery in high-risk early-stage cancer of the cervix. *J Clin Oncol* 2000;18:1606–1613, with permission.)

Randomized Studies in Other Countries

Lorvidhaya et al. (387) reported on 673 patients with predominantly stage IIB and IIIB disease randomized to receive either irradiation alone or combined with chemotherapy administered in either an adjuvant, concurrent, or adjuvant and concurrent schedule. Concomitant chemotherapy consisted of mitomycin C (10 mg/m²) given on days 1 and 30 and oral 5-FU (300 mg/m² per day) given on days 1 to 14 and 42 to 56. Adjuvant chemotherapy consisted of three cycles of oral 5-FU (200 mg per day) given for 4 weeks, with a 2-week rest every 6 weeks. With a median follow-up of 25 months, there was a statistically significant improvement in disease-free survival for all patients who received chemotherapy/RT, regardless of the timing of administration of the chemotherapy. However, the authors did not state the radiation dose delivered with brachytherapy, the total dose prescribed to point A, or the overall treatment time. In the absence of this information, the adequacy of the radiation therapy cannot be evaluated, and we cannot assume that the results of this study apply to all patients treated with irradiation.

On the other hand, Pearcey et al. (466) reported on a Canadian randomized study in which 127 patients with stage IB,

IIA >5 cm, or IIB carcinoma of the cervix were randomized to be treated with cisplatin (40 mg/m² weekly) and RT, and 126 patients were treated with RT alone (50.4 Gy to the pelvis combined with brachytherapy). With a median follow-up of 65 months, the 5-year survival rates were 59% and 56%, respectively ($p = 0.43$). There was a somewhat greater incidence of significant late morbidity in the RT alone group (12% vs. 6%; $p = 0.08$).

Possible explanations for the discrepancy in results between the five U.S. trials (436) and the NCI of Canada Study were analyzed by Lehman and Thomas (370).

Chemotherapy and Hyperfractionated Irradiation

Calkins et al. (66) assessed the toxicities of multiple–daily-fractionated (twice daily, 1.2-Gy fractions) whole pelvis radiation plus concurrent chemotherapy for locally advanced carcinoma of the cervix. In the first study (GOG 8801) of 38 patients, hydroxyurea was given orally (80 mg/kg to a maximum of 6 g) at least 2 hours before irradiation, twice every week. In the second

Table 66.29	FIVE RANDOMIZED STUDIES OF CONCURRENT CHEMOIRRADIATION IN CERVICAL CARCINOMA					

| | | | Survival | | | |
Author (Reference)	Drugs	No. of Patients	Chemotherapy/ Radiation Therapy (%)	Radiation Therapy (%)	p Value
Chemoirradiation versus Radiation Alone					
Eifel et al. (145) RTOG 9001[a]	CF	388	67	41	0.004
Keys et al. (312) GOG 123	C	369	84	68	0.008
Peters et al. (483) SWOG 8797	CF	243	81	63	0.01
Comparative Trials of Chemoirradiation Regimens					
Whitney et al. (653) GOG 85	CF vs. H	368	50.8 CF	39.8 H	0.018
Rose & Eifel (524) GOG 120	C vs. H	526	64 C	39 H	0.002
Rose & Eifel (524) GOG 120	CHF vs. H	526	66 CHF	39 H	0.002

C, cisplatin; F, 5-fluorouracil; GOG, Gynecologic Oncology Group; H, hydroxyurea; RTOG, Radiation Therapy Oncology Group; SWOG, Southwestern Oncology Group.
[a]Eight-year results.
Modified from Rose PG, Eifel PJ. Combined radiation therapy and chemotherapy for chemotherapy for carcinoma of the cervix. *Cancer J* 2001;7:86–94, with permission.

study (GOG 8901) of 30 patients, cisplatin and 5-FU were used concomitantly with RT. Acute toxicity was primarily enteric and appeared to be dose related. The maximum tolerated dose of whole pelvis radiation that could be delivered in a hyperfractionated setting with concomitant chemotherapy was 57.6 Gy in 48 fractions followed by brachytherapy.

Thomas et al. (607) conducted a four-arm study in which 234 women with bulky stage IB to IVA cervical cancer were randomized to receive either standard RT (EBRT and brachytherapy to deliver 90 Gy to point A) with or without a 4-day infusion of 5-FU (1 g/m^2) on days 1 to 5 and 22 to 25, or partially hyperfractionated RT with or without the same chemotherapy regimen. The partially hyperfractionated regimen delivered two fractions, 6 hours apart, on the first 4 days of treatment, coinciding with the infusion of 5-FU. The addition of 5-FU did not improve pelvic control, complications (42% vs. 46% at 5 years) or overall survival. However, this study closed without reaching target patient accrual.

Neoadjuvant Chemotherapy

Thomas (609) summarized the rationale and potential limitations of neoadjuvant chemotherapy in carcinoma of the cervix and pointed out that four randomized trials of neoadjuvant chemotherapy and irradiation had been reported. Although response rates to the chemotherapy are between 30% and 85%, none of the studies showed an advantage for pelvic tumor control or survival (33,70,77,244,341,361,587,593).

Colombo et al. (92), in a review of the literature, concluded that the role of neoadjuvant chemotherapy followed by radiation and by concomitant chemotherapy is controversial because high response rates are reported but no significant advantages in survival or local control have been shown.

Amifostine

De Los Santos and Small (110) reviewed the available data in several small phase I or II trials and concluded that this radioprotector may be beneficial in the treatment of patients with cervical cancer, particularly when using chemoradiation. Subcutaneous administration may facilitate the administration of the drug and decrease acute and late toxicity. RTOG conducted a phase I and II study (RTOG 0116) with subcutaneous amifostine in patients treated with extended field RT brachytherapy and chemotherapy without (Phase I) or with amifostine (Phase II). Phase I completed accrual with 27 patients and confirmed

the significant morbidity of this combination therapy. The phase II results have not been reported yet.

Hyperbaric Oxygen and Hypoxic Sensitizers

Several reports evaluated the efficacy of hyperbaric oxygen combined with irradiation in the treatment of a variety of human tumors, including carcinoma of the uterine cervix. Watson et al. (643), in a randomized clinical trial of 320 patients (stages III to IVA), reported a 5-year survival rate of 33% in the oxygen-treated group in contrast to 27% in the control group treated in normal air ($p = 0.08$). The local recurrence rate was 33% in the 161 patients treated with oxygen and 53% in 159 patients treated in normal air ($p < 0.001$). Morbidity in the patients treated with oxygen was greater (20 severe and 13 moderate complications) than in those treated in normal air (six severe and eight moderate complications, respectively). The difference was particularly striking in the bowel (13 and two severe complications, respectively).

Dische et al. (124) reviewed the data in a randomized study of patients with advanced carcinoma of the cervix treated with radiation therapy and hyperbaric oxygen or air and noted that the patients treated with oxygen had improved survival at Mount Vernon and Glasgow but not at Cape Town. Data from the three centers were merged, and analysis showed that local tumor control was significantly worse in patients treated in normal air who had a prior blood transfusion, but in the oxygen group this effect was reversed. The same interaction was noted in the survival results ($p = 0.042$).

A trial reported by Fletcher (161), in which 233 patients with stage IIB, III, and IV carcinoma of the cervix were randomized to be treated with irradiation in normal air or with hyperbaric oxygen, demonstrated no significant benefit in survival or tumor control (20/109 patients treated with oxygen failed in the pelvis, in contrast to 29/124 treated in normal air). Furthermore, morbidity was greater (26 complications) in patients treated with hyperbaric oxygen compared with the control group (15 complications).

Dische et al. (124) published results of a four-arm randomized trial of hyperbaric oxygen and radiation therapy of stage IIB and III carcinoma of the cervix in which 335 patients were randomized to treatment in 10 or 28 fractions, in hyperbaric oxygen or in normal air. Data of 327 cases were analyzed. There was no advantage in tumor control with the use of hyperbaric oxygen. There was an increase in late radiation morbidity when treatment was given in hyperbaric oxygen rather than in normal air, and when using 10 fractions, a total dose of 45 Gy rather than 40 Gy was administered.

No definite conclusions can be drawn concerning the use of hyperbaric oxygen in carcinoma of the cervix. It is possible that hyperbaric oxygen administered with fewer high-dose fractions may be more efficacious than when combined with conventional dose and fractionation schemes. The trials reported have not shown an increased incidence of distant metastasis, which has been observed in a clinical study and in some animal experiments (286).

Grigsby et al. (210) published results of an RTOG study in which 120 patients with carcinoma of the cervix were randomized to receive irradiation alone or combined with misonidazole. The 5-year progression-free survival was 22% and 29%, respectively. These findings are similar to those reported by Overgaard et al. (456), who, in a randomized study of 331 patients with carcinoma of the cervix treated with either misonidazole or a placebo and irradiation, found no significant difference in local tumor control (50% vs. 54%), disease-free survival (47% vs. 46%), or crude survival (39% vs. 45%).

Irradiation and Hyperthermia

Because of technical limitations in the delivery of adequate heat to large parts of the body such as the pelvis, the use of hyperthermia in the treatment of carcinoma of the uterine cervix has been sparse. Hornback et al. (260) described a nonrandomized study in which the combination of microwave hyperthermia (433 MHz) and irradiation resulted in improved pelvic tumor control (72%) in a group of 79 patients with stage IIIB carcinoma compared with previously irradiated historic control patients (53%). However, 5-year survival rates were comparable in both groups (22% to 30%).

Sharma et al. (552) reported a 70% disease-free survival rate at 18 months in 20 patients with stage IIB or III carcinoma of the uterine cervix treated with a combination of irradiation and hyperthermia (13.5 MHz, 42°C to 43°C, 30 minutes before irradiation), in comparison with a 50% disease-free survival rate in 22 patients treated with irradiation alone. The grade 3 complication rate (8%) was similar in both groups.

Dinges et al. (123) treated 18 patients with advanced carcinoma of the cervix with RT plus hyperthermia (in the first and fourth weeks, two regional hyperthermia treatments were applied). The acute toxicity was low and similar to that with RT alone. The local tumor control was 48% at 2 years.

Harima et al. (232) evaluated irradiation therapy or thermoirradiation (three sessions of hyperthermia) for stage IIIB cervical carcinoma; two groups of 20 patients each were randomly divided. A complete response was achieved in 50% (10/20) in the RT group versus 80% (16/20) in the thermoirradiation group ($p = 0.048$). The 3-year overall survival and disease-free survival rates for the patients who were treated with thermoirradiation (58.2% and 63.6%) were better than with RT (48.1% and 45%), but differences were not statistically significant. The 3-year local relapse-free survival rate of the patients who were treated with thermoirradiation (79.7%) was significantly better than that of the patients treated with irradiation alone (48.5%; $p = 0.048$). Thermoirradiation was well tolerated and did not add to either acute or long-term toxicity over radiation alone.

Vasanthan et al. (632) reported on 110 patients with locally advanced cervix cancer randomized to treatment with RT alone or combined with hyperthermia (minimum five sessions, 60 minutes each, once weekly). Overall 3-year pelvic tumor control was 68.5% and survival 73.2%, with no difference in either group, although survival was lower in the patients with stage IIB treated with hyperthermia. Acute toxicity was 18% (10/55) in the hyperthermia patients and 4% (2/55) with RT alone. Late toxicity was no different in the two arms.

Carcinoma of the Cervix and Pregnancy

The concurrent presence of carcinoma *in situ* or invasive carcinoma of the uterine cervix and pregnancy, although rare, poses a therapeutic dilemma to gynecologic and radiation oncologists. Reported incidence is one to 10 cases per 10,000 pregnancies (128). In the United States, the incidence has decreased with the less frequent diagnosis of invasive cervical cancer. Norstrom et al. (446), in Sweden, found cervical cancer was diagnosed in 33 women in association with pregnancy (incidence 11.1 cases per 100,000 deliveries and 7.5 per 100,000 pregnancies). Abnormal bleeding was the symptom that led to diagnosis in 54.5% of the women; 45.5% were asymptomatic but had an abnormal cervicovaginal cytologic test result (39.4%) or abnormal vaginal examination (6.1%) in association with pregnancy. During the follow-up, 1/12 women with cervix cancer in the first trimester, 4/12 in the third trimester, and 2/9 women postpartum died of the disease. Primary surgery was used more frequently than radiation therapy.

For carcinoma *in situ*, if the pregnancy is allowed to reach full term, confirmation of the diagnosis by colposcopy and conservative management with monthly Pap smears constitutes the best approach. Conization has frequently been performed. Punch biopsies can be obtained, but the diagnostic accuracy is less reliable. As many as 50% of the patients have residual carcinoma *in situ* after delivery.

In patients with invasive carcinoma, the lesion is usually clinically apparent. Multiple punch biopsies are adequate to confirm the diagnosis.

Management is individualized based on tumor size and stage, patient age, and desires of the patient (or couple) regarding the pregnancy. The majority of patients with cervical cancer diagnosed during pregnancy (approximately 75%) have stage I tumors (128,258,416). Occasionally in late pregnancy, if tumors are small, definitive therapy is postponed and delivery is allowed. In a review of the literature intentional treatment delay was associated with a recurrence rate of 4% (505). Sorosky et al. (572) reported on eight pregnant women with stage I carcinoma of the cervix who had declined immediate therapy and followed until the late third trimester; a cesarean section–radical hysterectomy was performed with delay in therapy ranging from 3 to 40 weeks during the pregnancies. There was no clinical progression of the disease with follow-up of 33 months.

Greer et al. (192) noted in 600 infants without congenital abnormalities, when stage IB cervical carcinoma was diagnosed during pregnancy and fetal survival was desired, the neonatal mortality rate decreased from 30% when the fetus was delivered at 26 to 27 weeks to 2.7% when the fetus was allowed to mature to 34 to 35 weeks.

Because there is a greater need to institute therapy as soon as possible that the accepted method of treatment in patients in the first 6 months of pregnancy is to carry out definitive surgery or radiation therapy, as indicated by the stage of the disease. In the third trimester of pregnancy, when the fetus may be salvaged, some gynecologic oncologists prefer a postpartum cesarean section, combined with a radical hysterectomy and lymphadenectomy or followed by definitive treatment. However, some authors report that vaginal delivery has no detrimental effect on the prognosis (100).

If a radical hysterectomy is performed and positive pelvic lymph nodes are found, the usual postoperative irradiation, including external beam with or without intracavitary insertion, should be carried out.

If it is decided to terminate the pregnancy and treat the patient with external irradiation, initially the whole pelvis is irradiated (40 Gy in 4 weeks). A spontaneous abortion occurs, and there is some involution of the uterus. However, in one series of 45 patients 27% did not abort spontaneously and surgical evacuation was required (568). After this dose of radiation, careful evacuation of the uterus and LDR (or equivalent dose HDR) brachytherapy may be performed under general anesthesia. Two intracavitary insertions for a total of 6,500 mgh (55 Gy to point A) and an additional 10 or 20 Gy are delivered to the parametria with a midline block. If surgery is to be carried out, approximately 4,000 mgh is given.

Patients who require high doses of pelvic irradiation (>40 Gy) should be counseled regarding the permanent loss of reproductive capability, not only because of ovarian ablation (which happens with doses of 8 Gy or higher), but as a consequence of radiation effects in the uterus (570).

Survival is the same regardless of the trimester of the pregnancy in which definitive treatment is instituted. Creasman et al. (100) reported on 48 patients treated by irradiation, 45 by irradiation followed by surgery, and five with radical hysterectomy alone. The survival was comparable with that of nonpregnant patients for similar stages. The survival rate for patients with stage I disease was comparable whether vaginal delivery was allowed or a cesarean section was performed (approximately 85% in stage I and 50% to 64% in stage II). Also, the percentage of infants surviving (>80%) was the same in both groups.

Sood et al. (570) performed a retrospective analysis of 26 women with cervical carcinoma diagnosed during pregnancy and treated primarily with radiation therapy (mean dose, 46.7 Gy) and LDR intracavitary radiation (mean dose, 56.5 Gy to point A). These cases were matched with 26 nonpregnant control patients based on age, histology, stage, treatment, and year of treatment. There were no statistically significant differences in recurrence rates or survival between the pregnant group and the control patients. Short-term toxicity was comparable in pregnant and nonpregnant patients. Long-term complication rates were 12% in pregnant patients and 27% in control patients, but this difference was not statistically significant. Most complications were likely related to radiation techniques (particularly the predominance of ^{60}Co).

Sood et al. (569) compared the prognosis of 56 women who had cervical cancer diagnosed during pregnancy and 27 who were diagnosed within 6 months after delivery. Control patients (cervical cancer diagnosed at least 5 years since last delivery) were matched one to one with cases based on age, histology, stage, treatment, and time of treatment. Among the postpartum women, 11 were treated with radical hysterectomies, 14 with radiation therapy, and two with stage IA1 disease were treated with vaginal hysterectomies. One of seven patients who had cesarean sections had a local and distant recurrence. In contrast, 10/17 (59%) who delivered vaginally had recurrences (*p* = 0.04). In multivariate analysis, vaginal delivery was the most significant predictor of recurrence, followed by high tumor stage. Survival for patients diagnosed in the postpartum period was significantly worse than for control patients and for those diagnosed during pregnancy. They concluded that pregnant women with cervical cancer should be delivered by cesarean section.

Jones et al. (288) published a survey by the American College of Surgeons that evaluated management of invasive cervical carcinoma in 161 pregnant patients; 86 were treated with surgery alone, 30 with radiation therapy alone, and 45 with a combination of the two modalities. Approximately one-third of patients were diagnosed in each trimester. The 5-year survival was 94.6% for patients diagnosed in the first trimester, 76.9% for the second, and 68.9% for the third trimester. The prognosis of patients with invasive carcinoma of the cervix associated with pregnancy was similar to that of nonpregnant patients. There was no significant difference in 5-year survival whether the patients delivered by cesarean section or normal vaginal delivery.

Senekjian et al. (549) reported no difference in survival or patterns of failure in 24 women who were pregnant at the time of diagnosis of clear-cell adenocarcinoma of the cervix and vagina compared with 408 who had never been pregnant. The 5- and 10-year actuarial survival rates were 86% and 68% for the pregnant patients and 87% and 79%, respectively, for patients who had not been pregnant.

Neoadjuvant chemotherapy for invasive squamous-cell carcinoma of the cervix in pregnancy has been considered in selected patients (604).

The practice popularized 30 years ago of administering a "restraining dose of radium" and deferring definitive radiation therapy until delivery is carried out should be strongly condemned. Strauss (583) reported 2/11 infants being born with microcephaly in addition to other complications such as alopecia, facial deformity, eye damage, and chromosomal abnormalities after this procedure.

Carcinoma of the Cervical Stump

Subtotal hysterectomy, a relatively popular procedure for benign conditions of the uterus in past years, is rarely performed today. These patients are, of course, at risk for development of carcinoma of the uterine cervix.

It is important to divide carcinoma of the cervical stump into *true*, when the first symptom occurs 3 or more years after subtotal hysterectomy, or *coincidental*, when the symptoms are noticed before the third postoperative year. This separation is important because the prognosis for carcinoma of the true stump is significantly better than for coincidental lesions, in which carcinoma was probably present when the hysterectomy was performed (478).

The natural history and patterns of spread of carcinoma of the cervical stump are similar to those of the cervix in the intact uterus. The diagnostic work-up, clinical staging, and basic principles of therapy are the same.

When surgery is performed for stage I tumors, it is somewhat more difficult because of the previous surgical procedures and the presence of adhesions in the pelvis. When irradiation is administered, the lack of uterine cavity into which to insert a tandem containing two or three sources makes intracavitary therapy more difficult. As many sources as technically feasible should be inserted in the remaining cervical canal. Occasionally, transvaginal irradiation may be used to boost the dose delivered to central disease in the stump. It is important to deliver higher whole pelvis irradiation. In general, patients with stage I disease are treated with a combination of 20 Gy to the whole pelvis and 30 Gy to the parametria with midline shielding combined with two intracavitary insertions. The dose of intracavitary therapy depends on the number of sources that can be placed in the cervical canal. More advanced stages should be treated with 40 Gy to the whole pelvis and 20 Gy to the parametria with midline shielding, combined with the same intracavitary doses. When there is no opportunity to insert any sources in the cervical canal, the whole pelvis dose must be increased to 60 Gy. Total dose (external and LDR intracavitary brachytherapy) to the upper vaginal mucosa should not exceed 150 Gy, and tolerance doses to small volumes of the bladder (80 Gy) or rectum (75 Gy) should be carefully monitored.

If there is bulky disease present in the cervix, parametrium, or vagina, additional interstitial therapy is advisable, if technically feasible. When intravaginal cones are used, a 30- to 40-Gy air dose is delivered in 2 to 3 weeks, in three to five weekly fractions.

The 5-year survival rate for carcinoma of the cervical stump treated with irradiation is similar to that reported for patients with carcinoma of the intact uterus (336,657). The anatomic sites of failure and the incidence of recurrences are similar to those of patients in whom the uterus is intact. Distant metastases also follow the same distribution.

In 253 patients with carcinoma of the cervical stump treated at M.D. Anderson Cancer Center, median survival was 203, 140, and 32 months for stages I, II, and III, respectively (411). Kovalic et al. (336) reported on 70 patients with carcinoma of the surgical stump treated with irradiation; 16 also underwent a surgical procedure. The 10-year disease-free survival was 79% for stage IB, 66% for stage IIB, and 39% for stage IIIB disease. The pelvic failure rates were 10%, 9%, and 50%, respectively. Major gastrointestinal complications were noted in 9% of patients, and urinary complications in 3.8%. The results are comparable with those seen in patients treated for invasive carcinoma of the cervix with intact uterus.

Hannoun-Levi et al. (229) published results in 77 patients treated for carcinoma of the cervical stump. Treatment consisted of a combination of EBRT and brachytherapy, and, in a few cases, patients underwent surgery or interstitial brachytherapy. Three-year pelvic tumor control was achieved in 59/77 patients (76.6%); tumor control probabilities were 77%, 73.7%, and 56% in patients with stage I, II, or III tumors, respectively. Late complications were grade 2 in five patients (6.5%); grade 3 in one patient (1.3%), and grade 4 in two patients (2.6%).

Hellstrom et al. (240) published a retrospective study of 145 patients treated for carcinoma of the cervical stump, representing 2.2% of all cervical cancers. Three control cases to each case were matched from the cohort of cases with cervical carcinoma with intact uterus. The dose of irradiation from the intracavitary application given to the stump cancers was lower than for comparable cases with intact uterus. Long-term prognosis for squamous-cell carcinoma of the uterine stump was comparable with that of the ordinary cervical carcinomas. Stump adenocarcinomas had a worse prognosis compared with adenocarcinoma of the intact uterus ($p < 0.07$) and with stump of the squamous-cell carcinoma ($p = 0.05$). The complication rate was higher for stump cancer cases compared with that for cervical cancers with intact uterus.

Because of the close proximity of the bladder, rectum, and small intestine to the intracavitary sources and owing to the often higher doses of external-beam irradiation given to the whole pelvis, complications are somewhat more frequent than in carcinoma of the cervix with intact uterus.

The use of concurrent chemotherapy with external-beam irradiation in patients with cervical stump carcinoma may be beneficial, especially because, as discussed, the brachytherapy dose is often compromised by anatomic constraints.

:: | Second Malignancy

The possible induction of secondary primary cancers by pelvic irradiation is controversial (616). Lee et al. (367) observed no significant increase in the incidence of second malignancies in patients irradiated for carcinoma of the cervix in comparison with the Connecticut Tumor Registry prevailing rates.

Boice et al. (43), in a review of 68,730 women with carcinoma of the cervix treated with radiation therapy, observed a second malignant tumor in 3,324, compared with 3,063 expected (4.8% increase; $p < 0.001$). The excess was concentrated in the lung, other genital organs, bladder, and rectum. In addition, in 10,817 women with invasive cervical cancer not treated with irradiation, 479 secondary malignant tumors were observed versus 435 expected (4.4%; $p = 0.02$). Thus, the incidence of secondary tumors in women treated for carcinoma of the cervix with or without irradiation is only slightly greater than in the general population. Pelvic organs receiving a high dose of irradiation appear to have a somewhat greater incidence of a second primary.

Storm (581), in a comprehensive analysis of the Danish Cancer Registry data of 24,970 women with invasive cervical cancer and 19,470 with carcinoma *in situ* of the cervix treated between 1943 and 1982, noted a small overall excess of secondary primary cancers in the lung, stomach, pancreas, rectum, and bladder and connective tissue sarcomas, although there was a decreased incidence of breast cancer in the irradiated patients compared with nonirradiated patients (attributable to ovarian ablation by radiation therapy). In the patients irradiated for invasive carcinoma, there was an excess of 64 cases per 10,000 women per year of tumors in organs close to or at an intermediate distance from the cervix, reaching a maximum after 30 years or longer of follow-up. A high risk for development of acute nonlymphatic leukemia was observed in irradiated patients with carcinoma *in situ*, but not in those with invasive lesions. This could be explained by the lower doses of irradiation delivered to the bone marrow in the *in situ* tumors treated with brachytherapy alone, with greater induction of mutations and less cell killing, which may be responsible for the leukemogenic effect. Decreased risk was noted for tumors of the brain, myeloma of the skin, and tumors of the colon other than rectal.

In a study of 117,830 women diagnosed with cervical carcinoma *in situ* and 17,556 with invasive cervical carcinoma in Sweden, treatment not specified and *in situ* lesions traditionally treated with surgery alone, there was an increased incidence (RR 2.3 to 3) of second primary tumors in the anus, rectum, urinary bladder, pancreas, esophagus, and lung compared with the standardized incidence rate for all women (241). The data showed consistent increases in suggested targets for HPV at tobacco-related sites. A contributing role for a depressed immune response was considered to play a role.

Werner-Wasik et al. (649), in an analysis of 125 women with stage I and II carcinoma of the cervix treated with radiation therapy, observed 11 secondary primary tumors in 10 patients (four breast, two lung, and one each of myeloma, non-Hodgkin's lymphoma, bladder, thyroid, and vulva). All secondary primary tumors were located outside the irradiation fields. The increased relative risk of breast cancer in these patients was 2.64, higher than reported by Boice et al. (43).

Mark et al. (401) identified 13/114 patients diagnosed with uterine sarcoma who had a prior history of pelvic irradiation (doses of 40 to 80 Gy). Criteria for radiation-induced sarcomas included

(a) Previous history of pelvic irradiation,

(b) Latent period of several years,

(c) Development of sarcoma within previously irradiated field, and

(d) Histologic confirmation of malignancy.

Histologic types of tumor were mixed müllerian in six, leiomyosarcoma in four, endometrial stroma sarcoma in one, fibrosarcoma in one, and angiosarcoma in one patient. Sarcoma developed in the uterus in 12 and at the vaginal cuff in one. Ten patients were treated with surgery and two with radiation therapy. The 5-year disease-free survival rate after salvage therapy was 17%.

:: | Cost of Care for Cervical Cancer

Wolstenholme and Whynes (660) carried out a detailed cost audit over 5 years on a sample of patients diagnosed in 1990 in one United Kingdom region. The mean costs of managing preinvasive carcinoma were found to be significantly lower than those of stage I invasive carcinoma, and both were lower than the costs of invasive cancer at stages II to IV.

References

1. Abe M, Shibamoto Y. The usefulness of intraoperative radiation therapy in the treatment of pelvic recurrence of cervical cancer. *Int J Radiat Oncol Biol Phys* 1996;34:513–514.
2. Abeler VM, Holm R, Nesland JM, et al. Small cell carcinoma of the cervix: a clinicopathologic study of 26 patients. *Cancer* 1994;73:672–677.
3. Abu-Rustum NR, Rajbhandari D, Glusman S, et al. Acute lower extremity paralysis following radiation therapy for cervical cancer. *Gynecol Oncol* 1999;75:152–154.
4. Adli M, Mayr NA, Kaiser HS, et al. Does prone positioning reduce small bowel dose in pelvic radiation with intensity-modulated radiotherapy for gynecologic cancer? *Int J Radiat Oncol Biol Phys* 2003;57:230–238.
5. Admad K, Kim YH, Ezzell G, et al. Reproducibility of multifractionated outpatient high dose rate brachytherapy in carcinoma of the cervix using the Ahmad-Kim positioner. *Endocuriether Hypertherm Oncol* 1992;8:171–173.
6. Agarwal SS, Sehgal A, Sardana S, et al. Role of male behavior in cervical carcinogenesis among women with one lifetime sexual partner. *Cancer* 1993;72:1666–1669.
7. Ahmed RS, Kim RY, Duan J, et al. IMRT dose escalation for positive para-aortic lymph nodes in patients with locally advanced cervical cancer while reducing dose to bone marrow and other organs at risk. *Int J Radiat Oncol Biol Phys* 2004;60:505–512.
8. Akine Y, Arimoto H, Ogino T, et al. High-dose rate intracavitary irradiation in the treatment of carcinoma of the uterine cervix: early experience with 84 patients. *Int J Radiat Oncol Biol Phys* 1988;14:893–898.
9. Akine Y, Hashida I, Kajiura Y, et al. Carcinoma of the uterine cervix treated with external irradiation alone. *Int J Radiat Oncol Biol Phys* 1986;12:1611–1616.
10. Alfsen GC, Kristensen GB, Skovlund E, et al. Histologic subtype has minor importance for overall survival in patients with adenocarcinoma of the uterine cervix: a population-based study of prognostic factors in 505 patients with nonsquamous cell carcinoma of the cervix. *Cancer* 2001;92:2471–2483.
11. Allt WEC. Supervoltage radiation treatment in advanced cancer of the uterine cervix. *CMAJ* 1969;100:792–797.
12. Alvarez RD, Soong SJ, Kinney WK, et al. Identification of prognostic factors and risk groups in patients found to have nodal metastasis at the time of radical hysterectomy for early stage squamous carcinoma of the cervix. *Gynecol Oncol* 1989;35:130–135.
13. American Association of Physicists in Medicine. *AAPM report no. 21: specification of brachytherapy source strength.* Report of Task Group 32. New York: American Institute of Physics, 1987.
14. Ampil F, Datta R, Datta S. Elective postoperative external radiotherapy after hysterectomy in early-stage carcinoma of the cervix: is additional vaginal cuff irradiation necessary? *Cancer* 1987;60:280–288.
15. Ampil FL, Apple S, Bell MC. Spinal epidural compression complicating cancer of the cervix: a review of seven cases. *Eur J Gynaecol Oncol* 1998;19:105–107.
16. An HJ, Kim KR, Kim IS, et al. Prevalence of human papillomavirus DNA in various histological subtypes of cervical adenocarcinoma: a population based study. *Mod Pathol* 2005;18:528–534.
17. Anders JC, Grigsby PW, Singh AK. Cisplatin chemotherapy (without erythropoietin) and risk of life-threatening thromboembolic events in carcinoma of the uterine cervix: the tip of the iceberg? A review of the literature. *Radiat Oncol* 2006;5:14.
18. Anderson B, LaPolla J, Turner D, et al. Ovarian transposition in cervical cancer. *Gynecol Oncol* 1993;49:206–214.
19. Andras EJ, Fletchor GH, Rutledge F. Radiotherapy of carcinoma of the cervix following simple hysterectomy. *Am J Obstet Gynecol* 1973;115:647–655.
20. Anson BJ, McVay CB. *Surgical anatomy,* vol. 2, 5th ed. Philadelphia: W.B. Saunders, 1971;800–835.
21. Arai T, Tohda H, Itoh H, Himeno H, et al. Radiation treatment of cervix cancer using the high dose rate remote afterloading intracavitary irradiation: an analysis of the correlation between optimal dose range and fractionation. *Jpn J Cancer Clin* 1979;25:605–612.
22. Arai T, Nakano T, Morita S, et al. High-dose rate remote afterloading intracavitary radiation therapy for cancer of the uterine cervix: a 20-year experience. *Cancer* 1992;69:175–180.
23. Arthur D, Kaufman N, Schmidt-Ullrich R, et al. Heuristically derived tumor burden score as a prognostic factor for stage IIIB carcinoma of the cervix. *Int J Radiat Oncol Biol Phys* 1995;31:743–751.
24. Ascher SM, Cooper C, Scoutt L, et al. Diagnostic imaging techniques in gynecologic cancer. In: Hoskins WJ, Perez CA, Young RC, eds. *Principles and practice of gynecologic oncology,* 4th ed. Philadelphia: Lippincott Williams & Wilkins, 2005;223–266.
25. Atkovar G, Uzel O, Ozsahin M, et al. Postoperative radiotherapy in carcinoma of the cervix: treatment results and prognostic factors. *Radiother Oncol* 1995;35:198–205.
26. Balega J, Michael H, Hurteau J, et al. The risk of nodal metastasis in early adenocarcinoma of the uterine cervix. *Int J Gynecol Cancer* 2004;14:104–109.
27. Barbera L, Paszat L, Thomas G, et al. The rapid uptake of concurrent chemotherapy for cervix cancer patients treated with curative radiation. *Int. J Radiat Oncol Biol Phys* 2006;64:1389–1394.
28. Barillot I, Horiot JC, Maingon P, et al. Impact on treatment outcome and late effects of customized treatment planning in cervix carcinomas: baseline results to compared new strategies. *Int J Radiat Oncol Biol Phys* 2000;48:189–200.
29. Barnes W, Waggoner S, Delgado G, et al. Manometric characterization of rectal dysfunction following radical hysterectomy. *Gynecol Oncol* 1991;42:116–119.
30. Barron BA, Richart RM. Statistical model of the natural history of cervical carcinoma: II. Estimates of the transition time from dysplasia to carcinoma in situ. *J Natl Cancer Inst* 1970;45:1025–1030.
31. Bastin K, Buchler D, Stitt J, et al. Resource utilization: high dose rate versus low dose rate brachytherapy for gynecology cancer. *Am J Clin Oncol* 1993;16:256–261.
32. Becker TM, Wheeler CM, McGough NS, et al. Sexually transmitted diseases and other risk factors for cervical dysplasia among Southwestern Hispanic and non-Hispanic white women. *JAMA* 1994;271:1181–1188.
33. Benedetti-Panici P, Greggi S, Colombo A, et al. Neoadjuvant chemotherapy and radical surgery versus exclusive radiotherapy in locally advanced squamous cell cervical cancer: results from the Italian multicenter randomized study. *J Clin Oncol* 2001;20:179–188.
34. Benedetti-Panici P, Maneschi F, Scambia G, et al. Lymphatic spread of cervical cancer: an anatomical and pathological study based on 225 radical hysterectomies with systematic pelvic and aortic lymphadenectomy. *Gynecol Oncol* 1996;62:19–24.
35. Benson WL, Norris HJ. A critical review of the frequency of lymph node metastasis and death from microinvasive carcinoma of the cervix. *Obstet Gynecol* 1977;49:632–638.
36. Berman ML, Keys H, Creasman W, et al. Survival and patterns of recurrence in cervical cancer metastatic to paraaortic lymph nodes: a Gynecologic Group study. *Gynecol Oncol* 1984;19:8–16.
37. Bianchi UA, Sartori E, Pecorelli S, et al. Treatment of primary invasive cervical cancer: considerations on 997 consecutive cases. *Eur J Gynaecol Oncol* 1988;9:47–53.
38. Biggs PJ, Russell MD. Effect of a femoral head prosthesis on megavoltage beam radiotherapy. *Int J Radiat Oncol Biol Phys* 1988;14:581–586.
39. Bjerre B, Eliasson G, Linell F, et al. Conization as only treatment of carcinoma in situ of the uterine cervix. *Am J Obstet Gynecol* 1976;125:143–152.
40. Blomlie V, Rofstad EK, Talle K, et al. Incidence of radiation-induced insufficiency fractures of the female pelvis: evaluation with MR imaging. *AJR Am J Roentgenol* 1996;167:1205–1210.
41. Bodurka-Bevers D, Morris M, Eifel PJ, et al. Posttherapy surveillance of women with cervical cancer: an outcomes analysis. *Gynecol Oncol* 2000;78:187–193.
42. Bohm JW, Krupp PJ, Lee FYL, et al. Lymph node metastases in microinvasive epidermoid cancer of the cervix. *Obstet Gynecol* 1976;48:65–67.
43. Boice JD, Day NE, Andersen A, et al. Second cancers following radiation treatment for cervical cancer: an international collaboration among cancer registries. *J Natl Cancer Inst* 1985;74:955–975.
44. Bolli JN, Doering DL, Bosscher JR, et al. Squamous cell carcinoma antigen: clinical utility in squamous cell carcinoma of the uterine cervix. *Gynecol Oncol* 1994;55:169–173.
45. Bonin SR, Lanciano RM, Corn BW, et al. Bony landmarks are not an adequate substitute for lymphangiography in defining pelvic lymph node location for the treatment of cervical cancer with radiotherapy. *Int J Radiat Oncol Biol Phys* 1996;34:167–172.
46. Bonomi P, Blessing JA, Ball H, et al. A phase II evaluation of cisplatin and 5-fluorouracil in patients with advanced squamous cell carcinoma of the cervix: a Gynecologic Oncology Group study. *Gynecol Oncol* 1989;34:357–359.
47. Boon ME, Susanti I, Tasche MJA, et al. Human papillomavirus (HPV)-associated male and female genital carcinomas in a Hindu population: the male as vector and victim. *Cancer* 1989;64:559–565.
48. Borras G, Molina R, Zercavins J, et al. Tumor antigen CA19-9, CA 125, and CEA in carcinoma of the uterine cervix. *Gynecol Oncol* 1995;57:205–211.
49. Boruta DM II, Schorge JO, Duska LA, et al. Multimodality therapy in early-stage neuroendocrine carcinoma of the uterine cervix. *Gynecol Oncol* 2001;81:82–87.
50. Bosch FX, Lorincz A, Munoz N, et al. The causal relation between human papilloma virus and cervical cancer. *J Clin Path* 2002;55:244–265.
51. Bosch FX, Manos MM, Muñoz N, et al. International Biological Study of Cervical Cancer (IBSCC) Study Group. Prevalence of human papillomavirus in cervical cancer: a worldwide perspective. *J Natl Cancer Inst* 1995;87:796–802.
52. Bouchard M, Nadeau S, Germain I, et al. Anatomy-based MLC field optimization for the treatment of gynecologic malignancies. *Int J Radiat Oncol Biol Phys* 2005;63:S344–S345.
53. Botsel EA, Ambekoglu C, Sertenk A, et al. Metachronous metastases from renal cell carcinoma to uterine cervix and vagina: case report and review of literature. *Gynecol Oncol* 2005;99:232–235.
54. Brewer CA, Blessing JA, Nagourney RA, et al. Cisplatin plus gemcitabine in previously treated squamous cell carcinoma of the cervix: a phase II study of the Gynecologic Oncology Group. *Gynecol Oncol* 2006;100:385–388.
55. Brixley CJ, Roeske JC, Lujan AE, et al. Impact of intensity-modulated radiotherapy on acute hematologic toxicity in women with gynecologic malignancies. *Int J Radiat Oncol Biol Phys* 2002;54:1388–1396.
56. Brooks SE, Chen TT, Ghosh A, et al. Cervical cancer outcomes analysis: impact of age, race, and comorbid illness on hospitalizations for invasive carcinoma of the cervix. *Gynecol Oncol* 2000;79:107–115.
57. Bruner DW, Lanciano R, Keegan M, et al. Vaginal stenosis and sexual function following intracavitary radiation for the treatment of cervical and endometrial carcinoma. *Int J Radiat Oncol Biol Phys* 1993;27:825–830.
58. Brunschwig A. The surgical treatment of cancer of the cervix stage I and II. *AJR Am J Roentgenol* 1968;102:147–151.
59. Buekers TE, Anderson B, Sorosky JI, et al. Ovarian function after surgical treatment for cervical cancer. *Gynecol Oncol* 2001;80:85–88.
60. Buglione M, Toninelli M, Pietta N, et al. Post-radiation pelvic disease and ureteral stenosis: physiopathology and evolution in the patient treated for cervical carcinoma. Review of the literature and experience of the Radium Institute. *Arch Ital Urol Androl* 2002;74:6–11.
61. Burger CW, van Leeuwen FE, Scheele F, et al. Hormone replacement therapy in women for gynaecological malignancy. *Maturitas* 1999;32:69–76.
62. Burnett AF, Coe FL, Klement V, et al. The use of a pelvic displacement prosthesis to exclude the small intestine from the radiation field following radical hysterectomy. *Gynecol Oncol* 2000;79:438–443.
63. Busch M, Rath W, Schaffer M, et al. Results of postoperative radiotherapy of cervix carcinoma after radical versus nonradical hysterectomy. *Radiol Med* 1997;93:110–114.
64. Bush RS. The significance of anemia in clinical radiation therapy. *Int J Radiat Oncol Biol Phys* 1986;12:2047–2050.
65. Bye A, Trope C, Loge JH, et al. Health-related quality of life and occurrence of intestinal side effects after pelvic radiotherapy: evaluation of long-term effects of diagnosis and treatment. *Acta Oncol* 2000;39:173–180.
66. Calkins AR, Harrison CR, Fowler WC Jr, et al. Hyperfractionated radiation therapy plus chemotherapy in local advanced cervical cancer: results of two phase I dose-escalation Gynecologic Oncology Group trials. *Gynecol Oncol* 1999;75:349–355.
67. Camilien L, Gordon D, Fruchter RG, et al. Predictive value of computerized tomography in the presurgical evaluation of primary carcinoma of the cervix. *Gynecol Oncol* 1988;30:209–215.

68. Campbell OB, Arowojolo AO, Adu FD, et al. Human immunodeficiency virus antibody in patients with cancer of the uterine cervix undergoing radiotherapy: clinical stages, histological grade and outcome of radiotherapy. *J Obstet Gynaecol* 1999;19:403–405.
69. Cerciello F, Hoffsteter B, Fatah SA, et al. G2/M cell cycle checkpoint is functional in cervical cancer patients after initiation of external beam radiotherapy. *Int J Radiat Oncol Biol Phys* 2005;62:1390–1398.
70. Chang TC, Lai CH, Hong JH, et al. Randomized trial of neoadjuvant cisplatin, vincristine, bleomycin, and radical hysterectomy versus radiation therapy for bulky stage IB and IIA cervical cancer. *J Clin Oncol* 2000;18:1740–1747.
71. Chao A, Wang TH, Lee YS, et al. Molecular characterization of adenocarcinoma and squamous carcinoma of the uterine cervix using microarray analysis of gene expression. *Int J Cancer* 2006;119:91–98.
72. Chao KS, Williamson JF, Grigsby PW, et al. Uterosacral space involvement in locally advanced carcinoma of the uterine cervix. *Int J Radiat Oncol Biol Phys* 1998;40:406–403.
73. Chao KSC, Grigsby PW, Mutch D, et al. Prognostic factors for distant metastasis in carcinoma of the cervix with endometrial extension. *J Brachyther Int* 2000;16:181–186.
74. Chatani M, Matayoshi Y, Masaki N, et al. A prospective randomized study concerning the point A dose in high-dose rate intracavitary therapy for carcinoma of the uterine cervix: the final results. *Strahlenther Onkol* 1994;170:636–642.
75. Chatani M, Matayoshi Y, Masaki N, et al. High-dose rate intracavitary irradiation for carcinoma of the uterine cervix: the adverse effect of treatment prolongation. *Strahlenther Onkol* 1997;173:379–384.
76. Chatani M, Nose T, Masaki N, et al. Adjuvant radiotherapy after radical hysterectomy of the cervical cancer: prognostic factors and complications. *Strahlenther Onkol* 1998;174:504–509.
77. Chauvergne J, Lhomme C, Rohart J, et al. Neoadjuvant chemotherapy of stage IIB and III cancers of the uterine cervix: long-term results of a multicenter randomized trial of 151 patients. *Bull Cancer* 1993;80:1069–1079.
78. Chen F, Trapido EJ, Davis K. Differences in stage at presentation of breast and gynecologic cancers among whites, blacks, and Hispanics. *Cancer* 1994;73:2838–2842.
79. Chen RJ, Change DY, Yen ML, et al. Prognostic factors of primary adenocarcinoma of the uterine cervix. *Gynecol Oncol* 1998;69:157–164.
80. Chiara S, Bruzzone M, Merlini L, et al. for the GONO (North-West Oncologic Cooperative Group). Randomized study comparing chemotherapy plus radiotherapy versus radiotherapy alone in FIGO stage IIB-III cervical carcinoma. *Am J Clin Oncol* 1994;17:294–297.
81. Choi P, Teo P, Foo W, et al. High-dose rate remote afterloading irradiation of carcinoma of the cervix in Hong Kong: unexpectedly high complication rate. *Clin Oncol* 1992;4:186–191.
82. Chou HH, Wang CC, Lai CH, et al. Isolated paraaortic lymph node recurrence after definitive irradiation for cervical carcinoma. *Int J Radiat Oncol Biol Phys* 2001;51:442–448.
83. Christie DRH, Bull CA, Gebski V, et al. Concurrent 5-fluorouracil, mitomycin C and irradiation in locally advanced cervix cancer. *Radiother Oncol* 1995;37:181–189.
84. Christopherson WM, Gray LA, Parker JE. Microinvasive carcinoma of the uterine cervix. *Cancer* 1976;38:629–632.
85. Christopherson WM, Parker JE. Relation of cervical cancer to early marriage and childbearing. *N Engl J Med* 1965;273:235–239.
86. Chung EJ, Seong J, Yang WI, et al. Spontaneous apoptosis as a predictor of radiotherapy in patients with stage IIB squamous cell carcinoma of the uterine cervix. *Acta Oncol* 1999;38:449–454.
87. Cikaric S. Radiation therapy of cervical carcinoma using either HDR or LDR afterloading: comparison of 5-year results and complications. *Strahlenther Onkol* 1988;82[Suppl]:119–122.
88. Clark BC, Souhami L, Roman TN, et al. Rectal complications in patients with carcinoma of the cervix treated with concomitant cisplatin and external beam irradiation with high dose rate brachytherapy: a dosimetric analysis. *Int J Radiat Oncol Biol Phys* 1994;28:1243–1250.
89. Clement PB, Zubovits JT, Young RH, et al. Malignant müllerian mixed tumors of the uterine cervix: a report of nine cases of a neoplasm with morphology often different from its counterpart in the corpus. *Int J Gynecol Pathol* 1998;17:211–222.
90. Coia L, Won M, Lanciano R, et al. The Patterns of Care Outcome Study for cancer of the uterine cervix: results of the Second National Practice Survey. *Cancer* 1990;66:2451–2456.
91. Coleman RL, Keeney ED, Freedman RS, et al. Radical hysterectomy for recurrent carcinoma of the uterine cervix after radiotherapy. *Gynecol Oncol* 1994;55:29–35.
92. Colombo A, Landoni F, Maneo A, et al. Neoadjuvant chemotherapy to radiation and concurrent chemoradiation for locally advanced squamous cell carcinoma of cervix: a review of the recent literature. *Tumori* 1998;84:229–237.
93. Contag SA, Gostout BS, Clayton AC, et al. Comparison of gene expression in squamous cell carcinoma and adenocarcinoma of the uterine cervix. *Gynecol Oncol* 2004;95:610–617.
94. Cooper RA, West CM, Logue JP, et al. Changes in oxygenation during radiotherapy in carcinoma of the cervix. *Int J Radiat Oncol Biol Phys* 1999;45:119–126.
95. Cooper RA, Wilks DP, Logue JP, et al. High tumor angiogenesis is associated with poorer survival in carcinoma of the cervix treated with radiotherapy. *Clin Cancer Res* 1998;4:2795–2800.
96. Corn BW, Schnall MD, Milestone B, et al. Signal characteristics of tumor shown by high-resolution endorectal coil magnetic resonance imaging may predict outcome among patients with cervical carcinoma treated with irradiation: a preliminary study. *Cancer* 1996;78:2535–2542.
97. Cosin JA, Fowler JM, Chen MD, et al. Pretreatment surgical staging of patients with cervical carcinoma: the case of lymph node debulking. *Cancer* 1998;82:2241–2248.
98. Coughlin CT, Richmond RC. Biologic and clinical developments of cisplatinum combined with radiation: concepts utilizing projection for new trials and the emergence of carboplatin. *Semin Oncol* 1989;16[Suppl 6]:31–43.
99. Crane CH, Schneider BF. Occult carcinoma discovered after simple hysterectomy treated with postoperative radiotherapy. *Int J Radiat Oncol Biol Phys* 1999;43:1049–1053.
100. Creasman WT, Rutledge FN, Fletcher GH. Carcinoma of the cervix associated with pregnancy. *Obstet Gynecol* 1970;36:495–501.
101. Crissman JD, Budhraja M, Aron BS, et al. Histopathologic prognostic factors in stage II and III squamous cell carcinoma of the uterine cervix. *Int J Gynecol Pathol* 1987;6:97–103.
102. Crozier M, Morris M, Levenback C, et al. Pelvic exenteration for adenocarcinoma of the uterine cervix. *Gynecol Oncol* 1995;58:74–78.
103. Cummings SR, Nevitt MC, Browner WS, et al. Study of Osteoporotic Fractures Research Group. Risk factors for hip fracture in white women. *N Engl J Med* 1995;332:767–773.
104. Curtin JP, Hoskins WJ, Venkatraman ES, et al. Adjuvant chemotherapy versus chemotherapy plus pelvic irradiation for high-risk cervical cancer patients after radical hysterectomy and pelvic lymphadenectomy (RH-PLND): a randomized phase III trial. *Gynecol Oncol* 1996;61:3–10.
105. D'Souza WD, Ahamad AA, Iyer RB, et al. Feasibility of dose escalation using intensity-modulated radiotherapy in posthysterectomy cervical cancer. *Int J Radiat Oncol Biol Phys* 2005;61:1062–1070.
106. Dargent DF, Plante M, Sonoda Y. Laparoscopic surgery in gynecologic cancer. In: Hoskins WJ, Perez CA, Young RC, eds. ***Principles and practice of gynecologic oncology***, 4th ed. Philadelphia: Lippincott Williams & Wilkins, 2005;333–373.
107. Daroca PJ Jr, Dhurandhar HN. Basaloid carcinoma of uterine cervix. *Am J Surg Pathol* 1980;4:235–239.
108. Dattoli MJ, Gretz HF III, Beller U, et al. Analysis of multiple prognostic factors in patients with stage IB cervical cancer: age as a major determinant. *Int J Radiat Oncol Biol Phys* 1989;17:41–47.
109. Davey DD, Zaleski S, Sattich M, et al. Prognostic significance of DNA cytometry of postirradiation cervicovaginal smears. *Cancer* 1998;84:11–16.
110. De Los Santos JF, Small W. The role of amifostine in the treatment of carcinoma of the uterine cervix: an update of RTOG-0116 and review of future directions. *Semin Oncol* 2004;31[Suppl 18]:37–41.
111. De Vuyst H, Claeys P, Njiru S, et al. Comparison of pap smear, visual inspection with acetic acid, human papillomavirus DNA-PCR testing and cervicography. *Int J Gynaecol Obstet* 2005;89:120–126.
112. Deckers PJ, Ketcham AS, Sugarbaker EV, et al. Pelvic exenteration for primary carcinoma of the uterine cervix. *Obstet Gynecol* 1971;37:647–659.
113. Del Regato JA, Cox JD. Transvaginal roentgenotherapy in the conservative management of carcinoma in situ of the uterine cervix. *Radiology* 1965;84:1090–1095.
114. Delaloge S, Pautier P, Kerbrat P, et al. Neuroendocrine small cell carcinoma of the uterine cervix: what disease? what treatment? Report of ten cases and a review of the literature. *Clin Oncol (R Coll Radiol)* 2000;12:357–362.
115. Delaloye JF, Coucke PA, Pampallona S, et al. Effect of total treatment time on event-free survival in carcinoma of the cervix. *Gynecol Oncol* 1996;60:42–48.
116. Delaloye JF, Pampallona S, Coucke PA, et al. Younger age as a bad prognostic factor in patients with carcinoma of the cervix. *Eur J Obstet Gynecol Reprod Biol* 1996;64:201–205.
117. Delgado G, Bundy BN, Fowler WC, et al. A prospective surgical pathological study of stage I squamous carcinoma of the cervix: a Gynecologic Oncology Group study. *Gynecol Oncol* 1989;35:314–320.
118. DePasquale SE, Mylonas I, Falkenberry SS. Fatal recurrent ureteroarterial fistulas after exenteration for cervical cancer. *Gynecol Oncol* 2001;82:192–196.
119. DeWitt KD, Hsu CJ, Speight J, et al. 3D inverse treatment planning for the tandem and ovoid applicator in cervical cancer. *Int J Radiat Oncol Biol Phys* 2005;63:1270–1274.
120. Di Stefano AB, Acquaviva G, Garozzo G, et al. Lymph node mapping and sentinel node detection in patients with cervical carcinoma: a 2-year experience. *Gynecol Oncol* 2005;99:671–679.
121. Dickson J, Davidson SE, Hunter RD, et al. Pretreatment plasma TGF beta 1 levels are prognostic for survival but not morbidity following radiation therapy of carcinoma of the cervix. *Int J Radiat Oncol Biol Phys* 2000;48:991–995.
122. Dimopoulos JCA, Schard G, Berger D, et al. Systematic evaluation of MRI findings in different stages of treatment of cervical cancer: potential of MRI on delineation of target, pathoanatomic structures and organs at risk. *Int J Radiat Oncol Biol Phys* 2006;64:1380–1388.
123. Dinges S, Harder C, Wurm R, et al. Combined treatment of inoperable carcinomas of the uterine cervix with radiotherapy and regional hyperthermia: results of a phase II trial. *Strahlenther Onkol* 1998;174:517–521.
124. Dische S, Saunders MI, Sealy R, et al. Carcinoma of the cervix and the use of hyperbaric oxygen with radiotherapy: a report of a randomised controlled trial. *Radiother Oncol* 1999;53:93–98.
125. Douple EB. Platinum-radiation interactions. *J Natl Cancer Inst Monogr* 1988;6:315–319.
126. Drescher CW, Hopkins MP, Roberts JA. Comparison of the pattern of metastatic spread of squamous cell cancer and adenocarcinoma of the uterine cervix. *Gynecol Oncol* 1989;33:340–343.
127. Drill VA. Oral contraceptives: relation to mammary cancer, benign breast lesions and cervical cancer. *Annu Rev Pharmacol* 1975;15:367–385.
128. Duggan B, Muderspach LI, Roman LK, et al. Cervical cancer in pregnancy: reporting on planned delay in therapy. *Obstet Gynecol* 1993;82:598–602.
129. Dunst J, Hansgen G, Lautenschlager C, et al. Oxygenation of cervical cancers during radiotherapy and radiotherapy plus cis-retinoic acid/interferon. *Int J Radiat Oncol Biol Phys* 1999;43:367–373.
130. Dunst J, Kuhnt T, Strauss HG, et al. Anemia in cervical cancers: impact on survival, patterns of relapse and association with hypoxia and angiogenesis. *Int J Radiat Oncol Biol Phys* 2003;56:778–787.
131. Durand RE, Aquino-Parsons C. Predicting response to treatment in human cancers of the uterine cervix: sequential biopsies during external beam radiotherapy. *Int J Radiat Oncol Biol Phys* 2004;58:555–560.
132. Dusenbery KE, Carson LF, Potish RA. Perioperative morbidity and mortality of gynecologic brachytherapy. *Cancer* 1991;67:2786–2790.
133. Dusenbery KE, McGuire WA, Holt PJ, et al. Erythropoietin increases hemoglobin during radiation therapy for cervical cancer. *Int J Radiat Oncol Biol Phys* 1994;29:1079–1084.
134. Earnest DL, Trier JS. Radiation enteritis and colitis. In: Sleisenger MH, Fordtran JS, Feldman M, et al., eds. *Gastrointestinal disease: athophysiology/diagnosis/management*, 5th ed. Philadelphia: W.B. Saunders, 1993.
135. Ebara T, Mitsuhashi N, Saito Y, et al. Prognostic significance of immunohistochemically detected p53 protein expression in stage IIIB squamous cell

carcinoma of the uterine cervix treated with radiation therapy alone. *Gynecol Oncol* 1996;63:216–218.

136. Ebner F, Kressel HY, Mintz MC, et al. Tumor recurrence versus fibrosis in the female pelvis: differentiation with MR imaging at 1.5 T. *Radiology* 1980;166:333–340.
137. Eich HT, Haverkamp U, Micke O, et al. Dosimetric analysis at ICRU reference points in HDR-brachytherapy of cervical carcinoma. *Rontgenpraxis* 2000;53:62–66.
138. Eifel PJ, Burke TW, Morris M, et al. Adenocarcinoma as an independent risk factor for disease recurrence in patients with stage IB cervical carcinoma. *Gynecol Oncol* 1995;59:38–44.
139. Eifel PJ, Jhingran A, Coleman R, et al. Is anemia a cause of radiation therapy failure in patients with squamous cell carcinoma of the cervix? *Int J Radiat Oncol Biol Phys* 2005;63:S64(abstr 157).
140. Eifel PJ, Levenback C, Wharton JT, et al. Time course and incidence of late complications in patients treated with radiation therapy for FIGO stage IB carcinoma of the uterine cervix. *Int J Radiat Oncol Biol Phys* 1995;32:1289–1300.
141. Eifel PJ, Morris MJ, Oswald MJ, et al. Adenocarcinoma of the uterine cervix: prognosis and patterns of failure in 367 cases treated at the M.D. Anderson Cancer Center between 1965 and 1985. *Cancer* 1990;65:2507–2514.
142. Eifel PJ, Morris M, Wharton JT, et al. The influence of tumor size and morphology on the outcome of patients with FIGO stage IB squamous cell carcinoma of the uterine cervix. *Int J Radiat Oncol Biol Phys* 1994;29:9–16.
143. Eifel PJ, Moughan J, Erickson B, et al. Patterns of radiotherapy practice for patients with carcinoma of the uterine cervix: a pattern of care study. *Int J Radiat Oncol Biol Phys* 2004;60:1144–1153.
144. Eifel PJ, Thoms WW Jr, Smith TL, et al. The relationship between brachytherapy dose and outcome in patients with bulky endocervical tumors treated with radiation dose. *Int J Radiat Oncol Biol Phys* 1994;28:113–118.
145. Eifel PJ, Winter K, Morris M, et al. Pelvic irradiation with concurrent chemotherapy versus pelvic and para-aortic irradiation for high risk cervical cancer: an update of radiation therapy oncology group trial (RTOG) 90-01. *J Clin Oncol* 2004;22:872–880.
146. Eifel PJ. The importance of locoregional control of cervical cancer: why is it still controversial? *Cancer J Sci Am* 1996;2:253.
147. Einhorn N, Patek E, Sjöberg B. Outcome of different treatment modifications in cervix carcinoma, stage IB and IIA: observation in a well-defined Swedish population. *Cancer* 1985;55:949–955.
148. el Omari-Alaoui H, Kebdani T, Benjaafar N, et al. Non-Hodgkin's lymphoma of the uterus: apropos of 4 cases and review of the literature. *Cancer Radiother* 2002;6:39–45.
149. el-Baradie M, Inoue T, Inoue T, et al. HDR and MDR intracavitary treatment for carcinoma of the uterine cervix: a prospective randomized study. *Strahlenther Onkol* 1997;173:155–162.
150. Esthappan J, Mutic S, Malyapa RS, et al. Treatment planning guidelines regarding the use of CT/PET guided IMRT for cervical carcinoma with positive paraaortic nodes. *Int J Rad Oncol Biol Phys* 2004;58:1289–1297.
151. Fagundes H, Perez CA, Grigsby PW, et al. Distant metastases after irradiation alone in carcinoma of the uterine cervix. *Int J Radiat Oncol Biol Phys* 1992;24:197–204.
152. Feeney DD, Moore DH, Look KY, et al. The fate of the ovaries after radical hysterectomy and ovarian transposition. *Gynecol Oncol* 1995;56:3–7.
153. Fellner C, Potter R, Knocke TH, et al. Comparison of radiography- and computed tomography-based treatment planning in cervix cancer in brachytherapy with specific attention to some quality assurance aspects. *Radiother Oncol* 2001;58:53–62.
154. Ferrigno R, Nishimoto IN, Novaes PE, et al. Comparison of low and high dose rate brachytherapy in the treatment of uterine cervix cancer. Retrospective analysis of two sequential series. *Int J Radiat Oncol Biol Phys* 2005;62:1108–1116.
155. Finan MA, DeCesare S, Fiorica JV, et al. Radical hysterectomy for stage IB1 vs IB2 carcinoma of the cervix: does the new staging system predict morbidity and survival? *Gynecol Oncol* 1996;62:139–147.
156. Fine RO, Hempling RE, Piver MS, et al. Severe radiation morbidity in carcinoma of the cervix: Impact of pretherapy surgical staging and previous surgery. *Int J Radiat Oncol Biol Phys* 1995;31:717–723.
157. Finlay MH, Ackerman I, Tirona RG, et al. Use of CT simulation for treatment of cervical cancer to assess the adequacy of lymph node coverage of conventional pelvic fields based on bony landmarks. *Int J Radiat Oncol Biol Phys* 2006;64:205–209.
158. Fiorica JV, Roberts WS, Greenberg H, et al. Morbidity and survival patterns in patients after radical hysterectomy and postoperative adjuvant pelvic radiotherapy. *Gynecol Oncol* 1990;36:343–347.
159. Flay LD, Matthews JHL. The effects of radiotherapy and surgery on the sexual function of women treated for cervical cancer. *Int J Radiat Oncol Biol Phys* 1995;31:399–404.
160. Fletcher GH, ed. *Textbook of radiotherapy*, 3rd ed. Philadelphia: Lea & Febiger, 1980;720–773, 812–828.
161. Fletcher GH. Cancer of the uterine cervix: Janeway lecture. *AJR Am J Roentgenol Radium Ther Nucl Med* 1971;111:225–242.
162. Fowler JF. Dose reduction factors when increasing dose rate in LDR and MDR brachytherapy of carcinoma of the cervix. *Radiother Oncol* 1997;45:49–54.
163. Fowler JF. The radiobiology of brachytherapy. In: Martinez AA, Orton CG, Mould RF, eds. *Brachytherapy HDR and LDR*. Leersum, the Netherlands: Nucletron International BV, 1990;121–137.
164. Fowler JM, Carter JR, Carlson JW, et al. Lymph node yield from laparoscopic lymphadenectomy in cervical cancer: a comparative study. *Gynecol Oncol* 1993;51:187–192.
165. Fu KK, Phillips TL. High-dose rate versus low-dose rate intracavitary brachytherapy for carcinoma of the cervix. *Int J Radiat Oncol Biol Phys* 1990;19:791–796.
166. Fujikawa K, Yamamichi F, Nonomura M, et al. Spontaneous rupture of the urinary bladder is not a rare complication of radiotherapy for cervical cancer: report of six cases. *Gynecol Oncol* 1999;73:439–442.
167. Fyles A, Keane TJ, Barton M, et al. The effect of treatment duration in the local control of cervix cancer. *Radiother Oncol* 1992;25:273–279.
168. Fyles AW, Milosevic M, Pintilie M, et al. Anemia, hypoxia and transfusion in patients with cervix cancer: a review. *Radiother Oncol* 2000;57:13–19.
169. Fyles AW, Milosevic M, Pintilie M, et al. Cervix cancer oxygenation measured following external radiation therapy. *Int J Radiat Oncol Biol Phys* 1998;42:751–753.
170. Fyles AW, Pintilie M, Kirkbride P, et al. Prognostic factors in patients with cervix cancer treated by radiation therapy: results of a multiple regression analysis. *Radiother Oncol* 1995;35:107–117.
171. Gadducci A, Sartori E, Maggino T, et al. The clinical outcome of patients with stage Ia1 and Ia2 squamous cell carcinoma of the uterine cervix: a Cooperation Task Force (CTF) study. *Eur J Gynaecol Oncol* 2003;24:513–516.
172. Gaffney DK, Holden J, Davis M, et al. Elevated cyclooxygenase-2 expression correlates with diminished survival in carcinoma of the cervix treated with radiotherapy. *Int J Radiat Oncol Biol Phys* 2001;49:1213–1217.
173. Garipagaoglu M, Tulunay G, Kose MF, et al. Prognostic factors in stage IB-IIA cervical carcinoma treated with postoperative radiotherapy. *Eur J Gynaecol Oncol* 1999;20:131–135.
174. Garton FG, Gunderson LL, Webb MJ, et al. Intraoperative radiation therapy in gynecologic cancer: the Mayo Clinic experience. *Gynecol Oncol* 1993;48:328–332.
175. Gebara WJ, Weeks KJ, Jones EL, et al. Carcinoma of the uterine cervix: a 3D-CT analysis of dose to the internal, external and common iliac nodes in tandem and ovoid applications. *Radiother Oncol* 2000;56:43–48.
176. Georgiou A, Grigsby PW, Perez CA. Radiation induced lumbosacral plexopathy in gynecologic tumors: clinical findings and dosimetric analysis. *Int J Radiat Oncol Biol Phys* 1993;26:479–482.
177. Gersell DJ, Mazoujian G, Mutch DG, et al. Small-cell undifferentiated carcinoma of the cervix: a clinicopathologic, ultrastructural, and immunocytochemical study of 15 cases. *Am J Surg Pathol* 1988;12:684–698.
178. Girardi F, Lichtenegger W, Tamussino K, et al. The importance of parametrial lymph nodes in the treatment of cervical cancer. *Gynecol Oncol* 1989;34:206–211.
179. Girinsky T, Rey A, Roche B, et al. Overall treatment time in advanced cervical carcinomas: a critical parameter in treatment outcome. *Int J Radiat Oncol Biol Phys* 1993;27:1051–1056.
180. Glaser FH. Comparison of HDR afterloading with 192Ir versus conventional radium therapy in cervix cancer: 5-year results and complications. *Strahlenther Onkol* 1988;82[Suppl]:106–113.
181. Gong QY, Brunt JN, Romaniuk CS, et al. Contrast enhanced dynamic MRI of cervical carcinoma during radiotherapy: early prediction of tumour regression rate. *Br J Radiol* 1999;72:1177–1184.
182. Gonzalez D, Kotting BW, van Dunningen B, et al. Carcinoma of the uterine cervix stage IB and IIA: results of postoperative irradiation in patients with microscopic infiltration in the parametrium and/or lymph node metastasis. *Int J Radiat Oncol Biol Phys* 1989;16:389–395.
183. Goodman HM, Niloff JM, Nelson JR, et al. Cervical malignancies. In: Knapp RC, Berkowitz RS, eds. *Gynecologic oncology*. New York: Macmillan, 1986;225–273.
184. Gordon HW. Adenoid cystic (cylindromatous) carcinoma of the uterine cervix: report of two cases. *Am J Clin Pathol* 1972;58:51–57.
185. Grace VM, Shalini JV, lekha TT, et al. Co-overexpression of p53 and bcl-2 proteins in HPV-induced squamous cell carcinoma of the uterine cervix. *Gynaecol Oncol* 2003;91:51–58.
186. Graeber TG, Osmanian C, Jacks T, et al. Hypoxia-mediated selection of cells with diminished apoptotic potential in solid tumors. *Nature* 1996;379:88–91.
187. Gram IT, Austin H, Stalsberg H. Cigarette smoking and the incidence of cervical intraepithelial neoplasia, grade III, and cancer of the cervix uteri. *Am J Epidemiol* 1992;135:341.
188. Green J, Barrington DG, Smith JS, et al. Human papillomavirus infection and use of oral contraceptives. *Br J Cancer* 2003;88:1713–1720.
189. Green JA, Tierney JM, Symonds RP, et al. Survival and recurrence after concomitant chemotherapy and radiotherapy for cancer of the uterine cervix: a systematic review and meta-analysis. *Lancet* 2001;358:781–786.
190. Green TH, Morse WJ. Management of invasive cervical cancer following inadvertent simple hysterectomy. *Obstet Gynecol* 1969;33:763–769.
191. Greene FL, Page DL, Flemming ID, et al., eds. *AJCC cancer staging manual*, 6th ed. New York: Springer, 2002.
192. Greer BE, Easterling TR, McLennan DA, et al. Fetal and maternal considerations in the management of stage IB cervical cancer during pregnancy. *Gynecol Oncol* 1989;34:61–65.
193. Greer BE, Koh W-J, Figge DC, et al. Gynecologic radiotherapy fields defined by intraoperative measurements. *Gynecol Oncol* 1990;38:421–424.
194. Greer BE, Koh WJ, Stelzer KJ, et al. Expanded pelvic radiotherapy fields for treatment of local-regionally advanced carcinoma of the cervix: outcome and complications. *Am J Obstet Gynecol* 1996;174:1141–1149.
195. Grigsby PW, Hall-Daniels L, Baker S, et al. Comparison of clinical outcome in black and white women treated with radiotherapy for cervical carcinoma. *Gynecol Oncol* 2000;79:357–361.
196. Grigsby PW, Lu JD, Mutch DG, et al. Twice-daily fractionation of external irradiation with brachytherapy and chemotherapy in carcinoma of the cervix with positive para-aortic nodes: phase II study of the Radiation Therapy Oncology Group 92-10. *Int J Radiat Oncol Biol Phys* 1998;41:817–822.
197. Grigsby PW, Mutch DG, Rader J, et al. Lack of benefit of concurrent chemotherapy in patients with cervical cancer and negative nodes by FDG-PET. *Int J Radiat Oncol Biol Phys* 2005;61:444–449.
198. Grigsby PW, Perez CA, Chao KS, et al. Lack of effect of tumor size on the prognosis of carcinoma of the uterine cervix stage IB and IIA treated with preoperative irradiation and surgery. *Int J Radiat Oncol Biol Phys* 1999;45:645–651.
199. Grigsby PW, Perez CA, Chao KS, et al. Radiation therapy for carcinoma of the cervix with biopsy-proven positive paraaortic lymph nodes. *Int J Radiat Oncol Biol Phys* 2001;49:733–738.
200. Grigsby PW, Perez CA, Kuske RR, et al. Adenocarcinoma of the uterine cervix: lack of evidence for a poor prognosis. *Radiother Oncol* 1988;12:289–296.
201. Grigsby PW, Perez CA. Radiotherapy alone for medically inoperable carcinoma of the cervix: stage IA and carcinoma in situ. *Int J Radiat Oncol Biol Phys* 1991;21:375–378.
202. Grigsby PW, Portelance L, Williamson JF. HDR cervical ring applicator to control bleeding from cervical cancer. *Int J Gynecol Oncol* 2002;12:18–21.
203. Grigsby PW, Roberts HL, Perez CA. Femoral neck fracture following groin irradiation. *Int J Radiat Oncol Biol Phys* 1995;32:63–67.
204. Grigsby PW, Russell A, Bruner D, et al. Late injury of cancer therapy on the female reproductive tract. *Int J Radiat Oncol Biol Phys* 1995;31:1281–1299.

205. Grigsby PW, Siegel BA, Dehdashti F, et al. Posttherapy [F18] fluorodeoxyglucose positron emmission tomography in carcinoma of the cervix: response and outcome. *J Clin Oncol* 2004;22:2167–2171.
206. Grigsby PW, Siegel BA, Dehdashti F, et al. Posttherapy surveillance of cervical cancer by FDG-PET. *Int J Radiat Oncol Biol Phys* 2003;55:907–913.
207. Grigsby PW, Siegel BA, Dehdashti F. Lymph node staging by positron emission tomography in patients with carcinoma of the cervix. *J Clin Oncol* 2001;19:3745–3749.
208. Grigsby PW, Singh AK, Siegel BA, et al. Lymph node control in cervical cancer. *Int J Radiat Oncol Biol Phys* 2004;59:706–712.
209. Grigsby PW, Winter K, Komaki R, et al. Long-term follow-up of RTOG 88-05: twice-daily external irradiation with brachytherapy for carcinoma of the cervix. *Int J Radiat Oncol Biol Phys* 2001;51[Suppl 1]:62.
210. Grigsby PW, Winter K, Wasserman TH, et al. Irradiation with or without misonidazole for patients with stages IIIB and IVA carcinoma of the cervix: final results of RTOG 80-05. Radiation Therapy Oncology Group. *Int J Radiat Oncol Biol Phys* 1999;44:513–517.
211. Grimard L, Genest P, Girard A, et al. Prognostic significance of endometrial extension in carcinoma of the cervix. *Gynecol Oncol* 1988;31:301–309.
212. Grogan M, Thomas GM, Melamed I, et al. The importance of hemoglobin levels during radiotherapy for carcinoma of the cervix. *Cancer* 1999;86:1528–1536.
213. Gruber G, Hess J, Stiefel C, et al. Correlation between tumoral expression of beta3-integrin and outcome in cervical cancer patients who had undergone radiotherapy. *Br J Cancer* 2005;92:41–46.
214. Guerrero M, Li XA, Ma L, et al. Simultaneous integrated intensity-modulated radiotherapy boost for locally advanced gynecological cancer: radiobiological and dosimetric considerations. *Int J Radiat Oncol Biol Phys* 2005;62:933–939.
215. Gupta BD, Ayyagari S, Sharma SC, et al. Carcinoma of the cervix: optimal time-dose-fractionation of HDR brachytherapy and comparison with conventional dose-rate brachytherapy. In: Mould RF, ed. *Brachytherapy 2*. Leersum, the Netherlands: Nucletron International BV, 1989:307–308.
216. Hacker NF, Wain GV, Nicklin JL. Resection of bulky positive lymph nodes in patients with cervical carcinoma. *Int J Gynecol Cancer* 1995;5:250–256.
217. Haensgen G, Krause U, Becker A, et al. Tumor hypoxia, p53, and prognosis in cervical cancers. *Int J Radiat Oncol Biol Phys* 2001;50:865–872.
218. Haider MA, Patlas M, Jhaveri K, et al. Adenocarcinomas involving the uterine cervix: magnetic resonance imaging findings in tumors of endometrial compared with cervical origin. *Can Assoc Radiol J* 2006;57:43–48.
219. Haie C, Pejovic MH, Gerbaulet A, et al. Is prophylactic para-aortic irradiation worthwhile in the treatment of advanced cervical carcinoma? Results of a controlled clinical trial of the EORTC radiotherapy group. *Radiother Oncol* 1988;11:101–112.
220. Haie-Meder C, Kramar A, Lambin P, et al. Analysis of complications in a prospective randomized trial comparing two brachytherapy low dose rates in cervical cancer. *Int J Radiat Oncol Biol Phys* 1994;29:953–960.
221. Haie-Meder C, Lhomme C, de Crevoisier R, et al. Concomitant radiochemotherapy in cancer of the cervix uteri: modifications of the standards. *Cancer Radiother* 2000;4:134S–140S.
222. Haie-Meder C, Potter R, Van Limbergen E, et al. Recommendations from Gynecological (Gyn) GEC ESTRO Working Group (I): concepts in terms of 3D-image based 3D treatment planning in cervix cancer brachytherapy with emphasis on MRI assessment of GTV and CTV. *Radiother Oncol* 2005;74:235–245.
223. Hall EJ, Brenner DJ. The dose-rate effect revisited: radiobiological considerations of importance in radiotherapy. *Int J Radiat Oncol Biol Phys* 1991;21:1403–1414.
224. Hall EJ. Intensity-modulated radiation therapy, protons and the risk of second cancers. *Int J Radiat Oncol Biol Phys* 2006;65:1–7.
225. Hama Y, Uematsu M, Nagata I, et al. Carcinoma of the uterine cervix: twice-versus once-weekly high-dose-rate brachytherapy. *Radiology* 2001;219:207–212.
226. Hamberger AD, Fletcher GH, Wharton JT. Results of treatment of early stage I carcinoma of the uterine cervix with intracavitary radium alone. *Cancer* 1978;41:980–985.
227. Han Y, Shin EH, Huh SJ, et al. Interfractional dose variation during intensity-modulated radiation therapy for cervical cancer assessed by weekly CT evaluation. *Int J Radiat Oncol Biol Phys* 2006;65:617–623.
228. Hanks GE, Herring DF, Kramer S. Patterns of Care Outcome Studies: results of the National Practice in Cancer of the Cervix. *Cancer* 1983;51:959–967.
229. Hannoun-Levi JM, Peiffert D, Hoffstetter S, et al. Carcinoma of the cervical stump: retrospective analysis of 77 cases. *Radiother Oncol* 1997;43:147–153.
230. Hansen MA, Pedersen PH, Andreasson B, et al. Staging uterine cervical carcinoma with low-field MR imaging. *Acta Radiol* 2000;41:647–652.
231. Hareyama M, Sakata K, Oouchi A, et al. High dose-rate versus low dose-rate intracavitary therapy for carcinoma of the uterine cervix: a randomized trial. *Cancer* 2002;94:117–124.
232. Harima Y, Nagata K, Harima K, et al. A randomized clinical trial of radiation therapy versus thermoradiotherapy in stage IIIB cervical carcinoma. *Int J Hyperthermia* 2001;17:97–105.
233. Harima Y, Nagata K, Harima K, et al. Bax and Bcl-2 protein expression following radiation therapy versus radiation plus thermoradiotherapy in stage IIIB cervical carcinoma. *Cancer* 2000;88:132–138.
234. Hart K, Han I, Deppe G, et al. Postoperative radiation for cervical cancer with pathologic risk factors. *Int J Radiat Oncol Biol Phys* 1997;37:833–838.
235. Hatano K, Sekiya Y, Araki H, et al. Evaluation of the therapeutic effect of radiotherapy on cervical cancer using magnetic resonance imaging. *Int J Radiat Oncol Biol Phys* 1999;45:639–644.
236. Hawnaur JM, Johnson RJ, Carrington BM, et al. Predictive value of clinical examination, transrectal ultrasound, and magnetic resonance imaging prior to radiotherapy in carcinoma off the cervix. *Br J Radiol* 1998;71:819–827.
237. Hayashi Y, Hachisuga T, Iwasaka T, et al. Expression of ras oncogene product and EGF receptor in cervical squamous cell carcinomas and its relationship to lymph node involvement. *Gynecol Oncol* 1991;40:147–151.
238. Hazelbag S, Kenter GG, Gorte A, et al. Prognostic relevance of TGF-beta1 and PAI-1 in cervical cancer. *Int J Cancer* 2004;112:1020–1028.
239. Heller PB, Malfetano JH, Bundy BN. Clinical pathologic study of stages IIB, III, and IVA carcinoma of the cervix: extended diagnostic evaluation for paraaortic node metastasis (a GOG study). *Gynecol Oncol* 1990;38:425–430.
240. Hellstrom AC, Sigurjonson T, Pettersson F. Carcinoma of the cervical stump. The Radiumhemmet series 1959–1987: treatment and prognosis. *Acta Obstet Gynecol Scand* 2001;80:152–157.
241. Hemminki K, Dong C, Vaittinen P. Second primary cancer after in situ and invasive cervical cancer. *Epidemiology* 2000;11:457–461.
242. Henriksen E. The lymphatic spread of carcinoma of the cervix and of the body of the uterus: a study of 420 necropsies. *Am J Obstet Gynecol* 1949;58:924–942.
243. Herbst AL, Cole PL. Epidemiologic and clinical aspects of clear cell adenocarcinoma in young women. In: Herbt AL, ed. *Intrauterine exposure to diethylstilbestrol in the human*. American College of Obstetrics and Gynecology, 1978;2–7.
244. Herold J, Burton A, Buxton J, et al. A randomised, prospective, phase III clinical trial of primary bleomycin, ifosfamide and cisplatin (BIP) chemotherapy followed by radiotherapy versus radiotherapy alone in inoperable cancer of the cervix. *Ann Oncol* 2000;11:1175–1181.
245. Heron DE, Gerszten K, Selvaraj RN, et al. Conventional and conformal versus intensity-modulated radiotherapy for the adjuvant treatment of gynecologic malignancies: a comparative dosimetric study of dose-volume histograms small star, filled. *Gynecol Oncol* 2003;91:39–45.
246. Hille A, Weiss E, Hess CF. Therapeutic outcome and prognostic factors in the radiotherapy of recurrences of cervical carcinoma following surgery. *Strahlenther Onkol* 2003;179:742–747.
247. Himmelmann A, Holmberg E, Oden A, et al. Intracavitary irradiation of carcinoma of the cervix stage IB and IIA: a clinical comparison between a remote high dose rate afterloading system and a low dose rate manual system. *Acta Radiol Oncol* 1985;24:139–144.
248. Hintz BL, Kagan AR, Chan P, et al. Radiation tolerance of the vaginal mucosa. *Int J Radiat Oncol Biol Phys* 1980;6:711–716.
249. Hirst DG. Anemia: a problem or an opportunity in radiotherapy? *Int J Radiat Oncol Biol Phys* 1986;12:2009–2017.
250. Hochman A, Ratzkowski E, Schrieber H. Incidence of carcinoma of cervix in Jewish women in Israel. *Br J Cancer* 1955;9:358–364.
251. Höckel M, Schlenger K, Mitze M, et al. Hypoxia and radiation response in human tumors. *Semin Radiat Oncol* 1996;6:3–9.
252. Hoffman M, Kalter C, Roberts W, et al. Early cervical cancer coexistent with idiopathic inflammatory bowel disease. *South Med J* 1989;82:905–906.
253. Holcomb K, Gabbur N, Tucker T, et al. ^{60}Cobalt vs. linear accelerator in the treatment of locally advanced cervix carcinoma: a comparison of survival and recurrence patterns. *Eur J Gynaecol Oncol* 2001;22:16–19.
254. Hong JH, Tsai CS, Change JT, et al. The prognostic significance of pre- and posttreatment SCC levels in patients with squamous cell carcinoma of the cervix treated by radiotherapy. *Int J Radiat Oncol Biol Phys* 1998;41:823–830.
255. Hong JH, Tsai CS, Lai CH, et al. Postoperative low-pelvic irradiation for stage I-IIA cervical cancer patients with risk factors other than pelvic node metastasis. *Int J Radiat Oncol Biol Phys* 2002;53:1284–1290.
256. Hong JH, Tsai CS, Lai CH, et al. Risk stratification of patients with advanced squamous cell carcinoma of cervix treated by radiotherapy alone. *Int J Radiat Oncol Biol Phys* 2005;63:492–499.
257. Hope AJ, Grigsby PW. FDG-PET in carcinoma of the uterine cervix with endometrial extension. *Cancer* 2006;106:196–200.
258. Hopkins MP, Morley GW. The prognosis and management of cervical cancer associated with pregnancy. *Obstet Gynecol* 1992;80:9–13.
259. Horiot J-C, Pigneux J, Pourquier H, et al. Radiotherapy alone in carcinoma of the intact uterine cervix according to GH Fletcher guidelines: a French Cooperative study of 1383 cases. *Int J Radiat Oncol Biol Phys* 1988;14:605–611.
260. Hornback NB, Shupe RE, Shidnia H, et al. Advanced stage IIIB cancer of the cervix: treatment by hyperthermia and radiation. *Gynecol Oncol* 1986;23:160–167.
261. Hoskins PJ, Wong F, Swenerton KD, et al. Small cell carcinoma of the cervix treated with concurrent radiotherapy, cisplatin, and etoposide. *Gynecol Oncol* 1995;56:218–225.
262. Hoskins WC, Perez CA, Young RC, eds. *Principles and practice of gynecologic oncology*, 4th ed. Philadelphia: Lippincott Williams & Wilkins, 2005.
263. Hreshchyshyn MM, Aron BS, Boronow RC, et al. Hydroxyurea or placebo combined with radiation to treat stages IIIB and IV cervical cancer confined to the pelvis. *Int J Radiat Oncol Biol Phys* 1979;5:317–322.
264. Hricak H, Hu KK. Radiology in invasive cervical cancer. *AJR Am Roentgenol* 1996;167:1101.
265. Hricak H, Powell B, Yu KK, et al. Invasive cervical carcinoma: role of MR imaging in pretreatment work-up: cost minimization and diagnostic efficacy analysis. *Radiology* 1996;198:403–409.
266. Hsu WL, Wu DJ, Jen YM, et al. Twice-per-day fractionated high versus continuous low dose rate intracavitary therapy in the radical treatment of cervical cancer: a nonrandomized comparison of treatment results. *Int J Radiat Oncol Biol Phys* 1995;32:1425–1431.
267. Huerta BJ, Labastida AS, Cortez AH, et al. Postoperative radiotherapy in patients with invasive uterine cervix cancer treated previously with simple hysterectomy. Results from the Hospital de Oncologia, Centro Medico Nacional SXXI. *Ginecol Obstet Mex* 2003;71:304–311.
268. Ijaz T, Eifel PJ, Burke T, et al. Radiation therapy of pelvic recurrence after radical hysterectomy for cervical carcinoma. *Gynecol Oncol* 1998;70:241–246.
269. Inoue T, Morita K. Long-term observation of patients treated by postoperative extended-field irradiation for nodal metastases from cervical carcinoma stages IB, IIA, and IIB. *Gynecol Oncol* 1995;58:4–10.
270. Inoue T, Okumura M. Prognostic significance of parametrial extension in patients with cervical carcinoma, stages IB, IIA and IIB: a study of 628 cases treated by radical hysterectomy and lymphadenectomy with or without postoperative irradiation. *Cancer* 1984;54:1714–1719.
271. International Commission on Radiation Units and Measurements. *Dose and volume specification for reporting intracavitary therapy in gynecology*. ICRU report 38. Bethesda, MD: ICRU, 1985;1–16.
272. International Federation of Gynecologists and Obstetricians (FIGO). Staging announcement: FIGO staging of gynecologic cancers: cervical and vulva. *Int J Gynecol Cancer* 1995;5:319.
273. Ishida GM, Kato N, Hayasaka T, et al. Small cell neuroendocrine carcinomas of the uterine cervix: a histological, immunohistochemistry and molecular genetic study. *Int J Gynecol Pathol* 2004;23:366–372.
274. Iversen T, Tretli S, Johansen A, et al. Squamous cell carcinoma of the penis and of the cervix, vulva and vagina in spouses: is there any relationship? An epidemiological study from Norway, 1960–1992. *Br J Cancer* 1997;76:658–660.

275. Iwasaka T, Yokoyama M, Oh-Uehida M, et al. Detection of human papillomavirus genome and analysis of expression of c-myc and Ha-ras oncogenes in invasive cervical cancers. *Gynecol Oncol* 1992;46:298–303.

276. Jacobs AJ, Perez CA, Camel HM, et al. Complications in patients receiving both irradiation and radical hysterectomy for carcinoma of the uterine cervix. *Gynecol Oncol* 1985;22:273–280.

277. Jain D, Srinivasan R, Patel FD, et al. Evaluation of p53 and Bcl-2 expression as prognostic markers in invasive cervical carcinoma stage IIb/III patients treated by radiotherapy. *Gynecol Oncol* 2003;88:22–28.

278. Jeffries SA, Robinson JW, Craighead PS, et al. An effective group psychoeducational intervention for improving compliance with vaginal dilation: a randomized controlled trial. *Int J Radiat Oncol Biol Phys* 2006;65:404–411.

279. Jemal A, Siegel R, Ward E, et al. Cancer statistics, 2006. *CA Cancer J Clin* 2006;56:106–130.

280. Jenkin RDT, Stryker JA. The influence of the blood pressure on survival in cancer of the cervix. *Br J Radiol* 1968;41:913–920.

281. Jensen PT, Groenvold M, Klee MC, et al. Longitudinal study of sexual function and vaginal changes after radiotherapy for cervical cancer. *Int J Radiat Oncol Biol Phys* 2003;56:937–949.

282. Jhingran A, Eifel PJ. Perioperative and postoperative complications of intracavitary radiation for FIGO stage I-III carcinoma of the cervix. *Int J Radiat Oncol Biol Phys* 2000;46:1177–1183.

283. Jhingran A, Yom SS, Zang X, et al. Recurrence above the radiotherapy field after definitive treatment of cervix cancer. *Int J Radiat Oncol Biol Phys* 2005;63:S217–S218.

284. Jobson VW, Girtanner RE, Averette HE. Therapy and survival of early invasive carcinoma of the cervix uteri with metastases to the pelvic nodes. *Surg Gynecol Obstet* 1980;151:27–29.

285. Johns HE. Optimization of energy and equipment. In: Kramer S, Suntharalingam N, Zinninger GF, eds. *High-energy photons and electrons: clinical applications in cancer management.* New York: John Wiley, 1976;333–345.

286. Johnson RJR, Walton RJ. Sequential study on the effect of the addition of hyperbaric oxygen on the 5-year survival rates of carcinoma of the cervix treated with conventional fractional irradiations. *AJR Am J Roentgenol Radium Ther Nucl Med* 1974;120:111–117.

287. Joneja MG, Coulson DB. Histopathology and cytogenetics of tumors induced by application of 7,12-dimethylbenz(a)anthracene (DMBA) in mouse cervix. *Eur J Cancer* 1973;9:367–374.

288. Jones WB, Shingleton HM, Russell A, et al. Cervical carcinoma and pregnancy: a national Patterns of Care Study of the American College of Surgeons. *Cancer* 1996;77:1479–1488.

289. Joslin CAF. High-activity source afterloading in gynecologic cancer and its future prospects. *Endocuriether Hypertherm Oncol* 1989;5:69–81.

290. Kagei K, Shirato H, Nishioka T, et al. High-dose rate intracavitary irradiation using linear source arrangement for stage II and III squamous cell carcinoma of the uterine cervix. *Radiother Oncol* 1998;47:207–213.

291. Kahousen M, Haas J, Pickel H, et al. Chemotherapy versus radiotherapy versus observation for high-cervical carcinoma after radical hysterectomy: a randomized, prospective, multicenter trial. *Gynecol Oncol* 1999;73:196–201.

292. Kainz C, Kohlberger P, Gitsch G, et al. Mutant p53 in patients with invasive cervical cancer stages IB to IIB. *Gynecol Oncol* 1995;57:212–214.

293. Kaminski PF, Maier RC. Clear cell adenocarcinoma of the cervix unrelated to diethylstilbestrol exposure. *Obstet Gynecol* 1983;62:720–727.

294. Kang S, Kim MH, Park IA, et al. Elevation of cyclooxygenase-2 is related to lymph node metastasis in adenocarcinoma of uterine cervix. *Cancer Lett* 2006;237:305–311.

295. Kapp DS, Glatcla AJ. New directions for radiation biology research in cancer of the uterine cervix. *J Natl Cancer Inst Monogr* 1996;21:131–139.

296. Kapp DS, Lawrence R. Temperature elevation during brachytherapy for carcinoma of the uterine cervix: adverse effect on survival and enhancement of distant metastases. *Int J Radiat Oncol Biol Phys* 1984;10:2281–2292.

297. Kapp KS, Poschauko J, Geyer E, et al. Evaluation of the effect of routine packed red cell transfusion in anemic cervix cancer patients treated with radical radiotherapy. *Int J Radiat Oncol Bio Phys* 2002;54:58–66.

298. Kapp KS, Stuecklschweiger GF, Kapp DS, et al. Dosimetry of intracavitary placements for uterine and cervical carcinoma: results of orthogonal film, TLD, and CT-assisted techniques. *Radiother Oncol* 1992;24:137–146.

299. Kapp KS, Stuecklschweiger GF, Kapp DS, et al. Prognostic factors in patients with carcinoma of the uterine cervix treated with external beam irradiation and Ir-192 high-dose rate brachytherapy. *Int J Radiat Oncol Biol Phys* 1998;42:531–540.

300. Kasibhatla M, Clough RW, Montana GS, et al. Predictors of severe gastrointestinal toxicity after external beam radiotherapy and interstitial brachytherapy for advanced or recurrent gynecologic malignancies. *Int J Radiat Oncol Biol Phys* 2006;65:398.

301. Kastritis E, Bamias A, Efstathiou E, et al. The outcome of advanced or recurrent non-squamous carcinoma of the uterine cervix after platinum-based combination chemotherapy. *Gynecol Oncol* 2005;99:376–382.

302. Kato S, Ohno T, Tsujii H, et al. Dose escalation study of carbon ion radiotherapy for locally advanced carcinoma of the uterine cervix. *Int J Radiat Oncol Biol Phys* 2006;65:388–397.

303. Katz A, Eifel PJ, Moughan J, et al. Socioeconomic characteristics of patients with squamous cell carcinoma of the uterine cervix treated with radiotherapy in the 1992 to 1994 patterns of care study. *Int J Radiat Oncol Biol Phys* 2000;47:443–450.

304. Katz A, Eifel PJ. Quantification of intracavitary brachytherapy parameters and correlation with outcome in patients with carcinoma of the cervix. *Int J Radiat Oncol Biol Phys* 2000;48:1417–1425.

305. Kavanagh BD, Fischer BA, Segreti EM, et al. A cost analysis of erythropoietin versus blood transfusions for cervix cancer patients receiving chemoradiotherapy. *Int J Radiat Oncol Biol Phys* 2001;51:435–441.

306. Kavanagh BD, Gieschen HL, Schmidt-Ullrich RK, et al. A pilot study of concomitant boost accelerated superfractionated radiotherapy for stage III cancer of the uterine cervix. *Int J Radiat Oncol Biol Phys* 1997;38:561–568.

307. Kavanagh BD, Schefter TE, Wu Q, et al. Clinical application of intensity-modulated radiotherapy for locally advanced cervical cancer. *Semin Radiat Oncol* 2002;12:260–271.

308. Kavanagh BD, Secomb TW, Hsu R, et al. A theoretical model for the effects of reduced hemoglobin-oxygen affinity on tumor oxygenation. *Int J Radiat Oncol Biol Phys* 2002;53:172–179.

309. Keighley E. Carcinoma of the cervix among prostitutes in a women's prison. *Br J Venereal Dis* 1968;44:254–255.

310. Ketcham AS, Sindelar WF, Felix EL, et al. Diagnostic scalene node biopsy in the preoperative evaluation of the surgical cancer patient. *Cancer* 1976;38:948–952.

311. Keys H, Bundy B, Stehman F, et al. Adjuvant hysterectomy after radiation therapy reduces detection of local recurrences in "bulky" stage IB cervical without improving survival: results of a prospective randomized GOG trial. *Cancer J Sci Am* 1997;3:117(abstr).

312. Keys H, Bundy B, Stehman F, et al. Cisplatin, radiation, and adjuvant hysterectomy compared with radiation and adjuvant hysterectomy for bulky stage IB cervical carcinoma. *N Engl J Med* 1999;340:1154–1161.

313. Kielbinska S, Ludwika T, Fraczek O. Studies of mortality and health status in women cured of cancer of the cervix uteri: comparison of long-term results of radiotherapy and combined surgery and radiotherapy. *Cancer* 1973;32:245–252.

314. Kilcheski T, Arger P, Mikuta J. Role of computed tomography in the presurgical evaluation of carcinoma of the cervix. *J Comput Assist Tomogr* 1981;5:378–383.

315. Kilgore LC, Soong S-J, Gore H, et al. Analysis of prognostic features in adenocarcinoma of the cervix. *Gynecol Oncol* 1988;31:137–148.

316. Kim CR, Eaton BA, Stevens KR Jr. Localization of the apex of the vagina: implications for radiation therapy planning. *Radiology* 1999;212:155–158.

317. Kim GE, Lim JJ, Park W, et al. Sensory and motor dysfunction assessed by anorectal manometry in uterine cervical carcinoma patients with radiation-induced late rectal complications. *Int J Radiat Oncol Biol Phys* 1998;41:835–841.

318. Kim HK, Silver B, Berkowitz R, et al. Bulky, barrel-shaped cervical carcinoma (stages IB, IIA, IIB): the prognostic factors for pelvic control and treatment income. *Am J Clin Oncol* 1999;22:232–235.

319. Kim JS, Kim JS, Kim SY, et al. Hyperfractionated radiotherapy with concurrent chemotherapy for para-aortic lymph node recurrence in carcinoma of the cervix. *Int J Radiat Oncol Biol Phys* 2003;55:1247–1253.

320. Kim RY, Trotti A, Wu C-J, et al. Radiation alone in the treatment of cancer of the uterine cervix: analysis of pelvic failure and dose response relationship. *Int J Radiat Oncol Biol Phys* 1989;17:973–978.

321. Kim SH, Han JK. Invasion of the urinary bladder by uterine cervical carcinoma: evaluation with MR imaging. *AJR Am J Roentgenol* 1997;168:393–406.

322. Kim YB, Kim GE, Pyo HR, et al. Differential cyclooxygenase 2 expression in squamous cell carcinoma ans adenocarcinoma of the uterine cervix. *Int J Radiat Oncol Biol Phys* 2004;60:822–829.

323. Kinney WK, Alvarez RD, Reid GC, et al. Value of adjuvant whole-pelvis irradiation after Wertheim hysterectomy for early-stage squamous carcinoma of the cervix with pelvic nodal metastasis: a matched-control study. *Gynecol Oncol* 1989;34:258–262.

324. Kinney WK, Hodge DO, Egorshin EV, et al. Surgical treatment of patients with stages IB and IIA carcinoma of the cervix and palpably positive pelvic lymph nodes. *Gynecol Oncol* 1995;57:145–149.

325. Kirisits C, Lang S, Dimopoulos J, et al. The Vienna applicator for combined intracavitary and interstitial brachytherapy of cervical cancer: design, application, treatment planning and dosimetric results. *Int J Radiat Oncol Biol Phys* 2006;65:624–630.

326. Kitano Y, Fujisaki S, Nakamura N, et al. Immunological disorder against the Epstein-Barr virus infection and prognosis in patients with cervical carcinoma. *Gynecol Oncol* 1995;57:150–157.

327. Kjorstad KE, Martinbeau PW, Iversen T. Stage IB carcinoma of the cervix: the Norwegian Radium Hospital: results and complications: III. Urinary and gastrointestinal complications. *Gynecol Oncol* 1983;15:42–47.

328. Klevens RM, Fleming PL, Mays MA, et al. Characteristics of women with AIDS and invasive cervical cancer. *Obstet Gynecol* 1996;88:169–273.

329. Knocke TH, Pokrajac B, Fellner C, et al. A comparison of CT-supported 3D planning with standard planning in the pelvic irradiation of primary cervical carcinoma. *Strahlenther Onkol* 1999;175:68–73.

330. Knocke TH, Weitmann HD, Feldmann HJ, et al. Intratumoral p02 measurements as predictive assay in the treatment of carcinoma of the uterine cervix. *Radiother Oncol* 1999;53:99–104.

331. Kodaira T, Fuwa N, Kamata M, et al. Clinical assessment by MRI for patients with stage II cervical carcinoma treated by radiation alone in multicenter analysis: are all patients with stage II disease suitable candidates for chemoradiotherapy? *Int J Radiat Oncol Biol Phys* 2002;52:627–636.

332. Kodaira T, Karasawa K, Shimizu T, et al. Clinical efficacy of applying four-field portals to paraaortic irradiation in the treatment of cervical carcinoma. *Radiat Oncol Invest* 1999;7:170–177.

333. Kolstad P. Follow-up study of 232 patients with stage Ia1 and 411 patients with stage Ia2 squamous cell carcinoma of the cervix (microinvasive carcinoma). *Gynecol Oncol* 1989;33:265–272.

334. Komaki R, Brickner TJ, Hanlon AL, et al. Long-term results of treatment of cervical carcinoma in the United States in 1973, 1978, and 1983: Patterns of Care Study. *Int J Radiat Oncol Biol Phys* 1995;31:973–982.

335. Koulos J, Wright TC, Follen MM, et al. Relationships between cKi-ras mutations, HPV types and prognostic indicators in invasive endocervical adenocarcinomas. *Gynecol Oncol* 1993;48:364–369.

336. Kovalic JJ, Grigsby PW, Perez CA, et al. Cervical stump carcinoma. *Int J Radiat Oncol Biol Phys* 1991;20:933–938.

337. Kramer C, Peschel RE, Goldberg N, et al. Radiation treatment of FIGO stage IVA carcinoma of the cervix. *Gynecol Oncol* 1989;32:323–326.

338. Kraus FT, Perez-Mesa C. Verrucous carcinoma: clinical and pathologic study of 105 cases involving oral cavity, larynx, and genitalia. *Cancer* 1966;19:26–38.

339. Kristensen GB, Kaern J, Abeler VM, et al. No prognostic impact of flow-cytometric measured DNA ploidy and S-phase fraction in cancer of the uterine cervix: a prospective study of 465 patients. *Gynecol Oncol* 1995;57:79–85.

339a. Kuipers T. High dose rate intracavety irradiation: results of treatment. In: Mould RF, ed. *Brachytherapy 2.* Leersum, the Netherlands: Nucletron International BV, 1984;169–175.

340. Kuipers T, Hoekstra CJ, van't Riet A, et al. HDR brachytherapy applied to cervical carcinoma with moderate lateral expansion: modified principles of treatment. *Radiother Oncol* 2001;58:25–30.

341. Kumar L, Grover R, Pokharel YH, et al. Neoadjuvant chemotherapy in locally advanced cervical cancer: two randomized studies. *Aust N Z J Med* 1998;28:387–390.

342. Kumar L, Kaushal R, Nandy M, et al. Chemotherapy followed by radiotherapy versus radiotherapy alone in locally advanced cervical cancer: a randomized study. *Gynecol Oncol* 1994;54:307–315.
343. Kupets R, Thomas GM, Covens A. Is there a role for pelvic lymph node debulking in advanced cervical cancer? *Gynecol Oncol* 2002;87:163–170.
344. Kuske RR, Perez CA, Jacobs AJ, et al. Mini-colpostats in the treatment of carcinoma of the uterine cervix. *Int J Radiat Oncol Biol Phys* 1988;14:899–906.
345. Lacava JA, Leone BA, Machiavelli M, et al. Vinorelbine as neoadjuvant chemotherapy in advanced cervical carcinoma. *J Clin Oncol* 1997;15:604–609.
346. Lagasse LD, Creasman WT, Shingleton HM, et al. Results and complications of operative staging in cervical cancer: experience of the Gynecologic Oncology Group. *Gynecol Oncol* 1980;9:90–98.
347. Lanciano R, Calkins A, Bundy BN, et al. Randomized comparison of weekly cisplatin or protracted venous infusion of fluorouracil in combination with pelvic irradiation in advanced cervix cancer: a Gynecologic Oncology Group study. *J Clin Oncol* 2005;23:8289–8295.
348. Lanciano R, Corn B, Martin E, et al. Perioperative morbidity of intracavitary gynecologic brachytherapy. *Int J Radiat Oncol Biol Phys* 1994;29:969–974.
349. Lanciano RM, Martz K, Montana GS, et al. Influence of age, prior abdominal surgery, fraction size, and dose on complications after radiation therapy for squamous cell cancer of the uterine cervix. *Cancer* 1992;69:2124–2130.
350. Lanciano RM, Pajak TF, Martz K, et al. The influence of treatment time on outcome for squamous cell cancer of the uterine cervix treated with radiation: a Patterns of Care Study. *Int J Radiat Oncol Biol Phys* 1993;25:391–406.
351. Landoni F, Bocciolone L, Perego P, et al. Cancer of the cervix, FIGO stages IB and IIA: patterns of local growth and paracervical extension. *Int J Gynecol Cancer* 1995;5:329–334.
352. Landoni F, Maneo A, Colombo A, et al. Randomised study of radical surgery versus radiotherapy for stage Ib-Iia cervical cancer. *Lancet* 1997;350:535–540.
353. Lang S, Nulens A, Briot E, et al. Intercomparison of treatment concepts for MR image assisted brachytherapy of cervical carcinoma based on GYN GEC-ESTRO recommendations. *Radiother Oncol* 2006;78:185–193.
354. Larson DM, Copeland LJ, Stringer CA, et al. Recurrent cervical carcinoma after radical hysterectomy. *Gynecol Oncol* 1988;30:381–387.
355. Larson DM, Stringer CA, Copeland LJ, et al. Stage IB cervical carcinoma treated with radical hysterectomy and pelvic lymphadenectomy: role of adjuvant radiotherapy. *Obstet Gynecol* 1987;69:378–381.
356. Lavey RS, Dempsey WH. Erythropoietin increases hemoglobin in cancer patients during radiation therapy. *Int J Radiat Oncol Biol Phys* 1993;27:1147–1152.
357. Lawhead RA Jr, Clark DGC, Smith DH, et al. Pelvic exenteration for recurrent or persistent gynecologic malignancies: a 10-year review of the Memorial Sloan-Kettering Cancer Center experience (1972–1981). *Gynecol Oncol* 1989;33:279–282.
358. Layton-Henry J, Scurry J, Planner R, et al. Cervical adenoid basal carcinoma: five cases and literature review. *Int J Gynecol Cancer* 1996;6:193–199.
359. Le Pechoux C, Akine Y, Sumi M, et al. High dose rate brachytherapy for carcinoma of the uterine cervix: comparison of two different fractionation regimens. *Int J Radiat Oncol Biol Phys* 1995;31:735–741.
360. Leborgne F, Fowler JF, Leborgne JH, et al. Fractionation in medium dose-rate brachytherapy of cancer of the uterus. *Int J Radiat Oncol Biol Phys* 1996;35:907–914.
361. Leborgne F, Leborgne JH, Doldan R, et al. Induction chemotherapy and radiotherapy of advanced cancer of the cervix: a pilot study and phase III randomized trial. *Int J Radiat Oncol Biol Phys* 1997;37:343–350.
362. Leborgne F, Leborgne JH, Zubizarreta E, et al. High-dose-rate brachytherapy at 14 Gy per hour to point A: preliminary results of a prospectively designed schedule for cancer of the cervix based on the linear-quadratic model. *Int J Gynecol Cancer* 2001;11:445–453.
363. LeBouedec G, Rabishong B, Canis M, et al. Ovarian transposition by laparoscopy in young women before curietherapy for cervical cancer. *J Gynecol Obstet Biol Reprod (Paris)* 2000;29:564–570.
364. Lee HC, Liu CS, Chiao C, et al. Hyperbaric oxygen therapy in hemorrhagic radiation cystitis: a report of 20 cases. *Undersea Hyperb Med* 1994;21:321–327.
365. Lee J-H, Lee S-K, Yang M-H, et al. Expression and mutation of H-ras in uterine cervical cancer. *Gynecol Oncol* 1996;62:49–54.
366. Lee JW, Kim BG, Lee SJ, et al. Preliminary results of consolidation chemotherapy following concurrent chemoradiation after radical surgery in hig-risk early-stage carcinoma of the uterine cervix. *Clin Oncol (R Coll Radiol)* 2005;17:412–417.
367. Lee JY, Perez CA, Ettinger N, et al. The risk of second primaries subsequent to irradiation for cervix cancer. *Int J Radiat Oncol Biol Phys* 1982;8:207–211.
368. Lee KC, Kim TH, Choi MS, et al. Use of the rectal retractor to reduce the rectal dose in high dose rate intracavitary brachytherapy for a carcinoma of the uterine cervix. *Yonsei Med J* 2004;45:113–122.
369. Lee SW, Suh CO, Chung EJ, et al. Dose optimization of fractionated external radiation and high-dose-rate brachytherapy for FIGO stage IB uterine cervical cancer. *Int J Radiat Oncol Biol Phys* 2002;52:1338–1344.
370. Lehman M, Thomas G. Is concurrent chemotherapy and radiotherapy the new standard of care for locally advanced cervical cancer? *Int J Gynecol Oncol* 2001;11:87–99.
371. Leibel S, Bauer M, Wasserman T, et al. Radiotherapy with or without misonidazole for patients with stage IIIB or stage IVA squamous cell carcinoma of the uterine cervix: preliminary report of a Radiation Therapy Oncology Group randomized trial. *Int J Radiat Oncol Biol Phys* 1987;13:541–549.
372. Lemus JF, Abdulhay G, Sobolewski C, et al. Cardiac metastasis from carcinoma of the cervix: report of two cases. *Gynecol Oncol* 1998;69:264–268.
373. Lertsanguansinchai P, Lertbutsayanukul C, Shotelersuk K, et al. Phase III randomized trial comparing LDR and HDR brachytherapy in treatment of caervical carcinoma. *Int J Radiat Oncol Biol Phys* 2004;59:1424–1431.
374. Levenback C, Eifel PJ, Burke TW, et al. Hemorrhagic cystitis following radiotherapy for stage IB cancer of the cervix. *Gynecol Oncol* 1994;55:206–210.
375. Leveque J, Laurent JF, Burtin F, et al. Prognostic factors of the uterine cervix adenocarcinoma. *Eur J Obstet Gynecol Reprod Biol* 1998;80:209–214.
376. Lin HH, Cheng WF, Chan KW, et al. Risk factors for recurrence in patients with stage IB, IIA, and IIB cervical carcinoma after radical hysterectomy and postoperative pelvic irradiation. *Obstet Gynecol* 1996;88:274–279.
377. Lin LL, Mutic S, Malyapa RS, et al. Sequential FDG-PET brachytherapy treatment planning in carcinoma of the cervix. *Int J Radiat Oncol Biol Phys* 2005;63:1494–1501.
378. Lin LL, Yang Z, Mutic S, et al. FDG-PET imaging for the assessment of physiologic volume response during radiotherapy in cervix cancer. *Int J Radiat Oncol Biol Phys* 2006;65:177–181.
379. Littman P, Clement PB, Henriksen B, et al. Glassy cell carcinoma of the cervix. *Cancer* 1976;37:2238–2246.
380. Liu W, Meigs JV. Radical hysterectomy and pelvic lymphadenectomy: a review of 473 cases including 244 for primary invasive carcinoma of the cervix. *Am J Obstet Gynecol* 1955;69:1–32.
381. Liu W-S, Yen S-H, Chang C-H, et al. Determination of the appropriate fraction number and size of the HDR brachytherapy for cervical cancer. *Gynecol Oncol* 1996;60:295–300.
382. Logsdon MD, Eifel PJ. FIGO IIIB squamous cell carcinoma of the cervix: an analysis of prognostic factors emphasizing the balance between external beam and intracavitary radiation therapy. *Int J Radiat Oncol Biol Phys* 1999;43:763–775.
383. Loncaster JA, Cooper RA, Logue JP, et al. Vascular endothelial growth factor (VEGF) expression is a prognostic factor for radiotherapy outcome in advanced carcinoma of the cervix. *Br J Cancer* 2000;83:620–625.
384. Long HJ, Bundy BN, Grendys EC, et al. Randomized phase III trial of cisplatin with or without topotecan in carcinoma of the uterine cervix: a Gynecologic Onclogy Group study. *J Clin Oncol* 2005;23:4626–4633.
385. Look KY, Brunetto VL, Clarke-Pearson DL, et al. An analysis of cell type in patients with surgically staged stage IB carcinoma of the cervix: a Gynecologic Oncology Group study. *Gynecol Oncol* 1996;63:304–311.
386. Lorvidhaya V, Tonusin A, Changwiwit W, et al. High-dose-rate afterloading brachytherapy in carcinoma of the cervix: an experience of 1992 patients. *Int J Radiat Oncol Biol Phys* 2000;46:1185–1191.
387. Lorvidhaya V, Tonusin A, Sukthomya W, et al. Induction chemotherapy and irradiation in advanced carcinoma of the cervix. *Gan Kagaku Ryoho* 1995;22[Suppl III]:244–251.
388. Lovecchio JL, Averette HE, Doinato D, et al. 5-year survival of patients with paraaortic nodal metastases in clinical stage IB and IIA cervical carcinoma. *Gynecol Oncol* 1989;34:43–45.
389. Lujan AE, Mundt AJ, Yamada SD, et al. Intensity-modulated radiotherapy as a means of reducing dose to bone marrow in gynecological patients receiving whole pelvic radiotherapy. *Int J Radiat Oncol Biol Phys* 2003;57:516–521.
390. Lynch HT, Rubinstein WS, Locker GY. Cancer in Jews: introduction and overview. *Fam Cancer* 2004;3:177–192.
391. MacLeod C, Bernshaw D, Leung S, et al. Accelerated hyperfractionated radiotherapy for locally advanced cervix cancer. *Int J Radiat Oncol Biol Phys* 2000;46:1082–1983.
392. Magrina JF, Goodrich MA, Weaver AL, et al. Modified radical hysterectomy: morbidity and mortality. *Gynecol Oncol* 1995;59:277–282.
393. Mahé M-A, Gérard J-P, Dubois J-B, et al. Intraoperative radiation therapy in recurrent carcinoma of the uterine cervix: report of the French Intraoperative Group on 70 patients. *Int J Radiat Oncol Biol Phys* 1996;34:21–26.
394. Mahmoud-Ahmed AS, Suh JH, Barnett GH, et al. Tumor distribution and survival in six patients with brain metastases from cervical carcinoma. *Gynecol Oncol* 2001;81:196–200.
395. Malfetano JH, Keys H, Cunningham MJ, et al. Extended field radiation and cisplatin for stage IIB and IIIB cervical carcinoma. *Gynecol Oncol* 1997;67:203–207.
396. Mandai M, Konishi I, Koshiyama M, et al. Altered expression of nm34-H1 and c-erbB-2 proteins have prognostic significance in adenocarcinoma but not in squamous cell carcinoma of the uterine cervix. *Cancer* 1995;75:2523–2529.
397. Manetta A, Podczaski ES, Larson JE, et al. Scalene lymph node biopsy in the preoperative evaluation of patients with recurrent cervical cancer. *Gynecol Oncol* 1989;33:332–334.
398. Maor MH, Gillespie BW, Peters LJ, et al. Neutron therapy in cervical cancer: results of a phase III RTOG study. *Int J Radiat Oncol Biol Phys* 1988;14:883–891.
399. Marcial VA, Amato D, Marks RD, et al. Split-course versus continuous pelvis irradiation in carcinoma of the uterine cervix: a prospective randomized clinical trial of the Radiation Therapy Oncology Group. *Int J Radiat Oncol Biol Phys* 1983;9:431–436.
400. Marcial VA, Blanco MS, DeLeon E. Persistent tumor cells in the vaginal smear during the first year after radiation therapy of carcinoma of the uterine cervix: prognostic significance. *AJR Am J Roentgenol Radium Ther Nucl Med* 1968;102:170–175.
401. Mark RJ, Poen J, Tran LM, et al. Postirradiation sarcoma of the gynecologic tract: a report of 13 cases and a discussion of the risk of radiation-induced gynecologic malignancies. *Am J Clin Oncol* 1996;19:59–64.
402. Martinez A, Edmundson GK, Cox RS, et al. Combination of external beam irradiation and multiple-site perineal applicator (MUPIT) for treatment of locally advanced or recurrent prostatic, anorectal, and gynecologic malignancies. *Int J Radiat Oncol Biol Phys* 1985;11:391–398.
403. Martinez-Monge R, Jurado M, Azinovic I, et al. Intraoperative radiotherapy in recurrent gynecological cancer. *Radiother Oncol* 1993;28:127–133.
404. Maruyama Y, Muir W. Human cervical cancer clearance after ^{252}Cf neutron brachytherapy versus conventional photon brachytherapy. *Am J Clin Oncol* 1984;7:347–352.
405. Mayer A, Nemeskeri C, Petnehazi C, et al. Primary radiotherapy of stage IIA/B-IIIB cervical carcinoma. A comparison of continuous versus sequential regimens. *Strahlenther Onkol* 2004;180:209–215.
406. McIntyre JF, Eifel PJ, Levenback C, et al. Ureteral stricture as a late complication of radiotherapy for stage IB carcinoma of the uterine cervix. *Cancer* 1995;75:836–843.
407. Meanwell CA, Kelly KA, Wilson S, et al. Young age as a prognostic factor in cervical cancer: analysis of population based on data from 10,022 cases. *BMJ* 1998;296:386–391.
408. Mendenhall WM, McCarty PJ, Morgan LS, et al. Stage IB-IIA-B carcinoma of the intact uterine cervix $\geq$ 6 cm diameter: is adjuvant extrafascial hysterectomy beneficial? *Int J Radiat Oncol Biol Phys* 1991;21:899–904.
409. Micke O, Proff FJ, Schafer U, et al. The impact of squamous cell carcinoma (SCC) antigen in patients with advanced cancer of uterine cervix treated with (chemo-) radiotherapy. *Anticancer Res* 2005;25:1663–1666.
410. Miller B, Dockter M, el Torky M, et al. Small cell carcinoma of the cervix: a clinical and flow-cytometric study. *Gynecol Oncol* 1991;42:27–33.
411. Miller BE, Copeland LJ, Hamberger AD, et al. Carcinoma of the cervical stump. *Gynecol Oncol* 1984;18:100–108.

412. Million RR, Fletcher GH, Rutledge F. Stage IV carcinoma of the cervix with bladder invasion. *Am J Obstet Gynecol* 1972;113:239–246.

413. Mitchell PA, Waggoner S, Rotmensch J, et al. Cervical cancer in the elderly treated with radiation therapy. *Gynecol Oncol* 1998;71:291–298.

414. Mitsuhashi N, Takahashi M, Yamakawa M, et al. Results of postoperative radiation therapy for patients with carcinoma of the uterine cervix: evaluation of intravaginal cone boost with an electron beam. *Gynecol Oncol* 1995;57:321–326.

415. Molla M, Escude L, Nouet P, et al. Fractionated stereotactic radiotherapy boost for gynecologic tumors: an alternative to brachytherapy? *Int J Radiat Oncol Biol Phys* 2005;62:118–124.

416. Monk BJ, Montz FJ. Invasive cervical cancer complicating intrauterine pregnancy: treatment with radical hysterectomy. *Obstet Gynecol* 1992;80:199–203.

417. Montana GS, Fowler WC, Varia MA, et al. Carcinoma of the cervix, stage III: results of radiation therapy. *Cancer* 1986;57:148–154.

418. Montana GS, Hanlon AL, Brickner TJ, et al. Carcinoma of the cervix: Patterns of Care studies review of 1978, 1983, 1988–1989 surveys. *Int J Radiat Oncol Biol Phys* 1995;32:1481–1486.

419. Montz FJ, Holschneider CH, Solh S, et al. Small bowel obstruction following radical hysterectomy: risk factors, incidence, and operative findings. *Gynecol Oncol* 1994;53:114–120.

420. Moreno A, Clemente J, Crespo C, et al. Pelvic insufficiency fractures in patients with pelvic irradiation. *Int J Radiat Oncol Biol Phys* 1999;44:61–66.

421. Morice P, Juncker L, Rey A, et al. Ovarian transposition for patients with cervical carcinoma. *Fertil Steril* 2000;74:743–748.

422. Morris M, Brador K, Levenback C, et al. Phase II study of vinorelbine in advanced and recurrent squamous cell carcinoma of the cervix. *J Clin Oncol* 1998;16:1094–1098.

423. Morris M, Eifel PJ, Burke TW, et al. Treatment of locally advanced cervical cancer with concurrent radiation and intra-arterial chemotherapy. *Gynecol Oncol* 1995;57:72–78.

424. Morris M, Gershenson DM, Eifel P, et al. Treatment of small cell carcinoma of the cervix with cisplatin, doxorubicin, and etoposide. *Gynecol Oncol* 1992;47:62–65.

425. Mukherjee G, Freeman A, Moore R, et al. Biologic factors and response to radiotherapy in carcinoma of the cervix. *Int J Gynecol Cancer* 2001;11:187–193.

426. Mundstedt K, Johnson P, Bohlmann MK, et al. Adjuvant radiotherapy in carcinomas of the uterine cervix: the prognostic value of hemoglobin levels. *Int J Gynecol Cancer* 2005;15:285–291.

427. Mundt AJ, Connell PP, Campbell T, et al. Race and clinical outcome in patients with carcinoma of the uterine cervix treated with radiation therapy. *Gynecol Oncol* 1998;71:151–158.

428. Munstedt K, Johnson P, Von Georgi R, et al. Consequences of inadvertent, suboptimal primary surgery in carcinoma of the uterine cervix. *Gynecol Oncol* 2004; 94:515–520.

429. Nag S, Erickson B, Thomadsen B, et al. The American Brachytherapy Society recommendations for high-dose-rate brachytherapy for carcinoma of the cervix. *Int J Radiat Oncol Biol Phys* 2000;48:201–211.

430. Nag S, Martinez-Monge R, Selman AE, et al. Interstitial brachytherapy in the management of primary carcinoma of the cervix and vagina. *Gynecol Oncol* 1998;70:27–32.

431. Nag S, Orton C, Young D, et al. The American Brachytherapy Society survey of brachytherapy practice for carcinoma of the cervix in the United States. *Gynecol Oncol* 1999;73:11–118.

432. Nahmias AJ, Naib ZM, Josey WE. Epidemiological studies relating genital herpetic infection to cervical carcinoma. *Cancer Res* 1974;34:1111–1117.

433. Nakano T, Arai T, Morita S, et al. Radiation therapy alone for adenocarcinoma of the uterine cervix. *Int J Radiat Oncol Biol Phys* 1995;32:1331–1336.

434. Nakano T, Kato S, Ohno T, et al. Long-term results of high-dose rate intracavitary brachytherapy for squamous cell carcinoma of the uterine cervix. *Cancer* 2005;103:92–101.

435. Nam TK, Ahn SJ. A prospective randomized study on two dose fractionation regimens of high-dose-rate brachytherapy for carcinoma of the uterine cervix: comparison of efficacies and toxicities between two regimens. *J Korean Med Sci* 2004;19:87–94.

436. National Cancer Institute. *Concurrent chemoradiation for cervical cancer.* Clinical announcement. Bethesda, MD: National Cancer Institute, 1999.

437. Nelson JH, Boyce J, Macasaet M, et al. Incidence, significance and follow up of para-aortic lymph nod metastases in late invasive carcinoma of the cervix. *Am J Obstet Gynecol* 1977;128:336–340.

438. Nelson R, Norton N, Cautley E, et al. Community-based prevalence of anal incontinence. *JAMA* 1995;274:559–561.

439. Netter FH. *The CIBA collection of medical illustrations,* vol. 2: *Reproductive system.* Summit, NJ: Ciba Pharmaceutical, 1972.

440. Newman G. Increased morbidity following the introduction of remote afterloading with increased dose rate, for cancer of the cervix. *Radiother Oncol* 1996;39:97–103.

441. Newton M. Radical hysterectomy or radiotherapy for stage I cervical cancer. *Am J Obstet Gynecol* 1975;123:535–542.

442. Ngan HYS, Cheng GTS, Cheng D, et al. Post-treatment serial serum squamous cell carcinoma antigen (SCC) in the monitoring of squamous cell carcinoma of the cervix. *Int J Gynecol Cancer* 1996;6:115–119.

443. Niibe Y, Hayakawa K, Kanai T, et al. Optimal dose for stage IIIB adenocarcinoma of the uterine cervix on the basis of biological effective dose. *Eur J Gynaecol Oncol* 2006;27:47–49.

444. Nishida M, Nasu K, Takai N, et al. Adenoid cystic carcinoma of the uterine cervix. *Int J Clin Oncol* 2005;10:198–200.

445. Noguchi H, Shiozawa I, Kitahara T, et al. Uterine body invasion of carcinoma of the uterine cervix as seen from surgical specimens. *Gynecol Oncol* 1988;30:173–182.

446. Norstrom A, Jansson I, Andersson H. Carcinoma of the uterine cervix in pregnancy: a study of the incidence and treatment in the western region of Sweden 1973 to 1992. *Acta Obstet Gynecol Scand* 1997;76:583–589.

447. Novak ER, Jones GS, Jones HW, eds. *Novak's textbook of gynecology.* Philadelphia: Williams & Wilkins, 1970.

448. Obermair A, Wanner C, Gilbi S, et al. Tumor angiogenesis in stage IB cervical cancer: correlation of microvessel density with survival. *Am J Obstet Gynecol* 1998;178:314–319.

449. Ogino I, Kitamura T, Okaima H, et al. High-dose-rate brachytherapy in the management of cervical and vaginal intraepithelial neoplasia. *Int J Radiat Oncol Biol Phys* 1998;40:881–887.

450. Ogino I, Kitamura T, Okamoto N, et al. Late rectal complication following high dose rate intracavitary brachytherapy in cancer of the cervix. *Int J Radiat Oncol Biol Phys* 1995;31:725–734.

451. Oguchi M, Ikeda H, Watanabe T, et al. Experiences of 23 patients ≥ 90 years of age treated with radiation therapy. *Int J Radiat Oncol Biol Phys* 1998;41:407–413.

452. Ohno T, Nakano T, Niibe Y, et al. Bax protein expression correlates with radiation-induced apoptosis in radiation therapy for cervical carcinoma. *Cancer* 1998;83:103–110.

453. Oka K, Suzuki Y, Nakano T. Expression of p27 and p53 in cervical squamous cell carcinoma patients treated with radiotherapy alone: radiotherapeutic effect and prognosis. *Cancer* 2000;88:2766–2773.

454. Onishi H, Yamaguchi M, Kuriyama K, et al. Effect of concurrent intra-arterial infusion of platinum drugs for patients with stage III or IV uterine cervical cancer treated with radical radiation therapy. *Cancer J Sci Am* 2000;6:40–45.

455. Orton CG, Seyedsadr M, Somnay A. Comparison of high and low dose rate remote afterloading for cervix cancer and the importance of fractionation. *Int J Radiat Oncol Biol Phys* 1991;21:1425–1434.

456. Overgaard J, Bentzen SM, Kolstad P, et al. Misonidazole combined with radiotherapy in the treatment of carcinoma of the uterine cervix. *Int J Radiat Oncol Biol Phys* 1989;16:1069–1072.

457. Palefsky JM, Minkoff H, Kalish LA, et al. Cervicovaginal human papillomavirus infection in human immunodeficiency virus-1 (HIV)-positive and high-risk HIV-negative women. *J Natl Cancer Inst* 1999;91:226–235.

458. Paley PJ, Goff BA, Minudri R, et al. The prognostic significance of radiation dose and residual tumor in the treatment of barrel-shaped endophytic cervical carcinoma. *Gynecol Oncol* 2000;76:373–379.

459. Park TK, Choi DH, Kim SN, et al. Role of induction chemotherapy in invasive cervical cancer. *Gynecol Oncol* 1991;41:107–112.

460. Park TK, Lee SK, Kim SN, et al. Comparison of concurrent and sequential regimens. *Gynecol Oncol* 1993;50:196–201.

461. Parker M, Bosscher J, Barnhill D, et al. Ovarian management during radical hysterectomy in the premenopausal patients. *Obstet Gynecol* 1993;82:187–190.

462. Parkin DE, Davis JA, Symonds RP. Urodynamic findings following radiotherapy for cervical carcinoma. *Br J Urol* 1988;61:213–217.

463. Patel PD, Sharma SC, Negi PS, et al. Low dose rate vs. high dose rate brachytherapy in the treatment of carcinoma of the uterine cervix: a clinical trial. *Int J Radiat Oncol Biol Phys* 1994;28:335–341.

464. Pauer HU, Viereck V, Burfeind P, et al. Uterine cervical metastasis of breast cancer: a rare complication that may be overlooked. *Onkologie* 2003;26:58–60.

465. Paxton JR, Bolger BS, Armour A, et al. Apoptosis in cervical squamous carcinoma: predictive value for survival following radiotherapy. *J Clin Pathol* 2000;53:197–200.

466. Pearcey RG, Brundage MD, Drouin P, et al. A clinical trial comparing concurrent cisplatin and radiation therapy versus radiation alone for locally advanced squamous cell carcinoma of the cervix carried out by the National Cancer Institute of Canada Clinical Trials Group. *Proc Am Soc Clin Oncol* 2000;19:3782.

467. Pedersen D, Bentzen SM, Overgaard J. Early and late radiotherapeutic morbidity in 442 consecutive patients with locally advanced carcinoma of the uterine cervix. *Int J Radiat Oncol Biol Phys* 1994;29:941–952.

468. Pelloski CE, Palmer M, Chronowski GM, et al. Comparison between CT-based volumetric calculations and ICRU reference-point estimates of radiation doses delivered to the bladder and rectum during intracavitary radiotherapy for cervical cancer. *Int J Radiat Oncol Biol Phys* 2005;62:131–137.

469. Perez CA, Breaux S, Bedwinek JM, et al. Radiation therapy alone in treatment of carcinoma of the uterine cervix: II. Analysis of complications. *Cancer* 1984;54:235–246.

470. Perez CA, Camel HM, Askin F, et al. Endometrial extension of carcinoma of the uterine cervix: a prognostic factor that may modify staging. *Cancer* 1981;48:170–180.

471. Perez CA, Camel HM, Kao MS, et al. Randomized study of preoperative radiation and surgery or irradiation in the treatment of stage IB and IIA carcinoma of the uterine cervix: final report. *Gynecol Oncol* 1987;27:129–140.

472. Perez CA, Grigsby PW, Camel HM, et al. Irradiation alone or combined with surgery in stage IB, IIA, and IIB carcinoma of uterine cervix: update of a non-randomized comparison. *Int J Radiat Oncol Biol Phys* 1995;31:703–716.

473. Perez CA, Grigsby PW, Castro-Vita H, et al. Carcinoma of the uterine cervix: I. Impact of prolongation of treatment time and timing of brachytherapy on outcome of radiation therapy. *Int J Radiat Oncol Biol Phys* 1995;32:1275–1288.

474. Perez CA, Grigsby PW, Chao KSC, et al. Tumor size, irradiation dose, and long-term outcome of carcinoma of the uterine cervix. *Int J Radiat Oncol Biol Phys* 1998;41:307–317.

475. Perez CA, Grigsby PW, Lockett MA, et al. Radiation therapy morbidity in carcinoma of the uterine cervix: dosimetric and clinical correlation. *Int J Radiat Oncol Biol Phys* 1999;44:855–866.

476. Perez CA, Grigsby PW, Nene SM, et al. Effect of tumor size on the prognosis of carcinoma of the uterine cervix treated with irradiation alone. *Cancer* 1992;69:2796–2806.

477. Perez CA, Grigsby PW. Adjuvant chemotherapy and irradiation in locally advanced squamous cell carcinoma of the uterine cervix. *PPGO Updates* 1993;1(4):1–20.

478. Perez CA, Kavanagh BD. Uterine cervix. In: Perez CA, Brady LW, Halperin EC, et al., eds. *Principles and practice of radiation oncology.* Philadelphia: Lippincott Williams & Wilkins, 2004;1800–1915.

479. Perez-Mesa C, Spratt JS. Scalene node biopsy in the pretreatment staging of carcinoma of the cervix uteri. *Am J Obstet Gynecol* 1976;125:93–95.

480. Petereit DG, Pearcey R. Literature analysis of high dose brachytherapy fractionation schedules in the treatment of cervical cancer: is there an optimal fractionation schedule? *Int J Radiat Oncol Biol Phys* 1999;43:359–366.

481. Petereit DG, Sarkaria JN, Chappell RJ. Perioperative morbidity and mortality of high-dose-rate gynecologic brachytherapy. *Int J Radiat Oncol Biol Phys* 1998;42:1025–1031.

482. Petereit DG, Sarkaria JN, Potter DM, et al. High-dose-rate versus low-dose-rate brachytherapy in the treatment of cervical cancer: analysis of tumor recurrence—the University of Wisconsin experience. *Int J Radiat Oncol Biol Phys* 1999;45:1267–1274.

483. Peters WA III, Liu PY, Barrett RJ, et al. Concurrent chemotherapy and pelvic radiation therapy compared with pelvic radiation therapy alone as adjuvant therapy after radical surgery in high-risk early-stage cancer of the cervix. *J Clin Oncol* 2000;18:1606–1613.
484. Pierquin B, Marinello G, Mege J-P, et al. Intracavitary irradiation of carcinomas of the uterus and cervix: the Creteil method. *Int J Radiat Oncol Biol Phys* 1988;15:1465–1473.
485. Piura B, Rabinovich A, Meirovitz M, et al. Glassy cell carcinoma of the uterine cervix. *J Surg Oncol* 1999;72:206–210.
486. Piver MS, Barlow JJ, Krishnamsetty R. Five-year survival (with no evidence of disease) in patients with biopsy-confirmed aortic node metastasis from cervical carcinoma. *Am J Obstet Gynecol* 1981;139:575–578.
487. Piver MS, Barlow JJ, Vongtama V, et al. Hydroxyurea as a radiation sensitizer in women with carcinoma of the uterine cervix. *Am J Obstet Gynecol* 1977;129:379–383.
488. Piver MS, Chung WS. Prognostic significance of cervical lesion size and pelvic node metastases in cervical carcinoma. *Obstet Gynecol* 1975;46:507–510.
489. Piver MS, Marchetti DL, Patton T, et al. Radical hysterectomy and pelvic lymphadenectomy versus radiation therapy for small (≤3 cm) stage IB cervical carcinoma. *Am J Clin Oncol* 1988;11:21–24.
490. Piver MS, Rutledge F, Smith JP. Five classes of extended hysterectomy for women with cervical cancer. *Obstet Gynecol* 1974;44:265–272.
491. Ploch E. Hormonal replacement therapy in patients after cervical cancer treatment. *Gynecol Oncol* 1987;26:169–177.
492. Podczaski E, Stryker JA, Kaminski P, et al. Extended field radiotherapy for carcinoma of the cervix. *Cancer* 1990;66:251–258.
493. Portelance L, Chao KSC, Grigsby PW, et al. Intensity-modulated radiation therapy (IMRT) reduces small bowel, rectum, and bladder doses in patients with cervical cancer receiving pelvic and para-aortic irradiation. *Int J Radiat Oncol Biol Phys* 2001;51:261–266.
494. Postema S, Pattynama PM, van den Berg-Huysmans A, et al. Effect of MRI on therapeutic decisions in invasive cervical carcinoma: direct comparison with the pelvic examination as a preoperative test. *Gynecol Oncol* 2000;79:485–489.
495. Potish RA, Deibel FC Jr, Khan FM. The relationship between milligram-hours and dose to point A in carcinoma of the cervix. *Radiology* 1982;145:479–483.
496. Potish RA, Downey GO, Adcock LL, et al. The role of surgical debulking in cancer of the uterine cervix. *Int J Radiat Oncol Biol Phys* 1989;17:979–984.
497. Potish RA. Surgical staging, extended field radiation, and enteric morbidity in the treatment of cervix cancer. *Int J Radiat Oncol Biol Phys* 1995;31:1009–1010.
498. Potter R, Haie-Meder C, Limbergen EV, et al. Recommendations from gynaecological (GYN) GEC ESTRO working group (II): Concepts and terms in 3D image-based treatment planning in cervix brachytherapy-3D dose volume parameters and aspects of 3D image-based anatomy, radiation physics, radiobiology. *Radiother Oncol* 2006;78:67–77.
499. Potter R, Knocke TH, Fellner C, et al. Definitive radiotherapy base on HDR brachytherapy with iridium 192 in uterine cervix carcinoma: report of the Vienna University Hospital findings (1993–1997) compared to the preceding period in the context of ICRU 38 recommendations. *Cancer Radiother* 2000;4:159–172.
500. Pourquier H, Dubois JB, Deland R. Cancer of the uterine cervix: dosimetric guidelines for prevention of late rectal and rectosigmoid complications as a result of radiotherapeutic treatment. *Int J Radiat Oncol Biol Phys* 1982;8:1887–1895.
501. Prasad KN, Pradhan S, Datta NR. Urinary tract infection in patients of gynecological malignancies undergoing external pelvic radiotherapy. *Gynecol Oncol* 1995;57:380–382.
502. Prempree T. Parametrial implant in stage IIIB cancer of the cervix: III. A 5-year study. *Cancer* 1983;52:748–750.
503. Pyo H, Kim YB, Cho NH, et al. Coexpression of cyclooxygenase 2 and thymidine phosphorylase as a prognostic indicator in patients with FIGO stage IIB squamous cell carcinoma of the cervix treated with radiotherapy and concurrent chemotherapy. *Int J Radiat Oncol Biol Phys* 2005;62:725–732.
504. Quilty PM. A report of late rectosigmoid morbidity in patients with advanced cancer of the cervix, treated with a 6-week pelvic brick technique. *Clin Radiol* 1988;39:297–300.
505. Randall ME, Michael H, Ver Morken J, et al. Uterine cervix. In: Hoskins WJ, Perez CA, Young RC, et al., eds. *Principles and practice of gynecologic oncology*. Philadelphia: Lippincott Williams & Wilkins, 2005;4:743–822.
506. Raspagliesi F, Ditto A, Quattrone P, et al. Prognostic factors in microinvasive cervical squamoous cell cencer: long-term results. *Int J Gynecol Cancer* 2005;15:88–93.
507. Reagan JW, Fu YS. Histologic types and prognosis of cancers of the uterine cervix. *Int J Radiat Oncol Biol Phys* 1979;5:1015–1020.
508. Recio FO, Piver MS, Hempling RE, et al. Laparoscopic-assisted application of interstitial brachytherapy for locally advanced cervical carcinoma: results of a pilot study. *Int J Radiat Oncol Biol Phys* 1998;40:411–414.
509. Reeves WC, Brinton LA, Garcia M, et al. Human papillomavirus infection and cervical cancer in Latin America. *N Engl J Med* 1989;320:1437–1441.
510. Resbeut M, Alzieu C, Gonzague-Casabianca L, et al. Combined brachytherapy and surgery for early carcinoma of the uterine cervix: analysis of extent of surgery on outcome. *Int J Radiat Oncol Biol Phys* 2001;50:873–881.
511. Rintala MA, Rantanen VT, Salmi TA, et al. PAP smear after radiation therapy for cervical cancer. *Anticancer Res* 1997;17:3747–3750.
512. Riou GF, Le MG, LeDoussal V, et al. c-Myc protooncogene expression and prognosis in early carcinoma of the uterine cervix. *Lancet* 1988;2:761–763.
513. Roberts KB, Urdaneta N, Vera R, et al. Interim results of a randomized trial of mitomycin C as an adjunct to radical radiotherapy in the treatment of locally advanced squamous-cell carcinoma of the cervix. *Int J Cancer* 2000;90:206–223.
514. Robinson JW, Faris PD, Scott CB. Psychoeducational group increases vaginal dilation for younger women and reduces sexual fears for women of all ages with gynecological carcinoma treated with radiotherapy. *Int J Radiat Oncol Biol Phys* 1999;44:497–506.
515. Roche B, Chautems R, Marti MC. Application of formaldehyde for treatment of hemorrhagic radiation-induced proctitis. *World J Surg* 1996;20:1092–1094.
516. Roddick JW Jr, Greenlaw RH. Treatment of cervical cancer. *Am J Obstet Gynecol* 1971;19:754–764.
517. Rodrigus P, DeWinter K, Venselaar J, et al. Evaluation of late morbidity in patients with carcinoma of the uterine cervix following a dose rate change. *Radiother Oncol* 1997;42:137–141.
518. Rofstad EK, Sundfr EK, Lyng H, et al. Hypoxia-induced treatment failure in advanced squamous cell carcinoma of the uterine cervix is primarily due to hypoxia-induced radiation resistance rather than hypoxia-induced metastasis. *Br J Cancer* 2000;83:354–359.
519. Rogers CL, Freel JH, Speiser BL. Pulsed low dose rate brachytherapy for uterine cervix carcinoma. *Int J Radiat Oncol Biol Phys* 1999;43:95–100.
520. Roman TN, Souhami L, Freeman CR. High dose rate afterloading intracavitary therapy in carcinoma of the cervix. *Int J Radiat Oncol Biol Phys* 1991;20:921–926.
521. Rose PG, Adler LB, Rodriguez M, et al. Positron emission tomography for evaluating para-aortic lymph node metastasis in locally advanced cervical cancer before surgical staging: a surgico-pathologic study. *J Clin Oncol* 1999;17:41–45.
522. Rose PG, Blessing JA, Gershenson DM, et al. Paclitaxel and cisplatin as first-line therapy in recurrent or advanced carcinoma of the cervix: a Gynecologic Oncology Group study. *J Clin Oncol* 1999;17:2676–2680.
523. Rose PG, Bundy BN, Watkins EB, et al. Concurrent cisplatin-based radiotherapy and chemotherapy for locally advanced cervical cancer. *N Engl J Med* 1999;340:1144–1153.
524. Rose PG, Eifel PJ. Combined radiation therapy and chemotherapy for carcinoma of the cervix. *Cancer J* 2001;7:86–94.
525. Rosseau J, Fenton J, Debertrand P, et al. Carcinoma of the cervix: a 7-year study on 1212 cases treated at Foundation Curie, Paris. *Radiology* 1972;103:413–418.
526. Rotman M, Aziz H, Boyce J. Postoperative irradiation in stage IB carcinoma of cervix. *Int J Radiat Oncol Biol Phys* 1988;15:1045–1046.
527. Rotman M, Pajak TF, Choi K, et al. Prophylactic extended-field irradiation of para-aortic lymph nodes in stages IIB and bulky IB and IIA cervical carcinoma: ten-year treatment results of RTOG 79-20. *JAMA* 1995;274:387–393.
528. Rotman M, Sedlis A, Piedmonte MR, et al. A phase III randomized trial of postoperative pelvic irradiation in stage IB cervical carcinoma with poor prognostic features: follow up of a gynecologic oncology group study. *Int J Radiat Oncol Biol Phys* 2006;65:169–176.
529. Rotman MZ. Chemoirradiation: a new initiative in cancer treatment: 1991 RSNA Annual Oration in Radiation Oncology. *Radiology* 1992;184:319–327.
530. Rotmensch J, Connell PP, Yamada D, et al. One versus two intracavitary brachytherapy applications in early-stage cervical cancer patients undergoing definitive radiation therapy. *Gynecol Oncol* 2000;78:32–38.
531. Rubinstein E, Ibsen T, Rasmussen RB, et al. Formalin treatment of radiation-induced hemorrhagic proctitis. *Am J Gastroenterol* 1986;81:44–45.
532. Russell AH, Jones DC, Russell KJ, et al. High dose paraaortic lymph node irradiation for gynecologic cancer: technique, toxicity, and results. *Int J Radiat Oncol Biol Phys* 1987;13:267–271.
533. Russell AH, Koh WJ, Markette K, et al. Radical re-irradiation for recurrent or second primary carcinoma of the female reproductive tract. *Gynecol Oncol* 1987;27:226–232.
534. Russell AH, Shingleton HM, Jones WB, et al. Trends in the use of radiation and chemotherapy in the initial management of patients with carcinoma of the uterine cervix. *Int J Radiat Oncol Biol Phys* 1998;40:605–613.
535. Russell AH, Walter JP, Anderson MW, et al. Sagittal magnetic resonance imaging in the design of lateral radiation treatment portals for patients with locally advanced squamous cancer of the cervix. *Int J Radiat Oncol Biol Phys* 1992;23:449–455.
536. Rutledge FN, Galakatos AE, Wharton JT, et al. Adenocarcinoma of the uterine cervix. *Am J Obstet Gynecol* 1975;122:235–245.
537. Rutledge FN, Mitchell MF, Nunsell S, et al. Youth as a prognostic factor in carcinoma of the cervix: a matched analysis. *Gynecol Oncol* 1992;44:123–130.
538. Sadan O, Frohlich RP, Driscoll JA, et al. Is it safe to prescribe hormonal contraception and replacement therapy to patients with premalignant and malignant uterine cervices? *Gynecol Oncol* 1989;34:159–163.
539. Saibishkumar EP, Patel FD, Ghoshal S, et al. Results of salvage radiotherapy after inadequate surgery in invasive cervical carcinoma patients: a retrospective analysis. *Int J Radiat Oncol Biol Phys* 2005;63:828–833.
540. Saibishkumar EP, Patel FD, Sharma SC, et al. Results of external-beam radiotherapy alone in invasive cancer of the uterine cervix: a retrospective analysis. *Clin Radio (R Coll Radiol)* 2006;18:46–51.
541. Saibishkumar EP, Patel FD, Sharma SC. Results of radiotherapy alone in the treatment of carcinoma of the uterine cervix: a retrospective analysis of 1069 patients. *Int J Gynecol Cancer* 2005;15:890–897.
542. Salama JK, Mundt AJ, Roeke J, et al. Preliminary outcome and toxicity report of extended-field intensity-modulated radiation therapy for gynecologic malignancies. *Int J Radiat Oncol Biol Phys* 2006;65:1170–1176.
543. Santucci MA, Barbieri E, Frezza G, et al. Radiation-induced gadd45 expression correlates with clinical response to radiotherapy of cervical carcinoma. *Int J Radiat Oncol Biol Phys* 2000;46:411–416.
544. Sardi JE, Giaroli A, Sananes C, et al. Long-term follow-up of the first randomized trial using neoadjuvant chemotherapy in stage IB squamous carcinoma of the cervix: the final results. *Gynecol Oncol* 1997;67:61–69.
545. Sarkaria JN, Peterett DG, Stitt JA, et al. A comparison of the efficacy and complication rates of low dose-rate versus high dose-rate brachytherapy in the treatment of uterine cervical carcinoma. *Int J Radiat Oncol Biol Phys* 1994;30:75–82.
546. Schilder RJ, Blessing J, Cohn DE. Evaluation of gemcitabine in previously treated patients with non-squamous cell carcinoma of the cervix: a phase II study of the Gynecology Oncology Group. *Gynecol Oncol* 2005;96:103–107.
547. Seidenfeld J, Piper M, Flamm C, et al. Epoetin treatment of anemia associated with cancer therapy: a systematic review and meta-analysis of controlled clinical trials. *J Natl Cancer Inst* 2001;93:1204–1214.
548. Selke P, Roman TN, Souhami L, et al. Treatment results of high dose rate brachytherapy in patients with carcinoma of the cervix. *Int J Radiat Oncol Biol Phys* 1993;27:803–809.
549. Senekjian EK, Hubby M, Bell DA, et al. Clear cell adenocarcinoma (CCA) of the vagina and cervix in association with pregnancy. *Gynecol Oncol* 1986;24:207–219.
550. Seow-Choen F, Goh H, Eu K, et al. A simple and effective treatment for hemorrhagic radiation proctitis using formalin. *Dis Colon Rectum* 1993;36:135–138.
551. Sevin B-U, Method MW, Nadji M, et al. Efficacy of radical hysterectomy as treatment for patients with small cell carcinoma of the cervix. *Cancer* 1996;77:1489–1493.
552. Sharma S, Patel FD, Sandhu APS, et al. A prospective randomized study of local hyperthermia as a supplement and radiosensitizer in the treatment of carcinoma

of the cervix with radiotherapy. *Endocuriether Hypertherm Oncol* 1989;5:151–159.

553. Shepherd JH. Staging announcement FIGO staging of gynecologic cancers: cervical and vulva. *Int J Gynecol Cancer* 1995;5:319.

554. Shepherd SF, Collins CD, Fryatt IJ, et al. Computerized axial tomographic scan measurements as prognostic indicators in patients with cervical carcinoma. *Br J Radiol* 1995;68:600–603.

555. Sheridan MT, Cooper RA, West CM. A high ratio of apoptosis to proliferation correlated with improved survival after radiotherapy for cervical adenocarcinoma. *Int J Radiat Oncol Biol Phys* 1999;44:507–512.

556. Shigematsu Y, Nishiiyama K, Masaki N, et al. Treatment of carcinoma of the uterine cervix by remotely controlled afterloading intracavitary radiotherapy with high-dose rate: a comparative study with a low-dose rate system. *Int J Radiat Oncol Biol Phys* 1983;9:351–356.

557. Shimada M, Kigawa J, Nishimura R, et al. Ovarian metastasis in carcinoma of the uterine cervix. *Gynecol Oncol* 2006;101:234–237.

558. Silver DF, Hempling RE, Piver MS, et al. Stage I adenocarcinoma of the cervix: does lesion size affect treatment options and prognosis? *Am J Clin Oncol* 1998;21:431–435.

559. Silverberg SG, Hurt WG. Minimal deviation adenocarcinoma ("adenoma malignum") of the cervix: a reappraisal. *Am J Obstet Gynecol* 1975;121:971–975.

560. Singh AK, Grigsby PW, Rader JS, et al. Cervix carcinoma, concurrent chemoradiotherapy, and salvage of isolated paraaortic lymph node recurrence. *Int J Radiat Oncol Biol Phys* 2005;61:450–455.

561. Sironi S, Belloni C, Taccagni GL, et al. Carcinoma of the cervix: value of MR in detecting parametrial involvement. *AJR Am J Roentgenol* 1991;156:753–756.

562. Smith HO, Jiang CS, Weiss GR, et al. Tirapazamine plus cisplatin in advanced or recurrent carcinoma of the uterine cervix: a Southwest Oncology Group study. *Int J Gynecol Cancer* 2006;16:298–305.

563. Snijders-Keilholtz A, Hellebrekers BW, Zwinderman AH, et al. Adjuvant radiotherapy following radical hysterectomy for patients with early-stage cervical carcinoma (1984–1996). *Radiother Oncol* 1999;51:161–167.

564. Soisson AP, Geszler G, Soper JT, et al. A comparison of symptomatology, physical examination, and vaginal cytology in the detection of recurrent cervical carcinoma after radical hysterectomy. *Obstet Gynecol* 1990;76:106–109.

565. Solomon D, Davey D, Kurman R, et al. The 2001 Bethesda system: terminology for reporting results of cervical cytology consensus statement. *JAMA* 2002;287:2114–2119.

566. Sommers G, Grigsby PW, Perez CA, et al. Outcome of recurrent cervical carcinoma following definitive irradiation. *Gynecol Oncol* 1989;35:150–155.

567. Song DY, Lawrie WT, Abrams RA, et al. Acute and late radiotherapy toxicity in patients with inflammatory bowel disease. *Int J Radiat Oncol Biol Phys* 2001;51:455–459.

568. Sood AK, Sorosky JI, Krogman S, et al. Surgical management of cervical cancer complicating pregnancy: a case-control study. *Gynecol Oncol* 1996;63:294–298.

569. Sood AK, Sorosky JI, Mayr N, et al. Cervical cancer diagnosed shortly after pregnancy: prognostic variables and delivery routes. *Obstet Gynecol* 2000;95:832–838.

570. Sood AK, Sorosky JI, Mayr N, et al. Radiotherapeutic management of cervical carcinoma that complicated pregnancy. *Cancer* 1997;80:1073–1078.

571. Sood BM, Gorla GR, Garg M, et al. Extended-field radiotherapy and high dose-rate brachytherapy in carcinoma of the uterine cervix: clinical experience with and without chemotherapy. *Cancer* 2003;97:1781–1788.

572. Sorosky JI, Squatrito R, Udubisi BU, et al. Stage I squamous cell cervical carcinoma in pregnancy: planned delay in therapy awaiting fetal maturity. *Gynecol Oncol* 1995;59:207–210.

573. Souhami L, Gil RA, Allan SE, et al. A randomized trial of chemotherapy followed by pelvic radiation therapy in stage IIIB carcinoma of the cervix. *J Clin Oncol* 1991;9:970–977.

574. Souhami L, Seymour R, Roman TN, et al. Weekly cisplatin plus external beam radiotherapy and high dose rate brachytherapy in patients with locally advanced carcinoma of the cervix. *Int J Radiat Oncol Biol Phys* 1993;27:871–878.

575. Spanos WJ, Clery M, Perez CA, et al. Late effect of multiple daily fraction palliation schedule for advanced pelvic malignancies (RTOG 8502). *Int J Radiat Oncol Biol Phys* 1994;29:961–967.

576. Spanos WJ, Guse C, Perez CA, et al. Phase I study of multiple daily fractionations in the palliation of advanced pelvic malignancies: preliminary report of RTOG 8502. *Int J Radiat Oncol Biol Phys* 1989;17:659–661.

577. Spanos WJ, Perez CA, Marcus S, et al. Effect of rest interval on tumor and normal tissue response: a report of phase III study of accelerated split course palliative radiation for advanced pelvic malignancies (RTOG 8502). *Int J Radiat Oncol Biol Phys* 1993;25:399–403.

578. Stehman FR, Bundy BN, DiSaia PH, et al. Carcinoma of the cervix treated with radiation therapy: I. A multivariate analysis of prognostic variables in the Gynecologic Oncology Group. *Cancer* 1991;67:2776–2785.

579. Stehman FR, Bundy EN, Thomas G, et al. Hydroxyurea versus misonidazole with radiation in cervical carcinoma: long-term follow-up of a Gynecologic Oncology Group trial. *J Clin Oncol* 1993;11:1523–1528.

580. Stockle E, Verdier G, Thomas L, et al. Functional outcome of laparoscopically transposed ovaries in the multidisciplinary treatment of cervical cancers: analysis of risk factors. *J Gynecol Obstet Biol Reprod (Paris)* 1996;25:244–252.

581. Storm HH. Second primary cancer after treatment for cervical cancer: late effects after radiotherapy. *Cancer* 1988;61:679–688.

582. Strang P, Eklund GM, Stendahl U, et al. S-phase rate as a predictor of early recurrences in carcinoma of the uterine cervix. *Anticancer Res* 1987;7:807–810.

583. Strauss A. Irradiation of carcinoma of the cervix uteri in pregnancy. *AJR Am J Roentgenol Radium Ther Nucl Med* 1940;43:552–566.

584. Stryker JA, Bartholomew M, Velkley DE, et al. Bladder and rectal complications following radiotherapy for cervix cancer. *Gynecol Oncol* 1988;29:1–11.

585. Stryker JA, Mortel R. Survival following extended field irradiation in carcinoma of cervix metastatic to para-aortic lymph nodes. *Gynecol Oncol* 2000;79:399–405.

586. Sundfør K, Lyng H, Kongsgard U, et al. Polarographic measurement of pO2 in cervix carcinoma. *Gynecol Oncol* 1997;64:230–235.

587. Sundfør K, Tropé CG, Högberg T, et al. Radiotherapy and neoadjuvant chemotherapy for cervical carcinoma: a randomized multicenter study of sequential cisplatin and 5-fluorouracil and radiotherapy in advanced cervical carcinoma stage IIIB and IVA. *Cancer* 1996;77:2371–2378.

588. Sundfør K, Trope CG, Kjorstad KE. Radical radiotherapy versus brachytherapy plus surgery in carcinoma of the cervix 2A and 2B: long-term results from a randomized study 1968–1980. *Acta Oncol* 1996;35[Suppl 8]:99–107.

589. Suyama S, Nakaguchi T, Kawakami K, et al. Computed tomography analysis of causes of local failure in radiotherapy for cervical carcinoma. *Cancer* 1998;83:1956–1965.

590. Suzuki Y, Nakano T, Arai T, et al. Progesterone receptor is a favorable prognostic factor of radiation therapy for adenocarcinoma of the uterine cervix. *Int J Radiat Oncol Biol Phys* 2000;47:1229–1234.

591. Syed AMN, Feder BH. Techniques of afterloading interstitial implants. *Radiol Clin* 1977;46:458–475.

592. Symonds P, Collingwood M, Kirwan J, et al. Concomitant hydroxyurea plus radiotherapy versus radiotherapy for carcinoma of the uterine cervix. *Cancer Treat Rev* 2004;30:405–414.

593. Symonds RP, Habeshaw AT, Reed NS, et al. The Scottish and Manchester randomised trial of neo-adjuvant chemotherapy for advanced cervical cancer. *Eur J Cancer* 2000;36:994–1001.

594. Szarewski A. Smoking and cervical neoplasia: a review of the evidence. *J Epidemiol Biostat* 1998;3:229–256.

595. Takeshi K, Katsuyuki K, Yoshiaki T, et al. Definitive radiotherapy combined with high-dose-rate brachytherapy for stage III carcinoma of the uterine cervix: retrospective analysis of prognostic factors concerning patient characteristics and treatment parameters. *Int J Radiat Oncol Biol Phys* 1998;41:319–327.

596. Tanaka E, Suzuki O, Oh RJ, et al. Intracavitary brachytherapy for carcinoma of the uterine cervix-comparison of HDR (Ir-192) and MDR (Cs-137). *Radiat Med* 2006;24:50–57.

597. Tanaka Y, Sawada S, Murata T. Relationship between lymph node metastases and prognosis in patients irradiated postoperatively for carcinoma of the uterine cervix. *Acta Radiol Oncol* 1984;23:455–459.

598. Tattersall MH, Loorvidhaya V, Vootiprux V, et al. Randomized trial of epirubicin and cisplatin chemotherapy followed by pelvic radiation in locally advanced cervical cancer: Cervical Cancer Study Group of the Asian Oceanian Clinical Oncology Association. *J Clin Oncol* 1995;13:444–451.

599. Tattersall MHN, Ramirez C, Coppleson M. A randomized trial comparing platinum-based chemotherapy followed by radiotherapy vs. radiotherapy alone in patients with locally advanced cervical cancer. *Int J Gynecol Oncol* 1992;2:244–251.

600. Tattersall MHN, Ramirez C, Coppleson M. A randomized trial of adjuvant chemotherapy and radical hysterectomy in stage IB-IIA cervical cancer patients with pelvic lymph node metastases. *Gynecol Oncol* 1992;46:176–181.

601. Taylor A, Rockall AG, Reznek RH, et al. Mapping pelvic lymph nodes: guidelines for delineation in intensity-modulated radiotherapy. *Int J Radiat Oncol Biol Phys* 2005;63:1604–1612.

602. Terris M, Wilson F, Nelson JH Jr. Relation of circumcision to cancer of the cervix. *Am J Obstet Gynecol* 1973;117:1056–1066.

603. Teshima T, Inoue T, Ikeda H, et al. High-dose rate and low-dose rate intracavitary therapy for carcinoma of the uterine cervix: final results of Osaka University Hospital. *Cancer* 1993;72:2409–2414.

604. Tewari K, Cappuccini F, Gambino A, et al. Neoadjuvant chemotherapy in the treatment of locally advanced cervical carcinoma in pregnancy: a report of two cases and review of issues specific to the management of cervical carcinoma in pregnancy including planned delay of therapy. *Cancer* 1998;82:1529–1534.

605. Thomadsen BR, Shahabi S, Stitt JA. High dose rate brachytherapy in carcinoma of the cervix: physics and dosimetry considerations. *Int J Radiat Oncol Biol Phys* 1992;24:349–357.

606. Thomas G. The effect of hemoglobin level on radiotherapy outcomes: the Canadian experience. *Semin Oncol* 2001;28[Suppl 8]:60–65.

607. Thomas GM, Dembo AJ, Ackerman I, et al. A randomized trial of standard versus partially hyperfractionated radiation with or without concurrent 5-fluorouracil in locally advanced cervical cancer. *Gynecol Oncol* 1998;69:137–145.

608. Thomas GM, Dembo AJ. Is there a role for adjuvant pelvic radiotherapy after radical hysterectomy in early stage cervical cancer? *Int J Gynecol Cancer* 1991;1:1–8.

609. Thomas GM. Is neoadjuvant chemotherapy a useful strategy for the treatment of stage IB cervix cancer [editorial]. *Gynecol Oncol* 1993;49:153–155.

610. Thomas JE, Cascino TL, Earle JD. Differential diagnosis between radiation and tumor plexopathy of the pelvis. *Neurology* 1985;35:1–7.

611. Thoms WW, Eifel PJ, Smith TL, et al. Bulky endocervical carcinoma of the uterine cervix: a 23-year experience. *Int J Radiat Oncol Biol Phys* 1992;23:491–499.

612. Tiersten A, Saltz L. Influence of inflammatory bowel disease on the ability of patients to tolerate system fluorouracil-based chemotherapy. *J Clin Oncol* 1996;14:2043–2046.

613. Tinker AV, Bhagat K, Swenerton KD, et al. Carboplatin and paclitaxel for advanced cervical carcinoma: the British Columbia Cancer Agency experience. *Gynecol Oncol* 2005;98:54–58.

614. Toita T, Nakano M, Higashi M, et al. Prognostic value of cervical size and pelvic lymph node status assessed by computed tomography for patients with uterine cervical cancer treated by radical radiation therapy. *Int J Radiat Oncol Biol Phys* 1995;33:843–849.

615. Tokoshima M, Okamura C, Niikura H, et al. Epitheloid leiomyosarcoma of the uterine cervix: a case report and review of the literature. *Gynecol Oncol* 2005;97:957–960.

616. Tominaga Y, Koyama Y, Sasagawa M, et al. A follow-up study of patients with cervical cancer after resection, with special emphasis on the incidence of second primary cancers. *Gynecol Oncol* 1995;56:71–74.

617. Tsai CC, Lin H, Huang EY, et al. The role of preoperative serum carcinoembryonic antigen level in early-stage adenocarcinoma of the cervix. *Gyenecol Oncol* 2004;94:363–367.

618. Tsai CC, Liu YS, Huang SC, et al. Value of preoperative serum CA 125 in early-stage adenocarcinoma of the uterine cervixwithout pelvic lymph node metastasis. *Gynecol Oncol* 2006;100:591–595.

619. Tsang RW, Wong CS, Fyles AW, et al. Tumour proliferation and apoptosis in human uterine cervix carcinoma: II. Correlations with clinical outcome. *Radiother Oncol* 1999;50:93–101.

620. Tseng CJ, Chang CT, Lai CH, et al. A randomized trial of concurrent chemoradiotherapy versus radiotherapy in advanced carcinoma of the uterine cervix. *Gynecol Oncol* 1997;66:52–58.

621. Tsukamoto N, Kaku T, Matsukuma K, et al. The problem of stage Ia (FIGO, 1985) carcinoma of the uterine cervix. *Gynecol Oncol* 1989;34:1–6.

622. Ulbright TM, Gersell DJ. Glassy cell carcinoma of the uterine cervix: a light and electron microscopic study of five cases. *Cancer* 1983;51:2255–2263.

623. Umesaki N, Fujii T, Nishimura R, et al. Plase II study of irinotecan combined with mitomycin-C for advanced or recurrent squamous cell carcinoma of the uterine cervix: the JGOG study. *Gynecol Oncol* 2004;95:127–132.

624. Uno T, Ito H, Itami J, et al. Postoperative radiation therapy for stage IB-IIB carcinoma of the cervix with poor prognostic factors. *Anticancer Res* 2000;20:2235–2239.

625. Upadhyay SK, Symonds RP, Haelterman M, et al. The treatment of stage IV carcinoma of cervix by radical dose radiotherapy. *Radiother Oncol* 1988;11:15–19.

626. van Bommel PFJ, Kenemans P, Helmerhorst TJM, et al. Expression of cytokeratin 10, 13, and involucrin as prognostic factors in low stage squamous cell carcinoma of the uterine cervix. *Cancer* 1994;74:2314–2320.

627. van der Heide UK, Ketelaars M, et al. Conventional, conformal, and intensity-modulated radiation therapy treatment planning of external radiotherapy for cervical cancer: the impact of tumor regression. *Int J Radiat Oncol Biol Phys* 2006;64:189–196.

628. van den Berg HA, Olofsen-van Acht MJ, van Santvoort JP, et al. Definition and validation of a reference target volume in early stage node-positive cervical carcinoma, based on lymphangiograms and CT-scans. *Radiother Oncol* 2000;54:163–179.

629. Van Nagell JR Jr, Powell DE, Gallion HH, et al. Small cell carcinoma of the uterine cervix. *Cancer* 1988;62:1586–1593.

630. VanDyke AH, Van Nagell JR Jr. The prognostic significance of ureteral obstruction in patients with recurrent carcinoma of the cervix uteri. *Surg Gynecol Obstet* 1975;141:371–373.

631. Varia MA, Bundy DN, Deppe G, et al. Cervical carcinoma metastatic to paraaortic nodes: extended field radiation therapy with concomitant 5-fluorouracil and cisplatin chemotherapy: a Gynecologic Oncology Group study. *Int J Radiat Oncol Biol Phys* 1998;42:1015–1023.

632. Vasanthan A, Mitsumori M, Park JH, et al. Regional hyperthermia combined with radiotherapy for uterine cancers: a multi-institutional prospective randomized trial of the international atomic energy agency. *Int J Radiat Oncol Biol Phys* 2005;61:145–153.

633. Vaupel P, Mayer A, Hockel M. Impact of hemoglobin levels on tumor oxygenation: the higher, the better? *Strahlenther Onkol* 2006;182:63–71.

634. Vernooij CB, Kruifwagen RF, Rodriqus P, et al. Hematometra after radiotherapy for cervical carcinoma. *Gynecol Oncol* 1997;67:325–327.

635. Verschraegen CF, Levy T, Kudelka AP, et al. Phase II study of irinotecan in prior chemotherapy-treated squamous cell carcinoma of the cervix. *J Clin Oncol* 1997;15:625.

636. Vieira SC, Silva BB, Pinto GA, et al. CD34 as a marker for evaluating angiogenesis in cervical cancer. *Pathol Res Pract* 2005;201:313–318.

637. Vijayakumar S, Roach M III, Wara W, et al. Effect of subcutaneous recombinant human erythropoietin in cancer patients receiving radiotherapy: preliminary results of a randomized, open-labeled, phase II trial. *Int J Radiat Oncol Biol Phys* 1993;26:721–729.

638. Viswanathan FR, Varghese C, Peedicayil A, et al. Hyperfractionation in carcinoma of the cervix: tumor control and late bowel complications. *Int J Radiat Oncol Biol Phys* 1999;45:653–656.

639. Volterrani F, Lombardi F. Long-term results of radium therapy in cervical cancer. *Int J Radiat Oncol Biol Phys* 1980;6:565–570.

640. Waldenstrom AC, Horvath G. Survival of patients with adenocarcinoma of the uterine cervix in Western Sweden. *Int J Gynecol Cancer* 1999;9:18–23.

641. Wang CJ, Leung SW, Chen HC, et al. High-dose rate intracavitary brachytherapy (HDR-IC) in treatment of cervical carcinoma: 5-year results and implication of increased s-w grade rectal complication on initiation of an HDR-IC fractionation scheme. *Int J Radiat Oncol Biol Phys* 1997;38:391–398.

642. Warmelink C, Ezzell G, Orton C. Use of a time-dose-fractionation model to design high-dose-rate fractionation schemes. In: Mould RF, ed. *Brachytherapy 2.* Leersum, the Netherlands: Nucletron International BV, 1989;41–48.

643. Watson ER, Halnan KE, Dische S, et al. Hyperbaric oxygen and radiotherapy: a Medical Research Council trial in carcinoma of the cervix. *Br J Radiol* 1978;51:879–887.

644. Webb JC, Key CR, Qualls CR, et al. Population-based study of microinvasive adenocarcinoma of the uterine cervix. *Obstet Gynecol* 2001;97:701–706.

645. Weiser EB, Bundy BN, Hoskins WJ, et al. Extraperitoneal versus transperitoneal selective paraaortic lymphadenectomy in the pretreatment surgical staging of advanced cervical carcinoma (a Gynecologic Oncology Group study). *Gynecol Oncol* 1989;33:283–289.

646. Weiss E, Richter S, Krauss T, et al. Conformal radiotherapy planning of cervic carcinoma: differences in the delineation of the clinical target volume. A comparison between gynaecologic and radiation oncologists. *Radiother Oncol* 2003;67:87–95.

647. Weiss JP, Mattei DM, Neville EC, et al. Primary treatment of radiation-induced hemorrhagic cystitis with hyperbaric oxygen: 10-year experience. *J Urol* 1994;151:1514–1517.

648. Weiss LK, Kau TY, Sparks BT, et al. Trends in cervical cancer incidence among young black and white women in metropolitan Detroit. *Cancer* 1994;73:1849–1854.

649. Werner-Wasik M, Schmid CH, Bornstein LE, et al. Increased risk of second malignant neoplasms outside radiation fields in patients with cervical carcinoma. *Cancer* 1995;75:2281–2285.

650. West CM, Davidson SE, Burt PA, et al. The intrinsic radiosensitivity of cervical carcinoma: correlations with clinical data. *Int J Radiat Oncol Biol Phys* 1995;31:841–846.

651. Wharton JT, Jones HW III, Day TG Jr, et al. Preirradiation celiotomy and extended field irradiation for invasive carcinoma of the cervix. *Obstet Gynecol* 1977;49:333–338.

652. Wheeler JA, Stephens LC, Tornos C, et al. ASTRO Research Fellowship: apoptosis as a predictor of tumor response to radiation in stage IB cervical carcinoma. *Int J Radiat Oncol Biol Phys* 1995;32:1487–1493.

653. Whitney CW, Sause W, Bundy BN, et al. Randomized comparison of fluorouracil plus cisplatin versus hydroxyurea as an adjunct to radiation therapy in stage IIB-IVA carcinoma of the cervix with negative paraaortic lymph nodes: a Gynecologic Oncology Group and Southwest Oncology Group study. *J Clin Oncol* 1999;17:1339–1348.

654. Whitney CW, Stehman FB. The abandoned radical hysterectomy: a Gynecologic Oncology Group study. *Gynecol Oncol* 2000;79:350–356.

655. Willett CG, Ooi C-J, Zietman AL, et al. Acute and late toxicity of patients with inflammatory bowel disease undergoing irradiation for abdominal and pelvic neoplasms. *Int J Radiat Oncol Biol Phys* 2000;46:995–998.

656. Williamson JF, Anderson LL, Grigsby PW, et al. American Endocurietherapy Society recommendations for specification of brachytherapy source strength. *Endocuriether Hypertherm Oncol* 1993;9:1–7.

657. Wolff JP, Lacour J, Chassagne D, et al. Cancer of the cervical stump: a study of 173 patients. *Obstet Gynecol* 1972;39:10–16.

658. Wolfson AH, Abdel-Wahab M, Markoe AM, et al. A quantitative assessment of standard vs. customized midline shield construction for invasive cervical carcinoma. *Int J Radiat Oncol Biol Phys* 1997;37:237–242.

659. Wollschlaeger K, Connell PP, Waggoner S, et al. Acute problems during low-dose-rate intracavitary brachytherapy for cervical carcinoma. *Gynecol Oncol* 2000;76:67–72.

660. Wolstenholme JL, Whynes DK. Stage specific treatment cost of care for cervical cancer in the United Kingdom. *Eur J Cancer* 1998;34:1889–1893.

661. Wong F, Bhimji S. The usefulness of ultrasonography in intracavitary radiotherapy using Selectron applications. *Int J Radiat Oncol Biol Phys* 1990;19:477–482.

662. Wong LC, Ngan HYS, Cheung ANY, et al. Chemoradiation and adjuvant chemotherapy in cervical cancer. *J Clin Oncol* 1999;17:2055–2060.

663. Wootipoom V, Lekhyananda N, Phungrassami T, et al. Prognostic significance of Bax, Bcl-2, and p53 expressions in cervical squamous cell carcinoma treated by radiotherapy. *Gynecol Oncol* 2004;94:636–642.

664. Wright J, Jones G, Whelan T, et al. Patient preference for high or low dose rate brachytherapy in carcinoma of the cervix. *Radiother Oncol* 1994;33:187–194.

665. Wright TC, Ellerbrock TV, Chiasson MA, et al. Cervical intraepithelial neoplasia in women infected with human immunodeficiency virus: prevalence, risk factors, and validity of Papanicolaou smears. *Obstet Gynecol* 1994;84:591–597.

666. Wun T, Law L, Harvey D, et al. Increased incidence of symptomatic venous thrombosis in patients with cervical carcinoma treated with concurrent chemotherapy, radiation and erythropoietin. *Cancer* 2003;98:1514–1520.

667. Yamazaki A, Shirato H, Nishioka T, et al. Reduction of late complications after irregularly shaped four-field whole pelvic radiotherapy using computed tomographic simulation compared with parallel-opposed whole pelvic radiotherapy. *Jpn J Clin Oncol* 2000;30:180–184.

668. Zhang J, Rose BR, Thompson CH, et al. Associations between oncogenic human papillomaviruses and local invasive patterns in cervical cancer. *Gynecol Oncol* 1995;57:170–177.

669. Zhang JM, Hashimoto M, Kawai K, et al. CD109 expression in squamous cell carcinoma of the uterine cervix. *Pathol Int* 2005;55:165–169.

670. Zola P, Volpe T, Castelli G, et al. Is the published literature a reliable guide for deciding between alternative treatments for patients with early cervical cancer? *Int J Radiat Oncol Biol Phys* 1989;16:785–797.

671. Zunino S, Rosato O, Lucino S, et al. Anatomic study of the pelvis in carcinoma of the uterine cervix as related to the box technique. *Int J Radiat Oncol Biol Phys* 1999;44:53–59.

Clinical Radiation Oncology

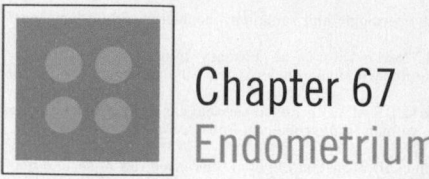

Chapter 67
Endometrium

Higinia R. Cardenes, Katherine Look, Helen Michael, Laura Cerezo

Anatomy

The uterus is a muscular organ located in the midplane of the true pelvis. It is divided into the body (corpus) and the cervix, separated by the isthmus. The superior portion of the corpus, the fundus, is pierced at each cornu by the fallopian tubes. The uterine surface is partially covered by peritoneum. The uterine cavity is lined by endometrium, made up of columnar cells forming many tubular glands; the wall of the uterus is composed of myometrium, consisting of smooth muscle fibers. The major supports of the uterus are the uterosacral and cardinal ligaments. Other nonsupporting attachments include broad and round ligaments. The major blood supply to the uterus is the uterine artery, which enters the uterus at the isthmus after it crosses over the ureter. The uterine lymphatic network components drain laterally along the parametrium into the paracervical lymph nodes, obturator nodes, and from there to the external iliac nodes and hypogastric nodes; subsequently, the pelvic lymphatics drain into the common iliac and periaortic lymph nodes. The lymphatics from the upper corpus and fundus pass through the infundibulopelvic and broad ligaments directly into the periaortic and upper abdominal lymph nodes. There are additional lymphatic channels that drain along the round ligaments to the femoral nodes.

Epidemiology and Risk Factors

Endometrial cancer (EC) is the most common gynecologic malignancy in the United States and will likely remain so, given current demographic trends of an aging population and increasing obesity. The National Cancer Institute's Surveillance, Epidemiology and End Results (SEER) Program estimated there would be 40,880 new cases of EC and 7,310 deaths in 2005 (91). In about 75% of the cases, the disease is confined to the uterus and cervix at the time of diagnosis, and uncorrected survival rates of ≥75% are expected (42).

EC is primarily a disease of postmenopausal women. The median age at diagnosis is 61 years. Approximately 25% of cases occur in premenopausal patients, including 5% that are diagnosed in patients younger than 40 years of age (102,190). Risk factors for EC include obesity, diabetes, early menarche and/or late menopause, unopposed estrogen therapy or tamoxifen, anovulatory cycles, and nulliparity (23). Among normal-weight premenopausal women with EC there is an increased incidence of infertility, irregular menstrual cycles, history of polycystic ovarian syndrome, and synchronous tumors of the endometrium and ovary (177).

Traditionally, EC has been divided into type I and type II categories characterized by distinct biologic and clinical behavior, with different causes (20). Type I carcinomas account for approximately 85% of all EC and are associated with a hyperestrogenic state and generally are low-grade, indolent tumors of endometrioid histology. In contrast, type II tumors are estrogen-independent and arise in the setting of uterine atrophy and generally consist of poorly differentiated, uterine papillary serous carcinoma (UPSC) or clear cell carcinoma (CCC) and malignant mixed müllerian tumor (MMMT). They represent approximately 15% of all ECs. Type II patients are more often multiparous, older, and less likely to be obese (184). Molecular genetic studies over the past decade have shown that the two tumor types evolve via distinct pathogenetic pathways (107).

Familial or genetical predisposition has been associated with increased risk of EC in the setting of the hereditary nonpolyposis colorectal cancer syndrome (HNPCC) or Lynch syndrome II. Germline mutations in mismatch repair genes (MLH1, MSH2 or MSH6) account for the majority of families with HNPCC. Women with this syndrome have a 40% to 60% lifetime risk of developing EC by age 70 and a similar risk for colon cancer (3).

Clinical Presentation and Natural History

Endometrial adenocarcinoma most commonly (75%) presents with postmenopausal vaginal bleeding or discharge, which should prompt endometrial sampling. The majority of cases (72%) will be diagnosed with stage I disease confined to the corpus, and these patients have excellent survival following surgery (44). More advanced disease may present with urinary or rectal bleeding, constipation, pain, lower extremity lymphedema, abdominal distension due to ascites, and cough and/or or hemoptysis (44). Patients with regional and distant metastases will have lower survival despite the use of modern multimodality therapy (91).

Malignant mesenchymal tumors of the uterus (carcinosarcomas or MMMT) commonly present in menopausal patients with vaginal bleeding, cramping, and a mass prolapsing through the cervix (90). Leiomyosarcomas are more commonly discovered incidentally in the pathologic specimen after simple hysterectomy for presumed uterine leiomyomata (18). Nodal metastases will be found in approximately 14% of carcinosarcomas at time of surgical staging but are rarely (<5%) seen in leiomyosarcoma unless there is obvious extrauterine disease (109,118). Lung metastases are frequently encountered in leiomyosarcoma patients. Any extrauterine extension from a uterine sarcoma portends poor survival (71).

There is no recognized screening program for the asymptomatic general population. However, screening has been recommended by the American Cancer Society for women who carry, or are related to carriers of, the HNPCC mutation, starting at age 35 (188).

Diagnostic Work-Up

Pathologic examination remains the gold standard by which the diagnosis of corpus cancer, whether glandular or mesenchymal type, is established. Endometrial tissue sampling can be easily performed in the office with a Pipelle or similar device (51). The occasional patient may have a stenotic os because of nulliparous status or prior cervical surgery and require dilatation and curettage under anesthesia in order to reach the endometrial cavity. Transvaginal ultrasonography may be useful to assess endometrial cavity thickness in those with bleeding but who are not amenable to office biopsy. If the thickness is <5 mm, the risk of EC is so minimal that endometrial sampling may be foregone in women with no further bleeding (187). Some surgeons have used hysteroscopy to effect the dilatation and curettage; however, there have been reports that the insufflation of the distending medium into the canal has been associated with an increase in positive peritoneal cytology, although the prognostic implications are unclear of such positive cytology "induced" by sampling (21). Even the most experienced pathologist may have difficulty differentiating between atypical hyperplasia and well-differentiated adenocarcinoma such that pathologic review may be very helpful before surgery or other therapy is undertaken (217).

Once the diagnosis of malignant disease is established, some have used radiologic imaging (e.g., sonography, computed tomography [CT] scan, magnetic resonance imaging [MRI]) and/or elevated serum CA 125 levels to predict which patients are most likely to deeply invasive or have extrauterine disease, and hence will benefit from extended surgical staging (ESS) (97,191). Kim et al. (97) reported that MRI yielded superior accuracy (89%), sensitivity (90%), and specificity (88%) regarding prediction of deep myometrial invasion when compared with transvaginal sonography or CT scans.

However, the International Federation of Gynecology and Obstetrics (FIGO) considers surgical staging (42); thus, preoperative imaging studies, in the absence of symptoms suspicious for extrauterine or metastatic disease, will add to the expense of the work-up, will not alter adjuvant therapy recommendations, and should *not* routinely be employed. Serum levels of CA 125 are elevated in most patients with advanced or metastatic EC. Preoperative levels >40 U/mL can be considered an indication for full pelvic and periaortic lymphadenectomy at the time of surgical staging, in the absence of metastatic disease (87). The experience of clinical application of positron emission tomography scan in EC has been very limited, although it seems to be useful in determining the extent of the regional disease or at the time of recurrence (86).

Pathologic Classification

The World Health Organization (WHO) classifies tumors of the uterine corpus as epithelial, mesenchymal, and mixed neoplasms (205). This chapter addresses both malignant tumors and lesions associated with endometrial malignancies (endometrial hyperplasia) and is written according to the 2003 WHO classification (205) (Table 67.1, A and B).

Endometrial Hyperplasia

Endometrial hyperplasia is an estrogen-dependent lesion that displays crowding and abnormal contours of endometrial glands lined by pseudostratified or stratified columnar epithelium with mitotic activity (102). Atypical hyperplasia refers to atypical nuclei in either simple or complex hyperplasia. Endometrial hyperplasia is associated with concomitant or subsequent endometrial adenocarcinoma, with the greatest risk associated with atypical hyperplasia.

Carcinoma of the Endometrium

Gross examination of the uterus removed for carcinoma may reveal a polypoid lesion protruding into the endometrium, generalized thickening of the endometrium, a lesion infiltrating the myometrium, or no abnormalities on gross examination (especially if most or all of the neoplasm was removed in a previous curettage).

Endometrioid Carcinoma

Eighty percent of ECs are endometrioid carcinomas. Endometrioid carcinomas are estrogen-dependent neoplasms. They are frequently associated with endometrial hyperplasia and they arise in association with unopposed estrogen stimulation of the endometrium. Endometrioid carcinomas of the endometrium (type I carcinoma) are often discovered at an early stage and have a better prognosis than the type II carcinomas, discussed later. Prolonged tamoxifen therapy is associated with endometrial carcinoma in some patients (89).

Typical endometrioid carcinoma (Fig. 67.1A) is composed of cribriform, racemose glands with varying amounts of a solid cellular component; there is usually no stroma between glands in carcinoma. These tumors are graded by the amount of glandular and solid areas present: grade 1 carcinomas have no more than 5% solid areas, grade 2 tumors have 6% to 50% solid areas, and grade 3 endometrioid carcinomas have >50% solid areas. High nuclear grade results in designation of one grade higher than it would be based on an architectural basis alone (227). Higher grade tumors tend to be more deeply invasive so that there is some correlation between grade and stage in many of these neoplasms.

Variants of endometrioid carcinoma in the recent WHO classification include endometrioid carcinoma with squamous differentiation, villoglandular endometrioid carcinoma, secretory carcinoma, and a ciliated cell variant (205). It is extremely important to distinguish villoglandular endometrioid carcinomas from the much more aggressive papillary serous carcinomas of the endometrium.

Nonendometrioid Carcinomas

Nonendometrioid carcinomas account for about 10% of endometrial carcinomas (37). Serous, clear cell, mucinous, and undifferentiated carcinomas are the most common types. Squamous, transitional cell, and other very rare tumor types also occur in the uterus (205). Serous and clear cell carcinomas represent type 2 tumors that are most often seen in older women with atrophic endometria.

Serous carcinoma accounts for 5% to 10% of all carcinomas of the endometrium (37). These neoplasms are not estrogen-dependent and they are not associated with endometrial hyperplasia. The endometrium associated with serous carcinoma is usually atrophic. Endometrial intraepithelial carcinoma may be a precursor lesion (8). Serous carcinomas are often associated with widespread lymphatic invasion even when they are superficial. They sometimes occur in polyps (136). Small fragments of these friable neoplasms may break off the main tumor and spread via the fallopian tube. Serous carcinoma of the endometrium is a highly aggressive neoplasm (78) that must be distinguished from villoglandular and poorly differentiated endometrioid carcinoma. Serous carcinoma (Fig. 67.1B) often has at least some papillary component, although it may be predominantly solid. Papillae may have fibrous stroma, but they display characteristic tufting of tumor cells without stroma. Nuclei are large with marked atypia. Mitoses are numerous. Psammoma bodies are seen in a minority of the cases. In contrast to villoglandular endometrioid carcinoma, the papillae and glandular spaces in serous carcinoma have irregular, uneven luminal borders caused by tufting of neoplastic cells and protrusion of large, atypical nuclei. Lymphatic invasion is usually widespread, and even occurs in the absence of myometrial invasion (220). All uterine serous tumors are considered high-grade neoplasms.

CCCs of the endometrium are uncommon neoplasms. They may display glandular, papillary, or solid patterns. Tumor cells usually have abundant clear cytoplasm, but oxyphilic cells can also be present. All CCCs of the endometrium are high-grade neoplasms. Although this type of tumor has a better prognosis

Table 67.1	PATHOLOGIC CLASSIFICATON OF ENDOMETRIAL CANCERS[a]

International Society of Gynecologic Pathologists (ISGP) and the World Health Organization (WHO) Classification of Uterine Tumors

Pathologic Subtypes	Incidence (%)
Endometrioid adenocarcinoma	75–80
Villoglandular	
Secretory adenocarcinoma	
Ciliated carcinoma	
Adenocarcinoma with squamous differentiation	
Uterine papillary serous	10
Clear cell carcinoma	4
Mucinous carcinoma	1
Squamous cell carcinoma	Rare
Transitional cell carcinoma	Rare
Mixed cell type	~10
Undifferentiated carcinoma	Rare
Metastatic Carcinoma to the Endometrium	Rare

Histopathology. Degree of differentiation: International Federation of Gynecology and Obstetrics and ISGP-WHO definitions

Histologic Grade	Definition
1: Well differentiated	≤5% of a nonsquamous or nonmorular solid growth pattern
2: Moderately differentiated	6%–50% of a nonsquamous or nonmorular solid growth pattern
3: Poorly differentiated	>50% of a nonsquamous or nonmorular solid growth pattern

[a]Notes on pathologic grading. Significant nuclear atypia, inappropriate for the architectural grade, raises the grade of 1 or 2 tumor by 1. Serous and clear cell carcinomas are all considered high-grade neoplasms. Adenocarcinomas with squamous differentiation are graded according to the glandular component only, without consideration of the squamous epithelium. Data derived from Silverberg S, Kurman R. *Tumors of the uterine corpus and gestational trophoblastic diseases.* Washington, DC: Armed Forces Institute of Pathology (ref. 180), and Tavassoli (ref. 205).

than serous carcinoma of the endometrium, CCC is the type of endometrial carcinoma most likely to recur outside the pelvis (4,119).

Mixed Cell Type Adenocarcinomas

Mixed adenocarcinomas of the endometrium have more than one type of carcinoma, with each type comprising at least 10% of the tumor. Some components, such as serous carcinoma, may adversely affect prognosis even when they represent a minority of the neoplasm.

Histologic and Molecular Features of Prognostic Significance

Studies performed by the Gynecologic Oncology Group (142) showed that the following histologic features of endometrial carcinoma have prognostic significance: tumor type, grade, depth of myometrial invasion, lymphovascular space invasion (LVSI), extension to the cervix (stromal invasion), and tumor extension outside the uterus (162). Endometrial carcinomas that are associated with endometrial hyperplasia tend to be lower grade tumors and therefore have a better prognosis than other

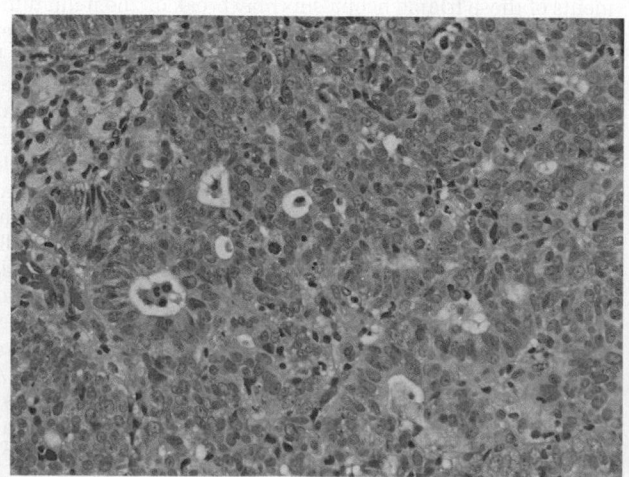
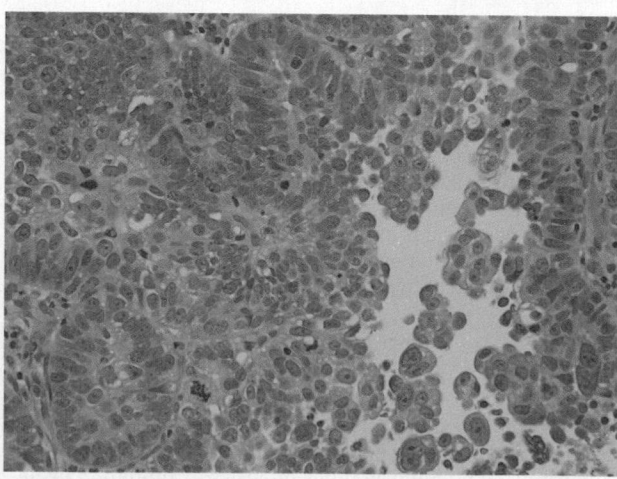

FIGURE 67.1. A: Endometrioid adenocarcinoma of the uterus. Cribriform glands and some solid areas are present. **B:** Serous carcinoma of the endometrium. Some papillary structures are present. Nuclei are very atypical.

carcinomas. The histologic subtype of endometrial carcinoma is an important prognostic factor. Histologic variants of endometrioid carcinoma (adenocarcinoma with squamous differentiation, villoglandular carcinoma, tumors with secretory or ciliated differentiation) have the same prognosis of other endometrioid carcinomas (162). Mucinous carcinomas of the endometrium are usually low-grade neoplasms with little myometrial invasion and they generally have a favorable prognosis. Serous, clear cell, and undifferentiated carcinomas of the endometrium are associated with a worse prognosis than endometrioid carcinoma. The presence of very small foci of serous carcinoma in endometrioid carcinomas is not clear, but any neoplasm with a 10% or greater serous component (37) should be placed in the mixed cell type category with the amount of serous carcinoma stated in the diagnosis.

There is evidence that endometrioid and serous carcinomas of the endometrium evolve by different pathways. Some endometrioid carcinomas are associated with microsatellite instability (30) in DNA mismatch repair genes. Microsatellite instability is associated with a better prognosis (134). In contrast to the microsatellite instability seen in endometrioid tumors, serous carcinomas display loss of heterozygosity on several chromosomes (215). In some cases, serous tumors may evolve from dedifferentiation of a poorly differentiated endometrioid carcinoma; those tumors show immunohistochemical and molecular features of both types of neoplasm (133).

Many well and moderately differentiated endometrioid carcinomas are diploid. The frequency of aneuploid type increases with the grade of tumor. Serous carcinomas are aneuploid (163). Aneuploid DNA content is an independent adverse prognostic factor and is associated with advanced stage, high-grade and serous histology, and higher probability of recurrence and death from EC (130,163,182,228). Most endometrioid carcinomas have a low Ki-67 proliferation index, in contrast to serous tumors (162). Serous carcinomas typically have p53 mutations, and accumulation of the abnormal p53 product can be demonstrated by immunostains (13). Endometrioid carcinomas do not usually display staining for p53 unless they are poorly differentiated or in the presence of extensive extrauterine disease; in these cases, p53 mutation confers significantly worse outcome (130,174,182). Mutations in K-ras and the tumor suppressor gene PTEN (28) occur in endometrioid neoplasms and β-catenin mutations may occur in less-aggressive neoplasms (173). Serous carcinomas also have lower frequencies of PTEN and K-ras mutations and less expression of bcl-2, E-cadherin, β-cadherin, and estrogen and progesterone receptors than do endometrioid carcinomas. In contrast to endometrioid neoplasms, serous carcinomas overexpressed C-myc, C-erbB-2 and Her2-neu (163,175). CCCs have a high Ki-67 index but, in contrast to serous carcinomas, they display low p53 immunostaining (106). Cyclooxygenase-2 expression in EC correlates with tumor aggressiveness and worse prognosis (63). Among the biochemical factors, expression of estrogen and progesterone receptors is associated with clinically less-aggressive behavior (62,183).

Uterine Sarcomas

Uterine sarcomas are much less frequent than endometrial carcinomas. The WHO classification includes endometrial stromal tumors, smooth muscle tumors, and miscellaneous mesenchymal tumors (205). Miscellaneous tumors are not included in this discussion because of their rarity. Tumor stage is the most important prognostic factor for all uterine sarcomas.

Endometrial stromal sarcomas are invasive tumors that have histologic features resembling normal proliferative-type endometrial stroma. These neoplasms invade the myometrium as serpiginous cords of tan-yellow tumor. Microscopically, they display small blood vessels reminiscent of those seen in the normal endometrium. Nuclei do not show marked atypia. The mi-

totic rate may vary, but it is usually low. In contrast, high-grade endometrial sarcomas do not resemble endometrial stroma. They contain pleomorphic, atypical nuclei, and numerous mitoses.

Leiomyosarcomas of the uterus are single myometrial masses that have a fleshy appearance, often with areas of necrosis. They are solitary lesions. They display nuclear atypia, high mitotic rates, and areas of coagulative tumor necrosis (17). All three of these histologic features should usually be present in order to diagnose a leiomyosarcoma.

Mixed Epithelial and Mesenchymal Tumors

Malignant tumors in this WHO category of uterine neoplasms include adenosarcomas and MMMTs (205). *Adenosarcomas* of the uterus have benign glands surrounded by malignant stroma. Neoplasms containing both malignant epithelium (carcinoma) and stroma (sarcoma) are called *malignant mixed müllerian tumors*. The MMMTs probably represent dedifferentiation of endometrial carcinoma that is most often the serous type (135). These neoplasms are often bulky, necrotic, and deeply invasive. Homologous tumors have stroma that contains cell types normally seen in the uterus, in contrast to heterologous tumors that may contain cartilage, bone, and striated muscle cells. Tumor metastases usually contain the epithelial component of the neoplasm. These are poorly differentiated, aggressive neoplasms. Disease stage is the most important prognostic factor.

Clinical and Pathologic Staging

Prior to 1988, patients with EC were clinically staged (Table 67.2), and many with apparent extrauterine disease or cervical

Table 67.2	ENDOMETRIAL CANCER CLINICAL STAGING SYSTEM: 1971 CLASSIFICATION OF INTERNATIONAL FEDERATION OF GYNECOLOGY AND OBSTETRICS
Stages/Grades	**Definition**
Stage 0	Atypical endometrial hyperplasia, carcinoma *in situ*. Histologic findings are suspicious of malignancy. Cases of stage 0 should not be included in any therapeutic statistics
Stage I	Tumor confined to the uterus
IA	Length of the uterine cavity ≤8 cm
IB	Length of the uterine cavity >8 cm
Histologic subtypes of adenocarcinoma	
Grade 1	Highly differentiated adenomatous carcinoma
Grade 2	Differentiated adenomatous carcinoma with partly solid areas
Grade 3	Predominantly solid or entirely undifferentiated carcinoma
Stage II	Extension to the cervix but not beyond the uterus
Stage III	Extension outside of the uterus/cervix but not outside of the true pelvis
Stage IVA	Extension outside of the true pelvis or involvement of the bladder and/or rectum Tumor invades bladder and/or bowel mucosa
Stage IVB	Distant metastasis including intra-abdominal and/or inguinal lymph nodes

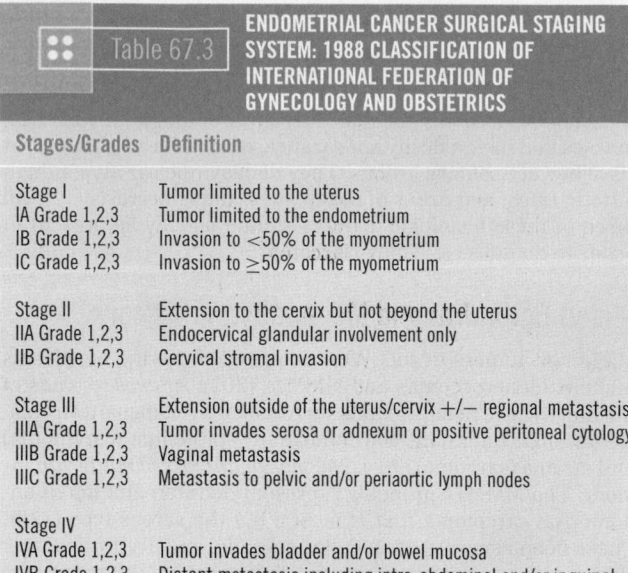

Table 67.3 ENDOMETRIAL CANCER SURGICAL STAGING SYSTEM: 1988 CLASSIFICATION OF INTERNATIONAL FEDERATION OF GYNECOLOGY AND OBSTETRICS

Stages/Grades	Definition
Stage I	Tumor limited to the uterus
IA Grade 1,2,3	Tumor limited to the endometrium
IB Grade 1,2,3	Invasion to <50% of the myometrium
IC Grade 1,2,3	Invasion to ≥50% of the myometrium
Stage II	Extension to the cervix but not beyond the uterus
IIA Grade 1,2,3	Endocervical glandular involvement only
IIB Grade 1,2,3	Cervical stromal invasion
Stage III	Extension outside of the uterus/cervix +/− regional metastasis
IIIA Grade 1,2,3	Tumor invades serosa or adnexum or positive peritoneal cytology
IIIB Grade 1,2,3	Vaginal metastasis
IIIC Grade 1,2,3	Metastasis to pelvic and/or periaortic lymph nodes
Stage IV	
IVA Grade 1,2,3	Tumor invades bladder and/or bowel mucosa
IVB Grade 1,2,3	Distant metastasis including intra-abdominal and/or inguinal lymph nodes

extension received radiation prior to hysterectomy and removal of the adnexum (26). Data from the Gynecologic Oncology Group surgical staging study made apparent deficiencies in the accuracy of clinical staging in that approximately 23% of the patients being upstaged after complete surgical staging (43). Pelvic node metastases were found in <3% of patients with grade 1 endometrium-confined disease, but in >30% when grade 3 disease penetrated the outer-third of the myometrium (43). Aortic nodal disease, although rare in grade 1 disease or in the absence of pelvic node metastasis, was seen in 14% and 23% of patients with deeply invasive grade 2 or 3 disease, respectively (43). Hence, FIGO promoted adoption of surgical staging for corpus carcinoma (Table 67.3) in order to better estimate 5-year prognoses for patients and to better tailor adjuvant therapy to those patients most likely to benefit from it (42).

Although many embraced the FIGO endorsed surgical staging as standard, there has not been universal adoption of routine surgical staging. Morrow et al. (142) reported that of 895 surgically staged patients, only 48 were found to have positive para-aortic nodes and 47/48 had either suspicious para-aortic nodes, grossly positive pelvic nodes, involved adnexa, or deep myometrial invasion. It was concluded that, "it is logical to limit the surgical evaluation of aortic nodes to those patients with suspicious aortic nodes on palpation or high risk factors such as grossly positive pelvic nodes, gross adnexal masses or outer-third myometrial invasion" (142). Such high-risk factors were seen in only 25% of patients, but accounted for 98% of those with positive para-aortic nodes (142). Despite the controversy as to the utility of *routine* surgical staging, the Society of Gynecologic Oncology, in collaboration with the American College of Obstetricians and Gynecologists, indicated that the standard of care should be comprehensive surgical staging in all patients when feasible (1).

According to GOG, ESS for endometrioid corpus carcinoma should include the following: excision or biopsy of any enlarged or suspicious pelvic or para-aortic nodes; in the absence of enlarged nodes, nodal tissues should be removed from over the distal vena cava below the inferior mesentery artery, between the aorta and the left ureter from the inferior mesentery artery to midleft common iliac artery, distal half of each common iliac artery, the anterior and medial aspect of proximal half of external iliac artery and vein, the distal half of the obturator fat pad anterior to the obturator nerve (221). In addition, generous omental sampling is indicated in those with papillary serous

or clear cell histology because such cell types have a known propensity to for upper abdominal spread (70).

Prognostic Factors

Pathologic stage is the most significant predictor of outcome (43). Pelvic and/or para-aortic node metastases influence patterns of recurrences and adversely impact recurrence-free and overall survival. In the absence of nodal metastases, the following histopathologic factors adversely impact local control and overall survival: cell type, grade, depth of invasion, and LVSI (142,162). Patient age has been found to be an important prognostic factor in multiple trials (2,45,95).

Nodal metastases are more commonly seen in patients with high-grade, atypical cell type, deeply invasive, cervical stroma invasion, positive LVSI, and older age (43,142). Deep myometrial invasion has been found to be the strongest predictor of hematogenous recurrence, whereas cervical stromal invasion and positive nodes are associated with lymphatic recurrence (128). Stage IV or stage I-III with at least two risk factors (i.e., cervical stroma invasion, positive peritoneal cytology, positive nodes, nonendometrioid histologies) were the strongest predictors for peritoneal recurrence (125).

The presence of LVSI has been extensively recognized as an unfavorable prognostic factor for recurrence and risk of nodal metastasis (22,95,123–125,142), and its presence, primarily in patients with deep myometrial invasion, independently of the grade, is associated with a significantly increased risk for pelvic nodal metastasis, indicating the need for adjuvant pelvic irradiation or lymphadenectomy in this group (38).

General Management: Results of Therapy in Endometrial Cancer

Surgery

The two current therapeutic paradigms in the surgical management of EC are (a) total abdominal hysterectomy and bilateral salpingo-oophorectomy (TAH-BSO), without lymph node dissection followed by a more liberal use of postoperative radiotherapy (RT) based on uterine histopathologic parameters, and (b) routine ESS followed by a more restricted use of postoperative RT. Proponents of ESS emphasize that it can be accomplished with acceptable morbidity, facilitates more accurate identification of disease extent, may be therapeutic even in those without nodal metastases, and can be cost-saving in that adjuvant therapy is limited to patients who are expected to benefit (16,40,82,96,126,156,196).

Although most of the experienced gynecologic oncologists have reported acceptable morbidity outcomes following ESS (58,82,105,156), others noted increased risks of vascular injuries, deep vein thromboses, and pulmonary emboli (36,68). The risk of postoperative complications may be somewhat higher in the elderly, frequently obese EC population, with the common antecedent comorbid medical conditions of hypertension, diabetes mellitus, coronary artery disease, and chronic obstructive pulmonary disease. Lymphocysts are uncommon (<2%) after ESS (156). ESS followed by radiation is accompanied by a higher rate of chronic enteric morbidity, necessitating surgical correction, when compared with the rate seen following simple hysterectomy and pelvic RT (110).

Originally, ESS was accomplished via open laparotomy via midline incision (43). It can be achieved in the obese, and in some morbidly obese patients by experienced gynecologic oncologists (58,157). Panniculectomy may improve access to the para-aortic nodes in morbidly obese patients, although it remains unclear as to whether improved para-aortic nodes yield improved 5-year survival (224). Subsequently, laparoscopy innovations have allowed many committed gynecologic oncologists to achieve excellent node yields and comprehensive staging with less morbidity and shorter duration of hospitalization (56,179).

Some patients are not candidates for ESS because of body habitus and/or significant comorbidities; they may have short-term quality of life issues and may be adequately treated with a vaginal hysterectomy and achieve reasonable 10-year disease-specific survival rates of 83% if the disease is confined to the corpus (197). On the other hand, not all oncologists have been convinced of the value-added utility of ESS (14,103). Excellent results have been achieved for an intermediate-risk group of EC patients by the Post Operative Radiation Therapy in Endometrial Carcinoma (PORTEC) investigators without ESS (45). Preliminary results from the ASTEC study, which randomized more than 1,400 patients to routine node sampling versus biopsy/debulking of suspicious node only, has failed to show a 3-year survival difference, with 88% and 89% observed in those with and without routine node sampling, respectively (167). Mature results from a study in endometrial carcinoma (ASTEC) trial are pending.

Improvements in median disease-free survival have been achieved in patients with advanced stage III and IV disease after maximal surgical cytoreduction efforts to achieve optimal debulking (24,35,104). In those with stage IIIC disease, complete resection of clinically involved nodes with no evidence of gross residual disease increased median survival from 8.8 to 37.5 months (24).

Adjuvant Therapy—Radiation Therapy

In order to minimize morbidity, it is imperative to tailor adjuvant RT to sites at significant risk for recurrence based on nodal status or, in the absence of nodal information, on the histopathologic factors found in the uterine specimen (137,142) (Table 67.4) shows the proposed classification of risk groups in EC.

Early Stage (FIGO I-II)

External-Beam Irradiation: Randomized Trials
Three randomized clinical trials, only one of which included surgical staging, have reported improved locoregional tumor control and progression-free survival (PFS) with the addition of postoperative external-beam radiotherapy (EBRT) in patients with intermediate-risk EC. However, none of them were able to document an improvement in overall survival (2,45,95). Table 67.5 shows eligibility criteria, randomization, and a comparison of outcomes for each trial.

A *subset* analysis of the trial by Aalders et al. (2) showed a cause-specific survival advantage with the addition of pelvic RT in the group of patients with stage IC or grade 3 disease. In the PORTEC trial, a *subset* analysis defined a group of patients at intermediate to high risk (>15%) of recurrence when at least two of the three following major risk factors present: age 60 or greater, deep (outer, 50%) myometrial invasion if grade 1–2, or superficially invasive grade 3 histology. Adjuvant pelvic RT given to this intermediate- to high-risk group lessened local relapse from 21.7% to 7.5% (178).

The GOG 99 trial *subset* analysis defined the "high-intermediate-risk" subgroup as those patients with grade 2–3 tumors, presence of LVSI, and deep myometrial involvement (95). Patients younger than 50 years with all three risk factors, or older than 50 but younger than 70 with two factors, or those older than 70 with any one of the risk factors, were most likely to benefit from EBRT. The 4-year cumulative locoregional recurrence rates were 13% in the RT arm and 27% in the observation arm, respectively (95).

In the PORTEC and GOG trials, the majority (approximately 70%) of the first site recurrences in the observation arm were in the vagina. The success of salvage therapy for vaginal relapses in the PORTEC study was 49% overall, with 61% achieving durable *local* tumor control (46).

Neither the PORTEC nor the GOG trial demonstrated an overall survival benefit with adjuvant pelvic RT. In the PORTEC trial, 8-year actuarial survivals were 71% for the RT and 77% for the no further therapy arms, respectively (46). In the GOG 99 trial (95), the estimated 4-year survival was 92% in the RT arm and 86% in the observation arm, respectively. The high-intermediate risk group accounted for nearly two thirds of the recurrences and cancer-related deaths. It has been postulated that the lack of survival benefit potentially could be to the result of the insufficient number of high-risk patients accrued and, therefore, lack of power to detect such a difference. A recently reported population analysis including >21,000 patients (approximately one third had nodal sampling), of which almost 20% received adjuvant RT (90% EBRT with or without brachytherapy; 10% brachytherapy alone), demonstrated improved survival in patients with stage IC disease, any grade, with the use of adjuvant RT (108).

A higher incidence of treatment-related complications was reported in those who received EBRT: 25% compared with 6% in the control group in the PORTEC trial, mostly grade 1–2 (68%) gastrointestinal and genitourinary toxicity, and 2% grade 3–4 (45). Similar results were reported in the GOG-99 trial (95), with a 3% grade 3–4 gastrointestinal toxicity in the pelvic RT arm. Of note, surgical staging did change the toxicity profile in the GOG study; patients in both the surgery and RT arms were noted to have lymphatic complications (primarily chronic

Table 67.4	**RISK GROUPS IN ENDOMETRIAL CANCER**		
Low Risk	**Intermediate-Low Risk**	**Intermediate-High Risk**	**High Risk**
Stage IA, Grade 1-2 Stage IB, Grade 1	Stage IA, grade 3 Stage IB, grade 2 Stage IIA, grade 1-2, <50% MI	Stage IB, grade 3 Stage IIA, grade 3, <50% MI Stage IC, grade 1-2 Stage IIA, grade 1-2, ≥50% MI +/-+LVSI 1/3 above w/ age ≥70 2/3 above w/ age <50–69 3/3 above w/age <50	Stage IC, grade 3 Stage IIA, grade 3, ≤50% MI Stage IIB, any grade UPSC CCC Stage III-IV

MI, myometrial invasion; LVSI, lymphovascular space invasion; UPSC, uterine papillary serous carcinoma; CCC, clear cell carcinoma.

	Aalders et al. (2) N = 540	PORTEC All patients[a] N = 714 5-year Actuarial	PORTEC HR[a] ∅	GOG-99 All Patients[b] N = 392 4-Year Cumulative	GOG 99 HR[b] δ	GOG 99 LR
Eligibility	cSt I	cSt I, G1, ≥50% MI G2, any MI G3, <50% MI	—	cSt IB-II (occult)	—	—
LRR—RT	1.9%	4%	5%	2%	5%	0%
LRR—no RT	6.9%	14%	18%	7%	13%	5%
DM—RT	9.9%	8%	6%	5%	10%	2%
DM—no RT	5.4%	7%	5%	8%	19%	3%
Any—RT	—	9.4%		6%	13%	2%
Any—no RT		17.2%		13%	27%	6%
EC Death—RT	—	9%	—	8%	12%	6%
EC Death—no RT		6%		14%	26%	8%
Survival	5-year	5-year	—	4-year		
RT	89%	81%		92%		
NFT	91%	85%		86%		
LRC	σ[c]	σ	—	σ	—	—
RT	98%	96%		97%		
NFT	93%	86%		88%		

PORTEC, Post Operative Radiation Therapy in Endometrial Carcinoma group; HR, high-Intermediate risk group; GOG, Gynecologic Oncology Group; LR, low risk group; cSt, cancer stage; MI, myometrial invasion; LRR, locoregional recurrence; RT, radiation therapy; DM, distant metastasis; EC, endometrial cancer; LRC, locoregional control.
[a]PORTEC: Vaginal recurrences, 73% of LRR in the observation arm. HR (∅) defined as ≥60 years old, deeply invasive (≥50% MI) grade 1-2 or superficially invasive (<50% MI) grade 3.
[b]GOG-99: Vaginal recurrences, 72% of LRR in the observation arm. HR (δ) defined as those with grade 2-3 tumors, presence of lymphovascular space invasion, and deep myometrial involvement; patients younger than 50 years old with the three risk factors, older than 50 years with two factors, or older than 70 years with any of those risk factors.
[c]σ, Statistically significant.

lymphedema, occurring in 2.5% of the control patients and 5% of the RT patients) (95). This complication was not noted in patients from the PORTEC study, in which lymph node dissection was not done.

Given the results from the randomized trials, it seems prudent to limit the use of postoperative pelvic RT to those patients with sufficiently high risk of locoregional recurrence (>15%). As 70% to 75% of the local recurrences in both randomized trials were vaginal, the PORTEC-2 investigators initiated a trial comparing vaginal brachytherapy with EBRT radiotherapy.

Although ESS was not employed in the PORTEC trial (45), the subset of stage IC grade 3 identified in a subsequent reanalysis of the PORTEC found as high a distant metastatic rate as 31% and only 58% overall survival after pelvic RT (47). It is speculated that having had ESS, this group would have been expected to have at least 30% risk of positive nodes and, as such, might have been expected to benefit from more aggressive adjuvant therapy than pelvic RT alone.

Intracavitary Vaginal Brachytherapy (IVB) Alone

The use of adjuvant IVB alone for patients with low and intermediate risk has yielded survival and low (≤4%) recurrence rates in vagina or pelvis whether or not ESS was done (Tables 67.6, A and B) (7,9,31,32,57,60,85,99,117,149,150,158,170,219). In addition, IVB has been shown to be cost-effective (61,85,158).

Risk Groups in Early-Stage Endometrial Cancer: Treatment Recommendations

Table 67.7 presents a synopsis of the treatment recommendations for all risk groups of patients with early EAC, with or without ESS.

Low-Risk Group

Patients with *stage IA disease, grade 1–2*, and *stage IB, grade 1*, without evidence of LVSI, have such a low risk of nodal metastases and recurrence that excellent results have been achieved with TAH BSO alone (43,126,142). In the presence of LVSI, IVB should be considered (129).

Intermediate-Low Risk Group

1. Stage IA, grade 3, represents a small group of patients for whom the incidence of pelvic nodal metastasis is low (3% in GOG-33) (43).
   (a) *ESS done:* IVB alone may be appropriate, given the higher incidence of vaginal relapses in patients with grade 3 disease (129). Of note, patients with stage IA disease were not included in the GOG-99 trial, the only one requiring surgical staging (95).
   (b) *ESS not done:* Pelvic EBRT should be considered, particularly in patients older than 60 years (2,45) with evidence of LVSI, as this represents an intermediate- to high-risk group. IVB alone versus observation should be discussed with younger patients (46). IVB is favored by the authors in the presence of LVSI.
2. Stage IB, grade 2, and Stage IIA (with <50% myometrial invasion), grade 1–2.
   (a) *ESS done*: In the absence of LVSI, patients could be offered IVB alone (mainly in older patients) versus observation (younger patients) (196). Patients older than 70 with LVSI are considered a high-risk group (95); therefore, EBRT is recommended, although IVB is an option (7).
   (b) *ESS not done:* The risk of nodal metastasis was found to be 6% in GOG-33 (43). IVB could be recommended in younger patients, mainly if LVSI is present (7,45,129). EBRT versus IVB alone should be considered primarily in patients >60 years old (46).

Table 67.6 USE OF INTRACAVITARY VAGINAL BRACHYTHERAPY ALONE

Evidence To Support Intracavitary Vaginal Brachytherapy (IVB) Alone in Incompletely Staged Patients

Study	No. of Patients	Pathologic Stage	Type of Adjuvant RT	Recurrence Rate (%)	Survival (%)
Sorbe & Smeds, 1990 (193)	404	93%, St I, G1-2 90% <1/3 MI	100% IVRT	3.7 overall 1.7 pelvis + vagina 0.7 vagina only	92 5-y OS
Kucera et al. 1990 (99)	376	348 pts St I, G1-3, ≤1/3 MI 28 pts St I, G1, 2/3 ≤MI>1/3	100% IVRT	0.8 overall 0.2 vagina only 0.6 pelvis + distant mets	91 OS 100 5-y OS
Eltabbakh et al., 1997 (57)	332	303 St I, G1-2, ≤50% MI, neg. peritoneal cytology 29 pts: positive peritoneal cytology	100% IVRT If peritoneal cytology: IVRT + Megace	2 overall 0.06 in pelvis 0 in vagina	99 5-y DFS
MacLeod et al., 1998 (117)	143	St I-IIA	100% IVRT	1.4 vagina 0.7 pelvis	98–100 5-y RFS 86–100 5-y OS
Weiss et al., 1998 (219)[a]	122	78 pts St IB, G1-2 44 pts St IC or G3	100% IVRT	3.8 20.5	94 5-y RFS 74 5-y RFS
Petereit et al., 1999 (158)	191	St I A-B, G1-2	100% IVRT	0.5 pelvis 1 upper abdomen	95 5-y OS 98 5-y DFS
Alektiar et al., 2005 (7)	382	St IB, G1-3 St IIB, G1-2 20% had surgical staging	100% IVRT	2 vaginal, 3% pelvis, 3 distant 5-y vaginal control 98 5-y pelvic control 95 St IBG3-IIB no CSS pelvic control 86 vs. 97 if CSS	93 5-y DFS 93 5y OS

IVRT, intravaginal brachytherapy; RT, external-beam radiation therapy; St, stage; G, grade; MI, myometrial invasion; OS, overall survival; pts, patients; mets, metastases; DFS, disease-free survival; RFS, relapse-free survival; SS, surgical staging.

Evidence To Support Intracavitary Vaginal Brachytherapy Alone in Completely Staged Patients

Study	No. of Patients	Pathologic Stage	Type of Adjuvant RT	Recurrence Rate (%)	Survival (%)
Berclaz et al., 1999 (19)	56	St I-II 19 pts, ≥50% MI, peritoneal cytology or G3	100% IVRT	0.02 pelvic or vaginal	—
Chadha et al., 1999 (32)	38	St IB, G3 St IC, any grade	100% IVRT	0 pelvic or vagina 8 upper abdomen	87 5-y DFS 93 5-y OS
Ng et al., 2000 (149)	77	St IB, G3 Any St IC	100% IVRT	14 overall 9 vagina, (6 were distal 2/3) 1 pelvis	82 5-y DFS 94 5-y OS
Anderson et al., 2000 (9)	102	St IB-C, any grade	100% IVRT	0.2 pelvis 0.15 vagina	93 5-y DFS 84 5-y OS
Fanning, 2001 (60)	66	St I G3, IC and II	100% IVRT	3 distant mets 0 pelvic or vaginal recurrences	97 5-y PFS 84 5-y OS
Ng et al., 2001 (150)	15	St II (occult)	100% IVRT	0	
Touboul, 2001 (214)	196	St IA, G3 St IB, IC, II	100% IVRT	4 overall 2 in vagina or pelvis	86 10-y DFS
Horowitz et al., 2002 (85)	164	St IB-II	100% IVRT	8.5 overall 1.2 vagina, 0.6 pelvis, 6 distant	90 5-y DFS 87 5-y OS
Rittenberg et al., 2003 (170)	53	St IC	100% IVRT	5.7 overall 0 vagina 1.9 pelvis 3.8 distant	91 5-y OS
Jolly et al., 2005 (93)	50	St I-II (occult), G1-3	100% IVRT	4 overall 2 vagina, 2 vagina + pelvis, 0 distant	97 5-y DFS 97 5-y OS
Solhjem et al., 2005 (189)	100	St IA-C, G1-3	100% IVRT	0 vaginal or pelvic 3 distant	93 3-y DFS 98,3-y OS

See footnote to part A. Also, PFS, progress-free survival.
[a]The Weiss series had 20% recurrence risk when IVB alone was used for those with grade 3 IC disease.

| | TABLE 67.7 | TREATMENT RECOMMENDATIONS FOR RISK GROUPS IN EARLY EAC WITH OR WITHOUT EXTENSIVE SURGICAL STAGING (ESS): LOW-RISK; INTERMEDIATE LOW-RISK; INTERMEDIATE HIGH-RISK; HIGH-RISK GROUPS[a] | | | |

Pathologic Stage	Age <60 years LVSI (−)	Age <60 years LVSI (+)	Age ≥60 years LVSI (−)	Age ≥60 years LVSI (+)
Stage IA, Grade 1-2 / Stage IB, Grade 1 / ESS done	NFT	NFT or IVB	NFT	IVB or NFT
Stage IA, Grade 1-2 / Stage IB, Grade 1 / ESS not done	NFT	NFT or IVB	NFT	IVB
Stage IA, Grade 3 / ESS done	NFT or IVB	IVB	IVB	IVB
Stage IA, Grade 3 / ESS not done	IVB	IVB	IVB or EBRT	IVB or EBRT (***)
Stage IB, Grade 2 / Stage IIA (<50% MI), Grade 1-2 / ESS done	NFT or IVB	IVB or NFT	IVB	IVB or EBRT
Stage IB, Grade 2 / Stage IIA (<50% MI), Grade 1-2 / ESS not done	IVB (IIA) NFT (IB)	IVB	IVB	IVB or EBRT
Stage IB, Grade 3 / Stage IIA (<50% MI), Grade 3 / ESS done	IVB	IVB	IVB or EBRT	EBRT
Stage IB, Grade 3 / Stage IIA (<50% MI), Grade 3 / ESS not done	IVB or EBRT	EBRT or IVB	EBRT	EBRT +/−
Stage IC, Grade 1-2 / Stage IIA (<50% MI), Grade 1-2 / ESS done	IVB	IVB or EBRT	EBRT	EBRT+/−IVB
Stage IC, Grade 1-2 / Stage IIA (<50% MI), Grade 1-2 / ESS not done	EBRT or IVB	EBRT	EBRT+/−IVB boost	EBRT+/−IVB
Stage IC, Grade 3 / Stage IIA (<50% MI), Grade 3 / ESS done	EBRT or IVB	EBRT	EBRT+/−IVB boost	EBRT+/−IVB boostIVB
Stage IC, Grade 3 / Stage IIA (<50% MI), Grade 3 / ESS not done	EBRT or IVB	EBRT+/−IVB boost	EBRT+/−IVB boost	EBRT+/−IVB boost
Stage IIB		EBRT+/−IVB boost		

LVSI, lymphovascular space invasion; ESS, extensive surgical staging; NFT, no further therapy; IVB, intracavitary vaginal brachytherapy; EBRT, external-beam radiation therapy; MI, myometrial invasion.

[a]Note: When there were two possible treatment options, the one sited first represents the authors' preference.

(***): High-risk group as per the Post Operative Radiation Therapy in Endometrial Carcinoma (PORTEC) trial (45).

Intermediate-High Risk Group

1. Stage IB, grade 3.
   (a) *ESS done:* Vaginal brachytherapy alone is recommended as these patients seem to be at similar risk of local and distant failures (7,95,196), primarily in the presence of LVSI (129). Patients age 60 and older, with evidence of LVSI, should be presented the option of EBRT versus IVB (95).
   (b) *ESS not done*: In patients with negative LVSI, given the incidence of positive pelvic nodes (10% to 15%%) (43), pelvic EBRT should be recommended, mainly in patients age 60 or older (2,7,45). In younger patients, IVB alone may suffice (46). In patients with positive LVSI, pelvic EBRT with or without IVB boost is recommended (121,126,129,130).
2. Stage IC and IIA (≥50% myometrial invasion), grade 1–2. Patients with deep myometrial invasion have >15% risk of positive pelvic nodes (43) and a recurrence rate of 15% to 20% (142).
   (a) *ESS done:* Patients with stage IC, grade 1–2 disease, without LVSI, can be treated with IVB alone (7,31,32,85,95).

Patients with LVSI, independently of the age, and grade 1–2 disease, should be considered for EBRT with or without IVB boost (95) versus IVB alone in the presence of comorbidities
   (b) *ESS not done:* EBRT is recommended in patients with stage IC, grade 1–2 disease, and who are older than 60 (2,45,46,196). Younger patients, with grade 1–2 disease, mainly in the presence of LVSI, should be offered at least IVB (45–47,129), although EBRT should be discussed with the patient as well.

Investigations continue as to the preferred adjuvant radiation modality for the intermediate- and high-risk group patients. The PORTEC-2 trial randomizes patients after TAH-BSO without ESS, stage IB grade 3, stage IC grades 1-2, age 60 or over, and stage IIA, grades 1-2 or grade 3 (<50% myometrial invasion), any age, to receive pelvic EBRT versus vaginal brachytherapy alone. The National Cancer Institute of Canada trial randomizes patients after TAH-BSO, without requiring ESS, with grade 3, any depth of myometrial invasion, and grade 2 lesions with >50% myometrial invasion to RT (EBRT with or without brachytherapy) versus observation. Similarly, the Medical Research Council Trial, ASTEC trial, is evaluating the role of ESS and adjuvant RT in patients with stage IC-IIA or grade 3 disease, including UPSC and CCC histologies.

High-Risk Group

Patients with *stage IC, grade 3* disease have been included in the high-risk groups and should receive EBRT with or without IVB boost (2,45,47). Unfortunately, these patients are at high risk of locoregional recurrence, distant failures, and death even after pelvic EBRT (47,128); therefore, new strategies are needed to improve outcome in this group, such as combined modality approach with systemic chemotherapy and volume-directed EBRT.

Stage IIA (>50% myometrial invasion), grade 3 disease and *stage IIB* disease, any grade, should be offered EBRT in addition to vaginal brachytherapy. Unfortunately, these groups (grade 3 and stage IIB, any grade) represented <10% of patients included in GOG-99. These patients may benefit from EBRT with or without vaginal brachytherapy, primarily in younger patients with evidence of LVSI.

Patients with unfavorable histologies, UPSC and CCC, are at high risk for recurrence and require adjuvant therapy, which will be discussed later in the chapter.

Advanced Stage (FIGO III-IV)

Patients with advanced EC represent a very heterogeneous group, with survival rates ranging from about 10% for patients with stage IVB to >90% for those patients with stage IIIA, with positive cytology only (122,127,165). Other favorable stage III subsets with relatively good prognosis include those patients with isolated adnexal involvement (39) or only positive pelvic nodes with pathologically confirmed negative paraaortic (periaortic) nodes (122,127,138,148). Such favorable subset patients do generally well with adjuvant pelvic RT or EFRT, with survival rates between 65% and 85%. However, patients with positive para-aortic nodes, gross residual disease, serosal involvement, or multiple sites of extrauterine disease have an unfavorable outcome, with survival rates of 40% or lower (11,122,127,128, 144,165).

Patients with advanced EC have been treated with different approaches in the adjuvant setting, including pelvic RT, extended fields RT (pelvic plus periaortic RT), whole abdominal irradiation (WAI), and chemotherapy (52,132,199,200). WAI has been used in the past for the adjuvant treatment of advanced EC, pathologic stages III-IVA, as well as all stages with unfavorable histologies such as UPSC and CCC with somewhat favorable results (52,132,199,200). However, WAI has fallen from favor given the unacceptable risk of high intra-abdominal failures (199) and the results of GOG-122, which demonstrated superior PFS and overall survival for patients treated with doxorubicin and cisplatin (166).

Randomized Trials in Advanced Stage (FIGO III-IV)

GOG-122 randomized 396 eligible patients with stage III-IV disease (without evidence of distant metastasis) after surgical staging and optimal surgical debulking to <2 cm residual, to receive WAI versus adjuvant doxorubicin and cisplatin (AP) (166). Nearly 25% of the patients in GOG-122 had high-risk papillary serous or clear cell histologies. The 5-year PFS and overall survival were 42% and 53%, respectively, in the AP arm compared with 38% and 42%, respectively, in the WAI arm. Unfortunately, the recurrence rates were quite high in both groups, 54% in the WAI and 50% in the AP arms, and the grade 3-4 toxicity (particularly hematologic, gastrointestinal, cardiac, and neurologic) were significantly more common in the AP arm (166).

GOG-184, investigating volume-directed RT given to all patients, followed by randomization to one of two cytotoxic regimens either doxorubicin, cisplatin, or the same with the addition of paclitaxel. The trial completed accrual in September 2004 and data analysis is pending.

Adjuvant Systemic Therapy

Chemotherapy with or without Radiotherapy

The GOG conducted a randomized trial on the role of adjuvant doxorubicin at 60 mg/m^2 versus no further therapy following surgical staging and RT for patients who were found to have >50% myometrial invasion, cervical involvement, pelvic or periaortic positive nodes, or adnexal metastasis. No difference was found in terms of disease-free survival, overall survival, or patterns of failure between the two arms; however the study was likely underpowered (141).

The RTOG conducted a phase I clinical trial investigating the role of adjuvant RT concurrently with cisplatin (days 1 and 28) followed by four cycles of cisplatin and Taxol. Sixty-six percent of the patients had stage III disease confined to the pelvis; 34% were high-risk stage I patients with grade 2–3 tumors with >50% myometrial invasion or stage IIB disease. The toxicity profile was acceptable; the low 5% locoregional recurrence rate and the 2-year overall and disease-free survival of 90% and 83%, respectively, makes the strategy attractive (74). However, at present, adjuvant cytotoxic therapy cannot be recommended for completely resected early-stage disease outside a clinical trial.

The GOG has conducted a series of phase II studies investigating the combination of WAI concurrently with a low dose of cisplatin (169) or followed by doxorubicin and cisplatin (192) in patients with stage III-IV EC; however, significant hematologic toxicity was noted and further development is not planned. Another potential strategy of alternating chemotherapy and limited pelvic irradiation to obtain both local and distant control in advanced EC has proved feasible, with acceptable toxicity and encouraging preliminary survival data (53).

Although the use of adjuvant chemotherapy for advanced disease is expected to increase following publication of GOG-122 (166), it must be acknowledged that patients with cervical, adnexal, and/or deep myometrial will remain at significant increased risk (>60%) to have pelvic failure if RT is not used (144).

Hormonotherapy

Endometrioid adenocarcinoma cells possess steroid receptors (50). Multiple randomized controlled trials of adjuvant progestational therapy following surgery for endometrioid adenocarcinoma have been conducted; however, none have shown a statistically significant improvement in disease-free survival or overall survival (131,218). As progestins have been implicated in non-EC deaths from cardiovascular events (172), their use in the adjuvant setting cannot be supported.

▪▪ | Radiation Therapy Techniques

Intracavitary brachytherapy (ICB) and EBRT can be used alone or in combination in the management of EC. During the last four decades there has been a shift from preoperative RT (EBRT with or without ICB) to postoperative EBRT with or without intravaginal brachytherapy (2), to EBRT alone in the early 1990s (45,95). Following the widespread, although not universal, adoption of ESS (42) there has been increased use of postoperative IVB alone, mostly for intermediate-risk patients (60,156), as well as a tendency toward "more tailored" adjuvant therapy based on the histopathologic features of the surgical specimen (128,137).

Preoperative Irradiation

Although preoperative irradiation is less commonly used in an era of ESS, it may still have a role for those patients with gross involvement of the cervix or vagina (FIGO clinical stages IIB and III, respectively). ICB alone or in combination with pelvic EBRT may be used. Patients with gross pelvic or retroperitoneal nodal disease, in the absence of distant metastasis, could be considered for preoperative extended-field RT (EFRT) and brachytherapy to be followed by surgical staging. Patients undergoing ICB only in the preoperative setting could undergo extrafascial hysterectomy as soon as 1 to 3 days from completion of the implant. If EBRT is required, surgery should be done no sooner than 4 to 6 weeks after completion of therapy to allow radiation-associated inflammation to subside (76).

Preoperative Intracavitary Brachytherapy

The Mallinckrodt Institute of Radiology has endorsed packing the uterine cavity with afterloading Heyman-Simon capsules. In the absence of Simon-Heyman capsules, one or two intrauterine tandems can be used in combination with vaginal ovoids. If there is tumor extension into the vagina, the entire length of the vagina should be treated with Delclos vaginal cylinders, if tumor infiltration is <5 mm thickness, or Syed-Nebblett interstitial implant, for thicker tumors (76). Grigsby et al. (76) reported on 858 patients with clinical stage I EC treated with preoperative RT (2,500 to 4,000 mghRaEq to the uterus with Heyman capsules and intrauterine tandem, and 6,500 cGy surface dose to the upper vagina) followed by TAH-BSO done within 3 days to 6 weeks following completion of the RT. When deep myometrial invasion was present, patients received postoperative EBRT, 2,000 cGy to the whole pelvis and an additional 3,000 cGy to the parametrium with a midline step wedge. The 5-year survival rate for all patients was 84%, with a 5-year PFS of 92% and 86% for FIGO clinical stages IA and IB, respectively.

Preoperative External-Beam Radiation Therapy

Patients with gross cervical involvement or disease that is more advanced could potentially benefit from EBRT to the pelvis in addition to ICB. CT scan simulation with oral and intravenous contrast is encouraged. A vaginal marker should be placed in the vagina in addition to seed markers at the most distal tumor extent in the vagina. The gross tumor volume (GTV) includes the entire uterus and cervix as well, and vaginal extension as well as any gross regional lymphadenopathy. The clinical target volume (CTV) includes the GTV as well as the pelvic lymph node areas potentially harboring microscopic disease; this is the obturator, external, and internal iliacs as well as the lower common iliacs. Careful attention should be paid to include the external iliac anteriorly as well as the presacral nodes posteriorly (S2–S3 level) in the lateral fields as these nodal areas are at high risk in the presence of gross cervical involvement (79). Generally, patients will receive a dose between 20 and 40 Gy (180 cGy/fraction), with a four-field technique (anteroposterior/posteroanterior and lateral fields). At Indiana University for those selected patients with clinical stage IIB uterine cancer with gross cervical infiltration, we have used a combination of EBRT, 4,500 cGy in 25 fractions, followed by a single ICB implant using intrauterine tandem and vaginal ovoids to deliver a dose of 3,500 cGy to classic point A.

Postoperative Irradiation

Adjuvant EBRT in early stage EC, either after TAH-BSO alone or after ESS, has been shown to improve pelvic tumor control and disease-free survival, when compared with observation, without impact in overall survival (2,45,46,95). However, EBRT is associated with acute and long-term toxicity, primarily gastrointestinal and urinary, which must be balanced against the absolute benefit derived from its use. Furthermore, 70% to 75% of recurrences are in the vagina, which can be successfully salvaged in a high proportion of cases (46,92).

EBRT is still recommended in those patients with deeply invasive tumors (stage IC), poorly differentiated histologies, and in patients with pathologic stage IIB primarily in the absence of ESS (7), or if there is evidence of LVSI (38). Whether some of these high-risk patients can be managed with vaginal brachytherapy alone, primarily after complete surgical staging, is unknown. Patients with advanced disease, pathological stages III-IVA have been treated in the past, depending upon the extent of the disease, presence of positive nodes, and after optimal surgical debulking, with a variety of approaches including pelvic EBRT with or without EFRT to cover the periaortic nodes in patients with positive nodes, whole abdominal irradiation (WAI), or even intraperitoneal radioisotopes (32p), the latter one in patients with only positive peritoneal citology.

Postoperative Intracavitary Brachytherapy

In the last decade there has been a tendency toward increasing use of vaginal brachytherapy alone or even observation for the majority of patients with low-to-intermediate risk of EC. Potential advantages of IVB when compared with EBRT include lower costs, lower morbidity, and patient convenience; the main disadvantage being that it does not address the pelvis and therefore should be limited to patients in whom it is estimated that the pelvic failure rate is small and the vagina represents the organ at risk for recurrence. In the Mayo Clinic series, grade 3 and presence of LVSI were found to be significant predictors of vaginal relapse (129). Traditionally, vaginal ovoids (6,500 cGy with low dose rate (LDR) brachytherapy, prescribed to the vaginal surface) have been used; however, high dose rate (HDR) techniques have become increasingly more common in the United Stated (185) and worldwide. However, there are not standardized treatment recommendations; generally, one to three insertions are performed at 1-week intervals, with vaginal ovoids or, more commonly, vaginal cylinders, 700 cGy per fraction per week, prescribed to a depth of 0.5 cm from the vaginal surface, to treat the proximal 3 to 5 cm of the vagina (147). At our institution, the entire length of the vagina is treated only in those patients with unfavorable histologies, such as UPSC and CCC, with special attention being paid to avoid protruding a source at the introitus.

When used in conjunction with EBRT, the most common IVB fractionation used at our institution is two fractions of 500 to 550 cGy prescribed at a depth of 0.5 cm, or three fractions of 600 cGy prescribed to the surface of the vagina. We generally use this regimen in higher risk patients with stage IIB, presence of LVSI, poorly differentiated histology, and/or lower uterine segment involvement. Alternative schedules have been published by Nag et al. (147).

Occasionally, at Indiana University, patients with stage III disease are given a single fraction of HDR IVB, delivering a dose of 700 cGy prescribed to a depth of 0.5 cm from the vaginal surface following 50.4 Gy of EBRT.

Postoperative EBRT Techniques

The postoperative EBRT technique is similar to that described for the preoperative RT technique. Because pelvic lymph nodes are poorly visualized by CT when normal, they should be defined by encompassing the contrast-enhanced blood vessels with an expansion of 7 mm (206). The whole pelvis is treated only in patients with negative pelvic and periaortic nodes, or positive pelvic nodes with negative sampled periaortic nodes, to a dose between 45 and 50.4 Gy with conventional fractionation.

EFRT, encompassing the pelvis and para-aortic areas, should be used for those patients with positive periaortic nodes, or when pelvic nodes are positive and no periaortic lymph node sampling has been performed, or in patients without ESS with positive pelvic nodes by CT scan. CT simulation is even more crucial when treating extended fields for accurate delineation of the kidneys, small bowel, and liver as well the CTV. This should include, in addition to the pelvic CTV, the pericaval, interaortocaval and para-aortic areas, defined by contrast-enhanced blood vessels with a modified 7- to 10-mm margin; the PTV will be created by expanding the CTV by 5 to 10 mm for microscopic disease or 10 to 15 mm for gross residual disease. Generally, the EFRT will receive 45 Gy when treating electively microscopic disease. If there are positive resected periaortic nodes, an additional boost of 500 cGy or higher, depending on the volume of disease and normal organ constraints, could be delivered to the high-risk area, generally using three-dimensional conformal RT or intensity-modulated radiation therapy (IMRT) techniques. The placement of intraoperative vascular clips in the areas of gross disease could be very helpful in delineating the boost areas.

More recently, IMRT is being incorporated in the adjuvant treatment of EC, for those patients requiring EBRT, in an attempt to minimize acute and long-term gastrointestinal and genitourinary toxicity (6,143) (Fig. 67.2). In addition, IMRT or intensity-modulated arc therapy allows significant reduction in dose to the bone marrow, which could potentially result in better hematologic tolerance in high-risk patients undergoing pelvic (with or without para-aortic) irradiation in combination with systemic chemotherapy (25,115,223). However, this technique requires accurate target delineation (CT simulation with intravenous and gastrointestinal contrast required), highly reproducible patient immobilization, and a clear understanding of internal organ motion in order to achieve optimal advantage in the use of IMRT over conventional methods of posthysterectomy pelvic radiation therapy (6,145,223).

Whole Abdominal Irradiation

The ability of WAI to alter failure patterns by decreasing upper abdominal relapse is determined by the adequacy of the technique, emphasizing the necessity of covering the diaphragm with adequate margin during all phases of normal respiration; this requires that liver shielding be limited or absent. In addition, appropriate kidney localization and blocking should be undertaken to keep total doses within tolerance. WAI dose is generally 2,500 to 3,000 cGy (at 150 cGy/fraction). The periaortic region generally receives a boost to 4,200 to 4,500 cGy and the pelvis is treated to 5,040 to 5,100 cGy. The kidney dose should be limited to ≤2,000 cGy via a 100% posterior transmission block. Martinez et al. (132) advocate the use of a liver transmission block to keep the total liver dose to 2,250 cGy. This is not universally accepted and it was not required in the GOG-122 trial. Most of the toxicity encountered with WAI is gastrointestinal, up to 10% to 15% grade 3-4, in some series (52,132,166,199,200). In addition, grade 3 renal and/or liver toxicity has been reported in about 2% of patients (132,199). Hematologic toxicity has been reported in 4% to 15% of patients undergoing WAI (166,199,200). IMRT and tomotherapy may allow higher and more uniform doses to be delivered with less toxicity and decreased rates of intra-abdominal failures (54,83).

Medically Inoperable Early-Stage Endometrial Cancer

Although surgery, including TAH-BSO with lymphadenectomy, remains the standard of care in the management of EC (1), approximately 3% to 10% of patients present with significant medical comorbidities, including morbid obesity and/or severe cardiovascular problems that preclude surgery. In these nonoperable cases, primary RT alone has been used, with success varying with the stage of disease and the individual experience of the treating institution, using a combination of brachytherapy with or without pelvic irradiation (34,66,100,151,152). The American Brachytherapy Society (ABS) (147) recommends determining the thickening of the myometrial wall and depth of infiltration, preferably using MRI (10).

Patients with clinical stage IA, and some selected stage IB, with well or moderately differentiated tumors, without evidence of myometrial infiltration or lymph node metastasis by CT or MRI scan, can be treated with ICB alone (147). This is generally performed with Fletcher-Suit applicators, with one or two tandems depending on the uterus size, and/or Simon-Heyman capsules in combination with vaginal ovoids, using a technique similar to the previously described preoperative ICB technique. There is no consensus regarding optimal dose or prescription points. In some institutions, one or two applications are performed to deliver a dose of 7,000 to 7,500 cGy to point A when using LDR ICB. The loading of the tandem(s) is different from that with cervical cancer in order to provide adequate dose distribution laterally and superiorly. Image-based brachytherapy, although not routinely employed, may potentially provide a more accurate understanding of the dosed received by the gross tumor (as delineated by MRI) and CTVs (defined as the entire uterus, cervix, and proximal 2 to 3 cm of the vagina). However,

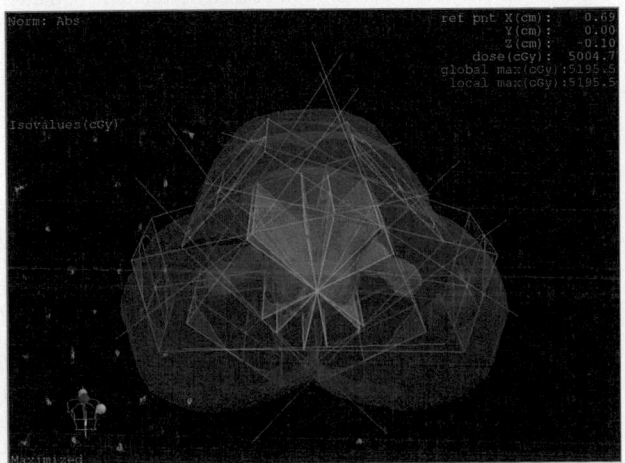
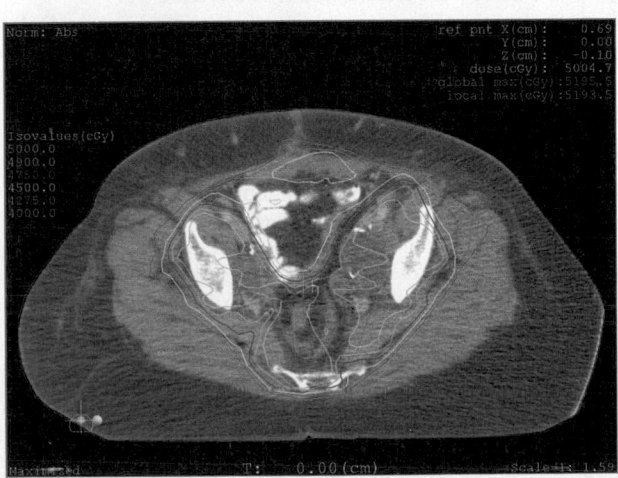

FIGURE 67.2. Adjuvant pelvic irradiation: intensity-modulated radiation therapy. **A:** Beam arrangement. **B:** Isodose distribution.

in the Mallinckrodt Institute system the prescription dose is made such that the total activity/exposure from the intrauterine sources (generally Simon-Heyman capsules and intrauterine tandem) would be around 5,000 mghrRaEq, and from the vaginal ovoids, approximately 3,000 mghrRaEq, with pelvic control rates of 100% for patients with stage IA with ICB alone, and 88% for patients with stage IB disease, generally with a combination of EBRT and ICB (34,75). Chao et al. (34) demonstrated a reasonable mortality of 2.1% and life-threatening complication rate of 4.2% with this approach.

Excellent disease-free survival rates of about 80% for stage IA and 55% to 60% for stage IB (98,100,151,152) have been reported using HDR ICB for EC, although the long-term toxicity was as high as 24%, probably related to overdosing the uterus and subsequently delivering high doses to the rectum and small bowel (100,151). The ABS recommendations regarding HDR ICB alone or in combination with EBRT in terms of prescription point (2 cm from the central axis at the midpoint along the intrauterine sources), number of fractions, dose per fraction, combination with EBRT, and optimization have been extensively reviewed by Nag et al. (147). A careful review of their guidelines is strongly recommended prior to implementation of such approach.

Patients with stage I disease, poorly differentiated or deeply invasive tumors, as well as patients with inoperable stage II disease, should be treated with a combination of EBRT (45 to 50 Gy) and ICB. When there is clinical involvement of the uterine cervix, FIGO clinical stage II, most series show disease-free survival outcomes with definitive RT to be 10% to 20% worse than those for clinical stage I disease (152,204).

Advanced stage EC is more difficult to definitively control with RT alone, as the risk for systemic spread dramatically increases and the local bulk of disease is usually significant. However, multiple series have shown long-term freedom from EC relapse in a significant proportion of patients, with disease-specific survival rates in up to 50% of patients at 5 years (101). Indeed, many clinical stage III patients are so staged on the basis of small vaginal nodules, which can be adequately treated with the ICB. Patients with inoperable stage III disease potentially could be treated to the pelvis only, followed by ICB in the absence of nodal pelvic or retroperitoneal metastasis, or with EFRT and ICB in those patients with nodal disease, followed by chemotherapy or enrollment in a clinical trial, if the patient has adequate performance status. This situation is very uncommon and, generally, patients with advanced pelvic and retroperitoneal disease present with multiple comorbidities that preclude them from such an aggressive approach, often being considered for palliative therapy only.

Recurrent Endometrial Cancer: Salvage Therapy

Localized Disease

After Surgery Alone

The rates of pelvic recurrence in patients with early-stage disease after surgery alone range between 5% and 15%, and 70% to 75% are isolated vaginal recurrences (2,45,46,95). Factors determining the prognosis after treatment of relapse are the size, location (vaginal versus regional/pelvic disease), the initial histology and grade, interval between the diagnosis and recurrence, initial treatment, RT dose, and the use of brachytherapy (77,92,112,146,186,225). The reported salvage rate with radical irradiation is 65% to 80% in patients with isolated vaginal relapses (as high as 80% to 90% in patients with lesions confined to the vaginal mucosa) compared with 25% to 60% salvage rate in patients with pelvic and/or regional recurrences

(5,46,77,92,112,146,159). However, the 5-year survival rate is 30% to 60%, given the high incidence of regional recurrences and/or distant failures (46,77,92,112,146,186), indicating the need for more aggressive salvage therapy, probably using a combined modality approach.

The treatment of recurrent EC after surgery generally requires a combination of EBRT and brachytherapy and higher doses of RT when compared with those delivered in the adjuvant setting, mainly when only IVB is used, which translates into higher toxicity (15% to 20% grade 3–4 toxicity) (92,112,146,159,186,225).

The EBRT volume will include the GTV locally and regionally, as per CT simulation, and the lymphatic regions (obturator, hypogastric, external, and internal iliac lymph nodes). A margin of 2 to 3 cm should be given around the GTV and 1.5 to 2 cm around uninvolved lymph nodes. Generally, the pelvis is treated to a dose of 45 to 50 Gy with EBRT followed by brachytherapy (20 to 25 Gy), using a combination of interstitial with or without intracavitary techniques. Patients with lesions involving the distal third of the vagina often require the inclusion of vulva or perineum in the EBRT fields. Inclusion of the inguinofemoral lymph node regions is highly recommended (see Chapter 70 for details regarding the technique for treating inguinofemoral nodes).

At our institution, the entire surface of the vagina receives a dose of 60 Gy with LDR brachytherapy (including the dose from EBRT). The GTV, as defined by physical examination and/or CT scan, will receive a total dose between 75 and 80 Gy, including the EBRT and the LDR brachytherapy. Intracavitary brachytherapy alone (LDR or HDR) will be allowed in patients with vaginal lesions <5 mm thickness. If so, dose should be prescribed to a depth of 0.5 cm unless only superficial mucosal infiltration is present. Interstitial brachytherapy should be used for lesions ≥5 mm thickness. The interstitial techniques used in the management of isolated vaginal recurrences from EC are similar to those described in Chapter 70.

Pelvic/regional recurrences that are nonamenable to brachytherapy implant should receive additional boost using conformal techniques (we prefer the use of multiple coplanar or noncoplanar beam arrangement) or IMRT techniques in order to deliver a total dose to the gross disease of around 6,500 cGy, providing the small bowel can be spared doses exceeding 4,500 cGy. Patients with extensive pelvic lymphadenopathy extending to the common iliacs and/or periaortic nodal disease, in the absence of distant metastasis, should be considered for EFRT with or without brachytherapy, if there is associated vaginal recurrence. These patients are at very high risk for distant failures. Although the data regarding combined modality therapy in this setting are limited, there is some indication that it may offer improved outcome (186). Similarly, patients with residual disease after completion of EFRT should be considered to be enrolled in clinical trials for advanced/recurrent disease, rather than waiting until progression, given the high rates of distant failures. An alternative approach will be a combination of "tailored EBRT" followed by systemic therapy similar to that investigated in the GOG-184 clinical trial.

After Surgery and Radiation: Role of Salvage Surgery

As most recurrences of EC following surgery and adjuvant RT have been outside the pelvis, exenteration series even from large institutions have been small and have accrued during several decades (15,140). Five-year survival rates have ranged from 20% to 45% in this highly selected series and such surgery is fraught with high complication rate of 60% to 80% (15,140). Advocates of aggressive surgical debulking of recurrent extrapelvic disease report improved local control and 60% 5-year survival rates if the patients can be debulked to no residual disease; however, such surgery carries a perioperative mortality risk of 8% to 10%, so should only be undertaken by those who are experienced in techniques and the intensive perioperative care required by such patients (29,176).

Regional and Metastatic Disease

The presence of steroid receptors in endometrioid adenocarcinoma (50) has prompted phase II investigations into the role of progestins, both oral and intramuscular forms, in recurrent disease with response rates of 20% to 30% (160,161,164). In a GOG randomized trial of low-dose (200 mg) versus high-dose (1,000 mg) of oral daily medroxyprogesterone, there was no advantage to higher dose (212). Tamoxifen has been noted to abrogate the down-regulation of the steroid receptor (153), and hence was integrated into hormonal regimens. Whitney et al. (222) reported a 33% response rate with 200 mg of oral daily medroxyprogesterone MPA for 1 week, alternating with tamoxifen 20 mg orally, twice daily, for 1 week. The combination of tamoxifen 20 mg orally, twice daily for 3 weeks alternating with megestrol acetate 80 mg orally, twice daily for 3 weeks yielded a 27% response rate (95% confidence interval [CI]: 17–38) and, of note, 53% of the responses were >20 months' duration (65). Paradoxically, only a 10% response rate was seen with tamoxifen as a single agent; hence, its use alone is not recommended (213). Aromatase inhibitors, despite their ability to lower serum estrogen levels by inhibiting peripheral conversion, have been associated with disappointing response rates of <10% and are not recommended outside a clinical trial (116,171).

Single cytotoxic agents with documented activity–response rates of 20% to 35% include cisplatin, carboplatin, doxorubicin, and paclitaxel (12,27,207,209). The GOG has run a series of randomized trials comparing doxorubicin-based combinations (67,69,210,211). The addition of cyclophosphamide to doxorubicin did not improve outcomes (210); however, the combination of doxorubicin and cisplatin (AC) improved response rates and median PFS (211). Circadian-timed AC was equivalent to standard AC regimen (69). Fleming et al. (67) reported that the addition of paclitaxel to AC (ACT or TAP) when compared to AC alone led to improved response rates (34% to 57%), median PFS (5.3 to 8.3 months), and median overall survival (12.3 to 15.3 months). However, it must be noted that the triplet regimen was more neurotoxic and did require the administration of colony-stimulating factors (67). The GOG opened a trial in 2003 comparing ACT to combination of carboplatin and paclitaxel to determine if it will be possible to drop out the doxorubicin and limit the myelosuppression and need for cytokines as well as lessen the risk of neurotoxicity by substituting carboplatin for cisplatin.

Palliative Therapy

Surgery

The role of surgery in the palliative setting in EC involves primarily (a) debulking large masses in an attempt to improve patients' symptoms and quality of life, and (b) an attempt to relieve intestinal obstruction generally related to a mechanical obstruction from recurrent masses. Careful preoperative evaluation is indicated before any surgical intervention, including assessment of patient's performance and nutritional status and history of prior RT. Imaging studies may help to delineate the number and location of obstructions as well as the extent of intra-abdominal disease in order to guide the surgical decision-making process. Patients with recurrent disease and short life expectancy are unlikely to benefit from exploration. It is important to exercise good judgment and expertise to maximize

outcome for these patients with short life expectancy in order to improve their quality of life.

Radiation Therapy

Patients with grossly recurrent and metastatic EC following surgery and RT often have significant symptoms unresponsive to further systemic therapy. Symptoms may be due to recurrent disease in the pelvis, causing pain and/or bleeding. Distant recurrence in the brain, chest, groin, and other areas may require palliation as well. The selection of treatment modality and doses of RT in the palliative setting depend primarily on the extent of the disease in the pelvis, prior RT, patient's performance status, and estimated length of survival. Patients with poor performance status and/or extensive distant disease should be treated using shorter RT regimens. If vaginal bleeding is the main concern, brachytherapy, using endocavitary and/or interstitial techniques, when feasible, often offers good symptom control with relatively low morbidity. For patients who have received prior RT, intracavitary doses in the range of 35 to 40 Gy tumor dose may suffice to palliate symptoms. For those patients who may not be candidates for brachytherapy, a short course of EBRT using high-dose fractionation schedules have been used (194,195).

Uterine Papillary Serous and Clear Cell Carcinoma

UPSC and CCC are aggressive histologic subtypes that differ from typical ECs by their poor prognosis, even in early-stage disease, and a propensity for peritoneal as well as lymphatic and systemic spread (78). Therefore, it is imperative to perform a complete surgical staging because of the expected high rate of surgical upstaging (70,72). The rarity of these subtypes makes prospective studies, and thus definitive treatment recommendations, difficult. Published adjuvant therapeutic approaches in patients with stage I and II disease, after complete surgical staging, include observation (33,41,88), systemic chemotherapy, and vaginal cuff brachytherapy (94,216), and limited-fields EBRT with (114) or without chemotherapy (139) or intraperitoneal ^{32}P in combination with IVB (59). Most clinicians will recommend some form of adjuvant therapy for these patients who have *not* undergone comprehensive staging, but at present there is not a standardized approach based on level I evidence.

The incidence of abdominal recurrences has led some investigators to study the impact of adjuvant WAI on these subtypes, with mixed results in single-institution series. In a relatively large retrospective series of patients treated in the British Columbia Cancer Agency, 78 patients underwent hysterectomy and were found to have uterine-confined disease or positive washings only (stages I-IIIA). Fifty-eight patients were treated with adjuvant WAI with a 5-year disease-specific survival of 74.9%, compared with 41.3% in 20 patients receiving less than WAI (111). Martinez et al. (132) have as well reported similar results with "high-dose WAI" in patients with UPSC and CCC, with 5-year cause-specific survival of 80%, whereas the 5-year disease-free survival was only 49%, given the high recurrence rates of intra-abdominal as well as distant failures. Sutton et al. (200) published the results of a phase II trial conducted by the GOG, in which all stages of UPSC and CCC underwent surgical staging with optimal cytoreduction to <2 cm residual disease and subsequently received adjuvant WAI (30 Gy) followed by a periaortic boost to 45 Gy and 49.8 Gy boost to the pelvis. The 5-year PFS for patients with stages I-II was 38% for patients with UPSC and 54% for those with CCC, respectively; more than half of the treatment failures were within the radiation field, indicating the need for other treatment approaches, namely chemotherapy or chemoradiotherapy. In patients with stage III and IV, WAI is associated with poor outcome; the 3-year recurrence-free survival and overall survival for this group was 27% and 35%, respectively, for these high-risk histologies (199). The role of adjuvant RT is probably best viewed using the principles of volume-directed EBRT and/or vaginal brachytherapy in combination with chemotherapy, a concept supported by several single-institutions limited series (94,114, 191).

In patients with negative nodes, comprehensively staged, without residual disease, the potential risk for peritoneal spread can be addressed with less toxicity using intraperitoneal treatment with radioactive colloids. Intraperitoneal radioactive phosphorus (^{32}P) has been used for similar adjuvant therapy in the ovarian counterpart of UPSC with low morbidity (226). Likewise, the vaginal cuff recurrence pattern can be addressed with IVB with acceptably low toxicity (7). Such a combined approach has been prospectively studied at Indiana University School of Medicine by the Hoosier Oncology Group (59) in 22 node-negative patients undergoing extensive surgical staging with maximal surgical debulking (<3 mm residual disease). The majority of patients (17) had stage I or II disease. The treatment consisted of intraperitoneal administration of 15 mCi of ^{32}P followed by three HDR vaginal brachytherapy procedures. The results from this experience were encouraging as acute toxicity was limited to grade 1, and no late toxicity was observed. In addition, with a median follow-up of 39.6 months, the disease-free survival data compare favorably with only five patients (20.3%) suffering recurrence (59). Of note, two recurrences were in the distal vagina early in the experience when we routinely treated the proximal vagina only. After these recurrences, the protocol was altered to treat the entire vaginal length, and thereafter no vaginal recurrences have been seen.

As the atypical endometrial histologies of UPSC and CCC are less likely to possess steroid receptors (50), the role of adjuvant progestins has not been investigated. Some have advocated adjuvant cytotoxic therapy in these patients because of their increased risk of peritoneal and distant failures, even after surgical staging (94,114,191). Doxorubicin and cisplatin were associated with superior PFS and overall survival when compared to WAI in advanced stage EC in the GOG 122 trial in which 25% of the patients had UPSC/CCC histology (114). In addition, some preliminary data have shown encouraging results when combining sequential chemotherapy (Taxol plus cisplatin) and pelvic EBRT (64). This role of adjuvant therapy cytotoxic chemotherapy or radiation or some combination thereof represents an area in which further investigation is needed; however, the rarity of these cell types make such clinical trials challenging to design.

Uterine Sarcoma (Adults Only) Management

Because of their rarity, it is difficult for a single institution to accrue large numbers of patients with uterine sarcomas, and prospective randomized trials have been limited. In addition, the interpretation of the results of treatments efficacy is complicated by the frequent inclusion of MMMTs along with leiomyosarcomas and endometrial stromal sarcomas as a generic group of uterine sarcomas (118,155).

Surgery

Mixed müllerian tumors of the uterus and endometrial stromal sarcoma require the same ESS as is done for adenocarcinomas of the uterus. Approximately 15% of such sarcomas will be found to harbor node metastases and those with deep myometrial invasion, LVSI, or isthmocervical junction involvement are at particularly high risk for nodal metastases (181). Leiomyosarcomas are more likely to disseminate hematogenously, seldom (<5%) spread to pelvic nodes, and hence ESS is not required for uterine leiomyo sarcoma (LMS) (73).

Radiation Therapy

There are not clear guidelines for recommending adjuvant RT for uterine sarcomas, given the conflicting data and lack of prospective randomized trial demonstrating a survival benefit for adjuvant RT. In general, RT should be recommended in those patients with substantial risk of locoregional recurrence: higher grade tumors, positive nodes (more common in MMMT), positive margins, or evidence of gross residual disease. A GOG clinicopathologic study (118) of 453 patients with uterine sarcomas reported a 53% recurrence rate in MMMT and 71% in leiomyosarcoma, with the site of first recurrence being the pelvis in 21% of MMMT (19% in homologous and 24% in heterologous types) and 14% of leiomyosarcoma, respectively. Distant failure, as the first site, occurred in 14% of MMMT and 41% of leiomyosarcoma patients, respectively. Forty percent of patients with MMMT received adjuvant pelvic RT compared with 22% of leiomyosarcoma patients. The pelvic failure was 17% in patients receiving RT compared with 24% for those that did not (118).

Neither adjuvant doxorubicin (155) nor RT (84) has been found to be associated with improvement in overall survival for patients with uterine sarcoma, although a benefit in local control has been shown only for patients with MMMT (84). The European Organization for Research and Treatment of Cancer completed a phase III trial to evaluate the role of adjuvant pelvic RT in the treatment of stages I–II uterine sarcomas. In their early report, there were 14% relapses in the adjuvant group versus 24% in the control group ($p = .004$), without impact in overall survival or PFS (168). Again, an impact on pelvic tumor control was seen only in patients with MMMT (168).

Major et al. (118) noted that almost 60% of the MMMT patients who failed did so in the abdomen with or without pelvic evidence of distant metastasis, indicating that WAI might impact on patterns of failure for this subset of uterine sarcomas. GOG-150, a phase III randomized study of whole abdominal RT versus combination ifosfamide-mesna with cisplatin in optimally debulked stage I–IV carcinosarcoma of the uterus has been conducted. The data have been analyzed but results have not yet been published by Dr. Wolfson. There were 207 evaluable patients, including 43.5% of whom with early-stage I-II disease and the remainder with stage III and IV disease. The cumulative incidence of recurrence for all patients was approximately 50%. Statistical analysis estimated that adjuvant chemotherapy reduced the recurrence rate 28.5% relative to adjunctive irradiation (hazard ratio: 0.715, 95% CI: 0.474–1.077; $p = .107$, two-tail test). Seven-year overall survival for all patients was approximately 40%. Overall survival at 7 years for the chemotherapy and WAI arms was 45% and 35%, respectively. Statistical analysis estimated that adjuvant chemotherapy reduced the death rate 32.8% relative to adjunctive RT (hazard ratio: 0.672, 95% CI: 0.458–0.986; $p = .042$). Because of the poor overall survival for all patients within this malignant class, new adjuvant therapeutic strategies should be investigated.

Given the high rates of locoregional and distant failures, a multimodality approach with tailored radiation therapy and chemotherapy has been evaluated with encouraging results (120) and deserves further investigation.

The role of adjuvant therapy in leiomyosarcoma is undefined. Adjuvant RT appears to modestly improve local control without significant impact in survival (71,84,118).

Chemotherapy

Prognosis is poor for those patients with unresectable disease, and chemotherapy should be considered palliative. Single cytotoxic agents with significant activity in uterine LMS include doxorubicin, ifosfamide, and gemcitabine (113,154,202). Multiagent combinations of ifosfamide with doxorubicin, hydroxyurea with dacarbazine and etoposide, and mitomycin with doxorubicin and cisplatin have achieved response rates of 18% to 30% (48,55,198). The best response rate (53%) for metastatic leiomyosarcoma was seen with gemcitabine and docetaxel (80). Uterine LMS is so rare that randomized trials are not feasible. Uterine sarcomas of the mixed müllerian variety have been noted to respond to cisplatin, ifosfamide, and paclitaxel alone or in combination (49,201,203,208). In a phase III trial, the combination of ifosfamide with or without cisplatin was found to improve response rates from 36% to 54% and median PFS from 4 to 6 months; however, there was no improvement in median overall survival (201). A subsequent phase III trial that compared ifosfamide alone to combination ifosfamide/paclitaxel for patients with advanced or recurrent uterine carcinosarcoma showed that the combination improved PFS (hazard ratio, 0.71 [95% CI: 0.51–0.97]; $p = .03$] and overall survival (hazard ratio 0.69 [95% CI: 0.49–0.97]; $p = .03$) (81).

References

1. American College of Obstetricians Gynecologists Practice Bulletin No. 65: Management of endometrial cancer. *Obstet Gynecol* 2005;106:413–425.
2. Aalders J, Abeler V, Kolstad P, et al. Postoperative external irradiation and prognostic parameters in stage I endometrial carcinoma: clinical and histopathologic study of 540 patients. *Obstet Gynecology* 1980;56:419–427.
3. Aarnio M, Mecklin JP, Aaltonen LA, et al. Life-time risk of different cancers in hereditary non-polyposis colorectal cancer (HNPCC) syndrome. *Int J Cancer* 1995;64:430–433.
4. Abeler VM, Vergote IB, Kjorstad KE, et al. Clear cell carcinoma of the endometrium. Prognosis and metastatic pattern. *Cancer* 1996;78:1740–1747.
5. Ackerman I, Malone S, Thomas G, et al. Endometrial carcinoma–relative effectiveness of adjuvant irradiation vs therapy reserved for relapse. *Gynecol Oncol* 1996;60:177–183.
6. Ahamad A, D'Souza W, Salehpour M, et al. Intensity-modulated radiation therapy after hysterectomy: comparison with conventional treatment and sensitivity of the normal-tissue-sparing effect to margin size. *Int J Radiat Oncol Biol Phys* 2005;62:1117–1124.
7. Alektiar KM, Venkatraman E, Chi DS, et al. Intravaginal brachytherapy alone for intermediate-risk endometrial cancer. *Int J Radiat Oncol Biol Phys* 2005;62:111–117.
8. Ambros RA, Sherman ME, Zahn CM, et al. Endometrial intraepithelial carcinoma: a distinctive lesion specifically associated with tumors displaying serous differentiation. *Hum Pathol* 1995;26:1260–1267.
9. Anderson JM, Stea B, Hallum AV, et al. High-dose-rate postoperative vaginal cuff irradiation alone for stage IB and IC endometrial cancer. *Int J Radiat Oncol Biol Phys* 2000;46:417–425.
10. Ascher SM, Reinhold C. Imaging of cancer of the endometrium. *Radiol Clin North Am* 2002;40:563–576.
11. Ashman JB, Connell PP, Yamada D, et al. Outcome of endometrial carcinoma patients with involvement of the uterine serosa. *Gynecol Oncol* 2001;82:338–343.
12. Ball HG, Blessing JA, Lentz SS, et al. A phase II trial of paclitaxel in patients with advanced or recurrent adenocarcinoma of the endometrium: a Gynecologic Oncology Group study. *Gynecol Oncol* 1996;62:278–281.
13. Bancher-Todesca D, Gitsch G, Williams KE, et al. p53 protein overexpression: a strong prognostic factor in uterine papillary serous carcinoma. *Gynecol Oncol* 1998;71:59–63.
14. Bar-Am A, Ron IG, Kuperminc M, et al. The role of routine pelvic lymph node sampling in patients with stage I endometrial carcinoma: second thoughts. *Acta Obstet Gynecol Scand* 1998;77:347–350.
15. Barakat RR, Goldman NA, Patel DA, et al. Pelvic exenteration for recurrent endometrial cancer. *Gynecol Oncol* 1999;75:99–102.
16. Barnes MN, Roland PY, Straughn M, et al. A comparison of treatment strategies for endometrial adenocarcinoma: analysis of financial impact. *Gynecol Oncol* 1999;74:443–447.
17. Bell SW, Kempson RL, Hendrickson MR. Problematic uterine smooth muscle neoplasms. A clinicopathologic study of 213 cases. *Am J Surg Pathol* 1994;18:535–558.
18. Berchuck A, Rubin SC, Hoskins WJ, et al. Treatment of uterine leiomyosarcoma. *Obstet Gynecol* 1988;71:845–850.
19. Berclaz G, Hanggi W, Kratzer-Berger A, et al. Lymphadenectomy in high risk endometrial carcinoma stage I and II: no more morbidity and no need for external pelvic radiation. *Int J Gynecol Cancer* 1999;9:322–328.
20. Bokhman JV. Two pathogenetic types of endometrial carcinoma. *Gynecol Oncol* 1983;15:10–17.
21. Bradley WH, Boente MP, Brooker D, et al. Hysteroscopy and cytology in endometrial cancer. *Obstet Gynecol* 2004;104:1030–1033.
22. Briet JM, Hollema H, Reesink N, et al. Lymphvascular space involvement: an independent prognostic factor in endometrial cancer. *Gynecol Oncol* 2005;96:799–804.
23. Brinton LA, Berman ML, Mortel R, et al. Reproductive, menstrual, and medical risk factors for endometrial cancer: results from a case-control study. *Am J Obstet Gynecol* 1992;167:1317–1325.
24. Bristow RE, Zahurak ML, Alexander CJ, et al. FIGO stage IIIC endometrial carcinoma: resection of macroscopic nodal disease and other determinants of survival. *Int J Gynecol Cancer* 2003;13:664–672.
25. Brixey CJ, Roeske JC, Lujan AE, et al. Impact of intensity-modulated radiotherapy on acute hematologic toxicity in women with gynecologic malignancies. *Int J Radiat Oncol Biol Phys* 2002;54:1388–1396.
26. Bruckman JE, Goodman RL, Murthy A, et al. Combined irradiation and surgery in the treatment of stage II carcinoma of the endometrium. *Cancer* 1978;42:1146–1151.
27. Burke TW, Munkarah A, Kavanagh JJ, et al. Treatment of advanced or recurrent endometrial carcinoma with single-agent carboplatin. *Gynecol Oncol* 1993;51:397–400.
28. Bussaglia E, del Rio E, Matias-Guiu X, et al. PTEN mutations in endometrial carcinomas: a molecular and clinicopathologic analysis of 38 cases. *Hum Pathol* 2000;31:312–317.
29. Campagnutta E, Giorda G, De Piero G, et al. Surgical treatment of recurrent endometrial carcinoma. *Cancer* 2004;100:89–96.
30. Catasus L, Machin P, Matias-Guiu X, et al. Microsatellite instability in endometrial carcinomas: clinicopathologic correlations in a series of 42 cases. *Hum Pathol* 1998;29:1160–1164.
31. Cengiz M, Singh AK, Grigsby PW. Postoperative vaginal brachytherapy alone is the treatment of choice for grade 1–2, stage IC endometrial cancer. *Int J Gynecol Cancer* 2005;15:926–931.
32. Chadha M, Nanavati PJ, Liu P, et al. Patterns of failure in endometrial carcinoma stage IB grade 3 and IC patients treated with postoperative vaginal vault brachytherapy. *Gynecol Oncol* 1999;75:103–107.
33. Chan JK, Loizzi V, Youssef M, et al. Significance of comprehensive surgical staging in noninvasive papillary serous carcinoma of the endometrium. *Gynecol Oncol* 2003;90:181–185.
34. Chao CK, Grigsby PW, Perez CA, et al. Medically inoperable stage I endometrial carcinoma: a few dilemmas in radiotherapeutic management. *Int J Radiat Oncol Biol Phys* 1996;34:27–31.
35. Chi DS, Welshinger M, Venkatraman ES, et al. The role of surgical cytoreduction in Stage IV endometrial carcinoma. *Gynecol Oncol* 1997;67:56–60.
36. Cilby W, Clarke-Pearson DL, Dodge R, et al. Acute morbidity and mortality associated with selective pelvic and para-aortic lymphadenectomy in the surgical staging of endometrial adenocarcinoma. *J Gynecol Tech* 1995;1:19.
37. Clement PB, Young RH. Non-endometrioid carcinomas of the uterine corpus: a review of their pathology with emphasis on recent advances and problematic aspects. *Adv Anat Pathol* 2004;11:117–142.
38. Cohn DE, Horowitz NS, Mutch DG, et al. Should the presence of lymphvascular space involvement be used to assign patients to adjuvant therapy following hysterectomy for unstaged endometrial cancer? *Gynecol Oncol* 2002;87:243–246.
39. Connell PP, Rotmensch J, Waggoner S, et al. The significance of adnexal involvement in endometrial carcinoma. *Gynecol Oncol* 1999;74:74–79.
40. Cragun JM, Havrilesky LJ, Calingaert B, et al. Retrospective analysis of selective lymphadenectomy in apparent early-stage endometrial cancer. *J Clin Oncol* 2005;23:3668–3675.
41. Craighead PS, Sait K, Stuart GC, et al. Management of aggressive histologic variants of endometrial carcinoma at the Tom Baker Cancer Centre between 1984 and 1994. *Gynecol Oncol* 2000;77:248–253.
42. Creasman W. FIGO Stages. *Gynecol Oncol* 1989;35:125–127.
43. Creasman WT, Morrow CP, Bundy BN, et al. Surgical pathologic spread patterns of endometrial cancer. A Gynecologic Oncology Group Study. *Cancer* 1987;60:2035–2041.
44. Creasman WT, Odicino F, Maisonneuve P, et al. Carcinoma of the corpus uteri. *Int J Gynaecol Obstet* 2003;83[Suppl 1]:79–118.
45. Creutzberg CL, van Putten WL, Koper PC, et al. Surgery and postoperative radiotherapy versus surgery alone for patients with stage-1 endometrial carcinoma: multicentre randomised trial. PORTEC Study Group. Post Operative Radiation Therapy in Endometrial Carcinoma. *Lancet* 2000;355:1404–1411.
46. Creutzberg CL, van Putten WL, Koper PC, et al. Survival after relapse in patients with endometrial cancer: results from a randomized trial. *Gynecol Oncol* 2003;89:201–209.
47. Creutzberg CL, van Putten WL, Warlam-Rodenhuis CC, et al. Outcome of high-risk stage IC, grade 3, compared with stage I endometrial carcinoma patients: the Postoperative Radiation Therapy in Endometrial Carcinoma Trial. *J Clin Oncol* 2004;22:1234–1241.
48. Currie J, Blessing JA, Muss HB, et al. Combination chemotherapy with hydroxyurea, dacarbazine (DTIC), and etoposide in the treatment of uterine leiomyosarcoma: a Gynecologic Oncology Group study. *Gynecol Oncol* 1996;61:27–30.
49. Curtin JP, Blessing JA, Soper JT, et al. Paclitaxel in the treatment of carcinosarcoma of the uterus: a gynecologic oncology group study. *Gynecol Oncol* 2001;83:268–270.
50. Deligdisch L, Holinka CF. Progesterone receptors in two groups of endometrial carcinoma. *Cancer* 1986;57:1385–1388.
51. Dijkhuizen FP, Mol BW, Brolmann HA, et al. The accuracy of endometrial sampling in the diagnosis of patients with endometrial carcinoma and hyperplasia: a meta-analysis. *Cancer* 2000;89:1765–1772.
52. Dusenbery KE, Potish RA, Gold DG, et al. Utility and limitations of abdominal radiotherapy in the management of endometrial carcinomas. *Gynecol Oncol* 2005;96:635–642.
53. Duska LR, Berkowitz R, Matulonis U, et al. A pilot trial of TAC (paclitaxel, doxorubicin, and carboplatin) chemotherapy with filgastrim (r-metHuG-CSF) support followed by radiotherapy in patients with "high-risk" endometrial cancer. *Gynecol Oncol* 2005;96:198–203.
54. Duthoy W, De Gersem W, Vergote K, et al. Whole abdominopelvic radiotherapy (WAPRT) using intensity-modulated arc therapy (IMAT): first clinical experience. *Int J Radiat Oncol Biol Phys* 2003;57:1019–1032.
55. Edmonson JH, Blessing JA, Cosin JA, et al. Phase II study of mitomycin, doxorubicin, and cisplatin in the treatment of advanced uterine leiomyosarcoma: a Gynecologic Oncology Group study. *Gynecol Oncol* 2002;85:507–510.
56. Eltabbakh GH. Analysis of survival after laparoscopy in women with endometrial carcinoma. *Cancer* 2002;95:1894–1901.

Clinical Radiation Oncology

57. Eltabbakh GH, Piver MS, Hempling RE, et al. Excellent long-term survival and absence of vaginal recurrences in 332 patients with low-risk stage I endometrial adenocarcinoma treated with hysterectomy and vaginal brachytherapy without formal staging lymph node sampling: report of a prospective trial. *Int J Radiat Oncol Biol Phys* 1997;38:373–380.

58. Everett E, Tamimi H, Greer B, et al. The effect of body mass index on clinical/pathologic features, surgical morbidity, and outcome in patients with endometrial cancer. *Gynecol Oncol* 2003;90:150–157.

59. Fakiris AJ, Moore DH, Reddy SR, et al. Intraperitoneal radioactive phosphorus (32P) and vaginal brachytherapy as adjuvant treatment for uterine papillary serous carcinoma and clear cell carcinoma: a phase II Hoosier Oncology Group (HOG 97-01) study. *Gynecol Oncol* 2005;96:818–823.

60. Fanning J. Long-term survival of intermediate risk endometrial cancer (stage IG3, IC, II) treated with full lymphadenectomy and brachytherapy without teletherapy. *Gynecol Oncol* 2001;82:371–374.

61. Fanning J, Hoffman ML, Andrews SJ, et al. Cost-effectiveness analysis of the treatment for intermediate risk endometrial cancer: postoperative brachytherapy vs. observation. *Gynecol Oncol* 2004;93:632–636.

62. Ferrandina G, Ranelletti FO, Gallotta V, et al. Expression of cyclooxygenase-2 (COX-2), receptors for estrogen (ER), and progesterone (PR), p53, ki67, and neu protein in endometrial cancer. *Gynecol Oncol* 2005;98:383–389.

63. Ferrandina G, Legge F, Ranelletti FO, et al. Cyclooxygenase-2 expression in endometrial carcinoma: correlation with clinicopathologic parameters and clinical outcome. *Cancer* 2002;95:801–807.

64. Fields A, Gebb J, Einstein M, et al. Pilot phase II Trial of radiation "sandwiched" in combination paclitaxel/platinum chemotherapy in patients with uterine papillary serous carcinoma. *Gynecol Oncol* 2006;101. Abstract 16.

65. Fiorica JV, Brunetto VL, Hanjani P, et al. Phase II trial of alternating courses of megestrol acetate and tamoxifen in advanced endometrial carcinoma: a Gynecologic Oncology Group study. *Gynecol Oncol* 2004;92:10–14.

66. Fishman DA, Roberts KB, Chambers JT, et al. Radiation therapy as exclusive treatment for medically inoperable patients with stage I and II endometrioid carcinoma with endometrium. *Gynecol Oncol* 1996;61:189–196.

67. Fleming GF, Brunetto VL, Cella D, et al. Phase III trial of doxorubicin plus cisplatin with or without paclitaxel plus filgrastim in advanced endometrial carcinoma: a Gynecologic Oncology Group Study. *J Clin Oncol* 2004;22:2159–2166.

68. Franchi M, Ghezzi F, Riva C, et al. Postoperative complications after pelvic lymphadenectomy for the surgical staging of endometrial cancer. *J Surg Oncol* 2001;78:232–240.

69. Gallion HH, Brunetto VL, Cibull M, et al. Randomized phase III trial of standard timed doxorubicin plus cisplatin versus circadian timed doxorubicin plus cisplatin in stage III and IV or recurrent endometrial carcinoma: a Gynecologic Oncology Group Study. *J Clin Oncol* 2003;21:3808–3813.

70. Geisler JP, Geisler HE, Melton ME, et al. What staging surgery should be performed on patients with uterine papillary serous carcinoma? *Gynecol Oncol* 1999;74:465–467.

71. Giuntoli RL, 2nd, Metzinger DS, DiMarco CS, et al. Retrospective review of 208 patients with leiomyosarcoma of the uterus: prognostic indicators, surgical management, and adjuvant therapy. *Gynecol Oncol* 2003;89:460–469.

72. Goff BA, Goodman A, Muntz HG, et al. Surgical stage IV endometrial carcinoma: a study of 47 cases. *Gynecol Oncol* 1994;52:237–240.

73. Goff BA, Rice LW, Fleischhacker D, et al. Uterine leiomyosarcoma and endometrial stromal sarcoma: lymph node metastases and sites of recurrence. *Gynecol Oncol* 1993;50:105–109.

74. Greven K, Winter K, Underhill K, et al. Preliminary analysis of RTOG 9708: Adjuvant postoperative radiotherapy combined with cisplatin/paclitaxel chemotherapy after surgery for patients with high-risk endometrial cancer. *Int J Radiat Oncol Biol Phys* 2004;59:168–173.

75. Grigsby PW, Kuske RR, Perez CA, et al. Medically inoperable stage I adenocarcinoma of the endometrium treated with radiotherapy alone. *Int J Radiat Oncol Biol Phys* 1987;13:483–488.

76. Grigsby PW, Perez CA, Kuten A, et al. Clinical stage I endometrial cancer: prognostic factors for local control and distant metastasis and implications of the new FIGO surgical staging system. *Int J Radiat Oncol Biol Phys* 1992;22:905–911.

77. Hasbini A, Haie-Meder C, Morice P, et al. Outcome after salvage radiotherapy (brachytherapy +/– external) in patients with a vaginal recurrence from endometrial carcinomas. *Radiother Oncol* 2002;65:23–28.

78. Hendrickson M, Ross J, Eifel P, et al. Uterine papillary serous carcinoma: a highly malignant form of endometrial adenocarcinoma. *Am J Surg Pathol* 1982;6:93–108.

79. Henriksen. The lymphatic spread of carcinoma of the cervix and the body of the uterus: a study of 420 necropsies. *Am J Obstet Gynecol* 1949;58:924.

80. Hensley ML, Maki R, Venkatraman E, et al. Gemcitabine and docetaxel in patients with unresectable leiomyosarcoma: results of a phase II trial. *J Clin Oncol* 2002;20:2824–2831.

81. Homesley H, Filiaci VL, Bitterman P, et al. Phase III trial of ifosfamide versus ifosfamide plus paclitaxel as first-line treatment of advanced or recurrent uterine carcinosarcoma (mixed mesodermal tumors): a Gynecologic Oncology Group study. *Gynecol Oncol* 2006;101:S31.

82. Homesley HD, Kadar N, Barrett RJ, et al. Selective pelvic and periaortic lymphadenectomy does not increase morbidity in surgical staging of endometrial carcinoma. *Am J Obstet Gynecol* 1992;167:1225–1230.

83. Hong L, Alektiar K, Chui C, et al. IMRT of large fields: whole-abdomen irradiation. *Int J Radiat Oncol Biol Phys* 2002;54:278–289.

84. Hornback NB, Omura G, Major FJ. Observations on the use of adjuvant radiation therapy in patients with stage I and II uterine sarcoma. *Int J Radiat Oncol Biol Phys* 1986;12:2127–2130.

85. Horowitz NS, Peters WA 3rd, Smith MR, et al. Adjuvant high dose rate vaginal brachytherapy as treatment of stage I and II endometrial carcinoma. *Obstet Gynecol* 2002;99:235–240.

86. Horowitz NS, Dehdashti F, Herzog TJ, et al. Prospective evaluation of FDG-PET for detecting pelvic and para-aortic lymph node metastasis in uterine corpus cancer. *Gynecol Oncol* 2004;95:546–551.

87. Hsieh CH, ChangChien CC, Lin H, et al. Can a preoperative CA 125 level be a criterion for full pelvic lymphadenectomy in surgical staging of endometrial cancer? *Gynecol Oncol* 2002;86:28–33.

88. Huh WK, Powell M, Leath CA, 3rd, et al. Uterine papillary serous carcinoma: comparisons of outcomes in surgical Stage I patients with and without adjuvant therapy. *Gynecol Oncol* 2003;91:470–475.

89. Ismail S. Endometrial pathology associated with prolonged tamoxifen therapy: a review. *Adv Anat Path* 1996;3:266–271.

90. Iwasa Y, Haga H, Konishi I, et al. Prognostic factors in uterine carcinosarcoma: a clinicopathologic study of 25 patients. *Cancer* 1998;82:512–519.

91. Jemal A, Murray T, Ward E, et al. Cancer statistics, 2005 [erratum appears in *CA Cancer J Clin* 2005;55:259]. *CA: Cancer J Clin* 2005;55:10–30.

92. Jhingran A, Burke TW, Eifel PJ. Definitive radiotherapy for patients with isolated vaginal recurrence of endometrial carcinoma after hysterectomy. *Int J Radiat Oncol Biol Phys* 2003;56:1366–1372.

93. Jolly S, Vargas C, Kumar T, et al. Vaginal brachytherapy alone: an alternative to adjuvant whole pelvis radiation for early stage endometrial cancer. *Gynecol Oncol* 2005;97:887–892.

94. Kelly MG, O'Malley D M, Hui P, et al. Improved survival in surgical stage I patients with uterine papillary serous carcinoma (UPSC) treated with adjuvant platinum-based chemotherapy. *Gynecol Oncol* 2005;98:353–359.

95. Keys HM, Roberts JA, Brunetto VL, et al. A phase III trial of surgery with or without adjunctive external pelvic radiation therapy in intermediate risk endometrial adenocarcinoma: a Gynecologic Oncology Group study[erratum appears in *Gynecol Oncol* 2004;94:241–242]. *Gynecol Oncol* 2004;92:744–751.

96. Kilgore LC, Partridge EE, Alvarez RD, et al. Adenocarcinoma of the endometrium: survival comparisons of patients with and without pelvic node sampling. *Gynecol Oncol* 1995;56:29–33.

97. Kim SH, Kim HD, Song YS, et al. Detection of deep myometrial invasion in endometrial carcinoma: comparison of transvaginal ultrasound, CT, and MRI. *J Comput Assist Tomogr* 1995;19:766–772.

98. Knocke TH, Kucera H, Weidinger B, et al. Primary treatment of endometrial carcinoma with high-dose-rate brachytherapy: results of 12 years of experience with 280 patients. *Int J Radiat Oncol Biol Phys* 1997;37:359–365.

99. Kucera H, Vavra N, Weghaupt K. Benefit of external irradiation in pathologic stage I endometrial carcinoma: a prospective clinical trial of 605 patients who received postoperative vaginal irradiation and additional pelvic irradiation in the presence of unfavorable prognostic factors. *Gynecol Oncol* 1990;38:99–104.

100. Kucera H, Knocke TH, Kucera E, et al. Treatment of endometrial carcinoma with high-dose-rate brachytherapy alone in medically inoperable stage I patients. *Acta Obstet Gynecol Scand* 1998;77:1008–1012.

101. Kupelian PA, Eifel PJ, Tornos C, et al. Treatment of endometrial carcinoma with radiation therapy alone. *Int J Radiat Oncol Biol Phys* 1993;27:817–824.

102. Kurman RJ, Kaminski PF, Norris HJ. The behavior of endometrial hyperplasia. A long-term study of "untreated" hyperplasia in 170 patients. *Cancer* 1985;56:403–412.

103. Kwon JS, Bryson P, Liu G, et al. A comparison of endometrial cancer outcomes in Ontario. *J Obstet Gynaecol Canada* 2004;26:793–798.

104. Lambrou NC, Gomez-Marin O, Mirhashemi R, et al. Optimal surgical cytoreduction in patients with Stage III and Stage IV endometrial carcinoma: a study of morbidity and survival. *Gynecol Oncol* 2004;93:653–658.

105. Larson DM, Johnson K, Olson KA. Pelvic and para-aortic lymphadenectomy for surgical staging of endometrial cancer: morbidity and mortality. *Obstet Gynecol* 1992;79:998–1001.

106. Lax SF, Pizer ES, Ronnett BM, et al. Clear cell carcinoma of the endometrium is characterized by a distinctive profile of p53, Ki-67, estrogen, and progesterone receptor expression. *Hum Pathol* 1998;29:551–558.

107. Lax SF, Kendall B, Tashiro H, et al. The frequency of p53, K-ras mutations, and microsatellite instability differs in uterine endometrioid and serous carcinoma: evidence of distinct molecular genetic pathways. *Cancer* 2000;88:814–824.

108. Lee CM, Szabo A, Shrieve DC, et al. Frequency and effect of adjuvant radiation therapy among women with stage I endometrial adenocarcinoma. *JAMA* 2006;295:389–397.

109. Tanan Mn, Simma Y, Krannan MP, et al. incidence of lymph node and ovarian metastases in leiomyosarcoma of the uterus. *Gynecol Oncol* 2003;71:417–421.

110. Lewandowski G, Torrisi J, Potkul RK, et al. Hysterectomy with extended surgical staging and radiotherapy versus hysterectomy alone and radiotherapy in stage I endometrial cancer: a comparison of complication rates. *Gynecol Oncol* 1990;36:401–404.

111. Lim P, Al Kushi A, Gilks B, et al. Early stage uterine papillary serous carcinoma of the endometrium: effect of adjuvant whole abdominal radiotherapy and pathologic parameters on outcome. *Cancer* 2001;91:752–757.

112. Lin LL, Grigsby PW, Powell MA, et al. Definitive radiotherapy in the management of isolated vaginal recurrences of endometrial cancer. *Int J Radiat Oncol Biol Phys* 2005;63:500–504.

113. Look KY, Sandler A, Blessing JA, et al. Phase II trial of gemcitabine as second-line chemotherapy of uterine leiomyosarcoma: a Gynecologic Oncology Group (GOG) Study. *Gynecol Oncol* 2004;92:644–647.

114. Low JS, Wong EH, Tan HS, et al. Adjuvant sequential chemotherapy and radiotherapy in uterine papillary serous carcinoma. *Gynecol Oncol* 2005;97:171–177.

115. Lujan AE, Mundt AJ, Yamada SD, et al. Intensity-modulated radiotherapy as a means of reducing dose to bone marrow in gynecologic patients receiving whole pelvic radiotherapy. *Int J Radiat Oncol Biol Phys* 2003;57:516–521.

116. Ma BB, Oza A, Eisenhauer E, et al. The activity of letrozole in patients with advanced or recurrent endometrial cancer and correlation with biological markers—a study of the National Cancer Institute of Canada Clinical Trials Group. *Int J Gynecol Cancer* 2004;14:650–658.

117. MacLeod C, Fowler A, Duval P, et al. High-dose-rate brachytherapy alone post-hysterectomy for endometrial cancer. *Int J Radiat Oncol Biol Phys* 1998;42:1033–1039.

118. Major FJ, Blessing JA, Silverberg SG, et al. Prognostic factors in early-stage uterine sarcoma. A Gynecologic Oncology Group study. *Cancer* 1993;71:1702–1709.

119. Malpica A, Tornos C, Burke TW, et al. Low-stage clear-cell carcinoma of the endometrium. *Am J Surg Pathol* 1995;19:769–774.

120. Manolitsas TP, Wain GV, Williams KE, et al. Multimodality therapy for patients with clinical Stage I and II malignant mixed Mullerian tumors of the uterus. *Cancer* 2001;91:1437–1443.

121. Mariani A, Webb MJ, Galli L, et al. Potential therapeutic role of para-aortic lymphadenectomy in node-positive endometrial cancer. *Gynecol Oncol* 2000;76:348–356.

122. Mariani A, Webb MJ, Keeney GL, et al. Surgical stage I endometrial cancer: predictors of distant failure and death. *Gynecol Oncol* 2002;87:274–280.

123. Mariani A, Webb MJ, Keeney GL, et al. Predictors of lymphatic failure in endometrial cancer. *Gynecol Oncol* 2002;84:437–442.

124. Mariani A, Webb MJ, Keeney GL, et al. Assessment of prognostic factors in stage IIIA endometrial cancer. *Gynecol Oncol* 2002;86:38–44.

125. Mariani A, Webb MJ, Keeney GL, et al. Endometrial cancer: predictors of peritoneal failure. *Gynecol Oncol* 2003;89:236–242.

126. Mariani A, Webb MJ, Keeney GL, et al. Low-risk corpus cancer: is lymphadenectomy or radiotherapy necessary? *Am J Obstet Gynecol* 2000;182:1506–1519.

127. Mariani A, Webb MJ, Keeney GL, et al. Stage IIIC endometrioid corpus cancer includes distinct subgroups. *Gynecol Oncol* 2002;87:112–117.

128. Mariani A, Dowdy SC, Keeney GL, et al. High-risk endometrial cancer subgroups: candidates for target-based adjuvant therapy. *Gynecol Oncol* 2004;95:120–126.

129. Mariani A, Dowdy SC, Keeney GL, et al. Predictors of vaginal relapse in stage I endometrial cancer. *Gynecol Oncol* 2005;97:820–827.

130. Mariani A, Sebo TJ, Katzmann JA, et al. Pretreatment assessment of prognostic indicators in endometrial cancer. *Am J Obstet Gynecol* 2000;182:1535–1544.

131. Martin-Hirsch PL, Jarvis G, Kitchener H, et al. Progestagens for endometrial cancer. *Cochrane Database Syst Rev* 2000:CD001040.

132. Martinez AA, Weiner S, Podratz K, et al. Improved outcome at 10 years for serous-papillary/clear cell or high-risk endometrial cancer patients treated by adjuvant high-dose whole abdomino-pelvic irradiation. *Gynecol Oncol* 2003;90:537–546.

133. Matias-guiu X, Catasus L, Bussaglia E, et al. Molecular pathology of endometrial hyperplasia and carcinoma. *Hum Pathol* 2001;32:569–577.

134. Maxwell GL, Risinger JI, Alvarez AA, et al. Favorable survival associated with microsatellite instability in endometrioid endometrial cancers. *Obstet Gynecol* 2001;97:417–422.

135. McCluggage WG. Uterine carcinosarcomas (malignant mixed Mullerian tumors) are metaplastic carcinomas. *Int J Gynecol Cancer* 2002;12:687–690.

136. McCluggage WG, Sumathi VP, McManus DT. Uterine serous carcinoma and endometrial intraepithelial carcinoma arising in endometrial polyps: report of 5 cases, including 2 associated with tamoxifen therapy. *Hum Pathol* 2003;34:939–943.

137. McCormick TC, Cardenes H, Randall ME. Early-stage endometrial cancer: is intravaginal radiation therapy alone sufficient therapy? *Brachytherapy* 2002;1:61–65.

138. McMeekin DS, Lashbrook D, Gold M, et al. Analysis of FIGO Stage IIIc endometrial cancer patients. *Gynecol Oncol* 2001;81:273–278.

139. Mehta N, Yamada SD, Rotmensch J, et al. Outcome and pattern of failure in pathologic stage I-II papillary serous carcinoma of the endometrium: implications for adjuvant radiation therapy. *Int J Radiat Oncol Biol Phys* 2003;57:1004–1009.

140. Morris M, Alvarez RD, Kinney WK, et al. Treatment of recurrent adenocarcinoma of the endometrium with pelvic exenteration. *Gynecol Oncol* 1996;60:288–291.

141. Morrow CP, Bundy BN, Homesley HD, et al. Doxorubicin as an adjuvant following surgery and radiation therapy in patients with high-risk endometrial carcinoma, stage I and occult stage II: a Gynecologic Oncology Group Study. *Gynecol Oncol* 1990;36:166–171.

142. Morrow CP, Bundy BN, Kurman RJ, et al. Relationship between surgical-pathological risk factors and outcome in clinical stage I and II carcinoma of the endometrium: a Gynecologic Oncology Group study. *Gynecol Oncol* 1991;40:55–65.

143. Mundt AJ, Mell LK, Roeske JC. Preliminary analysis of chronic gastrointestinal toxicity in gynecology patients treated with intensity-modulated whole pelvic radiation therapy. *Int J Radiat Oncol Biol Phys* 2003;56:1354–1360.

144. Mundt AJ, McBride R, Rotmensch J, et al. Significant pelvic recurrence in high-risk pathologic stage I–IV endometrial carcinoma patients after adjuvant chemotherapy alone: implications for adjuvant radiation therapy. *Int J Radiat Oncol Biol Phys* 2001;50:1145–1153.

145. Mundt AJ, Lujan AE, Rotmensch J, et al. Intensity-modulated whole pelvic radiotherapy in women with gynecologic malignancies. *Int J Radiat Oncol Biol Phys* 2002;52:1330–1337.

146. Nag S, Yacoub S, Copeland LJ, et al. Interstitial brachytherapy for salvage treatment of vaginal recurrences in previously unirradiated endometrial cancer patients. *Int J Radiat Oncol Biol Phys* 2002;54:1153–1159.

147. Nag S, Erickson B, Parikh S, et al. The American Brachytherapy Society recommendations for high-dose-rate brachytherapy for carcinoma of the endometrium. *Int J Radiat Oncol Biol Phys* 2000;48:779–790.

148. Nelson G, Randall M, Sutton G, et al. FIGO stage IIIC endometrial carcinoma with metastases confined to pelvic lymph nodes: analysis of treatment outcomes, prognostic variables, and failure patterns following adjuvant radiation therapy. *Gynecol Oncol* 1999;75:211–214.

149. Ng TY, Perrin LC, Nicklin JL, et al. Local recurrence in high-risk node-negative stage I endometrial carcinoma treated with postoperative vaginal vault brachytherapy. *Gynecol Oncol* 2000;79:490–494.

150. Ng TY, Nicklin JL, Perrin LC, et al. Postoperative vaginal vault brachytherapy for node-negative Stage II (occult) endometrial carcinoma. *Gynecol Oncol* 2001;81:193–195.

151. Nguyen TV, Petereit DG. High-dose-rate brachytherapy for medically inoperable stage I endometrial cancer. *Gynecol Oncol* 1998;71:196–203.

152. Niazi TM, Souhami L, Portelance L, et al. Long-term results of high-dose-rate brachytherapy in the primary treatment of medically inoperable stage I-II endometrial carcinoma. *Int J Radiat Oncol Biol Phys* 2005;63:1108–1113.

153. Nola M, Jukic S, Ilic-Forko J, et al. Effects of tamoxifen on steroid hormone receptors and hormone concentration and the results of DNA analysis by flow cytometry in endometrial carcinoma. *Gynecol Oncol* 1999;72:331–336.

154. Omura GA, Major FJ, Blessing JA, et al. A randomized study of adriamycin with and without dimethyl triazenoimidazole carboxamide in advanced uterine sarcomas. *Cancer* 1983;52:626–632.

155. Omura GA, Blessing JA, Major F, et al. A randomized clinical trial of adjuvant adriamycin in uterine sarcomas: a Gynecologic Oncology Group Study. *J Clin Oncol* 1985;3:1240–1245.

156. Orr JW, Jr., Holimon JL, Orr PF. Stage I corpus cancer: is teletherapy necessary? *Am J Obstet Gynecol* 1997;176:777–779.

157. Pavelka JC, Ben Shachar I, Fowler JM, et al. Morbid obesity and endometrial cancer: surgical, clinical, and pathologic outcomes in surgically managed patients. *Gynecol Oncol* 2004;95:588–592.

158. Petereit DG, Tannehill SP, Grosen EA, et al. Outpatient vaginal cuff brachytherapy for endometrial cancer. *Int J Gynecol Cancer* 1999;9:456–462.

159. Petignat P, Jolicoeur M, Alobaid A, et al. Salvage treatment with high-dose-rate brachytherapy for isolated vaginal endometrial cancer recurrence. *Gynecol Oncol* 2006;101(3):445–449.

160. Piver MS, Barlow JJ, Lurain JR, et al. Medroxyprogesterone acetate (Depo-Provera) vs. hydroxyprogesterone caproate (Delalutin) in women with metastatic endometrial adenocarcinoma. *Cancer* 1980;45:268–272.

161. Podratz KC, O'Brien PC, Malkasian GD, Jr., et al. Effects of progestational agents in treatment of endometrial carcinoma. *Obstet Gynecol* 1985;66:106–110.

162. Prat J. Prognostic parameters of endometrial carcinoma. *Hum Pathol* 2004;35:649–662.

163. Prat J, Oliva E, Lerma E, et al. Uterine papillary serous adenocarcinoma. A 10-case study of p53 and c-erbB-2 expression and DNA content. *Cancer* 1994;74:1778–1783.

164. Quinn MA, Cauchi M, Fortune D. Endometrial carcinoma: steroid receptors and response to medroxyprogesterone acetate. *Gynecol Oncol* 1985;21:314–319.

165. Randall ME, Reisinger S. Radiation therapy and combined chemo-irradiation in advanced and recurrent endometrial carcinoma. *Semin Oncol* 1994;21:91–99.

166. Randall ME, Filiaci VL, Muss H, et al. Randomized phase III trial of whole-abdominal irradiation versus doxorubicin and cisplatin chemotherapy in advanced endometrial carcinoma: a Gynecologic Oncology Group Study. *J Clin Oncol* 2006;24:36–44.

167. Redman C, Swart A, Amos C. ASTEC (surgery component): a study in the treatment of endometrial cancer: a randomized trial of lymphadenectomy in the treatment of endometrial cancer (ISRCTN 16571884). *Int J Gynecol Cancer* 2005;15:77.

168. Reed N, Mangioni C, Malmstrom H, et al. First results of a randomized trial comparing radiotherapy versus observation postoperatively in patients with uterine sarcoas: an EORTCGcG study. *Int J Gynecol Cancer* 2003;13:4.

169. Reisinger SA, Asbury R, Liao SY, et al. A phase I study of weekly cisplatin and whole abdominal radiation for the treatment of stage III and IV endometrial carcinoma: a Gynecologic Oncology Group pilot study. *Gynecol Oncol* 1996;63:299–303.

170. Rittenberg PV, Lotocki RJ, Heywood MS, et al. Stage II endometrial carcinoma: limiting post-operative radiotherapy to the vaginal vault in node-negative tumors. *Gynecol Oncol* 2005;98:434–438.

171. Rose PG, Brunetto VL, VanLe L, et al. A phase II trial of anastrozole in advanced recurrent or persistent endometrial carcinoma: a Gynecologic Oncology Group study. *Gynecol Oncol* 2000;78:212–216.

172. Rossouw JE, Anderson GL, Prentice RL, et al. Risks and benefits of estrogen plus progestin in healthy postmenopausal women: principal results From the Women's Health Initiative randomized controlled trial. *JAMA* 2002;288:321–333.

173. Saegusa M, Hashimura M, Yoshida T, et al. beta-Catenin mutations and aberrant nuclear expression during endometrial tumorigenesis. *Br J Cancer* 2001;84:209–217.

174. Saffari B, Bernstein L, Hong DC, et al. Association of p53 mutations and a codon 72 single nucleotide polymorphism with lower overall survival and responsiveness to adjuvant radiotherapy in endometrioid endometrial carcinomas. *Int J Gynecol Cancer* 2005;15:952–963.

175. Santin AD, Bellone S, Van Stedum S, et al. Amplification of c-erbB2 oncogene: a major prognostic indicator in uterine serous papillary carcinoma. *Cancer* 2005;104:1391–1397.

176. Scarabelli C, Campagnutta E, Giorda G, et al. Maximal cytoreductive surgery as a reasonable therapeutic alternative for recurrent endometrial carcinoma. *Gynecol Oncol* 1998;70:90–93.

177. Schmeler KM, Soliman PT, Sun CC, et al. Endometrial cancer in young, normal-weight women. *Gynecol Oncol* 2005;99:388–392.

178. Scholten AN, van Putten WL, Beerman H, et al. Postoperative radiotherapy for Stage 1 endometrial carcinoma: long-term outcome of the randomized PORTEC trial with central pathology review. *Int J Radiat Oncol Biol Phys* 2005;63:834–838.

179. Scribner DR, Jr., Walker JL, Johnson GA, et al. Laparoscopic pelvic and paraaortic lymph node dissection in the obese. *Gynecol Oncol* 2002;84:426–430.

180. Silverberg S, Kurman R. *Tumors of the uterine corpus and gestational trophoblastic diseases*. Washington, DC: Armed Forces Institute of Pathology; 1991.

181. Silverberg SG, Major FJ, Blessing JA, et al. Carcinosarcoma (malignant mixed mesodermal tumor) of the uterus. A Gynecologic Oncology Group pathologic study of 203 cases. *Int J Gynecol Pathol* 1990;9:1–19.

182. Silverman MB, Roche PC, Kho RM, et al. Molecular and cytokinetic pretreatment risk assessment in endometrial carcinoma. *Gynecol Oncol* 2000;77:1–7.

183. Sivridis E, Giatromanolaki A, Koukourakis M, et al. Endometrial carcinoma: association of steroid hormone receptor expression with low angiogenesis and bcl-2 expression. *Virch Archiv* 2001;438:470–477.

184. Slomovitz BM, Burke TW, Eifel PJ, et al. Uterine papillary serous carcinoma (UPSC): a single institution review of 129 cases. *Gynecol Oncol* 2003;91:463–469.

185. Small W, Jr., Erickson B, Kwakwa F. American Brachytherapy Society survey regarding practice patterns of postoperative irradiation for endometrial cancer: current status of vaginal brachytherapy. *Int J Radiat Oncol Biol Phys* 2005;63:1502–1507.

186. Smaniotto D, D'Agostino G, Luzi S, et al. Concurrent 5-fluorouracil, mitomycin C and radiation, with or without brachytherapy, in recurrent endometrial cancer: a scoring system to predict clinical response and outcome. *Tumori* 2005;91:215–220.

187. Smith-Bindman R, Kerlikowske K, Feldstein VA, et al. Endovaginal ultrasound to exclude endometrial cancer and other endometrial abnormalities. *JAMA* 1998;280:1510–1517.

188. Smith RA, von Eschenbach AC, Wender R, et al. American Cancer Society guidelines for the early detection of cancer: update of early detection guidelines for prostate, colorectal, and endometrial cancers. Also: update 2001—testing for early lung cancer detection [erratum appears in *CA Cancer J Clin* 2001;51):150]. *CA: Cancer J Clin* 2001;51:38–75; quiz 77–80.

189. Solhjem MC, Petersen IA, Haddock MG. Vaginal brachytherapy alone is sufficient adjuvant treatment of surgical stage I endometrial cancer. *Int J Radiat Oncol Biol Phys* 2005;62:1379–1384.

190. Soliman PT, Oh JC, Schmeler KM, et al. Risk factors for young premenopausal women with endometrial cancer. *Obstet Gynecol* 2005;105:575–580.

191. Sood BM, Jones J, Gupta S, et al. Patterns of failure after the multimodality treatment of uterine papillary serous carcinoma. *Int J Radiat Oncol Biol Phys* 2003;57:208–216.

192. Soper JT, Reisinger SA, Ashbury R, et al. Feasibility study of concurrent weekly cisplatin and whole abdominopelvic irradiation followed by doxorubicin/cisplatin

chemotherapy for advanced stage endometrial carcinoma: a Gynecologic Oncology Group trial. *Gynecol Oncol* 2004;95:95–100.

193. Sorbe BG, Smeds AC. Postoperative vaginal irradiation with high dose rate after-loading technique in endometrial carcinoma stage I. *Int J Radiat Oncol Biol Phys* 1990;18:305–314.

194. Spanos W, Jr., Guse C, Perez C, et al. Phase II study of multiple daily fractionations in the palliation of advanced pelvic malignancies: preliminary report of RTOG 8502. *Int J Radiat Oncol Biol Phys* 1989;17:659–661.

195. Spanos WJ, Jr., Perez CA, Marcus S, et al. Effect of rest interval on tumor and normal tissue response–a report of phase III study of accelerated split course palliative radiation for advanced pelvic malignancies (RTOG-8502). *Int J Radiat Oncol Biol Phys* 1993;25:399–403.

196. Straughn JM, Jr., Huh WK, Kelly FJ, et al. Conservative management of stage I endometrial carcinoma after surgical staging. *Gynecol Oncol* 2002;84:194–200.

197. Susini T, Massi G, Amunni G, et al. Vaginal hysterectomy and abdominal hysterectomy for treatment of endometrial cancer in the elderly. *Gynecol Oncol* 2005;96:362–367.

198. Sutton G, Blessing JA, Malfetano JH. Ifosfamide and doxorubicin in the treatment of advanced leiomyosarcomas of the uterus: a Gynecologic Oncology Group study. *Gynecol Oncol* 1996;62:226–229.

199. Sutton G, Axelrod JH, Bundy BN, et al. Whole abdominal radiotherapy in the adjuvant treatment of patients with stage III and IV endometrial cancer: a gynecologic oncology group study. *Gynecol Oncol* 2005;97:755–763.

200. Sutton G, Axelrod JH, Bundy BN, et al. Adjuvant whole abdominal irradiation in clinical stages I and II papillary serous or clear cell carcinoma of the endometrium: a phase II study of the Gynecologic Oncology Group. *Gynecol Oncol* 2006;100:349–354.

201. Sutton G, Brunetto VL, Kilgore L, et al. A phase III trial of ifosfamide with or without cisplatin in carcinosarcoma of the uterus: a Gynecologic Oncology Group Study. *Gynecol Oncol* 2000;79:147–153.

202. Sutton GP, Blessing JA, Barrett RJ, et al. Phase II trial of ifosfamide and mesna in leiomyosarcoma of the uterus: a Gynecologic Oncology Group study. *Am J Obstet Gynecol* 1992;166:556–559.

203. Sutton GP, Blessing JA, Rosenshein N, et al. Phase II trial of ifosfamide and mesna in mixed mesodermal tumors of the uterus (a Gynecologic Oncology Group study). *Am J Obstet Gynecol* 1989;161:309–312.

204. Taghian A, Pernot M, Hoffstetter S, et al. Radiation therapy alone for medically inoperable patients with adenocarcinoma of the endometrium. *Int J Radiat Biol Phys* 1988;15:1135–1140.

205. Tavassoli F, Devilee P. *Pathology and genetics of tumours of the breast and female genital organs*. Lyon, France: IARC Press; 2003.

206. Taylor A, Rockall AG, Reznek RH, et al. Mapping pelvic lymph nodes: guidelines for delineation in intensity-modulated radiotherapy. *Int J Radiat Oncol Biol Phys* 2005;63:1604–1612.

207. Thigpen JT, Buchsbaum HJ, Mangan C, et al. Phase II trial of adriamycin in the treatment of advanced or recurrent endometrial carcinoma: a Gynecologic Oncology Group study. *Cancer Treat Rep* 1979;63:21–27.

208. Thigpen JT, Blessing JA, Orr JW Jr, et al. Phase II trial of cisplatin in the treatment of patients with advanced or recurrent mixed mesodermal sarcomas of the uterus: a Gynecologic Oncology Group Study. *Cancer Treat Rep* 1986;70:271–274.

209. Thigpen JT, Blessing JA, Homesley H, et al. Phase II trial of cisplatin as first-line chemotherapy in patients with advanced or recurrent endometrial carcinoma: a Gynecologic Oncology Group Study. *Gynecol Oncol* 1989;33:68–70.

210. Thigpen JT, Blessing JA, DiSaia PJ, et al. A randomized comparison of doxorubicin alone versus doxorubicin plus cyclophosphamide in the management of advanced or recurrent endometrial carcinoma: a Gynecologic Oncology Group study. *J Clin Oncol* 1994;12:1408–1414.

211. Thigpen JT, Brady MF, Homesley HD, et al. Phase III trial of doxorubicin with or without cisplatin in advanced endometrial carcinoma: a gynecologic oncology group study. *J Clin Oncol* 2004;22:3902–3908.

212. Thigpen JT, Brady MF, Alvarez RD, et al. Oral medroxyprogesterone acetate in the treatment of advanced or recurrent endometrial carcinoma: a dose-response study by the Gynecologic Oncology Group. *J Clin Oncol* 1999;17:1736–1744.

213. Thigpen T, Brady MF, Homesley HD, et al. Tamoxifen in the treatment of advanced or recurrent endometrial carcinoma: a Gynecologic Oncology Group study. *J Clin Oncol* 2001;19:364–367.

214. Touboul E, Belkacemi Y, Buffat L, et al. Adenocarcinoma of the endometrium treated with combined irradiation and surgery: study of 437 patients. *Int J Radiat Oncol Biol Phys* 2001;50:81–97.

215. Tritz D, Pieretti M, Turner S, et al. Loss of heterozygosity in usual and special variant carcinomas of the endometrium. *Hum Pathol* 1997;28:607–612.

216. Turner BC, Knisely JP, Kacinski BM, et al. Effective treatment of stage I uterine papillary serous carcinoma with high dose-rate vaginal apex radiation (192Ir) and chemotherapy. *Int J Radiat Oncol Biol Phys* 1998;40:77–84.

217. Ventura KC, Popiolek D, Mittal K. Endometrial adenocarcinoma in situ in complex atypical hyperplasia: correlation with findings in subsequent hysterectomy specimen. *Int J Surg Pathol* 2004;12:225–230.

218. von Minckwitz G, Loibl S, Brunnert K, et al. Adjuvant endocrine treatment with medroxyprogesterone acetate or tamoxifen in stage I and II endometrial cancer–a multicentre, open, controlled, prospectively randomised trial. *Eur J Cancer* 2002;38:2265–2271.

219. Weiss E, Hirnle P, Arnold-Bofinger H, et al. Adjuvant vaginal high-dose-rate afterloading alone in endometrial carcinoma: patterns of relapse and side effects following low-dose therapy. *Gynecol Oncol* 1998;71:72–76.

220. Wheeler DT, Bell KA, Kurman RJ, et al. Minimal uterine serous carcinoma: diagnosis and clinicopathologic correlation. *Am J Surg Pathol* 2000;24:797–806.

221. Whitney CW. *Gynecologic Oncology Group surgical procedures manual*. 2005.

222. Whitney CW, Brunetto VL, Zaino RJ, et al. Phase II study of medroxyprogesterone acetate plus tamoxifen in advanced endometrial carcinoma: a Gynecologic Oncology Group study. *Gynecol Oncol* 2004;92:4–9.

223. Wong E, D'Souza DP, Chen JZ, et al. Intensity-modulated arc therapy for treatment of high-risk endometrial malignancies. *Int J Radiat Oncol Biol Phys* 2005;61:830–841.

224. Wright JD, Powell MA, Herzog TJ, et al. Panniculectomy: improving lymph node yield in morbidly obese patients with endometrial neoplasms. *Gynecol Oncol* 2004;94:436–441.

225. Wylie J, Irwin C, Pintilie M, et al. Results of radical radiotherapy for recurrent endometrial cancer. *Gynecol Oncol* 2000;77:66–72.

226. Young RC, Walton LA, Ellenberg SS, et al. Adjuvant therapy in stage I and stage II epithelial ovarian cancer. Results of two prospective randomized trials. *New Engl J Med* 1990;322:1021–1027.

227. Zaino RJ, Kurman RJ, Diana KL, et al. The utility of the revised International Federation of Gynecology and Obstetrics histologic grading of endometrial adenocarcinoma using a defined nuclear grading system. A Gynecologic Oncology Group study. *Cancer* 1995;75:81–86.

228. Zaino RJ, Davis AT, Ohlsson-Wilhelm BM, et al. DNA content is an independent prognostic indicator in endometrial adenocarcinoma. A Gynecologic Oncology Group study. *Int J Gynecol Pathol* 1998;17:312–319.

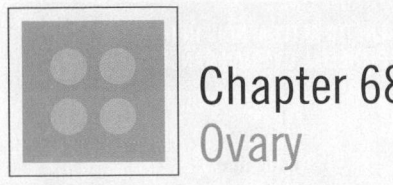

Chapter 68
Ovary

Paola A. Gehrig, Mahesh Varia, Smith Apisarnthanarax, Ruth Lininger, Michael D. Stambaugh

Ovarian neoplasms encompass a wide array of benign and malignant tumors with diverse histologic cell types, clinical features, and hormone-secreting tumors. Primary malignant tumors of the ovary include the epithelial cancers, germ cell tumors, and the sex cord tumors. Low-malignant potential (LMP) tumors of the ovary are noninvasive epithelial tumors usually confined to the ovary but paradoxically can have tumor implants outside the ovary. Metastases to the ovary occur from other cancers that include uterine, gastrointestinal (Krukenberg tumors), and breast cancers. Primary lymphoma, sarcoma, and melanoma of the ovary are rare. Relative to its incidence, epithelial cancers have substantially high mortality as effective screening tests are lacking; only 25% are found to be stage I at diagnosis, and current therapies for advanced cancer, although improving, have limited efficacy (Table 68.1). Surgery for diagnosis, staging, and initial treatment followed by chemotherapy are the major current therapeutic modalities. Radiation therapy has a limited role in management of ovarian cancer.

Anatomy

Ovaries are almond-shaped, grayish-pink, mostly solid organs measuring approximately 4 × 2.5 × 1 cm, with an average weight of approximately 4 to 5 g in premenopausal women, and atrophy through menopause becoming nonfunctional. When "normally" positioned, the ovary is attached by meso-ovarium to the broad ligament that covers the uterus and fallopian tubes. *Broad ligament* arises in development from an invagination of the urogenital fold and constitutes one of three ligaments offering stability to the reproductive organs. The ovary protrudes from posterior border of this broad ligament, the mesovarium. Suspensory ligament is a band of fibromuscular tissue that extends through the broad ligament from the fundus of the uterus to the lower, medial pole of the ovary. The infundibular pelvic ligament extends from the superior and lateral surface of the ovary to the lateral pelvic wall forming the superior and lateral aspect of the broad ligament, and contains the blood supply for the ovary.

Ovarian arteries stem directly from the aorta, immediately below the renal artery, and follow the peritoneum through the infundibular pelvic ligament to the ovary. The venous return and the lymphatic drainage travel to the renal vein on the left and directly to the vena cava on the right. Secondary lymphatic flow may pass through the inguinal canal and to the iliac nodal system (74). The sensory and autonomic nerves arise from the ovarian, hypogastric, and aortic plexuses as well as the celiac and mesenteric ganglia (44).

Histologically, the outer cortex is covered by a layer of pseudocolumnar or cuboidal epithelium, termed the *germinal epithelium of Waldeyer*. The inner medulla consists of dense stromal tissue filled with dense blood vessels and spindled, "muscle-like" connective tissue. The medulla also contains a tunica albuginea superficially and various degrees of maturing follicles throughout the various layers, to the center of the ovary.

Epidemiology

Approximately 22,400 women in the United States will be diagnosed with epithelial ovarian cancer in 2007, and 15,300 women will die of the disease (7). Ovarian cancer is the eighth most common cancer and the fourth leading cause of cancer-related death in women, following lung, breast, and colon cancers (7). The lifetime risk of ovarian cancer is approximately 1 in 70, the median age at diagnosis is 63 years, and >80% of ovarian cancer occurs after the age of 40 in the United States. The majority of ovarian cancers are sporadic, with about 10% ovarian cancers being hereditary. Hereditary ovarian cancers occur about 10 years earlier. Epithelial ovarian cancers are the most common of the ovarian malignancies, but germ cell tumors predominate in younger women.

Risk Factors

Little is known about the etiology or development of ovarian cancer. Numerous epidemiologic studies demonstrate an increase in the rates of disease in industrialized countries, suggesting an environmental effect. The incidence in African American women is slightly lower than in white women (10 vs. 13 cases per 100,000 women, respectively) and is more common in North American and northern European women compared with Japanese women. Overall, the mechanisms of ovarian carcinogenesis are poorly understood and are likely multifactorial and associated with patient-related and environmental factors (Table 68.2).

Patient-Related

Ovarian cancer incidence increases with advancing age and is associated with low parity and infertility giving rise to the "incessant ovulation hypothesis." This hypothesis proposes that ovarian cancer develops from an aberrant repair process of the surface epithelium as a result of repeated rupture of this epithelium during each ovulatory cycle, thought to produce inflammation and scarring that serves as a nidus for carcinogenesis (49). Suppression of ovulatory events from pregnancy, breast feeding, and oral contraceptive use may explain diminished risk of ovarian cancer, and nulliparity, infertility, early menarche, first childbirth after age 35, and late menopause that are associated with higher frequency of ovulatory events all may increase the risk of epithelial ovarian cancer. The risk of ovarian cancer is reduced by 40%, 53%, and 60% with oral contraceptive use for 4, 8, and 12 years, respectively (122). No correlation between unruptured, persistent ovarian cysts and epithelial cancers has been uncovered (35).

Although heredity tumors account for <5% to 10% of all ovarian cancers, family history is the strongest risk factor, after increasing age. The risk of developing ovarian cancer in the general population is 1.8%, but the risk for a woman with one first-degree family member affected by this disease has a lifetime risk of 5%, and with two first-degree relatives, the lifetime risk climbs to 25% to 50%. Three distinct autosomal dominant

Table 68.1	EPITHELIAL OVARIAN CANCER STAGE DISTRIBUTION AND SURVIVAL BY STAGE	
FIGO Stage	**Patients (n = 4,825) (%)**	**5-year Overall Survival (%)**
IA	13	90
IB	1	86
IC	14	83
IIA	2	71
IIB	2	66
IIC	5	71
IIIA	3	47
IIIB	6	42
IIIC	42	33
IV	13	19

FIGO, International Federation of Gynecology and Obstetrics.
Adapted from Heintz APM, Odicino F, Maisonneuve P, et al.
Carcinoma of the ovary. FIGO 6th Annual Report on the Results of Treatment in Gynecological Cancer. *International Journal of Gynecology and Obstetrics* 2006;95 (Suppl 1):S161–S192, with permission.

Table 68.3	GENETIC ALTERATIONS IN INVASIVE EPITHELIAL OVARIAN CANCERS		
	Class	**Activation**	**Approximate Frequency (%)**
Hereditary			
BRCA1	DS DNA repair	Mutation/deletion	5
BRCA2	DS DNA repair	Mutation/deletion	3
MSH2	DNA mismatch repair	Mutation	1
Sporadic			
Oncogenes			
HER-2/*neu*	Tyrosine kinase	Overexpression	10
K-*ras*	G protein	Mutation	5
AKT2	Serine/threonine kinase	Amplification	10
c-*myc*	Transcription factor	Overexpression	20
Tumor suppressor genes			
p53	Tumor suppressor Transcription factor	Mutation/deletion Overexpression	60
p16	Tumor suppressor cdk inhibitor	Homozygous deletion	15

Available at: www.cancer.gov/cancertopics/factsheet/Therapy/targeted. Accessed June 6, 2007.

syndromes, linked to an increased risk for disease development, have been reported (85,86). BRCA1 and BRCA2 mutations are the most common mutations, with up to 90% of all hereditary cases of ovarian cancer being associated with a mutation of the BRCA1 gene, located on chromosome 17q21, and the BRCA2 gene, located on chromosome 13q22. The lifetime risk of ovarian cancer is approximately 45% in BRCA 1 mutation carriers and 25% in BRCA2 mutation carriers; therefore, oral contraceptives may serve as an effective chemopreventive strategy until prophylactic surgery can be performed (2). Stage, grade, histology, and results of primary surgery have been observed to be similar between the hereditary and sporadic groups, but the hereditary group has a significantly longer recurrence-free and overall survival after chemotherapy compared with the sporadic group (16).

Hereditary nonpolyposis colorectal syndrome, or Lynch type II cancer syndrome, is responsible for the remaining 10% of hereditary ovarian cancers. In this syndrome, mutations of DNA mismatch repair genes lead to an increased risk of colorectal cancer, stomach cancer, endometrial cancer, and ovarian cancer (87).

The recent discovery of the genetic mutations, BRCA1, BRCA2, HER-2/*neu*, c-*myc*, k-*ras*, and *p53*, have also been implicated in the development of many "hormone-dependent" tumors such as breast, ovarian, and other gynecologic malignancies (Table 68.3). Other genetic disorders have been linked with nonepithelial ovarian cancers. Peutz-Jeghers syndrome is associated with an increased risk of sex cord-stromal tumors; gonadal dysgenesis is associated with dysgerminomas and gonadoblastomas; and multiple nevoid basal cell carcinoma is associated with ovarian fibroma.

Exposure-Related

Environmental or physical causes of ovarian cancer have been investigated through case-control studies. Surveys of women in underdeveloped countries with low exposure to carcinogens have shown that they have a lower rate of development of ovarian cancers than those living in industrialized nations (63). To date, no specific chemical carcinogens have been directly linked to ovarian cancer. Chronic exposure to asbestos-related products, including talc products, have long been implicated in the development of ovarian cancer (76). Dietary and metabolic issues have also been raised as a possible contributory factor in disease development. Obesity, diets high in fat (especially saturated fats), and consumption of milk or meat products have shown a weak positive correlation to ovarian cancer. However, in a recent Swedish population-based cohort study of the effect of body mass index on cancer risk in more than 35,000 women, a 36% higher risk of cancer was observed in obese women (body mass index $\geq$30) relative to women with body mass index in the normal range (18.5 to 25); cancer sites most strongly related to obesity were endometrium, ovary (risk for top quartile 2.09, 1.13–4.13), and colon (83).

There has been no evidence to show that other previously suggested environmental factors, such as exposure to radiation (natural or iatrogenic), tranquilizing and hypnotic drugs, or infection, directly increase the risk of ovarian cancer. To date, there have been no consistent associations of coffee, tobacco,

Table 68.2	FACTORS INFLUENCING THE RISK FOR OVARIAN CANCER	
Factor	**Estimated Risk (%)**	**Estimated Relative Risk**
Baseline lifetime risk	1.4 to 1.8	1
Race		
White	13 per 100,000	—
African American	10 per 100,000	—
Risk factors		
Family history	9.4	5–7
BRCA1 mutation	30–40	18–29
BRCA2 mutation	27	16–19
Lynch II/HPNCC	10	6–7
Infertility	—	2–5
Nulliparity	—	2–3
Late menopause	—	1.5–2
Early menarche	—	1–1.5
Protective factors		
Multiparity	—	0.4–0.6
Oral contraceptive use		
X 4 yr	—	0.6
X 8 yr	—	0.5
X 12 yr	—	0.4
Hysterectomy or tubal ligation	—	0.4–0.6

HPNCC, hereditary nonpolyposis colorectal cancer.
Modified from Holschneider CH, Berek JS. Ovarian cancer: epidemiology, biology, and prognostic factors. *Semin Surg Oncol* 2000;19(1):3–10, requested from Wiley 6/6/07.

or alcohol consumption with an increased risk (141). Specifically, medications such as medroxyprogesterone acetate and tamoxifen have not conclusively been shown to be associated with an increased risk, although some have suggested that infertility agents, which increase the number of ovulations, may increase the risk (30).

Screening

The high mortality rate of ovarian cancer can be directly attributed to the fact that 75% of women will have stage III and IV disease at the time of diagnosis, which is associated with poor survival rates. This is compared with an 80% to 90% 5-year survival with stage I disease (Table 68.1). No routine screening test for ovarian cancer is currently recommended for the general population. Lack of a known premalignant condition, the low sensitivity and specificity of the available tests, and the low prevalence of the disease in the general population leads to a low positive predictive value.

Chu and Rubin (28) have provided a comprehensive review of screening for ovarian cancer in the general population. The screening armamentarium includes serum CA 125 and transvaginal ultrasound (TVUS) as the two major tests, either alone or in combination. CA 125 is a high-molecular mucin that can be expressed by tissues derived from coelomic epithelium (pleura, pericardium, peritoneum) and müllerian epithelium (endometrial, cervical, tubal). CA 125 >35 U/mL was observed in 80% of patients with epithelial ovarian cancer and 90% of patients with advanced stage, but in only 50% of early-stage patients. CA 125 is nonspecific for ovarian cancer as it can be elevated in benign gynecologic and nongynecologic conditions as well as nongynecologic cancers.

In the University of Kentucky Ovarian Cancer Screening Program of 13,000 women 25 to 91 years of age undergoing annual TVUS, Pavlik et al. (105) observed that ovarian volume persistently >20 cm^3 in premenopausal women and 10 cm^3 in postmenopausal women warrants further investigation. In a study of more than 9,000 women for whom two or more serial samples were available from a large prospective ovarian cancer screening study, Skates et al. (128) noted that calculation of the risk of ovarian cancer from serial CA 125 significantly improves screening performance compared with a fixed cutoff for CA 125 for preclinical detection in postmenopausal women. Results from two large screening trials designed to assess reduction in mortality with early detection of ovarian cancer are awaiting long-term follow-up. The Prostate, Lung, Colorectal, and Ovarian Cancer (PLCO) Screening trial in United States has accrued 74,000 women. A CA 125 level elevation and an abnormal ultrasound improved the positive predictive value to 23.5% (22). A second trial, United Kingdom Collaborative Trial of Ovarian Cancer Screening, testing the value of TVUS and serum CA 125 compared with a control group without these screening tests, had accrued 200,000 postmenopausal women from the general population, with the results pending follow-up during the next 7 years (73).

Present data do not support routine screening for the general population. Women at high risk for ovarian cancer with BRCA 1 or 2 mutations, or hereditary nonpolyposis colorectal syndrome, could potentially benefit from chemoprevention, screening with annual pelvic examinations, TVUS, and CA 125 on a biannual or annual basis or prophylactic surgery; however, efficacy of such measures is unknown (19).

Natural History

Ovarian tissue is composed of embryonic yolk sac cells that give rise to the ova or germ cells, stromal cells that produce the steroid hormones, and the mesothelium that provides the epithelial covering for the follicle cysts. These respectively give rise to germ cell tumors, sex cord stromal tumors, and the epithelial tumors of the ovary. Ovarian cancer is an insidious disease with no early symptoms from its growth, nonspecific abdominal complaints during the early stages, leading to >70% of ovarian cancer patients presenting with advanced stage disease (Table 68.1).

Primary mode of spread is transperitoneal metastases as malignant cells exfoliate in the peritoneal cavity. Intraperitoneal spread is favored by intestinal peristalsis, negative hydrostatic pressure below the diaphragm, and the passage of exfoliated tumor cells that follow the intra-abdominal fluid stream passing along the paracolic gutters toward the diaphragm, more so on the right side (109,142). The lymphatic capillaries of the ovary converge on the hilus and follow the ovarian blood vessels to drain to the lumbar para-aortic nodes and also drain along the broad ligament to the hypogastric and external iliac nodes in the pelvis. Less frequently, the spread can occur to the inguinal nodes via the round ligament. Transdiaphragmatic spread occurs to the pleural cavity (142).

Autopsy findings have revealed involvement of pelvic nodes in 80% of all cases, para-aortic nodes in 78%, inguinal nodes in 40%, mediastinal nodes in 50%, and supraclavicular nodes in 48% (12). Metastases can be found in the uterus or contralateral ovary from peritoneal spread or flow through the fallopian tubes. Tumor can adhere to any surface of the peritoneum and dense tumor "caking" can cause infiltration into all abdominal organs and a mass effect on the omentum, ureter, bowel, liver, pancreas, spleen, and adrenals, resulting in advanced disease stages at presentation with associated ascites. Extra-abdominal spread is less common. Reed et al. (113) have noted a change in the pattern of disease spread at autopsy in patients treated after 1972 in that there was a higher proportion of patients with disease found in liver parenchyma, lung pleura, and the pericardium and a higher incidence of metastases to the adrenal glands, thoracic nodes, bladder, and liver parenchyma in patients who had received cisplatin as part of their initial treatment regimen.

Clinical Presentation

As ovarian cancer has insidious growth and is asymptomatic in the early stage, most women do not present for diagnosis until symptoms arise from disease progression to stage III or IV disease (Table 68.1). Vague gastrointestinal complaints of dyspepsia, nausea, early satiety, bloating, constipation, or obstipation are common presenting symptoms, as are genitourinary symptoms including frequency, urgency, or incontinence. These nonspecific symptoms can be present for several months but do not trigger diagnostic evaluation until after the symptoms fail to clear with other medical therapy (154). Detection of early-stage disease can occur by palpation of an asymptomatic adnexal mass on routine examination. However, most adnexal masses require moderate size for palpation. In premenopausal women, most of these masses are not malignant, and ovarian cancer represents fewer than 5% of adnexal neoplasms. An adnexal mass in a postmenopausal woman has a higher likelihood of malignancy, and surgical exploration is usually indicated (1).

Diagnostic Work-Up

Evaluation of a pelvic mass will be influenced by patient's age, clinical presentation, and imaging features. Ovarian mass is more likely to be a malignant neoplasm in the pediatric, peri-, and postmenopausal age groups, and benign during the reproductive years. Ultrasound supplements the pelvic examination in the initial evaluation of pelvic mass. PLCO trial guidelines recommend further evaluation for any ovary or cyst with volume $>10 \text{ cm}^3$, any solid area, or papillary projection extending into the cavity of cystic ovarian tumor of any size, and any mixed solid/cystic component within a cystic ovarian tumor of any size (22).

CA 125 is elevated in approximately 80% of all epithelial ovarian tumors and has a half-life of approximately 20 days. More than 90% of advanced ovarian cancer will have elevated CA 125 and 50% of stage I patients may have normal CA 125. Higher levels may suggest more advanced or greater bulk of disease, but CA 125 level is a weak predictor of surgical resection (95). Although limited as a screening tool, rising CA 125 can serve as an early marker of disease recurrence. CA 125 half-life and CA 125 nadir during induction chemotherapy are independent predictors of epithelial ovarian cancer outcome (114). Human chorionic gonadotropin (β-hCG), α-fetoprotein (AFP), total inhibin and lactate dehydrogenase levels may aid in the diagnosis and treatment of nonepithelial ovarian tumors.

Thus, in a patient suspected to have ovarian malignancy, a thorough history and full physical and pelvic examination, serologic (complete blood count, chemistries, CA 125, carcinoembryonic antigen, CA 19-9), and imaging evaluations (abdominal computed tomography/magnetic resonance imaging, directed ultrasound, chest x-ray) should be considered. Further evaluations with mammography, upper gastrointestinal endoscopy, or colonoscopy are frequently indicated. Comorbid conditions may prompt additional evaluations, including cardiac risk assessment, pulmonary function testing, and nutritional evaluation.

Other conditions can mimic ovarian cancer in their presentation, including colon, gastric, and appendicial carcinomas as well as metastatic breast cancer and primary lymphoma. Although it would be to be able to determine the primary site of disease in the preoperative setting, the diagnosis often cannot be made accurately until the time of surgery, and frozen section pathologic evaluation can guide surgical approach.

Pathologic Classification

The World Health Organization and International Federation of Gynecologists and Obstetricians (FIGO) adopted a unified classification of the common epithelial, germ cell, sex cord, and stromal tumors (Table 68.4) (123). The majority of ovarian malignancies, 65% to 70%, are epithelial, with germ cell tumors (25%), sex cord stromal (5%), and metastases to the ovary (5%) accounting for the remainder.

Serous tumors are most common, comprising 40% to 50% of epithelial tumors. The other subtypes include mucinous carcinoma, 10% to 15%; endometrioid carcinoma, 15%; undifferentiated carcinoma, 15% to 20%; clear cell carcinoma, 3% to 5%; and transitional 3% to 5%. Clinically, the mucinous tumors can be very large and can be associated with mucinous tumors of the appendix; therefore, appendectomy is recommended, particularly if the tumor is right-sided. The transitional cell tumors, Brenner tumors, are benign in the majority of cases (98%) with favorable prognosis. Conversely, clear cell carcinoma patients are noted to have a different clinical behavior compared with those with serous adenocarcinoma. Although more likely to be stage I, clear cell carcinoma histology is associated with lower response rate to platinum-based chemotherapy, higher recurrence rate, and poorer survival (136).

Serous tumors appear nodular with multiple papillary projections and contain cysts filled with clear serous fluid. Mucinous cancers are usually filled with large pockets of thick, often necrotic, mucinous debris. These closely resemble mucin-secreting tumors originating from other areas of the body.

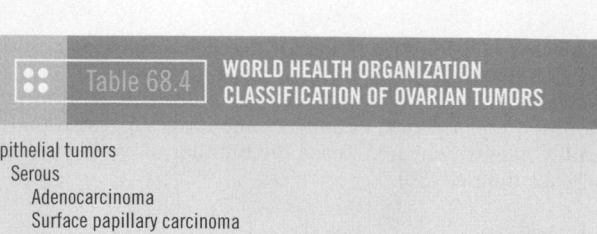

Table 68.4 WORLD HEALTH ORGANIZATION CLASSIFICATION OF OVARIAN TUMORS

Epithelial tumors
  Serous
    Adenocarcinoma
    Surface papillary carcinoma
    Adenocarcinofibroma (malignant adenofibroma)
  Mucinous
    Adenocarcinoma
    Adenocarcinofibroma (malignant adenofibroma)
    Mucinous cystic tumor with mural nodules
    Mucinous cystic tumor with pseudomyxoma peritonei
  Endometroid
    Adenocarcinoma NOS
    Adenocarcinofibroma (malignant adenofibroma)
    Malignant mullerian mixed tumor (carcinosarcoma)
    Adenosarcoma
    Endometroid stromal sarcoma
    Undifferentiated ovarian carcinoma
  Clear cell carcinoma
    Adenocarcinoma
    Adenocarcinofibroma (malignant adenofibroma)
  Transitional cell carcinoma
  Squamous cell tumors
  Mixed epithelial tumors
  Undifferentiated and unclassified tumors
Germ Cell Tumors
  Dysgerminoma
  Endodermal sinus tumor
  Embryonal carcinoma
  Polyembryoma
  Choriocarcinoma
  Teratoma
    Immature
    Mature
      Solid
      Cystic
      Dermoid cyst with malignant transformation
      Monodermal
  Mixed
Tumors composed of germ cells and sex cord-stromal derivative
  Gonadoblastoma
  Mixed germ cell-sex cord-stromal tumor
Sex cord tumors
  Granulosa-stromal cell tumors
    Granulosa cell tumor
    Adult type
    Juvenile type
    Thecoma-fibroma group
    Thecoma
    Fibroma-fibrosarcoma
    Sclerosing stromal tumor
  Sertoli-stromal cell tumors
    Sertoli-cell tumor
    Leydig-cell tumor
    Sertoli-Leydig cell tumor
Sex cord tumor with annular tubules
Steroid-cell tumors
  Stromal luteoma
  Leydig-cell tumor
  Steroid-cell tumor not otherwise specified
Unclassified
Gynandroblastoma

NOS, not otherwise specified.

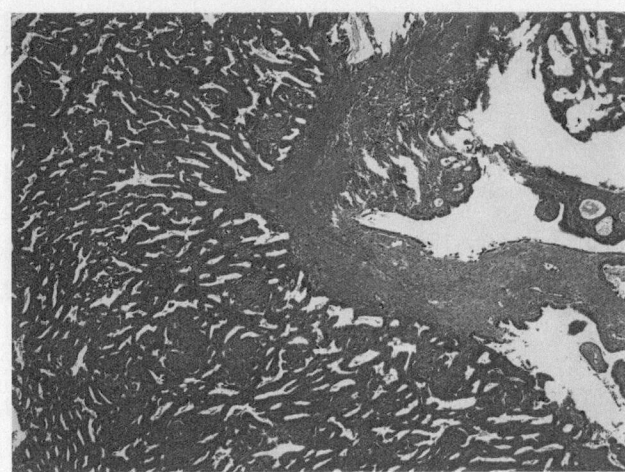

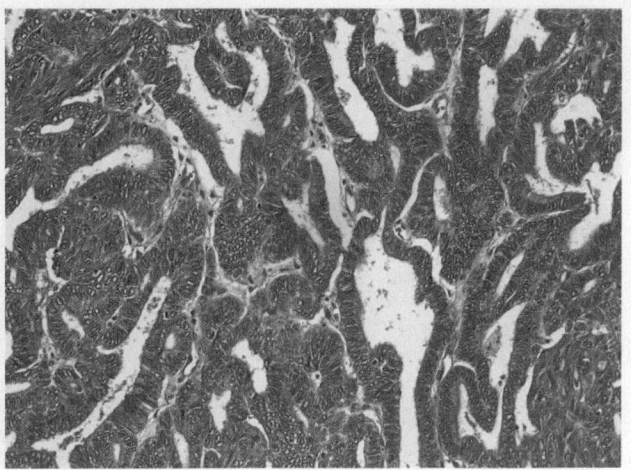

FIGURE 68.1. Endometrioid adenocarcinoma of the ovary. **A:** At low power, note the presence of a tumor composed of back-to-back endometrioid glands. **B:** At high power, note the presence of squamous metaplasia, commonly present in this epithelial variant. Assignment of tumor grade is based on similar criteria as for carcinomas arising in the endometrium. This tumor would qualify as well differentiated or grade 1.

Pseudomyxoma peritonei almost never results from a ruptured primary ovarian mucinous neoplasm, but often produces secondary borderlinelike ovarian tumors with prominent pseudomyxoma ovarii (66). Clear cell carcinoma is characterized by clear and hobnail cells. Bilateral presentation occurs frequently in epithelial tumors, 30% for serous tumors, 5% to 10% for mucinous tumors, and 15% for endometrioid tumors.

Synchronous primary cancers of the endometrium and ovary are found in 10% of women with ovarian cancer and 5% of women with endometrial cancer (131). They have a good prognosis, particularly when the disease is microscopically limited to the uterus and ovary or is of low histologic grade (158).

Tumors are graded on the basis of their degree of differentiation, and grade is independently associated with prognosis, as the 5-year survival for grade 1 tumors exceeds 90% and it is 70% for grade 3 tumors. Grade 1 tumors are well differentiated, resembling the normal tissues and retaining their glandular appearance, while the grade 2 and 3 tumors have increasing components of solid tumor areas and less glandular areas (Fig. 68.1).

LMP or borderline tumors have nuclear abnormalities and mitotic activity intermediate between benign and malignant tumors of similar cell type, but lack stromal invasion; they are a subcategory of ovarian malignancies that account for 15% to 20% of all epithelial neoplasms (Fig. 68.2) (64). The prognosis, surgical approach, and postoperative treatment recommendations are vastly different as compared with those of their invasive counterparts. The majority of LMPs (75%) present with stage I disease, which directly contrasts with the 75% advanced stages in the invasive epithelial tumors. The 5- and 10-year survival rates for women with LMP tumors were >95%. Nonlocalized LMP tumors of the ovary have decreased survival compared with the localized LMP tumors, but is similar to the survival of women with localized, well-differentiated epithelial ovarian carcinoma (127).

Ovarian germ cell tumors comprise fewer than 5% of ovarian malignancies and are classified by the World Health Organization (Table 68.4). Dysgerminoma are the most common of the germ cell tumors and occurs bilaterally in 10% to 20% of cases, and the other germ cell tumors are typically unilateral. Endodermal sinus tumors, also known as *yolk sac tumors,* are characterized by Schiller-Duvall bodies (Fig. 68.3). Embryonal carcinomas are rare and tend to occur in a younger populations; they can be seen with nongestational choriocarcinomas

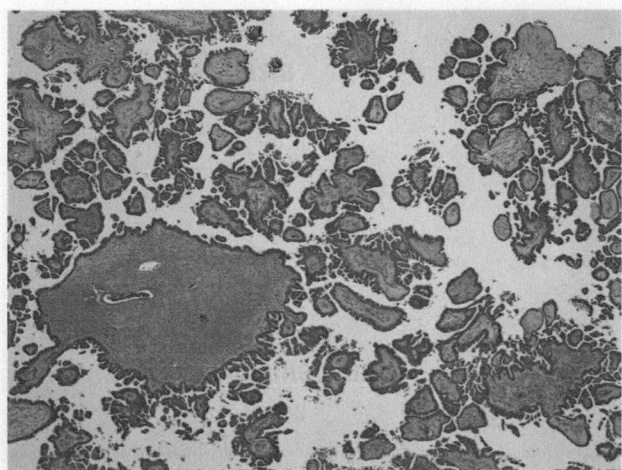

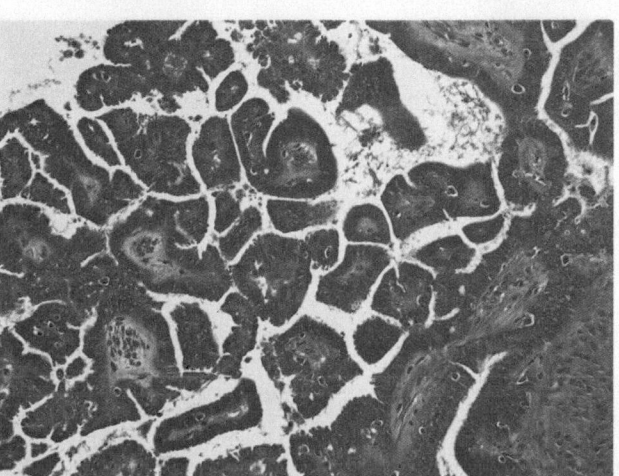

FIGURE 68.2. Serous tumor of low malignant potential of the ovary at **(A)** low power and **(B)** high power. At low power, note the presence of the progressively branching papillary fronds with fibrovascular support and detached papillary clusters; at high power note the serous epithelium with nuclear hyperchromasia and cytologic atypia. By definition, there is no destructive stromal invasion present.

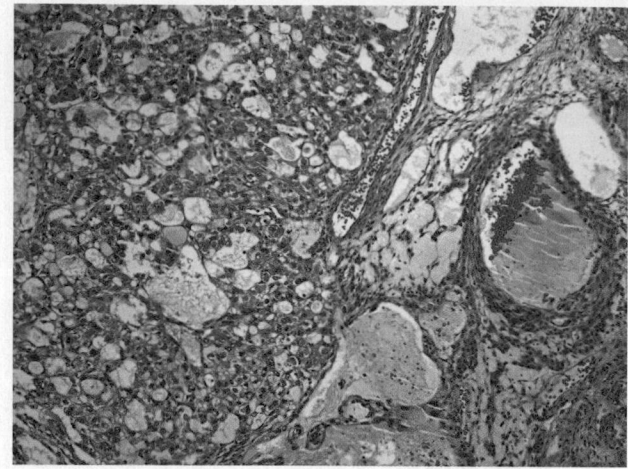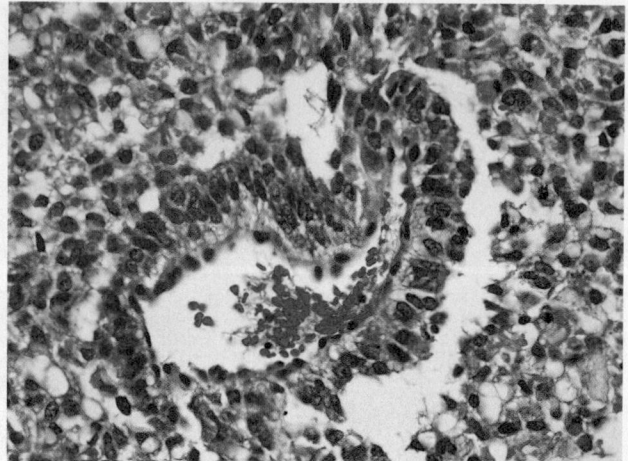

FIGURE 68.3. Yolk sac (endodermal sinus) tumor of the ovary at **(A)** low power and **(B)** high power. Yolk sac tumors are primitive germ cell tumors that may manifest any of a number of architectural patterns. In this example, note, at low power, the reticular pattern, and at high power, the presence of endodermal sinus structures (Schiller-Duval bodies) as well as prominent intracytoplasmic eosinophilic globules. These tumors are characteristically immunoreactive for α-fetoprotein.

as part of a mixed germ cell tumors (10% of all germ cell tumors). Immature teratomas are characterized by immature elements form the germ layers. The grade, treatment recommendations, and outcome are directed by the amount of immature neural elements (Fig. 68.4).

Sex cord-stromal tumors are also classified by the World Health Organization (Table 68.4), with granulosa cell tumors being the most common (70%). Histologically, the granulosa cell tumors are composed of granulosa cells that have a pale, grooved, "coffee bean" nuclei (Fig. 68.4) or a rosette of cells surrounding eosinophilic fluid, a Call-Exner body (Fig. 68.4). Thecomas (hormonally active) and fibromas (hormonally inactive) are both clinically benign tumors and are most common in middle-age women.

Metastases to the ovary pose a challenge in distinguishing them from primary ovarian cancer (65). Most commonly, the primary site is from the digestive organs, uterus, or breast. Krukenberg tumors are metastases to the ovary from gastric cancer and typically have signet ring cells. In addition to the intraoperative findings, immunohistochemical methods can be helpful in identifying the likely primary for further evaluation.

⁑ Treatment

Surgical advances in staging and therapeutic benefit of maximum resection of tumor burden, response to platinum-based, multiagent chemotherapy that includes taxanes, intraperitoneal (IP) delivery mode, and development of chemotherapy for recurrent cancer have improved progression-free and overall survival of patients with ovarian cancer in the past 2 decades.

Surgical Staging and Debulking

Traditional staging for ovarian cancer is based on the FIGO staging system (Table 68.5) (4). A parallel American Joint Committee on Cancer system of TNM staging also exists, with strong correlations between stage and prognostic value of these substages (69).

For both early- and advanced-stage ovarian cancer, surgery is the mainstay of diagnosis and initial treatment and this can be accomplished via laparotomy or via minimally invasive techniques (laparoscopy, robotic assistance). Gynecologic Cancer Intergroup Ovarian Cancer Consensus Conference (2004)

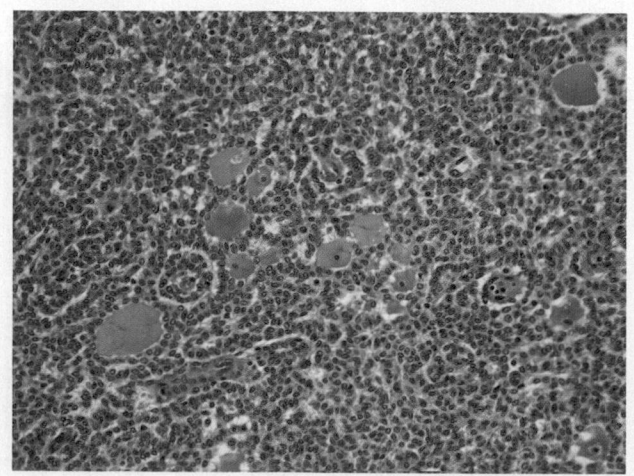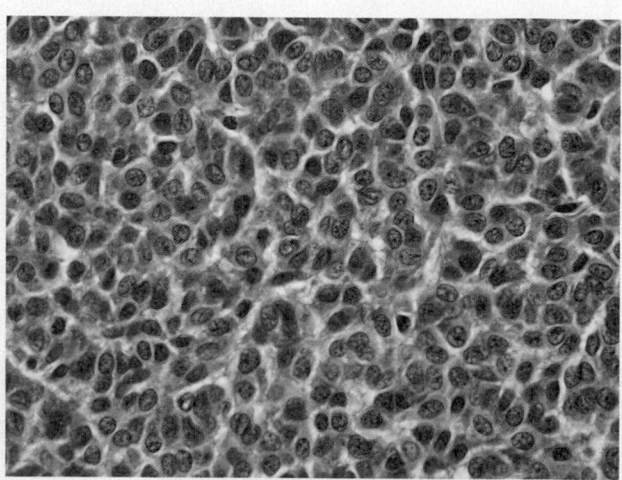

FIGURE 68.4. Granulosa cell tumor of the ovary. **A:** At low power, note a proliferation of sex cord (gonadal) stromal cells forming solid and microfollicular patterns with Call-Exner bodies containing hyaline material. **B:** At high power, the cells show a high nuclear: cytoplasmic ratio, with a degree of optical clearing of the nuclei and presence of nuclear grooves ("coffee bean" nuclei).

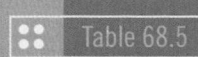

Table 68.5	FIGO STAGING FOR OVARIAN CARCINOMA

Stage I Growth limited to the ovaries
  Ia Growth limited to one ovary; no ascites present containing malignant cells. No tumor on the external surface; capsule intact
  Ib Growth limited to both ovaries; no ascites present containing malignant cells. No tumor on the external surfaces; capsules intact
  Ic Tumor either stage Ia or Ib, but with tumor on surface of one or both ovaries, or with capsule ruptured, or with ascites present containing malignant cells, or with positive peritoneal washings

Stage II Growth involving one or both ovaries with pelvic extension
  IIa Extension and/or metastases to the uterus and/or tubes
  IIb Extension to other pelvic tissues
  IIc Tumor either stage IIa or IIb, but with tumor on surface of one or both ovaries, or with ascites present containing malignant cells, or with positive peritoneal washings

Stage III Tumor involving one or both ovaries with histologically confirmed peritoneal implants outside the pelvis and/or positive retroperitoneal or inguinal nodes. Superficial liver metastases equals stage III. Tumor is limited to the true pelvis, but with histologically proven malignant extension to small bowel or omentum
  IIIa Tumor grossly limited to the true pelvis, with negative nodes, but with histologically confirmed microscopic seeding of abdominal peritoneal surfaces, or histologically proven extension to small bowel or mesentery
  IIIb Tumor of one or both ovaries with histologically confirmed implants, peritoneal metastases of abdominal peritoneal surfaces none exceeding 2 cm in diameter; nodes are negative
  IIIc Peritoneal metastases beyond the pelvis >2 cm in diameter and/or positive retroperitoneal or inguinal nodes

Stage IV Growth involving one or both ovaries with distant metastases. If pleural effusion is present, there must be positive cytology to allot a case to stage IV. Parenchymal liver metastases equals stage IV.

FIGO, International Federation of Gynecology and Obstetrics.
Available at http://www.figo.org/docs/staging_booklet_pdf. Accessed June 6, 2007.

recommends that tissue should be obtained for histopathologic diagnosis, staging should follow the FIGO guidelines, upfront maximal cytoreduction with the goal of no residual disease should be undertaken, and when primary cytoreductive surgery is not possible, it should be considered after three to five cycles of chemotherapy in patients who do not have progressive disease (46). Recommendation was also made for the surgery to be undertaken by an appropriately trained surgeon with experience in management of ovarian cancer.

The goals of surgery are complete staging and maximal cytoreduction of advanced stage disease (optimal, <1 cm residual; suboptimal, >1 cm residual). In select cases, preservation of the contralateral "unaffected" ovary and the uterus can be achieved in young women wishing to retain fertility and who have the germ cell and sex cord-stromal tumors. Surgical staging includes peritoneal washings and collection of any ascitic fluid for cytology, total hysterectomy, bilateral salpingo-oophorectomy, systematic biopsies (bladder serosa, anterior and posterior cul de sac, paracolic gutters, diaphragm scraping, omentectomy, and any suspicious adhesions or tissues), and performance of pelvic and para-aortic nodal dissection. Optimal cytoreduction has been correlated with survival (25). Bowel resection, diaphragm stripping, splenectomy, nodal dissection, and radical resection of peritoneal tumor nodules are often necessary to achieve the desired surgical outcome. Even in cases of unilateral disease, bilateral lymph node dissection should be carried out because contralateral nodal involvement can be present. Recently, the role of routine appendectomy has been questioned and is not recommended in the absence of visible pathology (112). Surgical advances and experience have led to an increase in the rates of laparoscopy for staging and therapy and a decrease in the morbidity associated with these procedures (121).

Prognostic Factors

Table 68.1 shows the poor survival rates with increasing stage. Volume of residual tumor after primary surgery strongly correlates with survival (69,70). It is unclear whether the degree of debulking that can be achieved depends on the intrinsic biologic behavior of the tumor or is truly an independent prognostic factor. Histologic grade is of a particular importance for early-stage

disease. Survival rates for stage I disease with grade 1, 2, or 3 tumors are 96%, 78%, and 62%, respectively (24).

The prognostic significance of histologic subtype of malignant epithelial ovarian neoplasms has not been definitively demonstrated. Histology does reflect degrees of differentiation, tumor burden, and stage at presentation. Patients with mucinous and endometrioid cancers are reported to have a higher survival rate. This may be because of an earlier stage at diagnosis and more frequent presentation with a well-differentiated histologic type. Clear cell carcinomas appear to be more aggressive than other epithelial malignancies. The 5-year survival rate for stage I clear cell carcinoma is 60%, and for other stages it is <15% (136).

Extent of successful cytoreductive surgery is considered one of the major prognostic indicators in ovarian cancer therapy (25).

Management of Epithelial Tumors

Treatments for ovarian cancer depend largely on the stage and grade of disease at presentation. Table 68.6 presents a general

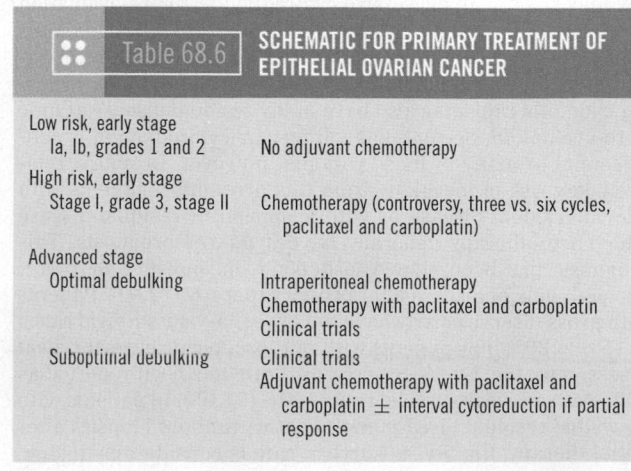

Table 68.6	SCHEMATIC FOR PRIMARY TREATMENT OF EPITHELIAL OVARIAN CANCER
Low risk, early stage	
Ia, Ib, grades 1 and 2	No adjuvant chemotherapy
High risk, early stage	
Stage I, grade 3, stage II	Chemotherapy (controversy, three vs. six cycles, paclitaxel and carboplatin)
Advanced stage	
Optimal debulking	Intraperitoneal chemotherapy
	Chemotherapy with paclitaxel and carboplatin
	Clinical trials
Suboptimal debulking	Clinical trials
	Adjuvant chemotherapy with paclitaxel and carboplatin ± interval cytoreduction if partial response

schematic for treatment recommendations for women with epithelial ovarian cancer.

Cytoreductive Surgery

For the majority of patients, conservative or limited surgery is not an option. Aggressive and thorough debulking of a primary tumor mass or diffuse disease in the abdominal cavity directly corresponds with patient outcome. Cytoreduction can be performed at various times in the treatment course. Surgical debulking may occur during initial management before adjuvant therapy (primary cytoreduction), after several cycles of chemotherapy (interval cytoreduction), or after all adjuvant therapy is completed (secondary cytoreduction).

As a basic premise of adjuvant chemotherapy, treatment of the smallest tumor volume possible is ideal. Several studies support the optimization of tumor cytoreduction in the clinical setting. In a report by Griffiths et al. (60), patients who had surgical cytoreduction before adjuvant therapy were found to have survival rates identical to those who presented with low volumes of disease at surgical staging. A randomized study by Young et al. (156) confirmed that optimally debulked tumors were more likely to attain a complete clinical response with postoperative chemotherapy. Residual disease larger than 2 cm was the only independent adverse prognostic factor, confirming indirectly that debulking alone can affect survival, independent of adjuvant therapy (70). Gynecologic Oncology Group (GOG) 52 and GOG 97 re-examined the impact of residual tumor diameter on survival in various stages of disease. In these reports, only the ability to surgically to reduce residual tumor volume below 2 cm in diameter affected overall survival (69,70).

Secondary Surgery

Failure to achieve optimal cytoreduction at initial surgery may be overcome with interval cytoreduction. A randomized trial by the European Organization for Research and Treatment of Cancer showed an increase in median and overall survival when the primary debulking procedure was performed after three cycles of platinum-based chemotherapy, and followed by three additional cycles of chemotherapy (143). However, a large GOG trial including 550 women who were randomized to either surgery or additional chemotherapy (paclitaxel and cisplatin) if there were no progression after three cycles of chemotherapy, failed to show a benefit in the cohort who underwent interval cytoreduction. This maybe secondary to the chemotherapy agents used, in that the GOG trial used a taxane and the European Organization for Research and Treatment of Cancer trial used cyclophosphamide, which is not as effective an agent.

Second-look laparotomy after definitive systemic chemotherapy may require an aggressive cytoreduction. On re-evaluation after chemotherapy, reports suggest that 20% to 50% of patients may have residual disease undetectable on physical examination and clinical evaluation. Up to one third of patients receiving chemotherapy may also have bulky residual disease at time of re-evaluation. Second-look surgery or cytoreduction is controversial in many of these patients, however. Despite a relatively low risk of morbidity from this procedure, patients with known residual disease or with suspicion of residual disease after chemotherapy generally have a poorer prognosis. This prognosis has been shown to depend on and directly correlate with bulk of disease after primary therapy (72,91). Patients with gross disease clearly have the lowest 5-year survival rates, at 15% to 20%. For patients with microscopic disease at repeat assessment, the 2- to 3-year survival rate has been reported as 60%, with a 5-year survival rate of 50% (31,68). In patients with no visible residual disease and negative random biopsies after initial therapy, the 5-year survival rate is considerably higher,

but as many as one-third relapse within that 60-month interval (69). Podratz and Cliby (110) found no difference in survival rates between patients with disease smaller or larger than 0.5 cm. Thus, based on the limited utility of this procedure, "second-look" evaluations for the purposes of determining therapy (not for the purposes of interval cytoreduction) should be reserved for women in clinical trials that mandate this procedure.

Clearly, time to recurrence and "platinum and taxane" sensitivity have been used to determine the potential response to subsequent therapy and survival, and this needs to be weighed when considering "debulking" in a woman with recurrent disease.

Intravenous Chemotherapy for Epithelial Ovarian Carcinoma

Numerous studies suggest that patients with low-risk, low-grade, early-stage disease do not require adjuvant therapy after definitive surgery has been performed. However, this is a small percent of the women who present with epithelial ovarian cancer, and in all other women, surgery alone is not curative. Current chemotherapy has evolved following clinical trials with multiple single agents, combinations, and schedules, leading to current use of platinum-based chemotherapy and taxanes.

Cisplatin has been used extensively in both single-agent and multidrug trials. In multiple trials, the cisplatin and cyclophosphamide combination has demonstrated clinical response rates of approximately 40% to 60%. A meta-analysis of 45 trials comparing platinum-based chemotherapy programs after initial surgery for advanced disease concluded that platinum compounds offer improved survival rates over nonplatinum regimens (3). This review also incorporated data from 11 trials that directly compared carboplatin and cisplatin, either as single agents or in combinations with other drugs, that suggested no difference in efficacy between the two agents. The Southwest Oncology Group and the National Cancer Institute of Canada both published randomized trials directly comparing cisplatin with carboplatin, each with cyclophosphamide. No difference in survival was seen between the agents in either study, but carboplatin clearly has lower treatment-related side effects including less nephrotoxicity, neurotoxicity and emetogenic potential (6,45). However, carboplatin does have more associated myelosuppression, primarily thrombocytopenia.

Dose-escalation trials of platinum-based agents have also been examined. The Scottish Trial randomly assigned patients with stage IC to IV disease to receive either standard cisplatin (50 mg/m^2) and cyclophosphamide (750 mg/m^2) or high-dose cisplatin (100 mg/m^2) and cyclophosphamide. The increased dosing offered a significant improvement in survival over the standard dosing regimen (75). The GOG randomly assigned standard or high-intensity cisplatin and cyclophosphamide to patients with stage III and IV disease (93). Each arm received the same total dose with no significant difference in complete response rate or survival. A significantly higher rate of toxicity was reported in the modified dosing arm. Other trials discount an increasing dose intensity for patients with advanced disease (93). However, one prospective trial in platinum pretreated women showed no improvement in survival for women in the higher paclitaxel (225 mg/m^2) group as compared with the standard (175 mg/m^2) group (89,103).

◆◆ Early-Stage Disease

In a GOG study, patients with grade 3 tumors and extension beyond the ovarian capsule or into the abdominal wall or peritoneum (stage IC or II) demonstrated a relapse rate of 20%

to 40%. In addition, Memorial Sloan-Kettering Cancer Center reviewed 62 patients with high-risk stage I disease randomized to receive platinum-based adjuvant chemotherapy. They reported that 24% of patients had relapsed by 40 months. Patients with grade 3 tumors had a relapse rate of 40% compared with 8% for those with grades 1 or 2 disease (11,90). For these reasons, patients with stage IC disease and high-risk features (i.e., high grade, clear cell histology, dense adherence, ruptured capsule, intraoperative rupture, large-volume ascites, positive peritoneal washings, or tumor on the ovarian surface) are recommended for adjuvant therapy to improve treatment response.

Bolis et al. (14) investigated role of cisplatin in stage I ovarian cancer patients. Trial I compared cisplatin with no further therapy in FIGO stage Ia and b, grade II-III patients; trial II compared cisplatin to ^{32}phosporous (^{32}P) in Ia2 and b2, and Ic patients. Cisplatin significantly reduced the relapse rate by 65% in trial I and 61% in trial II. Survival was not significantly different. International Collaborative Ovarian Neoplasm 1 and Adjuvant ChemoTherapy in Ovarian Neoplasm in early-stage ovarian cancer compared platinum-based adjuvant chemotherapy with observation following surgery. Overall survival at 5 years was 82% in the chemotherapy arm and 74% in the observation arm (140).

The GOG is currently conducting trials to determine the length of time that women with surgical stage I disease need to remain taking chemotherapy. A randomized prospective trial showed no benefits to six cycles of taxane and platinum-based chemotherapy as opposed to three cycles (97,104). A consolidation trial is being conducted in women with early-stage disease (GOG 175).

Advanced-Stage Disease

In addition to platinum, taxanes have become a cornerstone of the treatment schemas designed for women with epithelial ovarian cancer. McGuire et al. (94) reported a 30% response rate with paclitaxel in patients with advanced disease. The GOG randomized trial (GOG 111) comparing cisplatin and paclitaxel with cisplatin and cyclophosphamide reported a response rate of 59% versus 40%, respectively (93). Complete clinical response rates were 51% and 31%, respectively. An increase in the progression-free interval was seen in the paclitaxel arm of 18 versus 13 months. The GOG study for advanced stage III or IV disease with suboptimal resection compared cisplatin (100 mg/m^2), 24-hour infusion of paclitaxel (200 mg/m^2), or paclitaxel (135 mg/m^2) and cisplatin (75 mg/m^2) in 614 patients (100). Combined therapy produced improved results over either single-agent arm (67% vs. 42% overall response rate), with lower cumulative toxicity.

Currently, the cooperative groups are evaluating different regimens of intravenous chemotherapy, including sequential doublets, triplets, combining standard chemotherapeutics agents with biologics (bevacizumab) and consolidative strategies.

Intraperitoneal Chemotherapy

Because of the unique IP dissemination of epithelial ovarian cancer, there has been a significant interest in evaluating IP administration of chemotherapy. The National Cancer Institute published a consensus statement in 2006 stating that IP chemotherapy should be offered to every women with optimally debulked advanced-stage ovarian cancer based on the GOG study published by Armstrong et al. (9) showing a progression-free and overall survival benefit to IP chemotherapy as compared with intravenous therapy alone (23.6 vs. 18.3 months, and 65.6 vs. 49.7 months, respectively).

Recurrent Ovarian Cancer

Chemotherapy

Recurrent ovarian cancer can be subdivided into two broad categories, early or late. Patients who experience an early recurrence are those who either progress during initial induction chemotherapy or who recur <6 months after the completion of their initial chemotherapy and are considered "platinum- and taxane-resistant," with low likelihood of cure. Women who suffer an early recurrence do have options, including several Food and Drug Administration-approved "second-line" agents (topotecan, liposomal doxorubicin, gemcitabine, hexamethylmelamine, ifosfamide, docetaxel), hormonal therapies, targeted therapeutics (antiangiogenics), and the opportunity to participate in clinical trials. For women with a late recurrence, retreatment with platinum and taxanes is a reasonable option, and the longer the disease-free interval, the higher the response rate to the agents. Women with platinum-sensitive disease may also be offered treatment with second-line agents, with higher response rates being seen as compared with those women with platinum-resistant disease. With the exception of those women who have a prolonged disease-free interval, the opportunity for a meaningful second remission is low, and one needs to carefully balance quality of life, chemotherapy-related toxicity, cost, and patient wishes.

Palliative Surgery

There are controversies surrounding the benefits of secondary surgery as one needs to weigh the risks of the procedures against the potential gains. Secondary debulking procedures with intent at prolonging disease-free interval and survival needs to be considered in a different category than truly palliative surgery. Because ovarian cancer typically recurs in the peritoneal cavity with low propensity for metastatic disease in other areas, women will often experience bowel complications while otherwise enjoying a reasonable quality of life. The most common site of intestinal obstruction is the small intestine (44%), followed by the large intestine (33%) and a combination of both areas in 22% of women (118). If surgery cannot be performed (patient performance status, patient medical condition, extent of disease), percutaneous decompression and intravenous hydration with consideration of palliative chemotherapy and/or hospice referral may be appropriate.

Adjuvant Radiation Therapy Studies for Epithelial Ovarian Carcinoma

Radiation therapy is not currently used in the adjuvant treatment of epithelial ovarian carcinomas, but may have a role in salvage or palliative treatment in select cases. Early studies by GOG and others (5,41,77,146,156) have identified a small subgroup of early-disease patients with *stage IA-B with grade 1 or 2 tumors* who have a low risk of relapse and do not require adjuvant therapy. A study by the Ovarian Tumor Study Group showed no significant differences in relapse or survival rates at 7 years between 81 patients with stages IA-B, grade 1 or 2 disease, who received either oral melphalan or no postoperative treatment (156).

A statement at the National Institutes of Health Consensus Conference in 1995 stated that high-risk patients with stage I and poorly differentiated, stage IC, and II tumors have

| Table 68.7 | RANDOMIZED STUDIES OF ADJUVANT WHOLE ABDOMINAL RADIATION IN HIGH-RISK EARLY STAGE OVARIAN CANCER |

Trial	Stage	Study Design	N	5-Yr OS%		Bowel Obstruction%		Notes
				WAI	CTX	WAI	CTX	
WAI versus CTX + pelvic RT								
PMH (2,14)	IB, II, III asymptomatic	WAI	76	58 overall	41 overall	–	–	No complete surgical staging, benefit seen only in gross total resection patients
		Pelvic RT +/- chlorambucil	71	78[a] GTR	51 GTR			
NCIC (3)	I, IIA-B, IIIO	Melphalan WAI	106 107	62	61	15 overall 12 required surgery	10 overall 7 required surgery	*All received prior pelvic RT*
		^{32}P	44[b]					
DACOVA (15)	IB-C, II	WAI	60	63 (4-yr)	55 (4-yr)	8 required surgery	5 required surgery	More stage I in WAI group
		Pelvic RT + cyclophosphamide	58					
WAI versus CTX								
MDACC (17)	I-III < 2 cm residual disease	WAI Melphalan	51 57	71	72	14 required surgery	–	No complete surgical staging, WAI moving strip technique + pelvic boost, more advanced stage pts in WAI
NOCGI (16)	IA-BG3, IC, II	WAI Cisplatin + cyclophosphamide	34 36	53	71	3 required surgery	–	Closed prematurely due to poor compliance

OS, overall survival; WAI, whole abdominal irradiation; CTX, chemotherapy; RT, radiation therapy; GTR, gross total resection; PMH, Princess Margaret Hospital; NCIC, National Cancer Institute of Canada; DACOVA, Danish Cancer Ovarian Group; MDACC, M.D. Anderson Cancer Center; NOCGI, Northwest Oncologic Cooperative Group of Italy.
[a]Statistically significant.
[b]See Table 68.8 for data.

long-term prognoses similar to those with more advanced disease (5). It is in these high-risk, early-stage patients that adjuvant treatment has been proposed to improve clinical outcomes.

After complete primary surgical staging and cytoreduction, three treatment modalities have historically been employed as adjuvant treatment in early ovarian cancer: chemotherapy, external-beam radiation to the abdomen and pelvis, and IP instillation of radioisotopes.

Adjuvant Whole-Abdominal Radiation

Whole-abdominal irradiation (WAI) has been used as adjuvant postoperative treatment for completely resected ovarian cancer in the past. Patients with gross residual disease have not been traditionally treated with WAI radiation doses that are needed to adequately treat gross disease because of radiation dose tolerances of other organs in the region, including small bowel, kidneys, and liver. Early studies established the inadequacy of treating the pelvis alone with radiation for adjuvant treatment. Dembo et al. (40) reported that, although limited pelvic radiation therapy alone improved in-field local control, it offered little survival benefit for patients with stage I and II disease compared with observation or melphalan, the most commonly used chemotherapy agent at that time.

In studies comparing WAI to observation, WAI was not shown to reduce recurrence rates (42,71,125). Hreshchyshyn et al. (71) randomized 86 stage I patients to observation, chemotherapy, or WAI, and reported recurrence rates of 17% and 30% for observation and WAI, respectively. Similarly, Dembo et al. (42) analyzed predictive factors for relapse in 519 stage I patients from Princess Margaret Hospital and Norwegian Radium Hospital and found no significant differences between those who received adjuvant therapy and those who did not.

Randomized trials have compared adjuvant WAI with other adjuvant therapies including chemotherapy combined with pelvic radiation (21,39,40,77,124) or chemotherapy alone (26,130) in early-stage ovarian cancers (stage I-II predominantly) at high risk for recurrence (Table 68.7).

Studies by Dembo and the Princess Margaret Hospital prospectively compared limited pelvic radiation therapy with WAI with and without chlorambucil in stage IB-II and asymptomatic III patients (39,40). WAI modestly improved 10 year survival rates over limited pelvic therapy and chemotherapy (64% vs. 40%, respectively), but only in those with gross total resection after debulking surgery. No significant benefit was seen in patients with extensive residual tumor.

Multiple other randomized studies, however, have not shown WAI to be superior to other adjuvant treatments, with 5-year survival rates ranging from 53% to 71% (26,77,124,130). A randomized trial by the National Cancer Institute of Canada group assigned 257 high-risk stage I or optimally debulked stage II or III patients to receive melphalan, WAI, or ^{32}P (77). All patients had previously received 22.5 Gy to the pelvis prior to study entry. The WAI arm was given 22.5 Gy to the abdomen in 2.25-Gy fractions. Actuarial 5-year survival rates failed to demonstrate a statistically significant difference among all groups.

WAI has also been shown to be comparable to single or combination chemotherapy in the adjuvant setting (26,130). A prospective study from the M.D. Anderson Cancer Center randomized 129 stage I-III patients with no or <2 cm residual disease to WAI or melphalan (130). A moving strip technique for WAI plus a pelvic boost was employed. Five-year overall survival was nearly identical in the WAI and melphalan groups (71% and 72%, respectively). Late bowel toxicity was significant in this study: 14% required surgery for bowel obstruction. This study has been criticized for incomplete surgical staging of patients and an unequal balance of more advanced-stage patients in the WAI arm.

| Table 68.8 | RANDOMIZED STUDIES OF ADJUVANT INTRAPERITONEAL ^{32}P IN HIGH-RISK EARLY STAGE OVARIAN CANCER |

Trial	Stage	Study Design	N	5-Yr DFS% ^{32}P	5-Yr DFS% CTX	5-Yr OS% ^{32}P	5-Yr OS% CTX	Bowel Obstruction% ^{32}P	Bowel Obstruction% CTX	Notes
NCIC (3)	I, IIA-B, IIIO	Melphalan WAI ^{32}P	106 107^a 44	–	–	66	61	25 overall 19 required surgery	10 overall 7 required surgery	*All received prior pelvic RT*, ^{32}P accrual stopped early due to toxicity
GOG 7602 (5)	IC, II IA-B high grade	^{32}P Melphalan	44 68	80	80	78	81	6 overall	–	^{32}P not given in 7% due to technical difficulties
NRH (8)	I-III	^{32}P or WAI Cisplatin	169 171	81	75	83	81	9 overall 4.5 ^{32}P, 11 WAI required surgery	2 overall 1 required surgery	28 in ^{32}P group received WAI due to adhesions, IP ^{32}P distribution not assessed
GICOG (21)	IA-Bii, IC	^{32}P Cisplatin	75 77	65	85^b	79	81	1.3 overall	–	^{32}P not given in 20% due to adhesions
GOG 95 (22)	IA-BG3, IC, II	^{32}P CP	110 171	Recurrence 35 (10-yr)	Recurrence 28 (10-yr)	64 (10-yr)	69 (10-yr)	4 G3–4 GI toxicity 3 bowel perforation	12 G3–4 GI toxicity 0 bowel perforation	Inadequate ^{32}P distribution in 7%

DFS, disease-free survival; OS, overall survival; CTX, chemotherapy; NCIC, National Cancer Institute of Canada; WAI, whole abdominal radiation; GOG, Gynecologic Oncology Group; NRH, Norwegian Radium Hospital; IP, intraperitoneal; GICOG, Gruppo Interregionale Collaborativo in Ginecologia Oncologica; CP, cyclophosphamide + cisplatin.
^{a}Statistically significant.
^{b}See Table 68.7 for data.

A recent meta-analysis of 5 trials with 862 ovarian cancer patients compared the outcomes of adjuvant chemotherapy (4 trials with cisplatin and 1 with melphalan) and radiation therapy (2 trials with WAI and 3 with ^{32}P) (152). No significant differences were found between chemotherapy and WAI or ^{32}P. These data taken together must be interpreted with caution, however, as these trials contain a considerable amount of patient heterogeneity with small numbers of patients.

Adjuvant Intraperitoneal ^{32}Phosphorous

As an alternative to external-beam therapy, IP instillation of radioisotopes, such as gold (^{198}Au) and ^{32}P, has been extensively studied. These isotopes were initially considered attractive for their potential ability to cover all surfaces of the peritoneal cavity in the abdomen and pelvis; thus, allowing for complete coverage of all areas at high risk for disease dissemination, while minimizing toxicity to normal abdominal organs such as the kidneys. During the past few decades, ^{32}P has become the preferred and most frequently administered radioisotope. However, ^{32}P instillation has been shown to be limited by its ability to effectively treat bulky or gross residual disease. Patients with larger tumor volumes, disease beyond the abdomen, or nodal involvement after surgery are less likely to benefit from single-agent ^{32}P therapy (18). Soper et al. (132) reported a high rate of pelvic and para-aortic nodal failure (42%) in stage I and II patients treated with postoperative ^{32}P, suggesting that ^{32}P is inadequate in sterilizing micrometastatic disease in lymphatic sites.

Although no randomized data exist that compares adjuvant IP ^{32}P to observation after primary surgery, multiple cooperative groups have randomized high-risk, early-stage ovarian cancer patients to adjuvant IP ^{32}P versus chemotherapy (Table 68.8). Five-year disease-free survival ranged from 65% to 80%, and 5-year overall survival rates from 78% to 83% (50,126,147,156). The GOG randomized patients with stage IA-B with high-grade tumors, IC, and completely resected stage II disease to receive

postoperative ^{32}P or melphalan (156). The 5-year disease-free survival rate was 80% in both arms, with no significant difference in overall survival or patterns of failure. Greater toxicity, including a high rate of leukemia, was noted in the melphalan arm. The Norwegian Radium Hospital randomly assigned 240 patients with the same subsets of disease (except completely resected stage III patients were included in 5% to 10%) to receive ^{32}P or cisplatin (147). Again, there was no significant difference in the 5-year disease-free or overall survival rates (81% vs. 75% and 83% vs. 81%, respectively).

The most recent published randomized trial evaluating adjuvant ^{32}P, GOG 95, reported the longest term data to date for 281 patients with stage IA-B, grade 3, IC, and II disease who received ^{32}P (15 mCi) or cisplatin plus cyclophosphamide (155). At 10 years, no significant difference was seen in recurrence rates (35% and 28%, respectively) or overall survival rates (64% and 69%, respectively). Multiple studies cite limitations in administering ^{32}P, including higher incidence of bowel obstruction or perforation (6% to 9% vs. 0–2%), inadequate radioisotope distribution in the peritoneal cavity in 7% of patients (155), and inability to instill ^{32}P because of abdominal adhesions in up to 17% of patients (14,147). Thus, these studies indicate that instillation of IP ^{32}P has comparable recurrence and survival rates to chemotherapy after primary resection, but is associated with a higher incidence of bowel toxicity and may be hampered by heterogeneous dose distributions to target tissues.

Development of platinum- and taxane-based chemotherapy have replaced WAI and ^{32}P as adjuvant therapy for both early-stage, high-risk and advanced ovarian cancer.

Consolidative Therapy for Epithelial Ovarian Cancer

Second-look laparotomy (SLL) was introduced in the 1970s and 1980s as a method of assessing response to chemotherapy for asymptomatic patients in complete clinical remission to determine whether further chemotherapy could be discontinued in those with negative findings (120). Overall, approximately 50% patients with a complete remission will have no evidence of disease at SLL. However, subclinical residual disease remains a significant problem despite negative findings at SLL as recurrence rates were still high in these patients. Approximately 5% to 62% of these patients will experience relapse, with higher rates of failure at 42% to 62% in more advanced (stage III-IV), high-grade disease (15,55,111,119,129,137,150).

Similar to recurrence patterns after primary therapy, the most common sites of recurrence after negative SLL are in the pelvis and upper abdomen (58,119). Rubin et al. (58) reported that 44% of patients relapsed, predominantly in the abdomen, pelvis, or retroperitoneal nodes. Stage III and IV patients had a high risk of relapse (50% to 54%), and early-stage patients had a relatively low risk (stage I, 10%, and stage II, 28%). Patients most commonly recurred within 2 years, and nearly all patients (80%) relapsed within 3 years. This study reinforced the assertion that a negative SLL was not necessarily equivalent with long-term cure and represented an opportunity for consolidation therapy ^{32}P to improve outcomes.

Consolidative Whole-Abdominal Radiation

In the adjuvant setting, Dembo (38,39) previously demonstrated that WAI was effective against small residual disease (<2 cm) but not against residual disease >2 cm when compared with pelvic radiation with or without chemotherapy. WAI has been applied as consolidative therapy in several nonrandomized studies (20,27,51,57,58,80,88,96,97). The majority of these studies suggested that WAI did not have any advantage over additional chemotherapy (20,27,51,58,88,96,97). However, firm conclusions cannot be drawn from these studies because of the small number of patients and nonrandomized nature of the studies.

A few early, prospective randomized trials have evaluated the impact of consolidative WAI against that of extended chemotherapy in patients with advanced stage disease (stage III–IV) after initial surgical cytoreduction, adjuvant chemotherapy, and SLL (Table 68.9). Disease free and overall survival rates were not found to be significantly different between WAI and chemotherapy arms in all of these trials (17,81,82). Patients with minimal macroscopic residual disease after SLL, however, were included in these trials. A review by Thomas and Dembo (138) of 28 studies with 713 patients treated with consolidative WAI as a component of their therapy indicated that the volume of residual disease before radiation therapy was a significant factor in outcomes. The disease-free survival rate at variable times after treatment was 17%, 49%, and 76% for patients with macroscopic residual disease, microscopic or <5 mm disease, and no residual disease, respectively. It was suggested that a potential benefit with consolidative radiation may be seen in a small, select group of patients with no or minimal microscopic residual disease.

Two recent trials have evaluated consolidative WAI in this specific subgroup of patients and have had encouraging results (108,133). Pickel et al. (108) randomized 64 patients with stage IC-IV disease (majority with stage III) to WAI versus observation after primary comprehensive surgical staging and debulking and adjuvant chemotherapy. All patients had no clinical evidence of residual disease by clinical examination, imaging, or tumor markers, and no SLL was performed. The abdomen was treated to 30 Gy in 1.5-Gy fractions, the pelvis to 51.6 Gy, and para-aortic nodes to 42 Gy. WAI significantly improved disease-free survival from 26% to 49% and overall survival from 33% to 59% at 5 years compared with no further therapy. The greatest benefit was seen in stage III patients, with a disease-free survival of 45% and overall survival of 59% compared with 19% and 26% in the observation arm, respectively. The use of WAI was also found to be a positive prognostic factor on multivariate analysis.

The Swedish-Norwegian Ovarian Cancer Study Group recently reported their long-term results from a randomized trial limited to stage III only patients (133). Patients with complete pathological remission at SLL were randomized to WAI, chemotherapy (cisplatin, doxorubicin, or epirubicin), or observation. Those with microscopic residual disease received WAI or chemotherapy. The WAI arm was treated with 20 Gy in 1-Gy fractions to the abdomen in addition to a 20.4 Gy boost to the pelvis. In the subgroup with complete pathologic remission, patients treated with WAI had significantly superior 5-year progression-free survival compared with chemotherapy or no further therapy (56%, 36%, and 35%, respectively). Overall survival, however, was not statistically different. Analysis of relapse patterns showed that WAI reduced pelvic and distant failures in this subgroup. No significant differences between WAI and chemotherapy were seen in patients with microscopic residual disease. This study suggests that WAI may add a therapeutic benefit over observation and the chemotherapy regimen used in this trial after a negative SLL. It is unclear whether WAI would be equally advantageous compared with standard chemotherapy agents that are currently used.

The only published study to date to evaluate consolidative WAI after current standard chemotherapy for ovarian cancer, carboplatin and paclitaxel, has recently been reported from the Princess Margaret Hospital (43). Toxicity and clinical outcomes of 29 stage I-III patients (the majority were stage III with high-grade tumors) with no evidence of disease after primary surgery and carboplatin and paclitaxel, were assessed after consolidative WAI. At 4 years, 41% of patients relapsed, with disease-free and overall survival rates of 57% and 92%, respectively. Nearly all patients (92%) that relapsed were able to undergo subsequent salvage chemotherapy, which was well tolerated. This study suggests that, in the setting of currently used chemotherapy regimens, WAI does not appear to compromise the ability for patients to receive and tolerate salvage chemotherapy for those who relapse after WAI.

More recently, a retrospective study reported on long-term outcomes (median follow-up 14 years) of 105 stage III patients with minimal residual disease (<1 cm) after primary surgical debulking who received platinum-based chemotherapy and SLL (the majority had microscopic residual disease) followed by consolidative WAI (107). Patients with residual pelvic disease were given an additional pelvic boost to 44.5 Gy. Overall survival at 5 and 10 years was 53% and 36%, respectively. Late symptomatic enteritis occurred in 20% of patients, with 8% requiring surgical intervention for bowel obstruction. Deaths related to bowel complications were reported in 4%, all of which occurred in patients who received pelvic boosts.

Consolidative Intraperitoneal ^{32}Phosphorous

The value of IP ^{32}P over observation alone has been retrospectively studied in several trials in patients with no evidence of disease at SLL prior to ^{32}P instillation (Table 68.10). Disease-free survival rates ranged from 40% to 100% and overall survival rates ranged from 64% to 90% (106,116,135,144). The largest retrospective study was from the University of North Carolina by Varia et al. (144), with an update by Rogers et al. (116), which evaluated consolidative ^{32}P in 69 stage I-III patients with clinically and histologically negative disease at SLL following comprehensive surgical staging and cytoreduction and adjuvant chemotherapy. Patients receiving ^{32}P had a trend toward improved disease-free survival (86% vs. 67%) and overall survival (90% vs. 78%) rates compared with those observed.

Table 68.9   RANDOMIZED STUDIES OF CONSOLIDATIVE WHOLE ABDOMINAL RADIATION IN OVARIAN CANCER

Trial	Stage	Study Design	N	5-Yr DFS%			5-Yr OS%			Bowel Obstruction %[a]
				WAI	CTX	NFT	WAI	CTX	NFT	WAI
WAI versus CTX										
West Midlands, '44	IIB residual, III-IV	WAI Chlorambucil S + CTX + SLL	56 56	—	—	—	25 overall (2-yr) 40 < 2 cm residual	42 overall (2-yr) 68 < 2 cm residual	—	9
Italy (42)	III-IV	WAI PAC, CAC, PC S + CTX + SLL Minimal residual disease	20 21	45	71	—	55	85	—	5
NTOG (43)	IIB-IV	WAI Carboplatin S + CTX + SLL < 2 cm residual disease	58 59	NSD	NSD	—	NSD	32	—	1.7
Swedish-Norwegian, '47	III	WAI CTX[b] NFT S + CTX + SLL pCR: WAI, CTX, NFT Micro residual: WAI, CTX	32 35 31	56[c] pCR 17 micro	36 pCR 25 micro	35 pCR	69 pCR 32 micro	57 pCR 41 micro	pCR 65	6
WAI versus NFT										
Germany (46)	IC-IV	WAI NFT S + CTX (no SLL) Clinically negative	32 32	49[c] overall 45[c] stage III	—	26 overall 19 stage III	59[c] overall 59[c] stage III	—	33 overall 26 stage III	3

DFS, disease-free survival; OS, overall survival; WAI, whole abdominal radiation; CTX, chemotherapy; NFT, no further therapy; S, surgery; SLL, second-look laparotomy; PAC, cisplatin + adriamycin + cyclophosphamide; CAC, carboplatin + adriamycin + cyclophosphamide; PC, cisplatin + cyclophosphamide; NTOG, North Thames Ovary Group; NSD, no significant difference; pCR, pathologic complete remission.
[a]Requiring surgical intervention.
[b]Cisplatin + doxorubicin or epirubicin.
[c]Statistically significant.

Table 68.10 TRIALS OF CONSOLIDATIVE ^{32}P AFTER NEGATIVE SECOND-LOOK LAPAROTOMY IN OVARIAN CANCER

Study	Stage	Study Design	N	5-Yr DF %		5-Yr OS%		Bowel Obstruction %		Notes
				^{32}P	NFT	^{32}P	NFT	^{32}P	NFT	
Nonrandomized studies										
UNC (51,53)	I–III	^{32}P	51	86 DFS	DF, p = .05	90	78, p = .05	4 required surgery	6 required surgery	—
		NFT	18	14 recurrence	recurrence					
MUSC (52)	I–IV	^{32}P	14	100		86	76	7 overall	—	—
		NFT	17					0 required surgery		
University of Wash (50)	IC^{a} II–III	^{32}P	34	40	—	64	—	9 overall	—	22% bowel toxicity in first 23 patients, 0% after dose change from 15 mCi to 12 mCi
Randomized studies										
NRH (32)	IAG2–3, IB–III	^{32}P	25	84		—	—	7 overall	—	—
		NFT	25					4 required surgery		
GOG 93 (55)	III	^{32}P	104	42		67	63	3 required surgery	—	15% in ^{32}P did not receive treatment due to inadequate peritoneal radioisotope distribution
		NFT	98				63			

DFS, disease-free survival; OS, overall survival; NFT, no further therapy; UNC, University of North Carolina; MUSC, Medical University of South Carolina; NRH, Norwegian Radium Hospital; GOG, Gynecologic Oncology Group.
^{a}IC with incomplete surgical staging at laparotomy.

Randomized data evaluating consolidative ^{32}P are limited (Table 68.10). The Norwegian Radium Hospital randomized 50 patients with stage IA high-grade and IB-III disease to ^{32}P versus observation and found no significant difference between the arms (148). The GOG recently reported on a prospective randomized trial of 202 stage III patients with complete clinical remission and microscopically negative disease at SLL after initial surgery and adjuvant platinum-based chemotherapy (145). Compared with those patients who received no further therapy, those who received ^{32}P (15 mCi) within 10 days of the SLL did not have improved 5-year disease-free survival (36% vs. 42%, respectively) or overall survival (63% vs. 67%, respectively). Furthermore, there was no significant difference in site of first relapse (peritoneal, 33%, and extraperitoneal, 26%).

Palliative Radiation Treatment

Several retrospective studies have demonstrated the usefulness of local radiation therapy in providing palliation for recurrent and metastatic disease (33,48,53,90,139). Palliative radiation therapy has been most commonly employed for bleeding, pain, or obstructive symptoms, but other indications have included dyspnea, lymphedema, and brain metastasis. The median dose used varied from 30 to 38 Gy. Overall response rate ranged from 73% to 100%, with complete responses from 28% to 70%. The median duration was reported to be from 5 to 11 months. According to one study, the duration of response extended to >6 months in 70% of patients and >12 months in 40% (53). Radiation therapy was most effective for controlling vaginal or rectal bleeding. Virtually all patients experienced an improvement in bleeding, and 80% to 89% attained complete resolution of bleeding (48,53,90,139). It was also effective in relieving pain in 77% to 100% of patients, with 40% to 65% achieving complete pain relief. Symptoms stemming from bowel or ureteral obstruction were improved in 64% to 75% of patients (90,139). These responses have been compared favorably to results of recent salvage chemotherapy regimens published in the literature (139). Radiation therapy delivered locally to symptomatic sites appears to be of significant and durable benefit and should be considered for palliative purposes in select patients with symptomatic relapses, particularly in those that are refractory to chemotherapy.

Stereotactic Radiosurgery for Brain Metastases from Ovarian Cancer

Ovarian cancer metastatic to the brain is a rare occurrence (0.9% to 1.4% of cases), but the incidence has been reported to be rising as high as 11.6% in one report as chemotherapy regimens become more effective (8,29,62). Long-term prognosis is poor, with a median survival time of <12 months (32), although one study cited extended survival to 16.5 months with combined modality treatment of surgical resection, radiation, and chemotherapy (115).

Two retrospective studies have reported results on a combined total of eight patients treated with stereotactic radiosurgery (SRS) with or without whole-brain radiation (34,98). In a study of five highly selected patients treated with a median dose of 15 Gy, the majority of patients had a symptomatic and objective radiographic response. When compared with a small cohort of patients treated with whole-brain radiation alone, more patients treated with SRS experienced a complete radiographic response (29% and 40%, respectively). Two-year overall survival was 60% in the SRS group versus 15% in the whole-brain radiation group. Although no firm conclusions can be drawn from these small retrospective studies, SRS for brain metastases from ovarian cancer may be of clinical benefit to a subgroup of patients, and additional investigation is warranted.

Radiation Therapy Techniques

Whole-Abdominal Radiation Therapy

The clinical target volume includes the entire peritoneum from the diaphragm to the pelvic floor, encompassing both the visceral and parietal surfaces, which can harbor both tumor implants and microscopic disease and the pelvic and para-aortic nodes. Organs at risk that are dose-limiting include the kidneys, liver, small and large bowel, and bone marrow.

Conventionally, large anterior and posterior fields have been used. This requires attention to the excursion of the diaphragm at the superior margin during respiration to ensure appropriate coverage, inclusion of the pouch of Douglas inferiorly, and ensuring the coverage of the lateral extent of the peritoneal margins, especially in obese patients. Fluoroscopy helps to assess the range of quiet respiratory motion. Alternatively, image fusion of computed tomography scans obtained in inspiration and expiration can be used to design the treatment fields. Extended source to skin distance may be required in some patients to ensure adequate coverage.

Kidney and whole liver are limited to 15 Gy and 30 Gy. Daily dose fractions of 1.2 to 1.5 Gy can be delivered. The total dose to the whole abdomen is limited to 30 Gy. Additional dose to the pelvis and para-aortic lymph node regions to 50 Gy may be delivered, depending on the clinical requirements. Patients will need to be monitored for acute gastrointestinal and hematologic toxicity as well as nutritional support.

Intensity-Modulated Radiation Therapy for Whole-Abdominal Irradiation

The use of intensity-modulated radiation therapy (IMRT) in delivering WAI has been proposed as a means to reduce the radiation dose to the bone marrow and kidneys in order to decrease the incidence of myelotoxicity and renal damage, respectively (47,68). One recent study demonstrated improved planning target volume (PTV) dose coverage and significant dose reductions to bones with the same level of kidney sparing using dynamic multi-leaf collimator IMRT when compared with conventional fields (68). The PTV receiving 95% of the prescribed dose improved from 72% to 84%, and the volume of pelvic bones receiving more than 21 Gy was reduced by a relative 60% from 86% to 35%. Dose inhomogeneity, however, increased slightly, with small regions of underdosing near the kidneys. Similar improvements in PTV dose coverage were reported in a study using IMRT arc therapy (47). It remains to be seen whether the dosimetric advantages gained from WAI-IMRT will translate to a significant and clinically relevant benefit. Furthermore, technical considerations must be considered with great care given the complex anatomy and delineation of the peritoneal cavity boundaries. Patient breathing motion and setup uncertainties will also need to be addressed.

Intraoperative Radiation for Ovarian Cancer

Several studies have suggested that intraoperative radiation therapy (IORT) as part of salvage surgery for locally recurrent gynecologic cancers, including ovarian cancer, may improve locoregional control and overall survival (37,52,61,67,79,153). A total of 46 ovarian cancer cases have been reported in the literature. The largest IORT retrospective study to date that reported results of 22 ovarian cancer patients treated with IORT (median dose, 12 Gy; range, 9 to 14 Gy) suggests that the addition of IORT to cytoreductive surgery may potentially improve locoregional control and achieve palliation in highly selected patients with locally recurrent ovarian cancer (153). Various sites were treated, but the pelvic sidewalls was the most commonly treated site. Nearly all of the patients also received additional therapy after IORT including WAI, pelvic and/or inguinal radiation, and chemotherapy. Locoregional control was achieved in 68% of patients, with a median time to recurrence of 14 months and 5-year disease-free survival of 18% and overall survival of 22%. Overall treatment-related grade 3 toxicities occurred in 41%. Bowel obstruction occurred in seven patients, all of whom received postoperative WAI and two of whom also had a component of locoregional relapse. No long-term neurologic sequelae were reported.

Intraperitoneal Instillation of ^{32}P

The use of radiopharmaceuticals in the treatment of ovarian cancer was first described by Müller (102) in 1945. He initially used ^{63}Zn, but later instilled ^{198}Au. Radioisotopes were initially employed in the palliative treatment of malignant ascites. In the late 1950s and early 1960s, retrospective studies indicated a role for IP radioisotopes in the management of microscopic ovarian cancer (23,36). Since 1955, ^{32}P has been the preferred radioisotope for IP administration for several reasons, including lack of γ radiation emittance, greater ease of handling, and higher β energy, which results in greater tissue penetrance (23,78,117).

Radioactive ^{32}P, with a physical half-life of 14.3 days, decays by pure β emission with mean energy of 695 keV. The biologic effect of the isotope in colloid suspension remains within 4 mm, thus primarily treating the peritoneal surface. The absence of gamma decay limits the radiation dose to other intra-abdominal organs such as the liver, kidneys, and intestines, and permits safe treatment of large peritoneal surfaces. The ^{32}P colloid preparation is not absorbed into the systemic circulation and has no hematologic toxicity associated with other ^{32}P compounds.

Instillation of ^{32}P is typically prepared as a chromic phosphate suspension with concentrations of up to 5 mCi/mL. It is recommended that two IP catheters be placed at the time of the SLL, with the right IP catheter positioned along the right paracolic gutter toward the right hemidiaphragm, and the left IP catheter along the left paracolic gutter toward the pelvis. If IP catheters are not placed at the time of SLL, a multiperforated peritoneal dialysis catheter can be inserted under local anesthesia into the peritoneal cavity. Normal saline (250 mL) is then infused into the peritoneal cavity via the IP catheters to verify that there is no fluid leakage outside the peritoneal cavity. Peritoneal distribution can be assessed by several techniques, including anterior and lateral scans of the abdominal cavity after IP injection of technetium-99 m (^{99m}Tc), to confirm that loculation has not occurred. If the IP fluid distribution is acceptable, 15 mCi of chromic phosphate suspension mixed in 500 mL of normal saline is typically infused into the peritoneal cavity via the IP catheters. It is recommended that patients with inadequate distribution of ^{99m}Tc in the peritoneal cavity not be administered the ^{32}P suspension. After the ^{32}P infusion, the IP catheters are flushed with 250 mL of normal saline and the IP catheters are removed. To facilitate wide distribution of IP ^{32}P in the peritoneal cavity, the patient should be turned every 10 minutes for 2 hours, to the left lateral supine, Trendelenburg, reverse Trendelenburg, and right lateral positions as tolerated by the patient.

Intraperitoneal Radioimmunotherapy

The use of radiolabeled monoclonal antibodies has been proposed as a new potential method of molecularly targeting ovarian cancer to help control disseminated IP disease. Selective targeting of malignant cells in the peritoneal cavity using monoclonal antibodies labeled with radioisotopes such as ^{131}I, ^{125}I, or ^{90}Y has been of recent interest. *MUC1*, a glycosylated mucin protein differentially overexpressed on the surface of ovarian cancer and other adenocarcinoma cells (54,101), has been investigated as a potential therapeutic target in ovarian cancer. A large phase III trial recently reported results on the use of radiolabeled murine HMFG1 (^{90}Y-muHMFG1), an antibody directed against a specific epitope of *MUC1*, for consolidative therapy in patients with a complete clinical remission after cytoreductive surgery and platinum-based chemotherapy (149). Unfortunately, a single IP dose of ^{90}Y-muHMFG1 plus standard therapy did not improve recurrence or survival rates compared with standard therapy alone.

∷ Sequelae of Treatment

Acute Toxicity

Acute toxicity from WAI is common, but rarely severe. The use of large radiation fields that incorporate multiple abdominal organs contributes to the development of predictable side effects. Included in most abdominal or pelvic fields are whole or partial organ systems such as the liver, kidneys, gastrointestinal tract, bladder, spleen, lungs, and pancreas. Gastrointestinal side effects are the most common acute and subacute problems encountered with WAI. This is the result of the large amount of bowel tissue included in the radiation fields. Up to 75% of patients treated with abdominal and pelvic fields experience mild-to-moderate diarrhea. Limiting bowel exposure through the use of shielding or appropriately timed field reductions can minimize or prevent this toxicity. Approximately 60% to 70% may also experience nausea, particularly early during treatment, but emesis occurs infrequently. Appetite loss accompanied by weight loss is a frequent concern. It is thus essential to closely monitor and ensure proper nutrition to avoid malnourishment and dehydration.

Clinically significant liver damage is extremely rare with appropriate shielding (84). Approximately 50% of patients will develop transiently elevated alkaline phosphatase levels, but symptomatic hepatitis occurs in fewer than 1% (138). Hematologic toxicity is infrequent and significant drops in blood counts causing treatment interruption are rare. Splenic damage may occur even at low radiation doses because of the exquisite radiosensitivity of the spleen, resulting in transient reduction in platelet counts.

Urethritis and bladder spasm from pelvic irradiation may occur and should be treated symptomatically. Adequate and careful shielding of the kidneys at some point in WAI is critical to minimize renal damage and failure. Stricture of the ureters or urethra is rare, occurring in <1% of cases and is usually not seen until 3 to 6 months postradiation. Because treatment of the entire peritoneal cavity with adequate margins requires extension of fields above the diaphragm, inclusion of the lung bases bilaterally is required. Chest radiographs can show fibrosis or bibasilar pneumonitis in 5% to 20% of patients, but is generally self-limited and rarely symptomatic.

Late Toxicity

Late toxicities were more common with the moving strip technique than with the open-field technique, primarily because of the higher doses and hot spots that are generated. High radiation doses can exceed normal organ tolerances, leading to permanent organ damage and failure. Chronic gastrointestinal damage (i.e., bloating, intermittent diarrhea), occurs in <5% of treated patients. The overall incidence of bowel obstruction has been reported to be 5% to 10% at 5 years in cases in which IP ^{32}P or WAI is used independently (Tables 68.7 and 68.9). Approximately 50% of these patients who develop bowel obstructions will require surgical intervention (incidence, 3% to 5%); however, recent data suggest that this incidence may be higher and closer to 10% in long-term survivors at 10 years (107). These occur more frequently with doses above 45 Gy and in patients with gapped or abutted split fields. In addition, the presence of adhesions in the peritoneal cavity and the combination of additional pelvic radiation to ^{32}P or WAI have been shown to approximately double the risk of significant bowel complications (up to 20% to 25%) (77,147).

As with most anatomic sites, escalating doses of radiation do come with an increase in rate and degree of toxicity. Major bowel complications from 10 pooled series of 1,098 patients reported an incidence of 1.4% with abdominal dose of 22.5 Gy compared with 14% with 30 Gy (138). Furthermore, the timing of ^{32}P instillation may be an important factor in the development of late bowel toxicities. Spanos et al. (134) reported a significant difference in bowel complications between delayed instillation of ^{32}P (>12 hours) compared with immediately after surgery (21% to 4%, respectively) (134).

Management of Germ Cell Tumors

Presentation and management of nonepithelial tumors is, in general, similar to those of their epithelial counterparts, as patients usually experience vaginal bleeding, abdominal bloating, or pain and typically require surgical intervention and chemotherapy. On presentation, routine work-up is identical to that for other ovarian cancers, as previously outlined. Pretreatment AFP and β-hCG levels are of particular importance in diagnosis and treatment. For example, an elevated β-hCG with a normal AFP is strongly suggestive of dysgerminoma. Lactate dehydrogenase and CA 125 samples should also be drawn, as the germ cell tumors may have several tumor markers that can be followed (Table 68.11). Variations in surgical management and adjuvant chemotherapy and radiation do exist among the nonepithelial tumors. Treatments should consider the patient's desire to maintain fertility while offering the greatest chance for cure.

Most ovarian neoplasms diagnosed in children and adolescents are germ cell tumors, with approximately two thirds of these tumors being malignant at the time of diagnosis. Germ cell tumors comprise 20% of all ovarian neoplasms and 2% to 5% of all ovarian malignancies. The most common germ cell tumor is the mature cystic teratoma (also the most common

ovarian neoplasm), but fortunately only the minority contain a malignancy or contain immature elements.

Dysgerminoma

Dysgerminoma is the most common of the malignant germ cell tumors and also have the highest bilaterality rate (20%), with 10% of the ovaries being grossly involved and 10% being microscopically involved. Eighty percent of women with dysgerminomas present before the age of 30 years. As shown in Table 68.10, dysgerminomas may secrete lactate dehydrogenase and have elevated HCG levels. Approximately 75% to 80%, however, have early-stage disease at presentation. In many instances, the young women affected by this disease wish to maintain fertility after therapy. For some patients with early-stage disease, this may be possible. The high rate of contralateral disease does confer a greater risk with conservative surgical therapy.

Postoperative therapy for patients with dysgerminoma can be separated into those women with stage I disease and those with a more advanced of stage disease. Women with stage IA disease can be monitored closely and there is no need for adjuvant therapy. However, up to 15% to 25% of these women will experience a recurrence. For women with more advanced-stage disease, chemotherapy with BEP (bleomycin, etoposide, and cisplatin) is recommended. In trials reported by the GOG and M.D. Anderson Cancer Center in patients with stage III or IV disease and bulky residual disease, nearly all patients experienced a 5-year disease-free interval (56).

Dysgerminomas are unique in that they are radiosensitive tumors and radiotherapy has been used in those women who were not thought to be candidates for chemotherapy. Radiation dose of 25 Gy in 12 to 14 fractions may be used. However, radiotherapy will affect fertility, so this must be taken into consideration when recommending adjuvant therapy.

Other Germ Cell Tumors

Nondysgerminomas are almost always unilateral. For apparent early-stage disease, unilateral salpingo-oophorectomy appears to be as effective as more extensive surgery. Patients with stage I, grade 1 immature teratomas usually require no further therapy after unilateral salpingo-oophorectomy. All others, including stage I, grade 2 and 3 immature teratoma will require three cycles of BEP. Because of the low number of diagnosed cases, large-scale studies comparing adjuvant therapy are uncommon.

Extrapolation of data regarding the efficacy of chemotherapeutic regimens for the treatment of nonseminomatous testicular germ cell tumors has had a great impact on the treatment of patients with nondysgerminoma ovarian germ cell tumors. Patients with less well-differentiated tumors and all those with endodermal sinus tumor, embryonal carcinoma, choriocarcinoma, or mixed germ cell tumors should receive adjuvant postoperative chemotherapy. Various regimens have been used, including VAC (vincristine, dactinomycin, and cyclophosphamide), PVC (cisplatin, vincristine, and cyclophosphamide), and CVB (cyclophosphamide, vincristine, and bleomycin). The BEP regimen was prospectively randomized in patients with completely resected, surgically staged I, II, and III disease, and resulted in a 96% disease-free survival rate (151). Three courses of BEP as the standard treatment for well-staged patients with resected ovarian germ cell tumors were recommended.

Management of Sex Cord-Stromal Tumors

Sex cord-stromal tumors arrive from the intraovarian matrix that supports the germ cells. These tumors are responsible for

Table 68.11	SERUM MARKERS FOR OVARIAN GERM CELL TUMORS		
Tumor Type	AFP	hCG	LDH
Dysgerminoma	—	+/−	+
Choriocarcinoma	—	+	—
Endodermal sinus tumor	+	—	—
Immature teratoma	+/−	—	—
Mixed germ cell tumor	+/−	+/−	+/−
Embryonal carcinoma	+/−	+	—
Polyembryoma	+/−	+	—

AFP, α-fetoprotein; hCG, human chorionic gonadotrophin; LDH, lactate dehydrogenase.

<5% of all ovarian malignancies, but they account for 90% of all functioning ovarian neoplasms. One third of the tumors will produce estrogen, progesterone, testosterone, or other androgens. This hormonal expression may lead to its presenting signs and symptoms, including precocious puberty, postmenopausal bleeding, hirsutism or virilization. Sex cord-stromal tumors can develop in women of any age (with the granulosa cell tumors having a bimodal age distribution) but the peak incidence is in postmenopausal women around 50 years of age. These tumors typically behave in a benign fashion or have LMP. Surgery remains the mainstay of treatment, but occasionally postoperative therapy is required, although these tumors are relatively insensitive to chemotherapy.

The most common tumors are the granulosa cell tumors, which, like the Sertoli cell tumors, are derived from the sex cord cells, whereas the thecal cell tumors, Leydig cell tumor, and fibromas arise from the mesenchymal cells. These tumors are fairly uncommon. Granulosa cell tumors, which do have malignant potential and are also the most common, comprise 70% of the ovarian sex cord-stromal tumors. Most of these tumors are unilateral and can be treated with fertility-preserving therapy consisting of unilateral salpingo-oophorectomy and appropriate staging. In addition, endometrial sampling should be performed in women retaining their uterus because many tumors will be associated with concomitant hyperplasia or adenocarcinoma. In women not wishing to preserve fertility or those who are postmenopausal, complete hysterectomy with bilateral salpingo-oophorectomy would be the procedure of choice. Surgery alone is typically curative. However, risk factors that should be taken into consideration include histology, large tumor size, mitotic index, tumor rupture, and incomplete staging. In women with these risk factors who are thought to be at a higher risk for recurrence, BEP chemotherapy may be considered.

Adult Granulosa Cell Tumors

Adult granulosa cell tumors account for 95% of all granulose cell tumors. The majority of women are diagnosed after 30 years of age, with the median age being 52. Abdominal pain and distention and vaginal bleeding are the most common signs and symptoms. Because of the relative state of estrogen excess produced by these tumors, 25% of women will also have concomitant endometrial pathology, such as hyperplasia or adenocarcinoma (99). These tumors tend to be large, with the average diameter being 12 cm. If a granulose cell tumor is suspected preoperatively, inhibin A and B levels can help with the differential diagnosis. Once a granulosa cell tumor is diagnosed, rising inhibin levels can predate symptoms or clinical evidence of disease recurrence (13).

The majority of granulose cell tumors behave in a benign fashion. Ninety percent of patients present with stage I disease and the tumors are typically unilateral in 90% of cases. Therefore, in the young woman, fertility-sparing surgery can be an option. Stage is the most important prognostic factor for granulosa cell tumors; there are other factors such as tumor size, mitotic atypia, tumor rupture, but stage remains the most important. The 10-year survival for women with stage I disease is approximately 90%, with 15% to 25% of stage I patients ultimately suffering a disease recurrence. The 10-year survival for women with advanced stage disease is 26% to 49%.

Juvenile Granulosa Cell Tumors

Juvenile granulosa cell tumors are rare; however, they account for 90% of the granulosa cell tumors that occur in prepubertal

girls and women younger than 30 years of age (157). Similar to the adult form, the juvenile tumors may also secrete estrogen; therefore, the prepubertal girls may present with isosexual precocious puberty. This may be the most dramatic presentation, but the most common presentation is that of an abdominal mass. As with the adult variant, the juvenile variant is rarely bilateral, with bilaterality occurring in only 5% of cases. More than 90% of cases will be stage I at the time of diagnosis, but other prognostic factors apply as with the adult variant. The 5-year survival rate is 95%, and the prognosis remains poor with advanced-stage or recurrent disease.

Future Directions

Ovarian cancer remains a challenge for prevention, early detection, and treatment of advanced stages and recurrent disease. Vaccines may have a role for prevention of several different cancers (10). Breast and ovarian cancers express mucins that could serve as targets for vaccines to prevent both cancers. Results from two large screening trials of postmenopausal women (UKCTOCS, with 200,000 women, and USA-PLCO, with 39,000 women) using CA 125 and transvaginal ultrasound are pending long-term follow-up to assess reduction in ovarian cancer mortality (22,73).

Radiation therapy has a limited role in the current management of ovarian cancer. The future of radiation therapy for ovarian cancer can be expected to involve targeted delivery of radiation using radiolabeled antibodies and combined-modality protocols with chemotherapy or other novel molecular targeted agents that act as radiosensitizers, particularly with novel radiation-delivery methods such as IMRT and image-guided radiation therapy for localized disease. Functional and molecular imaging will advance diagnostic and staging therapeutic approaches, and radiation therapy targeting.

Genomic and proteomic research hold great promise for discovery of efficient screening tests and effective targeted therapies based on the molecular signatures of individual tumors. Principal component analysis and clustering analysis based on protein expression profiles and subtype-specific biomarker candidates of ovarian cancers can be identified (159). Xiao et al. (10) note that more than 30 serum markers have been evaluated alone and in combination with CA 125 and promising candidates include HE4, mesothelin, macrophage colony stimulating factor, osteopontin, kallikrein(s), and soluble epidermal growth factor receptors (10). Proteomic approaches have been used to define a distinctive pattern of peaks on mass spectroscopy or to identify a limited number of critical markers that can be assayed by more conventional methods. Although prevention of ovarian cancer awaits detailed understanding of the etiology of these tumors and factors that identify high-risk groups, early diagnosis and systemic therapies with novel chemotherapy and targeted biologics, optimal doses, delivery methods, and schedules based on patient selection factors will significantly improve survival outcomes for both early- and advanced-stage ovarian cancers. Development of less toxic therapies and research in ameliorating such toxicities can be expected to enhance the quality of life. Fertility-sparing approaches in nonepithelial cancers are already addressing this important aspect of ovarian cancer management (89).

References

1. ACOG Committee Opinion: number 280, December 2002. The role of the generalist obstetrician-gynecologist in the early detection of ovarian cancer. *Obstet Gynecol* 2002;100:1413–1416.
2. Cancer risks in BRCA2 mutation carriers. The Breast Cancer Linkage Consortium. *J Natl Cancer Inst* 1999;91:1310–1316.

3. Chemotherapy in advanced ovarian cancer: an overview of randomised clinical trials. Advanced Ovarian Cancer Trialists Group. *BMJ* 1991;303(6807):884–893.

4. FIGO (International Federation of Gynecology and Obstetrics) annual report on the results of treatment in gynecological cancer. *Int J Gynaecol Obstet* 2003;83[Suppl 1]:1–229.

5. NIH consensus conference. Ovarian cancer. Screening, treatment, and follow-up. NIH Consensus Development Panel on Ovarian Cancer. *JAMA* 1995;273(6):491–497.

6. Alberts, DS, Carboplatin versus cisplatin in ovarian cancer. *Semin Oncol* 1995;22[5 Suppl 12]:88–90.

7. American Cancer Society, Cancer Facts and Figures.http://www.cancer.org/downloads/STT/CAFF2007PWSecured.pdf.

8. Anupol, N, Ghamande, S, Odunsi, K, et al., Evaluation of prognostic factors and treatment modalities in ovarian cancer patients with brain metastases. *Gynecol Oncol* 2002;85(3):487–492.

9. Armstrong, DK, Bundy, B, Wenzel, L, et al., Intraperitoneal cisplatin and paclitaxel in ovarian cancer. *N Engl J Med* 2006;354(1):34–43.

10. Bast, RC, Jr., Brewer, M, Zou, C, et al., Prevention and early detection of ovarian cancer: mission impossible? *Recent Results Cancer Res* 2007;174:91–100.

11. Benjamin, I, Rubin, SC, Management of early-stage epithelial ovarian cancer. *Obstet Gynecol Clin North Am* 1994;21(1):107–119.

12. Bergman, F, Carcinoma of the ovary. A clinicopathological study of 86 autopsied cases with special reference to mode of spread. *Acta Obstet Gynecol Scand* 1966;45(2):211–231.

13. Boggess, JF, Soules, MR, Goff, BA, et al., Serum inhibin and disease status in women with ovarian granulosa cell tumors. *Gynecol Oncol* 1997;64(1):64–69.

14. Bolis, G, Colombo, N, Pecorelli, S, et al., Adjuvant treatment for early epithelial ovarian cancer: results of two randomised clinical trials comparing cisplatin to no further treatment or chromic phosphate (32P). G.I.C.O.G.: Gruppo Interregionale Collaborativo in Ginecologia Oncologica. *Ann Oncol* 1995;6(9):887–893.

15. Bolis, G, Villa, A, Guarnerio, P, et al., Survival of women with advanced ovarian cancer and complete pathologic response at second-look laparotomy. *Cancer* 1996;77(1):128–131.

16. Boyd, J, Specific keynote: hereditary ovarian cancer: what we know. *Gynecol Oncol* 2003;88(1 Pt 2):S8–1013.

17. Bruzzone, M, Repetto, L, Chiara, S, et al., Chemotherapy versus radiotherapy in the management of ovarian cancer patients with pathological complete response or minimal residual disease at second look. *Gynecol Oncol* 1990;38(3):392–395.

18. Buller, RE, Berman, ML, Bloss, JD, et al., CA 125 regression: a model for epithelial ovarian cancer response. *Am J Obstet Gynecol* 1991;165(2):360–367.

19. Burke, W, Daly, M, Garber, J, et al., Recommendations for follow-up care of individuals with an inherited predisposition to cancer. II. BRCA1 and BRCA2. Cancer Genetics Studies Consortium. *JAMA* 1997;277(12):997–1003.

20. Buser, K, Bacchi, M, Goldhirsch, A, et al., Treatment of ovarian cancer with surgery, short-course chemotherapy and whole abdominal radiation. *Ann Oncol* 1996;7(1):65–70.

21. Bush, RS, Allt, WE, Beale, FA, et al., Treatment of epithelial carcinoma of the ovary: operation, irradiation, and chemotherapy. *Am J Obstet Gynecol* 1977;127(7):692–704.

22. Buys, SS, Partridge, E, Greene, MH, et al., Ovarian cancer screening in the Prostate, Lung, Colorectal and Ovarian (PLCO) cancer screening trial: findings from the initial screen of a randomized trial. *Am J Obstet Gynecol* 2005;193(5):1630–1639.

23. Card, RY, Cole, DR, Henschke, UK, Summary of ten years of the use of radioactive colloids in intracavitary therapy. *J Nucl Med* 1960;1:195–198.

24. Carey, MS, Dembo, AJ, Simm, JE, et al., Testing the validity of a prognostic classification in patients with surgically optimal ovarian carcinoma: a 15-year review. *Int J Gynecol Cancer* 1993;3(1):24–35.

25. Chi, DS, Eisenhauer, EL, Lang, J, et al., What is the optimal goal of primary cytoreductive surgery for bulky stage IIIC epithelial ovarian carcinoma (EOC)? *Gynecol Oncol* 2006;103(2):559–564.

26. Chiara, S, Conte, P, Franzone, P, et al., High-risk early-stage ovarian cancer. Randomized clinical trial comparing cisplatin plus cyclophosphamide versus whole abdominal radiotherapy. *Am J Clin Oncol* 1994;17(1):72–76.

27. Chiara, S, Orsatti, M, Franzone, P, et al., Abdominopelvic radiotherapy following surgery and chemotherapy in advanced ovarian cancer. *Clin Oncol (R Coll Radiol)*, 1991;3(6):340–344.

28. Chu, CS and Rubin, SC, Screening for ovarian cancer in the general population. *Best Pract Res Clin Obstet Gynaecol* 2006;20(2):307–320.

29. Cohen, ZR, Suki, D, Weinberg, JS, et al., Brain metastases in patients with ovarian carcinoma: prognostic factors and outcome. *J Neurooncol* 2004;66(3):313–325.

30. Cook, LS, Weiss, NS, Schwartz, SM, et al., Population-based study of tamoxifen therapy and subsequent ovarian, endometrial, and breast cancers. *J Natl Cancer Inst* 1995;87(18):1359–1364.

31. Copeland, LJ, Vaccarello, L and Lewandowski, GS, Second-look laparotomy in epithelial ovarian cancer. *Obstet Gynecol Clin North Am* 1994;21(1):155–166.

32. Cormio, G, Gabriele, A, Maneo, A, et al., Complete remission of brain metastases from ovarian carcinoma with carboplatin. *Eur J Obstet Gynecol Reprod Biol* 1998;78(1):91–93.

33. Corn, BW, Lanciano, RM, Boente, M, et al., Recurrent ovarian cancer. Effective radiotherapeutic palliation after chemotherapy failure. *Cancer* 1994;74(11):2979–2983.

34. Corn, BW, Mehta, MP, Buatti, JM, et al., Stereotactic Irradiation: potential new treatment method for brain metastases resulting from ovarian cancer. *Am J Clin Oncol* 1999;22(2):143–146.

35. Crayford, TJ, Campbell, S, Bourne, TH, et al., Benign ovarian cysts and ovarian cancer: a cohort study with implications for screening. *Lancet* 2000;355(9209):1060–1063.

36. Decker, DG, Webb, MJ and Holbrook, MA, Radiogold treatment of epithelial cancer of ovary: late results. *Am J Obstet Gynecol* 1973;115(6):751–758.

37. del Carmen, M.G., McIntyre, JF, Fuller, AF, et al., Intraoperative radiation therapy in the treatment of pelvic gynecologic malignancies: a review of fifteen cases. *Gynecol Oncol* 2000;79(3):457–462.

38. Dembo, AJ, Epithelial ovarian cancer: the role of radiotherapy. *Int J Radiat Oncol Biol Phys* 1992;22(5):835–845.

39. Dembo, AJ, Radiotherapeutic management of ovarian cancer. *Semin Oncol* 1984; 11(3):238–250.

40. Dembo, AJ, Bush, RS, Beale, FA, et al., Ovarian carcinoma: improved survival following abdominopelvic irradiation in patients with a completed pelvic operation. *Am J Obstet Gynecol* 1979;134(7):793–800.

41. Dembo, AJ, Bush, RS, Beale, FA, et al., The Princess Margaret Hospital study of ovarian cancer: stages I, II, and asymptomatic III presentations. *Cancer Treat Rep* 1979;63(2):249–254.

42. Dembo, AJ, Davy, M, Stenwig, AE, et al., Prognostic factors in patients with stage I epithelial ovarian cancer. *Obstet Gynecol* 1990;75(2):263–273.

43. Dinniwell, R, Lock, M, Pintilie, M, et al., Consolidative abdominopelvic radiotherapy after surgery and carboplatin/paclitaxel chemotherapy for epithelial ovarian cancer. *Int J Radiat Oncol Biol Phys* 2005;62(1):104–110.

44. Droegmueller, W, In: Droegmueller W, Herbst I, Mishell DR, et al, eds. *Comprehensive Gynecology*. St. Louis, MO: CV Mosby; 1987.

45. du Bois, A, Luck, HJ, Meier, W, et al., A randomized clinical trial of cisplatin/paclitaxel versus carboplatin/paclitaxel as first-line treatment of ovarian cancer. *J Natl Cancer Inst* 2003;95(17):1320–1329.

46. du Bois, A, Quinn, M, Thigpen, T, et al., 2004 consensus statements on the management of ovarian cancer: final document of the 3rd International Gynecologic Cancer Intergroup Ovarian Cancer Consensus Conference (GCIG OCCC 2004). *Ann Oncol* 2005;16 [Suppl 8]:viii7–viii12.

47. Duthoy, W, De Gersem, W, Vergote, K, et al., Whole abdominopelvic radiotherapy (WAPRT) using intensity-modulated arc therapy (IMAT): first clinical experience. *Int J Radiat Oncol Biol Phys* 2003;57(4):1019–1032.

48. Choan, E, Samant, R, Fung, MF, et al., Palliative radiotherapy for recurrent granulosa cell tumor of the ovary: a report of 3 cases with radiological evidence of response. *Gynecol Oncol* 2006;102(2):406–410.

49. Fathalla, MF, Incessant ovulation—a factor in ovarian neoplasia? *Lancet* 1971; 2(7716):163.

50. Francis, P, Rowinsky, E, Schneider, J, et al., Phase I feasibility and pharmacologic study of weekly intraperitoneal paclitaxel: a Gynecologic Oncology Group pilot Study. *J Clin Oncol* 1995;13(12):2961–2967.

51. Fuks, Z, Rizel, S and Biran, S, Chemotherapeutic and surgical induction of pathological complete remission and whole abdominal irradiation for consolidation does not enhance the cure of stage III ovarian carcinoma. *J Clin Oncol* 1988;6(3):509–516.

52. Garton, GR, Gunderson, LL, Webb, MJ, et al., Intraoperative radiation therapy in gynecologic cancer: update of the experience at a single institution. *Int J Radiat Oncol Biol Phys* 1997;37(4):839–843.

53. Gelblum, D, Mychalczak, B, Almadrones, L, et al., Palliative benefit of external-beam radiation in the management of platinum refractory epithelial ovarian carcinoma. *Gynecol Oncol* 1998;69(1):36–41.

54. Gendler, SJ, MUC1, the renaissance molecule. *J Mammary Gland Biol Neoplasia* 2001;6(3):339–353.

55. Gershenson, DM, Copeland, LJ, Wharton, JT, et al., Prognosis of surgically determined complete responders in advanced ovarian cancer. *Cancer* 1985;55(5):1129–1135.

56. Gershenson, DM, Morris, M, Cangir, A, et al., Treatment of malignant germ cell tumors of the ovary with bleomycin, etoposide, and cisplatin. *J Clin Oncol* 1990;8(4):715–720.

57. Goldberg, H, Stein, ME, Steiner, M, et al., Consolidation radiation therapy following cytoreductive surgery, chemotherapy and second-look laparotomy for epithelial ovarian carcinoma: long-term follow-up. *Tumori* 2001;87(4):248–251.

58. Goldhirsch, A, Greiner, R, Dreher, E, et al., Treatment of advanced ovarian cancer with surgery, chemotherapy, and consolidation of response by whole-abdominal radiotherapy. *Cancer* 1988;62(1):40–47.

59. Greene, F, Page, D, Flemming, I, et al., in American Joint Committee on Cancer (AJCC): AJCC Cancer Staging Manual. 6th ed. New York: Springer-Verlag; 2002,

60. Griffiths, CT, Parker, LM and Fuller, AF, Jr., Role of cytoreductive surgical treatment in the management of advanced ovarian cancer. *Cancer Treat Rep* 1979; 63(2):235–240.

61. Haddock, MG, Petersen, IA, Webb, MJ, et al., IORT for locally advanced gynecological malignancies. *Front Radiat Ther Oncol* 1997;31:256–259.

62. Hardy, JR and Harvey, VJ, Cerebral metastases in patients with ovarian cancer treated with chemotherapy. *Gynecol Oncol* 1989;33(3):296–300.

63. Harlow, BL and Hartge, PA, A review of perineal talc exposure and risk of ovarian cancer. *Regul Toxicol Pharmacol* 1995;21(2):254–260.

64. Hart, WR, Borderline epithelial tumors of the ovary. *Mod Pathol* 2005;18[Suppl 2]:S33–50.

65. Hart, WR, Diagnostic challenge of secondary (metastatic) ovarian tumors simulating primary endometrioid and mucinous neoplasms. *Pathol Int* 2005;55(5):231–243.

66. Hart, WR, Mucinous tumors of the ovary: a review. *Int J Gynecol Pathol* 2005; 24(1):4–25.

67. Hicks, ML, Piver, MS, Mas, E, et al., Intraoperative orthovoltage radiation therapy in the treatment of recurrent gynecologic malignancies. *Am J Clin Oncol* 1993; 16(6):497–500.

68. Hong, L, Alektiar, K, Chui, C, et al., IMRT of large fields: whole-abdomen irradiation. *Int J Radiat Oncol Biol Phys* 2002;54(1):278–289.

69. Hoskins, WJ, Bundy, BN, Thigpen, JT, et al., The influence of cytoreductive surgery on recurrence-free interval and survival in small-volume stage III epithelial ovarian cancer: a Gynecologic Oncology Group study. *Gynecol Oncol* 1992;47(2):159–166.

70. Hoskins, WJ, McGuire, WP, Brady, MF, et al., The effect of diameter of largest residual disease on survival after primary cytoreductive surgery in patients with suboptimal residual epithelial ovarian carcinoma. *Am J Obstet Gynecol* 1994;170(4):974–980.

71. Hreshchyshyn, MM, Park, RC, Blessing, JA, et al., The role of adjuvant therapy in stage I ovarian cancer. *Am J Obstet Gynecol* 1980;138(2):139–145.

72. Husain, A, Chi, DS, Prasad, M, et al., The role of laparoscopy in second-look evaluations for ovarian cancer. *Gynecol Oncol* 2001;80(1):44–47.

73. Jacobs I, MU, Parmar M, Beveridge H, et al. UK Collaborative Trial of Ovarian Cancer Screening. 2000; United Kingdom Ovarian Cancer Screening Trial with transvaginal ultrasound and serum CA 125]. Available at: http://www.ukctocs.org.uk. Accessed January 2007.

74. Janovski, NA, Paramanandhar, TL. Ovarian tumors. Tumors and tumor-like conditions of the ovaries, fallopian tubes, and ligaments of the uterus. *Major Probl Obstet Gynecol* 1973;4:1–245.

75. Kaye, SB, Lewis, CR, Paul, J, et al., Randomised study of two doses of cisplatin with cyclophosphamide in epithelial ovarian cancer. *Lancet* 1992;340(8815): 329–333.
76. Keal, EE, Asbestosis and abdominal neoplasms. *Lancet* 1960;2:1211–1216.
77. Klaassen, D, Shelley, W, Starreveld, A, et al., Early stage ovarian cancer: a randomized clinical trial comparing whole abdominal radiotherapy, melphalan, and intraperitoneal chromic phosphate: a National Cancer Institute of Canada Clinical Trials Group report. *J Clin Oncol* 1988;6(8):1254–1263.
78. Kolstad, P, Davy, M and Hoeg, K, Individualized treatment of ovarian cancer. *Am J Obstet Gynecol* 1977;128(6):617–625.
79. Konski, AA, Neisler, J, Phibbs, G, et al., A pilot study investigating intraoperative electron beam irradiation in the treatment of ovarian malignancies. *Gynecol Oncol* 1990;38(1):121–124.
80. Kuten, A, Stein, M, Steiner, M, et al., Whole abdominal irradiation following chemotherapy in advanced ovarian carcinoma. *Int J Radiat Oncol Biol Phys* 1988; 14(2):273–279.
81. Lambert, HE, Rustin, GJ, Gregory, WM, et al., A randomized trial comparing single-agent carboplatin with carboplatin followed by radiotherapy for advanced ovarian cancer: a North Thames Ovary Group study. *J Clin Oncol* 1993;11(3):440–448.
82. Lawton, F, Luesley, D, Blackledge, G, et al., A randomized trial comparing whole abdominal radiotherapy with chemotherapy following cisplatinum cytoreduction in epithelial ovarian cancer. West Midlands Ovarian Cancer Group Trial II. *Clin Oncol (R Coll Radiol)* 1990;2(1):4–9.
83. Lukanova, A, Bjor, O, Kaaks, R, et al., Body mass index and cancer: results from the Northern Sweden Health and Disease Cohort. *Int J Cancer* 2006;118(2):458–466.
84. Lund, B, Hansen, M, Lundvall, F, et al., Intestinal obstruction in patients with advanced carcinoma of the ovaries treated with combination chemotherapy. *Surg Gynecol Obstet* 1989;169(3):213–218.
85. Lynch, HT, Bewtra, C and Lynch, JF, Familial ovarian carcinoma. Clinical nuances. *Am J Med* 1986;81(6):1073–1076.
86. Lynch, HT, Fitzsimmons, ML, Conway, TA, et al., Hereditary carcinoma of the ovary and associated cancers: a study of two families. *Gynecol Oncol* 1990;36(1): 48–55.
87. Lynch, HT and Smyrk, T, Hereditary nonpolyposis colorectal cancer (Lynch syndrome). An updated review. *Cancer* 1996;78(6):1149–1167.
88. MacGibbon, A, Bucci, J, MacLeod, C, et al., Whole abdominal radiotherapy following second-look laparotomy for ovarian carcinoma. *Gynecol Oncol* 1999;75(1): 62–67.
89. Marhhom, E and Cohen, I, Fertility preservation options for women with malignancies. *Obstet Gynecol Surv* 2007;62(1):58–72.
90. May, LF, Belinson, JL and Roland, TA, Palliative benefit of radiation therapy in advanced ovarian cancer. *Gynecol Oncol* 1990;37(3):408–411.
91. McCreath, WA and Chi, DS, Surgical cytoreduction in ovarian cancer. Oncology (Williston Park), 2004;18(5):645–654.
92. McGuire, WP, Hoskins, WJ, Brady, MF, et al., Assessment of dose-intensive therapy in suboptimally debulked ovarian cancer: a Gynecologic Oncology Group study. *J Clin Oncol* 1995;13(7):1589–1599.
93. McGuire, WP, Hoskins, WJ, Brady, MF, et al., Cyclophosphamide and cisplatin compared with paclitaxel and cisplatin in patients with stage III and stage IV ovarian cancer. *N Engl J Med* 1996;334(1):1–6.
94. McGuire, WP, Rowinsky, EK, Rosenshein, NB, et al., Taxol: a unique antineoplastic agent with significant activity in advanced ovarian epithelial neoplasms. *Ann Intern Med* 1989;111(4):273–279.
95. Memarzadeh, S, Lee, SB, Berek, JS, et al., CA125 levels are a weak predictor of optimal cytoreductive surgery in patients with advanced epithelial ovarian cancer. *Int J Gynecol Cancer* 2003;13(2):120–124.
96. Menczer, J, Ben-Baruch, G, Modan, M, et al., Intraperitoneal cisplatin chemotherapy versus abdominopelvic irradiation in ovarian carcinoma patients after second-look laparotomy. *Cancer* 1989;63(8):1509–1513.
97. Menczer, J, Modan, M, Brenner, J, et al., Abdominopelvic irradiation for stage II–IV ovarian carcinoma patients with limited or no residual disease at second-look laparotomy after completion of cisplatinum-based combination chemotherapy. *Gynecol Oncol* 1986;24(2):149–154.
98. Micha, JP, Goldstein, BH, Mattison, JA, et al., Experience with single-agent paclitaxel consolidation following primary chemotherapy with carboplatin, paclitaxel, and gemcitabine in advanced ovarian cancer. *Gynecol Oncol* 2005;96(1): 132–135.
99. Miller, BE, Barron, BA, Wan, JY, et al., Prognostic factors in adult granulosa cell tumor of the ovary. *Cancer* 1997;79(10):1951–1955.
100. Muggia, FM, Braly, PS, Brady, MF, et al., Phase III randomized study of cisplatin versus paclitaxel versus cisplatin and paclitaxel in patients with suboptimal stage III or IV ovarian cancer: a gynecologic oncology group study. *J Clin Oncol* 2000; 18(1):106–115.
101. Mukherjee, P, Madsen, CS, Ginardi, AR, et al., Mucin 1-specific immunotherapy in a mouse model of spontaneous breast cancer. *J Immunother* 2003;26(1): 47–62.
102. Muller, JH, [Further progress in treatment of peritoneal carcinosis in ovarian cancer with artificial radioactivity; Au198.]. *Gynaecologia* 1950;129(5):289–294.
103. Omura, GA, Brady, MF, Look, KY, et al., Phase III trial of paclitaxel at two dose levels, the higher dose accompanied by filgrastim at two dose levels in platinum-pretreated epithelial ovarian cancer: an intergroup study. *J Clin Oncol* 2003;21(15):2843–2848.
104. Ozols, RF, Update on Gynecologic Oncology Group (GOG) trials in ovarian cancer. *Cancer Invest* 2004;22[Suppl 2]:11–20.
105. Pavlik, EJ, DePriest, PD, Gallion, HH, et al., Ovarian volume related to age. *Gynecol Oncol* 2000;77(3):410–412.
106. Peters, WA, 3rd, Smith, MR, Cain, JM, et al., Intraperitoneal P-32 is not an effective consolidation therapy after a negative second-look laparotomy for epithelial carcinoma of the ovary. *Gynecol Oncol* 1992;47(2):146–149.
107. Petit, T, Velten, M, d'Hombres, A, et al., Long-term survival of 106 stage III ovarian cancer patients with minimal residual disease after second-look laparotomy and consolidation radiotherapy. *Gynecol Oncol* 2007;104(1):104–108.
108. Pickel, H, Lahousen, M, Petru, E, et al., Consolidation radiotherapy after carboplatin-based chemotherapy in radically operated advanced ovarian cancer. *Gynecol Oncol* 1999;72(2):215–219.
109. Pickel, H, Lahousen, M, Stettner, H, et al., The spread of ovarian cancer. *Baillieres Clin Obstet Gynaecol* 1989;3(1):3–12.
110. Podratz, KC and Cliby, WA, Second-look surgery in the management of epithelial ovarian carcinoma. *Gynecol Oncol* 1994;55(3 Pt 2):S128–133.
111. Podratz, KC, Malkasian, GD., Jr., Wieand, HS., et al., Recurrent disease after negative second-look laparotomy in stages III and IV ovarian carcinoma. *Gynecol Oncol* 1988;29(3):274–282.
112. Ramirez, PT, Slomovitz, BM, McQuinn, L, et al., Role of appendectomy at the time of primary surgery in patients with early-stage ovarian cancer. *Gynecol Oncol* 2006;103(3):888–890.
113. Reed, E, Zerbe, CS, Brawley, OW, et al., Analysis of autopsy evaluations of ovarian cancer patients treated at the National Cancer Institute, 1972–1988. *Am J Clin Oncol* 2000;23(2):107–116.
114. Riedinger, JM, Wafflart, J, Ricolleau, G, et al., CA 125 half-life and CA 125 nadir during induction chemotherapy are independent predictors of epithelial ovarian cancer outcome: results of a French multicentric study. *Ann Oncol* 2006;17(8):1234–1238.
115. Rodriguez, GC, Soper, JT, Berchuck, A, et al., Improved palliation of cerebral metastases in epithelial ovarian cancer using a combined modality approach including radiation therapy, chemotherapy, and surgery. *J Clin Oncol* 1992;10(10):1553–1560.
116. Rogers, L, Varia, M, Halle, J, et al., 32P following negative second-look laparotomy for epithelial ovarian cancer. *Gynecol Oncol* 1993;50(2):141–146.
117. Rosenshein, NB, Radioisotopes in the treatment of ovarian cancer. *Clin Obstet Gynaecol* 1983;10(2):279–295.
118. Rubin, SC, Hoskins, WJ, Benjamin, I, et al., Palliative surgery for intestinal obstruction in advanced ovarian cancer. *Gynecol Oncol* 1989;34(1):16–19.
119. Rubin, SC, Hoskins, WJ, Saigo, PE, et al., Prognostic factors for recurrence following negative second-look laparotomy in ovarian cancer patients treated with platinum-based chemotherapy. *Gynecol Oncol* 1991;42(2):137–141.
120. Rutledge, F and Burns, BC, Chemotherapy for advanced ovarian cancer. *Am J Obstet Gynecol* 1966;96(6):761–772.
121. Schlaerth, AC and Abu-Rustum, NR, Role of minimally invasive surgery in gynecologic cancers. *Oncologist* 2006;11(8):895–901.
122. Schlesselman, JJ, Net effect of oral contraceptive use on the risk of cancer in women in the United States. *Obstet Gynecol* 1995;85(5 Pt 1):793–801.
123. Scully, R, Young, RH and Clement, PB, Tumors of the ovary, maldeveloped gonads, fallopian tube, and broad ligament. In: Atlas of tumor pathology, 3rd Series, fasc. 23. Washington, DC: Armed Forces Institute of Pathology; 1998.
124. Sell, A, Bertelsen, K, Andersen, JE, et al., Randomized study of whole abdomen irradiation versus pelvic irradiation plus cyclophosphamide in treatment of early ovarian cancer. *Gynecol Oncol* 1990;37(3):367–373.
125. Ŝevelda, P, Gitsch, E, Dittrich, C, et al., [Therapeutic and prognostic results of a prospective multicenter ovarian cancer study of FIGO stages I and II]. *Geburtshilfe Frauenheilkd* 1987;47(3):179–185.
126. Shaw, MC, Wolfe, CD, Devaja, O, et al., Development of an evidence-based algorithm for the management of ovarian cancer. *Eur J Gynaecol Oncol* 2003;24(2): 117–125.
127. Sherman, ME, Mink, PJ, Curtis, R, et al., Survival among women with borderline ovarian tumors and ovarian carcinoma: a population-based analysis. *Cancer* 2004;100(5):1045–1052.
128. Skates, SJ, Menon, U, MacDonald, N, et al., Calculation of the risk of ovarian cancer from serial CA-125 values for preclinical detection in postmenopausal women. *J Clin Oncol* 2003;21[10 Suppl]:206–210.
129. Smith, JP, Delgado, G and Rutledge, F, Second-look operation in ovarian carcinoma: postchemotherapy. *Cancer* 1976;38(3):1438–1442.
130. Smith, JP, Rutledge, FN and Delclos, L, Postoperative treatment of early cancer of the ovary: a random trial between postoperative irradiation and chemotherapy. *Natl Cancer Inst Monogr* 1975;42:149–153.
131. Soliman, PT, Slomovitz, BM, Broaddus, RR, et al., Synchronous primary cancers of the endometrium and ovary: a single institution review of 84 cases. *Gynecol Oncol* 2004;94(2):456–462.
132. Soper, JT, Berchuck, A and Clarke-Pearson, DL, Adjuvant intraperitoneal chromic phosphate therapy for women with apparent early ovarian carcinoma who have not undergone comprehensive surgical staging. *Cancer* 1991;68(4):725–729.
133. Sorbe, B, Consolidation treatment of advanced ovarian carcinoma with radiotherapy after induction chemotherapy. *Int J Gynecol Cancer* 2003;13[Suppl 2]: 192–5.
134. Spanos, WJ, Jr., Day, T, Jr., Jose, B, et al., Use of P-32 in stage III epithelial carcinoma of the ovary. *Gynecol Oncol* 1994;54(1):35–39.
135. Spencer, TR, Jr., Marks, RD, Jr., Fenn, JO, et al., Intraperitoneal P-32 after negative second-look laparotomy in ovarian carcinoma. *Cancer* 1989;63(12):2434–2437.
136. Sugiyama, T, Kamura, T, Kigawa, J, et al., Clinical characteristics of clear cell carcinoma of the ovary: a distinct histologic type with poor prognosis and resistance to platinum-based chemotherapy. *Cancer* 2000;88(11):2584–2589.
137. Sutton, GP, Stehman, FB, Einhorn, LH, et al., Ten-year follow-up of patients receiving cisplatin, doxorubicin, and cyclophosphamide chemotherapy for advanced epithelial ovarian carcinoma. *J Clin Oncol* 1989;7(2):223–229.
138. Thomas, GM and Dembo, AJ, Integrating radiation therapy into the management of ovarian cancer. *Cancer* 1993;71[4 Suppl]:1710–1718.
139. Tinger, A, Waldron, T, Peluso, N, et al., Effective palliative radiation therapy in advanced and recurrent ovarian carcinoma. *Int J Radiat Oncol Biol Phys* 2001; 51(5):1256–1263.
140. Trimbos, JB, Parmar, M, Vergote, I, et al., International Collaborative Ovarian Neoplasm trial 1 and Adjuvant ChemoTherapy In Ovarian Neoplasm trial: two parallel randomized phase III trials of adjuvant chemotherapy in patients with early-stage ovarian carcinoma. *J Natl Cancer Inst* 2003;95(2):105–112.
141. Tzonou, A, Polychronopoulou, A, Hsieh, CC, et al., Hair dyes, analgesics, tranquilizers and perineal talc application as risk factors for ovarian cancer. *Int J Cancer* 1993;55(3):408–410.
142. Vahrson, H, Nitz, U and Bender, HG, Malignancies of the Ovaries, In: Vahrson, H, ed. Radiation Oncology of Gynecological Cancers. Berlin: Springer; 1997: 297–396.
143. van der Burg, ME and Vergote, I, The role of interval debulking surgery in ovarian cancer. *Curr Oncol Rep* 2003;5(6):473–481.
144. Varia, M, Rosenman, J, Venkatraman, S, et al., Intraperitoneal chromic phosphate therapy after second-look laparotomy for ovarian cancer. *Cancer* 1988; 61(5):919–927.
145. Varia, MA, Stehman, FB, Bundy, BN, et al., Intraperitoneal radioactive phosphorus (32P) versus observation after negative second-look laparotomy for stage III

ovarian carcinoma: a randomized trial of the Gynecologic Oncology Group. *J Clin Oncol* 2003;21(15):2849–2855.

146. Vergote, I, De Brabanter, J, Fyles, A, et al., Prognostic importance of degree of differentiation and cyst rupture in stage I invasive epithelial ovarian carcinoma. *Lancet* 2001;357(9251):176–182.

147. Vergote, IB, Vergote-De Vos, LN, Abeler, VM, et al., Randomized trial comparing cisplatin with radioactive phosphorus or whole-abdomen irradiation as adjuvant treatment of ovarian cancer. *Cancer* 1992;69(3):741–749.

148. Vergote, IB, Winderen, M, De Vos, LN, et al., Intraperitoneal radioactive phosphorus therapy in ovarian carcinoma. Analysis of 313 patients treated primarily or at second-look laparotomy. *Cancer* 1993;71(7):2250–2260.

149. Verheijen, RH, Massuger, LF, Benigno, BB, et al., Phase III trial of intraperitoneal therapy with yttrium-90-labeled HMFG1 murine monoclonal antibody in patients with epithelial ovarian cancer after a surgically defined complete remission. *J Clin Oncol* 2006;24(4):571–578.

150. Webb, MJ, Snyder, JA, Jr., Williams, TJ, et al., Second-look laparotomy in ovarian cancer. *Gynecol Oncol* 1982;14(3):285–293.

151. Williams, SD, Blessing, JA, Moore, DH, et al., Cisplatin, vinblastine, and bleomycin in advanced and recurrent ovarian germ-cell tumors. A trial of the Gynecologic Oncology Group. *Ann Intern Med* 1989;111(1):22–27.

152. Winter-Roach, B, Hooper, L and Kitchener, H, Systematic review of adjuvant therapy for early stage (epithelial) ovarian cancer. *Int J Gynecol Cancer* 2003; 13(4):395–404.

153. Yap, OW, Kapp, DS, Teng, NN, et al., Intraoperative radiation therapy in recurrent ovarian cancer. *Int J Radiat Oncol Biol Phys* 2005;63(4):1114–1121.

154. Yawn, BP, Barrette, BA and Wollan, PC, Ovarian cancer: the neglected diagnosis. *Mayo Clin Proc* 2004;79(10):1277–1282.

155. Young, RC, Brady, MF, Nieberg, RK, et al., Adjuvant treatment for early ovarian cancer: a randomized phase III trial of intraperitoneal 32P or intravenous cyclophosphamide and cisplatin—a gynecologic oncology group study. *J Clin Oncol* 2003;21(23):4350–4355.

156. Young, RC, Walton, LA, Ellenberg, SS, et al., Adjuvant therapy in stage I and stage II epithelial ovarian cancer. Results of two prospective randomized trials. *N Engl J Med* 1990;322(15):1021–1027.

157. Young, RH, Dickersin, GR and Scully, RE, Juvenile granulosa cell tumor of the ovary. A clinicopathological analysis of 125 cases. *Am J Surg Pathol* 1984; 8(8):575–596.

158. Zaino, R, Whitney, C, Brady, MF, et al., Simultaneously detected endometrial and ovarian carcinomas—a prospective clinicopathologic study of 74 cases: a gynecologic oncology group study. *Gynecol Oncol* 2001;83(2):355–362.

159. Zhu, Y, Wu, R, Sangha, N, et al., Classifications of ovarian cancer tissues by proteomic patterns. *Proteomics* 2006;6(21):5846–5856.

Clinical Radiation Oncology

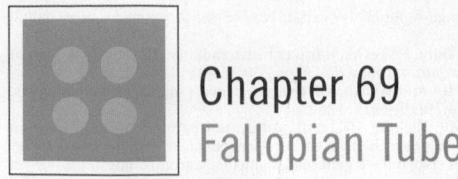

Chapter 69
Fallopian Tube

Patrizia Guerrieri, Luther W. Brady

Anatomy

The fallopian tubes are hollow, muscular viscera positioned horizontally within the superior part of the broad ligament. Each tube extends from its own ovary in communication with the peritoneal cavity. They project outward, backward, and then downward to open into the superior posterior part of the uterine fundus, where they communicate with the endometrial cavity. Histologically, the tubal wall consists of four separate layers: the mucosa, the submucosa, the muscularis (external longitudinal and inner circular layers), and the outer serosal layer, which is continuous with the visceral peritoneum of the uterus.

The mucosa is intricately folded, with the number of folds increasing from the interstitial portion to the ampulla. The epithelium is composed mainly of ciliated cells and secretory cells. Cyclic changes are evident in the tubal epithelium, similar to those of the endometrium, in response to estrogen and progesterone. The epithelium is the origin of most malignancies; its changes during the menstrual years and after menopause may play a role in tumorigenesis.

The arterial supply of the fallopian tube is derived from the ovarian artery, which anastomoses with the uterine artery. Venous drainage is through the pampiniform plexus to the ovarian vein along with the uterine plexus. The lymphatics, richly anastomosed with those of the adjacent organs, drain into the ovarian lymphatics and lumbar lymph nodes (28). These lymphatics course along the folds of the tubal mucosa, where they form a network of intercommunicating lymphatic sinusoids (28). From this area, they drain into the para-aortic and iliac nodes.

Epidemiology

The first descriptions of a primary malignancy of the fallopian tube are attributed to Renaud and Ricci (55) in 1845 and to Orthmann in 1866 and 1888. Since that time, there have been fewer than 1,500 cases reported. This is the rarest of the female genital tract malignancies, making up only 0.15% to 1.8% of all gynecologic malignancies (16,38,49,61), with an average of 0.3% (16). The theoretic incidence is 3 to 3.6 cases per 1 million women per year (62). There is a reported 14% higher incidence in white people than in black people (62).

The age range of this disease has been reported to be from 18 to 87 years, with most occurrences in the fifth and sixth decades of life. In the literature a mean age of 55 years is described. This is consistent with the mean age of 56.7 years in a meta-analysis of 577 patients computed in 1991 (43). The clinical profile of these patients reveals a relative low parity rate (35,67), with a mean parity of 1 to 1.7 (35,43). By virtue of the mean age of incidence, most patients are postmenopausal.

Pelvic inflammatory disease and tuberculous salpingitis once were believed to be causative factors in the development of fallopian tube malignancies. No study to date has proven this theory.

Natural History

The primary spread of disease is similar to that of ovarian cancers in that there is local extension of tumor to adjacent structures to involve the peritoneum, omentum, bowel, and ovaries (56,66). However, 70% of patients with fallopian tube tumors have disease confined to the pelvis at presentation, compared with 48% of patients with ovarian malignancies (56), and up to 50% of patients are diagnosed with stage I disease. This is probably a result of the early presentation of abnormal bleeding and pain with distention of a small tubal lumen, which is absent in the anatomy of the ovary.

With the advent of improved surgical resections with sampling or radical lymphadenectomy, early lymphatic invasion has been discovered to have a prominent role in disease progression (27). Lymph node positivity has been found to be 75% at autopsy. In a review of 67 patients, Sedlis (67) reported that tubal musculature rarely was involved when lymphatic metastases were present.

Transcoelomic spread has an impact on survival, with a decrease in survival rates as the depth of wall invasion increases (65). Although the fallopian tubes are derived from the same embryonic structure as the uterus, their malignant lesions behave, histologically and clinically, more like ovarian tumors, with one exception resulting from their particular anatomic structure. Unlike ovarian tumors, 50% of fallopian tube tumors are stage I and II and, similar to endometrial cancer, tubal wall penetration has been discovered to have a great impact on 5-year survival in early stages (41,44).

Far less common in fallopian tube cancer are distant metastases to liver and lung, which occur most often by local extension outside the peritoneal cavity by means of nodal versus transdiaphragmatic and hematogenous spread (66). Even though single cases of hematogenous spread to spleen, bone, and brain have been described in the literature, distant metastases are more important as a site of treatment failure in ovarian cancer, in which more than 50% of recurrences occur outside the peritoneal cavity along with intraperitoneal disease (8,30,40). With this difference between ovarian and fallopian tube cancer, and because of the frequency of lymphatic spread in fallopian tube cancer also in early stages, aggressive postsurgical adjuvant treatment with intensified use of chemotherapy today represents standard care in fallopian tube carcinoma (3,27,73).

Clinical Presentation

Unlike ovarian malignancies, tumors of the fallopian tube may cause early clinical signs and symptoms. Although the triads of pelvic pain, pelvic mass, and leukorrhea or vaginal bleeding, vaginal discharge, and lower abdominal pain have been described as pathognomonic, the highest percentage of patients presenting with such a triad of symptoms has been only 11% (16). Another classic sign, hydrops tubae profluens, which is a sudden emptying of accumulated fluid in the distended fallopian tube that causes profuse, watery, serosanguinous discharge to be released from the vagina, accompanied by a decrease in pelvic mass size on physical examination, was attributed to only 9% in a meta-analysis of 122 patients (43). In many other series it has been reported specifically that neither a triad nor hydrops tubae profluens was present in any of the patients reviewed (56,67).

Despite these inconsistencies in symptoms, the most common presenting sign is metrorrhagia (36,48,67), followed by pain and vaginal discharge (67). The most common physical sign is a pelvic mass, which occurs in 12% to 66% of patients (16).

Diagnostic Work-Up

Because of the rarity of primary malignancies of the fallopian tube and because the presenting signs are similar to those of salpingitis, ovarian abscess or tumor, pelvic inflammatory disease, and even ectopic pregnancy, it has been difficult to diagnose most cases before surgical exploration. Many series have reported missing the correct diagnosis entirely in their working differential (36,53,56).

Many different modalities for use in the detection of fallopian tube cancers are presently under investigation. Some of these have had promising results, including various nuclear medicine imaging techniques with radioactive nucleotides, magnetic resonance imaging (MRI), ultrasound, and tumor markers.

Radiologic Imaging

Ultrasonography

Ultrasonography, performed with a vaginal transducer, has added more accurate assessment of adnexal pathology than pelvic ultrasound alone (15,28).

In combination with other screening techniques and modalities, transvaginal sonography (TVS) can be made more effective as a screening tool for diagnosis of primary fallopian tube carcinoma. Kol et al. (28) described a case in which TVS was used to aid in the preoperative diagnosis in conjunction with elevated CA 125 levels. The addition of color flow and Doppler waveform measurements has increased the sensitivity of TVS (31,51). In malignant masses, there is typically a decreased amount of muscle in the lining of the tumor vessels, which, combined with increased arteriovenous shunting within the tumor, increases flow and results in abnormal pulsatile and resistance indices compared with those of normal vessels (51). Color flow alone in imaging of postmenopausal adnexal masses has a reported specificity of only 65%, assuming that flow is visible (31). Kurjak et al. (31) found that the differences in vessel resistance indices between benign and malignant tumors yielded a sensitivity of 96% and a specificity of 95% ($p < .001$). The drawbacks to TVS with color flow Doppler imaging lie in the experience of the operator, the quality of instrumentation used, and the change in imaging characteristics of tumors depending on stage (51).

Computed Tomography and Magnetic Resonance Imaging

Some authors report that MRI is superior to ultrasound and computed tomography in that it can better differentiate the fallopian tube from other pelvic organs (23,69). However, the separation of benign from malignant processes is difficult, and ultrasound was concluded to be superior to MRI as a screening modality in the evaluation of adnexal tumors (69).

Nuclear Scan Imaging

Radioimaging with a combination of immunolymphoscintigraphy and immunoscintigraphy with ^{131}I-labeled F(ab')$_2$ fragments of monoclonal OC 125 antibodies improved detection

of retroperitoneal lymph node metastases, with a sensitivity of 90% and a specificity of 83% (32). These findings were correlated with abnormally elevated levels of CA 125, which would indicate that women with high circulating levels of this tumor marker are at a higher risk of having metastatic disease.

As well as in other high malignancy tumors whole-body fluorodeoxy-2-glucose-positron emission tomography scanning has clearly shown its role in staging, biologic target definition, and follow-up of fallopian tube carcinomas *as well* (22).

Tumor Markers

CA 125

CA 125 is an antigen expressed by epithelial ovarian tumors as well as other cells derived from the müllerian duct and coelomic tissues. It is used chiefly for detection and surveillance of patients with ovarian malignancies.

CA 125 was first described as a tumor marker abnormally elevated in patients with recurrence of fallopian tube carcinoma (42). Within the next several years, numerous authors reported its use as a marker during treatment to monitor response to therapy (28,70).

Levels >65 U/mL are seen in about 50% of all new malignant fallopian tube carcinoma, with a specificity of 98% and a sensitivity of 75% (3,28). However, serum antigen levels are elevated in benign as well as malignant conditions, including endometriosis, pelvic inflammatory disease, and early pregnancy. Levels below the upper limit were noted in two patients who had disease recurrence at second-look laparotomy (70).

Recent reports suggest that screening with this tumor marker would be more effective if used in combination with ultrasound, specifically TVS plus serial levels of CA 125 (51). It also may have a role as a prognostic and monitoring marker in patients surgically treated. In a multicentric study the serum levels of CA 125 were measured in 403 samples from 53 patients affected by primary fallopian tube tumors. The pretreatment median serum CA 125 level was 183. Tumor stage and CA 125 were significantly associated with lower disease-free and overall survival in a univariate Cox regression model; the serum level during chemotherapy was correlated with the Gynecologic Oncology Group (GOG) response criteria to chemotherapy and had high specificity, sensitivity, and negative predictive value during follow-up with a median lead time of 3 months (3,18). It has been suggested that elevated levels of CA 125 in supposed early-stage disease, in conjunction with the use of CA 125 immunoscintigraphy, may be predictive of metastatic disease (13,32).

CA 19-9

CA 19-9 is a glycoprotein of normal cells, part of the Lewis blood group of antigens. It is expressed only by patients with a positive Lewis phenotype. CA 19-9 has been used in monitoring of malignancies of the gastrointestinal tract. Most recently, in 1991, it was screened for possible expression in gynecologic malignancies (64). Although it was found to be expressed in müllerian tissue-derived tumors, its sensitivity is low because it is not released well into the bloodstream and is expressed more overtly in less-differentiated or anaplastic tumors (64). Scharl et al. (64) concluded that CA 19-9 may have a role in surveillance of patients whose tumors do not express CA 125.

Staging

Because carcinoma of the fallopian tube is one of the rarest of all gynecologic malignancies and has both close proximity to the ovary and similarities in histopathology, diagnostic criteria

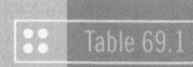

Table 69.1   CRITERIA FOR DIAGNOSIS OF PRIMARY CARCINOMA OF THE FALLOPIAN TUBE

1. Grossly, the main tumor is in the tube.
2. Microscopically, chiefly the mucosa should be involved and should show a papillary pattern.
3. If the tubal wall is involved to a great extent, the transition between benign and malignant tissue should be demonstrable.

were established by Hu et al. (21) in 1950. The guidelines that help to differentiate fallopian tube malignancies from those of the ovary and other primary sites are given in Table 69.1.

In spite of numerous staging classifications, inconsistent and poorly documented staging procedures have been reported in the literature through the years. Modern staging is based on the International Federation of Gynecology and Obstetrics (FIGO) staging for ovarian carcinoma and demonstrated a direct relation between stage of disease and survival. In 1991 an official staging system for carcinoma of the fallopian tube was established by FIGO (Table 69.2). This staging system follows the main directives set for ovarian carcinomas, with the addition of guidelines for carcinoma in situ or stage 0 based on involvement of the interface of the mucosal basement membrane and the tubal stroma (47). Within stage I the presence or absence of invasion of the tubal wall, the depth of invasion, *and* the location of the tumor in the fimbrial versus the nonfimbrial portion and the presence or absence of intraoperative tumor rupture seem to be significantly important for prognosis (1,3). Several reviews of patients with stage 0 and invasive stage I disease

Table 69.2   INTERNATIONAL FEDERATION OF GYNECOLOGY AND OBSTETRICS (FIGO) FALLOPIAN TUBE STAGING

Stage	Description
0	Carcinoma *in situ* (limited to tubal mucosa)
I	Growth limited to the fallopian tubes
IA	Growth limited to one tube with extension into the submucosa and/or muscularis but not penetrating the serosal surface; no ascites
IB	Growth limited to both tubes with extension into the submucosa and/or muscularis but not penetrating the serosal surgal surface; no ascites
IC	Tumor either stage IA or IB with tumor extension through or onto the tubal serosa; or with ascites present containing malignant cells or positive peritoneal washings
II	Growth involving one or both fallopian tubes with pelvic extension
IIA	Extension and/or metastasis to the uterus and/or ovaries
IIB	Extension to other pelvic tissues
IIC	Tumor either stage IIA or IIB with ascites present containing malignant cells or with positive peritoneal washings
III	Tumor involves one or both fallopian tubes with peritoneal implants outside the pelvis and/or positive retroperitoneal or inguinal nodes. Superficial liver metastasis equals stage III. Tumor appears limited to the true pelvis but with histologically proven malignant extension to the small bowel or omentum
IIIA	Tumor grossly limited to the true pelvis with negative nodes but with histologically confirmed microscopic seeding of abdominal peritoneal surfaces
IIIB	Tumor involving one or both tubes with histologically confirmed implants of abdominal peritoneal surfaces, none exceeding 2 cm in diameter; lymph nodes are negative
IIIC	Abdominal implants >2 cm in diameter and/or positive retroperitoneal or inguinal nodes
IV	Growth involving one or both fallopian tubes with distant metastasis. If pleural effusion is present, there must be positive cytology to be stage IV. Parenchymal liver metastases equal stage IV

Table 69.3   MODIFIED INTERNATIONAL FEDERATION OF GYNECOLOGY AND OBSTETRICS (FIGO) FALLOPIAN TUBE STAGING

Stage	Description
0	Carcinoma *in situ* (limited to tubal epithelium)
I	Growth limited to the fallopian tubes
IA	Growth limited to one tube with extension into the submucosa and/or muscularis but not penetrating the serosal surface; no ascites containing malignant cells, or positive peritoneal washings
0b	Growth limited to one tube, with no extension into lamina propria
1b	Growth limited to one tube with extension into lamina propria, but no extension into muscularis
2b	Growth limited to one tube with extension into muscularis
IB	Growth limited to both tubes with extension into the submucosa and/or muscularis but not penetrating the serosal sursal surface; no ascites containing malignant cells, or positive peritoneal washings
0b	Growth limited to both tubes, with no extension into lamina propria
1b	Growth limited to both tubes with extension into lamina propria, but no extension into muscularis
2b	Growth limited to both tubes with extension into muscularis
IC	Tumor either stage IA or IB with tumor extension through or onto the tubal serosa; or with ascites present containing malignant cells or positive peritoneal washings
I (F)	Tumor limited to fimbriated end of fallopian tube(s), without invasion of tubal wall
II	Growth involving one or both fallopian tubes with pelvic extension
IIA	Extension and/or metastasis to the uterus and/or ovaries
IIB	Extension to other pelvic tissues
IIC	Tumor either stage IIA or IIB with ascites present containing malignant cells or with positive peritoneal washings
III	Tumor involves one or both fallopian tubes with peritoneal implants outside the pelvis and/or positive retroperitoneal or inguinal nodes. Superficial liver metastasis equals stage III. Tumor appears limited to the true pelvis but with histologically proven malignant extension to the small bowel or omentum
IIIA	Tumor grossly limited to the true pelvis with negative nodes but with histologically confirmed microscopic seeding of abdominal peritoneal surfaces
IIIB	Tumor involving one or both tubes with grossly visible histologically confirmed implants of abdominal peritoneal surfaces, none exceeding 2 cm in diameter; lymph nodes are negative
IIIC	Abdominal implants >2 cm in diameter and/or positive retroperitoneal or inguinal nodes
IV	Growth involving one or both fallopian tubes with distant metastasis. If pleural effusion is present, there must be positive cytology to be stage IV. Parenchymal liver metastases equal stage IV

illustrate the prognostic implications of a well-weighted selection of adjuvant therapy in early-stage disease in achieving an overall improved survival (26,27). In 1998, a multi-institutional study by Wolfson et al. (73) demonstrated the importance of FIGO staging in all fallopian tube stages.

In 1999 Alvarado-Cabrero et al. (1) proposed expanding the staging system to permit staging of noninvasive tubal carcinomas and fimbrial carcinomas, and posed the basis for a substaging based on depth of invasion. The modified FIGO staging is reported in Table 69.3.

Pathologic Classification

The most common histopathology of fallopian tube malignancies is serous papillary adenocarcinoma, similar to that found in the ovary. Benign tumors are found even less frequently than malignant neoplasms. Rare histologic subtypes are found: endometrioid, clear cell, transitional cell, squamous cell, malignant mixed müllerian tumors, teratomas, and leiomyosarcomas. Tumors previously graded as papillary (pure), papillary–alveolar, and alveolar–medullary (21) now routinely are classified as well, moderately, and poorly differentiated (grades I, II, and III, respectively) (14).

Disease is bilateral in approximately 5% to 30% of patients at the time of initial diagnosis. This is considered to be a multicentric primary. Malignancies are distributed equally between the left and right fallopian tubes.

The gross appearance of a fallopian tube with a primary adenocarcinoma without invasion of the serosal lining usually is enlarged, deformed, fusiform, or sausagelike because of the large intraluminal growth of the tumor. It may mimic the appearance of more benign pathologic processes such as hydrosalpinx, pyosalpinx, or hematosalpinx (2). In more advanced disease with tubal wall invasion, cells may form nodules on the peritoneal surface, mimicking a tubo-ovarian abscess and making the diagnosis of primary organ involvement difficult. Multiple adhesions to surrounding tissue may be found; the most frequent site is the ampulla, followed by the infundibulum, and the lumen is closed approximately 50% of the time (74). Microscopically, the papillary configuration of epithelium usually is preserved, and diagnosis usually follows the criteria set by Hu et al. (21).

Prognostic Factors

According to various reports from the literature, statistically significant prognostic factors with a median p value ≤ 0.05 in univariate analyses are stage at presentation, age, presence of ascites, amount of residual tumor after primary surgical resection, depth of tubal wall infiltration, vascular space invasion, lymphatic spread, hydrosalpinxlike appearance and, to a lesser degree, serous versus nonserous histology (1,3), and aggressiveness of treatment. Although different than thought in earlier reports, the amount of histologic dedifferentiation and the presence of clinical symptoms at diagnosis have not been proven to be of statistical relevance (1,3,16,21,38,61,66). Some authors have shown that the closure of the fimbrial ostium of the tube or the presence of its pathologic effects, such as the appearance of hydrosalpinx, pyosalpinx or hematosalpinx and the associated history of infertility, are determinants of a good prognosis (1,3). The presence of vascular space invasion is strongly correlated with the depth of tubal wall infiltration and the presence of lymphonodal metastasis, whereas the depth of infiltration itself is strongly correlated with stage and presence of residual disease (1,3,27). Stromal invasion is associated with a significantly decreased 5-year survival (50% to 54%) compared with mucosal invasion (87.5% to 100%) (3,26,65).

In multivariate analyses performed by Baekelandt et al. (3) in 151 patients and by Rosen et al. (60) in 143 patients with fallopian tube carcinoma, the strongest independent prognostic factors were disease stage at diagnosis and residual tumor status after surgery, while a hydrosalpinxlike appearance was a marginally significant variable. In Rosen report, p-53 expression did not show a statistical significance in predicting disease stage nor survival. When a subgroup analysis examined the 41 stage I patients only, depth of infiltration and tumor rupture were retained as independent prognostic factors (3,60).

As previously stated, CA 125 serum level is a useful tumor marker and correlate with stage distribution also in fallopian tube carcinomas (1,3,18).

Molecular Genetics

By genomic hybridization performed on 20 primary fallopian tube carcinoma specimens, Pere et al. (46) found that the most frequent genomic changes, in decreasing order, were gains at 3q, 8q, 1q,5p, 7q, 12p, and 20q and losses at 18q, 8p, 4q, and 5q. This is similar to those observed in serous ovarian and uterus carcinomas.

In terms of altered gene expression, several studies report the overexpression of p53, c-myc, c-erbB-2, and p21 genes (6,19,52,59). It is interesting that two of them, p53 and c-erbB-2, recently have been found to be often correlated with the histopathologic aggressiveness of breast cancer. Also, the germline mutations present in breast–ovarian cancer families, BCRA 1 and BCRA 2, have been found in several cases of primary fallopian tube carcinoma, suggesting a common tumorigenesis pattern (58,75).

General Management

The early lymphogenous spread, reported as high as 50% of all cases of fallopian tube cancer, and the specific lymphatic situation that makes metastases to spread simultaneously into pelvic and para-aortic regions have to be taken into for a primary treatment that is surgical in principle. Extensive surgical resection, and staging, should therefore be carried out through total abdominal hysterectomy, omentectomy, and bilateral salpingectomy, radical pelvic and para-aortic lymphadenectomy as well as sampling of ascitic fluid or peritoneal washings and peritoneal sampling of diaphragm, bladder, and bowel (3,27,66). Numerous authors have observed that the amount of residual tumor left behind at primary resection (>2 cm) has major prognostic implications. Some investigators have reported satisfactory results with a more conservative treatment in selected stage 0–I fallopian tube carcinomas. After comprehensive surgical staging and treatment, patients without lymph node metastasis, without intraoperative tumor rupture and with tumor not invading beyond the mucosa (26), may be followed with close observation only (3). Most patients, however, require some form of adjuvant treatment postoperatively to combat bulky residual disease or to treat assumed microscopic involvement.

Deciphering the literature in search of the most favorable treatment regimens is fraught with difficulties. Most studies reporting results of adjuvant therapy for fallopian tube carcinomas cover the time span of several decades without prospective randomization of patients. More recently, to evaluate the results of different schemes of adjuvant chemotherapy, advanced fallopian tube cancers have been treated in pilot or phase I-II studies together with ovarian or peritoneal cancer, following the recommendation that the same principles for the treatment of patients with advanced ovarian cancer be applied to patients with more advanced diseases than favorable stage 0-I fallopian tube cancers (3,5,12,27,29,33,37,50,73).

Chemotherapy

Based on the results of phase II and III studies conducted during the 1980s, cisplatin-based combination chemotherapy today represents standard treatment also for fallopian tube carcinoma as first-line chemotherapy, in both localized and disseminated disease, with carboplatin being a valid cisplatin substitute (3,4,17,20,24,27,39,45,59,72,73). The usual combinations with cyclophosphamide and Adriamycin or with paclitaxel result in overall clinical response rates (complete plus partial) equal to 70% to 80% (3,4,7,17).

A phase I study of paclitaxel, carboplatin, and oral etoposide designed by GOG has been the basis for a second-line chemotherapy in platinum-resistant ovarian and tubal carcinoma (57). Verschraegen et al. (71) reported an overall 23% response rate by crossing to a different taxane in patients who had a long taxane-free interval. Liposomal doxorubicin, topotecan,

Table 69.4	FIVE-YEAR SURVIVAL IN FALLOPIAN TUBE CARCINOMA

Study	No. of Cases	Postoperative Treatment						Survival (%)
		Observation	Pelvic XRT	Abd XRT	Single CTX	Combo CTX	XRT + CTX	
Stages I and II								
Schray et al. (66)	21	—	10	7	—	—	4	42–78
Klein et al. (27)	63	25	32	—	—	31	—	83 vs. 58[a]
McMurray et al. (36)	20	3	6	1	—	6	4	27–56
Baekelandt et al. (3)								
Stage 0-I	49							87.5
Stage II	33	74	22	11	109			73
Stage III-IV	69							37
								29
								12
Stages III and IV								
Schray et al. (73)	12	6[b]	3	1	—	—	2	33
McMurray et al. (36)	10	—	—	4	2	4	4	0–14

XRT, irradiation; Abd XRT, abdominal external-beam irradiation or intraperitoneal ^{32}P; CTX, chemotherapy; NOS, not otherwise specified.
[a]Survival differences seen in patients treated with total abdominal hysterectomy and bilateral salpingo-oophorectomy with or without radical lymphadenectomy, respectively.
[b]Only six patients treated with curative intent.

docetaxel, and gemcitabine are currently under investigation as second- or third-line chemotherapy in platinum-refractory tubal carcinomas or in advanced-stage epithelial gynecologic cancers (5,9,33,34,37,68).

Table 69.4 shows the treatment variabilities for fallopian tube carcinomas over time. In a recent study, Baekelandt et al. (3) reports 14 different chemotherapeutic schemes at the Norwegian Radium Hospital and 3 different radiation protocols over a period of time spanning from January 1963 to June 1998.

Radiation Therapy

Postoperative radiation therapy was a traditional form of therapy for fallopian tube carcinoma dissemination and recurrence up to the 1980s. It has been recommended by some authors and questioned by others (16,38). It is difficult to evaluate results in the past literature because of variability in staging, surgical staging techniques, treatment volume, dose fractionation, and type of radiation used. All reported studies are retrospective and usually involve small numbers of patients treated over long periods.

Several early, small studies observed promising results with techniques similar to those used in treatment of ovarian carcinoma (see Chapter 63). These authors suggested that use of whole-abdomen external-beam irradiation or intraperitoneal administration of radioactive colloids (^{32}P, ^{198}Au) results in better survival rates than does surgery alone (49,66). Some investigators observed that there are too few data to support the use of radioactive colloids and that there is no role in patients with bulky disease (49).

The best results are achieved when total doses >50 Gy in 5 to 6 weeks were used with megavoltage as opposed to orthovoltage therapy (10,13,16,36). McMurray et al. (36) stated that recurrence of early-stage disease (I and II) was likely to be in the upper abdomen if only pelvic irradiation was performed and that areas at risk, such as the abdomen and para-aortic areas, should be included within the initial treatment volume. A 50% relapse rate was reported when early-stage disease was treated with surgery alone or with surgery plus pelvic irradiation, compared with a >50% 5-year survival rate when the abdomen and para-aortic areas were treated (36).

The issue arising between whole abdominal irradiation versus irradiation limited to the pelvic content does not seem to have a clear-cut answer and it has to be limited to specific clinical conditions. Comparable studies in ovarian cancer suggest that adjuvant whole abdominal irradiation can cure only when the postoperative residual tumor is <1 to 2 cm in the pelvis and there is no microscopic disease in the upper abdomen; in spite of the relative sensitivity of fallopian tube carcinoma to radiation, in fact, the tolerance dose to the abdomen can only cure microscopic disease. As radiotherapy was the treatment of choice up to the early 1980s, it has been gradually substituted by chemotherapy, even though there are no randomized studies comparing the efficacy of abdominopelvic radiotherapy and cisplatin containing chemotherapy or more sophisticated chemotherapeutic schemes, given the rarity of this tumor.

Wolfson et al. (73) reported on 72 patients with carcinoma of the fallopian tube (24 stage I, 20 stage II, 24 stage III, and 4 stage IV) treated at six medical centers. Adjuvant chemotherapy was administered to 54 patients, and postoperative irradiation was administered to 22 patients. Of the latter group, 14 received whole-pelvis external irradiation, 5 received whole-abdomen irradiation, 2 received ^{32}P instillation, and 1 received vaginal brachytherapy only. The 5-, 8-, and 15-year survival rates were 44%, 24%, and 19%, respectively, for patients treated with chemotherapy, and 27%, 17%, and 14%, respectively, for those treated with irradiation. Significant prognostic factors included stage I versus more advanced stage and age at diagnosis (younger or older than 60 years). Patterns of failure included 2 vaginal, 5 pelvic, 24 abdominal, and 15 distant metastases. There were 21% abdominal failures in patients with stage I disease versus 79% in stages II, III, and IV. Patients experiencing abdominal relapse were more likely to die (83%) than those without abdominal relapse (39%).

A study published by Klein et al. (26) in 1994 using the 1991 FIGO staging system compared the outcome in carcinoma in situ versus stage I with use of either irradiation or cisplatin-based chemotherapy; tumor penetration through the basement membrane (invasive carcinoma) reduced survival by 50%. The finding in this study that stage I patients treated by irradiation showed a significantly better prognosis than patients treated by chemotherapy ($p = .017$) is claimed to be confounded by the difference in staging of disease that has been carried out over the

Table 69.5	TREATMENT ALGORITHM OF PRIMARY FALLOPIAN TUBE CARCINOMA[a]			
Stage 0-I Negative cytology	Stage 0-I Positive cytology	Stage II-III-IV No residual disease Node negative	Stage II-III-IV Bulky residual disease (>2 cm) Node positive	Stage II-III-IV Residual disease in pelvis (≤1 cm)
No further therapy	Intraperitoneal ^{32}P or short-term CDDP or whole abdominal radiation therapy	Intraperitoneal ^{32}P or short-term CDDP or pelvic (for stage II)/whole abdominal radiation therapy	CDDP containing regimens	CDDP containing regimens followed by whole abdominal radiation or whole abdominal radiation therapy with pelvic boost

CDDP
[a]Staging laparotomy, total abdominal hysterectomy, bilateral salpingo-oophorectomy, omentectomy, and selective or therapeutic pelvic and aortic lymphadenectomy.
Modified by Paulson JD. Malignant lesions of the fallopian tube and broad ligament. Available at: www.emedicine.com. Accessed

years for fallopian tube carcinoma. A more recent retrospective study published in 1999 demonstrated no significant difference in survival between patients treated with adjuvantly radiation versus chemotherapy (60). However, patients in this study were assigned nonrandomly to treatment, and there was no stratification for amount of residual disease among the two groups of patients. Furthermore, many studies show frequent inconsistencies in terms of surgical or radiation therapy treatments (14,26,52,53). When comparing the effectiveness of chemotherapy or radiation therapy in an adjuvant setting for early-stage diseases like stage I and II, no statistical significant difference was found in several recent retrospective studies with a relatively large patients population (3,27,54).

A possible future direction for treating patients with more advanced disease is the exploitation of the cytotoxic activity of both chemotherapy and radiation by using both modalities either sequentially or concurrently. One report of sequential therapy from Toronto in 1991 suggested that it was superior to whole abdominal irradiation alone, with 5-year survival of 84% in the sequential treatment, compared with 37% for the historic cohort treated with irradiation alone ($p = .0006$) (54). A randomized, prospective study might be of help in this regard.

Table 69.5 reports a possible algorithm for the treatment of fallopian tube carcinoma, according to the most recent literature.

For a complete review about radiation therapy techniques, see Chapter 63.

Sequelae of Treatment

Although there have been reports of treatment complications with the use of irradiation (25), most have been small in number and minor in severity. With proper planning and shielding of vital structures during critical portions of treatment, the sequelae should be minimal. However, patients who have undergone multiple surgical explorations and have extensive disease involving bowel, bladder, and other vital structures, or who undergo sequential or concomitant chemotherapy, are always at increased risk for development of complications in any treatment regimen.

Second-Look Laparotomy

Second-look laparotomy is controversial in the treatment of fallopian tube carcinoma, although it generally has been accepted as a tool for management of ovarian cancer. The likelihood of being free of disease at second-look laparotomy is related to the initial stage and amount of residual disease remaining after initial surgery (63). The predictive value in remaining disease-free appears to be limited. Several authors have reported re-

lapse rates of 19% to 40% after a negative second-look operation (4,63).

Future Directions

There is an obvious need for randomized, controlled trials in determining the management of fallopian tube cancer, which, because of its rarity, will require a larger national or international cooperative effort. Presently, there is only one phase II trial acquiring patients with recurrent, persistent advanced ovarian cancer, fallopian tube, or primary peritoneal carcinoma after initial chemotherapy conducted by GOG-National Cancer Institute, to study the effectiveness of low-dose radiation therapy to the abdomen in combination with docetaxel (11).

References

1. Alvarado-Cabrero I, Young RH, Vanvakas EC, et al. Carcinoma of the fallopian tube: a clinicopathological study of 105 cases with observation on staging and prognostic factors. *Gynecol Oncol* 1999;72:367–379.
2. Anbrokh YM. Macroscopic characteristics of cancer of the fallopian tube. *Neoplasma* 1970;17:557–564.
3. Baekelandt M, Nesbakken AJ, Kristensen GB, et al. Carcinoma of the fallopian tube. Clinicopathologic study of 151 patients treated at the Norwegian Radium Hospital. *Cancer* 2000;89:2076–2084.
4. Barakat R, Rubin S, Saigo P, et al. Cisplatin-based combination chemotherapy in carcinoma of the fallopian tube. *Gynecol Oncol* 1990;42:156–160.
5. Chen MD, Fleming GF, Mitchell S, et al. A phase I trial of gemcitabine and topotecan in previously treated ovarian or peritoneal cancer: a GOG study. *Gynecol Oncol* 1006;100:111–115.
6. Chung TK, Cheung TH, To KF, et al. Overexpression of p53 and HER-2neu and c-myc in primary fallopian tube carcinoma. *Gynecol Obstet Invest* 2000;49:47–51.
7. Cormio G, Maneo A, Gabriele A, et al. Treatment of fallopian tube carcinoma with Cyclophosphamide, Adriamycin, and cisplatin. *Am J Clin Oncol* 1997;20:143–145.
8. Courville XF, Cortes Z, Katzman PJ, et al. Case report: Bone metastases from fallopian tube carcinoma. *Clin. Orthop Relat Res* 2005;434:278–281.
9. Dunton CJ, Neufeld J. Complete response to topotecan of recurrent fallopian tube carcinoma. *Gynecol Oncol* 2000;76:128–129.
10. Fogh IB. Primary carcinoma of the fallopian tube. *Cancer* 1961;23:1332–1335.
11. Fracasso PM, Look KY, Kryscio R, et al. Radiation therapy to the abdomen plus docetaxel in treating patients with recurrent or persistent advanced ovarian, peritoneal, or fallopian tube cancer. Ongoing Gynecologic Oncology Group-National Cancer Institute study. Available at: www.clinicaltrials.gov. Accessed May 2007.
12. Fujiwara K, Suzuki S, Ishikawa H, et al. Preliminary toxicity analysis of intraperitoneal carboplatin in combination with intravenous paclitaxel chemotherapy for patients with carcinoma of the ovary, peritoneum or fallopian tube. *Int J Gynecol Cancer* 2005;15:426–431.
13. Gadducci A, Madrigali A, Ciancia EM, et al. The clinical, serological, pathological and immunocytochemical features of a case of primary carcinoma of the fallopian tube. *Eur J Gynaecol Oncol* 1993;14:374–379.
14. Gompel C, Silverberg SG, eds. *Pathology in gynecology and obstetrics*, 4th ed. Philadelphia: JB Lippincott; 1994.
15. Granberg S, Jansson I. Early detection of primary carcinoma of the fallopian tube by endovaginal ultrasound. *Acta Obstet Gynecol Scand* 1990;69:667–668.
16. Hanton E, Malkasian G, Dahlin D, et al. Primary carcinoma of the fallopian tube. *Am J Obstet Gynecol* 1966;94:832–839.
17. Harries M, Moss C, Perren T, et al. A phase II feasibility study of carboplatin followed by sequential weekly paclitaxel and gemcitabine as first-line treatment for ovarian cancer. *Br J Cancer* 2004;91:627–632.
18. Hefler LA, Rosen AC, Graf AH, et al. The clinical value of serum concentrations of cancer antigen 125 in patients with primary fallopian tube carcinoma: a multicenter study. *Cancer* 2000;89:1555–1560.
19. Hellstrom AC, Blegen H, Malec M, et al. Recurrent fallopian tube carcinoma: TP53 mutation and clinical course. *Int J Gynecol Pathol* 2000;19:145–151.
20. Hertig AT, Mansell IT. *Tumors of the female sex organs. Atlas of tumor pathology*, part 1, series 1, fascicle 33. Washington, DC: Armed Forces Institute of Pathology; 1956:62–63.

21. Hu CT, Taymon MZ, Hertig AT. Primary carcinoma of the fallopian tube. *Am J Obstet Gynecol* 1950;59:58–67.
22. Karlan B, Hoh C, Tse N, et al. Whole body positron emission tomography with (fluorine-18)-2 deoxy-glucose can detect metastatic carcinoma of the fallopian tube. *Gynecol Oncol* 1993;49:383–388.
23. Kawakami S, Togashi K, Kimura I, et al. Primary malignant tumor of the fallopian tube: appearance at CT and MI imaging. *Radiology* 1993;186:503–508.
24. Kietpeerakool C, Suprasert P, Srisomboon J. Adverse effect of paclitaxel and carboplatin combination in epithelial gynecologic cancer. *J Med Assoc Thai* 2005;88:301–306.
25. Kinzel GE. Primary carcinoma of the fallopian tube. *Am J Obstet Gynecol* 1976;125:816–820.
26. Klein M, Rosen A, Graf A, et al. Primary fallopian tube carcinoma: a retrospective survey of 51 cases. *Arch Gynecol Obstet* 1994;255:141–146.
27. Klein M, Rosen A, Lahousen M, et al. The relevance of adjuvant therapy in primary carcinoma of the fallopian tube, stages I and II: Irradiation vs. chemotherapy. *Int J Radiat Oncol Biol Phys* 2000;48:1427–1431.
28. Kol S, Gal D, Friedman M, et al. Preoperative diagnosis of fallopian tube carcinoma by transvaginal sonography and CA-125. *Gynecol Oncol* 1990;37:129–131.
29. Komiyama S, Tsuji H, Asai S, et al. A pilot study of weekly docetaxel therapy for recurrent ovarian cancer, tubal cancer, and primary peritoneal cancer. *Eur J Gynaecol Oncol* 2005;26:299–302.
30. Kouame J, Vanlemmel M. Splenic metastasis of a fallopian tube carcinoma. *Acta Chir Belg* 1998;98:225–227.
31. Kurjak A, Schulman H, Sosic A, et al. Transvaginal ultrasound: color flow and Doppler wave form of the postmenopausal adnexal mass. *Obstet Gynecol* 1992;80:917–921.
32. Lehtovirta P, Kaisemo KJ, Liewendahl K, et al. Immunolymphoscintigraphy and immunoscintigraphy of ovarian and fallopian tube cancer using F(ab)^2 fragments of monoclonal OC125. *Cancer Res* 1990;50:937–940.
33. Markman M, Glass T, Smith HO, et al. Phase II trial of single agent carboplatin followed by dose-intense palcitaxel, followed by maintenance paclitaxel therapy in stage IV ovarian, fallopian tube, and peritoneal cancers: a SWOG trial. *Gynecol Oncol* 2003;88:282–288.
34. Markman M, Kennedy A, Webster K, et al. Phase 2 trial of liposomal doxorubicin (40 mg m(2)) in platinum/paclitaxel-refractory ovarian and fallopian tube cancers and primary carcinoma of the peritoneum. *Gynecol Oncol* 2000;78:369–373.
35. Markman M, Zaino RJ, Busowski JD, et al. Fallopian tube. In: Hoskins WJ, Perez CA, Young RC, eds. *Principles and practice of gynecologic oncology*. Philadelphia: JB Lippincott; 1992:783–794.
36. McMurray EH, Jacobs AJ, Perez CA, et al. Carcinoma of the fallopian tube: management and sites of failure. *Cancer* 1986;58:2070–2075.
37. Micha JP, Goldstein BH, Rettenmeier MA, et al. Pilot study of outpatient paclitaxel, carboplatin and gemcitabine for advanced stage epithelial ovarian, peritoneal, and fallopian tube cancer. *Gynecol Oncol* 2004;94:719–724.
38. Momtazee S, Kempson RL. Primary adenocarcinoma of the fallopian tube. *Obstet Gynecol* 1968;32:649–656.
39. Muntz IT, Tarraza H, Golf B, et al. Combination chemotherapy in advanced adenocarcinoma of the fallopian tube. *Gynecol Oncol* 1991;40:268–273.
40. Newton HB, Stevens C, Santi M. Brain Metastases from fallopian tube carcinoma responsive to intra-arterial carboplatin and intravenous etoposide: a case report. *J Neurooncol* 2001;55:179–184.
41. Ng P, Lawton F. Fallopian tube carcinoma. A review. *Ann Acad Med Singapore* 1998;27:693–697.
42. Niloff JM, Klu TZ, Schaatzel E, et al. Elevation of CA-125 in carcinomas of the fallopian tube, endometrium and endocervix. *Am J Obstet Gynecol* 1984;148:1057.
43. Nordin A. Primary carcinoma of the fallopian tube: a 20 year literature review. *Obstet Gynecol Surv* 1994;49:349–361.
44. Paulson JD. Malignant lesions of the fallopian tube and broad ligament. Available at: www.emedicine.com. Accessed October 2006.
45. Pectasides D, Sintila B, Varthalitis S, et al. Treatment of primary fallopian tube carcinoma with cisplatin containing chemotherapy. *Am J Clin Oncol* 1994;17:68–71.
46. Pere H, Tepper J, Seppala M, et al. Genomic alterations in fallopian tube carcinoma: comparison to serous uterine and ovarian carcinomas reveals similarity suggesting likeness in molecular pathogenesis. *Cancer Res* 1998;58:4274–4276.
47. Petterson F. Staging rules for gestational trophoblastic tumors and fallopian tube cancer. *Acta Obstet Gynecol Scand* 1992;71:224–225.
48. Pfeiffer P, Mogensen H, Amtrup F, et al. Primary carcinoma of the fallopian tube: a retrospective study of patients reported to the Danish Cancer Registry in a 5-year period. *Acta Oncol* 1989;28:7–11.
49. Phelps H, Chapman K. Role of radiation therapy in treatment of primary carcinoma of the uterine tube. *Obstet Gynecol* 1974;43:669–673.
50. Piura B, Rabinovich A. Primary carcinoma of the fallopian tube: study of 11 cases. *Eur J Obstet Gynecol Reprod Biol* 2000;91:169–175.
51. Podobnik M, Singer Z, Ciglar S, et al. Preoperative diagnosis of primary fallopian tube carcinoma by transvaginal ultrasound, cytological findings and CA-125. *Ultrasound Med Biol* 1993;19:587–591.
52. Rabczynski J, Ziolkowski P. Primary endometrioid carcinoma of fallopian tube. Clinomorphologic study (Review). *Pathol Oncol Res* 1999;5:61–66.
53. Raghavan S, Chadaya R, Rani R, et al. A review of fallopian tube carcinoma over 20 years (1971–90). *Pondicherry* 1991;28:188–195.
54. Rawlings G, Bush R, Dembo A, et al. Fallopian tube cancer: survival following radiation and chemotherapy. *International Proceedings, Gynecologic Cancer Society. Third Biennial Meeting,* 1999; Cairns, Australia.
55. Renaud F, Ricci JV. *One hundred years of gynecology*. Philadelphia: Blakiston; 1845.
56. Roberts J, Lifshitz S. Primary adenocarcinoma of the fallopian tube. *Gynecol Oncol* 1982;13:301–308.
57. Rose PG, Rodriguez M, Waggoner S, et al. Phase I study of paclitaxel, carboplatin, and increasing days of prolonged oral etoposide in ovarian, peritoneal and tubal carcinoma: a gynecology oncology group study. *J Clin Oncol* 2000;18:2957–2962.
58. Rose PG, Shrigley R, Wieser GL. Germline mutation in a patient with fallopian tube carcinoma: a case report. *Gyn Oncol* 2000;77:310–320.
59. Rosen AC, Ausch C, Hafner E, et al. A 15-year overview of management and prognosis in primary fallopian tube carcinoma. Austrian Cooperative Study Group for Fallopian Tube Carcinoma. *Eur J Cancer* 1998;34:1725–1729.
60. Rosen AC, Ausch C, Hafner E, et al. Management and prognosis of primary fallopian tube carcinoma. *Gynaecol Obstet Invest* 1999;47:45–51.
61. Rosen AC, Swelda P, Klein M, et al. A comparative analysis of management and prognosis in stage I and II fallopian tube carcinoma and epithelial ovarian cancer. *Br J Cancer* 1940;69:577–579.
62. Rosenblatt KA, Weiss NS, Schwartz SM. Incidence of malignant fallopian tube tumors. *Gynecol Oncol* 1989;35:236–239.
63. Rubin S, Hoskins W, Lewis J, et al. Recurrence after negative second-look laparotomy for ovarian cancer: analysis of risk factors. *Am J Obstet Gynecol* 1988;159:1094–1098.
64. Scharl A, Crombach G, Vorbuchen M, et al. Antigen CA 19-9 presence in mucosa of nondiseased müllerian duct derivatives and marker for differentiation in their carcinomas. *Obstet Gynecol* 1991;77:580–585.
65. Schiller HM, Silverberg SG. Staging and prognosis in primary carcinoma of the fallopian tube. *Cancer* 1971;28:389–395.
66. Schray MF, Podratz KC, Malkasian GD. Fallopian tube cancer: the role of radiation therapy. *Radiother Oncol* 1987;10:267–275.
67. Sedlis A. Carcinoma of the fallopian tube. *Surg Clin North Am* 1978;58:121.
68. Silver DF, Piver MS. Gemcitabine salvage chemotherapy for patients with gynecologic malignancies of the ovary, fallopian tube and peritoneum. *Am J Clin Oncol* 1999;22:450–452.
69. Thurner S, Hodler J, Baer S, et al. Gadolinium-DOTA enhanced MR imaging of adnexal tumors. *J Comput Assist Tomogr* 1990;14:939–949.
70. Tokunaga T, Miyazaki K, Matsuyama S, et al. Serial measurements of CA-125 in patients with primary carcinoma of the fallopian tube. *Gynecol Oncol* 1990;36:335–337.
71. Verschraegen CF, Sittisomwong T, Kudelka AP, et al. Docetaxel for patients with paclitaxel-resistant Müllerian carcinoma. *J Clin Oncol* 2000;18:2733–2739.
72. Wang PH, Yuan CC, Juang CM, et al. Prognosis of primary fallopian tube carcinoma: report of 25 patients. *Eur J Gynaecol Oncol* 1999;19:571–574.
73. Wolfson AH, Tralins KS, Green KM, et al. Adenocarcinoma of the fallopian tube: results of a multi-institutional retrospective analysis of 72 patients. *Int J Radiat Oncol Biol Phys* 1998;40:71–76.
74. Woodruff JD, Pauerstein CJ. *The fallopian tube*. Baltimore: Williams & Wilkins; 1969.
75. Zweemer RP, van Diest PJ, Verheijen RH, et al. Molecular evidence linking cancer of the fallopian tube to BCRA1 germline mutations. *Gynecol Oncol* 2000;76:45–50.

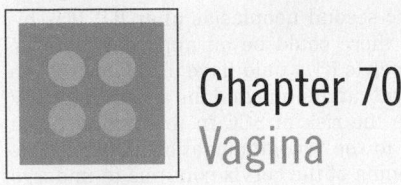

Chapter 70
Vagina

Higinia R. Cardenes, Carlos A. Perez

Anatomy

The vagina is a muscular dilatable tubular structure averaging 7.5 cm in length that extends from the cervix to the vulva. It is located dorsal to the base of the bladder and urethra and ventral to the rectum. The vagina forms from the upward spread of the epithelium from the urogenital sinus. The fused müllerian ducts meet the urogenital sinus at the müllerian tubercle. The hymen marks where the tubercle later opens up to establish the vaginal orifice. The upper portion of the posterior wall is separated from the rectum by a reflection of peritoneum, the pouch of Douglas. At its uppermost extent, the vaginal wall attaches to the uterine cervix at a higher point on the posterior wall than on the anterior wall. During embryonic development, there is no obvious demarcation between the portion of the fused müllerian ducts destined to form the uterus and those destined to form the upper vagina. In the later part of the third month of development, the uterine wall begins to be set off from the upper vagina at the cervical portion. A groove begins to form. This circular groove, formed at the juncture of the vagina and the cervix, is called the *fornix*.

The vaginal wall is composed of three layers: the mucosa, muscularis, and adventitia. The inner mucosal layer is formed by a thick, nonkeratinizing, stratified squamous epithelium overlying a basement membrane containing many papillae. The epithelium normally contains no glands but is lubricated by mucous secretions originating in the cervix. The epithelium changes little in response to the reproductive cycle. Beneath the mucosa lies a submucosal layer of elastin and a double muscularis layer, highly vascularized with a rich innervation and lymphatic drainage. The muscularis layer is composed of smooth muscle fibers, arranged circularly on the inner portion and longitudinally in the outer portion. A vaginal sphincter is formed by skeletal muscle at the introitus. The adventitia is a thin, outer connective tissue layer that merges with that of adjacent organs.

The proximal vagina is supplied by the vaginal artery branch from the uterine or cervical branch of the uterine artery. It runs along the lateral wall of the vagina and anastomoses with the inferior vesical and middle rectal arteries from the surrounding viscera. The accompanying venous plexus, running parallel to the arteries, ultimately drains into the internal iliac vein. The lumbar plexus and pudendal nerve, with branches from the sacral roots 2 to 4, provide innervation to the vaginal vault.

The lymphatic drainage of the vagina is complex, consisting of an extensive intercommunicating network. Fine lymphatic vessels coursing through the submucosa and muscularis coalesce into small trunks running laterally along the walls of the vagina. The lymphatics in the upper portion of the vagina drain primarily via the lymphatics of the cervix; the upper anterior vagina drains along cervical channels to the interiliac and parametrial nodes; the posterior vagina drains into the inferior gluteal, presacral, and anorectal nodes (Fig. 70.1). The distal vagina lymphatics follow drainage patterns of the vulva into the inguinal and femoral nodes and from there to the pelvic nodes. Lymphatic flow from lesions in the mid-vagina may drain either way (11). However, because of the presence of intercommunicating lymphatics along the terminal branches of the vaginal artery and near the vaginal wall, the external iliac nodes are at high risk, even in lesions of the lower third of the vagina. Such a complex lymphatic drainage pattern has significant implications for therapeutic planning. Therefore, bilateral pelvic nodes should be considered at risk in any invasive vaginal carcinoma, and bilateral groin nodes considered at risk in those lesions involving the distal third of the vagina.

Epidemiology and Etiological Risk Factors

Primary vaginal cancer, defined as a lesion arising in the vagina without involvement of the cervix or vulva, is a rare entity, representing only 1% to 2% of all female genital neoplasias. Most of vaginal neoplasms, 80% to 90%, are metastatic from other primary gynecologic (cervix or vulva) and nongynecologic sites, involving the vagina by direct extension or lymphatic or hematogenous routes. In the National Cancer Data Base (NCDB) report (33) based on 4885 patients with primary vaginal cancer, approximately 92% of the patients had in situ or invasive squamous cell carcinomas (SCC) or adenocarcinomas; 4% melanomas; 3% sarcomas; and 1% other or unspecified types of cancer. In situ carcinomas accounted for 28%; SCC represented 79% of invasive vaginal carcinomas; and adenocarcinomas represented 14%. Adenocarcinomas represent nearly all the carcinomas in patients younger than 20 years of age and are seen less frequently with advanced age (33).

Carcinoma of the vagina incidence peaks in the sixth and seventh decades of life (77). However, vaginal cancer is increasingly seen in younger women, possibly due to human papillomavirus (HPV) infection or other sexually transmitted disease. Only about 10% of patients are 40 years of age or younger (42). In the NCDB report (33), only 1% of the carcinoma patients were <20 years old at the time of diagnosis, and over 80% of those patients had in situ lesions. As patient age increased, the number of invasive tumors increased, reaching a peak in patients' ages 70 to 79 years, whereas the percentage of in situ carcinomas decreased to only 11% in patients over 80 years. A decrease in the incidence of primary vaginal tumors has been noted in recent years, possibly because of early detection with cervical cytology or more rigid diagnostic criteria, which have eliminated from this category primary cancers arising from adjacent organs, such as the cervix, vulva, or endometrium.

Vaginal Intraepithelial Neoplasia and Squamous Cell Carcinoma

Potential risk factors for SCC include prior history of HPV infection, cervical intraepithelial neoplasia (CIN), immunosuppression, and possibly previous pelvic irradiation. HPV is the likely etiologic agent of SCC and its precursor lesion, vaginal intraepithelial neoplasia (VAIN) (34,138,187,222). The process most commonly occurs primarily in sexually active women in the reproductive age, generally involves the upper vagina, and

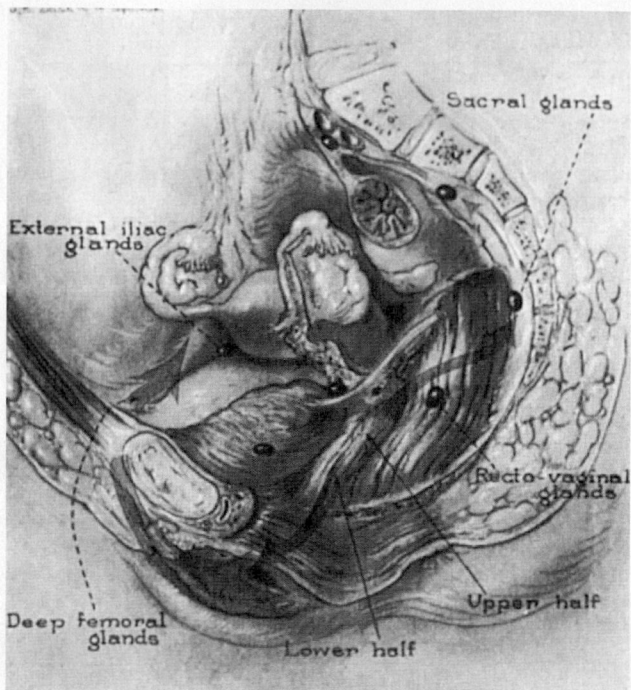

FIGURE 70.1. Lymphatic spread in carcinoma of the vagina. Lesions in the upper half drain to the same lymph node groups as do carcinomas of the uterine cervix. Tumors in the lower half tend to involve the inguinal and femoral nodes preferentially and may also drain into the deep pelvic lymph nodes. (From Benson RC. Cancer of the female genital tract. *CA Cancer J Clin* 1968;18:2, with permission.)

frequently is multifocal. Approximately one-half of the lesions are associated with concomitant CIN or vulvar intraepithelial neoplasia (2,138).

Brinton et al. (19) in a case-control study of 41 women with carcinoma in situ VAIN or invasive carcinoma of the vagina and 97 community control subjects, identified with low socioeconomic status, history of genital warts, vaginal discharge or irritation, a previous abnormal cytology, prior hysterectomy, and, less significant, vaginal trauma as potential risk factors. Weiderpass et al. (216), in a population-based study of 36,856 women, found that alcoholic women had an excess risk for cancer of the vagina, probably related with higher incidence of HPV infection associated to lifestyle factors such as promiscuity, smoking, use of contraceptive hormones, and dietary deficiencies. Iversen et al. (99) found no positive correlation between cancer of the penis in husbands and gynecologic cancer in their wives.

Patients with previous cervical carcinoma have a substantial risk of developing vaginal carcinoma, presumably because these sites share exposure and/or susceptibility to endogenous or exogenous carcinogenic stimuli. Ten percent to 50% of patients with VAIN-CIS or invasive carcinoma of the vagina have undergone prior hysterectomy or radiotherapy (RT) for CIS or invasive carcinoma of the cervix (10,29,54,107,116, 147,189,192,193,210). The interval from therapy for cervical cancer or preinvasive disease to the development of carcinoma of the vagina averages nearly 14 years, but there have been cases with the vaginal primary manifesting 50 years after therapy for cervical cancer (38,54).

It is controversial as to whether prior pelvic RT is a risk factor. Boice et al. (14) reported a 14-fold increase risk of cancer of the vagina in previously irradiated women before the age of 45 years, and a dose-response relationship was found to be significant. However, Lee et al. (114) in an analysis of 1,200 patients treated over a 20-year period at Washington University for carcinoma of the cervix failed to demonstrate an increase

in the incidence of pelvic second neoplasias after RT. It is biologically plausible that there could be an apparent increase in risk, given that prior pelvic RT would have likely been given for HPV-associated cervical carcinoma, and the antecedent HPV infection would increase the risk of SCC in the vagina. Such an association has lead to the recommendation that patients treated for CIN or carcinoma of the cervix continue to undergo lifelong surveillance with vaginal cytology, even after hysterectomy (122).

Clear-Cell Adenocarcinoma

An increased incidence of clear-cell adenocarcinoma (CCA) of the vagina in young women related to in utero exposure to diethylstilbestrol (DES) during the first 16 weeks of pregnancy was first reported in 1971 (82). Specific suggested mechanisms of carcinogenesis focus on the retention of nests of abnormal cells of müllerian duct origin, which, after stimulation by endogenous hormones during puberty, are promoted into adenocarcinomas (159). Herbst and Anderson (76) in 1990, indicated that there were 547 cases of CCA of the vagina and cervix recorded in the Registry for Research on Hormonal Transplacental Carcinogenesis. Hicks and Piver (84) noted that 60% of registered patients had been exposed to DES or similar agents in utero and that most cases involved the anterior upper-third of the vaginal wall. They also observed that the age at diagnosis ranged from 7 to 34 years (median, 19 years) and estimated the incidence of CCA in the exposed female population from birth to 34 years to be between 0.14 and 1.4 per 1,000. Approximately 90% of the patients had stage I or II disease at diagnosis (76). Fortunately, the incidence of this tumor has decreased in recent years, and may decrease even more since the practice of prescribing DES during pregnancy has been discontinued.

Bornstein et al. (16) reported an incidence of cervical and vaginal intraepithelial neoplasia in DES-exposed donors twice as high as in unexposed women, a finding not confirmed by others (73). Palmer et al. (142) assessed the influence of postnatal factors on the development of CCA in women exposed to DES in 244 cases compared with 244 age-matched non–DES-exposed women. Neither oral contraceptive use nor pregnancy was associated with risk of CCA.

Pathology

Epithelial Neoplasms

VAIN is a precursor of SCC and is graded from I to III, depending on the degree of nuclear atypia and crowding and the proportion of the epithelium involved. VAIN I typically involves the lower third to one-half of the epithelium, VAIN II one-half to two-thirds of the thickness of the epithelium, and VAIN III more than three fourths of the thickness. Alternatively, VAIN can be classified as low or high grade. High-grade lesions indicate involvement of the outer third of the mucosa, and include carcinoma in situ, which encompasses the entire thickness of the epithelium. The true incidence of VAIN and its rate of progression to invasive carcinoma are unknown, ranging in several series from 9% to 28% (2,19,92).

SCC represents 80% to 90% of primary malignant vaginal neoplasms. It may be difficult or impossible histologically to distinguish a primary vaginal SCC from recurrent cervical or vulvar disease. According to the recommendations of the International Federation of Gynecology and Obstetrics (FIGO), a tumor of the vagina that involves the cervix or vulva should be classified as a primary cervical or vulvar cancer, respectively. Additionally, for a neoplasm to be considered vaginal primary, there must not have been a cervical cancer for 5 years prior to the diagnosis (226).

Histologically, keratinizing, nonkeratinizing, basaloid, warty, and verrucous variants have been described. Tumors may also be graded as well, moderately, or poorly differentiated, based on a combination of cytologic and histologic features. However, there is little correlation between tumor grade and survival (77,144). Most cases are moderately differentiated and nonkeratinizing. Well-differentiated tumors show prominent keratin or squamous pearl formation and intercellular bridges. Rarely, poorly differentiated tumors have a spindle cell appearance. Warty SCC has a papillary appearance with hyperkeratosis and koilocytosis.

Verrucous carcinoma is a rare, distinct variant of well-differentiated SCC (213), usually with the appearance of a relatively large, well-circumscribed, soft, cauliflowerlike mass. Microscopically, the tumor exhibits a papillary growth pattern, pushing borders, bulbous pegs of acanthotic epithelium with little or no atypia, and surface maturation in the form of parakeratosis and hyperkeratosis, without koilocytosis. Because of its well-differentiated character, the microscopic diagnosis of verrucous carcinoma may be difficult, especially if the biopsy is superficial (213). Verrucous carcinoma may recur locally after surgery, but rarely, if ever, metastasizes. This behavioral difference justifies separating verrucous carcinoma as a distinct tumor entity.

Vaginal Adenosis and Clear-Cell Adenocarcinoma

Vaginal adenosis is a condition in which müllerian-type glandular epithelium is present after vaginal development is complete. Although adenosis is the most common histological abnormality in women exposed to DES in utero, it is not strictly confined to this population (169). The classic gross appearance of adenosis is red, velvety, grapelike clusters in the vagina. The process may involve the surface epithelium or glands in the superficial stroma. Microscopically, the glandular epithelium may be composed of any of the müllerian epithelial cell types. Tuboendometrial epithelium is present in approximately 25% of cases and is found more frequently in biopsies from the lower vagina (70). Adenosis is associated with 97% of vaginal and 52% of cervical CCA. The glandular epithelium may replace the surface epithelium, and undergoes progressive squamous metaplasia (70) and ultimately, only stromal nodules or pegs of immature squamous epithelium containing small mucin droplets may remain (170). A few CCA have been detected among women under surveillance for adenosis (104). Atypical adenosis of tuboendometrial type appears to be a precursor lesion of CCA. Whether immature squamous metaplasia in adenosis is associated with an increased risk of vaginal intraepithelial neoplasia or SCC is controversial.

DES-associated CCA (80,104) has a predilection for the upper third of the vagina and the ectocervix. It is frequently located at or near the lower margin of the zone of glandular tissue in the vagina or cervix. Most are exophytic and superficially invasive (80). Ninety-seven percent will be associated with mucosal adenosis (80). Microscopically, they exhibit three basic histologic patterns—tubulocystic (most common), solid, papillary, or mixed cell patterns—and are mainly composed of clear and hobnail-shaped cells. The clear cells are cuboidal or columnar, with abundant glycogen-rich cytoplasm and distinct cell membranes. The hobnail cells have large atypical protruding nuclei, rimmed by a small amount of cytoplasm (80). The major determinant of outcome in CCA is stage, but some pathologic features are statistically associated with better outcome, including a tubulocystic growth pattern, size <3 cm^2, and <3 mm of stromal invasion (80).

Other Adenocarcinomas

Primary adenocarcinoma of the vagina is rare and occurs predominantly in postmenopausal women. Reported histologic subtypes have included endometrioid, mucinous, mesonephric, and papillary serous adenocarcinomas. Only a few cases of mucinous adenocarcinoma have been described (47). Histologically, the tumors may resemble typical endocervical (30) or intestinal (51) adenocarcinoma. Some cases may be related to DES exposure (41). Rare cases of mucinous adenocarcinoma have been described in neovaginas (89). Endometrioid adenocarcinoma of the vagina usually arises in endometriosis (72). Mesonephric adenocarcinoma is a rare variant that may arise from mesonephric duct remnants that are mostly situated deep in the lateral walls of the vagina (87). Primary papillary serous adenocarcinoma of the vagina has rarely been reported (167).

Vaginal metastases from adenocarcinoma of the breast, other gynecological primaries, or renal cell carcinomas have been described (197).

Melanocytic Tumors

Malignant melanoma is the second most common cancer of the vagina, accounting for 2.8% to 5% of all vaginal neoplasms (28). Trimble's examination of the Surveillance, Epidemiology, and End Results (SEER) data on 30,295 melanomas found 51 vaginal melanomas (0.3% of all melanomas), with an annual incidence of 0.026 per 100,000 and a median age at diagnosis of 66.3 years (205). In the NCDB report by Creasman et al. (33), vaginal melanomas represented 4% of primary vaginal cancers. The most common location is the lower third and the anterior vaginal wall, although oftentimes it is multifocal (28). Grossly, these tumors are typically pigmented and show considerable variation in size, color, and growth patterns, being polypoid or nodular in the majority of cases. Microscopically, they are composed of epithelioid cells, spindle cells, or nevuslike cells; melanin pigment is often present. Junctional activity is usually present. Poorly differentiated tumors may be difficult to distinguish from sarcoma or SCC. Premelanosomes may be identified by electron microscopy. Immunohistochemical stains are frequently positive for S-100 protein, HMB-45, and melan A. Tyrosinase and MART-1 are useful markers when S-100 is negative or only focally positive. Tumor thickness correlates with prognosis and may be measured by the methods of Breslow (18).

Nonepithelial Tumors

Sarcomas represent 3% of primary vaginal cancers and are most common in adults, with leiomyosarcoma representing 50% to 65% of vaginal sarcomas (33). Malignant mixed müllerian tumor (MMMT-carcinosarcoma), endometrial stromal sarcoma, and angiosarcoma are less common. Embryonal rhabdomyosarcoma/sarcoma botryoides is a rare pediatric tumor. Prior pelvic RT is a risk factor, particularly for mixed mesodermal tumors and vaginal angiosarcomas (162). Unfortunately, most of the sarcomas are diagnosed at an advanced stage. Histopathological grade appears to be the most important predictor of outcome.

Smooth muscle tumors, although rare, are reported to be the most common benign and malignant mesenchymal tumors in adult women, and leiomyosarcoma is the most common vaginal sarcoma in adult women (153). The frequency and behavior are uncertain because of the variable histological criteria used to distinguish benign and malignant smooth muscle tumors. It is currently recommended that smooth muscle tumors >3 cm in diameter, with five or greater mitoses per 10 high-power fields (HPF), moderate or marked cytologic atypia, and infiltrating margins be classified as leiomyosarcoma (199).

Although they may originate in any part of the vagina, most are submucosal. The gross appearance varies greatly, depending on cellularity, type, and extent of degenerative change, and the amount of necrosis and hemorrhage (199). Microscopically, smooth muscle tumors are composed of interlacing bundles of spindle-shaped cells, with blunt-ended nuclei and fibrillar cytoplasm. An epithelioid pattern or extensive myxoid changes occurs uncommonly (199). Because smooth muscle tumors vary from area to area, adequate sampling (1 block per 1 to 2 cm of tumor diameter) is essential for accurate diagnosis.

Embryonal rhabdomyosarcoma (RMS) is a rare pediatric tumor. The botryoid variant, or sarcoma botryoides, is the most common malignant vaginal tumor in infants and children. Ninety percent of cases occur in children younger than 5 years of age. Sarcoma botryoides has a characteristic gross appearance consisting of multiple gray-red, translucent, edematous, grapelike masses that fill the vagina, and may protrude from it. Microscopically, there is a zone of condensed round, or spindle, cells (the cambium layer) immediately beneath the intact vaginal epithelium. Elsewhere, the tumor is composed of small, dark, spindle-shaped cells, sparsely distributed in a myxoid stroma. Some cells may show skeletal muscle differentiation, evidenced by intensely eosinophilic cytoplasm with cross striations. Immunohistochemical stains with antibodies directed against actin, desmin, or myoglobin facilitate the recognition of striated muscle differentiation.

Other sarcomas that may occur in the vagina include endometrioid stromal sarcoma, which may arise in endometriosis (208); alveolar soft part sarcoma (135); malignant fibrous histiocytoma (215), a biphasic tumor interpreted as resembling synovial sarcoma (138) or malignant mixed tumor (185); angiosarcoma (162); malignant peripheral nerve sheath tumor; and hemangiopericytoma (23).

Malignant Lymphoma and Leukemia

Malignant lymphoma may be localized to the female genital tract or occur there as part of a widespread disease process (68). The majority of primary lymphomas involving the vagina are of the diffuse large B-cell type, but follicular lymphomas also occur. The histologic diagnosis depends on the identification of monomorphous, cytologically atypical, mitotically active lymphoid cells, deeply penetrating the stroma. Characteristically the mucosa is intact. The tumors typically express CD20. Patients with vaginal lymphomas characteristically present with vaginal bleeding. Those with primary lymphomas also have a mass on clinical examination. Leukemic infiltrates, especially granulocytic sarcoma, can be impossible to distinguish from lymphoma. Chloroacetate esterase or myeloperoxidase stains may be helpful in some cases.

Uncommon Vaginal Tumors

Neuroendocrine small-cell carcinoma may occur in the vagina, either in pure form or associated with squamous or glandular elements (103,209). They are rare and very aggressive tumors. A high proportion shows immunohistochemical or ultrastructural evidence of neuroendocrine differentiation (209). Electron microscopy demonstrates neuroendocrine granules in the cytoplasm. Tumor cells strongly stain for cytokeratin, neuron-specific enolase, chromogranin A, and serotonin (209).

Adenosquamous carcinoma is an uncommon neoplasm of the vagina composed of an admixture of glandular and squamous elements. Tumors diagnosed as carcinosarcomas of the female genital tract appear to be metaplastic carcinomas and should be treated as epithelial neoplasms, but the prognosis is poor. This tumor is rare in the vagina, and typically occurs in postmenopausal women (186). Uncommonly, yolk sac tumors have been reported in the vagina (67).

Benign epithelial and mixed tumors of the vagina are rare and include müllerian papilloma, squamous papilloma, mixed tumor, and Brenner's tumor (207).

Natural History

The majority (57% to 83%) of vaginal primaries occur in the upper third or at the apex of the vault, most commonly in the posterior wall; the lower third may be involved in as many as 31% of patients (54,177,192). Location of the vaginal carcinoma is an important consideration in planning therapy and determining prognosis. Vaginal tumors may spread along the vaginal walls to involve the cervix or the vulva. However, if biopsies of the cervix or the vulva are positive at the time of initial diagnosis, the tumor cannot be considered a primary vaginal lesion. Because of the absence of anatomic barriers, vaginal tumors readily extend into surrounding tissues, such that a lesion on the anterior wall may infiltrate the vesicovaginal septum or the urethra; those on the posterior wall may eventually involve the rectovaginal septum, and subsequently infiltrate the rectal mucosa. Lateral extension toward the parametrium and paracolpal tissues is not uncommon in more advanced stages of the disease, extending into the obturator fossa, cardinal ligaments, lateral pelvic walls, and uterosacral ligaments.

The issue of regional nodal metastasis, both the incidence of occult nodal disease and the anatomic pathways of lymphatic spread, are somewhat controversial. The incidence of positive pelvic nodes at diagnosis varies with the stage and location of the primary tumor. Because the lymphatic system of the vagina is so complex, any of the nodal groups may be involved, regardless of the location of the lesion. Involvement of inguinal nodes is most common when the lesion is located in the lower third of the vagina.

Although data on staging lymphadenectomy are sparse, two studies reported a significant incidence of nodal disease in early stage vaginal carcinoma. In Al-Kurdi and Monaghan's (5) series, the incidence of pelvic nodal metastasis was 14% and 32% for stage I and II, respectively, whereas in the series of Davis et al. (38) the incidence was 6% and 26% for stage I and II, respectively. The incidence is expected to be higher for stage III, although no substantial data are available. Chyle et al. (29) noted a 10-year actuarial pelvic nodal failure rate of 30% and a 16% inguinal failure rate in patients who had local recurrence, in contrast to 4% and 2%, respectively, in the group without local recurrence (p <0.001). The incidence of clinically positive inguinal nodes at diagnosis reported by several authors ranges from 5.3% to 20% (Table 70.1) (29,147,218).

Distant metastasis may occur, primarily in patients with advanced disease at presentation, or those who recurred after primary therapy. In the series by Perez et al. (147), the incidence of distant metastasis was 16% in stage I, 31% in stage IIA, 46% in stage IIB, 62% in stage III, and 50% in stage IV. Robboy et al. (168) reported that metastases to the lungs or supraclavicular lymph nodes represented 35% of recurrences in young women with CCA, a proportion much greater than found with squamous cell carcinoma of the cervix or vagina.

Clinical Presentation

Vaginal Intraepithelial Neoplasia–Carcinoma In Situ

VAIN most often is asymptomatic and it is usually detected by cytology performed following hysterectomy in patients with a history of CIN or invasive cervical carcinoma. In these cases, VAIN has a predilection for involvement of the upper vagina,

Table 70.1	CLINICALLY POSITIVE PELVIC NODES AT DIAGNOSIS IN CARCINOMA OF THE VAGINA		
Study (Reference)	No. of Patients Reported	No. with Clinically Positive Nodes	Percentage with Clinically Positive Nodes
Plentl and Friedman (160)	679	141	20.8
Whelton and Kottmeier (218)	117	8[a]	6.8
Brown et al. (20)	76	5	6.6
Chyle et al. (29)	301	14 (pelvic)	5.0
		10 (inguinal)	3.0
Perez et al. (147)	113	6	5.3

[a]Four had presence of tumor confirmed by biopsy.

likely secondary to a "field effect." A discharge may be present, but is likely secondary to superimposed vaginal infections.

Invasive Carcinoma

In patients with invasive disease, irregular vaginal bleeding, often postcoital, is the most common presenting symptom followed by vaginal discharge and dysuria. Pelvic pain is a relatively late symptom, generally related to tumor extent beyond the vagina (54,177,203). Primary vaginal squamous cell carcinoma arising from the posterior vaginal wall can present as a cystic pelvic mass resembling an ovarian neoplasm. In 10% to 20% of the patients no symptoms are reported, and the diagnosis is made by cytological examination (203).

Diagnostic Work-Up

In patients with suspected vaginal malignancy, in addition to a complete history and physical examination, a thorough pelvic exam with detailed speculum inspection, digital palpation, colposcopic and cytologic evaluation, and biopsy constitutes the most effective procedure for diagnosing primary, metastatic, or recurrent carcinoma of the vagina. In symptomatic patients, biopsy of any abnormal exophytic or endophytic lesion noted at the time of the examination is indicated. Bimanual pelvic and rectal examinations are integral elements in the clinical evaluation. Examination under anesthesia is recommended for the thoroughness of evaluation of all of the vaginal walls and local extent of the disease, primarily if the patient is in great discomfort because of advanced disease, in order to obtain a biopsy. Biopsies of the cervix, if present, are recommended to rule out primary cervical tumor. The speculum must be rotated as it is slowly withdrawn from the vaginal fornix, so that the total vaginal mucosa may be visualized, and, in particular, posterior wall lesions, which occur frequently, are not overlooked.

The patient with a history of preinvasive or invasive carcinoma of the cervix found to have abnormal cytology following prior hysterectomy or RT should be offered colposcopy with application of acetic acid to the entire vault, followed by biopsies as indicated by areas of white epithelium, mosaicism, punctation, or atypical vascularity. It can be very helpful for the menopausal patient or the patient previously irradiated to use a short course of topical estrogen into the vault once or twice a week for 1 month prior to the colposcopy, in order to foster epithelial maturation. Another method of identifying the area(s) most in need of biopsy would be, after application of the acetic acid, to place half-strength Schiller's iodine to determine if the Schiller positive (nonstaining) areas correspond with the involved areas identified after acetic acid application.

Staging

At present, primary malignancies of the vagina are staged clinically. In addition to a complete history and physical examination, routine laboratory evaluations including complete blood cell (CBC) count with differential and platelets and assessment of renal and hepatic function should be undertaken. In order to determine the extent of disease, the following tests are allowed by FIGO criteria: chest x-ray, a thorough bimanual and rectovaginal examination, cystoscopy, proctoscopy, and intravenous pyelogram. Cystoscopy or proctosigmoidoscopy should be performed on patients with symptoms suggestive of bladder or rectal infiltration. If the patient is in significant discomfort, the examination should be conducted under anesthesia, preferably by a radiation oncologist and gynecologic oncologist who will be involved in the patient's ongoing care. However, it can be difficult even for the experienced examiner to differentiate between disease confined to the mucosa (stage I) and disease spread to the submucosa (stage II) (10,177).

Pelvic computed tomography (CT) scan is generally performed to evaluate inguinofemoral or pelvic lymph nodes, as well as extent of local disease. In patients with vaginal melanoma or sarcoma, chest, abdomen, and pelvis CT scans are often part of the work-up. Magnetic resonance imaging (MRI) has emerged as a potentially important imaging modality in the evaluation of vaginal cancers, predominantly the T1-weighted with contrast and T2-weighted images (94). Chang et al. (25) reported the results of pelvic MRI in 87 women: 51 with normal vagina, two with benign cysts, and 34 with vaginal carcinoma (eight primary, 22 metastatic, and eight recurrent). These findings were correlated with surgical-pathologic findings. The positive predictive value of MRI for primary and metastatic tumors was 84% and the negative predictive value 97%. The accuracy of MRI in detection of recurrent vaginal carcinoma was 82%, compared with clinical or surgical findings. An additional role of MRI is differentiation of tumor from fibrotic tissue in patients with suspected recurrent vaginal carcinoma (25,46,58). Positron emission tomography (PET) is evolving as a modality of potential use in the evaluation of vaginal cancer that allows detection of the extent of the primary as well as abnormal lymph nodes more often than does CT scan (60).

In modern practice, for the majority of patients with disease volume or location requiring definitive RT to achieve cure, therapeutic planning will be guided by disease volume assessment utilizing CT or MRI, even though such radiologic modalities are not "allowed" for purposes of staging.

The two commonly used staging systems for carcinoma of the vagina are the International FIGO (143) (Table 70.2) and the American Joint Commission on Cancer (tumor, node, metastasis [TNM]) classifications (3) (Table 70.3). According to FIGO guidelines, patients with tumor involvement of the cervix or vulva

Table 70.2	INTERNATIONAL FEDERATION OF GYNECOLOGY AND OBSTETRICS STAGING SYSTEM FOR CARCINOMA OF THE VAGINA

Stage	Description
Stage 0	Carcinoma in situ, intraepithelial neoplasia grade III
Stage I	Limited to the vaginal wall
Stage II	Involvement of the subvaginal tissue but without extension to the pelvic side wall
	Extension to the pelvic side wall
Stage III	Extension beyond the true pelvis or involvement of the bladder or rectal mucosa. Bullous edema as such
Stage IV	does not permit a case to be allotted to Stage IV.
Stage IVA	Spread to adjacent organs and/or direct extension beyond the true pelvis
Stage IVB	Spread to distant organs

From Pecorelli S, Beller U, Heintz AP, et al. FIGO annual report on the results of treatment in gynecological cancer. *J Epidemiol Biostat* 2000;24:56.

should be classified as primary cervical or vulvar cancers, respectively. Therefore, multiple biopsies of the cervix are mandatory to rule out a cervical primary. Perez et al. (144) proposed in 1973 that FIGO stage II vaginal cancer should be subdivided into stage IIA (tumor infiltrating the subvaginal tissues but not extending into the parametrium) and stage IIB (tumor infiltrating the parametrium but not extending to pelvic side walls) (Fig. 70.2). However, most authors do not use this classification, and there are limited published data to support it (147,161).

▪▪ Prognostic Factors Influencing
▪▪ Choice of Treatment

Invasive Squamous Cell Carcinoma

The stage of disease is the most significant prognostic factor regarding ultimate outcome (29,33,36,45,107,116,147,149,154). In the Perez et al. (147) series, including 165 patients with pri-

mary vaginal carcinomas treated with definitive RT, the 10-year actuarial disease-free survival (DFS) was 94% for stage 0, 75% for stage I, 55% for stage IIA, 43% for stage IIB, 32% for stage III, and 0% for those with stage IV.

The prognostic importance of lesion size has been controversial, with an adverse impact noted by Tjalma et al. (203) and Chyle et al. (29), contrary to the Perez et al. (146) findings. In the Chyle et al. (29) series, lesions measuring <5 cm in maximum diameter had a 20% 10-year local recurrence rate, compared to 40% for those lesions larger than 5 cm. Similarly, in the Princess Margaret Hospital (PMH) experience, tumors larger than 4 cm in diameter fared significantly worse than smaller lesions (107). In the Perez et al. (149) series, stage was an important predictor of pelvic tumor control and 5-year DFS, but the size of the tumor in stage I patients was not a significant prognostic factor. However, in stage IIA disease, lower pelvic tumor control and survival were noted with tumors larger than 4 cm. In stages IIB to III, tumor size was not a significant prognostic factor, probably related to the difficulty in assessing size, and the fact that higher doses of RT were delivered for larger tumors. Stock et al. (192) reported that disease volume, a likely surrogate for stage or lesion size, adversely impacted survival, as well as local control.

The impact of lesion location has been controversial. Several authors have shown better survival and decreased recurrence rates for patients with cancers involving the proximal half of the vagina when compared with those in the distal half, or those involving the entire length of the vagina (4,29,111,198,210). Chyle et al. (29) observed a 17% rate of pelvic relapse in patients with upper vaginal tumors, 36% in those with middle or lower vaginal tumors, and 42% with whole vaginal involvement. However, a larger series failed to note any difference in site of recurrence based on primary lesion location (147). In addition, lesions of the posterior wall have worse prognosis than those involving other vaginal walls (29), which probably reflects the greater difficulty of performing adequate brachytherapy procedures in this location.

With regard to the histological type and grade, several series have shown the histological grade to be an independent, significant predictor of survival (107,111,210). Chyle et al. (29) noted a higher incidence of local recurrence in patients with adenocarcinoma compared with squamous cell carcinoma (52% and 20%, respectively, at 10 years), as well as a higher incidence of distant metastases (48% and 10%, respectively), and lower 10-year survival rate (20% vs. 50%).

Overexpression of HER-2/neu oncogenes in squamous cancer of the lower genital tract is a rare event that may be associated with aggressive biologic behavior (12). Waggoner et al. (214), in a group of 21 women with CCA of the vagina and cervix, observed a more favorable prognosis in gynecologic tumors with an overexpression of wild-type p53 protein than in tumors containing mutated p53 genes.

Table 70.3	AMERICAN JOINT COMMISSION ON CANCER STAGING OF VAGINAL CANCER

Primary Tumor (T)

Tx	Primary tumor cannot be assessed
T0	No evidence of primary tumor
Tis/0	Carcinoma in situ
T1/I	Tumor confined to the vagina
T2/II	Tumor invades paravaginal tissues but not to the pelvic wall
	Tumor extends to the pelvic wall
T3/III	Tumor invades mucosa of the bladder or rectum and/or extends
T4/IVA	beyond the pelvis (Bullous edema is not sufficient to classify a tumor as T4)

Regional Lymph Nodes (N)

Nx	Regional lymph nodes cannot be assessed
N0	No regional lymph nodes
N1/IVB	Pelvic or inguinal lymph node metastasis

Distant Metastasis (M)

Mx	Distant metastasis cannot be assessed
M0	No distant metastasis
M1/IVB	Distant metastasis

Stage Groupings

Stage 0	Tis N0 M0
Stage I	T1 N0 M0
Stage II	T2 N0 M0
Stage III	T1-3 N1 M0, T3 N0 M0
Stage IVA	T4, any N, M0
Stage IVB	Any T, any N, M1

From American Joint Committee on Cancer (AJCC). Vagina. In: Greene FL, Page DL, Fleming ID, et al., eds. *AJCC Cancer Staging Manual*, 6th ed. New York: Springer-Verlag, 2002; 251–257.

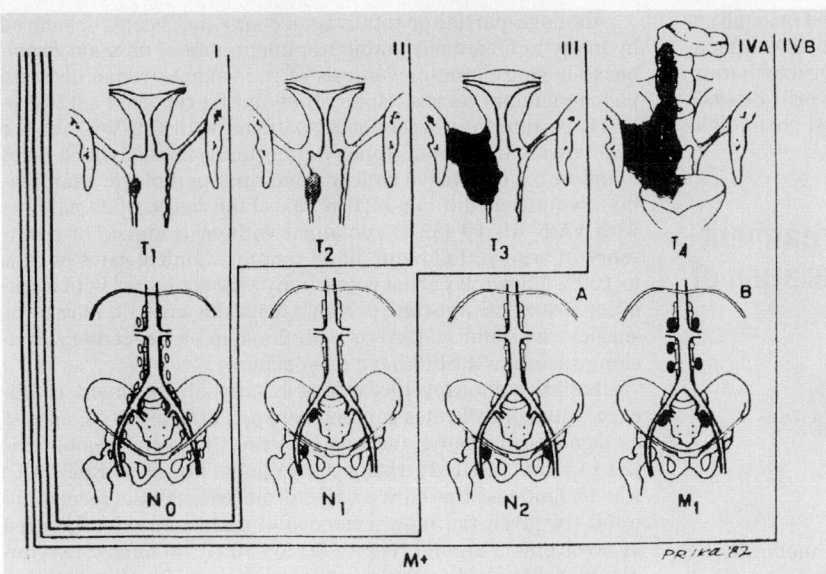

FIGURE 70.2. International Federation of Gynecology and Obstetrics clinical staging for carcinoma of the vagina. (From Perez CA, Grigsby PW, Mutch DG, et al. Gynecologic tumors. In: Rubin P, ed. *Clinical oncology: a multidisciplinary approach for primary care physicians and students,* 8th ed. Philadelphia: WB Saunders, 2001, with permission.)

Age was a significant prognostic factor in the series by Urbanski et al. (210), with 5-year survival of 63.2% for patients below the age of 60, compared with 25% for those over 60 years of age (*p* <0.001). However, most of these series do not correct for death secondary to intercurrent disease in the elderly population. No statistical significance of age to survival was found in the series of Dixit et al. (45) and Perez et al. (149).

Other Histologies

An increased propensity for distant metastases to the lung and supraclavicular nodes has been reported in patients with CCA (168). Stage, tubulocystic pattern, size <3 cm, and depth of invasion <3 mm were all noted to be associated with superior survival (80).

Vaginal melanoma has a higher propensity for development of distant metastases, and they do more poorly than patients SCC. A review by Reid et al. (166) of 115 vaginal melanoma patients noted that depth of invasion and size of lesion (>3 cm) adversely impacted survival, but stage did not, perhaps because it was known for only 42 of the 115 patients in the series.

Patients with malignant mesenchymal tumors of the vagina do less well than those with invasive SCC. Specific, adverse prognostic factors for vaginal sarcoma identified by Tavassoli and Norris (199) included infiltrative versus pushing borders, high mitotic rate ≥5 mitoses per 10 HPF, size >3 cm in diameter, and cytologic atypia.

Squamous Cell Carcinoma: General Management, Treatment Options, and Outcome

Vaginal cancer is a rare disease and, therefore, data concerning the natural history, prognostic factors, and treatment of vaginal carcinoma derive from small, retrospective series. Most of the currently available literature refers to primary SCC of the vagina. It is important to recognize the complexity of the management of patients with carcinoma of the vagina and the need for individualized approach after careful assessment by the gynecologic oncologist and radiation oncologist. With adequate therapy, the survival rates of patients with carcinoma of the vagina are comparable with those reported for carcinoma of the cervix, which range from 20% to 80% at 5 years, depend-

ing on stage of the disease (54,109,150,161,177,189). Perez et al. (147) noted a somewhat higher incidence of pelvic failures in patients with carcinoma of the vagina compared with 1,054 patients with invasive cervical carcinoma, although the differences are not statistically significant.

Creasman et al. (33) in the NCDB report based on 4,885 patients with primary vaginal cancer found the survival rate at 5 years to be 96% for stage 0, 73% for stage I, 58% for stage II, and 36% for stages III and IV. In addition, survival was better in the younger patients (90% vs. 30% in the older patients).

In most patients, the primary treatment modality for invasive vaginal cancer is RT, as reported by the Society of Gynecologist Oncologists (SGO) in practice guidelines published in 1998 (33). Several considerations may favor treating selected patients with surgery. There is evidence that patients with CIS-VAIN and early stage I, primarily with lesion located in the upper or distal third of the vagina and highly selected young women with stage II can be successfully treated with surgery alone (10,38,91,177,192,203). In addition, surgery could be considered in younger patients with a desire to preserve ovarian function or a functional vagina (192), patients with verrucous carcinoma (213), those with nonepithelial tumors, and patients with localized pelvic failures after radiation.

For the most part, surgical resection often requires a radical approach, resulting in urinary and fecal diversion in order to secure adequate margins (10,177). Even in patients with early stage I invasive tumors involving the middle or upper third of the vagina, surgical treatment requires radical hysterovaginectomy and pelvic lymph node dissection. Lindeque (119) pointed out that most tumors require removal of the full length of the vagina, although in localized lesions a partial colpectomy may be performed. Although radical surgery in the past precluded vaginal function, this has improved significantly by the use of split-thickness grafts, intestinal segments, and myocutaneous flap reconstruction (121).

Given the potentially devastating functional results often associated with radical surgery, definitive RT has largely replaced surgery as the primary therapeutic modality in patients with vaginal cancer, in order to maximize cure and improve quality of life. Furthermore, most patients are elderly, and a radical surgical approach is often not feasible. Despite the acceptance of RT as the treatment of choice for this disease, the optimal approach for each stage is not well defined in the literature. A combination of limited surgery and RT has been suggested to improve outcome, although the complication rates may increase (17).

Intracavitary or interstitial irradiation alone is used in small superficial stage I disease. External beam RT (EBRT) in combination with intracavitary (ICB), and/or interstitial brachytherapy (ITB) is generally used for more extensive stage I or II disease. Data regarding the use of combined radiation and chemotherapy in vaginal cancer are evolving.

Squamous Cell Carcinoma: Treatment Options and Outcome by Federation of Gynecology and Obstetrics Stages

Federation of Gynecology and Obstetrics Stage 0: Vaginal Intraepithelial Neoplasia–Carcinoma *In Situ*

VAIN has been approached both surgically and medically by multiple investigators. Treatment options range from partial or complete vaginectomy to more conservative approaches such as local excision, electrocoagulation, laser vaporization, topical 5% fluorouracil () administration, or ICB alone. For patients in whom invasive disease cannot be ruled out, as well as for those who fail conservative therapy, surgical resection remains the treatment of choice. Overall, the reported control rates are very similar among the different approaches, ranging from 48% to 100% for laser (92,190,204) 52% to 100% for colpectomy (33,91); 75% to 100% for topical 5-FU (108,156,159,221), and 83% to 100% for RT (62). Table 70.4 summarizes the results in the management of VAIN-CIS with different treatment approaches.

Although partial or total vaginectomy has been considered by many to be an acceptable treatment, one of its main drawbacks is shortening or stenosis of the vagina, frequently with poor functional results. Hoffman et al. (91) reported a 17% recurrence rate in a series of 32 patients with CIS-VAIN of the vagina who underwent upper vaginectomy, 28% of which were found to have invasive cancer upon final pathologic examination, requiring additional RT in 50% of the cases. Of 23 patients with VAIN-III, 19 (83%) remained without evidence of recurrence at a mean follow-up of 38 months. Control rates of 66% to 100% following partial colpectomy affected either with a traditional surgical approach (91,97), with the cavitron ultrasonic surgical aspirator (CUSA) or with the loop electrocautery excision procedure (LEEP) have been achieved.

Radiation therapy has a long history of documented efficacy, with control rates ranging between 80% to 100%, as well as significantly better therapeutic ratio than other modalities (29,115,116,149,161). Using conventional low–dose rate (LDR) ICB techniques, the entire vaginal mucosa should receive 50 to 60 Gy, given the high incidence of multicentricity; the area of involvement should receive 70 to –80 Gy, in one or two implants, prescribed to the mucosal surface (150). Higher doses may cause significant vaginal fibrosis and stenosis. Perez et al. (148,150) reported only one distal local failure in the 20 patients treated for CIS. Pelvic recurrences or distant failures have not been observed in the absence of invasive component, after ICB.

There have been some reports in the literature regarding the use of high–dose rate (HDR) ICB for patients with VAIN-3. Ogino et al. (136) reported six patients treated with HDR to a mean dose of 23.3 Gy (range 15 to 30 Gy), none of whom developed recurrent disease. Limited rectal bleeding and moderate to severe vaginal mucosa reactions were noted in patients treated to the entire length of the vagina. MacLeod et al. (120) reported on

Table 70.4	VAGINAL INTRAEPITHELIAL NEOPLASIA CARCINOMA IN SITU: TREATMENT APPROACH AND RESULTS		
Treatment Modality **Author (Reference)**	**No.** **Patients**	**Comments**	**Outcome** **Control (%)**
Laser Therapy			
Stafl et al. (190)	6	Depth to 1.5–2 mm	83
Townsend et al. (204)	36	32% had >1 treatment	92
Jobson and Homesly (100)	15	26% required 2nd treatment	100
Julian et al. (101)	10	Used to effect colpectomy	80
Hoffman et al. (92)	26	3/11 failures had invasive disease. Recommended excision. Not ideal.	58
Topical 5-FU			
Woodruff et al. (221)	9	1%–2% 5-FU q mo	88
Piver et al. (159)	8	20% 5-FU q d x 5 Could use 5% or 10%	75
Petrilli et al. (156)	15	5% 5-FU b.i.d. x 5 d Repeat in 12 wk	80
Krebs (108)	31	1/3 applicator q wk x 10 wk	81
Surgical Excision			
Creasman et al. (NCDB) (33)	23		96
Fanning et al. (49)	15	Used LEEP, 1 part had cancer	100
Robinson et al. (172)	46	CUSA—29 primaries CUSA—17 recurrent	66 52
Hoffman et al. (91)	32	28% invasive cancer out of 23 with VAIN	83
Indermaur et al. (97)	105	Upper vaginectomy 12% invasive cancer	88
Irradiation			
Chyle et al. (29)	37		83
Kirkbride et al. (107)	14		100
Perez et al. (150)	20		94

CUSA, cavitron ultrasonic surgical aspirator; 5-FU, 5-fluorouracil; LEEP, loop electrocautery excision procedure; VAIN, vaginal intraepithelial neoplasia.

14 patients with VAIN treated with HDR-ICB (34 to 45 Gy in 4.5- to 8.5-Gy fractions). With a median follow-up of 46 months, one patient had persistent tumor and another showed progression of tumor with an overall local control of 78.5%. Two patients had moderate or permanent vaginal atrophy and stenosis. Mock et al. (125) reported 100% recurrence-free survival in six patients with CIS treated with HDR intracavitary brachytherapy.

Estrogen therapy should be considered in women who are postmenopausal or have undergone radiation therapy, provided the possibility of invasive disease has been eliminated. The effect of irradiation on ovarian function, as well as occasional fibrosis of the vaginal vault, makes this treatment currently unacceptable except in cases resistant to conservative therapy.

Invasive Squamous Cell Carcinoma

Surgical Approach: Outcomes

In general, SCC of the vagina has been treated with RT. However, several surgical series have reported acceptable to excellent outcomes in well-selected patients, with survival rates after radical surgery for stage I disease ranging from 75% to 90% (10,33,38,177,192,203). Cases in which surgery may be the preferred treatment include selected stage I or II patients, with lesions at the apex and upper third of the posterior or lateral vagina that could be approached with radical hysterectomy, upper vaginectomy, and pelvic lymphadenectomy providing adequate margins (10,38,54,177,192) and very superficial lesions that may be removed with wide local excision. Lesions in the mid-lower vagina may require vulvovaginectomy, in addition to dissection of inguinofemoral nodes or even exenteration to achieve negative margins (10,54,177,192). If the margins are found to be close or positive after resection, adjuvant RT is recommended. However, for lesions requiring extensive resection, definitive RT is the treatment of choice since it offers excellent results (147), with isolated central failures offered exenteration (177).

Creasman et al. (33), in a review of the NCDB for cancers of the vagina, noted superior survival in those undergoing surgery. However, Creasman et al. and Tjalma et al. (203) recognized that there may be bias in surgical series, such that younger, healthier patients with better performance status are more likely to be offered radical surgery, whereas older patients with multiple comorbid medical conditions are offered RT.

In the largest single institution series reported to date by Stock et al. (192), of 100 patients with carcinoma of the vagina (including 85 with SCC), a 47% 5-year survival rate was achieved. In this series, 40 patients were treated with surgery alone, 47 with radiation alone, and 13 with combination therapy. Overall, 5-year survival was 47%. Survival for stage I patients was 56% when treated with surgery, versus 80% for those who received RT, whereas for stage II patients, the survival rates were 68% and 31% after surgery and RT, respectively. Stock et al. acknowledged that the apparent surgical superiority for stage II patients may have been due to selection bias in that those treated with RT alone were more likely to have had stage IIB disease with extensive paracolpos involvement, and those with lesser involvement were preferentially offered surgery. Stock et al. advocated RT for stage II patients with extensive paracolpos. They concluded that for upper-third vault lesions, radical hysterectomy pelvic lymphadenectomy with upper vaginectomy be offered to those with stage I lesions, with a consideration for wide local excision, and postoperative RT for patients with small lesions.

Tjalma et al. (203) reported on 55 cases of SCC of the vagina, including 27 cases stage I, and 12 with stage II disease, with a median follow-up of 45 months. Of the 27 cases with stage I disease, 26 underwent surgery, and four of these 26 patients received some form of postoperative RT; a 91% 5-year survival rate was achieved for stage I disease.

Although several series have reported on primary surgical approaches, including exenterations for patients with advanced stage III or IV squamous cell carcinoma, achieving control rates as high as 50% for highly selected patients (10,54,177,192), the number of patients treated in any single series is so small that in modern practice, primary exenteration for advanced disease would not be recommended as the preferred approach. Therefore, advanced stage patients should receive definitive RT, probably in combination with concurrent chemotherapy, although the role of combined modality therapy is unknown.

Radiation Approach: Outcomes

Stage I

In patients with stage I lesions, usually 0.5- to 1-cm thick, that may involve one or more vaginal walls, it is important to individualize radiation therapy techniques to obtain optimal functional results. Most authors emphasize that brachytherapy alone is adequate for superficial stage I patients, with 95% to 100% local control rates when using ICB and ITB techniques (111,116,147,155,165,192,210). Superficial lesions can be adequately treated with LDR-ICB alone using after-loading vaginal cylinders. The entire length of the vagina is generally treated to a mucosal dose of 60 Gy, and an additional mucosal dose of 20 to 30 Gy is delivered to the area of tumor involvement (150). For lesions thicker than 0.5 cm and involving one wall, it is advisable to combine ICB and ITB with a single-plane implant to increase the depth dose and limit excessive irradiation to the vaginal mucosa. With LDR-ICB, a dose of 60 to 65 Gy is delivered to the entire vaginal mucosa; a dose to 0.5-cm depth from the ICB should be calculated; an additional 15 to 20 Gy at a depth of 0.5 cm beyond the plane of the implant will be delivered with the ITB such that the base of the tumor receives between 65 to 70 Gy, with the involved vaginal mucosa receiving an estimated 80 to 100 Gy.

There are no well-established criteria regarding the use of EBRT in patients with stage I disease. Perez et al. (147,149) did not find a significant correlation between the technique of irradiation used and the probability of local or pelvic recurrence, probably since the treatment technique varied based on tumor-related factors. There is general consensus that EBRT is advisable for larger, more infiltrating, or poorly differentiated tumors that may have a higher risk of lymph node metastasis. The whole pelvis is treated with 10 or 20 Gy; an additional parametrial dose should be delivered with a midline block 5 half-value layer (HVL) to give a total of 45 to 50 Gy to the parametria and pelvic side walls. The 5-year survival for patients with stage I disease treated with RT alone ranges from 70% to 95% (29,33,38,107,111,149,192,210) (Table 70.5). Sites of recurrence by stage are shown in Table 70.6.

Stage II

Patients with stage IIA tumors have more advanced paravaginal disease without extensive parametrial infiltration. These patients are uniformly treated with EBRT, followed either by ICB or ITB. Generally, the whole pelvis receives 20 Gy followed by an additional parametrial dose with a midline 2- to 4-cm-wide (5 HVL) block, depending on the width of the implant, to deliver a total of 45 to 50 Gy to the pelvic side walls. A combination of LDR interstitial and intracavitary therapy may also be used to deliver a minimum of 50 to 60 Gy 0.5 cm beyond the deep margin of the tumor (in addition to the whole-pelvis dose). Double-plane or volume implants may be necessary for more

Table 70.5	INTERNATIONAL FEDERATION OF GYNECOLOGY AND OBSTETRICS STAGE I AND II VAGINAL CANCER: TREATMENT APPROACH AND RESULTS

Treatment Modality/Author (Reference)	No. Patients	Outcome/Survival (Reference)
Irradiation +/− Surgery		
Chyle et al. (29)	59 St I	10 y 76%
	104 St II	10 y 69%
Creasman et al. (33) (NCDB)	169 St I	5 y survival: 73%; 79% S+RT (47), 63% RT (122)
	175 St II	5 y survival: 58%; 58% S+RT (39), 57% RT (136)
Davis et al. (38)	19 St I	5 y survival: 100% S+RT (5), 65% RT (14)
	18 St II	5 y survival: 69% S+RT (9), 50% RT (9)
Kirkbride et al. (107)	40 St I	5 y 72%
	38 St II	5 y 70%
Kucera and Vavra (111)	16 St I	5 y 81%
	23 St II	5 y 43.5%
Perez et al. (149)	59 St I	10 y 80%
	63 St IIA	10 y 55%
	34 St IIB	10 y 35%
Stock et al. (192)	8 St I	5 y 100% S + RT, 80% RT
	35 St II	5 y 69% S + RT, 31% RT
Urbanski et al. (210)	33 St I	5 y 73%
	37 St II	5 y 54%
Frank et al. (52)	50 St I	5 y DSS 85%
	97 St II	5 y DSS 78%
Radical Surgery		5-Year Survival
Ball and Berman (10)	19 St I	84%
	8 St II	63%
Creasman et al. (33) (NCDB)	76 St I	90%
	34 St II	70%
Davis et al. (38)	25 St I	85%
	27 St II	49%
Rubin et al. (177)	5 St I	80%
	3 St II	33%
Stock et al. (192)	17 St I	56%
	23 St II	68%
Tjalma et al. (203)	26[a] St I	91%

St, stage.
[a]Four patients received adjuvant irradiation.

extensive disease (Fig. 70.3). Perez et al. (149) showed that in stage IIA, the local tumor control was 70% (37/53) in patients receiving brachytherapy combined with EBRT, compared with 40% (4/10) in patients treated with either brachytherapy or EBRT alone. The superiority of the combination of EBRT and brachytherapy over EBRT or brachytherapy alone has been shown in other series as well (29,192).

Patients with stage IIB, with more extensive parametrial infiltration, should receive 40 to 50 Gy, whole pelvis and 55- to 60-Gy total parametrial dose (with midline shielding). An additional boost of 30 to 35 Gy will be given with LDR interstitial and intracavitary brachytherapy, to deliver a total tumor dose of 75 to 80 Gy to the vaginal tumor (29,149,189) and 65 Gy to parametrial and paravaginal extensions (92). The local-regional control in patients with stage IIB, in the series by Perez et al. (149,150), was also superior with combined EBRT and brachytherapy (61% vs. 50%, respectively).

The 5-year survival for patients with stage II disease treated with RT alone ranges between 35% to 70% for stage IIA, and 35% to 60% for stage IIB (29,149,192). The results of several series published in the literature using different treatment approaches for the treatment of stage I and II vaginal cancer are shown in Table 70.5 (10,29,33,38,107,111,177,192,203,210). Sites of recurrence by stage are shown in Table 70.6.

Stages III and IVA

Generally, patients with stage III and IVA disease will receive 45 to 50 Gy EBRT to the pelvis, and in some cases, additional parametrial dose with midline shielding to deliver up to 60 Gy to the pelvic side walls. Ideally, ITB brachytherapy boost is performed, if technically feasible, to deliver a minimum tumor dose of 75 to 80 Gy. If brachytherapy is not feasible, a shrinking-field technique can be used, with fields defined using the three-dimensional treatment planning capabilities to deliver a tumor dose around 65 Gy. An alternative approach is intensity-modulated RT (IMRT), using multiple beams of varying intensity that conform the high-dose region to the shape of the target tissues, with more adequate sparing of the surrounding normal tissues, primarily the bladder, rectum, and small bowel (130,131) (Fig. 70.4).

Boronow et al. (17) proposed an alternative to exenterative procedure for locally advanced vulvovaginal carcinoma, using RT to treat the pelvic disease and a radical vulvectomy with bilateral inguinal node dissection to treat the vulvar extension of the tumor. External irradiation to the pelvis and inguinal nodes consisted of 45 to 50 Gy, combined with LDR intracavitary insertions to deliver maximal doses of 80 to 85 Gy to the vaginal mucosa with both modalities.

Table 70.6 SITES OF RECURRENCE

Author (Reference)	No. Patients	Percentage of Recurrence	Local-Regional Recurrence	Distant Recurrence	Local + Distant
Chyle et al. (29)	301	35% (overall)	21%[a] St 0 (17%) St I (15%) St II (18%) St III (35%) St IV (60%)	11%[a] St I (7%) St II (18%) St III (38%) St IV (38%)	3%[a]
Davis et al. (38)	89	St I (23%) St II (36%)	16% 16%	5% 20%	Not shown
Kirkbride et al. (107)	153	42%	32%	7%	3%
Kucera and Vavra (111)	110	24.5%	21%	4%	0.5%
Perez et al. (149)	212	St 0 (5%) St I (22%) St IIA (47%) St IIB (71%) St III (55%) St IVA (73%) TOTAL: 42%	5% 9% 17% 19% 5% 26% 13%	0 8% 13% 27% 20% 0 12%	0 5% 17% 25% 30% 47% 17%
Tabata et al. (196)	51	St 0–II (36%) St III–IV (92%)	36% 50%	0% 42%	Not shown
Urbanski et al. (210)	125	53%	41%	8%	4%
Frank et al. (52)	193 147, St I–II 46, St III–IV	25.3% St I–II (21%) St III–IVA (39%)	12.4% St I–II (9%) St III–IV (24%)	6.7% St I–II (6.8%) St III–IVA (6.5%)	6.2% St I–II (5.4%) St III–IVA (8.7%)

St, stage.
[a]Actuarial, 10 years.

The overall cure rate for patients with stage III disease is 30% to 50%. Stage IVA includes patients with rectal or bladder mucosa involvement, or in most series, positive inguinal nodes. Although some patients with stage IVA disease are curable, many patients are treated palliatively with EBRT only. Pelvic exenteration can also be curative in highly selected stage IV patients with small volume central disease. Table 70.7 (10,29,33,107,111,149,177,192,210) shows the treatment results with different therapeutic modalities, including four series that reported the use of primary surgery in highly selected patients with advanced disease. However, each of these series reported a far greater number of patients with similar stage disease treated with RT, which represents the preferred approach in contemporary practice (147,161). Sites of recurrence by stage are shown in Table 70.6.

Role of Chemotherapy and Radiation

The control rate in the pelvis for stages III and IV patients is relatively low, and about 70% to 80% of the patients have persistent disease or recurrent disease in the pelvis, in spite of high doses of external beam RT and brachytherapy. Failure in distant sites does occur in about 25% to 30% of the patients with locally advanced tumors, much less than pelvic recurrences. Therefore, there is a need for better approaches to the management of advanced disease such as the use of concomitant chemoradiotherapy. Agents such as 5-FU, mitomycin-C, and cisplatin have shown promise when combined with RT, with complete response rate as high as 60% to 85% (48,171), but long-term results of such therapy have been variable. In these small studies, many of the patients had advanced (stage III) disease at the initiation of combined modality therapy, perhaps explaining the lack of long-term disease control. Evans et al. (48) found no local recurrences, however, among patients achieving

a complete response with RT and 5-FU plus mitomycin-C (12 of 25 patients), with a median follow-up period of 28 months, suggesting that local control may be improved with combined modality therapy. The survival for the entire population was 56% (66% for patients with primary vaginal cancer). Only two patients had severe complications, although the authors recognize that the follow-up was short term. Roberts et al. (171) reported on a series of 67 patients with advanced cancers of the vagina, cervix, and vulva treated with concurrent 5-FU, cisplatin, and RT (seven patients with vaginal cancers of whom five had stage III and two recurrent disease). Although 85% experienced a complete response, 61% of them recurred, with a median time to recurrence of only 6 months, and an overall survival at 5 years of 22%. Further, nine of 67 patients (13%) developed severe late complications of which eight required surgeries. Kersh et al. (105) reported that five out of eight vaginal cancer patients achieved local control with combined modality therapy.

Dalrymple et al. (35) recently published a small study including 14 patients with primarily stages I and II SCC of the vagina treated with reduced doses of RT (median 63 Gy) concurrently with different 5FU-based chemotherapeutic regimens. They report a 93% control rate (four patients died of intercurrent disease with no evidence of tumor), probably reflecting a more favorable stage distribution. Interestingly, none of the patients required interstitial implants and no patients developed fistulas. The authors indicate that this approach, similar to the one used in the management of anal and vulvar cancer, would allow reducing the RT dose with the subsequent improvement in organ function and late toxicity.

Further investigation is needed to determine the therapeutic efficacy of the concurrent chemoradiotherapy and the optimal chemotherapy regimen. Recently published data on locally advanced cervical cancer have demonstrated an advantage

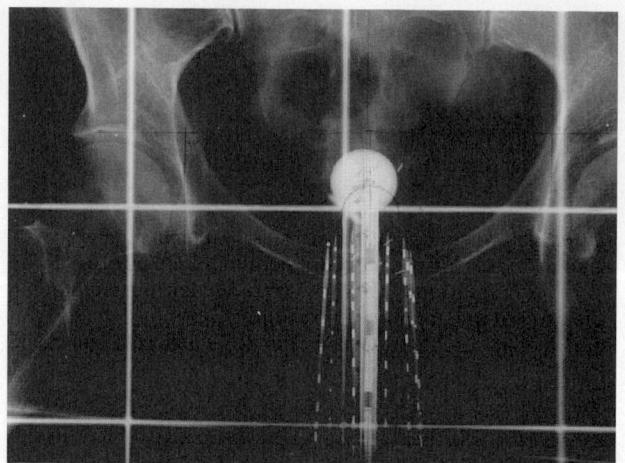

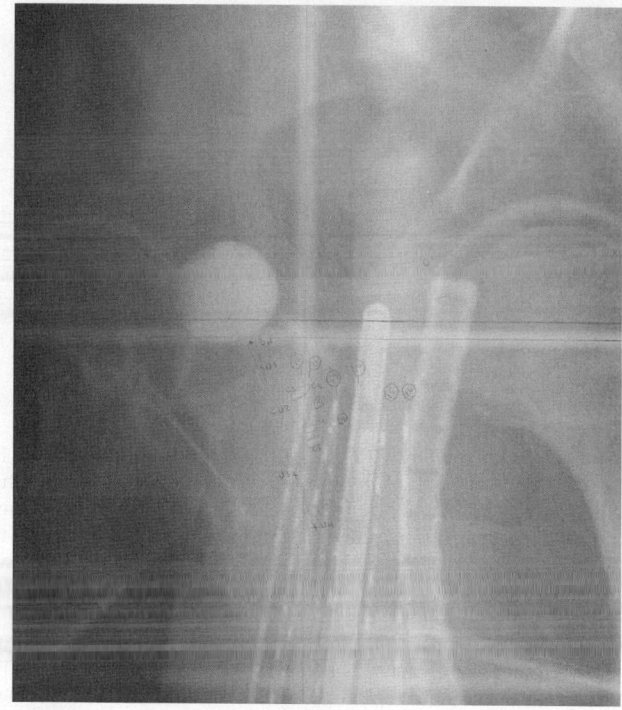

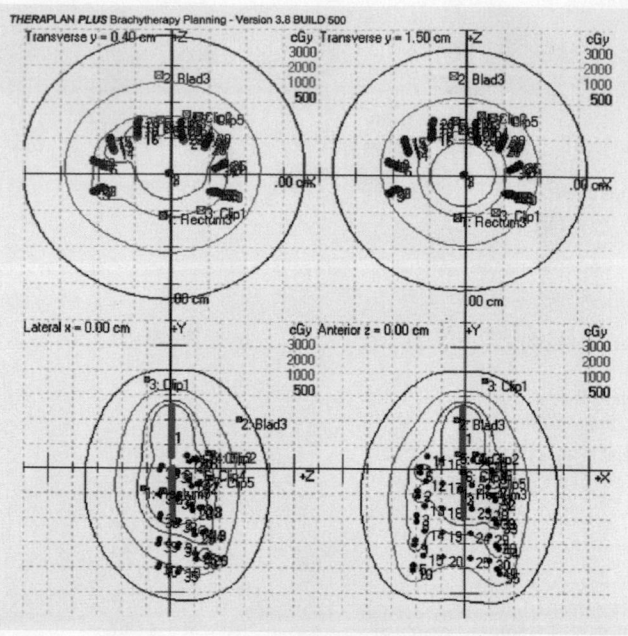

FIGURE 70.3. A: AP view interstitial and intracavitary implant in a patient with a lesion in the anterior wall of the vagina. **B:** Lateral view interstitial and intracavitary implant in a patient with a lesion in the anterior wall of the vagina. **C:** Isodose distribution interstitial and intracavitary implant in the anterior wall of the vagina.

in locoregional control, overall survival, and disease-free survival for patients receiving cisplatin-based chemotherapy concurrently with RT (106,127,175,219). The only drug common to all the studies was cisplatin, suggesting it may be the only agent needed to improve radiation sensitivity. Based on these data, as well as data on locoregionally advanced vulvar cancer (126), consideration should be given to a similar approach in patients with advanced vaginal cancer. Randomized trials comparing radiation therapy alone to chemoradiation therapy, however, are unlikely due to small patient population.

Radiotherapy Techniques

External Beam Radiotherapy

EBRT is advisable in patients with deeply infiltrating or poorly differentiated stage I lesions, and in all patients with stage II to IVA disease. The treatment is generally delivered using opposed anterior and posterior fields (AP/PA). The pelvis receives between 20 to 45 Gy, depending on the stage of the disease. This

will be followed, in some cases, by bilateral parametrial boost of 50 to 55 Gy. The distal margin of the tumor should be identified with a radiopaque marker or bead at the time of the simulation. High-energy photons (>10 MV) are usually preferred. CT simulation is highly encouraged since it allows a more accurate delineation of the regional lymph node areas, rather than relying on pelvic bony anatomy (200). Treatment portals cover at least the true pelvis with 1.5- to −2-cm margin beyond the pelvic rim. Superiorly, the field extends to either L4 or L5 or L5 to S1 to cover the pelvic lymph nodes up to the common iliacs, and extends distally to the introitus to include the entire vagina. Lateral fields, if used, should extend anteriorly to adequately include the external iliac nodes, anterior to the pubic symphysis, and at least to the junction of S2 or S3 posteriorly.

In patients with tumors involving the middle and lower vagina with clinically negative groins, the bilateral inguinofemoral lymph node regions should be treated electively to 45 to 50 Gy (149). Planning CT is recommended to adequately determine the depth of the inguinofemoral nodes. A number of techniques have been used to treat the areas at risk without overtreating the femoral necks. Some of the most commonly used techniques include the use of unequal loading (2:1, AP/PA),

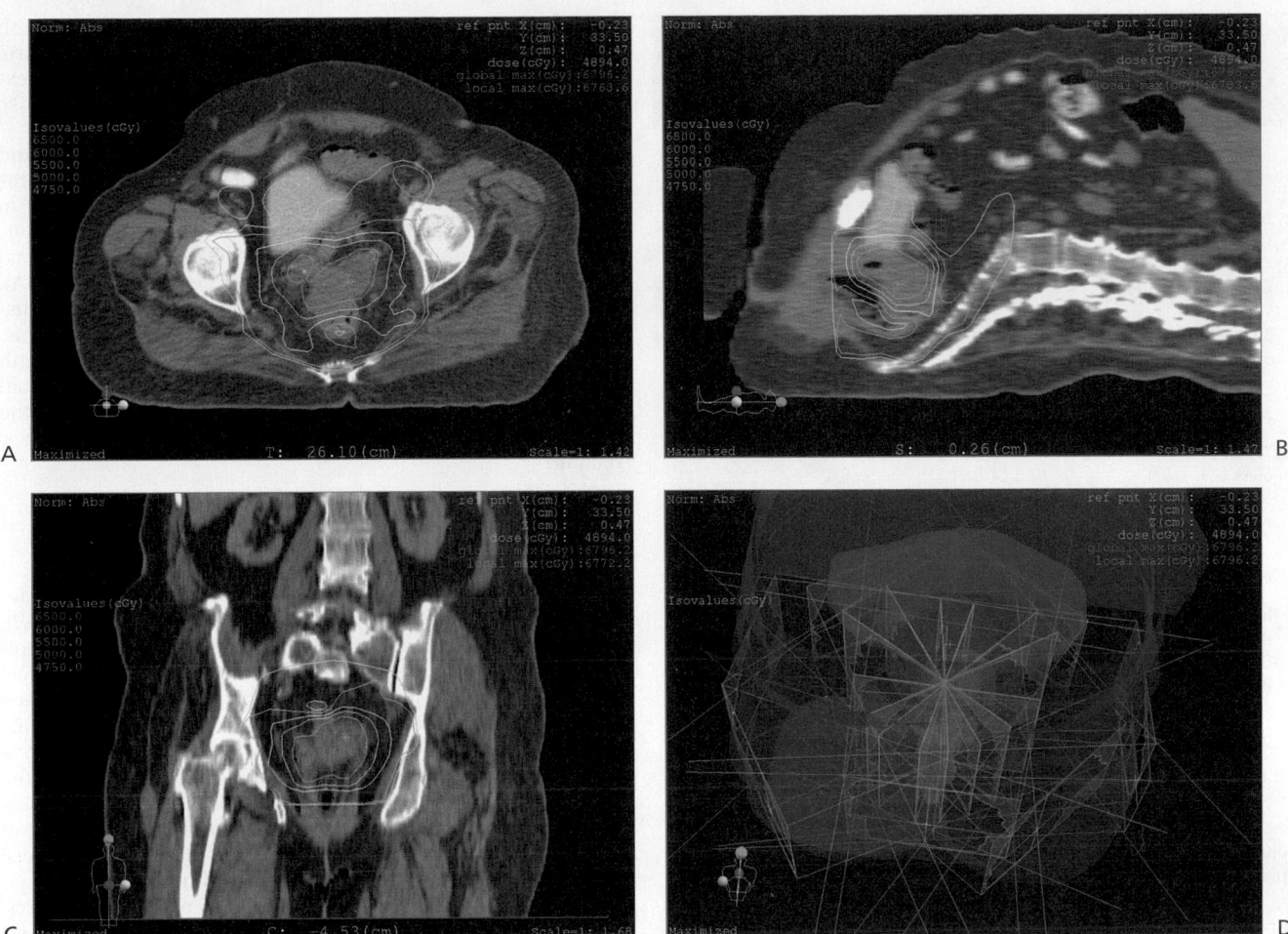

FIGURE 70.4. A: Axial dose distribution intensity-modulated radiation therapy (IMRT) plan for vaginal cancer. **B:** Saggital dose distribution IMRT plan for vaginal cancer. **C:** Coronal dose distribution IMRT plan for vaginal cancer. **D:** Beam arrangement IMRT plan for vaginal cancer.

a combination of low- and high-energy photons (4 to 6 MV, AP, and 15 to –18 MV, PA), or equally weighted beams with a transmission block in the central AP field, utilizing small AP photon or electron beams to deliver a daily boost to the inguinofemoral nodes (43). Special attention is needed to avoid areas of overlap. A technique has been developed and implemented at Indiana University that uses a narrow PA field to treat the pelvis, and a wider AP field encompassing the pelvis and inguinofemoral nodes, with daily AP photon boost to the inguinal nodes being delivered using the asymmetric collimators jaws (44). Advantages of this technique include simplicity of setup and treatment (single isocenter, no need for transmission block), dose homogeneity, reduced dose to the femoral necks, low potential risk of nodal under dose, and elimination of dosimetric difficulties inherent in electron boosts (Fig. 70.5).

For patients with positive pelvic nodes or those patients with advanced disease not amenable to interstitial implant, additional boost to the areas of gross disease, as defined by CT scan, should be given using conformal therapy to deliver a total dose between 65 to 70 Gy, when feasible, with high-energy photons. Boost to the gross pelvic nodes after brachytherapy should be given using small fields (similar to the parametrial boost with midline shielding) to deliver a total dose between 60 to 65 Gy with high-energy photons. In patients with clinically palpable inguinal nodes, additional doses of 15 to 20 Gy (calculated at a depth determined by CT scan) are necessary with reduced portals. This is generally achieved by using low-energy photons or electron beam (12 to 18 MeV). IMRT techniques are now avail-

able to deliver higher doses to the gross disease while reducing the dose to the bladder and rectum (130,173).

Overall treatment time (7 to 9 weeks) has been found to be a significant treatment factor predicting tumor control (115,158), although this has not been universally recognized (149).

Low–Dose Rate (LDR) Intracavitary Brachytherapy (LDR-ICB)

VAIN and small T1 lesions with <0.5 cm depth can be adequately treated with ICB alone. Low–dose rate intracavitary brachytherapy (LDR-ICB) is performed using vaginal cylinders such as Burnett, Bloedorn, Delclos (40) or MIRALVA (151,188) loaded with cesium-137 (^{137}Cs) radioactive sources. Delclos afterloading vaginal cylinders have a central hollow metallic cylinder in which the sources are placed, and plastic rings of varying diameter (2.5 to 4 cm), 2.5 cm in length, which are inserted over the cylinder (40). Domed cylinders are used to irradiate the vaginal cuff homogeneously, when indicated. Delclos et al. (40) recommended a short ^{137}Cs source to be used at the top to obtain a uniform dose around the dome, because a lower dose occurs at the end of the linear cilium source. Some cylinders have a lead shielding to protect selected portions of the vagina, the bladder, and the rectum. The largest possible diameter that can be comfortably accommodated by the patient should be used to improve the ratio of mucosa to tumor dose and eliminate vaginal rogation. In general, the vulva is sutured

Table 70.7	INTERNATIONAL FEDERATION OF GYNECOLOGY AND OBSTETRICS STAGE III AND IV VAGINAL CANCER: OUTCOME WITH RADIATION THERAPY WITH/WITHOUT SURGERY	
Treatment Modality **Author (Reference)**	**No. Patients**	**Outcome/Survival**
Irradiation +/− Surgery		
Chyle et al. (29)	55 St III	10 y 47%
	16 St IV	10 y 27%
Creasman et al. (NCDB) (33)	St III–IV, 180	5 y survival 36%; 60%-S + RT (36), 35%-RT (144)
Kirkbride et al. (107)	42[a] St III–IV	5 y 53%
Kucera and Vavra (111)	46 St III	5 y 35%
	19 St IVA	5 y 32%
Perez et al. (149)	20 St III	10 y 38%
	15 St IV	0%
Stock et al. (192)	9 St III	5 y 0%
	8 St IV	0%
Urbanski et al. (210)	40 St III	5 y 22.5%
	15 St IVA	0%
Frank et al. (52)	46 St III–IVA	5 y DSS 58%
Radical Surgery		5-Year Survival
Ball and Berman (10)	2 St III	50%
Creasman et al. (NCDB) (33)	St III–IV, 21	47%
Rubin et al. (177)	2 St III	50%

DSS, disease-specific survival; RT, radiotherapy; S, surgery; St, stage
[a]Twenty patients with St III–IV were treated with chemotherapy (5-FU +/− mitomycin-C) and radiotherapy.

closed for the duration of the implant in order to secure the position of the applicators.

In patients with upper vagina lesions with <0.5 cm depth of invasion, vaginal colpostats alone (after hysterectomy) or in combination with intrauterine tandem, loaded with ^{137}Cs sources similar to that used in treatment of cervical cancer, can be used to treat the proximal vagina to a minimum dose of 65- to 70-Gy, estimated to 0.5-cm depth, including the contribution of LDR, if given. When indicated, the remainder of the vagina can be treated by performing a subsequent implant using vaginal cylinders (generally 50 to 60 Gy, prescribed to the vaginal surface). It is important to avoid the placement of a protruding source over the vulva, with the subsequent increased risk of complications. When appropriate dose specification points are

chosen, a very uniform dose distribution over the entire length of the vagina can be obtained. The use of LDR remote control afterloading technology allows the reduction of radiation exposure to hospital personnel and optimization of the isodose distribution.

Perez et al. (151) and Slessinger et al. (188) designed and constructed a vaginal applicator, MIRALVA, which incorporates two ovoid sources and a central tandem that can be used to treat the entire vagina (alone, or in combination with the uterine cervix). The applicator has vaginal apex caps and additional cylinder sleeves to allow for increased dimensions (Fig. 70.5A). A tandem in the uterus can be used if clinically indicated, using standard loadings, depending on the depth of the uterus. When the tandem and vaginal cylinder are used, the strength of the sources in the ovoids should be 15 mgRaEq. The vaginal cylinder or uterine tandem never carries an active source at the level of the ovoids to prevent excessive doses to the bladder or rectum.

High–Dose Rate Intracavitary Brachytherapy

The International Commission of Radiation Units (ICRU) defines HDR brachytherapy as exceeding 12 Gy per hour (149). High–dose rate intracavitary brachytherapy (HDR-ICB) is typically performed with a 10 Ci single iridium-192 (^{192}Ir) source. The applicators are similar to those described for LDR. Limited information regarding HDR-ICB in the treatment of primary carcinoma of the vagina is available (133,193). Fewer patients have been treated when compared with LDR-ICB, follow-up for the most series is short term, publication bias is likely, and there is no agreement on treatment regimen. Generally, the number of insertions ranges from one to six (median three), with the dose per fraction ranging from 300 to 800 cGy (median 700 cGy).

Stock et al. (193) described results in 15 patients with carcinoma of the vagina treated with HDR brachytherapy; dose per treatment ranged from 3 to 8 Gy, with a median dose of 7 Gy, for a total median dose of 21 Gy. The median interval between fractions was 2 weeks. Brachytherapy was combined with EBRT (30 to 63 Gy, with a median dose of 42 Gy, 1.8 to 2.92 Gy per fraction). The median total tumor dose from both components was 63 Gy. The 5-year actuarial survival rate was 50% with brachytherapy, compared with 9% in the EBRT-alone patients (p <0.001), although a larger percentage of stage IV lesions (36%) were in the EBRT-alone group than in the brachytherapy group (5%). Local tumor control rates were 50% for stage I, 47%

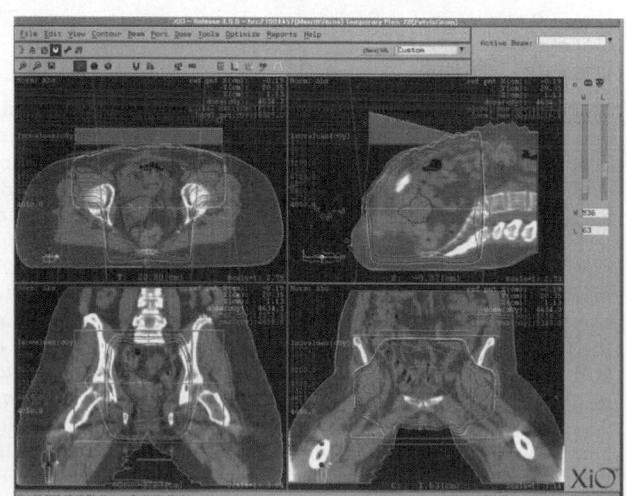
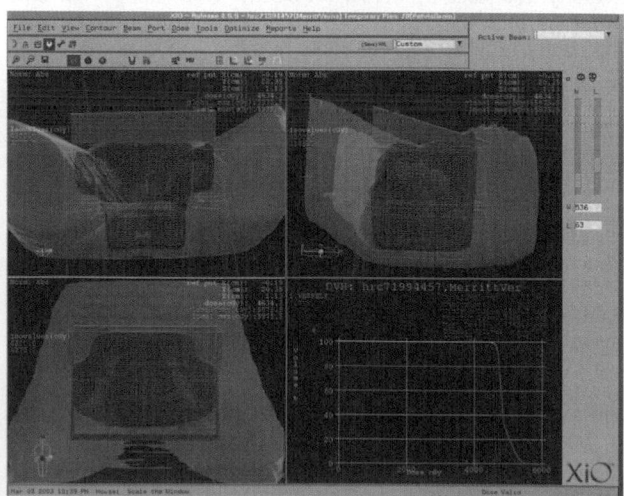

FIGURE 70.5. A: Beam arrangement external beam radiation therapy (EBRT) to the pelvis and inguinofemoral lymph node regions. **B:** Iodose distribution of EBRT to the pelvis and inguinofemoral lymph node regions.

for stage II, and 40% for stage III. Survival closely paralleled tumor control. There was no significant difference in outcome in the LDR or HDR groups. Acceptable morbidity of therapy was noted for all 49 patients, but no comment was made comparing LDR with HDR.

Nanavati et al. (133) reported 13 patients with primary vaginal cancer (five stage I, four stage IIA, and four stage IIB) treated with external beam RT (45 Gy) and HDR-ICB (20 to 28 Gy in three to four fractions, calculated at 0.5 cm from the surface of the applicator). All 13 patients had a complete response, and local control was achieved in 92% of the patients with a median follow-up of only 2.6 years (range 0.7 to 5.2 years). They did not observe any acute or chronic intestinal or bladder grade 3 or 4 toxicity. However, moderate to severe vaginal stenosis occurred in 46% of the patients. The authors recognize that "late-occurring toxicity could be missed at a medium follow-up of 2.6 years" (133). Kucera et al. (110) reported on 190 patients with invasive carcinoma of the vagina staged according to the FIGO system. Eighty were treated with intracavitary HDR ^{192}Ir brachytherapy with or without EBRT. These patients were compared with a historical group of 110 patients treated with intracavitary LDR brachytherapy with or without EBRT. No significant differences were found for stages, tumor grade, or location between the two groups. The crude 5-year survival rates for all patients were 41% in the LDR group, 81% in stage I, and 43% in stage II. Overall actuarial 3-year survival and disease-specific survival rates for all patients in the HDR series were 51% and 66%, respectively. Disease-specific 3-year survival rates were 83% in stage I and 66% in stage II. There were no significant differences in local and distant recurrences between the treatment modalities. Complications analysis showed no significant differences between the HDR and LDR series.

Kushner et al. (112) described a 15.8% of serious/late complications in 19 patients with vaginal cancer treated with different combinations of EBRT, intracavitary and interstitial HDR brachytherapy, with a low 39.3% 2-year progression-free survival.

Many aspects remain unknown or not well understood in the use of HDR-ICB. These include the radiobiologic equivalency of HDR to LDR, fractionation schedule, total dose, specification of dose prescription, and how to combine HDR with EBRT or LDR brachytherapy. In addition, optimization approaches and methods of dose calculation, such as the inclusion of anisotropic corrections, are not well described in the sparse literature available to date (59,118). These factors could result in an increased incidence of severe complications, such as vaginal necrosis and rectovaginal or vesicovaginal fistulas (112,179,206).

Interstitial Brachytherapy

ITB is an important component in the treatment of advanced vaginal cancer, typically in combination with EBRT or ICB. When performing ITB a careful definition of the "target volume," gross tumor volume (based on clinical, radiologic, and operative findings) and a margin of adjoining normal tissue, is required. Other considerations include whether a permanent (gold-198 or iodine-125) or temporary implant (^{192}Ir) is optimal, the geometry of the implant (e.g., single or double plane or volume implant) depending on the extent and thickness of the volume to be implanted, source distribution, dose rate, and total dose, based on tumor size, location, local extent, and proximity of normal structures (85). The principal advantages of temporary implants are readily controlled distribution of the radioactive sources and easier modification of the dose distribution. The main advantages of a permanent seed implant include relative safety/simplicity, easy applicability, cost-effectiveness, and ability, in most cases, to be performed using local anesthesia. As a general rule, temporary implants are more commonly used in the curative treatment of larger gynecological malignancies,

whereas permanent implants are usually performed for smaller volume disease.

Freehand implants or template systems designed to assist in preplanning and to guide and secure the position of the needles in the target volume can be employed. Commercially available templates include the Syed-Neblett template (SNIT) (Alpha Omega Services, Bellflower, CA) (195), the modified Syed-Neblett, and the MUPIT (Martinez Universal Perineal Interstitial Template) (123). These templates generally consist of a perineal template, vaginal obturator, and 17-gauge hollow guides of various lengths that can be afterloaded with ^{192}Ir sources. The vaginal obturator is 2 cm in diameter, and 12 or 15 cm in length, with six or seven grooves on its surface for the placement of guide needles. It is centrally drilled so that it can allow the placement of a tandem to be loaded with ^{137}Cs sources. This makes it possible to combine an interstitial and intracavitary application simultaneously. Improved dose-rate distributions are obtained by means of computer-assisted optimization of the source placement and strength during the planning and loading phase.

Due to the inaccuracies of pelvic examination and close proximity of the rectum and bladder to the target volume, there exists a serious risk of either underdosing the target volume or causing bladder and rectal morbidity. In order to improve the accuracy of target localization and needle placement, several investigators have explored performing ITI under transrectal ultrasound (TRUS), CT, MRI-planned implants with endorectal coil, laparotomy, and laparoscopic guidance (191). Although laparotomy facilitates the displacement of bowel during the procedure by using slings or tissue expanders or lysis of adherent bowel, there is some degree of associated morbidity, such as ileus, bleeding, and increased operative time. Laparoscopy is a shorter and less invasive procedure. Real-time TRUS-guided Syed-Neblett template implantation technique was reported by Stock et al. (191). With this technique, invasive laparotomy/laparoscopy can often be avoided, providing an interactive, noninvasive technique allowing for highly accurate needle placement.

An open retropubic approach allows direct visualization of the bladder and urethra during interstitial implantation of anterior vaginal malignancies and facilitates negotiation of the pubic arch. Paley et al. (141) described a technique using an open retropubic approach for Syed-Neblett template interstitial implants in anterior vaginal tumors under direct visualization. Complete response was noted in five of six patients, but persistent local control of disease was achieved in only one of five complete responses. Complications included paravaginal abscess ($n = 1$), postoperative deep venous thrombosis ($n = 1$), abdominal incision cellulitis ($n = 1$), and radiation enteritis ($n = 1$).

Tewari et al. (201) described results in 71 patients who underwent ITI with (61 patients) or without (10 patients) EBRT. Patients included those with stage I (10 patients), Perez modification stage IIA (14 patients), Perez modification stage IIB (25 patients), stage III (15 patients), and stage IV (seven patients) disease. Each implant delivered a total tumor dose reaching 80 Gy integrated with EBRT. Local control was achieved in 53 patients (75%), and with a median follow-up of 66 months the 5- and 10-year actuarial disease-free survival rates were both 58%. By stage, 5-year disease-free survival rates included stage I, 100%; stage IIA, 60%; stage IIB, 61%; stage III, 30%; and stage IV, 0%. Stage and primary lesion size independently influenced the survival rates. Significant complications occurred in nine patients (13%) including necrosis ($n = 4$), fistulas ($n = 4$), and small bowel obstruction ($n = 1$).

Stryker (194) treated 40 patients with vaginal carcinoma; 14 had a history of prior hysterectomy. There were four treatment groups: EBRT and intracavitary brachytherapy (group WPIC; $n = 15$); EBRT and interstitial brachytherapy (group WPIS; $n = 10$); EBRT alone (group WP; $n = 7$); and brachytherapy alone (group BA; $n = 2$). The 5-year disease-specific survival rates were 68% for 28 patients with squamous cell carcinoma and 50% for six patients with adenocarcinoma. The 5-year survival rates were 78% for stage I disease, 63% for stage II, 33% for stage III, and 50% for stage IV ($p = 0.2$). Local failure occurred in two patients (13%) in the WPIC group, two (20%) in WPIS, three (43%) in WP, and one (50%) in BA. Nine patients (26%) had late small/large intestine or bladder morbidity. Vaginal morbidity occurred in 15 patients (44%) (9/15 [60%] in the WPIC and 3/10 [30%] in the WPIS groups, respectively). When combining EBRT with brachytherapy, we prefers interstitial over intracavitary techniques.

Muench and Nath (129) described a shielded vaginal applicator used with encapsulated Americium-241 (^{241}Am). A few patients with recurrent pelvic, including vaginal, tumors have been treated with this applicator with significant reduction of bladder and rectal doses because of the profound effect of the shielding on the 16-keV photons. The HVL of ^{241}Am is only 0.125 mm of lead (compared with 6 mm for ^{137}Cs photons).

Clear Cell Carcinoma of the Vagina: General Management, Treatment Options, and Outcome

Since Herbst and Scully's (81) first report of seven adenocarcinomas arising in the vagina of adolescent females after in utero exposure to DES, there have been several reports limited to DES-related vaginal CCA (76,78,79,82). In 1979, Herbst et al. (79) reported 142 cases of stage I CCA of the vagina. An 8% risk of recurrence was seen after radical surgery ($n = 117$), and an 87% survival was achieved. There was a 36% risk of recurrence after RT for stage I lesions; however, the authors acknowledged that in general, RT was reserved for large stage I lesions that involved more of the vault and were less amenable to surgical resection. Surgery for stage I CCA may have the advantage of ovarian preservation and, after skin graft, better vaginal function. As the majority of CCA occur in the upper third of the vault, the largest series (79,182,183) addressing the surgical approach to these lesions have advocated radical hysterectomy, pelvic and para-aortic lymphadenectomy, and sufficient colpectomy to achieve negative margins. Senekjian et al. (181) have also reported a series of exenterations done for CCA. However, there have been efforts to also attempt fertility-sparing radical resections (95) or more limited wide local excisions followed by some form of radiation (182). Wharton et al. (217) advocate intracavitary or transvaginal irradiation for the treatment of small tumors because this may yield excellent tumor control with a functional vagina and preservation of ovarian function.

Senekjian et al. (182) reported a series of 219 stage I CCA cases of which 176 had conventional therapy and 43 underwent local therapy. The two groups appear to be similar with respect to symptoms, stage, location of the lesion in the vagina, greatest tumor diameter, surface area, depth of invasion, predominant histologic pattern, grade, and number of mitoses. Actuarial survival rates at 5 and 10 years for the local therapy group (92% and 88%, respectively) were essentially equivalent to those for the conventional therapy group (92% and 90%, respectively). However, the recurrence experience after local therapy was less favorable; at 10 years, the actuarial recurrence rate for the local excision subgroup was 45%, in comparison with only 13% for patients treated with more radical surgery. Local therapy consisted of vaginectomy in nine cases, local excision alone in 17 cases, and local irradiation (with or without local excision) in 17 cases. The subgroup of patients receiving local irradiation had a recurrence rate of 27%, similar to that of the conventional therapy group and more favorable than that of either the subgroup treated with vaginectomy or local excision alone. Re-

currences were more frequently noted in patients with tumors >2 cm, with invasion of ≥ 3 mm, and with a predominant histologic pattern other than tubulocystic. Pelvic lymph node metastases were noted at death in 12% of patients. They advocated a combination of wide local excision and extraperitoneal node dissection followed by brachytherapy for patients desirous of fertility preservation.

In a subsequent report, Senekjian et al. (183) reviewed the experience with 76 cases with stage II CCA from the Registry for Research on Hormonal Transplacental Carcinogenesis, which were subdivided into three substages according to the classification proposed by Perez et al. (145). The overall 5- and 10-year survival rates were 83% and 65%, respectively. Of the 76 patients, 22 received surgery exclusively (either radical hysterectomy with vaginectomy, 13 patients, or exenterative type procedure, nine patients), 38 received RT alone, 12 received combination therapy, and four underwent other approaches. Patients treated with primary RT achieved an 87% 5-year survival rate, versus 80% for those treated with surgery, and 85% for those receiving both treatments. The recurrence and survival experiences for the three substage groups were similar. The data available do not suggest any clinical benefit to categorizing cases of stage II vaginal clear cell adenocarcinoma into substages. The authors concluded that most patients with stage II vaginal CCA should be treated with combination EBRT and brachytherapy; however, small, easily resectable lesions in the upper fornix might undergo resection, allowing better preservation of coital and ovarian function (183).

In 1989, Senekjian et al. (181) reported their experience of 20 pelvic exenterations for CCA of the vagina, including 13 for primary lesions and seven for recurrent disease. The nine patients with stage II disease treated with primary exenteration were compared with the 67 who had other modalities of therapy; no significant difference in the survival experience was noted between the two groups. They reported a 72% success rate if the exenterations were done as part of primary therapy. The authors advocated reserving exenterative approaches for those who have failed RT in order to maximize quality of life for the greatest number of patients.

Noncpithelial Tumors of the Vagina: General Management, Treatment Options, and Outcome

Melanoma of the Vagina

Vaginal melanoma is an exceedingly rare entity; therefore, the number of patients is too small to permit prospective controlled trials. Melanoma of the vagina, with its propensity to develop distant metastases, possibly because only 5% of the patients had lesions <2 mm thick (28), and its lack of a recognized precursor lesion, has presented therapeutic challenges for surgeons. Authors have reported small series with generally disappointing results, irrespective of treatment modality (21,28,56,98,117,212). Because of the reputation of melanoma as a radioresistant tumor, it is not surprising that radical surgery has been considered the treatment of choice in operable patients. However, limited data are available to validate its efficacy. Although 75% 2-year survival has been achieved after radical excision in small series (212), most series report 5-year survival rates of 5% to 30%, regardless of radicality of surgery (28,166,212).

Morrow and DiSaia (128), in their review of all genital melanoma, noted no long-term survivors after isolated wide local excision for vaginal melanoma; however, 3/19 patients survived following exenteration. In the series by Chung et al. (28), of 19 patients, seven were treated with radical surgery, including one exenteration and six radical vaginectomies, with or without hysterectomy, with an overall survival of 21%. All patients treated with wide local excision developed recurrences. On the other hand, Levitan et al. (117), in their review of the literature, argued that although the 2-year survival following radical surgery was better (20% to 40%) than with any other therapy, the 5-year survival rates were equally poor (average 8%), regardless of type of therapy. Furthermore, the incidence of distant recurrence was not influenced by the extent of surgical resection. Geisler et al. (56) published the Indiana University experience using pelvic exenteration for malignant melanomas of the vagina or urethra with more than 3 mm of invasion. None of the four patients included in this study recurred, and three patients remained alive, with a minimum follow-up of 31 months. Conversely, Bonner et al. (15) reported nine cases of vaginal melanoma: three received wide local excisions, and six underwent radical surgery (including exenterations, and radical vaginectomies with or without hysterectomies), with a 29% actuarial 5-year survival rate. All nine patients suffered locoregional recurrence. Bonner et al. (15) advocated that surgery alone was ineffective in obtaining local control, and that preoperative RT should be considered.

Reid et al. (166) reported an overall 17% 5-year survival rate in a report of 15 patients, including 13 who underwent surgery. In addition, they reviewed the literature, summarizing the results achieved in 115 patients with vaginal melanoma, and compared outcomes for the 55 patients who underwent some form of surgery, including the 24 treated conservatively with wide local excision or partial vaginectomy to the 31 treated with more radical excisions. No difference in survival or DFS was found among the different surgical procedures. In a meta-analyses of essentially the same patient population ($n = 119$), Van Nostrand et al. (212), after adding eight of his own cases, concluded that radical surgery is recommended for patients with primary vaginal melanomas of <10 cm^2. In his own series of eight patients with vaginal melanoma, including four treated conservatively and four undergoing radical surgery, the only long-term survivor was in the radical surgery group. In his review of the literature, comprising a total of 119 patients, there was 48% 2-year survival rate if treated with radical surgery (50 patients), versus only 20% if treated conservatively (69 patients) ($p < 0.005$). Therefore, radical excision was advocated for those vaginal melanomas <10 cm^2 in area.

Not all authors support a radical resection approach. Buchanan et al. (21) performed a literature review of 66 cases reported since the publication of Reid et al. (166). Survival was influenced by tumor size, with a median survival time of 41 months of those with lesions <3 cm, and 21 months in those with larger lesions. However, there was no statistically significant difference in median survival, 2- and 5-year survival among the various surgical strategies. Hence, many investigators have adopted the suggestion of Irvin et al. (98) that if distant failure and death are expected, quality of life should be optimized by wide excision followed by RT to affect local control, while obviating the need for disfiguring radical surgery. In the series by Irvin et al. (98), all patients treated with wide local excision or brachytherapy alone recurred locally, whereas those patients treated with radical surgical resection or with wide local excision followed by high-dose per fraction EBRT maintained locoregional control until death.

Recent retrospective data suggest that vaginal melanoma is reasonably radio responsive, and possibly radiocurable (98,157). Volumes and doses of irradiation are similar to those used for epithelial tumors, ranging from 50 Gy for subclinical disease to 75 Gy for gross tumors. Retrospective analysis suggested a dose response curve of melanoma to external beam irradiation as the dose per fraction is increased and fractions of 3.5 Gy three times weekly to 5 Gy twice weekly have been used to treat melanoma because of a large D$_q$ observed in *in vitro*

studies (140). However, the Radiation Therapy Oncology Group conducted a prospective randomized study (RTOG 83-05) (180) evaluating the effectiveness of high dose per fraction irradiation in the treatment of melanoma. Patients with measurable lesions were randomized to four doses of 8.0 Gy in 21 days once weekly to 20 doses 2.5 Gy in 26 to 28 days, 5 days a week. One hundred thirty-seven patients were randomized and 126 patients were evaluable; stratification was performed on lesions <5 cm or ≥ 5 cm. There was no difference between the two arms in terms of response rate (complete responses 24.2% and 23.4% in the four-dose 8.0 Gy and in the 20-dose 2.5 Gy arms, respectively).

Chung et al. (28) reported on 16 cases of primary vaginal melanoma, eight from the Memorial Sloan-Kettering Cancer Center and eight from the Connecticut Tumor Registry. Local tumor control was obtained by primary radical surgery in five of seven patients, three of whom later died of disseminated disease. Six of eight patients treated primarily with radiation therapy died with metastatic melanoma; another died after pelvic exenteration for persistent local disease. Only one patient showed evidence of transient control after radiation therapy, but this patient had a local recurrence 36 months later and died with metastases. The overall 5-year survival rate for these 16 patients was 21%.

Harwood and Cummings (71) described a complete response in four patients with vaginal melanoma treated with irradiation, although two subsequently relapsed; complete response to irradiation was seen in one patient who was alive and well 10 months after treatment. Harrison et al. (69) reported that one of three patients with vaginal melanoma treated with irradiation survived 7.5 years; the other two died with distant metastases but had local tumor control.

Rogo et al. (174) reported on 22 cases of vulvovaginal melanoma treated with conservation surgery or irradiation, or both. Eleven patients had stage I, six had stage II, three had stage III, and two had stage IV tumors. Eight patients (36%) were alive 5 years and four 10 years after treatment. Inguinal lymph node recurrences and distant metastases were the most common modes of failure. Results were comparable with those obtained with radical surgery.

In the series by Petru et al. (157) of 14 patients, the three long-term survivors received either primary RT after biopsy only or adjuvantly after local excision. Tumor size was found to be prognostically important, with 43% of patients with tumors ≤ 3 cm surviving longer than 5 years, compared with 0% in patients with tumors >3 cm. The median overall survival was 10 months, and the 5-year DFS and overall survival rates were 14% and 21%, respectively. The authors concluded that prolonged local control could be obtained with RT as an adjunct to more limited surgery, or even with RT alone, primarily in patients with lesions ≤ 3 cm in diameter.

In summary, given that the high incidence of distant metastasis remains a major factor in limiting curability, a more conservative treatment approach might be more reasonable in selected patients. Patients with vaginal melanoma should probably be managed in a manner similar to that recommended for cutaneous lesions. Wide local excision with 1 to 2 cm margins should be the surgical treatment of choice for most primary vaginal melanomas, since radical surgery has failed to improve long-term survival. The role of adjuvant RT is unclear, but it appears to improve local control and even survival in some series. The role of systemic chemotherapy or immunotherapy has been very disappointing in the limited published data.

Sarcomas of the Vagina

Sarcomas represent 3% of vaginal primaries (33) with leiomyosarcoma representing 50% to 65% of vaginal sarcomas. Unfortunately, most of the sarcomas are diagnosed at an advanced stage. Histopathological grade appears to be the most important predictor of outcome.

Radical surgical resection, such as posterior pelvic exenteration, offers the best chance for cure for vaginal leiomyosarcomas (33,64). The largest series on vaginal sarcomas reported to date included 17 cases (10 leiomyosarcomas, four MMMT, and three other sarcoma types), of which 35% had received prior RT. These results underscore the importance of local therapy because in all 14 treatment failures, the tumor first recurred in the pelvis, and in seven of 14 this location was the only site of recurrence. There were only three survivors seen, and all had undergone exenterative surgery. The 5-year survival rate was 36% in patients with leiomyosarcoma, and 17% in those with MMMT (153).

Vaginal MMMT occurs more commonly in postmenopausal women. In approximately half of the cases there is a history of prior pelvic RT (134,153). Despite surgery and adjuvant RT, patients usually do poorly with a high incidence of local and distant recurrence. The treatment of choice is complete surgical resection, followed by EBRT and intracavitary brachytherapy, in an attempt to decrease local recurrence rate.

The role of adjuvant chemotherapy and RT in vaginal sarcomas has not been clearly defined, primarily due to limited patients numbers and even fewer data where chemotherapy was used as the primary treatment rather than as salvage therapy at recurrence. Adjuvant RT seems indicated in patients with high-grade tumors and locally recurrent low-grade sarcomas. According to Peters et al. (153), the most common site of failure is the pelvis. In 50% of patients with recurrence, it is the only site of failure. Extrapolating data from Gynecologic Oncology Group for uterine sarcomas and considering patterns of failure, patients with localized MMMT would be appropriately treated with pelvic exenteration, or with more limited surgical resection followed by postoperative RT, unless the patient has received prior pelvic RT (93). Since patterns of failure suggest that local therapies only reduce local recurrence rate and do not improve survival, consideration should be given to adjuvant treatments with agents that are active in similar tumors arising in the uterus. Agents found to be active in MMMT of the uterus include ifosfamide, cisplatin, and paclitaxel, although it remains unclear whether any combination of these agents is better than ifosfamide alone, which has produced the highest response rate among these agents (202), and doxorubicin remains the standard therapy for leiomyosarcoma (132).

Embryonal rhabdomyosarcoma (RMS) of the vagina is the most common pediatric vaginal tumor. The Intergroup Rhabdomyosarcoma Study Group (IRSG) through numerous clinical trials has demonstrated that the use of multimodality therapy with wide local excision and cytotoxic chemotherapy with or without RT makes it possible to avoid exenterative surgery used in the past (75,86) and optimizes quality of life and survival for these young patients (7,74,124,164), compared with previous data with surgery alone (75). After complete resection, irradiation of the entire pelvis is not required, thus avoiding its adverse effects. In addition, in a series of reports from the IRSG, survival rates in excess of 85% have been achieved utilizing vincristine, actinomycin-D, and cyclophosphamide (VAC) chemotherapy and wide excision with or without adjuvant RT (7,50,53,74,164). Andrassy et al. (8) summarized the outcome of 72 patients with embryonal RMS of the vagina treated on four IRSG trials indicating that the need for radical resection decreased from 100% to 13%, with continued improvement in disease-free survival. They suggested that after biopsy to document RMS, multiagent induction chemotherapy with doxorubicin, cisplatin, vincristine, actinomycin-D, and cyclophosphamide should be utilized, then local resection undertaken, with more radical surgery being reserved for those with persistent or recurrent disease. In addition, several non-IRSG series

have shown that combination chemotherapy with or without RT leads to sufficient tumor shrinkage, and that less radical resections can become feasible (50,53), allowing preservation of anatomy and function.

Flamant et al. (50) reported 11 cases of vaginal RMS (eight stage I, two stage II, one stage III), in whom 100% survival was achieved with multimodality therapy. Eight received neoadjuvant chemotherapy, generally VAC regimen, and all patients underwent brachytherapy (doses of 26 to 75 Gy), followed by maintenance chemotherapy, and VAC alternating with VAD (vincristine, doxorubicin, dacarbazine). Seven underwent ovarian transposition in an attempt to preserve function. They noted partial ovarian insufficiency in one of those without ovarian transposition, and recommended brachytherapy total dose around 50 to 60 Gy.

Lymphomas of the Vagina

Lymphoma of the vagina most often represents metastatic spread from another primary site. Although surgery including radical hysterectomy, pelvic lymphadenectomy, vaginectomy, and even exenteration has been performed in the past, more recent reports suggest that combination radiation and chemotherapy can achieve excellent results, and, therefore, radical surgery should be avoided. The most often used chemotherapy regimen is cyclophosphamide, doxorubicin, vincristine, and prednisone (CHOP) or bleomycin and CHOP (BACOP), usually six cycles.

Following biopsy, patients with lymphoma should be managed with combined chemoradiation. Extrapolation from patients with similar tumors arising in extranodal sites would suggest that radiation therapy has its primary role in preventing local recurrence in patients who present with bulky disease. In some patients who have a rapid and complete response to multiagent chemotherapy, radiation therapy may not be indicated since the combination of both modalities increases the risk of second malignancies. Harris and Scully (68) noted in a clinicopathologic series of 25 lower genital tract lymphomas, including four vaginal lymphomas, that definitive local therapy prevented relapse (68). Perren et al. (152) also advocated the use of less extensive surgery, with radiation plus appropriate multiagent chemotherapy such as CHOP or BACOP for six cycles to affect local control with better preservation of fertility in patients with stage IE and nonbulky tumors of low and intermediate grade.

Yolk Sac (Endodermal Sinus) Tumors of the Vagina

Yolk sac tumors (YST) produce α-fetoprotein, a tumor marker that allows earlier detection and treatment of persistent or recurrent disease. Prior to the use of multiagent cytotoxic chemotherapy, <25% of patients with YST of the vagina survived. However, Young and Scully (225) noted 100% survival in a small series of six patients who received chemotherapy. Similar results were published by Andersen et al. (6). The largest chemotherapy experience is with the VAC regimen. This combination has been administered to patients as an adjunct to surgery or radiation therapy (31) or in the treatment of metastatic disease and appears to have a major impact on survival. The VAC regimen in conjunction with surgery or RT was advocated by Copeland et al. (32). Collins et al. (31) reported on the use of combination bleomycin, vinblastine, and platinum (BVP) for patients with YST of the vagina. Aartsen et al. (1) reported on a successful pregnancy following surgery and chemotherapy. Most recently, Hwang et al. (96) has reported two cases: one of which did well with partial vaginectomy followed by 2 years of VAC; however, the second one developed a central persistence following wide local excision and VAC, but was salvaged with bleomycin, etoposide, and platinum (BEP). Given the excellent results that three to four cycles of BEP has achieved in malignant germ cell neoplasms of the ovary (220), it is likely that BEP will become the preferred regimen for YST of the vagina used in conjunction with partial vaginectomy, as it requires less prolonged administration and is less oophorotoxic than VAC (37). It appears that routine use of combination chemotherapy in the management of endodermal sinus tumor allows conservative surgery with preservation of sexual function in young patients, with excellent prospects for long-term survival.

The role of radiation in this disease is limited because of the younger age at presentation and preservation of ovarian function is desired; in addition, RT would potentially increase the risk for secondary malignancies (137), which may be even more significant with the use of IMRT as the volume of irradiation receiving lower doses are generally larger (66). Brachytherapy may occasionally be used, and in one instance, preservation of hormonal function and subsequent pregnancy were reported (1).

Patients with History of Previously Treated Uterine Tumors

Several authors have described the appearance of vaginal carcinoma after successful treatment of primary carcinoma of the cervix (27). Treatment outcome in patients with a second lower genital tract carcinoma is less satisfactory because of the difficulties in completing another definite treatment after previous radical surgery or radiation therapy. Senkus et al. (184) reported on 46 patients with second lower genital tract epidermoid cancers after previous treatment for invasive cervical carcinoma. There were four cases (9%) of synchronous cancers. The time between metachronous malignancies ranged from 66 to 406 months (median, 206 months). In 32 cases (70%), the second lesion was located in the vagina and in 14 (30%), in the vulva. Of 35 previously irradiated patients, the second tumor was located in the high-dose volume in 24 (69%). Treatment of the second cancer consisted of surgery in 12 patients (26%), radiation therapy in 23 (50%), combined surgery and radiation therapy in five (11%), chemotherapy in four (9%), and surgery plus chemotherapy in one case. The median survival was 52 months, and the 5-year survival rate from the diagnosis of second malignancy was 47.5%.

Kalogirou et al. (102) noted that in 993 women who had been treated with a hysterectomy for carcinoma in situ of the cervix, 41 subsequently had VAIN, 27 (65%) in the upper half and eight (19%) in the lower half. The authors recommended continued screening over a 5-year period for patients treated for carcinoma in situ of the cervix, including colposcopy. Of the 41 patients, 26 (63%) were treated with partial vaginectomy, eight with local incision and intracavitary irradiation, four with biopsy and intracavitary irradiation, and three with total vaginectomy.

These patients are preferentially treated with irradiation alone, as described for *de novo* primary vaginal carcinoma. Perez and Camel (147,148) reported that patients with carcinoma of the vagina who had a history of previously treated primary carcinoma of the cervix or endometrium (irradiation, hysterectomy, or combination of both) and received treatment more than 5 years before the diagnosis of vaginal carcinoma had survival and tumor control rates equal to those of patients with *de novo* primary vaginal carcinoma. The possibility of the vaginal lesion being a local recurrence or metastasis was considered unlikely because 95% of recurrences after treatment of primary carcinoma of the cervix or endometrium occur within 5 years after therapy. It is concluded that these lesions are most

likely second primary lesions that should be treated with definitive radiation therapy and a curative aim.

Hoffman et al. (91) described results in 32 women, 31 of whom had previous hysterectomy with upper vaginectomy for carcinoma in situ or occult, superficially invasive carcinoma of the vagina. Fourteen patients had undergone previous treatment for VAIN; nine had invasive cancer on final pathologic examination. Among the remaining 23 patients, a recurrence of vaginal neoplasia developed in four (17%) after surgical treatment, with a mean time to recurrence of 78 weeks. Nineteen patients were alive with no evidence of recurrent tumor at a mean follow-up of 152 weeks.

Stock et al. (192) reported on 100 cases of vaginal carcinoma; 50% of patients had hysterectomy before the diagnosis of vaginal cancer. Treatment consisted of surgery in 40 patients, radiation therapy in 47, and surgery plus irradiation in 13. With a median follow-up of 11.2 years, the 5-year disease-free survival rates were 67% for stage I (23 patients), 53% for stage II (58 patients), 0% for stage III (nine patients), and 15% for stage IV disease (10 patients). On univariate and multivariate analysis, treatment with surgery, disease limited to one-third of the vaginal canal, and FIGO stage I and II disease were significantly favorable prognostic factors for disease-free survival. Treatment with surgery was superior to radiation therapy alone in patients with stage II disease ($p = 0.00004$), but there was a selection bias because the patients with a more unfavorable prognosis were treated with radiation therapy.

Xiang-E et al. (224) reported on 73 patients with late recurrent vaginal malignancy after initial radiation therapy for carcinoma of the uterine cervix treated with additional brachytherapy (30 to 40 Gy in three to five fractions to the tumor base within 3 to 4 weeks) or with HDR brachytherapy (20 to 35 Gy in three to five fractions in 3 to 4 weeks); when necessary, a supplemental dose of 20 to 30 Gy was delivered at 0.5 cm below the surface of the vaginal mucosa in four to six fractions in 2 to 3 weeks in addition to 30- to 40-Gy EBRT (Cobalt-60 or electrons). Of these patients, 61 received irradiation alone, and 11 were treated with irradiation combined with chemotherapy. One patient was treated with hysterectomy after reirradiation. The 5-year survival rate was 40% (21/52). The 5-year survival rate for patients with upper-third tumors was 82%, compared with 33% for the upper-middle and 25% for upper-lower locations. The local tumor control rate was 86.5% for tumors <4 cm (32/37) and 26.6% for larger lesions (4/15; p <0.01). Moderate and severe rectal radiation sequelae were noted in 10 of 73 patients (13.6%), hematuria in 9 (12.3%), rectovaginal fistula in eight (11%), and vesicovaginal fistula in one (1.4%).

Squamous Cell Carcinoma of the Neovagina

In situ and invasive carcinomas arising in the neovagina are rare, and the type of malignancy seems to be related to the transplanted tissue. A few cases of squamous cell carcinoma have been described after split-thickness skin graft vaginoplasty in patients with vaginal agenesis (13), as well as after radical vulvovaginal resection for known malignancy (63). Mucinous adenocarcinoma has been described arising in the sigmoid colon used for the reconstruction of the neovagina (89). Neovaginal malignant melanoma following surgery and radiation therapy for vulvovaginal malignancies, although extremely rare, has been reported (113), suggesting the potential role on radiation-induced melanoma in non–sun-exposed areas such as the genital tract.

Malignant transformation occurs in the neovaginal epithelium, in relation with local carcinogenic environmental factors as well as possible viral infection, with the subsequent risk of malignancy. Therefore, it is important to emphasize the need for regular follow-up visits with Papanicolaou (Pap) smears. The elapsed time between the construction of the neovagina and the development of malignancy ranges between 10 to 30 years. The optimal treatment is not well defined. Radical surgery resection whenever possible should be the treatment of choice, since definitive RT seems to be associated with higher failure rates. Adjuvant RT could be considered in patients with positive margins or positive nodes (89).

Carcinoma in Episiotomy Scar

Episiotomy scar tumor implantation from a cervical or vulvar carcinoma is a very rare event. Van Dam et al. (211) reported on three cases of primary or metastatic carcinoma in an episiotomy scar. One patient had a primary squamous cell carcinoma of the vulva in an episiotomy scar; a second patient was diagnosed with cervical carcinoma 6 months postpartum and was found to have a metastatic deposit in the episiotomy scar during the staging of her disease; the third patient developed adenocarcinoma metastatic from an endocervical primary in an episiotomy scar that presented as a small nodule at the introitus. These cases exemplify the need for careful inspection and biopsy of any nodular lesions in episiotomy scars as part of the initial assessment and follow-up of patients with premalignant or malignant lesions of the lower genital track. Early initial stage, small-size lesion, and early therapy appear to improve prognosis. Treatment needs to be individualized given the rarity of this entity. Patients with limited recurrent disease at the episiotomy site without any other evidence of locoregional recurrence could be treated with surgical resection followed by tailored radiation therapy. Patients with more advanced disease may be offered radiation with or without chemotherapy followed by surgical resection when feasible (83).

Salvage Therapy

Patients with isolated pelvic or regional recurrences after definitive surgery who have not received prior RT are managed with EBRT, generally in combination with brachytherapy. Concurrent cisplatin-based chemotherapy may also be recommended. Salvage options for patients with central recurrence after definitive or adjuvant RT are limited to radical surgery, usually exenterative; or, in selected patients with small-volume disease, reirradiation using interstitial radiation implants or highly conformal three-dimensional EBRT. Response rates with chemotherapy are low and the impact on survival limited. Further, response to chemotherapy in central pelvic recurrences

following radiation therapy tends to be less common than response at distant sites. Additionally, prior high-dose radiation therapy compromises bone marrow tolerance of many agents that are active in this tumor (e.g., ifosfamide and doxorubicin). However, chemotherapy-responsive patients can obtain meaningful palliation in many cases.

Radiotherapy Considerations

Those patients who have not received prior RT should receive whole-pelvis EBRT followed when feasible by brachytherapy. Generally, the whole pelvis receives a dose of 40 to 50 Gy. Inguinofemoral lymph node regions should be included in patients with involvement of the distal third of the vagina or with vulvar recurrences. The gross tumor volume in the vagina, paravaginal tissues, or parametrium should receive an additional boost, preferably with an interstitial implant, to bring the total tumor dose to 75 to 80 Gy. The role of combined chemoradiotherapy in the management of patients with recurrent disease is unknown. Given the rarity of vaginal carcinoma and the heterogeneity within the population with recurrent disease, large randomized studies intended to answer this question will probably never be conducted. However, by extrapolation from the available data for locally advanced cervical and vulvar cancer (126,127,175,219), it seems that combined modality approach may improve the locoregional control and survival in patients with isolated pelvic recurrences.

Adequately selected patients who are medically inoperable, technically unresectable, or refuse to undergo exenterative surgery are appropriately considered for reirradiation to limited volumes, but this must be undertaken with extreme caution. A variety of techniques are available, and the choice is based on patient and tumor-related factors, as well as the experience of the radiation oncologist. When using EBRT, multiple beam arrangements utilizing three-dimensional treatment planning or IMRT are favored. Only limited doses are possible, and the physician might consider a hyperfractionated regimen in an attempt to decrease the incidence of late toxicity.

In patients with small, well-defined vulvovaginal or pelvic recurrences, reirradiation using primarily interstitial techniques has been attempted with control rates between 50% to 75%, and grade 3 or higher complication rates between 7% to 15% (26,62,139,163,178,224). The rationale, logistics, and selection of implant technique when performing an ITI have been reviewed earlier in the chapter. Permanent radioactive seed implants (e.g., ^{198}Gold) in patients with small vaginal recurrences often provides long-lasting tumor control in elderly or medically debilitated patients previously treated with definitive doses of RT (Fig. 70.6).

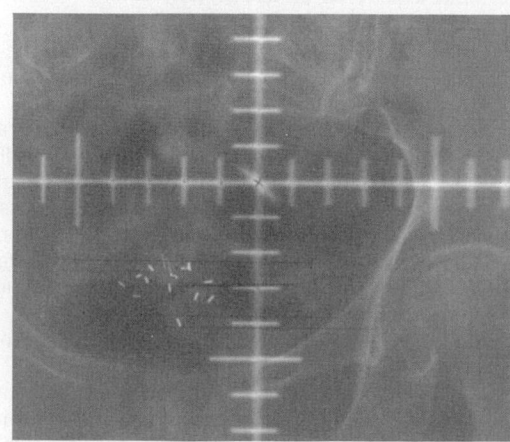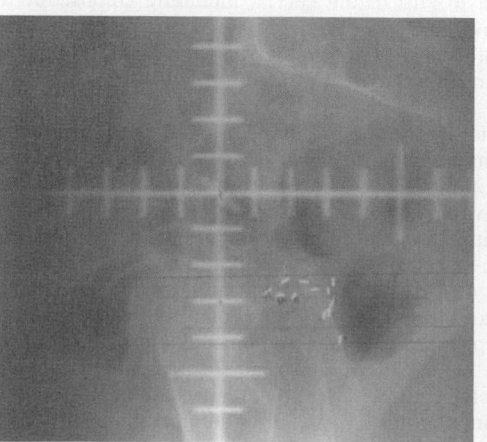

FIGURE 70.6. Salvage Gold-189 implant for local recurrence after definitive RT. **A:** Antero-posterior and **B:** Lateral simulation films.

Other potential treatment options include the use of surgery and intraoperative RT (IORT) with either intraoperative electron beam (55,65) or laparotomy or laparoscopically guided placement of HDR catheters (57,65,90,139). The locoregional recurrence and distant metastasis rates after IORT vary between 20% to 60% and 20% to 58%, respectively. The 3- to 5-year actuarial survival is poor, ranging from 8% to 25%. Grade 3 or higher toxicity has been reported in about 35% of patients (55,65). In the Memorial Sloan-Kettering Cancer Center experience using radical surgical resection and HDR-IORT, patients with complete gross resection had a 3-year local control rate of 83%, compared to 25% in patients with gross residual disease. Interestingly, most of the failures in the microscopic group were distant, perhaps indicating a potential role for adjuvant chemotherapy (57).

Stereotactic body radiotherapy (SBRT) is a novel treatment paradigm that delivers a small number of high-dose fractions to extracranial targets using a linear accelerator with highly precise, accurate, and reproducible target localization, based on the same principles as that of the gamma-knife therapy. Encouraging results have been published when using SBRT for patients with pelvic recurrences (223).

Treatment Complications and Their Management

Although in most of the retrospective series the authors comment on the nature of the complications encountered, little information is typically given regarding their prevention or management (10,54,91,154,177,192). The knowledge of common acute and late complications with standard RT and consideration of risk factors may improve the therapeutic ratio of RT for gynecological malignancies in general and for vaginal cancer in particular (24).

The incidence of $\geq$grade 2 complications has been reported to be 15% to 25%, with the average of severe complications (those requiring surgery for correction or necessitating hospitalization) around 8% to 10%. Table 70.8 (29,52,107,111, 149,154,177,192,210) shows the incidence of complications greater than grade 2 in several large series of vaginal cancer patients. Perez et al. (147) reported grade 2 or 3 complications in approximately 5% of patients treated for stage 0 and I disease and in approximately 15% of patients with stage II lesions. No complications were reported in stages III and IV disease, probably because few patients lived long enough to manifest complications of treatment. The most common major complications were proctitis (two patients), rectovesicovaginal fistula (three patients), and vesicovaginal fistula (two patients). The most common minor complications were fibrosis of the vagina

and small areas of mucosal necrosis, which were noted in approximately 10% of patients.

Lee et al. (115) showed that the total dose to the primary site was the most significant factor predicting the development of a severe complication (9% in patients receiving $\leq$80 Gy as compared with 25% in those receiving higher doses). Perez et al. (147) reported an increase in the rate of severe complications with higher clinical stage, probably reflecting the higher doses delivered with EBRT and brachytherapy.

Ball and Berman (10) reported on 58 patients with carcinoma of the vagina, including 30 who underwent surgery. There were four rectovaginal fistulae (one following RT, and three after exenterative surgery) and two vesicovaginal fistulae (one following radical vaginectomy and the other following a recurrence, being managed with cystectomy and diversion). The single ureterovaginal fistula occurred after radical vaginectomy and partial cystectomy and was managed with ureteroneocystostomy.

In the report of Peters et al. (154), of 86 vaginal primaries, there were two fistulae in 57 patients who received primary RT. However, there was a 44% rate of fistulae formation in the nine patients who underwent reirradiation after having previously received RT for an earlier cancer. Rubin et al. (177) reported a 23% incidence of complications after RT, including a 13% rate of fistula formation and a 10% rate of cystitis/proctitis. Although two patients developed fistulae following combination therapy, the authors did not think that the rate of complications following combination therapy was greater than that seen following RT alone.

In the series of Stock et al. (192), of 100 patients with vaginal carcinoma, there was a 16% actuarial complication rate at 10 years. All patients undergoing vaginectomies or exenterations lost vaginal function. None of the patients were offered vaginal reconstruction in this series. Stock et al. emphasized that therapeutic options needed to be individualized such that surgery is offered only to those most likely to benefit, and least likely to suffer complications.

Chyle et al. (29) in a study of 301 patients noted that 39 (13%) had 48 grade 2 or greater sequelae, including rectal ulceration or proctitis in 10 (three requiring colostomy), small bowel obstruction in seven, rectovaginal fistula in six, vesicovaginal fistula in four, vaginoperitoneal/cutaneous fistula in two, and vaginal ulceration or necrosis in eight patients. Fewer complications developed in patients with stage 0 or I tumors (8% to 9%) than with more advanced stages (14% to 40%). Vaginal ulceration occurred in eight of 206 patients (4%) treated with brachytherapy but in none of 95 patients who received no brachytherapy ($p = 0.06$).

Frank et al. (52) reported 10% and 17% 5- and 10-year cumulative rates of major (greater than grade 2) complications in a series of 193 patients treated with definitive RT with or without chemotherapy. They found FIGO stage and history of smoking to be the two factors significantly correlated with subsequent complications. Other clinical dosimetric factors or the addition of chemotherapy did not correlate with the likelihood of complications. However, 73% of patients with major complications had tumors involving the posterior vaginal wall.

The RT tolerance limits of the entire vagina are ill defined, given the variety of techniques employed for the treatment of vaginal cancers. An irradiation tolerance level of the proximal vagina was suggested by Hintz et al. (88) based on a study of 16 patients who received a maximum surface dose of 140 Gy, none of whom developed severe complications or necrosis of the upper vagina. Based on their previous observation of a patient who developed a vesicovaginal fistula after receiving a dose of 150 Gy mucosal dose to the anterior vaginal wall, they recommended a tolerance dose level of 140 Gy (direct summation of EBRT dose and ICB) to the anterior upper vaginal mucosa. They advocated dose rates of <0.8 Gy per hour. These authors cautioned against placing radioactive needles on the surface of

Author	No. Patients	Percentage of Complications (>Grade 2)
Chyle[44]	310	19% actuarial @ 20 years
Kirkbride[140]	153	10%
Kucera[144]	110	5.5%
Perez[193]	212	13%
Peters[197]	86	7 (8%)
Rubin[227]	75	15 (23%)
Stock[248]	100	16% actuarial @ 10 years
Urbanski[271]	125	13%
Frank[77]	193	10%, 5 y actuarial
		17%, 10 y actuarial

Table 70.8 **COMPLICATIONS OF THERAPY (>GRADE 2)**

the vaginal cylinder because this may increase the frequency of vaginal necrosis. They also recommended keeping the total dose to the distal vagina <98 Gy. In addition, it was also observed that the posterior wall of the vagina is more prone to radiation injury than the anterior or lateral walls, and that the dose should be kept below 80 Gy in order to minimize the risk of rectovaginal fistula. Rubin (176) suggested that the tolerance of the vaginal mucosa (TD 5/5: 5% necrosis within 5 years) is around 90 Gy for ulceration, and more than 100 Gy for fistula formation. This tolerance limit has been specified as a direct summation of dosage given by LDR-ICB and EBRT in the treatment of cervical cancer. Within the low–dose-rate range, whether a correction for brachytherapy dose rate is necessary remains controversial. In a more recent series from Washington University, the traditional LDR tolerance dose of 150 Gy to the mucosa of the proximal vagina was shown to yield a nominal 11% and 4% grades 1 or 2 and 3 sequela, respectively (9).

Host factors that may increase the risk of complications include prior pelvic surgery, pelvic inflammatory disease, immunosuppression status, collagen vascular disease, low body weight, patient age, significant smoking history, and comorbid illness (e.g., diabetes, hypertension, and cardiovascular disease) (147,149).

Treatment options for acute radiation vaginitis include daily vaginal douching with a diluted hydrogen peroxide/water mixture (61). This should continue for 2 to 3 months, or until the mucosal reactions have subsided. Patients are then advised to continue douching once or twice per week for several months. Regular vaginal dilation is recommended as a way for patients to maintain vaginal health and good sexual function, although the compliance rate is low. The lack of resolution of vaginal ulceration or necrosis after several months of adequate therapy must be appropriately evaluated, considering the possibility of recurrent tumor. The use of topical estrogens following completion of RT appears to stimulate epithelial regeneration more than systemic estrogens.

Some patients with severe radiation sequelae, such as fistula formation, will respond to conservative treatment with antibiotics and periodic limited debridement of necrotic tissue. More recently, Delanian et al. (39) published a randomized trial demonstrating the effectiveness of the combination of pentoxifylline and vitamin E in the regression of radiation-induced fibrosis.

Patients with more severe gastrointestinal or urinary late effects will require urinary or fecal diversion with possible delayed reanastomosis. Occasionally, repair of the fistula may be attempted by employing a myocutaneous graft, in which the skin, subcutaneous fat, and muscle are mobilized using a vascular pedicle to maintain the blood supply to the pedicled graft (Martius flap), or by excision of the necrotic tissue with reestablishment of organ continuity (such as in the treatment of high rectovaginal fistula). A detailed review of the pathogenesis and management of potential late effects of treatment is out of the scope of this chapter but may be found elsewhere in this book.

It is likely that improvements in modern practice such as advancements in surgical techniques (such as more generous use of myocutaneous flaps) (22,121), improved supportive care during the immediate postoperative stay, use of more sophisticated RT field setting (three-dimensional conformal therapy) and treatment delivery, more accurate brachytherapy techniques, and dose calculations have potential to lessen complication rates posttherapy, regardless of which modality is used.

References

1. Aartsen EJ, Delemarre JF, Gerretsen G. Endodermal sinus tumor of the vagina: radiation therapy and progeny. *Obstet Gynecol* 1993;81:893–895.
2. Aho M, Vesterinen E, Meyer B, et al. Natural history of vaginal intraepithelial neoplasia. *Cancer* 1991;68:195–197.
3. AJCC. *AJCC cancer staging manual.* 6th ed. New York: Springer-Verlag, 2002.
4. Ali MM, Huang DT, Goplerud DR, et al. Radiation alone for carcinoma of the vagina: variation in response related to the location of the primary tumor. *Cancer* 1996;77:1934–1939.
5. Al-Kurdi M, Monaghan JM. Thirty-two years experience in management of primary tumours of the vagina. *Br J Obstet Gynaecol* 1981;88:1145–1150.
6. Andersen WA, Sabio H, Durso N, et al. Endodermal sinus tumor of the vagina. The role of primary chemotherapy. *Cancer* 1985;56:1025–1027.
7. Andrassy RJ, Hays DM, Raney RB, et al. Conservative surgical management of vaginal and vulvar pediatric rhabdomyosarcoma: a report from the Intergroup Rhabdomyosarcoma Study III. *J Pediatr Surg* 1995;30:1034–1036; discussion 1036–1037.
8. Andrassy RJ, Wiener ES, Raney RB, et al. Progress in the surgical management of vaginal rhabdomyosarcoma: a 25-year review from the Intergroup Rhabdomyosarcoma Study Group. *J Pediatr Surg* 1999;34:731–734; discussion 734–735.
9. Au SP, Grigsby PW. The irradiation tolerance dose of the proximal vagina. *Radiother Oncol* 2003;67:77–85.
10. Ball HG, Berman ML. Management of primary vaginal carcinoma. *Gynecol Oncol* 1982;14:154–163.
11. Benson RC. Cancer of the female genital tract. *CA: Cancer J Clin* 1968;18:2–13.
12. Berchuck A, Rodriguez G, Kamel A, et al. Expression of epidermal growth factor receptor and HER-2/neu in normal and neoplastic cervix, vulva, and vagina. *Obstet Gynecol* 1990;76:381–387.
13. Bobin JY, Zinzindohoue C, Naba T, et al. Primary squamous cell carcinoma in a patient with vaginal agenesis. *Gynecol Oncol* 1999;74:293–297.
14. Boice JD Jr., Engholm G, Kleinerman RA, et al. Radiation dose and second cancer risk in patients treated for cancer of the cervix. *Radiat Res* 1988;116:3–55.
15. Bonner JA, Perez-Tamayo C, Reid GC, et al. The management of vaginal melanoma. *Cancer* 1988;62:2066–2072.
16. Bornstein J, Adam E, Adler-Storthz K, et al. Development of cervical and vaginal squamous cell neoplasia as a late consequence of in utero exposure to diethylstilbestrol. *Obstet Gynecol Surv* 1988;43:15–21.
17. Boronow RC, Hickman BT, Reagan MT, et al. Combined therapy as an alternative to exenteration for locally advanced vulvovaginal cancer. II. Results, complications, and dosimetric and surgical considerations. *Am J Clin Oncol* 1987;10:171–181.
18. Breslow A. Tumor thickness, level of invasion and node dissection in stage I cutaneous melanoma. *Ann Surg* 1975;182:572–575.
19. Brinton LA, Nasca PC, Mallin K, et al. Case-control study of in situ and invasive carcinoma of the vagina. *Gynecol Oncol* 1990;38:49–54.
20. Brown GR, Fletcher GH, Rutledge FN. Irradiation of in-situ and invasive squamous cell carcinomas of the vagina. *Cancer* 1971;28:1278–1283.
21. Buchanan DJ, Schlaerth J, Kurosaki T. Primary vaginal melanoma: thirteen-year disease-free survival after wide local excision and review of recent literature. *Am J Obstet Gynecol* 1998;178:1177–1184.
22. Burke TW, Morris M, Roh MS, et al. Perineal reconstruction using single gracilis myocutaneous flaps. *Gynecol Oncol* 1995;57:221–225.
23. Buscema J, Rosenshein NB, Taqi F, et al. Vaginal hemangiopericytoma: a histopathologic and ultrastructural evaluation. *Obstet Gynecol* 1985;66:82S–85S.
24. Cardenes H, Song G, Randall M. Late Sequelae of radiation therapy in the management of gynaecological malignancies. *Curr Med Lit Gynaecol Obstet* 2001;7:57–66.
25. Chang YC, Hricak H, Thurnher S, et al. Vagina: evaluation with MR imaging. Part II. Neoplasms. *Radiology* 1988;169:175–179.
26. Charra C, Roy P, Coquard R, et al. Outcome of treatment of upper third vaginal recurrences of cervical and endometrial carcinomas with interstitial brachytherapy. *Int J Radiat Oncol Biol Phys* 1998;40:421–426.
27. Choo YC, Anderson DG. Neoplasms of the vagina following cervical carcinoma. *Gynecol Oncol* 1982;11:125–132.
28. Chung AF, Casey MJ, Flannery JT, et al. Malignant melanoma of the vagina—report of 19 cases. *Obstet Gynecol* 1980;55:720–727.
29. Chyle V, Zagars GK, Wheeler JA, et al. Definitive radiotherapy for carcinoma of the vagina: outcome and prognostic factors. *Int J Radiat Oncol Biol Phys* 1996;35:891–905.
30. Clement PB, Benedet JL. Adenocarcinoma in situ of the vagina: a case report. *Cancer* 1979;43:2479–2485.
31. Collins HS, Burke TW, Heller PB, et al. Endodermal sinus tumor of the infant vagina treated exclusively by chemotherapy. *Obstet Gynecol* 1989;73:507–509.
32. Copeland LJ, Sneige N, Ordonez NG, et al. Endodermal sinus tumor of the vagina and cervix. *Cancer* 1985;55:2558–2565.
33. Creasman WT, Phillips JL, Menck HR. The National Cancer Data Base report on cancer of the vagina. *Cancer* 1998;83:1033–1040.
34. Daling JR, Madeleine MM, Schwartz SM, et al. A population-based study of squamous cell vaginal cancer: HPV and cofactors. *Gynecol Oncol* 2002;84:263–270.
35. Dalrymple JL, Russell AH, Lee SW, et al. Chemoradiation for primary invasive squamous carcinoma of the vagina. *Int J Gynecol Cancer* 2004;14:110–117.
36. Dancuart F, Delclos L, Wharton JT, et al. Primary squamous cell carcinoma of the vagina treated by radiotherapy: a failures analysis—the M.D. Anderson Hospital experience 1955–1982. *Int J Radiat Oncol Biol Phys* 1988;14:745–749.
37. Davidoff AM, Hebra A, Bunin N, et al. Endodermal sinus tumor in children. *J Pediatr Surg* 1996;31:1075–1078; discussion 1078–1079.
38. Davis KP, Stanhope CR, Garton GR, et al. Invasive vaginal carcinoma: analysis of early-stage disease. *Gynecol Oncol* 1991;42:131–136.
39. Delanian S, Porcher R, Balla-Mekias S, et al. Randomized, placebo-controlled trial of combined pentoxifylline and tocopherol for regression of superficial radiation-induced fibrosis. *J Clin Oncol* 2003;21:2545–2550.
40. Delclos L, Fletcher GH, Moore EB, et al. Minicolpostats, dome cylinders, other additions and improvements of the Fletcher-suit afterloadable system: indications and limitations of their use. *Int J Radiat Oncol Biol Phys* 1980;6:1195–1206.
41. DeMars LR, Van Le L, Huang I, et al. Primary non-clear-cell adenocarcinomas of the vagina in older DES-exposed women. *Gynecol Oncol* 1995;58:389–392.
42. Di Domenico A. Primary vaginal squamous cell carcinoma in the young patient. *Gynecol Oncol* 1989;35:181–187.
43. Digel CA, Lastner GM, Zinreich ES. The use of transmission block in the radiation therapy portal treatment of the inguinal nodes in late stage pelvic malignancies. *Radiol Tech* 1987;58:227–231.

44. Dittmer PH, Randall ME. A technique for inguinal node boost using photon fields defined by asymmetric collimator jaws. *Radiother Oncol* 2001;59:61–64.
45. Dixit S, Singhal S, Baboo HA. Squamous cell carcinoma of the vagina: a review of 70 cases. *Gynecol Oncol* 1993;48:80–87.
46. Ebner F, Kressel HY, Mintz MC, et al. Tumor recurrence versus fibrosis in the female pelvis: differentiation with MR imaging at 1.5T. *Radiology* 1988;166:333–340. [Erratum appears in *Radiology* 1988;168(1):286.]
47. Ebrahim S, Daponte A, Smith TH, et al. Primary mucinous adenocarcinoma of the vagina. *Gynecol Oncol* 2001;80:89–92.
48. Evans LS, Kersh CR, Constable WC, et al. Concomitant 5-fluorouracil, mitomycin-C, and radiotherapy for advanced gynecologic malignancies. *Int J Radiat Oncol Biol Phys* 1988;15:901–906.
49. Fanning J, Manahan KJ, McLean SA. Loop electrosurgical excision procedure for partial upper vaginectomy. *Am J Obstetr Gynecol* 1999;181:1382–1385.
50. Flamant F, Gerbaulet A, Nihoul-Fekete C, et al. Long-term sequelae of conservative treatment by surgery, brachytherapy, and chemotherapy for vulval and vaginal rhabdomyosarcoma in children. *J Clin Oncol* 1990;8:1847–1853.
51. Fox H, Wells M, Harris M, et al. Enteric tumours of the lower female genital tract: a report of three cases. *Histopathology* 1988;12:167–176.
52. Frank SJ, Jhingran A, Levenback C, et al. Definitive radiation therapy for squamous cell carcinoma of the vagina. *Int J Radiat Oncol Biol Phys* 2005;62:138–147.
53. Friedman M, Peretz BA, Nissenbaum M, et al. Modern treatment of vaginal embryonal rhabdomyosarcoma. *Obstetr Gynecol Surv* 1986;41:614–618.
54. Gallup DG, Talledo OE, Shah KJ, et al. Invasive squamous cell carcinoma of the vagina: a 14-year study. *Obstetr Gynecol* 1987;69:782–785.
55. Garton GR, Gunderson LL, Webb MJ, et al. Intraoperative radiation therapy in gynecologic cancer: update of the experience at a single institution. *Int J Radiat Oncol Biol Phys* 1997;37:839–843.
56. Geisler JP, Look KY, Moore DA, et al. Pelvic exenteration for malignant melanomas of the vagina or urethra with over 3 mm of invasion. *Gynecol Oncol* 1995;59:338–341.
57. Gemignani ML, Alektiar KM, Leitao M, et al. Radical surgical resection and high-dose intraoperative radiation therapy (HDR-IORT) in patients with recurrent gynecologic cancers. *Int J Radiat Oncol Biol Phys* 2001;50:687–694.
58. Glazer HS, Lee JK, Levitt RG, et al. Radiation fibrosis: differentiation from recurrent tumor by MR imaging. *Radiology* 1985;156:721–726.
59. Gore E, Gillin MT, Albano K, et al. Comparison of high dose-rate and low dose-rate dose distributions for vaginal cylinders. *Int J Radiat Oncol Biol Phys* 1995;31:165–170.
60. Grigsby PW, Mutch DG, Rader J, et al. Lack of benefit of concurrent chemotherapy in patients with cervical cancer and negative lymph nodes by FDG-PET. *Int J Radiat Oncol Biol Phys* 2005;61:444–449.
61. Grigsby PW, Russell A, Bruner D, et al. Late injury of cancer therapy on the female reproductive tract. *Int J Radiat Oncol Biol Phys* 1995;31:1281–1299.
62. Gupta AK, Vicini FA, Frazier AJ, et al. Iridium-192 transperineal interstitial brachytherapy for locally advanced or recurrent gynecological malignancies. *Int J Radiat Oncol Biol Phys* 1999;43:1055–1060.
63. Guven S, Guvendag Guven ES, Ayhan A, et al. Recurrence of high-grade squamous intraepithelial neoplasia in neovagina: case report and review of the literature. *Int J Gynecol Cancer* 2005;15:1179–1182.
64. Hachi H, Ottmany A, Bougtab A, et al. Le leiomyosarcome du vagin: une observation rare. *Bull Cancer* 1997;84:215–217.
65. Haddock M, Martinez-Monge R, Petersen I, et al. *Locally advanced primary and recurrent gynecologic malignancies. EBRT with or without IORT or HDR-IORT.* Totowa, NJ: Humana Press, 1999.
66. Hall EJ, Wuu CS. Radiation-induced second cancers: the impact of 3D-CRT and IMRT. *Int J Radiat Oncol Biol Phys* 2003;56:83–88.
67. Handel LN, Scott SM, Giller RH, et al. New perspectives on therapy for vaginal endodermal sinus tumors. *J Urol* 2002;168:687–690.
68. Harris NL, Scully RE. Malignant lymphoma and granulocytic sarcoma of the uterus and vagina. A clinicopathologic analysis of 27 cases. *Cancer* 1984;53:2530–2545.
69. Harrison LB, Fogel T, Peschel R. Primary vaginal cancer and vaginal melanoma: a review of therapy with external beam radiation and a simple intracavitary brachytherapy system. *Endocuriethe/Hyperther Oncol* 1987;3:67.
70. Hart WR, Townsend DE, Aldrich JO, et al. Histopathologic spectrum of vaginal adenosis and related changes in stilbestrol-exposed females. *Cancer* 1976;37:763–775.
71. Harwood AR, Cummings BJ. Radiotherapy for mucosal melanomas. *Int J Radiat Oncol Biol Phys* 1982;8:1121–1126.
72. Haskel S, Chen SS, Spiegel G. Vaginal endometrioid adenocarcinoma arising in vaginal endometriosis: a case report and literature review. *Gynecol Oncol* 1989;34:232–236.
73. Hatch EE, Palmer JR, Titus-Ernstoff L, et al. Cancer risk in women exposed to diethylstilbestrol in utero. *JAMA* 1998;280:630–634.
74. Hays DM, Shimada H, Raney RB Jr., et al. Sarcomas of the vagina and uterus: the Intergroup Rhabdomyosarcoma Study. *J Pediatr Surg* 1985;20:718–724.
75. Helders R, Malkasian G, Soule E. Embryonal rhabdomyosarcoma of the vagina. *Am J Obstetr Gynecol* 1972;197:484–502.
76. Herbst AL, Anderson D. Clear cell adenocarcinoma of the vagina and cervix secondary to intrauterine exposure to diethylstilbestrol. *Sem Surg Oncol* 1990;6:343–346.
77. Herbst AL, Green TH Jr. , Ulfelder H. Primary carcinoma of the vagina. An analysis of 68 cases. *Am J Obstetr Gynecol* 1970;106:210–218.
78. Herbst AL, Kurman RJ, Scully RE, et al. Clear-cell adenocarcinoma of the genital tract in young females. Registry report. *N Engl J Med* 1972;287:1259–1264.
79. Herbst AL, Norusis MJ, Rosenow PJ, et al. An analysis of 346 cases of clear cell adenocarcinoma of the vagina and cervix with emphasis on recurrence and survival. *Gynecol Oncol* 1979;7:111–122.
80. Herbst AL, Robboy SJ, Scully RE, et al. Clear-cell adenocarcinoma of the vagina and cervix in girls: analysis of 170 registry cases. *Am J Obstetr Gynecol* 1974;119:713–724.
81. Herbst AL, Scully RE. Adenocarcinoma of the vagina in adolescence. A report of 7 cases including 6 clear-cell carcinomas (so-called mesonephromas). *Cancer* 1970;25:745–757.
82. Herbst AL, Ulfelder H, Poskanzer DC. Adenocarcinoma of the vagina. Association of maternal stilbestrol therapy with tumor appearance in young women. *N Engl J Med* 1971;284:878–881.
83. Heron DE, Axtel A, Gerszten K, et al. Villoglandular adenocarcinoma of the cervix recurrent in an episiotomy scar: a case report in a 32-year-old female. *Int J Gynecol Cancer* 2005;15:366–371.
84. Hicks ML, Piver MS. Conservative surgery plus adjuvant therapy for vulvovaginal rhabdomyosarcoma, diethylstilbestrol clear cell adenocarcinoma of the vagina, and unilateral germ cell tumors of the ovary. *Obstetr Gynecol Clin North Am* 1992;19:219–233.
85. Hilaris BS, Nori D, Anderson LL. Brachytherapy treatment planning. *Front Radiat Ther Oncol* 1987;21:94–106.
86. Hilgers RD. Pelvic exenteration for vaginal embryonal rhabdomyosarcoma: a review. *Obstetr Gynecol* 1975;45:175–180.
87. Hinchey WW, Silva EG, Guarda LA, et al. Paravaginal wolffian duct (mesonephros) adenocarcinoma: a light and electron microscopic study. *Am J Clin Pathol* 1983;80:539–544.
88. Hintz BL, Kagan AR, Chan P, et al. Radiation tolerance of the vaginal mucosa. *Int J Radiat Oncol Biol Phys* 1980;6:711–716.
89. Hiroi H, Yasugi T, Matsumoto K, et al. Mucinous adenocarcinoma arising in a neovagina using the sigmoid colon thirty years after operation: a case report. *J Surg Oncol* 2001;77:61–64.
90. Hockel M, Sclenger K, Hamm H, et al. Five-year experience with combined operative and radiotherapeutic treatment of recurrent gynecologic tumors infiltrating the pelvic wall. *Cancer* 1996;77:1918–1933.
91. Hoffman MS, DeCesare SL, Roberts WS, et al. Upper vaginectomy for in situ and occult, superficially invasive carcinoma of the vagina. *Am J Obstetr Gynecol* 1992;166:30–33.
92. Hoffman MS, Roberts WS, LaPolla JP, et al. Laser vaporization of grade 3 vaginal intraepithelial neoplasia. *Am J Obstetr Gynecol* 1991;165:1342–1344.
93. Hornback NB, Omura G, Major FJ. Observations on the use of adjuvant radiation therapy in patients with stage I and II uterine sarcoma. *Int J Radiat Oncol Biol Phys* 1986;12:2127–2130.
94. Hricak H, Lacey CG, Sandles LG, et al. Invasive cervical carcinoma: comparison of MR imaging and surgical findings. *Radiology* 1988;166:623–631.
95. Hudson CN, Findlay WS, Roberts H. Successful pregnancy after radical surgery for diethylstilboestrol (DES)-related vaginal adenocarcinoma. Case report. *Br J Obstetr Gynaecol* 1988;95:818–819.
96. Hwang EH, Han SJ, Lee MK, et al. Clinical experience with conservative surgery for vaginal endodermal sinus tumor. *J Pediatr Surg* 1996;31:219–222.
97. Indermaur MD, Martino MA, Fiorica JV, et al. Upper vaginectomy for the treatment of vaginal intraepithelial neoplasia. *Am J Obstetr Gynecol* 2005;193:577–580; discussion 580–571.
98. Irvin WP Jr., Bliss SA, Rice LW, et al. Malignant melanoma of the vagina and locoregional control: radical surgery revisited. *Gynecol Oncol* 1998;71:476–480.
99. Iversen T, Tretli S, Johansen A, et al. Squamous cell carcinoma of the penis and of the cervix, vulva and vagina in spouses: is there any relationship? An epidemiological study from Norway, 1960–92. *Br J Cancer* 1997;76:658–660.
100. Jobson VW, Homesley HD. Treatment of vaginal intraepithelial neoplasia with the carbon dioxide laser. *Obstetr Gynecol* 1983;62:90–93.
101. Julian TM, O'Connell BJ, Gosewehr JA. Indications, techniques, and advantages of partial laser vaginectomy. *Obstetr Gynecol* 1992;80:140–143.
102. Kalogirou D, Antoniou G, Karakitsos P, et al. Predictive factors used to justify hysterectomy after loop conization: increasing age and severity of disease. *Eur J Gynaecol Oncol* 1997;18:113–116.
103. Kaminski JM, Anderson PR, Han AC, et al. Primary small cell carcinoma of the vagina. *Gynecol Oncol* 2003;88:451–455.
104. Kaufman RH, Korhonen MO, Strama T, et al. Development of clear cell adenocarcinoma in DES-exposed offspring under observation. *Obstetr Gynecol* 1982;59:68S–72S.
105. Kersh CR, Constable WC, Spaulding CA, et al. A phase I-II trial of multimodality management of bulky gynecologic malignancy. Combined chemoradiosensitization and radiotherapy. *Cancer* 1990;66:30–34.
106. Keys HM, Bundy BN, Stehman FB, et al. Cisplatin, radiation, and adjuvant hysterectomy compared with radiation and adjuvant hysterectomy for bulky stage IB cervical carcinoma. *N Engl J Med* 1999;340:1154–1161. [Erratum appears in *N Engl J Med* 1999;341(9):708.]
107. Kirkbride P, Fyles A, Rawlings GA, et al. Carcinoma of the vagina—experience at the Princess Margaret Hospital (1974–1989). *Gynecol Oncol* 1995;56:435–443.
108. Krebs HB. Treatment of vaginal intraepithelial neoplasia with laser and topical 5-fluorouracil. *Obstetr Gynecol* 1989;73:657–660.
109. Kucera H, Langer M, Smekal G, et al. Radiotherapy of primary carcinoma of the vagina: management and results of different therapy schemes. *Gynecol Oncol* 1985;21:87–93.
110. Kucera H, Mock U, Knocke TH, et al. Radiotherapy alone for invasive vaginal cancer: outcome with intracavitary high dose rate brachytherapy versus conventional low dose rate brachytherapy. *Acta Obstet Gynecol Scand* 2001;80:355–360.
111. Kucera H, Vavra N. Radiation management of primary carcinoma of the vagina: clinical and histopathological variables associated with survival. *Gynecol Oncol* 1991;40:12–16.
112. Kushner DM, Fleming PA, Kennedy AW, et al. High dose rate (192)Ir afterloading brachytherapy for cancer of the vagina. *Br J Radiol* 2003;76:719–725.
113. Lara PN Jr., Hearn E, Leigh B. Neovaginal malignant melanoma following surgery and radiation for vulvar squamous cell carcinoma. *Gynecol Oncol* 1997;65:520–522.
114. Lee JY, Perez CA, Ettinger N, et al. The risk of second primaries subsequent to irradiation for cervix cancer. *Int J Radiat Oncol Biol Phys* 1982;8:207–211.
115. Lee WR, Marcus RB Jr., Sombeck MD, et al. Radiotherapy alone for carcinoma of the vagina: the importance of overall treatment time. *Int J Radiat Oncol Biol Phys* 1994;29:983–988.
116. Leung S, Sexton M. Radical radiation therapy for carcinoma of the vagina—impact of treatment modalities on outcome: Peter MacCallum Cancer Institute experience 1970–1990. *Int J Radiat Oncol Biol Phys* 1993;25:413–418.
117. Levitan Z, Gordon AN, Kaplan AL, et al. Primary malignant melanoma of the vagina: report of four cases and review of the literature. *Gynecol Oncol* 1989;33:85–90.
118. Li Z, Liu C, Palta JR. Optimized dose distribution of a high dose rate vaginal cylinder. *Int J Radiat Oncol Biol Phys* 1998;41:239–244.
119. Lindeque BG. The role of surgery in the management of carcinoma of the vagina. *Baillieres Clin Obstet Gynaecol* 1987;1:319–329.

120. MacLeod C, Fowler A, Dalrymple C, et al. High-dose-rate brachytherapy in the management of high-grade intraepithelial neoplasia of the vagina. *Gynecol Oncol* 1997;65:74–77.
121. Magrina JF, Masterson BJ. Vaginal reconstruction in gynecological oncology: a review of techniques. *Obstetr Gynecol Surv* 1981;36:1–10.
122. Manetta A, Gutrecht EL, Berman ML, et al. Primary invasive carcinoma of the vagina. *Obstetr Gynecol* 1990;76:639–642.
123. Martinez A, Cox RS, Edmundson GK. A multiple-site perineal applicator (MUPIT) for treatment of prostatic, anorectal, and gynecologic malignancies. *Int J Radiat Oncol Biol Phys* 1984;10:297–305.
124. Maurer HM, Beltangady M, Gehan EA, et al. The Intergroup Rhabdomyosarcoma Study-I. A final report. *Cancer* 1988;61:209–220.
125. Mock U, Kucera H, Fellner C, et al. High-dose-rate (HDR) brachytherapy with or without external beam radiotherapy in the treatment of primary vaginal carcinoma: long-term results and side effects. *Int J Radiat Oncol Biol Phys* 2003;56:950–957.
126. Moore DH, Thomas GM, Montana GS, et al. Preoperative chemoradiation for advanced vulvar cancer: a phase II study of the Gynecologic Oncology Group. *Int J Radiat Oncol Biol Phys* 1998;42:79–85.
127. Morris M, Eifel PJ, Lu J, et al. Pelvic radiation with concurrent chemotherapy compared with pelvic and para-aortic radiation for high-risk cervical cancer. *N Engl J Med* 1999;340:1137–1143.
128. Morrow CP, DiSaia PJ. Malignant melanoma of the female genitalia: a clinical analysis. *Obstetr Gynecol Surv* 1976;31:233–271.
129. Muench PJ, Nath R. Dose distributions produced by shielded applicators using 241Am for intracavitary irradiation of tumors in the vagina. *Med Phys* 1992;19:1299–1306.
130. Mundt AJ, Lujan AE, Rotmensch J, et al. Intensity-modulated whole pelvic radiotherapy in women with gynecologic malignancies. *Int J Radiat Oncol Biol Phys* 2002;52:1330–1337.
131. Mundt AJ, Mell LK, Roeske JC. Preliminary analysis of chronic gastrointestinal toxicity in gynecology patients treated with intensity-modulated whole pelvic radiation therapy. *Int J Radiat Oncol Biol Phys* 2003;56:1354–1360.
132. Muss HB, Bundy B, DiSaia PJ, et al. Treatment of recurrent or advanced uterine sarcoma. A randomized trial of doxorubicin versus doxorubicin and cyclophosphamide (a phase III trial of the Gynecologic Oncology Group). *Cancer* 1985;55:1648–1653.
133. Nanavati PJ, Fanning J, Hilgers RD, et al. High-dose-rate brachytherapy in primary stage I and II vaginal cancer. *Gynecol Oncol* 1993;51:67–71.
134. Neesham D, Kerdemelidis P, Scurry J. Primary malignant mixed Mullerian tumor of the vagina. *Gynecol Oncol* 1998;70:303–307.
135. O'Toole RV, Tuttle SE, Lucas JG, et al. Alveolar soft part sarcoma of the vagina: an immunohistochemical and electron microscopic study. *Int J Gynecol Pathol* 1985;4:258–265.
136. Ogino I, Kitamura T, Okajima H, et al. High-dose-rate intracavitary brachytherapy in the management of cervical and vaginal intraepithelial neoplasia. *Int J Radiat Oncol Biol Phys* 1998;40:881–887.
137. Ohno T, Kakinuma S, Kato S, et al. Risk of second cancers after radiotherapy for cervical cancer. *Expert Rev Anticancer Ther* 2006;6:49–57.
138. Okagaki T, Twiggs LB, Zachow KR, et al. Identification of human papillomavirus DNA in cervical and vaginal intraepithelial neoplasia with molecularly cloned virus-specific DNA probes. *Int J Gynecol Pathol* 1983;2:153–159.
139. Orr JW Jr., Dosoretz DD, Mahoney D, et al. Surgically (laparotomy/laparoscopy) guided placement of high dose rate interstitial irradiation catheters (LG-HDRT): technique and outcome. *Gynecol Oncol* 2006;100:145–148.
140. Overgaard J, Overgaard M, Hansen PV, et al. Some factors of importance in the radiation treatment of malignant melanoma. *Radiother Oncol* 1986;5:183–192.
141. Paley PJ, Koh WJ, Stelzer KJ, et al. A new technique for performing Syed template interstitial implants for anterior vaginal tumors using an open retropubic approach. *Gynecol Oncol* 1999;73:121–125.
142. Palmer JR, Anderson D, Helmrich SP, et al. Risk factors for diethylstilbestrol-associated clear cell adenocarcinoma. *Obstetr Gynecol* 2000;95:814–820.
143. Pecorelli S, Beller U, Heintz A, et al. FIGO annual report on the results of treatment in gynecological cancer. *J Epidemiol Biostat* 2000;24:56.
144. Perez CA, Arneson AN, Dehner LP, et al. Radiation therapy in carcinoma of the vagina. *Obstetr Gynecol* 1974;44:862–872.
145. Perez CA, Arneson AN, Galakatos A, et al. Malignant tumors of the vagina. *Cancer* 1973;31:36–44.
146. Perez CA, Bedwinek J, Breaux S. Patterns of failure after treatment of gynecologic tumors. *Cancer Treat Rep* 1983;2:217.
147. Perez CA, Camel HM, Galakatos AE, et al. Definitive irradiation in carcinoma of the vagina: long-term evaluation of results. *Int J Radiat Oncol Biol Phys* 1988;15:1283–1290.
148. Perez CA, Camel HM. Long-term follow-up in radiation therapy of carcinoma of the vagina. *Cancer* 1982;49:1308–1315.
149. Perez CA, Grigsby PW, Garipagaoglu M, et al. Factors affecting long-term outcome of irradiation in carcinoma of the vagina. *Int J Radiat Oncol Biol Phys* 1999;44:37–45.
150. Perez CA, Korba A, Sharma S. Dosimetric considerations in irradiation of carcinoma of the vagina. *Int J Radiat Oncol Biol Phys* 1977;2:639–649.
151. Perez CA, Slessinger E, Grigsby PW. Design of an afterloading vaginal applicator (MIRALVA). *Int J Radiat Oncol Biol Phys* 1990;18:1503–1508.
152. Perren T, Farrant M, McCarthy K, et al. Lymphomas of the cervix and upper vagina: a report of five cases and a review of the literature. *Gynecol Oncol* 1992;44:87–95.
153. Peters WA 3rd, Kumar NB, Andersen WA, et al. Primary sarcoma of the adult vagina: a clinicopathologic study. *Obstetr Gynecol* 1985;65:699–704.
154. Peters WA 3rd, Kumar NB, Morley GW. Carcinoma of the vagina. Factors influencing treatment outcome. *Cancer* 1985;55:892–897.
155. Peters WA 3rd, Kumar NB, Morley GW. Microinvasive carcinoma of the vagina: a distinct clinical entity? *Am J Obstetr Gynecol* 1985;153:505–507.
156. Petrilli ES, Townsend DE, Morrow CP, et al. Vaginal intraepithelial neoplasia: Biologic aspects and treatment with topical 5-fluorouracil and the carbon dioxide laser. *Am J Obstetr Gynecol* 1980;138:321–328.
157. Petru E, Nagele F, Czerwenka K, et al. Primary malignant melanoma of the vagina: long-term remission following radiation therapy. *Gynecol Oncol* 1998;70:23–26.
158. Pingley S, Shrivastava SK, Sarin R, et al. Primary carcinoma of the vagina: Tata Memorial Hospital experience. *Int J Radiat Oncol Biol Phys* 2000;46:101–108.
159. Piver MS, Barlow JJ, Tsukada Y, et al. Postirradiation squamous cell carcinoma in situ of the vagina: treatment by topical 20 percent 5-fluorouracil cream. *Am J Obstetr Gynecol* 1979;135:377–380.
160. Plentl AA, Friedman EA. Lymphatic system of the female genitalia. The morphologic basis of oncologic diagnosis and therapy. *Major Prob Obstetr Gynecol* 1971;2:1–223.
161. Prempree T, Amornmarn R. Radiation treatment of primary carcinoma of the vagina. Patterns of failures after definitive therapy. *Acta Radiol Oncol* 1985;24:51–56.
162. Prempree T, Tang CK, Hatef A, et al. Angiosarcoma of the vagina: a clinicopathologic report. A reappraisal of the radiation treatment of angiosarcomas of the female genital tract. *Cancer* 1983;51:618–622.
163. Randall ME, Evans L, Greven KM, et al. Interstitial reirradiation for recurrent gynecologic malignancies: results and analysis of prognostic factors. *Gynecol Oncol* 1993;48:23–31.
164. Raney RB Jr., Gehan EA, Hays DM, et al. Primary chemotherapy with or without radiation therapy and/or surgery for children with localized sarcoma of the bladder, prostate, vagina, uterus, and cervix. A comparison of the results in Intergroup Rhabdomyosarcoma Studies I and II. *Cancer* 1990;66:2072–2081.
165. Reddy S, Saxena VS, Reddy S, et al. Results of radiotherapeutic management of primary carcinoma of the vagina. *Int J Radiat Oncol Biol Phys* 1991;21:1041–1044.
166. Reid GC, Schmidt RW, Roberts JA, et al. Primary melanoma of the vagina: a clinicopathologic analysis. *Obstetrics & Gynecology* 1989;74:190–199.
167. Riva C, Fabbri A, Facco C, et al. Primary serous papillary adenocarcinoma of the vagina: a case report. *Int J Gynecol Pathol* 1997;16:286–290.
168. Robboy SJ, Herbst AL, Scully RE. Clear-cell adenocarcinoma of the vagina and cervix in young females: analysis of 37 tumors that persisted or recurred after primary therapy. *Cancer* 1974;34:606–614.
169. Robboy SJ, Hill EC, Sandberg EC, et al. Vaginal adenosis in women born prior to the diethylstilbestrol era. *Hum Pathol* 1986;17:488–492.
170. Robboy SJ, Szyfelbein WM, Goellner JR, et al. Dysplasia and cytologic findings in 4,589 young women enrolled in diethylstilbestrol-adenosis (DESAD) project. *Am J Obstetr Gynecol* 1981;140:579–586.
171. Roberts WS, Hoffman MS, Kavanagh JJ, et al. Further experience with radiation therapy and concomitant intravenous chemotherapy in advanced carcinoma of the lower female genital tract. *Gynecol Oncol* 1991;43:233–236.
172. Robinson JB, Sun CC, Bodurka-Bevers D, et al. Cavitational ultrasonic surgical aspiration for the treatment of vaginal intraepithelial neoplasia. *Gynecol Oncol* 2000;78:235–241.
173. Roeske JC, Lujan A, Rotmensch J, et al. Intensity modulated whole pelvic radiation therapy in patients with gynecologic malignancies. *Int J Radiat Oncol Biol Phys* 2000;48:1613–1621.
174. Rogo KO, Andersson R, Edbom G, et al. Conservative surgery for vulvovaginal melanoma. *Eur J Gynaecol Oncol* 1991;12:113–119.
175. Rose PG, Bundy BN, Watkins EB, et al. Concurrent cisplatin-based radiotherapy and chemotherapy for locally advanced cervical cancer [see comment]. *N Engl J Med* 1999;340:1144–1153. [Erratum appears in *N Engl J Med* 1999;341(9):708.]
176. Rubin P. *The female genital tract.* Philadelphia: Saunders, 1968.
177. Rubin SC, Young J, Mikuta JJ. Squamous carcinoma of the vagina: treatment, complications, and long-term follow-up. *Gynecol Oncol* 1985;20:346–353.
178. Russell AH, Koh WJ, Markette K, et al. Radical reirradiation for recurrent or second primary carcinoma of the female reproductive tract. *Gynecol Oncol* 1987;27:226–232.
179. Rutkowski T, Bialas B, Rembielak A, et al. Efficacy and toxicity of MDR versus HDR brachytherapy for primary vaginal cancer. *Neoplasma* 2002;49:197–200.
180. Sause WT, Cooper JS, Rush S, et al. Fraction size in external beam radiation therapy in the treatment of melanoma. *Int J Radiat Oncol Biol Phys* 1991;20:429–432.
181. [illegible] of the vagina and cervix. *Gynecol Oncol* 1989;34:413–416.
182. Senekjian EK, Frey KW, Anderson D, et al. Local therapy in stage I clear cell adenocarcinoma of the vagina. *Cancer* 1987;60:1319–1324.
183. Senekjian EK, Frey KW, Stone C, et al. An evaluation of stage II vaginal clear cell adenocarcinoma according to substages. *Gynecol Oncol* 1988;31:56–64.
184. Senkus E, Konefka T, Nowaczyk M, et al. Second lower genital tract squamous cell carcinoma following cervical cancer. A clinical study of 46 patients. *Acta Obstetr Gynecol Scand* 2000;79:765–770.
185. Shevchuk MM, Fenoglio CM, Lattes R, et al. Malignant mixed tumor of the vagina probably arising in mesonephric rests. *Cancer* 1978;42:214–223.
186. Shibata R, Umezawa A, Takehara K, et al. Primary carcinosarcoma of the vagina. *Pathol Int* 2003;53:106–110.
187. Sillman FH, Fruchter RG, Chen YS, et al. Vaginal intraepithelial neoplasia: risk factors for persistence, recurrence, and invasion and its management. *Am J Obstetr Gynecol* 1997;176:93–99.
188. Slessinger ED, Perez CA, Grigsby PW, et al. Dosimetry and dose specification for a new gynecological brachytherapy applicator. *Int J Radiat Oncol Biol Phys* 1992;22:1117–1124.
189. Spirtos NM, Doshi BP, Kapp DS, et al. Radiation therapy for primary squamous cell carcinoma of the vagina: Stanford University experience. *Gynecol Oncol* 1989;35:20–26.
190. Stafl A, Wilkinson EJ, Mattingly RF. Laser treatment of cervical and vaginal neoplasia. *Am J Obstetr Gynecol* 1977;128:128–136.
191. Stock RG, Chan K, Terk M, et al. A new technique for performing Syed-Neblett template interstitial implants for gynecologic malignancies using transrectal-ultrasound guidance. *Int J Radiat Oncol Biol Phys* 1997;37:819–825.
192. Stock RG, Chen AS, Seski J. A 30-year experience in the management of primary carcinoma of the vagina: analysis of prognostic factors and treatment modalities. *Gynecol Oncol* 1995;56:45–52.
193. Stock RG, Mychalczak B, Armstrong JG, et al. The importance of brachytherapy technique in the management of primary carcinoma of the vagina. *Int J Radiat Oncol Biol Phys* 1992;24:747–753.
194. Stryker JA. Radiotherapy for vaginal carcinoma: a 23-year review. *Br J Radiol* 2000;73:1200–1205.
195. Syed A, Puthawala A, Neblett D, et al. Transperineal interstitial-intracavitary "Syed-Neblett" applicator in the treatment of carcinoma of the uterine cervix. *Endocurieth/Hyperther Oncol* 1986;2:1–13.

196. Tabata T, Takeshima N, Nishida H, et al. Treatment failure in vaginal cancer. *Gynecol Oncol* 2002;84:309–314.
197. Tarraza HM Jr., Meltzer SE, DeCain M, et al. Vaginal metastases from renal cell carcinoma: report of four cases and review of the literature. *Eur J Gynaecol Oncol* 1998;19:14–18.
198. Tarraza MH Jr., Muntz H, Decain M, et al. Patterns of recurrence of primary carcinoma of the vagina. *Eur J Gynaecol Oncol* 1991;12:89–92.
199. Tavassoli FA, Norris HJ. Smooth muscle tumors of the vagina. *Obstetr Gynecol* 1979;53:689–693.
200. Taylor A, Rockall AG, Reznek RH, et al. Mapping pelvic lymph nodes: guidelines for delineation in intensity-modulated radiotherapy. *Int J Radiat Oncol Biol Phys* 2005;63:1604–1612.
201. Tewari KS, Cappuccini F, Puthawala AA, et al. Primary invasive carcinoma of the vagina: treatment with interstitial brachytherapy. *Cancer* 2001;91:758–770.
202. Thigpen JT, Blessing JA, Orr JW Jr. , et al. Phase II trial of cisplatin in the treatment of patients with advanced or recurrent mixed mesodermal sarcomas of the uterus: a Gynecologic Oncology Group Study. *Cancer Treat Rep* 1986;70:271–274.
203. Tjalma WA, Monaghan JM, de Barros Lopes A, et al. The role of surgery in invasive squamous carcinoma of the vagina. *Gynecol Oncol* 2001;81:360–365.
204. Townsend DE, Levine RU, Crum CP, et al. Treatment of vaginal carcinoma in situ with the carbon dioxide laser. *Am J Obstetr Gynecol* 1982;143:565–568.
205. Trimble EL. Melanomas of the vulva and vagina. *Oncology (Huntington)* 1996;10:1017–1023; discussion 1024.
206. Tyree WC, Cardenes H, Randall M, et al. High-dose-rate brachytherapy for vaginal cancer: learning from treatment complications. *Int J Gynecol Cancer* 2002;12:27–31.
207. Ulbright TM, Alexander RW, Kraus FT. Intramural papilloma of the vagina: evidence of Mullerian histogenesis. *Cancer* 1981;48:2260–2266.
208. Ulbright TM, Kraus FT. Endometrial stomal tumors of extra-uterine tissue. *Am J Clin Pathol* 1981;76:371–377.
209. Ulich TR, Liao SY, Layfield L, et al. Endocrine and tumor differentiation markers in poorly differentiated small-cell carcinoids of the cervix and vagina. *Arch Pathol Lab Med* 1986;110:1054–1057.
210. Urbanski K, Kojs Z, Reinfuss M, et al. Primary invasive vaginal carcinoma treated with radiotherapy: analysis of prognostic factors. *Gynecol Oncol* 1996;60:16–21.
211. Van Dam PA, Irvine L, Lowe DG, et al. Carcinoma in episiotomy scars. *Gynecol Oncol* 1992;44:96–100.
212. Van Nostrand KM, Lucci JA 3rd, Schell M, et al. Primary vaginal melanoma: improved survival with radical pelvic surgery. *Gynecol Oncol* 1994;55:234–237.
213. Vayrynen M, Romppanen T, Koskela E, et al. Verrucous squamous cell carcinoma of the female genital tract. Report of three cases and survey of the literature. *Int J Gynaecol Obstetr* 1981;19:351–356.
214. Waggoner SE, Anderson SM, Luce MC, et al. p53 protein expression and gene analysis in clear cell adenocarcinoma of the vagina and cervix. *Gynecol Oncol* 1996;60:339–344.
215. Webb MJ, Symmonds RE, Weiland LH. Malignant fibrous histiocytoma of the vagina. *Am J Obstetr Gynecol* 1974;119:190–192.
216. Weiderpass E, Ye W, Tamimi R, et al. Alcoholism and risk for cancer of the cervix uteri, vagina, and vulva. *Cancer Epidemiol Biomarkers Prev* 2001;10:899–901.
217. Wharton JT, Tortolero-Luna G, Linares AC, et al. Vaginal intraepithelial neoplasia and vaginal cancer. *Obstetr Gynecol Clin North Am* 1996;23:325–345.
218. Whelton J, Kottmeier H. Primary carcinoma of the vagina: a study of a Radiumhemmet series of 145 cases. *Acta Obstetr Gynecol Scand* 1962;41:22–40.
219. Whitney CW, Sause W, Bundy BN, et al. Randomized comparison of fluorouracil plus cisplatin versus hydroxyurea as an adjunct to radiation therapy in stage IIB-IVA carcinoma of the cervix with negative para-aortic lymph nodes: a Gynecologic Oncology Group and Southwest Oncology Group study. *J Clin Oncol* 1999;17:1339–1348.
220. Williams S, Blessing JA, Liao SY, et al. Adjuvant therapy of ovarian germ cell tumors with cisplatin, etoposide, and bleomycin: a trial of the Gynecologic Oncology Group. *J Clin Oncol* 1994;12:701–706.
221. Woodruff JD, Parmley TH, Julian CG. Topical 5-fluorouracil in the treatment of vaginal carcinoma-in-situ. *Gynecol Oncol* 1975;3:124–132.
222. Wright VC, Chapman W. Intraepithelial neoplasia of the lower female genital tract: etiology, investigation, and management. *Sem Surg Oncol* 1992;8:180–190.
223. Wulf J, Hadinger U, Oppitz U, et al. Stereotactic boost irradiation for targets in the abdomen and pelvis. *Radiother Oncol* 2004;70:31–36.
224. Xiang-E W, Shu-mo C, Ya-qin D, et al. Treatment of late recurrent vaginal malignancy after initial radiotherapy for carcinoma of the cervix: an analysis of 73 cases. *Gynecol Oncol* 1998;69:125–129.
225. Young RH, Scully RE. Endodermal sinus tumor of the vagina: a report of nine cases and review of the literature. *Gynecol Oncol* 1984;18:380–392.
226. Zaino R, Robboy S, Kurman R. *Diseases of the vagina*. 5th ed. New York: Springer, 2002.

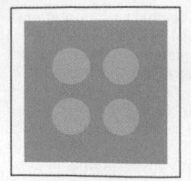

Chapter 71
Female Urethra

Tony Y. Eng

Urethral carcinoma is a rare tumor, accounting for less than 1% of all malignancies. Although the urethra in females is shorter than in males, urethral cancer is more common in females than in males. Female primary urethral carcinoma occurs primarily in elderly women. Optimal management of female urethral cancer depends on the clinical stage, tumor location, extent of nodal involvement, and the patient's health status.

Anatomy

The female urethra is approximately 3 to 4 cm long and 0.6 cm in resting diameter. It is embedded in the anterior vaginal wall behind the pubis symphysis, extending inferiorly and anteriorly from the urinary bladder through the urogenital diaphragm to the vestibule, where it forms the urethral meatus. Because of the proximity of the symphysis pubis, a small curve is formed with an anterior concavity. Figure 71.1 illustrates the urethra and adjacent organs in the female pelvis.

The wall of the urethra consists of three layers. The muscular layer is continuous with that of the bladder. At the vesicular end of the urethra, this muscular wall forms the internal sphincter. The voluntary urethral sphincter is at the plane of the urogenital diaphragm. A thin layer of erectile tissue consisting of a plexus of veins and muscle fibers forms the middle layer of the wall. The inner layer is the mucous membrane, which is continuous with the bladder proximally and with the vulva distally. This membrane consists of transitional epithelium near the bladder but distally changes to nonkeratinizing stratified squamous epithelium and pseudostratified columnar epithelium. The distal urethra also contains small mucous recesses and periurethral or Skene's glands, most of which are in the region of the meatus.

The lymphatic drainage of the distal urethra and urethral meatus parallels that of the vulva to the superficial and deep inguinal and external iliac lymph nodes. The primary drainage of the posterior or entire urethra is mainly to the obturator, and internal and external iliac nodes.

Epidemiology and Etiology

Approximately 1,800 cases of urethral carcinoma have been reported in the literature. Although urethral cancer occurs more frequently in white women than men, carcinoma of the urethra is rare in women. Only a few cases are seen annually at major cancer centers (33,39,57,62). Carcinoma of the female urethra makes up 0.02% of all cancers in women and accounts for approximately 0.1% of all gynecologic cancers (34,68). The average patient age at the time of diagnosis is 60 years, with most patients between 50 and 80 years of age (26,53,66). The incidence appears to be higher in white women than in black women (21).

Although chronic infection and local irritation have been proposed, the etiology of female urethral cancer remains obscure. Weiner and Walther (69) analyzed archival surgical specimens of women with urethral carcinoma. Human papilloma virus (HPV) was detected in 10 of 17 patients with invasive disease. HPV type 16 was found in eight patients. Eight women with squamous cell carcinoma and two with transitional cell carcinoma had HPV. Female urethral cancer may also be associated with urethral diverticula (48,49). Patients with transitional cell carcinoma of the bladder, especially the bladder neck, may have a higher risk of developing urethral cancer either synchronously or metachronously (6,11).

Natural History

Most urethral cancers are clinically aggressive. During the later stages, cancers of the middle or posterior urethra tend to extend upward into the urinary bladder, downward to invade the remainder of the urethra, and posteriorly into the vaginal mucosa. Lesions involving the anterior urethra account for approximately 30% of all cases (26,63).

Regional lymph node involvement is uncommon in early tumors (stage 0) of the urethral meatus. Advanced tumors (stages II and III) of the urethra have been associated with a 35% to 50% incidence of inguinal or pelvic lymph node involvement (7,25,37,53,68). Bilateral nodal involvement occurs in approximately one-third of patients with positive nodes. Grabstald (26) confirmed nodal involvement in 24 of 25 patients with clinically palpable nodes. In his series of patients with advanced disease, 26 underwent pelvic lymph node sampling and 13 (50%) had nodal involvement.

Distant metastases are found in approximately 10% of patients at presentation, and approximately 30% to 50% ultimately die of distant disease. The most common sites of metastasis are lung, liver, bone, and brain (26,52).

Clinical Presentation

A majority of patients with urethral cancer present with some degree of irritative or obstructive urethral symptoms (14). Bleeding (hematuria) or spotting is the prevailing presenting sign in 50% to 60% of patients (9,29,46). Approximately 30% to 50% of patients experience pain or irritative symptoms, difficulty urinating, and frequent micturition. Urinary retention and overflow incontinence may occur in advanced cases. Less frequently cited signs and symptoms are a mass in the introitus (10% to 20% of patients), dyspareunia, perineal pain, and inguinal lymphadenopathy (12,25,52). Urethrovaginal and vesicovaginal fistulas may develop in advanced, neglected cases.

Small tumors involving the urethral meatus are often mistakenly diagnosed as urethral caruncle, a benign, inflammatory lesion, or a prolapse of the mucosa through the urethral orifice. As the lesion progresses, it enlarges and eventually ulcerates (52). Tumors may arise in a urethral diverticulum (56,59). Larger lesions of the distal urethra are readily identified on inspection (Fig. 71.2). Tumors occupying the proximal urethra may produce a fusiform enlargement that can be palpated during pelvic examination.

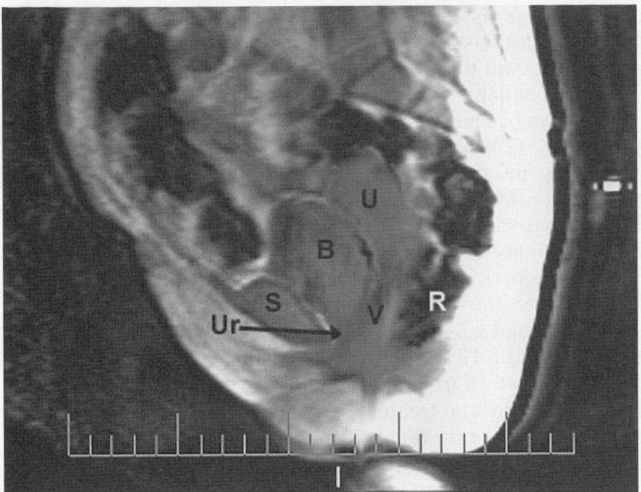

FIGURE 71.1. Sagittal magnetic resonance image of the female pelvis: U, uterus; B, bladder; S, symphysis pubis; Ur, urethra; V, vagina; R, rectum.

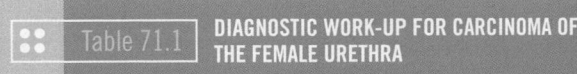

| Table 71.1 | DIAGNOSTIC WORK-UP FOR CARCINOMA OF THE FEMALE URETHRA |

General
History
Physical examination, including detailed pelvic examination under anesthesia
Special procedures
  Punch biopsy
  Urethroscopy
  Cystoscopy
  Rectosigmoidoscopy (advanced stages or if symptomatic)
Radiographic evaluation
  Standard
  Chest radiographs
  Intravenous urography
  Computed tomography scan (abdomen and pelvis)
  Bone scan (if symptomatic or elevated alkaline phosphatase)
  Barium enema (if symptomatic or advanced stages)
  Complementary
  Magnetic resonance imaging
  Ultrasound
  Urethrography
Laboratory evaluation
  Complete blood count
  Chemistry profile
  Urinalysis

Diagnostic Work-Up

An outline for the diagnostic work-up for carcinoma of the female urethra is presented in Table 71.1. A routine history and general physical examination should be performed for all patients. A detailed pelvic examination under anesthesia is necessary to fully evaluate the clinical extent of the disease. This examination can be performed at the time of urethroscopy and cystoscopy. Urine cytologic analyses have a high false-negative rate (65). The definitive diagnosis is made by punch or incisional biopsy.

Routine radiographic evaluation should include chest radiographs, an intravenous urogram, and a computed tomography (CT) scan of the abdomen and pelvis (47,59) (Fig. 71.3). Complementary studies include a barium enema for patients with symptoms of advanced disease, urethrography, and lymphangiography. Magnetic resonance imaging of the pelvis may be very helpful in delineating the tumor extent, especially when an endourethral coil is used. It provides a discrete view of the muscular layers of the urethra (18,55).

Staging Systems

Clinical staging is based on findings on physical examination, chest x-ray, and CT scan of the abdomen and pelvis. Many attempts have been made to formulate a staging system for carcinoma of the urethra. Urethral tumors can be classified in two groups: Those involving the distal half of the urethra and those located in the proximal or entire urethra. Most authors have found that this classification correctly depicts the feasibility of treatment and the prognosis. A staging system based on location has been proposed by Prempree et al. (54) (Table 71.2). The TNM staging system of the American Joint Committee on Cancer is shown in Table 71.3 (27).

Pathologic Classification

As the urethra is lined by transitional cells proximally and stratified squamous cells distally, transitional cell carcinoma occurs

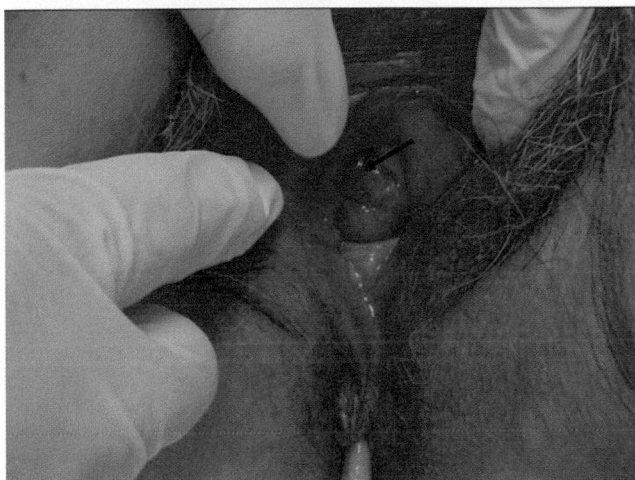

FIGURE 71.2. A meatal carcinoma of the urethra (*arrow*) in a 63-year-old white woman.

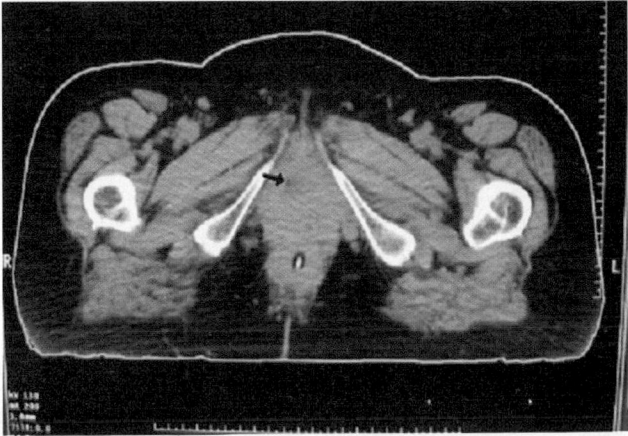

FIGURE 71.3. Transaxial computed tomography image of a patient with urethral cancer illustrating the periurethral and anterior vaginal wall expansion and deviation of the urethra (*arrow*).

Table 71.2 PROPOSED CLINICAL STAGING SYSTEM FOR CARCINOMA OF THE FEMALE URETHRA

Tumor Stage	Characteristics
I	Disease limited to distal one-half of urethra
II	Disease involving entire urethra, with extension to periurethral tissues, but not involving vulva or bladder neck
III	
A	Disease involving urethra and vulva
B	Disease invading vaginal mucosa
C	Disease involving urethra and bladder neck
IV	
A	Disease invading parametrium or paracolpium
B	Metastasis
B1	Inguinal lymph nodes
B2	Pelvic lymph nodes
B3	Paraaortic nodes
B4	Distant metastasis

From Prempree T, Amornmarn R, Patanaphan V. Radiation therapy in primary carcinoma of the female urethra: II. An update on results. *Cancer* 1984;54:729–733, with permission.

typically in the proximal urethra, whereas squamous cell carcinoma occurs frequently in the distal urethra. Squamous cell carcinoma is the most common histologic category in cancer of the female urethra, representing more than 50% of all cases (49). Transitional cell carcinoma and adenocarcinoma represent approximately 15% to 20% and 10% to 15%, respectively (43,50). The remainder of the histologic types include adenoid cystic carcinoma, melanoma, clear cell adenocarcinoma, anaplastic tumors, Kaposi's sarcoma, lymphomas, and metastatic lesions (1,2,4,15,36,41,44,51,57–59,67).

Prognostic Factors

Conventional prognostic factors such as grade and histology have not been consistently predictive for recurrence or survival. In the literature, some of the most important factors in determining prognosis and survival are depth of invasion, tumor size, and anatomic location (5,9,25,49). Lesions located in

Table 71.3 TNM CLASSIFICATION OF CARCINOMA OF THE URETHRA (MALE OR FEMALE)

Primary tumor (T)

TX	Primary tumor cannot be assessed
T0	No evidence of primary tumor
Ta	Noninvasive papillary, polypoid, or verrucous carcinoma
Tis	Carcinoma *in situ*
T1	Tumor invades subepithelial connective tissue
T2	Tumor invades corpus spongiosum or prostate or periurethral muscle
T3	Tumor invades corpus cavernosum or beyond the prostatic capsule or the anterior vagina or the bladder neck
T4	Tumor invades other adjacent organs

Regional lymph nodes (N)

NX	Regional lymph nodes cannot be assessed
N0	No regional lymph node metastasis
N1	Metastasis in a single lymph node, ≤2 cm in greatest dimension
N2	Metastasis in a single lymph node >2 cm or multiple lymph nodes

Distant metastasis (M)

MX	Presence of distant metastasis cannot be assessed
M0	No distant metastasis
M1	Distant metastasis

From Greene FL, Page DL, Fleming ID, et al., eds. *AJCC cancer staging manual*, 6th ed. Philadelphia: Lippincott-Raven; 2002.

the meatus or distal urethra tend to be superficial, with a better prognosis; lesions in the posterior urethra are often deeply invasive and tend to have a worse prognosis. Most investigators found that patients with advanced stage disease do poorly, often irrespective of their treatment (9,14,17,23).

Grigsby (29) and Grigsby and Corn (28) demonstrated a worsening prognosis with increased tumor size. The 5-year progression-free survival was 81% for patients with lesions <2 cm, compared with 37% for those with lesions 2 to 4 cm and 7% for patients with lesions >4 cm ($p = .0001$). For lesions confined to the proximal urethra, local control was observed in all four patients. However, patients with tumors involving the distal urethra had a 5-year progression-free survival rate of 69%, and there was a 12% survival rate for those with involvement of the entire urethra ($p = .0001$). Patients with meatal tumors, if diagnosed early and treated appropriately, can achieve an 80% to 90% survival rate (Figs. 71.4 and 71.5) (29). Bladder neck involvement, parametrial extension, and inguinal lymph node involvement have been identified as poor prognostic factors.

The histology of the primary lesion appears to be less important as a prognostic factor in determining response to therapy and survival. Patients with adenocarcinoma have been reported to have a good prognosis, but most studies have shown no difference in survival among patients with adenocarcinoma, squamous cell carcinoma, and transitional cell carcinoma (5,26,48,54). Grigsby (29) found a worse prognosis in patients with adenocarcinoma. Primary melanoma of the urethra, although rare, has a very poor prognosis (2,4).

General Management

Although various therapeutic approaches have been advocated in the management of carcinoma of the female urethra, there are no established therapeutic guidelines. The variety of treatments reflects the dimensions and locations of disease and the approaches of the treating physicians (20). In general, surgical resection is a primary mode of treatment. For patients with locally invasive urethral carcinoma, anterior exenteration may be required. Lesions of limited extent may be amenable to organ-sparing or conservative surgical management with or without adjuvant radiation therapy. Surgical approaches include neodymium:yttrium-aluminum-garnet (Nd:YAG) laser coagulation (10), Mohs' micrographic surgery, and partial or total urethrectomy (50). Radiation therapy may include external-beam radiation, interstitial brachytherapy, or a combination of these treatments. For patients who are medically nonsurgical candidates because of potential risks of anesthesia, outpatient high-dose-rate intracavitary and intraluminal brachytherapy may be an option (38).

Although most available data are insufficient, in patients with more advanced disease, some authors have advocated the use of combined irradiation and chemotherapy including 5-fluorouracil, cisplatin, vinblastine, epirubicin, carboplatin, bleomycin, methotrexate, or mitomycin C (16,31,35,40,61).

Anterior (Distal) Urethral Cancer

For stage 0 and I (Ta, Tis, or small T1) lesions, open excision, electroexcision, fulguration, and laser (Nd-YAG or CO_2) coagulation are possible for tumors at the meatus or with *in situ* involvement of the distal urethra (stage 0). For larger and more invasive lesions (stage T1 and T2), surgical resection of the distal third of the urethra is often adequate. Alternately, interstitial irradiation or a combination of interstitial and external-beam irradiation can be considered. For T3-T4 or recurrent anterior urethral lesions previously treated by local excision or radiation therapy, anterior exenteration and urinary diversion may be

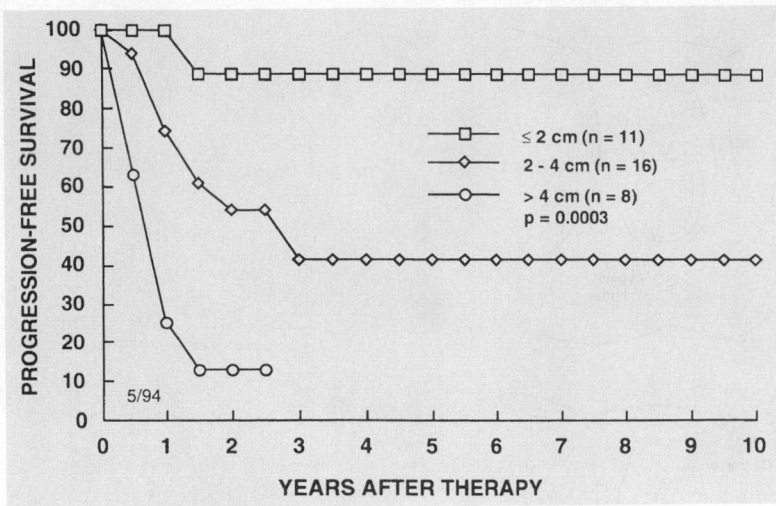

FIGURE 71.4. Progression-free survival correlated with tumor size. (From Grigsby PW, Herr HW. Urethral tumors. In: Vogelzang J, Scardino PT, Shipley WU, et al., eds. *Comprehensive textbook of genitourinary oncology.* Baltimore: Williams & Wilkins; 1996:1117–1123, with permission.)

curative. Adjuvant radiation therapy may be required, depending on surgical findings.

If a limited number of inguinal nodes are involved, ipsilateral node dissection or irradiation is indicated because cure is still achievable. If no inguinal adenopathy exists, node dissection is not recommended, but prophylactic groin irradiation is recommended for patients with invasive lesions (5,57).

Posterior (Proximal) Urethral Cancer

Cancers of the posterior or entire urethra are usually associated with invasion of the bladder, a high incidence of inguinal and pelvic lymph node metastases, and a worse prognosis. For lesions <2 cm, radical resection, definitive radiation therapy, or combined treatment may provide adequate control (28). However, for larger lesions or locally advanced disease, the best results have been achieved with preoperative irradiation, exenterative surgery, and urinary diversion. Pelvic lymphadenectomy is performed and inguinal node dissection may be indicated if the inguinal nodes are involved. In selected patients, it is possible to remove part of the pubic symphysis and the inferior pubic rami to maximize the surgical margin. A transpubic approach has been advocated by Golimbu et al. (24). Perineal closure and vaginal reconstruction can be accomplished with the use of myocutaneous flaps. Hedden et al. (32) have advocated the use of bladder-sparing surgery with or without irradiation.

Recurrent Urethral Cancer

In most cases, locally recurrent urethral cancer after radiation therapy should be treated by surgical excision. For those who are not surgical candidates, local reirradiation (i.e., hyperfractionated intensity-modulated radiation therapy or brachytherapy) may be considered if radiation tolerance has not been exceeded. Locally recurrent urethral cancer after surgery alone should be considered for combination radiation therapy and wider surgical resection. Patients with metastatic urethral cancer should be considered for investigational chemotherapy protocols. Radiation therapy may provide good symptomatic palliation.

Radiation Therapy Techniques

Small meatal or distal urethral lesions are curable with limited therapy. Interstitial implants have been the usual method for treating meatal carcinomas. Radioactive needles, forming a double-plane or a volume implant, have been used (Fig. 71.6). Afterloading implants using ^{192}Ir have replaced radium (34). For early localized disease without involvement of adjacent organs, a volume implant composed of 8 to 12 needles arranged in an arc around the urethral orifice is used (Fig. 71.7). Radiographs may be used to verify needle placement (Fig. 71.8).

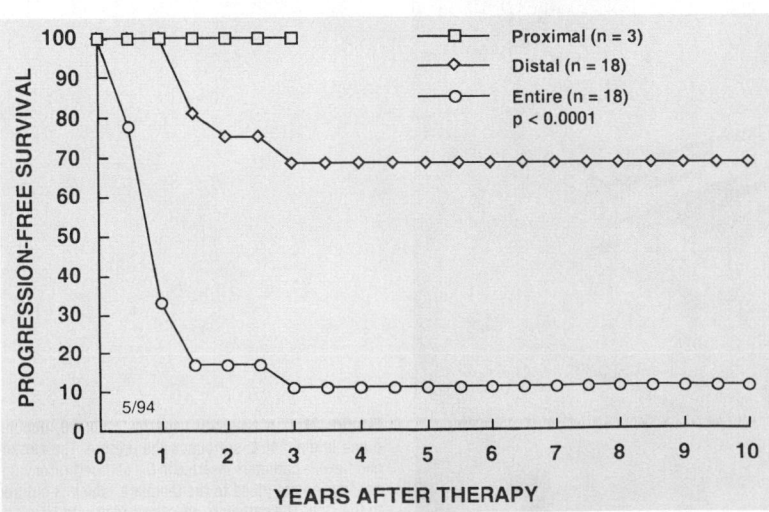

FIGURE 71.5. Progression-free survival correlated with tumor location. (From Grigsby PW, Herr HW. Urethral tumors. In: Vogelzang J, Scardino PT, Shipley WU, et al., eds. *Comprehensive textbook of genitourinary oncology.* Baltimore: Williams & Wilkins; 1996:1117–1123, with permission.)

Clinical Radiation Oncology

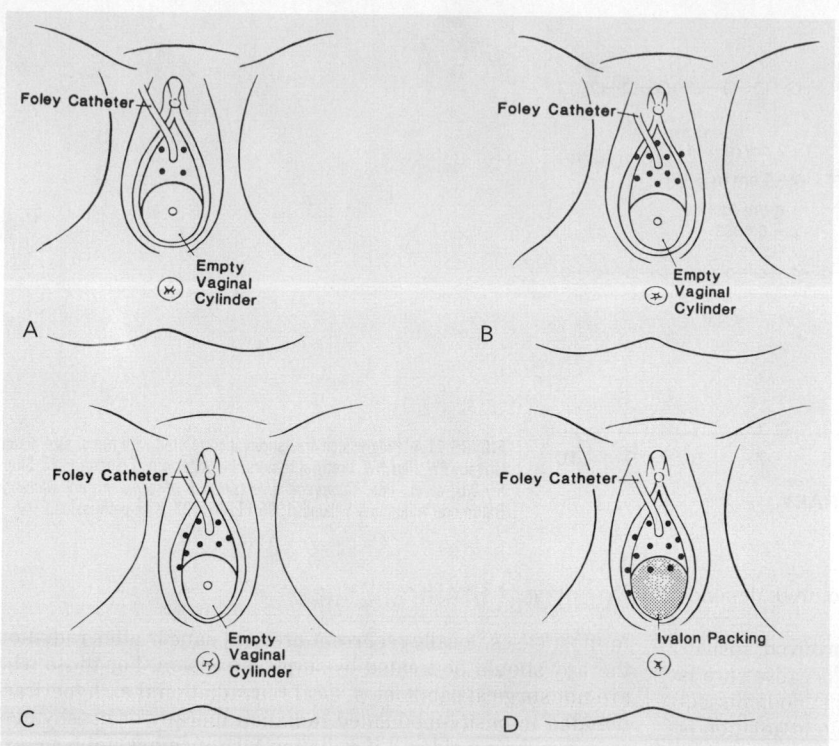

FIGURE 71.6. Diagrams of implants. **A:** Tumor limited to the urethra. **B:** Tumor extending to the periurethral tissues or originating in the periurethral glands. **C:** Tumor extending into the vagina or labia minora. **D:** Tumor involving the suburethral area. (From Delclos L. Carcinoma of the female urethra. In: Johnson DE, Boileau MA, eds. *Genitourinary tumors.* New York: Grune & Stratton; 1982:275–286, with permission.).

Computer planning with CT-based simulation should be the standard of care to spare the adjacent normal organs. A dose of 60 to 70 Gy should be given in 6 to 7 days (0.4 Gy/hour to the target volume) when an implant alone is used.

Advanced disease or large tumors extending into the labia, vagina, entire urethra, or base of the bladder cannot be treated with an implant alone. For these patients, a combination of external-beam irradiation and implant is recommended. The external-beam portal should flash the perineum to cover the entire urethra. The portal should be wide enough to cover the inguinal nodes and should extend cephalad to the L5-S1 interspace to include the pelvic nodes (Fig. 71.9) (19). A bolus, appro-

priate for the photon energy used, should be added to the groins when inguinal nodes are positive. This technique minimizes the hazard of groin failure due to underdosing of gross tumor. Hahn et al. (30) have demonstrated the importance of treating the inguinal lymph nodes in all patients. The whole pelvis is treated to a dose of 45 to 50 Gy. A boost of 10 to 15 Gy is delivered to positive groin nodes through reduced anteroposterior fields.

After pelvic radiation therapy, the primary tumor can be treated with a vaginal cylinder to bring the dose to the entire urethra to approximately 60 Gy. An interstitial implant is administered to raise the total tumor dose to 70 to 80 Gy. For patients undergoing postoperative therapy, the tumor bed is treated

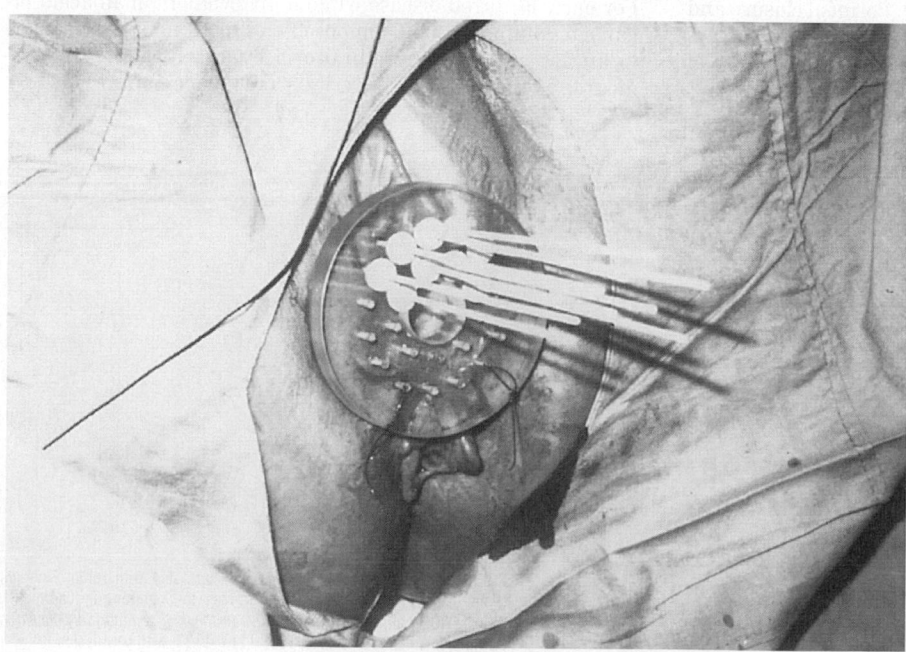

FIGURE 71.7. A template used for a curved, double-plane implant that surrounds the urethra. The closed-end flexible catheters inserted in the periurethral or vaginal tissues are glued to the template, which is sutured to the skin. The catheters are afterloaded with [192]Ir.

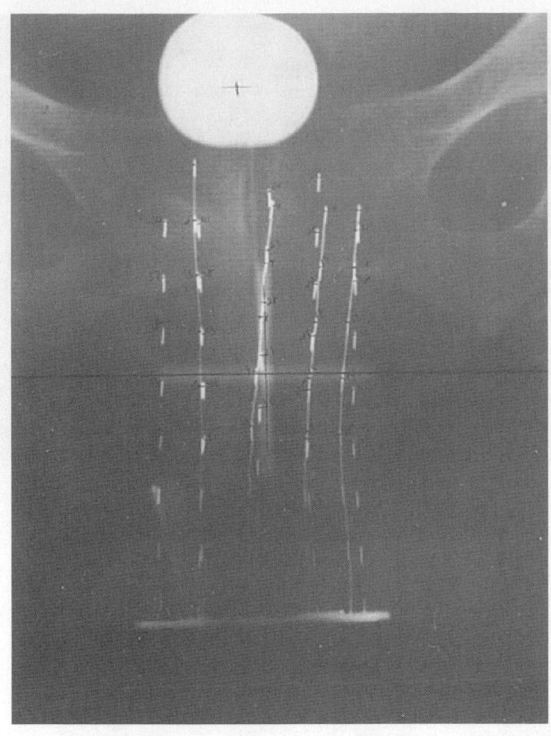
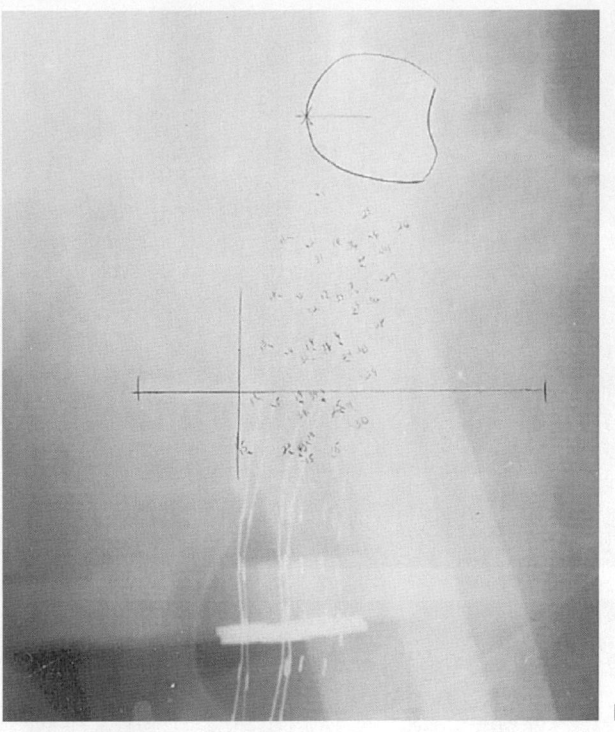

FIGURE 71.8. Anteroposterior **(A)** and lateral **(B)** simulation radiographs with dummy seeds in place. Contrast material is used to inflate the balloon of the urinary catheter, which is used to localize the bladder.

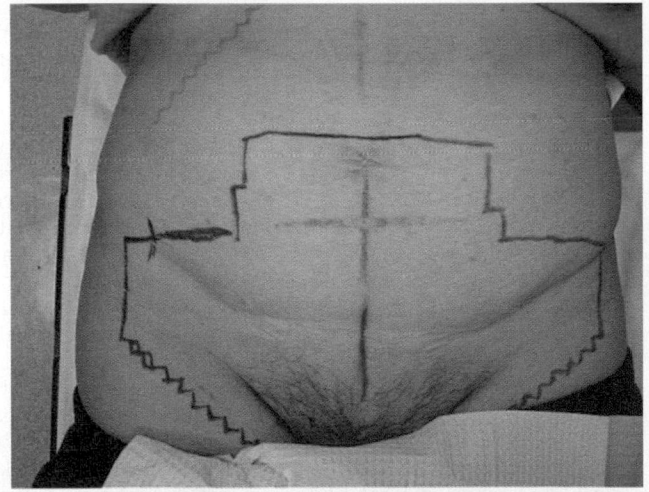
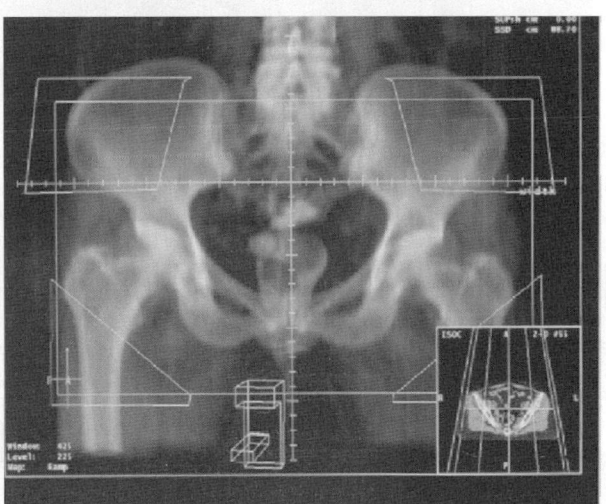
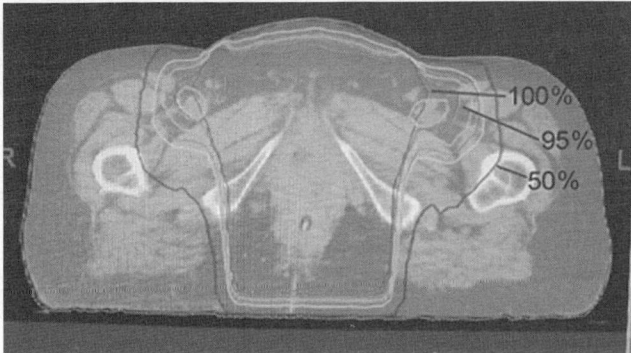

FIGURE 71.9. Whole pelvis and inguinal field. External skin marking **(A)** and anteroposterior simulation film **(B)** of a pelvic portal showing the lateral extension to cover the inguinal lymph nodes, and the isodose plan **(C)**.

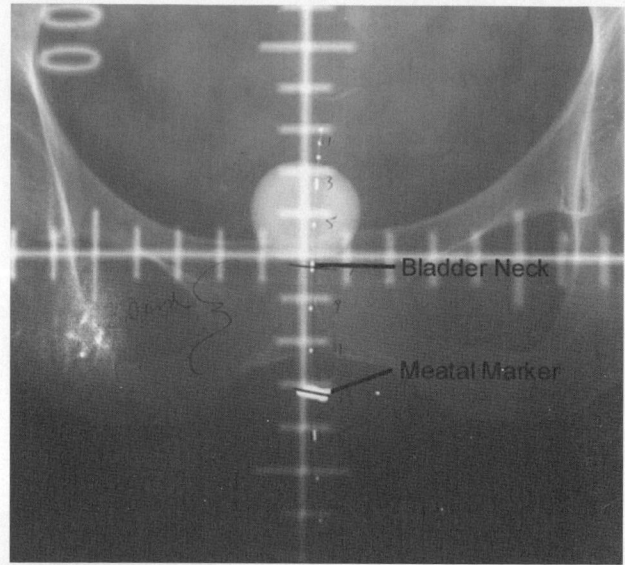

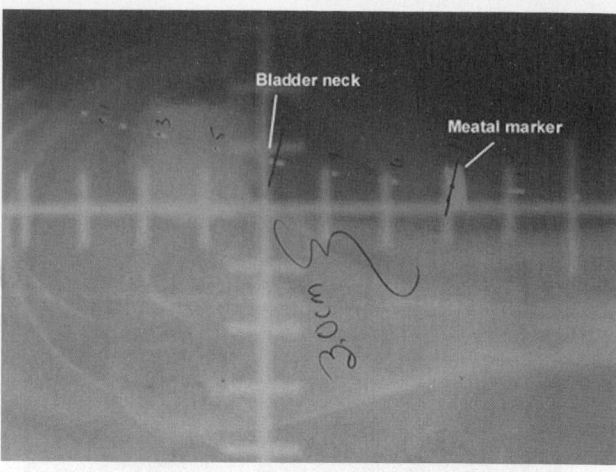

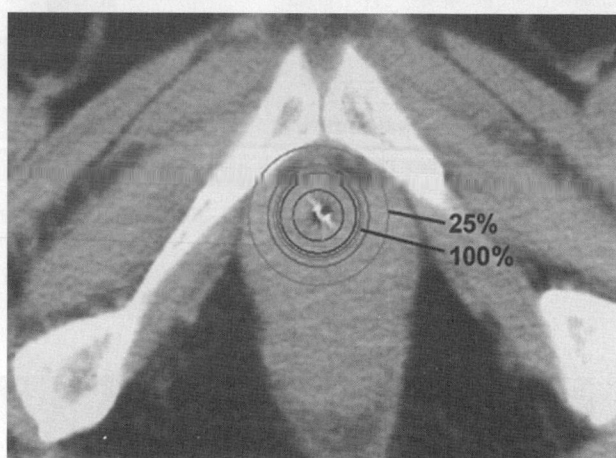

FIGURE 71.10. High-dose-rate brachytherapy with a Foley catheter. Anteroposterior **(A)** and lateral simulation **(B)** films, and transaxial computed tomography image with isodose plan **(C)**. The resultant uniformed, steep isodose lines cover the periurethral tissue well.

after pelvic radiation therapy with an additional 10 to 15 Gy using interstitial brachytherapy (8). Intracavitary irradiation with the vaginal cylinder and an interstitial implant are almost never used simultaneously because of the resultant high dose rate at the vaginal mucosa interface of the intracavitary and interstitial implant fields. A vaginal cylinder with partial shielding posteriorly can be used in selected patients. Gerbaulet et al. (22) have demonstrated the use of a catheter or a vaginal mold applicator for intraluminal/intracavitary brachytherapy and needles or guide gutters for interstitial brachytherapy.

In medically inoperable patients with small localized disease receiving radiation therapy alone, high-dose-rate brachytherapy without sedation or anesthesia after pelvic external beam radiation has been used (38) (Fig. 71.10).

One of the limiting factors in the use of external-beam irradiation is the tolerance of the perineal skin (i.e., confluent moist desquamation). Extensive disease combined with advanced age can be a formidable obstacle to completing the irradiation course. Diligent personal hygiene and individualized care are necessary if patients are to complete the course of treatment.

Results of Therapy

Surgery

There is a paucity of long-term outcome data. In general, female urethral cancers are clinically aggressive with high recurrence and poor survival rates (9,23,26,37,49,52).

DiMarco et al. (14) recently reviewed 59 female patients with primary urethral carcinoma undergoing partial urethrectomy or radical extirpation. The estimated 10-year cancer-specific survival was 60%. In a study of 72 patients treated at Memorial Sloan-Kettering Cancer Center between 1925 and 1994, the 5-year disease-specific survival was 89% for low-stage tumors and 33% for high-stage tumors (9). The overall survival was 78% and 22%, respectively, as shown in Table 71.4.

Five of seven patients with early meatal tumors were cured of disease in the series reported by Grabstald (26) after partial urethrectomy. In the remaining two patients, both local recurrences and distant metastases developed. Bracken et al. (5) reported local control in just one of four patients treated with local excision only for distal urethral lesions. Peterson et al. (52) reported on two patients in whom squamous cell carcinomas were excised successfully. In the same series, a patient with adenocarcinoma treated with local excision had a local recurrence and left inguinal adenopathy 4 years later.

Grabstald et al. (25) performed radical surgery on 15 patients with advanced disease; there were only 3 survivors at 5 years. Peterson et al. (52) performed radical surgery on seven patients, with three alive at 5 years. Primary radical cystectomy with anterior vaginectomy and total urethrectomy was performed on eight patients by Mayer et al. (42). Only three of these patients were free of disease at 1, 4, and 11 years.

Table 71.4 FEMALE URETHRA TREATMENT SUMMARY

Authors/Site/Years	Patients	Stage	Treatment	Radiation Dose (Gy)	Follow-Up	Results	Prognostic Factors
Thyavihally et al. Tata Memorial 2005 (64)	18	T1-4, N0-N+, M0 (stage I-IV)	2 LE/RT 4 exent 4 exent/RT 4 RT 4 Palliative/2 chemo	45-50 pelvis 20-25 boost	1.5-5.8	5-yr OS 33% (45%, distal vs. 16%, proximal; 50%, low vs. 0% high stage)	Stage Site (distal lesion do better)
DiMarco et al. Mayo Clinic 2004 (14)	53	pT1-3, N0-N+	26 Part urethrectomy 27 exent 20 adj RT/3 brachy 3 chemo (cis-platinum based)	20-60 (50, median)	12.8 (mean)	10-yr CSS 60% 10-yr CS 42% LR only 15 pts DM only 2 pts LR+DM 10 pts	Path stage and nodal status. Partial urethrectomy (LR 22%)
Eng et al. UTHSCSA 2003 (17)	10	Tis-3, N0-2, M0-1	5 Part urethrectomy 5 RT +/- chemo	30-68, primary 50 to nodes Brachy HDR 5 ×5	11 (mean)	OS 60% (4/5, low vs. 2/5, high stage)	Clinical stage
Dalbagni et al. MSKCC 1998 (9)	72	Tx-4, Nx-N+	42 exent/part urethrectomy 25 RT/brachy 10 pre-op RT	No details	7.1 (median)	5-yr OS 32% (78%, low vs. 22%, high stage) 5-yr DSS 46% (89%, low vs. 33%, high stage)	Stage, nodal status, surgery type, disease site
Grigsby MIR 1998 (29)	44	T1-4, N0-2	7 Surgery 25 RT 12 Surgery+RT	Adj 30-73.68 Gy (50.4 Gy median) RT 12-70 Gy (42.59 Gy median) Brachy 20-95 Gy (42.72 Gy median)	8.25 (mean)	5-yr OS 42% 5-yr DSS 40% (89%, 36%, 19% for <2, 2-4, >4 cm) LR 8 pts LR+DM 15 pts DM 4 pts	Size and histology
Gheiler et al. Wayne State U 1998 (23)	21 (11 were males)	Ta-4, N0-2	2 Urethrectomy 4 chemo+RT+exent 2 exent alone 2 chemoRT (5-FU, CDDP, MVAC)	45 Gy pelvis 25-30 Gy boost	3.5 (mean)	OS 62% (89%, low vs 42%, high stage)	Clinical stage
Garden et al. MDA 1993 (21)	97	T1-4, N0-N+	86 LE+RT : (35 RT + Brachy, 21 RT 30 Brachy) 11 preop RT/cyto-urethrectomy or exent	40-106 Gy (65 median) Brachy 45-75 Gy (60 median)	8.75 (median)	5-yr AS 41% 10-yr AS 31% 15-yr AS 22% LC 64% (RT only)	Local extension, fixation, and involvement of entire urethra

LE, local excision; RT, radiation therapy; exent, exenteration; chemo, chemotherapy; Part, partial; brachy, brachytherapy; CSS, cancer specific survival; CS, crude survival; LR, local recurrence; DM, distant metastasis; UTHSCSA, UTHSCSA, HDR, high-dose-rate; MSKCC, Memorial Sloan-Kettering Cancer Center; MIR, Mallinckrodt Institution of Radiology; preop, preoperative; adj, adjuvant; DSS, disease-specific survival; pts, patients; 5-FU, 5-fluorouacil; CDDP, cisplatin; MVAC, methotrexate, vinblastine, adriamycin, cisplatin; MDA, MD Anderson Cancer Center; AS, actuarial survival; LC, local control.

Radiation Therapy

Although DiMarco et al. (14) found that adjuvant radiation did not improve local control or survival in the study of 53 female patients urethral carcinoma,, treatment selection bias may have played a role as the higher stage tumors tended to receive adjuvant radiation therapy. Eng et a;. (17) reported only one of six patients with low-stage disease was referred for adjuvant radiation therapy, whereas four of five patients with advanced disease received radiation therapy. The one who did not receive radiation died 10 months after surgery.

Control of tumors of the urethral meatus or the distal urethra with irradiation alone is often satisfactory. Early meatal tumors have cure rates of 70% to 90% (54). Chu (7) reported a 5-year progression-free survival rate of 64% for 11 patients with tumor involvement of the anterior urethra treated with irradiation alone. Prempree et al. (54) treated three patients with stage I disease with interstitial irradiation alone (50 to 65 Gy) and achieved local control in all three. In the same series, two of four patients with stage II disease achieved local control and were alive 5 years after treatment. Weghaupt et al. (68) reported a 5-year survival rate of 71% for 42 patients with cancer of the anterior urethra. Their doses ranged from 55 to 70 Gy from intracavitary and external irradiation. Princess Margaret Hospital reported an 87% relapse-free survival rate in patients with stage I or II disease (45). The majority of patients with small primary tumors received brachytherapy as a component of their treatment. Patients receiving brachytherapy and external-beam radiation therapy had a median total dose of 65 Gy.

Tumors of the proximal urethra or the entire urethra are more difficult to treat. The overall local control rate is 20% to 30%. Bracken et al. (5) treated 81 patients, and the 5-year survival rate was approximately 25% for patients with stage III and 20% for those with stage IV disease. Princess Margaret Hospital reported stage III and IV tumors to have cause-specific survival rates of 26% and 16%, respectively (43). Weghaupt et al. (68) reported 20 patients with tumor involvement of the posterior urethra who received irradiation alone or preoperative irradiation and surgery. The 5-year survival rate for these patients was 50%. Garden et al. (21) treated 86 patients with irradiation only after excision or biopsy of the primary lesion. Radiation doses ranged from 40 to 106 Gy (median, 65 Gy). The 5-year disease-specific survival rate was 40%, and the 5-year local control rate was 64%. Preoperative irradiation combined with radical surgery is an approach used by Klein et al. (37). They treated five women in this manner and achieved a 5-year survival rate of 40%. Dalbagni et al. (8) used anterior pelvic exenteration with intraoperative tumor bed interstitial brachytherapy using ^{192}Ir, followed several weeks later by pelvic external beam radiation therapy. A variety of chemosensitizing agents were used. The median brachytherapy dose was 15 Gy and pelvic radiation therapy given was 45 Gy. Local control was achieved in four of six women with T2 and T4 disease.

Chemotherapy

Gheiler et al. (23) reported a disease-free survival rate of 60% in selected patients with advanced T3 or higher disease treated with a multimodality regimen consisting of neoadjuvant chemotherapy and radiation therapy. A phase 2 study has shown the combination of ifosfamide, paclitaxel, and cisplatin used in 45 patients with advanced transitional carcinoma of the urothelial tract is well tolerated and results in a median survival of 20 months (3). Similar encouraging results have been reported in patients with advanced urethral cancer receiving concomitant fluorouracil, mitomycin C, and radiation therapy (31,35,60).

Sequelae of Therapy

Complications as a result of surgery, irradiation, or combined-modality therapy vary greatly, from 0% to 42%, because of different tumor stages, the extent of surgery, and various irradiation doses (5,7,32,53). Garden et al. (21) reported that 27 of 55 patients (49%) achieving local control had complications, including urethral stenosis, fistula, necrosis, cystitis, and hemorrhage. Urethral strictures develop in some patients, necessitating dilatation or urinary diversion. Others may experience incontinence, cystitis, and vaginal stenosis. Severe complications include fistula formation, bowel obstruction, and, occasionally, operative death. In the case of advanced neoplasms, fistula formation may be unavoidable because of tumor erosion of adjacent organs and subsequent tumor necrosis. Unlike the male counterpart, the physical loss of the female urethra is not uniformly associated with sexual impotence; nevertheless, the associated treatment side effects and negative self-image may affect quality of life.

Future Direction

Most clinical information comes from retrospective case series accumulated over a long span of time using various treatment modalities. Clinical trials are needed to obtain prospective data. Improved knowledge of tumor and normal tissue radiobiology and continued technological advances in external-beam radiation therapy and brachytherapy delivery will minimize some of the treatment-related complications.

Acknowledgment

The author thanks Drs. David H. Hussey and Join Y. Luh (Department of Radiation Oncology, University of Texas Health Science Center at San Antonio) for their invaluable comments and suggestions.

References

1. Ali SZ, Smilari TF, Gal D, et al. Primary adenoid cystic carcinoma of Skene's glands. *Gynecol Oncol* 1995;57:257–261.
2. Aragona F, Maio G, Piazza R, et al. Primary malignant melanoma of the female urethra: A case report. *Int Urol Nephrol* 1995;27:107–111.
3. Bajorin DF, McCaffrey JA, Dodd PM, et al. Ifosfamide, paclitaxel and cisplatin for patients with advanced transitional cell carcinoma of the urothelial tract: Final report of a phase II trial evaluating two dose schedules. *Cancer* 2000;88:1671–1678.
4. Barbagli G, Natali A, Urso C, et al. Primary malignant melanoma of the female urethra: A case report with immunohistochemical findings. *Urol Int* 1988;43:110–112.
5. Bracken RB, Johnson DE, Miller JS, et al. Primary carcinoma of the female urethra. *J Urol* 1976;116:188–192.
6. Chen ME, Pisters LL, Malpica A, et al. Risk of urethral, vaginal and cervical involvement in patients undergoing radical cystectomy for bladder cancer: Results of a contemporary cystectomy series from M.D. Anderson Cancer Center. *J Urol* 1997;157:2120–2123.
7. Chu AM. Female urethral carcinoma. *Radiology* 1973;107:627–630.
8. Dalbagni G, Donat SM, Eschwege P, et al. Results of high dose rate brachytherapy, anterior pelvic exenteration, and external beam radiotherapy for carcinoma of the female urethra. *J Urol* 2001;166:1759–1761.
9. Dalbagni G, Zhang ZF, Lacombe L, et al. Female urethral carcinoma: An analysis of treatment outcome and a plea for a standardized management strategy. *Br J Urol* 1998;82:835–841.
10. Dann T, Schuller J, Schmeller NT, et al. Behandlung des distalen Urethrakarzinoms durch Laserkoagulation. *Urologe A* 1989;28:296.
11. De Paepe ME, Andre R, Mahadevia P. Urethral involvement in female patients with bladder cancer. A study of 22 cystectomy specimens. *Cancer* 1990;65:1237–1241.
12. Delcos L. Carcinoma of the female urethra. In: Johnson DE, Boileau MA, eds. *Genitourinary tumors*. New York: Grune & Stratton; 1982:275–286.
13. Desai S, Libertino JA, Zinman L. Primary carcinoma of the female urethra. *J Urol* 1973;110:693–695.
14. DiMarco DS, DiMarco CS, Zincke H, et al. Surgical treatment for local control of female urethral carcinoma. *Urol Oncol* 2004;22:404–409.

15. Ebisuno S, Miyai M, Nagareda T. Clear cell adenocarcinoma of the female urethra showing positive staining with antibodies to prostate-specific antigen and prostatic acid phosphatase. *Urology* 1995;45:682–685.
16. Eisenberger MA. Chemotherapy for carcinomas of the penis and urethra. *Urol Clin North Am* 1992;19:333–338.
17. Eng TY, Naguib M, Galang T, et al. Retrospective study of the treatment of urethral cancer. *Am J Clin Oncol* 2003;26:558–562.
18. Fisher M, Hricak H, Reinhold C, et al. Female urethral carcinoma: MRI staging. *Am J Radiol* 1985;144:603–604.
19. Foens CS, Hussey DH, Staples JJ, et al. A comparison of the roles of surgery and radiation therapy in the management of carcinoma of the female urethra. *Int J Radiat Oncol Biol Phys* 1991;21:961–968.
20. Forman JD, Lichter AS. The role of radiation therapy in the management of the male and female urethra. *Urol Clin North Am* 1992;19:383–389.
21. Garden AS, Zagars GK, Delclos L. Primary carcinoma of the female urethra: Results of radiation therapy. *Cancer* 1993;71:3102–3108.
22. Gerbaulet A, Haie-Meder C, Marsiglia H, et al. Brachytherapy in cancer of the urethra. *Ann Urol* 1994;28:312–317.
23. Gheiler EL, Tefilli MV, Tiguert R, et al. Management of primary urethral cancer. *Urol* 1998;52:487–493.
24. Golimbu M, Al-Askari S, Morales P. Transpubic approach for lower urinary tract surgery: A 15-year experience. *J Urol* 1990;143:72–76.
25. Grabstald H, Hilaris B, Henschke U, et al. Cancer of the female urethra. *JAMA* 1966;197:835–842.
26. Grabstald H. Tumors of the urethra in men and women. *Cancer* 1973;32:1236–1255.
27. Greene FL, Page DL, Fleming ID, et al., eds. *AJCC cancer staging manual*, 6th ed. Philadelphia: Lippincott-Raven; 2002.
28. Grigsby PW, Corn B. Localized urethral tumors in women: Indications for conservative versus exenterative therapies. *J Urol* 1992;147:1516–1520.
29. Grigsby PW. Carcinoma of the urethra in women. *Int J Radiat Oncol Biol Phys* 1998;41:535–541.
30. Hahn P, Krepart G, Malaker K. Carcinoma of the female urethra: Manitoba experience, 1958–1987. *Urol* 1991;37:106–109.
31. Hara I, Hikosaka S, Eto H, et al. Successful treatment for squamous cell carcinoma of the female urethra with combined radio- and chemotherapy. *Int J Urol* 2004;11:678–682.
32. Hedden RJ, Husseinzadeh N, Bracken RB. Bladder sparing surgery for locally advanced female urethral cancer. *J Urol* 1993;150:1135–1137.
33. Hopkins SC, Grabstald H. Benign and malignant tumors of the male and female urethra. In: Walsh PC, Gittes RF, Perlmutter AD, et al., eds. *Campbell's urology*, 5th ed. Philadelphia: WB Saunders; 1986:1441–1462.
34. Johnson DE, O'Connell JR. Primary carcinoma of the female urethra. *Urol* 1983;21:42–45.
35. Johnson DW, Kessler JF, Ferrigini RG, et al. Low dose combined chemotherapy/radiotherapy in the management of locally advanced urethral squamous cell carcinoma. *J Urol* 1989;141:615–616.
36. Kakizaki H, Nakada T, Sugano O, et al. Malignant lymphoma in the female urethra. *Int J Urol* 1994;1:281–282.
37. Klein FA, Whitmore WF, Herr HW, et al. Inferior pubic rami resection with en bloc radical excision for invasive proximal urethral carcinoma. *Cancer* 1983;51:1238–1242.
38. Kuettel MR, Parda DS, Harter KW, et al. Treatment of female urethral carcinoma in medically inoperable patients using external beam irradiation and high dose rate intracavitary brachytherapy. *J Urol* 1997;157:1669–1671.
39. Levine RL. Urethral cancer. *Cancer* 1980;45:1965–1972.
40. Licht MR, Klein EA, Bukowski R, et al. Combination radiation and chemotherapy for the treatment of squamous cell carcinoma of the male and female urethra. *J Urol* 1995;153:1918–1920.
41. Lopez AE, Latiff GA, Ciancio G, et al. Lymphoma of urethra in patient with acquired immune deficiency syndrome. *Urology* 1993;42:596–598.
42. Mayer R, Fowler JE Jr, Clayton M. Localized urethral cancer in women. *Cancer* 1987;60:1548–1551.
43. Meis JM, Ayala AG, Johnson DE. Adenocarcinoma of the urethra in women: A clinicopathologic study. *Cancer* 1987;60:1038–1052.
44. Millan-Rodriguez F, Montlleo-Gonzalez M, Rosales-Bordes A, et al. Kaposi's sarcoma of the urethral meatus: Management by urethral dilatation. *Br J Urol* 1995;75:558.
45. Milosevic MF, Warde PR, Banerjee D, et al. Urethral carcinoma in women: Results of treatment with primary radiotherapy. *Radiother Oncol* 2000;56:29–35.
46. Moinuddin Ali M, Klein FA, et al. Primary female urethral carcinoma: A retrospective comparison of different treatment techniques. *Cancer* 1988;62:54–57.
47. Morikawa K, Togashi K, Minami S, et al. MR and CT appearance of urethral clear cell adenocarcinoma in a woman. *J Comput Assist Tomogr* 1995;19:1001–1003.
48. Nakamura Y, Takahashi M, Suga A, et al. A case of adenocarcinoma arising within a urethral diverticulum diagnosed only by the surgical specimen. *Gynecol Obstet Invest* 1995;40:69–70.
49. Narayan P, Konety B. Surgical treatment of female urethral carcinoma. *Urol Clin North Am* 1992;19:373–382.
50. Nash PA, Bihrle R, Gleason PE, et al. Mohs' micrographic surgery and distal urethrectomy with immediate urethral reconstruction for glandular carcinoma in situ with significant urethral extension. *Urology* 1996;47:108–110.
51. Ohsawa M, Mishima K, Suzuki A, et al. Malignant lymphoma of the urethra: Report of a case with detection of Epstein-Barr virus genome in the tumour cells. *Histopathology* 1994;24:525–529.
52. Peterson DT, Dockerty MB, Utz DC, et al. The peril of primary carcinoma of the urethra in women. *J Urol* 1973;110:72–75.
53. Pointon RCS, Poole-Wilson DS. Primary carcinoma of the urethra. *Br J Urol* 1968;40:682–693.
54. Prempree T, Amornmarn R, Patanaphan V. Radiation therapy in primary carcinoma of the female urethra: II. An update on results. *Cancer* 1984;54:729–733.
55. Quick HH, Serfaty JM, Pannu HK, et al. Endourethral MRI. *Magn Reson Med* 2001;45:138–146.
56. Rajan N, Tucci P, Mallouh C, et al. Carcinoma in female urethral diverticulum: Case reports and review of management. *J Urol* 1993;150:1911–1914.
57. Sailer SL, Shipley WU, Wang CC. Carcinoma of the female urethra: A review of results with radiation therapy. *J Urol* 1988;140:1–5.
58. Seballos RM, Rich RR. Clear cell adenocarcinoma arising from a urethral diverticulum. *J Urol* 1995;153:1914–1915.
59. Selch MT, Mark RJ, Fu YS, et al. Primary lymphoma of female urethra: Long-term control by radiation therapy. *Urology* 1993;42:343–346.
60. Shah AB, Kalra JK, Silber L, et al. Squamous cell cancer of female urethra. Successful treatment with chemoradiotherapy. *Urol* 1985;25:284–286.
61. Skarlos DV, Aravantinos G, Linardou E, et al. Chemotherapy with methotrexate, vinblastine, epirubicin and carboplatin (Carbo-MVE) in transitional cell urothelial cancer. A Hellenic Co-Operative Oncology Group study. *Eur Urol* 1997;31:420–427.
62. Srinivas V, Khan SA. Female urethral cancer: An overview. *Int Urol Nephrol* 1987;19:423–427.
63. Taggart CG, Castro JR, Rutledge FN. Carcinoma of the female urethra. *AJR Am J Roentgenol* 1972;114:145–151.
64. Thyavihally YB, Wuntkal R, Bakshi G, et al. Primary carcinoma of the female urethra: Single center experience of 18 cases. *Jp J Clin Oncol* 2005;35:84–87.
65. Touijer AK, Dalbagni G. Role of voided urine cytology in diagnosing primary urethral carcinoma. *Urology* 2004;63:33–35.
66. Turner AG, Hendry WF. Primary carcinoma of the female urethra. *Br J Urol* 1980;52:549–554.
67. Vapnek JM, Turzan CW. Primary malignant lymphoma of the female urethra: A report of a case and review of the literature. *J Urol* 1992;147:701–703.
68. Weghaupt K, Gerstner GJ, Kucera H. Radiation therapy for primary carcinoma of the female urethra: A survey over 25 years. *Gynecol Oncol* 1984;17:58–63.
69. Weiner JS, Walther PJ. A high association of oncogenic human papillomaviruses with carcinomas of the female urethra: Polymerase chain reaction-based analysis of multiple histological types. *J Urol* 1994;151:49–53.

Clinical Radiation Oncology

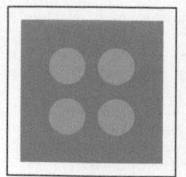

Chapter 72
Carcinoma of the Vulva

Gustavo S. Montana, Song K. Kang

Anatomy

The vulva is composed of the mons pubis, clitoris, labia majora and the minora, vaginal vestibule, and their supporting subcutaneous tissues. The vulva blends with the urinary meatus anteriorly and with the perineum and anus posteriorly. The mons pubis is a prominent mound of subcutaneous connective and adipose tissue located anteriorly to the pubic symphysis. After puberty the mons is covered with pubic hair. The labia majora are two elongated skin folds that course posteriorly from the mons pubis and blend into the perineal body. The skin of the labia majora is pigmented and contains hair follicles and sebaceous glands. The labia minora are a smaller pair of skin folds located between the labia majora; they extend posteriorly to form the margin of the vaginal vestibule. Anteriorly, the labia minora separates into two components that course above and below the clitoris, fusing with those of the opposite side to form the prepuce and frenulum, respectively. The skin of the labia minora contains numerous sebaceous glands but no hair follicles and has no underlying adipose tissue. The clitoris is 2 to 3 cm anterior to the urethral meatus and is supported externally by the fusion of the labia minora. The clitoris is composed of erectile tissue organized into the glans, body, and two crura, which course laterally, covered by the ischiocavernosus muscles and attach to the ischium.

The vaginal vestibule is in the center of the vulva and is demarcated laterally by the labia minora and posteriorly by the perineal body. Anteriorly, numerous small vestibular glands are located beneath the mucosa and open onto its surface adjacent to the urethral meatus. The Bartholin glands, two small mucous secreting glands, are situated within the subcutaneous tissue of the posterior labia majora. The ducts of the Bartholin glands open onto the posterolateral portion of the vestibule. The perineal body is a 3 to 4 cm band of skin that separates the vaginal vestibule from the anus and forms the posterior margin of the vulva (22).

The lymphatics of the labia drain into the superficial inguinal and femoral lymph nodes, located anteriorly to the cribriform fascia and fascia lata. The lymphatics then penetrate the cribriform fascia and reach the deep femoral nodes. The lymphatics of the fourchette, perineum, and prepuce follow the lymphatics of the labia. The lymph from the glans clitoris can drain not only to the superficial femoral nodes but also to the deep femoral and pelvic lymph nodes. Some lymphatics originating in the clitoris may enter the pelvis directly, bypassing the femoral nodes to connect with the obturator and external iliac lymph nodes (Fig. 72.1A). There are superficial inguinal lymph nodes that lie along the saphenous vein and its branches between Camper's fascia and the cribriform fascia overlying the femoral vessels. The superficial nodes are located within the triangle formed by the inguinal ligament superiorly, the border of the sartorius muscle laterally, and the border of the adductor longus muscle medially (Fig. 72.1B). There are usually three to five deep nodes, the most superior of which is located under the inguinal ligament and is known as Cloquet's node (22). From these nodes the lymph drains into the external and common iliac pelvic lymph nodes.

Epidemiology

Vulvar cancer is a rare malignancy that represents only about 1% to 2% of all the cancers diagnosed in women and about 3% to 4% of all gynecologic neoplasms (116). The incidence of this malignancy is 0.5 to 2 cases per 100,000 women, with a much higher incidence in women 70 years of age or older (53,137). Whereas this is true for invasive cancer, recent reports show a change in the incidence rates and peak age of *in situ* cancer (129). The annual incidence of carcinoma *in situ*, for all races combined, nearly doubled from the 1973–1976 period to that of 1985–1987. The largest proportional increase occurred in white women younger than 35 years of age, among whom the rate nearly tripled (129). At the same time, the incidence rate of invasive cancer remained stable in the periods of time studied. These changes in the incidence rates and age for carcinoma *in situ* are attributed, at least in part, to changes in sexual practices (21,124).

Patients with vulvar cancer, intraepithelial and invasive, have a higher incidence of nongenital second primary tumors than the general population (1,29). The majority of the secondary malignancies are tumors of the anogenital region, particularly of the cervix (30,52,76). In the series of Choo and Morley (30), the incidence of secondary carcinoma of the cervix was 33.5% for patients with intraepithelial neoplasia and 16% for patients with invasive carcinoma. There is no explanation for the increased incidence of nongynecologic tumors in patients with vulvar cancer. As for the increased incidence of second neoplasms of the anogenital region, some factors that can account for this are embryologic interrelation of the lower urogenital tract, infection with the human papilloma virus, and with herpes simplex virus (96,109).

Patients who are immunosuppressed, such as renal transplant patients, also have a higher incidence of cancer of the vulva (104). Other conditions that predispose patients to carcinoma of the vulva are leukoplakia, genital urinary cancer, and history of employment in the laundry and cleaning industries (92). Similar to carcinoma of the cervix, some observers have reported the incidence of vulvar cancer being up to three times higher in women of lower socioeconomic class. The increased frequency in patients afflicted with other gynecologic malignancies suggests common predisposing or etiologic factors.

Natural History

According to data collected by Plentl and Friedman (110), approximately 71% of the malignancies arise in the labia majora and minora, 14% in the clitoris, 5% in the perineum and fourchette, 5% in the prepuce Bartholin's glands and urethra, and 5% are too extensive at presentation to classify.

Carcinomas arising in the vulvar area ordinarily follow a predictable pattern of spread to the regional lymphatic nodes. The superficial inguinofemoral lymph nodes are usually involved first and then the disease may spread to the deep inguinofemoral nodes. For well-lateralized lesions, metastasis to the contralateral inguinal or pelvic lymph nodes is unusual in

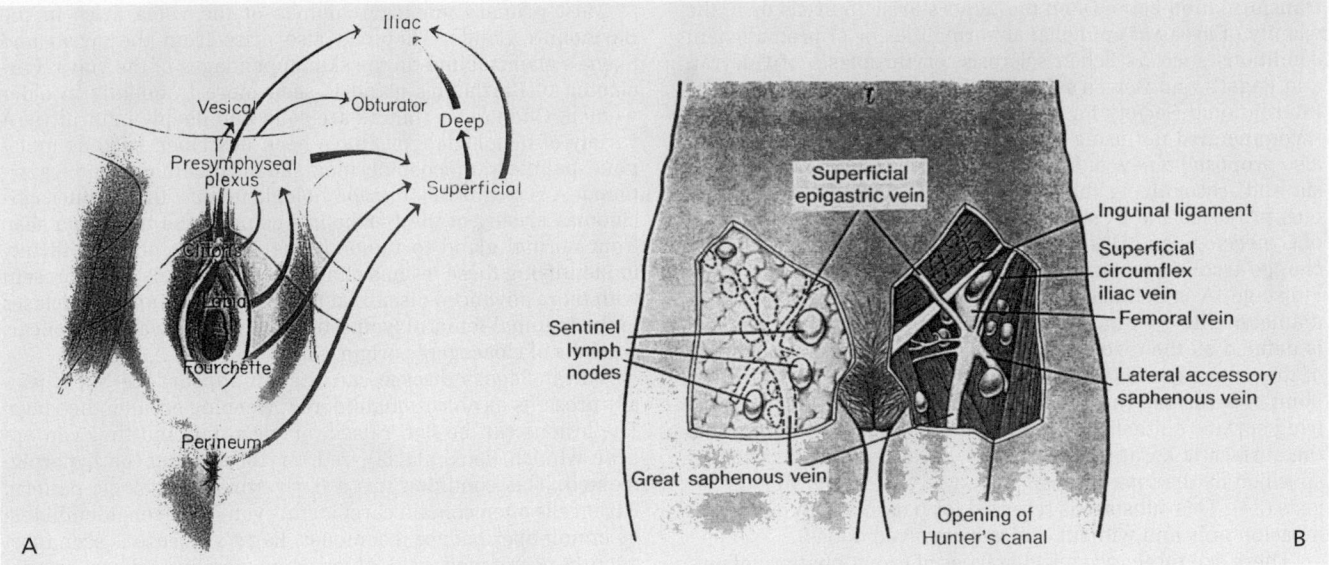

FIGURE 72.1. **A:** The lymphatic drainage of the vulva initially flows to the superficial inguinal nodes then to the deep femoral and iliac group. Drainage from midline structures may flow directly beneath the symphysis to the pelvic nodes. (Reprinted from Plentl AA, Friedman EA, eds. *Lymphatic system of the female genitalia.* Philadelphia: W.B. Saunders Co., 1971, with permission.) **B:** The superficial inguinal lymph nodes comprise 8 to 10 subcutaneous nodes located between Camper's fascia and the cribriform fascia. These nodes are immediately adjacent to the saphenous vein and its branches. (Reprinted from DiSaia PJ, Creasman WT, Rich WM. An alternative approach to early cancer of the vulva. *Am J Obstet Gynecol* 1979;133:825–832, with permission.)

the absence of ipsilateral inguinofemoral node involvement. Although lesions arising in or involving the glans clitoris or urethra theoretically can spread directly to pelvic lymph nodes, involvement of the pelvic nodes without involvement of the inguinal nodes is rare (53,84).

The frequency of inguinal lymph node metastasis in surgically staged patients ranges from 6% to 50%, depending on tumor invasion and extent of disease (19,42,61,67,103,120) (Table 72.1). Plentl and Friedman (110) reported a 62% incidence of lymph node metastases in patients with clinically palpable adenopathy and 35% in patients without clinically palpable adenopathy. In a review of clinical staging, Franklin (51) noted that approximately 75% of patients with clinically suspicious lymph nodes had nodal metastasis, and 11% to 43% of patients with clinically negative nodes had metastasis to the nodes. In a Gynecologic Oncology Group (GOG) study reported by Homesley et al. (70), 23.9% of the patients who had no palpable inguinal nodes, or had nodes that were considered normal, were found to have nodal metastasis in the surgical specimen.

When the lymph nodes were clinically suspicious, 76.2% of the patients had histologically positive nodes. In patients who have histologically positive inguinal nodes, the probability of having positive pelvic nodes is about 30% (32,70). Hematogenous dissemination generally occurs late in the natural history of the disease. The most common sites of metastatic disease are the lungs, liver, and bones.

Clinical Presentation

The diagnosis of invasive vulvar cancer is usually made because of patient's symptoms and rarely as an incidental finding. The symptoms are pruritus, spotting or bleeding, pain, and discharge. Often, the patients report having had symptoms for a long time and by the time they seek medical attention they have an obvious lesion. Depending on the extent and the location of the tumor, patients may also complain of dysuria, difficulty with defecation, and may also report difficulty or discomfort with intercourse. Most of the time, patients are not aware of or do not complain about the inguinal nodes until they become quite large. It is rare to have patients present with very advanced nodal disease or with edema of the lower extremities secondary to disease in the groins.

Pathology

Although a variety of tumors can develop in the vulvar area, most, about 85%, are squamous cell type (73). The remaining tumors are made up by melanomas, basaloid (cloacogenic), adenocarcinomas usually arising in the Bartholin's glands, neuroendocrine carcinomas (Merkel cell), and sarcomas.

Epidermoid Carcinoma

There are certain pathologic features that set epidermoid tumors apart from tumors in other parts of the female genital tract. Tumors of the vulva arise within squamous epithelium but, unlike tumors in the cervix, the vulva does not have a

Table 72.1	**INCIDENCE OF LYMPH NODE INVOLVEMENT CORRELATED WITH PRIMARY TUMOR SIZE AND EXTENT**	
Primary Tumor Size and Depth of Invasion	**No. of Patients**	**No. (%) of Patients with Positive Lymph Nodes**
Depth		
<1 mm	120	0 (0)
1.1–2 mm	121	8 (6.6)
2.1–3 mm	97	8 (8.2)
3.1–4 mm	50	11 (22)
4.1–5 mm	40	10 (25)
Size		
>5 mm	32	12 (37.5)
>2 cm	168	77 (45.8)
Any size primary tumor extending beyond the vulva	70	38 (54.2)

Adapted from Perez CA, Grigsby PW, Chao C. Vulva. In: Perez CA, Brady LW, eds. *Principles and practice of radiation oncology,* 3rd ed. Philadelphia: Lippincott-Raven; 1997.

transformation zone. Often the tumors arise in areas or in the vicinity of areas of epithelial abnormalities or of premalignant conditions such as lichen sclerosis, erythroplasia of Queyrat, and Paget's and Bowen's disease (26). To avoid confusion, the International Society for the Study of Vulvar Disease (ISSVD) recommended not using the term *dystrophy* (115). The ISSVD also proposed a new definition of vulvar intraepithelial neoplasia and, recognizing that the term *microinvasion* is ambiguous, proposed the IA substage in the International Federation of Gynecology and Obstetrics (FIGO) stage I classification. This change accounts for size of the tumor and depth of invasion (80). Substage IA is defined as a single lesion measuring ≤2 cm in diameter with ≤1 mm depth of invasion. The depth of invasion is defined as the distance from the epithelial stromal junction of the most superficial adjacent dermal papillae to the deepest point of invasion. Tumor thickness is measured from the overlying surface epithelium, or the bottom of the granular layer if the surface is keratinized, to the deepest point of invasion as specified by the International Society of Gynecological Pathologists (34). This substage is reserved for patients with one site of invasion only and without clinically involved nodes.

There are three recognizable types of growth pattern of epidermoid carcinoma: (a) confluent, (b) compact, and (c) fingerlike growth. Confluent growth is defined as a tumor mass composed of interconnected tumor exceeding 1 mm in dimension. This type of growth is characteristic for being deeply invasive, associated with stromal desmoplasia. Compact growth is a type of growth associated with well-differentiated tumors that maintain continuity with the overlying epithelium and infiltrate as a well-defined and circumscribed tumor mass, without separate islands of infiltrating tumor, away from the main tumor mass. This type of tumor rarely invades the vascular space. The cells in these tumors resemble the squamous cells of the adjacent and overlaying epithelium. The spray or fingerlike growth pattern is characterized by a trabecular appearance with small islands of poorly differentiated tumor cells found within the dermis or submucosa, deeper than the main tumor mass. These tumors are often associated with desmoplastic stromal response and a lymphocytic inflammatory infiltrate. Vascular space involvement is seen more commonly with this pattern of growth than with tumors with a compact pattern of growth (146). There are variants of squamous cell carcinoma of the vulva such as adenoid squamous cell carcinoma, squamous cell carcinoma with giant tumor cells, sebaceous cell carcinoma, spindle squamous cell carcinoma, and squamous carcinoma with sarcomalike stroma.

Uncommon Histologic Types

Malignant melanoma of the vulva is a very distinct entity and accounts for approximately 10% of all primary tumors of the vulva (31). These tumors are seen more often in white women with a peak incidence in the sixth and seventh decades. Sometimes the tumor arises in a pre-existing pigmented lesion and in the differential diagnosis vulvar melanosis needs to be considered. Vulvar melanomas can be subclassified into three specific categories: superficial spreading malignant melanoma, nodular melanoma, and acral lentiginous melanoma (11). As is the case for melanomas in other sites, the level of invasion and the tumor thickness are features that dictate the therapy and determine the prognosis (77). Like their counterparts in other parts of the body, vulvar melanomas can metastasize to other organs.

Merkle cell tumors can arise in the vulva. These tumors are rare and they carry a poor prognosis. Morphologically, they resemble the neuroendocrine tumors seen in other sites. These tumors contain neuron-specific enolase and low-molecular-weight keratin. The keratin stains as a distinct perinuclear cytoplasmic dot. The neurosecretory granules can be identified by electron microscopy.

Most primary adenocarcinomas of the vulva arise in the Bartholin's glands. They can also arise from the sweat and Skene's glands found on the skin appendages of the vulva. Carcinoma of Bartholin's gland is seen more frequently in older women. Often these tumors are solid and deeply infiltrative. A variety of histologic types have been described such as mucinous, papillary, mucoepidermoid, adenosquamous, and transitional. A recognizable histopathologic feature that defines carcinomas arising in the Bartholin's gland is the transition seen from normal gland to tumor tissue. Because of the difficulty in identifying these lesions clinically, the patients often present with more advanced disease at the primary site and metastases to the inguinal-femoral lymph nodes. There are also adenocarcinomas of cloacogenic origin.

Vulvar Paget's disease can vary in appearance but it usually presents as an eczematoid, red, weeping area on the vulva. The lesions can be flat, raised, or ulcerated and they can appear whitish (leukoplakia), red (erythroplastic), or hyperpigmented. This condition has a fairly typical histologic pattern. Paget cells often contain carcinoembryonic antigen, identifiable by immunoperoxidase techniques. Paget's disease is seen most often in postmenopausal, older white women and can be mistakenly diagnosed as eczema or contact dermatitis. Paget's disease in the vulvar region is analogous to that of the breast and is associated with invasive carcinoma in about 20% to 30% of the cases (66). Approximately 15% of the patients have an associated underlying adenocarcinoma of the apocrine or the Bartholin's glands.

Verrucous carcinomas of the vulva are rare and are usually found in patients in their fifth or sixth decade of life. These tumors may be well differentiated and have a relatively low incidence of lymph nodes, and in general they have a good prognosis (8), providing they can be treated surgically. Basal cell carcinomas arising in the vulva do occur but they are rare (9).

Transitional cell carcinomas have also been described in the vulva. In some instances they actually represent metastases from primary sites elsewhere in the lower urinary tract.

▪▪ | Prognostic Factors

Lymph node metastasis is the single most important prognostic factor in patients with vulvar cancer. The presence of inguinal node metastases results in about a 50% reduction in long-term survival (47,50). Determining the status of the nodes is extremely important as this has significant impact on the overall treatment approach and also has significant bearing on the prognosis. There are different ways to establish the status of the lymph nodes. These methods are complementary and sometimes more than one method is used. Surgical treatment of the nodes, particularly when combined with radiation, can cause morbidity that should be avoided if it is determined that the nodes are not involved or that the probability of nodal involvement is very low. Conversely, recurrence in the lymph node areas is almost always fatal. Clinical evaluation of the nodes by careful palpation should not be ignored but it can be misleading. As many as 23.9% of patients who are not overweight and do not have palpable nodes can be found to have positive nodes histologically (70). With computed tomography (CT) and magnetic resonance (MR) scans, enlarged or suspicious lymph nodes can be identified in the groins and pelvis and they can be biopsied, if they are accessible. Although both of these tests lack specificity, they can help with staging of the patients. The CT scan also provides information about the depth of the nodes in the inguinal area. This information may be useful for future radiation treatment planning. The CT and MR scans may reveal extension of the disease to adjacent organs like the bladder and the rectum. With these noninvasive methods it is possible to stage patients more accurately and to decide on a course of therapy. In the end, decisions about the management of the inguinal and pelvic nodes are made on the basis of the extent of the primary tumor and the evaluation of the groins.

Multiple clinical and histologic features of the primary tumor predict for nodal metastasis and determine prognosis. Some of these features are tumor thickness, histologic grade, capillary-like space involvement, depth of invasion, location of the tumor, and tumor size (15,123). Rutledge et al. (121) also described the adverse effect on local control and survival of tumor size, clinical stage, therapy aim, positive inguinal or pelvic nodes, and positive margins. When the tumor thickness is ≤1 mm, the probability of nodal metastasis is very small; 3.1% or less, but with tumor a tumor thickness ≥5 mm, the probability is about 33.3%. It should be noted that in the vulvar area the thickness of the epithelium varies significantly from one area to another, in some areas being as much as 0.77 mm thick, and this can influence the relative value given to tumor thickness and depth of invasion. Measuring tumor thickness in superficially ulcerated tumors can be misleading and may lead to underestimating the depth of invasion. Depth of invasion of 1, 2, and 3 mm corresponds to a 4.3%, 7.8%, and 17% incidence of nodal involvement, respectively. Perineural invasion is also strongly associated with lymph node metastasis (118).

Kurzl and Masserer (85) analyzed 124 patients with various stages of vulvar carcinoma treated with simple vulvectomy alone and local/inguinal irradiation. They found that age, disassociated growth, lymphatic spread, thickness, and ulceration of the primary tumor were important prognostic factors. Unfortunately, these features, except for ulceration, are not recognized clinically and cannot be incorporated in the clinical staging and thus taken into account when treatment is being planned.

In the detailed analysis of GOG Protocol No. 36, two significant risk factors were identified that predispose for recurrence in the vulva: (a) tumor size >4 cm, and (b) capillary lymphatic space involvement. If either of these factors was present, the risk of local recurrence after radical vulvectomy was 20.7% (30/184), but if neither factor was present, the risk of local recurrence was only 9.2% (37/404). In this study, the depth of invasion did not predict for vulvar failure (69).

In analysis of the GOG database on carcinoma of the vulva, several clinical and histologic tumor characteristics were identified as predictors of nodal involvement. In order of importance these are clinical node status (palpable vs. nonpalpable), GOG grade, capillary-lymphatic space involvement, tumor thickness, and patient's age (69,70,123). According to the size of the primary lesion, the incidence of inguinal node metastasis was 18.9% for patients with lesions ≤2 cm in diameter and 41.6% for patients with lesions >2 cm in diameter.

A significant effort is made now to identify patients without involvement of the inguinal nodes in whom node dissection can be avoided by considering the risk factors for nodal involvement.

Wharton (144) proposed not performing groin dissection for patients with small tumors with <5 mm of invasion. Later reports showed that 10% to 20% of these patients had occult groin metastases; thus, surgical evaluation of the nodes like with sentinel node biopsies may be indicated (16,39,42,60,79,88,99,103,114,134). Currently, the consensus is that lymph node dissection can be avoided in patients with tumors with <1 mm invasion (15,123). This is the rationale for the current staging system to assign tumors invading <1 mm to stage IA.

The incidence of lymph node involvement correlates with the size of the primary tumor (42,123). In the series of 66 patients reported by Donaldson et al. (42), the probability of having positive inguinal nodes rose from 18.9% for patients with lesions <3 cm to 72.4% for patients with primary tumors ≥3 cm. In a GOG study of 267 patients with superficial vulvar cancer reported by Sedlis et al. (123), the frequency of positive inguinal nodes was 18.1% for patients with lesions up to 3 cm in size

and 29.3% for patients with lesions ≥3 cm. There is also a correlation between the size of the primary tumor and the number and distribution of the nodes (69,70). Extension of the primary tumor to the urethra, vagina, and anal area is associated with an increased incidence of nodal involvement and worsening of prognosis. The significance of this is reflected in the stage assignment of the patients.

Extracapsular extension of the tumor in the lymph nodes has been noted in several series and it is know to have a negative effect on prognosis (102,138). Origoni et al. (102) studied both the size of the metastases in the lymph nodes, the number of positive lymph nodes, and extracapsular extension of the disease and found that the presence of any one of these factors worsened the prognosis. Extracapsular tumor extension as an adverse, independent prognostic factor on survival has been described also by van der Velden et al. (138).

In an analysis of formalin-fixed tissue specimens, Heaps et al. (64) demonstrated a sharp rise in the incidence of local recurrence for tumors with microscopic, surgical margins <8 mm. They suggested that this would correspond to a minimum margin of 1 cm in fresh, unfixed tissue. Although the frequency of local recurrences correlates with the adequacy of the margins of the surgical resection, when dealing with larger or thicker tumors, or when they involve midline structures, adequate surgical margins may be difficult to obtain.

It is evident that lymph node involvement is a very significant prognostic factor and that it is necessary to determine the status of the nodes to plan therapy and to provide a patient with prognostic information. The use of sentinel node biopsies to determine the pathologic status of the sentinel nodes, the first draining nodes of an anatomic region, that would also be representative of the pathology of the nonsentinel nodes in the region has been used for vulvar cancer successfully (39,79,88,99,114,134). The data on the studies conducted show that the sentinel node is identified in a very high percentage of patients, 97.5%. The sentinel node is involved in 13% to 41% of the cases, which maybe considered low; however, this reflects the early stage of the disease of the patients for whom this procedure is used. The false-negative rate is quite low, in the order of 6.5% (39,79,88,99,114,134).

Some surgeons routinely dissect the pelvis in patients with positive inguinal nodes; however, Curry et al. (37) noted that none of their patients with three or less positive, unilateral groin nodes had spread to the pelvic nodes. Similar findings have been reported by Hacker et al. (59). If both the superficial and the deep nodes are negative, the probability of pelvic node involvement is low. In the GOG study reported by Homesley et al. (68) of patients with positive inguinal nodes, the incidence of pelvic node involvement was 28.3% (15/23). In this study there was a correlation of pelvic node involvement with the extent of inguinal node involvement. The consensus is that the pelvic lymph nodes need not to be treated in patients without inguinal lymph node involvement; therefore, the status of the inguinal nodes determines the management of the pelvic nodes. Although deep pelvic node involvement is an ominous sign, one fourth to one third of the patients are still potentially curable, particularly if only a few nodes are involved (19,37,53).

⠿ | Staging

The staging system first adopted in 1983 was based on clinical findings. The system was modified in 1988, giving the clinical status of the nodes more importance. In 1997 the staging was revised again to create a separate category for minimally invasive lesions, stage IA (Table 72.2). In the current FIGO staging recommendations, all tumors >1 mm depth of invasion should have histologic assessment of the inguinal nodes. The status of the nodes bears on the prognosis and management of the

Table 72.2	**VULVAR CANCER STAGING**[a]		
2002 AJCC			**FIGO**
Tis	Carcinoma *in situ*.		0
T1a	Confined to vulva/perineum, size ≤2 cm, stromal invasion ≤1 mm.	N0	IA
T1b	Confined to vulva/perineum, size ≤2 cm, stromal invasion >1 mm.	N0	IB
T2	Confined to vulva/perineum, size >2 cm.	N0	II
T3	Adjacent spread to lower urethra and/or vagina or anus.		III
T4	Invades upper urethral mucosa, bladder mucosa, rectal mucosa, or it is fixed to pubic bone.		IVA
N1	Unilateral regional lymph node metastasis.		III
N2	Bilateral regional lymph node metastasis.		IVA
M1	Distant metastasis (Including pelvic lymph node metastasis).		IVB

The 2002 American Joint Committee on Cancer (AJCC) staging and corresponding International Federation of Gynecology and Obstetrics (FIGO) staging. According to the AJCC, femoral and inguinal nodes are considered regional spread, whereas iliac nodes are considered distant metastasis.

disease. For patients with advanced nodal disease, open biopsy of the nodes is not required for staging purposes; however, fine-needle aspiration is recommended as it is easy to perform and can provide documentation of the disease for therapeutic purposes and future reference. When the lesion is midline or when it involves both sides of the vulva, both inguinal regions need to be evaluated. Likewise, for lateralized lesions with positive inguinal nodes, evaluation of the contralateral side is recommended. In these cases, the status of the pelvic lymph nodes should be investigated, at least by noninvasive methods.

Diagnostic studies such as chest x-ray, CT and MR scans of the pelvis and abdomen and bone scans are not mandatory but are recommended based on the clinical stage of the disease. The CT and MR scans can identify enlarged nodes. These studies lack specificity but can help to identify suspicious nodes and or potential organ involvement so that biopsies can be directed to these sites. To complete the staging, procedures including cystoscopy and proctoscopy may be required, but the indications for these additional tests are determined by the location and extent of the primary lesion. The current staging system incorporates the lesion size and the clinical status of the lymph nodes as these variables are known to have bearing on prognosis. It also includes the recommendations of the ISSVD.

General Management

The treatment of carcinoma of the vulva is challenging for multiple reasons. In general, patients with this disease are older and have comorbidities. The tumor, by virtue of its location, can easily involve adjacent organs such as the bladder and the rectum and the frequency of nodal involvement is high. Because of its relatively low incidence, most published reports include rather small and heterogeneous groups of patients. Management of carcinoma of the vulva is further complicated by the major psychosexual impact that the treatment can have on the patients. For the aforementioned reasons, it has been difficult to study this disease and to develop treatment guidelines. In addition, the management of vulvar carcinoma has undergone very significant change in the last few decades. *En bloc* resection of the primary tumor and inguinal node dissection, which used to be the standard of care, has been replaced by multimodality therapy with the surgery being more tailored to the extent of the disease. This change follows the recognition of the morbidity associated with radical surgery, the improved results achieved with multimodality therapy, and the recognition of the negative impact that radical surgery can have on sexual function and body self-image (21,129,147). Although radical surgery retains an important place in the management of vulvar cancer,

surgery is no longer the mainstay of the treatment. If surgery is performed, it is not always necessary to perform a very radical procedure, as previously thought. The likelihood of controlling the primary tumor with surgery largely depends on the margins of resection rather than on the removal of the entire vulva. Clear margins of about 1 cm in all directions is sufficient to achieve high rate of local control of the primary tumor (64).

There have been refinements in the surgical technique that have made the procedures more tolerable. Examples of such improvements include primary closure of the perineal wound, the use of the sartorius muscle to close the surgical defect in the inguinal area, and the use of separate incisions for the resection of the primary tumor and the inguinal nodes. These developments have resulted in a decrease in the operative mortality and the complications and sequelae of surgery. In addition to these developments, the postoperative care of the patients has also improved.

In recent decades there have been also significant advances in all aspects of radiation therapy that apply to the treatment of carcinoma of the vulva. The technical resources at our disposal allow us to treat the vulvovaginal and inguinal regions effectively and with less morbidity and sequelae. With high photon energy units, well-collimated fields, compensators and electron beams of different energies, radiation can be delivered to the primary disease and lymph nodes, taking into account the differences in contour, tumor thickness, depth, and extent of the disease more precisely. It is possible to tailor the treatment to the specified treatment volume while the dose to the normal tissues is kept within limits of tolerance. With the improved and more refined dosimetry available, the dose delivered to a volume can be delivered with high degree of accuracy. Brachytherapy can also be used as primary treatment in very selected cases or in combination with external beam radiation therapy. With brachytherapy it is possible to deliver a high dose of radiation to a very limited volume of tissue.

Perhaps the most significant advance of recent decades in the management of cancer patients is the use of more than one treatment modality concurrently or sequentially. Chemotherapy, radiation, and surgery in sequence and/or in combination lessen the impact of any one modality and can achieve functional organ preservation with at least comparable or improved local tumor control and survival.

Early Invasive Disease

Surgery

In the past, early invasive vulvar cancer was considered a diffuse disease and patients were often subjected to radical vulvectomy, with 90% survival rates for stage I patients (64,112) but with considerable sequelae. Now it is accepted that small, favorable lesions (≤2 cm diameter, ≤5 mm depth) can be treated with radical, local excision rather than a radical vulvectomy in order to minimize surgical morbidity. The results are similar with either procedure with local recurrence ranging from 6% to 7%, and disease-free survival from 98% to 99% (62). Anterior lesions close to the clitoris may not be amenable to radical, local excision or may require a radical vulvectomy to obtain satisfactory margins.

Small, well-lateralized, T1 lesions with negative ipsilateral groin nodes have a low risk of contralateral groin involvement, <1% (62); therefore, treatment of the contralateral groin is not necessary if the ipsilateral nodes are negative. Patients with lesions with >5 mm invasion or with lesions with vascular space involvement, or poorly differentiated lesions, are at higher risk for inguinal node metastasis and should undergo bilateral groin dissections (70). Patients with centrally located lesions should undergo bilateral inguinal-femoral lymphadenectomies as both sides are at risk for metastatic disease. Tumors within 1 cm of the introitus are considered midline lesions and should undergo radical local excision, if possible (136). In addition, they should undergo bilateral, superficial lymph node dissection. A deep node dissection is also recommended if the superficial nodes are involved. Traditionally, primary tumors larger than 2 cm have been treated with radical vulvectomy and bilateral groin dissection because of the high risk of nodal involvement. Currently, the indications and extent of surgery for the inguinal nodes is subject of re-evaluation and specific guidelines cannot be given.

Radiation Therapy

In the setting of early invasive disease, radiation to the area of the primary may be advised to prevent local recurrence. Pathologic features associated with higher risk of local recurrence at the primary site include lymphatic-vascular invasion, depth of invasion >5 mm, margins <8 mm, and microscopically positive margins (64). However, it is unclear, if adjuvant radiation for these patients decreases the incidence of local recurrence. In a retrospective study by Faul et al. (48) of 62 patients with close surgical margins, ≤8 mm, or with positive margins, treated with postoperative radiation, the local recurrence rate was decreased. In this series, adjuvant, postoperative radiation improved survival in the group of patients with positive margins. Multivariate analysis also revealed an improvement in local control and survival when adjuvant radiation was given to patients with close or positive margins. Although local recurrence is decreased, it appears that survival is not affected because some patients with vulvar recurrences may be salvaged with surgery. In the absence of definitive data, patients with positive margins or patients with margins <8 mm and patients with deep invasion and/or lymphatic-vascular invasion should also be considered for adjuvant radiation. Preoperative radiation to the vulva should be offered also to patients with tumors close to the urethra, clitoris, or rectum. In these patients it is difficult to obtain a good margin.

The role of radiation in the management of the nodes was evaluated in a GOG trial reported in 1986 (68). In this trial, patients underwent bilateral inguinal lymphadenectomy and those with positive groin nodes were randomized to either pelvic lymphadenectomy or radiation to the pelvis and groins. The radiation group had significantly lower groin recurrence rate, 5.1% (3/59), compared with 23.6% (13/55) for the group that did not receive radiation. This translated into a significant survival benefit, 68% versus 54% ($p = .03$), at 2 years in favor of the group that received postoperative radiation (68). The benefit was limited to patients with more than one pathologically positive node. Based on this study, adjuvant radiation to the pelvis and both

groins is recommended for patients with pathologically involved groin nodes (68). Patients with extracapsular extension of tumor in the nodes or with residual disease in the inguinal areas should receive postoperative radiation to the pelvis, the groins, and the primary tumor bed area, as this predisposes them for recurrence at the primary and the lymph nodes areas (138) (Figs. 72.2 and 72.3).

Advanced Disease

The benefit of multimodality therapy for a number of malignancies, including vulvar cancer, has been established without doubt (35,54,117,139,145). For patients with vulvar cancer, this combination treatment has been used for nearly two decades (90). As experience with this treatment has evolved, different chemotherapy agents and schedules of chemotherapy and radiation have been tried. Most of the studies have been carried out on patients with advanced disease and/or recurrence postsurgery (13,36,45,82,91,97,119,132,141).

Surgery alone for patients with advanced disease has yielded disappointing results and this has led to the use of multimodality treatment for this type of patients (17,18,58,130,143). Another goal of this multimodality approach is to spare patients very radical surgical procedures such as exenterations. Extensive, radical surgery should be reserved for patients who fail initial therapy, who have no evidence of distant metastasis, and who are in good general condition and able to withstand this type of surgery. Exenterations have a very significant psychosexual impact on the patients, even when measures are taken to restore some sexual function (6). In selected patients, exenterations may have to be carried out when there is no other alternative. In these highly selected patients, the results can be acceptable in terms of the control of the disease (27,71,95,133). Algorithms summarizing the overall management of patients with different stages of disease are presented in Figures 72.2, 72.3, and 72.4.

Histologic Variants

Melanoma

Melanoma is the second most common malignancy of the vulva. The treatment should be surgery, if possible. The prognosis is worse in patients who have one or more of the following features: deep invasion, ulceration, nodular growth pattern versus superficially spreading, epithelioid cell type as opposed to spindle cell or mixed, high mitotic rate (20,111). The prognosis is worse in older patients. The extent of the surgery needed to achieve local control depends on the size of the lesion and the depth of invasion, and this is similar to melanomas in other parts of the body. The extent of surgery ranges from radical local resection with wide margins to radical vulvectomy. In a study of 32 patients treated at the Royal Marsden Hospital in London (38), there was no difference in the outcome between patients treated with local excision and those treated with more radical surgical procedures. Radiation plays a secondary role in the management of this disease. There is no proven role for radiation in the definitive management of patients with melanoma, but radiation is sometimes used for palliation of symptoms. Gynecologic melanomas, as with melanomas in other sites, are very difficult to control.

Bartholin's Gland Carcinoma

Carcinomas of the Bartholin's gland comprise 5% to 7% of all primary vulvar cancers. Histologically, these tumors are squamous or adenocarcinomas. The management consists of wide local excision and ipsilateral lymph node dissection. Contralateral groin dissection is reserved for patients with clinically

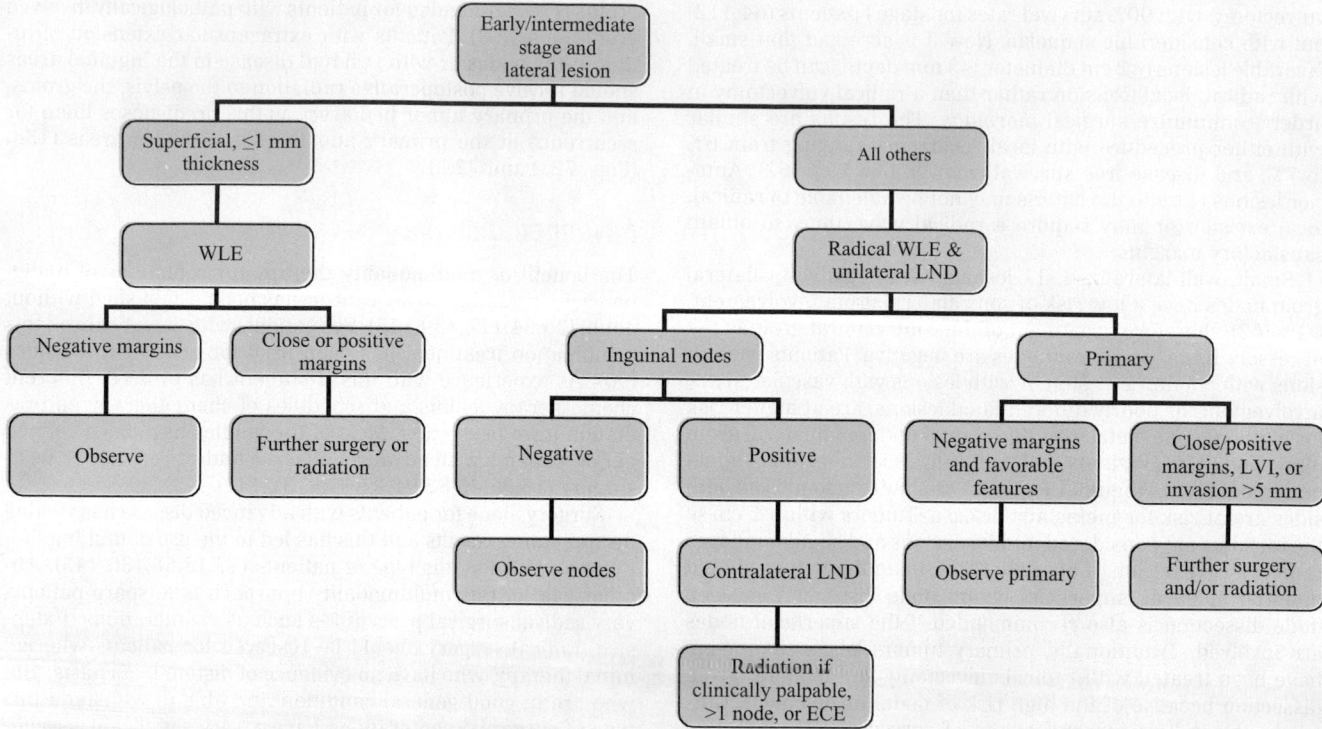

FIGURE 72.2. Treatment algorithm for well-lateralized, early/intermediate stage carcinoma of the vulva. WLE, wide local excision; LND, lymph node dissection; LVI, lymphatic-vascular invasion; ECE, extracapsular extension.

suspicious nodes or for patients with involvement of the ipsilateral nodes. Similar to other types of vulvar carcinoma, pelvic node dissections are not routinely recommended. Radiation to the pelvis is advised if involvement of the pelvic nodes is suspected. The role of radiation for these types of tumors was studied by Copeland et al. (33) and Leuchter et al. (87). These two series suggest that adjuvant radiation to the vulva and regional nodes, following conservative surgery, may decrease local recurrence. Five-year survival of 67% was obtained by Cardosi et al. (29) in patients who were found to have close margins

and who were treated with primary surgery and adjuvant radiation.

Verrucous Carcinoma

Verrucous carcinomas are locally invasive tumors that present as fungating, ulcerative masses. These lesions are usually treated by wide local excision. Node dissections are usually not performed because spread to the lymph nodes is uncommon. Most of the literature regarding vulvar verrucous carcinomas

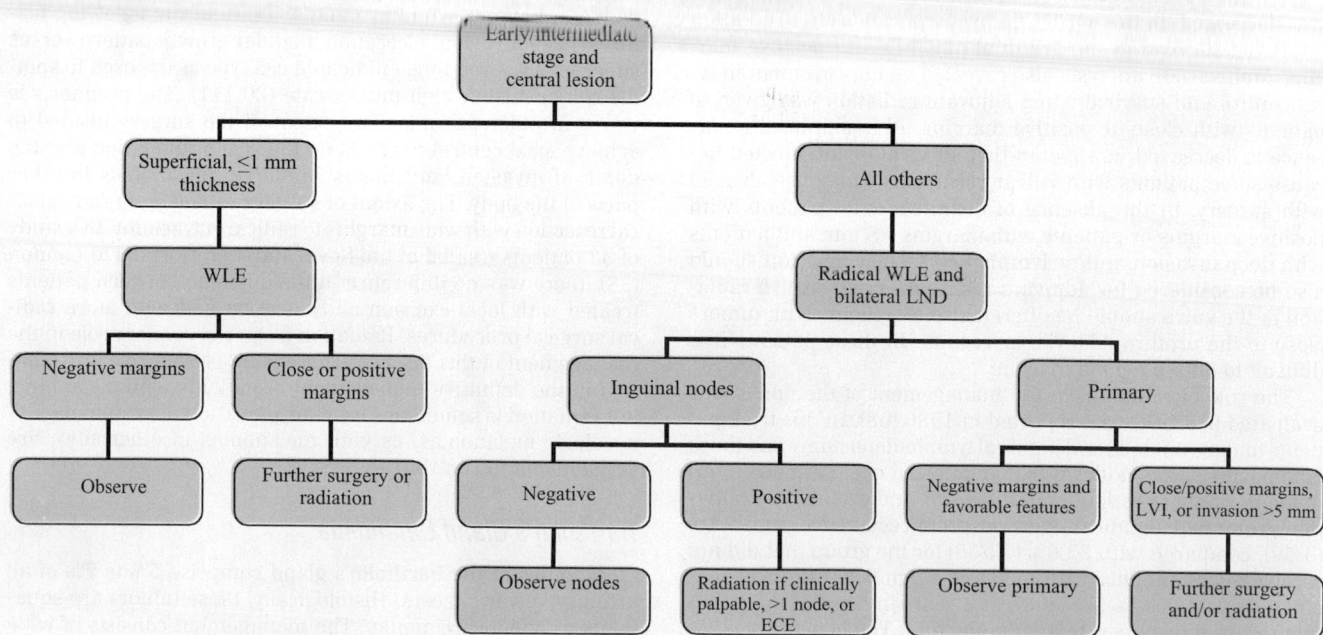

FIGURE 72.3. Treatment algorithm for central, early/intermediate stage carcinoma of the vulva. WLE, wide local excision; LND, lymph node dissection; LVI, lymphatic-vascular invasion; ECE, extracapsular extension.

Chapter 72   Carcinoma of the Vulva   **1699**

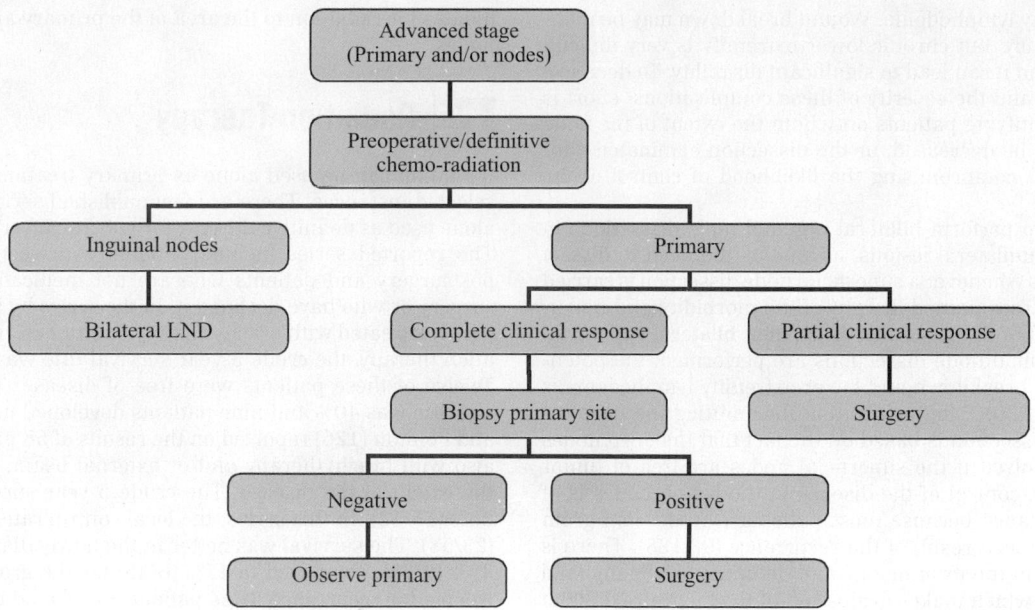

FIGURE 72.4. Treatment algorithm for advanced stage carcinoma of the vulva. LND, lymph node dissection.

Clinical Radiation Oncology

consists of case reports, with the exception of the series by Japaze et al. (75). This study is based on 24 patients, 17 of whom were treated with surgery only and 7 were treated with surgery and radiation. In the surgery group, only one patient developed recurrence and died as a result of it. In the radiation group, four patients developed recurrence and all died from the disease. Given the scarcity of literature on this subject, it is not possible to arrive at recommendations regarding the management of this type of tumor. It can be stated that there is no evidence that radiation is useful in the treatment for verrucous carcinomas of the vulvar area. As for radiation inducing anaplastic transformation and thus being detrimental, there is no sufficient evidence to support this assertion (83).

Surgery

Primary Tumor

The standard radical surgery for vulvar cancer used to consist of *en bloc* removal of the primary tumor and the superficial and deep groin nodes (143). The procedure was carried out through a large single incision extending from one anterior iliac spine to the other. Although acceptable local control and survival rates were achieved with this technique, postoperative wound breakdown was common. In 1955, Taussig (130) described a technique using a separate incision for the primary tumor and for each groin, thus leaving a "bridge" of normal tissue on each side. With this technique the incidence of wound breakdown was decreased by approximately one-half with comparable survival rates (61,65,72). Although bridge recurrences of up to 2% occur, the use of this surgical approach does not have a negative impact on survival (65,72).

The surgical approach to vulvar cancer has evolved from the traditional *en bloc* radical vulvectomy performed often on most patients, to a more individualized and less extensive surgery alone or in combination with radiation and chemotherapy. For small, limited lesions, a radical local excision (also referred to as wide local excision, radical wide excision, and modified radical vulvectomy) is recommended, if possible, instead of radical vulvectomy. At the time of surgery it is essential to obtain a minimum margin of 1 cm on the periphery of the tumor and to carry

the depth of the resection the perineal fascia to lower the risk of local recurrence (23,64). In a prospective GOG study of patients with stage I disease, with tumor thickness of ≤5 mm, who underwent modified radical hemivulvectomy, the local recurrence rate was 15.6% (19/21) (128). Ten of the recurrences were limited to the vulva (8.2%) and nine (7.3%) had a groin component. Two of these patients had vulvar and groin recurrence. Eight of the ten patients with vulvar recurrence only were salvaged with surgery. Five of the nine patients with groin recurrence died of disease. The survival in this group of patients was comparable to a historical group treated with radical vulvectomy (128). A review of other retrospective series reveals that there is a slightly higher risk of recurrence with radical local excision, but no appreciable difference in survival (62). Patients with multifocal lesions will usually require a radical vulvectomy because of the nature of the disease.

Patients with larger lesions, T2-T3, are best treated by radical vulvectomy. Selected patients with small T2 lesions, can be treated with radical local resection with acceptable results, depending on the location of the lesion (23,24). In general, patients with lesions in the posterior/lateral portions of the vulva are appropriate candidates for local excision in order to preserve the clitoris. If the tumor is close to the clitoris or rectum, <5 mm, preservation of these structures may not be possible. These patients should be evaluated for preoperative radiation in an attempt to sterilize microscopic tumor extension and to allow for a less radical resection.

When the rectum, vagina, or urethra are involved, extended radical vulvectomy and bilateral groin dissection or pelvic exenteration may be required (27,108). Because of the high morbidity and operative mortality and the major psychosexual impact this type of extensive surgery has, patients for whom this type of surgery is contemplated should be considered for preoperative radiation or combined preoperative chemoradiation to lessen the magnitude of the surgery.

Inguinofemoral Lymph Nodes

Attention to the risk factors for nodal involvement is very important as surgery for the lymph nodes, particularly for the inguinofemoral nodes, can lead to morbidity and sequelae. The main complications of groin surgery are wound breakdown and lower extremity lymphedema. Wound breakdown may be managed successfully, but chronic lower extremity is very difficult to deal with and it can lead to significant disability. To decrease the frequency and the severity of these complications, effort is placed on identifying patients on whom the extent of the node dissection can be decreased, or the dissection eliminated altogether without compromising the likelihood of control of the disease.

The need to perform bilateral inguinal node dissections in patients with unilateral lesions, as well as the need to dissect the deep nodes whenever a superficial node dissection is carried out, has been reexamined in light of the morbidity and potential for control of the groin disease. When bilateral superficial and deep inguinal node dissections are performed, the potential for wound breakdown and lower extremity lymphedema is increased (49,120). The justification for omitting the deep inguinal node dissection is based on the fact that the deep nodes are rarely involved if the superficial nodes are free of tumor (41). However, control of the disease in the lymph nodes is of utmost importance because most patients who develop groin failure will die as a result of the recurrence (93,128). There is inconsistency in the terminology and definition of the inguinal node surgery, which makes evaluation of the literature difficult (89). A clear distinction should be made between the superficial nodes and the deep nodes as the superficial nodes are the nodes found above the cribriform fascia along the femoral vein (94).

The standard surgical treatment of the groins nodes entails removal of the superficial and deep inguinal-femoral nodes, unless otherwise specified. Some investigators suggest that the superficial nodes may be regarded as sentinel nodes for the deep groin nodes (15,23,41). Patients with superficial primary tumors, with a depth of invasion ≤1 mm, have a very low risk of nodal involvement and the groin dissection may be omitted (74,93,103). A low incidence of groin recurrences is reported in patients with small (T1-T2), superficial (<5 mm deep) tumors treated with selective inguinal lymphadenectomy, sparing the deep lymph nodes if the superficial nodes are pathologically negative. The justification for this recommendation is based on a prospective study by the GOG that compared patients with similar prognostic features treated with an ipsilateral superficial inguinal lymphadenectomy to historical controls treated with bilateral inguinal-femoral lymphadenectomy (128). Groin recurrences occurred in 6% of patients treated with superficial lymphadenectomy, and most of the recurrences were in the ipsilateral, previously dissected groin. There were no groin recurrences in the control group. The risk of lymphedema following superficial and deep inguinal lymphadenectomy is substantial but it must be weighed against the risk of groin recurrence, which usually leads to death from uncontrolled disease (69,127).

Patients with advanced nodal disease, fixed or ulcerated inguinal nodes, are rarely curable (130). These patients should have a biopsy to document the nodal involvement and should be treated with combined radiation and chemotherapy, followed by surgery for the primary and the nodes if the response to the therapy has been good and the nodes are resectable (97).

Pelvic Lymph Nodes

Patients with clinically or pathologically positive groin nodes are at risk for having contralateral groin and pelvic nodal involvement. Thus, the status of the groin nodes is to be taken into consideration for the management of the pelvic nodes. The randomized GOG trial (68) of pelvic node dissection versus pelvic node radiation showed that control of the disease in the pelvis could be achieved with either form of therapy. Radiation to the pelvic nodes may be preferred over surgery because the treatment can be administered to the groins and pelvis at the same time, as patients in need of treatment to the pelvis may be candidates for radiation to the area of the primary and/or inguinal nodes.

Radiation Therapy

Radiation can be used alone as primary treatment in few and selected instances. There are few published series of radiation alone used as definitive therapy for vulvar cancer (46,113,126). The reported series include patients with recurrent disease postsurgery and patients who are not medically suitable for surgery or who have declined it. In the series by Ellis (46) of 65 patients treated with brachytherapy and/or external beam radiation therapy, the crude 5-year survival rate was 23% (15/65). Twelve of these patients were free of disease. The local control rate was 40% and nine patients developed necrosis. Slevin and Pointon (126) reported on the results of 58 patients treated also with brachytherapy and/or external beam, depending on the extent of the disease. The crude 5-year survival rate was 26% (15/58). In this series, the local control rate was also 40% (23/58). The survival was better in the newly diagnosed group, 39% (9/23), compared to 17% (6/35) for the group of patients treated for recurrence. Nine patients developed necrosis.

Brachytherapy has been used for inoperable vulvar cancer and as a boost to the primary tumor and/or to the lymph nodes (105). The efficacy of this treatment is difficult to evaluate because of the variability of the clinical situation in which this type of treatment may be employed. A high rate of necrosis, in up to one third of the patients, has been reported (46). A series from the Centre Alexis Vuitrin Institute in France describes 34 patients, 21 with primary and 13 with recurrent disease, treated with brachytherapy only (113). The median brachytherapy dose was 60 Gy, with a range of 53 to 88 Gy. In the group of 21 patients who underwent brachytherapy as primary treatment, 3 patients developed local recurrence and had regional recurrence. In this group of patients, the 5-year local control rate was 80%, with a disease-specific survival of 70%. In the group of 13 patients who were treated for recurrence, 8 developed local recurrence, with or without disease at other sites. With a median follow-up of 31 months, the local control for the two groups was 80% and 19% respectively. Five patients developed necrosis. This low complication rate most likely reflects that extensive experience and high quality of the brachytherapy carried out in this institution. The authors of this study advocate brachytherapy for primary vulvar cancer if the patient refuses surgery or if it is contraindicated. In this institution, patients with tumors >1.5 cm thick were treated with external beam and brachytherapy and are not part of this report.

The standard of care for early lesions is surgical resection; however, selected patients with small central lesions may be considered for definitive radiation, particularly when the lesions are in close proximity to the urethra, clitoris, or anus. More often, radiation is used in combination with surgery and or with chemotherapy. The objective of radiation is specific to the site in question, namely the lymph nodes or the primary tumor. For instance, in patients with advanced, unresectable nodes but less advanced primary tumor, complete control of the primary may be obtained with the combination of chemotherapy and radiation, obviating the need for surgery to the primary while making the nodes amenable to surgery (97,98). For patients with advanced primary tumors and limited nodal disease, it is possible to render the primary resectable while sterilizing the lymph nodes. Radiation can also play a significant role for palliation of symptoms.

Treatment Volume and Technique

The radiation target volume usually encompasses the vulva, both groins, and the lower pelvic nodes. When planning the treatment, careful attention should be given to the location and depth at which the dose is calculated for the inguinal area. The depth of the inguinal vessels can be highly variable, ranging from 2.0 to 18.5 cm (81). A CT or MR imaging scan of the pelvis is essential to obtain the depth of the inguinal nodes, as significant underdosing may occur if the radiation treatment factors are not properly selected. The imaging studies can also provide information about the pelvic nodes. If suspicious nodes are noted, a CT-directed biopsy can be performed, if the nodes are accessible. Patients with positive inguinal nodes have a 28% incidence of pelvic node involvement; consequently, the pelvic nodes should be treated in these patients (68). At the time of simulation, markers should be placed on the primary, the lymph nodes, and scars from previous surgery to document the extent of the disease. The location of the inguinofemoral nodes is depicted in Figure 72.5 (142).

The treatment is generally given with medium- or high-energy photon beams with anteroposterior/posteroanterior (AP/PA) fields with the patient in the supine position, with the thighs straight or in the "frog leg" position. The frog leg position has been used at some institutions to minimize the bolus effect from skin folds. Tattoos placed in certain points around the primary tumor, prior to therapy, can be used for objective evaluation of response to the treatment and for subsequent evaluation for boost therapy with reduced fields or with brachytherapy. The superior border of the pelvic field should extend to the middle of the sacroiliac joints to cover the external and internal iliac nodes. If a patient has suspected or proven internal or ex-

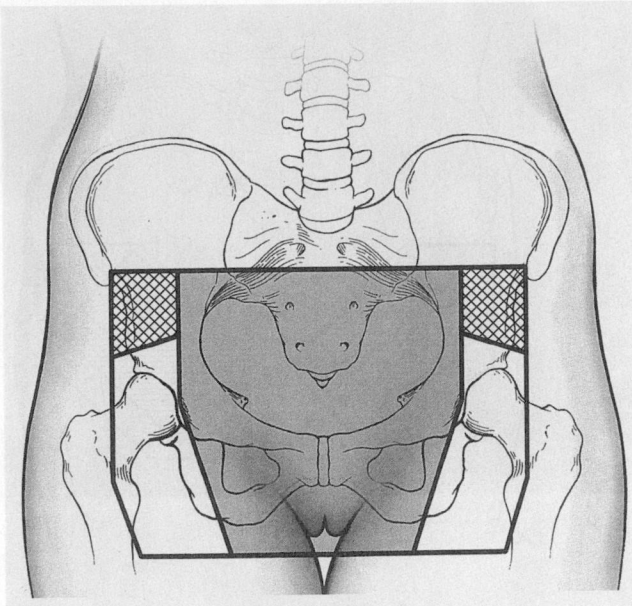

FIGURE 72.6. Treatment borders demonstrating the wide anterior field (*outer border*) and the narrow posterior field (*shaded region*).

ternal iliac node involvement, the superior border should be extended to the L3/4 interspace to cover the common iliac nodes. The inferior border should cover the entire vulva and the most superficial, inferior inguinal nodes. Laterally, the pelvic field extends 2 cm lateral to the widest point of the pelvic inlet. Although there are no data regarding scar recurrences, it is common practice to include the inguinal node dissection scars in the radiation field.

Depending on whether the inguinal/femoral lymph nodes and/or pelvic lymph nodes are to be included in the radiation volume, different field configurations may be used. To reduce the dose to the femoral heads while delivering an adequate dose to the inguinal nodes, various techniques are available. One approach is to use a wide AP field that includes the pelvic and inguinal areas, with a narrow posterior field covering only the pelvis and sparing the femoral heads. The photon fields are weighted equally, and the inguinal dose is supplemented by separate anterior electron fields matched to the pelvic field (Fig. 72.6). Bolus material should be used to ensure adequate dose to the superficial portions of the groin. An alternative method consists of using a wide AP field and narrow PA field, with a partial transmission block placed in the central portion of the AP field. The desired dose at a specified depth is delivered to the inguinal nodes through the AP field (78). The degree of central anterior beam attenuation is calculated so that the midpoint of the pelvis receives equal doses from the AP and PA beams. This technique eliminates the dosimetric problems of photon/electron field matching as well as the potential for daily setup variation, but the design of a precise partial transmission block is difficult. Another method consists of using matched AP/PA fields to include the primary and the pelvic nodes and treating the groins through separate anterior electron fields. This approach has the advantage of relatively easy setup, but the main drawback is ensuring an adequate dose at the match line, particularly when the match line is over gross disease. An example of an anteroposterior radiation field encompassing the inguinal/femoral and pelvic lymph nodes is shown in Figure 72.7.

Moran et al. (100) have described a modified segmental boost technique using multileaf collimators with a single isocenter technique and a wide AP field to cover the vulva, pelvis, and groins, and a narrow PA field to cover the vulva and pelvis. The

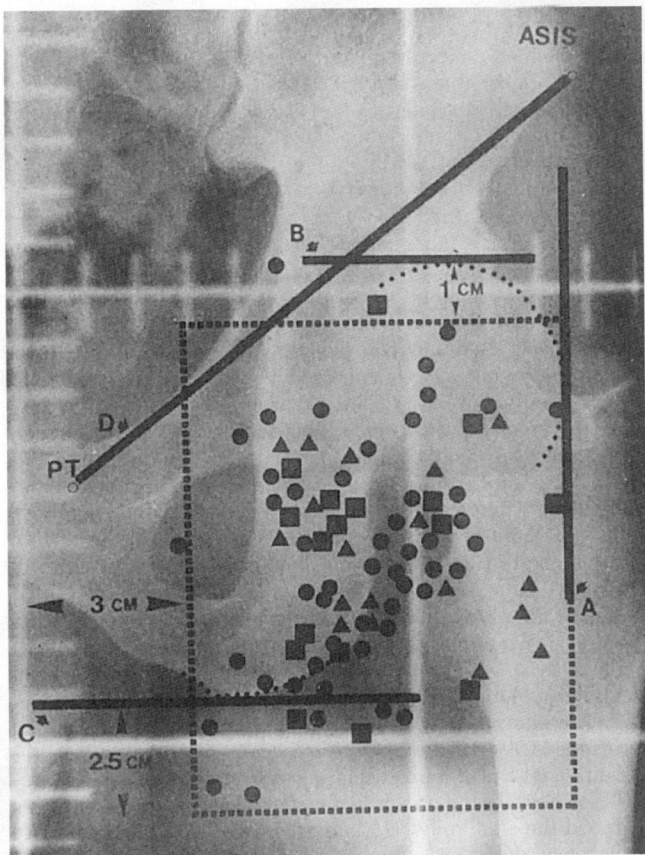

FIGURE 72.5. Topographic distribution of inguinal lymph node metastases in patients with carcinoma of the vulva-vagina-cervix (*triangles*), urethra (*squares*), or anus-low rectum (*circles*). (From Wang CJ, Chin YY, Leung SW, et al. Topographic distribution of inguinal lymph nodes metastasis: significance in determination of treatment margin for elective inguinal lymph nodes irradiation of low pelvic tumors. *Int J Radiat Oncol Biol Phys* 1996;35:133–136, with permission.)

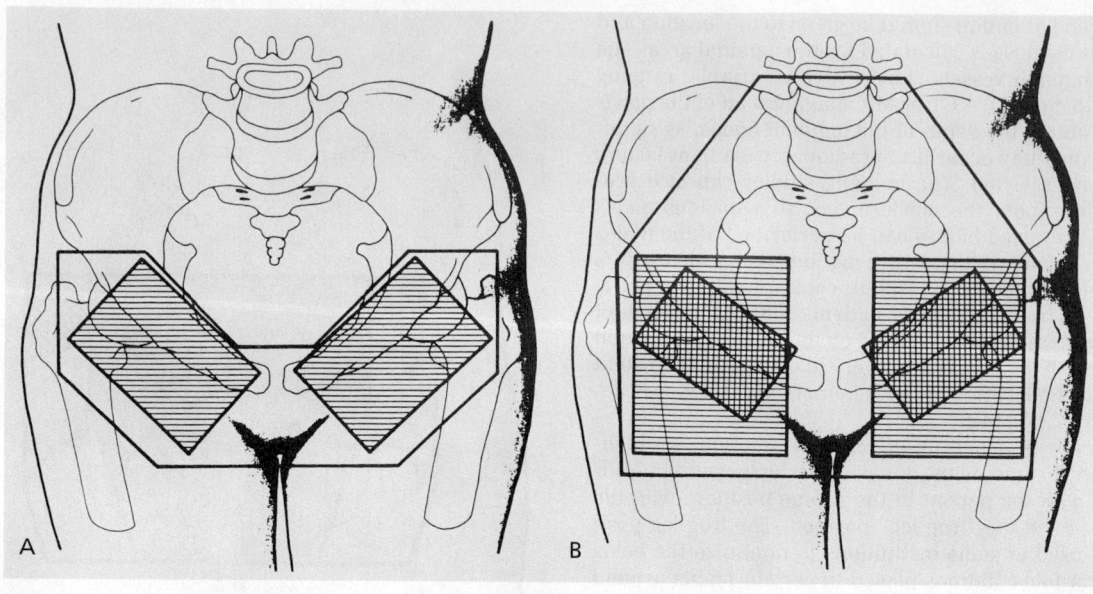

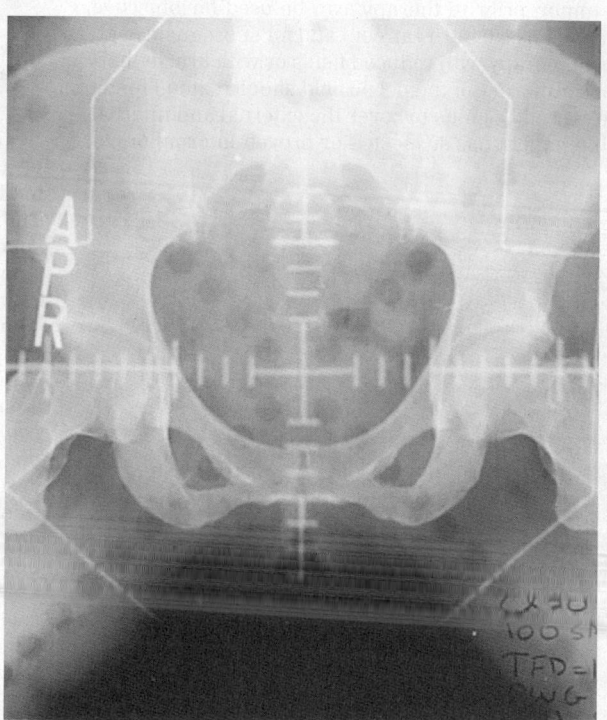

FIGURE 72.7. A: Portal for elective irradiation of regional lymphatics in patients with no clinical evidence of inguinal lymph node involvement. **B:** Portal for irradiation of pelvic and inguinofemoral lymph nodes and vulvar area. A final boost to the positive inguinal lymph nodes may be given with further field reduction. **C:** Simulation film of portal covering pelvic and inguinofemoral lymph nodes and vulva.

supplemental anterior photon groin fields are angled such that the central axis is coplanar with the divergence from the PA field. The medial blocking of the groin fields are designed to match the divergence from the PA field. This technique facilitates the reproducibility of the daily setup and provides a more homogeneous dose distribution (Fig. 72.8).

Intensity-modulated radiation therapy is now being used to treat the pelvis and inguinal nodes (3,14). Beriwal et al. (14) reported 15 patients treated with intensity-modulated radiation therapy using a median of seven fields. The clinical tumor volume (CTV) was defined as a 1- to 2-cm margin around bilateral external iliac, internal iliac, and inguinofemoral nodes, as well as a 1 cm margin around the entire vulvar region. Gross

tumor was also expanded by 1 cm for the CTV. The planning treatment volume (PTV) was defined as 1-cm margin beyond CTV. The plans were considered acceptable if <5% of the PTV received <100% of the prescribed dose, <10% of the PTV received >110% of the prescribed dose, and <1% of the PTV received >120% of the prescribed dose. Normal tissue constraints included the small bowel, bladder, and rectum (14). This early experience yielded reasonable clinical response with 13 of 15 patients having no evidence of disease at last follow-up (14), improved dose conformality (3), and resulted in lower doses to normal structures including rectum, bladder, small bowel (14), and femoral heads (3). This technique deserves further evaluation.

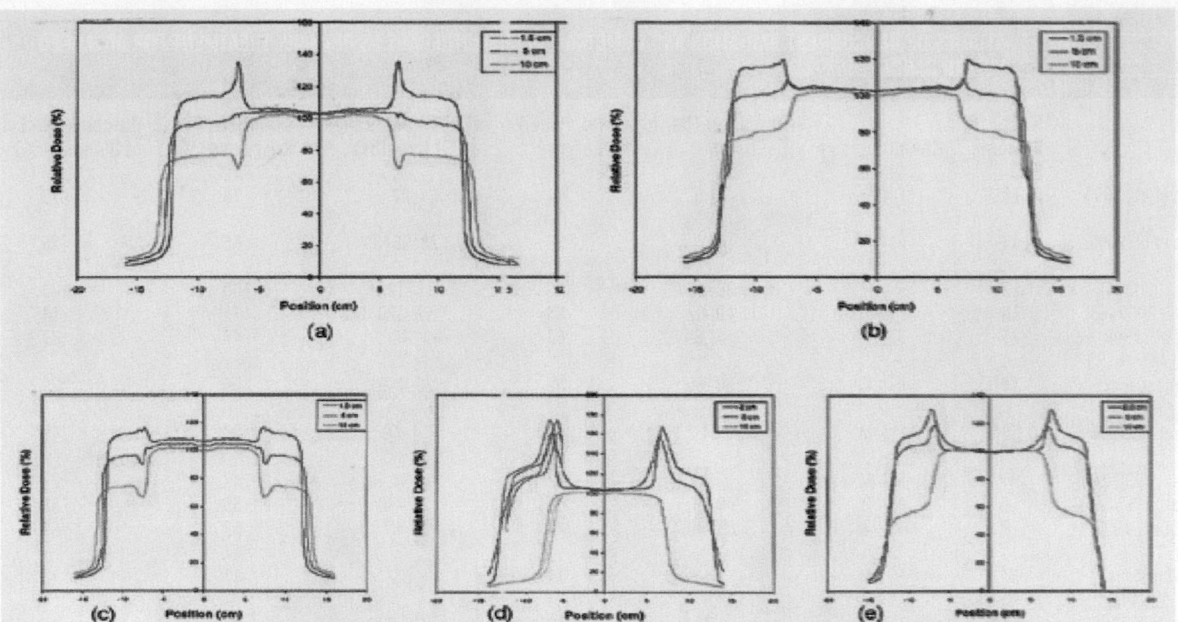

FIGURE 72.8. Dose profiles at three depths, in plastic water phantom, generated from digital axial images corresponding to five different treatment techniques. **(a)** Segmental boost technique. **(b)** Modified segmental boost technique. **(c)** Partial transmission block technique. **(d)** Photon with electron tag technique. **(e)** Photon with electron boost technique. (Adapted from Moran M, Lund MW, Ahmad M, et al. Improved treatment of pelvis and inguinal nodes using modified segmental boost technique: dosimetric evaluation. *Int J Radiat Oncol Biol Phys* 2004;59:1523–1530, with permission.)

Preoperative Radiation Therapy

As the treatment for vulvar cancer has evolved with the goal of decreasing the sequelae of surgery and to maximize functional outcome, preoperative radiation in addition to chemotherapy is now used more frequently. Patients with locally advanced lesions and/or clinically fixed/ulcerated lymph nodes may be best managed with preoperative chemoradiation or with preoperative radiation alone, if chemotherapy is contraindicated. This is to be followed by inguinal lymph node dissection and resection of residual disease at the primary site, depending on the extent of residual disease. In general it is recommended to carry out the inguinal node dissection whether or not there has been complete response of the lymph nodes as residual disease is often found in the lymph nodes (97). If there is complete regression of the disease at the site of the primary, an option can be to biopsy the site and if the biopsies are negative to forego resection of the primary site (98).

The preoperative radiation dose for the area of the primary and the lymph nodes should be 45 to 55 Gy (2,58). The most common chemotherapeutic agents used have been 5-fluorouracil, cisplatin, and mitomycin-C. Acute mucocutaneous toxicity from combined therapy can be severe, and a treatment break during the course of the treatment should be incorporated into the treatment plan (91,97,98,122). In the GOG trial for patients with advanced disease, nodal and/or at the primary site, the radiation treatment consisted of 170 cGy twice daily on days 1 to 4, and 170 cGy once a day on days 5 to 12, for a dose of 2,380 cGy (97,98). Cisplatin, 50 mg/m^2 was given on day 1, and 5-fluorouracil, 1,000 mg/m^2 by a 24-hour infusion, on days 1 to 4. The combined course was repeated after a 1.5 to 2.5 week break, for a total radiation dose of 4,760 cGy (97,98). The results of this trial are encouraging, but further investigation is needed to identify the best chemotherapy agents, the dose and schedule of administration, the radiation parameters, and patient selection to attain the most benefit of the treatment.

Definitive Chemoradiation Therapy

Definitive chemoradiation is used for patients with advanced tumors considered unresectable at presentation, or for patients who are medically inoperable (Table 72.3). In instances when the patient remains unresectable following the planned preoperative treatment, or is not a candidate for surgery, the treatment can be continued with curative intent. In these patients the chemotherapy should be continued throughout the course of radiation for the purpose of radiosensitization of the tumor in the treatment volume and possible eradication of subclinical disease outside the radiation field. With appropriate field reductions, the radiation dose should be brought up to 60 to 70 Gy. The total dose to certain areas depends on the location and extent or bulk of the disease, the response to the therapy, and the estimated tolerance of the area requiring the high radiation dose.

Some patients without clinically involved nodes and at low risk of having nodal involvement may be treated to the vulvar area only. The treatment can be delivered using electrons or low-energy photons. When the treatment is given with electrons only, a generous margin around the primary tumor should be used because the dose decreases toward the periphery of the field. Bolus material should also be used to avoid underdosing the surface of the tumor.

Postoperative Radiation Therapy

Adjuvant postoperative radiation can be used when limited surgery has been performed for organ conservation or when the surgical specimen reveals adverse pathologic features and local recurrence is likely to occur (107). Local recurrence is a major cause of failure in all patients irrespective of the stage (106). Patients with positive or close (<8 mm) margins, LVI, and depth of tumor invasion >5 mm, should undergo postoperative radiation as these are factors increase the likelihood of local recurrence (64). Patients with close margins may be

| Table 72.3 | STUDIES OF CONCURRENT RADIATION AND COMBINATION CHEMOTHERAPY AS PRIMARY TREATMENT FOR ADVANCED VULVAR CANCER |

Author, Year	No. of Patients	Chemotherapy	Radiation Therapy Dose (Gy)	No. Post-Tx Surgery	Median and Range of FU (months)	Complete Response (%)	Outcome, No Evidence of Disease (%)
Gerszten et al., 2005 (56)	18	F + P	44.6	14	27	78	72
Montana et al. 2000 (97)	46	F + P	47.6	38	78, 56–89	NS	26
Akl et al., 2000 (4)	12	F + M	30–36	NS	8–125	100	83
Han et al., 2000 (63)	10	F + F/M	40–62	NS	7–120	71[a]	54
Moore et al., 1998 (98)	71	F + P	47.6	64	45	47	67
Cunningham et al., 1997 (36)	14	F + P	50–65	NS	26, 1–81	64	29
Landoni et al., 1996 (86)	58*	F + M	54	42	4–48	27[a]	49[a]
Lupi et al., 1996 (91)	24	F + M	54	22	34	42	71
Eifel et al., 1995 (45)	11	F + P	40–50	8	17–30	55	58
Wahlen et al., 1995 (141)	19	F ± M	45–50	6	3–67	53	89
Sebag-Montefiore et al., 1994 (122)	37	F + M	45	14	NS	47	22
Koh et al., 1993 (82)	17	F ± M	30–70.4	10	(1–75)	53	47
Russell et al., 1992 (119)	18	F + P	46.8 72	1	24 (2–52)	89	75
Berek et al., 1991 (13)	12	F + P	44–54	4	37 (7–60)	67	83
Thomas et al., 1989 (132)	9*	F ± M	44–60	6	20 (5–43)	67	78

Post-Tx, posttreatment; FU, follow-up; F, 5-fluorouracil; P, cisplatin; M, mitomycin-C; NS, not stated.
[a]Includes patients treated for recurrent disease.

considered for repeat resection prior to radiation, particularly if the area in question is not in close proximity to the urethra, clitoris, or anus. Patients with more than one involved inguinal node, extracapsular extension, or gross residual nodal disease should receive adjuvant radiation to both groins and the pelvis. When the surgical margins are clear, and there is no pathologic indication to treat the vulva, a midline block can be used to avoid the reaction and the sequelae of the treatment to the vulvar area, although this practice raises the probability of local recurrence (44).

Adjuvant radiation to the primary area may be delivered with either photons or *en face* electrons with bolus. When treating a large area of the vulva and groins, AP/PA photon fields as previously described are appropriate. If the area of involvement is small, a direct electron field can be used and the groins are treated with separate fields. When it is indicated to treat the primary tumor bed area for possible residual microscopic disease, a dose of 50 Gy is recommended. If there is extracapsular extension of tumor in the lymph nodes, the dose to the groins should be carried to 50 to 60 Gy. If there is gross residual disease postsurgery, the dose to the area should be brought to 65 to 70 Gy.

Chemotherapy

Preoperative

The use of chemotherapy in the preoperative setting is usually reserved for patients who have advanced, inoperable, or recurrent disease. There is limited experience with single agents but among the agents used are cisplatin, piperazinedione, mitoxantrone, and etoposide, but the results with these single agents have been disappointing (101,125,131). Limited objective responses have been reported with Adriamycin (40) and bleomycin (135) used as single agents in a small number of pa-

tients. Some combination chemotherapy regimens (Table 72.4) have included bleomycin; however, this agent has been associated with pulmonary toxicity and fatality rates of 35% and 22%, respectively (28). The regimen of bleomycin, vincristine, mitomycin-C, and cisplatin (BOMP) has been effective for cervical carcinomas, but the results with carcinoma of the vulva are less encouraging (10). The Gynecological Cancer Cooperative Group of The European Organization for Radiation Therapy and Chemotherapy conducted phase II studies using a regimen of bleomycin, methotrexate, and CCNU and have reported better results (43). In this Gynecological Cancer Cooperative Group study, patients were treated with mitomycin, 5 mg intramuscularly, given on days 1 to 5; methotrexate, 15 mg orally on days 1 and 4; and CCNU, 40 mg orally on days 5 to 7 in the first week. For the next 5 subsequent weeks, patients received bleomycin, 5 mg intramuscularly, and methotrexate, 15 mg orally on days 1 and 4. The overall response rate was 64%, with a complete response rate of 10%. Of the 31 patients with inoperable or recurrent disease, 8 became resectable following chemotherapy. Unfortunately, the toxicity was high. The incidence of severe mucositis was in 21%, 13% had severe infections, and two patients developed severe pulmonary toxicity, one of which was fatal. Other severe toxicities included nausea/vomiting, hematologic, renal, and mucocutaneous reactions. Because of excessive toxicity, 33% of the patients did not complete the treatment. In an attempt to reduce toxicity, the dose of methotrexate was reduced and a 1-week break given between cycles (140). The response and toxicity rates were similar: 56% overall response rate and 40% grade 3-4 toxicity with two treatment-related deaths. In a small, recent report of neoadjuvant chemotherapy with cisplatin and 5-fluorouracil, at least a partial response was observed in all patients; however, three patients were treated with cisplatin alone with none showing any response (55).

In conclusion, single-agent chemotherapy is ineffective for advanced vulvar cancer except for bleomycin, but this agent causes significant toxicity. Combination chemotherapy regimens, particularly those including cisplatin and 5-fluorouracil,

Table 72.4	CHEMOTHERAPY FOR VULVAR CANCER			
Author, Year	No. of Patients	Regimen	PR (No. of Patients)	CR (No. of Patients)
Geisler et al., 2006 (55)	9	FP	5	4
Geisler et al., 2006 (55)	3	P	0	0
Wagenaar et al., 2001 (140)	25	BMC	12	2
Durrant et al., 1990 (43)	31	BMC	15	3
Benedetti-Panici et al., 1993 (12)	21	PBM	Tumor: 2 Node: 3	Tumor: 0 Node: 11
Belinson et al., 1985 (10)	3	BOMP	0	0

FP, 5-fluorouracil, cisplatin; P, cisplatin; BMC, bleomycin, methotrexate, CCNU; PBM, cisplatin, bleomycin, methotrexate; BOMP, bleomycin, vincristine, mitomycin-C, cisplatin.

yield improved response rates, but they are associated with significant toxicity. With recent studies using combined radiation and chemotherapy showing satisfactory response rates (97), preoperative chemotherapy alone is not recommended for patients with advanced vulvar cancer.

Adjuvant

In the postoperative setting, chemotherapy in combination with radiation may be justified for patients with high-risk pathologic features, such as close/positive margins, lymphatic space invasion, or involved nodes. These pathologic features portend a locoregional problem, for which radiation should be considered in addition to chemotherapy to address the problem of subclinical metastatic disease and to avert local recurrence. There are no outcome or toxicity data on adjuvant radiation alone compared with adjuvant chemoradiation. With 75% to 90% survival for early-stage vulvar cancer treated with surgery alone, the benefit of adding chemotherapy would not be detectable and the toxicity would be increased. If chemotherapy is given, it should be given concurrently with radiation to take advantage of the synergistic effect of the two modalities, although the morbidity of the treatment is enhanced.

Treatment Sequelae

The adverse effects of the treatment can be classified as acute and chronic, and depend on the treatment modality or modalities used and the magnitude of the treatment. Some of the adverse effects are specific to the type of therapy used and to the site treated, such as the primary or the lymph nodes.

When the disease is in early stage and the surgery is limited to the primary site, the acute surgical complications are relatively minor and essentially consist of wound infection and hematomas. With more extensive surgery, the frequency and degree of the complications can be far more significant. Before separate incisions for the inguinal lymphadenectomies and for the resection of the primary were performed, wound infection, necrosis, and breakdown occurred very frequently, in as many as 85% of the cases. Since the use of separate incisions was adopted, the incidence of groin wound infection, necrosis, and breakdown has decreased dramatically to a low of 15% (61,112). Other complications are wound infections, seromas, hemorrhage, deep vein thrombosis, pulmonary embolism, osteitis pubis, and anesthesia of the anterior aspect of the thigh secondary to femoral nerve injury.

The most significant chronic, surgical complication is edema of the lower extremities. Lymphedema is related to the extent of the lymphadenectomy and it is more likely to occur when a deep inguinal node dissection has been performed. The incidence of lymphedema may be as high as 69% (57,112). Lymphedema can be progressive and it can be very difficult to manage. Other chronic complications reported are chronic cellulitis of the inguinal areas, stenosis of the introitus, femoral hernias, and rectovaginal or rectoperineal fistulas.

The most significant acute morbidity of radiation alone or in combination with chemotherapy is the mucocutaneous reaction in the vulvar-perineal region and inguinal folds regions that can develop early during the course of the treatment. The severity of the reaction depends on the radiation fractionation schema used and the type of chemotherapy employed. Often the degree of reaction is such that a treatment interruption is advised if not mandatory. Acute hematologic toxicity is not uncommon and depends on the type and intensity of the chemotherapy used. This is managed well now with blood colony-stimulating factors, but in some instances blood transfusions are necessary. Chemotherapy dose adjustments or interruptions are often required. Severe hematologic toxicity can lead to septicemia, and in some instances this can lead to the demise of the patient (97,119).

The late complications of chemotherapy/radiation and surgery combined, trimodality therapy, include telangiectasis and atrophy of the skin and mucosa of the vulva, dryness of the mucosa of the vagina and vulva, and narrowing of the vaginal introitus aggravated by the inclusion of the vulvar area in the radiation field. Avascular necrosis of the femoral head has been reported in patients treated to the pelvis with radiation alone or radiation in combination with chemotherapy. In the GOG combined modality study for patients with advanced disease, only one patient developed avascular necrosis of the femoral head (97). In this study there were two instances of injury to the femoral artery. In one patient, the necrosis of the femoral artery occurred immediately following surgery and it was fatal. The other patient required femoral artery angioplasty.

Besides the generally recognized complications seen with surgery, radiation and/or chemotherapy, the treatment of carcinoma of the vulva has significant psychosexual consequences. This type of sequelae is, to some extent, related to the magnitude of the therapy, but in some instances it can be far greater than expected when considering the type and extent of the therapy given. The psychosexual impact of the treatment has been studied by some investigators (5), but thus far it has not received the attention that it merits, possibly because of the difficulty in the nature and the impact of it. In a study by Andersen et al. (7) of 42 patients, most of whom were treated with conservative surgery, wide local excision in 32 patients and simple vulvectomy in 10, there was a two- to threefold increase in the frequency of sexual dysfunction from the pretreatment level. In this study, 30% of the patients were sexually inactive at follow-up when compared with a match control. Andersen et al. (5) have also reported that vulvar surgery has a significant impact on sexual functioning and body image, even when intercourse remains possible. As might be expected, following pelvic exenteration, patients also experience significant sexual dysfunction, even when a neovagina is created (6). The concern for the significant impact of radical surgery on patients with carcinoma of the vulva has been one of the reasons for the use of multimodality therapy. With multimodality therapy organ preservation, maintenance of some organ function and improved body self-image is achieved in at least some patients.

References

1. Abell MR, Gosling JRG. Intraepithelial and infiltrative carcinoma of the vulva: Bowenoid type. *Cancer* 1961;14:318–329.
2. Acosta AA, Given FT, Frazier AB, et al. Preoperative radiation therapy in the management of squamous cell carcinoma of the vulva: preliminary report. *Am J Obstet Gynecol* 1978;132:198–206.
3. Ahmad M, Song H, Moran M, et al. IMRT of whole pelvis and inguinal nodes: evaluation of dose distributions produced by an inverse treatment planning system. *Int J Radiat Oncol Biol Phys* 2004;60[Suppl]:S484–485.
4. Akl A, Akl M, Boike G, et al. Preliminary results of chemoradiation as a primary treatment for vulvar carcinoma. *Int J Radiat Oncol Biol Phys* 2000;48:415–420.
5. Andersen BL, Hacker NF. Psychosexual adjustment after vulvar surgery. *Obstet Gynecol* 1983;62:457–462.
6. Andersen BL, Hacker NF. Psychosexual adjustment following pelvic exenteration. *Obstet Gynecol* 1983;61:331–338.
7. Andersen BL, Turnquist D, LaPolla J, et al. Sexual functioning after treatment of in situ vulvar cancer: preliminary report. *Obstet Gynecol* 1988;71:15–19.
8. Andersen ES, Sorensen IM. Verrucous carcinoma of the female genital tract: report of a case and review of the literature. *Obstet Gynecol* 1988;30:427–434.
9. Backstrom A, Edsmyr F, Wicklund H. Radiotherapy of carcinoma of the vulva. *Acta Obstet Gynecol* Scand 1972;51:109–115.
10. Belinson JL, Stewart JA, Richards AL, et al. Bleomycin, vincristine, mitomycin-C, and cisplatin in the management of gynecological squamous cell carcinomas. *Obstet Gynecol* 1985;20:387–390.
11. Benda JA, Platz CE, Anderson B. Malignant melanoma of the vulva: a clinical-pathologic review of 16 cases. *Int J Gynecol Pathol* 1986;5:202–216.
12. Benedetti-Panici P, Greggi S, Scambia G, et al. Cisplatin (P), bleomycin (B), and methotrexate (M) preoperative chemotherapy in locally advanced vulvar carcinoma. *Obstet Gynecol* 1993;50:49–53.
13. Berek JS, Heaps JM, Fu YS, et al. Concurrent cisplatin and 5-fluorouracil chemotherapy and radiation therapy for advanced-stage squamous carcinoma of the vulva. *Obstet Gynecol* 1991;42:197–201.
14. Beriwal S, Heron DE, Kim H, et al. Intensity-modulated radiotherapy for the treatment of vulvar carcinoma: a comparative dosimetric study with early clinical outcome. *Int J Radiat Oncol Biol Phys* 2006;64(5):1395–1400.
15. Berman ML, Soper JT, Creasman WT, et al. Conservative surgical management of superficially invasive stage I vulvar carcinoma. *Obstet Gynecol* 1989;35:352–357.
16. Binder SW, Huang I, Fu YS, et al. Risk factors for the development of lymph node metastasis in vulvar squamous cell carcinoma. *Obstet Gynecol* 1990;37:9–16.
17. Boronow RC. Combined therapy as an alternative to exenteration for locally advanced vulvo-vaginal cancer: rationale and results. *Cancer* 1982;49:1085–1091.
18. Boronow RC. Therapeutic alternative to primary exenteration for advanced vulvovaginal cancer. *Obstet Gynecol* 1973;1:233–255.
19. Boutselis JG. Radical vulvectomy for invasive squamous cell carcinoma of the vulva. *Obstet Gynecol* 1972;39:827–836.
20. Bradgate MG, Rollason TP, McConkey CC, et al. Malignant melanoma of the vulva: a clinicopathological study of 50 women. *Br J Obstet Gynaecol* 1990;97:124–133.
21. Brinton LA, Nasca PC, Mallin K, et al. Case-control study of cancer of the vulva. *Obstet Gynecol* 1990;75:859–866.
22. Burke TW, Eifel P, McGuire W, et al. Vulva. In: Hoskins WJ, Perez CA, Young RC, eds. *Principles and practice of gynecologic oncology.* Philadelphia: Lippincott-Raven; 1996:717–751.
23. Burke TW, Levenback C, Coleman RL, et al. Surgical therapy of T1 and T2 vulvar carcinoma: further experience with radical wide excision and selective inguinal lymphadenectomy. *Obstet Gynecol* 1995;57:215–220.
24. Burrell MO, Franklin EW 3rd, Campion MJ, et al. The modified radical vulvectomy with groin dissection: an eight-year experience. *Am J Obstet Gynecol* 1988;159:715–722.
25. Cardosi RJ, Speights A, Fiorica JV, et al. Bartholin's gland carcinoma: a 15-year experience. *Obstet Gynecol* 2001;82:247–251.
26. Carlson JA, Ambros R, Malfetano J, et al. Vulvar lichen sclerosus and squamous cell carcinoma: a cohort, case control, and investigational study with historical perspective; implications for chronic inflammation and sclerosis in the development of neoplasia. *Hum Pathol* 1998;29:932–948.
27. Cavanagh D, Shepherd JH. The place of pelvic exenteration in the primary management of advanced carcinoma of the vulva. *Obstet Gynecol* 1982;13:318–322.
28. Chambers SK, Flynn SD, Del Prete SA, et al. Bleomycin, vincristine, mitomycin C, and cis-platinum in gynecologic squamous cell carcinomas: a high incidence of pulmonary toxicity. *Obstet Gynecol* 1989;32:303–309.
29. Choo YC, Morley GW. Double primary epidermoid carcinoma of the vulva and cervix. *Obstet Gynecol* 1980;9:324–333.
30. Choo YC, Morley GW. Multiple primary neoplasms of the anogenital region. *Obstet Gynecol* 1980;56:365–369.
31. Chung AF, Woodruff JM, Lewis JL Jr. Malignant melanoma of the vulva: a report of 44 cases. *Obstet Gynecol* 1975;45:638–646.
32. Collins GC, Collins JH, Barclay DL, et al. Colon cancer involving the vulva. A report on 109 consecutive cases. *Am J Obstet Gynecol* 1963;87:762–772.
33. Copeland LJ, Sneige N, Gershenson DM, et al. Bartholin gland carcinoma. *Obstet Gynecol* 1986;67:794–801.
34. Creasman WT. New gynecologic cancer staging. *Obstet Gynecol* 1995;58:157–158.
35. Cummings BJ. Concomitant radiotherapy and chemotherapy for anal cancer. *Semin Oncol* 1992;19:102–108.
36. Cunningham MJ, Goyer RP, Gibbons SK, et al. Primary radiation, cisplatin, and 5-fluorouracil for advanced squamous carcinoma of the vulva. *Obstet Gynecol* 1997;66:258–261.
37. Curry SL, Wharton JT, Rutledge F. Positive lymph nodes in vulvar squamous carcinoma. *Obstet Gynecol* 1980;9:63–67.
38. Davidson T, Kissin M, Westbury G. Vulvo-vaginal melanoma—should radical surgery be abandoned? *Br J Obstet Gynaecol* 1987;94:473–476.
39. de Hullu JA, Hollema H, Piers DA, et al. Sentinel lymph node procedure is highly accurate in squamous cell carcinoma of the vulva. *J Clin Oncol* 2000;18:2811–2816.
40. Deppe G, Bruckner HW, Cohen CJ. Adriamycin treatment of advanced vulvar carcinoma. *Obstet Gynecol* 1977;50:13s–14s.
41. DiSaia PJ, Creasman WT, Rich WM. An alternate approach to early cancer of the vulva. *Am J Obstet Gynecol* 1979;133:825–832.
42. Donaldson ES, Powell DE, Hanson MB, et al. Prognostic parameters in invasive vulvar cancer. *Obstet Gynecol* 1981;11:184–190.
43. Durrant KR, Mangioni C, Lacave AJ, et al. Bleomycin, methotrexate, and CCNU in advanced inoperable squamous cell carcinoma of the vulva: a phase II study of the EORTC Gynaecological Cancer Cooperative Group (GCCG). *Obstet Gynecol* 1990;37:359–362.
44. Dusenbery KE, Carlson JW, LaPorte RM, et al. Radical vulvectomy with postoperative irradiation for vulvar cancer: therapeutic implications of a central block. *Int J Radiat Oncol Biol Phys* 1994;29:989–998.
45. Eifel PJ, Morris M, Burke TW, et al. Prolonged continuous infusion cisplatin and 5-fluorouracil with radiation for locally advanced carcinoma of the vulva. *Obstet Gynecol* 1995;59:51–56.
46. Ellis F. Cancer of the vulva treated by radiation. *Br J Radiol* 1949;22:513–520.
47. Farias-Eisner R, Cirisano FD, Grouse D, et al. Conservative and individualized surgery for early squamous carcinoma of the vulva: the treatment of choice for stage I and II (T1-2N0-1M0) disease. *Obstet Gynecol* 1994;53:55–58.
48. Faul CM, Mirmow D, Huang Q, et al. Adjuvant radiation for vulvar carcinoma: improved local control. *Int J Radiat Oncol Biol Phys* 1997;38:381–389.
49. Figge DC, Gaudenz R. Invasive carcinoma of the vulva. *Am J Obstet Gynecol* 1974;119:382–395.
50. Figge DC, Tamimi HK, Greer BE. Lymphatic spread in carcinoma of the vulva. *Am J Obstet Gynecol* 1985;152:387–394.
51. Franklin EW 3rd. Clinical staging of carcinoma of the vulva. *Obstet Gynecol* 1972;40:277–286.
52. Franklin EW, 3rd, Rutledge FD. Epidemiology of epidermoid carcinoma of the vulva. *Obstet Gynecol* 1972;39:165–172.
53. Franklin EW 3rd, Rutledge FD. Prognostic factors in epidermoid carcinoma of the vulva. *Obstet Gynecol* 1971;37:892–901.
54. Gage I, Recht A, Gelman R, et al. Long-term outcome following breast-conserving surgery and radiation therapy. *Int J Radiat Oncol Biol Phys* 1995;33:245–251.
55. Geisler JP, Manahan KJ, Buller RE. Neoadjuvant chemotherapy in vulvar cancer: avoiding primary exenteration. *Obstet Gynecol* 2006;100:53–57.
56. Gerszten K, Selvaraj RN, Kelley J, et al. Preoperative chemoradiation for locally advanced carcinoma of the vulva. *Obstet Gynecol* 2005;99:640–644.
57. Gould N, Kamelle S, Tillmanns T, et al. Predictors of complications after inguinal lymphadenectomy. *Obstet Gynecol* 2001;82:329–332.
58. Hacker NF, Berek JS, Juillard GJ, et al. Preoperative radiation therapy for locally advanced vulvar cancer. *Cancer* 1984;54:2056–2061.
59. Hacker NF, Berek JS, Lagasse LD, et al. Management of regional lymph nodes and their prognostic influence in vulvar cancer. *Obstet Gynecol* 1983;61:408–412.
60. Hacker NF, Berek JS, Lagasse LD, et al. Individualization of treatment for stage I squamous cell vulvar carcinoma. *Obstet Gynecol* 1984;63:155–162.
61. Hacker NF, Leuchter RS, Berek JS, et al. Radical vulvectomy and bilateral inguinal lymphadenectomy through separate groin incisions. *Obstet Gynecol* 1981;58:574–579.
62. Hacker NF, Van der Velden J. Conservative management of early vulvar cancer. *Cancer* 1993;71:1673–1677.
63. Han SC, Kim DH, Higgins SA, et al. Chemoradiation as primary or adjuvant treatment for locally advanced carcinoma of the vulva. *Int J Radiat Oncol Biol Phys* 2000;47:1235–1244.
64. Heaps JM, Fu YS, Montz FJ, et al. Surgical-pathologic variables predictive of local recurrence in squamous cell carcinoma of the vulva. *Obstet Gynecol* 1990;38:309–314.
65. Helm CW, Hatch K, Austin JM, et al. A matched comparison of single and triple incision techniques for the surgical treatment of carcinoma of the vulva. *Obstet Gynecol* 1992;46:150–156.
66. Helwig EB, Graham JH. Anogenital (extramammary) Paget's disease. *Cancer* 1963;16:387.
67. Hoffman MS, Roberts WS, Ruffolo EH. Basal cell carcinoma of the vulva with inguinal lymph node metastases. *Obstet Gynecol* 1988;29:113–119.
68. Homesley HD, Bundy BN, Sedlis A, et al. Radiation therapy versus pelvic node resection for carcinoma of the vulva with positive groin nodes. *Obstet Gynecol* 1986;68:733–740.
69. Homesley HD, Bundy BN, Sedlis A, et al. Assessment of current International Federation of Gynecology and Obstetrics staging of vulvar carcinoma relative to prognostic factors for survival (a Gynecologic Oncology Group study). *Am J Obstet Gynecol* 1991;164:997–1004.
70. Homesley HD, Bundy BN, Sedlis A, et al. Prognostic factors for groin node metastasis in squamous cell carcinoma of the vulva (a Gynecologic Oncology Group study). *Obstet Gynecol* 1993;49:279–283.
71. Hopkins MP, Morley GW. Pelvic exenteration for the treatment of vulvar cancer. *Cancer* 1992;70:2835–2838.
72. Hopkins MP, Reid GC, Morley GW. Radical vulvectomy. The decision for the incision. *Cancer* 1993;72:799–803.
73. Hunter DJ. Carcinoma of the vulva: a review of 361 patients. *Obstet Gynecol* 1975;3:117–123.
74. Iversen T, Abeler V, Aalders J. Individualized treatment of stage I carcinoma of the vulva. *Obstet Gynecol* 1981;57:85–89.
75. Japaze H, Van Dinh T, Woodruff JD. Verrucous carcinoma of the vulva: study of 24 cases. *Obstet Gynecol* 1982;60:462–466.

76. Jimerson GK, Merrill JA. Multicentric squamous malignancy involving both cervix and vulva. *Cancer* 1970;26:150–153.
77. Johnson TL, Kumar NB, White CD, et al. Prognostic features of vulvar melanoma: a clinicopathologic analysis. *Int J Gynecol Pathol* 1986;5:110–118.
78. Kalend AM, Park TL, Wu A, et al. Clinical use of a wing field with transmission block for the treatment of the pelvis including the inguinal node. *Int J Radiat Oncol Biol Phys* 1990;19:153–158.
79. Kim R, Rose PG. Surgical staging of gynecologic malignancies: the role of laparoscopy and sentinel node technology. *Surg Oncol Clin North Am* 2005;14:267–288.
80. Kneale BL. Microinvasive cancer of the vulva: report of the ISSVD task force. *J Reprod Med* 1984;454–456.
81. Koh WJ, Chiu M, Stelzer KJ, et al. Femoral vessel depth and the implications for groin node radiation. *Int J Radiat Oncol Biol Phys* 1993;27:969–974.
82. Koh WJ, Wallace HJ 3rd, Greer BE, et al. Combined radiotherapy and chemotherapy in the management of local-regionally advanced vulvar cancer. *Int J Radiat Oncol Biol Phys* 1993;26:809–816.
83. Kraus FT, Perezmesa C. Verrucous carcinoma. Clinical and pathologic study of 105 cases involving oral cavity, larynx and genitalia. *Cancer* 1966;19:26–38.
84. Krupp PJ, Bohm JW. Lymph gland metastases in invasive squamous cell cancer of the vulva. *Am J Obstet Gynecol* 1978;130:943–952.
85. Kurzl R, Messerer D. Prognostic factors in squamous cell carcinoma of the vulva: a multivariate analysis. *Obstet Gynecol* 1989;32:143–150.
86. Landoni F, Maneo A, Zanetta G, et al. Concurrent preoperative chemotherapy with 5-fluorouracil and mitomycin C and radiotherapy (FUMIR) followed by limited surgery in locally advanced and recurrent vulvar carcinoma. *Obstet Gynecol* 1996;61:321–327.
87. Leuchter RS, Hacker NF, Voet RL, et al. Primary carcinoma of the Bartholin gland: a report of 14 cases and review of the literature. *Obstet Gynecol* 1982;60:361–368.
88. Levenback C, Coleman RL, Burke TW, et al. Intraoperative lymphatic mapping and sentinel node identification with blue dye in patients with vulvar cancer. *Obstet Gynecol* 2001;83:276–281.
89. Levenback C, Morris M, Burke TW, et al. Groin dissection practices among gynecologic oncologists treating early vulvar cancer. *Obstet Gynecol* 1996;62:73–77.
90. Levin W, Goldberg G, Altaras M, et al. The use of concomitant chemotherapy and radiotherapy prior to surgery in advanced stage carcinoma of the vulva. *Obstet Gynecol* 1986;25:20–25.
91. Lupi G, Raspagliesi F, Zucali R, et al. Combined preoperative chemoradiotherapy followed by radical surgery in locally advanced vulvar carcinoma. A pilot study. *Cancer* 1996;77:1472–1478.
92. Mabuchi K, Bross DS, Kessler, II. Epidemiology of cancer of the vulva. A case-control study. *Cancer* 1985;55:1843–1848.
93. Magrina JF, Webb MJ, Gaffey TA, et al. Stage I squamous cell cancer of the vulva. *Am J Obstet Gynecol* 1979;134:453–459.
94. Micheletti L, Preti M, Zola P, et al. A proposed glossary of terminology related to the surgical treatment of vulvar carcinoma. *Cancer* 1998;83:1369–1375.
95. Miller B, Morris M, Levenback C, et al. Pelvic exenteration for primary and recurrent vulvar cancer. *Obstet Gynecol* 1995;58:202–205.
96. Monk BJ, Burger RA, Lin F, et al. Prognostic significance of human papillomavirus DNA in vulvar carcinoma. *Obstet Gynecol* 1995;85:709–715.
97. Montana GS, Thomas GM, Moore DH, et al. Preoperative chemo-radiation for carcinoma of the vulva with N2/N3 nodes: a gynecologic oncology group study. *Int J Radiat Oncol Biol Phys* 2000;48:1007–1013.
98. Moore DH, Thomas GM, Montana GS, et al. Preoperative chemoradiation for advanced vulvar cancer: a phase II study of the Gynecologic Oncology Group. *Int J Radiat Oncol Biol Phys* 1998;42:79–85.
99. Moore RG, DePasquale SE, Steinhoff MM, et al. Sentinel node identification and the ability to detect metastatic tumor to inguinal lymph nodes in squamous cell cancer of the vulva. *Obstet Gynecol* 2003;89:475–479.
100. Moran M, Lund MW, Ahmad M, et al. Improved treatment of pelvis and inguinal nodes using modified segmental boost technique: dosimetric evaluation. *Int J Radiat Oncol Biol Phys* 2004;59:1523–1530.
101. Muss HB, Bundy BN, Christopherson WA. Mitoxantrone in the treatment of advanced vulvar and vaginal carcinoma. A gynecologic oncology group study. *Am J Clin Oncol* 1989;12:142–144.
102. Origoni M, Sideri M, Garsia S, et al. Prognostic value of pathological patterns of lymph node positivity in squamous cell carcinoma of the vulva stage III and IVA FIGO. *Obstet Gynecol* 1992;45:313–316.
103. Parker RT, Duncan I, Rampone J, et al. Operative management of early invasive epidermoid carcinoma of the vulva. *Am J Obstet Gynecol* 1975;123:349–355.
104. Penn I. Cancers of the anogenital region in renal transplant recipients. Analysis of 65 cases. *Cancer* 1986;58:611–616.
105. Perez CA, Grigsby PW, Chao C. Vulva. In: Perez CA, Brady LW, eds. *Principles and practice of radiation oncology*. Philadelphia: Lippincott-Raven; 1997
106. Perez CA, Grigsby PW, Chao C, et al. Irradiation in carcinoma of the vulva: factors affecting outcome. *Int J Radiat Oncol Biol Phys* 1998;42:335–344.
107. Perez CA, Grigsby PW, Galakatos A, et al. Radiation therapy in management of carcinoma of the vulva with emphasis on conservation therapy. *Cancer* 1993;71:3707–3716.
108. Phillips B, Buchsbaum HJ, Lifshitz S. Pelvic exenteration for vulvovaginal carcinoma. *Am J Obstet Gynecol* 1981;141:1038–1044.
109. Pilotti S, Rotola A, D'Amato L, et al. Vulvar carcinomas: search for sequences homologous to human papillomavirus and herpes simplex virus DNA. *Mod Pathol* 1990;3:442–448.
110. Plentl AA, Friedman EA. *Lymphatic system of the female genitalia*. Philadelphia: W.B. Saunders; 1971.
111. Podratz KC, Gaffey TA, Symmonds RE, et al. Melanoma of the vulva: an update. *Obstet Gynecol* 1983;16:153–168.
112. Podratz KC, Symmonds RE, Taylor WF, et al. Carcinoma of the vulva: analysis of treatment and survival. *Obstet Gynecol* 1983;61:63–74.
113. Pohar S, Hoffstetter S, Peiffert D, et al. Effectiveness of brachytherapy in treating carcinoma of the vulva. *Int J Radiat Oncol Biol Phys* 1995;32:1455–1460.
114. Puig-Tintore LM, Ordi J, Vidal-Sicart S, et al. Further data on the usefulness of sentinel lymph node identification and ultrastaging in vulvar squamous cell carcinoma. *Obstet Gynecol* 2003;88:29–34.
115. Ridley CM. New nomenclature for vulvar disease: report of the Committee on Terminology, International Society for the Study of Vulvar Disease. *Int J Gynecol Pathol* 1989;8:83–84.
116. Ries LG, Pollack ES, Young JL Jr. Cancer patient survival: Surveillance, Epidemiology, and End Results Program, 1973–79. *J Natl Cancer Inst* 1983;70:693–707.
117. Rose PG, Bundy BN, Watkins EB, et al. Concurrent cisplatin-based radiotherapy and chemotherapy for locally advanced cervical cancer. *N Engl J Med* 1999;340:1144–1153.
118. Rowley KC, Gallion HH, Donaldson ES, et al. Prognostic factors in early vulvar cancer. *Obstet Gynecol* 1988;31:43–49.
119. Russell AH, Mesic JB, Scudder SA, et al. Synchronous radiation and cytotoxic chemotherapy for locally advanced or recurrent squamous cancer of the vulva. *Obstet Gynecol* 1992;47:14–20.
120. Rutledge F, Smith JP, Franklin EW. Carcinoma of the vulva. *Am J Obstet Gynecol* 1970;106:1117–1130.
121. Rutledge FN, Mitchell MF, Munsell MF, et al. Prognostic indicators for invasive carcinoma of the vulva. *Obstet Gynecol* 1991;42:239–244.
122. Sebag-Montefiore DJ, McLean C, Arnott SJ, et al. Treatment of advanced carcinoma of the vulva with chemoradiotherapy—can exenterative surgery be avoided? *Int J Gynecol Cancer* 1994;4:150–155.
123. Sedlis A, Homesley H, Bundy BN, et al. Positive groin lymph nodes in superficial squamous cell vulvar cancer. A Gynecologic Oncology Group Study. *Am J Obstet Gynecol* 1987;156:1159–1164.
124. Sherman KJ, Daling JR, Chu J, et al. Genital warts, other sexually transmitted diseases, and vulvar cancer. *Epidemiology* 1991;2:257–262.
125. Slayton RE, Blessing JA, Beecham J, et al. Phase II trial of etoposide in the management of advanced or recurrent squamous cell carcinoma of the vulva and carcinoma of the vagina: a Gynecologic Oncology Group Study. *Cancer Treat Rep* 1987;71:869–870.
126. Slevin NJ, Pointon RC. Radical radiotherapy for carcinoma of the vulva. *Br J Radiol* 1989;62:145–147.
127. Stehman FB, Bundy BN, Ball H, et al. Sites of failure and times to failure in carcinoma of the vulva treated conservatively: a Gynecologic Oncology Group study. *Am J Obstet Gynecol* 1996;174:1128–1132;discussion 1132–1123.
128. Stehman FB, Bundy BN, Dvoretsky PM, et al. Early stage I carcinoma of the vulva treated with ipsilateral superficial inguinal lymphadenectomy and modified radical hemivulvectomy: a prospective study of the Gynecologic Oncology Group. *Obstet Gynecol* 1992;79:490–497.
129. Sturgeon SR, Brinton LA, Devesa SS, et al. In situ and invasive vulvar cancer incidence trends (1973 to 1987). *Am J Obstet Gynecol* 1992;166:1482–1485.
130. Taussig FJ. Cancer of the vulva: an analysis of 155 cases (1911–1940). *Am J Obstet Gynecol* 1949;40:764–769.
131. Thigpen JT, Blessing JA, Homesley HD, et al. Phase II trials of cisplatin and piperazinedione in advanced or recurrent squamous cell carcinoma of the vulva: a Gynecologic Oncology Group Study. *Obstet Gynecol* 1986;23:358–363.
132. Thomas G, Dembo A, DePetrillo A, et al. Concurrent radiation and chemotherapy in vulvar carcinoma. *Obstet Gynecol* 1989;34:263–267.
133. Thornton WN Jr, Flanagan WC Jr. Pelvic exenteration in the treatment of advanced malignancy of the vulva. *Am J Obstet Gynecol* 1973;117:774–781.
134. Torne A, Puig-Tintore LM. The use of sentinel lymph nodes in gynaecological malignancies. *Curr Opin Obstet Gynecol* 2004;16:57–64.
135. Trope C, Johnsson JE, Larsson G, et al. Bleomycin alone or combined with mitomycin C in treatment of advanced or recurrent squamous cell carcinoma of the vulva. *Cancer Treat Rep* 1980;64:639–642.
136. van der Velden J. Surgery in the primary management of vulvar cancer. In: Luesley D, ed. *Cancer and pre-cancer of the vulva*. London: Arnold; 2000;106–119.
137. van der Velden J, van Lindert AC, Gimbrere CH, et al. Epidemiologic data on vulvar cancer: comparison of hospital with population-based data. *Obstet Gynecol* 1996;62:379–383.
138. van der Velden J, van Lindert AC, Lammes FB, et al. Extracapsular growth of lymph node metastases in squamous cell carcinoma of the vulva. The impact on recurrence and survival. *Cancer* 1995;75:2885–2890.
139. Veronesi U, Salvadori B, Luini A, et al. Conservative treatment of early breast cancer. Long-term results of 1232 cases treated with quadrantectomy, axillary dissection, and radiotherapy. *Ann Surg* 1990;211:250–259.
140. Wagenaar HC, Colombo N, Vergote I, et al. Bleomycin, methotrexate, and CCNU in locally advanced or recurrent, inoperable, squamous-cell carcinoma of the vulva: an EORTC Gynaecological Cancer Cooperative Group Study. European Organization for Research and Treatment of Cancer. *Obstet Gynecol* 2001;81:348–354.
141. Wahlen SA, Slater JD, Wagner RJ, et al. Concurrent radiation therapy and chemotherapy in the treatment of primary squamous cell carcinoma of the vulva. *Cancer* 1995;75:2289–2294.
142. Wang CJ, Chin YY, Leung SW, et al. Topographic distribution of inguinal lymph nodes metastasis: significance in determination of treatment margin for elective inguinal lymph nodes irradiation of low pelvic tumors. *Int J Radiat Oncol Biol Phys* 1996;35:133–136.
143. Way S. The anatomy of the lymphatic drainage of the vulva and its influence on the radical operation for carcinoma. *Ann R Coll Surg Engl* 1948;3:1159–1164.
144. Wharton JT. Microinvasive carcinoma of the vulva. *Am J Obstet Gynecol* 1974;118:159.
145. Whitney CW, Sause W, Bundy BN, et al. Randomized comparison of fluorouracil plus cisplatin versus hydroxyurea as an adjunct to radiation therapy in stage IIB-IVA carcinoma of the cervix with negative para-aortic lymph nodes: a Gynecologic Oncology Group and Southwest Oncology Group study. *J Clin Oncol* 1999;17:1339–1348.
146. Wilkinson EJ, Rico MJ, Pierson KK. Microinvasive carcinoma of the vulva. *Int J Gynecol Pathol* 1982;1:29–39.
147. Woodruff JD, Julian C, Puray T, et al. The contemporary challenge of carcinoma in situ of the vulva. *Am J Obstet Gynecol* 1973;115:677–686.

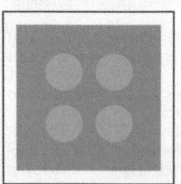

Chapter 73
Retroperitoneum

Brian D. Lawenda, Peter A.S. Johnstone

Primary tumors of the retroperitoneum are marked by widely disparate histologies and clinical presentations. The frequency of presentation in unselected series varies between 0.1% and 0.2% (4,7,35). The first report of a retroperitoneal lesion was a lipoma diagnosed at autopsy and credited to Morgagni in 1761 (37). In 1954, Pack and Tabah (35) surveyed the world's literature and quoted 750 prior reports, before adding 120 further from the Memorial Cancer Center experience. Although more recent series address lesions of specific histology (e.g., sarcomas), older series based on clinical presentations are composed of vastly different types of tumors. Thus, the most valuable data on presenting signs and symptoms are contained in these more historical analyses. However, as expected, this variety of different histologies led to widely disparate therapeutic recommendations based on the population reported. More recent data provide crucial information on radiographic interpretation. This chapter is concerned with lesions arising primarily from tissues of the retroperitoneum; lesions arising from organs that may have a retroperitoneal component (e.g., pancreas) are addressed elsewhere.

Anatomy

The retroperitoneal space is a potential space extending posterior to the abdominopelvic cavity (Fig. 73.1). In the abdomen, its superior border is the diaphragm and its inferior border is the superior aspect of the pelvic diaphragm. This includes the volume between the twelfth thoracic vertebra and distal coccyx. Bilaterally, the border was classically considered to be at the lateral edge of the quadratus lumborum, although Pack and Tabah (35) consider the lateral extent of the twelfth rib to be more valuable because this corresponds not only with the midiliac crest, but also with the origin of the transversus abdominus aponeurosis. The parietal peritoneum forms the anterior border with some aspects of the ascending and descending colon, the rectum, and a portion of the duodenum. The psoas and quadratus lumborum muscles of the abdominal wall form its posterior border.

In the pelvis, the posterior wall becomes the psoas and iliacus within the iliac fossa. In the true pelvis, the posterior musculature shifts to obturator internus and pyriformis. The pelvic diaphragm (levator ani and coccygeus muscles) represents the inferior portion of the pelvic retroperitoneum.

The tissue within this mixed potential and actual space is composed predominantly of lymphatics and loose connective tissue. Organs that are partially or completely retroperitoneal include the pancreas, kidney, adrenal glands, and ureters. Vascular structures include the aorta and inferior vena cava, and significant lumbar nerves traverse the space.

Surgical anatomy of the retroperitoneum has been recently well described by Nethercliffe et al. (30). In their extensive review, they describe the most commonly used surgical approaches to the retroperitoneum: (a) subcostal (below the twelfth rib); (b) supracostal (above the twelfth rib); (c) transcostal (removing the eleventh or twelfth rib); and (d) thoracoabdominal.

In this era of increasing use of laparoscopy, these approaches to the flank are often deferred for minimally invasive techniques that cause less postoperative morbidity.

Epidemiology

A frequency of about three per million persons has been quoted in two population-based studies (4,7). The age range of patients varied between 3 and 83 years, half were in the sixth, seventh, and eighth decades, with no difference in frequency between males and females (7).

Figure 73.2 reveals the age at diagnosis of several large series of patients with primary retroperitoneal tumors. There are two peak age periods: One during the first decade and the other during the sixth decade. These are due to vastly different histologies. Pediatric patients will generally have neuroblastoma or germ cell tumors; adults will generally have mesenchymal lesions. These histologies are outlined in Figure 73.3.

Natural History

The natural history of these lesions is obviously dependent on their histology. Because of the unique anatomic location involved, most lesions will have reached substantial size prior to presentation.

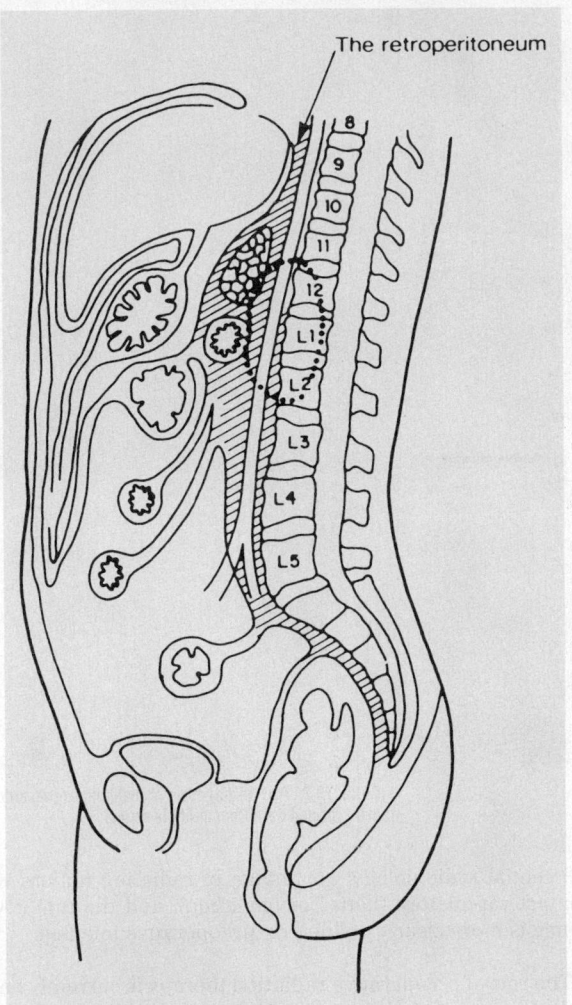

The retroperitoneum

8
9
10
11
12
L1
L2
L3
L4
L5

FIGURE 73.1. Sagittal view of trunk, showing the retroperitoneal space (*shaded area*). The kidney is outlined by dots. (From Wasserman TH, Tepper JE. Retroperitoneum. In: Perez CA, Brady LW, eds. *Principles and practice of radiation oncology*, 3rd ed. Philadelphia: Lippincott-Raven; 1997:1943–1956, with permission.)

Clinical Presentation

Table 73.1 outlines pooled data regarding signs and symptoms at presentation of retroperitoneal tumors. In general, presentation involves a mass or pain in the majority of cases.

Diagnostic Work-Up

Older series, as expected, focused on radiographic manifestations of patients presenting with clinically evident disease. Melicow (23) considered the ureter to be "the 'weather vane' of the retroperitoneum" on intravenous urography. Given the mobility of the kidney and ureter, hydroureter and hydronephrosis are considered to be late events due to retroperitoneal pathology. Abnormalities on these studies were noted in 80% of cases reported by Bose (7).

Oriana et al. (34) reported results of angiographic studies performed in 20 of their patients: Mass effect was noted in 85% of cases, and aberrant circulation was present in 70%. All of the patients undergoing angiography reported by Bose (7) had abnormal studies.

Neville and Herts (31) have recently published a comprehensive review of computed tomography (CT) appearance of primary retroperitoneal lesions. Large lesions with fatty components causing mass effect frequently represent liposarcomas. Teratomas often have fat, fluid, and calcified components. Paraspinal locations point to nerve sheath tumors or neurogenic derivation.

Magnetic resonance imaging (MRI) may demonstrate additional imaging details to further classify the lesion. In lieu of open or laparoscopic biopsy, CT-guided needle biopsy may be performed as the initial means of obtaining tissue for histologic diagnosis. PET scan can be helpful in evaluating the extent of distant metastases during the staging work-up.

Contemporary Population-Based Demographics

For this chapter, a comprehensive review of the Surveillance Epidemiology and End Results (SEER) public use registry was performed for the year 2002. The SEER system comprises 13 regional registries and provides in-depth cancer data on a significant minority of the population of the United States. Comprehensive results are provided in Table 73.2.

Retroperitoneal Sarcoma General Management

Whenever feasible, the primary treatment of retroperitoneal soft tissue sarcoma (STS) is to attempt a gross total resection. Criteria for unresectable tumors commonly include major vessel invasion and spinal cord or vertebral body involvement. Resectability has been reported in recent series to range from 65% to 85% (17,22,49). In order to obtain negative margins, involvement of adjacent structures may be necessary to accomplish *en bloc* resection of the primary tumor (16,49).

The extent of surgical resection is classified on margin status:

R0—macroscopically complete tumor resection with microscopically negative margins,

R1—macroscopically complete tumor resection with microscopically positive margins, and

R2—macroscopically incomplete tumor resection.

A macroscopically positive margin is one the most important prognostic features in determining local control and survival; however, the implications of microscopically involved margins are not as clearly defined (22,48). Nevertheless, even after a complete excision of RPS, local recurrence rates and overall survival rates are poor: 33% to 77% (local recurrence) and 35% to 63% (5-year overall survival) (9,22,49). Most patients who die of RPS die of local recurrence (16,49). Lewis et al. (22) reported that 75% of the patients with primary RPS in their series died in the absence of metastasis.

Although there are no randomized studies to support the use of postoperative radiation therapy compared to surgery alone for RPS, retrospective data demonstrate a decrease in local failure with adjuvant radiation therapy (9,49). The effect of postoperative radiation on survival is less certain. Preoperative or postoperative radiation therapy can be employed.

Postoperative radiation therapy is associated with increased treatment-related toxicity. This is primarily the consequence of radiating a substantial volume of normal tissue adjacent to the tumor bed. Preoperative radiation therapy may be advantageous for the following reasons:

1. Radiation fields are smaller (tumor volume alone) as they need not cover the entire operative site (e.g., operative bed, drains, incisions),

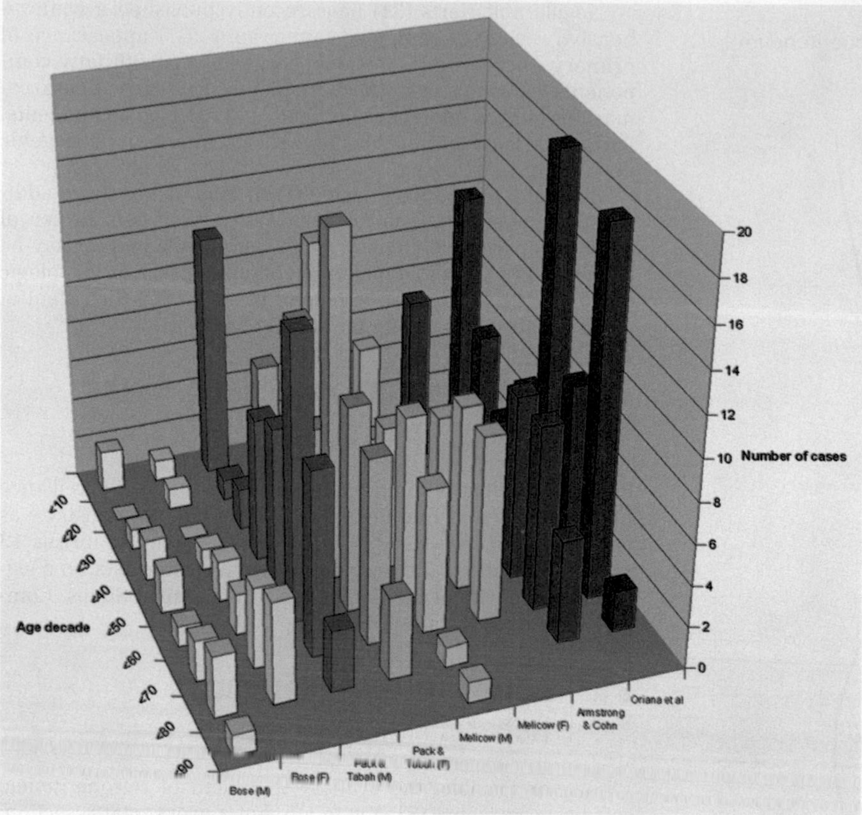

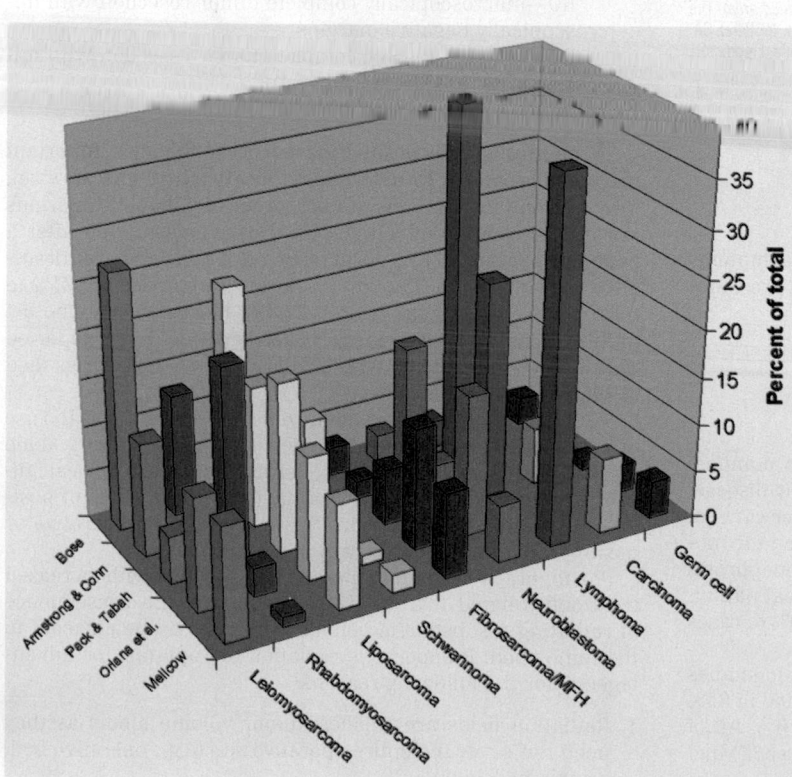

FIGURE 73.2. Age at diagnosis of malignant retroperitoneal tumors (pooled data from multiple series)

2. Less normal tissue volume in the field because of smaller fields and displacement of normal structures (e.g., bowel, kidney, liver) out of the field by the tumor mass itself,

3. Potential for reduction in risk of wound or peritoneal tumor seeding with preoperative radiation,

4. Potential radiobiologic advantage of radiating tumors with intact vasculature (better oxygenation), and the tumor volume is more clearly defined on preoperative imaging.

The role of preoperative radiation therapy is currently being studied in a prospective randomized trial, American College of

FIGURE 73.3. Percentage of retroperitoneal lesions by histology (pooled data from multiple published series).

Table 73.1	PRESENTING COMPLAINTS (%) OF PATIENTS WITH RETROPERITONEAL LESIONS (POOLED FROM LITERATURE SOURCES)		
Sign/ Symptom	Bose (7) (n = 30)	Pack and Tabah (35) (n = 120)	Oriana et al. (34) (n = 56)
Mass	83	31	42
Abdominal pain	60	51	42[a]
Back pain	20	7	
Weight loss	35	3	12
Anorexia	20	NS	9
Nausea/vomiting	20	20	8
Lower extremity edema	17	7	9

NS, data not stated.
[a]Indicates all patients with pain as presenting sign.

Surgeons Oncology Group protocol (ACOSOG) Z9031, a phase III randomized study of preoperative radiation plus surgery versus surgery alone for patients with retroperitoneal sarcomas (1).

Patients with unresectable disease may benefit from a course of preoperative radiotherapy or chemotherapy in attempt to shrink the tumor and make it resectable (24). The Massachusetts General Hospital reported a 60% 5-year local control rate in their series of unresected STS when using doses of 63 Gy or higher (20). Palliative debulking surgery may be offered to those patients with locally extensive tumors that are not amenable to complete resection (46).

Locally recurrent RPS is potentially salvageable with repeat resection, although the survival statistics are far from optimal (16). Longer disease-free intervals are associated with a better prognosis. Patients who have not received prior radiation to the tumor bed should be considered for either pre- or postoperative radiation therapy. Intraoperative radiation therapy (IORT) has been reported to increase local control after resection (2,15,38).

Patients who present or recur with distant metastases should be managed on a case-by-case basis, as there are no standard recommendations in this case. The National Comprehensive Cancer Network (NCCN) guidelines (V.2.2007) suggest that patients with solitary or limited metastases should be managed similarly to those with localized disease with consideration for preoperative radiation therapy and/or chemotherapy, metastasectomy, radiofrequency ablation, or cryotherapy of the metastatic lesions (28). Chemotherapy may be considered (most commonly, Doxorubicin-based regimens). Those patients with

Table 73.2	SURVEILLANCE, EPIDEMIOLOGY, AND END RESULTS DATA: RETROPERITONEAL MALIGNANCIES, 2002	
Patient Data (n = 162)	No.	%
Patient sex		
Male	78	48
Female	84	52
Patient race		
White	128	79
Black	16	9.9
Other	17	10.5
Unknown	1	0.06
Histologic derivation		
Soft tissue sarcoma	126	77.8
Sympathetic nervous system	14	8.6
Epithelial	7	4.3
Germ cell	5	3
Renal	1	0.06
Other (unspecified)	9	5.6

disseminated metastatic disease are treated with palliative intent (chemotherapy, radiation therapy, palliative surgery, ablative procedures, or best supportive care.) Chemotherapy use in patients with metastatic disease will be discussed in greater detail in Chapter 81.

Assessing response to therapy is challenging and is limited to either pathologic review of biopsy or resection specimens, or to serial imaging studies (i.e., CT or MRI with contrast enhancement). Based on the findings of a recently published meta-analysis, fluorodeoxyglucose positron emission tomography imaging may not accurately reflect response to radiation therapy (6).

Chemotherapy

Adjuvant chemotherapy is controversial in the management of adult patients with macroscopically completely resected retroperitoneal soft tissue sarcomas. In a National Cancer Institute trial, patients with STSs were randomized to chemotherapy or observation following resection; some patients had postoperative irradiation (42). Among patients who were assigned to chemotherapy, survival was favorably affected in those with extremity tumors. However, patients with head and neck and truncal lesions (including retroperitoneal sarcomas) did not benefit; the 5-year survival rate was approximately 40% in both arms. Similar findings were reported in a large meta-analysis of patients with STS (43).

The use of neoadjuvant or adjuvant chemotherapy is not standard in the management of nonmetastatic adult retroperitoneal STSs. Neoadjuvant chemotherapy has been primarily studied in the setting of high-grade, extremity STSs. Pisters et al. (39) demonstrated feasibility of using preoperative concurrent doxorubicin and external-beam radiotherapy (EBRT) (18 to 50.4 Gy), followed by resection and IORT (15 Gy) in patients with RPS. An R0 or R1 resection was possible in 90% of the patients who went to surgery (83%). Despite these promising results, concurrent neoadjuvant chemoradiotherapy is not recommended outside clinical protocols.

Radiation Therapy Techniques

Three-dimensional conformal radiation therapy (3DCRT) planning is preferable to conventional planning techniques to more clearly define target and nontarget tissues and to optimize field arrangements. Intensity-modulated radiation therapy and helical tomotherapy, proton beam therapy, and IORT have reported benefits over standard 3DCRT in enhancing the delivery of higher radiation doses to the target volume while minimizing doses to normal tissues (2,12,15,26,38).

We recommend preoperative radiation therapy for the reasons outlined previously. This usually requires that an initial procedure be done (CT-guided core needle biopsy, if adequate tissue can be obtained, or a small operative procedure) to obtain tissue for histologic study. Obtaining a contrast-enhanced CT scan or MRI prior to simulation will help to more clearly define tumor and normal tissues for planning purposes. The use of [F-18]FDG-PET in tumor localization has been reported, and may differentiate tumor versus surrounding normal tissues (45). Most cases of RPS will require irradiating the ipsilateral kidney. Therefore, a renal perfusion study should be ordered as part of the initial radiation planning process to ascertain the degree of functionality of each kidney.

Target volumes are defined as follows (preoperative volumes) (1).

1. The gross tumor volume (GTV) is the visualized GTV based on preradiotherapy imaging with CT and/or MRI.

2. The clinical target volume (CTV) is defined as the tissues adjacent to the GTV that have a potential for microscopic disease that are not visible on radiographic imaging. The CTV should be contoured at least 1.5 cm outside the GTV, but can be less in areas where there is minimal risk of direct invasion (i.e., peritoneum, bone, muscle).

3. The planning target volume (PTV) is an expansion volume outside the CTV that accounts for setup error and patient/organ movement.

This variable is institutionally dependent as well as patient-dependent. A minimum of 0.5 cm expansion outside the CTV should be used. Infraction organ-motion of retroperitoneal structures can be significant; that is, average movement between 11 and 19 mm (kidneys, normal breathing) and 18 and 22 mm (pancreas, normal breathing) (21). Stereotactic ultrasound-based image-guided targeting, cone beam CT imaging, active breathing control, and respiratory gating may be useful modalities in decreasing the required PTV expansion due to organ motion.

Critical normal structures should be contoured (i.e., liver, kidneys, spinal cord, bowel, stomach) and dose-volume histograms calculated. The spinal cord dose should be limited to 45 Gy in standard fractionation during 5 weeks. The current ACOSOG Z9031 trial limits liver doses: No more than 20% of the liver volume to receive >50 Gy, and no more than 50% should receive >25 Gy (1). At least two-thirds of the volume of one functioning kidney should receive <20 Gy. Stomach and bowel should be limited to a maximum dose of 45 Gy. Volume expansions should be minimized in regions where tolerance doses to critical structures will be reached.

Conventional anteroposterior/posteroanterior or slightly oblique fields often provide the best target coverage with the least amount of normal tissue in the beam. The use of lateral fields can result in irradiating a substantial volume of normal tissue (i.e., liver and kidneys) and should be used sparingly.

Preoperative radiation doses of 45 to 50 Gy (in 1.8 to 2.0 Gy per fraction per day) are recommended. Surgical resection usually is usually delayed until 3 to 8 weeks after completion of the radiation therapy. Radiographic restaging may be performed prior to resection to assess for metastases and response to therapy.

Intraoperative radiation therapy, with either brachytherapy or external-beam irradiation, may be used as a local boost to deliver additional radiation to areas of concern (i.e., close or positive margins.) The addition of an IORT boost has been shown to increase local control rates over resection and external-beam radiation therapy alone (15,47). Although not always possible, care should be taken to avoid including critical structures from the boost (i.e., bowel, ureters, nerves). A postoperative external-beam boost can also be delivered to an area of close or positive margin. We recommend asking the surgeon to place radio-opaque markers (i.e., clips, metallic seeds) at the borders of the resection cavity and in the areas where the margin may be close or positive. This will be helpful in defining these areas later if a postoperative boost is given. The boost dose is typically 10 to 15 Gy, and is delivered in either a single intraoperative dose (electron beam or brachytherapy) or in a once-daily, fractionated regimen (1.8 to 2.0 Gy per fraction) postoperatively.

High-dose-rate intraoperative brachytherapy has been described in the treatment of primary and locally recurrent retroperitoneal sarcomas. A Harrison-Anderson-Mick applicator (an array of catheters spaced 1 cm apart in a silicone rubber pad), or similar device, can be used to deliver an intraoperative dose of 12 to 15 Gy to the tumor bed, using ^{192}Ir sources (2).

Postoperative radiation therapy is recommended for patients who initially present after resection. These fields frequently are more extensive than preoperative fields and thus a larger volume of normal tissue is usually included. Normal tissues (i.e., stomach and bowel) that were previously displaced by the tumor mass will subsequently fill the resection cavity after the tumor has been removed, increasing the toxicity of the treatment and limiting the dose that can be delivered. Although not commonly employed, silicone-filled implants have been used to displace bowel and other tissues out of the radiation field (2). Postoperative radiation fields should include the preoperative GTV (as defined on the preoperative CT or MRI) and the entire resection cavity. Residual disease may be visible on postoperative scans; however, surgical clips placed at the time of the resection will remove much of the uncertainty of defining these areas. Boost fields can encompass areas of close margins or residual disease. Expansion volumes (CTV and PTV) should be limited in regions where the tumor did not violate fascial or peritoneal boundaries. A postoperative radiation dose of 45 Gy (1.8 Gy per fraction per day) is recommended. Limited boost fields (5.4 to 9 Gy per fraction) can be planned, but careful attention must be paid to the surrounding normal tissue tolerances.

Results of Therapy

Despite poor local control rates with resection alone, complete surgical resection remains the only curative treatment modality in patients with RPS (9). In patients with nonmetastatic, completely excised RPS, 5-year overall survival is 49% to 70% (9,14,48) (Table 73.3). Failure to achieve local control of disease is the major cause of death in patients with RPS (22). In a large, single institution report of retroperitoneal sarcomas, patients who successfully underwent a gross total resection (n = 185) had a median survival of 103 months versus 18 months (n = 46) for those who underwent an incomplete resection (22). Similarly, Stoeckle et al. (49) published actuarial 5-year overall survival rates of 62% versus 26% for patients who had a complete (n = 94) versus incomplete (n = 50) excision, respectively.

Retrospective studies demonstrate an improvement in local control with postoperative radiation therapy (Table 73.4). In the report by Stoeckle et al. (49), patients with complete excision had a significant reduction in local recurrence risk when they received postoperative radiation therapy (median dose = 50 Gy) than when they did not (relative risk 3.36; p = .0002); there was no improvement in overall survival in multivariate analysis. Catton et al. (9) found that adjuvant radiation therapy increased the time to locoregional relapse from 30 months (no radiation) to 103 months (p = 0.06). Similar to the trial by Stoeckle et al. (49), radiation did not exert an effect on survival.

The optimal dose for treating RPS after resection is not known. Fein et al. (13) reported improved local control rates with adjuvant radiation doses greater than 55 Gy (using shrinking photon fields and/or an IORT boost); 25% local failure with doses greater than 55 Gy versus 38% local failure with doses less than 55 Gy. The National Cancer Institute demonstrated higher locoregional control in patients who underwent a gross total resection followed by IORT (20 Gy) and EBRT (35 to 40 Gy) compared to postoperative EBRT alone (50 to 55 Gy); 60% versus 20%, respectively (47) (Table 73.5). Alektiar et al. (2) reported higher local control rates in patients who received IORT (12 to 15 Gy) and postoperative EBRT (45 to 50.4 Gy) compared to those who received IORT alone, 66% versus 50%.

In trials of preoperative radiation therapy, researchers from Princess Margaret Hospital published results using preoperative EBRT (median dose: 45 Gy) followed by resection and postoperative brachytherapy implant (low-dose rate, median dose: 25 Gy) (19). Local recurrence was 19.6% and overall survival at 2 years was 88% in the 46 patients resected with curative intent. In a Massachusetts General Hospital series, 35 patients received preoperative EBRT (45 to 50 Gy) followed by resection (79% complete resections, 11% partial resections, and 5%

Table 73.3	COMPLETE RESECTION AND SURVIVAL IN PATIENTS WITH NONMETASTATIC (M0) RETROPERITONEAL SARCOMA (RPS) AND SURVIVAL				
Study	Complete Resection (%)	Local Recurrence (%)	Overall Survival (%)	LR with Incomplete Excision (%)	Overall Survival with Incomplete Excision (%)
Ferrario and Karakousis (14)	95	Primary RPS: 41 Recurrent: 61	Primary RPS: 65 (5 yr), 56 (10 yr) Recurrent: 53 (5 yr), 34 (10 yr)		
Stoeckle et al. (49)	65	57 (5 yr)	49 (5 yr)		
Lewis et al. (22)	Primary RPS: 67		70 (5 yr); median, 103 mo		Median, 18 mo
Catton et al. (9)	43	50 (5 yr); 82 (10 yr)	55 (5 yr); 22 (10 yr)	86 (5 yr); 95 (10 yr)	15 (5 yr); 10 (10 yr)

LR, local recurrence.

unresectable) and IORT (n = 20/37) using 9- to 15-MeV electrons; 10 Gy (complete resection), 12.5 to 15 Gy (microscopically involved margins), and 15 to 20 Gy for macroscopic residual disease (15). In those patients who underwent a complete resection, there was a nonsignificant improvement for local control if they received IORT (83% vs. 61%; $p = 0.2$). Petersen et al. (38) reported the Mayo Clinic experience of primary and recurrent RPS or intrapelvic STS treated with preoperative EBRT (n = 53), postoperative EBRT (n = 12), or both (n = 12); the median EBRT dose was 47.6 Gy (38). IORT (median dose: 15 Gy, electron beam) was also employed. Local control at 5 years for patients with gross residual disease (n = 15) was 41%, for those with microscopic residual disease (n = 56), it was 60%, and for those with complete resections (n = 16) it was 100%. The 5-year overall survival rates were 37% (in patients with gross residual disease) and 52% (in patients with microscopic and no residual disease).

Treatment Sequelae

The most common acute symptoms from EBRT of tumors in the retroperitoneum are nausea, vomiting, diarrhea, skin redness, and fatigue. Anemia, neutropenia, and thrombocytopenia may occur, especially with large radiation fields that often involve the adjacent spine. Weekly monitoring of the patient's complete blood count and daily vital signs should be performed. Reported postoperative complications include bleeding, impaired wound healing or dehiscence, infection, myocardial infarction, and death (19,38).

The major long-term sequelae of surgery and radiation are small bowel enteritis, stricture, perforation, fistula, and obstruction. Development of nephritis is possible after radiation doses >30 Gy, with resultant hypertension. Late complications are associated with the number of laparotomies to which the patient has been subjected and to the radiation dose and volume (20). A lower incidence of enteritis has been reported with the use of EBRT and an IORT boost compared with EBRT alone as the bowel is subjected to lower radiation doses when it is able to

retracted out of the field (47) (Table 73.5). One must pay careful attention to potential areas of overlap when using abutting IORT boost fields to decrease the risk of neuropathy and ureteral injury (15,19,38). Studies of preoperative radiation therapy have demonstrated that this approach is well tolerated and appears to be less toxic than postoperative radiation therapy (15,19,38). As previously mentioned, the role of preoperative radiation therapy is the focus of a current phase III study (1).

Lymphomas

Lymphomas are the most common adult malignancy of the retroperitoneum. CT, MRI, and PET imaging can be used in the staging work-up of these tumors. CT-guided needle biopsy or fine-needle aspiration with flow cytometry (percutaneous or endoscopic ultrasound-guided) may be employed to obtain a tissue diagnosis when no other more easily accessible disease is obtainable. The diagnosis, staging, and management of retroperitoneal lymphoma are similar to that of other lymphoma sites, and is discussed elsewhere. As with all retroperitoneal tumors, radiation doses and fields are often limited by surrounding normal tissues.

Other Lesions

Neuroblastoma is the most common non–central nervous system solid tumor in children. The incidence is 2.26 per million person-years, with almost all cases diagnosed in children under the age of 10 years old. The incidence for adults, age 30 to 39 years, is 0.2 per million person-years (11). Most groups treat according to pediatric guidelines as there are no treatment recommendations for adults with neuroblastoma. Consultation with a pediatric oncologist is essential (see Chapter 84).

Wilms' tumor (WT) is the most common malignant renal tumor in children; however, there were only 300 reported cases of

Table 73.4	LOCAL RECURRENCE IN PATIENTS WITH OR WITHOUT POSTOPERATIVE RADIATION THERAPY (PORT) FOLLOWING A COMPLETE RESECTION		
Study	Local Recurrence with PORT (%)	Local Recurrence without PORT (%)	p Value
Ferrario and Karakousis (14)	38 (at 41 mo)	53 (at 41 mo)	0.16
Stoeckle et al. (49)	45 (5 yr)	77 (5 yr)	0.0021
Catton et al. (9)	103 mo to LRF	30 mo to LRF	0.02

LRF, locoregional failure.

Clinical Radiation Oncology

Table 73.5   OUTCOMES WITH EXTERNAL-BEAM RADIOTHERAPY (EBRT) + INTRAOPERATIVE RADIOTHERAPY (IORT) BOOST FOLLOWING RESECTION OF PRIMARY AND RECURRENT RETROPERITONEAL SARCOMA (RPS)

Study	Median EBRT Dose (Gy)	Median IORT Dose (Gy)	Local Recurrence (%)	Overall Survival (%)	Toxicity (%)
Petersen et al. (38)	Primary RPS: 48.6 (post-op) Recurrent: 45 (post-op)	Primary RPS: 12.5 Recurrent: 15	Primary RPS: 0 (CE), 8 (micro), 40 (gross); 5-yr LC Recurrent: 0 (CE), 64 (micro), 33 (gross)	Primary RPS: 62 (CE), 54 (micro), 29 (gross); 5 yr-OS Recurrent: 80 (CE), 44 (micro), 45 (gross)	Chronic enteritis (16); grade 3-4 GI complications (18); fistula formation (18); neuropathy (mild, 12; moderate/severe, 21)
Sindelar et al. (47)	IORT arm: 35–40 (post-op); EBRT alone arm: 50–55 (post-op)	20	IORT arm: time to in-field local recurrence: >127 mo EBRT alone arm: 38 mo (p <.05)	IORT arm: 45 mo EBRT alone arm: 52 (p = 0.39)	IORT arm: chronic enteritis (13); neuropathy (mild, 13; 47% moderate/severe, 47) EBRT alone arm: Chronic enteritis (50), fistula formation (25); neuropathy (mild, 6; moderate/severe, 0)
Gieschen et al. (15)	45–50.4 (pre-op)	10 (CE), 12.5–15 (micro), 15–20 (gross)	Complete excision: EBRT + IORT: 17 (5 yr); EBRT alone: 39 (5 yr)	Complete excision: EBRT + IORT: 74 (5 yr); EBRT alone: 30 (5 yr)	Neuropathy (19), hydronephrosis (19), vaginal fistula (6), ureteral fistula (6), small bowel obstruction (6)
Alektiar et al. (2)	45–50.4 (post-op)	12–15 (HDR, Ir-192)	Complete excision: EBRT + IORT: 29 (5 yr) primary RPS; 39 (5 yr) recurrent, 11% (5 yr) total IORT alone: NR (5 yr) primary RPS; 67 (5 yr) recurrent; 50% (5 yr) total	Primary RPS: 75 (5 yr) Recurrent: 30 (5 yr)	Bowel obstruction (18), fistula (9), neuropathy (mild, 6; moderate/severe, 0), ureteral injury (3)

CE, complete excision; micro, microscopic residual disease; gross, gross residual disease; LC, local control; OS, overall survival; GI, gastrointestinal; HDR, high-dose rate; NR, not reported.

adult and adolescent WT in the literature at the time of a 2004 review article (50). The main presenting symptom in adults is flank pain, which is different than in children, in whom the presentation of WT is usually painless abdominal swelling or is asymptomatic. Treatment in adults consists of nephrectomy followed by adjuvant chemotherapy with or without radiation therapy. The histologic subtype and staging determine which chemotherapy regimen will be used and whether or not radiation therapy will be added. A high percentage of adult patients with WT can be cured when treated with multimodality pediatric regimens. A recent European intergroup study of patients 16 to 62 years old with WT demonstrated an overall survival rate of 83% at a median follow-up of 4 years (40). The toxicities of treatment (severe acute neuropathy, 43%; grade 4 hematologic toxicity, 43%) were higher than in the pediatric studies, but thought to be reasonable in view of the high remission rate (see Chapter 83).

Schwannomas are the most common benign tumors in the retroperitoneum (27). They are associated with von Recklinghausen's disease in 5% to 18% of cases, and patients generally present between the ages of 20 and 50 years (3). They typically form large, well-circumscribed masses, and may display cystic degeneration, calcification, hemorrhage, and hyalinization. Benign schwannomas tend to displace, rather than invade, retroperitoneal structures and are frequently highly vascular. They can cause bony changes in the spine and extend through the intervertebral foramina, causing neurologic symptoms (i.e., paresthesias, weakness, and pain). MRI is the recommended imaging study to better visualize the extent of the mass and its vascular architecture, whereas CT imaging is useful in evaluating for bone involvement. Many investigators do not suggest

CT-guided biopsy or fine-needle aspiration for the diagnosis of retroperitoneal schwannomas because of the risk of hemorrhage (10). Whenever feasible, complete surgical resection with negative margins is the treatment of choice. The use of adjuvant radiation therapy has been reported for incompletely excised sacral schwannomas and malignant peripheral nerve sheath tumors (8).

Desmoid tumors (aggressive fibromatosis) are rare, benign neoplasms that arise from muscle fascia, aponeuroses, tendons, and scar tissue. They occur more commonly in females (female to male ratio, 1.5 to 2.5:1) and are associated with familial adenosis polyposis (41). Desmoid tumors tend to be locally aggressive and have a propensity to recur locally after resection. The recommended treatment is complete resection with a 2- to 3-cm margin, although this is often difficult to achieve (5). Whenever possible, a repeat resection is performed for local recurrences. Postoperative radiation therapy is used in cases with an unresectable primary, after multiple local recurrences, or when it is perceived that a recurrence would subject the patient to significant morbidity. Despite variable data on radiation dose-response and field margins, most studies recommend doses of 50 to 60 Gy and a 5- to 7-cm margin (25). A meta-analysis of 22 studies suggested that local control is improved with adjuvant radiation therapy compared to surgery alone; local control after surgery alone was 72% (R0) and 41% (R1 and R2) compared to 94% (R0) and 75% (R1 and R2) after surgery and adjuvant radiation (33). In patients with unresectable disease, radiation therapy alone is effective in providing long-term local control in up to 80% of patients (25,33). The use of systemic therapies (i.e., hormonal, chemotherapy, nonsteroidal anti-inflammatory drugs) is investigational.

Table 73.6 THE INTERNATIONAL GERM CELL CANCER COLLABORATIVE GROUP CLASSIFICATION SYSTEM FOR ASSESSING PROGNOSIS IN NSGCT AND SGCT[a]

Tumor	Good Prognosis	Intermediate Prognosis	Poor Prognosis
NSGCT	• Testis/retroperitoneal primary, no nonpulmonary visceral metastases, AFP <1,000 ng/mL, β-hCG <1,000 IU/L, and LDH <1.5 × upper limit of normal • 5-yr PFS, 89% • 5-yr survival rate, 92%	• Testis/retroperitoneal primary, no nonpulmonary visceral metastases, AFP >1,000 ng/mL and <10,000 ng/mL and/or β-hCG 5,000–50,000 IU/L and/or LDH >1.5 × normal to 10 × normal • 5-yr PFS, 75% • 5-yr survival rate, 92%	• Indicated by any of the following: Mediastinal primary, nonpulmonary visceral metastases or AFP >10,000 ng/mL, β-hCG >50,000 IU/L, or LDH >10 × normal • 5-yr PFS, 41% • 5-yr survival rate, 48%
Seminoma	• Any primary site, no nonpulmonary visceral metastases, normal AFP, any β-hCG, any LDH • 5-yr PFS, 92% • 5-yr survival rate, 88%	• Any primary site, nonpulmonary visceral metastases, normal AFP, any β-hCG, any LDH • 5-yr PFS, 67% • 5-yr survival rate, 72%	• No patients classified as having poor prognosis

NSGCT, nonseminomatous germ cell tumor; SGCT, seminomatous germ cell tumor (seminoma); AFP, alpha fetoprotein; β–hCG, beta-human chorionic gonadotropin; LDH, lactate dehydrogenase; PFS, progression-free survival.
[a]Data from International Germ Cell Cancer Collaborative Group. International Germ Cell Consensus Classification: A prognostic factor-based staging system for metastatic germ cell cancers. *J Clin Oncol* 1997;15:594–603.

Extragonadal germ cell tumors (GCTs) present in the retroperitoneum as the second most common extragonadal site after the mediastinum. Usually four cycles of BEP (bleomycin, etoposide, cisplatin) is the recommended primary treatment for nonseminomatous GCTs (NSGCTs). Residual masses on CT scan should be resected in patients with NSGCT (44). If residual NSGCT elements (yolk sac, embryonal, choriocarcinoma) are confirmed on pathologic review, additional platinum-based chemotherapy may be given. If necrosis or teratomatous elements only are found in the resection specimen, then observation is recommended (29). Patients with small (<5 cm) primary seminomatous GCT (SGCT or seminoma) can be treated with either radiotherapy alone or chemotherapy (three to four cycles of BEP) (32). SGCTs that are ≥5 cm should be treated with chemotherapy. Residual masses <3.0 cm are usually observed with serial imaging and tumor markers. An area of controversy exists in the management of SGCTs with 3 cm or larger residual masses; some groups favor surgical excision and others favor observation. Subsequent chemotherapy is recommended for patients with viable SGCT on resection. Pectasides et al. (36) reported their results on 16 cases of retroperitoneal GCTs (11 NSGCT and 5 SGCT) treated with a platin-based regimen (with or without surgical resection). A complete response was seen in 9 of 11 (82%) NSGCT and in 5 of 5 (100%) seminomas. The International Germ Cell Cancer Collaborative Group established a classification system for assessing prognosis in NSGCT and SGCT (18) (Table 73.6).

Conclusions

The retroperitoneum represents a unique anatomic site; a huge variety of different primary and metastatic lesions may occur there. Therapy should be guided by histology. Our ability to personalize radiation therapy with decreased normal tissue toxicity has vastly improved in the era of imaging-based target volumes and intensity-modulated radiation therapy.

References

1. ACOSOG Protocol Z9031. Available at: https://www.acosog.org/studies/synopses/Z9031_Synopsis.pdf. Accessed June, 2007.
2. Alektiar, KM, Hu, K, Anderson, L, et al. High-dose-rate intraoperative radiation therapy (HDR-IORT) for retroperitoneal sarcomas. *Int J Radiat Oncol Biol Phys* 2000;47:157–163.
3. Antiheimo J, Sankil R, Carpen O, et al. Population based analysis of sporadic and type 2 neurofibromatosis-associated meningiomas and schwannomas. *Neurology* 2000;54:71–76.
4. Armstrong JR, Cohn I Jr. Primary malignant retroperitoneal tumors. *Am J Surg* 1965;110:937–943.
5. Ballo MT, Zagars GK, Pollack A, et al. Desmoid tumor: Prognostic factors and outcome after surgery, radiation therapy, or combined surgery and radiation therapy. *J Clin Oncol* 1999;17:158–167.
6. Bastiaannet E, Groen H, Jager PL, et al. The value of FDG-PET in the detection, grading and response to therapy of soft tissue and bone sarcomas; a systematic review and meta-analysis. *Cancer Treat Rev* 2004;30:83–101.
7. Bose, B. Primary malignant retroperitoneal tumours: Analysis of 30 cases. *Can J Surg* 1979;22:215–220.
8. Carli M, Ferrari A, Mattke A, et al. Pediatric malignant peripheral nerve sheath tumor: The Italian and German soft tissue sarcoma cooperative group. *J Clin Oncol* 2005;23:8422–8430.
9. Catton, CN, O'Sullivan, B, Kotwall, C, et al. Outcome and prognosis in retroperitoneal soft tissue sarcoma. *Int J Radiat Oncol Biol Phys* 1994;29:1005–1010.
10. Daneshman S, Youssefzadeh D, Chamie K, et al. Benign retroperitoneal schwannoma: A case series and review of the literature. *Urology* 2003;62:993-997.
11. Davis S, Rogers M, Pendergrass T. The incidence and epidemiologic characteristics of neuroblastoma in the United States. *Am J Epidemiol* 1987;6:1063–1074.
12. DeLaney TF, Trofimov AV, Engelsman M, et al. Advanced-technology radiation therapy in the management of bone and soft tissue sarcomas. *Cancer Control* 2005;12:27–35.
13. Fein DA, Corn BW, Lanciano RM, et al. Management of retroperitoneal sarcomas: Does dose escalation impact on locoregional control? *Int J Radiat Oncol Biol Phys* 1995;31:129–134.
14. Ferrario T, Karakousis CP. Retroperitoneal sarcomas: Grade and survival. *Arch Surg* 2003;138:248–251.
15. Gieschen HL, Spiro IJ, Suit HD, et al. Long-term results of intraoperative electron beam radiotherapy for primary and recurrent retroperitoneal soft tissue sarcoma. *Int J Radiat Oncol Biol Phys* 2001;50:127–131.
16. Gronchi A, Casali PG, Fiore M, et al. Retroperitoneal soft tissue sarcomas: Patterns of recurrence in 167 patients treated at a single institution. *Cancer* 2004;100:2448–2455.
17. Hassan, I, Park, SZ, Donohue, JH, et al. Operative management of primary retroperitoneal sarcomas: A reappraisal of an institutional experience. *Ann Surg* 2004;239:244–250.
18. International Germ Cell Cancer Collaborative Group. International Germ Cell Consensus Classification: A prognostic factor-based staging system for metastatic germ cell cancers. *J Clin Oncol* 1997;15:594–603.
19. Jones JJ, Catton, CN, O'Sullivan, B, et al. Initial results of a trial of preoperative external-beam radiation therapy and postoperative brachytherapy for retroperitoneal sarcoma. *Ann Surg Oncol* 2002;9:346–354.
20. Kepka L, DeLaney TF, Suit HD, et al. Results of radiation therapy for unresected soft-tissue sarcomas. *Int J Radiat Oncol Biol Phys* 2005;63:852–859.
21. Langen KM, Jones DTL. Organ motion and its management. *Int J Radiat Oncol Biol Phys* 2001;50:265–278.
22. Lewis JJ, Leung D, Woodruff JM, et al. Retroperitoneal soft-tissue sarcoma: Analysis of 500 patients treated and followed at a single institution. *Ann Surg* 1998;228:355–365.
23. Melicow MM. Primary tumors of the retroperitoneum; a clinicopathologic analysis of 162 cases; review of the literature and tables of classification. *J Int Coll Surg* 1953;19:401–449.
24. Meric F, Milas M, Hunt KK, et al. Impact of neoadjuvant chemotherapy on postoperative morbidity in soft tissue sarcomas. *J Clin Oncol* 2000;18:3378–3383.
25. Micke O, Seegenschmiedt MH, and the German Cooperative Group on Radiotherapy for Benign Diseases. Radiation therapy for aggressive fibromatosis (desmoid tumors): Results of a national patterns of care study. *Int J Radiat Oncol Biol Phys* 2005;61:882–891.

26. Musat E, Kantor G, Caron J, et al. Comparison of intensity-modulated postoperative radiotherapy with conventional postoperative conformal radiotherapy for retroperitoneal sarcoma. *Cancer Radiother* 2004;8:255–261.

27. Nah YW, Suh JH, Choi DH, et al. Benign retroperitoneal schwannoma: Surgical consideration. *Hepatogastroenterology* 2005;52:1681–1684.

28. NCCN Practice Guidelines in Oncology—V.2.2007 (RETSARC: 1–4), www.nccn.org./professionals/physicians_gls/PDF/sarcoma.pdf. Accessed May 2007.

29. NCCN Practice Guidelines in Oncology—V.1.2007, (Test-10) www.nccn.org./professionals/physicians_gls/PDF/testicular.pdf. Accessed May 2007 .

30. Nethercliffe J, Wood DN, Andrich DE, et al. Retroperitoneal and transthoracic anatomy and surgical approaches. *BJU Int* 2004;94:705–718.

31. Neville A, Herts BR. CT characteristics of primary retroperitoneal neoplasms. *Crit Rev Comput Tomogr* 2004;45:247–270.

32. Nichols CR, Fox EP. Extragonadal and pediatric germ cell tumors. *Hematol Oncol Clin North Am* 1991;5:1189–1209.

33. Nuyttens JJ, Rust PF, Thomas CR, et al. Surgery versus radiation therapy for patients with aggressive fibromatosis or desmoid tumors: A comparative review of 22 articles. *Cancer* 2000;88:1517–1523.

34. Oriana S, Bonardi P, Preda F. Primary retroperitoneal tumors. *Tumori* 1977;63:397-405.

35. Pack GT, Tabah EJ. Primary retroperitoneal tumors: A study of 120 cases. *Int Abstr Surg* 1954;99:209–231.

36. Pectasides D, Aravantinos G, Visvikis A, et al. Platinum-based chemotherapy of primary extragonadal germ cell tumours: The Hellenic Cooperative Oncology Group experience. *Oncology* 1999;57:1–9.

37. Pemberton J de J., Whitlock ME. Large retroperitoneal lipoma. *Surg Clin North Am* 1934;14:601.

38. Petersen IA, Haddock MG, Donohue JH, et al. Use of intraoperative electron beam radiotherapy in the management of retroperitoneal soft tissue sarcomas. *Int J Radiat Oncol Biol Phys* 2002;52:469–475.

39. Pisters PW, Ball MT, Fenstermacher MJ, et al. Phase I trial of preoperative concurrent doxorubicin and radiation therapy, surgical resection, and intraoperative electron-beam radiation therapy for patients with localized retroperitoneal sarcoma. *J Clin Oncol* 2003;21:3092–3097.

40. Reinhard H, Aliani S, Ruebe C, et al. Wilms' tumor in adults: Results of the Society of Pediatric Oncology (SIOP) 93-01/Society for Pediatric Oncology and Hematology (GPOH) study. *J Clin Oncol* 2004;22:4500–4506.

41. Reitamo JJ, Scheinin TM, Hayry P. The desmoid syndrome. New aspects in the cause, pathogenesis and treatment of the desmoid tumor. *Am J Surg* 1986;151:230–237.

42. Rosenberg SA. Prospective randomized trials demonstrating the efficacy of adjuvant chemotherapy in adult patients with soft tissue sarcomas. *Cancer Treat Rep* 1984;9:1067–1078.

43. Sarcoma Meta-analysis Collaboration. Adjuvant chemotherapy for localized resectable soft-tissue sarcoma of adults: Meta-analysis of individual data. *Lancet* 1997;350:1647–1654.

44. Schneider BP, Kesler KA, Brooks JA, et al. Outcome of patients with residual germ cell or non-germ cell malignancy after resection of primary mediastinal nonseminomatous germ cell cancer. *J Clin Oncol* 2004;7:1195-1200.

45. Schwarzbach MH, Hinz U, Dimitrakopoulou-Strauss A, et al. Prognostic significance of preoperative [18-F] fluorodeoxyglucose (FDG) positron emission tomography (PET) imaging in patients with resectable soft tissue sarcomas. *Annals of Surgery* 2005;241:286–294.

46. Shibata, D, Lewis, JJ, Leung, DH, et al. Is there a role for incomplete resection in the management of retroperitoneal liposarcomas?. *J Am Coll Surg* 2001;193:373–379.

47. Sindelar WF, Kinsella TJ, Chen PW, et al. Intraoperative radiotherapy in retroperitoneal sarcomas. Final results of a prospective, randomized, clinical trial. *Arch Surg* 1993;128:402–410.

48. Singer S, Antonescu CR, Riedel E, et al. Histologic subtype and margin of resection predict pattern of recurrence and survival for retroperitoneal liposarcoma. *Ann Surg* 2003;238:358–370.

49. Stoeckle E, Coindre JM, Bonvalot S, et al. Prognostic factors in retroperitoneal sarcoma: A multivariate analysis of a series of 165 patients of the French Cancer Center Federation Sarcoma Group. *Cancer* 2001;92:359–368.

50. Terenziani M, Spreafico F, Collini P, et al. Adult Wilms' Tumor: A monoinstitutional experience and a review of the literature. *Cancer* 2004;101:289–293.

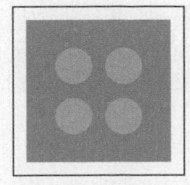

Chapter 74
Adrenal Gland

John J. Coen

Anatomy

The paired suprarenal (adrenal) glands are located between the superomedial aspects of the kidney and the diaphragmatic crura. They are surrounded by connective tissue containing perinephric fat. The glands are enclosed by renal fascia, but separated from the kidneys by fibrous tissue. The triangular right gland relates to the diaphragm posteriorly, and the inferior vena cava and liver anteriorly. The semilunar left adrenal gland is positioned in the middle of the left crux of the diaphragm. The omental bursa separates it from the stomach. It is also related to the spleen and pancreas (29).

The endocrine function of the adrenal glands necessitates an abundant blood supply. The superior suprarenal arteries are derived from the inferior phrenic artery, the middle suprarenal arteries from the abdominal aorta near the origin of the superior mesenteric artery, and the inferior suprarenal arteries from the renal artery. A large central vein leaves the anterior surface of the gland at the hilum. The shorter right suprarenal vein drains into the inferior vena cava and the longer left suprarenal vein drains into the left renal vein (29).

The lymphatic drainage follows the arterial supply and is predominantly to lumbar lymph nodes. The superior lymphatic trunks end in aortocaval lymph nodes located near the origin of the celiac plexus. The inferior lymphatic trunks end in lateroaortic nodes above the renal pedicle. Some trunks may pass through the diaphragm, following the splanchnic nerves, ending in retroaortic nodes in the posterior mediastinum. On the right, some lymphatic trunks may penetrate the liver (36).

The adrenal gland is composed of a central catecholamine-producing medulla enveloped by the steroid-secreting cortex. Although they are in intimate contact, they represent two functionally separate organs with different embryologic origins.

Epidemiology

Adrenal Cortical Tumors

Adrenocortical tumors are rare. Benign tumors are more common, occurring in 1% to 8% of the general population, and the incidence of carcinoma is approximately 1 per million population in the United States (12,26). There are approximately 75 to 115 new cases per year (39). Adrenal cortex carcinoma deaths account for 0.2% of all yearly cancer deaths. There is a bimodal age distribution with disease peaks before the age of 5 years and in the fourth to fifth decade of life.

Overall, adrenocortical carcinoma (ACC) is slightly more common in women than men. Nonfunctional carcinomas occur in an older age population (>30 years old) and are more common in men (3:2 male-to-female ratio), while functional tumors are more common in women (7:3 female-to-male ratio) and younger patients. As they frequently present with symptoms related to hormone production, functional tumors are detected at an earlier stage.

Although most cases of ACC are sporadic, it has been described as a component of several hereditary cancer syndromes including Li-Fraumeni syndrome (breast cancer, soft tissue and bone sarcoma, brain tumors, and ACC), Beckwith-Wiedemann syndrome (Wilms' tumor, neuroblastoma, hepatoblastoma, and ACC), multiple endocrine neoplasia type I (parathyroid, pituitary and pancreatic neuroendocrine tumors, and adrenal adenomas and carcinomas) and SBLA syndrome (sarcoma, breast, lung, ACC, and other tumors) (6–9). A role for p53 mutations in sporadic ACC is suspected.

Adrenal Medulla Tumors

Ganglioneuromas are rare, benign tumors of the adrenal medulla seen in children and young adults (11,14). Neuroblastoma is the most common malignant tumor of the adrenal gland in children, accounting for 90% of all cases (12,28).

Pheochromocytomas and functional ganglioneuromas (or extra-adrenal pheochromocytomas) are rare tumors that rise from chromaffin cells in the adrenal medulla and elsewhere. They secrete catecholamines and cause intermittent, episodic, or sustained hypertension. Pheochromocytomas have an estimated prevalence of 0.1% in hypertensive patients (4). In autopsy series, there is a 0.01% to 0.1% prevalence of unsuspected pheochromocytomas. Estimates of the incidence of malignancy in pheochromocytoma ranges from 5% to 46% in different series (5,10). Extra-adrenal tumors are more commonly malignant (27). Approximately 400 new cases of malignant pheochromocytomas are expected each year in the United States (15,32).

Pheochromocytomas may be associated with a variety of endocrine and nonendocrine inherited disorders. Bilateral pheochromocytomas are a component of multiple endocrine neoplasia type IIa (MEN IIA) syndrome (pheochromocytoma, medullary thyroid carcinoma, and parathyroid hyperplasia) or MEN IIB syndrome in which they are associated with marfanoid habitus, mucosal neuromas, and medullary thyroid carcinoma. Pheochromocytomas occur in 25% of patients with von Hippel-Lindau's disease and <1% of patients with neurofibromatosis and von Recklinghausen's disease (20,30).

Natural History

Fifty-nine percent of adrenal cortex tumors are functional, the left-to-right ratio is approximately 1:1, and 2.4% are bilateral (46). Diagnosis is frequently delayed because of the rarity of disease and the deep retroperitoneal location of the adrenal glands (13).

Nonfunctioning ACCs are typically larger tumors, >6 cm, while functioning tumors tend to be discovered at an earlier stage. (TNM staging; Table 74.1). Incidentally discovered adrenal masses <3 cm are rarely malignant. ACC is an aggressive malignancy that frequently violates the tumor capsule and invades surrounding tissues. It metastasizes to lungs, liver, brain, and regional lymph nodes. Many patients present with widespread metastasis; most of these patients die within 6 months of diagnosis. This situation is especially common in the pediatric population. For all stages, the 5-year overall survival is only 20% to 25% (13).

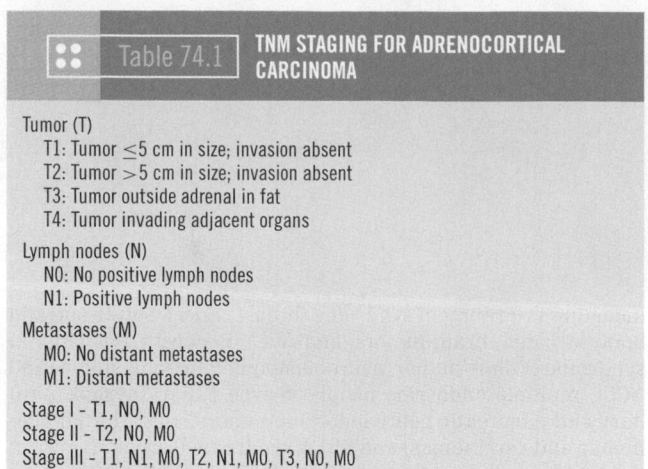

Table 74.1   TNM STAGING FOR ADRENOCORTICAL CARCINOMA

Tumor (T)
  T1: Tumor ≤5 cm in size; invasion absent
  T2: Tumor >5 cm in size; invasion absent
  T3: Tumor outside adrenal in fat
  T4: Tumor invading adjacent organs
Lymph nodes (N)
  N0: No positive lymph nodes
  N1: Positive lymph nodes
Metastases (M)
  M0: No distant metastases
  M1: Distant metastases

Stage I - T1, N0, M0
Stage II - T2, N0, M0
Stage III - T1, N1, M0, T2, N1, M0, T3, N0, M0
Stage IV - T3, N1, M0, T4, N1, M0, Any T, any N, M1

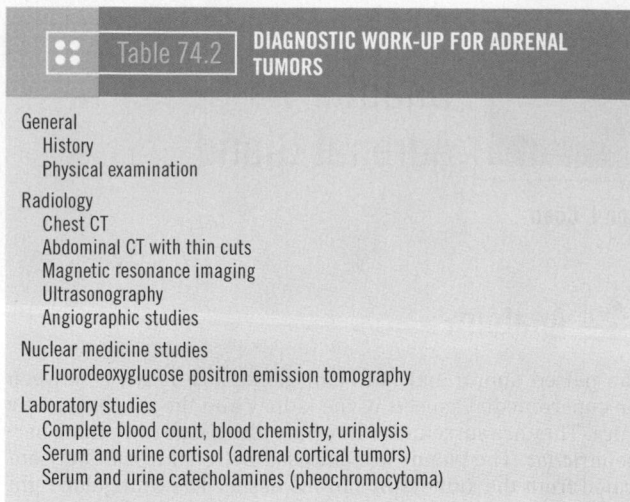

Table 74.2   DIAGNOSTIC WORK-UP FOR ADRENAL TUMORS

General
  History
  Physical examination
Radiology
  Chest CT
  Abdominal CT with thin cuts
  Magnetic resonance imaging
  Ultrasonography
  Angiographic studies
Nuclear medicine studies
  Fluorodeoxyglucose positron emission tomography
Laboratory studies
  Complete blood count, blood chemistry, urinalysis
  Serum and urine cortisol (adrenal cortical tumors)
  Serum and urine catecholamines (pheochromocytoma)

CT, computed tomography.

Malignant pheochromocytomas exhibit a similar pattern of spread but also metastasize to bone. They are equally common in men and women. The average age of presentation is 40 to 50 years old, but these carcinomas may also occur in children.

Clinical Presentation

Functional adrenocortical tumors most frequently secrete cortisol and androgens, resulting in Cushing's syndrome, virilization, and hypertension. Estrogen or aldosterone production is less common. Approximately 60% of ACCs are functional. In a child, virilization is the most common symptom of ACC and Cushing's syndrome is relatively uncommon. By contrast, adults usually present with either Cushing's syndrome alone or mixed with virilization. Patients with nonfunctioning tumors present with nonspecific symptoms related to tumor burden, including abdominal fullness, early satiety, pain, weight loss, weakness, fever, or an abdominal mass (1). Nonfunctional tumors ACCs are more common in older patients and tend to progress more rapidly. An increasing number of adrenal tumors are incidentally discovered during abdominal imaging in the absence of any symptoms.

Pheochromocytomas arising in the setting of an inherited disorder occur in the adrenal medulla in 90% of cases, as compared to 75% of sporadic pheochromocytomas. When associated with MEN II syndromes, 80% are bilateral. A tumor >5 cm more commonly has a malignant course than a smaller lesion. Serum catecholamines and urinary metanephrine and vanillylmandelic acid levels are elevated in 90% of pheochromocytomas. These patients present with a range of symptoms from mild labile hypertension to sudden cardiac death secondary to hypertensive crisis, myocardial infarction, or cerebrovascular accident. The classic triad of symptoms consists of episodic headaches, diaphoresis, and tachycardia (8,43). About half of patients have paroxysmal hypertension, and others have sustained hypertension. Pheochromocytomas may also present with normal blood pressure in 5% to 15%. Other symptoms may include pallor, palpitations, panic attack symptoms, or generalized weakness. Orthostatic hypertension may occur in association with hypovolemia.

Diagnostic Work-Up and Staging

Any patient with a suspected adrenal tumor should be screened for hormonal hypersecretion, including cortisol, aldosterone,

and catecholamine secretion. (Table 74.2) As hypercortisolism is the most frequent abnormality, serum cortisol, a 24-hour urinary cortisol, and an overnight dexamethasone suppression test should be obtained.

Computed tomography (CT) of the abdomen with thin cuts through the adrenal gland is the imaging test of choice for the evaluation of adrenal tumors. Carcinomas can mimic adenomas but are characterized by larger size, irregular margins, and heterogenous enhancement. They may also demonstrate tumor necrosis and cystic degeneration. Local invasion, tumor extension into the vena cava, as well as lymph node or other metastases, are often seen in advanced ACC. Magnetic resonance imaging (MRI) is useful in the evaluation of adrenal tumors (Fig. 74.1). ACC and pheochromocytomas are hyperintense on T2-weighted images and venous invasion is better imaged on MRI. If there is still question of vascular invasion, an angiographic study can be performed preoperatively, either selective arteriography or vena cavography. Fluorodeoxyglucose positron emission tomography may be useful in differentiating benign from malignant lesions. It may also serve as an additional staging study for patients with known ACC. A chest CT should also be performed.

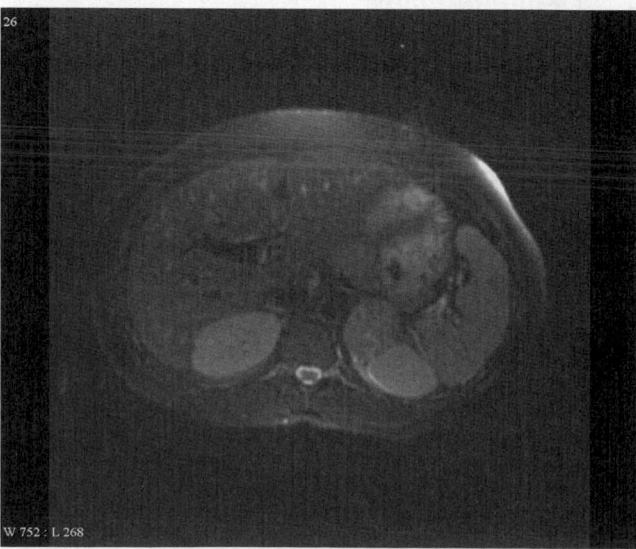

FIGURE 74.1. T2-weighted magnetic resonance image of a 35-year-old woman with a left adrenal carcinoma.

The diagnosis of pheochromocytoma is confirmed by measurements of urinary and plasma fractionated metanephrines and catecholamines. Biochemical confirmation of disease is followed by imaging to locate the tumor. Either CT or MRI of the abdomen will detect the majority of sporadic pheochromocytomas, which are generally >3 cm. A CT scan should be performed with thin cuts through the adrenal gland. On MRI, pheochromocytomas appear hyperintense on T2-weighted images as opposed to other lesions, which are frequently isointense with the liver on these images (7). Occasionally, CT or MRI may fail to reveal a lesion despite biochemical evidence of a pheochromocytoma. This is more common in the setting of an inherited disorder. In this case, ^{123}I-metaiodobenzylguanidine (MIBG), a radiolabeled analog of norepinephrine, scintigraphy may identify the location of the tumor (8). The major drawback of this study is that there is normal adrenal gland uptake of the compound. MIBG is also useful when there are multiple lesions or a high risk of metastasis (45). Additionally, it is used to follow patients after surgical resection.

Pathologic Classification

Tumors <6 cm are more likely adenomas, although some smaller tumors may be malignant (Table 74.3).

Hemorrhage and necrosis may be observed macroscopically in carcinomas. Numerous mitotic figures and cellular undifferentiation are common microscopic findings. Larger size, vascular invasion, or invasion of surrounding tissues and numerous mitotic figures are poor prognostic features (16).

Pheochromocytomas have malignant features in <10% of cases. Macroscopically, they tend to be encapsulated with areas of cystic change, hemorrhage, and necrosis. The capsule is frequently invaded, but that does not constitute malignant change. Benign and malignant pheochromocytomas may appear identical histologically. The only absolute criterion for malignancy is metastasis (9). Histologically, cell size, nuclear size, and arrangement of cells are variable. A twisted cell cord pattern, basophilic or cytophilic staining with fine intracytoplasmic pigment granules, and periodic acid-Schiff staining of secretory droplets aid in the diagnosis.

General Management

Surgery is the primary treatment for ACC. Complete resection is the only treatment that offers long-term disease-free survival, but is not always feasible. For patients with a macroscopically complete resection, a margin-free resection is a strong predictor for survival. Efforts to avoid tumor spillage are warranted and the tumor capsule should remain intact. Invasion or adherence of adjacent structures often necessitates *en bloc* resection of the kidney or spleen, partial hepatectomy, or pancreatectomy. The presence of tumor thrombus in the renal vein or vena cava does not preclude resection. A lymphadenectomy is often included. The role of tumor debulking in the presence of metastatic disease is not clear. Incomplete resection of the primary tumor or metastatic disease not amenable to surgery is associated with a poor prognosis. Still, tumor debulking may help control hormonal oversecretion or relieve local symptoms in certain cases. Even with a complete resection, local recurrence and metastatic disease are common.

The role of radiation in the management of ACC is not well defined. It has been proposed as adjuvant therapy after complete resection or as management of microscopic residual disease. One series reports a 10-year crude survival rate of 33% for surgical resection followed by adjuvant radiation (24). External radiation results in good response rates and effective palliation in patients with residual macroscopic disease or bone or nodal metastases (25,32).

Mitotane, a chemical congener of the insecticide DDT, is an adrenolytic compound with specific activity on the adrenal cortex. It is the chemotherapeutic agent most commonly used in the management of ACC. In patients with measurable disease, overall response rates of 14% to 36% have been reported, but most studies have reported no significant survival benefit (34). Responses are usually partial and transient, with only an occasional complete remission (46). The role of mitotane as adjuvant therapy after complete surgical resection is questionable (21,44). Despite limited supporting data, it is frequently employed in this setting, given the high rates of locoregional and distant recurrence. Serum levels of mitotane are monitored in order to optimize therapy because objective response in the metastatic setting was associated with higher serum levels (>14 mg/L). Unfortunately, increased toxicity is also associated with higher serum levels. Side effects are predominantly gastrointestinal, particularly nausea, but anorexia and diarrhea also occur. Although less common, CNS toxicity can include lethargy, somnolence, ataxia, dizziness, or confusion.

Single-agent chemotherapy has proven disappointing in the management of ACC. Doxorubicin and cisplatin have both been evaluated as single-agent therapy and in combination with mitotane. Neither drug was efficacious (1). Multiagent chemotherapy has shown more promise. A multicenter phase II study by the Italian Group for the Study of Adrenal Cancer demonstrated 49% overall response rate using a regimen of etoposide, doxorubicin, and cisplatin (EDP) in combination with mitotane. The regimen was well tolerated. The most common side effects were gastrointestinal. The time to progression in responding patients was 2 years (6). Inclusion of mitotane in a multidrug regimen is rational as ACCs are prone to multidrug resistance mediated by the multidrug resistance-1/P glycoprotein drug pump whose mechanism is inhibited by mitotane. This multidrug regimen is worthy of further study.

Surgical resection is the definitive management of pheochromocytoma, but it is a high-risk procedure. Cardiovascular and hemodynamic parameters must be monitored closely. Preoperative medical therapy is aimed at controlling hypertension and expanding intravascular volume. Preoperative pharmacologic preparation typically includes combined α- and β-adrenergic blockade.

In patients with undiagnosed pheochromocytomas who undergo surgery for other reasons, surgical mortality rates are high because of lethal hypertensive crisis and multiorgan failure (18). In the largest series of 147 patients undergoing surgery for pheochromocytoma, perioperative mortality and morbidity rates were 2.4% and 24%, respectively (33). Although it results in rapid symptomatic control, surgical removal of a

Table 74.3	CLASSIFICATION OF ADRENAL TUMORS

Adrenal cortex
  Adenoma
    Functioning
    Nonfunctioning
  Carcinoma
Adrenal medulla
  Ganglioneuroma
  Pheochromocytoma
  Neuroblastoma
  Mixed type (ganglioneuroblastoma)
Connective tissue tumors
  Myelolipomas
  Lipomas
  Myomas
  Angiomas
  Fibromas
  Fibrosarcoma

pheochromocytoma does not always lead to a long-time cure. In a large series of 176 patients, pheochromocytoma recurred in 16% of patients. Half of these recurrences were malignant (2). In patients with bilateral pheochromocytomas, usually in the setting of an inherited syndrome, bilateral adrenalectomy is recommended. Hormone replacement is required in this setting. Although not curative, debulking surgery for control of symptoms is the primary therapy for malignant pheochromocytoma.

The radioisotope ^{131}I-MIBG has been used a therapeutic agent in malignant pheochromocytomas which demonstrate avid uptake of the agent. Investigators have reported partial responses, based upon biochemical response as well as decreased tumor volume, ranging from 18 to 82% (40–43). Symptomatic improvement was observed in responding patients with regard to both painful metastases and manifestations of increased catecholamine levels. Partial remissions are usually temporary, with some patients relapsing between doses of MIBG. In other patients, sustained partial remissions have been noted with durable palliation extending 2 to 3 years (19,41). Prolonged survival has been associated with measurable responses and higher administered doses of MIBG (>500 mCi) (37). Toxicity includes bone marrow toxicity (particularly thrombocytopenia), nausea, and vomiting.

Combination chemotherapy with cyclophosphamide, vincristine, and dacarbazine has shown efficacy in a small study. In 14 treated patients, the clinical and biochemical response rates were 57% and 79%, respectively. Response was associated with objective improvement in performance status and blood pressure. Treatment was well tolerated (3).

Radiation Therapy Techniques

The role of radiation in the management of ACC is controversial. Locoregional disease control remains a major problem in this disease and some reports suggest that external radiation may reduce recurrence rates.

In the primary management of ACC, external radiation may play a role either preoperatively for unresectable tumors, postoperatively for patients with residual disease or high risk of local failure, or as definitive therapy for patients who are medically unfit for surgery. Radiation is also effective in the palliative setting for bone and local metastases.

For patients with macroscopic or unresectable disease, doses of 50 to 60 Gy delivered during 5 to 6 weeks should be considered. Initial fields should encompass the gross tumor with adequate margins as well as the regional lymph nodes, which should include the contralateral para-aortic lymph nodes. Dose to regional nodes can be limited to 45 Gy when they are not macroscopically involved. Care should be taken to limit dose to the spinal cord, kidneys, liver, and small bowel. For macroscopic disease for which high dose is desired, conformal techniques and intensity-modulated radiation should be considered. For patients receiving postoperative treatment for high-risk or microscopic disease, doses of 45 to 54 Gy are appropriate.

In the palliative setting, doses of 30 to 40 Gy given during the course of 2 to 3 weeks are reasonable. In patients with painful bone metastases, hypofractionated regimens should be considered for patients with poor performance status or otherwise limited life expectancy.

External-beam radiation is limited to a palliative role in the management of pheochromocytomas.

References

1. Ahlman H, Khorram-Manesh A, Jansson S, et al. Cytotoxic treatment of adrenocortical carcinoma. *World J Surg* 2001;25:927–933.
2. Amar L, Servais A, Gimenez-Roqueplo AP, et al. Year of diagnosis, features at presentation, and risk of recurrence in patients with pheochromocytoma or secreting paraganglioma. *J Clin Endocr Metab* 2005;90:2110–2116.
3. Averbuch SD, Steakley CS, Young RC, et al. Malignant pheochromocytoma: effective treatment with a combination of cyclophosphamide, vincristine, and dacarbazine. *Ann Intern Med* 1988;109:267–273.
4. Beard CM, Sheps SG, Kurland LT, et al. Occurrence of pheochromocytoma in Rochester, Minnesota, 1950 through 1979. *Mayo Clin Proc* 1983;58:802–4.
5. Beierwaltes WH, Sisson JC, Shapiro B. Malignant potential of pheochromocytoma. *Proceedings of the American Academy of Cancer Research* 1986;27:617.
6. Berruti A, Terzolo M, Sperone P, et al. Etoposide, doxorubicin and cisplatin plus mitotane in the treatment of advanced adrenocortical carcinoma: a large prospective phase II trial. *Endocr Relat Cancer* 2005;12:657–666.
7. Bravo EL. Evolving concepts in the pathophysiology, diagnosis, and treatment of pheochromocytoma. *Endocr Rev* 1994;15:356–368.
8. Bravo EL. Pheochromocytoma: new concepts and future trends. *Kidney Int* 1991;40:544–556.
9. Cotran A, Kumar V, Robbins SL. *Robbins Pathologic basis of disease*, 5th ed. Philadelphia: WB Saunders; 1994:1161–1164.
10. Cryer PE. Phaeochromocytoma. *Clin Endocrinol Metab* 1985;14:203–220.
11. De Maria M, Barbiera F, Bonadonna F, et al. Diseases of the adrenal medulla. *Rays* 1992;17:62–86.
12. Dunnick NR. Adrenal carcinoma. *Radiol Clin North Am* 1994;32:99–108.
13. Haak HR, Hermans J, van de Velde CJ, et al. Optimal treatment of adrenocortical carcinoma with mitotane: results in a consecutive series of 96 patients. *Br J Cancer* 1994;69:947–951.
14. Hubbard MM, Husami TW, Abumrad NN. Nonfunctioning adrenal tumors. Dilemmas in management. *Am Surg* 1989;55:516–522.
15. Javadpour N, Woltering EA, Brennan MF. Adrenal neoplasms. *Curr Probl Surg* 1980;17:1–52.
16. King DR, Lack EE. Adrenal cortical carcinoma: a clinical and pathologic study of 49 cases. *Cancer* 1979;44:239–244.
17. Koch CA, Pacak K, Chrousos GP. The molecular pathogenesis of hereditary and sporadic adrenocortical and adrenomedullary tumors. *J Clin Endocrinol Metab* 2002;87:5367–5384.
18. Lo CY, Lam KY, Wat MS, et al. Adrenal pheochromocytoma remains a frequently overlooked diagnosis. *Am J Surg* 2000;179:212–215.
19. Loh KC, Fitzgerald PA, Matthay KK, et al. The treatment of malignant pheochromocytoma with iodine-131 metaiodobenzylguanidine (131I-MIBG): a comprehensive review of 116 reported patients. *J Endocrinol Invest* 1997;20:648–658.
20. Loughlin KR, Gittes RF. Urological management of patients with von Hippel-Lindau's disease. *J Urol* 1986;136:789–791.
21. Luton JP, Cerdas S, Billaud L, et al. Clinical features of adrenocortical carcinoma, prognostic factors, and the effect of mitotane therapy. *N Engl J Med* 1990;322:1195–1201.
22. Lynch HT, Mulcahy GM, Harris RE, et al. Genetic and pathologic findings in a kindred with hereditary sarcoma, breast cancer, brain tumors, leukemia, lung, laryngeal, and adrenal cortical carcinoma. *Cancer* 1978;41:2055–2064.
23. Lynch HT, Radford B, Lynch JF. SBLA syndrome revisited. *Oncology* 1990;47:75–79.
24. Magee BJ, Gattamaneni HR, Pearson D. Adrenal cortical carcinoma: survival after radiotherapy. *Clin Radiol* 1987;38:587–588.
25. Markoe AM, Serber W, Micaily B, et al. Radiation therapy for adjunctive treatment of adrenal cortical carcinoma. *Am J Clin Oncol* 1991;14:170–174.
26. McClennan BL. Oncologic imaging. Staging and follow-up of renal and adrenal carcinoma. *Cancer* 1991; 67:1199–1208.
27. Melicow MM. One hundred cases of pheochromocytoma (107 tumors) at the Columbia-Presbyterian Medical Center, 1926–1976: a clinicopathological analysis. *Cancer* 1987;40:1987–2004.
28. Miller RW, Fraumeni JF Jr, Hill JA. Neuroblastoma: epidemiologic approach to its origin. *Am J Dis Child* 1968;115:253–261.
29. Moore K, Agur A. *Essential clinical anatomy*. Baltimore: Lippincott Williams & Wilkins; 2002:182–185.
30. Nakagawara A, Ikeda K, Tsuneyoshi M, et al. Malignant pheochromocytoma with ganglioneuroblastoma elements in a patient with von Recklinghausen's disease. *Cancer* 1985;55:2794–2798.
31. Thirlby J. Adrenal tumors. *Cancer: Principles & practice of oncology* 7th ed, Devita VT, Hellman S, Rosenberg SA, eds. Philadelphia: Lippincott Williams & Wilkins 2005;1528–1540.
32. Percarpio B, Knowlton AH. Radiation therapy of adrenal cortical carcinoma. *Acta Radiol Ther Phys Biol* 1976;15:288–292.
33. Plouin PF, Duclos JM, Soppelsa F, et al. Factors associated with perioperative morbidity and mortality in patients with pheochromocytoma: analysis of 165 operations at a single center. *J Clin Endocr Metab* 2001;86:1480–1486.
34. Pommier RF, Brennan MF. An eleven-year experience with adrenocortical carcinoma. *Surgery* 1992;112:963–971.
35. Rose B, Matthay KK, Price D, et al. High-dose 131I-metaiodobenzylguanidine therapy for 12 patients with malignant pheochromocytoma. *Cancer* 2003;98:239–248.
36. Rouvière H. *Anatomie des lymphatiques de l'homme*. Paris: Masson; 1932.
37. Safford SD, Coleman RE, Gockerman JP, et al. Iodine-131 metaiodobenzylguanidine is an effective treatment for malignant pheochromocytoma and paraganglioma. *Surgery* 2003;134:956–962.
38. Schlumberger M, Gicquel C, Lumbroso J, et al. Malignant pheochromocytoma: clinical, biological, histologic and therapeutic data in a series of 20 patients with distant metastases. *J Endocrinol Invest* 1992;15:631–642.
39. Shambaugh E, Ryan R. *Summary staging guide for the cancer surveillance, epidemiology and end results reporting (SEER) program*. Rockville, MD: US Dept of Health and Human Services, Public Health Service; 1977.
40. Shapiro B, Gross MD, Shulkin B. Radioisotope diagnosis and therapy of malignant pheochromocytoma. *Trends Endocrinol Metab* 2001;12:469–475.
41. Shapiro B, Sisson JC, Wieland DM, et al. Radiopharmaceutical therapy of malignant pheochromocytoma with [131I]metaiodobenzylguanidine: results from ten years of experience. *J Nucl Biol Med* 1991;35:269–276.
42. Sidhu S, Sywak M, Robinson B, et al. Adrenocortical cancer: recent clinical and molecular advances. *Curr Opin Oncol* 2004;16:13–18.
43. Stein PP, Black HR. A simplified diagnostic approach to pheochromocytoma. A review of the literature and report of one institution's experience. *Medicine* 1991;70:46–66.
44. Vassilopoulou-Sellin R, Guinee VF, Klein MJ, et al. Impact of adjuvant mitotane on the clinical course of patients with adrenocortical cancer. *Cancer* 1993;71:3119–3123.
45. Whalen RK, Althausen AF, Daniels GH. Extra-adrenal pheochromocytoma. *J Urol* 1992;147:1–10.
46. Wooten MD, King DK. Adrenal cortical carcinoma. Epidemiology and treatment with mitotane and a review of the literature. *Cancer* 1993;72:3145–3155.

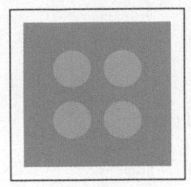

Chapter 75
Hodgkin Lymphoma

Richard T. Hoppe

The management of Hodgkin lymphoma continues to evolve. Since the last edition of this text, molecular imaging has taken on an expanded role in both initial staging and follow-up evaluations. Programs of combined-modality therapy have become the standard for early-stage disease and significant refinements have been introduced into the management of advanced disease based on prognostic factors. High-dose therapy programs for relapse have become safe and standard. Data regarding late effects continue to influence the development of new management approaches. Moreover, despite the excellent outcomes reported a decade ago, the results for treatment of this disease continue to improve.

Anatomy

Hodgkin lymphoma almost always begins in lymph nodes. More than 80% of patients with Hodgkin lymphoma present with cervical lymph node involvement, and more than 50% have mediastinal disease. Isolated extralymphatic involvement in the absence of nodal disease is rare.

Epidemiology and Risk Factors

Hodgkin lymphoma accounts for 0.58% of all cancers diagnosed and only 0.23% of all cancer deaths in the United States each year (54,129). The reported incidence is slightly less than 3 per 100,000 (162a). There is a slight male predominance (1.1:1). Hodgkin lymphoma is rare in children younger than 10 years of age; the median age of patients at the time of diagnosis is 26 years. The incidence of Hodgkin lymphoma has a bimodal peak as a function of age (123). The early peak, from ages 25 to 30 years, shows an incidence of approximately 5.5 per 100,000 per year. A second peak, from ages 75 to 80 years, shows a similar incidence. However, recent analysis suggests that this peak in older adults may be "contaminated" by cases that were actually anaplastic large cell or diffuse large cell lymphoma.

Geographic clusters of patients with Hodgkin lymphoma have been reported, but these are probably only coincidental

(55). A relation between Hodgkin lymphoma and previous infection with Epstein-Barr virus (EBV) has been proposed (3). Weiss et al. (181) identified components of the EBV genome in the cellular DNA of Reed-Sternberg cells in lymph nodes involved by Hodgkin lymphoma. In addition, Mueller et al. (128) identified elevated levels of immunoglobulin G and immunoglobulin A against the EBV capsid antigen and elevated levels of antibody against the EBV nuclear antigen, and early antigen D in the serum of patients with Hodgkin lymphoma 3 to 156 months *before* the diagnosis of Hodgkin lymphoma.

Finally, the risk for development of Hodgkin lymphoma is documented to be 2.55 times higher among individuals who have a history of infectious mononucleosis than among noninfected control subjects (69). Several series have demonstrated an association between EBV infection and mixed-cellularity Hodgkin lymphoma, especially in children in developing countries. An international analysis based on 1,546 patients with Hodgkin lymphoma shows an increased risk for EBV-associated Hodgkin lymphoma in Hispanics (vs. whites), those with the mixed-cellularity histologic subtype (vs. nodular sclerosis), children from economically less developed (vs. more developed) regions, and young adult men (vs. women) (50). Studies attempting to link occupational exposures or other etiologic factors with the development of Hodgkin lymphoma have been inconclusive or contradictory (55).

Natural History and Clinical Presentation

Patients with Hodgkin lymphoma usually present with painless lymphadenopathy. Some may note systemic symptoms such as unexplained fevers, drenching night sweats, weight loss, generalized pruritus, fatigue, and alcohol-induced pain in tissues involved by Hodgkin lymphoma. Still other patients are diagnosed after detection of a mediastinal mass on a routine chest radiograph.

If contiguity is assumed among the supraclavicular lymph nodes and upper paraaortic nodes/celiac axis/spleen, 90% of patients present with contiguous sites of involvement (99,149). In addition, disease spread after treatment with limited irradiation also occurs in a contiguous fashion in most instances (99). The theory of contiguity of spread and the development of treatment programs including presumptive treatment of uninvolved sites were important conceptual advances in the treatment of Hodgkin lymphoma (101).

Visceral involvement by Hodgkin lymphoma may be secondary to extension from adjacent lymph node regions, such as spread from enlarged mediastinal or bronchopulmonary (pulmonary hilar) lymph nodes directly into the pulmonary parenchyma, or it may be hematogenous, such as nodular disease in the liver or multiple bony sites. Involvement of the bones may cause blastic changes, especially in the vertebrae (creating the classic "ivory vertebra" on chest radiograph), pelvis, sternum, or ribs.

The mechanism of spread of disease to the spleen is unclear. However, the likelihood of disseminated disease, including bone marrow and liver involvement, increases as the extent of disease in the spleen increases (100). Nearly all patients with hepatic or bone marrow involvement by Hodgkin lymphoma have extensive involvement of the spleen (74).

Hodgkin lymphoma only rarely involves the gut-associated lymphoid tissues such as Waldeyer's ring and Peyer's patches. It also only rarely involves the upper aerodigestive tract, central nervous system, and skin (99).

The rapidity of Hodgkin lymphoma growth and spread is not predictable. Disease may evolve over a period of several years, demonstrated on serial radiographs or suspected by clinical history, and it is unusual to document progression during evaluation and staging.

The three so-called B symptoms are considered part of the staging system of Hodgkin lymphoma (see later discussion). They are fever, drenching night sweats, and significant weight loss. One third of patients present with one of these symptoms. Fevers may present in the classic waxing and waning Pel-Ebstein pattern. Night sweats may be drenching, and require a change of bedclothes. Night sweats may be a relatively unimportant B symptom, whereas patients who have both weight loss and fevers have a particularly poor prognosis (25). However, B symptoms may occur even in patients with relatively limited disease.

Historically, children have had a particularly good prognosis compared with adults, and therefore different treatment strategies have been developed for children (91,94,95,154,155,179). More recently, the results of treatment in young adults have improved to the same level enjoyed by children. In older adults (>60 years), the presence of intercurrent illness often affects the aggressiveness of staging and treatment and is likely to have a detrimental effect on outcome. However, older adults who have no significant intercurrent disease enjoy a high likelihood of cure (5,30).

Hodgkin lymphoma may be diagnosed during pregnancy, and many women become pregnant after successful treatment. However, no evidence exists that pregnancy per se has any effect on the natural history of the disease (96,108,145). Although patients infected with human immunodeficiency virus type 1 do not appear to be at increased risk for development of Hodgkin lymphoma, the disease tends to behave differently in infected persons (161,166,167).

Diagnostic Work-Up

Diagnostic and staging procedures commonly used for Hodgkin lymphoma are listed in Table 75.1. Patient age and the presence of intercurrent disease influence the selection of staging studies (52,70,172).

Hematologic evaluation may reveal anemia, leukopenia, lymphopenia, or thrombocytosis. This is often a paraneoplas-

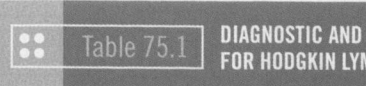

Table 75.1 — DIAGNOSTIC AND STAGING PROCEDURES FOR HODGKIN LYMPHOMA

History
  Systemic B symptoms: unexplained fever, drenching night sweats, weight loss >10% of body weight in the last 6 months
  Other symptoms: alcohol intolerance, pruritus, respiratory problems, fatigue
Physical examination
  Palpable nodes (note number, size, location, shape, consistency, mobility)
  Palpable viscera
Laboratory studies
  Complete blood count
  Platelet count
  Serum albumin
  Liver and renal function tests
  Blood chemistries
  Erythrocyte sedimentation rate
Radiographic studies
  Chest radiographs: posteroanterior and lateral
  Computed tomographic (CT) scan of thorax, abdomen, and pelvis
  CT scan of neck (if neck irradiation is indicated)
  Positron emission tomography scan, especially if equivocal CT scan
Additional biopsies, if indicated
  Bone marrow, needle biopsy (if subdiaphragmatic disease or B symptoms)
  Cytologic examination of effusions, if present
  Percutaneous liver biopsy if abnormal LFTs but normal CT

tic effect, but it may be indicative of bone marrow involvement. Anemia, lymphopenia, and hypoalbuminemia are adverse prognostic factors, especially for patients with advanced disease (stage III–IV) (65). The serum alkaline phosphatase level may serve as a nonspecific marker of tumor activity or hepatic, bone marrow, or bone disease. The erythrocyte sedimentation rate (ESR) may correlate with response to treatment and subsequent disease activity and is a prognostic factor for patients with limited disease (stage I–II) (67). Other useful markers may include the serum copper, lactate dehydrogenase, and β_2-microglobulin (162).

Radiographic evaluation should include posteroanterior and lateral chest radiographs. Mediastinal adenopathy may be quantified by a measurement of the maximum width of the mediastinal mass divided by the maximum intrathoracic diameter (near the level of the diaphragm) on a standing posteroanterior chest radiograph, as shown in Fig. 75.1. When this ratio exceeds 1:3, the disease is defined as bulky for assignment to many clinical trials. Other definitions of bulky mediastinal adenopathy include a mass >10 cm and a ratio of mediastinal mass to the chest diameter at T5-6 exceeding 0.35 (employed in European Organization for the Treatment of Cancer [EORTC] clinical trials). A computed tomography (CT) scan of the chest provides ancillary information regarding the extent of intrathoracic disease and assists in treatment planning (16,80).

An abdominal and pelvic CT scan should be obtained, with special attention paid to the presence of enlarged nodes in the retroperitoneal area, hepatosplenomegaly, or focal nodules in the spleen or liver. Lymph nodes are usually considered to be enlarged on CT if their short axis measurement exceeds 1 cm (20). Splenomegaly or hepatomegaly alone cannot be interpreted to represent involvement by Hodgkin lymphoma because enlarged spleens often are not involved at the time of splenectomy; however, the presence of focal nodules is usually indicative of involvement. The overall accuracy rate for detection of Hodgkin lymphoma in the spleen by CT is reported to be 58% (18).

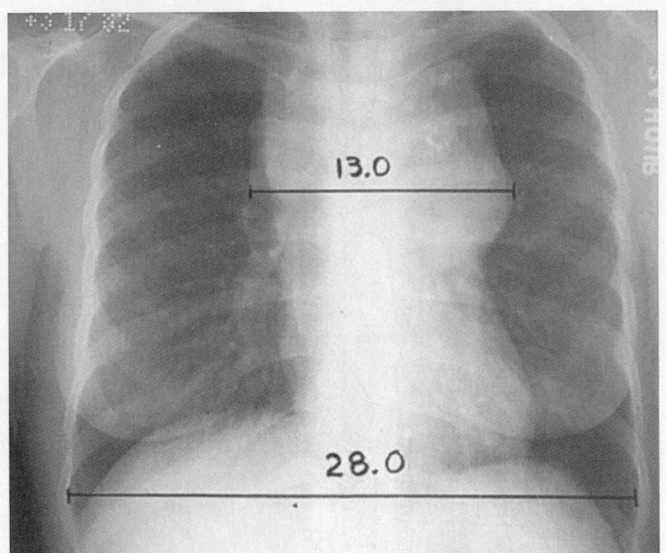

FIGURE 75.1. The mediastinal mass ratio (MMR). This ratio is defined as the maximum single horizontal mediastinal mass measurement divided by the maximum intrathoracic diameter, which is usually near the diaphragm. In this example, the MMR = 13.0/28.0 = 0.46.

The retroperitoneal nodes are generally evaluated by CT. The sensitivity, specificity, and overall accuracy of the CT in identifying nodal disease are 65%, 92%, and 87%, respectively (18). A CT scan of the neck may often be indicated, especially if irradiation to the cervical nodes is contemplated, in order to identify their precise location for treatment planning. Positron emission tomography using 2-fluoro-2-deoxy-D-glucose (FDG-PET) has become an important component of initial staging in Hodgkin lymphoma and it has largely replaced gallium imaging for that purpose. FDG-PET is more sensitive than CT (139) or gallium imaging (183) and is more convenient than gallium because of the shorter interval between injection and scanning (1 hour vs. 48 to 72 hours). It may be particularly useful as a follow-up study to evaluate residual masses detected by CT scanning (29).

Magnetic resonance imaging may be an alternative to chest or abdominal-pelvic CT scanning for initial staging, but has not been used widely (19). Its main value may be in the staging evaluation of women during pregnancy (145).

A needle biopsy of the posterior iliac crest bone marrow may be performed in selected patients. Because the yield is exceedingly low in asymptomatic patients with limited clinical disease, it should be restricted to patients with B symptoms or clinical evidence of subdiaphragmatic disease. The overall incidence of bone marrow involvement in Hodgkin lymphoma is only 5%.

Although staging laparotomy has been abandoned as a part of routine staging in Hodgkin lymphoma, its enduring value is the knowledge it provided regarding the patterns of initial involvement and spread of disease and the frequency of detection of occult subdiaphragmatic disease, despite negative imaging studies. Table 75.2 displays the yield of laparotomy in different clinical situations. These data were derived from an analysis of 915 patients with supradiaphragmatic clinical stage I or II Hodgkin lymphoma staged with a laparotomy at Stanford University (112). Subgroups of patients with a very low probability of disease identified below the diaphragm included the following:

(a) Patients with clinical disease limited to intrathoracic sites (yield 0%),
(b) Female patients with stage I disease (yield ~6%),
(c) Male patients with stage I disease and lymphocyte predominance or interfollicular histology (yield ~4%), and
(d) Female patients with stage II disease who have three or fewer sites of clinical involvement and are younger than 27 years (yield ~9%).

For all other clinical groups, the yield of laparotomy was ≥20%. Overall, the rate of detection of subdiaphragmatic disease was 28%, an observation that has had important implications for the design of treatment programs.

Staging

The Ann Arbor staging system for Hodgkin lymphoma, used since 1971, is outlined in Table 75.3 (13). The lymphoid

Table 75.2	YIELD OF LAPAROTOMY CORRELATED WITH MAJOR CLINICAL CHARACTERISTICS: RESULTS IN 915 PATIENTS STAGED AT STANFORD UNIVERSITY		
Characteristic	No. of Patients	Positive Laparotomy	Percentage Yield
Sex			
Male	519	174	36
Female	396	82	21
Symptoms			
A	841	217	26
B	174	57	33
Histology			
LPHD, NSHD	769	194	25
MCHD	128	58	45
Clinical stage I			
Right neck	43	8	19
Left neck	61	15	25
Mediastinum	12	0	0
Axilla (unilateral)	18	4	22
Clinical stage			
I	137	27	20
II	778	229	29
Total group	915	256	28

LPHD, lymphocyte predominance Hodgkin lymphoma; NSHD, nodular sclerosis Hodgkin lymphoma; MCHD, mixed-cellularity Hodgkin lymphoma.
Modified from Leibenhaut MH, Hoppe RT, Efron B, et al. Prognostic indicators of laparotomy findings in clinical stage I–II supradiaphragmatic Hodgkin disease. *J Clin Oncol* 1989;7:81–91, with permission.

::	Table 75.3	ANN ARBOR STAGING CLASSIFICATION[a]

Stage I	Involvement of a single lymph node region
Stage II	Involvement of two or more lymph node regions on the same side of the diaphragm (II), or localized involvement of an extralymphatic organ or site and one or more lymph node regions on the same side of the diaphragm (IIE)
Stage III	Involvement of lymph node regions on both sides of the diaphragm (III), which may also be accompanied by involvement of the spleen (IIIS) or by localized involvement of an extralymphatic organ or site (IIIE) or by both (IIISE)
Stage IV	Diffuse or disseminated involvement of one or more extralymphatic organs or tissues, with or without associated lymph node involvement

[a]The absence or presence of fever, night sweats, and/or unexplained loss of 10% or more of body weight in the 6 months before diagnosis is denoted by the suffix letters A or B, respectively. Patients are assigned a clinical stage based on the initial biopsy and all subsequent nonsurgical staging studies. A pathologic stage is assigned based on all clinical studies and subsequent surgical staging procedures such as bone marrow biopsy, staging laparotomy, and splenectomy.
Modified from Carbone PP, Kaplan HS, Musshof K, et al. Report of the Committee on Hodgkin Disease Staging Classification. *Cancer Res* 1971;31:1860–1861, with permission.

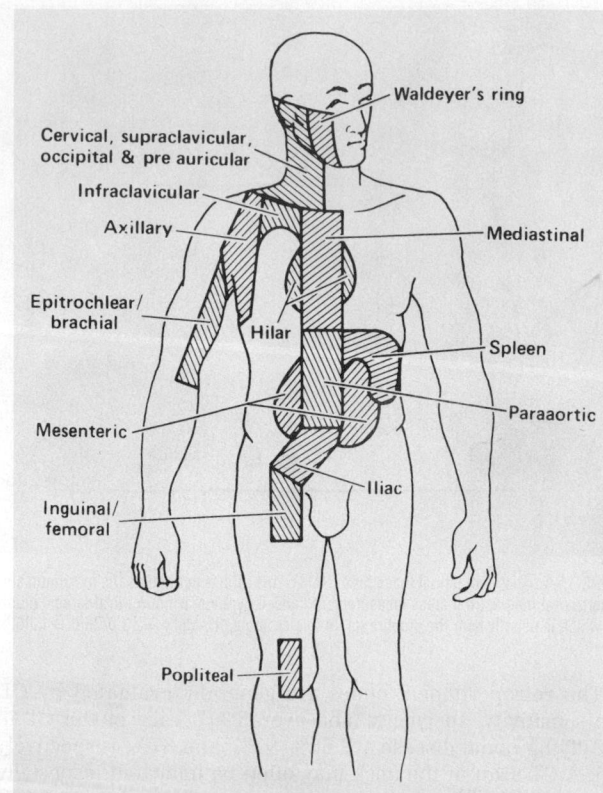

FIGURE 75.2. The lymph node regions as defined in the Ann Arbor staging system. Note that the ipsilateral supraclavicular, cervical, preauricular, and occipital nodes are defined as a single region. The mediastinum and pulmonary hila are defined as separate regions. (From Hoppe RT. The non-Hodgkin lymphomas: pathology, staging, treatment. *Current Problems in Cancer* 1987;11:363–447, with permission).

regions defined in this system are shown in Figure 75.2. The Ann Arbor system includes designation of a clinical stage, based on the results of the initial biopsy and clinical staging studies, and a pathologic stage, based on the results of any subsequent biopsies including bone marrow biopsy and those obtained at staging laparotomy. With the abandonment of staging laparotomy, the generic term *stage* (implying final stage designation after completion of all appropriate staging studies) is now usually employed, as opposed to clinical stage and pathologic stage. Deficiencies of the Ann Arbor system include its failure to consider bulk of disease and its lack of a more precise definition of the E-lesion (extralymphatic involvement) (22). However, the Cotswolds modification of the Ann Arbor system employs the subscript "x" to designate large mediastinal adenopathy (114).

:: | Pathologic Classification

The neoplastic cell of classical Hodgkin lymphoma is the Reed-Sternberg cell. It is typically binucleate, with a prominent, centrally located nucleolus in each nucleus, a well-demarcated nuclear membrane, and eosinophilic cytoplasm with a perinuclear halo. However, these cells usually account for <1% of the cells in a lymph node involved by Hodgkin lymphoma. The majority are lymphoid cells, eosinophils, plasma cells, and other normal cells (180).

Reed-Sternberg cells probably originate from B-lineage cells at various stages of development, including pre–B-cell and germinal center B-cell origin (107,108). In most instances, the Reed-Sternberg cells stain positively with the lymphocyte activation marker CD30 (Ki-1), the antigranulocyte monoclonal antibody CD15 (Leu-M1), the macrophage marker Leu-M3, and the Ki-67 marker for actively proliferating cells; they also express the interleukin-2 receptor and human leukocyte antigen DR antigens. They stain negatively with pan–B-cell markers such as B-1 and the leukocyte common antigen CD45 (21,37,182). Occasionally, they are CD20-positive, a marker of mature B cells (189).

There are five histologic subtypes of Hodgkin lymphoma as defined by the World Health Organization modification of the Lukes and Butler system. These include nodular lym-

phocyte predominance Hodgkin lymphoma and four subtypes of classical Hodgkin lymphoma: nodular sclerosis, lymphocyte rich, mixed cellularity, and lymphocyte depletion (64,118) (Table 75.4).

Nodular lymphocyte predominance Hodgkin lymphoma (nLPHD) is characterized by an abundance of normal-appearing lymphocytes and a scarcity of abnormal cells. Unlike the other subtypes of Hodgkin lymphoma, the abnormal cells ("L and H cells" or "popcorn cells") in nLPHD are strongly reactive for CD20 and CD45 and negative for CD15 and CD30 (142,180). nLPHD is often diagnosed in young people. Patients frequently present with early-stage disease, often in a solitary peripheral node, and systemic symptoms are uncommon (<10%). The natural history is the most favorable of the histologic subtypes. Occasional patients demonstrate a pattern of late relapse but good survival, similar to that observed in the follicular (B-cell) lymphomas (156). Some investigators suggest that nLPHD would more accurately be considered to be a form of non-Hodgkin B-cell lymphoma (142,144,146). A reactive process, termed

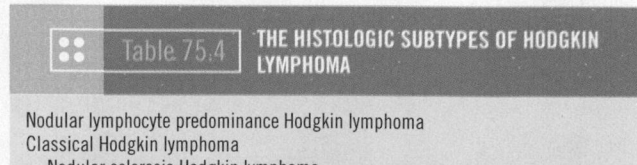

::	Table 75.4	THE HISTOLOGIC SUBTYPES OF HODGKIN LYMPHOMA

Nodular lymphocyte predominance Hodgkin lymphoma
Classical Hodgkin lymphoma
   Nodular sclerosis Hodgkin lymphoma
   Lymphocyte-rich classical Hodgkin lymphoma
   Mixed-cellularity Hodgkin lymphoma
   Lymphocyte depletion Hodgkin lymphoma

progressive transformation of germinal centers, may be observed in conjunction with nLPHD (63).

The other four histologic subtypes of Hodgkin lymphoma are termed *variants of classical Hodgkin lymphoma*. The Reed-Sternberg cells in these cases are CD15+, CD30+, and only occasionally CD20+. *Nodular sclerosis Hodgkin lymphoma* is the most common histologic subtype diagnosed in the United States. Involved nodes are traversed by broad bands of birefringent collagen that surround nodules of cells consisting of lymphocytes, eosinophils, plasma cells, and tissue histiocytes, intermixed with a variable proportion of atypical mononuclear cells and Reed-Sternberg cells. These cells may be in empty (lacunar) spaces, artifacts of formalin fixation. The mediastinum is often involved. One third of patients have B symptoms. The natural history of nodular sclerosis is less favorable than that of nLPHD.

Mixed cellularity Hodgkin lymphoma is characterized by a diffuse effacement of lymph nodes by lymphocytes, eosinophils, plasma cells, and relatively abundant atypical mononuclear and Reed-Sternberg cells. Patients with mixed-cellularity Hodgkin lymphoma present more commonly with advanced disease and tend to be slightly older than those with nodular sclerosing Hodgkin lymphoma or nLPHD. The natural history of mixed-cellularity Hodgkin lymphoma is less favorable than that of nodular sclerosis Hodgkin lymphoma.

Lymphocyte depletion Hodgkin lymphoma is characterized by a paucity of normal-appearing cells and an abundance of abnormal mononuclear cells, Reed-Sternberg cells, and Reed-Sternberg variants. This subtype may be difficult to differentiate from anaplastic large cell lymphoma (64). It is an exceedingly uncommon subtype of Hodgkin lymphoma. It tends to occur in older patients and is more likely to be associated with advanced disease and B symptoms. It has the worst prognosis of all histologic subtypes of Hodgkin lymphoma.

In addition to these major subtypes, *interfollicular Hodgkin lymphoma* is an uncommon pattern of focal involvement of a lymph node in which there is reactive hyperplasia with a small focus of Hodgkin lymphoma in the interfollicular zone. It is easy to confuse these cases with reactive lymphoid hyperplasia (33).

Table 75.5 summarizes the characteristics of patients treated according to histologic subtype at Stanford University from 1968 to 2001. These characteristics are similar to those reported from many other large centers in the United States and western Europe. However, the distribution of histologic subtypes and clinical behavior reported from South America, Asia, Africa, Eastern Europe, and even some parts of the United States indicates a greater proportion of unfavorable histologic subtypes and more aggressive clinical behavior in these regions (89,97).

Prognostic Factors and Therapeutic Implications

Because most patients with Hodgkin lymphoma are cured, prognostic factors are more important for defining therapy than in predicting outcome. Historically, when treatment programs were less effective, prognostic factors did have more importance in predicting survival (158).

The Ann Arbor stage is the single most important factor influencing therapy. Data generated at a time when treatment programs were more limited show a marked impact of stage on prognosis. With current management programs, this distinction has been blurred.

The bulk of disease is important, especially in the mediastinum. Bulk may be defined by absolute measurements, ratios of mass to anatomic measurements, surface area on radiographs, or volumetric determinations. Most series report that the risk of relapse after treatment with single-modality therapy is greater in the presence of bulky mediastinal disease than in nonbulky disease (10,73,120). For this reason, combined-modality therapy has long been the standard approach for patients with bulky disease (78,113,115).

Other measurements of disease extent that may influence treatment selection for Hodgkin lymphoma are the presence of B symptoms, the number of sites of involvement, and the elevation of serum markers such as the ESR. Sophisticated assessments of total tumor burden correlate very well with prognosis (160).

The histologic subtype of Hodgkin lymphoma has a minor impact on therapy. Agreement among pathologists is not perfect (23). After the extent of disease has been determined, histologic subtype seems to have little additional impact on prognosis, especially within the general category of classical Hodgkin lymphoma.

Large series report a slightly worse outcome for men than for women (53). However, gender is more important because of its influence on the choice of treatment secondary to potential reproductive complications (see "Sequelae of Treatment").

An important international study evaluated a series of prognostic factors among 5,141 patients with advanced Hodgkin lymphoma. Seven factors were identified, each of which had

Table 75.5	HISTOLOGIC SUBTYPE CORRELATED WITH CLINICAL CHARACTERISTICS OF 2,116 PATIENTS TREATED FOR HODGKIN LYMPHOMA AT STANFORD UNIVERSITY (1968–2001)		
	LPHD	**NSHD**	**MCHD**
No. of patients (%)	129 (6)	1829 (86)	365 (17)
Age (yr)			
Range	4–77	1–82	2–81
Median	29	26	30
Male:female ratio	108:21	943:886	287:78
Stage			
I (%)	50 (39)	141 (8)	73 (20)
II (%)	57 (44)	1067 (58)	138 (38)
III (%)	21 (16)	453 (25)	122 (33)
IV (%)	1 (1)	168 (9)	32 (9)
B symptoms (%)	2 (2)	516 (28)	103 (28)

LPHD, lymphocyte predominance Hodgkin lymphoma; NSHD, nodular sclerosis Hodgkin lymphoma; MCHD, mixed-cellularity Hodgkin lymphoma.

Table 75.6	A PROGNOSTIC SCORE FOR ADVANCED HODGKIN LYMPHOMA
Factor	**Unfavorable Covariate**
Serum albumin	<4 g/dL
Hemoglobin	<10.5 g/dL
Sex	Male
Age	$\geq$45 yr
Stage	IV (Ann Arbor)
Leukocyte count	$\geq$15,000/mm^3
Lymphocyte count	<600/mm^3 or <8% of white count

From Hasenclever D, Diehl V. A prognostic score for advanced Hodgkin disease: International Prognostic Factors Project on Advanced Hodgkin Disease. *N Engl J Med* 1998;339:1506–1514, with permission.

a similar impact on prognosis. These included gender, age, Ann Arbor stage, hemoglobin, white cell count, lymphocyte count, and albumin (Table 75.6). This "International Prognostic Score" is now used for assignment of patients to clinical trials. Patients who have three or more adverse risk factors are often considered to be in an unfavorable prognostic group for advanced Hodgkin lymphoma.

Patients with stage I–II disease often have only one or two adverse factors using this index. Large clinical trials groups have found other factors, such as number of sites of disease, age, ESR, and presence of B symptoms to be helpful in stratifying patients according to prognosis. Unfortunately, the criteria for defining "unfavorable" presentations of stage I–II disease vary among clinical trial groups (Table 75.7).

General Management

Radiation Therapy

Radiation therapy is the most effective single therapeutic agent for treating Hodgkin lymphoma. Optimal irradiation technique includes pretreatment simulation and requires the use of megavoltage photon beams, fields individually contoured to the patient's anatomy and tumor configuration, an adequate dose, multifield fractionated treatment, and portal film verification during therapy. Careful attention must be paid to every detail of therapy in order to maximize outcome and minimize risks (185).

Chemotherapy

The initial successful drug combination for treating Hodgkin lymphoma was nitrogen mustard, vincristine, procarbazine,

and prednisone (MOPP), reported by DeVita et al. (28) from the National Cancer Institute. The acute toxicities of MOPP are nausea, vomiting, peripheral neuropathy, constipation, leukopenia, and thrombocytopenia. Late effects of concern included sterility (especially in men) and the risk for secondary myelodysplastic syndrome or leukemia). A number of MOPP-like programs, such as chlorambucil, vinblastine, procarbazine, and prednisone (ChlVPP) achieve comparable results with similar drugs and less toxicity (156).

With the introduction of doxorubicin (Adriamycin), completely novel drug combinations were developed. The most successful of these is ABVD, which includes doxorubicin, bleomycin, vinblastine, and dacarbazine (11). ABVD has replaced MOPP as the gold standard of chemotherapy for Hodgkin lymphoma. This is based largely on the results of the intergroup trial that compared MOPP, ABVD, and MOPP/ABVD (12a).

Different combinations of drugs have been combined in an alternating fashion to prevent the emergence of resistant clones of cells. Most notable among these alternating non–cross-resistant regimens is the MOPP/ABVD combination, in which monthly cycles of MOPP and ABVD are alternated (9). Another innovation is the MOPP-ABV hybrid program in which partial cycles of MOPP and ABV are included in a single month of treatment (104). Most recently, in an effort to reduce toxicity or improve efficacy, new drug programs have been developed. These include Stanford V (88) and BEACOPP (40).

Table 75.8 summarizes the dosages and scheduling of these drug combinations (58).

Combined-Modality Therapy

Combined-modality therapy has become the most common form of general management for patients with Hodgkin lymphoma. Important considerations in combined-modality therapy include the sequence of therapy, the selection of irradiation fields, the decision to irradiate all involved sites or only "bulky" sites, the prescription of dose, and potential overlapping toxicities. It is logical to initiate treatment with chemotherapy. This has the advantages of treating all sites of disease at the outset (especially important in stage III or IV) and reducing bulky disease to facilitate subsequent irradiation (especially in the mediastinum). The irradiation dose used in combined-modality studies in adults ranges from 20 to 36 Gy (41,88,153).

Radiation Therapy Techniques

The principal objective of radiation therapy in Hodgkin lymphoma is to treat involved and contiguous lymphatic chains to

Table 75.7	DEFINITION OF "UNFAVORABLE" STAGE I–II HODGKIN LYMPHOMA IN RECENT CLINICAL TRIALS[a]			
	EORTC	**GHSG**	**NCIC**	**Stanford**
Age (yr)	$\geq$50	—	$\geq$40	—
Histology	—	—	MC/LD	—
ESR/B symptoms	$\geq$30 mm with any B	$\geq$30 mm with any B	$\geq$50 mm or	any B
Mediastinal mass	$\geq$50 mm without B	$\geq$50 mm without B	any B sx	
No. of nodal sites	MMR $\geq$0.33	MTR >0.35	MMR >0.33	10 cm or MMR >0.33
E-lesion	$\geq$4	$\geq$3	$\geq$4	—
	—	Present	—	—

[a]Patients with one or more of these factors were considered unfavorable.
EORTC, European Organization for Research and Treatment of Cancer; GHSG, German Hodgkin Study Group; NCIC, National Cancer Institute, Canada; MC, mixed cellularity; LD, lymphocyte depleted; ESR, erythrocyte sedimentation rate; sx, symptoms; MTR, maximum mediastinal width/chest width at T5–T6 on chest x-ray; MMR, maximum mediastinal width/maximum chest width on chest x-ray; E, extralymphatic.

| Table 75.8 | COMMON DRUG COMBINATIONS USED IN THE TREATMENT OF HODGKIN LYMPHOMA |

Drug Combination	Agents	Dose (mg/m²)	Route	Treatment Days	Cycle Duration (Days)
ABVD	Doxorubicin[a]	25	IV	1, 15	28
	Bleomycin	10	IV	1, 15	
	Vinblastine	6	IV	1, 15	
	Dacarbazine	375	IV	1, 15	
MOPP/ABVD	MOPP	—	—	1–14	56
	ABVD	—	—	29, 43	
MOPP-ABV	MOPP	—	—	1–7	28
	Doxorubicin[a]	35	IV	8	
	Bleomycin	10	IV	8	
	Vinblastine	6	IV	8	
	Prednisone	40	PO	8–14	
Stanford V	Nitrogen mustard	6	IV	1	28
	Doxorubicin[a]	25	IV	1, 15	
	Vinblastine	6	IV	1, 15	
	Vincristine	1.4	IV	8, 22	
	Bleomycin	5	IV	8, 22	
	Etoposide	60	IV	15, 16	
	Prednisone	40	PO	qod	
BEACOPP	Bleomycin	10	IV	8	21
	Etoposide	100 (190)[b]	IV	1–3	
	Doxorubicin[a]	25 (29)[b]	IV	1	
	Cyclophosphamide	650[b]	IV	1	
	Vincristine[c]	1.4	IV	8	
	Procarbazine	100	PO	1–7	
	Prednisone	40	PO	1–14	

IV, intravenous; PO, oral; qod, every other day.
[a]Adriamycin.
[b]Higher doses for "BEACOPP-escalated."
[c]Maximum = 2 mg.

a dose associated with a high likelihood of tumor eradication (58,185). This requires a well-collimated megavoltage beam and minimal penumbra. For example, the use of a dual-energy linear accelerator that produces 6- and 15-MV photons permits the treatment of custom fields that include the neck, axillae, chest, abdomen, and pelvis and provides a modest amount of skin-sparing. If photon energies in excess of 6 MV are used, bolus should be applied to the supraclavicular and inguinal-femoral lymph nodes. Meticulous treatment planning, simulation, and frequent verification by portal imaging are crucial factors in the success of treatment (99,102).

The most common techniques for field blocking are with multileaf collimation, divergent Cerrobend (Cerro Metal Products, Bellefonte, PA) blocks attached to a Lucite (Lucite International, Southampton, UK) plate and mounted to the head of the machine, or a combination of both for complex-shaped fields. Treatment at an extended source–skin distance of 110 to 140 cm may be necessary to achieve the large field sizes required. This is facilitated by extended travel distance couches that permit opposed-field treatment without changing the patient's position. Use of body molds reduces body movement and rotation and may increase patient comfort. Intensity-modulated radiation therapy is only rarely employed in treating patients with Hodgkin lymphoma (48,51,116,117).

Large field size, treatment at an extended source–skin distance, irregular-shaped blocks, and the presence of slanting body contours produce an inhomogeneous dose distribution. Use of treatment planning computers facilitates dose calculations and should include the effects of both primary and scattered radiation to each point of calculation. The minimum dosimetry should include an irregular field point calculation for each important nodal region in the field. The dose variation determined by these calculations must be compensated by individually designed compensators or selective area blocking (93).

Routine field simulation and portal imaging provide for optimal field design and document that the proposed treatment is executed properly.

When patients require separate treatment to adjacent regions, the calculation of field separation (gap) is exceedingly important (119). Special additional cord blocking should be used, if possible, when adjacent fields overlie the spinal cord.

In the uncommon situations when radiation therapy alone is used for the treatment of Hodgkin lymphoma, the National Cancer Center Network (NCCN) guidelines recommend a dose of 30 to 44 Gy fractionated at a rate of 7.5 to 10 Gy per week to involved sites (72). Because this situation is most common with the lymphocyte predominance histology, a dose of 30 to 36 Gy is usually sufficient. Evenly weighted opposed-field treatments;, all fields treated daily with fractions of 1.5 to 1.8 Gy, depending on field size and patient tolerance, were the general treatment parameters. A study by the German Hodgkin Study Group (GHSG) concluded that 30 Gy was an adequate dose for prophylactic fields (39).

More commonly, radiation therapy is used in the combined-modality setting. Doses vary considerably in different trials, depending on the prognostic category of patients, bulk of disease, and type and duration of chemotherapy. The range of doses considered acceptable according to the NCCN guidelines is 20 to 30 Gy for nonbulky and 20 to 36 Gy for bulky sites of disease (72).

As the use of combined-modality therapy for the treatment of Hodgkin lymphoma has increased, field configurations such as classic mantle, inverted-Y, and Waldeyer have been used less frequently. Radiation therapy is often limited to "involved fields" in this setting. However, involved fields are really portions of the classic treatment fields for Hodgkin lymphoma, and understanding these classic fields makes the design of involved fields more logical.

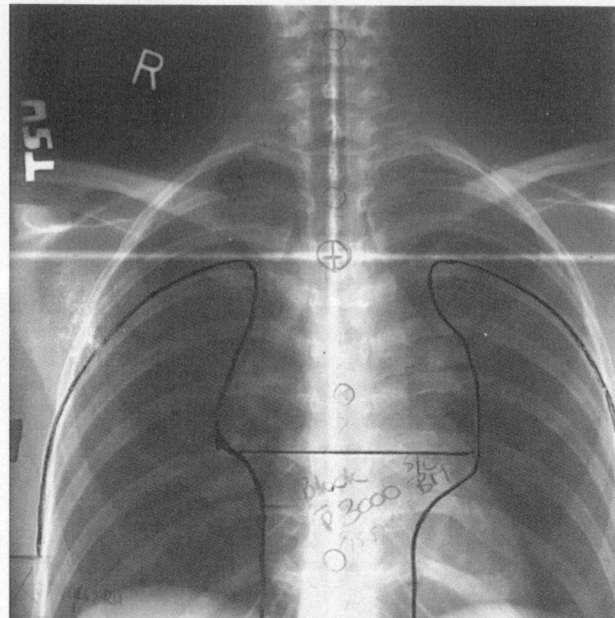

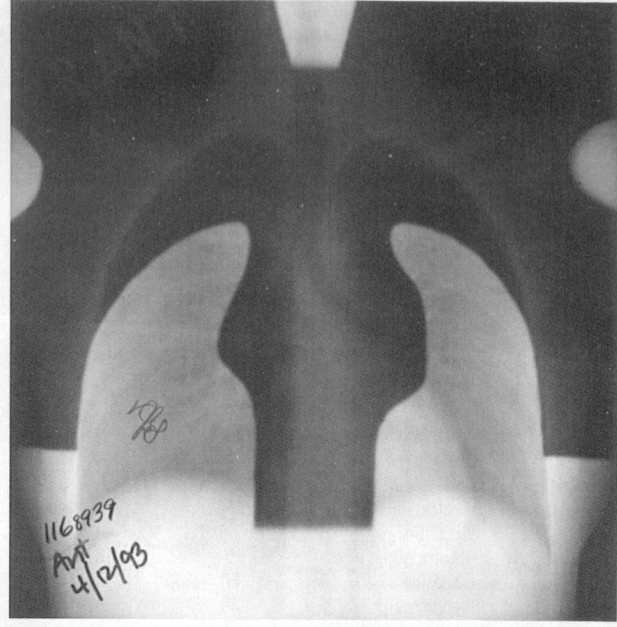

FIGURE 75.3. A classic mantle field anterior setup (**A**) and portal image (**B**) for a patient with a small mediastinal mass. (From Hoppe R. Hodgkin disease. In: Leibel S, Phillips T, eds. *Textbook of radiation oncology.* Philadelphia: WB Saunders; 2001, with permission).

The Mantle

The classic mantle included all of the major lymph node regions above the diaphragm considered to be at high risk for involvement in most patients with Hodgkin lymphoma. The field extended from the inferior portion of the mandible almost to the level of the insertion of the diaphragm. Individually contoured lung blocks conformed to the patient's anatomy and tumor localization. Patients were treated supine. An arms-up position pulled the axillary nodes further from the chest wall and thereby permitted more generous lung shielding. An arms-down or akimbo position permitted shielding of the humeral heads and minimized the effect of tissue folds in the supraclavicular/low neck regions.

An example of a classic mantle field is shown in Figure 75.3 (78,100). In addition to the lung blocks, blocks could be placed over the occipital region and spinal cord posteriorly, the larynx anteriorly, and the humeral heads both anteriorly and posteriorly. The use of these blocks depended on total dose planned and proximity of the adenopathy. For example, spinal cord shielding was not necessary with compensated fields if the prescribed tumor dose was ≤36 Gy, but was used when the calculated cord dose exceeded 40 Gy. A larynx block would be undesirable if there was very medially located cervical adenopathy.

In the classic two-dimensional planned mantle field, the patient was set up supine, with his or her head fully extended. The superior margin of the field bisected the mandible and passed through the mastoid process. The lateral margins were set to flash the axillae (with humeral head blocks if the arms were at sides or akimbo). The inferior axillary margins were at the level of the inferior tips of the scapulae. The inferior mediastinal border encompassed the initial inferior extent of the mediastinal disease with ~5 cm margin, usually at about the level of the T10-11 interspace. The lung blocks were designed to provide ~1 cm margin around the mediastinal contours and also encompass the pulmonary hilar lymph nodes. The superior most point of the lung blocks were no higher than the inferior tip of the head of the clavicle, with the tops of the lung blocks tapered laterally, often parallel to the projection of a posterior rib, in order to expose the high axillary/infraclavicular lymph nodes.

In contemporary management programs of combined-modality therapy, the full mantle is rarely treated. A more common configuration of fields includes just the mediastinum and supraclavicular areas. Cervical fields need not extend all the way to the mandible, unless there are involved high cervical nodes. The axillae are generally not treated unless they are involved. The two-dimensional design of these fields includes a superior border at the top or bottom of the larynx (depending on the extent of supraclavicular disease), lateral borders set at the coracoid processes of the scapulae (to include approximately two-thirds the length of the clavicle), and 1-cm margins beneath the clavicles. With three-dimensional (3D) treatment planning, now more commonly employed, the involved lymph nodes (gross tumor volume [GTV]), involved lymph node regions (clinical target volume [CTV]), and adjacent regions considered at risk (extended CTV) are outlined on cross-sectional images and blocking with multileaf collimators is employed, with isodose plan review to ensure a dose range of 95% to 105% to the planning target volume.

In the setting of a large mediastinal mass, the postchemotherapy treatment fields can usually conform to the width of the residual disease (unless there was pulmonary parenchymal extension), although the superior and inferior field margins should encompass the initial extent of disease. If a dose ≥36 Gy is planned, it is desirable to limit the dose to the subcarinal portion of the heart to 30 Gy in order to reduce the risk for pericarditis.

Subdiaphragmatic Fields

The classic subdiaphragmatic irradiation field for Hodgkin lymphoma is the inverted-Y, which includes the retroperitoneal and pelvic lymph nodes and spleen. With current management programs, a full inverted-Y is rarely treated. More commonly, portions of this field, such as the spleen with or without the para-aortic nodes, unilateral or bilateral pelvic fields are treated in the context of combined modality therapy. Sequential treatment to a mantle and inverted-Y field is referred to as *total lymphoid irradiation;* if the subdiaphragmatic field does not include the pelvis, the term *subtotal lymphoid irradiation* has been used.

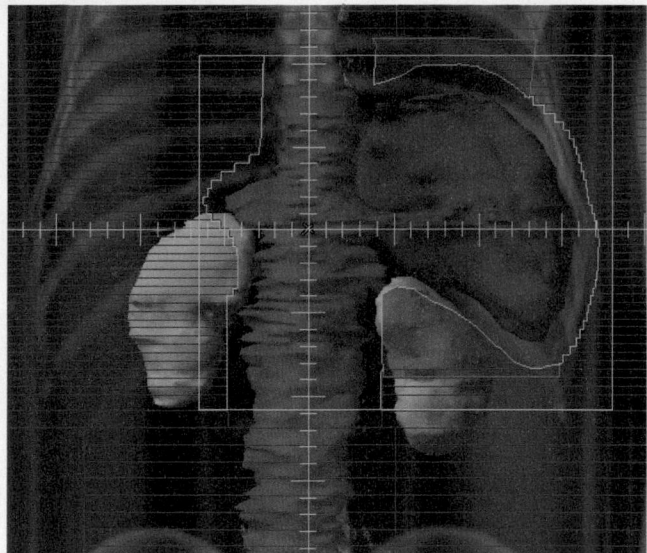

FIGURE 75.4. Example of a para-aortic-spleen field treated with respiratory gating. In this case, the inferior portion of the para-aortic field was at the bottom of L2 and was matched to another field that included the lower para-aortic, right iliac, and right inguinal-femoral nodes. The classic inferior margin of a para-aortic field would be at the bottom of L4. The clinical target volume (involved lymph node region) defined on cross-sectional computed tomography images is highlighted in light red and the spleen is highlighted in red. Because of the complex shape of this field, it is defined with a combination of multileaf collimators (blue horizontal lines) and Cerrobend blocks (light orange) to shield the base of the left lung and upper half of the left kidney.

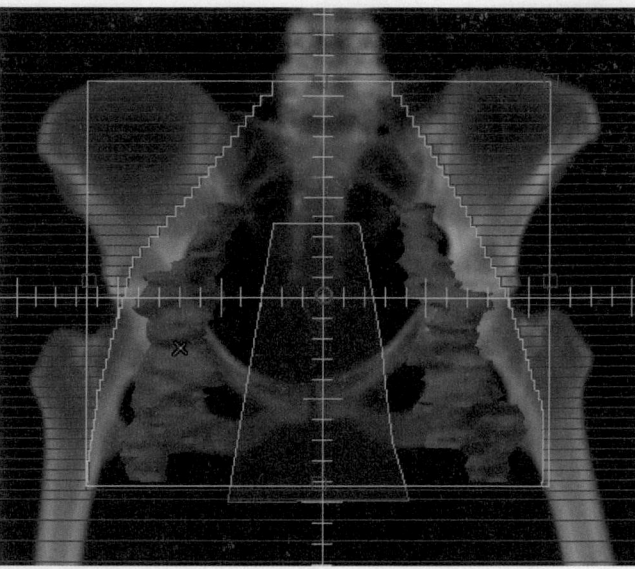

FIGURE 75.5. Example of a pelvic field. In a man, a gonadal shield would be used. In a woman, the ovaries would lie within this field unless they were transposed medially, behind the midline block or laterally, over the iliac crests. The field is defined with a combination of multileaf collimators (horizontal blue lines) and Cerrobend midline block (orange). The clinical target volume (involved lymph node regions) is highlighted in light red.

In the two-dimensional design of a para-aortic field, the width of the field generally corresponds to the width of the transverse processes. The spleen may be treated in contiguity with this field. The design of the splenic field requires consideration of respiration and the use of generous superior and inferior margins or respiratory gating. Three-dimensional planning for this field, especially if the spleen is being irradiated, is preferable, in order to more accurately localize the spleen and evaluate dose-volume histograms for the kidneys (Fig. 75.4).

Careful blocking considerations are required when the pelvic region is treated. Because the volume of marrow in the pelvis is substantial, the fields must be shaped carefully to minimize the amount of marrow treated (Fig. 75.5). With two-dimensional planning, the lateral margins are set 1.5 to 2 cm lateral to the widest point of the bony pelvis. Inferiorly, the pelvis field should extend to at least the lesser trochanters, unless there is disease that extends further inferiorly. Gonadal toxicity may also be an issue. In women, the ovaries normally overlie the iliac lymph nodes. To avoid irradiation-induced amenorrhea, an oophoropexy must be performed. This procedure is done by medial or lateral transposition of the ovaries via laparoscopy. The surgeon marks the ovaries with radiopaque sutures or clips and relocates them medially and as low as possible behind the uterine body. A double-thickness (10 half-value layers) midline block is then used; its location is guided by the position of the opacified nodes and transposed ovaries. When the ovaries are at least 2 cm from the edge of this block, the dose is decreased to 8% of that delivered to the iliac nodes (111). Alternatively, one or both of the ovaries can be transposed laterally to a position overlying the iliac wings.

In men, if no special blocking is provided for the testes, the testicular dose may be as high as 10% of the dose delivered to the inguinal-femoral nodes. Use of a double-thickness midline block and a specially constructed testicular shield can reduce this dose to 0.75% to 3.0%, most of which results from internal scatter. The precise dose depends on the position of the testes in relation to the inferior margin of the inguinal-femoral field.

Involved Fields

As noted previously, involved fields are simply portions of the classic radiation treatment fields. Although involved field treatment has generally implied treatment to the entirety of an involved lymphoid region (as displayed in Fig. 75.2) when any portion of that region was involved, that definition was derived at a time when irradiation alone was used for the management of Hodgkin lymphoma. Logical considerations mandate modification of these strict definitions in the context of combined-modality therapy. For example, if only the supraclavicular nodes are involved it is not necessary to treat the entire neck. On the other hand, the supraclavicular region is often included when the superior mediastinum is involved and portions of the iliac nodes may be irradiated when the inguinal-femoral nodes are involved (185).

3D Planning

The introduction of 3D simulation and treatment planning has permitted refinement in design of the radiation fields for Hodgkin lymphoma. Involved or "at-risk" lymph nodes may now be more precisely localized. 3D planning facilitates design of the axillary and pelvic fields and is essential in the design of a splenic field. In conjunction with the evolution of combined-modality therapy programs for all stages of Hodgkin lymphoma, the recognition that late effects may be limited by using smaller radiation fields, and the introduction of sensitive functional imaging techniques, there has been a conscious effort to reduce radiation fields from large fields such as the mantle to regional or involved fields. More recently, there even has developed an interest in "involved node" irradiation.

Using contemporary terminology for "involved field treatment," the *GTV* may be defined as all individual nodes or extranodal sites of disease that are palpable, enlarged on CT, or avid on FDG-PET. The *CTV* would be defined as the GTV plus the entire involved lymphoid region(s) (Fig. 75.2). An *extended CTV* may be defined as the inclusion of any portion of an uninvolved lymph node region. The *planning target volume* would include the CTV (or extended CTV) plus a 1- to 1.5-cm margin. In defining the concept of involved node treatment, the CTV includes

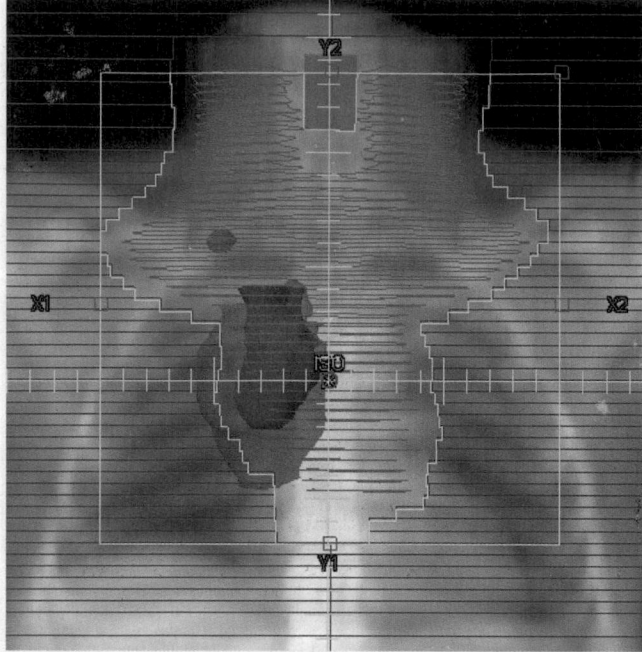

FIGURE 75.6. Example of a mediastinal/supraclavicular field. This patient had large mediastinal adenopathy and a right supraclavicular node at presentation (positron emission tomograph [PET]-positive volumes highlighted in light red). She was treated with 12 weeks of chemotherapy and the residual computed tomography abnormality in the mediastinum is highlighted in red (PET was negative). The radiation field was designed to encompass a clinical target volume (CTV) that included the bilateral supraclavicular, mediastinal, and bilateral hilar nodes (light red wire contour). Note that the CTV includes only the postchemotherapy extent of disease laterally, but extends 2 cm below the initial extent of disease. An anterior larynx block (Cerrobend) has been inserted. The remainder of the field shape is defined by multileaf collimators (horizontal blue lines).

the initial location and extent of the nodal disease, excluding normal structures displaced by the enlarged nodes, plus an additional ~1-cm margin for the planning target volume (49).

In the setting of a large mediastinal mass, the postchemotherapy treatment fields can usually conform to the width of the residual disease (unless there was pulmonary parenchymal extension), although the superior and inferior field margins should encompass the initial extent of disease (Fig. 75.6). If a dose 36 Gy is planned, it is desirable to limit the dose to the subcarinal portion of the heart to 30 Gy in order to reduce the risk for pericarditis.

:: | Results of Therapy

Hodgkin lymphoma is responsive to both irradiation and chemotherapy, and a variety of programs may achieve similar survival rates. However, there may be significant differences in freedom from relapse and potential complications of therapy. The results described in the following sections emphasize treatment programs that have been identified as appropriate ac-

cording to the guidelines of the NCCN (72). The results achieved at Stanford University with current combined-modality therapy protocols are displayed in Table 75.9.

Favorable Prognosis Stage I to IIA (Supradiaphragmatic) Classical Hodgkin Lymphoma

Favorable presentations of stage I–II include patients with stage I–II who do not have systemic symptoms or large mediastinal adenopathy. In some series from Europe and Canada, patients with an elevated ESR (50), extralymphatic extension (E-lesion), numerous sites of disease (more than two or three), older age (>50 years), or unfavorable histology (mixed cellularity or lymphocyte-depleted) are also excluded and treated according to algorithms for intermediate prognosis (Table 75.7) (122).

Historically, patients with favorable presentations of stage I–II Hodgkin lymphoma were candidates for treatment with radiation therapy alone, with curative intent and expectations. The treatment volume generally included the mantle and para-aortic fields, as well as the spleen. Results in single-institution and cooperative group trials included 10-year survival rates of 90% and freedom from relapse of 80% (73). These results are excellent, but the appearance of late risks of radiation therapy has resulted in a shift of management to the use of combined-modality therapy. The major concerns include the risks of secondary neoplasia, especially breast cancer in women, and an increased risk of cardiovascular disease after mediastinal irradiation (76).

The current treatment of choice for these patients is abbreviated chemotherapy plus limited (involved field) irradiation. Representative trials have included the Milan trial of Adriamycin, bleomycin, vinblastine, and dacarbazine (ABVD) times four plus 36 Gy involved field irradiation (IFRT) (8); the British trial of vinblastine, Adriamycin, prednisone, etoposide, cyclophosphamide, and bleomycin (VAPEC-B) for 4 weeks, followed by 30 to 40 Gy IFRT (126); and the Stanford University trial of 8 weeks of Stanford V chemotherapy followed by 30 Gy IFRT (82).

Important issues that have been addressed in clinical trials include the duration of chemotherapy and the dose of irradiation. In the HD10 trial of the GHSG, patients with favorable characteristics (normal ESR, no E lesions, less than three involved regions) were randomized to two versus four cycles of ABVD and 20 versus 30 Gy IFRT (91). Only preliminary results of this study have been presented, with recent suggestions that the 20-Gy dose may be associated with a higher risk for relapse than 30 Gy. Longer follow-up is required.

Trials that have eliminated radiation therapy entirely have been inconclusive. The National Cancer Institute Canada HD6 trial included arms of ABVD alone, but the comparison arms included subtotal lymphoid irradiation *alone* for the favorable patients (age <40 years, lymphocyte predominance or nodular sclerosis histology, ESR <50, and fewer than four involved regions) and 2 months of ABVD followed by subtotal

		Overall Survival (%)			Freedom from Progression (%)		
Stage	**Number**	**4-Yr**	**8-Yr**	**12-Yr**	**4-Yr**	**8-Yr**	**12-Yr**
I–II, Favorable	87	98	98		96	96	
I–II, large mediastinal mass	61	98	98	92	92	92	92
III–IV	108	95	95	95	86	86	83
Total	256	97	95	95	91	91	89

Table 75.9   RESULTS OF COMBINED MODALITY THERAPY FOR HODGKIN LYMPHOMA AT STANFORD UNIVERSITY (1989–2001) (82)

lymphoid irradiation for patients with any unfavorable characteristics. Although neither radiation therapy-containing arm would currently be considered appropriate management, the freedom from progression in the two radiation-containing arms of the trial was superior to that of ABVD alone (93% vs. 87%; $p = .006$) (125). There were no survival differences. In addition, the EORTC H9 trial treated patients with epirubicin, bleomycin, vinblastine, and prednisone (EBVP) chemotherapy and randomized those who achieved a complete response to no further therapy or IFRT (20 vs. 36 Gy). This study included patients who were younger than 50 years, had an ESR <50 (or <30 in the presence of B symptoms), and fewer than four sites of involvement. The 4-year event-free survival among patients treated with EBVP *alone* was an unacceptably low 70% and that arm of the study was closed early (138). Based on this trial, the EORTC has concluded that there is no role for EBVP in the management of even favorable presentations of Hodgkin lymphoma.

Based on consensus data, the most commonly employed treatment for favorable presentations of stage I–IIA Hodgkin lymphoma is combined-modality therapy with chemotherapy plus involved field irradiation. The expected freedom-from progression is 90% to 95%. Selected patients may be treated with chemotherapy alone if radiation therapy is contraindicated and the increased risk for relapse is acceptable.

The use of radiation therapy alone has a long history in the successful treatment of early-stage Hodgkin lymphoma, but has largely been abandoned because of the long-term risks of treatment, as noted here. However, it remains a good option for patients in whom there is a contraindication to chemotherapy.

Favorable Prognosis Stage I to IIA (Subdiaphragmatic) Classical Hodgkin Lymphoma

Fewer than 10% of patients with stage I or II Hodgkin lymphoma present with involvement limited to subdiaphragmatic sites. The same general treatment principles apply to the management of these patients as for those with supradiaphragmatic presentations. The most reasonable approach is to use combined-modality therapy, as outlined previously. In general, the outcome of treatment for patients with subdiaphragmatic disease is equivalent to that for patients with supradiaphragmatic disease (27,175).

Limited Presentations of Stage I to IIA Nodular Lymphocyte Predominance Hodgkin lymphoma

Contrary to the experience with classic Hodgkin lymphoma, it has been noted that patients with limited presentations of nLPHD may achieve long-term disease-free survival after treatment with involved or slightly extended field irradiation alone (132,137,152,163,184). For example, for a high cervical stage IA presentation, treatment may be limited to the ipsilateral neck. For a femoral node presentation, treatment may be limited to the inguinal-femoral region with or without the ipsilateral iliac region. The usual dose is 30 to 36 Gy. There does not appear to be any benefit from the addition of chemotherapy in this setting.

Unfavorable Prognosis Stage I to II (Supradiaphragmatic) Classical Hodgkin Lymphoma

Patients who have unfavorable prognosis stage I–II disease usually have B symptoms or a large mediastinal mass. Patients with bulky mediastinal Hodgkin lymphoma (mediastinal mass greater than one-third of maximum intrathoracic diameter) are difficult to categorize by the Ann Arbor staging criteria and have a poor outcome when treated with single-modality therapy (76). Early reports confirmed that these patients are best treated with combined-modality therapy (73).

When the choice of chemotherapy is made for these patients, the potential overlapping toxicities of doxorubicin and bleomycin with irradiation (cardiac and pulmonary effects) should be considered. The recommended radiation dose in this situation varies from 20 to 36 Gy, but most data cite doses of at least 30 Gy for this cohort (6,8,88). Doses in the higher part of the range should be used when the response to chemotherapy is incomplete, PET imaging remains positive after chemotherapy, or the chemotherapy course is abbreviated. The use of lower doses (as low as 20 Gy) should be restricted to clinical trials. Treatment may be to all initially involved sites or simply to the area of initial bulk (mediastinum). When treatment is limited to the mediastinum, it is reasonable to include the adjacent bilateral supraclavicular areas. The irradiation fields should conform to the area of residual disease with adequate margins laterally, not to the initial width of disease before chemotherapy. However, the fields usually extend inferiorly at least to the original extent of disease plus a reasonable margin (~2 cm.) (Fig. 75.6). Similar issues remain unanswered as for the favorable presentations, that is, the duration of chemotherapy and the dose of radiation therapy. The GHSG HD11 trial for patients with intermediate prognosis, which included patients with large mediastinal adenopathy, an elevated ESR, the presence of extranodal disease, or more than two sites of involvement, randomized the chemotherapy to BEACOPP versus ABVD and the radiation therapy dose to 20 versus 30 Gy. Thus far, no difference in outcome has been seen, but an analysis restricted to patients with large mediastinal masses has not been reported (103). Based on consensus data, the most commonly employed treatment for stage I–II Hodgkin lymphoma in the presence of large mediastinal adenopathy is combined-modality therapy with chemotherapy plus involved field irradiation. The expected freedom from progression is 80% to 90%.

Stage IB or IIB Hodgkin Lymphoma

Approximately 15% to 20% of patients with stage I or II disease have B symptoms. In general, these patients are managed in a fashion analogous to those with stage III to IV disease. However, given the limited anatomic extent of disease in stage I to II, one can make a strong argument to include consolidative involved field irradiation for these patients.

Stage III to IV Disease

Systemic chemotherapy is the mainstay of treatment for patients with advanced-stage Hodgkin lymphoma (32). Although early clinical trials of systemic therapy for Hodgkin lymphoma often excluded patients with stage IIIA, these patients are now included as patients with "advanced Hodgkin lymphoma" in most clinical trials.

With respect to the choice of chemotherapy for advanced stage Hodgkin lymphoma, the landmark study was the prospective, randomized clinical trial conducted by the Cancer and Leukemia Group B. Patients with stage III$_2$A, IIIB, or IV Hodgkin lymphoma were randomly assigned to treatment with either MOPP (six to eight cycles), MOPP/ABVD (12 months), or ABVD (six to eight cycles). The results of treatment with MOPP/ABVD and ABVD were equivalent, and both were superior to MOPP alone. Among the 115 patients treated with ABVD chemotherapy, the complete response rate was 82%, the 5-year failure-free survival was 61%, and the 5-year survival rate was 73% (12a,12b).

Several large series of combined-modality therapy for advanced disease have suggested an improvement in outcome compared with what would be expected with chemotherapy alone (77,153,186). Five-year survival rates of 70% to 80% and 5-year relapse-free rates of 63% to 75% have been reported. The use of combined-modality therapy is a rational approach because most patients who relapse after treatment with chemotherapy alone do so in sites of initial disease (187). However, many of the early trials intended to resolve this issue were poorly designed, used chemotherapy programs that are no longer considered to be optimal, or had inadequate accruals.

The most definitive trial to address the question is the EORTC-GPMC (Groupe Pierre-et-Marie Curie) H34 (20884) trial (2). In this trial, patients were treated with six to eight cycles of nitrogen mustard, vincristine, procarbazine, prednisone, Adriamycin, bleomycin, vinblastine (MOPP-ABV) chemotherapy and those who achieved a complete response were randomized to no further therapy versus 25 Gy IFRT. No differences in freedom from treatment failure or overall survival were identified. However, in that same trial, patients who achieved only a partial response all received 30 Gy IFRT. The subsequent freedom from treatment failure and survival for this group closely paralleled the outcome for patients who had achieved a complete response, suggesting a value to adding IFRT after only a partial response has been achieved (2a).

Although the EORTC 20884 trial failed to support the routine use of IFRT after patients achieved a complete response to a full course of conventional chemotherapy, there are programs of attenuated chemotherapy in which radiation therapy is retained. The Stanford V program includes only 12 weeks of chemotherapy, with very attenuated total doses of some of the drugs. Compared with six cycles of ABVD, there is only 50% of the cumulative dose of doxorubicin (Adriamycin) and 25% of the cumulative dose of bleomycin. Radiation therapy (36 Gy) is routinely added to initially bulky (>5 cm) sites of disease, as well as to macroscopic splenic involvement and commences 1 to 3 weeks after completion of chemotherapy. The results of this approach have been excellent (81). The 12-year freedom from progression is 83% and the 12-year survival is 95% (Table 75.9), with only minimal late complications of therapy. However, the radiation therapy component is essential as a study that did not employ the same planning for radiation therapy resulted in a much worse outcome (42). The Stanford V program has just been compared with treatment with ABVD chemotherapy alone in a phase 3 intergroup trial (see "Current Clinical Trials").

A general conclusion regarding the role of combined-modality therapy compared with chemotherapy alone for patients with stage III-IV disease is that patients who achieve a complete response to a full course of conventional chemotherapy have no proved benefit from the addition of chemotherapy. However, patients who achieve only a partial response may have an improved outcome. Ultimately, improved imaging and evaluation of early response to chemotherapy with FDG-PET imaging may help to identify a subset of patients who would truly benefit from consolidative irradiation.

Pediatric Patients

Most contemporary programs for the management of pediatric Hodgkin lymphoma are based on clinical staging and use chemotherapy alone or combined-modality therapy, with low-dose irradiation, as higher doses of irradiation are associated with unacceptable risks for growth impairment and late effects (90). To limit growth effects, irradiation doses should not exceed 15 to 25 Gy. Children treated with these programs, all stages combined, are reported to achieve 5-year survival rates of approximately 90% and relapse-free rates of at least 80% (34,92,131,141,151,155).

Older Adult Patients

The treatment of Hodgkin lymphoma in older patients (>60 years) also poses a challenge (5,30,56). These patients more likely have intercurrent disease that compromises the aggressive management programs used for younger people. Chemotherapy programs may often be modified to minimize cardiac or pulmonary toxicity and the hematologic reserve in elderly patients more often results in dose reductions or premature discontinuation compared with younger patients (40a). Drug combinations that seem to be more tolerable for older adults include ChlVPP (156), PAVe (procarbazine, Alkeran, and vinblastine) (83), and VBM (vinblastine, bleomycin, and methotrexate; used primarily for stage I to II) (87,188). With respect to the radiation therapy, patients may need to be treated with slower fractionation programs and observed carefully for signs of weight loss or general decline in performance status.

Treatment for Relapse

Treatment for relapse must be individualized. Initial disease characteristics, initial treatment and response duration, relapse sites, and general patient status must be considered in developing an effective secondary treatment program.

In general, patients who were treated initially with irradiation alone for stage I to II disease should receive chemotherapy as the primary salvage treatment (136,148,159). The efficacy of combination chemotherapy in this setting is similar to that achieved when chemotherapy is used in the primary management of advanced disease (long-term freedom from relapse rate of 60% or better). The role of irradiation in combination with salvage chemotherapy has not been defined, but it is advocated by some (148). After the completion of chemotherapy, 15 to 25 Gy may be delivered to previously irradiated sites and 30 to 36 Gy to previously nonirradiated regions.

For patients who presented initially with stage III to IV disease and who relapse after achieving a complete response to chemotherapy or combined-modality therapy, the standard salvage therapy is to use high-dose chemotherapy with autologous hematopoietic cell rescue (4). The long-term progression-free survival rate for these patients is expected to be approximately 50% (110). Favorable prognostic factors in this group include a longer duration of response to primary therapy and absence of extranodal disease (112,104).

More problematic is the management approach to patients who present initially with stage I to II disease and are treated with chemotherapy alone, a group for whom consensus best treatment has not been reached (73). In these patients, relapse may occur in initial sites of disease and be quite limited. It is possible that programs using irradiation alone, or at least emphasizing the use of radiation, may be safe and effective, especially given the success in treating some patients with initially advanced disease and limited relapse using this approach (147).

The Role of Radiation Therapy in High-Dose Chemotherapy Programs and Hematopoietic Cell Transplantation for Relapse, Partial Response, or Disease Progression

Radiation therapy may be incorporated into high-dose therapy programs as involved field, total lymphoid, or total-body irradiation (TBI) (4). Fractionated TBI is incorporated into a number of transplantation programs. Its value is debatable, and series that have used regimens with or without fractionated TBI report similar outcomes for both (132). TBI is probably not the most efficacious way to use irradiation in these patients. Recurrent Hodgkin lymphoma is often a locoregional problem rather than a systemic one. In addition, data suggest that irradiation doses in the range used in TBI programs (12 to 15 Gy) are likely to eradicate disease in only about 20% of treated sites (98). It is more logical to limit irradiation to sites of failure or those at high risk for disease, that is, initial sites of disease, especially bulky sites.

Important issues related to radiation therapy include timing (pre- or posttransplant), extent of fields, and dose. The advantages of using radiation therapy as cytoreductive treatment prior to high-dose therapy are that it can effectively reduce the tumor burden before high-dose treatment and the risk of interruption or delay of the locoregional radiation therapy is minimal. The primary disadvantages include potential delay of the high-dose therapy and the potential overlapping toxicities of the locoregional irradiation and high-dose therapy, including mucositis and pneumonitis (171). Cytoreductive radiation treatment may include all sites of relapse, the bulky sites of relapse, sites with an incomplete response, or even more extensive treatment, such as total lymphoid irradiation.

Many large published series of high-dose therapy for Hodgkin lymphoma have included locoregional irradiation in at least selected patients. In some series, irradiation is given pretransplant, although in the majority of reports, it is given after transplant (43). The range of intervals from transplant to irradiation varies from 1 to 4 months. Often, the fields treated include sites of bulky disease (variably defined) at the time of relapse or areas of residual disease after high-dose therapy has been administered. Some have included all sites involved at the time of relapse.

The range of radiation doses employed varies substantially in these series, from 18 to 40 Gy. In general, lower doses are employed in situations in which initially nonbulky disease is included in the treatment, or if there has been a complete response to high-dose therapy.

The use of locoregional irradiation in high-dose therapy programs has the potential for altering the patterns of failure and perhaps reducing the risk of failure. For example, at Stanford University 49 patients with relapsed stage I–III disease who underwent high-dose therapy for relapse of Hodgkin lymphoma had involved field irradiation as a component of their salvage treatment. Their 3-year freedom from relapse, survival, and EFS rates of 100%, 85%, and 85%, respectively, compared with only 67%, 60%, and 54%, respectively, for another group of patients who received high-dose chemotherapy alone (143). The difference in freedom from relapse was statistically significant ($p = .04$). A similar impact of local irradiation has been reported in cohorts of patients transplanted at the University of Chicago (131) and the University of Rochester (109).

Moskowitz et al. (127) at Memorial Sloan-Kettering Cancer Center reported the use of more extensive irradiation for these patients. Prior to high-dose chemotherapy and hematopoietic cell transplantation, patients who had not received previous irradiation were treated with involved field irradiation to 18 Gy and total lymphoid irradiation to 18 Gy (both with twice-daily fractionation). Patients who had prior irradiation were treated with involved field irradiation, if organ tolerance would not be exceeded, to a dose of 18 to 36 Gy in 5 to 10 days (twice-daily fractionation) depending on the prior doses received by the involved sites. The EFS rate was 68% and the overall survival rate was 81% for the 56 patients who underwent transplantation. Only three (18%) treatment failures occurred in a site that was irradiated during the salvage program.

Follow-Up

Patients should be monitored carefully after the completion of therapy for Hodgkin lymphoma, although the frequency of visits can decrease as the risk of relapse diminishes. Typical follow-up intervals include every 2 to 4 months during the first 2 years, every 4 to 6 months during the third and fourth years, and annually thereafter. As a rule of thumb, all studies that initially gave abnormal results (e.g., chest radiograph, CT scan, PET scan) should be repeated at the time of completion of therapy to document the completeness of response (70).

The most important component of subsequent follow-up is an interim history and physical examination, which leads to identification of two-thirds of relapses (38,168). The chest radiograph is the second most productive examination, detecting one quarter of relapses. Hematologic evaluation at each follow-up visit usually includes a complete blood count with platelet count and alkaline phosphatase level. The ESR, serum albumin, or other serum marker studies should be obtained if these markers were abnormal at presentation. Serum thyroxine (T_4) and sensitive thyroid-stimulating hormone (TSH) levels should be obtained at least annually in patients who received irradiation to the neck to detect subclinical hypothyroidism.

The frequency with which imaging studies should be repeated after the completion of therapy is not well defined. Chest radiographs may be obtained every 3 or 4 months during the first 2 years and annually beyond 3 years, especially if chest irradiation was included as a component of therapy. The value of more extensive imaging evaluation in the absence of symptoms or abnormalities on simple screening studies is questionable.

A challenging problem in follow-up evaluation has been the interpretation of residual mediastinal abnormality on chest radiograph or chest CT scan. In the absence of other clinical suspicion, it is reasonable to follow these patients carefully as long as the abnormality remains stable or regresses, with additional diagnostic procedures reserved for patients who appear to have progression of disease. However, this problem has been ameliorated somewhat by the introduction of FDG-PET scanning as a posttreatment assessment tool, where residual PET activity gives cause for concern (1,29,133,178).

In most instances, the first suspicion of relapse should be documented by biopsy. Reactive hyperplasia is especially common in nonirradiated lymph nodes just outside the previous irradiation portals, justifying biopsy documentation before initiation of any therapy (15). Progressive transformation of germinal center or the rebound growth of the thymus in young patients are other reactive processes that can be confused with recurrent Hodgkin lymphoma (63). All of these processes may be FDG-avid on PET scanning.

Sequelae of Treatment

Depending on the fields treated, the acute side effects of radiation therapy may include occipital hair loss, mild skin reaction, sore throat, an altered sense of taste, dysphagia, reflux symptoms, dry cough, nausea, occasional vomiting, diarrhea, and blood count suppression. Most of these sequelae can be managed symptomatically. Complications that may arise in the early phase of the follow-up program are mild radiation pneumonitis, radiation pericarditis, hypothyroidism, herpes zoster, Lhermitte's sign, and xerostomia.

Radiation pneumonitis may develop within 6 to 12 weeks after completion of mantle irradiation (177). Following classic "mantle" therapy, fewer than 5% of patients have symptomatic pneumonitis, manifested by cough, fever, pleuritic chest pain, and an infiltrate on chest radiography that usually conforms to the irradiation fields (14). Symptomatic management is usually sufficient; however, a small proportion of patients require treatment with corticosteroids, usually beginning with a daily dosage of 40 to 60 mg of prednisone (or other corticosteroid equivalent). The initiation of corticosteroid therapy commits one to a course of at least 4 to 6 weeks with slow, careful tapering to avoid exacerbation of symptoms. The risk is related to volume of lung irradiated, total dose, and fraction size. For example, one recent study identified a higher risk for Radiation Therapy Oncology Group grade 2 pneumonitis when the mean lung dose exceeds 14 Gy or the V_{20} exceeds 35% (105). The likelihood of radiation-related pulmonary complications may be increased by the use of bleomycin (24), and the impact that different drug combinations with variable doses of bleomycin may have on acceptable mean lung dose or V_{20} values is not known.

Radiation pericarditis is a potential risk primarily if the entire cardiac silhouette is treated, an uncommon scenario with current management programs. It presents as an acute febrile syndrome associated with chest pain and friction rub, an asymptomatic pericardial effusion diagnosed by chest radiograph or echocardiogram, or constrictive pericarditis or tamponade. The first of these syndromes is usually managed with conservative medical treatment that includes analgesics and nonsteroidal anti-inflammatory agents; it usually clears within a few weeks. The syndrome of tamponade or constrictive pericarditis is the most serious. It is seen only rarely in this era and may require surgical correction. It is important to differentiate this syndrome from recurrent Hodgkin lymphoma. Cardiopulmonary changes that represent a latent radiation injury may occur following steroid withdrawal used incidentally for the management of other disorders, even in long-term follow-up (17).

Subclinical hypothyroidism develops in at least half of patients with Hodgkin lymphoma, often as a late effect (60). It can be detected by an elevation of TSH even with a normal T_4 level. Thyroid replacement therapy with L-thyroxine is recommended, with an initial dose of up to 0.1 mg/day The T_4 and TSH values are monitored regularly to make adjustments in the dose. Evidence suggests that thyroid replacement therapy in this setting reduces the risk for development of benign thyroid nodules (46). Herpes zoster can occur during treatment for Hodgkin lymphoma or within the first few years after treatment in 10% to 15% of patients (57). The outbreak is usually limited to one or two contiguous dermatomes. Cutaneous dissemination is uncommon, and visceral involvement is extremely rare. If the cutaneous eruption is identified within 72 hours of its onset, treatment with acyclovir (800 mg five times per day for 7 to 10 days or other antiviral equivalent) can be initiated. This may limit the duration and intensity of infection and decrease the likelihood of cutaneous or visceral dissemination.

Lhermitte's sign develops in approximately 10% to 15% of patients after radiation therapy that includes a significant length of the spine. It is marked by paresthesias extending into the arms and legs on neck flexion and may be related to transient demyelinization of the spinal cord. Its onset is usually 1 to 2 months after completion of mantle therapy and it generally resolves spontaneously after 2 to 6 months. This sequela is more prominent if patients have received recent treatment with vinca alkaloids (vincristine and vinblastine), and it is not related to the more serious problem of transverse myelitis.

Significant xerostomia may follow irradiation of the Waldeyer lymphoid region, which is uncommonly required, and permanent attention to dental care is required for these patients. Frequent dental prophylaxis and use of fluoride supplements are recommended.

An uncommon but potentially serious complication is overwhelming sepsis following splenectomy or splenic irradiation (26,35). The most serious infections occur with Gram-positive organisms, including *Streptococcus pneumoniae*, meningococci, and *Haemophilus* strains. This risk can be minimized by immunization against these organisms. It is reasonable to immunize patients as soon as a diagnosis of Hodgkin lymphoma has been made (157). Recommendations for immunization of patients who have been treated previously but not immunized before therapy vary. Recent data suggest that if at least 2 years have passed since treatment, patients can develop adequate antibody titers to *H. influenzae* type b-conjugate, 4-valent meningococcal polysaccharide vaccine, and 23-valent pneumococcal polysaccharide vaccine (125). Reimmunization is currently recommended every 5 to 7 years.

An important concern of many patients with Hodgkin lymphoma is the possible effect of treatment on reproductive potential. In men, pelvic irradiation may be followed by azoospermia if no special precautions are taken to shield the testes. However, with appropriate testicular shielding, azoospermia is usually only transient, with subsequent recovery of sperm counts to fertile levels (140). Chemotherapy programs such as MOPP, MOPP-like combinations that include alkylating agents and procarbazine or BEACOPP may cause sterility in most men. However, the ABVD and Stanford V regimens seem to spare male fertility (85,176). Among women, the risk for infertility is influenced by patient age. With respect to the irradiation component, even with a proper oophoropexy and well-planned treatment fields, the scattered dose of irradiation may be sufficient to affect ovarian function and cause menopausal symptoms in women older than 30 years who receive pelvic irradiation (86). Younger women may not have an immediate effect, but may enter a premature menopause later in life. Similarly, with respect to chemotherapy that contains alkylating agents, normal menstrual function usually continues in women younger than 25 years but is altered in women older than 30 years (7,86). Again, younger women may later experience an earlier than normal onset of menopause. In contrast to MOPP and BEACOPP, the ABVD and Stanford V combinations appear to spare female fertility (85,176).

Long-term follow-up is essential to identify potential long-term complications of treatment (61,68,76,121,134,135). The most important long-term hazards are secondary malignancies (173) and cardiovascular disease (59).

Secondary malignancies include leukemia, lymphoma, and solid tumors. In large series, the relative risk for development of a second malignancy after treatment for Hodgkin lymphoma is 2.3 to 2.9, and the absolute excess risk is 44.5 to 47.2 (i.e., 44.5 excess cases per 10,000 patients per year) (36,165).

Leukemia may develop after treatment with chemotherapy programs that include alkylating agents or procarbazine (e.g., MOPP or BEACOPP) after a latent period of 3 to 7 years. The relative risk for this complication was 9.9 to 14.6 and absolute excess risk 8.8 to 8.9 during the era when alkylating agent chemotherapy was commonly used (36,166). The occurrence of leukemia after treatment with irradiation alone is unusual. It remains controversial whether the risk is greater after combined modality therapy or after chemotherapy alone.

Secondary lymphomas are usually of the diffuse large cell non-Hodgkin type. The latent interval is usually at least 5 years. The relative risk is 5.5 to 14.0 and the absolute excess risk is 5.2 to 9.9 (36,165). The development of secondary lymphomas does not seem to be related to any specific component of therapy but may be related to underlying immunosuppression.

Secondary solid tumors are related largely to radiation therapy, although recent analyses indicate an increased risk from chemotherapy as well, and an enhanced risk after combined-modality therapy (61,165,174). Secondary solid tumors usually have a longer latent period (at least 7 to 10 years) than is seen with leukemia. The greatest risks are for lung cancer (absolute excess risk 9.7 to 11.7) and female breast cancer (absolute excess risk 3.1 to 10.5) (36,165). Other sites at increased risk reported in different studies include mouth and pharynx, esophagus, stomach, pancreas, liver, colon, bone and soft tissue, melanoma, thyroid, central nervous system, bladder, and female genital organs.

The secondary breast cancer risk has been defined more clearly recently to be greater for younger women. An international study reported the relative risk to be 14.2 for women treated before age 21, 3.7 for women 21 to 30 years old at the time of treatment, and 1.2 (not statistically significant) for women 31 to 40 years old (36). In addition, the risk is related to radiation dose to the affected site. Travis et al. (170) reported that doses up to 7 Gy were not associated with a significant increase in risk when compared with the referent dose of 0 to 3.9 Gy. The range of relative risk was 2.0 to 6.8 for doses 7.0 to 40.4 Gy. This escalated risk for breast cancer mandates that women should begin mammographic screening as soon as 5 to 7 years after completion of mantle irradiation.

The lung cancer risk after irradiation exposure is also dose-related. Gilbert et al. (47) reported that doses up to 30 Gy were not associated with a significant increase in risk for lung cancer, but for doses >30 Gy the relative risk was 6.3 to 8.5. In addition, it has been clearly demonstrated that the lung cancer risk is extraordinarily high among irradiated patients who continue to smoke after treatment (169). Because of this inordinately high risk for lung cancer, patients who continue to smoke after treatment should be urged to stop and be entered into smoking-cessation programs.

Long-term cardiovascular sequelae include coronary artery disease, pericarditis, pancarditis, and valvular disease (62). The relative risk of death from cardiac disease is 3.1 among patients treated for Hodgkin lymphoma (61). The risk is greatest for coronary artery disease and appears to be related primarily to mediastinal irradiation; however, the anthracyclines are also potentially cardiotoxic. The data relevant to dose effects of irradiation are limited; however, in one study a threshold effect at 30 Gy was suggested (62). Screening studies have shown a significant risk of asymptomatic coronary artery disease, although optimal screening guidelines for patients after mediastinal irradiation have not yet been defined (66).

Another group of sequelae involves psychosocial problems, fatigue, marital difficulties, and employment issues (44,45,150). Identification of these problems may promote the development of rehabilitation programs to anticipate and deal with these issues early in the course of treatment.

Current Clinical Trials

The thrust of current clinical trials in Hodgkin lymphoma is to decrease the intensity of therapy in the majority of patients who have a good prognosis in order to reduce the risk for long-term complications. At the same time, there has been an intensification of treatment for patients with advanced disease who have a very unfavorable prognostic score.

For patients with favorable-prognosis stage I to II disease, current trials attempt to define the minimal combination of chemotherapy and irradiation that will maintain excellent treatment results (122). The HD13 trial of the GHSG retains a dose of 30 Gy for involved field treatment, but the chemotherapy is randomized among ABVD, ABV, ABD, and AV. The current nonrandomized Stanford G5 study includes only 8 weeks of Stanford V chemotherapy followed by 20 Gy involved field irradiation (a decrease from the 30 Gy on the G4 study). The EORTC is studying the reduction of radiation field size even more profoundly, defining the involved field as the involved node(s) (49).

For patients with unfavorable-prognosis stage I to II disease, optimal combinations of chemotherapy and radiation are being explored (75). In the GHSG HD14 trial, patients are randomized between four cycles of ABVD and two cycles of BEACOPP escalated plus two ABVD. Both arms are followed by involved field irradiation (30 Gy) (32a). The Stanford G2 study includes 12 weeks of Stanford V chemotherapy followed by 36 Gy to sites of disease >5 cm. The recently closed Eastern Cooperative Oncology Group 2496 intergroup trial randomized patients who had stage I–II disease with a large mediastinal mass between Stanford V (12 weeks) and ABVD (six to eight cycles) followed by 36 Gy to sites of disease >5 cm.

In advanced-stage Hodgkin lymphoma, more intensive treatment programs are being explored to identify improved outcomes. The GHSG HD15 trial compares 8 BEACOPP-escalated, 6 BEACOPP escalated, and 8 BEACOPP-14. In each case, chemotherapy is followed by 30-Gy irradiation to PET-positive residual disease. In the United States and Canada, the Eastern Cooperative Oncology Group 2496 intergroup study, noted previously, has just completed accrual to its trial of ABVD versus Stanford V (including 36 Gy to initial sites >5 cm).

References

1. Advani R, Maeda L, Lavori P, et al. FDG-PET Status after Stanford V chemotherapy predicts outcome in Hodgkin disease. Submitted for publication. *Ann Oncol.*
2. Aleman BM, et al. Involved field radiotherapy for advanced Hodgkin lymphoma. *N Engl J Med* 2003;348:2396–2406.
2a. Aleman BMP, Raemaekers JMM, Tomsic R, et al. Involved field radiotherapy for patients in partial remission after chemotherapy for advanced Hogkin's lymphoma. *Intel Jour Rad Oncol Biol Phys* 2007;67:19–30.
3. Ambinder RA, Weiss LM. Association of Epstein-Barr virus with Hodgkin lymphoma. In: Hoppe RT, Armitage JA, Diehl V, et al., eds. *Hodgkin lymphoma.* Philadelphia: Lippincott Williams & Wilkins; 2007.
4. Armitage JO, Carella A, Schnitz N, et al. Role of hematopoietic stem-cell transplantation in Hodgkin lymphoma. In: Hoppe RT, Armitage JA, Diehl V, et al., eds. *Hodgkin lymphoma.* Philadelphia: Lippincott Williams & Wilkins; 2007; 281–292.
5. Austin-Seymour MM, Hoppe RT, Cox RS, et al. Hodgkin disease in patients over sixty years old. *Ann Intern Med* 1984;100:13–18.
6. Behar RA, Horning SJ, Hoppe RT. Hodgkin disease with bulky mediastinal involvement: effective management with combined modality therapy. *Int J Radiat Oncol Biol Physs* 1993;25:771–776.
7. Behringer K, Breuer K, Reineke T, et al. Secondary amenorrhea after Hodgkin lymphoma is influenced by age at treatment, stage of disease, chemotherapy regimen, and the use of oral contraceptives during therapy: a report from the German Hodgkin Lymphoma Study Group. *J Clin Oncol* 2005;23:7555–7564.
8. Bonadonna G, Bonfante V, Viviani S, et al. ABVD plus subtotal nodal versus involved-field radiotherapy in early-stage Hodgkin disease: long-term results. *J Clin Oncol* 2004;22:2835–2841.
9. Bonadonna G, Valagussa P, Santoro A. Alternating non-cross-resistant combination chemotherapy or MOPP in stage IV Hodgkin disease. A report of 8-year results. *Ann Intern Med* 1986;104:739–746.
10. Bonadonna G, Valagussa P, Santoro A. Prognosis of bulky Hodgkin disease treated with chemotherapy alone or combined with radiotherapy. *Cancer Surv* 1985;4:439–458.
11. Bonadonna G. Chemotherapy strategies to improve the control of Hodgkin disease: the Richard and Hinda Rosenthal Foundation Award Lecture. *Cancer Res* 1982;42:4309–4320.
12. Brice P, Bouabdallah R, Moreau P, et al. Prognostic factors for survival after high-dose therapy and autologous stem cell transplantation for patients with relapsing Hodgkin disease: analysis of 280 patients from the French registry. Societe Francaise de Greffe de Moelle. *Bone Marrow Transplant* 1997;20:21–26.
12a. Canellos GP, Anderson JR, Propert KJ, et al. Chemotherapy of advanced Hodgkin lymphoma with MOPP, ABVD, or MOPP alternating with ABVD. *N Engl J Med* 1992;327:1478–1484.
12b. Canellos G, Josting A. Management of recurrent Hodgkin lymphoma. In: Hoppe RT, Armitage JA, Diehl V, et al. eds. *Hodgkin lymphoma.* Philadelphia: Lippincott Williams & Wilkins; 2007.
13. Carbone PP, Kaplan HS, Musshoff K, et al. Report of the Committee on Hodgkin disease staging classification. *Cancer Res* 1971;31:1860–1861.
14. Carmel RJ, Kaplan HS. Mantle irradiation in Hodgkin disease. An analysis of technique, tumor eradication, and complications. *Cancer* 1976;37:2813–2825.
15. Castellino RA, Billingham M, Dorfman RF. Lymphographic accuracy in Hodgkin disease and malignant lymphoma with a note on the "reactive" lymph node as a cause of most false-positive lymphograms. *Invest Radiol* 1974;9:155–165.
16. Castellino RA, Blank N, Hoppe RT, et al. Hodgkin disease: contributions of chest CT in the initial staging evaluation. *Radiology* 1986;160:603–605.
17. Castellino RA, Glatstein E, Turbow MM, et al. Latent radiation injury of lungs or heart activated by steroid withdrawal. *Ann Intern Med* 1974;80:593–599.
18. Castellino RA, Hoppe RT, Blank N, et al. Computed tomography, lymphography, and staging laparotomy: correlations in initial staging of Hodgkin disease. *Am J Roentgenol* 1984;143:37–41.
19. Castellino RA. Diagnostic imaging evaluation of Hodgkin disease and non-Hodgkin lymphoma. *Cancer* 1991;67:1177–1180.
20. Cheson BD, Pfistner B, Juweid ME, et al. Revised response criteria for malignant lymphoma. *J Clin Oncol.*
21. Chittal SM, Caveriviere P, Schwarting R, et al. Monoclonal antibodies in the diagnosis of Hodgkin disease. The search for a rational panel. *Am J Surg Pathol* 1988;12:9–21.
22. Connors JM, Klimo P. Is it an E lesion or stage IV?. An unsettled issue in Hodgkin disease staging. *J Clin Oncol* 1984;2:1421–1423.
23. Coppleson LW, Factor RM, Strum SB, et al. Observer disagreement in the classification and histology of Hodgkin disease. *J Natl Cancer Inst* 1970;45:731–740.
24. Cosset JM, Henry-Amar M, Meerwaldt JH. Long-term toxicity of early stages of Hodgkin disease therapy: the EORTC experience. EORTC Lymphoma Cooperative Group. *Ann Oncol* 1991;2 Suppl 2:77–82.
25. Crnkovich MJ, Leopold K, Hoppe RT, et al. Stage I to IIB Hodgkin disease: the combined experience at Stanford University and the Joint Center for Radiation Therapy. *J Clin Oncol* 1987;5:1041–1049.
26. Dailey MO, Coleman CN, Kaplan HS. Radiation-induced splenic atrophy in patients with Hodgkin disease and non-Hodgkin lymphomas. *N Engl J Med* 1980;302:215–217.

27. Darabi K, Sieber M, Chaitowitz M, et al. Infradiaphragmatic versus supradiaphragmatic Hodgkin lymphoma: a retrospective review of 1,114 patients. *Leuk Lymphoma* 2005;46:1715–1720.
28. De Vita VT, Hubbard SM, Longo DL. The chemotherapy of lymphomas: looking back, moving forward. The Richard and Hinda Rosenthal Foundation Award Lecture. *Cancer Res* 1987;47:4810.
29. de Wit M, Bohuslavizki KH, Buchert R, et al. 18FDG-PET following treatment as valid predictor for disease-free survival in Hodgkin lymphoma. *Ann Oncol* 2001;12:29–37.
30. Diaz-Pavon JR, Cabanillas F, Majlis A, et al. Outcome of Hodgkin disease in elderly patients. *Hematol Oncol* 1995;13:19–27.
31. Diehl V, Brillant C, Engert A, et al. HD 10: Investigating reduction of combined modality treatment intensity in early stage Hodgkin lymphoma. Interim analysis of a randomized trial of the German Hodgkin Study Group (GHSG). 2005;23(165):6506.
32. Diehl V, Behringer K, Raemaekers J. Treatment of stage III–IV Hodgkin lymphoma. In: Hoppe RT, Armitage JA, Diehl V, et al., es. *Hodgkin lymphoma*. Philadelphia: Lippincott Williams & Wilkins; 2007;253–270.
32a. Diehl V, Klimm B, Re D. Hodgkin lymphoma: a curable disease: what comes next? *Eur J Haematol Suppl* 2005;6–13.
33. Doggett RS, Colby TV, Dorfman RF. Interfollicular Hodgkin disease. *Am J Surg Pathol* 1983;7:145–149.
34. Donaldson SS, Hudson MM, Lamborn KR, et al. VAMP and low-dose, involved-field radiation for children and adolescents with favorable, early-stage Hodgkin disease: results of a prospective clinical trial. *J Clin Oncol* 2002;20:3081–3087.
35. Donaldson SS, Moore MR, Rosenberg SA, et al. Characterization of postsplenectomy bacteremia among patients with and without lymphoma. *N Engl J Med* 1972;287:69–71.
36. Dores GM, Metayer C, Curtis RE, et al. Second malignant neoplasms among long-term survivors of Hodgkin disease: a population-based evaluation over 25 years. *J Clin Oncol* 2002;20:3484–3494.
37. Drexler HG, Leber BF. The nature of the Hodgkin cell. Report of the First International Symposium on Hodgkin Lymphoma, Koln, Federal Republic of Germany, October 2–3, 1987. *Blut* 1988;56:135–137.
38. Dryver ET, Jernstrom H, Tompkins K, et al. Follow-up of patients with Hodgkin disease following curative treatment: the routine CT scan is of little value. *Br J Cancer* 2003;89:482–486.
39. Duhmke E, Franklin J, Pfreundschuh M, et al. Low-dose radiation is sufficient for the noninvolved extended-field treatment in favorable early-stage Hodgkin disease: long-term results of a randomized trial of radiotherapy alone. *J Clin Oncol* 2001;19:2905–2914.
40. Engel C, Loeffler M, Schmitz S, et al. Acute hematologic toxicity and practicability of dose-intensified BEACOPP chemotherapy for advanced stage Hodgkin disease. German Hodgkin Lymphoma Study Group (GHSG). *Ann Oncol* 2000;11:1105–1114.
40a. Engert A, Ballova V, Haverkamp H, et al. Hodgkin lymphoma in elderly patients: a comprehensive retrospective analysis from the German Hodgkin study group. *J Clin Oncol* 2005;23:5052–5060.
41. Fabian CJ, Mansfield CM, Dahlberg S, et al. Low-dose involved field radiation after chemotherapy in advanced Hodgkin disease. A Southwest Oncology Group randomized study. *Ann Intern Med* 1994;120:903–912.
42. Federico M, Levis S, Luminari S, et al. ABVD vs Stanford V (SV) vs MOPP-EBV-CAD (MEC) in advanced Hodgkin lymphoma. Final results of the IIL HD9601 randomized trial. *J Clin Oncol* 2004;22:559s.
43. Ferme C, Mounier N, Divine M, et al. Intensive salvage therapy with high-dose chemotherapy for patients with advanced Hodgkin disease in relapse or failure after initial chemotherapy: results of the Groupe d'Etudes des Lymphomes de l'Adulte H89 Trial. *J Clin Oncol* 2002;20:467–475.
44. Flechtner H, Henry-Amar M, Fobair P, et al. Assessing quality of life in patients with Hodgkin lymphoma: Instruments and Clinical trials. In: Hoppe RT, Armitage JA, Diehl V, et al., eds. *Hodgkin lymphoma*. Philadelphia. Lippincott Williams & Wilkins; 2007;393–410.
45. Fobair P, Hoppe RT, Bloom J, et al. Psychosocial problems among survivors of Hodgkin disease. *J Clin Oncol* 1986;4:805–814.
46. Fogelfeld L, Wiviott MB, Shore-Freedman E, et al. Recurrence of thyroid nodules after surgical removal in patients irradiated in childhood for benign conditions. *N Engl J Med* 1989;320:835–840.
47. Gilbert ES, Stovall M, Gospodarowicz M, et al. Lung cancer after treatment for Hodgkin disease: focus on radiation effects. *Radiat Res* 2003;159:161–173.
48. Girinsky T, Pichenot C, Beaudre A, et al. Is intensity-modulated radiotherapy better than conventional radiation treatment and three-dimensional conformal radiotherapy for mediastinal masses in patients with Hodgkin disease, and is there a role for beam orientation optimization and dose constraints assigned to virtual volumes?. *Int J Radiat Oncol Biol Phys* 2006;64:218–226.
49. Girinsky T, van der Maazen R, Specht L, et al. Involved-node radiotherapy (INRT) in patients with early Hodgkin lymphoma: concepts and guidelines. *Radiother Oncol* 2006;79:270–277.
50. Glaser SL, Lin RJ, Stewart SL, et al. Epstein-Barr virus-associated Hodgkin disease: epidemiologic characteristics in international data. *Int J Cancer* 1997;70:375–382.
51. Goodman KA, Toner S, Hunt M, et al. Intensity-modulated radiotherapy for lymphoma involving the mediastinum. *Int J Radiat Oncol Biol Phys* 2005;62:198–206.
52. Gossmann A. Anatomic imaging in Hodgkin lymphoma. In: Hoppe RT, Armitage JA, Diehl V, et al., eds. *Hodgkin lymphoma*. Philadelphia: Lippincott Williams & Wilkins; 2007;133–142.
53. Greenlee RT, Hill-Harmon MB, Murray T, et al. Cancer statistics, 2001. *CA Cancer J Clin* 2001;51:15–36.
54. Greenlee RT, Hill-Harmon, Murray T, et al. Cancer Statistics 2001. *CA Cancer J Clin 2001* 2001;51.
55. Grufferman S, Delzell E. Epidemiology of Hodgkin disease. *Epidemiol Rev* 1984;6:76–106.
56. Guinee VF, Bjorkholm JM, Monfardini S. Hodgkin disease in the elderly. In: Mauch P, Armitage JO, Diehl V, et al., eds. *Hodgkin disease*. Philadelphia: Lippincott Williams & Wilkins; 1999:713–726.
57. Guinee VF, Guido JJ, Pfalzgraf KA, et al. The incidence of herpes zoster in patients with Hodgkin disease. An analysis of prognostic factors. *Cancer* 1985;56:642–648.
58. Hancock BW. Principles of chemotherapy in Hodgkin lymphoma. In: Hough RE, Hoppe RT, Armitage JA, Diehl V, et al., eds. *Hodgkin lymphoma*. Philadelphia: Lippincott Williams & Wilkins; 2007;177–178.
59. Hancock S. Cardiovascular late effects after treatment of Hodgkin lymphoma. In: Hoppe RT, Armitage JA, Diehl V, et al., eds. *Hodgkin lymphoma*. Philadelphia: Lippincott Williams & Wilkins; 2007;371–382.
60. Hancock SL, Cox RS, McDougall IR. Thyroid diseases after treatment of Hodgkin disease. *N Engl J Med* 1991;325:599–605.
61. Hancock SL, Hoppe RT. Long-term complications of treatment and causes of mortality after Hodgkin disease. *Semin Radiat Oncol* 1996;6:225–242.
62. Hancock SL, Tucker MA, Hoppe RT. Factors affecting late mortality from heart disease after treatment of Hodgkin disease. *JAMA* 1993;270:1949–1955.
63. Hansmann ML, Fellbaum C, Hui PK, et al. Progressive transformation of germinal centers with and without association to Hodgkin disease. *Am J Clin Pathol* 1990;93:219–226.
64. Harris NL, Jaffe ES, Diebold J, et al. World Health Organization classification of neoplastic diseases of the hematopoietic and lymphoid tissues: report of the Clinical Advisory Committee meeting-Airlie House, Virginia, November 1997. *J Clin Oncol* 1999;17:3835–3849.
65. Hasenclever D, Diehl V. A prognostic score for advanced Hodgkin disease. International Prognostic Factors Project on Advanced Hodgkin Disease. *N Engl J Med* 1998;339:1506–1514.
66. Heidenreich PA, Schnittger I, Strauss HW, et al. Screening for coronary artery disease after mediastinal irradiation for Hodgkin disease. *J Clin Oncol* 2007;25:43–49.
67. Henry-Amar M, Friedman S, Hayat M, et al. Erythrocyte sedimentation rate predicts early relapse and survival in early-stage Hodgkin disease. The EORTC Lymphoma Cooperative Group. *Ann Intern Med* 1991;114:361–365.
68. Henry-Amar M, Hayat M, Meerwaldt JH, et al. Causes of death after therapy for early stage Hodgkin disease entered on EORTC protocols. EORTC Lymphoma Cooperative Group. *Int J Radiat Oncol Biol Phys* 1990;19:1155–1157.
69. Hjalgrim H, Askling J, Sorensen P, et al. Risk of Hodgkin disease and other cancers after infectious mononucleosis. *J Natl Cancer Inst* 2000;92:1522–1528.
70. Hodgson DC, Gospodarowicz M. Clinical evaluation and staging of Hodgkin lymphoma. In: Hoppe RT, Armitage JA, Diehl V, et al., eds. *Hodgkin lymphoma*. Philadelphia: Lippincott Williams & Wilkins; 2007.
71. Hoppe R. Hodgkin disease. In: Leibel S, Phillips T, eds. *Textbook of radiation oncology*. Philadelphia: WB Saunders; 2001.
72. Hoppe RT, Advani RH, Bierman PJ, et al. Hodgkin disease/lymphoma. Clinical practice guidelines in oncology *J Natl Compr Canc Netw* 2006;4:210–230.
73. Hoppe RT, Coleman CN, Cox RS, et al. The management of stage I–II Hodgkin disease with irradiation alone or combined modality therapy: the Stanford experience. *Blood* 1982;59:455–465.
74. Hoppe RT, Cox RS, Rosenberg SA, et al. Prognostic factors in pathologic stage III Hodgkin disease. *Cancer Treat Rep* 1982;66:743–749.
75. Hoppe RT, Engert A, Noordijk EM. Treatment of unfavorable prognosis stage I–II Hodgkin lymphoma. In: Hoppe RT, Armitage JA, Diehl V, et al., eds. *Hodgkin lymphoma*. Philadelphia: Lippincott Williams & Wilkins; 2007.
76. Hoppe RT. Hodgkin disease: complications of therapy and excess mortality. *Ann Oncol* 1997;8[Suppl 1]:115–118.
77. Hoppe RT. Radiation therapy in the management of Hodgkin disease. *Semin Oncol* 1990;17:704–715.
78. Hoppe RT. The management of bulky mediastinal Hodgkin disease. *Hematol Oncol Clin North Am* 1989;3:265–276.
79. Hoppe RT. The non-Hodgkin lymphomas: pathology, staging, treatment. *Current Problems in Cancer* 1987;11:363–447.
80. Hopper KD, Diehl LF, Lesar M, et al. Hodgkin disease: clinical utility of CT in initial staging and treatment. *Radiology* 1988;169:17.
81. Horning S, Hoppe R, Advani R, et al. Efficacy and late effects of Stanford V chemotherapy and radiotherapy in untreated Hodgkin disease: mature data in early and advanced stage patients. *Blood* 2001;104:308
82. Horning S. abstract. *Blood* 2000.
83. Horning SJ, Ang PT, Hoppe RT, et al. The Stanford experience with combined procarbazine, Alkeran and vinblastine (PAVe) and radiotherapy for locally extensive and advanced stage Hodgkin disease. *Ann Oncol* 1992;3:747–754.
84. Horning SJ, Hoppe RT, Advani R, et al. Efficacy and late effects of Stanford V chemotherapy and radiotherapy in untreated Hodgkin disease: Mature data in early and advanced stage patients [abstract 308]. *Blood* 2004;104:92a.
85. Horning SJ, Hoppe RT, Breslin S, et al. Stanford V and radiotherapy for locally extensive and advanced Hodgkin disease: mature results of a prospective clinical trial. *J Clin Oncol* 2002;20:630–637.
86. Horning SJ, Hoppe RT, Hancock SL, et al. Vinblastine, bleomycin, and methotrexate: an effective adjuvant in favorable Hodgkin disease. *J Clin Oncol* 1988;6:1822–1831.
87. Horning SJ, Hoppe RT, Mason J, et al. Stanford-Kaiser Permanente G1 study for clinical stage I to IIA Hodgkin disease: subtotal lymphoid irradiation versus vinblastine, methotrexate, and bleomycin chemotherapy and regional irradiation. *J Clin Oncol* 1997;15:1736–1744.
88. Horning SJ, Williams J, Bartlett NL, et al. Assessment of the stanford V regimen and consolidative radiotherapy for bulky and advanced Hodgkin disease: Eastern Cooperative Oncology Group pilot study E1492. *J Clin Oncol* 2000;18:972–980.
89. Hu E, Hufford S, Lukes R, et al. Third-World Hodgkin disease at Los Angeles County-University of Southern California Medical Center. *J Clin Oncol* 1988;6:1285–1292.
90. Hudson M, Korholz D, Donaldson SS. Pediatric Hodgkin lymphoma. In: Hoppe RT, Armitage JA, Diehl V, et al., eds. *Hodgkin lymphoma*. Philadelphia: Lippincott Williams & Wilkins; 2007;293–318.
91. Hudson MM, Greenwald C, Thompson E, et al. Efficacy and toxicity of multiagent chemotherapy and low-dose involved- field radiotherapy in children and adolescents with Hodgkin disease. *J Clin Oncol* 1993;11:100–108.
92. Hudson MM, Krasin M, Link MP, et al. Risk-adapted, combined-modality therapy with VAMP/COP and response-based, involved-field radiation for unfavorable pediatric Hodgkin disease. *J Clin Oncol* 2004;22:4541–4550.
93. Hughes DB, Smith AR, Hoppe R, et al. Treatment planning for Hodgkin disease: a Pattern of Care Study. *Intl J Radiat Oncol Biol Phys* 1995;33:519–524.
94. Hunger SP, Link MP, Donaldson SS. ABVD/MOPP and low-dose involved-field

radiotherapy in pediatric Hodgkin disease: the Stanford experience. *J Clin Oncol* 1994;12:2160–2166.
95. Hutchinson RJ, Fryer CJ, Davis PC, et al. MOPP or radiation in addition to ABVD in the treatment of pathologically staged advanced Hodgkin disease in children: results of the Children's Cancer Group Phase III Trial. *J Clin Oncol* 1998;16:897–906.
96. Jacobs C, Donaldson SS, Rosenberg SA, et al. Management of the pregnant patient with Hodgkin disease. *Ann Intern Med* 1981;95:669–675.
97. Jacobs P. Hodgkin lymphoma in developing countries: An African perspective with a note on Asia and Latin America. In: Hoppe RT, Armitage JA, Diehl V, et al., eds. *Hodgkin lymphoma*. Philadelphia: Lippincott Williams & Wilkins; 2007.
98. Kaplan HS. Evidence for a tumoricidal dose level in the radiotherapy of Hodgkin disease. *Cancer Res* 1966;26:1221–1224.
99. Kaplan HS. *Hodgkin disease*, Cambridge, MA: Harvard University Press; 1980.
100. Kaplan HS. On the natural history, treatment, and prognosis of Hodgkin disease. *Harvey Lect* 1968;64:215–259.
101. Kaplan HS. The radical radiotherapy of regionally localized Hodgkin disease. *Radiology* 1962;78:553.
102. Kinzie JJ, Hanks GE, MacLean CJ, et al. Patterns of care study: Hodgkin disease relapse rates and adequacy of portals. *Cancer* 1983;52:2223–2226.
103. Klimm BD, Engert A, Brillant C, et al. Comparison of BEACOPP and ABVD chemotherapy in intermediate stage Hodgkin lymphoma: results of the fourth interim analysis of the HD 11 trial of GHSG. *J Clin Oncol Proc* ASCO 2005; 23(16s):6507.
104. Klimo P, Connors JM. MOPP/ABV hybrid program: combination chemotherapy based on early introduction of seven effective drugs for advanced Hodgkin disease. *J Clin Oncol* 1985;3:1174–1182.
105. Koh ES, Sun A, Tran TH, et al. Clinical dose-volume histogram analysis in predicting radiation pneumonitis in Hodgkin lymphoma. *Int J Radiat Oncol Biol Phys* 2006;66:223–228.
106. Kuppers R, Rajewsky K, Zhao M, et al. Hodgkin disease: Hodgkin and Reed-Sternberg cells picked from histological sections show clonal immunoglobulin gene rearrangements and appear to be derived from B cells at various stages of development. *Proc Natl Acad Sci U S A* 1994;91:10962–10966.
107. Kuppers R, Re D. Nature of Reed-Sternberg and L & H cells, and their molecular biology in Hodgkin lymophoma. In: Hoppe RT, Armitage JA, Diehl V, et al., eds. *Hodgkin lymphoma*. Philadelphia: Lippincott Williams & Wilkins; 2007;73–86.
108. Lambe M, Hsieh CC, Tsaih SW, et al. Childbearing and the risk of Hodgkin disease. *Cancer Epidemiol Biomarkers Prev* 1998;7:831–834.
109. Lancet JE, Rapoport AP, Brasacchio R, et al. Autotransplantation for relapsed or refractory Hodgkin disease: long- term follow-up and analysis of prognostic factors. *Bone Marrow Transplant* 1998;22:265–271.
110. Lavoie JC, Connors JM, Phillips GL, et al. High-dose chemotherapy and autologous stem cell transplantation for primary refractory or relapsed Hodgkin lymphoma: long-term outcome in the first 100 patients treated in Vancouver. *Blood* 2005;106:1473–1478.
111. Le Floch O, Donaldson SS, Kaplan HS. Pregnancy following oophoropexy and total nodal irradiation in women with Hodgkin disease. *Cancer* 1976;38:2263–2268.
112. Leibenhaut MH, Hoppe RT, Efron B, et al. Prognostic indicators of laparotomy findings in clinical stage I–II supradiaphragmatic Hodgkin disease. *J Clin Oncol* 1989;7:81–91.
113. Leopold KA, Canellos GP, Rosenthal D, et al. Stage IA–IIB Hodgkin disease: staging and treatment of patients with large mediastinal adenopathy. *J Clin Oncol* 1989;7:1059–1065.
114. Lister TA, Crowther D, Sutcliffe SB, et al. Report of a committee convened to discuss the evaluation and staging of patients with Hodgkin disease: Cotswolds meeting. *J Clin Oncol* 1989;7:1630–1636.
115. Longo DL, Russo A, Duffey PL, et al. Treatment of advanced-stage massive mediastinal Hodgkin disease: the case for combined modality treatment. *J Clin Oncol* 1991;9:227–235.
116. Loo B, Hoppe RT. Hodgkin disease: case study. In: Mundt A, Roeske J, eds. *Intensity modulated radiation therapy: a clinical perspective*. Hamilton, Ontario: BC Decker, Inc; 2005:547–552.
117. Loo B, Hoppe RT. Lymphoma: overview. In: Mundt AJ RJ, ed. *Intensity modulated radiation therapy*. Hamilton, Ontario: BC Decker, Inc; 2005:535–546.
118. Lukes RJ, Butler JJ. The pathology and nomenclature of Hodgkin disease. *Cancer Res* 1966;26:1063–1083.
119. Lutz WR, Larsen RD. Technique to match mantle and para-aortic fields. *Int J Radiat Oncol Biol Phys* 1983;9:1753–1756.
120. Mauch P, Goodman R, Hellman S. The significance of mediastinal involvement in early stage Hodgkin disease. *Cancer* 1978;42:1039–1045.
121. Mauch P, Kalish LA, Marcus K. Longterm survival in Hodgkin disease: relative impact of mortality, second tumors, infection, and cardiovascular disease. *Cancer J Sci Am* 1995;1:33–42.
122. Mauch P. Treatment of favorable prognosis stage I–II Hodgkin lymphoma. In: Hoppe RT, Armitage JA, Diehl V, et al., eds. *Hodgkin lymphoma*. Philadelphia: Lippincott Williams & Wilkins; 2007.
123. Medeiros LJ, Greiner TC. Hodgkin disease. *Cancer* 1995;75:357–369.
124. Meyer RM, Gospodarowicz M, Connors JM, et al. Randomized comparison of ABVD chemotherapy with a strategy that includes radiation therapy in patients with limited-stage Hodgkin lymphoma: National Cancer Institute of Canada Trials Group and the Eastern Cooperative Oncology Group. *J Clin Oncol* 2005.
125. Molrine DC, George S, Tarbell N, et al. Antibody responses to polysaccharide and polysaccharide-conjugate vaccines after treatment of Hodgkin disease. *Ann Intern Med* 1995;123:828–834.
126. Moody AM, Pratt J, Hudson GV, et al. British National Lymphoma Investigation: pilot studies of neoadjuvant chemotherapy in clinical stage Ia and IIa Hodgkin disease. *Clin Oncol (R Coll Radiol)* 2001;13:262–268.
127. Moskowitz CH, Nimer SD, Zelenetz AD, et al. A 2–step comprehensive high-dose chemoradiotherapy second-line program for relapsed and refractory Hodgkin disease: analysis by intent to treat and development of a prognostic model. *Blood* 2001;97:616–623.
128. Mueller N, Evans A, Harris NL, et al. Hodgkin disease and Epstein-Barr virus. Altered antibody pattern before diagnosis. *N Engl J Med* 1989;320:689–695.
129. Mueller NE, Grufferman S, Chang ET. The epidemiology of Hodgkin lymphoma. In: Hoppe RT, Armitage JA, Diehl V, et al., eds. *Hodgkin lymphoma*. Philadelphia: Lippincott Williams & Wilkins; 2007:7–24.
130. Mundt AJ, Sibley G, Williams S, et al. Patterns of failure following high-dose chemotherapy and autologous bone marrow transplantation with involved field radiotherapy for relapsed/refractory Hodgkin disease. *Int J Radiat Oncol Biol Phys* 1995;33:261–270.
131. Nachman JB, Sposto R, Herzog P, et al. Randomized comparison of low-dose involved-field radiotherapy and no radiotherapy for children with Hodgkin disease who achieve a complete response to chemotherapy. *J Clin Oncol* 2002;20:3765–3771.
132. Nademanee A, O'Donnell MR, Snyder DS, et al. High dose chemotherapy with or without total body irradiation followed by autologous bone marrow and/or peripheral blood stem cell transplantation for patients with relapsed and refractory Hodgkin disease: results in 85 patients with analysis of prognostic factors. *Blood* 1995;85:1381–1390.
133. Naumann R, Vaic A, Beuthien-Baumann B, et al. Prognostic value of positron emission tomography in the evaluation of post-treatment residual mass in patients with Hodgkin disease and non-Hodgkin lymphoma. *Br J Haematol* 2001;115:793–800.
134. Ng A, Mauch P, Hoppe R. Life expectancy in Hodgkin lymphoma. In: Hoppe RT, Armitage JA, Diehl V, et al., eds. *Hodgkin lymphoma*. Philadelphia: Lippincott Williams & Wilkins; 2007.
135. Ng AK, Bernardo MP, Weller E, et al. Long-term survival and competing causes of death in patients with early-stage Hodgkin disease treated at age 50 or younger. *J Clin Oncol* 2002;20:2101–2108.
136. Ng AK, Li S, Neuberg D, et al. Comparison of MOPP versus ABVD as salvage therapy in patients who relapse after radiation therapy alone for Hodgkin disease. *Ann Oncol* 2004;15:270–275.
137. Nogova L, Reineke T, Eich HT, et al. Extended field radiotherapy, combined modality treatment or involved field radiotherapy for patients with stage IA lymphocyte-predominant Hodgkin lymphoma: a retrospective analysis from the German Hodgkin Study Group (GHSG). *Ann Oncol* 2005;16:1683–1687.
138. Noordijk EM, Thomas J, Ferme C, et al. First results of the EORTC-GELA H9 randomized trials: the H9–F trial (comparing 3 radiation dose levels) and H9–U trial (comparing 3 chemotherapy schemes) in patients with favorable or unfavorable early stage Hodgkin lymphoma. *J Clin Oncol Proc* ASCO 2005;23(16s):6505.
139. Partridge S, Timothy A, O'Doherty MJ, et al. 2–Fluorine-18–fluoro-2-deoxy-D glucose positron emission tomography in the pretreatment staging of Hodgkin disease: influence on patient management in a single institution. *Ann Oncol* 2000;11:1273–1279.
140. Pedrick TJ, Hoppe RT. Recovery of spermatogenesis following pelvic irradiation for Hodgkin disease. *Int J Radiat Oncol Biol Phys* 1986;12:117–121.
141. Pellegrino B, Terrier-Lacombe MJ, Oberlin O, et al. Lymphocyte-predominant Hodgkin lymphoma in children: therapeutic abstention after initial lymph node resection: a study of the French Society of Pediatric Oncology. *J Clin Oncol* 2003;21:2948–2952.
142. Pinkus GS, Said JW. Hodgkin disease, lymphocyte predominance type, nodular—a distinct entity?. Unique staining profile for L&H variants of Reed-Sternberg cells defined by monoclonal antibodies to leukocyte common antigen, granulocyte-specific antigen, and B-cell-specific antigen. *Am J Pathol* 1985; 118:1–6.
143. Poen JC, Hoppe RT, Horning SJ. High-dose therapy and autologous bone marrow transplantation for relapsed/refractory Hodgkin disease: the impact of involved field radiotherapy on patterns of failure and survival. *Int J Radiat Oncol Biol Phys* 1996;36:3–12.
144. Poppema S, Timens W, Visser L. Nodular lymphocyte predominance type of Hodgkin disease is a B cell lymphoma. *Adv Exp Med Biol* 1985;186:963–969.
145. Portlock CS, Yahalom J. The management of Hodgkin lymphoma during pregnancy. In: Hoppe RT, Armitage JA, Diehl V, et al., edrs. *Hodgkin lymphoma*. Philadelphia: Lippincott Williams & Wilkins; 2007;419–426.
146. Regula DP, Jr., Hoppe RT, Weiss LM. Nodular and diffuse types of lymphocyte predominance Hodgkin disease. *N Engl J Med* 1988;318:214–219.
147. Roach M, Kapp DS, Rosenberg SA, et al. Radiotherapy with curative intent: an option in selected patients relapsing after chemotherapy for advanced Hodgkin disease. *J Clin Oncol* 1987;5:550–555.
148. Roach MD, Brophy N, Cox R, et al. Prognostic factors for patients relapsing after radiotherapy for early-stage Hodgkin disease. *J Clin Oncol* 1990;8:623–629.
149. Rosenberg S, Kaplan HS. Evidence for an orderly progression in the spread of Hodgkin disease. *Cancer Res* 1966;26:1225–1231.
150. Ruffer JU, Flechtner H, Tralls P, et al. Fatigue in long-term survivors of Hodgkin lymphoma; a report from the German Hodgkin Lymphoma Study Group (GHSG). *Eur J Cancer* 2003;39:2179–2186.
151. Ruhl U, Albrecht M, Dieckmann K, et al. Response-adapted radiotherapy in the treatment of pediatric Hodgkin disease: an interim report at 5 years of the German GPOH-HD 95 trial. *Int J Radiat Oncol Biol Phys* 2001;51:1209–1218.
152. Russell KJ, Hoppe RT, Colby TV, et al. Lymphocyte predominant Hodgkin disease: clinical presentation and results of treatment. *Radiother Oncol* 1984;1:197–205.
153. Salloum E, Doria R, Farber LR, et al. Combined modality therapy in previously untreated patients with advanced Hodgkin disease: a 24-year followup study. *Cancer J Sci Am* 1995;1:267–273.
154. Schellong G. The balance between cure and late effects in childhood Hodgkin lymphoma: the experience of the German-Austrian Study-Group since 1978. German-Austrian Pediatric Hodgkin Disease Study Group. *Ann Oncol* 1996;7: 67–72.
155. Schellong G, Potter R, Bramswig JH, et al. High cure rates and reduced long-term toxicity in pediatric Hodgkin disease: the German-Austrian Multicenter Trial DAL-HD-90. *Clin Oncol* 1999;17:3736–3744.
156. Selby P, Patel P, Milan S, et al. Ch1VPP combination chemotherapy for Hodgkin disease: Longterm results. *Br J Cancer* 1990;62:279–285.
157. Siber GR, Gorham C, Martin P, et al. Antibody response to pretreatment immunization and post-treatment boosting with bacterial polysaccharide vaccines in patients with Hodgkin disease. *Ann Intern Med* 1986;104:467–475.
158. Specht L, Hasenclever D. Prognostic factors in Hodgkin lymphoma. In: Hoppe RT, Armitage JA, Diehl V, et al., eds. *Hodgkin lymphoma*. Philadelphia: Lippincott Williams & Wilkins; 2007;157–176.
159. Specht L, Horwich A, Ashley S. Salvage of relapse of patients with Hodgkin disease in clinical stages I or II who were staged with laparotomy and initially treated with radiotherapy alone. A report from the international database on Hodgkin disease. *Int J Radiat Oncol Biol Phys* 1994;30:805–811.

160. Specht L. Tumour burden as the main indicator of prognosis in Hodgkin disease. *Eur J Cancer* 1992;12:1982–1985.
161. Spina M, Vaccher E, Nasti G, et al. Human immunodeficiency virus-associated Hodgkin disease. *Semin Oncol* 2000;27:480–488.
162. Straus DJ, Gaynor JJ, Myers J, et al. Prognostic factors among 185 adults with newly diagnosed advanced Hodgkin disease treated with alternating potentially noncross-resistant chemotherapy and intermediate-dose radiation therapy. *J Clin Oncol* 1990;8:1173–1186.
162a. Stat Bite. *JNCL*; 2998:352.
163. Sutcliffe SB, Gospodarowicz MK, Bergsagel DE, et al. Prognostic groups for management of localized Hodgkin disease. *J Clin Oncol* 1985;3:393–401.
164. Sweetenham JW, Taghipour G, Milligan D, et al. High-dose therapy and autologous stem cell rescue for patients with Hodgkin disease in first relapse after chemotherapy: results from the EBMT. Lymphoma Working Party of the European Group for Blood and Marrow Transplantation. *Bone Marrow Transplant* 1997;20:745–752.
165. Swerdlow AJ, Barber JA, Hudson GV, et al. Risk of second malignancy after Hodgkin disease in a collaborative British cohort: the relation to age at treatment. *J Clin Oncol* 2000;18:498–509.
166. Tirelli U, Carbone A, Straus DJ. HIV-related Hodgkin disease. In: Mauch PM, Armitage JO, Diehl V, et al., eds. *Hodgkin disease*. Philadelphia: Lippincott Williams & Wilkins; 1999:701–712.
167. Tirelli U, Errante D, Dolcetti R, et al. Hodgkin disease and human immunodeficiency virus infection: clinicopathologic and virologic features of 114 patients from the Italian Cooperative Group on AIDS and Tumors. *J Clin Oncol* 1995;13:1758–1767.
168. Torrey MJ, Poen JC, Hoppe RT. Detection of relapse in early-stage Hodgkin disease: role of routine follow-up studies. *J Clin Oncol* 1997;15:1123–1130.
169. Travis LB, Gilbert E. Lung cancer after Hodgkin lymphoma: the roles of chemotherapy, radiotherapy and tobacco use. *Radiat Res* 2005;163:695–696.
170. Travis LB, Hill DA, Dores GM, et al. Breast cancer following radiotherapy and chemotherapy among young women with Hodgkin disease. *JAMA* 2003;290:465–475.
171. Tsang RW, Gospodarowicz MK, Sutcliffe SB, et al. Thoracic radiation therapy before autologous bone marrow transplantation in relapsed or refractory Hodgkin disease. PMH Lymphoma Group, and the Toronto Autologous BMT Group. *Eur J Cancer* 1999;35:73–78.
172. Ng AK, van denAbbecle AK. Functional imaging in Hodgkin lymphoma. In: Hoppe RT, Armitage JA, Diehl V, et al., eds. *Hodgkin lymphoma*. Philadelphia: Lippincott Williams & Wilkins, 2007;143–156.
173. van Leeuwen FA, Swerdlow AJ, Travis LB. Second cancers after treatment of Hodgkin lymphoma. In: Hoppe RT, Armitage JA, Diehl V, et al., eds. *Hodgkin lymphoma*. Philadelphia: Lippincott Williams & Wilkins; 2007;347–370.
174. van Leeuwen FE, Klokman WJ, Veer MB, et al. Long-term risk of second malignancy in survivors of Hodgkin disease treated during adolescence or young adulthood. *J Clin Oncol* 2000;18:487–497.
175. Vassilakopoulos TP, Angelopoulou MK, Siakantaris MP, et al. Pure infradiaphragmatic Hodgkin lymphoma. Clinical features, prognostic factor and comparison with supradiaphragmatic disease. *Haematologica* 2006;91:32–39.
176. Viviani S, Santoro A, Ragni G, et al. Gonadal toxicity after combination chemotherapy for Hodgkin disease. Comparative results of MOPP vs ABVD. *Eur J Cancer Clin Oncol* 1985;21:601–605.
177. Vose JM, Constine LS, Sutcliffe SB. Other Complications of the treatment of Hodgkin Lymphoma. In: Hoppe RT, Armitage JA, Diehl V, et al., eds. *Hodgkin lymphoma*. Philadelphia: Lippincott Williams & Wilkins; 2007;383–392.
178. Weihrauch MR, Re D, Scheidhauer K, et al. Thoracic positron emission tomography using 18F-fluorodeoxyglucose for the evaluation of residual mediastinal Hodgkin disease. *Blood* 2001;98:2930–2934.
179. Weiner MA, Leventhal B, Brecher ML, et al. Randomized study of intensive MOPP-ABVD with or without low-dose total- nodal radiation therapy in the treatment of stages IIB, IIIA2, IIIB, and IV Hodgkin disease in pediatric patients: a Pediatric Oncology Group study. *J Clin Oncol* 1997;15:2769–2779.
180. Weiss LM, Warnke R, Hansmann ML, et al. Pathology of Hodgkin lymphoma. In: Hoppe RT, Armitage JA, Diehl V, et al., eds. *Hodgkin lymphoma*. Philadelphia: Lippincott Williams & Wilkins; 2007;43–72.
181. Weiss LM, Movahed LA, Warnke RA, et al. Detection of Epstein-Barr viral genomes in Reed-Sternberg cells of Hodgkin disease. *N Engl J Med* 1989;320:502–506.
182. Weiss LM, Strickler JG, Hu E, et al. Immunoglobulin gene rearrangements in Hodgkin disease. *Hum Pathol* 1986;17:1009–1014.
183. Wirth A, Seymour JF, Hicks RJ, et al. Fluorine-18 fluorodeoxyglucose positron emission tomography, gallium-67 scintigraphy, and conventional staging for Hodgkin disease and non-Hodgkin lymphoma. *Am J Med* 2002;112:262–268.
184. Wirth A, Yuen K, Barton M, et al. Long-term outcome after radiotherapy alone for lymphocyte-predominant Hodgkin lymphoma: a retrospective multicenter study of the Australasian Radiation Oncology Lymphoma Group. *Cancer* 2005;104:1221–1229.
185. Yahalom J, Hoppe RT, Mauch PM. Principles and techniques of radiation therapy for Hodgkin lymphoma. In: Hoppe RT, Armitage JA, Diehl V, et al., eds. *Hodgkin lymphoma*. Philadelphia: Lippincott Williams & Wilkins; 2007;177–188.
186. Yahalom J, Ryu J, Straus DJ, et al. Impact of adjuvant radiation on the patterns and rate of relapse in advanced-stage Hodgkin disease treated with alternating chemotherapy combinations. *J Clin Oncol* 1991;9:2193–2201.
187. Young RC, Canellos GP, Chabner BA, et al. Patterns of relapse in advanced Hodgkin disease treated with combination chemotherapy. *Cancer* 1978;42:1001–1007.
188. Zinzani PL, Magagnoli M, Bendandi M, et al. Efficacy of the VBM regimen in the treatment of elderly patients with Hodgkin disease. *Haematologica* 2000;85:729–732.
189. Zukerberg LR, Collins AB, Ferry JA, et al. Coexpression of CD15 and CD20 by Reed-Sternberg cells in Hodgkin disease. *Am J Pathol* 1991;139:475–483.

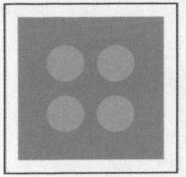

Chapter 76
Non-Hodgkin's Lymphoma

Leonard R. Prosnitz, Andrea Ng

Non-Hodgkin's lymphoma (NHL) is a heterogeneous group of malignancies of the lymphoid system characterized by an abnormal clonal proliferation of B cells, T cells, or both. Scientific knowledge regarding NHL has increased dramatically in the last decade, resulting in very specific advances in the spheres of molecular biology and immunobiology and leading to new histopathologic classifications as well as therapies.

Epidemiology

The U.S. age-adjusted incidence rate for NHL was 19.1 per 100,000 between 2000 and 2003, according to the Surveillance, Epidemiology, and End Results (SEER) Program of the National Cancer Institute (242). In 2006, the estimated number of new NHL cases in the United States was 59,000; deaths from NHL were 19,000 (152). International NHL incidence rates vary, with the highest reported incidence rates being in the United States, Europe, and Australia, whereas the lowest rates have been reported in Asia (8,218,235,267). NHL is primarily a disease of older populations, with a median age at diagnosis of 65 years (112)

There has been a striking increase in NHL incidence rates during the last four decades, with a doubling between 1970 and 1990. There is some evidence that the rate of increase has slowed since 1990, with a modest increase in incidence from 18.5/100,000 to 19.5/100,000 between 1990 and 2000 (242). The mortality rate for NHL has also risen steadily during the last four decades, albeit more slowly than the incidence. The U.S. mortality rate rose from 4.7 per 100,000 to 7.7 per 100,000 between 1973 and 2003 (242). Similar increases have been noted in international cancer registries (211). The change in incidence over time has varied substantially among lymphoid neoplasm subtypes (209).

The increased incidence of NHL has been partly attributed to advances in molecular diagnostic techniques, the aging of the population, the acquired immune deficiency syndrome (AIDS) epidemic, other infectious agents, and occupational exposures (96). There are other likely additional contributing factors, although they remain unknown at this time.

Etiology

Several genetic diseases, environmental agents, and infectious agents have been associated with the development of lymphoma. Familial clustering of NHL has been described. However, it is not clear whether the familial aggregations are the result of hereditary factors and/or shared environmental exposures (43).

Immunodeficiency

The frequency of NHL is greatly increased in immunocompromised patients. The two most common clinical circumstances are AIDS and patients undergoing prolonged immunosuppression, such as after organ transplantation (24,117). In patients with AIDS, NHL is the second most common malignancy. The introduction of highly active antiretroviral therapy, however, has resulted in a decline in the incidence as well as improved treatment outcome of NHL in this population (298).

Patients with autoimmune and chronic inflammatory disorders, including Sjogren's syndrome, Hashimoto's thyroiditis, systemic lupus erythematosus, and less commonly, celiac sprue, also have an increased risk of NHL (75,330).

Several rare inherited disorders are associated with as much as a 25% lifetime risk for development of lymphoma (88). These include severe combined immunodeficiency, hypogammaglobulinemia, common variable immunodeficiency, Wiskott-Aldrich syndrome, Chediak-Higashi syndrome, and ataxia-telangiectasia. Lymphomas associated with these disorders are often Epstein-Barr Virus (EBV)-related and usually highly aggressive in their behavior.

Infectious Agents

A number of infectious agents are implicated in the pathogenesis of NHL. EBV is associated with Burkitt's lymphoma, post-transplantation lymphoproliferative disorders, AIDS-associated primary central nervous system lymphoma (PCNSL), lymphomas associated with congenital immunodeficiency, and T/NK cell lymphomas (102). The human T-cell lymphotropic virus type 1 (HTLV-1) is an RNA virus that is responsible for adult T-cell leukemia/lymphoma (238). In endemic areas, more than 50% of all NHL cases are adult T-cell leukemia/lymphoma, although the risk for development of disease is only approximately 5% in infected patients. Human herpes virus 8, the causative agent for Kaposi's sarcoma, is also associated with several rare lymphoproliferative diseases, including primary effusion lymphoma (265). The hepatitis C virus is linked with NHL, particularly splenic marginal zone lymphoma (282).

The strongest association between infectious agents and NHL is seen in marginal zone lymphomas (MZL). The bacterium *Helicobacter pylori* has been linked to gastric mucosa-associated lymphoid tissue (MALT) lymphomas (322). It has been suggested that several other bacteria, including *Borrelia burgdorferi, Campylobacter jejuni,* and *Chlamydia psittaci,* may also play a role in the pathogenesis of MALT lymphoma of other sites (85,120,282).

Environmental and Occupational Exposures

Occupations associated with a higher risk include farmers, forestry workers, welders, and agricultural workers (224). Several studies have shown an increased risk of NHL in relation to herbicide exposure, especially phenoxy herbicides (201). The development of NHL has also been linked to hair dyes, organic solvents, high levels of nitrates in drinking water, arsenic, pesticides, fungicides, lead, vinyl chloride, and asbestos (201). Radiation has been suggested as a causative agent because of the increased lymphoma incidence in survivors of nuclear explosions or atomic reactor accidents. NHL is also observed as a late effect of prior radiation therapy or chemotherapy (253).

Dietary factors and tobacco and alcohol use may affect the risk of developing NHL (210).

Pathology and Immunobiology

NHL is a group of many different disease entities, often difficult to diagnosis, with a correspondingly complex histopathologic classification that has changed relatively frequently over the years. The changing classifications reflect new knowledge gained as well as difficulties with older systems that were recognized with the passage of time, such as interobserver variability and difficulties with reproducibility and a somewhat confusing picture with respect to clinical–pathologic correlates. In 1994, the Revised European American Lymphoma (REAL) classification was reported by the International Lymphoma Study Group (ILSG) (130). The REAL classification was subsequently modified by the Society for Hematopathology and the European Association of Hematopathologists, principally by the inclusion of myeloid neoplasms, to form the World Health Organization (WHO) classification. The latter is known variously as the REAL/WHO classification, or simply the WHO classification (151).

The predecessor system to the WHO classification was the Working Formulation (215). It subdivided NHL into groups by biologic behavior, that is low-grade, intermediate- and high-grade, and indolent/aggressive behavior groups. That characterization has been abandoned in the new WHO classification. The argument was that although such groupings were convenient and appeared clinically useful, they represented an oversimplification and did not account for several distinct clinical pathologic entities.

The WHO classification divides NHL into B-cell neoplasms and T-cell neoplasms, with 31 different and distinct lymphomas delineated. The neoplasms are shown in Table 76.1. These specific entities are distinguished on the basis of morphologic, immunologic, and genetic characteristics and are thought to be reproducibly identifiable.

The specific diseases described may be either indolent or aggressive in their behavior or, sometimes within a given disease, there may be a range of behaviors (e.g., anaplastic large cell lymphoma [ALCL]). Similarly, the histologic grade as well as the biologic behavior may vary within a specific disease entity (e.g., follicular lymphoma [FL]). In addition, the WHO classification describes some important new disease categories not clearly recognized in the Working Formulation, notably MZL, mantle cell lymphoma (MCL), peripheral T-cell lymphomas (PTCL), ALCL, and primary mediastinal large B-cell lymphoma.

A description of all 31 varieties of NHL is not practical and is beyond the scope of this chapter. We focus on the most common ones in order of decreasing frequency, namely diffuse large B-cell lymphoma (DLBCL), FL, MZL, MCL, PTCL, and small lymphocytic lymphoma B-cell/chronic lymphocytic leukemia (SLLB-CLL). Incidence data are derived largely from the non-Hodgkin's Lymphoma Classification Project (11), which evaluated 1,403 cases of NHL at nine study sites around the world, thus establishing the frequency of the different types, geographic variation in incidence, and clinical correlates.

It must be emphasized that lymphoma pathology is difficult and complex with a long history of interobserver disagreement as to the exact diagnosis. National Comprehensive Cancer Network (NCCN) guidelines describe as "essential" specialized hematopathology review of all slides and adequate immunophenotyping to establish the diagnosis (NCCN Practice Guidelines in Oncology 2006). Fine-needle aspiration alone is usually not acceptable for the initial diagnosis of lymphoma (132).

Diffuse Large B-Cell Lymphoma

DLBCL is a neoplasm of large, transformed B cells with a diffuse growth pattern and a high (>40%) proliferation fraction. The

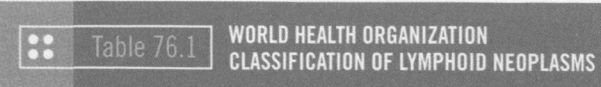

Table 76.1 WORLD HEALTH ORGANIZATION CLASSIFICATION OF LYMPHOID NEOPLASMS

B-cell neoplasms
Precursor B-cell neoplasm
Precursor B-lymphocytic leukemia/lymphoma (precursor B-cell acute lymphoblastic leukemia)

Mature (peripheral) B-cell neoplasms$^\alpha$
B-cell chronic lymphocytic leukemia/small lymphocytic lymphoma
B-cell prolymphocytic leukemia
Lymphoplasmacytic lymphoma
Splenic marginal zone B-cell lymphoma (± villous lymphocytes)
Hairy cell leukemia
Plasma cell myeloma/plasmacytoma
Extranodal marginal zone B-cell lymphoma of mucosa-associated lymphoid tissue type
Nodal marginal zone B-cell lymphoma (± monocytoid B cells)
Follicular lymphoma
Mantle cell lymphoma
Diffuse large B-cell lymphoma
Mediastinal large B-cell lymphoma
Primary effusion lymphoma
   Burkitt's lymphoma/Burkitt cell leukemia

T-cell and cell neoplasms
Precursor T-cell neoplasm
Precursor T-lymphoblastic lymphoma/leukemia (precursor T-cell auto lymphoblastic leukemia)

Mature (peripheral) T-cell neoplasms$^\alpha$
   T-cell prolymphocytic leukemia
   T-cell granular lymphocytic leukemia
   Aggressive NK cell leukemia
   Adult T-cell lymphoma/leukemia (human T cell leukemia virus type 1 positive)
   Extranodal NK/T-cell lymphoma, nasal type
   Enteropathy-type T-cell lymphoma
   Hepatosplenic gamma-delta T-cell lymphoma
   Subcutaneous panniculitislike T-cell lymphoma
   Mycosis fungoides/Sezary's syndrome
   Anaplastic large cell lymphoma, T-/null cell, primary cutaneous type
   Peripheral T-cell lymphoma, not otherwise characterized
   Angioimmunoblastic T-cell lymphoma
   Anaplastic large cell lymphoma, T-/null cell, primary systemic type

Hodgkin's lymphoma (Hodgkin's disease)
Nodular lymphocyte-redominant Hodgkin's lymphoma
Classic Hodgkin's lymphoma
   Nodular sclerosis Hodgkin's lymphoma (grades 1 and 2)
   Lymphocyte-rich classic Hodgkin's lymphoma
   Mixed cellularity Hodgkin's lymphoma

Lymphocyte-depletion Hodgkin's lymphoma

NK, natural killer.
$^\alpha$B-cell and T-/NK cell neoplasms are grouped according to major clinical presentations (predominantly disseminated/leukemic, primary extranodal, predominantly nodal).
From Jaffe ES, Harris NL, Stein H, Vardiman JW, eds. *Pathology and genetics of tumours of hematoporetic and lymphoid tissue.* World Health Organization Classification of Tumours. Lyon, France: IARC Press, 2001.

cells may resemble centroblasts, immunoblasts, multilobated cells, or anaplastic large cells. It is the most common type of NHL (31% of all cases, 33% if primary DLBCL of the mediastinum is included) (11). DLBCL is a heterogeneous group of neoplasms, with six morphologic variants described as well as three clinical subtypes (151). DNA microarrays (oligonucleotides or cDNA probes) show that different subtypes of DLBCL with varying prognosis can be distinguished based on the mRNA expression (5). Models predictive of clinical outcome using gene expression data have also been developed (189,251,272). Treatment tailored to molecular subclassification of this disease may become part of future routine clinical practice.

DLBCL express one or more B-cell–associated antigens (CD19, CD20), as well as CD45, and often surface immunoglobulin SIg

(33). Twenty-five percent to 80% in various studies express bcl-2 protein (190). Approximately 70% express bcl-6 protein, consistent with a germinal center origin (190,318). Most cases of DLBCL have somatic mutations in the immunoglobulin variable region genes, suggesting they have progressed through the germinal center where immunoglobulin affinity maturation occurs. The *bcl-2* gene is rearranged in 15% to 30% of cases, the c-*myc* gene is rearranged in 5% to 15%, and the *bcl-6* gene is rearranged in 20% to 40% of cases (190).

Follicular Lymphoma

The next most common type of NLH is follicular lymphoma (22% of all cases). In the working formulation it was described as low grade or indolent. It has also been referred to as *follicle center cell lymphoma* (11). In North America, the frequency is somewhat higher at 31% versus 14% at other geographic sites (8). Thus, in North America, FL and DLBCL are approximately equal in frequency.

FL is a tumor of follicle center B cells (centrocytes and centroblasts) with a follicular (nodular) pattern that morphologically is similar to normal germinal centers (151). The neoplastic follicles may be present in the entire tumor, or the lymphoma may contain a diffuse component as well. FLs are graded based on morphology. There is either a predominance of small cleaved cells (grade 1), a mixture of small cleaved and large cells (grade 2), or predominantly large cells (grade 3). In the WHO classification, the number of large cells per high-power field (0 to 5, 5 to 15, >15) is used to assign grades (1 to 3, respectively).

Clinically, grades 1 and 2 are closely related with no apparent differences in biologic behavior or response to therapy. FL grade 3 tends to have a somewhat higher relapse rate with an outlook favorably influenced by anthracycline-containing chemotherapy. Although grade 3 FL is not the same as DLBCL, it may contain areas of the latter, which further suggests the need for more aggressive therapy.

The tumor cells of FL are usually SIg-positive, express pan-B-cell–associated antigens (CD19, CD20) CD21, CD10 (60% of the time), but lack CD5. Most cases are *bcl-2*-positive; nuclear *bcl-6* is expressed by at least some of the neoplastic cells. T(14;18) and *bcl-2* gene rearrangement are present in the majority of the cases (85%). BCL-2 protein is expressed in most cases, ranging from 100% in grade 1 to 75% in grade 3 FL (67).

Marginal Zone Lymphomas

MALT was first described as a distinct clinical pathologic type of lymphoma in 1983 (147). MZL is now recognized as a distinctive subtype of NHL in the WHO classification, accounting for approximately 10% of all cases of NHL including extranodal MZL (MALT), nodal MZL, and splenic MZL.

Extranodal MZL is characterized by a polymorphous infiltrate of small lymphocytes, marginal zone (centrocyte-like) B cells, monocytoid B cells, and plasma cells, as well as rare large basophilic blast cells (centroblastlike or immunoblastlike). In epithelial tissues, the marginal zone B cells typically infiltrate the epithelium forming so-called lymphoepithelial lesions. Although transformed large cells are typically present, they are in the minority. If present in large numbers, a diagnosis of DLBCL is warranted.

The tumor cells express SIg and lack immunoglobulin D (IgD). Forty percent to 60% have monotypic cytoplasmic immunoglobulin, indicating plasmacytoid differentiation. They express B-cell–associated antigens (CD19, CD20, CD22, CD79a) and are usually negative for CD5 and CD10. Immunophenotyping studies are useful in confirming malignancy (light chain restriction) and in excluding B-cell chronic lymphocytic leukemia (B-CLL; CD5+), mantle cell (CD5 +) and follicular center (CD10+) lymphomas (78).

Immunoglobulin genes are rearranged; the variable region has a high degree of somatic mutation, as well as intraclonal diversity consistent with a postgerminal center stage of B-cell development (234). The most common reported cytogenetic abnormalities are trisomy 3, seen in 60%, and t(11;18), seen in 25% to 40% of patients (78,321). These changes are characteristically found in extranodal but not nodal MZL.

The most common site of MALT is the stomach. Lymphoid tissue is not normally present in the stomach, but in response to an antigenic stimulus brought about by *H. pylori,* normally present T cells in the gastric mucosa attract a B-cell population, giving rise to lymphoid follicles and, after prolonged antigenic stimulation, lymphomas (145).

Peripheral T-Cell Lymphomas

The PTCLs are the group most confusing to clinicians. They were not a separate entity in the Working Formulation but were frequently classified as either diffuse poorly differentiated lymphocytic lymphoma or diffuse mixed lymphocytic-histiocytic lymphoma. The term *PTCL* is often misinterpreted. It does not refer to the anatomic distribution of the lymphomas but rather to their origin from so-called peripheral or mature T cells outside the thymus, as opposed to thymic (precursor) T lymphocytes. The T-cell lymphomas collectively make up approximately 10% of all NHL (252). They are a diverse group that includes 13 different entities (Table 76.1).

PTCLs constitute the most frequently occurring variety of T-cell lymphoma. In the ILSG report, they were 7% of total cases, making them approximately equal in frequency to MALT lymphomas, small lymphocytic lymphoma (SLL), and MCL (252). Their frequency is quite different, however, by geographic locale. ILSG data showed a roughly 3% incidence of PTCL in North America compared with 9% in South Africa, Hong Kong, and London (8). EBV may be associated with T-cell lymphomas originating in the nasal cavity (65).

PTCLs typically contain a mixture of small and large atypical cells. The architectural pattern is diffuse. T-cell–associated antigens (CD2, CD3, CD4) are variably expressed, with some tumors expressing CD8. Sometimes the T-cell antigens CD5 and CD7 are lost. B-cell–associated antigens are lacking. The T-cell receptor genes (*TCR*) are usually but not always rearranged. No specific cytogenetic or oncogene abnormality has been reported.

A special variant of PTCL is anaplastic large T/null cell lymphoma (ALCL) (175,278). In the ILSG project, this comprised 2% of all NHLs (11). The tumor is usually composed of large cells with round, pleomorphic, or horseshoe-shaped nuclei with single or multiple prominent nucleoli and abundant cytoplasm, giving the cells an epithelial- or histiocytelike appearance. The cells express Ki-1 (CD30) and usually express CD25 and either T-cell– or null lineage–specific antigens (278). CD30 was originally recognized on Hodgkin's disease (HD) cells. In some cases, there may be confusion between ALCL and HD, but distinction between the two on the basis of immunophenotyping and morphology is usually possible.

Another characteristic feature of ALCL is the overexpression of a novel tyrosine kinase gene on chromosome 2 known as anaplastic lymphoma kinase (ALK) (278). Approximately 60% of cases overexpress the ALK protein; such cases have a better prognosis than ALK-negative cases, except for skin cases. ALCL in children is usually ALK-positive.

Small Lymphocytic Lymphoma/B-Cell Chronic Lymphocytic Leukemia

SLL is the nodal equivalent of B-cell chronic lymphocytic leukemia (151). It is a neoplasm composed predominantly of small lymphocytes with condensed chromatin and round nuclei.

Larger lymphoid cells (prolymphocytes and paraimmunoblasts) with more prominent nucleoli and dispersed chromatin are always present, usually clustered in pseudo follicles. SLL comprises approximately 7% of all NHL.

The tumor cells of SLL are phenotypically nearly identical to B-CLL. The cells express human leukocyte antigen (HLA)-DR, B-cell–associated antigens (CD19, CD20, CD22, CD79a), and both CD5 and CD23, and have faint surface immunoglobulin. CD23 is particularly useful in distinguishing B-CLL/SLL from MCL.

Approximately 50% of cases have abnormal karyotypes (153). Trisomy 12 is reported in one-third of cases with cytogenetic abnormalities, and correlates with atypical histology and an aggressive clinical course (153). Abnormalities of 13q are reported in no more than 25% of the cases and are associated with long survival. SLL/B-CLL can transform to DLBCL (Richter's syndrome) (296).

Mantle Cell Lymphoma

MCL was first distinguished in the 1980s by Weisenburger et al. (309), who described a type of FL in which there were wide mantles of malignant cells around apparently benign germinal centers. The term *mantle zone lymphoma* was proposed, subsequently modified to *mantle cell*. It was thought to represent a variant of FL and was classified under the Working Formulation as a low-grade lymphoma. Most of the cases of diffuse small cleaved cell lymphoma in the Working Formulation terminology were MCL.

Since the original description by Weisenburger et al. (309), additional features of this disease have been recognized. It is a neoplasm of small to medium-sized B cells with irregular nuclei that resemble the cleaved cells (centrocytes) of germinal centers. The morphologic pattern may be diffuse, nodular, a mantle zone, or some combination thereof. Tumor cells are typically CD5-positive, CD23-negative, CD20-positive, and CD10-negative. A characteristic cytogenetic abnormality is t(11;14) involving the *bcl-1* gene and resulting in the overexpression of cyclin D1. The product of the cyclin D1 gene can be detected in paraffin-embedded tissue sections with the immunoperoxidase technique and is very useful in distinguishing MCL from other lymphoma variants (79,308).

⠿ | Clinical Features

Nodal Versus Extranodal Disease

NHL is primarily a disease of older adults (in contrast to HD), with a median age at presentation from 55 to 65 years (60,248,281). There is a slight male over female preponderance (55% to 60% male). NHL may involve lymph nodes in almost any area of the body but may also present in extranodal sites, presumably arising from lymphoid tissue widely distributed throughout the body. Approximately two-thirds of NHL is nodal at presentation and one-third is extranodal, again in contrast to HD, where extranodal presentation is rare (60,116).

Patients with primarily nodal disease usually present with an asymptomatic lump in the neck or inguinal area; systemic symptoms (fever, night sweats, weight loss, B symptoms) may be present in 20% to 30% of patients. There is often a history of some spontaneous regression and then regrowth of the nodes.

The most frequent sites of nodal involvement are the neck in approximately 70% of patients, the groin in approximately 60%, and the axilla in approximately half (248,281). Although patients with nodal presentations may appear to have localized disease initially, full staging evaluation results in assignment to a more advanced stage in two-thirds (41).

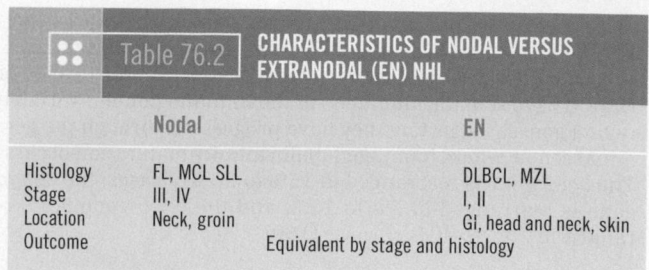

	Nodal	EN
Histology	FL, MCL SLL	DLBCL, MZL
Stage	III, IV	I, II
Location	Neck, groin	GI, head and neck, skin
Outcome	Equivalent by stage and histology	

Table 76.2 CHARACTERISTICS OF NODAL VERSUS EXTRANODAL (EN) NHL

FL, follicular lymphoma; MCL, mantle cell lymphoma; SLL, small lymphocytic lymphoma; DLBCL, diffuse large B-cell lymphoma; MZL, marginal zone lymphoma; GI, gastrointestinal.

Patients presenting with extranodal lymphoma, on the other hand, usually have localized disease. The symptoms relate to the site of involvement. The gastrointestinal (GI) tract is the most common (25% to 35% of extranodal disease), followed closely by Waldeyer's ring and other head and neck sites (18% to 28%) and skin (116). Epigastric discomfort, abdominal pain or bleeding, and sore throat or difficulty swallowing are among the usual symptoms for these locations.

The histologic picture of most primary ENLs is that of DLBCL. Nodal presentations conversely are more commonly FL. Nodal and extranodal disease of similar histologic type, stage, and other prognostic variables are treated in an equivalent fashion and have a similar outcome (285). For example, DLBCL stage IA in the neck treated with combination chemotherapy and radiotherapy would have the same outcome as stage IA DLBCL in the stomach treated similarly. These characteristics are summarized in Table 76.2.

Evaluation and Staging

A careful history and physical examination are required. All peripheral nodal areas should be examined clinically and inspection of the oral cavity and tonsils performed. Patients with suspected or established head and neck lymphoma or GI tract involvement should undergo direct fiberoptic laryngoscopy and/or endoscopy (Table 76.3).

The use of functional imaging, initially with gallium, now largely with positron emission tomography (PET) using ^{18}F-fluorodooxyglucose (FDG) has increased dramatically in the last decade (73,154,160,172,263). Clinical experience with the former is greater than with the latter PET, however, is largely replacing gallium because of greater accuracy, particularly in the abdomen, convenience and the ability to perform at one examination an integrated PET/computed tomography (CT) scan (172). The fused images obtainable from an integrated PET/CT increase the accuracy of diagnosis by more precisely localizing

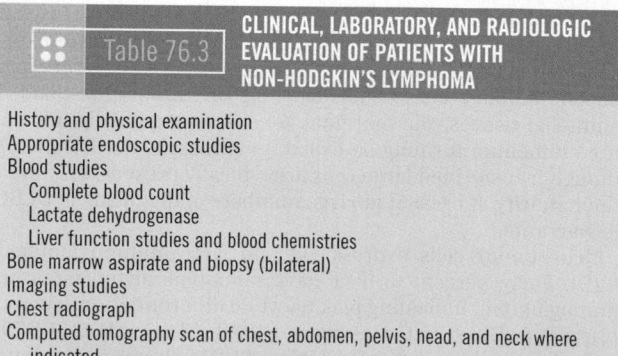

Table 76.3 CLINICAL, LABORATORY, AND RADIOLOGIC EVALUATION OF PATIENTS WITH NON-HODGKIN'S LYMPHOMA

History and physical examination
Appropriate endoscopic studies
Blood studies
   Complete blood count
   Lactate dehydrogenase
   Liver function studies and blood chemistries
Bone marrow aspirate and biopsy (bilateral)
Imaging studies
Chest radiograph
Computed tomography scan of chest, abdomen, pelvis, head, and neck where indicated
Positron emission tomography/gallium scanning
Upper gastrointestinal series/small bowel where indicated

anatomically areas of increased isotope uptake. The fused images are also very helpful to the radiation oncologist in planning radiation fields. A number of authors in relatively small series have suggested that PET imaging is the most sensitive indicator of disease present initially, surpassing CT scans in this regard with a sensitivity exceeding 90%, compared with 60% to 70% for conventional imaging (154,263)

PET/gallium scanning is particularly useful after therapy, where residual anatomic abnormalities on CT scan are common (53,155,178,297). Positive functional imaging studies after therapy are a poor prognostic sign, predicting for early relapse and suggesting that minimal cell kill has been accomplished by the therapy, because enough viable cells remain to take up the isotope in question. In contrast, patients with residual anatomic abnormalities as imaged on CT who have negative PET/gallium studies enjoy an outlook comparable with PET- and/or gallium-negative patients without residual anatomic abnormalities on CT scan. A positive PET scan following salvage chemotherapy for relapsing DLBCL (in preparation for high-dose chemotherapy) has also been reported as a poor prognostic sign and a relative contraindication to proceeding with transplant (277).

Other important staging studies include bilateral bone marrow aspirate and biopsy and routine blood studies, including particularly lactate dehydrogenase (LDH) because this is an important prognostic factor. Patients should be evaluated for the presence of hepatitis B antigen because of concerns of reactivation of this virus with chemotherapy and particularly if rituximab is administered (327).

The most widely used staging system is the anatomically based Ann Arbor system (Table 76.4), originally devised at a conference in Rye, New York, in 1965 (249) and modified at Ann Arbor, Michigan, in 1970 (40) and again at the Cotswolds conference in England in 1988 (186). The principal changes introduced at Cotswolds were the use of the subscript "x" to designate "bulky" disease, that is, a mass of ≥ 10 cm in maximum diameter, and the definition of criteria for liver or spleen involvement as evidence of focal defects with two or more imaging modalities. Abnormal liver function study results were to be ignored for staging purposes.

The Cotswolds conference and a subsequent workshop (46) also discussed categories of response to treatment. It was recognized that many patients had good clinical responses with improvement but not complete disappearance of disease on follow-up imaging studies such as CT scans. The category complete response—uncertain (CR_u)—was designated to describe this. Complete response (CR) and partial response (PR) categories were maintained. Results of functional imaging studies were not considered at the Cotswolds conference. Subsequent studies, however, have demonstrated that integration of information from PET scans can improve accuracy of response assessment (155).

Prognostic Factors

Anatomic stage of disease, tumor bulk, and systemic symptoms are important prognostic indicators. Other prognostic variables investigated have included patient age, performance status, histologic type of lymphoma, tumor size, number of nodal or extranodal sites, tumor phenotype (B or T cell), LDH, β_2-microglobulin levels, serum albumin, hemoglobin, and proliferation indices (207,279). Many of these variables were shown to be significant in univariate and multivariate analyses but in small series from individual institutions.

In an attempt to develop a better prognostic model, the International Non-Hodgkin's Lymphoma Prognostic Factors project examined data on 2,031 patients, all with aggressive histology NHL (2,273). Two indices were developed, the International Prognostic Index (IPI) and the Age Adjusted International Prognostic Index, because age was found to be a highly significant prognostic variable (>60 years vs. ≤60 years). For both indices, four risk groups were identified: low, low intermediate, high intermediate, and high, depending on the number of risk factors present in a given patient. Five prognostic variables were found to be significant: age, performance status, stage (I/II vs III/IV), number of extranodal sites, and LDH (Table 76.5). When patients were divided by age, three factors remained independently significant: performance status, stage, and LDH.

The IPI was developed primarily for patients with DLBCL. It has also been successfully applied with some modifications to patients with PTCL (101,276,311).

There were initial attempts to apply the IPI to FL, but here it was less useful because most patients fell into a favorable prognostic category. A recent international effort has addressed this problem, however (275). Patient characteristics were collected from 4,167 patients with FL diagnosed between 1985 and 1992. Five adverse prognostic factors were identified on multivariate analysis including age (>60 years vs. <60 years), stage (I/II

:: Table 76.4	THE ANN ARBOR/COTSWOLDS STAGING CLASSIFICATION FOR HODGKIN'S DISEASE AND NON-HODGKIN'S LYMPHOMA
Stage I	Involvement of a single lymph node region (215) or single extralymphatic organ or site (I_E)
Stage II	Involvement of two or more lymph node regions on the same side of the diaphragm (II) or localized involvement of an extralymphatic organ or site (II_E) and one lymph node region on the same side of the diaphragm. The number of anatomic regions involved is indicated by a subscript (e.g., II_3).
Stage III	Involvement of lymph node regions on both sides of the diaphragm (109), which may also be accompanied by involvement of the spleen (III_S) or by localized contiguous involvement of only one extranodal organ site (III_E), or both (III_{SE}).
III_1	With or without involvement of splenic hilar, celiac, or portal nodes
III_2	With involvement of para-aortic, iliac, and mesenteric nodes
Stage IV	Diffuse or disseminated involvement of one or more extranodal organs or tissues, with or without associated lymph node involvement
Designations applicable to any disease state	
A	No symptoms
B	Fever (temperature >38°C), drenching night sweats, unexplained loss of >10% body weight within the preceding 6 mo
X	Bulky disease (a widening of the mediastinum by more than one-third or the presence of a nodal mass with a maximal dimension >10 cm)
E	Involvement of a single extranodal site that is contiguous or proximal to the known nodal site
CS	Clinical stage
PS	Pathologic stage (as determined by a laparotomy)

From Lister TA, Crowther D, Sutcliffe SB, et al. Report of a committee convened to discuss the evaluation and staging of patients with Hodgkin's disease: Cotswolds meeting. *J Clin Oncol* 1989;7:1630–1636, with permission.

:: Table 76.5	INTERNATIONAL PROGNOSTIC INDEX FOR DIFFUSE LARGE B-CELL LYMPHOMA[a]	
Adverse Factors	Risk Groups	5-Year Survival (%)
Age >60	Low (none to one factor)	73
PS	Low intermediate (two factors)	51
Stage III-IV	High intermediate (three factors)	43
LDH	High (four to five factors)	26
Number of extranodal sites		

PS, pathologic stage; LDH, lactate dehydrogenase.
[a]Number of extranodal sites.

Table 76.6	FOLLICULAR LYMPHOMA INTERNATIONAL PROGNOSTIC INDEX	
Adverse Factors	Risk Groups	10-Year Survival (%)
Age >60	Low (none to one factor)	70.7
PS	Intermediate (two factors)	50.9
LDH	High (three or more factors)	35.5
Stage III-IV		
Hgb <120		

PS, pathologic stage; LDH, lactate dehydrogenase.

vs. III/IV) performance status (3-4 vs. 1-2), hemoglobin level (<120 g/L vs. ≥120 g/L), number of nodal areas (>4 vs. ≤4), and serum LDH. Three risk groups were identified: low risk (none to one adverse factor), intermediate risk (two factors), and poor risk (three or more adverse factors). Patients were approximately equally divided between the three groups. There was good separation between the groups in terms of survival (Table 76.6). The resulting index is known as the *follicular lymphoma international prognostic index* or FLIPI.

The molecular features of DLBCL have been examined using gene expression profiling as assessed by DNA microarrays or polymerase chain reaction. These studies have involved patients receiving chemotherapy for DLBCL and who had been classified according to the IPI risk categories (272). One study used 13 key genes, another 17 to divide patients into 2 or 4 groups, respectively, with markedly different survival rates, accounting for IPI risk categories (251,272).

Gene expression profiling has also been investigated in FL (63,111). These two reports differed significantly in that one examined the molecular features of tumor infiltrating cells, the other the actual lymphoma cells. The study by Dave et al. (63) was able to group the patients into four quartiles with widely disparate median lengths of survival depending on two gene expression signatures. This trial controlled for clinical features as determined by the IPI but not by the FLIPI. Similarly, the study by Glas et al. (111) used gene expression profiling to predicate clinical behavior. Again, the IPI was the clinical classification used rather than the FLIPI. Further investigations will be needed to determine the value of gene expression profiling in FL if patients are subdivided according to the FLIPI rather than the IPI. Additionally, it remains to be determined whether the tumor-infiltrating immune cells are the appropriate targets for gene expression profiling or the tumor itself. In general, gene expression profiling is not widely available clinically and must still be considered investigational at this writing.

Clinical–Histopathologic Correlates

The pathology and immunobiology of the most frequently encountered varieties of NHL have already been discussed. In this section, we describe the clinical features of the most commonly encountered NHLs. Data from the NHL classification project are invaluable in this regard (1,11).

Diffuse Large B-Cell Lymphoma

Patients most often present with an enlarging peripheral nodal mass or with symptoms related to a primary extranodal site of involvement, such as abdominal or epigastric pain. DLBCL is primarily a disease of older adults, with a median age of 64 years and a slight preponderance of men (55%). B symptoms are present in approximately one-third of patients. Just over half the patients (55%) have localized disease (stages I or II) at onset. Just over half the patients with stage I or II disease have

extranodal presentations. When subdivided according to IPI score, one-third of patients have a score of 0/1, one-half a score of 2/3, and the remainder a score of 4/5 (1,11). Lymphomas that present extranodally are most commonly DLBCL (285).

Some specific subtypes of DLBCL are recognized. The most notable is primary DLBCL of the mediastinum. This entity, believed to arise from thymic medullary B cells, has some distinct clinical pathologic and genetic features. Recent microarray studies have revealed a unique molecular signature for primary DLBCL of the mediastinum with a resemblance to nodular sclerosing HD. There are characteristic genetic changes, notably absence of BCL2 and BCL6 rearrangements, as well as consistent increases in chromosome 9P and 2P, the former being rather specific for primary mediastinal DLBCL and observed in up to 75% of cases.

Primary mediastinal DLBCL comprises about 2.4% of all NHL, about 7% of all DLBCL. The disease affects primarily young women (median age, 37). Two-thirds of patients have their disease confined to the mediastinum. Relapses tend to be extranodal, however. When grouped according to the IPI, the prognosis is similar to that of DLBCL generally, perhaps a bit more favorable (257,259).

Follicular Lymphoma

FL affects primarily older adults (median age, 59 years). There is a slight female preponderance. In contrast to DLBCL, approximately 70% of patients present with generalized disease, most with stage IV disease. The bone marrow is the principal extranodal organ involved. Localized extranodal presentation is uncommon, reported in only 6% of the ILSG series, again in contrast to DLBCL (1).

FL, in general, has a favorable outcome in the intermediate term, with 5- to 8-year survival rates from 70% to 80%. The failure-free survival (FFS) rate is considerably less, however, at approximately 40% (136,140,305). Furthermore, there is little evidence of flattening of the survival curves with time, suggesting that relapse occurs continually over the course of many years. An exception may be the small percentage of patients who present with localized disease and are treated curatively with radiotherapy, a significant number of whom may be cured with that treatment (200,312).

Marginal Zone Lymphoma

MZL includes both nodal and extranodal varieties and the unique entity of splenic MZL. The more familiar image for extranodal MZL is *MALT lymphoma*. Two-thirds to three-fourths of patients have stage I or II disease, the former more common than the latter.

Extranodal MALT lymphoma occurs primarily in the stomach, but a number of other anatomic sites are commonly seen, including the thyroid, parotid glands, orbit, and skin. Recently, association with bacterial infection for MALT at sites other than the stomach has been described (282). *Chlamydia psittaci* has been found in some cases of ocular adnexal lymphoma; antibiotic treatment has been shown to result in lymphoma regression (86). Additionally, *B. burgdorferi* and *C. jejuni* have been associated with MZLs arising in the skin and small intestine (6,282). The standard treatment for these conditions, however, remains local radiotherapy with very high rates of complete response and local control in excess of 90%, similar to what has been reported for gastric MALTs (293).

Two other distinct varieties of MZL have been recognized, namely nodal and splenic in origin (214,332). These lymphomas have also been termed *monocytoid B-cell* lymphomas. In contrast to MALT lymphomas, nodal MZLs are most often generalized at the time of diagnosis. Four types of MZL are identified:

nodal, splenic, splenic and nodal, and leukemic (26). The median survival of all patients was 9 years. The survival curves resembled those of FL with no flattening. The influence of a variety of therapies on outcome was not clear, similar to the situation in FL.

Splenic MZL patients usually present with splenomegaly (42,289). Most have stage IV disease, principally because of bone marrow involvement. The disease is relatively indolent with two-thirds to three-quarters of patients alive at 5 years, but a more aggressive subset does exist. The most effective therapy appears to be splenectomy. Indeed, the diagnosis is usually not clearly established until this time. Radiotherapy to the spleen has infrequently been used.

Peripheral T-Cell Lymphoma

This is a disease of older adults with a median age of 61 years (1,10,252,258). Slightly more than half of the affected patients are men. Most patients present with nodal disease in a similar fashion to B-cell lymphoma. In contrast to DLBCL, however, the great majority of patients have stage III or IV disease at diagnosis, 80% in the ILSG series and 72% in a reported series from three U.S. centers (10). Approximately half of the patients have B symptoms. The IPI also tends to be more advanced, with 52% of patients having a score of 2 or 3 and 31% with a score of 4 or 5. Many patients have some preceding disorder of the immune system (27% in the U.S. combined series) such as angioimmunoblastic lymphadenopathy, mononucleosis, lymphomatoid granulomatosis, or papulosis (10).

Extranodal NK/T-cell disease is a T-cell lymphoma of special interest. This lymphoma has a variety of names in the older literature, including *angiocentric lymphoma, midline malignant reticulosis, polymorphic reticulosis*, and *lethal midline granuloma* (143,166,185,241). It is much more frequent in Asia and Latin America than in the United States. It is associated with EBV (219). In contrast to most lymphomas, tissue destruction of the nasal/facial area is common. The response to chemotherapy and radiotherapy is variable and slow, in contrast to the usual rapid response observed in most other lymphomas (49).

ALCL is another T-cell lymphoma. Two forms may be distinguished, a systemic illness with widespread involvement of lymph nodes and extranodal sites and a type primarily limited to the skin (25,156,274,278,307,331). The systemic type may in turn be separated into those patients who are ALK-positive and those who do not overexpress this protein. The clinical features and prognosis differ widely among these two categories. Patients with ALK-positive ALCL are predominantly young men and, despite advanced-stage disease, respond well to combination chemotherapy with survival rates in the range of 75% to 90%. Patients who are ALK-negative, in contrast, tend to be older with a more nearly equal male-to-female ratio. Their response to chemotherapy is much worse, with survival rates reported in the 20% range.

Cutaneous ALCL constitutes a special situation (25). It is almost invariably ALK-negative but carries an excellent prognosis. It is often difficult to distinguish from benign lymphomatoid papulosis (LYP). The latter may spontaneously remit and tends to run a benign clinical course over many years. ALCL is quite responsive to localized radiotherapy (161) (see also "Cutaneous Lymphomas").

Overall, ALCL has one of the best survival rates of any lymphoma, approximately 75% at 5 years in the ILSG study, despite its aggressive appearance under the microscope. The heterogeneity and complexity of this particular variant of NHL well illustrates past difficulties of attempting to group lymphomas in categories of low grade, intermediate, and high grade, indolent or aggressive, favorable or unfavorable.

Small Lymphocytic Lymphoma

In the ILSG project, SLL accounted for approximately 7% of all NHL cases (1). The median age is 65 years, the oldest for any lymphoma. The male-to-female ratio is approximately even. Ninety percent of cases are generalized (i.e., stages III or IV), with 90% of those being stage IV (or 80% of the total). This is truly an indolent lymphoma. Survival may be prolonged even in the absence of therapy. In the ILSG project, the overall survival (OS) rate was approximately 50% at 5 years; the FFS rate was considerably less, however, at 25%.

Mantle Cell Lymphoma

MCL has a 74% male preponderance and a median age of 63 years (1,319). Eighty percent of patients have stage III or IV disease at onset. IPI scores are high, with 23% of patients with a score of 4 or 5, 54% 2 or 3, and only 23% with a score of 0 or 1. In common with FL, the organ most likely to be involved is the bone marrow, which is positive in two-thirds of patients at the time of diagnosis.

Although originally classified among the low-grade/indolent tumors, the clinical course for MCL is unfavorable in the great majority of patients. The 5-year survival rate in the ILSG project was only 27%, with an FFS rate of 11% (1). This FFS rate is, in fact, among the worst for virtually any type of lymphoma. The poor overall 5-year survival rate is matched only by PTCL and lymphoblastic lymphoma. The shape of the survival curve is continually negative, with no plateau to suggest cure in any significant percentage of patients. Thus, although tumor shrinkage is observed with systemic therapy, survival does not appear to be influenced with currently available agents. The situation is somewhat analogous to FL, but the latter usually has a much more prolonged natural history.

▪▪ Principles of Treatment

Surgery

Before modern radiotherapy and chemotherapy, surgical resection constituted the only potentially curative treatment for NHL. It was commonly used for extranodal sites such as the stomach or head and neck and was curative in a significant percentage of patients when the disease was truly localized. Similarly, patients with nodal presentations and localized disease were managed by radical surgical procedures. The surgical approach subsided rapidly with the development of radiotherapy and chemotherapy and the recognition of the unique radiosensitivity and chemotherapy responsiveness of lymphomas.

Surgery, however, is still widely used to establish a diagnosis by biopsy. That may involve a major surgical operation, such as exploratory laparotomy for the diagnosis of stomach, intestinal, retroperitoneal, or mesenteric lymphoma. This is becoming less common, however, with the use of endoscopic and laparoscopic techniques.

Radiation Therapy (RT)

Dose of Radiation Therapy When Used Alone

Malignant lymphomas are, in general, uniquely sensitive to ionizing radiation. For the great majority of anatomic locations, the sensitivity of the tumor is greater than that of the corresponding normal tissue, usually by a considerable amount, a luxury not available when treating most solid tumors. As a consequence, radiation fields can often be somewhat larger to cover potential microscopic areas of spread. Three-dimensional treatment planning and intensity-modulated RT may be less important for

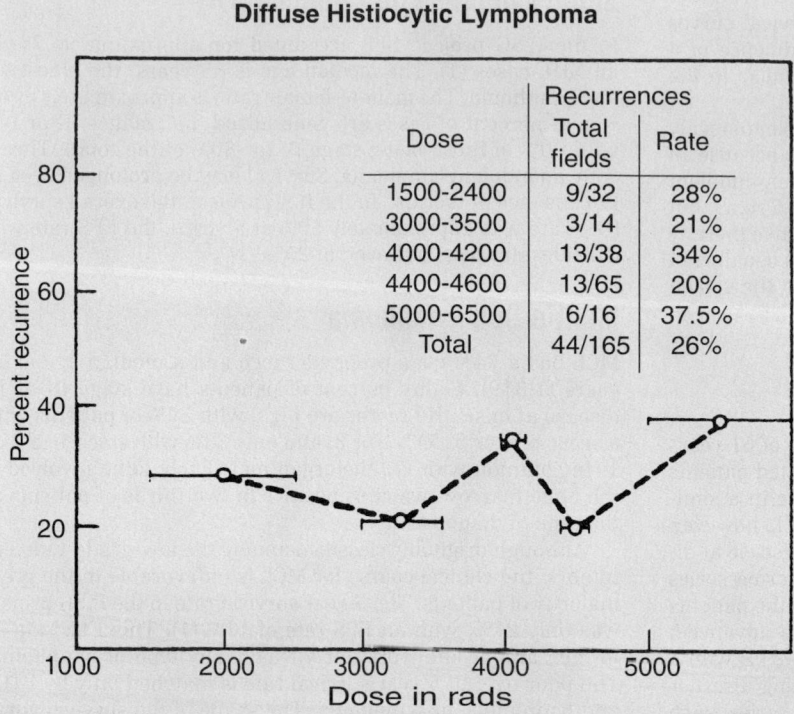

FIGURE 76.1. Local control as a function of radiation dose for patients with diffuse histiocytic lymphoma (mostly diffuse large B-cell lymphoma). (From Fuks Z, Kaplan HS. Recurrence rates following radiation therapy of nodular and diffuse malignant lymphomas. *Radiology* 1973;108:675–684, with permission.)

lymphomas than for solid tumors, but they have a role in specific situations.

Dose-response data for RT of NHL are sparse. To our knowledge, no prospective phase III trials address this question. Most data come from phase II retrospective analyses; almost all of these analyses were carried out years ago, well before the latest WHO pathologic classification. The diseases most often studied were what we now know as DLBCL and FL, with a reasonable amount of information also available for MALT lymphomas. On the other hand, diseases such as PTCL, MCL, and ALCL have never been analyzed separately, so one is forced to extrapolate from the data for DLBCL and FL.

The classic articles in this regard are from Stanford University and Princess Margaret Hospital. Fuks and Kaplan (99) in 1973 reported that doses in the range of 44 Gy achieved local control of FL in more than 95% of instances. For diffuse histiocytic lymphoma (corresponding roughly to DLBCL), local failure rates, however, were in the range of 20% to 30% regardless of the dose of RT delivered (Fig. 76.1). These data have been widely misinterpreted as suggesting or justifying a dose of 50 Gy for DLBCL. In fact, they suggest a subset of resistant disease in the range of 20%, regardless of the dose of RT delivered.

A series of articles from Princess Margaret Hospital (37,38, 286) has also addressed this issue. Dose-response curves were constructed for both diffuse histiocytic lymphoma (DLBCL) and FL. For patients with medium- or large-bulk disease, defined as 2.5 to 5 cm in size and more than 5 cm, respectively, an approximately 50% local control rate was achieved with a dose of 20 Gy, rising to 70% at 30 Gy and 80% at 40 Gy with a plateau thereafter, and no apparent improvement with additional dose (Fig. 76.2). For patients with small-volume (<2.5 cm) DLBCL, a local control rate >90% was achieved regardless of dose.

For patients with nodular (follicular) disease, doses in the range of 25 to 35 Gy produced a local control rate >90% (114).

Similar data were reported in a more contemporary series from the University of Florida (157). For patients with low-grade lymphomas treated with RT alone (mostly FL), doses of 30 Gy achieved local control in >90% of patients. For those with intermediate-/high-grade disease, doses of 30 to 50 Gy also achieved local control in >95% of instances.

There was a suggestion that tumor bulk appeared to influence the outcome. Patients with tumor size >6 cm were treated with combined modality therapy (CMT). It was suggested that doses of at least 40 Gy were necessary in these circumstances for optimal local control, although the data demonstrate local failure in 1 of 51 patients treated with more than 40 Gy as part of a CMT program versus 4 of 70 patients treated with doses of 30 to 40 Gy.

For MZL, particularly MALT of the stomach, high local control rates are achieved with doses of approximately 30 Gy. Data from Princess Margaret Hospital demonstrated a 96% CR with 4% PR and an overall local control rate of 95% (293–295). In a smaller series of patients from Memorial Sloan-Kettering Cancer Center, the response and local control rates were 100% with similar doses (30 Gy) (261). Similar data, although in smaller numbers, are available for MZL at sites other than the stomach.

It is unclear if tumor size affects the dose required for local control in FL and MZL. Smaller tumors may do well with <30 Gy.

Dose of Radiation Therapy in a Combined Modality Therapy Program

For DLCBL, almost all patients, including those with localized disease, are treated with CMT, now typically R-CHOP (rituximab, cyclophosphamide, doxorubicin, vincristine, prednisone) chemotherapy followed by RT. Thus, a more relevant question than the dose of RT required for local control in patients treated with RT alone is the required dose in a CMT program.

There are many reports in the literature of CMT for DLBCL with rather widely varying doses of RT used. The Vancouver group reported 308 patients with stage I and II DLBCL treated with CHOP (and related combinations) followed by involved field

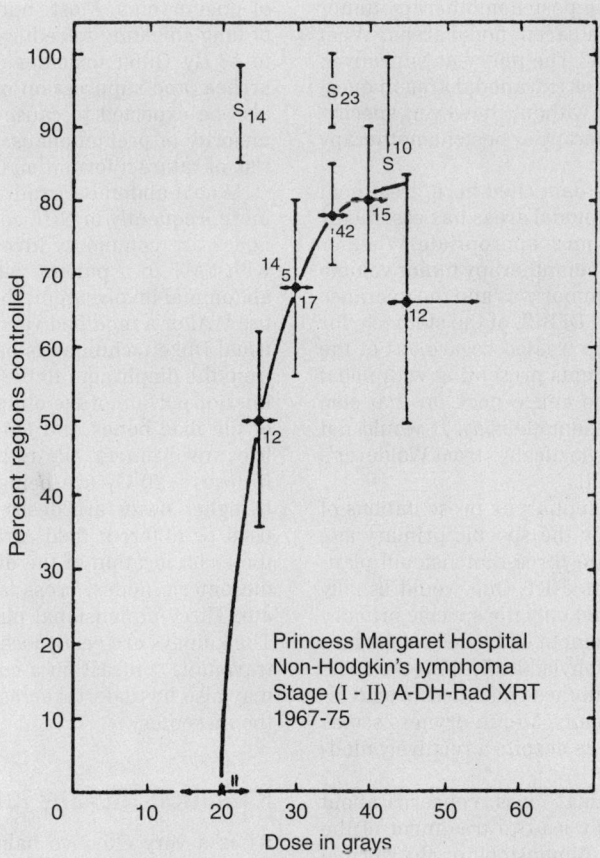

FIGURE 76.2. Local control as a function of radiation dose for diffuse histiocytic lymphoma (mostly diffuse large B-cell lymphoma). (Adapted from Bush RS, Gospodarowicz M. The place of radiation therapy in the management of patients with localized non-Hodgkin's lymphoma. In: Rosenberg SA, Kaplan HS, eds. *Malignant lymphomas: etiology, immunology, pathology, treatment.* New York: Academic Press;1982, with permission.)

radiotherapy (IFRT) to doses of 30 to 35 Gy (200 to 300 cGy per fraction) (270). The 10-year cause-specific survival rate was 82%. In-field local failures occurred in 3% of patients.

Investigators at the M.D. Anderson Cancer Center examined local control in 294 patients with stages I to IV DLBCL after CHOP-based chemotherapy in a retrospective review (314,315). Because of varying dose fractionation schemes, radiation doses were converted using the linear quadratic model to biologically equivalent doses given at 1.8 Gy per fraction. Patients were then grouped in the 30- to 40-Gy range and 40- to 50-Gy range. Patients were also divided by the size of the primary tumor: <3.5 cm, 3.5 to 10 cm, and >10 cm. For the smallest tumors, doses in the lower dose range provided excellent local control (96%), whereas those patients with tumors from 3.5 to 10 cm at onset had a local control rate of 40% with the lower doses compared with 98% with higher doses. Patients with tumors >10 cm at onset and a CR to chemotherapy had a 5-year local control rate of only 70% with a dose of 40 Gy. The authors suggested that doses >40 Gy might be needed for large tumors. The assumption in this study that fraction size and treatment time are important in the treatment of lymphomas may be questioned.

Krol et al. (173) at the Daniel den Hoed Cancer Center in Rotterdam looked at 26 Gy versus 40 Gy for patients with stage I DLBCL who had experienced a CR to CHOP. There was no difference in outcome for the two doses in this retrospective analysis.

At Duke University, we examined 45 patients with stage I and II DLBCL treated with CHOP who experienced a CR, defined by anatomic imaging and the presence of a negative gallium scan at the completion of therapy. Doses of RT ranged from 10 to 50 Gy but were clustered largely around 30 Gy. Durable local control was achieved in 92% of patients.

The issue of the dose of RT for FL or MZL in CMT programs has usually not been considered because of the lack of efficacy of such programs for localized FL or MZL.

Thus, the optimal RT dose in CMT programs is unsettled. Experience with solid tumors and HD suggests the dose of RT can be reduced in the presence of effective chemotherapy. For patients with stage I/II DLBCL achieving CR (PET negative) with chemotherapy, 30 Gy seems reasonable. Definitive resolution of this question awaits phase III trials.

Field Size/Treatment Volume

The optimal treatment volume or field size for RT of localized NHL is also a matter of some controversy because, as is the case for dose-response information, definitive phase III trials to resolve the issues are not available. Many of the conclusions regarding appropriate field size are extrapolated from information regarding patterns of failure.

For DLBCL, the pattern of failure after CMT is usually disseminated disease, with a small percentage with local failure (202). After chemotherapy alone, more local failure occurs (202,203). Failure in nodal areas adjacent to the original disease is uncommon. This suggests local radiation is sufficient.

The question frequently arises as to the appropriate treatment volume/field size when the patient with DLBCL has experienced CR to chemotherapy. Should one treat the original tumor volume prechemotherapy, the postchemotherapy tumor volume, or the original volume plus adjacent nodal areas? What kind of margin should be employed? The policy at Vancouver, for example, was to cover the nodal or extranodal area in question with a margin of about 5 cm, without, however, specifying whether to treat the prechemotherapy or postchemotherapy volume (270).

In view of the patterns of failure data cited here, treatment of the original volume plus adjacent nodal areas has essentially been abandoned. Thus, IFRT seems most appropriate. Whether the involved field is the pre- or postchemotherapy tumor volume depends a lot on where the original tumor was and the tolerance of surrounding normal tissues. With DLBCL of the stomach, for example, the entire organ would be treated regardless of the response to chemotherapy. For patients presenting with nodal disease in the neck unilaterally, the entire neck on that side would generally receive RT after chemotherapy. It would not be necessary or desirable to "prophylactically" treat Waldeyer's ring for neck presentations of DLBCL.

For tonsil, base of tongue, or nasopharynx presentations of DLBCL, after a CR to chemotherapy the specific primary site should be radiated with appropriate three-dimensional planning and perhaps intensity-modulated RT. One would usually not irradiate all of Waldeyer's ring but only the specific primary site. In the absence of clinical involvement of the neck at diagnosis, it would not be necessary to prophylactically treat the neck. Indeed, omission of neck radiation in these instances would facilitate parotid-sparing treatment plans. Mouth dryness seems to be a real problem for these patients despite a relatively modest dose of radiation.

Conversely, for a large mediastinal mass, concerns about excessive pulmonary toxicity usually lead to treatment of the reduced tumor mass in the lateral dimensions or the normal mediastinal and hilar structures, not the original tumor volume.

For FL, a number of authors have reported on patterns of failure and appropriate field sizes for patients with stage I or II disease (45,114). For patients presenting with nodal disease, most studies have suggested that FFS is improved with the use of total lymphoid irradiation (TLI), as opposed to IFRT (157,191,286,312). None of these studies has shown an improvement in OS, however, leading most centers to conclude that the morbidity and expense (of TLI) are not justified.

RT may be used alone to treat stage IIIA FL, although this is seldom done currently (212). In this instance, TLI would be required. The techniques of TLI (i.e., the mantle, para-aortic nodes, spleen, and pelvis) are discussed in Chapter 70.

Two additional specialized techniques may be applicable to NHL. Total-body irradiation (TBI) was used years ago for palliation of advanced FL but has largely been supplanted in this regard by a variety of newer systemic agents. It is still used, however, as a part of various regimens of high-dose chemotherapy (HDC) used in conjunction with stem cell transplantation (29). When used as part of a transplant program, TBI is typically administered in a dose of 1,200 to 1,500 cGy, 120 to 200 cGy per fraction, once or twice daily, all depending on institutional preference. One randomized trial of single-dose (10 Gy) TBI (dose rate, 0.125 Gy/min) versus 14.85 Gy in 11 fractions during 5 days (dose rate, 0.25 Gy/min) revealed similar therapeutic efficacy but a lesser degree of veno-occlusive disease in the fractionated group (109). Both groups had the lungs shielded after 8 to 9 Gy.

Patients are treated at an extended source-to-skin distance, the exact arrangement depending on the geometry of the treatment room. At Duke University, patients typically sit on a stretcher with the knees drawn up. Treatment is administered from each side. Unlike TBI for acute leukemia, a testicular boost is not used. The arms are crossed over the chest to provide some self-shielding of the lungs. Dose to the lungs is usually about 10 Gy for a 1,350-cGy overall dose, to reduce the risk

of pneumonitis. Most, but not all, institutions use some type of lung shielding to reduce the lung dose to approximately 10 to 12 Gy. Other toxicities of TBI include nausea, vomiting, diarrhea, and suppression of the blood counts. This dose would also be expected to cause permanent ovarian ablation in the majority of premenopausal women and carries the long-term risk of cataract formation (246,268).

Whole-abdomen irradiation (WAI) may also be undertaken more frequently in NHL compared with HD. Mesenteric lymph nodes are commonly involved in NHL, unlike HD. If treating with CMT in a patient with stage II disease and widespread abdominal involvement, the radiation oncologist might wish to use WAI or a modified version excluding the pelvis or liver. The usual Duke technique is opposed anterior and posterior fields from the diaphragm to the superior portion of the pelvis or the inferior portion of the obturator foramen with partial shielding of the iliac bones and femoral heads. Unless there is known liver involvement, the right lobe of the liver is also shielded. If doses <20 Gy are being used, kidney blocks are not used. If higher doses are desired, either kidney blocks need to be used or different field arrangements made. This depends on the exact location of the disease to be treated. If treating only mesenteric nodes, cross-table lateral fields may be appropriate. Three-dimensional planning is done in selected patients. The kidneys are easily localized with CT/simulation or with intravenous contrast on a conventional simulator. Modified WAI may also be undertaken as single treatment modality for FL of the mesentery.

Radiation Therapy for Palliation

RT is a very effective palliative agent and should be considered more often in patients not responding to multiple courses of drug treatment. Often, relatively small doses of radiation in brief courses can be quite effective. A Dutch trial described 304 sites treated in 109 patients with indolent lymphomas (mostly FL) (123). Patients received 4 Gy, either in one or two fractions, to the symptomatic areas. The overall response rate was 92% with a CR in 61% of patients and a PR in 31%. A French trial had similar results (110). The median time to local progression was 25 months. In this study, the number of prior chemotherapy regimens did not influence the response rate. Patients with FL that is behaving in an indolent fashion may sometimes be managed with judicious palliative irradiation for many years without systemic therapy (110,200). For critical local problems occurring in the palliative setting, such as spinal cord compression, RT is the treatment of choice. In this instance, where the goal is to maximize the chances of long-term freedom from local progression, doses of 30 Gy (2 Gy per day) would achieve that objective in 90% to 95% of instances.

For the more aggressive NHL histologies, responses to such low doses would not be predicted. However, doses that have been cited here as necessary for long-term local control are well in excess of those required for palliation. The latter is usually about two-thirds to three-quarters of the curative dose. Thus, doses of 20 to 30 Gy often provide excellent palliation for patients with DLBCL.

Chemotherapy

Chemotherapy forms the mainstay of treatment for the great majority of patients with NHL because these diseases are most often generalized. As with radiation, malignant lymphomas are, in general, very responsive to chemotherapy. This responsiveness, unfortunately, does not translate to cure of the patient in most instances. Of all the pathologic variants of NHL in the WHO classification, consistent curability is seen only in patients with DLBCL and to a lesser extent in some patients with PTCL and

ALCL. Some of the more "indolent" lymphomas such as FL do not appear curable with conventional chemotherapy.

A large variety of drugs are available for the treatment of malignant lymphomas including alkylating agents such as cyclophosphamide, corticosteroids, vinca alkyloids, purine analogs, and anthracyclines. They are typically used in combination in order to circumvent problems of drug resistance. The most widely used combination for the treatment of DLBCL has been CHOP (cyclophosphamide, doxorubicin, vincristine, prednisone) (92). For patients with advanced DLBCL, this combination produces an approximate 50% to 60% CR rate, just over half of which are durable responses, for an overall cure rate of approximately 30% to 40%. Results are significantly improved by the addition of the anti-CD antibody rituximab, so that R-CHOP has rapidly become the new standard (87,227).

Similarly, R-CHOP is probably the most widely used combination in the United States for the treatment of FL (58), although its superiority to other less-aggressive combinations has not been established in phase III studies. These data are discussed in greater detail in the sections dealing with the specific types of NHL.

Stem Cell Transplantation/High-Dose Chemotherapy

Because of the less than satisfactory cure rates obtained with conventional chemotherapy (even with the addition of rituximab), there has been a great interest in the application of HDC with stem cell rescue in the treatment of malignant lymphomas. The underlying concept is that larger doses of conventional chemotherapy will result in greater tumor cell kill and increased cure rates. The doses involved are so large that they would be lethal to the normal hematopoietic system without a rescue strategy. Accordingly, hematopoietic progenitor cells are harvested before the HDC, either from the bone marrow itself or, more often, mobilized from the patient's peripheral blood and then reinfused to re-establish marrow function (autologous stem cell transplantation [ASCT]).

Alternatively, an allogeneic transplant may be carried out in individuals with a suitable matched donor in whom the stem cells are harvested from the donor. In this procedure, it is hoped that the infused donor stem cells will additionally mount an immunologic attack on the tumor. Allogeneic transplantation may be preceded by full-dose myeloablative chemotherapy designed to have not only an antitumor effect, but also to condition the patient for the infusion of the donor cells, or it may be preceded by a nonmyeloablative or reduced-intensity conditioning program designed primarily to enable the recipient to accept the donor stem cells. In this latter situation, the major antitumor effect is postulated to derive from the infused donor stem cells. Nonmyeloablative allogeneic transplants are associated with a much lower treatment-related mortality (10% to 20%) compared with myeloablative allogeneic transplants (40% to 50%) (21,69). TBI is often a component of the conditioning program with doses varying quite widely from 200 to 1350 cGy (see "Principles of Treatment: Radiation Therapy").

Studies of stem cell transplantation (SCT) have been carried out in many varieties of NHL but primarily in DLBCL. Numerous phase I, II, and III trials have been reported.

In general SCT is used in three types of situations:

1. Patients who have been treated with conventional chemotherapy and then relapsed.
2. Patients who failed conventional chemotherapy from the onset (so-called primary refractory disease).
3. Patients who have responded well to primary chemotherapy but are considered at high risk for relapse.

The most widely accepted use is for the treatment of patients with DLBCL who have relapsed following initial CHOP or R-CHOP chemotherapy. In a phase III trial from the Parma group, patients with DLBCL who had relapsed following initial CHOP chemotherapy and who were responsive to a salvage program, DHAP (dexamethasone, cisplatin, cytarabine) were then randomly assigned to receive either four additional cycles of DHAP or a HDC program (229). Those patients receiving the HDC program had a markedly improved FFS and OS, compared with those getting conventional chemotherapy (46% FFS vs. 12%, 53% OS vs. 32%). Note that in both arms of this trial, IFRT to original bulky sites of disease (≥5 cm) was used, dose of 35 Gy in 20 fractions in the conventional chemotherapy arm and 26 Gy in 1.3 Gy fractions twice daily in the HDC arm.

All patients in the Parma trial were younger than 60 years of age. Patients with a favorable IPI score of 0 did not benefit (30). Those with a short remission after initial chemotherapy had a worse outcome (119). The Parma trial and associated phase II studies have led to the adaptation of ASCT as standard of care for patients <60 years of age with DLBCL relapsing after initial chemotherapy.

It is also important to note that in this, as well as almost all other trials, patients who do not respond to the initial salvage program do poorly with subsequent HDC and are not considered good candidates. PET scanning has also been used to define response: those with a persistently positive PET after a salvage program do poorly with HDC (277).

A number of groups have explored the incorporation of HDC programs into initial therapy. Eleven such trials done mostly in Europe were recently reviewed by Villanueva and Vose (302). The results have been conflicting, with some trials demonstrating benefit and others not showing benefit. Further, all of the trials published to date were carried out before the incorporation of rituximab into chemotherapy programs for DLBCL. Thus, additional studies are necessary to define the role of HDC as part of initial therapy in high-risk patients.

The final issue addressed by ASCT studies is the role of this procedure in patients with primary refractory DLBCL (i.e., those who failed chemotherapy induction). This group, in general, has a very poor prognosis. Several studies have attempted to assess the role of HDC, none of them phase III trials. An initial report from Nebraska indicated no patients with primary refractory disease were disease-free beyond 1 year after HDC (228,306). These patients were not sensitive, however, to second-line chemotherapy. Other trials suggested better results could be obtained in patients responsive to second-line salvage programs (163,164,204,280).

The role of radiotherapy in patients undergoing HDC with SCT, either autologous or allogeneic, is undefined. As previously mentioned, consolidation RT was employed in the landmark Parma trial. It is also commonly used at a number of institutions, usually directed at bulk disease sites present before the start of salvage chemotherapy, but with considerable interinstitutional variation and without a clear definition of what constitutes bulk disease. There are no phase III trials addressing this issue. Additionally, reported HDC trials usually do not indicate patterns of relapse, so it is even harder to determine the potential benefits of radiation. Prospective trials examining this issue would be of value.

HDC has also been studied in FL. The long natural history of this disease, the marked tendency for involvement of the bone marrow, and the advanced age of many patients with FL has resulted in a fairly select population entered into such trials. Nonetheless, there have been a number of phase I and II reports, as well as phase III trials (71,98,141,182,246, 264,299,302). Stem cell transplants have included both conventional ASCT, myeloablative allogeneic transplants, as well as reduced intensity allogeneic transplants. As with DLBCL, all reported trials were initiated in the era before rituximab. The trials have generally shown an improvement in progression-free and event-free survival. The effect on survival has been less clear. Late relapses do occur and in most instances FFS and OS do not plateau. In contrast, there does appear to be a plateau to FFS in some of the allogeneic transplant studies. That is counterbalanced, however, by a treatment-related mortality in excess of 30%, so that OS is not improved (299).

As with DLBCL, it appears as though patients whose disease is no longer chemosensitive (i.e., responsive to a salvage program) do very poorly with an HDC/stem cell program. Additionally a 5% incidence of myelodysplastic syndrome/acute leukemia has been reported. (181).

Immunotherapy

Perhaps the most promising new approach to the treatment of NHL has been the recent development of effective immunotherapy. The malignant lymphomas express a variety of surface antigens, most notably the B-cell antigen CD-20. The ubiquitous presence of the CD-20 antigen in many varieties of B-cell lymphomas led to the genetic engineering of a human chimeric anti CD-20 antibody, rituximab. In contrast to prior murine-derived monoclonal antibodies, rituximab is quite well tolerated in humans. Rituximab was the first antibody of any type approved by the Food and Drug Administration for the treatment of any human malignancy. Numerous trials of rituximab have been carried out in virtually all B-cell lymphomas (106,107,126,142,193,266,304). Responses as a single agent are seen frequently in FL, CLL, MCL, and MZL. Although responses are infrequent in DLBCL, the addition of rituximab to the standard CHOP program significantly improves outcome (87,227). Rituximab is also employed frequently in combination with chemotherapy for FL and significantly improves both response rate and duration of response. It has also been used for maintenance therapy in FL and combined with chemotherapy for MCL (108,109,136,183,247).

In parallel with the development of rituximab, efforts were undertaken to link radioactive isotopes to anti CD-20 antibodies, in view of the known radiosensitivity of lymphomas. Currently, two such radiolabeled anti-CD antibodies have been successfully developed: I-131 tositumomab (Bexxar) and 90-Y Ibritu-momab (Zevalin). Both of these agents were approved by the Food and Drug Administration in 2002 and 2003. Both demonstrate significant antilymphoma activity, either alone or in combination with other chemotherapeutic regimens (48,232).

Most of the experience has been gained with FL. The overall response rates are in the range of 80%, with approximately one-third of patients achieving a complete response. In relapsed large cell lymphoma patients, response rates are somewhat lower (approximately 40%). In one trial of untreated FL patients, very high response rates of 95% overall with 75% CR were achieved (159). The optimal time for the use of radioimmunotherapy in patients with lymphoma has not been established, nor has the optimal integration into other available therapeutic modalities.

Treatment of Specific Lymphomas

Diffuse Large B-Cell Lymphoma, Stage I/II

Historically in the prechemotherapy era, early-stage DLBCL was treated with RT alone (38,45,157,158,300,301,324). Ten-year FFS and OS in these series ranged from 30% to 60%, depending on the mix of patients and prognostic variables. The doses of RT varied widely from 30 to 60 Gy. The CR rate was high, usually >80%. No clear evidence exists for improved local control with

doses exceeding 40 Gy. Field sizes and arrangements also varied widely but, in general, IFRT was used.

The pattern of failure in these series was primarily distal, either organ involvement or nodal sites remote from the primary site. Patients with both nodal and extranodal disease were included in these series and appear to have equivalent prognoses. Stage II had a long-term FFS and OS in the range of 25%, in contrast to patients with stage I disease in whom the FFS and OS were in the 50% to 60% range.

In the late 1970s and early 1980s, efforts to improve on these results by the addition of combination chemotherapy were begun. The phase III trials in many instances antedated the phase II trials, but the former were typically carried out with older combinations such as CVP (cyclophosphamide, vincristine, prednisone) with results not as good as the more modern phase II studies incorporating CHOP (207,220). These latter trials demonstrated a substantial improvement in both FFS and OS with CMT compared to RT alone. CR rates of approximately 90% are reported with FFS and OS in the range of 70% to 85% (233,270).

These studies differed widely in their design. The number of cycles of CHOP varied between two and eight. The radiation dose ranged from 20 to 60 Gy, with the larger doses of radiation generally for patients not experiencing a CR. There has been, however, no standardization of response criteria. Virtually none of the reports used functional imaging for assessment of response. Radiotherapy fields were generally involved fields (IF) only, although the latter were vaguely, if at all, defined in most reports. Usually, they covered the original site of disease before chemotherapy with a margin.

It may be more appropriate, however, to restrict IFRT to the postchemotherapy volume in situations where excessive dose to normal tissue might result, such as with primary DLBCL of the mediastinum. For RT of the mediastinum, the field reduction would typically be in the lateral dimensions to spare normal lung, but superior inferior margins may be more generous.

One of the more recent and highest quality phase II trials is that from the British Columbia Cancer Center (270). In this trial, 308 patients with stage I or II disease were treated with CHOP chemotherapy or closely related combinations followed by IFRT. The CR rate was 97%, the FFS was 74% at 10 years, and OS was 63% at 10 years. Radiation doses were 30 to 35 Gy.

Two large cooperative trials from Southwest Oncology Group (SWOG) and Eastern Oncology Group (ECOG) have examined whether chemotherapy alone would suffice for early stage disease (138,202). The SWOG trial compared eight cycles of CHOP with three cycles followed by IFRT. Four hundred one patients were entered and approximately evenly divided between the two arms. The great majority of patients had a low IPI score. Patients were randomized to receive eight cycles of CHOP or three cycles followed by IFRT. After CHOP, the CR rate was 74% in both arms. Doses of RT ranged from 40 to 55 Gy at the discretion of the treating radiation oncologist, with most patients receiving between 45 and 50 Gy at a rate of 180 to 200 cGy/day. RT fields were usually the prechemotherapy tumor volume. The results favored the CMT arm. FFS and OS in the chemotherapy alone arm were 64% and 72%, respectively, compared with 77% and 82% in the CMT group, both differences being statistically significant. Additionally, toxicity was greater in the chemotherapy alone arm.

The ECOG trial compared eight cycles of CHOP with or without IFRT in 352 patients. Patients were randomized before initiation of chemotherapy. Patients with CR received either 30 Gy of radiotherapy to the involved sites or were observed. Patients in PR all received 40 Gy. The 6-year FFS was 73% for the CMT group versus 56% for chemotherapy alone ($p = .05$). There was a tendency for improved survival in the CMT arm (82% vs. 71%), but the differences were not statistically significant.

These two trials have led to a general acceptance of treatment with CMT therapy for early-stage DLBCL. Their results must be interpreted in the light of rituximab not having been used. A recent French study, however, suggested that more aggressive chemotherapy was superior to CHOP plus radiotherapy for localized aggressive lymphoma (240).

Treatment of Stage III-IV Diffuse Large B-Cell Lymphoma

The mainstay of treatment of disseminated DLBCL is clearly systemic chemotherapy. RT has been thought to play little, if any, role (271). A re-examination, however, may be in order, given some trials that do suggest benefit (13,18,262). The standard chemotherapeutic combination has been CHOP, first introduced in the late 1970s (196). With this combination, CR in the range of 60% to 70% were reported with most of these (approximately 60%) being durable, for a long-term cure rate of 35% to 40% (92,94).

Although these results were better than the past, they were far from optimal. During the next several decades, there were numerous attempts to improve on the CHOP program with promising phase II trials of new combinations, but unfortunately, that promise was unsupported by follow-up phase III studies. The best known of the latter was the Intergroup/SWOG trial comparing CHOP, M-BACOD, Pro-MACE-CYTABOM (prednisone, methotrexate, doxorubicin, cyclophosphamide, etoposide, cytarabine, bleomycin, and vincristine) and MACOP-B (CHOP plus methotrexate and bleomycin) (92). This trial analyzed approximately 900 patients. Three-year survival rates were 50%, with 3-year FFS rates 41%, with no differences between the four drug combinations (Fig. 76.3). The least toxic combination, CHOP, thus became the standard treatment.

A recently published overview of chemotherapy for "aggressive" NHL histologic type reviewed 111 scientific reports, including 35 randomized trials with a total of approximately 22,000 patients. The overview concluded that in unselected patients with advanced-stage disease, CHOP was curative in approximately one-third of the patients (168).

A major improvement in the outcome for patients with DLBCL has come with the introduction of rituximab. Several phase III trials have now demonstrated the value of adding rituximab to standard CHOP. The GELA study (Groupe d'Etudes des Lymphomes de l'Adulte) compared CHOP alone with rituximab and CHOP in 399 patients >60 years old (87). FFS improved from 30% to 54% and 5-year OS from 45% to 58%. Similarly, a European cooperative trial compared R-CHOP and CHOP in 824 patients age 18 to 60 years with stages II-IV DLBCL (227). Three-year FFS was 79% in the R-CHOP group compared with 59% in the CHOP group. Three-year OS rates were 93% and 84%, respectively. In this trial, unlike the GELA trial, RT was given to select patients with bulky disease and/or extranodal disease. These studies have led to the rapid adaptation of R-CHOP as standard initial therapy of DLBCL for all stages of disease.

There have also been attempts to improve on the CHOP combination by the introduction of HDC and ASCT for patients with a poor prognosis in first remission, as mentioned in the ASCT/HDC section. Results have been variable with no consensus as to the value of this treatment approach. The use of HDC/ASCT for DLBLL patients in first remission has not been explored in patients treated with R-CHOP.

A comparatively unexplored approach is the use of consolidation RT in combination with chemotherapy for advanced DLBCL. One rationale for the use of such RT is the tendency of patients with advanced lymphoma to relapse at sites of disease present at diagnosis and, in particular, sites of bulky disease present at diagnosis (127,313,314). This observation is somewhat controversial (271). In view of the efficacy, however, of CMT in localized disease, the exploration of its value in more advanced disease appears worthwhile. There have been a few reports regarding its use. Aviles et al. (15,18) performed a phase III trial in which patients with DLBCL who experienced a CR with CHOP and who had preexisting bulky disease were randomized to receive RT (40 to 50 Gy) or not to prior sites of bulky disease. The FFS rate was 72% in those receiving CMT compared with 35% in those treated with chemotherapy alone. Corresponding OS rates were 81% and 55%, all differences being statistically significant.

A retrospective analysis at M.D. Anderson Cancer Center compared a group of patients with stage III/IV DLBCL treated with chemotherapy only with a similar group treated with CMT (262). RT dramatically improved local control (89% vs. 52%) and freedom from progression (85% 5-year FFS rate vs. 51%), but not OS (87% vs. 81%, respectively).

A similar analysis from Milan examined 94 patients with stage III/IV DLBCL and bulky disease (tumor mass ≥6 cm) (84). Forty patients received consolidation RT, whereas 54 did not. Doses and field sizes varied between 30 and 46 Gy. Improvements were noted in OS as well as FFS. These reports raise the issue of additional phase III trials to further evaluate this concept (262).

Follicular Lymphoma: Stages I/II

The treatment historically for stage I/II FL has been RT alone. Representative series are shown in Table 76.7 (38,45,157, 174,191,197,223,239,301,312). The largest experiences are from the Princess Margaret Hospital (38), British National Lymphoma Investigation (301), and Stanford University (191). The reported series were accumulated over a long period, with patients staged in different ways and treated with differing doses and fields of radiation. Although these series are grouped as FL, most of them included patients with other histologic types classified as low-grade lymphoma in older pathologic classifications.

Despite the heterogeneity of the patient population and the lack of uniformity in data reporting, certain conclusions may be drawn:

1. Five- and 10-year OS is high, in the range of 75% to 90%, particularly if cause-specific survival is the quantity measured. Early deaths from lymphoma in this group are quite uncommon.

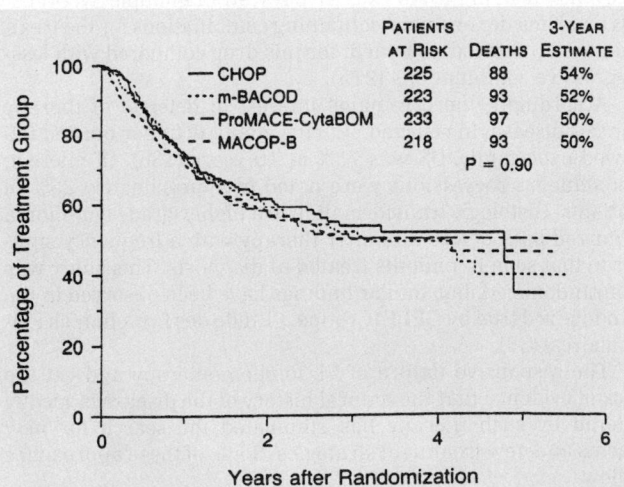

	PATIENTS AT RISK	DEATHS	3-YEAR ESTIMATE
CHOP	225	88	54%
m-BACOD	223	93	52%
ProMACE-CytaBOM	233	97	50%
MACOP-B	218	93	50%
			P = 0.90

FIGURE 76.3. Overall survival rate in patients with diffuse large B-cell lymphoma treated with CHOP (cyclophosphamide, doxorubicin, vincristine, prednisone) versus three other combinations. (From Fisher RI, Gaynor ER, Dahlberg S, et al. Comparison of a standard regimen [CHOP] with three intensive chemotherapy regimens for advanced non-Hodgkin's lymphoma. *N Engl J Med* 1993;328:1002–1006, with permission.)

Clinical Radiation Oncology

Table 76.7 | RADIATION THERAPY OF STAGE I/II FOLLICULAR LYMPHOMA SELECTED PHASE II TRIALS

Study	Year	No. of Patients	Stage	Radiation Dose (Gy)	Complete Response Rate (%)	Failure-Free Survival (%)	Survival (%) (Years)
Bush et al. (37)	1982	130	I/IIA	25–40	—	53	72 (10)
Chen et al. (45)	1979	25	I/IIA	35–40	—	83	100(5)
Kamath et al. (157)	1999	72	I/II	30–50	—	59	46(10)
Krol et al. (174)	1998	56	I	—	87	75	73(5)
MacManus and Hoppe (191)	1996	177	I/II	35–50	—	43	65(10)
McLaughlin et al. (197)	1986	50	I/II	30–40	—	35	72(5)
Pendlebury et al. (223)	1995	40	I	30–54	—	43	82(10)
		18	II			42	76 (10)
Readdy et al. (239)	1989	14	I	—		82	90 (10)
		24	II	—	—	46	54(10)
Vaughan Hudson et al. (301)	1994	208	I	~35	98	49	71(64)
Wilder et al. (315)	2001	33	I	26–50		66	87(15)

2. The FFS rate is less, with wide variability from 40% to 80%. Most series report much better FFS rates for patients with stage I versus stage II disease. Most series also suggest few relapses beyond 10 years.

3. Radiation doses varied widely. The local control rate was greater than 90% in almost all instances when reported, with no dose response demonstrated above 30 Gy.

4. Radiation field sizes varied widely as well, with no evidence for improved survival with increasing field size.

There have been a few attempts to improve on these results with the use of CMT. Two phase III trials published in the early 1980s that showed positive results for the effects of CMT compared with RT alone for DLBCL, showed no benefit for the use of CMT in FL (206,220). Very small numbers of patients were included, however, so the studies were grossly underpowered to detect meaningful differences. Two additional phase III trials were published in the 1990s (162,326). The Memorial Sloan-Kettering Cancer Center trial similarly contained very small numbers of patients with FL. The British National Lymphoma Investigation had by far the largest number of patients. Single-agent chlorambucil was the chemotherapy; the trial was negative.

This lack of enthusiasm for CMT for stage I/II disease no doubt mirrors the general attitude toward advanced disease, where, to date, combination chemotherapy has not shown curative potential (47,133,140). As with DLBCL, all these series antedate rituximab, which has a profound effect in FL. Additionally, they antedate the introduction of the FLIPI, so whether certain prognostic groups might benefit from CMT is unknown.

The predominant pattern of failure for patients with stage I/II disease treated with RT alone is distant. Local failure of any type, either alone or combined with distant failure, occurs in <10% of patients. Nodal extension is an uncommon pattern of failure, seen in perhaps 20% of patients.

The question frequently arises as to whether patients with localized FL who respond well to RT and experience a prolonged disease-free survival are truly cured of their disease. Although the OS and FFS curves appear to flatten beyond 10 years, concern has been raised by reports of persistent molecular abnormalities in such patients. In particular, circulating t(14:18)-positive cells were noted in one-third of patients with FL in prolonged remission in one report (89). On the other hand, such cells were also found in 23% of healthy individuals (284). Thus, the issue of molecular cure remains unsettled. Additionally, one Stanford University study suggests an equivalent outcome with a watch-and-wait policy for early-stage disease (3).

Majority opinion, however, would support involved field RT for patients with early-stage FL.

Follicular Lymphoma: Stages III/IV

The treatment of advanced-stage FL is a special challenge. The disease has a long natural history (47,133,136,231). Median survivals ranging from 6 to 11 years have been described with or without treatment. FL is quite responsive to a variety of systemic agents, including alkylating agents, anthracyclines, purine analogs, vinca alkaloids, corticosteroids, and monoclonal antibodies. Examination of published survival curves after a whole variety of therapeutic approaches, however, demonstrates a continuing pattern of relapse and death, albeit over a long period, with no evidence for flattening of the survival curve, the pattern usually associated with cure. There is also no clear evidence for the superiority of any one drug or combinations of drugs in the treatment of this disease. Studied agents have ranged from single-agent chlorambucil or cyclophosphamide to aggressive combinations such as ProMACE/MOPP (prednisone, methotrexate, doxorubicin, cyclophosphamide, etoposide, mustargen, vincristine, procarbazine). As would be expected, the CHOP combination has been extensively studied in FL. Although superior to less-aggressive therapies for DLBCL, CHOP has no proven benefit in FL. An extensive review of multiple SWOG trials involving doxorubicin-containing combinations for the treatment of FL showed no benefit for this drug compared with less-aggressive combinations (225).

Accordingly, there remains interest in deferral of therapy for this disease. In selected patients with low tumor burden followed expectantly, OS was 73% at 10 years (136). Of interest, spontaneous regressions were noted in approximately 25% of patients. Histologic transformation to a higher-grade lymphoma occurred both before and after therapy with a frequency similar to that seen in patients treated at diagnosis. This study was nonrandomized, but similar findings have been observed in the randomized trial by GELF (Groupe d'Etude des Lymphomes Folliculaires) (35).

The responsive nature of FL to chemotherapy and yet the lack of evidence that the natural history of the disease is greatly altered by such therapy has stimulated the search for new agents and new treatment strategies. Some of these approaches follow.

Immunotherapy: Rituximab produces responses in about 50% of relapsed FL patients as a single agent. As first-line therapy, the response rate is about 70%. More often, however, rituximab has been combined with chemotherapy. A number of phase II, as well as phase III trials have been conducted using a variety of drug combinations with rituximab (108,125,134,194,333). These studies have consistently shown benefit for the addition of rituximab. To which chemotherapy program one should add rituximab, however, is not clear. In the United States, the most popular combination has been R-CHOP (58).

Radioimmunotherapy has also been extensively investigated in FL, both for the treatment of relapsed disease as well as initial therapy. The two agents in wide use are 90_y ibritumomab (Zevalin) and ^{131}I-tositumomab (Bexxar), the former a pure beta emitter, the latter a gamma and beta emitter. Both agents demonstrate comparable activity with response rates of 60% to 80% in relapsed FL patients (64,93,139). In a select group of previously untreated patients, a 95% response rate was obtained with ^{131}I-tositumomab (75% CR), with half of patients in continuous CR at 4 years (159). These radiolabeled antibodies have been cautiously combined with chemotherapy as their primary toxicity is myelosuppression. In a recent SWOG phase II trial of CHOP followed by ^{131}I-tositumomab, 5-year FFS was 67% and OS was 87% (232). To our knowledge, there are no studies combining radioimmunoconjugates with external-beam radiotherapy.

Interferon: A large number of trials have been conducted examining the effect of this agent, both as a part of induction therapy and as maintenance after chemotherapy. A recent meta-analysis concluded that when given in the context of relatively intensive initial chemotherapy interferon-α prolongs both remission duration and survival (245). Nonetheless, its toxicity has inhibited widespread use, and further, all those trials preceded the rituximab era.

Stem cell transplantation: A number of studies have examined the role of transplantation, either autologous preceded by HDC or allogeneic with or without accompanying HDC (71,144,182,264,299). These studies have looked at transplant for both relapsing FL and FL in first remission following induction chemotherapy. Although a number of phase II trials looked promising, most phase III trials do not show OS benefit for patients with relapsing disease. For patients treated in first remission, the data are more suggestive of benefit. FFS was significantly improved in three European phase III trials, but results on OS are still pending (71,182).

The use of full-dose myeloablative allogeneic transplants has been inhibited by treatment-related mortality of 40% to 50%. Reduced-intensity allogeneic transplant may have curative potential with less toxicity (144,299).

Role of Radiation Therapy in Advanced Follicular Lymphoma

The curative potential of RT for localized FL together with the early HD experience led to the initiation of trials of TLI for patients with stage III FL, primarily by the Stanford group (212). Sixty-six patients with stage III FL were treated either with TLI (61 patients) or TBI (5 patients). The FFS rate was 35% at 15 years, the CSS was 58%, and the OS was 35%, reflecting additional mortality from nonlymphoma causes. A small cohort of eight patients with a lower tumor burden, so-called limited stage III disease, defined as fewer than five disease sites and no tumor mass >10 cm, had an FFS of 88% and CSS of 100% at 15 years. Doses of RT used were 40 to 48 Gy, much greater than would be considered optimal currently. There were few relapses occurring beyond the 10th year. Similar data have been reported from the University of Florida, the Medical College of Wisconsin, and M.D. Anderson Cancer Center (68,122,150).

RT has also been advocated as consolidation therapy after chemotherapy in patients with advanced-stage FL. A phase III trial by Aviles et al. (17) randomized 118 untreated patients with stage III or IV FL to receive CVP chemotherapy alone or the same

chemotherapy followed by IFRT to initially involved nodal sites, at doses of 35 to 45 Gy. The 7-year FFS was 33% in the group treated by chemotherapy alone and 66% in those receiving CMT. The 7-year OS was also doubled from approximately 40% to 80%. The improvement in FFS was highly significant, and the survival improvement of borderline statistical significance (p = .06). There have been no additional studies attempting to replicate these results.

Follicular Lymphoma, Grade 3

Follicular large cell lymphoma, or FL grade 3 in the WHO classification, is an uncommon but distinct variety of FL. Follicular large cell lymphoma comprises approximately 15% of all cases of FL or approximately 5% of all cases of NHL (9,128,137,243). The biologic behavior of this specific type of lymphoma is somewhat controversial because of its infrequency and the relatively small number of patients reported in various retrospective series in the literature.

Initial reports suggested an unfavorable outlook; a median survival >10 years was reported in the Stanford series, but only 22% of patients were disease-free at that time (137). The advent of anthracycline-based chemotherapy appears to have resulted in some improvement in that prognosis and perhaps a plateauing of the FFS curve. The Nebraska group reported 3-year survival rates of 76% and 61% for patients with stage I/II disease and III/IV disease, respectively, but FFS rates of only 61% and 34%, respectively, results not that different from those seen with other FLs (9). On the other hand, the M.D. Anderson group reported 5-year survival rates of 72% in a series of 100 patients with stage I to IV disease and an FFS rate of 67%, with a "possible plateau in the FFS curve for patients with stage I–III disease" (243). In both series, patients received anthracycline-containing combination chemotherapy, with the patients with earlier-stage disease receiving IFRT as well in varying dosages. The aforementioned, as well as other, series have led to a consensus that patients with FL grade 3 should be treated similarly to patients with DLBCL in terms of chemotherapy (128,310). The prognosis, in general, is better than DLBCL, but median survivals are shorter than that of FL.

Data regarding dose-response information for RT are lacking. Because virtually all patients are receiving chemotherapy, however, we consolidate patients with early-stage disease with 30 to 35 Gy IFRT in a fashion similar to that for early-stage DLBCL.

Marginal Zone Lymphomas

Extranodal MZL or MALT lymphomas are the most common variant, and the most common location is the stomach. The treatment of MALT lymphoma of the stomach is discussed in the section on Primary Extranodal Lymphomas (ENLs). MALT lymphoma involving sites other than the stomach and GI tract behaves similarly, but there is no association with *H. pylori.* The disease is very responsive to RT. Doses of approximately 30 Gy produce long-term control in more than 90% of patients. In one large series combining MALT of all sites, the overall local control rate was 97%, the OS was 96%, and FFS at 5 years was 76% (293,294). When MALT lymphoma relapses, it tends to have a prolonged clinical course.

Occasionally, patients with MALT lymphoma present with isolated organ involvement that is, however, bilateral (e.g., involvement of the salivary glands or conjunctivae). This behavior, referred to as *lymphocyte homing,* is not well understood. Such patients may be treated with local RT to both paired sites with apparent long-term FFS observed (113).

MALT lymphoma is responsive to chemotherapy in a high percentage of patients. With single-agent chlorambucil, a 75% CR rate was observed in one series (129). A large SWOG analysis, however, indicated that FFS and OS rates were similar to those observed in FL, with no plateauing of the survival curve (91). Thus, chemotherapy is palliative and reserved for patients with generalized disease who are symptomatic. Asymptomatic individuals with generalized disease may be considered for observation, similar to patients with generalized FL.

Nodal and splenic MZL have been discussed previously in the section "Clinical-Histopathologic Correlates." Both are most often generalized and managed similarly to advanced FL.

Peripheral T-Cell Lymphomas

PTCL of nodal type, not otherwise specified, resembles DL-BCL in its clinical characteristics and presentation (1,11,12,39, 188,230,252,258). Overall, there is a worse outlook. PTCL is more often generalized, the IPI tends to be worse, and approximately half of patients have B symptoms. The treatment for PTCL is similar to that used for DLBCL. Rituximab, however, has no role, as this is a T-cell lymphoma.

Patients who present with localized PTCL should be treated with CHOP (three to six cycles) and IFRT. Doses and field sizes of RT are comparable with those used for DLBCL, given the lack of specific dose-response data for PTCL. Little data exist regarding the role of RT for advanced disease. As for DLBCL, the concept may warrant further exploration.

In contrast to most patients with PTCL, those with ALCL have a much better prognosis, among the best of any of the lymphoma categories and certainly the best of the ostensibly "aggressive" histologic types. The presence of the ALK gene distinguishes prognostic groups. ALK-positive patients have a good prognosis when treated with CHOP. OS is around 70% at 10 years (77,104). ALK-negative patients have a considerably worse outlook, with OS from 14% to 40% following CHOP therapy. ALCL of the skin is discussed in the section "Primary Extranodal Lymphomas."

Small Lymphocytic Lymphoma

Treatment for SLL is essentially that of B-CLL. The purine analogs appear to be the most active agents (50,52). The disease is also responsive to alkylating agent chemotherapy such as chlorambucil or combination chemotherapy, with CHOP, for example. Rituximab also plays a major role as with FL, and that, there is neither evidence for a plateauing of the survival curve nor definite benefit from combination chemotherapy, as opposed to single-agent treatment (61,244). In that rare situation in which the disease is localized (i.e., stage I or II nodal only), one would predict RT might achieve long-term FFS for some patients with doses and field sizes similar to those used for FL, namely, approximately 30 Gy in 3 weeks to a generous involved field.

Mantle Cell Lymphoma

The treatment of MCL is unsatisfactory. This recently designated disease is distinguished by one of the worst outlooks for any lymphoma. For example, the SWOG data describe a 10-year FFS rate of only 6% and a 10-year OS of 8% (95). Another way of describing the survival pattern of MCL is that it resembles FL in its response to therapy and FFS (i.e., no plateauing of the FFS curve and thus no indication of cure), but DLBCL in its OS (i.e., much shorter than FL) (135).

The therapy of MCL has been explored in a number of retrospective analyses as well as prospective phase II trials using a variety of chemotherapy programs (319). Chemotherapy programs can be generally grouped as CHOP-like, now usually including rituximab, which does have activity in MCL, purine analog-containing programs (e.g. R-FCM [fludarabine, cyclophosphamide, mitoxantrone]) or more intensive programs

such as hyper-CVAD (cyclophosphamide, vincristine, doxorubicin decadron, cytarabine, and methotrexate). High response rates are seen (80% to 90%), but relapse usually occurs with no plateauing of FFS. There is no evidence for superiority of one regimen to another, although the addition of rituximab does seem beneficial (107,180).

HDC and SCT have also been employed, both autologous as well as allogeneic, both in first remission and for relapse (103,165,319). One phase III trial did demonstrate improved FFS for SCT in first remission, but no survival benefit as yet (74). Thus, SCT must still be considered unproven. NCCN guidelines indicate no standard therapy for MCL (216). Entry into clinical trial is recommended.

Patients with localized MCL (stage I or II) are seldom encountered. One small series from British Columbia has been reported, however (179). Seventeen patients treated with RT (30 to 35 Gy) with or without chemotherapy had a 5-year FFS of 68% and OS of 71%. Adjuvant chemotherapy did not seem to influence the outcome. Thus, RT appears to have an important role for those few patients with limited-stage MCL. RT is also very effective palliation for patients with advanced disease (250).

▒▒ | Primary Extranodal Lymphomas

Thus far we have considered NHL primarily from the standpoint of the histopathologic classification. NHL may also be clinically divided, however, on the basis of origin from nodal or extranodal tissue; the latter may be further subdivided as to site of origin. The frequency of extranodal lymphoma (ENL) and certain characteristic clinical entities associated with lymphoma in various extranodal sites makes the discussion of ENL as such appropriate.

It is important to re-emphasize certain principles that recur in this section: localized disease, whether presenting nodally or extranodally, seems to have the same prognosis. The management strategy for localized nodal lymphoma of a given histologic type applies as well to that same histologic type when presenting extranodally.

Extranodal disease accounts for approximately 35% to 40% of all patients with NHL and approximately half of those with stage I and II NHL (221,285). The most common sites of involvement are the GI tract, accounting for approximately 25% to 35% of all ENL, the head and neck region, which accounts for approximately 20% to 30% (including Waldeyer's ring and other head and neck sites, but excluding brain), and skin, with a variety of miscellaneous sites accounting for the rest. PCNSL, which accounts for approximately 10% of all ENL, is discussed separately.

Histopathologically, ENLs are classified in much the same fashion as nodal lymphomas. The extranodal location may cause difficulties in histopathologic diagnosis. Immunophenotyping as well as cellular morphology may be helpful in this respect. Establishing the diagnosis of ENL on the basis of fine-needle aspirate or similarly sized biopsy, however, is an unwise practice. Accurate histopathologic classification is essential for proper management and almost always requires at least a core of tissue (132).

Gastrointestinal Lymphoma

The stomach is the most common site of involvement (50% to 80% of all cases of GI lymphoma) (59,121,169,285). The remaining GI lymphomas occur in the small and large intestine, primarily ileum, followed by colon and rectum, but lymphomas may arise in any of the GI tissues. Histopathologically, 90% to 95% of stomach lymphomas are MALT or DLBCL, the two being approximately equal in frequency (7,66,169).

Patients with gastric lymphoma usually present with symptoms of abdominal pain (~80% [171]). Other common complaints are loss of appetite (~50%), weight loss (25%), and bleeding (20%). B symptoms are uncommon, (10% of patients). In this regard, only fever and night sweats are significant because weight loss is so often a function of direct effects on the stomach. Perforation as an initial symptom is very uncommon, occurring in <2% of patients.

The diagnosis of stomach lymphoma is usually established endoscopically, although in past years laparotomy was often necessary (287). Surgical resection has traditionally been the cornerstone of treatment, followed by adjuvant RT and/or chemotherapy. This approach at the Princess Margaret Hospital, for example, resulted in an FFS of 81% and CSS of 88% in 149 patients treated between 1967 and 1996 (57). Other surgical series have been extensively reviewed by Bozzetti et al. (34) and Thirlby (290) with OS of 60% to 100% in stage I patients and 40% to 80% for stage II disease.

Beginning in the 1980s, however, some authors began to question the necessity for surgery in a disease that is usually quite responsive to RT or chemotherapy. Subsequently, a number of reports showed equivalent outcomes when patients were treated with RT and chemotherapy without surgery (51,83,146,169,170). A large series of gastric lymphomas reported by a German GI multicenter group is representative (170,171). They reported on 398 stage I and II patients with primary gastric lymphoma about equally divided between MALT and DLBCL. Three hundred thirty-five patients were managed conservatively without surgical resection; 63 had subtotal gastrectomy. Outcomes were essentially identical with an 80% 5-year survival.

Gastric Diffuse Large B-Cell Lymphoma

The historical experience with the treatment of localized DLBCL of the stomach without systemic therapy demonstrated OS in the range of 25% to 50%, as with DLBCL generally. The use of systemic chemotherapy has resulted in considerable improvement. Multiple centers now report 5-year OS in the range of 70% to 80% for patients with localized disease treated with chemotherapy with or without RT (169,237,256,291). Although some authors have suggested that chemotherapy alone is adequate treatment (237,291), most studies have used CMT.

Although these studies mostly used CHOP, treatment should be initiated with R-CHOP. The risk of chemotherapy-induced gastric perforation is very low, 1% to 2%. The number of cycles is not well defined; three to six have been most often used, with the precise number depending on the rapidity of response, initial volume of disease, and investigator preference, as with stage I and II disease in general (202,270). The response to chemotherapy should be assessed with appropriate imaging studies, usually a repetition of those studies that were positive before the onset of chemotherapy. Repeat endoscopic evaluation and biopsy are particularly useful for assessing the completeness of response.

Radiation doses and field sizes to be used for gastric DLBCL are not well defined. Excellent results have been reported in patients treated with 25 Gy after surgical resection (115). For patients treated without resection, a wide variety of radiation doses have been reported, ranging from 30 to 50 Gy, similar to what has been described for the treatment of nodal DLBCL. Treatment fields have also varied considerably from whole abdomen to involved field. There is no apparent correlation between field size or dose and outcome. Local control in almost all the reported series has been high, in the range of 90%. FFS and OS for patients with stage I and II disease have also ranged from 70% to 80% (7,57,113,146,170,208,256).

The radiation field should probably encompass the entire stomach, immediately adjacent celiac axis nodes, and any other involved areas with a margin of several centimeters. The stomach and kidneys should be opacified with oral and intravenous contrast, respectively, so that the former can be adequately encompassed and the latter excluded from the field as much as possible. Intravenous contrast for the kidneys is not necessary if a CT simulator is used. Patients should be fasting for several hours prior to simulation and treatment. The typical field arrangement is parallel-opposed anterior and posterior fields. More complex field arrangements may be necessary to exclude most of the left kidney. In the event the patient has responded completely to chemotherapy by negative endoscopic examination and biopsy, doses in the range of 30 to 35 Gy seem reasonable, similar to what would be done for nodal disease. Our preference is for 30 Gy, given the unusual ability to assess accurately the response to chemotherapy in the stomach and the radiosensitivity of intra-abdominal organs. If there is persistent biopsy-documented disease after chemotherapy, other systemic therapy should be considered or higher doses of radiation must be used, in the range of 40 Gy.

Gastric Lymphoma, Mucosa-Associated Lymphoid Tissue Type

MALT lymphoma is a distinct clinical-pathologic entity first described by Isaacson and Wright (147) and occurring most often in the stomach. A unique feature of gastric MALT is the association with *H. pylori* infection, initially reported by Wothespoon et al. (320,322). *H. pylori* can be identified in up to 92% of patients (322).

Accordingly, treatment with appropriate antibiotics has been used. A frequently recommended combination is omeprazole, metronidazole, and clarithromycin (254). More than 300 patients with gastric MALT treated with antibiotics have been reported. The complete remission rate is approximately 75%. Approximately two-thirds of complete responders remain in remission at 5 years (44,90,323) for an overall 5-year FFS of about 50%. The 5-year OS is much higher at 90%, with most deaths resulting from causes other than lymphoma (323). Response of *H. pylori*-negative cases to antibiotics has also been reported (236).

The t(11:18) translocation is predictive of resistance to antibiotics (183). Additionally, some patients in CR will have persistent B-cell monoclonality on polymerase chain reaction analysis and are at higher risk of relapse (323).

These results appear inferior to those achieved with radiation therapy where the CR rate exceeds 95% and the relapse rate is <10% with doses of 30 Gy (293), although no direct comparison has even been done. Nonetheless, NCCN guidelines call for initial therapy with antibiotics and close follow-up because of the simplicity of this approach and the slow growth of MALT lymphomas (216). RT is reserved for patients failing antibiotic therapy. The same techniques used for gastric DLBCL apply. Doses are less, no more than 30 Gy. There is no apparent role for adjuvant chemotherapy. Rituximab has been used in patients who are not suitable for RT with promising but very short-term results (195).

Intestinal Lymphomas

Small intestinal lymphomas may comprise 20% to 50% of all GI lymphomas (59,62,169,208). Three different types of lymphomas may be found. The first, B-cell lymphomas, comprise about two-thirds of intestinal lymphoma. The majority of these appear to be DLBCL (59,72). DLBCL of the intestine is seen primarily in Western countries and resembles primary DLBCL of the stomach. The clinical presentation is usually with abdominal pain, anorexia, and weight loss. However, ileus or perforation is much more common than in gastric lymphoma, occurring in approximately 40% of the patients in the German series (169). Most patients have localized disease at onset, but the usual staging work-up is appropriate. CT scans of chest, abdomen, and pelvis or, better, PET/CT should be performed, primarily for delineation of disease outside the intestinal tract and determination of the size of mass lesions in the intestinal tract. Intraluminal disease is probably better visualized with conventional barium studies.

Because of the frequent presentation with obstructive signs and symptoms, along with the increased complexity of establishing a diagnosis endoscopically, surgery is more commonly used, both for diagnosis and for therapy, than it is for gastric lymphoma. For surgically resected, localized intestinal lymphoma of the DLBCL type, anthracycline-based chemotherapy should be given after surgery, as for localized DLBCL of other sites. For completely resected disease, postoperative RT is probably not necessary. In the case of localized disease incompletely resected, some authorities recommend the addition of WAI (57).

From 20% to 30% of patients with B-cell lymphomas of the intestine have low-grade disease. Most of this is of the MALT variety. A smaller percentage is MCL (72,170). MALT intestinal lymphomas are not thought to be *H. pylori*-related. They are managed primarily with RT. The role of chemotherapy is limited. Crump et al. (57) recommend WAI for intestinal MALT after surgical resection with a dose of 20 to 25 Gy in 1- to 1.25-Gy fractions. Most of the liver may be shielded from the onset but should definitely be excluded after 15 to 18 Gy. The kidneys should be shielded after 15 to 18 Gy. Depending on the segment of intestine involved and the extent, less WAI may also be used. The technique of cross-table laterals previously mentioned for treatment of mesenteric adenopathy may be applicable. In this technique, both the small bowel and kidneys are outlined with contrast (oral and intravenous, respectively) and the lateral fields shaped to include the former and exclude the latter. Even with less than WAI, the dose of RT should not exceed 25 to 30 Gy.

Precise data as to the prognosis of localized intestinal B-cell lymphoma are lacking. In the large German series, intestinal lymphomas had a somewhat worse outlook than gastric lymphomas, with an approximately 50% long-term survival rate. The authors distinguish other small bowel sites from lymphoma of the ileocecal region, which had a greater tendency to be localized and an outlook similar to that of gastric lymphoma, namely long-term survival rates of 75% to 80%.

The second type of intestinal lymphoma encountered is intestinal T-cell lymphoma, also referred to as *enteropathy-associated T-cell lymphoma*. This has also been described as malignant histiocytosis of the intestine, but it is now known to represent a T-cell lymphoma (148). T-cell lymphomas account for approximately one-third of all intestinal lymphomas. Patients with celiac disease have an approximately 200-fold increased risk for development of intestinal T-cell lymphoma (285).

The clinical presentation is similar to that described for B-cell intestinal lymphomas. Diarrhea is prominent, reported in approximately 40% of patients. Presentation with perforation or obstruction occurred in approximately 40% of patients (100). There is a greater tendency for these patients to have widespread bowel involvement. The diagnosis is usually established with laparotomy. After surgical resection, treatment has usually consisted of anthracycline-based chemotherapy. The outcome, however, has been poor, with 5-year survivals of 20% to 25%. (72,100). These patients usually have a worse performance status and tolerate chemotherapy poorly. Intestinal perforation after chemotherapy is not unusual.

There are no reported results for RT. For patients with residual disease after surgery, it is possible that a protracted course of RT with small fractions followed by chemotherapy might reduce the frequency of intestinal perforation reported after conventional doses of CHOP. Field sizes and arrangements would be similar to those described for intestinal MALT. More dosage is presumably required (30 to 40 Gy) but would be difficult to administer because of tolerance problems.

The third type of intestinal lymphoma is *immunoproliferative small intestinal disease* (IPSID), also referred to as *Mediterranean lymphoma*. This disease occurs mainly in young adults in the Middle East and North Africa (255). In Western series, it is quite uncommon. Immunoproliferative small intestinal disease is a B-cell lymphoma, believed to arise from the clonal proliferation of B lymphocytes that produce immunoglobulin-A (IgA heavy chain). *Campylobacter jejuni* has recently been shown to have an etiologic role. In its early stages, the disease responds to antibiotic therapy. The disease frequently affects the entire small intestine. Symptoms of malabsorption predominate. Treatment has usually consisted of chemotherapy (4,255). The prognosis has been poor, with survival rates not exceeding 20%. WAI has been reported to be useful in selected patients (255).

Head and Neck Lymphomas

Head and neck lymphomas are the second most frequent variant of ENL after those of the GI tract, representing approximately 20% of all ENL (116,213,221,285,328). They occur in a variety of sites, including Waldeyer's ring, the thyroid, salivary glands, nasal cavity, paranasal sinuses, and orbit, with differing histologic types and clinical characteristics depending on the site of origin. Most appear to be of B-cell origin and most of those are DLBCL. MZL is less common but constitutes a majority of salivary gland lymphomas. A special entity is that of nasal NK/T-cell lymphoma (143,166,167,185). This disease for a number of years was of uncertain cause but is now believed to represent a T-cell lymphoma. It went by many names in the past, including angiocentric lymphoma, lethal midline granuloma, midline malignant reticulosis, and polymorphic reticulosis, reflecting its uncertain etiology. The preferred terminology, however, is *NK* or *NK/T cell lymphoma*.

Lymphomas presenting in Waldeyer's ring typically involve tonsil, base of tongue, or nasopharynx. The clinical symptoms are those associated with epithelial tumors in those sites, such as dysphagia, sore throat, nasal congestion, and eustachian tube blockage. The lesions are frequently clinically apparent on thorough head and neck examination. Neck adenopathy is common.

The usual lymphoma staging studies are appropriate including CT or PET/CT scans of head and neck, chest, and abdomen and bone marrow examination. There is a predilection for Waldeyer's ring lymphomas to have GI tract involvement as well, so direct imaging (i.e., upper GI series or endoscopy) is indicated. Most cases are stage I or II after full staging evaluation.

The pathologic type is usually DLBCL. The treatment guidelines are those for nodal stage I and II DLBCL. Older series report results of RT alone: 50% survival rates in patients with stage I disease and 25% to 50% in stage II, but more often the former number, results clearly suboptimal (149,213). Consequently, almost all centers now report the use of CMT, three to six cycles of CHOP followed by IFRT. Again, R-CHOP would now be the preferred combination. Retrospective analyses show an improvement in survival rates to approximately 80% for patients with stage I disease and 50% for those with stage II disease after CMT (76,213). The one phase III study is that of Aviles et al. (16), who randomized 316 patients to RT alone, CMT, or chemotherapy alone. Although a CR was achieved in >90% of patients in all three groups, relapses were frequent for the single-modality arms. The 5-year survival rate was approximately 90% in the CMT arm versus approximately 50% for the chemotherapy- and RT-alone arms.

Paranasal sinus and nasal cavity lymphomas are often grouped together but in reality appear to have a different prognosis and should be discussed separately. Most paranasal sinus tumors are B cell in origin and usually present in men in the sixth or seventh decade. The outlook when treated with RT alone seems to be particularly poor for both stage I and II disease, with 12% long-term survival in the Stanford University series and approximately 30% in an M.D. Anderson Cancer Center report (131,187). Some authors have described a predilection for CNS spread (131); others have not found this to be the case (185,187). In any event, the outlook improves markedly when patients are treated with CMT. In the M.D. Anderson Cancer Center report, FFS approximately doubled from 34% to 63% at 10 years with the addition of chemotherapy to RT (187). With CMT, survival rates in the range of 70% to 80% are expected, similar to those seen in other sites.

Nasal cavity lymphomas, on the other hand, appear to be of predominantly T-cell origin and fall into the category of NK/T-cell lymphomas. They are seen more commonly in Asia. The disease affects primarily men, mostly in the fifth decade. It often presents as a destructive necrotizing process. Because of this, histologic diagnosis may be difficult. The disease appears to progress primarily locally with only a small predilection for regional or systemic failure (166). Treatment approaches have consisted of RT alone, chemotherapy alone, and the two combined. With RT alone, approximately two-thirds of patients achieved CR (166,167,185), but half of these will relapse. The prognosis appears somewhat worse for stage II than stage I (185).

The contribution of chemotherapy to the management of NK/T-cell lymphoma is unclear. When treated initially with chemotherapy, CR occurs in only a minority of patients (49,184,185,241), in contrast to the results seen with most other head and neck lymphomas. Nonetheless, the suboptimal results with RT alone argue for further exploration of the combined modality approach despite discouraging results to date (49,184). Ribrag et al. (241) suggested that a different sequencing of CMT might be more useful; that is, chemotherapy after RT or the use of an alternating schedule of RT and chemotherapy, as opposed to the more usual pattern of induction chemotherapy followed by RT. Alternatively, different agents other than the standard CHOP combination may prove to be more effective.

In contrast to most other head and neck lymphomas, salivary gland lymphomas are frequently of a more benign histologic type (i.e., MZL) (199). In Asian countries, the percentage of MZL may be lower. These patients usually present with painless enlargement of the parotid gland. There is an association with previous Sjögren's syndrome (328). Treatment usually consists of RT alone. The prognosis is excellent, with survival >90% (199,328). One small randomized trial explored the use of chemotherapy in addition to RT (14). In this trial, 5-year survival rates of 90% were achieved with RT alone or with CMT. These data are consistent with the lack of improvement shown for the addition of chemotherapy to RT for MZL in other sites, as well as the lack of benefit for chemotherapy in addition to RT in localized FL.

There are occasional patients with salivary gland lymphomas presenting with bilateral paired organ involvement (e.g., both parotid glands). When the histologic type is MZL, such patients, although not stage II in the conventional sense, appear to do quite well, with localized RT directed to both parotids.

Little information is available regarding appropriate dose or field size in head and neck lymphomas. General principles of lymphoma management apply. For DLBCL in which induction chemotherapy with R-CHOP is used, patients achieving CR should be treated with doses in the range of 30 to 40 Gy to the site of initial involvement with a generous margin. Our tendency is to use doses at the lower end of this range. These patients seem unusually susceptible to xerostomia, which is lessened with reduced doses. Prophylactic treatment of clinically uninvolved areas is probably not necessary. Intensity-modulated RT may be appropriate to maximize parotid sparing. For salivary gland tumors that are MZL histologically, the appropriate dose is 30 Gy directed to the parotid and covering the immediately adjacent upper neck nodes if the latter are clinically uninvolved, with more extensive neck fields if there is clinical adenopathy. Dose response data are lacking regarding NK/T-cell nasal cavity lymphoma. In view of the questionable activity of chemotherapy, a dose of at least 40 Gy is suggested.

Cutaneous Lymphomas

The term *primary cutaneous lymphoma* (PCL) is used to define those lymphomas that present in and are confined to the skin without evidence of extracutaneous disease. Including mycosis fungoides (discussed in Chapter 72), PCL is the third most common ENL, closely following GI and head and neck lymphomas. PCL is a relatively unique type of lymphoma whose clinical behavior seems to be governed more by presentation in the skin than by its histologic appearance, in contrast to the situation with most other lymphomas, in which the histopathologic appearance predicts the clinical behavior. To complicate matters further, the location in the skin where the disease originates may have a significant bearing on outcome. DLBCL originating on the legs has a much worse outlook than that originating on skin surfaces elsewhere (25,118). The biologic explanation for this phenomenon is unknown.

PCL is an uncommon entity, with an overall incidence of 1 in 1.5/100,000. Separate pathologic classifications were devised by the EORTC (317) and WHO (151) but have recently been reconciled (316) (Table 76.8). About 75% of all PCL is of T-cell origin, and 25% are of B-cell origin. Most cutaneous T-cell lymphomas are mycosis fungoides.

Most other cutaneous T-cell lymphomas consist of the closely related categories of LYP and ALCL. LYP and ALCL have overlapping clinical, histologic, and immunophenotypical characteristics. The largest reported experience is from the Dutch Cutaneous Lymphoma Group (25). These authors described 219 patients in the period 1983 through 1998, approximately equally divided between LYP and ALCL. The distinction between the two was often difficult, but both had an excellent prognosis. Only 2% of patients with LYP and 4% of those with ALCL died of lymphoma. LYP is often generalized, and spontaneous remissions are common and are an important clue as to diagnosis.

Cutaneous ALCL, on the other hand, is localized or regional in approximately 80% of cases.

We have mentioned previously the difference between ALCL arising in the skin and ALCL that originates elsewhere. The latter has a highly variable course depending on whether the ALK

| Table 76.8 | WORLD HEALTH ORGANIZATION—EUROPEAN ORGANISATION FOR RESEARCH AND TREATMENT OF CANCER CLASSIFICATION OF CUTANEOUS LYMPHOMAS |

Type	Frequency (%)	5-Year CSS (%)
Cutaneous T Cell		
MF	44	88
LYP	12	100
ALCL	8	95
Cutaneous B Cell		
MZL	7	99
Follicle center	11	95
DLBCL—leg	4	55

CSS, cause-specific survival; MF, mycosis fungoides; LYP, lymphomatoid papulosis; ALCL, anaplastic large cell lymphoma; MZL, marginal zone lymphoma; DLBCL, diffuse large B-cell lymphoma.

protein is overexpressed. ALK-negative patients have a worse outlook. ALCL in the skin, however, is ALK-negative, with the determining factor in biologic behavior the site of origin.

Cutaneous B-cell lymphoma comprises about 25% of skin lymphomas. In the new WHO-EORTC classification, it is divided into primary cutaneous follicle center lymphoma (PCFCL), primary cutaneous marginal zone lymphoma (PCMZL), and primary cutaneous large cell lymphoma, leg type (316). DLBCL of the skin not in the leg is now included in the PCFCL group, which also contains FL of the skin. An unusual feature of a minority of cases of PCMZL is the association with *B. burgdorferi* infection, in which case the disease may respond to antibiotics (282).

Both PCFCL and PCMZL have an excellent prognosis. The treatment of choice is RT, dose of 40 Gy for the former and 30 Gy for the latter, as for MZL elsewhere. The 5-year disease-specific survival for both conditions exceeds 95% (118,316). Adjuvant chemotherapy is not recommended.

PCLBCL of the leg, however, has a much worse prognosis, with a cause-specific survival of about 50% at 5 years. Chemotherapy with R-CHOP followed by RT is usually recommended, although it is not clear if this favorably influences outcome (118).

Orbital Lymphomas

Lymphomas of the eye may involve either the extraocular orbital tissues such as the conjunctiva, retrobulbar region, or lacrimal gland, or may be primary in the tissues of the eye itself. The latter condition is referred to as *primary intraocular lymphoma* and is, in essence, a subset of PCNSL in which lymphoma cells are initially present only in the eyes, without evidence of disease in the brain or other CNS tissues (36). Its management is essentially that of PCNSL, which is discussed later.

Orbital lymphomas comprise approximately 4% of all ENLs. They typically arise in superficial tissues such as conjunctiva and eyelids and are most commonly seen in an older population, with a median age of approximately 60 years (285). Histopathologically, approximately two-thirds of these tumors are MZL. Most of the remainder of the tumors are DLBCL.

Patients typically present with mass lesions in the conjunctivae or lids, described in the literature as "salmon pink" in color. Tumors of the retrobulbar region may present with swelling and proptosis and associated disturbances in function of the extraocular muscles. Bilaterality is not unusual, occurring in 10% to 15% of cases. Similar to salivary gland and skin tumors this does not adversely affect prognosis.

The usual staging studies for systemic disease should be performed. Magnetic resonance imaging of the orbit should be done to delineate precisely the anatomic extent of disease for RT planning purposes.

The treatment principles for lymphomas generally apply. MZL is treated with RT alone. No more than 30 Gy is required for local control. Doses of 20 to 30 Gy have been reported as equally effective (226,283,329). Local control exceeds 95%, as does 5-year cause-specific survival. Most series report about 20% of patients relapsing, almost always at distant sites.

Field arrangements are somewhat controversial. Some authors suggest the entire orbit be treated to avoid marginal misses (226,329). This may be done with a single anterior field or a wedged pair. Three-dimensional planning may be helpful. A lens shield is often used to prevent cataracts, but may increase marginal misses. With whole-orbital doses of 20 to 30 Gy, cataract formation is the principal risk, occurring in 20% to 30% of patients (329). Some dryness may result from inclusion in the field of a portion of the lacrimal gland. As mentioned, orbital MZL may involve both eyes at presentation. Under these circumstances, RT alone remains the treatment of choice, with careful attention to treatment planning and prescribed dose to avoid eye complications.

Orbital MZL has recently joined the group of MZLs associated with infectious agents, in this instance *C. psittaci* (85). A trial of antibiotic therapy has been suggested for patients in whom this organism is identified (86). It has also been suggested that observation only is a reasonable strategy. In a Japanese series of 36 patients, 70% did not require treatment with a median follow-up of 7 years (288).

A much smaller percentage of patients (10% to 30%) presents with orbital disease that is DLBCL. The prognosis in the literature in the past has been poor—a 33% survival rate in Florida and 50% at the Royal Marsden Hospital (27,32) with RT alone. The treatment of choice is CMT, R-CHOP followed by IFRT. After CR to chemotherapy, we limit RT to approximately 30 Gy to minimize complications. With this program, cure rates of 80% would be expected and have been reported (222).

Extranodal Lymphomas of Other Sites

In addition to the areas previously described, NHL may arise in almost any organ or tissue of the body, including but not limited to bone, testis, ovary, kidney, bladder, female genital tract, breasts, and lung. Lymphoma in any of these sites is quite uncommon. General principles of evaluation and management apply. Accurate histopathologic diagnosis is essential, followed by full staging work-up with treatment decisions governed by stage and histopathologic diagnosis.

A few brief comments regarding the special features of testicular, bone, and lung lymphomas are appropriate. Testicular lymphoma is rare, accounting for approximately 2% to 3% of all ENLs and less than 1% of all NHLs (56,205,269). It presents typically in elderly men in their seventh and eighth decades. Most patients have stage I or II disease. The histologic type is typically DLBCL. Approximately one-fourth of patients have stage IV disease at presentation, with a predilection for unusual sites of involvement such as CNS, skin, and lung. In most reported series, patients have been treated in a variety of ways because of the rarity of the disease and the long period over which cases are collected from any one institution.

The disease is typically diagnosed by orchiectomy. In the past, that was frequently followed by RT to pelvic and para-aortic nodes in a fashion similar to that for testicular carcinoma. Such treatment programs were notably unsuccessful, with probably <20% OS (269). The introduction of CHOP combined with RT and surgery did not improve matters much. Treatment programs of surgery, CHOP, and RT have still resulted in only an approximately 30% long term survival (269,303). There is a high predilection for both contralateral testis relapse as well as CNS relapse, with some 30% to 40% of patients failing in these sites as well as other generalized sites (176,269,334). Accordingly, more recent treatment programs have advocated the use of CNS prophylaxis with intrathecal methotrexate as well as systemic high-dose methotrexate coupled with prophylactic RT to the contralateral testis and sometimes pelvic and para-aortic nodes. RT doses have ranged from 10 to 40 Gy. One report demonstrated a 5-year FFS rate of 91% with this program, compared with 30% with CHOP and RT alone (303). There is no reported experience with R-CHOP.

ENL of bone is another uncommon entity, representing less than 5% of all ENLs (19,20,23). Patients tend to be somewhat younger, with a median age in the fifth decade. The long bones are primarily affected. The presenting signs and symptoms are usually local bone pain, with or without soft tissue swelling, and occasionally a palpable mass lesion or a pathologic fracture. Approximately two-thirds to three-fourths of patients have stage I and II disease at presentation, with the remainder having stage IV disease. Histopathologically, 70% to 90% of patients have DLBCL (19).

The disease is managed similarly to stage I or II NHL of other sites. Thus, for DLBCL, therapy is initiated with R-CHOP followed by IFRT. Although a dose of 30 Gy is appropriate for patients achieving CR, that determination may be difficult in bone disease. The normal reparative processes may cloud the imaging determination of a CR. Therefore, we often use 40 Gy consolidative RT but try and avoid this dose to entire joints because of the risk of avascular necrosis. Treatment volume should include the original tumor with a margin of several centimeters. Radiation of the entire bone is probably unnecessary. FFS and OS are high, 85% to 95% in a recent series (23).

Another quite uncommon variety of ENL is that arising in the lung (80,124). Although secondary involvement in the lung in NHL is common, primary involvement in the lung represents approximately 1% of all ENL presentations. The prognosis of primary lung lymphoma is good, as these are primarily MZL. They are known as *BALT tumors* because they arise from bronchus-associated lymphoid tissue. Five-year survival rates in the range of 90% have been reported from the Mayo Clinic and a large French series (54,80).

Patients usually present with an asymptomatic abnormality on chest radiograph. It is difficult to obtain sufficient tissue at bronchoscopy with bronchial washings or with fine-needle aspirate to establish the diagnosis. An open procedure, either thoracoscopy or thoracotomy, is usually required. Most of the reported patients in the literature have been treated with surgical resection, sometimes followed by chemotherapy. There are very few patients reported treated with radiation, either alone or in combination with surgery and chemotherapy. Excellent local tumor control would be predicted for RT, however, in modest doses typical for MZL. It is therefore the treatment of choice in unresectable BALT lymphoma or where the extent of pulmonary resection would significantly compromise lung function. If only a small amount of lung needs to be surgically removed to encompass the tumor, surgical resection may carry less morbidity than RT.

The role of chemotherapy in BALT lymphoma is not well studied but would be predicted to be quite similar to that in MALT or FL; that is, the disease is chemotherapy-responsive, with no data to suggest that the natural history is altered or survival prolonged by initiation of chemotherapy at diagnosis.

A small percentage of pulmonary lymphomas are DLBCL. These should be managed in accordance with the accepted principles of management of DLBCL, namely R-CHOP. If the disease has been completely resected to establish the diagnosis, no additional RT appears necessary. If resection has not been accomplished, R-CHOP should be followed by RT, with the dose chosen reflecting the adequacy of response to R-CHOP. The treatment volume is problematic. A balance should be struck between treatment of the original tumor volume, which could conceivably involve a large amount of normal lung, and treatment of the postchemotherapy tumor volume, where the disease may all have disappeared (124).

Primary Central Nervous System Lymphoma

PCNSL is a rare type of NHL but one that is increasing rapidly in frequency. From 1973 to 1992, it is estimated that the frequency of brain lymphoma increased more than 10-fold, from 2.5 to 30 cases per 10 million population (55). Part of this increase is attributable to human immunodeficiency virus (HIV)-associated cases, but most of it has occurred in immunocompetent patients. The median age at presentation is 55 years for immunocompetent patients and 31 years for patients with AIDS. Neurologic symptoms are usually of brief duration, ≤3 months, and may include specific neurologic deficits depending on the location of the tumor, generalized symptoms such as altered mental status, seizures, and symptoms of increased intracranial pressure such as headache, nausea, and vomiting. Immunocompetent patients are more likely to have specific neurologic deficits compared with patients with AIDS, who more often have diffuse disease leading to altered mental status and more generalized signs (22,192).

Radiologic imaging often suggests a diagnosis. PCNSL is usually isodense or hyperdense on nonenhanced CT scans, in contradistinction to other primary brain tumors or metastatic lesions. The location of the lesion may also suggest the diagnosis because the majority occur in a periventricular distribution, usually involving the corpus callosum, thalamus, or basal ganglia. In patients with HIV infection, disease is often multifocal in the brain and may be quite difficult to distinguish from CNS infections (22).

In the immunocompetent patient, the histologic appearance is typically that of DLBCL. Further, immunophenotyping suggests the tumor is the same as DLBCL occurring outside the nervous system, raising the question as to why it responds so differently to therapy, a question that remains unanswered.

In HIV-positive patients, aggressive or high-grade histopathologic pictures are common. In addition, the tumor is virtually always associated with EBV (260). EBV is rare in immunocompetent patients with PCNSL.

At the time of diagnosis, although most patients with PCNSL have a solitary brain lesion, the leptomeninges may be involved in approximately one-third of cases and the eye in 20%. Therefore, evaluation of these two areas is indicated, including a lumbar puncture (if the intracranial pressure is not increased and it can be done safely) and full ophthalmologic evaluation of the eye. It is very common to perform staging studies to look for lymphoma outside the CNS, but this is rarely found (22,70). In the absence of specific signs or symptoms suggesting disease outside the CNS, such staging procedures are probably not worthwhile.

The management of PCNSL has evolved considerably over recent years. Historically, the treatment was RT alone. Results were poor, however, despite the known radiosensitivity of NHL outside the CNS. Two representative series from RTOG and Princess Margaret Hospital report median survivals of 12.2 months and 17 months, respectively, and 5-year survivals of 10% to 20% (177,217). Although the tumor initially responds to RT, regrowth is common and uncontrolled disease in the brain the primary cause of death.

These and virtually all subsequent studies have emphasized the prognostic importance of age and performance status. Patients younger 60 years had a 42% survival in the Princess Margaret series compared with 9% for those older than 60. The International Extranodal Lymphoma Study Group has also reported elevated LDH, increased CSF protein, and tumor location within the deep regions of the brain as significant prognostic variables (81,82).

The role of surgery in the management of PCNSL is limited to establishing the diagnosis, preferably by means of stereotactic biopsy. The tumor is usually not amenable to surgical resection because of its deep location and involvement of critical structures. Occasionally, surgical decompression and shunt placement is necessary for relief of increased intracranial pressure.

Corticosteroids serve to reduce intracranial pressure but also have a direct antitumor effect (70). Tumor regression may lead to difficulties in establishing the diagnosis histologically. Accordingly, steroids should be withheld if possible until after biopsy, if the diagnosis is suspected.

Given the poor results achieved with RT alone and the chemoresponsiveness of lymphomas generally, evaluation of systemic chemotherapy for PCNSL was soon undertaken. Initial programs consisted of CHOP and variations on that combination. Despite the efficacy of this combination in NHL outside the CNS, the results in PCNSL have been quite disappointing. A randomized trial by the Medical Research Council showed no benefit for CHOP added to RT (198). Other studies have come to similar conclusions. This lack of efficacy may be due to failure to penetrate the blood–brain barrier.

Methotrexate, particularly in high doses, is known to penetrate the blood–brain barrier. It was first used for treatment of PCNSL in 1980 (22). Subsequently, its use has become widespread. The approach has been variable in terms of dosage, scheduling, and combinations with intrathecal methotrexate or other drugs such as cytarabine, vincristine, or thiotepa. The infrequency of PCNSL has precluded phase III trials to resolve these and many other issues. Nonetheless, methotrexate appears to represent an important advance. For example, an RTOG study treated patients with combination chemotherapy, including high-dose methotrexate and whole-brain radiotherapy (WBRT). The 5-year OS was 32%, the FFS was 25%, which were results much better than those historically obtained with RT alone. Another study from Memorial Sloan-Kettering Cancer Center demonstrated 5-year OS of 45% and FFS of 50% with a similar program (105).

Considerable toxicity, however, has been reported with the combination of high-dose methotrexate and WBRT to a dose of 45 Gy (conventional fractionation). Both leukoencephalopathy and/or dementia have been frequently reported. It is difficult to determine the precise incidence because actuarial complication rates are seldom reported. One study described 26% severe neurotoxicity at 6 years (31). The problem is much worse in the population older than 60 years. DeAngelis (70) suggests the frequency approaches 100% in the older age group; current policy at Memorial Sloan-Kettering Cancer Center is to treat patients >60 years old with chemotherapy alone with RT reserved for relapsing patients. A number of centers have suggested that all patients be treated with chemotherapy alone, but numbers of patients treated are small and follow-up was short.

To alleviate neurotoxicity, Bessell et al. (28) reduced RT dose to 30 Gy in 26 patients who had achieved CR to chemotherapy. The 3-year risk of relapse increased to 83% compared with 25% in a prior series of 31 patients treated with 45 Gy. The series of Bessell et al., however, used eight drugs, with a methotrexate dose of 1.5 g/m^2 and delivered the 30 Gy of RT during 5 weeks.

Treatment of PCNSL is therefore unsettled. High-dose methotrexate, probably >3 g/m^2 every 2 to 4 weeks, is the cornerstone of therapy. Other drugs and schedules remain controversial. Most authorities recommend WBRT in younger patients to 45 Gy. Recently, the Memorial Sloan-Kettering Cancer Center group has reduced the dose to 2,340 cGy for patients achieving CR to chemotherapy with promising short term results (325). WBRT is not recommended for patients >60 years old. The role of stereotactic radiosurgery for patients with isolated lesions, alone or in combination with WBRT, is unknown.

References

1. A clinical evaluation of the International Lymphoma Study Group classification of non-Hodgkin's lymphoma. The Non-Hodgkin's Lymphoma Classification Project. *Blood* 1997;89:3909–3918.
2. A predictive model for aggressive non-Hodgkin's lymphoma. The International Non-Hodgkin's Lymphoma Prognostic Factors Project. *N Engl J Med* 1993;329:987–994.
3. Advani R, Rosenberg SA, Horning SJ. Stage I and II follicular non-Hodgkin's lymphoma: long-term follow-up of no initial therapy. *J Clin Oncol* 2004;22: 1454–1459.
4. Al-Bahrani ZR, Al-Mondhiry H, Bakir F, Al-Saleem T. Clinical and pathologic subtypes of primary intestinal lymphoma. Experience with 132 patients over a 14-year period. *Cancer* 1983;52:1666–1672.
5. Alizadeh AA, Eisen MB, Davis RE, et al. Distinct types of diffuse large B-cell lymphoma identified by gene expression profiling. *Nature* 2000;403:503–511.
6. Al-Saleem T, Al-Mondhiry H. Immunoproliferative small intestinal disease (IPSID): a model for mature B-cell neoplasms. *Blood* 2005;105:2274–2280.
7. Amer MH, el-Akkad S. Gastrointestinal lymphoma in adults: clinical features and management of 300 cases. *Gastroenterology* 1994;106:846–858.
8. Anderson JR, Armitage JO, Weisenburger DD. Epidemiology of the non-Hodgkin's lymphomas: distributions of the major subtypes differ by geographic locations. Non-Hodgkin's Lymphoma Classification Project. *Ann Oncol* 1998;9:717–720.
9. Anderson JR, Vose JM, Bierman PJ, et al. Clinical features and prognosis of follicular large-cell lymphoma: a report from the Nebraska Lymphoma Study Group. *J Clin Oncol* 1993;11:218–224.
10. Armitage JO, Greer JP, Levine AM, et al. Peripheral T-cell lymphoma. *Cancer* 1989;63:158–163.
11. Armitage JO, Weisenburger DD. New approach to classifying non-Hodgkin's lymphomas: clinical features of the major histologic subtypes. Non-Hodgkin's Lymphoma Classification Project. *J Clin Oncol* 1998;16:2780–2795.
12. Arrowsmith ER, Macon WR, Kinney MC, et al. Peripheral T-cell lymphomas: clinical features and prognostic factors of 92 cases defined by the revised European American lymphoma classification. *Leuk Lymphoma* 2003;44:241–249.
13. Aviles A, Delgado S, Fernandez E. Combined therapy in advanced stages (III and IV) of follicular lymphoma increases the possibility of cure: results of a large controlled clinical trial. *Eur J Haematol* 2002;68:144–149.
14. Aviles A, Delgado S, Huerta-Guzman J. Marginal zone B cell lymphoma of the parotid glands: results of a randomised trial comparing radiotherapy to combined therapy. *Eur J Cancer B Oral Oncol* 1996;32B:420–422.
15. Aviles A, Delgado S, Nambo MJ, et al. Adjuvant radiotherapy to sites of previous bulky disease in patients stage IV diffuse large cell lymphoma. *Int J Radiat Oncol Biol Phys* 1994;30:799–803.
16. Aviles A, Delgado S, Ruiz H, et al. Treatment of non-Hodgkin's lymphoma of Waldeyer's ring: radiotherapy versus chemotherapy versus combined therapy. *Eur J Cancer B Oral Oncol* 1996;32B:19–23.
17. Aviles A, Diaz-Maqueo JC, Sanchez E, et al. Long-term results in patients with low-grade nodular non-Hodgkin's lymphoma. A randomized trial comparing chemotherapy plus radiotherapy with chemotherapy alone. *Acta Oncol* 1991;30:329–333.
18. Aviles A, Fernandezb R, Perez F, et al. Adjuvant radiotherapy in stage IV diffuse large cell lymphoma improves outcome. *Leuk Lymphoma* 2004;45:1385–1389.
19. Baar J, Burkes RL, Gospodarowicz M. Primary non-Hodgkin's lymphoma of bone. *Semin Oncol* 1999;26:270–275.
20. Barbieri E, Cammelli S, Mauro F, et al. Primary non-Hodgkin's lymphoma of the bone: treatment and analysis of prognostic factors for Stage I and Stage II. *Int J Radiat Oncol Biol Phys* 2004;59:760–764.
21. Baron F, Maris MB, Sandmaier BM, et al. Graft-versus-tumor effects after allogeneic hematopoietic cell transplantation with nonmyeloablative conditioning. *J Clin Oncol* 2005;23:1993–2003.
22. Batchelor T, Loeffler JS. Primary CNS lymphoma. *J Clin Oncol* 2006;24:1281–1288.
23. Beal K, Allen L, Yahalom J. Primary bone lymphoma: treatment results and prognostic factors with long-term follow-up of 82 patients. *Cancer* 2006;106:2652–2656.
24. Behler CM, Kaplan LD. Advances in the management of HIV-related non-Hodgkin lymphoma. *Curr Opin Oncol* 2006;18:437–443.
25. Bekkenk MW, Geelen FA, van Voorst Vader PC, et al. Primary and secondary cutaneous CD30(+) lymphoproliferative disorders: a report from the Dutch Cutaneous Lymphoma Group on the long-term follow-up data of 219 patients and guidelines for diagnosis and treatment. *Blood* 2000;95:3653–3661.
26. Berger F, Felman P, Thieblemont C, et al. Non-MALT marginal zone B-cell lymphomas: a description of clinical presentation and outcome in 124 patients. *Blood* 2000;95:1950–1956.
27. Bessell EM, Henk JM, Wright JE, et al. Orbital and conjunctival lymphoma treatment and prognosis. *Radiother Oncol* 1988;13:237–244.
28. Bessell EM, Lopez-Guillermo A, Villa S, et al. Importance of radiotherapy in the outcome of patients with primary CNS lymphoma: an analysis of the CHOD/BVAM regimen followed by two different radiotherapy treatments. *J Clin Oncol* 2002;20:231–236.
29. Bierman P, Armitage JO. Salvage therapy for patients with relapsed or refractory aggressive non-Hodgkin's lymphoma. *Oncology (Huntingt)* 1987;1:11–21.
30. Blay J, Gomez F, Sebban C, et al. The International Prognostic Index correlates to survival in patients with aggressive lymphoma in relapse: analysis of the PARMA trial. Parma Group. *Blood* 1998;92:3562–3568.
31. Blay JY, Conroy T, Chevreau C, et al. High-dose methotrexate for the treatment of primary cerebral lymphomas: analysis of survival and late neurologic toxicity in a retrospective series. *J Clin Oncol* 1998;16:864–871.
32. Bolek TW, Moyses HM, Marcus RB Jr, et al. Radiotherapy in the management of orbital lymphoma. *Int J Radiat Oncol Biol Phys* 1999;44:31–36.
33. Borowitz MJ, Bray R, Gascoyne R, et al. U.S.-Canadian consensus recommendations on the immunophenotypic analysis of hematologic neoplasia by flow cytometry: data analysis and interpretation. *Cytometry* 1997;30:236–244.
34. Bozzetti F, Audisio RA, Chiavoni R, et al. Role of surgery in patients with primary non-Hodgkin's lymphoma of the stomach: an old problem revisited. *Br J Surg* 1993;80:1101–1106.
35. Brice P, Bastion Y, Lepage E, et al. Comparison in low-tumor-burden follicular lymphomas between an initial no-treatment policy, prednimustine, or interferon alfa: a randomized study from the Groupe d'Etude des Lymphomes Folliculaires. Groupe d'Etude des Lymphomes de l'Adulte. *J Clin Oncol* 1997;15:1110–1117.
36. Buggage RR, Chan CC, Nussenblatt RB. Ocular manifestations of central nervous system lymphoma. *Curr Opin Oncol* 2001;13:137–142.
37. Bush RS, Gospodarowicz M, Sturgeon J, et al. Radiation therapy of localized non-Hodgkin's lymphoma. *Cancer Treat Rep* 1977;61:1129–1136.
38. Bush RS, Gospodarowicz M. The place of radiation therapy in the management of patients with localized non-Hodgkin's lymphoma. In: Rosenberg SA, Kaplan HS, eds. *Malignant lymphomas: etiology, immunology, pathology, treatment.* New York: Academic Press; 1982.
39. Campo E, Gaulard P, Zucca E, et al. Report of the European Task Force on Lymphomas: workshop on peripheral T-cell lymphomas. *Ann Oncol* 1998;9:835–843.
40. Carbone PP, Kaplan HS, Musshoff K, et al. Report of the Committee on Hodgkin's Disease Staging Classification. *Cancer Res* 1971;31:1860–1861.
41. Chabner BA, Fisher RI, Young RC, et al. Staging of non-Hodgkin's lymphoma. *Semin Oncol* 1980;7:285–291.
42. Chacon JI, Mollejo M, Munoz E, et al. Splenic marginal zone lymphoma: clinical characteristics and prognostic factors in a series of 60 patients. *Blood* 2002;100:1648–1654.
43. Chang ET, Smedby KE, Hjalgrim H, et al. Family history of hematopoietic malignancy and risk of lymphoma. *J Natl Cancer Inst* 2005;97:1466–1474.
44. Chen LT, Lin JT, Tai JJ, et al. Long-term results of anti-*Helicobacter pylori* therapy in early-stage gastric high-grade transformed MALT lymphoma. *J Natl Cancer Inst* 2005;97:1345–1353.
45. Chen MG, Prosnitz LR, Gonzalez-Serva A, et al. Results of radiotherapy in control of stage I and II non-Hodgkin's lymphoma. *Cancer* 1979;43:1245–1254.
46. Cheson BD, Horning SJ, Coiffier B, et al. Report of an international workshop to standardize response criteria for non-Hodgkin's lymphomas. NCI Sponsored International Working Group. *J Clin Oncol* 1999;17:1244.

47. Cheson BD. Current approaches to therapy for indolent non-Hodgkin's lymphoma. *Oncology (Huntingt)* 1998;12[10 Suppl 8]:25–34.
48. Cheson BD. Radioimmunotherapy of non-Hodgkin lymphomas. *Blood* 2003;101:391–398.
49. Cheung MM, Chan JK, Lau WH, et al. Early stage nasal NK/T-cell lymphoma: clinical outcome, prognostic factors, and the effect of treatment modality. *Int J Radiat Oncol Biol Phys* 2002;54:182–190.
50. Coiffier B, Neidhardt-Berard EM, Tilly H, et al. Fludarabine alone compared to CHVP plus interferon in elderly patients with follicular lymphoma and adverse prognostic parameters: a GELA study. Groupe d'Etudes des Lymphomes de l'Adulte. *Ann Oncol* 1999;10:1191–1197.
51. Coiffier B, Salles G. Does surgery belong to medical history for gastric lymphomas? *Ann Oncol* 1997;8:419–421.
52. Coiffier B, Thieblemont C, Felman P, et al. Indolent nonfollicular lymphomas: characteristics, treatment, and outcome. *Semin Hematol* 1999;36:198–208.
53. Coiffier B. How to interpret the radiological abnormalities that persist after treatment in non-Hodgkin's lymphoma patients? *Ann Oncol* 1999;10:1141–1143.
54. Cordier JF, Chailleux E, Lauque D, et al. Primary pulmonary lymphomas. A clinical study of 70 cases in nonimmunocompromised patients. *Chest* 1993;103:201–208.
55. Corn BW, Marcus SM, Topham A, et al. Will primary central nervous system lymphoma be the most frequent brain tumor diagnosed in the year 2000? *Cancer* 1997;79:2409–2413.
56. Crellin AM, Hudson BV, Bennett MH, et al. Non-Hodgkin's lymphoma of the testis. *Radiother Oncol* 1993;27:99–106.
57. Crump M, Gospodarowicz M, Shepherd FA. Lymphoma of the gastrointestinal tract. *Semin Oncol* 1999;26:324–337.
58. Czuczman M, Weaver RL, Akluzweny B, et al. Prolonged clinical and molecular remission in patients with low-grade or follicular non-Hodgkin's lymphoma treated with Rituximab plus CHOP chemotherapy: 9-year follow-up. *J Clin Oncol* 2004;22:4659–4664.
59. d'Amore F, Brincker H, Gronbaek K, et al. Non-Hodgkin's lymphoma of the gastrointestinal tract: a population-based analysis of incidence, geographic distribution, clinicopathologic presentation features, and prognosis. Danish Lymphoma Study Group. *J Clin Oncol* 1994;12:1673–1684.
60. d'Amore F, Christensen BE, Brincker H, et al. Clinicopathological features and prognostic factors in extranodal non-Hodgkin lymphomas. Danish LYFO Study Group. *Eur J Cancer* 1991;27:1201–1208.
61. Dana BW, Dahlberg S, Nathwani BN, et al. Long-term follow-up of patients with low-grade malignant lymphomas treated with doxorubicin-based chemotherapy or chemoimmunotherapy. *J Clin Oncol* 1993;11:644–651.
62. Daum S, Ullrich R, Heise W, et al. Intestinal non-Hodgkin's lymphoma: a multicenter prospective clinical study from the German Study Group on Intestinal non-Hodgkin's Lymphoma. *J Clin Oncol* 2003;21:2740–2746.
63. Dave SS, Wright G, Tan B, et al. Prediction of survival in follicular lymphoma based on molecular features of tumor-infiltrating immune cells. *N Engl J Med* 2004;351:2159–2169.
64. Davies AJ, Rohatiner AZ, Howell S, et al. Tositumomab and iodine I 131 tositumomab for recurrent indolent and transformed B-cell non-Hodgkin's lymphoma. *J Clin Oncol* 2004;22:1469–1479.
65. de Bruin PC, Jiwa M, Oudejans JJ, et al. Presence of Epstein-Barr virus in extranodal T-cell lymphomas: differences in relation to site. *Blood* 1994;83:1612–1618.
66. de Jong D, Boot H, van Heerde P, et al. Histological grading in gastric lymphoma: pretreatment criteria and clinical relevance. *Gastroenterology* 1997;112:1466–1474.
67. de Jong D. Molecular pathogenesis of follicular lymphoma: a cross talk of genetic and immunologic factors. *J Clin Oncol* 2005;23:6358–6363.
68. De Los Santos JF, Mendenhall NP, Lynch JW Jr. Is comprehensive lymphatic irradiation for low-grade non-Hodgkin's lymphoma curative therapy? Long-term experience at a single institution. *Int J Radiat Oncol Biol Phys* 1997;38:3–8.
69. Dean RM, Bishop MR. Allogeneic hematopoietic stem cell transplantation for lymphoma. *Clin Lymphoma* 2004;4:238–249.
70. DeAngelis LM. Primary CNS lymphoma: treatment with combined chemotherapy and radiotherapy. *J Neurooncol* 1999;43:249–257.
71. Deconinck E, Foussard C, Milpied N, et al. High-dose therapy followed by autologous purged stem-cell transplantation and doxorubicin-based chemotherapy in patients with advanced follicular lymphoma: a randomized multicenter study by GOELAMS. *Blood* 2005;105:3817–3823.
72. Domizio P, Owen RA, Shepherd NA, et al. Primary lymphoma of the small intestine. A clinicopathological study of 119 cases. *Am J Surg Pathol* 1993;17:429–442.
73. Draisma A, Maffioli L, Gasparini M, et al. Gallium-67 as a tumor-seeking agent in lymphomas–a review. *Tumori* 1998;84:434–441.
74. Dreyling M, Lenz G, Hoster E, et al. Early consolidation by myeloablative radiochemotherapy followed by autologous stem cell transplantation in first remission significantly prolongs progression-free survival in mantle-cell lymphoma: results of a prospective randomized trial of the European MCL Network. *Blood* 2005;105:2677–2684.
75. Engels EA, Cerhan JR, Linet MS, et al. Immune-related conditions and immune-modulating medications as risk factors for non-Hodgkin's lymphoma: a case-control study. *Am J Epidemiol* 2005;162:1153–1161.
76. Ezzat AA, Ibrahim EM, El Weshi AN, et al. Localized non-Hodgkin's lymphoma of Waldeyer's ring: clinical features, management, and prognosis of 130 adult patients. *Head Neck* 2001;23:547–558.
77. Falini B, Pileri S, Zinzani PL, et al. ALK+ lymphoma: clinico-pathological findings and outcome. *Blood* 1999;93:2697–2706.
78. Farinha P, Gascoyne RD. Molecular pathogenesis of mucosa-associated lymphoid tissue lymphoma. *J Clin Oncol* 2005;23:6370–6378.
79. Fernandez V, Hartmann E, Ott G, et al. Pathogenesis of mantle-cell lymphoma: all oncogenic roads lead to dysregulation of cell cycle and DNA damage response pathways. *J Clin Oncol* 2005;23:6364–6369.
80. Ferraro P, Trastek VF, Adlakha H, et al. Primary non-Hodgkin's lymphoma of the lung. *Ann Thorac Surg* 2000;69:993–997.
81. Ferreri AJ, Abrey LE, Blay JY, et al. Summary statement on primary central nervous system lymphomas from the Eighth International Conference on Malignant Lymphoma, Lugano, Switzerland, June 12 to 15, 2002. *J Clin Oncol* 2003;21:2407–2414.
82. Ferreri AJ, Blay JY, Reni M, et al. Prognostic scoring system for primary CNS lymphomas: the International Extranodal Lymphoma Study Group experience. *J Clin Oncol* 2003;21:266–272.
83. Ferreri AJ, Cordio S, Ponzoni M, Villa E. Non-surgical treatment with primary chemotherapy, with or without radiation therapy, of stage I-II high-grade gastric lymphoma. *Leuk Lymphoma* 1999;33:531–541.
84. Ferreri AJ, Dell'Oro S, Reni M, et al. Consolidation radiotherapy to bulky or semibulky lesions in the management of stage III-IV diffuse large B cell lymphomas. *Oncology* 2000;58:219–226.
85. Ferreri AJ, Ponzoni M, Guidoboni M, et al. Regression of ocular adnexal lymphoma after Chlamydia psittaci-eradicating antibiotic therapy. *J Clin Oncol* 2005;23:5067–5073.
86. Ferreri AJ, Guidoboni M, Ponzoni M, et al. Evidence for an association between Chlamydia psittaci and ocular adnexal lymphomas. *J Natl Cancer Inst* 2004;96:586–594.
87. Feugier P, Van Hoof A, Sebban C, et al. Long-term results of the R–CHOP study in the treatment of elderly patients with diffuse large B-cell lymphoma: a study by the Groupe d'Etude des Lymphomes de l'Adulte. *J Clin Oncol* 2005;23:4117–4126.
88. Filipovich AH, Mathur A, Kamat D, et al. Primary immunodeficiencies: genetic risk factors for lymphoma. *Cancer Res* 1992;52[19 Suppl]:5465s–5467s.
89. Finke J, Slanina J, Lange W, et al. Persistence of circulating t(14;18)-positive cells in long-term remission after radiation therapy for localized-stage follicular lymphoma. *J Clin Oncol* 1993;11:1668–1673.
90. Fischbach W, Goebeler-Kolve ME, Dragosics B, et al. Long term outcome of patients with gastric marginal zone B cell lymphoma of mucosa associated lymphoid tissue (MALT) following exclusive Helicobacter pylori eradication therapy: experience from a large prospective series. *Gut* 2004;53:34–37.
91. Fisher RI, Dahlberg S, Nathwani BN, et al. A clinical analysis of two indolent lymphoma entities: mantle cell lymphoma and marginal zone lymphoma (including the mucosa-associated lymphoid tissue and monocytoid B-cell subcategories): a Southwest Oncology Group study. *Blood* 1995;85:1075–1082.
92. Fisher RI, Gaynor ER, Dahlberg S, et al. Comparison of a standard regimen (CHOP) with three intensive chemotherapy regimens for advanced non-Hodgkin's lymphoma. *N Engl J Med* 1993;328:1002–1006.
93. Fisher RI, Kaminski MS, Wahl RL, et al. Tositumomab and iodine-131 tositumomab produces durable complete remissions in a subset of heavily pretreated patients with low-grade and transformed non-Hodgkin's lymphomas. *J Clin Oncol* 2005;23(30):7565–7573.
94. Fisher RI. Diffuse large-cell lymphoma. *Ann Oncol* 2000;11 Suppl 1:29–33.
95. Fisher RI. Mantle-cell lymphoma: classification and therapeutic implications. *Ann Oncol* 1996;7[Suppl]6:S35–S39.
96. Fisher SG, Fisher RI. The epidemiology of non-Hodgkin's lymphoma. *Oncogene* 2004;23:6524–6534.
97. Franco V, Florena AM, Iannitto E. Splenic marginal zone lymphoma. *Blood* 2003;101:2464–2472.
98. Freedman AS, Gribben JG, Nadler LM. High dose therapy and autologous stem cell transplantation in follicular non-Hodgkin's lymphoma. *Leuk Lymphoma* 1998;28:219–230.
99. Fuks Z, Kaplan HS. Recurrence rates following radiation therapy of nodular and diffuse malignant lymphomas. *Radiology* 1973;108:675–684.
100. Gale J, Simmonds PD, Mead GM, et al. Enteropathy-type intestinal T-cell lymphoma: clinical features and treatment of 31 patients in a single center. *J Clin Oncol* 2000;18:795–803.
101. Gallamini A, Stelitano C, Calvi R, et al. Peripheral T-cell lymphoma unspecified (PTCL-U): a new prognostic model from a retrospective multicentric clinical study. *Blood* 2004;103:2474–2479.
102. Gandhi MK. Epstein-Barr virus-associated lymphomas. *Expert Rev Anti Infect Ther* 2006;4:77–89.
103. Ganti AK, Bierman PJ, Lynch JC, et al. Hematopoietic stem cell transplantation in mantle cell lymphoma. *Ann Oncol* 2005;16:618–624.
104. Gascoyne RD, Aoun P, Wu D, et al. Prognostic significance of anaplastic lymphoma kinase (ALK) protein expression in adults with anaplastic large cell lymphoma. *Blood* 1999;93:3913–3921.
105. Gavrilovic IT, Hormigo A, Yahalom J, et al. Long-term follow-up of high-dose methotrexate-based therapy with and without whole brain irradiation for newly diagnosed primary CNS lymphoma. *J Clin Oncol* 2006;24:4570–4574.
106. Ghielmini M, Rufibach K, Salles G, et al. Single agent rituximab in patients with follicular or mantle cell lymphoma: clinical and biological factors that are predictive of response and event-free survival as well as the effect of rituximab on the immune system: a study of the Swiss Group for Clinical Cancer Research (SAKK). *Ann Oncol* 2005;16:1675–1682.
107. Ghielmini M, Schmitz SF, Cogliatti S, et al. Effect of single-agent rituximab given at the standard schedule or as prolonged treatment in patients with mantle cell lymphoma: a study of the Swiss Group for Clinical Cancer Research (SAKK). *J Clin Oncol* 2005;23:705–711.
108. Ghielmini M, Schmitz SF, Cogliatti SB, et al. Prolonged treatment with rituximab in patients with follicular lymphoma significantly increases event-free survival and response duration compared with the standard weekly x 4 schedule. *Blood* 2004;103:4416–4423.
109. Girinsky T, Benhamou E, Bourhis JH, et al. Prospective randomized comparison of single-dose versus hyperfractionated total-body irradiation in patients with hematologic malignancies. *J Clin Oncol* 2000;18:981–986.
110. Girinsky T, Guillot-Vals D, Koscielny S, et al. A high and sustained response rate in refractory or relapsing low-grade lymphoma masses after low-dose radiation: analysis of predictive parameters of response to treatment. *Int J Radiat Oncol Biol Phys* 2001;51:148–155.
111. Glas AM, Kersten MJ, Delahaye LJ, et al. Gene expression profiling in follicular lymphoma to assess clinical aggressiveness and to guide the choice of treatment. *Blood* 2005;105:301–307.
112. Glass AG, Karnell LH, Menck HR. The National Cancer Data Base report on non-Hodgkin's lymphoma. *Cancer* 1997;80:2311–2320.
113. Gospodarowicz M, Tsang R. Mucosa-associated lymphoid tissue lymphomas. *Curr Oncol Rep* 2000;2:192–198.
114. Gospodarowicz MK, Bush RS, Brown TC, et al. Prognostic factors in nodular lymphomas: a multivariate analysis based on the Princess Margaret Hospital experience. *Int J Radiat Oncol Biol Phys* 1984;10:489–497.
115. Gospodarowicz MK, Sutcliffe SB, Clark RM, et al. Outcome analysis of localized gastrointestinal lymphoma treated with surgery and postoperative irradiation. *Int J Radiat Oncol Biol Phys* 1990;19:1351–1355.

116. Gospodarowicz MK, Sutcliffe SB. The extranodal lymphomas. *Semin Radiat Oncol* 1995;5:281–300.
117. Gottschalk S, Rooney CM, Heslop HE. Post-transplant lymphoproliferative disorders. *Annu Rev Med* 2005;56:29–44.
118. Grange F, Bekkenk MW, Wechsler J, et al. Prognostic factors in primary cutaneous large B-cell lymphomas: a European multicenter study. *J Clin Oncol* 2001;19:3602–3610.
119. Guglielmi C, Gomez F, Philip T, et al. Time to relapse has prognostic value in patients with aggressive lymphoma enrolled onto the Parma trial. *J Clin Oncol* 1998;16:3264–3269.
120. Guidoboni M, Ferreri AJ, Ponzoni M, et al. Infectious agents in mucosa-associated lymphoid tissue-type lymphomas: pathogenic role and therapeutic perspectives. *Clin Lymphoma Myeloma* 2006;6:289–300.
121. Gurney KA, Cartwright RA, Gilman EA. Descriptive epidemiology of gastrointestinal non-Hodgkin's lymphoma in a population-based registry. *Br J Cancer* 1999;79:1929–1934.
122. Ha CS, Kong JS, Tucker SL, et al. Central lymphatic irradiation for stage I-III follicular lymphoma: report from a single-institutional prospective study. *Int J Radiat Oncol Biol Phys* 2003;57:316–320.
123. Haas RL, Poortmans P, de Jong D, et al. High response rates and lasting remissions after low-dose involved field radiotherapy in indolent lymphomas. *J Clin Oncol* 2003;21:2474–2480.
124. Habermann TM, Ryu JH, Inwards DJ, et al. Primary pulmonary lymphoma. *Semin Oncol* 1999;26:307–315.
125. Hagenbeek A, Eghbali H, Monfardini S, et al. Phase III intergroup study of fludarabine phosphate compared with cyclophosphamide, vincristine, and prednisone chemotherapy in newly diagnosed patients with stage III and IV low-grade malignant non-Hodgkin's lymphoma. *J Clin Oncol* 2006;24:1590–1596.
126. Hainsworth JD, Litchy S, Burris HA 3rd, et al. Rituximab as first-line and maintenance therapy for patients with indolent non-Hodgkin's lymphoma. *J Clin Oncol* 2002;20:4261–4267.
127. Hallahan DE, Farah R, Vokes EE, et al. The patterns of failure in patients with pathological stage I and II diffuse histiocytic lymphoma treated with radiation therapy alone. *Int J Radiat Oncol Biol Phys* 1989;17:767–771.
128. Hans CP, Weisenburger DD, Vose JM, et al. A significant diffuse component predicts for inferior survival in grade 3 follicular lymphoma, but cytologic subtypes do not predict survival. *Blood* 2003;101:2363–2367.
129. Harris NL, Jaffe ES, Diebold J, et al. Lymphoma classification–from controversy to consensus: the R.E.A.L. and WHO Classification of lymphoid neoplasms. *Ann Oncol* 2000;11 [Suppl 1]:3–10.
130. Harris NL, Jaffe ES, Stein H, et al. A revised European-American classification of lymphoid neoplasms: a proposal from the International Lymphoma Study Group. *Blood* 1994;84:1361–1392.
131. Hausdorff J, Davis E, Long G, et al. Non-Hodgkin's lymphoma of the paranasal sinuses: clinical and pathological features, and response to combined-modality therapy. *Cancer J Sci Am* 1997;3:303–311.
132. Hehn ST, Grogan TM, Miller TP. Utility of fine-needle aspiration as a diagnostic technique in lymphoma. *J Clin Oncol* 2004;22:3046–3052.
133. Hiddemann W, Buske C, Dreyling M, et al. Treatment strategies in follicular lymphomas: current status and future perspectives. *J Clin Oncol* 2005;23:6394–6399.
134. Hiddemann W, Kneba M, Dreyling M, et al. Frontline therapy with rituximab added to the combination of cyclophosphamide, doxorubicin, vincristine, and prednisone (CHOP) significantly improves the outcome for patients with advanced-stage follicular lymphoma compared with therapy with CHOP alone: results of a prospective randomized study of the German Low-Grade Lymphoma Study Group. *Blood* 2005;106:3725–3732.
135. Hiddemann W, Unterhalt M, Herrmann R, et al. Mantle-cell lymphomas have more widespread disease and a slower response to chemotherapy compared with follicle-center lymphomas: results of a prospective comparative analysis of the German Low Grade Lymphoma Study Group. *J Clin Oncol* 1998;16:1922–1930.
136. Horning SJ, Rosenberg SA. The natural history of initially untreated low grade non-Hodgkin's lymphomas. *N Engl J Med* 1984;311:1471–1475.
137. Horning SJ, Weiss LM, Nevitt JB, et al. Clinical and pathologic features of follicular large cell (nodular histiocytic) lymphoma. *Cancer* 1987;59:1470–1474.
138. Horning SJ, Weller E, Kim K, et al. Chemotherapy with or without radiotherapy in limited-stage diffuse aggressive non-Hodgkin's lymphoma: Eastern Cooperative Oncology Group study 1484. *J Clin Oncol* 2004;22:3032–3038.
139. Horning SJ, Younes A, Jain V, et al. Efficacy and safety of tositumomab and iodine-131 tositumomab (Bexxar) in B-cell lymphoma, progressive after rituximab. *J Clin Oncol* 2005;23:712–719.
140. Horning SJ. Follicular lymphoma: have we made any progress? *Ann Oncol* 2000;11 [Suppl 1]:23–27.
141. Horning SJ. High-dose therapy and transplantation for low-grade lymphoma. *Hematol Oncol Clin North Am* 1997;11:919–935.
142. Horning SJ. Optimizing rituximab in B-cell lymphoma. *J Clin Oncol* 2005;23:1056–1058.
143. Hu W, Chen M, Sun Y, et al. Multivariate prognostic analysis of stage I(E) primary non-Hodgkin's lymphomas of the nasal cavity. *Am J Clin Oncol* 2001;24:286–289.
144. Hunault-Berger M, Ifrah N, Solal-Celigny P. Intensive therapies in follicular non-Hodgkin lymphomas. *Blood* 2002;100:1141–1152.
145. Hussell T, Isaacson PG, Crabtree JE, et al. The response of cells from low-grade B-cell gastric lymphomas of mucosa-associated lymphoid tissue to Helicobacter pylori. *Lancet* 1993;342:571–574.
146. Ibrahim EM, Ezzat AA, Raja MA, et al. Primary gastric non-Hodgkin's lymphoma: clinical features, management, and prognosis of 185 patients with diffuse large B-cell lymphoma. *Ann Oncol* 1999;10:1441–1449.
147. Isaacson P, Wright DH. Malignant lymphoma of mucosa-associated lymphoid tissue. A distinctive type of B-cell lymphoma. *Cancer* 1983;52:1410–1416.
148. Isaacson PG, O'Connor NT, Spencer J, et al. Malignant histiocytosis of the intestine: a T-cell lymphoma. *Lancet* 1985;2:688–691.
149. Jacobs C, Hoppe RT. Non-Hodgkin's lymphomas of head and neck extranodal sites. *Int J Radiat Oncol Biol Phys* 1985;11:357–364.
150. Jacobs JP, Murray KJ, Schultz CJ, et al. Central lymphatic irradiation for stage III nodular malignant lymphoma: long-term results. *J Clin Oncol* 1993;11:233–238.
151. Jaffe E, Haris NL, Stein H, et al. *Pathology and genetics of tumours of hematoporetic and lymphoid tissue*. World Health Organization Classification of Tumours. Lyon, France: IARC Press; 2001.
152. Jemal A, Siegel R, Ward E, et al. Cancer statistics, 2006. *CA Cancer J Clin* 2006;56:106–130.
153. Juliusson G, Merup M. Cytogenetics in chronic lymphocytic leukemia. *Semin Oncol* 1998;25:19–26.
154. Juweid ME, Cheson BD. Role of positron emission tomography in lymphoma. *J Clin Oncol* 2005;23:4577–4580.
155. Juweid ME, Wiseman GA, Vose JM, et al. Response assessment of aggressive non-Hodgkin's lymphoma by integrated International Workshop Criteria and fluorine-18-fluorodeoxyglucose positron emission tomography. *J Clin Oncol* 2005;23:4652–4661.
156. Kadin ME, Carpenter C. Systemic and primary cutaneous anaplastic large cell lymphomas. *Semin Hematol* 2003;40:244–256.
157. Kamath SS, Marcus RB Jr, Lynch JW, et al. The impact of radiotherapy dose and other treatment-related and clinical factors on in-field control in stage I and II non-Hodgkin's lymphoma. *Int J Radiat Oncol Biol Phys* 1999;44:563–568.
158. Kaminski MS, Coleman CN, Colby TV, et al. Factors predicting survival in adults with stage I and II large-cell lymphoma treated with primary radiation therapy. *Ann Intern Med* 1986;104:747–756.
159. Kaminski MS, Tuck M, Estes J, et al. 131I-tositumomab therapy as initial treatment for follicular lymphoma. *N Engl J Med* 2005;352:441–449.
160. Karam M, Novak L, Cyriac J, et al. Role of fluorine-18 fluoro-deoxyglucose positron emission tomography scan in the evaluation and follow-up of patients with low-grade lymphomas. *Cancer* 2006;107:175–183.
161. Kaufmann TP, Coleman M, Nisce LZ. Ki-1 skin lymphoproliferative disorders: management with radiation therapy. *Cancer Invest* 1997;15:91–97.
162. Kelsey SM, Newland AC, Hudson GV, et al. A British National Lymphoma Investigation randomised trial of single agent chlorambucil plus radiotherapy versus radiotherapy alone in low grade, localised non-Hodgkins lymphoma. *Med Oncol* 1994;11:19–25.
163. Kewalramani T, Zelenetz AD, Hedrick EE, et al. High-dose chemoradiotherapy and autologous stem cell transplantation for patients with primary refractory aggressive non-Hodgkin lymphoma: an intention-to-treat analysis. *Blood* 2000;96:2399–2404.
164. Kewalramani T, Zelenetz AD, Nimer SD, et al. Rituximab and ICE as second-line therapy before autologous stem cell transplantation for relapsed or primary refractory diffuse large B-cell lymphoma. *Blood* 2004;103:3684–3688.
165. Khouri IF, Lee MS, Saliba RM, et al. Nonablative allogeneic stem-cell transplantation for advanced/recurrent mantle-cell lymphoma. *J Clin Oncol* 2003;21:4407–4412.
166. Kim GE, Cho JH, Yang WI, et al. Angiocentric lymphoma of the head and neck: patterns of systemic failure after radiation treatment. *J Clin Oncol* 2000;18:54–63.
167. Kim WS, Song SY, Ahn YC, et al. CHOP followed by involved field radiation: is it optimal for localized nasal natural killer/T-cell lymphoma? *Ann Oncol* 2001;12:349–352.
168. Kimby E, Brandt L, Nygren P, et al. A systematic overview of chemotherapy effects in aggressive non-Hodgkin's lymphoma. *Acta Oncol* 2001;40:198–212.
169. Koch P, del Valle F, Berdel WE, et al. Primary gastrointestinal non-Hodgkin's lymphoma: I. Anatomic and histologic distribution, clinical features, and survival data of 371 patients registered in the German Multicenter Study GIT NHL 01/92. *J Clin Oncol* 2001;19:3861–3873.
170. Koch P, del Valle F, Berdel WE, et al. Primary gastrointestinal non-Hodgkin's lymphoma: II. Combined surgical and conservative or conservative management only in localized gastric lymphoma–results of the prospective German Multicenter Study GIT NHL 01/92. *J Clin Oncol* 2001;19:3874–3883.
171. Koch P, Probst A, Berdel WE, et al. Treatment results in localized primary gastric lymphoma: data of patients registered within the German multicenter study (GIT NHL 02/96). *J Clin Oncol* 2005;23:7050–7059.
172. Kostakoglu L, Leonard JP, Kuji I, et al. Comparison of fluorine-18 fluorodeoxyglucose positron emission tomography and G1-67 scintigraphy in evaluation of lymphoma. *Cancer* 2002;94:879–888.
173. Krol AD, Berenschot HW, Doekharan D, et al. Cyclophosphamide, doxorubicin, vincristine and prednisone chemotherapy and radiotherapy for stage I intermediate or high grade non-Hodgkin's lymphomas: results of a strategy that adapts radiotherapy dose to the response after chemotherapy. *Radiother Oncol* 2001;58:251–255.
174. Krol AD, Hermans J, Dawson L, et al. Treatment, patterns of failure, and survival of patients with Stage I nodal and extranodal non-Hodgkin's lymphomas, according to data in the population-based registry of the Comprehensive Cancer Centre West. *Cancer* 1998;83:1612–1619.
175. Kutok JL, Aster JC. Molecular biology of anaplastic lymphoma kinase-positive anaplastic large-cell lymphoma. *J Clin Oncol* 2002;20:3691–3702.
176. Lagrange JL, Ramaioli A, Theodore CH, et al. Non-Hodgkin's lymphoma of the testis: a retrospective study of 84 patients treated in the French anticancer centres. *Ann Oncol* 2001;12:1313–1319.
177. Laperriere NJ, Cerezo L, Milosevic MF, et al. Primary lymphoma of brain: results of management of a modern cohort with radiation therapy. *Radiother Oncol* 1997;43:247–252.
178. Lavely WC, Delbeke D, Greer JP, et al. FDG PET in the follow-up management of patients with newly diagnosed Hodgkin and non-Hodgkin lymphoma after first-line chemotherapy. *Int J Radiat Oncol Biol Phys* 2003;57:307–315.
179. Leitch HA, Gascoyne RD, Chhanabhai M, Voss NJ, Klasa R, Connors JM. Limited-stage mantle-cell lymphoma. *Ann Oncol* 2003;14:1555–1561.
180. Lenz G, Dreyling M, Hoster E, et al. Immunochemotherapy with rituximab and cyclophosphamide, doxorubicin, vincristine, and prednisone significantly improves response and time to treatment failure, but not long-term outcome in patients with previously untreated mantle cell lymphoma: results of a prospective randomized trial of the German Low Grade Lymphoma Study Group (GLSG). *J Clin Oncol* 2005;23(9):1984–1992.
181. Lenz G, Dreyling M, Schiegnitz E, et al. Moderate increase of secondary hematologic malignancies after myeloablative radiochemotherapy and autologous stem-cell transplantation in patients with indolent lymphoma: results of a prospective randomized trial of the German Low Grade Lymphoma Study Group. *J Clin Oncol* 2004;22:4926–4933.
182. Lenz G, Dreyling M, Schiegnitz E, et al. Myeloablative radiochemotherapy followed by autologous stem cell transplantation in first remission prolongs progression-free survival in follicular lymphoma: results of a prospective, randomized trial of the German Low-Grade Lymphoma Study Group. *Blood* 2004;104:2667–2674.
183. Levy M, Copie-Bergman C, Gameiro C, et al. Prognostic value of translocation

t(11;18) in tumoral response of low-grade gastric lymphoma of mucosa-associated lymphoid tissue type to oral chemotherapy. *J Clin Oncol* 2005;23:5061–5066.

184. Li YX, Yao B, Jin J, et al. Radiotherapy as primary treatment for stage IE and IIE nasal natural killer/T-cell lymphoma. *J Clin Oncol* 2006;24:181–189.

185. Liang R, Todd D, Chan TK, et al. Treatment outcome and prognostic factors for primary nasal lymphoma. *J Clin Oncol* 1995;13:666–670.

186. Lister TA, Crowther D, Sutcliffe SB, et al. Report of a committee convened to discuss the evaluation and staging of patients with Hodgkin's disease: Cotswolds meeting. *J Clin Oncol* 1989;7:1630–1636.

187. Logsdon MD, Ha CS, Kavadi VS, et al. Lymphoma of the nasal cavity and paranasal sinuses: improved outcome and altered prognostic factors with combined modality therapy. *Cancer* 1997;80:477–488.

188. Lopez-Guillermo A, Cid J, Salar A, et al. Peripheral T-cell lymphomas: initial features, natural history, and prognostic factors in a series of 174 patients diagnosed according to the R.E.A.L. Classification. *Ann Oncol* 1998;9:849–855.

189. Lossos IS, Czerwinski DK, Alizadeh AA, et al. Prediction of survival in diffuse large-B-cell lymphoma based on the expression of six genes. *N Engl J Med* 2004;350:1828–1837.

190. Lossos IS, Morgensztern D. Prognostic biomarkers in diffuse large B-cell lymphoma. *J Clin Oncol* 2006;24:995–1007.

191. MacManus MP, Hoppe RT. Is radiotherapy curative for stage I and II low-grade follicular lymphoma? Results of a long-term follow-up study of patients treated at Stanford University. *J Clin Oncol* 1996;14:1282–1290.

192. Maher EA, Fine HA. Primary CNS lymphoma. *Semin Oncol* 1999;26:346–356.

193. Maloney DG. Immunotherapy for non-Hodgkin's lymphoma: monoclonal antibodies and vaccines. *J Clin Oncol* 2005;23:6421–6428.

194. Marcus R, Imrie K, Belch A, et al. CVP chemotherapy plus rituximab compared with CVP as first-line treatment for advanced follicular lymphoma. *Blood* 2005;105:1417–1423.

195. Martinelli G, Laszlo D, Ferreri AJ, et al. Clinical activity of rituximab in gastric marginal zone non-Hodgkin's lymphoma resistant to or not eligible for anti-*Helicobacter pylori* therapy. *J Clin Oncol* 2005;23:1979–1983.

196. McKelvey EM, Gottlieb JA, Wilson HE, et al. Hydroxyldaunomycin (Adriamycin) combination chemotherapy in malignant lymphoma. *Cancer* 1976;38:1484–1493.

197. McLaughlin P, Fuller LM, Velasquez WS, et al. Stage I-II follicular lymphoma. Treatment results for 76 patients. *Cancer* 1986;58:1596–1602.

198. Mead GM, Bleehen NM, Gregor A, et al. A medical research council randomized trial in patients with primary cerebral non-Hodgkin lymphoma: cerebral radiotherapy with and without cyclophosphamide, doxorubicin, vincristine, and prednisone chemotherapy. *Cancer* 2000;89:1359–1370.

199. Mehle ME, Kraus DH, Wood BG, et al. Lymphoma of the parotid gland. *Laryngoscope* 1993;103:17–21.

200. Mendenhall NP, Lynch JW Jr. The low-grade lymphomas. *Semin Radiat Oncol* 1995;5:254–266.

201. Miligi L, Costantini AS, Benvenuti A, et al. Occupational Exposure to Solvents and the Risk of Lymphomas. *Epidemiology* 2006;17:552–561.

202. Miller TP, Dahlberg S, Cassady JR, et al. Chemotherapy alone compared with chemotherapy plus radiotherapy for localized intermediate- and high-grade non-Hodgkin's lymphoma. *N Engl J Med* 1998;339:21–26.

203. Miller TP, Jones SE. Initial chemotherapy for clinically localized lymphomas of unfavorable histology. *Blood* 1983;62:413–418.

204. Mills W, Chopra R, McMillan A, et al. BEAM chemotherapy and autologous bone marrow transplantation for patients with relapsed or refractory non-Hodgkin's lymphoma. *J Clin Oncol* 1995;13:588–595.

205. Moller MB, d'Amore F, Christensen BE. Testicular lymphoma: a population-based study of incidence, clinicopathological correlations and prognosis. The Danish Lymphoma Study Group, LYFO. *Eur J Cancer* 1994;30A:1760–1764.

206. Monfardini S, Banfi A, Bonadonna G, et al. Improved five year survival after combined radiotherapy-chemotherapy for stage I-II non-Hodgkin's lymphoma. *Int J Radiat Oncol Biol Phys* 1980;6:125–134.

207. Moore DF Jr., Cabanillas F. Overview of prognostic factors in non-Hodgkin's lymphoma. *Oncology (Huntingt)* 1998;12[10 Suppl 8]:17–24.

208. Morton JE, Leyland MJ, Vaughan Hudson G, et al. Primary gastrointestinal non-Hodgkin's lymphoma: a review of 175 British National Lymphoma Investigation cases. *Br J Cancer* 1993;67:776–782.

209. Morton LM, Wang SS, Devesa SS, et al. Lymphoma incidence patterns by WHO subtype in the United States, 1992–2001. *Blood* 2006;107:265–276.

210. Morton LM, Zheng T, Holford TR, et al. Alcohol consumption and risk of non-Hodgkin lymphoma: a pooled analysis. *Lancet Oncol* 2005;6:469–476.

211. Muller AM, Ihorst G, Mertelsmann R, et al. Epidemiology of non-Hodgkin's lymphoma (NHL): trends, geographic distribution, and etiology. *Ann Hematol* 2005;84:1–12.

212. Murtha AD, Knox SJ, Hoppe RT, et al. Long-term follow-up of patients with Stage III follicular lymphoma treated with primary radiotherapy at Stanford University. *Int J Radiat Oncol Biol Phys* 2001;49:3–15.

213. Nathu RM, Mendenhall NP, Almasri NM, et al. Non-Hodgkin's lymphoma of the head and neck: a 30-year experience at the University of Florida. *Head Neck* 1999;21:247–254.

214. Nathwani BN, Anderson JR, Armitage JO, et al. Marginal zone B-cell lymphoma: a clinical comparison of nodal and mucosa-associated lymphoid tissue types. Non-Hodgkin's Lymphoma Classification Project. *J Clin Oncol* 1999;17:2486–2492.

215. National Cancer Institute sponsored study of classifications of non-Hodgkin's lymphomas: summary and description of a working formulation for clinical usage. The Non-Hodgkin's Lymphoma Pathologic Classification Project. *Cancer* 1982;49:2112–2135.

216. National omprehensive Cancer Network. Non-Hodgkin's lymphoma clinical practice guidelines in Oncology. Available at: National Comprehensive Cancer Network Inc. http://www.nccn.org; 2.2006. Accessed

217. Nelson DF, Martz KL, Bonner H, et al. Non-Hodgkin's lymphoma of the brain: can high dose, large volume radiation therapy improve survival? Report on a prospective trial by the Radiation Therapy Oncology Group (RTOG): RTOG 8315. *Int J Radiat Oncol Biol Phys* 1992;23:9–17.

218. Newton R, Ferlay J, Beral V, et al. The epidemiology of non-Hodgkin's lymphoma: comparison of nodal and extra-nodal sites. *Int J Cancer* 1997;72:923–930.

219. Niedobitek G, Meru N, Delecluse HJ. Epstein-Barr virus infection and human malignancies. *Int J Exp Pathol* 2001;82:149–170.

220. Nissen NI, Ersboll J, Hansen HS, et al. A randomized study of radiotherapy versus radiotherapy plus chemotherapy in stage I-II non-Hodgkin's lymphomas. *Cancer* 1983;52:1–7.

221. Otter R, Gerrits WB, vd Sandt MM, et al. Primary extranodal and nodal non-Hodgkin's lymphoma. A survey of a population-based registry. *Eur J Cancer Clin Oncol* 1989;25:1203–1210.

222. Pelloski CE, Wilder RB, Ha CS, et al. Clinical stage IEA-IIEA orbital lymphomas: outcomes in the era of modern staging and treatment. *Radiother Oncol* 2001;59:145–151.

223. Pendlebury S, el Awadi M, Ashley S, et al. Radiotherapy results in early stage low grade nodal non-Hodgkin's lymphoma. *Radiother Oncol* 1995;36:167–171.

224. Persson B, Fredrikson M. Some risk factors for non-Hodgkin's lymphoma. *Int J Occup Med Environ Health* 1999;12:135–142.

225. Peterson BA, Petroni GR, Frizzera G, et al. Prolonged single-agent versus combination chemotherapy in indolent follicular lymphomas: a study of the cancer and leukemia group B. *J Clin Oncol* 2003;21:5–15.

226. Pfeffer MR, Rabin T, Tsvang L, et al. Orbital lymphoma: is it necessary to treat the entire orbit? *Int J Radiat Oncol Biol Phys* 2004;60:527–530.

227. Pfreundschuh M, Trumper L, Osterborg A, et al. CHOP-like chemotherapy plus rituximab versus CHOP-like chemotherapy alone in young patients with good-prognosis diffuse large-B-cell lymphoma: a randomised controlled trial by the MabThera International Trial (MInT) Group. *Lancet Oncol* 2006;7:379–391.

228. Philip T, Armitage JO, Spitzer G, et al. High-dose therapy and autologous bone marrow transplantation after failure of conventional chemotherapy in adults with intermediate-grade or high-grade non-Hodgkin's lymphoma. *N Engl J Med* 1987;316:1493–1498.

229. Philip T, Guglielmi C, Hagenbeek A, et al. Autologous bone marrow transplantation as compared with salvage chemotherapy in relapses of chemotherapy-sensitive non-Hodgkin's lymphoma. *N Engl J Med* 1995;333:1540–1545.

230. Pileri SA, Ascani S, Sabattini E, Falini B. Peripheral T-cell lymphoma: a developing concept. *Ann Oncol* 1998;9:797–801.

231. Portlock CS, Rosenberg SA. No initial therapy for stage III and IV non-Hodgkin's lymphomas of favorable histologic types. *Ann Intern Med* 1979;90:10–13.

232. Press OW, Unger JM, Braziel RM, et al. Phase II trial of CHOP chemotherapy followed by tositumomab/iodine I-131 tositumomab for previously untreated follicular non-Hodgkin's lymphoma: five-year follow-up of Southwest Oncology Group Protocol S9911. *J Clin Oncol* 2006;24:4143–4149.

233. Prestidge BR, Horning SJ, Hoppe RT. Combined modality therapy for stage I-II large cell lymphoma. *Int J Radiat Oncol Biol Phys* 1988;15:633–639.

234. Qin Y, Greiner A, Trunk MJ, et al. Somatic hypermutation in low-grade mucosa-associated lymphoid tissue-type B-cell lymphoma. *Blood* 1995;86:3528–3534.

235. Rabkin CS, Devesa SS, Zahm SH, et al. Increasing incidence of non-Hodgkin's lymphoma. *Semin Hematol* 1993;30:286–296.

236. Raderer M, Streubel B, Wohrer S, et al. Successful antibiotic treatment of *Helicobacter pylori* negative gastric mucosa associated lymphoid tissue lymphomas. *Gut* 2006;55:616–618.

237. Raderer M, Valencak J, Osterreicher C, et al. Chemotherapy for the treatment of patients with primary high grade gastric B-cell lymphoma of modified Ann Arbor Stages IE and IIE. *Cancer* 2000;88:1979–1985.

238. Ratner L. Human T cell lymphotropic virus-associated leukemia/lymphoma. *Curr Opin Oncol* 2005;17:469–473.

239. Reddy S, Saxena VS, Pellettiere EV, et al. Stage I and II non-Hodgkin's lymphomas: long-term results of radiation therapy. *Int J Radiat Oncol Biol Phys* 1989;16:687–692.

240. Reyes F, Lepage E, Ganem G, et al. ACVBP versus CHOP plus radiotherapy for localized aggressive lymphoma. *N Engl J Med* 2005;352:1197–1205.

241. Ribrag V, Ell Hajj M, Janot F, et al. Early locoregional high-dose radiotherapy is associated with long-term disease control in localized primary angiocentric lymphoma of the nose and nasopharynx. *Leukemia* 2001;15:1123–1126.

242. Ries L, Harkins D, Krapcho M, et al. SEER Cancer Statistics Review, 1975–2003, National Cancer Institute. Bethesda, MD. Available at: http://seercancergov/csr/1975_2003/2005. Accessed November 2005.

243. Rodriguez J, McLaughlin P, Hagemeister FB, et al. Follicular large cell lymphoma: an aggressive lymphoma that often presents with favorable prognostic features. *Blood* 1999;93:2202–2207.

244. Rohatiner A, Lister TA. "Diffuse" low-grade B-cell lymphomas. In: Canellos G, Lister TA, Sklar JL, eds. *The lymphomas.* Philadelphia: W.B. Saunders; 1998:389–398.

245. Rohatiner AZ, Gregory WM, Peterson B, et al. Meta-analysis to evaluate the role of interferon in follicular lymphoma. *J Clin Oncol* 2005;23:2215–2223.

246. Rohatiner AZ, Johnson PW, Price CG, et al. Myeloablative therapy with autologous bone marrow transplantation as consolidation therapy for recurrent follicular lymphoma. *J Clin Oncol* 1994;12:1177–1184.

247. Romaguera JE, Fayad L, Rodriguez MA, et al. High rate of durable remissions after treatment of newly diagnosed aggressive mantle-cell lymphoma with rituximab plus hyper-CVAD alternating with rituximab plus high-dose methotrexate and cytarabine. *J Clin Oncol* 2005;23:7013–7023.

248. Rosenberg SA, Diamond HD, Jaslowitz B, et al. Lymphosarcoma: a review of 1269 cases. *Medicine* 1961;40:31–84.

249. Rosenberg SA. Report of the Committee on the Staging of Hodgkin's Disease. *Ca Res* 1966;20:1310.

250. Rosenbluth BD, Yahalom J. Highly effective local control and palliation of mantle cell lymphoma with involved-field radiation therapy (IFRT). *Int J Radiat Oncol Biol Phys* 2006;65:1185–1191.

251. Rosenwald A, Wright G, Chan WC, et al. The use of molecular profiling to predict survival after chemotherapy for diffuse large-B-cell lymphoma. *N Engl J Med* 2002;346:1937–1947.

252. Rudiger T, Weisenburger DD, Anderson JR, et al. Peripheral T-cell lymphoma (excluding anaplastic large-cell lymphoma): results from the Non-Hodgkin's Lymphoma Classification Project. *Ann Oncol* 2002;13:140–149.

253. Rueffer U, Josting A, Franklin J, et al. Non-Hodgkin's lymphoma after primary Hodgkin's disease in the German Hodgkin's Lymphoma Study Group: incidence, treatment, and prognosis. *J Clin Oncol* 2001;19:2026–2032.

254. Salcedo JA, Al Kawas F. Treatment of *Helicobacter pylori* infection. *Arch Intern Med* 1998;158:842–851.

255. Salem PA, Estephan FF. Immunoproliferative small intestinal disease: current concepts. *Cancer J* 2005;11:374–382.

256. Salvagno L, Soraru M, Busetto M, et al. Gastric non-Hodgkin's lymphoma: analysis of 252 patients from a multicenter study. *Tumori* 1999;85:113–121.

257. Savage KJ, Al-Rajhi N, Voss N, et al. Favorable outcome of primary mediastinal large B-cell lymphoma in a single institution: the British Columbia experience. *Ann Oncol* 2006;17:123–130.

258. Savage KJ, Chhanabhai M, Gascoyne RD, et al. Characterization of peripheral T-cell lymphomas in a single North American institution by the WHO classification. *Ann Oncol* 2004;15:1467–1475.

259. Savage KJ, Monti S, Kutok JL, et al. The molecular signature of mediastinal large B-cell lymphoma differs from that of other diffuse large B-cell lymphomas and shares features with classical Hodgkin lymphoma. *Blood* 2003;102:3871–3879.

260. Scadden DT. Epstein-Barr virus, the CNS, and AIDS-related lymphomas: as close as flame to smoke. *J Clin Oncol* 2000;18:3323–3324.

261. Schechter NR, Portlock CS, Yahalom J. Treatment of mucosa-associated lymphoid tissue lymphoma of the stomach with radiation alone. *J Clin Oncol* 1998;16:1916–1921.

262. Schlembach PJ, Wilder RB, Tucker SL, et al. Impact of involved field radiotherapy after CHOP-based chemotherapy on stage III-IV, intermediate grade and large-cell immunoblastic lymphomas. *Int J Radiat Oncol Biol Phys* 2000;48:1107–1110.

263. Schoder H, Meta J, Yap C, et al. Effect of whole-body (18)F-FDG PET imaging on clinical staging and management of patients with malignant lymphoma. *J Nucl Med* 2001;42:1139–1143.

264. Schouten HC, Qian W, Kvaloy S, et al. High-dose therapy improves progression-free survival and survival in relapsed follicular non-Hodgkin's lymphoma: results from the randomized European CUP trial. *J Clin Oncol* 2003;21:3918–3927.

265. Schulz TF. The pleiotropic effects of Kaposi's sarcoma herpesvirus. *J Pathol* 2006;208:187–198.

266. Sehn LH, Donaldson J, Chhanabhai M, et al. Introduction of combined CHOP plus rituximab therapy dramatically improved outcome of diffuse large B-cell lymphoma in British Columbia. *J Clin Oncol* 2005;23:5027–5033.

267. Seow A, Lee J, Sng I, et al. Non-Hodgkin's lymphoma in an Asian population: 1968–1992 time trends and ethnic differences in Singapore. *Cancer* 1996;77:1899–1904.

268. Seyfarth B, Kuse R, Sonnen R, et al. Autologous stem cell transplantation for follicular lymphoma: no benefit for early transplant? *Ann Hematol* 2001;80:398–405.

269. Shahab N, Doll DC. Testicular lymphoma. *Semin Oncol* 1999;26:259–269.

270. Shenkier TN, Voss N, Fairey R, et al. Brief chemotherapy and involved-region irradiation for limited-stage diffuse large-cell lymphoma: an 18-year experience from the British Columbia Cancer Agency. *J Clin Oncol* 2002;20:197–204.

271. Shipp MA, Klatt MM, Yeap B, et al. Patterns of relapse in large-cell lymphoma patients with bulk disease: implications for the use of adjuvant radiation therapy. *J Clin Oncol* 1989;7:613–618.

272. Shipp MA, Ross KN, Tamayo P, et al. Diffuse large B-cell lymphoma outcome prediction by gene-expression profiling and supervised machine learning. *Nat Med* 2002;8:68–74.

273. Shipp MA. Prognostic factors in aggressive non-Hodgkin's lymphoma: who has "high-risk" disease? *Blood* 1994;83:1165–1173.

274. Shulman LN, Frisard B, Antin JH, et al. Primary Ki-1 anaplastic large-cell lymphoma in adults: clinical characteristics and therapeutic outcome. *J Clin Oncol* 1993;11:937–942.

275. Solal-Celigny P, Roy P, Colombat P, et al. Follicular lymphoma international prognostic index. *Blood* 2004;104:1258–1265.

276. Sonnen R, Schmidt WP, Muller-Hermelink HK, et al. The International Prognostic Index determines the outcome of patients with nodal mature T-cell lymphomas. *Br J Haematol* 2005;129:366–372.

277. Spaepen K, Stroobants S, Dupont P, et al. Prognostic value of pretransplantation positron emission tomography using fluorine 18-fluorodeoxyglucose in patients with aggressive lymphoma treated with high-dose chemotherapy and stem cell transplantation. *Blood* 2003;102:53–59.

278. Stein H, Mason DY, Gerdes J, et al. The expression of the Hodgkin's disease associated antigen Ki-1 in reactive and neoplastic lymphoid tissue: evidence that Reed-Sternberg cells and histiocytic malignancies are derived from activated lymphoid cells. *Blood* 1985;66:848–858. CD30(+) anaplastic large cell lymphomas 3695.

279. Stein RS, Greer JP, Flexner JM, et al. Large-cell lymphomas: clinical and prognostic features. *J Clin Oncol* 1990;8:1370–1379.

280. Stiff PJ, Dahlberg S, Forman SJ, et al. Autologous bone marrow transplantation for patients with relapsed or refractory diffuse aggressive non-Hodgkin's lymphoma: value of augmented preparative regimens—a Southwest Oncology Group trial. *J Clin Oncol* 1998;16:48–55.

281. Straus DJ, Filippa DA, Lieberman PH, et al. The non-Hodgkin's lymphomas. I. A retrospective clinical and pathologic analysis of 499 cases diagnosed between 1958 and 1969. *Cancer* 1983;51:101–109.

282. Suarez F, Lortholary O, Hermine O, et al. Infection-associated lymphomas derived from marginal zone B cells: a model of antigen-driven lymphoproliferation. *Blood* 2006;107:3034–3044.

283. Suh CO, Shim SJ, Lee SW, et al. Orbital marginal zone B-cell lymphoma of MALT: radiotherapy results and clinical behavior. *Int J Radiat Oncol Biol Phys* 2006;65:228–233.

284. Summers KE, Goff LK, Wilson AG, et al. Frequency of the Bcl-2/IgH rearrangement in normal individuals: implications for the monitoring of disease in patients with follicular lymphoma. *J Clin Oncol* 2001;19:420–424.

285. Sutcliffe S, Gospodarowicz MK. Primary extranodal lymphomas. In: Canellos GP, Lister TA, Sklar JF, eds. *The lymphomas.* Philadelphia: W.B. Saunders Company; 1998:449–479.

286. Sutcliffe SB, Gospodarowicz MK, Bush RS, et al. Role of radiation therapy in localized non-Hodgkin's lymphoma. *Radiother Oncol* 1985;4:211–223.

287. Taal BG, Burgers JM, van Heerde P, et al. The clinical spectrum and treatment of primary non-Hodgkin's lymphoma of the stomach. *Ann Oncol* 1993;4:839–846.

288. Tanimoto K, Kaneko A, Suzuki S, et al. Long-term follow-up results of no initial therapy for ocular adnexal MALT lymphoma. *Ann Oncol* 2006;17:135–140.

289. Thieblemont C, Felman P, Berger F, et al. Treatment of splenic marginal zone B-cell lymphoma: an analysis of 81 patients. *Clin Lymphoma* 2002;3:41–47.

290. Thirlby RC. Gastrointestinal lymphoma: a surgical perspective. *Oncology (Huntingt)* 1993;7:29–34; discussion 4:7;7–8.

291. Tondini C, Balzarotti M, Santoro A, et al. Initial chemotherapy for primary resectable large-cell lymphoma of the stomach. *Ann Oncol* 1997;8:497–499.

292. Tondini C, Ferreri AJ, Siracusano L, et al. Diffuse large-cell lymphoma of the testis. *J Clin Oncol* 1999;17:2854–2858.

293. Tsang RW, Gospodarowicz MK, Pintilie M, et al. Localized mucosa-associated lymphoid tissue lymphoma treated with radiation therapy has excellent clinical outcome. *J Clin Oncol* 2003;21:4157–4164.

294. Tsang RW, Gospodarowicz MK, Pintilie M, et al. Stage I and II MALT lymphoma: results of treatment with radiotherapy. *Int J Radiat Oncol Biol Phys* 2001;50:1258–1264.

295. Tsang RW, Gospodarowicz MK. Radiation therapy for localized low-grade non-Hodgkin's lymphomas. *Hematol Oncol* 2005;23:10–17.

296. Tsimberidou AM, Keating MJ. Richter's transformation in chronic lymphocytic leukemia. *Semin Oncol* 2006;33:250–256.

297. Ulusakarya A, Lumbroso J, Casiraghi O, et al. Gallium scan in the evaluation of post chemotherapy mediastinal residual masses of aggressive non-Hodgkin's lymphoma. *Leuk Lymphoma* 1999;35:579–586.

298. Valencia ME. AIDS-related lymphomas—potentially curable in the HAART era. *AIDS Rev* 2006;8:108–110.

299. van Besien K, Loberiza FR Jr, Bajorunaite R, et al. Comparison of autologous and allogeneic hematopoietic stem cell transplantation for follicular lymphoma. *Blood* 2003;102:3521–3529.

300. van der Maazen RW, Noordijk EM, Thomas J, et al. Combined modality treatment is the treatment of choice for stage I/IE intermediate and high grade non-Hodgkin's lymphomas. *Radiother Oncol* 1998;49:1–7.

301. Vaughan Hudson B, Vaughan Hudson G, MacLennan KA, Anderson L, Linch DC. Clinical stage 1 non-Hodgkin's lymphoma: long-term follow-up of patients treated by the British National Lymphoma Investigation with radiotherapy alone as initial therapy. *Br J Cancer* 1994;69:1088–1093.

302. Villanueva M, Vose J. The role of hematopoietic stem cell transplantation in non-Hodgkin lymphoma. *Clin Advances Hemat Oncol* 2006;4:521–530.

303. Visco C, Medeiros LJ, Mesina OM, et al. Non-Hodgkin's lymphoma affecting the testis: is it curable with doxorubicin-based therapy? *Clin Lymphoma* 2001;2:40–46.

304. Vose J. Immunotherapy for non-Hodgkin's lymphoma. *Clin Oncol updates* 2004;5:1–11.

305. Vose JM. Classification and clinical course of low-grade non-Hodgkin's lymphomas with overview of therapy. *Ann Oncol* 1996;7[Suppl 6]:S13–S19.

306. Vose JM. High-dose chemotherapy and hematopoietic stem cell transplantation for relapsed or refractory diffuse large-cell non-Hodgkin's lymphoma. *Ann Oncol* 1998;9 [Suppl 1]:S1–S3.

307. Weisenburger DD, Anderson JR, Diebold J, et al. Systemic anaplastic large-cell lymphoma: results from the non-Hodgkin's lymphoma classification project. *Am J Hematol* 2001;67:172–178.

308. Weisenburger DD, Armitage JO. Mantle cell lymphoma—an entity comes of age. *Blood* 1996;87:4483–4494.

309. Weisenburger DD, Kim H, Rappaport H. Mantle-zone lymphoma: a follicular variant of intermediate lymphocytic lymphoma. *Cancer* 1982;49:1429–1438.

310. Wendum D, Sebban C, Gaulard P, et al. Follicular large-cell lymphoma treated with intensive chemotherapy: an analysis of 89 cases included in the LNH87 trial and comparison with the outcome of diffuse large B-cell lymphoma. Groupe d'Etude des Lymphomes de l'Adulte. *J Clin Oncol* 1997;15:1654–1663.

311. Went P, Agostinelli C, Gallamini A, et al. Marker expression in peripheral T-cell lymphoma: a proposed clinical-pathologic prognostic score. *J Clin Oncol* 2006;24:2472–2479.

312. Wilder RB, Jones D, Tucker SL, et al. Long-term results with radiotherapy for Stage I-II follicular lymphomas. *Int J Radiat Oncol Biol Phys* 2001;51:1219–1227.

313. Wilder RB, Rodriguez MA, Ha CS, et al. Bulky disease is an adverse prognostic factor in patients treated with chemotherapy comprised of cyclophosphamide, doxorubicin, vincristine, and prednisone with or without radiotherapy for aggressive lymphomas. *Cancer* 2001;91:2440–2446.

314. Wilder RB, Rodriguez MA, Tucker SL, et al. Radiation therapy after a partial response to CHOP chemotherapy for aggressive lymphomas. *Int J Radiat Oncol Biol Phys* 2001;50:743–749.

315. Wilder RB, Tucker SL, Ha CS, et al. Dose-response analysis for radiotherapy delivered to patients with intermediate-grade and large-cell immunoblastic lymphomas that have completely responded to CHOP-based induction chemotherapy. *Int J Radiat Oncol Biol Phys* 2001;49:17–22.

316. Willemze R, Jaffe ES, Burg G, et al. WHO-EORTC classification for cutaneous lymphomas. *Blood* 2005;105:3768–3785.

317. Willemze R, Meijer CJ. EORTC classification for primary cutaneous lymphomas: a comparison with the R.E.A.L. Classification and the proposed WHO Classification. *Ann Oncol* 2000;11[Suppl 1]:11–15.

318. Winter JN, Weller EA, Horning SJ, et al. Prognostic significance of Bcl-6 protein expression in DLBCL treated with CHOP or R-CHOP: a prospective correlative study. *Blood* 2006;107:4207–4213.

319. Witzig TE. Current treatment approaches for mantle-cell lymphoma. *J Clin Oncol* 2005;23:6409–6414.

320. Wotherspoon AC, Doglioni C, Diss TC, et al. Regression of primary low-grade B-cell gastric lymphoma of mucosa-associated lymphoid tissue type after eradication of *Helicobacter pylori.* *Lancet* 1993;342:575–577.

321. Wotherspoon AC, Finn TM, Isaacson PG. Trisomy 3 in low-grade B-cell lymphomas of mucosa-associated lymphoid tissue. *Blood* 1995;85:2000–2004.

322. Wotherspoon AC, Ortiz-Hidalgo C, Falzon MR, et al. Helicobacter pylori-associated gastritis and primary B-cell gastric lymphoma. *Lancet* 1991;338:1175–1176.

323. Wundisch T, Thiede C, Morgner A, et al. Long-term follow-up of gastric MALT lymphoma after *Helicobacter pylori* eradication. *J Clin Oncol* 2005;23:8018–8024.

324. Wylie JP, Cowan RA, Deakin DP. The role of radiotherapy in the treatment of localised intermediate and high grade non-Hodgkin's lymphoma in elderly patients. *Radiother Oncol* 1998;49:9–14.

325. Yahalom J, Shah GD, Lai RK, et al. Reduced-dose whole brain radiotherapy (WBRT) following complete response to immuno-chemotherapy in patients with priamry CNS lymphoma (PCNSL). *Int J Radiat Oncol Biol Phys* 2006;66 [Suppl 3]:584.

326. Yahalom J, Varsos G, Fuks Z, et al. Adjuvant cyclophosphamide, doxorubicin, vincristine, and prednisone chemotherapy after radiation therapy in stage I low-grade and intermediate-grade non-Hodgkin lymphoma. Results of a prospective randomized study. *Cancer* 1993;71:2342–2350.

327. Yeo W, Johnson PJ. Diagnosis, prevention and management of hepatitis B virus reactivation during anticancer therapy. *Hepatology* 2006;43:209–220.

328. Yuen A, Jacobs C. Lymphomas of the head and neck. *Semin Oncol* 1999;26:338–345.

329. Zhou P, Ng AK, Silver B, et al. Radiation therapy for orbital lymphoma. *Int J Radiat Oncol Biol Phys* 2005;63:866–871.

330. Zintzaras E, Voulgarelis M, Moutsopoulos HM. The risk of lymphoma development in autoimmune diseases: a meta-analysis. *Arch Intern Med* 2005;165:2337–2344.

331. Zinzani PL, Bendandi M, Martelli M, et al. Anaplastic large-cell lymphoma: clinical and prognostic evaluation of 90 adult patients. *J Clin Oncol* 1996;14:955–962.

332. Zinzani PL, Magagnoli M, Galieni P, et al. Nongastrointestinal low-grade mucosa-associated lymphoid tissue lymphoma: analysis of 75 patients. *J Clin Oncol* 1999;17:1254.

333. Zinzani PL, Pulsoni A, Perrotti A, et al. Fludarabine plus mitoxantrone with and without rituximab versus CHOP with and without rituximab as front–line treatment for patients with follicular lymphoma. *J Clin Oncol* 2004;22:2654–2661.

334. Zucca E, Conconi A, Mughal TI, et al. Patterns of outcome and prognostic factors in primary large-cell lymphoma of the testis in a survey by the International Extranodal Lymphoma Study Group. *J Clin Oncol* 2003;21:20–27.

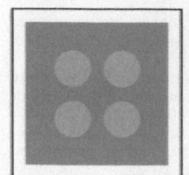

Chapter 77
Cutaneous T-Cell Lymphoma

Curt Heese, Sushil Beriwal, Luther W. Brady, Eric C. Vonderheid

Cutaneous T-cell lymphoma (CTCL) refers to a spectrum of closely related malignant T-cell lymphoproliferative disorders in which the predominant clinical manifestations involve the skin (89,172). There are two major subgroups within the CTCL spectrum: mycosis fungoides (MF) and Sézary's syndrome, in which the malignant cells have an immunophenotype characteristic of mature T cells, usually with CD4 positivity, and show a propensity to infiltrate the epidermis (epidermotropism) (9,16,17,26,63,66,79,95,106,121,131,167,176). The malignant nature of CTCL has been established by autopsy findings showing widespread infiltration of almost every organ system by malignant T cells in advanced disease (18,42,87,144) and by DNA cytophotometric and cytogenetic studies of the abnormal cells (15,21,30,60,90,109,167).

The etiology of CTCL is still unknown. Its relationship to occupational or environmental factors has been stressed in several studies (27,45). Cohen et al. (27) compared patients with age- and sex-matched control subjects and found a statistically significant correlation between industrial exposure and MF. Genetic factors are implicated by reports of MF occurring in families (55,128,136) and an increased incidence of the human leukocyte antigens Aw31 and Aw32 (32) or DR5 (126) in MF and B8 and Bw35 in Sézary's syndrome (125). Finally, a viral cause has been suggested because of clinical similarities between CTCL and adult T-cell lymphoma, a disease caused by a type C retrovirus, designated *human T-cell lymphotrophic virus type 1* (HTLV-1) (13), and the demonstration of type C viruslike particles in skin and lymph node biopsies from patients with MF (137,151). However, screening of blood samples for antibodies against HTLV-1 antigens (52) and molecular studies on DNA extracted from cells of patients with CTCL for HTLV-1 viral sequences (40) argue against a pathologic role for HTLV-1 in classic CTCL. The possibility that a different virus may be the cause has not been excluded (93).

Epidemiology

According to data from the Surveillance, Epidemiology and End Results Program of the National Cancer Institute (NCI) (164), the incidence of CTCL in the United States has increased 3.2-fold during the period 1973 to 1984 and currently exceeds 0.4 new cases per 100,000 population. This reported increase was probably the result of improved and earlier diagnosis (48,163). CTCL occurs more frequently in men than in women by a ratio of approximately 2:1, and blacks are twice as likely to be affected as whites. As with other lymphomas, the incidence of CTCL increases sharply with age.

Natural History

Mycosis Fungoides

Most cases of MF evolve slowly and progressively through three clinical phases: patch or premycotic phase, infiltrated plaques or mycotic phase, and tumor or fungoid phase. This typical evolution is referred to as the *classic* or *Alibert-Bazin form*.

The patch phase of classic MF is the most variable in clinical appearance and duration. These early lesions are frequently mistaken for other dermatoses, particularly eczema, superficial fungal infections, pityriasis rosea, psoriasis, parapsoriasis en plaques, or skin eruption caused by a drug. In some patients, the patch phase of MF manifests as chronic poikilodermatous patches that traditionally have been diagnosed as poikiloderma atrophicans vasculare, retiform parapsoriasis (parakeratosis variegata, parapsoriasis lichenoides), or prereticulotic parapsoriasis (96,97) (Fig. 77.1). After many years, these lesions ultimately can develop into the superimposed infiltrative plaques or tumors more typical of MF (127).

The plaque and tumor phases of classic MF are characterized by clinically perceptible accumulations of atypical lymphoid cells in the skin to produce palpable lesions. Individual lesions tend to regress spontaneously in areas and merge with adjacent lesions to form lesions with irregular shapes. The magnitude of infiltration varies from lesion to lesion, which, with the characteristic configurations, produces a virtually diagnostic clinical appearance (Fig. 77.2). Tumorous lesions may develop gradually from preexisting plaques or may appear suddenly in an eruptive manner, indicating a biologically more aggressive clone of malignant cells. Cutaneous ulceration and secondary infections are frequently encountered in this phase (118).

In 1885, Vidal and Brocq (157) described several patients with MF on whom cutaneous tumors appeared *de novo* without being preceded by patch or plaque lesions. This sequence of evolution is referred to as *MF fungoides tumeurs d'emblée* (*d'emblée,* French for "at the very onset"). This variant is controversial because many cases described as *MF fungoides tumeurs d'emblée* in the past were examples of other lymphomas with secondary involvement of the skin (7). The histopathologic diagnosis of MF in this circumstance may be more difficult to establish on a skin biopsy specimen because the malignant T cells may not invade the epidermis (nonepidermotropic form of CTCL). In our experience, only approximately 1% of patients with CTCL present with *MF fungoides tumeurs d'emblée.*

Erythrodermic Cutaneous T-Cell Lymphoma, Including Sézary's Syndrome

In 1892, Besnier and Hallopeau (4) described cases of MF in which erythroderma developed during the course of disease, either before or after the appearance of tumors (erythrodermic MF). Later, from 1938 to 1949, Sézary (135) observed the presence of large mononuclear cells with peculiar cerebriform nuclei (Sézary cells) in the skin and peripheral blood in four patients with chronic pruritic erythroderma. Lutzner et al. (90) extended the definition of Sézary's syndrome to include erythrodermas and other extensive dermatoses with hyperconvoluted mononuclear cells in the blood (small cell variant). Because of its histopathologic and cytologic similarities to MF, most investigators consider Sézary's syndrome to be an erythrodermic and leukemic expression of CTCL (130). The distinction between Sézary's syndrome and the erythrodermic form of MF is based

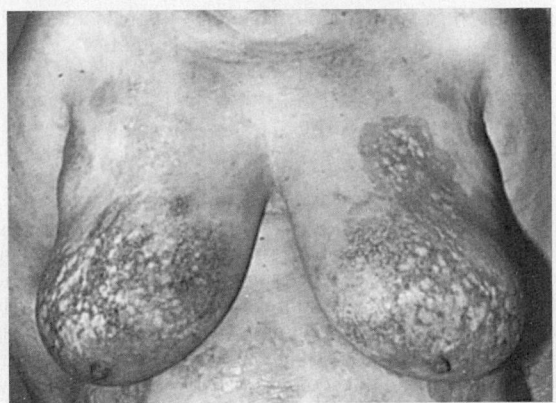

FIGURE 77.1. Classic mycosis fungoides, premycotic phase, presenting as poikiloderma.

solely on the presence or absence of malignant T cells in the peripheral blood (14,90,158). In our experience, approximately 17% of patients with CTCL present with generalized erythroderma, and approximately 50% of these have clear-cut Sézary's syndrome.

Course of Disease

The median duration from the onset of skin lesions to histologic diagnosis of CTCL is approximately 8 to 10 years, with considerable variation from patient to patient. After the histologic diagnosis is established, the median survival for all patients has been reported to be <5 years (27,42,51). However, more recent series record a median survival after histopathologic confirmation of approximately 10 years, which may reflect earlier diagnosis or improvement in treatment approaches (69,160).

Extracutaneous involvement is present in >80% of cases of CTCL at autopsy (42,87,123). Skin-associated peripheral lymph nodes are involved preferentially, if not initially, during the process of dissemination (145) and are considered a poor barrier against further spread. Any organ system can be infiltrated by

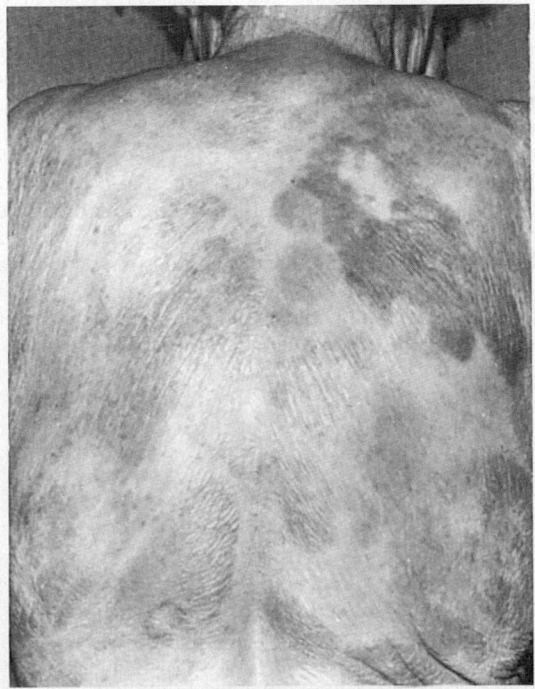

FIGURE 77.2. Classic mycosis fungoides, plaque phase.

malignant lymphocytes in advanced CTCL, but the most common extracutaneous sites at autopsy are the lymph nodes (68%), spleen (56%), liver (49%), lungs (50%), and bone marrow (42%) (42,87,123). The median survival of patients with histopathologically confirmed lymph node involvement is <2 years. Patients with visceral disease have a more ominous prognosis, with median survival of <1 year (19,27,42,69,160).

Diagnostic Work-Up

With clinical data alone, the physician has considerable information about the likely stage, biologic aggressiveness of disease, and prognosis of the patient (80). Several punch biopsy specimens should be taken from the most infiltrated lesions for routine and immunopathologic processing to establish the diagnosis and define the characteristics of the malignant infiltrate.

The status of lymph nodes in the cervical, axillary, and inguinal regions in the staging and evaluation of patients is of primary importance (Table 77.1). If lymph nodes are palpable, a biopsy should be obtained. If the nodes are nonpalpable, it is less certain that a lymph node biopsy should be performed at random. We perform a biopsy of a nonpalpable lymph node only when the patient presents with extensive cutaneous involvement or when radiographic or laboratory evidence of systemic disease is present.

If abnormalities are detected clinically or by tests, an effort should be made to confirm the presence of extracutaneous involvement by histopathologic means. Staging laparotomies have been performed in patients with CTCL, but their usefulness relative to the morbidity of the procedure is uncertain (35,56).

Staging Systems

The staging system proposed originally by Fuks and Bagshaw (50) and Fuks et al. (51) at Stanford has particular significance to the radiation oncologist because it concerns data generated from patients treated with total-skin electron beam (TSEB) irradiation (Table 77.2). A unifying staging system based on the tumor–node–metastasis (TNM) format was proposed initially at a Mycosis Fungoides Cooperative Group workshop on CTCL (20) at the NCI (Tables 77.3 and 77.4). Both the Stanford (70) and Mycosis Fungoides Cooperative Group staging systems

Table 77.1	**EVALUATION OF CUTANEOUS T-CELL LYMPHOMA**

General
  History (attention to pace of disease evolution)
  Dermatologic examination to assess degree of lesion infiltration and surface
    involvement
  Routine physical examination, including palpation for lymphadenopathy,
    hepatosplenomegaly, other visceral abnormalities

Radiographic studies
  Chest radiograph
  Computed tomography of abdomen and pelvis
  Bone scan (when clinically indicated)

Laboratory studies
  Complete blood count, blood chemistry
  Blood smear for presence and quantitation of atypical mononuclear
    (Sézary) cells
  Biopsy studies
  Punch biopsy samples from most infiltrated lesions
  Biopsy of palpable lymph nodes
  Bone marrow biopsy

Table 77.2	STANFORD STAGING SYSTEM

Stage	Description
I	Mycosis fungoides limited to the skin; no tumors, ulcers, significant adenopathy, or visceral involvement (clinical or pathologic)
Ia	Eczematous or limited plaque disease with involvement of <25% of the total skin surface
Ib	Involvement of >25% of the total skin surface; includes the generalized plaque, lichenoid, and generalized erythroderma variants
II	The presence of skin tumors or biopsy-proven dermatopathic lymphadenopathy; no extracutaneous involvement
III	Mycosis fungoides involving the skin with biopsy-proven involvement of the lymph nodes or spleen; no other visceral involvement
IV	Cutaneous and extracutaneous mycosis fungoides with documented visceral involvement

From Hoppe RT, Fuks Z, Bagshaw MA. The rationale for curative radiotherapy in mycosis fungoides. *Int J Radiat Oncol Biol Phys* 1977;2:843–851, with permission.

Table 77.3	TNM CLASSIFICATION OF CUTANEOUS T-CELL LYMPHOMA

Magnitude of skin involvement (T)[a]

T0	Clinically or pathologically suspect lesions
T1	Premycotic lesions, papules, or plaques involving <10% of the skin
T2	Premycotic lesions, papules, or plaques involving >10% of the skin
T3	One or more tumors on the skin
T4	Extensive, often generalized erythroderma

Status of peripheral lymph nodes (N)[b]

N0	Clinically normal; pathologically not involved
N1	Clinically abnormal; pathologically not involved
N2	Clinically normal; pathologically involved
N3	Clinically abnormal; pathologically involved

Status of peripheral blood (B)

B0	Atypical circulating cells not present (<1,000 Sézary cells [CD4+ CD7−/ml])
B1	Atypical circulating cells present (>1,000 Sézary cells [CD4+ CD7−/ml])

Status of visceral organs (M)

M0	Pathologically not involved
M1	Pathologically involved

[a]T1–T4 require pathologic confirmation. When more than one classification applies, indicate both ratings and use highest for staging (e.g., T3 [T2]).
[b]Record sites of abnormal nodes (e.g., axillary [L + R]).

Table 77.4	MYCOSIS FUNGOIDES COOPERATIVE GROUP STAGING SYSTEM FOR CUTANEOUS T-CELL LYMPHOMAS

Stage	T	N	M
Ia	T1	N0	M0
Ib	T2	N0	M0
IIa	T1–2	N1	M0
IIb	T3	N0–1	M0
III	T4	N0–1	M0
IVa	T1–4	N2–3	M0
IVb	T1–4	N0–3	M1

recognize the prognostic importance of cutaneous tumors, lymphadenopathy, and extracutaneous involvement.

Pathologic Classification

The cellular infiltrate of CTCL consists of malignant T cells admixed with varying numbers of normal lymphocytes, histiocytes, eosinophils, plasma cells, and other cells (a polymorphous cellular infiltrate) (61,82). If cellular atypism is not pronounced, the diagnosis of CTCL often cannot be established definitively by histopathologic means. The cytomorphology of the atypical lymphoid cells varies from small cells with hyperchromatic, convoluted nuclei (referred to as *cerebriform cells*), to large cells with pale-staining vesicular nuclei and prominent nucleoli (12,159). Many intermediary cellular forms with pleomorphic nuclei may occur, including the so-called mycosis cell, a mononuclear cell with a large, hyperchromatic nucleus. In some instances, lymphocytoid or histiocytoid lymphoma cells may predominate in the infiltrate to such an extent that a diagnosis of a monomorphous lymphoma is suggested.

In patch, plaque, and erythrodermic lesions of CTCL, the cellular infiltrate is located predominantly in the superficial part of the dermis, often arranged in a bandlike distribution immediately beneath the epidermis. However, it may extend into deeper regions around hair follicles and eccrine glands. With tumor formation, the infiltrate penetrates between the collagen bundles of the reticular dermis and into the subcutaneous fat; the depth may range from a few millimeters to several centimeters, an important factor in treatment planning. Characteristically, atypical lymphoid cells in classic MF and Sézary's syndrome invade the epidermis and follicular epithelium to form small groups surrounded by a haInlike clear space (Pautrier's microabscess). The appreciation of functional interactions between keratinocytes, Langerhans' cells, and normal T lymphocytes provides the rationale that accounts for the observed homing properties of malignant T cells (115,132).

The histopathologic appearance of CTCL in organ systems other than the skin may be confused with that of other lymphomas. The presence of clusters and sheets of mononuclear cells with convoluted nuclei is highly suggestive of CTCL (123). Lymph node involvement is underestimated by routine methods because early nodal involvement cannot be easily differentiated from dermatopathic lymphadenitis or other nonspecific changes. Malignant T cells frequently can be demonstrated in lymph nodes, otherwise diagnosed as dermatopathic lymphadenitis, using special techniques such as quantitative morphometry of nuclear shapes (150), DNA cytophotometry (21,156), cytogenetic analysis (43,166), demonstration of tumor-associated antigens on the cell membrane with monoclonal antibodies (3), and molecular studies to show clonal rearrangement of T-cell receptor genes (165). The T-cell characteristics of the malignant cells explain the early localization of the infiltrate in the paracortical regions of lymph nodes and periarteriolar regions of the spleen.

Prognostic Factors

Age of Patient

Several studies have implicated age as a prognostic variable (42,54,62,147). Patients >60 years of age at diagnosis have a significantly shortened survival compared with younger patients, even when the survival data are corrected for deaths related to CTCL only. When subjected to multivariate analysis in the presence of staging information, age no longer retains its prognostic significance (54), which indicates that older patients more often present with advanced disease.

Stage of Disease

Parameters having prognostic implications include type and extent of skin involvement, lymph node enlargement, and overt visceral organ involvement. The probability of 5-year survival is 90% for patients with limited patch–plaque disease (T1), 67% for extensive patch–plaque disease (T2), 35% for tumorous disease (T3), and 40% for erythrodermic disease (T4) (23,80,172). These survival data reflect the refractoriness of CTCL to therapy, especially in the advanced and late stages. Likewise, lymph node enlargement *per se* connotes an unfavorable prognosis. Histopathologic documentation of lymph node involvement (effacement of nodal architecture by malignant T cells) is associated with a median survival of <2 years (19,28,42). Despite the higher response rates with current therapies, successful treatment of CTCL has not yet translated into improved long-term survival. In the National Mycosis Fungoides Cooperative Group study, the 3-year survival rates were 85% for patients without nodal enlargement, 68% for patients with enlarged nodes located in only one region, and 60% for patients with enlarged nodes in more than one region (80). Multivariate analysis indicates that, although skin and lymph node parameters are highly correlated findings, more prognostic information is provided when both variables are used independently in staging (54).

Clinical evidence of visceral involvement by CTCL (liver, spleen, or lung abnormalities) is associated with median survival of <1 year (19,27,42,161). These prognostic variables have been incorporated into the Mycosis Fungoides Cooperative Group staging system based on the TNM format (Tables 77.3 and 77.4).

Laboratory Studies

The demonstration of malignant T cells (Sézary cells) in the peripheral blood is associated with an unfavorable prognosis (27,42,105,108,155,161). Median survival intervals have ranged from <1 year to approximately 3 years, depending on the criteria used for the definition of blood involvement (158). The presence of markedly aneuploid cells by DNA cytophotometry or cytogenetic studies signifies an even shorter survival interval (21,109,120). This observation may explain why the presence of Sézary cells with diameters >14 μm on blood smears from patients with Sézary's syndrome was found to correlate more significantly with survival patterns than did absolute numbers of Sézary cells (158).

Other laboratory studies that may have prognostic importance include immunopathologic findings (loss of maturation antigens or expression of antigens of activation by malignant T cells) (16,67,79), responsiveness of peripheral lymphocytes to various mitogens and antigens (99), and proliferation kinetics of the malignant T cells (11,39,134,143). Relevant immunophenotypic studies should include CD2, CD3, CD4, CD8, CD20, CD30, CD52, CD68, CD56, p53, and T-cell internal antigen 1 (129).

⠿ | General Management

Staging procedures define two general situations based on the localization of CTCL: patients with disease apparently limited to the skin and those with pathologic evidence of extracutaneous involvement. Current evidence indicates that malignant cells readily circulate between the skin and extracutaneous tissues, particularly the so-called skin-associated lymph nodes and spleen (145,146); therefore, separation of CTCL into these two groups is arbitrary.

Because CTCL may originate in the skin, intensive therapy directed at the skin alone seems to offer the possibility of cure mostly for patients with early, limited involvement (stage Ia). The goal of therapy in early disease is to induce complete remission, reduce tumor burden, reduce symptoms, and prevent disease progression. Frequent remissions and sustained long-term disease-free intervals have occurred in such patients treated with TSEB irradiation (69,71,98,120,122,147), topically applied solutions of mechlorethamine (76,160), photochemotherapy using oral methoxsalen (8-methoxypsoralen) followed by intensive exposure to long-wave ultraviolet light (65,68), and ultraviolet B (UVB) phototherapy using either broadband or narrowband UVB without oral methoxsalen (33). The determination of "cure" requires considerable follow-up intervals because of the characteristically indolent time course of early MF. At present, sufficient numbers of patients have been observed after treatment with TSEB irradiation, topical mechlorethamine chemotherapy, and methoxsalen photochemotherapy to indicate a long-term remission rate approaching 40%, largely in patients with limited intracutaneous CTCL (70). Patients with stage IIB disease have T3 tumor involvement and tend to have aggressive disease with poor prognosis, despite being free of visceral or nodal disease. Most patients with this stage require more aggressive therapy to clear tumors. TSEB therapy, oral bexarotene, and the recombinant fusion protein denileukin diftitox are relatively well tolerated and effective options, although systemic treatment may be required in patients with disease refractory to treatment. Oral bexarotene, which is a retinoid, and denileukin diftitox, which is a fusion toxin protein, have been approved by U.S. Food and Drug Administration for treatment of CTCL in patients who have disease that is refractory or resistant to treatment or who are unable to tolerate other therapies (36–38,111).

Patients with stage III disease or Sézary's syndrome who have leukemic involvement are often best treated with extracorporeal photopheresis with addition of biologic response modifiers as needed (39,40,110,169). Another option in these patients is oral low-dose methotrexate, which is also active in erythrodermic CTCL (129,182). Alemtuzumab is a humanized recombinant monoclonal antibody specific for the CD52 cell surface glycoprotein, found on normal and malignant B and T cells. A phase 2 trial has shown some potential efficacy of this antibody, although severe neutropenia was seen and severe cardiac toxicity may be a significant complication of treatment (88).

For patients with widespread intracutaneous CTCL, particularly in the presence of cutaneous tumors, long-lasting complete remissions are uncommon after therapies with cutaneous effects only, regardless of the treatment modality. The current trend is to administer systemic therapy for these inapparent foci of extracutaneous disease (172). For patients treated with TSEB irradiation, this treatment may consist of administering concomitant multiagent systemic chemotherapy (18,57,91) or total lymph node irradiation (99) if the treatment is being provided with curative intent. However, if treatment is being administered for palliation alone, patients should be placed on maintenance therapy with topical mechlorethamine chemotherapy or well-tolerated systemic drugs after a course of TSEB irradiation.

Pathologically confirmed extracutaneous involvement usually means that systemic chemotherapy must be provided to control CTCL. Several single agents produce beneficial, albeit temporary, responses in most patients. These include several alkylating agents (mechlorethamine [34,41,74,147], cyclophosphamide [1,41,88,146], chlorambucil [22,41,165,171], and temozolomide), antimetabolites (methotrexate [41,67,170,171, 174,181], gemcitabine [174], and pentostatin), and antitumor antibiotics (bleomycin [31,43,135,149,172] and doxorubicin [81,168,175,182]). Attention also has been directed to combinations of drugs, and preliminary results have been encouraging (24,42,58,59,81,91,103,148,180). CHOP (cyclophosphamide, doxorubicin, vincristine, prednisone) has been the most frequently used multiagent regimen in advanced CTCL, and can produce a complete response in up to 38% of patients (46). However, most cytotoxic chemotherapy with either single or multiple drugs results in complete responses in only 20% to 25% of patients with advanced CTCL, and there are no long-term disease-free survivors who underwent chemotherapy alone (172).

Failure of systemic drugs to control advanced CTCL usually is the result of incomplete responses of cutaneous lesions, whereas extracutaneous foci of disease often respond completely. For this reason, additional treatment for cutaneous lesions (e.g., topical mechlorethamine chemotherapy or TSEB irradiation) would be expected to have additive beneficial effects for patients treated primarily with systemic drugs and should be considered for every patient.

Autologous bone marrow transplantation as an adjunct to systemic therapy has been tried in treatment of advanced CTCL (72,116) without achieving sustained response because not all malignant T cells are eradicated from the marrow. The use of allogenic transplantation has higher potential for success in the treatment of CTCL, especially if the prevention and treatment of graft-versus-host disease can be improved (112). Depsipeptide, a histone deacetylase inhibitor, has been used in a small number of CTCL patients with some success (117). Systemic drugs, denileukin diftitox, and serotherapy with ^{90}Y-tagged murine monoclonal anti–T-cell antibodies against CD5 antigen are potential additional therapeutic measures that can be used in advanced CTCL (2,47,107).

Radiation Therapy Techniques

The overall thickness of normal skin varies from <0.5 mm (eyelids) to ≥5 mm (back); the average thickness is 2 to 3 mm. The cellular infiltration of CTCL tends to localize primarily in the superficial portion of the skin but often extend into deeper regions around hair follicles and eccrine glands, even in minimally infiltrated lesions (82,123). The cellular infiltration associated with tumor formation usually extends into the subcutaneous tissue to a depth of ≥15 mm. Ionizing radiation is the most effective treatment for CTCL. Doses as low as 2 to 7 Gy could result in complete clearance of the infiltrative process in the treatment volume. The quality of radiation must be chosen to provide an adequate dose to the lowest margins of the lesion. Several types of ionizing radiation are used in the treatment of CTCL. Grenz-ray radiation is not recommended because of poor penetration. Soft radiation from beryllium-windowed tubes in the 40- to 60-kV range (53,173) and β-rays emitted from ^{90}Sr sources (10) are suitable for superficial lesions and have been used successfully for treatment of extensive skin involvement, primarily in Europe. In the United States, with the development of the modern linear accelerator, the major radiotherapeutic approach for extensive CTCL is TSEB irradiation. A number of technical modifications have been made with the goals of optimizing dose distribution and improving clinical outcome. Emerging evidence from recent studies suggests an association between TSEB techniques and efficacy in the treatment of MF. Based on this evidence, the European Organization for Research and Treatment of Cancer Cutaneous Lymphoma Project Group, in association with experts from radiation therapy centers in North America, has reached a consensus on acceptable methods and clinical indications for TSEB in the treatment of MF (74) (Table 77.5). Superficial, orthovoltage, or supervoltage irradiation also may be used for individual infiltrated lesions.

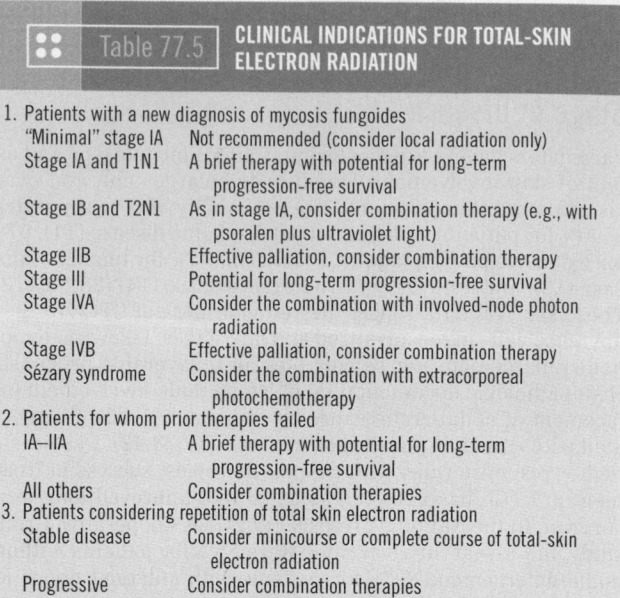

Table 77.5	CLINICAL INDICATIONS FOR TOTAL-SKIN ELECTRON RADIATION

1. Patients with a new diagnosis of mycosis fungoides

"Minimal" stage IA	Not recommended (consider local radiation only)
Stage IA and T1N1	A brief therapy with potential for long-term progression-free survival
Stage IB and T2N1	As in stage IA, consider combination therapy (e.g., with psoralen plus ultraviolet light)
Stage IIB	Effective palliation, consider combination therapy
Stage III	Potential for long-term progression-free survival
Stage IVA	Consider the combination with involved-node photon radiation
Stage IVB	Effective palliation, consider combination therapy
Sézary syndrome	Consider the combination with extracorporeal photochemotherapy

2. Patients for whom prior therapies failed

IA–IIA	A brief therapy with potential for long-term progression-free survival
All others	Consider combination therapies

3. Patients considering repetition of total skin electron radiation

Stable disease	Consider minicourse or complete course of total-skin electron radiation
Progressive	Consider combination therapies

Conventional Radiation Therapy

Superficial irradiation (80 to 140 kVp) with a half-value layer of 0.7 to 1 mm aluminum and a target–skin distance of 15 to 30 cm can be used for most infiltrated plaques. For markedly infiltrated plaques and tumors, higher-energy orthovoltage irradiation (200 to 280 kVp) or local-field electron beam irradiation (10 to 15 MeV) is recommended. Discrete lesions may be treated satisfactorily with a variety of protraction–fractionation schedules, ranging from 10 to 12 Gy in three or four treatment fractions during a 3- to 4-day period, up to 20 to 30 Gy in 10 to 15 fractions during 2 to 3 weeks. Generous portals should be used to cover defined anatomic areas. Because of the possible need for subsequent treatment in adjacent areas, it is important to document the treated areas with photographs, accurate portal drawings, and, if feasible, tattooing of the corners of the fields with India ink (100,101).

Cotter et al. (29) reported on 20 patients (110 lesions) who underwent palliative radiation therapy for cutaneous MF. The modalities for treatment included superficial x-rays, ^{60}Co, and electron-beam irradiation. The total tumor doses ranged from 6 to 40 Gy. Fifty-three percent of the lesions were classified as plaques, 20% as tumors ≤3 cm in diameter, and 27% as tumors >3 cm in diameter. Complete response to treatment was observed in 95% of plaque lesions, 95% of tumors ≤3 cm in diameter, and 93% of tumors >3 cm in diameter. A complete response occurred in all lesions receiving >20 Gy. In the total population of lesions having a complete response, a local in-field recurrence rate of 42% was noted in the group receiving up to 10 Gy, 32% in those receiving 10 to 20 Gy, 21% in those receiving 20 to 30 Gy, and 0% in the group receiving >30 Gy (Tables 77.6 and 77.7, Fig. 77.3). Of the 30 recurrences, 83% occurred within 1 year of treatment, and all occurred within 2 years. The data from this study indicate that tumor doses equivalent to at least 30 Gy, 2 Gy per fraction, five fractions per week (total dose fraction of ≤40 Gy) are needed for adequate local control of cutaneous MF lesions. Our experience at Hahnemann University, based on more than 1,000 individual lesions treated, indicates excellent local control with modest doses of fractionated radiation (10 to 20 Gy administered during 1 to 2 weeks). Bulky tumors and lesions in locations where retreatment could compromise functional or cosmetic outcome should be treated to a full dose (30 Gy during 3 to 3.5 weeks) for optimal control. In most patients, the lesions do not clear during or at the

Table 77.6	**LOCAL RESPONSE TO TREATMENT AS A FUNCTION OF IRRADIATION DOSE (110 TOTAL LESIONS)**			
	$\leq$10 Gy	10.01–20 Gy	20.01–30 Gy	30.01–40 Gy
No. of lesions	27	46	28	9
Complete response	26 (96%)	41 (89%)	28	9
Partial response	1	5	0	0
Recurrence after complete response	11/26 (42%)	13/41 (32%)	6/28 (21%)	0/9
Mean time to recurrence	5 mo	10 mo	16 mo	No failures
Treatment failures (persistent or recurrent lesions)	12/27 (44%)	18/46 (39%)	6/28 (21%)	0/9

From Cotter GW, Baglan RJ, Wasserman TH, et al. Palliative radiation treatment of cutaneous mycosis fungoides: a dose response. *Int J Radiat Oncol Biol Phys* 1983;9:1477–1480, with permission.

completion of irradiation, and it may take up to 6 to 8 weeks for complete response.

Patients with unilesional MF can be treated and potentially cured with local electron beam radiation only. Micaily et al. (100) have reported results of 18 patients of unilesional CTCL treated with local electron radiation to a median dose of 30.6 Gy. The 10-year actuarial relapse-free and overall survival rates were 86% and 100%, respectively. TSEB is not indicated for these patients.

Total-Skin Electron-Beam Irradiation

Various treatment techniques have been used since the introduction of TSEB therapy in the early 1950s. Initially, treatment was administered to the anterior and posterior skin surfaces by passing patients on a moving couch under a narrow radiation beam (149). More recent techniques have used stationary two-, four-, six-, and eight-field positions, as well as rotational techniques. In general, the uniformity of dose distribution improves as the number of fields increases, but at the expense of complexity and increased machine time for the treatment of each patient (6). The optimal technique with reasonable uniformity of dose appears to be a six–dual-field technique refined by Page et al. (113). The electron beam with an effective central axis energy of 3 to 6 MeV and, rarely, 9 MeV is used to treat three anterior and three posterior stationary treatment fields, each having a superior and inferior portal with beam angulation 20 degrees above and 20 degrees below the horizontal axis (Fig. 77.4). The patient is placed in front of the beam in six positions during treatment (Fig. 77.5). The straight anterior, right posterior oblique, and left posterior oblique fields are treated on the first day of each treatment cycle, and the straight posterior, right anterior oblique, and left anterior oblique fields are treated on the second day of each cycle. The entire wide-field skin surface receives 1.5 to 2 Gy each 2-day cycle. The majority of patients can tolerate 2 Gy per cycle. However, patients with previous course of TSEB irradiation or atrophic skin tolerate 1.5 Gy per cycle better. Irradiation usually is administered on a

4-day/week dose schedule; the total dose depends on the intent (curative versus palliative). Doses of 30 to 40 Gy are delivered during an 8- to 10-week interval with a 1- to 2-week break at 18 to 20 Gy for patients treated with curative intent; 10 to 20 Gy is administered for palliation. The average skin dose is calculated as the product of the dose delivered to the center of the treatment plane for one of the dual fields multiplied by a correction factor (F). Factor F represents the fact that any given point on the surface receives some radiation from at least two of the six dual-exposure fields and is calculated from phantom measurements. The percentage of photon contamination for a single dual-field cycle should not exceed 0.3%. Machine calibration is performed daily, as are point-of-dose prescription and side-to-side flatness. Verification of delivered doses should be performed routinely using thermoluminescent dosimeters placed on skin surfaces.

During wide-field skin irradiation, internal or external eye shields are used routinely to protect the cornea and lens. The globe of the eye must not receive more than 15% of the prescribed skin surface dose. If internal eye shields are used, the energy build-up at the surface of the eye shields (if metallic uncoated shields are used) could result in significant overdosage of the eyelids. Shielding of the digits and lateral surfaces of the hands or feet may be necessary because of local skin reaction from overlapping treatment fields in these areas. In palliative setups, shielding of uninvolved skin is recommended.

Areas not directly exposed to the path of the electron beam (soles of feet, perineum, medial upper thighs, axillae, posterior auricular areas, inframammary regions, vertex of scalp, and areas under the skin folds) are treated with separate electron beam fields (with appropriate energy) or individual 100-kV orthovoltage x-rays (0.4-mm aluminum filtration), usually at a rate of 1 Gy daily to a total dose of 20 Gy. Markedly infiltrated tumors may be treated with supplemental orthovoltage irradiation or higher-energy electrons to bring the total dose to 36 to 40 Gy. A comparison of published 10-year data from Yale, Stanford, and Hamilton suggests that progression-free survival might be improved by 10% to 20% by applying patch treatments.

Table 77.7	**LOCAL RESPONSE TO TREATMENT AS A FUNCTION OF IRRADIATION DOSE FOR RECURRENT MYCOSIS FUNGOIDES LESIONS (N = 28)**			
	$\leq$10 Gy	10.01–20 Gy	20.01–30 Gy	30.01–40 Gy
No. of lesions	7	16	5	0
Complete response	7 (100%)	13 (81%)	5	0
Partial response	0	3	0	0
Recurrence after complete response	3/7 (43%)	7/13 (54%)	1/5	0
Treatment failures (persistent or recurrent lesions)	3/7 (43%)	10/16 (63%)	1/5	0

From Cotter GW, Baglan RJ, Wasserman TH, et al. Palliative radiation treatment of cutaneous mycosis fungoides: a dose response. *Int J Radiat Oncol Biol Phys* 1983;9:1477–1480, with permission.

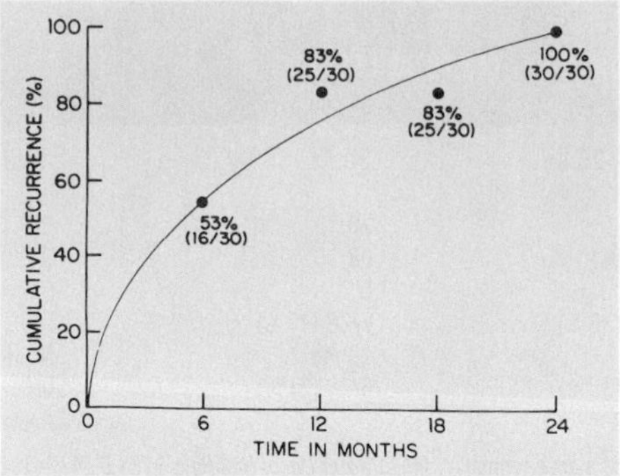

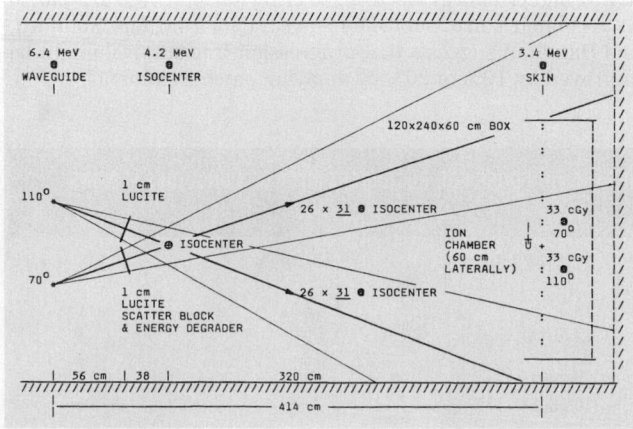

FIGURE 77.3. Cumulative percentage of recurrences as a function of time after complete response to radiation therapy. (From Cotter GW, Baglan RJ, Wasserman TH, et al. Palliative radiation treatment of cutaneous mycosis fungoides: a dose response. *Int J Radiat Oncol Biol Phys* 1983;9:1477, with permission. Copyright 1983 by Elsevier Science, Inc.)

Results of Radiation Therapy

Historical Aspects

Scholtz (133) reported use of ionizing radiation in the treatment of MF in 1902. In 1939, Sommerville (139,140) suggested an "x-ray bath" to large cutaneous areas, but this technique was limited by adverse side effects, particularly bone marrow suppression. Other investigators also reported severe bone marrow suppression in patients treated with superficial radiation therapy to many treatment fields (114).

Total-Skin Electron-Beam Irradiation

In 1951, Trump et al. (149) used a modified Van de Graff accelerator to treat disseminated MF with a beam of 2.5-MeV electrons to a total dose of 6 to 8 Gy during an 8- to 10-day interval, and then repeated the treatment course as needed for recurrent disease. Of 220 patients with MF (50% in the tumor-ulcerative phase) treated in this fashion during the next 10 years, 90 (40%) survived 2 to 7 years, but detailed actuarial survival rates are unavailable (138). In 1971, Fuks and Bagshaw (50) presented therapeutic results in 107 patients treated with 2.5-MeV electrons at Stanford University. They increased the total dose to 30 Gy and presented evidence indicating that the posttreatment disease-free intervals justified a more aggressive

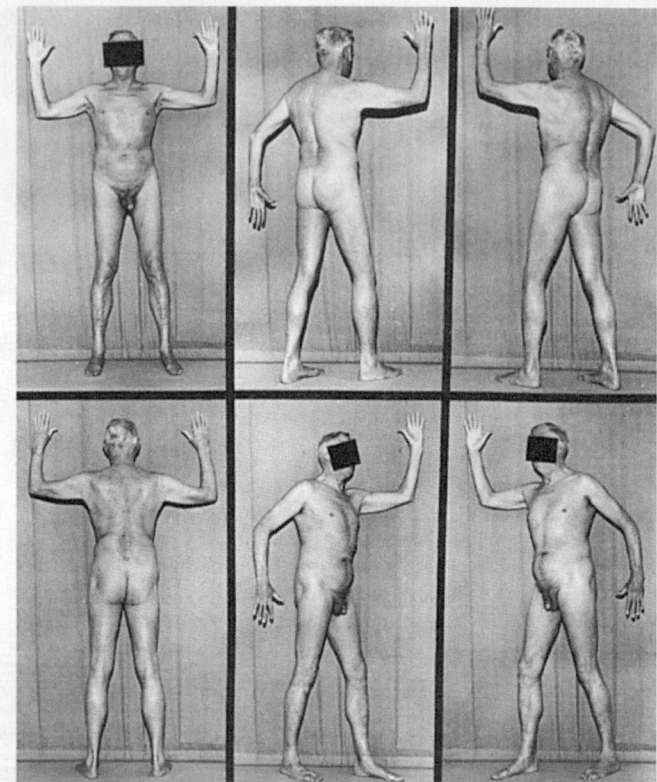

FIGURE 77.5. Positions assumed by the patient for total-skin electron-beam irradiation, six-field technique.

therapeutic approach than that used previously, particularly in patients with early manifestations of disease.

A 1979 Stanford University report concerning TSEB irradiation described patients who had been treated with 4-MeV electrons to doses up to 40 Gy (69). A complete response occurred in 47%, 67%, and 94% of patients treated with low doses (8 to 19.99 Gy), moderate doses (20 to 29.99 Gy), and high doses (30 to 40 Gy), respectively. With initial doses exceeding 20 Gy, 118 of 110 patients (84%) achieved complete remission of disease overall, with clearance rates of 96%, 87%, 72%, and 71% for patients with limited plaque, generalized plaque, tumors, or erythrodermic disease, respectively. The actuarial 5-year survival rates for these patients were approximately 96% for those with limited plaque disease, 75% for those with generalized plaque disease, 28% for those with tumorous disease, and 54% those with for erythrodermic disease. Up to 40% of patients with early CTCL (stages Ia and Ib) who are treated with high-dose TSEB irradiation remain relapse-free for long intervals after treatment, a strong argument for the administration of TSEB irradiation for cure rather than for palliation in the management of early CTCL.

An update reported the outcome of 226 patients with MF limited to the skin treated with TSEB irradiation (>20 Gy) at Stanford University between 1966 and 1989 (71). The median follow-up for all the patients was 9 years. The overall survival of all the patients calculated from the time of electron-beam irradiation was 10 years. Twenty-one of 44 patients (48%) with limited plaques, 14 of 105 (13%) with generalized plaques, 3 of 47 (7%) with tumors, and 2 of 30 (7%) with erythroderma have remained disease-free without any relapse since the completion of electron-beam irradiation. The median follow-up for patients with limited plaque was not stated (71).

The high frequency of initial clearing after high-dose electron-beam irradiation has been confirmed by other groups (8, 25,73,98,108,147,154,162,168,171), but most have reported

FIGURE 77.4. The portal geometry of total-skin electron-beam therapy, as administered at Hahnemann University.

a somewhat lower continuous disease-free survival rate for early CTCL (up to 30% in some series) (98,147). Moreover, not all investigators agree that administration of high-dose TSEB irradiation is the method of choice (86,142). Lo et al. (86) at the Leahy Clinic found that the prognosis of patients with widespread CTCL who were treated with high-dose TSEB irradiation was not significantly different from that of patients treated with lower doses, and that long-term disease-free survival can be achieved with small-field megavoltage irradiation in patients with localized disease (85).

Several radiation oncology groups have used more aggressive radiotherapeutic approaches for advanced CTCL. Micaily et al. (99) treated 19 patients with rapidly progressing plaque- or tumor-phase MF with high-dose TSEB irradiation (36 to 40 Gy during 8 to 10 weeks) and total nodal irradiation (25 to 30 Gy in 4 to 5 weeks). Fourteen patients had disease apparently confined to the skin (stages Ib, IIa, and IIb), and five patients had proven lymph node involvement (stage IVa). Although a complete response was recorded in nearly all instances, sustained disease-free intervals were recorded primarily for patients with stage Ib or IIa disease. These patients had an overall survival rate of 100% and a disease-free survival rate of 44% at 6 years. The acute effects of this treatment approach were well tolerated, but in three patients a second malignancy developed and one patient had myelodysplasia, possibly the result of radiation therapy.

Total-body photon irradiation (TBI) may play an important role in the management of advanced CTCL. Horriot JC, et al. have achieved promising results with low-dose, fractionated TBI (92). Five of 10 patients with extracutaneous CTCL have remained disease-free for >12 to 56 months after treatment. Bigler et al. (5) from Hahnemann University reported results in six patients with advanced CTCL treated with the combination of TSEB irradiation and TBI (one patient); TSEB irradiation, TBI, and high-dose cyclophosphamide (Cytoxan; one patient); TSEB irradiation and high-dose cyclophosphamide, BCNU (carmustine), and VP16 (etoposide; one patient); and TSEB irradiation and high-dose BCNU, etoposide, and cisplatin (two patients) supported by autologous bone marrow transplantation. There were no treatment-related deaths, and the two patients treated with TSEB irradiation and BCNU, etoposide, and cisplatin (BVP) were relapse-free 14 and 13 months after completion of treatment (5).

Sequelae of Treatment

The cutaneous complications of total-skin irradiation for CTCL depend primarily on the total dose of irradiation administered (74) (Table 77.8).

Table 77.8	EXPECTED ADVERSE EFFECTS WITH TOTAL-SKIN ELECTRON RADIATION

Mild erythema in some normal regions of skin with greater skin reaction in areas of prior ultraviolet exposure; the lesions of mycosis fungoides become erythematous, then pigmented

- Complete, temporary scalp alopecia (100%)
- Temporary nail stasis (100%)
- Some edema of hands and feet (<50%)
- Minor nosebleeds (<10%)
- Blisters on fingers and feet (<5%)
- Self-limiting anhidrosis, minor parotiditis, and gynecomastia in men (<3% each)
- Corneal tears from internal eye shields (<1%)
- Chronic nail dystrophy, chronic xerosis, partial but permanent alopecia of the scalp, and fingertip dysesthesias that persist for more than a year (<1% each)
- Acute or late mortality attributable to total-skin electron-beam irradiation (0%)

Short-Term Radiation Therapy Sequelae

The skin of patients treated with TSEB irradiation at doses >10 Gy usually develops mild erythema and dry desquamation that may become uncomfortably symptomatic. Lesions frequently become more erythematous than clinically normal areas during the early phase of treatment and may later become hyperpigmented. At higher doses (>25 Gy), some patients experience transient swelling of the hands, edema of the ankles, and occasionally large blisters that may necessitate local shielding or temporary discontinuation of therapy (119).

Unless hair and nails are shielded, loss of these skin appendages invariably occurs by the end of treatment, but they regenerate within 4 to 6 months (unless previously destroyed by the disease process). Gynecomastia also may develop; the mechanism for this is unknown.

With current methods, a mild leukopenia may develop during treatment in patients treated with TSEB irradiation, but they no longer are subject to severe bone marrow suppression from contaminating photon radiation. Other reported systemic sequelae such as arthralgias and nausea have not been observed in our patients.

Long-Term Radiation Therapy Sequelae

Chronic cutaneous damage from TSEB irradiation is unusual at doses of <10 Gy and is acceptably mild through 25 Gy (119). Superficial atrophy with wrinkling, telangiectases, xerosis, and uneven pigmentation are the most common changes. With higher total doses, frank poikiloderma, permanent alopecia, skin fragility, and subcutaneous fibrosis are more likely to occur but are uncommon. An increased incidence of radiation-induced cutaneous neoplasia has been noticed in patients receiving additional therapy along with TSEB (84). In general, the nature and severity of acute and chronic radiation effects are a function of technique, fractionation scheme, total dose, concomitant use of topical or systemic cytotoxic drugs, previous treatments, and the condition of the skin before irradiation (102).

Summary of Clinical Trials

Total-Skin Electron-Beam Irradiation versus Topical Mechlorethamine Chemotherapy

In 1975, a multi-institutional Mycosis Fungoides Cooperative Group was organized to evaluate uniformly patients with MF and to compare therapeutic results in patients randomly selected for TSEB irradiation, topically applied mechlorethamine, or a combination of both (41). However, the number of patients registered was insufficient to show statistically meaningful results. Nevertheless, one randomized, prospective study (61) and one retrospective study (161) compared TSEB irradiation and mechlorethamine chemotherapy and found no difference in overall survival patterns.

Aggressive versus Conservative Treatment of CTCL

Several groups have reported on the feasibility of combining TSEB irradiation with concomitant or sequential administration of cytotoxic chemotherapy for CTCL (18,57,171).

The response rates usually exceed 90%, with complete responses occurring in most patients; however, no survival advantage has been shown. An NCI randomized study was conducted to compare the "aggressive" combined-modality approach with traditional "conservative" management, consisting of various topical treatments and single-agent systemic drugs administered sequentially as needed (75). The results indicate no significant differences in survival patterns between the two groups (77). The median duration of complete responses after combined-modality therapy for advanced disease was <2 years.

References

1. Abele DC, Dobson RL. The treatment of mycosis fungoides with a new agent, cyclophosphamide (Cytoxan). *Arch Dermatol* 1960;82:725.
2. Bast RC Jr, Ritz J, Lipton JM, et al. Elimination of leukemia cells from human bone marrow using monoclonal antibody and complement. *Cancer Res* 1983;43:1389.
3. Berger CL, Morrison S, Chu A, et al. Diagnosis of cutaneous T-cell lymphoma by use of monoclonal antibodies reactive with tumor-associated antigens. *J Clin Invest* 1982;70:1205.
4. Besnier E, Hallopeau H. On the erythroderma of mycosis fungoides. *J Cutan Genitourin Dis* 1892;10:453.
5. Bigler RD, Crilley P, Micaily B, et al. Autologous bone marrow transplant in advanced CTCL. *Bone Marrow Transplant* 1991;7:133.
6. Bjarngard BE, Chen GTY, Piontek RW, et al. Analysis of dose distributions in whole body superficial electron therapy. *Int J Radiat Oncol Biol Phys* 1977;2:319.
7. Blasik LG, Newkirk RE, Dimond RL, et al. Mycosis fungoides d'emblée: a rare presentation of cutaneous T-cell lymphoma. *Cancer* 1982;49:742.
8. Blasko J, Becker L, Griffin TW, et al. Electron beam therapy of mycosis fungoides. *Acta Radiol Oncol* 1979;18:321.
9. Boumsell L, Bernard A, Reinherz EL, et al. Surface antigens on malignant Sézary and T-CLL cells correspond to those mature T-cells. *Blood* 1982;57:526.
10. Bratherton DG. Strontium beam therapy. *Mod Trends Radiother* 1982;2:176.
11. Braylan RC, Fowlkes BJ, Jaffe ES, et al. Cell volumes and DNA distributions of normal and neoplastic human lymphoid cells. *Cancer* 1987;41:201.
12. Brehmer-Andersson E. Mycosis fungoides and its relation to Sézary's syndrome, lymphomatoid papulosis, and primary cutaneous Hodgkin's disease. *Acta Derm Venereol Suppl (Stockh)* 1976;57:75.
13. Broder S, Bunn PA Jr, Jaffe ES, et al. T-cell lymphoproliferative syndrome associated with human T-cell leukemia/lymphoma virus. *Ann Intern Med* 1984;100:543.
14. Broder S, Edelson RL, Lutzner MA, et al. The Sézary syndrome: a malignant proliferation of helper T-cells. *J Clin Invest* 1976;58:1297.
15. Brouet JC, Flandrin G, Seligmann M. Indications of the thymus-derived nature of the proliferating cells in six patients with Sézary's syndrome. *N Engl J Med* 1973;289:341.
16. Buechner SA, Winkelmann RK, Banks PM. T cells in cutaneous lesions of Sézary's syndrome and T-cell leukemia. *Arch Dermatol* 1983;119:895.
17. Buechner SA, Winkelmann RK, Banks PM. T-cells and T-cell subsets in mycosis fungoides and parapsoriasis. *Arch Dermatol* 1984;120:897.
18. Bunn PA Jr, Fischmann AB, Schechter GP, et al. Combined modality therapy with electron beam irradiation and systemic chemotherapy for cutaneous T-cell lymphomas. *Cancer Treat Rep* 1979;63:713.
19. Bunn PA Jr, Huberman MS, Whang-Peng J, et al. Prospective staging evaluation of patients with cutaneous T-cell lymphoma. *Ann Intern Med* 1980;93:223.
20. Bunn PA Jr, Lamberg SI. Report of the committee on staging and classification of cutaneous T-cell lymphomas. *Cancer Treat Rep* 1979;63:725.
21. Bunn PA, Whang-Peng J, Carney DN, et al. DNA content analysis by flow cytometry and cytogenetic analysis in mycosis fungoides and Sézary syndrome. *J Clin Invest* 1980;65:1440.
22. Campbell EW, Fromer JL. Adjunct chemotherapy in the treatment of cutaneous malignancies. *Surg Clin North Am* 1959;39:585.
23. Carney DN, Bunn PA Jr. Manifestations of cutaneous T-cell lymphomas. *J Dermatol Surg Oncol* 1980;6:369.
24. Case DC Jr. Combination chemotherapy for mycosis fungoides with cyclophosphamide, vincristine, methotrexate, and prednisone. *Am J Clin Oncol* 1984;7:453.
25. Chinn DM, Chow S, Kim YH, et al. Total skin electron beam therapy with or without adjuvant topical nitrogen mustard or nitrogen mustard alone as initial treatment of T2 and T3 mycosis fungoides. *Int J Radiat Oncol Biol Phys* 1999;43:951.
26. Chu A, Patterson J, Berger C, et al. In situ study of T-cell subpopulations in cutaneous T-cell lymphoma. *Cancer* 1984;54:2414.
27. Cohen SR, Stenn KS, Braverman IM, et al. Mycosis fungoides: clinicopathologic relationships, survival, and therapy in 59 patients with observations on occupation as a new prognostic factor. *Cancer* 1980;46:2654–2666.
28. Colby TV, Burke JS, Hoppe RT. Lymph node biopsy in mycosis fungoides. *Cancer* 1981;47:351.
29. Cotter GW, Baglan RJ, Wasserman TH, et al. Palliative radiation treatment of cutaneous mycosis fungoides: a dose response. *Int J Radiat Oncol Biol Phys* 1983;9:1477.
30. Crossen PE, Mellor JEL, Finley AG, et al. The Sézary syndrome: cytogenetic studies and identification of the Sézary cell as an abnormal lymphocyte. *Am J Med* 1971;50:24.
31. de Bast C, Moriame N, Wanet J, et al. Bleomycin in mycosis fungoides and reticulum cell lymphoma. *Arch Dermatol* 1971;104:508.
32. Dick HM, Mackie R. Distribution of HLA antigens in patients with mycosis fungoides. *Dermatologica* 1977;155:275.
33. Dierderen PV, van Weelden H, Sanders CJ, et al. Narrowband UVB and psoralen-UVA in the treatment of early-stage mycosis fungoides: a retrospective study. *J Am Acad Dermatol* 2003;48:215–219.
34. Dolan ME, McRac BI, Ferries-Rowe E, et al. 06-Alkylguanine-DNA alkyltransferase in cutaneous T-cell lymphoma:implications for treatment with alkylating agents. *Clin Cancer Res* 1999;5:2059.
35. Doyle JA, Winkelmann RK. Staging laparotomy in cutaneous T-cell disease. *Arch Dermatol* 1981;117:543.
36. Duvic M, Cather J. Immunotoxin DAB389-interleukin2 (Ontak) in the management of cutaneous T cell lymphoma. *Curr Pract Med* 1999;2:7.
37. Duvic M, Hymes K, Herald P, et al. Bexarotene is effective and safe for treatment of refractory advanced stage cutaneous T cell lymphoma: multinational phase II–III trials results. *J Clin Oncol* 2001;19:2456.
38. Duvic M, Martin A, Kim Y, et al. Phase 2 and 3 clinical trial of oral bexarotene for the treatment of refractory or persistent early stage cutaneous T cell lymphoma. *Arch Dermatol* 2001;137:581.
39. Edelson RL. Efficacy of leukopheresis procedures in the management of cutaneous "T" cell lymphoma: leukemic phase. *Proc Adv Blood Compon Semin* 1977;4:1.
40. Edelson RL. Sezary syndrome, cutaneous T-cell lymphoma, and extracorporeal photopheresis. *Arch Dermatol* 1999;135:600.
41. Editorial. The Mycosis Fungoides Cooperative Study Group Steering Committee: Mycosis Fungoides Cooperative Study. *Arch Dermatol* 1975;111:457.
42. Epstein EH Jr, Levin DL, Croft JD, et al. Mycosis fungoides: survival, prognostic features, response to therapy and autopsy findings. *Medicine (Baltimore)* 1972;15:61.
43. Erkman-Balis B, Rappaport H. Cytogenetic studies in mycosis fungoides. *Cancer* 1974;34:626.
44. European Organization for Research and Treatment of Cancer. Co-operative Group for Leukaemia and Reticulocytoses: bleomycin in the reticuloses. *BMJ* 1972;1:285–286.
45. Fischmann AB, Bunn PA Jr, Guccion JG, et al. Exposure to chemicals, physical agents, and biologic agents in mycosis fungoides and the Sézary syndrome. *Cancer Treat Rep* 1979;63:591.
46. Fisher RI, Gaynor ER, Dahlberg, S, et al. Comparison of a standard regimen (CHOP) with three intensive chemotherapy regimens for advanced non-Hodgkin's lymphoma. *N Engl J Med* 1993;328:1002–1006.
47. Foss FM, Raubitscheck A, Mulshine JL, et al. Phase 1 study of the pharmacokinetics of radioimmunoconjugate, 90Y-T101 in patients with CD5-expressing leukemia and lymphoma. *Clin Cancer Res* 1998;4:2691.
48. Foss FM, Weinstock MA, Gardstein B. Twenty-year trends in the reported incidence of mycosis fungoides and associated mortality. *Am J Public Health* 1999;89:1240–1244.
49. Franchini G, Wong-Staal F, Gallo RC. Molecular studies of human T-cell leukemia virus and adult T-cell leukemia. *J Invest Dermatol* 1984;83:635.
50. Fuks Z, Bagshaw MA. Total-skin electron treatment of mycosis fungoides. *Radiology* 1971;100:145.
51. Fuks ZY, Bagshaw MA, Farber EM. Prognostic signs and the management of the mycosis fungoides. *Cancer* 1973;32:1385.
52. Gallo RC, Kalyanaraman VS, Sarngadharan MG, et al. Association of the human type C retrovirus with a subset of adult T-cell cancers. *Cancer Res* 1983;43:3892.
53. Goldschmidt H, Lukacs S, Schoefinius HH. Teleroentgentherapy for mycosis fungoides. *J Dermatol Surg Oncol* 1978;4:600.
54. Green SB, Byar DP, Lamberg SI. Prognostic variables in mycosis fungoides. *Cancer* 1981;47:2671.
55. Greene MH, Pinto HA, Kant JA, et al. Lymphomas and leukemias in the relatives of patients with mycosis fungoides. *Cancer* 1982;49:737.
56. Griem ML, Moran EM, Ferguson DJ, et al. Staging procedures in mycosis fungoides. *Br J Cancer* 1975;31[Suppl II]:362.
57. Griem ML, Tokars RP, Petras V, et al. Combined therapy for patients with mycosis fungoides. *Cancer Treat Rep* 1979;63:655.
58. Groth O, Molin L, Thomsen K, et al. Tumour stage of mycosis fungoides treated by bleomycin and methotrexate: report from Scandinavian Mycosis Fungoides Study Group. *Acta Derm Venereol (Stockh)* 1979;59:59.
59. Grozea PN, Jones SE, McKelvey EM, et al. Combination chemotherapy for mycosis fungoides: a Southwest Oncology Group study. *Cancer Treat Rep* 1979;63:647.
60. Hagedorn M, Kiefer G. DNA content of mycosis fungoides cells. *Arch Dermatol Res* 1977;258:127.
61. Hamminga B, Noordijk EM, van Vloten WA. Treatment of mycosis fungoides: total-skin electron-beam irradiation versus topical mechlorethamine therapy. *Arch Dermatol* 1982;118:150.
62. Hamminga L, Hermans J, Noordijk EM, et al. Cutaneous T-cell lymphoma: clinicopathologic relationships, therapy, and survival in 92 patients. *Br J Dermatol* 1982;107:145.
63. Haynes BF, Metzger RS, Minna JD, et al. Phenotype characterization of cutaneous T-cell lymphoma: use of monoclonal antibodies to compare with other malignant T-cells. *N Engl J Med* 1981;[illegible].
64. Haynes HA, Van Scott EJ. Therapy of mycosis fungoides. *Prog Dermatol* [illegible];3:1.
65. Herrmann JJ, Roenigk HH Jr, Hurria A, et al. Treatment of mycosis fungoides with photochemotherapy (PUVA): long-term follow up. *J Am Acad Dermatol* 1995;33:234–242.
66. Holden CA, Morgan EW, MacDonald DM. The cell population in the cutaneous infiltrate of mycosis fungoides: in situ studies using monoclonal antisera. *Br J Dermatol* 1982;106:385.
67. Holden CA, Staughton RCD, Campbell M-A, et al. Differential loss of T-cell lymphocyte marker in advanced cutaneous T-cell lymphoma. *J Am Acad Dermatol* 1982;6:507.
68. Honigsmann H, Brenner W, Rauschmeier W, et al. Photochemotherapy for cutaneous T-cell lymphoma. *J Am Acad Dermatol* 1984;10:238.
69. Hoppe RT, Cox RS, Fuks Z, et al. Electron-beam therapy for mycosis fungoides: the Stanford experience. *Cancer Treat Rep* 1979;63:691.
70. Hoppe RT, Fuks Z, Bagshaw MA. The rationale for curative radiotherapy in mycosis fungoides. *Int J Radiat Oncol Biol Phys* 1977;2:843.
71. Hoppe RT, Wood GS, Abel EA. Mycosis fungoides and the Sézary syndrome: pathology, staging and treatment. *Curr Prob Cancer* 1990;14:293.
72. Johnston L, Horning SJ. Autologous hematopoietic cell transplantation in non-Hodgkin's lymphoma. *Hematol Oncol Clin North Am* 1999;13:889–916.
73. Jones GW, Hoppe RT, Glatstein E. Electron beam treatment for cutaneous T-cell lymphoma. *Hematol Oncol Clin North Am* 1995;9:1057.
74. Jones GW, Kacinski BM, Wilson LD, et al. Total skin electron radiation in the management of mycosis fungoides: consensus of the European Organization for Research and Treatment of Cancer (EORTC) Cutaneous Lymphoma Project Group. *J Am Acad Dermatol* 2002;47:364–370.
75. Kaye F, Bunn PA Jr, Steinberg SM, et al. A randomized trial comparing combination electron-beam radiation and chemotherapy with topical therapy in the initial treatment of mycosis fungoides. *N Engl J Med* 1989;321:1784.
76. Kierland RR, Watkins CH, Shullenberger CC. The use of nitrogen mustard in the treatment of mycosis fungoides. *J Invest Dermatol* 1947;9:195.
77. Kim JH, Nisce LZ, D Angio GJ. Dose-time fractionation study in patients with mycosis fungoides and lymphoma cutis. *Radiology* 1976;119:439.
78. Kirova YM, Piedbois Y, Haddad E, et al. Radiotherapy in the management of mycosis fungoides: indications, results, prognosis: twenty years experience. *Radiother Oncol* 1999;51:147–151.

79. Kung PC, Berger CL, Goldstein G, et al. Cutaneous T-cell lymphoma: characterization by monoclonal antibodies. *Blood* 1981;57:261.
80. Lamberg SI, Green SB, Byar DP, et al. Clinical staging for cutaneous T-cell lymphoma. *Ann Intern Med* 1984;100:187.
81. Leavell UW Jr, DeSimone P. Combined chemotherapy (COP) in treatment of mycosis fungoides: report of four cases. *South Med J* 1976;69:915.
82. Lever WF, Schaubburg Lever G. *Histopathology of the skin*, 5th ed. Philadelphia: JB Lippincott; 1975: 696.
83. Levi JA, Diggs CH, Wiernik PH. Adriamycin therapy in advanced mycosis fungoides. *Cancer* 1977;39:1967.
84. Licata AG, Wilson LD, Braverman IM, et al. Malignant melanoma and other second cutaneous malignancies in cutaneous T-cell lymphoma: the influence of additional therapy after total skin electron beam radiation. *Arch Dermatol* 1995;131:432–435.
85. Lo TCM, Salzman FA, Costey GE, et al. Megavolt electron irradiation for localized mycosis fungoides. *Acta Radiol Oncol* 1981;20:71.
86. Lo TCM, Salzman FA, Moschella SL, et al. Whole body surface electron irradiation in the treatment of mycosis fungoides. *Radiology* 1979;130:453.
87. Long JC, Mihm MC. Mycosis fungoides with extracutaneous dissemination: a distinct clinicopathologic entity. *Cancer* 1974;34:1745.
88. Lundin J, Hagberg H, Repp R, et al. Phase 2 study of alemtuzumab (anti-CD52 monoclonal antibody) in patients with advanced mycosis fungoides/Sezary syndrome. *Blood* 2003;101:4267–4272.
89. Lutzner M, Edelson R, Schein P, et al. Cutaneous T-cell lymphomas: the Sézary syndrome, mycosis fungoides, and related disorders. *Ann Intern Med* 1975;83:534.
90. Lutzner MA, Emerit I, Durepaire R, et al. Cytogenetic, cytophotometric, and ultrastructural study of large cerebriform cells of the Sézary syndrome and description of a small-cell variant. *J Natl Cancer Inst* 1973;50:1145.
91. Maguire A. Treatment of mycosis fungoides with cyclophosphamide and chlorpromazine. *Br J Dermatol* 1968;80:54.
92. Maingon P, Truc G, Dalac S, et al. Radiotherapy of advanced mycosis fungoides: indications and results of total skin electron beam and photon beam irradiation. *Radiother Oncol* 2000;54:73–78.
93. Manzari V, Gismondi A, Barillari G, et al. A new human retrovirus isolated in a Tac-negative T cell lymphoma/leukemia. *Science* 1987;238:1581.
94. McDonald CJ, Bertino JR. Treatment of mycosis fungoides lymphoma: effectiveness of infusion of methotrexate followed by oral citrovorum factor. *Cancer Treat Rep* 1978;62:1009.
95. McMillan EM, Wasik R, Beeman K, et al. In situ immunologic phenotyping of mycosis fungoides. *J Am Acad Dermatol* 1982;6:888.
96. McMillan EM, Wasik R, Everett MA. HLA DR-positive cells in large plaque (atrophic) parapsoriasis. *J Am Acad Dermatol* 1981;5:444.
97. McMillan EM, Wasik R, Peters S, et al. OKT 9, reactivity in mycosis fungoides and large plaque (atrophic) parapsoriasis. *Cancer* 1983;51:403.
98. Meyler TS, Blumberg AL, Purser P. Total skin electron beam therapy in mycosis fungoides. *Cancer* 1978;42:1171.
99. Micaily B, Campbell O, Moser C, et al. Total-skin electron beam and total nodal irradiation of cutaneous T-cell lymphoma. *Int J Radiat Oncol Biol Phys* 1991;20:809.
100. Micaily B, Miyamoto C, Kantor G, et al. Radiotherapy for unilesional mycosis fungoides. *Int J Radiat Oncol Biol Phys* 1998;42:361–364.
101. Micaily B, Moser C, Vonderheid EC, et al. The radiation therapy of early stage mycosis fungoides. *Int J Radiat Oncol Biol Phys* 1990;18:1333.
102. Micaily B, Vonderheid EC, Brady LW. Combined moderate dose electron beam radiation and topical chemotherapy for cutaneous T-cell lymphoma. *Int J Radiat Oncol Biol Phys* 1983;9:475.
103. Molin L, Thomsen K, Volden G, et al. Combination chemotherapy in the tumour stage of mycosis fungoides with cyclophosphamide, vincristine, VP-16, Adriamycin and prednisone (COP, CHOP, CAVOP): a report from the Scandinavian Mycosis Fungoides Study Group. *Acta Derm Venereol (Stockh)* 1980;60:542.
104. Molina A, Arber D, et al. Clinical, cytogenetic and molecular remissions after allogenic hematopoietic stem cell transplantation (HSCT) for refractory Sezary syndrome and tumor-stage mycosis fungoides. In: *Proceedings of the 43rd Annual Meeting of the American Society of Hematology;* December 7–11, 2001; Orlando, Fla. Abstract 1715.
105. Moran EM, Walther JR, Aronson IK, et al. Clinical significance of circulating Sézary cells in mycosis fungoides. *Proc Am Soc Clin Oncol* 1977;18:276.
106. Nasu K, Said J, Vonderheid EC, et al. Immunopathology of cutaneous T cell lymphomas. *Am J Pathol* 1985;119:436.
107. Nickoloff BJ. Role of interferon-gamma in cutaneous trafficking of lymphocytes with emphasis on molecular and cellular adhesion events. *Arch Dermatol* 1988;124:1835.
108. Nisce IZ, Safai B, Kim JH. Effectiveness of once-weekly total skin electron beam therapy in mycosis fungoides and Sézary syndrome. *Cancer* 1981;47:870.
109. Nowell PC, Finan JB, Vonderheid EC. Clonal characteristics of cutaneous T cell lymphomas: cytogenetic evidence from blood, lymph nodes, and skin. *J Invest Dermatol* 1982;78:69.
110. Olsen E, Bunn PA. Interferon in the treatment of cutaneous T-cell lymphoma, *Hematol Oncol Clin North Am* 1995;9:1089–1107.
111. Olsen EA, Duvic M, Frankel A, et al. Pivotal phase 111 trial of two dose levels of denileukin diftitox for the treatment of cutaneous T-cell lymphoma. *J Clin Oncol* 2001;68:376–361.
112. Oyama Y, Guitart J, Kuzel TM, et al. High-dose therapy and bone marrow transplantation in cutaneous T-cell lymphoma. *Hematol Oncol Clin North Am* 2003;17:1475–1483.
113. Page V, Gardner A, Karzmark CJ. Patient dosimetry in the electron treatment of large superficial lesions. *Radiology* 1970;94:635.
114. Pascher F, Kanee B. Reactions of the hemopoietic system to agents used in the treatment of dermatoses: effects of low-voltage roentgen ray therapy. *Arch Dermatol* 1946;53:1.
115. Patterson JAK, Edelson RL. Interactions of T cells with the epidermis. *Br J Dermatol* 1982;107:117.
116. Phillips GL, Herzig RH, Lazarus HM, et al. Treatment of resistant malignant lymphoma with cyclophosphamide, total body irradiation, and transplantation of cryopreserved autologous marrow. *N Engl J Med* 1984;310:1557.
117. Piekarz RL, Robey R, Sandor V, et al. Inhibitor of histone deacetylation, depsipeptide (FR901228), in the treatment of peripheral and cutaneous T-cell lymphoma: a case report. *Blood* 2001;98:2865–2868.
118. Posner LE, Fossieck BE Jr, Eddy JL, et al. Septicemic complications of the cutaneous T-cell lymphomas. *Am J Med* 1981;71:210.
119. Price NM. Radiation dermatitis following electron beam therapy. *Arch Dermatol* 1978;114:63.
120. Quiros PA, Jones GW, Kacinski BM, et al. Total skin electron beam therapy followed by adjuvant psoralen/ultraviolet—A light in the management of patients with T1 and T2 cutaneous T-cell lymphoma (mycosis fungoides). *Int J Radiat Oncol Biol Phys* 1997;38:1027–1035.
121. Ralfkiaer E, Lange Wantzin G, et al. Phenotypic characterization of lymphocyte subsets in mycosis fungoides. *Am J Clin Pathol* 1985;84:610.
122. Rampino M, Ragona R, Monetti U, et al. Total skin electron beam therapy in mycosis fungoides: our experience from 1985 to 1999. *Radiol Med* 2002;103:108–114.
123. Rappaport H, Thomas LB. Mycosis fungoides: the pathology of extracutaneous involvement. *Cancer* 1974;34:1198.
124. Rook AH, Suchin KR, Kao DMF, et al. Photopheresis: clinical applications and mechanism of action. *J Invest Dermatol Symp Proc* 1999;4:85–90.
125. Rosen ST, Radvany R, Roenigk J Jr, et al. Human leukocyte antigens in cutaneous T-cell lymphomas. *J Am Acad Dermatol* 1985;12:531.
126. Safai B, Myskowski PL, Dupont B, et al. Association of HLA-DR5 with mycosis fungoides. *J Invest Dermatol* 1983;80:395.
127. Samman PD. Mycosis fungoides and other cutaneous reticuloses. *Clin Exp Dermatol* 1976;1:197.
128. Sandbank M, Katzenellenbogen I. Mycosis fungoides of prolonged duration in siblings. *Arch Dermatol* 1968;98:620.
129. Scarisbruck J. Staging and management of cutaneous T-cell lymphoma. *Clin Exp Dermatology* 2006;31:181–186.
130. Schein PS, MacDonald JS, Edelson R. Cutaneous T-cell lymphoma. *Cancer* 1976;38:1859.
131. Schmitt D, Souteyrand P, Brochier J, et al. Phenotype of cells involved in mycosis fungoides and Sézary syndrome (blood and skin lesions): immunomorphological study with monoclonal antibodies. *Acta Derm Venereol (Stockh)* 1982;62:193.
132. Schmitt D, Thivolet J. Lymphocyte-epidermis interactions in malignant epidermotrophic lymphomas: I. Ultrastructural aspects. *Acta Derm Venereol (Stockh)* 1980;60:1.
133. Scholtz W. Ueber den einfluee der roentgenstrahlen auf die haut in gesunden und krankein zustande. *Arch Dermatol Syphil (Berlin)* 1902;59:421.
134. Schwarzmeier JD, Paietta E, Radaszkiewicz T, et al. Proliferation kinetics of Sézary cells. *Blood* 1981;57:1049.
135. Sézary A. Une nouvelle réticulose cutanée. La réticulose maligne leucémique a histiomonocytes monstreux et a forme d'érythrodermie oedémateuse et pigmentée. *Ann Dermatol Venereol (Paris)* 1949;9:5.
136. Shelley WB. Familial mycosis fungoides revisited. *Arch Dermatol* 1980;116:1177.
137. Slater D, Bleehan S, Rooney N, et al. Type C retrovirus-like particles in mycosis fungoides. *Br J Dermatol* 1983;109:120.
138. Smedal MI, Johnston DO, Salzman FA, et al. Ten-year experience with low megavolt electron therapy. *AJR Am J Roentgenol* 1962;88:215.
139. Sommerville J. General x-ray baths in generalized dermatoses. *Br J Dermatol* 1942;54:234.
140. Sommerville J. Mycosis fungoides treated with general x-ray bath. *Br J Dermatol* 1939;51:323.
141. Spigel SC, Coltman CA Jr. Therapy of mycosis fungoides with bleomycin. *Cancer* 1973;32:767.
142. Spittle MF. Electron-beam therapy in England. *Cancer Treat Rep* 1979;63:639.
143. Sterry W, Pullmann H, Steigleder G-K. Proliferation kinetics of the dermal infiltrate in cutaneous malignant lymphomas. *Arch Dermatol Res* 1981;270:285.
144. Stokar LM, Vonderheid EC, Abell MB, et al. The antemortem clinical manifestations of intrathoracic cutaneous T-cell lymphoma. *Cancer* 1985;56:2694.
145. Streilein JW. Lymphocyte traffic, T-cell malignancies and the skin. *J Invest Dermatol* 1978;71:167.
146. Streilein JW. Skin-associated lymphoid tissues (SALT): Origins and functions. *J Invest Dermatol* 1983;80:125.
147. Tadros AAM, Tepperman BS, Hryniuk WM, et al. Total skin electron irradiation for mycosis fungoides: failure analysis and prognostic factors. *Int J Radiat Oncol Biol Phys* 1981;9:1279.
148. Tirelli U, Carbone A, Veronesi A, et al. Combination chemotherapy with cyclophosphamide, vincristine and prednisone (CVP) in TNM-classified stage IV mycosis fungoides. *Cancer Treat Rep* 1982;66:167.
149. Trump JG, Wright KA, Evans WW, et al. High energy electrons for the treatment of extensive superficial malignant lesions. *AJR Am J Roentgenol* 1953;69:623.
150. Van der Loo EM, Meijer CJLM, Scheffer E, et al. The prognostic value of membrane markers and morphometric characteristics of lymphoid cells in blood and lymph nodes from patients with mycosis fungoides. *Cancer* 1981;48:738.
151. Van der Loo EM, van Muijen GNP, van Vloten WA, et al. C-type virus-like particles specifically localized in Langerhans cells and related cells of skin and lymph nodes of patients with mycosis fungoides and Sézary syndrome. *Virchows Arch [B]* 1979;31:193.
152. Van Scott EJ, Auerbach R, Clendenning WE. Treatment of mycosis fungoides with cyclophosphamide. *Arch Dermatol* 1962;85:499.
153. Van Scott EJ, Grekin DA, Kalmanson JD, et al. Frequent low doses of intravenous mechlorethamine for late-stage mycosis fungoides lymphoma. *Cancer* 1975;36:1613.
154. Van Vloten WA, de Vroome H, Noordijk FM. Total skin electron beam irradiation for cutaneous T-cell lymphoma (mycosis fungoides). *Br J Dermatol* 1985;112:697.
155. Van Vloten WA, Polano MK. Bleomycin therapy in mycosis fungoides. *Dermatologica* 1975;150:50.
156. Van Vloten WA, Scheffer E, Meijer CJLM. DNA cytophotometry of lymph node imprints from patients with mycosis fungoides. *J Invest Dermatol* 1979;73:275.
157. Vidal E, Brocq L. Etude sur le mycosis fungoide. *France Med* 1885;2:946,957,969, 983,993,1005,1019.
158. Vonderheid EC, Sobel EL, Nowell PC, et al. Diagnostic and prognostic significance of Sézary cells in peripheral blood smears from patients with cutaneous T-cell lymphoma. *Blood* 1985;66:358.
159. Vonderheid EC, Tam DW, Johnson WC, et al. Prognostic significance of cytomorphology in cutaneous T-cell lymphomas. *Cancer* 1981;47:119.
160. Vonderheid EC, Tan ET, Kantor AF, et al. Long-term efficacy, curative potential, and carcinogenicity of topical mechlorethamine chemotherapy in cutaneous T-cell lymphoma. *J Am Acad Dermatol* 1989;20:416.

161. Vonderheid EC, Van Scott EJ, Wallner PE, et al. A 10-year experience with topical mechlorethamine for mycosis fungoides: comparison with patients treated by total-skin electron beam radiation therapy. *Cancer Treat Rep* 1979;63:681.

162. Wallner PE, Vonderheid EC, Brady LW, et al. Evaluation and recommendations for therapy of advanced mycosis fungoides lymphoma. *Int J Radiat Oncol Biol Phys* 1979;5:23.

163. Weinstock MA, Gardstein B. Twenty-year trend in the reported incidence of mycosis fungoides and associated mortality. *Am J Public Health* 1999;89:1240–1244.

164. Weinstock MA, Horm JW. Mycosis fungoides in the United States. *JAMA* 1988;260:42.

165. Weiss LM, Hu E, Wood GS, et al. Clonal rearrangements of T-cell receptor genes in mycosis fungoides and dermatolopathic lymphadenopathy. *N Engl J Med* 1985;313:539.

166. Whang-Peng J, Bunn PA Jr, Knutsen T, et al. Clinical implications of cytogenetic studies in cutaneous T-cell lymphoma (CTCL). *Cancer* 1982;50:1539.

167. Willemze R, De Graaff-Reitsma CB, Cnossen J, et al. Characterization of T-cell subpopulations in skin and peripheral blood of patients with cutaneous T-cell lymphomas and benign inflammatory dermatoses. *J Invest Dermatol* 1983;80:60.

168. Williams PC, Hunter RD, Jackson SM. Whole body electron therapy in mycosis fungoides: a successful translational technique achieved by modification of an established linear accelerator. *Br J Radiol* 1979;52:302.

169. Wilson LD, Jones GW, Kim D, et al. Experience with total skin electron beam therapy in combination with extracorporeal photopheresis in the management of patients with erythrodermic (T4) mycosis fungoides. *J Am Acad Dermatol* 2000;43:54–60.

170. Wilson LD, Jones GW, Kim D, et al. Experience with total skin electron beam therapy in combination with extracorporeal photopheresis in the management of patients with erythrodermic (T4) mycosis fungoides. *J Am Acad Dermatol* 2000;43:54–60.

171. Wilson LD, Licata AL, Braverman IM, et al. Systemic chemotherapy and extracorporal photochemotherapy for T3 and T4 cutaneous T-cell lymphoma patients who have achieved complete response to total skin electron beam radiation. *Int J Radiat Oncol Biol Phys* 1995;32:987.

172. Winkelmann RK, Diaz-Perez JL, Buechner SA. The treatment of Sézary syndrome. *J Am Acad Dermatol* 1984;10:1000.

173. Winkler CF, Bunn PA Jr. Cutaneous T-cell lymphoma: a review. *CRC Crit Rev Oncol Hematol* 1983;1:49.

174. Wiskemann A, Buck C. Radiotherapy of mycosis fungoides: twenty years of experience with teleroentgen and low voltage x-ray therapy. *J Dermatol Surg Oncol* 1978;4:606.

175. Wollina U, Dummer R, Brockmeyer NH, et al. Multicenter study of pegylated liposomal doxorubicin in patients with cutaneous T-cell lymphoma. *Cancer* 2003;98:993–1001.

176. Wollina U, Graefe T, Kaatz M. Pegylated doxorubicin for primary cutaneous T cell lymphoma. *Ann N Y Acad Sci* 2001;941:214–216.

177. Wood GS, Deneau DG, Miller RA, et al. Subtypes of cutaneous T-cell lymphoma defined by expression of Leu-1 and 1a. *Blood* 1982;59:876.

178. Wright JC, Gumport SL, Golomb FM. Remissions produced with the use of methotrexate in patients with mycosis fungoides. *Cancer Chemother Rep* 1960;9:11.

179. Wright JC, Lyons MM, Walker DG, et al. Observations on the use of cancer chemotherapeutic agents in patients with mycosis fungoides. *Cancer* 1964;17:1045.

180. Yagoda A, Mukherji B, Young C, et al. Bleomycin: an antitumor antibiotic. *Ann Intern Med* 1972;77:861.

181. Zachariae H, Grunnet E, Thestrup-Pederson K, et al. Oral retinoid in combination with bleomycin, cyclophosphamide, prednisone, and transfer factor in mycosis fungoides. *Acta Derm Venereol (Stockh)* 1982;62:162.

182. Zackheim HS, Kashani-Sabet M, McMillan A. Low-dose methotrexate to treat mycosis fungoides: a retrospective study in 69 patients. *J Am Acad Dermatol* 2003;49:873–878.

183. Zinzani PL, Baliva G, Magagnoli M, et al. Gemcitabine treatment in pretreated cutaneous T-cell lymphoma: experience in 44 patients. *J Clin Oncol* 2000;18:2603–2606.

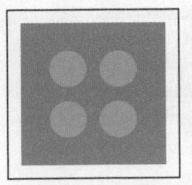

Chapter 78
Leukemia

Kenneth B. Roberts, Stuart Seropian

The leukemias are a neoplastic disorder of the hematopoietic system, characterized by aberrant or arrested differentiation. The role of radiotherapy in curative treatment is largely to deliver central nervous system (CNS) treatment in combination with systemic therapy for patients with acute lymphocytic leukemia (ALL). Although the role of CNS prophylaxis has declined during the last 15 years because of toxicity concerns, it remains an important component of therapy for high-risk patients. Radiation oncologists must also be familiar with certain palliative situations unique to leukemias as well as total body irradiation (discussed in Chapter 14) as the latter is often part of a stem cell transplant program.

Childhood ALL can now be cured in approximately 86% of cases, with initial remissions generally occurring in 90% (54,93). In adults, ALL remission rates are equally high, but cure rates are only in the 30% to 45% range (65). Pediatric acute myelocytic leukemia (AML) generally also fairs poorly with 50% cure rates, although this represents a marked improvement since the 1970s when cure rates were roughly 20% (54). Adult AML cures are less frequent, in good part a reflection that this disease principally afflicts the elderly. In the United States, the estimated annual incidence and mortality from AML are 11,930 cases and 9,040 deaths (54). Allogeneic stem cell transplantation has specifically targeted AML or refractory/recurrent ALL. Reduced-intensity transplants are being investigated to address the needs of high-risk or elderly patients with acute leukemia.

Chronic myelogenous leukemia (CML) and chronic lymphocytic leukemia (CLL) have natural histories measured in years to decades. Both have the ability to transform to more aggressive diseases, although CML in particular, reliably progresses to a more acute disease or blast crisis in its terminal phase. Allogeneic stem cell transplantation is associated with a high cure rate for patients with CML if conducted early in the chronic phase of the disease.

Anatomic Considerations

The radiation oncologist must be knowledgeable about the anatomy of the CNS, particularly the meninges (dura mater, arachnoid, and pia mater) and subarachnoid space for the proper design of CNS-directed radiation treatments. The epidural space lies between periosteum and the dura, and the potential space between the dura and arachnoid is called the *subdural space*. The pia and arachnoid are often described as a combined membrane called the *leptomeninges*. Between the arachnoid and pia is the subarachnoid space, which is filled with cerebrospinal fluid (CSF). The pia hugs the surface of the brain extending into sulci, fissures, and the internal cavities or ventricles, and the bulk of the arachnoid follows along the dura except for the fine trabeculations and into some of the major fissures of the brain. Arachnoid sheathes both nerves and blood vessels penetrating the pia and exiting the CNS creating relatively short segments of subarachnoid space, which is of particular anatomic importance in the vertebral column. In the design of the inferior aspect of craniospinal radiation fields, the subarachnoid space extends laterally to the spinal ganglia, which

are located within the intervertebral foramina (48,49). Thus, coverage of the entire sacroiliac joints in such spinal field design is excessive. The caudad extent of the subarachnoid space is variable within the sacrum (32). Clinically, the end of the thecal sac is now routinely determined on magnetic resonance image scanning. Pathologically, CNS leukemia originates as a perivascular infiltrate along the subpial blood vessels. As this infiltrate progresses, the leukemia permeates preferentially into the subarachnoid space, but also into the brain parenchyma (92).

Base of skull anatomy is also of importance to the radiation oncologist in the design of lateral cranial fields. The middle cranial fossa and temporal lobe project over the sphenoid sinuses on lateral radiographs. The cribriform plate projects along the roof of the orbit along an imaginary line that connects to the inferior aspect of the frontal sinuses. Several radiologic-anatomic studies have pointed out how the eye's lens in this "beam's-eye view" is <1 cm away from the cribriform plate, having implications in field design. Ensuring coverage of the entire subarachnoid space should supersede the concerns of radiation-induced cataracts (57,133). Moreover, as subarachnoid space extends as a sheath along the optic nerve, it is standard to include the posterior half of the eye globes within cranial radiation fields by using the anterolateral aspect of the bony orbit as an anatomic landmark, as it typically lies along a line that roughly bisects the eye (133) (Figs. 78.1 and 78.2).

To compensate for the blood–brain barrier, certain drugs are administered directly into the subarachnoid space either via lumbar puncture or an intraventricular reservoir (e.g., an Ommaya reservoir). Intrathecal (IT) drugs distribute unevenly, however, throughout the subarachnoid space (102,110). This is not surprising, given the knowledge of brain anatomy and CSF circulation. CSF is mainly formed in the brain ventricles by the choroid plexuses, which are specialized capillary-rich tufted structures. This fluid then flows through the intraventricular foramina and the cerebral aqueduct of the midbrain into the fourth ventricle, from where it communicates with the rest of the subarachnoid space. CSF is resorbed principally in the dural sinuses via buttonlike projections called *arachnoid villi*. Thus, IT therapy theoretically undertreats the ventricular spaces and cerebral/cerebellar sulci as well as any gross disease extending into the brain substance. This concern has led to the concept of combining cranial radiotherapy with IT chemotherapy, the latter to cover the spinal subarachnoid space. Similarly, when craniospinal irradiation (CSI) is needed to treat a higher burden of CNS leukemia, IT therapy allows the spine to be treated to a lower dose than the brain.

Acute Leukemias

Classification Systems, Pathology, and Risk Stratification

Acute leukemias have traditionally been classified using the French-American-British (FAB) morphologic and cytologic criteria of classification. AML and its subtypes can most often be

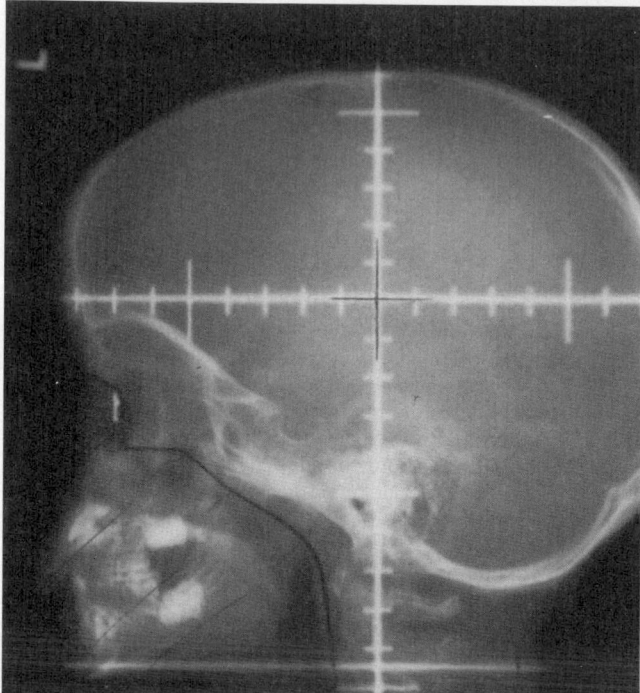

FIGURE 78.1. Cranial irradiation field outlining treatment that encompasses the entire cranial subarachnoid space. The radio-opaque markers outline the anterior aspect of the bony orbit so as to demarcate inclusion of the posterior aspect of the eye within the treatment fields. (From Halperin EC, et al., eds., *Pediatric Radiation Oncology*, 4th ed. Leukemia chapter, Philadelphia: Lippincott Williams & Wilkins, p. 22, with permission.)

Table 78.1	CORRELATION OF FRENCH-AMERICAN-BRITISH (FAB) CLASSIFICATION OF ACUTE MYELOGENOUS LEUKEMIA (AML) WITH COMMON CYTOGENETIC ABNORMALITIES
FAB Type	**Cytogenetic Finding**
M0, M1 (Undifferentiated AML)	trisomy 11, t(10;11)
M2 (Acute myeloid leukemia)	t(8;21)
M3 (Acute promyelocytic leukemia)	t(15;17), t(11;17), t(5;17)
M4Eo (Acute myelomonocytic leukemia with eosinophilia)	inv(16)
M5 (Acute monocytic leukemia)	t(11;23)
M6 (Acute erythroleukemia)	t(3;5)
M7 (Acute megakaryocytic leukemia)	t(3;3), t(3;12)

differentiated AML subtypes M2-M6 are usually recognizable by morphology and cytochemistry.

Recently, the World Health Organization (WHO) proposed a new classification scheme for myeloid neoplasms (127). The WHO classification creates three new subgroups based on the presence of recurring genetic abnormalities, dysplastic features, or history of alkylator or topoisomerase therapy. Leukemias bearing none of these features are grouped according to maturation features, similar to the traditional FAB classification, in a fourth subgroup termed *AML, not otherwise categorized*. The new subgroups are meant to highlight meaningful biologic and genetic differences between disease entities with differing prognosis and clinical behavior. In addition, in the new WHO scheme the number of blasts in the blood or bone marrow required to confirm a diagnosis of AML was lowered from 30% to 20%.

The FAB classification for ALL has three subtypes based on morphology. L1 is the predominant type in 85% of childhood ALL. It is characterized by small cells with scanty cytoplasm and inconspicuous nucleoli. L2 is common in ALL of adults and is identified morphologically by blasts that show prominent nucleoli, abundant cytoplasm and more variability in size.

identified microscopically by the presence of Auer rods, staining for myeloperoxidase or monocyte-associated esterases, and other cytologic features of differentiation. Certain chromosome translocations are common to each AML subtype, as also shown in Table 78.1. AML with minimal or no myeloid differentiation (M1 and M0 subtypes) can be confused with ALL but for flow cytometric identification of early myeloid antigens. The more

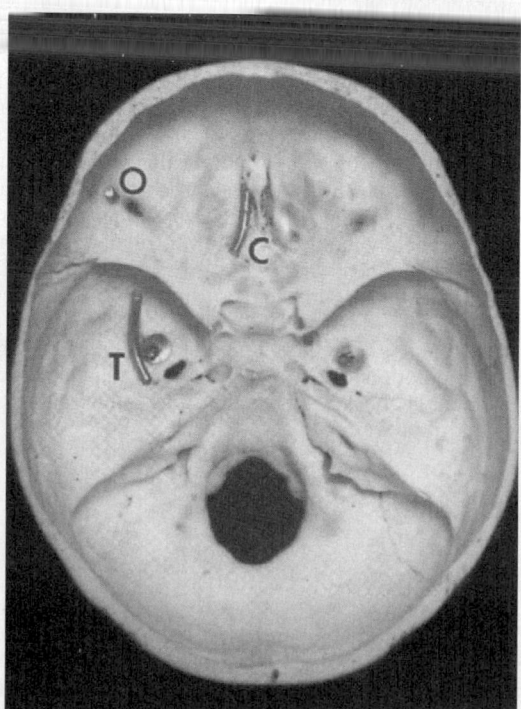

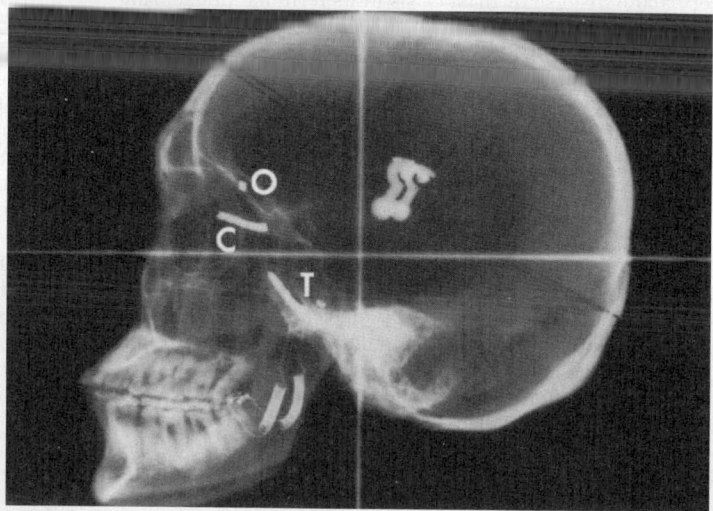

FIGURE 78.2. Skull views outlining anatomic limits of the base of skull for inclusion of the cranial subarachnoid space. **A:** Radio-opaque markers have been placed at the cribriform plate (C), roof of the orbit (O), and the temporal fossa (T). **B:** Plain lateral radiograph shows the projection of the cribriform plate, orbital roof, and temporal fossa. (From Halperin EC, et al., eds., *Pediatric Radiation Oncology*, 4th ed., Leukemia chapter, Philadelphia: Lippincott Williams & Wilkins, p. 22, with permission.)

L3 lymphoblasts are large cells with cytoplasmic basophilia and vacuolization, similar to Burkitt's lymphoma cells. The common ALL antigen is expressed in about 85% of ALL cases. At least with childhood ALL, this FAB system has not proved to be terribly useful, with high interobserver variability and a lack of correlation with the more prognostically important immunologic and genetic features for ALL (94).

Immunophenotyping is a cornerstone in classifying ALL and some forms of AML. Flow cytometry using specific monoclonal antibodies can be used to assay for a panel of antigens, often known as *cluster of differentiation (CD) molecules,* that define leukocyte maturation. For instance, CD19 and cytoplasmic CD79a define B-cell lineage and CD7 and CD3 define T-cell lineage. Myeloid cells are correlated with positivity for CD13, CD33, and cytoplasmic myeloperoxidase. With other markers defining different degrees of differentiation and maturation, ALL is now conventionally divided into T-cell and B-cell lineage. B-cell leukemia has four distinct subclasses: early pre-B, pre-B, transitional pre-B, and the more mature B-cell. The transitional pre-B subclass is relatively new and is associated with a relatively good prognosis in children (60).

Cytogenetic or chromosomal abnormalities occur in up to 90% of ALL cases. Of these, roughly two-thirds are nonrandom, falling into distinct patterns. Some of these have distinct prognostic and therapeutic implications. Adult and childhood forms of ALL have distinctly different patterns of genetic abnormalities as well as immunophenotyping (Table 78.2). This may partially explain the poorer prognosis in older patients. For example, the Philadelphia chromosome or bcr/abl gene fusion/t(9;22) translocation in precursor B-cell ALL is associated with a poorer prognosis. It occurs in 4% of childhood ALL cases compared with 25% in adults. Abnormal DNA ploidy is extremely common, but two patterns seem to be clinically important. Hyperdiploidy with >50 chromosomes per cell (or DNA index >1.6) occurs in 25% of children with ALL. Although there is some association with favorable clinical factors (age >10 years and low presenting leukocyte counts), hyperdiploidy is an independent favorable factor, except in adults with ALL, in which outcomes are poor.

The aforementioned laboratory assessment and clinical disease features have led to distinct risk stratification categories, at least as far as childhood ALL is concerned. Clinical prognostic features of B-cell leukemias have been commonly used to place patients into risk groups. Standard risk has been generally understood to include patients whose age at diagnosis is between 1 and 10 years as well as a presenting leukocyte count of <50,000/μL, in the absence of CNS involvement (114). T-cell phenotype occurs in 15% of pediatric ALL cases and was once thought to convey a relatively poorer prognosis. This prejudice has been due to numerous unfavorable clinical correlations including older age, male sex, elevated white blood cell (WBC) count, extensive extramedullary disease including mediastinal and peripheral adenopathy or hepatosplenomegaly, and a higher tendency for relapse in the CNS and testes in males (125). Current clinical practice is for T-cell leukemias to be treated on different protocols than B-cell lineage ALL. Nevertheless, when one factors out unfavorable clinical features, the prognostic difference between T- and B-cell ALL is difficult to discern. In regard to B-cell ALL, current protocols assign patients to low, standard, and high risk. Low-risk patients are operationally defined by standard risk features along with a rapid early response to induction chemotherapy (39). Age is also an important prognostic factor. Apart from this, the intensity of the treatment program is of importance, as shown by the fact that adolescents treated with pediatric leukemia regimens have had better outcomes than those treated with adult programs (28).

Assessment of CNS involvement at diagnosis in acute leukemia is critical as to risk stratification, which is, of course, of particular importance to the radiation oncologist. Unfortunately, a traumatic lumbar puncture has been noted to be associated with a worse prognosis (37). Regardless, CNS involvement has been unequivocally defined by a CSF leukocyte count of 5 or more WBC per microliter along with either blast cells on cytospin or the presence of cranial nerve palsy. By convention, this is now classified as CNS-3. CNS-1 is defined as no blast cells on CSF cytology and CNS-2 is <5 WBC per microliter with blast cells present. Clinical data are conflicting as to the prognostic importance of CNS-2, reflecting the fact that CNS involvement is not simply a distinction of being present or absent, but also has been associated with improved control with more intensive systemic and IT therapies (41,71). Patients with CNS-3 disease who have more intensive IT chemotherapy along with cranial radiation within the first year of therapy have a similar event-free survival as CNS-2 patients. For patients in remission who undergo surveillance lumbar punctures, there is even controversy regarding the prognostic importance of finding low numbers of blast or atypical cells in the CSF (86,123).

Radiotherapeutic Emergencies

The radiation oncologist will be called on to assist with certain emergencies when the patient first presents with leukemia or at the time of relapse. Mediastinal adenopathy causing airway compression or spinal cord compression from epidural disease are clear indications for emergent radiotherapy. Generally, only one to three 1.5 to 2.0 Gy fractions are required while the diagnosis is being established and systemic therapy is being

	Table 78.2	**FREQUENCY AND DISEASE CONTROL ASSOCIATED WITH IMMUNOPHENOTYPES AND CYTOGENETIC ABNORMALITIES AND SURVIVAL IN ACUTE LYMPHOBLASTIC LEUKEMIA IN CHILDREN (AGES 1–18) VERSUS ADULTS (AGES 18 AND OLDER)**			
	Frequency (%)		**5-Year Disease-Free Survival (%)**		
Pattern	**Children**	**Adults**	**Children**	**Adults**	
Pre B cell	80–85	75–80	80	30–40	
B cell	2	3–5	45–85	45–65	
T cell	15	20–25	65–75	40–60	
TEL/AML1 t(12;21)	20–25	1–3	90	rare	
MLL/AF4 t(4;11)	2	5–7	20	20	
BCR/ABL t(9;22)	5	25–30	20–40	<10	
Hyperdiploid	25	5	80–90	10–40	
Normal karyotype	9–37	30	70–87	40	

Adapted from DeAngelo DJ. The treatment of adolescents and young adults with acute lymphoblastic leukemia. *Hematology* 2005;1:123–130.

Clinical Radiation Oncology

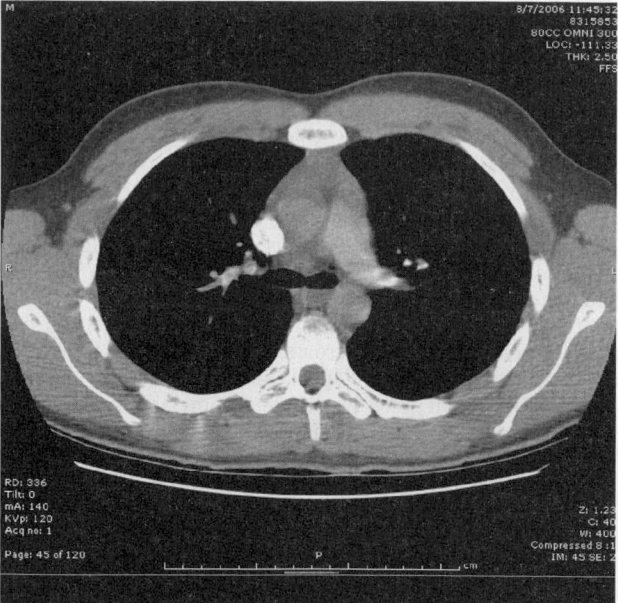

FIGURE 78.3. Computed tomography scans of chest before **(A)** and after **(B)** palliative radiotherapy for mediastinal mass associated with T-cell acute lymphocytic leukemia. A 16-year-old male presented with dyspnea and chest pain. A chest x-ray showed a mediastinal mass while blood counts revealed a lymphocytosis. Diagnosis was established by flow cytometry of blood. Initial treatment with steroids, doxorubicin, vincristine, and methotrexate failed to produce immediate response. Megavoltage radiotherapy with anterior and posterior opposed beams for 6 Gy in three fractions was administered, subsequently relieving acute symptoms and allowing for general anesthesia to take place without risk for complete airway obstruction in order for central line placement and lumbar puncture to be performed.

initiated (Fig. 78.3). Glucocorticoids are an important adjunct to CNS radiotherapy but can produce rapid lysis of some lymphoblastic lymphomas/leukemias, which may hamper diagnostic evaluation. In the presence of cranial nerve palsies at diagnosis, some radiation oncologists recommend 10 to 15 Gy to the base of skull early in the treatment course to try and reverse the neurologic deficits (53,89). Extreme leukocytosis with blood counts >100,000/μL is a concern with myeloid, but usually not lymphoid, leukemias, when neurologic deficits may result from leukostasis. In decades past, radiotherapy directed at the whole brain was employed using low doses on the order of 6 to 10 Gy in various fractionations. However, the role of radiotherapy in this setting has been questioned (17,81,94), but may be considered when leukophoresis or exchange transfusion is contraindicated or unavailable.

Treatment of Acute Myelocytic Leukemias

Classic induction therapy for AML is an anthracycline on days 1 to 3 with cytosine arabinoside (ara-C) for 7 days. Daunomycin has been commonly used, but other anthracyclines such as mitoxantrone and idarubicin have shown some improved response rates in comparison. A meta-analysis of multiple trials suggests that idarubicin has a higher complete response (CR) rate and survival over daunomycin (135). Remission rates vary from 50% to 80% depending on patient age, karyotype, and subtype of AML. Patients ≤60 years of age have CR rates of 70% to 80% and older patients tend to have lower CR rates of 50% to 60%. Patients who develop secondary AML following chemotherapy for other cancers have CR rates in the 40% to 60% range. Some induction regimens in children have added other drugs such as etoposide.

Once remission is achieved, the need for additional therapy has been well documented in large randomized trials. Current data suggest that optimal postremission consolidative therapy begins with high-dose ara-C for up to four cycles. Lumping all types of AML together as one group, the roughly 10% to 20% of patients who then remain in remission for 3 years have a high likelihood of being cured. High-dose ara-C has considerable CNS toxicity in elderly patients and has also been avoided in pediatric protocols. Other drugs used for consolidative treatment or for second-line induction therapy include etoposide, 6-mercaptopurine, amsacrine, 5-azacytidine, and methotrexate (MTX), but no one regimen is clearly advantageous.

The role of CNS prophylaxis is not well defined for AML, particularly as CNS relapse rates are relatively infrequent (at about 5% to 10%). Some studies show no difference in relapse rates with cranial radiation. Nevertheless, many pediatric regimens employ IT drugs such as ara-C. Patients with a high WBC count at diagnosis or monocytic variants of AML are believed to have a higher risk for CNS relapse, which may justify both IT chemotherapy and cranial radiation in this setting. At least one study of childhood AML demonstrated a lower systemic relapse rate after cranial radiation (26).

Leukemia-free survival rates vary widely from 15% to 80% in AML and depend on risk stratification. Younger patients with standard risk M2 AML or with favorable cytogenetic abnormalities have relatively better prognoses, and those with older age, induction failure, adverse cytogenetic abnormalities or other FAB subtypes of AML do worse (18,43). An exception is acute promyelocytic leukemia, which is among the curable types of AML thanks to the efficacy of all transretinoic acid in the management of this leukemic subtype. Postremission therapy for AML patients with adverse features may include transplantation with autologous or allogeneic stem cells.

Treatment of Acute Lymphoblastic Leukemia

The four components of specific ALL therapy are (a) induction of remission, (b) intensification and/or consolidation, (c) maintenance therapy, and (d) CNS prophylaxis. In the 1960s, the problem of CNS recurrence was addressed with CNS radiation and IT chemotherapy. Subsequent improvements in ALL cure rates during the last 2 to 3 decades has resulted from improved risk stratification of patients with more effective, tailored multidrug regimens. As discussed later, the late sequela of 24-Gy cranial irradiation were recognized in the 1980s and 1990s, leading to the elimination of cranial RT in favor of intermediate- or high-dose MTX in all but high-risk patients or those with CNS-3 disease. In addition, with the improvements in systemic therapy, testicular relapse in males has become a rare event (35). Testicular irradiation is rarely necessary except in the setting of testicular relapse or bone marrow transplantation.

Induction therapy for ALL as a minimum typically includes a glucocorticoid, vincristine, and L-asparaginase. Higher-risk patients often receive additional drugs such as an anthracycline, especially for adult ALL. Other four or greater multidrug regimens have been used, all of which has resulted in initial remission rates of 95% to 99% in children and 75% to 90% in adults. Dexamethasone may be the preferred systemic steroid treatment as suggested in two clinical reports comparing it with prednisone (14,55). This may be related to the better penetration of dexamethasone into the CSF and longer half-life, providing enhanced protection against CNS relapse (4).

Following induction and achieving CR, patients then receive intensification therapies that have been developed by cooperative groups in the United States and Europe (99,107). This may consist of high doses of antimetabolites such as MTX, ara-C, or L-asparaginase. Additional anthracycline therapy is beneficial in high-risk patients (108). High-dose MTX is believed to help control CNS disease, which has allowed for less use of cranial radiation in some pediatric programs.

Following intensification therapy, patients undergo a phase of maintenance treatment. In all but mature B-cell ALL, maintenance therapy during 2 to 3 years with agents such as weekly low-dose MTX and mercaptopurine appears to be quite important, albeit for unclear reasons. In high-risk patients, cooperative group studies have demonstrated a benefit to an additional "delayed" intensification after a period of maintenance therapy (23,107).

For ALL in adults, particularly those with the L3 subtype, patients have experienced improved remission rates with multiagent induction regimens that include high-dose MTX, cyclophosphamide, and sometimes ara-C. These drugs in combination with vincristine, steroids, L-asparaginase, and sometimes doxorubicin have been associated with 68% to 85% CR rates.

For relapsed ALL, a second induction generally consists of multiple drugs including vincristine, prednisone, L-asparaginase, an anthracycline with or without MTX, VP-16, or teniposide, and ara-C. If the CNS is involved, IT treatment is given along with radiotherapy (104). If testicular relapse occurs, bilateral testicular irradiation is administered. When isolated CNS or testicular relapse develops, systemic therapy is indicated along with local radiotherapy (138).

If a second remission develops, as occurs in 70% to 90% of cases, subsequent treatment includes either allogeneic transplantation or consolidative chemotherapy (122,138). There are no randomized trials to indicate which is better, but comparative analysis suggests that survival is improved with allogeneic transplantation, particularly in ALL patients who had brief initial remissions (5,122).

CNS Prophylaxis of Acute Leukemia and the Role of Cranial Radiotherapy

Historically, as multiagent chemotherapy proved to be highly effective in producing remissions in childhood ALL, numerous investigators noted a significant increase in CNS relapses. The CNS was recognized as a sanctuary site, protected from chemotherapy by the blood–brain barrier. In addition, CNS recurrences invariably led to systemic recurrence, suggesting that CNS disease was capable of reseeding the blood and marrow.

This observation led to a long series of CNS preventive therapy trials, which initially used CSI. For instance, studies V and VI in 1962–1967 from St. Jude's Cancer Research Hospital (SJCRH), established that CSI to 24 Gy in 15 to 16 fractions reduced the isolated CNS relapse rate from 67% to 4% (2,27). CSI doses of 12 Gy did not appear to be effective with the early chemotherapy regimens from this time (52). Concerns that full spinal radiotherapy would be associated with more acute myelosuppression, late musculoskeletal hypoplasia, as well as the technical difficulties of CSI, led the SJCRH investigators to compare CSI with cranial radiation plus IT MTX in study VII (111). Here, the two CNS preventive regimens were found to be equivalent with about an 8% risk of CNS relapse.

In SJCRH study VIII (1972–1975), all patients received 24-Gy cranial radiation plus IT MTX. Patients were randomized to one of four maintenance regimens: (a) weekly intravenous (IV) MTX begun during cranial radiation, (b) oral MTX and 6-mercaptopurine, (c) oral MTX, mercaptopurine, and cyclophosphamide, and (d) same three drugs plus ara-C (3). The incidence of CNS relapse was 5.0%, 1.5%, 20%, and 11.4% respectively. More troublesome, however, was the development in some patients of leukoencephalopathy, a disabling syndrome of lethargy, seizures, spasticity, paresis, and ataxia. The incidence of leukoencephalopathy in the four randomization groups was 55%, 0%, 7.1%, and 1.4%, respectively. Thus, standard maintenance with oral MTX and mercaptopurine following CNS treatment with cranial radiation along with IT MTX to treat the spinal subarachnoid space was found to have the lowest CNS relapse rate and the least toxicity. The major lesson learned was that IV MTX and cranial radiation in close temporal proximity should be avoided.

In the 1970s and 1980s, additional phase III trials further defined appropriate preventative CNS therapy for childhood ALL. The Children's Cancer Study Group (CCSG) trial no. 101 compared: (a) 24-Gy CSI plus extended field RT encompassing the liver, spleen, and gonads; (b) 24-Gy CSI alone; (c) 24-Gy cranial RT plus IT MTX; and (d) IT MTX alone. Overall, the different radiation regimens were comparable in preventing CNS relapse while statistically superior to IT chemotherapy alone (83). This finding was further confirmed in a cross-study comparison (45) as well as a Cancer and Leukemia Group B trial (35). CCSG further compared cranial RT plus IT MTX with CSI in high risk patients, defined by a WBC at diagnosis of >50,000/μL; cranial irradiation and IT MTX proved to be significantly superior with respect to both CNS and systemic relapse rates.

Further cooperative group trials have refined the efficacy of CNS-directed therapies within patient groups stratified by risk. Several trials have compared cranial RT with intermediate- or high-dose IV MTX along with IT chemotherapy (some with the addition of IT hydrocortisone and ara-C to MTX know as "triple" IT therapy) (35,61,118). The essential findings have been that in patients with low or standard risk ALL, CNS relapse rates have been about 5% regardless of CNS-specific therapy. Additionally, with triple IT chemotherapy, there was a trend toward fewer systemic failures as well as excellent CNS control when given throughout consolidation and maintenance therapy. This may be at the expense of increased neurotoxicity, however, when given in conjunction with intermediate-dose IV MTX (72).

Within the United States, the collective wisdom among many pediatric and adult oncologists has been to avoid cranial radiation in all but high-risk patients, even if that requires more intensive chemotherapy. This treatment philosophy stems from the recognition of several long-term risks of cranial radiation, particularly in children, which includes learning disabilities and other cognitive defects, growth retardation, hypopituitarism, secondary malignancies, and the aforementioned leukoencephalopathy. (One should note, however, these long-term toxicity data stem from a radiation prescription dose of 24 Gy during 2.5 weeks, and more recent radiation dose prescriptions have been lowered.) Several cooperative group trials have demonstrated that low-risk ALL (e.g., age 3 to 6 years and WBC count <10,000/μL) could be effectively managed without cranial radiation, substituting IT MTX throughout induction, consolidation, and maintenance therapy in place of cranial radiation (16,24,72).

In CCG-105, 1,388 patients with intermediate-risk ALL (defined by a complex matrix of patient age, presenting WBC count, and FAB subtype) were randomly assigned to receive either IT MTX alone or cranial radiation for CNS treatment (124). A secondary complex randomization scheme allocated patients to standard or intensive chemotherapy. Intensive chemotherapy included either more drugs for induction or the addition of a delayed intensification chemotherapy phase after consolidative and CNS therapies. CNS recurrence rates were comparable in all groups at about 5% to 7% except in those patients receiving standard chemotherapy without cranial radiation, in whom the CNS recurrence was 20%. Thus, more intensive systemic therapy does have an impact on lower CNS recurrence rates.

High-risk ALL patients have generally continued to receive cranial radiation. An analysis of T-cell ALL patients (generally with other poor risk features) treated within several Pediatric Oncology Group (POG) protocols suggested that omitting cranial radiation had an adverse impact on CNS relapse rates (67). Specifically, the 3-year CNS relapse rate was 18% for those who did not receive radiation therapy (RT) compared with 7% of who did. On the other hand, a European report looking at a subgroup of favorable T-cell ALL patients suggests that it may be safe to omit cranial radiation (24).

In order to reduce the toxicity of prophylactic cranial radiation, several investigations have explored a reduction in radiation dose. The use of 18 Gy in 9 or 10 fractions along with IT MTX yields comparable disease control rates as 24 Gy (82). Although there were some initial reports of reduced cognitive dysfunction even with such a dose reduction (47), this issue is by no means settled (25,70,105). Nevertheless, a dose of 18 Gy for prophylactic cranial irradiation has become more or less standard for pediatric ALL. For adults with ALL, various protocols have used 24 Gy and others employ 18 Gy (25,66).

The German-Austrian-Swiss ALL-BFM ("Berlin-Frankfurt-Munich") Study Group has further reduced the radiation dose to 12 Gy initially in a selected group of standard-risk pediatric patients (16). With modern chemotherapy regimens as opposed to the older ALL-BFM regimens, this further reduction in radiation dose was associated with excellent CNS control. In fact, the most recent ALL-BFM 90 protocol has both the medium- and high-risk patients receiving 12 Gy prophylactic cranial radiation resulting in CNS recurrence rates <5% (108). Further follow-up and additional experience within the Children's Oncology Group with this lower radiation dose will be required to see if also results in a reduction in late toxicity without compromising efficacy.

The Dana Farber Cancer Institute ALL Consortium has been studying the role of hyperfractionated cranial radiation (0.9 Gy twice daily) compared with standard daily fractionated treatments (1.8 Gy daily) to 18 Gy in high-risk patients (68,128). Preliminary results show excellent CNS control rates with both the standard or hyperfractionated treatments. Thus far, few late neurocognitive sequelae have been reported with systemic therapy that emphasizes L-asparaginase and omits high-dose MTX.

In summary, cranial radiotherapy may be used to prevent CNS relapse of leukemia. From a historical perspective, its use has been well documented for ALL. With concerns about late sequelae and improvements in systemic therapy including agents that can better penetrate the blood–brain barrier, prophylactic cranial radiotherapy is used less frequently. In current practice, cranial radiation is employed selectively in high-risk ALL patients, with a general trend toward decreasing radiation dosage to address toxicity concerns. High-risk ALL is a shifting defini-

tion and must take into account the intensity and specifics of chemotherapy, but includes older age (e.g., >6 to 7 years old), T-cell phenotype, and CNS 2 or 3 CSF findings. All adults with ALL may be considered to be at high risk for CNS relapse. Patients with AML, except for specific subtypes such as monocytic variants, are not generally treated with prophylactic cranial radiation at the present as the risk for CNS relapse is <5%. Unless indicated otherwise in a specific treatment protocol, the radiation prescription for prophylactic cranial radiation to prevent ALL relapse is 18 Gy in 9 or 10 fractions. The spinal region is specifically treated by IT chemotherapy.

Meningeal Leukemia at Diagnosis

At the time of diagnosis of ALL, approximately 3% to 5% of patients will present with clinically detectable CNS involvement (i.e., CNS-3 disease). Meningeal leukemia at diagnosis is managed as high-risk leukemia with cranial radiotherapy, but there are no set recommendations as to dose and whether the spine needs to be irradiated as the various chemotherapy programs include dose-intensive therapy with agents that penetrate the blood–brain barrier as well as IT therapy. Nevertheless, cranial radiation doses may vary from 18 to 25 Gy, and the spine doses vary from zero to 15 Gy. In children with ALL, meningeal involvement is no longer a poor prognostic factor, with 5-year disease-free survival rates approaching 70% (21).

Within the CCSG clinical trials for ALL, CSI has been consistently used in the management of CNS-3 disease. Until 1983, the cranial and spinal doses were 24 Gy and 12 Gy, respectively. Subsequent trials through 1989 used more intensive consolidation chemotherapy with a decrease in spinal radiation doses to 6 Gy. This allowed for a nonrandomized comparison of 6 and 12 Gy doses to the spine (in 2-Gy fractions). Interestingly, the patients who received a reduced spinal dose did just as well as those who received 12 Gy with less intensive chemotherapy. The 5-year event-free survival rate for patients with CNS-3 disease was 69% compared with 67% for patients enrolled in all CCG ALL protocols in 1983–1989 who were without CNS-3 disease (21).

Delay in radiotherapy up to 12 months has been found to be safe as long as intensive chemotherapy is being given first (73,103). This avoids the marrow compromise that could potentially occur with early spine irradiation. In addition, with doses <16 Gy to the spine, myelosuppression has not been a major problem. Musculoskeletal hypoplasia would not be expected to be a significant problem for long-term survivors. The sequencing of radiotherapy *after* rather than *before* potentially neurotoxic drug therapy such as MTX may theoretically result in a lower incidence of cognitive dysfunction or encephalopathy. Some pediatric protocols will also tailor the dose to the brain based on patient age. For instance, the ALL-BFM 90 protocol, which uses cranial rather than CSI, avoids any radiotherapy for those <1 year of age, 18 Gy for age 1 to 2 years, and 24 Gy for older patients. In this large multicenter trial, 54 patients presented with CNS-3 disease and achieved a 48% 6-year event-free survival (108). Arguably, this is inferior to protocols that use CSI, such as those reported by the CCG (21).

Therapeutic CNS Irradiation for Meningeal Relapse

With modern chemotherapy programs incorporating CNS-directed treatment, CNS relapse rates are typically <10%. As in overt CNS leukemia at diagnosis, radiotherapy has a central role. Formally, CNS relapse was thought to have a poor prognosis. Studies in the 1970s and 1980s describe disease control rates of 25% to 50% (6,40,63,87,90,134,136). Later trials, however, using more intensive chemotherapy as well as CNS directed radiotherapy have reported 5-year survival rates in the 50% to 70% range (62,64,100,103,137). Almost all trials have employed radiotherapy; the debate has been between cranial RT alone or CSI. Doses used have generally been approximately 24 Gy to the brain and 10 to 15 Gy to the spine. Most comparisons have not been randomized, but superior outcomes seem to be achieved with CSI (62,64,100,103,108,137). One small phase III trial did show superiority for CSI compared with cranial RT (64).

Although CNS relapse may ostensibly occur without overt systemic disease, the latter is viewed as inevitable without additional systemic therapy. Therefore, intensive chemotherapy is an essential component of the treatment of meningeal relapse (34).

Several prognostic factors have been found to be of importance in the setting of CNS relapse (10–12). Patients who were originally deemed at diagnosis to be at low risk for CNS relapse by virtue of a low initial leukocyte count ($<20,000/\mu$L), who originally did not receive cranial irradiation, or whose CNS relapse occurred at a relatively long period after the original diagnosis, have a better prognosis after CNS recurrence. An isolated CNS relapse has generally had a more favorable prognosis compared with combined CNS and systemic relapse. After completing chemotherapy, those children with CNS relapse have better outcomes with longer disease-free intervals. For instance, experience within the POG with isolated CNS relapse of ALL in which RT used a cranial dose of 24 Gy and a spine dose of 15 Gy. The four year event free survival was 71%. Those patients who presented with greater than an 18 month disease-free interval prior to CNS relapse had a four year event-free survival of 83% compared to 46% for those with shorter initial remission durations (103). This has lead to more recent POG trials that omit radiotherapy to the spine if there is a long disease free interval. Whether or not the omission of spinal RT in this favorable subgroup is detrimental is unclear.

As for adults with CNS leukemia, most of the published experience and commentary from medical oncologists has been opposed to the use of CSI mainly for fear of excessive myelosuppression (25). Cranial irradiation is relatively standard, however. Quite possibly, the avoidance in treating the entire CNS is detrimental, although admittedly this is not a settled issue.

Selected high-risk patients with CNS relapse may be candidates for allogeneic transplants. TBI is often a component of the preparative regimen. One function of the TBI is to specifically treat the CNS burden of disease. Because doses on the order of 12 to 15 Gy are employed here, it makes sense to boost the head prior to TBI to bring total doses to the cranium to 18 to 25 Gy.

Testicular Relapse

In boys with ALL, particularly those with T-cell subtype, testicular involvement was once a common problem. Overt testicular involvement by leukemia at diagnosis occurs in approximately 2% of males with ALL, and is a particularly poor prognostic situation. Microscopic burden in the testes is estimated to be higher at 5% to 15% based on biopsy data and the historic risk for testicular relapse. With modern chemotherapy, especially the use of intermediate- to high-dose MTX, this is now rare. Similar to the experience with CNS relapse, there once was speculation as to whether the testes acted as a sanctuary site because of a physiologic blood–testes barrier. A trial in 1980 of prophylactic testicular irradiation significantly reduced the risk of testicular relapse, but did not improve survival (120).

In cases of testicular relapse, systemic and/or CNS relapse usually follows (119). Both intensive systemic therapy and local radiotherapy are indicated. Doses <12 Gy are generally thought to be suboptimal, and doses of 24 to 26 Gy over 2.5 to 3.5 weeks are considered standard. Case reports of local recurrences despite adequate radiotherapy have led some to suggest higher doses. When only one testis is clinically involved, imaging or biopsy of the contralateral testis frequently reveals bilateral dis-

ease. Similarly, unilateral irradiation or orchiectomy as local management is thought to be associated with a significant risk of contralateral testicular relapse, justifying treatment directed at both testes for leukemia management, despite the expectation of infertility from RT. Data from CCG and POG studies suggests that local irradiation and intensive systemic therapy results in prolonged event-free survival in about 50% to 65% of patients (79,138). Where allogeneic transplantation is indicated, TBI is often part of the conditioning regimen. One retrospective series from the Memorial Sloan-Kettering Cancer Center suggests that for TBI/cyclophosphamide preparative regimens, the risk of testicular relapse is significantly reduced with a local boost to the scrotum of 4 Gy to bring the total testicular dose to 16 to 20 Gy (109). Regardless, there is not universal agreement about the need for a testicular boost in this setting.

The Chronic Leukemias

Chronic Myelogenous Leukemia

CML is a chronic myeloproliferative disorder arising from clonal expansion of the primitive hematopoietic stem cell. It involves myeloid, erythroid, megakaryocytic, and sometimes lymphoid elements. It is the first neoplastic process to be characterized by a specific cytogenetic marker, the Philadelphia chromosome (Ph+), t(9;22) described in 1960 (84). This is detectable by cytogenetics in 90% to 95% of patients, and in most other patients by molecular analysis (29). This translocation results in a fusion protein that has tyrosine kinase activity critical for leukemic transformation.

Clinically, the disease manifests several phases: an initial chronic indolent phase of 3 to 4 years with progression to an accelerated phase and finally an acute transformation to blast phase, which occurs in 75% to 85% of patients, with a survival of 3 to 6 months. As the disease advances, the accelerated phase is characterized by increasing difficulty in controlling the peripheral WBC count, increasing splenomegaly, increasing blasts in the peripheral blood and bone marrow, increasing basophilia and eosinophilia. The blast crisis resembles acute leukemia with >30% blasts in blood or bone marrow with symptoms such as bone pain, sweats, fever, anorexia, or weight loss. Anemia, thrombopenia, and extramedullary disease involving bones, skin, CNS, and lymph nodes are common. In about 20% of cases, blasts are lymphoid by phenotype.

Prognostic factors have been identified in CML and include age, splenic size, platelet count, percent of basophils in blood, and marrow. Poor prognosis factors are age >60 years, spleen >10 cm below the costal margin, blasts >3% in blood or marrow, basophilia >7% in blood or marrow, and platelets >700,000/μL (106,116). A poor response to therapy and a short duration of remission also are considered unfavorable, as well as failure to achieve significant cytogenetic remission (56).

Therapy of CML

The first effective therapy for chronic leukemias was radiotherapy to the spleen and sometimes the liver, initiated in 1902 by Pusey (95) and assessed in 1924 by Minot et al. (76). Now radiotherapy is primarily used in a palliative setting to relieve painful splenomegaly or other extramedullary sites when indicated. In some centers, TBI plays an important role in allogeneic transplantation.

There is a long history of treating CML in chronic phase with alkylating agents, hydroxyurea, ara-C, and interferon alpha, which is beyond the scope of this chapter. What had been standard therapy with interferon and ara-C has given way in recent years to therapy with the specific bcr-abl tyrosine kinase inhibitor imatinib (85). Imatinib is a relatively nontoxic oral medication that has been shown to be effective in inducing remissions of CML in chronic and accelerated phases (30,31). This agent has been a paradigm for molecularly targeted therapies and is now used as upfront therapy for CML, having successfully changed the natural history of this disease and delaying the need for stem cell transplantation. Allogeneic transplantation can cure a substantial proportion of patients with CML (38,121). About 70% of good-risk patients achieve long-term disease-free survival (33). Allotransplantation and TBI are further discussed in Chapter 14. Increasing experience has also demonstrated the potential for leukemic drug resistance to imatinib through a number of mechanisms that include critical point mutations and gene amplification of the bcr/abl tyrosine kinase (44). Alternate tyrosine kinase inhibitors for imatinib-resistant CML are in development.

Palliative radiotherapy may be of benefit in those patients with massive splenomegaly (see later discussion). In addition, chloromas (which may also occur with AML) are responsive to modest doses of radiotherapy. The name derives from the fact that myeloid cells contain myeloperoxidase, which manifests a greenish color on gross inspection. Extramedullary leukemic tumors have also been called *granulocytic sarcomas*. Based on various case reports in the literature, symptomatic problems from chloromas or leukemic infiltration of the spleen may be readily relieved with doses of 10 to 20 Gy. The fractionation and total dose needs to take into consideration any normal tissue toxicities and the potential for future TBI, should the patient be a potential candidate for an allotransplant.

Chronic Lymphocytic Leukemia

About 95% of cases of CLL are B cell in origin, with the remainder having a T-cell origin. The course of the disease demonstrates marked variability. Many patients live a normal lifespan, never require therapy, and die of unrelated causes. The disease of others progresses within a few years despite treatment. The usual course is characterized by gradual progression from no significant physical findings to lymphadenopathy, gradual increase in peripheral blood count with increasing splenomegaly, sometimes massive in size. Nonlymphoid organ involvement may occur with advanced stage of disease. As disease progression occurs, anemia and thrombocytopenia occur.

An occasional patient with CLL demonstrates transformation to an aggressive large B-cell lymphoma referred to as *Richter's syndrome* (101). Its incidence ranges from 3% to 5% of CLL cases (42). It may arise in the setting of active disease or during a CR. It is characterized by an abrupt onset of asymmetric adenopathy, fever, and elevated lactate dehydrogenase. Other transformations include evolution to prolymphocytic leukemia with development of progressive refractory disease and a majority of prolymphocytes in the blood. Rarely, ALL or myeloma develop in the course of CLL (15,91).

The clinical diagnosis is based on the blood lymphocyte count, which must be at least $5 \times 10^3/\mu$L in an adult, the typical phenotype, a monoclonal cell population, and at least 30% lymphocytes in a normocellular or hypercellular marrow (22). There have been many staging systems proposed, but the most widely used are those modified by Rai et al. (98) and Binet et al. (7), the former used in the United States and the latter in Europe. These systems are shown in Table 78.3. Clinical stage is the most important predictor of survival in patients with CLL. Other factors reported to have an impact on survival include age (older patients have a worse prognosis), sex (women have a better survival), the rate of increase in blood lymphocytes (a progressive increase connotes a poor outcome), and pattern of marrow involvement (the degrees and nodularity versus mixed pattern, the latter conferring a worse outcome). β-2 microglobulin levels, immunophenotype, lymphocyte doubling time, and

Table 78.3	CHRONIC LYMPHOCYTIC LEUKEMIA STAGING SYSTEMS	
Staging System	**Clinical Features**	**Median Survival (yr)**
Rai staging		
Low risk		>10
0	Lymphocytosis of blood and marrow	
Intermediate risk		7
I	Lymphadenopathy	
II	Splenomegaly	
High risk		2–4
III	Anemia, hgb <10 g/dL (unrelated to hemolysis)	
IV	Thrombocytopenia <100,000 platelets/μL	
Binet staging		
A	<3 Areas of lymphadenopathy	12
B	≥3 Involved nodal areas	7
C	Anemia and/or thrombocytopenia	2

cytogenetic and molecular abnormalities also may have prognostic implications in CLL (139).

Asymptomatic early-stage patients may be followed without therapy. About 20% of such patients will have an indolent course indefinitely. Of the remaining patients, the decision to intervene therapeutically is often challenging. The NCI has established guidelines for the initiation of treatment, which include constitutional symptoms due to CLL, symptomatic lymphadenopathy and/or hepatosplenomegaly, anemia (hemoglobin <10 g/dL), thrombocytopenia (platelets <100,000/μL), and refractory autoimmune disease (22). A controversial indication includes a WBC count >300,000/μL.

Until recently, the standard treatment for CLL has been single-agent chlorambucil, with or without prednisone (20). The newer purine analogs, 2-deoxycoformycin, fludarabine, and 2-chloro-2′-deoxy-β-D-adenosine (cladribine or 2-CDA) have been tested in CLL and, of these, fludarabine has shown a high response rate (19). In a phase III trial comparing fludarabine with chlorambucil, the CR rate with chlorambucil was 3% and with fludarabine it was 37% (97). Overall response rates were 10% with chlorambucil and 70% with fludarabine. The survival was 33 months (fludarabine) versus 17 months. Fludarabine as compared to combination therapy (CAP or CHOP) has also shown a favorable outcome (8). For these reasons, fludarabine is now accepted as a standard therapy for CLL. Recently, a combination of fludarabine, cyclophosphamide, and the anti-CD20 antibody, rituximab, has resulted in a very high complete remission rate of 70% in patients with CLL, with a progression-free survival of 69% at 4 years (58).

Allogeneic transplantation is being used in younger patients (<55 years of age) with CLL. The 3-year survival rate was 45% among 60 patients in a European study with 46% treatment-related complications. Follow-up at 12 months is reported in the U.S. studies (59,75,96). In both groups, conditioning included cyclophosphamide with TBI. Patients included in these studies were either in remission, had minimal residual disease, or had disease documented to be refractory to fludarabine. It is not clear whether survival advantage will occur with stem cell transplantation as there are no controlled trials.

Newer approaches to the treatment of CLL involve vaccines, cell cycle inhibitors, differentiating agents, and monoclonal antibodies (20). The anti-CD52 antibody, alemtuzumab, has established single-agent activity in patients refractory to fludarabine and is under investigation in a variety of combination regimens (88). Rituximab, initially considered ineffective, has been studied in innovative regimens with some evidence of benefit when administered three times weekly (19).

Radiotherapy, once the initial effective therapy for CLL, is now used in the management of painful splenomegaly or occasionally for cytopenias associated with splenomegaly when splenectomy is not an option. It is also indicated in instances of unresponsive disease to alleviate symptomatic adenopathy or nonlymphoid organ involvement. Historically, low-dose TBI without stem cell support was used to control CLL. Remarkably, low doses on the order of several Gray can be effective for palliation, although fractionated doses up to 20 Gy are also reasonable.

:: | Irradiation Techniques

Cranial Radiation

The volume of treatment must include the subarachnoid space within the cranial vault. The inferior margin has by convention extended to the bottom of either the first or second cervical vertebra and includes the whole vertebral body. This may facilitate matching of potential future treatment fields to the spine. Other field boundaries typically involve "flashing" over the scalp. With regard to blocking the anterior facial structures, attention must be given to the base of skull anatomy to adequately cover the cribriform plate and the middle cranial fossa. The cribriform plate is somewhat variable as a function of the age of the patient but is generally in line with the bottom of the frontal sinuses extending posteriorly for several centimeters. The middle cranial or temporal fossa projects on lateral radiographs over the sphenoid sinuses. Figure 78.1 shows a plain radiograph of an adult skull with radio-opaque markers at various anatomic landmarks. The posterior globe of the eye is typically included, given concerns of leukemic relapse in the posterior retina near where there is subarachnoid space extending alone the optic nerves. Radio-opaque markers on the anterior aspect of the bony orbit are generally a good anatomic landmark that bifurcates the globe. (See Fig. 78.1, an example of lateral fields used to treat a patient with ALL.)

Head immobilization with aquaplast or similar thermoplastic material facilitates a high degree of treatment position reproducibility. Accounting for setup variation and beam penumbra leads to field design that clearly must encroach on the eye. With forward gaze of the eyes, this would imply that the superior half of the lens is within the dose build-up region of the treatment fields. With the exception of very young children who cannot cooperate, voluntary rotation of the eye downward ("looking toward one's toes") would theoretically reduce the risk of cataracts. Another important caveat in treatment technique to minimize dose to the anterior portion of the eyes is the alignment of the anterior beam edge divergence. Figure 78.4 depicts this concept of angling the gantry 3 to 5 degrees to achieve a parallel anterior beam margin at the back of the eye. The simple trigonometric equation to determine the proper gantry rotation is:

$$\tan A = D/SAD$$

where A is the desired rotation angle, D is the anterior-posterior distance between the central axis (i.e., isocenter) and the projection of the anterior aspect of the bony orbit at midplane, and SAD is the source to axis (or isocenter) distance (which is generally 100 cm for most linear accelerator geometries). Since tan $A \cong A$ (in radians) for small angles and the conversion factor for radians to degrees is approximately 57 (i.e., 180 degrees per π radians), this further simplifies to:

$$A = (D)(0.57) \text{ for a source to axis/isocenter distance of 100 cm}$$

Some radiation oncologists prefer to simply place the isocenter of the treatment beam just posterior to the lens so that the anterior eye is protected by a modified "half-beam block." This is a fine technique for linear accelerators equipped with independent primary collimators so that block trays are not excessively heavy. With the advent of CT simulators, alignment of beam divergence can be performed graphically without the need for trigonometric calculations. The standard radiation dose for prophylactic cranial radiation in pediatric ALL is 18 Gy in 9 to 10 fractions. Although this is a reasonable dose for adults, some protocols still continue to utilize 24 Gy in 12 fractions. Photon energies >6 MV should not be used so that the dose build-up region at initial depths is superficial to the meninges.

Craniospinal Radiation and Therapeutic Cranial Radiation for CNS Leukemia

The techniques of cranio-spinal radiation involve precise matching of beam divergence between a posteroanterior spine field and lateral parallel opposed cranial fields. It is recommended that there be minimal or no gap between the spine and cranial fields. The field junction may be shifted or "feathered" by 1 to 2 cm once or twice to avoid any excessive overlap of dose over the cervical spine. Some physicians prefer to place the beam isocenter at the inferior or caudad border of the initial craniocervical field so as to avoid the complexity of a couch rotation in the treatment setup. A gantry rotation to align the anterior beam divergence near the eye may still be performed. Other physicians place the isocenter near the eye to avoid divergence into the anterior globe, which can be done in conjunction with an appropriate couch rotation to match divergence with the posteroanterior spine field.

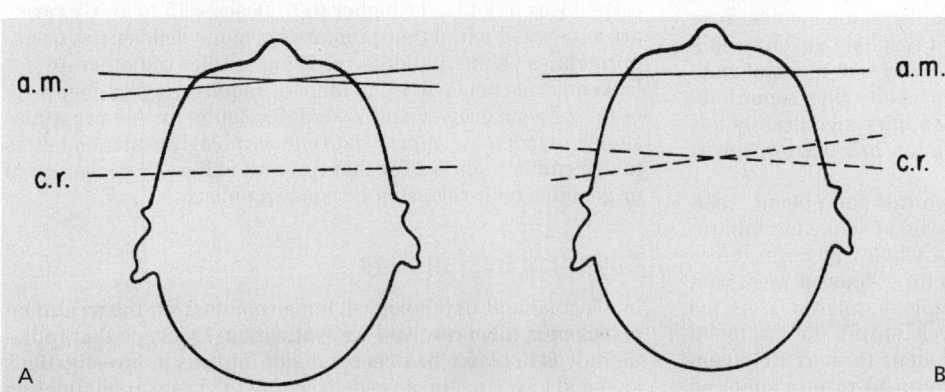

FIGURE 78.4. Illustration of beam divergence of lateral cranial fields showing anterior margin (a.m.) at level of the eyes and central ray (c.r.). **A:** Parallel opposed fields result in exit dose from each field Into region of contralateral anterior eye. **B.** Gantry angle of 3 to 5 degrees results in alignment of anterior margin beam divergence from lateral fields. (Shown with permission.)

Maximum beam energy of 6 MV is recommended. Radiation doses for overt CNS leukemia are 18 to 30 Gy to the cranium in 1.5- to 1.8-Gy fractions. Spine doses have been variable from 6 to 24 Gy with some advocates for 0 Gy. The authors recommend that overt CNS leukemia, including that for adults, be treated with true craniospinal fields with the spine being treated to 6 to 15 Gy depending on individual circumstances. Plans for possible TBI must be taken into account. This part of the preparative regimen for an allogeneic transplant can be conceptualized as being in part CNS therapy.

Testicular Irradiation

For the management of leukemic infiltration of the testes, both gonads and the scrotum can be irradiated with either electrons or photons. With the patient in a "frog-leg" position and the penile shaft taped onto the abdomen, an anterior inferior oblique photon field works well. Attention to the cremaster reflex and potential ascent of the testes into the inguinal canal is important so as to avoid a geographic miss. For megavoltage photon beams, bolus may be required to avoid superficial underdosing. In young boys in whom the scrotum/testes thickness is under 2 cm, 250 kV orthovoltage x-rays may also be used. Alternatively, direct *en face* electron beams of appropriate energy work adequately. Although there are considerable dose inhomogeneities in treating such a curved surface with electrons, the relatively low doses employed in this setting translates into relatively low risks related to skin and subcutaneous soft tissue reactions. Radiation doses typically used are 24 to 26 Gy in 1.5- to 2.0-Gy fractions. When a testicular boost is given in conjunction with TBI for a hematopoietic stem cell transplant, the dose is either 4 Gy × one fraction or 2 Gy two fractions.

Splenic Irradiation

Massive splenomegaly may be seen with CML, CLL, hairy cell leukemia, and splenic marginal zone lymphomas, where the spleen can extend into the pelvis. Significant splenomegaly may also occur with prolymphocytic leukemia, myeloproliferative disorders such as polycythemia vera or essential thrombocytosis, or myelofibrosis. One type of myelofibrosis called *agnogenic myeloid metaplasia* is characterized by progressive bone marrow failure, splenomegaly, and extramedullary hematopoiesis. It is therapeutically important to recognize which conditions of splenomegaly are due to extramedullary hematopoiesis rather than leukemic infiltration as whole spleen radiotherapy with modest radiation doses can result in severe, long-lasting pancytopenia when the spleen is the primary hematopoiesis site. Splenic hematopoiesis can also occur with late stages of CML, myeloproliferative disorders, and hairy cell leukemia.

Historically, splenic radiotherapy was commonly employed for palliation, but it is now uncommon, as more effective systemic treatments have been developed. Nevertheless, the radiation oncologist is called on to assist with the management of symptomatic splenomegaly from these hematologic disorders from time to time, often with excellent results. Leukemic infiltration of the spleen responds to relatively low doses of radiation. Particularly in an elderly patient with other comorbidities, palliative splenic radiotherapy can offer significantly less risk than splenectomy. Splenic irradiation has been reviewed by Weinmann et al. (132).

Anterior and posterior opposed portals for photon treatments are generally employed. In cases of leukemic infiltration, standard practice is to treat the whole spleen in 0.5 to 1.0 Gy fractions either daily or two to three times a week with doses titrated to response and hematologic tolerance. As the spleen responds, one may progressively shrink the treatment fields accordingly. Generally, it is prudent to start treatment very conservatively. Blood counts may need to be monitored

several times a week. Total radiation dose delivered is determined clinically by when palliation is achieved. Total doses are typically in the range of 4 to 10 Gy with usually no more than 20 Gy required. Occasionally, a large spleen that is extensively fibrotic will not respond to radiotherapy. CLL and prolymphocytic leukemia are particularly radiosensitive, with occasional abscopal effects seen with splenic irradiation.

In patients with extramedullary hematopoiesis, the potential for severe neutropenia or thrombocytopenia is very high with even modest radiation doses. Dose per fraction may need to be as low as 0.1 to 0.5 Gy treating several times a week to avoid severe and protracted myelosuppression. Another strategy in this situation is to treat only half of the spleen. For myelodysplastic conditions or extramedullary/intrasplenic hematopoiesis, total doses of 1 to 9 Gy are usually adequate.

With splenic irradiation, nausea is uncommon with these low-dose fractions, but can be readily managed with antiemetics if necessary. As there can be rapid cell lysis, allopurinol to prevent uric acid nephropathy is advised. Cumulative dose to the left kidney should be monitored, especially as retreatment in the future may be required; but it is rare for doses beyond 20 Gy to be required.

Sequelae of Therapy

Somnolence Syndrome

Approximately 1 month following cranial radiation, up to 40% to 50% of patients may develop lethargy, irritability, anorexia, and even fevers. This condition has been termed *somnolence syndrome*. It has been associated with electroencephalographic abnormalities and CSF pleocytosis (1,36). This syndrome is self-limited and typically reverses within 1 to 3 weeks. Glucocorticoids in acute management may be helpful. There are two reports that suggest that the incidence of this syndrome is reduced if patients receive steroids during cranial radiotherapy (74,126).

Pituitary Dysfunction

Hypothalamic pituitary irradiation can impact endocrine function in a dose and age-dependent manner. For the doses used in leukemia management, growth hormone (GH) deficiency is the most common abnormality observed. Age <5 years at the time of radiotherapy is associated with particular susceptibility to the development of GH deficiency. Higher radiation doses as well as younger age correlate with an increased incidence of GH deficiency and a shorter time period for its clinical manifestations (9). It is more common after 24 Gy than 18 Gy (112,117). Precocious puberty has been reported with radiation doses to the hypothalamic-pituitary region as low as 18 Gy, although it seems to be more prevalent in females who receive doses of 24 Gy or higher (69). Doses <35 to 40 Gy rarely are associated with other pituitary hormone deficiencies or abnormalities. Thus, patients receiving cranial radiotherapy for leukemia, particularly in childhood, require regular follow-up of their linear growth and sexual development. Abnormalities should then lead to appropriate endocrinologic evaluation so as to determine the need for therapy with either GH replacement or gonadotropin-releasing hormone agonists.

Cognitive Dysfunction

Intellectual and psychological impairments from the treatment of leukemia have received wide attention. Evidence that radiotherapy is to blame has been a major impetus in investigations aimed at lowering the dose delivered to the brain or eliminating it completely. Increasingly, however, there is evidence that chemotherapy may also be causing similar detriments. Objective measures of cognitive function and social functioning are inherently difficult. Nevertheless, a variety of assessment tools, intelligence quotients (IQs), or scales have been verified as useful measures of language, reasoning, and performance skills. Other descriptive measures of lowered school achievement have also been reported. Cognitive dysfunction is thought to be the result of white matter injury causing deficits in the speed of information processing (50). These effects are most pronounced in children <5 years of age and probably most pronounced in those <3 years of age when the brain is still undergoing growth and development, especially with myelinization.

Some reports have suggested a gender difference in susceptibility to radiation injury, with females more likely than males to develop intellectual impairments, although this has not been consistently reported (77,130). The Dana Farber group has suggested that the reduction in IQ seen in girls was the result of an interaction between high-dose MTX and cranial radiation (129). Moreover, impairment in verbal memory observed in both boys and girls was independent of cranial radiation, suggesting toxicity from systemic therapy (129).

A reduction in radiation dose from 24 Gy to 18 Gy has not consistently reported to result in a lower cognitive difficulties (47,70,105). Further reduction to 12 Gy is under study. Overall, for these radiation doses the cognitive deficits have been arguably small, with average full-scale IQ measures decreasing by no more than 10% while other studies fail to show measurable changes. Perhaps a more important statistic is the proportion of patients with significant reductions, say >15 points in IQ scales; the SJCRH group has reported that up to 22% to 30% of children have such deficits after 18 Gy, 24 Gy, or no cranial radiotherapy (77). One hypothesis is that a component of cognitive difficulties is related to chemotherapy rather than radiotherapy. Regardless, a recent report from the Dana Farber group suggests that in high-risk ALL patients receiving 18 Gy cranial radiation, neurocognitive function many years after therapy is not significantly different from that of the general population (128). Importantly, this was a group of patients who experienced a favorable 5-year disease-free survival of 75% with a 1% CNS relapse rate. The Dana Farber group has been investigating hyperfractionated cranial radiation for CNS prophylaxis (0.9 Gy twice daily vs. 1.8 Gy daily to a total dose of 18 Gy). There are no obvious differences between standard or hyperfractionated radiotherapy in terms of late neurotoxicity reported thus far, although there are numerous method problems inherent in such a comparison (68,128). An emerging experience suggests that stimulants such as methylphenidate may be of help in managing treatment-related cognitive problems, particularly some attentional or social deficits (78).

Leukoencephalopathy

Some early prophylactic cranial radiation studies for childhood ALL showed an significant incidence of profound encephalopathy occurring months after irradiation (13,34). The highest incidence was seen when cranial radiation with doses as low as 24 Gy combined with IV MTX. Leukoencephalopathy is thought to represent a demyelinating condition that may be initiated by endothelial damage and a subsequent cytokine cascade with ischemic microinfarcts (51). Concomitant IV MTX seems to be a significant synergistic factor, but leukoencephalopathy has been observed at low incidence rates with radiotherapy alone at doses >30 to 35 Gy, with IT MTX, or in conjunction with other chemotherapy agents. High-dose chemotherapy alone is becoming increasingly recognized as causing similar dementialike syndromes. One should also remember that after cranial radiotherapy, the blood–brain barrier is thought to be more permeable, which may contribute to chemotherapy effects on cog-

nitive function (46). Regardless, the risk of leukoencephalopathy is decidedly rare after doses of <20 Gy.

Secondary Malignancies

In a report from the CCSG of 9,720 patients treated for ALL, 43 secondary cancers were observed after a mean follow-up of 6 years (131). Of these, 24 were CNS tumors in patients who had previously received 24-Gy cranial radiotherapy. All but one of these patients with CNS tumors had been <5 years of age at diagnosis of their acute leukemia. A report from the SJCRH documented 15 brain tumors in 1,705 children followed long-term aftertreatment for ALL (80). The types of secondary brain tumors tend to be evenly split between meningiomas and high-grade gliomas. In a review of 3,182 children treated by an allogeneic bone marrow transplant, 25 solid tumors were observed, compared with an expected incidence of one case (115). A majority of these cancers originated in the CNS or thyroid gland. Moreover, most of these patients had received TBI as part of their preparative regimen before transplant.

Testicular Effects from Radiotherapy

Gonadal dysfunction is quite rare from cranial radiotherapy for leukemia management unless patients undergo retreatment that results in high cumulative doses. Direct effects from testicular irradiation, however, are very common. Doses as low as 1 Gy, even from scattered dose from adjacent external-beam fields, will cause transient oligospermia or azospermia. Higher doses, particularly those used in TBI or therapeutic testicular radiation, would be expected to cause permanent infertility. Leydig cell function on the other hand is more radioresistant (113). Low serum testosterone levels or delayed puberty are unusual with doses <29 Gy to the testes. One report of 60 male survivors of ALL showed significant germ cell dysfunction as manifested by increased follicle-stimulating hormone levels and testicular atrophy in 55% of patients treated with testicular radiotherapy and in 17% treated with craniospinal radiotherapy. The incidence of Leydig cell dysfunction was very low (113).

References

1. Aronson S, Elmquist D, Garwicz S. Somnolence in children with acute leukaemia [letter]. *Br Med J* 1974;3:344.
2. Aur RJ, Hustu HO, Verzosa MS, et al. Comparison of two methods of preventing central nervous system leukemia. *Blood* 1973;42:349–357.
3. Aur RJ, Simone JV, Hustu HO, et al. A comparative study of central nervous system irradiation and intensive chemotherapy early in remission of childhood acute lymphocytic leukemia. *Cancer* 1972;29:381–391.
4. Balis FM, Lester CM, Chrousos GP, et al. Differences in cerebrospinal fluid penetration of corticosteroids: possible relationship to the prevention of meningeal leukemia. *J Clin Oncol* 1987;5:202–207.
5. Barrett AJ, Horowitz MM, Pollock BH, et al. Bone marrow transplants from HLA-identical siblings as compared with chemotherapy for children with acute lymphoblastic leukemia in a second remission. *N Engl J Med* 1994;331:1253–1258.
6. Behrendt H, van Leeuwen EF, Schuwirth C, et al. The significance of an isolated central nervous system relapse, occurring as first relapse in children with acute lymphoblastic leukemia. *Cancer* 1989;63:2066–2072.
7. Binet JL, Auquier A, Dighiero G, et al. A new prognostic classification of chronic lymphocytic leukemia derived from a multivariate survival analysis. *Cancer* 1981;48:198–206.
8. Binet JL, Chastang C, Chevret S. Comparison of fludarabine, CAP and CHOP in advanced previously untreated chronic lymphocytic leukemia. *Blood* 1993; 82:140(abstr).
9. Birkebaek NH, Fisker S, Clausen N, et al. Growth and endocrinological disorders up to 21 years after treatment for acute lymphoblastic leukemia in childhood. *Med Pediatr Oncol* 1998;30:351–356.
10. Bleyer WA, Poplack DG. Prophylaxis and treatment of leukemia in the central nervous system and other sanctuaries. *Semin Oncol* 1985;12:131–148.
11. Bleyer WA, Sather H, Hammond GD. Prognosis and treatment after relapse of acute lymphocytic leukemia and non-Hodgkin's lymphoma: 1985. A report from the Childrens Cancer Study Group. *Cancer* 1986;58:590–594.
12. Bleyer WA. Central nervous system leukemia. *Pediatr Clin North Am* 1988; 35:789–814.
13. Bleyer WA. Neurologic sequelae of methotrexate and ionizing radiation: a new classification. *Cancer Treat Rep* 1981;65 Suppl 1:89–98.
14. Bostrom B, Gaynon PS, Sather H. Dexamethasone (DEX) decreases central nervous system (CNS) relapse and improves event-free survival (EFS) in lower risk acute lymphoblastic leukemia (ALL).1998;17:527(abstr).

15. Brouet JC, Fermand JP, Laurent G, et al. The association of chronic lymphocytic leukaemia and multiple myeloma: a study of eleven patients. *Br J Haematol* 1985;59:55–66.

16. Buhrer C, Henze G, Hofmann J, et al. Central nervous system relapse prevention in 1165 standard-risk children with acute lymphoblastic leukemia in five BFM trials. *Hamatol Bluttransfus* 1990;33:500–503.

17. Bunin NJ, Pui CH. Differing complications of hyperleukocytosis in children with acute lymphoblastic or acute nonlymphoblastic leukemia. *J Clin Oncol* 1985;3:1590–1595.

18. Burnett AK, Goldstone AH, Stevens RM, et al. Randomised comparison of addition of autologous bone-marrow transplantation to intensive chemotherapy for acute myeloid leukaemia in first remission: results of MRC AML 10 trial. UK Medical Research Council Adult and Children's Leukaemia Working Parties. *Lancet* 1998;351:700–708.

19. Byrd JC, Murphy T, Lucas MS. Thrice weekly rituximab demonstrates significant activity in chronic lymphocytic leukemia. *Blood* 2000;96:837(abstr).

20. Byrd JC, Rai KR, Sausville EA, et al. Old and new therapies in chronic lymphocytic leukemia: now is the time for a reassessment of therapeutic goals. *Semin Oncol* 1998;25:65–74.

21. Cherlow JM, Sather H, Steinherz P, et al. Craniospinal irradiation for acute lymphoblastic leukemia with central nervous system disease at diagnosis: a report from the Children's Cancer Group. *Int J Radiat Oncol Biol Phys* 1996;36:19–27.

22. Cheson BD, Bennett JM, Grever M, et al. National Cancer Institute-sponsored Working Group guidelines for chronic lymphocytic leukemia: revised guidelines for diagnosis and treatment. *Blood* 1996;87:4990–4997.

23. Clavell LA, Gelber RD, Cohen HJ, et al. Four-agent induction and intensive asparaginase therapy for treatment of childhood acute lymphoblastic leukemia. *N Engl J Med* 1986;315:657–663.

24. Conter V, Schrappe M, Arico M, et al. Role of cranial radiotherapy for childhood T-cell acute lymphoblastic leukemia with high WBC count and good response to prednisone. Associazione Italiana Ematologia Oncologia Pediatrica and the Berlin-Frankfurt-Munster groups. *J Clin Oncol* 1997;15:2786–2791.

25. Cortes J. Central nervous system involvement in adult acute lymphocytic leukemia. *Hematol Oncol Clin North Am* 2001;15:145–162.

26. Creutzig U, Ritter J, Zimmermann M, et al. Does cranial irradiation reduce the risk for bone marrow relapse in acute myelogenous leukemia? Unexpected results of the Childhood Acute Myelogenous Leukemia Study BFM-87. *J Clin Oncol* 1993;11:279–286.

27. Dahl GV, Simone JV, Hustu HO, et al. Preventive central nervous system irradiation in children with acute nonlymphocytic leukemia. *Cancer* 1978;42:2187–2192.

28. DeAngelo DJ. The treatment of adolescents and young adults with acute lymphoblastic leukemia. *Hematology* 2005;2005:123–130.

29. Dobrovic A, Morley AA, Seshadri R, et al. Molecular diagnosis of Philadelphia negative CML using the polymerase chain reaction and DNA analysis: clinical features and course of M-bcr negative and M-bcr positive CML. *Leukemia* 1991;5:187–190.

30. Druker BJ, Sawyers CL, Kantarjian H, et al. Activity of a specific inhibitor of the BCR-ABL tyrosine kinase in the blast crisis of chronic myeloid leukemia and acute lymphoblastic leukemia with the Philadelphia chromosome. *N Engl J Med* 2001;344:1038–1042.

31. Druker BJ, Talpaz M, Resta DJ, et al. Efficacy and safety of a specific inhibitor of the BCR-ABL tyrosine kinase in chronic myeloid leukemia. *N Engl J Med* 2001;344:1031–1037.

32. Dunbar SF, Barnes PD, Tarbell NJ. Radiologic determination of the caudal border of the spinal field in cranial spinal irradiation. *Int J Radiat Oncol Biol Phys* 1993;26:669–673.

33. Enright H, Daniels K, Arthur DC, et al. Related donor marrow transplant for chronic myeloid leukemia: patient characteristics predictive of outcome. *Bone Marrow Transplant* 1996;17:537–542.

34. Evans AE. Central nervous system workshop. *Cancer Clin Trials* 1981;4[Suppl]:31–35.

35. Freeman AI, Weinberg V, Brecher ML, et al. Comparison of intermediate dose methotrexate with cranial irradiation for the post induction treatment of acute lymphocytic leukemia in children. *N Engl J Med* 1983;308:477–484.

36. Freeman JE, Johnston PG, Voke JM. Somnolence after prophylactic cranial irradiation in children with acute lymphoblastic leukemia. *Br Med J* 1973;4:523–525.

37. Gajjar A, Harrison PL, Sandlund JT, et al. Traumatic lumbar puncture at diagnosis adversely affects outcome in childhood acute lymphoblastic leukemia. *Blood* 2000;96:3381–3384.

38. Gale RP, Hehlmann R, Zhang MJ, et al. Survival with bone marrow transplantation versus hydroxyurea or interferon for chronic myelogenous leukemia. The German CML Study Group. *Blood* 1998;91:1810–1819.

39. Gaynon PS, Desai AA, Bostrom BC, et al. Early response to therapy and outcome in childhood acute lymphoblastic leukemia: a review. *Cancer* 1997;80:1717–1726.

40. George SL, Ochs JJ, Mauer AM, et al. The importance of an isolated central nervous system relapse in children with acute lymphoblastic leukemia. *J Clin Oncol* 1985;3:776–781.

41. Gilchrist GS, Tubergen DG, Sather HN, et al. Low numbers of CSF blasts at diagnosis do not predict for the development of CNS leukemia in children with intermediate-risk acute lymphoblastic leukemia: a Childrens Cancer Group report. *J Clin Oncol* 1994;12:2594–2600.

42. Giles FJ, O'Brien SM, Keating MJ. Chronic lymphocytic leukemia in (Richter's) transformation. *Semin Oncol* 1998;25:117–125.

43. Goldstone AH, Burnett AK, Wheatley K, et al. Attempts to improve treatment outcomes in acute myeloid leukemia (AML) in older patients: the results of the United Kingdom Medical Research Council AML11 trial. *Blood* 2001;98:1302–1311.

44. Gorre ME, Mohammed M, Ellwood K, et al. Clinical resistance to STI-571 cancer therapy caused by BCR-ABL gene mutation or amplification. *Science* 2001;293:876–880.

45. Green DM, Freeman AI, Sather HN, et al. Comparison of three methods of central-nervous-system prophylaxis in childhood acute lymphoblastic leukaemia. *Lancet* 1980;1:1398–1402.

46. Griffin TW, Rasey JS, Bleyer WA. The effect of photon irradiation on blood-brain barrier permeability to methotrexate in mice. *Cancer* 1977;40: UNKNOWN.

47. Halberg FE, Kramer JH, Moore IM, et al. Prophylactic cranial irradiation dose effects on late cognitive function in children treated for acute lymphoblastic leukemia. *Int J Radiat Oncol Biol Phys* 1992;22:13–16.

48. Halperin EC. Concerning the inferior portion of the spinal radiotherapy field for malignancies that disseminate via the cerebrospinal fluid. *Int J Radiat Oncol Biol Phys* 1993;26:357–362.

49. Halperin EC. Impact of radiation technique upon the outcome of treatment for medulloblastoma. *Int J Radiat Oncol Biol Phys* 1996;36:233–239.

50. Hill JM, Kornblith AB, Jones D, et al. A comparative study of the long term psychosocial functioning of childhood acute lymphoblastic leukemia survivors treated by intrathecal methotrexate with or without cranial radiation. *Cancer* 1998;82:208–218.

51. Hong JH, Chiang CS, Campbell IL, et al. Induction of acute phase gene expression by brain irradiation. *Int J Radiat Oncol Biol Phys* 1995;33:619–626.

52. Hustu HO, Aur RJ. Extramedullary leukaemia. *Clin Haematol* 1978;7:313–337.

53. Ingram LC, Fairclough DL, Furman WL, et al. Cranial nerve palsy in childhood acute lymphoblastic leukemia and non-Hodgkin's lymphoma. *Cancer* 1991;67:2262–2268.

54. Jemal A, Siegel R, Ward E, et al. Cancer Statistics, 2006. *CA Cancer J Clin* 2006;56:106–130.

55. Jones B, Shuster JJ, Holland JF. Lower incidence of meningeal leukemia when dexamethasone is substituted for prednisone in the treatment of acute lymphocytic leukemia– a late follow-up.1984;3:204.

56. Kantarjian HM, Smith TL, McCredie KB, et al. Chronic myelogenous leukemia: a multivariate analysis of the associations of patient characteristics and therapy with survival. *Blood* 1985;66:1326–1335.

57. Karlsson U, Kirby T, Orrison W, et al. Ocular globe topography in radiotherapy. *Int J Radiat Oncol Biol Phys* 1995;33:705–712.

58. Keating MJ, O'Brien S, Albitar M, et al. Early results of a chemoimmunotherapy regimen of fludarabine, cyclophosphamide, and rituximab as initial therapy for chronic lymphocytic leukemia. *J Clin Oncol* 2005;23:4079–4088.

59. Khouri IF, Keating MJ, Vriesendorp HM, et al. Autologous and allogeneic bone marrow transplantation for chronic lymphocytic leukemia: preliminary results. *J Clin Oncol* 1994;12:748–758.

60. Koehler M, Behm FG, Shuster J, et al. Transitional pre-B-cell acute lymphoblastic leukemia of childhood is associated with favorable prognostic clinical features and an excellent outcome: a Pediatric Oncology Group study. *Leukemia* 1993;7:2064–2068.

61. Komp DM, Fernandez CH, Falletta JM, et al. CNS prophylaxis in acute lymphoblastic leukemia: comparison of two methods a Southwest Oncology Group study. *Cancer* 1982;50:1031–1036.

62. Kumar P, Kun LE, Hustu HO, et al. Survival outcome following isolated central nervous system relapse treated with additional chemotherapy and craniospinal irradiation in childhood acute lymphoblastic leukemia. *Int J Radiat Oncol Biol Phys* 1995;31:477–483.

63. Kun LE, Camitta BM, Mulhern RK, et al. Treatment of meningeal relapse in childhood acute lymphoblastic leukemia. I. Results of craniospinal irradiation. *J Clin Oncol* 1984;2:359–364.

64. Land VJ, Thomas PR, Boyett JM, et al. Comparison of maintenance treatment regimens for first central nervous system relapse in children with acute lymphocytic leukemia. A Pediatric Oncology Group study. *Cancer* 1985;56:81–87.

65. Laport GF, Larson RA. Treatment of adult acute lymphoblastic leukemia. *Semin Oncol* 1997;24:70–82.

66. Larson RA, Dodge RK, Burns CP, et al. A five-drug remission induction regimen with intensive consolidation for adults with acute lymphoblastic leukemia: cancer and leukemia group B study 8811. *Blood* 1995;85:2025–2037.

67. Laver JH, Barredo JC, Amylon M, et al. Effects of cranial radiation in children with high risk T cell acute lymphoblastic leukemia: a Pediatric Oncology Group report. *Leukemia* 2000;14:369–373.

68. LeClerc JM, Billett AL, Gelber RD, et al. Treatment of childhood acute lymphoblastic leukemia: results of Dana-Farber ALL Consortium Protocol 87-01. *J Clin Oncol* 2002;20:237–246.

69. Leiper AD, Stanhope R, Kitching P, et al. Precocious and premature puberty associated with treatment of acute lymphoblastic leukaemia. *Arch Dis Child* 1987;62:1107–1112.

70. MacLean WE, Jr., Noll RB, Stehbens JA, et al. Neuropsychological effects of cranial irradiation in young children with acute lymphoblastic leukemia 9 months after diagnosis. The Children's Cancer Group. *Arch Neurol* 1995;52:156–160.

71. Mahmoud HH, Rivera GK, Hancock ML, et al. Low leukocyte counts with blast cells in cerebrospinal fluid of children with newly diagnosed acute lymphoblastic leukemia. *N Engl J Med* 1993;329:314–319.

72. Mahoney DH, Jr., Shuster J, Nitschke R, et al. Intermediate-dose intravenous methotrexate with intravenous mercaptopurine is superior to repetitive low-dose oral methotrexate with intravenous mercaptopurine for children with lower-risk B-lineage acute lymphoblastic leukemia: a Pediatric Oncology Group phase III trial. *J Clin Oncol* 1998;16:246–254.

73. Mandell LR, Steinherz P, Fuks Z. Delayed central nervous system (CNS) radiation in childhood CNS acute lymphoblastic leukemia. Results of a pilot trial. *Cancer* 1990;66:447–450.

74. Mandell LR, Walker RW, Steinherz P, et al. Reduced incidence of the somnolence syndrome in leukemic children with steroid coverage during prophylactic cranial radiation therapy. Results of a pilot study. *Cancer* 1989;63:1975–1978.

75. Michallet M, Archimbaud E, Bandini G, et al. HLA-identical sibling bone marrow transplantation in younger patients with chronic lymphocytic leukemia. European Group for Blood and Marrow Transplantation and the International Bone Marrow Transplant Registry. *Ann Intern Med* 1996;124:311–315.

76. Minot GR, Buckman TE, Isaacs R. Chronic myelogenous leukemia: age incidence, duration and benefit derived from irradiation. *JAMA* 1924;82:1489.

77. Mulhern RK, Fairclough D, Ochs J. A prospective comparison of neuropsychologic performance of children surviving leukemia who received 18-Gy, 24-Gy, or no cranial irradiation. *J Clin Oncol* 1991;9:1348–1356.

78. Mulhern RK, Khan RB, Kaplan S, et al. Short-term efficacy of methylphenidate: a randomized, double-blind, placebo-controlled trial among survivors of childhood cancer. *J Clin Oncol* 2004;22:4795–4803.

79. Nachman J, Palmer NF, Sather HN, et al. Open-wedge testicular biopsy in childhood acute lymphoblastic leukemia after two years of maintenance therapy: diagnostic accuracy and influence on outcome–a report from Children's Cancer Study Group. *Blood* 1990;75:1051–1055.

80. Neglia JP, Meadows AT, Robison LL, et al. Second neoplasms after acute lymphoblastic leukemia in childhood. *N Engl J Med* 1991;325:1330–1336.

81. Nelson SC, Bruggers CS, Kurtzberg J, et al. Management of leukemic hyper-

leukocytosis with hydration, urinary alkalinization, and allopurinol. Are cranial irradiation and invasive cytoreduction necessary? *Am J Pediatr Hematol Oncol* 1993;15:351–355.

82. Nesbit ME Jr, Sather HN, Robison LL, et al. Presymptomatic central nervous system therapy in previously untreated childhood acute lymphoblastic leukaemia: comparison of 1800 rad and 2400 rad. A report for Children's Cancer Study Group. *Lancet* 1981;1:461–466.

83. Nesbit ME, Sather H, Robison LL, et al. Sanctuary therapy: a randomized trial of 724 children with previously untreated acute lymphoblastic leukemia: a report from Children's Cancer Study Group. *Cancer Res* 1982;42:674–680.

84. Nowell P, Hungerford D. A minute chromosome in human chronic granulocytic leukemia. *Science* 1960;132:1497.

85. O'Brien SG, Guilhot F, Larson RA, et al. Imatinib compared with interferon and low-dose cytarabine for newly diagnosed chronic-phase chronic myeloid leukemia. *N Engl J Med* 2003;348:994–1004.

86. Odom LF, Wilson H, Cullen J, et al. Significance of blasts in low-cell-count cerebrospinal fluid specimens from children with acute lymphoblastic leukemia. *Cancer* 1990;66:1748–1754.

87. Ortega JA, Nesbit ME, Sather HN, et al. Long-term evaluation of a CNS prophylaxis trial–treatment comparisons and outcome after CNS relapse in childhood ALL: a report from the Children's Cancer Study Group. *J Clin Oncol* 1987;5:1646–1654.

88. Osterborg A, Dyer MJ, Bunjes D, et al. Phase II multicenter study of human CD52 antibody in previously treated chronic lymphocytic leukemia. European Study Group of CAMPATH-1H Treatment in Chronic Lymphocytic Leukemia. *J Clin Oncol* 1997;15:1567–1574.

89. Paryani SB, Donaldson SS, Amylon MD, et al. Cranial nerve involvement in children with leukemia and lymphoma. *J Clin Oncol* 1983;1:542–545.

90. Pinkerton CR, Chessells JM. Failed central nervous system prophylaxis in children with acute lymphoblastic leukaemia: treatment and outcome. *Br J Haematol* 1984;57:553–561.

91. Preudhomme C, Lepelley P, Lovi V, et al. T-cell acute lymphoblastic leukemia occurring in the course of B cell chronic lymphocytic leukemia: a case report. *Leuk Lymphoma* 1995;18:361–364.

92. Price RA, Johnson WW. The central nervous system in childhood leukemia. I. The arachnoid. *Cancer* 1973;31:520–533.

93. Pui CH, Evans WE. Acute lymphoblastic leukemia. *N Engl J Med* 1998;339:605–615.

94. Pui CH. Childhood leukemias. *N Engl J Med* 1995;332:1618–1630.

95. Pusey WA. Report of cases treated with roentgen rays. *JAMA* 1902;38:911.

96. Rabinowe SN, Soiffer RJ, Gribben JG, et al. Autologous and allogeneic bone marrow transplantation for poor prognosis patients with B-cell chronic lymphocytic leukemia. *Blood* 1993;82:1366–1376.

97. Rai KR, Peterson B, Kolitz J. A randomized comparison of fludarabine and chlorambucil for patients with previously untreated chronic lymphocytic leukemia. A CALGB, SWOG, CTG/NCI-C, and ECOG Inter Group Study. *Blood* 1996;88:141(abstr).

98. Rai KR, Sawitsky A, Cronkite EP, et al. Clinical staging of chronic lymphocytic leukemia. *Blood* 1975;46:219–234.

99. Reiter A, Schrappe M, Ludwig WD, et al. Chemotherapy in 998 unselected childhood acute lymphoblastic leukemia patients. Results and conclusions of the multicenter trial ALL-BFM 86. *Blood* 1994;84:3122–3133.

100. Ribeiro RC, Rivera GK, Hudson M, et al. An intensive re-treatment protocol for children with an isolated CNS relapse of acute lymphoblastic leukemia. *J Clin Oncol* 1995;13:333–338.

101. Richter MN. Generalized reticular cell sarcoma of lymph nodes associated with lymphocytic leukemia. *Am J Pathol* 1928;4:285–292.

102. Rieselback RE, DiChiro, Freireich EJ, et al. Subarachnoid distribution of drugs after lumbar puncture. *N Engl J Med* 1962;267:1273–1278.

103. Ritchey AK, Pollock BH, Lauer SJ, et al. Improved survival of children with isolated CNS relapse of acute lymphoblastic leukemia: a pediatric oncology group study. *J Clin Oncol* 1999;17:3745–3752.

104. Rivera G, George SL, Bowman WP, et al. Second central nervous system prophylaxis in children with acute lymphoblastic leukemia who relapse after elective cessation of therapy. *J Clin Oncol* 1983;1:471–476.

105. Roman DD, Sperduto PW. Neuropsychological effects of cranial radiation: current knowledge and future directions. *Int J Radiat Oncol Biol Phys* 1995;31:983–998.

106. Savage DG, Szydlo RM, Goldman JM. Clinical features at diagnosis in 430 patients with chronic myeloid leukaemia seen at a referral centre over a 16-year period. *Br J Haematol* 1997;96:111–116.

107. Schorin MA, Blattner S, Gelber RD, et al. Treatment of childhood acute lymphoblastic leukemia: results of Dana-Farber Cancer Institute/Children's Hospital Acute Lymphoblastic Leukemia Consortium Protocol 85-01. *J Clin Oncol* 1994;12:740–747.

108. Schrappe M, Reiter A, Ludwig WD, et al. Improved outcome in childhood acute lymphoblastic leukemia despite reduced use of anthracyclines and cranial radiotherapy: results of trial ALL-BFM 90. German-Austrian-Swiss ALL-BFM Study Group. *Blood* 2000;95:3310–3322.

109. Shank B, Chu FC, Dinsmore R, et al. Hyperfractionated total body irradiation for bone marrow transplantation. Results in seventy leukemia patients with allogeneic transplants. *Int J Radiat Oncol Biol Phys* 1983;9:1607–1611.

110. Shapiro WR, Young DF, Mehta BM. Methotrexate: distribution in cerebrospinal fluid after intravenous, ventricular and lumbar injections. *N Engl J Med* 1975;293:161–166.

111. Simone JV. Leukaemia remission and survival. *Lancet* 1981;2:531.

112. Sklar C, Mertens A, Walter A, et al. Final height after treatment for childhood acute lymphoblastic leukemia: comparison of no cranial irradiation with 1800 and 2400 centigrays of cranial irradiation. *J Pediatr* 1993;123:59–64.

113. Sklar CA, Robison LL, Nesbit ME, et al. Effects of radiation on testicular function in long-term survivors of childhood acute lymphoblastic leukemia: a report from the Children's Cancer Study Group. *J Clin Oncol* 1990;8:1981–1987.

114. Smith M, Arthur D, Camitta B, et al. Uniform approach to risk classification and treatment assignment for children with acute lymphoblastic leukemia. *J Clin Oncol* 1996;14:18–24.

115. Socie G, Curtis RE, Deeg HJ, et al. New malignant diseases after allogeneic marrow transplantation for childhood acute leukemia. *J Clin Oncol* 2000;18:348–357.

116. Sokal JE, Cox EB, Baccarani M, et al. Prognostic discrimination in "good-risk" chronic granulocytic leukemia. *Blood* 1984;63:789–799.

117. Stubberfield TG, Byrne GC, Jones TW. Growth and growth hormone secretion after treatment for acute lymphoblastic leukemia in childhood. 18-Gy versus 24-Gy cranial irradiation. *J Pediatr Hematol Oncol* 1995;17:167–171.

118. Sullivan MP, Chen T, Dyment PG, et al. Equivalence of intrathecal chemotherapy and radiotherapy as central nervous system prophylaxis in children with acute lymphatic leukemia: a pediatric oncology group study. *Blood* 1982;60:948–958.

119. Sullivan MP, Perez CA, Herson J, et al. Radiotherapy (2500 rad) for testicular leukemia: local control and subsequent clinical events: a Southwest Oncology Group study. *Cancer* 1980;46:508–515.

120. Testicular disease in acute lymphoblastic leukaemia in childhood. Report on behalf of the Medical Research Council's Working Party on leukaemia in childhood. *Br Med J* 1978;1:334–338.

121. Thomas ED, Clift RA, Fefer A, et al. Marrow transplantation for the treatment of chronic myelogenous leukemia. *Ann Intern Med* 1986;104:155–163.

122. Torres A, Martinez F, Gomez P, et al. Allogeneic bone marrow transplantation versus chemotherapy in the treatment of childhood acute lymphoblastic leukemia in second complete remission. *Bone Marrow Transplant* 1989;4:609–612.

123. Tubergen DG, Cullen JW, Boyett JM, et al. Blasts in CSF with a normal cell count do not justify alteration of therapy for acute lymphoblastic leukemia in remission: a Children's Cancer Group study. *J Clin Oncol* 1994;12:273–278.

124. Tubergen DG, Gilchrist GS, O'Brien RT, et al. Prevention of CNS disease in intermediate-risk acute lymphoblastic leukemia: comparison of cranial radiation and intrathecal methotrexate and the importance of systemic therapy: a Children's Cancer Group report. *J Clin Oncol* 1993;11:520–526.

125. Uckun FM, Sensel MG, Sun L, et al. Biology and treatment of childhood T-lineage acute lymphoblastic leukemia. *Blood* 1998;91:735–746.

126. Uzal D, Ozyar E, Hayran M, et al. Reduced incidence of the somnolence syndrome after prophylactic cranial irradiation in children with acute lymphoblastic leukemia. *Radiother Oncol* 1998;48:29–32.

127. Vardiman JW, Harris NL, Brunning RD. The World Health Organization (WHO) classification of the myeloid neoplasms. *Blood* 2002;100:2292–2302.

128. Waber DP, Shapiro BL, Carpentieri SC, et al. Excellent therapeutic efficacy and minimal late neurotoxicity in children treated with 18 grays of cranial radiation therapy for high-risk acute lymphoblastic leukemia: a 7-year follow-up study of the Dana-Farber Cancer Institute Consortium Protocol 87-01. *Cancer* 2001;92:15–22.

129. Waber DP, Tarbell NJ, Fairclough D, et al. Cognitive sequelae of treatment in childhood acute lymphoblastic leukemia: cranial radiation requires an accomplice. *J Clin Oncol* 1995;13:2490–2496.

130. Waber DP, Tarbell NJ, Kahn CM, et al. The relationship of sex and treatment modality to neuropsychologic outcome in childhood acute lymphoblastic leukemia. *J Clin Oncol* 1992;10:810–817.

131. Walter AW, Hancock ML, Pui CH, et al. Secondary brain tumors in children treated for acute lymphoblastic leukemia at St Jude Children's Research Hospital. *J Clin Oncol* 1998;16:3761–3767.

132. Weinmann M, Becker G, Einsele H, et al. Clinical indications and biological mechanisms of splenic irradiation in chronic leukemias and myeloproliferative disorders. *Radiother Oncol* 2001;58:235–246.

133. Weiss E, Krebeck M, Kohler B, et al. Does the standardized helmet technique lead to adequate coverage of the cribriform plate? An analysis of current practice with respect to the ICRU 50 report. *Int J Radiat Oncol Biol Phys* 2001;49:1475–1480.

134. Wells RJ, Weetman RM, Baehner RL. The impact of isolated central nervous system relapse following initially complete remission in childhood acute lymphocytic leukemia. *J Pediatr* 1980;97:429–432.

135. Wheatley K. The AML Collaborative Group: Meta-analysis of randomized trials of idarubicin (IDAR) or mitoxantrone (MITO) versus daunomycin (DNR) as induction therapy for acute myeloid leukemia (AML). *Blood* 1995;86:434(abstr).

136. Willoughby ML. Treatment of overt meningeal leukaemia in children: results of second MRC meningeal leukaemia trial. *Br Med J* 1976;1:864–867.

137. Winick NJ, Smith SD, Shuster J, et al. Treatment of CNS relapse in children with acute lymphoblastic leukemia: a Pediatric Oncology Group study. *J Clin Oncol* 1993;11:271–278.

138. Wofford MM, Smith SD, Shuster JJ, et al. Treatment of occult or late overt testicular relapse in children with acute lymphoblastic leukemia: a Pediatric Oncology Group study. *J Clin Oncol* 1992;10:624–630.

139. Zwiebel JA, Cheson BD. Chronic lymphocytic leukemia: staging and prognostic factors. *Semin Oncol* 1998;25:42–59.

Clinical Radiation Oncology

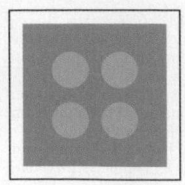

Chapter 79
Plasma Cell Myeloma and Plasmacytoma

David C. Hodgson, Joseph Mikhael, Richard W. Tsang

Epidemiology and Etiology

Plasma cell neoplasms account for 22% of all mature B-cell neoplasms in the Surveillance, Epidemiology, and End Results (SEER) program in the United States (85). The majority of plasma cell neoplasms are multiple myeloma, with solitary plasmacytoma accounting for ≤6% of cases and rarely plasma cell leukemia. Although the incidence of multiple myeloma has gradually increased in the 1970s through the 1990s (100), recently there has been a downward trend, with an annual decrease of 0.3% from 1992 to 2002 (101). Data from SEER indicate an incidence rate of 5.5/100,000 per year and mortality rate of 3.8/100,000 per year during the period 1998 to 2002 (101). For 2007, it is estimated that there will be 19,900 new cases and 10,790 deaths due to multiple myeloma in the United States (5). The incidence rate exceeds that of Hodgkin's lymphoma and is about one-quarter that of non-Hodgkin's lymphoma. The incidence rate rises with advancing age, with a median age at diagnosis of 70 years (101), and <1% of cases are diagnosed in persons <35. Nonregistry studies usually report a lower median age ranging from 60 to 66 years (50,68). There is a slight male predominance, and for black Americans, the incidence and mortality rates are approximately double that of whites. The 5-year relative survival rates have increased, from 26% in 1975 to 1977, to 33% in 1996 to 2002 (p <.05) (5). The etiology of multiple myeloma is not known, but there are studies reporting association with prior exposure to radiation (e.g., atomic bomb survivors in Hiroshima) (88), certain chemicals such as petroleum products (18,29) and monoclonal gammopathy of unknown significance (MGUS) (69). The previously reported association with herpes simplex virus type 8 does not appear to be causally related (113).

Natural History, Genetic Mechanisms

Multiple myeloma is a disease with a wide clinical spectrum, ranging from the condition known as MGUS to the most aggressive form, plasma cell leukemia (Table 79.1). In all cases, a plasma cell clone exists but to varying degrees. The secretion of a monoclonal protein by these plasma cells, along with their interaction with the bone marrow environment, is the source of organ damage in patients with this illness (54). These concepts have become particularly important as the molecular mechanisms by which the disease progresses through these "stages" provide essential information that may help to better understand the disease and its potential therapies.

Monoclonal Gammopathy of Unknown Significance

MGUS has traditionally been considered a benign or a premalignant condition in which only a small proportion of patients will progress to multiple myeloma or related diseases (see Table 79.1). In MGUS, the monoclonal protein is ≤3 g/dL and the bone marrow clonal plasma cells are <10% with no related organ damage. This condition is likely much more common than initially thought, as it has been documented in 3% of the overall population and 5% in those over the age of 70 (70). The risk of transformation to myeloma and related diseases (such as amyloidosis or Waldenstrom's macroglobulinemia) has been estimated at 1% per year, based on a 30-year follow-up of 1,384 patients at the Mayo Clinic (69).

Asymptomatic Multiple Myeloma (Smoldering Myeloma)

Asymptomatic multiple myeloma represents an intermediate form of myeloma whereby patients meet serological monoclonal protein and bone marrow criteria for the diagnosis of myeloma (in excess of 10% clonal plasmacytosis) but have yet to develop evidence of end organ damage (see Table 79.1). These patients are not significantly anemic, do not have renal insufficiency, and do not have bony disease. Although the risk of transformation to multiple myeloma is much higher than in MGUS (5–10% per year), some patients may "smolder" for many years. These patients generally do not require therapy but should be followed closely to monitor for progression.

Pathophysiology

Multiple myeloma arises from malignant transformation of a late-state B cell. Although the seminal event has yet to be defined, one of the earliest genetic events is the illegitimate switch recombination of partner oncogenes into the immunoglobulin heavy (IgH) chain (65). Other events may occur such as cytogenetic hyperploidy and upregulation of cell cycle control genes. The result of these genetic abnormalities is the development and propagation of a clonal population of B cells within the bone marrow; this, however, is common and can be seen in up to 5% of the general population over the age of 70 (70). Most of these will not go on to develop myeloma, so there must be additional events to create the malignant phenotype of multiple myeloma. These secondary events may include mutations of kinases, deletions of chromosomes, and up-regulation of enzymes such as c-myc (43). Having sustained a secondary event, the malignant plasma cells begin to proliferate in the bone marrow microenvironment, producing monoclonal proteins and causing osteolytic bone disease. The slow accumulation of these malignant cells gradually results in the characteristic clinical features of myeloma of anemia, bone resorption, hypercalcemia, renal failure, and immunodeficiency. Established myeloma is dependent and sustained on a number of microenvironment features, including the bone marrow stroma itself and the cytokines interleukin-6 and insulinlike growth factor-1 (54). The bone disease that arises in myeloma appears to be mediated in part by RANK ligand/osteoprotegerin and the Wnt-signaling antagonist dickkopf 1 (DKK1) (114).

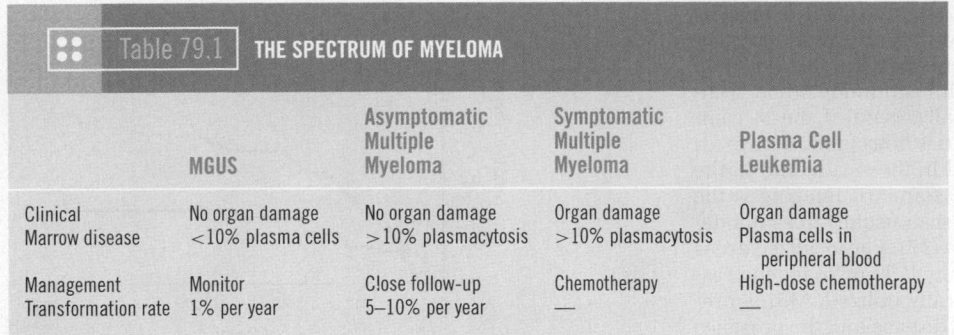

	MGUS	Asymptomatic Multiple Myeloma	Symptomatic Multiple Myeloma	Plasma Cell Leukemia
Clinical Marrow disease	No organ damage <10% plasma cells	No organ damage >10% plasmacytosis	Organ damage >10% plasmacytosis	Organ damage Plasma cells in peripheral blood
Management Transformation rate	Monitor 1% per year	Close follow-up 5–10% per year	Chemotherapy —	High-dose chemotherapy —

MGUS, monoclonal gammopathy of unknown significance

Clinical Presentation

Solitary Plasmacytomas

The median age at diagnosis of solitary plasmacytoma (SP) is 55 to 65 years, on average about 10 years younger than patients with multiple myeloma (90,110,117). Males are affected predominately (male:female ratio 2:1) (90). A diagnosis of SP is made if all the following criteria are satisfied at presentation: a histologically confirmed single lesion with negative skeletal imaging outside the primary site, normal bone marrow biopsy (<10% monoclonal plasma cells), and no myeloma-related organ dysfunction (37). A monoclonal protein is present in 30% to 75% of cases (particularly for an osseous presentation), the level is usually minimally elevated (IgG <3.5 g/dL, IgA <2.0 g/dL, and urine monoclonal kappa or lambda <1.0 g per 24 hours) (37,121).

The disease more commonly presents in bone (80%). Such cases are considered stage I multiple myeloma according to the Durie and Salmon (38) staging system. The most common location is the vertebra (90). Patients with bone involvement often present with pain, neurologic compromise, and occasionally pathologic fracture. A lytic lesion is typical, with or without adjacent soft tissue mass. Less commonly SP presents in an extramedullary site (20%), usually as a mass in the upper aerorespiratory passages that produces local compressive symptoms (4,90,110,116). The histologic diagnosis of extramedullary plasmacytoma (EMP) can be difficult, with the main differential diagnosis being extranodal marginal zone lymphoma (MALT type), where there can be extensive infiltration by plasmacytoid cells (4,58).

Multiple Myeloma

Bone pain and symptoms due to anemia, such as easy fatigability, are the most common (68). Because of the myriad effects of the disease, other insidious symptoms can result from a combination of hypercalcemia, renal impairment, infection, neurologic compression, and occasionally, hyperviscosity. Bone disease manifesting as generalized osteopenia and multiple lytic bone lesions can frequently lead to pathologic fractures. In the vertebral column, this often results in a diminished height. Sclerotic lesions at presentation are rare.

Laboratory evaluation generally confirms anemia, high erythrocyte sedimentation rate, and a variable degree of granulocytopenia and thrombocytopenia. An abnormal monoclonal immunoglobulin (M-protein) in the blood and/or urine is characteristic (68), most commonly immunoglobulin G (IgG) or immunoglobulin A (IgA). Biclonal disease is also recognized, and, rarely, nonsecretary disease. Occasionally only monoclonal light chains are detected. It is important to assess for hypercalcemia, renal dysfunction, and integrity of the skele-

ton because these complications require appropriate management. A constellation of polyneuropathy, organomegaly, endocrinopathy, M-protein, and skin changes characterize a rare plasma cell dyscrasia known as polyneuropathy, organomegaly, endocrinopathy, monoclonal gammopathy, and skin changes (POEMS) syndrome (33,89).

Plasma Cell Leukemia

Plasma cell leukemia is a very rare variant of multiple myeloma, where the proliferation of plasma cells is not confined to the bone marrow but may be detected in the peripheral blood. It carries a very poor prognosis with median survival of only 3 to 6 months (123). There is currently no standard therapy for this condition, but patients are usually treated with high-dose, multiagent chemotherapeutic regimens or with experimental therapies.

Diagnostic Work-Up and Staging

The recommended tests for the diagnosis of plasma cell neoplasms are outlined in Table 79.2. The most important components relate to the measurement and quantification of the M-protein, bone marrow examination with ancillary

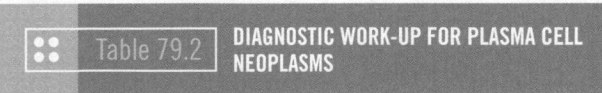

Table 79.2   DIAGNOSTIC WORK-UP FOR PLASMA CELL NEOPLASMS

General
  History and physical examination
  Complete blood count, and blood smear, chemistry panel including calcium and creatinine

Standard laboratory tests
  Bone marrow aspirate and trephine biopsy, or biopsy of mass if solitary lesion (clonality, immunophenotype and cytogenetic studies, plasma cell labeling index)
  Serum β_2 microglobulin, albumin, C-reactive protein, and lactate dehydrogenase

M-component measurement:
  • serum protein electrophoresis (SPEP) and immunofixation for quantification of immunoglobulins
  • Urine protein electrophoresis
  • Free light chain measurements

Imaging studies
  Skeletal survey
  Computed tomography and magnetic resonance imaging where indicated (e.g., to visualize soft tissue tumor, detailed assessment of local disease extent and bulk, assessing vertebral column osteopenia and compression fractures, and spinal cord compression)
  ^{18}F-fluorodeoxyglucose positron emission tomography or magnetic resonance imaging may be ordered to detect occult disease if clinically indicated

Clinical Radiation Oncology

studies, serum β_2 microglobulin and albumin, and diagnostic imaging of involved bony sites. The M-protein should be measured with serum protein electrophoresis (SPEP). Quantification of the monoclonal immunoglobin with immunofixation techniques is also acceptable and especially useful if the M component is at a low level. If no M-protein is detectable, assays for free light chains should be performed in the serum and in the urine (Bence-Jones proteinuria). The standard imaging is the skeletal survey, as radionuclide bone scan usually does not detect lytic disease and has limited value (37). For localized areas of concern, both computed tomography (CT) or magnetic resonance imaging (MRI) should be liberally utilized. MRI is preferred to assess the extent of vertebral disease and the presence of spinal cord or nerve root compression. With advances in diagnostic imaging, it is likely that "stage migration" has occurred (41). It has been documented that some patients with presumed solitary plasmacytoma of bone will be upstaged following the detection of multiple vertebral lesions or bone marrow disease by MRI (74,76,118) or by ^{18}F-fluorodeoxyglucose positron emission tomography (FDG-PET) (105). The staging criteria for the widely used Durie and Salmon staging system are detailed in Table 79.3 (38). The newer International Myeloma staging system is simple, validated, and of importance particularly for present and future clinical trials (see Table 79.3) (50). Criteria for the diagnosis of MGUS and asymptomatic (smoldering) myeloma are also well established (37,51).

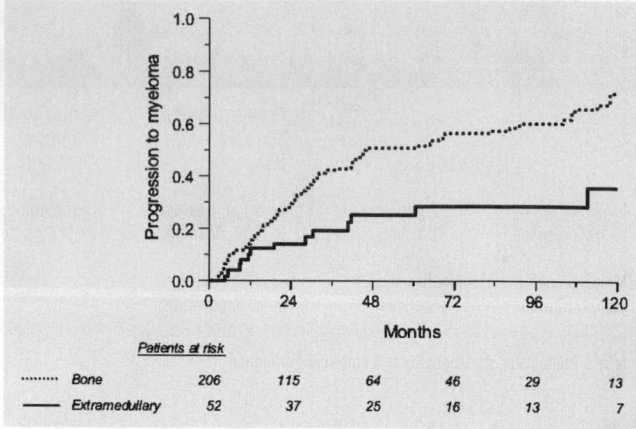

FIGURE 79.1. Probability of progression to multiple myeloma according to bone (*dotted line*) versus extramedullary (*solid line*) solitary plasmacytoma in 258 patients ($p = .0009$). (From Ozsahin M, Tsang RW, Poortmans P, et al. Outcomes and patterns of failure in solitary plasmacytoma: a multicenter Rare Cancer Network study of 258 patients. *Int J Radiat Oncol Biol Phys* 2006;64:210–217, with permission from Elsevier Inc.)

Prognostic Factors

Solitary Plasmacytoma

Age is a factor affecting the risk of progression to myeloma in some series (14,24,117) but not in others (20,56,77,90,106). A bony presentation has been consistently demonstrated to have a significantly higher risk of subsequent development of myeloma with a 10-year rate of 76%, compared with an extramedullary presentation where the 10-year rate was 36% (Fig. 79.1) (90). Subclinical bone disease, either detected as generalized osteopenia (45) or through abnormal MRI scan of the spine (76,86,118), predicts for rapid progression to symptomatic multiple myeloma. A suppression of the normal immunoglobulin classes, also known as immunoparesis, has been shown to correlate with a higher risk of progressing to myeloma (45,59). Where there was an elevation of M-protein pretreatment, the persistent of the M-protein following radiation therapy (RT) promotes for progression to myeloma (71,101). Many of these factors reflect the presence of occult myeloma. Therefore, it is not surprising that generalized disease becomes manifest once the local disease is controlled. Pathologic factors have been examined in some studies, with the finding that anaplastic plasmacytomas (those with a higher histologic grade) (112), and those tumors expressing a high level of angiogenesis (67) are associated with a poor outcome. Anaplastic plasmacytomas share some common pathologic and clinical features with aggressive B-cell lymphomas (plasmablastic type) and can arise in the context of immunosuppression and Epstein-Barr virus infection (28,42).

With respect to local control, tumor bulk appears to be an important unfavorable factor. Tumors <5 cm achieved a high level of local control with 35 Gy, whereas those >5 cm had a local failure rate of 58% (7/12 patients, total dose range 25 to 50 Gy) (117). The importance of tumor bulk is also supported by other studies (56,77,90).

Multiple Myeloma

Univariate analysis of over 1,000 patients evaluated at the Mayo Clinic revealed the following adverse prognostic risk factors: Eastern Cooperative Oncology Group performance status 3 or 4, serum albumin <3 g/dL, serum creatinine ≥2 mg/dL, platelet count <150,000/μL, age ≥70 years, β_2 microglobulin >4 mg/L,

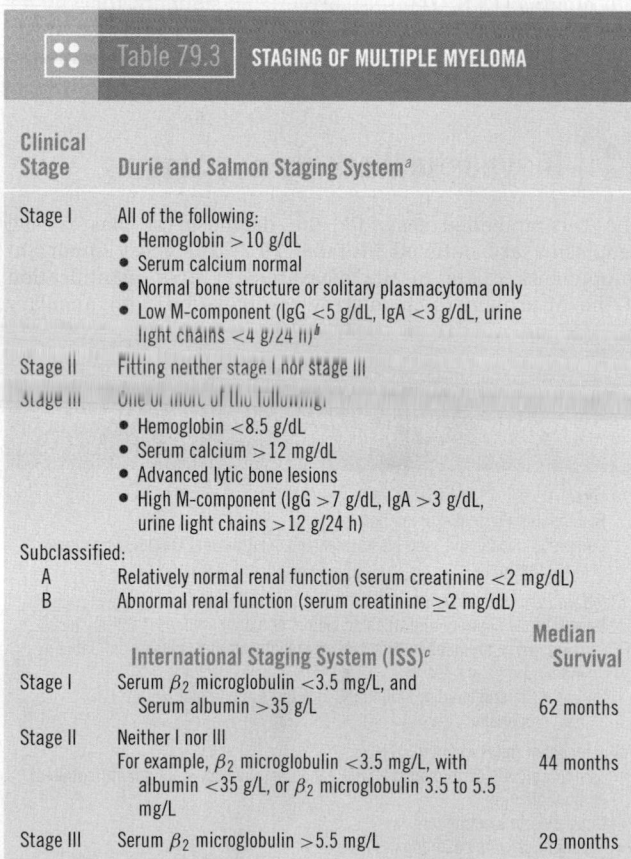

Table 79.3	**STAGING OF MULTIPLE MYELOMA**

Clinical Stage	Durie and Salmon Staging System[a]
Stage I	All of the following: • Hemoglobin >10 g/dL • Serum calcium normal • Normal bone structure or solitary plasmacytoma only • Low M-component (IgG <5 g/dL, IgA <3 g/dL, urine light chains <4 g/24 h)[b]
Stage II	Fitting neither stage I nor stage III
Stage III	One or more of the following: • Hemoglobin <8.5 g/dL • Serum calcium >12 mg/dL • Advanced lytic bone lesions • High M-component (IgG >7 g/dL, IgA >3 g/dL, urine light chains >12 g/24 h)
Subclassified: A B	Relatively normal renal function (serum creatinine <2 mg/dL) Abnormal renal function (serum creatinine ≥2 mg/dL)

International Staging System (ISS)[c]		Median Survival
Stage I	Serum β_2 microglobulin <3.5 mg/L, and Serum albumin >35 g/L	62 months
Stage II	Neither I nor III For example, β_2 microglobulin <3.5 mg/L, with albumin <35 g/L, or β_2 microglobulin 3.5 to 5.5 mg/L	44 months
Stage III	Serum β_2 microglobulin >5.5 mg/L	29 months

[a]From Durie BG, Salmon SE. A clinical staging system for multiple myeloma. Correlation of measured myeloma cell mass with presenting clinical features, response to treatment, and survival. *Cancer* 1975;36:842–854.

[b]For solitary plasmacytoma, current recommendations are IgG <3.5 g/dL, IgA <2 g/dL. (See Durie BG, Kyle RA, Belch A, et al. Myeloma management guidelines: a consensus report from the scientific advisors of the International Myeloma Foundation. *Hematol J* 2003;4:379–398.)

[c]From Greipp PR, San Miguel J, Durie BG, et al. International staging system for multiple myeloma. *J Clin Oncol* 2005;23:3412–3420.

plasma cell labeling index $\geq 1\%$, serum calcium ≥ 11 mg/dL, hemoglobin <10 g/dL, and bone marrow plasma cell $\geq 50\%$ (68).

A new International Staging System has been validated to assist in prognostication (50). Over 10,000 patients were evaluated, and the three-stage system was developed based on two variables: serum albumin and β_2 microglobulin (see Table 79.3). In addition to stage, the other area emerging as important to prognosis is cytogenetics. Much like acute leukemia, cytogenetic and molecular features are influencing treatment options. Some abnormalities demonstrated to carry a poorer prognosis include: deletion of chromosome 13 (39), presence of the t(4;14) translocation (25), and p53 deletion (92). It is expected that additional cytogenetic and molecular features of prognostic significance will be identified, especially with enhanced techniques such as fluorescence *in situ* hybridization and gene microarray analysis.

Management of Solitary Plasmacytoma

RT is the standard treatment for solitary plasmacytoma. Surgery should be considered for structural instability of bone or rapidly progressive neurologic compromise such as spinal cord compression (37,109,111). For patients treated with gross tumor excision, RT is still indicated due to a high likelihood of microscopic residual disease. Surgery alone without RT leads to an unacceptably high local recurrence rate (90). A review of the literature for solitary bone plasmacytoma in Table 79.4 indicates a high local control rate with RT (79% to 95%), yet a modest overall survival of approximately 50% at 10 years. This is due to a high rate of progression to multiple myeloma in the bone plasmacytomas, a finding consistently reported from all series (see Fig. 79.1) (14,24,44,45,56,59,63,90,117,121). As shown in Table 79.4, over 60% of patients with solitary bone tumor progressed to myeloma, at a median of 2 to 3 years after treatment. When actuarial methods were not used, the progression rate is slightly lower (crude rates ranges 53% to 54%) (44,56). Therefore, solitary plasmacytoma of the bone appears to be an early form of multiple myeloma. Studies have doc-

umented about 29% to 50% of patients with apparent solitary plasmacytoma will have multiple asymptomatic lesions detected in the spine on MRI (76,87,118). Provided that all the other diagnostic criteria for solitary plasmacytoma are satisfied, it is still appropriate to treat with local RT to the presenting site (109). For these patients the risk of developing symptomatic myeloma in a short time is high (76,86,118). Chemotherapy can be started at the time of symptomatic progression. The presence of low level M-protein preradiation is extremely common and is not associated with a higher risk of progression to multiple myeloma. However, its persistence following radiation is highly predictive of subsequent systemic failure (31,45,74,121), attesting to the importance of monitoring this as part of posttreatment follow-up.

The addition of adjuvant chemotherapy is theoretically attractive, both in enhancing local control and eradicating subclinical disease to prevent the development of myeloma. One randomized trial suggested a benefit with adjuvant melphalan and prednisone given for 3 years after RT (10). With a median follow up of 8.9 years, those treated with chemotherapy had a myeloma progression rate of 12%, whereas with RT alone it was 54% (10). However, this was a small study and the concerns regarding prolonged use of alkylating agents on the bone marrow (negative effect on stem cell reserve and risk of leukemia) do not justify its routine use.

It has been observed that some patients recur with plasmacytoma(s) of bone or soft tissues, without bone marrow involvement (14,56,64). This is infrequent and the subsequent development of multiple myeloma is high, 75% in one series (14).

In the management of EMP, while complete surgical excision may be curative for small lesions, most patients with larger lesions or those with tumor location not amenable to complete excision should receive local RT. Postoperative RT is indicated for incompletely excised lesions. In contrast to bone plasmacytoma, EMPs are frequently controlled with local radiation (Table 79.5), with a lower rate of progression to myeloma, ranging from 8% to 44% (22,27,46,61,64,75,90,108,110, 112,116,122), indicating a significant proportion of patients are cured of their disease. Although the 10-year survival varies widely in the reported literature (range 31% to 90%), the two largest series report 10-year survival rates of 72% (90) and 78% (46). The issue of dose will be discussed later.

| Table 79.4 | SOLITARY PLASMACYTOMA OF BONE: REPRESENTATIVE TREATMENT RESULTS | | | | |

Author (Reference)	Institution	No. of Patients (Median f/u)[a]	Local Control (%)	Progression to Myeloma (10-Year Rate) (%)	Overall Survival (10-Year Rate) (%)
Bataille and Sany (14)	Hospital St. Eloi, France	114 (>10 y)	88	58	68[b]
Chak et al. (24)	Stanford[c]	65[c] (87 mo)	95	77	52
Frassica et al. (44)	Mayo Clinic	46 (90 mo)	89	54[b]	45
Jackson and Scarffe (59)	Christie Hospital	32 (101 mo)	97*	~76	~45
Holland et al. (56)	Mallinckrodt	32 (66 mo)	94	53[b]	—
Galieni et al. (45)	Siena, Italy[c]	32[c] (69 mo)	91[b]	~68	49
Tsang et al. (117)	Princess Margaret Hospital	32 (95 mo)	87	64 (8-year rate)	65 (8-year rate)
Wilder et al. (121)	M.D. Anderson Cancer Center	60 (94 mo)	90	62	59
Ozsahin et al. (90)	RARE Cancer Network[c]	206[c] (56 mo)	79 (10-year rate)	72	52

mo, months
[a]Series including more than 30 patients.
[b]Crude rate.
[c]Multiple institutions.

Table 79.5 SOLITARY EXTRAMEDULLARY PLASMACYTOMA: REPRESENTATIVE TREATMENT RESULTS

Author (Reference)	Institution	No. of Patients[a] (Median f/u)	Local Control (%)	Progression to Myeloma (10-Year Rate) (%)	Overall Survival (10-Year Rate) (%)
Wiltshaw (122)	Royal Marsden	44	70	41[b]	40
Kapadia et al. (61)	U. Pittsburgh	17 (62 mo)	85	31[b]	31[b] (5-year rate)
Knowling et al. (64)	Princess Margaret Hospital	25 (71 mo)	88	28	43
Brinch et al. (22)	Oslo	18	—	—	90
Soeson et al. (108)	Padua, Italy	25 (44 mo)	88	—	~50
Susnerwala et al. (112)	Christie Hospital	25 (73 mo)	79	8[b]	59 (5-year rate)
Liebross et al. (75)	M.D. Anderson Cancer Center	22	95	44 (5-year rate)	50
Galieni et al. (46)	Siena, Italy[c]	46[c] (118 mo)	92	15[b]	78 (15 years)
Strojan et al. (110)	Slovenia Cancer Registry	26 (61 mo)	87	8	61
Chao et al. (27)	Australia[c]	16 (66 mo)	100	31	54
Ozsahin et al. (90)	RARE Cancer Network[c]	52[c] (56 mo)	74 (10-year rate)	36	72
Tournier-Rangeard et al. (116)	Centre Alexis Vautrin, France	17 (80.5 mo)	73 (10-year rate)	36	63

mo, months
[a]Series including more than 15 patients.
[b]Crude rate.
[c]Multiple institutions.

Management of Multiple Myeloma

A description of therapy of myeloma would not be complete without addressing the need to treat not only the disease itself, but the complications of this disease. Patients often present with both bony disease and anemia—both of these complications are treatable, allowing an improved quality of life. Erythropoietic agents have become the mainstay of anemia management, as have bisphosphonates (15–17,35) and local RT for bony disease. Newer surgical techniques such as vertebroplasty and kyphoplasty are also being used to improve back pain and spinal symptoms. Other supportive care interventions being addressed include diet, exercise, and patient support groups.

Initial Treatment of Symptomatic Multiple Myeloma

Patients who have symptomatic multiple myeloma require treatment of the malignant plasma cell clone. Once the decision is made to treat, however, the first step is to determine candidacy for autologous stem cell transplantation (ASCT) (Fig. 79.2). As this modality has become the standard of care for eligible patients, it is necessary to stratify patients initially so that the ability to collect stem cells is not compromised by induction therapy (49).

Patients Eligible for Autologous Stem Cell Transplantation

In patients who are candidates for ASCT, various regimens can be used to induce response prior to stem cell collection. Historically most regimens are high dose and steroid based, either with high-dose dexamethasone alone (3) or with vincristine, adriamycin, and dexamethasone (VAD) (104). An alternative induction is the combination of thalidomide and dexamethasone. Rajkumar et al. (95) demonstrated in 50 patients that this com-

bination yields a response rate of 64% (similar to VAD), without compromising the ability to collect stem cells, but with a rate of deep vein thrombosis of 12% (95). Newer agents that have been validated in the relapse setting, such as bortezomib and lenalidomide, are now being tested as initial therapy with impressive results. Early studies with bortezomib, a first-in-class proteosome inhibitor, have produced response rates of 75% to 100%, with complete remission rates of 20% to 30% (97). Lenalidomide, a derivative of thalidomide, has also been tested in newly diagnosed patients. Rajkumar et al. (96) evaluated the combination of lenalidomide with dexamethasone in 34 patients, with a response rate of 91%.

Patients Not Eligible for Autologous Stem Cell Transplantation

In patients who will not be undergoing a transplant, there are various options available for initial therapy. Most will receive alkylator-based therapy, commonly melphalan and prednisone (MP) (94). This regimen yields partial remissions in approximately 55% of patients, with the occasional complete response. Recent trials have evaluated the addition of thalidomide to melphalan and prednisone (MPT). For patients aged 60 to 85, Palumbo et al. (91) demonstrated a 76% response rate with MPT, superior to the 48% in the MP arm; however, thromboses were more common with thalidomide with an incidence of 12% (vs. 2% in the MP group). Newer agents are now being incorporated into trials in this population as well, including bortezomib and lenalidomide. The precise role of these agents in older patients has yet to be determined.

Autologous Stem Cell Transplantation

ASCT has become the standard of care for eligible patients, as it has been demonstrated in multiple trials to improve the likelihood of complete response, prolong disease-free survival, and

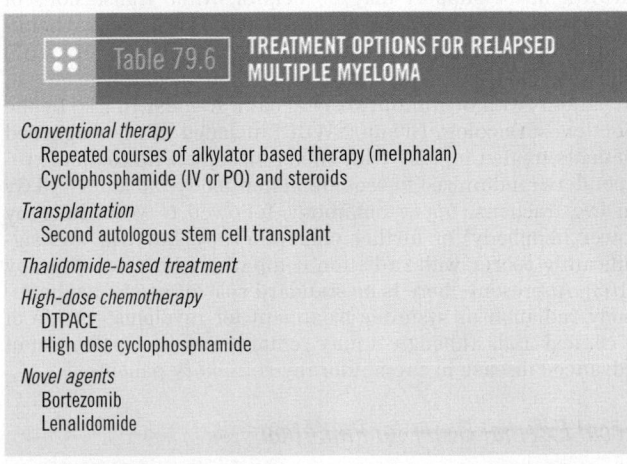

Symptomatic Multiple Myeloma: Approach to Initial Therapy

Eligible for transplantation
↓
High-dose dexamethasone-based therapy or VAD or investigational therapy
↓
Stem cell harvest
↓
ASCT
↓
No treatment or investigational therapy

Not eligible for transplantation
↓
Melphalan + prednisone
or
other alkylator-based therapy
or
Thalidomide based therapy
↓
No treatment or investigational therapy

VAD = vincristine, adriamycin (doxorubicin), and dexamethasone
ASCT = Autologous stem cell transplant

FIGURE 79.2. Treatment algorithm for symptomatic multiple myeloma, according to the patient's candidacy for autologous stem cell transplantation. ASCT, autologous stem cell transplantation; VAD, vincristine, adriamycin, and dexamethasone

extend overall survival (9,19,66). Treatment-related mortality rates are now <2%, and often the transplant can be performed entirely as an outpatient. Melphalan 200 mg/m^2 is the most commonly used conditioning regimen, although it may be reduced in elderly patients or patients with renal insufficiency.

Tandem Transplantation

Tandem or double transplantation refers to a planned second ASCT after the patient has recovered from the first. A phase III trial in France evaluated tandem transplant versus single ASCT and demonstrated superior overall survival in the tandem group (8); however, when further analyzed, the patients who benefited most from the second transplant were those who did not achieve a 90% reduction in their disease after the first ASCT. Therefore, it may be more prudent to consider tandem transplantation only in patients whose response to the first ASCT is suboptimal.

Allogeneic Stem Cell Transplantation

Myeloablative stem cell transplant is perhaps the only current potential cure for patients with myeloma, as the graft is not contaminated with tumor cells and may produce a profound graft versus myeloma effect (79). However, its use is very limited due to the lack of donors, age restriction, high treatment-related mortality, and graft versus host disease.

Novel Therapies

The general approach to myeloma is to provide sequential therapies to patients, knowing each will not be curative but will prolong the period of disease control. The goal is to convert the disease into a chronic illness. Whereas there used to be very limited treatment options, the armamentarium available has grown considerably over the past few years. This has contributed to a prolongation of the median survival of patients with myeloma. Patients will relapse after a median of 2 years after first ASCT (81), and several options may be pursued for treatment (Table 79.6). The most exciting is the development and availability of novel, biological agents. Bortezomib is the first proteosome inhibitor to be used in clinical trials. Various phase I and II studies have been completed, and a large multicenter phase III trial compared bortezomib to high-dose dexamethasone (99). The updated results of 669 patients revealed time to progression of 6.2 months in the bortezomib arm and 3.5 months in the dexamethasone arm, along with a superior 1-year overall survival (80% vs. 67%) favoring bortezomib (98).

Side effects included peripheral neuropathy, cyclical thrombocytopenia, and diarrhea.

Lenalidomide is an immunomodulatory drug derived from thalidomide and is currently undergoing extensive clinical investigation worldwide. Its role has been established for relapsed disease based on a large phase III trial comparing the combination of lenalidomide and dexamethasone with dexamethasone alone (32). The trial was stopped prematurely due to a large difference between the treatment groups favoring the lenalidomide combination arm. Time to progression was 4.7 months with dexamethasone alone and 11.3 months in the combination arm. Overall response rates were 24% (4% complete response [CR] and 20% partial response [PR]) with dexamethasone alone and 59% (17% CR and 42% PR) in the combination group. There was also an overall survival advantage, with median overall survival of 104 weeks in the dexamethasone alone arm, but this end point had not been reached yet in the lenalidomide arm (32). Side effects included neutropenia, thrombocytopenia, and constipation.

Radiation Therapy of Multiple Myeloma

Total Body Irradiation

Some high dose chemotherapy protocols for multiple myeloma incorporate total body irradiation (TBI) into the conditioning regimen. Because of toxicity concerns (mucosal and

Table 79.6	**TREATMENT OPTIONS FOR RELAPSED MULTIPLE MYELOMA**

Conventional therapy
  Repeated courses of alkylator based therapy (melphalan)
  Cyclophosphamide (IV or PO) and steroids
Transplantation
  Second autologous stem cell transplant
Thalidomide-based treatment
High-dose chemotherapy
  DTPACE
  High dose cyclophosphamide
Novel agents
  Bortezomib
  Lenalidomide

DTPACE: dexamethasone, thalidomide, cisplatin, doxorubicin, cyclophosphamide, and etoposide; IV, intravenous; PO, orally

Clinical Radiation Oncology

hematologic) with TBI, many programs use chemotherapy alone, most commonly melphalan. A phase III French study (Intergroupe Francophone du Myelome [IFM] trial 9502) examined melphalan, 200 mg/m² alone (M200) versus melphalan 140 mg/m² with TBI, 8 Gy in four fractions (M140/TBI) (84) and found that patients in the TBI-containing arm suffered more grade 3 or 4 mucosal toxicity, heavier transfusion requirement, and longer hospitalization stay. There was a higher toxic death rate in the M140/TBI arm (3.6% vs. 0% for the M200 arm). The event-free survival was no different between the two treatments, but the 45-month overall survival favored the M200 arm (M200: 65.8%, M140/TBI: 45.5%; $p = .05$) (84).

Similarly, another IFM protocol tested TBI in the tandem transplant setting by intensifying the conditioning regimen for the second transplant to melphalan 200 mg/m² without TBI and comparing with the standard tandem regimen (M140 for the first, M140/TBI for the second). There was no benefit with TBI, and increased toxicity was again observed. Therefore, all subsequent IFM trials abandoned the use of TBI (52). Another study from the Spanish bone marrow transplant registry compared M140/TBI with three other chemotherapy conditioning regimens (71). There were no significant differences in the hospitalization duration, hematologic recovery, event-free survival, and overall survival among the four regimens. The authors concluded that no one regimen was clearly superior to another.

The Toronto protocol with intensification of the conditioning regimen to melphalan 140 mg/m², etoposide 60 mg/kg, and fractionated TBI (12 Gy in six fractions over 3 days, with a high dose rate) was used in 100 patients. The main toxicity was interstitial pneumonitis (28% of patients) of whom seven died (1), leading to discontinuation of the TBI in the subsequent protocol. Presently, the use of TBI is based on institutional experience and the specific drug regimen used for conditioning. The tandem transplant program at the University of Arkansas (11,12,30) and the Memorial Sloan-Kettering Cancer Center (57) continue to use TBI in their ASCT programs for specific indications.

Hemibody Radiation

Diffuse bone pain involving wide areas of the skeleton can be effectively palliated by half body radiation with single doses of 5 to 8 Gy (21,78,115), although this is rarely used now. The bone marrow in the unirradiated half body serves as a stem cell reserve and will slowly repopulate the irradiated marrow after treatment. The dose for upper half body should not exceed 8 Gy due to lung tolerance (119). The main toxicity is myelosuppression. The use of hemibody radiation must be carefully considered in patients heavily pretreated with chemotherapy. Growth factor support may be helpful, while transfusions of blood products should be given as needed. The sequential hemibody radiation technique has been used in phase II (102,107) and phase III trials as "systemic" treatment to control myeloma, in patients with or without skeletal pain. A phase III trial by the Southwest Oncology Group (SWOG) included newly diagnosed patients treated initially with chemotherapy, with complete responders randomized to sequential hemibody radiation (7.5 Gy in five fractions, upper hemibody, followed 6 weeks later by lower hemibody) or further chemotherapy. Survival was significantly poorer with radiation compared with chemotherapy (103). At present, there is no standard role for sequential hemibody radiation as systemic treatment for myeloma outside of a clinical trial, although it may remain useful for palliation of advanced disease in chemotherapy-refractory patients.

Local External Beam for Palliation

The most common use of RT in the management of plasma cell tumors is for palliative treatment of bony disease (2,21,73), relief of compression of spinal cord (6,93,120), cranial nerves, or peripheral nerves. It has been estimated that approximately 40% of patients with multiple myeloma will require palliative RT for bone pain at some time during the course of their disease (40). In practice the actual proportion is lower than estimated varying from 24% to 34%, leading investigators in Australia to suggest that this potentially useful modality of treatment has been underutilized, even taking into account the beneficial effect of bisphosphonates, particularly for the elderly (40). Palliative RT to the spine reduces the incidence of future vertebral fractures or appearance of new lesions (72). However, the role of RT in preventing impending pathologic fracture is unclear. In general, lesions at high risk for pathologic fracture should be referred for surgical stabilization, and RT can be administered after surgery for control of residual disease at the local site.

When RT is given for pain due to disease involving a long bone, a local field suffices. It is unnecessary to treat the entire bone (23). Doses of 10 to 20 Gy (in five to 10 fractions) are effective, although the pain relief is often partial (82). With an average dose of 25 Gy given to 306 sites in 101 patients, Leigh et al. (73) found a symptomatic response rate of 97% (complete pain relief in 26%, and partial relief in 71%). There was no dose-response relationship above 10 Gy. Recurrence of symptoms requiring further treatment was seen in 6% of sites after a median of 16 months.

It is not clear if pain relief is better if RT is given concurrently with chemotherapy. A study by Adamietz et al. (2) reported complete pain relief in 80% of patients receiving RT with chemotherapy, compared with 40% among those receiving RT alone. In contrast, Leigh et al. (73) found no significant difference in pain relief when RT was given with or without concurrent chemotherapy. For spinal cord compression, motor improvement is expected in approximately 50% of irradiated patients. A multicenter study suggested that a longer fractionated regimen (30 Gy in 10 fractions or higher) was associated with better neurologic recovery than 20 Gy in five fractions or a single 8 Gy fraction (93). With the availability of newer drugs, the advantage of radiation sensitizing efforts with drug-radiation combinations requires continued investigation, both in terms of enhancing local control (48) and possible toxicity. Bortezomib and spinal radiation given concurrently was reported to result in severe enteritis (83). The use of bisphosphonates (e.g., pamidronate) has been shown to reduce skeletal complications and pain (15,17,85) with a reduction of the use of RT from 50% to 34% in one study (16).

Radioimmunotherapy Approaches

Bone seeking radiopharmaceuticals targeting the bone marrow have been studied as an alternative to TBI. Typically a β-emitting isotope is conjugated to a phosphonate complex, such as ^{153}Samarium-ethylene diamine tetramethylene phosphonate (^{153}Sm-EDTMP). The isotope also emits a γ-ray permitting scanning to locate areas of uptake. This agent has been used for palliation of bone metastasis (7,13). The feasibility of this approach in a small number of myeloma patients has been reported for stem cell transplantation both in the autologous (34,55) and allogeneic settings (62). Another bone-seeking pharmaceutical is ^{166}Holmium-DOTMP (1,4,7,10-tetraazacyclododecane-1,4,7,10-tetramethylene-phosphonic acid), with a higher energy β-emission (maximum energy 1.85 MeV) than ^{153}Sm, and a shorter $T_{1/2}$ of 26.8 hours. It also has a γ-emission (81 KeV) suitable for imaging. A phase I/II study incorporating ^{166}Holmium-DOTMP into a transplant regimen has been performed at the M.D. Anderson Cancer Center with encouraging results (47). With the ability to deliver much higher doses to the bone marrow than TBI, in the range of 30 to 60 Gy, yet sparing the dose-limiting normal tissues such as lung, mucosa, and kidneys, the concept of targeted radiation therapy is tantalizing.

However, there remains a problem of heterogeneity of uptake in the skeleton, and the dosimetric variation may be even larger at a microscopic level due to the limited range of the β particle. Whether this approach will have a more favorable therapeutic ratio than standard conditioning regimens in the transplant setting awaits larger scale phase II and phase III trials.

Radiation Therapy Techniques

Radical Radiation Therapy for Local Control of Solitary Plasmacytoma

Accurate evaluation of tumor extent is an important feature of radical RT for solitary plasmacytoma. MRI is useful to evaluate the extent of disease both within and beyond bone. This is particularly true for the paranasal sinuses, where inflammatory changes may be difficult to distinguish from tumor on CT imaging. Currently, the accuracy of FDG-PET in the evaluation of tumor extent is uncertain.

There are few data to support specific guidelines regarding RT treatment volumes. CT and MRI imaging should be used to determine gross tumor volumes (GTV). Clinical target volumes (CTV) should encompass probable routes of microscopic spread, recognizing that barriers to the extension of local disease will vary according to anatomic location, as will the morbidity of treating adjacent normal tissues (Fig. 79.3). For the spine, inclusion of two vertebral bodies above and below the grossly involved vertebra(e) is a common practice. As this is based on relapse patterns seen following RT for spinal metastases for solid tumors rather than plasmacytomas, it may not be directly applicable to solitary plasmacytoma.

For RT of long bone lesions, while coverage of the entire involved bone has been recommended by some authors, a study of palliative RT to only the symptomatic area for multiple myeloma found that recurrence in the untreated portion of the involved bone was rare (23), and similarly, no marginal recurrences were

seen among 30 patients with solitary plasmacytoma treated with RT that encompassed only the tumor with a margin (60). Prophylactic regional nodal coverage is not necessary in solitary plasmacytoma of bone as multiple studies have found a very low risk of regional nodal failure after involved-field radiation without intentional coverage of adjacent nodes (i.e., 0% to 4%) (60,75,112,117). For extramedullary plasmacytoma, nodal involvement at presentation is observed in 10% to 20%, and occasional nodal failure in the literature led to a common practice of extending the RT coverage to the draining lymph node region (20,57,110). Some authors specifically recommend this practice if the primary disease involves a lymphatic structure (e.g., lymph nodes, or Waldeyer's ring) (53,64,117). However, this is controversial as some series reported a low incidence of regional nodal failure without routine prophylactic nodal irradiation (53,64,77), leading to variation in practice between centers (110). After reviewing their own series of 26 patients with EMP and contrasting the results with the literature, Strojan et al. (110) concluded that prophylactic nodal radiation is probably unnecessary.

Planning target volumes (PTV) should account for day-to-day setup variation and will typically add 5 to 10 mm around CTV volumes depending on the immobilization technique employed (see Fig. 79.3). Overall, RT field edges are typically 2 to 3 cm from gross tumor seen on imaging. Although parallel-opposed fields are commonly adequate to encompass disease without significant irradiation of normal tissues, CT-based planning, and the use of conformal techniques, including intensity modulated radiation therapy, should be employed when needed to treat the PTV adjacent to critical structures. This can be particularly important in extramedullary disease involving the paranasal sinuses, where avoidance of the optic structures and salivary glands is desirable.

Radiation Therapy Dose

Studies evaluating RT dose response in plasmacytoma have produced differing results. Most studies have found response rates

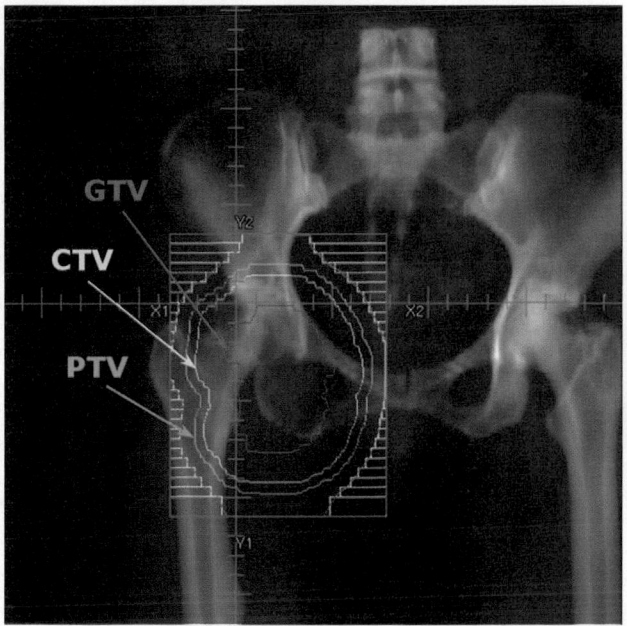

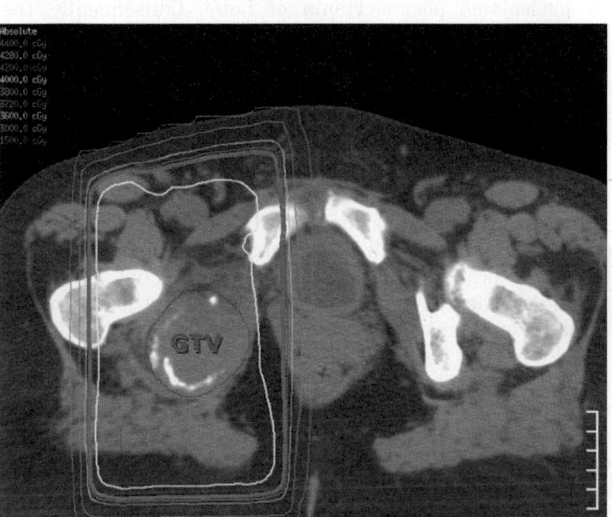

FIGURE 79.3. Radiation treatment plan for a solitary plasmacytoma of the right iliac bone involving the acetabulum down to the ischial tuberosity, with associated soft tissue mass, 40 Gy in 20 fractions, anterior posterior/posterior-anterior fields with 18 MV photons. **A:** Digital reconstructed radiograph displaying GTV, CTV, and PTV. Note that the entire iliac bone need not be covered, and regional lymph nodes were not intentionally treated. **B:** Isodose distribution in the axial perspective. The objective is to cover the PTV with 40 Gy +/− 5%. CTV, clinical target volumes; GTV, gross tumor volume; PTV, planning target volumes.

>85% among patients treated with ≥35 Gy; some investigators have found better local control following doses ≥45 Gy (44,116), while others have found no indication of improved outcome with higher doses (60,90). Based on a dose–response analysis of 81 patients by Mendenhall et al. (80) reported in 1980, a minimum dose of 40 Gy was recommended, including osseous and extramedullary lesions. A total dose of 40 Gy and above resulted in a local failure rate of 6% versus 31% for lower doses. Therefore, the usual practice is to administer a dose of 40 to 45 Gy or even higher for bulky tumors. However, in the largest of these studies (n = 258), there was no evidence of improved local control with RT doses ranging from 30 to 50 Gy, including a subset of patients with tumors >4 cm (90). In fact there was a worse local control rate for the group receiving total dose ≥50 Gy, although not statistically significant (90). It should be noted, however, that retrospective studies of dose response are typically confounded by selection bias, as higher doses are prescribed to larger tumors with worse prognosis. Several studies have demonstrated durable local control in >85% of tumors <5 cm with 35 to 40 Gy, and there is little evidence that higher doses are necessary for small tumors, regardless of bone or EMP locations. In contrast, plasmacytomas >5 cm have worse local control (90,117), and doses of 45 to 50 Gy are recommended in these bulkier tumors, which also tend to be EMPs. However, one should be aware that the quality of evidence supporting the use of higher RT doses is limited, and local failures are occasionally observed even after doses exceeding 50 Gy (80,90, 117).

Assessment of Response and Follow-Up

Reimaging is of greatest value in the response assessment of extramedullary plasmacytoma. Repeat imaging, preferably MRI, should be done approximately 6 to 8 weeks following completion of treatment. It is rare to have symptoms suggestive of local progression that necessitate reimaging prior to this. It is common for a residual soft-tissue abnormality to persist on follow-up imaging, and periodic reimaging may be required every 4 to 6 months until any residual mass disappears or remains stable on consecutive scans. It is generally not beneficial to continue to reimage a stable abnormality.

Bone destruction caused by tumor can produce permanent abnormalities on imaging following either painful bone metastases or isolated plasmacytoma of bone. Consequently, repeat imaging is of less value in establishing response in such cases.

With a high risk of recurrence of disease as multiple myeloma, the occurrence of new bone pain requires further investigations, including imaging as appropriate. Repeat measurement of the M-protein often detects the onset of systemic disease prior to the development of symptoms and can be used as an indicator of disease burden (26,121). Complete blood counts should be taken periodically to evaluate bone marrow function. A team of international investigators have recently developed recommendations for uniform response criteria for assessing the treatment of multiple myeloma (36).

RT doses used for myeloma are rarely associated with significant delayed side effects. Treatment of significant volumes of the parotid or submandibular glands may result in prolonged xerostomia and should be avoided. As noted previously, TBI has been associated with significant toxicity and is not widely used. Evaluation of renal function should be undertaken prior to initiating RT that may include the kidneys, and blood counts should be evaluated prior to treating a large volume of bone marrow in the spine or pelvis. Reirradiation of vertebral metastases is possible, but careful evaluation of all prior RT records is required to ensure that the tolerance of the spinal cord is not exceeded.

References

1. Abraham R, Chen C, Tsang R, et al. Intensification of the stem cell transplant induction regimen results in increased treatment-related mortality without improved outcome in multiple myeloma. *Bone Marrow Transplant* 1999;24:1291–1297.
2. Adamietz IA, Schober C, Schulte RW, et al. Palliative radiotherapy in plasma cell myeloma. *Radiother Oncol* 1991;20:111–116.
3. Alexanian R, Dimopoulos MA, Delasalle K, et al. Primary dexamethasone treatment of multiple myeloma. *Blood* 1992;80:887–890.
4. Alexiou C, Kau RJ, Dietzfelbinger H, et al. Extramedullary plasmacytoma: tumor occurrence and therapeutic concepts. *Cancer* 1999;85:2305–2314.
5. American Cancer Society. Cancer facts and figures, 2006. Available at: http://www.cancer.org/docroot/home/index.asp. Accessed July 19, 2007.
6. Ampil FL, Chin HW. Radiotherapy alone for extradural compression by spinal myeloma. *Radiat Med* 1995;13:129–131.
7. Anderson PM, Wiseman GA, Dispenzieri A, et al. High-dose samarium-153 ethylene diamine tetramethylene phosphonate: low toxicity of skeletal irradiation in patients with osteosarcoma and bone metastases. *J Clin Oncol* 2002;20:189–196.
8. Attal M, Harousseau JL, Facon T, et al. Single versus double autologous stem-cell transplantation for multiple myeloma. *N Engl J Med* 2003;349:2495–2502.
9. Attal M, Harousseau JL, Stoppa AM, et al. A prospective, randomized trial of autologous bone marrow transplantation and chemotherapy in multiple myeloma. *N Engl J Med* 1996;335:91–97.
10. Aviles A, Huerta-Guzman J, Delgado S, et al. Improved outcome in solitary bone plasmacytomata with combined therapy. *Hematol Oncol* 1996;14:111–117.
11. Barlogie B, Jagannath S, Desikan KR, et al. Total therapy with tandem transplants for newly diagnosed multiple myeloma. *Blood* 1999;93:55–65.
12. Barlogie B, Jagannath S, Vesole DH, et al. Superiority of tandem autologous transplantation over standard therapy for previously untreated multiple myeloma. *Blood* 1997;89:789–793.
13. Bartlett ML, Webb M, Durrant S, et al. Dosimetry and toxicity of Quadramet for bone marrow ablation in multiple myeloma and other haematological malignancies. *Eur J Nucl Med Mol Imaging* 2002;29:1470–1477.
14. Bataille R, Sany J. Solitary myeloma: clinical and prognostic features of a review of 114 cases. *Cancer* 1981;48:845–851.
15. Berenson JR, Hillner BE, Kyle RA, et al. American Society of Clinical Oncology clinical practice guidelines: the role of bisphosphonates in multiple myeloma. *J Clin Oncol* 2002;20:3719–3736.
16. Berenson JR, Lichtenstein A, Porter L, et al. Efficacy of pamidronate in reducing skeletal events in patients with advanced multiple myeloma. Myeloma Aredia Study Group. *N Engl J Med* 1996;334:488–493.
17. Berenson JR, Lichtenstein A, Porter L, et al. Long-term pamidronate treatment of advanced multiple myeloma patients reduces skeletal events. Myeloma Aredia Study Group. *J Clin Oncol* 1998;16:593–602.
18. Bergsagel DE, Wong O, Bergsagel PL, et al. Benzene and multiple myeloma: appraisal of the scientific evidence. *Blood* 1999;94:1174–1182.
19. Blade J, Vesole DH, Gertz M. High-dose therapy in multiple myeloma. *Blood* 2003;102:3469–3470.
20. Bolek TW, Marcus RB, Mendenhall NP. Solitary plasmacytoma of bone and soft tissue. *Int J Radiat Oncol Biol Phys* 1996;36:329–333.
21. Bosch A, Frias Z. Radiotherapy in the treatment of multiple myeloma. *Int J Radiat Oncol Biol Phys* 1988;15:1363–1369.
22. Brinch L, Hannisdal E, Abrahamsen AF, et al. Extramedullary plasmacytomas and solitary myeloma cell tumours of bone. *Eur. J. Haematol.* 1990;44:131–134.
23. Catell D, Kogen Z, Donahue B, et al. Multiple myeloma of an extremity: must the entire bone be treated? *Int J Radiat Oncol Biol Phys* 1998;40:117–119.
24. Clark IY, Cox RS, Bagtwick DG, et al. Solitary plasmacytoma of bone: treatment, progression, and survival. *J Clin Oncol* 1987;5:1811–1815.
25. Chang H, et al. ... is associated with poor prognosis in myeloma patients undergoing autologous stem cell transplant. *Br J Haematol* ...
26. Chang MY, Shih LY, Dunn P, et al. Solitary plasmacytoma of bone. *J Formos Med Assoc* 1994;93:397–402.
27. Chao MW, Gibbs P, Wirth A, et al. Radiotherapy in the management of solitary extramedullary plasmacytoma. *Intern Med J* 2005;35:211–215.
28. Colomo L, Loong F, Rives S, et al. Diffuse large B-cell lymphomas with plasmablastic differentiation represent a heterogeneous group of disease entities. *Am J Surg Pathol* 2004;28:736–747.
29. Correa A, Jackson L, Mohan A, et al. Use of hair dyes, hematopoietic neoplasms, and lymphomas: a literature review. II. Lymphomas and multiple myeloma. *Cancer Invest* 2000;18:467–479.
30. Desikan R, Barlogie B, Sawyer J, et al. Results of high-dose therapy for 1000 patients with multiple myeloma: durable complete remissions and superior survival in the absence of chromosome 13 abnormalities. *Blood* 2000;95:4008–4010.
31. Dimopoulos MA, Goldstein J, Fuller L, et al. Curability of solitary bone plasmacytoma. *J Clin Oncol* 1992;10:587–590.
32. Dimopoulos MA, Spencer A, Attal M, et al. Study of lenalidomide plus dexamethasone versus dexamethasone alone in relapsed or refractory multiple myeloma (MM): results of a phase 3 study (MM-010). *Blood* 2005;106:6a.
33. Dispenzieri A, Kyle RA, Lacy MQ, et al. POEMS syndrome: definitions and long-term outcome. *Blood* 2003;101:2496–2506.
34. Dispenzieri A, Wiseman GA, Lacy MQ, et al. A phase I study of ^{153}Sm-EDTMP with fixed high-dose melphalan as a peripheral blood stem cell conditioning regimen in patients with multiple myeloma. *Leukemia* 2005;19:118–125.
35. Djulbegovic B, Wheatley K, Ross J, et al. Bisphosphonates in multiple myeloma (Cochrane Review). *Cochrane Database Syst Rev* 2002: CD003188.
36. Durie BG, Harousseau JL, Miguel JS, et al. International uniform response criteria for multiple myeloma. *Leukemia* 2006;9:1467–1473.
37. Durie BG, Kyle RA, Belch A, et al. Myeloma management guidelines: a consensus report from the scientific advisors of the International Myeloma Foundation. *Hematol J* 2003;4:379–398.
38. Durie BG, Salmon SE. A clinical staging system for multiple myeloma. Correlation of measured myeloma cell mass with presenting clinical features, response to treatment, and survival. *Cancer* 1975;36:842–854.
39. Facon T, Avet-Loiseau H, Guillerm G, et al. Chromosome 13 abnormalities identified by FISH analysis and serum β_2-microglobulin produce a powerful myeloma

staging system for patients receiving high-dose therapy. *Blood* 2001;97:1566–1571.
40. Featherstone C, Delaney G, Jacob S, et al. Estimating the optimal utilization rates of radiotherapy for hematologic malignancies from a review of the evidence: part II-leukemia and myeloma. *Cancer* 2005;103:393–401.
41. Feinstein AR, Sosin DM, Wells CK. The Will Rogers phenomenon. Stage migration and new diagnostic techniques as a source of misleading statistics for survival in cancer. *N Engl J Med* 1985;312:1604–1608.
42. Folk GS, Abbondanzo SL, Childers EL, et al. Plasmablastic lymphoma: a clinicopathologic correlation. *Ann Diagn Pathol* 2006;10:8–12.
43. Fonseca R, Barlogie B, Bataille R, et al. Genetics and cytogenetics of multiple myeloma: a workshop report. *Cancer Res* 2004;64:1546–1558.
44. Frassica DA, Frassica FJ, Schray MF, et al. Solitary plasmacytoma of bone: Mayo Clinic experience. *Int J Radiat Oncol Biol Phys* 1989;16:43–48.
45. Galieni P, Cavo M, Avvisati G, et al. Solitary plasmacytoma of bone and extramedullary plasmacytoma: two different entities? *Ann Oncol* 1995;6: 687–691.
46. Galieni P, Cavo M, Pulsoni A, et al. Clinical outcome of extramedullary plasmacytoma. *Haematologica* 2000;85:47–51.
47. Giralt S, Bensinger W, Goodman M, et al. ^{166}Ho-DOTMP plus melphalan followed by peripheral blood stem cell transplantation in patients with multiple myeloma: results of two phase 1/2 trials. *Blood* 2003;102:2684–2691.
48. Goel A, Dispenzieri A, Greipp PR, et al. PS-341-mediated selective targeting of multiple myeloma cells by synergistic increase in ionizing radiation-induced apoptosis. *Exp Hematol* 2005;33:784–795.
49. Goldschmidt H, Hegenbart U, Wallmeier M, et al. Factors influencing collection of peripheral blood progenitor cells following high-dose cyclophosphamide and granulocyte colony-stimulating factor in patients with multiple myeloma. *Br J Haematol* 1997;98:736–744.
50. Greipp PR, San Miguel J, Durie BG, et al. International staging system for multiple myeloma. *J Clin Oncol* 2005;23:3412–3420.
51. Group TIMW. Criteria for the classification of monoclonal gammopathies, multiple myeloma and related disorders: a report of the International Myeloma Working Group. *Br J Haematol* 2003;121:749–757.
52. Harousseau JL, Attal M. The role of stem cell transplantation in multiple myeloma. *Blood Rev* 2002;16:245–253.
53. Harwood AR, Knowling MA, Bergsagel DE. Radiotherapy of extramedullary plasmacytoma of the head and neck. *Clin Radiol* 1981;32:31–36.
54. Hideshima T, Bergsagel PL, Kuehl WM, et al. Advances in biology of multiple myeloma: clinical applications. *Blood* 2004;104:607–618.
55. Hogan WJ, Lacy MQ, Wiseman GA, et al. Successful treatment of POEMS syndrome with autologous hematopoietic progenitor cell transplantation. *Bone Marrow Transplant* 2001;28:305–309.
56. Holland J, Trenkner DA, Wasserman TH, et al. Plasmacytoma. Treatment results and conversion to myeloma. *Cancer* 1992;69:1513–1517.
57. Hu K, Yahalom J. Radiotherapy in the management of plasma cell tumors. *Oncology* 2000;14:101–111.
58. Hussong JW, Perkins SL, Schnitzer B, et al. Extramedullary plasmacytoma. A form of marginal zone cell lymphoma?. *Am J Clin Pathol* 1999;111:111–116.
59. Jackson A, Scarffe JH. Prognostic significance of osteopenia and immunoparesis at presentation in patients with solitary myeloma of bone. *Eur J Cancer* 1990;26:363–371.
60. Jyothirmayi R, Gangadharan VP, Nair MK, et al. Radiotherapy in the treatment of solitary plasmacytoma. *Br J Radiol* 1997;70:511–516.
61. Kapadia SB, Desai U, Cheng VS. Extramedullary plasmacytoma of the head and neck. *Medicine* 1982;61:317–329.
62. Kennedy GA, Durrant S, Butler J, et al. Outcome of myeloablative allogeneic stem cell transplantation in multiple myeloma with a ^{153}Sm-EDTMP-based preparative regimen. *Leukemia* 2005;19:879–880.
63. Knobel D, Zouhair A, Tsang RW, et al. Prognostic factors in solitary plasmacytoma of the bone: a multicenter Rare Cancer Network study. *BMC Cancer* 2006;6: 118.
64. Knowling MA, Harwood AR, Bergsagel DE. Comparison of extramedullary plasmacytomas with solitary and multiple plasma cell tumors of bone. *J Clin Oncol* 1983;1:255–262.
65. Kuehl WM, Bergsagel PL. Multiple myeloma: evolving genetic events and host interactions. *Nat Rev Cancer* 2002;2:175–187.
66. Kumar A, Loughran T, Alsina M, et al. Management of multiple myeloma: a systematic review and critical appraisal of published studies. *Lancet Oncol* 2003;4:293–304.
67. Kumar S, Fonseca R, Dispenzieri A, et al. Prognostic value of angiogenesis in solitary bone plasmacytoma. *Blood* 2003;101:1715–1717.
68. Kyle RA, Gertz MA, Witzig TE, et al. Review of 1,027 patients with newly diagnosed multiple myeloma. *Mayo Clin Proc* 2003;78:21–33.
69. Kyle RA, Therneau TM, Rajkumar SV, et al. A long-term study of prognosis in monoclonal gammopathy of undetermined significance. *N Engl J Med* 2002; 346:564–569.
70. Kyle RA, Therneau TM, Rajkumar SV, et al. Long-term follow-up of IgM monoclonal gammopathy of undetermined significance. *Blood* 2003;102:3759–3764.
71. Lahuerta JJ, Grande C, Blade J, et al. Myeloablative treatments for multiple myeloma: update of a comparative study of different regimens used in patients from the Spanish registry for transplantation in multiple myeloma. *Leuk Lymphoma* 2002;43:67–74.
72. Lecouvet F, Richard F, Vande Berg B, et al. Long-term effects of localized spinal radiation therapy on vertebral fractures and focal lesions appearance in patients with multiple myeloma. *Br J Haematol* 1997;96:743–745.
73. Leigh BR, Kurtts TA, Mack CF, et al. Radiation therapy for the palliation of multiple myeloma. *Int J Radiat Oncol Biol Phys* 1993;25:801–804.
74. Liebross RH, Ha CS, Cox JD, et al. Solitary bone plasmacytoma: outcome and prognostic factors following radiotherapy. *Int J Radiat Oncol Biol Phys* 1998;41:1063–1067.
75. Liebross RH, Ha CS, Cox JD, et al. Clinical course of solitary extramedullary plasmacytoma. *Radiother Oncol* 1999;52:245–249.
76. Mariette X, Zagdanski AM, Guermazi A, et al. Prognostic value of vertebral lesions detected by magnetic resonance imaging in patients with stage I multiple myeloma. *Br J Haematol* 1999;104:723–729.
77. Mayr NA, Wen BC, Hussey DH, et al. The role of radiation therapy in the treatment of solitary plasmacytomas. *Radiother Oncol* 1990;17:293–303.
78. McSweeney EN, Tobias JS, Blackman G, et al. Double hemibody irradiation (DHBI) in the management of relapsed and primary chemoresistant multiple myeloma. *Clin Oncol (R Coll Radiol)* 1993;5:378–383.
79. Mehta J, Singhal S. Graft-versus-myeloma. *Bone Marrow Transplant* 1998;22: 835–843.
80. Mendenhall CM, Thar TL, Million RR. Solitary plasmacytoma of bone and soft tissue. *Int J Radiat Oncol Biol Phys* 1980;6:1497–1501.
81. Mikhael J, Samiee S, Stewart AK, et al. Second autologous stem cell transplantation as salvage therapy in patients with relapsed multiple myeloma: Improved outcomes in patients with longer disease free interval after first autologous stem cell transplantation. *Biol Blood Marrow Transplant* 2006;12[Suppl 1]:117.
82. Mill WB, Griffith R. The role of radiation therapy in the management of plasma cell tumors. *Cancer* 1980;45:647–652.
83. Mohiuddin MM, Harmon DC, Delaney TF. Severe acute enteritis in a multiple myeloma patient receiving bortezomib and spinal radiotherapy: case report. *J Chemother* 2005;17:343–346.
84. Moreau P, Facon T, Attal M, et al. Comparison of 200 mg/m^2 melphalan and 8 Gy total body irradiation plus 140 mg/m^2 melphalan as conditioning regimens for peripheral blood stem cell transplantation in patients with newly diagnosed multiple myeloma: final analysis of the Intergroupe Francophone du Myelome 9502 randomized trial. *Blood* 2002;99:731–735.
85. Morton LM, Wang SS, Devesa SS, et al. Lymphoma incidence patterns by WHO subtype in the United States, 1992–2001. *Blood* 2006;107:265–276.
86. Moulopoulos LA, Dimopoulos MA, Smith TL, et al. Prognostic significance of magnetic resonance imaging in patients with asymptomatic multiple myeloma. *J Clin Oncol* 1995;13:251–256.
87. Moulopoulos LA, Dimopoulos MA, Weber D, et al. Magnetic resonance imaging in the staging of solitary plasmacytoma of bone. *J Clin Oncol* 1993;11:1311–1315.
88. Nishiyama H, Anderson RE, Ishimaru T, et al. The incidence of malignant lymphoma and multiple myeloma in Hiroshima and Nagasaki atomic bomb survivors, 1945–1965. *Cancer* 1973;32:1301–1309.
89. Ofran Y, Elinav E. POEMS syndrome: failure of newly suggested diagnostic criteria to anticipate the development of the syndrome. *Am J Hematol* 2005;79: 316–318.
90. Ozsahin M, Tsang RW, Poortmans P, et al. Outcomes and patterns of failure in solitary plasmacytoma: a multicenter Rare Cancer Network study of 258 patients. *Int J Radiat Oncol Biol Phys* 2006;64:210–217.
91. Palumbo A, Bringhen S, Caravita T, et al. Oral melphalan and prednisone chemotherapy plus thalidomide compared with melphalan and prednisone alone in elderly patients with multiple myeloma: randomised controlled trial. *Lancet* 2006;367:825–831.
92. Pruneri G, Carboni N, Baldini L, et al. Cell cycle regulators in multiple myeloma: prognostic implications of p53 nuclear accumulation. *Hum Pathol* 2003;34: 41–47.
93. Rades D, Hoskin PJ, Stalpers LJ, et al. Short-course radiotherapy is not optimal for spinal cord compression due to myeloma. *Int J Radiat Oncol Biol Phys* 2006; 64:1452–1457.
94. Rajkumar SV, Gertz MA, Kyle RA, et al. Current therapy for multiple myeloma. *Mayo Clin Proc* 2002;77:813–822.
95. Rajkumar SV, Hayman S, Gertz MA, et al. Combination therapy with thalidomide plus dexamethasone for newly diagnosed myeloma. *J Clin Oncol* 2002;20:4319–4323.
96. Rajkumar SV, Hayman SR, Lacy MQ, et al. Combination therapy with lenalidomide plus dexamethasone (Rev/Dex) for newly diagnosed myeloma. *Blood* 2005;106:4050–4053.
97. Reece DE. An update of the management of multiple myeloma: the changing landscape. *Hematology (Am Soc Hematol Educ Program)* 2005; :353–359.
98. Richardson P, Sonneveld P, Schuster M, et al. Bortezomib continues demonstrates superior efficacy compared with high-dose dexamethasone in relapsed multiple myeloma: updated results of the APEX trial. *Blood* 2005;106:2547a.
99. Richardson PG, Sonneveld P, Schuster MW, et al. Bortezomib or high-dose dexamethasone for relapsed multiple myeloma. *N Engl J Med* 2005;352:2487–2498.
100. Ries LAG, Eisner MP, Kosary CL, et al., eds. *SEER statistics review, 1973–1997*. Bethesda, MD: National Cancer Institute, 2000.
101. Ries LAG, Eisner MP, Kosary CL, et al., eds. *SEER cancer statistics review, 1975–2002*. Bethesda, MD: National Cancer Institute, 2005.
102. Rowland CG, Garrett MJ, Crowley FA. Half body radiation in plasma cell myeloma. *Clin Radiol* 1983;34:507–510.
103. Salmon SE, Tesh D, Crowley J, et al. Chemotherapy is superior to sequential hemibody irradiation for remission consolidation in multiple myeloma: a Southwest Oncology Group study. *J Clin Oncol* 1990;8:1575–1584.
104. Samson D, Gaminara E, Newland A, et al. Infusion of vincristine and doxorubicin with oral dexamethasone as first-line therapy for multiple myeloma. *Lancet* 1989;2:882–885.
105. Schirrmeister H, Buck AK, Bergmann L, et al. Positron emission tomography (PET) for staging of solitary plasmacytoma. *Cancer Biother Radiopharm* 2003;18:841–845.
106. Shih LY, Dunn P, Leung WM, et al. Localised plasmacytomas in Taiwan: comparison between extramedullary plasmacytoma and solitary plasmacytoma of bone. *Br J Cancer* 1995;71:128–133.
107. Singer CR, Tobias JS, Giles F, et al. Hemibody irradiation. An effective second-line therapy in drug-resistance multiple myeloma. *Cancer* 1989;63:2446–2451.
108. Soesan M, Paccagnella A, Chiarion-Sileni V, et al. Extramedullary plasmacytoma: clinical behaviour and response to treatment. *Ann Oncol* 1992;3:51–57.
109. Soutar R, Lucraft H, Jackson G, et al. Guidelines on the diagnosis and management of solitary plasmacytoma of bone and solitary extramedullary plasmacytoma. *Clin Oncol (R Coll Radiol)* 2004;16:405–413.
110. Strojan P, Soba E, Lamovec J, et al. Extramedullary plasmacytoma: clinical and histopathologic study. *Int J Radiat Oncol Biol Phys* 2002;53:692–701.
111. Sundaresan N, Steinberger AA, Moore F, et al. Indications and results of combined anterior-posterior approaches for spine tumor surgery. *J Neurosurg* 1996;85:438–446.
112. Susnerwala SS, Shanks JH, Banerjee SS, et al. Extramedullary plasmacytoma of the head and neck region: clinicopathological correlation in 25 cases. *Br J Cancer* 1997;75:921–927.
113. Tarte K, Chang Y, Klein B. Kaposi's sarcoma-associated herpesvirus and multiple myeloma: lack of criteria for causality. *Blood* 1999;93:3159–3163; discussion 3163–3154.

114. Tian E, Zhan F, Walker R, et al. The role of the Wnt-signaling antagonist DKK1 in the development of osteolytic lesions in multiple myeloma. *N Engl J Med* 2003;349:2483–2494.

115. Tobias JS, Richards JD, Blackman GM, et al. Hemibody irradiation in multiple myeloma. *Radiother Oncol* 1985;3:11–16.

116. Tournier-Rangeard L, Lapeyre M, Graff-Caillaud P, et al. Radiotherapy for solitary extramedullary plasmacytoma in the head-and-neck region: a dose greater than 45 Gy to the target volume improves the local control. *Int J Radiat Oncol Biol Phys* 2006;64:1013–1017.

117. Tsang RW, Gospodarowicz MK, Pintilie M, et al. Solitary plasmacytoma treated with radiotherapy: impact of tumor size on outcome. *Int J Radiat Oncol Biol Phys* 2001;50:113–120.

118. Van de Berg BC, Lecouvet FE, Michaux L, et al. Stage I multiple myeloma: value of MR imaging of the bone marrow in the determination of prognosis. *Radiology* 1996;201:243–246.

119. van Dyk J, Keane TJ, Kan S, et al. Radiation pneumonitis following large single dose irradiation: a re-evaluation based on absolute dose to lung. *Int J Radiat Oncol Biol Phys* 1981;7:461–467.

120. Wallington M, Mendis S, Premawardhana U, et al. Local control and survival in spinal cord compression from lymphoma and myeloma. *Radiother Oncol* 1997;42:43–47.

121. Wilder RB, Ha CS, Cox JD, et al. Persistence of myeloma protein for more than one year after radiotherapy is an adverse prognostic factor in solitary plasmacytoma of bone. *Cancer* 2002;94:1532–1537.

122. Wiltshaw E. The natural history of extramedullary plasmacytoma and its relation to solitary myeloma of bone and myelomatosis. *Medicine* 1976;55:217–238.

123. Wohrer S, Ackermann J, Baldia C, et al. Effective treatment of primary plasma cell leukemia with thalidomide and dexamethasone—a case report. *Hematol J* 2004;5:361–363.

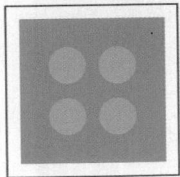

Chapter 80
Osteosarcoma

Nicole A. Larrier

Epidemiology and Risk Factors

Osteosarcoma is the most common malignant bone tumor in childhood, representing approximately 50% of newly diagnosed malignant pediatric bone tumors or 700 new U.S. cases annually (27). The annual incidence is 4.5 per million in girls and 5.5 per million in boys (27). This incidence peaks in those ages 10 to 19 years (40). There does not appear to be a difference in incidence among African Americans and whites.

The etiology of osteosarcoma is unknown in most cases. The incidence does correlate with the growth spurt in teenagers. However, specific pathways associated with this finding are elusive. For a minority of patients, a specific risk factor is identified. These risk factors include, prior radiotherapy (58), and specific genetic syndrome. Survivors of hereditary retinoblastoma carry a risk of osteosarcoma of 6% at 18 years (20), Li-Fraumeni syndrome (6), and in older adults, there is an association between Paget's.

Clinical Presentation

Most patients present with pain in the affected limb or region and soft tissue swelling. In some patients, trauma and a subsequent pathologic fracture brings the individual to medical attention.

Approximately 90% present in the diaphysis of the extremities, with the distal femur and proximal tibia being the most common sites. Other sites such as the pelvis and head and neck represent significant minority of the locations (27).

Diagnostic Evaluation

Radiologic investigation begins with a plain radiograph (Fig. 80.1A). Classic findings include an ill-defined zone of transition, Codman's triangle (defined as osteoid formation under the periosteum), and bone formation in the adjacent soft tissue. The lesion itself may be sclerotic (Fig. 80.2), lytic (Fig. 80.1A), or mixed. Most lesions are subsequently evaluated by magnetic resonance imaging (Fig. 80.1B). This will show the proximal and distal extent of involvement, evaluate any soft tissue component, and establish the proximity of nerves, vessels, and the joint space. Skip metastases are a well-defined but uncommon entity in osteosarcoma. Modern series place the incidence of isolated skip metastases at diagnosis at <5% (33,51).

At diagnosis, approximately 15% of patients have detectable distant metastases. More than 80% of metastases are pulmonary, followed by metastases at bony sites (5). Therefore, chest computed tomography and radionuclide bone scan are needed to complete staging.

Positron emission tomography is being investigated as a part of the initial staging work-up and as a modality to evaluate response to chemotherapy (8). However, to date, it is not a part of the recommended work-up.

Staging Systems

There are two major staging systems for this disease: the Enneking system (22) and the American Joint Committee on Cancer system (1) (Table 80.1). However, most practitioners usually classify the disease state as nonmetastatic or metastatic, based on the presence or absence of distant metastases.

Pathology

The commonly accepted histologic description of osteosarcoma is based on the World Health Organization classification (53). This divides osteosarcomas into intramedullary and surface subtypes. The most commonly encountered subtype is the conventional category of medullary tumors. These are further subclassified into osteoblastic, chondroblastic, fibroblastic, and mixed types based on the pathologist's visualization of the specific elements. Other categories of medullary (or conventional) osteosarcoma are small cell, telangiectatic, and well-differentiated (or low-grade) types.

Surface osteosarcomas are divided into parosteal (juxtacortical), periosteal, and high grade.

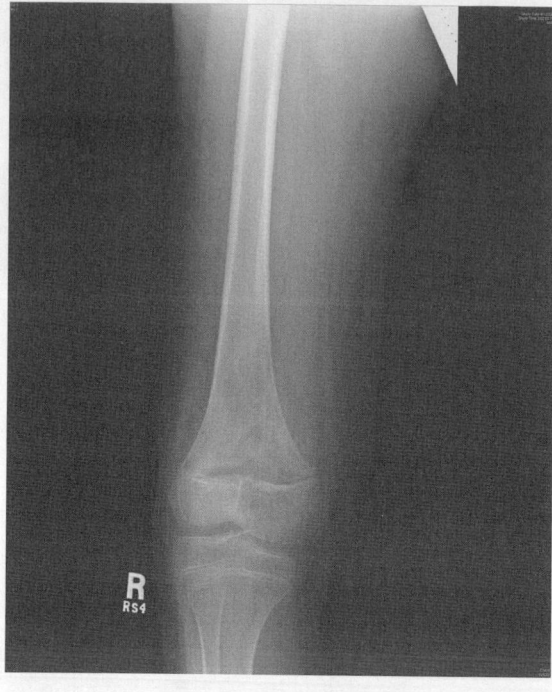
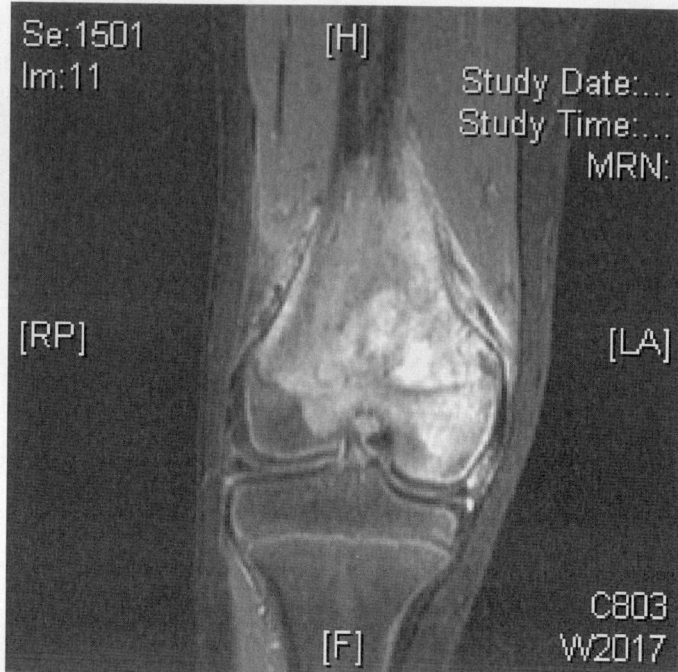

FIGURE 80.1. A: Plain radiograph of a distal femur osteosarcoma showing a lytic region and Codman's triangle in the medial distal femur. **B:** Magnetic resonance image scan of the same lesion.

Overall Management

Chemotherapy is essential for cure. In the nonmetastatic setting, the overall schema consists of chemotherapy followed by resection of the primary tumor, and adjuvant chemotherapy.

In patients with pulmonary metastatic disease, the treatment program is the same as for nonmetastatic disease, with the addition of possible resection of any pulmonary nodules remaining after the completion of chemotherapy.

Low-grade osteosarcomas are usually managed with surgery alone.

Surgical Management

Resection of the primary tumor is part of the standard management. Subsequent to an *en bloc* resection of the tumor, re-

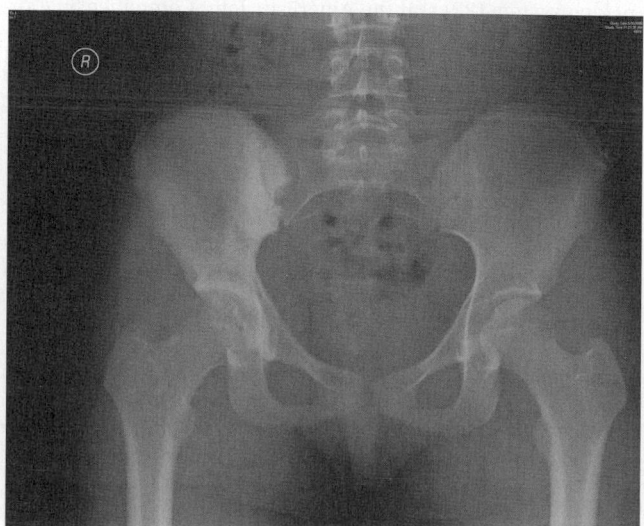

FIGURE 80.2. Plain radiograph of a sclerotic pelvic osteosarcoma.

construction is usually required. The goal of the surgical intervention is to remove the tumor *en bloc* and achieve adequate negative margins.

Presurgical planning includes careful evaluation of the pre- and postneoadjuvant chemotherapy imaging and determination of the anticipated reconstruction. For extremity tumors, imaging will often show a decrease in the soft tissue component of the tumor and allows visualization of the neurovascular structure, muscle groups, and fascial planes; the relationship of the tumor to the epiphysis and articular surface; and provides an estimate of the length of bone to be removed.

There are several options for surgery. Amputation should be recommended if the patient will be left with a nonfunctioning limb (39). Most individuals will undergo some type of limb sparing procedure. Reconstruction options include autologous bone grafts, allografts, and endoprosthetics. Less commonly, rotationplasty or arthrodesis is employed. In the current era, 80% to 90% of patients will undergo a limb salvage (39).

Reconstructions can suffer infections, nonunion, and fracture, depending on the technique. Endoprosthetics are prone to infection. Allografts can fracture up to 20% of the time (37). However, the functional outcome of various reconstructive techniques can be good in 60% to 90% of cases (24,37).

Traditionally, pelvic osteosarcomas present a challenge to the orthopaedic oncologist. Small tumors may be adequately resected with or without reconstruction. Resection of large tumors may mean not only the loss of the ipsilateral lower extremity, but compromising of bowel and bladder function.

Chemotherapy

Systemic chemotherapy is standard of care for all patients who are able to tolerate the intensive regimens.

Two randomized studies demonstrated the efficacy of adjuvant chemotherapy (21,29). Table 80.2 shows various randomized trials of adjuvant chemotherapy. Notably, an early randomized trial had negative findings (36). The standard agents used are methotrexate, cisplatin, and doxorubicin, all of these with or without ifosfamide.

Table 80.1   STAGING OF OSTEOSARCOMA

A. Enneking Staging System

Stage	Grade	Site	Metastases
I A	Low	Intracompartmental	No
I B	Low	Extracompartmental	No
II A	High	Intracompartmental	No
II B	High	Extracompartmental	No
III	Any	Any	Yes

B. AJCC Staging System

Stage	Grade	Local Extent (cm)	Metastases
I A	Low	≤ 8	None
I B	Low	>8	None
II A	High	≤ 8	None
II B	High	>8	None
III	Any	Any	Skip metastases
IV A	Any	Any	Pulmonary metastases
IV B	Any	Any	Other metastases

American Joint Committee on Cancer.

Subsequent studies investigated neoadjuvant chemotherapy as a way to evaluate tumor response. A randomized Pediatric Oncology Group study showed no difference in outcome whether preoperative or postoperative chemotherapy was administered (26) Advantages of neoadjuvant chemotherapy include the determination of the pathologic response, early treatment of micrometastatic disease, and allowing adequate time for surgical planning and ordering of a custom prosthesis.

The percent necrosis after neoadjuvant chemotherapy is a prognostic factor (5,32). The classification scheme is according to the Huvos grade. The overall survival of patients with nonmetastatic disease with >90% necrosis is near 70%, compared with 50% in those with <90% necrosis (31). Therefore, the next therapeutic question was whether the survival of poor responders could be improved by altering and/or intensifying chemotherapy administered after surgery. Several studies have investigated this, but no improvement in survival has been demonstrated (3,61). Likewise, attempts to intensify the chemotherapy regimen delivered preoperatively have failed to show an increase in survival despite a small increase in the percentage of good responders (41,48).

Radiotherapy

Historically, radiotherapy has been used in the treatment of osteosarcoma. Prior to effective chemotherapy, Cade (13) pioneered a technique of radiotherapy with delayed amputation in those who did not develop distant metastases. Subsequently, others questioned the need for amputation. The radiotherapy doses employed were 5,000 to 8,000 R. Of note, in these series many patients did have resolution of their symptoms (pain and swelling) soon after starting radiation. Beck et al. (4) report only 1 of 21 survivors in a group treated with definitive radiotherapy. However, prior to death, three patients had local recurrences. deMoor (18) describes a cohort treated with "radical radiotherapy." Of the 27 initial patients, 9 had survived at least 5 years and 3 had local recurrences.

Table 80.2   RANDOMIZED TRIALS OF ADJUVANT CHEMOTHERAPY IN OSTEOSARCOMA

Study	No. of Patients	Adjuvant Treatment Arms	Chemotherapy Agents	DFS (%)	Overall Survival (%)
Edmonson (17)	18	None	Methotrexate, vincristine, doxorubicin	42 (5 yr)	55 (5 yr)
	20	Chemotherapy		40 (NS)	50 (NS)
Eilber et al. (21)	27	None	Methotrexate, vincristine, Adriamycin, bleomycin, Cytoxan, actinomycin D	20 (2 yr)	48 (2 yr)
	32	Chemotherapy		55 (SS)	80 (SS)
Link et al. (36)	18	None	Methotrexate, bleomycin, cyclophosphamide, doxorubicin, cisplatin	11 (6 yr)	50 (6 yr)
	18	Chemotherapy		66 (SS)	71 (SS)

NS, not statistically significant; SS, statistically significant.

Table 80.3	MODERN RADIOTHERAPY FOR OSTEOSARCOMA					
Study	No. of Patients	Location	Regimen	Modality	Dose (Gy)	Outcome
Dincbas et al. (19)	46	Extremity	CT → RT → S → CT	Photons	36–46	5-yr LC = 97.5%
Delaney et al. (17)	41	Mixed	CT → RT +/−S → CT	Photons and/or protons	10–80	5-yr LC: Overall, 68%; GTR, 74%; STR, 74%; biopsy, 22%
Machak et al. (38)	31	Extremity	CT → RT → CT	Photons	40–68	5-yr OS = 61%; 5-yr local PFS = 56%

CT, chemotherapy; RT, radiotherapy; S, surgery; LC, local control; GTR, gross total resection; STR, subtotal resection; PFS, progression-free survival.

With the advent of chemotherapy, Caceres et al. (12) reported on a group of 16 patients who were treated with chemotherapy and definitive radiotherapy. Tumors and surrounding tissue received 6,000 rad after one cycle of chemotherapy. Chemotherapy was then continued for 1 year. Biopsies were performed at the primary site in 15 of 16 patients every 3 months after the initiation of treatment. Results of this study showed that 80% of patients had a complete pathologic response. Complications included soft tissue fibrosis in nine patients, fracture in four, infection in two, and necrosis in two.

The role of radiotherapy in osteosarcoma therapy in the 21st century is now limited to select situations. Specifically, irradiation is considered in patients who refuse surgery, those with positive margins after resection, those with sites that are not amenable to resection and reconstruction, and palliation.

Modern External-beam Radiotherapy

Table 80.3 gives an overview of modern radiotherapy treatment. In recent years, contemporary chemotherapy and definitive radiotherapy in dose relative accumulation has been reported by Machak et al. (38). A median of 60 Gy was given using conventional fractionation. The 5-year local progression-free survival was 56%, with an overall survival of 61%. Those with a good response to neoadjuvant chemotherapy had an overall survival of 90%, compared with 35% in those who were poor responders. This phenomenon was also paralleled in local control. There were no local failures in good responders, but nearly one third of poor responders failed locally.

Conversely, Delaney et al. (17) reported only a 22% local control rate in patients who were treated with chemotherapy and local radiotherapy. For the group of patients receiving radiotherapy adjuvantly after surgery, the local control rate was 74%, with a gross total resection or a subtotal resection.

Dincbas et al. (19) recently reported preoperative radiotherapy integrated in the usual osteosarcoma treatment protocol. Local control was excellent at 97% with good limb salvage. However, this is similar to what would be expected in the cooperative group trials. Therefore, it is not clear that radiotherapy added to the overall outcome.

Extracorporeal and Definitive Intraoperative Radiotherapy

The techniques of extracorporeal and definitive intraoperative radiotherapy (IORT) have been investigated in bone tumors (Table 80.4) (9,15,28,44,58,59). The extracorporeal technique includes *en bloc* resection of the tumor and surrounding soft tissues, irradiation of the specimen, and reimplantation, often with the aid of prostheses. With definitive IORT, the operative field is exposed and radiotherapy is administered. No resection of the tumor is performed.

Extracorporeal irradiation is associated with a low rate of local recurrence (<5%). Chen et al. (15) noted a higher rate of complications (62%) in their initial series. The events included fractures, nonunions, wound infections, and loss of cartilage. Subsequently, they incorporated the use of prostheses placed at the time of reimplantation. Their local recurrence rate

Table 80.4	EXTRACORPOREAL AND DEFINITIVE INTRAOPERATIVE RADIOTHERAPY (IORT) FOR OSTEOSARCOMA			
Study	N	Dose (Gy)	LR	Comments
Extracorporeal				
Bohm et al. (7)	6	250	1/6	
Chen et al. (15)	13	300	1/13	1991–1994: complication rate = 62%
	7	300	0/7	1995–1998: fewer complications with prosthetic and ECIR
Hong et al. (28)	4	50	0/4	—
Uyttendaele et al. (59)	10	300	2/10	—
Definitive IORT				
Oya et al. (44)	39	45–80	9/39	—
Tsuboyama et al. (57)	21	45–70	5/21	—

LR, local relapse; ECIR, extracorporeal irradiation.

Clinical Radiation Oncology

Table 80.5	**PARTICLE THERAPY FOR OSTEOSARCOMA**	
Study	**Modality**	**Local Control**
Laramore et al. (35)	Neutrons	40/73 (55%)
Oda et al. (43)	Neutrons	1/2
Carrie et al. (14)	Neutrons/photons	4/4
Hug et al. (30)	Protons/photons	59% (n = 15)

continued to be low and there was only one complication (a nerve palsy) in their series of 14 patients (15).

The reported local control rate for definitive IORT is 20% to 25% (44,57). The complication rate is >50% as reported by Tsuboyama et al. (57), but minimal in the hands of Oya et al. (44).

Particle Therapy

Because of the difficulty of achieving adequate local control with photons, neutrons and protons have been employed in the treatment of osteosarcoma (Table 80.5). Neutrons are thought to have a higher relative biologic effectiveness and oxygen-enhancement ratio, making them radiobiologically more effective against osteosarcomas. The advantage of protons is in the physical properties of the Bragg peak, which falls off rapidly and spares adjacent tissue.

The earliest studies of particle therapy are with neutrons in the 1970s and 1980s, prior to optimal chemotherapy and surgical reconstruction. The review of the early data by Laramore et al. (35) shows an overall local control rate of 55% in 73 patients pooled from seven institutions worldwide.

In a more recent review of head and neck sarcomas, Oda et al. (43) report local control in a patient treated with chemotherapy, surgery, and neutron irradiation. One other patient who received only surgery and neutron therapy had local failure. Carrie et al. (14) describe local control in 4/4 pelvic osteosarcomas treated with modern chemotherapy and a combination of photons and neutrons.

The major complications surrounding neutron therapy are severe fibrosis and scarring of the soft tissues and adjacent organs (35).

The largest proton experience is at the Massachusetts General Hospital (30). Fifteen patients with osteosarcoma of the base of skull or vertebra were treated by this form of therapy. The 5-year local control is reported at 59%.

Whole-lung Irradiation

Prophylactic lung irradiation has been investigated in osteosarcoma. Three randomized trials were conducted in the 1970s and 1980s (Table 80.6) (9,11,49). The Mayo Clinic and first European Organisation for Research and Treatment of Cancer studies were conducted prior to the routine use of chemotherapy (9,49). They both showed trends toward improved survival with whole-lung irradiation. However, a three-arm EORTC/SIOP study that compared chemotherapy, whole-lung irradiation, or a combination of both, showed the same disease-free survival and overall survival in both arms (43% and 24%) (11). Therefore, with the recognition of the other advantages of systemic therapy, prophylactic lung irradiation has fallen out of favor (60).

Radionuclide Therapy

Several investigators have used radionuclides in the treatment of bony metastatic osteosarcoma (Table 80.7). There are case reports of the use of rhenium (52), strontium (25), and samarium (10). The major toxicity is decreased in the platelet and white blood cell counts.

Anderson et al. (2) conducted a phase I dose-escalation study of samarium-153 in metastatic osteosarcoma. The goal was to evaluate the toxicity of increasing doses of radionuclide using hematopoietic stem cells to decrease the bone marrow toxicity. Bone marrow toxicity and transient hypocalcemia were seen at the highest dose level. The authors report good pain relief.

Results of Radiotherapy in Specific Disease Sites

Pelvis

The management of large pelvic osteosarcomas continues to present a challenge. Definitive surgery often includes a hemipelvectomy. Despite being the most common nonextremity site of osteosarcomas, the percentage is <10%. The overall local failure rate in the 22 patients with spinal primaries was 70% in the Cooperative Osteosarcoma Study Group (45). Eleven of 67 patients received radiotherapy. Seven patients were treated definitively and four were treated in a postoperative fashion. The definitive dose was 56 to 68 Gy and the postoperative dose was 45 to 51 Gy. The majority of those patients receiving radiotherapy failed locally (6/7 treated definitively, and three of four treated after an intralesional surgery).

In the St. Jude Children's Research Hospital experience, local control was achieved in three-fourths of the patients using 50 to

Table 80.6	**RANDOMIZED TRIALS OF WHOLE-LUNG IRRADIATION (WLI) FOR OSTEOSARCOMA**		
Study	**No. of Patients**	**Dose (Gy)**	**Outcome (Control vs. WLI)**
Mayo Clinic (Rab et al. 49)	53	15	Median survival: 25 vs. 42 months (NS)
EORTC-02 (Breur et al. 9)	86	17.5	3-yr DFS: 28% vs. 43% (NS) 5-yr OS: 40% vs. 55% (NS)
EORTC/SIOP-03 (Burgers et al. 11) Group 1: chemotherapy Group 2: WLI Group 3: chemotherapy/WLI	240	20	Same OS and DFS (43% and 24%)

NS, not significant; EORTC, European Organisation for Research and Treatment of Cancer; SIOP, International Society of Pediatric Oncology; DFS, disease-free survival; OS, overall survival.

Table 80.7	RADIONUCLIDE THERAPY FOR OSTEOSARCOMA				
Study	Isotope	No. of Patients	EBRT	Outcome	Comments
Anderson et al. (2)	Sm-153	20	No	"Most able to discontinue opiates"	Phase I dose-escalation study using peripheral stem cell rescue
Sawyer et al. (52)	Re-186	1	Yes	Disease-free at 3 yr. Negative biopsy at 3 and 15 months.	—
Gompakis et al. (25)	S-89	1	No	DOD at 6 weeks. Pain relieved.	—
Bruland e al. (10)	Sm-153	1	No	Pain relief for 6 months	—

DOD, dead of disease.

98 Gy and modern chemotherapy (50). Promising local control was achieved in the University of South Florida series of five patients treated with intra-arterial cisplatin and radiotherapy (23).

Spine

Fewer than 2% of patients present with spinal primaries. Within the Cooperative Osteosarcoma Study (COSS) studies, overall survival for patients with spinal primaries is <2 years and the local failure rate was near 70% in the 22 patients studied (46). Seven of the 17 patients who underwent an intralesional procedure or biopsy received radiotherapy only as part of their care. Radiotherapy doses ranged from 20 to 60 Gy. Five of seven patients had local recurrences.

When the group from Memorial Sloan-Kettering Cancer Center analyzed their series, 5 of 11 patients in the cohort treated with resection, external-beam radiotherapy, and chemotherapy were long-term survivors (56).

Head and Neck

Most head and neck osteosarcomas present in the mandible or maxilla. The age of presentation tends to be somewhat older than that of patients with extremity lesions (55). The review by Kassir et al. (34) finds an overall local control rate of 50% at these sites. Almost 40% of the patients received radiotherapy (external-beam or brachytherapy), but no comment is made on the effect of irradiation on local control. Those receiving radiotherapy did have a lower survival rate than those treated with surgery and chemotherapy.

St. Jude Children's Research Hospital researchers reported on four children who received 31 to 74 Gy postoperatively (21). The two who received 31 Gy and 40 Gy both had local failure. In the University of Washington experience, five patients received postoperative radiotherapy (49). The three who received chemotherapy have maintained local control. However, the two who did not receive chemotherapy died, but no comment was made regarding the status of the primary site.

Late Effects

Late complications are largely related to chemotherapy and surgical interventions. Doxorubicin can cause cardiomyopathy (47) and cisplatin results in high-frequency hearing loss in about half of patients (54). Some patients will exhibit transient changes in renal function, but late complications are unusual. Second malignancies, with a minimum 5-year follow-up, were reported in 7% (42).

Nicholson et al. (42) report long-term survivors having more difficulty climbing stairs; the patients had similar employment and marital status as sibling controls.

With respect to radiotherapy, the data are limited. This is largely because this modality is used in patients with unfavorable prognoses, with a low chance of long-term survival. Laramore et al. (35) report a 25% to 40% complication rate of study results gleaned from reviewing the literature for neutron therapy, which is often related to dense fibrotic reactions. Delaney et al. (17) report a 24% complication rate in a proton/photon cohort. In a definitive external-beam radiotherapy series, Machak et al. (38) describe three-quarters of the patients as having good limb function. Three of the 31 patients had pathologic fractures and 1 had skin necrosis.

References

1. American Joint Committee on Cancer. *Cancer Staging manual,* 6th ed. New York: Springer-Verlag; 2002.
2. Anderson PM, Wiseman GA, Dispenzieri, A, et al. High dose samarium-153 ethylene diamine tetra methylene phosphonate: low toxicity in skeletal irradiation in patients with osteosarcoma and bone metastases. *J Clin Oncol* 2002;20:189–196.
3. Bacci G, Bertoni F, Longhi A, et al. Neoadjuvant chemotherapy for high-grade central osteosarcoma of the extremity. Histologic response to preoperative chemotherapy correlates with histologic subtype of the tumor. *Cancer* 2003;97:3068–3075.
4. Beck JC, Wara WM, Bovill EG, et al. The role of radiation therapy in the therapy of osteosarcoma. *Radiology* 1976;120:163–165.
5. Bielack SS, Kempf-Bielack B, Delling G, et al. Prognostic factors in high-grade osteosarcoma of the extremities and trunk: an analysis of 1702 patients treated with neoadjuvant Cooperative Osteosarcoma Study Group Protocols. *J Clin Oncol* 2002;20:776–790.
6. Birch JM, Alston RD, McNally RJQ, et al. Relative frequency and morphology of cancers in carriers of germline TP53 mutations. *Oncogene* 2001;20:4621–4628.
7. Bohm P, Fritz J, Thiede S, et al. Reimplantation of extracorporeal irradiated bone segments in musculoskeletal tumor surgery: clinical experience in eight patients and review of the literature. *Langerbecks Arch Surg* 2003;387:355–365.
8. Brenner W, Bohuslavizki K, Eary J. PET imaging in osteosarcoma. *J Nucl Med* 2003;44:930–942.
9. Breur K, Cohen P, Schweisguh O, et al. Irradiation of the lungs of an adjuvant therapy in the treatment of osteosarcoma of the limbs. An EORTC randomized study. *Eur J Cancer* 1978;14:461–471.
10. Bruland OS, Skretting A, Solheim OP, et al. Targeted radiotherapy of osteosarcoma using 153Sm-EDTMP. *Acta Oncol* 1996;35:381–384.
11. Burgers JM, van Glabbeke M, Busson A, et al. Osteosarcoma of the limbs. Report of the EORTC-SIOP o3 trial 20781 investigating the value of adjuvant therapy with chemotherapy and /or prophylactic lung irradiation. *Cancer* 1988;61:1024–1031.
12. Caceres E, Zaharia M, Valdivia S, et al. Local control of osteogenic sarcoma by radiation and chemotherapy. *IJROBP* 1984;10:35–39.
13. Cade S. Osteogenic sarcoma. A study based on 133 patients. *Clin Orthop Rel Res* 1991;264:4–9.
14. Carrie C, Breteau N, Negrier S, et al. The role of fast neutron therapy in unresectable pelvic osteosarcoma: preliminary report. *Med Pediatr Oncol* 1994;22:355–357.
15. Chen WM, Chen TH, Huang CK, et al. Treatment of malignant bone tumors by extracorporeal irradiated autograft-prosthetic composite arthroplasty. *J Bone Joint Surg* 2002;84:1156–1161.
16. Daw NC, Mahmoud HH, Meyer WH, et al. Bone sarcomas in the head and neck in children. The St. Jude Children's Research Hospital experience. *Cancer* 2000;88:2173–2180.
17. Delaney TF, Park L, Goldberg S, et al. Radiotherapy for local control of osteosarcoma. *IJROBP* 2005;61:492–498.

18. deMoor NG. Osteosarcoma. A review of 72 cases treated by megavoltage radiation therapy with or without surgery. *S Afr J Surg* 1975;12:137–146.

19. Dincbas FO, Koca S, Mandel NM, et al. The role of preoperative radiotherapy in nonmetastatic high-grade osteosarcoma of the extremities for limb-sparing surgery. *IJOBP* 2005;62:820–828.

20. Draper GJ, Sanders BM, Kingston JE. Second primary neoplasms in patients with retinoblastoma. *Br J Cancer* 1986;53:661–671.

21. Eilber F, Giuliano A, Eckardt J, et al. Adjuvant chemotherapy for osteosarcoma: a randomized prospective trial. *J Clin Oncol* 1987;5:21–26.

22. Enneking WF, Spanie SS, Goodman MA. A system for the surgical staging of musculoskeletal sarcoma. *Clin Orthop Rel Res* 2003;415:4–18.

23. Estrada-Aguilar J, Greenberg H, Walling A, et al. Primary treatment of pelvic osteosarcoma. Report of five cases. *Cancer* 1992;69:1137–1145.

24. Gebhardt M, Roth YF, Mankin HJ. The use of bone allografts for limb salvage in high grad extremity osteosarcoma. *Clin Orthop* 1991;270:181–196.

25. Gompakis N, Sidi B, Salem N, et al. Strontium-89 for palliation of bone pain. *Med Ped Oncol* 2003;40:136.

26. Goorin AM, Schwartzentruber DJ, Devidas M, et al. Presurgical chemotherapy compared with immediate surgery and adjuvant chemotherapy for nonmetastatic osteosarcoma: Pediatric Oncology Group POG-8651. *J Clin Oncol* 2003;21:1574–1580.

27. Gurney JG, Swensen AR, Bulterys M. SEER Pediatric Monograph. Available at: http://seer.cancer.gov/publications/childhood/bone.pdf. Accessed

28. Hong A, Stevens G, Stalley P, et al. Extracorporeal irradiation for malignant bone tumors. *IJROBP* 2001;50:441–447.

29. Horowitz SM, Glasser DB, Lane DB, et al. Prosthetic and extremity survivorship after limb salvage for sarcoma. How long do the reconstructions last?. *Clin Orthop* 1993;293:280–286.

30. Hug EB, Fitzek MM, Liebsch NJ, et al. Locally challenging osteo- and chondrogenic tumors of the axial skeleton: results of combined proton and photon radiation therapy using three dimensional treatment planning. *IJROBP* 1995;31:467–476.

31. Huvos A. *Bone tumors: diagnosis, treatment and prognosis,* 2nd Ed. Philadelphia: WB Saunders; 1991.

32. Juergens H, Kosloff C, Nirenberg A, et al. Prognostic factors in the response of primary osteogenic sarcoma to preoperative chemotherapy (high-dose methotrexate with citrovorum factor). *NCI Monogr* 1981;56:221–226.

33. Kager L, Soubek A, Kastner U, et al. Skip metastases in osteosarcoma: experience of the Cooperative Osteosarcoma Study Group. *J Clin Oncol* 2006;24:1535–1541.

34. Kassir RR, Rassekh CH, Kinsella JB, et al. Osteosarcoma of the head and neck: meta-analysis of nonrandomized studies. *Laryngoscope* 1997;107:56–61.

35. Laramore GE, Griffith JT, Boespflug M, et al. Fast neutron radiotherapy for sarcomas of soft tissue, bone and cartilage. *Am J Clin Oncol* 1989;12:320–326.

36. Link MP, Goorin AM, Horowitz M, et al. Adjuvant chemotherapy of high-grade osteosarcoma of the extremity. Updated results of the Multi-Institutional Osteosarcoma Study. *Clin Orthop* 1991;270:8–14.

37. Longhi A, Errani C, DePaolis M, et al. Primary bone osteosarcoma in the pediatric age: state of the art. *Cancer Treat Rev* 2006;32:423–436.

38. Machak GN, Tkachev SI, Solovyev YN, et al. Neoadjuvant chemotherapy and local radiotherapy for high-grade osteosarcoma of the extremities. *Mayo Clin Proc* 2003;78:147–155.

39. Marina N, Gebhardt M, Leot L, et al. Biology and therapeutic advances for pediatric osteosarcoma. *Oncologist* 2004;9:422–441.

40. Mascarenhas L, Siegel S, Spector L et al; SEER AYA Monograph. Available at: http://www.seer.cancer.gov/publications/aya/. Accessed October 2006.

41. Meyers PA, Gorlick R, Heller G, et al. Intensification of preoperative chemotherapy for osteogenic sarcoma: results of the Memorial Sloan-Kettering (T12) protocol. *J Clin Oncol* 1998;16:2452–2458.

42. Nicholson HS, Mulvihill JJ, Byrne J. Late effects in adult survivors of osteosarcoma and Ewing's sarcoma. *Med Pediatr Oncol* 1992;20:6–12.

43. Oda D, Bavisotto LM, Schmidt RA, et al. Head and neck osteosarcoma at the University of Washington. *Head Neck* 1997;19:513–523.

44. Oya N, Kobubo M, Mizowaki T, et al. Definitive intraoperative very high dose radiotherapy for localized osteosarcoma in the extremities. 2001;51:878–893.

45. Ozaki T, Flege S, Kevric M, et al. Osteosarcoma of the pelvis: experience of the Cooperative Osteosarcoma Study Group. *J Clin Oncol* 2003;21:334–341.

46. Ozaki T, Flege S, Liljenqvist U, et al. Osteosarcoma of the spine: experience of the Cooperative Osteosarcoma Study Group. *Cancer* 2002;94;1069–1077.

47. Paulides M, Kremers A, Stohr W, et al. Prospective longitudinal evaluation of doxorubicin-induced cardiomyopathy in sarcoma patients. *Pediatr Blood Cancer* 2006;46:489–495.

48. Provisor AJ, Ettinger LJ, Nachman JB, et al. Treatment of non-metastatic osteosarcoma of the extremity with preoperative and postoperative chemotherapy: a report from the Children's Cancer Group. *J Clin Oncol* 1997;15:76–84.

49. Rab GT, Ivins JC, Childs DS, et al. Elective whole lung irradiation in the treatment of osteogenic sarcoma. *Cancer* 1976;38:939–942.

50. Saab R, Rao BN, Rodriguez-Galindo C, et al. Osteosarcoma of the pelvis in children and young adults: the St. Jude Children's Research Hospital experience. *Cancer* 2005;103:1468–1474.

51. Sajadi KR, Heck RK, Neal MD. The incidence and prognosis of osteosarcoma skip metastases. *Clin Orthop Rel Res* 2004;426:92–96.

52. Sawyer EJ, Cassoni AM, Waddington W, et al. Rhenium-186 HEDP as a boost to external beam irradiation in osteosarcoma. *Br J Radiol* 1999;72:1225–1229.

53. Schajowicz F, Sissons HA, Sobin LH. The World Health Organization's histologic classification of bone tumors. A commentary on the second edition. *Cancer* 1995;75:1208–1214.

54. Stohr W, Langer T, Kremers A, et al. Cisplatin-induced ototoxicity in osteosarcoma patients: a report from the late effects surveillance system. *Cancer Invest* 2005;23:201–207.

55. Sturgis EM, Potter BO. Sarcomas of the head and neck region. *Current Opin Oncol* 2003;15:239–252.

56. Sundaresan N, Rosen G, Huvos AG, et al. Combined treatment of osteosarcoma of the spine. *Neurosurgery* 1998;23:714–719.

57. Tsuboyama T, Toguchida J, Kotoura Y, et al. Intra-operative radiation therapy for osteosarcoma in the extremities. *Int Orthop* 2000;24:202–207.

58. Tucker MA, D'Angio GJ, Boice JD, et al. Bone cancer linked to radiotherapy and chemotherapy in children. *N Engl J Med* 1987;317:588–593.

59. Uyttendaele D, DeSchryver A, Claessens H, et al. Limb conservation in primary bone tumors by resection, extracorporeal irradiation and re-implantation. *J Bone Joint Surg* 1988;70:348–353.

60. Whelan JS, Burcombe RJ, Janinis J, et al. A systematic review of the role of pulmonary irradiation in the management of primary bone tumors. *Ann Oncol* 2002;13:23–30.

61. Winkler K, Beron G, Delling G, et al. Neoadjuvant chemotherapy of osteosarcoma: results of a randomized cooperative trial (COSS_82) with salvage chemotherapy based on histological tumor response. *J Clin Oncol* 1988;6:329–337.

Clinical Radiation Oncology

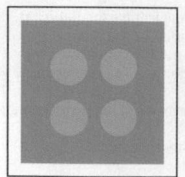

Chapter 81
Soft Tissue Sarcomas (Excluding Retroperitoneum)

Michael E. Ray, Cornelius J. McGinn

Sarcomas are rare malignancies that arise from the connective tissues in any organ or at any anatomic location of the body. This chapter addresses sarcomas that arise in the extraskeletal, nonvisceral connective tissues of adults, excluding the retroperitoneum. Despite the diversity of tissues and locations of origin, these soft tissue sarcomas are grouped together because of overall similarities in natural history and treatment. Retroperitoneal sarcomas, pediatric sarcomas, osteosarcomas, sarcomas arising in visceral organs, Kaposi's sarcoma, and sarcomas arising in the vasculature are discussed elsewhere in this textbook.

Anatomy

The majority of soft tissue sarcomas occur in the muscle groups of the extremities (Table 81.1). These tumors often remain confined to the muscle compartment of origin. The thigh is the most common subsite of origin and is partitioned into three compartments (37). The muscle compartments of the arm, forearm, and leg are similarly defined (4) (Fig. 81.1). Anatomic knowledge is essential for the radiation oncologist because it allows appropriate positioning of the limb to encompass the portion of the compartment at risk, while avoiding compartments that are not involved.

Epidemiology, Genetics, and Risk Factors

Approximately 9,100 cases of soft tissue sarcoma are diagnosed yearly in the United States, accounting for 0.7% of cancers and an estimated 3,500 deaths (68). Men are more frequently affected than women, and rates are higher among African Americans than whites. Most sarcomas arise in a sporadic fashion, without identifiable etiology. Sarcomas do not appear to develop from pre-existing benign lesions. Associated factors can be identified in certain subsets of sarcomas, including predisposing genetic mutations, previous ionizing radiation or chemical exposures, and chronic soft tissue injury or lymphedema.

The Li-Fraumeni syndrome is an autosomal dominant familial cancer predisposition syndrome in which the risk of breast and other invasive cancers, including sarcomas, by age 35 years is almost 50% (88). A germline mutation in the *p53* tumor suppressor gene is identifiable in most of the affected families (91). The *p53* gene is central in modulating a cell's response to DNA damage by arresting the cell cycle and inducing apoptosis (81). Somatic mutations of *p53* are among the most common genetic alterations seen in mesenchymal tumors, occurring in nearly 60% of sarcomas (26). The activity of *p53* can also be disrupted by amplification of the *MDM2* gene, located at chromosome 12q13-q14 and coding for a nuclear phosphoprotein that inactivates wild type *p53*. *MDM2* amplification has been demonstrated in 10% to 30% of sarcomas (43).

Patients with hereditary retinoblastoma inherit a germline mutation in the *RB* gene, and a "second hit" in the remaining allele results in malignancy. The RB protein regulates the cell cycle, governing the entrance into the DNA synthesis (S) phase of the cell cycle. In addition to malignant retinoblastomas of the eye, these patients are at increased risk of developing osteosarcomas and soft tissue sarcomas later in life, particularly after exposure to therapeutic radiation (145). Genetic disruption of the RB pathway is observed in over 50% of sarcomas (22).

Patients with neurofibromatosis type 1 (NF1, von Recklinghausen's neurofibromatosis) develop multiple neurofibromas and are at increased risk for gliomas and malignant peripheral nerve sheath tumors (MPNSTs) (155). As in heritable retinoblastoma, a germline mutation in *NF1*, followed by somatic mutation of the remaining allele, results in malignant degeneration (59).

Ionizing radiation exposure produces a small but detectable risk of both bone and soft tissue sarcoma. Radiation-induced sarcomas were first reported in the 1920s among workers painting radium watch dials (48). Sarcomas arising after therapeutic irradiation, reported since the 1930s (16), develop after a latency period (between 2 and 25 years) within the radiation portal and are histologically distinct from the primary malignancy (17). In one review, 3.3% of 1,089 sarcoma patients met these criteria (94). The median latency period was 14 years, and risk was increased after high radiation doses. In a large Finnish cohort study, the absolute risk of postirradiation sarcoma with long-term follow-up was 0.03% (140). The most commonly observed radiation-induced sarcomas arise after radiation therapy for breast cancer. These aggressive malignancies often involve a large portion of the breast (Fig. 81.2). Among 194,798 women diagnosed with localized or regional invasive breast cancer between 1973 and 1995, the relative risks of angiosarcoma and other sarcoma subtypes were 15.9 and 2.2 for irradiated patients compared with unirradiated patients (66). Despite high relative risks, the absolute risk of developing radiation-induced sarcomas is small, 0.28% and 0.48% at 15 years after in two large series (78,116). Angiosarcoma is also observed in patients with chronic lymphedema (Stewart-Treves syndrome), which may or may not be associated with radiation therapy (73).

Epidemiologic studies of industrial chemical exposures and sarcoma risk are limited by the small numbers of individuals exposed to a variety of different agents. Studies have suggested links between vinyl chloride and hepatic angiosarcoma (36), as well as phenoxy herbicides, particularly those contaminated with chlorinated dioxins, and soft tissue sarcomas (38). Studies of United States veterans exposed to Agent Orange, a dioxin-containing herbicide used extensively during the Vietnam War, have shown no evidence of increased sarcoma risk (133).

Natural History

Extremity soft tissue sarcomas spread directly by local extension along the longitudinal axis of muscular compartments. Fascial planes and bone are rarely violated and constitute barriers

Table 81.1	OCCURRENCE OF SOFT TISSUE SARCOMAS BY SITE, BASED ON AMERICAN COLLEGE OF SURGEONS PATTERNS OF CARE SUMMARY					
No. of Patients	Head and Neck (%)	Trunk (%)	Upper Extremity (%)	Lower Extremity (%)	Retroperitoneum (%)	Mediastinum (%)
4,550	8.9	17.9	13.1	46.4	12.5	1.3

From Lawrence W, Donegan WL, Natarajan N, et al. Adult soft tissue sarcomas. *Ann Surg* 1987;205:349–359, with permission.

to local spread. Grossly, lesions appear encapsulated; however, this is a pseudocapsule, representing compressed normal tissue and reactive fibrosis (37). Subclinical disease can infiltrate adjacent tissues, extending 5 to 10 cm beyond the pseudocapsule, "skipping" areas that appear uninvolved. Biopsy procedures can potentially change the pattern of spread if they violate an uninvolved compartment or if an extensive hematoma results (4). In the trunk or head and neck regions, the disease more commonly invades adjacent structures.

High-grade sarcomas have the potential to metastasize. Because lymph nodes are involved in <10% of sarcoma cases, routine lymph node sampling is usually not performed. Clear cell sarcoma, epithelioid sarcoma, angiosarcoma, rhabdomyosarcoma, and synovial cell sarcoma have higher rates of nodal spread (44), and sampling should be considered for these histologies. Hematogenous metastases occur frequently in patients with high-grade sarcomas; most occur in the lungs (111), with less frequent metastasis to other soft tissue sites, bone, liver or skin (139). The median time to metastasis is approximately 1 year (107). However, metastasis >5 years after initial diagnosis is not uncommon (87).

Clinical Presentation

Soft tissue sarcoma classically presents as a growing, painless mass. Several-month delays in presentation to a physician, establishment of a sarcoma diagnosis, and referral to a sarcoma center are not uncommon (21). Numbness, pain, or edema may be caused by tumor-induced neurovascular compromise. Deep tumors may attain an enormous size before coming to clinical attention. Metastases are noted at the time of diagnosis in <10% of patients (118).

Clinical Evaluation

The history should detail family history and previous radiation exposure. The physical examination must detail the size, location, and depth (superficial or deep) of the mass, as well as its proximity to joints. Evidence of neurovascular compromise and fixation to bone should be sought because the ability to perform a limb-sparing procedure in a patient with these findings is greatly decreased. A careful lymph node examination should always be performed.

Obtaining diagnostic imaging before an attempt to obtain tissue diagnosis may be advantageous because it provides images devoid of biopsy-related changes, and may provide guidance for appropriate biopsy technique. Plain radiographs and ultrasound of the affected area are underused, and often provide valuable information including the presence of a solid versus cystic mass, calcification, or bony invasion. Magnetic resonance imaging (MRI) is increasingly preferred as an imaging modality for soft tissue masses and provides excellent soft tissue detail (Fig. 81.3). Computed tomography (CT) supplements MRI and is particularly helpful in identifying bony invasion or destruction. Although certain soft tissue neoplasms may have

characteristic radiographic features, no imaging modality has sufficient specificity to specifically distinguish benign from malignant masses (27). Because the lungs are the predominant site of distant metastasis for soft tissue sarcomas, chest imaging by posterior and lateral chest x-ray or CT is appropriate at initial evaluation and subsequent surveillance for distant metastases, particularly for patients with high-grade disease.

The clinical role of positron emission tomography (PET) in the evaluation of soft tissue sarcomas is an active area of investigation. Uptake of [F-18]-fluorodeoxy-D-glucose (FDG) is somewhat variable in soft tissue neoplasms, but is generally increased in malignant compared with benign, and in high-grade compared with low-grade neoplasms (12). FDG-PET activity may have prognostic significance and may have promise for predicting treatment response (121,123).

A biopsy should be performed on any soft tissue mass that persists or grows, with the exception of subcutaneous lesions that have remained unchanged for years. Ideally, biopsy of a soft tissue mass should be performed by an experienced surgeon. Consideration should be given to biopsy technique and selection of biopsy site, given that all potentially contaminated tissue may need to be removed in a subsequent definitive resection and included in radiation therapy target volumes. Excisional biopsies should be avoided in all but the smallest superficial lesions. Fine-needle aspiration is used by experienced groups for the diagnosis of soft tissue tumors (6), but does not allow for the examination of tissue architecture and is not preferred for diagnosis by most pathologists. Fine-needle aspiration may be most useful to diagnose recurrence or metastasis in patients with an established histologic diagnosis (135). Sufficient tissue for diagnosis is more easily obtained by incisional biopsy or core needle (TruCut) biopsy. The incision for biopsy should be oriented along the longitudinal axis of the extremity such that it can be encompassed in a subsequent resection. Core needle biopsy is minimally invasive as well as easier and cheaper to perform. Although less volume of tissue is obtained by core needle biopsy, it has become standard practice and has been proven to be accurate for diagnosis in the majority of cases (62).

Staging

The American Joint Committee on Cancer staging system (2002 edition) emphasizes grade (G) as the most important prognostic factor for soft tissue sarcoma (Table 81.2) (54). A three- or four-tier system of histologic grading may be used. The prognostic importance of tumor size and depth of invasion is incorporated in the primary tumor (T) stage. The presence of either nodal (N) or distant (M) metastases constitutes stage IV disease. The primary anatomic site of disease is not considered. Comparisons with alternate staging systems developed by investigators at Memorial Sloan-Kettering Cancer Center (MSKCC) and other institutions confirm that tumor depth, grade, and size are the most predictive of systemic relapse (147). However, most systems provide little prognostic information relevant to local recurrence.

Clinical Radiation Oncology

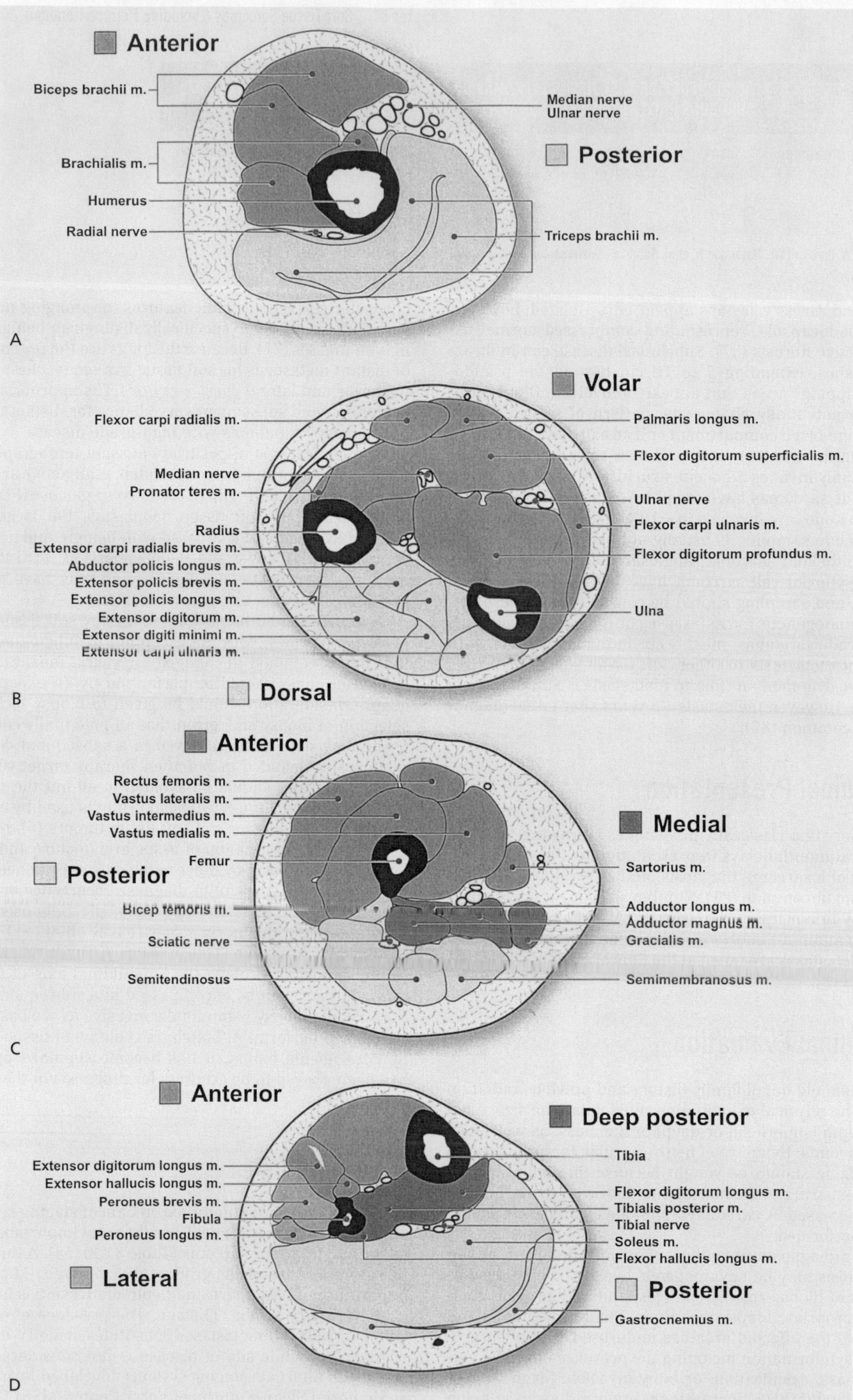

FIGURE 81.1. Cross-sectional diagram of the midarm showing the contents of the anterior and posterior compartments **(A)**; midforearm showing the contents of the volar and dorsal compartments **(B)**; midthigh showing the contents of the anterior, medial, and posterior compartments **(C)**; and midleg showing the contents of the anterior, lateral, posterior, and deep posterior compartments **(D)**. (Redrawn from Anderson MW, Temple HT, Dussault RG, et al. Compartmental anatomy: Relevance to staging and biopsy of musculoskeletal tumors. *AJR Am J Roentgenol* 1999;173:1663–1671, with permission.)

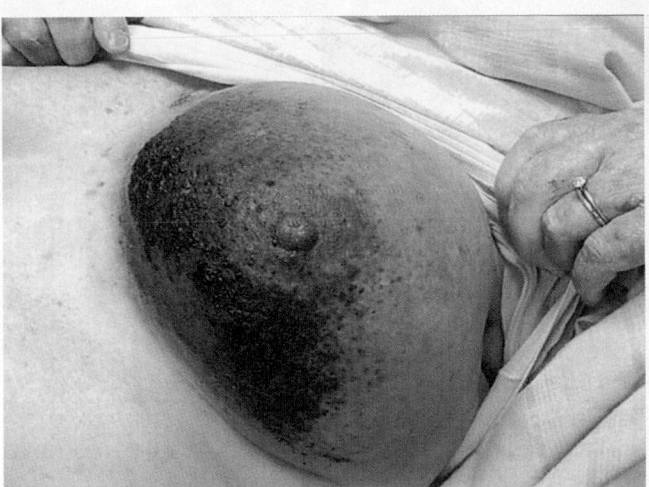

FIGURE 81.2. Angiosarcoma of the breast 3 years after lumpectomy and adjuvant radiation therapy for stage I breast cancer.

Pathologic Classification

Soft tissue sarcomas are classified according to their presumed tissue of origin, using histologic designations such as liposarcoma (adipose tissue), leiomyosarcoma (smooth muscle), or angiosarcoma (vascular tissue) (41). Tumors without identifiable histogenesis are designated according to morphologic appearance or the presumed "line of differentiation" of the tumor cells. Changes in histologic classification have occurred over time. For example, the category of malignant fibrous histiocytoma (MFH) was established in the 1970s, but subsequently became the most common histologic diagnosis for adult soft tissue sarcomas, coinciding with a reduction in the number of cases classified as pleomorphic rhabdomyosarcoma (Table 81.3). The MFH classification is controversial because neither the tissue of origin nor the line of differentiation is clear. In a review, a specific line of differentiation could be identified in the majority of MFH specimens when reanalyzed histologically, immunohisto-

chemically, or ultrastructurally (40), suggesting that the MFH designation is overused.

Pathologic grading is subjective, but the significance of grade as a predictor of metastasis has been demonstrated repeatedly (41). No grading system is uniformly accepted, but most assign tumors to one of three or four categories. The grading system developed by the French Federation Nationale des Centres de Lutte Contre le Cancer assigns a tumor to grade 1 through 3 based on differentiation, mitotic rate, and degree of necrosis (24). The National Cancer Institute system uses histologic type, cellularity, nuclear pleomorphism, frequency of mitoses, and degree of necrosis. There was 34.6% discordance in grading between the two systems in a study of 410 nonmetastatic soft tissue sarcoma cases (58). Although both systems were prognostic, the French Federation Nationale des Centres de Lutte Contre le Cancer system yielded the best correlation with distant metastasis and overall survival. In our current practice, every attempt is made to assign a given tumor into either a high- or low-grade category in order to facilitate clinical decision-making.

Two immunohistochemical stains that are useful for distinguishing sarcomas from more common carcinomas are vimentin (positive in almost all sarcomas, and negative in most carcinomas) and cytokeratin (positive in almost all carcinomas, and negative in most sarcomas). S100 and HMB-45 are positive in melanoma, but may also be positive in specific soft tissue sarcomas. Sarcoma subclassification can be aided by desmin or myoD1 (positive in myogenic tumors), vascular markers (positive in angiosarcomas), and MIC2 (positive in peripheral neuroectodermal tumors). These stains may confirm a diagnosis already considered on morphologic grounds or may raise the possibility of a diagnosis not previously considered.

Metaphase cytogenetics or polymerase chain reaction-based molecular testing may be useful for the identification of chromosomal rearrangements and gene fusions specific to particular subtypes of soft tissue sarcomas (153), such as the t(12;16)(q13;p11) translocation that creates a fusion between adipocyte differentiation gene *CHOP* and nuclear RNA-binding protein *TLS* (28), t(X;18)(p11.2;q11.2) that results in a fusion between the *SYT* gene and either the *SSX1* or *SSX2* genes in synovial cell sarcoma (20), t(12;22)(q13;q12) (*ATF1-EWS*) in clear cell sarcoma (42), t(11;22)(p13;q12) (*WT1-EWS*) in desmoplastic small round cell tumor (50), t(9;22)(q22;q12) (*CHN-EWS*) in

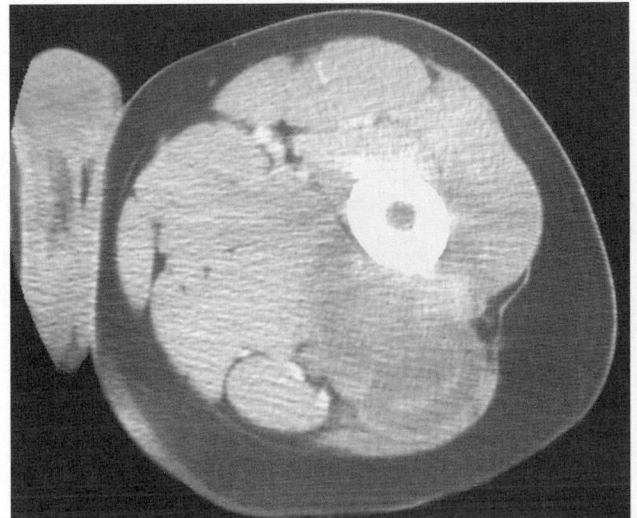

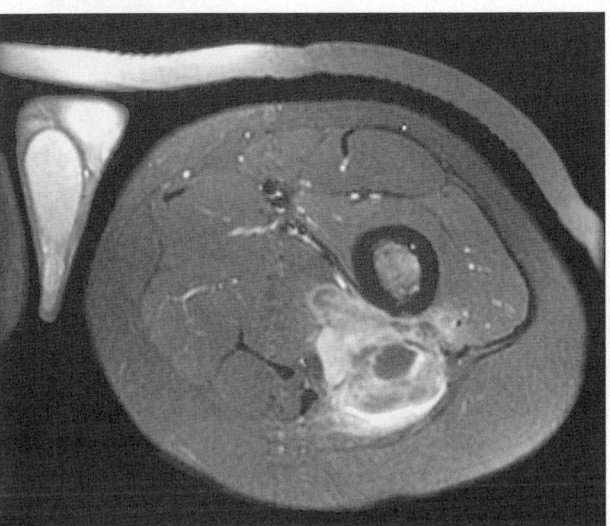

FIGURE 81.3. Radiographic evaluation of a large high-grade soft tissue sarcoma involving the posterior compartment of the left thigh. **A:** Computed tomography scan in the axial plane. **B:** T1-weighted magnetic resonance image (with fat saturation) after contrast enhancement in the same axial plane reveals hypervascular characteristics with multiple areas of necrosis as well as hemorrhage, and also allows greater definition of the tumor margin, which may involve the vastus lateralis, adductor magnus, and gluteus maximus, as well as the hamstring muscles.

Table 81.2 TNM STAGING FOR SOFT TISSUE SARCOMAS

Primary tumor (T)

TX	Primary tumor cannot be assessed
T0	No evidence of primary tumor
T1	Tumor ≤5 cm in greatest diameter
T1a	Superficial tumor
T1b	Deep tumor
T2	Tumor >5 cm in greatest diameter
T2a	Superficial tumor
T2b	Deep tumor

Nodal involvement (N)

NX	Regional nodes cannot be assessed
N0	No regional lymph node metastasis
N1	Regional lymph node metastasis

Distant metastasis (M)

MX	Presence of distant metastasis cannot be assessed
M0	No distant metastasis
M1	Distant metastasis

Histologic grade (G)

GX	Grade cannot be assessed
G1	Well differentiated
G2	Moderately differentiated
G3	Poorly differentiated
G4	Poorly differentiated or undifferentiated (four-tiered systems only)

Stage Grouping				Four-Tier System	Three-Tier System	
I	T1a, 1b, 2a, 2b	N0	M0	G1–G2	G1	Low
II	T1a, 1b, T2b	N0	M0	G3–G4	G2–G3	High
III	T2b	N0	M0	G3–G4	G2–G3	High
IV	Any T	N1	M0	Any G	Any G	High or low
	Any T	N0	M1	Any G	Any G	High or low

Adapted from Greene FL, Page DL, Fleming ID, et al. *AJCC cancer staging manual,* 6th ed. New York: Springer-Verlag; 2002.

Table 81.3 FREQUENCY OF HISTOLOGIC SUBTYPES OF SOFT TISSUE SARCOMA

Histologic Type	American College of Surgeons Patterns of Care Summary		French Federation Sarcoma Group
	1977–1978 (N = 2,355) (%)	1983–1984 (N = 3,457) (%)	1980–1994 (N = 1240) (%)
Malignant fibrous histiocytoma	14.9	25.9	28.2
Liposarcoma	23.2	17.7	15.2
Leiomyosarcoma	13.8	14.8	11.9
Fibrosarcoma	11.1	6.6	
Sarcoma, not otherwise specified	5.4	5.4	11.3
Malignant schwannoma/MPNST	3.2	4.0	5.8
Rhabdomyosarcoma	7.1	3.6	4.8
Synovial sarcoma	3.7	3.6	10.1
Angiosarcoma	2.0	2.9	
Extraskeletal chondrosarcoma	1.2	1.2	
Malignant mesenchymoma	1.4	1.0	
Extraskeletal osteosarcoma	0.4	0.6	
Alveolar soft part sarcoma	0.4	0.6	
Other	14.1	12.8	12.7

MPNST, malignant peripheral nerve sheath tumor.

Data adapted from Lawrence W, Donegan WL, Natarajan N, et al. Adult soft tissue sarcomas. *Ann Surg* 1987;205:349–359; and Coindre J-M, Terrier P, Guillou L, et al. Predictive value of grade for metastasis development in the main histologic types of adult soft tissue sarcomas. *Cancer* 2001;91:1914–1926.

extraskeletal myxoid chondrosarcoma (64), t(17;22)(q22;q13) (*COL1A1-PDGFB*) in dermatofibrosarcoma protuberans (105), or t(X;17)(p11;q25) (*ASPL-TFE3*) in alveolar soft parts sarcoma (70). Chromosomal and molecular analyses such as gene expression profiling can subclassify sarcomas based on molecular biology, providing insight into tumor biology and identifying potential therapeutic targets (60). Molecular classification may supplement or even supplant traditional histologic classification in the future.

Prognostic Factors

The most important prognostic factor for distant metastasis and survival is grade (24,107,152). For low-grade tumors, the risk of distant metastases at 5 years is <10%, compared with almost 50% for high-grade tumors. Tumor size and depth are also prognostic with respect to distant metastasis. Certain histologic subtypes such as MPNST or leiomyosarcoma may be associated with increased distant metastasis and worse survival (24,107). Nomograms predicting disease-specific survival after resection of localized soft tissue sarcoma have been developed (74,93).

Risk factors for local recurrence are distinct from those for distant metastasis and survival. Multiple prospective and retrospective studies have demonstrated that the presence of tumor cells at the surgical margin and inadequate surgical excision are the most important adverse risk factors for local recurrence (23,56,107,115,119,130,134,143,152). Age >50 years, locally recurrent disease, MPNST or fibrosarcoma histology, the presence of symptoms at presentation, deep location, and withholding of radiation therapy have also been associated with increased local recurrence risk.

No conclusive link has been demonstrated between local control and survival in soft tissue sarcoma. Randomized trials have not detected a survival difference between patient groups with disparate local control (108,112,149). However, Gronchi et al. (56) found that the 10-year rates of distant metastasis and cause-specific mortality were higher for patients with positive margins, compared with patients with negative margins. Although these differences were not large, several studies have suggested this trend (23,35,63,134,142,152). Interestingly, Gronchi et al. reported a cause-specific mortality hazard ratio of 0.7 (*p* = .032) in favor of patients receiving adjunctive radiation therapy. Whether local recurrence seeds distant metastasis to impact survival, or it is simply a reflection of biologically aggressive disease, remains controversial.

A variety of molecular pathologic factors have been evaluated for prognostic significance. Proliferative activity as assessed by Ki-67 (MIB-1) immunohistochemistry has been shown to be prognostic (61). Increased expression of *p53* and *MDM2* has been associated with a poor prognosis in some studies (148), but not others (61). In synovial sarcomas, the presence of the fusion gene *SYT-SSX2* was shown to associate with higher metastasis-free survival than *SYT-SSX1* (75). Despite these preliminary data, routine application of molecular prognostic biomarkers awaits prospective validation in larger patient cohorts. These molecular markers may be most useful for selecting high-risk patients for future trials of adjuvant chemotherapy.

General Management

The majority of soft tissue sarcoma patients require multimodality treatment. Treatment is optimally delivered by a multidisciplinary team of dedicated surgical, orthopaedic, medical and radiation oncologists, plastic and reconstructive surgeons, pathologists, and radiologists with specific interest and expertise in mesenchymal malignancies (51). Given the rarity of soft tissue sarcomas, it is understandable that treatment results are optimized at specialized sarcoma centers.

Surgery

Surgical resection is the primary and only potentially curative treatment for soft tissue sarcomas. The primary goals of sarcoma surgery are to achieve optimal oncologic resection while preserving maximal function with minimal morbidity. Surgical specimens, including all surgical margins, should be thoroughly assessed by expert pathologists. For an optimal oncologic resection, negative surgical margins should be obtained if at all feasible, and often may require re-resection. If these goals cannot be anticipated with primary surgery, strong consideration should be given to preoperative treatment with chemotherapy and/or radiation therapy.

Four categories of surgical procedures have been described, based on the surgical plane of dissection (37). An *intralesional procedure* results in partial tumor removal with violation of the pseudocapsule. Although appropriate for a planned incisional diagnostic biopsy, it is not an appropriate therapeutic procedure. A *marginal procedure* (simple excision or "shellout") removes the tumor within the confines of the pseudocapsule with a high likelihood of local recurrence due to residual subclinical disease (156). In *wide local excision*, the tumor is removed with a margin of normal tissue from within the same muscle compartment without removal of the entire structure of origin. *Radical excisions*, including compartmental resections and most amputations, remove the entire tumor and the structure of origin (entire anatomic compartment) *en bloc*. Local recurrence rates after surgery alone range from <10% after radical excision to ≥80% after marginal excision.

Historically, radical resections were performed to maximize local control, but also severely compromised limb function (143). Subsequently, more conservative, limb-sparing surgical procedures have become standard. Surgery alone may be sufficient for selected, small soft tissue sarcomas excised with wide (>1 cm) margins (49,72). However, conservative surgery with adjunctive radiation therapy is required in the majority of cases and results in local control comparable to amputation (89,111,127,144) with superior functional and cosmetic results (114,126). Amputations are now applied to <5% of patients at major sarcoma centers, and are reserved for massive disease in which functional limb-preservation is not feasible. Amputation may also be used for salvage of patients with local recurrence after previous conservative resection and radiation therapy, although limb salvage may still be possible in these cases (18).

Multidisciplinary communication regarding surgical technique can influence the effectiveness of postoperative radiation therapy as well as the incidence of late complications. Surgical scars and drain sites, which are at risk for subclinical disease, should be positioned and oriented such that their inclusion in the radiation treatment portal avoids circumferential (or near-circumferential) limb irradiation. Surgical clip placement at the boundaries of the tumor bed facilitates radiation treatment planning (131). Prophylactic bone stabilization in anticipation of circumferential bone irradiation may reduce risk of subsequent fracture.

Chemotherapy

The efficacy of chemotherapy for soft tissue sarcoma is difficult to assess because of the heterogeneity of patients and drugs studied and the small sizes of individual trials. There remains no uniform consensus regarding the value of chemotherapy in patients with soft tissue sarcoma. Anthracyclines (doxorubicin and epirubicin) achieve response rates of 15% to 25% in patients with metastatic disease (98). Single-agent ifosfamide achieves similar response rates at conventional doses, and may be more active at higher doses (84). Combination chemotherapy regimens may be more active than single-agent regimens, although with increased toxicity (120). Regimens combining ifosfamide with an anthracycline appear to result in higher response rates than those without ifosfamide (146).

Early randomized trials of adjuvant chemotherapy in patients with localized disease showed no significant benefit for treatment (5); however, a meta-analysis found that patients receiving adjuvant doxorubicin had significantly improved local and distant recurrence-free survival (1). A 4% absolute benefit in overall survival at 10 years was not statistically significant, although for patients with extremity sarcomas, an absolute overall survival benefit of 7% at 10 years was statistically significant. Criticisms have centered on the inclusion of patients with visceral soft tissue sarcoma and the lack of central pathology review in this analysis (138). A recent randomized Italian trial randomized 104 patients with ≥5 cm or locally recurrent high-grade extremity sarcomas to five cycles of adjuvant epirubicin and ifosfamide or observation (47). With an updated median follow-up of 90 months, the 5-year survival for the chemotherapy group was 66% compared with 46% for the control group ($p = .04$) (46). A retrospective analysis of 245 patients with resected high-grade liposarcomas of the extremity treated with or without adjuvant chemotherapy suggested improved disease-specific survival with ifosfamide-based chemotherapy but not doxorubicin-based chemotherapy (34). In 215 patients with resected synovial cell sarcoma, distant metastasis-free survival was improved in patients receiving adjuvant chemotherapy (39). However, when 674 patients treated with neoadjuvant or adjuvant doxorubicin-containing chemotherapy at the MSKCC and the M.D. Anderson Cancer Center were combined for a retrospective analysis, the benefit of chemotherapy in improved disease-free survival was only sustained for 1 year after treatment (25), emphasizing the importance of sufficient follow-up in clinical studies of adjuvant chemotherapy for soft tissue sarcomas.

Chemotherapy given in the neoadjuvant setting allows investigators to judge clinical and pathologic response to treatment, and may provide a basis for identifying patients for whom additional chemotherapy may provide a benefit (106). A retrospective study of patients treated with surgery alone versus those receiving neoadjuvant doxorubicin and ifosfamide before surgery showed improved disease-specific survival for those receiving neoadjuvant chemotherapy, with the benefit mainly seen in patients with tumors >10 cm (55). However, a prospective randomized phase II trial of surgery alone versus neoadjuvant doxorubicin and ifosfamide followed by surgery failed to demonstrate a survival benefit (53). For many institutions, including our own, clinical trials of neoadjuvant and adjuvant chemotherapy in selected patients with high-grade extremity sarcomas are ongoing.

The next generation of systemic treatment strategies for soft tissue sarcoma may arise from current translational research that has identified specific molecular targets for therapy. The development and use of the imatinib mesylate (STI 571) in patients with gastrointestinal stromal tumor provides proof of principle for this type of approach (69). Molecular agents designed to modulate various receptor tyrosine kinases and their downstream signaling pathways governing growth and differentiation, survival and apoptosis, normal and aberrant transcription, invasion and metastasis, and angiogenesis are all being investigated in soft tissue sarcoma (14).

Radiation Therapy

Radiation therapy plays a central role in the treatment of soft tissue sarcoma. Although historically considered to be "radioresistant," sarcomas have similar radiosensitivity to epithelial neoplasms (117). Multimodality treatment combining conservative

surgery and radiation therapy achieves excellent local control rates while minimizing morbidity and maximizing long-term extremity function in comparison to radical surgery. Radiation therapy may be delivered using external beam, brachytherapy, or intraoperative electron beam techniques, and advancing technologies such as intensity-modulated radiation therapy (IMRT) and proton or other charged particle radiation therapy are also being applied to sarcomas (31,108,149).

Adjunctive radiation therapy may be effectively and safely delivered either before or after surgery. Postoperative radiation therapy allows for examination of resected specimen, including assessment of the surgical margins, to aid in treatment planning. Preoperative radiation therapy may allow for smaller radiation treatment volumes and may reduce the risk of local and distant dissemination at the time of resection. A phase III Canadian trial randomized 190 patients to preoperative (50 Gy preoperative radiation therapy with 16 to 20 Gy postoperative boost for positive margins) versus postoperative radiation therapy (50 Gy to large field and 16 to 20 Gy cone down boost) with a primary end point of acute wound complications (102). At a median follow-up of 3.3 years, there was a 35% incidence of wound complications in patients treated with preoperative radiation therapy, compared with 17% of patients treated with postoperative radiation therapy ($p = .001$). Interestingly, increased wound complications were only observed for lower extremity tumors. Updated results with a median follow-up of 6.9 years reveal that local and distant control rates as well as survival are equivalent between the two arms; however, a higher rate of late complications including fibrosis was observed with postoperative radiation therapy (29,103).

Preoperative radiation therapy (44 Gy in split-course) interdigitated with MAID chemotherapy (mesna, doxorubicin, ifosfamide, and dacarbazine) was developed as a strategy to enhance local control and limb preservation (30). Of the 66 patients treated with this regimen as part of a Radiation Therapy Oncology Group trial, 83% experienced grade 4 toxicities and there were three treatment-related deaths (79). Only 22% of patients had partial responses; however, 91% of patients were able to have complete tumor resection, and 27% of resected tumors showed no residual viable tumor. Regional delivery of intraarterial doxorubicin with concurrent preoperative radiation therapy has been shown to result in excellent local control rates, but was also associated with a substantial incidence of wound complications (90,141).

Although many sarcoma centers use preoperative radiation as standard treatment, at our own institution we use mainly postoperative radiation therapy because of concerns about acute wound complications and the fact that many patients are treated on clinical trials of neoadjuvant chemotherapy. If attempted resection will clearly result in gross residual disease and limb-sparing treatment is still desired, preoperative radiation therapy should be considered in an attempt to avoid amputation. The current National Comprehensive Cancer Network practice guidelines include each radiation treatment strategy (preoperative external beam, brachytherapy, and postoperative external beam) because all are effective at achieving excellent local control rates, and there are no data to suggest that one approach has greater efficacy (33). The optimal sequencing for surgery, radiation therapy, and chemotherapy remains unknown.

Retrospective series of highly selected soft tissue sarcoma patients treated with wide local excision with generous margins alone have reported high local control rates (3,7). Interestingly, size and depth were not associated with local relapse in these series. The subset of patients that may be adequately treated with radiation therapy alone has not been well defined; however, for lesions that have been properly excised with wide negative margins (all margins >1 cm), it is reasonable to consider observation, particularly if local recurrence in the tumor bed could be re-excised with preservation of function. These criteria are met in fewer than 10% of patients. Current strategies place less emphasis on grade because data from randomized trials of adjuvant brachytherapy (108) and external-beam irradiation (149) show similar incidence of local recurrence for both low- and high-grade tumors. Adjuvant radiation therapy appears to improve local control for both low- and high-grade tumors.

Radiation therapy can also be delivered with radical intent for patients who refuse surgery or have unresectable sarcomas (124,132). However, the local failure rate remains unacceptably high. Several alternative approaches have been investigated for these patients, including preoperative radiation therapy with concurrent chemotherapy (discussed earlier), preoperative radiation therapy with concurrent hyperthermia (113), the use of iododeoxyuridine or other radiosensitizers (125), high linear energy transfer radiation (fast neutrons) (122), and isolated limb perfusion with tumor necrosis factor-α, melphalan, and interferon-γ (86). If these strategies or others could improve local control rates in patients with unresectable disease, consideration could then be given to limb-sparing procedures in the 5% to 10% of patients with extremity sarcomas who otherwise would still require amputation to achieve clear proximal margins.

:: | Radiation Therapy Techniques

Radiation therapy techniques for treatment of sarcomas of the extremity, trunk, and head and neck are described here; retroperitoneal sarcomas are discussed in Chapter 73.

Compartmental Nature of Soft Tissue Sarcomas

Before commencing a course of radiation therapy, the radiation oncologist must evaluate the extent of tumor involvement in the muscle compartment, understand the anatomy of the compartment, and be able to assess the risk of extracompartmental involvement based on MRI and CT imaging. For patients treated in the postoperative setting, attendance in the operating room at the time of resection and surgical clip placement is invaluable in this regard.

Volume at Risk

The radiation target volume is determined based on physical examination, radiologic studies, and knowledge of anatomy and the natural history of sarcomas. Normal structures and organs

in proximity to the targeted region must be identified, and appropriate dose constraints for each must be considered. In the postoperative setting, details from the surgeon regarding the extent of dissection or observations from the resection itself must be considered. Some authorities recommend treating the entire compartment (origin to insertion) because hematoma can theoretically track cells to the farthest reaches of a muscle compartment (150). Others recommend margins around the tumor or tumor bed ranging from less than 5 cm up to 15 cm (in the long axis of the extremity), based on the grade and size of the tumor (128). One retrospective analysis of patients treated with postoperative radiation therapy demonstrated that an initial margin of <5 cm was associated with a significantly higher rate of local failure, compared with ≥5 cm (99). Our general practice is to include the resection bed with a 5-cm margin, the incision, and any drain sites in the initial treatment volume. However, the MSKCC brachytherapy experience calls this into question because excellent local control is achieved with a technique that does not cover the surgical scar, the drain sites, or the wide margins discussed previously (108). Clearly, margins should not extend beyond natural barriers of spread (i.e., fascial planes, bone). Regional lymph nodes are rarely at risk in extremity sarcomas, and there are no convincing data that prophylactic lymph node irradiation is beneficial.

Positioning the Extremity

The extremity should be positioned so as to treat the region of the affected compartment with minimal treatment of uninvolved tissue. The anterior compartment of the thigh can be treated in the "frog-leg" position, with external hip rotation, separating the anterior compartment from the medial and posterior compartments. A lateral decubitus position, with the affected thigh closest to the couch with flexion of the uninvolved extremity, allows treatment of the posterior compartment (Fig. 81.4A). The anterior compartment of the arm (biceps) can be treated by having the shoulder abducted approximately 90 degrees and maximally internally rotated (Fig. 81.4B). Positioning of extremities can be difficult for patients because of effects of tumor or surgery. If the extremity is placed at too extreme an angle, CT scanning may be more difficult. It is often necessary to assess multiple limb positions to discover the optimal setup. The body part must be immobilized with a device such as a foam cradle, plaster mold, or thermoplastic cast (Fig. 81.4), with the limb secured above and below the treatment area to reduce the possibility of rotation in the cradle. Cradle material can be removed from the region to be treated, if it will not compromise the immobilization, to reduce skin toxicity due to bolus effect.

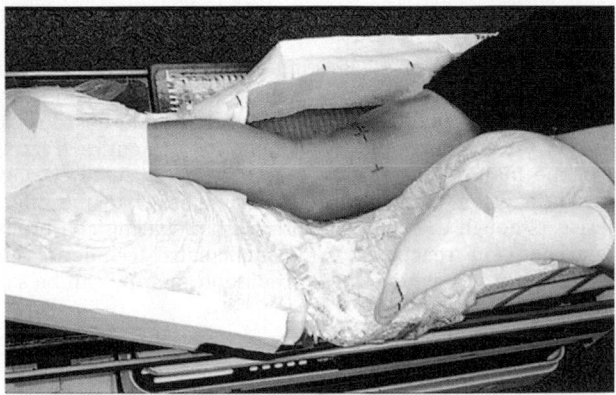
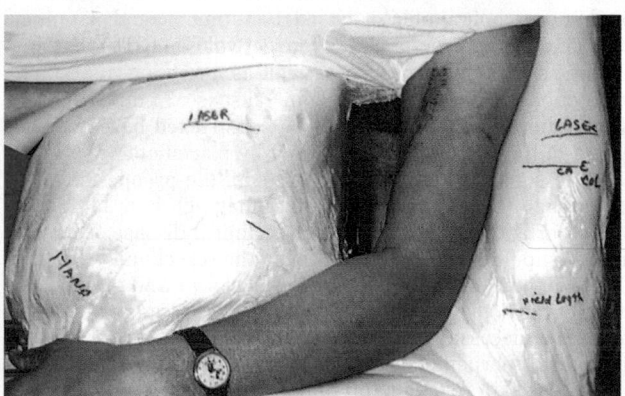

FIGURE 81.4. A: A custom-made foam cast immobilization with the patient in a lateral decubitus position demonstrates positioning that is frequently used for patients with posterior thigh or leg sarcoma. **B:** A custom-made foam cast immobilization with the patient's shoulder abducted approximately 90 degrees and maximally internally rotated (with the elbow flexed) is frequently used for patients with biceps sarcoma.

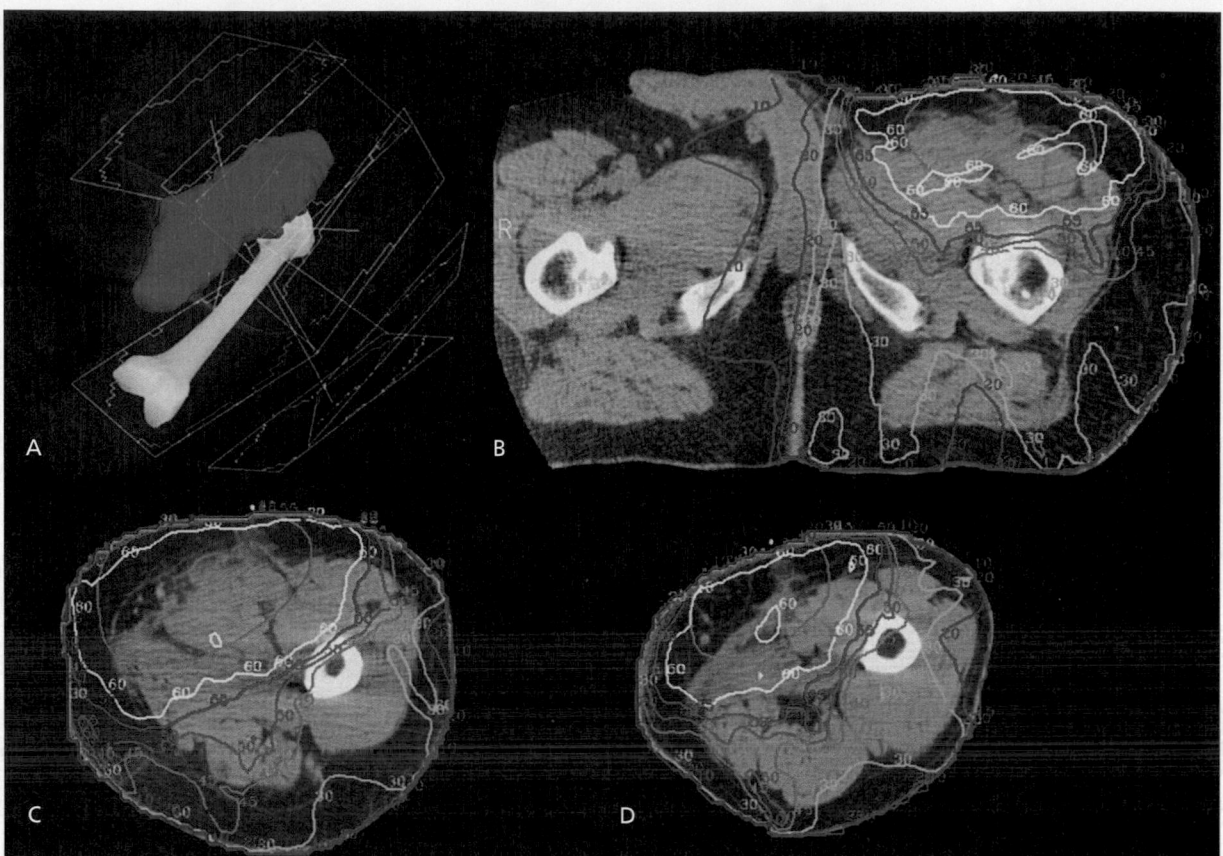

FIGURE 81.5. A large target volume extended from the left inguinal region inferiorly and medially along the thigh in a patient after resection of a high-grade soft tissue sarcoma of the sartorius muscle. **A:** Six gantry angles were selected for intensity-modulated radiation therapy treatment planning to achieve the desired target coverage while limiting dose to uninvolved bone and soft tissue. The isodose distributions of the intensity-modulated radiation therapy plan are shown from superior (**B**) and more inferior axial slices of the planning scan (**C** and **D**).

Treatment Planning

It is common practice to use a "shrinking-field technique" for treatment of sarcomas. For postoperative radiation therapy, the initial treatment fields are designed to encompass the resection bed with generous margins. Subsequently, reduced fields encompassing the preoperative tumor volume can be boosted with smaller margins. For preoperative radiation therapy, the gross tumor itself with a margin is treated. Usually, no field reduction is made prior to surgery, but a postoperative boost can be delivered in case of a positive margin.

For either CT-based, three-dimensional planning, or conventional fluoroscopic simulator-based, two-dimensional planning, it is useful to construct a clinical target volume (CTV) that encompasses any gross disease as well as a volume to account for potential subclinical (microscopic) disease. In the postoperative setting, the initial CTV can be constructed based on the volume of the resection bed (defined by placement of surgical clips and consultation with the surgeon), the preoperative tumor volume (based on preoperative imaging), and additional volume for extension of potential subclinical disease. This initial CTV should be generous, covering the resection bed with a 3- to 6-cm margin, as well as the surgical scar and drain sites. If the scar is being struck tangentially by the irradiation fields, no bolus is necessary. However, if the scar is being irradiated with a direct perpendicular field, bolus should be applied to ensure a brisk skin reaction and full dose over the scar itself. The "boost" CTV usually is limited to the preoperative tumor volume only with smaller 2- to 3-cm margins. In preoperative cases, the CTV can be derived by expansion of the visible gross tumor volume, again with generous 3- to 6-cm margins. The planning target volume should be an expansion of the CTV accounting for potential variation in daily setup, easily 1 cm or more for extremity targets.

A ≥1 cm strip of soft tissue in the circumference of the extremity should be spared to avoid subsequent edema. Attempts should be made to avoid circumferential bone radiation, if possible, to reduce fracture risk, and to minimize joint irradiation, if possible. Three-dimensional conformal radiation therapy and IMRT treatment planning may be useful in achieving the desired dose distribution in selected extremity cases (Fig. 81.5). Although these techniques are useful to spare normal tissues and bone to reduce morbidity (65), extra caution must be used with steep dose gradients to ensure adequate dose coverage of target volumes.

Treatment of thin regions of anatomy (e.g., hand, foot, and forearm) presents additional technical concerns. Skin-sparing by high-energy photon beams can produce underdosed regions inside the tumor volume, and bolus to the entire treatment volume may be necessary. Treatment of the involved region inside a water bath ensures uniform dosage to the affected area, although the complete loss of skin-sparing can produce marked skin reactions. With meticulous technique, limb-sparing surgery with adjuvant radiation therapy can be safely applied (95,129).

Radiation Energy and Dose

Lower energy (6-MV) photons are usually used because higher energies could potentially spare too much superficial tissue. However, higher energy (10- to 16-MV) photons are occasionally required for thigh or buttock lesions to produce reasonable dose homogeneity. Sarcomas are usually treated to high doses, even in the adjuvant setting. In postoperative therapy, the initial volume is usually treated to 45 to 50 Gy, with subsequent cone downs to a final dose of 60 to 66 Gy, using 1.8- or 2.0-Gy daily fractions. For preoperative irradiation, 45 to 50 Gy is often delivered 2 to 4 weeks before resection with an intraoperative or postoperative boost as indicated by the surgical margin. Brachytherapy or intraoperative radiation therapy may be used in combination with either preoperative or postoperative external-beam radiation therapy. Doses of 12 to 25 Gy may be given by intraoperative electron beam, or perioperative low dose rate (LDR) or high dose rate (HDR) afterloading brachytherapy, with 36 to 50 Gy external beam (2,19,32,80). Brachytherapy may be used as the sole radiation therapy mode of treatment, using doses of 42 to 50 Gy. For unresectable sarcomas, doses above 70 Gy are used, limiting the high-dose volume to the tumor plus a minimal margin.

Truncal and Head and Neck Sarcomas

Tumors arising in the trunk are usually more superficial than extremity sarcomas, but have similar clinical behavior (57). Tumors on the chest wall and abdominal wall often can be treated with oblique tangential fields. After 45 Gy of photon irradiation, a direct electron boost to the surgical bed can be use to minimize dose to underlying lung or bowel.

In the head and neck, target volumes and sensitive normal tissues are often in close proximity, and toxicity is a significant concern. Treatment planning techniques with three-dimensional conformal radiation therapy and IMRT are particularly useful in these locations. Treatment planning must account for the different patterns of spread that distinguish sarcomas from squamous cell carcinomas in the head and neck region, including the substantially lower risk of nodal spread for sarcomas. Several techniques for entire scalp irradiation have been described, and may be used for the treatment of angiosarcomas, which are infiltrative and prone to local recurrence after surgery alone (77,96,136).

Interstitial Brachytherapy

Interstitial brachytherapy can be used to deliver all or part of the radiation dose (8). After surgical excision of the tumor, hollow plastic afterloading catheters are inserted using sharp metal trocars in a single plane at approximately 1-cm intervals within the tumor bed (Fig. 81.6). Surgical clips placed at the margin of the tumor bed permit the target volume to be delineated for planning purposes, and the catheters are secured in place. Orthogonal localization films are obtained 2 to 4 days after surgery, and catheter positions may be digitally recorded into a radiation therapy planning system. In contrast to the wide margins typically employed for external-beam irradiation, the MSKCC experience demonstrates that a brachytherapy CTV encompassing only the clipped tumor bed with a 2-cm margin resulted in adequate local control (108). The dose is prescribed to 5 to 10 mm from the implant plane. Catheters are loaded with wired LDR ^{192}Ir seeds or connected for HDR treatments no sooner than the sixth postoperative day to reduce the risk of wound complications. After completion of the treatment, sources are removed and catheters are cut at one end for removal by pulling through the skin.

For LDR implants, a dose of 42 to 45 Gy has been shown to be adequate adjuvant treatment when used alone for high-grade lesions (108). If brachytherapy is to be used in combination with external-beam radiation therapy, a dose of 15 to 25 Gy is used with 45 to 50 Gy external beam (2,32). HDR implants allow for more customization of the treatment plan because the dwell times of the single HDR source at each position can be

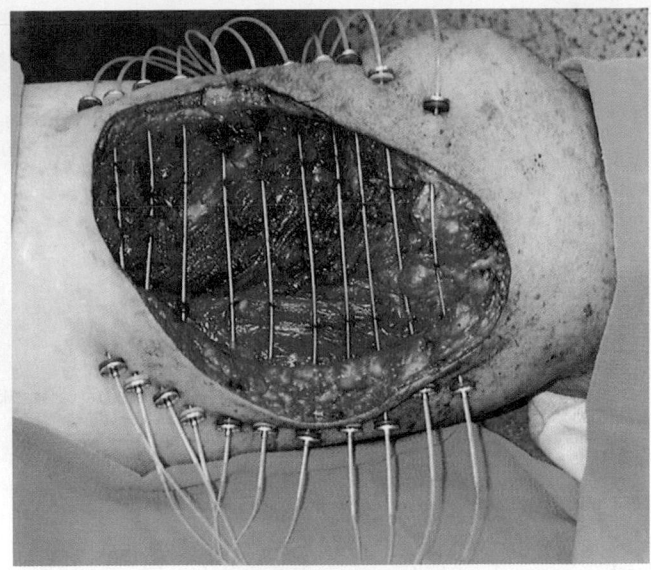

FIGURE 81.6. Demonstration of brachytherapy catheter placement after resection of soft tissue sarcoma involving the medial and distal thigh, which had recurred after resection alone.

manipulated. HDR treatments are usually given twice daily at 2 to 5 Gy per fraction to 35 to 50 Gy when used alone, or 15 to 20 Gy when to be used with postoperative external beam (19). HDR treatments can be delivered using conventional interstitial catheters as already described; a technique for intraoperative HDR treatment has also been described (80). A detailed list of recommendations for brachytherapy has recently been published by the American Brachytherapy Society (100).

Results of Standard Treatment

Retrospective reports and a prospective randomized trial have demonstrated conclusively that limb-sparing surgery plus adjunctive radiation therapy produces local control and survival rates similar to those achieved with amputation (89,112,115,127,151). The value of adjuvant radiation therapy after limb-sparing surgery has been demonstrated in randomized trials (108,149). Local control rates for patients with intermediate and high-grade sarcomas treated with surgical resection and adjunctive radiation therapy are generally in the 80% to 90% range, and representative series are presented in Table 81.4. The brachytherapy literature is limited in comparison to the extensive literature supporting the local control benefits of external-beam radiation therapy. Nonetheless, investigators from MSKCC and a limited number of other institutions have demonstrated that brachytherapy achieves comparable local control benefits for intermediate and high-grade disease when used alone or in combination with external irradiation (2,32,108). That these different techniques produce similar and excellent local control further validates the basic concept that radical treatment can be achieved with limb preservation. Even for patients with large high-grade lesions, a local control rate of approximately 85% can be achieved with the use of limb-sparing, wide local excision, and meticulous radiation therapy techniques.

Local control rates for low-grade lesions are also excellent with either postoperative or preoperative external-beam irradiation. In a series of patients treated at the National Cancer Institute, adjuvant external-beam irradiation significantly decreased local recurrence rates, primarily in patients with positive margins (92). Importantly, a randomized trial from MSKCC revealed

Table 81.4	LOCAL CONTROL AFTER RADIATION THERAPY FOR INTERMEDIATE- AND HIGH-GRADE SARCOMAS, SELECTED SERIES			
Institution/Study	No. of Patients	Median Follow-Up (ys)	Local Control at 5 Years[a] (%)	Radiation Therapy[b]
MGH (127)	132	9.0	94	Preoperative
M.D. Anderson (151)	271	6.4	85	Preoperative
NCI Canada (103)	94	6.9	93	Preoperative
MSKCC (108)	56	6.3	89	Brachytherapy
NCI Canada (103)	96	6.9	92	Postoperative
M.D. Anderson (151)	246	9.1	75	Postoperative
NCI (149)	47	9.6	100	Postoperative

MGH, Massachusetts General Hospital; NCI Canada, National Cancer Institute of Canada; MSKCC, Memorial Sloan-Kettering Cancer Center; NCI, National Cancer Institute of the National Institutes of Health, United States.
[a]Percentage of all patients.
[b]In all series, doxorubicin-based chemotherapy was used in selected patients as well.

that brachytherapy does not improve local control compared with surgery alone in low-grade lesions (109). Therefore, external beam is preferred over brachytherapy for treatment of low-grade soft tissue sarcoma. Unlike the high- and intermediate-grade lesions, low-grade tumors have almost no metastatic potential. Therefore, local control is tantamount to cure in this group.

Despite the increased technical demands, similar local control rates with limb-sparing procedures have been described for sarcomas of the distal extremities. Local recurrences can be salvaged with additional surgery (amputation) with no apparent decrement in survival (15,95,129). Although the head and neck represents another technically challenging site because of the difficulty obtaining negative margins, local control rates have been reported in the 75% to 90% range when radiation therapy is combined with wide local excision (11,85, 104).

Overall survival for patients with soft tissue sarcoma closely relates to the development of distant metastases. This is related to the current American Joint Committee on Cancer stage, as can be seen in Fig. 81.7.

Unresectable Sarcomas

In patients who are not eligible for surgical resection, radiation therapy alone can be considered but results in relatively low rates of durable local control. In one series, local control was related to radiation dose and tumor size (76). Neutron radiation, carbon ion beam or photon radiation in combination with radiosensitizing iododeoxyuridine, or isolated limb perfusion with tumor necrosis factor-α, melphalan, and interferon-γ have also been used (52,71,122,124,125,132). Although the optimal treatment of sarcomas clearly involves complete excision, high-dose irradiation may at least achieve palliative benefits.

Treatment of Metastatic Disease

For patients with metastatic disease and controlled primary tumors, complete surgical resection of pulmonary metastases may be potentially curative and can result in disease-free survival rates of 40% at 3 years (13,137). The role of radiation therapy in treatment of metastatic disease is mainly limited to palliation of sites of disease causing local symptoms, although the possibility of using extracranial stereotactic radiation techniques for patients with solitary or oligometastasic disease in unresectable locations may be an area for future investigation.

Aggressive Fibromatosis and Dermatofibrosarcoma Protuberans

Aggressive fibromatosis (desmoid tumor) and dermatofibrosarcoma protuberans (DFSP) are soft tissue neoplasms that almost never metastasize but can be very invasive locally. Desmoids arise within the muscle or its fascial coverings, and DFSPs arise within the dermis. Microscopically, bundles of spindle-shaped fibroblasts are surrounded by abundant fibrous stoma devoid of mitotic figures. Complete surgical excision alone is usually curative for these tumors, but is not always possible because of their size and location. Local recurrence is common. For desmoid tumors, postoperative radiation therapy improved local control for patients with positive margins or gross residual disease (10,97,101,154). It should be noted that some authorities prefer to observe surgically resected patients with microscopically positive margins if the disease site can be readily followed and a local recurrence could be re-excised with minimal morbidity. Primary radiation therapy achieves high rates of local control when surgery is not feasible. Little evidence exists for a dose–response relation, and doses of 50 to 55 Gy are used for either subclinical or gross disease. Tumor responses are rarely seen in <6 months, but can occur after 1 to 2 years. Nonsteroidal antiinflammatory agents, hormonal agents, cytotoxic chemotherapy, and imatinib have activity against desmoid tumors (67). For

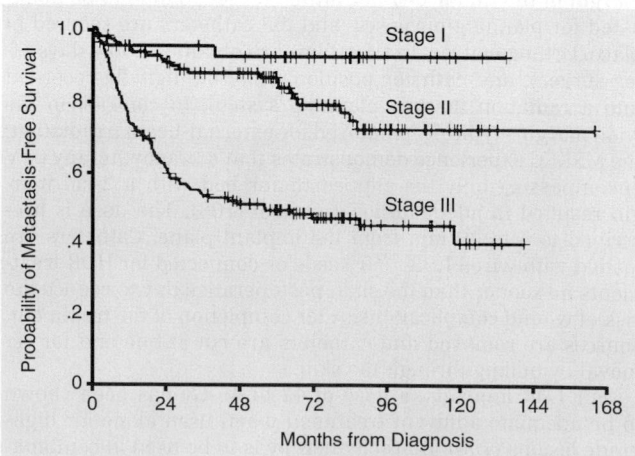

FIGURE 81.7. Metastasis-free survival in a cohort of 300 patients treated between 1982 and 1989, based on the 5th edition of the American Joint Committee on Cancer staging system. (From Wunder JS, Healey JH, Davis AM, et al. A comparison of staging systems for localized extremity soft tissue sarcoma. *Cancer* 2000;88:2721–2730, with permission.)

DFSP, radiation therapy enhances local control in patients with positive margins after surgery, or as sole treatment (9).

Sequelae of Treatment

The most significant short-term toxicity of radiation therapy for sarcomas is usually moist desquamation in the high-dose volume. This can be very uncomfortable in patients with proximal thigh tumors who receive significant dose to the perineum. Patients treated for truncal and head and neck sarcomas experience toxicity similar to breast cancer and head and neck squamous cell carcinoma patients. Major wound complications (delayed wound healing or need for surgical intervention) occur in approximately 5% to 15% of patients after surgical resection with postoperative irradiation, and perhaps more commonly with preoperative irradiation.

The long-term sequelae after conservative surgery and irradiation for extremity lesions must always be considered because they may significantly limit the function of the preserved limb. They include decrease in range of motion related to fibrosis, contracture of the joint, edema, pain, and bone fracture. In centers treating high volumes of patients with soft tissue sarcoma, the incidence of moderate-to-severe late effects is <10% (110). The risk of these complications may be reduced by sparing a strip of normal tissue (to allow lymphatic drainage from the extremity) and a portion of the circumference of uninvolved bone. If possible, joint spaces should be excluded after a dose of 40 to 45 Gy to avoid fibrotic constriction of joint capsules. Collaboration with physical therapy specialists is essential in minimizing disabilities after treatment of soft tissue sarcomas. Mobility of the extremity should be stressed, and patients should be on an exercise and range-of-motion program early in the course of therapy. In the treatment of patients with truncal sarcomas, it is particularly important to use cone down fields to limit the dose to normal tissues deep to the target volume (e.g., lung and bowel). In contrast to acute wound complications, late limb morbidity may be reduced with preoperative radiation, likely due to the lower doses and smaller volumes used with preoperative treatment (29). With attention to these details, a high local control rate can be achieved with minimum sequelae.

High-dose irradiation does not appear to compromise the viability of skin grafts used to repair defects after sarcoma surgery if adequate time is allotted for healing (at least 3 weeks) (83). Fertility can be preserved in men undergoing irradiation for lower extremity sarcomas through the use of a gonadal shield to decrease testicular dose (45). The risk of a second malignancy associated with adjuvant irradiation must also be considered, particularly in young patients with low-grade tumors in which an otherwise normal life expectancy is anticipated.

Future Directions

The most significant challenge in the management of soft tissue sarcomas is to reduce the mortality related to systemic disease in patients who present with M0 disease. Further investigation into the benefits of conventional cytotoxic chemotherapy, as well as new molecularly targeted agents, will ultimately determine whether mortality rates can be reduced. Molecular characterization of individual patients and tumors will improve patient selection in future trials. Many clinical trials in soft tissue sarcoma currently use neoadjuvant chemotherapy. Earlier systemic treatment may have a greater capacity to influence occult micrometastases, and allows the assessment of *in vivo* response. Unfortunately, given the rarity of the disease and the small size of many trials, statistical power will continue to be limited in power to resolve the current controversies regarding

the value of chemotherapy. Ultimately, these questions must be addressed in multi-institutional cooperative group studies.

The local treatment of soft tissue sarcomas is markedly different today than it was 25 years ago. Most patients with extremity lesions are now treated with limb-preserving methods, achieving local control rates of $\geq 90\%$. Although we prefer wide local excision followed by postoperative irradiation for resectable extremity tumors, excellent results can be obtained with preoperative irradiation or brachytherapy. Wide local excision and meticulous shrinking-field radiation therapy given either before or after surgery have improved the local control rates for patients with truncal and head and neck sarcomas almost to that of extremity lesions. Because wide local excision alone would lead to approximately a 50% local failure rate, radiation therapy appears to permit organ preservation without a significant sacrifice in control rates.

Several issues remain important with respect to local control. Although it has become less common, some patients with advanced extremity sarcomas still require amputation to achieve clear proximal margins, or have unresectable tumors. Continued innovations in the use of combined-modality therapy or radiosensitizers may lead to further improvements in this area. The Radiation Therapy Oncology Group is building on its previous study of preoperative chemotherapy and radiation therapy with another phase II trial investigating interdigitated MAID with combined thalidomide and radiation therapy for high-grade disease, and combined thalidomide and radiation therapy for low-grade disease (see http://www.clinicaltrials. gov/ct/show/NCT00089544). The issues of acute and late treatment morbidity also remain active areas of investigation. The results of the Canadian trial comparing preoperative and postoperative irradiation have further emphasized the relation between field size and radiation dose to toxicity. The necessity of large 5- to 7-cm margins compared with the more conservative 2- to 3-cm margins successfully used in brachytherapy may be an area for randomized study. Currently, Canadian investigators are running a prospective trial investigating the potential benefit of IMRT in reducing wound complications (see http://www.clinicaltrials.gov/ct/show/NCT00188175). Finally, it will be important to develop methods to prospectively identify those patients who may be managed adequately with wide local excision alone. Although adjuvant irradiation can often be delivered without significant acute or late toxicity, selective elimination of its use without loss of local control would represent an additional success in the management of these patients.

References

1. Adjuvant chemotherapy for localised resectable soft-tissue sarcoma of adults: Meta-analysis of individual data. Sarcoma Meta-analysis Collaboration. *Lancet* 1997;350:1647–1654.
2. Alekhteyar KM, Leung DH, Brennan MF, et al. The effect of combined external beam radiotherapy and brachytherapy on local control and wound complications in patients with high-grade soft tissue sarcomas of the extremity with positive microscopic margin. *Int J Radiat Oncol Biol Phys* 1996;36:321–324.
3. Alektiar KM, Leung D, Zelefsky MJ, et al. Adjuvant radiation for stage II-B soft tissue sarcoma of the extremity. *J Clin Oncol* 2002;20:1643–1650.
4. Anderson MW, Temple HT, Dussault RG, et al. Compartmental anatomy: Relevance to staging and biopsy of musculoskeletal tumors. *AJR* 1999;173:1663–1671.
5. Antman KH. Adjuvant therapy of sarcomas of soft tissue. *Semin Oncol* 1997;24:556–560.
6. Ayala AG, Ro JY, Fanning CV, et al. Core needle biopsy and fine-needle aspiration in the diagnosis of bone and soft-tissue lesions. *Hematol Oncol Clin North Am* 1995;9:633–651.
7. Baldini EH, Goldberg J, Jenner C, et al. Long-term outcomes after function-sparing surgery without radiotherapy for soft tissue sarcoma of the extremities and trunk. *J Clin Oncol* 1999;17:3252–3259.
8. Ballo MT, Lee AK. Current results of brachytherapy for soft tissue sarcoma. *Curr Opin Oncol* 2003;15:313–318.
9. Ballo MT, Zagars GK, Pisters P, et al. The role of radiation therapy in the management of dermatofibrosarcoma protuberans. *Int J Radiat Oncol Biol Phys* 1998;40:823–827.
10. Ballo MT, Zagars GK, Pollack A, et al. Desmoid tumor: Prognostic factors and outcome after surgery, radiation therapy, or combined surgery and radiation therapy. *J Clin Oncol* 1999;17:158–167.

11. Barker JL Jr, Paulino AC, Feeney S, et al. Locoregional treatment for adult soft tissue sarcomas of the head and neck: An institutional review. *Cancer J* 2003;9:49–57.
12. Bastiaannet E, Groen H, Jager PL, et al. The value of FDG-PET in the detection, grading and response to therapy of soft tissue and bone sarcomas; a systematic review and meta-analysis. *Cancer Treat Rev* 2004;30:83–101.
13. Billingsley KG, Burt ME, Jara E, et al. Pulmonary metastases from soft tissue sarcoma: Analysis of patterns of diseases and postmetastasis survival. *Ann Surg* 1999;229:602–610.
14. Borden EC, Baker LH, Bell RS, et al. Soft tissue sarcomas of adults: State of the translational science. *Clin Cancer Res* 2003;9:1941–1956.
15. Brien EW, Terek RM, Geer RJ, et al. Treatment of soft-tissue sarcomas of the hand. *J Bone Joint Surg Am* 1995;77:564–571.
16. Cade S. Radiation induced cancer in man. *Br J Radiol* 1957;30:393–402.
17. Cahan WG, Woodward HQ, Higinbothan NL, et al. Sarcoma arising in irradiated bone: Report of 11 cases. *Cancer* 1948;1:3–29.
18. Catton C, Davis A, Bell R, et al. Soft tissue sarcoma of the extremity. Limb salvage after failure of combined conservative therapy. *Radiother Oncol* 1996;41:209–214.
19. Chun M, Kang S, Kim BS, et al. High dose rate interstitial brachytherapy in soft tissue sarcoma: Technical aspects and results. *Jpn J Clin Oncol* 2001;31:279–283.
20. Clark J, Rocques PJ, Crew AJ, et al. Identification of novel genes, SYT and SSX, involved in the t(X;18)(p11.2;q11.2) translocation found in human synovial sarcoma. *Nature Genet* 1994;7:502–508.
21. Clark MA, Thomas JM. Delay in referral to a specialist soft-tissue sarcoma unit. *Eur J Surg Oncol* 2005;31:443–448.
22. Cohen JA, Geradts J. Loss of RB and MTS1/CDKN2 (p16) expression in human sarcomas. *Hum Pathol* 1997;28:893–898.
23. Coindre JM, Terrier P, Bui NB, et al. Prognostic factors in adult patients with locally controlled soft tissue sarcoma. A study of 546 patients from the French Federation of Cancer Centers Sarcoma Group. *J Clin Oncol* 1996;14:869–877.
24. Coindre JM, Terrier P, Guillou L, et al. Predictive value of grade for metastasis development in the main histologic types of adult soft tissue sarcomas: A study of 1240 patients from the French Federation of Cancer Centers Sarcoma Group. *Cancer* 2001;91:1914–1926.
25. Cormier JN, Huang X, Xing Y, et al. Cohort analysis of patients with localized, high-risk, extremity soft tissue sarcoma treated at two cancer centers: Chemotherapy-associated outcomes. *J Clin Oncol* 2004;22:4567–4574.
26. Creager AJ, Cohen JA, Geradts J. Aberrant expression of cell-cycle regulatory proteins in human mesenchymal neoplasia. *Cancer Detect Prev* 2001;25:123–131.
27. Crim JR, Seeger LL, Yao L, et al. Diagnosis of soft-tissue masses with MR imaging: Can benign masses be differentiated from malignant ones? *Radiology* 1992;185:581–586.
28. Crozat A, Aman P, Mandahi N, et al. Fusion of CHOP to a novel RNA-binding protein in human myxoid liposarcoma. *Nature* 1993;363:640–644.
29. Davis AM, O'Sullivan B, Turcotte R, et al. Late radiation morbidity following randomization to preoperative versus postoperative radiotherapy in extremity soft tissue sarcoma. *Radiother Oncol* 2005;75:48–53.
30. DeLaney TF, Spiro IJ, Suit HD, et al. Neoadjuvant chemotherapy and radiotherapy for large extremity soft-tissue sarcomas. *Int J Radiat Oncol Biol Phys* 2003;56:1117–1127.
31. DeLaney TF, Trofimov AV, Engelsman M, et al. Advanced-technology radiation therapy in the management of bone and soft tissue sarcomas. *Cancer Control* 2005;12:27–35.
32. Delannes M, Thomas L, Martel P, et al. Low-dose-rate intraoperative brachytherapy combined with external beam irradiation in the conservative treatment of soft tissue sarcoma. *Intl J Radiat Oncol Biol Phys* 2000;47:165–169.
33. Demetri GD, Baker LH, Beech D, et al. Soft tissue sarcoma: Clinical practice guidelines in oncology. *J Natl Compr Canc Netw* 2005;3:158–194.
34. Eilber FC, Eilber FR, Eckardt J, et al. The impact of chemotherapy on the survival of patients with high-grade primary extremity liposarcoma. *Ann Surg* 2004;240:686–695.
35. Eilber FC, Rosen G, Nelson SD, et al. High-grade extremity soft tissue sarcomas: Factors predictive of local recurrence and its effect on morbidity and mortality. *Ann Surg* 2003;237:218–226.
36. Elliott P, Kleinschmidt I. Angiosarcoma of the liver in Great Britain in proximity to vinyl chloride sites. *Occup Environ Med* 1997;54:14–18.
37. Enneking WF, Spanier SS, Malawer MM. The effect of the anatomic setting on the results of surgical procedures for soft parts sarcoma of the thigh. *Cancer* 1981;47:1005–1022.
38. Eriksson M, Hardell L, Adami H-O. Exposure to dioxins as a risk factor for soft tissue sarcoma: A population-based case-control study. *J Natl Cancer Inst* 1990;82:486–490.
39. Ferrari A, Gronchi A, Casanova M, et al. Synovial sarcoma: A retrospective analysis of 271 patients of all ages treated at a single institution. *Cancer* 2004;101:627–634.
40. Fletcher CD, Gustafson P, Rydholm A, et al. Clinicopathologic re-evaluation of 100 malignant fibrous histiocytomas: Prognostic relevance of subclassification. *J Clin Oncol* 2001;19:3045–3050.
41. Fletcher CDM, Unni KK, Mertens F, eds. *Pathology and genetics of tumours of soft tissue and bone* Lyon, France: IARC Press; 2002
42. Fletcher JA. Translocation (12;22)(q13-14;q12) is a nonrandom aberration in soft-tissue clear-cell sarcoma. *Genes Chromosom Cancer* 1992;5:184.
43. Florenes VA, Maelandsmo GM, Forus A, et al. MDM2 gene amplification and transcript levels in human sarcomas: Relationship to TP53 gene status. *J Natl Cancer Inst* 1994;86:1297–1302.
44. Fong Y, Goit DG, Wooodruff JM, et al. Lymph node metastasis from soft tissue sarcoma in adults. *Ann Surg* 1993;217:72–77.
45. Fraass BA, Kinsella TJ, Harrington FS, et al. Peripheral dose to the testes: The design and clinical use of a practical and effective gonadal shield. *Int J Radiat Oncol Biol Phys* 1985;11:609–615.
46. Frustaci S, De Paoli A, Bidoli E, et al. Ifosfamide in the adjuvant therapy of soft tissue sarcomas. *Oncology* 2003;65[Suppl 2]:80–84.
47. Frustaci S, Gherlinzoni F, De Paoli A, et al. Adjuvant chemotherapy for adult soft tissue sarcomas of the extremities and girdles: Results of the Italian randomized cooperative trial. *J Clin Oncol* 2001;19:1238–1247.
48. Fry SA. Studies of U.S. radium dial workers: An epidemiological classic. *Radiat Res* 1998;150(S5):21–29.
49. Geer RJ, Woodruff J, Casper ES, et al. Management of small soft-tissue sarcoma of the extremity in adults. *Arch Surg* 1992;127:1285–1289.
50. Gerald WL, Rosai J, Ladanyi M. Characterization of the genomic breakpoint and chimeric transcripts in the EWS-WT1 gene fusion of desmoplastic small round cell tumor. *Proc Natl Acad Sci U S A* 1995;92:1028–1032.
51. Glencross J, Balasubramanian SP, Bacon J, et al. An audit of the management of soft tissue sarcoma within a health region in the UK. *Eur J Surg Oncol* 2003;29:670–675.
52. Goffman T, Tochner Z, Glatstein E. Primary treatment of large and massive adult sarcomas with iododeoxyuridine and aggressive hyperfractionated irradiation. *Cancer* 1991;67:572–576.
53. Gortzak E, Azzarelli A, Buesa J, et al. A randomised phase II study on neo-adjuvant chemotherapy for 'high-risk' adult soft-tissue sarcoma. *Eur J Cancer* 2001;37:1096–1103.
54. Greene FL, Page DL, Fleming ID, et al., eds. *AJCC cancer staging manual*, 6th ed. New York: Springer-Verlag; 2002.
55. Grobmyer SR, Maki RG, Demetri GD, et al. Neo-adjuvant chemotherapy for primary high-grade extremity soft tissue sarcoma. *Ann Oncol* 2004;15:1667–1672.
56. Gronchi A, Casali PG, Mariani L, et al. Status of surgical margins and prognosis in adult soft tissue sarcomas of the extremities: A series of patients treated at a single institution. *J Clin Oncol* 2005;23:96–104.
57. Gross JL, Younes RN, Haddad FJ, et al. Soft-tissue sarcomas of the chest wall: Prognostic factors. *Chest* 2005;127:902–908.
58. Guillou L, Coindre JM, Bonichon F, et al. Comparative study of the National Cancer Institute and French Federation of Cancer Centers Sarcoma Group grading systems in a population of 410 adult patients with soft tissue sarcoma. *J Clin Oncol* 1997;15:350–362.
59. Gutmann DH, Collins FS. Recent progress toward understanding the molecular biology of Von Recklinghausen neurofibromatosis. *Ann Neurol* 1992;31:555–561.
60. Helman LJ, Meltzer P. Mechanisms of sarcoma development. *Nature Rev Cancer* 2003;3:685–694.
61. Heslin MJ, Cordon-Cardo C, Lewis JJ, et al. Ki-67 detected by MIB-1 predicts distant metastasis and tumor mortality in primary, high grade extremity soft tissue sarcoma. *Cancer* 1998;83:490–497.
62. Heslin MJ, Lewis JJ, Woodruff JM, et al. Core needle biopsy for diagnosis of extremity soft tissue sarcoma. *Ann Surg Onc* 1997;4:423–431.
63. Heslin MJ, Woodruff J, Brennan MF. Prognostic significance of a positive microscopic margin in high-risk extremity soft tissue sarcoma: Implications for management. *J Clin Oncol* 1996;14:473–478.
64. Hirabayashi Y, Ishida T, Yoshida MA, et al. Translocation (9;22)(q22;q12). A recurrent chromosome abnormality in extraskeletal myxoid chondrosarcoma. *Cancer Genet Cytogenet* 1995;81:33–37.
65. Hong L, Alektiar KM, Hunt M, et al. Intensity-modulated radiotherapy for soft tissue sarcoma of the thigh. *Int J Radiat Oncol Biol Phys* 2004;59:752–759.
66. Huang J, Mackillop WJ. Increased risk of soft tissue sarcoma after radiotherapy in women with breast carcinoma. *Cancer* 2001;92:172–180.
67. Janinis J, Patriki M, Vini L, et al. The pharmacological treatment of aggressive fibromatosis: A systematic review. *Ann Oncol* 2003;14:181–190.
68. Jemal A, Murray T, Ward E, et al. Cancer statistics, 2005. *CA Cancer J Clin* 2005;55:10–30.
69. Joensuu H, Roberts PJ, Sarlomo-Rikala M, et al. Effect of the tyrosine kinase inhibitor STI571 in a patient with a metastatic gastrointestinal stromal tumor. *N Engl J Med* 2001;344:1052–1056.
70. Joyama S, Ueda T, Shimizu K, et al. Chromosome rearrangement at 17q25 and xp11.2 in alveolar soft-part sarcoma: A case report and review of the literature. *Cancer* 1999;86:1246–50.
71. Kamada T, Tsujii H, Tsuji H, et al. Efficacy and safety of carbon ion radiotherapy in bone and soft tissue sarcomas. *J Clin Oncol* 2002;20:4466–4471.
72. Karakousis CP, Emrich LJ, Rao U, et al. Limb salvage in soft tissue sarcomas with selective combination of modalities. *Eur J Surg Oncol* 1991;17:71–80.
73. Karlsson P, Holmberg E, Samuelsson A, et al. Soft tissue sarcoma after treatment for breast cancer: A Sweedish population-based study. *Eur J Cancer* 1998;34:2068–2075.
74. Kattan MW, Leung DH, Brennan MF. Postoperative nomogram for 12-year sarcoma-specific death. *J Clin Oncol* 2002;20:791–796.
75. Kawai A, Woodruff J, Healy JH, et al. SYT-SSX gene fusion as a determinant of morphology and prognosis in synovial sarcoma. *N Engl J Med* 1998;338:153–160.
76. Kepka L, DeLaney TF, Suit HD, et al. Results of radiation therapy for unresected soft-tissue sarcomas. *Int J Radiat Oncol Biol Phys* 2005;63:852–859.
77. Kinard JD, Zwicker RD, Schmidt-Ulrich RK, et al. Short communication: Total craniofacial photon shell technique for radiotherapy of extensive angiosarcomas of the head. *Br J Radiol* 1996;69:351–355.
78. Kirova YM, Vilcoq JR, Asselain B, et al. Radiation-induced sarcomas after radiotherapy for breast carcinoma: A large-scale single-institution review. *Cancer* 2005;104:856–63.
79. Kraybill WG, Harris J, Spiro IJ, et al. Phase II study of neoadjuvant chemotherapy and radiation therapy in the management of high-risk, high-grade, soft tissue sarcomas of the extremities and body wall: Radiation Therapy Oncology Group Trial 9514. *J Clin Oncol* 2006;24:619–625.
80. Kretzler A, Molls M, Gradinger R, et al. Intraoperative radiotherapy of soft tissue sarcoma of the extremity. *Strahlenther Onkol* 2004;180:365–370.
81. Lane DP. Cancer. p53, guardian of the genome. *Nature* 1992;358:15–16.
82. Lawrence W, Donegan WL, Natarajan N, et al. Adult soft tissue sarcomas. *Ann Surg* 1987;205:349–359.
83. Lawrence WT, Zabell A, McDonald HD. The tolerance of skin grafts to postoperative radiation therapy in patients with soft-tissue sarcoma. *Ann Plast Surg* 1986;16:204–210.
84. Le Cesne A, Antoine E, Spielmann M, et al. High-dose ifosfamide: Circumvention of resistance to standard-dose ifosfamide in advanced soft tissue sarcomas. *J Clin Oncol* 1995;13:1600–1608.
85. Le QT, Fu KK, Kroll S, et al. Prognostic factors in adult soft-tissue sarcomas of the head and neck. *Int J Radiat Oncol Biol Phys* 1997;37:975–984.
86. Lejeune FJ, Pujol N, Lienard D, et al. Limb salvage by neoadjuvant isolated perfusion with TNFalpha and melphalan for non-resectable soft tissue sarcoma of the extremities. *Eur J Sur Oncol* 2000;26:669–678.
87. Lewis JJ, Leung D, Casper ES, et al. Multifactorial analysis of long-term follow-up (more than 5 years) of primary extremity sarcoma. *Arch Surgery* 1999;134:190–194.

88. Li FP, Fraumeni JF, Mulvihill JJ, et al. A cancer family syndrome in twenty-four kindreds. *Cancer Res* 1988;48:5358–5362.
89. Lindberg RD, Martin RG, Romsdahl MM, et al. Conservative surgery and postoperative radiotherapy in 300 adults with soft-tissue sarcomas. *Cancer* 1981;47:2391–2397.
90. Mack LA, Crowe PJ, Yang JL, et al. Preoperative chemoradiotherapy (modified Eilber protocol) provides maximum local control and minimal morbidity in patients with soft tissue sarcoma. *Ann Surg Oncol* 2005;12:646–653.
91. Malkin D, Li FP, Strong LC, et al. Germ line p53 mutations in a familial syndrome of breast cancer, sarcomas, and other neoplasms. *Science* 1990;250:1233–1238.
92. Marcus SG, Merino MJ, Glatstein E, et al. Long-term outcome in 87 patients with low-grade soft-tissue sarcoma. *Arch Surg* 1993;128:1336–1343.
93. Mariani L, Miceli R, Kattan MW, et al. Validation and adaptation of a nomogram for predicting the survival of patients with extremity soft tissue sarcoma using a three-grade system. *Cancer* 2005;103:402–408.
94. Mark SJ, Poen J, Tran LM, et al. Postirradiation sarcomas. *Cancer* 1994;73:2653–2662.
95. McPhee M, McGrath BE, Zhang P, et al. Soft tissue sarcoma of the hand. *J Hand Surg* 1999;24:1001–1007.
96. Mellenberg DE, Schoeppel SL. Total scalp treatment of mycosis fungoides: The 4 × 4 technique. *Int J Radiat Oncol Biol Phys* 1993;27:953–958.
97. Micke O, Seegenschmiedt MH. Radiation therapy for aggressive fibromatosis (desmoid tumors): Results of a national Patterns of Care Study. *Int J Radiat Oncol Biol Phys* 2005;61:882–891.
98. Mouridsen HT, Bastholt L, Somers R, et al. Adriamycin versus epirubicin in advanced soft tissue sarcomas. A randomized phase II/phase III study of the EORTC Soft Tissue and Bone Sarcoma Group. *Eur J Cancer Clin Oncol* 1987;23:1477–1483.
99. Mundt AJ, Awan A, Sibley GS, et al. Conservative surgery and adjuvant radiation therapy in the management of adult soft tissue sarcoma of the extremities: Clinical and radiobiological results. *Int J Radiat Oncol Biol Phys* 1995;32:977–985.
100. Nag S, Shasha D, Janjan N, et al. The American Brachytherapy Society recommendations for brachytherapy of soft tissue sarcomas. *Int J Radiat Oncol Biol Phys* 2001;49:1033–1043.
101. Nuyttens JJ, Rust PF, Thomas CR Jr, et al. Surgery versus radiation therapy for patients with aggressive fibromatosis or desmoid tumors: A comparative review of 22 articles. *Cancer* 2000;88:1517–1523.
102. O'Sullivan B, Davis AM, Turcotte R, et al. Preoperative versus postoperative radiotherapy in soft-tissue sarcoma of the limbs: A randomised trial. *Lancet* 2002;359:2235–2241.
103. O'Sullivan B, Davis AM, Turcotte R, et al. Five-year results of a randomized phase III trial of pre-operative vs post-operative radiotherapy in extremity soft tissue sarcoma. *Proc Am Soc Clin Oncol* 2004;815a.
104. O'Sullivan B, Gullane P, Irish J, et al. Preoperative radiotherapy for adult head and neck soft tissue sarcoma: Assessment of wound complication rates and cancer outcome in a prospective series. *World J Surg* 2003;27:875–883.
105. Pedeutour F, Simon MP, Minoletti F, et al. Translocation, t(17;22)(q22;q13), in dermatofibrosarcoma protuberans: A new tumor-associated chromosome rearrangement. *Cytogenet Cell Genet* 1996;72:171–174.
106. Pezzi CM, Pollock RE, Evans HL, et al. Preoperative chemotherapy for soft-tissue sarcomas of the extremities. *Ann Surg* 1990;211:476–81.
107. Pisters PW, Leung DH, Woodruff J, et al. Analysis of prognostic factors in 1,041 patients with localized soft tissue sarcomas of the extremities. *J Clin Oncol* 1996;14:1679–89.
108. Pisters WT, Harrison LB, Leung DHY, et al. Long-term results of a prospective randomized trial of adjuvant brachytherapy in soft tissue sarcoma. *J Clin Oncol* 1996;14:859–868.
109. Pisters WT, Harrison LB, Woodruff JM, et al. A prospective randomized trial of adjuvant brachtherapy in the management of low-grade soft tissue sarcomas of the extremity and superficial trunk. *J Clin Oncol* 1994;12:1150–1155.
110. Pollack A, Zagars GK, Goswitz MS, et al. Preoperative vs. postoperative radiotherapy in the treatment of soft tissue sarcomas: A matter of presentation. *Int J Radiat Oncol Biol Phys* 1998;42:563–572.
111. Potter DA, Glenn J, Kinsella TJ, et al. Patterns of recurrence in patients with high-grade soft-tissue sarcomas. *J Clin Oncol* 1985;3:353–356.
112. Potter DA, Kinsella T, Glatstein E, et al. High-grade soft tissue sarcomas of the extremities. *Cancer* 1986;58:190–205.
113. Prosnitz LR, Maguire P, Anderson JM, et al. The treatment of high-grade soft tissue sarcomas with preoperative thermoradiotherapy. *Int J Radiat Oncol Biol Phys* 1999;45:941–949.
114. Robinson MH, Spruce L, Eeles R, et al. Limb function following conservation treatment of adult soft tissue sarcoma. *Eur J Cancer* 1991;27:1567–1574.
115. Rosenberg SA, Tepper J, Glatstein E, et al. The treatment of soft-tissue sarcomas of the extremities: Prospective randomized evaluations of (1) limb-sparing surgery plus radiation therapy compared with amputation and (2) the role of adjuvant chemotherapy. *Ann Surg* 1982;196:305–315.
116. Rubino C, Shamsaldin A, Le MG, et al. Radiation dose and risk of soft tissue and bone sarcoma after breast cancer treatment. *Breast Cancer Res Treat* 2005;89:277–288.
117. Ruka W, Taghian A, Gioioso D, et al. Comparison between the in vitro intrinsic radiation sensitivity of human soft tissue sarcoma and breast cancer cell lines. *J Surg Oncol* 1996;61:290–294.
118. Rydholm A, Berg NO, Gullberg B, et al. Epidemiology of soft-tissue sarcoma in the locomotor system. A retrospective population-based study of the interrelationships between clinical and morphologic variables. *Acta Pathol Microbiol Immunol Scand* 1984;92:363–374.
119. Sadoski C, Suit HD, Rosenberg A, et al. Preoperative radiation, surgical margins, and local control of extremity sarcomas of soft tissues. *J Surg Oncol* 1993;52:223–230.
120. Santoro A, Tursz T, Mouridsen H, et al. Doxorubicin versus CYVADIC versus doxorubicin plus ifosfamide in first-line treatment of advanced soft tissue sarcomas: A randomized study of the European Organization for Research and Treatment of Cancer Soft Tissue and Bone Sarcoma Group. *J Clin Oncol* 1995;13:1537–1545.
121. Schuetze SM, Rubin BP, Vernon C, et al. Use of positron emission tomography in localized extremity soft tissue sarcoma treated with neoadjuvant chemotherapy. *Cancer* 2005;103:339–348.
122. Schwartz DL, Einck J, Bellon J, et al. Fast neutron radiotherapy for soft tissue and cartilaginous sarcomas at high risk for local recurrence. *Int J Radiat Oncol Biol Phys* 2001;50:449–456.
123. Schwarzbach MH, Hinz U, Dimitrakopoulou-Strauss A, et al. Prognostic significance of preoperative [18-F] fluorodeoxyglucose (FDG) positron emission tomography (PET) imaging in patients with resectable soft tissue sarcomas. *Ann Surg* 2005;241:286–294.
124. Slater JD, McNeese MD, Peters LJ. Radiation therapy for unresectable soft tissue sarcomas. *Int J Radiat Oncol Biol Phys* 1986;12:1729–1734.
125. Sondak VK, Robertson JM, Sussman JJ, et al. Preoperative idoxuridine and radiation for large soft tissue sarcomas: Clinical results with five-year follow-up. *Ann Surg Oncol* 1998;5:106–112.
126. Stinson SF, DeLaney TF, Greenberg J, et al. Acute and long-term effects on limb function of combined modality limb sparing therapy for extremity soft tissue sarcoma. *Int J Radiat Oncol Bio Phys* 1991;21:1492–1499.
127. Suit HD, Mankin HJ, Wood WC, et al. Treatment of the patient with stage M0 soft tissue sarcoma. *J Clin Oncol* 1988;6:854–862.
128. Suit HD, Spiro I. Role of radiation in the management of adult patients with sarcoma of soft tissue. *Semin Surg Oncol* 1994;10:347–356.
129. Talbert ML, Zagars GK, Sherman NE, et al. Conservative surgery and radiation therapy for soft tissue sarcoma of the wrist, hand, ankle, and foot. *Cancer* 1990;66:2482–2491.
130. Tanabe KK, Pollock RE, Ellis LM, et al. Influence of surgical margins on outcome in patients with preoperatively irradiated extremity soft tissue sarcomas. *Cancer* 1994;73:1652–1659.
131. Tepper JE, Rosenberg SA, Glatstein E. Radiation therapy in soft tissue sarcomas of the extremity: Policies of treatment at the National Cancer Institute. *Int J Radiat Oncol Biol Phys* 1982;8:263–273.
132. Tepper JE, Suit HD. Radiation therapy alone for sarcoma of soft tissue. *Cancer* 1985;56:475–479.
133. The association of selected cancers with service in the US military in Vietnam. II. Soft-tissue and other sarcomas. The Selected Cancers Cooperative Study Group. *Arch Intern Med* 1990;150:2485–2492.
134. Trovik CS, Bauer HC, Alvegard TA, et al. Surgical margins, local recurrence and metastasis in soft tissue sarcomas: 559 surgically-treated patients from the Scandinavian Sarcoma Group Register. *Eur J Cancer* 2000;36:710–716.
135. Trovik CS, Bauer HC, Brosjo O, et al. Fine needle aspiration (FNA) cytology in the diagnosis of recurrent soft tissue sarcoma. *Cytopathology* 1998;9:320–328.
136. Tung SS, Shiu AS, Starkschall G, et al. Dosimetric evaluation of total scalp irradiation using a lateral electron-photon technique. *Int J Radiat Oncol Biol Phys* 1993;27:153–160.
137. van Geel AN, Pastorino U, Jauch KW, et al. Surgical treatment of lung metastases: The European Organization for Research and Treatment of Cancer-Soft Tissue and Bone Sarcoma Group study of 255 patients. *Cancer* 1996;77:675–682.
138. Verweij J, Seynaeve C. The reason for confining the use of adjuvant chemotherapy in soft tissue sarcoma to the investigational setting. *Semin Radiat Oncol* 1999;9:352–359.
139. Vezeridis MP, Moore R, Karakousis CP. Metastatic patterns in soft-tissue sarcomas. *Arch Surg* 1983;118:915–918.
140. Virtanen A, Pukkala E, Auvinen A. Incidence of bone and soft tissue sarcoma after radiotherapy: A cohort study of 295,712 Finnish cancer patients. *Int J Cancer* 2006;118:1017–1021.
141. Wanebo HJ, Temple WJ, Popp MB, et al. Preoperative regional therapy for extremity sarcoma. A tricenter update. *Cancer* 1995;75:2299–2306.
142. Weitz J, Antonescu CR, Brennan MF. Localized extremity soft tissue sarcoma: Improved knowledge with unchanged survival over time. *J Clin Oncol* 2003;21:2719–2725.
143. Williard WC, Hajdu SI, Casper ES, et al. Comparison of amputation with limb-sparing operations for adult soft tissue sarcoma of the extremity. *Ann Surg* 1992;215:269–275.
144. Wilson AN, Davis A, Bell RS, et al. Local control of soft tissue sarcoma of the extremity: The experience of a multidisciplinary sarcoma group with definitive surgery and radiotherapy. *Eur J Cancer* 1994;30A:746–751.
145. Wong FL, Boice JD Jr, Abramson DH, et al. Cancer incidence after retinoblastoma. Radiation dose and sarcoma risk. *JAMA* 1997;278:1262–1267.
146. Worden FP, Taylor JM, Biermann JS, et al. Randomized phase II evaluation of 6 g/m2 of ifosfamide plus doxorubicin and granulocyte colony-stimulating factor (G-CSF) compared with 12 g/m2 of ifosfamide plus doxorubicin and G-CSF in the treatment of poor-prognosis soft tissue sarcoma. *J Clin Oncol* 2005;23:105–112.
147. Wunder JS, Healey JH, Davis AM, et al. A comparison of staging systems for localized extremity soft tissue sarcoma. *Cancer* 2000;88:2721–2730.
148. Wurl P, Meye A, Schmidt H, et al. High prognostic significance of Mdm2/p53 co-overexpression in soft tissue sarcomas of the extremities. *Oncogene* 1998;16:1183–1185.
149. Yang JC, Chang AE, Baker AR, et al. Randomized prospective study of the benefit of adjuvant radiation therapy in the treatment of soft tissue sarcomas of the extremity. *J Clin Oncol* 1998;16:197–203.
150. Yang JC, Rosenberg SA, Glatstein EJ, et al. Sarcomas of soft tissues. In: Devita VT, Hellman S, Rosenberg SA, eds. *Cancer: Principles and practice of oncology*, 4th ed. Philadelphia: JB Lippincott; 1993:1436–1488.
151. Zagars GK, Ballo MT, Pisters PW, et al. Preoperative vs. postoperative radiation therapy for soft tissue sarcoma: A retrospective comparative evaluation of disease outcome. *Int J Radiat Oncol Biol Phys* 2003;56:482–488.
152. Zagars GK, Ballo MT, Pisters PW, et al. Prognostic factors for patients with localized soft-tissue sarcoma treated with conservation surgery and radiation therapy: An analysis of 225 patients. *Cancer* 2003;97:2530–2543.
153. Zhang P, Brooks JS. Modern pathological evaluation of soft tissue sarcoma specimens and its potential role in soft tissue sarcoma research. *Curr Treat Options Oncol* 2004;5:441–450.
154. Zlotecki RA, Scarborough MT, Morris CG, et al. External beam radiotherapy for primary and adjuvant management of aggressive fibromatosis. *Int J Radiat Oncol Biol Phys* 2002;54:177–181.
155. Zoller ME, Rembeck B, Oden A, et al. Malignant and benign tumors in patients with neurofibromatosis type 1 in a defined Swedish population. *Cancer* 1997;79:2125–2131.
156. Zornig C, Peiper M, Schroder S. Re-excision of soft tissue sarcoma after inadequate initial operation. *Br J Surg* 1995;82:278–279.

Clinical Radiation Oncology

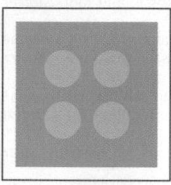

Chapter 82
Central Nervous System Tumors in Children

Carolyn R. Freeman, Jean-Pierre Farmer, Roger E. Taylor

Central nervous system (CNS) tumors account for 20% to 25% of all malignancies that occur in childhood. According to the Central Brain Tumor Registry of the United States, the age adjusted incidence rate in the 0 to 19 year age group for the period 1997 to 2001 is four per 100,000 person-years (36). The increase in comparison with previous periods in North America as well as elsewhere has been attributed partly to changes in tumor classification and coding and partly to increased detection—particularly of low-grade astrocytomas and brainstem gliomas—as a result of the availability of improved neuroimaging modalities over the past two decades (217). The incidence is highest among children 0 to 4 years (4.6 per 100,000 person-years) and lowest among 10- to 19-year-olds (3.7 per 100,000 person-years).

The etiology of pediatric CNS tumors remains largely unknown. Only 3% to 5% can be ascribed to a genetic predisposition (14,101,256,285), included in this category are those developing in patients with neurofibromatosis types 1 and 2, tuberous sclerosis, nevoid basal cell (Gorlin's) syndrome, the adenomatous polyposis syndromes, and Li-Fraumeni syndrome. An even smaller percentage can be attributed to ionizing radiation used for diagnostic or therapeutic purposes. For the majority of patients, no predisposing factors can be identified, although many have been suggested, including viral agents, pre- and postnatal environmental exposures, and birth characteristics, such as weight and head circumference (14,256,285).

The management of children with CNS tumors has changed greatly over the past three decades. Improved imaging, especially MRI, and now functional imaging as well, together with improved techniques for pathologic examination have contributed to a better understanding of the natural history of the different tumor types. Improved neurosurgical techniques and perioperative care permit greater degrees of surgical resection, even for tumors previously considered inoperable because of their location in eloquent areas of the brain. Better understanding of the risks and benefits of adjuvant treatment, namely radiotherapy and chemotherapy, and interdisciplinary collaborations at local, national, and international levels have also resulted in more judicious integration of all treatment modalities. These factors may have contributed to the substantial decrease in mortality observed over this period; currently, the 5-year relative survival rate is estimated at 72% for all CNS tumors occurring in the 0- to 19-year age group (256).

Radiotherapy is an important component of treatment for many children with CNS tumors and recent developments in radiotherapy treatment planning and delivery offer considerable opportunities for therapeutic gain. Indeed, improved targeting and newer technologies and techniques for treatment may be particularly beneficial for children with CNS tumors who have a high probability of long-term survival and are at significant risk for the development of long-term sequelae.

Radiotherapy for Pediatric Central Nervous System Tumors: General Principles

The planning and delivery of radiotherapy for children with CNS tumors is technically challenging, not only for the radiation oncologist but for the entire multiprofessional team, often requiring the expertise of specialist personnel such as pediatric nurses and play therapists. The role of these professionals can be pivotal in encouraging a young child to comply with and to lie still for the making of a head shell or other immobilization device, for complex radiotherapy planning procedures, and for treatment itself. For children younger than age 4 or 5 years, daily anesthesia will almost always be necessary, and this will require a skilled pediatric anesthetist because anesthesia will be administered in a different environment without all of the support normally available in an operating room. The treatment of children with radiotherapy is labor intensive and time consuming, but the extra effort is essential to ensure precision in treatment planning and delivery.

Long-Term Effects of Radiotherapy for Central Nervous System Tumors

The quality of survival of children with brain tumors may be compromised by long-term sequelae. Although some patients (e.g., patients with neurofibromatosis type 1 [NF-1]) may be at particular risk and some sequelae (e.g., neurologic deficits) are more often due to the tumor and/or surgery, it is clear that radiotherapy is directly, alone or modulated by other factors, responsible for many late effects. A review by Kortmann et al. (137) gives an excellent account of radiation-related sequelae in children treated for low-grade glioma, including effects on brain parenchyma, neurological deficits, neurocognitive and behavioral effects, endocrine dysfunction, vasculopathy, and the development of second tumors.

The neurocognitive sequelae of radiotherapy have become much better characterized over recent years. It is now known that myelinization and functional maturation of the CNS continue until well into adolescence and even into young adulthood. Radiotherapy causes white matter changes (178). Patients fail to acquire new knowledge and skills at an age-appropriate rate and show a progressive decline in IQ over time (191). The magnitude of the deficit depends most importantly on age at treatment, but many other host (e.g., NF-1 or not), tumor (e.g., location, hydrocephalus or not), and treatment factors (e.g., radiotherapy volume and dose [95,175,177], use of chemotherapy [218,262]) play a role. Moreover, the development of other deficits, such as behavioral difficulties related to the location of the tumor and/or surgery and hearing impairment due to cisplatin, may have a modulating effect. The end result is impaired school and social performance that deteriorates over time. There is increasing evidence that intervention using cognitive or behavioral therapy or pharmacotherapy may be useful, and that this should start soon after treatment for best results (29,154). Mathematic models have been described that may help identify patients particularly at risk for neurocognitive damage who could be targeted for such intervention (167,168).

Endocrine deficits are very common after radiotherapy (163). Although a substantial proportion of patients may have had deficits prior to radiotherapy (98,172), it is clear that radiotherapy plays a major role, for example, in the development of growth hormone deficiency that correlates with the dose of radiotherapy delivered to the hypothalamic–pituitary axis (1,240,251), and primary hypothyroidism seen after craniospinal radiotherapy with photons. There may be direct and indirect effects on musculoskeletal development. Osteopenia is a rather common finding (98,139) that may put patients with residual neurological deficits at significant risk for fracture.

Radiotherapy can be implicated as well in the development of cardiovascular complications including cerebrovascular events and coronary heart disease (98,118). Although, again, the etiology is likely multifactorial, it is important to be cognizant of the risks and to minimize the dose to vascular structures and the heart.

A number of strategies have been devised in an attempt to minimize the long-term effects of treatment for pediatric brain tumors. These include the following:

- Avoidance of radiotherapy altogether (e.g., in patients with low-grade astrocytoma for whom surgery alone may be a good option),
- Delay to radiotherapy for young children (i.e., those younger than age 3 to 8 years) by the use of chemotherapy,
- Use of focal rather than extended-field radiotherapy when evidence suggests that extended field (whole-brain, craniospinal) radiotherapy does not influence survival (e.g., ependymoma),
- Use of daily anesthesia and of improved immobilization techniques (e.g., rigid casts or a stereotactic frame for small-volume focal radiotherapy for all or part of the treatment) that allow the use of reduced margins around the target volume,
- Use of image-based treatment planning using CT–magnetic resonance imaging (MRI) or CT–MRI–positron emission tomography (PET) coregistration and better treatment-planning techniques that result in greater sparing of normal brain tissue (e.g., three-dimensional conformal radiation therapy [3DCRT] and intensity-modulated radiation therapy [IMRT]),

- Use of new radiation modalities (e.g., proton beams that allow even greater sparing of the surrounding normal brain and organs at risk),
- Reduction of the dose of radiotherapy (e.g., in patients with standard risk medulloblastoma for whom in the North American studies the dose for craniospinal irradiation has been reduced progressively from 35 to 36 Gy to 23.4 Gy and, in current studies, to 18 Gy),
- Use of smaller fraction sizes where appropriate (e.g., a fraction size of 1.5 Gy each day for patients with radiosensitive tumors such as germinoma),
- Use of hyperfractionated radiotherapy (HFRT) (e.g., as in the current European studies for standard risk medulloblastoma).

All of these options will be discussed later in the context of the relevant clinical situation.

Radiation Dose and Dose-Fractionation Regimens

The conventional daily fraction size for the treatment of most pediatric CNS tumors is 1.8 Gy. For the majority of tumors it is necessary to deliver a total dose that is close to normal tissue tolerance. Thus, a typical dose-fractionation regimen is 54 Gy in 30 daily fractions of 1.8 Gy, which carries a very low risk of radionecrosis. When treating a primary tumor of the spinal cord it is conventional to use a lower total dose (e.g., 50.4 Gy). It is also usual to reduce the radiotherapy dose for children younger than age 3 years to reduce the risk of neurocognitive deficits. When treating radiosensitive tumors such as intracranial germinoma, radiotherapy may be delivered using a lower dose per fraction (e.g., 1.5 Gy) and lower total doses of 30 to 50 Gy.

Many pediatric brain tumors exhibit a dose–response relationship for tumor control, and in some cases local progression is not prevented by the use of a CNS tolerance radiation dose. When the target contains only a small volume of normal brain tissue, dose escalation may be feasible. This is more likely to be the case now than in the past because of improvements in treatment planning and delivery. HFRT may be a useful strategy in situations where dose escalation cannot be achieved safely using conventional fractionation.

Follow-Up During and After Radiotherapy

An excellent review by Donahue (48) describes in detail the acute reactions seen during treatment with radiotherapy and provides guidelines for their management. These days nausea and vomiting secondary to treatment almost always can be prevented by the use of the 5HT-3 antagonists. Headache is not common in children and should be investigated by physical examination for signs of raised intracranial pressure and by imaging as appropriate. Steroids, if used, usually can be tapered by the third or fourth week of treatment. Fatigue is a rather common symptom and is cumulative. The neurologic status of the patient, especially coordination and gait disorders, may appear to worsen during the last weeks of treatment because of this. Children usually recover relatively quickly, however, and often can get back to their usual routine by 6 weeks to 2 months following completion of treatment.

Other predictable effects of treatment include hormonal deficits, especially growth-hormone deficit secondary to inclusion of the hypothalamic–pituitary axis and primary hypothyroidism when craniospinal irradiation (CSI) is delivered using photons. Patients should be monitored closely in follow-up, and treatment should be instituted as appropriate.

Extra pedagogic support may be necessary. Patients should have ready access to a neuropsychologist for evaluation of any

Tumors of Neuroepithelial Tissue
Astrocytic tumors ★   Oligodendroglial   Mixed gliomas   Ependymal tumors ★   Choroid plexus tumors ★   Glial tumors of uncertain origin   Neuronal and mixed neuronal-glial tumors ★   Neuroblastic tumors   Pineal parenchymal tumors ★   Embryonal tumors ★
Tumors of the Meninges
Lymphomas and Hematopoietic Neoplasms
Germ Cell Tumors ★
Tumors of the Sellar Region ★
Metastatic Tumors
★ *Topics addressed in this chapter; the remainder are uncommon in the pediatric*

FIGURE 82.1. World Health Organization classification of tumors of the central nervous system (133).

special needs, and in the long term they may require vocational assessment and counseling.

Specific Tumor Types

The World Health Organization (WHO) classification of tumors of the nervous system (133) is given in Fig. 82.1 and the distribution by tumor type and location in Fig. 82.2. There are important differences between tumors seen in childhood and those occurring in adults. In children, almost half of all tumors arise in the infratentorial compartment. Low-grade astrocytic tumors as a group account for approximately one third to half of all CNS tumors, but medulloblastoma is the most common distinct entity. High-grade gliomas, which account for the majority of primary brain tumors seen in adults, are much less common in children.

This chapter will follow the order of the WHO classification. Although in the past, tumors arising in infants and very young children were grouped together and managed similarly with chemotherapy, they increasingly are managed according to the specific tumor type and so will be discussed here in each relevant section.

Astrocytic Tumors

According to the WHO classification of tumors of the nervous system, astrocytic tumors comprise the following clinicopathologic entities:

- Diffusely infiltrating astrocytomas,
  - Diffuse astrocytomas (WHO grade II),
  - Anaplastic astrocytoma (WHO grade III),
  - Glioblastoma multiforme (WHO grade IV) and variants,
- Pilocytic astrocytoma (WHO grade I),
- Pleomorphic xanthoastrocytoma,
- Desmoplastic cerebral astrocytoma of infancy,
- Subependymal giant cell astrocytoma.

These tumors are heterogeneous with respect to clinical presentation (age, gender, location in the CNS, imaging findings) as well as to growth potential and rate of progression, and their management will depend on the specific tumor type. The last three tumors in this category (pleomorphic xanthoastrocytoma, desmoplastic cerebral astrocytoma of infancy, and subependymal giant cell astrocytoma) are rare tumors. Their clinical presentation and imaging findings are quite characteristic, and surgery is usually curative. They will not be discussed further here.

Low-Grade Astrocytomas (WHO Grades I and II)

So-called benign or low-grade astrocytomas (LGA) comprise a heterogeneous group of tumors whose principal common characteristic is that of an indolent clinical course with overall survival rates at 10 and 15 years as high as 80% to 100%. LGA can be grouped according to their anatomic location:

- Cerebellar astrocytomas (15% to 20% of all CNS tumors),
- Hemispheric astrocytomas (10% to 15% of all CNS tumors),
- Midline supratentorial tumors, including the corpus callosum, lateral and third ventricles, and the hypothalamus and thalamus (10% to 15% of all CNS tumors),
- Optic pathway tumors (approximately 5% of all CNS tumors),
- Brainstem LGA (brainstem tumors account for 10% to 15% of all CNS tumors; 20% to 30% of these are LGA),
- LGA of the spinal cord (spinal cord tumors account for 3% to 6% of all CNS tumors; approximately 60% of these are LGA).

Most LGA occurring in childhood are of one of two types: pilocytic astrocytoma and low-grade astrocytoma of diffuse or fibrillary type. According to the WHO classification, pilocytic astrocytomas are designated as grade I regardless of any specific histologic characteristic that in other classification systems would lead to their designation as higher-grade lesions. All other low-grade astrocytomas are designated as grade II. That these two groups of LGA should be regarded as distinct clinicopathologic entities is supported by molecular studies that show genetic alterations including TP53 mutations and loss of heterozygosity on chromosome 17p in the diffuse or fibrillary astrocytomas (in common with high grade astrocytomas) but not in pilocytic astrocytomas (133).

Pilocytic astrocytomas are the most common type in the pediatric age group, accounting for almost all of the LGA at certain sites (e.g., the anterior optic pathway, the cerebellum). They account for a smaller proportion of those arising in the deep midline structures and in the cerebral hemispheres. Macroscopically, pilocytic astrocytomas appear well circumscribed and frequently have an associated cystic component. Pilocytic astrocytomas are characterized histologically by a biphasic pattern with a varying proportion of compacted bipolar cells with Rosenthal fibers and loose-textured multipolar cells with microcysts and granular bodies. Rare mitoses, occasional hyperchromatic nuclei, microvascular proliferation, and even infiltration of the meninges are compatible with a diagnosis of pilocytic astrocytoma and not a sign of malignancy (133). A variant, pilomyxoid astrocytoma, first described in infants and young children with chiasmatic/hypothalamic tumors, is characterized by more frequent mitoses and lack of the typical biphasic pattern and appears to be associated with more aggressive behavior that may include leptomeningeal seeding (134).

Diffuse, or fibrillary, low-grade astrocytomas account for only approximately 15% of all LGA in children but for a relatively higher proportion of those seen in infants and adolescents. Most intrinsic pontine tumors and a large proportion of astrocytomas arising in the cerebral hemispheres are diffuse astrocytomas. Diffuse astrocytomas grow by infiltration rather

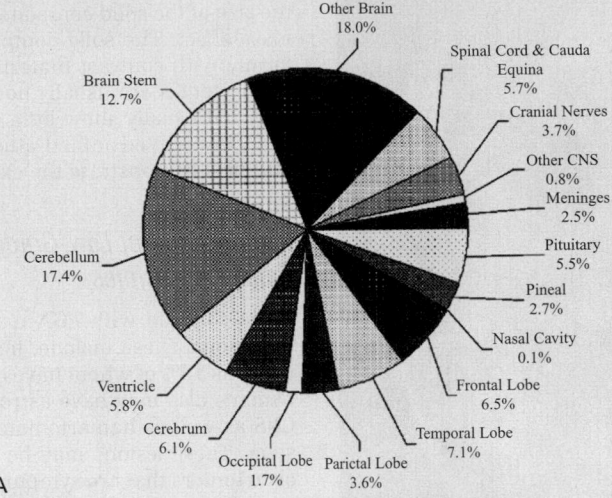

Distribution of All Childhood Primary Brain and CNS Tumors (0–19 yr) by Site CBTRUS 1998–2002 (n = 5,455)

A

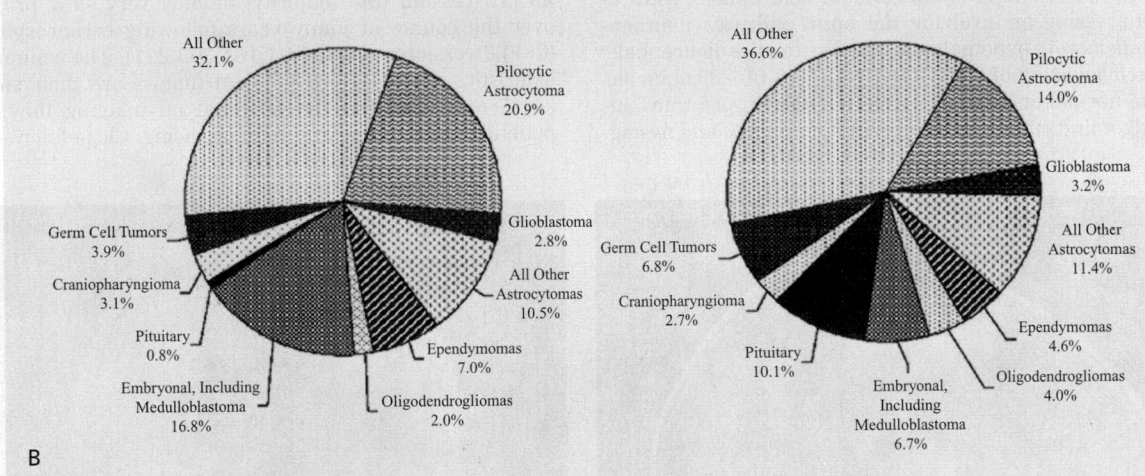

Distribution of Childhood Primary Brain and CNS Tumors by Histology CBTRUS 1998–2002

Ages 0–14 (n = 4,214)   Ages 15–19 (n = 1,241)

B

FIGURE 82.2. Distribution of central nervous system (CNS) tumors by site (**A**) and histology (**B**) (From CBTRUS: Central Brain Tumor Registry of the United States. CBTRUS. 2004.) www.cbtrus.org

than destruction of anatomic structures and are usually not well circumscribed. Microscopically, they are composed of well-differentiated fibrillary or gemistocytic neoplastic astrocytes on a background of loosely structured, often microcystic, tumor matrix. Cellularity is moderately increased. The presence of nuclear atypia is a diagnostic criterion, but mitotic activity, necrosis, and microvascular proliferation are absent. The growth fraction as determined by Ki-67 and MIB-1 labeling indices is usually low. There is some evidence that higher labeling indices, even in tumors with otherwise similar histologic features, are associated with a worse outcome. Diffuse astrocytomas, particularly those with a significant fraction of gemistocytes, may undergo malignant progression, although this is not common

in the pediatric age group with the notable exception of tumors arising in the pons.

Patients with LGA typically present with a long history of nonspecific and nonlocalizing symptoms. Symptoms and signs of raised intracranial pressure may be seen in patients with midline and cerebellar tumors. Patients with posterior fossa tumors may present with neck stiffness and a head tilt as a manifestation of raised intracranial pressure, causing tonsillar herniation, altitudinal diplopia, or spinal-accessory nerve irritation. Seizures are present in as many as three quarters of patients with hemispheric lesions. Other symptoms, relatively less frequent and usually of more recent onset, relate to the location of the tumor. These may include, for example, focal motor

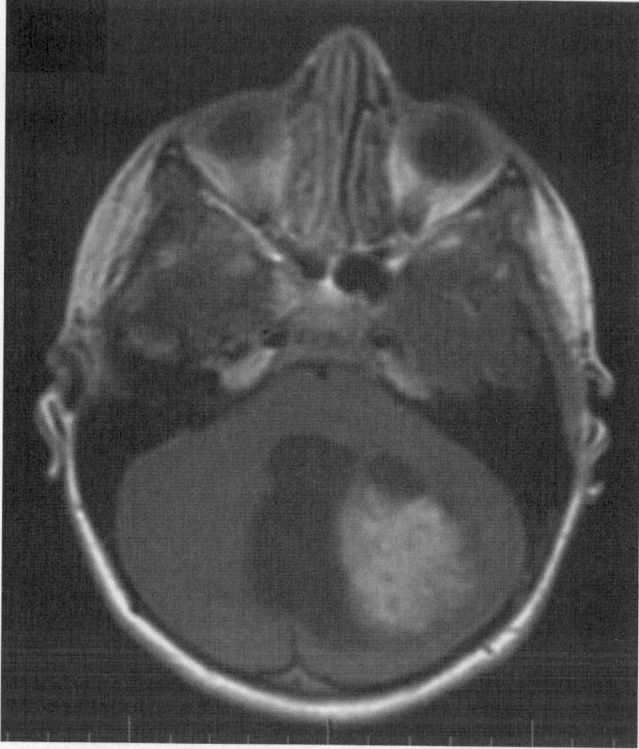

FIGURE 82.3. Typical appearance of pilocytic astrocytoma of the cerebellum with a large cystic component. The solid component enhances brightly after injection of contrast material, while the wall of the cyst, as is usually the case, does not.

deficits with hemispheric tumors, visual field deficits with tumors compressing or involving the optic pathway, neuroendocrine deficits with hypothalamic tumors, and the diencephalic syndrome (consisting of emaciation with loss of subcutaneous fat despite normal or increased appetite, alert appearance, increased vigor and euphoria, pallor without anemia, and nystag-

moid movements of the eyes) seen in very young children with chiasmatic/hypothalamic tumors.

Neuroimaging findings are usually quite characteristic. Typically, pilocytic astrocytomas are well circumscribed. They often have a cystic component that may be large in comparison with the size of the solid component. There is usually little edema or mass effect. The solid component enhances brightly and uniformly with contrast material (Fig. 82.3). Diffuse or fibrillary astrocytomas are usually not well seen on nonenhanced CT or MRI and usually show little enhancement with contrast material. T2-weighted or fluid-attenuated inversion recovery (FLAIR) MRI best demonstrate the extent of the disease (Fig. 82.4).

Management of Low-Grade Astrocytomas: General Principles

Some children with LGA may not require any tumor-specific treatment. These include, for example, patients with NF-1, as many as 15% of whom have optic pathway tumors (149). These patients also may have astrocytic tumors in other parts of the CNS as well as hamartomatous lesions, typically in the brainstem. These lesions may be detected on routine imaging, but even tumors that are symptomatic may remain stable over long periods so that surveillance is appropriate initial management (59,132,206). Active intervention is reserved for patients who develop progressive disease that is symptomatic.

Progression-free survival without treatment may be very good as well for patients with tectal lesions who present with hydrocephalus without localizing brainstem signs. Some of these lesions are probably also hamartomatous. However, even LGA in this region may be very indolent; several groups have reported their experience with such tumors and shown either no progression (the majority) or only very slow progression over the course of many years following cerebrospinal fluid (CSF) diversion alone (64,91,161,205,221). The common characteristics of these very indolent tumors are their small size (<1.5 or 2 cm) and the fact that on imaging they are hypodense/hypointense and nonenhancing. Close follow-up with

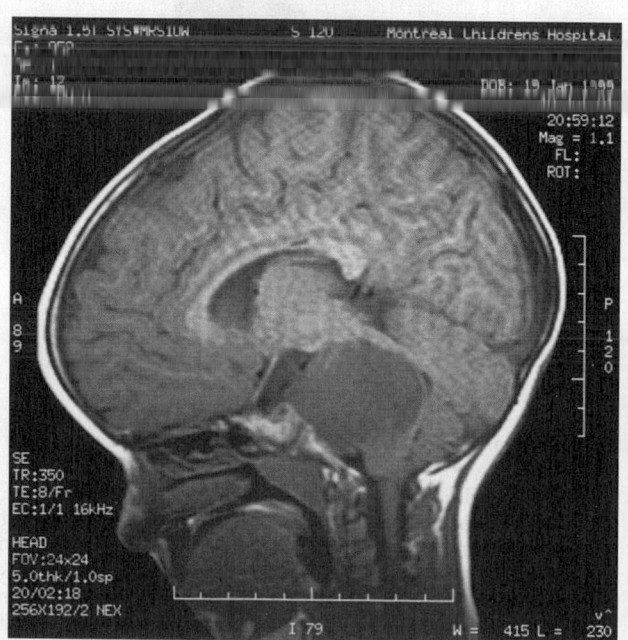

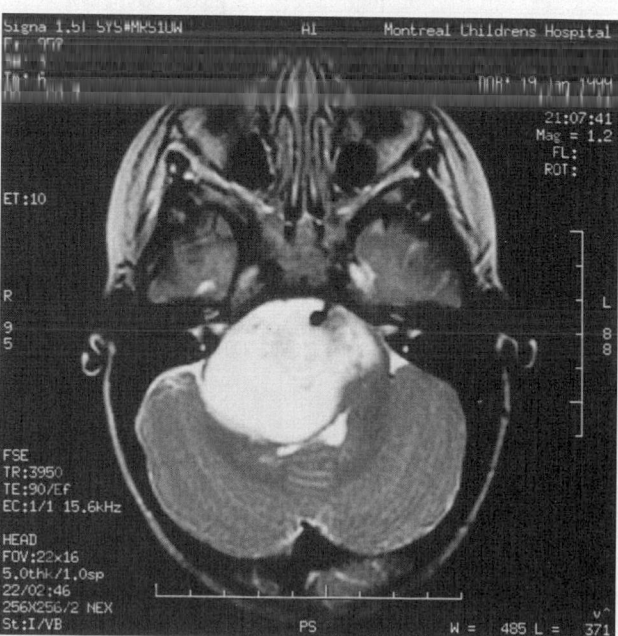

FIGURE 82.4. Typical appearance of a diffuse or fibrillary astrocytoma located in the pons in a 2-year-old girl who presented with multiple bilateral cranial nerve deficits and a left hemiparesis. **A:** The tumor is hypointense on T1-weighted magnetic resonance imaging (MRI) and does not enhance after injection of contrast material. As for diffuse or fibrillary low-grade astrocytoma in other locations, the extent of disease is best demonstrated on T2-weighted or fluid-attenuated inversion recovery (FLAIR) MRI (**B**), and these are the images that should be used for target volume definition for radiotherapy.

regular MRI is essential to identify patients with progressive lesions as manifested by increasing size and/or enhancement with gadolinium. Treatment (usually radiotherapy but sometimes now surgery) at the time of progression is associated with a high probability of long-term tumor control.

These special situations underscore the need for careful evaluation and individualization of management of patients with LGA depending on the specific clinical situation and tumor type. If in doubt, a period of surveillance generally will be an acceptable initial approach.

Surgery is the mainstay of treatment for LGA. Complete resection is more likely to be accomplished in patients with smaller tumors and those arising in noneloquent parts of the brain as well as in patients with the generally well-circumscribed pilocytic tumors. Modern surgical techniques that include, for example, computer-assisted resections (neuronavigation) aided by preoperative functional MRI and intraoperative electrophysiologic mapping of eloquent areas permit greater degrees of resection in larger proportions of patients, including many who in the past would have been considered to have inoperable lesions. Currently, complete resection is achieved in approximately 80% of cerebral, cerebellar, and spinal-cord tumors and 40% of diencephalic tumors.

Children with LGA who undergo complete resection fare very well, with long-term disease-free and overall survival rates of 80% to 100% (62,79,110,202,247). In most series, results are better (close to 100%) for patients with pilocytic astrocytomas than for those with diffuse or fibrillary LGA, although some have disputed this, showing equally satisfactory results for both. In either type, postoperative adjuvant therapy is clearly not indicated.

For children who undergo less than complete resection, the progression-free survival rate after surgery alone is less satisfactory. In a joint Children's Cancer Group (CCG)–Pediatric Oncology Group (POG) study in which patients who had undergone subtotal resection (<1.5 cm³ residual tumor) were observed without adjuvant treatment, the 5-year progression-free survival rate was only 65%. However, the majority of patients can be salvaged with a second surgical resection and/or radiotherapy; in the CCG–POG study, overall survival at 5 years was 95% (Sanford, personal communication, June 2006). Consequently, the usual recommendation following subtotal resection will be close follow-up.

The role of postoperative radiotherapy following lesser degrees of tumor resection remains unclear. In most series, the use of radiotherapy in this situation results in improved disease-free survival without any benefit in terms of overall survival. Since only approximately half of all patients who have undergone incomplete resections will develop progressive disease and given the concerns with regard to the use of radiotherapy in young children, the usual recommendation for a patient who has undergone incomplete resection and who is neurologically stable will also be surveillance, with MRI performed at least every 6 months for the first 3 years (232). A second surgical procedure would be considered at time of progression, and radiotherapy is reserved for patients with progressive, inoperable disease (Fig. 82.5).

Traditionally, patients with deep midline and other tumors previously considered surgically inaccessible were treated with radiotherapy, often without histologic confirmation of diagnosis. Outcome is not as good as for hemispheric lesions, with overall survival rates in the 35% to 75% range (21,79,279). Using modern neurosurgical techniques it is feasible to resect surgically about 40% of these lesions, and the overall strategy for these patients should now be as for patients with LGA at other locations.

When adjuvant therapy is indicated because of residual symptomatic or progressive disease, the options include chemotherapy, particularly for infants and young children and

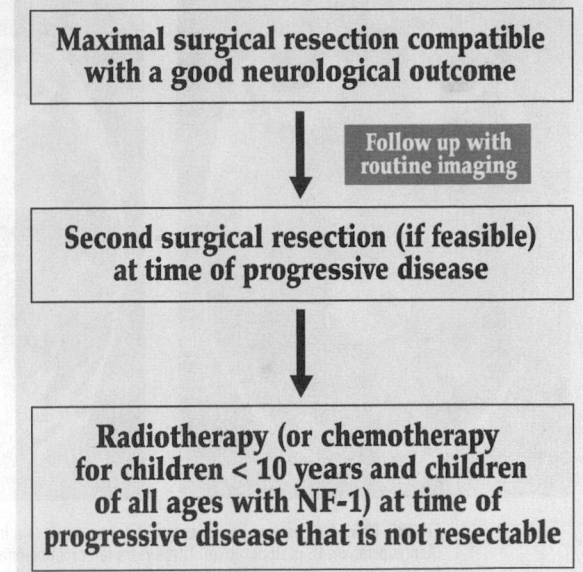

FIGURE 82.5. An algorithm for the management of patients with low-grade astrocytoma. NF-1, neurofibromatosis type 1.

for patients of all ages with NF-1 who are at greatest risk of developing neurocognitive and neuroendocrine sequelae of treatment. Complete responses to chemotherapy are not common but overall response rates that include stable disease range from 70% to 100% and the use of chemotherapy has been shown to permit delay of radiotherapy by 2 to as much as 4 or more years (68,86,143,214). The age limit below which chemotherapy should be used is controversial. It is very likely that delaying radiotherapy for 2 to 3 years will be of significant benefit for a child younger than age 5. However, the benefit from a similar delay for a child age 10 is less clear, particularly when any benefit may be offset by the risk of neurologic compromise from further tumor progression and/or the need for a larger radiotherapy target volume. Recent advances in radiotherapy practice (100,117,136,156,173,230,242,261) that have the potential to reduce the risks of radiotherapy have led to a reassessment of the role of radiotherapy in LGA and better acceptance of its earlier use even in very young children.

Radiotherapy in Low-Grade Astrocytomas

Indications for Radiotherapy

To summarize:

- Radiotherapy is not indicated after complete resection.
- Radiotherapy may be indicated following incomplete resection in situations when tumor progression would compromise neurologic function (e.g., "threat to vision").
- The clearest indication for radiotherapy is in patients with progressive and/or symptomatic disease that is unresectable.

Radiotherapy Target Volume

The radiotherapy target volume (the gross tumor volume or GTV) consists of the tumor bed and any macroscopic disease seen on MRI prior to treatment (173) (Fig. 82.6). The resulting treatment volume usually will be considerably smaller than one based on preoperative imaging, which until now would have constituted standard practice. Similarly, margins that were considered standard practice (i.e., 2 to 3 cm) are overly generous, particularly for the well-circumscribed pilocytic tumors; margins of 0.5 cm around the GTV as seen on T1 weighted

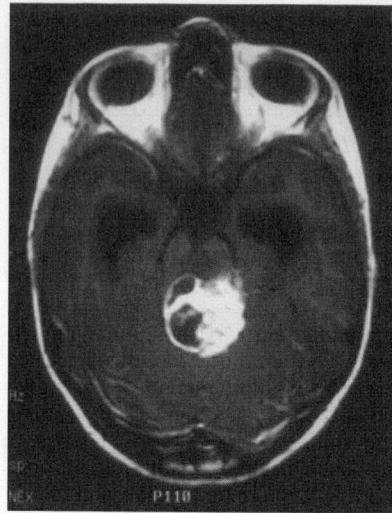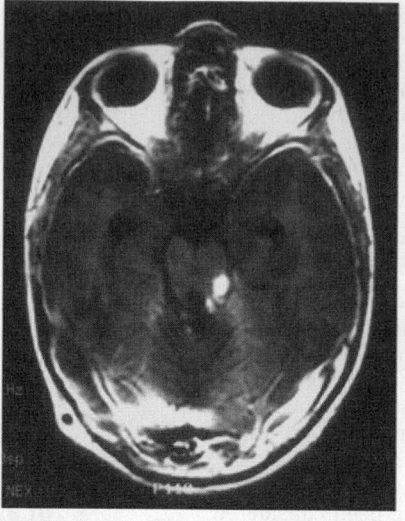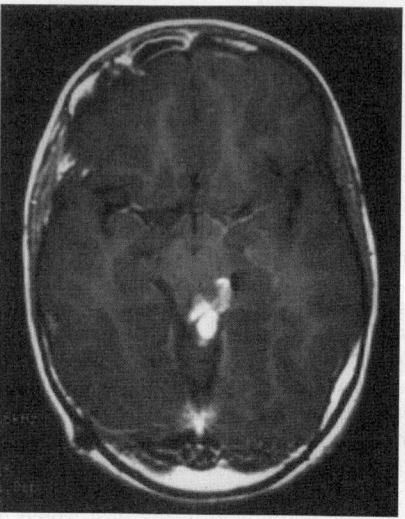

A, B   **C**

FIGURE 82.6. This patient underwent subtotal resection of a low-grade astrocytoma of the left cerebellar peduncle at the age of 8 years (**A:** preoperative, **B:** postoperative). Three years later routine imaging showed evidence of progressive disease (**C**). The gross tumor volume for radiotherapy consists of the tumor as seen on T1-weighted gadolinium-enhanced magnetic resonance imaging at the time of treatment (**C**).

gadolinium-enhanced images probably represent an adequate clinical target volume (CTV) for such tumors. More generous margins of 1 to 1.5 cm around the GTV as seen on T2 weighted or FLAIR images are more appropriate for the more infiltrative diffuse fibrillary tumors. Prospective studies under way in North America and in Europe are testing the safety of these reduced volumes.

The use of smaller margins mandates optimal imaging for target-volume definition as well as optimal immobilization. With thermoplastic masks it will be necessary to add an additional 3 to 4 mm around the CTV to arrive at the planning target volume (PTV), but the use of rigid or stereotactic localization systems may require an additional margin of only 1 to 2 mm (136).

Radiotherapy Dose

Evidence for a dose response correlation in LGA in children is scant. Although the European Organisation for Research and Treatment in Cancer (EORTC) study that randomized adult patients with LGA between low-dose (45 Gy) and high-dose (59.4 Gy) radiotherapy failed to demonstrate any advantage for the higher dose (124), it may be unwise to extrapolate that in children doses of 45 to 50 Gy are as effective as the higher doses of 54 to 55 Gy that until now have constituted standard practice. Adult patients treated on the EORTC study were treated soon after diagnosis. Children who have progressed on chemotherapy given prior to radiotherapy may have tumors that are less sensitive. As well, there are known biologic differences between LGA in children and in adults. For now, the recommendation for children with LGA would be a "standard" dose of 50 to 54 Gy depending on the age of the child and the location of the tumor and its relationship to critical normal structures, such as the optic chiasm.

Radiotherapy Technique

The radiotherapy technique to be used is that which provides homogeneous irradiation of the CTV and spares the greatest volume of normal tissue. This is best accomplished using CT-simulation, CT–MRI, or even CT–MRI–PET image coregistration and 3D treatment planning. Tools such as dose-volume histograms, which allow quantitative comparison of treatment plans, as well as radiotherapy treatment equipment that allows the use of multiple, often noncoplanar, field arrangements, automated field shaping, and intensity modulation of the radiation

beam, make it easier to achieve conformity of the treated volume to the target than ever before.

Radiosurgery has also been used and preliminary results of single-fraction treatment using the Gamma knife or fractionated treatment using linear accelerator-based techniques are promising (19,89,261). However, the use of one fraction, typically of 10 to 20 Gy to the periphery of the lesion (89), or a small number of large treatment fractions, such as the McGill schedule of 42 Gy in six fractions over 2 weeks (19), may not be optimal for slowly growing tumors, particularly those comprised of tumor cells embedded in rather than displacing normal brain, as is the case for diffuse or fibrillary LGA. Although such treatment may be of interest for part or even all of the treatment for pilocytic astrocytomas, which are often small even at the time of progression, conventional dose fractionation schedules would be more appropriate for most patients and feasible now using modern linear accelerators and accessories.

Other options for treatment include brachytherapy, which has been used with some success particularly in European centers (138,179,235), and instillation of radioactive solutions such as phosphorus-32 (^{32}P), yttrium-90 (^{90}Y), gold-198 (^{198}Au), and rhenium-186 (^{186}Re). As for radiosurgery or stereotactic irradiation, the principal limitation with respect to the use of brachytherapy is the size of the target volume. Brachytherapy series necessarily select for smaller tumors, and there is no evidence that brachytherapy is a better treatment option than external-beam radiotherapy. Radioactive solutions may be useful in cystic LGA, particularly for patients with recurrent disease after radiotherapy in whom symptoms not infrequently relate more to the cyst than to the solid component of tumor. Simple aspiration with or without placement of an internal shunt usually will alleviate symptoms for protracted periods. In some cases, particularly those in which the cyst wall enhances and is felt to be biologically active, control of the cyst fluid may be difficult, and the use of radioactive solutions could be considered. However, this is not a procedure without risks and special care has to be taken to avoid leakage.

High-Grade Astrocytomas (WHO Grades III and IV)

According to the WHO classification, anaplastic astrocytoma (AA) is a diffusely infiltrating astrocytoma with focal or dispersed anaplasia and marked proliferative potential. Glioblastoma multiforme (GBM) is the most malignant astrocytic tumor, composed of poorly differentiated neoplastic astrocytes. Histopathologic features include cellular pleomorphism, nuclear atypia, brisk mitotic activity, vascular thrombosis, microvascular proliferation, and necrosis. Both AA and GBM may develop from diffuse or fibrillary astrocytomas (WHO grade II). However, with the exception of tumors that arise in the pons that show genetic alterations such as a high frequency of TP-53 mutations that suggest malignant progression of a lower grade lesion, they arise more frequently in the pediatric age group *de novo* without evidence of a less malignant precursor lesion.

High-grade astrocytomas (HGA) account for 5% of all CNS tumors in the pediatric age group. They are the most common tumor type in older adolescents. Two thirds of HGA are located in the cerebral hemispheres, and the remainder are approximately equally divided between the deep midline structures (thalamus and basal ganglia) and cerebellum. Patients with HGA usually present with symptoms of short duration (<6 months) that relate to the location of the lesion.

Surgery is an important component of treatment. Since most studies show a survival advantage for patients who have undergone complete resection (32,63,108,280), maximal surgical resection compatible with a good neurologic outcome should be the goal for all patients, regardless of tumor location or histology. A second surgical procedure should be considered if there is significant residual tumor after the first (280). Postoperative radiotherapy is always indicated. Although leptomeningeal seeding is seen in a substantial minority (10% to 30%) of patients, the predominant failure pattern is local (108) and the radiotherapy target volume is local with a GTV that consists of the tumor bed and any macroscopic residual disease plus a margin for the CTV of 1.5 to 2 cm. Because these are often large tumors and high doses are required, it is usual to consider a field-size reduction at 50 to 54 Gy to a CTV that consists of the tumor bed and any macroscopic residual disease plus a margin of 1 to 1.5 cm. PET and CT–MRI–PET coregistration may prove to be useful in defining the target volumes by revealing biologically more active areas of the tumor that can be treated to higher doses. The dose to the CTV should be at least 54 Gy given over 6 weeks, but a dose of 59 to 60 Gy is more usual if feasible. There is no evidence that higher doses, as delivered using radiosurgery or stereotactic boosts, boosts with brachytherapy, or HFRT, result in improved outcomes, but newer approaches such as IMRT, which allows accelerated treatment to a component of the target volume (such as the GTV), may be of interest if only to decrease the overall treatment time.

The role of chemotherapy remains to be defined. There have been few phase III randomized trials of chemotherapy in HGA in children and only one, CCG-943, that included a radiotherapy alone arm. In this study, event-free and overall survival were significantly better for patients who received chemotherapy using a CCNU (lomustine)-based regimen (252). In the follow-up study (CCG-945), results using the same regimen were not as good, and no advantage was seen with the more aggressive experimental regimen (63). Although responses are seen to many different agents and regimens (200), results have often been difficult to interpret because of small patient numbers, inconsistent inclusion criteria with respect to pathology, and confounding variables such as tumor location and extent of surgical resection. The cooperative groups in North America and Europe are investigating a number of approaches that include newer chemotherapeutic and biologic agents, some of which have radiosensitizing properties. Whenever possible, patients should be treated on such protocols. Off study it may be difficult to make a recommendation with respect to adjuvant chemotherapy, although the poor prognosis, particularly for patients with macroscopic residual disease following surgery, usually is given as an argument for the use of the "current best" regimen (200).

The prognosis for children with HGA is poor, with a median time to progression of 10 to 11 months, and an overall survival for patients 0 to 19 years diagnosed between 1973 and 2001 of only 19% at 5 years according to the SEER registry (256). Several factors correlate with outcome. Patients with lesions in the cerebral hemispheres fare better than those with tumors in other locations, apparently independent of extent of surgical resection. The prognosis for children with bithalamic lesions is particularly poor (8), and these patients are managed similarly to patients with diffuse intrinsic pontine tumors (see below). Age also may be an important factor. In contrast to most other tumor types, infants with HGA appear to fare somewhat better than older children with overall survival at 3 to 5 years in the 33% to 50% range in the North American infant studies (52,83,84). Histologic grade (AA versus GBM) has not been shown consistently to affect outcome, but p53 overexpression and a high MIB-1 labeling index appear to identify patients with a particularly adverse prognosis who might be appropriate candidates for novel therapeutic approaches (201).

Astrocytic Tumors in Specific Locations

Optic Pathway Gliomas

Optic pathway gliomas collectively account for approximately 5% of all CNS tumors in the pediatric age group. These are tumors of young children: the peak age incidence is between 2 and 6 years, and 75% of all patients are <10. One third of patients have NF-1. They may be divided into three clinicopathologic entities: tumors confined to the optic nerve(s), tumors of the optic chiasm with or without optic nerve involvement (collectively "anterior" tumors), and tumors that involve the hypothalamus or adjacent structures ("chiasmatic/hypothalamic" or "posterior" tumors). Management of patients with optic pathway gliomas is often said to be controversial but is really not, provided that the differences in behavior between these different tumor types and between patients with and without NF-1 are taken into consideration.

Optic nerve gliomas may involve one or both optic nerves. Bilateral involvement is pathognomonic of NF-1. In a substantial proportion of cases, the optic nerve tumors are incidental findings on routine imaging, and patients may remain asymptomatic with nonprogressive lesions over long periods; even spontaneous regressions are well documented. The frequency of progression is difficult to establish, ranging from lows of <10% among patients followed in NF-1 clinics to 40% to 50% in series reported by oncology centers. Even in patients with symptomatic tumors, the course can be quite variable, and only 30% to 60% of such patients will develop progressive disease that requires treatment (92,132). Thus, management of patients with optic nerve tumors will usually consist initially of close follow-up with regular ophthalmologic examinations and MRI, with active intervention, usually chemotherapy, reserved for patients with clear evidence of progression that is symptomatic (41,92,122).

Patients with unilateral optic nerve involvement may not have NF-1. They present most frequently with proptosis that may be relatively long standing. Findings on examination may include optic atrophy and impaired visual acuity. On MRI, optic nerve tumors are usually relatively small and well circumscribed, with bright enhancement typical for pilocytic astrocytoma. Biopsy is not necessary to make a diagnosis. Treatment usually, although not always, will be necessary, and the approach will depend on whether there is useful vision. If not, then surgical resection will be the treatment of choice. If useful vision is preserved, chemotherapy would be the preferred option for infants, very young children up to the age of 3 to 5 years, and for patients of all ages with NF-1. Radiotherapy could be considered for older children. Overall, the prognosis is very good. Visual acuity remains stable or improves in the majority of cases following chemotherapy or radiotherapy. Long-term tumor control approaches 100% with either modality (41,127).

Chiasmatic gliomas are tumors that involve the optic chiasm and sometimes one or both optic nerves as well. Patients typically present with loss of visual acuity and temporal field defects. On imaging, the tumors are usually relatively small and well circumscribed and enhance uniformly and brightly with contrast material, suggestive of pilocytic histology. Biopsy is usually not necessary.

A period of surveillance is appropriate initial management, particularly for patients with NF-1. For patients without NF-1, especially those who present before the age of 5, there is a high probability of early progression and the majority of patients will require treatment within a few months following diagnosis. Surgery is rarely an option for tumors in this location. As for optic nerve tumors, chemotherapy usually will be the treatment of choice for infants and young children and for patients with NF-1. Radiotherapy is reserved for salvage postchemotherapy and for definitive treatment of older children without NF-1, providing a reasonable expectation that vision will not deteriorate further and a probability of long-term progression-free survival in the 60% to 90% range (17,90,116,122,259). Overall survival for patients with chiasmatic tumors is in the 90% to 100% range.

Posterior, or *chiasmatic/hypothalamic, gliomas* account for approximately 70% of all optic pathway gliomas in children. They are typically rather large lesions that probably arise in the optic chiasm and extend to involve the hypothalamus. They may extend posteriorly along the optic tracts as well. They often fill the third ventricle, eventually causing hydrocephalus. Early findings consist of nystagmus, impaired visual acuity, and visual field deficits; only later do patients present with increasing head circumference and/or symptoms and signs of raised intracranial pressure.

Treatment consists of CSF diversion, if necessary, and surgical resection particularly if tumor is growing exophytically into the basal cisterns, since this may provide rapid relief of symptoms. In most patients, however, resection will be incomplete. As for LGA at other locations, a period of surveillance is reasonable, although most patients will require adjuvant therapy (68,127). The treatment of choice for children younger than 5 and those with NF-1 usually will be chemotherapy, most often now using a carboplatin-based regimen. Progression-free survival at 3 to 5 years is rather low at 20% to at best 60% (68,86,121,143). However, some patients will need no further treatment, and for those who do, the use of chemotherapy allows radiotherapy to be deferred by a median of 2 to 4 or more years without jeopardizing overall survival.

The indications for radiotherapy are (a) progressive disease on chemotherapy for children younger than 10 years and (b) progressive disease at diagnosis or after surgery for older patients. Radiotherapy in this situation, given to local fields to a dose of 45 to 50 Gy for younger children and of 50 to 54 Gy for those older than 5 years, can be expected to result in local tumor control in 70% to 80% of cases according to the recent literature (18,43,68,90,127). Overall, however, the results of treatment are less satisfactory for this group of patients than for those with anterior tumors. Long-term survival is in the 50% to 80% range, and many patients will be left with significant neuroendocrine and neuropsychologic sequelae. Patients with NF-1 are particularly at risk. They may have subnormal IQ even without chemotherapy and/or radiotherapy (142). They are also at greater risk for Moyamoya syndrome, a progressive vaso-occlusive process involving the circle of Willis. This may be seen without radiotherapy, but when radiotherapy is used in patients with NF-1 it is important to include MR angiography as part of the regular follow-up imaging protocol and to intervene surgically if necessary to avoid a cerebrovascular accident.

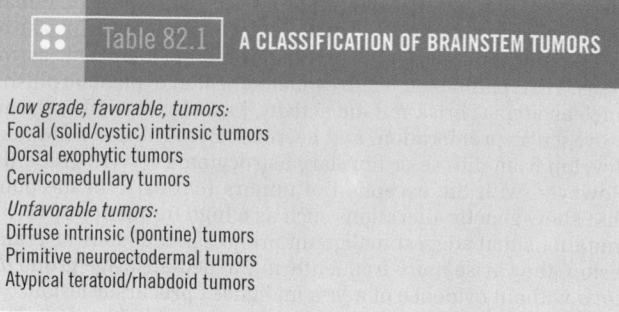

Table 82.1	A CLASSIFICATION OF BRAINSTEM TUMORS

Low grade, favorable, tumors:
Focal (solid/cystic) intrinsic tumors
Dorsal exophytic tumors
Cervicomedullary tumors

Unfavorable tumors:
Diffuse intrinsic (pontine) tumors
Primitive neuroectodermal tumors
Atypical teratoid/rhabdoid tumors

Brainstem Gliomas

Tumors arising in the midbrain, pons, and medulla oblongata account for 10% to 15% of all CNS tumors in the pediatric age group. Historically, tumors arising in this location were regarded as single entity and treated without histologic confirmation of diagnosis with radiotherapy alone. Results of treatment were poor, with 5-year survival rates commonly in the 20% to 30% range. As a result of advances in neuroimaging and particularly with the advent of MRI, it has become clear that tumors arising in the brainstem are of several distinct types that can be broadly grouped as the more favorable low-grade focal, dorsal exophytic, and cervicomedullary tumors and the much more aggressive diffuse intrinsic tumors (Table 82.1) (55,64,71). Over the same period, improvements in neurosurgical techniques and perioperative care have made surgery not only feasible but the treatment of choice for all except the diffuse intrinsic tumors (54).

Focal tumors by definition are tumors of limited size (smaller than 2 cm) that on MRI are well circumscribed, without evidence of infiltration, and without edema. They may be cystic, and, as with cystic tumors at other sites, the cystic component may be large relative to the solid, biologically active, component. Focal tumors may occur at any level in the brainstem but are most frequently seen in the midbrain and medulla. They usually present with a long history of localizing findings such as an isolated cranial nerve deficit and a contralateral hemiparesis. Signs and symptoms of raised intracranial pressure are uncommon except in patients with tumors arising in the tectal region that may cause aqueduct stenosis while still small.

The management depends on the location of the tumor in the brainstem and the specific imaging characteristics of the tumor (Fig. 82.7). As noted previously, patients with nonenhancing focal tumors in the tectal region who present with only hydrocephalus may do well without any treatment other than CSF diversionary procedures. Active intervention, including biopsy, is reserved for patients with clinical and radiologic evidence of progressive tumor (25,54,91). This is important because surgery for tumors in this location is associated with a substantial risk of morbidity even when using modern techniques.

Surgery is the treatment of choice for focal tumors at other locations that are surgically accessible (meaning either that they extend toward the surface of the brainstem laterally or at the floor of the fourth ventricle) and have imaging characteristics suggestive of low-grade histology. In this regard, uniform bright enhancement with contrast material, which correlates with pilocytic histology, and the absence of peritumoral hypodensity are of particular importance. In experienced hands, the risk of morbidity for well-selected patients is acceptable and, as with completely or subtotally resected LGA at other sites, results may be excellent with freedom from progression in a high percentage of cases (60,146). Results are less satisfactory for patients

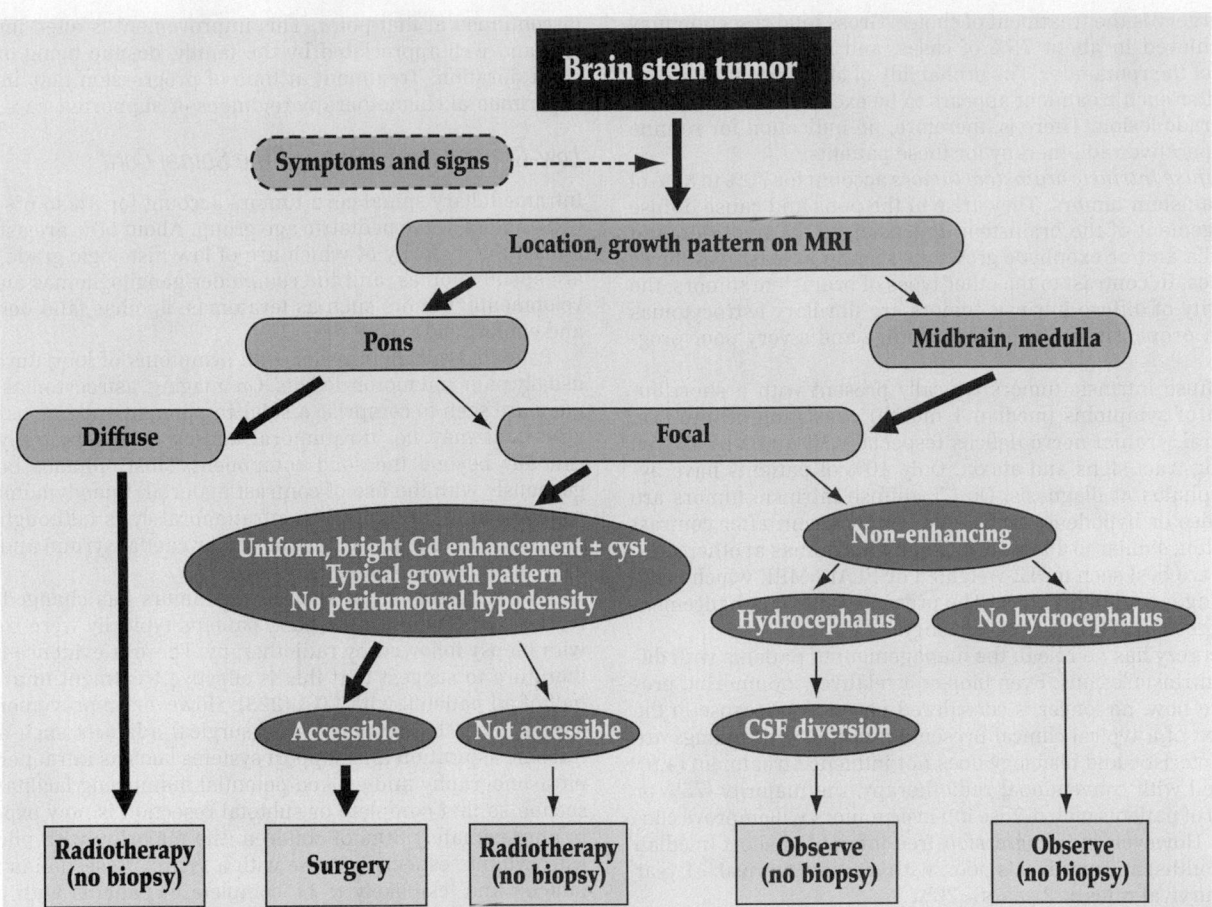

FIGURE 82.7. An algorithm for the management of patients with brainstem tumors. The heavier arrows represent the more frequent clinical situations. CSF, cerebrospinal fluid; Gd, gadolinium; MRI, magnetic resonance imaging.

with bulky tumors and for patients with tumors in the medulla with lower cranial nerve deficits who are at high risk of developing postoperative complications.

There are several treatment options for patients with surgically inaccessible focal lesions. By extrapolation from series reporting results of treatment using conventional radiotherapy in brainstem tumors in which outcome correlates with location (pons vs. other), imaging appearance (tumor volume, density on CT, enhancement pattern), and histology (malignant vs. benign), it is reasonable to assume that at least 50% to 70% of focal lesions may be permanently controlled with such treatment. Similar results have been obtained in small numbers of patients treated with HFRT and with interstitial irradiation using iodine-125 (138,179). There is also some experience with the use of radiosurgery and stereotactic irradiation. However, with the advent of improved treatment planning and conformal radiotherapy treatment techniques, standard treatment for these lesions should be considered to be external-beam radiotherapy, using limited treatment volumes with a margin for the CTV of 0.5 cm, to a total dose of the order of 54 Gy given over 6 weeks, as for LGA at other locations. The risks of HFRT, stereotactic irradiation with large fraction sizes, or interstitial irradiation in inexperienced hands cannot be justified in the absence of any established superiority.

Dorsal exophytic tumors arise from the floor of the fourth ventricle. They are usually large, filling the fourth ventricle, but do not invade the brainstem to any significant extent. They present insidiously with failure to thrive in younger children and symptoms and signs of raised intracranial pressure in older patients. Cranial nerve deficits are seen in about half of the patients, but long tract signs are distinctly unusual. On MRI,

they are sharply delineated from surrounding structures. They are hypointense on T1-weighted images, hyperintense on T2-weighted images, and enhance uniformly and brightly after gadolinium injection. Most are pilocytic astrocytomas.

Surgery is the treatment of choice for dorsal exophytic tumors. Ultrasound guidance is essential to achieve a maximal degree of tumor resection. However, because there is usually no definite tumor–brainstem interface, even an optimal resection will leave a thin layer of tumor on the floor of the fourth ventricle. Nonetheless, the majority of children do well following surgery, and routine postoperative adjuvant therapy is not indicated. Radiotherapy should be considered for the rare patient who is found to have a high-grade lesion or for patients with low-grade tumors who are found to have progressive disease in the early (0 to 9 months) postoperative period. For patients whose tumors recur later, further surgery should be considered and radiotherapy should be reserved for those with inoperable disease. The radiotherapy volume and dose should be similar to those used for LGA in other locations. The literature suggests that salvage is possible in the majority of cases, and overall the prognosis for patients with dorsal exophytic tumors is excellent (112,129,204).

Cervicomedullary tumors arise in the upper cervical cord and grow rostrally beyond the foramen magnum. Most are low-grade lesions whose axial growth is limited by the pyramidal decussations located ventrally at the junction of the cervical cord and medulla. At this point, the tumor grows posteriorly, causing a bulge in the dorsal aspect of the medulla, toward the fourth ventricle (55). These tumors typically present with lower cranial nerve deficits, long tract signs, and sometimes torticollis. Hydrocephalus is unusual.

Surgery is the treatment of choice. Gross total resection may be achieved in about 75% of cases, and subtotal removal in most of the remainder. The probability of long-term tumor control after such treatment appears to be excellent for the typical low-grade lesion. There is, therefore, no indication for routine postoperative radiotherapy for these patients.

Diffuse intrinsic brainstem tumors account for 70% to 80% of all brainstem tumors. They arise in the pons and cause diffuse enlargement of the brainstem. Extension to the midbrain and medulla and/or exophytic growth is seen in at least two thirds of cases. In contrast to the other types of brainstem tumors, the majority of diffuse intrinsic tumors are fibrillary astrocytomas with a propensity for malignant change and a very poor prognosis.

Diffuse intrinsic tumors typically present with a short duration of symptoms (median 1 month) consisting of multiple, bilateral, cranial nerve deficits (especially VI and VII) as well as long tract signs and ataxia. Only 10% of patients have hydrocephalus at diagnosis. On CT, diffuse intrinsic tumors are isodense or hypodense, with little enhancement after contrast injection, similar to diffuse fibrillary astrocytomas at other sites. They are best seen on T2-weighted or FLAIR MRI, which is the imaging modality of choice. The presence of ring enhancement is suggestive of high-grade histology.

Surgery has no role in the management of patients with diffuse intrinsic lesions. Even biopsy, a relatively nonmorbid procedure now, no longer is considered necessary because in the context of a typical clinical presentation, the MRI findings are characteristic and histology does not influence treatment (4,6). Treated with conventional radiotherapy, the majority (75% or more) of patients with diffuse intrinsic tumors will improve clinically. However, the progression-free interval is short (median <6 months) and survival is poor, with median survival <1 year and survival rates at 2 years <20%.

So far, all attempts to improve the outcome for children with diffuse intrinsic tumors have proved futile. HFRT was tested in a series of phase I or II studies using doses ranging from 64.8 to 78 Gy. Time to progression and overall survival were not improved in comparison with conventional radiotherapy (72,75). Moreover, at the higher doses of HFRT of 75.6 Gy and 78 Gy morbidity was considerable. This included steroid dependency, vascular events, and white matter changes outside the radiation field, as well as hearing loss, hormone deficiencies, and late-developing seizure disorders in the small number of long-term survivors (70,73,187,207). Accelerated radiotherapy was explored in a study in the United Kingdom in which patients were treated to a total dose of 50.4 Gy given in 28 twice-daily fractions of 1.8 Gy over 3 weeks. Progression-free and overall survival rates were similar to those seen in the HFRT studies (147).

Alternative approaches that use chemotherapy in combination with radiotherapy also have been disappointing (74). None of the many single-agent and multiagent regimens that have been tested in this patient population have been shown to provide a survival advantage compared with conventional radiotherapy alone. New agents and novel chemotherapy–radiotherapy combinations are under investigation by the pediatric cooperative groups in North America and Europe (27).

Currently, standard treatment for diffuse intrinsic brainstem tumors consists of radiotherapy given to the GTV as demonstrated by T2-weighted or FLAIR MRI with a margin for the CTV of 1 to 1.5 cm to a dose of 54 Gy given in 30 daily fractions over 6 weeks. Because of the initial rapid progression of neurologic deficit and the need to achieve a prompt symptomatic response, a lateral opposed field arrangement generally will be used. The use of a more complex conformal technique that reduces the dose to the auditory apparatus and temporal lobes may be considered as long as treatment will not be delayed. A worthwhile improvement in clinical status is usually evident as early as 2 to 3 weeks into treatment, and steroids, if used, usually can be discontinued at that point. This improvement is often impressive and well appreciated by the family, despite being of only short duration. Treatment at time of progression may include experimental chemotherapy regimens or supportive care.

Low-Grade Astrocytomas of the Spinal Cord

Intramedullary spinal cord tumors account for 3% to 6% of all CNS tumors in the pediatric age group. About 60% are astrocytomas, the majority of which are of low histologic grade, 30% are ependymomas, and the remainder gangliogliomas and developmental tumors such as teratomas, lipomas, and dermoid and epidermoid cysts.

Patients typically present with symptoms of long duration, usually pain and motor deficits. On imaging, astrocytomas most often are seen to comprise a solid component and one or more cysts that may be intratumoral and/or extend rostrally and caudally beyond the solid component. Most enhance heterogeneously with the use of contrast material. Ependymomas, in contrast, only rarely harbor intratumoral cysts (although they may have an associated rostral and/or caudal syrinx) and usually enhance homogeneously.

The management of spinal cord tumors has changed over recent years (180). In the past, patients typically were treated with biopsy followed by radiotherapy. There is evidence in the literature to suggest that this is effective treatment in at least half of all patients with LGA (223). However, improvements in surgery and the routine use of surgical adjuncts such as ultrasonic aspiration and support systems such as intraoperative ultrasonography and evoked potential monitoring facilitate resection so that complete or subtotal resection is now expected in approximately 80% of children (the majority) with pilocytic astrocytoma, especially those with a syrinx. Resection is more difficult and less likely to be complete in patients with grade II astrocytoma because of the more infiltrative nature of those tumors and the absence of a plane of cleavage (180). Since outcome following complete or subtotal resection for LGA is very good, with long-term progression-free survival in the 70% to 90% range (44,120,169), routine postoperative adjuvant therapy is not indicated.

For children in whom complete or subtotal resection is not possible, options will be as for patients with LGA in other locations, that is, early second surgery or close follow-up with second surgery and/or radiotherapy at the time of progression. As for LGA in other locations, chemotherapy may be an alternative to radiotherapy for infants and very young children in this situation (47,151). Immediate treatment would be indicated for patients with a high-grade astrocytoma.

The radiotherapy target volume for LGA usually will consist only of the solid portion of the tumor (including intratumoral cysts) with a margin for the CTV of 0.5 to 1 cm around the GTV. The usual dose would be 50.4 Gy given in 28 daily fractions over approximately 6 weeks. The CTV should be larger for patients with high-grade lesions, most of whom will have had only a biopsy; a margin beyond the entire lesion of 1.5 cm would be more appropriate. The dose prescription usually will be as for low-grade lesions because of a substantial risk of morbidity at higher doses, but often chemotherapy will be given as well. There is evidence from the literature that some of these patients, perhaps as many as 30% (44,223), will survive following such treatment, in contrast to the situation for patients with high-grade gliomas at other locations in the CNS who have macroscopic disease at time of treatment with radiotherapy.

▪▪ | Ependymal Tumors

Ependymal tumors arise from the ependymal lining of the cerebral ventricles and from the remnants of the central canal of the spinal cord. The following types are seen in children:

- Ependymoma (WHO grade II),
- Anaplastic ependymoma (WHO grade III),
- Myxopapillary ependymoma (WHO grade I).

These tumors, even when histologically similar, have been shown to have distinct genetic profiles that correlate with location within the CNS.

Ependymomas

Ependymomas account for 5% to 10% of all brain tumors in the pediatric age group, with a predilection for infants and children younger than age 5 years. They can occur at any site in the ventricular system or in the spinal canal, but in children approximately two-thirds arise in the ependymal lining of the fourth ventricle. Tumors in this location typically present with symptoms and signs of raised intracranial pressure. On imaging the tumor is usually large but relatively well circumscribed, with displacement rather than invasion of adjacent structures. Extension through the foramen magnum into the upper cervical region is not uncommon (Fig. 82.8). Tumors that arise in the supratentorial compartment, some of which arise outside the ventricular system, present with focal neurologic deficits. Intramedullary ependymomas, which account for approximately 30% of all spinal cord tumors arising in childhood, usually present initially with dysesthesia and sensory deficits due to their central location in the cord and only later with pain and motor deficits.

Spread of ependymoma is primarily local. Although gadolinium-enhanced MRI of the whole CNS and CSF cytology are essential components of the work-up for all patients, the risk of leptomeningeal seeding at diagnosis is at most 5% to 10%.

Management of Ependymoma

The completeness of the surgical resection is the factor that has the greatest impact on the outcome of children with ependymoma, regardless of tumor location (67,107,115,170,195,

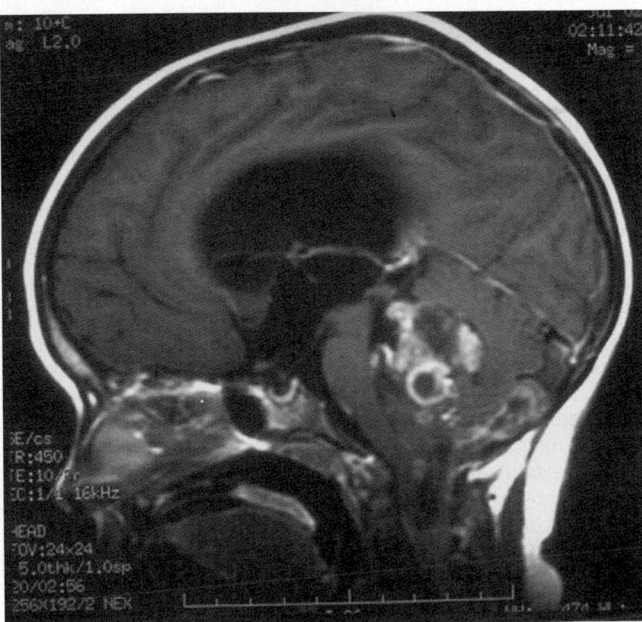

FIGURE 82.8. Typical appearance of an ependymoma that fills the fourth ventricle, causing hydrocephalus, and extends inferiorly below the foramen magnum over the dorsal aspect of the spinal cord to the level of C4. Care is necessary to ensure that the inferior extent of disease is included in the radiotherapy target volume.

203,222,224,276,277). Currently, it is estimated that complete resection is possible in 70% to 85% of supratentorial ependymomas and in a similar percentage of spinal ependymomas. The rate of complete resection is lower in patients with infratentorial ependymomas, particularly in those in whom tumor extends through the foramen of Magendie or Luschka and in infants and very young children who often have very large tumors at presentation. Most commonly, residual tumor is left behind on the floor of the fourth ventricle or laterally at the cerebellopontine angle where tumor protruding through the foramen of Luschka encircles lower cranial nerves and vessels. Since residual disease is associated with a much worse outcome, "second-look" surgery should be considered, if feasible, either after the realignment of structures that takes place following resection of an initially bulky tumor or after chemotherapy.

Postoperative radiotherapy is the standard of care for all children with ependymoma. Some have questioned the need for such treatment for patients who have undergone complete resection (115,182,190). However, recent reports (224) as well as evidence from studies in infants in which the goal was to delay or avoid altogether radiotherapy (53,93,276) suggest that such a strategy results in worse disease-free and perhaps also overall survival and therefore can be considered acceptable only for (a) patients with ependymoma of the spinal cord who have undergone complete resection for whom disease-free survival in contemporary series approaches 100% (88,105,148,150) and (b) selected patients with supratentorial ependymoma, such as those with intraventricular tumors or with extraventricular tumors that are solid and located in noneloquent areas and can be resected with a wider margin (190).

For the majority of patients who will need postoperative radiotherapy, there are important questions with respect to the optimal radiotherapy target volume, dose, and dose-fractionation schedule. In the past, CSI was recommended for treatment of infratentorial ependymoma. However, there is no evidence that the use of CSI affects outcome, and because the predominant pattern of failure is local, local radiotherapy is now accepted as the standard of care (163,265), using a GTV that is a composite of the tumor bed, based on preoperative imaging, taking into account any anatomic changes that have resulted from the surgery, and including any macroscopic residual disease, with a margin for the CTV of 1 cm (163,170). Results are excellent with event-free survival rates at 3 years as high as 90% (170). Although controversial, the literature provides evidence for improved tumor control with radiotherapy doses >45 to 50 Gy (265). Although such doses are the maximum possible for spinal ependymomas, the current standard is a dose of at least 54 to 55 Gy for lesions in the brain. However, because failure most often occurs at the site of macroscopic residual disease, even higher doses may be desirable. HFRT has been explored in ependymoma for this reason. Pilot data from a POG study (POG 9132) that used a dose of 69.6 Gy given in 58 fractions over 6 weeks (105) and from the Children's Hospital of Philadelphia in which the majority of patients received HFRT to a mean dose of 70.7 Gy (183) were promising, but a larger study of the Italian Pediatric Oncology Group showed no evidence of benefit for HFRT (157). Moreover, it is now feasible using stereotactic radiosurgery (2) or conformal treatment techniques (170) to safely deliver higher doses, and the current COG study uses 59.4 Gy for all patients over 18 months of age.

The role of chemotherapy in ependymoma remains to be defined. Response rates to chemotherapy are quite poor, and there is little evidence that chemotherapy is effective in this type tumor (24,56,93). Nonetheless, there is some rationale to continue to investigate chemotherapy in two situations. In infants and very young children chemotherapy has been used because of the desire to delay or even avoid altogether radiotherapy (53,93). However, because prolonged use of chemotherapy and delay to radiotherapy of more than 1 year may be associated with a worse survival (53), the current COG protocol uses radiotherapy for all children older than 12 months. In patients with macroscopic residual disease, chemotherapy has been justified because of the poor prognosis; it may in addition facilitate complete resection of residual disease at "second-look" surgery, and the current North American and Société Internationale d'Oncologie Pédiatrique (SIOP) trials are both testing chemotherapy in this setting.

Anaplastic Ependymomas

By definition, an anaplastic ependymoma is a malignant glioma of ependymal origin. Anaplastic ependymomas exhibit high mitotic activity, often accompanied by microvascular proliferation and pseudopalisading necrosis. There are no histopathologic features that can reliably differentiate anaplastic ependymomas from the more slowly growing and more favorable ependymomas, which probably explains the controversy in the literature with respect to the prognostic significance of tumor grade (67,82,133,222). Proliferation markers such as MIB-I may prove to be more useful in this regard.

Management of anaplastic ependymoma begins with maximum surgical resection consistent with a good neurologic outcome and a work-up consisting of a gadolinium-enhanced MRI of the spinal axis and CSF cytology to rule out leptomeningeal seeding, which is only slightly more frequent than in ependymoma. Postoperatively all patients receive radiotherapy and chemotherapy. The sequence depends on the age of the child, with younger children receiving chemotherapy first to delay the use of radiotherapy.

The radiotherapy target volume is more controversial than for ependymoma. CSI has been the standard of care, but several institutional studies, a careful retrospective review, and prospective studies by the POG all suggest that there is no survival advantage for CSI as compared with local fields (87,164,237,269,271,277). Thus, local treatment consisting of the tumor bed and any macroscopic residual disease with a margin for the CTV of 1.5 cm is used for patients with localized disease; only patients with leptomeningeal seeding at diagnosis receive CSI. As for ependymomas, the dose should be 54 to 55 Gy, with a boost to macroscopic residual disease, if feasible, to 59 to 60 Gy.

In contemporary series, disease-free survival for patients with anaplastic ependymoma is still only in the 20% to 45% range at 3 to 5 years (147,170,271). As for ependymomas, the prognosis is significantly better for patients in whom complete resection has been achieved than for those with residual disease (269,271). Patients with leptomeningeal dissemination at diagnosis fare extremely poorly despite aggressive treatment with craniospinal radiotherapy and systemic chemotherapy.

Myxopapillary Ependymoma

Myxopapillary ependymomas are slowly growing lesions almost always located in the conus-filum terminale region of the spinal cord. They are the most common spinal cord tumor in this location. They usually present with back pain that may be of long duration. On imaging, myxopapillary ependymomas are well circumscribed and usually enhance brightly with contrast material.

Surgical resection is the treatment of choice. If the tumor is contained within the filum, complete resection is usually possible after mobilization of the filum. If the tumor is in continuity with the conus, resection is more difficult and more likely to result in significant neurologic sequelae so that there frequently will be macroscopic residual tumor. If the tumor is not resected *en bloc* or if there is macroscopic residual tumor, postoperative radiotherapy should be used since outcome appears to be significantly worse in these situations (62,217). The radiother-

apy target volume is local (macroscopic disease plus a margin cephalad and caudad of 1.5 cm for the CTV) and the dose, 50.4 Gy. Leptomeningeal seeding at diagnosis may not be as uncommon as previously believed nor the prognosis in this situation as bleak (61,169), and patients should therefore be treated with curative intent with CSI followed by a boost to the primary site.

Choroid Plexus Tumors

Choroid plexus tumors arise from the epithelium of the choroid plexus of the cerebral ventricles. The WHO classification lists two different entities: choroid plexus papilloma (WHO grade I) and choroid plexus carcinoma (WHO grade III).

Choroid plexus tumors account for only 2% to 4% of all brain tumors that occur in children, but as many as 20% of those seen in the first year of life. Choroid plexus papillomas, which account for two thirds or more of choroid plexus tumors in children, are composed of delicate fibrovascular connective tissue fronds covered by a single layer of uniform cuboidal columnar epithelial cells with round or oval basally situated monomorphic nuclei. In contrast, choroid plexus carcinomas are solid tumors that show frank evidence of malignancy including nuclear pleomorphism, frequent mitoses, high nucleus/cytoplasm ratio, increased cell density, blurring of the papillary pattern with poorly structured sheets of tumor cells, necrotic areas, and brain invasion. The distinction between choroid plexus papilloma and choroid plexus carcinoma is not always clear because some tumors show only one or a few histologic features of malignancy. Such tumors have been called atypical choroid plexus papillomas, but clear diagnostic criteria for such an entity have not been established (133).

In children, most choroid plexus tumors arise in the lateral ventricles causing obstruction to CSF flow. Infants commonly present with increasing head circumference. Older children present with symptoms and signs of raised intracranial pressure. On neuroimaging, choroid plexus tumors are usually hyperdense, contrast-enhancing masses. Even papillomas seed into the CSF space, and work-up for both benign and malignant lesions should include a gadolinium-enhanced MRI of the spinal axis and CSF cytology.

Management of Choroid Plexus Tumors

Surgery is the treatment of choice for choroid plexus papillomas both for the primary lesion and for microscopic metastatic deposits, if feasible. Blood loss may be considerable, however, and staged procedures may be necessary to obtain maximal resection. Following complete resection, outcome is excellent with survival rates that approach 100% (140,194). The role of radiotherapy following incomplete resection is unclear; not all patients will progress (140) so that close follow-up would seem reasonable, with consideration of a second surgical procedure, if feasible, and/or radiotherapy at the time of progression.

Results are much less satisfactory for patients with choroid plexus carcinomas. Surgery is an important component of treatment. Results are best for patients who have undergone complete surgical resection (20,40,66,174,189,194,197,282,283,284). The need for adjuvant therapy in this situation is not clearly established. In one series of pooled data, survival was significantly better when radiotherapy had been given postoperatively, despite a probable bias toward the use of radiotherapy in patients considered to have more unfavorable disease (283,284). Others have reported excellent results following complete resection, in some cases with chemotherapy, but without radiotherapy (20,66,189,197). In contrast, patients who have residual disease fare very poorly. Postoperative radiotherapy appears to be useful (66,282), but the desire to avoid radiotherapy in infants and very young children may mean that chemotherapy is used instead, despite less convincing evidence of efficacy (20,51,84).

An international effort is under way to evaluate prospectively the value of radiotherapy and chemotherapy in choroid plexus tumors, including atypical lesions. In this study, local fields are recommended for patients with choroid plexus papillomas with postoperative residual (including metastatic sites) as well as for patients with atypical lesions or choroid plexus carcinomas without evidence of leptomeningeal seeding. Patients with atypical lesions or choroid plexus carcinomas with leptomeningeal seeding receive craniospinal radiotherapy. Radiotherapy is delivered following two cycles of chemotherapy with the exception of infants and very young children in whom radiotherapy is delayed until age 3 years.

Neuronal and Mixed Neuronal-Glial Tumors

Neuronal and mixed neuronal-glial tumors are uncommon tumors that are characterized by the presence of both neuronal and glial elements in variable amount. They include entities such as desmoplastic infantile astrocytoma and dysembryoplastic neuroepithelial tumor. Most will be cured by surgery, but radiotherapy may be indicated in two tumor types: ganglioglioma and anaplastic ganglioglioma, and central neurocytoma.

Ganglioglioma and Anaplastic Ganglioglioma

Gangliogliomas are well-differentiated, slowly growing tumors composed of mature ganglion cells in combination with neoplastic glial cells WHO grade I or II. Tumors in which the glial component shows anaplastic features (WHO grade III) are called anaplastic gangliogliomas.

Although these tumors can arise anywhere within the CNS, most in children arise in the temporal region and typically present with seizures. Surgery is the treatment of choice. When resection is complete, the probability of long-term tumor control in patients with ganglioglioma is excellent (144,153). The indications for radiotherapy would be as for patients with LGA, that is, for patients with progressive or recurrent disease that is not resectable, and likewise for the radiotherapy target volume and dose. The significance of a high proliferation index or of the presence of anaplasia in patients with ganglioglioma has been controversial. Although it seems clear that the risk of recurrence is higher in patients with these features (144,153,226), the indications for postoperative radiotherapy remain undefined except for patients with anaplastic gangliogliomas who have undergone less than complete resection for whom the use of radiotherapy has been shown to result in improved progression-free survival (246).

Central Neurocytoma

Central neurocytoma is a neoplasm composed of uniform round cells with neuronal differentiation that arises in the lateral or third ventricles, typically the former, that is seen predominantly in adolescents and young adults. Patients usually present with symptoms and signs of raised intracranial pressure. Surgery is the treatment of choice, and when complete resection is achieved, long-term tumor control is excellent without adjuvant treatment (210). Patients in whom complete resection cannot be achieved, as well as those with tumors with atypical histology or an MIB-1 labeling index >3%, fare less well and postoperative radiotherapy should be considered in these situations. Although a dose of 50 Gy appears adequate for patients with typical neurocytomas (209), there is evidence of improved tumor control

at doses of at least 54 Gy in patients with atypical neurocytoma (208).

Pineal Parenchymal Tumors

Pineal region tumors account for 2% to 8% of intracranial tumors in children. Approximately half are germ-cell tumors, one-fourth to one-third are pineal parenchymal tumors, and most of the remainder are astrocytic tumors.

Pineal parenchymal tumors are derived from pinocytes, which are cells with photosensory and neuroendocrine functions, or their embryonal precursors. They range from tumors composed of mature elements to ones consisting of primitive cells. Intermediate degrees of differentiation are seen, as are tumors that are biphasic with fully differentiated as well as immature cells. According to the WHO classification, the following entities can be distinguished: pineoblastoma (WHO grade IV), pineocytoma (WHO grade II), and pineal parenchymal tumor of intermediate differentiation.

Pineoblastoma

Pineoblastoma is a highly malignant primitive embryonal tumor composed of patternless sheets of densely packed small cells with round to irregular nuclei and scant cytoplasm. Pineocytomatous rosettes are lacking, but Homer-Wright and Flexner-Wintersteiner rosettes may be seen.

Pineoblastomas most frequently affect infants and young children, who typically present with an enlarged head circumference or symptoms and signs of short duration of raised intracranial pressure. On MRI, pineoblastomas are usually multilobulated and often enhance heterogeneously, with areas of necrosis and/or hemorrhage. Infiltration of surrounding structures is common. Leptomeningeal spread is seen in as many as 50% of patients at diagnosis.

Surgery for lesions in the pineal region is particularly delicate, and complete resection is often not possible. Postoperatively, older children are treated with CSI and chemotherapy, as for medulloblastoma and supratentorial primitive neuroectodermal tumor (S-PNETs) (see below). The outcome of treatment in this age group is reasonably satisfactory, with 5-year survival in the 50% to 70% range (42,119,239). However, infants who are treated with chemotherapy without radiotherapy fare extremely poorly; in prospective studies of POG and CCG, all patients developed progressive disease within the first 11 months (POG) and 1.2 years (CCG) and all patients died of the disease (50,85). Thus, more aggressive treatment, possibly consisting of chemotherapy dose intensification and/or high-dose chemotherapy with stem cell rescue, is necessary. The other group of patients with an extremely poor prognosis comprises patients with familial bilateral retinoblastoma with pineoblastoma (trilateral retinoblastoma), most of whom die less than a year following diagnosis.

Pineocytoma

Pineocytoma is a slow-growing tumor composed of small uniform mature cells resembling pinocytes, with occasional large pineocytomatous rosettes. They account for approximately half of pineal parenchymal tumors and in childhood most commonly occur in the teenage years. Patients typically present with symptoms and signs of raised intracranial pressure. Some will have symptoms of upper mesencephalic tegmental dysfunction (Parinaud's syndrome), consisting of limitation of upward gaze, lid retraction, retraction nystagmus, and pupils that react more poorly to light than to accommodation. On MRI, pineocytomas are usually spherical, well-circumscribed masses, hypointense on T1- and hyperintense on T2-weighted images, with homogeneous contrast enhancement. Leptomeningeal spread has been described in pineocytoma (45), but it is probable that the explanation for this lies in sampling error. With better imaging and more extensive surgery and with more complete histologic evaluation of the tumor it seems that leptomeningeal spread can be considered to be an uncommon event (239).

Treatment consists of surgical resection where feasible using either an occipital transtentorial or an infratentorial supracerebellar approach. If complete or subtotal resection is accomplished, the outcome is probably quite favorable even without any adjuvant treatment (123). Following lesser degrees of resection, postoperative radiotherapy usually is recommended using local fields consisting of macroscopic residual disease, with a margin of 1 to 1.5 cm and a dose of 50 to 55 Gy over 6 weeks. The outcome following such treatment appears to be very good; in one study, no patient developed leptomeningeal spread and 5-year survival was 86% (238).

Pineal Parenchymal Tumor of Intermediate Differentiation

Pineal parenchymal tumors of intermediate differentiation are monomorphous tumors characterized by moderately high cellularity, mild nuclear atypia, occasional mitoses, and the absence of large pineocytomatous rosettes. They are rare tumors, accounting for only 10% of pineal parenchymal tumors, and optimal management remains to be defined. In one series, three patients treated with surgery alone survived free of disease (123). At the other extreme, another group considers these to be tumors "with seeding potential" and recommends postoperative treatment with CSI as for pineoblastomas (239).

⠿ | Embryonal Tumors

Embryonal tumors as a group are the second most common type of CNS tumor in the pediatric age group. There is ongoing controversy with regard to their cell(s) of origin. Most fall into the category of PNETs—undifferentiated round cell tumors with divergent patterns of differentiation as follows:

- Ependymoblastoma,
- Medulloblastoma,
  - Desmoplastic medulloblastoma
  - Large cell medulloblastoma
- Supratentorial PNET.

Two tumor types with distinctly different histologies that appear to evolve by different genetic pathways also are included in the category of embryonal tumors:

- Medulloepithelioma,
- Atypical teratoid/rhabdoid tumor.

Medulloblastoma

Medulloblastoma accounts for 15% to 20% of all CNS tumors in the pediatric age group. The median age at presentation is 6 years. In the majority of cases the tumor arises in the cerebellar vermis and projects into the fourth ventricle. Patients typically present with symptoms and signs of raised intracranial pressure, that is, headache and morning vomiting. On CT and MRI medulloblastomas appear as solid masses that enhance usually fairly homogeneously with contrast material (Fig. 82.9). The frequency of spinal seeding at diagnosis is approximately 30% to 35%, and investigation at diagnosis must include a gadolinium-enhanced MRI of the spinal axis and CSF cytology. The former should be obtained whenever possible preoperatively or else at least 2 to 3 weeks postoperatively to avoid misinterpretation resulting from artifactual changes seen in the later postoperative period. CSF cytology, which should be obtained by lumbar puncture, often cannot be obtained preoperatively because of the presence of raised intracranial pressure and more commonly is obtained at approximately 3 weeks postoperatively, again to avoid the risk of misinterpretation of the findings in the early postoperative period. Medulloblastoma is one of the few CNS tumors to spread outside the CNS (to lymph nodes, bone), although this is an uncommon event.

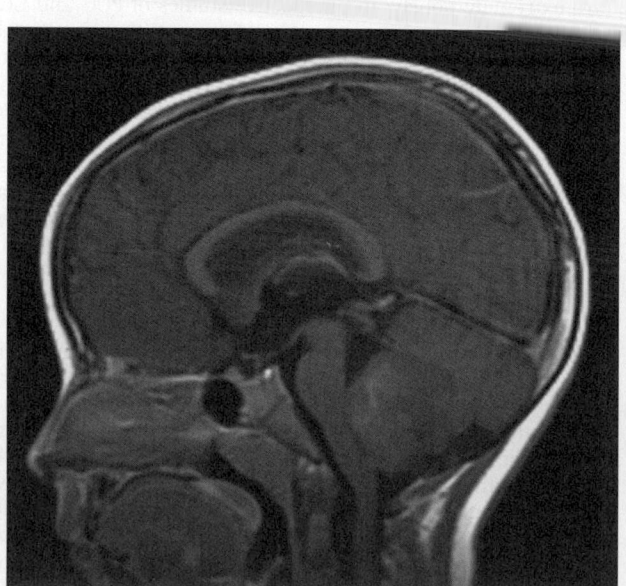
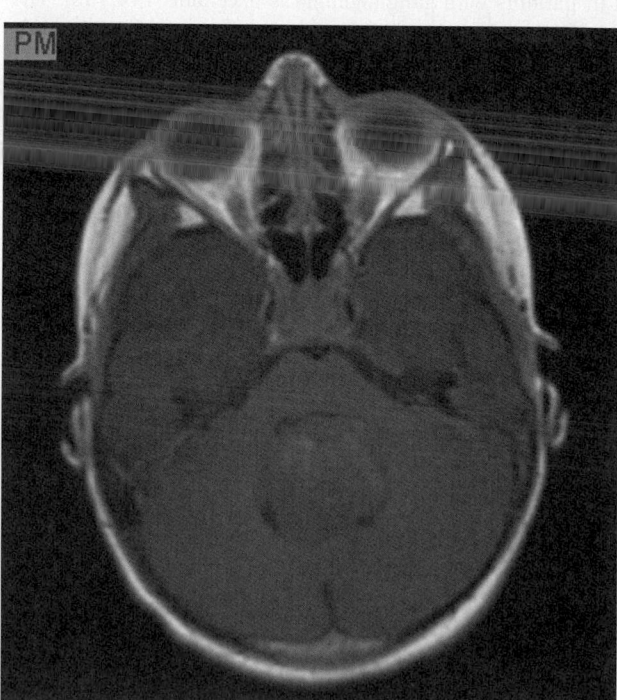

FIGURE 82.9. Sagittal (**A**) and axial (**B**) magnetic resonance images of a medulloblastoma in a 3-year-old girl. Note the typical midline location of the tumor that is causing ventricular outlet obstruction with dilatation of the third and lateral ventricles.

Table 82.2	**CHANG STAGING SYSTEM FOR METASTASES IN PATIENTS WITH MEDULLOBLASTOMA**
M0	No metastases
M1	Tumor cells found in cerebrospinal fluid
M2	Gross nodular seeding in the cerebellar, cerebral subarachnoid space, or in the third or lateral ventricles
M3	Gross nodular seeding in the spinal subarachnoid space
M4	Metastases outside the central nervous system

Modified from Chang CH, Housepian EM, Herbert C, Jr. An operative staging system and a megavoltage radiotherapeutic technic for cerebellar medulloblastomas. *Radiology* 1969;93:1351–1359.

Factors that correlate with outcome include age at diagnosis, the presence or absence of leptomeningeal spread at diagnosis, and the completeness of the surgical resection. Patients are allocated to one of two risk categories: standard and high risk. Those who have undergone complete or subtotal resection with <1.5 cm^2 of residual tumor and no evidence of CSF dissemination (M0) (37) (Table 82.2) are considered to have "standard-risk" disease, whereas patients who have larger volume residual tumor and those with evidence of CSF dissemination at diagnosis are characterized as "high risk." With contemporary neurosurgical techniques, complete or near-total resection is accomplished in approximately 80% of cases. Overall, two thirds of patients will be "standard risk" and one third will be "high risk."

Management of Standard-Risk Medulloblastoma

Until relatively recently, the standard of care for patients older than 3 years with standard-risk disease consisted of postoperative radiotherapy to the craniospinal axis to a dose of 35 to 36 Gy followed by a boost to the whole posterior fossa to a total dose of 54 to 55.8 Gy. In multi-institution studies, such treatment results in long-term event-free survival in 60% to 65% of patients (13,262,267). Sequelae of treatment include hormonal deficits, decreased bone growth, and neurocognitive deficits that correlate with the age of the child and the radiation dose (177).

Several treatment strategies designed to reduce the morbidity associated with the use of radiotherapy have been tested. An attempt by the French cooperative group Société Française d' Oncologie Pédiatrique (SFOP) to reduce the radiotherapy target volume to avoid supratentorial radiation produced disastrous results (23), and CSI remains the standard of care. The use of reduced-dose CSI (23.4 Gy) alone (without chemotherapy) in the North American intergroup study (CCG-923/POG 8631) resulted in a significantly increased risk of isolated neuraxis failure and an event-free survival at 5 and 8 years of only 52% (267). HFRT may be more promising. In a SFOP pilot study that tested HFRT to a CSI dose of 36 Gy without chemotherapy, early toxicity was reduced and progression-free survival at 3 years was 81% (35). HFRT is being tested in the current European SIOP PNET-4 study in which patients are randomized to HFRT or conventional radiotherapy.

An alternative strategy consists of reduced-dose CSI followed by a boost to the posterior fossa to a total dose of 55.8 Gy in combination with systemic chemotherapy. Progression-free survival was 79% (±7%) at 5 years in a CCG pilot study that used reduced-dose (23.4 Gy) CSI in combination with weekly vincristine, followed by adjuvant systemic chemotherapy consisting of vincristine 1.5 mg/m^2, CCNU 75 mg/m^2, and cisplatin 75 mg/m^2 (188). In the joint CCG/POG phase III randomized study (A9961) that followed, this regimen was compared to a regimen in which the CCNU was replaced by cyclophosphamide. Event-free survival at 4 years was approximately 85% in both arms (Packer, personal communication, May 2006), and such an ap-

proach is now considered to be the standard of care for children with standard-risk medulloblastoma in North America. Current studies are testing the safety of an even lower dose of CSI (18 Gy) in children aged 3 to 8 years and of a reduced-volume posterior fossa boost in children of all ages (see below).

Management of High-Risk Medulloblastoma

Patients with residual disease >1.5 cm^2 and/or those with evidence of leptomeningeal seeding (M+) are considered to have high-risk disease. This is the group of patients in which the use of chemotherapy was shown in the prospective randomized phase III studies conducted in the 1970s to result in significant improvement in disease-free survival (57,258). Consequently, all such patients receive chemotherapy and research efforts since then have largely focused on the chemotherapy regimens, including changes in scheduling in relation to radiotherapy and in doses and routes of delivery of chemotherapy (78,81,96,135,141,176,254,264,286). Some have used higher dose CSI or altered radiotherapy fractionation schedules (7).

It is important to note that the definition of risk factors has evolved considerably over the past two decades, making comparison of published data quite problematic. Better postoperative imaging and more complete staging as well as identification of unfavorable pathological features (e.g., large cell anaplastic histology) has led to transfer of patients from the standard-risk to the high-risk category, which may partly explain the improving results for both standard-risk and high-risk disease. The category of high-risk disease is heterogeneous and includes more favorable subsets such as patients with postoperative residual disease without leptomeningeal spread and even those with M1 disease, for whom it may be appropriate to consider a treatment approach different from that for patients with M2–3 disease. For example, for patients with residual disease, M0, it would be logical to consider using a radiotherapy dose to residual disease in the posterior fossa higher than the standard 55.8 Gy, and this may be feasible using stereotactic radiotherapy or 3D conformal techniques. Patients with M1 disease may do well using a standard CSI dose of 35 to 36 Gy; in the POG 9031 study, event-free survival at 5 years was 65% (Tarbell, personal communication, June 2006). In contrast, results for patients with M2–3 disease remain quite poor, although the use of a higher radiotherapy dose (40 Gy CSI plus a boost of 5 Gy to macroscopic disease) produced excellent early results in POG 9031, approaching those for patients with less advanced disease. The hyperfractionated accelerated radiotherapy (HART) regimen under investigation by the U.K. group may prove to be an equally efficacious and safer way to deliver high dose CSI.

Preradiotherapy chemotherapy may also be of interest in this group of patients. Response to preradiotherapy chemotherapy appears to correlate with outcome (141), so the use of preradiotherapy chemotherapy may allow identification of patients who do not respond and who might benefit from more aggressive chemotherapy, such as high-dose chemotherapy with stem cell rescue in combination with conventional radiotherapy, HFRT, or HART.

Management of Medulloblastoma in Infants

Medulloblastoma accounts for 20% to 40% of all CNS tumors in infants and carries a worse prognosis than in older children. The explanation for this is likely multifactorial. The rate of complete resection is lower in this age group, and the frequency of leptomeningeal seeding at diagnosis is higher (as much as 50%), but as well many patients do not receive optimal treatment (231). Because of the significant risks with respect to neurocognitive function associated with the use of radiotherapy in infants and very young children, chemotherapy has been used in an attempt to either delay or avoid radiotherapy altogether. Infants with M0 disease who have undergone total resection may do well with chemotherapy alone, with a 5-year overall survival of 69% in the first POG infant study (51) and of 93% in the German study (227), although it is noteworthy that treatment in the latter included intraventricular methotrexate for which there are also concerns about the risk of neurocognitive sequelae. In other studies results were less satisfactory, in some because of the need for aggressive salvage regimens that were associated with significant long-term sequelae (94). In fact, evidence suggests that radiotherapy is an important component of treatment (83), and because in the North American studies recurrences were generally early (within 6 months) and local (51,83,114), the current North American study uses early radiotherapy to a limited treatment volume consisting of the tumor bed plus a margin for the CTV of 1 cm for patients without leptomeningeal seeding. Infants with M2–3 disease fare poorly and require more aggressive treatment such as high-dose chemotherapy with stem cell rescue and/or chemotherapy given using alternative routes of administration, such as intrathecal or intraventricular, with or without radiotherapy.

Radiotherapy for Medulloblastoma

Craniospinal radiotherapy is one of the more complex techniques delivered in most radiotherapy departments. The CTV for CSI has an irregular shape that consists of the whole of the brain and spinal cord and overlying meninges. The majority of centers use techniques in which the lower borders of lateral whole-brain fields are matched to the cephalad border of a posterior spine field. Most use a "moving junction" between the brain and spine fields to minimize the risk of underdose or overdose in the cervical spinal cord (131,275). Compensators may be needed to achieve dose homogeneity throughout the target volume.

Patient Positioning and Immobilization

Patients have traditionally received CSI in the prone position, but modern technology allows safe treatment in the supine position that in general is more comfortable and, if anesthesia is required, allows better control of the airway. In either case, immobilization is essential and involves the use of a head shell or full-body immobilization. Careful attention to positioning at the time of simulation is critical to minimize or even eliminate the risk of certain long-term effects. For example, using neck extension together with careful selection of the level for the junction of the brain and spine fields it is possible to avoid including the dentition in the exit from the superior aspect of the spinal field, and thus any damage to developing teeth that may result in stunted tooth growth, impaction, incomplete calcification, delayed development, and caries.

Target Volume Definition

Careful attention to coverage of the entire target volume is critical. In the SFOP M-7 protocol, 50% of relapses could be correlated with targeting deviations. In the subsequent studies (MSFOP-93 and MSFOP-98) the relapse rate was 17% in patients who had inadequate coverage of only one part of the CTV (a typical example being the cribriform plate), 28% for patients who had inadequate coverage at two sites, and 67% for patients who had inadequate coverage at three or more sites (33,34). In a SFOP pilot study that tested reduced-dose CSI for standard-risk disease, overall survival at 5 years was significantly worse for patients with inadequate coverage at two or more sites as compared with no or only one major deviation (54.4% vs. 79.3%) (186). In the most recent North American and French cooperative group studies, the frequency of major deviations is still approximately 30%.

CT simulation is invaluable for target volume definition for patients with medulloblastoma. Adequate coverage of the CTV

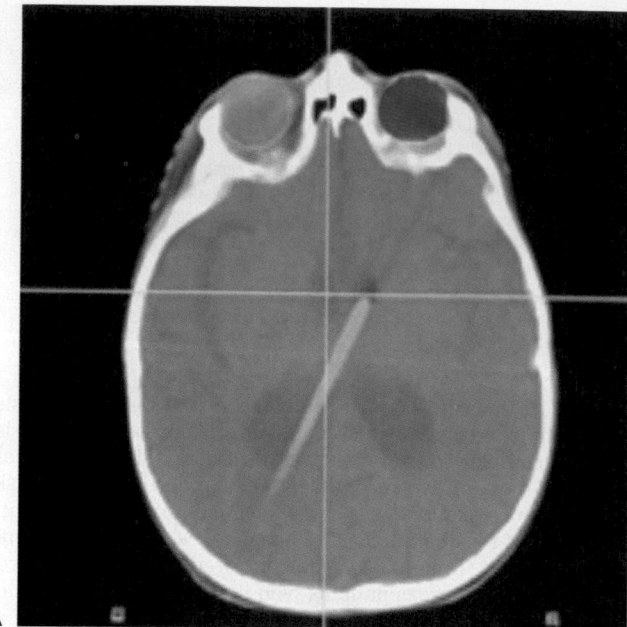

A

	Margin to block edge 0mm	Margin to block edge 5mm	Margin to block edge 7mm	Margin to block edge 10mm
Minimum dose to cribriform plate	56.7%	91.2%	96.1%	98.3%
Maximum dose to lens	36.8%	80.5%	90.7%	98.6%

B

FIGURE 82.10. The use of computed tomography (CT) simulation is superior to conventional radiographs for determination of the clinical target volume for craniospinal irradiation and ensures coverage of the meninges in the subfrontal region (**A**). Dosimetric evaluation for a patient treated with 6 MV photons shows that, as is usually the case, the minimum margin to block edge is 7 mm, which precludes significant sparing of the lens (**B**).

in the subfrontal region at the cribriform plate is much more easily ensured than with conventional radiographs (97). Traditionally, blocks have been used in the lateral fields to shield not only the facial structures and teeth but also the lens to minimize the risk of cataract. However, it is impossible to adequately irradiate the cribriform plate and shield the lenses in most children (Fig. 82.10). With current cataract surgical techniques, it is preferable to cover the target volume, keeping shielding of the lenses a secondary objective.

CT simulation is helpful, too, in identifying the lateral aspect of CTV for the spine field that includes the extensions of the meninges along the nerve roots to the lateral aspects of the spinal ganglia. The field, which must be wide enough to encompass the intervertebral foramina in the lumbar region, can be blocked laterally in the dorsal region to avoid unnecessary irradiation of the heart and lungs (Fig. 82.11). In the lumbar region, it is important to avoid an excessively wide field that will result in unnecessary irradiation of the bone marrow and gonads.

MRI is required to determine the lower limit of CTV for the spine field. Traditionally the lower border of the spine field was placed at the lower border of the second sacral vertebra, but it is well documented that the lower border of the thecal sac can be as high as L5 or as low as S3. It is below S2 in 7% of children (104). In the interest of both CTV coverage and normal tissue sparing it is important that the lower border be individualized according to the MRI findings.

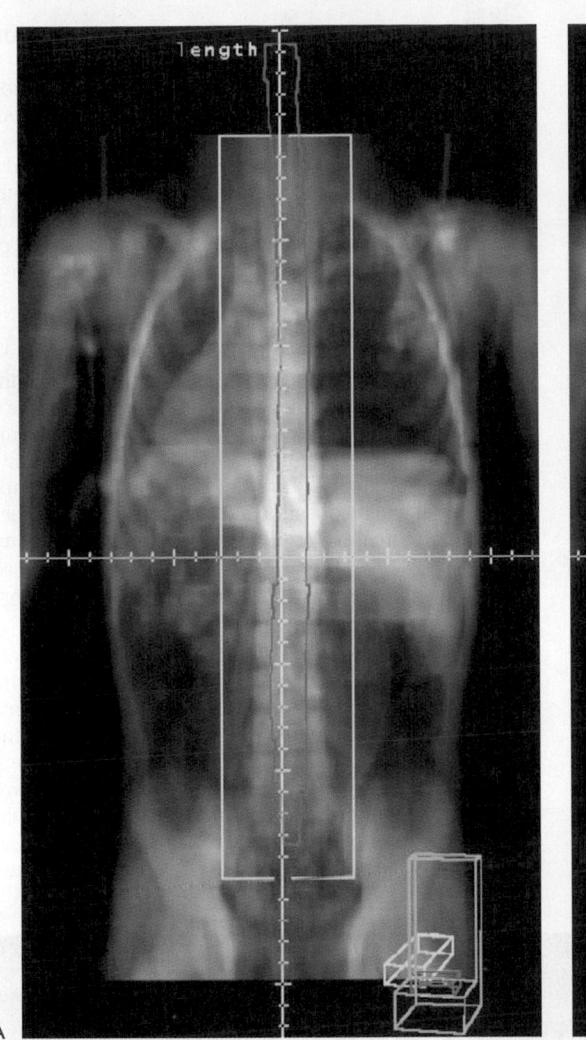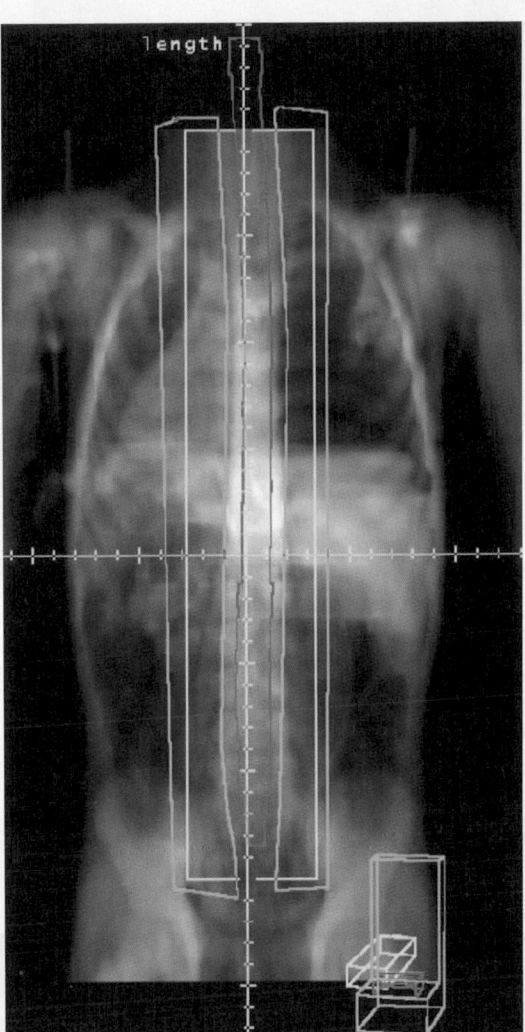

A   B

FIGURE 82.11. A: The use of computed tomography simulation with contouring of the cord and overlying meninges that extend laterally to the lateral aspect of the spinal ganglia results in a field width that is narrower than one based on bony anatomy. **B:** The addition of shielding reduces even further the volume of normal tissues included in the treated volume.

CT simulation with CT–MRI coregistration is required for accurate determination of the target volume for the posterior fossa boost, both for definition of the target volume and for contouring of critical normal structures such as the cochlea, pituitary/hypothalamus, and brain that will allow accurate estimation of the dose to these structures.

Treatment Planning and Delivery

There are many issues that need to be addressed in designing a CSI technique (Table 82.3). Many of the different solutions (275) add further complexity. Using modern tools for treatment planning and delivery it is possible to greatly simplify the technique and substantially reduce planning and delivery times. One such technique is shown in Fig. 82.12 (192). In general, photons in the 6 to 10 MV range provide satisfactory coverage of the PTV. A variation of dose along the spinal axis of >10% will require the use of dose compensation that can be achieved using dynamic multileaf collimator (MLC).

Care is required if using electrons to treat the spinal axis. In addition to targeting deviations discussed earlier, outcome in the French studies correlated with the electron-beam energy used to treat the spinal axis. Despite a dose distribution that appeared appropriate, the relapse rate among patients treated with electron-beam energies of <18 MeV was 78% (34). A possible explanation for this is underdosage resulting from inac-

curate corrections for tissue heterogeneity. The use of electrons to treat the spinal axis most often is justified by reduced acute gastrointestinal toxicity. Because available data regarding late effects suggest that there may be little or no advantage to the use of electrons (80), one might question the use of electrons, particularly now with the availability of effective antiemetic medication. Late injury to other organs (i.e., the heart and gonads) is of much greater concern (98,118). Newer treatment planning and delivery methods such as IMRT may allow much improved dosimetry with photons.

The Posterior Fossa Boost

Another issue of current interest in treatment for medulloblastoma is the volume for the posterior fossa boost. Traditionally, the entire posterior fossa has been treated to a total dose of 54 to 55.8 Gy. Using conformal treatment techniques it is possible to reduce the dose to the inner ear, which is important in children who will also be receiving chemotherapy with cisplatin, but there will be little sparing of other structures such as, and most especially, supratentorial brain. Better sparing can be achieved using a reduced target volume for the boost (Fig. 82.13). Fukunaga-Johnson et al. (76) found a low risk of isolated failure outside the tumor bed in the posterior fossa in a cohort of 114 patients, and data from several other centers, as well as a SFOP pilot study that used a conformal boost

Table 82.3	**TECHNICAL CONSIDERATIONS FOR CRANIOSPINAL IRRADIATION**
Problem	**Possible Solutions**
Target volume definition may be difficult using conventional simulation	Use CT simulation with CT-MRI co registration
Prone position uncomfortable, difficult to monitor airway	Supine position preferred
Field matching over cervical spine, risk of over- or underdosage	Angle brain fields Use half beam block for brain fields Use couch rotation or match line wedge
Choice of extended SSD or second field for treatment of spinal axis	Two fields preferred
Inhomogeneity along spinal axis	Use compensator, MLC
Irradiation of normal tissues: Mandible/teeth	Neck extension Care with level of junction
Thyroid	Use lower junction
Heart	Care with width of spine field Use electrons, IMRT, protons
GI tract	Use electrons, IMRT, protons
Gonads	Care with lower limit and width of spine field

GI, gastrointestinal; IMRT, intensity-modulated radiation therapy; MLC, multileaf collimator; SSD, source-skin distance.

limited to the tumor bed, similarly support such an approach (35,49,166,281).

The optimal CTV for a reduced-volume posterior fossa remains to be defined, although it probably consists of a composite of any macroscopic residual tumor and the surgical bed plus a margin of 1 to 1.5 cm. The use of a reduced target volume for the boost offers potentially significant benefits in terms of greater sparing of the cochlea (77), pituitary and hypothalamus, and the temporal lobes. Care is necessary to ensure that doses to structures outside the CNS such as the thyroid gland remain acceptable.

New Treatment Modalities for CSI
A few centers have reported their results using protons for treatment of medulloblastoma. Although protons provide a dose distribution that cannot yet be achieved by the most sophisticated photon beam treatment planning (253), the major disadvantages of proton therapy are the restricted access and high cost. Hopefully, it will be possible in the future, using better dosimetry and IMRT, to achieve equivalent results with photons.

Scheduling of Radiotherapy in Relation to Chemotherapy and Time–Dose Considerations
Delay to radiotherapy may be associated with poorer outcomes and CSI ideally should start within 28 days following surgery. There is evidence, too, that it is important to deliver radiotherapy in a timely fashion, avoiding unnecessary gaps in treatment resulting from machine servicing, holidays, and the like. In the SIOP PNET-3 study event-free and overall survival were significantly worse when the duration of treatment exceeded 50 days as compared with the results for children treated as planned over 45 to 47 days (263). When CSI has to be interrupted for

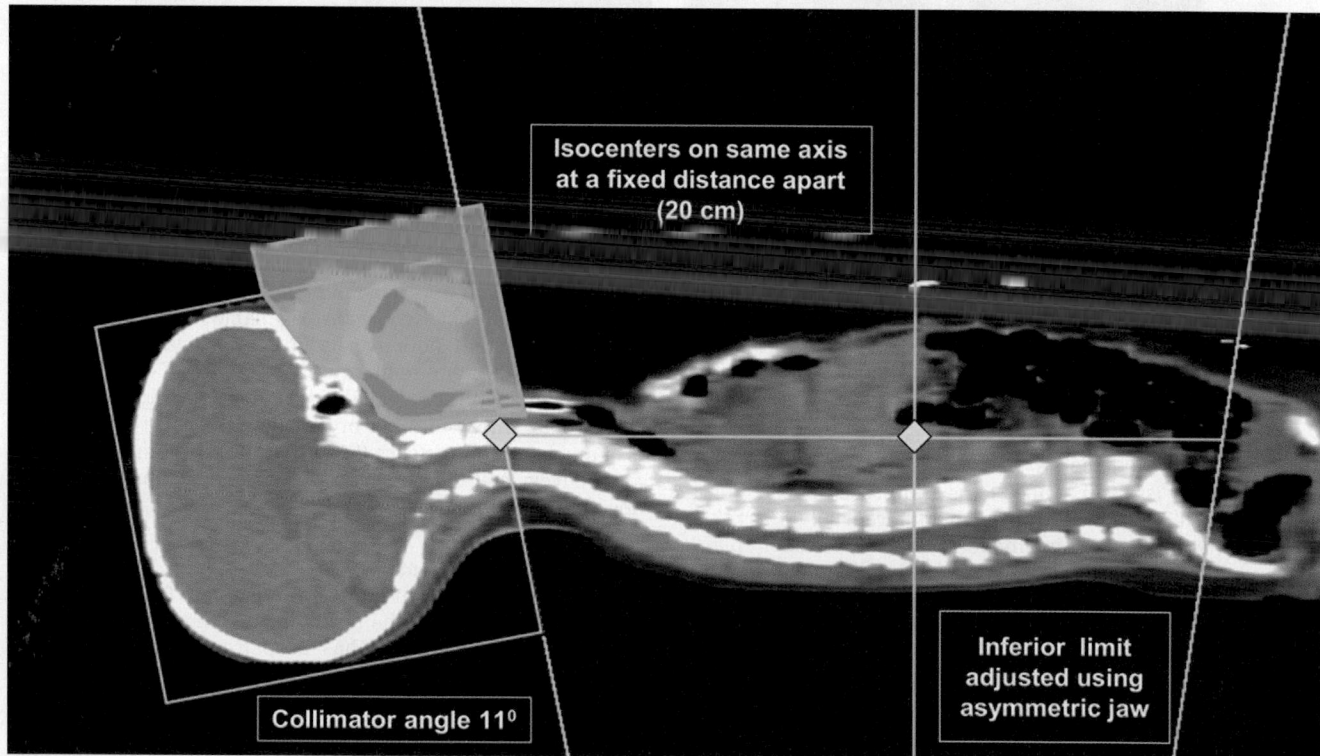

FIGURE 82.12. To cover the clinical target volume for craniospinal irradiation, lateral opposed fields are used to treat the brain and a direct posterior field is used to cover the spinal axis. Correlation with magnetic resonance imaging is necessary to identify the caudal extent of the thecal sac. The field junction, which is over the cervical cord at a level that avoids the inclusion of the teeth in the exit of the spinal field, usually is moved weekly to avoid over- or underdosage. The supine position is more comfortable for the patient and safer if sedation or anesthesia is required. In the technique shown, fixed field parameters are used, which greatly facilitates treatment planning and delivery. (From Parker WA, Freeman CR. A simple technique for craniospinal radiotherapy in the supine position. *Radiother Oncol* 2006;78:217–222, with permission.)

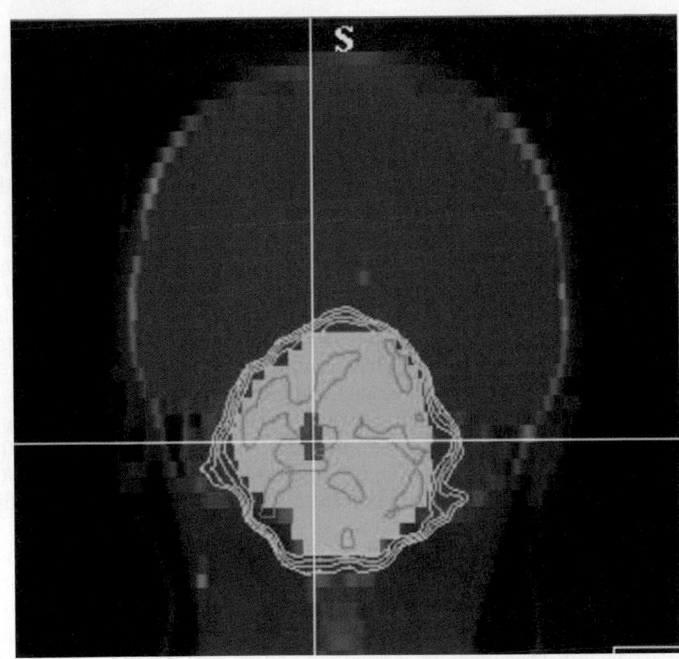 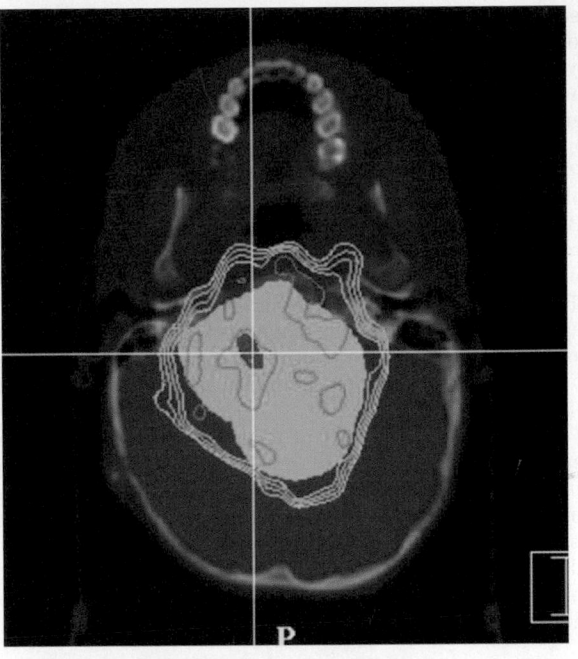

FIGURE 82.13. Coronal (**A**) and axial (**B**) views of a reduced volume posterior fossa boost comprising the tumor bed plus a margin for the CTV of 1 cm that results in greater sparing of supratentorial brain compared with traditional whole posterior fossa treatment.

example, because of hematologic toxicity with a neutrophil count of <0.5 times 10⁹/L, treatment should continue to the posterior fossa boost volume while waiting for the blood counts to recover. Granulocyte colony-stimulating factor may be used to hasten recovery of the counts.

Supratentorial Primitive Neuroectodermal Tumor

By definition, a S-PNET is an embryonal tumor arising in the supratentorial compartment, most commonly in the cerebral hemispheres, composed of undifferentiated or poorly differentiated neuroepithelial cells that have the capacity for or display differentiation along neuronal, astrocytic, ependymal, muscular, or melanocytic lines. Tumors with a distinct neuronal differentiation are termed cerebral neuroblastoma or, if ganglion cells are also present, ganglioneuroblastoma. S-PNET arising in the pineal region (pineoblastoma) was discussed earlier in the section on pineal parenchymal tumors.

S-PNETs account for <5% of all CNS tumors in the pediatric age group. The median age at presentation is 3 years. Patients characteristically present with symptoms and signs of short duration, typically of raised intracranial pressure. Tumors arising in the cerebral hemispheres in particular are often very large at diagnosis (Fig. 82.14). On imaging they are often quite heterogeneous with cystic or necrotic areas and areas of hemorrhage. Leptomeningeal seeding is present at diagnosis in up to 40% of patients, and MRI of the spinal axis and CSF cytology are mandatory prior to treatment.

In the past, the results of treatment of S-PNETs were dismal. Results have been better since treatment has consisted more routinely of postoperative radiotherapy using CSI and chemotherapy, often using the same protocols as for high-risk medulloblastoma. Even so, in contemporary series, progression-free survival is still only in the range of 40% to 55% for patients M0 and 0% to 30% for patients M+ at diagnosis (42,113,193,213,270). The prognosis is worse still for younger patients (51,84,272). With respect to treatment, the importance of the extent of tumor resection is unclear, although there is some evidence that patients who have undergone complete resection fare better than those who have undergone less

extensive resection (5,51,213). The use of radiotherapy has been shown to be associated with a better outcome even in infants and very young children (272), and radiotherapy treatment factors appear to be very important. Patients treated with CSI fare better than those who are treated using reduced volumes (whole brain or local) (46,193,270). In the German experience, other factors such as the timing of radiotherapy (i.e., its

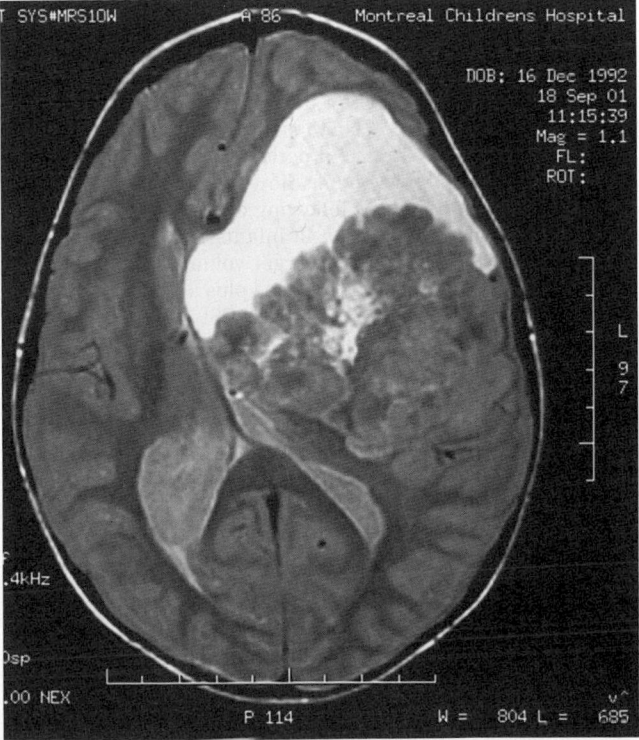

FIGURE 82.14. A supratentorial primitive neuroectodermal tumor in an 8-year-old boy. The tumor, as is often the case, is huge.

use immediately postoperatively rather than following completion of chemotherapy) and the radiotherapy dose (CSI dose >35 Gy and dose to the primary site >54 Gy) also correlated significantly with an improved outcome (270). Even in contemporary series, however, failure at both the primary site and in the leptomeninges is a significant problem: local failure was seen in 42% of patients with M0 disease treated on the CCG 921 protocol, and failure in the leptomeninges as a first site of failure in 43% of M+ patients (113). HFRT and hyperfractionated accelerated radiotherapy have been tested as a means to more safely deliver higher radiotherapy doses. Of five patients treated with HFRT at Duke University, four survived without evidence of disease 4.3 to 8 years following diagnosis (103). Preliminary results from the Italian cooperative group using HART were interpreted as promising with a progression-free survival at 3 years of 54% (158).

For now, the standard of care for children older than 3 years with S-PNETs without leptomeningeal spread consists of maximal surgical resection followed by postoperative radiotherapy (CSI plus a boost to doses similar to those used for high-risk medulloblastoma) followed by chemotherapy. Experimental regimens such as preradiotherapy chemotherapy and high-dose chemotherapy with rescue are used in infants and young children and in patients with M2–3 disease.

Atypical Teratoid/Rhabdoid Tumor

Atypical teratoid/rhabdoid tumor (AT/RT) is an uncommon, highly malignant embryonal tumor unique to childhood. It is composed of rhabdoid cells with or without fields resembling a classical PNET and is diagnosed on the basis of the characteristic molecular findings, namely loss of one copy of chromosome 22 or a deletion or translocation involving the INI1 gene that maps to chromosome band 22q11.2. AT/RT can arise at any location within the CNS, although in children it most commonly arises in the posterior fossa (cerebellopontine angle and/or brainstem).

In the past AT/RT often was misdiagnosed as medulloblastoma and treated as such, but outcome was very poor and the majority of patients died within 1 year of diagnosis (28,225). It is important, therefore, to identify AT/RT as a separate entity and to administer aggressive multimodality therapy (109). Radiotherapy is an important component of treatment (39,215,266,278), and since leptomeningeal seeding is seen in as many as a third of patients, CSI would be the logical radiotherapy target volume. However, because failure occurs early (within 6 months following diagnosis), radiotherapy should be delivered early even in infants, and this may mean using a modified radiotherapy target volume (i.e., tumor bed and any macroscopic residual disease plus a margin). Children older than 3 years should receive early CSI.

Germ Cell Tumors

Germ cell tumors of the CNS constitute a unique class of rare tumors that are morphologic homologues of germinal neoplasms arising in the gonads and at other extragonadal sites. They include the following entities, although in many cases more than one tumor type is present:

- Germinoma,
- Embryonal carcinoma,
- Yolk sac tumor (endodermal sinus tumor),
- Choriocarcinoma,
- Mature teratoma,
- Immature teratoma,
- Teratoma with malignant transformation,
- Mixed germ cell tumors.

A teratoma is a tumor composed of an admixture of different tissue types representative of ectoderm, endoderm, and mesoderm. A mature teratoma is composed exclusively of fully differentiated tissues, sometimes arranged in such a manner as to resemble normal tissue relationships. Mitoses are absent or rare. An immature teratoma is composed of incompletely differentiated tissues resembling those of the fetus. Mitoses typically are present.

In the West, CNS germ cell tumors are relatively rare, accounting for 3% to 5% of all CNS tumors in the pediatric age group. They are more common in Asia, where they account for as many as 15% to 18% of all CNS tumors occurring in childhood. The peak age incidence is 10 to 12 years. Boys are affected more frequently than girls, with a ratio of approximately 3:1. CNS germ cell tumors arise from primordial germ cells in structures about the third ventricle, with the region of the pineal gland being the most common site of origin, followed by the suprasellar region. Nongerminomatous germ cell tumors (NGGCT) are the most common tumor type in the former area, and germinomas in the latter.

The presenting symptoms and signs depend on the tumor type and the location of the tumor. Tumors in the pineal region cause obstruction to CSF flow at the aqueduct of Sylvius, which results in hydrocephalus, and most patients with tumors in this region present with a relatively short history with symptoms and signs of raised intracranial pressure. Another characteristic presentation of tumors in this region is Parinaud's syndrome as a result of dorsal midbrain compression. In contrast, patients with tumors in the suprasellar region usually present with a longer history initially of neuroendocrine deficits, especially diabetes insipidus, growth failure, and precocious puberty, and only later of visual-field deficits and, later still, of hydrocephalus. On imaging, most germ cell tumors appear as solid masses. Teratomas are more heterogeneous with cysts, areas of calcification, and sometimes fat, whereas choriocarcinomas commonly contain areas of hemorrhage. Bi- or multifocal disease around the third ventricle is seen in approximately 10% of patients with germinomas. Gadolinium-enhanced MRI of the spinal axis is an essential part of the work-up to exclude leptomeningeal dissemination, which is found at diagnosis in <10% of patients with germinomas and 10% to 15% of patients with NGGCT. Measurement of serum and CSF tumor markers is another essential part of the initial work-up. Modest elevation of beta human chorionic gonadotropin (β-hCG (+) < 100 IU/mL) may be seen with pure germinomas that often contain syncytiotrophoblastic cells. Higher levels of β-hCG are more suggestive of a choriocarcinoma. An elevated α-fetoprotein (AFP) is diagnostic of a yolk sac tumor.

In the past, many lesions arising in or about the third ventricle were treated without histologic confirmation of diagnosis. This is no longer considered acceptable practice because the differential diagnosis includes many disparate entities (such as Langerhans cell histiocytosis, astrocytoma, and ependymoma), and all patients should undergo biopsy unless CSF and/or serum markers confirm the presence of a NGGCT (elevated AFP and/or β-hCG >100 IU/mL) or unless a histologic diagnosis is made by other means (e.g., CSF cytology). For tumors in the pineal region with hydrocephalus, the usual surgical approach is an endoscopic third ventriculostomy, which allows access to the lesion for biopsy purposes. Intraventricular lesions have to be biopsied with care, however, because hemorrhage, which is not infrequent, may be difficult to manage endoscopically. A stereotactic approach is also possible, but this may be quite challenging because of the proximity of deep cerebral veins and, moreover, may be suboptimal for diagnosis because of the potential for sampling error. Occasionally complete resection will be possible; this would be a reasonable strategy for patients with NGGCT, particularly for mature teratomas if it can be accomplished without major morbidity because in that situation it would obviate the need for adjuvant treatment.

Germinoma

In the past, standard treatment for patients with germinoma was radiotherapy alone. Results of treatment using craniospinal radiotherapy followed by a boost to the primary site are excellent, with long-term disease-free survival rates of 100% in some series (99,155,171,241,250). For patients with unifocal disease and without leptomeningeal spread, radiotherapy alone to more limited volumes, that is, whole brain (102,184) or whole ventricle (99,248,250), results in a high probability of control in the brain and a low (0% to 5%) risk of failure in the spinal axis. Experience with local radiotherapy (tumor plus a margin) alone generally has been less satisfactory (10,102,184,249), although some have reported excellent results (248). Because of the success of treatment with chemotherapy for analogous tumors outside the CNS and a desire to reduce the risk of morbidity associated with radiotherapy, chemotherapy has been considered another option either alone or in combination with reduced volume and/or dose radiotherapy. Several studies have shown clearly that the former, that is, the use of chemotherapy alone, is not acceptable. Only 40% to 50% of patients remain disease free, and although salvage using further chemotherapy together with radiotherapy is possible in most cases and overall survival is high, this is achieved at the expense of considerable toxicity (16,125,160). In contrast, a combined approach using platinum-based chemotherapy followed by reduced-volume, reduced-dose radiotherapy is a very attractive option that is being investigated by many groups, with disease-free survival rates in the 90% to 96% range (9,22,160,234).

There are, therefore, a number of reasonable options for patients with unifocal germinoma without evidence of leptomeningeal dissemination. These include craniospinal radiotherapy, limited volume (whole-ventricle) radiotherapy alone, and chemotherapy followed by whole ventricle or local radiotherapy. Given that the best results in terms of tumor control are seen following CSI, the decision to use other approaches has to be based on other considerations. Whole ventricle irradiation alone may be acceptable for a patient with a unifocal lesion with no evidence of leptomeningeal dissemination. In children younger than the median age of presentation (i.e., younger than 10 to 12 years of age), the risk of neurocognitive and neuroendocrine sequelae may justify a combined-modality approach of chemotherapy plus reduced-dose whole ventricle or local radiotherapy, although the available data would suggest that this is not a valid concern for patients with germinoma (130,171,184,228,257). Extracranial metastases are seen in a small percentage of patients treated with CSI alone but appear to be rare in patients treated with a combination of chemotherapy and radiotherapy, regardless of the target volume so that patients at increased risk for systemic failure (e.g., those with ventriculoperitoneal shunts) may be best treated with a combined chemotherapy–radiotherapy approach. These various approaches are currently under investigation by cooperative groups in Europe, North America, and Asia.

For patients with bi- or multifocal disease by imaging or by inference (for example, in a patient with a pineal region primary who has diabetes insipidus) and those with leptomeningeal spread at diagnosis, radiotherapy alone using CSI with boosts to macroscopic disease is certainly an option, although in North America a combination chemotherapy–radiotherapy regimen consisting of two cycles of chemotherapy followed by CSI followed by a boost to all sites of involvement would be the more usual approach.

It is necessary to comment on several issues that pertain to radiotherapy target-volume definition in patients with germinoma. CSI has been described in detail elsewhere. CT simulation is also a prerequisite for whole ventricular irradiation. Because subependymal spread is common, such treatment logically would include the lateral, third, and fourth ventricles with

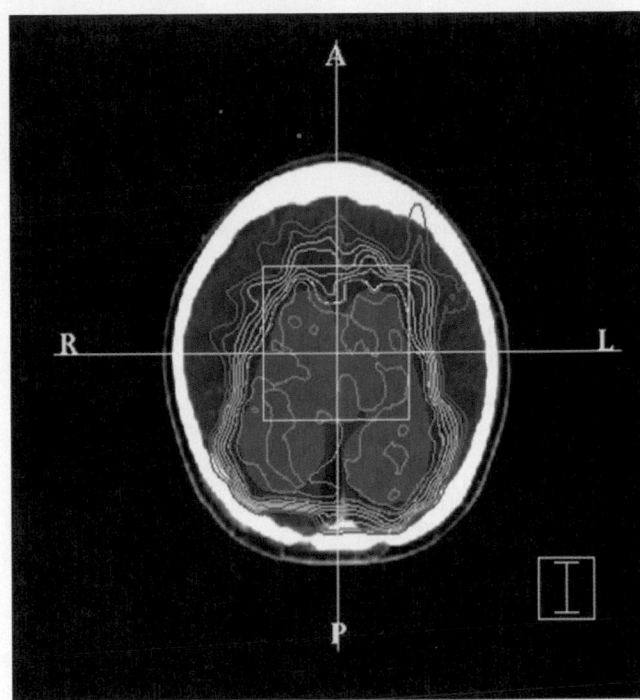

FIGURE 82.15. Intensity-modulated radiation therapy (IMRT) for whole ventricular irradiation. The use of a four-field technique or IMRT reduces the volume of brain in the treated volume compared with lateral opposed fields. (From Roberge D, Kun LE, Freeman CR. Intracranial germinoma: on whole-ventricular irradiation. *Pediatr Blood Cancer* 2005;44:358–362, with permission.)

a margin of 1 to 1.5 cm. If lateral opposed fields are used, the volume of brain spared in comparison with whole brain irradiation will be quite small. Better sparing can be achieved using CT planning and a four-field arrangement (Fig. 82.15) (219). Treatment planning for a local target volume requires CT simulation with MRI coregistration. The CTV consists of the preoperative, prechemotherapy volume with a margin of 1.5 cm, taking into account any shifts that may have taken place, for example, as a result of CSF decompression, surgical resection, and/or tumor shrinkage due to chemotherapy. This usually will be more of an issue for tumors arising in the pineal region than for suprasellar lesions.

There is less controversy now than a decade ago with regard to the radiotherapy dose and dose-fractionation schedule for germinoma. Results are excellent with a CSI dose as low as 21 Gy even in patients with leptomeningeal spread. The total dose to the primary site has typically been 40 to 45 Gy but probably can be reduced to 30 Gy in patients who have undergone complete resection or those who have been treated with a combined chemotherapy–radiotherapy regimen with a complete response to chemotherapy. These are the doses that are used in the current COG study. Finally, because germinoma is a very radiosensitive tumor, a fraction size of 1.5 Gy can be used, which, in theory, would further reduce the risk of injury to normal structures.

Nongerminomatous Germ Cell Tumors

For NGGCTs the diagnosis can be made in as many as one third of all patients on the basis of imaging findings (location, appearance) plus tumor markers. As noted, NGGCTs are of several different histopathological types that carry different prognoses (Table 82.4). Patients with mature teratomas without any associated malignant elements can be managed with surgery alone, while those with mature teratoma with germinomatous elements will be treated as germinomas. All other patients

Table 82.4	CLASSIFICATION OF NONGERMINOMATOUS GERM CELL TUMORS

Good prognosis
Mature teratoma

Intermediate prognosis
Immature teratoma
Mixed germ cell tumors consisting of germinoma with either mature or immature teratoma

Poor prognosis
Teratoma with malignant transformation
Embryonal carcinoma
Yolk sac tumor
Choriocarcinoma
Mixed germ cell tumors including a component of embryonal carcinoma, yolk sac tumor, choriocarcinoma, or teratoma with malignant transformation

Adapted from Sawamura Y, Ikeda J, Shirato H, et al. Germ cell tumours of the central nervous system: treatment consideration based on 111 cases and their long-term clinical outcomes. *Eur J Cancer* 1998;34:104–110.

with intermediate and poor prognosis tumor types (233) require more aggressive treatment. The results of treatment using radiotherapy alone are very poor, with overall survival in the 10% to 30% range. Results are better with chemotherapy alone, although 40% to 60% of patients relapse following chemotherapy and will be subjected to aggressive salvage regimens (15,16,126). A multimodality approach that includes both chemotherapy and radiotherapy appears to be associated with the best outcome. Event-free survival was 81% in the German/Italian pilot study that led to the current SIOP CNS GCT study (30). The current standard of care therefore consists of platinum-based chemotherapy followed by radiotherapy.

There is controversy with respect to the radiotherapy target volume for NGGCT. Although good results have been reported by some groups using chemotherapy followed by local radiotherapy (236), others show a high rate of failure outside the primary site (11,31,126,159,185,220). In the current North American study, CSI is used for all patients with NGGCT. A dose of 36 Gy is used, followed by a boost to the primary site to a total dose of 54 Gy.

Patients who have less than a complete response to chemotherapy fare so poorly that current studies are exploring other options. Second-look surgery may be useful to both exclude the possibility that the residual imaging abnormality represents mature teratoma and/or resect residual viable tumor. If the latter, this would be followed by CSI and then more aggressive chemotherapy, such as high-dose chemotherapy with stem cell rescue.

Tumors of the Sellar Region

Tumors arising in the sellar region in children include the following:

* Craniopharyngioma,
  — Adamantinomatous craniopharyngioma
  — Papillary craniopharyngioma
* Xanthogranuloma,
* Pituitary adenomas.

Craniopharyngioma

By definition, craniopharyngiomas are benign partly cystic epithelial tumors that arise in the sellar region from remnants of Rathke's pouch. In children, most are of the adamantinomatous type. They account for approximately 5% of intracranial tumors

in the pediatric age group, with a peak incidence between the ages of 5 and 14 years.

In the majority of patients, craniopharyngiomas have both suprasellar and intrasellar components. Children typically present with neuroendocrine deficits, especially diabetes insipidus and growth failure. Visual-field deficits often go unnoticed initially. Cognitive and behavioral changes are not uncommon. Compression of the third ventricle may lead to hydrocephalus and symptoms and signs of raised intracranial pressure. On neuroimaging, the findings are very typical, with solid and cystic areas in varying proportions; calcification is seen in the majority of cases. The solid portion(s) and the cyst capsule usually enhance with the use of contrast material.

Treatment of craniopharyngiomas has long been a controversial issue (26). Complete surgical resection, as confirmed on postoperative imaging, is associated with long-term tumor control in 85% to 100% of patients (274). Visual deficits, if present, improve after surgery in the majority of cases. However, new neuroendocrine deficits are very common after surgery, as well as hypothalamic damage, particularly in patients with supradiaphragmatic tumors that grow retrochiasmatically to involve the floor of the third ventricle (198,229). The transsphenoidal approach that has been used more frequently in recent years, even in younger children and in patients with tumors with a supradiaphragmatic component, is associated with fewer complications. Most important of all, however, is the now more widely accepted need to tailor management according to specific characteristics. Thus, patients with tumors that are smaller and/or subdiaphragmatic in location and without hypothalamic symptoms would be managed surgically, while other patients at higher risk for complications secondary to surgery would be managed with biopsy, cyst decompression, if necessary, and radiotherapy (3,12,101,245,268,273).

Radiotherapy may, therefore, be given as the sole therapeutic option, after incomplete surgery, or at the time of progression/recurrence after surgery, and the heterogeneity of tumor types and situations means that one of several approaches may be used. A lesion with a small solid component and a simple cyst, for example, may be treated with intracavitary injection of liquid radioactive material. Most contemporary experience is with β-emitters such as ^{32}P and ^{90}Y delivering a high dose (i.e., 200 Gy) to the cyst wall. Intracavitary injection of radioactive material is not always easy (199). Sometimes the cyst fluid is very thick in consistency, and there may be little or no communication between multiple cysts. It is essential to use contrast material to ensure that the catheter is well placed in the cavity and that there is no leakage of material outside the cyst before injecting radioactive material. This could be combined with radiosurgery or fractionated stereotactic irradiation to the associated solid component, although it may be reasonable to do so only later and only if there is evidence of progressive disease. Special care is needed if, as is usually the case, the tumor is in close proximity to the optic chiasm or optic nerves (152). Tumor control rates using this approach are good for carefully selected patients (106). However, conventionally fractionated external-beam irradiation using modern techniques may be a better option with a lower risk of morbidity for all except very small tumors (26,260).

External-beam radiotherapy also will be the treatment of choice for patients with residual disease following surgery who are at high risk for progressive disease even relatively early following surgery (58,65,111,128) or for those in whom surgical resection is not feasible. The target volume is local. The GTV consists of the whole lesion (i.e., both the solid and cystic components). The margin used for the CTV in one recent study was 0 cm and in another 1 cm (166,243). A margin of 0.5 cm seems reasonable using contemporary planning and delivery techniques. A dose of 54 to 55 Gy given in 30 daily fractions over 6 weeks appears to be necessary to achieve a high probability of tumor control. Cystic enlargement during treatment or within the first 2 to 3 months after completion of radiotherapy is not uncommon. Early recognition and appropriate management, usually consisting of cyst decompression, is essential to avoid further neurologic compromise or even death (212). The long-term prognosis is good, with event-free survival of 80% to 100% in most recent series (166,211,243,244).

In summary, the choice of treatment for patients with craniopharyngioma will depend on the specific characteristics of the tumor and the availability of the necessary expertise. It is clear that surgical resection is an excellent option when feasible. When complete resection is not feasible, biopsy, subtotal resection, or simply cyst decompression followed by external-beam radiotherapy is a better choice. There is equal if not better probability of tumor control in this situation with a lower risk of potentially devastating sequelae than with "heroic" surgery, particularly in less-experienced hands.

Pituitary Adenomas

Pituitary adenomas are rare in childhood. Almost all cases arise in adolescence. Most are functioning adenomas that present with endocrine dysfunction, most often menstrual irregularities and galactorrhea in girls and delayed puberty in boys. They may be quite large, with extrasellar extension, and appear to be more invasive than those seen in adults (38,69,145). Visual loss, when present, may be more severe and more likely to be associated with optic atrophy (145).

The therapeutic approach will, in general, parallel that for adult patients. Transphenoidal surgery appears to be feasible and safe in children, even in those with poor pneumatization of the sphenoid sinus, using neuronavigational tools (38,69). Radiotherapy is indicated if surgical resection is not possible or if hormone levels remain elevated following surgery. Conformal fields with a margin of 0.5 cm beyond macroscopic residual disease (the GTV) are used. Optimal sparing of normal brain is achieved using a four- to six-field arrangement (196). The usual dose, as in the adult population, will be 45 to 50 Gy over 5 to 6 weeks. Close follow-up by an endocrinologist is essential to ensure appropriate management of hormone deficits. Prolactin- and growth–hormone-secreting adenomas are managed medically as in adults.

References

1. Adan L, Trivin C, Sainte-Rose C, et al. GH deficiency caused by cranial irradiation during childhood: factors and markers in young adults. *J Clin Endocrinol Metab* 2001;86:5245–5251.
2. Aggarwal R, Yeung D, Kumar P, et al. Efficacy and feasibility of stereotactic radiosurgery in the primary management of unfavorable pediatric ependymoma. *Radiother Oncol* 1997;43:269–273.
3. Albright AL, Hadjipanayis CG, Lunsford LD, et al. Individualized treatment of pediatric craniopharyngiomas. *Childs Nerv Syst* 2005;21:649–654.
4. Albright AL, Packer RJ, Zimmerman R, et al. Magnetic resonance scans should replace biopsies for the diagnosis of diffuse brain stem gliomas: a report from the Children's Cancer Group. *Neurosurgery* 1993;33:1026–1029.
5. Albright AL, Wisoff JH, Zeltzer P, et al. Prognostic factors in children with supratentorial (nonpineal) primitive neuroectodermal tumors. A neurosurgical perspective from the Children's Cancer Group. *Pediatr Neurosurg* 1995;22:1–7.
6. Albright AL. Diffuse brainstem tumors: when is a biopsy necessary?. *Pediatr Neurosurg* 1996;24:252–255.
7. Allen JC, Donahue B, DaRosso R, et al. Hyperfractionated craniospinal radiotherapy and adjuvant chemotherapy for children with newly diagnosed medulloblastoma and other primitive neuroectodermal tumors. *Int J Radiat Oncol Biol Phys* 1996;36:1155–1161.
8. Allen JC. Initial management of children with hypothalamic and thalamic tumors and the modifying role of neurofibromatosis-1. *Pediatr Neurosurg* 2000;32:154–162.
9. Aoyama H, Shirato H, Ikeda J, et al. Induction chemotherapy followed by low-dose involved-field radiotherapy for intracranial germ cell tumors. *J Clin Oncol* 2002;20:857–865.
10. Aoyama H, Shirato H, Kakuto Y, et al. Pathologically-proven intracranial germinoma treated with radiation therapy. *Radiother Oncol* 1998;47:201–205.
11. Aoyama H, Shirato H, Yoshida H, et al. Retrospective multi-institutional study of radiotherapy for intracranial non-germinomatous germ cell tumors. *Radiother Oncol* 1998;49:55–59.
12. Backlund EO. Treatment of craniopharyngiomas: the multimodality approach. *Pediatr Neurosurg* 1994;21[Suppl 1]:82–89.
13. Bailey CC, Gnekow A, Wellek S, et al. Prospective randomised trial of chemotherapy given before radiotherapy in childhood medulloblastoma. International Society of Paediatric Oncology (SIOP) and the (German) Society of Paediatric Oncology (GPO): SIOP II. *Med Pediatr Oncol* 1995;25:166–178.
14. Baldwin RT, Preston-Martin S. Epidemiology of brain tumors in childhood—a review. *Toxicol Appl Pharmacol* 2004;199:118–131.
15. Balmaceda C, Heller G, Rosenblum M, et al. Chemotherapy without irradiation—a novel approach for newly diagnosed CNS germ cell tumors: results of an international cooperative trial. The First International Central Nervous System Germ Cell Tumor Study. *J Clin Oncol* 1996;14:2908–2915.
16. Baranzelli MC, Patte C, Bouffet E, et al. An attempt to treat pediatric intracranial alpha FP and beta HCG secreting germ cell tumors with chemotherapy alone. SFOP experience with 18 cases. Societe Francaise d'Oncologie Pediatrique. *J Neurooncol* 1998;37:229–39.
17. Bataini JP, Delanian S, Ponvert D. Chiasmal gliomas: results of irradiation management in 57 patients and review of literature. *Int J Radiat Oncol Biol Phys* 1991;21:615–623.
18. Benesch M, Lackner H, Sovinz P, et al. Late sequela after treatment of childhood low-grade gliomas: a retrospective analysis of 69 long-term survivors treated between 1983 and 2003. *J Neurooncol* 2006;.
19. Benk V, Clark BG, Souhami L, et al. Stereotactic radiation in primary brain tumors in children and adolescents. *Pediatr Neurosurg* 1999;31:59–64.
20. Berger C, Thiesse P, Lellouch-Tubiana A, et al. Choroid plexus carcinomas in childhood: clinical features and prognostic factors. *Neurosurgery* 1998;42:470–475.
21. Bloom HJ, Glees J, Bell J, et al. The treatment and long-term prognosis of children with intracranial tumors: a study of 610 cases, 1950-1981. *Int J Radiat Oncol Biol Phys* 1990;18:723–745.
22. Bouffet E, Baranzelli MC, Patte C, et al. Combined treatment modality for intracranial germinomas: results of a multicentre SFOP experience. Societe Francaise d'Oncologie Pediatrique. *Br J Cancer* 1999;79:1199–1204.
23. Bouffet E, Bernard JL, Frappaz D, et al. M4 protocol for cerebellar medulloblastoma: supratentorial radiotherapy may not be avoided. *Int J Radiat Oncol Biol Phys* 1992;24:79–85.
24. Bouffet E, Foreman N. Chemotherapy for intracranial ependymomas. *Childs Nerv Syst* 1999;15:563–570.
25. Bowers DC, Georgiades C, Aronson LJ, et al. Tectal gliomas: natural history of an indolent lesion in pediatric patients. *Pediatr Neurosurg* 2000;32:24–29.
26. Brada M, Thomas DG. Craniopharyngioma revisited. *Int J Radiat Oncol Biol Phys* 1993;27:471–475.
27. Broniscer A, Gajjar A. Supratentorial high-grade astrocytoma and diffuse brainstem glioma: two challenges for the pediatric oncologist. *Oncologist* 2004;9:197–206.
28. Burger PC, Yu IT, Tihan T, et al. Atypical teratoid/rhabdoid tumor of the central nervous system: a highly malignant tumor of infancy and childhood frequently mistaken for medulloblastoma: a Pediatric Oncology Group study. *Am J Surg Pathol* 1998;22:1083–1092.
29. Butler RW, Mulhern RK. Neurocognitive interventions for children and adolescents surviving cancer. *J Pediatr Psychol* 2005;30:65–78.
30. Calaminus G, Andreussi L, Garre ML, et al. Secreting germ cell tumors of the central nervous system (CNS). First results of the cooperative German/Italian pilot study (CNS sGCT). *Klin Padiatr* 1997;209:222–227.
31. Calaminus G, Bamberg M, Jurgens H, et al. Impact of surgery, chemotherapy and irradiation on long term outcome of intracranial malignant non-germinomatous germ cell tumors: results of the German Cooperative Trial MAKEI 89. *Klin Padiatr* 2004;216:141–149.
32. Campbell JW, Pollack IF, Martinez AJ, et al. High-grade astrocytomas in children: radiologically complete resection is associated with an excellent long-term prognosis. *Neurosurgery* 1996;38:258–264.
33. Carrie C, Alapetite C, Mere P, et al. Quality control of radiotherapeutic treatment of medulloblastoma in a multicentric study: the contribution of radiotherapy technique to tumour relapse. The French Medulloblastoma Group. *Radiother Oncol* 1992;24:77–81.
34. Carrie C, Hoffstetter S, Gomez F, et al. Impact of targeting deviations on outcome in medulloblastoma: study of the French Society of Pediatric Oncology (SFOP). *Int J Radiat Oncol Biol Phys* 1999;45:435–439.
35. Carrie C, Muracciole X, Gomez F, et al. Conformal radiotherapy, reduced boost volume, hyperfractionated radiotherapy, and online quality control in standard-risk medulloblastoma without chemotherapy: results of the French M-SFOP 98 protocol. *Int J Radiat Oncol Biol Phys* 2005;63:711–716.
36. Central Brain Tumor Registry of the United States. CBTRUS.2004. www.cbtrus.org
37. Chang CH, Housepian EM, Herbert C Jr. An operative staging system and a megavoltage radiotherapeutic technic for cerebellar medulloblastomas. *Radiology* 1969;93:1351–1359.
38. Chang CZ, Wang CJ, Howng SL. Pituitary adenomas in adolescence-ten-year experience and literature review. *Kaohsiung J Med Sci* 1999;15:691–696.
39. Chen YW, Wong TT, Ho DM, et al. Impact of radiotherapy for pediatric CNS atypical teratoid/rhabdoid tumor (single institute experience). *Int J Radiat Oncol Biol Phys* 2006;64:1038–1043.
40. Chow E, Reardon DA, Shah AB, et al. Pediatric choroid plexus neoplasms. *Int J Radiat Oncol Biol Phys* 1999;44:249–254.
41. Cohen BH, Kaplan AM, Packer RJ. Management of intracranial neoplasms in children with neurofibromatosis type 1 and 2. The Children's Cancer Study Group. *Pediatr Neurosurg* 1990;16:66–72.
42. Cohen BH, Zeltzer PM, Boyett JM, et al. Prognostic factors and treatment results for supratentorial primitive neuroectodermal tumors in children using radiation and chemotherapy: a Children's Cancer Group randomized trial. *J Clin Oncol* 1995;13:1687–1696.
43. Combs SE, Schulz-Ertner D, Moschos D, et al. Fractionated stereotactic radiotherapy of optic pathway gliomas: tolerance and long-term outcome. *Int J Radiat Oncol Biol Phys* 2005;62:814–819.
44. Constantini S, Miller DC, Allen JC, et al. Radical excision of intramedullary spinal cord tumors: surgical morbidity and long-term follow-up evaluation in 164 children and young adults. *J Neurosurg* 2000;93:183–193.
45. D'Andrea AD, Packer RJ, Rorke LB, et al. Pineocytomas of childhood. A reappraisal of natural history and response to therapy. *Cancer* 1987;59:1353–1357.
46. Dirks PB, Harris L, Hoffman HJ, et al. Supratentorial primitive neuroectodermal tumors in children. *J Neurooncol* 1996;29:75–84.

47. Doireau V, Grill J, Zerah M, et al. Chemotherapy for unresectable and recurrent intramedullary glial tumours in children. Brain Tumours Subcommittee of the French Society of Paediatric Oncology (SFOP). *Br J Cancer* 1999;81:835–840.
48. Donahue B. Short- and long-term complications of radiation therapy for pediatric brain tumors. *Pediatr Neurosurg* 1992;18:207–217.
49. Douglas JG, Barker JL, Ellenbogen RG, et al. Concurrent chemotherapy and reduced-dose cranial spinal irradiation followed by conformal posterior fossa tumor bed boost for average-risk medulloblastoma: efficacy and patterns of failure. *Int J Radiat Oncol Biol Phys* 2004;58:1161–1164.
50. Duffner PK, Cohen ME, Sanford RA, et al. Lack of efficacy of postoperative chemotherapy and delayed radiation in very young children with pineoblastoma. Pediatric Oncology Group. *Med Pediatr Oncol* 1995;25:38–44.
51. Duffner PK, Horowitz ME, Krischer JP, et al. The treatment of malignant brain tumors in infants and very young children: an update of the Pediatric Oncology Group experience. *Neurooncology* 1999;1:152–161.
52. Duffner PK, Krischer JP, Burger PC, et al. Treatment of infants with malignant gliomas: the Pediatric Oncology Group experience. *J Neurooncol* 1996;28:245–256.
53. Duffner PK, Krischer JP, Sanford RA, et al. Prognostic factors in infants and very young children with intracranial ependymomas. *Pediatr Neurosurg* 1998;28:215–222.
54. Epstein F, Constantini S. Practical decisions in the treatment of pediatric brain stem tumors. *Pediatr Neurosurg* 1996;24:24–34.
55. Epstein FJ, Farmer JP. Brain-stem glioma growth patterns. *J Neurosurg* 1993;78:408–412.
56. Evans AE, Anderson JR, Lefkowitz-Boudreaux IB, et al. Adjuvant chemotherapy of childhood posterior fossa ependymoma: cranio-spinal irradiation with or without adjuvant CCNU, vincristine, and prednisone: a Children's Cancer Group study. *Med Pediatr Oncol* 1996;27:8–14.
57. Evans AE, Jenkin RD, Sposto R, et al. The treatment of medulloblastoma. Results of a prospective randomized trial of radiation therapy with and without CCNU, vincristine, and prednisone. *J Neurosurg* 1990;72:572–582.
58. Fahlbusch R, Honegger J, Paulus W, et al. Surgical treatment of craniopharyngiomas: experience with 168 patients. *J Neurosurg* 1999;90:237–250.
59. Farmer JP, Khan S, Khan A, et al. Neurofibromatosis type 1 and the pediatric neurosurgeon: a 20-year institutional review. *Pediatr Neurosurg* 2002;37:122–136.
60. Farmer JP, Montes JL, Freeman CR, et al. Brainstem gliomas. A 10-year institutional review. *Pediatr Neurosurg* 2001;34:206–214.
61. Fassett DR, Pingree J, Kestle JR. The high incidence of tumor dissemination in myxopapillary ependymoma in pediatric patients. Report of five cases and review of the literature. *J Neurosurg* 2005;102:59–64.
62. Fernandez C, Figarella-Branger D, Girard N, et al. Pilocytic astrocytomas in children: prognostic factors—a retrospective study of 80 cases. *Neurosurgery* 2003;53:544–553.
63. Finlay JL, Boyett JM, Yates AJ, et al. Randomized phase III trial in childhood high-grade astrocytoma comparing vincristine, lomustine, and prednisone with the eight-drugs-in-1-day regimen. Children's Cancer Group. *J Clin Oncol* 1995;13:112–123.
64. Fisher PG, Breiter SN, Carson BS, et al. A clinicopathologic reappraisal of brain stem tumor classification. Identification of pilocystic astrocytoma and fibrillary astrocytoma as distinct entities. *Cancer* 2000;89:1569–1576.
65. Fisher PG, Jenab J, Goldthwaite PT, et al. Outcomes and failure patterns in childhood craniopharyngiomas. *Childs Nerv Syst* 1998;14:558–563.
66. Fitzpatrick LK, Aronson LJ, Cohen KJ. Is there a requirement for adjuvant therapy for choroid plexus carcinoma that has been completely resected?. *J Neurooncol* 2002;57:123–126.
67. Foreman NK, Love S, Thorne R. Intracranial ependymomas: analysis of prognostic factors in a population-based series. *Pediatr Neurosurg* 1996;24:119–125.
68. Fouladi M, Wallace D, Langston JW, et al. Survival and functional outcome of children with hypothalamic/chiasmatic tumors. *Cancer* 2003;97:1084–1092.
69. Fraioli B, Ferrante L, Celli P. Pituitary adenomas with onset during puberty. Features and treatment. *J Neurosurg* 1983;59:590–595.
70. Freeman CR, Bourgouin PM, Sanford RA, et al. Long term survivors of childhood brain stem gliomas treated with hyperfractionated radiotherapy. Clinical characteristics and treatment related toxicities. The Pediatric Oncology Group. *Cancer* 1996;77:555–562.
71. Freeman CR, Farmer JP. Pediatric brain stem gliomas: a review. *Int J Radiat Oncol Biol Phys* 1998;40:265–271.
72. Freeman CR, Kepner J, Kun LE, et al. A detrimental effect of a combined chemotherapy-radiotherapy approach in children with diffuse intrinsic brain stem gliomas?. *Int J Radiat Oncol Biol Phys* 2000;47:561–564.
73. Freeman CR, Krischer JP, Sanford RA, et al. Final results of a study of escalating doses of hyperfractionated radiotherapy in brain stem tumors in children: a Pediatric Oncology Group study. *Int J Radiat Oncol Biol Phys* 1993;27:197–206.
74. Freeman CR, Perilongo G. Chemotherapy for brain stem gliomas. *Childs Nerv Syst* 1999;15:545–553.
75. Freeman CR. Hyperfractionated radiotherapy for diffuse intrinsic brain stem tumors in children. *Pediatr Neurosurg* 1996;24:103–110.
76. Fukunaga-Johnson N, Lee JH, Sandler HM, et al. Patterns of failure following treatment for medulloblastoma: is it necessary to treat the entire posterior fossa?. *Int J Radiat Oncol Biol Phys* 1998;42:143–146.
77. Fukunaga-Johnson N, Sandler HM, Marsh R, et al. The use of 3D conformal radiotherapy (3DCRT) to spare the cochlea in patients with medulloblastoma. *Int J Radiat Oncol Biol Phys* 1998;41:77–82.
78. Gajjar A, Kuhl J, Epelman S, et al. Chemotherapy of medulloblastoma. *Childs Nerv Syst* 1999;15:554–562.
79. Gajjar A, Sanford RA, Heideman R, et al. Low-grade astrocytoma: a decade of experience at St. Jude Children's Research Hospital. *J Clin Oncol* 1997;15:2792–2799.
80. Gaspar LE, Dawson DJ, Tilley-Gulliford SA, et al. Medulloblastoma: long-term follow-up of patients treated with electron irradiation of the spinal field. *Radiology* 1991;180:867–870.
81. Gentet JC, Bouffet E, Doz F, et al. Preirradiation chemotherapy including "eight drugs in 1 day" regimen and high-dose methotrexate in childhood medulloblastoma: results of the M7 French Cooperative Study. *J Neurosurg* 1995;82:608–614.
82. Gerszten PC, Pollack IF, Martinez AJ, et al. Intracranial ependymomas of childhood. Lack of correlation of histopathology and clinical outcome. *Pathol Res Pract* 1996;192:515–522.
83. Geyer JR, Finlay JL, Boyett JM, et al. Survival of infants with malignant astrocytomas. A Report from the Children's Cancer Group. *Cancer* 1995;75:1045–1050.
84. Geyer JR, Sposto R, Jennings M, et al. Multiagent chemotherapy and deferred radiotherapy in infants with malignant brain tumors: a report from the Children's Cancer Group. *J Clin Oncol* 2005;23:7621–7631.
85. Geyer JR, Zeltzer PM, Boyett JM, et al. Survival of infants with primitive neuroectodermal tumors or malignant ependymomas of the CNS treated with eight drugs in 1 day: a report from the Children's Cancer Group. *J Clin Oncol* 1994;12:1607–1615.
86. Gnekow AK, Kortmann RD, Pietsch T, et al. Low grade chiasmatic-hypothalamic glioma-carboplatin and vincristine chemotherapy effectively defers radiotherapy within a comprehensive treatment strategy—report from the multicenter treatment study for children and adolescents with a low grade glioma—HIT-LGG 1996—of the Society of Pediatric Oncology and Hematology (GPOH). *Klin Padiatr* 2004;216:331–342.
87. Goldwein JW, Corn BW, Finlay JL, et al. Is craniospinal irradiation required to cure children with malignant (anaplastic) intracranial ependymomas?. *Cancer* 1991;67:2766–2771.
88. Gomez DR, Missett BT, Wara WM, et al. High failure rate in spinal ependymomas with long-term follow-up. *Neurooncology* 2005;7:254–259.
89. Grabb PA, Lunsford LD, Albright AL, et al. Stereotactic radiosurgery for glial neoplasms of childhood. *Neurosurgery* 1996;38:696–701.
90. Grabenbauer GG, Schuchardt U, Buchfelder M, et al. Radiation therapy of optico-hypothalamic gliomas (OHG)—radiographic response, vision and late toxicity. *Radiother Oncol* 2000;54:239–245.
91. Grant GA, Avellino AM, Loeser JD, et al. Management of intrinsic gliomas of the tectal plate in children. A ten-year review. *Pediatr Neurosurg* 1999;31:170–176.
92. Grill J, Laithier V, Rodriguez D, et al. When do children with optic pathway tumours need treatment? An oncological perspective in 106 patients treated in a single centre. *Eur J Pediatr* 2000;159:692–696.
93. Grill J, Le Deley MC, Gambarelli D, et al. Postoperative chemotherapy without irradiation for ependymoma in children under 5 years of age: a multicenter trial of the French Society of Pediatric Oncology. *J Clin Oncol* 2001;19:1288–1296.
94. Grill J, Lellouch-Tubiana A, Elouahdani S, et al. Preoperative chemotherapy in children with high-risk medulloblastomas: a feasibility study. *J Neurosurg* 2005;103:312–318.
95. Grill J, Renaux VK, Bulteau C, et al. Long-term intellectual outcome in children with posterior fossa tumors according to radiation doses and volumes. *Int J Radiat Oncol Biol Phys* 1999;45:137–145.
96. Grill J, Sainte-Rose C, Jouvet A, et al. Treatment of medulloblastoma with postoperative chemotherapy alone: an SFOP prospective trial in young children. *Lancet Oncol* 2005;6;573–580.
97. Gripp S, Kambergs J, Wittkamp M, et al. Coverage of anterior fossa in whole-brain irradiation. *Int J Radiat Oncol Biol Phys* 2004;59:515–520.
98. Gurney JG, Kadan-Lottick NS, Packer RJ, et al. Endocrine and cardiovascular late effects among adult survivors of childhood brain tumors: Childhood Cancer Survivor study. *Cancer* 2003;97:663–673.
99. Haas-Kogan DA, Missett BT, Wara WM, et al. Radiation therapy for intracranial germ cell tumors. *Int J Radiat Oncol Biol Phys* 2003;56:511–518.
100. Habrand JL, de Crevoisier CR. Radiation therapy in the management of childhood brain tumors. *Childs Nerv Syst* 2001;17:121–133.
101. Habrand JL, Saran F, Alapetite C, et al. Radiation therapy in the management of craniopharyngioma: current concepts and future developments. *J Pediatr Endocrinol Metab* 2006;19[Suppl 1]:389–394.
102. Haddock MG, Schild SE, Scheithauer BW, et al. Radiation therapy for histologically confirmed primary central nervous system germinoma. *Int J Radiat Oncol Biol Phys* 1997;38:915–923.
103. Halperin EC, Friedman HS, Schold SC Jr., et al. Surgery, hyperfractionated craniospinal irradiation, and adjuvant chemotherapy in the management of supratentorial embryonal neuroepithelial neoplasms in children. *Surg Neurol* 1993;40:278–283.
104. Halperin EC. Concerning the inferior portion of the spinal radiotherapy field for malignancies that disseminate via the cerebrospinal fluid. *Int J Radiat Oncol Biol Phys* 1993;26:357–362.
105. Hanbali F, Fourney DR, Marmor E, et al. Spinal cord ependymoma: radical surgical resection and outcome. *Neurosurgery* 2002;51:1162–1172.
106. Hasegawa T, Kondziolka D, Hadjipanayis CG, et al. Management of cystic craniopharyngiomas with phosphorus-32 intracavitary irradiation. *Neurosurgery* 2004;54:813–820.
107. Healey EA, Barnes PD, Kupsky WJ, et al. The prognostic significance of postoperative residual tumor in ependymoma. *Neurosurgery* 1991;28:666–671.
108. Heideman RL, Kuttesch J Jr., Gajjar AJ, et al. Supratentorial malignant gliomas in childhood: a single institution perspective. *Cancer* 1997;80:497–504.
109. Hilden JM, Watterson J, Longee DC, et al. Central nervous system atypical teratoid tumor/rhabdoid tumor: response to intensive therapy and review of the literature. *J Neurooncol* 1998;40:265–275.
110. Hirsch JF, Sainte RC, Pierre-Kahn A, et al. Benign astrocytic and oligodendrocytic tumors of the cerebral hemispheres in children. *J Neurosurg* 1989;70:568–572.
111. Hoffman HJ, De SM, Humphreys RP, et al. Aggressive surgical management of craniopharyngiomas in children. *J Neurosurg* 1992;76:47–52.
112. Hoffman HJ. Dorsally exophytic brain stem tumors and midbrain tumors. *Pediatr Neurosurg* 1996;24:256–262.
113. Hong TS, Mehta MP, Boyett JM, et al. Patterns of failure in supratentorial primitive neuroectodermal tumors treated in Children's Cancer Group Study 921, a phase III combined modality study. *Int J Radiat Oncol Biol Phys* 2004;60:204–213.
114. Hong TS, Mehta MP, Boyett JM, et al. Patterns of treatment failure in infants with primitive neuroectodermal tumors who were treated on CCG-921: a phase III combined modality study. *Pediatr Blood Cancer* 2005;45:676–682.
115. Horn B, Heideman R, Geyer R, et al. A multi-institutional retrospective study of intracranial ependymoma in children: identification of risk factors. *J Pediatr Hematol Oncol* 1999;21:203–211.
116. Horwich A, Bloom HJ. Optic gliomas: radiation therapy and prognosis. *Int J Radiat Oncol Biol Phys* 1985;11:1067–1079.
117. Hug EB, Muenter MW, Archambeau JO, et al. Conformal proton radiation therapy for pediatric low-grade astrocytomas. *Strahlenther Onkol* 2002;178:10–17.

118. Jakacki RI, Goldwein JW, Larsen RL, et al. Cardiac dysfunction following spinal irradiation during childhood. *J Clin Oncol* 1993;11:1033–1038.

119. Jakacki RI, Zeltzer PM, Boyett JM, et al. Survival and prognostic factors following radiation and/or chemotherapy for primitive neuroectodermal tumors of the pineal region in infants and children: a report of the Children's Cancer Group. *J Clin Oncol* 1995;13:1377–1383.

120. Jallo GI, Freed D, Epstein F. Intramedullary spinal cord tumors in children. *Childs Nerv Syst* 2003;19:641–649.

121. Janss AJ, Grundy R, Cnaan A, et al. Optic pathway and hypothalamic/chiasmatic gliomas in children younger than age 5 years with a 6-year follow-up. *Cancer* 1995;75:1051–1059.

122. Jenkin D, Angyalfi S, Becker L, et al. Optic glioma in children: surveillance, resection, or irradiation?. *Int J Radiat Oncol Biol Phys* 1993;25:215–225.

123. Jouvet A, Fevre-Montange M, Besancon R, et al. Structural and ultrastructural characteristics of human pineal gland, and pineal parenchymal tumors. *Acta Neuropathol (Berl)* 1994;88:334–348.

124. Karim AB, Maat B, Hatlevoll R, et al. A randomized trial on dose-response in radiation therapy of low-grade cerebral glioma: European Organization for Research and Treatment of Cancer (EORTC) Study 22844. *Int J Radiat Oncol Biol Phys* 1996;36:549–556.

125. Kellie SJ, Boyce H, Dunkel IJ, et al. Intensive cisplatin and cyclophosphamide-based chemotherapy without radiotherapy for intracranial germinomas: failure of a primary chemotherapy approach. *Pediatr Blood Cancer* 2004;43:126–133.

126. Kellie SJ, Boyce H, Dunkel IJ, et al. Primary chemotherapy for intracranial nongerminomatous germ cell tumors: results of the second international CNS germ cell study group protocol. *J Clin Oncol* 2004;22:846–853.

127. Khafaga Y, Hassounah M, Kandil A, et al. Optic gliomas: a retrospective analysis of 50 cases. *Int J Radiat Oncol Biol Phys* 2003;56:807–812.

128. Khafaga Y, Jenkin D, Kanaan I, et al. Craniopharyngioma in children. *Int J Radiat Oncol Biol Phys* 1998;42:601–606.

129. Khatib ZA, Heideman RL, Kovnar EH, et al. Predominance of pilocytic histology in dorsally exophytic brain stem tumors. *Pediatr Neurosurg* 1994;20:2–10.

130. Kiltie AE, Gattamaneni HR. Survival and quality of life of paediatric intracranial germ cell tumour patients treated at the Christie Hospital, 1972-1993. *Med Pediatr Oncol* 1995;25:450–456.

131. Kiltie AE, Povall JM, Taylor RE. The need for the moving junction in craniospinal irradiation. *Br J Radiol* 2000;73:650–654.

132. King A, Listernick R, Charrow J, et al. Optic pathway gliomas in neurofibromatosis type 1: the effect of presenting symptoms on outcome. *Am J Med Genet* 2003;122:95–99.

133. Kleihues P, Cavanee WK, eds. *Pathology and genetics tumours of the nervous system.* Lyon: IARC Press, 2006.

134. Komotar RJ, Burger PC, Carson BS, et al. Pilocytic and pilomyxoid hypothalamic/chiasmatic astrocytomas. *Neurosurgery* 2004;54:72–79.

135. Kortmann RD, Kuhl J, Timmermann B, et al. Postoperative neoadjuvant chemotherapy before radiotherapy as compared to immediate radiotherapy followed by maintenance chemotherapy in the treatment of medulloblastoma in childhood: results of the German prospective randomized trial HIT 91. *Int J Radiat Oncol Biol Phys* 2000;46:269–279.

136. Kortmann RD, Timmermann B, Becker G, et al. Advances in treatment techniques and time/dose schedules in external radiation therapy of brain tumours in childhood. *Klin Padiatr* 1998;210:220–226.

137. Kortmann RD, Timmermann B, Taylor RE, et al. Current and future strategies in radiotherapy of childhood low-grade glioma of the brain. Part II: Treatment-related late toxicity. *Strahlenther Onkol* 2003;179:585–597.

138. Kreth FW, Faist M, Warnke PC, et al. Interstitial radiosurgery of low-grade gliomas. *J Neurosurg* 1995;82:418–429.

139. Krishnamoorthy P, Freeman C, Bernstein ML, et al. Osteopenia in children who have undergone posterior fossa or craniospinal irradiation for brain tumors. *Arch Pediatr Adolesc Med* 2004;158:491–496.

140. Krishnan S, Brown PD, Scheithauer BW, et al. Choroid plexus papillomas: a single institutional experience. *J Neurooncol* 2004;68:49–55.

141. Kuhl J, Muller HL, Berthold F, et al. Preradiation chemotherapy of children and young adults with malignant brain tumors: results of the German pilot trial HIT 88/89. *Klin Padiatr* 1998;210:227–233.

142. Lacaze E, Kieffer V, Streri A, et al. Neuropsychological outcome in children with optic pathway tumours when first-line treatment is chemotherapy. *Br J Cancer* 2003;89:2038–2044.

143. Laithier V, Grill J, Le Deley MC, et al. Progression-free survival in children with optic pathway tumors: dependence on age and the quality of the response to chemotherapy—results of the first French prospective study for the French Society of Pediatric Oncology. *J Clin Oncol* 2003;21:4572–4578.

144. Lang FF, Epstein FJ, Ransohoff J, et al. Central nervous system gangliogliomas. Part 2: Clinical outcome. *J Neurosurg* 1993;79:867–873.

145. Lee AG, Sforza PD, Fard AK, et al. Pituitary adenoma in children. *J Neuroophthalmol* 1998;18:102–105.

146. Lesniak MS, Klem JM, Weingart J, et al. Surgical outcome following resection of contrast-enhanced pediatric brainstem gliomas. *Pediatr Neurosurg* 2003;39:314–322.

147. Lewis J, Lucraft H, Gholkar A. UKCCSG study of accelerated radiotherapy for pediatric brain stem gliomas. United Kingdom Childhood Cancer Study Group. *Int J Radiat Oncol Biol Phys* 1997;38:925–929.

148. Lin YH, Huang CI, Wong TT, et al. Treatment of spinal cord ependymomas by surgery with or without postoperative radiotherapy. *J Neurooncol* 2005;71:205–210.

149. Listernick R, Charrow J, Greenwald M, et al. Natural history of optic pathway tumors in children with neurofibromatosis type 1: a longitudinal study. *J Pediatr* 1994;125:63–66.

150. Lonjon M, Goh KY, Epstein FJ. Intramedullary spinal cord ependymomas in children: treatment, results and follow-up. *Pediatr Neurosurg* 1998;29:178–183.

151. Lowis SP, Pizer BL, Coakham H, et al. Chemotherapy for spinal cord astrocytoma: can natural history be modified?. *Childs Nerv Syst* 1998;14:317–321.

152. Lunsford LD, Pollock BE, Kondziolka DS, et al. Stereotactic options in the management of craniopharyngioma. *Pediatr Neurosurg* 1994;21[Suppl 1]:90–97.

153. Luyken C, Blumcke I, Fimmers R, et al. Supratentorial gangliogliomas: histopathologic grading and tumor recurrence in 184 patients with a median follow-up of 8 years. *Cancer* 2004;101:146–155.

154. Mabbott DJ, Spiegler BJ, Greenberg ML, et al. Serial evaluation of academic and behavioral outcome after treatment with cranial radiation in childhood. *J Clin Oncol* 2005;23:2256–2263.

155. Maity A, Shu HK, Janss A, et al. Craniospinal radiation in the treatment of biopsy-proven intracranial germinomas: twenty-five years' experience in a single center. *Int J Radiat Oncol Biol Phys* 2004;58:1165–1170.

156. Marcus KJ, Goumnerova L, Billett AL, et al. Stereotactic radiotherapy for localized low-grade gliomas in children: final results of a prospective trial. *Int J Radiat Oncol Biol Phys* 2005;61:374–379.

157. Massimino M, Gandola L, Giangaspero F, et al. Hyperfractionated radiotherapy and chemotherapy for childhood ependymoma: final results of the first prospective AIEOP (Associazione Italiana di Ematologia-Oncologia Pediatrica) study. *Int J Radiat Oncol Biol Phys* 2004;58:1336–1345.

158. Massimino M, Gandola L, Spreafico F, et al. Supratentorial primitive neuroectodermal tumors (S-PNET) in children: a prospective experience with adjuvant intensive chemotherapy and hyperfractionated accelerated radiotherapy. *Int J Radiat Oncol Biol Phys* 2006;64:1031–1037.

159. Matsutani M, Sano K, Takakura K, et al. Primary intracranial germ cell tumors: a clinical analysis of 153 histologically verified cases. *J Neurosurg* 1997;86:446–455.

160. Matsutani M. Combined chemotherapy and radiation therapy for CNS germ cell tumors-the Japanese experience. *J Neurooncol* 2001;54:311–316.

161. May PL, Blaser SI, Hoffman HJ, et al. Benign intrinsic tectal "tumors" in children. *J Neurosurg* 1991;74:867–871.

162. Meacham L. Endocrine late effects of childhood cancer therapy. *Curr Probl Pediatr Adolesc Health Care* 2003;33:217–242.

163. Merchant TE, Fouladi M. Ependymoma: new therapeutic approaches including radiation and chemotherapy. *J Neurooncol* 2005;75:287–299.

164. Merchant TE, Haida T, Wang MH, et al. Anaplastic ependymoma: treatment of pediatric patients with or without craniospinal radiation therapy. *J Neurosurg* 1997;86:943–949.

165. Merchant TE, Happersett L, Finlay JL, et al. Preliminary results of conformal radiation therapy for medulloblastoma. *Neurooncology* 1999;1:177–187.

166. Merchant TE, Kiehna EN, Kun LE, et al. Phase II trial of conformal radiation therapy for pediatric patients with craniopharyngioma and correlation of surgical factors and radiation dosimetry with change in cognitive function. *J Neurosurg* 2006;104:94–102.

167. Merchant TE, Kiehna EN, Li C, et al. Modeling radiation dosimetry to predict cognitive outcomes in pediatric patients with CNS embryonal tumors including medulloblastoma. *Int J Radiat Oncol Biol Phys* 2006;65:210–221.

168. Merchant TE, Kiehna EN, Li C, et al. Radiation dosimetry predicts IQ after conformal radiation therapy in pediatric patients with localized ependymoma. *Int J Radiat Oncol Biol Phys* 2005;63:1546–1554.

169. Merchant TE, Kiehna EN, Thompson SJ, et al. Pediatric low-grade and ependymal spinal cord tumors. *Pediatr Neurosurg* 2000;32:30–36.

170. Merchant TE, Mulhern RK, Krasin MJ, et al. Preliminary results from a phase II trial of conformal radiation therapy and evaluation of radiation-related CNS effects for pediatric patients with localized ependymoma. *J Clin Oncol* 2004;22:3156–3162.

171. Merchant TE, Sherwood SH, Mulhern RK, et al. CNS germinoma: disease control and long-term functional outcome for 12 children treated with craniospinal irradiation. *Int J Radiat Oncol Biol Phys* 2000;46:1171–1176.

172. Merchant TE, Williams T, Smith JM, et al. Preirradiation endocrinopathies in pediatric brain tumor patients determined by dynamic tests of endocrine function. *Int J Radiat Oncol Biol Phys* 2002;54:45–50.

173. Merchant TE, Zhu Y, Thompson SJ, et al. Preliminary results from a phase II trail of conformal radiation therapy for pediatric patients with localised low-grade astrocytoma and ependymoma. *Int J Radiat Oncol Biol Phys* 2002;52:325–332.

174. Meyers SP, Khademian ZP, Chuang SH, et al. Choroid plexus carcinomas in children: MRI features and patient outcomes. *Neuroradiology* 2004;46:770–780.

175. Miralbell R, Lomax A, Bortfeld T, et al. Potential role of proton therapy in the treatment of pediatric medulloblastoma/primitive neuroectodermal tumors: reduction of the supratentorial target volume. *Int J Radiat Oncol Biol Phys* 1997;38:477–484.

176. Mosijczuk AD, Nigro MA, Thomas PR, et al. Preradiation chemotherapy in advanced medulloblastoma. A Pediatric Oncology Group pilot study. *Cancer* 1993;72:2755–2762.

177. Mulhern RK, Kepner JL, Thomas PR, et al. Neuropsychologic functioning of survivors of childhood medulloblastoma randomized to receive conventional or reduced-dose craniospinal irradiation: a Pediatric Oncology Group study. *J Clin Oncol* 1998;16:1723–1728.

178. Mulhern RK, Palmer SL, Reddick WE, et al. Risks of young age for selected neurocognitive deficits in medulloblastoma are associated with white matter loss. *J Clin Oncol* 2001;19:472–479.

179. Mundinger F, Braus DF, Krauss JK, et al. Long-term outcome of 89 low-grade brain-stem gliomas after interstitial radiation therapy. *J Neurosurg* 1991;75:740–746.

180. Nadkarni TD, Rekate HL. Pediatric intramedullary spinal cord tumors. Critical review of the literature. *Childs Nerv Syst* 1999;15:17–28.

181. Narod SA, Stiller C, Lenoir GM. An estimate of the heritable fraction of childhood cancer. *Br J Cancer* 1991;63:993–999.

182. Nazar GB, Hoffman HJ, Becker LE, et al. Infratentorial ependymomas in childhood: prognostic factors and treatment. *J Neurosurg* 1990;72:408–417.

183. Needle MN, Goldwein JW, Grass J, et al. Adjuvant chemotherapy for the treatment of intracranial ependymoma of childhood. *Cancer* 1997;80:341–347.

184. Ogawa K, Shikama N, Toita T, et al. Long-term results of radiotherapy for intracranial germinoma: a multi-institutional retrospective review of 126 patients. *Int J Radiat Oncol Biol Phys* 2004;58:705–713.

185. Ogawa K, Toita T, Nakamura K, et al. Treatment and prognosis of patients with intracranial nongerminomatous malignant germ cell tumors: a multi-institutional retrospective analysis of 41 patients. *Cancer* 2003;98:369–376.

186. Oyharcabal-Bourden V, Kalifa C, Gentet JC, et al. Standard-risk medulloblastoma treated by adjuvant chemotherapy followed by reduced-dose craniospinal radiation therapy: a French Society of Pediatric Oncology study. *J Clin Oncol* 2005;23:4726–4734.

187. Packer RJ, Boyett JM, Zimmerman RA, et al. Outcome of children with brain stem gliomas after treatment with 7800 cGy of hyperfractionated radiotherapy. A Children's Cancer Group phase I/II trial. *Cancer* 1994;74:1827–1834.

188. Packer RJ, Goldwein J, Nicholson HS, et al. Treatment of children with

medulloblastomas with reduced-dose craniospinal radiation therapy and adjuvant chemotherapy: a Children's Cancer Group study. *J Clin Oncol* 1999;17:2127–2136.
189. Packer RJ, Perilongo G, Johnson D, et al. Choroid plexus carcinoma of childhood. *Cancer* 1992;69:580–585.
190. Palma L, Celli P, Mariottini A, et al. The importance of surgery in supratentorial ependymomas. Long-term survival in a series of 23 cases. *Childs Nerv Syst* 2000;16:170–175.
191. Palmer SL, Goloubeva O, Reddick WE, et al. Patterns of intellectual development among survivors of pediatric medulloblastoma: a longitudinal analysis. *J Clin Oncol* 2001;19:2302–2308.
192. Parker WA, Freeman CR. A simple technique for craniospinal radiotherapy in the supine position. *Radiother Oncol* 2006;78:217–222.
193. Paulino AC, Cha DT, Barker JL Jr., et al. Patterns of failure in relation to radiotherapy fields in supratentorial primitive neuroectodermal tumor. *Int J Radiat Oncol Biol Phys* 2004;58:1171–1176.
194. Pencalet P, Sainte-Rose C, Lellouch-Tubiana A, et al. Papillomas and carcinomas of the choroid plexus in children. *J Neurosurg* 1998;88:521–528.
195. Perilongo G, Massimino M, Sotti G, et al. Analyses of prognostic factors in a retrospective review of 92 children with ependymoma: Italian Pediatric Neuro-oncology Group. *Med Pediatr Oncol* 1997;29:79–85.
196. Perks JR, Jalali R, Cosgrove VP, et al. Optimization of stereotactically-guided conformal treatment planning of sellar and parasellar tumors, based on normal brain dose volume histograms. *Int J Radiat Oncol Biol Phys* 1999;45:507–513.
197. Pierga JY, Kalifa C, Terrier-Lacombe MJ, et al. Carcinoma of the choroid plexus: a pediatric experience. *Med Pediatr Oncol* 1993;21:480–487.
198. Pierre-Kahn A, Recassens C, Pinto G, et al. Social and psycho-intellectual outcome following radical removal of craniopharyngiomas in childhood. A prospective series. *Childs Nerv Syst* 2005;21:817–824.
199. Pollack BE, Lunsford LD, Kondziolka D, et al. Phosphorus-32 intracavitary irradiation of cystic craniopharyngiomas: current technique and long-term results. *Int J Radiat Oncol Biol Phys* 1995;33:437–446.
200. Pollack IF, Boyett JM, Finlay JL. Chemotherapy for high-grade gliomas of childhood. *Childs Nerv Syst* 1999;15:529–544.
201. Pollack IF, Boyett JM, Yates AJ, et al. The influence of central review on outcome associations in childhood malignant gliomas: results from the CCG-945 experience. *Neurooncology* 2003;5:197–207.
202. Pollack IF, Claassen D, al-Shboul Q, et al. Low-grade gliomas of the cerebral hemispheres in children: an analysis of 71 cases. *J Neurosurg* 1995;82:536–547.
203. Pollack IF, Gerszten PC, Martinez AJ, et al. Intracranial ependymomas of childhood: long-term outcome and prognostic factors. *Neurosurgery* 1995;37:655–666.
204. Pollack IF, Hoffman HJ, Humphreys RP, et al. The long-term outcome after surgical treatment of dorsally exophytic brain-stem gliomas. *J Neurosurg* 1993;78:859–863.
205. Pollack IF, Pang D, Albright AL. The long-term outcome in children with late-onset aqueductal stenosis resulting from benign intrinsic tectal tumors. *J Neurosurg* 1994;80:681–688.
206. Pollack IF, Shultz B, Mulvihill JJ. The management of brainstem gliomas in patients with neurofibromatosis 1. *Neurology* 1996;46:1652–1660.
207. Prados MD, Wara WM, Edwards MS, et al. The treatment of brain stem and thalamic gliomas with 78 Gy of hyperfractionated radiation therapy. *Int J Radiat Oncol Biol Phys* 1995;32:85–91.
208. Rades D, Fehlauer F, Ikezaki K, et al. Dose-effect relationship for radiotherapy after incomplete resection of atypical neurocytomas. *Radiother Oncol* 2005;74:67–69.
209. Rades D, Schild SE. Is 50 Gy sufficient to achieve long-term local control after incomplete resection of typical neurocytomas?. *Strahlenther Onkol* 2006;182:415–418.
210. Rades D, Schild SE. Treatment recommendations for the various subgroups of neurocytomas. *J Neurooncol* 2006;77:305–309.
211. Rajan B, Ashley S, Gorman C, et al. Craniopharyngioma—a long-term results following limited surgery and radiotherapy. *Radiother Oncol* 1993;26:1–10.
212. Rajan B, Ashley S, Thomas DG, et al. Craniopharyngioma: improving outcome by early recognition and treatment of acute complications. *Int J Radiat Oncol Biol Phys* 1997;37:517–521.
213. Reddy AT, Janss AJ, Phillips PC, et al. Outcome for children with supratentorial primitive neuroectodermal tumors treated with surgery, radiation, and chemotherapy. *Cancer* 2000;88:2189–2193.
214. Reddy AT, Packer RJ. Chemotherapy for low-grade gliomas. *Childs Nerv Syst* 1999;15:506–513.
215. Reddy AT. Atypical teratoid/rhabdoid tumors of the central nervous system. *J Neurooncol* 2005;75:309–313.
216. Rezai AR, Woo HH, Lee M, et al. Disseminated ependymomas of the central nervous system. *J Neurosurg* 1996;85:618–624.
217. Rickert CH, Paulus W. Epidemiology of central nervous system tumors in childhood and adolescence based on the new WHO classification. *Childs Nerv Syst* 2001;17:503–511.
218. Ris MD, Packer R, Goldwein J, et al. Intellectual outcome after reduced-dose radiation therapy plus adjuvant chemotherapy for medulloblastoma: a Children's Cancer Group study. *J Clin Oncol* 2001;19:3470–3476.
219. Roberge D, Kun LE, Freeman CR. Intracranial germinoma: on whole-ventricular irradiation. *Pediatr Blood Cancer* 2005;44:358–362.
220. Robertson PL, DaRosso RC, Allen JC. Improved prognosis of intracranial non-germinoma germ cell tumors with multimodality therapy. *J Neurooncol* 1997;32:71–80.
221. Robertson PL, Muraszko KM, Brunberg JA, et al. Pediatric midbrain tumors: a benign subgroup of brainstem gliomas. *Pediatr Neurosurg* 1995;22:65–73.
222. Robertson PL, Zeltzer PM, Boyett JM, et al. Survival and prognostic factors following radiation therapy and chemotherapy for ependymomas in children: a report of the Children's Cancer Group. *J Neurosurg* 1998;88:695–703.
223. Rodrigues GB, Waldron JN, Wong CS, et al. A retrospective analysis of 52 cases of spinal cord glioma managed with radiation therapy. *Int J Radiat Oncol Biol Phys* 2000;48:837–842.
224. Rogers L, Pueschel J, Spetzler R, et al. Is gross-total resection sufficient treatment for posterior fossa ependymomas?. *J Neurosurg* 2005;102:629–636.
225. Rorke LB, Packer RJ, Biegel JA. Central nervous system atypical teratoid/rhabdoid tumors of infancy and childhood: definition of an entity. *J Neurosurg* 1996;85:56–65.
226. Rumana CS, Valadka AB, Contant CF. Prognostic factors in supratentorial ganglioglioma. *Acta Neurochir (Wien)* 1999;141:63–68.
227. Rutkowski S, Bode U, Deinlein F, et al. Treatment of early childhood medulloblastoma by postoperative chemotherapy alone. *N Engl J Med* 2005;352:978–986.
228. Sands SA, Kellie SJ, Davidow AL, et al. Long-term quality of life and neuropsychologic functioning for patients with CNS germ-cell tumors: from the First International CNS Germ-Cell Tumor Study. *Neurooncology* 2001;3:174–183.
229. Sands SA, Milner JS, Goldberg J, et al. Quality of life and behavioral follow-up study of pediatric survivors of craniopharyngioma. *J Neurosurg* 2005;103:302–311.
230. Saran FH, Baumert BG, Khoo VS, et al. Stereotactically guided conformal radiotherapy for progressive low-grade gliomas of childhood. *Int J Radiat Oncol Biol Phys* 2002;53:43–51.
231. Saran FH, Driever PH, Thilmann C, et al. Survival of very young children with medulloblastoma (primitive neuroectodermal tumor of the posterior fossa) treated with craniospinal irradiation. *Int J Radiat Oncol Biol Phys* 1998;42:959–967.
232. Saunders DE, Phipps KP, Wade AM, et al. Surveillance imaging strategies following surgery and/or radiotherapy for childhood cerebellar low-grade astrocytoma. *J Neurosurg* 2005;102:172–178.
233. Sawamura Y, Ikeda J, Shirato H, et al. Germ cell tumours of the central nervous system: treatment consideration based on 111 cases and their long-term clinical outcomes. *Eur J Cancer* 1998;34:104–110.
234. Sawamura Y, Shirato H, Ikeda J, et al. Induction chemotherapy followed by reduced-volume radiation therapy for newly diagnosed central nervous system germinoma. *J Neurosurg* 1998;88:66–72.
235. Scerrati M, Montemaggi P, Iacoangeli M, et al. Interstitial brachytherapy for low-grade cerebral gliomas: analysis of results in a series of 36 cases. *Acta Neurochir (Wien)* 1994;131:97–105.
236. Schild SE, Haddock MG, Scheithauer BW, et al. Nongerminomatous germ cell tumors of the brain. *Int J Radiat Oncol Biol Phys* 1996;36:557–563.
237. Schild SE, Nisi K, Scheithauer BW, et al. The results of radiotherapy for ependymomas: the Mayo Clinic experience. *Int J Radiat Oncol Biol Phys* 1998;42:953–958.
238. Schild SE, Scheithauer BW, Haddock MG, et al. Histologically confirmed pineal tumors and other germ cell tumors of the brain. *Cancer* 1996;78:2564–2571.
239. Schild SE, Scheithauer BW, Schomberg PJ, et al. Pineal parenchymal tumors. Clinical, pathologic, and therapeutic aspects. *Cancer* 1993;72:870–880.
240. Schmiegelow M, Lassen S, Weber L,. Dosimetry and growth hormone deficiency following cranial irradiation of childhood brain tumors. *Med Pediatr Oncol* 1999;33:564–571.
241. Schoenfeld GO, Amdur RJ, Schmalfuss IM, et al. Low-dose prophylactic craniospinal radiotherapy for intracranial germinoma. *Int J Radiat Oncol Biol Phys* 2006;65:481–485.
242. Schulz-Ertner D, Debus J, Lohr F, et al. Fractionated stereotactic conformal radiation therapy of brain stem gliomas: outcome and prognostic factors. *Radiother Oncol* 2000;57:215–223.
243. Schulz-Ertner D, Frank C, Herfarth KK, et al. Fractionated stereotactic radiotherapy for craniopharyngiomas. *Int J Radiat Oncol Biol Phys* 2002;54:1114–1120.
244. Scott RM, Hetelekidis S, Barnes PD, et al. Surgery, radiation, and combination therapy in the treatment of childhood craniopharyngioma—a 20-year experience. *Pediatr Neurosurg* 1994;21[Suppl 1]:75–81.
245. Scott RM. Craniopharyngioma: a personal (Boston) experience. *Childs Nerv Syst* 2005;21:773–777.
246. Selch MT, Goy BW, Lee SP, et al. Gangliogliomas: experience with 34 patients and review of the literature. *Am J Clin Oncol* 1998;21:557–564.
247. Sgouros S, Fineron PW, Hockley AD. Cerebellar astrocytoma of childhood: long-term follow-up. *Childs Nerv Syst* 1995;11:89–96.
248. Shibamoto Y, Sasai K, Oya N, et al. Intracranial germinoma: radiation therapy with tumor volume-based dose selection. *Radiology* 2001;218:452–456.
249. Shirato H, Aoyama H, Ikeda J, et al. Impact of margin for target volume in low-dose involved field radiotherapy after induction chemotherapy for intracranial germinoma. *Int J Radiat Oncol Biol Phys* 2004;60:214–217.
250. Shirato H, Nishio M, Sawamura Y, et al. Analysis of long-term treatment of intracranial germinoma. *Int J Radiat Oncol Biol Phys* 1997;37:511–515.
251. Sklar CA, Constine LS. Chronic neuroendocrinological sequelae of radiation therapy. *Int J Radiat Oncol Biol Phys* 1995;31:1113–1121.
252. Sposto R, Ertel IJ, Jenkin RD, et al. The effectiveness of chemotherapy for treatment of high grade astrocytoma in children: results of a randomized trial. A report from the Children's Cancer study group. *J Neurooncol* 1989;7:165–177.
253. St. Clair WH, Adams JA, Bues M, et al. Advantage of protons compared to conventional x-ray or IMRT in the treatment of a pediatric patient with medulloblastoma. *Int J Radiat Oncol Biol Phys* 2004;58:727–734.
254. Strother D, Ashley D, Kellie SJ, et al. Feasibility of four consecutive high-dose chemotherapy cycles with stem-cell rescue for patients with newly diagnosed medulloblastoma or supratentorial primitive neuroectodermal tumor after craniospinal radiotherapy: results of a collaborative study. *J Clin Oncol* 2001;19:2696–2704.
255. Strother D. Atypical teratoid rhabdoid tumors of childhood: diagnosis, treatment and challenges. *Expert Rev Anticancer Ther* 2005;5:907–915.
256. Surveillance Epidemiology and End Results.SEER 2006. http://seer.cancer.gov/publications
257. Sutton LN, Radcliffe J, Goldwein JW, et al. Quality of life of adult survivors of germinomas treated with craniospinal irradiation. *Neurosurgery* 1999;45:1292–1297.
258. Tait DM, Thornton-Jones H, Bloom HJ, et al. Adjuvant chemotherapy for medulloblastoma: the first multi-centre control trial of the International Society of Paediatric Oncology (SIOP I). *Eur J Cancer* 1990;26:464–469.
259. Tao ML, Barnes PD, Billett AL, et al. Childhood optic chiasm gliomas: radiographic response following radiotherapy and long-term clinical outcome. *Int J Radiat Oncol Biol Phys* 1997;39:579–587.
260. Tarbell NJ, Barnes P, Scott RM, et al. Advances in radiation therapy for craniopharyngiomas. *Pediatr Neurosurg* 1994;21[Suppl 1]:101–107.
261. Tarbell NJ, Loeffler JS. Recent trends in the radiotherapy of pediatric gliomas. *J Neurooncol* 1996;28:233–244.
262. Taylor RE, Bailey CC, Robinson K, et al. Results of a randomized study of preradiation chemotherapy versus radiotherapy alone for nonmetastatic medulloblastoma: the International Society of Paediatric Oncology/United Kingdom Children's Cancer Study Group PNET-3 study. *J Clin Oncol* 2003;21:1581–1591.
263. Taylor RE, Bailey CC, Robinson KJ, et al. Impact of radiotherapy parameters on outcome in the International Society of Paediatric Oncology/United Kingdom

Children's Cancer Study Group PNET-3 study of preradiotherapy chemotherapy for M0-M1 medulloblastoma. *Int J Radiat Oncol Biol Phys* 2004;58:1184–1193.

264. Taylor RE, Bailey CC, Robinson KJ, et al. Outcome for patients with metastatic (M2-3) medulloblastoma treated with SIOP/UKCCSG PNET-3 chemotherapy. *Eur J Cancer* 2005;41:727–734.

265. Taylor RE. Review of radiotherapy dose and volume for intracranial ependymoma. *Pediatr Blood Cancer* 2004;42:287–460.

266. Tekautz TM, Fuller CE, Blaney S, et al. Atypical teratoid/rhabdoid tumors (ATRT): improved survival in children 3 years of age and older with radiation therapy and high-dose alkylator-based chemotherapy. *J Clin Oncol* 2005;23:1491–1499.

267. Thomas PR, Deutsch M, Kepner JL, et al. Low-stage medulloblastoma: final analysis of trial comparing standard-dose with reduced-dose neuraxis irradiation. *J Clin Oncol* 2000;18:3004–3011.

268. Thompson D, Phipps K, Hayward R. Craniopharyngioma in childhood: our evidence-based approach to management. *Childs Nerv Syst* 2005;21:660–668.

269. Timmermann B, Kortmann RD, Kuhl J, et al. Combined postoperative irradiation and chemotherapy for anaplastic ependymomas in childhood: results of the German prospective trials HIT 88/89 and HIT 91. *Int J Radiat Oncol Biol Phys* 2000;46:287–295.

270. Timmermann B, Kortmann RD, Kuhl J, et al. Role of radiotherapy in the treatment of supratentorial primitive neuroectodermal tumors in childhood: results of the prospective German brain tumor trials HIT 88/89 and 91. *J Clin Oncol* 2002;20:842–849.

271. Timmermann B, Kortmann RD, Kuhl J, et al. Role of radiotherapy in anaplastic ependymoma in children under age of 3 years: results of the prospective German brain tumor trials HIT-SKK 87 and 92. *Radiother Oncol* 2005;77:278–285.

272. Timmermann B, Kortmann RD, Kuhl J, et al. Role of radiotherapy in supratentorial primitive neuroectodermal tumor in young children: results of the German HIT-SKK87 and HIT-SKK92 trials. *J Clin Oncol* 2006;24:1554–1560.

273. Tomita T, Bowman RM. Craniopharyngiomas in children: surgical experience at Children's Memorial Hospital. *Childs Nerv Syst* 2005;21:729–746.

274. Tomita T, McLone DG. Radical resections of childhood craniopharyngiomas. *Pediatr Neurosurg* 1993;19:6–14.

275. Urie M, FitzGerald TJ, Followill D, et al. Current calibration, treatment, and treatment planning techniques among institutions participating in the Children's Oncology Group. *Int J Radiat Oncol Biol Phys* 2003;55:245–260.

276. van Veelen-Vincent ML, Pierre-Kahn A, Kalifa C, et al. Ependymoma in childhood: prognostic factors, extent of surgery, and adjuvant therapy. *J Neurosurg* 2002;97:827–835.

277. Vanuytsel LJ, Bessell EM, Ashley SE, et al. Intracranial ependymoma: long-term results of a policy of surgery and radiotherapy. *Int J Radiat Oncol Biol Phys* 1992;23:313–319.

278. Weiss E, Behring B, Behnke J, et al. Treatment of primary malignant rhabdoid tumor of the brain: report of three cases and review of the literature. *Int J Radiat Oncol Biol Phys* 1998;41:1013–1019.

279. West CG, Gattamaneni R, Blair V. Radiotherapy in the treatment of low-grade astrocytomas. I. A survival analysis. *Childs Nerv Syst* 1995;11:438–442.

280. Wisoff JH, Boyett JM, Berger MS, et al. Current neurosurgical management and the impact of the extent of resection in the treatment of malignant gliomas of childhood: a report of the Children's Cancer Group trial no. CCG-945. *J Neurosurg* 1998;89:52–59.

281. Wolden SL, Dunkel IJ, Souweidane MM, et al. Patterns of failure using a conformal radiation therapy tumor bed boost for medulloblastoma. *J Clin Oncol* 2003;21:3079–3083.

282. Wolff JE, Sajedi M, Brant R, et al. Choroid plexus tumours. *Br J Cancer* 2002;87:1086–1091.

283. Wolff JE, Sajedi M, Coppes MJ, et al. Radiation therapy and survival in choroid plexus carcinoma. *Lancet* 1999;353:2126.

284. Wrede B, Liu P, Ater J, et al. Second surgery and the prognosis of choroid plexus carcinoma—results of a meta-analysis of individual cases. *Anticancer Res* 2005;25:4429–4433.

285. Wrensch M, Minn Y, Chew T, et al. Epidemiology of primary brain tumors: current concepts and review of the literature. *Neurooncology* 2002;4:278–299.

286. Zeltzer PM, Boyett JM, Finlay JL, et al. Metastasis stage, adjuvant treatment, and residual tumor are prognostic factors for medulloblastoma in children: conclusions from the Children's Cancer Group 921 randomized phase III study. *J Clin Oncol* 1999;17:832–845.

Chapter 83
Wilms' Tumor

John A. Kalapurakal, Patrick R.M. Thomas

Wilms' tumor (WT, nephroblastoma) is a highly curable childhood neoplasm. The prognosis of children with WT has considerably improved from a very high mortality rate at the beginning of the 20th century to the current cure rate of >90% (21). The management of WT is a paradigm for successful interdisciplinary treatment of solid tumors of childhood to maximize cure rates and minimize treatment-related complications.

Epidemiology

WT is the most common malignant renal tumor of childhood. It occurs with an annual incidence of 7 cases per million children <15 years of age. Approximately 450 new cases are diagnosed each year in North America. The peak incidence is between 3 and 4 years of age. WT may arise as sporadic or hereditary tumors, or in the setting of specific genetic disorders (8). Most WTs are solitary lesions, multifocal within a single kidney in 12% and bilateral in 7% (11). The clinical syndromes associated with WT include WAGR syndrome (WT, aniridia, genitourinary malformations, mental retardation), Denys-Drash syndrome (pseudohermaphroditism, mesangial sclerosis, renal failure, and WT), and overgrowth syndromes like Beckwith-Wiedemann syndrome (somatic gigantism, omphalocele, macroglossia, genitourinary abnormalities, ear creases, hypoglycemia, hemihypertrophy, and a predisposition to WT and other malignancies) and Simpson-Golabi-Behmel syndrome (15,20).

Biology

Among the various genetic changes implicated in the development of WT, the most widely studied involves *WT1*. *WT1* is a tumor suppressor gene at chromosome 11p13 that was isolated from a child with WAGR syndrome (17). *WT1* is likely to play a specific role in glomerular and gonadal development (66). *WT1* can also act as a dominant negative oncogene resulting in abnormal cell growth such as in Denys-Drash syndrome (64). Germline *WT1* mutations are observed in approximately 82% of WT patients who have genitourinary anomalies or renal failure. The frequency of *WT1* mutations in sporadic and familial WT is much lower at ~20% and ~4%, respectively (47). Beckwith-Wiedemann syndrome maps to chromosome 11p15.5; this locus is also referred to as "*WT2*" (53). Patients with loss of heterozygosity (LOH) on 16q and 1p have been shown to have higher relapse and mortality rates (43). A primary objective of the National Wilms' Tumor Study-5 (NWTS-5) was to prospectively evaluate the prognostic significance of LOH on 16q and 1p. In this study, the frequency of LOH in favorable histology (FH), anaplasia, clear cell sarcoma of kidney (CCSK), and rhabdoid tumor of kidney (RTK) was 11%, 16%, 4% and 0% respectively. Patients with tumor-specific LOH at 1p or 16q had a significantly increased relative risk (RR) of relapse of 1.56 and 1.49, respectively. For stage I/II patients with no LOH, the 4-year relapse-free survival (RFS) and overall survival (OS) rates were 91% and 98%, respectively. For these patients

who had LOH at 1p only or 16q only or LOH at both 1p and 16q, their OS rates were 91% (*p* = .02), 98% (*p* = .6), and 91% (*p* = .01), respectively. In children with LOH at both loci, the RR for relapse and death were 2.9 (*p* = .001) and 4.3 (*p* = .01), respectively. Among advanced stage (stage III/IV) patients, those with LOH at both 1p and 16q had a higher risk of relapse (RR, 2.4; *p* = .01) and death (RR, 2.7; *p* = .04). LOH at either locus did not correlate with relapse or death in these patients. It was postulated that, in the advanced-stage patients, the use of doxorubicin and radiation therapy (RT) may have overcome the adverse effects caused by the loss of the putative tumor suppressor genes located within these chromosomal regions. Based on these results, it was proposed that in future WT trials, the therapy for children with LOH at both 1p and 16q be augmented by the addition of doxorubicin to regimen EE4A for early-stage (stage I/II) tumors and cyclophosphamide/etoposide to regimen DD4A for advanced-stage tumors (stage III/IV) (42) (see Tables 83.3 and 83.4).

Pathologic Classification

Although histopathologists had attempted to relate appearance to prognosis, no generally acceptable classification was available until the report of Beckwith and Palmer (2) from the National Wilms' Tumor Study-1 (NWTS-1). The NWTS classifies all tumors as having either FH or unfavorable histology (UH). The UH tumors include anaplastic tumors, clear cell sarcoma, and rhabdoid tumor of kidney (2). Of 1,465 patients randomly assigned on NWTS-3, 163 (11.1%) had UH (23). WT are usually sharply demarcated, spherical masses with a "pushing" border and a surrounding distinct intrarenal pseudocapsule. Histologically, WT reflects the development of the normal kidney, consisting of three components, blastemal, epithelial (tubules), and stromal elements, in varying proportions (2). The proportion of the different components has prognostic significance (3).

Nephrogenic rests consist of embryonal nephroblastic tissue and are found in 35% of kidneys with unilateral WT and in nearly 100% of kidneys with bilateral WT (6). Nephrogenic rests may be intralobar or perilobar based on their location within the kidney (5). Most nephrogenic rests undergo spontaneous regression, and only a small proportion (1% to 5%) transform into WT (19).

The histologic feature of greatest clinical significance in WT is anaplasia (10). Anaplasia may be focal (FA) or diffuse (DA). The definition of FA and DA has been revised to reflect the distribution of anaplastic cells in the tumor rather than their quantitative density. This revised definition is of prognostic significance. The 4-year survival rates for patients with stage II, III, and IV FA disease were 90%, 100%, and 100%, compared with 55%, 45%, and 4%, respectively, for patients with similar-stage DA disease (31).

CCSK and malignant RTK are no longer considered true WT, but have been included in NWTS protocols (2). CCSK has a propensity to metastasize to bone, and a skeletal survey and bone scan should be performed. RTK is the most lethal renal neoplasm in children. Primitive neuroepithelial tumors of the cerebellum or pineal region may be seen in 10% to 15% of patients with RTK (71).

Clinical Presentation

The classic presentation for WT is that of a healthy child in whom abdominal swelling is discovered by the child's mother or by a physician during a routine physical examination. A smooth, firm, nontender mass on one side of the abdomen is felt. Gross hematuria occurs in as many as 25% of these cases (55). The child may be hypertensive or have nonspecific symptoms such as malaise or fever (74). Only rarely does a patient present with symptomatic metastases.

Diagnostic Work-Up

The differential diagnosis of WT includes other malignant childhood lesions of the kidney, neuroblastoma, and benign conditions such as hydronephrosis, polycystic disease, and splenomegaly in left-sided tumors. Plain films of the abdomen may demonstrate calcifications, which occur in 60% to 70% of neuroblastomas but in only 5% to 10% of WT. Excretory urography (intravenous pyelography) was once the mainstay of imaging in WT and now has largely been replaced by ultrasonography and computed tomography (CT) scanning. Ultrasonography is very useful because it is readily available and is cost-effective (45). A specific advantage of ultrasonography is its ability to assess vessels for flow and tumor thrombus with duplex and color Doppler (67). Abdominal CT scans can demonstrate gross extrarenal spread, lymph node involvement, liver metastases, and the status of the opposite kidney (68) (Fig. 83.1). Magnetic resonance imaging has several advantages over CT scans, especially in identifying renal origin and vascular extension of the tumor (7). CT and magnetic resonance imaging are useful in the detection and follow-up of patients with nephrogenic rests (44). Clinical and imaging impressions do not, however, obviate the need for inspection at laparotomy (69).

Plain chest radiography and chest CT are also essential because asymptomatic pulmonary metastases are common (18).

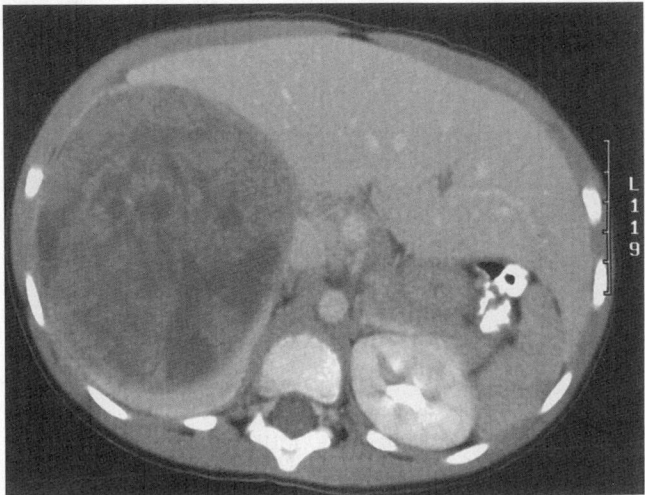

FIGURE 83.1. Computed tomography scan of a 4-year-old girl with a large right-sided Wilms' tumor measuring 10.5 × 8.4 × 13.5 cm. The left kidney did not show any lesions. At laparotomy, the tumor was found to invade the diaphragm. She underwent a right radical nephrectomy. Surgical margins of resection were positive and she had metastases in the para-aortic lymph nodes. The tumor was classified as stage III favorable histology and received 10.8 Gy to the right flank and chemotherapy with vincristine, dactinomycin, and doxorubicin.

In children enrolled in NWTS-3 and NWTS-4, with FH tumors, negative chest radiographs, and CT scans positive for pulmonary metastases, the 4-year event-free survival rates with and without irradiation were similar at 89% and 80%, respectively (58).

A complete blood cell count and urinalysis should be performed. Patients with WT can be anemic from hematuria. Serum blood urea nitrogen and creatinine levels and liver function tests are routine. If neuroblastoma is not ruled out, a test for urinary catecholamines should be performed. Table 83.1 outlines the pretreatment investigations recommended in NWTS-5.

Natural History

The disease is often localized at diagnosis, as evidenced by the fact that surgery and radiation therapy is curative in almost 50% of cases (40). The first signs of local tumor spread beyond the pseudocapsule are invasion into the renal sinus or the intrarenal blood and lymphatic vessels. Spread throughout the peritoneal cavity may also occur, especially if there has been preoperative rupture or the disease has been spilled at surgery (24,30). The most common sites of metastases of WT are in the lungs, lymph nodes, and liver. Among patients with stage IV disease, lungs were the only metastatic site in approximately 80% of patients (12). The NWTS-2 study demonstrated the prognostic importance of lymph node involvement. The 2-year RFS rate was 82% without lymph node involvement, compared with 54% with positive lymph nodes (24).

Staging

Tumor staging is performed after examining the radiologic, operative, and histopathologic findings. In NWTS-1 and NWTS-2, a tumor grouping system was used for tumor staging and treatment stratification. After analyzing the prognostic significance of several clinicopathologic factors in NWTS-1 and NWTS-2, a new staging system was adopted in NWTS-3. The presence of lymph node involvement was upstaged as stage III instead of group II, and local tumor spill was downstaged from group III to stage II (30). For NWTS-5, the most significant change was the distinction between stages I and II. Criteria for stage I were refined to accommodate an important subset of WT that is being managed by nephrectomy alone. Before NWTS-5, the distinction between stages I and II in the renal sinus was established by the hilar plane, which was an imaginary plane connecting the most medial aspects of the upper and lower poles of the kidney. This criterion was difficult to apply because of tumor distortion, and thus the hilar plane criterion has been replaced with renal sinus vascular or lymphatic invasion. This definition includes not only the involvement of vessels within the hilar soft tissue, but of vessels located in the radial extensions of the renal sinus into the renal parenchyma (4,79). The Children's Oncology Group (COG) staging guidelines for WT are shown in Table 83.2. The major change from NWTS-5 is that children with tumor spillage are upstaged from stage II to stage III because of the higher risk for relapse with two-drug chemotherapy alone (49). The COG risk group classification for treatment assignment in the new generation of WT protocols are shown in Table 83.3. In addition to tumor stage, this classification will also consider patient's age, tumor weight, presence or absence of LOH at 1p and 16q, and response to chemotherapy in children with FH tumors and lung metastases (Table 83.4).

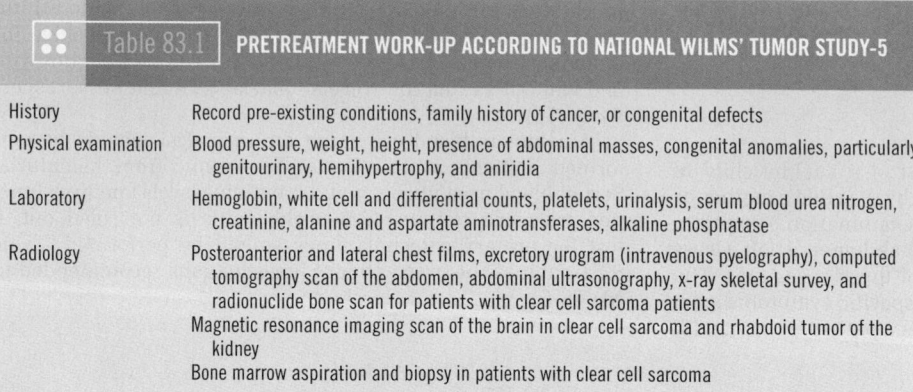

Table 83.1	PRETREATMENT WORK-UP ACCORDING TO NATIONAL WILMS' TUMOR STUDY-5
History	Record pre-existing conditions, family history of cancer, or congenital defects
Physical examination	Blood pressure, weight, height, presence of abdominal masses, congenital anomalies, particularly genitourinary, hemihypertrophy, and aniridia
Laboratory	Hemoglobin, white cell and differential counts, platelets, urinalysis, serum blood urea nitrogen, creatinine, alanine and aspartate aminotransferases, alkaline phosphatase
Radiology	Posteroanterior and lateral chest films, excretory urogram (intravenous pyelography), computed tomography scan of the abdomen, abdominal ultrasonography, x-ray skeletal survey, and radionuclide bone scan for patients with clear cell sarcoma patients
	Magnetic resonance imaging scan of the brain in clear cell sarcoma and rhabdoid tumor of the kidney
	Bone marrow aspiration and biopsy in patients with clear cell sarcoma

Table 83.2	CHILDREN'S ONCOLOGY GROUP STAGING OF WILMS TUMOR, RHABDOID TUMOR AND CLEAR CELL SARCOMA OF THE KIDNEY

Stage I—Tumor limited to kidney, completely resected. The renal capsule is intact. The tumor was not ruptured or biopsied prior to removal. The vessels of the renal sinus are not involved. There is no evidence of tumor at or beyond the margins of resection. Note: For a tumor to quality for certain therapeutic protocols as stage I, regional lymph nodes must be examined microscopically.

Stage II—The tumor is completely resected and there is no evidence of tumor at or beyond the margins of resection. The tumor extends beyond kidney, as is evidenced by any one of the following criteria:

- There is regional extension of the tumor (i.e., penetration of the renal capsule or extensive invasion of the soft tissue of the renal sinus, as discussed later)
- Blood vessels within the nephrectomy specimen outside the renal parenchyma, including those of the renal sinus, contain tumor.

Note: Rupture of spillage confined to the flank, including biopsy of the tumor, is no longer included in stage II and is now included in stage III.

Stage III—Residual nonhematogenous tumor present following surgery, and confined to abdomen. Any one of the following may occur:

- Lymph nodes within the abdomen or pelvis are involved by tumor. (Lymph node involvement in the thorax, or other extra-abdominal sites is a criterion for stage IV.)
- The tumor has penetrated through the peritoneal surface
- Tumor implants are found on the peritoneal surface
- Gross or microscopic tumor remains postoperatively (e.g., tumor cells are found at the margin of surgical resection on microscopic examination)
- The tumor is not completely resectable because of local infiltration into vital structures
- Tumor spillage occurring either before or during surgery
- The tumor was biopsied (whether tru-cut, open, or fine-needle aspiration) before removal
- Tumor is removed in more than one piece (e.g., tumor cells are found in a separately excised adrenal gland; a tumor thrombus within the renal vein is removed separately from the nephrectomy specimen)

Stage IV—Hematogenous metastases (ouch or lung, liver, bone, brain) or lymph node metastases outside the abdominopelvic region are present. (The presence of tumor within the adrenal gland is not interpreted as metastasis and staging depends on all other staging parameters present.)

Stage V—Bilateral renal involvement by tumor is present at diagnosis. An attempt should be made to stage each side according to the criteria here on the basis of the extent of disease.

Table 83.3	CHILDREN'S ONCOLOGY GROUP (COG) RISK GROUP CLASSIFICATION FOR FAVORABLE HISTOLOGY WILMS TUMORS

Age	Tumor Weight	Stage	LOH (both 1p and 16q)	Rapid Response No.	Risk Group	COG Study	Treatment
<2 yr	<550 g	I	Any	N/A	Very Low	AREN0532	Surgery only
Any	≥550 g	I	None	N/A	Low	AREN0532	EE4A
≥2 yr	Any	I	None	N/A	Low	AREN0532	EE4A
Any	Any	II	None	N/A	Low	AREN0532	EE4A
≥2 yr	Any	I	Yes	N/A	Standard	AREN0532	DD4A
Any	≥550 g	I	Yes	N/A	Standard	AREN0532	DD4A
Any	Any	II	Yes	N/A	Standard	AREN0532	DD4A
Any	Any	III	None	Any	Standard	AREN0532	DD4A
Any	Any	III	Yes	Any	Higher	AREN0533	M
Any	Any	IV	Yes	Any	Higher	AREN0533	M
Any	Any	IV	None	Yes	Standard	AREN0533	DD4A
Any	Any	IV	None	No	Higher	AREN0533	M

LOH, loss of heterozygosity; N/A, not applicable; AREN, DD4A (V [vincristine] A [dactinomycin] D [doxorubicin]); M (VAD/Cy [cyclophosphamide] E [etoposide]), EE4A (VA)

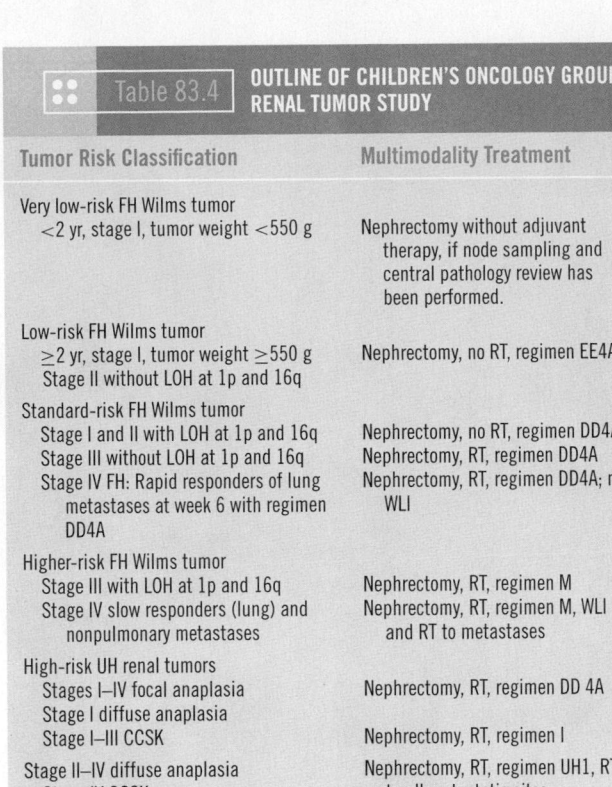

Table 83.4 OUTLINE OF CHILDREN'S ONCOLOGY GROUP RENAL TUMOR STUDY

Tumor Risk Classification	Multimodality Treatment
Very low-risk FH Wilms tumor <2 yr, stage I, tumor weight <550 g	Nephrectomy without adjuvant therapy, if node sampling and central pathology review has been performed.
Low-risk FH Wilms tumor ≥2 yr, stage I, tumor weight ≥550 g Stage II without LOH at 1p and 16q	Nephrectomy, no RT, regimen EE4A
Standard-risk FH Wilms tumor Stage I and II with LOH at 1p and 16q Stage III without LOH at 1p and 16q Stage IV FH: Rapid responders of lung metastases at week 6 with regimen DD4A	Nephrectomy, no RT, regimen DD4A Nephrectomy, RT, regimen DD4A Nephrectomy, RT, regimen DD4A; no WLI
Higher-risk FH Wilms tumor Stage III with LOH at 1p and 16q Stage IV slow responders (lung) and nonpulmonary metastases	Nephrectomy, RT, regimen M Nephrectomy, RT, regimen M, WLI and RT to metastases
High-risk UH renal tumors Stages I–IV focal anaplasia Stage I diffuse anaplasia Stage I–III CCSK	Nephrectomy, RT, regimen DD 4A Nephrectomy, RT, regimen I
Stage II–IV diffuse anaplasia Stage IV CCSK Stage I–IV RTK	Nephrectomy, RT, regimen UH1, RT to all metastatic sites

FH, favorable histology; LOH, loss of heterozygosity; RT, flank or abdominal irradiation; regimen EE4A (VA); regimen DD 4A (V [vincristine] A [dactinomycin] D [doxorubicin]); WLI, whole-lung irradiation; regimen M (VAD/Cy [cyclophosphamide] E [etoposide]); UH, unfavorable histology; CCSK, clear cell sarcoma of kidney; RTK, rhabdoid tumor of kidney; regimen I (alternating VDCy/CyE); regimen UH1 (alternating VDCy/CyC [carboplatin] E).

General Management

The diagnosis of WT is usually made before surgery and confirmed at surgery. A transverse transabdominal, transperitoneal incision is recommended for adequate exposure and thorough abdominal exploration. The contralateral kidney should be palpated and visualized to rule out bilateral WT before nephrectomy (54). The surgeon must excise all tumor without spillage, if possible. Lymph node sampling from the para-aortic, celiac, and iliac areas must be performed. The use of titanium clips to identify residual tumor and margins of resection is also recommended.

Radiation Therapy Techniques

Radiation therapy guidelines used for primary and recurrent WT in the COG protocols are shown in Table 83.5.

Timing of Radiation Therapy

The NWTS has shown that, although irradiation does not need to be given immediately after surgery (40), a delay of ≥10 days after surgery was associated with a significantly higher abdominal relapse rate, particularly among patients with UH tumors (25,26,76,77). Because the pathologist cannot always rule out UH quickly, all patients with WT should be scheduled to start RT not later than day 9, the day of surgery being day 0. Although most patients may not be irradiated, it is easier to cancel than to make arrangements to start irradiation for a small child on short notice. The influence of RT delay on abdominal tumor recurrence in patients with FH tumors treated on NWTS-3 and

NWTS-4 have been reported. The mean RT delay was 10.9 days. Although univariate and multivariate analysis did not reveal RT delay of ≥10 days to adversely influence flank and abdominal recurrence, it is important to note that in 59% of children the RT delay ranged from 8 to 12 days (50). For the COG protocols it is recommended that RT be given preferably by day 9 but no later than day 14 after surgery (Table 83.5).

Radiation Therapy Dose

In NWTS-1 and NWTS-2, radiation dosages to the operative bed were given according to the age of the patient, and no significant dose-response association was detected (26,77). In NWTS-3, there was a randomization for patients with FH tumors that resulted in elimination of radiation therapy for stage II FH, and a dose of 10 Gy for stage III and 12 Gy for lung irradiation in stage IV (23,76). NWTS-3 and NWTS-4 data showed no radiation dose response for CCSK and anaplastic tumors (33). Therefore, it was decided to treat all abdominal disease with 10 Gy. In the COG protocols, children with stage III anaplastic tumors and RTK will receive a higher dose of 19.8 Gy (29,78) (Table 83.5).

Table 83.5 CHILDREN'S ONCOLOGY GROUP RENAL TUMOR PROTOCOL RADIATION THERAPY GUIDELINES

Abdominal Tumor Stage and Histology	RT Dose/RT Field[a]
Stage I and II FH Wilms tumor	None
Stage III FH, stage I–III focal anaplasia, stage I–II diffuse anaplasia, stage I–III CCSK[c]	10.8 Gy to the flank[b]
Stage III diffuse anaplasia, stage I–III RTK	19.8 Gy (infants 10.8 Gy) flank[b] RT
Recurrent abdominal Wilms tumor	12.6–18 Gy (<12 months of age)[b] or 21.6 Gy (older children) if previous radiation dose is ≤10.8 Gy. Boost dose of up to 9 Gy to gross residual tumor after surgery
Lung metastases (favorable histology)	12 Gy WLI in 8 fractions[d]
Lung metastases (unfavorable histology)	12 Gy WLI in 8 fractions
Brain metastases	30.6 Gy whole brain in 17 fractions, or 21.6 Gy whole brain + 10.8 Gy IMRT or stereotactic boost
Liver metastases	19.8 Gy whole liver in 11 fractions
Bone metastases	25.2 Gy to the lesion plus 3-cm margin
Unresected lymph node metastases	19.8 Gy

RT radiation therapy; FH, favorable histology; CCSK, clear cell sarcoma of the kidney; RTK, rhabdoid tumor of kidney; WLI, whole-lung irradiation; IMRT, intensity-modulated RT.
[a]Timing of RT (RT delay): RT should begin as close to the beginning of chemotherapy as possible, preferably by day 9 (surgery is day 0), but no later than day 14, unless medically contraindicated or when there is a delay in central pathology review.
[b]Whole-abdomen irradiation (WAI) is indicated when there is diffuse tumor spillage, preoperative or intraperitoneal tumor rupture, peritoneal tumor seeding, and cytology positive ascites. When WAI dose is >10 Gy, renal shielding is required to limit the dose to the remaining kidney to <14.4 Gy. Gross residual disease after surgery should receive a boost of 10 Gy.
[c]Children's Oncology Group (COG) protocol (AREN0321) is studying the possibility of eliminating RT in children with stage I CCSK tumors after central pathology review and lymph node sampling.
[d]COG protocol (AREN0533) is studying the possibility of eliminating WLI in children with lung metastases who are rapid responders (complete response of lung metastasis after three-drug chemotherapy on central review of computed tomography [CT] scans at week 6). Tumor size, number of lesions, and CT or x-ray detectability are not considered indications for WLI in FH tumors.

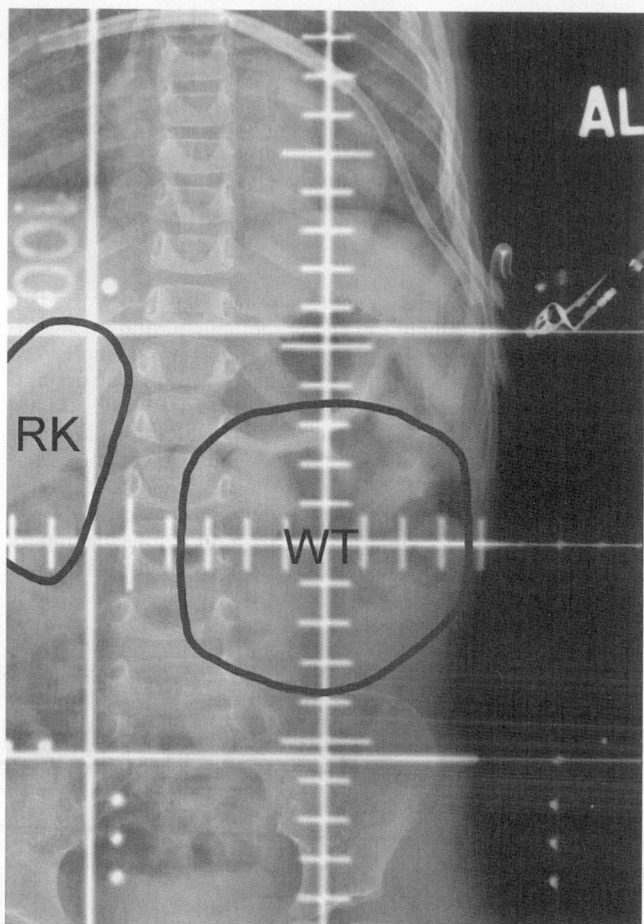

FIGURE 83.2. Simulation film of an anteroposterior portal of the flank in a 2-year-old child with a left-sided stage III favorable-histology Wilms' tumor (WT), showing inclusion of the entire width of the vertebral body in the irradiated volume. The outline of the right kidney (RK) and the WT from the preoperative computed tomography scan is shown.

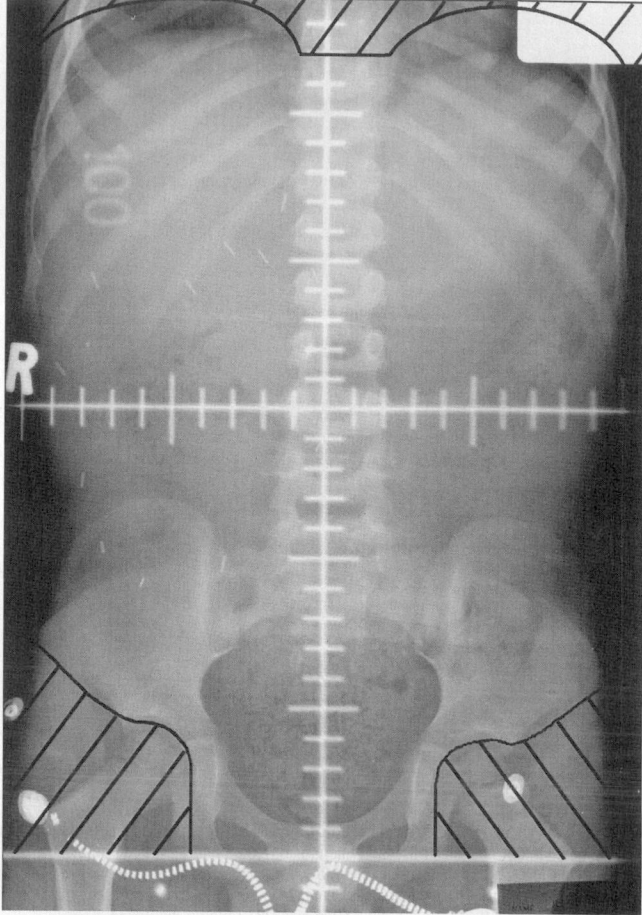

FIGURE 83.3. Anteroposterior portal for the whole abdomen used in irradiation of patients with stage III Wilms' tumor and diffuse peritoneal tumor spillage. The upper margin of the abdominal field must include the diaphragm. The acetabulum and femoral head should be excluded from the irradiated volume to decrease the probability of slipped femoral capital epiphysis. The pants zipper can be seen low on the hips. In general, it is advisable to remove the trousers completely to ensure a reproducible setup.

Radiation Therapy Volume

Parallel opposed fields using 4- or 6-MV photons are preferred. The treatment portals should encompass the tumor bed and the site of the excised kidney with a 2- to 3-cm margin. The medial border must cross the midline to include the entire width of the vertebrae so as to minimize growth disturbances. A tangential abdominal wall shield may be used. An example of a portal used for flank irradiation is presented in Figure 83.2 (26). When whole-abdomen irradiation is administered, shaped portals must be used, and the femoral heads and acetabulum must be shielded (Fig. 83.3). Whole-lung irradiation portals are shown in Figure 83.4.

Results of Therapy

The major advances in its treatment have come from randomized clinical trials. Single-institution studies have not had a major impact.

Summary of Clinical Trials

No tumor has been studied by clinical trials as thoroughly and effectively as WT. The NWTS has been active in North America since 1969. There have also been successful studies run by the

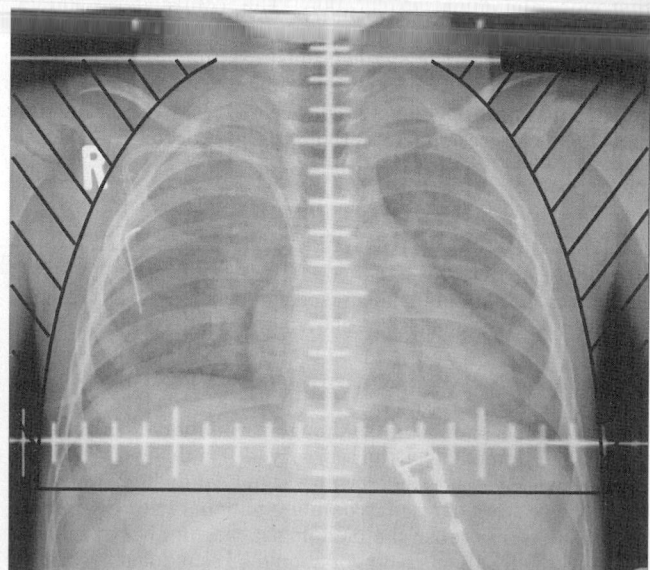

FIGURE 83.4. Simulation film of a patient with stage IV favorable histology Wilms' tumor receiving whole-lung irradiation. A lateral radiograph of the chest should be obtained at simulation to ascertain inclusion of the anterior and posterior costophrenic angles at the inferior edge of the treatment volume.

Table 83.6	LONG-TERM RESULTS OF NATIONAL WILMS' TUMOR STUDIES 3 AND 4[a]		
Category	No. of Patients	10-Year Relapse–Free Survival Rate (%)	10-Year Survival Rate (%)
Stage I FH	1,582	91.4	96.6
Stage II FH	1,006	85.5	93.4
Stage III FH	1,038	84.2	89.5
Stage IV FH	592	75.2	80.7
Stage V FH	344	65.1	77.9
All FH	4,562	84.4	90.8
Clear cell sarcoma	170	67.1	77.1
Stage II–III anaplasia	128	43.0	49.2
Stage IV anaplasia	55	18.2	18.2
Rhabdoid tumor	88	27.3	28.4

FH, favorable histology.
[a]National Wilms' Tumor Study unpublished data.

International Society for Pediatric Oncology (SIOP). The long-term results of NWTS-3 and NWTS-4 are shown in Table 83.6.

First National Wilms' Tumor Study (1969–1974)

NWTS-1 showed that postoperative irradiation was not necessary for children younger than 2 years of age with group I tumors, and that combined dactinomycin and vincristine for irradiated patients with group II and III tumors was better than therapy with either agent alone. The disease-free survival rates with and without irradiation among patients with group I tumors younger than 2 years of age were 90% and 88%, respectively (25).

Second National Wilms' Tumor Study (1974–1979)

This study showed that in patients with group I tumors there was no survival difference between 6 months or 15 months of dactinomycin plus vincristine. Patients with group II to IV tumors had a superior 2-year RFS rate of 77% with doxorubicin, dactinomycin, and vincristine compared with 63% with dactinomycin and vincristine alone (24).

Third National Wilms' Tumor Study (1979–1985)

The overall objective of NWTS-3 was to reduce therapy for low-risk patients (stages I to III FH) and to intensify treatment by adding a fourth drug, cyclophosphamide, for stage IV tumors with FH and all UH tumors. The results of this study demonstrated that RT and doxorubicin could be eliminated in children with stage II FH tumors. Patients with stage III FH tumors who received doxorubicin or 20 Gy had fewer abdominal relapses than those receiving 10 Gy without doxorubicin (76). The addition of cyclophosphamide in high-risk patients did not improve outcome (23) (Table 83.7).

Fourth National Wilms' Tumor Study (1986–1994)

By the conclusion of NWTS-3, it was clear that the treatment of WT had been refined for the majority of patients; 62% of patients with WT have stage I or II FH disease and therefore require neither flank irradiation nor the potentially cardiotoxic doxorubicin. NWTS-4 was designed with cost containment in mind. The results proved that the survival was similar among patients who received standard-course (5 days) or single-dose, pulse-intensive dactinomycin chemotherapy. Further, pulse-intensive therapy was associated with less hematologic toxicity and marked reduction of treatment costs (34,36).

Other Recent National Wilms' Tumor Study Results

Bilateral Wilms' Tumor

The goals of treatment in bilateral WT are to maximize cure rates and to preserve functional renal parenchyma; thus, the role of radical nephrectomy and irradiation has been restricted. Using an approach that emphasizes nephron-sparing surgery and chemotherapy, nephrectomy can be avoided in almost 50% of patients undergoing initial biopsy. Initial surgical resections should be performed only if more than two-thirds of each kidney can be preserved (9). Flank irradiation is indicated in patients with stage I/II FH only if there is unresectable disease after three-drug chemotherapy, residual tumor, or positive margins after surgery. In other stages for FH and UH disease, radiation therapy indications are as shown in Table 83.4. In NWTS-4, complete removal of all gross tumor was accomplished in 88% of kidneys after either partial nephrectomy or tumor enucleation. The OS rate was 92% at 2 years and 82% at 4 years (46). The incidence of renal failure has also steadily decreased from 16% in NWTS-1 and NWTS-2, to 10% and 4% in NWTS-3 and NWTS-4, respectively (70,73).

Table 83.7	RESULTS OF NATIONAL WILMS' TUMOR STUDY-3		
Stage	Regimen	No. of Patients	Relapse-Free Survival Rate at 4 Years (%)
I FH	AMD + VCR 10 wk vs. 6 mo	607	89 vs. 92
II FH	AMD + VCR + ADR vs. AMD + VCR	278	87 vs. 89
II FH	20 Gy vs. no RT	278	89 vs. 88
III FH	AMD + VCR + ADR vs. AMD + VCR	275	84 vs. 74
III FH	20 Gy vs. 10 Gy	275	81 vs. 77
IV FH	AMD + VCR + ADR vs. AMD + VCR + ADR + CY	120	72 vs. 78
All UH	AMD + VCR + ADR vs. AMD + VCR + ADR + CY	159	64 vs. 60

FH, favorable histology; AMD, dactinomycin; VCR, vincristine; ADR, doxorubicin; RT, radiation therapy; CY, cyclophosphamide; UH, unfavorable histology. Reference (23).

Clinical Radiation Oncology

Effect of Tumor Spillage on Outcome in Patients with Stage II and III Disease

Operative tumor spillage was identified in 24% of patients in NWTS-3 and NWTS-4, and 22% of the spills were classified as diffuse (13,72). An analysis was undertaken to determine the influence of RT and chemotherapy on abdominal tumor recurrence caused by spilled cells in abdominal stage II and III FH WT. The odds ratio for the risk of recurrence relative to no RT was 0.35 for 10 Gy ($p = .01$) and 0.08 for 20 Gy ($p = .01$). Thus RT (10 Gy or 20 Gy) significantly reduced abdominal tumor recurrence rates following tumor spillage. After adjusting for RT, the effect of doxorubicin on tumor recurrence was not significant. For stage II patients (NWTS-4), the 8 year RFS and OS rates with and without spillage were 74% and 85% ($p = .02$) and 90% and 94% ($p = .4$), respectively. The higher relapse rate among stage II children with spillage was the reason behind the decision of COG to upstage those patients with spillage to stage III. These patients will now receive three drugs and RT (Table 83.2) (49).

Nephrectomy Only for Patients with Stage I FH Wilms' Tumor

In NWTS-5, a single-arm study was conducted to evaluate the efficacy of nephrectomy alone in children younger than 24 months of age with small (<550 g) stage I FH WT. A total of 75 children were enrolled, the 2-year disease-free survival rate was 87%, and the 2-year OS rate was 100%. This study was stopped because of stringent stopping rules (35). The COG will again examine the possibility of avoiding any chemotherapy or RT in these children. However, only those children (<24 months, tumors <550 g) who have stage I FH tumors after central pathology review, lymph nodes sampling, and CT scan staging will be eligible for the surgery-only therapy.

Clear Cell Sarcoma

In the NWTS-1 through NWTS-4 experience comprising of 351 patients with CCSK, the overall survival rate was 69%. Multivariate analysis revealed four independent prognostic factors for survival: treatment with doxorubicin, tumor stage, age at diagnosis, and tumor necrosis (1).

Rhabdoid Tumor of Kidney

A total of 142 children with RTK were enrolled in NWTS 1–5 trials. The OS at 4 years was 23%. The survival rate for children with stage I/II tumors (42%) was significantly higher than those with stage II/III tumors (16%; $p = .014$). The survival rate in infants <6 months of age was 9% compared with 41% in children >2 years of age ($p < .001$). Children who received a higher dose of RT (>25 Gy) had a significantly better outcome. However, the dose of RT was not an independent predictor or survival (78).

Anaplastic Wilms' Tumor

In NWTS-5 among 2,596 patients who were enrolled, 281 (11%) had anaplastic WT. The 4-year RFS and OS rates for patients with stage I anaplasia who were treated with vincristine and dactinomycin without RT were 70% and 83%, respectively. The 4-year RFS for anaplastic tumor patients who underwent immediate nephrectomy and regimen-I chemotherapy, with stages II, III, and IV tumors were 83%, 65%, and 33%, respectively. The 4-year RFS and OS rates for stage V tumors were 44% and 55%, respectively. Based on these results, the therapy for stage I, III and IV tumors will be augmented in the new COG protocol (Tables 83.4 and 83.5) (29).

Recurrent Wilms' Tumor

Successful retreatment of children with recurrent WT remains a challenge. In a report from NWTS-2 and NWTS-3, the 3-year survival rate was 30%. The prognosis of children with relapsed WT depends on tumor histology, initial stage, site of relapse, previous therapy, and time from initial diagnosis to relapse. Among FH tumors, the 3-year postrelapse survival rates were 44%, 28%, and 11% when the relapse was confined to the lungs, abdomen, or other sites, respectively (41). The salvage rate of patients with recurrent WT has improved with the use of ifosfamide-, carboplatin-, and etoposide-based chemotherapy regimens (59). Encouraging results have been reported with high-dose chemotherapy and stem cell transplantation (63). Among relapsed WT patients treated on stratum B of the NWTS-5 relapse study, the 4-year RFS and OS rates were 71% and 82%, respectively. These children were initially treated with vincristine and actinomycin-D and did not receive doxorubicin or irradiation. The salvage regiment consisted of surgery when feasible, RT, and alternating courses of vincristine, doxorubicin, cyclophosphamide, and etoposide/cyclophosphamide (regimen I) (37).

Wilms' Tumor in Older Patients

WT is rarely seen in patients ≥ 16 years of age. Their survival is similar to that of children and they should be treated similarly (51).

International Society of Pediatric Oncology Trials

The SIOP studies have primarily used preoperative therapy. The goals of administering preoperative therapy are to facilitate surgical removal of the tumor without rupture, to allow for early treatment of micrometastases, and to stratify patients for postoperative therapy based on pathologic tumor response at the time of surgery. The first SIOP trial found that preoperative irradiation reduced the incidence of tumor spillage but did not increase survival (57). SIOP-5, reported in 1983, showed that preoperative chemotherapy with vincristine and dactinomycin was as effective as preoperative irradiation plus dactinomycin in preventing tumor rupture (56). In SIOP-6, patients with stage I disease were randomly assigned to either 17 or 38 weeks of vincristine and dactinomycin, and showed no difference in survival. Among patients with stage II disease and negative lymph nodes (SIOP staging is not identical to NWTS staging) who were randomly assigned not to receive RT, there was a higher recurrence rate (48). In SIOP-9, there was a randomization as to the length of prenephrectomy therapy with vincristine and dactinomycin (4 vs. 8 weeks). No advantage was noted for 8 weeks of therapy. Among patients with stage II disease with negative lymph nodes, the rate of abdominal relapse was reduced to 7% by the addition of epirubicin (28). SIOP-93–01 further stratifies treatment according to the pathologic response to preoperative chemotherapy. The recommended dose of irradiation in SIOP-9 and SIOP-93–01 is 15 Gy in patients with low- and intermediate-risk stage III disease and 30 Gy in high-risk patients (32). SIOP protocol 93–01 showed that the amount of postoperative chemotherapy of stage I patients with either intermediate-risk histology or anaplasia could be reduced to four doses of vincristine and one course of dactinomycin with a 5-year RFS and OS rates of 87% and 95%, respectively (27).

United Kingdom Children's Cancer Study Group

The first United Kingdom Children's Cancer Study Group (UKCCSG) Wilms' tumor study (UKW1) showed that vincristine could be used alone in patients with stage I FH disease. Among patients with lung metastases, the 6-year survival rate of 65% was significantly worse than the 4-year survival rate of 82% on NWTS-3, probably because of the inclusion of routine lung irradiation in the NWTS (65). In the second UKCCSG WT study (UKW2), patients with stage I FH disease treated with 10 weekly doses of vincristine had survival rates similar to those in patients with NWTS stage I disease. The 4-year survival rate in patients with stage IV disease was higher than in UKW1, at 75%, probably owing to the greater use of whole-lung irradiation. The irradiation doses used for stage III FH and UH tumors are 20 Gy and 30 Gy, respectively (60). The UKW3 trial conducted a randomized comparison of a primary nephrectomy followed by adjuvant therapy based on surgical stage (NWTS approach) and a preoperative chemotherapy followed by nephrectomy and adjuvant therapy (SIOP approach). The 4-year RFS and OS rates were equivalent between the two arms at 80% and 85%, respectively, for the primary nephrectomy arm, and 79% and 95% for the preoperative chemotherapy arm. The preoperative chemotherapy arm had fewer surgical tumor ruptures and other surgical complications. The UKCCSG has now joined the current SIOP 20001 clinical study (61).

Late Effects of Treatment

The study of late effects is of paramount importance to prevent survivors of childhood cancer from becoming chronically sick adults.

Scoliosis

A series from Washington University showed a high incidence of scoliosis in 54% of patients who were treated with a median dose of 30 Gy. However, there was minimal functional disability (75). In another report, the incidences of scoliosis after 10 to 12 Gy, 12.1 to 23.9 Gy, and 24 to 40 Gy were 8%, 46%, and 63%, respectively (62). Thus, at present, with the use of megavoltage x-rays, lower doses, and coverage of the entire width of the vertebra, the incidence of scoliosis should be low.

Congestive Heart Failure

The cumulative frequency of congestive heart failure among patients on NWTS-1 through NWTS-4 was 4.4% at 20 years among patients treated initially with doxorubicin and 17.4% among patients treated with doxorubicin for their first or subsequent relapse. The factors that were significantly associated with the incidence of heart failure were female sex, cumulative doxorubicin dose, lung irradiation, and left abdominal irradiation (38).

Pregnancy Outcome in Wilms' Tumor Survivors

As a part of the NWTS Long-Term Follow-up Study, the pregnancy outcomes among WT survivors were analyzed. Malposition of the fetus and premature labor were significantly more frequent among previously irradiated women. The offspring of female patients who received flank irradiation were more likely to be of low birth weight (<2,500 g) and premature (<36 weeks of gestation), and to have congenital malformations. A radiation dose response was identified, with higher complication rates at doses >25 Gy to the flank. A number of radiation-induced side effects involving the spine, uterus, and ovaries may all have been responsible (22,39). The pregnancy outcomes in childhood WT survivors who received abdominal RT in NWTS protocols were also analyzed. Fertility could be preserved in children with upper abdominal RT that did not include the pelvis. In rare instances, fertility could be preserved after whole-abdominal RT

to 10.5 Gy. However, higher doses to the abdomen and pelvis resulted in miscarriages and fetal deaths (52).

Second Malignant Neoplasm

The cumulative 15-year risk of second malignant neoplasm was 1.6% among patients enrolled on the NWTS, after a mean follow-up of 7.5 years per patient. Higher doses of abdominal irradiation and doxorubicin increased the risk of second malignant neoplasm (16).

End Stage Renal Disease

In a report from the NWTS of WT survivors who had unilateral WT, the 20-year cumulative incidence of end stage renal disease was 74% for children with Denys-Drash syndrome, 36% for children with WAGR syndrome, 7% for children with genitourinary anomalies, and 0.6% for patients with none of these conditions. The importance of long-term screening for high-risk children to facilitate early detection and treatment of impaired renal function was emphasized (14).

References

1. Argani P, Perlman EJ, Breslow NE, et al. Clear cell sarcoma of the kidney: a review of 351 cases from the National Wilms' Tumor Study Group Pathology Center. *Am J Surg Pathol* 2000;24:4–18.
2. Beckwith JB, Palmer NJ. Histopathology and prognosis of Wilms' tumor: results from the first National Wilms' Tumor Study. *Cancer* 1978;41:1937–1948.
3. Beckwith JB, Zuppan CE, Browning NG, et al. Histological analysis of aggressiveness and responsiveness in Wilms' tumor. *Med Pediatr Oncol* 1996;27:422–428.
4. Beckwith JB. National Wilms' Tumor Study: an update for pathologists. *Pediatr Dev Pathol* 1998;1:79–84.
5. Beckwith JB. Nephrogenic rests and the pathogenesis of Wilms' tumor: developmental and clinical considerations. *Am J Med Genet* 1998;79:268–273.
6. Beckwith JB. Precursor lesions of Wilms' tumor: clinical and biological implications. *Med Pediatr Oncol* 1993;21:158–168.
7. Belt TG, Cohen MD, Smith JA, et al. MRI of Wilms' tumor: promise as the primary imaging modality. *AJR Am J Roentgenol* 1986;146:955–961.
8. Birch JM, Breslow N. Epidemiologic features of Wilms' tumor. *Hematol Oncol Clin North Am* 1995;9:1157–1178.
9. Blute ML, Kelalis PP, Offord KP, et al. Bilateral Wilms' tumor. *J Urol* 1987;138:968–973.
10. Bonadio JF, Storer B, Norkool P, et al. Anaplastic Wilms' tumor: clinical and pathologic studies. *J Clin Oncol* 1985;3:513–520.
11. Breslow N, Beckwith JB, Ciol M, et al. Age distribution of Wilms' tumor: report from the National Wilms' Tumor Study. *Cancer Res* 1988;48:1653–1657.
12. Breslow N, Churchill G, Nesmith B, et al. Clinicopathologic features and prognosis for Wilms' tumor patients with metastases at diagnosis. *Cancer* 1986;58:2501–2511.
13. Breslow NE, Beckwith JB, Haase GM et al. Radiation therapy for favorable histology Wilms' tumor: prevention of flank recurrence did not improve survival on National Wilms Tumor Studies 3 and 4. *Int J Radiat Oncol Biol Phys* 2006;65:203–209.
14. Breslow NE, Collins AJ, Ritchey ML et al. End stage renal disease in patients with Wilms tumor: results from the National Wilms Tumor Study Group and the United States renal data system. *J Urol* 2005;174:1972–1975.
15. Breslow NE, Olshan A, Beckwith JB, et al. Epidemiology of Wilms' tumor. *Med Pediatr Oncol* 1983;21:172–181.
16. Breslow NE, Takashima JR, Whitton JA, et al. Second malignant neoplasms following treatment for Wilms' tumor: a report from the National Wilms' Tumor Study Group. *J Clin Oncol* 1995;13:1851–1859.
17. Call KM, Glaser T, Ito CY, et al. Isolation and characterization of a zinc finger polypeptide gene at the human chromosome 11 Wilms' tumor locus. *Cell* 1990;60:509–520.
18. Cohen MD. Current controversy: is computed tomography scan of the chest needed in patients with Wilms' tumor? *Am J Pediatr Hematol Oncol* 1994;16:191–193.
19. Coppes MJ, Arnold M, Beckwith JB, et al. Factors affecting the risk of contralateral Wilms' tumor development: a report from the National Wilms' Tumor Study Group. *Cancer* 1999;85:1616–1625.
20. Coppes MJ, Egeler RM. Genetics of Wilms' tumor. *Semin Urol Oncol* 1999;17:2–10.
21. Coppes MJ, Ritchey ML, D'Angio GJ. Preface: the path to progress in medical science: a Wilms' tumor conspectus. *Hematol Oncol Clin North Am* 1995;9:xiii–xviii.
22. Critchley HOD. Factors of importance for implantation and problems after treatment for childhood cancer. *Med Pediatr Oncol* 1999;33:9–14.
23. D'Angio GJ, Breslow N, Beckwith JB, et al. The treatment of Wilms' tumor: results of the Third National Wilms' Tumor Study. *Cancer* 1989;64:349–360.
24. D'Angio GJ, Evans AE, Breslow NE, et al. The treatment of Wilms' tumor: results of the Second National Wilms' Tumor Study. *Cancer* 1981;47:2302–2311.
25. D'Angio GJ, Evans AE, Breslow NE, et al. The treatment of Wilms' tumor: results of the National Wilms' Tumor Study. *Cancer* 1976;38:633–646.
26. D'Angio GJ, Tefft M, Breslow NE, et al. Radiation therapy of Wilms' tumor: results according to dose, field, postoperative timing and histology. *Int J Radiat Oncol Biol Phys* 1978;4:769–780.

27. De Kraker J, Graf N, van Tinteren H et al. Reduction of postoperative chemotherapy in children with stage I intermediate-risk and anaplastic Wilms tumor (SIOP-93-01): a randomized trial. *Lancet* 2004;364:1229–1235.
28. DeKraker J, Weitzman S, Vote PA. Preoperative strategies in the management of Wilms' tumor. *Hematol Oncol Clin North Am* 1995;9:1275–1285.
29. Dome JS, Cotton CA, Perlman EJ et al. Treatment of anaplastic histology Wilms tumor: results from the fifth National Wilms Tumor Study. *J Clin Oncol* 2006;24:2352–2358.
30. Farewell VT, D'Angio GJ, Breslow N, et al. Retrospective validation of a new staging system for Wilms' tumor. *Cancer Clin Trials* 1981;4:167–171.
31. Faria P, Beckwith JB, Mishra K, et al. Focal versus diffuse anaplasia in Wilms' tumor: new definitions with prognostic significance. A report from the National Wilms' Tumor Study Group. *Am J Surg Pathol* 1996;20:909–920.
32. Graf N, Tournade MF, de Kraker J. The role of preoperative chemo-therapy in the management of Wilms' tumor. The SIOP studies. *Urol Clin North Am* 2000;27:443–454.
33. Green DM, Beckwith JB, Breslow NE, et al. The treatment of children with stages II–IV anaplastic Wilms' tumor: a report from the National Wilms' Tumor Study Group. *J Clin Oncol* 1994;12:2126–2131.
34. Green DM, Breslow NE, Beckwith JB, et al. Comparison between single-dose and divided-dose administration of dactinomycin and doxorubicin for patients with Wilms' tumor: a report from the National Wilms' Tumor Study Group. *J Clin Oncol* 1998;16:237–245.
35. Green DM, Breslow NE, Beckwith JB, et al. Treatment with nephrectomy only for small, stage I/favorable histology Wilms' tumor: a report from the National Wilms' Tumor Study Group. *J Clin Oncol* 2001;19:3719–3724.
36. Green DM, Breslow NE, Evans I, et al. The effect of chemotherapy dose intensity on the hematological toxicity of the treatment for Wilms' tumor: a report from the National Wilms' Tumor Study Group. *Am J Pediatr Hematol Oncol* 1994;16:207–212.
37. Green DM, Cotton CA, Malogolowkin M et al. Treatment of Wilms tumor relapsing after initial therapy with vincristine and actinomycin D. A report from the National Wilms Tumor Study Group. *Pediatric Blood Cancer* In press.
38. Green DM, Grigoriev YA, Nan B, et al. Congestive heart failure after treatment for Wilms' tumor: a report from the National Wilms' Tumor Study Group. *J Clin Oncol* 2001;19:1926–1934.
39. Green DM, Peabody EM, Nan B, et al. Pregnancy outcome after treatment for Wilms' tumor. *J Clin Oncol* 2002;20:2506–2513.
40. Gross RE, Neuhauser EBD. Treatment of mixed tumors of the kidney in childhood. *Pediatrics* 1950;6:843.
41. Grundy P, Breslow N, Green DM, et al. Prognostic factors for children with recurrent Wilms' tumor: results from the second and third National Wilms Tumor Study. *J Clin Oncol* 1989;7:638–647.
42. Grundy PE, Breslow NE, Li S et al. Loss of heterozygosity for chromosomes 1p and 16q is an adverse prognostic factor in favorable histology Wilms tumor: a report from the National Wilms Tumor Study Group. *J Clin Oncol* 2005;23:7312–7321.
43. Grundy PE, Telzerow PE, Breslow N, et al. Loss of heterozygosity for chromosomes 16q and 1p in Wilms' tumors predicts an adverse outcome. *Cancer Res* 1994;54:2331–2333.
44. Gylys-Morin V, Hoffer FA, Kozakewich H, et al. Wilms' tumor and nephroblastomatosis: imaging characteristics at gadolinium-enhanced MR imaging. *Radiology* 1993;188:517–521.
45. Hartman DS, Sanders RC. Wilms' tumor versus neuroblastoma: usefulness of ultrasound in differentiation. *J Ultrasound Med* 1982;1:117–122.
46. Horwitz JR, Ritchey ML, Moksness J, et al. Renal salvage procedures in patients with synchronous bilateral Wilms' tumors: a report from the National Wilms' Tumor Study Group. *J Pediatr Surg* 1996;31:1020–1025.
47. Huff V. Wilms' tumor genetics. *Am J Hum Genet* 1998;79:260–267.
48. Jereb B, Burgers MV, Tournade M-F, et al. Radiotherapy in the SIOP (International Society of Paediatric Oncology) nephroblastoma studies: a review. *Med Pediatr Oncol* 1994;22:221–227.
49. Kalapurakal JA, Li SM, Breslow NE et al. Influence of irradiation and doxorubicin on abdominal recurrence caused by spilled tumor cells in abdominal stage II and III favorable histology Wilms tumor in NWTS-3 and -4: a report from the National Wilms Tumor Study. *Int J Radiat Oncol Biol Phys* 2003;57:477.
50. Kalapurakal JA, Li SM, Breslow NE et al. Influence of radiation therapy delay on abdominal tumor recurrence in patients with favorable histology Wilms tumor treated on NWTS-3 and -4: a report from the National Wilms Tumor Study Group. *Int J Radiat Oncol Biol Phys* 2003;57:495–499.
51. Kalapurakal JA, Nan B, Norkool P et al. Treatment outcomes in adults with favorable histologic type Wilms tumor: an update from the National Wilms Tumor Study Group. *Int J Radiat Oncol Biol Phys* 2004;60:1379–1384.
52. Kalapurakal JA, Peterson S, Peabody EM et al. Pregnancy outcomes after abdominal irradiation that included or excluded the pelvis in childhood Wilms tumor survivors: a report of the National Wilms Tumor Study. *Int J Radiat Oncol Biol Phys* 2004;58:1364–1368.
53. Koufos A, Grundy P, Morgan K, et al. Familial Wiedemann-Beckwith syndrome and a second Wilms' tumor locus both map to 11p15.5. *Am J Hum Genet* 1989;44:711–719.
54. Leape LL, Breslow NE, Bishop HC. The surgical treatment of Wilms' tumor: results of the National Wilms' Tumor Study. *Ann Surg* 1978;187:351–356.
55. Ledlie EM, Mynors LS, Draper GJ, et al. Natural history and treatment of Wilms' tumor: an analysis of 335 cases occurring in England and Wales 1962–1966. *BMJ* 1970;4:195–200.
56. Lemerle J, Vote PA, Tournade MF, et al. Effectiveness of preoperative chemotherapy in Wilms' tumor: results of an International Society of Pediatric Oncology (SIOP) trial. *J Clin Oncol* 1983;1:604–609.
57. Lemerle J, Vote PA, Tournade MF, et al. Preoperative versus postoperative radiotherapy, single versus multiple courses of actinomycin D in the treatment of Wilms' tumor. *Cancer* 1976;38:647–654.
58. Meisel JA, Guthrie KA, Breslow NE, et al. Significance and management of computed tomography detected pulmonary nodules: a report from the National Wilms' Tumor Study Group. *Int J Radiat Oncol Biol Phys* 1999;44:579–585.
59. Miser JS, Tournade MF. The management of relapsed Wilms' tumor. *Hematol Oncol Clin North Am* 1995;9:1287–1302.
60. Mitchell C, Jones PM, Kelsey A, et al. The treatment of Wilms' tumor: results of the United Kingdom Children's Cancer Study Group (UKCCSG) second Wilms' tumor study. *Br J Cancer* 2000;83:602–608.
61. Mitchell C, Shannon R, Vujanic GM et al. The treatment of Wilms tumor: Results of the United Kingdom Children's Cancer Study group Third Wilms Tumor Study. *Med Pediatr Oncol* 2003;41:289.
62. Paulino AC, Wen BC, Brown CK, et al. Late effects in children treated with radiation therapy for Wilms' tumor. *Int J Radiat Oncol Biol Phys* 2000;46:1239–1246.
63. Pein F, Michon J, Valteau-Couanet D, et al. High-dose melphalan, etoposide and carboplatin followed by autologous stem-cell rescue in pediatric high-risk recurrent Wilms' tumor: a French Society of Pediatric Oncology Study. *J Clin Oncol* 1998;16:3295–3301.
64. Pelletier J, Bruening W, Kashtan CE, et al. Germline mutations in the Wilms' tumor suppressor gene are associated with abnormal urogenital development in Denys-Drash syndrome. *Cell* 1991;67:437–447.
65. Pritchard J, Imeson J, Barnes J, et al. Results of the United Kingdom Children's Cancer Study Group First Wilms' Tumor Study. *J Clin Oncol* 1995;13:124–133.
66. Pritchard-Jones K, Fleming S, Davidson D, et al. The candidate Wilms' tumor gene is involved in genitourinary development. *Nature* 1990;346:194–197.
67. Ramos IM, Taylor KJW, Kier R, et al. Tumor vascular signals in renal masses: detection with Doppler US. *Radiology* 1988;168:633.
68. Reiman TAH, Siegel MJ, Shackelford GD. Wilms' tumor in children: abdominal CT and US evaluation. *Radiology* 1986;160:501–505.
69. Ritchey ML, Green DM, Breslow NB. Accuracy of current imaging modalities in the diagnosis of synchronous bilateral Wilms' tumor: a report from the National Wilms' Tumor Study Group. *Cancer* 1995;75:600–604.
70. Ritchey ML, Green DM, Thomas PR, et al. Renal failure in Wilms' tumor patients: a report from the National Wilms' Tumor Study Group. *Med Pediatr Oncol* 1996;26:75–80.
71. Schmidt D, Beckwith JB. Histopathology of childhood renal tumors. *Hematol Oncol Clin North Am* 1995;9:1179–1200.
72. Shamberger RC, Guthrie KA, Ritchey ML, et al. Surgery-related factors and local recurrence of Wilms' tumor in National Wilms' Tumor Study 4. *Ann Surg* 1999;229:292–297.
73. Smith GR, Thomas PRM, Ritchey M, et al. Long-term renal function in patients with irradiated bilateral Wilms' tumor. *Am J Clin Oncol* 1998;21:58–63.
74. Sukarochana K, Tolentino W, Kiesewetter WB. Wilms' tumor and hypertension. *J Pediatr Surg* 1972;7:573–576.
75. Thomas PRM, Griffith KD, Fineberg BB, et al. Late effects of treatment for Wilms' tumor. *Int J Radiat Oncol Biol Phys* 1983;9:651–657.
76. Thomas PRM, Tefft M, Compaan PJ, et al. Results of two radiotherapy randomizations in the third National Wilms' Tumor Study (NWTS-3). *Cancer* 1991;68:1703–1707.
77. Thomas PRM, Tefft M, Farewell VT, et al. Abdominal relapses in the second National Wilms' Tumor Study patients. *J Clin Oncol* 1984;2:1098–1101.
78. Tomlinson GE, Breslow NE, Dome J et al. Rhabdoid tumor of the kidney in the National Wilms Tumor Study: age at diagnosis as a prognostic factor. *J Clin Oncol* 2005;23:7641–7645.
79. Weeks DA, Beckwith JB, Luckey DW. Relapse-associated variables in stage I favorable histology Wilms' tumor: a report of the National Wilms' Tumor Study. *Cancer* 1987;60:1204–1212.

Chapter 84
Neuroblastoma

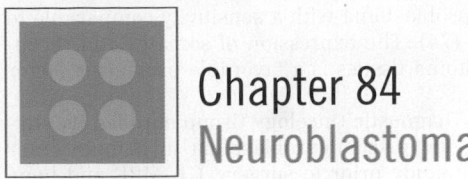

David B. Mansur, Jeff M. Michalski

Neuroblastoma is an enigmatic malignant neoplasm. In its early stages it can be readily cured with surgery or, in some circumstances, can even spontaneously regress or mature to a benign ganglioneuroma. In the more common advanced stages, the disease is often fatal. The unique biology of neuroblastoma has attracted the interest of many prominent scientists and is one of the first malignancies in which molecular biologic assays have influenced treatment and prognosis.

Epidemiology

After brain tumors and leukemia, neuroblastoma is the third most common malignancy diagnosed in children, with an annual incidence of nine new cases per 1 million children in the United States. It is the most common cancer diagnosed before the age of 12 months, accounting for almost half of all cancers in infants. The median age at diagnosis is 2 years. The relatively good prognosis of infants diagnosed with early stage neuroblastoma prompted the initiation of infant-screening studies (113).

Screening of infants for neuroblastoma has been studied systematically in large clinical trials conducted in Japan, North America, and Europe (89,90,112,115). Excretion of catecholamine metabolites in the urine of children with neuroblastoma has served as the basis of these screening tests. Urine samples were collected and dried on filter paper and returned to screening centers where they would be tested qualitatively for vanillylmandelic acid (VMA) levels or quantitatively for VMA and homovanillic acid (HVA) measured by high-performance liquid chromatography and normalized to urinary creatinine levels. Children with elevated levels of these metabolites subsequently were referred for further diagnostic evaluation. The incidences of the diagnosis and death rates from neuroblastoma in the screened populations were compared to control populations in the same country or continent. The study populations generally were chosen because of access to an existing screening infrastructure that could readily be adapted to neuroblastoma. The Japanese study screened children at 6 months of age. The Quebec study screened children at 3 weeks and 6 months of age. The German study tested children at their first year's birthday.

The results and conclusions of these three large screening trials on three continents are remarkably similar. In Japan, 1,142,519 children were screened using a qualitative test and another 550,331 were screened with the quantitative test; they all were compared to 713,025 children in a control population. The incidence rates per 100,000 were 1.12 in the control group compared to 5.69 in the qualitative group and 17.81 in the quantitative group. Despite this increased incidence in the screened group, the neuroblastoma mortality rates were unchanged by the screening (115). In Germany, 1,475,773 children were screened between 1994 and 1999. Screening detected neuroblastoma in 149 children, three of whom died. Despite the screening at 12 months, another 55 children subsequently developed neuroblastoma, 14 of whom died. Compared to the control group, the incidence of stage 4 neuroblastoma was

similar. The death rate from neuroblastoma was unaffected by the screening (90). In Quebec, a total of 425,838 children were enrolled in the neuroblastoma screening trial (89% of births during a 5-year study period from 1989 to 1994). The standardized incidence ratios of neuroblastoma death in the Quebec cohort were nearly identical to control groups in Ontario, Minnesota, Florida, and the Greater Delaware Valley (112). In summary, each of these trials demonstrates that screening does not affect the mortality rate of neuroblastoma. Furthermore, the overdiagnosis of clinically insignificant disease may lead to significant financial, emotional, and physical burdens on the children and their families. This tumor has a high frequency of spontaneous regression in infancy. The mass screening programs have led to the diagnosis of biologically favorable and clinically insignificant tumors (67,114).

Natural History

Neuroblastoma, along with ganglioneuroma and ganglioneuroblastoma, may arise from any site in the sympathetic nervous system. The most common site of origin is the adrenal medulla (30% to 40%) or paraspinal ganglia in the abdomen or pelvis (25%). Thoracic (15%) and head and neck primary tumors (5%) are slightly more common in infants than in older children. More than 70% of patients have metastatic disease at presentation. The most frequent metastatic sites are lymph nodes, bone, bone marrow, skin (or subcutaneous tissues), and liver (28). The lung and central nervous system are rare sites of involvement.

Neuroblastoma has the highest spontaneous remission rate of any human neoplasm, usually by maturation to ganglioneuroma (32). Microscopic neuroblastomas have been found in the autopsy material of the adrenal glands of young infants at more than 40 times the expected rate. It has been suggested that most potential neuroblastomas are never clinically manifested because of spontaneous regression (1). Despite these peculiarities, clinically obvious neuroblastoma is frequently a progressive and relentless disease.

Clinical Presentation

Pain is the most common presenting symptom. This frequently is caused by bone, liver, or bone marrow metastases or local visceral invasion by the primary tumor. Other constitutional symptoms may include weight loss, anorexia, malaise, and fever. Respiratory distress may accompany massive hepatomegaly, especially in infants with stage IV-S disease (28). Horner's syndrome can accompany a primary tumor originating in the neck. Spinal cord compression with paralysis of the lower extremities can accompany the so-called dumbbell-shaped tumor that extends from its origin along the sympathetic ganglia through the adjacent neural foramina. Orbital metastases are not uncommon and can cause proptosis and ecchymosis. Skin metastases may have a bluish tinge, giving the classic "blueberry muffin" sign. When pressed, the release of catecholamine into the tissue causes transient blanching of the adjacent skin. An unusual presentation of localized neuroblastoma is the opsoclonus–myoclonus syndrome, manifested by truncal ataxia and cerebellar encephalopathy. This syndrome typically indicates a favorable prognosis from the tumor, but the patients may have persistent neurologic sequelae after successful tumor therapy (6,85).

Diagnostic Work-Up

As in the case of any suspected malignant neoplasm in children, the diagnosis of neuroblastoma must be established by pathologic evaluation. Tumor tissue may be obtained from the suspected primary tumor site or from involved lymph nodes by excision (if the tumor is resectable) or incisional biopsy. Bone marrow aspirate and biopsy frequently show metastatic tumor deposits that can establish the diagnosis. Pathologic evaluation of bone marrow is also a requirement for staging of neuroblastoma. Characteristically, neuroblastoma in bone marrow appears in clumps and pseudorosettes. The absence of pseudorosettes does not eliminate the possibility of neuroblastoma.

Laboratory studies should include measurement of urinary catecholamines and their metabolites. Either HVA or VMA, metabolites of dopa/norepinepherine and epinephrine, respectively, is elevated in more than 90% of patients with stage IV neuroblastoma. A ratio of VMA to HVA exceeding 1.5 is associated with a favorable prognosis in patients with metastatic neuroblastoma. An assay for urinary VMA is the basis for screening studies of infants in Japan, Europe, and North America. Anemia secondary to bone marrow involvement with tumor can be evaluated with a complete blood cell count. Serum ferritin, lactate dehydrogenase (LDH), and other liver function indicators should be assayed routinely.

Appropriate use of imaging studies assists in staging and in planning an approach to therapy. X-ray studies demonstrate intrinsic speckled calcifications in 85% of neuroblastomas. Computed tomography (CT) of the abdomen with intravenous contrast is more sensitive than intravenous pyelography and provides more information about lymph node or hepatic metastases as well as tumor resectability (4). Increasingly, high quality magnetic resonance imaging (MRI) scans are replacing the routine use of CT in evaluation of suspicious thoracic or abdominal masses in children. Although MRI cannot demonstrate intratumoral calcifications, it allows better evaluation of blood vessel encasement, intraspinal extension (dumbbell tumors), diffuse hepatic replacement, and bone marrow involvement (Fig. 84.1). Each of these findings improves staging accuracy and facilitates the decision-making process regarding appropriate surgical interventions (19,33,80, 100).

Nuclear medicine scans are helpful in determining the extent of metastatic disease. Because neuroblastoma has a predilection for bony metastases, a radionuclide bone scan is a mandatory investigation. It is more sensitive than a skeletal survey in detecting bone metastases (106). Metaiodobenzylguanidine (MIBG) is concentrated by neurosecretory granules of both normal and neoplastic tissues of neural crest origin and can be used to image primary and metastatic sites of neuroblastoma. MIBG labeled with either iodine-131 (^{131}I) or ^{123}I has a sensitivity of 85% to 90% and a specificity of almost 95% in the detection of metastatic neuroblastoma (94). Poor scintigraphic response on ^{123}I-MIBG scans following induction chemotherapy has been shown to predict for a poor event-free survival in patients undergoing high-dose chemotherapy with stem cell rescue (53). Like other neural crest–derived neoplasms, neuroblastoma can express somatostatin receptors. The long-acting somatostatin analog, octreotide, labeled with ^{123}I, has been used to image neuroblastoma with a sensitivity comparable to that of ^{131}I-MIBG (74). The expression of somatostatin receptors by neuroblastoma tissues is a favorable prognostic factor (66).

The Radiology Diagnostic Oncology Group enrolled 96 children with newly diagnosed neuroblastoma in a multicenter prospective cohort study prior to surgery. CT, MRI, and bone scintigraphy were used to evaluate tumor stage. The results show that MRI is more accurate than CT for detection of stage IV disease (sensitivities 0.83 and 0.43, respectively). When combined with bone scintigraphy, both imaging tests have high accuracy for the detection of metastases (Figs. 84.2–84.4). The prevalence of determinants of local disease was relatively low in this study because patients who had extensive disease at the time of entry underwent delayed surgery after induction chemotherapy. Although the numbers are small, the data suggest the following:

(a) In stage 1 tumor, abdominal extent was more likely to be staged correctly with CT than with MRI, which often overstaged tumor;

(b) For stage 2 and 3 tumors, both CT and MRI were more likely to understage than overstage tumor; and

(c) For stage 2 tumor, understaging was more likely with CT than MRI (99,101).

Staging

The most commonly used staging system is the International Neuroblastoma Staging System (INSS). It is based on clinical, radiographic, and surgical findings (8). The INSS integrates many of the concepts of previous staging systems promoted by the Children's Cancer Group (CCG) and Pediatric Oncology Group (POG) (30,72) and unifies them into a single system (Table 84.1).

Pathologic Classification

Neuroblastomas are derived from primitive neural-crest cells arising from within sympathetic ganglia. Three types of tumors, representing different degrees of differentiation, are recognized. *Ganglioneuroma* consists of mature ganglion cells, Schwann cells, and nerve bundles and is benign in appearance and nature. It frequently is calcified and may represent a matured neuroblastoma (110). Cases of maturation of proven neuroblastomas to ganglioneuromas, either spontaneously or after therapy, have been reported (32). *Ganglioneuroblastoma* is the intermediate form between ganglioneuroma and neuroblastoma. Both mature ganglion cells and undifferentiated neuroblasts are evident.

Neuroblastoma is at the undifferentiated end of the spectrum of neural-crest tumors. It is a small, round, blue cell tumor composed of dense nests of hyperchromatic cells. Homer Wright rosettes with a central fibrillary core can be present. Areas of necrosis, hemorrhage, and calcium are frequently present. Immunohistochemical stains may help distinguish neuroblastoma from other undifferentiated malignant neoplasms of childhood. Neuroblastoma characteristically stains positive for neurofilaments, neuron-specific enolase (NSE), synaptophysin, and chromogranin A and negative for muscle and leukocyte common antigens. The use of electron microscopy to demonstrate neurosecretory granules is required infrequently to establish the diagnosis.

A grading system has been proposed by Shimada et al. (95), and its significance has been confirmed by the CCG (16,52). This clinicopathologic staging system evaluates tumor specimens for stromal development (i.e., stromal-rich and stromal-poor

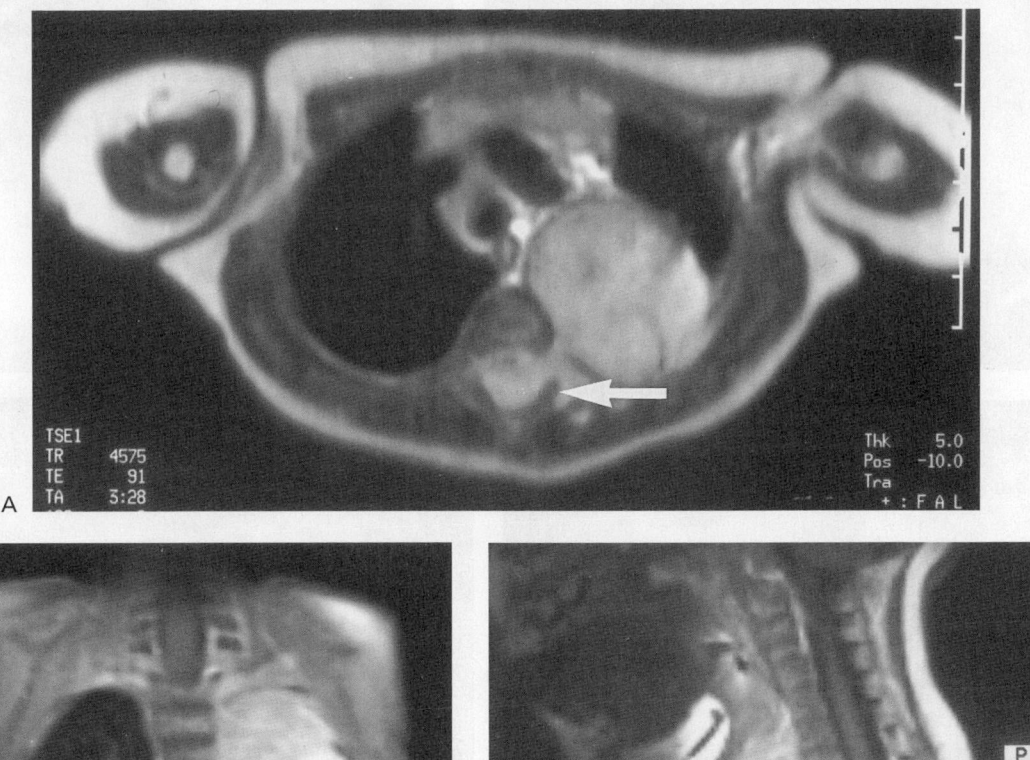

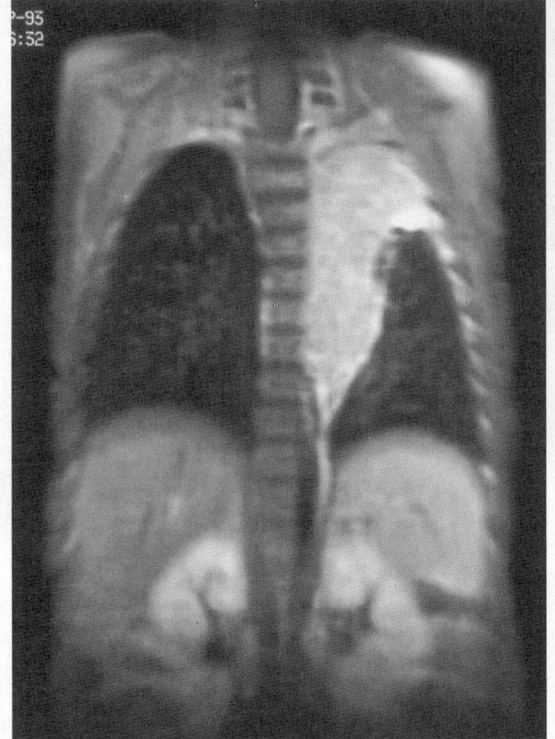

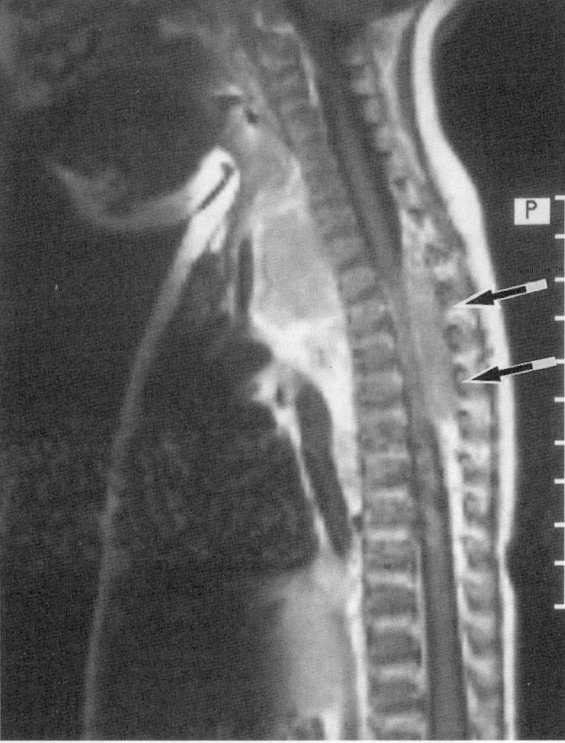

FIGURE 84.1. Magnetic resonance imaging scans of a 4-month-old child with a thoracic neuroblastoma. The dumbbell shape of the paraspinal mass can be appreciated on axial (**A**), coronal (**B**), and sagittal (**C**) images. The intraspinal component is indicated by arrows. The three views of this child's tumor are helpful in radiation-therapy field design.

tumors), neuroblastic differentiation, and mitosis-karyorrhexis index of neuroblastic cells. These three histologic features and the patient's age at diagnosis divide children into favorable and unfavorable prognostic groups. The stroma-rich tumors are characterized by an extensive Schwann cell stroma. The well-differentiated stroma-rich tumors may correspond to ganglioneuroma, and the "intermixed" stroma-rich tumors may correspond to the ganglioneuroblastomas. To be reliable, the Shimada classification requires pretreatment evaluation of the entire primary tumor specimen. However, primary tumors often are not completely resectable, or the presence of widespread metastases makes thorough tumor resection inappropriate before introduction of initial systemic therapy, thereby limiting the usefulness of this system.

Prognostic Factors

Patient age and stage at initial presentation remain the two most important factors that influence outcome (Table 84.2). In general more than 75% of infants and children younger than 2 years old survive, as do 90% to 100% of children with INSS stages 1 and 2 (10,18,29,31,36,44,46,48,70,88,102). The presence of tumor in regional lymph nodes is a poor prognostic factor and was recognized as such by the POG in their staging system (47). Infants younger than 12 months old with metastatic disease confined to the liver, bone marrow (not bone), or skin (stage IV-S) have a remarkably good prognosis; more than 75% of these

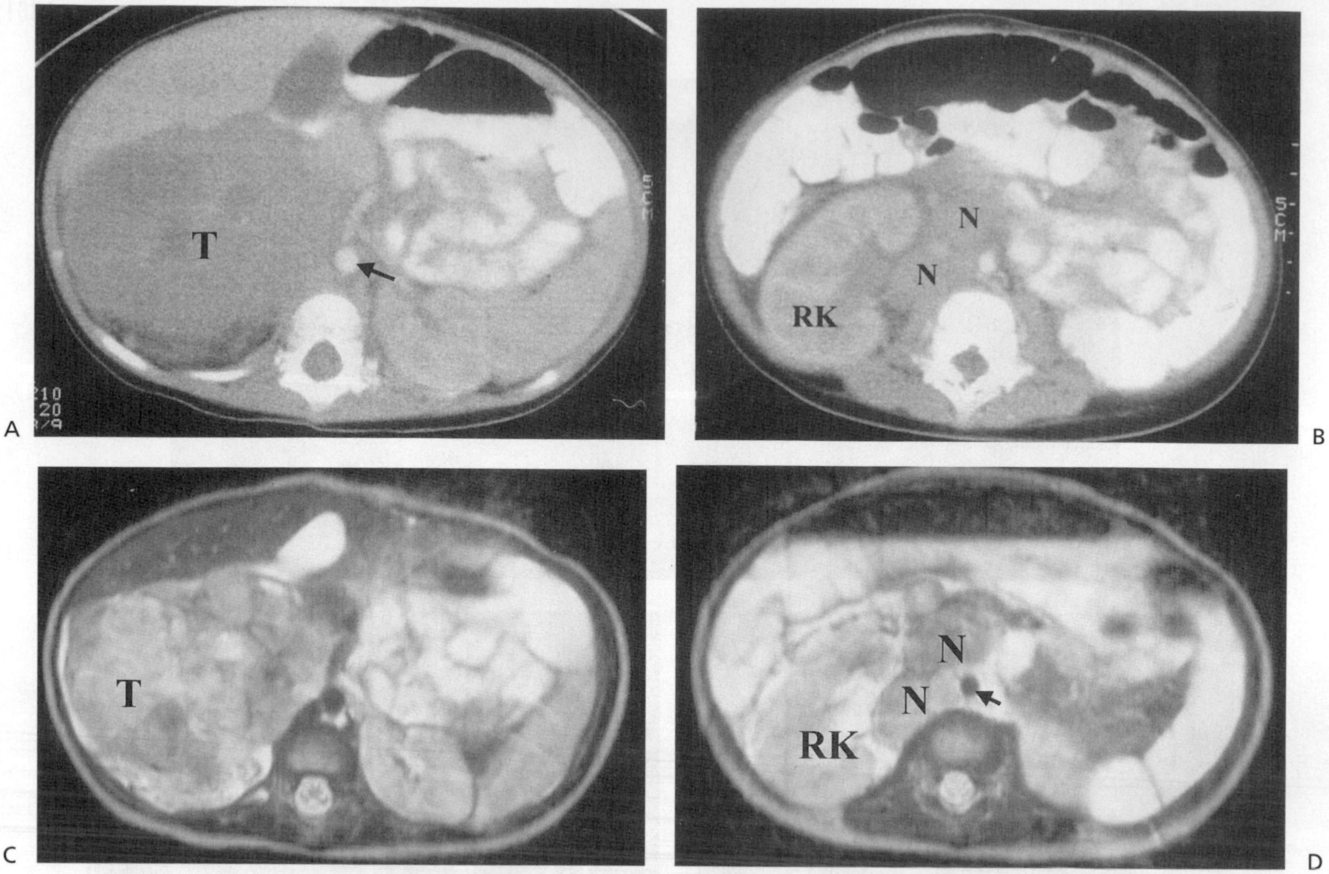

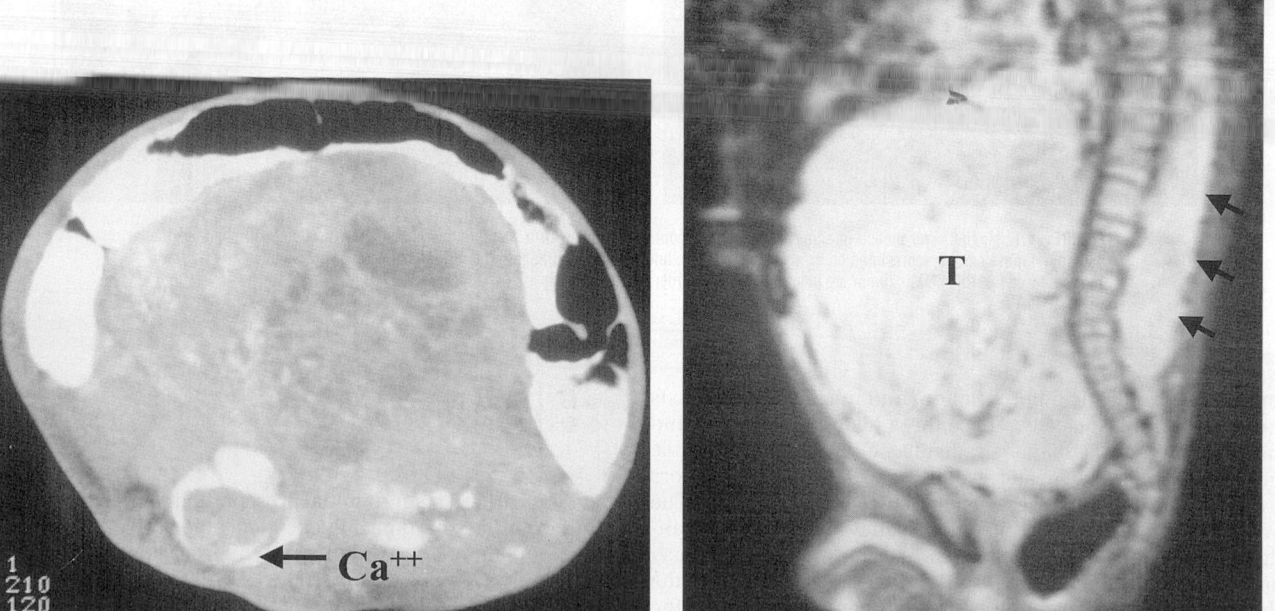

FIGURE 84.2. Neuroblastoma with nodal involvement, 3-year-old boy. **A:** Computed tomography (CT) through the upper abdomen shows a large soft-tissue mass (*T*) arising in the right adrenal gland and extending to the midline (*arrow indicates aorta*). **B:** A CT scan several centimeters lower shows several small nodes (*N*) in the right pararenal area. (*RK indicates right kidney.*) **C:** T_2-weighted axial image shows a high signal-intensity tumor (*T*) in the right suprarenal area. **D:** T_2-weighted image at a lower level shows enlarged, mildly enhancing paracaval lymph nodes (*N*). (*RK indicates right kidney; arrow indicates aorta.*) (Courtesy of Dr. Marilyn Siegel, Mallinckrodt Institute of Radiology, St. Louis, MO.)

FIGURE 84.3. 1-year-old child with constipation and a palpable mass. Also noted to have lower leg weakness. **A:** Computed tomography shows a large soft tissue mass with calcifications and necrosis filling the retroperitoneum. Tumor calcification (*arrow*) is noted in the spinal cord. **B:** Sagittal, STIR image shows the large prevertebral mass displacing bowel loops superiorly. Intraspinal tumor extends from the lower thoracic level through the lumbar level. The patient underwent emergent resection of the intraspinal tumor (*arrows*). (Courtesy of Dr. Marilyn Siegel, Mallinckrodt Institute of Radiology, St. Louis, MO.)

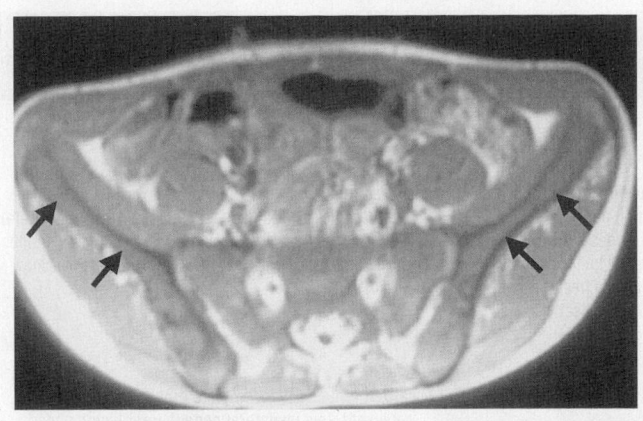
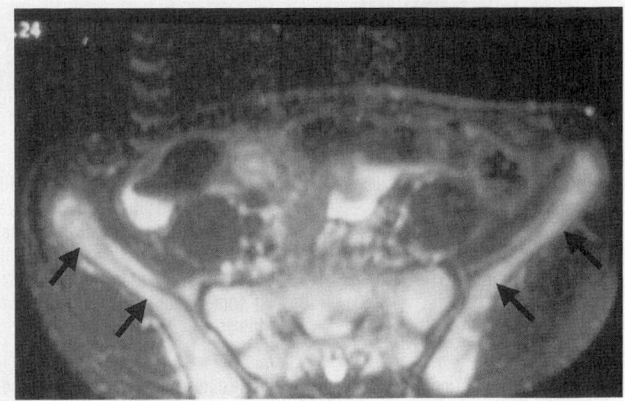
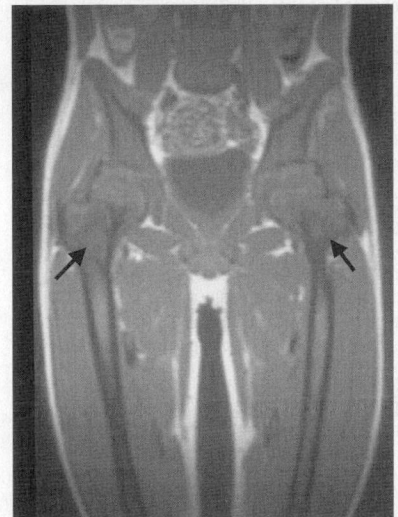
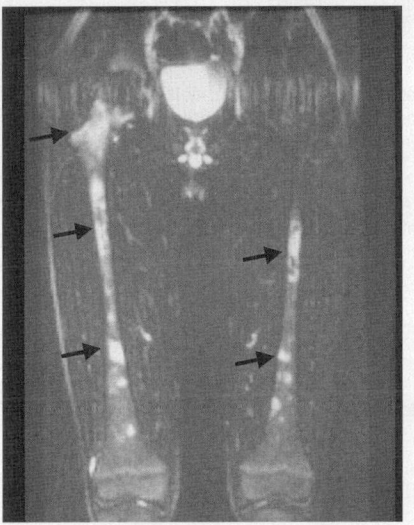

FIGURE 84.4. A 6-year-old boy who presented with bone pain. Axial (**A**) and coronal (**B**) T_1-weighted image of the pelvis and femurs show diffusely low signal–intensity marrow from metastases (*arrows*). **C:** Fat-saturated T_2-weighted image of the pelvis. The involved marrow has increased in signal intensity and is now hyperintense to adjacent fat and soft tissue (*arrows*). **D:** Fat-saturated T_2-weighted coronal image of the pelvis and femurs. Multiple high-signal foci are noted throughout the long bones (*arrows*). By comparison, normal marrow has a signal intensity similar to that of muscle on fat-saturated images. (Courtesy of Dr. Marilyn Siegel, Mallinckrodt Institute of Radiology, St. Louis, MO.)

children survive with little or no treatment (26,28). Treatment should be directed at relief of the acute presenting event (often respiratory distress secondary to hepatomegaly), and the temptation to aggressively treat these patients in the absence of other bad prognostic factors should be avoided.

Patients with more differentiated tumors (e.g., ganglioneuroma, ganglioneuroblastoma) fare better than children with poorly differentiated or undifferentiated neuroblastomas. A favorable Shimada stage is associated with 90% survival, compared with 22% with unfavorable Shimada stages. Elevated serum ferritin (>142 ng/mL), NSE (>100 ng/mL), and LDH (>1,500 IU) are all associated with advanced disease and a poor prognosis (3,7,29,97).

MYCN (N-*myc*) is a proto-oncogene that resides on the short arm of chromosome 2. An increased number of *MYCN* gene copies is associated with an extremely poor prognosis (5% survival) (9,92). *MYCN* amplification has been associated with the multidrug-resistance gene and may account for this tumor's notorious resistance to therapy (73). A tumor with a DNA index of 1 (diploid or near diploid) paradoxically gives a worse prognosis than tumors that are aneuploid (59). Hyperdiploid tumors occur more often in lower stages and are associated with better chemotherapy responsiveness. Allelic loss of the short arm of chromosome 1 represents a loss of heterozygosity of a tumor suppressor gene and is also associated with a poor prognosis

independent of age and stage. It reliably identifies patients with stage I, II, or IV-S disease who have a high risk of relapse and require aggressive therapy (11).

General Management

Because of the biologic heterogeneity of neuroblastoma, the following treatment recommendations should be considered as guidelines. The prognostic implications of a tumor's biologic indices, such as *MYCN* amplification and DNA index, may warrant more aggressive therapy in otherwise young patients with a favorable stage. There are three risk groups that allow protocol assignment by prognosis (Table 84.3).

Low-Risk Disease

This category includes all patients with INSS stage 1, infants with stage 4S disease with favorable histology, nonamplified *MYCN,* and aneuploid tumors. Low-stage, resectable tumors (INSS stage 1, 2, or 3 with negative nodes) have an excellent prognosis after complete gross surgical excision. Adjuvant chemotherapy or irradiation has not improved the outcome in children with completely resected tumors with favorable biologic features (27,55,62,70,71). Positive surgical margins or

Table 84.1 NEUROBLASTOMA STAGING SYSTEMS[a]

Evans and D'Angio	Pediatric Oncology Group	International Staging System
Stage I Tumor confined to the organ or structure of origin.	*Stage A* Complete gross resection of primary tumor, with or without microscopic residual. Intracavitary lymph nodes, not adhered to and removed with primary (nodes adhered to or within tumor resection may be positive for tumor without upstaging patient to stage C), histologically free of tumor. If primary in abdomen or pelvis, liver histologically free of tumor.	*Stage 1* Localized tumor with complete gross excision, without microscopic residual disease; representative ipsilateral lymph nodes negative for tumor microscopically (nodes attached to and removed with the primary tumor may be positive).
Stage II Tumor extending in continuity beyond the organ midline. Regional lymph nodes on the ipsilateral side may be involved.	*Stage B* Grossly unresected primary tumor. Nodes and liver same as stage A.	*Stage 2A* Localized tumor with incomplete gross excision; representative ipsilateral nonadherent lymph nodes negative for tumor microscopically.
Stage III Tumor extending in continuity beyond the midline. Regional lymph nodes may be involved bilaterally.	*Stage C* Complete or incomplete resection of primary. Intracavitary nodes not adhered to primary histologically positive for tumor. Liver as in stage A.	*Stage 2B* Localized tumor with or without complete gross excision, with ipsilateral nonadherent lymph nodes positive for tumor. Enlarged contralateral lymph nodes must be negative microscopically.
Stage IV Remote disease involving skeleton, bone marrow, soft tissue, distant lymph node groups, etc. (See stage IV-S.)	*Stage D* Any dissemination of disease beyond intracavitary nodes (i.e., extracavitary nodes, liver, skin, bone marrow, bone).	*Stage 3* Unresectable unilateral tumor infiltrating across the midline,[b] with or without regional lymph node involvement; or localized unilateral tumor with contralateral regional lymph node involvement; or midline tumor with bilateral extension by infiltration (unresectable) or by lymph node involvement.
Stage IV-S Patients who would otherwise be stage I or II but who have remote disease confined to liver, skin, or bone marrow (without radiographic evidence of bone metastases on complete skeletal survey).	*Stage DS* Infants <1 year of age with stage IV-S disease (see Evans and D'Angio).	*Stage 4* Any primary tumor with dissemination to distant lymph nodes, bone, bone marrow, liver, skin, and/or other organs (except as defined for stage 4S).
		Stage 4S Localized primary tumor as defined for stage 1, 2A, or 2B with dissemination limited to skin, liver, and/or bone marrow[c] (limited to infants <1 year of age).

[a]Multifocal primary tumors (e.g., bilateral adrenal primary tumors) should be staged according to the greatest extent of disease, as defined in the table, and followed by a subscript letter M (e.g., 3_M).
[b]The midline is defined as the vertebral column. Tumors originating on one side and crossing the midline must infiltrate to or beyond the opposite side of the vertebral column.
[c]Marrow involvement in stage 4S should be minimal—that is, <10% of total nucleated cells identified as malignant on bone marrow biopsy or on marrow aspirate. More extensive marrow involvement would be considered to be stage 4. The *meta*-iodobenzylguanidine (MIBG) scan (if performed) should be negative in the marrow.
(Modified from Halperin EC, Constine LS, Tarbell NJ, et al., eds. *Pediatric radiation oncology.* Baltimore: Lippincott Williams & Wilkins, 2005;189–190, with permission.)

Table 84.2 PROGNOSTIC VARIABLES IN NEUROBLASTOMA

Prognostic Factor	Favorable	Unfavorable	Survival (%) Favorable	Unfavorable
Age	<2 y	>2 y	77	38
Stage	I, II, IVS	III, IV	90–100	50, 30
Pathology (Shimada)	Favorable	Unfavorable	90	23
Ferritin	<143 ng/mL	>143 ng/mL	83	19
Neuron-specific enolase	<100	>100	79	10
Chromogranin	<190 ng/mL	>190 ng/mL	69	30
GD2 ganglioside	<103 pmol/mL	>568 pmol/mL	70	24
Urine VMA/HVA	<1	>1	84	44
gp 140TRK-A	High expression	Low expression	78	14
N-*myc*	Single copy	Amplified	70	5
DNA index	>1.1	1	100	10
1p deletion	No 1p deletion	1p deletion	90	10

HVA, homovanillic acid; VMA, vanillylmandelic acid
Adapted from Matthay KK. Neuroblastoma: a clinical challenge and biologic puzzle. *CA Cancer J Clin* 1995;45:179–192, with permission.

Table 84.3 PROTOCOL ASSIGNMENT BY RISK GROUP

INSS Stage	Age	MYCN Status	Shimada Histology	DNA Ploidy[a]	Risk Group
1	0–21 y	Any	Any	Any	Low
2A/2B	<365 d	Any	Any	Any	Low
	≤365 d–21 y	Nonamp	Any	—	Low
	≥365 d–21 y	Amp	Fav	—	Low
	≥365 d–21 y	Amp	Unfav	—	High
3	<365 d	Nonamp	Any	Any	Intermediate
	<365 d	Amp	Any	Any	High
	≥365 d–21 y	Nonamp	Fav	—	Intermediate
	≥365 d–21 y	Nonamp	Unfav	—	High
	≥365 d–21 y	Amp	Fav	—	High
4	<365 d	Nonamp	Any	Any	Intermediate
	<365 d	Amp	Any	Any	High
	≥365 d–21 y	Any	Any	—	High
4S	<365 d	Nonamp	Fav	>1	Low
	<365 d	Nonamp	Any	=1	Intermediate
	<365 d	Nonamp	Unfav	Any	Intermediate
	<365 d	Amp	Any	Any	High

Amp, amplified; Fav, Favorable; INSS, International Neuroblastoma Staging System; Nonamp, nonamplified; Unfav, unfavorable
[a]DNA ploidy: DNA index (DI) >1 or = 1; hypodiploid tumors (with DI<1) will be treated as a tumor with a DI >1. (DNA index <1 [hypodiploid] to be considered favorable ploidy.) Asymptomatic low- and intermediate-risk group patients will not be registered on a neuroblastoma study until central lab biology results are known.

microscopic residual disease does not uniformly require more aggressive therapy. Patients with *MYCN* amplification or low DNA index may require adjuvant therapy and should be enrolled in clinical trials (59).

Unresectable tumors that are otherwise of low stage (INSS stages 1, 2, and 3 with negative lymph nodes) may require preoperative chemotherapy and occasionally radiation therapy to convert them to a resectable status. Second-look surgery is performed to remove a previously unresectable primary tumor and achieve a complete remission after induction chemotherapy. Complete resection can be achieved in almost two thirds of previously unresectable stage III to IV primary tumors (41). The CCG has reported that eventual complete resection of the primary tumor in advanced disease may have a favorable impact on outcome (41). The benefit to complete resection in patients with advanced disease has not been uniformly established. Patients with biologically favorable tumors may be more amenable to surgery after chemotherapy, and the apparent benefit of complete resection may be a result of patient selection (96). POG-8104 enrolled patients with INSS stage 1 (POG stage A) disease. In that trial, *MYCN* amplification and DNA index were not evaluated uniformly. Treatment was surgery only. Regardless of the presence of residual microscopic disease, the 2-year disease-free survival rate was 89% (72). In the CCG experience (CCG trial 3881) with stage 1 disease, the 4-year event-free and overall survival rates for children treated initially with surgery alone are 93% and 99%, respectively. For patients with stage 2 disease, the event-free and overall survival rates were 81% and 98%, respectively. In that trial, only 13% of patients with stage 2 disease received any chemotherapy or radiotherapy, despite the fact that 104 patients had INSS stage 2B disease. The authors ascribe the favorable results to improved surgical management and better staging with MIBG scanning (79).

Intermediate-Risk Disease

The intermediate-risk category includes all stage 2A/2B disease except patients with amplified *MYCN* and unfavorable histology unless they are younger than age 1 year. Locally ad-

vanced and regionally metastatic tumors (INSS stage 2B to 3 with positive lymph nodes) require more intensive therapy. Infants younger than 1 year of age should undergo complete resection of the primary tumor and receive adjuvant chemotherapy (5,14,37,96). In unresectable cases, chemotherapy may be administered initially, and surgery can be performed after response to systemic treatment. In older children with lymph node metastases, adjuvant radiation therapy to the primary and regional lymph nodes has improved the disease-free and overall survival rates. A prospective randomized trial of postoperative chemotherapy or chemotherapy plus regional irradiation demonstrated 31% disease-free survival in children treated with chemotherapy, compared with 58% in those who also received radiation therapy (13). However, the value of radiation therapy in intermediate-risk patients is not universally accepted. De Bernardi et al. (21) failed to demonstrate a benefit from the addition of radiotherapy in 29 children older than 1 year with postoperative residual tumor or positive regional lymph nodes. Children in that randomized study received two cycles of peptichemio with or without radiation. Progression-free survival was 64% in the radiotherapy arm and 73% in the arm without radiotherapy (21). Coupled with the risk of late effects from even moderate radiotherapy doses, this small trial has provided an argument that systematic radiation therapy, even for POG stage C patients, may not be necessary. Current COG trials reflect this bias as the use of radiation therapy is decreasing.

Patients with intraspinal extension of neuroblastoma pose a unique problem. They frequently have severe neurologic compromise resulting from spinal cord compression. Historically, these patients were treated with laminectomy and surgical debulking with or without radiation therapy and chemotherapy (84). Because the morbidity of this approach is significant, with a high rate of spinal growth deformity, a number of investigators have proceeded with treatment of these patients using primary chemotherapy (41). A prospective series of 42 patients treated with primary chemotherapy demonstrated a 92% improvement in neurologic deficits, allowing children to avoid neurosurgical decompression in more than 60% of cases when receiving courses of carboplatin and etoposide alternating with cyclophosphamide, vincristine, and doxorubicin.

The POG experience (POG trials 8742 and 9244) with stages 2B to 3 disease demonstrates an 85% event-free survival with completely resected tumors at diagnosis, compared to 70% with incomplete resection at diagnosis ($p = .259$). On both of these studies, patients underwent maximum safe tumor resection followed by five courses of induction chemotherapy. On POG-8742 they received cisplatin and etoposide alternating with cyclophosphamide and doxorubicin. On POG-9244 they received alternating cycles of OPEC (vincristine, cisplatin, etoposide, cyclophosphamide) and OJEC (vincristine, carboplatin, etoposide, cyclophosphamide). After a second-look surgery the same chemotherapy was given as maintenance. Radiotherapy was given to patients with viable residual tumor discovered at the time of the second-look operation. Children age 12 to 24 months at the time of radiation therapy received 24 Gy in 1.5-Gy fractions to the primary tumor site. Older children received 30 Gy in 1.5 Gy fractions. Of the 37 patients on these two protocols that survived "event free," 11 (30%) received radiotherapy. Patients with favorable Shimada histology tumors had a 92% event-free survival, compared with 58% with unfavorable tumors ($p = .009$). Patients with *MYCN* amplification did poorly, with outcomes comparable to stage D patients (95).

Based on CCG and POG data, patients with intermediate-risk neuroblastoma have an estimated 3-year survival of between 75% to 98%. Cyclophosphamide, doxorubicin, carboplatin, and etoposide are the four most active agents (12,25,81). The COG now is evaluating the role of chemotherapy dose intensity and duration for children based on tumor biology.

Surgery plays a critical role in the primary management of neuroblastoma. The goals of surgery are to establish a diagnosis; provide tissue for evaluation of prognostic biologic markers; stage the disease according to INSS criteria; and attempt to totally excise the primary, if feasible. The extent of surgery has an important impact on outcome. O'Neill et al. (75) reported that 55/59 patients with a complete or near-complete resection were alive and free of disease 2 years after surgery, compared to only 13/24 cases with a subtotal resection. Just as Haase et al. have reported (41), Grosfield and Baehner (36) found evidence for improved outcome in stage 4 patients attaining complete resection of primary tumor at delayed second-look procedures (36).

High-Risk Disease

The high-risk disease category includes older children with INSS stages 2 to 3 and unfavorable Shimada histology and/or amplified *MYCN* and those with metastatic disease (INSS stage 4). The majority of patients with neuroblastoma present with metastatic disease. With the exception of infants with favorable biologic disease confined to the skin, bone marrow, or liver, the outcome is poor. Aggressive treatment regimens have been used in these patients. Intensive high-dose chemotherapy regimens appear to be superior to less intensive regimens. Active drugs in advanced neuroblastoma include cyclophosphamide, cisplatin, doxorubicin, etoposide, and teniposide (17).

Many recent clinical trials have sought to intensify treatment of metastatic neuroblastoma through the use of high-dose myeloablative chemotherapy with stem cell rescue or bone marrow transplantation (BMT). The French Lyon-Marseille-Curie East (LMCE) group reported a 40% progression-free survival at 2 years and 20% at 5 years in 62 patients proceeding to autologous bone marrow transplant (ABMT) (82). The CCG reported a 43% 2-year event-free survival in 43 children undergoing consolidation melphalan, cisplatin, teniposide, doxorubicin, and total body irradiation (TBI) to 1,000 cGy in three fractions of 330 cGy per day. The toxic death rate was 22% (93). Australian in-

vestigators tested a less intense preparative regimen with a TBI regimen consisting of 12 Gy in six twice daily fractions (64). Of 28 patients registered, 19 achieved complete remission following induction chemotherapy. Seventeen of these 19 patients underwent ABMT and 15 (87%) remain free of disease at 5 years from ABMT. Of the 28 patients registered, 50% have survived 5 years.

Uncertain that ABMT could be studied successfully in a cooperative group, the CCG conducted two pilot studies for children with stage 4 disease. In CCG-321, patients received induction chemotherapy consisting of cisplatin, etoposide, doxorubicin, and cyclophosphamide. Of 207 patients, 159 remained disease free during induction chemotherapy. Of these patients, 67 received myeloablative chemotherapy and ABMT, whereas 74 continued conventional chemotherapy for a total of 13 cycles. The patients receiving the ABMT had a higher event-free survival than patients continuing standard chemotherapy (40% vs. 19%; $p = .019$) (103). Because they are not randomized trials, these studies potentially may have allowed a biased allocation of patients to one arm based on clinical concerns or prognostic risk factors. The POG failed to show a benefit to BMT in high-risk metastatic neuroblastoma (POG 8340) (97).

The European Neuroblastoma Study Group studied the role of consolidative ABMT with high-dose melphalan versus no further treatment following induction chemotherapy with the OPEC regimen in patients with stage 3 and 4 disease (83,86). With a median follow-up of 14.3 years for surviving children, they report an improvement in event free survival (38% vs. 27%) and overall survival (47% and 30%) for the high-dose melphalan arm, but those differences did not reach statistical significance. The subset of patients with stage IV disease who were >1 year of age, however, did show statistically significant improvement in event-free survival (33% vs. 17%; $p = .01$) and overall survival (46% vs. 21%; $p = .03$).

In a randomized trial completed in 1996, patients with high-risk neuroblastoma were treated initially with cisplatin (60 mg/m^2 of body-surface area administered intravenously over a period of 6 hours on day 0), doxorubicin (30 mg/m^2 intravenously on day 2), etoposide (100 mg/m^2 intravenously on days 2 and 5), and cyclophosphamide (1,000 mg/m^2 intravenously on days 3 and 4) for five cycles at 28-day intervals, plus surgery and radiotherapy for gross residual disease (63). The patients then were randomized to receive either myeloablative therapy and purged ADMT or three further cycles of intensive chemotherapy. The ABMT conditioning regimen consisted of high-dose carboplatin, etoposide, and melphalan followed by three daily fractions of TBI (333 cGy per fraction). Purged autologous marrow was infused with granulocyte macrophage colony stimulating factor (GM-CSF). The mean event-free survival rate 3 years after the first randomization was significantly better among the 189 patients who were assigned to undergo transplantation than among the 190 patients assigned to receive continuation chemotherapy (34% vs. 22%; $p = .034$). Overall survival was not significantly different between the randomized groups. All patients who completed cytotoxic therapy without disease progression were then randomly assigned to receive a 6-month course of 13-cis-retinoic acid (RA), versus observation. Retinoic acid has been shown to promote differentiation and growth arrest of neuroblastoma *in vitro* and may decrease *MYCN* expression in cells with amplified *MYCN* (87). The RA was given as 160 mg/m^2/day, 2 weeks per month for 6 months and began approximately 3 months following ABMT. The 3-year event-free survival from the time of the second randomization was 47% for the 130 patients who received RA, as compared to 30% for the 128 patients randomized to no further therapy ($p = .027$). There was no difference in overall survival among the randomized groups. The benefit of RA appeared to be limited to patients with no residual or minimal residual disease. Patients who did not achieve a complete response to induction chemotherapy did not benefit from the administration of RA.

Berthold et al. (2) reported results of a prospective randomized trial in children with high-risk neuroblastoma comparing myeloablative therapy with melphalan, etoposide, and carboplatin and autologous stem cell rescue, with maintenance chemotherapy with cyclophosphamide. When analyzed as treated, a statistically significantly improved 3-year event-free survival (53% vs. 30%) and overall survival (68% vs. 53%) was seen with myeloablative therapy.

Local control of the primary tumor in stage 4 neuroblastoma is an important element of patient management. The role of surgical resection in metastatic disease remains controversial. Many authors have reported more favorable outcomes in patients undergoing complete resection (15,56). There is a strong association between chemotherapy dose intensity and surgical respectability, which diminishes the significance that aggressive resection is an independent favorable factor. It can be assumed that tumors amenable to resection may have an inherently less aggressive biology.

In the CCG-321-P3 pilot there was a 33% rate of local relapse in patients not undergoing a complete resection at their initial surgery, irrespective of their ultimate surgical resection status, including second-look operations (61). This high local failure rate suggests there is a role for local radiation therapy. In that pilot study, patients received radiotherapy if they had gross residual disease after second-look surgery. Although the local control in patients receiving radiotherapy was the same as in unirradiated patients, it should be noted that only patients with gross residual disease received this local treatment, suggesting that the radiotherapy was beneficial.

In a reanalysis of CCG-3891, Hass-Kogan et al. (39) compared locoregional control rates in those patients on the non-ABMT arm who received 10 to 20 Gy to gross residual disease following induction therapy to those patients in the ABMT arm who received similar RT to residual disease, but also received 10 Gy TBI in 3.33-Gy daily fractions in their conditioning regimens. The patients in the ABMT arm had an lower locoregional recurrence rate (33% vs. 51%; $p = .004$). Although this affect may be due to the higher dose of RT delivered in this group of patients, it is not possible to separate the RT effect from that of the more intense systemic therapy also given to these patients in the ABMT arm.

Laprie et al. (57) analyzed locoregional control in MYCN amplified INSS stage 2 and 3 patients treated with different regimens over different eras. Their approach varied from conventional chemotherapy and RT only to gross residual disease after surgery in patients older than 1 year, to high-dose chemotherapy with ABMT, and local radiation therapy to all patients. They note an improvement in EFS with ABMT and RT (83% vs. 25%; $p = .001$). Again, conclusions regarding the effect of RT independent of the intensified systemic therapy are difficult to make since this was not a randomized comparison.

Local therapy to the primary tumor and metastatic sites may be beneficial in the curative therapy of children with disseminated disease. Surgical resection of the primary tumor has been associated with improved survival and local control after aggressive systemic therapy (41,61). There is a predilection for recurrence in previous sites of disease, and it is conceivable that additional local therapy with irradiation to the primary tumor site and distant metastases may enhance tumor control and cure rates (61,98).

The POG reported that patients with persistent disease at primary or metastatic sites received boost irradiation of 12 Gy prior to TBI for bone marrow transplant. Only 2/27 patients relapsed at irradiated sites. Six of 10 first remission patients given local radiation remained in remission, compared to only 13/40 who were not irradiated, despite the fact that irradiated patients had residual disease (35).

Radiation therapy plays an extremely important role in the palliative management of patients with end-stage symptomatic neuroblastoma. Pain from bone or other visceral metastases often can be relieved with external-beam radiation therapy. Mass effect from a rapidly enlarging tumor can respond dramatically to radiation therapy. In a series of 10 patients with symptomatic liver metastases treated at Duke University Medical Center, Halperin (42) reported seven complete responses to radiation therapy, either alone or in conjunction with chemotherapy. Radiation doses ranged from 4 to 24.4 Gy at a rate of 1 to 1.5 Gy per fraction. The seven patients with complete response survived without recurrence.

Systemic radionuclide therapy with ^{131}I-MIBG has been tested in several European and U.S. centers with early encouraging results. This radioactive agent produced objective responses in previously treated and chemoresistant stage 4 neuroblastoma (51,58). These early positive results have prompted some investigators to test this agent in previously untreated metastatic neuroblastoma. DeKraker et al. (22) reported that a combination of ^{131}I-MIBG and second-look surgery produced response rates comparable to those of multidrug chemotherapy. Preliminary research on the combination of ^{131}I-MIBG with systemic chemotherapy and/or TBI with BMT has demonstrated that this is a safe treatment and worthy of more investigation (34,60,116).

A recent COG protocol utilizes targeted therapy and immunotherapy for patients following ABMT and RA therapy. The human-mouse chimeric monoclonal antibody ch14.18 targets a tumor associated antigen, GD2 (91). This therapy has resulted in reasonable response rates in preliminary clinical trials (45,117). The current phase III protocol will randomize high-risk patients following initial response to intensive therapy to treatment with ch14.18, interleukin-2, and GM-CSF along with RA, or treatment with RA alone.

⬛⬛ | Radiation-Therapy Techniques

Treatment Planning and Field Design

Significant reductions in irradiation-associated morbidity have accompanied technologic advancements. The transition from orthovoltage to megavoltage x-rays has decreased the risk of severe growth-related skeletal defects (105). CT-assisted simulation and three-dimensional radiation-therapy treatment planning have the potential to decrease the volume of normal tissues irradiated and thereby decrease the incidence of late effects (Fig. 84.5). The radiation oncologist must be aware of the increased risk of spinal deformity or other skeletal anomalies if symmetric irradiation of the bone is not administered. The clinician needs to balance the treatment of disease and normal tissues to maximize tumor coverage while not sacrificing the growing tissues.

Radiation therapy portals to a primary tumor site should treat the gross residual tumor remaining after chemotherapy, with at least a 2-cm margin from the tumor to the block edge. This margin usually ensures adequate dosimetric coverage of the residual tumor, taking into account treatment-related positional uncertainties and beam penumbra. Children who are not sedated may require more margin if they tend to shift or move on the treatment table. Regional lymph node sites should be covered if nodes were radiographically or pathologically involved at any time during the disease course. The POG study that demonstrated an advantage to radiation therapy for POG stage C disease included extended-field radiation therapy to adjacent lymph node sites (i.e., elective mediastinal irradiation for abdominal primary tumors) (13). It is not clear that this extended-field treatment contributed to the beneficial effect of radiation

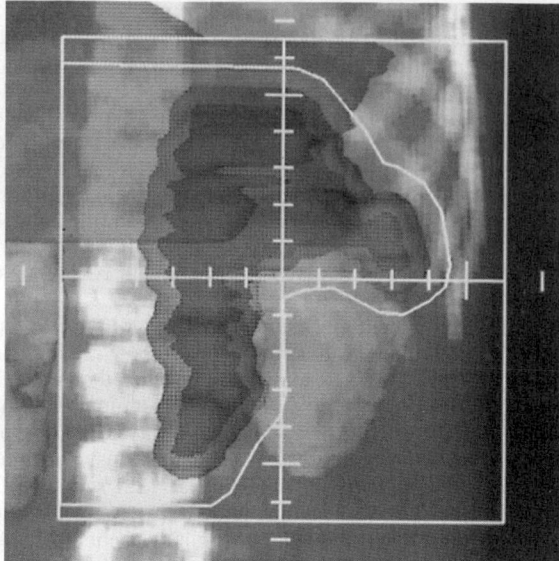

FIGURE 84.5. Radiation-therapy treatment field for a child with a left adrenal primary neuroblastoma and para-aortic lymph node metastases. The beam's eye-view display with a digital reconstructed radiograph allows for adequate coverage of the target volume and lymph node region with sparing of the ipsilateral kidney and liver while homogeneously irradiating the adjacent spine.

therapy, and current COG trials do not include it. Halperin (43) reviewed the patterns of failure in 13 children with stage C neuroblastoma treated with systemic therapy and radiation therapy directed to the primary tumor and without "prophylactic" irradiation of contiguous lymph node regions. Of the seven patients who failed, two of them developed a recurrence in contiguous lymph node regions. In both of these circumstances the regional failures were accompanied by local or distant failure. Considering the morbidity associated with the additional radiation volume and its impact on the tolerance to subsequent chemotherapy, he recommended against this prophylactic regional irradiation.

CT or MRI scans should be used to define the full extent of disease when a radiation therapy portal is designed. In many instances parallel opposed anterior and posterior portals may suffice for tumor coverage. They have the added advantage of allowing homogenous irradiation of the spine in paraspinal tumors. In cases with larger tumors more intimately associated with critical structures, advances in technology have the potential to improve the therapeutic ratio. The use of intensity-modulated radiation therapy can offer a dosimetric advantage in select patients (78). Likewise, the use of proton beam radiation may offer improved dose distribution compared to photon radiation therapy (50).

Radiation therapy of metastatic sites should include generous margins. Bony metastases often are more extensive than a plain radiograph may suggest. Orbital metastases may require treatment of the entire orbit. Hepatic metastases do not require whole liver irradiation, but adequate margins must be used to account for respiratory motion during treatment. The patient's life expectancy should influence the selection of radiation-therapy portals, field shaping, and dose fractionation. Children who have end-stage disease with tumors that are resistant to most chemotherapy drugs should be treated with wide fields and a rapid fractionation schedule. Complex field design and prolonged fractionation schedules may prevent the terminal child from spending quality time off therapy. The exception is infants with stage 4S disease. These children frequently have a very good prognosis, and sparing of normal tissues is an important goal.

Low-dose TBI has been used with variable success in the curative management of children with metastatic neuroblastoma (20,54). More important has been the use of TBI as part of the preparative regimen for patients undergoing BMT for high-risk metastatic disease. It is not clear if TBI is essential in the preoperative program for a transplant. Patterns of failure after BMT are predominately in sites of prior disease, including the original primary tumor and previously documented metastatic sites (61,98). These data suggest that involved-field boost irradiation, before or after BMT with TBI, may be beneficial.

The appropriate radiation dose is debatable. Laboratory data suggest that neuroblastoma is very radiosensitive and that neuroblasts exhibit very little repair capacity between fractions (109). This makes hyperfractionated radiation therapy an attractive option because comparable tumoricidal doses can be achieved with minimization of the risk of late effects (23,24). However, despite irradiation doses that approach normal tissue tolerance in the young, local recurrences after radiation therapy still occur. The irradiation dose required to control gross disease may be age dependent (52,65,88). In infants <1 year of age, a dose of 12 Gy appears sufficient for durable local control (52,65). Tumors in children aged 12 to 48 months may require doses of at least 25 Gy. Children older than 4 years of age frequently develop local failures even with doses of >25 Gy. Local control of the primary tumor site in patients with high-risk disease may be improved with the use of local radiation to the primary site and regional lymph nodes. Kushner et al. (55) updated the experience from Memorial Sloan-Kettering Cancer Center, reporting that 21 Gy of hyperfractionated radiation therapy resulted in 90% primary-site local control at 5 years. Radiation was delivered after all chemotherapy with a minimum interval of 4 hours between fractions. No TBI was administered in this group of patients. If patients had a gross total resection, the local control was 100%, whereas in seven patients with gross disease three had recurrence (55,111). In the series by Kushner et al., 92% of metastatic sites were controlled with 21 Gy of hyperfractionated radiation therapy at 36 months.

The use of intraoperative radiation therapy has been reported by several investigators (76,118). Haas-Kogan et al. (38) described the results of intraoperative radiation therapy (IORT) in 23 patients with high-risk disease. Seven patients received additional external beam radiation therapy (either to the primary site or from total body irradiation). A single fraction of 7 to 16 Gy (median 10 Gy) to the primary tumor bed was associated with a local control rate of 100% in patients who had gross total resection, whereas IORT was unable to control any patients with gross residual disease.

Children treated palliatively for symptomatic metastatic disease should receive adequate irradiation doses for durable tumor control if they have a reasonable expectation of long survival. Total dose and fractionation regimens similar to those used for curative therapy should be considered. Low-dose, short-fractionation schedules are appropriate if the child is not expected to live beyond 6 to 12 months. In these instances, minimizing a child's visits to the radiation-therapy facility while rapidly relieving symptoms is a worthwhile goal. If the likelihood of long survival is small, 5 to 20 Gy in one to five daily fractions can allow rapid palliation.

⬢⬢ | Results of Therapy

Low-Risk Disease

Survival rates after surgery alone of 85% to 90% or better can be expected (27,40,71,72,79). Additional therapy usually is not indicated unless unfavorable biologic features are present.

Intermediate-Risk Disease

Children with large, initially unresectable tumors often respond to primary chemotherapy with combinations of drugs including cyclophosphamide, vincristine, cisplatin, etoposide, doxorubicin, or teniposide. Children with unresponsive, unresectable gross residual disease may require external-beam irradiation. Frequently, these children can undergo resection of the tumor at a second-look operation (41) and achieve a survival rate of 60% to 90% (40,71).

The presence of lymph node metastases, even with a localized primary tumor, negatively affects prognosis. These children have a 50% to 75% survival rate even with aggressive systemic therapy and adjuvant radiation therapy (13,40). Infants with lymph node–positive disease have a more favorable outcome, with a 3-year disease-free survival rate of 93% after treatment with cyclophosphamide and doxorubicin and complete resection without irradiation (14).

High-Risk Disease

Children >1 year of age with metastatic neuroblastoma continue to have a poor prognosis, with expected 3- or 4-year survival rates of <10% to 30%. The addition of cisplatin and teniposide to the chemotherapy armamentarium improved the expected 4-year survival rate from 7% to 28% in a series of trials conducted from 1962 to 1988 at St. Jude Children's Research Hospital (5). The CCG has reported that ABMT can improve outcome in selected patients with metastatic neuroblastoma. With this aggressive therapy, the 3-year event-free survival was 34%. The addition of cis-retinoic acid was associated with a 47% event-free survival (63). The COG is investigating even more intensive systemic therapy with tandem stem cell transplant.

Infants with metastatic disease have a uniquely favorable outcome. In stage 4S, survival rates can be as high as 75% to 90% (69,104). In these patients, the goal of therapy should be limited to the relief of acute presenting symptoms. Local-field, fractionated, low-dose irradiation (<12 Gy), minimal chemotherapy, or supportive care may be sufficient to achieve high survival rates. Infants with metastases to other sites (brain, bone, or lung) or who have tumors with poor biologic features (DNA index of 1, *MYCN* amplification) should be managed with more aggressive regimens (59,77).

:: | Sequelae of Treatment

Early Complications

Acute side effects of radiation therapy depend on tumor site and fields of treatment. The short-term effects are those that can be expected for any patient receiving radiation therapy. Acute effects, especially skin reactions and mucositis, may be enhanced if concurrent chemotherapy or a hyperfractionated irradiation schedule is used.

Late Effects

Long-term effects depend on the site irradiated and the total dose of both radiation and chemotherapy agents used. Age at the time of treatment may influence the risk and severity of skeletal anomalies (107), which may include spinal deformities such as kyphosis, scoliosis, or limb shortening. Generally, younger children are more prone to late radiation injury than older children. Fortunately, in neuroblastoma, the youngest children require radiation therapy infrequently or at lower total doses (Table 84.4). Chemotherapy may increase the risk of irradiation sequelae, and the expected tolerance may be reduced (108).

Table 84.4	WASHINGTON UNIVERSITY NEUROBLASTOMA STUDY OF LONG-TERM SEQUELAE RELATED TO RADIATION THERAPY	
Complication	**No. of Patients**	**Dose (Gy)**
Scoliosis (mild)	6	8–30
Scoliosis (severe)	6	16–37
Muscle hypoplasia	3	28–30
Bone hypoplasia	4	28–30
Breast hypoplasia	5	28–30
Kidney hypoplasia	2	30–33
Pulmonary hypoplasia	3	28–30
Lung fibrosis	1	48 (possibly fatal)
Liver fibrosis	1	39.5 (fatal)
Rib necrosis	1	48
Thyroid adenocarcinoma	1	20
Chondrosarcoma	1	20
Cataracts	1	20
Hypopituitarism	1	20
Urinary tract infection	1	20
Thyroid adenoma	1	18
Total	38	—

Neve et al. (68) reported a high rate of pulmonary function impairment in children receiving TBI as part of their conditioning regimen for ABMT. The impairment was most severe in younger children or those patients requiring more chemotherapy. TBI was fractionated: a total of 12 Gy were given in six fractions over 3 days, with a dose rate of 50 cGy per minute with lung shielding at 10 Gy. TBI also has been associated with poor growth in survivors of neuroblastoma treated with ABMT. Hovi et al. (49) described a series of 31 children, 15 who were treated with high-dose chemotherapy and no TBI and 16 who received TBI of 10 to 12 Gy in five or six fractions over 3 days. After 10 years of follow-up, the height standard deviation score of the TBI group was –2.0 compared to –0.7 to –0.9 for the nonirradiated group. This loss of height may have been related to growth-hormone deficiency. The majority of patients in both groups responded to growth-hormone deficiency with a mean increase in their height standard deviation score of 0.8 at 3 years.

References

1. Beckwith JB, Perrin EV. *In situ* neuroblastomas: a contribution to the natural history of neural crest tumors. *Am J Pathol* 1963;43:1089–1104.
2. Berthold F, Boos J, Burdach S, et al. Myeloablative megatherapy with autologous stem-cell rescue versus oral maintenance chemotherapy as consolidation treatment in patients with high-risk neuroblastoma: a randomised controlled trial. *Lancet Oncol* 2005;6:649–658.
3. Berthold F, Trechow R, Utsch S, et al. Prognostic factors in metastatic neuroblastoma: a multivariate analysis of 182 cases. *Am J Pediatr Hematol Oncol* 1992;14:207–215.
4. Boechat MI, Ortega J, Hoffman AD, et al. Computed tomography in stage III neuroblastoma. *AJR Am J Roentgenol* 1985;145:1283–1287.
5. Bowman LC, Hancock ML, Santana VM, et al. Impact of intensified therapy on clinical outcome in infants and children with neuroblastoma: the St. Jude Children's Research Hospital experience, 1962–1988. *J Clin Oncol* 1991;9:1599–1608.
6. Bray PF, Ziter FA, Lahey ME, et al. The coincidence of neuroblastoma and acute cerebellar encephalopathy. *J Pediatr* 1969;75:983–990.
7. Brodeur G, Castleberry R. Neuroblastoma. In: Pizzo P, Poplack D, eds. *Principles and practice of pediatric oncology.* Philadelphia: J.B. Lippincott, 1993;.
8. Brodeur GM, Seeger RC, Barrett A, et al. International criteria for diagnosis, staging and response to treatment in patients with neuroblastoma. *J Clin Oncol* 1988;6:1874–1881.
9. Brodeur GM, Seeger RC, Schwab M, et al. Amplification of N-*myc* in untreated human neuroblastomas correlates with advanced disease stage. *Science* 1984;224:1121–1124.
10. Carlsen NL, Christensen IJ, Schroeder H, et al. Prognostic factors in neuroblastoma treated in Denmark from 1943 to 1980: a statistical estimate of prognosis based on 253 cases. *Cancer* 1986;58:2726–2735.
11. Caron H, van Sluis P, De Kraker J, et al. Allelic loss of chromosome 1p as a predictor of unfavorable outcome in patients with neuroblastoma. *N Engl J Med* 1996;334:225–230.
12. Castleberry RP, Cantor AB, Green AA, et al. Phase II investigational window using carboplatin, iproplatin, ifosfamide, and epirubicin in children with untreated

disseminated neuroblastoma: a Pediatric Oncology Group study. *J Clin Oncol* 1994;12:1616–1620.
13. Castleberry RP, Kun LE, Shuster JJ, et al. Radiotherapy improves the outlook for patients older than 1 year with Pediatric Oncology Group stage C neuroblastoma. *J Clin Oncol* 1991;9:789–795.
14. Castleberry RP, Shuster JJ, Altshuler G, et al. Infants with neuroblastoma and regional lymph node metastases have a favorable outlook after limited postoperative chemotherapy: a Pediatric Oncology Group study. *J Clin Oncol* 1992;10:1299–1304.
15. Cecchetto G, Luzzatto C, Carli M, et al. The role of surgery in non-localized neuroblastoma. Analysis of 59 cases. *Tumori* 1983;69:327–329.
16. Chatten J, Shimada H, Sather HN, et al. Prognostic value of histopathology in advanced neuroblastoma: a report from the Children's Cancer Study Group. *Human Pathol* 1988;19:11887–1198.
17. Cheung NV, Heller G. Chemotherapy dose intensity correlates strongly with response, median survival, and median progression-free survival in metastatic neuroblastoma (review). *J Clin Oncol* 1991;9:1050–1058.
18. Coldman AJ, Fryer CJH, Elwood JM, et al. Neuroblastoma: influence of age at diagnosis, stage, tumor site, and sex on prognosis. *Cancer* 1980;46:1896–1901.
19. Couanet D, Geoffray A, Hartmann O, et al. Bone marrow metastases in children's neuroblastoma studies by magnetic resonance imaging. *Prog Clin Biol Res* 1988;271:547–555.
20. D'Angio GJ, Evans A. Cyclic low-dose total body irradiation for metastatic neuroblastoma. *Int J Radiat Oncol Biol Phys* 1983;9:1961.
21. de Bernardi B, Rogers D, Carli M, et al. Localized neuroblastoma; surgical and pathologic staging. *Cancer* 1987;60:1066–1072.
22. DeKraker J, Hoefnagel CA, Caron H, et al. First line targeted radiotherapy: a new concept in the treatment of advanced stage neuroblastoma. *Eur J Cancer* 1995;31A:600–602.
23. Eifel PJ. Decreased bone growth arrest in weanling rats with multiple radiation fractions per day. *Int J Radiat Oncol Biol Phys* 1988;15:141–145.
24. Eifel PJ, Sampson CM, Tucker SL. Radiation fractionation sensitivity of epiphyseal cartilage in a weanling rat model. *Int J Radiat Oncol Biol Phys* 1990;19:661–664.
25. Ettinger LJ, Gaynon PS, Krailo MD, et al. A phase II study of carboplatin in children with recurrent or progressive solid tumors. A report from the Children's Cancer Group. *Cancer* 1994;73:1297–1301.
26. Evans AE, Baum E, Chard R. Do infants with stage IV-S neuroblastoma need treatment?. *Arch Dis Child* 1981;56:271–274.
27. Evans AE, Brand W, de Lorimier A, et al. Results in children with local and regional neuroblastoma managed with and without vincristine, cyclophosphamide, and imidazole carboxamide: a report from the Children's Cancer Study Group. *Am J Clin Oncol* 1984;6:3.
28. Evans AE, Chatten J,D'Angio GJ, et al. A review of 17-IV-S neuroblastoma patients at the Children's Hospital of Philadelphia. *Cancer* 1980;45:833–839.
29. Evans AE, D'Angio GJ, Propert K, et al. Prognostic factors in neuroblastoma. *Cancer* 1987;59:1853–1859.
30. Evans AE, D'Angio GJ, Randolph J. A proposed staging for children with neuroblastoma. Children's Cancer Study Group A. *Cancer* 1971;27:374–378.
31. Evans AE, D'Angio GJ, Sather HN, et al. A comparison of four staging systems for localized and regional neuroblastoma: A report from the Children's Cancer Study Group. *J Clin Oncol* 1990;8:678–688.
32. Everson EC, Cole WH. *Spontaneous regression of cancer*. Philadelphia: W.B. Saunders, 1966.
33. Fletcher BD, Kopiwoda SY, Strandjord SE, et al. Abdominal neuroblastoma: magnetic resonance imaging and tissue characterization. *Radiology* 1985;155:699–703.
34. Gaze MN, Wheldon TE, O'Donoghue JA, et al. Multi-modality megatherapy with [131I]*meta*-iodobenzylguanidine, high dose melphalan and total body irradiation with bone marrow rescue: Feasibility study of a new strategy for advanced neuroblastoma. *Eur J Cancer* 1995;31A:252–256.
35. [illegible] High-dose chemoradiotherapy supported by marrow infusions for advanced neuroblastoma: a Pediatric Oncology Group study. [illegible] 1991;[illegible]
36. Grosfeld JL, Baehner RL. Neuroblastoma: an analysis of 160 cases. *World J Surg* 1980;4:29–37.
37. Guglielmi M, DeBernardi B, Rizzo A, et al. Resection of primary tumor at diagnosis in stage IV-S neuroblastoma: Does it affect the clinical course?. *J Clin Oncol* 1996;14:1537–1544.
38. Haas-Kogan DA, Fisch BM, Wara WM, et al. Intraoperative radiation therapy for high-risk pediatric neuroblastoma. *Int J Radiat Oncol Biol Phys* 2000;47:985–992.
39. Haas-Kogan DA, Swift PS, Selch M, et al. Impact of radiotherapy for high-risk neuroblastoma: a Children's Cancer Group study. *Int J Radiat Oncol Biol Phys* 2003;56:28–39.
40. Haase GM, Atkinson JB, Stram DO, et al. Surgical management and outcome of locoregional neuroblastoma: comparison of the Children's Cancer Group and the International Staging Systems. *J Pediatr Surg* 1995;30:289–294.
41. Haase GM, O'Leary MC, Ramsay NKC, et al. Aggressive surgery combined with intensive chemotherapy improves survival in poor-risk neuroblastoma. *J Pediatr Surg* 1991;26:1119–1123.
42. Halperin EC. Hepatic metastasis from neuroblastoma. *South Med J* 1987;80:1370–1373.
43. Halperin EC. Long-term results of therapy for stage C neuroblastoma. *J Surg Oncol Suppl* 1996;63:172–178.
44. Halperin EC, Cox EB. Radiation therapy in the management of neuroblastoma: the Duke University Medical Center experience, 1967–1984. *Int J Radiat Oncol Biol Phys* 1986;12:1829–1837.
45. Handgretinger R, Anderson K, Lang P, et al. A phase I study of human/mouse chimeric antiganglioside GD2 antibody ch14.18 in patients with neuroblastoma. *Eur J Cancer* 1995;31A:261–267.
46. Hayes FA, Green AA. Neuroblastoma. *Pediatr Ann* 1983;12:366–367.
47. Hayes FA, Green AA, Hustu HO, et al: Surgicopathologic staging of neuroblastoma: prognostic significance of regional lymph node metastases. *J Pediatr* 1983;102:59–62.
48. Hayes FA, Thompson EI, Huizdala E, et al. Chemotherapy as an alternative to laminectomy and radiation in the management of epidural tumor. *J Pediatr* 1984;104:221–224.
49. Hovi L, Saarinen-Pihkala UM, Vettenranta K, et al. Growth in children with poor-risk neuroblastoma after regimens with or without total body irradiation in preparation for autologous bone marrow transplantation. *Bone Marrow Transplant* 1999;24:1131–1136.
50. Hug EB, Nevinny-Stickel M, Fuss M, et al. Conformal proton radiation treatment for retroperitoneal neuroblastoma: introduction of a novel technique. *Med Ped Oncol* 2001;37:36–41.
51. Hutchinson RJ, Sisson JC, Shapiro B, et al. 131-I-metaiodobenzylguanidine treatment in patients with refractory advanced neuroblastoma. *Am J Clin Oncol* 1992;15:226–232.
52. Jacobson GM, Sause WT, O'Brien RT. Dose response analysis of pediatric neuroblastoma to megavoltage radiation. *Am J Clin Oncol* 1984;7:693–697.
53. Katzenstein HM, Cohn SL, Shore RM, et al. Scintigraphic response by 123I-metaiodobenzylguanidine scan correlates with event-free survival in high-risk neuroblastoma. *J Clin Oncol* 2004;22:3909–3915.
54. Kun LE, Casper JT, Kline RW, et al. Fractionated total body irradiation for metastatic neuroblastoma. *Int J Radiat Oncol Biol Phys* 1981;7:1599–1602, 1981.
55. Kushner BH, Cheung N-K, LaQuaglia MP, et al. International neuroblastoma staging system stage 1 neuroblastoma: a prospective study and literature review. *J Clin Oncol* 1996;14:2174–2180.
56. La Quaglia MP, Kushner BH, Heller G, et al. Stage 4 neuroblastoma diagnosed at more than 1 year of age: gross total resection and clinical outcome. *J Pediatr Surg* 1994;29:1162–1165.
57. Laprie A, Michon J, Hartmann O, et al. High-dose chemotherapy followed by locoregional irradiation improves the outcome of patients with international neuroblastoma staging system stage II and III neuroblastoma with *MYCN* amplification. *Cancer* 2004;101:1081–1089.
58. Lashford LS, Lewis IJ, Fielding SL, et al. Phase I/II study of iodine 131 metaiodobenzylguanidine in chemoresistant neuroblastoma: a United Kingdom Children's Cancer Study Group investigation. *J Clin Oncol* 1992;10:1889–1896.
59. Look A, Hayes FA, Shuster J, et al. Clinical relevance of tumor cell ploidy and N-*myc* gene amplification in childhood neuroblastoma: a Pediatric Oncology Group study. *J Clin Oncol* 1991;9:581–591.
60. Mastrangelo R, Tornesello A, Riccardi R, et al. A new approach in the treatment of stage IV neuroblastoma using a combination of [131I]meta-iodobenzylguanidine (MIBG) and cisplatin. *Eur J Cancer* 1995;31A:606–611.
61. Matthay KK, Atkinson JB, Stram DO, et al. Patterns of relapse after autologous purged bone marrow transplantation for neuroblastoma: a Children's Cancer Group pilot study. *J Clin Oncol* 1993;11:2226–2233.
62. Matthay KK, Sather HN, Seeger RC, et al. Excellent outcome of stage II neuroblastoma is independent of residual disease and radiation therapy. *J Clin Oncol* 1989;7:236–244.
63. Matthay KK, Villablanca JG, Seeger RC, et al. Treatment of high-risk neuroblastoma with intensive chemotherapy, radiotherapy, autologous bone marrow transplantation, and 13-cis-retinoic acid. Children's Cancer Group. *New Engl J Med* 1999;341:1165–1173.
64. McCowage GB, Vowels MR, Shaw PJ, et al. Autologous bone marrow transplantation for advanced neuroblastoma using teniposide, doxorubicin, melphalan, cisplatin, and total body irradiation. *J Clin Oncol* 1995;13:2789–2795.
65. Michalski JM, Ratheesan K, Grigsby PW. *Neuroblastoma: treatment and patient factors influencing local tumor control by radiotherapy. Proceedings of the American Radium Society 7th Annual Meeting*. 1995.
66. Moertel CL, Reubi JC, Scheithaur BS. Expression of somatostatin receptors in childhood neuroblastoma. *Am J Clin Pathol* 1994;102:752–756.
67. Murphy SB, Cohn SL, Craft AW, et al. Do children benefit from mass screening for neuroblastoma?: consensus statement from the American Cancer Society Workshop on Neuroblastoma Screening. *Lancet* 1991;337:344–346.
68. Neve V, Foot AB, Michon J, et al. Longitudinal clinical and functional pulmonary follow-up after megatherapy, fractionated total body irradiation, and autologous bone marrow transplantation for metastatic neuroblastoma. *Med Pediatr Oncol* 1999;32:170–176.
69. Nickerson HJ, Nesbit ME, Grosfeld JL, et al. Comparison of stage IV and IV-S neuroblastoma in the first year of life. *Med Pediatr Oncol* 1985;13:261–268.
70. Ninane J, Wese FX. Treatment of localized neuroblastoma. *Am J Pediatr Hematol Oncol* [illegible]
71. Nitschke R, Smith EI, Altshuler G, et al. Postoperative treatment of nonmetastatic visible residual neuroblastoma: a Pediatric Oncology Group study. *J Clin Oncol* 1991;9:1181–1188.
72. Nitschke R, Smith EI, Shochat S, et al. Localized neuroblastoma treated by surgery: a Pediatric Oncology Group study. *J Clin Oncol* 1988;6:1271–1279.
73. Norris MD, Bordow SB, Marshall GM, et al. Expression of the gene for multidrug-resistance-associated protein and outcome in patients with neuroblastoma. *N Engl J Med* 1996;334:231–238.
74. O'dorisio MS, Hauger M, Cecalupo AJ. Somatostatin receptors in neuroblastoma: diagnosis and therapeutic implications. *Semin Oncol* 1994;21:33–37.
75. O'Neill JA, Littman P, Blitzer P, et al. The role of surgery in localized neuroblastoma. *J Pediatr Surg* 1985;20:708–712.
76. Oertel S, Niethammer AG, Krempien R, et al. Combination of external-beam radiotherapy with intraoperative electron-beam therapy is effective in incompletely resected pediatric malignancies. *Int J Radiat Oncol Biol Phys* 2006;64:235–241.
77. Paul SR, Tarbell NJ, Korf B, et al. Stage IV neuroblastoma in infants: long-term survival. *Cancer* 1991;67:1493–1497.
78. Paulino AC, Ferenci MS, Chiang KY, et al. Comparison of conventional to intensity modulated radiation therapy for abdominal neuroblastoma. *Pediatr Blood Cancer* 2006;46:739–744.
79. Perez CA, Matthay KK, Atkinson JB, et al. Biologic variables in the outcome of stages I and II neuroblastoma treated with surgery as primary therapy: a Children's Cancer Group study. *J Clin Oncol* 2000;18:18–26.
80. Petrus LV, Hall TR, Boechat MI, et al. The pediatric patient with suspected adrenal neoplasm: which radiological test to use? *Med Pediatr Oncol* 1992;20:53–57.
81. Philip T, Gentet JC, Carrie C, et al. Phase II studies of combinations of drugs with high dose carboplatin in neuroblastoma (800 mg/m^2 to 1 g 250/m^2): a report from the LMCE group. *Prog Clin Biol Res* 1988;271:573–582.
82. Philip T, Zucker JM, Bernard JL, et al. Improved survival at 2 and 5 years in the LMCE1 unselected group of 72 children with stage IV neuroblastoma older than 1 year of age at diagnosis: is cure possible in a small subgroup? *J Clin Oncol* 1991;9:1037–1044.
83. Pinkerton CR. ENSG 1-randomized study of high-dose melphalan in neuroblastoma. *Bone Marrow Transplant* 1991;7:112–113.

84. Plantaz D, Rubie H, Michon J, et al. The treatment of neuroblastoma with intraspinal extension with chemotherapy followed by surgical removal of residual disease. *Cancer* 1996;78:311–319.
85. Pranzatelli MR. The neurobiology of the opsoclonus-myoclonus syndrome. *Clin Neuropharmacol* 1992;19:1–47.
86. Pritchard J, Cotterill SJ, Germond SM, et al. High dose melphalan in the treatment of advanced neuroblastoma: results of a randomised trial (ENSG-1) by the European Neuroblastoma Study Group. *Pediatr Blood Cancer* 2005;44:348–357.
87. Reynolds CP, Kane DJ, Einhorn PA, et al. Response of neuroblastoma to retinoic acid in vitro and in vivo. *Prog Clin Biol Med* 1991;366:203–211.
88. Rosen EM, Cassady JR, Frantz CN, et al. Neuroblastoma: the Joint Center for Radiation Therapy/Dana Farber Cancer Institute/Children's Hospital experience. *J Clin Oncol* 1984;2:719–732.
89. Schilling FH, Berthold F, Erttmann R, et al. Population-based and controlled study to evaluate neuroblastoma screening at one year of age in Germany: interim results. *Med Ped Oncol* 2000;35:701–704.
90. Schilling FH, Spix C, Berthold F, et al. Neuroblastoma screening at one year of age. *N Engl J Med* 2002;346:1047–1053.
91. Schulz G, Cheresh DA, Varki NM, et al. Detection of ganglioside GD2 in tumor tissues and sera of neuroblastoma patients. *Cancer Res* 1984;44:5914–5920.
92. Seeger RC, Brodeur GM, Sather H, et al. Association of multiple copies of the N-*myc* oncogene with rapid progression of neuroblastomas. *N Engl J Med* 1985;313:1111–1116.
93. Seeger RC, Villablanca JG, Matthay KK, et al. Intensive chemoradiotherapy and autologous bone marrow transplantation for poor prognosis neuroblastoma. *Prog Clin Biol Res* 1991;366:527–533.
94. Shapiro B. Imaging of catecholamine-secreting tumors: uses of MIBG in diagnosis and treatment. *Ballieres Clin Endocrinol Metab* 1993;7:491–507.
95. Shimada H, Chatten J, Newton WA, et al. Histopathologic prognostic factors in neuroblastic tumors: definition of subtypes of ganglioneuroblastoma and an age-linked classification of neuroblastomas. *J Natl Cancer Inst* 1984;73:405–416.
96. Shorter NA, Davidoff AM, Evans AE, et al. The role of surgery in the management of stage IV neuroblastoma: a single institution study. *Med Pediatr Oncol* 1995;24:287–291.
97. Shuster J, McWilliams N, Castleberry R, et al. Serum lactate dehydrogenase in childhood neuroblastoma: a Pediatric Oncology Group recursive partitioning study. *Am J Clin Oncol* 1992;15:295–303.
98. Sibley GS, Mundt AJ, Goldman S, et al. Patterns of failure following total body irradiation and bone marrow transplantation with or without a radiotherapy boost for advanced neuroblastoma. *Int J Radiat Oncol Biol Phys* 1995;32:1127–1135.
99. Siegel M. RDOG for pediatric solid tumors. National Institute of Health NIH Grant No. 51001CA59403.
100. Siegel M, Jamroz GA, Glazer HS, et al. MR imaging of intraspinal extension of neuroblastoma. *J Comput Assist Tomogr* 1986;10:593–595.
101. Siegel MJ, Ishwaran H, Fletcher BD, et al. Staging of neuroblastoma by imaging: report of the Radiology Diagnostic Oncology Group. *Radiology* 2002;223:168–175.
102. Simone JV. The treatment of neuroblastoma. *J Clin Oncol* 1984;2:717–718.
103. Stram DO, Matthay KK, O'Leary M, et al. Consolidation chemoradiotherapy and autologous bone marrow transplantation versus continued chemotherapy for metastatic neuroblastoma: a report of two concurrent Children's Cancer Group studies. *J Clin Oncol* 1996;14:2417–2426.
104. Strother D, Shuster JJ, McWilliams N, et al. Results of Pediatric Oncology Group 8104 for infants with stages D and DS neuroblastoma. *J Pediatr Hematol Oncol* 1995;17:254–259.
105. Thomas PR, Griffith KD, Fineberg BB, et al. Late effects of treatment for Wilms' tumor. *Int J Radiat Oncol Biol Phys* 1983;9:651–657.
106. Turba E, Fagioli G, Mancini AF, et al. Evaluation of stage 4 neuroblastoma patients by means of MIBG and 99mTc-MDP scintigraphy. *J Nucl Biol Med* 1993;37:107–114.
107. Wallace WH, Shalet SM. Chemotherapy with actinomycin D influences the growth of the spine following abdominal irradiation. *Med Pediatr Oncol* 1992;20:177.
108. Wallace WHB, Shalet SM, Morris-Jones PH, et al. Effect of abdominal irradiation on growth in boys treated for a Wilms' tumor. *Med Pediatr Oncol* 1990;18:441–446.
109. Wheldon TE, Wilson L, Livingstone A, et al. Radiation studies on multicellular tumor spheroids derived from human neuroblastoma: absence of sparing effect of dose fractionation. *Eur J Cancer Clin Oncol* 1986;22:563–566.
110. Willis RA. *The pathology of tumors in children*. Springfield, IL: Charles C. Thomas, 1962.
111. Wolden SL, Gollamudi SV, Kushner BH, et al. Local control with multimodality therapy for stage 4 neuroblastoma. *Int J Radiat Oncol Biol Phys* 2000;46:969–974.
112. Woods WG, Gao RN, Shuster JJ, et al. Screening of infants and mortality due to neuroblastoma. *N Engl J Med* 2002;346:1041–1046.
113. Woods WG, Tuchman M, Bernstein ML, et al. Screening for neuroblastoma in North America: 2-year results from the Quebec Project. *Am J Pediatr Hematol Oncol* 1992;14:312–319.
114. Yamamoto K, Hayaski Y, Hanada R, et al. Mass screening and age-specific incidence of neuroblastoma in Suitama Prefecture, Japan. *J Clin Oncol* 1995;13:2033–2038.
115. Yamamoto K, Ohta S, Ito E, et al. Marginal decrease in mortality and marked increase in incidence as a result of neuroblastoma screening at 6 months of age: cohort study in seven prefectures in Japan. *J Clin Oncol* 2002;20:1209–214.
116. Yanik GA, Levine JE, Matthay KK, et al. Pilot study of iodine-131-metaiodobenzylguanidine in combination with myeloablative chemotherapy and autologous stem-cell support for the treatment of neuroblastoma. *J Clin Oncol* 2002;20:2142–2149.
117. Yu AL, Uttenreuther-Fischer MM, Huang CS, et al. Phase I trial of a human-mouse chimeric anti-disialoganglioside monoclonal antibody ch14.18 in patients with refractory neuroblastoma and osteosarcoma. *J Clin Oncol* 1998;16:2169–2180.
118. Zachariou Z, Sieverts H, Eble MJ, et al. IORT (intraoperative radiotherapy) in neuroblastoma: experience and first results. *Eur J Pediatr Surg* 2002;12:251–254.

Clinical Radiation Oncology

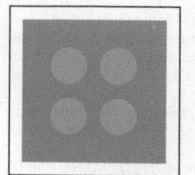

Chapter 85
Rhabdomyosarcoma

John C. Breneman, Sarah S. Donaldson

:: | Anatomy

Rhabdomyosarcoma is a highly malignant soft tissue sarcoma that arises from unsegmented, undifferentiated mesoderm or myotome-derived skeletal muscle. It may occur at any site in the body, but the most frequently involved sites are the orbit, 9%; head and neck (excluding parameningeal tumors), 7%; parameningeal, 25%; genitourinary 31%; extremity, 13%; trunk, 5%; retroperitoneum, 7%, and other sites 3% (24).

:: | Epidemiology and Risk Factors

Rhabdomyosarcoma is the most common of the childhood soft tissue sarcomas, with an annual incidence of 4.4 per 1 million whites and 1.3 per 1 million blacks. The male-to-female ratio is ~1.5:1. Gender does not appear to carry prognostic significance.

Diagnosis is most common in the childhood and adolescent years, with two peak age frequencies, at ages 2 to 6 and in adolescence. The great majority of patients are <10 years of age at the time of diagnosis, and approximately 5% are infants, <1 year of age. Tumors in this younger age group are likely to be of embryonal histology (or one of its subtypes). About 25% of patients are ≥10 years at diagnosis and their tumors are more commonly of alveolar histology. Age has been identified as an independent predictor of prognosis, with children <1 year and >10 years having inferior survival (51). Adults with rhabdomyosarcoma have been reported to have poor outcomes, although there is evidence that when treated aggressively using pediatric-type protocols, the prognosis may be similar to that of younger patients (36).

The cause of rhabdomyosarcoma is unknown, however, it is associated with disorders in development, including central nervous system, genitourinary, gastrointestinal, and cardiovascular anomalies. Rhabdomyosarcoma has been reported in association with several congenital disorders, including congenital pulmonary cysts, Gorlin's basal cell nevus syndrome, and neurofibromatosis.

Groups of families have been described in which relatives of children with rhabdomyosarcoma have an increased frequency of breast cancer. The relative risk of breast cancer was 3.74 among a cohort of 177 mothers of children with embryonal rhabdomyosarcoma (12). Multiple tumors can occur in siblings and relatives of children with rhabdomyosarcoma, including adrenocortical carcinoma, brain tumors (particularly glioblastoma), lung cancer, breast cancer, and other sarcomas. This occurrence is termed the *Li-Fraumeni syndrome*.

Recent developments in cytogenetics and molecular genetics now provide a more comprehensive understanding of the origin and biologic behavior of rhabdomyosarcoma. These are discussed in more detail later.

:: | Natural History and Patterns of Spread

There are unexplained associations of site of primary tumor with age at diagnosis and tumor histology. For example, tumors arising in the urinary bladder and vagina occur primarily in infants and often are of the embryonal or botryoid histologic type. Tumors arising in the trunk and extremity occur in adolescents and are often alveolar or undifferentiated type. Tumors of the head and neck area occur throughout childhood and are commonly of the embryonal type.

Rhabdomyosarcoma, a locally invasive tumor often with a pseudocapsule, has the potential for local spread along fascial or muscle planes, lymphatic extension, and hematogenous dissemination. The overall risk of regional lymphatic spread is approximately 15%, but varies with the site of the primary lesion. Lymph node metastases are rare in orbital tumors, but they occur in approximately 15% of tumors at other head and neck sites, most commonly the nasopharynx. Accounting for staging inaccuracies, regional lymph node extension occurs in approximately 25% of children with paratesticular tumors and in 20% of patients with extremity and truncal tumors. The risk for lymph node involvement also correlates with primary tumor invasiveness and large tumor size.

Hematogenous metastases are detected at the time of presentation in approximately 15% of patients, particularly those with truncal and extremity primary tumors. The most common sites of hematogenous dissemination are lungs, bone marrow, and bone. Malignant pleural and peritoneal effusions may also accompany tumors primary to the chest and abdomen/pelvis, respectively (18).

:: | Clinical Presentation

Because rhabdomyosarcoma occurs in multiple primary sites, there are many site-specific clinical signs and symptoms. It usually presents, however, as an asymptomatic mass. When symptoms are present, they relate to mass effect on associated organs and tissues. Tumors of the orbit may cause proptosis and ophthalmoplegia. Patients with parameningeal tumors often present with nasal, aural, or sinus obstruction, cranial nerve palsy, and headache. Genitourinary tumors may cause hematuria, urinary obstruction, or constipation.

:: | Diagnostic Work-Up

Determination of tumor extent is best done with a multidisciplinary approach by a radiation oncologist, pediatric oncologist, and appropriate subspecialty surgeon. An expeditious local and systemic work-up is essential because these tumors have the potential to grow rapidly. Early experience with positron emission tomography scanning indicates this modality may also be a valuable component of staging (66). Some children whose tumors exhibit characteristic fusion transcripts can be shown to have micrometastatic disease using reverse-transcriptase polymerase chain reaction techniques, even when there is no evidence of metastases from routine diagnostic procedures. The clinical significance of this is, however, unknown (52). The initial assessment by all members of the team permits accurate staging and the formation of a uniform treatment plan.

Table 85.1	RECOMMENDED WORK-UP FOR TUMORS AT VARIOUS SITES	

All Patients	Optional
All sites	
History	
Physical examination by several observers	Examination under anesthesia for infants and youngsters
Laboratory studies	Plain films of bones abnormal on scans
Complete blood count	
Liver function tests	Abdomen-pelvis CT, MRI, or ultrasound
Renal function tests	
Urinalysis	
Imaging studies	
Chest radiograph	
Thoracic CT scan	
Bone scan	
MRI or CT of primary tumor	
Bone marrow biopsy and aspirate	
PET scan (investigational)	
Head and neck	
MRI or CT of primary tumor (with contrast)	Plain films of area
	Dental films
Lumbar puncture with cytologic examination of fluid in parameningeal primary tumors	Paranasal sinus and skull films
	MRI of spine if cerebrospinal fluid is positive or patient is symptomatic
Genitourinary	
CT of MRI of abdomen-pelvis (with contrast)	Ultrasound of pelvis
	Cystoscopy
Pelvic examination under anesthesia	
Extremity and truncal lesions	
MRI or CT of primary lesion (with contrast)	Plain films of primary site
	Ultrasound
	Barium gastrointestinal contrast studies

CT, computed tomography; MRI, magnetic resonance imaging; PET, positron emission tomography.

Table 85.1 provides recommendation for diagnostic work-up at various sites.

Staging Systems

The clinical grouping classification used extensively by the Intergroup Rhabdomyosarcoma Study Group (now known as the Soft Tissue Sarcoma Committee of the Children's Oncology Group) investigators is somewhat of a misnomer because it actually requires surgical-pathologic evaluation (Table 85.2). This system does not accurately reflect the biology of the disease; rather, it is affected by the surgical procedure selected for an individual patient. A more valid pretreatment staging system uses a TNM (tumor-node-metastasis) approach, which emphasizes characteristics of the primary tumor, size and invasiveness, nodal status, and systemic spread. Noninvasiveness, small size, and absence of metastases have been shown to influence prognosis (58,76). The site of primary tumor also has a significant impact on survival (26,58,87). The Intergroup Rhabdomyosarcoma Study (IRS) IV has prospectively demonstrated the validity of a staging system incorporating TNM classification along with primary tumor site (Table 85.3). Three-year failure-free survival was 86% for stage 1 tumors, 80% for stage 2, 68% for stage 3, and 25% for stage 4 (18,24). Of note, the clinical grouping did not correlate as well with survival. In fact, failure-free survival for clinical group II patients was superior to clinical group I (86%

Table 85.2	INTERGROUP RHABDOMYOSARCOMA STUDY CLINICAL GROUPING CLASSIFICATION	

Group I	Localized disease, completely resected
A	Confined to organ or muscle of origin
B	Infiltration outside organ or muscle of origin; regional nodes not involved
Group II	Compromised or regional resection
A	Grossly resected tumor with microscopic residual disease
B	Regional disease, completely resected, in which nodes may be involved or extension of tumor into adjacent organ may exist
C	Regional disease with involved nodes, grossly resected, but with evidence of microscopic residual disease
Group III	Incomplete resection or biopsy with gross residual disease
Group IV	Distant metastases at diagnosis

Mauer HM. The Intergroup Rhabdomyosarcoma Study: objectives and clinical staging classification. *J Pediatr Surg* 1980;15:371–372.

vs. 83%), probably reflecting the routine use of radiotherapy for group II patients.

Pathologic Classification

The histogenesis of rhabdomyosarcoma can be traced from mesoderm to mesenchyme and ultimately to striated muscle tissue. The classic classification of rhabdomyosarcoma used by the IRS investigators consists of four histologic subtypes: embryonal, botryoid subtype of embryonal, alveolar, and pleomorphic. Other variants including a "solid" alveolar pattern, considered a subtype of alveolar rhabdomyosarcoma, a spindle cell subtype of embryonal rhabdomyosarcoma, and a diffuse anaplastic variant have also been described (79,108). To improve reproducibility of pathologic subtyping and prognostic utility, pediatric pathologists developed a classification system: the International Classification of Rhabdomyosarcoma. This system is based on a review of IRS-II data. It groups pathologic subtypes into distinct prognostic groups (Table 85.4). The International Classification of Rhabdomyosarcoma system appears to be predictive of outcome and has been reproduced by several reference pediatric pathologists (6,79). The superior-prognosis group, made up of two subsets (botryoid and spindle cell), carries a projected 5-year survival rate of 88% to 95% (6). The botryoid subtype, a polypoid variant of embryonal rhabdomyosarcoma, has a grapelike appearance. The stroma consists of loose cellular tissue with a myxoid appearance. Under the superficial stroma is a condensed tumor cell or cambium layer of Nicholson. The botryoid tumors are usually noninvasive and localized and occur in mucosal-lined organs such as the vagina, urinary bladder, middle ear, biliary tree, and nasopharynx.

The spindle cell subtype of embryonal rhabdomyosarcoma has a spindled appearance, often with a storiform pattern. It is frequently found in paratesticular sites (19,59).

Patients with embryonal rhabdomyosarcoma have intermediate outcome, with an 83% failure-free survival at 3 years (24). The embryonal type consists of blastemal mesenchymal cells that tend to differentiate into cross-striated muscle cells. There is often a considerable variation in degree of cytoplasmic development, ranging from primitive mesenchymal to highly differentiated muscle tumor cells. Most of the tumor cells have eosinophilic cytoplasm, which is positive by periodic acid-Schiff staining. Immunohistochemistry may demonstrate actin- or desmin-positive reactions. Ultrastructural studies exhibit evidence of myogenesis with the presence of thick and thin cytoplasmic intermediate filaments or Z-band material. Ribbon or strap-shaped cells and tadpole cells are characteristic. The

Table 85.3	INTERGROUP RHABDOMYOSARCOMA STUDY IRS PRETREATMENT STAGING SYSTEM[a]				
Stage	Site[b]	Invasiveness	Size	Nodal Status	Metastases
I	Favorable	T1 or T2	a or b	N0 or N1	M0
II	Unfavorable	T1 or T2	a	N0	M0
III	Unfavorable	T1 or T2	b	N0	M0
			a or b	N1	M0
IV	Any site		T1 or T2	N0 or N1	M1

[a]T1, tumor confined to site or organ of origin; T2, regional extension beyond the site or organ of origin; a, ≤5 cm; b, >5 cm; N0, no evidence of regional node involvement; N1, evidence of regional node involvement (enlargement of nodes on radiographic imaging is considered evidence of involvement, although histologic confirmation is recommended when possible); M0, no distant metastasis; M1, evidence of distant metastasis.
[b]Favorable sites: orbit, head and neck (nonparameningeal), genitourinary (non–bladder-prostate); unfavorable sites: genitourinary (bladder-prostate), extremity, parameningeal, other.

presence of cross-striations confirms the diagnosis. The embryonal form may be distinguished from the other subtypes by specific structural abnormalities. A consistent loss of heterozygosity at the chromosome 11p15.5 locus suggests that this site is specific for the embryonal subtype (74) although, unlike alveolar histology, no characteristic translocation has been identified. Immunohistochemical presence of epidermal growth factor receptor and fibrillin-2 appears to be highly specific for this subtype, and is predictive of a favorable outcome (112). The embryonal histology occurs in 60% of cases and is found most commonly in the orbit, head and neck, and genitourinary sites.

The group with poor prognosis includes alveolar, diffuse anaplastic, and undifferentiated sarcomas. With routine use of immunohistochemistry and molecular genetic analysis, 40% of rhabdomyosarcomas are now classified as alveolar; it is most commonly found in adolescents with truncal, retroperitoneal, and extremity tumors. The alveolar subtype is characterized by a pseudoalveolar pattern of connective tissue trabeculae, lined by large rhabdomyoblasts and multinucleated giant cells. The "solid" variant of alveolar rhabdomyosarcoma grows as solid nests of closely aggregated tumor cells with less alveolar pattern. Alveolar histology is strongly associated with hyperdiploid content (95). Approximately 80% of children with alveolar rhabdomyosarcoma exhibit a characteristic translocation involving chromosomes 2 and 13, t(2,13)(q35,q14), and occasionally a 1,13 translocation (74,97,100,114). These translocations correspond to abnormal fusion genes involving PAX3-FKHR and PAX7-FKHR, respectively, and are probably the initial oncogenic events in these tumors (93,110). Immunohistochemical presence of AP2-beta and P-cadherin is also highly specific for alveolar histology (112). The projected 3-year failure-free survival for children with the alveolar subtype is 66% (24).

Undifferentiated sarcoma is largely a diagnosis of exclusion; it consists of a diffuse cell population of primitive, noncommitted mesenchymal cells. The 3-year failure-free survival rate of patients with undifferentiated sarcoma is 55% (24).

The pleomorphic type is extremely rare; many cases formerly classified as pleomorphic rhabdomyosarcoma are currently considered to be malignant fibrous histiocytoma.

Previously, tumors classified as extraosseous Ewing sarcoma were treated using guidelines for rhabdomyosarcoma. These are now believed to be more appropriately considered in the Ewing family of tumors and are managed as such.

Prognostic Factors and Therapeutic Considerations

Because rhabdomyosarcoma is protean in presentation, factors such as age, site, stage, extent of disease, and pathologic characteristics of the tumor influence therapeutic decisions. These prognostic factors are interrelated and are best discussed as a function of the specific site (Fig. 85.1). Although most treatment failures occur within 3 years of diagnosis, about 10% of children who are free of disease at 5 years will subsequently experience disease recurrence (102).

Orbit

The orbit has long been recognized as a favorable prognostic site. In addition to prompt recognition of the tumor, the paucity of lymphatics in this area means that lymphatic extension is rare. Most tumors in this site have embryonal histology, and hematogenous metastasis at the time of diagnosis is uncommon. Approximately 10% are alveolar histology, however, and the prognosis for these children is more guarded (53).

When treatment for orbital tumors is individualized, it is generally agreed that no surgical procedure should be used that may compromise vision. In most patients, this means that biopsy only should be performed to provide the diagnosis. Primary treatment usually consists of vincristine, actinomycin D, and Cytoxan (VAC) chemotherapy with local radiotherapy beginning between the 3rd and 12th week of treatment. Radiation doses of approximately 50 Gy are often used, although early results from the IRS-V study suggest that 45 Gy may be sufficient (113). Using this approach, cure rates of >90% can be achieved (25,26,115). Chemotherapy without irradiation has resulted in local relapse and inferior event-free survival (89). Although salvage radiotherapy for these patients can still be curative, functional vision in this setting is often poor (70). Orbital exenteration should be reserved for salvage treatment and enucleation for management of post-treatment ocular complications.

Historically, when radiation therapy alone was used, the entire orbit was considered to be at risk, and it was recommended that the entire orbit be included in the treated volume. However,

Table 85.4	INTERNATIONAL CLASSIFICATION OF RHABDOMYOSARCOMA

I. Superior prognosis
  a. Botryoid rhabdomyosarcoma
  b. Spindle cell rhabdomyosarcoma
II. Intermediate prognosis
  a. Embryonal rhabdomyosarcoma
III. Poor prognosis
  a. Alveolar rhabdomyosarcoma
  b. Undifferentiated sarcoma
  c. Anaplastic rhabdomyosarcoma
IV. Subtypes whose prognosis is not presently evaluable
  a. Rhabdomyosarcoma with rhabdoid features

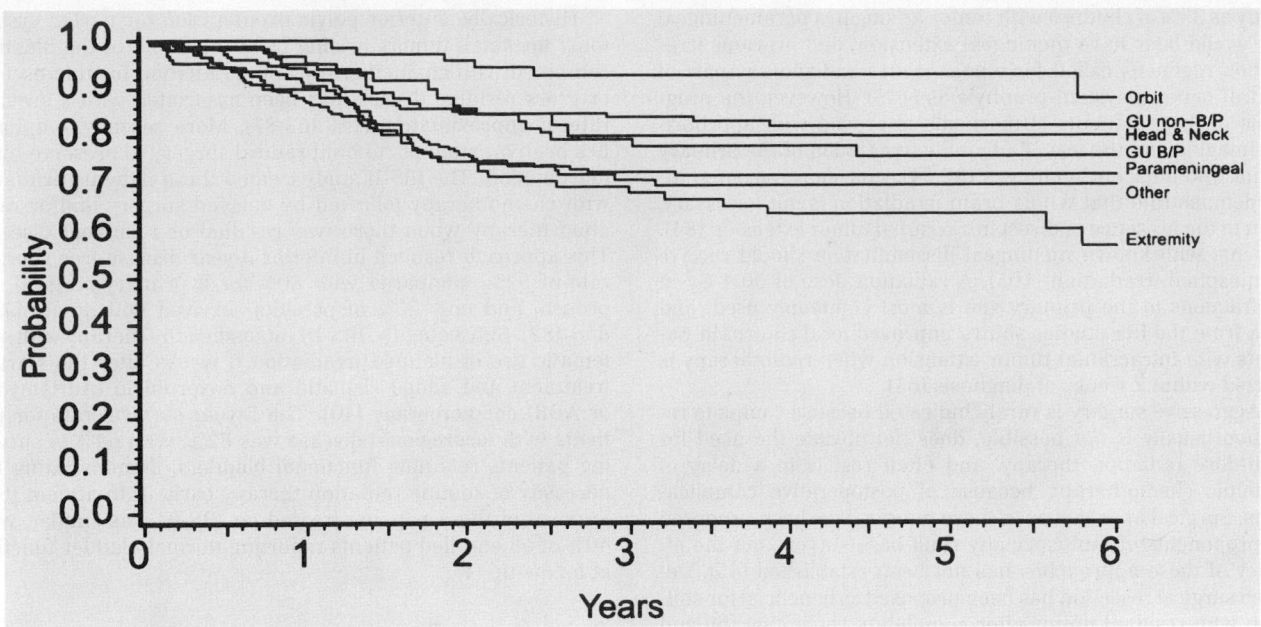

FIGURE 85.1. Survival curves for 883 children with nonmetastatic disease entered onto the Fourth Intergroup Rhabdomyosarcoma Study are shown by anatomic site of the primary tumor. GU, genitourinary; B/P, bladder-prostate. (Redrawn from Crist WM, Anderson JR, Meza JL, et al. The Intergroup Rhabdomyosarcoma Study-IV: results for patients with non-metastatic disease. *J Clin Oncol* 2001;19:3091–3102, with permission.)

with a combined-modality approach, radiotherapy can be directed to the tumor plus a margin without necessarily irradiating the entire orbit. Technique is very important for minimizing corneal and lacrimal gland dose and for preserving useful vision in the treated eye. Photon irradiation with the eyelid open minimizes corneal dose when an anterior field is used and may be associated with improved long-term functional outcome (90). Techniques using beam-shaping devices and corneal and lens protection are also of benefit (Figs. 85.2 and 85.3). Three-dimensional conformal or intensity-modulated radiotherapy technique is optimal for treating the target volume and sparing normal structures, and proton radiation has also been used successfully (127).

Head and Neck: Parameningeal Sites

Nonorbital rhabdomyosarcomas of the head and neck are grouped into parameningeal sites (nasopharynx, nasal cavity, paranasal sinuses, middle ear, pterygopalatine fossa, and infratemporal fossa) and nonparameningeal sites based on differences in natural history, treatment, and prognosis. Parameningeal rhabdomyosarcomas represent the majority of nonorbital head and neck rhabdomyosarcomas and radiotherapy is essential for maximizing the chance of cure (10,26,64). These tumors have a propensity for invading the base of the skull, creating a potential for cranial nerve palsy and direct extension into the central nervous system, a pattern of spread that is seen in as many as 41% of these patients (65). Historically, as

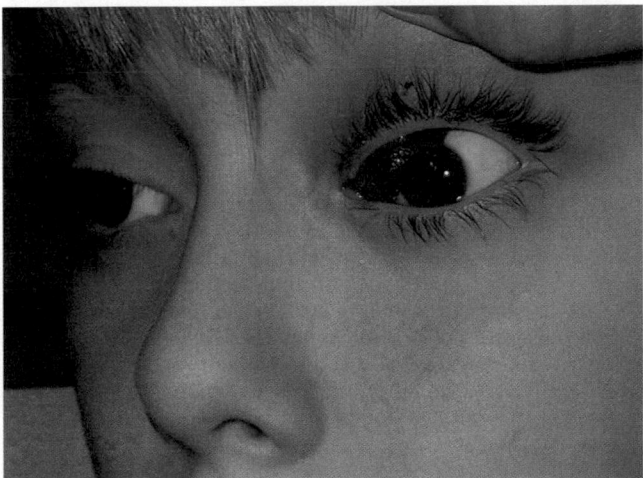

FIGURE 85.2. A 7-year-old girl with an embryonal rhabdomyosarcoma involving the orbit and eyelid. The child had a 3-week history of a lesion obstructing vision without any associated discomfort.

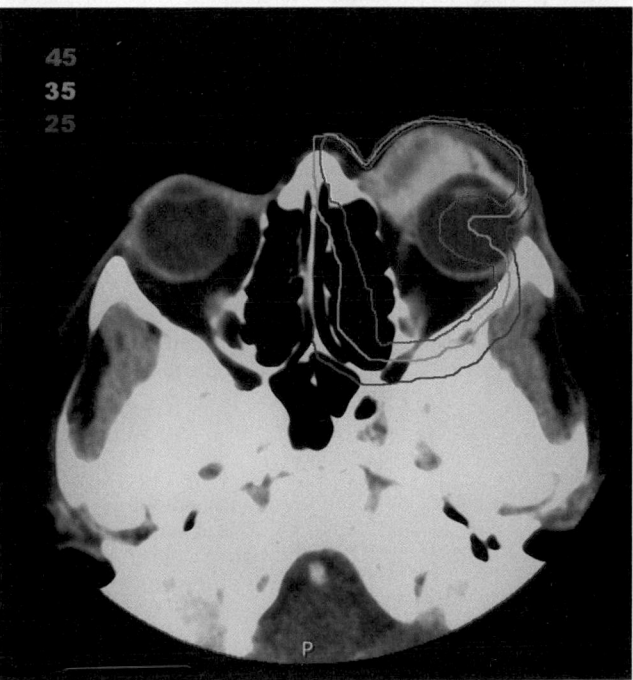

FIGURE 85.3. Isodose distribution from the treatment of the child in Figure 85.2 (doses in Gy). The technique of intensity-modulated radiotherapy was used to shape the radiation dose distribution around the globe, excluding much of the lens and retina. Five years following treatment, she is free of disease with intact vision.

many as 35% of children with tumor arising in a parameningeal site would later have meningeal extension, and previous irradiation regimens called for whole-brain irradiation as part of central nervous system prophylaxis (105). However, the prognosis of these patients is markedly improved with appropriate imaging and the use of adequate irradiation of the primary tumor and adjacent meninges (37,84), and more recent studies demonstrate that whole-brain irradiation is not necessary, even in the presence of direct intracranial tumor extension (84). Patients with known meningeal dissemination should receive craniospinal irradiation (105). A radiation dose of 50.4 Gy in 28 fractions to the primary site is most commonly used, and data from the IRS studies shows improved local control in patients with intracranial tumor extension when radiotherapy is started within 2 weeks of diagnosis (65).

Aggressive surgery is rarely indicated because complete resection usually is not possible, does not obviate the need for high-dose radiation therapy, and often results in a delay of systemic chemotherapy because of postoperative complications. Surgical approaches to these tumors have been proposed by proponents of multispecialty skull-base surgery but the efficacy of these approaches has not been established (45). Delayed surgical resection has been proposed as beneficial for children with residual tumor after completing chemotherapy and radiotherapy (13). The role of postradiation surgical resection is being investigated in select intermediate-risk patients enrolled onto IRS-V.

Five-year survival for patients with parameningeal rhabdomyosarcoma patients is approximately 75% with adequate radiotherapy (10). For the subset of parameningeal tumors arising in the nasopharynx/nasal cavity, middle ear and parapharyngeal locations, survival may be even higher (84).

Head and Neck: Non-Parameningeal Sites

Children with tumors in nonparameningeal head and neck sites tend to have a better outcome than their parameningeal counterparts (80% 5-year failure-free survival in IRS-IV) and require less-intensive chemotherapy (24,26). These sites include the scalp, parotid, oral cavity, larynx, oropharynx, and cheek. These tumors may be more amenable to complete gross surgical excision than their parameningeal counterparts. Approximately 15% of these patients present with regional lymph node metastases. Radiotherapeutic management is based on the amount of residual tumor after surgery. Draining regional lymph nodes are not routinely irradiated unless they contain metastatic tumor.

Pelvis

Pelvic tumors usually are divided into anatomic subgroups because the natural history, treatment, and prognosis are different for each site. Some children present with locally advanced pelvic tumors for which an exact site of origin cannot be determined. These large tumors are associated with an unfavorable prognosis (81).

Bladder and Prostate Tumors

Bladder and prostate primary tumors account for about half of all pelvic rhabdomyosarcomas (64); 75% of patients are age <5 years at presentation, and there is a strong male predominance. More than 90% of these tumors are of the embryonal histologic subtype, with approximately one-third having a botryoid morphology. In boys, it is often difficult to differentiate a tumor of prostatic origin from one of bladder origin because disease usually involves both structures. However, patients with tumors arising in the prostate have significantly inferior survival than those with tumor confined to the bladder (57).

Historically, anterior pelvic exenteration (or partial cystectomy for small tumors arising from the dome of the bladder) combined with chemotherapy and irradiation for microscopic or gross residual disease has been associated with a survival rate of approximately 70% (63,87). More recently, emphasis has been on attempts to limit radical surgery to preserve bladder function. The IRS-II study treated these patients primarily with chemotherapy followed by delayed surgery and/or radiation therapy when there was residual or recurrent disease. This approach resulted in inferior 3-year disease-free survival rate of 52%, compared with 80% for a primary surgical approach, and only 22% of patients survived with intact bladders (82). Subsequently, IRS-III intensified the therapy with systematic use of planned irradiation 6 weeks after the start of treatment and added cisplatin and doxorubicin (Adriamycin, or ADR) chemotherapy (40). The 5-year survival rate for patients with locoregional disease was 82%, with 64% of surviving patients retaining functional bladders, demonstrating the necessity of routine radiation therapy early in treatment (60). Survival of these patients treated on IRS-IV was similar, with 40% of all enrolled patients reporting normal bladder function at follow-up (4).

Paratesticular Tumors

Paratesticular tumors represent approximately 7% of all rhabdomyosarcomas and may arise anywhere along the spermatic cord, from the intrascrotal area through the inguinal canal (119). At presentation, the tumor usually is a painless scrotal or inguinal mass that does not transilluminate. Most boys with paratesticular rhabdomyosarcoma present with early-stage disease that is amenable to complete resection and is associated with cure rates approaching 90%. As with prostatic primary tumors, the lymphatic network is rich, draining directly to the retroperitoneal nodes along the external iliac and spermatic vessels, the aorta, and the vena cava. The incidence of retroperitoneal lymph node involvement varies with the age of the patient and method of staging (surgical vs. nonsurgical). In the IRS-III study, retroperitoneal lymph node sampling was done in most patients, showing a 14% incidence of node involvement for children <10 years of age, and a 47% incidence for those ≥10 years. In IRS-IV, thin-cut computerized tomography without surgical sampling was used for staging, and the incidence of detected nodes dropped to 4% and 13% for the two age groups, respectively (119).

The recommended surgical procedure for the primary tumor is inguinal orchiectomy. If there is no evidence of invasion into the scrotum and the proximal spermatic cord is free of tumor, this procedure is considered equivalent to an amputation, and no further local therapy is necessary. Surgical staging of retroperitoneal lymph nodes is controversial (71,119). European investigators do not recommend retroperitoneal lymph node sampling for these patients, preferring to treat with intensified chemotherapy in high-risk patients and salvage radiotherapy, if necessary (71,101). In the IRS, the high risk of nodal involvement in certain subsets of these patients has led to the recommendation for ipsilateral retroperitoneal nerve-sparing node dissection for staging of all children ≥10 years of age (119,120). In the absence of histologic documentation, enlargement of retroperitoneal lymph nodes on thin-section computed tomographic imaging is considered evidence of tumor involvement.

Patients with nodal disease have a 5-year survival rate of 69%, compared with 96% for those without regional nodal disease ($p < .001$). Regional lymph node irradiation to the periaortic and ipsilateral iliac nodes is recommended when there is nodal involvement (122). Surgical violation of the scrotum or tumor extension to the structure is an indication for hemiscrotectomy or, less commonly, scrotal irradiation. If scrotal irradiation is used, orchiopexy should be considered prior to treatment to protect the remaining testes. Treatment programs must be planned to reduce morbidity, particularly among this group with high likelihood of cure (47).

Gynecologic Tumors

Tumors arising in the vulva, vagina, cervix, and uterus are about one-third as common as bladder and prostate primary tumors and account for 4% of all rhabdomyosarcomas (5). Within this group, the vagina is the most common site of origin (42). Patients with vaginal tumors are often much younger than those with other pelvic rhabdomyosarcomas, with most girls diagnosed before the age of 3 years. Most present with a vaginal mass or discharge; botryoid morphology is common.

Initial surgery is used primarily for diagnosis, although gross tumor resection is occasionally possible without cosmetic or functional deformity. These tumors are often quite sensitive to chemotherapy, and many may not require radical surgery or radiation therapy for local tumor control (3,5,62). Even when surgery is used for persistent tumor after chemotherapy, preservation of bladder and sexual function is often possible with vaginal tumors. However, vulvar and uterine tumors may not be as amenable to organ-preserving therapy when surgery is necessary for local control (42). Radiation therapy usually is reserved for patients with residual disease after resection or as part of a preoperative treatment regimen to help limit the extent of surgery. Intracavitary and interstitial brachytherapy are useful irradiation techniques in these (39). Data are limited, but with proper patient selection, disease control is excellent and late normal tissue effects are often significantly less than is seen with external-beam techniques (39,44,68). Permanent implants with iodine-125, temporary low-dose-rate, and high-dose-rate brachytherapy have all been used, and there are no clear differences between these techniques in terms of disease control or late effects. When temporary implants are used, high-dose-rate brachytherapy has the practical advantage of minimizing radiation exposure to the family and medical personnel caring for the child.

Survival after treatment is excellent. Children ages 1 to 9 years have a 98% 5-year survival. Survival for infants and adolescents approaches 90%, although these patients may require more intensive systemic therapy for cure (5).

Other Pelvic Sites

These tumors include perianal, perirectal, and perineal primary sites. Regional lymph node involvement may be high. The location of these primary tumors creates surgical and irradiation challenges. Combined chemotherapy and radiation therapy programs are favored over primary surgical procedures, if excision demands exenteration with urinary and fecal diversion procedures.

Extremity

Tumors arising in the extremity are often of the alveolar or undifferentiated subtypes, large, deeply invasive, and associated with a high probability of lymphatic and hematogenous metastasis (61). However, several series show that when combined-modality treatment is given, these patients have an outcome approximating that for other tumor sites of similar TNM stage (76,85). Complete surgical resection is difficult to achieve, usually requires extensive dissection, and is associated with a high risk of residual disease. Children with extremity tumors subjected to amputation and chemotherapy may have a relapse rate of more than 83% (43). Because radiation therapy and multiagent chemotherapy have been shown to provide excellent local control, it is advisable to avoid disfiguring and mutilating surgical procedures, with their attendant functional disabilities, and

to recommend limb-salvage procedures including irradiation and chemotherapy.

No data show that lymph node dissection offers a therapeutic advantage. However, patients with lymph node involvement have a particularly poor prognosis (61). If lymph node dissection is performed, it is for the purpose of staging, not for treatment. Sentinel lymph node mapping and biopsy are being investigated for their diagnostic and prognostic value (67).

Radiation therapy for extremity primary tumors requires careful immobilization techniques, sparing of nonirradiated skin for lymphatic drainage, and use of shrinking fields. Routine physical therapy during and after radiation therapy is important for obtaining an optimal functional result.

Overall survival at 3 years for these patients is about 70%, although failure-free survival is only 55% (69).

Other Sites

Patients with tumors arising in sites such as a paraspinal, retroperitoneal, or intrathoracic location have a poor outcome compared with other patients (26,64).

Most patients with tumors in these locations are unable to undergo complete resection of the tumor. Both local and distant relapse are common. These patients should be treated aggressively with high-dose radiation therapy and multiagent chemotherapy.

Metastatic Disease

Hematogenous or distant lymph node metastases at the time of diagnosis are ominous findings, although not all these children do poorly. The subset only one or two of patients who are <10 years of age and have sites of metastatic disease may have long-term survival chances of >50% (18). Intensive multiagent chemotherapy plays a major role in the treatment of these patients, although marrow ablative techniques have not improved efficacy compared with conventional chemotherapy approaches (48). Local control of the primary tumor is site specific, as previously described. Metastatic sites should be treated with radiotherapy when feasible.

General Management

A multidisciplinary approach using surgery, irradiation, and chemotherapy is important in the management of rhabdomyosarcoma; however, the optimal sequence and specific application of each modality continue to be investigated. Although the primary goal remains long-term cure, improvement in therapeutic results necessitates considerations of quality of life, with particular attention to maximization of functional and cosmetic results.

Surgery

Before the era of multidisciplinary therapy, surgical ablation resulted in a long-term survival rate of approximately 20% of those patients able to undergo resection (56). Certain primary sites represented exceptions to these data; for example, approximately 50% of those with localized disease of the orbit survived after orbital exenteration (50). However, with the introduction of effective adjunctive treatment, preservation of function and appearance became major goals. The concept of reasonable surgery evolved; it involves removal of the bulk of tumor with maximal conservation of anatomic structures, including preservation of bladder, bowel, and sexual function in patients with tumors of genitourinary origin, limb function in patients with extremity tumors, and vision, voice, deglutition, and appearance in patients with head and neck tumors.

Resection of rhabdomyosarcoma from normal surrounding tissues is often technically challenging. Only 20% of tumors are located in sites where complete excision can readily be accomplished without an undesirable loss of function or cosmesis (26). An additional 20% of patients have compromised surgical procedures, leaving microscopic residual disease. Sixty percent of patients have tumors amenable to biopsy only or present with metastatic disease and are not candidates for primary resection. When the IRS surgical grouping system is used, patients with tumor amenable to complete excision fare better than those who have subtotal resection or biopsy alone. However, the tumors that are most accessible to surgical excision are small and non-invasive and are confined to the organ or structure of origin. Assessment using a TNM system demonstrates that prognosis is dictated by tumor size and invasiveness rather than by the initial surgical approach (76).Furthermore, combined-modality therapy provides good local control of the primary tumor even after subtotal excision (29,49). For these reasons, the trend in recent years has been toward less-aggressive surgical resection, with more reliance on radiation therapy and chemotherapy to provide local control (26).

In cases of suspected rhabdomyosarcoma, the initial surgical procedure should be an incisional biopsy. Surgical excision is indicated if it can be done without compromise of function or cosmesis. Normal tissue margins of at least 5 mm around the tumor are usually required to consider the resection "complete" (IRS group I). If microscopic disease remains after initial resection, a "primary re-excision" can be considered prior to beginning chemotherapy. Those children who can be rendered microscopically free of disease by this procedure have an improved outcome, compared with children who remain in clinical group II following initial surgery (21,41). Amputation of an extremity, orbital exenteration, mutilating surgery of the head and neck area, therapeutic lymphadenectomy, and radical neck dissection are procedures reserved in case initial therapy fails (45).

Second-look operations may be useful for converting partial responses after chemotherapy into complete responses. To investigate if this might allow a reduction in the amount of radiotherapy that is necessary to provide local tumor control, the IRS-V study evaluated this approach; results are currently pending. Some investigators have used second-look operations in an attempt to eliminate radiotherapy, although this approach has resulted in inferior local control and survival (20). Second-look operations may be used to evaluate therapeutic response after chemotherapy and/or radiation therapy (118). In the IRS-III study, 28% of patients categorized as having clinical partial response and 43% of those scored as having no response to induction chemotherapy were reclassified as having pathologic complete response after second-look operation (121). These children enjoyed a survival rate similar to that of children who were able to undergo complete surgical excision at the time of initial diagnosis. Therefore, a clinical and/or radiographic evaluation indicating residual tumor after initial therapy may be misleading.

Chemotherapy

Chemotherapy is necessary in all cases. Several drugs have demonstrated single-agent activity measured as percent response rate, including vincristine (59%), dactinomycin (24%), cyclophosphamide (54%), cisplatin (15% to 21%), dacarbazine (11%), mitomycin C (36%), etoposide (15% to 21%), ifosfamide (86%), irinotecan (23) and topotecan (46%) (72,73,77). Agents with known activity against central nervous system tumors, such as the nitrosoureas and methotrexate, have not shown activity against rhabdomyosarcomas.

The most extensive experience in combination chemotherapy is with VAC (vincristine, dactinomycin, cyclophosphamide) or VAC plus Adriamycin (VACA). Patients with embryonal histology tumors in favorable sites who have no gross residual disease or lymph node involvement after the initial surgical resection appear to be adequately treated with VA (vincristine and dactinomycin) for 1 year, provided that irradiation is given for microscopic residual disease. Cyclophosphamide and Adriamycin do not improve survival in this patient group (26,63,64). Patients with unresectable pelvic tumors may benefit from the addition of Adriamycin and cisplatin to VAC, but tumors in other sites do not seem to benefit from the addition of these drugs compared with an intensive regimen of VAC alone.

Some subsets of patients, such as those with tumors of unfavorable histology or unfavorable site and those with extensive tumor burden, continue to fare poorly. Some of these patients with embryonal histology may benefit from intensification of the cyclophosphamide or ifosfamide component of their chemotherapy, although there are conflicting data regarding this (8,99). Patients with metastatic rhabdomyosarcoma benefit from the addition of ifosfamide and etoposide to the standard VAC regimen (17). High-dose chemotherapy with total-body irradiation and autologous bone marrow transplantation has not improved the outcome in these high-risk patients (48).

Initial intensive chemotherapy is now being used as a means of pharmacologic debulking, potentially allowing for a more conservative surgical approach or less aggressive radiation therapy (55,82,86). However, response to induction chemotherapy—whether complete, partial, or no response—does not predict ultimate outcome (15). When chemotherapy alone is used for tumors in sites such as the head and neck or pelvis, most children require radiation therapy or a follow-up surgical procedure because of incomplete response or local recurrence (87,89,100,115), and omission of radiotherapy may result in inferior survival (20,30). Even patients with only microscopic disease after initial resection (group II) require radiotherapy to achieve optimal local control (94). In patients with group II disease, who routinely receive radiotherapy, local control is 92% (98). The approach of initial chemotherapy followed by limited irradiation or less radical surgery may be appropriate in the management of infants and very young children, in whom late effects of aggressive surgery or high-dose, large-volume irradiation are particularly severe.

Radiation Therapy

Adequate irradiation implies careful attention to volume and dose. It is essential to evaluate the soft tissue extent of the primary lesion by computed tomography scan or magnetic resonance imaging. Because rhabdomyosarcoma tends to infiltrate tissue planes widely, tumors often extend beyond a fascial compartment and beyond the obvious visible margins. Careful examination by a radiation oncologist at the time of initial diagnosis, even if the treatment plan calls for neoadjuvant chemotherapy, is essential to establish the appropriate tumor volume.

Treatment portals usually are designed to encompass the involved region at the time of presentation (before chemotherapy) with margins that encompass surgical sites and biopsy tracts. Some have used modified radiation treatment volumes in cases of histologically proven response to neoadjuvant chemotherapy, although the efficacy of this approach has not been firmly established (55). A biopsy should be performed of clinically suspicious lymph nodes, or they should be included in the radiation therapy portal. Prophylactic lymph node irradiation is not necessary in children with clinically negative findings who will be receiving combination chemotherapy.

Patients with tumors at parameningeal sites (middle ear, paranasal sinuses, nasopharynx, nasal cavity, infratemporal fossa, and parapharyngeal area) have developed meningeal extension of tumor when inadequate irradiation portals were used (84). Radiation therapy portals that cover the adjacent meninges in these patients can prevent meningeal relapse

(26,64,65). Even patients with advanced parameningeal tumors presenting with cranial nerve palsies, base of skull erosion, or intracranial extension do not have significantly decreased 5-year survival rates, compared with those with less advanced parameningeal tumors, if appropriate irradiation portals are used (11).

High-dose irradiation is necessary to ensure local tumor control in patients who are unable to undergo complete surgical resection, even if concomitant multiagent chemotherapy is given. Local control of gross disease requires doses of at least 50 to 55 Gy, but microscopic disease can often be controlled with somewhat lower doses (49). IRS investigators have been unable to generate a strict dose-response curve but have observed an association with age that suggests that lower doses, often given to infants and youngsters, are associated with high relapse rates (80). They also suggest that local tumor control is greater for tumors <5 cm in diameter than for larger lesions, supporting the adult experience with soft tissue sarcomas (106,116,117). As part of a multimodality treatment program, radiation doses of 40 to 41.4 Gy given in 4.5 weeks provide a 90% likelihood of local control of microscopic disease, with 50.4 to 55.8 Gy in 5.5 to 6 weeks recommended for gross residual disease (11,49,106). Early results of IRS-V data suggest that 36 Gy may be sufficient for microscopic residual, and in orbital primaries, 45 Gy may be sufficient for gross disease (113). Results of the IRS-I study had indicated that radiotherapy was not needed for patients whose tumors were completely resected at diagnosis (group I). However, a reanalysis of data from the IRS-I to III studies indicates that the subset of group I patients with alveolar or undifferentiated histology had improved overall and failure-free survival when radiotherapy was given to the primary tumor site (124). Current recommendations are to deliver 36 to 41.4 Gy to the operative bed of completely resected patients with alveolar or undifferentiated histology.

In the IRS-IV study, investigators studied the efficacy of a higher radiation dose, 59.4 Gy, given in 1.1-Gy fractions twice daily at 6-hour intervals for children with gross residual disease (28,31). This hyperfractionated regimen was compared in a prospective, randomized fashion to a standard radiotherapy regimen consisting of 50.4 Gy given as 1.8 Gy once daily. There was no difference in locoregional disease control, failure-free survival, or overall survival between the two groups. Therefore, the standard of care for group III rhabdomyosarcoma continues to be conventionally fractionated radiation with chemotherapy.

Three-dimensional conformal and intensity-modulated radiotherapy treatment planning techniques are valuable for ensuring adequate treatment of the tumor volume and minimizing acute and chronic toxicity from the irradiation of uninvolved, adjacent structures (Fig. 85.4) (65,125,126). The gross tumor volume is defined as the prechemotherapy extent of disease. The clinical target volume includes the gross tumor volume and any involved regional nodal chain, plus a 1-cm margin. This clinical target volume can at times be further modified to account for anatomic barriers to tumor spread (such as the bony orbit in primary orbital tumors), or to account for regression of "pushing" tumor border after chemotherapy such as may occur in large pelvic tumors that initially displace contents of the peritoneal cavity. The planning target volume adds a patient-specific margin, which is typically about 5 mm. Proton beam radiotherapy has also been used successfully in certain sites (127). Immobilization techniques that ensure reproducible portals are essential. Sedation or anesthesia may be necessary to ensure adequate implementation of the treatment plan. These complex programs are best conducted in regional centers by an experienced team of physicians including a pediatric surgeon, pediatric anesthesiologist, pediatric oncologist, and radiation oncologist.

Interstitial radiation therapy may play an important role as primary treatment or as a boost after external-beam ther-

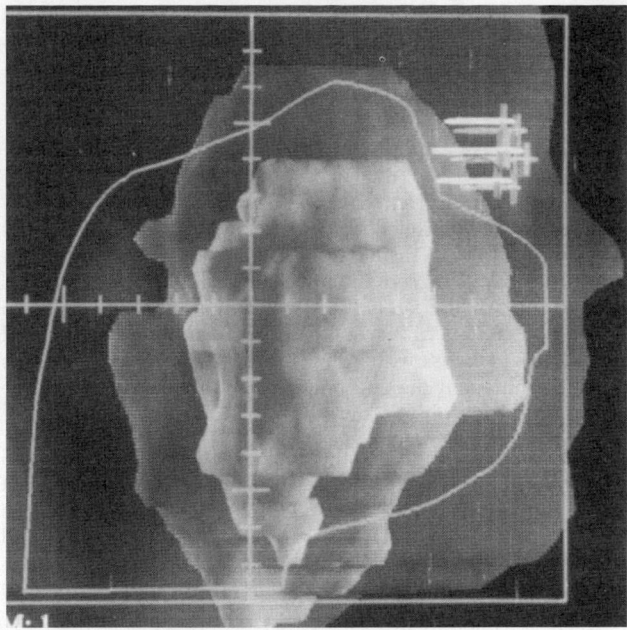

FIGURE 85.4. Three-dimensional treatment planning image shows the gross tumor (central, solid) and planning target (outer, transparent) volumes for a child with an infratemporal rhabdomyosarcoma. The portal aperture was designed using conventional two-dimensional techniques, demonstrating the inadequate coverage of both the gross tumor and target volumes with this approach. (Reprinted from Michalski JM, Sur RK, Harms WB, et al. Three dimensional conformal radiation therapy in pediatric parameningeal rhabdomyosarcomas. *Int J Radiat Oncol Biol Phys* 1995;33:985–991, with permission.)

apy for selected sites (44,68). The advantages of precise shaping of the dose distribution, sharp fall-off of radiation dose, and shortening of overall treatment time are especially attractive in dealing with infants and youngsters. Some investigators report a decrease in late normal tissue effects when compared with external-beam techniques (39). There are no data regarding comparative efficacy or toxicity between high-dose-rate and low-dose-rate techniques. However, high-dose-rate remote brachytherapy may be particularly attractive in this patient population for logistical reasons. These children often require extensive care from family members and medical personnel during their treatment, and high-dose-rate techniques can eliminate radiation exposure to these caregivers.

The timing of radiation therapy must be carefully coordinated with planned surgical intervention and combination-chemotherapy scheduling to optimize local control and ensure optimization of drug doses and unimpaired postoperative healing. Although radiation therapy is often delayed for several weeks to allow administration of neoadjuvant chemotherapy, some data suggest that earlier irradiation, particularly in high-risk patients, may provide better local tumor control and survival (26,55,64,65). Interaction between radiation and some of the commonly used chemotherapeutic drugs can produce undesirable early and late effects. This is particularly true of dactinomycin and Adriamycin. Radiation therapy given concurrently with these agents is usually avoided. In contrast, systemic treatment with drugs such as vincristine and cyclophosphamide can often be continued concurrently with the administration of irradiation.

Results of Therapy: Summary of Clinical Trials

Owing to the low incidence of rhabdomyosarcoma, much of what has been learned about its treatment has come from co-operative group trials performed in North America and Europe.

Various cooperative groups have used different philosophies of treatment. In general, the North American IRS studies have emphasized the role of local control measures and European studies have focused more on chemotherapeutic approaches.

Intergroup Rhabdomyosarcoma Studies

The IRS began intergroup clinical trials for rhabdomyosarcoma in 1972 and has enrolled several thousand children with this disease since then. A primary goal has been to test the efficacy of chemotherapy and radiation therapy as a function of surgical stage. In the first IRS study (IRS-I), radiation therapy was given initially for patients with group I and II disease and was delayed until week 6 for those with group III and IV disease. All patients received multiagent chemotherapy for 2 years. This study made several important observations (63):

i. For localized tumors amenable to complete resection (IRS group I), postoperative radiation therapy is unnecessary if the patient is given 2 years of VAC. For these patients, the relapse-free survival rate in IRS-I at 5 years was 80%, and the 5-year survival rate was 81% to 93%. Subsequent analysis has shown a benefit to postoperative radiation therapy for patients with group I tumors of alveolar or undifferentiated histology (124).

ii. VAC failed to improve results obtained with intensive VA for patients with group II disease if postoperative radiation therapy was given. For these patients, the relapse-free survival rate at 5 years was 65% to 72%, and the overall 5-year survival rate was 72%.

iii. VACA provided no advantage over VAC for patients with group III disease (gross residual) or group IV disease (metastasis) if routine radiation therapy was used in addition. The complete remission rate for group III patients was 69%, and for group IV patients it was 50%. Those who achieved complete remission had a 60% chance of staying in remission for 5 years in group III and a 30% chance in group IV. The survival rate at 5 years was 52% for group III and 20% for group IV patients.

iv. The 5-year survival rate for the entire group was 55%.

v. Survival after relapse was poor—32% at 1 year and 17% at 2 years.

vi. The risk of distant metastasis was much greater than the risk of local recurrence.

vii. Primary tumors of the orbit and genitourinary tract carried the best prognoses, and tumors of the retroperitoneum had the worst.

viii. The alveolar histologic subset had a poor prognosis, especially in extremity lesions.

A second IRS study (IRS-II) was built on the findings of IRS-I (64). The results from this study include:

i. The 5-year survival rate for the IRS-II group was 62%, a 7% improvement over the IRS-I rate.

ii. Patients in group I (excluding alveolar extremity patients) had better disease-free status with VAC (82%) than those who received only VA (68%), but they had similar survival rates (82% and 88%) at 5 years. Cyclophosphamide could not be withdrawn safely from the standard VAC regimen if irradiation was omitted from patients with group I disease.

iii. Intensive (cyclic-sequential) VA therapy was as effective as repetitive pulse VAC therapy for patients with group II disease, if all patients received postoperative irradiation. At 5 years, 68% to 75% remained disease free and 77% to 90% were alive, with no differences between the two therapy groups.

iv. Repetitive pulse chemotherapy for 2 years increased survival in children with group III disease but not in those

with group IV disease; Adriamycin and dactinomycin had comparable efficacy in the pulse regimens used. The complete remission rates were 72%. At 5 years, 70% remained in complete remission, and 64% were surviving.

v. In IRS-I, patients having tumors in parameningeal sites with high-risk factors (cranial nerve palsy, erosion of the base of the skull, or intracranial extension) had a high incidence of CNS relapse. In IRS-II, whole-brain radiotherapy irradiation, with or without intrathecal chemotherapy, was introduced. This prevented meningeal recurrence and increased survival in these patients with high-risk parameningeal primary tumors.

vi. Primary repetitive pulse VAC for patients with special pelvic primary tumors (i.e., bladder, prostate, uterus, vagina) did not reduce the frequency of total cystectomy or produce durable bladder salvage, although survival was not compromised.

vii. Survival after relapse was only 17% at 5 years.

The third IRS study (IRS-III) covered the period 1984 to 1991. This study revealed the following (26):

i. The 5-year survival rate for the IRS-III group was 71%, an 8% improvement over the IRS-II rate. The 5-year progression-free survival rate was 65%, a 10% improvement over IRS-II.

ii. Patients with group I favorable-histology tumors fared as well on a 1-year regimen of VA as did a comparable group treated with VA plus cyclophosphamide. The 5-year progression-free survival rates were 83% and 76%, respectively ($p = .18$).

iii. Results for patients with group II favorable-histology tumors, excluding orbit, head, and paratesticular sites, were not improved with the addition of Adriamycin over VA chemotherapy × 1 year and radiation therapy.

iv. Patients with group III tumors, excluding those in special pelvic, orbit, and other selected head sites (scalp, parotid, oral cavity, larynx, oropharynx, and cheek), fared better on the more intensive regimens of IRS-III than on pulsed VAC or VAC-VADR in IRS-II; the 5-year progression-free survival rates were 62% and 52%, respectively. The intensive regimen from IRS-III included multiple agents (VAC + Adriamycin + cisplatin + etoposide) plus radiation therapy plus second-look surgery. There were no differences in outcome among the three chemotherapy programs on IRS-III.

v. Patients with group IV tumors did not benefit from the aggressive therapy of IRS-III.

vi. Patients with tumors in the bladder, vagina, and central pelvis in clinical group III had significantly improved outcome as compared with IRS-II patients, primarily because of the routine administration of early radiation therapy, which improved the bladder salvage rate from 25% in IRS-II to 60% in IRS-III.

vii. Patients with unfavorable histology, in clinical groups I and II, who received VADR-VAC + cisplatin and radiation therapy had improved outcome over patients in IRS-II receiving VA or VAC and irradiation.

viii. Patients with favorable-histology group II paratesticular tumors and those with favorable-histology orbit and head tumors in groups II and III do not require cyclophosphamide when VA × 1 year plus radiation therapy is used.

ix. Whole-brain radiotherapy was omitted for patients with parameningeal primary tumors and cranial nerve palsy or base of skull erosion (although patients with intracranial extension of tumor still received this treatment). Risk of CNS relapse and survival were not compromised by this change if adequate local fields were used.

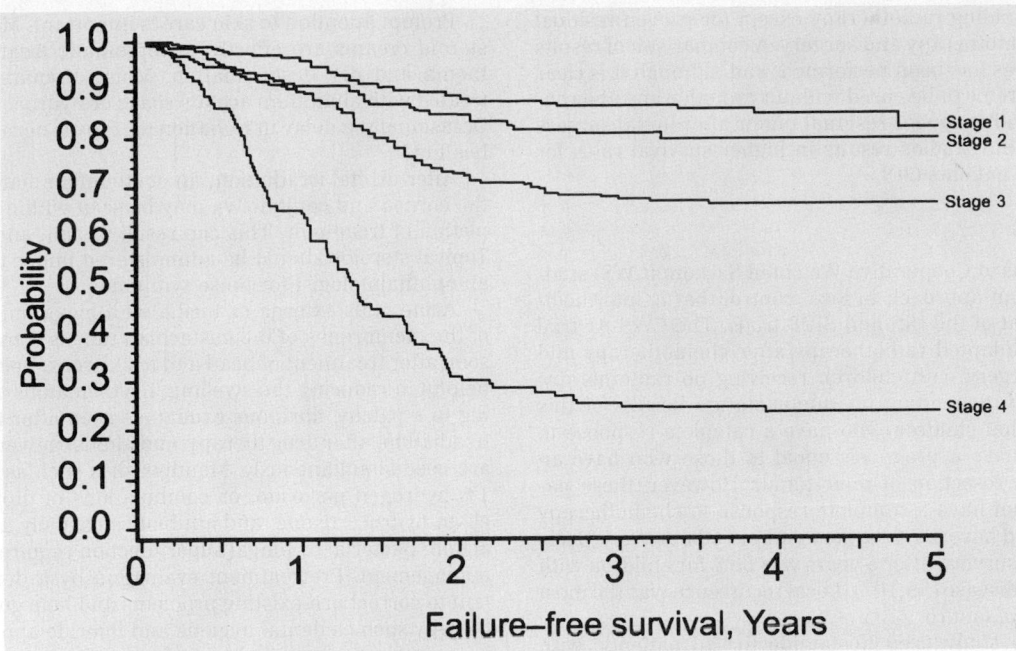

FIGURE 85.5. Survival curves of 1,010 children with rhabdomyosarcoma entered onto the Fourth Intergroup Rhabdomyosarcoma Study are shown by stage. (Adapted from Breneman JC, Lyden E, Pappo AS, et al. Prognostic factors and outcome in children with metastatic rhabdomyosarcoma: a report from the Intergroup Rhabdomyosarcoma Study IV. *J Clin Oncol* 2003;21:78–84; and from Crist WM, Anderson JR, Meza JL, et al. The Intergroup Rhabdomyosarcoma Study-IV: results for patients with non-metastatic disease. *J Clin Oncol* 2001;19:3091–3102, with permission.)

The fourth IRS study (IRS-IV) was conducted from 1991 to 1997 (Fig. 85.5) (24). Results from this study are as follows:

i. For patients with group III tumors, hyperfractionated radiotherapy was no more effective than conventional radiotherapy for tumor control and survival.

ii. There was no difference in survival between VAC versus vincristine/actinomycin/ifosfamide versus vincristine/ifosfamide/etoposide in children with nonmetastatic disease.

iii. Failure-free survival at 3 years for patients with embryonal histology was superior to results seen in IRS-III (83% vs. 74%) but no difference was seen for alveolar or undifferentiated subtypes.

iv. Survival for patients with group I or II orbit/eyelid tumors was excellent when treated with VA and radiotherapy for group II disease.

v. Prognostic subsets of patients based on histologic subtype, stage and group could be identified as follows: Low-risk patients had embryonal histology and were stage 1 (all groups), or stage 2/3 and group I or II. All other patients with locoregional disease were intermediate-risk.

vi. Survival for patients with metastatic disease was superior with the drug pair ifosfamide/etoposide when compared with vincristine/melphalan. (16)

vii. Whole-brain radiotherapy was omitted for all patients with parameningeal primary tumors except when there was cytologic evidence of cerebrospinal fluid involvement. Survival was not compromised by this approach.

The fifth IRS studies (IRS-V) were conducted from 1997 to 2005. They studied a number of questions that included:

i. Can a subset of the most favorable patients be treated without alkylating agents?

ii. Can radiation dose be reduced to 36 Gy for microscopic disease, and 45 Gy for gross tumor in the subset of patients with orbital primaries?

iii. Can radiation dose be reduced for group III patients after induction chemotherapy and second-look operation?

iv. What is the activity of topotecan and irinotecan in the treatment of rhabdomyosarcoma?

Early results from the IRS-V studies support the elimination of alkylating agents from chemotherapy regimens for patients with a favorable prognosis, and the reduction of radiation dose to 36 Gy and 45 Gy for microscopic tumor and group III orbital primaries, respectively (113).

SIOP Studies

SIOP (the French acronym for the International Society of Pediatric Oncology) began multi-institutional trials for rhabdomyosarcoma in 1975, and has reported results from three studies to date (38,88,100). The focus of these studies has been to minimize local therapy by using risk-adapted intensification of chemotherapy, with attempted salvage of patients who fail locally.

The first SIOP study (RMS 75) used VAC chemotherapy plus Adriamycin. Group III patients were randomized to early local therapy versus response-based delayed local therapy (surgery preferred over radiotherapy) after maximal chemotherapy response. No survival difference was seen between these arms, although overall survival was only 40%.

The second SIOP study, MMT 84, used a similar strategy of limited radiotherapy only when there was residual tumor after chemotherapy and surgery. Overall survival at 5 years was 68%, although event free survival was only 53% and 29% of patients had isolated local relapse.

The third SIOP study, MMT 89, concluded that alkylating agents can be omitted for the patients with the most favorable prognosis. The use of radiotherapy was again limited, resulting in a local failure rate of 34%.

The SIOP and IRS studies differ significantly in their use of local therapy, with IRS studies emphasizing early introduction of radiotherapy for patients with residual tumor after surgery, and

SIOP studies avoiding radiotherapy except for proven residual tumor after chemotherapy and surgery. A comparison of results of the two studies has been performed, and although it is clear that some children can be cured without radiotherapy, the routine use of radiotherapy for residual tumor after initial surgery as used in the IRS studies results in higher survival rates for most subsets of patients (30).

CWS Studies

The German-based Cooperative Weichteil Sarkom (CWS) studies have taken an approach to local control that is intermediate between that of the IRS and SIOP trials. The CWS-81 trial used response-adapted radiotherapy after chemotherapy and second-look surgery with children receiving no radiotherapy, 40 Gy or 50 Gy depending on tumor status. Results of this study showed that children who have a complete response to chemotherapy have a prognosis equal to those who have an initial complete resection of their tumor. However, those patients who do not have a complete response to chemotherapy by week 9 should have early surgery and/or radiotherapy. Overall disease-free survival after 5 years was 68% for children with non-metastatic disease (55,107). Local recurrence was the most common cause of failure.

The CWS-86 study used ifosfamide for all patients, with an abbreviated course of chemotherapy for favorable patients with early-stage disease, and altered the way radiotherapy was given (54). Patients who had an early complete response to chemotherapy did not receive radiotherapy. Most received hyperfractionated accelerated radiotherapy of 1.6 Gy twice daily concurrent with ifosfamide and Adriamycin containing chemotherapy, using 32 Gy after a good response and 54.4 Gy after a poor response. Conclusions from this study were:

i. Duration of chemotherapy can be reduced to as little as 16 weeks for the most favorable patients.

ii. Ifosfamide gives improved response rates compared with cyclophosphamide.

iii. Hyperfractionated accelerated radiotherapy concurrent with chemotherapy as used in the study is tolerable and provided acceptable local control.

Like CWS-81, the majority of failures in this study were local, with an especially high local recurrence rate in those group II and III patients who did not receive radiotherapy.

Sequelae of Treatment

Acute Effects

Acute side effects from surgery are primarily postoperative complications that are usually reversible and not serious. The acute toxicity from chemotherapy includes nausea, vomiting, mucositis, alopecia, and hematopoietic suppression. Drug-induced granulocytopenia significantly increases the risk of fever and infection, although the routine use of granulocyte colony-stimulating factor has lessened these risks. Newer protocols using more aggressive therapy including topoisomerase inhibitors, ifosfamide, etoposide, and other agents have other acute side effects, including renal and electrolyte imbalance, which demand close monitoring.

Acute radiation toxicity is related to the regions irradiated and the dose administered. It can be especially pronounced for tumors of the head and neck, abdomen, and pelvis. The synergistic effect of chemotherapeutic drugs such as dactinomycin and Adriamycin can be severe and may require modification of the treatment plan. Both dactinomycin and Adriamycin are known to accentuate a "recall" of radiation injury if given during or immediately after the course of radiation therapy.

Prompt attention to skin care is important. Moisturizers and steroid creams are effective symptomatic treatments for erythema and dry desquamation. Moist desquamation may be treated with aluminum acetate soaks or hydrocolloid dressings. Occasionally, a delay in radiation therapy is necessary to permit healing.

After orbital irradiation, an acute inflammatory reaction of the cornea and conjunctiva may be seen within weeks of completion of treatment. This can result in pain and photophobia. Topical steroids should be administered under the direction of an ophthalmologist for these symptoms.

Acute otitis externa or media with hyperemia and swelling of the membranes of the eustachian tube is common during or soon after treatment of head and neck areas. Decongestants are helpful in reducing the swelling. Erythematous mucositis leading to a patchy, fibrinous exudate is seen after head and neck irradiation, after drug therapy, and almost universally if the two are used simultaneously. Mouthwashes such as salt and soda, 1% hydrogen peroxide, or combinations of diphenhydramine elixir, hydrocortisone, and antibiotics partially alleviate the reaction. Bacterial or fungal superinfection requires specific drug management. Pretreatment evaluation by a dentist is important to correct pre-existing problems and help guide preventive therapy such as dental hygiene and fluoride applications.

Acute gastrointestinal sequelae, such as vomiting and diarrhea, are usually managed by supportive care. Parenteral nutritional support may be necessary to prevent protein/calorie malnutrition.

Late Effects

Long-term sequelae related to specific chemotherapy drugs are usually site-specific, and the morbidity may be accentuated by radiation therapy. Cyclophosphamide may induce hemorrhagic cystitis, and Adriamycin is implicated in late myocardiopathies (78). Cisplatin carries a high incidence of hearing impairment. Alkylating agents and topoisomerase inhibitors are associated with the development of secondary neoplasms, particularly acute myeloid leukemia (46,91).

Late radiation effects are related to the irradiated site, the dose of radiation, and the age of the child at the time of treatment. Effects include bone and soft tissue growth disturbances, dental abnormalities, cataract, hypopituitarism, gonadal dysfunction, induction of second malignant tumors (particularly bone sarcomas), and chronic organ dysfunction (1,46,75,83). Long-term follow-up and treatment is important to minimize the impact of these, particularly for endocrine and dental complications (34). Combined-modality treatment programs are significantly implicated in many of these complications.

Late surgical complications depend mainly on the choice of surgical procedure for primary treatment of the tumor. They include disfigurement and loss of function. Serious late effects of surgical treatment include the consequences of fecal and urinary diversion as well as ejaculatory impotence after retroperitoneal lymph node dissection.

Future Directions and Research

Advances in molecular biology are now providing a more comprehensive understanding of the biologic behavior of rhabdomyosarcoma and direct new research initiatives.

Chromosome aberrations are common in rhabdomyosarcoma. A consistent loss of heterozygosity at 11p15.5 is seen in embryonal rhabdomyosarcoma. Cytogenetic studies of alveolar rhabdomyosarcomas often demonstrate a translocation involving chromosomes 2 and 13, which affects the *PAX3* gene in band 2q35 and the *FKHR* gene in band 13q14 (9,96). The reciprocal translocation of the t(2;13) fuses *PAX3* to the *FKHR* gene, resulting in a chimeric structure that functions as an oncoprotein, resulting in dysregulation of cell growth and transformation (32). Similarly, t(1;13) juxtaposes the *PAX7* gene on chromosome 1p36 with the *FKHR* gene on chromosome 13q14, again producing a chimeric transcript. These findings suggest that there may be a set of target genes involved in the pathogenesis of rhabdomyosarcoma, and work is currently underway to engineer vaccines against the resulting fusion proteins (110). The identification of genes in alveolar rhabdomyosarcoma has permitted the development of molecular diagnostic assays including reverse-transcriptase polymerase chain reaction and fluorescence *in situ* hybridization for improved detection of alveolar rhabdomyosarcoma cells (2).

Studies of the genetic control of myogenesis now help establish the diagnosis of rhabdomyosarcoma as opposed to other small, round, blue cell tumors, and present opportunities for targeted drug therapy (14,111). The presence of MyoD protein expression represents a commitment to myogenic lineage and serves as a useful marker to skeletal muscle precursor cells (27). The availability of MyoD monoclonal antibodies also facilitates the differential diagnosis of the small round cell tumor of childhood and may assist in the detection of minimal disseminated disease (27,92). The MyoD gene products not only drive cells toward myogenesis but also halt cell cycling, thus producing differentiation along with cessation of cell replication (103).

Proto-oncogene research has focused on nuclear transcription factors. Embryonal rhabdomyosarcoma does not reveal amplification of either N-*myc* or c-*myc;* however, the majority of alveolar cases do have N-*myc* amplification. Survival among N-*myc*–amplified patients is poor (33). In addition, evaluation of insulinlike growth factor-2 reveals abnormalities and overproduction (128). Studies are ongoing in this area with respect to treatment (42). Flow cytology analyses of cell proliferation in rhabdomyosarcoma suggest that improved prognosis correlates with low (<15%) S-phase fraction (123).

Alteration of tumor suppressor genes is described in rhabdomyosarcoma, although their significance is unclear. Investigators have reported that >50% of both alveolar and embryonal rhabdomyosarcomas in established cell lines contain a mutant *p53* tumor suppressor gene (35). However, more recent data indicate that the actual incidence of mutant p53 in tissue derived directly from patient biopsies is much lower, and data regarding its predictive value for survival are mixed (7,104). Studies of multiple-drug resistance genes, which encode P-glycoprotein, suggest that in rhabdomyosarcoma, high levels of P-glycoprotein lead to tumor resistance. In these tumors, there appears to be a correlation between P-glycoprotein positivity and poor outcome (22).

The next generation of IRS studies, now named *Soft Tissue Sarcoma studies*, will test a number a clinical hypothesis. These include testing the ability to reduce the duration of chemotherapy for favorable prognosis tumors, studying the effect of delivering radiotherapy early in the course of treatment (week 4) concurrently with irinotecan for intermediate-risk patients, and evaluating the prognostic value of early treatment response as assessed by positron emission tomography imaging.

Future directions and research in rhabdomyosarcoma are being driven by many exciting molecular biologic and technologic advances. Such new findings provide hope for more refined risk-based therapy in rhabdomyosarcoma and potentially for gene therapy to be added to the therapeutic armamentarium.

References

1. Abramson DH, Notis CM. Visual acuity after radiation for orbital rhabdomyosarcoma. *Am J Opthalmol* 1994;118:808–809.
2. Anderson J, Gordon T, McManus A, et al. Detection of the PAX3–FKHR fusion gene in paediatric rhabdomyosarcoma: a reproducible predictor of outcome? *Br J Cancer* 2001;85:831–835.
3. Andrassy RJ, Wiener ES, Raney RB, et al. Progress in the surgical management of vaginal rhabdomyosarcoma: a 25-year review from the Intergroup Rhabdomyosarcoma Study Group. *J Pediatr Surg* 1999;34:731–734.
4. Arndt C, Rodeberg D, Breitfeld PP, et al. Does bladder preservation (as a surgical principle) lead to retaining bladder function in bladder/prostate rhabdomyosarcoma? Results from Intergroup Rhabdomyosarcoma Study IV *J Urol* 2004;171:2396–403.
5. Arndt CA, Donaldson SS, Anderson JR, et al. What constitutes optimal therapy for patients with rhabdomyosarcoma of the female genital tract? *Cancer* 2001;91:2454–2468.
6. Asmar L, Gehan EM, Newton WA, et al. Agreement among and within groups of pathologists in the classification of rhabdomyosarcoma and related childhood sarcomas: Report of an international study of four pathology classifications. *Cancer* 1994;74:2579–2588.
7. Ayan I, Dogan O, Kebudi R, et al. Immunohistochemical detection of p53 protein in rhabdomyosarcoma: association with clinicopathological features and outcome. *J Pediatr Hematol Oncol* 1997;19:48–53.
8. Baker KS, Anderson JR, Link MP, et al. Benefit of intensified therapy for patients with local or regional embryoneal rhabdomyosarcoma: results from the Intergroup Rhabdomyosarcoma Study IV. *J Clin Oncol* 2000;18:2427–2434.
9. Barr FG, Galili N, Holick J, et al. Rearrangement of the *PAX 3* paired box gene in the pediatric solid tumor alveolar rhabdomyosarcoma. *Nature Genet* 1993;3:113–117.
10. Benk V, Rodary C, Donaldson SS, et al. Parameningeal rhabdomyosarcoma: results of an international workshop. *Int J Radiat Oncol Biol Phys* 1996;36:533–540.
11. Berry MD, Jenkin RP: Parameningeal rhabdomyosarcoma in the young. *Cancer* 1981;48[Suppl 2]:281–288.
12. Birch JM, Hartley AL, Blair V, et al. Identification of factors associated with high cancer risk in the mothers of children with soft tissue sarcoma. *J Clin Oncol* 1990: 8:583–590.
13. Blatt J, Snyderman C, Wollman MR, et al. Delayed resection in the management of non-orbital rhabdomyosarcoma of the head and neck in childhood. *Med Pediatr Oncol* 1997;28:294–299.
14. Bortoluzzi S, Bisognin A, Romualdi C, et al: Novel genes, possibly relevant for molecular diagnosis or therapy of human rhabdomyosarcoma, detected by genomic expression profiling. *Gene* 2005;348:65–71.
15. Breitfeld P, Anderson J, Kao S, et al. Assessment of response to induction therapy and its influence on 5-year failure-free survival (FFS) in Group III rhabdomyosarcoma (RMS): Intergroup Rhabdomyosarcoma Study (IRS)-IV experience. Annual Proceedings of the American Society of Clinical Oncology, Abstract 8513, New Orleans, LA, June 2004.
16. Breitfeld PP, Lyden E, Raney BR, et al. Ifosfamide and Etoposide are superior to vincristine and melphalan for pediatric metastatic rhabdomyosarcoma when administered with irradiation and combination chemotherapy: a report from the Intergroup Rhabdomyosarcoma Study Group. *Am J Pediatr Hematol Oncol* 2001;23:225–233.
17. Breitfeld PP, Lyden E, Raney RB, et al. Ifosfamide and etoposide are superior to vincristine and melphalan for pediatric metastatic rhabdomyosarcoma when administered with irradiation and combination chemotherapy: a report from the Intergroup Rhabdomyosarcoma Study Group. *J Pediatr Hematol Oncol* 2001;23:334–337.
18. Breneman JC, Lyden E, Pappo AS, et al. Prognostic factors and outcome in children with metastatic rhabdomyosarcoma: a report from the Intergroup Rhabdomyosarcoma Study IV. *J Clin Oncol* 2003;21:78–84.
19. Carazzana AO, Schmidt D, Ninfo V, et al. Spindle cell rhabdomyosarcoma: A clinicopathologically favorable variant of rhabdomyosarcoma. *Am J Surg Pathol* 1992;16:229–235.
20. Carretto E, Scarzello G, Bisogno B, et al. IRS Group III non-alveolar rhabdomyosarcomas (RMS): Is complete delayed surgery sufficient to avoid radiotherapy? *Pediatr Blood Cancer* 2005;45:387.
21. Cecchetto G, Carli M, Sotti G, et al. Importance of local treatment in pediatric soft tissue sarcomas with microscopic residual after primary surgery: results of the Italian cooperative study RMS-88. *Med Pediatr Oncol* 2000;34:97–101.
22. Chan HSL, Thorner PS, Haddad G, et al. Immunohistochemic detection of p-glycoprotein: Prognostic correlation in soft tissue sarcoma of childhood. *J Clin Oncol* 1990;8:689–704.
23. Cosetti M, Wexler LH, Calleja E, et al. Irinotecan for pediatric solid tumors: the Memorial Sloan-Kettering experience. *J Pediatr Hematol Oncol* 2002;24:84–85.
24. Crist WM, Anderson JR, Meza JL, et al. The Intergroup Rhabdomyosarcoma Study-IV: results for patients with non-metastatic disease. *J Clin Oncol* 2001;19:3091–3102.
25. Crist WM, Garnsey L, Beltangady MS, et al. Prognosis in children with rhabdomyosarcoma: a report of the Intergroup Rhabdomyosarcoma Studies I and II. *J Clin Oncol* 1990;8:443–452.
26. Crist W, Gehan EA, Ragab AH, et al. The third Intergroup Rhabdomyosarcoma Study. *J Clin Oncol* 1995;13:610–630, 1995.
27. Dias P, Parham DM, Shapiro DN, et al. Monoclonal antibodies to the myogenic regulatory protein MyoD 1: Epitope mapping and diagnostic utility. *Cancer Res* 1992;52:6431–6439.
28. Donaldson SS, Asmar L, Breneman J, et al. Hyperfractionated radiation in children with rhabdomyosarcoma: results of an Intergroup Rhabdomyosarcoma Pilot Study. *Int J Radiat Oncol Biol Phys* 1995;32:903–911.
29. Donaldson SS, Castro JR, Wilbur JR, et al. Rhabdomyosarcoma of the head and neck in children: combination treatment by surgery, irradiation and chemotherapy. *Cancer* 1973;31:26–35.
30. Donaldson SS, Anderson JR: Rhabdomyosarcoma: many similarities, a few philosophical differences. *J Clin Oncol* 2005;23:2586–2587.
31. Donaldson SS, Meza J, Breneman JC, et al. Results from the IRS-IV randomized trial of hyperfractionated radiation in children with rhabdomyosarcoma: a report from the IRSG. *Int J Radiat Oncol Biol Phys* 2001;51:718–728.
32. Douglass E, Shapiro D, Valentine M, et al. Alveolar rhabdomyosarcoma with the t(2;13): cytogenetic findings and clinicopathologic correlations. *Med Pediatr Oncol* 1993;21:83–87.
33. Driman D, Thorner P, Greenberg M, et al. *MYCN* gene amplification in rhabdomyosarcoma. *Cancer* 1994;73:2231–2237.
34. Estilo CL, Huryn JM, Kraus DH, et al. Effects of therapy on dentofacial development in long-term survivors of head and neck rhabdomyosarcoma: the Memorial Sloan–Kettering Cancer Center experience. *J Pediatr Hematol Oncol* 2003;25:215–222.

35. Felix CA, Kappel CC, Mitsudomi T, et al. Frequency and diversity of *p53* mutations in childhood rhabdomyosarcoma. *Cancer Res* 1992;52:2243–2247.
36. Ferrari A, Dileo P, Casanova M, et al. Rhabdomyosarcoma in adults. A retrospective analysis of 171 patients treated at a single institution. *Cancer* 2003;98:571–580.
37. Flamant F, Hill C: The improvement in survival in childhood rhabdomyosarcoma: a historical comparison of 345 patients in the same center. *Cancer* 1984;53:2417–2421.
38. Flamant F, Rodary C, Rey A, et al. Treatment of non-metastatic rhabdomyosarcomas in childhood and adolescence. Results of the second study of the international society of paediatric oncology: MMT84. *Eur J Cancer* 1998;34:1050–1062.
39. Gerbaulet A, Panis X, Flamant F, et al. Iridium afterloading curietherapy in the treatment of pediatric malignancies: the Institut Gustave-Roussy experience. *Cancer* 1985;56:1274–1279.
40. Hays DM: Bladder/prostate rhabdomyosarcoma: results of the multi-institutional trials of the Intergroup Rhabdomyosarcoma Study. *Semin Surg Oncol* 1993;9:520–523.
41. Hays DM, Lawrence W Jr, Wharam M, et al. Primary reexcision for patients with 'microscopic residual' tumor following initial excision of sarcomas of trunk and extremity sites. *J Pediatr Surg* 1989;24:5–10.
42. Hays DM, Shimada H, Raney RB, et al. Clinical staging and treatment results in rhabdomyosarcoma of the female genital tract among children and adolescents. *Cancer* 1988;61:1893–1903.
43. Hays DM, Soule EH, Lawrence W, et al. Extremity lesions in the Intergroup Rhabdomyosarcoma Study (IRS-I): a preliminary report. *Cancer* 1982;49:1–8.
44. Healey EA, Shamberger RC, Grier HE, et al. A 10-year experience of pediatric brachytherapy. *Int J Radiat Oncol Biol Phys* 1995;32:451–455.
45. Healy GB, Upton J, Mc Black P, et al. The role of surgery in rhabdomyosarcoma of the head and neck in children. *Arch Otolaryngol Head Neck Surg* 1991;117:1185–1188.
46. Heyn R, Haeberlen V, Newton WA, et al. Second malignant neoplasms in children treated for rhabdomyosarcoma. *J Clin Oncol* 1993;11:262–270.
47. Heyn R, Raney RB, Hays DM, et al. Late effects of therapy in patients with paratesticular rhabdomyosarcoma. *J Clin Oncol* 1992;10:614–623.
48. Horowitz ME, Kinsella TJ, Wexler LH, et al. Total-body irradiation and autologous bone marrow transplant in the treatment of high-risk Ewing's sarcoma and rhabdomyosarcoma. *J Clin Oncol* 1993;11:1911–1918.
49. Jereb B, Cham W, Lattin P, et al. Local control of embryonal rhabdomyosarcoma in children by radiation therapy when combined with concomitant chemotherapy. *Int J Radiat Oncol Biol Phys* 1976;1:217–225.
50. Jones IS, Reese AB, Krout J: Orbital rhabdomyosarcoma: an analysis of sixty-two cases. *Trans Am Ophthalmol Soc* 1965;63:223–255.
51. Joshi D, Anderson J, Paidas C, et al. Age is an independent prognostic factor in rhabdomyosarcoma: a report from the Soft Tissue Sarcoma Committee of the Children's Oncology Group. *Pediatr Blood Cancer* 2004;42:64–73.
52. Kelly KM, Womer RB, Barr FG: Minimal disease detection in patients with alveolar rhabdomyosarcoma using a reverse transcriptase-polymerase chain reaction method. *Cancer* 1996;78:1320–1327.
53. Kodet R, Newton WA, Hamoudi AB, et al. Orbital rhabdomyosarcomas and related tumors in childhood: relationship of morphology to prognosis—an Intergroup Rhabdomyosarcoma study. *Med Pediatr Oncol* 1997;29:51–60.
54. Koscielniak E, Harms D, Henze G, et al. Results of treatment for soft tissue sarcoma in childhood and adolescence: a final report of the German Cooperative Soft Tissue Sarcoma Study CWS-86. *J Clin Oncol* 1999;17:3706–3719.
55. Koscielniak E, Jurgens H, Winkler K, et al. Treatment of soft tissue sarcoma in childhood and adolescence. *Cancer* 1992;70:2557–2567.
56. Lacey SR, Jewett TC JR, Karp MP, et al. Advances in the treatment of rhabdomyosarcoma. *Semin Surg Oncol* 1986;2:139–146.
57. LaQuaglia MP, Ghavimi F, Herr H, et al. Prognostic factors in bladder and bladder/prostate rhabdomyosarcoma. *J Pediatr Surg* 1990;25:1066–1072.
58. Lawrence W, Gehan EA, Hays DM, et al. Prognostic significance of staging factors of the UICC system in childhood rhabdomyosarcoma: a report from the Intergroup Rhabdomyosarcoma Study (IRS-II). *J Clin Oncol* 1987;5:46–54.
59. Leuschner I, Newton WA, Schmidt D, et al. Spindle cell variants of embryonal rhabdomyosarcoma in the paratesticular region: a report of the Intergroup Rhabdomyosarcoma Study. *Am J Surg Pathol* 1993;17:221–230.
60. Lobe TE, Wiener E, Andrassy RJ, et al. The argument for conservative, delayed surgery in the management of prostatic rhabdomyosarcoma. *J Pediatr Surg* 1996;31:1084–1087.
61. Mandell L, Ghavimi F, LaQuaglia M, et al. Prognostic significance of regional lymph node involvement in childhood extremity rhabdomyosarcoma. *Med Pediatr Oncol* 1990;18:466–471.
62. Martelli H, Oberlin O, Rey A, et al. Conservative treatment for girls with nonmetastatic rhabdomyosarcoma of the genital tract: a report from the study committee of the International Society of Pediatric Oncology. *J Clin Oncol* 1999;17:2117–2122.
63. Maurer HM, Beltangady M, Gehan EA, et al. The Intergroup Rhabdomyosarcoma Study-I: a final report. *Cancer* 1988;61:209–220.
64. Maurer HM, Gehan EA, Beltangady M, et al. The Intergroup Rhabdomyosarcoma Study-II. *Cancer* 1993;71:1904–1922.
65. Michalski JM, Meza J, Breneman JC, et al. Influence of radiation therapy parameters on outcome in children treated with radiation therapy for localized parameningeal rhabdomyosarcoma in intergroup rhabdomyosarcoma study group trials II through IV. *J Radiat Oncol Biol Phys* 2004;59:1027–1038.
66. McCarville MB, Christie R, Daw NC, et al. PET/CT in the evaluation of childhood sarcomas. *Am J Roentgenol* 2005;184:1293–1304.
67. McMulkin HM, Yanchar NL, Fernandez CV, et al: Sentinel lymph node mapping and biopsy: a potentially valuable tool in the management of childhood extremity rhabdomyosarcoma. *Pediatr Surg Int* 2003;19:452–456.
68. Nag S, Tippin D, Ruymann FB. Intraoperative high-dose-rate brachytherapy for the treatment of pediatric tumors: the Ohio State University experience. *Int J Radiat Oncol Biol Phys* 2001;51:729–735.
69. Neville HL, Andrassy RJ, Lobe TE, et al. Preoperative staging, prognostic factors, and outcome for extremity rhabdomyosarcoma: a preliminary report from the Intergroup Rhabdomyosarcoma Study IV (1991–1997). *J Pediatr Surg* 2000;35:317–321.
70. Oberlin O, Rey A, Anderson J, et al. Treatment of orbital rhabdomyosarcoma: survival and late effects of treatment. Results of an International Workshop. *J Clin Oncol* 2001;19:197–204.
71. Olive D, Flamant F, Zucker JM, et al. Paraaortic lymphadenectomy is not necessary in the treatment of localized paratesticular rhabdomyosarcoma. *Cancer* 1984;54:1283–1287.
72. Pappo AS, Etcubanas E, Santana VM, et al. A phase II trial of ifosfamide in previously untreated children and adolescents with unresectable rhabdomyosarcoma. *Cancer* 1993;71:2119–2125.
73. Pappo AS, Lyden E, Breneman J, et al. Up–front window trial of topotecan in previously untreated children and adolescents with metastatic rhabdomyosarcoma: an Intergroup Rhabdomyosarcoma Study. *J Clin Oncol* 2001;19:213–219.
74. Pappo AS, Shapiro DN, Crist WM, et al. Biology and therapy of pediatric rhabdomyosarcoma. *J Clin Oncol* 1995;13:2123–2139.
75. Paulino AC, Simon JH, Zhen W, et al. Long-term effects in children treated with radiotherapy for head and neck rhabdomyosarcoma. *Int J Radiat Oncol Biol Phys* 2000;48:1489–1495.
76. Pedrick TJ, Donaldson SS, Cox RS. Rhabdomyosarcoma: the Stanford experience utilizing a TNM staging system. *J Clin Oncol* 1986;4:370–378.
77. Pratt CB, Stewart C, Santana VM, et al. Phase I study of topotecan for pediatric patients with malignant solid tumors. *J Clin Oncol* 1994;12:539–543.
78. Punyko JA, Mertens AC, Gurney JG, et al. Long-term effects of childhood and adolescent rhabdomyosarcoma: a report from the Childhood Cancer Survivor Study. *Pediatr Blood Cancer* 2005;44:643–653.
79. Qualman SJ, Coffin CM, Newton WA, et al. Intergroup Rhabdomyosarcoma Study: Update for pathologist. *Pediatr Devel Pathol* 1998;1:550–561.
80. Ragab A, Heyn R, Tefft M, et al. Infants younger than 1 year of age with rhabdomyosarcoma. *Cancer* 1986;58:2606–2610.
81. Raney B, Carey A, Snyder HM, et al. Primary site as a prognostic variable for children with pelvic soft tissue sarcoma. *J Urol* 1986;136:874–878.
82. Raney RB, Gehan EA, Hays DM, et al. Primary chemotherapy with or without radiation therapy and/or surgery for children with localized sarcoma of the bladder, prostate, vagina, uterus, and cervix: a comparison of the results in Intergroup Rhabdomyosarcoma Studies I and II. *Cancer* 1990;66:2072–2081.
83. Raney B, Heyn R, Hays DM, et al. Sequelae of treatment in 109 patients followed for 5 to 15 years after diagnosis of sarcoma of the bladder and prostate. *Cancer* 1993;71:2387–2394.
84. Raney RB, Meza J, Anderson JR, et al. Treatment of children and adolsescents with localized parameningeal sarcoma: experience of the Intergroup Rhabdomyosarcoma Study Group protocols IRS-II through –IV, 1978–1997. *Med Pediatr Oncol* 2002;38:22–32.
85. Ransom JL, Pratt CB, Shanks E: Childhood rhabdomyosarcoma of the extremity: Results of combined modality therapy. *Cancer* 1977;40:2810–2816.
86. Regine WF, Fontanesi J, Kumar P, et al. Local tumor control in rhabdomyosarcoma following low-dose irradiation: comparison of group II and select group III patients. *Int J Radiat Oncol Biol Phys* 1995;31:485–491.
87. Rodary C, Gehan EA, Flamant F, et al. Prognostic factors in 951 nonmetastatic rhabdomyosarcoma in children: a report from the International Rhabdomyosarcoma Workshop. *Med Pediatr Oncol* 1991;19:89–95.
88. Rodary C, Rey A, Olive D, et al. Prognostic factors at diagnosis in 281 children with nonmetastatic rhabdomyosarcoma (RMS) at diagnosis. *Med Pediatr Oncol* 1988;16:71–77.
89. Rousseau P, Flamant F, Quintana E, et al. Primary chemotherapy in rhabdomyosarcoma and other malignant mesenchymal tumors of the orbit: results of the International Society of Pediatric Oncology MMT 84 Study. *J Clin Oncol* 1994;12:516–521.
90. Sagerman RH: Orbital rhabdomyosarcoma: a paradigm for irradiation. *Radiology* 1993;187:605–607.
91. Sandoval C, Pui CH, Bowman LC, et al. Secondary acute myeloid leukemia in children previously treated with alkylating agents, intercalating topoisomerase II inhibitors, and irradiation. *J Clin Oncol* 1993;11:1039–1045.
92. Sartori F, Alaggio R, Zanazzo G, et al. Results of a prospective minial disseminated disease study in human rhabdomyosarcoma using three different molecular markers. *Cancer* 2006;106:1766–1775.
93. Scheidler S, Fredericks WJ, Rauscher FJ, et al. The hybrid PAX3-FKHR fusion protein of alveolar rhabdomyosarcoma transforms fibroblasts in culture. *Proc Natl Acad Sci* 1996;93:9805–9809.
94. Schuck A, Matke A, Schmidt B, et al. Group II rhabdomyosarcoma and rhabdomyosarcoma-like tumors: is radiotherapy necessary? *J Clin Oncol* 2004;22:143–149.
95. Shapiro DN, Parham DM, Douglass EC, et al. Relationship of tumor cell ploidy to histologic subtype and treatment outcome in children and adolescents with unresectable rhabdomyosarcoma. *J Clin Oncol* 1991;9:159–166.
96. Shapiro DN, Sublett JE, Li B, et al. Fusion of PAX 3 to a member of the forkhead family of transcription factors in human alveolar rhabdomyosarcoma. *Cancer Res* 1993;53:5108–5112.
97. Shapiro DN, Valentine MB, Sublett JE, et al. Chromosomal sublocalization of the (2;13) translocation breakpoint in alveolar rhabdomyosarcoma. *Genes Chromosomes Cancer* 1991;4:241–249.
98. Smith LM, Anderson JR, Qualman SJ, et al. Which patients with rhabdomyosarcoma (RMS) and microscopic residual tumor (group II) fail therapy? A report from the Soft Tissue Sarcoma Committee of the Children's Oncology Group. *J Clin Oncol* 2001;19:4058–4064.
99. Spunt SL, Smith LM, Ruymann FB, et al. Cyclophosphamide dose intensification during induction therapy for intermediate–risk pediatric rhabdomyosarcoma is feasible but does not improve outcome: a report from the Soft Tissue Sarcoma Committee of the Children's Oncology Group. *Clin Cancer Res* 2004;10:6072–6079.
100. Stevens M, Rey A, Bouvet N, et al. Treatment of nonmetastatic rhabdomyosarcoma in childhood and adolescence: third study of the International Society of Paediatric Oncology—SIOP Malignant Mesenchymal Tumor 89. *J Clin Oncol* 2005;23:2618–2628.
101. Stewart RJ, Marelli H, Oberlin O, et al. Treatment of children with nonmetastatic paratesticular rhabdomyosarcoma: results of the Malignant Mesenchymal Tumors Studies (MMT 84 and MMT 89) of the International Society of Pediatric Oncology. *J Clin Oncol* 2003;21:793–798.
102. Sung L, Anderson JR, Donaldson SS, et al. Late events occurring five years or more after successful therapy for childhood rhabdomyosarcoma: a report from the Soft Tissue Sarcoma Committee of the Children's Oncology Group. *Eur J Cancer* 2004;40:1878–1885.

103. Tapscott SJ, Thayer MJ, Weintraub H: Deficiency in rhabdomyosarcomas of a factor required for MyoD activity and myogenesis. *Science* 1993;259:1450–1453.

104. Taylor AC, Shu L, Danks MK, et al. P53 mutation and MDM2 amplification frequency in pediatric rhabdomyosarcoma tumors and cell lines. *Med Pediatr Oncol* 2000;35:96–103.

105. Tefft M, Fernandez CH, Donaldson MH, et al. Incidence of meningeal involvement by rhabdomyosarcoma of the head and neck in children: a report of the Intergroup Rhabdomyosarcoma Study (IRS). *Cancer* 1978;48[suppl 2]:253–258.

106. Tefft M, Lindberg RD, Gehan EA: Radiation therapy combined with systemic chemotherapy of rhabdomyosarcoma in children: local control in patients enrolled in the Intergroup Rhabdomyosarcoma Study. *J Natl Cancer Inst Monogr* 1981;56:75–81.

107. Truener J, Kuhl J, Beck J, et al. New aspects in the treatment of childhood rhabdomyosarcoma: results of the German Cooperative Soft-Tissue Sarcoma Study (CWS-81). *Prog Pediatr Surg* 1989;22:162–173.

108. Tsokos M, Webber B, Parham D, et al. Rhabdomyosarcoma: a new classification scheme related to prognosis. *Arch Pathol Lab Med* 1992;116:847–855.

109. Valentine M, Douglass EC, Look AT. Closely linked loci on the long arm of chromosome 13 flank a specific 2;13 translocation breakpoint in childhood rhabdomyosarcoma. *Cytogenet Cell Genet* 1989;52:128–132.

110. van den Broeke LT, Pendleton CD, Mackall C, et al. Identification and epitope enhancement of a PAX-FKHR fusion protein breakpoint epitope in alveolar rhabdomyosarcoma cells created by a tumorigenic chromosomal translocation inducing CTL capable of lysing human tumors. *Cancer Res* 2006;66:1818–1823.

111. Wachtel M, Dettling M, Koscielniak E, et al. Gene expression signatures identify rhabdomyosarcoma subtypes and detect a novel t(2;2)(q35;p23) translocation fusing PAX3 to NCOA1. *Cancer Res* 2004;64:5539–5545.

112. Wachtel M, Runge T, Leuschner I, et al. Subtype and prognostic classification of rhabdomyosarcoma by immunohistochemistry. *J Clin Oncol* 2006;24:816–822.

113. Walterhouse DO, Meza JL, Raney RB, et al. Dactinomycin (A) and vincristine (V) with or without cyclophosphamide (C) and radiation therapy (RT) for newly diagnosed patients with low-risk embryonal/botryoid rhabdomyosarcoma (RMS). An IRS-V report from the Soft Tissue Sarcoma Committee of the Children's Oncology Group (STS COG). In press.

114. Whang-Peng J, Knutsen T, Theil K, et al. Cytogenetic studies in subgroups of rhabdomyosarcoma. *Genes Chromosomes Cancer* 1993;5:299–310.

115. Wharam MD, Beltangady M, Hays D, et al. Localized orbital rhabdomyosarcoma: an interim report of the Intergroup Rhabdomyosarcoma Study Committee. *Ophthalmology* 1987;94:251–254.

116. Wharam MD, Hanfelt JJ, Tefft MC, et al. Radiation therapy for rhabdomyosarcoma: local failure risk for clinical group III patients on Intergroup Rhabdomyosarcoma Study II. *Int J Radiat Oncol Biol Phys* 1997;38:797–804.

117. Wharam MD, Meza J, Anderson J, et al. Failure pattern and factors predictive of local failure in rhabdomyosarcoma: a report of group III patients on the third Intergroup Rhabdomyosarcoma Study. *J Clin Oncol* 2004;22:1902–1908.

118. Wiener ES: Rhabdomyosarcoma: New dimensions in management. *Semin Pediatr Surg* 1993;2:47–58.

119. Wiener ES, Anderson JR, Ojimba JI, et al. Is staging retroperitoneal lymph node dissection necessary for adolescents with resected paratesticular rhabdomyosarcoma? *Sem Pediatr Surg.* In press.

120. Wiener ES, Anderson JR, Ojimba JI, et al. Controversies in the management of paratesticular rhabdomyosarcoma: is staging retroperitoneal lymph node dissection necessary for adolescents with resected paratesticular rhabdomyosarcoma? *Semin Pediatr Surg* 2001;10:146–152.

121. Wiener E, Lawrence W, Hays D, et al. Survival is improved in clinical group III children with complete response established by second look operations in the Intergroup Rhabdomyosarcoma Study (IRS) III. *Med Pediatr Oncol* 1991;19:399.

122. Wiener ES, Lawrence W, Hays D, et al. Retroperitoneal node biopsy in paratesticular rhabdomyosarcoma. *J Pediatr Surg* 1994;29:171–177.

123. Wijnaendts LC, van der Linden JC, van Diest P, et al. Prognostic importance of DNA flow cytometric variables in rhabdomyosarcomas. *J Clin Pathol* 1993;46:948–953.

124. Wolden SL, Anderson JR, Crist WM, et al. Indications for radiotherapy and chemotherapy after complete resection in rhabdomyosarcoma: a report from the Intergroup Rhabdomyosarcoma Studies I to III. *J Clin Oncol* 1999;17:3468–3475.

125. Wolden SL, La TH, LaQuaglia MP, et al. Long-term results of three-dimensional conformal radiation therapy for patients with rhabdomyosarcoma. *Cancer* 2003;97:179–185.

126. Wolden SL, Wexler LH, Draus DH, et al. Intensity-modulated radiotherapy for head and neck rhabdomyosarcoma. *Int J Radiat Oncol Biol Phys* 2005;61:1432–1438.

127. Yock T, Schneider R, Friedmann A, et al. Proton radiotherapy for orbital rhabdomyosarcoma: clinical outcome and a dosimetric comparison with photons. *Int J Radiat Oncol Biol Phys* 2005;63:1161–1168.

128. Zhan S, Shapiro DN, Helman LJ. Activation of an imprinted allele of the insulin-like growth factor II gene implicated in rhabdomyosarcoma. *J Clin Invest* 1994;94:445–448.

Chapter 86
Ewing Tumor

Robert B. Marcus, Jr.

Epidemiology

Ewing tumor is the second most common primary tumor of bone in childhood, and also occurs in soft tissues. Ewing tumor is uncommon before 8 years of age and after 25 years of age (11). In the European Intergroup Cooperative Ewing Sarcoma Study group (EICESS), the median age was 14 years, with 57% of the patients male and 43% female, although a majority of the patients <10 years of age were female (11). The malignancy is rare in African Americans (37). In the EICESS, 24.7% of lesions presented in the pelvis, 16.4% in the femur, 16.7% below the knee, 12.1% in the ribs, 8.0% in the spine, and 4.8% in the humerus (11).

Pathology and Cytogenetics

Light microscopy shows a tumor of small, round, blue cells that lack markers for lymphoma, neuroblastoma, or rhabdomyosarcoma. Cytogenetics has shown that Ewing tumor of bone and soft tissue is the most undifferentiated member of a family of tumors that share a common neuroectodermal precursor cell, arrested at different stages of differentiation (63,76). Approximately 95% of Ewing tumors have a translocation between the EWS gene on chromosome 22 and the FLI1 gene on chromosome 11 (t[11:22][q24:q12]) or the ERG gene on chromosome 21 (t[21;22][q22;q12]) (64,72). The translocations are present only in tumor cells and occur in bone and soft tissue Ewing tumor, primitive neuroectodermal tumors of bone and soft tissue, peripheral primitive neuroectodermal tumors, Askin tumors, some esthesioneuroblastomas in children, and some CNS tumors (30). Intra-abdominal desmoplastic small round cell tumor appears to have a different translocation t(11;22)(p13;q12), indicating it is not one of these neoplasms (64). The proto-oncogene c-myc, not seen in neuroblastoma, is expressed in the Ewing family of tumors, whereas n-myc is not amplified (64).

Clinical Presentation

The most frequent presenting symptoms are pain and swelling. Pain can wax and wane as the tumor progresses. Symptoms of systemic disease occur at times, including low-grade fevers, malaise, and weakness. Ewing tumor patients exhibit a mean lag time of 146 days between the onset of symptoms and diagnosis, the longest lag time of any pediatric solid tumor (60). Both patients and physicians contribute to this delay.

Diagnostic Work-Up

In Ewing tumor of bone, plain films usually reveal a mottled or moth-eaten lesion. Lytic and blastic areas may be present; lytic areas are more commonly seen. Subperiosteal reactive new bone may be present, producing an "onion skin" appearance. Like an osteosarcoma, Ewing tumors may produce spicules radiating from the cortex of the involved bone, or expansion of the bone may produce a cystic-appearing tumor. Occasionally, the tumor may appear to arise on the surface of the bone, producing a saucerlike indentation of the surface (19). A magnetic resonance imaging (MRI) scan of the primary lesion will show the extent of bone marrow involvement and soft tissue invasion, whereas bone destruction is best seen using computed tomography (CT). The radiographic differential includes osteosarcoma, osteomyelitis, eosinophilic granuloma, primary lymphoma of the bone, and even an occasional metastatic malignancy.

The systemic work-up should include blood studies, a chest roentgenogram, a CT scan of the chest, a bone scan, and a bone marrow biopsy. Fluorodeoxyglucose positron emission tomography (PET) scans have been shown to detect considerably more bone metastases than traditional bone scans, both at diagnosis and recurrence. Because few lesions <8 mm are detectable using PET imaging, CT scans are still more accurate for the screening of lung metastases (29). Whole-body MRI has also been reported to be superior to bone scan in detecting bone metastases in patients with Ewing tumor (47).

Approximately 20% of patients present with metastatic disease. Of these patients, 44% present with lung metastases only; 51% have bone or bone marrow involvement (with or without lung metastases); and 5% present with metastases in other organs (11).

Prognostic Features

Metastases at diagnosis, a large or pelvic or truncal primary tumor, the presence of a large soft tissue mass, an older age at diagnosis, a poor response to induction chemotherapy, not using surgery as part of the treatment of the primary lesion, and a filigree histologic pattern have all been proposed as poor prognostic factors (1,3,5,6,11,22,46,65,77). These factors are interrelated; 90% of tumors in the pelvis and femur are usually large and have a large soft tissue mass, and occur more often in older adolescents and adults (33). The presence of necrosis on pretreatment MRI scans has been linked to an increased risk of metastases at diagnosis (15).

The radiologic or histologic response of the soft tissue mass to induction chemotherapy is an extremely good prognostic indicator (11,44,77). Ewing tumors with p53, p16/p14ARF alterations or the presence of vascular endothelial growth factor respond poorly to chemotherapy and have a poor prognosis (23,35). Overall, patients with the EWS-FLI1 fusion have a similar clinical presentation and prognosis to those with the less common EWS-ERG fusion (26). The EWS-FLI1 transcript can be detected in the peripheral blood or bone marrow, where it may indicate residual occult disease (4).

General Management

Effective local *and* systemic therapy is necessary for the cure of Ewing tumor. Most chemotherapy regimens are a combination of cyclophosphamide, doxorubicin HCl (Adriamycin), vincristine, dactinomycin, ifosfamide, and etoposide

(5,9,21,22,28,34,52,77). Induction chemotherapy is preferred over starting the systemic therapy and local therapy concomitantly. The advantages of this approach are several:

i. Giving the chemotherapy first allows an evaluation of the effectiveness of the regimen for each patient;

ii. Shrinkage of the soft tissue mass may help the surgeon or radiation oncologist decrease the volume of the local therapy; and

iii. Some bone healing takes place during the chemotherapy, which may diminish the risk of pathologic fracture if radiation therapy is used to treat the primary lesion.

Response rates to induction chemotherapy are high, with radiologic complete response and partial response rates of up to 90% reported (32,44,53). For institutions that use surgery for the treatment of the primary lesion, excellent necrosis rates have been reported in many patients (1,77). Almost all patients die whose lesions show a poor response either radiologically or histologically (1,44,77).

The biopsy should be performed in the same institution in which the treatment will be performed, and the biopsy specimen should only be taken from the soft tissue component, if present. Enough tissue should be collected for light and electron microscopy, as well as cytogenetics. In experienced hands, a large needle biopsy may be sufficient, although usually a larger sample is preferred.

For definitive therapy, limb-salvage surgery is preferable over amputation, but amputation may be an option for younger patients with lesions of the fibula, tibia, and foot. In older patients, lesions of the proximal fibula, ribs, scapula, clavicle, and wing of the ilium are easier to resect than other sites. Lesions of the bones of the hands and feet may be resectable with a ray resection. Other sites may be resectable with major reconstructive procedures and significant morbidity (70).

Radiotherapy Techniques

For gross disease, standard treatment is a total dose of 55.8 Gy at 1.8 Gy per day, with a field reduction at 45 Gy, although 36 Gy may be adequate for the initial field (7,13,45). Local control rates of 53% to 93% have been reported with these doses (Table 86.1). Local control at doses <40 Gy is significantly worse, even for small lesions (38).

Twice-a-day irradiation has been used in several trials. The University of Florida used 1.2 Gy twice a day to a total dose of 50.4 Gy, 55.2 Gy, or 60 Gy, depending on the tumor response to induction chemotherapy, and showed that late effects could be decreased, while maintaining good local control, even for large primary tumors (7,45). In CESS-86, doses of 1.6 Gy twice a day to a total of 60 Gy were given, although not in a continuous course. The Italian SE-91 trial also used 1.6 Gy twice a day to a total of 60.8 Gy, but in a continuous course. The CESS-86 trial showed no advantage for the accelerated hyperfractionated approach, but the early results of SE-91 are promising with regard to local control (16,62). Both of the latter regimens would be theoretically expected to increase late effects.

The Pediatric Oncology Group trial (POG 8346) showed in a randomized fashion that the traditional approach of irradiating the entire marrow cavity was not necessary (14). Although "tailored" fields are the standard of care today, attention to the requisite volume is critical to obtaining maximal control rates; geographic miss has been a frequent source of failure in cooperative group studies (14,65). Three-dimensional treatment planning is essential. The initial field should include the prechemotherapy tumor volume with a 2- to 4-cm margin. The boost should be to the residual tumor volume at the time of radiotherapy plus a 1.5- to 2.0-cm margin. PET-CT may be helpful for planning.

Extremity lesions require sparing at least a 1- to 2-cm strip of tissue to prevent lymphedema. This can be very difficult at times, particularly in arm lesions, although the arm is less likely to develop lymphedema than the leg. It may be necessary to consider surgery as an alternative if a strip of tissue cannot be spared. It is more important to cover the tumor adequately than to spare adjacent growth plates and joints.

With the high doses of cyclophosphamide or ifosfamide given in chemotherapy regimens for Ewing tumor, it is important to minimize the dose to the bladder. Radiation cystitis can be a significant risk even at doses as low as 20 Gy. Because pelvic lesions rarely infiltrate into the tissues around the bladder, but instead tend to push aside those structures, neoadjuvant chemotherapy allows additional bladder to be spared if good shrinkage is obtained. A 2-cm medial margin on the residual disease at the time of treatment is adequate from the beginning of radiation therapy.

Rib lesions should be treated conformally with a minimum of lung and heart in the high-dose field. However, rib primary tumors often present with pleural effusions, and in the EICESS and Children's Oncology Group (COG) trials hemithorax

		Local Control (%)			5-Year Survival (%)			
Trial	Years Open	RT	Surgery	Both	RT	Surgery	Both	Overall
IESS-1 (52)	1973–1978	—	—	—	—	—	—	50[a]
IESS-2 (9)	1978–1982	—	—	—	—	—	—	70[a]
IESS-2 (pelvic) (21)	1978–1982	85	91	100	59	73	62	63
CESS-81 (65)	1981–1985	53	91	80	44	55	67	50
CESS-86 (16)	1986–1991	86	100	95	70	66	74	70
UKCCSG ET-2 (12)	1987–1993	82	71	100	—	—	—	62
CCG/POG Intergroup I (27)	1988–1992	—	—	—	—	—	—	66[a]
CESS-81, 86, EICESS 92[b] (67)	1981–1999	74	96	92	—	—	—	—
SE 91-CNR (85)[c]	1991–1997	93	93	94	75[a]	77[a]	87[a]	—
CCG/POG Intergroup II (28)	1995–1998	—	—	—	—	—	—	79

Table 86.1 SURVIVAL AND LOCAL CONTROL BY METHOD OF TREATMENT TO PRIMARY LESIONS IN MAJOR COOPERATIVE GROUP TRIALS (LOCALIZED LESIONS ONLY)

RT, radiotherapy; IESS, Intergroup Ewing's Sarcoma Study; CESS, Cooperative Ewing's Sarcoma Study; UKCCSG, United Kingdom Children's Cancer Study Group; ET, Ewing tumor; SE 91-CNR, Italian Cooperative Study of Ewing Sarcoma; EICESS, European Intergroup Cooperative Ewing Sarcoma Study; CCG/POG, Children's Cancer Group and Pediatric Oncology Group.
[a]Estimated from results of individual arms.
[b]Combined; data for EICESS 92 alone not available.
[c]Only 3-year survival available.

irradiation was used, even for surgically resected lesions. A dose of 15 Gy for patients younger than 14 years and 20 Gy for older patients was given, corrected for lung transmission. In the EICESS 92 trial, the 7-year rate of event-free survival was 63% with hemithorax irradiation versus 46% without (66).

The standard dose for vertebral lesions in the United States is 45 Gy; it is not clear whether this decreases local control and survival rates. The average dose used in the CESS 81, CESS 86, and EICESS 92 trials was 49.6 Gy, although sometimes spinal shielding was used (68,74). In these trials, neurologic late effects were seen in 1 of 47 patients irradiated, occurring at a dose of 44.8 Gy at 1.6 Gy twice a day. Sacral lesions should be treated to full dose.

Doxorubicin and dactinomycin given during the course of radiation therapy will often cause moist desquamation, particularly with beams of 6 MV or less, tangential irradiation, or skin folds. These drugs may also cause a "recall" phenomenon of the dry or moist desquamation when given after the end of radiation therapy.

The indications for adjuvant radiotherapy with surgery are not completely defined. Jereb et al. (36) found that the local recurrence rate after conservative surgery was high without irradiation. Ozaki et al. (54) also reported a slight advantage for adding postoperative irradiation for patients with inadequate margins. Dunst and Schuck (18) reported that patients with a wide resection alone but a poor histologic response had a local failure rate of 12%, in comparison with 6% for similar patients who received postoperative radiotherapy. With present data, postoperative radiotherapy should probably be given to all patients with marginal margins and all with a poor histologic response. Intralesional surgery is not indicated as the EICESS trials showed no improvement in local control in patients with intralesional surgery plus radiotherapy versus radiotherapy alone (18).

In the COG trials, a dose of 50.4 Gy at 1.8 Gy once a day is given if postoperative radiotherapy is indicated. Doses in the range of 30 to 44.8 Gy at 1.8 Gy a day have also been reported to be effective for subclinical disease (48,54). Intralesional resections should be treated to the same dose as in patients receiving radiotherapy alone. Table 86.2 lists the recommended doses and fields for different clinical situations.

In a review of 153 patients treated with surgery followed by postoperative radiotherapy from CESS-86 and EICESS 92, Schuck et al. (69) showed that the interval between surgery and radiotherapy did not influence survival, although there was a slight trend for improved local control in patients receiving radiotherapy <90 days postoperatively.

Good results have also been reported with preoperative radiotherapy for patients with a poor response (<50% reduction of the evaluable soft tissue mass) after two cycles of chemotherapy (54,67). Doses of 36 to 63 Gy have been used (54).

Results of Therapy

The majority of studies reported in the literature reflect the results of therapy only for Ewing tumor of bone, since before 1991 soft-tissue Ewing tumors were treated on Intergroup Rhabdomyosarcoma Study protocols. The addition of chemotherapy to local therapy increased the survival for Ewing tumor of bone from <10% to >40% at 5 years for patients with localized disease at diagnosis (10). Modern protocols show better results, and Surveillance Epidemiology and End Results (SEER) data confirm this gradual improvement in survival rates over time. Five-year survival improved from 36% for patients treated from 1973 to 1977 to 59% for patients treated from 1993 to 1997 (20). However, late recurrences and deaths from complications continue to occur for years, yielding 10- and 15-year survival rates 10% to 15% lower than 5-year rates (25,44).

Local control and survival rates are shown in Table 86.1 for patients treated with different local control strategies in cooperative group trials that reported appropriate data. Surgery has become the treatment of choice for the primary lesion at most centers, and many series report superior local control for patients receiving surgery as a component of their local treatment, particularly if radiotherapy compliance was poor (14,65). The influence of different local control strategies on survival is less certain. In CESS-86, with good radiotherapy compliance, survival rates were not influenced by the method of therapy to the primary tumor (16). Other trials show an advantage for surgery or a combination of surgery and radiotherapy. With no

Table 86.2	**RECOMMENDATIONS FOR RADIATION THERAPY FIELDS AND DOSES**				
Clinical Situation		**Total Dose (%)**	**Dose Per Fraction (%)**	**Volume**	**Margin (cm)**
Gross disease (after biopsy only or intralesional resection)					
Treatment once a day	Initial field	45	1.8 q.d.	Original bone and soft tissue mass	2–4
	Boost field	10.8	1.8 q.d.	Original bone and *residual* soft tissue mass	2
Treatment twice a day	Initial field	36	1.2 b.i.d.	Original bone and soft tissue mass	2–4
	Boost field	19.2	1.2 b.i.d.	Original bone and *residual* soft tissue mass	2
After marginal resection or poor histologic response at surgery		41.4–45	1.8 q.d.	Original bone and soft tissue mass plus surgical scars and drains if feasible	2–4
Preoperative radiotherapy:		45	1.8 q.d.	Original bone and soft tissue mass	2–4
consider for patients with poor clinical response (<50% shrinkage of soft tissue mass) to induction chemotherapy		(doses as low as 35 have been successful)			

q.d., once a day; b.i.d., twice a day.

randomized studies addressing this question, and considerable selection going into the choice of local treatment, conclusions regarding the relative influence of different local therapies on survival are based more on opinion than fact (65).

However, systemic therapy does influence the rate of detectable local relapse. The first Intergroup Ewing's Sarcoma Study (IESS-I) reported that the addition of doxorubicin improved local control (58). The first Children's Cancer Group/Pediatric Oncology (CCG/POG) Group intergroup study showed an improvement in survival in the intensified arm for patients with localized disease and large primary or pelvic tumors. The improvement with the more intensive regimen was due to a decrease in the rate of local relapse; the rate of distant metastases was similar in both arms (28). The time interval between initiation of chemotherapy and start of radiotherapy has also been reported to influence survival (local control was not evaluated), with early radiotherapy preferable to late radiotherapy (18).

It is difficult to salvage patients who relapse, particularly those who relapse within the first 2 years after the beginning of therapy (11). Relapse occurring only at the local site warrants aggressive attempts at salvage (31). Patients who relapse only with lung metastases can sometimes be salvaged with additional chemotherapy and lung irradiation. Resecting the lung metastases if there are fewer than four lesions may also be beneficial (42). Patients with late pulmonary relapses fare better than those with early relapses (12). Patients who relapse with bone metastases, however, are essentially incurable with standard therapy.

Results of Clinical Trials for Patients with Localized Disease at Diagnosis

IESS-I showed that VACA chemotherapy (vincristine, dactinomycin, cyclophosphamide, and doxorubicin) produced superior 5-year relapse-free survival rates over a VAC (vincristine, dactinomycin, and cyclophosphamide) regimen alone. The third arm combined bilateral whole-lung irradiation (WLI) with VAC and produced survival rates better than VAC alone but less than VACA, indicating that bilateral WLI is an effective adjuvant, although it has not been studied in any subsequent trial except in patients with lung metastases at diagnosis (52). IESS-I also showed poorer survival rates in all arms for patients with pelvic tumors, and intensifying systemic therapy in IESS-II improved the results for pelvic tumors. IESS-II also showed that induction chemotherapy was a viable option (21). A trial at St. Jude Children's Research Hospital confirmed this approach, and it has since been the standard of care (32).

Based on data from previous trials (46), both the University of Florida and the German Cooperative Ewing Sarcoma Study stratified by tumor size and intensified treatment for large localized tumors. Although neither approach was randomized, both the University of Florida studies and CESS-86 found that intensifying treatment improved survival closer to the level as achieved with smaller primary lesions and less aggressive chemotherapy (44,45,57).

In the first CCG/POG intergroup study starting in 1988, a randomization between VACA chemotherapy alone versus VACA alternating with etoposide and ifosfamide showed that the addition of etoposide–ifosfamide improved the survival rates, particularly for patients with primary tumors of the pelvis (28). The United Kingdom Children's Cancer Study Group trials ET-1 and ET-2 showed a better survival rate in the ET-2 trial if ifosfamide was substituted for most of the cyclophosphamide used in ET-1. However, the dose intensity in ET-2 was also higher (12).

The second POG and CCG intergroup trial, accruing 483 eligible patients between 1995 and 1998, built on the previous

intergroup protocol. The 48-week vincristine, doxorubicin, cyclophosphamide, ifosfamide, and etoposide regimen was used as the standard arm, compared with the same drugs given in fewer cycles but with higher drug doses per cycle. There was no significant difference in survival rates in the two arms, with a 5-year event-free survival of 71% and an overall survival of 79% (27).

Raney et al. (61) reported the results of treating extraosseous Ewing tumors on the Intergroup Rhabdomyosarcoma Study until 1991. Long-term survival of these patients was probably better than for patients with bony primaries, with 10-year survival of 62%, 61%, and 77% for IRS-I, IRS-II, and IRS-III therapeutic protocols. Survival rates were better for patients with primary lesions of the head and neck, extremities, and trunk and for those with gross tumor removal.

Results of Clinical Trials for Patients with Metastatic Disease at Diagnosis

The prognosis of the patients with metastatic disease at diagnosis is poor. In a report from the EICESS, the 5-year relapse-free survival for patients with lung metastases only was 29%; for patients with bone and bone marrow metastases, it was 19%; and for patients with both lung and bone metastases at diagnosis, it was only 8% (11).

Although there was an improvement in survival rates in patients with localized disease treated on the first intergroup POG/CCG trial, the addition of ifosfamide-etoposide did not improve survival for patients with metastatic disease at diagnosis (50).

WLI improved survival on the CESS 81, CESS 86, and EICESS 92 trials for patients with lung metastases as the only site of metastatic disease at diagnosis (56). The CESS 81 and 86 studies also showed increasing survival rates with an increasing radiation dose to the lung fields, particularly with a dose of >18 Gy (corrected for lung transmission) at either 1.5 Gy once a day or 1.25 Gy twice a day. The dose to individual residual lesions was boosted (17). Bone metastases are usually irradiated if there are not too many. It is acceptable to delay the radiotherapy until close to the end of chemotherapy if a significant amount of bone marrow would be treated.

High-Dose Therapy with Stem Cell Rescue

End-intensification with megatherapy and stem cell rescue has been investigated by a large number of institutions, using high-dose chemotherapy with and without total-body irradiation. Patients with metastatic disease treated on EICESS studies between 1990 and 1995 had a superior 4-year event-free survival when megatherapy was added to the end of therapy, but CCG-7951 showed no improvement with this approach over a matched cohort from other Ewing tumor studies for patients with bone or bone marrow metastases (49,56). Some institutional pilot studies without strict selection criteria show promising but not conclusive results (34,39,44,59). The use of two sequential transplants (tandem transplants) has produced early promising results (41). Total-body irradiation has been reported to add to toxicity but not improve event-free survival (8,41).

A few institutions have used a single transplant to treat high-risk patients (large primary tumors or tumors of the pelvis or trunk) with localized disease. Five-year survival rates of 48% to 71% have been reported (34,41,43,44). Although the results are clearly better than standard treatment for similar high-risk groups treated historically, recent intensified regimens without end-intensification appear to give similar results

(1,27,28,44), showing that intensifying systemic therapy for patients with high-risk localized disease has improved survival rates, whether the intensification is with an ablative approach or more intensive conventional chemotherapy.

Sequelae of Treatment

Ewing tumor has been reported to have an actuarial complication rate of 70% at 35 years (24). Paulino et al. (55) reported that 10 (53%) of 19 patients receiving radiotherapy alone, four (25%) of 16 receiving surgery alone, and two (40%) of five who underwent combined surgery and radiation therapy had significant late effects (55). Neither study included loss of function related to planned surgical resection as a complication.

The most common skeletal complication of radiotherapy is abnormal growth and development of the irradiated tissues. Radiation can cause premature closure of active epiphyses, producing growth deficits and limb length discrepancies. The degree of discrepancy depends on radiation dose, patient's age, and the epiphysis radiated. Because 65% of leg growth is from the distal femoral (37%) and proximal tibial (28%) epiphyses, typical radiotherapy doses to the knee in boys younger than 14 years of age and girls younger than 12 years of age will usually cause a severe enough leg-length discrepancy to require intervention (2). Deficits of 2 to 6 cm can usually be managed by a shoe lift; larger deficits require surgical treatment (51).

Approximately 15% of long-bone lesions develop pathologic fractures at some time in their course, 5% at diagnosis and 10% after radiation therapy, although approximately one-third of the latter are caused by tumor recurrence or occasionally a secondary malignancy (75). Whether the fracture is disease- or treatment-related, the most common site is the femur, particularly the proximal femur. Radiotherapy-related fractures usually occur within 24 months after treatment, but can be much later. Doses below 40 Gy using once-a-day doses of 1.8 to 2.0 Gy appear to have a very low risk, as does a hyperfractionated approach using 1.2 Gy twice a day from 50.4 to 55.2 Gy (7,75).

Extremity weakness, decreased range of motion secondary to fibrosis, pain in the extremity (particularly in the early morning), discoloration of the skin, and lymphedema can also occur after radiotherapy, even with careful planning and sparing of an adequate strip of tissue.

The risk of secondary neoplasia at the site of the primary lesion is related to radiation therapy dose, with an increased risk at doses >60 Gy (40). Sarcomas, often osteosarcoma, are the most common second tumor, and the risk for megavoltage treatment has been reported as 1% to 4% at 20 years (40,52,71). With more intensive chemotherapy regimens and the increased use of etoposide, the risk of secondary leukemia is about 2% (27).

Future Considerations

Although the 5-year survival rate of patients with Ewing tumor appears to have improved since 1970, almost half of all patients diagnosed with Ewing tumor die of it within 10 years (20). Intensifying systemic treatment appears to improve survival, but the limits of intensification have probably been reached with the presently available drugs and the recently completed (in 2005) Children's Oncology Group Trial evaluating the role of interval compression chemotherapy, with each cycle given as soon as the counts recovered. No results have been released yet. The final results of the EICESS trial, assessing the role of etoposide, among other questions, have not been published either.

Topotecan is the most promising drug being tested (28). The combination of ifosfamide, carboplatin, and etoposide (ICE) appears to be useful for recurrent disease, but has not been thoroughly explored for newly diagnosed patients (73). In addition,

a number of institutions and cooperative groups continue to explore the use of megatherapy with stem cell rescue.

With regard to local therapy, the focus should be on improving function and decreasing the incidence of long-term sequelae. It is unlikely that refinements in local therapy with radiotherapy or surgery will significantly improve the cure rate. Metastases remain the primary mechanism of failure, and major improvements in the long-term survival rates will probably not occur until the development of better systemic agents or genetic therapy targeted at the unique translocations that produce these malignancies.

References

1. Ahrens S, Hoffmann C, Jabar S, et al. Evaluation of prognostic factors in a tumor volume-adapted treatment strategy for localized Ewing sarcoma of bone: the CESS 86 experience. *Med Pediatr Oncol* 1999;32:186–195.
2. Anderson M, Green WT, Messner MB. Growth and predictions of growth in the lower extremities. *J Bone Joint Surg* 1963;45A:1–14.
3. Aparicio J, Munarriz B, Pastor M, et al. Long-term follow-up and prognostic factors in Ewing's sarcoma. A multivariate analysis of 116 patients from a single institution. *Oncology* 1998;55:20–26.
4. Avigad S, Cohen IJ, Zilberstein J, et al. The predictive potential of molecular detection in the nonmetastatic Ewing family of tumors. *Cancer* 2004;100:1053–1058.
5. Bacci G, Picci P, Mercuri M, et al. Predictive factors of histological response to primary chemotherapy in Ewing's sarcoma. *Acta Oncol* 1998;37:671–676.
6. Barbieri E, Emiliani E, Zini G, et al. Combined therapy of localized Ewing's sarcoma of bone: analysis of results in 100 patients. *Int J Radiat Oncol Biol Phys* 1990;19:1165–1170.
7. Bolek TW, Marcus RB Jr, Mendenhall NP, et al. Local control and functional results after twice-daily radiotherapy for Ewing's sarcoma of the extremities. *Int J Radiat Oncol Biol Phys* 1996;35:687–692.
8. Burdach S, Meyer-Bahlburg A, Laws HJ, et al. High-dose therapy for patients with primary multifocal and early relapsed Ewing's tumors: results of two consecutive regimens assessing the role of total-body irradiation. *J Clin Oncol* 2003;21:3072–3078.
9. Burgert EO Jr, Nesbit ME, Garnsey LA, et al. Multimodal therapy for the management of nonpelvic, localized Ewing's sarcoma of bone: intergroup study IESS-II. *J Clin Oncol* 1990;8:1514–1524.
10. Chan RC, Sutow WW, Lindberg RD, et al. Management and results of localized Ewing's sarcoma. *Cancer* 1979;43:1001–1006.
11. Cotterill SJ, Ahrens S, Paulussen M, et al. Prognostic factors in Ewing's tumor of bone: analysis of 975 patients from the European Intergroup Cooperative Ewing's Sarcoma Study group. *J Clin Oncol* 2000;18:3108–3114.
12. Craft A, Cotterill S, Malcolm A, et al. Ifosfamide-containing chemotherapy in Ewing's sarcoma: the Second United Kingdom Children's Cancer Study Group and the Medical Research Council Ewing's Tumor Study. *J Clin Oncol* 1998;16:3628–3633.
13. Donaldson SS. Ewing sarcoma: radiation dose and volume. *Pediatr Blood Cancer* 2004;42:471–476.
14. Donaldson SS, Torrey M, Link MP, et al. A multidisciplinary study investigating radiotherapy in Ewing's sarcoma: end results of POG #8346. Pediatric Oncology Group. *Int J Radiat Oncol Biol Phys* 1998;42:125–135.
15. Dunst J, Ahrens S, Paulussen M, et al. Prognostic impact of tumor perfusion in MR-imaging studies in Ewing tumors. *Strahlenther Onkol* 2001;177:153–159.
16. Dunst J, Jurgens H, Sauer R, et al. Radiation therapy in Ewing's sarcoma: an update of the CESS 86 trial. *Int J Radiat Oncol Biol Phys* 1995;32:919–930.
17. Dunst J, Paulussen M, Jurgens H. Lung irradiation for Ewing's sarcoma with pulmonary metastases at diagnosis: results of the CESS-studies. *Strahlenther Onkol* 1993;169:621–623.
18. Dunst J, Schuck A. Role of radiotherapy in Ewing tumors. *Pediatr Blood Cancer* 2004;42:465–470.
19. Edeiken J, Karasick D. Imaging in bone cancer. *CA Cancer J Clin* 1987;37:239–245.
20. Esiashvili N, Goodman M, Marcus RB Jr. Incidence and survival of patients with Ewing sarcoma of bone over the past three decades based on surveillance epidemiology and end results data. 38th Annual Congress of International Society of Pediatric Oncology (SIOP), Geneva, Switzerland, 2006.
21. Evans RG, Nesbit ME, Gehan EA, et al. Multimodal therapy for the management of localized Ewing's sarcoma of pelvic and sacral bones: a report from the second intergroup study. *J Clin Oncol* 1991;9:1173–1180.
22. Fizazi K, Dohollou N, Blay JY, et al. Ewing's family of tumors in adults: multivariate analysis of survival and long-term results of multimodality therapy in 182 patients. *J Clin Oncol* 1998;16:3736–3743.
23. Fuchs B, Inwards CY, Janknecht R. Vascular endothelial growth factor expression is up-regulated by EWS-ETS oncoproteins and Sp1 and may represent an independent predictor of survival in Ewing's sarcoma. *Clin Cancer Res* 2004;10:1344–1353.
24. Fuchs B, Valenzuela RG, Inwards C, et al. Complications in long-term survivors of Ewing sarcoma. *Cancer* 2003;98:2687–2692.
25. Gasparini M, Lombardi F, Ballerini E, et al. Long-term outcome of patients with monostotic Ewing's sarcoma treated with combine modality. *Med Pediatr Oncol* 1994;23:406–412.
26. Ginsberg JP, de Alava E, Ladanyi M, et al. EWS-FLI1 and EWS-ERG gene fusions are associated with similar clinical phenotypes in Ewing's sarcoma. *J Clin Oncol* 1999;17:1809–1814.
27. Granowetter L. COG Public Report, 8/29/01. Available from: COG Statistical Center, 440 E Huntington Drive, Suite 300, Arcadia, CA 91006.
28. Grier HE, Krailo MD, Tarbell NJ, et al. Addition of ifosfamide and etoposide to standard chemotherapy for Ewing's sarcoma and primitive neuroectodermal tumor of bone. *N Engl J Med* 2003;348:694–701.
29. Gyorke T, Zajic T, Lange A, et al. Impact of FDG PET for staging of Ewing sarcomas and primitive neuroectodermal tumours. *Nucl Med Commun* 2006;27:17–24.

30. Hadfield MG, Quezado MM, Williams RL, et al. Ewing's family of tumors involving structures related to the central nervous system: a review. *Pediatr Dev Pathol* 2000;3:203–210.
31. Hayes FA, Thompson EI, Kumar M, et al. Long-term survival in patients with Ewing's sarcoma relapsing after completing therapy. *Med Pediatr Oncol* 1987;15:254–256.
32. Hayes FA, Thompson EI, Meyer WH, et al. Therapy for localized Ewing's sarcoma of bone. *J Clin Oncol* 1989;7:208–213.
33. Hense HW, Ahrens S, Paulussen M, et al. Factors associated with tumor volume and primary metastases in Ewing tumors; results from (EI)CESS studies. *Ann Oncol* 1999;10:1073–1077.
34. Horowitz ME, Kinsella TJ, Wexler LH, et al. Total-body irradiation and autologous bone marrow transplant in the treatment of high-risk Ewing's sarcoma and rhabdomyosarcoma. *J Clin Oncol* 1993;11:1911–1918.
35. Huang HY, Illei PB, Zhao Z, et al. Ewing sarcomas with p53 mutation or p16/p14ARF homozygous deletion: a highly lethal subset associated with poor chemoresponse. *J Clin Oncol* 2005;23:548–558.
36. Jereb B, Ong RL, Mohan M, et al. Redefined role of radiation in combined treatment of Ewing's sarcoma. *Pediatr Hematol Oncol* 1986;3:111–118.
37. Kissane JM, Askin FB, Foulkes M, et al. Ewing's sarcoma of bone: clinicopathologic aspects of 303 cases from the Intergroup Ewing's Sarcoma Study. *Hum Pathol* 1983;14:773–779.
38. Krasin MJ, Rodriguez-Galindo C, Billups CA, et al. Definitive irradiation in multidisciplinary management of localized Ewing sarcoma family of tumors in pediatric patients: outcome and prognostic factors. *Int J Radiat Oncol Biol Phys* 2004;60:830–838.
39. Kushner BH, Meyers PA. How effective is dose-intensive/myeloablative therapy against Ewing's sarcoma/primitive neuroectodermal tumor metastatic to bone or bone marrow? The Memorial Sloan-Kettering experience and a literature review. *J Clin Oncol* 2001;19:870–880.
40. Kuttesch JF Jr, Wexler LH, Marcus RB Jr, et al. Second malignancies after Ewing's sarcoma: radiation dose-dependency of secondary sarcomas. *J Clin Oncol* 1996;14:2818–2825.
41. Ladenstein R, Hartmann O, Pinkerton R, et al. A multivariate and match pair analysis on high risk Ewing tumor patients treated by megatherapy and stem cell reinfusion in Europe. In: Proceedings of the Annual Meeting of the American Society of Clinical Oncology, ASCO Meeting, Atlanta, GA, 1999;18:555(abstr).
42. Lanza LA, Miser JS, Pass HI, et al. The role of resection in the treatment of pulmonary metastases from Ewing's sarcoma. *J Thorac Cardiovasc Surg* 1987;94:181–187.
43. Madero L, Munoz A, Sanchez de Toledo J, et al. Megatherapy in children with high-risk Ewing sarcoma in first complete remission. *Bone Marrow Transplant* 1998;21:795–799.
44. Marcus RB Jr, Berrey BH, Graham-Pole J, et al. The treatment of Ewing's sarcoma of bone at the University of Florida: 1969 to 1998. *Clin Orthop Relat Res* 2002;397:290–297.
45. Marcus RB Jr, Cantor A, Heare TC, et al. Local control and function after twice-a-day radiotherapy for Ewing's sarcoma of bone. *Int J Radiat Oncol Biol Phys* 1991;21:1509–1515.
46. Marcus RB Jr, Million RR. The effect of primary tumor size on the prognosis of Ewing's sarcoma. *Int J Radiat Oncol Biol Phys* 1984;10[suppl 2]:88(abstr 24).
47. Mentzel HJ, Kentouche K, Sauner D, et al. Comparison of whole-body STIR-MRI and ^{99m}Tc-methylene-diphosphonate scintigraphy in children with suspected multifocal bone lesions. *Eur Radiol* 2004;14:2297–2302.
48. Merchant TE, Kushner BH, Sheldon JM, et al. Effect of low-dose radiation therapy when combined with surgical resection for Ewing sarcoma. *Med Pediatr Oncol* 1999;33:65–70.
49. Meyers PA, Krailo MD, Ladanyi M, et al. High-dose melphalan, etoposide, total-body irradiation, and autologous stem-cell reconstitution as consolidation therapy for high-risk Ewing's sarcoma does not improve prognosis. *J Clin Oncol* 2001;19:2812–2820.
50. Miser JS, Krailo MD, Tarbell NJ, et al. Treatment of metastatic Ewing's sarcoma or primitive neuroectodermal tumor of bone: evaluation of combination ifosfamide and etoposide—a Children's Cancer Group and Pediatric Oncology Group study. *Clin Oncol* 2004;22:2873–2876.
51. Moseley CF. Leg-length discrepancy. In: Morrissy RT, ed. *Lovell and Winter's pediatric orthopaedics*, 3rd ed, vol 2. Philadelphia: Lippincott; 1990: 767–813.
52. Nesbit ME Jr, Gehan EA, Burgert EO Jr, et al. Multimodal therapy for the management of primary, nonmetastatic Ewing's sarcoma of bone: a long-term follow-up of the first intergroup study. *J Clin Oncol* 1990;8:1664–1674.

53. Oberlin O, Patte C, Demeocq F, et al. The response to initial chemotherapy as a prognostic factor in localized Ewing's sarcoma. *Eur J Cancer Clin Oncol* 1985;21:463–467.
54. Ozaki T, Hillman A, Hoffmann C, et al. Significance of surgical margin on the prognosis of patients with Ewing's sarcoma. A report from the Cooperative Ewing's Sarcoma Study. *Cancer* 1996;78:892–900.
55. Paulino AC, Nguyen TX, Mai WY. An analysis of primary site control and late effects according to local control modality in non-metastatic Ewing sarcoma. *Pediatr Blood Cancer* 2007;48(4):423–429.
56. Paulussen M, Ahrens S, Craft AW, et al. Ewing's tumors with primary lung metastases: survival analysis of 114 (European Intergroup) Cooperative Ewing's Sarcoma Studies patients. *J Clin Oncol* 1998;16:3044–3052.
57. Paulussen M, Ahrens S, Dunst W, et al. Localized Ewing tumor of bone: final results of the Cooperative Ewing's Sarcoma Study CESS 86. *J Clin Oncol* 2001;19:1818–1829.
58. Perez CA, Tefft M, Nesbit ME Jr, et al. Radiation therapy in the multimodal management of Ewing's sarcoma of bone: report of the Intergroup Ewing's Sarcoma Study. *Nat Cancer Inst Monogr* 1981;56:263–271.
59. Pinkerton CR, Bataillard A, Guillo S, et al. Treatment strategies for metastatic Ewing's sarcoma. *Eur J Cancer* 2001;37:1338–1344.
60. Pollock BH, Krischer JP, Vietti TJ. Interval between symptom onset and diagnosis of pediatric solid tumors. *J Pediatr* 1991;119:725–732.
61. Raney RB, Asmar L, Newton WA Jr, et al. Ewing's sarcoma of soft tissues in childhood: a report from the Intergroup Rhabdomyosarcoma Study, 1972 to 1991. *J Clin Oncol* 1997;15:574–582.
62. Rosito P, Mancini AF, Rondelli R, et al. Italian Cooperative Study for the treatment of children and young adults with localized Ewing sarcoma of bone: a preliminary report of 6 years of experience [published correction appears in *Cancer* 2005;104:667]. *Cancer* 1999;86:421–428.
63. Sandberg AA, Bridge JA. *The cytogenetics of bone and soft tissue tumors*. Austin, TX: R.G. Landes Company; 1994: 303.
64. Sandberg AA, Bridge JA. Updates on the cytogenetics and molecular genetics of bone and soft tissue tumors: Ewing sarcoma and peripheral primitive neuroectodermal tumors. *Cancer Genet Cytogenet* 2000;123:1–26.
65. Sauer R, Jürgens H, Burgers JMV, et al. Prognostic factors in the treatment of Ewing's sarcoma. The Ewing's Sarcoma Study Group of the German Society of Paediatric Oncology CESS 81. *Radiother Oncol* 1987;10:101–110.
66. Schuck A, Ahrens S, Konarzewska A, et al. Hemithorax irradiation for Ewing tumors of the chest wall. *Int J Radiat Oncol Biol Phys* 2002;54:830–838.
67. Schuck A, Ahrens S, Paulussen M, et al. Local therapy in localized Ewing tumors: results of 1058 patients treated in the CESS 81, CESS 86, and EICESS 92 trials. *Int J Radiat Oncol Biol Phys* 2003;55:168–177.
68. Schuck A, Ahrens S, von Schorlemer I, et al. Radiotherapy in Ewing tumors of the vertebrae: treatment results and local relapse analysis of the CESS 81/86 and EICESS 92 trials. *Int J Radiat Oncol Biol Phys* 2005;63:1562–1567.
69. Schuck A, Rube C, Konemann S, et al. Postoperative radiotherapy in the treatment of Ewing tumors: influence of the interval between surgery and radiation. *Strahlenther Onkol* 2002;178:25–31.
70. Scully SP, Temple HT, O'Keefe RJ, et al. Role of surgical resection in pelvic Ewing's sarcoma. *J Clin Oncol* 1995;13:2336–2341.
71. Tucker MA, D'Angio GJ, Boice JD Jr, et al. Bone sarcomas linked to radiotherapy and chemotherapy in children. *N Engl J Med* 1987;317:588–593.
72. Turc-Carel C, Aurias A, Mugneret F, et al. Chromosomes in Ewing's sarcoma: I. An evaluation of 85 cases and remarkable consistency of t(11; 22)(q24;q12). *Cancer Genet Cytogenet* 1988;32:229–238.
73. Van Winkle P, Angiolillo A, Krailo M, et al. Ifosfamide, carboplatin, and etoposide (ICE) reinduction chemotherapy in a large cohort of children and adolescents with recurrent/refractory sarcoma: the Children's Cancer Group Experience. *Pediatr Blood Cancer* 2005;44:338–347.
74. Venkateswaran L, Rodriguez-Galindo C, Merchant TE, et al. Primary Ewing tumor of the vertebrae: clinical characteristics, prognostic factors, and outcome. *Med Pediatr Oncol* 2001;37:30–35.
75. Wagner LM, Neel MD, Pappo AS, et al. Fractures in pediatric Ewing sarcoma. *J Pediatr Hematol Oncol* 2001;23:568–571.
76. Whang-Peng J, Freter CE, Knutsen T, et al. Translocation t(11;22) in esthesioneuroblastoma. *Cancer Genet Cytogenet* 1987;29:155–157.
77. Wunder JS, Paulian G, Huvos A, et al. The histological response to chemotherapy as a predictor of the oncological outcome of operative treatment of Ewing sarcoma. *J Bone Joint Surg Am* 1998;80:1020–1033.

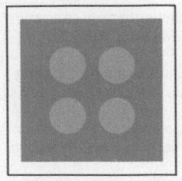

Chapter 87
Lymphomas in Children

Melissa M. Hudson, Barbara L. Asselin, Louis S. Constine

The childhood lymphomas are gratifying to treat because of their curability. Central to this progress has been single and multi-institutional clinical trials that, in turn, have benefited from advances in our understanding of the normal immune system and in diagnostic imaging and pathology. The primary focus of pediatric trials in the past decade has been stratification of patients into risk groups to refine treatment as follows: (a) less morbid therapy in children with a favorable prognosis, and (b) intensification of therapy in children with an unfavorable prognosis.

Commensurate with the increasingly effective use of chemotherapy has been a more restrictive role for radiotherapy. Our recognition of the long-term sequelae of therapy has, of course, played a prominent role in the development of effective treatment strategies.

Hodgkin's Disease

Historically, children with Hodgkin's disease (HD) were thought to have a worse prognosis than adults—a misconception relating to treatment approaches initially used for children (88). In fact, the converse may be true (32,42,92,156,177). Moreover, when irradiation techniques and doses used in adults were administered to children, substantial morbidities (primarily musculoskeletal growth inhibition) were produced (43,119). Contemporary treatment programs use a risk-adapted approach in which patients receive varying intensities of multiagent chemotherapy and low-dose involved field irradiation (11,13, 14,17,50,53,54,77,79,81,85,99,106,131,133,156,158,166,169, 179,187,194,195,199,200,202,203). It is now clear that the vast majority of children with HD can be cured, prompting increased attention to devising nonmorbid therapy for these patients. Considering the excellent outcome for the majority of children and adolescents diagnosed with HD, the identification of biologic factors predicting very good or very poor outcome is critical to direct future refinements in therapy.

Epidemiology

Lymphomas are the third most common form of childhood cancer, comprising 15% of cancer diagnoses in individuals younger than age 20 years. Overall, pediatric HD is more common than non-Hodgkin's lymphoma, with an annual incidence rate of 12.8 per 1 million children (≤19 years old) (142).

Childhood HD has unique epidemiologic presentations that vary geographically:

- The childhood form occurs in patients age 14 years or younger. It is rare in children <4 years of age, usually occurring in children >10 years. The childhood form of HD is associated with increasing family size and decreasing socioeconomic status. Early and intense exposure to an infectious agent has been speculated to increase the risk for the childhood form of HD (30,56).
- The young adult form affects patients aged 15 to 34 years and has a roughly equal incidence between older adolescent males and females. In contrast to childhood HD,

young adult HD is associated with a higher socioeconomic status, as found in developed countries. The risk for young adult HD also decreases significantly with increased sibship size and later birth order (204). Delayed exposure to an infectious agent has been proposed as a risk factor for the development of young adult HD because its epidemiologic features are similar to that seen with paralytic poliomyelitis (56). However, Chang et al. (30) demonstrated that early exposure to other children at nursery school and day care seems to decrease the risk of young adult HD, most likely by facilitating childhood exposure to common infections and promoting maturation of cellular immunity.

Biology

HD is unique among the lymphomas because the malignant Hodgkin and Reed-Sternberg (HRS) cells, lymphocytic and histiocytic (L&H) cells, and their variants account for <1% of the tumor cell population. Identical immunologic gene rearrangements in HRS and L&H cells support their origin from a single transformed B-cell that subsequently undergoes monoclonal expansion (66,97,144). Two distinct immunophenotypes of HD exist. The first immunophenotype, characteristic of L&H cells, consistently expresses CD20 and J chain and does not express CD30 and CD15 (117,144). The second immunophenotype, characteristic of HRS cells, consistently expresses CD30, frequently expresses CD15, and does not express J chain. These immunophenotypes differentiate lymphocyte-predominant HD from classical HD, as outlined in the revised European–American classification of lymphoid neoplasms (70). Substantial data exist to support a strong association between HD and the Epstein-Barr virus (EBV) (3,57). The incidence of EBV-associated HD varies by age, gender, ethnicity, histologic subtype, and regional economic level (57). EBV-positive tumor genomes are more frequent in children younger than 10 years of age and in those who live in developing countries (see Chapter 75). HD is also associated with congenital (e.g., ataxia telangiectasia) and acquired (e.g., human immunodeficiency virus [HIV]) immunodeficiency states (52). Familial cases of HD suggest a genetic predisposition to the disease or a common environmental exposure. Concordance of HD has been observed in first-degree relatives (particularly of the same gender) and in parent–child pairs (109).

Pathologic Classification

The Rye classification subcategorizes HD into four pathologic subtypes: nodular sclerosing (NS), mixed cellularity (MC), lymphocyte predominance (LP), and lymphocyte depletion (LD). With modern treatment, the prognostic significance of these subtypes has diminished. The presenting characteristics and natural history remain evident, particularly for the nodular subtype of LPHD (nLPHD). The importance of distinguishing nLPHD from the other types has led to the Revised European–American classification (REAL), in which nLPHD is separated from "classic disease," which includes lymphocyte-rich classic disease, NS, MC, and LD (70). The pathologic characteristics are the same as in adults and are described in Chapter 75. The relative

Table 87.1	DISTRIBUTION OF PATHOLOGIC SUBTYPES OF HODGKIN'S DISEASE ACCORDING TO PATIENT AGE		
	Age =10 Years	11–16 Years	= 17 Years
Number of patients	91 (4%)	235 (11%)	1,912 (85%)
Male-to-female ratio	4:1	1:1	3:2
Histology			
Nodular sclerosing	44%	77%	72%
Mixed cellularity	33%	11%	17%
Lymphocyte predominance	13%	8%	5%
Lymphocyte depletion	0%	1%	1%
Unclassified/interfollicular	10%	3%	5%

From Cleary S, Link M, Donaldson S. Hodgkin's disease in the very young. *Int J Radiat Oncol Biol Phys* 1994;28:77–84, with permission. Copyright 1994 by Elsevier Science, Inc.

distribution of the subtypes differs in younger children, compared with adolescents and adults, as shown in an analysis of 2,238 patients treated at Stanford University (32). LP is relatively more common (13%) in children younger than age 10, whereas LD is exceedingly rare. Although NS is the most common subtype in all age groups, it is more frequent in adolescents (77%) and adults (72%) than in younger children (44%). Conversely, MC is more common in younger children (33%) than in adolescents (11%) or adults (17%) (Table 87.1) (32).

Clinical Presentation

Most children (80%) present with cervical lymphadenopathy. Mediastinal involvement is present in 76% of adolescents but only in 33% of children aged 1 to 10 years (88). Occasionally patients are diagnosed after the onset of respiratory distress, although isolated mediastinal disease is rare as is isolated infradiaphragmatic HD, both occurring in <5% of patients. One third of patients have one or more of the so-called B symptoms at diagnosis (unexplained fever >38°C and recurrent during the previous month, night sweats recurrent during the previous month, and/or weight loss of more than 10% in the 6 months preceding diagnosis) (36,88). Cytokine production induced by the HRS cells are responsible for a variety of other clinical and pathologic features of HD including anorexia, pruritus, fibrosis, eosinophilia, thrombocytosis, plasmacytosis, and immunodeficiency (87).

Diagnostic Work-Up

The diagnosis of HD is made by lymph node biopsy and is confirmed pathologically by the presence of HRS cells and their mononuclear variants. The diagnosis is facilitated through an excisional lymph node biopsy, which enables evaluation of the malignant HRS cells within the characteristic architectural changes associated with the specific histologic subtypes. The recommended procedures for pretreatment evaluation of the child with HD are similar to those for the adult. Because bone marrow involvement at initial presentation is uncommon and rarely occurs as an isolated site of extranodal disease, bone marrow biopsy can be restricted to patients with B symptoms or stage III or IV disease.

Imaging studies of the thorax include a chest radiograph and a computed tomography (CT) scan, which alters treatment decisions in at least 10% of patients through delineation of radiographically inapparent disease involving subcarinal, hilar, or cardiophrenic angle nodes, and in extranodal sites (pleura, chest wall, or pericardium). Using the ratio of the measurement of the mediastinal mass to the maximum diameter of the thoracic cavity on an upright chest radiograph is a standard

method to assess mediastinal bulk. Patients with bulky disease, as defined by a mediastinal ratio of ≥33%, may benefit from a combined-modality treatment approach. Nuclear imaging studies such as positron emission tomography (PET) scanning are helpful in staging and monitoring treatment response, particularly in cases with persistent radiographic abnormalities or "rebound" thymic growth after completion of therapy (153).

Abdominopelvic CT scanning, magnetic resonance imaging (MRI), or lymphography (LAG) can be used to assess infradiaphragmatic disease. The optimal CT evaluation requires oral and intravenous contrast agents to distinguish lymphadenopathy from other infradiaphragmatic structures. CT evaluation of abdominopelvic disease may be compromised in suboptimally contrasted studies and in children who lack retroperitoneal fat. In these cases, MRI may provide better assessment of disease involvement in the retroperitoneal lymph nodes (69). LAG, which is the only imaging modality that assesses internal nodal architecture, can differentiate large normal reactive nodes and small lymphomatous nodes. However, the procedure has largely been abandoned because it is invasive and requires specific expertise to interpret and perform.

Splenic and hepatic involvement by HD is suggested by the presence of enlarged organs with areas of abnormal density on CT or MRI scans. The degree of lymphomatous involvement of the spleen and liver may not correlate with organ size because tumor deposits may be <1 cm and not visualized by diagnostic imaging modalities. Liver function studies are also unreliable indicators of hepatic disease. Histologic assessment is required to unequivocally diagnose involvement in the liver and spleen. However, because of the common use of chemotherapy in contemporary pediatric treatment regimens, surgical staging of these organs currently has limited indications.

Surgical staging, based on the histologic findings of a laparotomy with retroperitoneal nodal sampling and splenectomy, was used routinely from 1970 to 1990 at many centers. The benefits of staging laparotomy were emphasized after the appreciation of subclinical splenic disease at presentation in an unexpectedly high number of patients. However, by the end of the 1980s, several factors motivated the change from surgical to clinical staging at most pediatric centers:

(a) Newer diagnostic imaging modalities provided more accurate assessment of the retroperitoneal lymphatics,
(b) Histologic confirmation of microscopic retroperitoneal disease became unnecessary with the increasing use of chemotherapy, and
(c) Appreciation of long-term infectious and neoplastic complications after splenectomy motivated the desire to maintain intact splenic function.

Consequently, staging laparotomy has been abandoned as a standard modality in staging pediatric HD, although limited nodal sampling without splenectomy may be pursued if findings will significantly affect treatment planning.

Staging Systems

As for adults, children with HD are staged according to the system devised at the Ann Arbor Staging Conference in 1970. This was revised most recently at the Cotswolds Meeting. Refer to Chapter 75 for complete staging information.

The distribution of stages observed in children is different from that in adults. Among 2,238 consecutive patients with HD treated at Stanford, stage I or II disease was present in about 60%. Stage I disease was slightly more common in younger children (18%) than in adolescents (8%); stage II disease occurred in 40% to 50% of all age groups, and stage IV disease was less common in younger children (3%) than in adolescents (15%). B symptoms occurred in 19% of younger children and in 30% of adolescents (32).

Prognostic Factors

As the treatment of HD has improved, the factors that influenced outcome have diminished in importance. However, several factors continue to influence the choice and success of therapy. These factors are interrelated in that disease stage, bulk, and biologic aggressiveness are frequently codependent (183,185). A further complication in the determination of prognostic factors is that relevant variables often depend on staging evaluation and treatment. Thus, the prognostic variables for clinically staged patients are different from those for pathologically staged patients. Similarly, patients with early stage disease have different prognosticators than patients with advanced stage disease (185). Illustrating the complexity of this subject are data from Stanford University that specifically address prognostic factors in 320 children with clinical stage I to IV disease treated with combined-modality therapy at three institutions in the past decade. On univariate analysis stage IV, nodular sclerosing Hodgkin's disease, B symptoms, white blood cell count (WBC) of $\geq 11,500/mm^3$, hemoglobin ≤ 11.0 g/dL, bulky mediastinal disease, extranodal disease, and erythrocyte sedimentation rate (ESR) ≥ 50 mm per hour were significant for inferior disease-free survival (DFS) and overall survival (OS). By multivariate analysis, male gender; stage IIB, IIIB, or IV disease; WBC $\geq 11,500/mm^3$; and hemoglobin ≤ 11.0 g/dL were significant for inferior DFS and OS. Prognosis was associated with the number of adverse factors (181).

We list here some generalizations regarding prognostic variables derived from both adult and pediatric data:

- *Stage of disease* is the most significant prognosticator of treatment outcome. Stage IV disease with multiple organ involvement confers an exceptionally poor prognosis when managed with conventional therapy (10,181).
- *Bulk of disease* is reflected in the disease stage but more specifically is determined by the volume of distinct areas of involvement and the number of disease sites. Large mediastinal adenopathy (LMA), defined as a mass of more than one third of the thoracic diameter, is associated with an increased risk of disease recurrence particularly when managed with radiation therapy alone (16,88,114,118,184). However, overall survival remains high because of the effectiveness of salvage chemotherapy (16,114,184). Clinically (but not pathologically) staged patients with multiple sites of involvement (usually defined as three or more sites) have an inferior freedom from relapse and survival in some but not all reports (59,74,118,184).
- *Presence of systemic symptoms* (B disease), which result from cytokine secretion, reflects biologic aggressiveness and correlates with an increased risk of relapse compared with the absence of such symptoms (A disease) (36,181). The constellation of symptoms appears to be relevant to this observation; that is, patients with night sweats only (at least among patients with PSI-II disease) appear to fare as well as PSI-IIA patients, whereas those with both fever and weight loss have the worst prognosis (36).
- *Abnormally high levels of certain serum markers* have been reported to be prognosticators of a negative outcome (130). Whether the elevated levels are caused by more malignant biology of disease or by increased tumor volume is unclear. Recent data from Stanford support an association between anemia and an elevated WBC with prognosis (181). In most reports, independent prognostic significance for serum markers is unproven except in select clinical scenarios (e.g., decreased serum albumin CSI-IIB disease) (185).
- *Histologic subtype* may correlate with prognosis. LD histology confers a worse outcome than do the other subtypes, but it is exceedingly rare (184). MC disease is asso-

ciated with an increased risk of subdiaphragmatic relapse in pathologically staged patients who have disease apparently confined to supradiaphragmatic areas. Patients with LP histology are more commonly early stage (22). However, in a 1997 report from the United Kingdom Children's Cancer Study Group (UKCCSG) assessing the relevance of histology in 331 children, no associations with outcome were seen (179).
- Finally, *patient age* appears to be a determinant of patient outcome (32,95). Children younger than 10 years of age have been observed to fare better than older patients (32). Younger children are more likely to have early stage or A disease, which may, in part, explain their superior prognosis (32).

The use of these prognostic factors is reflected in the risk grouping that various pediatric trials employ for assignment of therapy. Such stratification is discussed below in the "Risk-adapted Therapy" section and are reflected in the summary treatment recommendations.

General Management

Although HD is one of the few pediatric malignancies that has an adult counterpart with similar natural history and biology, determination of the optimal therapeutic approach for children with this disease is complicated by their increased risk for adverse treatment-related side effects. In particular, radiation therapy doses and fields used in adults can produce significant musculoskeletal growth retardation, described later in this chapter (43,119). Consequently, the various successful approaches to treatment of HD in children (Tables 87.2, 87.3, and 87.4) must be considered in terms of efficacy and morbidity, and this is influenced by the developmental status of the patient.

Radiation Therapy

The establishment of a curative dose range (33 to 44 Gy) and standardized anatomic treatment fields produced the first cures in patients with HD. Appreciation of the contiguous pattern of nodal spread in the disease promoted the concept of extended radiation treatment volumes. Initially, treatment programs were similar for adults and children. Surgical staging was routinely recommended at most centers because of concern about undertreating patients with occult abdominal disease. Five-year DFS rates following standard-dose radiation therapy in pathologically staged children with early stage disease ranged from 60% to 80% (Table 87.4) (13,14,45,54). However, with longer follow-up, pediatric investigators began to appreciate the morbidity associated with standard-dose irradiation in the prepubertal child (43).

Growth impairment of irradiated skeletal and soft tissues was the initial impetus for the development of combined-modality treatment programs prescribing non–cross-resistant chemotherapy and reduced radiation doses in pediatric patients. These regimens reduced the dose-related toxicity of both chemotherapeutic agents and radiation therapy and improved DFS in advanced stage patients (43,53,77,79,81,202,203). Treatment with standard-dose radiation therapy alone was reserved for physically mature adolescents who presented with localized disease. Following the observation of radiation-associated cardiovascular disease and solid tumor malignancies in aging survivors of childhood HD (16,60,67,68), advances in radiation technology and diagnostic imaging led to further modifications of radiation therapy permitting involved-field treatment approaches and more effective shielding of normal tissues. Even in full-grown adolescents, treatment with standard-dose radiation therapy alone has been largely abandoned by most

Table 87.2 | TREATMENT RESULTS OF COMBINED-MODALITY TRIALS OF PEDIATRIC HODGKIN'S DISEASE

Chemotherapy/ Study (Reference)	Radiation Therapy	Stage	No. of Patients	EFS	DFS	RFS/FFP	Survival
Stanford							
3 MOPP/3 ABVD (79)	15–25.5 Gy, IF	CS/PS I–IV	57	96 (10)	—	—	93 (10)
6 MOPP (43)	15–25.5 Gy, IF	PS I–IV	55	—	—	90 (15)	89 (15)
St. Jude							
4–5 COP(P)/3–4 ABVD (77)	20 Gy, IF	CS II–IV	85	—	93 (5)	—	93 (5)
Toronto							
6 MOPP (85)	20–30 Gy, EF	CS IIA–IV	57	—	—	80 (10)	85 (10)
Children's Cancer Group							
6 ABVD (81)	21 Gy, EF	PS III–IV	54	87 (4)	—	—	90 (4)
12 ABVD (53)	21 Gy, R	PS III–IV	64	87 (3)	—	—	89 (3)
4 COPP/ABV (129)	21 Gy, IF	CS IA/IB,IIA	294	100	—	—	100
6 COPP/ABV (129)	+/– 21 Gy, IF	CS I/II adverse, CS IIB, III	394	88 (IF)	—	—	95 (IF)
COPP/ABV, CHOP, Ara-C/VP-16 (129)	+/– 21 Gy, IF	CS IV	141	91 (IF)	—	—	100 (IF)
Pediatric Oncology Group							
4 MOPP/4 ABVD (202)	21 Gy, EF	CS/PS IIB, IIIA$_2$, IIIB–IV	80	80 (5)	—	—	87 (5)
4 MOPP/4 ABVD (203)	21 Gy, TLI	CS/PS IIB, IIIA$_2$, IIIB, IV	62	77 (3)	—	—	91 (3)
DBVE (191)	25.5 Gy, IF	CS/PS I/II/IIIA	51	91	—	—	98
Intergroup Hodgkin's							
6 MOPP (54)	=35 Gy, IF	PS I–II	97	—	—	95 (5)	90 (5)
Gustave-Roussy (131)							
			60	—	—	86% (5)	93 (5)
3 MOPP	40 Gy, IF	All stages	40	—	—	—	—
6 MOPP	40 Gy, IF	—	20	—	—	—	—
SFOP MDH-82 (132)							
			238	—	86 (6)	—	92 (6)
4 ABVD	20–40 Gy, IF	CS I–IIA	79	—	89 (6)	90 (6)	—
2 MOPP/2 ABVD	20–40 Gy, IF	CS I–IIA	67	—	89 (6)	87 (6)	—
3 MOPP/3 ABVD	20–40 Gy, EF	CS IB–IIB	31	—	89 (6)	—	—
3 MOPP/3 ABVD	20–40 Gy, EF	CS III	40	—	82 (6)	—	—
3 MOPP/3 ABVD	20–40 Gy, EF	CS IV	21	—	62 (6)	—	—
SFOP MDH-90 (99)							
	—	—	202	1 (5)	—	—	98 (5)
4 VBVP, good responders	20 Gy, IF	I–II	171	91	—	—	—
4 VBVP + 1–2 OPPA, poor responders	20 Gy, IF	I–II	27	78	—	—	—
AEIOP-MH-83 (199)							
			215	—	—	82 (7)	86 (7)
Group A			83			95	—
3 ABVD	20–40 Gy, IF	IA	—	—	—	—	—
3 ABVD	20–40 Gy, R	IIA (M/T <0.33)	—	—	—	—	—
Group B			83			81	
3 MOPP/3 ABVD	20–40 Gy, R	IIA (M/T = 0.33)	—	—	—	—	—
3 MOPP/3 ABVD	20–40 Gy, EF	IIIA	—	—	—	—	—
Group C							
5 MOPP/5 ABVD	20–40 Gy, EF	IIIB–IV	49	—	—	60	—
Germany-Austria							
HD-82							
2 OPPA (167)	35 Gy, IF	IA/IB–IIA	100	98 (9)	—	—	100 (9)
2 OPPA/2 COPP	30 Gy, IF	IIB–IIIA	53	94	—	—	96
2 OPPA/4 COPP	25 Gy, IF	IIIB–IV	50	86	—	—	85
HD-85							
2 OPA (167)	35 Gy, IF	IA/IB–IIA	53	85 (6)	—	—	98 (6)
2 OPA/2 COMP	30 Gy, IF	IIB–IIIA	21	55	—	—	95
2 OPA/4 COMP	25 Gy, IF	IIIB–IV	24	49	—	—	100
HD-90							
2 OEPA/OPPA (165)	25 Gy, IF	IA/IB–IIA	275	94/95 (5)	—	—	99 (5)
2 OEPA/OPPA + 2 COPP	25 Gy, IF	IIB–IIIA	124	90/96	—	—	97
2 OEPA/OPPA + 4 COPP	20 Gy, IF	IIIB–IV	179	84/89	—	—	94

(Continued)

Clinical Radiation Oncology

| Table 87.2 | TREATMENT RESULTS OF COMBINED-MODALITY TRIALS OF PEDIATRIC HODGKIN'S DISEASE (*Continued*) |

Chemotherapy/ Study (Reference)	Radiation Therapy	Stage	No. of Patients	Outcome (Years) EFS	DFS	RFS/FFP	Survival
GPOH-HD95 (155)			830	90 (3)			97 (3)
	0 Gy for CR	TG1, TG2, or TG3	185	—	—	89 (3)	—
	20–35 Gy, IF for PR	—	611	—	—	93	—
2 OEPA/OPPA	TG1: IA/B, IIA	—	326	94 (3)	—	—	—
2 OPEA/OPPA + 2 COPP	TG2: IIEA, IIB, IIIA	—	224	91 (3)	—	—	—
2 OEPA/OPPA + 4 COPP	TG3: IIEB, IIIEA/B, IIIB, IVA/B	—	280	84 (3)	—	—	—
United Kingdom Children's Cancer Study Group							
6–10 ChIVPP (179)	35 Gy, IF	II	125	—	—	85 (10)	92 (10)
6–10 ChIVPP	35 Gy, IF	III	80	—	—	73	84
6–10 ChIVPP	35 Gy, IF	IV	27	—	—	38	71
Argentina (GATLA) (158)			64				81 (5)
Intermediate[a]							
6 CVPP	30–40 Gy, IF	I–IV	43	—	—	87 (5)	—
6 AOPE	30–40 Gy, IF	I–IV	21	—	—	67	—
Unfavorable[a]							
CCOPP/CAPTe	30–40 Gy, IF	I–IVV	24	—	—	83	—

EFS, event-free survival; DFS, disease-free survival; RFS, relapse-free survival; FFP, freedom from progression; MOPP, mustargen, Oncovin, procarbazine, prednisone; ABVD, Adriamycin, bleomycin, vinblastine, dacarbazine; IF, involved field; CS, clinical stage; PS, pathologic stage; COPP, cyclophosphamide, Oncovin, Procarbazine, prednisone; EF, extended field; R, regional; TLI, total lymphoid Irradiation; VBVP, vinblastine bleomycin etoposide (VP16) prednisone; M/T, mediastinal mass/thoracic ration; OPPA, Oncovin, prednisone, procarbazine, Adriamycin; OPA, Oncovine, prednisone, Adriamycine; COMP, cyclophosphamide, Oncovin, methotrexate, prednisone; OEPA, Oncovin, etoposide, prednisone, Adriamycin; PR, partial response; ChiVPP, chlorambucii, vinblastine, procarbazine, prednisone; GATLA, The Grupo Argentino de Tratamiento de Leucemia Aguda; CVPP, cyclophosphamide, vincristine, prednisone, procarbazine; AOPE, Adriamycin, Oncovin, prednisone, etoposide; CCOPP/CAPTe, CCNU, vincristine, procarbazine, prednisone/ cyclophosphamide, Adriamycin, prednisone, teniposide.
[a]Intermediate and unfavorable prognostic group determined on the basis of age, symptoms, stage, and number of nodal regions.

pediatric centers because of its strong association with solid tumor carcinogenesis and other morbidities. However, low-dose (15 to 25.5 Gy), involved-field radiation remains a critical component of primary combined-modality regimens and as salvage therapy for patients with refractory or relapsed disease.

Combination Chemotherapy

The development of non–cross-resistant chemotherapy combinations provided the first effective therapy for advanced HD and formed the cornerstone for contemporary risk-adapted therapy. The specific chemotherapeutic combinations have changed as their morbidities have become better understood, but most treatment regimens include MOPP (mechlorethamine, vincristine, procarbazine, and prednisone), ABVD (doxorubicin, bleomycin, vinblastine, and dacarbazine), or therapies derived from one of the combinations (see Table 87.3).

Despite the excellent disease control with ABVD (17,68, 81,113), bleomycin and doxorubicin cause pulmonary and cardiovascular damage, respectively. To reduce the treatment-related toxicities associated with six cycles of either MOPP or ABVD, regimens alternating the two combinations, and using fewer cycles of each, have been developed. The combined ABVD and MOPP regimens used for children have produced excellent disease control with apparent diminished toxicity (77,79,201).

Combined-Modality Therapy versus Chemotherapy Alone

Contemporary therapy for pediatric HD using chemotherapy alone or combined-modality therapy produces long-term DFS in 85% to 100% of patients with localized disease and 70% to 90% of patients with advanced disease (11,17,44,46,49,50, 53,77,79,81,96,99,106,129,131–133,156,158,165,169,173, 187,194,195,199,200,202,203). Single-modality chemotherapy

treatment usually involves more cycles of chemotherapy, whereas combined-modality therapies prescribe low-dose, involved-field radiation in lieu of several chemotherapy cycles. Although early treatment results appear comparable with results of more mature trials of combined-modality therapy, the long-term efficacy and treatment toxicities associated with chemotherapy alone have not been reported. Earlier randomized pediatric trials prospectively comparing outcomes in patients treated with chemotherapy alone to those treated with combined-modality therapy have not definitively established the superiority of one treatment approach over the other (81,202). However, other trials suggest a better outcome in patients with unfavorable localized or advanced disease treated with combined-modality therapy (202). Children's Cancer Group investigators closed enrollment into a randomized controlled trial comparing outcomes in patients treated with contemporary risk-adapted combined-modality therapy with COPP/ABV (cyclophosphamide, vincristine, prednisone, procarbazine/doxorubicin, bleomycin, vinblastine) hybrid chemotherapy and low-dose, involved-field radiation to those treated with COPP/ABV chemotherapy alone based on a significantly higher 3-year event-free survival in patients randomized to receive combined-modality therapy (129). However, early follow-up did not demonstrate a significant difference in overall survival among the groups due to the successful retrieval of relapsed patients following salvage therapy. Similarly, the German HD-DAL 90 protocol treated intermediate- and high-risk patients with two cycles of OPPA (vincristine, prednisone, procarbazine, doxorubicin), or OEPA (vincristine, etoposide, prednisone, doxorubicin) (females and males, respectively), followed by two to four cycles of COPP. All patients received 20 to 35 Gy involved-field radiation therapy (IFRT), including those with stage III and IV disease. Five-year EFS in the intermediate- and high-risk groups was 93% and

Table 87.3 TREATMENT RESULTS OF CHEMOTHERAPY ALONE IN PEDIATRIC HODGKIN'S TRIALS

Chemotherapy/Study (Reference)	Stage	No. of Patients	Outcome (Years)			
			EFS	DFS	RFS/FFP	Survival
Children's Cancer Group (81)		111	82 (4)			
6 MOPP/6 ABVD	PS III/IV	57	77 (4)	—	—	87 (4)
Pediatric Oncology Group (202)						
4 MOPP/4 ABVD	CS IIB, IIA2, IIIB, IV	81	79 (5)	—	—	96 (5)
Australia/New Zealand						
5–6 VEEP (49)	All stages	53	59 (3)	78 (5)		92 (5)
3 EVAP/ABV (48)	CS IA–IVA	25	—	—	79 (3)	100
6–8 MOPP or 6 ChlVPP (50)	CS I–IV	38	—	—	98 (4)	94 (4)
Costa Rica (106)						
6 CVPP	CS I–IIIA	52	—	—	90 (5)	100 (5)
6 CVPP/EBO	CS IIIB/IV	24	—	—	60 (5)	81 (5)
Argentina (GATLA) (158)						
3 CVPP	CS IA, IIA	10	86 (6.7)	—	—	—
6 CVPP	CS IB, IIB	16	87 (6.7)	—	—	—
Nicaragua (11)						
6 COPP	CS I, IIA	14	100 (3)	—	—	100 (3)
8–10 COPP-ABV	CS IIB, III, IV	34	75 (3)	—	—	—
Madras, India						
6 COPP/ABV (187)	CS I–IIA	10	89 (5)	—	—	—
6 COPP/ABV (187)	CS IIB–IVB	43	90 (5)	—	—	—
4 COPP/4 ABVD (8)	CS I–IV	133	87.9	—	—	91
The Netherlands (195)						
6 MOPP	CS I–IV (lymph nodes <4 cm)	21	91 (10)	—	—	100 (10)
6 ABVD	CS I–IV (lymph nodes <4 cm)	17	70 (10)	—	—	94 (10)
6 ABVD/MOPP	CS I–IV	21		91 (10)	—	91 (10)
Uganda (133)						
6 MOPP	CS I–IIIA	38		—	75 (5)	—
6 MOPP	CS IIIB–IV	10		—	60 (5)	—

ABVD, Doxorubicin, bleomycin, vinblastine, dacarbazine; ChlVPP, vinblastine, procarbazine, prednisone; COPP, cyclophosphamide, Vincristine, procarbazine, prednisone; CS, clinical stage; CVPP, cyclophosphamide, vincristine, procarbazine, prednisone; DFS, disease-free survival; EBO, epirubicin, bleomycin, Vincristine; EFS, event-free survival; EVAP, etoposide, vinblastine, cytosine arabinoside, cisplatium; FFP, freedom from progression; GATLA, The Grupo Argentino de Tratamiento de Leucemia Aguda; MOPP, Mustargen, Vincristine, procarbazine, prednisone; PS, pathologic stage; RFS, relapse-free survival; VEEP, vincristine, etoposide, epirubicin, prednisone.

86%, respectively, which was comparable to that seen in the low-risk group. Overall survival (5-year) for all three risk groups was ≥94% (155,156,169). In the subsequent HD-95 trial, which employed the same chemotherapy but omitted IFRT in complete responders, the EFS for intermediate- and high-risk patients was 91% and 84%, respectively (156).

Currently, consensus regarding the optimal therapy for children and adolescents with HD has not been established. Treatment with chemotherapy alone is preferred by many investigators desiring to avoid long-term sequelae of radiation, including musculoskeletal growth impairment, cardiovascular dysfunction, and solid tumor carcinogenesis. However, single modality

Table 87.4 TREATMENT RESULTS IN CHILDREN WITH HODGKIN'S DISEASE WITH RADIATION THERAPY

Group/Institution and Study (Reference)	No. of Patients	Stage	% Survival (Years)	
			Overall	Relapse-Free
Children's Hospital of Philadelphia (67)	31	PS IA, IIA	83	64
Joint Center/Harvard (119, 190)	50	PS I, IIA	97 (5)	82 (5)
St. Bartholomew's Great Ormond St. (45)	28	CS I, II	95.5 (10)	79 (10)
Stanford University (45)	48	PS I, II	86 (10)	82 (10)
Intergroup Hodgkin's Study (54)	39 (IF)	PS I, II	95 (5)	41 (5)
	58 (EF)	PS I, II	96 (5)	67 (5)
University of Toronto (85)	8 (EF) 23 (IF)	CS, PS I	95	87
	42 (EF)	PS IIA, IIIA	85	45
Gustave-Roussy (14)	33 (EF)	PS I	80 (5)	33 (5)
Royal Marsden Hospital (179)	99	CS I	92 (10)	70 (10)

PS, pathologic stage; CS, clinical stage; EF, extended field; IF, involved field.

chemotherapy protocols typically use higher cumulative doses of chemotherapeutic agents with dose-related toxicity, especially alkylating agents. Moreover, low-dose involved-field radiation therapy has substantially reduced all the undesirable radiation-associated sequelae.

Risk-Adapted Therapy

Ongoing risk-adapted trials aim to identify patients who require radiation to optimize DFS and those who can be cured by limited chemotherapy alone. For example, the ongoing Children's Oncology Group (COG) Intermediate Risk HD study treats patients with stage IA/IIA bulky disease, IB, IIB, IIIA, or IVA disease with two cycles of ABVE-PC (doxorubicin, bleomycin, vincristine, etoposide, prednisone, cyclophosphamide) prior to response evaluation. Those with a rapid response to therapy (>60% reduction in the tumor dimension), and those who achieve complete recovery after an additional two cycles of the same chemotherapy, are randomized to 21 Gy IFRT or no additional treatment. Patients with slow response to two cycles of chemotherapy are randomized to either standard therapy (an additional two cycles of ABVE-PC + 21 Gy IFRT) or intensified therapy (two cycles of ABVE-PC, two cycles of DECA [dexamethasone, etoposide, cisplatin, cytarabine] + 21 Gy IFRT). This trial will provide useful data regarding the selection of patients who may avoid radiation therapy (RT), and the value of chemotherapy intensification among those with slow early response (SER).

Favorable Early Stage Disease

In the 1990s, pediatric Hodgkin's investigations evaluated risk-adapted therapies using fewer cycles of combination chemotherapy and lower radiation doses and treatment volumes in clinically staged patients with favorable disease presentations. Favorable disease presentations were characterized by localized nodal involvement in the absence of B symptoms and bulky mediastinal lymphadenopathy. The number of involved nodal regions, the presence of extranodal extension, hilar lymphadenopathy, and peripheral nodal bulk comprised other risk factors considered in some of these studies. Most treatment regimens prescribed two to four cycles of novel chemotherapy combinations that limited or omitted alkylating agent and anthracycline chemotherapy and bleomycin. The results of these trials demonstrated that excellent treatment outcomes could be maintained in patients with favorable presentations of localized HD using minimal therapy (44,46,99,129,132,156,166,167,169, 191,200).

Unfavorable Localized and Advanced Disease

Localized (stage I or II) and advanced (stage III or IV) disease associated with B symptoms, bulky lymphadenopathy, or extranodal extension are considered unfavorable presentations in the era of risk-adapted therapy. Two treatment approaches are used for unfavorable disease, both of which include chemotherapy regimens derived from the original MOPP and ABVD combinations. MOPP has largely been replaced by COPP because cyclophosphamide is less myelosuppressive and leukemogenic than mechlorethamine (170).

In the conventional treatment approach, combination chemotherapy is administered on a twice monthly schedule for 6 to 8 months (46,53,77,79,81,129,156,166,167,169,202,203). More recent trials are evaluating the second treatment approach, which has been used successfully in adults with HD. These protocols prescribe dose-intensive, multiagent chemotherapy in an abbreviated schedule over a period of 3 to 5 months. Prototypes of the dose-intensive therapy include the MOPP/ABV hybrid, Stanford V, or BEACOPP (bleomycin, etoposide, doxorubicin, cyclophosphamide, vincristine, procarbazine, prednisone) regimens (40,75,76,91,129).

These treatments alternate myelosuppressive and non-myelosuppressive chemotherapy combinations in a weekly schedule with the aim of reducing the development of resistant disease. Growth factor support is required to facilitate bone marrow recovery and maintain the compacted treatment schedule. Low-dose, involved-field radiation therapy generally is used to consolidate remission after completion of chemotherapy. In ongoing pediatric trials, the response to chemotherapy influences the ultimate amount of therapy. For example, in the Stanford/St.Jude/Dana Farber protocols, rapid early responders to chemotherapy, defined by complete response after two to three cycles of chemotherapy, are being targeted for reduced treatment (less or no radiation therapy, depending on the risk group). In the COG Intermediate Risk protocol (previously discussed), patients who are rapid responders (>60% tumor reduction) and then completely respond to chemotherapy are randomized to either receive or not receive RT. In the German studies mentioned earlier, complete responders do not receive chemotherapy. Early treatment outcomes appear comparable for both treatment approaches. However, long-term follow-up is needed to assess the acute and late toxicity of dose-intensive therapy and to determine if this treatment approach is more effective than conventional therapy.

Sequence of Therapy

The most effective sequence of therapy in the setting of combined chemotherapy and irradiation is not unequivocally established. However, chemotherapy is usually the first modality. This allows assessment of drug response, maximization of the amount of drug treatment, and shrinkage of disease and more limited fields of irradiation. Occasionally, focal irradiation prior to chemotherapy will be necessary because of airway obstruction.

Refractory or Relapsed Disease

Treatment failures in pediatric HD patients typically develop within the first 3 years, although late relapses have been reported, particularly in patients with lymphocyte-predominant HD. The pattern of relapse following newer risk-adapted therapies has not been established. Because of the excellent outcome for the majority of children and adolescents with HD, investigations of salvage therapy have been limited. Prognosis following relapse is dependent on the primary therapy. Salvage rates range from 50% to 80% in patients initially treated with standard-dose radiation therapy alone following another treatment with chemotherapy or combined-modality therapy. Standard multiagent chemotherapy and radiation therapy may salvage 40% to 50% of patients who relapse one or more years after primary therapy, but treatment complications such as second malignancies may reduce long-term survival. More aggressive salvage chemotherapy short of stem cell transplant has recently been shown to provide satisfactory outcome for patients with late relapses (168). Patients with primary refractory disease (i.e., those unresponsive to initial therapy or who relapse within 1 year of primary therapy) have a very poor prognosis. Intensive cytoreductive chemotherapy followed by myeloablation and hematopoietic stem cell transplantation is reported to salvage 30% to 60% of these patients, but relapses after 5 years have been observed, and long-term treatment complications may predispose to early mortality (12,103,123,148,168,188,205).

Historically, because of higher treatment-related mortality, allogeneic transplantation has not provided a survival advantage compared with autologous stem cell transplantation. However, allogeneic bone marrow transplantation may be a useful treatment in healthy patients who have failed or cannot have an autologous transplant and have an HLA-matched sibling. The lower relapse rates in these cases have been attributed to an immune-mediated graft-versus-lymphoma effect. Newer, less toxic, nonmyeloablative approaches to allogeneic transplantation are currently under investigation and may increase the use of allogeneic grafting in the future (7,171,189).

Techniques of Radiation Therapy

As discussed above, most children with HD will be treated with combined chemotherapy and low-dose involved-field radiation using a risk-adapted approach. The use of radiation therapy in isolation has been largely abandoned. A possible exception is the fully grown child with localized nLPHD, where involved field RT is a consideration. The Patterns of Care studies document the relationship between technique and outcome (74). The HD-DAL 90 trial (German-Austrian pediatric multicenter trial) showed that up-front centralized review of patients entered into the study altered the treatment approach in a large number of children (39). Unpublished data from the Pediatric Oncology Group (POG) also support the superior outcome of children treated with appropriate radiation fields and doses, in contrast to those in whom protocol violations occurred. Because technique is discussed in Chapter 75, only select points applicable to children will be discussed here. An example of definitions for IFRT are in Table 87.5.

In a child <5 years, consideration has historically been given to treating bilateral areas (e.g., both sides of the neck) to avoid growth asymmetry. However, this is less of a concern with low radiation doses and thus unilateral fields are usually appropriate if the disease is unilateral. Other considerations relate to the risk of second malignant neoplasms. For example, a child with isolated mediastinal disease receiving combined-modality therapy can be treated with shielding of the axilla and thus the breast tissue and perhaps the thyroid gland. Clearly, careful planning and judgment are necessary. Most difficult is the treatment of involved supradiaphragmatic fields or a mantle field, which requires precision because of the distribution of lymph nodes and the critical adjacent normal tissues. These fields can be simulated with the arms up over the head or down with hands on the hips. The former pulls the axillary lymph nodes away from the lungs, allowing greater lung shielding. However, the axillary lymph nodes then move into the vicinity of the humeral heads, which should be blocked in growing children. Thus, the position chosen involves weighing concerns regarding lymph nodes, lung, and humeral heads. Attempts should be made to exclude or position breast tissue under the lung/axillary blocking. Radiation doses are also dependent on choice of therapy because combined radiation and chemotherapy generally entails low-dose radiation. This is also variously

defined and often protocol specific. In general, doses of 15 to 25 Gy are used, with modifications based on patient age, the presence of bulk or residual (postchemotherapy) disease, and normal tissue concerns. In some situations, a boost of 5 Gy is appropriate. Although IFRT remains as the standard when patients are treated with combined-modality therapy, restricting RT to areas of initial bulk disease (generally defined as ≥5 cm at the time of disease presentation), or postchemotherapy residual disease (generally defined as 2 cm or more, or residual PET avidity), is under investigation. An example of definitions for IFRT are in Table 87.5.

An approach being studied in Europe (European Organisation for Research and Treatment Center-Groupe d Etudes des Lymphomes de l Adulte [EORTC-GELA]) is the use of involved node RT (INRT), which restricts RT to the initially involved lymph node (55). This is based on the premise that chemotherapy can effectively eliminate microscopic disease that may exist within adjacent but clinically uninvolved nodes. This concept is supported by the observation that among patients treated with chemotherapy alone, initially involved lymph nodes are the most common site of recurrence (178). In contrast to conventional IFRT, uninvolved hila are not included in the clinical target volume (CTV) for mediastinal presentations, and the length of the treated volume is not routinely extended beyond 1 cm for the planning target volume (Fig. 87.1). Clearly, successive reduction in treatment volume may reduce the toxicity of therapy.

Results of Therapy

The actuarial 10-year survival rate for children with early stage disease ranges from 85% to 97%, and for those with advanced-stage disease it ranges from 70% to 90% (Tables 87.2, 87.3 and 87.4). One of the few reports that assessed treatment in pathologically versus clinically staged disease was by Donaldson et al. (45), who compared results in early stage disease from Stanford (pathologic staging, extended-field irradiation alone, or combined chemotherapy and involved-field irradiation) with those from the St. Bartholomew's/Great Ormond Street study (clinical staging, involved-field, and regional-field full-dose irradiation). Overall survival from each institution was 91% at 10 years, although the DFS rate for stage I patients at St. Bartholomew's was somewhat lower than at Stanford (83% vs. 90%; *p* =.18). There is a similar OS for patients treated with full-dose radiation therapy, combined full-dose irradiation and chemotherapy, or low-dose radiation therapy and chemotherapy. However, the toxicities vary greatly (Tables 87.2, 87.3, 87.4, 87.6).

The overall relapse-free survival rate is 53% for patients with LMA treated with irradiation alone, in contrast to 86% for those with small or no mediastinal disease. Overall survival rates are not significantly different (88% and 93%, respectively) because of the use of salvage chemotherapy. The high rate of relapse, however, makes the use of initial chemotherapy with consolidative irradiation a more rational approach in patients with LMA.

Although relapse-free and overall survival rates remain excellent for patients with advanced disease when all are analyzed together, patients with stage IV disease continue to fare poorly (see Tables 87.2–87.4) (10,32). Overall survival is compromised by death resulting from second malignancy and toxicity, as well as recurrent HD (20,60,61,78,122).

Complications of Radiation Therapy

Acute Effects

Acute side effects most often associated with mantle irradiation include temporary loss or change in taste, xerostomia, sore throat, esophagitis, low posterior scalp epilation, skin erythema, and occasionally dyspepsia and nausea and vomiting.

Table 87.5	**INVOLVED FIELD RADIATION GUIDELINES**
Involved Node(s)	**Radiation Field**
Unilateral neck	Unilateral neck[a] + ipsilateral supraclavicular
Supraclavicular	Supraclavicular + mid/low neck + infraclavicular
Axilla	Axilla +/− infraclavicular/supraclavicular
Mediastinum	Mediastinum + hila + infraclavicular/supraclavicular[b]
Hila	Hila +/− mediastinum
Spleen	Spleen +/− adjacent para-aortics
Para-aortics	Para-aortics +/− spleen
Iliac	Iliacs + inguinal/femoral

[a]Upper neck region not treated if supraclavicular involvement is extension of the mediastinal disease.
[b]Clinical target volume (CTV) encompasses postchemotherapy mediastinal width laterally and prechemotherapy extent in superior-inferior direction.

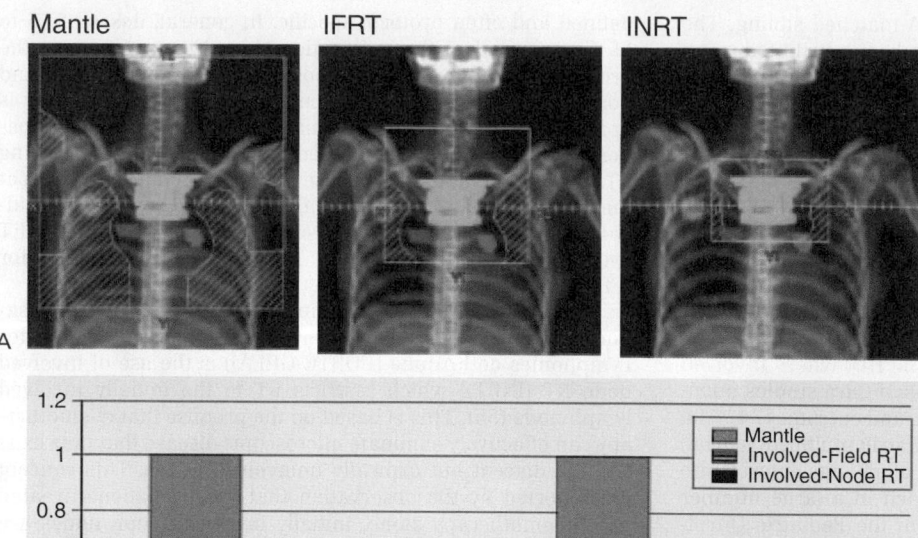

FIGURE 87.1. A: Digitally reconstructed radiographs demonstrating typical radiation therapy (RT) fields for historic mantle RT, contemporary involved-field RT (IFRT), and involved node RT (INRT) for a patient with stage I disease involving the upper mediastinum. The postchemotherapy volume of initially involved mediastinal nodes is shown in green. Hila are shown in blue and violet. **B:** Reduction in dose to breast and lung for the female patient shown in (A). For each volume the prescribed dose to the CTV is the same. The resulting mean dose to breast and lung tissue with mantle RT is a set value equal 1. The proportional reduction in normal tissue dose occurs as a result of the reduction in treated volume with IFRT and INRT. (Reprinted from Hodgkin D, Hudson M, Constine L. Pediatric Hodgkin Lymphoma; Maximizing efficacy, minimizing morbidity. *Sem Radiat Oncol*, in press, with permission from Elsevier.)

Table 87.6 | GUIDELINES FOR TREATMENT SELECTION IN PEDIATRIC HODGKIN'S DISEASE

Stage	Clinical Presentation	Therapy Considerations
IA, IIA	*Favorable* Without bulk No extranodal extension 3 or less involved nodal regions	*Recommended therapy* 2–4 cycles non–cross-resistant chemotherapy without alkylators (ABVD or derivative) plus low-dose, involved-field radiation (1,500–2,550 cGy) *Other considerations* 6 cycles non–cross-resistant chemotherapy alone (alternating COPP or MOPP/ABVD or derivative) In clinical trial setting only, 4 cycles of chemotherapy alone
IA, IIA, IIIA Selected IIB sweats only without bulk	*Unfavorable localized* Bulky lymphadenopathy Mediastinal ratio ≥33% Peripheral nodes ≥6–10 cm More than 3 involved nodal regions	*Recommended therapy* 4–6 cycles of non–cross-resistant chemotherapy (ABVD or alternating COPP or MOPP/ABVD or derivative) plus low-dose, involved-field radiation (1,500–2,550 cGy) -or- 3–5 cycles compacted chemotherapy (COPP or MOPP/ABCD or derivative ± etoposide) plus low-dose, involved-field radiation (1,500–2,550 cGy) *Other considerations* 6–8 cycles non–cross-resistant chemotherapy alone (alternating COPP or MOPP/ABVD or derivative) 5 cycles compacted chemotherapy (COPP or MOPP/ABVD or derivative ± etoposide) alone
IIB, IIIB, IVA/B	*Unfavorable advanced*	*Recommended therapy* 6–8 cycles non–cross-resistant chemotherapy alone (alternating COPP or MOPP/ABVD or derivative ± etoposide) plus low-dose, involved-field radiation (1,500–2,550 cGy) -or- 5 cycles compacted chemotherapy (COPP or MOPP/ABVD or derivative ± etoposide) plus low-dose, involved-field radiation (1,500–2,550 cGy) *Other considerations* 8 cycles non–cross-resistant chemotherapy alone (alternating COPP or MOPP/ABVD or derivative ± etoposide) -or- 5–7 cycles compacted chemotherapy (COPP or MOPP/ABVD or derivative ± etoposide) alone

ABVD, Doxorubicin, bleomycin, vinblastine, dacarbazine; COPP, cyclophosphamide, Vincristine, procarbazine, prednisone; MOPP, Mustargen, Vincristine, procarbazine, prednisone.

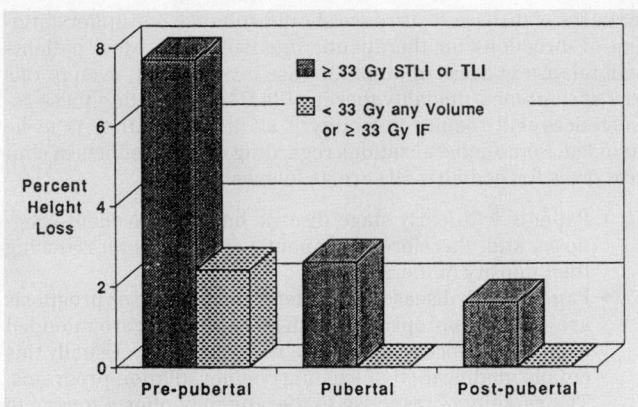

FIGURE 87.2. Relative height impairment for different age and treatment groups in pediatric Hodgkin's disease. (From Willman K, Cox K, Donaldson S. Radiation induced height impairment in pediatric Hodgkin's disease. *Int J Radiat Oncol Biol Phys* 1994;28:85–92 with permission. Copyright 1994 by Elsevier Science, Inc.)

Acute effects of para-aortic irradiation include early onset nausea and vomiting, which usually abates after the second or third treatment without antiemetic therapy.

Long-Term Effects

Musculoskeletal

Height reduction is most severe in prepubertal children treated with full-dose irradiation, but it is modest following the low doses currently used (Fig. 87.2) (41,119,206). Interclavicular shortening and hypoplasia of the neck muscles occur in most children irradiated before puberty; the severity of these complications is more pronounced in children <5 years of age at the time of irradiation. Slipped capital femoral epiphysis occurs in ≤50% of young children whose femoral heads have been irradiated. Avascular necrosis of the femoral or humeral heads is rare if appropriate shielding is provided. Radiation doses of 20 to 40 Gy to the mandible may result in dental abnormalities, such as stunted tooth development, incomplete calcification, premature apical closure or eruption, and root tapering with apical constriction if the tooth germ tissue is in the irradiated field (112).

Cardiovascular

Radiation-associated pericardial and myocardial disease are related to dose (including fraction size) and volume and are complicated by the use of anthracyclines. Of concern is that progressive cardiovascular deterioration is now becoming evident in aging survivors. Conversely, modern treatment approaches based on tailored low-dose radiation and less cardiotoxic chemotherapy, sometimes including cardioprotectants, will optimistically reduce such effects. Cardiac sequelae, including pericarditis and effusion, valvular thickening, biventricular dysfunction, and coronary artery disease, all are observed with irradiation to the heart (2,43,68,93,191). Radiation doses of <30 Gy and techniques that use adequate cardiac shielding and avoid anterior weighting of the treatment fields appear to reduce the risk of cardiac complications, particularly pericarditis and myocarditis (2,68). Although the proximal coronary arteries are not shielded by a central cardiac block, the 45-fold excess mortality risk from acute myocardial infarction associated with higher radiation doses has diminished substantially with current approaches (78).

Pulmonary

Pulmonary complications, most typically pneumonitis, occur in 5% of patients treated with standard-dose irradiation. With doses of 25 Gy (43), the incidence is low except when used in combination with pulmonary toxic chemotherapeutic agents (e.g., bleomycin). In a report from the Children's Cancer Group (CCG), 9% of children treated with ABVD and 21 Gy of mantle irradiation exhibited clinically significant pulmonary damage (53). Through serial evaluation of pulmonary function during and after completion of therapy in a cohort treated with alternating cycles of COP(P) and ABVD chemotherapy and involved-field radiation, St. Jude investigators demonstrated improvement in vital capacity and diffusing capacity with increasing time from diagnosis. Clinical compromise of pulmonary function was minimal in this group who routinely had bleomycin withheld when diffusing capacity declined to 50% predicted during therapy (115).

Thyroid

Thyroid dysfunction may result from neck, mediastinal, or mantle field irradiation and most often is manifested by an elevated serum concentration of thyroid-stimulating hormone (TSH). The incidence of hypothyroidism varies, but it appears to be directly related to irradiation dose. Constine et al. (35) noted an increased serum TSH in 4/24 children (17%) who received mantle irradiation of ≤26 Gy and in 74/95 (78%) who received >26 Gy. Approximately one fourth of these children had a concomitant low thyroxine level. In this series, 36% of children experienced spontaneous improvement in thyroid function. In a recent Childhood Cancer Survivor Study, thyroid abnormalities were self-reported by 34% of patients surveyed. Hypothyroidism was the most common thyroid disturbance, with a relative risk of 17.1 (*p* <.0001) compared to sibling controls. Risk factors for hypothyroidism included increasing dose of radiation, older age at diagnosis of HD, and female sex. The estimated actuarial risk of hypothyroidism for survivors treated with ≥4,500 cGy was 50% at 20 years from diagnosis. Other thyroid abnormalities identified in excess from sibling controls included hyperthyroidism (eightfold excess risk), thyroid nodules (27-fold excess risk), and thyroid cancer (18-fold excess risk) (180).

Gonad

Gonadal injuries, including infertility and impaired secretion of sex hormones, are potential complications of pelvic irradiation (102). Oophoropexy in girls may allow preservation of ovarian function (102). Of 86 girls treated at Stanford, 87% demonstrated normal menstrual function on prolonged follow-up. Those who underwent pelvic irradiation without prior oophoropexy failed to maintain ovarian function. In childhood cancer survivors who continued to have spontaneous menses more than 5 years after their cancer diagnosis, the cumulative incidence of nonsurgical menopause was 8% by age 40 years, representing a 13-fold higher risk compared to a sibling control group. Risk factors for premature menopause include attained age, exposure to increasing doses of ovarian radiation, increasing alkylating agent score (based on number of agents and cumulative dose), and diagnosis of HD (180). Normal pregnancies, without increased risk of fetal wastage, spontaneous abortion, or birth defects, have been reported after pelvic irradiation (102).

In boys irradiated to the pelvis, oligospermia is common, but it is reversible (usually by 18 to 24 months) in most cases if the radiation dose scattered to the shielded testes is small (119,135,140). Permanent oligospermia may occur, however, after full-dose pelvic irradiation (140). Several investigations have demonstrated that fertility is compromised in boys treated with gonadotoxic combinations like COPP even when cycles of alkylating agent chemotherapy are limited (23,73).

Small Bowel

Small bowel obstruction may be observed in surgically staged patients who receive para-aortic irradiation. Obstruction requiring surgical intervention is rare and appears to be related to the total radiation dose given: 1% for <35 Gy and 3% for doses higher than 35 Gy.

Second Malignant Neoplasm

The 15-year actuarial risk of second malignant neoplasms ranges from 8% to 15% (15,19,20,60,78,121,122,154, 163,192,196–198,208). Although the absolute risk of solid tumors increases with time, the ratio of observed to expected incidence ultimately stabilizes because of the increasing background incidence of neoplasia (31,33). The risk of leukemia, which plateaus after 10 to 15 years, is associated primarily with the use of alkylating agents (15,20). Several studies reveal an increased ratio of observed to expected risk of second tumors for girls compared with boys, with median follow-up of 10 to 16 years (15,190). A portion of this risk results from breast cancer, which is the most common solid second malignant neoplasm following the treatment of children. Adolescents and women treated with more than 20 to 40 Gy are at greatest risk (20,192).

Recommendations for the screening of chronic effects of therapy are presented in Figure 87.3.

Future Investigations

Development of new strategies for the treatment of children with HD is problematic because of the overall success of current treatment regimens. The ability to conduct clinical trials in which the differences in survival among the treatment arms are likely to be small is compromised by the large patient numbers necessary to detect such differences. Analyzing patterns of disease recurrence should enhance our understanding of directions for therapeutic intensification. Most patients will relapse in areas of initial disease involvement, even in this era of combined-modality therapy (34,94). Preventing these recurrences will require ingenuity if additional toxicity is to be avoided. Some generalizations regarding ongoing efforts in clinical trials for pediatric HD are as follows:

- Patients with early stage disease have an excellent prognosis, and, therefore, therapeutic aims focus on reducing the intensity of therapy.
- Patients with disease of an intermediate stage or prognosis are studied appropriately with questions that are intended to increase efficacy without increasing toxicity. Usually this entails modification of existing chemoradiation programs. The rapidity of response to therapy may offer a means to risk-adapt subsequent treatment and is under investigation.
- Patients with advanced-stage disease require more effective treatment regimens. This may be attainable by increasing the dose intensity or the rate of drug delivery or by combining agents into new regimens. The use of hemopoietic growth factors may assist in drug delivery. The definition of the role of radiation therapy in such trials will continue to be important.

Of interest will be immunotherapeutic approaches under development that are based on recent experiences in adult HD, such as the use of antiferritin antibody jointed with yttrium-90 (21) and EBV-specific T lymphocytes (154). Current approaches under investigation for relapsed/refractory HD aim to evaluate

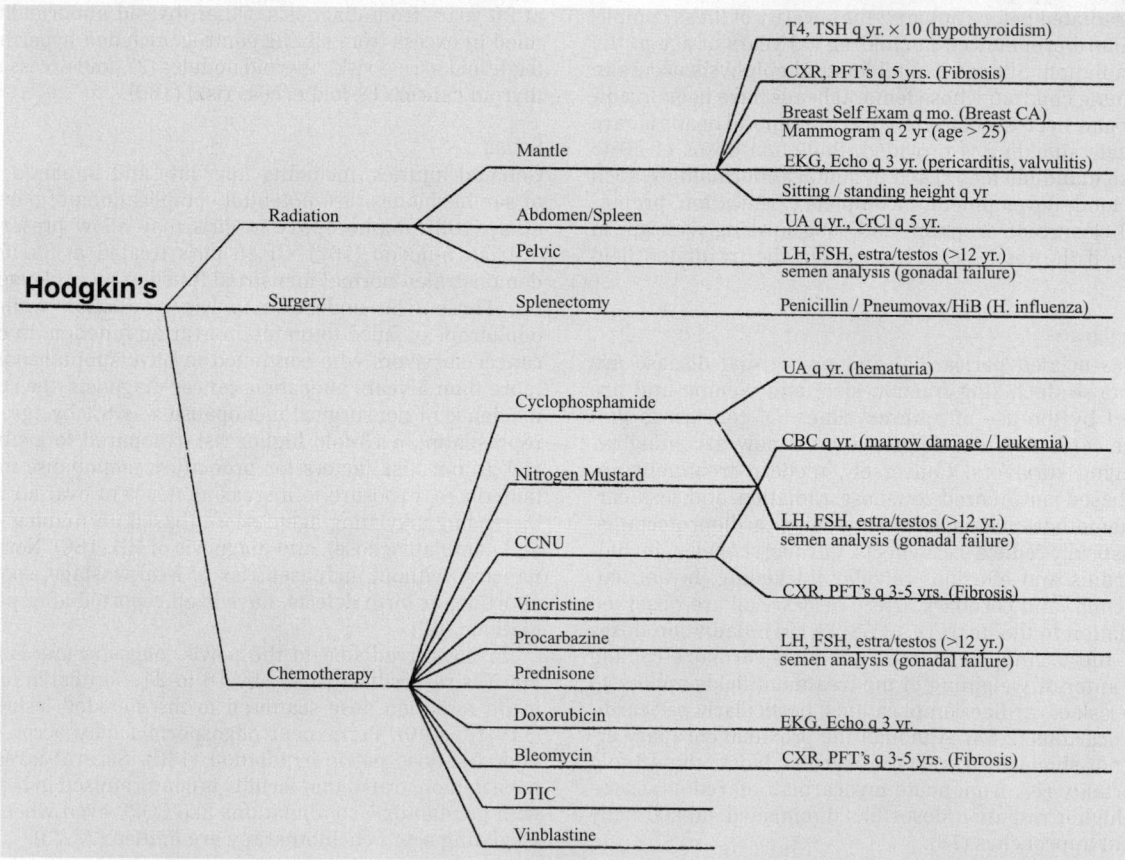

FIGURE 87.3. Late effects screening recommendations for childhood Hodgkin's disease. CA, contrast angiography; CBC, complete blood count; CCNU,; CrCl,; CXR, Echo, echocardiogram; EKG, electrocardiogram; FSH, follicle-stimulating hormone; LH, luteinizing hormone; PFT, TSH, thyroid-stimulating hormone; UA, urine analysis. (From Constine L, Hobbie W, Schwartz C. Facilitated assessment of chronic treatment by symptom and organ systems. In: Schwartz C, Constine L, Hobbie W, et al., eds. *Survivors of childhood cancer: assessment and management.* St Louis: Mosby Year Book, 1994;21–80, with permission.)

Clinical Radiation Oncology

Table 87.7	BIOLOGIC CHARACTERISTICS OF THE FOUR MAJOR SUBTYPES OF CHILDHOOD NON-HODGKIN'S LYMPHOMA AS DEFINED BY HISTOLOGY AND IMMUNOPHENOTYPE			
Histology	**Immunophenotype**	**Cytogenetics**[a]	**Molecular Genetics**
Small noncleaved cell (Burkitt's and Burkitt-like)	B-cell	T(8;14), t(8;22) t(2;8)	IgH/c-myc, Igkappa/c-myc, Iglambda/c-myc
Lymphoblastic lymphoma	Immature T-cell (80%)	T(10;14), t(11;14) T(1;14), t(1;19) and others	TCR/TAL1 TCR/RHOMB2 TCR/LCK
	Precursor-B-cell (20%)	Hyperdiploid	Ig gene rearrangement
Large cell lymphoma (LCL) Anaplastic LCL (Ki-1+)	T-cell or null	T(2;5), t(1;5)	TCR rearrangements NPM/ALK
DB-LCL	B-cell	T(8;14)	Ig gene rearrangement

[a]Not all tumors in each category contain one of the translocations or molecular lesions described.
Modified from Shad A, Magrath I. Non-Hodgkin's lymphoma. *Pediatr Clin North Am* 1997;44(4):863–890, with permission.

therapeutic strategies that directly or indirectly inhibit NF-κB, a nuclear transcription factor that regulates the expression of a variety of genes that play a crucial role in viral replication, tumorigenesis, apoptosis, various autoimmune diseases, and inflammation (210).

Non-Hodgkin's Lymphoma

Childhood non-Hodgkin's lymphomas (NHLs) are a heterogeneous group of malignancies with variable histopathology, site of origin, and clinical manifestations. Childhood NHLs are diffuse, high-grade, and poorly differentiated; extranodal involvement is common and dissemination occurs early and often (110). This is in striking contrast to the adult NHL where low- and intermediate-grade nodal disease predominates (126). These differences in pathology and clinical behavior observed between adults and children explain the markedly different presentations, staging practices, and treatment strategies.

Epidemiology

In the United States, approximately 800 children and adolescents <20 years of age are diagnosed with NHL each year. According to the Surveillance Epidemiology and End Results (SEER) program of the National Cancer Institute, NHL accounts for about 8% of all cases of childhood cancer (142). The incidence increases with age, being rare in the child <3 years of age, higher in males than females (3:1), and higher in whites than African Americans (1.5:1). In younger children, NHL is more frequent than HD, whereas the reverse is true for adolescents.

Although NHL is related to several genetic and environmental factors, its cause and pathogenesis remain unclear (110, 159). A small proportion of cases are seen in association with inherited immunodeficiencies (e.g., Wiskott-Aldrich syndrome, X-linked lymphoproliferative disease, ataxia-telangiectasia) (51) as well as acquired immunodeficiency syndromes (e.g., HIV infection, immunosuppressive therapy in patients receiving solid organ, or bone marrow transplants) (120,141). Evidence of EBV infection has been demonstrated in the majority of endemic (i.e., African) Burkitt's tumors and in about 15% of sporadic cases (United States), suggesting a significant role for this virus in lymphomagenesis (64,110), although the mechanisms have not yet been elucidated. EBV infection has also been associated with development of posttransplant lymphoproliferative disease (PTLD), a B-cell lymphoproliferative disorder seen in patients following solid organ or hematopoietic transplantation (72,146). With the increasing use of transplantation, the inci-

dence of PTLD in children has increased to over 150 new cases per year among children and adolescents in the United States, making it one of the most common types of NHL in pediatrics (108,145).

Pathologic Classification

Pediatric NHLs are divided into four major histopathologic subtypes based on morphology and immunophenotype: (a) small, noncleaved cell (SNCC) lymphoma (Burkitt's and non-Burkitt's subtypes), (b) lymphoblastic lymphoma, (c) diffuse large B-cell lymphoma, and (d) anaplastic large cell lymphoma (27,143, 162). Identification of large numbers of monoclonal antibodies directed against surface antigens has allowed subclassification of the NHLs according to immunophenotype (see Chapter 76) (84). Thorough evaluation of histology and immunophenotype is key to the determination of diagnosis, prognosis, and appropriate course of treatment. Cytogenetic analysis and identification of molecular markers provide a more precise means of characterization of these tumors, and in the future will likely contribute toward the understanding of the pathogenesis as well as the development of novel therapeutic approaches (Table 87.7) (27,71,87,98,111,147,176).

Clinical Presentation

The signs and symptoms that present in the child with NHL correlate with the disease site(s), histologic subtype, and extent of involvement (Table 87.8). Children with NHL usually present

Table 87.8	CLINICAL CHARACTERISTICS OF CHILDHOOD NON-HODGKIN'S LYMPHOMA	
Histologic Subtype	**Proportion of Cases (%)**	**Most Common Sites of Presentation**
Small noncleaved cell (Burkitt's and Burkitt-like)	40	Abdomen or head and neck
Lymphoblastic lymphoma	30	Mediastinum or head and neck
Anaplastic LCL (T- and null-cell phenotypes)	10	Mediastinum, abdomen, head and neck including orbits, or skin
DB-LCL	20	Mediastinum and abdomen

Modified from Sandlund JT. Childhood Lymphoma. In: Abeloff MD, Armitage JO, Lichter AS, et al., eds. *Clinical Oncology*, 2nd ed. New York: Churchill Livingstone 2000;2438, with permission.

with extranodal disease, most frequently involving the abdomen (35% of cases), the mediastinum (26% of cases), or head and neck region (25% of cases) (128). Almost two-thirds of the children have widespread disease at the time of diagnosis that may involve the bone marrow, central nervous system (CNS), or both (110). Some patients with lymphoblastic or Burkitt's subtype present with isolated bone marrow involvement without any other lymphomatous features or the replacement of more than 25% of the bone marrow by tumor cells associated with a primary tumor elsewhere. This is usually designated and treated as acute lymphoblastic leukemia, T-cell or mature B-cell (Burkitt's) phenotype. CNS involvement may present with cranial nerve palsies, headache, nausea and vomiting, and vision changes (160). Systemic symptoms are relatively rare in childhood NHL except in anaplastic large cell lymphoma.

Diagnostic Evaluation

Tissue diagnosis and investigation to determine the clinical extent of disease should be completed expeditiously. It is important that appropriate therapy be initiated promptly because of the extremely rapid growth rate of pediatric NHL. Although histology and immunophenotype remain the primary means of establishing the definitive diagnosis, karyotype and molecular studies will be vital for implementation of an optimal treatment plan. Thus, it is critical that an adequate amount of tissue be obtained at biopsy, using either open biopsy or core needle biopsy. If the patient's condition does not permit an open biopsy (e.g., a large mediastinal mass is causing airway obstruction), less invasive means of sampling tumor cells, such as percutaneous fine-needle aspiration, or examination of pleural fluid, ascites, peripheral blood, or bone marrow can be diagnostic (Table 87.9).

Bilateral bone marrow biopsies are superior to a single aspirate or biopsy in identifying bone marrow involvement, which is often patchy in distribution in the NHLs (52). Omitting this procedure may result in understaging. Gallium scans can be helpful, particularly in following residual masses that were gallium-avid at diagnosis (89). Positron emission tomography imaging with fluorodeoxyglucose (FDG-PET scan) is now widely available and has established value in adults with HD or NHL (86,211); however, its usefulness in childhood NHL is under investigation. PET imaging will likely replace gallium scans in the future as part of assessment of extent of disease at diagnosis, speed of response to therapy, and posttherapy remission status (38,182). Laparotomy is not performed routinely for staging purposes because combination chemotherapy is part of the primary treatment. This procedure rarely may be necessary in select cases for diagnostic purposes, but aggressive debulking procedures are not advised. MRI may be helpful in detecting disease at specific sites, particularly the nervous system, but it is not routinely used.

Staging Systems

The Ann Arbor staging system (commonly used in adult NHL) has proved of limited use in pediatric NHL because of the unique clinical presentation and course of the disease in children. These special features of childhood NHL include the preponderance of extranodal presentations, the noncontiguous pattern of disease spread, and a tendency to evolve into leukemia and to involve the CNS. To address the uniqueness of childhood NHL, staging systems specific for pediatric NHL have been developed. The St. Jude Children's Research Hospital staging system (126) is used most widely (Table 87.10). Of interest, several of the clinical cooperative groups have adopted the designation of limited disease (including stages I and II) versus advanced disease (stages III and IV) for the purposes of determination of appropriate treatment strategies. European investigators have developed a clinical grouping system in the B-cell lymphomas (Burkitts, non-Burkitts, and large cell subtypes) that is based on extent of disease, modified St. Jude staging criteria, and relative risk of relapse (136). Treatment intensity is based on designation of group A, B, or C disease, which correlates to low, intermediate, or high risk disease, respectively. This strategy has proven very effective in recent ongoing B-NHL treatment trials of the Children's Oncology Group (26,28,29).

Table 87.9 **INVESTIGATIONS REQUIRED FOR ACCURATE STAGING OF CHILDHOOD LYMPHOMAS**

Essential studies
History and physical examination
Complete blood count
Chemistry panel
    Serum electrolytes with calcium, phosphorus, and magnesium
    Liver enzymes with bilirubin
    BUN, serum creatinine, LDH, and uric acid
Imaging studies
    Chest radiograph
    Chest and abdominal CT scan
    Gallium[57] scan
    [F[18]] FDG-PET imaging
Bone-marrow examination (bilateral aspirates and biopsies)
Cerebrospinal fluid examination (cell counts and cytology)

Optional studies
Abdominal ultrasound examination (helpful in young children where the lack of intra-abdominal fat makes CT less sensitive)
Bone scan (if symptoms or Gallium suggest bone involvement)
Serum lactate, IL2-R, bcl-2
MR imaging for bone marrow involvement

BUN, blood urea nitrogen; CT, computed tomography; FDG-PET, fluorodeoxyglucose positron emission tomography; IL, interleukin; LDH, lactate dehydrogenase; MR magnetic resonance
Modified from Shad A, Magrath I. Non-Hodgkin's lymphoma. *Pediatr Clin North Am* 1997;44(4):863–890, with permission.

Table 87.10 **THE ST. JUDE STAGING SYSTEM FOR CHILDHOOD NON-HODGKIN'S LYMPHOMA**

Stage	Description
I	A single tumor (extranodal) or single anatomic area (nodal), excluding the mediastinum or abdomen
II	A single tumor (extranodal) with regional lymph node involvement on same side of the diaphragm: (a) Two or more nodal areas (b) Two single (extranodal) tumors with or without regional node involvement A primary gastrointestinal tract tumor (usually ileocecal) with or without associated mesenteric node involvement, grossly completely resected
III	On both sides of the diaphragm: (a) Two single tumors (extranodal) (b) Two or more nodal areas All primary intrathoracic tumors (mediastinal, pleural, thymic) All extensive primary intra-abdominal disease; unresectable All primary paraspinal or epidural tumors regardless of other sites
IV	Any of the above with initial central nervous system or bone marrow involvement (<25% blasts)

From Murphy SB. Classification, staging and end results of treatment of childhood non-Hodgkin's lymphomas: dissimilarities from lymphomas in adults. *Semin Oncol* 1980;7:332–339, with permission.)

Prognostic Factors

The most important factor in determining prognosis in childhood NHL is stage, which takes into account other known prognostic variables such as tumor burden, site, and extent of involvement (128). The fact that most cases of pediatric NHL are of the diffuse, high-grade, and aggressive subtypes may have obscured the prognostic value of histology; few reports support its role as a prognostic factor (82,162). The clinical relevance of genetic abnormalities such as the translocation t(2;5)(p23;q35) nonrandomly expressed in Ki-1-positive anaplastic large cell lymphomas, *c-myc* rearrangements in diffuse B large cell and small noncleaved B cell lymphomas and the translocation t(8;14) characteristic of Burkitt's cells, have only recently been elucidated in childhood lymphomas (71). In pediatric anaplastic large cell lymphomas, there is almost always an ALK rearrangement, and the presence of anaplastic lymphoma kinase (ALK) rearrangements is associated with a favorable prognosis. This is in contrast to adult cases of anaplastic large cell lymphoma where ALK rearrangements are less common and are associated with poor prognosis. Similarly, *c-myc* gene rearrangements are almost always present in pediatric cases of Burkitts and non-Burkitts and are associated with favorable response to therapy, whereas in adult cases *c-myc* rearrangement is uncommon but the outcomes are poor (71).

Treatment and Results

The overall survival of children with NHL was poor before the advent of multiagent chemotherapy in the mid-1970s (128). Even in cases in which the disease apparently was localized, cure rates as low as 20% were reported. Failure in most cases was caused by early systemic dissemination of disease. In modern regimens, chemotherapy is the primary therapeutic modality for all histologies and stages of childhood NHLs. The dramatic improvement in the overall rate of survival in childhood NHLs can be attributed not only to the development of highly effective, multiagent chemotherapy regimens, but also to the systematic evaluation of these diseases and their treatment by the pediatric cooperative group clinical trials (Fig. 87.4). Cure rates of 85% to 90% in patients with limited disease and 60% to 80% in those with extensive involvement have been reported.

Surgery is indicated only for diagnostic purposes or in the case of an abdominal emergency such as intussusception or acute appendicitis due to abdominal mass effect at presentation. Patients with extensive NHLs may present with a number of life-threatening complications that require urgent intervention including respiratory distress from airway obstruction, superior vena cava syndrome, spinal cord compression, intestinal

TABLE 87.11   TREATMENT OUTCOMES FOR LIMITED STAGE NON-HODGKIN'S LYMPHOMA

Protocol (Reference)	Stage	No. of Patients	Event-Free Survival
POG 1983–1991 (105)	I/II	138/202	5 y = 89, 86, 88% for 3 treatment groups
Small non cleaved cell (SNCC)	I/II	185	5 y = 89%
Lymphoblastic lymphoma	I/II	50	5 y = 63%
Large cell lymphoma (LCL)[a][b]	I/II	81	5 y = 88%
SFOP LMB 89* (136)	I/II	119	5 y = 98%
NHL-BFM 90* (152)	I/II	164	6 y = 98%
CCG[a]-COMP (nonlymphoblastic) (121)	I/II	104	5 y >95%
CCG–lymphoblastic lymphoma (121)	I/II	15	5 y = 67%

[a]Includes B-cell lymphomas with SNCC, Burkitt, and LCL subtypes.

obstruction, hydronephrosis, renal insufficiency, or tumor lysis syndrome. The priority in these situations is to maximize supportive care and initiate specific chemotherapy as soon as a diagnosis has been established.

Chemotherapy

The importance of tailoring therapy to address the inherent biologic differences of the various histologic subtypes became evident early in the evolution of NHL therapy (Tables 87.11 and 87.12). The results of the landmark CCG randomized trial (Study 551) (6) confirmed the efficacy of COMP (cyclophosphamide, vincristine, methotrexate, prednisone) chemotherapy for localized NHL, regardless of histology. In contrast, among children with advanced-stage disease, outcome varied with histology and therapy. Children with SNCC NHL had a better outcome with the COMP regimen. For advanced-stage lymphoblastic NHL, the results were significantly superior with the 10-drug LSA$_2$L$_2$ therapy (cyclophosphamide, vincristine, prednisone, daunomycin, methotrexate, cytarabine, thioguanine, asparaginase, carmustine [BCNU], and hydroxyurea)—a regimen designed for treatment of acute lymphoblastic leukemia (ALL). In this trial, neither regimen was superior for children with advanced-stage large cell lymphoma. An update confirmed the early findings (Fig. 87.5) (5). Although some investigators

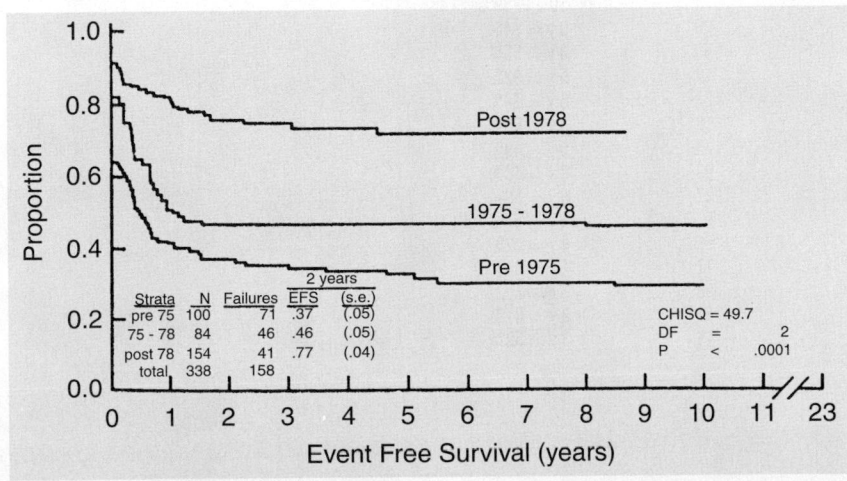

FIGURE 87.4. The overall event-free survival (EFS) of pediatric non-Hodgkin's lymphoma as a function of the treatment eras for all cases. There is a successive and significant increase in the proportion of patients who are event free ($p < .0001$). (From Murphy SB, Fairclough DL, Hutchison RE, et al. Non-Hodgkin's lymphomas of childhood: an analysis of the histology, staging, and response to treatment of 338 cases at a single institution. *J Clin Oncol* 1989;7:186–193, with permission.)

Table 87.12	TREATMENT OUTCOMES FOR ADVANCED STAGE NON-HODGKIN'S LYMPHOMA BASED ON HISTOLOGICAL SUBTYPE

Protocol (Reference)	Stage	No. of Patients	Event-Free Survival
A. Small non-cleaved cell (Burkitt's and Burkitt-like) lymphoma			
CCG 551–LSA$_2$L$_2$	III/IV/B-ALL	44	5 y = 29%
vs. COMP (6)	III/IV/B-ALL	93	5 y = 50%
POG 8616–Comparison 8106	III	65	2 y = 64%
vs. SJCRH Total B (24)	III	58	2 y = 79%
POG 9317–8617 vs. Total B (175)	III/IV/B-ALL	327	2 y = 83% (all)
SFOP LMB 89[a] (136)	I–II	119	5 y = 98%
	III	278	5 y = 91%
	IV	62	5 y = 87%
	B-ALL	102	5 y = 87%
	Burkitt (SNCC)	420	5 y = 92%
	DB-LCL	63	5 y = 89%
NHL-BFM 90[a] (136)	I, II,	164	6 y = 98%
(152)	III	169	6 y = 88%
	IV	24	6 y = 73%
	B-ALL	56	6 y = 74%
NHL-BFM 95[a] (207)	All	505	3 y = 89%
	I/II	172	3 y = 98%
	III	221	3 y = 87%
	IV	33	3 y = 81%
	B-ALL	79	3 y = 77%
Burkitt (SNCC)	All	283	3 y = 93%
CCG 5911–Orange/French (29)	III/IV/B-ALL	46	4 y = 80%
vs. 552 (CHOP-AraC/VP/Mtx)	III/IV/B-ALL	52	4 y = 58%
vs. 503 (COMP,D-COMP)	III/IV/B-ALL	241	4 y = 60%
B. Lymphoblastic lymphoma			
CCG 551-LSA$_2$L$_2$	III/IV	124	5 y = 64%
vs. COMP (6)	III/IV	40	5 y = 35%
MSKCC–LSA2L2 (modified) (124)	III	41	5 y = 85%
	IV/ALL	19/27	5 y = 73%/70%
BFM 86 (150)	III/IV	73	7 y = 82%
BFM 90 (152)	III/IV/T-ALL	101	5 y = 90%
DFCI 81, 85, 87, 91–01 (58)	III/IV	15	5 y = 87%
	T-ALL	125	5 y = 75%
POG 8704–with ASP intensification (4)	III/IV	84	4 y (CCR) = 78%
	T-ALL	160	4 y (CCR) = 68%
POG 9404–with HDMtx (9)	III/IV/T-ALL	220	3 y = 86%
CCG 5941 (1)	III/IV	86	3 y = 79%
C. Large cell lymphoma			
CCG 551 - LSA$_2$L$_2$	III/IV	18	5 y = 43%
vs. COMP (6)	III/IV	42	5 y = 52%
MSKCC–LSA2L2, LSA4 (125)	III/IV	19	5 y = 56% (OS 84%)
SJCRH 1975–1990 (161)	I/II	4	5 y = 75%
	III/IV	14	5 y = 57%
BFM 83, 86, 90 (151)	I/II	4/16	5 y = 75%/ 68%
	III/IV	35/7	5 y = 86%/ 86%
CCG 503 – COMP vs D-COMP (186)	I–III	106	10 y = 48%
	IV	14	10 y = 39%
SFOP HM-89, HM-91 (25)	I/II	23	3 y = 94%
	III/IV	59	3 y = 55%
CCG 5911 Orange (CCG hybrid) (26)	III/IV	12	5 y = 92%
	III/IV	27[b]	5 y = 70%
CCG 5911 (Orange/French) (28)	Disseminated	18	5 y = 65%
vs. pre-5911 (1983–1990)	Disseminated	173	5 y = 49%
POG 8615–APO vs. ACOP+[a] (101)	III	93	8 y = 68%
	IV	27	8 y = 59%
POG 9315–APO vs. IDM/HiDAC (100)	III/IV	85/90	4 y = 67% (all)
Anaplastic LCL	III/IV	86	4 y = 72%
Diffuse B-cell LCL	III/IV	71	4 y = 64%
NHL-BFM 90–diffuse B-cell LCL (152)	All	56	3 events
NHL-BFM 95–diffuse B-cell LCL (207)	All	81	3 y = 81%
Primary mediastinal B-cell LCL	III	15	3 y = 53%

[a]Includes patients with B-cell large cell non-Hodgkin's lymphoma.
[b]Median observation time 4.3 years.

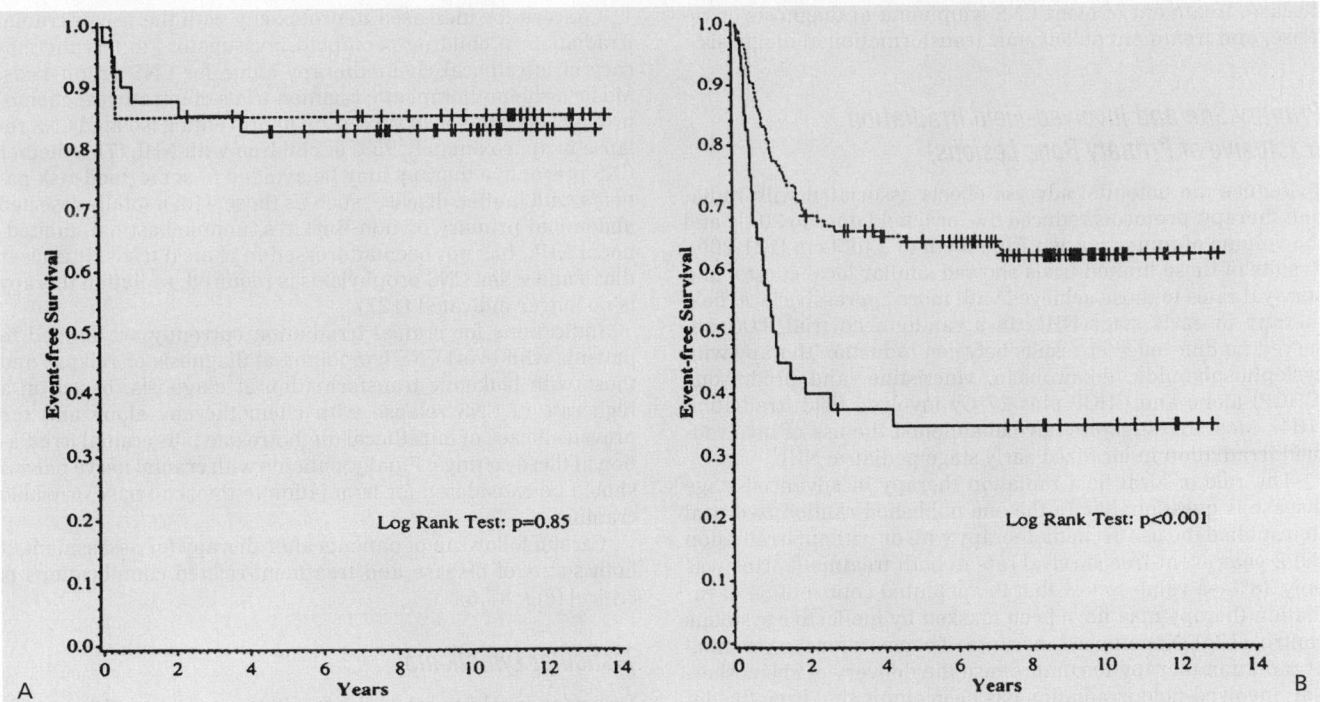

FIGURE 87.5. A: Event-free survival for 68 non-Hodgkin's lymphoma patients with localized disease by treatment group (*solid line,* COMP [41 patients]; *dotted line,* LSA$_2$L$_2$ [27 patients]). **B:** Event-free survival for patients with disseminated lymphoblastic lymphoma by treatment group (*solid line,* COMP [40 patients]; *dotted line,* LSA$_2$-L$_2$ [124 patients]). COMP, cyclophosphamide, vincristine, methotrexate, and prednisone; LSA, cyclophosphamide, vincristine, prednisone, daunomycin, methotrexate, cytarabine, thioguanine, asparaginase, carmustine [BCNU], and hydroxyurea (From Anderson JR, Jenkin RDT, Wilson JF, et al. Long-term follow-up of patients treated with COMP or LSA$_2$L$_2$ therapy for childhood non-Hodgkin's lymphoma: a report of CCG-551 from the Children's Cancer Group. *J Clin Oncol* 1993;11:1024–1032, with permission.)

have failed to show significant differences in response for lymphoblastic versus nonlymphoblastic subgroups, most modern protocols have been designed to account for differences in not only stage of disease but also histologic subtype. In contrast to this stage- and histology-directed approach common in the United States, the European approach has been stage and immunophenotype directed with significant success (138,139, 149,150). Recent studies suggest that the immunophenotype-directed approach has advantages for treating children with advanced-stage large cell lymphomas (80).

Children with early stage NHL have an excellent prognosis (see Table 87.11) (104,105,121,139). Recent studies have been designed to maintain high cure rates while reducing the intensity and duration of therapy, thus sparing young patients from acute and long-term side effects. This strategy was successfully used by POG investigators in two serial trials that demonstrated that a 9-week chemotherapy regimen without irradiation of the primary sites of involvement is adequate therapy for >90% of children with early stage nonlymphoblastic NHL (104,105). Children with limited-stage lymphoblastic NHL did not fare as well even on the longer 34-week treatment arm, although salvage therapy was successful for the majority of patients who suffered a recurrence. Most investigators advocate treatment regimens for lymphoblastic NHL similar to those used for ALL or advanced-stage disease featuring prolonged maintenance therapy for 2 years (137,149,150,172,193).

Improvements in the treatment outcome of patients with advanced-stage NHL have resulted from strategies of increased treatment intensity by dose intensification and inclusion of additional agents. Regimens successful in treatment of advanced-stage SNCC are characterized by intensive cyclophosphamide-based combinations including high-dose methotrexate and cytarabine given over 2 to 4 months (see Table 87.12A).

Advanced-stage lymphoblastic lymphoma has been treated successfully with the same treatment regimens used for high-risk or T-cell ALL (see Table 87.12B).

The optimal approach for children with advanced-stage large cell NHL remains controversial. In the United States, the traditional approach (see Table 87.12C) has been histology directed with regimens incorporating a basic backbone of cyclophosphamide, vincristine, prednisone, and doxorubicin with additional agents such as etoposide, ifosfamide, and high-dose methotrexate being evaluated. This histology directed approach is being re-evaluated because of the excellent results of European investigators in treating children with B-cell large cell lymphoma according to SNCC treatment regimens (137–139,172); those with T-cell large cell lymphoma according to T-ALL protocols (149,150,172); and those with CD 30+ anaplastic lymphomas according to a variety of approaches (151,164). A recent study by POG demonstrated that children with large cell lymphoma of the B-cell immunophenotype had a better outcome than those with a non–B-cell immunophenotype (80). Immunophenotype-directed therapies for pediatric large cell lymphoma are under way in the United States through the Children's Oncology Group.

Role of Radiation Therapy

With the development of effective multiagent chemotherapy regimens, radiation therapy for local control of primary disease (exclusive of bone) or for CNS prophylaxis has been virtually eliminated. It is reserved for emergency treatment of mediastinal disease or spinal cord compression, treatment for patients who fail to obtain a complete remission after induction chemotherapy, palliation of pain or mass effect, consolidation before bone marrow transplantation in patients with recurrent disease, treatment of overt CNS lymphoma at diagnosis or relapse, and treatment of leukemic transformation at diagnosis.

Primary Site and Involved-Field Irradiation (Exclusive of Primary Bone Lesions)

To reduce the potential adverse effects associated with radiation therapy, protocols reduced the local field dose to 20 Gy and the volume of tumor margin from 5 cm to 2 to 3 cm (121,209). Results of these limited trials showed similar local control and survival rates to those achieved with more aggressive local field therapy in early stage NHL. In a randomized trial, POG observed no difference in results between induction therapy with cyclophosphamide, doxorubicin, vincristine, and prednisone (CHOP) alone and CHOP plus 27 Gy involved field irradiation (104). Most investigators have abandoned the use of involved-field irradiation in localized early stage pediatric NHL.

The role of local field radiation therapy in advanced-stage disease is questionable. In the one published randomized trial that studied the use of chemotherapy with or without irradiation the 2-year event-free survival rate in both treatment arms was only 38%—a value so low that the potential contribution of radiation therapy may have been masked by ineffective systemic control (126). Nonetheless, because of concern for the potential of radiation therapy to compromise the delivery of chemotherapy, involved-field irradiation has been eliminated from the design of advanced-stage pediatric NHL trials. Recent results of chemotherapy-alone trials tend to support this practice (174).

Local residual disease, after induction chemotherapy or as relapse after a complete remission, often most is managed with local field irradiation in doses ranging from 30 Gy for the small cell lymphocyte/lymphoblastic to 45 Gy for the large cell histiocytic subtypes. The data concerning dose–response relationships, by histology, in adult NHL are reviewed in detail in Chapter 76. The potential benefit of radiation therapy as consolidative therapy for high-risk patients in bone marrow transplantation is being addressed in current study trials. For palliation, radiation therapy at total doses as low as 10 Gy (given as conventional fractionation) often results in rapid relief from symptoms associated with such conditions as superior vena cava syndrome, acute respiratory distress, spinal cord compression, and orbital proptosis. Palliation of cranial nerve deficits, however, requires higher total doses of local field irradiation (20 to 30 Gy) (83).

Primary Non-Hodgkin's Lymphoma of Bone

Primary NHL of bone (PBL) is a disseminated disease at diagnosis, as evidenced by its high rate of systemic spread in patients with clinically apparent early stage presentation. Local field irradiation to the involved bone was included in the early chemotherapy trials. Total doses used for PBL (45 to 55 Gy) were typically higher than for nodal disease. However, because of the increased incidence of second primary bone tumors observed with the combined-modality therapy and the potential for increased morbidity in growing children, studies attempting to reduce the risk of late morbidity by eliminating irradiation are under way (107).

Prophylaxis and Overt Central Nervous System Disease

In the only published randomized trial of CNS presymptomatic therapy in pediatric NHL, 1/18 (6%) children randomly assigned to cranial irradiation and intrathecal methotrexate developed an isolated CNS relapse, compared with 4/16 (25%) of those who did not receive any specific form of CNS prophylactic therapy (126).

Concern for increased neurotoxicity with the use of cranial irradiation in children prompted investigators to test the efficacy of intrathecal chemotherapy alone for CNS prophylaxis. Modern chemotherapeutic regimen trials of intrathecal chemoprophylaxis have been successful in preventing isolated CNS relapse in approximately 95% of children with NHL (7). Whether CNS preventive therapy may be avoided in some good-risk patients with limited disease, such as those with a totally resected abdominal primary or non-Burkitt's, nonmediastinal, limited-nodal NHL, has not been addressed in clinical trials. It is clear that if and when CNS prophylaxis is required, radiation therapy is no longer indicated (127).

Indications for cranial irradiation currently are limited to patients with overt CNS lymphoma at diagnosis or relapse and those with leukemic transformation at diagnosis, based on a high rate of CNS relapse with chemotherapy alone and the proven efficacy of intrathecal methotrexate plus cranial irradiation in these settings. Finally, patients with cranial nerve palsies should be considered for irradiation to the skull base or whole cranium.

Careful follow-up of patients after therapy for assessment of both status of disease and treatment-related complications is critical (Fig. 87.6).

Testicular Lymphoma

Testicular involvement at diagnosis is uncommon (5% to 10% of children with disseminated SNCC NHL). Most of these patients undergo orchiectomy, and the efficacy of scrotal irradiation is unclear. Although the prolonged remissions seen in children with chemosensitive disease suggest that scrotal irradiation may not be necessary, the poor prognosis of patients with testicular involvement and the occurrence of relapses in the testes argue in favor of local therapy with orchiectomy or irradiation as a component of therapy (65,90,116). Testicular relapse on therapy appears to indicate drug-resistant disease and a poor prognosis, despite testicular irradiation and chemotherapy.

Posttransplant Lymphoproliferative Disorder

PTLD encompasses a spectrum of abnormal B-cell lymphoid proliferation that occurs following transplant in the setting of compromised T-cell immunity, antirejection immunosuppressive therapy, and is almost always associated with EBV infection (18,37,47,72,108). Although their efficacy is not proven, antiviral agents such as acyclovir and ganciclovir along with high doses of intravenous immunoglobulin, are commonly used as prophylaxis and treatment of PTLD (62,63). Historically, removal of immune suppression has been the mainstay of therapy, but this approach is unsuccessful in the majority of patients due to poor response with refractory disease or development of graft rejection (146). Other strategies include cytotoxic chemotherapy similar to other NHL regimens (e.g., cyclophosphamide, prednisone), cytokine therapy (e.g., α-interferon), cellular immunotherapy, and anti-B-cell antibody therapy. The use of rituximab, a humanized anti-CD 20 monoclonal antibody, has shown promise in early studies and is under investigation in both adults and children (134).

Future Investigations

In children with localized disease (stages I and II), the excellent survival rates achieved with reduced therapy support the practice of minimizing treatment to potentially reduce the incidence and severity of adverse late effects. For the small number of children who do suffer a relapse, secondary treatment with salvage chemotherapy regimens is highly successful. In children with advanced stage NHL (stages III and IV) in whom survival

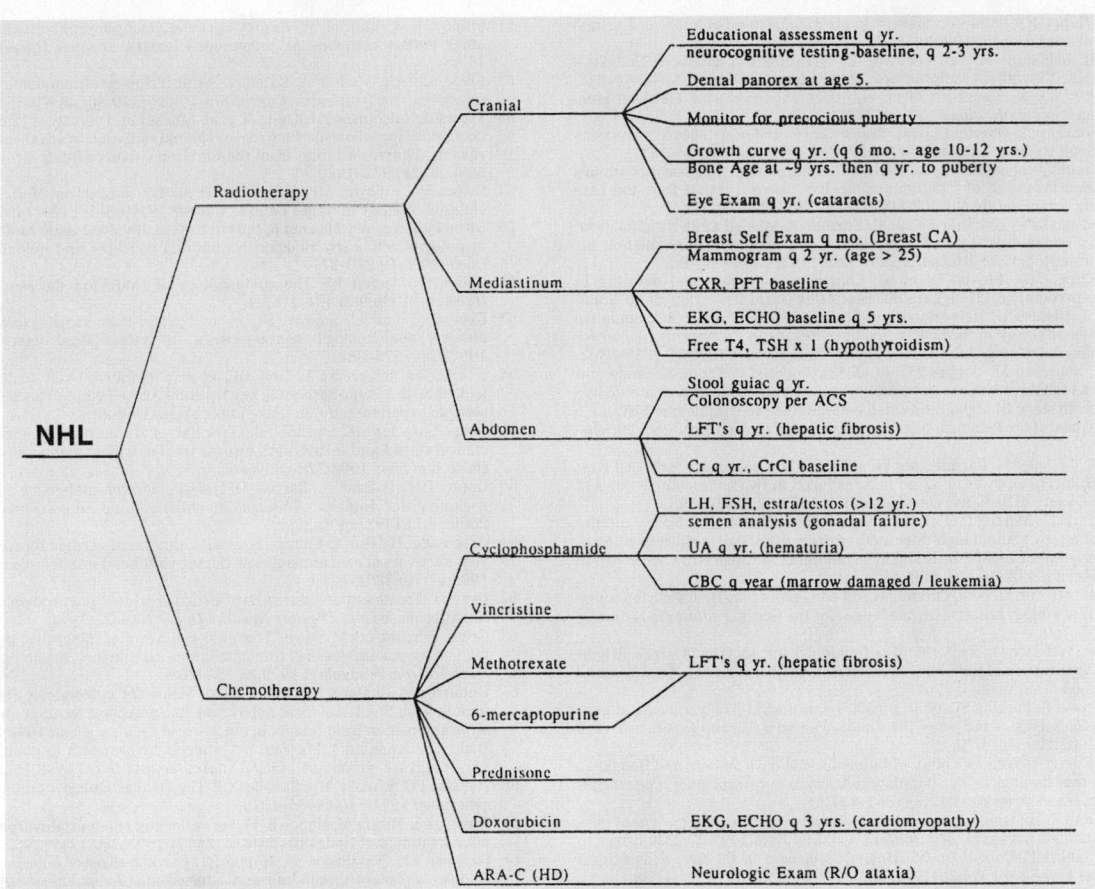

FIGURE 87.6. Late effects screening recommendations for childhood non-Hodgkin's lymphoma. ACS,; ARA-C,; CBC, complete blood count; CA,; Cr,; Crcl,; CXR,; ECHO, echocardiogram; EKG, electrocardiogram; FSH, follicle-stimulating hormone; LFTs,; LH,; NHL, non-Hodgkin's lymphoma; PFT,; R/O,; TSH, thyroid-stimulating hormone; UA, urine analysis. (From Constine L, Hobbie W, Schwartz C. Facilitated assessment of chronic treatment by symptom and organ systems. In: Schwartz C, Constine L, Hobbie W, et al., eds. *Survivors of childhood cancer: assessment and management.* St Louis: Mosby Year Book, 1994;21–80, with permission.)

rates remain poor, future trials are aimed at the development of more effective therapeutic regimens that include new types of active chemical agents, hematopoietic growth factors to allow for dose intensification of chemotherapy, biologic response modifiers (e.g., interleukin-2, interferon, monoclonal antibodies), and stem cell transplantation. The goal in developing modern therapies such as immunotherapy (e.g., rituximab, the anti-CD 20 antibody) is to increase cure rates for those patients at higher risk of failure without increasing morbidity, toxicity, or late effects. New diagnostic strategies such as PET scan may contribute to improved outcomes through more accurate staging and response monitoring, thus allowing early intervention when primary treatments fail. Detection of minimal residual disease, which has proven to be an effective end point of therapeutic efficacy in children with leukemia, is being evaluated in childhood NHL (157). The challenges lie in utilizing new technologies to investigate the cytogenetic and molecular subtypes of pediatric NHL, understand the key events in lymphomagenesis, identify critical genes that can be used for targeted therapy, develop techniques for assessment of minimal residual disease, and ultimately to develop better therapeutic strategies that are more effective, but less toxic.

References

1. Abromowitch M, Sposto R, Perkins S, et al. Outcome of Children's Cancer Group (CCG) 5941: a pilot study for the treatment of newly diagnosed pediatric patients with disseminated lymphoblastic lymphoma. ASCO. *J Clin Oncol* 2000;19:583a(abstr).

2. Adams MJ, Hardenbergh PH, Constine LS, et al. Radiation-associated cardiovascular disease. *Crit Rev Oncol Hematol* 2003;45(1):55–75.

3. Ambinder RF, Browning PJ, Lorenzana I, et al. Epstein-Barr virus and childhood Hodgkin's disease in Honduras and the United States. *Blood* 1993;81(2):462–467.

4. Amylon M, Shuster J, Pullen J, et al. Intensive high-dose asparaginase consolidation improves survival for pediatric patients with T cell acute lymphoblastic leukemia and advanced stage lymphoblastic lymphoma: a Pediatric Oncology Group study. *Leukemia* 1999;13:335–342.

5. Anderson J, Jenkin R, Wilson J, et al. Long-term follow-up of patients treated with COMP or LSA2-L2 therapy for childhood non-Hodgkin's lymphoma: a report of CCG-551 from the Children's Cancer Group. *J Clin Oncol* 1993;11:1024–1032.

6. Anderson J, Wilson J, Jenkin R, et al. Childhood non-Hodgkin's lymphoma: the results of a randomized trial comparing a 4-drug regimen (COMP) with a 10-drug regimen (LSA2-L2). *N Engl J Med* 1983;308:559–565.

7. Anderson JE, Litzow MR, Appelbaum FR, et al. Allogeneic, syngeneic, and autologous marrow transplantation for Hodgkin's disease: the 21-year Seattle experience. *J Clin Oncol* 1993;11(12):2342–2350.

8. Arya LS, Dinand V, Thavaraj V, et al. Hodgkin's disease in Indian children: outcome with chemotherapy alone. *Pediatr Blood Cancer* 2006;46(1):26–34.

9. Asselin B, Shuster J, Amylon M, et al. Improved event-free survival (EFS) with high dose methotrexate in T-cell acute lymphoblastic leukemia (T-ALL) and advanced stage lymphoblastic lymphoma (T-NHL): a Pediatric Oncology Group (POG) study. ASCO. *J Clin Oncol* 2001;20:367a(abstr).

10. Bader SB, Weinstein H, Mauch P, et al. Pediatric stage IV Hodgkin disease. Long-term survival. *Cancer* 1993;72(1):249–255.

11. Baez F, Ocampo E, Conter V, et al. Treatment of childhood Hodgkin's disease with COPP or COPP-ABV (hybrid) without radiotherapy in Nicaragua. *Ann Oncol* 1997;8(3):247–250.

12. Baker KS, Gordon BG, Gross TG, et al. Autologous hematopoietic stem-cell transplantation for relapsed or refractory Hodgkin's disease in children and adolescents. *J Clin Oncol* 1999;17(3):825–831.

13. Barrett A, Crennan E, Barnes J, et al. Treatment of clinical stage I Hodgkin's disease by local radiation therapy alone. A United Kingdom Childrens Cancer Study Group study. *Cancer* 1990;66(4):670–674.

14. Bayle-Weisgerber C, Lemercier N, Teillet F, et al. Hodgkin's disease in children. Results of therapy in a mixed group of 178 clinical and pathologically staged patients over 13 years. *Cancer* 1984;54(2):215–222.

15. Beaty O 3rd, Hudson MM, Greenwald C, et al. Subsequent malignancies in children and adolescents after treatment for Hodgkin's disease. *J Clin Oncol* 1995;13(3):603–609.

16. Behar RA, Hoppe RT. Radiation therapy in the management of bulky mediastinal Hodgkin's disease. *Cancer* 1990;66(1):75–79.
17. Behrendt H, Brinkhuis M, van Leeuwen EF. Treatment of childhood Hodgkin's disease with ABVD without radiotherapy. *Med Pediatr Oncol* 1996;26(4):244–248.
18. Bhatia S, Ramsay N, Steinbuch M, et al. Malignant neoplasms following bone marrow transplantation. *Blood* 1996;87:3633–3639.
19. Bhatia S, Robison LL, Oberlin O, et al. Breast cancer and other second neoplasms after childhood Hodgkin's disease. *N Engl J Med* 1996;334(12):745–751.
20. Bhatia S, Yasui Y, Robison LL, et al. High risk of subsequent neoplasms continues with extended follow-up of childhood Hodgkin's disease: report from the Late Effects Study Group. *J Clin Oncol* 2003;21(23):4386–4394.
21. Bierman PJ, Vose JM, Leichner PK, et al. Yttrium 90-labeled antiferritin followed by high-dose chemotherapy and autologous bone marrow transplantation for poor-prognosis Hodgkin's disease. *J Clin Oncol* 1993;11(4):698–703.
22. Bodis S, Kraus MD, Pinkus G, et al. Clinical presentation and outcome in lymphocyte-predominant Hodgkin's disease. *J Clin Oncol* 1997;15(9):3060–3066.
23. Bramswig J, Heimes U, Heierman E, et al. The effects of different cumulative doses of chemotherapy on testicular function. Results in 75 patients treated for Hodgkin's disease during childhood or adolescence. *Cancer* 1990;65:1298–1302.
24. Brecher M, Schwenn M, Coppes MJ, et al. Fractionated cyclophosphamide and back to back high dose methotrexate and cytosine arabinoside improves outcome in patients with stage III high grade small non-cleaved cell lymphomas (SNCCL): a randomized trial of the Pediatric Oncology Group. *Med Pediat Oncol* 1997;29:526–533.
25. Brugieres L, LeDeley M, Pacquement H, et al. CD 30+ anaplastic large-cell lymphoma in children: analysis of 82 patients enrolled in two consecutive studies of the French Society of Pediatric Oncology. *Blood* 1998;92:3591–3598.
26. Cairo M, Krailo M, Morse M, et al. Long-term follow-up of short intensive multiagent chemotherapy without high-dose methotrexate ('Orange') in children with advanced non-lymphoblastic non-Hodgkin's lymphoma: a Children's Cancer Group report. *Leukemia* 2002;16:594–600.
27. Cairo M, Raetz E, Lim M, et al. Childhood and adolescent non-Hodgkin lymphoma: new insights in biology and critical challenges for the future. *Pediatr Blood Cancer* 2005;45:753–769.
28. Cairo M, Sposto R, Hoover-Regan M, et al. Childhood and adolescent large-cell lymphoma (LCL): a review of the Children's Cancer Group experience. *Am J Hematol* 2003;72:53–63.
29. Cairo M, Sposto R, Perkins SL, et al. Burkitt's and Burkitt-like lymphoma in children and adolescents: a review of the Children's Cancer Group experience. *Br J Haematol* 2003;120:660–670.
30. Chang ET, Zheng T, Weir EG, et al. Childhood social environment and Hodgkin's lymphoma: new findings from a population-based case-control study. *Cancer Epidemiol Biomarkers Prev* 2004;13(8):1361–1370.
31. Clark D, Rubin P, Hudson A, et al. Increased incidence of second malignant neoplasms in Hodgkin's disease. *In J Radiat Oncol Biol Phys* 1993;27:233(abstr).
32. Cleary SF, Link MP, Donaldson SS. Hodgkin's disease in the very young. *Int J Radiat Oncol Biol Phys* 1994;28(1):77–83.
33. Constine L, Clark D, Schwartz C, et al. Second malignant neoplasms in children irradiated for Hodgkin's disease. *Med Pediat Oncol* 1993;21:611(abstr).
34. Constine L, Marcus R, Chauvenet A, et al. Patterns of failure after response-based, dose-dense therapy for intermediate/high risk pediatric Hodgkin's disease (POG 9425). *Int J Radiat Oncol Biol Phys* 2005;63:S21–22.
35. Constine LS, Donaldson SS, McDougall IR, et al. Thyroid dysfunction after radiotherapy in children with Hodgkin's disease. *Cancer* 1984;53(4):878–883.
36. Crnkovich MJ, Leopold K, Hoppe RT, et al. Stage I to IIB Hodgkin's disease: the combined experience at Stanford University and the Joint Center for Radiation Therapy. *J Clin Oncol* 1987;5(7):1041–1049.
37. DeMario M, Liebowitz D. Lymphomas in the immunocompromised patient. *Sem Oncol* 1998;4:492–502.
38. DeWit M, Bumann D, Beyer W, et al. Whole body positron emission tomography (PET) for diagnosis of residual mass in patients with lymphoma. *Ann Oncol* 1997; 8[Suppl 1]:S57–S60.
39. Dieckmann K, Potter R, Wagner W, et al. Up-front centralized data review and individualized treatment proposals in a multicenter pediatric Hodgkin's disease trial with 71 participating hospitals: the experience of the German-Austrian pediatric multicenter trial DAL-HD-90. *Radiother Oncol* 2002;62(2):191–200.
40. Diehl V, Franklin J, Hasenclever D, et al. BEACOPP, a new dose-escalated and accelerated regimen, is at least as effective as COPP/ABVD in patients with advanced-stage Hodgkin's lymphoma: interim report from a trial of the German Hodgkin's Lymphoma Study Group. *J Clin Oncol* 1998;16(12):3810–3821.
41. Donaldson SS. Effects of irradiation on skeletal growth and development. In: Green DMD'Angio GJ, eds. *Late effects of treatment for childhood cancer*. New York: Wiley-Liss, 1992;.
42. Donaldson SS, Hancock SL, Hoppe RT. The Janeway lecture. Hodgkin's disease—finding the balance between cure and late effects. *Cancer J Sci Am* 1999;5(6):325–333.
43. Donaldson SS, Kaplan HS. Complications of treatment of Hodgkin's disease in children. *Cancer Treat Rep* 1982;66(4):977–989.
44. Donaldson SS, Hudson MM, Lamborn KR, et al. VAMP and low-dose, involved-field radiation for children and adolescents with favorable, early-stage Hodgkin's disease: results of a prospective clinical trial. *J Clin Oncol* 2002;20(14):3081–3087.
45. Donaldson SS, Whitaker SJ, Plowman PN, et al. Stage I-II pediatric Hodgkin's disease: long-term follow-up demonstrates equivalent survival rates following different management schemes. *J Clin Oncol* 1990;8(7):1128–1137.
46. Dorffel W, Luders H, Ruhl U, et al. Preliminary results of the multicenter trial GPOH-HD 95 for the treatment of Hodgkin's disease in children and adolescents: analysis and outlook. *Klin Padiatr* 2003;215(3):139–145.
47. Dror Y, Greenberg M, Taylor G, et al. Lymphoproliferative disorders after organ transplantation in children. *Transplantation* 1999;67:990–998.
48. Ekert H, Fok T, Dalla-Pozza L, et al. A pilot study of EVAP/ABV chemotherapy in 25 newly diagnosed children with Hodgkin's disease. *Br J Cancer* 1993;67(1):159–162.
49. Ekert H, Toogood I, Downie P, et al. High incidence of treatment failure with vincristine, etoposide, epirubicin, and prednisolone chemotherapy with successful salvage in childhood Hodgkin disease. *Med Pediatr Oncol* 1999;32(4):255–258.
50. Ekert H, Waters KD, Smith PJ, et al. Treatment with MOPP or ChlVPP chemotherapy only for all stages of childhood Hodgkin's disease. *J Clin Oncol* 1988;6(12):1845–1850.
51. Filipovich A, Mathur A, Kamat D, et al. Lymphoproliferative disorders and other tumors complicating immunodeficiencies. *Immunodeficiency* 1994;5:91–112.
52. Filipovich AH, Mathur A, Kamat D, et al. Primary immunodeficiencies: genetic risk factors for lymphoma. *Cancer Res* 1992;52[19 Suppl]:5465S–5467S.
53. Fryer CJ, Hutchinson RJ, Krailo M, et al. Efficacy and toxicity of 12 courses of ABVD chemotherapy followed by low-dose regional radiation in advanced Hodgkin's disease in children: a report from the Children's Cancer Study Group. *J Clin Oncol* 1990;8(12):1971–1980.
54. Gehan EA, Sullivan MP, Fuller LM, et al. The intergroup Hodgkin's disease in children. A study of stages I and II. *Cancer* 1990;65(6):1429–1437.
55. Girinsky T, van der Maazen R, Specht L, et al. Involved-node radiotherapy (INRT) in patients with early Hodgkin lymphoma: concepts and guidelines. *Radiother Oncol* 2006;79:270–277.
56. Glaser SL, Jarrett RF. The epidemiology of Hodgkin's disease. *Baillieres Clin Haematol* 1996;9(3):401–416.
57. Glaser SL, Lin RJ, Stewart SL, et al. Epstein-Barr virus-associated Hodgkin's disease: epidemiologic characteristics in international data. *Int J Cancer* 1997;70(4):375–382.
58. Goldberg J, Silverman L, Levy DE, et al. Childhood T-cell acute lymphoblastic leukemia: the Dana-Farber Cancer Institute Acute Lymphoblastic Leukemia Consortium experience. *J Clin Oncol* 2003;21:3616–3622.
59. Gospodarowicz MK, Sutcliffe SB, Clark RM, et al. Analysis of supradiaphragmatic clinical stage I and II Hodgkin's disease treated with radiation alone. *Int J Radiat Oncol Biol Phys* 1992;22(5):859–865.
60. Green DM, Hyland A, Barcos MP, et al. Second malignant neoplasms after treatment for Hodgkin's disease in childhood or adolescence. *J Clin Oncol* 2000;18(7):1492–1499.
61. Green DM, Hyland A, Chung CS, et al. Cancer and cardiac mortality among 15-year survivors of cancer diagnosed during childhood or adolescence. *J Clin Oncol* 1999;17(10):3207–3215.
62. Gross T. Treatment of Epstein-Barr virus-associated post transplant lymphoproliferative disorders. *J Pediatr Hematol Oncol* 2001;23:7–9.
63. Gross T, Steinbuch M, DeFor T, et al. B-cell lymphoproliferative disorders following hematopoietic stem cell transplantation: risk factors, treatment and outcome. *Bone Marrow Transplant* 1999;23:251–258.
64. Guiterrez M, Bhatia K, Barriga R, et al. Molecular epidemiology of Burkitt's lymphoma from South America: differences in breakpoint location and Epstein-Barr virus association from tumors in other world regions. *Blood* 1992;79:3261–3266.
65. Haddy T, Sandlund J, Magrath I. Testicular involvement in young patients with non-Hodgkin's lymphoma. *Am J Pediatr Hematol Oncol* 1988;10:224–229.
66. Haluska FG, Brufsky AM, Canellos GP. The cellular biology of the Reed-Sternberg cell. *Blood* 1994;84(4):1005–1019.
67. Hancock S, Tucker M, Hoppe R. Factors affecting late mortality from heart disease after treatment of Hodgkin's disease. *JAMA* 1993;270:1949–1955.
68. Hancock SL, Donaldson SS, Hoppe RT. Cardiac disease following treatment of Hodgkin's disease in children and adolescents. *J Clin Oncol* 1993;11(7):1208–1215.
69. Hanna SL, Fletcher BD, Boulden TF, et al. MR imaging of infradiaphragmatic lymphadenopathy in children and adolescents with Hodgkin disease: comparison with lymphography and CT. *J Magn Reson Imaging* 1993;3(3):461–470.
70. Harris NL, Jaffe ES, Stein H, et al. A revised European-American classification of lymphoid neoplasms: a proposal from the International Lymphoma Study Group. *Blood* 1994;84(5):1361–1392.
71. Heerema N, Bernheim A, Lim M, et al. State of the art and future needs in cytogenetic/molecular genetics/arrays in childhood lymphoma: summary report of workshop at the First International Symposium on childhood and adolescent non-Hodgkin lymphoma. *Pediatr Blood Cancer* 2005;45:616–622.
72. Ho M, Jaffe R, Miller G, et al. The frequency of Epstein-Barr virus infection and associated lymphoproliferative syndrome after transplantation and its manifestations in children. *Transplantation* 1988;45:719–727.
73. Hobbie WL, Ginsberg JP, Ogle SK, et al. Fertility in males treated for Hodgkins disease with COPP/ABV hybrid. *Pediatr Blood Cancer* 2005;44(2):193–196.
74. Hoppe RT, Hanlon AL, Hanks GE, et al. Progress in the treatment of Hodgkin's disease in the United States, 1973 versus 1983. The Patterns of Care Study. *Cancer* 1994;74(12):3198–3203.
75. Horning SJ, Hoppe RT, Breslin S, et al. Stanford V and radiotherapy for locally extensive and advanced Hodgkin's disease: mature results of a prospective clinical trial. *J Clin Oncol* 2002;20(3):630–637.
76. Horning SJ, Williams J, Bartlett NL, et al. Assessment of the Stanford V regimen and consolidative radiotherapy for bulky and advanced Hodgkin's disease: Eastern Cooperative Oncology Group pilot study E1492. *J Clin Oncol* 2000;18(5):972–980.
77. Hudson MM, Greenwald C, Thompson E, et al. Efficacy and toxicity of multiagent chemotherapy and low-dose involved-field radiotherapy in children and adolescents with Hodgkin's disease. *J Clin Oncol* 1993;11(1):100–108.
78. Hudson MM, Poquette CA, Lee J, et al. Increased mortality after successful treatment for Hodgkin's disease. *J Clin Oncol* 1998;16(11):3592–3600.
79. Hunger SP, Link MP, Donaldson SS. ABVD/MOPP and low-dose involved-field radiotherapy in pediatric Hodgkin's disease: the Stanford experience. *J Clin Oncol* 1994;12(10):2160–2166.
80. Hutchison R, Berard C, Shuster J. B-cell lineage confers a favorable outcome among children and adolescents with large-cell lymphoma: a Pediatric Oncology Group study. *J Clin Oncol* 1995;13:2023–2032.
81. Hutchinson RJ, Fryer CJ, Davis PC, et al. MOPP or radiation in addition to ABVD in the treatment of pathologically staged advanced Hodgkin's disease in children: results of the Children's Cancer Group phase III trial. *J Clin Oncol* 1998;16(3):897–906.
82. Hvizdala E, Berard C, Callihan T, et al. Non-lymphoblastic lymphoma in children: histology and stage-related response to therapy. A Pediatric Oncology Group study. *J Clin Oncol* 1991;9:1889–1895.
83. Ingram L, Fairclough D, Furman W, et al. Cranial nerve palsy in childhood acute lymphoblastic leukemia and non-Hodgkin's lymphoma. *Cancer* 1991;67:2262–2268.
84. Jaffe E. The role of immunophenotypic markers in the classification of non-Hodgkin's lymphomas. *Semin Oncol* 1990;17:11–19.
85. Jenkin D, Doyle J, Berry M, et al. Hodgkin's disease in children: treatment with MOPP and low-dose, extended field irradiation without laparotomy. Late results and toxicity. *Med Pediatr Oncol* 1990;18(4):265–272.

86. Jerusalem G, Beguin Y, Fassotte M, et al. Whole-body positron emission tomography using fluorine-18-fluorodeoxyglucose for post-treatment evaluation in Hodgkin's disease and non-Hodgkin's lymphoma has a higher diagnostic and prognostic value than classical computed tomography scan imaging. *Blood* 1999;94:429–433.
87. Kadin ME, Liebowitz DN. Cytokine and cytokine receptors in Hodgkin's disease. In: Mauch PM, et al., eds. *Hodgkin's disease*. Philadelphia: Lippincott Williams & Wilkins, 1999;139–157.
88. Kaplan H. *Hodgkin's disease*. Cambridge: Harvard University Press, 1980.
89. Kaplan W, Jochelson M, Herman T, et al. Gallium-67 imaging: a predictor of residual tumor viability and clinical outcome in patients with diffuse large-cell lymphoma. *J Clin Oncol* 1990;8:1966–1970.
90. Kellie S, Pui C, Murphy S. Childhood non-Hodgkin's lymphoma involving the testis: clinical features and treatment outcome. *J Clin Oncol* 1989;7:1066–1070.
91. Kelly KM, Hutchinson RJ, Sposto R, et al. Feasibility of upfront dose-intensive chemotherapy in children with advanced-stage Hodgkin's lymphoma: preliminary results from the Children's Cancer Group Study CCG-59704. *Ann Oncol* 2002;13[Suppl 1]:107–111.
92. Kennedy BJ, Loeb V Jr., Peterson V, et al. Survival in Hodgkin's disease by stage and age. *Med Pediatr Oncol* 1992;20(2):100–104.
93. King V, Constine LS, Clark D, et al. Symptomatic coronary artery disease after mantle irradiation for Hodgkin's disease. *Int J Radiat Oncol Biol Phys* 1996;36(4):881–889.
94. Krasin M, Rai S, Kun L, et al. Patterns of treatment failure in pediatric and young adult patients with Hodgkin's disease: local disease control with combined-modality therapy. *J Clin Oncol* 2005;23:8406–8413.
95. Kung FH. Hodgkin's disease in children 4 years of age or younger. *Cancer* 1991;67(5):1428–1430.
96. Kung FH, Schwartz CL, Ferree CR, et al. POG 8625: a randomized trial comparing chemotherapy with chemoradiotherapy for children and adolescents with stages I, IIA, IIIA1 Hodgkin disease: a report from the Children's Oncology Group. *J Pediatr Hematol Oncol* 2006;28(6):362–368.
97. Kuppers R, Rajewsky K. The origin of Hodgkin and Reed/Sternberg cells in Hodgkin's disease. *Ann Rev Immunol* 1998;16:471–493.
98. Kurtzberg J, Graham M. Non-Hodgkin's lymphoma: biologic classification and implications of therapy. *Pediatr Clin North Am* 1991;38:443–456.
99. Landman-Parker J, Pacquement H, Leblanc T, et al. Localized childhood Hodgkin's disease: response-adapted chemotherapy with etoposide, bleomycin, vinblastine, and prednisone before low-dose radiation therapy-results of the French Society of Pediatric Oncology Study MDH90. *J Clin Oncol* 2000;18(7):1500–1507.
100. Laver J, Kraveka J, Hutchison R, et al. Advanced-stage large-cell lymphoma in children and adolescents: results of a randomized trial incorporating intermediate-dose methotrexate and high-dose cytarabine in the maintenance phase of the APO regimen: a Pediatric Oncology Group phase III trial. *J Clin Oncol* 2005;23: 541–547.
101. Laver J, Mahmoud H, Pick T, et al. Results of a randomized phase III trial in children and adolescents with advanced stage diffuse large cell non-Hodgkin's lymphoma: a Pediatric Oncology Group study. *Leuk Lymphoma* 2002;43:105–109.
102. Le Floch O, Donaldson SS, Kaplan HS. Pregnancy following oophoropexy and total nodal irradiation in women with Hodgkin's disease. *Cancer* 1976;38(6):2263–2268.
103. Lieskovsky YE, Donaldson SS, Torres MA, et al. High-dose therapy and autologous hematopoietic stem-cell transplantation for recurrent or refractory pediatric Hodgkin's disease: results and prognostic indices. *J Clin Oncol* 2004;22(22):4532–4540.
104. Link M, Donaldson S, Berard C, et al. Results of treatment of childhood localized non-Hodgkin's lymphoma with combination chemotherapy with or without radiotherapy. *N Engl J Med* 1990;322:1169–1174.
105. Link M, Shuster J, Donaldson S, et al. Treatment of children and young adults with early-stage non-Hodgkin's lymphoma. *N Engl J Med* 1997;337:1259–1266.
106. Lobo-Sanahuja F, Garcia I, Barrantes JC, et al. Pediatric Hodgkin's disease in Costa Rica: twelve years' experience of primary treatment by chemotherapy alone, without staging laparotomy. *Med Pediatr Oncol* 1994;22(6):398–403.
107. Lones M, Perkins S, Sposto R, et al. Non-Hodgkin's lymphoma arising in the bone in children and adolescents is associated with an excellent outcome: a Children's Cancer Group report. *J Clin Oncol* 2002;20:2293–2301.
108. Loren A, Porter D, Stadtmauer E, et al. Post-transplant lymphoproliferative disorder: a review. *Bone Marrow Transplant* 2003;31:145–155.
109. Mack TM, Cozen W, Shibata DK, et al. Concordance for Hodgkin's disease in identical twins suggesting genetic susceptibility to the young-adult form of the disease. *N Engl J Med* 1995;332(7):413–418.
110. Magrath I. In: Pizzo P, Poplack D, eds. *Principles and practice of pediatric oncology*, 4th ed. Malignant Non-Hodgkin's Lymphomas in Children. Philadelphia: Lippincott Williams & Wilkins, 2002;661–705.
111. Magrath I, Bhatia K. Pathogenesis of small noncleaved cell lymphomas (Burkitt's lymphoma). In Magrath I, ed. The Non-Hodgkin's Lymphomas, 2nd ed. London: Arnold, 1997;385–409.
112. Maguire A, Craft AW, Evans RG, et al. The long-term effects of treatment on the dental condition of children surviving malignant disease. *Cancer* 1987;60(10):2570–2575.
113. Maity A, Goldwein JW, Lange B, et al. Comparison of high-dose and low-dose radiation with and without chemotherapy for children with Hodgkin's disease: an analysis of the experience at the Children's Hospital of Philadelphia and the Hospital of the University of Pennsylvania. *J Clin Oncol* 1992;10(6):929–935.
114. Maity A, Goldwein JW, Lange B, et al. Mediastinal masses in children with Hodgkin's disease. An analysis of the Children's Hospital of Philadelphia and the Hospital of the University of Pennsylvania experience. *Cancer* 1992;69(11):2755–2760.
115. Marina N, Greenwald C, Fairclough D, et al. Serial pulmonary function studies in children treated for newly diagnosed Hodgkin's disease with mantle radiotherapy plus cycles of cyclophosphamide, vincristine, and procarbazine alternating with cycles of doxorubicin, bleomycin, vinblastine, and decarbazine. *Cancer* 1995;75:1706–1711.
116. Martenson J, Buskirk S, Listrup D, et al. Patterns of failure in primary testicular non-Hodgkin's lymphoma. *J Clin Oncol* 1988;6:297–302.
117. Mason DY, Banks PM, Chan J, et al. Nodular lymphocyte predominance Hodgkin's disease. A distinct clinicopathological entity. *Am J Surg Pathol* 1994;18(5):526–530.
118. Mauch PM. Controversies in the management of early stage Hodgkin's disease. *Blood* 1994;83(2):318–329.
119. Mauch PM, Weinstein H, Botnick L, et al. An evaluation of long-term survival and treatment complications in children with Hodgkin's disease. *Cancer* 1983;51(5):925–932.
120. McClain K, Joshi V, Murphy S. Cancers in children with HIV infection. *Hematol Oncol* 1996;10:1189–1201.
121. Meadows A, Sposto R, Jenkin R, et al. Similar efficacy of 6 and 18 months of therapy with four drugs (COMP) for localized non-Hodgkin's lymphoma of children: a report from the Children's Cancer Study Group. *J Clin Oncol* 1989;7:92–99.
122. Mertens AC, Yasui Y, Neglia JP, et al. Late mortality experience in five-year survivors of childhood and adolescent cancer: the Childhood Cancer Survivor Study. *J Clin Oncol* 2001;19(13):3163–3172.
123. Mink SA, Armitage JO. High-dose therapy in lymphomas: a review of the current status of allogeneic and autologous stem cell transplantation in Hodgkin's disease and non-Hodgkin's lymphoma. *Oncologist* 2001;6(3):247–256.
124. Mora J, Filippa D, Qin J, et al. Lymphoblastic lymphoma of childhood and the LSA2-L2 protocol: the 30-year experience at Memorial Sloan-Kettering Cancer Center. *Cancer* 2003;98:1283–1291.
125. Mora J, Filippa D, Thaler H, et al. Large cell non-Hodgkin lymphoma of childhood: analysis of 78 consecutive patients enrolled in 2 consecutive protocols at the Memorial Sloan-Kettering Cancer Center. *Cancer* 2000;88:186–197.
126. Murphy S. Classification, staging and end results of treatment of childhood non-Hodgkin's lymphomas: dissimilarities from lymphoma in adults. *Semin Oncol* 1980;7:332–339.
127. Murphy S, Bleyer W. Cranial irradiation is not necessary for central nervous system prophylaxis in pediatric non-Hodgkin's lymphoma. *Int J Radiat Oncol Biol Phys* 1987;13:467–468.
128. Murphy S, Fairclough D, Hutchison R, et al. Non-Hodgkin's lymphomas of childhood: an analysis of the histology, staging, and response to treatment of 338 cases at a single institution. *J Clin Oncol* 1989;7:186–193.
129. Nachman JB, Sposto R, Herzog P, et al. Randomized comparison of low-dose involved-field radiotherapy and no radiotherapy for children with Hodgkin's disease who achieve a complete response to chemotherapy. *J Clin Oncol* 2002;20(18):3765–3771.
130. Nadali G, Vinante F, Ambrosetti A, et al. Serum levels of soluble CD30 are elevated in the majority of untreated patients with Hodgkin's disease and correlate with clinical features and prognosis. *J Clin Oncol* 1994;12(4):793–797.
131. Oberlin O, Boilletot A, Leverger G, et al. Clinical staging, primary chemotherapy and involved field radiotherapy in childhood Hodgkin's disease. *Eur Paediatr Haematol Oncol* 1985;2:65–70.
132. Oberlin O, Leverger G, Pacquement H, et al. Low-dose radiation therapy and reduced chemotherapy in childhood Hodgkin's disease: the experience of the French Society of Pediatric Oncology. *J Clin Oncol* 1992;10(10):1602–1608.
133. Olweny CL, Katongole-Mbidde E, Kiire C, et al. Childhood Hodgkin's disease in Uganda: a ten year experience. *Cancer* 1978;42(2):787–792.
134. Orjuela M, Gross T, Cheung Y-K, et al. Pilot study of chemoimmunotherapy (Cyt, Pred, Ritux) in patients with post transplant lymphoproliferative disorder (PTLD) following solid organ transplant. *Clin Cancer Res* 2003;9[Suppl]:3945S–3952S.
135. Ortin TT, Shostak CA, Donaldson SS. Gonadal status and reproductive function following treatment for Hodgkin's disease in childhood: the Stanford experience. *Int J Radiat Oncol Biol Phys* 1990;19(4):873–880.
136. Patte C, Auperin A, Michon J, et al. The Societe Francaise d'Oncologie Pediatrique LMB89 protocol: highly effective multiagent chemotherapy tailored to the tumor burden and initial response in 561 unselected children with B-cell lymphomas and L3 leukemia. *Blood* 2001;97:3370–3379.
137. Patte C, Kalifa C, Flamant F, et al. Results of the LMB81 protocol a modified LSA2L2 protocol with high dose methotrexate in 84 children with non-B-cell (lymphoblastic) lymphoma. *Med Pediat Oncol* 1992;20:105–113.
138. Patte C, Leverger G, Perel Y, et al. Updated results of the LMB 86 protocol of the French Pediatric Oncology Society (SFOP) for B-cell non-Hodgkin's lymphomas (B-NHL) with CNS involvement (CNS+) and B-ALL. *Med Pediat Oncol* 1990;18: 397.
139. Patte C, Michon J, Behrendt H, et al. Results of the LMB 89 protocol for childhood B-cell lymphoma and leukemia (ALL). SIOP XXIX. *Med Pediat Oncol* 1997;29:358.
140. Pedrick TJ, Hoppe RT. Recovery of spermatogenesis following pelvic irradiation for Hodgkin's disease. *Int J Radiat Oncol Biol Phys* 1986;12(1):117–121.
141. Penn I. De novo malignancies in pediatric organ transplant recipients. *Pediatr Transplant* 1998;2:56–63.
142. Percy CL, Smith MA, Linet M, et al. Lymphomas and reticuloendothelial neoplasms. In: Ries LAG, et al., eds. *Cancer incidence and survival among children and adolescents: United States SEER program, 1975–1995,* Bethesda, MD: National Cancer Institute, SEER Program, 1999;.
143. Perkins S, Segal G, Kjeldsberg C. Classification of non-Hodgkin's lymphomas in children. *Sem Diag Pathol* 1995;12:303–313.
144. Pileri SA, Ascani S, Leoncini L, et al. Hodgkin's lymphoma: the pathologist's viewpoint. *J Clin Pathol* 2002;55(3):162–176.
145. Pinkerton C. Continuing challenges in childhood non-Hodgkin's lymphoma. *Br J Haematol* 2005;130:480–488.
146. Pinkerton C, Hann I, Weston C, et al. Immunodeficiency-related lymphoproliferative disorders: prospective data from the United Kingdom Children's Cancer Study Group registry. *Br J Haematol* 2002;118:456–461.
147. Raetz E, Perkins S, Bhojwani D, et al. Gene expression profiling reveals intrinsic differences between T-cell acute lymphoblastic leukemia and T-cell acute lymphoblastic lymphoma. *Pediatr Blood Cancer* 2006;47:130–140.
148. Rapoport AP, Rowe JM, Kouides PA, et al. One hundred autotransplants for relapsed or refractory Hodgkin's disease and lymphoma: value of pretransplant disease status for predicting outcome. *J Clin Oncol* 1993;11(12):2351–2361.
149. Reiter A, Schrappe M, Ludwig W, et al. Intensive ALL-type therapy without local radiotherapy provides a 90% event-free survival of children with T-cell lymphoblastic lymphoma: a BFM group report. *Blood* 1994;95:416–421.
150. Reiter A, Schrappe M, Parwaresch R, et al. Non-Hodgkin's lymphomas of childhood and adolescence: results of a treatment stratified for biologic subtypes and stage a report of the Berlin-Frankfurt-Munster Group. *J Clin Oncol* 1995;13:359–372.
151. Reiter A, Schrappe M, Tiemann M, et al. Successful treatment strategy for Ki-1 anaplastic large cell lymphomas of childhood: a prospective analysis of 62 patients enrolled in three consecutive Berlin-Frankfurt-Munster group studies. *J Clin Oncol* 1994;12:899–908.

152. Reiter A, Schrappe M, Tiemann M, et al. Improved treatment results in childhood B-cell neoplasms with tailored intensification of therapy: a report of the Berlin-Frankfurt-Munster Group trial NHL-BFM 90. *Blood* 1999;94:3294–3306.
153. Rhodes MM, Delbeke D, Whitlock JA, et al. Utility of FDG-PET/CT in follow-up of children treated for Hodgkin and non-Hodgkin lymphoma. *J Pediatr Hematol Oncol* 2006;28(5):300–306.
154. Rooney CM, Smith CA, Ng CY, et al. Use of gene-modified virus-specific T lymphocytes to control Epstein-Barr-virus-related lymphoproliferation. *Lancet* 1995;345(8941):9–13.
155. Ruhl U, Albrecht M. The German multinational GPOH-HD 95 trial: treatment results and analysis of failures in pediatric Hodgkin's disease using combination chemotherapy with and without radiation. *Int J Radiat Oncol Biol Phys* 2004;60(1):S131.
156. Ruhl U, Albrecht M, Dieckmann K, et al. Response-adapted radiotherapy in the treatment of pediatric Hodgkin's disease: an interim report at 5 years of the German GPOH-HD 95 trial. *Int J Radiat Oncol Biol Phys* 2001;51(5):1209–1218.
157. Sabesan V, Cairo M, Lones M, et al. Assessment of minimal residual disease in childhood non-Hodgkin lymphoma by polymerase chain reaction using patient-specific primers. *J Pediatr Hematol Oncol* 2003;25:109–113.
158. Sackmann-Muriel F, Zubizarreta P, Gallo G, et al. Hodgkin disease in children: results of a prospective randomized trial in a single institution in Argentina. *Med Pediatr Oncol* 1997;29(6):544–552.
159. Sandlund J, Downing J, Crist W. Non-Hodgkin's lymphoma in childhood. *N Engl J Med* 1996;331:1238–1248.
160. Sandlund J, Murphy S, Santana V, et al. CNS involvement in children with newly diagnosed non-Hodgkin's lymphoma. *J Clin Oncol* 2000;12:895–898.
161. Sandlund J, Pui C-H, Santana V, et al. Clinical features and treatment outcome for children with CD 30+ large-cell non-Hodgkin's lymphoma. *J Clin Oncol* 1994;12:895–898.
162. Sandlund J, Santana V, Abromowitch M, et al. Large cell non-Hodgkin lymphoma of childhood: clinical characteristics and outcome. *Leukemia* 1994;8:30–34.
163. Sankila R, Garwicz S, Olsen JH, et al. Risk of subsequent malignant neoplasms among 1,641 Hodgkin's disease patients diagnosed in childhood and adolescence: a population-based cohort study in the five Nordic countries. Association of the Nordic Cancer Registries and the Nordic Society of Pediatric Hematology and Oncology. *J Clin Oncol* 1996;14(5):1442–1446.
164. Santana V, Abromowitch M, Sandlund J, et al. MACOP-B treatment in children and adolescents with advanced diffuse large-cell non-Hodgkin's lymphoma. *Leukemia* 1993;7:187–191.
165. Schellong G. Treatment of children and adolescents with Hodgkin's disease: the experience of the German-Austrian Paediatric Study Group. *Baillieres Clin Haematol* 1996;9(3):619–634.
166. Schellong G. The balance between cure and late effects in childhood Hodgkin's lymphoma: the experience of the German-Austrian Study-Group since 1978. German-Austrian Pediatric Hodgkin's Disease Study Group. *Ann Oncol* 1996;7[Suppl 4]:67–72.
167. Schellong G, Bramswig JH, Hornig-Franz I. Treatment of children with Hodgkin's disease—results of the German Pediatric Oncology Group. *Ann Oncol* 1992;3[Suppl 4]:73–76.
168. Schellong G, Dorffel W, Claviez A, et al. Salvage therapy of progressive and recurrent Hodgkin's disease: results from a multicenter study of the pediatric DAL/GPOH-HD study group. *J Clin Oncol* 2005;23(25):6181–6189.
169. Schellong G, Potter R, Bramswig J, et al. High cure rates and reduced long-term toxicity in pediatric Hodgkin's disease: the German-Austrian multicenter trial DAL-HD-90. The German-Austrian Pediatric Hodgkin's Disease Study Group. *J Clin Oncol* 1999;17(12):3736–3744.
170. Schellong G, Riepenhausen M, Creutzig U, et al. Low risk of secondary leukemias after chemotherapy without mechlorethamine in childhood Hodgkin's disease. German-Austrian Pediatric Hodgkin's Disease Group. *J Clin Oncol* 1997;15:2247–2253.
171. Schmitz N, Sureda A. The role of allogeneic stem-cell transplantation in Hodgkin's disease. *Eur J Haematol Suppl* 2005;66:146–149.
172. Schrappe M, Tiemann M, Ludwig W, et al. Risk-adapted therapy for lymphoblastic T-cell lymphomas: results from trials NHL-BFM 86 and 90. SIOP XXIX. *Med Pediat Oncol* 1997;29:356.
173. Schwartz CL. The management of Hodgkin disease in the young child. *Curr Opin Pediatr* 2003;15(1):10–16.
174. Schwenn M, Blattner S, Lynch E, et al. A 2-month intensive chemotherapy regimen for children with stage III and IV Burkitt's lymphoma and B-cell acute lymphoblastic leukemia. *J Clin Oncol* 1991;9:133–138.
175. Schwenn M, Mahmoud H, Bowman W, et al. Successful treatment of small non-cleaved cell (SNCC) lymphoma and B cell acute lymphoblastic leukemia (B-ALL) with central nervous system (CNS) involvement: a Pediatric Oncology Group (POG) study. *ASCO*.2000;19:580a(abstr).
176. Shad A, Magrath I. Non-Hodgkin's lymphoma. *Pediatr Clin North Am* 1997; 44:863–890.
177. Shah AB, Hudson MM, Poquette CA, et al. Long-term follow-up of patients treated with primary radiotherapy for supradiaphragmatic Hodgkin's disease at St. Jude Children's Research Hospital. *Int J Radiat Oncol Biol Phys* 1999;44(4):867–877.
178. Shahidi M, Kamangari N, Ashley S, et al. Site of relapse after chemotherapy alone for stage I and II Hodgkin's disease. *Radiother Oncol* 2006;78(1):1–5.
179. Shankar AG, Ashley S, Radford M, et al. Does histology influence outcome in childhood Hodgkin's disease? Results from the United Kingdom Children's Cancer Study Group. *J Clin Oncol* 1997;15(7):2622–2630.
180. Sklar CA, Mertens AC, Mitby P, et al. Premature menopause in survivors of childhood cancer: a report from the childhood cancer survivor study. *J Natl Cancer Inst* 2006;98(13):890–896.
181. Smith RS, Chen Q, Hudson MM, et al. Prognostic factors for children with Hodgkin's disease treated with combined-modality therapy. *J Clin Oncol* 2003;21(10):2026–2033.
182. Spaepen K, Stroobants S, Dupont P, et al. Early restaging positron emission tomography with 18F-fluorodeoxyglucose predicts outcome in patients with aggressive non-Hodgkin's lymphoma. *Annal Oncol* 2002;13:1356–1363.
183. Specht L. Prognostic factors in Hodgkin's disease. *Semin Radiat Oncol* 1996;6(3):146–161.
184. Specht L, Nordentoft AM, Cold S, et al. Tumor burden as the most important prognostic factor in early stage Hodgkin's disease. Relations to other prognostic factors and implications for choice of treatment. *Cancer* 1988;61(8):1719–1727.
185. Specht LK, Hasenclever D. Prognostic factors of Hodgkin's disease. In: Mauch PM, et al., eds. *Hodgkin's disease*. Philadelphia: Lippincott Williams & Wilkins, 1999;295–325.
186. Sposto R, Meadows A, Chilcote R, et al. Comparison of long-term outcome of children and adolescents with disseminated non-lymphoblastic non-Hodgkin lymphoma treated with COMP or daunomycin-COMP: a report from the Children's Cancer Group. *Med Pediat Oncol* 2001;37:432–441.
187. Sripada PV, Tenali SG, Vasudevan M, et al. Hybrid (COPP/ABV) therapy in childhood Hodgkin's disease: a study of 53 cases during 1989–1993 at the Cancer Institute, Madras. *Pediatr Hematol Oncol* 1995;12(4):333–341.
188. Sureda A, Arranz R, Iriondo A, et al. Autologous stem-cell transplantation for Hodgkin's disease: results and prognostic factors in 494 patients from the Grupo Espanol de Linfomas/Transplante Autologo de Medula Osea Spanish Cooperative Group. *J Clin Oncol* 2001;19(5):1395–1404.
189. Sureda A, Schmitz N. Role of allogeneic stem cell transplantation in relapsed or refractory Hodgkin's disease. *Ann Oncol* 2002;13[Suppl 1]:128–132.
190. Tarbell NJ, Gelber RD, Weinstein HJ, et al. Sex differences in risk of second malignant tumours after Hodgkin's disease in childhood. *Lancet* 1993;341(8858):1428–1432.
191. Tebbi CK, Mendenhall N, London WB, et al. Treatment of stage I, IIA, IIIA1 pediatric Hodgkin disease with doxorubicin, bleomycin, vincristine and etoposide (DBVE) and radiation: a Pediatric Oncology Group (POG) study. *Pediatr Blood Cancer* 2006;46(2):198–202.
192. Travis LB, Hill DA, Dores GM, et al. Breast cancer following radiotherapy and chemotherapy among young women with Hodgkin disease. *JAMA* 2003;290(4):465–475.
193. Tubergen D, Krailo M, Meadows A, et al. Comparison of treatment regimens for pediatric lymphoblastic non-Hodgkin's lymphoma: a Children's Cancer Group study. *J Clin Oncol* 1995;13:1368–1376.
194. van den Berg H, Stuve W, Behrendt H. Treatment of Hodgkin's disease in children with alternating mechlorethamine, vincristine, procarbazine, and prednisone (MOPP) and adriamycin, bleomycin, vinblastine, and dacarbazine (ABVD) courses without radiotherapy. *Med Pediatr Oncol* 1997;29(1):23–27.
195. van den Berg H, Zsiros J, Behrendt H. Treatment of childhood Hodgkin's disease without radiotherapy. *Ann Oncol* 1997;8[Suppl 1]:15–17.
196. van Leeuwen FE, Klokman WJ, Hagenbeek A, et al. Second cancer risk following Hodgkin's disease: a 20-year follow-up study. *J Clin Oncol* 1994;12(2): 312–325.
197. van Leeuwen FE, Klokman WJ, Stovall M, et al. Roles of radiation dose, chemotherapy, and hormonal factors in breast cancer following Hodgkin's disease. *J Natl Cancer Inst* 2003;95(13):971–980.
198. van Leeuwen FE, Klokman WJ, Veer MB, et al. Long-term risk of second malignancy in survivors of Hodgkin's disease treated during adolescence or young adulthood. *J Clin Oncol* 2000;18(3):487–497.
199. Vecchi V. Childhood Hodgkin's disease: results of the Italian Multicentric Study AIEOP-MH89-CNR. *Med Pediatr Oncol* 1997;29:434.
200. Vecchi V, Pileri S, Burnelli R, et al. Treatment of pediatric Hodgkin disease tailored to stage, mediastinal mass, and age. An Italian (AIEOP) multicenter study on 215 patients. *Cancer* 1993;72(6):2049–2057.
201. Weiner M, Leventhal B, Cantor A, et al. Gallium-67 scans as an adjunct to computed tomography scans for the assessment of a residual mediastinal mass in pediatric patients with Hodgkin's disease. A Pediatric Oncology Group study. *Cancer* 1991;68(11):2478–2480.
202. Weiner MA, Leventhal B, Brecher ML, et al. Randomized study of intensive MOPP-ABVD with or without low-dose total-nodal radiation therapy in the treatment of stages IIB, IIIA2, IIIB, and IV Hodgkin's disease in pediatric patients: a Pediatric Oncology Group study. *J Clin Oncol* 1997;15(8):2769–2779.
203. Weiner MA, Leventhal BG, Marcus R, et al. Intensive chemotherapy and low-dose radiotherapy for the treatment of advanced-stage Hodgkin's disease in pediatric patients: a Pediatric Oncology Group study. *J Clin Oncol* 1991;9(9):1591–1598.
204. Westergaard T, Melbye M, Pedersen JB, et al. Birth order, sibship size and risk of Hodgkin's disease in children and young adults: a population-based study of 31 million person-years. *Int J Cancer* 1997;72(6):977–981.
205. Williams CD, Goldstone AH, Pearce R, et al. Autologous bone marrow transplantation for pediatric Hodgkin's disease: a case-matched comparison with adult patients by the European Bone Marrow Transplant Group Lymphoma Registry. *J Clin Oncol* 1993;11(11):2243–2249.
206. Willman KY, Cox RS, Donaldson SS. Radiation induced height impairment in pediatric Hodgkin's disease. *Int J Radiat Oncol Biol Phys* 1994;28(1):85–92.
207. Woessmann W, Seidemann K, Mann G, et al. The impact of the methotrexate administration schedule and dose in the treatment of children and adolescents with B-cell neoplasms: a report of the BFM Group Study NHL-BFM 95. *Blood* 2005;105:948–958.
208. Wolden SL, Lamborn KR, Cleary SF, et al. Second cancers following pediatric Hodgkin's disease. *J Clin Oncol* 1998;16(2):536–544.
209. Wollner N, Mandell L, Filippa D, et al. Primary nasal-paranasal oropharyngeal lymphoma in the pediatric age group. *Cancer* 1990;65:1438–1444.
210. Younes A, Garg A, Aggarwal B. Nuclear transcription factor-kappaB in Hodgkin's disease. *Leuk Lymphoma* 2003;44:929–935.
211. Zinzani P, Magagnoli M, Chierichetti F, et al. The role of positron emission tomography (PET) in the management of lymphoma patients. *Ann Oncol* 1999;10:1181–1184.

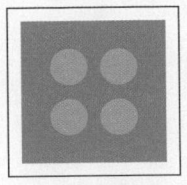

Chapter 88
Unusual Tumors in Childhood

Christian Carrie, Abraham Kuten

Some unusual and rare childhood tumors are comparable to those that occur in the adult population and require the same therapeutic strategy, with particular attention given to late sequelae. Some of these tumors are more characteristic of children and require specific radiotherapeutic strategies.

Nasopharyngeal Carcinoma in Childhood

Nasopharyngeal carcinoma (NPC) is a rare malignant tumor in childhood and adolescence (<1% of pediatric malignancies). The frequency differs greatly by geographic area: 1 case per 100,000 in Europe, the United States, and Australia; 10 in 100,000 in North Africa; and 80 in 100,000 in South China, Malaysia, and Greenland. According to the World Health Organization there are three distinct classification groups: type I, keratinizing squamous cell carcinoma; type II, nonkeratinizing carcinoma; and type III, undifferentiated carcinoma. Most pediatric NPC cases are type III (289). As in older patients, Epstein-Barr virus is associated with this type of NPC. The virus is found in the tumoral cells and not in the surrounding lymphocytes. Antibody and antigen titers are useful for both diagnosis and follow-up (234) (Table 88.1).

Clinical Presentation

The mean age at presentation is 14 years; boys are more often affected than girls (288). The tumor usually originates in the fossa of Rosenmuller followed early on by locoregional extension including extensive pharyngeal involvement, and often bone, lung, and cervical lymph node metastases. The most frequent clinical symptoms are nasal obstruction, epistaxis, otitis, and neck and facial pain.

On clinical examination, bilateral lymphadenopathy and cranial nerve palsies are found; a nasopharyngeal mass can be seen by direct or indirect nasopharyngoscopy and sometimes a protruding mass can be seen in the oral cavity.

The diagnostic work-up must include a cranial and neck computed tomography (CT) scan and magnetic resonance imaging (MRI), a thorax CT scan, and bone scintigraphy. Pathologic confirmation is obtained by biopsy. Commonly used staging systems are the TNM/AJC, Kyoto, and Ho classifications. Ho and Kyoto are based on topographic extension; the more commonly used TNM/AJC classification is based on tumor volume and CT information (10).

Treatment

In adult NPC, concomitant radiotherapy and chemotherapy (cisplatinum and 5-fluorouracil) is standard of care (6,48). Because of the scarcity of pediatric NPC cases, it is not feasible to perform randomized studies in this age group. Based on adult trials, multimodality treatment is generally accepted as standard of care for children. Usually two courses of 5-fluorouracil/CDDP (cisplatin, [*cis*-diamminedichloroplatinum II]) are given on week 1 and week 5 of radiotherapy (341). Others have used neoadjuvant cisplatinum-based chemotherapy, followed by radiation (21).

Radiation Therapy

A dose-response relationship for local control with a threshold at 60 Gy has been reported in a number of series (288,321,341). However, more recently Habrand et al. (120) have reported interesting results with lower doses of radiation therapy (50 Gy) in patients with good response to chemotherapy. These results are in accordance with the report of Polychronopoulou et al. (258). In this series, 70% of children achieved local control with doses <60 Gy (50% received only 52 Gy). Techniques include CT for dosimetric purposes, three-dimensional (3D) dosimetry, customized blocking and, if possible, MRI/CT scan image fusion for intensity-modulated radiotherapy (IMRT). Proton beam therapy is appropriate where available.

The target volume encompasses the tumor site and the neck (even in N_0 disease) with traditional opposed fields. After 45 Gy, more sophisticated planning (three-field technique, arc rotation, 3D planning, IMRT) is used to administer an additional boost of 20 Gy to the tumor bed and involved nodal areas. High-dose-rate, pulsed low-dose-rate, or conventional low-dose-rate intraluminal brachytherapy are used for the boost at some institutions. For some physicians, hyperfractionated radiotherapy is believed to be standard of care. A recent publication concerning hyperfractionated radiotherapy shows an increased rate of neurologic complication (315). The overall survival for T1-T2 disease is 70% to 90%. The survival for T3-T4 disease using combined modality is 50% to 60%. For advanced stage, innovative targeted therapies are in the development process. These include induction of the lytic viral cycle with ganciclovir, gene therapy, or antitumor vaccination against the viral protein LMP2 (90,192).

Late Effects

Xerostomia is the main side effect of treatment followed by dental caries, trismus, muscular atrophy, nerve palsies, and endocrine dysfunction resulting from pituitary irradiation. Significant auditory late toxicity and sporadic cases of visual morbidity, secondary to radiotherapy, with or without cisplatin-based chemotherapy, have been reported (274).

New techniques such as IMRT or radioprotective drugs such as amifostine may be able to decrease late sequelae.

Other Head and Neck Tumors

Carcinoma of the Oropharynx and Salivary Glands

Schwaab et al. (282) reported the largest pediatric series, with only 2% squamous cell carcinoma among 380 head and neck tumors. The more frequent sites of disease are the tongue, lip, tonsil palate, and salivary glands. Cigarette smoking or use of smokeless tobacco have been shown to be the etiologic factors

Table 88.1	ANTIGEN AND ANTIBODY EBV TITERS					
	IgG VCA	Ig EA	IgM VCA	IgA VCA	IgA EA	EBNA
Naive patient	0	0	0	0	0	0
Immune patient	Mild	0	0	0	0	Mild
Burkitt lymphoma	Raised	Raised	0	0	0	Raised
AIDS	Very raised	Raised	0	0	0	0
NC	Very raised	Very raised	Mild	Raised	Raised	Very raised

EBV, Epstein-Barr virus; Ig, immunoglobulin; VCA, vision capsid antigen (immune status); EA, early antigen (active disease); EBNA, EBV-associated nuclear antigen (cellular immunity); AIDS, acquired immunodeficiency syndrome; NC, nasopharynx carcinoma.

for adolescent tongue carcinoma (153). For other sites, passive smoking, poor oral hygiene, or genetic predispositions (xeroderma pigmentosam or retinoblastoma) have been suggested.

Special attention must be paid to larynx carcinoma as some of the cases may develop from juvenile papillomatisis, a benign condition of the aerodigestive tract that may undergo malignant degeneration. Guidelines for surgery and radiation therapy are the same as those for adults. Combined chemotherapy and radiation can be attempted for organ conservation (317).

Psychological support and rehabilitation programs are an essential part of the comprehensive treatment for children who undergo major surgical resection.

Esthesioneuroblastoma

Esthesioneuroblastoma is a malignant tumor arising from the olfactory nerve in the upper nasal cavity. Intracranial extension is common at the time of diagnosis. Esthesioneuroblastoma is mostly seen in patients in their 20s or their 60s. Positive S-100 and neuron-specific enolase stains combined with negative epithelial markers strongly suggest a neurogenic origin (156). The clinical presentation includes nasal obstruction, loss of smell, epistaxis, and sometimes enlarged cervical lymph nodes. Bony structures are often involved, as well as the ethmoid and maxillary sinuses. The most commonly used staging/grouping system is by Kadish et al. (156) and is based on degree of local tumor extension.

Standard treatment has not yet been defined. Localized tumors are often treated by surgery alone but local relapse is very frequent. Therefore, postoperative radiotherapy is often proposed. In patients treated by combined surgery and irradiation, local control can be obtained in >75% of cases (93). Eich et al. (80) and Broich et al. (41) recommend combined surgery and ra-

diotherapy in all stages. The recommended dose is 50 to 60 Gy. Elective neck irradiation or dissection is not advocated because <10% of early-stage cases exhibit nodal involvement. However, node metastases are frequent if the tumor extends beyond the paranasal sinuses. In this case, lymph node dissection or prophylactic irradiation should be considered. Chemotherapy has not yet been accepted as part of routine first-line treatment, although responses to chemotherapy have been reported (291). Chemotherapy can be employed to reduce tumor volume prior to surgery or radiotherapy, as well as for palliative purposes in advanced cases. Promising results with cyclophosphamide, doxorubicin, vincristine, cisplatinum, and etoposide, combined with radiotherapy and stem cell support have been reported recently by Mishima et al. (221). They obtained 8 complete responses in 12 Kadish stage C and D patients.

Juvenile Nasopharyngeal Angiofibroma (JNA)

JNA is a malignant vascular tumor most often arising from the posterior lateral wall of the nasopharynx. The lesion tends to extend into the nasal cavities, maxillary and sphenoid sinuses, orbit, and infratemporal fossa. Several classifications have been proposed but the classification of Radkowski et al. (264) appears to be the most appropriate, at least for the surgical purposes (Table 88.2). Common symptoms are epistaxis, cheek swelling, a visible orbital tumor, and cranial nerve palsies. JNA is more frequent in familial adenomatous polyposis patients. A mutation in the cluster region of the APC gene was reported in several studies, suggesting that JNA is perhaps a familial adenomatous polyposis tumor (2,323).

Treatment consists of surgery for small lesions, often with preoperative embolization or hormone therapy. Surgery carries a risk of significant operative blood loss. For localized JNA, the

Table 88.2	STAGING CLASSIFICATION FOR JUVENILE NASOPHARYNGEAL ANGIOFIBROMA[a]

Stage	Description
Ia	Limited to the nose and/or nasopharynx
Ib	Same as Ia but with extension into one or more paranasal sinuses
IIa	Minimal extension through the sphenopalatine foramen, into and including a minimal part of the medial-most part of pterygomaxillary fossa
IIb	Full occupation of the pterygomaxillary fossa, displacing the posterior wall of the maxillary antrum forward. Lateral and/or anterior displacement of branches of the maxillary artery. Superior extension may occur, eroding orbital bones
IIc	Extension through the pterygomaxillary fossa into the cheek and temporal fossa or posterior to the pterygoid plates
IIIa	Erosion of the skull base with minimal intracranial extension
IIIb	Erosion of the skull base with extensive intracranial extension with or without cavernous sinus invasion

[a]Based on the classification of Radkowski D, McGill T, Healy GB, et al. Angiofibroma. Changes in staging and treatment. *Arch Otolaryngol Head Neck Surg* 1996;122:122–129.

cure rate obtained by surgery alone can be as high as 90%. Resection with negative margins is required as inadequate margins will result in a high local failure rate (60). Minimally invasive endoscopic resection has recently been proposed for early-stage JNA. Lesions limited to the nasal cavity and/or nasopharynx or lesions with minimal extension through the sphenopalatine foramen are suitable for this procedure. A craniofacial approach is recommended for lesions extending into the pterygoid plates (83,342). Radiation therapy is used either as adjuvant treatment or as sole treatment in locally advanced lesions. Modern techniques such as IMRT have been successfully applied in unresectable and recurrent tumors (173). A wide range of doses have been used but there is no proof that doses >36 Gy are advantageous. There is no role for cytotoxic chemotherapy in JNA. The role of antiangiogenesis agents is speculative.

Lung Cancer

Bronchogenic Carcinoma

Pediatric bronchogenic carcinoma is extremely rare and its management does not differ from that of adults. Most of the tumors occur during adolescence. Histology is more frequently undifferentiated adenocarcinoma or carcinoid tumors rather than squamous cell carcinoma (178).

Of 230 cases of primary pulmonary neoplasms of childhood reviewed by Hartman and Shochat (134), <25% were bronchogenic carcinoma. The survival rate was very similar to that of adults, stage for stage.

Pleuropulmonary Blastoma (PPB)

Fewer than 100 cases of PPB have been reported. This tumor can occur from the neonatal period up to 12 years of age (262). PPB was often mixed with pulmonary blastoma until it was accepted that PPB is purely a pediatric tumor. The main histologic difference between pulmonary blastoma and PPB is the absence of epithelial carcinomatous components in PPB; PPB consists of mesenchymal stroma only. The tumor usually begins in pulmonary tissue but it can also originate in the pleura or mediastinum (273). According to the Dehner et al. (68) classification, three pathologic features can occur: cystic, mixed, and solid. However, it seems that this subdivision has neither prognostic nor therapeutic value (68,203). Some reports have also described PPB associated with pre-existing pulmonary cyst (71). It is unclear if PPB arises in pre-existing malformation or whether PPB induced cystic lesion formation.

Clinically, PPB exhibits no specific symptoms. The usual presentation is cough, thoracic pain, and fever. Respiratory impairment is unusual. Radiologic findings depend on the extent of the cystic component (Fig. 88.1). The standard treatment is surgery, which can be curative in early-stage disease, but the prognosis is often poor even after complete excision, especially if the size of tumor exceeds 5 cm (287).

Priest (262) reported only 8% survival rate at 5 years among 50 patients (15). Postoperative radiation therapy can be offered for a positive margin resection or in recurrent disease. The recommended dose is 50 Gy to the tumor bed and, because most of the relapses are local or metastatic, it is our opinion that lymphatic irradiation is not necessary. The value of chemotherapy is controversial. There are, however, long-term survivals reported with multiagent combinations such as actinomycin D, cyclophosphamide, cisplatin, etoposide, Adriamycin, and vincristine (148,170,244,246,273). Multimodal therapy with surgery followed by chemotherapy and radiotherapy (10.5 Gy) has been reported with good results at 3 years (254).

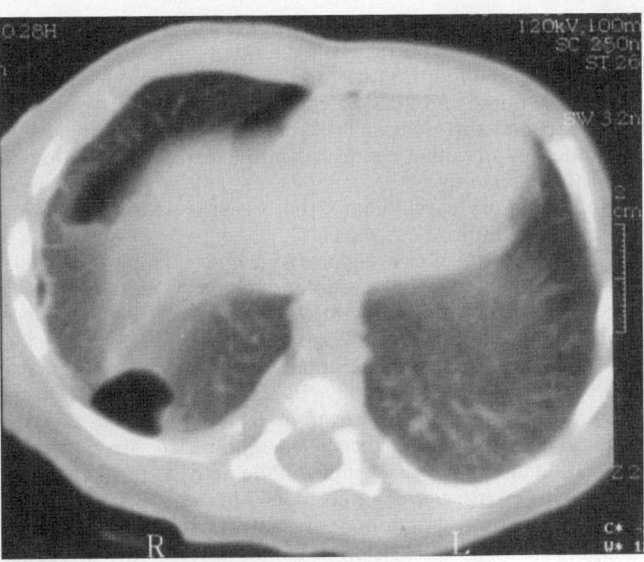

FIGURE 88.1. Pleuropneumoblastoma in a 1-year-old girl.

Breast Tumors

Malignant breast tumors account for <1% of all childhood cancers and <0.1% of all breast cancers (8,65,88,118).

A review of adolescents seen at the M.D. Anderson Cancer Center during a 40-year period identified breast cancer in 16 patients younger than 20 years of age. Ten patients had primary adenocarcinoma of the breast, four had cystosarcoma phylloides, and two had breast metastases from other primary tumors. Four of the 16 patients had a family history of *Breast Disease* (55). Roisman et al. (272) reported seven female patients, ages 14 to 17 years, who were treated in various hospitals in Israel for malignancy of the breast during 1967 to 1989. There were two cases of undifferentiated carcinoma with positive axillary lymph nodes, two cases of cystosarcoma phylloides, one case of rhabdomyosarcoma, and two cases of malignant lymphoma, one of them Burkitt's type.

Breast self-examination is recommended for girls who carry the BRCA1 or BRCA2 gene, beginning at age 18 to 21 years (78,82). Ultrasonography is the most appropriate initial investigation in any adolescent patient with a breast mass, owing to dense breast tissue adversely affecting the quality of mammography (313). MRI is recommended for diagnosing breast cancer when conventional imaging is complex and indeterminate, especially in young patients with dense mammographies.

Juvenile secretory carcinoma of the breast is rare and was first described by McDivitt and Stewart (212) in 1966 in seven girls ages 3 to 15 years, all of whom had a benign clinical course. The tumor cells are characterized by abundant mucin and mucopolysaccharide containing materials (75). Hormonal receptors are generally negative (85). Local tumor excision alone may be adequate therapy, although simple and radical mastectomies have also been used (34,75,85,285).

The histology and patterns of spread of adenocarcinoma of the breast in children and adolescents are similar to those in adults. As most publications refer to isolated cases, neither a consensus of opinion nor specific guidelines exist with regard to treatment. In general, principles of clinical management established for adults should be adopted. Because recurrences were found in 25% of patients treated with excisional biopsy alone, this seems inadequate, and a simple mastectomy with axillary lymph node dissection should probably be performed (157). Sentinel lymph node biopsy offers an approach to stage the axillary lymphatic drainage with a lower complication rate than formal dissection (31). On the other hand, McDivitt and Stuart (212) thought that the disease tends to run a relatively favorable course and that radical therapy is therefore unnecessary. Hartman and Magrish (133) consider it important to avoid radiotherapy in young children, and instead they recommend radical mastectomy.

Inflammatory carcinoma of the breast is extremely rare in children (46,236).

There have been case reports of primary lymphoma, rhabdomyosarcoma, adenoid cystic carcinoma, radiation-induced sarcoma, and cystosarcoma phylloides of the breast in children (30,213,219,226,237,297).

Cystosarcoma phylloides appears as a large breast mass; in 25% of cases it is bilateral. Norris and Taylor (237) were the first to separate benign from malignant lesions in this disorder. The distinction is based on tumor size, stromal invasion, cellular atypia, degree of mitotic activity, focal calcification, and/or patterns of infiltration. Metastases occur in the lungs and bones. Lymph node metastases are extremely rare. Simple or wide local excision or simple mastectomy, with rare local recurrences, may adequately treat histologically benign lesions. In malignant cystosarcoma phylloides some authors recommend radical mastectomy with or without axillary lymph node dissection, and others are in favor of simple mastectomy (127,196,279,319,336). The use of radiotherapy and postoperative chemotherapy in cystosarcoma phylloides is controversial. These modalities should be reserved for locally advanced, palliative, and disseminated cases.

Rhabdomyosarcoma of the breast, either primary or metastatic, is rare. Billroth (27) reported the first case of primary rhabdomyosarcoma in a 16-year-old girl in 1860. In a series of 108 patients under the age of 20 years with this malignancy, Howarth et al. (143) reported seven patients who had metastatic tumors to the breast with primary rhabdomyosarcoma located on an extremity or buttock. Six of the seven patients had alveolar histology. Rhabdomyosarcoma of the breast and other sarcomas of the breast are treated primarily by surgery followed, in most cases, by adjuvant radiation and chemotherapy.

Breast metastases in the pediatric age group include hepatocarcinoma, non-Hodgkin's lymphoma, rhabdomyosarcoma Hodgkin's disease, neuroblastoma, and adenocarcinoma (271).

Gastrointestinal Tumors of Childhood

Gastrointestinal tract malignant tumors are relatively rare in children. Carcinoid and hepatobiliary tumors are the most common (99). Others are adenocarcinoma, lymphoma, and leiomyosarcoma. More common are benign tumors such as hamartoma, leiomyoma, neurofibroma, and hemangioma.

Esophagus

In most cases, an esophageal tumor is of an epithelial origin, either squamous cell carcinoma or adenocarcinoma. Rarely, sarcomas may develop in the esophagus (leiomyosarcoma, carcinosarcoma, malignant schwannoma). Malignization of a chemical injury to the esophagus has been described (278). Carcinoma of the esophagus may develop in association with Barretts's esophagus and Cornelia de Lange syndrome (77,136). The most common benign tumor of the esophagus in the pediatric age group is leiomyoma; desmoid and teratoma may also occur (32,261,322). The management of esophageal cancer in the pediatric age group follows the same guidelines of treatment as in adults (37).

Stomach

Non-Hodgkins' lymphoma is the most frequent gastric malignancy in the pediatric age group, followed by leiomyosarcoma and leiomyoblastoma (151,163,186,201). Adenocarcinoma is extremely rare; it may arise in association with Peutz-Jeghers syndrome (132,215,318).

The management of non-Hodgkin's lymphoma follows the treatment guidelines of non-Hodgkin's lymphoma in adults (113,122,205,316).

Leiomyosarcoma of the stomach is treated primarily with surgery. Postoperative irradiation is given to patients with high risk of local recurrence (such as positive surgical margins, extension into the retroperitoneum).

As in the adult age group, subtotal gastrectomy with resection of associated lymph nodes is the treatment of choice for children with gastric carcinoma. No data are available on adjuvant radiation–chemotherapy in the pediatric age group. However, based on the results of a randomized study in adult patients with locoregionally advanced gastric carcinoma (198), one could assume that the use of combined irradiation and chemotherapy (5-fluorouracil and leucovorin) after surgery could be beneficial.

Radiotherapy guidelines are similar to the adult age group. At the time of radiotherapy planning, attention should be given to vital structures such as spinal cord, kidneys, small bowel, and liver. During treatment, acute side effects may occur, such as nausea, weight loss, and fatigue.

Several combination chemotherapy regimens have been used in the adjuvant setting and for locally advanced or metastatic gastric carcinoma. Numerous phase II and phase III studies were reported in the adult age group (123,162,306,339).

Small Bowel

According to the SEER (Surveillance, Epidemiology, and End Results) data, the incidence of malignant small intestine tumors is low in patients younger than 30 years of age (334). The most common malignancy of the small intestine in children is non-Hodgkin's lymphoma (16). Sarcomas of the small bowel and carcinoids may also develop in children. Small intestine adenocarcinoma may develop spontaneously or in association with Peutz-Jeghers syndrome (318)

Treatment guidelines are similar to those of the adult age group. Adjuvant irradiation can be given following surgery for duodenal sarcomas or adenocarcinomas arising in the segment fixed to the retroperitoneum, or for palliative purposes such as pain or bleeding.

Colorectal Cancer

Carcinoma of the rectum and the large bowel is rare in children and adolescents. According to the SEER data, only 80 cases of colorectal carcinoma in patients younger than 20 years of age occur annually in the United States, compared with 145,000 new cases per annum of colorectal carcinoma in adults (9). Young patients with long-standing ulcerative colitis have an increased risk of developing colorectal cancer (140). Several genetic conditions may be associated with colorectal carcinoma in childhood and adolescence. These include familial polyposis, Turcot's syndrome, Oldfield's syndrome, and Gardner's syndrome (50,100,129,240). The genetic events associated with the development of colorectal carcinoma in familial adenomatous polyposis syndrome, from epithelial proliferation, through formation of adenomas, to the sequential development of colorectal malignancy, have been described by Vogelstein et al. (327).

Similar to the adult age group, signs and symptoms of colorectal cancer are related to the segment of the large bowel where the tumor is located. Because of its rarity in the pediatric and adolescent age groups, diagnosis of colorectal carcinoma is often delayed and patients usually present with acute symptoms that necessitate urgent laparotomy. Colorectal cancer in the young is usually diagnosed at an advanced stage with metastases involving the omentum, peritoneum, mesenteric lymph nodes, liver, ovaries, and sometimes lungs, brain, and bones, and, therefore, carries a poor prognosis.

Colorectal carcinoma is diagnosed by direct fiberoptic colonoscopy. Radiographic studies include barium enema with air contrast, CT scan and radioisotope studies (fluorodeoxyglucose positron emission tomography [FDG-PET]) to determine metastatic spread. Preoperative carcinoembryonic antigen (CEA) level is important both as a prognosticator and for follow-up purposes. CA19-9 essay has been less valuable, although some tumors produce CA19-9 without CEA production.

Adenocarcinoma of the colorectum may be well, moderately, or poorly differentiated. The mucinous variety and signet cell types are associated with extremely poor prognosis. Unlike adult patients, in whom 60% of colonic cancers are located within 25 cm of the anus and in whom the rectum and sigmoid are also common sites for mucinous adenocarcinoma, tumors in children are probably more evenly distributed in all parts of the colon (47,261,309). In a series reported by Andersson and Bergdahl (12), the most common area was the transverse colon (39%). In a series of 20 patients reported by Karnak et al. (158) from Turkey, the rectosigmoid area was the most frequent site of location of the primary tumor (65%, the same as in adults).

Surgery is the primary and most effective treatment for colorectal carcinoma. Because of late diagnosis, the rate of complete resection has been less than optimal in children. In the series of Karnak et al. (158), complete resection was possible in only 6 of 20 patients. The surgical guidelines are similar to those of adult patients. Similarly, the use of chemotherapy and radiotherapy follows the guidelines of the adult age group. Special attention should be given to radiochemotherapy sequelae on the reproductive system.

Appendix

The most frequent malignant tumors of the appendix in the pediatric age group are carcinoids. These tumors are usually diagnosed incidentally during surgery for acute appendicitis or during other abdominal surgery. Complete surgical removal is the treatment of choice (91,223).

Pancreas

Pancreatic tumors are rare in children. The most important types are the functional tumors, pancreatoblastomas, and solid papillary epithelial neoplasms (230,293). The adult form of pancreatic adenocarcinoma rarely occurs in children.

Functional islet cell tumors are characterized by their hormonal activity. The diagnostic procedures and management follow the same guidelines set for adults.

The pediatric type of carcinoma of the pancreas, pancreatoblastoma, is a rare tumor; a few more than 50 cases have been reported in literature. It is characterized by adenocarcinomatous tissue with ductal cells, acinar cells, squamoid corpuscles and sometimes islet cell differentiation. These tumors stain positively by periodic acid-Schiff, α-trypsin, and α-keratin,

and in many cases can be associated with increased levels of α-fetoprotein (AFP) (49,167,340).

In most cases the tumor is located in the head of the pancreas. In patients with a solitary noninfiltrative tumor, complete local resection without radical pancreatoduodenectomy is recommended. Unlike patients with local disease, in whom local resection can be curative, in many other cases the tumor is clearly malignant with invasion, local recurrences, and nodal and disseminated metastases. The prognosis for these patients is very poor (200,218,325).

Radiation therapy is used in the postoperative setting, in locoregional recurrences, and in the neoadjuvant setting. A dose of 40 to 50 Gy is recommended (229,340). Technical guidelines of radiotherapy planning are similar to those of the adults. Intraoperative radiotherapy for recurrent disease has also been used.

Chemotherapy has been used for unresectable tumors, to treat metastatic disease, or in the adjuvant setting. 5-Fluorouracil, cyclophosphamide, actinomycin D, vincristine, vinblastine, mitomycin c, bleomycin, ifosfamide, etoposide, cisplatin, doxorubicin, gemcitabine, alone or in combination, have been used with very modest results (67,79,128,238,292,320, 325,328). Because the disease is so rare, it is impossible to set firm guidelines and treatment policies for chemotherapy in pediatric pancreatoblastoma.

Papillary cystic tumors of the pancreas, also known as Frantz tumors, are usually encapsulated lesions that can develop throughout the pancreas. They are characterized by cystic or pseudocystic spaces surrounded by residual solid tissue. Only 15% of these tumors are malignant and they usually occur in female patients at a mean age of 24 years at diagnosis (204).

These tumors usually present as an upper abdominal mass. Unlike other malignant pancreatic tumors, their prognosis is excellent after complete surgical excision (165).

The adult type of pancreatic adenocarcinoma is extremely rare in the pediatric and adolescent age groups. Signs and symptoms are similar to those of adult carcinoma of the pancreas (229). These tumors are managed according to guidelines of treatment set for adult patients.

Hepatobiliary Tumors

Hepatobiliary tumors are the most common neoplasms of the gastrointestinal tract to occur in children. They constitute 0.5% to 2% of pediatric cancer in Europe and in the United States. Hepatocellular carcinoma (HCC) occurs more frequently in Saharan Africa and the Orient (105,228,245,257,332,333). This geographic clustering may be explained by the high rates of hepatitis B infection and the hepatitis B serum antigen (HBsAg) positivity (191).

Benign hepatic tumors are more frequent than malignant tumors in young children. In older children, malignant tumors become more common. Benign tumors are classified according to the cell of origin: mesenchymal (hemangioma, hemangioendothelioma, hamartoma, peliosis hepatis) or epithelial (cysts, focal nodal hyperplasia, adenoma) (311). On rare occasions, radiation therapy may be used for the treatment of hemangiomas.

Malignant tumors of the liver are classified according to the tissue of origin with hepatocellular tumors (hepatoblastoma [HBL] and HCC) most common, constituting 75% to 90% of primary hepatic malignant tumors of childhood. Other tumors include malignant mesenchymoma, undifferentiated embryonal sarcoma, primary hepatic malignant tumors with rhabdoid features, leiomyosarcoma, angiosarcoma, hepatic sinusoid tumors, carcinoid, and non-Hodgkin's lymphoma.

Bile duct adenocarcinoma (cholangiocarcinoma) is extremely rare before the age of 30. This tumor has been associated with certain rare congenital biliary anomalies, ulcerated

▪▪ Table 88.3	HISTOLOGIC CLASSIFICATION OF HEPATOBLASTOMA
Epithelial type (56%)	Mixed epithelial and mesenchymal type (44%)
Fetal pattern (31%)	Without teratoid features (34%)
Embryonal and fetal pattern (19%)	With teratoid features (10%)
Macrotrabecular pattern (3%)	
Small cell undifferentiated pattern (3%)	

Modified from Stocker JT. Hepatoblastoma. *Semin Diagn Pathol* 1994;11:136–143, with permission.

colitis, cystic fibrosis, and sclerosing cholangitis (125,311). The liver is also a common site for metastatic disease.

Of the malignant tumors of the liver in childhood, HBL is the most common. HBL occurs almost exclusively in small infants, although isolated instances in older children and in young adolescents have been reported. These tumors occur more frequently among males.

HBL is associated with Beckwith-Wiedemann syndrome, familial adenomatous polyposis, and congenital anomalies like hemihypertrophy and cleft palate, Wilm's tumor, and glycogen storage diseases (26,149,166,188). Although the association between HBL and Beckwith-Wiedemann syndrome indicates abnormalities on chromosome 11 and loss of heterozygosity on chromosome 11p, increased incidence of HBL in families with familial adenomatous polyposis indicates a possible significance for abnormalities of chromosome 5q (166,171).

The presenting signs and symptoms are distention of the abdomen, anorexia, vomiting, anemia, fever, and jaundice. Isosexual precocity secondary to human chorionic gonadotropin (HCG) secretion by the tumor can be seen in some cases (188).

Serum AFP produced by the embryonal endoderm is increased in 84% to 90% of patients with HBL (332). HCG and cystathionase may also serve as tumor markers (329). Histologically, hepatoblastomas are classified into five subtypes (Table 88.3). These subtypes can occur together in varying properties, but present definitions do not take this into account, which makes it difficult to relate a specific histologic subtype with prognosis. Pure fetal histology has a better outcome, but the definition of "pure fetal" is not clear. The prognosis of the rare (3%) small cell undifferentiated subtype is poor. In long-term survivors of HBL, the most common histologic variant is the conventional type with predominantly fetal cell patterns. A trial performed by the Pediatric Oncology Group (POG) and the Children's Cancer Study Group (CCSG) demonstrated the importance of the distinction between fetal hepatoblastoma and the other histologic subtypes in stage I disease (1). A German study (HB 89–94) (256) identified several poor prognostic factors in HBL: metastatic disease, AFP >1,000,000 ng/mL, extra- and intrahepatic vascular invasion, multifocal disease, involvement of both liver lobes, stage (TNM), and poorly differentiated epithelial histology.

HCC is the second most common primary malignant liver tumor in the pediatric age group and accounts for about one-fourth to one-third of hepatic malignancies. Although reported in children as young as 21 months, most reports indicate that HCC usually develops in early adolescence (86,235). This is in contrast to HBL, which occurs primarily in infancy and is seldom seen in children older than 3 years. Similar to HBL, HCC occurs mainly in males (70,163). The fibrolamellar carcinoma variant of HCC occurs mainly in young adults around the age of 20 years but has also been reported in childhood (58,180).

Approximately 25% of HCC cases in childhood are associated with cirrhosis secondary to biliary atresia, Fanconi's anemia, glucose-6-phosphatase deficiency, and hereditary tyrosinemia

▪▪ Table 88.4	CHILDREN'S CANCER STUDY GROUP STAGING SYSTEM FOR PRIMARY MALIGNANT LIVER TUMORS	
Stage		**Description**
I		Complete excision
	A	Favorable histology (fetal HBL)
	B	Unfavorable histology (embryonal HBL, HCC)
II		Microscopic residual disease
	A	In liver
	B	Extrahepatic
III		Gross residual disease ± node involvement ± spilled tumor
	A	Tumor completely removed; tumor spilled, residual gross disease in nodes, or both
	B	Gross tumor not completely removed ± positive nodes ± spill
IV		Metastatic disease
	A	Primary tumor completely excised
	B	Primary tumor not completely excised

HBL, hepatoblastoma; HCC, hepatocellular carcinoma.
Data derived from Cohen MD, Bugaieski EM, Haliloglu M, et al. Visual presentation of the staging of pediatric tumors. *Radiographics* 1996;16:523–545; and from Perilango G, Sinniah D, Meadows AT, et al. Liver tumors. In: D'Angio GJ, Sinniah D, Meadows AT, et al., eds. *Practical pediatric oncology.* New York: Wiley-Liss; 1992;233–337, with permission.

(179). The most important known etiologic factor for HCC is the high incidence of maternal transmission of the hepatitis B surface antigen in Africa and the Orient (94,135). Other etiologic factors include exposure to aflatoxins, hepatic fibrosis, anabolic steroids, inherited disorders of metabolism, membranous obstruction of the inferior vena cava, and possibly ethanol abuse (11,163,333). However, these etiologic factors apply mostly to HCC in the adult age group. In adult black South African patients, deletions of alleles on chromosome 17p and P53 (codon 249) have been identified (38,144); the exact molecular mechanisms responsible for the development of HCC are still not known.

Similar to HBL, two thirds of children with HCC have an elevated AFP (109). AFP levels are high in the healthy newborn and drop rapidly by the age of 1 month and should not be detectable by age 2 years (295). Initial AFP level is a significant prognostic factor: In a study performed by the Radiation Therapy Oncology Group (301), the mortality in HCC was 1.8 times higher in patients with strongly positive AFP. AFP is an indicator of tumor growth and can serve as a valuable marker of response to therapy. Following complete tumor resection, AFP level should return to normal within 2 months (103). Increasing levels of AFP during the follow-up period after surgery indicate local recurrence or metastatic disease (109).

The CCSG intergroup and POG staging systems for primary malignant liver tumors are based on resectability and on the histologic subtype (Table 88.4 [ref 53,252] and Table 88.5 [ref 35]).

▪▪ Table 88.5	PEDIATRIC ONCOLOGY GROUP STAGING SYSTEM FOR PRIMARY MALIGNANT LIVER TUMORS
Stage	**Description**
I	Complete resection achieved
II	Microscopic residual tumor remaining
III	Gross residual tumor remaining
IV	Metastatic disease present at diagnosis

Modified from Bowman LC, Riely CA. Management of pediatric liver tumors. *Surg Oncol Clin North Am* 1996;5:451–459, with permission.

Successful therapy of localized HBL or HCC depends mainly on the feasibility of complete surgical excision (256). Up to two thirds of HBL patients have resectable tumors at presentation because these tumors are usually unifocal and encapsulated. Cure can be achieved in one third of the successfully operated patients, typically those with fetal HBL (1,26,231). In contrast, only 30% of the cases of HCC are suitable for complete resection at the time of diagnosis because of the multifocal involvement or size. Fifty percent to 75% of the fibrolamellar variant of HCC are amenable to complete resection at the time of presentation (121,280). In principle, tumor resectability is determined by the tumor size, the existence of bilobar involvement necessitating the resection of more than three liver segments, vascular invasion, or metastatic spread. Patients with advanced disease who are not suitable for primary surgery may be considered for neoadjuvant preoperative cytoreductive chemotherapy. In these cases, the diagnosis of can either be based on clinical presentation, imaging findings, including FDG-PET scan (222) and tumor markers, or on tissue diagnosis obtained via open biopsy or CT/ultrasound-guided needle biopsy, although there are some concerns that a needle biopsy may cause a significant hemorrhage. Preoperative cytoreductive chemotherapy can reduce the size of the tumor in the majority of HBL patients and in a significant percentage of HCC patients, rendering them resectable. Chemotherapy regimens include combinations of cisplatin, vincristine, 5-fluorouracil (269), ifosfamide, cisplatin, doxorubicin (96), vincristine, doxorubicin, cyclophosphamide or vincristine, cyclophosphamide, and cisplatin (44,121). It has been shown that carboplatin-based chemotherapy is effective, and can probably replace cisplatin-based regimens. New agents that were recently introduced include camptothecin analogues topotecan and irinotecan; a novel platinum derivative, oxaliplatin; and liposomal doxorubicin (Doxil) (256). If resectability cannot be achieved using chemotherapy, there is still a chance to render unresectable tumors resectable by radiotherapy (121). The perioperative mortality of hepatic lobectomy is in the order of 5% to 10% in specialized centers applying improved surgical techniques, modern methods of anesthesia, and state-of-the-art postoperative intensive care (117).

Surgical resection of pulmonary metastases can be attempted if they persist after chemotherapy and if the primary tumor can be completely resected. Patients who are successfully operated on for stage I disease and later develop a solitary lung metastasis are also suitable for metastasectomy.

Total hepatectomy and liver transplantation can be attempted in unresectable HBL (about 10% after chemotherapy) and HCC (>50% are unresectable at diagnosis) with tumor confined to the liver without penetration of the capsule and in the absence of lymph node and distant metastases. The overall survival is between 50% and 83%, with a minimum follow-up of 2 years. The best outcome was achieved in patients with a good response to chemotherapy who had a "first-line transplant" (i.e., not after an unsuccessful attempt at resection) (139,256, 307,310).

Although it has been used preoperatively and postoperatively in children with HBL and HCC, radiation therapy has a limited role in curative management.

Preoperative radiation was given to children who remained unresectable after initial chemotherapy (24,51,121). In the postoperative setting, it has been shown that patients with residual disease after surgery may benefit from postoperative irradiation. In a combined POG-CCSG protocol (1), patients with microscopic residual disease after surgery received postoperative chemotherapy and limited field irradiation, 45 Gy to the tumor bed. Their 3-year progression-free survival was 60%. Patients who were unable to undergo complete resection following preoperative chemotherapy received whole-liver irradiation, 30 Gy. Their 3-year progression-free survival was 22%.

According to the Institut Gustave Roussy protocol (121), children were treated with preoperative chemotherapy followed by surgery. If there was evidence for microscopic or gross persistent tumor at surgery, more chemotherapy was given and limited field irradiation was administered to the site of residual tumor, 25 to 45 Gy. Fifteen patients were reported by Habrand et al. (121), 11 with HBL, 2 with HCC, and 2 without tissue diagnosis. Nine patients who underwent surgical resection of the primary tumor, received either pre- or postoperative chemotherapy consisting of vincristine, doxorubicin, and cyclophosphamide, alternating with vincristine, cyclophosphamide, and cis-platinum. Radiotherapy with a median dose of 40 Gy was given to eight incompletely resected patients. Six of eight patients were alive at a median of 45 months from the time of diagnosis. One inoperable patient was rendered operable by whole-liver irradiation (24 Gy) and concurrent 5-fluorouracil and cis-platinum. This patient was alive at 68 months following radiation therapy. Of four unresectable primaries, one was controlled by radiotherapy. Two children received whole-lung irradiation, 18 to 20 Gy, for pulmonary metastases; neither of them was controlled. One of these two patients underwent pulmonary metastasectomy and was alive without evidence of disease 41 months after surgery.

When radiotherapy is given to children with HBL or HCC, careful assessment of the tumor volume is essential to reduce the amount of normal liver tissue irradiated. Parallel opposed high-energy beams or multiple-field techniques, using 3D treatment-planning systems should be employed. When limited irradiation volume is administered, a dose of 35 to 45 Gy is appropriate for bulky disease and 25 to 45 Gy for microscopic residual disease. For children treated with a palliative intent, whole-liver irradiation, 20 to 25 Gy in 2 to 2.5 weeks is adequate.

The results of whole-lung irradiation for macroscopic pulmonary metastases are discouraging. A total dose of 12 to 13 Gy whole-lung irradiation might be considered in patients with microscopic residual pulmonary metastatic disease, after chemotherapy or following surgery and chemotherapy.

A number of multicenter trials have been performed by cooperative study groups, to test the value of preoperative and postoperative combination chemotherapy in HBL and HCC. In some of the studies, radiotherapy was included as part of the treatment protocol. It has been demonstrated that a significant number of initially unresected tumors could be surgically removed following chemotherapy, and that complete resection followed by adjuvant chemotherapy was superior to surgery alone.

In CCG trial 831 (248), patients with residual disease in one lobe after surgery received actinomycin D, vincristine, and cyclophosphamide combination chemotherapy and involved-field irradiation. Patients with disseminated tumors received chemotherapy alone. Of 40 children entered into the study, there were only 7 long-term survivors: those with either stage I disease or minor residual tumor who received irradiation.

In CCG trial 881 (248), doxorubicin and 5-fluorouracil were added to the actinomycin D, vincristine, and cyclophosphamide combination used in CCG 831. A response rate of 44% was observed in patients with measurable disease, and 83% of patients receiving the drug combination as an adjuvant treatment were disease-free at 30 months.

In CCG trial 823F (248), patients with HBL (33 children) or HCC (14 children), confined to the liver received doxorubicin and cisplatin prior to definitive surgery. Although only 2 of 14 HCC patients survived, 78% of 25 HBL patients who completed chemotherapy and were eligible for surgery were alive without evidence of disease. In 16 patients, complete resection was performed, and no viable tumor was found in 9 of them at the time of surgery. Fifteen of these patients were alive and disease-free. It was found that for children with unresectable or metastatic

HBL entered into this study, early changes in AFP levels were a reliable predictor of outcome and could identify poor responders to therapy. The authors suggested, that if the AFP level failed to decrease by two logs prior to surgery, a surgical approach should probably not be attempted (324).

In a trial performed by the Pediatric Hepatoma Study Intergroup (CCG 8881/POG 8945) (243), patients were allocated to receive either cisplatin, vincristine, and 5-fluorouracil or cisplatin and doxorubicin. Both chemotherapy regimens were equally effective in terms of overall and disease-free survival; however, the cisplatin plus doxorubicin combination was significantly more toxic.

POG study 8679 (72) enrolled children with stage I-IV HBL. Children with stage I favorable histology received surgery alone. Children with stage I unfavorable histology or stage II disease received surgery and adjuvant cisplatin, vincristine, and 5-fluorouracil. Children with stage III-IV disease received five cycles of chemotherapy, following which they were evaluated for surgery. Unresectable patients received limited field irradiation, 33 to 39 Gy, and additional chemotherapy. The 3-year disease-free survival for stage I unfavorable histology and stage II patients was 91, for stage III it was 67, and for stage IV patients it was 13. Three of five irradiated patients underwent complete resection and were free of disease.

The International Society of Pediatric Oncology (SIOP) designed a series of clinical trials based on a risk adapted treatment approach philosophy. In the SIOPEL I trial patients received preoperative cisplatin-doxorubicin (PLADO) regimen (62). The investigators concluded that the extent of pretreatment hepatic disease and the presence of pulmonary metastases were significant prognosticators of 5-year event-free survival. Survival for HCC patients was significantly inferior to that of children with HBL, and complete tumor excision remained the only realistic chance of cure. A novel staging system was developed, called *PRETEXT* (pretreatment extent of disease), and two risk clusters for treatment failure were identified: a "standard risk" group, comprising patients with disease confined to the liver and involving up to three hepatic sectors, and "high-risk" group, with disease extending to all four hepatic sectors or with extrahepatic spread. It was suggested that PLADO chemotherapy followed by delayed surgery and a short course of postoperative chemotherapy used in the SIOPEL I trial should be regarded as best treatment for children with HBL, and that other future treatment programs should be measured against this standard (211,263).

In the SIOPEL II trial, patients were stratified according to standard and high-risk groups. For high-risk HBL patients, treatment was intensified by adding carboplatin to the cisplatin/doxorubicin regimen used in the SIOPEL I trial, in a rapidly alternating sequence of administration.

For standard-risk HBL patients, 3-year overall and progression-free survivals were 91% and 89%, and for the high-risk HBL group, 53% and 48%, respectively. Despite chemotherapy intensification, only half of the high-risk HBL patients were long-term survivors (251). For standard-risk HBL patients, the efficacy of cisplatin monotherapy and cisplatin/doxorubicin combination are now being compared in a prospective SIOPEL III randomized trial (256).

Investigators from the United States analyzed the effectiveness of intrahepatic chemotherapy (108) and intrahepatic chemoembolization (14). They concluded that these treatment modalities can halt the progression and possibly downstage advanced hepatic malignancies.

Japanese investigators used transarterial chemoembolization with Lipiodol and cisplatin/etoposide and concluded that this treatment modality was particularly useful in potentiating the cytoreductive effect of antitumor drugs and was also useful in reducing toxicities (239).

Other Japanese investigators analyzed the survival outcome for patients with HBL treated by preoperative and/or postoperative chemotherapy using a combination of cisplatin and tetrahydropyranyl–Adriamycin. They concluded that preoperative chemotherapy resulted in an improved resectability of the tumor, whereas postoperative chemotherapy played an important role in the increased cure rate of patients with an incomplete tumor resection or metastasis (305).

In a prospective, multicenter, single-arm German Liver Tumor Study HB94, children undergoing primary surgery received IPA (ifosfamide, cisplatin, Adriamycin) chemotherapy and or etoposide and carboplatin. Treatment was risk-stratified according to stage: stage I patients receive IPA ×2; stage II, IPA ×2 to 3; stage III-IV, carboplatin/etoposide plus IPA. Growth pattern of the liver tumor, vascular tumor invasion, occurrence of distant metastases, initial AFP level, and surgical radicality were found to be pretreatment prognostic factors (97).

In an interim analysis of the German Liver Tumor Study HB 99, it was shown that adding high-dose carboplatin and etoposide to high-risk HBL patients was highly efficient and induced a remission in the majority of patients with advanced and metastasized high-risk HBL (119).

Innovative radiotherapeutic approaches include intraoperative irradiation, intra-arterial Yttrium-90 microspheres (112,185,194), and intraluminal iridium-192 with or without regional hyperthermia (56,147,227).

Langerhans Cell Histiocytosis

Pathology

Histiocytosis results from dysregulation of the mononuclear cell line. Usually, after maturation in the bone marrow, monocytes migrate to the liver (Kupffer cells), bone marrow (macrophages), or connective tissue and skin (histiocytes). The Langerhans cell is characterized by the presence of the intracytoplasmic Birbeck granule of unknown origin but which develops only after an antigenic stimulation. Langerhans cell histiocytosis (LCH) is a proliferative disorder in which infiltration by Langerhans cells leads to tissue damage. The pathogenesis is not completely understood but excessive production of interleukin 1 and prostaglandin E_2 have been demonstrated in affected bone. These factors can play a major role in osteoclast activation.

In the past, three subentities of LCH were recognized. In 1893, Hand was the first to describe the *craniohypophysis xanthomatoses* (130). This was followed by reports by Christian and Schuller. The Hand-Schuller-Christian disease is characterized by skull lesions, exophthalmos, and diabetes insipidus and occurs in children older than age 2.

Twenty years later, Letterer and Siwe described an entity in children younger than age 2, with splenomegaly, hepatomegaly, anemia, and hemorrhagic diathesis.

Twenty years after this, Otani and Erblich described the solitary eosinophilic granuloma in children older than 2 years, with a characteristic bony site (33,99,103). Lichtenstein (193) merged the variants into one entity, which he called *histiocytosis X*. It should be emphasized that it is not yet clear whether LCH is a malignant disorder. The finding of monoclonality has been described but is not sufficient to establish the existence of malignancy. Moreover, Langerhans cells are not aneuploid, and LCH has been reported with Hodgkin's disease.

Clinical Presentation

The annual incidence of LCH is 0.5 to 2 cases per 100,000 children (126). The clinical presentation is age-related. In children younger than 2 years old, the disseminated form (Letterer-Siwe) is more frequent, with wasting, hepatosplenomegaly, pancytopenia, and sometimes with massive seborrheic dermatitis on the groin and scalp. The infant is often irritable and fails to thrive (40,141).

In children older than 2 years, the disease is less aggressive, with widespread bone granulomas causing pain, otitis, diabetes insipidus (42%), and exophthalmos. Eosinophilic granuloma is characterized by bone involvement only and with symptoms related to the location of the granuloma.

Central nervous system involvement is possible; most frequently, meningeal and pituitary lesions occur, but intraparenchymal lesions, especially hypothalamic and cerebellar, can also be encountered.

Whatever the clinical presentation, the definitive diagnosis is made by biopsy confirming the presence of the Birbeck granule in a Langerhans cell. Staging procedures include a skeletal survey (rather than isotopic bone scan). Many prognostic scores have been proposed, all based on the extent of disease, age at diagnosis, and demonstrable organ dysfunction (126). As suggested by Halperin et al. (126), patients are classified into three groups:

i. very favorable, with unifocal lesion requiring minimal therapy,
ii. very unfavorable, with organ dysfunction necessitating intensive therapy, and
iii. all others, not well defined, for which treatment by surgery, steroids, chemotherapy and/or radiotherapy may be required.

Treatment

Many cases of LCH are indolent or resolve spontaneously. Aggressive treatment therefore should not be given if there is no organ dysfunction.

Surgery

The POG 8047 study demonstrated that a similar control rate can be achieved (70% to 90%) with biopsy, curettage, or tumor excision (25). Wide excision is recommended for expendable bones (clavicle, ribs) and biopsy for other sites. Curettage is not indicated if there is a risk of instability (cervical vertebra, femoral neck) or if a poor cosmetic or orthopaedic outcome is likely.

Radiation Therapy

There is no indication for postoperative radiotherapy except in cases in which local healing has not been achieved by surgery. Radiation therapy is indicated for local relapse, in patients with medical contraindications to surgery, with nerve compression (optic nerve, spinal cord), and for pain relief (especially in cases of multifocal LCH and for persistent pain despite steroids, intralesional injections, or chemotherapy).

Special attention must be paid to patients with diabetes insipidus. Radiotherapy should be initiated shortly after the onset of symptoms (116).

There seems to be no relationship between dose of radiation and local control. The recommended dose is usually 10 Gy with conventional fractionation; the local control rate is in the order of 80% (116).

Medical Treatment

In Situ *Injection of Steroids*

The procedure is performed under general anesthesia and fluoroscopic guidance. Methylprednisolone is injected directly into the granuloma (52). It has not been proven whether the steroids or the local trauma are responsible for the effects.

Chemotherapy

The exact point in the course of the disease at which chemotherapy should be considered is controversial. There is little agreement on the factors that should be considered as bad prognostic signs. Only organ dysfunction and/or multiorgan disease have been generally accepted as indications for chemotherapy. Initially, high-dose steroids are used and followed, when necessary, by vinblastine or etoposide. There is no proof that a multidrug regimen is more effective than single-agent chemotherapy as first-line therapy. Furthermore, it is still unknown if early treatment prevents the development of diabetes insipidus at a later stage (76,101). Recently, promising results were reported using thalidomide for treatment of disseminated LCH (208).

For resistant disease (especially in infants), a more aggressive approach, including cyclosporine, liver transplantation, *Bone Marrow Transplant*ation, and/or monoclonal antibody therapy, is under investigation (5,95). Pamidronate has been shown to be effective in reducing bone pain secondary to skeletal involvement by LCH (87).

⠿ | Endocrine Tumors

Adrenocortical Carcinoma

Adrenocortical carcinoma (ACC) accounts for 0.2% of childhood cancer and occurs, in 75% of the cases, in children younger than 5 years, more commonly in females (3,36,142,146,154,217,275). ACC is sometimes associated with Beckwith-Wiedemann syndrome and with hemihypertrophy (187).

Children with ACC may present with abdominal pain and a palpable mass. More than 75% of the tumors are functional, secreting one or more hormones: androgens, cortisol, aldosterone, or estrogens. The most common presenting sign is virilization with deepening of the voice, hirsutism, premature pubic hair, clitoromegaly, phallomegaly, excessive muscular development, and advanced bone age. Pure Cushing syndrome (moon face, plethora, hypertension, striae, weight gain, acne, and "buffalo hump") is rare in children. Feminization or aldosterone-secreting tumors is also rare (217).

Urinary 17-ketocorticosteroids and 17-hydroxycorticosteroids are usually elevated, with steroid production not influenced by adrenocorticotropic hormone suppression.

Diagnostic imaging studies include CT and/or MRI. It is sometimes difficult to separate ACC from adenoma. However, at presentation, most carcinomas are larger than 6 cm and calcified, and benign adenomas are small and nonfunctional. A characteristic echogenic star pattern can be seen on ultrasonography, and CT scan shows an inhomogeneous tumor with irregular contrast material. Recently, the use of [18]FDG-PET has been shown to be effective in discriminating between benign and malignant adrenal lesions (314,346) As both benign adenomas and ACC may exhibit abnormal mitoses and cellular and nuclear pleomorphism, malignancy is determined by the finding of capsular penetration, invasion of the inferior vena cava up to the right atrium, lymph node, and distant metastases (3).

Generally, the prognosis of ACC is poor (20,59,111) Small, well-encapsulated, and easily excised tumors can be cured by surgery alone. In locally advanced cases, there is a significant risk of locoregional and metastatic relapse (217,275). Repeat complete resection of local recurrences and discrete metastatic lesions can improve survival (281).

The literature on adjuvant radiation therapy following resection of ACC is scarce, relatively old, and consists of small series or case reports. Postoperative whole-abdominal irradiation (15 to 30 Gy) was administered by Stewart et al. (300). Three of four irradiated patients were long-term survivors. Percarpio and Knowlton (249) used preoperative irradiation, 45 to 50 Gy to treat two patients and postoperative irradiation to treat four patients with unresectable tumors or spillage at the time of surgery. One patient who was treated preoperatively was rendered operable; three of four postoperatively treated patients relapsed in the field of radiation and one outside the field.

Magee et al. (199) reported a series of 15 patients with ACC, 9 of whom received postoperative irradiation. Three of the irradiated patients were girls under the age of 2 years, who received 30 Gy in 4 weeks. Two of these girls died as the result of a second malignancy arising in the irradiated volume.

Based on these results and the results of similar small retrospective series (36,159,207,348), it is difficult to make any firm recommendations on the role of radiotherapy in ACC. Investigators from the United Kingdom reported a relatively high frequency of second, fatal, primary tumors, especially if radiotherapy was part of the treatment protocol (74).

Mitotane (o,p-DDD) is the most frequently used chemotherapeutic agent for recurrent or metastatic ACC, with a response rate of approximately 20%. Other agents include suramin, doxorubicin, 5-fluorouracil, streptozotocin, cisplatin, and etoposide, alone or in combination, with response rates of 20% to 30% (150). The administration of adjuvant chemotherapy is controversial. Some investigators advocate the use of adjuvant mitotane following surgery (160); however, the administration of this drug is associated with significant gastrointestinal, neuromuscular, and skin toxicity as well as with abnormal platelet aggregation and prolongation of bleeding time. There is also a significant decrease in urinary 17-hydroxysteroids and 17-ketosteroids. The response rates to mitotane are highly dependent on obtaining adequate serum levels (>10 to 14 mcg/mL) and the therapeutic window between toxicity and efficacy is quite narrow. Hence, most authorities agree that, in the absence of solid data based on randomized well-controlled clinical trials, it is difficult to justify the administration of radiation or chemotherapy in the adjuvant setting (70,74,197).

Pheochromocytoma and Paraganglioma

Pheochromocytoma and paraganglioma are rare tumors of childhood and adolescence (45,66,161,164,250,298). Pediatric pheochromocytoma occurs usually between 8 and 14 years of age, more frequently in males. More than 90% of all pheochromocytomas in adults, and 70% of pheochromocytomas in children, originate in the adrenal gland, but the tumor can occur at any site in the sympathetic chain, most commonly below the diaphragm. The most common sites of occurrence of extra-adrenal pheochromocytoma are the superior para-aortic region, between the diaphragm and the lower renal poles, in the paraganglia, the organs of Zuckerkandl, and the bladder. Extra-abdominal tumors may develop in the brain, thorax, and the bladder (45,92,250,338). Approximately 10% of all patients with pheochromocytoma are children, but several characteristics distinguish them from their adult counterparts. Unlike pheochromocytomas of the adult age group, children with pheochromocytoma have a higher incidence of bilaterality, a higher association with the multiple endocrine neoplasia (MEN) syndromes, and a lower incidence of malignant neoplasms (45,92,283,290,312).

Familial pheochromocytoma is associated with other endocrine tumors in the MEN IIa-IIb syndromes (89,92,98,110).

In addition to the familial syndrome of isolated pheochromocytomas, pheochromocytomas in the pediatric age group can be associated with other inherited diseases, such as von Hippel-Lindau (retinocerebral angiomatosis), tuberous sclerosis, and von Recklinghausen's neurofibromatosis.

Malignant pheochromocytomas occur in 10% of the pediatric cases of pheochromocytoma. The definition of malignancy is based on biologic and clinical behavior and not on histologic features alone.

Pheochromocytoma is responsible for 1% of cases of childhood hypertension, which, unlike adults, is sustained and not paroxysmal. Other signs and symptoms include diaphoresis, flushing, fatigue, headache, and convulsions (210).

Adrenal pheochromocytomas produce epinephrine and norepinephrine, but most extra-adrenal pheochromocytomas produce only norepinephrine.

Urinary epinephrine, norepinephrine, metanephrine, and vanillylmandelic acid values remain the gold standard for biochemical screening of pheochromocytoma. On some occasions, urinary catecholamine levels may be normal while serum levels are elevated. Imaging studies include ultrasonography, CT scan, and/or MRI. Iodine-131 MIBG (metaiodobenzylguanidine) scan provides the most accurate and direct method of diagnosing adrenal, extra-adrenal, or metastatic pheochromocytoma because MIBG, which has a molecular structure similar to that of norepinephrine, is actively concentrated and stored in catecholamine storage vesicles of pheochromocytoma cells (45,92,190,214,335).

Surgery is the definitive therapy. The most significant reduction in pre- and postoperative mortality has come from the control of perioperative hypertension using alpha and beta blockers (92,267).

External-beam irradiation is used for palliation of lymph node, bone, brain, and spinal cord metastases. High-dose Iodine-131 MIBG has been used with modest results in metastatic disease. Streptozotocin or cyclophosphamide, vincristine, and dacarbazine may produce modest decreases in catecholamine secretion in patients with malignant pheochromocytoma (150). Patients with malignant pheochromocytoma require chronic medical control of their elevated blood pressure by alpha and beta blockade or inhibition of catecholamine synthesis with α-methyl-para-tyrosine (57,183,265).

Thyroid Carcinoma

Thyroid carcinoma accounts for 1% to 1.5% of all cases of cancer in the pediatric and adolescent age groups, with between 0.4 and 1.5 cases per million, two to three times as frequent in girls as in boys (284,303). After the April 26, 1986, Chernobyl nuclear reactor accident, a remarkable increase of incidence was observed in children exposed to radioactive iodine (RAI) fallout (13,189). The incidence of thyroid cancer in Belarus and Ukraine began to rise sharply in 1989 to 1990: in adults, the number of new cases increased two to threefold, and in children younger than 20 years, and particularly during the first 5 years of life, the number of new cases increased 20- 30-fold (13,124). Almost all new pediatric cases were papillary tumors (94% to 98%), with a relatively high incidence of lymph node (65%) and lung (5%) metastases at presentation (124) (Table 88.6).

Follicular carcinoma is characterized by vascular invasion and accounts for 16% to 20% of cases.

Medullary carcinomas are rare. These tumors develop from the neural crest parafollicular or C cells and tend to be more aggressive than the differentiated carcinomas and can be fatal. They are associated with the immunoreactive thyrocalcitonin marker. Because of their aggressive clinical course, experts advocate genetic testing to identify affected individuals with

Table 88.6	HISTOLOGIC TYPES OF CHILDHOOD THYROID CANCER

Type	Frequency (%)	Characteristics
1. Differentiated carcinoma		
A Papillary carcinoma	70–80	Infiltrative and multicentric; lymph node metastases in 70%–90% of cases; hematogenous spread (mainly lung) in 5%–10% of cases
B Follicular carcinoma	16–20	Vascular invasion
2. Medullary carcinoma	Rare	Occurs in isolation, but more frequently associated with one of the MEN syndromes; usually aggressive and can be fatal
3. Undifferentiated carcinoma	Rare	Aggressive, usually fatal within 6 months of diagnosis
4. Insular carcinoma	Very rare	A variant of the poorly differentiated carcinoma; aggressive, poor prognosis

MEN, multiple endocrine neoplasia.

Clinical Radiation Oncology

specific mutations in the ret oncogene that predict for MEN syndromes. Those individuals could be candidates for prophylactic thyroidectomy at an earlier age than if the increase in serum calcitonin was used to identify C-cell hyperplasia or early carcinoma. At present, genetic testing should be performed at birth in children suspected of having the MEN IIa syndrome, and no later than 1 year of age for those with possible MEN IIb (7,104,177).

Children with thyroid cancer are commonly euthyroid and usually present with a thyroid nodule or palpable cervical lymph node. Conventional radiographs may show calcifications in the region of the thyroid gland (psammoma bodies). Iodine radionuclide scan may show a cold nodule.

Paradoxically, despite the fact that 70% to 80% of patients present with regional lymph node involvement and approximately 20% have distant metastases at diagnosis, the prognosis of differentiated thyroid cancer in children and adolescents is excellent (177,289,326,337). In the Mayo Clinic series, survival rates for children did not differ significantly from those of matched controls at 20 to 30 years (347). In the Royal Marsden series (182), the median overall survival was 53 years, and the median survival for patients who developed recurrence was 30 years. The only presenting feature predictive of poorer survival was the presence of metastases at diagnosis. According to a study reported by the Surgical Discipline Committee of the Children's Cancer Group, the overall survival for children presenting with distant metastases was 100% at 10 years. The progression-free survival rate was 76% at 5 years and 66% at 10 years. In a series of 14 children with papillary thyroid cancer and pulmonary metastases treated at the Mayo Clinic (39) by various surgical procedures, RAI, external-beam irradiation (one patient), and suppressive hormone therapy, at a mean follow-up time of 19.3 years 50% were alive completely free of disease and 50% were alive and asymptomatic with residual pulmonary disease.

Thyroid carcinoma is treated primarily by surgery. The extent of surgery for the primary tumor (subtotal lobectomy, lobectomy, total thyroidectomy) and involved lymph nodes (node picking, modified or radical neck dissection) is controversial (286).

The arguments in favor of total thyroidectomy include the multifocality of the tumor, decrease in neck recurrences, the ability to use serum thyroglobulin as a tumor marker after radical surgery, and the ability to detect pulmonary metastases by radioactive iodine scan earlier. The arguments for more limited surgery are mainly the increased complication rate of radical surgery, with apparently no clear survival advantage (104,168,176,177,182,195,242,289,326,331).

The use of RAI for routine ablation of remaining thyroid tissue after surgery in patients without any known metastatic disease is another area of controversy. Because the mortality rate of pediatric thyroid cancer is extremely low and recurrences can develop many years after surgery, it is impossible to perform randomized trials to answer therapeutic questions. However, most authorities support the administration of RAI in this setting because of the high incidence of nodal and systemic metastases of thyroid cancer in the young (124,343).

RAI is indicated in patients with cervical lymph node involvement or distant metastases. The radiopharmaceutical is taken up by 50% to 80% of well-differentiated tumors, and is able to deliver high focal doses of irradiation to any remaining thyroid tissue.

Side effects of RAI include nausea, glossalgia, hypogeusia, thyroiditis, and gastrointestinal discomfort. Potential and rare long-term complications include myelosuppression, leukemia, bladder cancer, salivary cancer, gastric cancer, breast cancer, and infertility. These complications were mainly reported in the past, when high, repetitive doses of RAI were used, and should not occur, or occur rarely, with today's treatment policies and dosages (124,343).

RAI concentrates in the salivary glands and is secreted into the saliva. Following the administration of high-dose RAI, salivary gland swelling and pain, usually involving the parotid gland, can be seen in conjunction with radiation sialadenitis. Secondary complications reported include xerostomia, taste alterations, increases in caries, stomatitis, and candidiasis (42,202).

Exogenous thyroid hormone is given to suppress thyroidstimulating hormone production and to decrease the probability of tumor recurrence. Exogenous thyroid hormone is also given as replacement therapy, to keep the patients euthyroid despite thyroidectomy (39,69,182).

External-beam irradiation in children with differentiated thyroid cancer is indicated for unresectable primary tumor or cervical or mediastinal lymph nodes that do not take up RAI. It also has a role in advanced locoregional disease, with extensive extrathyroid extension, or where there is gross residual tumor after attempted surgical excision, or when definitive resection has not been possible. Although external-beam irradiation is useful for palliative therapy of advanced or metastatic disease, the lack of randomized controlled studies makes its role as part of initial adjuvant treatment controversial and it is rarely indicated for microscopic residual disease. Radiotherapy, with or without chemotherapy, can be administered in children with anaplastic thyroid carcinoma (337).

External-beam irradiation for thyroid cancer requires careful and meticulous treatment planning in order to minimize acute toxicity and avoid serious long-term complications. The volume of irradiation is adjusted according to operative and pathological findings and can range from whole-neck and upper mediastinal irradiation to just treating the thyroid gland or thyroid bed.

The anatomy of the area causes significant technical difficulties, especially because the treatment volume curves around the vertebral bodies. CT-based planning, three-dimensional treatment planning, or IMRT is advocated to allow the administration of curative doses (in the range of 55 to 65 Gy) to the target volume, without compromising spinal cord tolerance. This can be achieved by a variety of techniques (17).

Germ Cell Tumors (GCTs)

Gonadal or extragonadal GCTs represent <2% of pediatric cancer. Their cure rate is high and strongly correlated with adherence to strict treatment guidelines.

Pathology

The tumor is the result of neoplastic transformation of primitive germ cells or totipotent embryonal cells (241) (Table 88.7). The site of the tumor depends on the site of arrest of the neoplastic cell during migration from the brain to the sacrococcygeal region in the fetal period. The most common sites are testis, ovary, sacrococcygeal region, retroperitoneum, and mediastinum. Aberrant migration can occur, which explains unusual tumor sites (23). The most frequent cytogenetic abnormality is the isochromosome 12p for both gonadal and extra-

gonadal GCT, except for children <3 years of age at diagnosis. Klinefelter syndrome can be associated with GCT in boys (13). Intracranial germ cell tumors are discussed in Chapter 11.

Clinical Presentation

Abdominal pain, abdominal distention, and saccrococcygeal or buttock swelling are the frequent presenting signs (259). Staging includes imaging both of the primary tumor and most frequent sites of metastatic dissemination (lungs, liver, brain, and bone). Serum AFP, β-HCG, lactate dehydrogenase, CEA, and placental alkaline phosphatase levels are mandatory prior to the initiation of any treatment. Serum AFP level must be interpreted according to patient age (level >1,000 mg/mL is normal until the age of 1 month). Clinical markers are strongly correlated with some histologic features (Table 88.8); however, high AFP levels can be detected in infectious diseases of the liver and increased β-HCG level can be associated with malignancies other than choriocarcinoma. The half-life time of AFP is 5 to 7 days and that of β-HCG is 24 to 36 hours. Both are very useful tools for predicting and monitoring treatment response, progression of disease, and relapse (63).

Treatment

Surgery is the standard treatment for mature teratomas and saccrococcygeal tumors (with complete removal of the tumor and the coccyx) but it may be combined with chemotherapy to limit the extent of irradiation. Surgery is often the first treatment for malignant gonadal GCT: orchiectomy with high inguinal ligation or ovariectomy with careful peritoneal cavity exploration. Lymph node dissection is not recommended in early-stage GCT, especially in germinomas. Second-look surgery can be

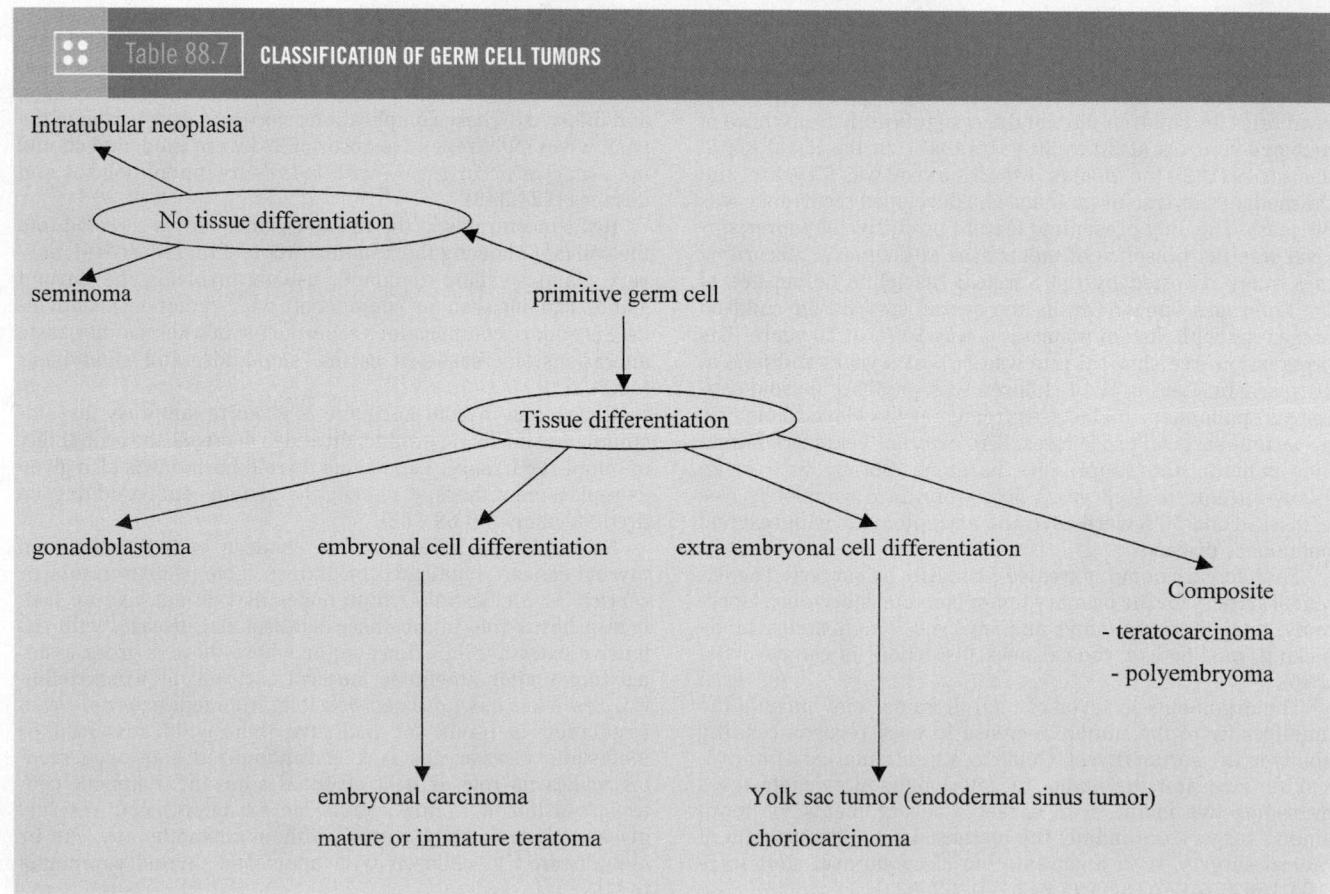

Table 88.7   CLASSIFICATION OF GERM CELL TUMORS

Table 88.8	GERM CELL TUMOR AND CLINICAL MARKERS				
Tumor Type	β-HCG	AFP	LDH	CEA	PLAP
Embryonal carcinoma	+	+		+	
Mature teratoma					
Immature teratoma	+	+	+	+	
Yolk sac tumor		+++	+	+	
Choriocarcinoma	+++		+		
Germinoma	+		+	+	+++

β-HCG, human chorionic gonadotropin; AFP, α-fetoprotein; LDH, lactate dehydrogenase; CEA, carcinoembryonic antigen; PLAP, placental alkaline phosphatase.

indicated in cases of residual disease (clinical or biochemical) after chemotherapy.

Since the introduction of cisplatin-based chemotherapy, the survival rate of GCT has risen from 60% to 90% (81) and regimens used are similar to those used in the adult age group. There is now a trend to use carboplatin in order to reduce late toxicities (255). The value of rate of decline of serum tumor markers has been proven to be of prognostic significance and must be used in the management of poor-risk patients (211). Radiotherapy is rarely indicated except for some cases of early-stage ovarian germinoma in adolescents (dose, 20 to 25 Gy). The use of radiotherapy for ovarian germinoma in the young, however, must be compared with salvage chemotherapy after surgery alone. In advanced cases of ovarian dysgerminoma, careful surgical staging followed by conservative resection and chemotherapy without radiotherapy results in an overall survival rate as high as 85% without compromising the possibility of future pregnancy (15). There is no indication for radiotherapy after complete response in extragonadal GCT. Radiotherapy, however, can be proposed in selected cases of extragonadal GCT with persistent disease after chemotherapy and surgery. A minimal dose of 45 Gy can be given, but has low rate of success (18).

Hemangiomas and Lymphangioma

Hemangiomas

Hemangiomas constitute a very common vascular abnormality of infancy. In some cases their development can be associated with adverse cosmetic effects, unacceptable symptoms, and organ compression that in certain cases could be life-threatening. Such cases require therapy. There are two distinct types of hemangiomas (247): dynamic lesions, which include cellular hemangiomas, capillary hemangiomas, and cavernous hemangiomas; and adynamic lesions, which include port wine stains, telangiectasias, and venous lakes. Radiation therapy is very rarely used in the treatment of hemangiomas. It is generally considered only for lesions that are not likely to spontaneously regress and when other therapies have been tried and failed. Second malignant neoplasms have been described in long-term survivors of radiotherapy for hemangioma. Steroids or interferon are considered first-line therapy. Only cavernous and capillary hemangiomas are suitable for radiotherapy. In infants, a total dose of 7.5 Gy in three fractions is often sufficient for capillary hemangioma. Higher doses (30 to 40 Gy) are used in older patients for large and progressive lesions. Special attention must be given to the Kasabach-Merritt syndrome (Fig. 88.2). Kasabach-Merritt syndrome is defined as combination of cutaneous vascular abnormalities with or without visceral involvement and thrombopenia due to intravascular coagulopathy. There are alarming hemangiomas with life-threatening lesions (mediastinum, lower extremities, abdomen) either due to compression or secondary to a thrombocytic coagulopathy or high-output cardiac failure. A dose of 10 Gy in 10 fractions can be given; it is not mandatory to encompass the whole hemangioma in the target volume (29,84).

Cavernous hemangiomas can be located in the epidural space and cause spinal cord compression. Surgical resection is the standard treatment (220).

Gamma-knife radiosurgery has been employed successfully for circumscribed choroidal hemangioma (232).

Lymphangiomas

Histologically, lymphangiomas are a benign proliferation of lymph vessels. Four types are recognized: (a) capillary lymphangiomas, (b) cavernous lymphangiomas, (c) cystic hygromas, and (d) lymphangeal hemangiomas. Surgery is the treatment of choice.

Special attention must be given to the Gorham syndrome, also known as the bone-vanishing syndrome or massive osteolysis of bone (225). Gorham syndrome is a bone hamartoma with various percentages of lymphangioma and hemangioma, characterized by well-margined osteolytic scattered lesions that progressively affect the cortex, with no respect for joint boundaries (Fig. 88.3). All bones can be affected (vertebrae, ribs, scapula). Progression is unpredictable, from spontaneous remission to bone absorption and sometimes even death. The prognosis is very poor when pleural or visceral involvement develops. Some encouraging results have been reported using antiresorptive therapy such as calcitonin or biphosphonates (224). Although radiotherapy is the last resort for the patient, encouraging results have been reported for patients with chylothorax and with patients with rib, thorax, and vertebral body involvement. The usual dose is ~18 Gy to the hemithorax and ~40 Gy to the affected bone (137). An encouraging response has been reported for base of the skull lesions with doses of 40 Gy (43,209).

Desmoplastic Small Round-Cell Tumor (DSRCT)

DSRCT was first described in 1989 (107). It is a rare aggressive neoplasm with typical clinical, histologic, karyotypic, and biologic characteristics. DSRCT mainly affects male adolescents and young adults, but sometimes occurs in young females. Clinically, patients present with a bulky abdominal or pelvic mass, but intracranial, testicular, renal soft tissue, or bone DSRCT have also been described (4,61,114,304).

The tumor is characterized by a desmoplastic stroma with circumscribed tumor cells and encased nests of primitive undifferentiated cells. The tumoral cells express epithelial (keratin, EMA), conjunctival (vimentin), muscular (desmin), and neuroendocrinal markers.

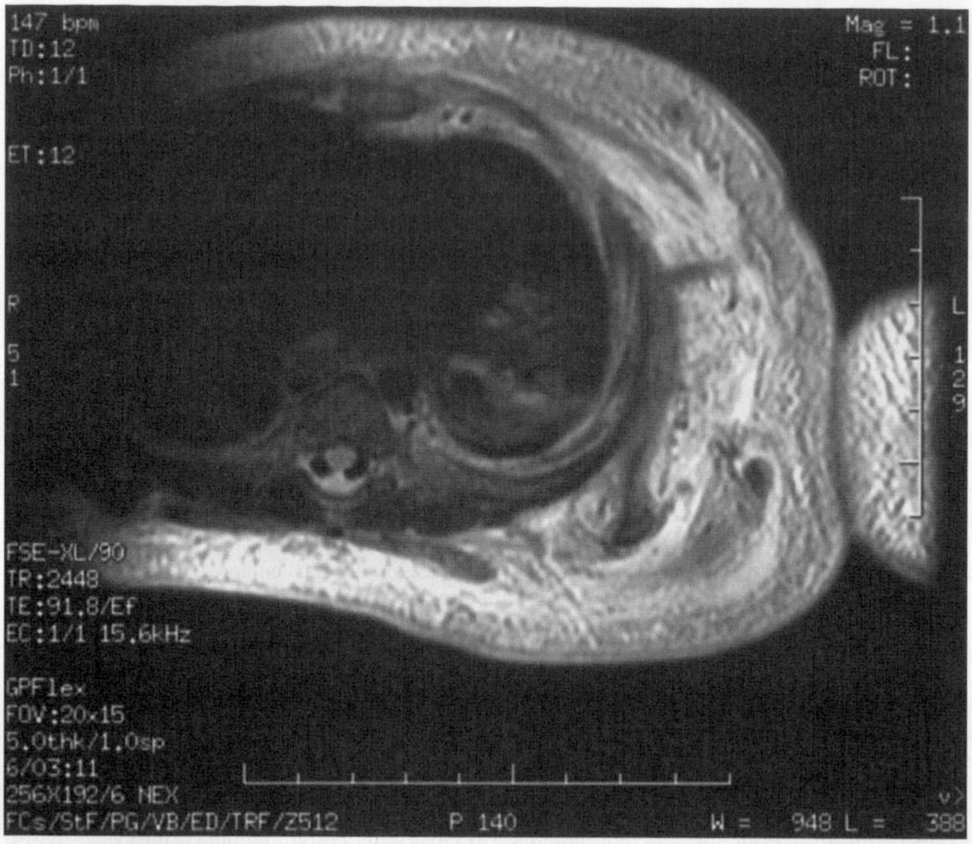

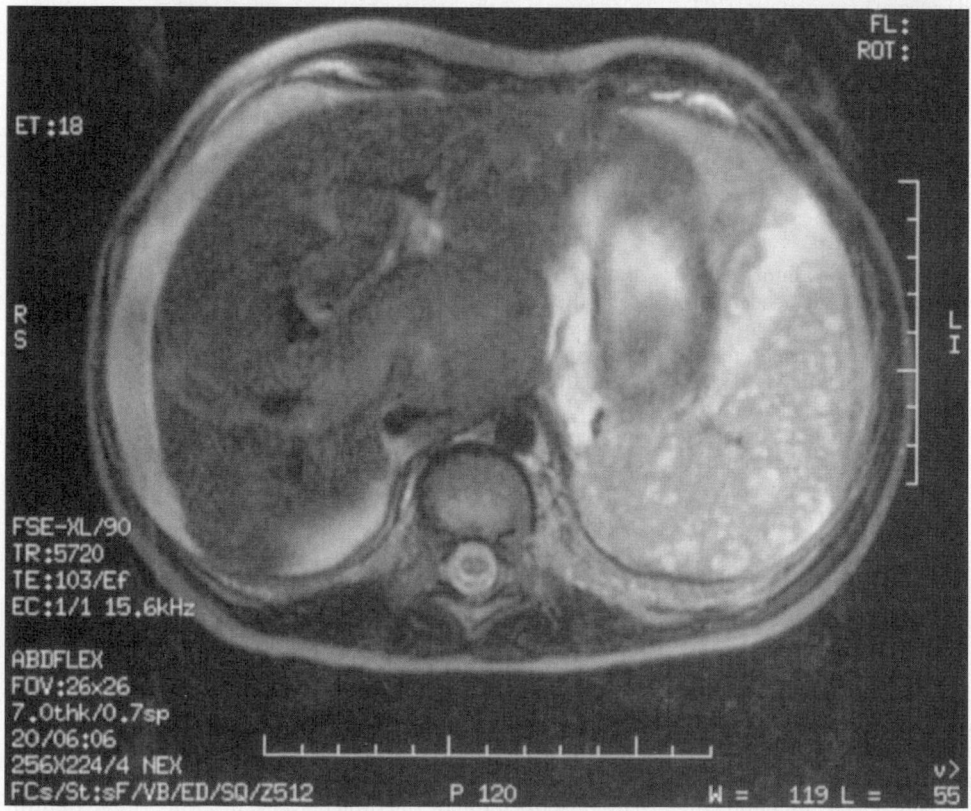

FIGURE 88.2. Kasabach-Merritt syndrome. Massive left hemithorax infiltration and involvement of the left arm.

FIGURE 88.3. Gorham disease in a 3-year-old girl. Diffuse lymphangiomatosis affecting pelvic bones, ribs, spleen, and liver.

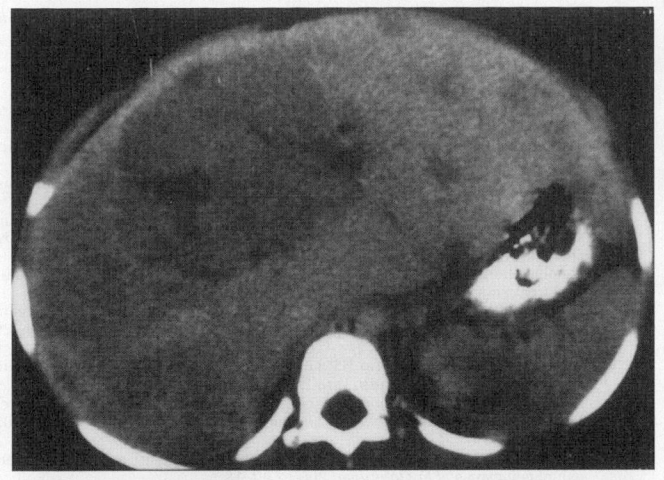

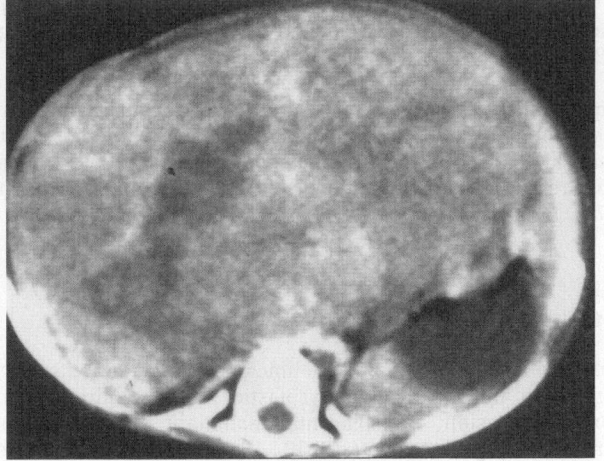

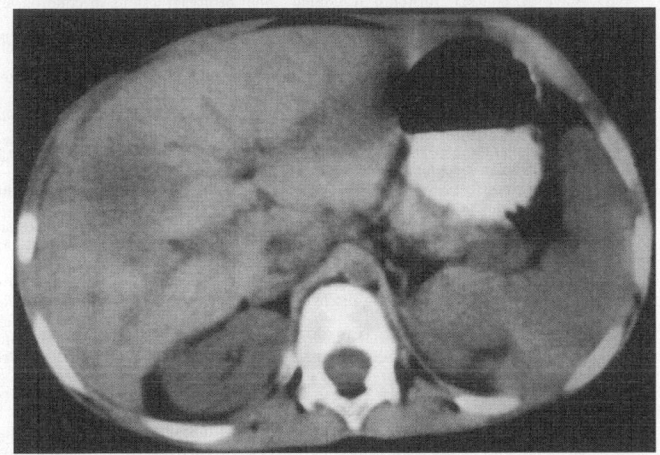

FIGURE 88.4. A 7-year-old girl with hepatoblastoma. **A:** at diagnosis, **B:** following one cycle of chemotherapy, and **C:** following four cycles of chemotherapy before right hepatic lobectomy.

Reciprocal translocation (11:22) (p13:q12) has been described, which results from a fusion between the terminal part of the Ewing's sarcoma gene (EWS) and the carboxy terminus part of the Wilm's tumor gene (WT1) (106).

The DSRCTs are highly chemosensitive but the prognosis is still poor. Kretschmar et al. (172) reviewed 101 cases of DSRCT: after 2 years only two patients were still alive and the median survival was 17 months.

More recently, investigators from the Memorial Sloan-Kettering Cancer Center reported a series of 66 patients treated with high-dose alkylating agents–based chemotherapy with autologous *Bone Marrow Transplant*ation, surgical debulking, and whole-abdominopelvic radiotherapy. The dose to the whole abdomen was 30 Gy (1.5 Gy twice daily) and patients with gross residual disease received a boost of 6 to 15 Gy. The 3-year overall survival was 48%, but the progression-free survival was only 35% in the first report (172). In a more recent publication, a slightly better survival rate at 3 years (55%) has been reported. Survival at 3 years was only 27% when the three modalities were not used, with only 10 patients surviving without evidence of disease at a median follow-up of 2.4 years (181).

:: | Skin Cancer

Basal and squamous cell carcinomas are rare in children and adolescents. When they occur in the pediatric and adolescent age groups, there is usually an underlying predisposing genetic disorder, such as basal cell nevus syndrome (BCNS), or Gorlin-Goltz syndrome and xeroderma pigmentosum. Basal and squamous carcinomas have also been reported to arise in nevus

sebaceous (145) and after radiation for benign or malignant conditions (277,344).

BCNS or Gorlin-Goltz syndrome (28,33,115,152) is an autosomal dominant disorder with variable penetration characterized by a "coarse face" with hypertelorism and frontal bossing, multiple basal cell carcinomas presenting at a young age, pits on the palms and soles, skeletal abnormalities (e.g., bifid ribs, hemivertebrae, fusion of vertebral bodies), jaw cysts, epidermic cysts and hamartomas, oculoneurologic abnormalities, and ectopic calcification of the falx cerebri and other structures. Skin lesions located in the head and neck tend to invade the deep structures. Several patients with BCNS have been reported to develop medulloblastoma at early childhood and ovarian fibromas (33,73,155,165,184,270,299,330).

Mutation of the human homologue of Drosophila Patched (PTC) gene is considered to be the molecular defect in BCNS (330,345). The Gorlin-Goltz syndrome is a unique example of the genetic-environmental interaction for the production of malignancies: children treated for medulloblastoma by craniospinal irradiation developed multiple skin cancers in the irradiated area, an unusual and special illustration of multihit mutagenesis, suggesting that radiotherapy should probably be omitted or limited in children with BCNS (330).

Xeroderma pigmentosum (XP) is an extremely rare, autosomal recessive inherited disease characterized by abnormal pigmentation and more than 1,000-fold increase in nonmelanoma skin cancer (basal cell carcinoma and squamous cell carcinoma) on sun-exposed skin. XP patients are also at a significant risk to develop melanoma (54,169). Neurologic abnormalities such as areflexia and mental retardation are sometimes associated with XP.

The genetic abnormality underlying XP leads to defects in nucleotide excision repair of ultraviolet-induced DNA damage (22,54,294).

Skin cancer in affected children is treated by standard techniques (such as surgery, cryosurgery, chemosurgery). There should not be any contraindication to using radiotherapy to treat skin cancer or any other malignancy in XP patients as ionizing radiation damage is normally repaired in these patients (276).

Malignant Melanoma

Childhood melanoma can sometimes be associated with large congenital nevocytic nevi, dysplastic nevus syndrome, immunosuppression, transplacental malignant melanoma, and xeroderma pigmentosum (102,131,216,233,260,268,308). Pediatric malignant melanoma should be distinguished from the juvenile melanoma or Spitz nevus characterized by a relatively benign course and long-term survival (19,138,296).

The management of childhood melanoma follows the guidelines set for adult patients (266). The prognosis is related to the Breslow's or Clark's thickness of the primary lesion and nodal status. Radiotherapy has a role mainly for palliation of metastatic disease or in locally advanced lesions.

References

1. Ablin A, Krailo M, Hass J, et al. Hepatoblastoma and hepatocellular carcinoma in children: a report from the Children's Cancer Study Group (CCG) and the Pediatric Oncology Group (POG). *Med Pediatr Oncol* 1988;16:417.
2. Abraham SC, Montgomery EA, Giardiello FM, et al. Frequent beta-catenin mutations in juvenile nasopharyngeal angiofibromas. *Am J Pathol* 2001;158:1073–1078.
3. Abramson MJ. Adrenal neoplasms in children. *Radiol Clin North Am* 1997; 35:1415–1453.
4. Adsay V, Cheng J, Athanasian E, et al. Primary desmoplastic small cell tumor of soft tissues and bone of the hand. *Am J Surg Pathol* 1999;23:1408–1413.
5. Akkari V, Donadieu J, Piguet C, et al. French Langerhans Cell Study Group. Hematopoietic stem cell transplantation in patients with severe Langerhans cell histiocytosis and hematological dysfunction: experience of the French Langerhans Cell Study Group. *Bone Marrow Transplant* 2003;31:1097–103.
6. Al Sarraf M, LeBlanc M, Giri PG, et al. Chemoradiotherapy versus radiotherapy in patients with advanced nasopharyngeal cancer: phase III randomized Intergroup study 0099. *J Clin Oncol* 1998;16:1310–1317.
7. Alsanea, Clark OH. Familial thyroid cancer. *Curr Opin Oncol* 2001;13:44–51.
8. Altman AJ, Schwartz AD. *Malignant diseases of infancy, childhood and adolescence.* 2nd ed. Philadelphia: W.B. Saunders; 1983:505.
9. American Cancer Society. *Cancer facts and figures–1995.* New York: American Cancer Society; 1995.
10. American Joint Committee for Cancer staging and end results reporting. *Manual for staging of cancer,* 4th ed. Philadelphia: JB Lippincott; 1992.
11. Ames BN, Durston WE, Yamaski E, et al. Carcinogens are mutagens: a simple screen test system combining liver homogenates for activation and bacteria for detection. *Proc Natl Acad Sci U S A* 1973;70:2281–2285.
12. Andersson A, Bergdahl L. Carcinoma of the colon in children: a report of six new cases and a review of the literature. *J Pediatr Surg* 1976;11:967–971.
13. Antonelli A, Miccoli P, Derzhitski VE, et al. Epidemiologic and clinical evaluation of thyroid cancer in children from the Gomel region. *World J Surg* 1996;20:867–871.
14. Arcement CM, Towbin RB, Meza MP, et al. Intrahepatic chemoembolization in unresectable pediatric liver malignancies. *Pediatr Radiol* 2000;30:779–85.
15. Ayhan A, Bildirici I, Gunalp S, et al. Pure dysgerminoma of the ovary: a review of 45 well staged cases. *Eur J Gynaecol Oncol* 2000;21:98–101.
16. Azab MB, Henry-Amar M, Rougier P, et al. Prognostic factors in primary gastrointestinal non-Hodgkin's lymphoma: a multivariate analysis, report of 106 cases and review of the literature. *Cancer* 1989;64:1208–1217.
17. Baker DL, Bonnin NJ. Germ cell tumors. In: D Angio GJ, Simiah D, Meadows AT, et al, eds. *Practical pediatric oncology.* New York: Wiley Liss; 1992:341.
18. Baranzelli MC, Flamant F, De Lumley L, et al. Treatment of non-metastatic, non-seminomatous malignant germ-cell tumours in childhood: experience of the "Societe Francaise d'Oncologie Pediatrique" MGCT 1985–1989 study. *Med Pediatr Oncol* 1993;21:395–401.
19. Barnhill RL, Flotte TJ, Fleischli M, et al. Cutaneous melanoma and atypical spitz tumors in childhood. *Cancer* 1995;76:1833–1845.
20. Bellantone R, Ferrante A, Boscherini M, et al. Role of reoperation in recurrence of adrenal cortical carcinoma: results from 188 cases collected in the Italian National Registry for Adrenal Cortical Carcinoma. *Surgery* 1997;1:212–1218.
21. Ben Arush M, Stein ME, Rosenblatt E, et al. Advanced nasopharyngeal carcinoma in the young: the Northern Israel Oncology Center experience. 1973–1991. *Pediatr Hematol Oncol* 1995;12:271–276.
22. Berneburg M, Lehmann AR. Xeroderma pigmentosum and related disorders: defects in DNA repair and transcription. *Adv Genet* 2001;43:71–102.
23. Berney DM, Lee A, Randle SJ, et al. The frequency of intratubular embryonal carcinoma: implications for the pathogenesis of germ cell tumours. *Histopathology* 2004;45:155–161.
24. Berry CL, Keeling JW. Hepatoblastoma. In: *Pediatriatric pathology.* Berlin: Springer-Verlag; 1981:660–662.
25. Berry DH, Gresik M, Maybee D, et al. Histiocytosis X in bone only. *Med Pediatr Oncol* 1990;18:292–294.
26. Bhattacharya S, Lobo FD, Pai PK. Hepatic neoplasms in childhood—a clinicopathologic study. *Pediatr Surg Int* 1998;14:51–54.
27. Billroth T. Untersuchungen uber den feineren Bau und die Entwicklung der Brustdrusengeschwulste. *Virchows Arch Pathol Anat Physiol* 1860;18:69.
28. Binkley GW, Johnson HH. Epithelioma adenoids cyticum: basal cell nevi Agenesis of the corpus callosum and dental cysts. A clinical and autopsy study. *Arch Dermatol* 1951;63:73–84.
29. Bistolfi F, Bonacci W, Zullino E, et al. Role of low dose radiotherapy on the multinodal treatment of Kasach-Merrith syndrome. *Radiol Med* 1995;90:162–166.
30. Blichert-Taft M, Hansen JPH, Hansen OH, et al. Clinical course of cysto-sarcoma phylloides related to histologic appearance. *Surg Gynecol Obstet* 1975;140:929–932.
31. Bond SJ, Buchino JJ, Nagaraj HS, et al. Sentinel lymph node biopsy in juvenile secretory carcinoma. *J Pediatr Surg* 2004;39:120–121.
32. Bourque MD, Spigland N, Bensoussan AL, et al. Esophageal leiomyoma in children: two case reports and reviews of the literature. *J Pediatr Surg* 1989;24:1103–1107.
33. Boutimzine N, Laghmari A, Karib H, et al. La phacomatose de Gorlin-Goltz: aspects ophtalmologiques. *J Fr Ophtalmol* 2000;23:2–18.
34. Bower R, Bell MJ, Ternberg JL. Management of breast lesions in children and adolescents. *J Surg* 1976;11:337–346.
35. Bowman LC, Riely CA. Management of pediatric liver tumors. *Surg Oncol Clin North Am* 1996;5:451–459.
36. Bradley EL III. Primary and adjunctive therapy in carcinoma of the adrenal cortex. *Surg Gynecol Obstet* 1975;141:507–511.
37. Brenner B, Ilson DH, Minsky BD. Treatment of localized esophageal cancer. *Semin Oncol* 2004;31:554–65.
38. Bressac B, Kew M, Wands J, et al. Selective G to T mutations of p53 gene in hepatocellular carcinoma from Southern Africa. *Nature* 1991;350:429–431.
39. Brink JS, van Heerden JA, McIver B, et al. Papillary thyroid cancer with pulmonary metasteses in children: long term prognosis. *Surgery* 2000;128:881–887.
40. Broadbent V, Chu AC. Langerhans' cell histiocytosis. In: Plowman PN, Pinkerson CR, eds. *Paediatric oncology: clinical practice and controversies.* London: Chapman and Hall; 1992:4322–4335.
41. Broich G, Pagliari A, Ottaviani F. Esthesioneuroblastoma: a general review of the cases published since the discovery of the tumour in 1924. *Anticancer Res* 1997;17:2683–2706.
42. Caglar M, Tuncel M, Alpar R. Scintigraphic evaluation of salivary gland dysfunction in patients with thyroid cancer after radioiodine treatment. *Clin Nucl Med.* 2002;27:767–771.
43. Carrie C, Bouffet E, Thiesse P, et al. Osseous hemolymphangiomatosis. *Medical and Pediatric Oncology* 1991;5:363 (abstr. 96).
44. Casanova M, Massimino M, Ferrari A, et al. Etoposide, cisplatin, epirubicin chemotherapy in the treatment of pediatric liver tumors. *Pediatr Hematol Oncol* 2005;22:189–198.
45. Caty MG, Coran AG, Geagen M, et al. Current diagnosis and treatment of pheochromocytoma in children. Experience with 22 consecutive tumors in 14 patients. *Arch Surg* 1990;125:978–981.
46. Chamadol W, Pesie M, Puapairoj A. Inflammatory carcinoma of the breast in a 12-year-old Thai girl. *J Med Assoc Thai* 1987;70:543–548.
47. Chen LK, Hwang SJ, Li AF, et al. Colorectal cancer in patients 20 years old or less in Taiwan. *South Med J* 2001;94:1202–1205.
48. Cheng SH, Jian JJ, Tsai SY, et al. Long-term survival of nasopharyngeal carcinoma following concomitant radiotherapy and chemotherapy. *Int J Radiat Oncol Biol Phys* 2000;48:1323–1330.
49. Chun Y, Kim W, Park K, et al. Pancreatoblastoma. *J Pediatr Surg* 1997;32:1612–1615.
50. Church J. M.,McGannon E, Burke C, et al. Teenagers with familial adenomatous polyposis: what is their risk for colorectal cancer. *Dis Colon Rectum* 2002;45:887–889.
51. Clatworth HW Jr, Schiller M, Grosfeld JL. Primary liver tumors in infancy and childhood: 41 cases variously treated. *Arch Surg* 1974;109:143–147.
52. Cohen M, Zornoza J, Cangir A, et al. Direct injection of methylprednisolone sodium succinate in the treatment of solitary eosinophilic granuloma of bone: a report of 9 cases. *Radiology* 1980;136:289–293.
53. Cohen MD, Bugaieski EM, Haliloglu M, et al. Visual presentation of the staging of pediatric tumors. *Radiographics* 1996;16:523–545.
54. Copeland NE, Hanke CW, Michalak JA. The molecular basis of xeroderma pigmentosum. *Dermatol Surg* 1997;23:447–455.
55. Corpron CA, Black CT, Singletary SE, et al. Breast cancer in adolescent females. *J Pediatr Surg* 1995;30:322–324.
56. Coughlin CT, Wang TZ, Ryan TP, et al. Interstitial microwave-induced hyperthermia and iridium brachytherapy for the treatment of obstructing biliary carcinomas. *Int J Hyperthermia* 1992;8:157–171.
57. Coutant R, Pein F, Adamsbaum C, et al. Prognosis of children with malignant pheochromocytoma. Report of 2 cases and review of the literature. *Horm Res* 1999;52:145–199.
58. Craig JR, Peters RL, Edmonson HA, et al. Fibrolamellar carcinoma of the liver. *Cancer* 1980;46:372–379.
59. Crucitti F, Bellantone R, Ferrante A, et al. The Italian registry for Adrenal Cortical carcinoma; analysis of a multiinstitutional series of 129 patients. The ACC Italian registry Study group. *Surgery* 1996;119:161–170.
60. Cummings BJ, Blend R, Keane T, et al. Primary radiation therapy for juvenile nasopharyngeal angiofibroma. *Laryngoscope* 1984;94:1599–1605.
61. Cummings OW, Ulbright TM, Young RH, et al. Desmoplastic small round cell tumors of the paratesticular region. A report of six cases. *Am J Surg Pathol* 1997;21:219–225.
62. Czauderna P, Mackinlay G, Perilongo G, et al. Liver Tumors Study Group of the International Society of Pediatric Oncology. Hepatocellular carcinoma in children: results of the first prospective study of the International Society of Pediatric Oncology group. *J Clin Oncol* 2002;15;20:2798–804.

63. D'Angio GJ. Yolk sac carcinoma. Tumor Board of the Children's Hospital of Philadelphia. *Med Pediatr Oncol* 1987;15:96–101.
64. Davidoff AM, Cirrincione C, Seigler HF. Malignant melanoma in children. *Ann Surg Oncol* 1994;1:278–282.
65. de Cholnoky T. Mammary cancer in youth. *Surg Gynecol Obstet* 1943;77:55–60.
66. Deal JE, Severs PS, Baratt TM, et al. Pheochromocytoma—investigation and management of 10 cases. *Arch Dis Child* 1990;65:269–274.
67. Defachelles AS, Martin De Lassalle E, Boutard P, et al. Pancreatoblastoma in childhood: clinical course and therapeutic management of seven patients. *Med Pediatr Oncol* 2001;37:47–52.
68. Dehner LP, Natterson J, Priest J. Pleuropulmonary blastoma. A unique intrathoracic pulmonary neoplasm of childhood. *Perspect Pediatr Pathol* 1995;18:214–216.
69. Desjardins JG, Bass J, Leboeuf G, et al. A twenty year experience with thyroid carcinoma in children. *J Pediatr Surg* 1988;23:709–713.
70. Dickstein G, Shechner C, Arad E, et al. Is there a role for low doses of mitotane as adjuvant therapy in ACC? *J Clin Endocrinol Metab* 1998;83:3100.
71. Dosios T, Stinios J, Nicolaides P, et al. Pleuropulmonary blastoma in childhood. A malignant degeneration of pulmonary cysts. *Pediatr Surg Int* 2004;20:863–865.
72. Douglass EC, Reynolds M, Finegold M, et al. Cisplatin, vincristine and fluorouracil therapy for hepatoblastoma: a pediatric oncology group study. *J Clin Oncol* 1993;11:96–99.
73. Dowling PA, Fleming P, Saunders ID, et al. Odontogenic keratocysts in a 5-year-old: initial manifestations of nevoid basal cell carcinoma syndrome. *Pediatr Dent* 2000;22:53–55.
74. Driver CP, Birch J, Gough DC, et al. Adrenal cortical tumors in childhood. *Pediatr Hematol Oncol* 1998;15:527–532.
75. Dugue G, Back G, Molho L, et al. Breast cancer in the young. *J Natl Med Assoc* 1989;81:1184–1187.
76. Dunger DB, Broadbent V, Yeoman E, et al. The frequency and natural history of diabetes insipidus in children with Langerhans-cell histiocytosis. *N Engl J Med* 1989;321:1157–1162.
77. DuVall GA, Wladen DT. Adenomcarcinoma of the esophagus complicating Cornelia de Lange Syndrome. *J. Clin Gastroenterol* 1996;22:131–133.
78. Easton DF, Ford D, Bishop DT, et al. Breast and ovarian cancer incidence in BRCA1 mutation carriers. *Am J Hum Genet* 1995;56:265–271.
79. Eden OB, Shaw MP. Chemotherapy for pancreaticoblastoma. *Med Pediatr Oncol* 1995;20:357–358.
80. Eich HT, Staar S, Micke O, et al. Radiotherapy of esthesioneuroblastoma. *Int J Radiat Oncol Biol Phys* 2001;49:155–160.
81. Einhorn LH, Williams SD, Loehrer PJ, et al. Evaluation of optimal duration of chemotherapy in favorable-prognosis disseminated germ cell tumors: a Southeastern Cancer Study Group protocol. *J Clin Oncol* 1989;7:387–391.
82. Ellis T, Davidson SA. Hereditary breast and ovarian cancer. Identifying and managing patients at risk. *OB Management* 1998;53–60.
83. Enepekides DJ. Recent advances in the treatment of juvenile angiofibroma. *Curr Opin Otolaryngol Head Neck Surg* 2004;12:495–499.
84. Enjolras O, Riche MC, Merland JJ, et al. Management of alarming hemangiomas in infants and children. A review of 25 cases. *Pediatrics* 1990;85:491–498.
85. Eskelinen M, Vainio J, Tuominen L, et al. Carcinoma of the breast in children. *Z Kinderchir* 1990;45:52–55.
86. Exelby P, Filler R, Grosfield JL. Liver tumors in children in particular reference to hepatoblastoma and hepatocellular carcinoma: American Academy of Pediatrics Surgical Survey system. *J Pediatr Surg* 1974;10:329–337.
87. Farran RP, Zaretski E, Egeler RM. Treatment of Langerhans cell histiocytosis with pamidronate. *J Pediatr Hematol Oncol* 2001;23:54–56.
88. Farrow JH, Ashikari H. Breast lesions in young girls. *Surg Clin North Am* 1969; 49:261–269.
89. Fassbender WJ, Krohn-Grimberghe B, Gortz B, et al. Multiple endocrine neoplasia (MEN): an overview and case report. Patient with sporadic bilateral pheochromocytoma, hyperparathyroidism and marfanoid habitus. *Anticancer Res* 2000;20:4877–4887.
90. Feng WH, Israel B, Raab-Traub N, et al. Chemotherapy induces lytic EBV replication and confers ganciclovir susceptibility to EBV-positive epithelial cell tumors. *Cancer Res* 2002;62:1920–1926.
91. Field JL, Adamson LF, Stoeckle HE. Review of carcinoids in children: functioning carcinoid in a 15-year-old male. *Pediatrics* 1962;29:953–960.
92. Fonkalsrud EW. Pheochromocytoma in childhood. In: Progress in pediatric surgery, Berlin: Springer-Verlag; 1991;26:101–111.
93. Foote RL, Morita A, Ebersold MJ, et al. Esthesioneuroblastoma: the role of adjuvant radiation therapy. *Int J Radiat Oncol Biol Phys* 1993;27:835–842.
94. Fossati Bellani F, Massimino M. Liver tumors in childhood: epidemiology and clinics. *J Surg Oncol* 1993;3[Suppl]:119–121.
95. Frost JD, Wiersma SR. Progressive Langerhans cell histiocytosis in an infant with Klinefelter syndrome successfully treated with allogeneic Bone Marrow Transplantation. *J Pediatr Hematol Oncol* 1996;18:396–400.
96. Fuchs J, Bode U, von Schweinitz D, Weinel, et al. Analysis of treatment efficiency of carboplatin and etoposide in combination with radical surgery in advanced and recurrent childhood hepatoblastoma: a report of the German Cooperative Pediatric Liver Tumor Study HB 89 and HB 94. *Klin Pediatr* 1999;211:305–309.
97. Fuchs J, Rydzynski J, Von Schweinitz D, et al. Study Committee of the Cooperative Pediatric Liver Tumor Study Hb 94 for the German Society for Pediatric Oncology and Hematology. Pretreatment prognostic factors and treatment results in children with hepatoblastoma: a report from the German Cooperative Pediatric Liver Tumor Study HB 94. *Cancer* 2002;95:172–182.
98. Gagel RF, Tashijian AH Jr, Cummings T, et al. The clinical outcome of prospective screening for multiple endocrine neoplasia type 2a: an 18-year experience. *N Engl J Med* 1988;318:478–484.
99. Garcia Marcilla JA, Sanchez Bueno F, Aguilar J, et al. Primary small bowel malignant tumors. *Eur J Surg Oncol* 1994;20:630–634.
100. Gardner EJ. Follow-up study of a family group exhibiting dominant inheritance for a syndrome including intestinal polyps osteomas, fibromas, and epidermal cysts. *Am J Hum Genet* 1962;14:376–390.
101. Gardner H, Heilger A, Groin N, et al. A treatment strategy for disseminated Langerhans cell histiocytosis. *Med Pediatr Oncol* 1994;23:72.
102. Gari LM, Rivers JK, Kopf AW. Melanomas arising in large congenital nevocytic nevi: a prospective study. *Pediatr Dermatol* 1988;5:151–158.
103. Gauthier F, Valayer J, Thai BL, et al. Hepatoblastoma and hepatocarcinoma in children: analysis of a series of 29 cases. *J Pediatr Surg* 1986;21:424–429.
104. Geiger JD, Thompson NW. Thyroid tumors in children. *Otolaryngol Clin North Am* 1996;29:711–719.
105. Gelfand M, Castle WM, Buchanan WM. Primary carcinoma of the liver (hepatoma) in Rhodesia. *S Afr Med J* 1972;46:527–532.
106. Gerald WL, Ladanyi M, de Alava E, et al. Clinical, pathologic, and molecular spectrum of tumors associated with t(11;22)(p13;q12): desmoplastic small round-cell tumor and its variants. *J Clin Oncol* 1998;16:3028–3036.
107. Gerald WL, Rosai J. Case 2. Desmoplastic small cell tumor with divergent differentiation. *Pediatr Pathol* 1989;9:177–183.
108. Gerber DA, Arcement C, Carr B, et al. Use of intrahepatic chemotherapy to treat advanced pediatric hepatic malignancies. *J Pediatr Gastroenterol Nutr* 2000;30:137–144.
109. Giacomantonio M, Ein SH, Mancer K, et al. 30 years experience with pediatric malignant liver tumors. *J Pediatr Surg* 1984;19:523–526.
110. Gifford RW, Manger WM, Bravo EL. Pheochromocytoma. *Endocrinol Metab Clin North Am* 1994;23:387–404.
111. Godine L, Berdon W, Brasch R, et al. Adrenocortical carcinoma with extension into inferior vena cava and right atrium: report of three cases in children. *Pediatr Radiol* 1990;20:166–168.
112. Goin JE, Salem R, Carr BI, et al. Treatment of unresectable hepatocellular carcinoma with intrahepatic yttrium 90 microspheres: a risk-stratification analysis. *J Vasc Interv Radiol* 2005;16:195–203.
113. Goldthorn JF, Canizaro PC. Gastrointestinal malignancies in infancy, childhood and adolescence. *Surg Clin North Am* 1986;66:845–861.
114. Goodman KA, Wolden SL, La Quaglia MP, et al. Whole abdominopelvic radiotherapy for desmoplastic small round-cell tumor. *Int J Radiat Oncol Biol Phys* 2002;54:170–176.
115. Gorlin RJ, Goltz RW. Multiple nevoid basal cell epithelioma. Jaw cysts and bifid rib: A syndrome. *N Engl J Med* 1960;262:908–912.
116. Greenberger JS, Cassady JR, Jaffe N. Radiation therapy in patients with histiocytosis: management of diabetes insipidus and bone lesions. *Int J Radiat Oncol Biol Phys* 1979;5:1749–1755.
117. Guglielmi M, Perilongo G, Cecchetto G, et al. Rationale and results of the international society of pediatric oncology (SIOP) Italian pilot study on childhood hepatoma:surgical resection d'emblee or after primary chemotherapy? *J Surg Oncol Suppl* 1993;3:122–126.
118. Haagensen CD. *The relation of age to the frequency of breast carcinoma in diseases of the breast,* 3rd ed. Philadelphia: WB Saunders; 1986:402.
119. Haberle B, Bode U, von Schweinitz D. Differentiated treatment protocols for high- and standard-risk hepatoblastoma—an interim report of the German Liver Tumor Study HB99 [in German]. *Klin Padiatr* 2003;215:159–165.
120. Habrand J, Guillot Valls D, Petras S, et al. Carcinoma of the nasopharynx in children and adolescents treated with initial chemotherapy (CT) followed by adapted doses of radiotherapy (RT).
121. Habrand J-L, Nehme D, Kalifa C, et al. Is there a place for radiation therapy in the management of hepatoblastoma and hepatocellular carcinomas in children. *Int J Radiat Oncol Biol Phys* 1992;23:525–531.
122. Haim N, Leviov M, Ben-Arieh Y, et al. Intermediate and high-grade gastric non-Hodgkin's lymphoma: a prospective study of non-surgical treatment with primary chemotherapy, with or without radiotherapy. *Leuk Lymphoma* 1995;17:321–326.
123. Haim N, Tsalik M, Robinson E. Treatment of Gastric Adenocarcinoma with the combination of Etoposide, Adriamycin and Cisplatin (EAP); Comparison between two Schedules. *Oncology* 1994;51:102–107.
124. Halperin EC, Constine L, Tarbell N, et al. Endocrine, aerodigestive tract and breast tumors. In: *Pediatric radiation oncology,* 3rd ed. Philadelphia: Lippincott, Williams & Wilkins; 1999;395:421.
125. Halperin EC, Constine L, Tarbell N, et al. Tumors of the liver and biliary tree. In: *Pediatric radiation oncology,* Nalperin E, Constine L, Tarbell, et al., eds. 3rd ed. Philadelphia: Lippincott, Williams & Wilkins; 1999;373:385.
126. Halperin EC, Constine LS, Tarbell NJ, et al. Langerhans' cell histiocytosis. In: *Pediatric radiative oncology.* Nalperin E, Constine L, Tarbell, et al., eds. New York: Raven Press; 1994:446–472.
127. Halverson JD, Hori-Rubaina JM. Cystosarcoma phylloides of the breast. *Am Surg* 1974;40:295–301.
128. Hamada Y, Sato M, Okamura S, et al. Pancreatoblastoma managed by pancreatoduodenectomy and extended lobectomy. *Pediatr Surg Int* 1995;10:391–393.
129. Hamilton SR, Liu B, Parsons RE, et al. The molecular basis of Turcot's syndrome. *N Engl J Med* 1995;332:839–847.
130. Hand A. Polyuria and tuberculosis. *Arch Pediatr* 1893;10:673–675.
131. Handerfield-Jones SE, Smith NP. Malignant melanoma in childhood. *Br J Dematol* 1996;134:607–616.
132. Harting MT, Blakely ML, Herzog CE, et al. Treatment issues in pediatric gastric adenocarcinoma. *J Pediatr Surg* 2004;39:8–10.
133. Hartman AW, Magrish P. Carcinoma of breast in children. Case report: *six-year-old* boy with adenocarcinoma. *Ann Surg* 1995;141:792–798.
134. Hartman GE, Shochat SJ. Primary pulmonary neoplasms of childhood: a review. *Ann Thorac Surg* 1983;36:108–119.
135. Harvey WJ, Woodfield DG, Probert JC. Maternal transmission of hepatocellular carcinoma. *Cancer* 1984;54:1360–1363.
136. Hassall E. Barrett's esophagus: new definitions and approaches in children. *J Pediatr Gastroenterol* 1993;16:345–364.
137. Helfre S, Fauroux B, Zucker JM, et al. Radiotherapy in Gorham's syndrome: a report on two cases in children. *Med Pediatr Oncol* 2000;35:318(abstr. P-393).
138. Helm KF, Schwartz RA, Janninger CK. Juvenile melanoma (Spitz nevus). *Cutis* 1996;57:35–39.
139. Hertl M, Cosimi AB. Liver transplantation for malignancy. *Oncologist* 2005;10: 269–281.
140. Hinton JM. Risk of malignant change in ulcerative colitis. *Gut* 1966;7:427–432.
141. Histiocytosis syndromes in children.Writing Group of the Histiocyte Society. *Lancet* 1987;1:208–209.
142. Honour JW, Price DA, Grant DB. Virilizing adrenocortical tumors in childhood. *Pediatrics* 1986;78:547.
143. Howarth CB, Cases JN, Pratt CB. Breast metasteses in children with rhabdomyosarcoma. *Cancer* 1980;46:2520–2524.
144. Hsu IC, Metcalf RA, Sun T, et al. Mutational hotspot in the p53 gene in human hepatocellular carcinoma. *Nature* 1991;350:427–428.

145. Hughes JR, O'Donnell PJ, Pembroke AC. Basal cell carcinoma arising in a naevus sebaceous in a 5-year-old girl. *Clin Exp Dermatol* 1995;20:177.
146. Humphrey GB, Pysher T, Holcombe J, et al. Overview of the management of adrenocortical carcinoma. In: Humphrey GB, Grindey GB, Dehner LP, et al, eds. *Adrenal and endocrine tumors in children.* Boston: Martinus Nijhoff Publishers; 1983:349–358.
147. Ii N, Yamakado K, Shoji K, et al. Advanced hepatocellular carcinoma—feasibility and clinical impact of high-dose-rate brachytherapy on the treatment of lesions growing into biliary trees, portal veins and the vena cava [in Japanese]. *Gan To Kagaku Ryoho* 2001;28:1498–500.
148. Indolfi P, Casale F, Carli M, et al. Pleuropulmonary blastoma: management and prognosis of 11 cases. *Cancer* 2000;89:1396–401.
149. Ito E, Sato Y, Kawanchi K, et al. Type 1 glycogen storage disease with hepatoblastoma in siblings. *Cancer* 1987;59:1776–1780.
150. Norton JA. Adrenal Tumors. Section 4 in Cancer Principles and Practice. 7th ed. DeVita V, Hellman S, Rosenberg S, eds. 2005;1528–1539.
151. Jaeger HJ, Schmitz-Stolbrink A, Albrecht M, et al. Gastric leiomyosarcoma in a child. *Eur J Radiol* 1996;23:111–114.
152. Jarisch W, Zur leher von den Hautgeschwulsten. *Arch Dermatol Syph* (Berl) 1984;28:163.
153. Johnson GK, Squier CA. Smokeless tobacco use by youth: a health concern. *Pediatr Dent* 1993;14:169–174.
154. Jones GS, Shah KJ, Mann JR. Adreno-cortical carcinoma in infancy and childhood; a radiological report of ten cases. *Clin Radiol* 1985;36:257—262.
155. Jose Tincani A, Santos Martins A, Gomes Andrade R, et al. Nevoid basal-cell syndrome: literature review and case report in a family. *Rev Paul Med* 1995;113:917–921.
156. Kadish S, Goodman M, Wang CC. Olfactory neuroblastoma. A clinical analysis of 17 cases. *Cancer* 1976;37:1571–1576.
157. Karl SR, Ballantine TVN, Zaino R. Juvenile secretory carcinoma of the breast. *J Pediatr Surg* 1985;20:368–371.
158. Karnak I, Ciftci AO, Senocak ME, et al. Colorectal carcinoma in children. *J Pediatr Surg* 1999;34:1499–1504.
159. Kasperlik-Zaluska AA, Migdalska BM, Zgliczyinski S, et al. Adrenocortical carcinoma: a clinical study and treatment results of 52 patients. *Cancer* 1995;75:2587–2591.
160. Kasperlik-Zaluska AA, Migdlska BM, Zgliczynski S, et al. Adrenal carcinoma; a clinical study and treatment results of 52 patients. *Cancer* 1995;75:2587–2591.
161. Kaufman BH, Telander RL, Van Heerden JA, et al. Pheochromocytoma in the pediatric age group. Current status. *J Pediatr Surg* 1983;18:879–884.
162. Kelsen D, Atiq OT, Saltz L, et al. FAMTX versus etoposide, doxorubicin and cisplatin: a random assignment trial in gastric cancer. *J Clin Oncol* 1992;10:541–548.
163. Kew MC. Hepatocellular carcinoma with and without cirrhosis. *Gastroenterology* 1989;97:136–139.
164. Khafagi FA, Shapiro B, Fischer M, et al. Pheochromocytoma and functioning paraganglioma in childhood and adolescence: role of iodine 131 metaiodobenzylguanidine. *Eur J Nucl Med* 1991;18:191–198.
165. Kimonis VE, Goldstein AM, Pastakia B, et al. Clinical manifestations in 105 persons with nevoid basal cell carcinoma syndrome. *Am J Med Genet* 1997;997:299–308.
166. Kingston JE, Herbert A, Draper GJ, et al. Association between hepatoblasoma and polyposis coli. *Arch Dis Child* 1983;58:953–958.
167. Klimstra DS, Wenig BM, Adair CF, et al. Pancreatoblastoma: a clinicopathologic study and review of the literature. *Am J Surg Pathol* 1995;19:1371–1389.
168. Klopp CT, Rosvoll RV, Winship T. Is destructive surgery ever necessary for treatment of thyroid cancer in children? *Ann Surg* 1967;165:745–750.
169. Kocabalkan O, Ozgur F, Erk Y, et al. Malignant melanoma in xeroderma pigmentosum patients; a report of five cases. *Eur J Surg Oncol* 1997;23:43–47.
170. Kotiloglu E, Kaya H, Guney I, et al. The Mckusick-Kaufman syndrome: report of a case with some associations. *Turk J Pediatr* 2002;44:156–159.
171. Koufos A, Hansen MF, Copeland NG, et al. Loss of heterozygosity in three embryonal tumors suggests a common pathogenetic mechanism. *Nature* 1985;316:330–334.
172. Kretschmar CS, Colbach C, Bhan I, et al. Desmoplastic small cell tumor: a report of three cases and a review of the literature. *J Pediatr Hematol Oncol* 1996;18:293–298.
173. Kuppersmith RB, Teh BS, Donovan DT, et al. The use of intensity modulated radiotherapy for the treatment of extensive and recurrent juvenile angiofibroma. *Int J Pediatr Otorhinolaryngol* 2000;52:261–268.
174. Kushner BH, LaQuaglia MP, Wollner N, et al. Desmoplastic small round-cell tumor: prolonged progression-free survival with aggressive multimodality therapy. *J Clin Oncol* 1996;14:1526–1531.
175. La Quaglia MP, Black T, Holcomb GW, et al. Differentiated thyroid cancer: clinical characteristics, treatment and outcome in patients under 21 years of age who present with distant metastases. A report from the Surgical Discipline Committee of the Children's Cancer Group. *J Pediatr Surg* 2000;35:955–960.
176. La Qualglia MP, Corbally MT, Heller G, et al. Recurrence and morbidity in differentiated thyroid carcinoma in children. *Surgery* 1988;104:1149–1156.
177. La Quaglia MP, Telander RL. Differentiated and medullary thyroid cancer in childhood and adolescence. *Semin Pediatr Surg* 1997;6:42–49.
178. La Salle AJ, Andrassy RJ, Stanford W. Bronchogenic squamous cell carcinoma in childhood; a case report. *J Pediatr Surg* 1977;12:519–521.
179. Lack EE, Neave C, Vawter GF. Hepatoblastoma: a clinical and pathologic study of 54 cases. *Am J Surg Pathol* 1982;6:693–705.
180. Lack EE, Neave C, Vawter GF. Hepatocellular carcinoma: review of 32 cases in childhood and adolescence. *Cancer* 1983;52:1510–1515.
181. Lal DR, Su WT, Wolden SL, et al. Results of multimodal treatment for desmoplastic small round cell tumors. *J Pediatr Surg* 2005;40:251–255.
182. Landau D, Vini L, A'Hern R, et al. Thyroid cancer in children: the Royal Marsden Hospital experience. *Eur J Cancer* 2000;36:214–220.
183. Laporte R, Godart F, Breviere GM, et al. Severe arterial hypertension and pheochromocytoma in childhood. Case report and review of the literature. *Arch Mal Coeur Vaiss* 2000;93:627–630.
184. Lasso JM, Garcia-Tutor E, Bazan A. Aggressive basal cell carcinoma of the temporal region in a patient with Gorlin-Goltz syndrome. *Ann Plast Surg* 2000;44:429–434.
185. Lau WY, Ho SK, Yu SC, et al. Salvage surgery following downstaging of unresectable hepatocellular carcinoma. *Ann Surg* 2004;240:299–305.
186. Lavin P, Hajdu SI, Foote FW Jr. Gastric and extragastric leiomysarcomas; clinicopathologic study of 44 cases. *Cancer* 1972;29:305–311.
187. Lee P, Winter R, Green O. Virulizing adrenocortical tumors in childhood: Eight cases and a review of the literature. *Pediatrics* 1985;76:437–444.
188. Lee RG. Neoplasms and other masses. In: *Diagnostic liver pathology.* St Louis: Mosby; 1994;450–455.
189. Leenhouts HP, Brugmans MJ, Chadwick KH. Analysis of thyroid cancer data from the Ukraine after 'Chernobyl' using a two-mutation carcinogenesis model. *Radiat Environ Biophys* 2000;39:89–98.
190. Leung A, Shapiro B, Hattner R, et al. Specifity of radioiodinated MIBG for neural crest tumors in childhood. *J Nucl Med* 1997;38:1352–1357.
191. Leuschner I, Harms D, Schmidt D. The association of hepatocellular carcinoma in childhood with hepatitis B virus infection. *Cancer* 1998;62:2363–2369.
192. Li JH, Shi W, Chia M, et al. Efficacy of targeted FasL in nasopharyngeal carcinoma. *Mol Ther* 2003;8:964–973.
193. Lichenstein L. Histiocytosis X: integration of eosinophilic granuloma of bone, Letterer Siwe disease and Schuller-Christian disease as related manifestation of a single nosologic entity. *Arch Pathol* 1953;56:84–102.
194. Liu MD, Uaje MB, Al-Ghazi MS, et al. Use of Yttrium-90 TheraSphere for the treatment of unresectable hepatocellular carcinoma. *Am Surg* 2004;70:947–953.
195. LoGerfo P, Chabot J, Gazetas P. The intraoperative incidence of detectable bilateral and multicentric disease in papillary cancer of the thyroid. *Surgery* 1990;108:958–963.
196. Long RTL, Hesker AE, Johnson RE. Surgical management of cystosarcoma phylloides: With a report of eight cases. *Missouri Med* 1962;59:1179–1181.
197. Luton JP, Cerdas S, Baillaud L, et al. Clinical features of adrenocortical carcinoma: prognostic factors and the effect of mitotane therapy. *N Engl J Med* 1990;322:1195–1201.
198. Macdonald JS, Smalley S, Bendedetti J, et al. Postoperative combined radiation and chemotherapy improves disease-free survival (DFS) and overall survival (OS) in resected adenocarcinoma of the stomach and G.E. junction. *N Engl J Med* 2001;345:725–730.
199. Magee BJ, Gattameneni HR, Pearson D. Adrenal cortical carcinoma: survival after radiotherapy. *Clin Radiol* 1987;38:587–588.
200. Mah PT, Loo DC, Tock EPC. Pancreatic acinar cell carcinoma in childhood. *Am J Dis Child* 1974;128:101–104.
201. Mahour GH, Isaacs H Jr, Cahnge L. Priamary malignant tumors of the stomach in children. *J Pediatr Surg* 1980;15:603–608.
202. Mandel SJ, Mandel L. Radioactive iodine and the salivary glands. *Thyroid* 2003;13:265–271.
203. Manivel JC, Priest JR, Watterson J, et al. Pleuropulmonary blastoma. The so-called pulmonary blastoma of childhood. *Cancer* 1988;62:1516–1526.
204. Mao C, Guvendi M, Domenico DR, et al. Papillary cystic and solid tumors of the pancreas. A pancreatic embryonic tumor? Studies of three cases and cumulative review of the world's literature. *Surgery* 1995;118:821–828.
205. Maor MH, Velasquez WS, Fuller LM, et al. Stomach conservation in stages IE and IIE gastric non-Hodgkin's lymphoma. *J Clin Oncol* 1990;8:266–271.
206. Marchetti G. Beitrag zur kenntniss der pathologischen Anatomie der nebennieren. *Arch Pathol Anat* 1904;177:227–231.
207. Markoe AM, Serber W, Micaily B, et al. Radiation therapy for adjunctive treatment of adrenal cortical carcinoma. *Am J Clin Oncol* 1991;14:170–174.
208. Mauro E, Fraulini C, Rigolin GM, et al. A case of disseminated Langerhans' cell histiocytosis treated with thalidomide. *Eur J Haematol* 2005;74:172–174.
209. Mawk JR, Obukhov SK, Nichols WD, et al. Successful conservative management of Gorham disease of the skull base and cervical spine. *Childs Nerv Syst* 1997;13:622–625.
210. Mayo CH. Paroxysmal hypertension with tumor of retroperitoneal nerve: report of a case. *JAMA* 1927;89:1047–1050.
211. Mazumdar M, Bajorin DF, Bacik J, et al. Predicting outcome to chemotherapy in patients with germ cell tumors: the value of the rate of decline of human chorionic gonadotrophin and alpha-fetoprotein during therapy. *J Clin Oncol* 2001;19:2534–2541.
212. McDivitt RW, Stewart FW. Breast carcinoma in children. *JAMA* 1966;195:388–390
213. McDivitt RW, Urban JA, Farrow JH. Cystosarcoma phylloides. *Johns Hopkins Med J* 1967;120:33–45.
214. McEwan AJ, Shapiro B, Sisson JC, et al. Radiodobenzyl-gaunidine for the scintigraphic location of therapy of adrenergenic tumors. *Semin Nucl Med* 1985;15:132–153.
215. McGill TW, Downey EC, Westbrook J, et al. Gastric carcinoma in children. *J Pediatr Surg* 1993;28:1620–1621.
216. McWhirter WR, Dobson C, Ring I. Childhood cancer in Australia. *Int J Cancer* 1996;65:34–38.
217. Michalkiewicz EL, Sandrini R, Bugg MF, et al. Clinical characteristics of small functioning adrenocortical tumors in children. *Med Pediatr Oncol* 1997;28:175–178.
218. Mielcarek PA. Primary adenocarcinoma of the pancreas in a 15-year-old boy. *Am J Pathol* 1935;11:527–533.
219. Miliauskas JR, Leong AS-Y. Adenoid cystic carcinoma in a juvenile male breast. *Pathology* 1991;23:298–301.
220. Minh NH. Cervicothoracic spinal epidural cavernous hemangioma: case report and review of the literature. *Surg Neurol* 2005;64:83–85.
221. Mishima Y, Nagasaki E, Terui Y, et al. Combination chemotherapy (cyclophosphamide, doxorubicin, and vincristine with continuous-infusion cisplatin and etoposide) and radiotherapy with stem cell support can be beneficial for adolescents and adults with estheisoneuroblastoma. *Cancer* 2004;101:1437–1444.
222. Mody RJ, Pohlen JA, Malde S, et al. FDG PET for the study of primary hepatic malignancies in children. *Pediatr Blood Cancer* 2006;47:51–55.
223. Moertel CG, Weiland LH, Nagorney DM, et al. Carcinoid tumor of the appendix: treatment and prognosis. *N Engl J Med* 1987;317:1699–1701.
224. Moller G, Gruber H, Priemel M, et al. [Gorham-Stout idiopathic osteolysis—a local osteoclastic hyperactivity?]. *Pathologe,* 1999;20:177–182.
225. Moller G, Priemel M, Amling M, et al. The Gorham-Stout syndrome (Gorham's massive osteolysis). A report of six cases with histopathological findings. *J Bone Joint Surg Br* 1999;81:501–506.
226. Mollit DL, Golladay ES, Gloster ES, et al. Cystosarcoma phylloides in the adolescent female. *J Pediatr Surg* 1987;22:907–910.
227. Molt P, Hopfan S, Watson RC, et al. Intraluminal radiation therapy in the management of malignant biliary obstruction. *Cancer* 1986;57:536–544.

228. Moore SW, Hesseling PB, Wessels G, et al. Hepatocellular carcinoma in children. *Pediatr Surg Int* 1997;12:266–270.
229. Murakami T, Ueki K, Kawakami H, et al. Pancreatoblastoma: case report and review of treatment in the literature. *Med Pediatr Oncol* 1996;27:193–197.
230. Nadler EP, Novikov A, Landzberg BR, et al. The use of endoscopic ultrasound in the diagnosis of solid pseudopapillary tumors of the pancreas in children. *J Pediatr Surg* 2002;37:1370–1373.
231. Nagasue M, Yakaya H, Chang Y-C, et al. Active uptake of testosterone by androgen receptors of hepatocellular carcinoma in humans. *Cancer* 1986;57:2162–2167.
232. Nam TK, Lee JI, Kang SW. Gamma knife radiosurgery for circumscribed choroidal hemangioma. *Acta Neurochir (Wien)* 2005;147:651–654.
233. Nassan A, Al-Nafussi A, Quaba A. Cutaneous malignant melanoma in children and adolescents in Scotland 1979–1991. *Plast Reconstr Surg* 1996;98:442–446.
234. Neel HB, III, Pearson GR, Taylor WF. Antibodies to Epstein-Barr virus in patients with nasopharyngeal carcinoma and in comparison groups. *Ann Otol Rhinol Laryngol* 1984;93:477–482.
235. Newman KD. Malignant liver tumors in childhood. *Semin Pediatr Surg* 1992;1:145–151.
236. Nichini FM, Goldman L, Lapayowker MS, et al. Inflammatory carcinoma of the breast in a 12-year-old girl. *Arch Surg* 1972;105:505–508.
237. Norris HJ, Taylor HB. Relationship of the histologic features to behavior of cystosarcoma phylloides: analysis of ninety-four cases. *Cancer* 1967;20:2090–2099.
238. Ogawa B, Okinaga K, Obana K, et al. Pancreatoblastoma treated by delayed operation after effective chemotherapy. *J Pediatr Surg* 2000;35:1663–1665.
239. Ogita S, Tokiwa K, Taniguchi H, et al. Intraarterial injection of anti-tumor drugs dispersed in lipid contrast medium: a choice for initially unresectable hepatoblastoma in infants. *J Pediatr Surg* 1987;22:412–414.
240. Oldfield MC. The association of familial polyposis of the colon with multiple sebaceous cysts. *Br J Surg* 1954;41:534–541.
241. Oliver RT, Leahy M, Ong J. Combined seminoma/non-seminoma should be considered as intermediate grade germ cell cancer (GCC). *Eur J Cancer* 1995;31A:1392–1394.
242. Ontai S, Straehley CJ. The surgical treatment of well-differentiated carcinoma of the thyroid. *Am Surg* 1985;51:653–657.
243. Ortego JA, Douglas EC, Feusner JH, et al. Randomized comparison of Cisplatin/Vineristine/Fluorouracil and Cisplatin/Continuous Infusion Doxorubicin for treatment of pediatric hepatoblastoma: a report from the Children's Cancer Group and the Pediatric Oncology Group. *J Clin Oncol* 2000;18:2665–2675.
244. Ozkaynak MF, Ortega JA, Laug W, et al. Role of chemotherapy in pediatric pulmonary blastoma. *Med Pediatr Oncol* 1990;18:53–56.
245. Parkin DM, Laara E, Muirs CS. Estimates of the worldwide frequency of sixteen major cancers in 1980. *Int J Cancer* 1998;41:184–197.
246. Parsons SK, Fishman SJ, Hoorntie LE, et al. Aggressive multimodal treatment of pleuropulmonary blastoma. *Ann Thorac Surg* 2001;72:939–942.
247. Pasyk KA. Classification and clinical and histopathological features of hemangiomas and other vascular malformation. In: Ryan TJ, Cherry GW, eds. Vascular birthmarks: pathogenesis and management, Oxford: Oxford University Press; 1987:1–55.
248. Pazdur R, Bready B, Cangir A. Pediatric hepatic tumors: clinical trials conducted in the United States. *J Surg Oncol* 1993;3:127–130.
249. Percarpio B, Knowlton AH. Radiation therapy for adrenal cortical carcinoma. *Acta Radiol Ther Phys Biol* 1976;1:288–292.
250. Perel Y, Schlumberger M, Marguerite G, et al. Pheochromocytoma and paraganglioma in children: a report of 24 cases of the French Society of Pediatric Oncology. *Pediatr Hematol Oncol* 1997;14:413–422.
251. Perilongo G, Shafford E, Maibach R, et al. Risk-adapted treatment for childhood hepatoblastoma. Final report of the second study of the International Society of Paediatric Oncology-SIOPEL 2. *Eur J Cancer* 2004;40:411–421.
252. Perilango G, Sinniah D, Meadows AT, et al. Liver tumors. In: D'Angio GJ, Sinniah D, Meadows AT, et al, eds. *Practical pediatric oncology*. New York: Wiley-Liss; 1992:233–337.
253. Pick L. Das Ganglioma Embryonale Sympathicum. *Klin Wochenschr* 1912;19:16–22.
254. Pinarli FG, Oguz A, Ceyda K, et al. Type II pleuropulmonary blastoma responsive to multimodal therapy. *Pediatr Hematol Oncol* 2005;22:71–76.
255. Pinkerton CR, Broadbent V, Horwich A, et al. 'JEB'—a carboplatin based regimen for malignant germ cell tumours in children. *Br J Cancer* 1990;62:257–262.
256. Plaschkes J. Proceedings of an International Research Workshop on Pediatric Liver Tumors—Into the Year 2000. *Med Pediatr Oncol* 2001;36:380–382.
257. Pochedly C, ed. *Neoplastic diseases of childhood*. Langhorne, PA: Harwood Academic Publications; 963–980.
258. Polychronopoulou S, Kostaridou S, Panagiotou JP, et al. Nasopharyngeal carcinoma in childhood and adolescence: a single institution's experience with treatment modalities during the last 15 years. *Pediatr Hematol Oncol* 2004;21:393–402.
259. Powles TB, Bhardwa J, Shamash J, et al. The changing presentation of germ cell tumours of the testis between 1983 and 2002. *BJU Int.* 2005;95:1197–1200.
260. Pratt CB, Palmer MK, Thatcher N, et al. Malignant melanoma in children and adolescents. *Cancer* 1981;47:392–397.
261. Pratt CB, Rivers G, Shanks E, et al. Colorectal carcinoma in adolescents—implications regarding etiology. *Cancer* 1997;40:2464–2472.
262. Priest JR, McDermott MB, Bhatia S, et al. Pleuropulmonary blastoma: a clinicopathologic study of 50 cases. *Cancer* 1997;80:147–161.
263. Pritchard J, Brown J, Shafford E, et al, Doxorubicin and delayed surgery for childhood hepatoblastoma: a successful approach—results of the first prospective study of the International Society of Pediatric Oncology. *J Clin Oncol* 2000;18:3819–3828.
264. Radkowski D, McGill T, Healy GB, et al. Angiofibroma. Changes in staging and treatment. *Arch Otolaryngol Head Neck Surg* 1996;122:122–129.
265. Ram CV. Pheochromocytoma. *Cardiol Clin* 1988;6:517–535.
266. Rao BN, Hayes FA, Prah CB, et al. Malignant melanoma in children; its management and prognosis. *J Pediatr Surg* 1990;25:198–203.
267. Raum WJ. Pheochromocytoma. *Curr Ther Endocrinol Metab* 1994;5:172–178
268. Reintgen DS, Vollmer R, Seigler HF. Juvenile malignant melanoma. *Surg Gynecol Obstet* 1989;168:249–253.
269. Reynolds M, Douglass EC, Finegold M, et al. Chemotherapy can convert unresectable hepatoblastoma. *J Pediatr Surg* 1992;27:1080–1084.
270. Rivet J, Servant J-M, Monteil J-P, et al. Syndrome de Gorlin-Goltz. *Rev Stomatol Chir Maxillofac* 2000;101:194–196.
271. Rogers DA, Lobe TE, Rao BN, et al. Breast malignancy in children. *J Pediatr Surg* 1994;24:48–51.
272. Roisman I, Barak V, Robinson E, et al. Breast malignancies in adolescents in Israel (1967–1989). *Breast Dis* 1992;5:149–168.
273. Romeo C, Impellizzeri P, Grosso M, et al. Pleuropulmonary blastoma: long-term survival and literature review. *Med Pediatr Oncol* 1999;33:372–376.
274. Rosenblatt E, Brook OR, Erlich N, et al. Late visual and auditory toxicity of radiotherapy for nasopharyngeal carcinoma. *Tumori* 2003;89:68–74.
275. Sabbaga C, Avilla S, Schulz C, et al. Adenocortical carcinoma in children: clinical aspects and prognosis. *J Pediatr Surg* 1993;28:841–843.
276. Sakata K, Aoki Y, Kumakura Y, et al. Radiation therapy for patients with xeroderma pigmentosum. *Radiat Med* 1996;14:87–90.
277. Scerri L, Navaratnam AE. Basal cell carcinoma presenting as a delayed complication of thorium X used for treating congenital hemangioma. *J Am Acad Dermatol* 1994;31:796–797.
278. Schettini ST, Ganc A, Saba L. Esophageal carcinoma secondary to a chemical injury in a child. *Pediatr Surg Int* 1998;13:519–520.
279. Schmidt B, Lantsberg L, Goldstein J, et al. Cystosarcoma phylloides. *Isr J Med Sci* 1981;17:895–898.
280. Schmidt D, Harms D, Lang W. Primary malignant hepatic tumors in childhood. *Virchows Arch* 1985;407:387–405.
281. Schulick RD, Brennan MF. Long term survival after complete resection and repeat resection in patient with adrenocortical carcinoma. *Ann Surg Oncol* 1999;6:719–726.
282. Schwaab G, Bouzouita K, Janot F, et al. [ORL cancer in the child. Histologic and topographic distribution. Therapeutic indications (apropos of 380 IGR cases 1975–1987)]. *Bull Cancer* 1989;76:757–762.
283. Schwartz DL, Gann DS, Haller JA. Endocrine surgery in children. *Surg Clin North Am* 1974;54:363–385.
284. Schweisguth O. *Solid tumors in children*. New York: John Wiley & Sons; 1982.
285. Sears JB, Chlesinger MJ. Carcinoma of the breast in a ten-year-old girl: report of a case. *N Engl J Med* 1940;223:760–761.
286. Segal K, Shvero J, Stern Y, et al. Surgery of thyroid cancer in children and adolescents. *Head Neck* 1998;20:293–297.
287. Senac MO Jr, Wood BP, Isaacs H, et al. Pulmonary blastoma: a rare childhood malignancy. *Radiology* 1991;179:743–746.
288. Serin M, Erkal HS, Elhan AH, et al. Nasopharyngeal carcinoma in childhood and adolescence. *Med Pediatr Oncol* 1998;31:498–505.
289. Shanmugartnam K, Sobin L. Histological typing of hyper-respiratory tract tumors n°19. Genova: World Health Organization; 1978:32.
290. Shapiro B, Fig L. Management of pheochromocytoma. *Endocrinol Metab Clin North Am* 1988;18:443–481.
291. Sheehan JM, Sheehan JP, Jane JA Sr, et al. Chemotherapy for esthesioneuroblastomas. *Neurosurg Clin North Am* 2000;11:693–701.
292. Sheng L, Weixia Z, Longhai Y, et al. Clinical and biologic analysis of pancreatoblastoma. *Pancreas* 2005;30:87–90.
293. Shorter NA, Glick RD, Klimstra DS, et al. Malignant pancreatic tumors in childhood and adolescence: the Memorial Sloan-Kettering experience, 1967 to present. *J Pediatr Surg* 2002;37:887–892.
294. Slor H, Batko S, Kahn SG, et al. Clinical, cellular and molecular features of an Israeli xeroderma pigmentosum family with a frame shift mutation in the XPC gene: sun protection prolongs life. *J Invest Dermatol* 2000;115:974–980.
295. Smith WL, Franken EA, Mitros FA. Liver tumors in children. *Semin Roentgenol* 1983;18:136–148.
296. Spitz S. Melanomas of childhood. *Am J Pathol* 1948;24:591–609.
297. Squire R, Bianchi A, Jakate SM. Radiation-induced sarcoma of the breast in a female adolescent. *Cancer* 1988;60:2444–2447.
298. Stackpole RH, Melicow MM, Uson AC. Pheochromocytoma in children: report of 3 cases and review of the first 100 published cases with follow-up studies. *J Pediatr* 1963;63:315–327.
299. Stavrou T, Dubovsky EC, Reaman GH, et al. Intracranial calcifications in childhood medulloblastoma: relation to nevoid basal cell carcinoma syndrome. *Am J Neuroradiol* 2000;21:790–794.
300. Stewart DR, Morris-Jones PH, Jolleys A. Carcinoma of the adrenal gland in children. *J Pediatr Surg* 1974;9:59–67.
301. Stilwagon G, Order SE, Guse C, et al. Prognostic factors in unresectable hepatocellular cancer. Radiation therapy oncology Group study. *Int J Radiat Oncol Biol Phys* 1991;20:65–71.
302. Stocker JT. Hepatoblastoma. *Semin Diagn Pathol* 1994;11:136–143.
303. Storm HH, Plesko I. Survival of children with thyroid cancer in Europe 1978–1989. *Eur J Cancer* 2001;37:775–779.
304. Su MC, Jeng YM, Chu YC. Desmoplastic small round cell tumor of the kidney. *Am J Surg Pathol* 2004;28:1379–1383.
305. Suita S, Tajiri T, Takamatsu H, et al; Committee for Pediatric Solid Malignant Tumors in the Kyushu Area, Japan. Improved survival outcome for hepatoblastoma based on an optimal chemotherapeutic regimen—a report from the study group for pediatric solid malignant tumors in the Kyushu area. *J Pediatr Surg* 2004;39:195–198.
306. Sulkes A. Chemotherapy in gastric cancer: a brief chronicle with emphasis on recent developments. *Isr Med Assoc J* 2004;6:415–419.
307. Superina R, Billik R. Results of liver transplantation in children with unresectable liver tumors. *J Pediatr Surg* 1996;31:835–839.
308. Swerdlow AJ. Epidemiology of cutaneous malignant melanoma. *Clin Oncol* 1984;3:407–437.
309. Symonds DA, Vickery AL Jr. Mucinous carcinoma of the colon and rectum. *Cancer* 1976;37:1891–1900.
310. Tagge EP, Tagee DU, Reyes J, et al. Resection, including transplantation for hepatoblastoma and hepatocellular carcinoma. Impact on survival. *J Pediatr Surg* 1992;27:292–296.
311. Takano H, Smith WL. Gastrointestinal tumors of childhood. *Radiol Clin North Am* 1997;35:1367–1389.
312. Telander RL, Zimmerman D, Kaufman BH, et al. Pediatric endocrine surgery. *Surg Clin North Am* 1985;65:1551–1572.
313. Templeman C, Paige Hertweck S. Breast disorders in the pediatric and adolescent patient. *Obstet Gynecol Clin North Am* 2000;27:19–34.

314. Tenenbaum F, Groussin L, Foehrenbach H, et al. 18F-fluorodeoxyglucose positron emission tomography as a diagnostic tool for malignancy of adrenocortical tumours. Preliminary results in 13 consecutive patients. *Eur J Endocrinol* 2004; 150:789–792.

315. Teo PM, Leung SF, Chan AT, et al. Final report of a randomized trial on altered-fractionated radiotherapy in nasopharyngeal carcinoma prematurely terminated by significant increase in neurologic complications. *Int J Radiat Oncol Biol Phys* 2000;48:1311–1322.

316. Tondini C, Zanini M, Lombardi F, et al. Combined modality treatment with primary CHOP chemotherapy followed by locoregional irradiation in stage I or II histologically aggressive non-Hodgkin's lymphomas. *J Clin Oncol* 1993;11:720–725.

317. Torossian JM, Beziat JL, Philip T, et al. Squamous cell carcinoma of the tongue in a 13 *year-old* boy. *J Oral Maxillofac Surg* 2000;58:1407–1410.

318. Tovar JA, Eizeguirre I, Albert A, et al. Peutz-Jeghers syndrome in children: report of two cases and review of the literature. *J Pediatr Surg* 1983;18:1–6.

319. Treves N, Sunderland DA. Cystosarcoma phylloides of the breast. A malignant and a benign tumor. A clinicopathological study of seventy-seven cases. *Cancer* 1951;4:1286–1332.

320. Tsukimoto I, Watanabe K, Lin JB, et al. Pancreatic carcinoma in children in Japan. *Cancer* 1973;31:1203–1207.

321. Uzel O, Yoruk SO, Sahinler I, et al. Nasopharyngeal carcinoma in childhood: long-term results of 32 patients. *Radiother Oncol* 2001;58:137–141.

322. Vade A, Nolan J. Posterior mediastinal teratoma involving the esophagus. *Gastrointest Radiol* 1989;14:106–108.

323. Valanzano R, Curia MC, Aceto G, et al. Genetic evidence that juvenile nasopharyngeal angiofibroma is an integral FAP tumour. *Gut* 2005;54:1046–1047.

324. Van Tornout JM, Buckley JD, Quinn JJ, et al. Timing and magnitude of decline in alpha-fetoprotein levels in treated children with unresectable or metastatic hepablastoma are predictors of outcome; a report from the Children's Cancer Group. *J Clin Oncol* 1997;15:1190–1197.

325. Vannier JP Flamant F, Hemet J, et al. Pancreatoblastoma: response to chemotherapy. *Med Pediatr Oncol* 1991;19:187–191.

326. Vassilopoulou-Sellin R, Goepfert H, Raney B, et al. Differentiated thyroid cancer in children and adolescents: clinical outcome and mortality after long-term follow-up. *Head Neck* 1998;20:549–555.

327. Vogelstein B, Fearon ER, Hamilton SR, et al. Genetic alterations during colorectal tumor development. *N Engl J Med* 1988;319:525–532.

328. Vossen S, Goretzki PE, Goebel U, et al. Therapeutic management of rare malignant pancreatic tumors in children. *World J Surg* 1998;22:879–882.

329. Voute PA, Penkerton R. Liver tumors. In: Peckham M, Pinedo H, Umberto V, eds. *Oxford textbook of oncology.* New York: Oxford Press; 1995;2036–2039.

330. Walter AW, Pivnik EK, Bale AE, et al. Complications of the nevoid basal cell carcinoma syndrome. *A case report. J Pediatr Hematol Oncol* 1997;19:258–262.

331. Webb AJ, Brewster S, Newington D. Problems in diagnosis and management of goiter in childhood and adolescence. *Br J Surg* 1996;83:1586–1590.

332. Weinberg AG, Finegold MJ. Primary hepatic tumors in childhood. In: Finegold MJ, Bennington JL, eds. *Pathology of neoplasia in children and adolescents.* Philadelphia: WB Saunders; 1986;333–372.

333. Weinberg AG, Finegold MJ. Primary hepatic tumors of childhood. *Hum Pathol* 1983;14:512–537.

334. Weiss NS, Yang C. Incidence of histologic types of cancer of the small instentine. *J Natl Cancer Inst* 1987;78:653–656.

335. Welbourn RB. Early surgical history of phaeochromocytoma. *Br J Surg* 1987;74: 594–596.

336. West TL, Weiland LH, Clagett OT. Cystosarcoma phylloides. *Ann Surg* 1971;173: 520–528.

337. Weyl Ben Arush M, Stein M, Perez Nahum M, et al. Pediatric thyroid carcinoma: 22 Years of experience at the Northern Israel Oncology Center (1973–1995). *Pediatr Hematol Oncol* 2000;17:1–8.

338. Whalen RK, Althausen AF, Daniels GH. Extra-adrenal pheochromocytoma. *J Urol* 1992;147:1–10.

339. Wilke H, Preusser P, Fink U, et al. New Development in the treatment of gastric carcinoma. *Semin Oncol* 1990;17:61–70.

340. Willnow U, Willberg B, Schwamborn D, et al. Pancreatoblastoma in children: case report and review of the literature. *Eur J Pediatr Surg* 1996;6:396–372.

341. Wolden SL, Steinherz PG, Kraus DH, et al. Improved long-term survival with combined modality therapy for pediatric nasopharynx cancer. *Int J Radiat Oncol Biol Phys* 2000;46:859–864.

342. Wormald PJ, Van Hasselt A. Endoscopic removal of juvenile angiofibromas. *Otolaryngol Head Neck Surg* 2003;129:684–691.

343. Yeh SD, La Quaglia MO. I-311 therapy for pediatric thyroid cancer. *Semin Pediatr Surg* 1997;6:128–133.

344. Yoshihara T, Ikuta H, Hibi S, et al. Second cutaneous neoplasms after acute lymphoblastic leukemia in childhood. *Int J Hematol* 1993;59:67–71.

345. Zedan W, Robinson PA, High AS. A novel polymorphism in the PTC gene allows easy identification of allelic loss in basal cell nevus syndrome lesions. *Diagn Mol Pathol* 2001;10:41–45.

346. Zettinig G, Mitterhauser M, Wadsak W, et al. Positron emission tomography imaging of adrenal masses: (18)F-fluorodeoxyglucose and the 11beta-hydroxylase tracer (11)C-metomidate. *Eur J Nucl Ed Mol Imaging* 2004;31: 1224–1230.

347. Zimmerman D, Hay ID, Gough IR, et al. Papillary thyroid carcinoma in children and adults: long term follow-up of 1039 patients conservatively treated at one institution during three decades. *Surgery* 1988;104:1157–1166.

348. Zografos GC, Driscoll DL, Karakousis CP, et al. Adrenal adenocarcinoma: a review of 53 cases. *J Surg Oncol* 1994;56:160–164.

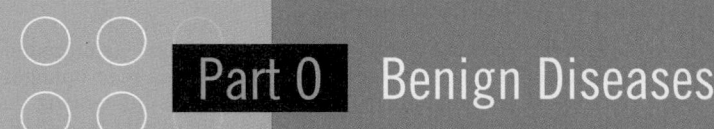

Part O   Benign Diseases

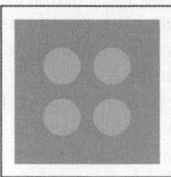

Chapter 89
Radiotherapy of Nonmalignant Diseases

Michael Heinrich Seegenschmiedt

General Aspects

Classification of Nonmalignant Diseases

Nonmalignant or "benign" diseases can be successfully treated with ionizing radiation. These diseases can be classified as inflammatory, degenerative, hyperproliferative, functional, or other disorders, but topography and morphology are more relevant. There are differences in practice between Anglo-American, European, and other geographic regions because of clinical traditions and differences in organization and training. Criteria of evidence-based medicine are relevant for the use of radiotherapy for nonmalignant diseases.

Justification and Indication for Radiotherapy

The use of radiotherapy (RT) for benign diseases can be justified for invasive and aggressive growth (e.g., by desmoids), for cosmetic disfiguration and functional loss (e.g., by keloids or endocrine orbitopathy [EO]), and for life-threatening complications (e.g., by hepatic hemangioma [Kasabach-Merritt Syndrome]) or juvenile angiofibroma in the face of children or adolescents. Because nonmalignant diseases may have a lasting effect on the quality of life by causing pain or other serious symptoms, there is also a sufficient indication for RT, if other methods are unavailable, have failed, or may induce more side effects. As RT in most nonmalignant diseases is classified as an elective measure, a thorough risk-benefit analysis is required. Organ-specific acute toxicity rates and chronic late effects including potential effects on reproduction (pelvic region) and possible induction of tumors and leukemia are potential risks that have to be explained to patients within the informed consent.

Long-Term Risk of Tumor Induction

Data about tumor and leukemia induction after whole-body radiation exposure (UNSCEAR, BEIR) allow calculation of possible risks on a gender- and age-related basis: the average lifetime risk is lower in men (9.5%) than women (11.5%). Apart from age and gender, the individual risk depends on individual sensitivity (e.g., genetically predisposed diseases), anatomic site, and technical parameters, such as single and total doses and radiation protection (e.g., use of protective shields, optimal beam direction).

Principles of Application

Principles of irradiation of nonmalignant diseases are adequately defined on an international basis and can be summarized in 10 statements (Table 89.1). Irradiation of nonmalignant diseases is carried out by a well-trained radiation therapist. Radiotherapists are familiar with all technical and clinical aspects of modern RT. Long-term follow-up has to be assured because of the responsibility for radiogenic late effects.

Evidence-based Medicine

Apart from some exceptions, today there are only a few prospective controlled clinical studies available that justify the use of RT. Controlled studies are required to validate the experience-based indications, compare RT with standard treatments, or improve radiation parameters (single/total dose and fractionation).

Phase 3 studies should be based on positive phase 1 and 2 studies. It is not appropriate to start a phase 3 study when there is still not a proven dose-effect relation. Phase 4 studies were introduced as patterns of care studies by the Radiation Therapy Oncology Group in order to verify quality and outcome after RT for specific tumors. Using this method, the German Cooperative Group "Radiotherapy of Benign Diseases" has conducted patterns of care studies for various benign diseases and developed generally accepted guidelines for RT of nonmalignant diseases. For rare benign diseases, well-organized national or international registries have to be implemented.

Validated criteria are required for evaluation of treatment success by the patient ($\rightarrow$ subjective criteria), by the physician, or an established examination ($\rightarrow$ objective criteria).

Radiobiological Aspects

Radiobiological mechanisms and deterministic radiation effects on proliferating target cells that are well known from cancer therapy are only partially applicable to nonmalignant diseases. Usually lower single (0.5 to 1 Gy) and total (5 to 10 Gy) doses

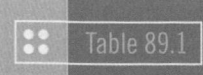

| Table 89.1 | PRINCIPLES OF APPLICATION OF RADIOTHERAPY FOR NONMALIGNANT DISEASES |

1. Estimate the *natural course of disease* without therapy.
2. Consider potential consequences of nontreatment of the patient.
3. Review data about *alternative therapies* and their therapeutic results.
4. Conduct a *risk-benefit analysis* compared with other possible measures.
5. Proof that the indication is justified: if *conventional therapies* have failed, if risks and consequences of other therapies are greater, and if nontreatment has more dramatic consequences than irradiation.
6. Consider the individual *potential long-term radiogenic risks*.
7. Inform *patient* about all details of radiotherapy: target volume, single/total dose, duration of session and series, relevant radiogenic risks, and side effects.
8. *Written consent* of the patient following *thorough patient education*.
9. Assurance of *long-term aftercare* in order to document result.
10. Request a competent *second opinion* in case of doubts and if the provided patient data or treatment decision are uncertain.

are used, which do not induce cell killing. Many other radiobiological principles are not applicable. Specific cells and cellular and functional mechanisms act as "other targets" for ionizing radiation depending on the specific disease. Ionizing radiation has proven effects on adhesion molecules on induction of apoptosis in selected target cells, on the expression of cytokines in macrophages, leukocytes, endothelial, and other cells. Radiation influences the inflammation cascade and progress of inflammation. Generally, RT does not work via one single or particular mechanism but rather through a complex interaction of different effects on many cell types.

Effects on Connective Tissue

Following trauma, acute or chronic inflammation, several cell systems regulate the repair process by which fibroblasts play a key role, particularly during the reparative phase, which is characterized by high cell proliferation and stimulation of growth factors. Ionizing radiation has a pivotal influence on cellular differentiation. In hyperproliferative disorders, fibroblast overreaction is responsible for the pathologic disease process, as in keloids. Radiation influences differentiation and suppresses cell proliferation.

Effects on Vascular System

Endothelial cells of capillaries and large arterial and venous blood vessels are the origin of cytokine-mediated cellular reactions and possess proliferative potential. Among other reactions, ICAM-1, a mediator of the leukocyte-endothelial interaction, is induced by low-dose irradiation. Selectins influence mononuclear blood cells to penetrate into interstitial space. Endothelial prostaglandin release is modulated by ionizing radiation. Cellular and membrane functions are modified by ionizing radiation. The radiation reaction of damaged and unaffected endothelial cells differs greatly, depending on the local tissue environment.

Large single or total doses cause endothelial damage, leading to sclerosis and obliteration of blood vessels. In vascular disorders such as hemangiomas or arteriovenous malformations (AVMs), high radiation doses may induce occlusion of pathologic vessels. Radiogenic effects depend on the dose concept and type of disease, which originates from blood vessels or is mediated by vascular endothelium. High fractionated or single doses are used for cerebral AVM or vertebral hemangioma, and low single or total doses are applied to reduce inflammation in heterotopic ossification (HO).

Effects on Inflammation

Low radiation doses exert anti-inflammatory effects on mononuclear cells of the immune system (lymphocytes, macrophages, monocytes) and endothelial cells of capillaries influencing the adhesion of inflammatory cells to the capillary surface and the capillary permeability and migration of inflammatory cells into inflamed tissue. Monocytes and macrophages are known to be radiosensitive; they express proinflammatory cytokines (e.g., interleukin-1, interleukin-6) or necrosis factors (e.g., tumor necrosis factor-α), which influence the complement cascade and enzymes of inflammatory reaction: interleukin-1 stimulates production and release of proinflammatory prostaglandins; there is a lasting change in synthesis of inducible nitric oxide synthetase. Radiation-induced changes in macrophage function can lead to modulation of the immune response and modification of the inflammatory process. Pain onset can be influenced directly via those mechanisms and cellular functions.

Low-dose irradiation can speed up local inflammation and lead to a rapid inflammation decline. Refractory nail bed inflammation (paronychia) and sweat gland abscesses (hidradenitis suppurativa) are typical examples for these beneficial radiogenic effects. Chronic inflammation processes are triggered by antigen-antibody reactions and mediated via mononuclear peripheral blood cells (e.g., lymphocytes, macrophages, monocytes) in the immune system. Ionizing radiation can help to suppress cell populations, such as T lymphocytes, in the inflammation process or modulate the effect such that the inflammation is stopped, as for EO.

Effects on Pain and Related Symptoms

Degenerative processes in hypotrophic tissues such as tendons, ligaments, and joints cause pain by chronic inflammation and trigger functional impairment of the musculoskeletal system. Although radiation does not influence the degenerative process, it may reduce the inflammation and provide partial or complete pain relief and, as a consequence, improve the function of affected joints. Radiotherapy affects degenerative processes on tendons, joints (osteoarthritis, synovitis), bursae (bursitis), and in soft tissues surrounding joints. A hardly proven analgetic effect on the autonomous nervous system was postulated in the context of neuralgiform pain (zoster/trigeminal neuralgia). It is not clear which cells are influenced and in which way, but the clinical effect is well established.

Summary of Dose Concepts

In summary, different dose concepts can be applied for nonmalignant diseases that differ greatly from each other because of different potential mechanisms of action (Table 89.2).

| Table 89.2 | RADIATION THERAPY MECHANISMS OF ACTION AND DOSE CONCEPTS |

Mechanisms of Action	Single Dose (Gy)	Total Dose (Gy)
Cellular gene and protein expression (e.g., eczemas)	<2.0	<2
Inhibition of inflammation in lymphocytes (e.g., in pseudotumor orbitae)	0.3–1.0	2–6
Inhibition of fibroblast proliferation (e.g., in keloids)	1.5–3.0	8–12
Inhibition of proliferation in benign tumors (e.g., in desmoids)	1.8–3,0	45–60

Radiophysical Aspects

Basic Principles of Radiation Planning

Radiotherapy of nonmalignant diseases is conducted according to the radiophysical principles and techniques applied for malignant tumors. In addition to histologic documentation and clinical diagnosis, imaging techniques are necessary within the scope of medical irradiation planning in order to determine the disease process in topographic and anatomic terms. Physical planning defines the target volume and dose prescription based on the International Commission on Radiation Units and Measurements 50/62 concept (reference point concept, specification of minimum and maximum dose at the target volume).

Near-Surface Lesions

For near-surface lesions, conventional x-rays (≤ 300 kV photon energy) with a focus-skin distance of 20 to 40 cm is used. With this technique, maximum doses are always in the skin. The dose profile of x-rays is variable depending on tube size and selected hardening filter, and can be modulated by bolus material of different thicknesses. The irradiated area can be collimated individually with flexible lead foils or elastic lead-rubber plates (1 to 3 mm thickness). Special lead or gold calottes are used for radiation of the oral or nasal cavity or close to the eye(lid). For small target volumes, bolus material is recommended in order to use the full tube area and avoid underdosage. Electrons with energies of ≤ 9 MeV are an alternative because of shortage of orthovoltage machines. Clinically, there is no difference in the efficacy of both methods. The skin dose is below 90% of the maximum dose. Bolus of 5 to 10 mm thickness is required if the maximum dose is required on the skin. For protection of healthy tissues, lead covers of 5 to 10 mm thickness are applied at the electron tube, and the gonads or thyroid gland are recommended to be shielded with a lead apron and collar. The lead thickness increases with the energy of the electrons used: per 1 MeV electron energy, about 0.5 mm lead must be mounted at the surface of the skin to reduce the transmission to about 0.5% per MeV.

Deep Lesions

Most deeply located lesions are irradiated with photons from linear accelerators. The maximum dose is situated up to several centimetres below the skin, depending on the energy used. Irradiation is usually done via an enface or isocentric opposing fields. In special occasions, coplanar multiple-field techniques are employed. For individual field collimation, lead blocks with five to six thicknesses of half-value layers are produced and employed, if no multileaf collimator is available.

Intracranial Lesions

Intracranial processes are treated with stereotactic techniques at dedicated linear accelerators or at the gamma knife. For selected indications, proton and heavy ion therapy are applied in specialized centers. In stereotactic RT, noncoplanar techniques and the use of several irradiation arcs or individually collimated stationary fields allow extremely steep dose gradients between target volume and critical structures (e.g., brainstem, cranial nerves). In one-time irradiation, a stereotactic ring is attached to the head to immobilize it, and this ring is fixed directly onto the irradiation desk; in fractionated irradiation, a very stable removable head mask is produced. Latest developments in stereotactic RT allow intensity-modulated RT (IMRT) with different dose profiles per single field and automatic adjustment of the individual collimation of the irradiation arcs (dynamic arc technique).

Disorders of the Head and Neck

Nonmalignant tumors of the central nervous system (CNS) can lead to severe, life-threatening symptoms due to local expansion and pressure on neighboring structures. Depending on their growth rate and location, the surrounding tissue may well adapt and delay the clinical diagnosis.

Meningioma

Background and Clinical Aspects

Meningiomas make up 15% to 20% of primary brain tumors and occur between the ages of 40 to 60 with a clear prevalence for women (1.8:1). Most tumors originate from the arachnoid cap cells, which occur anywhere within the skull, at the convexity and base of skull, where they sometimes grow infiltratively. Topographically, they are named *meningiomas of the sphenoid bone, clivus,* or *pars petrosa.* Olfactory meningiomas do not originate from the olfactoric tract but close to the olfactory nerve. According to the World Health Organization (WHO), most meningiomas are grade I tumors with a benign nature, but size and spread may bring about consequences, which are threatening as a malignant tumor. Less than 10% of patients have the aggressive and malignant form (WHO grade IV), which leads to extensive infiltrations, even metastases. Meningiomas and other benign tumors are distinguished from normal brain tissue by computed tomography (CT) and magnetic resonance imaging (MRI). Clinical symptoms depend on the location and are very similar to those of malignant tumors, which are characterized by headaches, vomiting, papillary edema, and focal cramp attacks.

Nonradiotherapeutic Treatment

For asymptomatic and elderly patients with minor symptoms and slow progression, a "wait and see" strategy is adequate (clinical examination, MRI every 6 months). Probability of local tumor control by surgery decreases with increasing Simpson classification (Table 89.3).

Radical surgical resection is the treatment of choice and depends on age and life expectancy, general condition, and neurologic conditions. After complete resection the relapse rate is low; after subtotal resection, additive RT improves long-term outcome. Local control after surgical intervention is 91%, 81%, 71%, and 56% for resections according to Simpson I through IV, respectively. After total resection, 5- and 10-year survival without recurrences is 93% and 80%, respectively, but these values decrease to 63% and 45% when subtotal resection was carried out.

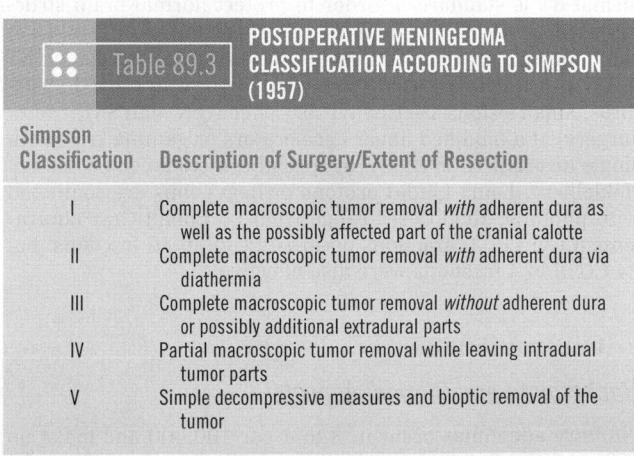

Table 89.3	POSTOPERATIVE MENINGEOMA CLASSIFICATION ACCORDING TO SIMPSON (1957)
Simpson Classification	**Description of Surgery/Extent of Resection**
I	Complete macroscopic tumor removal *with* adherent dura as well as the possibly affected part of the cranial calotte
II	Complete macroscopic tumor removal *with* adherent dura via diathermia
III	Complete macroscopic tumor removal *without* adherent dura or possibly additional extradural parts
IV	Partial macroscopic tumor removal while leaving intradural tumor parts
V	Simple decompressive measures and bioptic removal of the tumor

Clinical Radiation Oncology

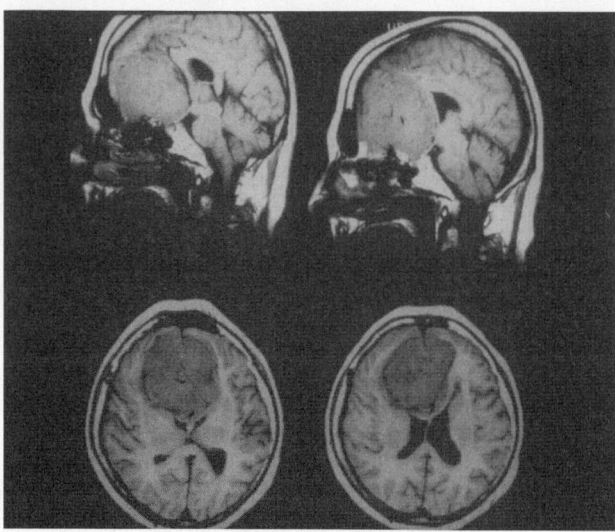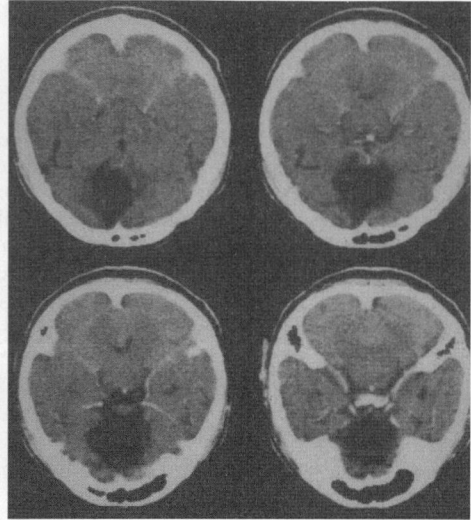

FIGURE 89.1. Frontobasal meningioma before (**left**) and after (**right**) microsurgical extirpation.

In some cases, *preoperative embolization* may be advantageous in order to reduce blood supply, but this procedure is not established and evaluated in long-term follow-up. Recurrent or aggressively growing meningiomas can also be treated with *cytostatic drugs* such as ifosfamide, doxorubicin, dacarbazine, and hydroxyurea. Hormonal therapy with tamoxifen or mefipristone has led to clinical regressions in individual cases.

Radiotherapeutic Options

RT is an effective alternative or supplement to surgery with following indications: (a) residual tumor after subtotal resection, (b) tumor relapse after previous surgery, (c) inoperability because of proximity of critical brain structures, or (d) different comorbidities prohibiting a surgical approach (Fig. 89.1). After incomplete resection, *additive RT* is carried out postoperatively, as the relapse is more difficult to control. For WHO grade II/III meningiomas, *adjuvant RT* is recommended. Postoperative RT improves local control significantly with 10-year progression-free survival of 90% in subtotally resected meningiomas. If surgery is impossible or refused, *primary RT* can reduce growth inhibition of most meningiomas. Remissions after RT occur slowly and are often insignificant, as with other benign intracranial tumors, but neurologic function(s) can be maintained or improved.

Benign meningiomas are irradiated with a safety margin of 1 cm and a total dose of 54 (50 to 58) Gy (single dose, 1.8 to 2 Gy). Today, three-dimensional (3D) CT- or MRI-planned conformal RT is standard in order to protect normal brain structures. More aggressive tumors are irradiated with 2 to 3 cm safety margin and a total dose of up to 68 Gy. Stereotactic RT (SRT) and IMRT are used to reduce RT dose to critical structures. Small lesions are treated very effectively with SRT (radiosurgery) at a modified linear accelerators or gamma knife with single doses of 15 to 25 Gy. In special centers (such as Boston, Heidelberg, Loma Linda) protons or heavy ions are combined with photons. Total doses range from 53 Cobalt-Gray equivalents (CGyE) in 27 fractions up to 74 CGyE in 16 fractions, but 24 CGyE in 4 fractions were also effective.

Pituitary Adenoma

Background and Clinical Aspects

Pituitary adenomas occur in 3 to 4 per 100,000 and make up 10% to 12% of all intracranial tumors. They originate from the adenohypophysis and grow slowly. In 70% of cases, hormone production is increased, mostly prolactin, adrenocorticotropic hormone (ACTH), or cortisol, rarely thyroid-stimulating hormone or gonadotropin. Large adenomas may exert pressure on the chiasm and lead to impaired vision (bitemporal hemianopsy) or insufficiency of the gland; about 20% suffer from headaches. Some tumors grow laterally and exert pressure on vascular structures (sinus-cavernous syndrome) and trigger ophthalmoplegia. Growth toward the hypothalamus often threatens hormone release of the adenohypophysis up to *panhypopituitarism*. Neurologic and ophthalmologic examinations, CT, MRI, and endocrinologic status lead to diagnosis.

Nonradiotherapeutic Treatment

Therapeutic options include surgery, drugs, and RT, and sometimes clinical surveillance. Primary therapy for all pituitary adenomas except for prolactinomas is the *transsphenoidal, selective adenectomy*. Microadenomas (≤10 mm) are removed radically and require no additional therapy. Residual tumor after surgery requires medical control of irregular hormone production. Macroadenomas (>10 mm) are operated because of the risk of compression of the optical chiasm. Surgery is also indicated in cases of autonomous hormone secretion. Prolactinomas are effectively treated with *dopamine agonists*, leading to reduction of tumor size within 24 hours.

Radiotherapeutic Options

The indication for RT is *always postoperatively* (a) after subtotal resection, (b) in clinically relevant persisting hormone secretion, and/or (c) in tumor recurrences after surgery.

For hormone inactive tumors like prolactinomas and with acromegaly, surveillance should always be considered; primary RT is an option for inoperable cases. Using fractionated RT and total doses of 45 to 50 Gy (single doses, 1.5 to 2 Gy), tumor control rates beyond 90% are reached.

In *hormone inactive adenomas*, 20% to 40% are resected incompletely. Postoperative RT is used for unfavorable tumor sites, spread toward the hypothalamus, or after subtotal removal or relapse.

More than 50% of endocrinally active adenomas are *prolactinomas* that induce the amenorrhea, galactorrhea syndrome in women and potency disfunction and infertility in men. Loss of libido and increased osteoporosis occurs in both sexes. Prolactinomas are treated with dopamine agonists (bromocriptine, cabergoline), leaving RT for inadequate surgical or medical incompatibility response.

Excessive growth hormones (such as STH) bring about the typical growth of forehead, chin, tongue, fingers, and toes in about 20% of pituitary adenomas RT is indicated in micro- and macroadenomas in postoperatively persisting hormonal secretion, but secondary surgery has to be evaluated before using RT. After RT, increased STH values decrease slowly and dopamine agonists (bromocriptine) or somatostatin analogs (octreotide) are still necessary for several years.

Increased ACTH, corticotropin-releasing hormone, and cortisol lead to *Cushing disease,* which is characterized by hypophyseal-hypothalamic dysfunction. After insufficient surgery bilateral adrenalectomy is performed, but if this intervention is not carried out, RT is indicated. After bilateral adrenalectomy, up to 40% of patients develop a *Nelson tumor* with extremely high ACTH serum levels and dark pigmentation due to increased melanocyte-stimulating hormone production, whereby there is an indication for RT at an early stage.

Rare TSH-secreting (macro)adenomas are primarily operated, but the recurrence rate of 30% to 50% is high. RT is indicated after incomplete resection or relapse and still-relevant hormone secretion or macroscopic recurrences. Gonadotrophinomas producing leutinizing hormone and/or follicle stimulating hormone are operated primarily, but postoperative RT is indicated for clinically relevant hormonal secretion or in the case of recurrence.

Radiotherapeutic Technique

MRI- or CT-based 3D planning (2- to 3-mm layers) and fractionated RT with 6 to 18 MV photons are mandatory for treatment. Total doses of 45 or 50Gy (single doses, 1.8 to 2 Gy) are applied for micro- and macroadenomas. Depending on tumor site and RT technique, 2- to 10-mm safety margins are applied. Protection of critical structures is important, but conventional masks have positioning inaccuracies of 5 to 7 mm, which usually are avoided with stereotactic RT (radiosurgery). Standard requirements for radiosurgery are well defined. Depending on applied RT technique, doses to the tumor region and critical structures are summarized in Table 89.4. Comparison of conventional RT with SRT and IMRT-SRT for an irregular target volume are shown in Figure 89.2. In case of compression of brainstem or temporal lobes, or short distance to chiasma/visual nerve, fractionated RT is favored. RT alone and as adjuvant modality in conjunction with surgery yields long-term control rates in the range of 90%, while radiogenic late effects are rare with fractionated modern RT techniques.

Craniopharyngioma

Background and Clinical Aspects

Craniopharyngiomas are dysontogenetic midline tumors originating from Rathke's pocket or the ductus craniopharyngicus.

They make up 6% to 10% of pediatric CNS tumors (age 5 to 15 years) and are located near the sella, with close connection to pituitary gland, hypothalamus, chiasma opticum, and visual nerves, but rarely involve the sella. Symptoms are vision loss or impairment (bitemporal hemianopsy), endocrine dysfunction (dwarfism, fat tissue disturbance, adrenal cortex insufficiency), signs of intracranial pressure, sella expansion (x-ray), typical calcifications (CT), and cystic or mixed solid and cystic components (MRI) (Fig. 89.3).

Nonradiotherapeutic Treatment

Primary therapy consists of complete resection, which is equivalent to permanent cure, but high sequelae (visual impairment, 20%; panhypopituitarism, ≤95%) following radical neurosurgery make less radical surgery with adjuvant 3D-conformal RT the preferred approach today. Ten-year control after complete tumor resection reaches 60% to 93%.

Radiotherapeutic Options

Indications for RT are (a) primary RT for inoperable tumors and (b) additive RT after subtotal resection; otherwise progression rate would be 90% after 3 years. After subtotal resection alone, the relapse rate is 30%, and postoperative RT improves control rates to 80% to 95% after 5 to 20 years. Thus, long-term control after primary RT or adjuvant RT with 50 to 54 Gy total dose (single dose, 1.8 to 2 Gy) is comparable with complete resection. After conformal RT, visual deterioration may reach up to 10%, but severe sequelae like necroses, cognitive changes, and secondary malignomas occur in <2%. Because of proximity to the optic chiasm and visual nerves, fractionated stereotactic RT (FSRT) should be the preferred RT technique. Using FSRT, a 10-year control rate of 100% is possible without radionecroses, secondary malignomas, or visual deteriorations. The hypophysial hormonal situation deteriorated in about 30%. Another option is the local application of radionuclides in the craniopharyngeomal cysts, which can bring tumor growth to a halt.

Acusticus Neurinomas (Schwannomas)

Background and Clinical Aspects

Acusticus neurinomas are benign neuroectodermal tumors originating from Schwann cells of the neurilemma at the vestibulocochlear nerve (CN IV) and make up 5% of primary brain tumors. With an incidence of 1 in 100,000, 5% of cases are affected by patients with neurofibromatosis type II (M. Recklinghausen). Growth in the cerebellopontine angle exerts pressure on the vestibularis and cochlear nerves, causing hearing impairment, tinnitus, and vertigo. Later facialis paresis (CN VII), trigeminus neuropathy (CN V), and brainstem symptoms occur. Diagnosis is made via high-resolution CT and MRI which show intra- or extrameatal location and size.

	Table 89.4	**RADIATION DOSE PLAN FOR PITUITARY ADENOMAS AND TOTAL DOSE 5/5**				
Radiation	**Dose at Target Volume**	**Chiasma and CN II**	**CN III–VI**	**Brain Tissue**	**Rest of Pituitary Gland/Hypothalamus**
Radiosurgery	≥12–13 Gy for STH-secreting and all inactive adenomas	≤8 Gy	CN V ≤12 Gy, otherwise ≤15 Gy	≤10 mL with dose of >10 Gy	≤20 Gy maximum protection
Single-dose RT	≥15 Gy for all other adenomas				
Fractionated RT	SD 1.8 Gy, TD 45.0 Gy (microadenoma), 50.4 Gy (macroadenoma)	≤50 Gy: maximum protection!	≤60 Gy: maximum protection!	≤50 Gy brainstem, ≤60 Gy rest of brain	≤50 Gy maximum protection

CN, cranial nerve; RT, radiotherapy; STH, SD, single dose; TD, total dose.

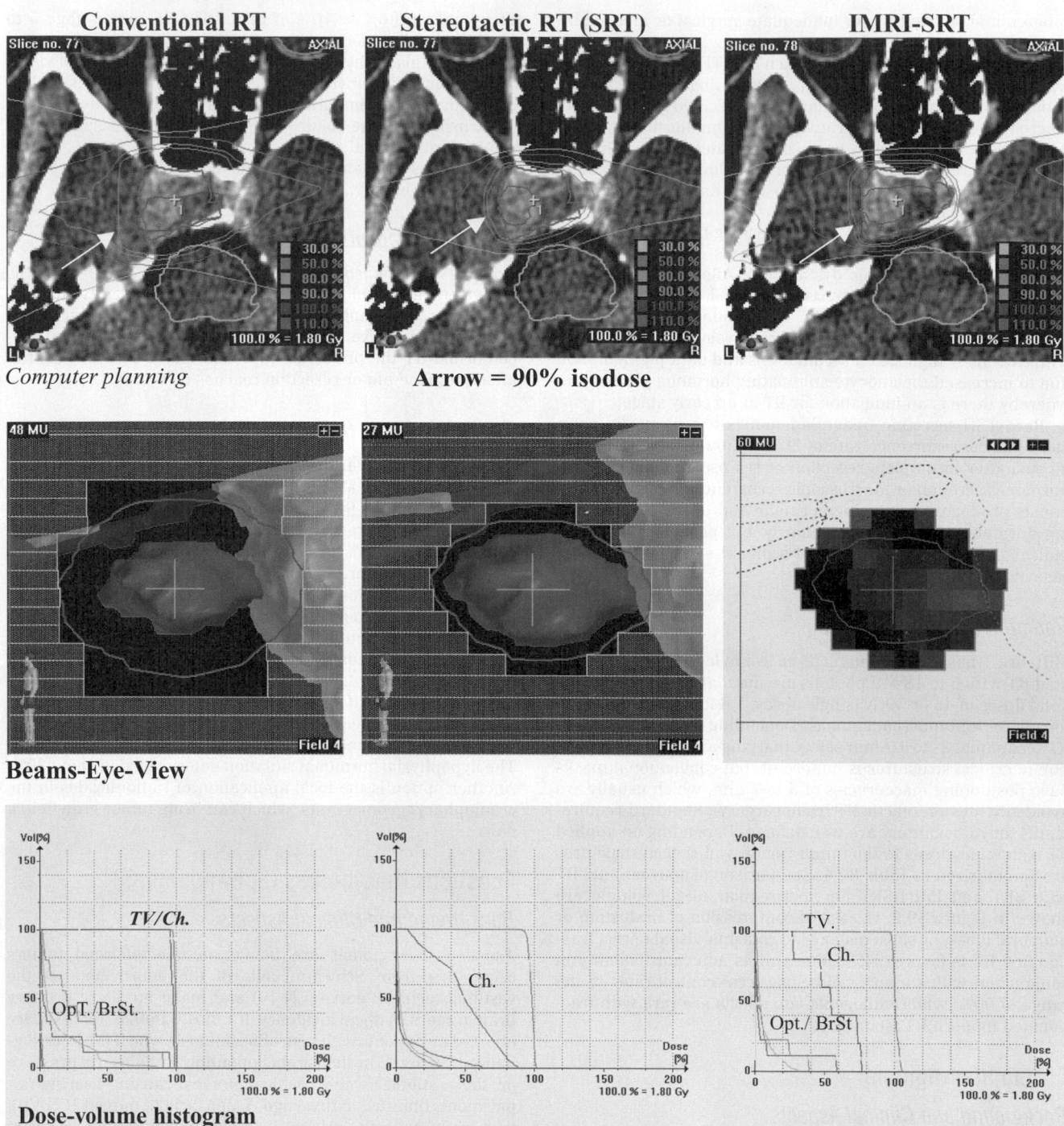

FIGURE 89.2. Comparison of conventional radiotherapy (RT) irradiation with stereotactic RT (SRT) and intensity-modulated SRT (IMRI-SRT) for an irregular target volume (TV).

Nonradiotherapeutic Treatment

Complete tumor resection is the standard therapy, particularly for large tumors (>25 mm). Nerve injury can be avoided intraoperatively by electrophysiological monitoring, but maintenance of hearing function is preserved in only 40%; 10% of cases develop liquor fistulas, 6% develop pareses of caudal cranial nerves, 2% hydrocephalus, and 1% meningitis or hemiparesis.

Radiotherapeutic Options

RT is indicated for progressive and symptomatic *primary or recurrent acusticus neurinoma* up to a size of 25 mm (Tos grade 0 to 2). *Stereotactic single-dose RT* with gamma knife or modified linear accelerator is the preferred RT technique. Besides direct damage of proliferating tumor cells, tumor vessels may slowly be occluded, and 40% to 70% of cases will develop a tumor remission. With larger tumor size, RT exposure of the

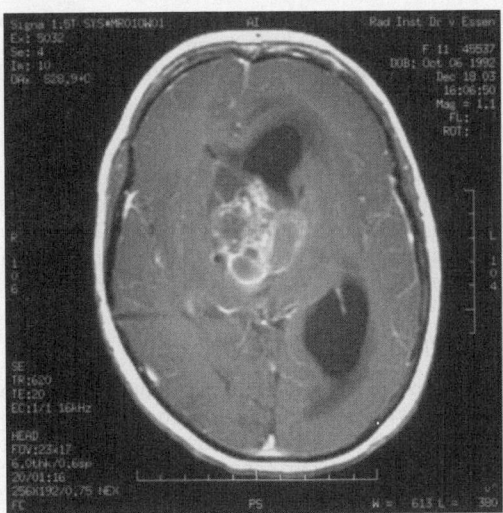 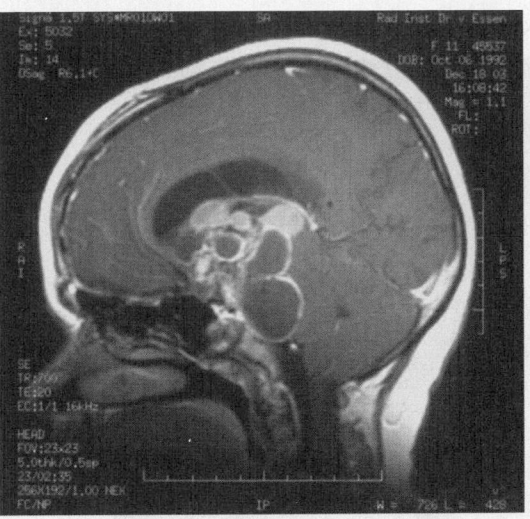

FIGURE 89.3. Magnetic resonance image of a cystic craniopharyngioma in an 11-year-old patient.

cranial nerves and brainstem and side effects increase. Aims of RT are disappearance of tumor and symptoms, prevention of tumor progression, and maintenance of the remaining hearing ability. The tolerance dose for vestibulocochlear, facial, and trigeminal nerves are known and depend on irradiated length, tumor size, and dose at tumor edge. With SRT techniques, radiogenic sequelae of cranial nerves occur rarely, but because the vestibulocochlear nerve goes right through the tumor, it is less protected.

With single doses of 12 to 14 Gy at tumor edge (depending on reference isodose 15 to 25 Gy centrally), local control reaches up to 95%. In order to decrease side effects, FSRT at linear accelerators has been preferred recently: RT concepts are 5×5 Gy, 10×3 Gy, 25×2 Gy, and 30×1.8 Gy. In a comparison between SRT, surgery, and monitoring alone, an overview showed that with monitoring, 50% of tumors progressed within 3 years and 20% of those needed surgery. With SRT, up to 8% relapsed after 3 years and only 5% had to be operated. After primary surgery, 2% relapse and 3% functional impairment are observed. Today, SRT is considered as effective as surgery, but less side effects.

Arteriovenous Malformation

Background and Clinical Aspects

Intracranial AVMs are vessel abnormalities consisting of widened arteries connected to the normal capillary bed. About 80% of AVMs are located supratentorially. The prevalence is low in the western hemisphere (about 0.01%; 18 in 100,000). Most AVMs are diagnosed at the age of 20 to 40 years. They extend to aneurysms and rupture in 2% to 5% per year Headaches, hemorrhage, cramp attacks, and sudden death through bleeding characterize the clinical course. AVMs have an annual bleeding risk of 2% to 4%, which increases to 2% to 18% after rupture, and is much higher in men than women. Large AVMs with deep arterial feeders or those located at basal ganglia or thalamus have an increased bleeding risk. After first bleeding, lethality is 30%, and 10% to 20% of survivors have neurologic defects.

For surgery and RT planning, precise knowledge about size, site, and arterial and venous drainage of the nidus is required. Five AVM categories are defined; the sixth group contains all inoperable AVMs, with high risk of morbidity and mortality. Further indicators of AVM are previous bleeding, atrophy, and gliosis of neighboring brain structures. The aim of therapy is the prevention of bleeding by complete obliteration of the nidus,

and if possible the improvement of neurologic malfunctions and the simultaneous prevention of therapy-induced side effects.

Nonradiotherapeutic Treatment

Treatment of choice is the elective *complete AVM excision*. Particularly with small AVMs in superficial, noneloquent regions of the brain, *microsurgery* reaches very high healing rates. *Endovascular embolization* is rarely curative, but part of a multimodal concept for large AVMs in order to decrease the initial lesion size, improving conditions for subsequent surgery or radiosurgery, but even then, recurrence of bleeding cannot be fully excluded.

Radiotherapeutic Options

AVMs are irradiated with single-dose SRT at linear accelerator or gamma knife. Fractionated RT with total doses of up to 60 Gy have produced inadequate results. Depending on AVM size and location, a single dose of 15 to 25 Gy is required in the periphery of the nidus, but the bleeding risk continues until complete obliteration is achieved. The obliteration rate after SRT is 65% to 95% (Table 89.5).

Radiogenic side effects are mostly chronic by nature: radionecrosis or leucoencephalopathy occur at 9 to 36 months after SRT, but may also appear after a few weeks. The risk correlates strongly with the irradiated brain volume and total SRT dose: the brain volume irradiated with >10 Gy is an important predictive factor.

Table 89.5	CLINICAL OBLITERATION RATE AND RADIOGENIC SIDE EFFECTS AFTER RADIOSURGERY			
Clinical Study (>200 Cases)	**N**	**Obliteration Rate (%)**	**Moderate Side Effects (%)**	**Severe Side Effects (%)**
Steiner et al., 1992 (160)	247	81	8	1
Engenhart et al., 1994 (282)	212	72	4	4
Flickinger et al., 1996, 1999 (38)	1255	72	5	3
Chang et al., 2000	254	79	3	2
Friedman et al., 2003	269	53	4	1

a) Axial T2w MRI

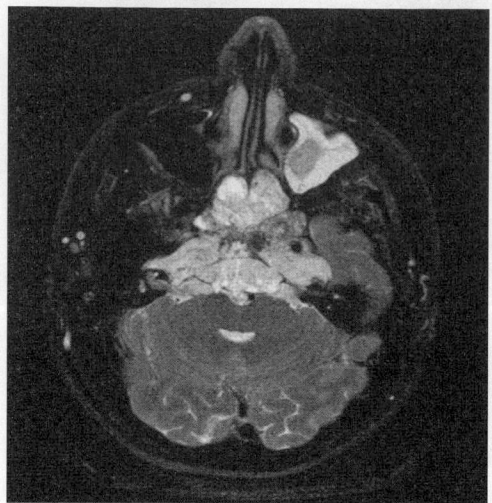

b) Sagittal T2w MRI

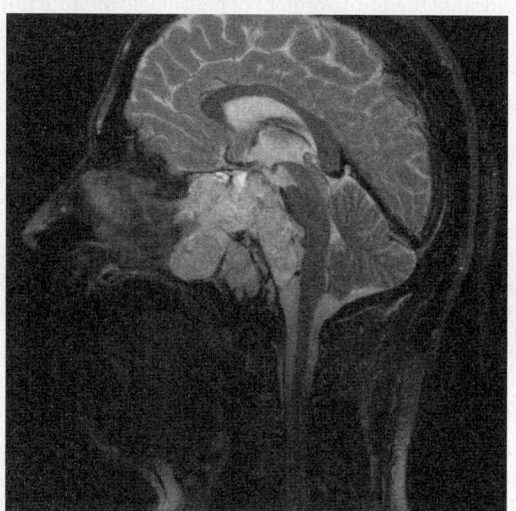

FIGURE 89.4. Magnetic resonance image (MRI) diagnosis of large chordoma of the skull base and clivus. **A:** Axial T2-weighted MRI. **B:** Sagittal T2-weighted MRI.

Chordomas

Background and Clinical Aspects

Chordomas are rare, slowly growing midline tumors originating from embryonal notochord rests in the base of the skull and clivus (35%), vertebral column (15%), or sacral region (50%).

They are distinguished immunohistochemically from *low-grade chondrosarcomas*, which have a more favorable prognosis. Neurologic symptoms and MRI lead to diagnosis (Fig. 89.4).

Nonradiotherapeutic Treatment

Complete tumor resection is the therapy of choice. Large tumor rests, bioptic evidence of tumor necroses in histology, and female gender are unfavorable prognosis factors. Because of the proximity of critical brain structures, complete removal is only rarely possible and relapse occurs in about 50%.

Radiotherapeutic Options

Indications for RT are (a) inoperability and (b) after incomplete resection. With total RT doses of more than 65 Gy, local control is significantly improved. Using fractionated photon RT doses of up to 60 Gy, 5-year control rates of 17% to 33% have been reached Higher total doses can be given when FSRT is used, but experiences are limited. In Heidelberg, 37 patients received a median total dose of 66.6 Gy. Local control rate after 5 years was 50%. Radiosurgery with gamma knife or modified linear accelerators are possible in small tumors and with sufficient distance to visual nerves, chiasma, and brainstem.

Concerning protons, total RT doses of 65 to 85 GyE have been applied and resulted in a local control rate of 73% after 5 years. Other centers have confirmed these results or have combined photon (about two-thirds dose) and proton therapy (about one-third dose) and total doses of 60 to 70 GyE (median, 67 GyE); the local 3-year control rate was about 70% (Table 89.6).

Glomus Tumor/Chemodectoma

Background and Clinical Aspects

Glomus tumors (chemodectomas, nonchromaffin paragangliomas) are rare benign tumors that occur in the following anatomic sites: (a) at the carotid glomus near the bifurcation, (b) near the jugular bulb, (c) near the tympanum, and (d) in other sites (larynx, near the aorta, pulmonary artery, orbital cavity). Most tumors are located near the skull base in the jugular fossa. Peak age is at 45 years, with no gender preference. Only 10% to 20% are bilateral or multiple. Growing slowly, they are rarely endocrinally active or show malignant transformation in 5% to 10%; they may infiltrate bone, vessels, middle ear, and cranial nerves. Symptoms are headache, cranial nerve failure (CN V–XII), dysphagia, pulsatile tinnitus, vertigo, hypoacusis, and large, pulsating swellings in the neck. Without treatment the risk of cranial nerve failure and chronic invalidization are high; the swelling may increase to life-threatening size, causing severe complications. Diagnosis is made clinically and with high-resolution CT, angiography, and MRI. For prognosis estimation, the classification according to Fisch and Mattox (1988) is used.

Table 89.6	CLINICAL RESULTS OF PHOTON AND PROTON RADIOTHERAPY OF CHORDOMA				
Selected Studies	N	Period	Technique	Dose (Gy)	Control Rate
Debus et al., Heidelberg (22)	37	1990–1997	Photons (FSRT)	66.6	50% / 5 y
Munzenrider and Leibsch, MGH Boston (115)	519	1975–1988	Prot. + Phot.	66–83 GyE	73% / 5 y
Hug et al., Loma Linda UMC (60)	58	1992–1998	Protons	70.7 GyE	67% / 3 y
Noel et al., Orsay (117)	49	1995–2000	Prot. + Phot.	67 GyE	71% / 3 y
Castro et al., LBL Berkeley (15)	53	1977–1992	He ions	65 GyE	63% / 5 y
Schulz-Ertner et al., Heidelberg (148)	44	1997–2001	C12 ions	60 GyE	81% / 3 y

FSRT, fractionated stereotactic radiotherapy; MGH, Massachusetts General Hospital; Prot. + Phot., protons plus photons; GyE, Gray equivalent; UMC, University Medical Center; LBL,

Table 89.7	CLINICAL RESULTS OF RADIOTHERAPY WITH OR WITHOUT SURGERY IN PARAGANGLIOMAS				
Study (Recent Series)	N	Dose (Gy)	Local Control (%)	Follow-Up (years)	Comments
Liscak et al., 1999 (93)	66	10–30	100	2	Gamma knife–RT
Foote et al., 2002 (43)	25	12–18	100	1–9	Gamma knife–RT
Eustacchio et al., 2002 (30)	19	12–20	95	1.5–10	Gamma knife–RT
Maarouf et al., 2003 (96)	12	11–20	100	0.8–9	Stereotactic radiosurgery
Pohl et al., 2003 (131)	12	60	100	2–14	Sx +/– RT, partly RT alone
Zabel et al., 2003 (192)	24	58	92	1.5–15.5	Fract. stereotactic RT

RT, radiotherapy; Sx, surgery; Fract., fractionated.

Nonradiotherapeutic Treatment

In the carotid region, primary tumor resection after previous embolization is the therapy of choice. At the skull base or at the tympanum, neurosurgical interventions are more risky, and fractionated RT is favored in those cases. In selected cases, primary surgery is already curative; after incomplete surgery, adjuvant treatment should be started only if the tumor starts to progress again.

Radiotherapeutic Options

Depending on size and location, indication for RT is either primary RT, in cases of inoperability (mostly jugular paragangliomas), or additive RT, for incomplete resection or salvage RT for relapse. 3D-conformal RT with 45 to 55 Gy total dose is applied. Here, wedged and angled fields, superior-inferior, and lateral angled fields and multifield plans can be employed using 4 to 6 MV photons and 15 to 18 MeV electrons for dose optimization.

Two overviews show that RT produces control rates that are as good as or even better than surgery. Even in large, diffusely growing, or multiple tumors, RT produces a local control rate of 88% to 93% and noticed a relapse rate of 22% with doses of ≤40 Gy, and relapse occurred in 1.4% with doses of >40 Gy. Total doses of 45 to 50 Gy do not compromise surgery that might become necessary later (Table 89.7). During the last decade, SRT and gamma knife were also used for the treatment of paragangliomas. FSRT will prevail in extensive lesions or relapse after prior RT.

Acute radiogenic side effects include pharyngeal mucositis and skin reactions in the external acoustic canal, resulting in tube ventilation dysfunction, reduced sound conduction, and salivary retention, requiring temporary paracentesis. Chronic side effects are fibrosis, dryness of pharyngeal mucosa, and, rarely, radiogenic consequences in the inner ear (2% to 3%), bone necroses (1.7%), and brain necroses or abscess formation (0.8%). In one case, a fibrosarcoma had developed 15 years after successful RT of a jugular glomus tumor.

Juvenile Nasopharyngeal Angiofibroma

Background and Clinical Aspects

Juvenile nasopharyngeal angiofibroma (JNA) is a rare, benign, vascularized tumor in the head and neck, affecting mainly male adolescents. JNAs develop in the sphenoethmoidal suture and spread from the epipharynx and nasal cavity to sphenopalatine foramen and into the pterygopalatine fossa. Beyond bony destruction, there is spread into the paranasal sinuses, infratemporal fossa, orbital space, and middle cranial fossa. Clinical features, high-resolution CT, MRI, and angiography lead to diagnosis. Topographic staging is done according to Chandler et al. (11). Intracranial spread occurs in 25%. Symptoms

are epistaxis, impaired nose breathing, and eventually facial swelling and orbital and intracranial symptoms (e.g., blindness, cranial nerve failure). As biopsies can cause massive bleeding, histologic proof is often lacking. Presence of hormone receptors shows the influence of androgenous hormones. Spontaneous remission after puberty is possible, but therapy is often urgently required when symptoms increase and complications are threatening.

Nonradiotherapeutic Treatment

Surgery combined with embolization is the preferred treatment. Through surgery, most JNA of stages I through III (without intracranial spread) can reach local control of up to 100% with only minimal toxicity; in advanced stages, complete resection is usually not possible.

Radiotherapeutic Options

Tumors with intracranial spread (stage IV) require primary RT. Other indications are as follows: (a) tumor rests, (b) inoperability, or (c) relapse after initial surgery. For optimal protection of risk organs, FSRT and stereotactic IMRT will help to protect the eyes, visual nerve, chiasma, brainstem, myelon, and salivary glands effectively.

Total RT doses of 30 to 55 Gy (single doses, 1.8 to 2 Gy) are effective. Relapses increase with total doses below 36 Gy; otherwise, local control rates reach 80% to 100% (Table 89.8). After RT, JNA remission is slow and recurrences may occur later. Subacute and chronic radiogenic side effects include mucositis, xerostomy, caries, pituitary gland dysfunction, cranial nerve failure, temporal lobe necrosis, osteoradionecrosis, growth impairment of the facial skull, cataract, glaucoma, and atrophic rhinitis. Radiogenic sequelae are limited by careful RT planning and high-conformal RT. Radiogenic tumors occur in up to 4%, particularly in younger patients. Secondary malignization of JNA has rarely been reported,

Disorders of Eye and Orbit

Pterygium

Background and Clinical Aspects

Pterygium is a wing-shaped, fibrovascular, proliferating tissue at the border between conjunctiva and cornea that extends from the medial (nasal) corner of the eye to the cornea and beyond. The highest geographic incidence occurs in hot, dusty, dry, and sun-exposed regions ("desert belts"). Symptoms include foreign body sensation and tearing and motility problems. Cornea affection cause reduced vision leading to blindness (Fig. 89.5).

Table 89.8	CLINICAL RESULTS OF RADIOTHERAPY (RT) IN JUVENILE NASOPHARYNGEAL ANGIOFIBROMA				
Study/Selected Institution	N	Period	Dose (Gy)	Local Control	Side Effects
Jereb et al., 1979 (69) Radiumhemmet, Stockholm, Sweden	69	1919–1966	20–60	47/63 (10 y) 10/63 (5 y) 6/47 (1 y)	No malignant tumor
Cummings et al., 1984 (20) Princess Margaret Hospital, Toronto, Canada	55	1956–1980	30–35	83% primary RT 69% recurrence RT	Thyroid carcinoma (1), basal cell carcinoma (1), cataract (2)
Fields et al., 1990 (31) Washington, USA	13	1962–1984	36–52	11/13 (85%)	Xerostomy, caries (2), no tumor formation
Million et al., 1994 (109) Univ. of Florida, USA	9	1980–1991	30–55	8/9 (89%)	
Reddy et al., 2001 (136) Univ. of Florida, USA	15	1975–1996	30–35	13/15 (86%)	Cataract (3), CNS (1), basal cell carcinoma (1)
Lee et al., 2002 (89) UCLA, USA	27	1960–2000	30–55	23/27 (85%)	15% Late toxicity

UCLA, University of California, Los Angeles.

Nonradiotherapeutic Treatment

Treatment is indicated if vision is threatened by growth toward the pupil and if aesthetics is subjectively affected. Complete surgical excision is the treatment of choice with several options, such as open wound defect, primary conjunctival occlusion, rotation flap, keratoplastics, or free transplant. Local control rate is 50% to 70%. For recurrent cases, adjuvant treatment is advised, including the use of local cytostatics (mitomycin C), which may lead to scleral ulceration, secondary glaucoma, corneal edema or perforation, iritis, and cataract.

Radiotherapeutic Options

RT is indicated after relapse and local resection of pterygium; a few centers have used primary or preoperative RT. Orthovolt therapy and strontium-90 brachytherapy applicators with effective diameter of 8 to 12 mm have been employed.

Results of postoperative RT for prophylaxis and, rarely, primary RT are unambiguously positive: Van den Brenk (178) observed 1.4% relapses in 1,300 cases of treated pterygia (1,064 patients); irradiation was carried out once a week (days 0, 7, and 14 postoperatively). Paryani et al. (127) had a relapse rate of 1.7% in 825 eyes using 6 × 10 Gy (1 time per week). Wilder et al. (186) observed 11% relapses in 244 eyes after 3 × 8 Gy (1 time per week). In a placebo-controlled study, 1 × 25 Gy had significantly lower relapse rates than the control group (70).

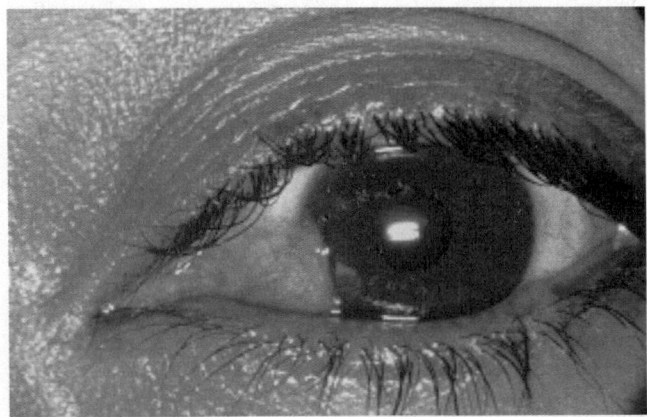

FIGURE 89.5. Pterygium of the left eye originating from the nasal angle.

Thus, today the level of evidence for the effectiveness of postoperative RT is very high (70); however, for the use of primary RT alone, there are still no controlled studies available. Radiogenic sequelae are not frequently observed, but may include scleromalacia and corneal ulcerations; they were detected in about 5% of cases after high total RT doses and with single-dose RT as high as 1 × 20 to 22 Gy.

Choroidal Hemangioma

Background and Clinical Aspects

Choroid membrane hemangiomas are slowly-growing benign tumors originating from vessels of the choroid. They can occur in congenital Sturge-Weber syndrome. Diffuse (at ages 5 to 10) and local types (at ages 30 to 50) can be distinguished. Hemangiomas are detected ophthalmoscopically and by clinical phenomena (e.g., glaucoma, retinal detachment). Further procedures are ultrasound, fluorescence angiography, CT, MRI, and scintigraphy (phosphorus-32).

Nonradiotherapeutic Treatment

Lesions outside the central area receive photodynamic therapy, photocoagulation, or transpapillary thermotherapy, but often vision deteriorates thereafter; in 40% to 52%, recurrent retinal detachment occurs. Lesions very close to the macula or papilla are not coagulated as there is a risk of central scotoma; the same holds for incomplete retinal detachment and the diffuse type (Sturge-Weber syndrome). Ophthalmologists favor photodynamic therapy with verteporfin. Subretinal edema disappears within a few weeks, hemangiomas shrink, and vision is improved in some patients; with subfoveal hemangiomas, the results are less favorable.

Radiotherapeutic Options

RT is indicated in nonresponding cases and particularly in lesions with proximity to the macula or papilla. Irradiation can be done with linear accelerator photons, protons, and brachytherapy. The earlier RT starts, the better are the long-term results: Schilling et al. (146) irradiated 36 localized and 15 diffuse lesions with 10 × 2 Gy; after 5 years, 23 (64%) eyes of localized type had a complete retinal reattachment; visual acuity was stable in 50% and improved in 50%; results were also favorable for the diffuse type. In advanced cases, RT cannot conserve the visual acuity but maintains the eye as a whole organ.

For percutaneous RT 18 to 20 Gy (local type) or 30 Gy (diffuse type) total dose (1.8 to 2 Gy single dose) is recommended. A head mask and vacuum contact lenses can be combined for better eye fixation. In localized lesions, brachytherapy is used with individually loaded eye plaques (iodine-125, ruthenium-106, cobalt-60). Plaque shape and size vary from 10 to 18 mm diameter. Iodine-125 seeds are prefered and deliver 30- to 240-Gy doses from the apex to base of lesion. Results are permanent resorption of subretinal edema, complete retinal attachment, and maintenance of vision. Radiogenic side effects are rare. Further RT options are fractionated protons with 20 to 30 CGyE. Zografos et al. (1998) reported on 48 localized and 6 diffuse lesions treated with 16.4 to 18.2 CGyE; in all cases, the retina reattached and visual acuity was improved in 70%. SRT with steep dose decrease is suitable for localized lesions in critical locations. Both procedures are only possible in specialized centers. Potential radiogenic side effects are retinopathy and papillopathy with doses >30 Gy; cataracts may also occasionally develop.

Age-Related Macular Degeneration

Background and Clinical Aspects

Macular degeneration is age-dependent and a leading cause of blindness in developed countries. Its prevalence rises from 20% in the 7th decade to 35% in the 8th decade of life. If one eye is affected, the risk for involvement of the other eye is 7% to 12% per year. An important risk factor is nicotine abuse. Typical signs are (a) drusen (yellowish depots of cellular detritus), (b) retinal pigment epithelium changes, (c) serous or hemorrhagic detachment of retinal pigment epithelium, and (d) choroidal neovascularization (CNV), partly combined with scars in the macular region (Fig. 89.6). In terms of progression, early and late forms and topographically foveal, extra- and subfoveal forms are to be distinguished, at the final stage dry (geographical) and wet (neovascular) forms can be differentiated. The classic age-related macular degeneration is well circumscribed in contrast to occult forms. The dry form exposes drusen, small atrophies, and slight loss of visual acuity appear frequently (80%), and 20% develop as wet (exudative) form with visual impairment up to blindness; in 90% CNV occurs together with edema and bleeding.

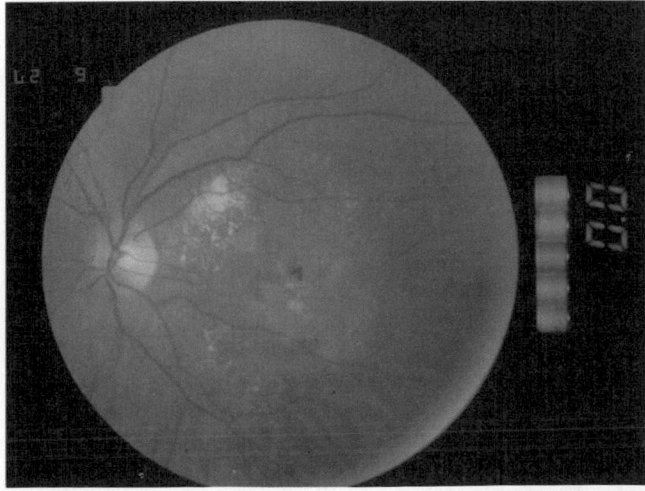

FIGURE 89.6. Macular degeneration with pigment changes and "Drusen formation."

Nonradiotherapeutic Treatment

Laser coagulation is suitable for selected lesions, while rare "classic" extrafoveal CNV is mostly treated with photocoagulation. For subfoveal CNV, antiangiogenic drugs and transpapillary thermotherapy are employed; photodynamic therapy with intravenous verteporfin causes selective photochemical vessel wall damage in classic CNV, which delays or prevents visual loss. Improvement of visual acuity in wet age-related macular degeneration is rare, but cases with classic (nonoccult) CNV benefit frequently.

Radiotherapeutic Options

Photons, protons, and brachytherapy have been used, but so far no comparative studies have been conducted. Photon therapy (with linear accelerator) was conducted with mask fixation via lateral semifield technique; the unaffected eye is spared by 10-degree posterior gantry inclination; anterior angled fields are applied with lens protection; rotational techniques are also suitable. Protons and brachytherapy with palladium-103 or strontium-90 and ruthenium-106 applicators may provide a better protection of normal eye structures.

Results of Radiotherapy

Use of RT was triggered by a dose-finding study that revealed stable or improved visual acuity in 63%; membranes degenerated in 77% after 1 year. This study, without outlining effective RT dose and appropriate indication, triggered many other studies. Some questioned RT, as positive outcome could not be comprehended only partially. In some retrospective analysis, total doses of 5 to 36 Gy achieved positive effects, while other studies had negative results were outnumbered. A possible explanation is, that the "therapeutic corridor" for antiangiogenetic effects is small; with increasing doses, neovascular membranes may regress, but risks of radiogenic sequelae (retinopathy) increases.

In a placebo-controlled study, after 1 year FRT with 8×2 Gy showed no improvement of visual acuity, and a clinically beneficial effect was excluded. Another study compared 1, 8, and 16 Gy total dose; after 12 to 18 months the corrected visual acuity was significantly better with 8 or 16 Gy than with 1 Gy, and patients with classic CNV or initial visual acuity of $\geq 20/100$ had the highest benefit; no difference in reading ability or CNV size was observed. Another study compared 5×2 Gy and 18×2 Gy with a control group; for classic CNV, higher RT dose stabilized visual acuity more frequently, but there was no difference in occult CNV. The study was discontinued because 25% of cases irradiated with 36 Gy developed retinopathy. A single dose of 7.5 Gy improved visual acuity compared with the control group and did not produce side effects (78% vs. 38%).

No firm data are available for protons: Yonemoto et al. (191) compared 8 and 14 GyE to find a dose-effect; higher dose and small initial lesion size were prognostically significant factors. There were no radiogenic side effects. Brachytherapy (12 to 23Gy in up to 28 hours) produced stable or improved visual acuity in 87% of subretinal CNV; one-third relapsed, and after 18 months, visual acuity remained stable or better in 61%. In another study 15 Gy within 0.9 hour produced a clinical response in 74% of patients with subfoveal CNV; visual acuity remained stable within two line pairs in 55% after 6 month and in 45% after 12 months.

Overall, the value of RT is not adequately defined, neither in terms of a precise indication nor in terms of ideal RT concepts for the respective disease stages. In primarily occult CNV, visual acuity appears to remain stable for a certain length of time. Clinical use of RT should be continued in selected refractory cases. However, there is only mixed evidence level of efficacy.

Table 89.9	MODIFIED NOSPECS CLASSIFICATION FOR ENDOCRINE ORBITOPATHY		
Stage/Clinical Features	Grade 1 (= 1 point)[a]	Grade 2 (= 2 points)[a]	Grade 3 (= 3 points)[a]
I **NO** = No objective eye symptoms	Minimal subjective eye symptoms	Moderate subjective eye symptoms	Severe subjective eye symptoms
II **S** = Soft tissue involvement of periorbital soft tissue	*Minimal* objective symptoms: redness, chemosis, slight periorbital oedema	*Moderate* objective symptoms: redness, chemosis; moderate periorbital edema	*Severe* objective symptoms: conjunctival exposition, prominent periorbital edema
III **P** = Proptosis, amount of exophthalmus	>20–23 mm	24–27 mm	>27 mm
IV **E** = Eye muscles, eye muscle dysfunction	Rarely, diplopy; none in primary position	Frequently, diplopy; moderate mobility impairment	Severe constant muscular dysfunction
V **C** = Cornea, corneal involvement	Slight corneal changes and clinical symptoms	Prominent corneal changes and moderate symptoms	Keratitis and other severe eye symptoms
VI **S** = Sight loss of vision due to nerve compression	20/25–20/40	20/45–20/100	>20/100

[a]Orbitopathy index = sum of points of all symptom categories; maximum, 18 points.

Endocrine Orbitopathy (Graves Disease)

Background and Clinical Aspects

Endocrine orbitopathy (EO) is an inflammatory fibrosing eye disease related to hyperthyroidism, toxic struma, and, rarely, Hashimoto thyroiditis. In this autoimmune disorder, autoantibodies are formed against TSH receptors of the eye muscles. The inflammation and fibrosis in the eye muscles and orbital space cause edema and proptosis. Other symptoms are tearing, photophobia, pressure sensation, and pain. The clinical signs are grouped in the NOSPECS system, which classifies six disease categories and three degrees of severity; the sum of parameters is the ophthalmopathy index (Table 89.9). The diagnosis is affirmed with ultrasound, CT or MRI, and thyroid diagnostics. Other orbital diseases (pseudotumor orbitae, malignoma, lymphoma, or metastases) have to be excluded, particularly for unilateral exophthalmus. Histologic proof is required in exceptional cases. The eye symptoms are carefully followed during the clinical course by the ophthalmologist, and the thyroid disorder is managed by the endocrinologist.

Nonradiotherapeutic Treatment

Many treatments have been used for Graves orbitopathy, including corticosteroids, cyclosporine, surgery, plasmapheresis, and RT, but the optimal therapy for individual patients has not been determined. Moreover, spontaneous remission is always possible. Euthyreosis in case of underlying thyroid disease is the most important precondition. Risk factors like nicotine abuse have to be eliminated. For mild but progressive EO, topical therapy alone is recommended. More severe EO requires sys-

temic glucocorticoids. Operative corrective measures on eyelids and muscles are undertaken in stable disease conditions when diplopy has not recurred. Rarely, orbital fatty tissue is resected for severe exophthalmus and cosmetic impairment. Emergency surgery aims to decompress the optic nerve by removal of one or several bony walls of the eye socket.

Radiotherapeutic Options

Ionizing radiation affects cellular reactions mediated either by T lymphocytes during the early stage or by fibroblasts during the later stages of EO, but different dose effects are required. The broad range of "effective RT concepts" probably reflects these different aspects. According to two studies, low-dose RT is very effective for early inflammatory EO, but efficacy of other measures is possible and spontaneous remission may also occur. Medium-dose RT is indicated in progressive and recurring disease in which combined measures are required. Modern treatment guidelines for RT of EO were compiled by Donaldson et al. (24) (Table 89.10).

Radiotherapeutic Technique

Both orbits are irradiated via lateral opposing fields in head mask fixation with 6- to 10-MV photons. CT planning is advised. Half-beam technique or lateral fields with 10-degree posterior angled fields are used for sparing lens and posterior eye chamber. Blocks are used to protect the paranasal sinuses and intracranial structures. The center beam or anterior field border, respectively, is controlled daily and adjusted to 5 to 6 mm behind the iris or pupil on both sides. The posterior field border covers the ring of Zinn at the superior orbital fissure and thus

Table 89.10	GUIDELINES FOR RADIOTHERAPY OF ENDOCRINE ORBITOPATHY (EO)		
Radiotherapy Goals	Precondition/Indications	Contraindications
1. Bring about clinical regression	*Pretherapeutic diagnostics:* evidence of autoimmune disease of the thyroid gland; CT/MRI	Stable EO without clinical Progression
2. Reduce/eliminate functional deficits	*Ophthalmologic diagnostics:* documented progression	Lack of euthyreosis
3. Improve cosmetics/esthetics	*Subjective/objective findings:* evidence of functional deficits and disorders	"Cosmetic" indication alone, without functional impairment
4. Avoid/decrease undesired effects of other measures	*Exclusion of risk factors:* no other eye disease (e.g., diabetic retinopathy)	No consent to planned therapy

| Table 89.11 | RADIATION RESPONSE IN TERMS OF NOSPECS CATEGORIES AND SYMPTOMS |

Study	No. of Patients	EO Duration (years) (range)	Relative Response for Each NOSPECS Category (%)						Comment
			Cat. II S	Cat. III P	Cat. IV E	Cat. V C	Cat. VI S	Total	
Bartalena et al., 1983 (4)	36 Ⓡ	2.3 (0.3–15)	97	56	93	– –	100	72	C + RT, 100%; versus C
	12		100	45	56		100	25	alone; eye-op, 3%
Friedrich et al., 1997 (45)	106 Ⓡ	0.8 (0.4–4)	56	62	70	——	——	78(26 Gy)	106, only RT; 142, C + RT;
	142		79	56	70			80 (13 Gy)	eye-op, 3%
Hurbli et al., 1985 (61)	62	0.6 (0.1–1.5)	—	23	74	23	57	56	C + RT, >23%; eye-op, 34%
Prummel et al., 1993 (133)	28 Ⓡ	NA	64	—	43	——	——	50	Only C
	28		38	—	85			46	C + RT
Petersen et al., 1990 (128)	311	0.9 average	80	51	56	71	65	—	C + RT, 32%; eye-op, 29%
Staar et al., 1997 (168)	225	0.7 (0.2–3)	80	64	69	—	—	68	C + RT, 100%; eye-op, 29%
Seegenschmiedt (156) et al., 1998	60	1.5 (0.5–20)	83	70	69	87	47	87	Failure after C; RT only; eye-op, 8%

Ⓡ, randomized study; C, corticosteroids; RT, radiotherapy; eye-op, operation (diplopy, lid correction, decompression); NA, no data available.

the entire length of the eye muscles. Adequate dose delivery to the target volume requires field sizes of 5 × 6 (12 for half-beam) centimeter.

Results of Radiotherapy

Clinical studies reporting "good clinical responses" are of limited value as stage-related analysis (including NOSPECS categories) and confounding variables were not analyzed. Response has to be analyzed for all EO categories and degrees of symptoms, and follow-up should be at least 6 to 12 months because clinical response may occur slowly. Adequate clinical studies using RT alone or in combination and meeting these criteria are shown in Table 89.11.

In a placebo-controlled randomized study, Mourits et al. (112) showed no additional symptomatic benefit of RT for EO categories I through III, but very good benefit for advanced EO categories IV and V. They concluded that RT is best indicated for EO categories IV through VI, nonrecurrent symptoms of grade 2–3 and in patients with orbitopathy index of >4. Short-term high-dose corticoid therapy may precede RT but is not a precondition for RT. A prospective randomized study found that orbital RT combined with corticosteroids was superior to corticosteroids alone, and another double-blind study showed that RT alone was more effective than RT with high-dose corticos-

teroids, but no stage-dependent analysis of those results was carried out.

Petersen et al. (128) reported results from 311 patients. The best response occurred in the NOSPECS categories "soft tissue" (II), "cornea" (V), and "loss of vision" (VI), but the condition of >50% patients with "proptosis" (III) and "eye muscle involvement" (IV) also improved after RT. They found several prognostic factors including age, gender, use of thyreostatic therapy, and functional thyroid status. About 30% required surgical correction of eye muscles or eyelids after RT, which does not reflect no effectiveness of RT! In individual cases, RT may replace eye surgery or corticosteroids when there is a relevant contraindication. Figure 89.7 shows a clinical example of the effectiveness of irradiation in combination with cortisone therapy.

Low-dose RT produces minor acute side effects. Cataract or retinopathy is triggered by inadequate RT technique or dosimetric mistakes. Existing eye diseases may be misinterpreted as radiation sequelae in advanced stages of EO. Using Monte-Carlo simulation for 10 × 2 Gy with 5 × 5 cm^2 opposing fields at a cobalt-60 machine, a theoretical tumor induction risk of 1.2% was calculated in a 20-year-old female patient; after optimization of RT technique, the radiation exposure and risk were reduced by 50%. Overall, appropriately indicated and delivered RT for advanced EO categories IV through VI offers a favorable risk-benefit ratio.

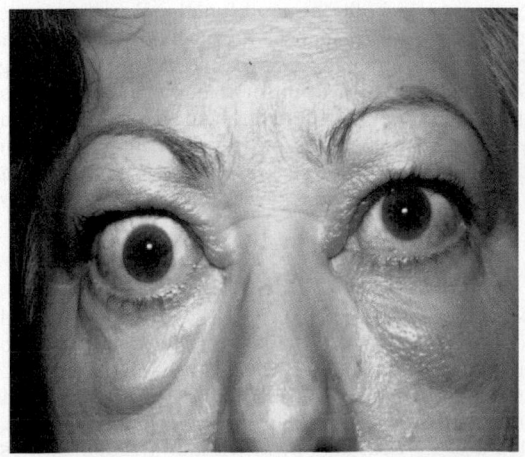
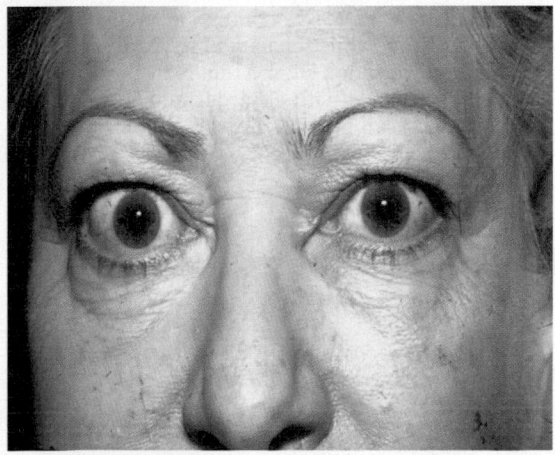

FIGURE 89.7. Percutaneous radiotherapy (RT) and corticoid therapy for eyelid edema and strabismus in a 50-year-old patient (before RT and 3 months after start of RT treatment).

Reactive Lymphoid Hyperplasia/ Pseudotumor Orbitae

Background and Clinical Aspects

Lymphoid orbital disease is rare and may include pseudotumor orbitae and malignant lymphomas. Pseudotumors of the orbit (PO) appear in up to 7% of all orbital tumors. The etiology is unclear with three possible causes: (a) infectious process (e.g., transmitted sinusitis), (b) autoimmune process (circulating antibodies against extraocular muscle proteins), and (c) fibroproliferative process. PO contains histologically fibrous, hypocellular chronic inflammatory foci. Other causes of orbital space requirement such as granulomatous diseases (e.g., sarcoidosis, Wegener granulomatosis), local infections, or autoimmune diseases have to be excluded.

Acute onset of symptoms, unilateral affection, and impaired eye motility points to PO. Retrobulbar pain, eyelid swelling, and exophthalmus appear most frequently (65% to 95%). Bilateral forms occur in up to 50%. CT and MRI reveal infiltrates in retrobulbar adipose tissue (up to 80%), enlarged eye muscles (up to 60%), optic nerve thickening (up to 40%), and proptosis bulbi (up to 70%) together with increased contrast agent uptake in 95%. Histologic backup is useful, as PO is a "chameleon" in terms of diagnostics and treatment, which is often unmasked as a malignant disease later.

Nonradiotherapeutic Treatment

Local excision is useful in accessible lesions, but relapses are frequent. Corticosteroids are the mainstay of treatment, but up to 50% of patients have no or insufficient response; others have to discontinue medication because of side effects or have contraindications for steroids. Without treatment, visual acuity can deteriorate permanently, but there is no correlation between duration of progression and irreversible loss of vision. Moreover, the potential of PO for malignant transformation is currently not clear.

Radiotherapeutic Options

The use of RT is indicated for recurrent, surgically not accessible, and medication-refractory lesions after histologic proof has been obtained. Adequately administered RT achieves long-term complete remission in 70% to 100% of cases (Table 89.12). Single doses vary between 0.5 to 3.0 Gy and 20 to 35 Gy total dose. Different adjustment techniques and application of certain radiation qualities, similar to the use for Graves orbitopathy, help to keep radiogenic side effects low.

A planning CT is mandatory to apply 4 to 6 MV photons via anterior and lateral fields with 1:3 weighting and wedged filters for dose homogenization while the patient's eyes are open. In unilateral disease and location of the tumor in the eyelid or conjunctiva, an anterior field with electrons and "hanging" lens block (diameter, 1 cm) can be used. Six to 9 MeV electrons are used in superficial lesions, and 16 to 20 MeV electrons in deeper lesions. In bilateral affection, parallel opposing lateral fields with semiblock technique or two anterior electron fields are used.

At onset, an attempt of low-dose RT with 2 × 0.5 Gy per week up to 5 Gy total dose (first series) is recommended: in acute or chronic inflammation, low-dose RT can initiate early response and may keep total dose as low as possible to minimize radiogenic side effects; if nonresponsive, daily fractionation is increased to 1.5 to 2 Gy single dose up to 30 to 40 Gy total dose (second series), a dose also effective for low-grade non-Hodgkin lymphoma. However, if total doses of 35 Gy are unsuccessful, other causes are likely, such as Wegener granulomatosis.

Few severe complications are observed. During RT, inflammatory signs may appear more intensely and require use of corticosteroids. With higher RT doses, there may be a hypolacrimation ("dry eye syndrome") and cataract formation in the long run. The theoretic risk of tumor induction has to be weighed against immediate eye dysfunction, loss of visual acuity, or eye enucleation.

Diseases of Joints and Tendons

General Aspects

Using RT for painful joint and tendon disorders is controversially discussed. Placebo-controlled studies have revealed no additional benefit for using RT compared with sham treatment, but from a modern perspective all studies had severe method deficiencies, which have to be substituted by modern study concepts and clear inclusion criteria. RT is a last-resort approach after failure of other noninvasive treatments, but before surgery is indicated. Recommended RT concepts use daily fraction doses of 0.5 Gy up to 3 Gy for acute inflammation, and 0.5 to 1.0 Gy are applied two to three times per week up to 6 Gy for chronic inflammatory reactions; in case of minor response, a second series is delivered after 6 weeks.

Numerous noninvasive measures are employed, often without better evidence for long-term response, including local or systemic pain medication (e.g., analgesics, antiphlogistics, corticoids, or local anesthetics). Physio- and electrophysical therapy (heat, cold, ultrasound) and immobilization of affected joints and tendons with casts or tapes or efforts to balance incorrect movements with orthoses (e.g., shoe inlays) are other applied measures without high evidence of results. After noninvasive measures have failed, surgery is the last option by using partial or total joint replacement.

Subjective and objective criteria are required for treatment evaluation, as both pain and functional performance are measures of clinical response. It is useful to evaluate pain symptoms in different categories (pain at strain, during night, during day time, at rest or at onset of motion) using a 1 to 10 visual analogue scale. Joint function can be evaluated quantitatively with established scores. In Germany, national guidelines and RT concepts were developed by professional associations over a decade using national surveys or patterns of care studies.

Degenerative Osteoarthritis

Degenerative osteoarthritis (OA) designates a painful joint process associated with cartilage destruction, bone modification, and structural changes of capsule and synovia. The typical arthralgia is caused by reactive inflammation of joint surface and joint capsule lining (synovia). Degenerative OA increases significantly with age: even without symptoms, most 60-year-old individuals show typical signs of arthrosis in plain radiographs (Table 89.13). Usually there is a disproportion of strain

Table 89.12			**RESPONSE TO RADIOTHERAPY (RT) OF PSEUDOTUMOUR ORBITAE**
Study	**N**	**Dose (Gy)**	**Results**
Lanciano et al., 1989 (88)	32	20	77% Local control, 53 Mte
Keleti et al., 1992 (77)	45	20–30	83% Local control
Wagner et al., 1992 (183)	18	8–18	67% Local control
Notter et al., 1997 (118)	10	2–3, >30	2–3 Gy: 50% NED, + 2nd RT series: 90% NED, 2–15 y

Mte, NED,

Table 89.13	RADIOLOGIC STAGING OF ARTHROSIS ACCORDING TO KELLGREN AND LAWRENCE (1957)	
Stage	**Description**
I	No osteophytes No narrowing of joint space Low subchondral sclerosis
II	Commencing formation of osteophytes Slight narrowing of joint space Moderate irregularities of joint contours and surfaces
III	Pronounced formation of osteophytes Clear narrowing of joint space Clear irregularities of joint contours and surfaces Subchondral cyst formation
IV	Pronounced narrowing of joint space up to the point of complete destruction Deformation and necrosis of the respective counterjoint

and "stress capacity" of the joint, causing wear and typical degeneration of the joint. The course is enhanced by congenital (dysplasia) and acquired (deformity, axial deviation, trauma) disorders. Some metabolic dysfunctions may favor development of arthrosis as well (e.g., diabetes mellitus or hyperuricemia).

Localized pain is the key symptom of reactive synovialitis caused by chronic stress through cartilage abrasion (activated arthrosis). This is followed by irritation of joint capsule and tendon attachment sites (periarthrosis) causing joint-dependent muscle tension. Subjective symptoms and radiographic findings are often incongruent. Functional loss has an impact on professional and leisure activities and reduces quality of life. Objective findings are joint reddening, hyperthermia, and swelling due to effusion, joint grinding, deformity, reduced mobility, and typical radiologic signs (Fig. 89.8).

Nonradiotherapeutic Treatment

Prevention and early recognition are crucial; prearthrotic changes (axial malposition, incongruent joint surfaces) are treated with corrective osteotomy. Noninvasive measures are described in 6.1. Invasive measures include arthroscopic lavage, debridement of inflammatory synovial changes, and smoothing of chondral joint surface. Autologous cartilage replacement to repair damaged chondral surfaces is possible in individual cases for small joint areas. Partial or total joint replacement with an artificial implant is the last option, but the patency rate of implants is only 10 to 15 years.

Radiotherapeutic Options

Low-dose RT is indicated if noninvasive measures have failed and surgery is not compulsory. It may reduce pain and pain-related dysfunction, but does not remove pathomorphologic changes. The affected joints of the upper (shoulder, elbow, thumb, fingers) and lower (hip, knee, ankle) extremity are irradiated via enface, lateromedial or ventrodorsal opposing fields using the orthovolt (150 to 200 kV/20 mA, 4-mm Al filter) or linear accelerator low-energy photons (<6 MV). The dose reference point is always located in the center of the joint (for opposing field setup)

RT can lead to primary freedom from pain and secondary to improved joint function. Numerous uncontrolled studies have been published and almost all have reported long-term pain relief and functional gain in 50% to 75%. A pain record of >2 years and objective findings like joint grinding, deformity, radiologic OA stage IV, are indicators of unfavorable prognosis.

In a monocenter study, 103 painful joints received 6 to 12 Gy low-dose RT after failing available conservative treatments. Established orthopaedic scores were applied for response evaluation. A total of 63% joints improved significantly in long-term follow-up (19% free of symptoms; 44% pain relief, and functional gain of >50%). It was concluded that RT is a very effective treatment option for pain reduction in refractory OA compared with other methods. Because of very low risk of side effects and low costs, RT provides an excellent alternative to conventional conservative treatments and in case of inoperability. Joint replacement surgery might be delayed or completely avoided in individual cases. Results of RT and a literature review have been provided by Keilholz et al. (76).

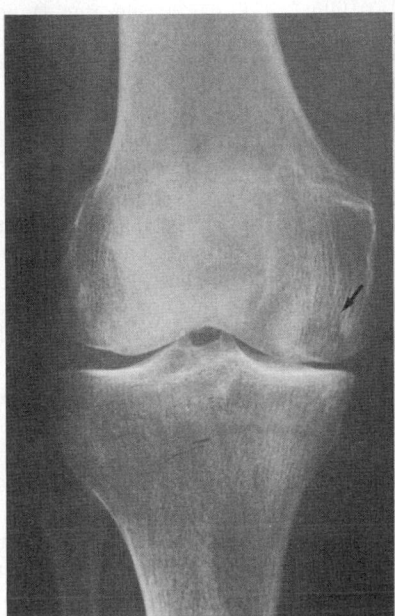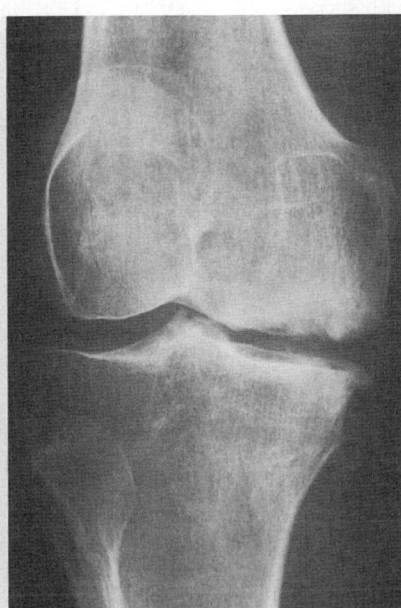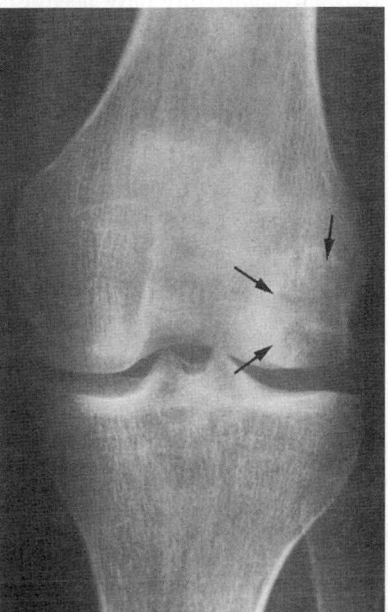

FIGURE 89.8. Typical signs of arthrosis: narrowing of joint space (**left**, *arrow*), incongruency and sclerosis of joint surfaces (**center**), and subchondral cysts (**right**, *arrows*).

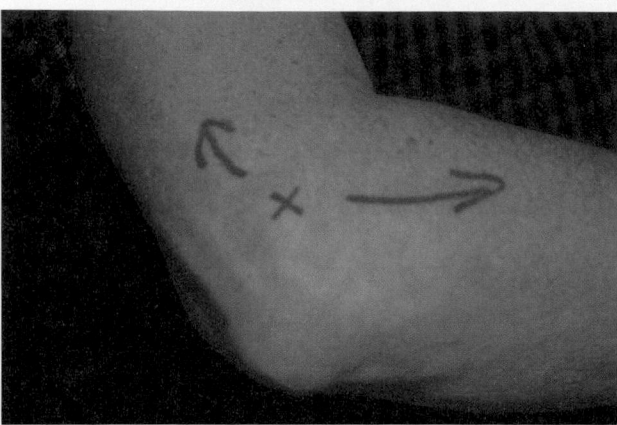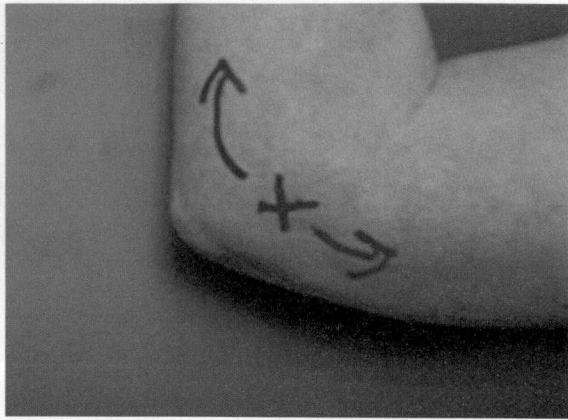

FIGURE 89.9. Typical pain pressure points and pain extension in radial or ulnar epicondylopathia humeri (EPH). **Left:** tennis elbow (EPH radialis). **Right:** golfer's elbow (EPH ulnaris).

Tendonitis and Bursitis

Acute and chronic strain together with macro- or micro-trauma at tendons and their attachment site can cause acute and chronic inflammation about the tendon (paratendonitis/tendonitis), at the attachment sites at the bones (insertion tendinopathy), and at the neighboring bursae. The local pain in tendon, tendon attachment, or bursa may radiate distally or proximally in the corresponding muscles and cause functional impairment. Particularly affected are the shoulder (peritendinopathia humeroscapularis), the elbow (epicondylopathia humeri or tennis/golfer's elbow), the ankle joint (plantar fasciitis), Achilles tendon (achillodynia), and the heel region (calcaneodynia), which are frequently associated with osseous changes close to the joint or bone (Fig. 89.9).

General management includes immobilization and protection of joint function during the acute inflammatory stage that often leads to spontaneous remission within weeks. As in degenerative OA, numerous conservative procedures have been employed, such as local cold or heat, administration of analgesics and antiphlogistics, local injections of anesthetics and corticosteroids; physiotherapy (stretching/deep friction technique) is a reasonable treatment; sometimes, shock wave therapy, electrotherapy, or acupuncture have been used with success, but the level of evidence is low because of lack of controlled clinical studies. Surgical measures are indicated in chronic-recurrent cases.

The indication for RT is given when conservative measures have failed and before use of surgery. Local and systemic medication can be continued during RT. Local response to irradiation is often preceded by short-term intensification of pain about the irradiated tendon or bursa. Depending on which region is affected, different technical adjustments are required for RT at the orthovolt machine (100 to 300 kV) or at the linear accelerator (6 to 10 MV), respectively.

Rotator Cuff Syndrome

Background and Clinical Aspects

Rotator cuff syndrome (periarthropathia humeroscapularis; subacromial syndrome) describes a condition of pain and functional loss of the shoulder joint. All muscular structures, tendons, and bursae of the shoulder region can be affected. The actual underlying cause remains unclear. Numerous conditions may trigger this problem: acute or chronic inflammation of the shoulder joint itself (arthritis, capsulitis), of the sheath tissue (bursitis), and of different tendons or tendon attachment sites

(tendonitis); local calcifications or ossifications are signs of a chronic reactive disease process.

Painful pressure points close to affected tendons and muscle attachment zones or about bursae are characteristic. Pain-related abduction and rotation impairment is typical. Lifting and carrying heavy objects and, particularly, overhead movements are difficult. Stress-related pain impairs professional and leisure activities. Radiologically, degenerative changes of the shoulder joint are seen, and soft tissue changes can be detected by MRI. A cervical spine syndrome has to be excluded.

Nonradiotherapeutic Treatment

As already described, local injections (corticoids, anesthetics), oral antiphlogistics and analgesic, and physical therapy and physical measures are frequently employed. In particular situations, surgical measures are also indicated, as in the case of tendon rupture. If the conservative measures fail, radiation therapy is indicated prior to any invasive procedure.

Radiotherapeutic Options

RT can be applied with an orthovolt machine (200 to 250 kV, 15 mA, 1-mm Cu filter) or linear accelerator. Opposing fields are applied for shoulder joint-related pain, and localized tendinopathies can be irradiated via direct single fields. The dose reference point is located in the center of the affected joint (5 to 8 cm) or at the depth of the tendon attachment site (1 to 2 cm). Field sizes range between 10×10 to 10×15 cm².

Pain relief and improved mobility has been reported in up to 80% of patients. The pain record (>2 years) and the extent of joint modifications (accompanying arthrosis) are determinants for prognosis. Short-term intensification of pain during the RT series is frequently a favorable sign for clinical response. In case of residual pain and functional deficit after one RT series of 6×1 Gy, a second series of RT is indicated. The clinical improvement is often long-lasting (Table 89.14).

Tennis/Golfer's Elbow

Background and Clinical Aspects

Tennis or golfer's elbow (epicondylitis humeri radialis or ulnaris) is a painful inflammation of the tendon attachment site of the finger and hand muscles of the radial (lateral) or ulnar (medial) epicondylus of the upper arm, impairing flexion and extension function of finger and hand muscles. The clinical situation is termed *tennis elbow* or golfer's elbow but has many causes, such as intensive fine and gross motor activity, extreme

Table 89.14	RADIOTHERAPY FOR REFRACTORY ROTATOR CUFF SYNDROME: SELECTED STUDIES				
Study	Year	No. of Cases	Pain-Free (CR) (%)	Pain Improved (PR/MR) (%)	Total Response (CR/PR/MR) (%)
Seegenschmiedt and Keilholz (156)	1998	89	49%	32	81
Zwicker et al. (195)	1998	77	33%	55	88
Adamietz and Sauer (2)	2003	107	65%	14	79

CR, complete freedom from pain; PR, clear of symptoms; MR, moderate improvement of symptoms.

strain of the arm or awkward movements during exercise, traumatic or mechanical irritation of the bursae at the radial head and articular constriction of the right deep radial nerve. Genders are equally affected; average age for either condition is 45 years.

First symptoms appear during stress, later also during night and day as constant pain, resting pain, and startup pain (in the morning). Affected people are impaired in professional work and leisure activities. Radiographs rarely demonstrate clear findings; MRI may uncover typical soft tissue modifications (edema of muscles and insertion zone). Cervical spine syndrome has to be excluded.

Nonradiotherapeutic Treatment

Spontaneous remission is often possible. During the acute stage, the elbow joint is relieved by bandages or immobilized with cast; antiphlogistic and analgesic medication is applied for relief; local measures include microwaves, ultrasound, friction physical therapy, underwater massage and warm packages; injections of cortisone and anesthetics complement the noninvasive therapeutic spectrum. In refractory cases, surgery is performed to relieve the aponeurosis of the extension or flexion muscles from stress; sensory cutaneous branches of radial or ulnar nerve in the elbow region are cut. The success rate after surgery is almost 80%.

Radiotherapeutic Options

If noninvasive treatments have failed, RT is indicated and applied using orthovoltage photons (100 to 150 kV, 20 mA, 4-mm Al filter) or linear accelerator low-energy photons (<6 MeV). A stationary field is targeted directly to the affected lateral or medial epicondylus. The dose reference point is calculated at a depth of 5 mm.

Even for chronic pain, RT achieves good pain reduction in up to 80% of cases, but for cases with >12 months pain record, the response is worse than for early RT. Relapses after therapeutic success are rare (5%). Disease record (>1 year), number of previous treatments, and long immobilization are unfavorable prognostic results; they are cofactors for the existence of a "chronic pain syndrome." If pain reappears after surgery, RT as "salvage therapy" is successful in about 50% of cases; the same holds true for response to surgery after RT.

Calcaneodynia/Achillodynia

Background and Clinical Aspects

Calcaneodynia (heel pain) and achillodynia (Achilles tendon pain) are pain syndromes of the heel region. Frequently, the entire osseous and tendinous system of the foot and legs is impaired in terms of statics and function (e.g., flatfoot, splayfoot, and skew foot deformities) or through genu varum or valgum

malposition. The chronic stress may lead to plantar and dorsal osseous spurs of up to 20 mm in length. Short-term vigorous forces or malpositions and minitrauma are triggering factors. Both genders are affected equally; the incidence increases with age. Running and sports with sudden or impulsive movements may lead to an earlier onset of disease. MRI frequently uncovers further modifications such as inflammatory changes of bursae or local irritation of the periosteum and bone edema of the calcaneum. In achillodynia, a painful lumpy or strandy thickening along the Achilles tendon is observed, originating from the peritendineum or directly within the tendon itself (Fig. 89.10).

Nonradiotherapeutic Treatment

Spontaneous remission may occur at any time. Potential anatomic malpositions are corrected to avoid further stress. The painful heel can be relieved by special cushion inlays. Local injections (with corticoids, anesthetics) and oral antiphlogistics or analgesics are used for immediate pain relief; physical therapy and physical measures (cold, ultrasound, microwaves, shock waves) have a supportive effect. Surgical incision of the plantar fascia is only done if conservative therapy fails because it is associated with several risks (infection, wound-healing defects, strong scar formation).

Radiotherapeutic Options

RT is indicated if noninvasive treatment fails. The affected plantar or dorsal region of the heel is irradiated using orthovolt photons (100 to 150 kV, 20 mA, 4-mm Al filter) or linear accelerator with low-energy photons (<6 MeV). A stationary 6 × 6 to 8 × 8 cm² field (plantar) or opposing fields (dorsal) are used to deliver a dose of 3 to 6 × 0.5 to 1 Gy to the dose reference point located at a depth of 5 mm (stationary field) or at the center of the joint (opposing fields) (Fig. 89.11).

RT achieves high response rates of 65% to 100%; about 50% become completely pain-free (Table 89.15). Pain threshold and pain type are other important prognostic factors for response. In contrast to the plantar heel syndrome, the response for dorsal heel syndrome and achillodynia are less favorable. Clinical response, if achieved, is usually long-lasting.

∷ | Diseases of Connective Tissue and Skin

Desmoid (Aggressive Fibromatosis)

Background and Clinical Aspects

Desmoids are benign connective tissue tumors of deep muscular-aponeurotic structures in the region of muscle fascias, aponeuroses, tendons, and scar tissue. The incidence is 2–4 per 1 million per year. The female gender is more frequently

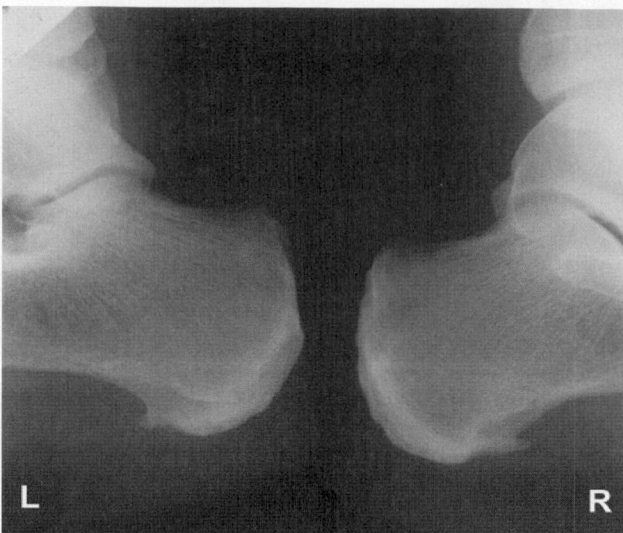 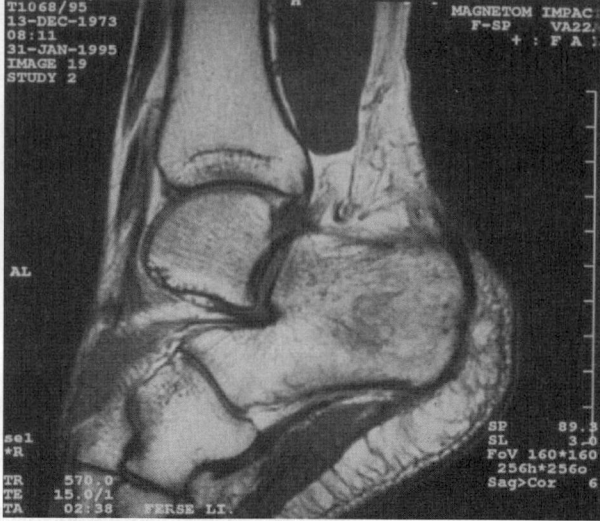

FIGURE 89.10. Radiologic and magnetic resonance tomographic imaging of plantar heel spur.

affected (1:1.5 to 2.5). Desmoids occur during the third and fourth decades of life, but also children can be affected. Extra- (70%) and intra-abdominal (10%) sites and abdominal wall (20%) are to be differentiated. The extra-abdominal type relapses more frequently, and the intra-abdominal type is associated with Gardner syndrome. Genetic factors, trauma, or surgical invention are considered to initiate the onset of desmoids. Pathohistologically, desmoids are similar to highly differentiated (G1) fibrosarcomas. The border to the surrounding tissue is mostly diffuse, which has led to the coining of the term *aggressive fibromatosis*. Diagnostics work-up with MRI helps to estimate size and infiltration into other organs and to prepare incision biopsy.

Nonradiotherapeutic Treatment

Desmoids may suspend spontaneously or grow fast, causing severe symptoms. Surgical removal with a safety margin of 2 to 5 cm is the "gold standard" and aims for R0 resection. After R0 resection, no therapy is required; in case of initial R1 resection, one may wait and treat the upcoming relapse. Depending on site and spread, long-term control can be achieved by resection alone, but up to 50% of patients require additional surgery and

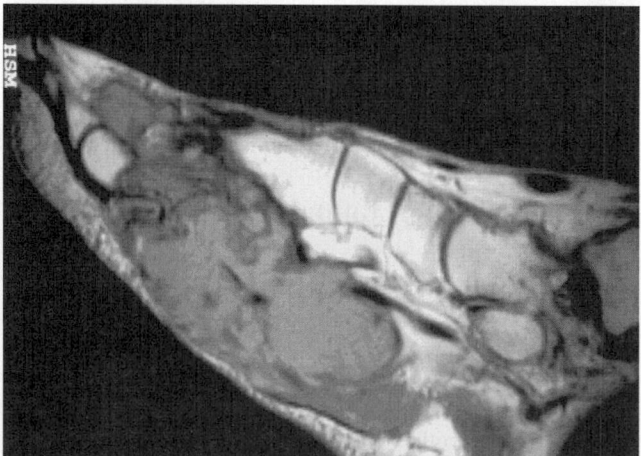

FIGURE 89.11. Desmoid of plantar region before starting primary radiotherapy.

other measures later because of local relapse. Tamoxifen and progesterone can exert growth inhibitory effects. Nonsteroidal antirheumatics and vitamin C and alkylating substances have been tested but are not yet established as treatment.

Radiotherapeutic Options

RT is indicated for inoperable cases, after R2 resection and R1 resection if repeated surgery was already applied. RT is often used as adjuvant or primary treatment; significantly reduced recurrence rates compared with surgery alone have been observed: with total doses of >50 Gy, recurrence rate decreased from 60% to 80% to 10% to 30%. Total dose of 50 to 55 Gy (single dose, 1.8 to 2.0 Gy) is recommended postoperatively; for inoperable or recurrent desmoids, the recommended total dose is 60 to 65 Gy. After primary RT, local control rate does not differ from those after adjuvant RT. In case of rest tumor or recurrence, 50 to 55 Gy achieve long-term local control in 70%.

In most studies, tumor size had no prognostic influence on local control. According to a meta-analysis (698 cases in 13 studies) local control after R0 resection and RT was improved by 17% compared with surgery alone; with macroscopic (R2) and microscopic (R1) tumor rests, patients with adjuvant RT had even better results than this. A patterns of care study on the treatment of desmoids was carried out in Germany collecting data on 345 patients. Location was in the extremities (81%), body trunk (14%), and head and neck region (5%). Fifty-nine percent of patients received primary RT for recurrent or unresectable lesions, and 41% received postoperative RT for high-risk situations (marginal or unclear resection). The median total dose was 60 Gy (range, 36 to 65 Gy) and the median single dose was 2 Gy (range, 1.6 to 2.2 Gy). The long-term local control rate was 81.4% after primary RT and 79.6% after resection and postoperative RT.

Induratio Penis Plastica (Morbus Peyronie)

Background and Clinical Aspects

Morbus Peyronie is a chronic, mostly progressive, inflammation and tissue proliferation of the penile tunica albuginea that affects men at 40 to 60 years. The cause is unknown, but diabetes mellitus and arterial and venous vascular disease are risk factors, along with an assumed genetic predisposition. Connective tissue disorders like Morbus Dupuytren(MD)/ Morbus

Table 89.15	RESULTS OF RADIOTHERAPY IN CALCANEODYNIA/ACHILLODYNIA/HEEL SPUR: SELECTED STUDIES				
Study	Year	No. of Cases	Pain-Free (CR) (%)	Improved (PR/MR) (%)	Total Response (CR/PR/MR) (%)
Seegenschmiedt et al.[a] (153)					
Group A	1996a	72	67	33	100
Group B	1996b	98	72	23	95
Oehler et al.	2000	258	81	7	88
Koeppen et al.	2000	673	13	65	78
Heyd et al. (58)	2001	127	46	42	88

CR, complete freedom from pain; PR, clear of symptoms; MR, moderate improvement of symptoms.
[a]Prospective controlled study: comparison of three different dosage groups.

Ledderhose (ML) are more frequent. First inflammatory changes occur at the tunica albuginea, followed by connective tissue reactions and formation of hard plaques, lumps, and cords (100%), which can either appear in herds or spread all the way from the penis root across the entire shaft. The strands lead to penile bending (80%), cause pain at erection (80%), and impair cohabitation (30% to 50%). Slow progression over several months is typical, but spontaneous remission may develop rarely.

Nonradiotherapeutic Treatment

So far there is no successful standard treatment. Vitamin E, para-aminobenzoate, and steroids have favorable influence during the early phase of morbus Peyronie. Local treatments are ultrasound or shock waves as well as treatment with corticoid, procaine, and hyaluronic acid injections, but their evidence is small. Resection and plastic surgery are associated with complications and are only carried out in advanced stages. RT may delay induration and lead to softening of lumps and strands, and may reduce pain, bending, and functional problems.

Radiotherapeutic Options

RT is best indicated during the early stages because in the later stages, there are hardly any radiosensitive fibroblasts and inflammatory cells remaining. RT is carried out with gonad protection (lead apron or capsule) and the glans penis is spared. With the orthovoltage machine, the nonerected penis is irradiated via a dorsal field; with the linear accelerator, electrons up to 6 MeV with 5 to 10 mm bolus are used. For extensive indurations, high dose rate brachytherapy is suitable.

Usually 20 Gy total dose with 2 Gy single dose and daily fractionation is recommended, but this may be extended to hypofractionation with 2 to 4 Gy single dose and two to four frac-

tions per week up to a total dose of 12 to 15 Gy. In case of nonresponse, it is recommended to repeat this regimen after 6 to 12 weeks up to a total dose of 30 Gy.

Within 1 to 2 years, RT leads to improvement of symptoms in two thirds of early-stage patients. Local pain and associated clinical symptoms decrease in up to 75%. Angulation (25% to 30%) and dysfunction of the penis (30% to 50%) show less response because these symptoms often indicate that the disease is already in a more advanced stage.

Morbus Dupuytren and Morbus Ledderhose

Background and Clinical Aspects

Morbus Dupuytren (MD) and Morbus Ledderhose (ML) are connective tissue disorders that affect the palmar or plantar aponeurosis and often bilateral affection. It is more common in the hands (MD) than in the feet (ML) and appears mostly between the ages of 40 and 70 years. The risk is increased with familial disposition, alcohol abuse, diabetes mellitus, epilepsy, and other conditions, but causes and pathogenesis are still not adequately determined. Initially, there is an inflammatory proliferative phase with fibroblast activity. Subcutaneous lumps with skin fixation appear; later, strands occur that may reach as far as to the periosteum. This is followed by the reparative phase with myofibroblast activity, which then moves on to the residual phase with strong scar formation (evidence of many collagen fibers). With increasing palmar (MD) or plantar (ML) connective tissue hardening, flexion contractures develop in the metacarpophalangeal or proximal interphalangeal joints, and grabbing (MD) or walking (ML) is impaired. Mostly, the fourth/fifth phalanges of the hand (MD) or the first/second toes of the foot (ML) are affected. The extent of the extension deficit determines the clinical staging in MD (Table 89.16; Fig. 89.12).

Table 89.16	CLASSIFICATION AND STAGING OF MORBUS DUPUYTREN (MD) ACCORDING TO TUBIANA ET AL. (1966)[a]	
Stage	Clinical Symptoms	Flexion Contraction/Extension Deficit (degree)
N	Clinical symptoms such as nodules, cords, skin retraction, and fixation without flexion contraction	
N/I[a]	Clinical symptoms plus total flexion contraction of fingers	1–10
I	Clinical symptoms plus total flexion contraction of fingers	11–45
II	Clinical symptoms plus total flexion contraction of fingers	46–90
III	Clinical symptoms plus total flexion contraction of fingers	91–135
IV	Clinical symptoms plus total flexion contraction of fingers	>135

[a]Modification by Keilholz et al., 1996 (175).

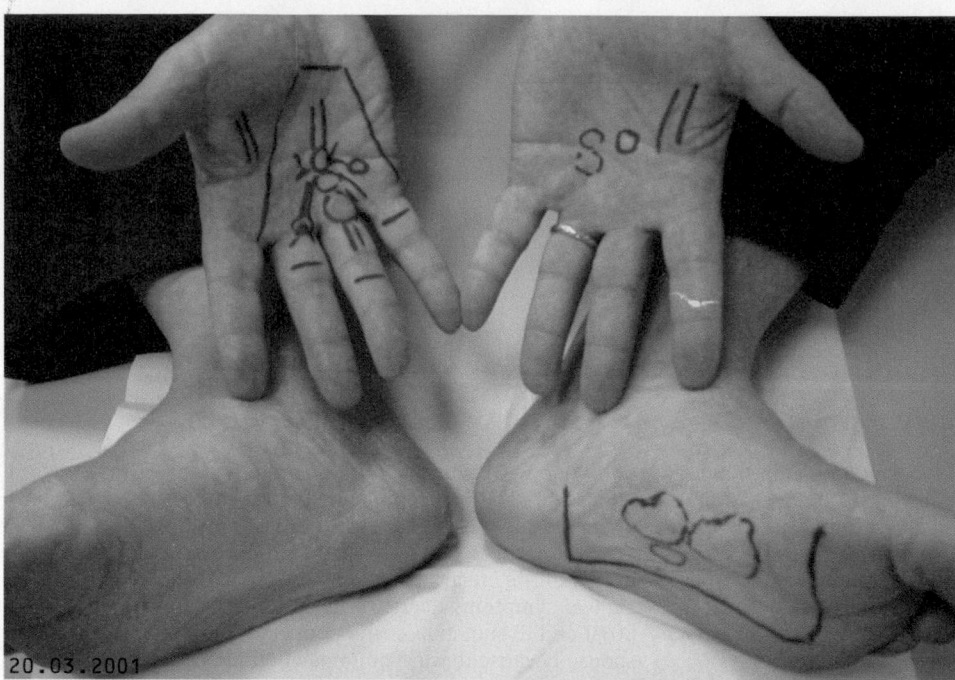

FIGURE 89.12. Morbus Dupuytren on both hands. Morbus Ledderhose on the left foot.

Nonradiotherapeutic Treatment

Without therapy, more than 50% of patients will have disease progression after 5 years. During the early stage, medication (steroids, allopurinol, nonsteroidal antiphlogistics, enzymes, vitamin E, and "softeners") are possible, but they are often without long-term effect. Surgery is indicated with functionally impairing flexion contractions of the fingers (>30 degrees) or in case of strong pain while walking. Local and total fasciectomy and limited or complete resection of palmar or plantar aponeurosis is carried out, but all surgical measures are burdened by complications (15% to 20%) and relapse in 30% to 50% of all cases at 3 years. Although spontaneous halt of progression is possible, a cure from the disease is not realistic at all; thus, preventive strategies become more important.

Radiotherapeutic Options

Because of the lack of alternatives, prophylactic use of RT during the early stages of MD and ML provide a good rationale and indication for RT. RT makes sense during the early stage (lumps, strands) with moderate extension deficit (≤10 degrees). The target cells are proliferating and radiosensitive fibroblasts and inflammatory cells. The goal of treatment is to avoid further progression or later surgery.

RT can be administered with orthovolt (100 to 150 kV photons) or linear accelerator with electrons (up to 6 MeV) via stationary field. Particular attention has to be paid to the protection of unaffected areas (individually adapted lead shields). A safety margin of 1 cm laterally and 2 cm proximally and distally is important to avoid recurrences at the edge of the field. Total dose of 20 to 30 Gy with fractionation of 2 to 3 Gy single dose were tested successfully. Repetition after 6 to 12 Wochen up to a total dose of 30 Gy is possible. Even single doses with 4 to 5 Gy every 1 to 2 months were clinically tried and tested with good results in the past. End points of therapy are permanent softening of lumps and strands, possibly improved function (in gripping and walking), and, primarily, avoiding potentially necessary surgery (Table 89.17).

Results of Radiotherapy

Many studies have shown good response to RT in terms of stabilization of the disease (70% to 80%). Regression of nodules and strands (20% to 30%) occurs in only a few early-stage patients. Disease progression in spite of previous irradiation occurs in 20% to 25%. Existing extension deficits are normally not improved; patients with extension deficits (stage I/II) have a significantly increased rate of recurrence or progression. Only a few studies have controlled long-term observation for >2 years or a controlled design for dose and therapy optimization.

In a phase II study, 25 patients (36 feet) received RT for symptomatic ML. Twelve patients had additional MD. The RT field involved all nodules and cords plus safety margin, and two RT series of 5 × 3 Gy up to a total dose of 30 Gy was applied. With a median follow-up of >3 years, none of the patients had experienced progression or underwent surgery and >50% experienced reduced symptoms and size of nodules and cords. Slight erythema (CTC 1) and dry skin was observed in three cases (11%) in long-term follow-up (>12 months). Thus, RT was very effective in treating ML and may have prevented otherwise necessary surgical interventions.

Keloids and Hypertrophic Scars

Background and Clinical Aspects

Keloids are an excessive tissue proliferation about scars after skin injury from surgery, heat, chemical burns, inflammation (e.g., acne), or even spontaneous proliferation. They differ from hypertrophic scars by their typical infiltrative growth pattern, causing local pain and inflammatory reactions, and sometimes long-term progression; hypertrophic scars show thickening without surrounding reaction and can flatten spontaneously. Keloids appear mostly in the upper body and in regions with high skin tension (e.g., sternum, earlobes). The cause is still unknown, although there is a genetic and race-specific predisposition that is already noted during adolescence. Keloids at the earlobe after piercing are typical. Disturbed cosmesis may be accompanied by pain, itching, and dysfunction (Fig. 89.13).

Table 89.17	CLINICAL RESULTS AND LONG-TERM OUTCOME AFTER RADIOTHERAPY OF KELOIDS					
Study	Year	No. of Cases	Total Dose (cGy)	Follow-Up (Months)	Control	%
Borok et al. (9)	1988	393	Variable doses (O)	Not stated	366	92
Kovalic and Perez (84)	1989	113	Variable doses (O)	12	82	73
Sallstrom et al. (142)	1989	117	18/3 Fx (O)	24	108	92
Lo et al. (95)	1990	168	8/15 (E)	1	146	87
Doornbos et al. (25)	1990	208	Variable doses	12	173	85
Escarmant et al. (29)	1993	570	8–30 (B) Iridium-192 implant	15; mean, 6.9 years	450 better; 53 stable; 52 worse; 120 recurrences	79 9 9 21
Rösler et al. (139)	1993	50	12–20	12	40	80
Guix et al. (50)	2001	169	12/18 (B) postop./primary RT Iridium-192 implant	24; mean, 4 years	147 better; 14 stable; 8 recurrences	87 8 5

O, orthovolt; Fx, fraction; E, electrons at the linear accelerator; B, brachytherapy iridium-192.

Nonradiotherapeutic Treatment

Besides surgical excision, it is possible to apply conservative measures by using pressure and silicon bandages, steroid injections, and application of plant extracts for small lesions. In >50% of patients, local relapse occurs that is not dependent on the type of resection (sharp excision, laser, cryotherapy).

Radiotherapeutic Options

Indications for RT are given for (repeated) recurrences postoperatively or high-risk situations (e.g., marginal resection, wider spread, unfavorable location). Primary RT is promising in cases of functional inoperability and in actively proliferating disorders within about 6 months after the triggering trauma. Proliferating fibroblasts and mesenchymal and inflammatory cells

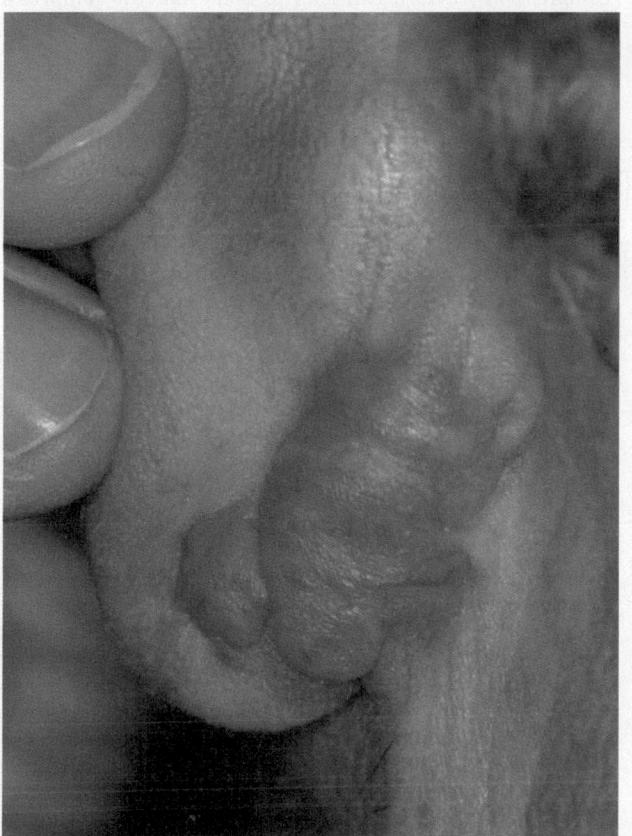
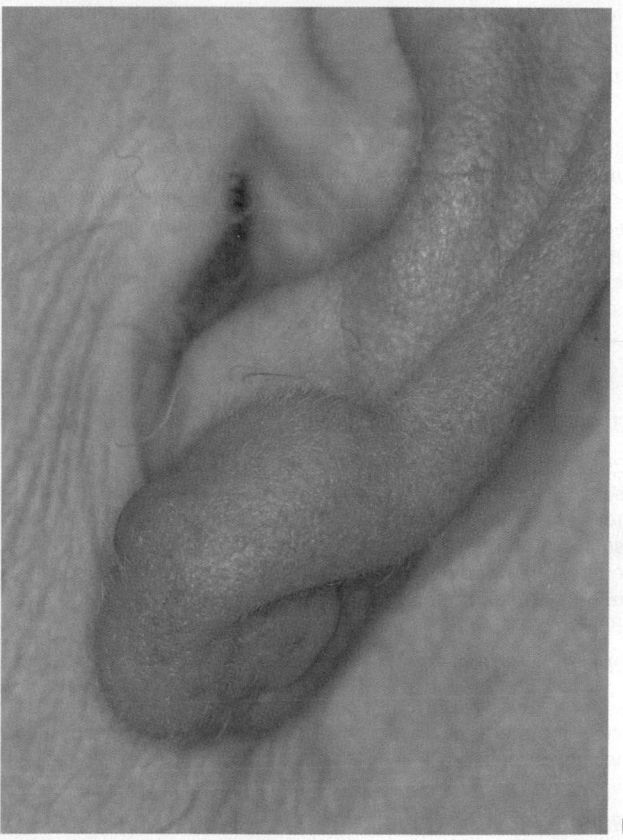

FIGURE 89.13. A: Keloid behind left earlobe. **B:** Status of keloid following resection plus 4 × 4 Gy radiotherapy.

are the target cells. Fully matured keloids hardly respond to primary RT; prophylactic RT immediately after excision of the recurrence is most effective. In only 20% to 25% of cases, recurrences occur after postoperative RT (Table 89.17).

RT is initiated 24 hours after surgery. Radiation quality has to be adapted to the local conditions. Conventional x-rays (70 to 150 kV), electrons (<6 MeV), and iridium-192 brachytherapy with implants or strontium-90 dermal plates are useful. The target volume is limited to the scar plus a 1-cm deep safety margin on both sides of the scar. Lead absorbers need to be prepared if required. The recommended total dose is 12 to 20 Gy; for example, 5 × 3 or 4 × 4 Gy within 1 week. Single-dose RT with 7.5 to 10 Gy is also effective. Clinical end points are long-term control, low relapse rate, and good cosmesis.

Diseases of Bony Tissues

Aneurysmatic Bone Cyst

Definition and Clinical Features

Aneurysmatic bone cysts are benign, vascular cystic lesions in the metaphase of bones, which cause functional impairment, pathologic fractures, and damage of neighboring structures. They can infiltrate into the surrounding soft tissue. In spite of their nonmalignant character, cysts can lead to bone destruction and evoke serious problems, which is why treatment is recommended once a cyst has been diagnosed, particularly if the vertebral column is affected.

Nonradiotherapeutic Measures

Surgery (resection or curettage) is the gold standard as long as this does not lead to a considerable functional impairment. Following curettage, recurrence occurs in up to 60% of patients. After complete resection, there is normally no recurrence.

Radiotherapeutic Options

RT is indicated if cysts cannot be treated by surgery or if curettage is difficult because of size or site of the lesion. Cyst progression or repeated recurrences are indications for RT. Inaccessible cysts of the vertebral column and the pelvis should be irradiated. Because >50% of patients are 10 to 19 years old, RT doses should be kept as low as possible. Ten to 20 Gy for 1 to 2 weeks seem to be an adequate dose to control the aneurysmatic bone cysts reliably.

Pigmented Villonodular Synovitis

Background and Clinical Aspects

Pigmented villonodulos synovitis (PVNS) is a rare proliferative disease affecting the synovia of joints and the tendon sheaths. There are two types of disease: the strictly localized and the diffuse affection of synovial membranes. In the majority of cases, the lesion is restricted to one joint and can spread to muscles, tendons, and skin membranes.

Nonradiotherapeutic Measures

Surgical excision normally consists of synovectomy, which is rarely complete, particularly in the large joints like the knee. Therefore, recurrences occur with a frequency of up to 45%.

Radiotherapeutic Options

RT can be applied with radionuclides for localized PVNS or with external-beam RT for diffuse PVNS. The most important study of external RT was conducted in Toronto when 41 patients with PVNS were reviewed retrospectively. After a mean follow-up of >8 years (range, 1 to 28 years), only 1 of 41 patients (98%) had residual disease. Most patients showed excellent functional results and only a few had fair function, but all patients were functionally better than before treatment. There was no RT toxicity and no amputation after combined treatment. The authors used 30 to 50 Gy in 15 to 20 fractions of 1.8 to 2.5 Gy as standard regimen for PVNS.

A recent German monocentric study reported on seven patients with diffuse PVNS who underwent radical surgery and postoperative RT with total doses of 30 to 50 Gy, depending on the resection status and estimated risk of relapse. With a mean follow-up of 29 months (range, 3 to 112 months), no evidence was found of recurrent or persistent disease in any patient. RT induced no acute adverse effects. The functional analysis revealed six patients with asymptomatic limb function and excellent quality of life, but there was one patient with persistent restriction of joint movement after repeated surgery. No radiogenic late effects were seen. The study concluded that combined treatment should be considered for all patients with suspected or proven residual D-PVNS.

Vertebral Hemangiomas

Background and Clinical Aspects

Vertebral hemangiomas (VHs) are benign lesions that can lead to a resorption of the affected bone. Usually only one vertebral body is affected. VHs are well diagnosed by their typical radiologic appearance: rarefied vertical, dense trabecles ("honeycomb pattern"). Most lesions are small and rare and require no therapy. In most cases, symptoms occur during the fourth or fifth decade of life. Women are more frequently affected than men. Spread of tumor into extradural space, hemorrhage, or compression fracture can lead to bone marrow compression and severe consequences.

Nonradiotherapeutic Measures

Transarterial embolization followed by laminectomy is a safe and effective procedure for treatment of cord compression by VH, causing stenosis without instability or deformity. Vertebrectomy preceded by embolization and followed by reconstruction can be used to treat cord compression from extraosseous extension. Transarterial embolization without decompression is effective for painful intraosseous hemangiomas. Vertebroplasty is useful for improving pain symptoms, especially when vertebral body compression fracture has occurred in patients without neurologic deficit, but is less effective in providing long-term pain relief. In most cases, only partial resection or occlusion of the lesion is possible and postoperative irradiation should be given.

Radiotherapeutic Options

Pain is the most frequent symptom; with bone marrow compression, motor deficits may occur as well. Heyd et al (58) and Rades et al. (134) reviewed the literature on the use of RT for symptomatic VH. They analyzed data of 339 patients with symptomatic VHs from publications of the last 50 years. However, 222 patients had to be excluded, either because surgery was part of the treatment or because the data were incomplete (n = 124). Of the remaining 117 patients, 54 patients received 36 to 44 Gy (group A) and 62 patients received 20 to 34 Gy (group B). After a median follow-up of 36 months (range, 6 to 312 months), 39% of group A and 82% of group B patients had complete pain relief, and the difference was highly significant (p = .003). Because no difference in toxicity was seen in either

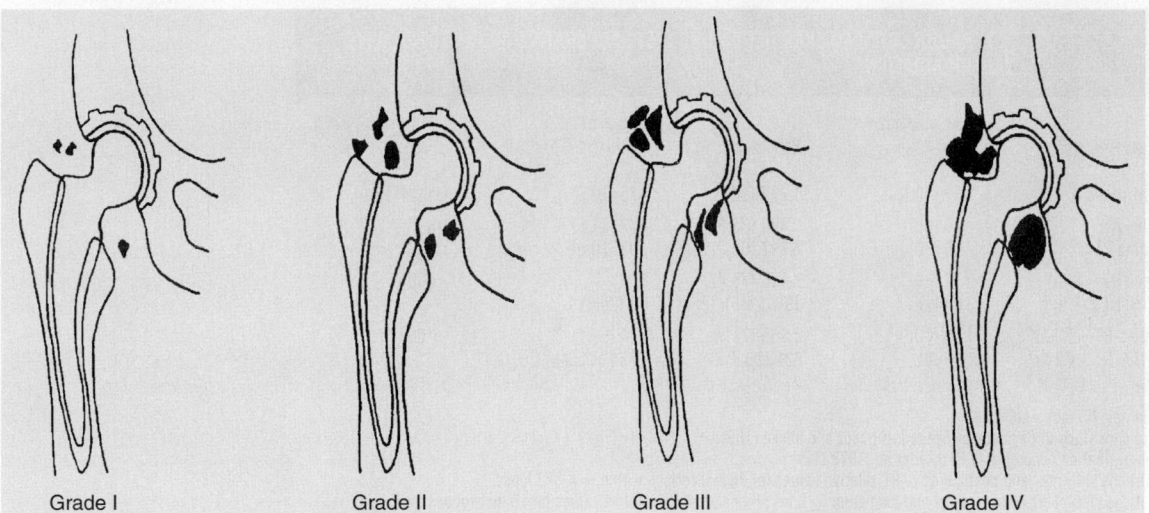

Grade I   Grade II   Grade III   Grade IV

FIGURE 89.14. Staging of heterotopic ossifications according to classification of Brooker et al. (1973). Grade I: Bone islands within soft tissue around hip. Grade II: Exophytes of pelvic or proximal femoral bone with a minimum distance of 1 cm. Grade III: Exophytes of pelvic or proximal femoral bone with a distance of <1 cm. Grade IV: Bony ankylosis between proximal femoral and pelvic bones.

group, treatment recommendation was a total dose of 40 Gy (single doses, 2 Gy).

Heterotopic Ossification

Background and Clinical Aspects

Heterotopic ossifications (HOs) develop in 10% to 80% of cases and with varying severity after trauma or surgery of the hip. They consist of real bone located in the periarticular soft tissue. About every third patient who has to face HO following total hip arthroplasty will develop pain and dysfunction resulting from extensive HO. Furthermore, HO jeopardizes functional outcome, impairs rehabilitation, and is costly because of secondary surgical procedures. The first pain symptoms start a few days after surgery; calcified structures with blurred contours are detectable by x-rays at 3 to 6 weeks postoperatively. The structures increase in size and density within a few weeks and develop to mature bone within 1 year. Predisposing factors for HO are skeletal diseases (Forestier disease, Bechterew disease) and severe trauma of the brain and spinal cord with comatous conditions and pareses.

The etiology of HO is not fully understood. It is assumed that pluripotent mesenchymal stem cells, which are present ubiquitously in periarticular soft tissue, under certain conditions develop into osteoblastic stem cells that finally form HOs. *In vivo* experiments showed that differentiation of osteoblastic stem cells reaches its maximum after 32 hours.

Patients with ipsi- or contralateral HO after a previous total hip arthroplasty carry the greatest risk to develop HO postoperatively (incidence, 90% to100%, high-risk group); patients with femoral or pelvic bone osteophytes >1 cm in length also carry an increased HO risk (incidence >50%; medium risk group). After acetabular or pelvic fractures, HO appears in 50% to 90%. Several interventions at the hip joint increase the risk of HO. Men are more likely to be affected than women. Ankylosing spondylitis and the (rare) disseminated idiopathic hyperosthosis of skeleton are predisposing factors.

Severe injuries of the skull and spinal cord with paraplegia may lead to HO in 11% to 76% of cases, where all large joints besides the hip can be affected. Severe injuries and diseases of the central nervous system, infections, or acute respiratory distress syndrome may also lead to massive HO about joints, although these joints had never previously been traumatized.

The literature provides a multitude of staging approaches. The most frequent one is the classification of HO according to

Brooker et al. (12; Fig. 89.14). According to Brooker et al., HO grades III and IV are designated severe or clinically relevant although there may not be any pain or mobility impairment, and some HO grades I and II may be already symptomatic.

Nonradiotherapeutic Treatment

Patients with symptomatic HO and those likely to develop clinically relevant postoperative HO because of individual risk factors are target groups for prophylactic treatment. Ethylhydroxydiphosphonates (EHDP) has been used for prevention of HO, but outcome was contradictory: EHDP inhibits the conversion of amorphous calcium phosphate to hydroxyapatite crystals and prevents mineralization of the bone matrix. Indomethacin, a prostaglandin synthesis inhibitor that inhibits inflammation reaction and suppresses proliferation of mesenchymal cells, is effective in patients at high risk. It is administered in different dosages immediately after surgery for about 3 to 6 weeks. Nevertheless, nonsteroidal anti-inflammatory drugs may trigger gastrointestinal or renal side effects.

Radiotherapeutic Options

Prophylactic RT to prevent HO has been employed since the late 1970s. Starting from initial dose concepts using 20 Gy in 10 fractions, effective regimens reduced total doses and fractions to as low as 7 Gy in 1 fraction or 6 Gy in 1 fraction, while 5 Gy in 2 fractions were insufficient. Higher total doses or more fractions provided no better outcome. Various studies pointed out that RT should be started no later than day 4 after surgery. It is important to keep the postoperative interval as short as possible (24 to 48 hours), particularly in high-risk patients with existing ipsi- or contralateral HO.

Preoperative RT with single fraction of 7 to 8 Gy has been successfully applied. There was no significant difference of clinically relevant HO compared with patients who were irradiated postoperatively, which was supported by experimental data. Finally, a prospective randomized study showed the equivalence of preoperative and postoperative RT for the prevention of HO after total hip arthroplasty, but with the exception of patients with preoperatively existing ipsi- or contralateral Broker grade III or IV HO, who should be irradiated exclusively postoperatively. The effect of timing was confirmed in a large patterns of care study involving 30 centers and 4,377 hips (Table 89.18).

Single dose pre- or postoperative RT is tolerated well. Neither RT concept has led to an increased frequency of perioperative bleeding, infection rate, or wound-healing disturbances.

Table 89.18	RADIOLOGIC FAILURES DEPENDING ON PREOPERATIVE OR POSTOPERATIVE IRRADIATION[a]			
Radiologic Result[b]	Institutions No. (%)	Hips No. (%)	Brooker Failures No. (%)	p Value
All RT institutions	30 (100)	4,377 (100)	475 (10.9)	Univariate
Preoperative RT[c]	19 (63)	1,480 (33.8)	172 (11.6)	NS
Postoperative RT[c]	15 (50)	2,897 (66.2)	303 (10.5)	
Preoperative RT ≤8 hr[d]	17 (89)	1,116 (75.4)	97 (8.7)	<.005
Preoperative RT >8 hr[d]	8 (42)	364 (24.6)	75 (20.6)	
Postoperative RT ≤72 hr[e]	15 (100)	2,065 (71.3)	124 (6.0)	<.001
Postoperative RT <72 hr[e]	9 (60)	832 (28.7%)	179 (21.5%)	

RT, radiotherapy; NS, not significant.
[a]Patterns of care study in Germany by Seegenschmiedt and Micke (159).
[b]Radiologic evaluation according to Brooker et al., 1973 (12).
[c]Two institutions with pre- and postoperative RT; relative values for 30 institutions with n = 4,377 hips.
[d]Six institutions with short-term (<8 hr) and long-term (≥8 hr) preoperative RT; relative values for 19 institutions with n = 1,480 hips.
[e]Nine institutions with short-term (<96 hr) and long-term (≥96 hr) postoperative RT; relative values for 15 institutions with n = 2,897 hips.

So far, none of the patients have developed a malignant tumor within the irradiation field postoperatively. Because radiation-induced tumors appear very rarely and only after latencies of 10 to 30 years, this risk is almost irrelevant as most patients are already in the fifth or sixth decade. For younger patients, medical prophylaxis appears to be more adequate.

With regard to the RT technique, the target volume should encompass the typical localizations of periarticular HO; the cranial field border is located approximately 3 cm above the acetabulum and includes about two thirds of the implant shaft. Thus, the usual field size is 14 × 14 cm. The dose reference point is the central beam at the center of the target volume (at about 8 to 12cm deep), HO prophylaxis can also be carried out in other body regions, such as the knee, elbow, shoulder, or jaw joints, or in paraplegic patients after CNS or spinal cord trauma.

Suggested Reading

1. Adamietz B, Keilholz L, Grünert J, Sauer R: Die Radiotherapie des Morbus Dupuytren im Frühstadium.Langzeitresuktate nach einer medianen Nachbeobachtungszeit von 10 Jahren. *Strahlenther Onkol*177:604–610(2001).
2. Adamietz B, Sauer R. Strahlentherapie beim Impingement-Syndrom des Schultergelenks. *Strahlenther Onkol* 2003;179(Sondernr. 1):1.
3. Augsburger JJ, Freire J, Brady LW. Radiation Therapy for Choroidal and Retinal Hemangiomas. In: Wiegel T, Bornfeld N, Foerster MH, Hinkelbein W (eds) Radiotherapy of Ocular Disease. *Front Radiat Ther Oncol. Basel, Karger, vol 30*, pp 265–280(1997)
4. Bartalena L, Marcocci C, Chiovato L, et al. Orbital cobalt irradiation combined with systemic corticosteroids for Graves' ophthalmopathy: comparison with systemic corticosteroids alone. *J Clin Endocrinol Metab* 1983;56:1139–1144.
5. Becker G et al. Radiation Therapy in the multimodal treatment approach of pituitary adenoma. *Strahlenth Onkol* 2002;4:173–186.
6. Becker G, Kortmann RD, Skaley M, et al. The role of radiotherapy in the treatment of craniopharyngioma—indications, results, side effects. *Front Radiat Ther Oncol* 1999;33:100–113.
7. Berger B, Ganswindt U, Bamberg M, et al. External beam radiotherapy as postoperative treatment of diffuse pigmented villonodular synovitis. *Int J Radiat Oncol Biol Phys* 67;(4):1130–1134.
8. Bloom HJ, Glees J, Bell J. The treatment and long-term prognosis of children with intracranial tumors: A study of 610 cases, 1950—1981. *Int J Radiol Oncol Biol Phys* 1990;18:723–745.
9. Borok TL, Bray M, Sinclair I, et al. Role of ionizing irradiation for 393 keloids. *Int J Radiol Oncol Biol Phys* 1988;15:865–870.
10. Bosse MJ, Poka A, Reinert CM, Ellwanger F, Slawson R, Mc Devitt ER: Heterotopic bone formation as a complication of acetabular fractures. *J Bone Joint Surg* 1988;70-A:1231–1237.
11. Bremnes RM, Hauge HN, Sagsveen R. Radiotherapy in the treatment of symptomatic vertebral hemangiomas: Technical case report. *Neurosurgery* 1996;39:1054–1058.
12. Brooker AF, Bowerman JW, Robinson RA, et al. Ectopic ossification following total hip replacement. *J Bone Joint Surg* 1973;55-A:1629–1632.
13. Bruns F, Kardels B, Schäfer U, et al. Strahlentherapie bei Induratio penis plastica. *Röntgenpraxis* 1999;52:33–37.
14. Burch HB, Wartofsky L. Graves' ophthalmopathy. Current concepts regarding pathogenesis and management. *Endocr Rev* 1993;146:747ff.
15. Castro JR, Linstadt DE, Bahary J-P, et al. Experience in charged particle irradiation of tumors of the skull base: 1977–1992. *Int J Radiat Oncol Biol Phys* 1994;29:647–655.
16. Chakravarty M, Gardiner TA, Archer DB, et al. Treatment of age-related subfoveal choroidal neovascular membranes by teletherapy: A pilot study. *Br J Ophthalmol* 1993;77:265–273.
17. Chandler JR, Goulding R, Moskowitz L, et al. Nasopharyngeal angiofibromas: Staging and management. *Ann Otol Rhinol Laryngol* 1984;93:322–329.
18. Char DH, Irvine AI, Posner MD et al. Randomized trial of radiation for age-related macular degeneration. *Am J Ophthalmol* 1999;127:574–578.
19. Ciric I, Rosenblatt S. Suprasellar meningiomas. *Neurosurgy* 2001;49:1372–1377.
20. Cummings BJ, Blend R, Keane T. Primary radiation therapy for juvenile nasopharyngeal angiofibroma. *Laryngoscope* 1984;94:1599–1605.
21. Debus J, Schulz-Ertner D, Schad L, et al. Stereotactic fractionated radiotherapy for chordomas and chondrosarcomas of the skull base. *Int J Radiat Oncol Biol Phys* 2000;47:591–596.
22. Debus J, Wuendrich M, Pirzkall A, et al. High efficacy of fractionated stereotactic radiotehrapy of large skull base meningiomas: Long-term results. *J Clin Oncol* 2001;19:3547–3553.
23. Dion JE, Mathis JM. Cranial arteriovenous malformations: The role of embolization and stereotactic surgery. *Neurosurg Clin North Am* 1994;5:459–474.
24. Donaldson SS, McDougall IR: Graves' Disease. Radiotherapy of intraocular and orbital tumors. In: Alberti WE, Sagerman RH (eds.): Radiotherapy of Intraocular and Orbital Tumors. Springer, Berlin (2nd edition), pp 145–152(2002)
25. Doornbos JF, Stoffel TJ, Hass AC, et al. The role of kilovoltage irradiation in the treatment of keloids. *Int J Radiat Oncol Biol Phys* 1990;18:833–839.
26. Doppman JL, Oldfield EH, Heiss JD. Symptomatic vertebral hemangiomas: Treatment by means of direct intralesional injection of ethanol. *Radiology* 2000;214:341–348.
27. Economou TS, Abemayor E, Ward PH. Juvenile nasopharyngeal angiofibroma: an update of the UCLA experience, 1960–1985. *Laryngoscope* 1988;13:40–47.
28. Engenhart R, Wowra B, Debus J, et al. The role of high-dose, single-fraction irradiation in small and large intracranial AVMs. *Int J Radiat Oncol Biol Phys* 1994;30:521–529.
29. Escarmant P, Zimmermann S, Amar A et al. The treatment of 783 keloid scars by Iridium 192 interstitial irradiation after surgical excision. *Int J Radiat Oncol Biol Phys* 1993;26:245–251.
30. Eustacchio S, Trummer M, Unger F, et al. The role of gamma knife radiosurgery in the management of glomus jugulare tumors. *Acta Neurochir Suppl* 2002;84:91ff.
31. Fields JN, Halverson KJ, Devineni VR, et al. Juvenile nasopharyngeal angiofibroma: efficacy of radiation therapy. *Radiology* 1990;176:263–265.
32. Fine SL, Maguire MG. It is not time to abandon radiotherapy for neovascular age-related macular degeneration. *Arch Ophthalmol* 2001;119:275–276.
33. Finger PT, Immonen I, Freire J, et al. Brachytherapy for macular degeneration associated with subretinal neovascularisation. In: Alberti WE, Richard G, Sagerman RH (eds.). Age-related Macular Degeneration. Current Treatment Concepts. Springer, Berlin: Springer; 2001: 167–173.
34. Fisch U, Mattox P. Microsurgery of the skull base. New York: Thieme; 1988.
35. Flanders AE, Mafee MF, Rao VM, et al. CT characteristics of orbital pseudotumors and other inflammatory orbital processes. *J Comput Assist Tomgr* 1989;13:40–47.
36. Fleetwood IG, Marcellus ML, Levy RP, et al. Deep arteriovenous malformations of the basal ganglia and thalamus: natural history. *J Neurosurg* 2003;98:747–750.
37. Flickinger JC, Kondziolka D, Lunsford L. Dose and diameter relationships for facial, trigeminal, and acoustic neuropathies following acoustic neuroma radiosurgery. *Radiother Oncol* 1996;41:215–219.
38. Flickinger JC, Kondziolka D, Lunsford LD et al. A multi-institutional analysis of complication outcomes after arteriovenous malformation radiosurgery. *Int J Radiat Oncol Biol Phys* 1999;44:67–74.
39. Flickinger JC, Kondziolka D, Maitz AH, et al. An analysis of the dose-response for arteriovenous malformation radiosurgery and other factors affecting obliteration. *Radiother Oncol* 2002;63:347–354.
40. Flickinger JC, Kondziolka D, Niranjan A, et al. Results of acoustic neuroma radiosurgery: An analysis of 5 years' experience using current methods. *J Neurosurg* 2001;94:1–6.
41. Flickinger JC, Pollock BE, Kondziolka D, et al. LD A dose-response analysis of arteriovenous malformation obliteration after radiosurgery. *Int J Radial Oncol Biol Phys* 1999;36:873–879.
42. Foote KD, Friedman WA, Buatti JM, et al. Analysis of risk factors associated with radiosurgery for vestibular schwannoma. *J Neurosurg* 2001;95:440–449.

43. Foote RL, Pollock BE, Gorman DA, et al. Glomus jugulare tumor: tumor control and complication after stereotactic radiosurgery. *Head Neck* 2002;24:332ff.
44. Frau E, Rumen F, Noel G, et al. Low-dose proton beam therapy for circumscribed choroidal hemangiomas. *Arch Ophthalmol* 2004;122:1471–1475.
45. Friedrich A, Kamprad F, Goldmann A, et al. Clinical importance of radiotherapy in the treatment of Graves' Disease. In: Wiegel T, Bornfeld N, Foerster MH, et al. (eds). Radiotherapy of ocular disease. *Front Radiat Ther Oncol Basel* 1997;30:206–217.
46. Gerling J, Kommerell G, Henne K, et al. Retrobulbar irradiation for thyroid-associated orbitopathy: double-blind comparison between 2.4 and 16Gy. *Int J Radiat Oncol Biol Phys* 2003;55(1):182–189.
47. Goldie I, Rosengren B, Moberg E, et al. Evaluation of radiation treatment of painful conditions of the locomotor system. *Acta Radiol Ther Phys* 1970;9:311–322.
48. Gregoritch S, Chadha M, Pellegrini V, et al. Preoperative irradiation for prevention of heterotopic ossification following prothetic total hip replacement. Preliminary results. *Int J Radiat Oncol Phys* 1993;27(Suppl 1):157–158.
49. Gudjonsson O, Blomquist E, Nyberg G, et al. Stereotactic irradiation of skull base meningiomas with high energy protons. *Acta Neurochir (Wien)* 1999;141:933–940.
50. Guix B, Henriquez I, Andres A, et al. Treatment of keloids by high-dose-rate brachytherapy : a seven-year-study. *Int J Radiat Oncol Biol Phys* 2001;50:167–172.
51. Habrand JL, Ganry O, Couanet D, et al. The role of radiation therapy in the management of craniopharyngioma: a 25-year experience and review of the literature. *Int J Radiat Oncol Biol Phys* 1999;44:255–263.
52. Han PP, Ponce FA, Spetzler RF. Intention-to-treat analysis of Spetzler-Martin grades IV and V AVMs: natural history and treatment paradigm. *J Neurosurg* 2003;98:3–7.
53. Hannouche D, Frau E, Desjardins L, et al. Efficacy of Proton therapy in circumscribed choroidal hemangiomas associated with serous retinal detachment. *Opthalmology* 1997;104:1780–1784.
54. Hart PM, Chakravarthy U, MacKenzie G, et al. Teletherapy for subfoveal choroidal neovascular-isation of age related macular degeneration: Results of follow up in a non-randomised study. *Br J Ophthalmol* 1996;80:1046–1050.
55. Hart PM, Chakravarthy U, Mackenzie G. et al. Visual outcomes in the subfoveal radiotherapy study. *Arch Ophthalmol* 2002;120:1029–1039.
56. Hauck EW, Weidner W. Francois de la Peyronie and the disease named after him. *Lancet* 2001;357:2049–2051.
57. Heyd R, Seegenschmiedt MH, Strassmann G, et al. Radiotherapy of Graves' Orbitopathy: results of a national survey. *Strahlenther Onkol* 2203;179:372–376.
58. Heyd R, Strassmann G, Filipowicz I, et al: [Radiotherapy in vertebral hemangioma] Rontgenpraxis. 2001;53:208–220.[Article in German]
59. Hildebrandt G, Jahns J, Hindemith M, et al. Effects of low dose radiation therapy on adjuvant induced arthritis in rats. *Int J Radiat Biol* 2000;76:1143–1153.
60. Hug EB, Loredo LN, Slater JD, et al. Proton radiation therapy for chordomas and chondro-sarcomas of the skull base. *J Neurosurg* 1999;91:432–439.
61. Hurbli T, Char DH, Harris J, et al. Radiation therapy for thyroid eye diseases. *Am J Ophthalmol* 1985;99:633–637.
62. Incrocci L, Wijnmaalen A, Slob AK et al. Low-dose radiotherapy in 179 patients with Peyronie's disease: treatment outcome and current sexual function. *Int J Radiat Oncol Biol Phys* 2000;47:1353–1356.
63. International Commission on Radiation Units. Prescribing, Recording, and Reporting Photon Beam Therapy, ICRU-Report 50. Bethesda, MD: International Commission on Radiation Units and Measurements; 1993.
64. International Commission on Radation Units. Prescribing, Recording, and Reporting Photon Beam Therapy, Supplement to ICRU Report 50, ICRU-Report 62. Bethesda, MD: International Commission on Radiation Units; 1999.
65. Isaacson PG,Norton AJ (eds). *Extranodal lymphomas: Chapter 7: Lymphomas of the ocular adnexa and eye. Chruchill Livingstone, Edinburgh,* (1st edition): 117–129, 1994
66. Jaakola A, Heikkonen J, Tarkkanen A, et al. Visual function after Strontium-90 plaque irradiation in patients with age-related subfoveal choroidal neovascularisation. *Acta Ophthalmol Scand* 1998;76:1–5.
67. Jansen JT, Broerse JJ, Zoetelief J, et al. Estimation of the carcinogenic risk of radiotherapy of benign diseases from shoulder to heel. *Radiother Oncol* 2005;76(3):270–277.
68. Jansen JTM, Broerse JJ, Zoetelief J, et al. Estimation of the carcinogenic risk of radiotherapy of benign diseases from shoulder to heel. *Radiother Oncol* 2005;76:270–277.
69. Jereb J, Anggard A, Baryd I. Juvenile nasopharyngeal angiofibroma. A clinical study of 69 cases. *Acta Radiol Ther Phys Biol* 1979;9:302–310.
70. Jurgenliemk-Schulz IM, Hartman LJ, Roesink JM, et al. Prevention of pterygium recurrence by postoperative single-dose beta-irradiation: a prospective randomized clinical double-blind trial. *Int J Radiat Oncol Biol Phys* 2004;59(4):1138–1147.
71. Kahaly GJ, Rösler HP, Pitz S, et al. Low- versus high-dose radiotherapy for Graves' ophthalmopathy: a randomized, single blind trial. *J Clin Endocrinol Metab* 2000;85(1):102–108.
72. Kamath SS, Parsons JT, Marcus RB. Radiotherapy for local control of aggressive fibromatosis. *Int J Radiat Oncol Biol Phys* 1996;36:325–328.
73. Kantorowitz DA, Miller GJ, Ferrara JA, et al. Preoperative versus postoperative irradiation in the prophylaxis of heterotopic bone formation in rats. *Int J Radiat Oncol Biol Phys* 1990;19:1431–1438.
74. Karpinos M, Teh BS, Zeck O, et al. Treatment of acoustic neuroma: stereotactic radiosurgery vs. microsurgery. *Int J Radiat Oncol Biol Phys* 2002;54:1410–1421.
75. Keilholz L, Seegenschmiedt MH, Sauer R. Radiotherapy in early stage Dupuytren's Contracture: Initial and Long-Term Results. *Int J Radiat Oncol Biol Phys* 1996;36:891–897.
76. Keilholz L, Seegenschmiedt MH, Sauer R: Radiotherapy of degenerative joint disorders. Indication, technique and clinical results. *Strahlenther Onkol* 1998;174:243–250.
77. Keleti D, Flickinger JC, Hobson SR, et al. Radiotherapy of lymphoproliferative diseases of the orbit: surveillance of 65 cases. *Am J Clin Oncol* 1992;15:422–427.
78. Kellgren JH, Lawrence JS. Radiological assessment of osteoarthrosis. *Annals of Rheum Dis* 1957;16:494–502.
79. Kern PM, Keilholz L, Forster C, et al. Low-dose radiotherapy selectively reduces adhesion of peripheral blood mononuclear cells to endothelium in vitro. *Radiother Oncol* 2000;54:273–282.
80. Kim JA, Elkon D, Lim ML, et al. Optimum dose of radiotherapy for chemodectomas in the middle ear. *Int J Radiat Oncol Biol Phys* 1980;6:815ff.
81. Kirschner MJ, Sauer R. Die Rolle der Radiotherapie bei der Behandlung von Desmoidtumoren. *Strahlenther Onkol* 1993;169:77–82.
82. Kivela T, Tenhunen M, Joensuu T, et al. Stereotactic radiotherapy of symptomatic circumscribed choroidal hemangiomas. *Opthalmology* 2003;110:1977–1982.
83. Kondziolka D, Levy EI, Niranjan A, et al. Long-term outcomes after meningioma radiosurgery: Physician and patient perspectives. *J Neurosurg* 1999;91:44–50.
84. Kovalic JJ, Perez CA: Radiation therapy following keloidectomy: A 20-year experience. *Int J Radiat Oncol Biol Phys* 1989;17:77–80.
85. Kuppersmith RB, Teh BS, Donovan DT, et al. The use of intensity modulated radiotherapy for the treatment of extensive and recurrent juvenile angiofibroma. *Int J Pediatr Otorhinolaryngol* 2000;52:261–268.
86. Lalwani AK, Jackler RK, Gutin PH. Lethal fibrosarcoma complicating radiation therapy for bening glomus jugulare tumor. *Am J Otol* 1993;14:398ff.
87. Lambo MJ, Brady LW, Shields CL. Lymphoid tumors of the orbit. In: Alberti WE, Sagerman RH (eds.). Radiotherapy of Intraocular and Orbital Tumors. Springer, Berlin; 1993: 205–216.
88. Lanciano R, Fowble B, Sergott R, et al. The results of radiotherapy for orbital pseudotumor. *Int J Radiat Oncol Biol Phys* 1989;18:407–411.
89. Lee JT, Chen P, Safa A, et al. The role of radiation in the treatment of advanced juvenile angio-fibroma. *Laryngoscope* 2002;112(7 Pt 1):1213–1220.
90. Leer JWH, van Houtte P, Davelaar J. Indications and treatment schedules for irradiation of benign diseases: a survey. *Radiother Oncol* 1998;48:249–257.
91. Leithner A, Schnack B, Katterschafka T, et al. Treatment of extra-abdominal desmoid tumors with interferon-alpha with or without retinoin. *J Surg Oncol* 2000;73:21–25.
92. Linskey ME, Martinez AJ, Kondziolka D, et al. The radiobiology of human acoustic schwannoma xenografts after stereotactic radiosurgery evaluated in the subrenal capsule of athymic mice. *J Neurosurg* 1993;78:645–653.
93. Liscak R, Vladyka V, Wowra B, et al. Gamma knife radiosurgery of the glomus jugulare tumor—early multicentre experience. *Acta Neurochir* 1999;141:1141ff.
94. Lloyd WC, Leone CR. Supervoltage orbital radiotherapy in 36 cases of Graves' disease. *Am J Ophthalmol* 1992;113:374–380.
95. Lo TCM, Seckel BR, Salzman FA, et al. Single-dose electron beam irradiation in treatment and prevention of keloids and hypertrophic scars. *Radiother Oncol* 1990;19:267–272.
96. Maarouf M, Voges J, Landwehr P, et al. Stereotactic linear accelerator based radiosurgery for the treatment of patients with glomus jugulare tumors. *Cancer* 2003;97:1093–1097.
97. MacKenzie FS, Hirst LW, Kynaston B, et al. Recurrence rate and complications after beta irradiation for pterygia. *Ophthalmology* 1991;98:1776–1780.
98. Madreperla SA. Choroidal hemangioma treated with photodynamic therapy using verteporfin. *Arch Ophthalmology* 2001;119:1606–1610.
99. Maeda M, Tateishi H, Takaiga, et al. High-energy, low-dose radiation therapy for aneurismal bone cyst. Report of a case. *Clin Orthop* 1989;243:200.
100. Makek MS, Andrews JC, Fisch U. Malignant transformation of a nasopharyngeal angiofibroma. *Laryngoscope* 1989;99:1088–1092.
101. Mashayekhi A, Shields CL. Circumscribed choroidal hemangioma. *Curr Opin Ophthalmol* 2003;14:142–149.
102. McCord MW et al. Radiotherapy for pituitary adenoma: long-term outcome and sequelae. *Int J Radiat Oncol Biol Phys* 1997;39:437–444.
103. Meijer OW, Vandertop WP, Baayen JC, et al. Single-fraction vs. fractionated linac-based stereotactic radiosurgery for vestibular schwannoma: a single-institution study. *Int J Radiat Oncol Biol Phys* 2003;56:1390–1396.
104. Mendenhall WM, Mendenhall CM, Reith JD, et al. *(2006)* Pigmented villonodular synovitis. *Am J Clin Oncol* 2006;29(6):548–550.
105. Micke O, Seegenschmiedt MH. The German Working Group guidelines for radiation therapy of benign diseases: a multicenter approach in Germany. *Int J Radiat Oncol Biol Phys* 2002;52:496–513.
106. Micke O, Seegenschmiedt MH; German Cooperative Group on Radiotherapy for Benign Diseases. Radiation therapy for aggressive fibromatosis (desmoid tumors): Results of a national Patterns of Care Study. *Int J Radiat Oncol Biol Phys* 2005;61(3):882–891.
107. Milker-Zabel S, et al. Fractionated stereotacally guided radiosurgery and radiotherapy for pituitary adenomas. *Int J Radiat Oncol Biol Phys* 2001;50:1279–1286.
108. Million RR, Cassisi NJ, Mancuso AA, et al. Chemodectomas (glomus body tumors). In: Million RR, Cassisi NJ (eds.). Management of Head and Neck Cancer. A Multidisciplinary Approach. 2nd ed. Philadelphia:; 1994: 765–783.
109. Million RR, Cassisi NJ, Mancuso AA, et al. Juvenile angiofibroma. In: Million RR, Cassisi NJ (eds.). Management of head and neck cancer. A multidisciplinary approach. 2nd ed. Philadelphia:; 1994: 627–641.
110. Milosevic M, Frost PJ, Laperriere NJ, et al. Radiotherapy for atypical or malignant intracranial meningioma. *Int J Radiat Oncol Biol Phys* 1996;34:817–822.
111. Monteiro-Grillo I, Gaspar L, Monteiro-Grillo M, et al. Post-operative irradiation of primary or recurrent pterygium: results and sequalae. *Int J Radiation Oncol Biol Phys* 2000;48:865–869.
112. Mourits MP, et al. Radiotherapy for Graves' orbitopathy: randomised placebo-controlled study. *Lancet* 2000;355:1505–1509.
113. Munzenrider JE, Liebsch NJ. Proton therapy for tumors of the skull base. *Strahlenther Onkol* 1999;175(Suppl II):57–63.
114. Nesbit RM. Congenital curvature of the phallus. Report of three cases with description of corrective operation. *J Urol* 1950;93:230–232.
115. Nishimura Y, Nakai A, Yoshimasu T, et al. Long-term results of fractionated strontium-90 therapy for pterygia. *Int J Radiat Oncol Biol Phys* 2000;46:137–141.
116. Nobler MP, Higinbotham ML, Phillips RF. The cure of aneurismal bone cyst. Irradiation superior to surgery in analysis of 33 cases. *Radiology* 1968;90:1185.
117. Noel G, Habrand JL, Jauffret E, et al. Radiation therapy for chordoma and chondrosarcoma of the skull base and the cervical spine. Prognostic factors and patterns of failure. *Strahlenther Onkol* 2003;179:241–248.
118. Notter M, Kern T, Forrer A, et al. Radiotherapy of pseudotumor orbitae. *Front Radiat Ther. Oncol* 1997;30:180–191.
119. Nutting C, Brada M, Brazil L, et al. Radiotherapy in the treatment of benign meningioma of the skull base. *J Neurosurg* 1999;90:823–827.
120. Nuyttens JJ, Rust PF, Thomas ChR, et al. Surgery versus radiation therapy for patients with aggressive fibromatosis or desmoid tumors. *Cancer* 2000;88:1517–1523.
121. O'Sullivan B, Griffin A, Wunder J, et al. Sustained remission following radiation treatment for high-risk pigmented villonodular synovitis (Abstract). *Int J Radiat Oncol Biol Phys* 2005;63:S50.

122. Order EO, Donaldson SS,eds. Radiation Therapy of Benign Diseases. 2nd Ed. Berlin: Springer Publishers; 1998.
123. Order S, Donaldson SS: Radiation Therapy of Benign Diseases, Medical Radiology, 2nd edition, Springer, BerlinHeidelberg New York (1999)
124. O'Sullivan B, Cummings B, Catton C et al. (1995) Outcome following radiation treatment for high-risk pigmented villonodular synovitis; *Int J Radiat Oncol Biol Phys*32 (3):777–786.
125. Paijc B, Pugnale-Verilotte N, Greiner RH, et al. Results of strontium-yttrium-90 for pterygia. *J Fr Ophthalmol* 2002;25:473–479.
126. Pajic B, Pallas A, Aebersold D, et al. Prospektive study about course of primary pterygia after exclusive treatment with Sr-/Y-90 irradiation. *Strahlenther Oncol* 2004;
127. Parayani SB, Scott WP, Wells JW Jr, et al. Management of pterygium with surgery and radiation therapy. The North Florida Pterygium Study Group. *Int J Radiat Oncol Biol Phys* 1994;28:101–103.
128. Petersen IA, Donaldson SS, McDougall IR, et al. Prognostic factors in the radiotherapy of Graves' ophthalmopathy. *Int J Radiat Oncol Biol Phys* 1990;19:259–264.
129. Plenk HP. Calcifying tendinitis of the shoulder. A critical study of the value of X-ray therapy. *Radiology* 1952;59:384–389.
130. Plowman PN, Hungerford JL. Radiotherapy for ocular angiomas. *Br J Ophthalmol* 1997;81:258–259.
131. Pohl F, Thile W, Koelbl O, et al. retrospective Analyse von 12 Patienten mit Glomus jugulare Tumoren nach Radiotherapie. *Strahlenther Onkol* 2003;179:3ff.
132. Prummel MF, Bakker A, Wiersinga WM, et al. Multi-center study on the characteristics and treatment strategies of patients with Graves' orbitopathy: first European Group on Graves' Orbitopathy experience. *Eur J Endocrinol* 2003;148:491–495.
133. Prummel MF, Mourits MP, Blank L, et al. Randomized double-blind trial of prednisone versus radiotherapy. In: Graves' Ophthalmopathy. *Lancet* 1993;342:949–954.
134. Rades D, Bajrovic A, Alberti A, et al. Is there a dose-effect relationship for the treatment of symptomatic vertebral hemangioma? *Int J Radiat Oncol Biol Phys* 2002;55:178–181.
135. Radiation Therapy for Age-related Macular Degeneration Study. A prospectiv, randomized, double-masked trial on radiation therapy for neovascular age-related degeneration. *Ophthalmology* 1999;106:2239–2247.
136. Reddy KA, Mendenhall WM, Amdur RJ, et al. Long-term results of radiation therapy for juvenile nasopharyngeal angiofibroma. *Am J Otolaryngol* 2001;22:172–175.
137. Rodemann HP, Bamberg M. Cellular basis of radiation-induced fibrosis. *Radiother Oncol* 1985;35:83–90.
138. Rodrigues CI, Hian Njo, Karim AB. Results of radiotherapy and vitamin E in the treatment of Peyronie's disease. *Int J Radiat Oncol Biol Phys* 1995;31:571–574.
139. Roesler HP, Zapf S, Kuffner HD, et al. Strahlentherapie beim Narbenkeloid. *Fortschritte der Medizin* 1993;111:46–49.
140. Rowe JG, Radatz MW, Walton L, et al. Gamma knife stereotactic radiosurgery for unilateral acoustic tumors. *J Neurol Neurosurg Psychiatry* 2003;74:1536–1542.
141. Rubin, P, Soni A, Williams JP. The molecular and cellular basis for the radiation treatment of benign proliferative diseases. *Semin Radiat Oncol* 1999;9:203–214.
142. Sallstrom KO, Larson O, Heden P, et al. Treatment of keloids with surgical excision and postoperative X-ray radiation. *Scand J Plast Reconstr Surg Hand Surg* 1989;23:211–214.
143. Samii M, Matthies C. Management of 1000 vestibular schwannomas (acoustic neuromas): Surgical management and results with an emphasis on complications and how to avoid them. *Neurosurg* 1997;40:11–21.
144. Sanford RA. Craniopharyngioma: Results of survey of the American Society of Pediatric Neurosurgery. *Pediatr Neurosurg* 1994;21(Suppl 1):39–43.
145. Sautter-Bihl ML, Liebermeister E, Heinze HG, et al. The radiotherapy of heterotopic ossifications in paraplegics. The preliminary results. *Strahlenther Onkol* 1995;171:454–459.
146. Schilling H, Sauerwein W, Lommatzsch A, et al. Longterm results after low dose ocular irradiation for choroidal hemangiomas. *Br J Ophthalmol* 1997;81:267–273.
147. Schulz-Ertner D, Frank C, Herfarth KK, et al. Fractionated stereotactic radiotherapy for craniopharyngiomas. *Int J Radiat Oncol Biol Phys* 2002;54:1114–1120.
148. Schulz-Ertner D, Nikoghosyan A, Thilmann C, et al. Carbon ion radiotherapy for chordomas and low-grade chondrosarcomas of the skull base. *Strahlenther Onkol* 2003;179:598–605.
149. Seegenschmiedt MH, Attassi M. [Radiation therapy for Morbus Ledderhose - indication and clinical results]. *Strahlenther Onkol* 2003;179(12):847–853.
150. Seegenschmiedt MH, Goldmann AR, Wölfel R, et al. Prevention of heterotopic ossification (HO) after total hip replacement: randomized high versus low dose radiotherapy. *Radioth Oncol* 1993;26:271–274.
151. Seegenschmiedt MH, Katalinic A, Makoski H, et al. Radiation therapy for benign diseases: patterns of care study in Germany. *Int J Radiat Oncol Biol Phys* 2000;47:195–202.
152. Seegenschmiedt MH, Keilholz L, Gusek-Schneider G, et al. Endokrine Orbitopathie: Vergleich der Langzeitergebnisse und Klassifikationen nach Radiotherapie. *Strahlenther Onkol* 1998;174:449–456.
153. Seegenschmiedt MH, Keilholz L, Katalinic A, et al: Heel spur: radiation therapy for refractory pain—results with three treatment concepts. *Radiology* 1996;200:271–276.
154. Seegenschmiedt MH, Keilholz L, Martus P, et al. Epicondylopathia humeri: Indication, technique and clinical results of radiotherapy. *Strahlenther Onkol* 1997;173:208–218.
155. Seegenschmiedt MH, Keilholz L, Martus P, et al. Prevention of heterotopic ossification about the hip: Final Results of two ran-domised trials in 410 patients using either preoperative or postoperative radiation therapy. *Int J Radiat Oncol Biol Phys* 1997;39:161–171.
156. Seegenschmiedt MH, Keilholz L. Epicondylopathia humeri and peritendinitis humeroscapularis: Evaluation of radiation therapy long-term results and literature review. *Radiother Oncol* 1998;47:17–28.
157. Seegenschmiedt MH, Makoski H-Br, Micke O. German cooperative group radiotherapy for benign diseases: benign diseases: radiation prophylaxis for heterotopic ossification about the hip joint—a multi-center study. *Int J Radiat Oncol Biol Phys* 2001;51:756–765.
158. Seegenschmiedt MH, Martus P, Goldmann AR, et al. Peroperative vesus postoperative radiotherapiy for prevention of heterotopic ossification: First results of a randomised trial in high-risk patients. *Int J Radiat Oncol Biol Phys* 1994;30:63–73.
159. Seegenschmiedt MH, Micke O, Willich N. Radiation therapy for non-malignant diseases in Germany—Current concepts and future perspectives. *Strahlenther Onkol* 2004;180:718–730.
160. Seegenschmiedt MH, Olschewski T, Guntrum F. Radiotherapy optimization in early-stage Dupuytren's contracture: first results of a randomized clinical study. *Int J Radiat Oncol Biol Phys* 2001;49:785–798.
161. Shaw E, et al. Radiation therapy oncology group: Radiosurgery quality assurance guidelines. *Int J Radiat Oncol Biol Phys* 1995;33:301–307.
162. Shields CL, Honavar SC, Shields JA, et al. Circumscribed choroidal hemangioma. Clinical mani-festations and factors predictive of visual outcome in 200 consecutive cases. *Ophthalmology* 2001;108:2237–2248.
163. Shields CL, Shields JA, Barrett J, et al. Vasoproliferative tumors of the ocular fundus. Classification and clinical manifestations in 103 patients. *Arch Ophthalmol.* 1995;113:615–623.
164. Shields JA, Shields CL, Materin MA, et al. Changing concepts in management of circumscribed choroidal hemangioma. The 2003 J. Howard Stokes Lecture (Part 1). *Oph Surg Lasers* 2004;35:383–393.
165. Simpson D. The recurrence of intracranial meningiomas after surgical treatment. *J Neurol Neurosurg Psyiatry* 1957;20:22–39.
166. Spetzler RF, Martin NA. A proposed grading system for arteriovenous malformations. *J Neurosurg* 1986;65:476–483.
167. Springate SC, Weichselbaum RR. Radiation or surgery for chemodectomas of the temporal bone: A review of local control and complications. *Head Neck* 1990;12:303ff.
168. Staar S, Müller RP, Hammer M, et al. Results and prognostic factors in retrobulbar radiotherapy combined with systemic corticosteroids for endocrine orbitopathy (Graves' Disease). In: Wiegel T, Bornfeld N, Foerster MH, et al. (eds.). Radiotherapy of ocular disease. Front Radiat Ther Oncol, Basel: Karger, 1997;30:206–217.
169. Steiner L, Lindquist C, Adler JR, et al. Clinical outcome of radiosurgery for cerebral arteriovenous malformations. *J Neurosurg* 1992;77:1–8.
170. Suit HD, Spiro I. Radiation treatment of benign mesenchymal disease. *Sem Radiat Oncol* 1999;9:171–178.
171. Thölen A, Meister A, Bernasconi PP, et al. Radiotherapie von subretinalen Neovaskularisations-membranen bei altersabhängiger Makuladegeneration. *Ophthalmologe* 1998;95:691–698.
172. Tomita T, McLone D. Radical resection of childhood craniopharyngiomas. *Pediatr Neurosurg* 1993;19:6–14.
173. Tos M, Thomsen J. Proposal of classification of tumor size in acoustic neuroma surgery. In: Tos M, Thomsen J (eds). *Proceedings of the First International Conference on Acoustic Neuroma*. Amsterdam: Kugler; 1992.
174. Treatment of Age-related Macular Degeneration with Photodynamic Therapy (TAP) Study Group: Photodynamic therapy of subfoveal choroidal neovascularisation in age-related macular degeneration with verteporfin. One-year results of two randomised clinical trials-TAP report. *I Arch Ophthalmol*117:1329–1345(1999)
175. Trott K-R, Kamprad F. Radiobiological mechanisms of anti-inflammatory radiotherapy. *Radiother Oncol* 1999;51:197–203.
176. Valmaggia C, Ries G, Ballinari P. Radiotherapy for subfoveal choroidal neovascularization in age-related macular degeneration: A randomized clinical trial. *Am J Ophthalmology* 2002;133:521–529.
177. Valtonen EJ, Lilius HG, Malmio K. The value of roentgen irradiation in the treatment of painful degene-rative and inflammatory musculo-skeletal conditions. *Scand J Rheumatol* 1975;4:247–249.
178. Van den Brenk HA. Results of prophylactic postoperative irradiation in 1300 cases of pterygium. *Am J Roentgenol* 1968;103:723–733
179. Vernimmen FJ, Harris JK, Wilson JA, et al. Stereotactic proton beam therapy of skull base meningiomas. *Int J Radiat Oncol Biol Phys* 2001;49:99–105.
180. Voges J, Treuer H, Sturm V, et al. Risk analysis of linear accelerator radiosurgery. *Int J Radiat Oncol Biol Phys* 1996;36:1055–1063.
181. von Pannewitz G. Degenerative Erkrankungen. In: Diethelm L, et al.. (eds). Handbuch der medizinischen Radiologie Band XVII. Berlin: Springer; 19970: 73–107.
182. Von Wangenheim KH, Petersen HP, Schwenke K. A major component of radiation action: interference with intracellular control of differentiation. *Int J Radiat Biol* 1995;68:369–388.
183. Wagner W, Gerding H, Busse H. Pseudotumor orbitae - ein Chamäleon in Diagnostik und Therapie? *Strahlenther Onkol* 1992;168:528–535.
184. Wenkel E, Thornton AF, Finkelstein D, et al. Benign meningioma: partially resected, biopsied, and recurrent intracranial tumors treated with combined proton and photon radiotherapy. *Int J Radiat Oncol Biol Phys* 2000;48:1363–1370.
185. Werner SC. Modification of the classification of the eye changes of Graves' disease: Recom-mendations of the Ad Hoc Committee of The American Thyroid Association. *J Clin Endocrinol Metab* 1977;44:203–204.
186. Wilder RB, Buatti JM, Kittelson JM, et al. Pterygium treated with excision and postoperative beta-irradiation. *Int J Radiation Oncol Biol Phys* 1992;23:533–537.
187. Willner J, Flentje M, Lieb W, et al. Soft X-ray therapy of recurrent pterygium-an alternative to Sr-90 eye applicators. *Strahlenther Oncol* 2001;177:404–409.
188. Wilms M, Kocher M, Makoski H-B, et al. Langzeitergebnisse der semistereotaktischen konventionell fraktionierten Strahlenbehandlung arterio-venöser Malformationen des Gehirns. *Strahlenther Onkol* 2003;179(Suppl):69.
189. Winkler C, Dornfeld S, Baumann M, et al. Effizienz der Strahlentherapie bei Wirbelhämangiomen. *Strahlenther Onkol* 1996;172:681–684.
190. Yamakami I, Uchino Y, Kobayashi E, et al. Conservative management, gammaknife radiosurgery, and microsurgery for acoustic neurinomas: a systematic review of outcome and risk of three therapeutic options. *Neurol Res* 2003;25:682–690.
191. Yonemoto LT, Slater JD, Blacharski PB, et al. Dose response in the treatment of subfoveal choroidal neovascularization in age-related macular degeneration: Results of a phase I/II dose escalation study using proton radiotherapy. *J Radiosurg* 2000;3:47–54.
192. Zabel A, Milker-Zabel S, Schulz-Erner D, et al. Fraktionierte stereotaktische Konformations-bestrahlung von Glomus jugulare Tumoren. *Strahlenther Oncol* 2003;179:67ff.
193. Zierhut D et al. External radiotherapy of pituitary adenomas. *Int J Radiat Oncol Biol Phys* 1995;33:307–314.
194. Zografos L, Egger E, Bercher L, et al. Proton beam irradiation of choroidal hemangiomas. *Am J Ophthalmol* 1998;126:261–268.
195. Zwicker C, Hering M, Brecht L, et al. [Radiotherapy of Periarthritis humeroscapularis with high-energy photons. Comparison of magnetic resonance tomograpy findings] *Radiologe* 1998;38:774–778.

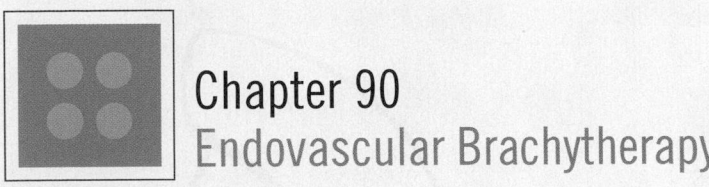

Chapter 90
Endovascular Brachytherapy

Ray Lin, Prabhakar Tripuraneni

Vascular brachytherapy (VBT) continues to have a role in the treatment of coronary in-stent restenosis and has a promising role in the treatment of restenosis following intervention of the peripheral arterial system.

There are more than 1.5 million coronary interventions performed worldwide each year for coronary stenosis (40). Coronary stenting with stainless steel stents has become a standard of care in treating patients with coronary stenosis. Restenosis has been the major complication of percutaneous transluminal coronary angioplasty since the introduction of balloon angioplasty by Gruentzig in the mid-1970s (27,35,43). This process has been thought to consist of three separate mechanisms: vascular recoil, neointimal hyperplasia, and negative remodeling.

Despite trials of various pharmacologic agents (18,20,55,107) such as heparin and the introduction of debulking techniques such as directional atherectomy, laser, and rotablation (38,110), the frequency of restenosis remained approximately 40% at 6 months. Prosthetic stent implantation, which eliminates the problem of vascular recoil and negative remodeling and creates a larger lumen with the initial procedure, initially appeared very promising with restenosis rates of 10% to 20% (19,68).

VBT has been shown in several double-blinded randomized trials to demonstrate its efficacy in reducing rates of in-stent restenosis. The potential usefulness of vascular radiation therapy to prevent restenosis emerged rapidly from positive preclinical studies carried out in animals in the late 1980s and early 1990s, to a large number of feasibility trials and randomized clinical trials in the mid-to-late 1990s, to U.S. Food and Drug Administration (FDA) approval of the first commercial devices in the last quarter of 2000. Although initial preclinical studies have included evaluation of both teletherapy and brachytherapy approaches, only vascular systems have been tested extensively in human coronary vessels.

Of the 1 million angioplasties expected in the United States annually, approximately 80% to 90% of these patients will undergo stenting. In-stent restenosis will develop in approximately 15% of these patients, and these patients present a considerable management problem to the interventional cardiologist. Restenosis rates approaching 80% for long, diffuse lesions in small vessels have been reported.

The role for VBT, however, has become less clear in recent years since the introduction of drug-eluting stents (DESs). Studies on DESs have now matured. DESs using antiproliferative agents such as paclitaxel (26) and immunosuppressive agents such as sirolimus (13,50,62,71) have been shown to be effective in treating in-stent restenosis. Furthermore, recently published randomized trials show DESs to be superior to VBT in treating in-stent restenosis (29,73). DESs will likely replace VBT as first-line therapy for coronary in-stent restenosis. Additionally, interventional cardiologists may simply prefer DESs over VBT in order to avoid the logistics and expense of having radiation oncology involved in the catheterization laboratory (13,62). However, adverse events such as acute stent thrombosis, aneurysm, and incomplete apposition do occur with DESs. Furthermore, restenosis still can occur following DESs at rates between 2% and 10% (14).

VBT will probably find a niche in treatment of patients who fail DESs. The Checkmate system (Cordis Corporation, Miami Lakes, FL) and the Galileo system (Guidant Corporation, Indianapolis, IN) are no longer commercially available. Currently, the Betacath system using ^{90}Sr is the only system clinically available for use in coronary artery in-stent restenosis following repeat intervention.

Approximately 400,000 peripheral vascular procedures are done each year in United States. The risk of restenosis after angioplasty and stent placement varies considerably in different parts of the peripheral arterial tree. Initial clinical trials of VBT in superficial femoral arteries and renal artery in-stent restenosis (31,94) show similar results as observed in the coronary system. VBT appears to be safe and effective in certain patients with restenosis in the peripheral vascular system.

Historical Perspective

VBT was empirically tried in Frankfurt, Germany by Liermann and colleagues on restenosed femoral popliteal arteries starting in 1990. A small cohort of patients has been followed for 10 years, and no long-term adverse events have been reported (65). The first coronary brachytherapy procedure was performed in Caracas, Venezuela, by Condado et al. (11) in 1994, and the results of their initial feasibility trial were reported in 1997. At 5-year follow-up, the data from this landmark study are durable and demonstrate the feasibility of brachytherapy for preventing coronary artery restenosis. The first randomized trial of VBT was carried out by investigators at the Scripps Clinic in 1995, and the positive results from this trial were subsequently published in the *New England Journal of Medicine* (79). That led to GAMMA I, the first multi-institutional, double-blind, randomized pivotal trial using ^{192}Ir, which led to the approval of the Checkmate system (Cordis Corporation, Miami Lakes, FL) for native coronary in-stent restenosis (42).

In the mid-1990s, a Geneva group and a second group at Emory University began testing the feasibility of intracoronary brachytherapy using beta-emitting sources (34,93). The Betacath system, which was piloted at Emory, became the focus of the START trial, the second pivotal trial. In November 2000, it was approved, along with the Checkmate system, for in-stent restenosis (41). The INHIBIT trial testing the Galileo system represents the third pivotal trial of VBT for in-stent restenosis and led to the approval of this device in November 2001 (102). The only randomized trial of VBT for *de novo* lesions in native coronary vessels used the Betacath system and was reported as a negative trial (39).

The approval of VBT is unique in radiation oncology in a number of ways. It is the first time that level I evidence supported by multi-institutional, randomized trials was required by FDA mandate before VBT became available in the routine clinical setting. Likewise, under FDA and Nuclear Regulatory Commission mandate, it was the first time that all specialists, including radiation oncologists (therapeutic radiologist and oncologist), interventional cardiologists, and medical physicists, were required to be part of the team delivering VBT. Since 1995, more than 6,000 patients have been enrolled in approximately 50 protocols testing the efficacy of VBT (86).

Coronary Anatomy

(This section is modified with permission from Windecker S, Meier B. Basics of interventional cardiology. In: Tripuraneni P, Jani S, Minar E, et al., eds. *Intravascular brachytherapy: from theory to practice.* London: Remedica; 2001:83–86.) The coronary arteries originate as the only branches of the ascending aorta from the aortic root (111). Coronary arteries usually have an epicardial course and terminate as arterioles in the capillary network. The left and right coronary arteries surround the epicardial surface as a ring-loop system in two orthogonal planes defined by the fibrous skeleton of the heart. Thus, the right coronary artery (RCA) and the left circumflex coronary artery (LCX) run around the atrioventricular groove and form a circle between the atria and ventricles at the base of the heart. Perpendicular to this plane, the left anterior descending coronary artery (LAD) and the posterior descending RCA constitute a semicircle around the interventricular groove and encircle the left ventricular apex.

Left Coronary Artery

The left coronary artery usually originates from a single ostium in the middle portion of the left sinus of Valsalva (Fig. 90.1). The vessel originating from the left ostium is termed the *left main coronary artery* (LM) if it subsequently gives rise to both the LAD and the LCX. The LM measures 3 to 10 mm in diameter and is usually <40 mm long. The LM has no side branches and divides into the LAD and the LCX, although in 20% to 40% of cases a trifurcation with an intermediate branch between LAD and LCX can be seen.

The LAD leads, in direct continuation of the LM, to the anterior interventricular groove toward the apex and supplies 40% to 60% of the left ventricular myocardium.

The LAD gives rise to septal branches, diagonal branches, and branches to the free right ventricular wall. The LCX originates at an almost vertical angle from the LM and courses posteriorly at variable length along the left atrioventricular groove, beneath the left atrial appendage and toward the crux of the heart. The LCX gives off one to three obtuse marginal branches, which supply the free lateral left ventricular wall and have the same course as the diagonal branches of the LAD.

Right Coronary Artery

Usually the RCA arises from the right sinus of Valsalva and runs in the right atrioventricular groove toward the crux of the heart. The segment from the ostium to the right-angled turn into the vertical part of the RCA is called the *proximal RCA*, the mid-RCA is defined as the vertical segment, and the distal RCA extends from the right-angled turn at the distal end of the vertical segment to the bifurcation into posterior descending coronary artery and posterolateral branches.

Percutaneous Coronary Intervention

(This section is modified with permission from Windecker S, Meier B. Basics of interventional cardiology. In: Tripuraneni P, Jani S, Minar E, et al., eds. *Intravascular brachytherapy: from theory to practice.* London: Remedica; 2001:88–100.) The indications for percutaneous coronary intervention (PCI) have expanded during the past 2 decades, and there is currently no

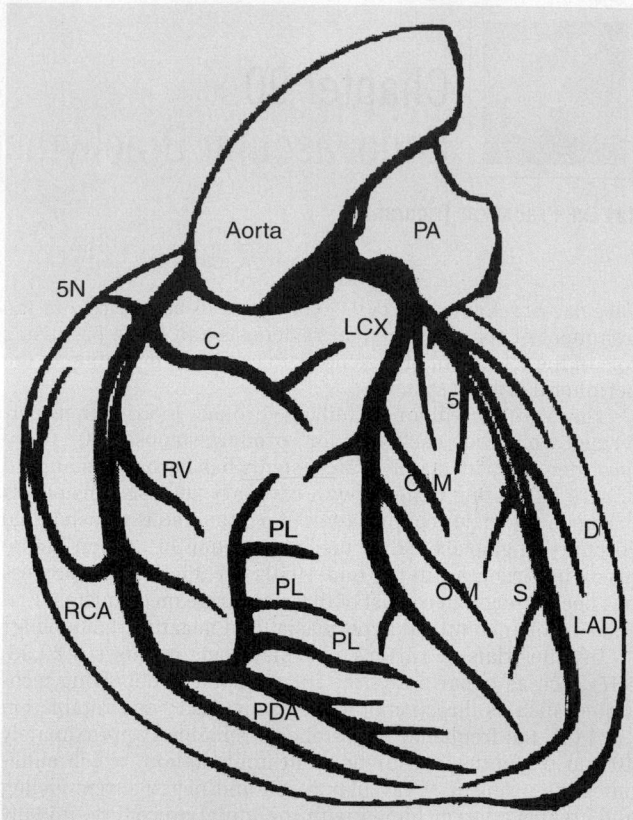

FIGURE 90.1. Schematic representation of the major epicardial coronary arteries as seen in an anteroposterior projection. The left coronary artery originates left and posterior from the cusp of the aortic root as the left main (LM) coronary artery. The LM coronary artery divides after a variable length into the left anterior descending (LAD) artery and the left circumflex (LCX) artery. The LAD runs as a direct continuation of the LM anteriorly along the interventricular groove to the ventricular apex. The LAD gives rise to the septal branches, which take off at a vertical angle and immediately become intramural in the interventricular septum. The LAD also gives rise to the diagonal branches, which course epicardially over the anterolateral free wall. The LCX originates at a nearly vertical angle from the LM and courses posteriorly along the left atrioventricular groove. It gives rise to the obtuse marginal branches, which course epicardially and supply the free lateral wall. The right coronary artery (RCA) takes off anteriorly from the right coronary cusp and follows the right atrioventricular groove. The first branch of the RCA is the conal or infundibular artery, followed by the sinus node artery as the second branch. In the vertical portion of the atrioventricular groove, the RCA gives rise to the right ventricular marginal branches, which supply the right ventricular free wall. The RCA then courses posteriorly and divides at the crux of the heart base into the posterior descending artery (PDA) and a variable number of posterolateral branches. The PDA courses along the posterior interventricular groove toward the left ventricular apex. It closes a loop with the LAD along with the interventricular groove, whereas the posterolateral branches of RCA close a second perpendicular loop of blood supply with the LCX along with the atrioventricular groove. C, conus branch; D, diagonal branch; OM, obtuse marginal branch; PA, pulmonary artery; PL, posterolateral branch; RV, right ventricular branch; S, septal branch; SN, sinus node artery.

absolute contraindication to this technique. Arterial access is usually gained through an anterior wall stick of the right femoral artery using the Seldinger technique. The coronary guidewire is advanced by the coronary guiding catheter into the coronary artery, and is cautiously navigated through the narrowing (stenosis) into the periphery of the vessel to be treated. It secures access to the coronary artery during the intervention and allows for the rapid exchange of balloons, stents, and other devices (Fig. 90.2).

The balloon catheter is not only central to balloon angioplasty but serves as a complementary instrument for other intracoronary interventions, such as delivery of stents, local drugs, or radiation sources. Balloon catheters consist of a shaft providing support when pushing the catheter through vessels, a central lumen for the coronary guidewire, and an inflation channel for balloon expansion.

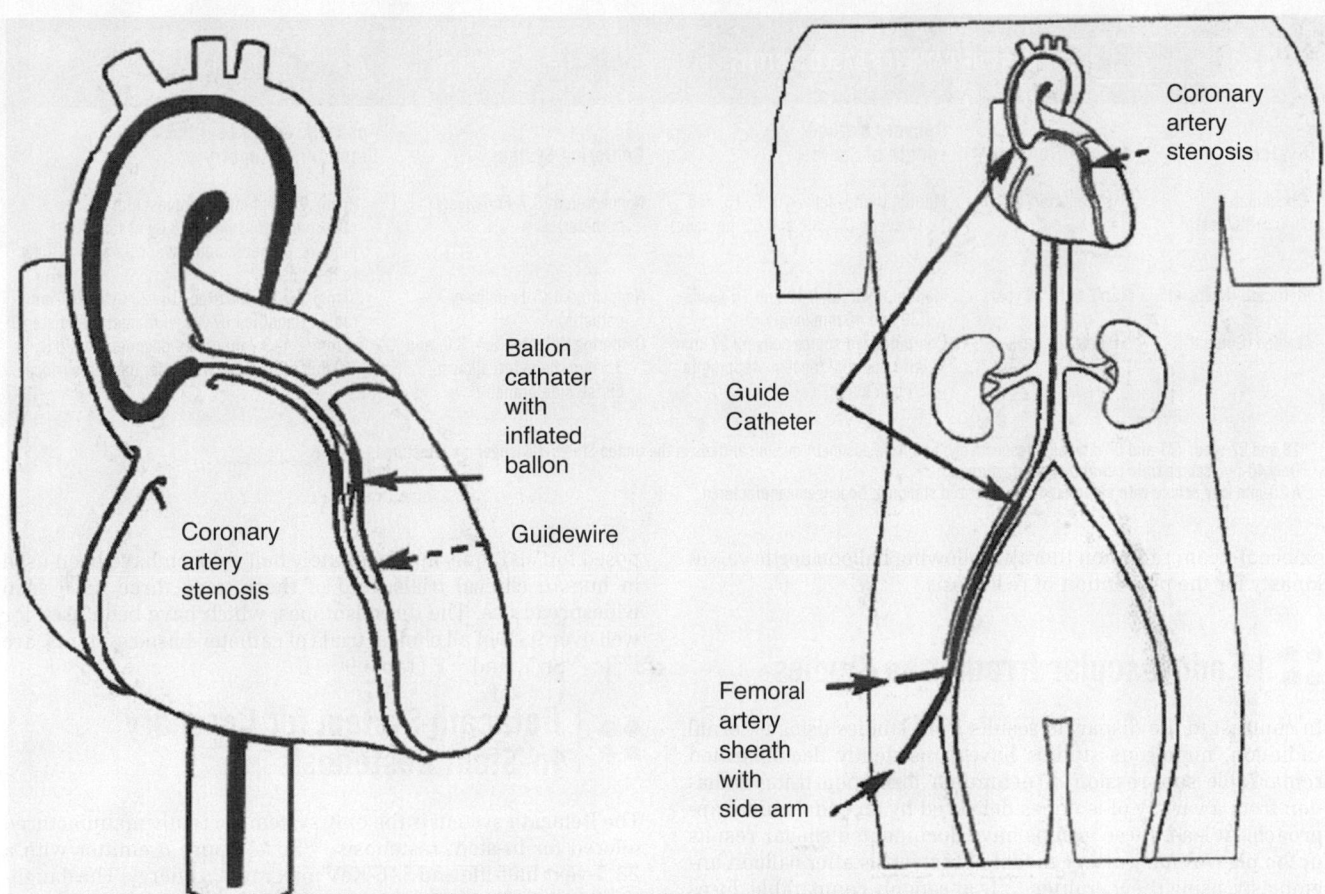

FIGURE 90.2. Schematic diagram of access to the coronary arteries during percutaneous coronary interventions. **A:** An introducer sheath with side arm is placed in the artery chosen for vascular access. A guiding catheter is introduced through the vascular access sheath and advanced to the coronary artery ostium chosen for the intervention. **B:** A guidewire is advanced through the guiding catheter into the coronary artery, navigated through the artery, and placed distal to the stenosis to be treated. A balloon catheter is then placed in the coronary stenosis for dilatation.

During conventional balloon angioplasty (percutaneous transluminal coronary angioplasty), a balloon catheter is advanced over the previously inserted coronary guidewire into the target stenosis and subsequently inflated until the balloon is fully expanded. The chief limitations to event-free survival after balloon angioplasty have been abrupt vessel closure (a short-term complication) and restenosis (a long-term complication) (40). Abrupt vessel closure, defined as the sudden occlusion of the target vessel during or after angioplasty, has been reported in 4% to 8% of cases. Restenosis, defined as stenosis >50% diameter at follow-up angiography, has been the most important long-term limitation of balloon angioplasty, with an incidence of 30% to 50% and with 20% to 30% of patients requiring target vessel revascularization. Most restenoses occur during the first 4 months after balloon angioplasty.

The therapeutic effect of arterial vessel enlargement through PCI is accompanied by various degrees of arterial injury with exposure of thrombogenic components. This may result in intracoronary thrombus formation with its subsequent ischemic sequelae. Therefore, inhibition of platelets and the coagulation system has always been a central focus of interventional investigations. In patients undergoing PCI, aspirin is recommended at a low dose (75 to 325 mg/day), ideally administered at least 1 day before the procedure and continued indefinitely thereafter. Ticlopidine and clopidogrel are typically administered in addition to aspirin for 2 to 4 weeks following stent placement under the discretion of the interventional cardiologist.

External-Beam Irradiation Studies

Results using external-beam irradiation have been mixed (1,44,67,69,74,91). Studies of external-beam irradiation in the pig coronary balloon angioplasty model, done at Emory University, revealed that when 14 Gy was administered immediately before or after, or 2 days after balloon injury, there was reduced neointima formation compared with controls, but the lumens were smaller owing to negative remodeling (contracture) of the vessel. Results from studies using 21 Gy after either angioplasty or stenting indicate a profound and consistent suppression of neointima formation (60,91). The lack of benefit seen with a 14-Gy external beam compared with 14 Gy delivered by VBT at a 2-mm radius from the source suggests that the minimum dose delivered to the vessel wall is not the only factor in determining outcome. Studies of 14- and 21-Gy external radiation treatment have shown focal myocardial necrosis, an effect never seen with endovascular irradiation at any dose. This suggests that sophisticated treatment techniques, limiting the dose to normal tissues, will be essential for external-beam therapy to be adopted.

External-beam radiation therapy, however, has a well-established role in the treatment of benign disorders outside the cardiac system, such as for the prevention of heterotopic ossification, pterygium, and scar formation. Currently, there is a single-institution trial looking into the role of fractionated

TABLE 90.1	**SUMMARY OF CATHETER BASED SYSTEMS**			
System	Isotope/Half-Life	Delivery Method/ Length of Source	Centering System	Approved Injury Length/ Diameter/Dosimetry
Checkmate (Cordis/Best)[a]	[192]Ir gamma/74 days	Manual (hand-delivered) 6, 10, and 14 seeds (23, 39, and 55 mm long)	Noncentered (3.7-Fr delivery catheter)	≤45 mm/2.75–4 mm/ intravascular ultrasonography based; 8 Gy at farthest junction of media and adventitia and <30 Gy to the closest
Betacath (Novoste)[b]	[90]Sr/Y beta/28 years	Manual (hydraulic) 12 and 16 seeds (30 and 40 mm long)	Noncentered (5-Fr delivery catheter)	≤20 mm/2.7–4 mm/fixed, 16–23 Gy at 2.0-mm radius (modified by vessel diameter and stent)
Galileo (Guidant)[c]	[32]P beta/14 days	Computerized source delivery 27-mm wire (manual tandem stepping to 54 mm long)	Centering catheter, 2.5, 3.0, and 3.5 mm diameter, allowing distal, side branch flow	≤47 mm/2.4–3.7 mm/fixed dosimetry of 20 Gy at 1.0 mm into vessel wall from balloon surface

[a]18 and 22 seeds (71 and 87 mm long, respectively) and fixed dosimetry in clinical trials in the United States. No longer manufactured.
[b]Only 40-mm source train currently manufactured.
[c]A 20-mm long source with automated computerized stepping. No longer manufactured.

external-beam radiation therapy following balloon aortic valvuloplasty for the prevention of restenosis.

Endovascular Irradiation Studies

In contrast to the disparate results from studies using external radiation, numerous studies have consistently demonstrated remarkable suppression of neointima formation using radiation from a variety of isotopes delivered by an endoluminal approach. At least three groups have documented similar results in the pig coronary artery model of restenosis after balloon angioplasty, using the γ emitter ^{192}Ir at roughly comparable doses (104,108,109).

VBT typically reduces the neointima formation and maintains the patency of the lumen. Scanning electron microscopy of arteries irradiated to 14 Gy showed no morphologic differences from controls at 2 weeks; a confluent layer of endothelial or endothelial-like cells was present throughout the region of the angioplasty injury. However, at 28 and 56 Gy, neointima formation was nearly eradicated and endothelial coverage was incomplete. Inadequate endothelial recovery of an irradiated artery after angioplasty might render its luminal surface prothrombotic and, in the setting of an appropriate physiologic stimulus, result in thrombotic occlusion. The problem of late thrombosis observed in clinical trials certainly is compatible with the delayed healing observed in the animal studies.

With stents playing an increasingly important role in the management of coronary stenosis, it became important to test whether radiation might prove a useful adjunct to coronary stenting. Studies carried out with β and γ emitters have demonstrated conclusively that the excess intimal hyperplasia occurring in a stent can be effectively eliminated by radiation delivered either before or after stenting (46).

Vascular Brachytherapy Physics and Devices

The initial evaluation of radiation therapy in animal models of restenosis focused on testing the effect of radiation with commercially available radiation sources. Testing has included both teletherapy and brachytherapy. Although occasional positive results have been reported with teletherapy in experimental models of restenosis, consistently positive results emerged from a variety of brachytherapy approaches. These approaches have included both temporary (VBT) and permanent implants (radioactive stents). Although many isotopes have been proposed for VBT, only approximately half a dozen have been used in human clinical trials, and of those, only three have seen widespread use. The three isotopes, which have been used for well over 95% of all clinical trials of catheter-based systems, are ^{192}Ir, ^{90}Sr/Y, and [32]P (Table 90.1).

Betacath System for Coronary In-Stent Restenosis

The Betacath system is the only system currently manufactured offered for in-stent restenosis. [90]Sr is a pure β emitter with a 28.5-year half-life and 546-KeV maximum β energy. The daughter isotope ^{90}Y is also a pure β emitter with a 64-hour half-life and 2.27-MeV maximum β energy. It is primarily the [90]Y β emissions that are used for therapy because the [90]Sr β particles are mostly absorbed by the stainless steel encapsulation and the surrounding catheter. The Betacath system contains sources that are 0.6 mm in diameter and 2.5 mm in length. Source trains of 12 seeds (30 mm), 16 seeds (40 mm), and 24 seeds (60 mm) are commercially available. A nonradioactive marker seed is located both proximally and distally to the radioactive sources (Fig. 90.3). This helps with fluoroscopic verification of the position of the radioactive seeds and allows verification of the return of the sources to the delivery device. For lesions longer than 60 mm, a "pullback technique" is used in which the most distal portion of the lesion is treated first, then the catheter is carefully pulled back to treat the more proximal lesion. The appropriate size of the source train should be used. For instance, a 40-mm source train can be used with a pullback technique to cover a distance of 80 mm. This technique could also be used for treatment of lesions at vessel bifurcations (12). Significant overlap or gaps between the treatment fields should be avoided. A careful review of the cine angiograms is pertinent when using this technique.

The Betacath system consists of four main components: the source train, transfer device, delivery catheter, and accessories. The sources are stored in a hand-held transfer device and are advanced by a closed-loop hydraulic system that uses sterile water to advance (and then retract) the sources. The advantage of the Betacath system is the relatively short treatment times (3 to 5 minutes) and the absence of radiation exposure to catheterization laboratory staff. The long half-life of the isotope permits the sources to be exchanged once every 6 months (4), with no need to change the treatment times during that 6-month period. A potential disadvantage of this system is the inferior depth–dose gradient compared with the γ source, attenuation by calcifications or stents, and the lack of utility in larger vessels (Fig. 90.4).

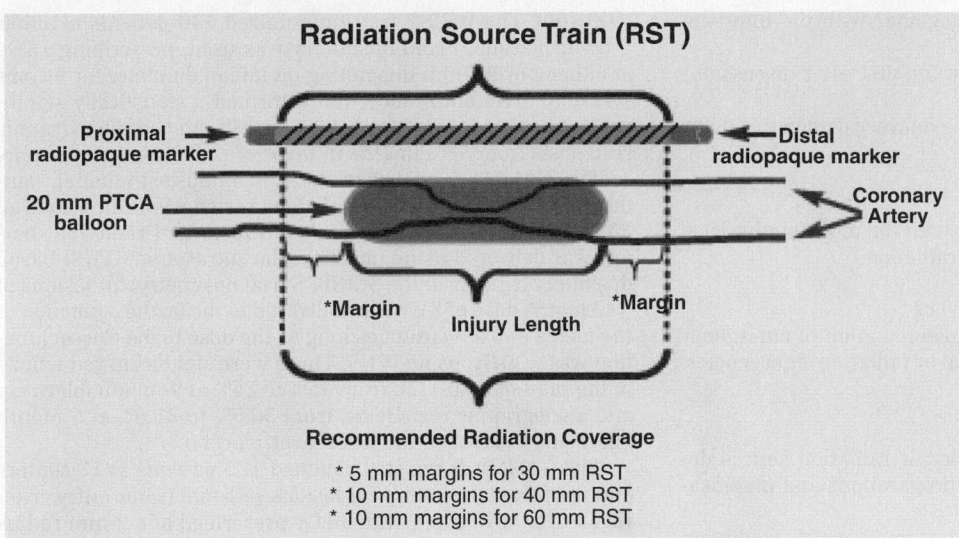

FIGURE 90.3. Radiation source train with proximal and distal radiopaque markers noted. (Courtesy of Novoste Corporation, Norcross, GA.)

A dose of 18.4 Gy is prescribed at 2-mm radius at the center of the source axis for vessels with a reference diameter between 2.7 and 3.3 mm. For reference diameters between 3.4 and 4 mm, a dose of 23 Gy is prescribed. The gross target volume is the stenotic area itself. The clinical target volume is the dilated part of the vessel. The planning target includes at least 5 mm proximal and distal to the clinical target volume (22,24,84).

Roles and Responsibilities

(This text is modified and printed with permission from Tripuraneni P. In: Tripuraneni P, Jani S, Minar E, et al., eds. *Intravascular brachytherapy: from theory to practice*. London: Remedica; 2001:272–274.) The FDA has mandated that VBT be carried out by a team consisting of an interventional cardiologist/radiologist, a radiation oncologist/therapeutic radiologist and oncologist, and a medical physicist. The roles and responsibilities of these specialists are listed in the following sections (86).

Interventional Cardiologist/Radiologist

1. Perform preprocedure evaluation and communicate patient's status (risk factors, interventions) with radiation oncologist.
2. Perform angioplasty with or without stenting, as necessary.
3. Define the anatomic location of diseased vessel amenable to intervention, length/volume of intervention, angioplasty and stenting, reference vessel diameter (including preintervention and postintervention vessel segment diameters), and communicate with radiation oncologist.
4. Determine the target volumes, jointly with the radiation oncologist and medical physicist.
5. Place delivery catheter and make final adjustment, in consultation with the radiation oncologist.
6. Advise the radiation oncologist of any changes in the delivery catheter position during the delivery of radiation.
7. Assist the radiation oncologist with any procedural details.
8. Assist the radiation oncologist in source removal as needed. In cases of medical or radiation emergencies, have procedures in place to ensure that radiation treatments are preplanned and nothing is left to chance.

Therapeutic Radiologist/Oncologist (Authorized User)

1. Review preprocedure evaluation, including patient's status (including risk factors and interventions), with interventional cardiologist for the advisability of using intravascular radiation.
2. Review the anatomic location of diseased vessels amenable to intervention, length/volume of intervention, angioplasty, and stenting, reference vessel diameter (including preintervention and postintervention vessel segment) with the interventional cardiologist.

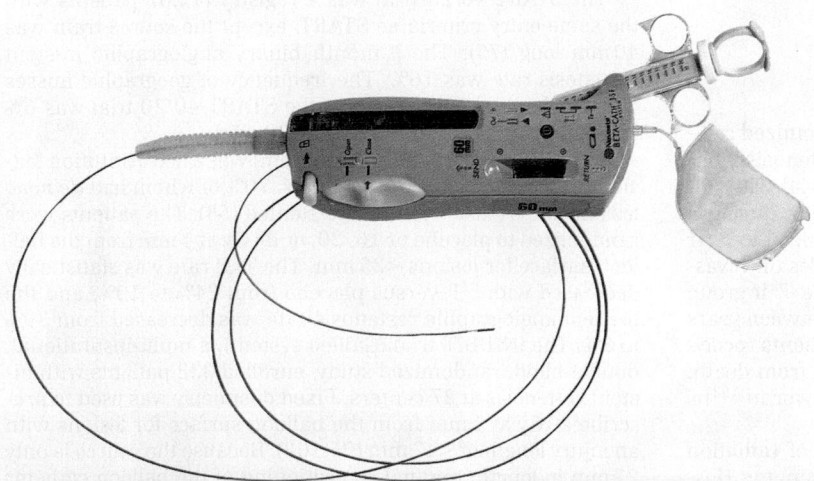

FIGURE 90.4. The Betacath system is a hydraulic delivery system with a noncentered, 5-Fr, closed, over-the-wire delivery catheter. ^{90}Sr seeds of 12, 16, and 22 source trains (30, 40, and 60 mm in length, respectively) are available. The delivery unit is shown. (Courtesy of Novoste Corporation, Norcross, GA.)

3. Determine the target volumes together with the interventional cardiologist.
4. Obtain proper informed consent for VBT after discussions with the patient.
5. Review the final placement of the delivery catheter and any adjustments as needed.
6. Prescribe radiation dose.
7. Insert radiation source.
8. Calculate treatment time, along with the medical physicist.
9. Ensure appropriate delivery of radiation.
10. Remove radiation source.
11. Supervise overall radiation delivery.
12. Participate in decisions and implementation of emergency source removal in case of medical or radiation emergencies.

Medical Physicist

1. Survey catheterization laboratory or radiation source delivery room, make appropriate preparations and modifications as needed.
2. Order radiation sources, under the direction of the radiation oncologist.
3. Calibrate sources on arrival.
4. Ensure safe-keeping of radiation sources.
5. Prepare sources for clinical use.
6. Calculate treatment-delivery times.
7. Assist radiation oncologist and interventional cardiologist in source removal in cases of radiation or medical emergencies.
8. Conduct radiation survey of patient after source removal.
9. In case of radiation or medical mishaps, inform appropriate regulatory authorities.
10. Participate in preparation of license application for medical use of VBT sources.
11. Develop and oversee quality assurance and improvement programs for efficacious and safe use of VBT sources in consultation with the radiation oncologist and interventional cardiologist as appropriate.

Clinical Trials of Coronary Brachytherapy

Nearly 5,000 patients have participated in clinical trials to determine the safety and efficacy of VBT (42,57,95). There have been seven double-blind randomized trials investigating the use of VBT on patients with in-stent restenosis (25,42,57,58,79,80,96,103,106). These trials led to the approval of one γ system using ^{192}Ir and two β systems using ^{32}P and ^{90}Sr/Y isotopes (42,70,90).

γ-Radiation In-Stent Coronary Artery Restenosis Trials

The SCRIPPS I trial was the first double-blind, randomized radiation trial for coronary in-stent restenosis and restenosis without stents (46,77–81). It was a single-institution trial with off-site analysis involving the treatment of 55 patients during a 9-month period. Twenty-six patients were randomized to ^{192}Ir and 29 to placebo. At 5-year follow-up, the target lesion revascularization (TLR) rate was significantly lower in the ^{192}Ir group (23.1% vs. 48.3%; $p = .05$). There were two TLRs between years 3 and 5 in the treated patients, but none in the patients receiving placebo. The event-free survival rate (freedom from death, myocardial infarction, or TLR) was significantly lower in ^{192}Ir-treated patients (34.5% vs. 61.5%; $p = .028$).

A second single-institution, randomized study of radiation for in-stent restenosis was carried out at the Washington Hospital Center in Washington, DC, and is known as the WRIST trial

(100,106). The WRIST trial randomized 130 patients to either ^{192}Ir or placebo. Fixed dosimetry was used, prescribing 15 Gy at either 2 or 2.4 mm depending on lumen diameter for lesions $\leq$47 mm. Six-month follow-up confirmed a statistically significant reduction in TLR from 63% to 14% and in angiographic restenosis from 58% to 19% in favor of radiation over placebo.

The GAMMA I trial was the first multi-institutional, randomized radiation trial for in-stent restenosis (42). A total of 252 patients at 12 centers were enrolled, and radiation therapy was delivered using intravascular ultrasound (IVUS)-based dosimetry (similar to the SCRIPPS trial dosimetry) for lesions of $\leq$45 mm. A dose of 8 Gy was delivered to the farthest junction of the media and adventitia as long as the dose to the closest junction was <30 Gy, using IVUS. There were significant reductions in the rates of both TLR, from 45% to 24% at 9-month follow-up and angiographic restenosis, from 50.5% to 21.6% at 6-month follow-up, in favor of radiation over placebo.

The GAMMA II registry included 125 patients at 12 centers and used fixed dosimetry for lesions $\leq$45 mm (same entry criteria as GAMMA I trial), with 14 Gy prescribed at a 2-mm radius for all patients (88). There was a TLR rate of 23% at the 9-month follow-up and an angiographic restenosis rate of 25% at the 6-month follow-up. This registry showed that the results with ^{192}Ir were reproducible and similar to those in the GAMMA I trial with simplified dosimetry (63).

The LONG WRIST trial was a two-institution, 120-patient randomized trial that used fixed dosimetry of 15 Gy at a 2- or 2.4-mm radius, for longer lesions of 36 to 80 mm. There was a statistically significant decrease in the 6-month angiographic restenosis rate (32% vs. 71%; $p = .0002$) in favor of radiation (47). The PLAVIX WRIST trial was a registry of 120 patients who received 6 months of clopidogrel. Six-month follow-up has demonstrated that extended antiplatelet therapy is able to eliminate the problem of late thrombosis observed in the WRIST and GAMMA studies (97) (Table 90.2).

β-Radiation In-Stent Coronary Artery Restenosis Trials

The START trial (Betacath system) was a 50-center multi-institutional, double-blind, randomized trial of 476 patients with in-stent restenosis (56). A 30-mm-long ^{90}Sr/Y source was used to treat lesions $\leq$20 mm; the dose prescribed was 18.4 Gy at a 2-mm radius for vessels $\geq$2.7 and $\leq$3.35 mm in diameter, and 23 Gy at a 2-mm radius for vessels $\geq$3.35 and $\leq$4 mm in diameter. At 8-month follow-up, the TLR rate was statistically decreased from 22% to 13% ($p <.008$), and the angiographic in-stent restenosis rate was also significantly decreased from 41% to 14% in favor of radiation over placebo.

The START 40/20 trial was a registry of 207 patients with the same entry criteria as START, except the source train was 40 mm long (75). The 8-month binary angiographic in-stent restenosis rate was 16%. The frequency of geographic misses with the longer source train in the START 40/20 trial was 6% compared with 15% in the START 30 trial.

The PREVENT trial (Galileo system) was a six-institution feasibility study involving 105 patients, 70% of whom had *de novo* lesions and 61% of whom were stented (58). The patients were randomized to placebo or 16, 20, or 24 Gy at 1 mm from the balloon surface for lesions $\leq$25 mm. The TLR rate was statistically decreased with ^{32}P versus placebo from 24% to 10%, and the in-stent angiographic restenosis rate was decreased from 39% to 8%. The INHIBIT trial (Galileo system), a multi-institutional, double-blind, randomized study, enrolled 332 patients with in-stent restenosis at 27 centers. Fixed dosimetry was used to prescribe 20 Gy at 1 mm from the balloon surface for lesions with an injury length of $\leq$47 mm (95,102). Because the source is only 27 mm in length, manual repositioning of the balloon catheter was used to treat the longer lesions. At 9-month follow-up, the

Table 90.2 SUMMARY OF PUBLISHED OR PRESENTED TRIAL RESULTS FOR CORONARY IN-STENT RESTENOSIS[a]

Study/System	Lesion Length (mm)/ Dose (Gy)	Percentage Target Lesion Revascularization (Radiation vs. Placebo)	Percentage Angiographic in-Stent Restenosis (Radiation vs. Placebo)
SCRIPPS I/Checkmate	≤30/<8 farthest EEM, <30 closest EEM	15 vs. 48	33 vs. 64
WRIST/Checkmate	≤47/15 at 2 or 2.4 mm	14 vs. 63	19 vs. 58
GAMMA I/Checkmate	≤45/<8 farthest EEM, <30 closest EEM	24 vs. 45	22 vs. 51
GAMMA II Registry/Checkmate	≤45/14 at 2 mm	23	25
Long WRIST/Checkmate	36–80/15 at 2 mm	30 vs. 60	32 vs. 71
Long WRIST HD Registry/Checkmate	36–80/18 at 2 mm	17	24
SVG WRIST/Checkmate[b]	≤80/15 at 2 or 2.4 mm	10 vs. 48	10 vs. 48
START/Betacath	≤20/18 or 23 at 2 mm	13 vs. 22	14 vs. 41
START 40/20 Registry/Betacath	≤20/18 or 23 at 2 mm	16	
INHIBIT/Galileo	<47/20 at 1 mm	11 vs. 29	16 vs. 49
BETA WRIST Registry/Schneider	≤47/20.6 at 1 mm	16	22

EEM, external elastic lamina.

[a]Some of the above results have not been published yet. The results may not be directly comparable because the enrollment and reporting criteria are sometimes different. All of the above trials statistically significantly positive in favor of radiation.

[b]Saphenous vein graft.

rate of major adverse cardiac events was decreased from 31% to 15% ($p = .0006$), and the rate of angiographic in-stent restenosis was also significantly decreased from 49% to 16% ($p < .0001$) in favor of radiation over placebo. Sixty-four patients in the radiation group and 76 patients from the placebo group were treated with pullback technique for lesions longer than 20 mm. No safety issues were identified in patients in whom there had been a significant overlap of active sources at the junction.

The BRITE (^{32}P balloon system trial) and BETTER trials (RDX system) have completed the feasibility phase (101). Seventy-six patients with in-stent restenosis were enrolled into these studies. A dose of 20 Gy at 1 mm into vessel wall was delivered to a treatment length of 33 mm. The mean dwell time was 7.9 minutes, with a procedure time of approximately 15 minutes. At 6-month follow-up, an 11% TLR rate was observed with an angiographic restenosis rate of 10%.

The Beta WRIST trial was a registry of 50 patients with in-stent restenosis treated with the Boston Scientific/Schneider system at the Washington Hospital Center using the same entry criteria as the WRIST trial (106). An angiographic restenosis rate of 22% and a TLR rate of 16% at 6 months were noted, which were similar to the results obtained in the radiation arm of the WRIST study (Tables 90.3 and 90.4).

Trials on Drug-eluting Stents for Coronary In-Stent Restenosis

The role of VBT in coronary in-stent restenosis has clearly changed with the introduction of effective DESs. The first trial

using DESs was a Brazilian study involving 31 patients. There was no incidence of restenosis reported on initial evaluation of patients at 4 months. No clinical events were reported at 8 months (71).

The RAVEL (Randomized Study with Sirolimus-eluting Velocity Balloon-Expandable Stent) involved 238 patients randomized to either DES or bare-metal stents (BMS) (50). At 3 years, event-free survival rates for target lesion revascularization was 93.7% in the DES arm versus 75% for the control group ($p < .001$) (17).

Paclitaxel-eluting stents have been investigated in the series of TAXUS trials I-IV (10,26,72,76). TAXUS I evaluated 61 patients randomized to 15-mm TAXUS NIRx paclitaxel-eluting stent (Boston Scientific, Natick, MA) or similar drug-free stent. At 6 months, there were no incidence of in-stent restenosis in the DES arm and three patients developed restenosis in the BMS arm ($p = .112$) (26). TAXUS II investigates two different drug formulations and compared them to BMS. No differences were noted between the two drug arms but a statistical advantage was noted in the DES arms compared with BMS (10). TAXUS IV randomized 1,314 patients to EXPRESS BMS or EXPRESS DES. Nine-month angiographic results were available in 559 patients. A relative risk of restenosis was reduced by 70% in the DES arm ($p < .001$) (72). The TAXUS V and VI trials evaluate the EXPRESS DES in patients with more complex diseases.

The two major trials comparing DESs to VBT have now been completed (85). The TAXUS V trial is a multicenter randomized trial with 396 patients enrolled. This study demonstrated that paclitaxel-eluting stents when compared to VBT significantly reduced the ischemic target lesion revascularization rate by 40%

Table 90.3 SUMMARY OF THE PIVOTAL MULTI-INSTITUTION RANDOMIZED TRIALS AND REGISTRIES FOR CORONARY IN-STENT RESTENOSIS

Trial	Isotope	Patients/ Centers	Randomization	Centering Balloon	Lesion Maximum Length/Diameter (mm)	Dose (Gy)
GAMMA I	[192]Ir	252/12	Yes	No	45/2.75–4.0	Intravascular ultrasonography-based 8–30
GAMMA II	[192]Ir	125/12	No	No	45/2.75–4.0	14 at 2-mm radius
START	Sr/[90]Y	476/50	Yes	No	20/2.7–4.0	18.4–23 at 2-mm radius
START 40/20	Sr/[90]Y	207/22	No	No	20/2.7–4.0	18.4–23 at 2-mm radius
INHIBIT	[32]P	332/27	Yes	Yes	47/2.4–3.7	20 at 1-mm radius from balloon surface

From Tripuraneni P, Teirstein P. Radiation therapy in coronary arteries: catheter based trials. In: Tripuraneni P, Janis P, Minar E, et al., eds. *Intravascular brachytherapy: from theory to practice*. London: Remedica; 2001:210, with permission.

Clinical Radiation Oncology

Table 90.4   RESULTS OF PIVOTAL TRIALS AND REGISTRIES FOR CORONARY IN-STENT RESTENOSIS[a]

Trial	Percentage Target Lesion Revascularization	Percentage Major Adverse Cardiac Events	Percentage In-Stent Restenosis	Percentage Analysis Restenosis	In-Stent Late Loss (mm)
GAMMA I	42 vs. 24	46 vs. 29	52 vs. 22	56 vs. 33[b]	1.14 vs. 073
GAMMA II	23	30	25	34[b]	0.61
START	22 vs. 13	26 vs. 18	41 vs. 14	45 vs. 29	0.67 vs. 0.21
START 40/20	Pending	Pending	16	22	0.20
INHIBIT	29 vs. 11	33 vs. 22	49 vs. 16	52 vs. 26	

[a]The results may not be directly comparable because the reporting criteria and enrollment criteria are sometimes different. GAMMA II and START 40/20 are single-arm registries with the same entry criteria as GAMMA I and START, respectively. Results are placebo versus radiation.
[b]In-lesion.
From Tripuraneni P, Teirstein P. Radiation therapy in coronary arteries: catheter based trials. In: Tripuraneni P, Janis P, Minar E, et al., eds. *Intravascular brachytherapy: from theory to practice.* London: Remedica; 2001:210, with permission.

at 9 months, 6.3% DES versus 13.9% VBT. Relative reductions in total target lesion (61%) and target vessel (49%) revascularization events were higher in patients treated with paclitaxel-eluting stents rather than those receiving VBT when considering only ischemic-related events. Additionally, the 9-month rate of major adverse coronary events was reduced by 43% in the DES arm versus the VBT arm (73). The SISR Trial is a prospective, multicenter randomized trial with 384 patients enrolled. Patients were randomized to sirolimus-eluting stents versus VBT for restenosis following BMS implantation. At 6 months, the DES arm had superior clinical and angiographic outcomes when compared with VBT. The publication of these trials will clearly change the role of VBT from first-line therapy to second-choice treatment for coronary in-stent restenosis.

Vascular Brachytherapy for In-Stent Restenosis Following DES

Up to 10% of patients develop restenosis following DES. The optimal treatment remains unclear for patients who fail DES. Options include balloon angioplasty, additional DES with either the same or a different drug, or VBT.

The RESCUE Registry is a multicenter international electronic registry for patients who receive VBT for recurrent restenosis following DES. The purpose of the registry is to evaluate the safety and efficacy of VBT following DES and to compare it to repeat DES following in-stenosis of DES.

Sixty-one patients received VBT following DES and were compared with 50 patients who received additional DES (Taxus or Cypher stents) after DES restenosis. The patient's demographic and angiographic characteristics were similar in both groups. Torguson et al. (83) presented the data at the 2005 American Heart Association Scientific Sessions. VBT appeared to be safe. At 6 months, VBT was associated with lower major adverse cardiac events compared with repeat DES (3.3% vs. 22%; $p = .02$). Additionally, target vessel revascularization rates were 3.3% versus 16% ($p = .04$) in favor of VBT. TLR rates were 3.3% versus 8% ($p = .24$) in favor of the VBT as well.

At Scripps Clinic, the clinical experience on the first five patients treated with VBT following DES has been reviewed. Median follow-up is 256 days. One episode of TLR is noted at 182 days and no episodes of nonfatal myocardial infarction or thrombosis have been observed.

Saphenous Vein Graft In-Stent Restenosis Clinical Trials

Saphenous vein grafts often are larger vessels with luminal diameters of >4 mm. Allowances must be made to deliver adequate doses when using IVUS-based or fixed dosimetry. All SCRIPPS trials included patients with saphenous vein grafts. However, the number of patients enrolled into SCRIPPS I was too small to reach any conclusions. Thirty of 130 patients in the WRIST trial were treated for in-stent restenosis of saphenous vein grafts. Subgroup analysis of WRIST suggests that radiation was as effective in saphenous vein grafts as in native coronary vessels. The more definitive study, SVG WRIST, a multi-institutional, randomized trial testing the efficacy of the Checkmate system with ^{192}Ir, enrolled 120 patients with lesions <47 mm in length (7). A dose of 15 Gy at a 2-mm radius for vessels of 2.5- to 4-mm radius and 18 Gy at a 2-mm radius for vessels of 4- to 5-mm radius was delivered. A statistically significant reduction in the rate of in-stent restenosis of 43% versus 15% ($p = .004$), in favor of radiation over placebo, was observed. Likewise, the TLR rate at 6 months was statistically significantly decreased (10% vs. 48%; $p < .01$) in favor of radiation over placebo. At 36 month follow-up, TLR rate was still in favor of the radiation arm (43% vs. 66%; $p = .02$) (59). With appropriate doses, the in-stent rate of saphenous vein grafts can be reduced with adjuvant brachytherapy after appropriate recanalization.

In summary, there are numerous multi-institutional, randomized trials confirming the efficacy of radiation in decreasing in-stent restenosis. The three pivotal trials, GAMMA I, START, and INHIBIT, led to the approval of VBT for use in native coronary in-stent restenosis after recanalization. The Betacath system, the only commercial system that is currently available, was approved based on the START trial. The system has been used successfully and has registry confirming that longer margins decrease edge restenosis. This system was initially approved for 20-mm long injured length with 2-mm radius prescription dosimetry. Doses would need to be adjusted for vessels with larger diameters between 3 and 5 mm (64).

De Novo Coronary Artery Stenosis Clinical Trials

There are no clear data supporting the use of routine radiation therapy to prevent restenosis for *de novo* coronary artery stenosis after recanalization. However, there are some data in the BETACATH trial indicating that radiation may indeed decrease the rate of restenosis in patients. This trial was a multi-institution, double-blind randomized study with 1,456 patients (39). After balloon angioplasty, patients received either radiation doses of 14 or 18 Gy depending on vessel diameter or no adjuvant radiation. The 8-month angiographic analysis showed statistically significant decrease in restenosis in favor of radiation (34.3% vs. 21.4%; $p = .003$). However, with edge failures, this did not translate into a clinical benefit. Likewise, the GENEVA dose-finding trial (16,92) confirmed the dose response with increasing doses, with the effect being more profound in the patients receiving angioplasty only without stenting. Nevertheless, with emerging data from the DES trials, it seems unlikely that VBT will be used routinely in *de novo* coronary artery stenosis. However, for special situations of high-risk *de novo* stenosis in which stents may not be optimal, such as small-diameter vessels, longer lesions, or branch vessels, VBT may possibly find a niche role.

Radioactive Stents

Currently, the majority of patients undergoing PCI receive coronary stents. Coupling the radiation delivery to the stent appears attractive in that it simplifies the delivery of treatment. Most clinical investigations have been undertaken with the ^{32}P β-emitting stent (2). Stents have been tested with activities ranging from 0.5 to 20 μCi. These stents are of extremely low activity and can be handled with the aid of a 1-cm acrylic shield. Unfortunately, clinical trials using the ^{32}P stent demonstrated restenosis rates of approximately 50%, largely owing to intimal proliferation at the stent edges. These are often called *candy wrapper* edge failures. These clinical failures have inspired recent investigation of variations of the ^{32}P-coated stent with "cold" ends, "hot" ends, low-pressure balloon deployment systems, and so forth, ^{103}Pd (a γ-emitting isotope), and ^{198}Au-emitting stents. Because studies to date indicate a lack of efficacy, currently there are no clinical trials evaluating the efficacy of radioactive-coated stents.

Peripheral Vascular Brachytherapy Trials

Peripheral vascular disease involves more organs than coronary artery disease (CAD), and hence there are more diverse clinical situations, manifestations, and end points (87). It is challenging to define measurable clinical end points for a diverse group of "host" organs (e. g., extremities, kidney, liver), that differ not only anatomically but in function. Unlike coronary vessels, most peripheral vessels have a diameter >3 mm, and, in fact, are typically approximately 7 to 10 mm. Peripheral vascular lesions tend to be much longer and are more likely to be multifocal. Because of the larger vessel diameter and increased thickness of the vessel wall, VBT in peripheral arteries is likely to require the use of either a more penetrating γ source (^{192}Ir) or a β source that is in direct contact with the vessel wall.

Most trials in peripheral vessels have used an HDR afterloader and treatment of the superficial femoral or popliteal artery. After successful percutaneous transluminal angioplasty (PTA) of these arteries, the restenotic rate at 6 months varies from 25% to 77% (32,51). In a Veterans Administration study, the actuarial restenosis rate was 41% at 36 months (110).

The feasibility of VBT for peripheral vascular system in humans was first documented in a study from Frankfurt, Germany (65). In this study, 30 patients with in-stent restenotic lesions in femoropopliteal arteries were treated with repeat PTA, stent implant, and VBT. A dose of 12 Gy at 3 mm was administered with a ^{192}Ir HDR afterloader through a 5-Fr, noncentered catheter. At last follow-up, the median follow-up time was 32.9 months for 28 patients (range, 7 to 84 months). There were no adverse effects from the brachytherapy. The 5-year vessel patency rate was 82% (23 of 28 patients) based on Doppler ultrasonography. Stenosis developed in the treated vessel in 3 of 28 patients (11%); 2 (7%) had complete occlusion of the vessel due to thrombosis after 16 and 37 months.

Investigators in Vienna, Austria, have mounted a series of trials exploring the use of VBT in similar patients (49,53). The Vienna II trial enrolled 107 patients with symptomatic *de novo*

or restenotic femoropopliteal lesions treated with angioplasty and then randomly assigned patients to either additional radiation therapy or no further treatment. A fixed dose of 12 Gy at a 3-mm radius from the source center and a margin of 1 cm at each end of the injured segment were delivered with a ^{192}Ir HDR afterloading system. At 6 months, the angiographic restenosis rate was significantly lower in the radiation group compared with the control group (28% vs. 54%; $p <.05$). The cumulative patency rate at 12 months was significantly higher in the radiation group than in the control group (64% vs. 35%; $p <.005$). Subgroup analysis demonstrated that restenotic lesions, occlusions, and long lesions benefit the most from VBT. Despite radiation, the recurrence rate in the radiation arm was 28%. It is postulated that this may be due to the relatively modest radiation dose and the absence of a centering catheter. This randomized trial demonstrated conclusively that radiation could have a significant impact on restenosis in peripheral vessels.

The Vienna III trial enrolled 134 patients. This double-blind study randomized patients following angioplasty to brachytherapy or placebo irradiation. Patients had either *de novo* lesions $\geq$5 cm or restenosis following femoropopliteal angioplasty. A dose of 18 Gy (γ-irradiation) was prescribed 2 mm from the surface of the centering balloons. At 24 months, patency rates based on intention to treat analysis was 54% in the brachytherapy arm and 27% in the placebo arm ($p <.005$) (54). VBT, however, reduced the restenosis rates for recurrent lesions only and not for *de novo* lesions.

Vienna V trial studied 88 patients with femoropopliteal lesions at high risk for restenosis (mean treatment length, 16.8 $\pm$ 7.3 cm). This double-blind study randomized patients to receive either brachytherapy with ^{192}Ir (14 Gy to 2 mm into arterial wall) or with nonradioactive seeds. In this trial, brachytherapy did not improve 6-month patency after femoropopliteal stent in high-risk patients mainly because of a high incidence of early and late thrombotic events (112).

The Peripheral Artery Radiation Investigational Study (PARIS) is the pivotal multi-institutional, randomized trial of VBT in superficial femoropopliteal arteries using the Nucletron HDR afterloader (Nucletron, The Netherlands). This study consists of two phases: an initial lead-in phase of 40 patients, followed by a second phase in which 300 patients were randomized to receive or not receive radiation after PTA. In the initial phase, 35 of 40 patients were successfully irradiated with no procedural complications (106). The angiographic restenosis rate at 6 months was 17.2%, which is very promising. The second phase started in early 1998 as the first multicenter, multinational, prospective, double-blind, randomized trial. Although initial results were promising at 6 months, the restenosis rates were similar in both groups (27.5% placebo and 28.6% brachytherapy) at 12 months (Table 90.5).

Recently, Krueger et al. (37) reported on 30 patients who underwent PTA for *de novo* femoropopliteal stenosis. Patients received either 14 Gy centered VBT or no radiation. Rates of restenosis were statistically significantly lower in the radiated group at 6 ($p = .006$) and 12 ($p = .042$) months.

Compared with the femoropopliteal arteries, the tibioperoneal arteries are smaller; hence, post-PTA restenosis tends to occur more frequently. Long-term success is limited mostly by neointimal hyperplasia. In a study of 55 PTA lesions in 40 patients, 44% remained patent at an average follow-up of 25.8 months (6). There are no clinical data reported on the use of radiation therapy for the tibial-peroneal vessels, but this remains a potentially fertile site for further investigation.

There are two types of stenosis in renal arteries: ostial (at the origin of the renal artery from the aorta) and nonostial (beyond the ostium). Ostial stenoses are more difficult to treat and tend to recur; hence, they are often treated with stenting. The restenosis rates as determined by angiography are somewhat lower, at 23%, for nonostial regions compared with 30% for

Table 90.5 | **DETAILS OF FEMORAL POPLITEAL ARTERY BRACHYTHERAPY TRIALS**[a]

Trial	No. of Patients	Randomization	Centering Catheter	Dose (Gy)	Dose (mm)	Patency
Frankfurt	40	No	No	12	3	82%
Vienna 01	10	No	No	12	3	60%
Vienna 02[b]	113	Yes	No	12	3	72%
						$p < .004$
Vienna 03	200	Yes	Yes	18	R +2	—
Vienna 04		Yes	Yes	14	R +2	—
Vienna 05	88	Yes	Yes	14	R +2	—
Swiss	320	Yes	No	14	R +2	—
Paris[c]	300	Yes	Yes	14	R +2	—

R, radius of the vessel.

[a]The general trend of more recent trials of peripheral artery brachytherapy is the use of a high–dose-rate remote afterloader with ^{192}Ir gamma source and centering catheter.

[b]Single-institution randomized trial for high-risk de novo and in stent restenosis lesions. Statistically significant improvement in patency at 12 months.

[c]Multi-institution randomized trial for high-risk de novo stenosis. Feasibility phase results encouraging. Completed enrollment of randomized phase and results expected in late 2002.

both ostial and nonstial lesions together (45,66). Renal artery stenosis also lends itself to exploration with VBT. In certain clinical subgroups, the prevalence of serious renal artery disease is as high as 43%, especially in the growing population of patients older than 50 years of age with multiple manifestations of atherosclerosis (28). Renal artery disease may account for up to 15% of patients with renal failure in the dialysis population older than 50 years of age. The morbidity and mortality among these patients are very high; hence, any potential benefit of VBT in the treatment of renal artery disease deserves investigation. In recent years, there have been some limited and selected cases published in the literature demonstrating the efficacy and safety of VBT for the treatment of renal artery in-stent restenosis (3,9,15,30).

There are more than 120,000 patients with end-stage renal disease in the United States who require vascular access for hemodialysis. The most common forms of vascular access are arteriovenous (AV) grafts and central venous canalization. AV grafts typically fail within 14 to 19 months, with a reported primary occlusion rate of 15% to 50% at 1 year (52). The most common cause of failure is stenosis at the anastomosis. The most common causes are thrombosis and intimal hyperplasia. Development of intimal hyperplasia at the site of venous anastomosis is due to several factors, including high-flow turbulence, compliance mismatch, vessel vibration, and platelet activation The restenosis rates for AV dialysis grafts after PTA are 9% at 3 months, 29% at 6 months, and 61% at 12 months; the restenosis rate for the subclavian vein after PTA alone is 71% at 6 months (5). The restenosis rate post-PTA and stenting for the subclavian vein is 30% to 53% at 1 year. An FDA-approved pilot study at New York Hospital used external-beam radiation (8 to 12 Gy, given in two equal fractions 48 hours apart) in a total of 10 patients to prevent restenosis. Unfortunately, all patients had restenosis by 18 months, suggesting no benefit from the therapy (48). A feasibility study involving a series of eight patients with restenosis of AV fistula in hemodialysis patients has been recently published (36). Although it appeared that radiation with ^{192}Ir after PTA of fistula stenosis appeared as a safe and feasible method in these patients, the radiation did not seem to decrease the incidence of restenosis. Different fractionation schemes are currently under investigation.

Compared with trials in CAD, peripheral vascular disease clinical trials testing the efficacy of VBT in reducing restenosis are in their early stages. VBT has now been tried in numerous sites outside the coronary arteries, including vein grafts,

renal artery in-stent restenosis, femoropopliteal arteries, and even the carotid arteries (8). The Vienna II and III trials, single-institution randomized trials, supported its efficacy in peripheral vascular disease. However, other trials have shown mixed results, particularly in high-risk patients. Certainly, there are many opportunities to explore the role of VBT in peripheral arterial disease.

Additional Clinical Considerations

Edge Restenosis

When restenosis occurs after VBT, the renarrowing is found at the treatment edges in one third to one half of patients. The etiology of edge failure is likely to be multifactorial, but most likely results from inadequate radiation dose delivered to injured lesion margins. Many factors can lead to higher-than-expected rates of edge failure. These include geographic miss, which arises from misalignment of the radioactive source in the injured segment of the vessel (33,61). In several studies using catheter-based radiation, careful, quantitative coronary angiographic measurements have documented a surprisingly high incidence of inadequate coverage of the injured region by the radioactive source. The balloon catheters used initially to open the stenotic segment can slip forward or backward ("watermelon seeding"), causing unintended injury to the lesion margins. Also, barotrauma from both angioplasty and stent deployment contributes to arterial wall injury beyond the nominal lengths of the balloons or stents (23). Longitudinal seed displacement may also contribute to higher-than-expected restenotic rates at lesion margins owing to the movement of the radioactive seeds relative to the coronary vessel during the cardiac cycle. In a seed movement analysis of 19 cineangiograms, proximal movement of 0 to 2 mm and distal movement of 1 to 5 mm was observed (21). In addition to more movement in the distal portion of arteries, the movement also varies with the particular artery (possibly more in the circumflex, for example). Uncertainty in target localization can arise because of the difficulty in visual estimation of proximal and distal lesion ends. This uncertainty is compounded by different magnifications and obliquity of various projections during fluoroscopy and cineangiography, and the relative lack of reference points available (branch vessels are commonly used as reference points for targeting). Last, the dose falloff and penumbra effect of the particular isotope used can contribute to marginal failure (89).

VBT cannot be effective in regions injured by angioplasty or atherectomy where radiation is not delivered. Although the causes of edge failure are still unclear and most likely multifactorial, several strategies have been used to decrease edge failures. First, careful cineangiographic documentation of injury to the vessel should be carried out at every balloon angioplasty or stent placement (discouraged to minimize late thrombosis). Second, the most proximal and distal extents of the injury to the vessel should be carefully determined, ideally with a side-branch reference point. Finally, a very wide margin (i.e., 4 to 10 mm) of the radiation source should be provided on either side of the injured vessel region. These measures will not eliminate edge failure, but will probably considerably reduce its occurrence (90).

Terminology

Based on the International Commission on Radiation Units and Measurements Report 50, terminology for VBT volumes was proposed that takes into consideration both radial and longitudinal dimensions (89). This terminology will help to define the target volume with attention to appropriate margins to decrease edge failures. The gross target volume (GTV) is the length of stenotic segment with an appropriate radius that may vary along the length. The clinical target volume (CTV) is the interventional length, which is delineated by the most proximal and distal extents of injury, is always larger than GTV. The planning target volume (PTV) is the CTV plus a margin to account for both heart and catheter movements and inaccuracies in the visual delineation of the ends of the CTV. The uncertainty or magnitude of the margin depends on the location of the target in the vessel, the delivery system (centered or noncentered), and the cardiac cycle. The target volume is the volume irradiated based on the PTV and the penumbra of the isotope's effect, which depends on the isotope, source design, and prescription distance. In practice, it is necessary to give at least a 4- to 8-mm margin to the longest injured length of the vessel (Table 90.6).

Subacute Thrombosis

Similar to the first attempts at stent implantation, initial enthusiasm for VBT was dampened by reports of target thrombosis, particularly thrombosis occurring late (>30 days) after treatment. In early trials, late thrombosis after VBT was observed in 3% to 10% of patients independent of the isotope and delivery system tested (97,98). The thrombotic episode usually manifested itself as a sudden target vessel occlusion resulting in myocardial infarction 1 to 9 months after radiation treatment. There is no uniform definition or criteria for subacute thrombosis. Total occlusions can be subdivided into two groups: (a) symptomatic late thrombosis, occurring more than 30 days after the index procedure and resulting in myocardial infarction, and confirmed by angiography; and (b) silent late occlusions, occurring more than 30 days after the index procedure. These total occlusions are seen on the protocol-required follow-up angiogram without clinical symptoms of myocardial infarction (99).

The emergence of this complication seriously jeopardized radiation as a viable treatment modality for CAD. Careful study, however, yielded two helpful clues that led to a dramatic reduction in radiation-associated late thrombosis: (a) the overwhelming majority of patients sustaining a late thrombosis had a new stent implanted at the time of the radiation procedure, and (b) almost all patients sustaining late thrombosis had discontinued antiplatelet therapy. Two strategies to prevent late thrombosis were initiated. First, the implantation of new stents during or immediately after treatment with brachytherapy was strongly discouraged. Second, antiplatelet therapy was extended for 6 to 12 months after the radiation therapy procedure. This strategy has now been tested with apparent success in several large series. In more recent trials using the aforementioned strategies, the incidence of late thrombosis was similar to that in placebo arm, in the range of 1% to 3%. In the ongoing SCRIPPS III trial, the late thrombosis rate is zero (82).

Stent placement at time of radiation delivery can cause both increased late thrombosis and possibly decreased efficacy of the brachytherapy itself. Pooled retrospective data from the SCRIPPS 1, WRIST, and GAMMA I trials for patients with in-stent restenosis show an even more pronounced effect of brachytherapy in patients without new stent placement than in patients with stent placement. The Geneva dose-finding study of *de novo* stenosis confirmed these results, with decreased restenosis rates with radiation after angioplasty-only compared with angioplasty and stenting

Summary

VBT is the first proven, clinically effective therapy in the management of in-stent restenosis. The Betacath system using ^{90}Sr/Y is currently the only available system used in the treatment of coronary in-stent restenosis. Despite its established efficacy, there is room for improvement. The optimum dose may not yet been established. It may be that the dose should be varied according to patient risk factors, much as is the dose is adjusted for the stage/volume of tumor in radiation oncology. However, the results of DES trials have decreased the need for VBT in coronary in-stent restenosis. The TAXUS V study and the SISR randomized trials demonstrate that DES may be superior to VBT in treating coronary in-stent restenosis (73). Nevertheless, there may be circumstances in which VBT continues to play a role, such as in drug-resistant in-stent restenosis, bifurcation lesions, small-diameter vessels, and for treatment of recurrent, multi-DES resistant restenosis.

Additionally, VBT may have an increased role in the treatment of vein graft in-stent restenosis and for peripheral vascular disease. The role of VBT for peripheral vascular disease will mainly be defined based on results of current clinical trials. The dose and volume to be treated will need to be refined to improve efficacy further.

Table 90.6	VASCULAR BRACHYTHERAPY TREATMENT TERMINOLOGY[a]
Target Volume Definition	**Description**
Gross target volume (GTV)	Stenotic or restenotic lesion
Clinical target volume (CTV)	Intervened or injured (angioplasty, stent, stent deployment, atherectomy) length
Planning target volume (PTV)	CTV + uncertainty for heart/catheter movement + uncertainty in target localization
Treatment volume (TV)	PTV + penumbra effect

[a]Volume includes the length and radius of the vessel. The target radius varies depending on the vessel, plaque in the vessel wall, and location of the delivery catheter in the lumen of the vessel. Intravascular ultrasonography may be helpful in determining target radius, but is not widely available and not widely used. It is common practice to accept a 2-mm radius for noncentered systems, and 1 mm into the vessel wall for the centered systems as the target radius.
Modified from Tripuraneni P, Parikh S, Giap H, et al. How long is enough? Defining the treatment length in endovascular brachytherapy. *Cathet Cardiovasc Intervent* 2000;51:147–153, with permission.

Finally, external-beam radiation therapy already has an established role in the treatment of benign diseases outside the cardiac system, such as for prevention of heterotopic ossification, pterygium, and scar formation. It will be interesting to see whether or not external-beam radiation therapy will find a role in the treatment of cardiac diseases, such as preventing restenosis following cardiac valvuloplasty.

References

1. Abbas MA, Afshari NA, Stadius ML, et al. External beam irradiation inhibits neointimal hyperplasia following balloon angioplasty. *Int J Cardiol* 1994;44:191–202.
2. Albiero R, Colombo A. Radiation therapy in coronary arteries: radioactive stent trials. In: Tripuraneni P, Jani S, Minar E, et al., eds. *Intravascular brachytherapy: from theory to practice.* London: Remedica; 2001:215–224.
3. Aslam, MS, Balasubramanian J, Greenspahn BR. Brachytherapy for renal artery in-stent restenosis. *Catheter Cardiovasc Interv* 2003;58:151–154.
4. Azeem T, Adlam D, Gershlick A. Evolution of vascular brachytherapy over time: data from the RENO-registry analysis. *Int J Cardiol* 2005;100:225–228.
5. Beathard GA. Percutaneous transvenous angioplasty in the treatment of vascular access stenosis. *Kidney Int* 1992;42:1390–1397.
6. Brown KT, Moore ED, Getrajdman GI, et al. Infrapopliteal angioplasty: long-term follow up. *J Vasc Intervent Radiol* 1993;4:139–144.
7. Castagna M, Mintz G, Weissman N, et al. Intravascular ultrasound analysis of the impact of gamma radiation on the treatment of saphenous vein graft in stent restenosis. *Am J Cardiol* 2002;90(12):1378–1381.
8. Chan AW, Roffi M, Mukherjee D, et al. Carotid brachytherapy for in-stent restenosis. *Catheter Cardiovasc Interv* 2003;58:86–92.
9. Chrysant GS, Goldstein JA, Casserly IP, et al. Endovascular brachytherapy for treatment of bilateral renal artery in-stent restenosis. *Catheter Cardiovasc Interv* 2003;59:251–254.
10. Colombo A, Drzewiecki J, Banning A, et al. Randomized study to assess the effectiveness of slow- and moderate-release polymer-based paclitaxel-eluting stent for coronary artery lesions. *Circulation* 2003;108:788–794.
11. Condado JA, Waksman R, Gurdiel O. Long-term angiographic and clinical outcome after percutaneous transluminal coronary angioplasty and intracoronary radiation therapy in humans. *Circulation* 1997;96:727–732.
12. Costa R, Joyal M, Harel F, et al. Treatment of bifurcation in-stent restenotic lesions with beta radiation using strontium 90 and sequential positioning pullback technique: procedural details and clinical outcomes. *J Invasive Cardiol* 15:469–473.
13. Degertekin M, Regar E, Tanabe K, et al. Sirolimus-eluting stent for treatment of complex in-stent restenosis: the first clinical experience. *J Am Coll Cardiol* 2003;41:184–189.
14. Dobesh PP, Stacy ZA, Ansara AJ, et al. Drug-eluting stents: a mechanical and pharmacologic approach to coronary artery disease. *Pharmacotherapy* 2004;24:1554–1577.
15. Ellis K, Murtagh B, Loghin C, et al. The use of brachytherapy to treat renal artery in-stent restenosis. *J Interv Cardiol* 2005;18:49–54.
16. Erbel R, Verin V, Popowski Y, et al. Intracoronary beta-irradiation to reduce restenosis after balloon angioplasty: results of a multicenter European dose-finding study (abstr). *Circulation* 1999;100:1–154.
17. Fajadet J, Morice MC, Bode C, et al. Maintenance of long-term clinical benefit with sirolimus-eluting coronary stents: three-year results of the RAVEL trail. *Circulation* 2005;111:958–960.
18. Faxon DP, and the ERA Investigators. Low molecular weight heparin in prevention of restenosis after angioplasty: results of the enoxaparin restenosis (ERA) trial. *Circulation* 1994;90:908–914.
19. Fischman DL, Leon MB, Baim DS, et al. A randomized comparison of coronary stent placement and balloon angioplasty in the treatment of coronary artery disease. *N Engl J Med* 1994;331:496–501.
20. Franklin SM, Faxon DP. Pharmacologic prevention of restenosis: review of the randomized clinical trials. *Coron Artery Dis* 1993;4:232–242.
21. Giap HB, Bendre DD, Huppe GB, et al. Source displacement during the cardiac cycle in coronary endovascular brachytherapy. *Int J Radiat Oncol Biol Phys* 2001;49:273–277.
22. Giap H, Massullo V, Teirstein P, et al. Theoretical assessment of late cardiac complication from endovascular brachytherapy for restenosis prevention. *Cardiovasc Radiat Med* 1999;1:233–238.
23. Giap H, Teirstein P, Massullo V, et al. Barotrauma due to stent deployment in endovascular brachytherapy for restenosis prevention. *Int J Radiat Oncol Biol Phys* 2000;47:1021–1024.
24. Giap H, Tripuraneni P, Teirstein P, et al. Theoretical assessment of dose-rate effect in endovascular brachytherapy. *Cardiovasc Radiat Med* 1999;1:227–232.
25. Grise MA, Massullo V, Jani S, et al. Five-year clinical follow-up after intracoronary radiation: results of a randomized clinical trial. *Circulation* 2002;105:2737–2740.
26. Grube E, Silber S, Hauptamann KE, et al. TAXUS I: six- and twelve-month results form a randomized double-blind trial on the slow release paclitaxel-eluting stent for de novo coronary lesions. *Circulation* 2003;107:38–42.
27. Hillegass WB, Ohman EM, Califf RM. Restenosis: the clinical issues. In: Topol EJ, ed. *Textbook of interventional cardiology,* vol 1, 2nd ed. Philadelphia: WB Saunders; 1994:415–435.
28. Holley KE, Hunt JC, Brown AL, et al. Renal artery stenosis: clinical pathologic study. *Am J Med* 1964;37:14–22.
29. Holmes DR, Teirstein P, Satler L, et al. Sirolimus-eluting stents vs vascular brachytherapy for in-stent restenosis within bare-metal stents. *JAMA* 2006;295:1264–1273.
30. Jahraus CD, Meigooni AS. Vascular brachytherapy: a new approach to renal artery in-stent restenosis. *J Invasive Cardiol* 2004;16:224–227.
31. Jahraus, CD, St Clair W, Gurley J, et al. Endovascular brachytherapy for the treatment of renal artery in-stent restenosis using a beta-emitting source: a report of five patients. *South Med J* 2003;96:1165–1168.

32. Johnston KW. Femoral and popliteal arteries: reanalysis of results of angioplasty. *Radiology* 1992;183:767–771.
33. Kim HS, Waksman R, Kollum M. Edge stenosis after intracoronary radiotherapy: angiographic, intravascular, and histological findings. *Circulation* 2001;103:2219–2220.
34. King SB, Williams DO, Prakash C, et al. Endovascular beta-radiation to reduce restenosis after coronary balloon angioplasty: results of the Beta Energy Restenosis Trial (BERT). *Circulation* 1998;97:2025–2030.
35. Klein LW, Rosenblum J. Restenosis after successful percutaneous transluminal coronary angioplasty. *Prog Cardiovasc Dis* 1990;32:365–382.
36. Krueger K, Bendel M, Zaehringer M, et al. Centered endovascular irradiation to prevent postangioplasty restenosis of arteriovenous fistula in hemodialysis patients; results of a feasibility study. *Cardiovasc Radiat Med* 2004;5:1–8.
37. Krueger K, Zaehringer M, Bendel M, et al. De novo femoropopliteal stenoses: endovascular gamma irradiation following angioplasty—angiographic and clinical follow-up in a prospective randomized controlled trial. *Radiology* 2004;231:546–551.
38. Kuntz RE, Gibson M, Nobuyoshi M, et al. Generalized model of restenosis after conventional balloon angioplasty, stenting and directional atherectomy. *J Am Coll Cardiol* 1993;21:15–25.
39. Kuntz RE, Speiser B, Joyal M, et al. Acute and midterm clinical outcomes after use of ^{90}Sr/^{90}Y beta radiation for the treatment of native coronary artery obstructions: acute results from the Novoste™ Beta-Cath™ System trial. Presented at the American College of Cardiology, 49th Annual Scientific Session, Anaheim, CA, March. 2000;12–16.
40. Landau C, Lange RA, Hillis LD. Percutaneous transluminal coronary angioplasty. *N Engl J Med* 1994;330:981–983.
41. Lansky A, Desai K, Costantino C, et al. Predictors of stent and stent-edge restenosis after Sr-90 radiation in the START trial. *J Am Coll Cardiol* 2001;37:54A.
42. Leon MB, Teirstein PS, Moses JW, et al. Localized intracoronary gamma-radiation therapy to inhibit the recurrence of restenosis after stenting. *N Engl J Med* 2001;344:250–256.
43. Ludbrook PA. Coronary restenosis: its mechanisms and modification—overview. *Coron Artery Dis* 1993;4:225–228.
44. Marijianowski M, Crocker I, Styles T, et al. Fibrocellular tissue responses to endovascular and external beam irradiation in the porcine model of restenosis. *Int J Radiat Oncol Biol Phys* 1999;44:633–641.
45. Martin LG, Rees CR, O'Bryant T. Percutaneous angioplasty of the renal arteries. In: Strandness DE, vanBreda A, eds. *Vascular diseases: surgical and interventional therapy.* New York: Churchill Livingstone; 1994:721–742.
46. Massullo VM, Teirstein PS, Jani SK, et al. Endovascular brachytherapy to inhibit coronary artery restenosis: an introduction to the Scripps Coronary Radiation to inhibit proliferation post stenting trial. *Int J Radiat Oncol Biol Phys* 1996;36:973–975.
47. Mehran R, Lansky A, Waksman R. Gamma radiation vs placebo in focal vs. diffuse in-stent restenosis: the length makes the difference. *J Am Coll Cardiol* 2001;35:82A.
48. Minar E, Parikh S. Peripheral trials of radiation therapy for prophylaxis of restenosis. In: Tripuraneni P, Jani S, Minar E, et al., eds. *Intravascular brachytherapy: from theory to practice.* London: Remedica; 2001:225–242.
49. Minar E, Pokrajac B, Maca T, et al. Endovascular brachytherapy for prophylaxis of restenosis after femoropopliteal angioplasty: results of a prospective randomized study. *Circulation* 2000;102:2694–2699.
50. Morice MC, Serruys PW, Sousa JE, et al. A randomized comparison of a sirolimus-eluting stent with a standard stent for coronary revascularization. *N Engl J Med* 2002;346:1315–1323.
51. Murray RRJ, Hewes RC, White RIJ, et al. Long-segment femoro-popliteal stenoses: is angioplasty a boon or a bust. *Radiology* 1987;162:473–476.
52. Palder SR, Kirkman RL, Whittermore AD, et al. Vascular access for hemodialysis: patency rates and results of revision. *Ann Surg* 1995;202:235–239.
53. Pokrajac B, Potter R, Maca T, et al. Intra arterial high dose rate brachytherapy for prophylaxis of restenosis after femoropopliteal percutaneous transluminal angioplasty: the prospective randomized Vienna 2 trial radiotherapy parameters and risk factor analysis. *Int J Radiat Oncol Biol Phys* 2000;48:923–931.
54. Pokrajac B, Potter R, Wolfram RM, et al. Endovascular brachytherapy prevents restenosis after femoropopliteal angioplasty: results of the Vienna-3 randomised multicenter study. *Radiother Oncol* 2005;74:1–2.
55. Popma JJ, Califf RM, Topol EJ. Clinical trials of restenosis after coronary angioplasty. *Circulation* 1994;84:1426–1436.
56. Popma J, Heuser R, Suntharalingam M, et al., for the START Investigators. Late clinical and angiographic outcomes after use of ^{90}Sr/Y beta radiation for the treatment of in-stent restenosis. *J Am Coll Cardiol* 2000;36:311–312.
57. Popma JJ, Suntharanlingam M, Lansky AJ, et al. Randomized trial of 90Sr/90Y b-radiation versus placebo control for treatment of in-stent restenosis. *Circulation* 2002;106:1090–1096.
58. Raizner AE, Oesterle SN, Waksman R, et al. Inhibition of restenosis with beta-emitting radiotherapy: report of the proliferation reduction with vascular energy trial. *Circulation* 2000;102:951–958.
59. Rha SW, Kuchulakanti P, Ajani AE, et al. Three-year follow-up after intravascular gamma-radiation for in-stent restenosis in saphenous vein grafts. *Catheter Cardiovasc Interv* 2005;65:257–262.
60. Robinson KA, Verheye S, Salame MY, et al. External radiation for restenosis. *J Intervent Cardiol* 1999;12:235–241.
61. Sabate M, Costa MA, Kozuma K, et al. Geographic miss: a cause of treatment failure in radio-oncology applied to intracoronary radiation therapy. *Circulation* 2000;101:2467–2471.
62. Saia F, Lemos PA, Sianos G, et al. Effectiveness of sirolimus-eluting stent implantation for recurrent in-stent restenosis after brachytherapy. *Am J Cardiol* 2003;41:184–189.
63. Sanfilippo NJ, Tripuraneni P. Intravascular brachytherapy trials for coronary heart disease using gamma sources. *Front Radiat Ther Oncol* 2001;35:202–210.
64. Schiele TM, Regar E, Silber S, et al. Clinical and angiographic acute and follow up results of intracoronary beta brachytherapy in saphenous vein bypass grafts: a subgroup analysis of multicentric European registry of intraluminal coronary beta brachytherapy (RENO). *Heart* 2003;89:640–644.
65. Schopohl B, et al. ^{192}Ir endovascular brachytherapy for avoidance of intimal hyperplasia after percutaneous transluminal angioplasty and stent implantation

in peripheral vessels: 6 years of experience. *Int J Radiat Oncol Biol Phys* 1996;36:835–840.

66. Schwarten DE. Percutaneous transluminal angioplasty of the renal arteries: intravenous digital subtraction angiography for follow-up. *Radiology* 1984;150:369–373.

67. Schwartz RS, Koval TM, Edwards WD, et al. Effect of external beam irradiation on neointimal hyperplasia after experimental coronary artery injury. *J Am Coll Cardiol* 1992;19:1106–1113.

68. Serruys PW, De Jaegere P, Kiemenij F, et al. A comparison of balloon-expandable stent implantation with balloon angioplasty in patients with coronary artery disease. *N Engl J Med* 1994;331:489–495.

69. Shimatokahara S, Mayberg MR. Gamma irradiation inhibits neointimal hyperplasia in rats after arterial injury. *Stroke* 1994;25:424–428.

70. Silber S, Popma JJ, Suntharalingam M, et al. Two-year clinical follow-up of 90 Sr/90 Y beta-radiation versus placebo control for the treatment of in-stent restenosis. *Am Heart J* 2005;149:689–694.

71. Sousa JE, Costa MA, Abizaid A, et al. Lack of neointimal proliferation after implantation of sirolimus-coated stents in human coronary arteries: a quantitative coronary angiography and three-dimensional intravascular ultrasound study. *Circulation* 2001;103:192–195.

72. Stone GW, Ellis SG, Cox DA, et al. A polymer-based, paclitaxel-eluting stent in patients with coronary artery disease. *N Engl J Med* 2004;350:221–231.

73. Stone GW, Ellis SC, O'Shaughnessy CD, et al. Paclitaxel-eluting stents versus vascular brachytherapy for in-stent restenosis within bare metal stents: the TAXUS V ISR randomized trial. *JAMA* 2006;295:1253–1263.

74. Styles T, Marijianowski MMH, Robinson KA, et al. Effects of external irradiation of the heart on the coronary artery response to balloon angioplasty injury in pigs. In: *Proceedings from Advances in Cardiovascular Radiation Therapy* 1997;:11.

75. Suntharalingam M, Laskey W, Lansky W, et al. Analysis of clinical outcomes from the START and START 40 trials:the efficacy of Sr-90 radiation in the treatment of long lesion in-stent restenosis. *Int J Radiat Oncol Biol Phys* 2001;51[Suppl 3]:142.

76. Tanabe K, Serruys PW, Grube E, et al. TAXUS III: in-stent restenosis treated with stent-based delivery of paclitaxel incorporated in a slow-release polymer formation. *Circulation* 2003;107:559–564.

77. Teirstein PS, Massullo V, Jani S. Radiation therapy to inhibit restenosis:early clinical results. *Mt Sinai J Med* 2001;68:192–196.

78. Teirstein PS, Masullo V, Jani S et al. A subgroup analysis of the Scripps Coronary Radiation to Inhibit Proliferation Poststenting Trial. *Int J Radiat Oncol Biol Phys* 1998;42:1097–1104.

79. Teirstein PS, Masullo V, Jani S, et al. Catheter-based radiotherapy to inhibit restenosis after coronary stenting. *N Engl J Med* 1997;336:1697–1703.

80. Teirstein PS, Masullo V, Jani S, et al. Three-year clinical and angiographic follow-up after coronary radiation: results of a randomized clinical trial. *Circulation* 2000;101:360–365.

81. Teirstein PS, Masullo V, Jani S, et al. Two-year follow-up after catheter based radiotherapy to inhibit coronary restenosis. *Circulation* 1999;99:243–247.

82. Teirstein PS, Moses JW, Casterella PJ, et al. Late thrombosis after coronary radiation may be eliminated by longer antiplatelet therapy and reduced stenting: the Scripps III results. *J Am Coll Cardiol* 2001;37[Suppl A]:60 A.

83. Torguson R, Sabate M, Okubagzi P, et al. Intravascular brachytherapy for the treatment of patients with drug-eluting stent restenosis: the RESCUE Registry. Presented at Annual Meeting of the American Heart Association, November 13–16, 2005; Dallas, Tex,.

84. Tripuraneni P. Coronary artery radiation therapy for the prevention of restenosis after percutaneous coronary angioplasty, II: outcomes of clinical trials. *Semin Radiat Oncol* 2002;12:17–30.

85. Tripuraneni P. The future of CART in the era of drug-eluting stents: "It's not over until it's over." Counterpoint. *Brachytherapy* 2003;2:74–76.

86. Tripuraneni P, Berger B. Summary and future of vascular brachytherapy in 2000. In: Meyer JL, ed. *Radiation therapy for benign diseases: current indications and techniques.* Basel: Karger; 2001:211–215.

87. Tripuraneni P, Giap H, Jani S. Endovascular brachytherapy for peripheral vascular disease. *Semin Radiat Oncol* 1999;9:190–202.

88. Tripuraneni P, Leon MB, Teirstein PS, et al. Gamma II, a prospective multicenter registry, with fixed dosing regimen compared to the gamma I trial, using Ir-192 in the treatment of coronary treatment of coronary in-stent restenosis. *Int J Radiat Oncol Biol Phys* 2000;48[Suppl 3]:183–184.

89. Tripuraneni P, Parikh S, Giap H, et al. How long is enough? Defining the treatment length in endovascular brachytherapy. *Cathet Cardiovasc Intervent* 2000;51:147–153.

90. Urban P, Serruys P, Baumgart D, et al. A multicentre European registry of intraluminal coronary beta brachytherapy. *Eur Heart J* 2003;24:604–612.

91. Verheye S, Salame M, Cui J, et al. High-dose external beam irradiation prevents lumen loss and inhibits neointima formation in stented pig coronary arteries. *Int J Radiat Oncol Biol Phys* 2001;51:820–827.

92. Verin V, Popowski Y, de Bruyne B. Endoluminal beta-radiation therapy for the prevention of coronary restenosis after balloon angioplasty: the Dose-Finding Study Group. *N Engl J Med* 2001;344:243–249.

93. Verin V, Urban P, Popowski Y, et al. Feasibility of intracoronary β-irradiation to reduce restenosis after balloon angioplasty. *Circulation* 1997;95:1138–1144.

94. Waksman, R. An update on peripheral brachytherapy. *Endovascular Today* 2004; October:43–52.

95. Waksman R, Ajani A, White RL, et al. Two year follow up after beta and gamma intracoronary radiation therapy for patients with diffuse in-stent restenosis. *Am J Cardiol* 2001;88:425–428.

96. Waksman R, Ajani AE, White RL, et al. Intravascular gamma radiation for in-stent restenosis in saphenous-vein bypass grafts. *N Engl J Med* 2002;346:1194–1199.

97. Waksman R, Ajani AE, White RL, et al. Prolonged antiplatelet therapy to prevent late thrombosis after intracoronary gamma-radiation in patients with in-stent restenosis: Washington Radiation for In-Stent Restenosis Trial Plus 6 Months of Clopidogrel (WRIST PLUS). *Circulation* 2001;103:2332–2335.

98. Waksman R, Bhargava B, Leon MB. Late thrombosis following intracoronary brachytherapy. *Cathet Cardiovasc Intervent* 2000;49:344–347.

99. Waksman R, Bhargava B, Mintz GS, et al. Late total occlusion after intracoronary brachytherapy for patients with in-stent restenosis. *J Am Coll Cardiol* 2000;36:65–68.

100. Waksman R, Bhargava B, White LR, et al. Intracoronary beta radiation therapy inhibits recurrence of in-stent restenosis. *Circulation* 2000;101:1895–1898.

101. Waksman R, Buchbinder M, Reisman M, et al. The "Brite" Trial: a feasibility study of a novel ^{32}P deployable balloon system for the treatment of in-stent restenosis. *Circulation* 2000;102[Suppl]:3235.

102. Waksman R, Raizner A, Chiu K, et al. Beta radiation to inhibit recurrence of in-stent restenosis: clinical and angiographic results of the multicenter, randomized double blind study. *Circulation Online* 2000;102:e9046

103. Waksman R, Raizer AE, Yeung AC, et al. Use of localized intracoronary β radiation in treatment of in-stent restenosis: the INHIBIT randomized controlled trial. *Lancet* 2002;350:551–557.

104. Waksman R, Robinson KA, Crocker IR, et al. Endovascular low dose irradiation inhibits neointima formation after coronary artery balloon injury in swine: a possible role for radiation therapy in restenosis prevention. *Circulation* 1995;91:1553–1539.

105. Waksman R, Laird JR, Jurkovitz CT, et al., for the Peripheral Artery Radiation Investigational Study (PARIS) Investigators. Intravascular radiation therapy after balloon angioplasty of narrowed femoropopliteal arteries to prevent restenosis: results of the PARIS feasibility clinical trial. *J Vasc Intervent Radiol* 2000;12:915–921.

106. Waksman R, White L, Chan RC, et al., for the Washington Radiation for In-Stent Restenosis Trial (WRIST) Investigators. Intracoronary γ-radiation therapy after angioplasty inhibits recurrence in patients with in-stent restenosis. *Circulation* 2000;101:2165–2171.s

107. Weintraub WS, and the LRT Study Group. Lack of effect of lovastatin on restenosis after coronary angioplasty. *N Engl J Med* 1994;331:1331–1337.

108. Wiedermann JG, Marboe C, Amols H, et al. Intracoronary irradiation markedly reduces neointimal proliferation after balloon angioplasty in swine: persistent benefit at 6-month follow-up. *J Am Coll Cardiol* 1995;25:1451–1456.

109. Wiedermann JG, Marboe C, Schwartz A, et al. Intracoronary irradiation reduces restenosis after balloon angioplasty in a porcine model. *J Am Coll Cardiol* 1994;23:1491–1498.

110. Wilson SE, Wolf GL, Cross AP. Percutaneous transluminal angioplasty versus operation for peripheral arteriosclerosis: report of a prospective randomized trial in a selected group of patients. *J Vasc Surg* 1989;9:1–9.

111. Windecker S, Meier B. Basics of interventional cardiology. In: Tripuraneni P, Jani S, Minar E, et al., eds. *Intravascular brachytherapy: from theory to practice.* London: Remedica; 2001:83–100.

112. Wolfram RM, Budinsky AC, Pokrajac B, et al. Endovascular brachytherapy: restenosis in de novo versus recurrent lesions of femoropopliteal artery—the Vienna experience. *Radiology* e-pub 2005;236:338–42.

Clinical Radiation Oncology

Chapter 91

Evaluation of Brain and Spinal Cord Metastases

Section IV

Palliative and Supportive Care

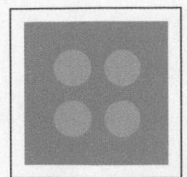

Chapter 91
Palliation of Brain and Spinal Cord Metastases

Young Kwok, Roy A. Patchell, William F. Regine

Brain Metastasis

Brain metastasis is very common, with an annual incidence of approximately 170,000 to 200,000. The rising incidence of brain metastasis is most likely from a combination of increasing survival from recent advances in systemic therapy, and a greater availability and use of magnetic resonance imaging (MRI). The most common primary site is the lung followed by breast. Metastatic brain tumors outnumber primary brain tumors by a factor of 10 to 1, with autopsy series demonstrating a 10% to 30% incidence rate for all patients with a diagnosis of cancer (Table 91.1) (33,74).

Clinical Presentation, Diagnosis, and Prognosis

The majority of patients present with neurologic signs and symptoms (Table 91.2) (51). Although differential diagnoses such as an abscess or a stroke must be considered, new-onset neurologic symptoms in a known cancer patient should always be presumed to be from brain metastasis until proven otherwise.

Given its ability to image in multiple orientations and sequences, including superior resolution and accuracy compared to computed tomography (CT), MRI has become the standard of care for imaging of the central nervous system (CNS) in cancer patients (9). MRI will frequently disclose smaller lesions not seen on CT scans, which can have a significant effect on the patient's prognosis and treatment course. Full systemic work-up (e.g., positron emission tomography and CT) should be promptly initiated if brain metastasis is the presenting event. The incidence of unknown primaries may subsequently decrease with the increasing popularity of integrated positron emission tomography/CT scans.

Performance status and extracranial disease status have consistently been shown to impact prognosis. Gaspar et al. (15) reported on the Radiation Oncology Therapy Group (RTOG) experience of 1,200 patients. This analysis revealed three recursive partitioning analysis (RPA) classes, with the RPA class I (Karnofsky Performance score [KPS] ≥70, controlled primary, age <65 years, brain metastasis only), II (not meeting requirements of classes I or III), and III (KPS <70) having median survivals of 7.1, 4.2, and 2.3 months, respectively (15).

Corticosteroids

The initial therapy should promptly start with corticosteroids (e.g., dexamethasone or methylprednisolone), which effectively improve edema and neurologic deficits in approximately two thirds of patients (58). The only randomized trial on the dosage question was reported by Vecht et al. (72). This trial included two successive groups of patients. The first group (n = 47) evaluated 8 mg/day versus 16 mg/day initial dexamethasone doses, with tapering schedules during 4 weeks. The second group (n = 49) evaluated 4 mg/day versus 16 mg/day of initial dexamethasone, with continuation of these doses for 28 days before tapering. The patients were scheduled for whole-brain radiotherapy (WBRT) and concurrent ranitidine. All arms had similar KPS improvements at 7 days (54% to 70%) and 28 days (50% to 81%). The study concludes that 4 mg/day of dexamethasone (with a taper during 4 weeks) is the preferable regimen. One should be cautious, however, in interpreting the results of this study. Patients in the 4-mg/day arm had to have the medication be reinstituted at a higher rate than the patients in the 8- or 16-mg/day arms. Furthermore, the arm with the greatest improvement in the KPS was the 16-mg/day arm when this was tapered during 4 weeks, compared to any of the other arms. It can be argued that higher KPS improvement arose from the maximal anti-inflammatory effects of the initial higher doses, with the 4-week taper minimizing the late toxicity associated with corticosteroids.

A reasonable corticosteroid regimen in patients with brain metastases is a 10-mg intravenous (IV) or oral bolus, followed by a 4 to 6 mg every 6 to 8 hours of dexamethasone-equivalent dose (with a concurrent proton-pump inhibitor) before this is tapered in a clinically cautious manner. In asymptomatic patients with little peritumoral edema or mass effect, initial corticosteroids may be reserved until the first sign of neurologic symptoms.

Whole-Brain Radiotherapy

WBRT continues to be the standard of care in patients with brain metastasis. In general, WBRT should be given soon after the diagnosis of brain metastasis. There has never been any evidence to suggest that delaying systemic chemotherapy for WBRT compromises overall survival, especially when one considers that progression in the brain frequently leads directly to the death of the patient.

There is still no agreement on the dose and fractionation schedule for WBRT despite numerous studies designed to determine the optimum delivery. Table 91.3 summarizes selected randomized fractionation studies (4,19,44,52). Typically, the radiographic and clinical response rates range from 50% to 75%. Most of these studies have been negative, and the overall survival has not improved appreciably during the last 25 to 30 years. A total of 30 Gy in 10 fractions continues to be the standard for most patients. In chemotherapy-refractory, RPA class III patients, a shorter fractionation scheme (e.g., 20 Gy in five fractions) should be considered. However, short fractionation schemes should be avoided in chemotherapy-naive patients with brain metastasis as the presenting event in the cancer diagnosis. The natural disease course of such patients can be frequently unpredictable, so they may live sufficiently long enough to experience late radiation toxicity posed by such short fractionation schedules (10).

Surgical Resection

Surgical resection can provide immediate relief of the tumor mass effect (Fig. 91.1). On the other hand, radiation typically takes several days to work. Radiobiologically, 30 Gy in 10 fractions to a solid tumor (excluding radiosensitive tumors) is not adequate to achieve long-term tumor control. This issue is especially germane since historically up to half of all patients died from neurologic causes after being treated with WBRT alone.

::	Table 91.1	**EPIDEMIOLOGY OF BRAIN METASTASIS**

Primary site

Lung	50%
Breast	15–20%
Other known primary	10–15%
Unknown primary	10–15%
Melanoma	10%
Colon	5%

Relevant facts

Median survival	<1 year
Mean age	60 years
Annual U. S. incidence	>170,000
Autopsy incidence	10–30%
Clinical incidence	15–30%
Metastatic/primary ratio	10:1

From Li KC, Poon PY. Sensitivity and specificity of MRI in detecting malignant spinal cord compression and in distinguishing malignant from benign compression fractures of vertebrae. *Magn Reson Imaging* 1998;6:547–556; Wen PY, McLaren BP, Loeffler JS. Treatment of metastatic cancer, in DeVita VT, Hellman S, Rosenberg SA, eds. *Cancer: principles and practice of oncology.* Philadelhpia: Lippincott Williams & Wilkins, 2001;2655–2670, with permission.

There have now been three phase III trials testing the hypothesis that surgical resection to single brain metastasis is potentially beneficial. All three trials were of patients with a single lesion, which is defined as the presence of only one lesion in the brain regardless of the extracranial disease status, while a solitary lesion is defined as the presence of the CNS metastasis as the only site of the metastatic disease burden. Table 91.4 summarizes the three trials (43,45,48). The studies by Patchell et al. (48) (KPS $\geq$70) and Noordijk et al. (45) (World Health Organization grade $\leq$2) included better performance status patients compared to the Mintz et al. (43) study (KPS $\geq$50) that mainly contributed to the differences in the survival outcomes between the studies. The results of these studies suggest that surgical resection should be reserved for lesions causing life-threatening complications or those patients with good performance status (i.e., KPS $\geq$70).

Radiosurgery Boost Trials

Radiosurgery provides a substitute or alternative to conventional surgery. The three randomized trials of surgical resection were performed before the widespread availability of stereotactic radiosurgery (SRS). Although no randomized trials have been performed comparing surgery with SRS, the latter appears to provide similar local control rates (in the order of 80% to 90% only when combined with WBRT). Unless the tumor causes significant edema and mass effect, with consequent hydrocephalus

::	Table 91.2	**CLINICAL PRESENTATION OF BRAIN METASTASIS**

Symptom	Percent of Patients	Sign	Percent of Patients
Headache	49	Hemiparesis	59
Mental problems	32	Cognitive deficits	58
Focal weakness	30	Sensory deficits	21
Ataxia	21	Papilledema	20
Seizures	18	Ataxia	19
Speech problems	12	Apraxia	18

From Posner JB. Brain metastases:1995. A brief review *J. Neurooncol* 1996;27:287–293, with permission.

or herniation requiring urgent surgical intervention, SRS can serve as a noninvasive alternative. Frequently, a patient may not be a craniotomy candidate because of tumor location in eloquent areas or existing medical contraindications. Although two of the three conventional surgery trials have shown a survival benefit in single brain metastasis, there have been no randomized trials addressing multiple lesions and the retrospective data available are contradictory. For SRS there have been three randomized trials assessing the efficacy of SRS in the treatment of multiple metastases (Table 91.5).

The first randomized trial was reported by Kondziolka et al. (30) from the University of Pittsburgh. This small study was stopped early at a planned interim analysis of 60% patient accrual because the authors reported to have found a large difference in the primary end point of local control in favor of SRS (92% vs. 0%; $p = .0016$). Unfortunately, the study used nonstandard end points to measure recurrence, defining it as *any* increase in the lesion size on MRI rather than the more usual 25% increase in product of the diameter. Furthermore, no attempt was made to control for steroid use, radiation changes, or other factors that might produce small fluctuations in the lesion size on MRI. Therefore, this study is difficult to interpret.

Chougule et al. (7) from Brown University reported the second trial, although this is published only in abstract form. This trial had three treatment arms and randomized patients to treatment with SRS alone with gamma-knife, SRS plus WBRT, or WBRT alone. This trial suffers from several serious method problems. Although the authors conclude that the survival times among the treatment arms were similar and that patients treated with SRS experienced superior local control and fewer brain metastases, no probability values are given. Furthermore, 51 of the patients had surgical resection for at least one symptomatic brain metastasis prior to entry into the study, and no attempt was made to stratify for previous surgery. The inclusion of the surgically resected patients effectively made this a six-arm trial and, therefore, the size of this trial was not large enough to support a meaningful analysis. Finally, the radiation doses used in the SRS arms cannot be considered conventional because the peripheral dose was not individualized based on the tumor size or volume.

In the third study, RTOG 95–08, the primary end point was overall survival, which was not statistically different between the WBRT plus SRS and WBRT alone arms (6.5 months and 5.7 months, respectively; $p = .1356$), although SRS boost favored the survival in the subgroup (planned analysis) of patients with single metastasis (1). For secondary end points, the local control and performance measures were higher in the SRS boost arm, but this did not translate into a lower death rate from neurologic progression. Multiple, unplanned subgroup analyses were made, and an overall survival benefit with the SRS boost was found in several subgroups that included patients with RPA class 1, tumor size $\geq$2 cm, and non-small cell lung cancer or metastatic squamous histology from any site. Unfortunately, these subset analyses were not planned or prespecified, and the p-values needed for significance should have been adjusted for inflation of the type I error. When this was done, none of these subgroup analyses showed a positive benefit for SRS (12). On the other hand, this trial did demonstrate that SRS is associated with lower edema and corticosteroid use, countering a commonly held notion that SRS actually increases the edema risk. However, with regard to the major end points for multiple metastases, this study should be considered a negative trial.

Although SRS boost is indicated (from RTOG 95–08 and from the extrapolation of surgical resection data) in patients with a single metastasis, it is difficult to justify its routine use in patients with multiple metastases in the light of the equivocal phase III SRS boost trials.

| Table 91.3 | SELECTED RANDOMIZED TRIALS EXAMINING VARIOUS FRACTIONATION SCHEDULES FOR BRAIN METASTASIS | | | |

Author/Study Group	Dose (Gy)/Fractions	N	Median Survival	P Value
Borgelt et al. (4)/RTOG				
First study				
(1971–1973)	30/10	233	21 wk	NS
	30/15	217	18 wk	
	40/15	233	18 wk	
	40/20	227	16 wk	
Second study				
(1973–1976)	20/5	447	15 wk	NS
	30/10	228	15 wk	
	40/15	227	18 wk	
Haie-Meder et al. (19)/French	25/10	110	4.2 mo	NS
(1986–1989)	36/6[a]	106	5.3 mo	
Priestman et al. (52)/Royal	30/10	263	84 d	0.04
College of Radiology	12/2	270	77 d	
(1990–1993)				
Murray et al. (44)/RTOG	30/10	213	4.5 mo	NS
91-04 (1991–1995)	54.4/34[b]	216	4.5 mo	

NS, not significant; RTOG, Radiation Therapy Oncology Group.
[a]18 Gy/three split course with another 18 Gy/three within 1 month.
[b]54.4 Gy in 1.6 Gy twice daily hyperfractionation for the entire course of therapy.

Postoperative Whole-Brain Radiotherapy

A controversy in the treatment of brain metastasis is the routine use of postoperative or post-SRS WBRT. In a multi-institutional retrospective SRS study, Sneed et al. (63) argue for the omission of upfront WBRT as this does not compromise overall survival. Unfortunately, only an overall survival analysis was performed, and no local control or retreatment data were given. In an earlier study by Sneed et al. (62) on the University of California, San Francisco SRS experience, patients who were initially treated with SRS alone without WBRT experienced worse freedom from new brain metastasis and overall brain freedom from progression despite the imbalance of the prognostic factors that favored the SRS alone group, although the overall survival was not different (62). Because of the equivalency of overall survival, many have advocated withholding upfront WBRT. They often use repeat SRS for the failures, which can be very expensive. Furthermore, brain failure can lead to unacceptable consequences. For example, Regine et al. (56) reported on 36 patients with planned observation after initial SRS alone. Even with close follow-up with examinations and high-resolution MRIs, 47% of patients experienced brain failure, with 71% and 59% experiencing symptomatic relapse and neurologic deficits, respectively.

The omission of upfront WBRT may have even more serious consequences for patients with more radioresistant tumors such as renal cell carcinoma (RCC). The SRS dose given is typically limited by tumor size and volume, and not by whether the patient received additional dose with WBRT. Therefore, a patient treated with WBRT plus SRS receives much higher tumor dose than SRS alone. It is then not a surprise that Eastern Cooperative Oncology Group Protocol E 6397 demonstrates very disappointing results (37). In this phase II trial that evaluated SRS alone in radioresistant tumors (RCC, melanoma, sarcoma), Manon et al. (37) reported a 6-month total brain failure rate of 48.3%. The authors correctly conclude that routine avoidance of WBRT should be approached judiciously.

Fortunately, there have been two phase III trials that have assessed the use of postoperative WBRT (Table 91.6). Patchell et al. (47) demonstrated that surgical resection without WBRT led to a failure rate at the original site and the entire brain of 46% and 70%, respectively. More importantly, 44% of the patients in the surgery alone arm died as a result of neurological sequalae from the brain failure. The results of this study have been frequently misinterpreted in the literature. Some have justified the withholding of upfront WBRT based on the fact that this study demonstrated equivalent survivals. In fact, this study was designed with brain tumor recurrence rate as the primary end point and not overall survival. To show an overall survival difference, this trial needed to enroll more than 2,000 patients. This study met its primary end point and confirmed the importance of postoperative WBRT in preventing brain failure and death from neurologic causes.

The results of the Japanese JROSG 99–1 have now been reported (3). In this phase III trial of one to four lesions, the SRS-only arm experienced worse 1-year total brain recurrence rate ($p < .001$) and more frequently required salvage therapy ($p < .001$). The main drawback of this study was the designation of overall survival as the primary end point. There is very little evidence that adjuvant WBRT after surgery is likely to improve overall survival. However, this study did demonstrate the importance of WBRT in decreasing brain failure, corroborating the findings of the study by Patchell et al. (47).

It is difficult to ignore the level I evidence provided by these two phase III trials. Adjuvant WBRT, therefore, should be considered the standard of care after local therapy with surgical resection or SRS.

Repeat Whole-Brain Radiotherapy

Occasionally, patients will fail in the brain with multiple lesions after initial WBRT. Repeat WBRT should strongly be considered. Wong et al. (75) reported on a series of 86 patients who underwent repeat WBRT. The median dose for the first course was 30 Gy, and the median dose for the second course was 20 Gy. A total of 70% experienced neurologic improvement, with 27% experiencing complete neurologic resolution and 43% had partial improvement after repeat WBRT. A retreatment dose of >20 Gy was associated with a significantly longer survival. Only one patient experienced dementia that was thought to be caused by radiation.

A: Pre-operative T1 axial MRI

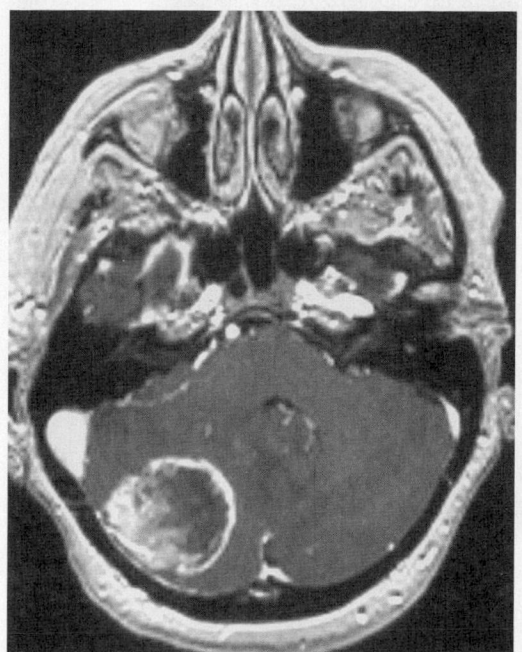

B: Pre-operative T2 axial MRI

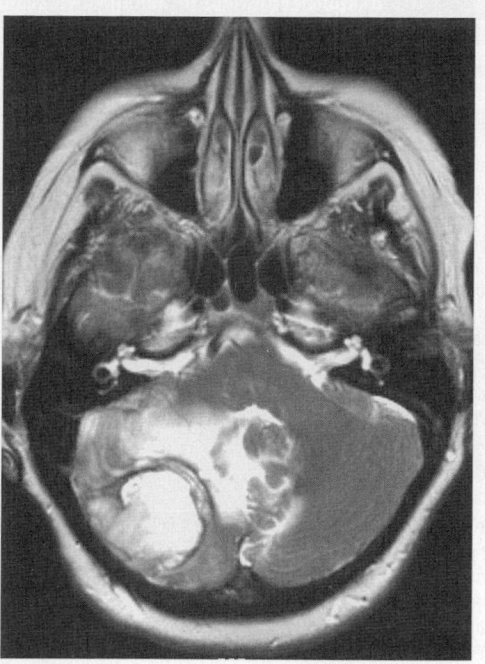

C: Pre-operative T1 axial MRI

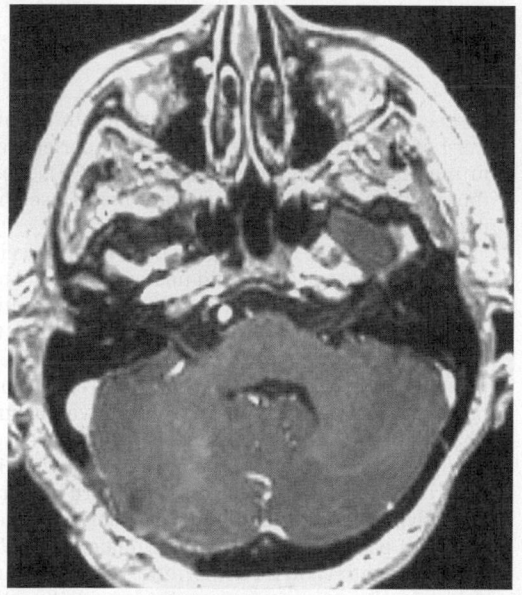

FIGURE 91.1. A: Six months after definitive therapy for stage IIIB non-small cell lung carcinoma (NSCLC), a patient presented with progressively worsening headache, nausea, vomiting, and coordination difficulties. T1 gadolinium-enhanced axial magnetic resonance image (MRI) demonstrates a large, necrotic right cerebellar mass. **B:** T2 axial MRI image reveals large area of vasogenic edema, with resultant mass effect causing fourth ventricular compression and hydrocephalus (not shown). **C:** Patient was taken immediately for a craniotomy and a gross total resection was achieved. Pathology revealed metastatic NSCLC. Postoperative T1 gadolinium-enhanced axial MRI image reveals no residual tumor, decompression of the mass effect and re-expansion of the fourth ventricle.

Repeat WBRT is relatively safe because most patients have limited survival with recurrent or progressive brain metastases after initial WBRT. A minimum of 20 Gy in 1.8 to 2 Gy fractions should be given.

Concurrent Radiosensitizers

Although a majority of patients with brain metastases ultimately succumb to the systemic progression, a significant percent will die from neurologic progression. Multiple randomized trials of concomitant radiosensitizers have been performed in an attempt to optimize brain control (Table 91.7) (2,18,29,41, 48,67,70,73). No trial has demonstrated a survival advantage although a few have demonstrated an increased response rate. The two trials with temozolomide show promise. Temozolo-

mide is an oral alkylating agent with excellent CNS penetration. However, the findings of these two relatively small trials need to be confirmed in a larger trial. Concurrent temozolomide with WBRT should be considered in a patient with bulky brain metastases burden who is unlikely to become a SRS candidate. Otherwise, a patient should be treated with a concomitant radiosensitizer only on a prospective trial.

Causes of Neurocognitive Decline in Brain Tumor Patients

Historically, brain radiation has been frequently cited as the major cause of neurocognitive decline in cancer patients. One of the most misinterpreted studies on this subject is the Memorial Sloan-Kettering experience reported by DeAngelis et al. (10). An

Table 91.4 | RANDOMIZED TRIALS OF SURGICAL RESECTION OF SINGLE BRAIN METASTASIS

Author/Study Group	Surgery + RT	RT Alone	P Value
Patchell et al. (48)/University of Kentucky (n = 48)			
Primary end point			
Overall survival	40 wk	(36 Gy/12 fx) 15 wk	<0.01
Secondary end points			
Local control			
Local failure	20%	52%	<0.02
Time to local failure	>59 wk	21 wk	<0.0001
Time to neurologic death	62 wk	26 wk	<0.0009
KPS ≥70 maintenance	38 wk	8 wk	<0.005
Noordijk et al. (45)/Dutch (n = 63)			
Primary end points			
Overall survival	10 mo	(40 Gy/20 fx)[a] 6 mo	0.04
FIS[b]	7.5 mo	3.5 mo	0.06
Mintz et al. (43)/Canadian (n = 84)			
Primary end point			
Overall survival	5.6 mo	(30 Gy/10 fx) 6.3 mo	NS
Secondary end points			
FIS (proportion of days, mean)[c]	32%	32%	NS
Quality of life (Spitzer score)			
1–3 months (mean)	6.38	5.36	NS
4–6 months (mean)	6.32	6.15	NS

RT, whole-brain radiotherapy; fx, fraction number; KPS, Karnofsky performance score; FIS, functionally independent survival; NS, not significant.
[a]40 Gy total in 2-Gy twice daily hyperfractionation for the entire course of therapy.
[b]FIS defined by World Health Organization performance status ≤1 and neurologic condition ≤1.
[c]FIS defined by KPS ≥70.

11% risk of radiation-induced dementia is reported in patients undergoing WBRT for brain metastasis. The 11% figure is very misleading. Of the 47 patients who survived 1-year after WBRT, 5 patients (11%) developed severe dementia. When these five patients are examined, all were treated in a fashion that would significantly increase the risk of late radiation toxicity (i.e., large daily fractions and concurrent radiosensitizer). Three patients received 5 Gy and 6 Gy daily fractions, and a fourth patient received 6 Gy fractions with concurrent adriamycin. Only one patient received what is considered a standard radiation fractionation scheme (i.e., 30 Gy in 10 fractions), but this patient received a concurrent radiosensitizer (lonidamine). No patient who received the standard 30 Gy in 10 fractions WBRT alone experienced dementia.

The accuracy of the 11% dementia rate is further questioned by the nature of the statistical interpretation used. Even though the study included 232 patients in the initial analysis, it only examined the 47 patients who survived at least 1 year. The principals of conditional probability dictate that the 11% risk is accurate only if a patient survives 1 year, which is significantly longer than most reported series. Therefore, a radiation-induced dementia risk of 2% (5/232) would reflect the true probability *ab initio* for patients presenting with brain metastasis. Indeed, in a separate study of a larger cohort, DeAngelis et al. (11) estimate the risk of radiation-induced dementia to be 1.9% to 5.2% for all patients presenting with brain metastasis. In the authors' opinion, this risk of dementia is not high enough to warrant withholding quality of life-prolonging WBRT.

Many have argued that the increased local control with adjuvant WBRT does not translate into a survival benefit, and that performing repeat SRS or deferring WBRT for recurrences are reasonable approaches. However, WBRT may actually improve neurocognition in a significant number of patients, and brain recurrence or progression is associated with decrease in neurocognitive function (68). In a neurocognitive analysis of RTOG 91–04, Regine et al. (57) demonstrated that approximately one third of patients treated with WBRT experienced improvement in minimental status examination (MMSE); most importantly, those who had uncontrolled brain metastases had an average decrement of 6 points on the MMSE.

The experience of DeAngelis et al. (11), as well as other studies that employed MMSE, did not use sophisticated neurocognitive testing. It is possible that subtle neurocognitive dysfunction may indeed result from WBRT. Recent studies that have used sophisticated neurocognitive testing are clearly demonstrating that the brain tumor (presence, recurrence, and progression) has the greatest effect on neurocognitive decline. In the large phase III motexafin gadolinium study, the neurocognitive battery examined memory recall, memory recognition, memory-delayed recalled, verbal fluency, pegboard hand coordinate, and executive function (42). This study demonstrated that 21% to 65.1% of patients had impaired functioning *at baseline* before treatment with WBRT. Furthermore, patients who progressed in the brain after treatment experienced significantly worse scores in all of these individual tests.

There are now strong data that other factors, such as anticonvulsants, benzodiazepines, opioids, chemotherapy, craniotomy and, most importantly, the brain tumor, contribute significantly to the neurocognitive decline of patients with brain tumor (5,26,27,64,78).

Anticonvulsants

Patients frequently present to the radiation oncologist who have already started taking prophylactic anticonvulsants. This represents one of the most preventable causes of neurocognitive decline in brain tumor patients. Anticonvulsants are clearly known to impact negatively on quality of life and neurocognition. In a study of 156 patients with low-grade glioma (85% experiencing a seizure), Klein et al. (27) correlated seizure-burden with quality

Table 91.5	RANDOMIZED TRIALS OF STEREOTACTIC RADIOSURGERY BOOST IN BRAIN METASTASES			
Author/Study Group	RT + SRS	RT Alone	SRS Alone	P Value
Andrews et al. (1)/RTOG 95-08 (n = 333; 1 to 3 lesions)				
Primary end point (overall survival)	(37.5 Gy/10 fx)			
1 to 3 lesions	5.7 mo	6.5 mo		NS
Single brain metastasis (planned subgroup analysis)	6.5 mo	4.9 mo		0.04
Secondary end points				
Local control (1 year)	82%	71%		0.01
Neurologic death rate	28%	31%		NS
Performance outcome				
KPS stable/improve				
at 3 mo	50%	33%		0.02
at 6 mo	43%	27%		0.03
Mental status				NS
Unplanned subgroup analysis (overall survival)				
Largest tumor >2 cm	6.5 mo	5.3 mo		0.04
RPA class I	11.6 mo	9.6 mo		0.05
Squamous/NSCLC	5.9 mo	3.9 mo		0.05
Other outcomes				
Response rate (3 mo)				
Tumor	73%	62%		0.04
Edema	70%	47%		0.002
Kondziolka et al. (30)/University of Pittsburgh (n = 27; 2 to 4 lesions)				
Primary end point	(30 Gy/12 fx)			
Local control (1 yr)	92%	0%		0.0016
Time to local failure	36 mo	6 mo		0.005
Time to any brain failure	34 mo	5 mo		0.002
Secondary end points				
Overall survival	11 mo	7.5 mo		NS
Treatment morbidity	0	0		
Progression-free survival	Not reported			
Need for retreatment	Not reported			
Chougule et al. (7)/Brown University (n = 109; 1 to 3 lesions)				
End points (abstract only)	(30 Gy + 20 Gy SRS)	(30 Gy/10 fx)	(30 Gy SRS)	
Overall survival	5 mo	9 mo	7 mo	Not reported
Local control	91%	62%	87%	Not reported
New brain lesions	19%	23%	43%	Not reported

RT, whole-brain radiotherapy; SRS, stereotactic radiosurgery; RTOG, Radiation Therapy Oncology Group; fx, fraction number; KPS, Karnofsky performance score; RPA, recursive partitioning analysis; NSCLC, non-small cell lung cancer.

of life and neurocognitive function. This study convincingly demonstrates the significant correlation between the increase in the number anticonvulsants (even with lack of seizures) with the decrease in quality of life and neurocognitive function.

Based on four negative randomized trials, the American Academy of Neurology recommends that prophylactic anticonvulsants not be initiated in newly diagnosed brain tumor patients who have not experienced a seizure (17). It is safe to taper a patient off of anticonvulsants provided that the patient has not experienced a seizure.

Spinal Cord Compression

In the United States, >20,000 cases of metastatic spinal cord compression (MSCC) are diagnosed annually and it is estimated to develop in approximately 5% to 14% of all cancer patients (6,53). MSCC is a devastating complication of cancer. It is considered a true medical emergency and immediate intervention is required. Even with aggressive therapy, results can often be unsatisfactory. Although most patients with MSCC have limited survival, up to one-third will survive beyond 1 year (23,38). Therefore, aggressive therapy should always be considered to preserve or improve the quality of life.

Pathophysiology

MSCC develops primarily in one of three ways:

(a) Continued growth and expansion of vertebral bone metastasis into the epidural space,
(b) Neural foramina extension by a paraspinal mass, and
(c) Destruction of vertebral cortical bone, causing vertebral body collapse with displacement of bony fragments into the epidural space. Although complex, the most significant damage caused by MSCC appears to be vascular in nature. Epidural tumor extension causes epidural venous plexus compression, which leads to edema of the spinal cord. This increase in vascular permeability and edema cause increased pressure on the small arterioles. Capillary blood flow diminishes as the disease progresses, leading to white matter ischemia. Prolonged ischemia eventually results in white matter infarction and permanent cord damage (25)

Clinical Presentation, Diagnosis, and Prognosis

Most patients with MSCC have a cancer diagnosis history. In a review by Fuller et al. (14) of >1,000 patients with MSCC, the most common tumor types are breast cancer (29%), lung cancer (17%), and prostate cancer (14%). This reflects the high

Table 91.6	RANDOMIZED TRIALS OF POST-OPERATIVE WHOLE BRAIN RADIOTHERAPY

Study	Surgery + RT	Surgery Only	P Value
Patchell et al. (47)/University of Kentucky (n = 95; single lesion)			
Primary end point	(50.4 Gy/28 fx)	Craniotomy	
Brain tumor recurrence			
Total brain recurrence	*18%*	*70%*	*<0.001*
Original site only	4%	33%	
Distant site only	8%	24%	
Original and distant	6%	13%	
Distant site total	14%	37%	<0.01
Original site total	10%	46%	<0.001
Secondary end points			
Cause of death			
Neurologic	14%	44%	0.003
Systemic	84%	46%	<0.001
Functional independence*	37 wk	35 wk	NS
Overall survival	48 wk	43 wk	NS
Aoyama et al. (3)/Japanese JROSG99-1 (n = 132; 1 to 4 lesions)			
Primary end point	(30 Gy/10 fx)	radiosurgery	
Overall survival			
1-year	39%	28%	NS
Median	7.5 mo	8.0 mo	NS
Secondary end points			
Brain recurrence (total)[a]	47%	76%	<0.001
Functional preservation[a,b]	34%	27%	NS
Neurologic death	23%	19%	NS
Need for salvage therapy	10 patients	29 patients	<0.001
Radiation morbidity			
Acute	4 patients	8 patients	NS
Late	7 patients	3 patients	NS

RT, whole-brain radiotherapy; fx, fraction number; NS, not significant.
[a]One-year actuarial rates.
[b]As defined by Karnofsky performance score $\geq$70 maintenance.

Table 91.7	SELECTED RANDOMIZED TRIALS OF RADIOSENSITIZERS IN BRAIN METASTASIS

Author/Study Group	Arms	Response Rate	P Value	Median Survival	P Value
Komarnicky et al. (29)/	RT (30 Gy/10 fx)	45%[a]		4.5 mo	
RTOG 79–16 (n = 859)	RT + misonidazole	42%[a]	NS	3.9 mo	NS
	RT (30 Gy/6 fx)	42%[a]		4.1 mo	
	RT + misonidazole	45%[a]	NS	3.1 mo	NS
Ushio et al. (70)/Japan[b]	RT (40 Gy/20 fx)	36%		27 wk	
(n = 88)	RT + nitrosurea	69%		31 wk	
	RT + nitrosurea + tegafur	74%	<0.05	29 wk	NS
Phillips et al. (49)/RTOG 89-05	RT (37.5/15 fx)	50%		6.1 mo	
(n = 72)	RT + BrdUrd	63%	NS	4.3 mo	NS
Guerrieri et al. (18)/Australia[b]	RT (20 Gy/5 fx)	10%		4.4 mo	
(n = 42)	RT+carboplatin	29%	NS	3.7 mo	NS
Antonadou et al. (2)/Greece	RT (40 Gy/20 fx)	67%		7.0 mo	
(n = 52)	RT+temozolomide	96%	0.017	8.6 mo	NS
Verger et al. (73)/Spain	RT (30 Gy/10 fx)	54%[c]		3.1 mo	
(n = 82)	RT + temozolomide	72%[c]	0.03	4.5 mo	NS
Mehta et al. (41)/9801 Trial	RT (30 Gy/10 fx)	51%		4.9 mo	
(n = 401)	RT + MGd	46%	NS	5.2 mo	NS
Suh et al. (67)/REACH Trial	RT (30 Gy/10 fx)	38%		4.4 mo	
(n = 515)	RT + efaproxiral	46%	NS	5.4 mo	NS

RTOG, Radiation Therapy and Oncology Group; RT, whole-brain radiotherapy; fx, fractions; NS, not significant; BrdUrd, bromodeoxyuridine; MGd, motexafin gadolinium.
[a]Percent of survival time in Karnofsky performance score 90–100 range.
[b]Only lung cancer patients.
[c]Ninety-day freedom from brain metastasis.

natural incidence of these tumors. New onset back pain in cancer patients needs to be taken seriously and investigated. Even without a prior cancer diagnosis, MSCC should be suspected in anyone who presents with progressively worsening back pain, incontinence, or paraplegia, especially in the high-risk population such as long-time smokers. The most common level of the MSCC involvement is in the thoracic spine (59% to 78%), followed by lumbar (16% to 33%) and cervical spine (4% to 15%), while multiple levels are involved in up to half of the patients (14,22,60). Back pain is the most common presenting symptom (88% to 96%), followed by weakness (76% to 86%), sensory deficits (51% to 80%), and autonomic dysfunction (40% to 64%) (16,22,39,40,69).

MRI is the standard modality for spine imaging. It has a very high sensitivity (93%), specificity (97%), and accuracy (95%) in diagnosing MSCC (34,36). Because patients can have synchronous, multifocal MSCC, an MRI of the entire spine, with and without contrast, should be promptly performed in anyone suspected of having MSCC (35). High-resolution CT scan or CT myelogram of the spine should be performed for those with contraindications to MRI.

Prognostic factors predicting survival are generally similar to patients with brain metastasis, as previously discussed. In terms of predicting ambulatory outcome, one of the most important factors is the rapidity of symptom onset. Other important prognostic factors include radiosensitive histology (e.g., multiple myeloma, germ cell tumors, small cell carcinoma) and pretherapy ambulatory function. In a prospective study of 98 patients with MSCC reported by Rades et al. (54), the single strongest predictor for ambulatory status after therapy on multivariate analysis was time to development of motor deficits before radiation ($p < .001$) from the start of any symptoms. This cohort was separated into three groups according to the time to motor deficits before radiation therapy: 1 to 7 days (group A), 8 to 14 days (group B), and >14 days (group C). The ambulatory rates after therapy for groups A, B, and C were 35%, 55%, and 86% ($p < .001$), respectively. The symptom improvement rates for groups A, B, and C were 10%, 29%, and 86% ($p = .026$), respectively. The other factor significant on the multivariate analysis for posttherapy ambulatory status was favorable histology ($p = .005$), and there was a trend regarding pretherapy ambulatory status ($p = 0.076$). Acute, rapid deterioration is predictive of irreversible spinal cord infarction. Only 10% of the patients in group A had symptom improvement; therefore, prompt diagnosis and treatment of MSCC is essential.

Corticosteroids

Corticosteroids must be administered as soon as possible in anyone suspected of having MSCC, even before radiographic diagnosis, as this can be rapidly discontinued with a negative diagnosis. They effectively decrease cord edema and serve as an effective bridge to definitive treatment. Although multiple retrospective studies have demonstrated its clinical efficacy, Sorensen et al. (65) reported the only randomized controlled study (n = 57) on the utility of high-dose corticosteroids before definitive radiotherapy in MSCC from solid tumors. The treatment arm consisted of 96 mg of IV bolus of dexamethasone followed by 96 mg oral per day for 3 days and a 10-day taper, versus no corticosteroid therapy. This study demonstrated 3-month and 6-month ambulatory rates of 81% versus 63% and 59% versus 33% ($p < .05$), respectively, in favor of high-dose dexamethasone.

The optimal maintenance dose of corticosteroids is unknown. Vecht et al. (71) reported the only randomized study (n = 37) comparing corticosteroid doses in patients with MSCC, but this study only evaluated the IV loading dose. It compared IV loading doses of 10 mg versus 100 mg, followed in both arms by the same oral regimen of 16 mg per day. Both arms demonstrated significant reductions in pain from baseline ($p < .001$); however, there was no difference between the two arms with respect to pain reduction, ambulation, or bladder function.

Very high doses of corticosteroids are associated with significant side effects. The Sorensen et al. (65) phase III study reported an 11% incidence of serious side effects for patients in the treatment arm, and Heimdal et al. (21) reported a 14.3% incidence of serious gastrointestinal (GI) side effects in 28 consecutive patients treated with 96 mg of IV dexamethasone per day. The toxicities in the report by Heimdal et al. included one fatal ulcer hemorrhage, one case of rectal bleeding, and two bowel perforations. Subsequently, the dexamethasone dose was decreased to 16 mg per day for the next 38 consecutive patients, and there was no incidence of serious side effects ($p < .05$). Most importantly, the ambulatory rates were not different between the two dexamethasone doses.

Based on these data, a loading of 10 mg of IV dexamethasone and followed by a maintenance dose of 4 to 6 mg every 6 to 8 hours should be sufficient before being tapered. Patients can be safely switched to an oral regimen after 24 to 48 hours as there is good oral bioavailability of corticosteroids. Furthermore, patients should be started on a proton pump inhibitor (PPI) for GI prophylaxis. Although here has been no randomized trial using PPIs in patients receiving corticosteroids, there have been multiple phase III studies demonstrating the protective effects of PPIs against peptic ulcers in patients receiving chronic nonsteroidal anti-inflammatory drugs (NSAIDS) (32). NSAIDS and corticosteroids both cause GI mucosal injury by decreasing mucosal-protective prostaglandin levels. Therefore, it is not an unreasonable extrapolation to assume that PPIs provide a similar mucosal protective effect with corticosteroids, especially considering that the morbidity of GI toxicity can be life-threatening. Chronic use of should be avoided because the short half-life of these agents requires a large amount to be ingested per day. Increased popularity of over-the-counter antacids as a means of calcium supplementation, which has been recognized as an important cause of the recent increase in milk-alkali syndrome and resultant hypercalcemia (61,79).

Surgery

Radiation for nonradiosensitive tumors typically takes several days to have an effect and does not stabilize the spine, while surgery allows for immediate cord decompression and provides an opportunity to stabilize the spine intraoperatively. At some institutions, surgery was used infrequently because several retrospective studies and one, small randomized study showed no benefit to surgery plus radiation over radiation alone. Young et al. (77) randomized 29 patients with MSCC to decompressive laminectomy followed by radiation versus radiation alone. Although this trial showed no benefit to surgery in terms of pain relief, ambulation, or sphincter function, it is difficult to draw any conclusion because of the small sample size. All of these studies used posterior laminectomy in conjunction with radiotherapy; however, most of the lesions in MSCC involve the anterior portion of the vertebral body (6). Therefore, a laminectomy does not effectively relieve the compression and may actually worsen the stability of the spine.

Recently, multiple authors have advocated the use of direct surgical decompression, tumor debulking, and spinal stabilization via instrumentation to improve on the results from radiation alone. Patchell et al. (46) reported the first phase III randomized trial testing the efficacy of direct decompressive surgery in patients with MSCC (Table 91.8). The study compared radiation alone (standard 30 Gy in 10 fractions) versus decompressive and stabilization surgery within 24 hours of diagnosis followed by the same radiotherapy (within 2 weeks of surgery). The trial was terminated early when early-stopping rules were met regarding the primary end point of ambulation

Table 91.8	KEY FINDINGS OF THE PATCHELL ET AL. (46) PHASE III STUDY OF PATIENTS WITH METASTATIC SPINAL CORD COMPRESSION		
	Surgery + Radiation Median (n = 50)	**Radiation Alone** Median (n = 51)	**P Value**
Primary end point			
Ability to walk			
Rate (%)	84 (42/50)	57 (29/51)	0.001
Time (days)	122	13	0.003
Secondary end points			
Maintenance of continence (days)	156	17	0.016
Maintenance of ASIA score[a] (days)	566	72	0.001
Maintenance of Frankel score[a]	566	72	0.0006
Overall survival (days)	126	100	0.033
Other end points			
Mean daily morphine[b] (mg)	0.4	4.8	0.002
Mean daily dexamethasone[b] (mg)	1.6	4.2	0.0093
In patients ambulatory at study entry			
Ability to walk (maintaining)			
Rate (%)	94 (32/34)	74 (26/34)	0.024
Time (days)	153	54	0.024
In patients nonambulatory at study entry			
Ability to walk (regaining)			
Rate (%)	62 (10/16)	19 (3/16)	0.012
Time (days)	59	0	0.04

ASIA, American Spinal Injury Association.
[a]Measures of spinal function after injury.
[b]Converted into equivalent doses.

after treatment. This trial definitively demonstrated an advantage to surgery for every end point at statistically significant levels. For nonambulatory patients, the combined treatment patients had a significant higher chance of regaining the ability to walk after therapy. Maintenance of continence, maintenance of American Spinal Cord Injury (ASIA) and Frankel scores (measures of spinal function after injury), median overall survival, and median mean daily dexamethasone and morphine-equivalent doses all favored the surgery arm.

If operable, patients should undergo surgical decompression and stabilization followed by radiotherapy. Even for radiosensitive tumors, surgery can often stabilize the spine. Therefore, all patients with MSCC should be evaluated by a surgeon. Effective multidisciplinary teamwork is critical to the rapid evaluation and management of patients with MSCC.

Radiotherapy

Palliative radiotherapy has been the standard of care in the treatment of patients with MSCC. Although a total of 30 Gy in 10 fractions is most frequently employed fractionation schedule, multiple fractionation schemes have been reported, which undoubtedly reflects the heterogeneity in the patient population and tumor histology (34). In one of the largest studies to date, Rades et al. (55) reported a retrospective series of 1,304 patients with MSCC. The patients were separated into five schedules: 8 Gy × 1 in 1 day (n = 261, group 1), 4 Gy × 5 in 1 week (n = 279, group 2), 3 Gy × 10 in 2 weeks (n = 274, group 3), 2.5 Gy × 15 in 3 weeks (n = 233, group 4), and 2 Gy × 20 in 4 weeks (n = 257, group 5). All of the groups had similar posttreatment ambulatory rates (63% to 74%) and motor function improvements (26% to 31%). However, in-field recurrence rates were much lower for the protracted schedules. The 2-year in-field recurrence rates for groups 1, 2, 3, 4, and 5 were 24%, 26%, 14%, 9%, and 7% (p <.001), respectively. They recommend that a single fraction of 8 Gy should be used in MSCC patients with limited survival

expectations, and that 30 Gy in 10 fractions should be used for all other patients.

Maranzano et al. (38) have reported the only randomized trial on radiation schedule for patients with MSCC. They compared two hypofractionation schemes, a short course (8 Gy × 1→6-day break→8 Gy × 1; 16 Gy total in 1 week) versus a split course (5 Gy × 3→4-day break→3 Gy × 5; 30 Gy total in 2 weeks). The study concludes that the treatment with short versus split courses of RT resulted in similar back pain relief (56% vs. 59%), ambulatory maintenance (68% vs. 71%), and good bladder function (90% vs. 89%) rates. Therefore, they recommend that an 8 Gy × 2 regimen should be used for patients with MSCC. Readers should be cautious before implementing this recommendation. When one limits the definition of response to regaining motor function and sphincter control, the rates of success decrease to 29% and 14%, respectively. Confounding variables included having patients with favorable histology, excellent performance status, and the use of nonstandard, large fraction sizes in both arms (31). It is conceivable that the 5% who progressed to paraplegia without in-field recurrence may have suffered from late radiation-induced toxicity, even if it was not scored by the authors.

For patients receiving radiotherapy for MSCC from solid tumors, 30 Gy in 10 fractions is considered the standard of care. Shorter fractionation schedules, such as 8 Gy × 1 or 4 Gy × 5, should only be reserved for those with clear evidence of progressive disease, refractory to systemic therapy. Furthermore, these short schedules should be avoided in newly diagnosed, chemotherapy-naive patients as the clinical course can be quite variable and unpredictable. Chemotherapy may be considered in select, newly diagnosed patients with excellent neurologic functional status and very chemosensitive tumors (e.g., lymphoma, multiple myeloma, germ cell tumors), but this is still considered outside the accepted standard. If the patient is found to have unresectable/inoperable tumor, and otherwise has good performance status, oligometastatic disease, and controlled primary disease, then consideration should be made to escalate

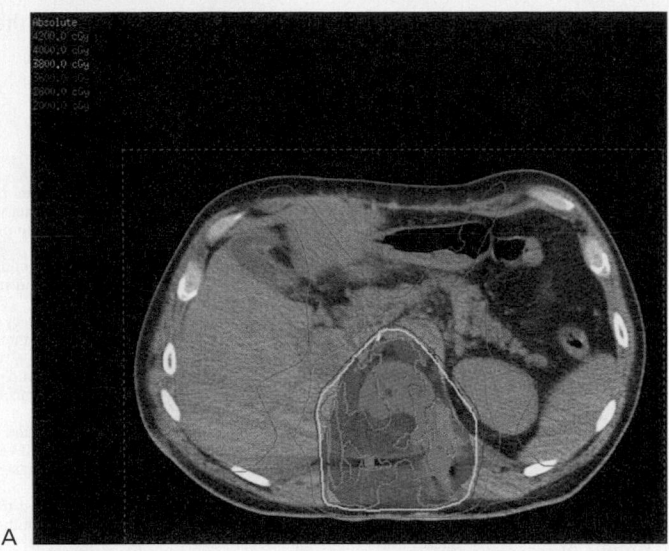

A

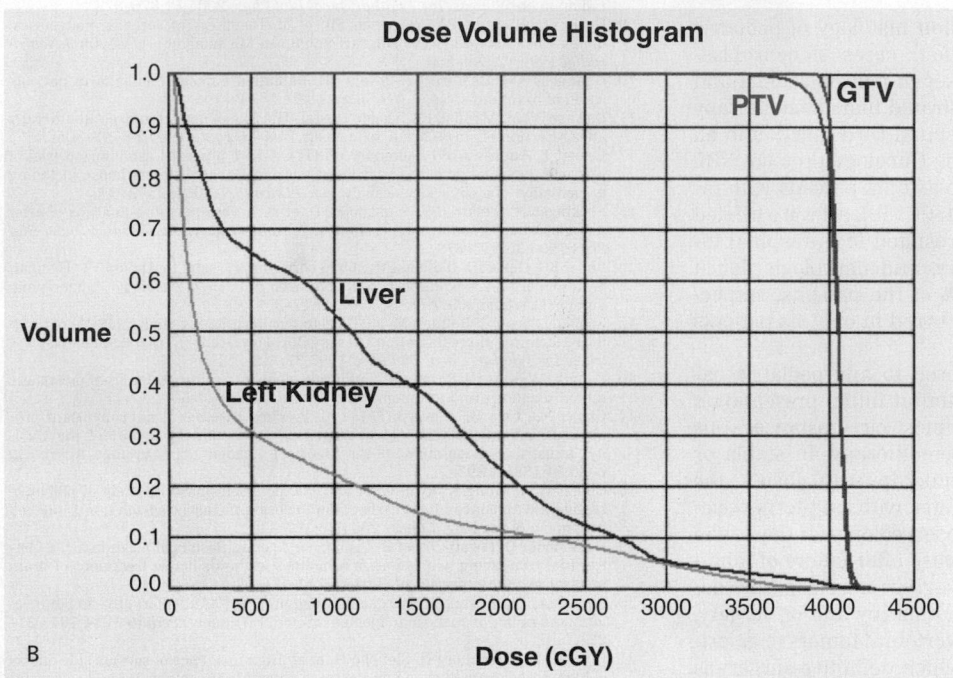

B

FIGURE 91.2. A: Five years after undergoing a right nephrectomy for a stage I renal call carcinoma (RCC), a patient presented with progressively worsening midback pain. Magnetic resonance image of the spine revealed a T11-T12 right-sided paraspinal mass invading the right lateral T12 vertebral body and neural foramina causing T12 spinal cord compression. Patient underwent a gross total resection and instrumentation to stabilize the spine. A full metastatic work-up revealed the vertebral disease as the solitary site of recurrent RCC. Chemistries revealed a mild chronic renal insufficiency, with creatinine level of 2.1 mg/dL. Intensity-modulated radiotherapy (IMRT) was used to minimize the dose to the left kidney. The figure shows an axial computed tomography image of the IMRT plan generated, with the red and blue color washes representing gross tumor volume (GTV) and planning target volume (PTV), respectively. **B:** The dose-volume histogram of the IMRT plan is shown. A total of 40 Gy in 20 fractions was delivered to the PTV (GTV + 1 cm). The PTV was modified so that the margin was decreased to 8 mm along the left lateral edge of the vertebral body next to the left kidney.

Palliative and Supportive Care

the total dose beyond 30 Gy as this will not be sufficient to achieve long-term gross tumor control. Special techniques such as intensity-modulated radiation therapy (IMRT) or fractionated stereotactic body radiation therapy should be considered to safely escalate the total dose (Fig. 91.2). However, the routine use of IMRT or stereotactic body radiation therapy cannot be recommended because the technology is expensive, and it has yet to show definite benefit over conventional delivery of radiation in a patient population that has a median survival of 6 months or less.

Caution Against Short, Hypofractionated Radiotherapy

A common mistake made by those who advocate a short hypofractionated regimen (e.g., 8 Gy × 2 or 4 Gy × 5) for MSCC is equating the safety and equivalency of these abbreviated schedules in bone and lung metastases trials as a justification for

the safety of such regimens in MSCC. The consequence of progression of a bone metastasis despite prior radiotherapy (i.e., 8 Gy × 1) is an increase in pain, which leads to an increased need for pain medications and usually reirradiation. By contrast, the consequences of MSCC progression despite prior radiotherapy are an increase in pain, paralysis, and incontinence, which usually contributes significantly to the direct demise of the patient. Because some studies, but not all, suggest that single-fraction radiotherapy for bone metastasis is associated with a higher retreatment rate than fractionated therapy, a note of caution is appropriate for single fraction radiotherapy for MSCC (76).

The predominant mechanism of cord injury by both MSCC and radiation-induced myelopathy is vascular damage leading to ischemia (66). There are many studies that have established the vascular effects of high fraction dose. Dose response to single dose of SRS for arteriovenous malformation obliteration starts at doses as low as 8 Gy and as soon as 6 months or earlier (13). It is possible that a compressed cord has a lower threshold for radiation-induced myelopathy when a short, hypofractionated schedule of radiation therapy is used. Chow et al. (8) demonstrated that oncologists are not accurate at all in predicting survival times. As systemic therapy improves for patients with metastatic disease, our ability to predict survival will undoubtedly become less accurate. Therefore, these abbreviated schedules should be routinely avoided unless the patient is chemotherapy-refractory, and has convincing evidence of progressive systemic disease with limited expected survival.

Pediatric Spinal Cord Compression

MSCC in the pediatric population differs from adult MSCC. Histologic subtypes commonly encountered in children (e.g., neuroblastoma, Wilms tumor, and Ewing sarcoma) rarely occur in adults. In adults, most cases of MSCC are caused by direct invasion into the epidural space by metastatic vertebral body tumors, while in children most are caused by direct neural foraminal invasion, causing the characteristic "dumbbell" tumor. Chemotherapy plays a central role in the treatment of pediatric MSCC (28).

Neuroblastoma is the most common histology of pediatric MSCC (49). Sanderson et al. (59) (four cases of neuroblastoma) and Hayes et al. (20) (nine cases of neuroblastoma and five cases of Ewing sarcoma) demonstrated that chemotherapy alone allowed complete recovery of spinal cord function in all cases. The French Society of Pediatric Oncology protocol NBL 90 included 42 nonmetastatic neuroblastoma patients with intraspinal extension and consequent MSCC (50). All were treated with initial chemotherapy, and this resulted in intraspinal tumor shrinkage, avoidance of surgery, and neurologic deficit improvement in 58%, 60%, and 92% of the patients, respectively. Severe neurologic sequelae occurred in only six patients (15%).

Emergent surgery should be offered to any pediatric patient with rapid neurologic progression at initial presentation or while receiving chemotherapy. In most circumstances, this should be followed by definitive chemotherapy. In stable or mildly symptomatic patients, chemotherapy can obviate the need for surgery, which is often associated with long-term skeletal deformities. Radiation should be reserved only for those who require palliation for progressive disease after failure of multiple systemic regimens, those who progress neurologically despite the initial treatment with chemotherapy and/or surgery, and those who present with primary vertebral tumors (e.g., primary vertebral Ewing sarcoma) in which definitive surgery is rarely feasible.

Intramedullary Spinal Cord Metastasis

Intramedullary spinal cord metastasis (ISCM) is rare, representing only 1% of all intramedullary tumors. According to a review by Kalayci et al. (24), ISCM is most commonly secondary to a lung primary (54%), followed by breast cancer (11%), in contrast to patients with MSCC. Although back pain is common in >90% of MSCC patients, back or neck pain was seen in only 38% with ISCM. However, high sensory deficits (79%), sphincter dysfunction (60%), and weakness (91%) are more common in ISCM. The most striking difference between ISCM and MSCC is the high incidence of synchronous brain metastasis (41%) in patients presenting with ISCM. This is not surprising when one considers the route of spread and the high incidence of lung primaries in patients with ISCM. An MRI of the brain should be obtained.

The treatment of ISCM should be approached very similarly to that of MSCC, save for the role of surgery. Most surgeons are reluctant to operate in ISCM because surgery carries a high morbidity rate. Only 32 cases of surgery in ISCM have ever been re-

ported (24). Corticosteroids as well as radiation therapy should be promptly initiated.

References

1. Andrews DW, Scott CB, Sperduto PW, et al. Whole brain radiation therapy with and without stereotactic radiosurgery boost for patients with one to three brain metastases: phase III results of the RTOG 9508 randomized trial. *Lancet* 2004;363:1665–1672.
2. Antonadou D, Paraskevaidis M, Sarris G, et al. Phase II randomized trial of temozolomide and concurrent radiotherapy in patients with brain metastases. *J Clin Oncol* 2002;20:3644–3650.
3. Aoyama H, Shirato H, Tago MK, et al. Stereotactic radiosurgery plus whole-brain radiation therapy vs stereotactic radiosurgery alone for treatment of brain metastases. *JAMA* 2006; 295:2483–2491.
4. Borgelt B, Gelber R, Kramer S, et al. The palliation of brain metastases: final results of the first two studies by the Radiation Therapy Oncology Group. *Int J Radiat Oncol Biol Phys* 1980;6:1–9.
5. Brezden CB, Phillips KA, Abdolell M, et al. Cognitive function in breast cancer patients receiving adjuvant chemotherapy. *J Clin Oncol* 2000;18:2695–2701.
6. Byrne TN: Spinal cord compression from epidural metastases. *N Engl J Med* 1992;327:614–619.
7. Chougule PB, Burton-Williams M, Saris S, et al. Randomized treatment of brain metastases with gamma knife radiosurgery, whole brain radiotherapy or both. *Int J Radiat Oncol Biol Phys* 2000;48:114.
8. Chow E, Davis L, Panzarella T, et al. Accuracy of survival prediction by palliative radiation oncologists. *Int J Radiat Oncol Biol Phys.* 2005;61:870–873.
9. Davis PC, Hudgins PA, Peterman SB, et al. Diagnosis of cerebral metastases: double-dose delayed CT vs contrast-enhanced MR imaging. *AJNR Am J Neuroradiol* 1991;12:293–300.
10. DeAngelis LM, Delattre JV, Posner JB. Radiation-induced dementia in patients cured of brain metastases. *Neurology* 1989;39:789–796.
11. DeAngelis LM, Mandell LR, Thaler T, et al. The role of postoperative radiotherapy after resection of single brain metastases. *Neurosurgery* 1989;24:798–805.
12. Elveen T, Andrews DW. Summary of RTOG 95-01 phase III randomized trial of whole brain radiation with and without stereotactic radiosurgery boost, including presentation of a clinical case study. *Am J Oncol Rev* 2004;3:592–600.
13. Flickinger JC, Pollock BE, Kondziolka D, et al. A dose-response analysis of arteriovenous malformation obliteration after radiosurgery. *Int J Radiat Oncol Biol Phys* 1996;36:873–879.
14. Fuller BG, Heiss JD, Oldfield EH. Spinal cord compression. In: DeVita VT, Hellman S, Rosenberg SA, eds. *Cancer: principles and practice of oncology.* Philadelphia: Lippincott Williams & Wilkins; 2001: 2617–2633.
15. Gaspar L, Scott C, Rotman M, et al. Recursive partitioning analysis (RPA) of prognostic factors in three Radiation Therapy Oncology Group (RTOG) brain metastases trials. *Int J Radiat Oncol Biol Phys* 1997;37:745–751.
16. Gilbert RW, Kim JH, Posner JB. Epidural spinal cord compression from metastatic tumor: diagnosis and treatment. *Ann Neurol* 1978;3:40–51.
17. Glantz MJ, Cole BF, Forsyth PA, et al. Practice parameter: anticonvulsant prophylaxis in patients with newly diagnosed brain tumors: report of the Quality Standards Subcommittee of the American Academy of Neurology. *Neurology* 2000;54:1886–1893.
18. Guerrieri M, Wong K, Ryan G, et al. A randomised phase III study of palliative radiation with concomitant carboplatin for brain metastases from non-small cell carcinoma of the lung. *Cancer* 2004;46:107–111.
19. Haie-Meder C, Pellae-Cosset B, Laplanche A, et al. Results of a randomized clinical trial comparing two radiation schedules in the palliative treatment of brain metastases. *Radiother Oncol* 1993;26:111–116.
20. Hayes FA, Thompson EI, Hvizdala E. Chemotherapy as an alternative to laminectomy and radiation in the management of epidural tumor. *J Pediatr* 1984;104:221–224
21. Heimdal K, Hirschberg H, Slettebo H, et al. High incidence of serious side effects of high-dose dexamethasone treatment in patients with epidural spinal cord compression. *J Neurooncol* 1992;12:141–144.
22. Heldmann U, Myschetzky PS, Thomsen HS. Frequency of unexpected multifocal metastasis in patients with acute spinal cord compression. Evaluation by low-field MR imaging in cancer patients. *Acta Radiol* 1997;38:372–375.
23. Helweg-Larsen S, Sorensen PS. Symptoms and sings in metastatic spinal cord compression: a study of progression from first symptom until diagnosis in 153 patients. *Eur J Cancer* 1994;30A:396–398.
24. Kalayci M, Cagavi F, Gul S, et al. Intramedullary spinal cord metastases: diagnosis and treatment - an illustrated review. *Acta Neurochir (Wien)* 2004;146:1347–1354.
25. Kato A, Ushio Y, Hayakawa T, et al. Circulatory disturbance of the spinal cord with epidural neoplasm in rats. *J Neurosurg* 1985;63:260–265.
26. Klein M, Engelberts NH, van der Ploeg HM, et al. Epilepsy in low-grade gliomas: the impact on cognitive function and quality of life. *Ann Neurol* 2003;54:514–520.
27. Klein M, Heimans JJ, Aaronson NK, et al. Effect of radiotherapy and other treatment-related factors on mid-term to long-term cognitive sequelae in low-grade gliomas: a comparative study. *Lancet* 2002;360:1361–1368.
28. Klein SL, Sanford RA, Muhlbauer MS. Pediatric spinal epidural metastases. *J Neurosurg* 1991;74:70–75.
29. Komarnicky LT, Phillips TL, Martz K, et al. A randomized phase III protocol for the evaluation of misonidazole combined with radiation in the treatment of patients with brain metastases (RTOG-7916). *Int J Radiat Oncol Biol Phys* 1991;20:53–58.
30. Kondzioka D, Patel A, Lunsford LD, et al. Stereotactic radiosurgery plus whole brain radiotherapy versus radiotherapy alone for patients with multiple brain metastases. *Int J Radiat Oncol Biol Phys* 1999;45:427–434.
31. Kwok Y, Regine WF, Patchell RA. Radiation therapy alone for spinal cord compression: time to improve upon a relatively ineffective status quo. *J Clin Oncol* 2005;23:3308–3310. Epub 2005 Feb 28.
32. Lai KC, Lam SK, Chu KM, et al. Lansoprazole for the prevention of recurrences of ulcer complications from long-term low-dose aspirin use. *N Engl J Med* 2002;346:2033–2038.

33. Li KC, Poon PY. Sensitivity and specificity of MRI in detecting malignant spinal cord compression and in distinguishing malignant from benign compression fractures of vertebrae. *Magn Reson Imaging* 1988;6:547–556.

34. Larson DA, Rubenstein JL, McDermott MW. Treatment of metastatic cancer. In: DeVita VT, Hellman S, Rosenberg SA, eds. *Cancer: principles and practice of oncology.* Philadelphia: Lippincott Williams & Wilkins; 2005: 2323–2336.

35. Loblaw DA, Laperriere NJ. Emergency treatment of malignant extradural spinal cord compression: an evidence-based guideline. *J Clin Oncol* 1998;16: 1613–1624.

36. Loughrey GJ, Collins CD, Todd SM, et al. Magnetic resonance imaging in the management of suspected spinal canal disease in patients with known malignancy. *Clin Radiol* 2000;55:849–855.

37. Manon R, O'Neill A, Knisely J, et al. Phase II trial of radiosurgery for one to three newly diagnosed brain metastases from renal cell carcinoma, melanoma, and sarcoma: an Eastern Cooperative Oncology Group study (E 6397). *J Clin Oncol* 2005;23:8870–8876.

38. Maranzano E, Bellavita R, Rossi R, et al. Short-course versus split-course radiotherapy in metastatic spinal cord compression: results of a phase III, randomized, multicenter trial. *J Clin Oncol* 2005;23:3358–3365.

39. Maranzano E, Latini P, Checcaglini F, et al: Radiation therapy in metastatic spinal cord compression: a prospective analysis of 105 consecutive patients. *Cancer* 1991;67:1311–1317.

40. Martenson JA, Evans RG, Lie MR, et al. Treatment outcome and complications in patients treated for malignant epidural spinal cord compression (SCC). *J Neurooncol* 1985;3:77–84.

41. Mehta MP, Rodrigus P, Terhaard CH, et al. Survival and neurologic outcomes in a randomized trial of motexafin gadolinium and whole-brain radiation therapy in brain metastases. *J Clin Oncol* 2003;21:2529–2536.

42. Meyers CA, Smith JA, Bezjak A, et al. Neurocognitive function and progression in patients with brain metastases treated with whole-brain radiation and motexafin gadolinium: results of a randomized phase III trial. *J Clin Oncol* 2004;22: 157–165.

43. Mintz AH, Kestle J, Rathbone MP, et al. A randomized trial to assess the efficacy of surgery in addition to radiotherapy in patients with a single cerebral metastasis. *Cancer* 1996;78:1470–1476.

44. Murray KJ, Scott C, Greenberg HM, et al. A randomized phase III study of accelerated hyperfractionation versus standard in patients with unresected brain metastases: a report of the Radiation Therapy Oncology Group (RTOG) 9104. *Int J Radiat Oncol Biol Phys* 1997;39:571–574.

45. Noordijk EM, Vecht CJ, Haaxma-Reiche H, et al. The choice of treatment of single brain metastasis should be based on extracranial tumor activity and age. *Int J Radiat Oncol Biol Phys* 1994;29:711–717.

46. Patchell RA, Tibbs PA, Regine WF, et al. Direct decompressive surgical resection in the treatment of spinal cord compression caused by metastatic cancer: a randomised trial. *Lancet* 2005;366:643–648.

47. Patchell RA, Tibbs PA, Regine WF, et al. Postoperative radiotherapy in the treatment of single metastases to the brain: a randomized trial. *JAMA* 1998;280:1485–1489.

48. Patchell RA, Tibbs PA, Walsh JW, et al. A randomized trial of surgery in the treatment of single metastases to the brain. *N Engl J Med* 1990;322:494–500.

49. Phillips TL, Scott CB, Leibel SA, et al. Results of a randomized comparison of radiotherapy and bromodeoxyuridine with radiotherapy alone for brain metastases: report of RTOG trial 89–05. *Int J Radiat Oncol Biol Phys* 1995;33:339–348.

50. Plantaz D, Rubie H, Michon J, et al. The treatment of neuroblastoma with intraspinal extension with chemotherapy followed by surgical removal of residual disease. A prospective study of 42 patients—results of the NBL 90 Study of the French Society of Pediatric Oncology. *Cancer* 1996;78:311–319

51. Posner JB. Brain metastases: 1995. A brief review. *J Neurooncol* 1996;27:287–293.

52. Priestman TJ, Dunn J, Brada M, et al. Final results of the Royal College of Radiologists' trial comparing two different radiotherapy schedules in the treatment of cerebral metastasis. *Clin Oncol (R Coll Radiol)* 1996;8:308–315.

53. Quinn JA, DeAngelis LM: Neurologic emergencies in the cancer patient. *Semin Oncol* 2000;27:311–321.

54. Rades D, Heidenreich F, Karstens JH. Final results of a prospective study of the prognostic value of the time to develop motor deficits before irradiation in metastatic spinal cord compression. *Int J Radiat Oncol Biol Phys* 2002;53:975–979.

55. Rades D, Stalpers LJ, Veninga T, et al. Evaluation of five radiation schedules and prognostic factors for metastatic spinal cord compression. *J Clin Oncol* 2005;23:3366–3375.

56. Regine WF, Huhn JL, Patchell RA, et al. Risk of symptomatic brain tumor recurrence and neurologic deficit after radiosurgery alone in patients with newly diagnosed brain metastases: results and implications [erratum appears in *Int J Radiat Oncol Biol Phys* 2002;53:259].*Int J Radiat Oncol Biol Phys* 2002;52:333–338.

57. Regine WF, Scott C, Murray K, et al. Neurocognitive outcome in brain metastases patients treated with accelerated-fractionation vs. accelerated-hyperfractionated radiotherapy: an analysis from Radiation Therapy Oncology Group Study 91-04. *Int J Radiat Oncol Biol Phys* 2001;51:711–717.

58. Ruderman NB, Hall TC. Use of glucocorticoids in the palliative treatment of metastatic brain tumors. *Cancer* 1965;18:298–306.

59. Sanderson IR, Pritchard J, Marsh HT. Chemotherapy as the initial treatment of spinal cord compression due to disseminated neuroblastoma. *J Neurosurg* 1989;70:688–690.

60. Schiff D, O'Neill BP, Wang CH, et al. Neuroimaging and treatment implications of patients with multiple epidural spinal metastases. *Cancer* 1998;83:1593–1601.

61. Scofield RH. Milk-alkali syndrome. In: Pourmotabbed G, Talavera F. Khardori, eds. Available at: http://www.emedicine.com/med/topic1477.htm. Updated June 13, 2006. Accessed July 3, 2006.

62. Sneed PK, Lamborn KR, Forstner JM, et al. Radiosurgery for brain metastases: is whole brain radiotherapy necessary? *Int J Radiat Oncol Biol Phys* 1999;43:549–558.

63. Sneed PK, Suh JH, Goetsch SJ, et al. A multi-institutional review of radiosurgery alone vs. radiosurgery with whole brain radiotherapy as the initial management of brain metastases. *Int J Radiat Oncol Biol Phys* 2002;53:519–526.

64. Sonderkaer S, Schmiegelow M, Carstensen H, et al. Long-term neurological outcome of childhood brain tumors treated by surgery only. *J Clin Oncol* 2003; 21:1347–1351.

65. Sorensen S, Helweg-Larsen S, Mouridsen H, et al. Effect of high-dose dexamethasone in carcinomatous metastatic spinal cord compression treated with radiotherapy: a randomised trial. *Eur J Cancer* 1994;30A:22–27

66. St Clair WH, Arnold SM, Sloan AE, et al. Spinal cord and peripheral nerve injury: current management and investigations. *Semin Radiat Oncol* 2003;13:322–332.

67. Suh JH, Stea B, Nabid A, et al. Phase III study of efaproxiral as an adjunct to whole-brain radiation therapy for brain metastases. *J Clin Oncol* 2006;24:106–114.

68. Taylor BV, Buckner JC, Cascino TL, et al. Effects of radiation and chemotherapy on cognitive function in patients with high-grade glioma. *J Clin Oncol* 1998;16:2195–2201.

69. Torma T. Malignant tumors of the spine and spinal epidural space: a study based on 250 histologically verified cases. *Acta Chir Scand* 1957;225:1–176.

70. Ushio Y, Arita N, Hayakawa T, et al. Chemotherapy of brain metastases from lung carcinoma: a controlled randomized study. *Neurosurgery* 1991;28:201–205.

71. Vecht CJ, Haaxma-Reiche H, van Putten WL, et al. Initial bolus of conventional versus high-dose dexamethasone in metastatic spinal cord compression. *Neurology* 1989;39:1255–1257.

72. Vecht CJ, Hovestadt A, Verbiest HB, et al. Dose-effect relationship of dexamethasone on Karnofsky performance in metastatic brain tumors: a randomized study of doses of 4, 8, and 16 mg per day. *Neurology* 1994;44:675–580.

73. Verger E, Gil M, Yaya R, et al. Temozolomide and concomitant whole brain radiotherapy in patients with brain metastases: a phase II randomized trial. *Int J Radiat Oncol Biol Phys* 2005;61:185–191.

74. Wen PY, McLaren Black P, Loeffler JS. Treatment of metastatic cancer. In: DeVita VT, Hellman S, Rosenberg SA, eds. *Cancer: principles and practice of oncology.* Philadelphia: Lippincott Williams & Wilkins; 2001: 2655–2670.

75. Wong WW, Schild SE, Sawyer TE, et al. Analysis of outcome in patients reirradiated for brain metastases. *Int J Radiat Oncol Biol Phys* 1996;34:585–590.

76. Wu JS, Wong R, Johnston M, et al. Meta-analysis of dose-fractionation radiotherapy trials for the palliation of painful bone metastases. *Int J Radiat Oncol Biol Phys* 2003;55:594–605.

77. Young RF, Post EM, King GA. Treatment of spinal epidural metastases: randomized prospective comparison of laminectomy and radiotherapy. *J Neurosurg* 1980;53:741–748.

78. Zacny JP, Gutierrez S. Characterizing the subjective, psychomotor, and physiological effects of oral oxycodone in non-drug-abusing volunteers. *Psychopharmacology (Berl)* 2003;170:242–254.

79. Ziegler R. Hypercalcemic crisis. *J Am Soc Nephrol* 2001;12:S3–9.

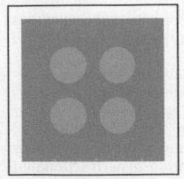

Chapter 92
Palliation of Bone Metastases

William F. Hartsell, Santosh Yajnik

Background and Incidence

Metastatic disease to the bone is a common cause of pain and other significant symptoms that are detrimental to quality of life. The exact incidence of bone metastases is difficult to determine, but estimates are that more than 100,000 people in the United States will develop osseous metastatic disease annually (59). The incidence of bone metastases varies significantly depending on the primary site, with breast and prostate cancer accounting for up to 70% of patients with metastatic disease (10). Bone metastases may be found in up to 85% of patients dying from breast, prostate, or lung cancer. Other primary sites with a propensity for bone metastases include thyroid, melanoma, and kidney. On the other hand, gastrointestinal sites of primary malignancy give rise to bone metastasis in only 3% to 15% of patients with metastatic disease (50). Some hematologic malignancies including myeloma and lymphoma can also cause significant pain and bone destruction.

The ultimate prognosis for patients with bone metastases is poor, with median survival typically measured in months rather than years. Overall survival depends on the primary site and the presence or absence of visceral metastases. Patients with bone metastases from lung cancer have short median survival durations of 6 months. However, patients with bone metastases from breast or prostate primary sites may have significantly longer survival times. In patients with bone-only metastatic prostate or breast cancer, median survivals of 2 to 4 years have been reported (10,11,79). Whether the survival time is only a few months or extends to multiple years, these patients will often require active treatment because of pain, difficulty with ambulation and immobility, hypercalcemia, pathologic fractures, neurologic deficits, anxiety, depression, spinal cord or nerve root compression, and general deterioration of quality of life (50).

The axial skeleton is the most common site of bone metastasis, with metastasis most frequently occurring in the spine, pelvis, and ribs. The lumbar spine is the single most frequent site of bone metastasis (1,27,40,82). In the appendicular skeleton, the proximal femurs are the most common site of metastatic disease, and humeral lesions also occur frequently. The acral sites (feet and hands) are rarely involved. Certain skeletal sites are associated with specific areas of bone metastases. For example, scapular metastases are seen more frequently from renal primaries (21). Involvement of the skull is more common with breast primaries. The distal appendicular skeleton (tibia, fibula) and acral sites (especially the hands) are more common with lung primaries, and involvement of the toes is seen more commonly with genitourinary primaries (Fig. 92.1).

The most common symptom of bone metastases is slowly progressive, insidious pain that is fairly well localized. The pain may be worse at night. Pain from the femur or acetabulum may worsen with weight bearing or ambulation. In contrast, pain from the inferior ischium or sacrum may be worse with sitting but less bothersome with ambulation. Although the pain is frequently localized, pain may radiate to other areas. This is most frequently seen with pain in the lower back, pelvis or hips that may radiate down the legs. Pain that radiates does not necessarily indicate nerve impingement because radicular pain can also be caused by spasm of muscles that originate or insert near the area of disease (e.g., pain in the hip radiating to the knee).

Pathophysiology

There are primarily three types of cells within mature bone: osteocytes, osteoblasts, and osteoclasts. Osteoblasts originate from osteogenic cells, found in the periosteum or endosteum. The osteogenic cells differentiate into osteoblasts when there is a mechanical or chemical stimulus for remodeling or repair. The osteoblasts build bone by depositing collagen type I into the extracellular space. An inorganic complex of calcium and phosphate (hydroxyapatite) is laid down within this organic matrix to provide the strength and density of the bone. The osteoblasts then mature into osteocytes, which maintain the bone structure. Osteoclasts are multinucleated giant cells that originate from pluripotent hematopoietic bone marrow cells and are adherent to the bone surface (62). These cells create an acidophilic environment that causes dissolution of the hydroxyapatite crystals and proteolysis of the bone matrix.

The differentiation and activation of osteoclasts occurs because of the effects of a group of proteins that are related to tumor necrosis factor, including osteoprotegerin, receptor activator of nuclear factor-κB (RANK), and the RANK ligand (RANKL). Osteoblasts and stromal cells express RANKL and activated T cells may also release RANKL. The RANKL binds to the RANK receptor on osteoclast precursors, which then induces the formation of mature osteoclasts. Osteoprotegerin is a decoy receptor for RANKL, and inhibits the differentiation and activation of osteoclasts (62). The destruction of bone by osteolytic metastases is mediated by the osteoclasts, not by the tumor cells. However, the factors that activate the osteoclasts are likely produced by the tumor cells including RANKL, interleukin-1, interleukin-6, and macrophage inflammatory protein 1α. The mechanisms for osteoblastic activation are not clearly delineated, but it appears that bone resorption occurs first even in osteoblastic metastases from prostate cancer (63).

Normal bone is constantly being remodeled in a cycle lasting about 120 days (3 to 6 months). For the first 20 days of the cycle, the bone is resorbed by osteoclasts. The bone is then rebuilt by osteoblasts during the next 100 days.

The structure of the bone changes during growth and development. All bones are immature, woven bone at the time of birth. Woven bone is more cellular, with no organized orientation to the collagen fibers of the bone. As the woven bone is absorbed, it is replaced by lamellar bone. The lamellar bone is organized circumferentially around neurovascular canals. This cylindrical structure provides much more strength than the haphazard orientation of woven bone. Most adult bone is lamellar.

The strength of bone is provided primarily by cortical bone, which is the dense, compact bone found in the diaphysis of long bones and along the exterior surfaces of cuboidal bones. Cortical bone comprises most of the mass of the skeletal system, and provides most of the strength of the skeleton. Trabecular bone is the spongy, cancellous bone found in the center of cuboidal bones, and in the center of the metaphysis and diaphysis of long bones. There is much more rapid remodeling of trabecular

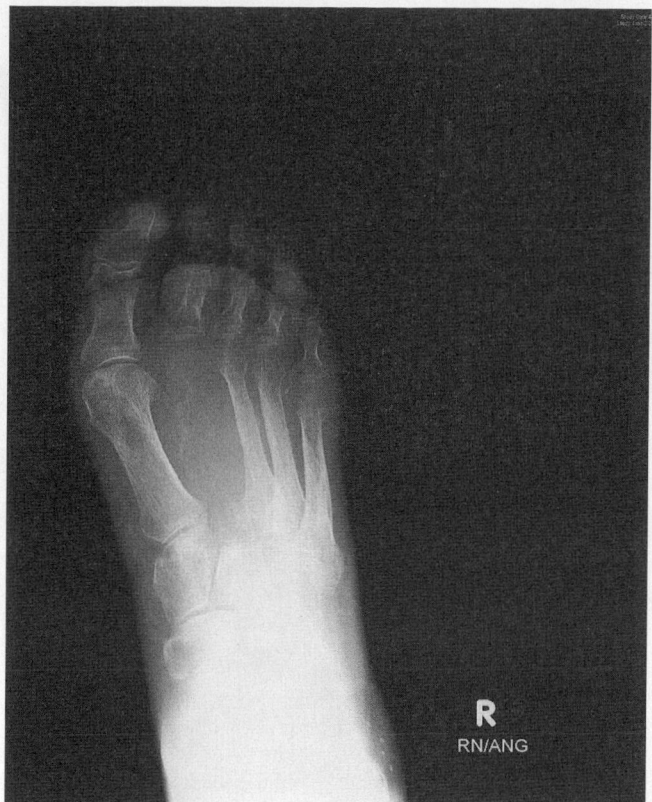

FIGURE 92.1. Radiograph of right foot of a patient with metastatic transitional cell carcinoma of the bladder. Note the destruction of the second metatarsal.

bone, with replacement of 25% of trabecular bone per year, compared with 3% of cortical bone (39).

Long bones consist of the epiphysis, metaphysis, and diaphysis. The diaphysis is the long shaft of the bone. The epiphyses are at the ends of the bone. These are composed of hyaline cartilage initially, which becomes ossified during puberty. The metaphysis is the area between the epiphysis and diaphysis. The metaphysis is an area of rapidly growing trabecular bone.

Metastases to the bone most often occur in the red marrow, which is found in highest concentration in the axial skeleton. This most often occurs by hematogenous spread, but may occur by direct extension as well. Involvement of adjacent bone by direct extension (e.g., mandibular involvement from an oral cavity cancer) does not necessarily imply that there is a higher likelihood of distant bone metastases, and its management is very different from that of bone metastases from hematogenous spread. The predilection of certain tumor sites to metastasize to bone may be related to local growth factors in the bone such as transforming growth factor-β, insulin-like growth factors I and II, fibroblastic growth factors, or platelet-derived growth factors, preferential adherence to endothelial surfaces in certain bones by cell adhesion molecules, or chemotactic attraction from bone cells by osteocalcin or type I collagen (50,60,62). The relatively high proportion of hematogenous metastasis to bone compared with other sites in the body cannot simply be explained by blood flow, which is more than 30 times greater in lung than in red bone marrow (92).

Bone metastases are often described as either osteolytic or osteoblastic, but these are different representations of abnormalities in the normal bone-remodeling process. Breast and lung cancers more commonly cause osteolytic-appearing lesions, and lesions caused by prostate and thyroid cancers more often have an osteoblastic appearance. However, only myeloma is associated with purely osteolytic lesions (62). Most other tumors have a combination of osteolytic and osteoblastic components. Even in osteoblastic-appearing prostate cancer metastases, increased bone resorption does occur.

The mechanism of pain from bone metastases is not clearly understood. Possible mechanisms include mechanical instability, irritation of periosteal stretch receptors, tumor-directed osteoclast-mediated osteolysis, tumor cells themselves, or tumor-induced nerve injury, production of nerve growth factor or stimulation of other cytokine receptors (10,19,30). Because the mechanisms of pain may be multifactorial, a combination of therapies may be superior to any one therapy alone (19).

Evaluation

The physical examination is an important step in evaluating a patient with bone metastases. The physical examination may help make decisions regarding appropriate subsequent imaging studies. Firm palpation will often elicit the specific area of pain, with "point tenderness" often pointing directly to the affected area in the bone. It is important to carefully evaluate the entire skeletal system with examination, as intense pain at one site often masks subjective reports of pain at other sites. A careful physical examination may reveal hidden pain in other locations. A thorough neurologic examination is also important, especially in patients with spinal metastases, to carefully evaluate for the possibility of spinal cord, cauda equina, or nerve root compression.

For symptomatic patients with point tenderness, plain radiographs are typically the most appropriate first imaging study. Such radiographs are easy to obtain and inexpensive. The appearance of bone metastases on x-rays varies depending on the primary site and histology. Most bone metastases from lung cancer and breast cancer appear osteolytic, whereas most from prostate cancer appear osteoblastic (Fig. 92.2). However, nearly all bone metastases have components of both osteolytic and osteoblastic processes. The primary disadvantage of plain radiographs is that small lesions are rarely seen. Approximately 30% to 50% of the bone mineral content must be lost before the lesion will be apparent on x-rays.

Technetium-99 m bone scintigraphy (nuclear medicine bone scan) is the best method for screening patients at risk for bone metastasis and is useful to evaluate the extent of metastatic disease in the bone. Bone scintigraphy is an indicator of osteoblastic activity. Because multiple myeloma is frequently purely osteolytic, bone scans are less useful for evaluating extent of disease in myeloma. Bone scintigraphy is not specific for metastatic disease, and positive findings must often be confirmed using other imaging studies. A confirmatory study is especially important in a weight-bearing bone such as the proximal femur. False-positive readings may be seen in areas of arthritis, trauma, or Paget's disease. In addition, the osteoblastic activity in healing bone after treatment may give the appearance of progressive disease. False-negative readings may occur in fast-growing, highly aggressive tumors, especially if these are mainly osteolytic.

Computed tomography (CT) scans are more sensitive than plain radiographs, and may be better able to localize the lesion within the bone. However, CT scans are more expensive, more time-consuming, and may not be useful as a screening tool for skeletal metastasis. The CT may be useful in defining the extent of cortical destruction and helping to assess the risk of a pathologic fracture (72). In addition, the CT scan may be used to guide needle biopsies to obtain a tissue diagnosis. CT scans have limited usefulness in detecting marrow involvement, but are much better than plain radiographs at evaluating soft tissue extension of disease.

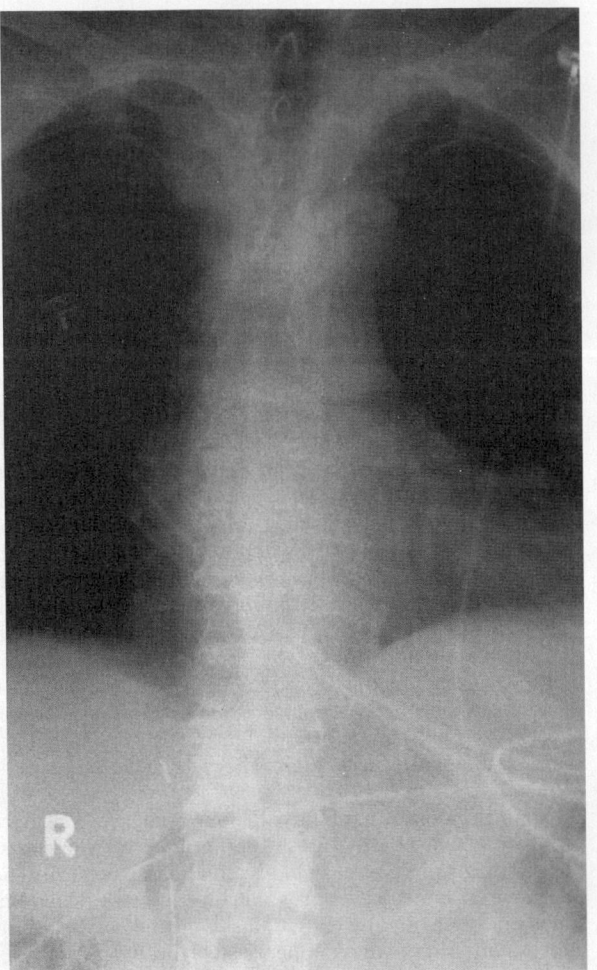
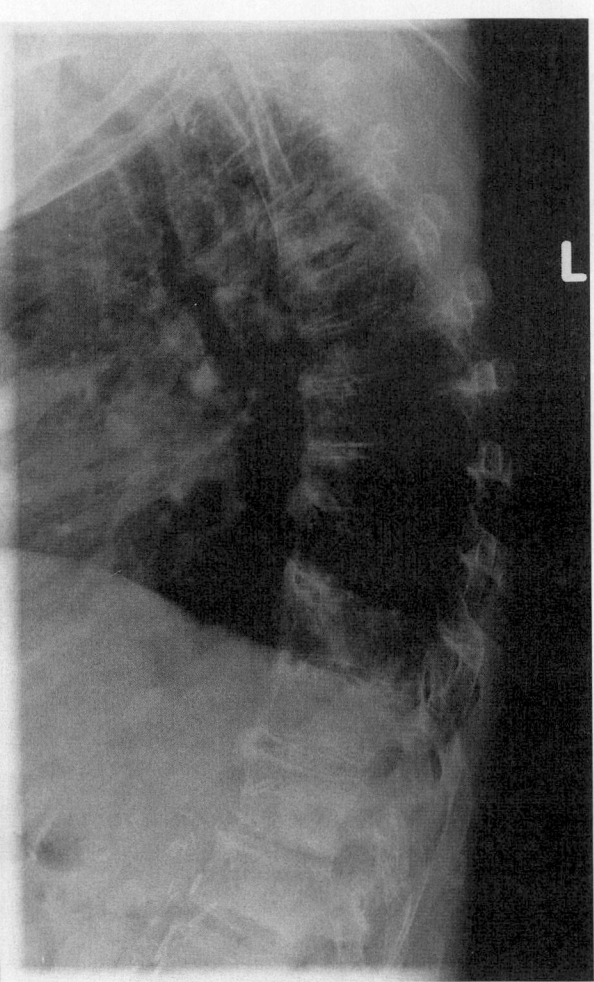

FIGURE 92.2. Anteroposterior **(A)** and lateral **(B)** spine radiographs from a patient with metastatic prostate cancer. There are osteoblastic lesions seen in T12 and L1.

Magnetic resonance imaging (MRI) is better than plain radiography or nuclear medicine bone scintigraphy at assessing the involvement of trabecular bone (red marrow), especially in the vertebral bodies. The findings are typically best seen on T1 contrast-enhanced images and short tau inversion recovery (STIR) images. Metastatic prostate cancer is visible as high-intensity lesions on the STIR images, and is visible prior to its appearance on bone scintigraphy (16). In addition, MRI scans are useful in determining the involvement of neurovascular structures. MRI scans are not useful as a screening tool for bone metastases. However, MRI scans may be more sensitive than bone scintigraphy in the vertebral body region (Fig. 92.3). The sensitivity of MRI scanning has been reported as 91% to 100%, compared with 62% to 85% for bone scintigraphy (16,22). In addition, MRI images can help distinguish whether a vertebral body compression fracture is from malignancy or from osteoporosis.

Positron emission tomography (PET) scanning evaluates areas of increased metabolic activity, most commonly using the 18-fluorodeoxyglucose (FDG) isotope. These scans are useful in detecting osteolytic bone metastases, but are less sensitive for osteoblastic metastases. In addition, precise determination of the location of lesions is difficult with PET scans, but the use of simultaneous CT scans allows for much better localization of the abnormal FDG uptake (14). PET scans may be useful as a whole-body screening tool (14,17). Comparative studies have shown PET scans to be more sensitive than Tc-99 m scintigraphy or whole-body MRI scans in detecting bone metastases (13,52).

There may be limitations in the sensitivity of PET scanning in certain areas such as the skull, where the intense physiologic uptake from the adjacent brain parenchyma may obscure small skull metastases.

Pain Management

The majority of patients with bone metastases will experience pain during their disease course, and pain control can significantly improve their quality of life. Pain management may be achieved either by debulking disease using cytotoxic therapy or by symptomatic control with pharmacologic interventions.

Despite increasing understanding about the effective treatment of pain, patients with pain from bone metastases frequently have inadequate pain management. Barriers to pain treatment include physician underestimation of the patient's pain and reluctance by the patient to report pain (8). There is a significant discrepancy between the physician estimate of pain and the pain level reported by the patient (9). The use of a validated pain scale, such as the Brief Pain Inventory, gives the patient an opportunity to describe the severity of pain and the interference of pain with function in a manner that can be understood both by the patient and the physician (8). This also allows for comparisons of pain levels over time, to better assess the effectiveness of treatments.

Pain control can be achieved in the majority of patients using the World Health Organization analgesic ladder. Step I uses

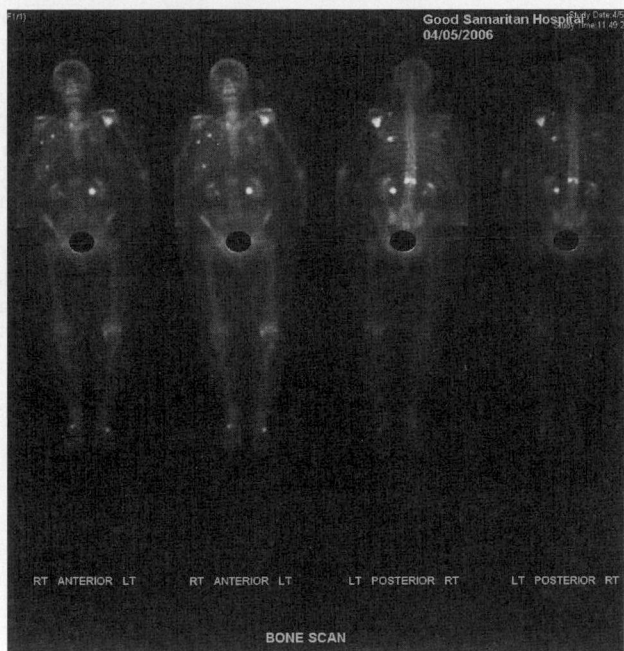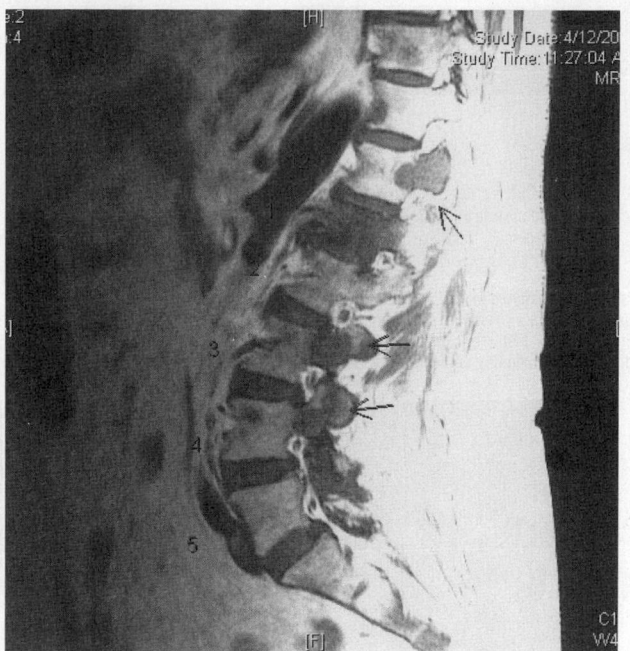

FIGURE 92.3. Nuclear medicine bone scan **(A)** and sagittal T1 magnetic resonance image (MRI) scan **(B)** from a woman with metastatic breast cancer. The bone scan shows the abnormality at L1, but the MR shows lesions at multiple levels including the pedicles of T12, L3, and L4 *(arrows)*.

nonopioid analgesics such as acetaminophen or nonsteroidal anti-inflammatory drugs; step II uses weak opioids such as codeine; step III uses strong opioids such as morphine. These medications are increased as necessary until the patient is free of pain. Typically, the medications are given on a routine schedule ("by the clock") rather than waiting until a certain level of pain ("on demand"). Using this schedule, 70% to 76% of patients will have good pain relief (44,91). Adjuvant medications such as gabapentin or amitriptyline may be added for neuropathic pain. Antianxiety or antidepressant medications may also be of benefit in selected patients.

The opioid-based pain medications frequently cause constipation and may cause nausea. Patients using opioid medications should routinely be administered a fiber medication with or without a stool softener to minimize constipation. Other side effects of the opioid analgesics may include sedation, mental status changes, and mood changes.

Surgical Management

Surgical management of bone metastases is performed primarily to prevent or treat pathologic fractures. The goals of surgical intervention are to prevent or relieve pain, improve motor function, and to improve overall quality of life. Treatment techniques are simpler and more effective when the procedure is performed prophylactically for an impending fracture rather than following the occurrence of a pathologic fracture. The risk of pathologic fracture depends on multiple factors including location and extent of the lesion; whether the lesion is osteolytic, osteoblastic or mixed; and the primary cancer site.

Fractures of the weight-bearing bones are the most likely to cause significant functional deficits. The proximal femur may have a higher propensity for fracture than other sites, but some authors have suggested that the fracture risk in upper limbs is similar to the risk in the femur. Whether or not there is a difference in the risk of fracture, the peritrochanteric femur is the site most likely to cause serious morbidity, and, therefore, the threshold for prophylactic intervention should be relatively low.

The femur accounts for 65% of pathologic fractures requiring surgical intervention (23). The humerus and vertebral bodies are also sites that require special attention because of the potential functional deficits from pathologic fractures.

The size of the bone metastasis is an important predictor of risk of fracture, especially with regard to the extent of cortical destruction. Various models have been used to predict the risk of pathologic fracture, based on the size of the lesion. In series using plain radiographs, lesions ≥ 2.5 cm in the cortex of the femur were significantly more likely to fracture (3). The proportion of cortical destruction is important as well. The risk of pathologic fracture of the femur begins to significantly increase when there is destruction of >50% of the cortex; the risk of fracture is 80% when >75% of the cortex is destroyed (15). The location within the bone is important as well. An experimental model has shown that the greatest reduction in strength of the femur occurs with lesions in the inferior and medial aspect of the femoral neck, and posterior lesions have the least impact (6). The use of CT scans may offer more accurate assessment of the bone strength. Femoral lesions with axial cortical destruction >30 mm had a 23% risk of pathologic fracture, compared with 3% risk of fracture for cortical destruction ≤30 mm (88).

A scoring system was proposed by Mirels (47) that had a 12-point scale based on the location of the lesion, pain, extent of cortical destruction, and radiographic appearance (Table 92.1). The risk of fracture was 15% for a score of 8 and 33% for a score of 9. He proposed that prophylactic fixation was indicated for a score of ≥9.

The decision to proceed with surgery should be based on a number of factors, which include but are not limited to the estimated risk of pathologic fracture. For patients with a very limited life span, surgery may not be indicated even if the risk of pathologic fracture is relatively high (23). Clinical prediction of survival may be more accurate than relying on specific parameters such as diagnosis (primary site), performance status, number of bone metastases, presence of visceral metastases, and hemoglobin level (48).

Fractures of the femoral neck can be managed either by total hip arthroplasty (which replaces both the femoral head

Table 92.1   **MIRELS' SCORING SYSTEM OF PREDICTION OF PATHOLOGIC FRACTURE RISK**[a]

Score	Pain	Location	Cortical Destruction	Radiographic Appearance
1	Mild	Upper limb	<1/3	Blastic
2	Moderate	Lower limb	1/3–2/3	Mixed
3	Severe	Peritrochanteric	>2/3	Lytic

[a]A score is assigned for each of the four categories, and the sum of those scores is used to estimate the risk of pathologic fracture.
From Mirels H. Metastatic disease in long bones: a proposed scoring system for diagnosing impending pathologic fractures. *Clin Orthop Relat Res* 1989;249:256–264.

and acetabulum) or by a proximal femoral endoprosthesis alone (23). Fractures of the intertrochanteric area may be managed by open reduction and internal fixation without the use of a prosthesis. This may allow for better long-term gait because of preservation of the hip flexor and adductor strength (23). Lytic disease that extends below the intertrochanteric area is treated with a long intramedullary rod that provides stability throughout the length of the femur (Fig. 92.4). If there is significant destruction of the greater trochanter and femoral neck or head in addition to subtrochanteric involvement, a prosthetic replacement would be more appropriate than a reconstruction nail (78). Fractures of the distal femur may be managed either with a plate and compression screw or with an intracondylar

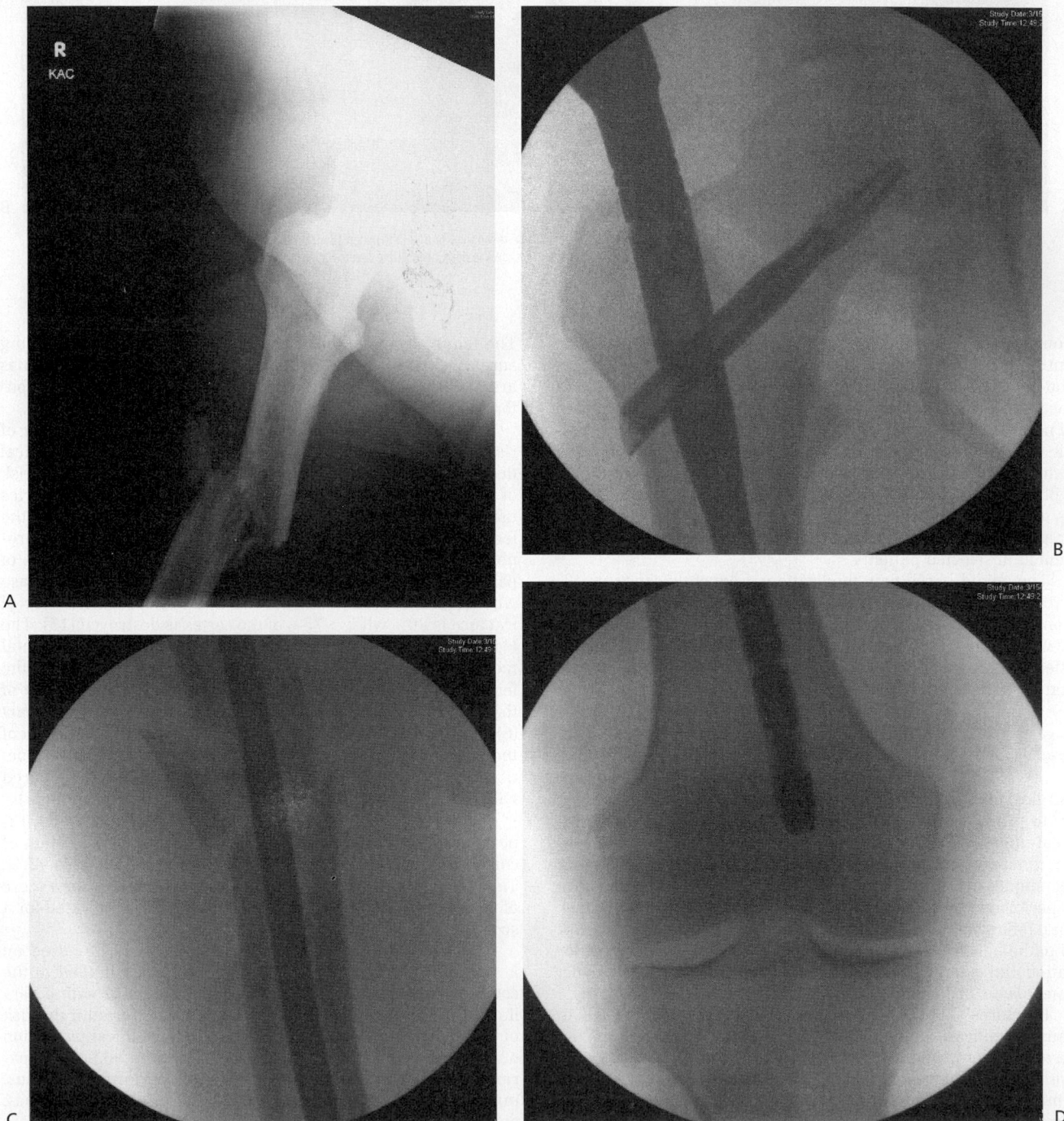

FIGURE 92.4. Anteroposterior radiograph **(A)** of a diaphyseal fracture of the femur in a patient with diffuse large cell lymphoma. Intraoperative fluoroscopic views of the proximal **(B)**, mid-shaft **(C)**, and distal **(D)** femur after internal fixation with a trochanter fixation nail (TFN) nail.

nail and screws augmented by intramedullary methylmethacrylate cement. The latter method may reduce the risk of late failure of the repair, especially in patients receiving postoperative radiation therapy (23).

Repair of pathologic fractures of the humerus may be more problematic because of the small intramedullary canal and because of the proximity of the radial nerve, which may require extensive dissection (23). Pathologic fractures of the proximal humerus will frequently require prosthetic replacement (23). Fractures in the diaphysis may be repaired with a compression plate and screws. An alternative is to use a segmental diaphyseal replacement prosthetic device, which involves a prosthetic device than can be cemented into an allograft (78). Supracondylar fractures are difficult to manage because the shape of the bone is not conducive to a plate and screws; these lesions may require intramedullary rods inserted retrograde through both the medial and lateral condyles, supplemented by intramedullary cement (23).

Most pathologic fractures of the pelvis do not require surgical intervention, except for those involving the acetabulum (23). Repair of acetabular fractures may involve the use of a total hip acetabular prosthesis, but more extensive lesions may require reconstruction that transfers the load-bearing stresses into more structurally intact bone in the iliac bone or sacroiliac joint (23).

Vertebroplasty is an effective method of palliating pain from vertebral body metastases, even in patients who have received prior radiotherapy (7). Most patients experience pain relief within 48 hours. The procedure involves percutaneous injection of methylmethacrylate under CT or fluoroscopic guidance. Retropulsion of bone, epidural tumor, or collapse of the bone to less than one-third of its original height are relative contraindications to percutaneous vertebroplasty because of the risk of extrusion of the cement into the spinal canal potentially causing neurologic complications. In some patients with epidural tumor, percutaneous vertebroplasty can be performed safely and effectively with a low risk of complications (25,76).

▪▪ | Systemic Treatment

The rationale for using systemic therapy in the management of bone metastasis is compelling. The pathophysiology of bone metastasis involves hematogenous dissemination and most patients with bone metastasis suffer from multiple synchronous sites of disease. In theory, administering a systemic cytotoxic therapy should deliver palliative benefit by simultaneously addressing all sites of bone metastasis. A localized therapy such as external-beam radiation may be most appropriate for palliation if symptoms are localized. On the other hand, systemic chemotherapy may offer palliative benefit if symptoms are diffuse or constitutional, and disease is widespread.

Measurement of response to systemic therapy has generally been with the same criteria used for solid metastatic tumors: a measurable radiographic change. This works well for lung and liver metastasis, but not as well for bone metastasis. For bone metastases, the definition of a complete response is complete disappearance of all lesions on radiographs for at least 4 weeks. This is unlikely to occur even if all tumor cells are eradicated. A partial response requires some recalcification of lytic lesions, which may not be evident for 6 months or more (31). PET scans may be more accurate at assessing response in a timely manner, but are too expensive to be used as a routine follow-up evaluation for bone metastases. Markers of bone resorption may be a good way to detect response to therapy, but are not clinically available at this time. Response to therapy for other modalities (i.e., radiotherapy, bisphosphonates) is measured in terms of pain relief and quality-of-life measures. Unfortunately, there is not much literature on accurate and reliable response criteria to palliative systemic therapy for bone

metastasis. Most of the studies of chemotherapy for metastatic disease involve patients with visceral as well as osseous metastases. The responses in terms of pain are typically reported for all patients, not just those with bone metastases. There is more information regarding response to chemotherapy for patients with metastatic prostate cancer as this more frequently involves bone-only metastatic disease. The chemotherapy drugs are frequently given with bisphosphonates or corticosteroids, which may impact on the response rates.

Tannock et al. (83) recommended using more relevant end points of palliation. They performed a randomized trial of mitoxantrone plus prednisone versus prednisone alone for patients with hormone-refractory prostate cancer and pain. Improvement in pain was seen in 29% of patients receiving the chemotherapy, compared with 12% of those who received prednisone alone. In a subsequent study, they compared mitoxantrone and prednisone plus or minus clodronate for a similar group of patients. Most had mild pain at study entry (160/209, 77%), and the remainder had moderate pain scores. The patients with moderate pain who received chemotherapy and clodronate had a 58% response rate (≥ 2 point improvement in pain score) compared with 26% for those who received chemotherapy alone. The median duration of pain response was 6 months.

In patients with bone metastasis, there is seldom reason to combine chemotherapy with concurrent radiation therapy because of the potential for increased toxicity when both modalities are delivered concurrently.

A number of hormonal therapies are available in the management of metastatic prostate and breast cancer. In properly selected patients, hormonal therapy has the potential for providing excellent palliation of metastatic disease with limited morbidity. In 1984, the Medical Research Council started a prospective, randomized trial in which 938 patients who either had asymptomatic metastatic prostate cancer or were not medical candidates for definitive therapy were randomized to immediate versus delayed hormone ablation therapy. Hormone ablation was achieved using either a leutinizing hormone-releasing hormone agonist or by orchiectomy. This study showed that immediate versus delayed initiation of hormone ablation therapy in the subset of patients with metastatic prostate cancer helped to prevent serious complications from metastatic disease. Serious complications including pathologic fracture, spinal cord compression, development of extraskeletal metastases, and ureteral obstruction were twofold more frequent in patients whose hormonal therapy was deferred compared with patients who received immediate hormone ablation therapy (42).

The bisphosphonates are pyrophosphate analogs that bind to calcium phosphate with high affinity and are potent agents affecting bone resorption (45). There is emerging evidence that the bisphosphonates also induce apoptosis in cancer cells (74). Clodronate is a first-generation, nonnitrogen-containing bisphosphonate. Clodronate has a high affinity for bone mineral and is subsequently taken up into activated osteoclasts during bone resorption, thereby ensuring high concentrations within osteoclasts (20). The nitrogen-containing bisphosphonates inhibit the key enzyme farnesyl diphosphonate synthase in the mevalonate pathway (65). This prevents the action of several additional enzymes required for bone resorption. The bisphosphonates include pamidronate, alendronate, ibandronate, risedronate, and zoledronic acid. Zoledronate is much more potent than the other bisphosphonates, in part because it also inhibits tumor cell adhesion to the extracellular matrix.

The initial studies of bisphosphonate usage were primarily in women with metastatic breast cancer. Pamidronate was evaluated in multiple randomized prospective studies of women with osteolytic bone metastases from breast cancer. The Aredia Breast Cancer Study Group Protocols 18 and 19 enrolled women receiving either chemotherapy (P19) or hormonal therapy (P18). In the P18 study, 372 women were randomized to receive either placebo or pamidronate 90 mg as a 2-hour infusion every 4 weeks for 24 cycles (84). The primary end point was the prevention of "skeletal-related complications" (pathologic fractures, spinal cord compression, hypercalcemia, or the requirement for surgery or radiation therapy on bone). There were fewer skeletal-related complications in the pamidronate arm (475 events vs. 648 in the placebo group), but the benefit in reducing pathologic fractures and hypercalcemia was not significant until 18 to 24 months of treatment. The primary difference was that twice as many placebo patients required radiation therapy for palliation of pain, most often in the first 6 to 12 months. There was no difference in survival, although pain levels and serum markers of bone resorption were significantly lower in the group receiving pamidronate.

In the P19 study, women with stage IV breast cancer who were receiving chemotherapy and had lytic bone metastasis were given placebo or pamidronate for 12 monthly cycles (28). Patients in the pamidronate arm suffered fewer overall skeletal complications and had a greater median time to first skeletal complication when compared with patients in the placebo arm of the study. Women treated with pamidronate maintained better performance status and had less bone pain secondary to metastasis.

Rosen et al. (64) evaluated 773 patients with bone metastases from solid tumors including lung cancer, renal cell carcinoma, head and neck cancers, thyroid, and other primaries sites (exclusive of breast and prostate cancer). They compared placebo with zoledronic acid in doses of either 4 or 8 mg given every 3 weeks for 9 months. The primary end point was proportion of patients developing a skeletal-related event (SRE), including pathologic fracture, spinal cord compression, or the need for surgery or radiation therapy. The proportion of patients developing an SRE was 44% in the placebo group compared with 38% in the 4-mg zoledronic acid group ($p = .127$) and 35% in the 8-mg group ($p = .023$). The time to development of an SRE was significantly longer with zoledronic acid compared with placebo (230 vs. 163 days; $p = .017$). The dose of the 8-mg group was reduced to 4 mg during the latter part of the study because of safety concerns, and thus 25% of patients in the 8-mg treatment arm actually received only 4 mg per dose. In addition, only 25% of patients received the full 9-month course of treatment because of death (27%), adverse events (21%), patient decision to discontinue (15%), or "insufficient efficacy (7%)." There was no improvement in two specific events—surgery to bone and spinal cord compression—in the patients receiving zoledronic acid compared with placebo. Additionally, the need for analgesics gradually increased and functional capacity decreased from baseline to month 9 in all groups, with no differences between zoledronic acid and placebo.

Complications of supportive therapy with bisphosphonates include osteoradionecrosis (particularly of the jaw) and renal insufficiency (43). The mechanism of bisphosphonate-induced osteoradionecrosis is not known. Risk factors include the intravenous use of pamidronate and zoledronic acid, duration of treatment of 36 months or longer, older age in patients with multiple myeloma, and need for periodontal procedures (46).

Bisphosphonates are not metabolized by the body and are excreted by the kidneys. Bisphosphonate therapy can lead to renal toxicity. The incidence of renal toxicity is 9% to 15% in trials when 4 mg of zoledronic acid is delivered intravenously during 15 minutes (43). Moreover, the rate of renal toxicity depends on underlying renal disease, dose of bisphosphonate used, and the duration of the infusion.

Radiation Therapy

Radiation therapy has been reported to be effective in palliating painful bone metastases, with partial pain relief seen in 80% to 90% of patients, and complete pain relief in 50% of patients (Fig. 92.5). These data are primarily from studies using physician evaluation of pain. When patient evaluation of pain is used, pain improvement is seen in 60% to 80% of patients and complete pain relief is seen in 15% to 40% of patients (90). The response to treatment depends on a large number of factors, including sex, primary site and histology, performance status, type of lesion (osteolytic vs. osteoblastic), location of the metastases, weight-bearing vs. non–weight-bearing site, extent of disease, number of painful sites, marital status, and level of pain prior to treatment. The effectiveness of the treatment also depends on the goal: palliation of pain, prevention of pathologic fracture, avoidance of future treatments, or local control of the disease. The doses required and volumes treated may be quite different for each of these goals.

Local-field external-beam radiation therapy is typically used for palliation of a few discrete areas of painful metastases. The first large randomized study evaluating different dose and fractionation schemes was the Radiation Therapy Oncology Group (RTOG) 74-02 trial (86). Patients with solitary bone metastases were randomized to 40.5 Gy in 15 fractions versus 20 Gy in 5 fractions. Patients with multiple painful metastases were allocated to one of four treatment schedules: 30 Gy in 10 fractions, 15 Gy in 5 fractions, 20 Gy in 5 fractions, or 25 Gy in 5 fractions. The initial analysis by Tong et al. (86) in 1982 showed no statistically significant difference in response rates between any of the treatment arms, with complete responses in 49% to 61% of patients. These results were questioned by Blitzer (4); he reanalyzed the data using different criteria for complete response, which excluded patients who received repeat treatment, and defined complete response as no pain and no analgesic usage. With this adjustment in response definition, there was a significant difference in response favoring the longer treatment courses: 40.5 Gy in 15 fractions for the solitary metastases and 30 Gy in 10 fractions for multiple metastases. This was touted as evidence that higher doses were necessary for optimal palliation, even though one of the highest biologic doses for multiple fractions (25 Gy in 5 fractions) had one of the lower response rates. This reanalysis highlighted the importance of retreatment in this group of patients, especially in those given lower total doses during the initial course of radiation therapy.

There have been multiple randomized prospective trials evaluating different dose and fractionation schemes (5,18, 24,26,33,34,36,38,49,51,58,81,86). Most of the earlier studies evaluated different multifraction treatment regimens (Table 92.2). No significant difference was seen between longer course treatments and the shorter duration, lower total dose treatment courses. Two randomized studies evaluated single doses of radiation therapy for palliation of bone metastases. Hoskin et al. (29) randomized patients to 4 versus 8 Gy, and Jeremic et al. (32) randomized patients to one of three dose levels, 4 versus 6 versus 8 Gy. In both of these studies, the 8-Gy arm was superior to 4 Gy, indicating that there is a threshold dose necessary to achieve adequate palliation. Most of the randomized trials during the past 15 years have used a multiple fraction treatment scheme as the control arm, and a single dose of 8 to 10 Gy as the study arm (Tables 92.3 and 92.4).

Two recent large studies have compared single-dose treatment to longer courses of radiation therapy. The Dutch trial evaluated patients with bone metastases from solid tumors, primarily breast (39%), prostate (23%), and lung (25%); metastatic melanoma and renal cell carcinomas were excluded (81). The primary end point was patient-assessed pain relief, evaluated on an 11-point scale (0 = no pain, 10 = worst imaginable pain). A total of 1,171 patients were randomized to either 8 Gy in a single fraction or 24 Gy in six fractions. The painful areas had to be included in a single treatment volume. The spine (36%) and pelvis (30%) were the two most common sites of treatment. The median pain score was 6.3, with a minimum

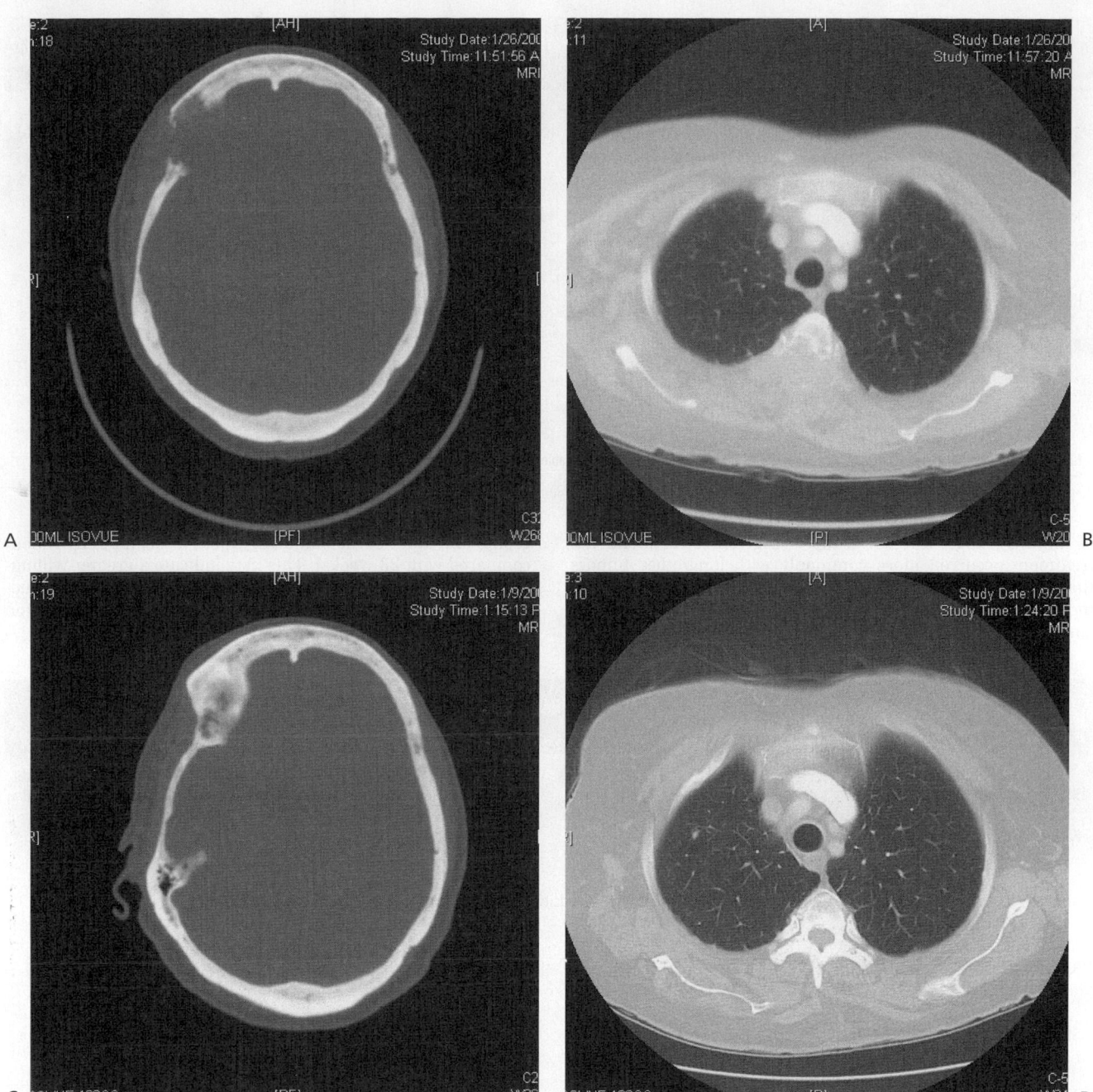

FIGURE 92.5. Axial computed tomography scans from a patient with metastatic breast cancer. Images through the frontal skull **(A)** and thoracic spine **(B)** show large, destructive, osseous lesions. Images 1 year later **(C,D)** after palliative external-beam radiation show significant healing of the bone.

score of 2. About half of the patient were receiving narcotic pain medications prior to randomization, and slightly more than half (53%) were receiving systemic therapy. The median survival after treatment was 30 weeks, with no difference between the two treatment groups. There was no difference in overall or complete response rates between the single dose versus longer course treatment arms. Overall, 71% of patients achieved a response to therapy during follow-up, with 35% achieving a complete response. Most of the responses occurred within the first 4 to 6 weeks following treatment. Complete response rates were higher for patients with breast and prostate primaries than with lung or other primary sites (44% and 41% vs. 21% and 16%).

There were two significant differences between the two treatment groups: retreatment rates and pathologic fracture rates. The rate of pathologic fracture in the treated area was 4% for the 8-Gy single-treatment arm compared with 2% for the 24 Gy/six fraction group. The median time to fracture was similar for the two groups, at 21 and 17 weeks. Although there was a significant difference in pathologic fracture between the two groups, these rates are still relatively low. There was also a significant difference in retreatment rates between the two arms of the study, with a much higher likelihood of a second course of treatment in the single treatment group. The group of patients receiving 24 Gy in six fractions initially was given a second course of treatment 7% of the time, while 25%

Table 92.2 RANDOMIZED TRIALS WITH ≥100 EVALUABLE PATIENTS COMPARING MULTIPLE FRACTION TREATMENTS FOR PALLIATION OF BONE METASTASES[a]

Study	No. of Patients (No. of Eval)	Dose (Gy)/ No. of Fractions	Complete Response (%)	Overall Response (%)	Path Fractures (%)
Tong et al., 1982, USA (solitary treatment site) (86)	266 (146)	20/5	53	82	4
		40/15	61	85	18
Tong et al., 1982, USA (multiple sites) (86)	750 (613)	15/5	49	87	5
		20/5	56	85	7
		25/5	49	83	9
		30/10	57	78	8
Hirokawa et al., 1988, Japan (26)	128 (128)	25/5	NA	75	NA
		30/10		75	
Rasmusson et al., 1995, Denmark (58)	217 (127)	15/3	NA	69	NA
		30/10		66	
Niewald et al., 1996, Germany (51)	100 (100)	20/5	33	77	8
		30/15	31	86	13

No. of Patients, number of patients entered on study; No. of Eval, number of patients evaluable for response; Path Fractures, proportion of patients with pathologic fractures after treatment; NA, not available from published report.
[a]Response rates listed are for pain relief.

of the 8-Gy single-fraction group was given retreatment. Retreatment occurred more commonly with lung/other tumors than with breast/prostate primaries. In addition, the retreatment was given at a lower pain score (median 6.8 for 8-Gy single-fraction compared with 7.5 for the multiple fraction group) and at an earlier time (14 weeks after initial treatment compared with 23 weeks). This may indicate a greater willingness to reirradiate after a single dose of 8 Gy or more reluctance to give retreatment after a higher initial dose of radiation therapy.

Table 92.3 RANDOMIZED TRIALS OF SINGLE VS MULTIPLE FRACTIONS WITH ≥100 EVALUABLE PATIENTS: DEMOGRAPHICS AND STUDY DESIGN

Study	No. of Patients (No. Eval)	1° End Point	2° End Points	Primary Sites	Treatment Site	Response Eval Time	% Severe Pain Pretreatment
Kaasa et al., 2006, Norway/Sweden (33)	376	Pain relief	Fatigue Quality of life	Prostate, 38% Breast, 30% Lung, 11%	Spine, 38% Pelvis, 35% Extrem, 20%	—	35–41
Hartsell et al., 2005, USA/Canada (24)	949 (898)	Pain relief	Analgesic usage, toxicity, path fracture rate, retreatment rate	Breast, 50% Prostate, 50%	C-spine, 5% T-spine, 19% L-spine, 27%	3 mo	72–73
Kirkbride et al., 2000, Canada (34)	398 (287)	Pain relief and analgesics	—	Breast, 40% Lung, 26% Prostate, 23%	Spine, 30% Pelvis, 29%	3 mo	—
Steenland et al., 1999, Netherlands (81)	1171 (1073)	Pain relief	Quality of life	Breast, 39% Lung, 25% Prostate, 23%	TL spine, 30% Pelvis, 36% Femur, 10% Ribs, 8% Humerus, 6%	During first year	Mean pain score 6.3 (moderate)
Bone Pain Working Group, 1999, UK/New Zealand (5)	765	Pain relief	Nausea and vomiting	Breast, 36% Prostate, 34% Lung, 12%	Pelvis/hip, 28% L spine, 20% Ribs, 11% T spine, 9% Femur, 6%	—	22–23
Koswig & Budach, 1999, Germany (36)	107	Pain relief	Recalcification	Breast, 58% Lung, 24% Prostate, 10% Kidney, 7%	Spine, 81% Extrem, 13%	6 wk	—
Nielsen et al., 1998, Denmark (49)	241 (239)	Pain relief	Quality of life Analgesic usage	Breast, 39% Prostate, 34% Lung, 13%	TL spine, 42% Pelvis, 21% Hips/femur, 18% Other, 19%	12 wk	—
Gaze et al., 1997, UK (18)	265 (240)	Pain relief	Side effects Quality of life	Any epithelial tumor	—	—	—

No. of Patients, number of patients entered on study; No. Eval, number of patients evaluable for response; 1° End Point, primary end point of study; 2° End Point, secondary end point(s) of study; Response Eval Time, time from study entry to assessment of response; % Severe Pain Pretreatment, proportion of patients with severe pain scores at the time of study entry; extrem, extremities, C-, T-, L-spine, cervical, thoracic, and lumbar spine; NA, not available from published report.

Table 92.4 RANDOMIZED TRIALS OF SINGLE VERSUS MULTIPLE FRACTIONS: RESULTS[a]

Study	No. of Patients (No. Eval)	Dose (Gy)/ Fractions	Median Survival (mo)	Complete Response	Overall Response	Retreat Rate (%)	Path Fractures (%)	Toxicity
Kaasa et al., 2006, Norway/Sweden (33)	376	8/1 vs. 30/10	9.6 7.9	NA	No difference	16 4	4 11	NA
Hartsell et al., 2005 USA/Canada (24)	949 (898)	8/1 vs. 30/10	9.1 9.3	15 18	65 66	18 9	5 4	10% grade 2–4 17% $p = .002$
Kirkbride et al., 2000, Canada (34)	398 (287)	8/1 vs. 20/5	NA	22 29	51 48	NA	NA	NA
Steenland et al., 1999, Netherlands (81)	1171 (1073)	8/1 vs. 20/5	7	37 33	72 69	25 7	4 2	No difference
Bone Pain Working Party, 1999, UK/New Zealand (5)	761 (681)	8/1 vs. 20/5[b]	NA	57 58	78 78	23 10	2 <1	No difference
Koswig & Budach, 1999, Germany (36)	107 (107)	8/1 vs. 30/10	NA	33 31	81 78	NA	NA	NA
Nielsen et al., 1998, Denmark (49)	241 (239)	8/1 vs. 20/5	NA	15 15	73 76	21 12	NA	No difference
Gaze et al., 1997, UK (18)	265 (240)	10/1 vs. 22.5/5	NA	37 47	81 76	NA	NA	21% $p =$ NS 26% emesis

No. of Patients, number of patients entered on study; No. Eval, number of patients evaluable for response; Path Fractures, proportion of patients with pathologic fractures after treatment; NA, not available from published report; NS, not statistically significant.
[a]Response rates listed are for pain relief
[b]30 Gy/10 was also allowed; 98% of patients received 20 Gy/5.

The second large study of single dose versus longer course treatment for palliation of bone metastases was the RTOG study 9714, which was conducted in the United States and Canada (24). This was limited to patients with painful bone metastases from breast or prostate primaries, with up to three painful sites allowed. Pain was evaluated using the Brief Pain Inventory, an 11-point scale. At the time of randomization, the patient was required to have a minimum pain score of 5 or a high narcotic pain medication requirement of the equivalent of >60 mg of morphine per day. More than 70% of the patients had severe pain at study entry (pain scores of 7 to 10). Patients were randomized to 8 Gy in a single fraction versus 30 Gy in 10 treatments. The median survival was 9.3 months. Overall toxicity rates were low, with fewer patients in the 8-Gy treatment group experiencing acute toxicity. There were no significant differences in complete (17%) and partial pain response rates (49%) between the two treatment groups. Complete pain and narcotic response (0 pain score and no narcotic pain medication use) was seen in 11%; these responses were all determined at the 3-month posttreatment evaluation. As in the Dutch trial, the rate of retreatment was higher in the 8-Gy treatment group, with 18% in that group receiving retreatment compared with 9% in the 30-Gy group. This disparity in the rate of retreatment occurred despite nearly identical rates of stable (26% vs. 24%) or progressive pain scores (9% vs. 10%), and similar rates of narcotic usage between the two groups.

In contrast to the Dutch trial, there was no difference in the rate of pathologic fractures between the two groups (5% for 8 Gy vs. 4% for 30 Gy). Further analysis of this study has shown that certain subgroups may benefit from the longer course of palliative radiation therapy. Konski et al. (35) showed that although married men and single and married women were more likely to receive retreatment after receiving 8 Gy versus 30 Gy of palliative radiation therapy, there was no difference in retreatment rates among single men (35). The authors suggest that social support factors may significantly impact the ability of some patients to access repeat therapies for painful bone metastasis, especially as their health declines. Such subgroups of patients may benefit from the longer 10-fraction course of therapy.

These two large, prospective, randomized trials comparing single fraction to multiple fraction palliative radiation therapy have similar results and help to clarify the role of palliative radiotherapy for bone metastases. The assessment of pain was performed by the patients rather than by physicians or other health care providers. The studies with the highest response rates have generally used physician assessment of pain response (e.g., the RTOG 7402 study). Even with patient assessment of response, the single-fraction treatment yields similar response rates to the longer course treatment. The patients in the Dutch trial were treated when their pain was in the moderate range, with only half on narcotic pain medications, compared with severe pain and high-dose narcotic pain medication for most of the patients entered on the RTOG trial. This may account for the higher rates of complete response on the Dutch trial. In the RTOG trial, the group of patients with a single area of pain or with moderate pain scores at the time of study entry had higher complete response rates. Thus, it appears that the outcome is much better if patients are treated with palliative radiotherapy earlier in the course of their bone metastases, rather than waiting until pain is severe or narcotic pain medication requirements are significant. The rates of pathologic fracture following treatment are relatively low, but it is not clear if higher doses provide greater protection from fractures. The rates of retreatment are significantly higher with the single-dose schedules, but there may be some physician bias partially accounting for this difference as the retreatment tends to be offered at an earlier time and at lower levels of pain following the single-dose treatment.

There have been multiple randomized prospective trials in the past 25 years comparing shorter-course, lower total-dose treatment to the more "standard" longer course, higher-dose treatment. Several conclusions are clear from these studies:

a. Single dose treatments of 8 Gy provide similar pain relief to longer treatment regimens (30 Gy in 10 fractions or 20 to 24 Gy in five to eight treatments).
b. The retreatment rates are higher after short course treatment, by a factor of 2 to 3.

c. Response rates are lower when scored by the patient instead of by the treating physician.

d. Response rates are better when the initial pain scores are lower, that is, when the patients are treated for moderate pain rather than severe pain.

e. There is no consistent dose response relationship for palliation of bone metastases.

The lack of a dose-response relationship suggests that the mechanism of initial pain relief is not a reduction in tumor burden, but more likely a change in the local environment that has caused activation of bone resorption by osteoclasts. This helps to explain the seeming paradox of similar pain improvement with single-dose treatment compared with higher total-dose, longer-course treatment. The treatment paradigm for bone metastases may be more analogous to treatments for certain benign conditions such as prevention of heterotopic ossification or keloid formation. In those conditions, a single or few treatments are given to diminish the activation of osteoblasts or fibroblasts.

This mechanism of pain relief may also help to explain the higher rates of retreatment after single-dose 8-Gy treatment as there will be less cell kill with this dose compared with 30 Gy in 10 fractions. Thus, for patients with a longer life span, there is a greater opportunity for regrowth of the tumor, which may again impact the local milieu, causing osteoclast activation.

For patients with a poor performance status, difficulty making multiple trips for treatment, extensive nonosseous metastases, and/or a short life expectancy, the most appropriate treatment is a single fraction of 8 Gy. For patients with a longer life expectancy, bone-only metastases, and good performance status, a longer course of treatment (30 Gy in 10 fractions) may be more appropriate to minimize the risk of retreatment. For selected patients with a solitary bone metastasis ("oligometastasis"), an even higher dose of treatment may be indicated, although this must be tempered by potential weakening of surrounding normal bone.

The single large fraction treatment may be more likely to cause a "flare" reaction, with a temporary increase in pain at the site of the metastases (37). The risk of this side effect may be diminished by the use of anti-inflammatory medications, either corticosteroids or nonsteroidal anti-inflammatory medications. Although the risk of significant acute toxicity has been low in the randomized trials, another potential concern is the risk of nausea or emesis if a significant portion of the stomach is within the treatment field (e.g., with a field covering the lower thoracic spine). It may be beneficial to give prophylactic antiemetics 1 to 2 hours prior to the treatment to minimize the possibility of this side effect.

The use of bisphosphonates with external-beam radiotherapy may further improve the outcome in terms of both pain and bone healing. A prospective trial by Vassiliou et al. (89) evaluated 45 patients who received both external-beam irradiation and monthly ibandronate for painful bone metastases from solid tumors. All of the patients had improvement in pain, with 57% complete responses and 43% partial responses when using the same response criteria as RTOG 9714. The average pain score decreased from 6.3 to 0.8, and opioid pain medication usage decreased from 84% of the patients prior to treatment to 24% after treatment. Bone density in the area of the metastases increased by 73% by 10 months following treatment. A similar study using pamidronate and 30 Gy of external-beam radiotherapy in women with painful bone metastases from breast cancer found that 88% of patients had complete radiographic response by International Union Against Cancer (UICC) criteria (33).

The majority of patients with osseous metastases have multiple lesions. Although radiation therapy is effective at palliating pain in a few sites, it cannot be used to treat widespread disease. Two techniques that have been used to treat more diffuse metastases are hemibody irradiation and intravenous radiopharmaceuticals.

Hemibody Radiation Therapy

Hemibody irradiation (HBI), or wide-field radiation therapy, refers to the technique of treating a large portion of the body with external-beam irradiation. Although the term *hemibody irradiation* is used, typically the field does not cover half of the body, but more accurately treats about one third of the body. The treatment has been used for palliation of symptoms and as an adjuvant to prevent the development of new bone metastases. The treatment for palliation of pain is most useful in patients who have diffuse, widespread bone metastases.

The treatment volumes have been divided into upper, middle, and lower HBI. The fields for upper HBI cover the thorax and abdomen from the neck to the top of the iliac crests. For midbody HBI, the fields include the abdomen and pelvis from the diaphragm to the ischial tuberosities, and for lower HBI treatment, the field borders are from the top of the pelvis to the inferior portion of the femurs. The toxicities from each of the fields depend on the critical structures included. The most problematic of these is the risk of radiation pneumonitis with upper HBI. This is the dose-limiting toxicity for upper HBI, and dose-inhomogeneity corrections for the lung are necessary to minimize the risk of fatal pneumonitis. A lower total dose can be given to the upper hemibody fields compared with the middle or lower hemibody areas.

RTOG 78-10 was a dose-searching prospective protocol evaluating the maximum tolerated dose (MTD) for single-dose HBI (66). The MTD for middle and lower hemibody treatment was 8 Gy. The MTD for the upper HBI was 6 Gy if the lung dose was uncorrected and 7 Gy if lung corrections were used. Improvement in pain was noted in 80% of patients with breast cancer and 90% of patients with prostate cancer. Overall, the response rate in terms of pain relief was 73%, with complete relief of symptoms seen in 19%. Pain relief was seen relatively rapidly, with 50% of responses occurring within 2 days and 95% of responses within 2 weeks. The subsequent study RTOG 82-06 evaluated the use of HBI in addition to local radiotherapy to determine if the HBI would prevent the development of new sites of disease (56). All of the patients received involved field irradiation to one or more painful sites, and half of the patients were randomly assigned to receive single-dose HBI as well. The median time to progression was 6.3 months in the local treatment only group compared with 12.6 months for those receiving HBI. Fewer patients receiving HBI required additional treatment. The incidence of severe hematologic toxicity was low and transitory, but was seen only in the group receiving HBI.

Both the RTOG and the International Atomic Energy Agency have performed trials evaluating multifraction courses of HBI (67,71). The doses per fraction have ranged from 2.5 to 4 Gy to a total of 8 to 20 Gy. The maximum tolerated dose on the RTOG 88-08 study was 17.5 Gy in seven fractions. On the International Atomic Energy Agency study, 3 Gy twice daily for 2 days (12 Gy total) or 3 Gy daily for 5 days (15 Gy total) was more effective than 4 Gy daily for 2 days. The primary toxicities were hematologic and gastrointestinal. The rationale for these doses was to decrease the acute toxicity. However, each of these regimens requires multiple treatments during several days, and the acute toxicities are not appreciably different than the single-dose treatment. With the use of appropriate antiemetic premedications and with cytokines to aid in hematologic recovery, there does not appear to be any appreciable benefit to the fractionated HBI compared with the single dose.

Premedication with antiemetics and anti-inflammatory medications will significantly reduce the acute side effects of treatment. Prior to the development of the 5-HT3 receptor antagonists, nausea was a significant side effect of treatment, even with pre- and posttreatment using steroids, prochlorperazine, and intravenous hydration. With the use of ondansetron, granisetron, or other 5-HT3 receptor antagonists, the incidence of acute nausea and emesis has been minimized and HBI is well tolerated (70). A typical premedication regimen consists of dexamethasone, 8 to 16 mg, and ondansetron, 8 to 16 mg, 1 hour before treatment with HBI (68).

Radiopharmaceuticals

The concept of radiopharmaceutical treatment is compelling (2). Calcium (and to a lesser extent phosphorous) analogs will preferentially accumulate in bone, especially in areas of active bone turnover. A radioactive isotope that is a β-emitter or low energy γ-source will allow localized treatment in the areas in which the radiopharmaceutical accumulates, thus minimizing side effects and giving an excellent therapeutic ratio. The radiopharmaceuticals are given in a single injection that is easily administered. The treatment can be combined with other modalities, including chemotherapy or external-beam radiation therapy.

The first radiopharmaceutical used for treatment of bone metastases was phosphorous-32 (P-32). Treatment with P-32 for diffuse bone metastases was successful in giving subjective pain relief, but with unacceptable bone marrow toxicity. Other radioisotopes have been used for the palliation of diffuse osseous metastases, with a better therapeutic ratio than P-32. Strontium-89 (Sr-89) is chemically similar to calcium, and is deposited in the bone matrix, preferentially in sites of active osteogenesis. Sr-89 is a pure β-emitter with an energy of 1.4 MeV and a half-life of 50.6 days (77). Samarium-153 (Sm-153) is primarily a β-emitter, but also has a component of gamma emission, which is useful for imaging purposes. The Sm-153 ethylenediaminetetra methylenephosphoric acid (EDTMP) is concentrated in areas of high bone turnover, accumulating in areas of hydroxyapatite. The physical half-life of Sr-153 is 46.3 hours, but the biologic half-life is much shorter because about half of the compound is excreted in the urine within 8 hours of injection (75). These two isotopes have been evaluated in multiple prospective trials. There are other newer isotopes that are being evaluated including rhenium-186, rhenium-188, and tin-117 m. All of these isotopes accumulate in areas of osteoblastic activity, especially in areas of increased uptake on bone scintigraphy; for this reason, most of the patients entered on prospective trials have metastatic prostate cancer.

Strontium-89

The first study of Sr-89 with substantial numbers of patients was a randomized prospective trial of Sr-89 versus placebo in 126 men with metastatic prostate cancer, reported by Porter and McEwan (55) in 1993. The patients were randomized following involved field radiation therapy in a double-blind fashion to 400 MBq of Sr-89 versus placebo. Although there was no statistically significant difference in the primary end point of pain relief, there were several secondary end points that were improved with the Sr-89. More patients were able to discontinue pain medications (17% vs. 2%), and there were fewer sites of new pain requiring additional radiotherapy in the patients who received Sr-89. Smeland et al. (80) reported on a similar study of Sr-89 versus placebo following involved field radiation therapy, which showed no difference in outcome between the two groups. In this study, the dose of Sr-89 was only 150 MBq.

There have been two randomized trials of Sr-89 versus external-beam radiation therapy. A study by Quilty et al. (57) from the United Kingdom evaluated Sr-89 given in a dose of 200 MBq, compared with external-beam radiotherapy. For the patients with a few bone metastases, the randomization was Sr-89 versus local field radiation therapy. Patients with more

widespread metastases were randomized to Sr-89 versus HBI of 8 Gy to the lower hemibody or 6 Gy to the upper hemibody. There was no difference in pain relief, toxicity, or median survival between the groups. In the patients with diffuse disease, there were fewer new pain sites following Sr-89 than HBI. The trial by Oosterhof et al. (54) evaluated 203 patients with hormone-refractory metastatic prostate cancer, randomly assigning patients to receive local-field radiation therapy or 150 MBq of intravenous Sr-89. There was no difference in pain relief or toxicity between the two treatment arms.

Sr-89 can be given concomitantly with chemotherapy. Two randomized prospective trials have evaluated concomitant chemotherapy with Sr-89 for patients with hormone-refractory metastatic prostate cancer. In the trial by Sciuto et al. (73), 70 patients received 148 MBq of Sr-89 on day 0. They were randomly assigned to receive cisplatin 18 mg/m^2 intravenously on day 0 and 16 mg/m^2 on days 10 and 11, or placebo on the same days. The group that received cisplatin and Sr-89 had significantly more patients with pain relief (91% vs. 63%), longer duration of pain palliation (120 days vs. 60 days), longer median survival (9 months vs. 6 months), and a significantly greater proportion of patients with improvement in performance status (66% vs. 26%), with no significant difference in toxicity. Tu et al. (87) performed a phase II randomized study of doxorubicin 20 mg/M^2 per week given intravenously, with randomization between 2.035 MBq/kg of intravenous Sr-89 versus placebo. Neutropenia and anemia were common in the combined Sr-89 plus doxorubicin group compared with doxorubicin alone, but the median survival was also significantly better (28 months vs. 17 months).

An economic evaluation of the Trans-Canada randomized study found Sr-89 treatment to be cost-effective (41). The patients who received the Sr-89 had significantly lower subsequent costs for palliative medications, hormonal therapy, and subsequent radiation therapy. However, Oosterhof et al. (54) found that Sr-89 was associated with higher costs than external-beam radiotherapy.

Samarium-153

Samarium-153 is chelated with ethylenediaminetetramethylenephosphoric acid to form Sm-153 EDTMP, a compound that is preferentially taken up in newly formed bone. The unbound remainder of the drug is rapidly cleared via urinary excretion. Phase I/II studies have shown that doses above 2.5 mCi/kg are associated with neutropenia. In a dose-escalation study, Collins et al. (12) evaluated doses from 0.5 to 3.0 mCi/kg. There was no significant difference in clinical response between 1.0 and 2.5 mCi. There have been at least five randomized prospective evaluations of Sm-153 for metastatic cancers (primarily for prostate cancers) (53,61,69,75,85). Two of these studies used a placebo arm in comparison to 1.0 mCi/kg (69) or 0.5 and 1.0 mCi/kg (75). In both of these studies, the 1.0 mCi/kg dose gave significant improvement in pain relief compared to placebo. The average opioid dose decreased for the patients receiving Sm-153, compared to an increase in the patients receiving placebo. Transient marrow suppression was seen, with a nadir at 4 to 6 weeks and recovery by 8 weeks; this was primarily manifest as grade ≥ 3 neutropenia (14% compared with 0% for placebo).

The other phase III study evaluated three dose levels of Sm-153 (0.5, 1.0, and 1.5 mCi/kg). Olea et al. (53) reported no difference in response rates among the different dose levels, with an overall pain relief response rate of 73%. Two randomized phase II studies compared doses of 0.5 mCi/kg with 1.0 mCi/kg, with no placebo arm (61,85). In these two studies, there was no significant difference between the two dose levels for response or toxicity. There was no difference in response by primary site, although the numbers of patients were small for each primary site. The study by Tian et al. (85) is the only one in which metastatic prostate cancer did not comprise the majority of patients included.

Patient Selection

Radiopharmaceuticals, specifically Sr-89 and Sm-153, are effective in providing pain relief for patients with diffuse osseous metastases. This is primarily true for metastases that have an osteoblastic component. In general, if a Tc-99 m nuclear medicine bone scan shows localized areas of increased uptake, then radiopharmaceutical treatment is likely to be of benefit. An advantage of radioisotope treatment is that it can be combined with other modalities, such as external-beam radiation therapy or chemotherapy. Because the targets of treatment are similar, treatment with bisphosphonates should not be given simultaneously with radioisotopes as this may reduce the efficacy of both medications. Relative contraindications to therapy would be impaired renal or hepatic function, or inadequate hematologic reserve.

Radiopharmaceuticals: Summary

The primary advantages of Sm-153 compared with Sr-89 are reduced radiation safety issues (because of the much shorter half-life) and the ability to image the distribution of the Sm-153. Although there has not been a randomized comparison of Sr-89 and Sm-153, there does not appear to be a significant difference in the incidence, severity, onset, or duration of hematologic toxicity, despite the short half-life of the Sm-153. Both radiopharmaceuticals appear equally effective at palliating pain from bone metastasis. These radiopharmaceuticals add to the growing armamentarium of therapies designed to palliate pain and improve the quality of life of patients with bone metastasis from cancer.

Conclusion

Palliative radiation therapy is of significant benefit to patients with painful bone metastasis, with most patients experiencing relief in the magnitude of pain following treatment. Response rates to palliative radiation therapy for localized sites of pain are consistently higher than response rates from palliative systemic therapy, and palliative external-beam radiation therapy remains the mainstay of treatment for clinically localized painful bone metastasis. Providing shorter, single fraction palliative treatment schedules (i.e., 800 cGy × one fraction) for properly selected patients with bone metastasis can help better integrate palliative radiation therapy into the multidisciplinary management of patients with metastatic cancer and offer equivalent palliation compared with longer courses of palliative radiation therapy. Systemic targeted therapies including Sm-153 and Sr-89 offer yet another means to target painful sites of blastic bone metastasis without limiting our ability to use localized external-beam radiation therapy and systemic chemotherapy.

References

1. Asdourian PL, Weidenbaum M, DeWald RL, et al. The pattern of vertebral involvement in metastatic vertebral breast cancer. *Clin Orthop Relat Res* 1990;250:164–170.
2. Bauman G, Charette M, Reid R, et al. Radiopharmaceuticals for the palliation of painful bone metastasis—a systemic review. *Radiother Oncol* 2005;75:258–270.
3. Beals RK, Lawton GD, Snell WE. Prophylactic internal fixation of the femur in metastatic breast cancer. *Cancer* 1971;28:1350–1354.
4. Blitzer P: Reanalysis of the RTOG study of the palliation of symptomatic osseous metastasis. *Cancer* 1985;55:1468–1472.
5. Bone Pain Trial Working Party. 8 Gy single fraction radiotherapy for the treatment of metastatic skeletal pain: randomised comparison with a multifraction schedule over 12 months of patient follow-up. *Radiother Oncol* 1999;52:111–121.
6. Cheal EJ, Hipp JA, Hayes WC. Evaluation of finite element analysis for prediction of the strength reduction due to metastatic lesions in the femoral neck. *J Biomech* 1993;26:251–264.
7. Chow E, Holden L, Danjoux C, at al. Successful salvage using percutaneous vertebroplasty in cancer patients with painful spinal metastases or osteoporotic compression fractures. *Radiother Oncol* 2004;70:265–267.
8. Cleeland CS. The measurement of pain from metastatic bone disease: capturing the patient's experience. *Clin Cancer Res* 2006;12:6236s–6242s.
9. Cleeland CS, Gonin R, Hatfield AK, et al. Pain and its treatment in outpatients with metastatic cancer. *N Engl J Med* 1994;330:592–596.
10. Coleman RE. Skeletal complications of malignancy. *Cancer* 1997;80[Suppl 8]:1588–1594.
11. Coleman RE, Rubens RD: The clinical course of bone metastases from breast cancer. *Br J Cancer* 1987;55:61–66.
12. Collins C, Eary JF, Donaldson G, et al. Samarium-153-EDTMP in bone metastases of hormone refractory prostate carcinoma: a phase I/II trial. *J Nucl Med* 1993;34:1839–1844.
13. Daldrup-Link HE, Franzius C, Link TM. Whole-body MR imaging for detection of bone metastases in children and young adults: comparison with skeletal scintigraphy and FDG PET. *Am J Roentgenol* 2001;177:229–236.
14. Evan-Sapr E, Mester U, Mishani E, et al. The detection of bone metastases in patients with high-risk prostate cancer: 99mTc-MDP Planar bone scintigraphy, single- and multi-field-of-view SPECT, 18F-fluoride PET, and 18F-fluoride PET/CT. *J Nucl Med* 2006;47:287–297.
15. Fidler M: Incidence of fracture through metastases in long bones. *Acta Orthop Scand* 1981;52:623–627.
16. Flickinger FW, Sanal SM. Bone marrow MRI: techniques and accuracy for detecting breast cancer metastases. *Magn Reson Imaging* 1994;12:829–835.
17. Fujimoto R, Higashi T, Nakamoto Y, et al. Diagnostic accuracy of bone metastases detection in cancer patients: comparison between bone scintigraphy and whole-body FDG-PET. *Ann Nucl Med* 2006.20:399–408.
18. Gaze MN, Kelly CG, Kerr GR, et al. Pain relief and quality of life following radiotherapy for bone metastases: a randomized trial of two fractionation schedules. *Radiother Oncol* 1997;45:109–116.
19. Goblirsch MJ, Zwolak PP, Clohisy DR. Biology of bone cancer pain. *Clin Cancer Res* 2006;12:6231s–6235s.
20. Green JR. Bisphosphonates: preclinical review. *Oncologist* 2004;9[Suppl]:3–13.
21. Gurney H, Larcos G, McKay M, et al. Bone metastases in hypernephroma. Frequency of scapular involvement. *Cancer* 1989;64:1429–1431.
22. Hamaoka T, Madewell JE, Podoloff DA, et al. Bone imaging in metastatic breast cancer. *J Clin Oncol* 2004;22:2942–2953.
23. Harrington KD: Orthopaedic management of extremity and pelvic lesions. *Clin Orthop Rel Res* 1995;312:136–147.
24. Hartsell WF, Scott CB, Bruner DW, et al. Randomized trial of short-versus long-course radiotherapy for palliation of painful bone metastases. *J Natl Cancer Inst* 2005;97:798–804.
25. Hentschel SJ, Burton AW, Fourney DR, et al. Percutaneous vertebroplasty and kyphoplasty performed at a cancer center: refuting proposed contraindications. *J Neurosurg Spine* 2005;2:436–440.
26. Hirokawa Y, Wadasaki K, Kashiwado K, et al. A multiinstitutional prospective randomized study of radiation therapy of bone metastases [in Japanese]. *Nippon Igaku Hoshasen Gakkai Zasshi* 1988;48:1425–1431.
27. Hitchins RN, Philip PA, Wignall B, et al. Bone disease in testicular and extragonadal germ cell tumours. *Br J Cancer* 1988;58:793–796.
28. Hortobagyi GN, Theriault RL, Porter L: Efficacy of pamidronate in reducing skeletal complications in patients with breast cancer and lytic bone metastases. Protocol 19 Aredia Breast Cancer Study Group. *N Engl J Med* 1996;335:1785–1791.
29. Hoskin PJ, Price P, Easton D, et al. A prospective randomized trial of 4 Gy or 8 Gy single doses in the treatment of metastatic bone pain. *Radiother Oncol* 1992;23:74–78.
30. Hoskin PJ, Stratford MRL, Folkes LK, et al. Effect of local radiotherapy for bone pain on urinary markers of osteoclast activity. *Lancet* 2000;355:1428–1429.
31. Houston SJ, Rubens RD. The systemic treatment of bone metastases. *Clin Orthop Rel Res* 1995;312:95–104.
32. Jeremic B, Shibamoto Y, Acimovic L, et al. A randomized trial of three single-dose radiation therapy regimens in the treatment of metastatic bone pain. *Int J Radiat Oncol Biol Phys* 1998;42:161–167.
33. Kaasa S, Brenne E, Lund JA, et al. Prospective randomized multicenter trial on single fraction radiotherapy (8 Gy × 1) versus multiple fractions (3 Gy × 10) in the treatment of painful bone metastases. *Radiother Oncol* 2006;79:278–284.
34. Kirkbride P, Warde RR, Panzarella T, et al. A randomized trial comparing the efficacy of a single radiation fraction with fractionated radiation therapy in the palliation of skeletal metastases. *Int J Radiat Oncol Biol Phys* 2000;48[Suppl 1]:185(abstr).
35. Konski A, DeSilvio M, Hartsell W, et al. Continuing evidence for poorer treatment outcomes for single male patients: retreatment data from RTOG 97 14. *Int J Radiat Oncol Biol Phys* 2006;66:229–233.
36. Koswig S, Budach V: Remineralization and pain relief in bone metastases after different radiotherapy fractions (10 time 3 Gy vs 1 time 8 Gy). A prospective study. *Strahlenther Onkol* 1999;175:500–508.
37. Loblaw DA, Wu JS, Kirkbride P, et al. Pain flare in patients with bone metastases after palliative radiotherapy—a nested randomized control trial. *Support Care Cancer* 2007;15:451–455
38. Madsen EL. Painful bone metastasis: Efficacy of radiotherapy assessed by the patients—a randomized trial comparing 4 Gy × 6 versus 10 Gy × 2. *Int J Radiat Oncol Biol Phys* 1983;9:1775–1779
39. Manolagas SC, Jilka RL. Bone marrow, cytokines and bone remodeling. Emerging insights into the pathophysiology of osteoporosis. *N Engl J Med* 1995;332:305–311.
40. Matsuyama T, Tsukamoto N, Imachi M, et al. Bone metastasis from cervix cancer. *Gynecol Oncol* 1989;32:72–75.
41. McEwan AJ, Amyotte GA, McGowan DG, et al. A retrospective analysis of the cost effectiveness of treatment with Metastron (89Sr-chloride) in patients with prostate cancer metastatic to bone. *Nucl Med Commun* 1994;15:499–504.
42. Medical Research Council Prostate Cancer Working Party Investigators Group: Immediate versus deferred treatment for advanced prostatic cancer: initial results of the MRC trial. *Br J Urol* 1997;79:235–246.

43. Mehrotra B, Ruggiero S. Bisphosphonate complications including osteonecrosis of the jaw. *Hematology* 2006;1:356–360.

44. Meuser T, Pietruck C, Radbruch L, et al. Symptoms during cancer pain treatment following WHO-guidelines: a longitudinal follow-up study of symptom prevalence, severity and etiology. *Pain* 2001;93:247–257.

45. Michaelson MD, Smith MR. Bisphosphonates for treatment and prevention of bone metastases. *J Clin Oncol* 2005;23:8219–8224.

46. Migliorati CA, Siegel MA, Elting LS. Bisphosphonate-associated osteonecrosis: a long-term complication of bisphosphonate treatment. *Lancet Oncol* 2006;7:508–514.

47. Mirels H. Metastatic disease in long bones: a proposed scoring system for diagnosing impending pathologic fractures. *Clin Orthop Relat Res* 1989;249:256–264.

48. Nathan SS, Healey JH, Mellano D, et al. Survival in patients operated on for pathologic fractures: implication for end-of-life orthopedic care. *J Clin Oncol* 2005;23:6072–6082.

49. Nielsen OS, Bentzen SM, Sandberg E, et al. Randomized trial of single dose versus fractionated palliative radiotherapy of bone metastases. *Radiother Oncol* 1998;47:233–240.

50. Nielsen OS, Munro AJ, Tannock IF. Bone metastases: Pathophysiology and Management Policy. *J Clin Oncol* 1991;9:509–524

51. Niewald M, Tkocz HJ, Abel U, et al. Rapid course radiation therapy vs. more standard treatment: a randomized trial for bone metastases. *Int J Radiat Oncol Biol Phys* 1996;36:1085–1089.

52. Ohta M, Tokuda Y, Suzuki Y, et al. Whole body PET for the evaluation of bony metastases in patients with breast cancer: comparison with 99Tcm-MDP bone scintigraphy. *Nucl Med Commun* 2001;22:875–879.

53. Olea E, Riccabona G, Tian J, et al. Efficacy and toxicity of 153Sm EDTMP in the palliative treatment of painful skeleton metastases: results of an IAEA international multicenter study. *J Nucl Med* 2000;51:146P(abstr).

54. Oosterhof GON, Roberts JT, De Reijke T, et al. Strontium89 chloride versus palliative local field radiotherapy in patients with hormonal escaped prostate cancer: a phase III study of the European organisation for research and treatment of cancer genitourinary group. *Eur Urol* 2003;44:519–526.

55. Porter AT, McEwan AJ. Strontium-89 as an adjuvant to external beam radiation improves pain relief and delays disease progression in advanced prostate cancer: results of a randomized controlled trial. *Semin Oncol* 1993;20:38–43.

56. Poulter C, Cosmatos D, Rubin P, et al. A report of RTOG 82-06: A phase III study of whether the addition of single dose hemibody irradiation is more effective than local field irradiation alone in the treatment of symptomatic osseous metastases. *Int Radiat Oncol Biol Phys* 1992;23:207–214.

57. Quilty PM, Kirk D, Bolger JJ, et al. A comparison of the palliative effects of strontium-89 and external beam radiotherapy in metastatic prostate cancer. *Radiother Oncol* 1994;31:33–40.

58. Rasmusson B, Vejborg I, Jensen AB, et al. Irradiation of bone metastases in breast cancer patients: A randomized study with 1 year follow-up. *Radiother Oncol* 1995;34:179–184.

59. Ratanatharathorn V, Powers WE, Moss WT, et al. Bone metastasis: Review and critical analysis of random allocation trials of local field treatment. *Int J Radiat Oncol Biol Phys* 1999;44:1–18.

60. Ratanatharathorn V, Powers WE, Temple HT. In: Perez CA, Brady LW, Halperin EC, et al., eds. *Principles and practice of radiation oncology*, 4th ed. Philadelphia: JB Lippincott; 2003: 2385–2404

61. Resche I, Chatal JF, Pecking A, et al. A dose-controlled study of 153Sm-ethylenediaminetetramethylenephosphonate (EDTMP) in the treatment of patients with painful bone metastases. *Eur J Cancer* 1997;33:1583–1591.

62. Roodman GD. Mechanisms of bone metastases. *N Engl J Med* 2004;350:1655–1664.

63. Roodman GD. Biology of osteoclast activation in cancer. *J Clin Oncol* 2001;19:3562–3571.

64. Rosen LS, Gordon L, Tchekmedyian NS, et al. Long-term efficacy and safety of zoledronic acid in the treatment of skeletal metastases in patients with nonsmall cell lung carcinoma and other solid tumors: a randomized, phase III, double-blind, placebo-controlled trial. *Cancer* 2004;100:2613–2621.

65. Russell RG, Rogers MJ, Frith JC, et al. The pharmacology of bisphosphonates and new insights into their mechanisms of action. *J Bone Miner Res* 1999;14[Suppl 2]:53–65.

66. Salazar OM, Rubin P, Hendrickson F, et al. Single dose half-body irradiation for palliation of multiple bone metastases from solid tumors: Final Radiation Therapy Oncology Group Report. *Cancer* 1986;58:29–36.

67. Salazar OM, Sandhu T, da Motta NW, et al. Fractionated half-body irradiation (HBI) for the rapid palliation of widespread, symptomatic, metastatic bone disease: a randomized Phase III trial of the International Atomic Energy Agency (IAEA). *Int J Radiat Oncol Biol Phys* 2001;50:765–775.

68. Sarin R, Budrukkar A. Efficacy, toxicity and cost-effectiveness of single-dose versus fractionated hemibody irradiation (HBI) [letter]. *Int J Radiat Oncol Biol Phys* 2002;52:1146.

69. Sartor O, Quick D, Reid R, et al. A double blind placebo controlled study of 153Samarium-EDTMP for palliation of bone pain in patients with hormone-refractory prostate cancer. *J Urol* 1997;157:321(abstr).

70. Scarantino C, Omitz, RD, Hoffman LG, et al. On the mechanism of radiation induced emesis: the role of serotonin. *Int J Radiat Oncol Biol Phys* 1994;30:825–830.

71. Scarantino CW, Caplan R, Rotman M, et al. A phase I/II study to evaluate the effect of fractionated hemibody irradiation in the treatment of osseous metastases—RTOG 88-22. *Int J Radiat Oncol Biol Phys* 1996;36:37–48.

72. Schmidt GP, Schoenberg SO, Reiser MF, et al. Whole-body MR imaging of bone marrow. *Eur J Radiol* 2005;55:33–40.

73. Sciuto R, Festa A, Rea S, et al. Effects of low-dose cisplatin on 89Sr therapy for painful bone metastases from prostate cancer: a randomized clinical trial. *J Nucl Med* 2002;43:79–86.

74. Senaratne SG, Pirianov G, Mansi JL, et al. Bisphosphonates induce apoptosis in human breast cancer cell lines. *Br J Cancer* 2000;82:1459–1468.

75. Serafini AN, Houston SJ, Resche I, et al. Palliation of pain associated with metastatic bone cancer using Samarium-153 Lexidronam: a double-blind placebo controlled clinical trial. *J Clin Oncol* 1998;16:1574–1581.

76. Shimony JS, Gilula LA, Zeller AJ, Brown DB. Percutaneous vertebroplasty for malignant compression fractures with epidural involvement. *Radiology* 2004;232:846–853.

77. Siegel HJ, Luck JV Jr, Siegel ME. Advances in radionuclide therapeutics in orthopaedics. *J Am Acad Orthop Surg* 2004;12:55–64.

78. Sim FH, Frassica FJ, Chao EYS: Orthopaedic management using new devices and prostheses. *Clin Orthop Rel Res* 1995;312:160–172.

79. Singh D, Yi WS, Brasacchio RA, et al. Is there a favorable subset of patients with prostate cancer who develop oligometeastases? *Int J Radiat Oncol Biol Phys* 2004;58:3–10.

80. Smeland S, Erikstein B, Aas M, et al. Role of Strontium-89 as adjuvant to palliative external beam radiotherapy is questionable: results of a double-blind randomized study. *Int J Radiat Oncol Biol Phys* 2003;56:1397–1404.

81. Steenland E, Leer JW, van Houwelingen H, et al. The effect of a single fraction compared to multiple fractions on painful bone metastases: a global analysis of the Dutch Bone Metastases Study. *Radiother Oncol* 1999;52:101–109.

82. Steinmetz MP, Mekhail A, Benzel EC. Management of metastatic tumors of the spine: strategies and operative indications. *Neurosurg Focus* 2001;11:e2.

83. Tannock IF, Osoba D, Stockler MR, et al. Chemotherapy with mitoxantrone plus prednisone or prednisone alone for symptomatic hormone-resistant prostate cancer: a Canadian randomized trial with palliative end points. *J Clin Oncol* 1996;14:1756–1764.

84. Theriault RL, Lipton A, Hortobagyi GN, et al. Pamidronate reduces skeletal morbidity in women with advanced breast cancer and lytic bone lesions: a randomized, placebo-controlled trial. Protocol 18 Aredia Breast Cancer Study Group. *J Clin Oncol* 1999;17:8464–8454.

85. Tian JH, Zhang JM, Hou QT, et al. Multicentre trial on the efficacy and toxicity of single-dose samarium-153-ethylene diamine tetramethylene phosphonate as a palliative treatment for painful skeletal metastases in China. *Eur J Nucl Med* 1999;26:2–7.

86. Tong D, Gillick L, Hendrickson FR. The palliation of symptomatic osseous metastases: final results of the study by the Radiation Therapy Oncology Group. *Cancer* 1982;50:893–899.

87. Tu S-M, Delpassand ES, Jones D, et al. Strontium-89 combined with doxorubicin in the treatment of patients with androgen independent prostate cancer. *Urol Oncol* 1996;2:191–197.

88. Van der Linden Y, Dijkstra PD, Kroon HM, et al. Comparative analysis of risk factors for pathological fracture with femoral metastases. *J Bone Joint Surg Br* 2004;86:566–573.

89. Vassiliou V, Kalogeropoulou G, Christopoulos C, et al. Combination ibandronate and radiotherapy for the treatment of bone metastases: Clinical evaluation and radiographic assessment. *Int J Radiat Oncol Biol Phys* 2007;67:264–272.

90. Wu JS, Wong R, Johnston M, et al. Meta-analysis of dose-fractionation radiotherapy trials for the palliation of painful bone metastases. *Int J Radiat Oncol Biol Phys* 2003;55:594–605.

91. Zech DF, Grond S, Lynch J, et al. Validation of World Health Organization guidelines for cancer pain relief: a 10-year prospective study. *Pain* 1995;63:65–76.

92. Zetter BR. The cellular basis of site-specific tumor metastasis. *N Engl J Med* 1990;322:605–612.

Palliative and Supportive Care

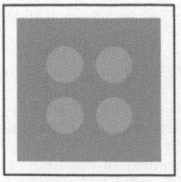

Chapter 93
Palliation of Visceral Recurrences and Metastases

Laurie E. Gaspar

In this era of complex treatment planning, high-dose reirradiation, or stereotactic body radiation, and so forth, it is often forgotten that a simple short course of radiation can lead to effective palliation of symptoms. This chapter reviews the literature regarding the palliative benefit of radiation therapy in the following situations:

- Liver metastases
- Biliary obstruction
- Adrenal metastases
- Splenic metastases
- Vaginal bleeding, discharge or pelvic pain due to gynecologic malignancies
- Recurrent rectal cancer

Liver Metastases

Liver metastases often cause pain, nausea, and vomiting and are a common cause of morbidity and mortality, particularly in colorectal cancer. Surgery, radiofrequency ablation, higher doses of radiation with respiratory gating, and other local modalities have been used when the goal of treatment is prolonged survival (2,9,10,11,13,16,19,28). Table 93.1 summarizes several prospective studies of radiation for the palliation of liver metastases from solid tumors (3,5,21,26). Eligibility criteria varied but there was usually an expected life survival of 3 months or more, although palliative benefit, when it occurred, was noted within several weeks of treatment (6,21). Radiation treatment was usually anterior-posterior fields to cover the whole liver, particularly in the planning era preceding computed tomography. Early studies used nuclear medicine liver scans for the detection, quantification, and radiation treatment planning of liver metastases. Excluding one third of the right kidney was required in the computed tomography era (26). Acute toxicity leading to discontinuation of treatment is uncommon, but approximately 20% of patients will experience some nausea. Some authors report premedicating with dexamethasone (6). Borgelt et al. (3) noted that patients most likely to achieve palliation were ambulatory, had a bilirubin level ≤1.5 mg/dL, and had more severe symptoms at the outset. Pain relief as a result of treatment was reasonably durable, with minimal-to-mild pain reported for 60% to 80% of remaining life. Leibel et al. (21) reported a randomized phase III study of whole-liver radiation with or without intravenous misonidazole and found no significant benefit in terms of survival or palliation. Although prolonging survival is not the primary goal with palliative treatment, one Radiation Therapy Oncology Group study found that survival of 6 months or more following hepatic radiation was significantly correlated with colorectal primary, good initial performance status, and lack of extrahepatic metastases (20). However, when these factors were built into the eligibility criteria of a subsequent dose-escalation study using twice-daily radiation, the median survival was only 4 to 4.5 months (26). Higher doses of radiation led to higher acute and delayed toxicity, with no significant improvement in survival.

There is no evidence that whole-liver radiation and concurrent chemotherapy is associated with a higher rate of palliation.

Mohiuddin et al. (24) reported a retrospective series of 45 patients with hepatic metastases from colorectal cancer treated with radiation and concurrent chemotherapy. The chemotherapy was usually 5-fluorouracil-based. The acute hematologic toxicity was moderate: 22% thrombocytopenia (platelets 50,000 or less), leading to discontinuation of treatment in two patients. Abdominal pain, jaundice, anorexia, and nausea/vomiting were improved in 67%, 33%, 39%, and 40% of affected patients, respectively.

Bydder et al. (5) conducted a prospective trial in 28 patients with liver metastases causing hepatic pain, abdominal distension, night sweats, and nausea and/or vomiting. Thirty-nine percent of the liver metastases were due to colorectal adenocarcinoma. Most of these patients had failed prior treatment such as chemotherapy or hormonal therapy. The median survival was just 10 weeks, consistent with the advanced stage of disease. For those patients alive at 6 weeks, pain, distension, night sweats, nausea, and vomiting were reported as improved in 63%, 30%, 63%, 44%, and 100%, respectively. The last 17 treated patients were asked whether they believed that the treatment had been helpful to them. Seventy-five percent reported a perceived overall benefit on at least one occasion of follow-up. The authors noted that although the short course of radiation therapy offered useful palliation to the majority of patients with little associated toxicity, few patients obtained a long-lasting or complete palliation of their hepatic symptoms.

Selective internal radiation therapy using radioactive yttrium-90 microspheres has been used in advanced nonresectable primary and metastatic liver cancer (14). This requires injecting radioactive yttrium spheres into the arterial blood supply of the liver. The hypothesis is that there is selective concentration of the radioactivity within the metastases as they are almost entirely supplied by the arterial system as opposed to the portal system. A randomized trial of radioactive spheres plus chemotherapy versus chemotherapy alone was conducted in patients with liver metastases from primary colon cancer (14). The combination therapy resulted in a higher rate of tumor response and progression-free survival but there was no significant difference in quality of life measures. Both treatments tended to provide an improvement in quality of life for approximately 18 months.

In summary, whole-liver radiation to doses of 20 to 30 Gy given once daily can provide rapid but temporary palliation of extensive liver metastases, particularly in patients experiencing abdominal pain. Figures 93.1 and 93.2 demonstrate possible techniques for external beam radiation.

Biliary Obstruction

Biliary obstruction due to primary tumors, pancreatic malignancies, or lymph nodes causing extrinsic compression can be the cause of considerable morbidity. Patients often complain of pruritus, jaundice, anorexia, and weight loss (1). Jaundice is most often the result of diffuse hepatic malignancy rather than focal extrahepatic lymphadenopathy or intraluminal obstruction. Intraluminal irradiation of the bile duct for extrahepatic

Table 93.1 | **PROSPECTIVE STUDIES OF RADIATION FOR THE PALLIATION OF LIVER METASTASES FROM SOLID TUMORS**

Study	No. of Patients	Radiation Therapy Dose (Gy)	Results
Borgelt et al., 1981 (3)	103; 38% colon 25% lung 8% solitary	Solitary: whole liver 30–30 in 15–19 qd Fx ± 20 boost Multiple: whole liver 20–30 in 7–15 qd Fx	3% Acute toxicity leading to discontinuation of RT Improvement at 4 wk in abdominal pain, 55%; nausea/vomiting, 49%; fever/night sweats, 45%; weakness/fatigue 19%
Russell et al., 1993 (26)	173	Whole liver: 27–33 in 18–22 Fx, 1.5 bid	11% Serious acute toxicity, 33% serious late toxicity at 33 Gy No survival advantage to higher doses. Median survival, 4.1–4.3 mo
Bydder et al., 2003 (5)	28; 39% colorectal 21% lung	Entire symptomatic portion: 10 in 2 Fx within 6–24 hr	Improvement at 6 wk in abdominal pain, 63%; distention, 30%; night sweats, 63%; nausea, 44%
Leibel et al., 1987 (21)	187; 60% colon 15% lung 23% single lobe	Whole liver: 21 in 7 Fx qd during 1.4 wk +/− misonidazole	No acute toxicity leading to discontinuation of RT Improvement at any time in abdominal pain, 80%; performance status, 28% No benefit to addition of misonidazole

qd, once daily; Fx, fractions; RT, radiation therapy; bid, twice daily.

obstruction has been used following relief of biliary obstruction, but there is no literature regarding its palliative benefit. Endoscopic stents, percutaneous transhepatic drainage procedures, and celiac plexus block constitute the preferred management in many patients (12).

In summary, the literature does not currently support the use of short-course, external-beam radiation for relief of biliary obstruction.

Adrenal Metastases

There is little published information regarding the role of radiation therapy in the palliation of symptomatic adrenal metastases. Anecdotal reports suggest that radiation therapy results in pain relief in most patients for long periods of time (27). Soffen et al. (29) reviewed the experience at two Philadelphia institutions with treating 16 patients treated between 1972 and 1988. Fifteen of the 16 patients had primary lung cancer. Pain in the back/flank or epigastric region was present in all patients.

Although a variety of techniques was used, the most common regimen was 30 Gy in 10 or 12 daily fractions using opposed anterior and posterior photon fields. The median field size was 10 × 12 cm. Thirteen of the 16 patients reported moderate or complete pain relief at 2 to 4 weeks following treatment. The most common acute treatment side effects were moderate nausea or transient diarrhea that was experienced by 44% and 19% of patients, respectively. No late toxicity data were reported in this group whose median survival was only 3 months.

Based on this small number of reports, there does appear to be some palliative benefit of a short course of radiation for adrenal metastases.

Splenic Metastases

Splenomegaly is associated with abdominal pain, anemia, and thrombocytopenia. Splenic radiation is occasionally done for patients with splenomegaly due to leukemias and myeloproliferative diseases resistant to standard chemotherapy or biologic

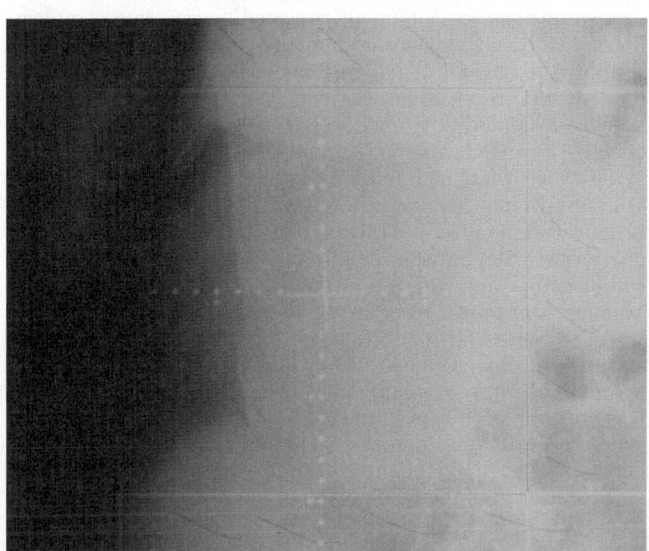

FIGURE 93.1. Anterior-posterior simulation film demonstrating simple field arrangement to cover massive hepatomegaly due to metastatic rectal cancer.

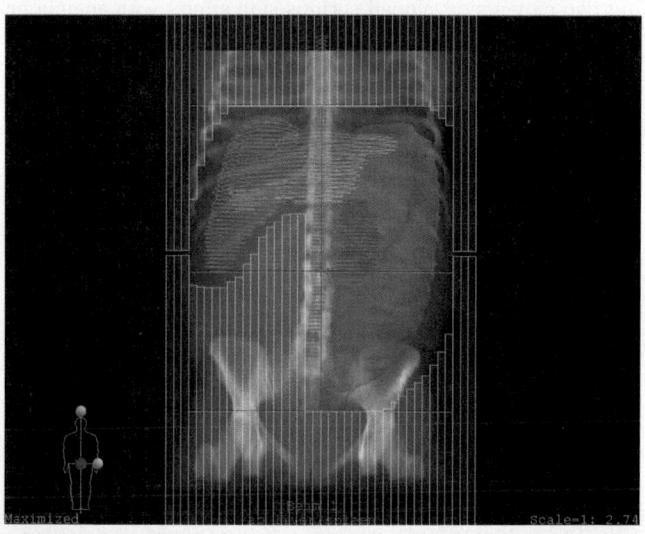

FIGURE 93.2. Digital-reconstructed rendering from computed tomography simulation. Target volumes demonstrate massive hepatomegaly and splenomegaly due to lymphomatous involvement. Multileaf collimators were used to shape the large anterior-posterior fields.

Table 93.2	RETROSPECTIVE SERIES OF PATIENTS TREATED WITH HYPOFRACTIONATED PELVIC RADIATION FOR ADVANCED GYNECOLOGIC CANCER			
Study	No. of Patients	Radiation Therapy Dose (Gy) per Fraction/No. of Fractions	Results	
Boulware et al., 1979 (4)	86	10/1–3 usually 4 wk apart	Reduction of bleeding: 10 Gy, 45%; 20 Gy, 85%; 30 Gy, 100% Pelvic pain: 10 Gy, 45%; 20 Gy, 59%; 30 Gy, 63% Serious complications:-none attributed to treatment	
Chafe et al., 1984 (7)	30	10/1–3 during 6 mo	Reduction of bleeding, 100% Serious complications, ~3%	
Halle et al., 1986 (15)	42	10/1–2 at monthly intervals	Total cessation of bleeding, 18/30 (60%); complete pain relief, 2/9 (22%); serious complications, 5/42 (12%)	
Onsrud et al., 2001 (25)	46	10/1–3 usually 4 wk apart	Reduction of bleeding, 79%; pain reduction, 0%; serious complications, ~5%[a]	

[a]Complications given for a larger group of patients.

therapy. The underlying biologic mechanisms to explain the response of splenomegaly to radiation is poorly understood (30). Possible underlying mechanisms include direction radiation-induced cell death, immune modulation, or cytokine induction (30). Splenic radiation for the palliation of painful splenomegaly due to chronic lymphocytic leukemia, prolymphocytic leukemia, is effective in >50% of patients (23,30). A common regimen would be 1 Gy given three times per week to a total dose of about 5 to 10 Gy, Splenomegaly due to hairy cell leukemia or chronic myeloproliferative syndromes such as polycythemia vera or essential thrombocytopenia, probably also respond to this regimen also. Radiation appears less effective in the treatment of splenomegaly-related anemia or thrombocytopenia (6,23).

McFarland et al. (23) reported the results of 16 patients treated between 1990 and 2001. Treatments were delivered using an anterior/posterior technique, biweekly with an increase in dose with each successive week. The first two treatments were 0.5 Gy, the second two were 0.75 Gy, and the third two were 1 Gy. A complete blood count was done prior to each treatment, and treatment was held if there were "worrisome values." Total treatment doses generally ranged from 3.5 to 6 Gy. Fourteen of the 16 patients had improvement in their symptoms. Twelve patients had a documented objective response in their splenomegaly. Retreatment was done in patients whose symptoms returned. Treatments were generally tolerated well, but two patients developed serious side effects with anemia or thrombocytopenia contributing to death. The authors therefore concluded that splenic radiation should be reserved for nonsurgical patients. Specific guidelines regarding when to hold radiation in the face of declining blood counts are not available.

In conclusion, there appears to be significant palliative benefit to a short course of low-dose radiation therapy for patients with splenic metastases related to leukemias and lymphomas. Patients must be observed very carefully for low blood counts, particularly thrombocytopenia, during palliative radiation.

Vaginal Bleeding, Discharge, or Pelvic Pain Related to Gynecologic Malignancies

Bleeding from a lesion on the vulva, vagina, or cervix is usually the result of venous ooze from the tumor. Pressure dressings or vaginal packing, often associated with hospitalization and bed rest coincident with beginning irradiation, are successful in most clinically emergent conditions. However, multiple retrospective experiences have shown that vaginal bleeding and mal-odorous discharge due to cervical or uterine cancer or ovarian cancer can be effectively palliated with 10 Gy whole-pelvis radiation given either once or repeated 1 month later (4,7,8,15,25). Several studies of hypofractionated radiation therapy are summarized in Table 93.2 (4,7,15,25). Reduction of bleeding occurs often within 24 to 48 hours of the first treatment. The selection criteria in these retrospective studies varied, with some studies differentiating between patients who were considered too ill or frail for aggressive treatment from other patients with symptomatic disease recurrence following definitive treatment. Patients were sometimes given antinausea medication prior to each treatment, although most series report low acute toxicity. The first or second radiation treatment was usually delivered to the whole pelvis using anterior and posterior fields. A field reduction was sometimes used for the third fraction.

In one relatively recent retrospective series, 46 patients with primary advanced or recurrent cervical or uterine cancer were treated with 10 Gy whole-pelvis radiation therapy. Another 10 Gy was given again 1 month later if there was no tumor progression and the patient's clinical condition was stable (25). Only two of these patients received a third fraction of 10 Gy 1 month later to a reduced field. Significant reduction or disappearance of bleeding was observed in 88% of patients; vaginal discharge improved in 36%. Unfortunately, six patients with pelvic pain did not report any reduction in pain following treatment. Acute side effects were tolerable, with mild-to-moderate nausea or diarrhea commonly reported. Severe late complications, including bowel perforation and rectal stenosis, occurred in approximately 5% of patients but only after 9 months in those patients who received at least two fractions of 10 Gy. The authors concluded that 10 Gy whole-pelvis radiation therapy is an effective means of palliating vaginal bleeding and discharge due to advanced or recurrent gynecologic cancer. However, because of excessive late toxicity, 20 to 30 Gy in two to three fractions is not recommended in patients in whom the life expectancy is greater than 9 months. Halle et al. (15) also noted a 12% serious complication rate, with most of these complications appearing 10 months or longer from radiation treatment.

A few series have suggested an association between radiation dose and probability of symptom improvement (4,25). Symptomatic improvement after only a single fraction of 10 Gy was uncommon. However, the decision to give a second or third fraction of radiation therapy was often based on observing a good objective or symptomatic response to the first fraction (7).

In summary, palliation of vaginal bleeding and discharge is frequently obtained using a palliative course of radiation. A simple treatment using anterior/posterior opposed fields can be used (Fig. 93.3). Unfortunately, improvement in pelvic pain is less likely to be palliated with radiation therapy.

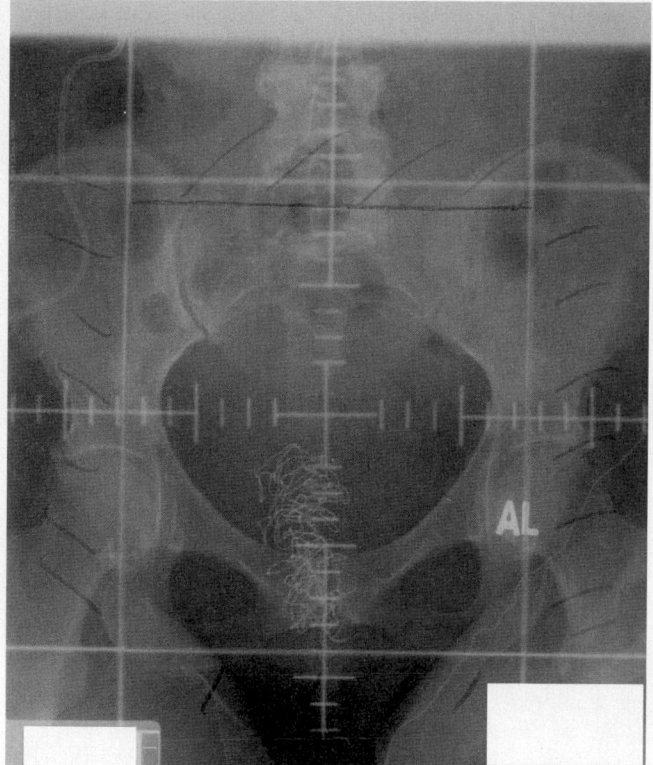

FIGURE 93.3. Simple simulation of anterior-posterior opposed pair to treat cervical cancer presenting with massive hemorrhage. Vaginal packing is in place. Lower border of field placed to cover extensive involvement of vagina.

patients, respectively. The incidence of late toxicity was significantly reduced in patients treated with the hyperfractionated regimen. Although toxicity was significant, there was complete or partial relief of symptoms reported in 100%, 98%, and 88% of patients with bleeding, pain, or mass effect, respectively. The median duration of palliation varied from 8 to 10 months and the median survival time was 12 months. Multivariate analysis revealed that increased median survival was associated with Karnofsky performance status of ≥70 and low initial low stage of cancer.

High-dose-rate intraluminal brachytherapy has also been described as a palliative treatment for advanced inoperable anal and rectal cancer (17). Cylindrical applicators that hold a single line source have been designed that have the option of treating all, or only part, of the rectal circumference. Hoskin et al. (17) described the results of treating 22 patients with advanced or metastatic rectal or anal cancer with a single dose of 10 Gy prescribed at 1 cm from the surface of the cylinder. Mucous drainage, bleeding, pain, and diarrhea responded (partially or completely) in 64%, 64%, 87%, and 100%, respectively, in the 65% of patients who were seen in follow-up. The median response duration was 4, 10, 7, and 7 months for mucous discharge, bleeding, pain, and diarrhea, respectively. There were no serious acute or late treatment-related toxicities reported. The authors believed that this was an effective method of palliating anal or rectal cancers that are within 10 cm of the anal verge. Prebrachytherapy insertion of radio-opaque clips made treatment planning easier and likely more accurate. Hoskin et al. recommended that the interval from clip placement to treatment be short because clip movement and migration were noted to occur after 2 to 3 weeks.

In summary, a hypofractionated course of radiation therapy frequently reduces vaginal bleeding and pelvic pain, and to a lesser extent, vaginal discharge.

Recurrent Rectal Cancer

Locally advanced or recurrent rectal cancer is a common cause of pelvic pain, rectal bleeding, and discharge. Wong et al. (31) reviewed the older literature (1956–1992) regarding radiation therapy for recurrent rectal cancer. These patients had not received prior radiation but the treatment intent was usually palliative. Chemotherapy was not generally part of the retreatment regimen. Total doses of radiation ranged from 8 to 70 Gy. Radiation resulted in symptom control for at least 6 months in up to 50% of patients. Although no strong recommendation was made regarding any particular dose/fractionation regimen, doses above 20 Gy were associated with increased local control and palliation. James et al. (18) analyzed the factors associated with an increased response to palliative radiation in 143 patients with locally recurrent rectal cancer. The only factor found to be associated with a statistically significant prolonged response was experiencing an initial good response. Other factors tending toward significance were an interval of at least 2 years from surgery and tumor volume of 100 mL or less.

Lingareddy et al. (22) reported the results of palliative reirradiation in 52 patients with recurrent rectal adenocarcinoma following previous pelvic radiation. The reirradiation dose was typically 30.0 to 30.6 Gy given in either single daily fractions of 1.8 to 2.0 Gy, or 1.2 Gy twice daily given at least 6 hours apart. Twenty patients received an additional boost dose of 6.0 to 20 Gy. The entire presacral region and gross disease with a 2–3-cm margin was treated. Ninety percent of patients received concurrent protracted venous infusion 5-fluorouracil. Acute toxicity such as diarrhea, mucositis, or perineal skin reaction required a treatment break in 31% of patients. Late toxicity such as bowel obstruction or fistula occurred in 17% and 8% of

References

1. Abraham NS, Barkun JS, Barkun AN. Palliation of malignant biliary obstruction: a prospective trial examining impact on quality of life. *Gastrointest Endosc* 2002;56:835–841.
2. Billingsley KG, Jarnagin WR, Fong Y, et al. Segment-oriented hepatic resection in the management of malignant neoplasms of the liver. *J Am Coll Surg* 1998;187:471–481.
3. Borgelt BB, Gelber R, Brady LW, et al. The palliation of hepatic metastases: results of the Radiation Therapy Oncology Group pilot study. *Int J Radiat Oncol Biol Phys* 1981;7:587–591.
4. Boulware RJ, Caderao JB, Delclos L, et al. Whole pelvis megavoltage irradiation with single doses of 1000 rad to palliate advanced gynecologic cancers. *Int J Radiat Oncol Biol Phys* 1979;5:333–338.
5. Bydder S, Spry NA, Christie DRH, et al. A prospective trial of short-fractionation radiotherapy for the palliation of liver metastases. *Aust Radiol* 2003;47:284–288.
6. Byhardt RW, Brace KC, Wiernik PH. The role of splenic irradiation in chronic lymphocytic leukemia. *Cancer* 1975;35:1621–1625.
7. Chafe W, Fowler WC, Currie JL, et al. Single-fraction palliative pelvic radiation therapy in gynecologic oncology: 1,000 rads. *Am J Obstet Gynecol* 1984;148:701–705.
8. Corn BW, Lanciano RM, Boente M, et al. Recurrent ovarian cancer. Effective radiotherapeutic palliation after chemotherapy failure. *Cancer* 1994;74:2979–2983.
9. Cummins ER, Vick KD, Poole GV. Incurable colorectal carcinoma: the role of surgical palliation. *Am Surg* 2004;70:433–437.
10. Dawson LA, Lawrence TS. The role of radiotherapy in the treatment of liver metastases. *Cancer J* 2004;10:139–144.
11. Fong Y, Cohen AM, Forter JG, et al. Liver resection for colorectal metastases. *J Clin Oncol* 1997;15:938–946.
12. Freeman ML, Sielaff TD. A modern approach to malignant hilar biliary obstruction. *Rev Gastroenterol Disord* 2003;3:187–201.
13. Gayowksi TJ, Iwatsuki S, Madariaga JR, et al. Experience in hepatic resection for metastatic colorectal cancer: analysis of clinical and pathological risk factors. *Surgery* 1994;116:703–711.
14. Gray B, Van Hazel G, Hope M, et al. Randomised trial of SIR-Spheres plus chemotherapy vs. chemotherapy alone for treating patients with liver metastases from primary large bowel cancer. *Ann Oncol* 2001;12:1711–1720.
15. Halle JS, Rosenman JG, Varia MA, et al. 1000 cGy single dose palliation for advanced carcinoma of the cervix or endometrium. *Int J Radiat Oncol Biol Phys* 1986;12:1947–1950.
16. Herfarth KK, Debus J, Wannenmacher M. Stereotactic radiation therapy of liver metastases: update of the initial phase-I/II trial. *Front Radiat Ther Oncol* 2004;38:100–105.
17. Hoskin PJ, de Canha SM, Bownes P, et al. High dose rate afterloading intraluminal brachytherapy for advanced inoperable rectal carcinoma. *Radiother Oncol* 2004;73:195–198.

18. James RD, Johnson RJ, Eddleston B, et al. Prognostic factors in locally recurrent rectal carcinoma treated by radiotherapy. *Br J Surg* 1983;70:469–472.

19. Khatri VP, McGahan J. Non-resection approaches for colorectal liver metastases. *Surg Clin North Am* 2004;84:587–606.

20. Leibel SA, Guse C, Order SE, et al. Accelerated fractionation radiation therapy for liver metastases: selection of an optimal patient population for the evaluation of late hepatic injury in RTOG studies. *Int J Radiat Oncol Biol Phys* 1990;18:523–528.

21. Leibel SA, Pajak TF, Massullo V, et al. A comparison of misonidazole sensitized radiation therapy to radiation therapy alone for the palliation of hepatic metastases: results of a Radiation Therapy Oncology Group randomized prospective trial. *Int J Radiat Oncol Biol Phys* 1987;13:1057–1064.

22. Lingareddy V, Ahmad NR, Mohiuddin M. Palliative reirradiation for recurrent rectal cancer. *Int J Radiat Oncol Biol Phys* 1997;38:785–790.

23. McFarland JT, Kuzma C, Millard FE, et al. Palliative irradiation of the spleen. *Am J Clin Oncol* 2003;26:178–183.

24. Mohiuddin M, Chen E, Ahmad N. Combined liver radiation and chemotherapy for palliation of hepatic metastases from colorectal cancer. *J Clin Oncol* 1996;14:722–728.

25. Onsrud M, Hagen B, Strickert T. 10-Gy single-fraction pelvic irradiation for palliation and life prolongation in patients with cancer of the cervix and corpus uteri. *Gynecol Oncol* 2001;82:167–171.

26. Russell AH, Clyde C, Wasserman TH, et al. Accelerated hyperfractionated hepatic irradiation in the management of patients with liver metastases: results of the RTOG dose escalating protocol. *Int J Radiat Oncol Biol Phys* 1993;27:117–123.

27. Short S, Chaturvedi A, Leslie MD. Palliation of symptomatic adrenal gland metastases by radiotherapy. *Clin Oncol* 1996;8:387–389.

28. Singletary AE, Walsh G, Vauthey JN, et al. A role for curative surgery in the treatment of selected patients with metastatic breast cancer. *Oncologist* 2003;8:241–251.

29. Soffen EM, Solin LJ, Rubenstein JH, et al. Palliative radiotherapy for symptomatic adrenal metastases. *Cancer* 1990;65:1318–1320.

30. Weinmann M, Becker G, Einsele H, et al. Clinical indications and biological mechanisms of splenic irradiation in chronic leukaemias and myeloproliferative disorders. *Radiother Oncol* 2001;58:235–246.

31. Wong R, Thomas G, Cummings B, et al. The role of radiotherapy in the management of pelvic recurrence of rectal cancer. *Can J Oncol* 1996;6:39–47.

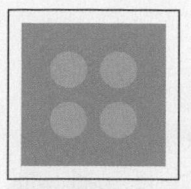

Chapter 94
Pain Management

Gary Deng, Amitabh Gulati, Barrie R. Cassileth

Pain can significantly decrease the patient's quality of life during and after radiotherapy. Yet, as in many other disciplines, appropriate and adequate management of pain syndromes remains imperfect. More than half of the patients undergoing treatment at a radiotherapy department may experience pain (43), and the majority of patients and physicians feel that patients' pain is inadequately treated (10).

Pain in radiotherapy may result from tissue damage by the tumor, such as bone destruction by a metastasis from prostate cancer or invasion of the celiac plexus by pancreatic cancer, or from radiotherapy per se. Irradiation of normal tissues, especially those with a rapid growth turnover rate, causes cell death and triggers a cascade of proinflammatory cytokines, thrombotic factors, and growth factors, propagating local painful reactions (8,18). Radiation oncologists must be knowledgeable about pain management during and after radiotherapy. In this chapter we discuss the pathophysiology of pain, treatment options, and practice guidelines for developing a stepwise, integrated treatment plan.

Radiotherapy is also a valuable modality in the treatment of cancer pain. It is commonly used in the palliative setting when a radiosensitive cancer invades bone, soft tissue, or nerves (15). Radiotherapy for palliation of pain caused by various types of cancer is covered in their respective chapters elsewhere in this book.

Types of Pain

Pain generally can be defined as either nociceptive or nonnociceptive. Nociceptive pain refers to the nervous system response that is proportionate to the tissue damage initiating the response. Nociceptive pain is divided into somatic pain and visceral pain, depending on the location and symptoms of the painful stimulus. Typically, somatic pain presents as a well-localized sharp, stabbing (knifelike), and achy pain as a response to skin, muscle, and connective tissue damage. On the other hand, patients have difficulty localizing visceral pain and often complain of cramping or a dull ache (5).

Non-nociceptive pain encompasses both neuropathic and psychogenic (or idiopathic) pain syndromes. In these cases, nervous system responses are atypical to the damage causing the response. In fact, responses may occur without tissue damage. Neuropathic pain involves abnormal pain processing by the peripheral or central nervous system. Patients may complain of burning, shooting, tingling, or numbness, which generally occurs along a nerve distribution (24). Patients may also experience pain that is out of proportion to their physical injury. Psychogenic causes (i.e., depression and anxiety) may exacerbate the perception of painful stimuli.

Understanding a patient's symptoms allows the physician to understand the pathophysiology of the pain syndrome. Each type of pain syndrome is amenable to treatment with different modalities. For example, somatic pain, localized sharp pain, may be better treated with opioid medications, whereas, anticonvulsants or antidepressants may be used to treat neuropathic pain.

Medical Management

Many national and international organizations have developed guidelines for pain management. Although there may be disagreement in the details, the principles and approaches are consistent across guidelines. The World Health Organization (WHO), American Pain Society (APS), and National Comprehensive Cancer Network (NCCN) guidelines are discussed here.

WHO Pain Ladder

The WHO guidelines for analgesic management of cancer pain, first described in the early 1980s (25,58), include a three-step approach that has been validated in recent trials (65). Despite some debate on its effectiveness (3), it provides for a widely practiced, stepwise approach in treating various levels of pain severity.

The first tier involves the use of nonopiate medications, primarily nonsteroidal anti-inflammatory drugs (NSAIDs) (Table 94.1). These medications include acetaminophen, nonspecific cyclooxygenase inhibitors (including ibuprofen, diclofenac, aspirin), and cyclooxygenase-2 inhibitors (celecoxib and meloxicam) (6). NSAIDS are considered the first group of medications to administer. If the patient's pain persists or worsens, a weak opiate can be initiated in addition to the nonopiate. Finally, continued treatment for worsening pain will involve the addition of a strong opiate to replace the weak opiate (Fig. 94.1).

Physicians using the WHO guidelines face difficulties deciding which medication (especially opiates) to begin and at which dosages to use when changing medications (Table 94.2). Often a patient may not respond to a weak opiate but may respond to a strong opiate. Once pain control becomes inadequate, the physician can use a higher tier for pain management (62). In light of advances in pharmacogenomics, it is increasingly clear that genetics plays a role in an individual patient's sensitivity to an analgesic (42,55). If a patient does not respond or develops tolerance to a particular agent, the current medical regimen should be increased to maximum tolerated dosing or the patient switched to a different agent.

APS and NCCN Guidelines

As the understanding of pain physiology and treatments expands, so do management strategies. Although the WHO guidelines are a good initial step in pain management, other organizations have modified and expanded these initial strategies to improve treatment for cancer pain. These references (and others) are good sources of information for the radiation oncologist to develop pain management skills. These guides provide initial medication dosages, the addition of adjuvant medications, and information on appropriate dose increases.

The 2005 APS *Guideline for the Management of Cancer Pain in Adults and Children* contains detailed discussions of cancer pain management algorithms, pharmacologic strategies, coanalgesics, psychological strategies, supportive therapy,

Table 94.1	GUIDE TO COMMON NONOPIATE MEDICATIONS AND STARTING DOSES FOR ADULTS	
Medication	**Starting Dose (Maximum Daily Dose in mg)**	
Acetaminophen	500, 3–4 × day (4,000)	
Nonsteroidal anti-inflammatory drugs		
Aspirin	325, 3–4 × day (4,000)	
Ibuprofen	200, 3 × day (2,400)	
Naproxen	250, 2 × day (1,250)	
Ketorolac	IV 15–30 up to 4 doses	
Diclofenac	50, 3 × day (150 mg)	
Specific COX-2 inhibitors		
Celecoxib	100, 2 × day (400–800)	
Meloxicam	7.5 every day (15)	

IV, intravenous; COX-2, cyclooxygenase 2.

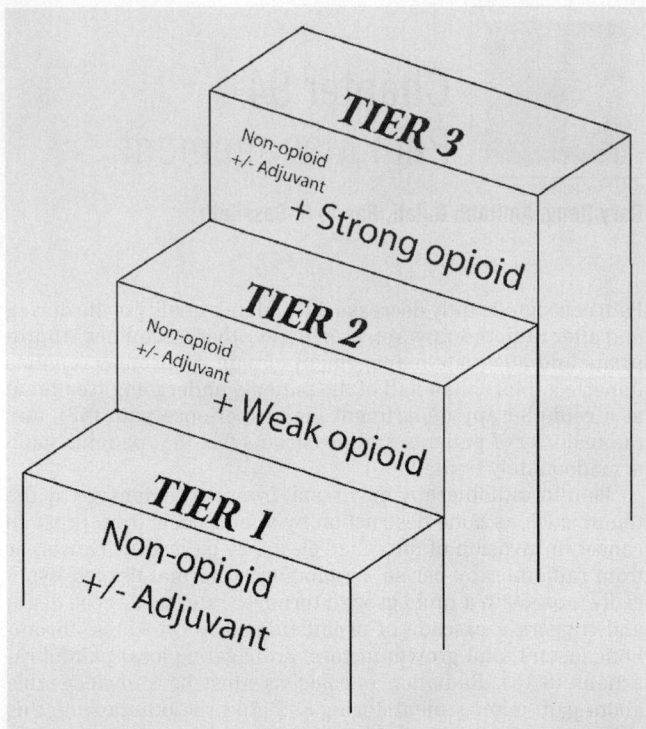

FIGURE 94.1. World Health Organization (WHO) guidelines for initial medical treatment for cancer pain. A three-tiered system broadly indicating the use of opiate medications for continued pain control is shown. As pain symptoms worsen, a physician may enter a higher tier of medications for pain control. (Adapted from World Health Organization. *WHO guidelines cancer pain relief*, 2nd ed. Geneva: World Health Organization; 1996, with permission.)

integration of nonpharmacologic and pharmacologic treatments, physical strategies, nerve blocks, surgical strategies, radiation therapy, chemotherapy, and pain management in special populations (39). It also discusses patient education and adherence to the pain management plan, as well as how to improve quality of care in pain management (18)

The NCCN guidelines recommend universal screening of pain in cancer patients, followed by a comprehensive assessment of the characteristics, underlying pathophysiology and etiology, psychosocial issues, and risk factors for undertreatment of pain. Patients' goals and expectations should be sought for any patient whose pain score is not zero. Patients are then stratified based on the urgency and severity of the pain and treated with escalating aggressiveness. Repeat reassessments are done frequently to adjust treatment plans until patient's goals and expectations in comfort and function are met. It is preferable to convert short-acting opioids to long-acting ones when the doses required to achieve adequate pain control is stabilized. Rescue dosing with short-acting agents should be provided for breakthrough pain during maintenance therapy.

Opiate Side Effects

Patients taking opioids should also be provided with a bowel regimen. Side effects may limit the maximal tolerable dose of opioid analgesics. Treating a patient's pain is a balance of maximizing analgesic effects and minimizing side effects (7). Common opioid side effects include gastrointestinal (constipation, nausea, and emesis), respiratory (decreased respiratory rate),

Table 94.2	GUIDE TO COMMON WEAK AND STRONG OPIOID MEDICATIONS AND POTENTIAL STARTING DOSES[a]		
Opioid	**PO Starting Dose (mg)**	**PO Conversion (mg)**	**IV Conversion (mg)**
Tramadol	50, 2–3 × day	—	—
Weak			
Codeine	30, 4–6 × day	—	—
Hydrocodone	5, 4–6 × day	—	—
Propoxyphene	65, 4–6 × day	—	—
Strong			
Morphine	15, 4–6 × day	30	10
Hydromorphone	2–4, 4–6 × day	8	2
Methadone	2.5–5, 2–3 × day	2	1
Fentanyl	Transdermal 25 μg/d	NA	0.2
Oxycodone	5–15, 4–6 × day	20	NA

PO, by mouth; IV, intravenous; NA, not applicable.
[a]Opiate medication must be titrated for adequate pain relief and minimal side effects. For the strong opiates, equivalent doses for conversion are given, with methadone IV as the base dose of 1 mg (31,41,54). The conversion factors can be used to change PO or IV doses among the different opiates (i.e., 2 mg of PO methadone is roughly equivalent to 30 mg of PO morphine). Similarly, 2 mg of PO methadone is equivalent to 1 mg of IV methadone. When changing from one opiate to another, a reduction factor is sometimes applied (usually 25% to 75% of the original medication's dose) because of less tolerance to the new medication. For example, if a patient is using 60 mg of PO morphine every 4 hours, an equivalent oxycodone dose may be 40 mg × a 50% reduction, leading to 20 mg every 4 hours.

dermatologic (pruritis and dry mouth), and central nervous system (sedation, hallucinations, and seizures) effects. Many strategies are implemented in balancing analgesic effects and side effects (9,34). Although no consensus exists, physicians can manage side effects by some of the following strategies:

a. Pharmacologic treatment of the side effects (laxative for constipation or psychostimulant for sedation),
b. Reducing opiate dose,
c. Addition of adjuvant for pain management (see following discussion), and opioid rotation.

Opioid rotation refers to drug-switching within a group, for example, changing hydrocodone to codeine because of nausea (45). Medications should be changed every 2 to 3 months so that the patient does not become tolerant to agent.

Adjuvant Therapy

Using the WHO ladder, most pain related to cancer can be managed with oral medications in 70% to 85% of patients (59,65). At any point of the WHO analgesic ladder, adjuvant therapy can be initiated to supplement NSAIDs and opioid treatment. Benefits of adjuvant therapy include use of medications tailored toward specific causes of nociceptive responses (i.e., neuropathic) and reduction of opiate side effects.

Neuropathic pain is generally not responsive to opiate medications, unless significantly high doses are used, so other classes of drugs are often prescribed (40). Anticonvulsants, such as gabapentin, carbamazepine, and pregabalin, have been shown to be effective in managing neuropathic symptoms (24). Both gabapentin and pregabalin are renally excreted and have minimal drug-drug interactions, making these medications effective first-line treatment for neuropathic pain (24).

Like anticonvulsants, antidepressants are another broad category of medications that stabilize neurons involved in neuropathic pain. Tricyclic antidepressants in low doses, such as amitriptyline, have been well studied for pain relief (20). Less well studied, but still prescribed for neuropathic pain, are serotonin reuptake inhibitors and newer classes of antidepressants, including selective serotonin and norepinephrine reuptake inhibitors (duloxetine and venlafaxine). Because many patients with neuropathic pain may have depressive or anxiety symptoms, antidepressants may have a dual role in treatment, resulting in improved efficacy (20).

When faced with a patient with neuropathic pain, the radiation oncologist may prescribe an anticonvulsant, such as gabapentin, at low doses and titrate the medication to improve analgesia while monitoring side effects. Some physicians may choose to initiate antidepressant treatment, especially if patients also exhibit signs of depression or anxiety, and then add the anticonvulsant as a secondary medication. In any case, both medications can be used synergistically to improve analgesia for neuropathic pain.

The NMDA (*N*-methyl-D-aspartate) receptor has received much attention for its role in modulating pain signals throughout the nervous system. Methadone is a long-acting opiate receptor antagonist, which may act as a NMDA receptor antagonist, preventing morphine tolerance and NMDA hyperalgesia effects (23). Pain-management specialists have also used ketamine, a specific NMDA receptor antagonist, to relieve cancer and neuropathic pain, especially refractory pain (30).

Other adjuvant analgesic drug classes used in cancer therapy include local anesthetics, steroids, muscle relaxants, benzodiazepines, α-adrenergic agonists, and bisphosphonates (30). Many of these medications are used in specific pain syndromes, which may be useful for the radiation oncologist (Table 94.3).

Nonoral Routes of Administration

Chemotherapy, surgery, and radiotherapy often produce significant side effects. Pain medications given by mouth may not be the most appropriate mode of delivery. When changing from oral to another mode of medication delivery, care must be taken to give equipotent analgesic doses. Conversion charts for opiates are readily available in the literature (9).

Some pain medications come in formulations that can be delivered rectally, intramuscularly, intravenously, and topically. NSAIDS and opiates are commercially available in suppository

Table 94.3	COMMON ADJUVANT MEDICATIONS WITH STARTING DOSAGES AND COMMON SIDE EFFECTS	
Medication	**Starting Dose (PO unless Otherwise Specified; mg)**	**Significant Side Effects**
Antidepressants		
Amitriptyline	10–25 at night	Cardiac, CNS
Nortriptyline	10–25 at night	Cardiac, CNS
Venlafaxine	37.5 every day	CNS
Duloxetine	60 every day	Nausea, somnolence
Anticonvulsants		
Gabapentin	100, 3 × day	CNS, sedation
Carbamazepine	100, 2 × day	Bone marrow, liver, CNS
Pregabalin	75 every day	CNS, sedation
Topicals		
Lidocaine 5%	1–3 patches for 12 hr	CNS, Cardiac
Capsaicin	0.025% Cream	Burning
Muscle relaxants		
Baclofen	5, 3 × day	CNS
Cyclobenzaprine	5, 3 × day	Drowsiness, dry mouth
Tizanidine	2 every night (4 mg tid)	Weakness, dry mouth
N-methyl-D-aspartate antagonist		
Ketamine	Intravenous infusion	Hallucinations, CNS

PO, by mouth; tid, three times a day.

form. Intramuscular forms of medications, such as morphine, have variable efficacy and are not recommended (35). Patient-controlled analgesia allows patients to regularly administer intravenous medications without nursing assistance, especially in the inpatient setting. Both fentanyl and lidocaine are available in a transdermal patch (44). Capsaicin cream has been shown to be effective for local treatment of neuropathic pain (48).

Interventional Management

Although most cancer pain can be managed medically, some patients require interventional procedures to achieve pain relief. Interventions include peripheral nerve block, neuroablation, and neuroaxial techniques.

During Radiotherapy Procedure

Most patients can tolerate the radiotherapy procedure, but occasionally a patient may not tolerate proper positioning secondary to pain. Most patients can be managed with oral or intravenous pain medications, primarily with opiates such as morphine or fentanyl. When these methods fail, the radiation oncologist may need the assistance of an anesthesiologist.

If the region of radiotherapy is an extremity, the specific nerves to an extremity may be anesthetized with local anesthetic or peripheral nerve block (32). For multiple-day procedures, a peripheral nerve catheter may be placed for delivery of continuous anesthetic (19). Patients with abdominal or thoracic pain may benefit with local anesthetic being delivered epidurally (61). If these methods are contraindicated, general anesthesia may be the only option.

Neuroablative Techniques

Although most pain symptoms can be managed with oral and intravenous medications, the regimen may become insufficient or side effects become intolerable. Pain management specialists offer a myriad of neurolytic procedures with the goal of reducing pain medication requirements.

Peripheral nerves, once leaving the spinal cord, can be visualized with magnetic resonance imaging or ultrasound and exposed to various types of neurolytic procedures. Common nerves that are neurolyzed include intercostal nerves (for thoracotomy pain), maxillary and mandibular nerves (for postherpetic neuralgia), and median branch nerves (for back pain) (56). Cryoanalgesia techniques involve the application of subzero temperatures to induce wallerian degeneration of neurons, but allowing normal regrowth of axons. Radiofrequency techniques apply heat to nerves to cause damage. Chemical neurolysis can be achieved with phenol or alcohol preparations.

Pain initiating from the perineal, pelvic, and abdominal regions are supplied by pain fibers following sympathetic fibers innervating the region. Along with the pain fibers, the sympathetic nerves coalesce at specific ganglia (impar, hypogastric, and celiac, respectively). At these sites, image-guided neurolytic procedures can be performed with alcohol or phenol (12). When pain fibers are destroyed in this process, the associated region is also sympathetically denervated.

Not all pain in the cancer population is mediated by pain fibers (C and Aδ nerve fibers). Sympathetically mediated pain, known as *complex regional pain syndromes I and II*, may present at an extremity with initial symptoms of swelling, redness and temperature change. Chronic skin changes, hair loss, and muscle atrophy and disuse may follow (2). Along with pharmacologic treatment, neuroablative techniques targeting sympathetic fibers to the upper extremity (stellate ganglion) and lower extremity (lumbar sympathetics) can be used to treat these syndromes (36).

Neuroaxial Techniques

Neuroaxial procedures involving drug-delivery systems are indicated when oral opiate regimen doses are escalating without significant pain relief or side effects are intolerable (38). Both semipermanent epidural systems and permanent intrathecal delivery systems can be used to deliver local anesthetic and opiate medications in low concentrations to appropriate spinal cord root levels (28). The benefits of these methods include the use of local anesthetics in concentrations that are not toxic but can provide analgesia at the spinal cord level and the use of adjuvants (such as clonidine), which should not be given at equivalent oral doses because of side effects.

Another technique of disrupting the flow of pain signals in the spinal cord involves electrostimulation techniques. Transcutaneous electrical nerve stimulation, spinal cord stimulators at thoracic and lumbar regions, and deep-brain stimulators at the thalamus or motor cortex can interfere with the conduction of pain signals (34). The stimulation of large motor fibers inhibits the conduction of pain signals by small nerve fibers and has shown efficacy for various pain syndromes (46).

Neurosurgical techniques are generally reserved for refractory pain and for specific indications. Plexus root avulsions may be responsive to dorsal root entry zone lesioning, but the indications and success rates are limited (52). More specific lesions at the spinal cord and central nervous system (e.g., thalamotomy and deep-brain stimulation) have also been used with variable success and significant side effects (53).

Complementary Therapies

Conventional medical regimens may not satisfactorily treat cancer-related pain syndromes. Several complementary medicine modalities such as hypnosis, massage, music therapy, mind-body exercises, and dietary supplementation have been shown to reduce anxiety and chronic pain (13).

Acupuncture is perhaps the most extensively studied method for pain control. Acupuncture relieves both acute (e.g., postoperative dental pain) and chronic (e.g., headache, osteoarthritis) pain (4,22,37). Acupuncture appears effective against cancer-related pain. A randomized, placebo-controlled trial performed in patients tested auricular acupuncture for patients with cancer pain despite stable medication. Pain intensity decreased by 36% at 2 months from baseline in the patients in the treatment group, a statistically significant difference compared with the patients in the two control groups, for whom little pain reduction was seen (1). Most patients in this study had neuropathic pain, which is often refractory to conventional treatment.

Neurophysiologic studies show that acupuncture-induced analgesic effects appear to be mediated by endogenous opioids and other neurotransmitters (21). Functional brain imaging studies suggest that acupuncture also modulates the affective-cognitive aspect of pain perception (64). Correlations between functional magnetic resonance imaging signal intensities and analgesic effects induced by acupuncture have been reported (66).

Specific Scenarios

The following section identifies specific pain syndromes that the radiation oncologist may commonly face.

Muscle Spasm

Muscle fibers, once thought to be radioresistant, may undergo significant changes, especially months after radiation exposure (17). One-time muscle exposures to 10 to 20 Gy or fractionated doses >55 Gy are associated with myokymia, pain, and decreased muscle strength and range of motion (17). Specific cancer locations susceptible to muscle complications include head and neck cancers and soft tissue cancers (e.g., Ewing's sarcoma) (17). Treatment regimen includes early physical therapy and orthopaedic exercises, and pharmacologic therapy such as muscle relaxants (e.g., baclofen). Novel treatments involve the use of botulinum toxin injected in small doses (15 to 25 units) into the muscle to relieve contracture or spasm (29,57).

Plexopathy

Similar to muscle fibers, nerve bundles exposed to a one-time dose of 28 Gy, or fractionated doses totaling 60 Gy, undergo significant decreases in large nerve fiber density (60). Although more common in neoplastic plexopathy, significant pain may ensue months to years after radiotherapy, especially in the brachial plexus distribution (16). Rates of radiation-induced plexopathy range from 1% to 5%, with 10% of this population with complicated pain syndromes, including causalgia, dysesthesias, and numbness (26). Treatments involve early physical and occupational therapy, multimodality pain regimens (opiate and neuropathic pain medications as previously discussed), neurolytic procedures (e.g., stellate ganglion), and electrical stimulation (transcutaneous electrical nerve stimulation or spinal cord stimulators) (49).

Mucositis and Proctitis

Pain associated with mucositis (up to 75% of patients treated with radiation) is debilitating and may result in dose limitations of radiotherapy (50). Pain-control strategies include NSAIDS and oral opiates, with patient-controlled analgesia providing good management of pain when patients are in the hospital. Topical analgesics, such as viscous lidocaine, ice chips, capsaicin, benzydamine (Gelclair, Sinclair Pharma Ltd, UK), and diphenhydramine, may provide relief prior to ingestion of food (51). Some helpful interventions include good oral hygiene, honey, hydrolytic enzymes, zinc, laser therapy, gelclair, and povidone (33,63). Management of radiation-induced alimentary tract mucositis is discussed in-depth in Chapter 90.

Similar to oral mucosa, the rectum is susceptible to late radiation damage and proctitis, with patients presenting with tenesmus and rectal pain. Medical treatments involve reducing inflammation with NSAIDs and steroids, such as hydrocortisone cream, and the use of sucralfate (14). Novel therapies, including hyperbaric oxygen and heat therapy (laser therapy), have also been used to heal rectal mucosa and reduce tenesmus (11,27).

References

1. Alimi D, Rubino C, Pichard-Leandri E, et al. Analgesic effect of auricular acupuncture for cancer pain: a randomized, blinded, controlled trial. *J Clin Oncol* 2003;21:4120–4126.
2. Aprile AE. Complex regional pain syndrome. *Aana J* 1997;65:557–560.
3. Azevedo Sao Leao Ferreira K, Kimura M, Jacobsen Teixeira M. The WHO analgesic ladder for cancer pain control, twenty years of use. How much pain relief does one get from using it? *Support Care Cancer* 2006.
4. Berman BM, Lao L, Langenberg P, et al. Effectiveness of acupuncture as adjunctive therapy in osteoarthritis of the knee: a randomized, controlled trial. *Ann Intern Med* 2004;141:901–910.
5. Besson JM, Chaouch A. Peripheral and spinal mechanisms of nociception. *Physiol Rev* 1987;67:67–186.
6. Bruera E. Mechanism of action of nonsteroidal anti-inflammatory drugs. *Cancer Invest* 1998;16:538–539.
7. Cherny NI. The management of cancer pain. *CA Cancer J Clin* 2000;50:70–116; quiz 117–120.
8. Cherny N, Ripamonti C, Pereira J, et al. Strategies to manage the adverse effects of oral morphine: an evidence-based report. *J Clin Oncol* 2001;19:2542–2554.
9. Cherny NI, Portenoy RK. Cancer pain management. Current strategy. *Cancer* 1993;72[11 suppl]:3393–3415.
10. Cleeland CS, Janjan NA, Scott CB, et al. Cancer pain management by radiotherapists: a survey of radiation therapy oncology group physicians. *Int J Radiat Oncol Biol Phys* 2000;47:203–208.
11. Colwell JC, Goldberg M. A review of radiation proctitis in the treatment of prostate cancer. *J Wound Ostomy Continence Nurs* 2000;27:179–187.
12. de Leon-Casasola OA. Critical evaluation of chemical neurolysis of the sympathetic axis for cancer pain. *Cancer Control* 2000;7:142–148.
13. Deng G, Cassileth BR. Integrative oncology: complementary therapies for pain, anxiety, and mood disturbance. *CA Cancer J Clin* 2005;55:109–116.
14. Denton AS, Andreyev HJ, Forbes A, et al. Systematic review for non-surgical interventions for the management of late radiation proctitis. *Br J Cancer* 2002;87:134–143.
15. Friedland J. Local and systemic radiation for palliation of metastatic disease. *Urol Clin North Am* 1999;26:391–402.
16. Galecki J, Hicer-Grzenkowicz J, Grudzien-Kowalska M, et al. Radiation-induced brachial plexopathy and hypofractionated regimens in adjuvant irradiation of patients with breast cancer—a review. *Acta Oncol* 2006;45:280–284.
17. Gillette EL, Mahler PA, Powers BE, et al. Late radiation injury to muscle and peripheral nerves. *Int J Radiat Oncol Biol Phys* 1995;31:1309–1318.
18. Gordon DB, Dahl JL, Miaskowski C, et al. American pain society recommendations for improving the quality of acute and cancer pain management: American Pain Society Quality of Care Task Force. *Arch Intern Med* 2005;165:1574–1580.
19. Grossi P, Allegri M. Continuous peripheral nerve blocks: state of the art. *Curr Opin Anaesthesiol* 2005;18:522–526.
20. Hainline B. Chronic pain: physiological, diagnostic, and management considerations. *Psychiatr Clin North Am* 2005;28:713–735.
21. Han JS. Acupuncture and endorphins. *Neurosci Lett* 2004;361:258–261.
22. Health NIO. NIH Consensus Conference. Acupuncture. *JAMA* 1998;280:1518–1524.
23. Inturrisi CE. Pharmacology of methadone and its isomers. *Minerva Anestesiol* 2005;71:435–437.
24. Irving GA. Contemporary assessment and management of neuropathic pain. *Neurology* 2005;64[12 Suppl 3]:S21–27.
25. Jadad AR, Browman GP. The WHO analgesic ladder for cancer pain management. Stepping up the quality of its evaluation. *JAMA* 1995;274:1870–1873.
26. Jaeckle KA. Neurological manifestations of neoplastic and radiation-induced plexopathies. *Semin Neurol* 2004;24:385–393.
27. Jones K, Evans AW, Bristow RG, et al. Treatment of radiation proctitis with hyperbaric oxygen. *Radiother Oncol* 2006;78:91–94.
28. Lordon SP. Interventional approach to cancer pain. *Curr Pain Headache Rep* 2002;6:202–206.
29. Lou JS, Pleninger P, Kurlan R. Botulinum toxin A is effective in treating trismus associated with postradiation myokymia and muscle spasm. *Mov Disord* 1995;10:680–681.
30. Lussier D, Huskey AG, Portenoy RK. Adjuvant analgesics in cancer pain management. *Oncologist* 2004;9:571–591.
31. Malhotra V, Moryl N. *Palliative cancer care.* Sudbury, MA: Jones and Bartlett Publishers, Inc.; 2006.
32. Marhofer P, Greher M, Kapral S. Ultrasound guidance in regional anaesthesia. *Br J Anaesth* 2005;94:7–17.
33. Marlow C, Johnson J. A guide to managing the pain of treatment-related oral mucositis. *Int J Palliat Nurs* 2005;11:338–345.
34. McNicol E, Horowicz-Mehler N, Fisk RA, et al. Management of opioid side effects in cancer-related and chronic noncancer pain: a systematic review. *J Pain* 2003;4:231–256.
35. McQuay HJ, Carroll D, Moore RA. Injected morphine in postoperative pain: a quantitative systematic review. *J Pain Symptom Manage* 1999;17:164–174.
36. Mekhail N, Kapural L. Complex regional pain syndrome type I in cancer patients. *Curr Rev Pain* 2000;4:227–233.
37. Melchart D, Linde K, Fischer P, et al. Acupuncture for recurrent headaches: a systematic review of randomized controlled trials. *Cephalalgia* 1999;19:779–786; discussion 765.
38. Mercadante S. Neuraxial techniques for cancer pain: an opinion about unresolved therapeutic dilemmas. *Reg Anesth Pain Med* 1999;24:74–83.
39. Miaskowski C, Cleary J. *Guideline for the management of cancer pain in adults and children.* Glenview, IL: American Pain Society; 2005.
40. Milch RA. Neuropathic pain: implications for the surgeon. *Surg Clin North Am* 2005;85:225–236.
41. National Comprehensive Cancer Network. *Practice guidelines in oncology: adult cancer pain* (ver 1). www.nccn.org. Accessed June 2007.
42. Palmer SN, Giesecke NM, Body SC, et al. Pharmacogenetics of anesthetic and analgesic agents. *Anesthesiology* 2005;102:663–671.
43. Pignon T, Fernandez L, Ayasso S, et al. Impact of radiation oncology practice on pain: a cross-sectional survey. *Int J Radiat Oncol Biol Phys* 2004;60:1204–1210.
44. Priano L, Gasco MR, Mauro A. Transdermal treatment options for neurological disorders: impact on the elderly. *Drugs Aging* 2006;23:357–375.
45. Quigley C. Opioid switching to improve pain relief and drug tolerability. *Cochrane Database Syst Rev* 2004;:CD004847.
46. Rushton DN. Electrical stimulation in the treatment of pain. *Disabil Rehabil* 2002;24:407–415.
47. Sachs CJ. Oral analgesics for acute nonspecific pain. *Am Fam Physician* 2005;71:913–918.
48. Sawynok J. Topical analgesics in neuropathic pain. *Curr Pharm Des* 2005;11:2995–3004.
49. Schierle C, Winograd JM. Radiation-induced brachial plexopathy: review. Complication without a cure. *J Reconstr Microsurg* 2004;20:149–152.
50. Scully C, Epstein J, Sonis S. Oral mucositis: a challenging complication of radiotherapy, chemotherapy, and radiochemotherapy: part 1, pathogenesis and prophylaxis of mucositis. *Head Neck* 2003;25:1057–1070.
51. Scully C, Epstein J, Sonis S. Oral mucositis: a challenging complication of radiotherapy, chemotherapy, and radiochemotherapy. Part 2: diagnosis and management of mucositis. *Head Neck* 2004;26:77–84.
52. Sindou M, Mertens P. Neurosurgical management of neuropathic pain. *Stereotact Funct Neurosurg* 2000;75:76–80.
53. Slavik E, Ivanovic S. Cancer pain (neurosurgical management). *Acta Chir Iugosl* 2004;51:15–23.
54. Society AP. *Principles of analgesic use in the treatment of acute pain and cancer pain.* Glenview, IL: International Association for the Study of Pain; 1999.
55. Stamer UM, Bayerer B, Stuber F. Genetics and variability in opioid response. *Eur J Pain* 2005;9:101–104.

56. Trescot AM. Cryoanalgesia in interventional pain management. *Pain Physician* 2003;6:345–360.

57. Van Daele DJ, Finnegan EM, Rodnitzky RL, et al. Head and neck muscle spasm after radiotherapy: management with botulinum toxin A injection. *Arch Otolaryngol Head Neck Surg* 2002;128:956–959.

58. Ventafridda V, Saita L, Ripamonti C, et al. WHO guidelines for the use of analgesics in cancer pain. *Int J Tissue React* 1985;7:93–96.

59. Ventafridda V, Tamburini M, Caraceni A, et al. A validation study of the WHO method for cancer pain relief. *Cancer* 1987;59:850–856.

60. Vujaskovic Z, Gillette SM, Powers BE, et al. Ultrastructural morphometric analysis of peripheral nerves after intraoperative irradiation. *Int J Radiat Biol* 1995;68:71–76.

61. Waurick R, Van Aken H. Update in thoracic epidural anaesthesia. *Best Pract Res Clin Anaesthesiol* 2005;19:201–213.

62. World Health Organization. *WHO guidelines cancer pain relief,* 2nd ed. Geneva: World Health Organization; 1996.

63. Worthington HV, Clarkson JE, Eden OB. Interventions for preventing oral mucositis for patients with cancer receiving treatment. *Cochrane Database Syst Rev* 2006;CD000978.

64. Wu MT, Hsieh JC, Xiong J, et al. Central nervous pathway for acupuncture stimulation: localization of processing with functional MR imaging of the brain—preliminary experience. *Radiology* 1999;212:133–141.

65. Zech DF, Grond S, Lynch J, et al. Validation of World Health Organization Guidelines for cancer pain relief: a 10-year prospective study. *Pain* 1995;63:65–76.

66. Zhang WT, Jin Z, Cui GH, et al. Relations between brain network activation and analgesic effect induced by low vs. high frequency electrical acupoint stimulation in different subjects: a functional magnetic resonance imaging study. *Brain Res* 2003;982:168–178.

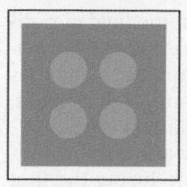

Chapter 95
Supportive Care and Quality of Life

Gary Deng, Barrie R. Cassileth

Overview: Basic Principles of Supportive Care and Quality of Life

"Quality of life" entered the medical lexicon for the first time in 1976 with the groundbreaking publication by Priestman and Baum (131). Attention to quality of life was paid increasingly through the 1980s, spurred in part by efforts to differentiate among numerous chemotherapeutic agents similar in their ability to treat malignancies. In 1989, the Institute of Medicine issued a *Quality of Life and Technology Assessment* document, supporting the importance of quality of life and its appropriate measurement with validated, patient-reported instruments (115). The Food and Drug Administration confirmed its interest in what was often termed *cancer-related side effects* (73). Today, it is widely recognized that existing cancer treatments, in addition to the disease itself, can negatively impact the patient's physical, psychosocial, cognitive, and other aspects of well-being, which, in the aggregate, we call *quality of life* (55).

As the current voluminous literature suggests (there were 20,160 MEDLINE hits for "cancer quality of life" as of this writing), understanding of what impairs cancer patients' well-being and new ways to identify and manage these problems have emerged. As it became widely recognized that cancer patients have multiple concurrent symptoms from comorbidities as well as from cancer and its treatment, a new focus on symptom clusters, rather than on individual symptoms, has been stressed (10,111). This important concept embodies a relationship among concurrent symptoms based on a common etiology or mechanism, or by producing outcomes different from those that would be produced by a single symptom alone. It also includes the idea of "symptom burden," the associated level of patient or survivor distress.

A joint report of the National Cancer Institutes of the United Kingdom, Canada, and the United States on supportive care emphasized the importance of assessing and treating multiple symptoms simultaneously. It indicates that some symptoms are more likely to cluster than others, and thus may share a common cause (e.g., pain, fatigue, and depression) (60). Research on this topic began relatively recently and much more is required, but some data are beginning to emerge. Examples include an analysis of 25 symptoms from 922 patients with advanced cancer that revealed seven clusters: (a) fatigue/anorexia-cachexia, (b) neuropsychological, (c) upper gastrointestinal, (d) nausea and vomiting, (e) aerodigestive, (f) debility, and (g) pain. Many symptoms are associated with site of radiotherapy (RT). For example, emesis is most likely with radiation to chest and upper abdomen, diarrhea, and other gastrointestinal (GI) symptoms tend to occur with RT to the lower digestive tract.

It is widely agreed that recognition of symptom clusters should lead to better understanding of symptom pathophysiology, to targeted therapies, and improved quality of life. Using this approach may also reduce polypharmacy, lessen drug side effects, and produce pharmacoeconomic benefits (168). A "cancer anorexia-cachexia syndrome" is described, consisting of a combination of anorexia, tissue wasting, malnutrition, weight loss, and loss of compensatory increase in feeding, the result of

complex interaction between cancer growth and host response (163). This is a growing and important area of work.

Constitutional Symptoms: Fatigue and Related Mood Dysfunction

Fatigue remains a major problem for cancer patients even after treatment for underlying anemia (68). RT-produced fatigue typically is short-lived and far less severe than chemotherapy-generated fatigue. This symptom is associated with depression and anxiety as well as with specific areas of the body treated. Although most surveys are careful to request information about "cancer-related" fatigue, it may not be possible for all patients to distinguish among various potential etiologies, including comorbidities or life problems.

It is necessary to bear in mind the complex, reciprocal relationship between physical dysfunction/distress, individual capacity to cope effectively, anxiety or depression, and fatigue. Moreover, the pathogenesis of fatigue, not yet well understood, is thought to play an important role. In most studies, fatigue returns to prediagnosis levels not long after completion of RT or chemotherapy. Prediagnosis levels are not necessarily minimal or no fatigue; rather, they reflect personality and coping characteristics as well as other life factors.

The Prevalence and Severity of Fatigue Associated with RT

In a prospective study of 28 men receiving radical external-beam RT for prostate cancer, the prevalence of moderate-severe fatigue increased from 7% at baseline to 32% at RT completion. Fatigue significantly interfered with walking ability, normal work, daily chores, and enjoyment of life, but only at the end of RT. Improvement occurred after completion of treatment, but at 6.5 weeks of follow-up remained higher than at baseline. Neither age, Gleason score, prostate-specific antigen, T-stage, hormone therapy duration, nor RT dose and fractions were significantly associated with fatigue scores (161). Similar results are seen in studies of breast cancer patients. In 38 women alive with no evidence of disease 2.5 years after adjuvant RT for localized breast cancer, there was no significant difference between chronic fatigue levels at 2.5 years after RT and pretreatment values. Neither age nor hormonal therapy was associated with fatigue levels, but cancer-related distress correlated closely with fatigue scores. Personality patterns tend to be stable over time and typically predictive of how patients will react to cancer diagnosis and treatment. Patients with pretreatment elevated fatigue, anxiety, or depression are at risk for chronic fatigue. RT did not contribute to posttreatment fatigue in this patient sample (52).

Compared with women who received adjuvant RT, women receiving adjuvant chemotherapy were more than twice as likely to develop fatigue during the course of therapy (3). In a typical study, during and for 3 months after primary RT for breast cancer, fatigue increased from 33% to 93%, and gradual improvement occurred during the following 3 months (84).

Among 115 Taiwanese nasopharyngeal carcinoma patients, significantly higher symptom distress was seen for patients undergoing RT compared with those who completed RT 1 to 3 years previously (91).

In patients with advanced cancer, fatigue levels initially worsened with RT, stabilized at week 8, and returned to baseline by week 27 (22). Patients with brain metastases who received whole-brain RT (69% of 104 patients) experienced severe fatigue and many problems with cognition, whereas only 34% of those receiving only radiosurgery reported side effects. Only 5% of radiosurgery patients reported fatigue (86).

Treatment

Treatment with an erythropoietic agent for fatigue related to anemia should be considered, although erythropoietins should not be used for prolonged periods as there are concerns that they may decrease survival by enhancing tumor growth [16428469]. Medication or referral for underlying depression, anxiety, or pain may be appropriate and should also be considered. However, the most promising intervention is exercise. Strong evidence increasingly indicates not only that exercise reduces fatigue and improves mood state (173), but also that it improves survival.

A 2005 study reported a significant protective relationship between increased physical activity after diagnosis and recurrence, cancer-related mortality, and overall mortality among 2,987 stage I-III breast cancer survivors in the Nurse's Health Study (66). Two additional, prospective studies published simultaneously in 2006 found the same results with colorectal cancer patients (109,110). These studies each found a protective association between postdiagnosis physical activity and survival. Data from these three observational studies suggest a rare 50% to 60% reduced risk of recurrence with postdiagnosis exercise.

Complementary therapies in addition to exercise also should be considered. They are appropriate because the risk is minimal and because most patients perceive a benefit. These noninvasive, self-directed therapies include massage therapy, meditation and other mind-body therapies, acupuncture, music therapy, yoga, and the like. In controlled studies, massage therapy was found superior to standard care for fatigue, anxiety, nausea, and general well-being {Ahles, 1999 284 /id}. Acupuncture reduced fatigue in an early-phase trial involving patients with chronic postchemotherapy fatigue, and multiple randomized trials document the value of mind-body therapies such as meditation, relaxation therapies, and yoga. In a typical study, 109 cancer patients with varying diagnoses and stages of disease were randomized to receive meditation classes and encouraged to practice at home. Anxiety and depression scores fell by nearly 50% in the meditation group with little change in controls. Relaxation training sessions in women with gynecologic cancers {Petersen, 2002 9856 /id} decreased mood disturbance about as effectively as did benzodiazepine (Alprazolam).

Although definitive effectiveness data are not always available, the National Comprehensive Cancer Network (NCCN) recommends relaxation techniques and restorative therapies such as meditation for stress management. These therapies should be considered for fatigue as well. They are safe and associated with other quality of life benefits, importantly the opportunity for proactive self-care, use of therapies to which patients are drawn and from which they derive comfort and relief, and the opportunity to play an active role in their well-being.

Salivary Gland Injury: Xerostomia

Xerostomia, the subjective experience of dry mouth, is among the most common complaints experienced by cancer patients treated with RT to the head and neck area. It is caused by salivary gland dysfunction as a result of damage in the field of radiation. Histologically, irradiated salivary glands demonstrate acinar atrophy and chronic inflammation. Inflammatory changes and fibrosis are observed in periductal and intralobular areas, whereas the ductal system remains relatively intact (16,58).

Salivary dysfunction develops immediately and predictably. A 50% to 60% decrease is salivary flow occurs during the first week. As RT continues and the total radiation dose increases, salivary function decreases accordingly in a dose-dependent fashion. After initial deterioration, a recovery phase may be seen, with patients reporting reduced xerostomia even though salivary flow remains depressed. This may result from adaptation to the sensation of xerostomia and compensatory response from surviving functional glandular tissues. However, salivary function usually continues to decline for 6 to 8 months after therapy, and many patients show no recovery even at 12 months (46,164). In some patients, xerostomia may be permanent.

In addition to oral discomfort, radiation-induced salivary gland injury contributes to systemic problems including loss of appetite, chronic esophagitis, gastroesophageal reflux, and sleep disruption due to the need for frequent mouth moistening and subsequent polyuria (165). The lubricating, buffering, and antimicrobial effects of saliva maintain the integrity of oral tissue (dental and mucosal). Saliva also assists in speech, taste perception, mastication, bolus formation, and swallowing (125). Decreased salivation can lead to dental caries, periodontal diseases, a shift of oral flora, poor tolerability to dental prosthesis and inflammation, and atrophy and ulceration of mucosa. As a result, radiation-induced xerostomia has a debilitating impact on health and overall quality of life in head and neck cancer patients and survivors (148).

Prevention

The extent of radiation-induced salivary dysfunction is influenced by radiation field, radiation dose, and initial volume and function of the salivary gland. Several approaches have been developed to prevent or minimize injury to salivary glands. They include salivary gland transplantation, intensity-modulated RT and amifostine therapy.

In several earlier studies, surgical transfer of submandibular glands into the submental space prior to radiation therapy resulted in prevention of xerostomia (1,72,134). A 2-year follow-up showed that 83% of patients reported normal amounts of saliva production (143). The Radiation Therapy Oncology Group is conducting an ongoing phase II study to further investigate the role of submandibular gland transfer in a multi-institutional setting. Advances in three-dimensional conformal radiation therapy and intensity-modulated RT technology make it possible to conduct gland-sparing RT. Several studies showed that both subjective and objective measures of salivatory function are preserved. Limiting the mean dose of the parotid glands to ≤ 26 Gy decreases the risk of long-term xerostomia. Local treatment failure rates are not affected by intensity-modulated RT (2,45,92,117,124).

Intravenous (IV) amifostine, a thiol-containing radioprotectant, administered at 200 mg/m(2) daily 15 to 30 minutes before irradiation reduced acute and chronic xerostomia in an open label phase III study. Antitumor treatment efficacy was preserved; however, mucositis was not reduced. Nausea, vomiting, hypotension, and allergic reactions were the most common side effects (21). Subcutaneous administration of amifostine has been explored for reduced side effects (4,88). A side-by-side comparison between IV and subcutaneous routes showed equivalent efficacy for reduction of xerostomia, fewer side effects and better compliance, at least in the short term. Long-term data are not available at this time (9). Other agents are less promising. Reports of prophylactic use of pilocarpine are limited to retrospective studies. Cevimeline, a muscarinic agonist, was evaluated in randomized controlled trial with conflicting results (32).

Treatment

Current treatment of RT-induced xerostomia includes dietary and oral hygiene, saliva substitution, or stimulation of salivation by moistening agents or medications (121). Cold, tepid, soft food and beverages are preferred. Hard, spicy foods should be avoided. In patients without residual salivary function, saliva substitutes are used to relieve xerostomia. Water is commonly used and preferred by patients. Other types of mouthwash such as saline, bicarbonate, glycerol, or commercial formulations are available. Artificial saliva has been designed to mimic natural saliva. It may contain carboxymethylcellulose, porcine and bovine mucin, or xanthan gum.

In patients with residual salivary function, increased flow of natural saliva can be achieved by stimulation with chewing gum, sucking ointment, sugarless candies, menthol, acid, vitamin C, or lozenges developed to provide antimicrobial enzymes.

Several sialogogues, defined as systemic salivary gland stimulants, have been tested with mixed results. They are typically muscarinic agonists such as pilocarpine, bethanechol, carbachol, or cevimeline. Other classes of agents include neostigmine, physostigmine, nicotinic acid, potassium iodide, bromhexine (a mucolytic), and anethole trithione (58). Current data are inconclusive except for pilocarpine.

The most extensively studied pharmacologic treatment for xerostomia is pilocarpine. Oral administration at 5 to 10 mg, three times daily is the standard regimen. Several randomized, double-blind, placebo-controlled trials have shown clinical efficacy and safety of pilocarpine in treating radiation-induced xerostomia (74,94,135). In a multicenter study, 54% of the 207 study subjects reported reduction in the overall severity of xerostomia. Only 25% of those receiving placebo reported improvement. Speaking ability improved in 33% of patients receiving pilocarpine versus 18% of those receiving placebo. Saliva production also improved, but this did not correlate with subjective symptom relief (74). In another multicenter trial that involved 162 patients, both subjective symptom and objective measurement of saliva flow improved significantly in those receiving pilocarpine versus placebo. Best results were obtained with continuous treatment for 8 to 12 weeks (94).

Some patients require pilocarpine treatment for 2 months or longer to achieve maximum effect. Sweating, the most common side effect, is experienced by 37% to 65% of patients. In one study, 6% and 29% of patients in the 5- and 10-mg groups, respectively, dropped out because of the adverse effects (74). Because of the cholinergic activity of pilocarpine, it is not recommended for patients with cardiovascular disease, and it is contraindicated in patients with narrow-angle glaucoma and uncontrolled asthma (174).

Acupuncture has been shown to stimulate saliva production (18,19,75). It even shows some benefit in pilocarpine-resistant xerostomia (76). Salivary flow also may be induced by an acupuncturelike transcutaneous nerve stimulator (175). Acupuncture appears to modulate the function of the autonomic nervous system, which may stimulate salivary gland function and induce salivary flow (61,82,97,112). The role of acupuncture as a treatment modality is under investigation (82,114).

:: Mucosal Injury: Oral Mucositis, Nausea and Vomiting, Diarrhea, and Other GI Toxicity

Radiation therapy causes mucosal injury. When such injury occurs in the oral cavity, as commonly seen in patients irradiated at the head and neck area, it is called *stomatitis* or *oral mucositis*. When the injury occurs in nonoral alimentary tract mucosa, it presents as esophagitis, gastritis, enteritis, colitis, or proctitis. These injuries manifest as pain, dysphagia, odynophagia, nausea, vomiting, and diarrhea, typically described as "GI toxicity." Mucosal injuries by radiation appear to share the same underlying molecular pathogenesis, regardless of anatomic location (44,78,152). Some favor the terminology of *alimentary mucositis* to describe the hierarchy and constellation of toxicity to the oral and GI mucosa (128). Depending on the site of irradiation, dosage, and fractionation, patients' risks of mucositis vary. More than 50% of patients receiving radiation to the head and neck, abdomen, or the pelvis will experience moderate-to-severe mucositis. Accelerated fractionation increases the risk. Stem cell transplant recipients who received total-body irradiation have more severe and prolonged symptoms (159). Graft-versus-host-disease further exacerbates mucosal injury.

Recent research indicates that the pathogenesis of mucositis is not simply the result of nonspecific epithelial cell death. Rather it may involve a more complex pan-tissue process (17,151,177). The complexity of the pathogenesis of mucositis reflects the dynamic interactions of all of the cell and tissue types that comprise the epithelium and submucosa. Gender, circadian variables, epithelial type and characteristics, and local microbial environment all play a role in determining the risk of mucosal injury (5,150). New therapies are being developed based on these new findings (150,153).

A practice guideline developed in 2004 by the Multinational Association of Supportive Care in Cancer and International Society of Oral Oncology was updated in 2005 (www.mascc.org) (139,151) Recommendations related to RT are summarized in Table 95.1.

Oral Mucositis Prevention

Midline mucosa-sparing blocks were shown to protect the aerodigestive tract and significantly reduce acute toxicity during RT for head and neck cancer without compromising tumor control (126). Another technique is three-dimensional treatment planning and conformational dose delivery. It reduces the volume of mucosa exposed to irradiation (147). Topical benzydamine, a drug with anti-inflammatory, analgesic, and antimicrobial effects, reduces the frequency and severity of oral ulcers and pain in several randomized controlled trial. It inhibits the production proinflammatory cytokines, including tumor necrosis factor-α (47,81). Chlorhexidine failed to prevent radiation-induced oral mucositis (Fig. 95.1) (50,141,154).

Basic oral care is the foundation of care for oral mucositis. There is a lack of evidence supporting one protocol over another. Therefore, feasibility, adherence, performance, and outcomes are more important than the use of specific agents. Three randomized and three nonrandomized trials, showed that implementation of a systematic protocol improved outcome (12,20,29,42, 79, 95). Protocols usually consist of tooth brushing, plaque removal, chlorhexidine rinse, iodopovidone, and nystatin.

Studies testing amifostine for oral mucositis have been disappointing. Although it appeared useful in the prevention of xerostomia, inconsistent results have been reported for its use for oral symptoms (13).

New classes of agents are being investigated. Recombinant human keratinocyte growth factor-1 (rhuKGF-1, palifermin) was shown to reduce mucositis in patients with hematologic malignancies receiving high-dose chemotherapy and total-body irradiation with autologous stem cell transplantation.

On the other hand, a local granulocyte macrophage colony-stimulating factor mouthwash should *not* be used in efforts to prevent oral mucositis in the transplant setting. Other growth factors and cytokines are in early stage of development,

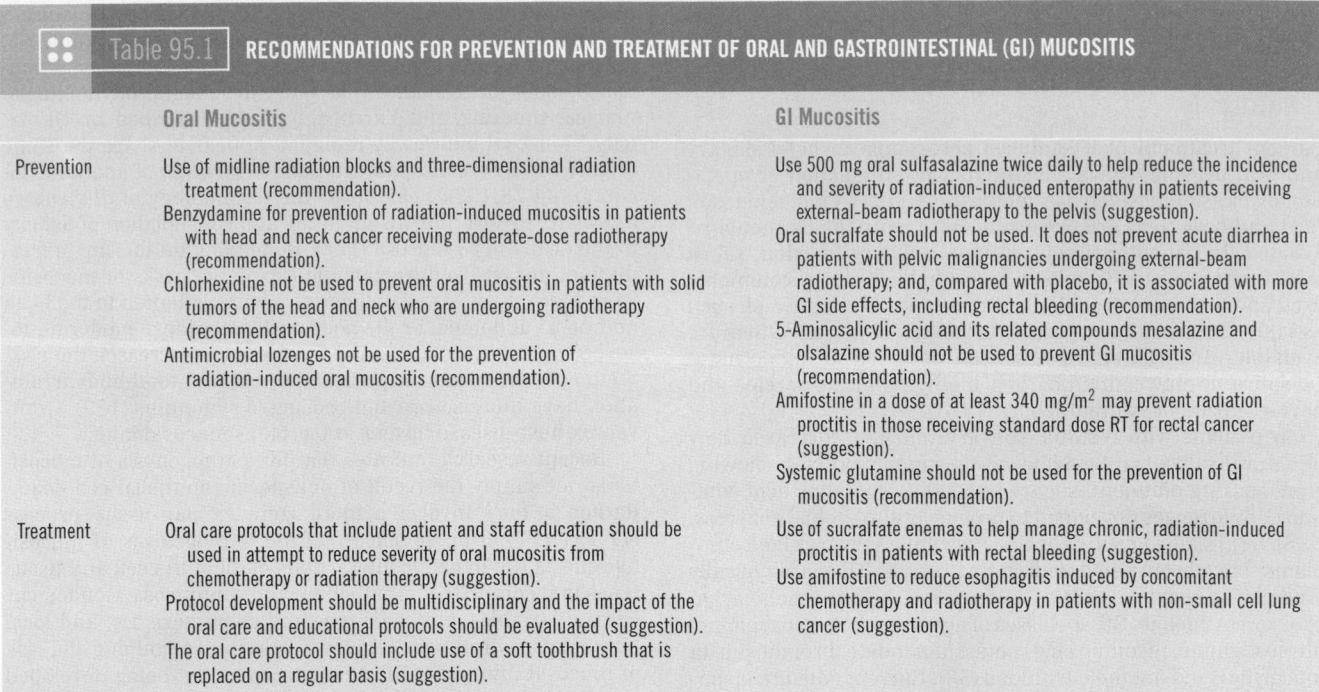

	Oral Mucositis	GI Mucositis
Prevention	Use of midline radiation blocks and three-dimensional radiation treatment (recommendation). Benzydamine for prevention of radiation-induced mucositis in patients with head and neck cancer receiving moderate-dose radiotherapy (recommendation). Chlorhexidine not be used to prevent oral mucositis in patients with solid tumors of the head and neck who are undergoing radiotherapy (recommendation). Antimicrobial lozenges not be used for the prevention of radiation-induced oral mucositis (recommendation).	Use 500 mg oral sulfasalazine twice daily to help reduce the incidence and severity of radiation-induced enteropathy in patients receiving external-beam radiotherapy to the pelvis (suggestion). Oral sucralfate should not be used. It does not prevent acute diarrhea in patients with pelvic malignancies undergoing external-beam radiotherapy; and, compared with placebo, it is associated with more GI side effects, including rectal bleeding (recommendation). 5-Aminosalicylic acid and its related compounds mesalazine and olsalazine should not be used to prevent GI mucositis (recommendation). Amifostine in a dose of at least 340 mg/m^2 may prevent radiation proctitis in those receiving standard dose RT for rectal cancer (suggestion). Systemic glutamine should not be used for the prevention of GI mucositis (recommendation).
Treatment	Oral care protocols that include patient and staff education should be used in attempt to reduce severity of oral mucositis from chemotherapy or radiation therapy (suggestion). Protocol development should be multidisciplinary and the impact of the oral care and educational protocols should be evaluated (suggestion). The oral care protocol should include use of a soft toothbrush that is replaced on a regular basis (suggestion).	Use of sucralfate enemas to help manage chronic, radiation-induced proctitis in patients with rectal bleeding (suggestion). Use amifostine to reduce esophagitis induced by concomitant chemotherapy and radiotherapy in patients with non-small cell lung cancer (suggestion).

Table 95.1   RECOMMENDATIONS FOR PREVENTION AND TREATMENT OF ORAL AND GASTROINTESTINAL (GI) MUCOSITIS

including epidermal growth factor, transforming growth factor-β, glucagonlike peptide-2, lactoferrin, anti-inflammatory amino acid decapeptide, recombinant human interleukin-11, and insulinlike growth factor-I (167). Natural product and dietary supplements such as glutamine, PV701 (milk-derived protein extract), several vitamins (A, B$_{12}$, E), folate, aloe vera (a plant extract), and curcumin, an extract from turmeric, were shown to hold promise in reducing radiation-induced mucositis. Most of the studies are not of sufficient quality to support a recommendation.

Oral Mucositis Treatment

Pain management is an important component of the management of oral mucositis. Most studies were done in the setting of chemotherapy-induced mucositis, instead of radiation-induced oral mucositis. Systemic and topical analgesics are used, as are coating agents. The use of opioids, nonopioids, and adjuvant medications is covered in more detail in Chapter 89. These agents can be given via oral, transmucosal, transdermal, or intravenous routes. Use of topical agents is widespread

in practice, with practices and institutions using their own favorite formulation. Typically, these are compounded mixtures with nicknames such as "magic mouth wash." Common ingredients include viscous lidocaine, milk of magnesia, chlorhexidine, and diphenhydramine. Despite their popularity, there is no significant evidence supporting their effectiveness or tolerability (27,30,38,39,137,155,162). A recent systematic review recommends against use of antibiotic lozenges or sucralfate for the prevention of radiation therapy-induced oral mucositis. Guidelines could not be generated because of conflicting data or insufficient evidence on topical anesthetics or analgesics (morphine, fentanyl) (8).

GI Mucositis Prevention

Several medications have been shown to significantly reduce the frequency and severity of radiation-induced GI mucositis, which usually presents as diarrhea and pain. Depending on the location, the GI mucositis may be termed *esophagitis, enteritis, colitis, proctosigmoiditis*, or *proctitis*. External-beam irradiation to the pelvis as part of treatment for prostate, rectal, or

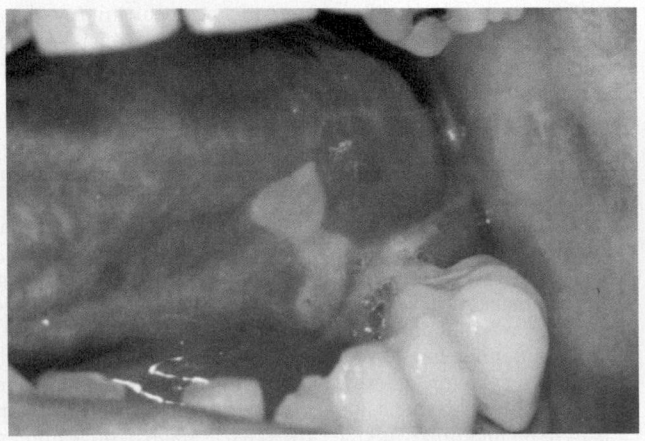
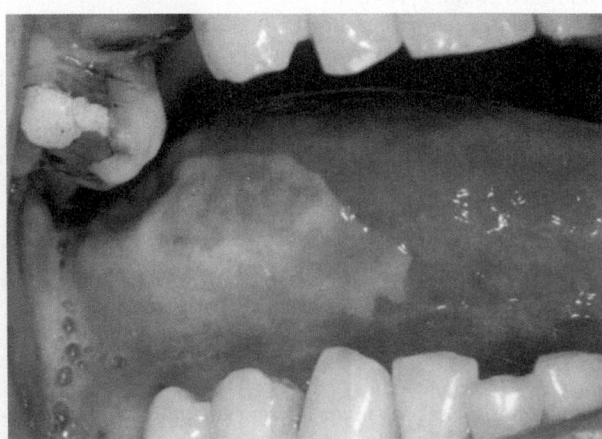

A   B

FIGURE 95.1. Radiotherapy-induced oral mucositis

cervical cancer produces lower GI injury in the majority of patients. In a randomized, controlled trial of pelvic irradiation, sulfasalazine, 1 g orally, twice daily, reduces GI toxicity from 93% to 80% and diarrhea from 86% to 55%, when compared with placebo. Grade 4 diarrhea was reduced from 16% of the patients to none (80).

Amifostine is an antioxidant that appears to protect normal cells from radiation injury preferentially to cancer cells (87). Amifostine was shown in several studies to prevent proctitis in patients receiving standard-dose RT for rectal cancer (13). The frequency, onset, and duration of acute rectal toxicity was reduced (6,89,118). When used in patients receiving combined chemoradiation for non-small cell lung cancer, amifostine significantly reduced the need for morphine to control pain from severe esophagitis (85) but its efficacy was mixed in other settings (6,93,116). IV amifostine is not without side effects. Other routes of administration that might reduce side effects are under study.

Other agents that did not show significant benefit include glutamine (93), oral sucralfate (83,103), rectal administration of sucralfate (123), and other anti-inflammatories commonly used in ulcerative colitis, such as 5-aminosalicylates (11), mesalazine (133), and olsalazine (104). They should not be used to prevent radiation GI toxicity.

GI Mucositis Treatment

Nausea and Vomiting

In addition to measures discussed here that aim to treat the underlying pathology of radiation-induced mucosal injury, symptomatic treatment should be provided. Radiation-induced nausea and emesis tend to be undertreated. Factors that influence radiation-induced emesis include single and total dose, dose rate; fractionation; field-size and irradiated volume; site of irradiation and organs included in the radiation field; patient positioning; radiation technique, energy, and beam quality; previous or simultaneous influencing therapy; and general health status of the patient (49). Evidence-based practice guidelines developed by national organizations differ in specific recommendations and in when recommendations apply, reflecting the limited amount of high-level evidence available to date. The 2006 updated guidelines from Multinational Association of Supportive Care in Cancer (48), American Society of Clinical Oncology (90), and NCCN (119,120) are summarized in Table 95.2.

Diarrhea

Symptomatic management of radiation-induced diarrhea is similar to that of chemotherapy-induced diarrhea but may not require hospitalization (59,122). Diarrhea usually occurs during the third week of fractionated abdomen or pelvic RT. Guidelines were developed by an expert panel and updated in 2004 (14).

For mild-to-moderate diarrhea, the initial management should include dietary modifications (157). Patients should eat small, frequent, protein-rich meals. Adequate fluid intake (35 mL/kg/day) is necessary. Liquids should be taken primarily between meals. Soluble fibers such as oats, pectin, guar, and psyllium help retain stool consistency. Spices, alcohol, caffeine, high-osmolar beverages, and high-lactose food should be avoided. Probiotics, guar extracts, and glutamine supplements are worthy of consideration (157).

Loperamide remains the mainstay of pharmacologic treatment. It should be started at 4 mg followed by 2 mg every 4 hours or after every unformed stool (maximum, 16 mg/d).

	Table 95.2	**GUIDELINES FOR PREVENTION AND TREATMENT OF RADIATION-INDUCED NAUSEA AND VOMITING**		
	Risk			
	High	**Moderate**	**Low**	**Minimal**
MASCC risk category	Total body	Upper abdomen	Lower thorax, pelvis, cranium (radiosurgery) and craniospinal	Head and neck, extremities, cranium and breast
MASCC recommendation	Prophylaxis with 5-HT$_3$ antagonists +/− dexamethasone	Prophylaxis or rescue with 5-HT$_3$ antagonists	Prophylaxis with 5-HT$_3$ antagonists	Rescue with dopamine receptor antagonists or 5-HT$_3$ antagonists
ASCO risk category	Total body	Upper abdomen hemibody irradiation, upper abdomen, abdominal-pelvic, mantle, craniospinal irradiation, and cranial radiosurgery	Lower thorax, cranium (radiosurgery), and craniospinal	Breast, head and neck, cranium, and extremities
ASCO recommendation	A 5-HT$_3$ serotonin receptor antagonist with or without a corticosteroid before each fraction and for at least 24 hr after	A 5-HT$_3$ serotonin receptor antagonist before each fraction	A 5-HT$_3$ serotonin receptor antagonist before each fraction	Dopamine or 5-HT$_3$ serotonin receptor antagonists as needed. Should be continued prophylactically for each remaining radiation treatment day
NCCN risk category	Total body	Upper abdomen	—	Other
NCCN recommendation for prevention	Ondansetron, 8 mg PO bid-tid or granisetron, 2 mg PO daily, or 3 mg IV daily (category 2B) ± dexamethasone, 2 mg PO tid	Ondansetron, 8 mg PO bid-tid or dexamethasone, 2 mg PO tid or granisetron, 2 mg PO daily	—	—
NCCN recommendation for breakthrough treatment	The same in chemo-induced nausea vomiting	The same in chemo-induced nausea vomiting	—	Start pretreatment for each day of RT treatment; ondansetron, 8 mg PO bid-tid

MASCC, Multinational Association of Supportive Care in Cancer; -5-HT$_3$, 5-hydroxytryptamine 3; ASCO, American Society of Clinical Oncology; NCCN, National Comprehensive Cancer Network; PO, orally; bid, twice a day; tid, three times a day; IV, intravenously.

Palliative and Supportive Care

Unlike in chemotherapy where loperamide may be discontinued after initial response, standard doses of loperamide should be continued for the duration of RT. This is because the long duration of fractionated radiation may cause repeated injury to the intestinal mucosa. The dose is increased to 2 mg every 2 hours if the diarrhea persists for more than 24 hours.

If diarrhea has not resolved after another 24 hours on the higher dose of loperamide, the drug should be continued and a second-line agent, such as tincture of opium (paregoric), an antimotility agent, can be added. Diphenoxylate and atropine can also be used, although they do not have as favorable a side effect profile as loperamide. The patient may require outpatient evaluation and IV fluid. Octreotide, antibiotics, and complete stool and blood work-up are usually not necessary in the absence of signs of dehydration or infection. If the diarrhea is severe, persistent, or complicated, hospitalization may be considered (14).

Skin Injury: Acute Dermatitis and Chronic Skin Changes

Radiation-induced skin injury can lead to acute dermatitis and/or chronic skin changes (69,170). These changes can occur at both the entrance and exit site of the irradiation beam. Severity is determined by the dose, fractionation, beam, volume, and surface area. Patient-specific factors also play a role, such as poor nutrition status, pre-existing vascular condition or connective tissue disease, excessive skin folds, or genetics (63). The pathophysiology is a combination of direct radiation injury and a subsequent inflammatory response. Free radicals from ionizing radiation cause alteration of DNA, proteins, lipids, and carbohydrates. Epithelial basal cells, vascular endothelial cells, and Langerhans cells are damaged. A cascade of proinflammatory cytokines, thrombotic factors, growth factors, and other molecules is activated (35).

Acute skin changes may become visible after 10 to 14 hours. They present as erythema, desquamation, edema, necrosis, or ulceration, depending on the dose and duration of radiation exposure. The symptoms usually peak at 1 to 2 weeks after the last dosing and resolve within the next 1 to 3 months, depending on the location. Sweat glands and hair follicles are also damaged. Alopecia may become permanent if there is follicular fibrosis (100). Chronic changes may develop months or years after the initial exposure. Postinflammatory hypo- or hyperpigmentation, textural changes (xerosis and hyperkeratosis), loss of hair follicles and sebaceous glands, atrophy, telangiectasia, or subcutaneous fibrosis are among the manifestations. Fibrosis can result in tissue retraction, pain, and limitation of movement. Scalp appears more tolerant to radiation injury than the skin of the face, neck, trunk, and extremities. Affected skin can be predisposed to ulcers and skin breakdown (43,105). In some patients, radiation recall dermatitis may occur. This happens when a patient who has completed RT encounters a drug and develops skin reaction similar to acute radiation dermatitis. The drugs are usually cytotoxic agents. It is probably due to local cutaneous immunologic responses to the challenging agent (Fig. 95.2) (26).

Mild acute dermatitis is treated symptomatically. Washing with water, gentle cleansing with a mild agent, wearing loose, nonbinding clothing, and avoidance of irritants and ultraviolet exposure all help. When erythema and dry desquamation occurs, creams or ointments (petrolatum-based, castor oil, balsam of Peru, trypsin, trolamine) can be used. Other topical agents such as aloe vera, D-panthenol, and chamomile can also be tried. The use of these agents is supported only by uncontrolled studies or anecdotal evidence (67).

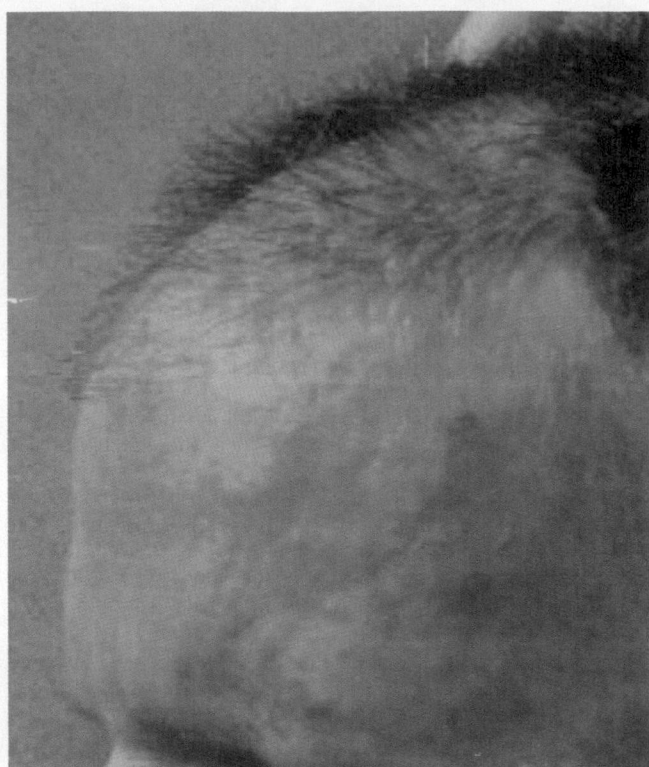

FIGURE 95.2. Acute dermatitis after whole-brain radiation.

The value of topical antioxidants is not established and topical steroids are controversial, with research producing conflicting results. There are concerns of infection and skin atrophy, known side effects of topical steroids. At best, steroids may ameliorate the symptoms, but they do not prevent the dermatitis (142). Topical ascorbic acid lotion (vitamin C) did not show discernible benefit for the prevention of radiation dermatitis (62). Topical sucralfate or hyaluronic acid was shown to be efficacious in some controlled studies (96,99). In a phase III study in breast cancer patients receiving postoperative RT, an extract from calendula plant significantly reduced the occurrence of moderate-to-severe acute dermatitis from 63% to 41% when compared with trolamine, a nonsteroidal agent (130).

When acute dermatitis becomes severe, usual wound care should be applied to the erosions and ulcerations. Key measures are keeping the site clean and moist, pain management, protection from contamination, debridement, and infection control (40,105). During radiation treatment, hydrogel dressings, hydrocolloid dressing, burn pads, or foam dressings can be applied. If the wound is infected, ionic silver powder, topical antibiotics, cadexomer iodine, or maltodextrin powder can be added. Referral to wound care specialists should be made (67). In recent years, more specific agents are being investigated. They include topical granulocyte-macrophage–colony-stimulating factor, tacrolimus, pimecrolimus, and platelet-derived growth factor (69).

Chronic skin changes from radiation injury are harder to treat. Chronic fibrosis is associated with high incidence of skin breakdown and infection. Pentoxifylline (Trental) appears to have an antifibrotic effect. Oral pentoxifylline (800 mg/d) and vitamin E (1,000 IU/d) for 6 months significantly reduce radiation-induced fibrosis (34). Prophylactic use of pentoxifylline significantly reduces late skin changes, fibrosis, and soft tissue necrosis in a randomized controlled study, possibly through its protective effect against vascular pathology (7). Intramuscular liposomal superoxide dismutase, subcutaneous interferon gamma, or hyperbaric oxygen therapy has also been used. A team approach should be adopted that includes wound care, physical therapy, deep massage, and pain management.

:: | Genitourinary Tract Injury

Urinary Symptoms

Irradiation to the pelvic region as part of treatment for cancer of the prostate, uterus, ovary, cervix rectum, or urinary bladder can cause urinary problems due to injury to mucosa, vasculature, and smooth muscles (77,102). Acute reactions occur within 3 to 6 months of treatment. Chronic changes occur later. Acute reactions present as dysuria, frequency, and urgency as a result of radiation cystitis. They are usually not as severe as some of the cystitis caused by chemotherapy. Strictures or fistula can develop during the years following RT (57,127).

If infection is ruled out, symptomatic relief with phenazopyridine (Pyridium) is usually the first-line treatment for acute symptoms. It is given at 200 mg orally, three times a day. Phenazopyridine accumulates in the urine essentially unchanged and acts as a topical analgesic within the bladder. Patients should be warned that phenazopyridine turns the urine into a bright orange color and can stain clothing. If the symptoms are not adequately relieved, antispasmodics can be added. Oxybutynin (Ditropan) or flavoxate (Urispas) help relax the smooth muscles and reduce urinary urgency and frequency (113). Tolterodine (Detrol) is a cholinergic antagonist that is also effective for overactive bladder. It causes less dry mouth but its response rate is lower (37). Trospium (Sanctura) is a new drug approved in the United States in 2004. It was documented to improve symptoms in radiation-induced cystitis and is significantly better tolerated than immediate-release oxybutynin (138). In patients with severe pain, aggressive pain control with opioids may be needed.

Symptomatic management of chronic changes is similar to that of acute reactions. Dilatation or placement of a permanent catheter may be required for significant obstruction. Patients not responding to less aggressive treatment may be candidates for reconstructive surgery to repair the stricture, sphincter failure, or fistula.

Female Sexuality

High-dose radiation to the pelvis causes varying degrees of sexual dysfunction related to injury to the ovaries and vagina (36,156). Ovarian failure as a result of pelvis irradiation leads to postmenopausal changes. Acute injury occurs during the course of RT and the following few months. It usually presents as vaginal and vulval mucositis, pain, and ulceration. Chronic changes are less frequent than acute changes, which can develop more than 3 months after the completion of treatment. Chronic changes include fibrosis, loss of elasticity and sensation, susceptibility to trauma and infection, postcoital bleeding, and dyspareunia (28,145,172).

Maintenance of local hygiene, aggressive treatment of infection, and regular dilatation of the vaginal canal help reduce the acute reaction. Hormone replacement therapy and application of lubricants for mucosal dryness can be used to treat acute injury. To prevent chronic changes, uses of vaginal dilators, lubricants, and supplemental estrogen were shown to be helpful. When fibrosis is established, treatment may require more drastic measures, such as hyperbaric oxygen therapy or surgical reconstruction. Although these are common options in clinical practice, the level of evidence supporting their use varies (36).

Most studies of topical estrogen showed benefit (65,129). Radiation causes damage to the epithelium, which may persist for another 3 to 6 months after therapy. Topical estrogen promotes epithelial regeneration. Benzydamine is an anti-inflammatory that also has analgesic, local anesthetic, and antimicrobial effects. It can be applied topically to achieve a higher local tissue concentration. It reduced both subjective symptoms and objective observation of vaginal mucositis (15,166). There have been several uncontrolled studies of hyperbaric oxygen therapy in the treatment of established necrotic wound resulting from perineal and vaginal radiation; the strength of evidence is modest (23,171). In women with severe radiation damage, such as perineal defect or obliteration of vagina, reconstructive surgery may be considered. All reported studies are retrospective (36).

Male Sexuality

When planning RT for prostate cancer, its effect on male sexual function must be considered and discussed with the patient. Although the rate of erectile dysfunction (ED) is lower in patients receiving RT versus radical prostatectomy, sexual dysfunctions remain one of the most important posttreatment quality of life issues (136). A survey showed that 68% of men aged 45 to 70 years were willing to trade off a 10% or greater advantage in 5-year survival to maintain sexual potency (149). Onset of ED is gradual, usually beginning about 6 months posttreatment and continuing to deteriorate for 4 years (51).

RT does not appear to reduce testosterone production or cause pelvic nerve injury (158). In addition to psychological reasons, vascular changes after RT appear to be the predominant cause of postradiation male sexual dysfunction. As such, smoking and hypertension as risk factors (53,178). With external-beam RT, the rates of ED vary from 7% to 72%, a wide range attributed to the study populations. Brachytherapy is associated with 2% to 89% of ED (70). Diminished sexual desire, decreased orgasmic pleasure, and a reduced ejaculation volume are other problems reported by patients (64).

Treatment of post-RT sexual dysfunction should take a multidisciplinary approach including psychosocial evaluation and counseling, pharmacologic intervention, and exploration of mechanical devices (70,108). The mainstay of pharmacologic treatment is phosphodiesterase inhibitors in patients with arteriogenic ED. In a single-arm study, sildenafil (Viagra) was found to improve erectile function in 77% of patients treated with external-beam RT. Its effect was less prominent in patients receiving concurrent hormonal therapy (169). In another single-arm study of a similar population, sildenafil was effective in 74% of patients. Patients with some residual erectile function responded better (179). For patients receiving brachytherapy, up to 85% responded favorably to sildenafil, comparable to those who underwent bilateral nerve-sparing radical prostatectomy and significantly better than patients who underwent unilateral nerve-sparing or nonnerve-sparing surgery. Diabetes is a risk factor for poor response (106,107). There is no study of tadalafil (Cialis) or vardenafil (Levitra) in these patient populations to date.

Intracavernosal injection of prostaglandins or phentolamine-papaverine is also effective. For patients who are refractory to pharmacologic intervention, implantation of a penile prosthesis can be considered. Minimal intraoperative and postoperative complications and an excellent patient satisfaction rate were reported (41). Vacuum devices are another option.

:: | Nutrition

Nutritional support is very important for patients undergoing RT. Patients may be malnourished when they come for initial treatment. Cancer creates a catabolic state. Anorexia, early satiety, nausea and vomiting, and involvement of the alimentary tract by cancer all contribute to impaired nutrition intake, digestion, and absorption. Once RT is started, a patient's nutritional status can deteriorate, especially in those with GI toxicity. A weight loss of more than 20% of total body weight is associated with poorer outcome. Nutritional support measures include prescription of appetite enhancers, provision of a high-quality diet, ensuring adequate enteral intake via tube feeding, and hyperalimentation with parenteral nutrition (71). A multidisciplinary approach should be taken with the involvement of GI physicians, nutritionists, and nursing staff.

A systematic review showed that only progestins (megestrol [Megace]) and corticosteroids (methylprednisolone, prednisolone, and dexamethasone) are supported by evidence for cancer-related anorexia. A number of other drugs have been tested. They include metoclopramide, cyproheptadine, pentoxifylline, melatonin, erythropoietin, eicosapentaenoic acid (fish oil), androgenic steroids (nandrolone or fluoxymesterone), ghrelin, interferon, and cannabinoid (dronabinol [Marinol]). Data are mixed. No strong recommendation can be made at this point regarding these agents (33,176).

Cancer patients tend to have a higher protein turnover. Adequate protein intake is critical in patients undergoing cancer treatment. Daily intake of 1.5 to 2.0 g of protein per kilogram of ideal body weight generally maintains a positive nitrogen balance. Caloric intake help maintain the weight. Between 30% and 90% of total calories can come from carbohydrates. Fat provides energy, serves as vehicle for other nutrients, and performs other important biological functions. It usually makes up around 30% of the content in enteral formulas. Vitamins, minerals, and other micronutrients should be included. Sufficient water intake is required to offset the 2.5-liter daily fluid loss. Dietary counseling improves outcomes in selected populations (132). Body weight and serum markers (albumin, transferrin, and prealbumin) can be monitored to assess whether the nutritional support is adequate (24,31,160).

In patients with moderate-to-severe radiation-induced oral mucositis or esophagitis, oral nutritional support can be challenging. Tube feeding bypasses the injured tissues and provides direct access to the absorption surface. Nasogastric or nasojejunal tubes enable short-term access. For longer term access (>30 days), gastrostomy, gastrojejunostomy, and jejunostomy tubes can be placed endoscopically, radiologically, or surgically. Percutaneous endoscopic gastrostomy is increasingly the method of choice, often placed prophylactically when severe upper GI toxicity is anticipated (25,54,101,144). Gastrostomy tube placement is not without risk. Some series suggest a 17% morbidity rate. In 3% of patients, serious complications such as peritonitis, sepsis, perforation, and dislodgement were reported (56,140). Metastasis to percutaneous endoscopic gastrostomy site has also been reported, likely due to direct implantation of cancer cells (175). For patients with reflux esophagitis, gastroparesis, aspiration pneumonia, or limited stomach volume, a jejunostomy tube may be placed instead. The feeding tube should be cared for properly to prevent displacement or malfunctioning such as clogging.

When adequate nutrition intake can be achieved, enteral intake is preferred over parenteral support because it uses and helps maintain the existing alimentary functions. It is less expensive, safer, and associated with fewer side effects. However, in patients without a functioning GI tract because of obstruction, poor GI motility, intractable vomiting, severe diarrhea, short bowel syndrome, or severe pancreatitis, total parenteral nutrition may be appropriate. Implementation of total parenteral nutrition requires special expertise and is done in a concerted manner between the cancer-treating team and the nutrition support team (98,146).

Acknowledgments

The authors thank Dr. Joseph Huryn, Chief, Dental Service, and Dr. Liang Deng, Dermatology Service, at Memorial Sloan-Kettering Cancer Center for providing the photographs for this chapter, and Jyothirmai Gubili for expert editorial assistance.

References

1. Al-Qahtani K, Hier MP, Sultanum K, et al. The role of submandibular salivary gland transfer in preventing xerostomia in the chemoradiotherapy patient. *Oral Surg Oral Med Oral Pathol Oral Radiol Endod* 2006;101:753–756.
2. Amosson CM, Teh BS, Van TJ, et al. Dosimetric predictors of xerostomia for head-and-neck cancer patients treated with the smart (simultaneous modulated accelerated radiation therapy) boost technique. *Int J Radiat Oncol Biol Phys* 2003;56:136–144.
3. Andrykowski MA, Schmidt JE, Salsman JM, et al. Use of a case definition approach to identify cancer-related fatigue in women undergoing adjuvant therapy for breast cancer. *J Clin Oncol* 2005;23:6613–6622.
4. Anne PR, Curran WJ, Jr. A phase II trial of subcutaneous amifostine and radiation therapy in patients with head and neck cancer. *Semin Radiat Oncol* 2002;12[1 Suppl 1]:18–19.
5. Anthony L, Bowen J, Garden A, et al. New thoughts on the pathobiology of regimen-related mucosal injury. *Support Care Cancer* 2006;14:516–518.
6. Athanassiou H, Antonadou D, Coliarakis N, et al. Protective effect of amifostine during fractionated radiotherapy in patients with pelvic carcinomas: results of a randomized trial. *Int J Radiat Oncol Biol Phys* 2003;56:1154–1160.
7. Aygenc E, Celikkanat S, Kaymakci M, et al. Prophylactic effect of pentoxifylline on radiotherapy complications: a clinical study. *Otolaryngol Head Neck Surg* 2004;130:351–356.
8. Barasch A, Elad S, Altman A, et al. Antimicrobials, mucosal coating agents, anesthetics, analgesics, and nutritional supplements for alimentary tract mucositis. *Support Care Cancer* 2006;14:528–532.
9. Bardet E, Martin L, Calais G, et al. Preliminary data of the GORTEC 2000-02 phase III trial comparing intravenous and subcutaneous administration of amifostine for head and neck tumors treated by external radiotherapy. *Semin Oncol* 2002;29[6 Suppl 19]:57–60.
10. Barsevick AM, Whitmer K, Nail LM, et al. Symptom cluster research: conceptual, design, measurement, and analysis issues. *J Pain Symptom Manage* 2006;31:85–95.
11. Baughan CA, Canney PA, Buchanan RB, et al. A randomized trial to assess the efficacy of 5-aminosalicylic acid for the prevention of radiation enteritis. *Clin Oncol (R Coll Radiol)* 1993;5:19–24.
12. Beck S. Impact of a systematic oral care protocol on stomatitis after chemotherapy. *Cancer Nurs* 1979;2:185–199.
13. Bensadoun RJ, Schubert MM, Lalla RV, et al. Amifostine in the management of radiation-induced and chemo-induced mucositis. *Support Care Cancer* 2006;14:566–572.
14. Benson AB 3rd, Ajani JA, Catalano RB, et al. Recommended guidelines for the treatment of cancer treatment-induced diarrhea. *J Clin Oncol* 2004;22:2918–2926.
15. Bentivoglio G, Diani F. Use of topical benzydamine in gynecology. *Clin Exp Obstet Gynecol* 1981;8:103–110.
16. Berk LB, Shivnani AT, Small W Jr. Pathophysiology and management of radiation-induced xerostomia. *J Support Oncol* 2005;3:191–200.
17. Blijlevens NM, Donnelly JP, De Pauw BE. Mucosal barrier injury: biology, pathology, clinical counterparts and consequences of intensive treatment for haematological malignancy: an overview. *Bone Marrow Transplant* 2000;25:1269–1278.
18. Blom M, Dawidson I, Fernberg JO, et al. Acupuncture treatment of patients with radiation-induced xerostomia. *Eur J Cancer B Oral Oncol* 1996;32B:182–190.
19. Blom M, Lundeberg T. Long-term follow-up of patients treated with acupuncture for xerostomia and the influence of additional treatment. *Oral Dis* 2000;6:15–24.
20. Borowski B, Benhamou E, Pico JL, et al. Prevention of oral mucositis in patients treated with high-dose chemotherapy and bone marrow transplantation: a randomised controlled trial comparing two protocols of dental care. *Eur J Cancer B Oral Oncol* 1994;30B:93–97.
21. Brizel DM, Wasserman TH, Henke M, et al. Phase III randomized trial of amifostine as a radioprotector in head and neck cancer. *J Clin Oncol* 2000;18:3339–3345.
22. Brown P, Clark MM, Atherton P, et al. Will improvement in quality of life (QOL) impact fatigue in patients receiving radiation therapy for advanced cancer? *Am J Clin Oncol* 2006;29:52–58.
23. Bui QC, Lieber M, Withers HR, et al. The efficacy of hyperbaric oxygen therapy in the treatment of radiation-induced late side effects. *Int J Radiat Oncol Biol Phys* 2004;60:871–878.
24. Buzby K. Overview: screening, assessing, and monitoring. In: Bloch A, ed. *Nutrition management of the cancer patient.* Rockville, MD: Aspen Publishers, Inc.; 1990:15–22.
25. Byrne KR, Fang JC. Endoscopic placement of enteral feeding catheters. *Curr Opin Gastroenterol* 2006;22:546–550.
26. Camidge R, Price A. Characterizing the phenomenon of radiation recall dermatitis. *Radiother Oncol* 2001;59:237–245.
27. Carnel SB, Blakeslee DB, Oswald SG, et al. Treatment of radiation- and chemotherapy-induced stomatitis. *Otolaryngol Head Neck Surg* 1990;102:326–330.
28. Cartwright-Alcarese F. Addressing sexual dysfunction following radiation therapy for a gynecologic malignancy. *Oncol Nurs Forum* 1995;22:1227–1232.
29. Cheng KK, Molassiotis A, Chang AM, et al. Evaluation of an oral care protocol intervention in the prevention of chemotherapy-induced oral mucositis in paediatric cancer patients. *Eur J Cancer* 2001;37:2056–2063.
30. Coetzee MJ, Boshoff B, Goedhals L, et al. Formula C—popular, cheap and readily available relief for radiation and cancer chemotherapy mucositis. *S Afr Med J* 1997;87:80–81.

31. Colasanto JM, Prasad P, Nash MA, et al. Nutritional support of patients undergoing radiation therapy for head and neck cancer. *Oncology (Williston Park)* 2005;19:371–382.

32. Conference CSO. New approaches to preventing xerostomia. *J Support Oncol* 2006;4:87–88.

33. Davis MP, Dreicer R, Walsh D, et al. Appetite and cancer-associated anorexia: a review. *J Clin Oncol* 2004;22:1510–1517.

34. Delanian S, Balla-Mekias S, Lefaix JL. Striking regression of chronic radiotherapy damage in a clinical trial of combined pentoxifylline and tocopherol. *J Clin Oncol* 1999;17:3283–3290.

35. Denham JW, Hauer-Jensen M. The radiotherapeutic injury—a complex 'wound.' *Radiother Oncol* 2002;63:129–145.

36. Denton AS, Maher EJ. Interventions for the physical aspects of sexual dysfunction in women following pelvic radiotherapy. *Cochrane Database Syst Rev* 2003;CD003750.

37. Diokno AC, Appell RA, Sand PK, et al. Prospective, randomized, double-blind study of the efficacy and tolerability of the extended-release formulations of oxybutynin and tolterodine for overactive bladder: results of the OPERA trial. *Mayo Clin Proc* 2003;78:687–695.

38. Dodd MJ, Dibble SL, Miaskowski C, et al. Randomized clinical trial of the effectiveness of 3 commonly used mouthwashes to treat chemotherapy-induced mucositis. *Oral Surg Oral Med Oral Pathol Oral Radiol Endod* 2000;90:39–47.

39. Dodd MJ, Larson PJ, Dibble SL, et al. Randomized clinical trial of chlorhexidine versus placebo for prevention of oral mucositis in patients receiving chemotherapy. *Oncol Nurs Forum* 1996;23:921–927.

40. Dormand EL, Banwell PE, Goodacre TE. Radiotherapy and wound healing. *Int Wound J* 2005;2:112–127.

41. Dubocq FM, Bianco FJ Jr, Maralani SJ, et al. Outcome analysis of penile implant surgery after external beam radiation for prostate cancer. *J Urol* 1997;158:1787–1790.

42. Dudjak LA. Mouth care for mucositis due to radiation therapy. *Cancer Nurs* 1987;10:131–140.

43. Dutreix J. Human skin: early and late reactions in relation to dose and its time distribution. *Br J Radiol Suppl* 1986;19:22–28.

44. Eilers J, Epstein JB. Assessment and measurement of oral mucositis. *Semin Oncol Nurs* 2004;20:22–29.

45. Eisbruch A, Dawson LA, Kim HM, et al. Conformal and intensity modulated irradiation of head and neck cancer: the potential for improved target irradiation, salivary gland function, and quality of life. *Acta Otorhinolaryngol Belg* 1999;53:271–275.

46. Eisbruch A, Kim HM, Terrell JE, et al. Xerostomia and its predictors following parotid-sparing irradiation of head-and-neck cancer. *Int J Radiat Oncol Biol Phys* 2001;50:695–704.

47. Epstein JB, Silverman S Jr, Paggiarino DA, et al. Benzydamine HCl for prophylaxis of radiation-induced oral mucositis: results from a multicenter, randomized, double-blind, placebo-controlled clinical trial. *Cancer* 2001;92:875–885.

48. Feyer P, Maranzano E, Molassiotis A, et al. Radiotherapy-induced nausea and vomiting (RINV): antiemetic guidelines. *Support Care Cancer* 2005;13:122–128.

49. Feyer PC, Stewart AL, Titlbach OJ. Aetiology and prevention of emesis induced by radiotherapy. *Support Care Cancer* 1998;6:253–260.

50. Foote RL, Loprinzi CL, Frank AR, et al. Randomized trial of a chlorhexidine mouthwash for alleviation of radiation-induced mucositis. *J Clin Oncol* 1994;12:2630–2633.

51. Fransson P, Widmark A. Self-assessed sexual function after pelvic irradiation for prostate carcinoma. Comparison with an age-matched control group. *Cancer* 1996;78:1066–1078.

52. Geinitz H, Zimmermann FB, Thamm R, et al. Fatigue in patients with adjuvant radiation therapy for breast cancer: long-term follow-up. *J Cancer Res Clin Oncol* 2004;130:327–333.

53. Goldstein I, Feldman MI, Deckers PJ, et al. Radiation-associated impotence. A clinical study of its mechanism. *JAMA* 1984;251:903–910.

54. Gopalan S, Khanna S. Enteral nutrition delivery technique. *Curr Opin Clin Nutr Metab Care* 2003;6:313–317.

55. Gralla RJ. Quality-of-life considerations in patients with advanced lung cancer: effect of topotecan on symptom palliation and quality of life. *Oncologist* 2004;[9 Suppl 6]:14–24.

56. Grant MD, Rudberg MA, Brody JA. Gastrostomy placement and mortality among hospitalized Medicare beneficiaries. *JAMA* 1998;279:1973–1976.

57. Greskovich FJ, Zagars GK, Sherman NE, et al. Complications following external beam radiation therapy for prostate cancer: an analysis of patients treated with and without staging pelvic lymphadenectomy. *J Urol* 1991;146:798–802.

58. Guchelaar HJ, Vermes A, Meerwaldt JH. Radiation-induced xerostomia: pathophysiology, clinical course and supportive treatment. *Support Care Cancer* 1997;5:281–288.

59. Gwede CK. Overview of radiation- and chemoradiation-induced diarrhea. *Semin Oncol Nurs* 2003;19[4 Suppl 3]:6–10.

60. Hagen NA, Addington-Hall J, Sharpe M, et al. The Birmingham International Workshop on Supportive, Palliative, and End-of-Life Care Research. *Cancer* 2006.

61. Haker E, Egekvist H, Bjerring P. Effect of sensory stimulation (acupuncture) on sympathetic and parasympathetic activities in healthy subjects. *J Auton Nerv Syst* 2000;79:52–59.

62. Halperin EC, Gaspar L, George S, et al. A double-blind, randomized, prospective trial to evaluate topical vitamin C solution for the prevention of radiation dermatitis. CNS Cancer Consortium. *Int J Radiat Oncol Biol Phys* 1993;26:413–416.

63. Harper JL, Franklin LE, Jenrette JM, et al. Skin toxicity during breast irradiation: pathophysiology and management. *South Med J* 2004;97:989–993.

64. Helgason AR, Fredrikson M, Adolfsson J, et al. Decreased sexual capacity after external radiation therapy for prostate cancer impairs quality of life. *Int J Radiat Oncol Biol Phys* 1995;32:33–39.

65. Hintz BL, Kagan AR, Gilbert HA, et al. Systemic absorption of conjugated estrogenic cream by the irradiated vagina. *Gynecol Oncol* 1981;12:75–82.

66. Holmes MD, Chen WY, Feskanich D, et al. Physical activity and survival after breast cancer diagnosis. *JAMA* 2005;293:2479–2486.

67. Hom DB, Adams G, Koreis M, et al. Choosing the optimal wound dressing for irradiated soft tissue wounds. *Otolaryngol Head Neck Surg* 1999;121:591–598.

68. Hudis CA, Van Belle S, Chang J, et al. rHuEPO and treatment outcomes: the clinical experience. *Oncologist* 2004;[9 Suppl 5]:55–69.

69. Hymes SR, Strom EA, Fife C. Radiation dermatitis: clinical presentation, pathophysiology, and treatment 2006. *J Am Acad Dermatol* 2006;54:28–46.

70. Incrocci L, Slob AK, Levendag PC. Sexual (dys)function after radiotherapy for prostate cancer: a review. *Int J Radiat Oncol Biol Phys* 2002;52:681–693.

71. Isenring EA, Capra S, Bauer JD. Nutrition intervention is beneficial in oncology outpatients receiving radiotherapy to the gastrointestinal or head and neck area. *Br J Cancer* 2004;91:447–452.

72. Jha N, Seikaly H, Harris J, et al. Prevention of radiation induced xerostomia by surgical transfer of submandibular salivary gland into the submental space. *Radiother Oncol* 2003;66:283–289.

73. Johnson JR, Williams G, Pazdur R. End points and United States Food and Drug Administration approval of oncology drugs. *J Clin Oncol* 2003;21:1404–1411.

74. Johnson JT, Ferretti GA, Nethery WJ, et al. Oral pilocarpine for post-irradiation xerostomia in patients with head and neck cancer. *N Engl J Med* 1993;329:390–395.

75. Johnstone PA, Niemtzow RC, Riffenburgh RH. Acupuncture for xerostomia: clinical update. *Cancer* 2002;94:1151–1156.

76. Johnstone PA, Peng YP, May BC, et al. Acupuncture for pilocarpine-resistant xerostomia following radiotherapy for head and neck malignancies. *Int J Radiat Oncol Biol Phys* 2001;50:353–357.

77. Kagan AR. Bladder, testicle, and prostate irradiation injury. *Front Radiat Ther Oncol* 1989;23:323–340.

78. Keefe DM. Gastrointestinal mucositis: a new biological model. *Support Care Cancer* 2004;12:6–9.

79. Kenny SA. Effect of two oral care protocols on the incidence of stomatitis in hematology patients. *Cancer Nurs* 1990;13:345–353.

80. Kilic D, Egehan I, Ozenirler S, et al. Double-blinded, randomized, placebo-controlled study to evaluate the effectiveness of sulphasalazine in preventing acute gastrointestinal complications due to radiotherapy. *Radiother Oncol* 2000;57:125–129.

81. Kim JH, Chu FC, Lakshmi V, et al. Benzydamine HCl, a new agent for the treatment of radiation mucositis of the oropharynx. *Am J Clin Oncol* 1986;9:132–134.

82. Kimura A, Sato A. Somatic regulation of autonomic functions in anesthetized animals—neural mechanisms of physical therapy including acupuncture. *Jpn J Vet Res* 1997;45:137–145.

83. Kneebone A, Mameghan H, Bolin T, et al. The effect of oral sucralfate on the acute proctitis associated with prostate radiotherapy: a double-blind, randomized trial. *Int J Radiat Oncol Biol Phys* 2001;51:628–635.

84. Knobf MT, Sun Y. A longitudinal study of symptoms and self-care activities in women treated with primary radiotherapy for breast cancer. *Cancer Nurs* 2005;28:210–218.

85. Komaki R, Lee JS, Kaplan B, et al. Randomized phase III study of chemoradiation with or without amifostine for patients with favorable performance status inoperable stage II–III non-small cell lung cancer: preliminary results. *Semin Radiat Oncol* 2002;12[1 Suppl 1]:46–49.

86. Kondziolka D, Niranjan A, Flickinger JC, et al. Radiosurgery with or without whole-brain radiotherapy for brain metastases: the patients' perspective regarding complications. *Am J Clin Oncol* 2005;28:173–179.

87. Koukourakis MI. Amifostine: is there evidence of tumor protection? *Semin Oncol* 2003;30[6 Suppl 18]:18–30.

88. Koukourakis MI, Kyrias G, Kakolyris S, et al. Subcutaneous administration of amifostine during fractionated radiotherapy: a randomized phase II study. *J Clin Oncol* 2000;18:2226–2233.

89. Kouvaris J, Kouloulias V, Malas E, et al. Amifostine as radioprotective agent for the rectal mucosa during irradiation of pelvic tumors. A phase II randomized study using various toxicity scales and rectosigmoidoscopy. *Strahlenther Onkol* 2003;179:167–174.

90. Kris MG, Hesketh PJ, Somerfield MR, et al. American Society of Clinical Oncology guideline for antiemetics in oncology: update 2006. *J Clin Oncol* 2006;24:2932–2947.

91. Lai YH, Chang JT, Keefe FJ, et al. Symptom distress, catastrophic thinking, and hope in nasopharyngeal carcinoma patients. *Cancer Nurs* 2003;26:485–493.

92. Lee N, Xia P, Fischbein NJ, et al. Intensity-modulated radiation therapy for head-and-neck cancer: the UCSF experience focusing on target volume delineation. *Int J Radiat Oncol Biol Phys* 2003;57:49–60.

93. Leong SS, Tan EH, Fong KW, et al. Randomized double-blind trial of combined modality treatment with or without amifostine in unresectable stage III non-small-cell lung cancer. *J Clin Oncol* 2003;21:1767–1774.

94. LeVeque FG, Montgomery M, Potter D, et al. A multicenter, randomized, double-blind, placebo-controlled, dose-titration study of oral pilocarpine for treatment of radiation-induced xerostomia in head and neck cancer patients. *J Clin Oncol* 1993;11:1124–1131.

95. Levy-Polack MP, Sebelli P, Polack NL. Incidence of oral complications and application of a preventive protocol in children with acute leukemia. *Spec Care Dentist* 1998;18:189–193.

96. Liguori V, Guillemin C, Pesce GF, et al. Double-blind, randomized clinical study comparing hyaluronic acid cream to placebo in patients treated with radiotherapy. *Radiother Oncol* 1997;42:155–161.

97. Loaiza LA, Yamaguchi S, Ito M, et al. Electro-acupuncture stimulation to muscle afferents in anesthetized rats modulates the blood flow to the knee joint through autonomic reflexes and nitric oxide. *Auton Neurosci* 2002;97:103–109.

98. Mahaffey SM, Copeland EM 3rd. Total parenteral nutrition in the cancer patient. *Adv Surg* 1987;20:47–67.

99. Maiche A, Isokangas OP, Grohn P. Skin protection by sucralfate cream during electron beam therapy. *Acta Oncol* 1994;33:201–203.

100. Malkinson FD, Keane JT. Radiobiology of the skin: review of some effects on epidermis and hair. *J Invest Dermatol* 1981;77:133–138.

101. Marcy PY, Magne N, Bensadoun RJ, et al. Systematic percutaneous fluoroscopic gastrostomy for concomitant radiochemotherapy of advanced head and neck cancer: optimization of therapy. *Support Care Cancer* 2000;8(5):410–413.

102. Marks LB, Carroll PR, Dugan TC, et al. The response of the urinary bladder, urethra, and ureter to radiation and chemotherapy. *Int J Radiat Oncol Biol Phys* 1995;31:1257–1280.

103. Martenson JA, Bollinger JW, Sloan JA, et al. Sucralfate in the prevention of treatment-induced diarrhea in patients receiving pelvic radiation therapy: a North Central Cancer Treatment Group phase III double-blind placebo-controlled trial. *J Clin Oncol* 2000;18:1239–1245.

104. Martenson JA Jr, Hyland G, Moertel CG, et al. Olsalazine is contraindicated during pelvic radiation therapy: results of a double-blind, randomized clinical trial. *Int J Radiat Oncol Biol Phys* 1996;35(2):299–303.
105. Mendelsohn FA, Divino CM, Reis ED, et al. Wound care after radiation therapy. *Adv Skin Wound Care* 2002;15:216–224.
106. Merrick GS, Butler WM, Galbreath RW, et al. Erectile function after permanent prostate brachytherapy. *Int J Radiat Oncol Biol Phys* 2002;52:893–902.
107. Merrick GS, Butler WM, Lief JH, et al. Efficacy of sildenafil citrate in prostate brachytherapy patients with erectile dysfunction. *Urology* 1999;53:1112–1116.
108. Merrick GS, Wallner KE, Butler WM. Management of sexual dysfunction after prostate brachytherapy. *Oncology (Williston Park)* 2003;17:52–62; discussion 62, 67–70,73.
109. Meyerhardt JA, Giovannucci EL, Holmes MD, et al. Physical activity and survival after colorectal cancer diagnosis. *J Clin Oncol* 2006;24:3527–3534.
110. Meyerhardt JA, Heseltine D, Niedzwiecki D, et al. Impact of physical activity on cancer recurrence and survival in patients with stage III colon cancer: findings from CALGB 89803. *J Clin Oncol* 2006;24:3535–3541.
111. Miaskowski C, Dodd M, Lee K. Symptom clusters: the new frontier in symptom management research. *J Natl Cancer Inst Monogr* 2004:17–21.
112. Middlekauff HR, Shah JB, Yu JL, et al. Acupuncture effects on autonomic responses to cold pressor and handgrip exercise in healthy humans. *Clin Auton Res* 2004;14:113–118.
113. Milani R, Scalambrino S, Carrera S, et al. Flavoxate hydrochloride for urinary urgency after pelvic radiotherapy: comparison of 600 mg versus 1200 mg daily dosages. *J Int Med Res* 1988;16:71–74.
114. Morganstein WM. Acupuncture in the treatment of xerostomia: clinical report. *Gen Dent* 2005;53(3):223–227.
115. Mosteller F, Falotico-Taylor J, eds, *Institute of medicine: quality of life and technology assessment*. Washington, DC: The National Academy Press; 1989.
116. Movsas B, Scott C, Langer C, et al. Randomized trial of amifostine in locally advanced non-small-cell lung cancer patients receiving chemotherapy and hyperfractionated radiation: radiation therapy oncology group trial 98-01. *J Clin Oncol* 2005;23(10):2145–2154.
117. Munter MW, Karger CP, Hoffner SG, et al. Evaluation of salivary gland function after treatment of head-and-neck tumors with intensity-modulated radiotherapy by quantitative pertechnetate scintigraphy. *Int J Radiat Oncol Biol Phys* 2004;58:175–184.
118. Myerson R, Zobeiri I, Birnbaum E, et al. Early results from a phase I/II radiation dose-escalation study with concurrent amifostine and infusional 5-fluorouracil chemotherapy for preoperative treatment of unresectable or locally recurrent rectal carcinoma. *Semin Oncol* 2002;29[6 Suppl 19]:29–33.
119. NCCN antiemesis practice guidelines. *Oncology (Williston Park)* 1997;11:57–89.
120. Network NCC. NCCN antiemesis guidelines emphasize 'delayed' emesis, new 5-HT3 inhibitors, and NK-1 blockers. *J Support Oncol* 2004;2:366.
121. Nieuw Amerongen AV, Veerman EC. Current therapies for xerostomia and salivary gland hypofunction associated with cancer therapies. *Support Care Cancer* 2003;11:226–231.
122. O'Brien BE, Kaklamani VG, Benson AB, 3rd. The assessment and management of cancer treatment-related diarrhea. *Clin Colorectal Cancer* 2005;4(6):375–381; discussion 382–383.
123. O'Brien PC, Franklin CI, Dear KB, et al. A phase III double-blind randomised study of rectal sucralfate suspension in the prevention of acute radiation proctitis. *Radiother Oncol* 1997;45:117–123.
124. Parliament MB, Scrimger RA, Anderson SG, et al. Preservation of oral health-related quality of life and salivary flow rates after inverse-planned intensity-modulated radiotherapy (IMRT) for head-and-neck cancer. *Int J Radiat Oncol Biol Phys* 2004;58:663–673.
125. Pedersen AM, Bardow A, Jensen SB, et al. Saliva and gastrointestinal functions of taste, mastication, swallowing and digestion. *Oral Dis* 2002;8:117–129.
126. Perch SJ, Machtay M, Markiewicz DA, et al. Decreased acute toxicity by using midline mucosa-sparing blocks during radiation therapy for carcinoma of the oral cavity, oropharynx, and nasopharynx. *Radiology* 1995;197:863–866.
127. Perez CA, Camel HM, Kuske RR, et al. Radiation therapy alone in the treatment of carcinoma of the uterine cervix: a 20-year experience. *Gynecol Oncol* 1986;23:127–140.
128. Peterson DE, Keefe DM, Hutchins RD, et al. Alimentary tract mucositis in cancer patients: impact of terminology and assessment on research and clinical practice. *Support Care Cancer* 2006;14:499–504.
129. Pitkin RM, VanVoorhis LW. Postirradiation vaginitis. An evaluation of prophylaxis with topical estrogen. *Radiology* 1971;99:417–421.
130. Pommier P, Gomez F, Sunyach MP, et al. Phase III randomized trial of Calendula officinalis compared with trolamine for the prevention of acute dermatitis during irradiation for breast cancer. *J Clin Oncol* 2004;22:1447–1453.
131. Priestman TJ, Baum M. Evaluation of quality of life in patients receiving treatment for advanced breast cancer. *Lancet* 1976;1:899–900.
132. Ravasco P, Monteiro-Grillo I, Vidal PM, et al. Dietary counseling improves patient outcomes: a prospective, randomized, controlled trial in colorectal cancer patients undergoing radiotherapy. *J Clin Oncol* 2005;23:1431–1438.
133. Resbeut M, Marteau P, Cowen D, et al. A randomized double blind placebo controlled multicenter study of mesalazine for the prevention of acute radiation enteritis. *Radiother Oncol* 1997;44:59–63.
134. Rieger J, Seikaly H, Jha N, et al. Submandibular gland transfer for prevention of xerostomia after radiation therapy: swallowing outcomes. *Arch Otolaryngol Head Neck Surg* 2005;131:140–145.
135. Rieke JW, Hafermann MD, Johnson JT, et al. Oral pilocarpine for radiation-induced xerostomia: integrated efficacy and safety results from two prospective randomized clinical trials. *Int J Radiat Oncol Biol Phys* 1995;31:661–669.
136. Robinson JW, Dufour MS, Fung TS. Erectile functioning of men treated for prostate carcinoma. *Cancer* 1997;79:538–544.
137. Rothwell BR, Spektor WS. Palliation of radiation-related mucositis. *Spec Care Dentist* 1990;10:21–25.
138. Rovner ES. Trospium chloride in the management of overactive bladder. *Drugs* 2004;64:2433–2446.
139. Rubenstein EB, Peterson DE, Schubert M, et al. Clinical practice guidelines for the prevention and treatment of cancer therapy-induced oral and gastrointestinal mucositis. *Cancer* 2004;100[9 Suppl]:2026–2046.
140. Safadi BY, Marks JM, Ponsky JL. Percutaneous endoscopic gastrostomy. *Gastrointest Endosc Clin North Am* 1998;8:551–568.
141. Samaranayake LP, Robertson AG, MacFarlane TW, et al. The effect of chlorhexidine and benzydamine mouthwashes on mucositis induced by therapeutic irradiation. *Clin Radiol* 1988;39:291–294.
142. Schmuth M, Wimmer MA, Hofer S, et al. Topical corticosteroid therapy for acute radiation dermatitis: a prospective, randomized, double-blind study. *Br J Dermatol* 2002;146:983–991.
143. Seikaly H, Jha N, Harris JR, et al. Long-term outcomes of submandibular gland transfer for prevention of postradiation xerostomia. *Arch Otolaryngol Head Neck Surg* 2004;130:956–961.
144. Senft M, Fietkau R, Iro H, et al. The influence of supportive nutritional therapy via percutaneous endoscopically guided gastrostomy on the quality of life of cancer patients. *Support Care Cancer* 1993;1:272–275.
145. Shell JA. Evidence-based practice for symptom management in adults with cancer: sexual dysfunction. *Oncol Nurs Forum* 2002;29:53–66.
146. Shike M. Nutrition therapy for the cancer patient. *Hematol Oncol Clin North Am* 1996;10:221–234.
147. Ship JA, Eisbruch A, D'Hondt E, et al. Parotid sparing study in head and neck cancer patients receiving bilateral radiation therapy: one-year results. *J Dent Res* 1997;76:807–813.
148. Ship JA, Hu K. Radiotherapy-induced salivary dysfunction. *Semin Oncol* 2004;31 [6 Suppl 18]:29–36.
149. Singer PA, Tasch ES, Stocking C, et al. Sex or survival: trade-offs between quality and quantity of life. *J Clin Oncol* 1991;9:328–334.
150. Sonis ST. The pathobiology of mucositis. *Nat Rev Cancer* 2004;4:277–284.
151. Sonis ST, Elting LS, Keefe D, et al. Perspectives on cancer therapy-induced mucosal injury: pathogenesis, measurement, epidemiology, and consequences for patients. *Cancer* 2004;100[9 Suppl]:1995–2025.
152. Sonis ST, Peterson DE, McGuire DB, et al. Prevention of mucositis in cancer patients. *J Natl Cancer Inst Monogr* 2001: 1–2.
153. Spielberger R, Stiff P, Bensinger W, et al. Palifermin for oral mucositis after intensive therapy for hematologic cancers. *N Engl J Med* 2004;351:2590–2598.
154. Spijkervet FK, Van Saene HK, Panders AK, et al. Effect of chlorhexidine rinsing on the oropharyngeal ecology in patients with head and neck cancer who have irradiation mucositis. *Oral Surg Oral Med Oral Pathol* 1989;67:154–161.
155. Spijkervet FK, Van Saene HK, Van Saene JJ, et al. Effect of selective elimination of the oral flora on mucositis in irradiated head and neck cancer patients. *J Surg Oncol* 1991;46:167–173.
156. Stead ML. Sexual function after treatment for gynecological malignancy. *Curr Opin Oncol* 2004;16:492–495.
157. Stern J, Ippoliti C. Management of acute cancer treatment-induced diarrhea. *Semin Oncol Nurs* 2003;19[4 Suppl 3]:11–16.
158. Tomic R. Some effects of orchiectomy, oestrogen treatment and radiation therapy in patients with prostatic carcinoma. *Scand J Urol Nephrol Suppl* 1983;77: 1–37.
159. Trotti A, Byhardt R, Stetz J, et al. Common toxicity criteria: version 2.0. an improved reference for grading the acute effects of cancer treatment: impact on radiotherapy. *Int J Radiat Oncol Biol Phys* 2000;47:13–47.
160. Trujillo E. Enteral nutrition: a comprehensive overview. In: Matarese L, Gottschlich M, eds. *Contemporary nutrition support practice: a clinical guide*. Philadelphia: WB Saunders; 1998:192–199.
161. Truong PT, Berthelet E, Lee JC, et al. Prospective evaluation of the prevalence and severity of fatigue in patients with prostate cancer undergoing radical external beam radiotherapy and neoadjuvant hormone therapy. *Can J Urol* 2006;13:3139–3146.
162. Turhal NS, Erdal S, Karacay S. Efficacy of treatment to relieve mucositis-induced discomfort. *Support Care Cancer* 2000;8:55–58.
163. Uomo G, Gallucci F, Rabitti PG. Anorexia-cachexia syndrome in pancreatic cancer: recent development in research and management. *JOP* 2006;7:157–162.
164. Valdez IH. Radiation-induced salivary dysfunction: clinical course and significance. *Spec Care Dentist* 1991;11:252–255.
165. Vissink A, Panders AK, Gravenmade EJ, et al. The causes and consequences of hyposalivation. *Ear Nose Throat J* 1988;67:166–168,173–176.
166. Volterrani F, Tana S, Trenti N. Topical benzydamine in the treatment of vaginal radiomucositis. *Int J Tissue React* 1987;9:169–171.
167. von Bultzingslowen I, Brennan MT, Spijkervet FK, et al. Growth factors and cytokines in the prevention and treatment of oral and gastrointestinal mucositis. *Support Care Cancer* 2006;14:519–527.
168. Walsh D, Rybicki L. Symptom clustering in advanced cancer. *Support Care Cancer* 2006;14:831–836.
169. Weber DC, Bieri S, Kurtz JM, et al. Prospective pilot study of sildenafil for treatment of postradiotherapy erectile dysfunction in patients with prostate cancer. *J Clin Oncol* 1999;17:3444–3449.
170. Wickline MM. Prevention and treatment of acute radiation dermatitis: a literature review. *Oncol Nurs Forum* 2004;31:237–247.
171. Williams JA, Jr., Clarke D, Dennis WA, et al. The treatment of pelvic soft tissue radiation necrosis with hyperbaric oxygen. *Am J Obstet Gynecol* 1992;167:412–416.
172. Wilmoth MC, Spinelli A. Sexual implications of gynecologic cancer treatments. *J Obstet Gynecol Neonatal Nurs* 2000;29:413–421.
173. Windsor PM, Nicol KF, Potter J. A randomized, controlled trial of aerobic exercise for treatment-related fatigue in men receiving radical external beam radiotherapy for localized prostate carcinoma. *Cancer* 2004;101:550–557.
174. Wiseman LR, Faulds D. Oral pilocarpine: a review of its pharmacological properties and clinical potential in xerostomia. *Drugs* 1995;49:143–155.
175. Wong RK, Jones GW, Sagar SM, et al. A Phase I-II study in the use of acupuncture-like transcutaneous nerve stimulation in the treatment of radiation-induced xerostomia in head-and-neck cancer patients treated with radical radiotherapy. *Int J Radiat Oncol Biol Phys* 2003;57:472–480.
176. Yavuzsen T, Davis MP, Walsh D, et al. Systematic review of the treatment of cancer-associated anorexia and weight loss. *J Clin Oncol* 2005;23(33):8500–8511.
177. Yeoh AS, Bowen JM, Gibson RJ, et al. Nuclear factor kappaB (NFkappaB) and cyclooxygenase-2 (Cox-2) expression in the irradiated colorectum is associated with subsequent histopathological changes. *Int J Radiat Oncol Biol Phys* 2005;63:1295–1303.
178. Zelefsky MJ, Eid JF. Elucidating the etiology of erectile dysfunction after definitive therapy for prostatic cancer. *Int J Radiat Oncol Biol Phys* 1998;40:129–133.
179. Zelefsky MJ, McKee AB, Lee H, et al. Efficacy of oral sildenafil in patients with erectile dysfunction after radiotherapy for carcinoma of the prostate. *Urology* 1999;53:775–778.

Section V

Economics, Ethics, and Technology Assessment

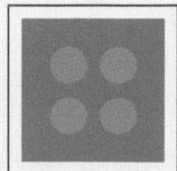

Chapter 96
Technology Assessment, Cost Benefit, Outcome Analysis Research and Evidence-Based Radiation Oncology

Carlos A. Perez, Edward C. Halperin

Rising medical costs are a concern worldwide. The problem is particularly acute in the United States. Health care expenditures constitute about 15% of the U.S. gross domestic product, compared to 6% to 10% for Canada, Germany, Japan, and the United Kingdom (23). Recent projections show an increase in U.S. health care costs to about 17% (gross domestic product) by 2007 (86).

Concern over the magnitude and continued growth of expenditures for health care in the United States has led to economic pressure on health service providers to contain costs. This change in market dynamics led to increased recognition of the need to understand cost structure and the economics of various treatment modalities. Economic assessment is now routinely becoming an important criterion for evaluation of therapeutic strategies (49).

The medical literature provides abundant guidelines for protocols comparing clinical outcomes of alternative treatment strategies. Unfortunately, consistent criteria are not followed for evaluation of the economics of treatment, which reduces the usefulness and credibility of comparative cost and other financial data/statistics across studies or over time (49).

In evaluating medical care, the term *efficacy* is not interchangeable with *effectiveness*. It is rare for a medical intervention to cure every patient. The maximum possible reduction in a disease due to the use of medical intervention is properly termed efficacy. We generally measure efficacy with randomized control trials, which will achieve the maximum possible benefit when patients are carefully selected and stratified, randomization arms are properly designed, compliance is high, and trial participants are often free of other diseases or conditions that might interfere with the intervention being evaluated (61). The benefits established in a randomized control trial are only partially applicable to day-to-day practice in a general population. The value of a medical intervention in the general population is termed effectiveness. The difference between efficacy and effectiveness can be very large, and obtaining a realistic measurement of effectiveness is often difficult (61).

There are three approaches to health economic evaluation for comparing two therapies:

(a) cost minimization, in which one assumes or observes no difference in effectiveness, (b) incremental cost-effectiveness, and (c) incremental net benefit. The latter can be expressed either in units of effectiveness or costs. When analyzing data from a clinical trial, expressing incremental net benefit in units of cost allows the investigator to examine all the approaches in a single graph, complete with the corresponding statistical inferences.

A computerized literature search of >14,000 articles published since 1994 having *cost* as a keyword was carried out. Criticisms of these costing studies focus on three areas:

(a) Costs are not measured correctly (15,24,64,82) because most studies use charge or reimbursement dollars as a proxy for cost. This is an incorrect measure because neither value is representative of the resources consumed or foregone in the process of providing a good service; hence, it is not a cost; the former figure is a construct and the latter is the result of a negotiation between a payer and a provider.

(b) Costs are not compiled using a proper perspective and scope (24,26,64,80). Most studies only tabulate the cost of the health care provider and not to the patient, their family, or society.

(c) There is a lack of consistency in reporting results (15,26,77,80,85,92), which prevents interstudy and interinstitutional comparison (92).

As a result of these problems, the data and conclusions from cost-based studies are suspect (80).

Clearly, a better costing method is required. Russell (79) emphasized that to serve its purpose a model must produce accurate predictions and low probability for substantial variation in the factors that influence costs and effects. He identified three aspects of modeling: validating effectiveness estimates, modeling costs, and the implications of common statistical forms. Validation procedures similar to those for effectiveness estimates are proposed for costs. Modelers need to pay more attention to ensuring that the events described by a model represent costs and effects. Modelers can also help improve the epidemiologic and clinical research on which cost-effectiveness analyses depend by showing the implications for resource allocation of the statistical forms conventionally used in these fields.

Technology assessment, cost-benefit outcome analysis, and clinical trials supported by evidence-based medicine together can enhance the rationale and quality of medical care provided to patients, at a competitive cost.

Technology Assessment

The purpose of technology assessment is to (a) determine the appropriateness of adopting a new procedure consistent with the health care organization's mission and strategic plan; (b) determine safety, efficacy, and cost-effectiveness of the new technology; (c) discriminate between appropriate and inappropriate use for the new technology; and (d) devise quality improvement methods to optimize the use of new technology (20). Technology assessment is a complex process that involves financial considerations, therapeutic outcome (locoregional tumor control, amelioration of symptoms survival), treatment-induced morbidity, and quality of life but impact on caregivers, family, and coworkers and lost-opportunity costs.

When new technology emerges and priorities for allocation of increasingly scarce resources are considered, it is imperative to carry out economic analyses and also to assess the positive effects to the population who will benefit from the new technology compared with standard treatment techniques. The United States Center for Medicare Management concluded that cost-effectiveness should be considered in approving reimbursement by Medicare for new technology procedures (52).

Technology has the promise to improve outcomes but usually increases costs of intervention by either premature adoption of the technology without adequate evidence that it improves outcome, or overuse of technology, regardless of value, to provide a competitive market advantage or to generate revenues (20). Glatstein (36) and Halperin (40) pointed out the importance of technology assessment in determining the merits of new devices or modalities and the impact they may have on the cost of health care.

Health care organizations use a variety of models to assess and acquire technology, some of which include outcome. Reliable data for such benchmarking is frequently scarce. Some compare new and emerging technology against existing technology, although again, reliable outcome data are rare. Most organizations buy what physicians, advocacy groups, philanthropists, or governing boards want and use manufacturers and physicians as the primary sources of technology information. Cowan and Berkowitz (20) pointed out several key mistakes that occur during the diffusion of technology:

a. Technologies are adopted simply because they are new, without assessing their impact on outcomes.
b. Equipment is replaced solely because of its age. Health care organizations must carefully match the capacity of existing technology with projected utilization in a world of limited resources, to avoid overuse of technology.
c. Applications of technology expand without adequate justification on outcome or cost considerations.
d. Numerous vendors are used and numerous models of products with duplicative specifications are purchased. Reducing the number of brands and models of devices used may provide an opportunity to reduce purchasing and inventory costs, as well as maintenance and repair costs. On the other hand, competitive pressures in the market place may provide downward pressure on equipment prices, and argue in favor of the existence of multiple vendors.
e. Economies of scale in regionalizing technology decisions are missed because of lack of consolidation of services. This is sometimes related to inadequate systems for patient transport to treatment centers.
f. Duplication of services sometimes adds cost without significant increase in work volume.

A number of studies on the costs of treating cancer patients with radiation therapy (19,35–37,41,69,71,73,78,91,94) used either relevant costs defined in a number of ways, or different proxies for actual costs (billed charges, revenue received, Medicare-allowable). Recent reviews illustrate the wide variety of cost information and cost methods used in the literature and call for a consistent method for estimating site- and intent-specific treatment costs (45,80,82,87,92). Luce et al. (56) provide a conceptual discussion of the theory and process of estimating costs of health care interventions. Several decision tools, including cost-analysis, cost-effective analysis, cost-utility analysis, and cost-benefit analysis, seek to define a unit of health outcome per unit input of cost.

Prior to employing any of these decision tools, proper calculation of cost is essential. Costs to the family or society can be substantial. These include the patient's travel costs, the patient's or care provider's time off from work, and the considerable strain on caregivers. There may also be "downstream" effects. If a caregiver is devoting time to an ill spouse, he or she is taking away from work or childcare responsibilities, for example.

Activity-based costing (ABC) is a system widely used in manufacturing industries but rarely in health care (30). ABC dissects the process of providing patient care into a series of microlevel tasks and assigns costs to these tasks. As a result, ABC directly identifies resources consumed by cost objects (treatments, patients, or health care providers) (44). Tabulating these tasks and resources consumed allows for comparison of cost values across institutions and time, in a consistent and credible way. From this, the economic impact of differences in operating policies can be quantified and the comparison of cost to health outcome will be improved.

Economic analyses are most valuable to health policy analysts and health care managers who must allocate resources and establish benefit packages. An economic health care analysis tries to directly relate the incremental cost of an intervention to its potential benefit. The intervention is always evaluated relative to an alternative form of treatment (45).

Forms of Economic Analysis

Cost minimization, which relates to a lower cost of an alternative treatment without regard to the efficacy. The major drawback of only using this approach to evaluate cancer treatment is the fact that complex oncology therapies almost never result in truly identical outcomes.

Cost effectiveness relates the additional costs of an intervention to its incremental impact on any clinically relevant measure of benefit. Because one of the primary uses of economic analysis is the allocation of limited resources among different choices, benefit is often measured in units that are universally applicable to all interventions. Years of life saved is the most commonly used measure (45). A nonmonetary unit for evaluation is the quality-adjusted life year (QALY). QALY measures the "usefulness" or "utility" of a health state and the length of life lived under those conditions. For example, is the value or quality of living a year as a paraplegic equal to half of a year of life without paralysis? One attempts to obtain values or utility measures by expert opinion, by using values derived in previous studies, and by surveys of patients. These surveys can be difficult to construct and may involve asking patients to make a "time tradeoff" or engage in a "rating scale" of various conditions or to assign a preference weight on a scale of 0 to 1 to a condition. A treatment cost-effectiveness ratio is calculated by dividing its incremental cost by the incremental impact on survival, as compared to the most reasonable alternative treatment. The intervention's cost-effectiveness ratio, expressed in units of dollars per year of lives saved, is compared to the standard intervention.

Cost benefit relates the additional cost of treatment to its incremental benefit, as compared to the most reasonable alternative treatment, where benefit is measured in a unit of currency such as dollars. Results of cost benefit analyses can also be reported as a ratio, where the additional cost of treatment is divided by its added benefit, again compared to the most reasonable alternative.

Cost utility relates the additional cost of treatment to its impact on both survival and quality of life, as well as productivity of the patient following treatment. The length of time spent in each outcome is multiplied by that outcome's weighting factor and the products are summed. A cost-utility analysis may be considered as a special form of a cost-effective analysis. In the cost-utility analysis, the health outcome of the denominator is valued in terms of utility or quality of life. The monetary units of evaluation include either the QALY or the disability-adjusted life year. It is common to express cost utility analyses as a total net cost per unit of utility or measure of quality; for example, a number of dollars cost or savings per QALY gained. A cost-utility ratio can be calculated by dividing its additional cost by its incremental change in QALYs, compared to a reasonable alternative. During the past decade it has become increasingly clear that, in addition to quantity of life, the impact of treatment on quality of life must be incorporated into measures of benefit.

Advantages of ABC versus Traditional Cost Accounting Systems

The traditional cost models that hospitals use are outdated and ill-equipped to provide accurate information on costs of a specific medical procedure or global cost of medical care for a patient. Cost models break organizations into departments for financial oversight and budgetary control; the focus of these cost models is departments and not a patient or a procedure, when it is really patients and procedures, not the department, triggering costs. For example, the accounting system of a hospital may be able to provide a fair assessment of the total budget (cost) of its radiation oncology department. However, the same system is of little help in assessing the actual cost of treating a patient with, for instance, prostate cancer using radiation therapy. This lack of applicability of cost information at the patient or the procedure level often leads to faulty decision-making because analysis of the whole (department) does not necessarily translate into conclusions about an individual patient.

ABC is concerned with measuring resource consumption by an individual patient. There are two general advantages of using ABC: increased accuracy of cost measurements and transparency of cost-incurring sections. The latter advantage, increased accounting transparency, means that there is a more lucid and readily apparent correlation between costs and actions. This allows managers to evaluate each step of the process, perceive inefficiencies in the system, and quantify economic benefits of process improvements.

The cost data of any technology should reflect the equipment, space costs, and recorded time and effort of all professional staff treating patients; for example, undergoing definitive radiation therapy (standard two-dimensional [2D], three-dimensional [3D] conformal radiation therapy [CRT] or intensity-modulated radiation therapy [IMRT]) for prostate cancer. Time and effort observations for multiple tasks must be recorded by the respective staff members as they take place. The numbers of observations provide a representative sample of treatment procedures.

Technical cost is defined as the actual expenditures recorded in hospital accounting records. The total technical cost of a course of therapy includes staff time and effort, compensation including fringe benefits, space, utilities, maintenance, equipment depreciation, supplies, support services, liability cost, and administrative overhead. A detailed description of the method to calculate all technical expenses is in preparation (30).

ABC method (4,17,18,29) was used to derive technical (hospital) resource utilization costs for the 2D and 3D treatment processes in treating localized prostate cancer (49,73). The same method applies to utilization costs for IMRT or image-guided radiation therapy (IGRT). The costing method consists of four major steps:

a. Creating a process flow map that identifies and defines all of the activities and steps associated with the treatment of patients with standard irradiation or with 3DCRT (Fig. 96.1).
b. Collecting and recording the staff time expended on each activity.
c. Identifying and accumulating all hospital costs from the general accounting ledger system related to the patients treated at a radiation oncology center in a given period.
d. Allocating actual cost to each activity to derive total specific costs of technical resource utilization for a course of 2D, 3D, IMRT, or IGRT.

Time and Effort Analysis

The first step in identifying process flow is to list each individual involved in the process and to record the actual amount of time spent to perform an activity by the staff, using electronic or paper daily activity logs. Determining the participant's task time should follow the monopolizing rule; timing begins when a specific patient requires the participant's attention and stops when he or she is no longer doing so. Whether or not the patient is still present in the activity area is immaterial. For example, for an office visit, the nurse's time to prepare the patient's paperwork should be attributed to the patient, even before the patient arrives or after he or she has left the office. The actual activity time may be adjusted upward to recognize some normal unproductive time of activity participants, such as time spent in work breaks. Tables are generated to show the time and effort involved in each one of the functions necessary to register, evaluate the patient, perform treatment planning, deliver external-beam irradiation, and supervise the management, as well as preparation of the appropriate records to document all information, including quality assurance requirements.

Times are collected for each activity in the treatment process beginning with the initial consultation through the first follow-up visit after full treatment. These data points are analyzed and used to generate average times for patients treated with a specific technique along with the standard deviation of times.

Resource Utilization

Four types of resources should be cataloged and measured for each task:

a. Activity participants (e.g., radiation oncologists, physicists, therapists, dosimetrists, nurses, receptionists),
b. Physical resources (e.g., space, equipment, machines),
c. Supplies (e.g., x-ray films, office supply), and
d. Support services (e.g., administration, centralized information system).

Direct patient-related expenses include salaries and fringe benefits of the staff, Social Security, retirement annuity, health, life disability and long-term care, dental insurance, tuition and childcare benefits, and disability insurance. Average hourly salary and related costs for each staff member are computed.

There are many supplies such as office paper and latex gloves for which the cost is trivial and it is not economically worthwhile to track their specific use by individual patients. An average cost rate can be computed for such supplies by dividing their total cost by the total number of patients, which is applied to each patient. However, supplies used only by patients with specific diseases or procedures (e. g., contrast material, immobilization devices) need to be recorded for individual patients.

For hospital-based departments, indirect operating costs are classified into general hospital operating expenses and administrative overhead, which includes hospital liability insurance and administrative costs such as shared activities (administrative personnel for purchasing and payroll functions, human resources, public relations, and financial operations). The allocation of indirect operating costs between different departments of the hospital is complex. Models include allocating them as a proportion of personnel costs and many others. The allocation of cost among various units in a hospital can also be the source of pitched battles between different units. In many hospitals allocation of costs is a mechanism of cross-subsidization between different departments (i.e., the surgery department subsidizing primary care). Administrative cost can be determined by computing prorated allocation, dividing the total hospital indirect expenses by the proportion of the radiation oncology center technical budget to the total hospital annual budget.

Technical equipment expenses for treatment of patients are included using American Hospital Association standard depreciation schedules.

The cost of depreciation of all equipment involved in the management of these patients, including treatment planning and delivery, should be accounted for on a prorated basis. Annual cost of space is prorated for the facilities and equipment involved in the management of the patients with a specific cancer, corresponding to approximately $70,914. The cost of all supplies should be prorated for the specific patients treated. The administrative and other overhead costs must be accounted for.

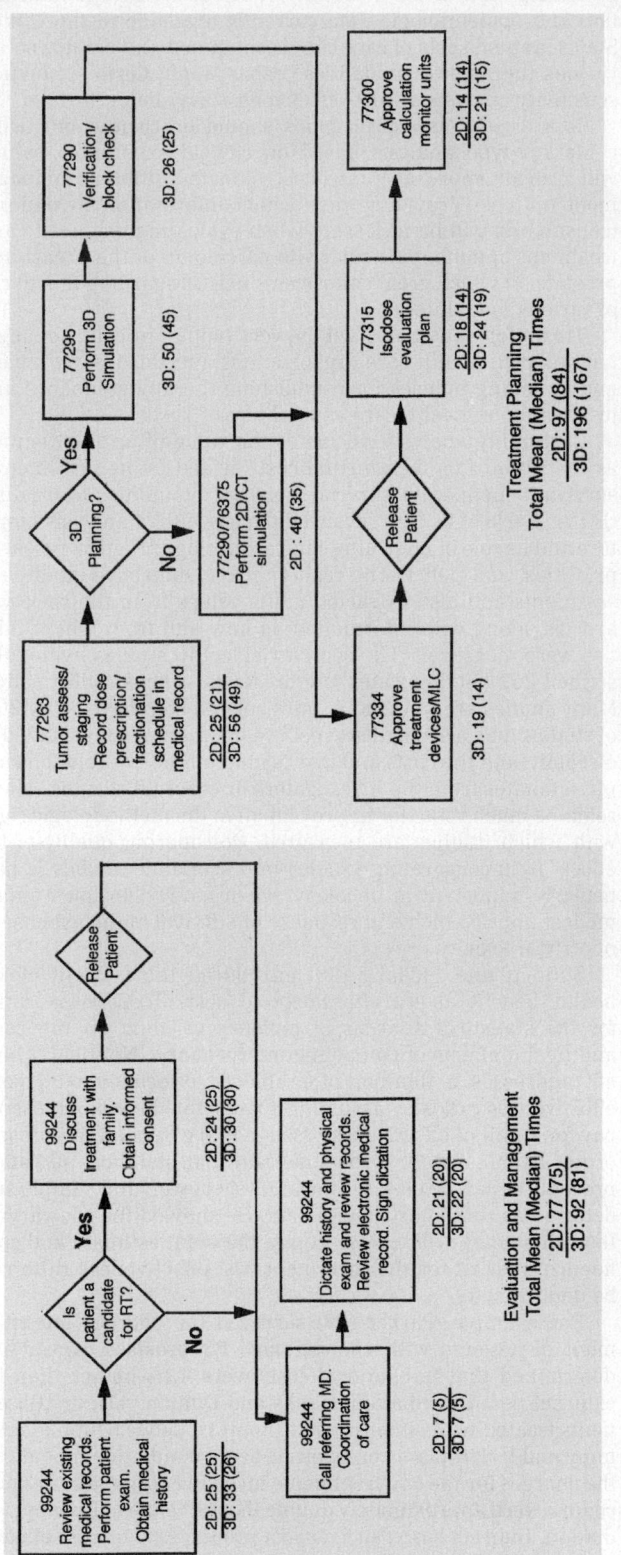

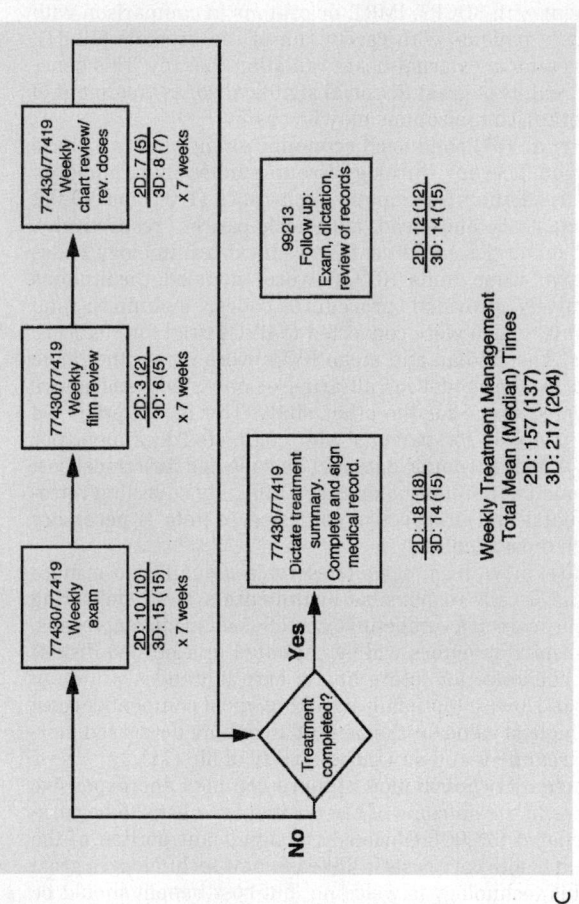

FIGURE 96.1. Process flow chart. Activity map and corresponding mean (median) times for definitive irradiation of cancer of prostate. **A:** Evaluation and management. **B:** Treatment planning. **C:** Weekly management.

Cost Benefit

If all that matters is minimizing expense, then the lowest-cost treatment (or no treatment) will be preferred. However, cost benefit, which incorporates the incremental impact of a new technology on outcome, and cost utility, which also relates additional costs to impact on survival as well as on the patient's quality of life and productivity, are important parameters in the assessment of new technology (45).

As a concomitant to an increasing proportion of the health insurance market being controlled by managed care, with its cost-cutting pressures, there may be a tendency to de-emphasize the importance of quality of care. However, it is critical, for instance, to document the alleged decreased morbidity of treatment with 3DCRT, IMRT, or protons in comparison with treatment of patients with carcinoma of the prostate (43,81), with conventional external-beam radiation therapy. This benefit, if it is real, is of great financial significance, as treatment of major therapy complications may be costly.

Owen et al. (67) conducted economic studies for two phase III Radiation Therapy Oncology Group studies that compared different irradiation fractionation schedules (1-04 and 90-03, brain metastasis and head and neck cancer, respectively). Expected quantities of current procedural terminology codes and relative value units (RVUs) were modeled. Institutions retrospectively provided procedure codes, quantities, and components, which were converted to RVUs used for Medicare payments. The median and mean RVUs were within the range predicted by the model for all arms of one study and above the predicted range for the other study. The model predicted resource use well for patients who completed treatment per protocol. Actual economic data can be collected for critical cost items. Some institutions experienced difficulty collecting retrospective data, and prospective collection of data is necessary to validate these studies.

We must move from a fee-for-service mentality to a more critical and fiscally responsible health care system, delivering high-quality care at a competitive cost. Based on current trends, 70% of hospital revenues will be capitated in a not-too-distant future. A challenge for future health care initiatives will be to strive for the lowest (optimally speaking, most competitive) cost with the highest value for the patient, including decreased morbidity of treatment and enhanced quality of life (11).

The potential contribution of more complex and expensive procedures to the outcome of cancer therapy needs to be carefully evaluated (31,90). Obviously, a significant portion of the increase in health care costs is linked to new technology; a great deal of this technology is welcome, but cost benefit should be demonstrated (32). Some technologic advances improve health care and can be justified economically if we document a positive impact on tumor control, patient survival, morbidity of treatment, and quality of life. The efficacy of diagnostic and therapeutic procedures can be related to outcome studies and costs should be carefully evaluated based on both monetary and health-related considerations (22). Doubilet et al. (22) cautioned against the indiscriminate use of "cost-effectiveness" as the criterion on which medical decisions should be made, and thus we must carefully define the end points on which these studies are based.

Models can be constructed using a marker model and available data on the natural history of a tumor, prognostic factors, efficacy and morbidity of a given therapeutic modality (based on outcome analysis), and reimbursement data for treating a specific patient population. When patterns of failure data are used, the cost differential can be calculated for a patient treated successfully in contrast to one who fails in a specific anatomic site (locoregional failure, distant metastasis, or combination), incorporating expenditures related to management of the treatment failure. The model can be made more complete (and complex)

by adding costs of the morbidity of therapy. With the information and epidemiologic data currently available in the United States, annual costs of care can be computed and compared for various therapeutic modalities. Using Monte Carlo simulation sensitivity analysis of cost-effectiveness may be performed.

Total cost-of-care projections should be carried out using a Markov-type analysis based on clinical experience, which will provide more accurate cost data for different management options. Providing cost-benefit information to patients (consumers) will be necessary when evaluating diagnostic and treatment options, particularly in carcinoma of the breast and prostate, in which great controversy exists regarding the merits of various modalities.

This information also will be very helpful in contract negotiations with health care organizations and third-party payers and in setting policies for establishing therapy guidelines and justification of health care expenditures.

Cost-utility analysis calculates the value of an intervention as the ratio of its incremental cost divided by its incremental survival benefit, with survival weighted by utilities to produce QALYs. Earle et al. (25) reviewed the cost-utility analysis literature and its role in informing clinical oncology practice, research priorities, and policy. The readers made subjective quality assessments and also extracted utility values from the reviewed articles, along with information on how and from whom utilities were measured. The search yielded 40 studies, which described 263 healing states and presented 89 cost-utility ratios. Many studies are at variance with current standards; only 20% of studies took a societal perspective, more than a third failed to discount both the costs and QALYs, and utilities were often simply estimates from the investigators or other physicians. There remains much room for improvement in the methodologic rigor with which utilities are measured. Considering quality-of-life effects by incorporating utilities into economic studies is particularly important in oncology, when many therapies obtain modest improvements in response or survival at the expense of nontrivial toxicity.

Stinnett and Mullahy (88) introduced the concept of net health benefit as an alternative to cost-effectiveness ratios for the statistical analysis of patient-level data on the costs and health effects of competing interventions. Net health benefit addresses a number of problems associated with cost-effectiveness ratios by assuming a value for the willingness-to-pay for a unit of effectiveness. Willan (93) extended the concept of net health benefit to demonstrate that standard statistical procedures can be used for the analysis power, and sample size determines cost-effectiveness data. He showed that by varying the value of the willingness-to-pay, the point estimate and confidence interval for the increment cost-effectiveness ratio can be determined.

For example, Parker (69) surveyed the charges for treatment of patients with clinical stage B1 prostate cancer and determined that the surgical costs were 42% higher than for external-beam irradiation. Hanks and Dunlap (41), in 105 patients treated with either prostatectomy or pelvic lymphadenectomy and ^{125}I implants or external-beam irradiation, noted that the charges for the two treatments involving either surgical procedure were approximately double those of external-beam irradiation. Indirect costs, such as lost productivity or cost of complications, were not taken into account.

On the other hand, one of the authors (75) documented that the reimbursement for initial treatment per patient in U.S. dollars at his institution for 3DCRT, SRT, or radical prostatectomy were $13,823, $10,864, and $12,250, respectively, which are fairly equivalent. Horwitz et al. (46) showed a cost benefit in treating patients with localized prostate cancer using 3DCRT in comparison with standard techniques. Although the initial costs were higher for 3DCRT, the mean total charges ranged from $17,259 to $24,250 for 3DCRT and from $9,800 to $59,635 for the patients treated with conventional technique. The projected cost of treating a patient who has control of the local tumor and no distant metastases is about one-third of that for a patient who develops a treatment failure (73).

The benefit of 3DCRT, IMRT, or IGRT is hypothetically linked to improved local tumor control because of better coverage of the target volume with a specific dose of irradiation, less acute and late morbidity, possibility of carrying out dose-escalation studies if morbidity is held to acceptable level, resulting in improved survival (73). Several institutions, the Radiation Therapy Oncology Group, and ten institutions under cooperative agreement with the National Cancer Institute conducted a phase I/II dose-escalation studies in carcinoma of the prostate and are carrying out a study on carcinoma of the lung. Depending on the results, the cost benefit of 3DCRT, IMRT, or IGRT must be further evaluated in dose-escalation and in larger multi-institutional phase III studies, comparing it with standard techniques to justify its somewhat higher initial cost (75). Cases that are most likely to benefit from 3DCRT, IMRT, or IGRT, include patients with (a) tumors in sites with complex anatomy, (b) irregular-shaped tumors, (c) tumors adjacent to radiation-sensitive normal structures, and (d) small-volume or high-dose treatment. Implementing new technologies in radiation oncology with advanced engineering, such as linear accelerators cone-beam tomotherapy, planning and delivery techniques, and accessories that enhance the efficiency and accuracy of operation, may decrease overall cost of treatment computed over the lifetime of the patient.

Costs of a procedure based on activity and resource use analysis can be realistically and accurately determined. A consistent method and terminology is needed to obtain and calculate actual costs of radiation therapy.

Evidence-Based Medicine

In the past 10 years there have been significant scientific advances in biologic sciences and health care. At the same time, there has been increased accountability and in some instances attempts to ration services; as a mechanism to accomplish this, arbitrary clinical practice guidelines have been promulgated. A more rational basis to define optimal heath care should be based on identification of innovative approaches, outcome analysis in properly designed clinical trials, and careful assessment of current practice; more importantly, we have a dire need for solid and credible clinical research and evidence-based decision making in medicine.

The growth in basic and translational research data to guide medical practice has made it critical for clinicians to appraise and use published evidence for medical decisions. Evidence-based medicine exemplifies the effort to teach clinicians to evaluate research data by methodologic standards, and to critically appraise published evidence from both a scientific and sociocultural perspective. It helps correct an imbalance in contemporary medicine in which clinicians are being trained to maintain high standards of critical consciousness in methodologic domains but not in the broader historic and sociocultural domains that surround them (8).

Practicing evidence-based medicine requires recognition that, in most encounters with patients, questions arise that should be answered to provide the patient with the best available medical care. Appropriate and relevant clinical questions contain four elements: (a) a patient or problem, (b) an intervention, (c) a comparison intervention (if necessary), and (d) an outcome. Important practical steps in practicing evidence-based medicine include:

(a) Formulation of the patient's clinical problem
(b) Search of literature for relevant and reliable data
(c) Evaluation of validity and usefulness of data

(d) Integrating critical evaluation of evidence with clinical judgment
(e) Implementation of useful information
(f) Assessment of outcome to improve medical practice

Once the right questions have been formulated, the best source for finding most types of best evidence is by searching Medline (National Library of Medicine), PubMed (National Library of Medicine), OVID, the Cochrane Database or a similar database by computer.

The quality (strength) of evidence is based on a hierarchy, proceeding from the most reliable results of systematic reviews of well-designed prospective clinical trials to results of one or more well-designed meta-analysis studies, results of large retrospective case series, expert opinion, and personal experience (Table 96.1). Once the best data have been found, the evidence-based medicine approach involves critically appraising the quality of the evidence, determining its magnitude and precision, and applying it to a specific patient (9,33). A hierarchal guide to treatment recommendations is illustrated in Table 96.2. Table 96.3 presents a scheme for classifying the methodologic quality of treatment recommendations, emphasizing consideration of all relevant options and outcomes, a systematic summary of the evidence, and explicit or quantitative consideration of societal or patient preferences (39).

Evidence-based medicine promotes rule-based behavior on the part of physicians in an effort, among other things, to eliminate variations in medical practice. But professionals do not follow rules per se; they intuit what is right in a situation, including, sometimes, that it is right to defer to a rule (89).

The practice of evidence-based medicine (careful clinical judgment in evaluating the "best available data") should be differentiated from the special collection of data regarded as "suitable evidence." The new collection of best available information has major constraints for the care of individual patients; derived almost exclusively from randomized trials and meta-analyses, the data do not include many types of treatments or patients seen in clinical practice, and the results show comparative efficacy of treatment for an "average" randomized

Table 96.1	LEVELS OF EVIDENCE AND GRADING OF EVIDENCE FOR RECOMMENDATIONS
	Type of Evidence
Level	
I	Evidence obtained from meta-analysis of multiple, well-designed, controlled studies or from high-power randomized, controlled clinical trial
II	Evidence obtained from at least one well-designed experimental study or low-power randomized, controlled clinical trial
III	Evidence obtained from well-designed, quasiexperimental studies such as nonrandomized, controlled single-group, pre/post, cohort, time, or matched case-control series
IV	Evidence from well-designed, nonexperimental studies, such as comparative and correlational descriptive and case studies
V	Evidence from case reports and clinical examples
Grade	
A	There is evidence of type I or consistent findings from multiple studies of types II, III, or IV
B	There is evidence of types II, III, or IV and findings are generally consistent
C	There is evidence of types II, III, or IV but findings are inconsistent
D	There is little or no systematic empirical evidence

From Canadian Medical Association. The Canadian Task Force on the Periodic Health Examination. *Can Med Assoc J* 1979;121:1193–1254, with permission.

Table 96.2   A HIERARCHY OF RIGOR IN MAKING TREATMENT RECOMMENDATIONS

Level of Rigor	Systematic Summary of Evidence	Considers All Relevant Options and Outcomes	Explicit Statement of Values	Example of Methods
High	Yes	Yes	Yes	Practice guidelines or decision analysis[a]
Intermediate	Yes	Yes or no	No	Systematic review[a]
Low	No	Yes or no	No	Traditional reviews; original articles

[a]Example of methods may not reflect the level of rigor shown. If a systematic review considers all relevant options and at least qualitatively considers values, it can produce recommendations approaching high rigor.
From Guyatt GH, Sinclair J, Cook DJ, et al. Users' guides to the medical literature: XVI. How to use a treatment recommendation. *JAMA* 1999;281:1836–1843, with permission.

patient, not for pertinent subgroups formed by such cogent clinical features as severity of symptoms, illness, comorbidity, and other clinical nuances. The intention-to-treat analyses in clinical trials reporting do not reflect important post randomization events leading to altered treatment, and the results seldom provide suitable background data when therapy is given prophylactically rather than remedially. Randomized trial information is also seldom available for issues in etiology, diagnosis, and prognosis and for clinical decisions that depend on pathophysiologic changes, psychosocial factors and support, person preferences of patients, and strategies for giving comfort and reassurance. The authoritative aura given to the "collection of data" may lead to abuses that produce inappropriate guidelines or poorly supported doctrinaire dogmas for clinical practice (28).

There are a variety of mechanisms to apply evidence-based medicine to clinical practice, including formulation of treatment pathways, practice guidelines, appropriateness criteria, consensus conferences, patterns of care, and institutional peer review. A fundamental part of evidence-based medicine is the filtering of evidence through the clinical skill of the clinician (38). It is not easy to determine which level of evidence is required, and it is estimated that only 20% of medical procedures currently in practice can be justified by evidence-based medical standards.

Outcome Research

Outcome research focuses on identifying variations in medical procedures and associated health outcomes (95). Figure 96.2 illustrates the interplay of outcome research and clinical trials with clinical and policy decision-making.

Table 96.3   METHODOLOGIC REQUIREMENTS FOR SYSTEMATIC, RIGOROUS RECOMMENDATIONS

1. Comprehensive statement of management options and possible outcomes.
2. Systematic review and summary of evidence linking options to outcomes. Examination of the magnitude of impact, in terms of both benefits and risks, in relative and absolute terms.
3. Consideration of different populations and the characteristics of these populations that may affect impact of intervention.
4. Examination of strength of evidence linking options to outcomes. Where evidence is weak, examine the implications of plausible differences in effects.
5. Explicit, appropriate specification of values of preferences associated with outcomes.

Guyatt GH, Sinclair J, Cook DJ, et al. Users' guides to the medical literature: XVI. How to use a treatment recommendation. *JAMA* 1999;281:1836–1843, with permission.

The term *outcome* is frequently used to describe a variety of end points or products of health care. Areas of specific focus of outcome analysis include:

a. Structure of care (such as features of health care facilities, staffing, equipment)
b. Process of care (such as type of studies performed, services provided)
c. Patient characteristics (gender, age, race, ethnic group)
d. Disease focus (such as location and type of tumor, histology, pathologic features)

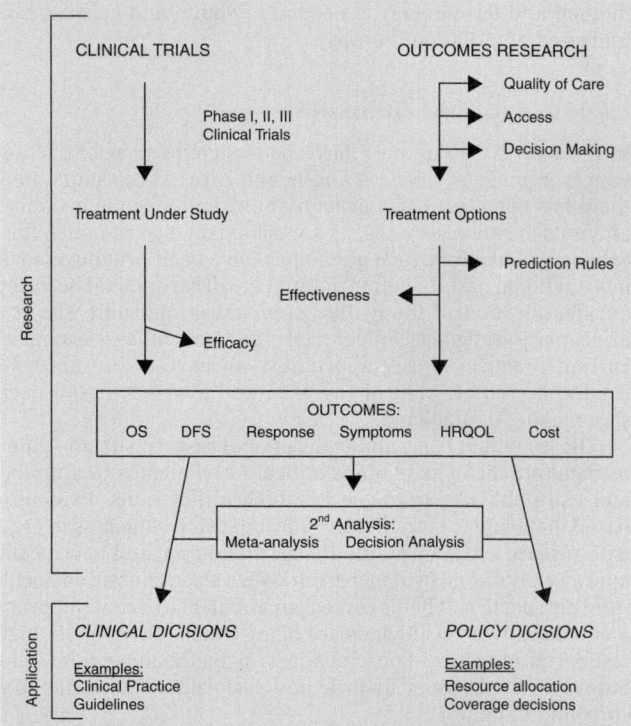

FIGURE 96.2. Conceptual framework of outcome research. Interaction is shown between research topics, end points, analytic techniques, and applications in defining outcomes research. Depicted in the *upper left corner* are the classic clinical trials and analytic techniques that are *not* outcomes research. In the *upper right corner* are shown the study topics, end points, and analytic techniques that are considered to be outcomes research. Outcomes depicted in the *center box* may or may not constitute outcomes research, depending on the context. For example, overall survival as measured in a phase III trial is not an outcomes study (efficacy), whereas it is if observed in a large community cohort (effectiveness). Symptoms have both efficacy and outcomes influences. Applications are indicated in italics and may emanate from either clinical trials or outcomes research. See text for further details (7,60). (From Lee SJ, Earle CC, Weeks JC. Outcomes research in oncology: history, conceptual framework, and trends in the literature. *J Natl Cancer Inst* 2000;92:195–204, with permission.)

e. Treatment-related factors (type of treatment, tumor response, disease-free survival, overall survival, morbidity of therapy)

f. Socioeconomics (such as cost benefit, quality of life, financial impact of the disease recovery and rehabilitation)

The principles of outcome research were emphasized in 1972 by Archie Cochrane, an epidemiologist in 1992, the Cochrane Centre opened in Oxford. In addition to the collaborative review and Cochrane method groups and centers, the Cochrane Library and *The Cochrane Database of Systematic Reviews* were established. The Cochrane Collaboration Controlled Clinical Trials Registry contains more than 190,000 controlled clinical trials and as part of an international effort to systematically search the world's health care journals and other sources of information to create an unbiased source of data for systematic reviews in medicine (16).

Meta-analysis is another mechanism to systematically research and collect published/unpublished randomized clinical trial data and quantitatively summarize results to obtain objective assessment of efficacy. The process should be: (a) hypothesis driven, (b) protocol based, and (c) reproducible and comprehensive.

However, meta-analysis has some potential shortcomings, such as uncontrolled testing conditions, sample heterogeneity, unrecorded interventions, ambiguous end points, lack of independence of determinant factors, synergistic interactions, and sometimes contradictory experimental results.

Efforts have intensified during the past 20 years to promote outcome research in oncology and there is a critical need to continue to support randomized controlled studies. Interventions must be practical, feasible, and easily disseminated to have an impact on the general population of patients with cancer. Goals should be to prevent the development of cancer, enhance screening and early diagnosis, design more effective therapeutic strategies to improve local tumor control and survival, and minimize morbidity of therapy to enhance quality of life, as well as carry out cost-benefit studies. Patient and physician acceptance of participation in outcome research studies must be improved, as only 10% to 20% of patients with newly diagnosed cancer participate in these important studies (65).

There is considerable variation in participation of patients in research studies as a function of patient age and disease site. In general, compliance with participation in studies is much higher among pediatric patients than adults. Also, when a specific effort is expended along with a concentration of resources, participation in studies can be improved as, for example, in the Collaborative Ocular Melanoma Study for choroidal melanoma sponsored by the National Eye Institute.

Among the most commonly used data are those of the Surveillance, Epidemiology, and End Result (SEER) program. SEER is a continuing project of the biometry branch of the United States National Cancer Institute. The program draws data from several population-based cancer reporting systems covering approximately 14% of the total population of the United States. When linked to Medicare and other insurance administrative files, it has been extremely valuable in assessing the quality of care of the elderly and other insured populations. Although an excellent data source, SEER has been criticized as being inadequate to represent the diversity of systems of care throughout the country.

The National Cancer Data Base, a joint project of the American College of Surgeons' Commission on Cancer and the American Cancer Society, now holds information on more than half of all newly diagnosed cases of cancer in the United States and includes many of the demographic, clinical, and health systems data elements necessary to assess quality of care. A serious limitation of the National Cancer Data Base is the absence of complete information on outpatient care; its data have not been widely used to assess quality of care, but it has great potential for doing so.

An effective national system to collect this type of information should be established in the U.S.A. to collect data about:

- Demographics of individuals with cancer (e. g., age, ethnic group, socioeconomic status, and insurance or health plan coverage)
- Type of cancer (stage, histologic type, grade, comorbid conditions)
- Treatment, including outcome of procedures, such as adjuvant chemotherapy, radiation therapy.
- Specialty training of care providers
- Site of care delivery (such as community hospital specialized cancer center)
- Type of care delivery system (such as managed care, fee for service, government agency)
- Outcomes (tumor control, survival, complications of treatment, quality of life, satisfaction with services provided)

Barriers to Progress in Cancer Outcome Research

Despite growing interest, there are numerous obstacles to overcome in health care outcome research, including the need to apply scientific disciplines that are different from the biomedical sciences (survey research, psychology, health services research, statistics, economics), the need for resources to collect additional data and information beyond that of standard clinical care, and limited coordination and collaboration among researchers working in the field. Other barriers are intrinsic to a specific cancer as a disease, including heterogeneity of patients, type of tumor, phases of the disease, and ethnic and socioeconomic characteristics. Further, many institutions do not give a high priority or adequately fund outcome research because this activity is considered a cost, not a revenue center, and there is a lack of conviction that this effort will reduce health care spending (84).

Efforts to educate the biomedical community in the scientific aspects of health care and outcome research may contribute substantially to elevating the quality and perception of relevance of this type of research. Data sharing and increased collaboration in data collection and analysis should be promoted among the various groups conducting outcome research. Creative approaches to educating providers and patients about outcome studies are needed, as well as mechanisms to ensure that patients and health professionals have ready access to the results of outcome research (13).

:: | Evidence-Based Oncology

Making a treatment selection involves defining the patient's condition, identifying management options and outcome, collecting and summarizing evidence, and applying value judgments or preferences to arrive at an optimal course of action (39). The randomized controlled clinical trial, the first of which was published in 1952, has become the "gold standard" for evaluating the efficacy of health care intervention. In the past 30 years, starting in 1966, more than 76,000 journal articles from randomized controlled trials results were registered in the Medline database. The first 5 years of that period contributed less than 1% of the total number of articles, whereas the last half-decade contributed more than the previous 25 years combined. Noteworthy, only 22 of 150 randomized trials (15%) in the treatment of lung cancer published between 1970 and 1987 were judged to apply adequate randomization methods (66). For more detailed review of the principles of design in clinical trials, the reader is referred to Bentzen (7). A proposal for structured reporting of randomized clinical trials was described in the consolidation of standards for reporting trials guidelines (5) that have been accepted by many medical journals. For instance, the journal *Radiotherapy and Oncology* has adopted a set of guidelines for reporting clinical research (Table 96.4). Linking management options to known outcomes in clinical trials or obtained through systematic reviews is becoming a common procedure (Fig. 96.2).

Clinical decisions are complex and based on many sources of information (Fig. 96.3) (63). Patient management decisions are always a function of both scientific evidence and individual preferences (physicians, health care providers, patients). A recent development to improve the basis for clinical decision-making is an international movement to improve the reporting of clinical research results, particularly in randomized controlled trials and method analyses. New data on current molecular biology and genetics investigation have broadened the scope of evidence-based oncology.

Hunt et al. (47) reported on an analysis of 68 controlled medical trials, 40 of which were published since 1992, to assess the effects of computer-based clinical decision support systems on physician performance and patient outcome. They observed that, in 43 of 65 studies (66%) on physician performance, a benefit was found, including drug-dosing systems, use of diagnostic aids, preventive care assistance, and other medical care procedures. Only 6 of 14 studies assessing patient outcome found a benefit, indicating that the impact of clinical decision support systems on patient outcome has been insufficiently studied. Furthermore, very few reports have dealt with cancer-related issues; most have centered on prevention, activities, and cancer screening (57–59,76).

Table 96.4	GUIDELINES FOR REPORTING CLINICAL OUTCOME STUDIES IN *RADIOTHERAPY AND ONCOLOGY*[a]			

Heading	Subheading	Item	Was It Reported? Yes/No/NA[b]	If Yes, on What Page No.?
Title		1. Identify the study as a randomized trial	_____	_____
Introduction		2. State the prospectively defined hypothesis, clinical objectives and planned subgroup or covariate analyses	_____	_____
Methods	Study design	3. Define the patient population, inclusion and exclusion criteria	_____	_____
		4. Planned treatments and their timing		
	Radiotherapy	5. Radiotherapy dose prescription method, dose-planning procedure		_____
		6. Target volume definition, critical organs considered, simulation and verification procedures	_____	_____
		7. Dose fractionation details	_____	_____
		8. Planned RT quality assurance procedures	_____	_____
	End points and analysis	9. Primary and secondary endpoints, specific follow-up procedures, the minimum clinically relevant difference, the target sample size and how it was decided	_____	_____
		10. Statistical analyses, their purpose and methods used, and whether the intention-to-treat principle was used.	_____	_____
		11. Trial monitoring, early stopping rules	_____	_____
	Randomization	12. Method used for randomization	_____	_____
		13. Method of concealment and time of randomization	_____	_____
		14. Method to separate the generator of random treatment assignments from the treating physician	_____	_____
Results	Masking patient flow and follow-up analysis	15. Describe any blinding procedures (if relevant)	_____	_____
		16. Provide an overview of number of patients randomized, compliance with treatment, RT quality assurance results	_____	_____
		17. State the effect of treatment on primary and secondary tumor outcome measures, including effect estimates with confidence intervals	_____	_____
		18. Describe the incidence and grade of treatment-induced early and late toxicity by treatment group	_____	_____
		19. State frequencies as absolute numbers when feasible (e.g., 10/20 and not just 50%)	_____	_____
		20. Present summary data with appropriate statistics to permit alternative analyses or interpretations and comparisons with other trials on the same problem	_____	_____
		21. Describe prognostic variables by treatment group, check, if they were balanced, and if not describe attempts to adjust for them	_____	_____
		22. Describe protocol deviations from the study as planned, together with reasons	_____	_____
Discussion		23. State the interpretation of the study findings, including sources of bias and imprecision, discuss how this trial compares with other similar studies	_____	_____
Conclusion		24. State the general interpretation of the trial in view of all available evidence in the literature	_____	_____

RT, radiation therapy.
[a]These guidelines meet the minimum criteria defined in the CONSORT statement for reporting of randomized clinical trials (5).
[b]NA, not applicable; certain items apply to randomized studies only.
From Bentzen SM. Towards evidence based radiation oncology: Improving the design, analysis, and reporting of clinical outcome studies in radiotherapy. *Radiother Oncol* 1998;46:5–18, with permission.

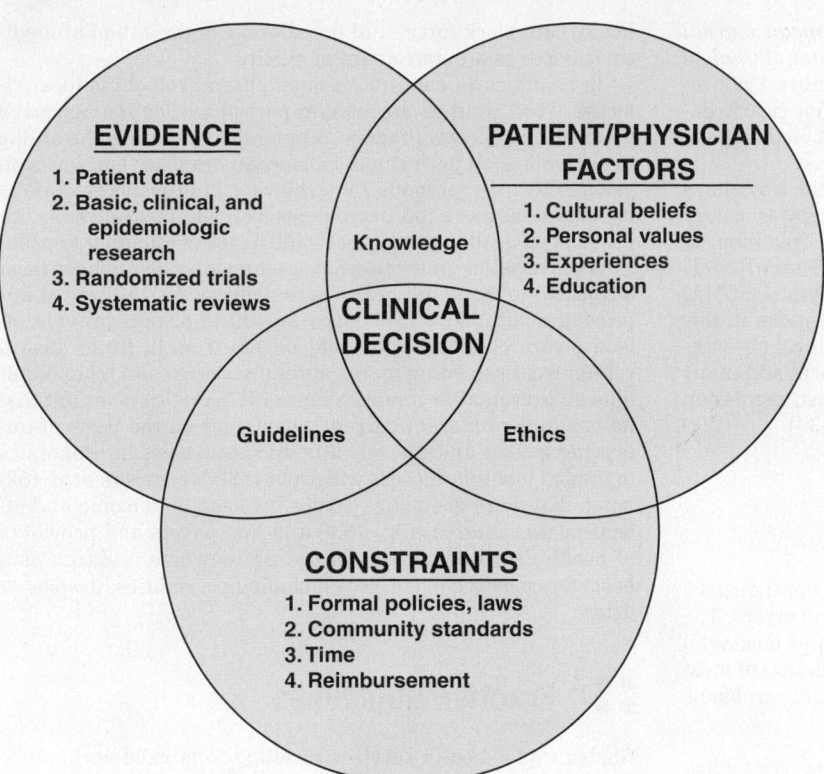

EVIDENCE
1. Patient data
2. Basic, clinical, and epidemiologic research
3. Randomized trials
4. Systematic reviews

PATIENT/PHYSICIAN FACTORS
1. Cultural beliefs
2. Personal values
3. Experiences
4. Education

Knowledge

CLINICAL DECISION

Guidelines

Ethics

CONSTRAINTS
1. Formal policies, laws
2. Community standards
3. Time
4. Reimbursement

FIGURE 96.3. Factors that enter into clinical decisions. (From Mulrow CD, Cook DJ, Davidoff F. Systematic reviews: critical links in the great chain of evidence. In: *Systematic reviews: synthesis of best evidence for health care decisions.* Philadelphia: American College of Physicians; 1998:1–4, with permission.)

Although oncologists, patients, and national organizations recognize that communication is very important in cancer care, evidence-based data on the subject is scarce. Oncologists should use a patient-centered interview approach, ask patients what level of involvement they want in medical decision-making, develop a caring attitude, and consider the patient-physician encounter as providing both cognitive data of patient understanding and emotional feelings (5).

Clinical Trials

Prospective randomized clinical trials have come to occupy a prominent role in clinical research in radiation oncology. The most commonly used clinical endpoints are summarized in Table 96.5. Unfortunately, many published reports have unclear definitions or lack some of the fundamental endpoints (96). Altman et al. (1) examined 132 articles containing survival

---

Table 96.5   MOST COMMONLY USED CLINICAL END POINTS IN RADIATION THERAPY TRIALS

End Point	Definition of Event	Comments
Local control	No evidence of disease at the primary site (T position)	Statistically this is the absence of an event (i.e., local recurrence). Estimated at a given time as the local-recurrence-free rate.
Local failure rate	Recurrence in T position	Estimated as 1 minus the local-recurrence-free rate
Locoregional control	No evidence of disease in T and N position	See above, but for T or N recurrence, whichever comes first. Sometimes defined as in-field control (i.e., control within the treated volume).
Survival or overall survival	Death irrespective of cause	
Cancer-specific survival or cause-specific survival	Death of cancer	Often defined as death of cancer or with active disease
Disease-free survival	Any recurrence or death from any cause, whichever comes first	A composite endpoint combining survival and disease control
Local recurrence-free survival	Local recurrence or death from any cause, whichever comes first	As above but with local recurrence as the relevant event
Disease-free rate	Any recurrence	Death without recurrence is a cause of censoring
Local relapse-free rate	Local recurrence	As above
Early reactions	Signs or symptoms of a specific early reaction. Defined by measuring scale.	Typically defined inside a time window. Actuarial methods normally not used.
Late reactions	Signs or symptoms of a specific late reaction. Defined by measuring scale.	Actuarial methods should be used.
Palliation	Typically defined by measuring scale.	May require special statistical considerations.
Quality of life	Typically defined by measuring scale.	May require special statistical considerations.

All definitions involving local recurrence are defined for nodal recurrence (N position) or distant recurrence (M) by analogy.
From Bentzen SM. Towards evidence based radiation oncology: Improving the design, analysis, and reporting of clinical outcome studies in radiotherapy. *Radiother Oncol* 1998;46:5–18, with permission.

analyses from the *British Journal of Cancer, European Journal of Cancer, Clinical Oncology,* and *American Journal of Clinical Oncology* published between October and December 1992. In 62% of the articles, at least one end point was not clearly defined, and in 39 (61%) it was unclear how it was included in the analysis of time to progression.

Measurement scales for the toxicity of therapy have been standardized through the Radiation Therapy Oncology Group/European Organization for Research and Treatment of Cancer system (21) and the Late Effects in Normal Tissue (LENT) and the Subjective, Objective, Management, Analytical (SOMA) criteria developed by these groups (70). Several items in this toxicity scale need to be validated with further clinical observations. Statistical validation of clinical data is critical and many methods are widely used, including chi-square test, regression analysis, probability values, and so forth (6,7,10,34).

Quality of Medical Care and Evidence-Based Medicine

Continuous quality improvement emerged from the industrial sector as an effective means of reducing production errors. The quality of health care can be precisely defined and measured with a degree of scientific accuracy comparable to that of most measures in clinical medicine (83). Health care quality problems may be classified into three categories:

(a) *Underuse* is the failure to provide a health care service when it would have produced a favorable outcome for a patient, such as not administering irradiation in breast-conserving therapy.
(b) *Overuse* occurs when a health care service is provided under circumstances in which its potential for harm exceeds the possible benefit, for example, prescribing postoperative pelvic irradiation to a patient with stage IA G1 endometrial carcinoma.
(c) *Misuse* takes place when an appropriate service has been selected but a preventable complication occurs and the patient does not received the full potential benefit of the service; avoidable complications of surgery, medications, or irradiation are important misuse problems (83).

Other issues influencing the inadequate use of services include geographic variation in the rate of use, training of general practice or specialist physicians, the makeup of the nonphysician health care work force, and the effect of organization of medical services as a determinant of quality.

In health care, continuous quality improvement is most effective when used as an integral part of a scientific approach to improving clinical practice. A potential strength is the ability to motivate good performers to excel and to place emphasis on generating new methods for achieving improvement. Among its limitations are a too-narrow focus on administrative (as opposed to clinical) aspects of care and a lack of attention to problems of overuse or underuse. Several major strategies have been advocated to move the health care delivery system toward improving quality. The challenges are (a) to always provide effective care of those who could benefit from it, (b) to always refrain from providing inappropriate services, and (c) to eliminate all preventable complications (14). Skeptics point out that no health care market currently competes on the basis of improving quality and there is little theoretic basis in economics to predict that this success will occur (83). Mendelson et al. (62) noted that there are many parties involved in outcome and effectiveness research (Fig. 96.4) and that payers and providers of health care may, in the future, use outcome research as a basis for coverage of services including procedures, devices or drugs.

Practice Guidelines

Guidelines for health services resulting from valid and appropriate outcome studies have the potential to promote consistency and quality of care. In the United States, clinical practice guidelines have been promulgated by the American Cancer Society, Association of Free Standing Cancer Centers, American College of Radiology, and other professional organizations (2,3,50,55). Sisk (84) observed that for such guidelines to be successful it is very important to involve local physicians in the process, to get their views and ultimately their support. The values of practice guidelines in medicine include minimizing inappropriate practice variations, providing reference points for education/practice, improving patient care and outcomes, providing criteria for self-evaluation, setting indicators for external quality review, assisting with service coverage and reimbursement, and decreasing overall cost of medical care. Perceived drawbacks to such guidelines include overregulation and loss of autonomy for both physicians and patients. The conflicting needs and motivations of physicians, patients, third-party

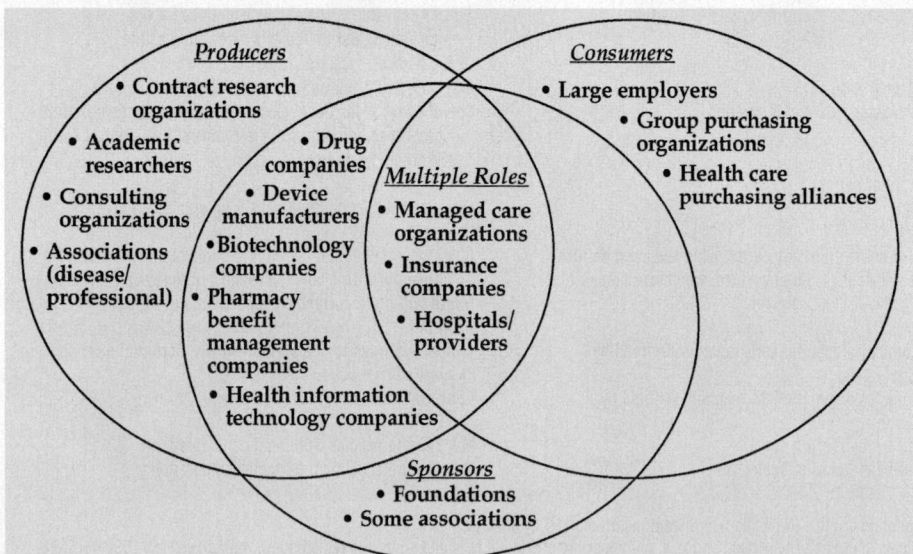

FIGURE 96.4. Stakeholders in outcomes and effectiveness research. (From Lewin Group. *Outcomes and effectiveness research in the private sector: final report.* Fairfax, VA: Lewin Group; 1997, with permission; and Mendelson DN, Goodman CS, Ahn R, et al. Outcomes and effectiveness research in the private sector. *Health Affairs* 75–90 Sep/Oct 1998:75–90, with permission.)

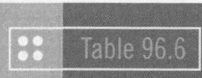

Table 96.6	AMERICAN COLLEGE OF RADIOLOGY APPROPRIATENESS GUIDELINES LITERATURE EVIDENCE TABLE KEY

Strength of Recommendation
(Quality of the study design)

- *Good* evidence to support recommendation that procedure be performed
- *Fair* evidence to support recommendation be performed
- *Poor* evidence to support recommendation, but it may be made on other grounds
- *Fair* evidence to support recommendation not be performed
- *Good* evidence to support recommendation not be performed

From Report of the US Preventative Services Task Force, Guide to Clinical Prevention Services: An Assessment of the Effectiveness of 169 Interventions (12).

carriers, and society bring into play a variety of ethical perspectives. Although contrasting ethical foundations likely will lead to significantly different solutions to the health care resource problem, it is only through educated and reasoned discussion that this problem can be tackled (68).

United States courts have ruled that guideline developers can be held liable for faulty guidelines and that doctors cannot pass off their liability by claiming that adherence to guidelines has corrupted clinical judgment. Protocols and guidelines provide the courts with examples of clinical standards across a wide range of medical practice. However, adherence to guidelines has not automatically been equated with reasonable practice, and the courts seem unlikely to follow the standards enunciated in clinical guidelines without critically evaluating their authority, flexibility, and scope of application (48).

Appropriateness Criteria Guidelines

This process to set radiology and radiation oncology practice guidelines, widely used by the American College of Radiology, consists of panels of academic and community practitioners who review published scientific information, critically assess evidence (for type and grade of validity). Based on specific clinical situations and using the Delphy method for grading evidence (1–3 = inappropriate, 4–6 = equivocal, 7–10 = acceptable) the panel of experts reaches a consensus, the data is tabulated, and reports are prepared. The strength of the recommendations are summarized in Table 96.6. In general, the appropriateness criteria documents are reviewed every 3 years and updates are published (55).

The Patterns of Care Study in the United States

The basic concepts of the Patterns of Care Study are based on analysis of structure, process, and outcome (51). Initially, all facilities in the United States that provided radiation therapy were identified, and a master list was developed; a statistically determined group of the facilities was selected to reflect the practice of radiation oncology throughout university hospitals, community hospitals, and free-standing facilities. The size and type of practice in each case were part of the evaluation process. Several surveys were conducted to define the structure of the facilities, including equipment, staffing, and prevailing standards of practice. More than 1,000 institutions were surveyed in each period of study, and thousands of patients have been included in the database.

Ten diseases were chosen in which curative radiation therapy played a major role. Through extensive discussions with appropriate physicians, a consensus of the best current management was developed for each disease, and decision trees were designed that logically led to the appropriate application

of radiation therapy (42). Process criteria were grouped into three categories, which included work-up, treatment, and auxiliary services (53). Data were collected on individual patients (with appropriate safeguard of privacy) and later the institutions were resurveyed to record the results of treatment including local/regional recurrence, disease outside the treated field, major complications of therapy, and so forth, leaving to publication of several reports correlating process with treatment outcome. An example is a recent report on practice of radiotherapy in carcinoma of the uterine cervix published by Eifel et al. (27).

Reports similar to those of the Patterns of Care studies in United States have been published in other countries, such as a recent one by Ringborg et al. (78) in Sweden.

Conclusions

Technology assessment, outcome analysis, cost benefit, and clinical trials supported by evidence-based medicine should be strengthened and fostered to enhance the rationale and quality of medical care provided to our patients at a competitive cost. Basic and translational laboratory research and properly designed, relevant, and timely prospective clinical trials should be strongly promoted, and patient participation must be increased to acquire more accurate information to develop innovative therapeutic strategies in oncology. Methods for accurate cost accounting of medical care and cost-benefit studies needs further development. Technology assessment will substantially contribute to better utilization of scarce health care resources and will be invaluable in determining the potential value of innovative therapeutic approaches.

References

1. Altman DG, De Stavola BL, Love SB, et al. Review of survival analyses published in cancer journals. *Br J Cancer* 1995;72:511–518.
2. American Society for Therapeutic Radiology and Oncology Consensus Panel. Consensus statement: guidelines for PSA following radiation therapy. *Int J Radiat Oncol Biol Phys* 1997;37:1035–1041.
3. American Society of Clinical Oncology. Recommended breast cancer surveillance guidelines. *J Clin Oncol* 1997;15:2149–2156.
4. Antos J, Brimson JA. *Activity-based management for service industries, government entities and nonprofit organizations.* New York: Wiley & Sons; 1994.
5. Back A. Patient-physician communication in oncology: what does the evidence show? *Oncology* 2006;20:67–74.
6. Begg C, Cho M, Eastwood S, et al. Improving the quality of reporting of randomized controlled trials. The CONSORT statement. *JAMA* 1996;276:637–639.
7. Bentzen SM. Towards evidence based radiation oncology: improving the design, analysis, and reporting of clinical outcome studies in radiotherapy. *Radiother Oncol* 1998;46:5–18.
8. Berkwits M. From practice to research: the case for criticism in an age of evidence. *Soc Sci Med* 1998;47:1539–1545.
9. Bigby M. Evidence-based medicine in a nutshell. A guide to finding and using the best evidence in caring for patients. *Arch Dermatol* 1998;134:1609–1618.
10. Borenstein M. The case for confidence intervals in controlled clinical trials. *Control Clin Trials* 1994;15:411–428.
11. Brook RH, Kamberg CJ, McGlynn EA. Health system reform and quality. *JAMA* 1996;276:476–480.
12. Canadian Medical Association: The Canadian Task Force on the Periodic Health Examination. *Can Med Assoc J* 1979;121:1193–1254.
13. Charting the course: Priorities for breast cancer research. In Breast Cancer Review Group Report, Bethesda, MD, National Cancer Institute, 1998.
14. Chassin MR, Galvin RW. The urgent need to improve health care quality. Institute of Medicine National Roundtable on Health Care Quality. *JAMA* 1998;280:1000–1005.
15. Clancy CM, Kamerow DB. Evidence-based medicine meets cost-effectiveness analysis. *JAMA* 1996;276:329–330.
16. Cochrane collaboration: preparing, maintaining, and promoting the accessibility of systemic reviews of the effects of healthcare interventions. Oxford: The Cochrane Collaboration; 1999.
17. Cooper R. *Elements of activity-based costing, emerging practices in cost management.* New York: Warren, Gorham & Lamont; 1990.
18. Cooper R, Kaplan RS. *The design of cost management systems.* Upper Saddle River, NJ: Prentice-Hall; 1991.
19. Cotter GW. Surgery or radiation therapy: a comparative cost analysis for early carcinoma of the prostate and breast. *Appl Radiol* 1990;19:25–28.
20. Cowan J, Berkowitz D. Technology assessment at work: part I—principles and a case study. *Physician Exec* 1996;22:5–6, 8–9.
21. Cox JD, Stetz J, Pajak TF. Toxicity criteria of the Radiation Therapy Oncology Group (RTOG) and the European Organization for Research and Treatment of Cancer (EORTC). *Int J Radiat Oncol Biol Phys* 1995;31:1341–1346.

Economics, Ethics, and Technology Assessment

22. Doubilet P, Weinstein MC, McNeil BJ. Use and misuse of the term "cost effective" in medicine. *N Engl J Med* 1986;314:253–256.

23. Doyle R. Health care costs. *Scientific America* 1999;280:36.

24. Drummond MF, Richardson WS. How to use an article on an economic analysis of clinical practice A. Are the results of the study valid. *JAMA* 1997;277:1552–1557.

25. Earle CC, Chapman RH, Baker CS, et al. Systematic overview of cost-utility assessments in oncology. *J Clin Oncol* 2000;18:3302–3317.

26. Eddy DC. Cost-effectiveness analysis, is it up to the task? *JAMA* 1992;267:3342–3348.

27. Eifel PJ, Moughan J, Erickson B, et al. Patterns of radiotherapy practice for patients with carcinoma of the uterine cervix: a pattern of care study. *Int J Radiat Oncol Biol Phys* 2004;60:1144–1153.

28. Feinstein AR, Horwitz RI. Problems in the "evidence" of "evidence-based medicine". *Am J Med* 1997;103:529–535.

29. Foster G, Gupta M. Activity accounting: an electronics industry implementation. In: Kaplan RS, ed. *Measures for manufacturing excellence.* Boston: Harvard Business School Press; 1990: 225–268.

30. Franklin E. Methodology for activity based costing in radiation oncology.

31. Fryback DG, Thornbury JR. The efficacy of diagnostic imaging. *Med Decis Making* 1991;11:88–94.

32. Fuchs VR, Garber AM. The new technology assessment. *N Engl J Med* 1990;323:673–677.

33. Gambrill E. Evidence-based clinical practice, [corrected] evidence-based medicine and the Cochrane collaboration. *J Behav Ther Exp Psychiatry* 1999;30:1–14.

34. Gardner MJ, Altman DG. Confidence intervals rather than P values: estimation rather than hypothesis testing. *Br Med J (Clin Res Ed)* 1986;292:746–750.

35. Giles K. Using clinical financial pathways to capitate cancer. *Oncology Issues* 1995;10:15–17.

36. Glatstein E. What is research? *Int J Radiat Oncol Biol Phys* 2001;51:288–290.

37. Goddard MK, Hutton J. What is the cost of radiotherapy? *Eur J Radiol* 1991;13:76–79.

38. Grimes DA, Atkins D. The U.S. Preventive Services Task Force: putting evidence-based medicine to work. *Clin Obstet Gynecol* 1998;41:332–342.

39. Guyatt GH, Sinclair J, Cook DJ, et al. Users' guides to the medical literature: XVI. How to use a treatment recommendation. Evidence-Based Medicine Working Group and the Cochrane Applicability Methods Working Group. *JAMA* 1999;281:1836–1843.

40. Halperin EC. Overpriced technology in radiation oncology. *Int J Radiat Oncol Biol Phys* 2000;48:917–918.

41. GE, Dunlap K. A comparison of the cost of various treatment methods for early cancer of the prostate. *Int J Radiat Oncol Biol Phys* 1986;12:1879–1881.

42. Hanks GE, Kramer S. Consensus of best current management: the starting point for clinical quality assessment. *Int J Radiat Oncol Biol Phys* 1984;10[Suppl 1]:87–97.

43. Hanks GE, Schultheiss TE, Hunt MA, et al. Factors influencing incidence of acute grade 2 morbidity in conformal and standard radiation treatment of prostate cancer. *Int J Radiat Oncol Biol Phys* 1995;31:25–29.

44. Harngren CT, Foster G, Datar SM. *Cost accounting. a managerial emphasis,* 9th ed. Upper Saddle River, NJ: Prentice Hall; 1996.

45. Hayman J, Weeks J, Mauch P. Economic analyses in health care: an introduction to the methodology with an emphasis on radiation therapy. *Int J Radiat Oncol Biol Phys* 1996;35:827–841.

46. Horwitz EM, Hanlon AL, Pinover WH, et al. The cost effectiveness of 3D conformal radiation therapy compared with conventional techniques for patients with clinically localized prostate cancer. *Int J Radiat Oncol Biol Phys* 1999;45:1219–1225.

47. Hunt DL, Haynes RB, Hanna SE, et al. Effects of computer-based clinical decision support systems on physician performance and patient outcomes: a systematic review. *JAMA* 1998;280:1339–1346.

48. Hurwitz B. Clinical guidelines and the law: advice, guidance or regulation? *J Eval Clin Pract* 1995;1:49–60.

49. Kobeissi BJ, Gupta M, Perez CA, et al. Physician resource utilization in radiation oncology: a model based on management of carcinoma of the prostate. *Int J Radiat Oncol Biol Phys* 1998;40:593–603.

50. Kotwall CA. Breast cancer treatment and chemoprevention. *Can Fam Physician* 1999;45:1917–1924.

51. Kramer S. An overview of process and outcome data in the patterns of care study. *Int J Radiat Oncol Biol Phys* 1981;7:795–800.

52. Kramer S, Herring DF. The patterns of care study: a nationwide evaluation of the practice of radiation therapy in cancer management. *Int J Radiat Oncol Biol Phys* 1976;1:1231–1236.

53. Leaf A. Cost effectiveness as a criterion for Medicare coverage. *N Engl J Med* 1989;321:898–900.

54. Lee SJ, Earle CC, Weeks JC. Outcomes research in oncology: history, conceptual framework, and trends in the literature. *J Natl Cancer Inst* 2000;92:195–204.

55. Leibel SA. ACR appropriateness criteria. Expert Panel on Radiation Oncology. American College of Radiology. *Int J Radiat Oncol Biol Phys* 1999;43:125–168.

56. Luce BR, Manning WG, Siegel JEea. Estimating costs in cost-effectiveness analysis. In: Gold MR, Siegel JE, Russell LB, et al., eds. *Cost-effectiveness in health and medicine.* New York: Oxford University Press; 1996:176–213.

57. McAlister FA, Straus SE, Guyatt GH, et al. Users' guides to the medical literature: XX. Integrating research evidence with the care of the individual patient. Evidence-Based Medicine Working Group. *JAMA* 2000;283:2829–2836.

58. McPhee SJ, Bird JA, Fordham D, et al. Promoting cancer prevention activities by primary care physicians. Results of a randomized, controlled trial. *JAMA* 1991;266:538–544.

59. McPhee SJ, Detmer WM. Office-based interventions to improve delivery of cancer prevention services by primary care physicians. *Cancer* 1993;72:1100–1112.

60. Meinert CL, Tonascia S. *Clinical trials: design, conduct, and analysis.* New York: Oxford University Press; 1986.

61. Meltzer MI. Introduction to health economics for physicians. *Lancet* 2001;358:993–998.

62. Mendelson DN, Goodman CS, Ahn R, et al. Outcomes and effectiveness research in the private sector. *Health Aff (Millwood)* 1998;17:75–90.

63. Mulrow CD, Cook DJ, Davidoff F. Systematic reviews; critical links in the great chain of evidence. In: *Systematic reviews: synthesis of best evidence for health care decisions.* American College of Physicians; Philadelphia, PA, 1998:1–4.

64. Neilson AR, Davies HT. Interpreting reported health-care costs. *Hosp Med* 1998;59:803–806.

65. Newman L, ed. *Medical outcomes & guidelines sourcebook,* 2000 New York: Faulkner & Gray; 1999.

66. Nicolucci A, Grilli R, Alexanian AA, et al. Quality, evolution, and clinical implications of randomized, controlled trials on the treatment of lung cancer. A lost opportunity for meta-analysis. *JAMA* 1989;262:2101–2107.

67. Owen JB, Grigsby PW, Caldwell TM, et al. Can costs be measured and predicted by modeling within a cooperative clinical trials group? Economic methodologic pilot studies of the radiation therapy oncology group (RTOG) studies 90-03 and 91-04. *Int J Radiat Oncol Biol Phys* 2001;49:633–639.

68. Panek WC. Ethical considerations related to outcome studies-based clinical practice guidelines. *J Glaucoma* 1999;8:267–272.

69. Parker RG. Varying charges for comparably effective cancer treatments. *Am J Clin Oncol* 1992;15:281–287.

70. Pavy JJ, Denekamp J, Letschert J, et al. EORTC Late Effects Working Group. Late effects toxicity scoring: the SOMA scale. *Radiother Oncol* 1995;35:11–15.

71. Penn CR. Megavoltage irradiation in a district general hospital remote from a main oncology centre: the Torbay experience reviewed. *Clin Oncol (R Coll Radiol)* 1992;4:108–113.

72. Perez CA. Methodology of research and practice for the third millennium: evidence-based medicine. *Rays* 2000;25:285–308. *Radiat Oncol Phys* 1993;25:895–906.

73. Perez CA, Kobeissi B, Smith BD, et al. Cost accounting in radiation oncology: a computer-based model for reimbursement. *Int J*

74. Perez CA, Kobeissi BJ, Chao KSC, et al. *3-D conformal and intensity modulated radiation therapy: physics & clinical applications.* Madison, WI: Advanced Medical Publishing, Inc.; 2001.

75. Pollack A, Zagars GK, Smith LG, et al. Preliminary results of a randomized radiotherapy dose-escalation study comparing 70 Gy with 78 Gy for prostate cancer. *J Clin Oncol* 2000;18:3904–3911.

76. Pringle M, Robins S, Brown G. Computer assisted screening: effects on the patient and his consultation. *Br Med J (Clin Res Ed)* 1990;290:1709–1712.

77. Rigby K, Silagy C, Crockett A. Health economic reviews. Are they compiled systematically? *Int J Technol Assess Health Care* 1996;12:450–459.

78. Ringborg U, Bergqvist D, Brorsson B, et al. The Swedish Council on Technology Assessment in Health Care (SBU) systematic overview of radiotherapy for cancer including a prospective survey of radiotherapy practice in Sweden 2001—summary and conclusions. *Acta Oncol* 2003;42:357–365.

79. Russell LB. Modelling for cost-effectiveness analysis. *Stat Med* 1999;18:3235–3244.

80. Russell LB, Gold MR, Siegel JE, et al. The role of cost-effectiveness analysis in health and medicine. Panel on Cost-Effectiveness in Health and Medicine. *JAMA* 1996;276:1172–1177.

81. Sackett DL, Straus S, Richardson S, et al. *Evidence-based medicine: how to practice and teach EBM,* 2nd ed. London: Churchill Livingston; 2000.

82. Siegel JE, Weinstein MC, Russell LB, et al. Recommendations for reporting cost-effectiveness analyses. Panel on Cost-Effectiveness in Health and Medicine. *JAMA* 1996;276:1339–1341.

83. Sisk JE. Increased competition and the quality of health care. *Milbank Q* 1998;76:687–707, 512.

84. Sisk JE. How are health care organizations using clinical guidelines? *Health Aff (Millwood)* 1998;17:91–109.

85. Sisk JM. Effectively costing out options. *JAMA* 1996;276:1180.

86. Smith S, Freeland M, Heffler S, et al. The next ten years of health spending: what does the future hold? The Health Expenditures Projection Team. *Health Aff (Millwood)* 1998;17:128–140.

87. Smith TJ, Hillner BE, Desch CE. Efficacy and cost-effectiveness of cancer treatment: rational allocation of resources based on decision analysis. *J Natl Cancer Inst* 1993;85:1460–1474.

88. Stinnett AA, Mullahy J. Net health benefits: a new framework for the analysis of uncertainty in cost-effectiveness analysis. *Med Decis Making* 1998;18:S68–80.

89. Tanenbaum SJ. Evidence and expertise: the challenge of the outcomes movement to medical professionalism. *Acad Med* 1999;74:757–763.

90. Thornbury JR. Eugene W. Caldwell Lecture. Clinical efficacy of diagnostic imaging: love it or leave it. *AJR Am J Roentgenol* 1994;162:1–8.

91. Walker QJ, Salkeld G, Hall J, et al. The management of oesophageal carcinoma: radiotherapy or surgery? Cost considerations. *Eur J Cancer Clin Oncol* 1989;25:1657–1662.

92. Weinstein MC, Siegel JE, Gold MR, et al. Recommendations of the Panel on Cost-effectiveness in Health and Medicine. *JAMA* 1996;276:1253–1258.

93. Willan AR. Analysis, sample size, and power for estimating incremental net health benefit from clinical trial data. *Control Clin Trials* 2001;22:228–237.

94. Wodinsky HB, Jenkin RD. The cost of radiation treatment at an Ontario regional cancer centre. *CMAJ* 1987;137:906–909.

95. Youngs MT, Wingerson L. *The 1996 medical outcomes & guidelines sourcebook.* New York: Faulkner & Gray; 1995.

96. Zola P, Volpe T, Castelli G, et al. Is the published literature a reliable guide for deciding between alternative treatments for patients with early cervical cancer? *Int J Radiat Oncol Biol Phys* 1989;16:785–797.

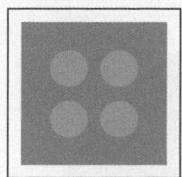

Chapter 97
Ethics, Professional Values, and Legal Considerations in Radiation Oncology

Brian D. Kavanagh, Laurie Lyckholm, Jeremy Sugarman

The medical profession experienced a rise in socioeconomic stature in the United States during the 20th century (43). Physicians began to receive higher wages for their services and enjoy greater personal respect as providers of health. Although progress in medical science has improved the quality and duration of life for some patients with cancer and other serious illnesses, technical expertise alone does not fully account for the upsurge in the societal standing of medical doctors during the last hundred years.

High regard for physicians is contingent on the trust that doctors act unselfishly in a patient's best interest, a role sometimes called *moral fiduciary* (10). Essential to this role are medical knowledge and a firm grasp of ethics. Derived from the Greek ηθοσ (*ethos*), meaning *character*, ethics refers to the process of applying values and principles in professional interactions and particularly in medical decision-making on behalf of patients. The curriculum of most medical schools now includes coursework in ethics, but many physicians practicing today completed their training without formal instruction in this topic. To foster an appreciation for the intellectual underpinnings of modern medical ethics, this chapter begins with an overview of scholarly approaches to ethics. Next is a discussion of selected proclamations and codes of ethics published by professional societies, federal commissions, and other authorities as guidelines for medical practice and research. Finally, common ethical issues in radiation oncology are addressed, including relevant medicolegal considerations.

Conceptual Approaches to Medical Ethics

The term *bioethics*, coined in the early 1970s, refers to the academic inquiry and public policy movement addressing the application of science and medicine from a humanistic perspective (39). Medical ethics may be most accurately viewed as a branch of bioethics, but the terms are commonly used interchangeably. Among the more influential theoretical approaches to ethics that are used in bioethics are *utilitarianism*, *deontology*, *casuistry*, *virtue theory*, and *principlism*.

Utilitarianism is based on the premise that, in any situation, the best course of action is the one that produces the maximum net positive value (or least negative value). Utilitarianism can be applied to an individual patient's case or to matters of health policy, in which decisions might be made to achieve the greatest overall benefit for the largest number of people.

Unlike utilitarianism, deontology is an ethical theory based on the morality of actions themselves rather than their net result. Deontology, sometimes called *Kantianism* in recognition of the influence of Immanuel Kant (6), calls for consistent standards of behavior at all times, regardless of the consequences. One simple example of the difference between utilitarianism and deontology is the issue of educating patients about their diagnosis, especially if the prognosis is very poor. Whereas a deontologist would always feel obliged to tell the truth even at the risk of causing distress, a utilitarian considers whether telling a patient the complete truth about the disease does or does not really benefit the patient. In practice, there is obviously a need to find the right balance between purely utilitarian and purely deontologic perspectives in a situation like this one. Respect for the patient's autonomy, for example, is one of the *prima facie* ethical principles discussed further in the next section. Truthtelling is an integral component, and overriding this principle requires justification.

Casuistry is an approach to ethics that emphasizes inductive reasoning based on established precedents, and it is a common practice in both law and medicine. The proper course of action in any individual case is decided by recalling decisions made in prior similar cases. The major weakness of casuistry is the lack of a reference benchmark or settled opinion on novel technologies.

Virtue theory focuses on the character of moral agents, in this case physicians and other health care providers, focusing less on actions or outcomes. As such, virtue theory captures the way in which correct moral actions occur. For example, it is not only important to tell patients the truth about their diagnoses, but it is also critical to do so in a compassionate manner. In this case, the virtue is compassion. Accordingly, while virtue is a critical part of assessing moral action, virtues themselves have little guiding force.

Principlism is a system of applied ethics through which core principles ideally govern behavior in the absence of compelling reasons to override them. Principlism can be integrated with the other philosophical approaches already mentioned and serves as a unifying influence. Key features of principlism are addressed in the next section.

Ethical Principles

A *prima facie* obligation may be defined as one that is "binding unless overridden or outweighed by competing moral obligations" (6). Four *prima facie* principles of bioethics are highlighted here: *respect for autonomy*, *beneficence*, *nonmaleficence*, and *justice*.

Respect for a patient's autonomy is based on respect for the right to individual liberty. A patient's voluntary decision to seek medical care or comply with referral to a specialist is the starting point of most patient–physician relationships, and competent patients should remain free to forego therapy or change physicians at any time. The responsibility to respect patients' autonomy is established not only in ethics but also in law. An example is the requirement to obtain a patient's informed consent for proposed medical therapy. In a landmark case involving postmastectomy chest wall radiation therapy, a patient who sustained soft tissue necrosis won a lawsuit against her radiation oncologist for negligence and for lack of proper disclosure regarding possible treatment-related toxicity. The Kansas Supreme Court ruled that doctors should explain "in language as simple as necessary" the side effects associated with any recommended therapy (32).

The principle of *beneficence* is intertwined with that of *nonmaleficence*. Some authors have offered nuanced distinctions between the two principles (6), but the key point is that physicians should act for the benefit of patients and should not harm their patients. Beneficence and nonmaleficence are typically concordant objectives, but sometimes an intervention that is helpful also entails a high risk of adverse treatment-induced sequelae. For example, administering high-dose morphine to a patient severely dyspneic from an incurable lung malignancy can relieve symptoms but at the same time risks fatally suppressing respiratory drive. Here the quality of remaining life might be improved by a measure that also hastens death. Such an action can sometimes be justified by the principle of double effect, the earliest expression of which is generally attributed to St. Thomas Aquinas (3). According to this concept, the benefit of an action might be valuable enough to outweigh a simultaneous significant risk of serious adverse event, as long as achieving benefit is the primary intent. High-dose chemotherapy, bone marrow transplant, and some high-complexity surgeries, such as Whipple procedures, are examples of cancer therapies in which potential burdens and risks might militate against potential benefits.

The principle of justice refers to fairness, typically the equitable distribution of health care resources. Justice-related questions often arise in regard to matters of public policy. Two examples are determining the means to allocate scarce organs for transplantation and selecting what types of research merit government funding. More globally relevant in the United States is the challenge of allocating federal dollars for health care. Distributive justice implies that persons ought to be afforded medical care according to their medical needs and the ability of the system to provide. The Center for Medicare Services applies a relative value unit method to compare the physician workload of different medical services and assign reimbursement values accordingly. However, the Center for Medicare Services relative value unit method does not address the much more complex challenge of weighting specific physician activities according to net value to society as a whole, which would be a more formidable task.

Formal Oaths and Codes of Ethics

There are many published declarations of medical ethics authored by physicians. Not surprisingly, the tone and language of each reflect the social mores and sometimes historical events of the era in which it was composed.

The Hippocratic Oath

"... I will prescribe regimen for the good of my patients according to my ability and my judgment and never do harm to anyone...."

The *Corpus Hippocraticum* is a collection of medical treatises dating from around the fifth century BCE, believed to be the work of philosopher–physicians from the Greek island of Cos (Fig. 97.1). Contained within the *Corpus* is the well-known oath of Hippocrates, an ancient physician's pledge of professionalism. Curiously, the oath is inconsistent with some other sections of the *Corpus*, perhaps because it was added later. Comments about abortion and surgery, for example, are at variance with teachings elsewhere in the collected works (29). Nevertheless, timeless themes are included, and the oath has survived in various modernized versions. The oath is often recited by medical students at the time of graduation—even if its contents are not always well remembered (19,31).

Percival's Medical Ethics

"Hospital physicians and surgeons should minister to the sick, with due impressions of the importance of their office, reflecting

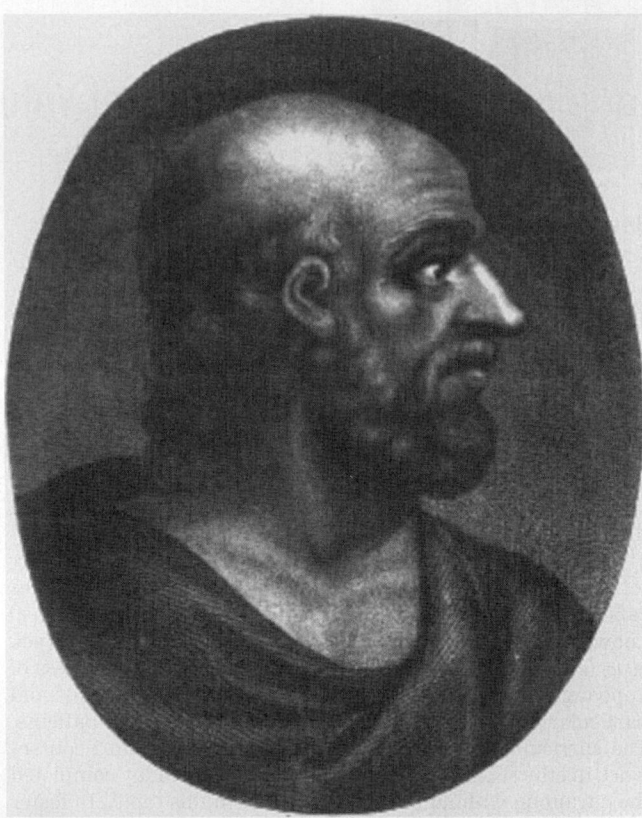

FIGURE 97.1. Early 19th century engraving depicting a likeness of Hippocrates, closely resembling images of ancient coins found on the island of Cos bearing his likeness. (Courtesy of the National Library of Medicine.)

that the ease, the health, and the lives of those committed to their charge depend on their skill, attention, and fidelity."

Thomas Percival (1740–1804) (Fig. 97.2) published *Medical Ethics* (26) at a time when there were considerable tensions among clinicians in his community. In the 1760s, Manchester, England, was a prosperous urban society that comfortably supported public health initiatives, including an infirmary serving as a charity hospital and teaching institution. But as the city grew and became crowded by the 1790s, tensions arose between rival groups in the medical community. Percival was prompted to draft a code of ethics after a contentious dispute about enlarging the infirmary's staff, a threat to the controlling physician faction (38).

When he began writing *Medical Ethics*, Percival was already a well-known writer and moralist whose *A Father's Instructions to His Children*, published in 1775, included essays promoting personal virtues and social awareness to young readers. While completing *Medical Ethics*, Percival suffered devastating personal tragedies, bereaving the untimely deaths of two of his own sons. The finished work was dedicated to a third son studying medicine at the time.

Ultimately, *Medical Ethics* provided a template for the codes of ethics adopted by the American Medical Association (AMA) and other societies in the 19th century. Early 20th century pundits criticized Percival's work as merely a book of medical *etiquette* rather than medical *ethics*. However, revisionist historians have subsequently argued that although Percival focused on interprofessional relationships, he also taught that a physician's duty toward the patient outweighs obligations of civility toward other health care professionals. Furthermore, Percival advanced the enlightened view that indigent patients should receive the same quality of care as affluent patients (4).

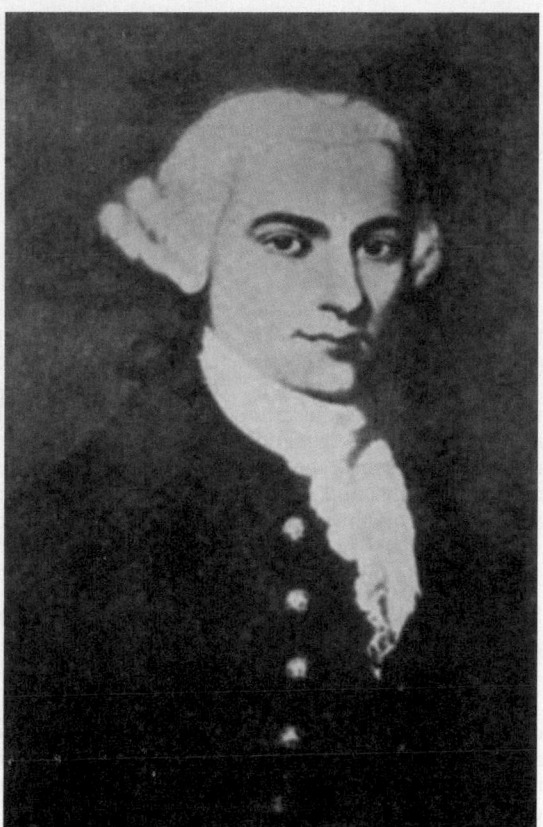

FIGURE 97.2. Thomas Percival (1740–1804). (From Brockbank EM. *Sketches of the lives and work of the honorary medical staff of the Manchester Infirmary , from its foundation in 1752 to 1830 when it became the Royal Infirmary .* Manchester, England: University Press; 1904, with permission.)

The American Medical Association Code of Ethics

The AMA first adopted a code of ethics at its inaugural meeting in 1847. The initial code was modeled on the work of Percival, but subsequent updates have reflected societal changes and technological progress. The most recently revised format (2) includes four components:

(a) *Principles of Medical Ethics;*
(b) *Fundamental Elements of the Patient–Physician Relationship;*
(c) *Current Opinions of the Council on Ethical and Judicial Affairs;* and
(d) *Reports of the Council on Ethical and Judicial Affairs.*

The seven *Principles* are general instructions for a physician to maintain competence and integrity in the context of individual patient care and also in the larger view toward enhancing the standard of care in the community. The *Fundamental Elements* expand the concept of a collaborative interaction between physicians and patients, specifically mentioning the need for good communication and the need to protect the patients' confidentiality. The AMA here advocates that all patients have a right to "necessary care" regardless of their ability to pay for that care, and that physicians should play a role in safeguarding this right. The *Current Opinions* and the *Reports of the Council on Ethical and Judicial Affairs* provide situational interpretations of the *Principles* and *Fundamental Elements,* and they are often referenced in legal proceedings.

The Nuremberg Code and the Declaration of Geneva

During World War II, odious crimes were committed by Nazi physicians who conducted horrific experiments on concentration camp prisoners who were coerced to submit. The Nuremberg Code was a formal response to these World War II era human rights atrocities disguised as medical investigation (48). Issued from the military tribunal that tried some of the Nazi doctors who conducted these experiments, the Nuremberg Code acknowledges that medical investigations are important. However, for a medical experiment to be morally permissible, it must meet 10 criteria, paraphrased as follows:

- Voluntary consent of the human subject
- Necessity to yield results helpful to society
- Appropriate design based on knowledge of the disease under study
- Avoidance of unnecessary physical and mental suffering and injury
- Absence of reason to believe that death or disabling injury will occur
- Overall degree of risk in proportion to the nature of the problem to be solved
- Adequate precautions against the possibility of the subject's injury, disability, or death
- Qualified persons conducting the study
- Unrestricted freedom of the subject to end the experiment if he or she reaches the physical or mental state where continuation of the experiment seems impossible
- Willingness of the investigator to discontinue the study at any time if there is reason to believe that continuing the experiment is likely to result in injury or death to the subject

In the aftermath of the war, the international medical community was especially sensitized to the need for universal adherence to high standards of ethical behavior. The Declaration of Geneva was adopted in 1948 by the World Medical Association and has been updated since then. The text includes the physician's vow to ignore "considerations of age, disease or disability, creed, ethnic origin, gender, nationality, political affiliation, race, sexual orientation, or social standing" in the treatment of a patient and to uphold "even under threat . . . the utmost respect for human life."

Case Study

Despite publicity about the Nuremberg Code and the Geneva declaration, controversial large-scale, government-sponsored medical studies took place in the years following World War II. Experimentation on the effects of radiation exposure on humans was conducted in the United States during the Cold War, when fears of nuclear warfare prompted inquiry into the carcinogenic and other adverse health effects of environmental exposure to ionizing radiation. In response to growing public concern about possibly unethical federally funded studies conducted from the 1940s through 1970s, in 1994 the U.S. Department of Energy established the Office of Human Radiation Experiments. A massive effort to identify and analyze more than 4,000 experiments culminated in the publication of *Human Radiation Experiments: The Department of Energy Roadmap to the Story and the Records,* available online through the Department of Energy web site (http://tis.eh.doe.gov/ohre/roadmap/index.html).

A federal advisory committee of ethicists, radiation oncologists, and others with relevant expertise was charged with evaluating the experiments' ethical and scientific standards and recommending actions to ensure that any mistakes of the past would not be repeated. This Advisory Committee on Human

Radiation Experiments reviewed all available documentation and also conducted an oral history project in which scientists described prevailing sentiments regarding human research ethics during the era of interest.

After sifting through studies of nontherapeutic research on children and intentional environmental releases of radiation, among others, Advisory Committee on Human Radiation Experiments found that government officials and investigators were in some cases culpable "for not having had policies and practices in place to protect the rights and interests of human subjects who ... could not possibly derive direct medical benefit" (1). One example was the observational study of uranium mine workers exposed to radon levels known to be hazardous, without warning and without efforts to reduce the radon levels by ventilating the mines. As a result, lung cancer developed in hundreds of workers, and appropriate compensation was recommended for the individuals affected.

The Belmont Report

In 1972 Jean Heller exposed the injustices of the United States Public Health Services (USPHS) Study of Untreated Syphilis in the Negro Male that was conducted in Tuskegee, Alabama (22). During a 40-year period beginning in the 1930s, 399 indigent African American sharecroppers with syphilis and 200 without syphilis were subjects in a natural history study of the disease. The men mistakenly believed that diagnostic blood tests and lumbar punctures composed treatment for their "bad blood" when in reality these were done solely to monitor the course of the infection. Moreover, years later when penicillin was discovered and found to be effective in the treatment of syphilis, it was withheld intentionally from the men. Public awareness of the USPHS study likely contributed to enduring reluctance among minority groups to participate in clinical trials (12,13), and the political backlash provoked action by the federal government.

The 1974 National Research Act established the National Commission for the Protection of Human Subjects of Biomedical and Behavioral Research. The Commission met at the Smithsonian Institution's Belmont Conference Center in Maryland to develop ethical guidelines for the conduct of biomedical and behavioral research. In 1979 the Commission published *Ethical Principles and Guidelines for the Protection of Human Subjects of Research,* commonly known as the Belmont Report.

In the Belmont Report, a clear distinction is made between medical research and clinical practice. The term *practice* describes interventions intended "to enhance the well-being of an individual patient ... that have a reasonable expectation of success," whereas *research* is "designed to test an hypothesis, permit conclusions to be drawn, and ... contribute to generalizable knowledge." Sometimes a clinician uses good judgment and departs from standard methods for the benefit of an individual patient in special circumstances. However, if major innovations are proposed as replacement for standard techniques, then a formal investigation should be conducted to assess safety and efficacy. Even quality-improvement initiatives such as patient satisfaction questionnaires might be classified as research activity in certain circumstances (9).

The National Commission embraced a principlist perspective in drafting the report, emphasizing in particular respect for persons, beneficence, and justice. The Belmont Report definition of respect for persons incorporates respect for autonomy and special concern for individuals with diminished capacity to exercise their autonomy. Involving prisoners in research activity is cited as an example. Although it is inappropriate to deny prisoners the possible benefit of experimental interventions, any direct or indirect pressure on prisoners to participate in clinical studies must be avoided. For instance, a promise of clemency in return for study enrollment is unacceptable. The report also addresses the nature of justice in medical research, emphasizing that the process of selecting subjects for a research study must be carefully examined. Investigators should minimize the chance that socioeconomically disadvantaged groups are represented disproportionately as a result of a vulnerability to manipulation in the health care environment.

The American College of Radiation Oncology Code of Ethics

The American College of Radiation Oncology (ACRO) has developed a code of ethics, available for review at the organization's web site (www.acro.org). The principles expressed are concordant with accepted ethical standards and include respect of patient autonomy, the expectation that a radiation oncologist should always act in the best interest of the patient, and respect of patient confidentiality. The ACRO code also forbids deceptive billing arrangements, and members of ACRO who do not comply with the code of ethics are subject to disciplinary action by the organization.

National Electrical Manufacturers Association Code of Ethics

The makers of equipment and software used in the practice of radiation oncology are not required to demonstrate clinical efficacy of a new device or software through the same sort of clinical testing that is required by the Food and Drug Administration (FDA) for approval of a new drug or implantable medical device. Rather, most treatment devices are approved after demonstration of safety and substantial equivalence to an approved device already commercially available. A company that wishes to sell a new device submits a premarket notification to the FDA at least 90 days before commercial distribution is to begin, in accordance with section 510(k) of the FDA Modernization Act of 1997. Because devices may be introduced into the market without proof of superiority in any given clinical situation, manufacturers may promote their products to physicians by emphasizing intuitively attractive features that might or might not provide meaningful clinical advantage to patients.

On January 1, 2005, members of the National Electrical Manufacturers Association (NEMA) adopted a code of ethics regarding interactions between makers of medical imaging and treatment equipment and physicians (www.nema.org). Individual sections of the NEMA code address member-sponsored product training and education, support for third-party educational conferences, sales and promotional meetings, arrangements with consultants, gifts, provision of reimbursement and other economic information, charitable donations, and research grants. The guidelines are essentially consistent with the AMA policy on gifts and applicable federal regulations. NEMA members are allowed to support educational conferences and advertise their wares in these venues, and also they may provide educational support for individual customers in the safe use of their products. However, hospitality provided by NEMA member at conferences and meeting should be "modest in value and ... subordinate in time and focus to the purpose of the meeting." When necessary to demonstrate nonportable equipment, members may pay for reasonable travel costs of attendees with a bona fide professional interest but not for their guests.

●● | Common Ethical Issues in Radiation Oncology

Doctors wear a lot of hats these days; besides the usual physician role, we are expected to be a researcher, financial counselor, administrator, gatekeeper, patient advocate in the medicolegal system, ethicist, and Lord knows what else.

Thomas J. Smith (42)

Financial Relationships with Hospitals and Referring Physicians

Reimbursement for radiation oncology services or other procedure-intensive subspecialties can be a major revenue source for hospitals. At the same time, subspecialists depend on other physicians to refer patients for evaluation and management. These situations can tempt hospital administrators to reward subspecialists for practicing in their facility and might tempt the subspecialists to induce referrals with financial incentives. In either case, a conflict of interest emerges: Treatment recommendations can be influenced not only appropriately by patient-centered beneficence but also inappropriately by the physician's interest in personal gain. In the United States, the Anti-Kickback Statute and the Stark Law make it illegal to engage in such unscrupulous medical business practices.

The Anti-Kickback Statute (42 U.S.C. §1320a-7b) describes criminal penalties for acts involving Medicare or state health care programs. Section (b) makes it a felony punishable by a fine up to $25,000 and up to 5 years in prison to solicit or receive "any remuneration (including any kickback, bribe, or rebate) directly or indirectly ... in return for referring an individual to a person for ... any item or service" reimbursed in whole or in part through Medicare or a state health care program. The Anti-Kickback Statute also bans other fraudulent transactions supported through the same funding sources.

Named for its leading congressional author, Rep. Pete Stark of California, the Stark Law (42 U.S.C. §1395nn; "Limitation on certain physician referrals") bans other misconduct involving Medicare and Medicaid patients. The Stark Law prohibits a physician from referring a patient for a "designated health service" to a clinic or other facility with which the physician or an immediate family member of the physician has a financial relationship. Radiation therapy is considered a designated health service, but it is clarified that a request by a radiation oncologist for radiation therapy is considered integral to the consultation request from the (nonradiation oncologist) referring physician and does not constitute a self-referral per se in most situations. Sanctions for violations of the numerous Stark Law regulations may include civil prosecution with fines of up to $100,000 per incident in certain cases.

Managed Care

By the early 1990s, more than 70% of Americans with health insurance were enrolled in some form of managed care plan (18) in which patients are restricted in their choices of physicians and medical services for the purpose of limiting the cost of the health care (40). The idea has existed in the United States at least since the time of the Great Depression of 1929, when Dr. Michael Shadid of Oklahoma organized a prepay and copay system for surgical, medical, and dental services. To maintain profitability, managed care organizations influence the behavior of patients and physicians through strategies to minimize expenditures. Tactics directed toward patients are promotion of preventive medicine, limitation of access to medical specialists unless approved by a "gatekeeper" primary care physician, and restricted selection of physicians to those willing to accept lower reimbursements. Physicians are prompted to lower costs by capitation-based compensation packages and financial rewards to avoid excess resource utilization.

Managed care is ethically defensible insofar as it can provide equal access for participants and promote well-being through an emphasis on preventive medicine. However, managed care

can also threaten the physician–patient relationship by undermining the patient's autonomy and creating a conflict of interest for the health care provider (16). If the physician gatekeeper shares financial risk with the managed care organization, a patient with a difficult medical problem might be less likely to be referred to a specialist where higher costs would be expected to result.

Physicians' attitudes about managed care reflect concern about ethics. A survey of primary care physicians revealed that most of them believed that managed care has a negative impact on the patient–physician relationships by interfering with patients' choices and compromising the physicians' ability to put the patients' interest first (17). Medical students and residents frequently receive negative messages about managed care from their faculty mentors (41).

Oncology services are often still provided by managed care organizations through fee-for-service contracts with independent practitioners. Although financial conflicts of interest can potentially be avoided for the specialists involved, there remain problematic patient management issues. Among the items identified as challenging with regard to delivering radiation therapy in the setting of managed care are the sometimes fragmented care and inconvenience for the patient, whose managed care organization might have contracted with several centers for various aspects of oncology care, and the administrative burdens associated with obtaining documentation of preapproval for patients' radiation treatments (15). A legislative solution proposed but not passed to date in the U.S. Congress is the Patients' Bill of Rights establishing the legal right to sue managed care organizations when profit-driven policies adversely affect access to needed services or lead to injury.

Electronic Record-Keeping and Billing Practices

The principles of respect for autonomy and nonmaleficence oblige confidentiality in physician-patient communications. Publicizing private details of a patient's condition can create social and economic harms for patients. With the advent of electronic medical records and Internet communication, there is a greater need for vigilance in this respect.

In the United States, the Health Insurance Portability and Accountability Act of 1996 (HIPAA) empowered the Department of Health and Human Services to codify standards for storage and transmission of an individual patient's health information. Penalties for violations vary in proportion to their severity. In the worst case of wrongful disclosure of information with intent to sell it, a fine of up to $250,000 and a prison term of up to 10 years can be imposed.

Submitting fraudulent claims to the government for reimbursement of health care services is illegal. The False Claims Act (31 U.S.C. §3729) provides that any person who knowingly presents fraudulent claims to the U.S. government may be fined $5,000 to $10,000 and may be liable for three times the amount of any damages sustained by the government.

Applications of New Technology

Innovative treatment-delivery technologies such as intensity-modulated radiation therapy and stereotactic body radiation therapy provide radiation oncologists freedom to exercise creativity in customizing treatment plans for individual patients. Ideally, it is best that such innovations are tested in formal research protocols in which a clinical problem is identified and the new technology is proposed as a solution so that toxicity and efficacy can be monitored closely. A prospective clinical trial approved and monitored by an institutional review board affords the opportunity to advance knowledge in the field with ethical oversight (14). It is inappropriate to apply a novel, more expensive technology to generate higher revenue in the absence

Economics, Ethics, and Technology Assessment

of a sound clinical rationale. The AMA Code of Ethics proscribes superfluous therapy of no benefit to the patient (36).

Clinical Trial Conduct

Instances of flagrantly improper clinical research taint the annals of medical history. The USPHS study of syphilis mentioned earlier and the many human radiation experiments conducted during the Cold War without the consent of the participants are dark reminders of the need for ethical oversight of research.

Obtaining a participant's informed consent is of paramount importance in conducting most clinical research. Despite the recognized importance of informed consent, precisely how much information should be conveyed to a potential clinical trial participant is debatable. The Belmont Report offers this criterion: "the extent and nature of information should be such that persons, knowing that the procedure is neither necessary for their care nor perhaps fully understood, can decide whether they wish to participate" in the study. In certain situations the nature of a study requires that there is incomplete disclosure of information to the participant to sustain the integrity of the study. The Belmont Report condones such research only when "i) incomplete disclosure is truly necessary to accomplish the goals of the research, ii) there are no undisclosed risks to subjects that are more than minimal, and iii) there is an adequate plan for debriefing subjects, when appropriate, and for dissemination of research results to them." The federal rules governing research (45 CFR 46) reflect these arguments.

Advances in the biosciences, such as stem cell research, cloning, and manipulations of the human genome, have been associated with contentious public debate. Federal government and professional policies on such matters have sometimes been constructed as a compromise between scientific opportunity and political ideology (30). Extra safeguards have been imposed in some settings; for example, the federal government requires an extra level of review for gene-transfer experiments (33).

At a professional level, the AMA Code of Ethics endorses clinical research into somatic cell gene-transfer experiments in which cells are genetically altered for therapeutic gain. However, the AMA has objected to intentional germline alterations, in which heritable traits are modified by integrating replacement genes into gametes (34). This position might change as scientists acquire more preclinical understanding of the effects of germline modification.

Relationships with Industry Sponsors

Incentives from industry representatives to prescribe pharmaceuticals or purchase equipment threaten the fiduciary obligations physicians have to their patients. The AMA Code of Ethics allows that gifts of modest value with direct or indirect benefit to patients are acceptable (35). Examples include textbooks or unrestricted educational grants for students or fellows. Subsidies for "modest meals or social events held as part of a conference" are permissible, as are honoraria for lectures or legitimate consulting services. However, cash or other valuable incentives intended to influence the decision to use a company's products are forbidden. Also unacceptable would be a blanket indemnification from liability for use of a product, except in special circumstances such as sponsored research activity. Advertising items such as patient education pamphlets and anatomic models bearing a sponsor's name are commonly found in radiation oncology clinics (24). Physicians should be aware of any real or perceived influence on the patient-physician relationships resulting from their tacit compliance with such marketing activities.

In recent years some pharmaceutical companies have been prosecuted for kickback schemes or other illegal enticements to physicians, and the civil and criminal penalties paid by the corporations held responsible have ranged up to hundreds of millions of dollars (44). Brennan et al. (8) contend that voluntary self-regulation by physicians, industry, and government is an insufficient safeguard against the conflict of interest nurtured by close relationships between practicing doctors and sellers of pharmaceuticals and medical products. These authors argue that academic medical centers should set an example for the rest of the medical community by establishing policies that forbid gifts to physicians, funds for travel, unjustified consulting fees, participation in speakers' bureaus, and the practice of "ghostwriting" medical articles, among other things. At least one medical school has come forth with a stringent policy prohibiting its faculty from receiving personal gifts or meals and mandating compliance with university policy on the resolution of conflicts of interest (11).

Case-Specific Dilemmas: the Role of an Ethics Consultant or Committee

The radiation oncology-related ethical issues discussed thus far relate primarily to general practice and research guidelines. However, individual cases can also pose uncertainties regarding the proper choice of action for a specific patient.

Case study: A 37-year-old woman undergoes modified radical mastectomy for a pathologic T3N2M0 breast cancer; postoperative chemotherapy and locoregional radiation therapy are recommended. The patient wishes to receive the therapy only if she can periodically interrupt it to alternate with what she calls a "natural herbal" therapy.

In this case, respect for a patient's autonomy conflicts with what is believed to be in the patient's best interest, but a physician cannot ethically abrogate the fiduciary responsibility to a patient simply for reasons of unfamiliarity with alternative medicine or prejudice against its worth (45). Similar situations may arise when patients are noncompliant with standard treatment recommendations because of a particular religious faith or cultural heritage. Although physicians must respect patients' choices, there is no strict obligation for a physician to accept a particular individual as a patient, especially if there are foreseeable personal conflicts that might adversely affect the patient–physician relationship (37).

Pediatric oncology also requires special considerations. Parents are the chief decision-makers, but sometimes their wishes can seem discordant with the best interests of the child. In a different context, what should be done if the adult children of a patient with a heritable trait for malignancy inquire of the patient's diagnosis, but the patient has instructed the physician not to reveal any information to them? The obligation to patient–physician confidentiality conflicts with a potentially overriding obligation toward the family members who might benefit from guidance toward screening.

In cases such as these in which it is difficult to choose between two defensible courses of action, individuals with experience in clinical medical ethics can provide the expertise needed to sort through the ethical, legal, and social issues involved (28).

∷ | Ethics and Medical Errors

Soon after the discovery of x-rays by Wilhelm Röntgen more than 100 years ago, the first cases of malpractice involving the clinical use of radiation therapy were tried in the U.S. court system (20). During the early 20th century, severe dermatitis was a frequent plaintiff's complaint—not surprising in view of the physical limitations of the low-energy machines available at the time.

In 1999, the Institute of Medicine published a report on medical errors, elevating the level of public awareness and stimulating inquiry into this topic (25,27). Estimates of the number of Americans who die each year as a result of medical error have ranged from 44,000 to 98,000 (7,46), and the annual cost of preventable adverse events has been projected to be $17 billion to $29 billion (47). In addition to encouraging efforts to improve patient safety, the Institute of Medicine recommended the development of confidential self-reporting programs and legislation to prevent voluntary reporting from legal discovery (25).

Physicians are often reluctant to discuss errors. It has been suggested that doctors and patients "harbor deep within themselves the expectation that the physician will be perfect" (23). Other reasons for reticence include uncertainty about whether an event really is an error, concern for the patient's well-being, and fear of litigation (5). Each of these items warrants comment.

First, if a patient has an undesirable treatment outcome, careful review of the case can help distinguish error from untoward but unsurprising occurrence. For example, severe pneumonitis after breast radiation therapy is uncommon but not necessarily proof of negligence. Second, concern that disclosing an error causes a patient undue anxiety is contradicted by studies revealing that patients prefer physicians to acknowledge errors (50) and might even sue for lack of apology (49). Finally, in cases of alleged or suspected error leading to injury, the institutional risk-management service should usually be contacted for advice. However, fear of litigation should be mitigated by the fact that a low overall percentage of patients who suffer negligent injuries actually file malpractice claims (5,21).

Nondisclosure of error can weaken the trust at the core of the patient–physician relationship. The argument for disclosure is especially strong when there is a specific preventive intervention that might lessen the severity of possible future injury. Nevertheless, the question still remains: Are physicians ethically obliged to disclose an error, even if there is no immediate harm to the patient?

Case study: A patient with T3N1M0 squamous cell carcinoma of the left retromolar trigone received concurrent cetuximab plus intensity-modulated radiation therapy to the gross disease, with elective coverage of adjacent nodal echelons. The intent was to give 54 Gy to adjacent uninvolved lymph nodes at a rate of 1.8 Gy per day and 66 Gy to the gross disease at a rate of 2.2 Gy per day using a synchronous integrated boost technique, with all treatment completed in 30 fractions. After the spinal cord was contoured as an organ at risk, the structure was inadvertently deleted on all planning computed tomography slices below the level of the gross disease. As a result, when the intensity-modulated radiation therapy inverse planning software optimized the dose distribution according to the constraint of limiting the maximum dose to the spinal cord to 50 Gy, the entire cross-section of a 6-cm length of cervical spinal cord received the full prescription dose, with some areas of the cord located in a "hot spot" region receiving more than 70 Gy. The error was not detected until 1 week after the patient completed treatment, during a routine quality assurance check.

In this example, no injury has yet occurred, but the patient is at increased risk for radiation myelitis. Although there is currently no available proven preventive measure, if the escalated risk of myelitis is unknown to the patient, he or she might later undergo misguided management by another physician if symptoms develop. For instance, if the patient develops arm and leg weakness, a magnetic resonance imaging scan showing nonspecific enhancement and edema in the cervical spinal cord might be interpreted as evidence of metastatic intramedullary or epidural tumor rather than radiation change. Unaware of the prior treatment error, the patient would be unable to inform the other physician involved about the high risk for radiation injury. As a result, the patient might be given only minimal supportive care on the assumption of incurable recurrent disease rather than appropriate efforts toward rehabilitation.

Conclusions

Society's view concerning medical ethics has shifted over time to adapt to the forces of advancing knowledge. Ethical guidelines have sometimes been constructed as formal documents or mandated as law, but no one system comprehensively predicts and resolves all situational dilemmas. The core central principles of medical ethics remain essential foundations for the practice of medicine.

References

1. Advisory Committee on Human Radiation Experiments. Final Report of the Advisory Committee on Human Radiation Experiments (stock number 061-000-00-848-9). Washington, D.C.: Government Printing Office; 1995.
2. American Medical Association Council on Ethical and Judicial Affairs. *Code of medical ethics: current opinions with annotations.* (Annotations prepared by the Southern Illinois University Schools of Medicine and Law). Chicago: AMA Press; 2004.
3. Aquinas T. *Summa Theologica* II-II, Q64, art. 7, "Of Killing." In: Baumgarth WP, Regan RJ, eds. On law, morality, and politics. Indianapolis, Ind: Hackett Publishing Co.; 1988:226–227.
4. Baker R. Deciphering Percival's code. In: Baker R, Porter D, Porter R, eds. *The codification of medical morality: historical and philosophical studies of the formalization of Western medical morality in the eighteenth and nineteenth centuries,* vol 1. *Medical ethics and etiquette in the eighteenth century (Philosophy and Medicine,* vol 45). Boston: Kluwer Academic; 1993.
5. Baylis F. Errors in medicine: nurturing truthfulness. *J Clin Ethics* 1997;8:336–340.
6. Beauchamp TL, Childress JF. *Principles of biomedical ethics,* 4th ed. New York: Oxford University Press; 1994.
7. Brennan TA, Leape LL, Laird NM, et al. Incidence of adverse events and negligence in hospitalized patients: results of the Harvard Medical Practice Study I. *N Engl J Med* 1991;324:370–376.
8. Brennan TA, Rothman DJ, Blank L, et al. Health industry practices that create conflicts of interest: a policy proposal for academic medical centers. *JAMA* 2006;295:429–433.
9. Casarett D, Karlawish JHT, Sugarman J. Determining when quality improvement initiatives should be considered research: proposed criteria and potential implications. *JAMA* 2000;283:2275–2280.
10. Chervenak FA, McCullough LB. The moral foundation of medical leadership: the professional virtues of the physician as fiduciary of the patient. *Am J Obstet Gynecol* 2001;184:875–879.
11. Coleman DL, Kazdin AE, Miller LA, et al. Guidelines for interactions between clinical faculty and the pharmaceutical industry: one medical school's approach. *Acad Med* 2006;81:154–160.
12. Corbie-Smith G, Thomas S, Williams M, et al. Attitudes and beliefs of African Americans toward participation in medical research. *J Gen Intern Med* 1999;14:537–546.
13. Corbie-Smith G. The continuing legacy of the Tuskegee Syphilis Study: Implications for Clinical Research. *Am J Med Sci* 1999;317:5–8.
14. Dunn CM, Chadwick G. *Protecting study volunteers in research: a manual for investigative sites.* Boston: CenterWatch; 1999.
15. Egan C, Jewler D. The impact of managed oncology care: integration or disintegration? *Oncol Issues* 1997;12:22–27.
16. Emanuel EJ, Dubler NN. Preserving the physician-patient relationship in the era of managed care. *JAMA* 1995;273:323–329.
17. Feldman DS, Novack DH, Gracely E. Effects of managed care on physician-patient relationships, quality of care, and the ethical practice of medicine. *Arch Intern Med* 1998;158:1626–1632.
18. Glied S. Managed care. National Bureau of Economic Research working paper no. W7205, 1999. Available at: http//www.nber.org/papers/w7205. Accessed
19. Halperin EC. Physician awareness of the contents of the Hippocratic Oath. *J Med Humanities* 1989;2:107–114.
20. Halperin EC. X-rays at the bar, 1896–1910. *Invest Radiol* 1988;23:639–646.
21. Harvard Medical Practice Study Group. *Patients, doctors, and lawyers: medical injury, malpractice litigation, and patient compensation in New York.* Cambridge, MA: Harvard Medical Practice Study Group; 1990.
22. Heller J. Syphilis victims in the U.S. study went untreated for 40 years. *The New York Times.* July 26, 1972:1, 8. The story was also reported in part in *The Evening Star and Washington Daily News.* July 25, 1972:A1.
23. Hilfiker D. Facing our mistakes. *N Engl J Med* 1984;310:118–122.
24. Hutchinson P, Halperin EC. The hidden persuaders: subtle advertising in radiation oncology. *Int J Rad Onc Biol Phys* 2002;54:989–991.
25. Kohn LT, Corrigan JM, Donaldson MS, eds. *To err is human: building a safer health system* Washington, DC: Institute of Medicine; 1999.
26. Leake CD, ed. *Percival's medical ethics.* Huntington, NY: Robert E. Krieger; 1975. (Reprint of the 1927 ed, published by Williams & Wilkins, Baltimore.)
27. Leape LL. Institute of medicine medical figures are not exaggerated. *JAMA* 2000;284:95–97.
28. Lo B. *Resolving ethical dilemmas: a guide for clinicians,* 2nd ed. Philadelphia: Lippincott Williams & Wilkins; 2000.
29. Lyons AS. Hippocrates. In: Lyons AS, Petrucelli RJ, eds. *Medicine: an illustrated history.* Hong Kong: Harry N. Abrams; 1987.
30. Marwick C. President Bush sidesteps critics in stem cell debate *BMJ* 2001;323:357.
31. Moffic HS, Coverdale J, Bayer T. The Hippocratic Oath and clinical ethics. *J Clin Ethics* 1992;1:287–289.
32. *Natanson v Kline,* 350 P. 2d 1093 (Kan 1960).
33. National Institutes of Health (NIH) Guidelines for Research Involving Recombinant DNA Molecules, Appendix M. Department of Health and Human Services, 2002. Available at: www4.od.nih.gov/oba/rac/guidelines_02/APPENDIX_M.htm. Accessed.
34. Opinion 2.11 "Gene therapy." AMA *Code of Medical Ethics* (ref. 2). Chicago: AMA Press; 2001:31–32.

35. Opinion 8.061 "Gifts to physicians from industry." AMA *Code of Medical Ethics* (ref. 2). Chicago: AMA Press; 2001:160–163.

36. Opinion 8.20 "Invalid medical treatment." AMA *Code of Medical Ethics* (ref. 2). Chicago: AMA Press; 2001:192.

37. Opinion 9.06 "Free choice." AMA *Code of Medical Ethics* (ref. 2). Chicago: AMA Press; 2001:207–209.

38. Pickstone JV. Thomas Percival and the production of medical ethics. In: Baker R, Porter D, Porter R, eds. *The codification of medical morality: historical and philosophical studies of the formalization of Western medical morality in the eighteenth and nineteenth centuries,* vol 1. *Medical ethics and etiquette in the eighteenth century (Philosophy and Medicine,* vol 45.) Boston: Kluwer Academic; 1993.

39. Reich WT. The word "bioethics": its birth and the legacies of those who shaped it. *Kennedy Inst Ethics J* 1994;4:319–335.

40. Rodwin MA. Conflicts in managed care. *N Engl J Med* 1995;332:604–607.

41. Simon SR, Pan RJD, Sullivan AM, et al. Views of managed care: a survey of students, residents, faculty, and deans at medical schools in the United States. *N Engl J Med* 1999;340:928–936.

42. Smith TJ. A piece of my mind: which hat do I wear? *JAMA* 1993;270:1657–1659.

43. Starr P. *The social transformation of American medicine.* New York: Basic Books; 1982.

44. Studdert DM, Mello MM, Brennan TA. Financial conflict of interest in physician relationships with the pharmaceutical industry: self-regulation in the shadow of federal prosecution. *N Engl J Med* 2004;351:1891–1900.

45. Sugarman J, Burk L. Physicians' ethical obligations regarding alternative medicine. *JAMA* 1998;280:1623–1625.

46. Thomas EJ, Studdert DM, Burstin HR, et al. Incidence and types of adverse events and negligent care in Utah and Colorado. *Med Care* 2000;38:261–271.

47. Thomas EJ, Studdert DM, Newhouse JP, et al. Costs of medical injuries in Utah and Colorado. *Inquiry* 1999;36:255–264.

48. Trials of War Criminals before the Nuremberg Military Tribunals under Control Council Law No. 10. Nuremberg, October 1946–April 1949. Washington, DC: U.S. Government Printing Office; 1949–1953.

49. Vincent C, Young M, Phillips A. Why do people sue doctors? A study of patients and relatives taking legal action. *Lancet* 1994;343:1609–1613.

50. Whitman AB, Park DM, Hardin SB. How do patients want physicians to handle mistakes? A survey of internal medicine patients in an academic setting. *Arch Intern Med* 1996;156:2565–2569.

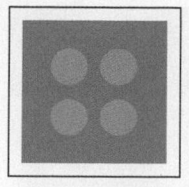

Chapter 98
The Economics of Radiation Oncology

Paul J. Schilling

Economics of Local and Regional Failure

In 2005 570,280 deaths from cancer were recorded (3). Of these, half had a component of local or regional failure. As systemic therapy improves, consequences of local failure become more pronounced (6,11). Improving systemic therapy may lead to a longer lifetime free of systemic metastasis during which local failure can occur. This is one of the principal reasons that postoperative radiation treatment improves survival in breast cancer, small cell lung cancer, prostate cancer, and rectal cancer. The cost of regional failure in terms of human life and tragedy is staggering.

Understanding Billing and Collections

For patients who have Medicare as their primary insurance (these are the majority of radiation oncology patients), Medicare has a set allowable fee that they pay for each medical procedure. Medicare pays 80% of this allowable fee, and the patient's secondary insurance pays the remaining 20%. Nearly all practices have electronic billing, so the charges are submitted by computer. The turnaround time to receive payment if billed electronically can be as few as 14 days. Some secondary insurance companies will take between 6 and 9 months to pay the final 20%. Many secondary insurance companies must be billed using a paper claim sent through the mail instead of an electronic claim, thus delaying payment for up to 6 months.

Hospital-owned, hospital-based radiation oncology practices usually bill under Medicare Part A. This provides for a technical component of radiation treatment delivery for the hospital. The professional component for physician services is billed separately, also under Medicare Part A. The basis on which the technical component is paid to the hospital is called an *ambulatory payment classification* (APC). APC groups have different payments based on the complexity of radiation treatment delivery. The payments under the APC classification compared with those paid to outpatient free-standing facilities vary widely. For example, radiation treatment delivery for intensity-modulated radiation treatment, code 77418, is paid to the hospital under Medicare Part A at considerably less than the rate paid to free-standing centers under Medicare Part B. Alternatively, code 77370, special medical physics consultation, is paid to the hospital at approximately twice that paid to a free-standing facility.

For a free-standing radiation oncology center, Medicare Part B is billed, and a global fee is paid. This includes both the professional fee to the physician and the technical fee to the equipment owner bundled into one payment. Some current procedural technology (CPT) codes have a professional component only, and some codes have a technical component only. Other codes have a professional and a technical component, indicating that the physician and the equipment owner split this code based on their investment of physician time or equipment ownership. Calculating the professional/technical "split" in an outpatient facility can be difficult and depends on the payer mix, as well as the complexity of patients treated. The professional/technical split is calculated using the relative value units assigned to each CPT code. The relative value units are units of work assigned by Medicare, with each unit of work having a standard reimbursement. The relative value units in professional/technical split are shown in Table 98.1 and, as can be seen, vary depending on the complexity and objective of treatment. Calculating the professional/technical split is often difficult for physicians who are in free-standing centers and eligible to receive a portion of the professional component. In general, the professional component of global collections is approximately 11% to 35%, depending on the payer mix. Table 98.1 shows the professional/technical split, which varies depending on the course and complexity of treatment delivered.

Appealing Denied Medicare Claims for Radiation Oncology

In January 2006 the Centers for Medicare and Medicaid Services (CMS) reduced the maximum time for adjudicating appeals for denied claims from a maximum of 1,000 days to 300 days. Nearly 20% of processed Medicare claims are denied. However, only 5% of denied Medicare claims are appealed (20, 22).

Physicians are successful in appealing payment denial in more than 60% of cases, indicating that the appeals process can be rewarding for you. If resubmitting the first rejection does not resolve the problem, the first level of appeal is called a *fair hearing*, and is usually conducted by telephone. You simply need to write a letter to the Medicare carrier requesting a fair hearing. The minimum denied amount needed to appeal a denied claim is $100. Multiple denied claims on different patients can be batched together as long as the appeal is greater than $100. Include the appropriate documentation with the appeal and CPT definitions to describe what medical care was rendered and why you should be paid. Much to your surprise, most of the reviewers are not familiar with radiation oncology coding or the CPT coding books.

For the carrier who habitually denies the same code, a previous favorable ruling will get the same code paid over and over again. In this situation, your goal is to use the last favorable ruling as evidence that the same denied code should be paid. This actually works, and sometimes the bill is just paid without the hearing, as described here (22).

For all fair hearings, the Medicare carrier is required to give you a written decision within 90 days. If the fair hearing process results in additional denial, the next step is a hearing before an administrative law judge. This is much more formal, and you likely should have legal representation. Above all, do not be afraid to try the appeals process if you believe the denial is inappropriate.

Table 98.1 — PROFESSIONAL VS. TECHNICAL R.V.U.S. FOR MODEL COURSES OF RADIATION TREATMENT

IMRT Prostate

CPT Code	Professional RVU's	Technical RVU's
99245	5.89	
77263	4.40	
76370	1.18	3.09
77280	1.94	7.24
77290	4.24	13.60
77417		8.82
77300	15.48	25.20
77336		24.96
77427	36.16	
77334	23.66	47.46
77470	2.85	11.64
77301	21.46	58.34
77418		754.32
	117.26	954.67
	10.93%	89.10%

3 Dimensional Conformal Treatment

CPT Code	Professional RVU's	Technical RVU's
99245	5.89	
77263	4.40	
76370	1.18	3.00
77280	0.97	3.60
77290	4.24	13.60
77295	6.22	29.17
77417		6.30
77300	5.16	8.40
77336		21.84
77427	31.64	
77334	8.45	16.95
77414		80.52
77470	2.85	11.64
77315	2.12	2.87
	73.12	197.80
	27.00%	73.00%

Palliative Treatment

CPT Code	Professional RVU's	Technical RVU's
99245	5.58	
77263	4.40	
76370	1.18	99245
77290	2.12	99245
77417		99245
77300	7.72	99245
77336		99245
77427	9.04	
77334	3.38	99245
77414		99245
77315	2.12	99245
	35.85	99245
	35.30%	99245

Radiation Oncology Negotiation with Managed Care Plans

In 1937, Dr. Sidney Garfield provided prepaid medical care for Henry J. Kiser's company in California. This was the beginning of managed care in the United States. Managed care proliferated with the objective to reduce health care costs for workers covered by health care plans paid for by their employers (17).

Many physicians have experience negotiating the rate of compensation for their contracts. However, a managed care company may be reluctant to disclose its fee schedule if other physicians in the area are contracted with them. The physician should begin the negotiation by making an inquiry for ten codes commonly used in radiation oncology. Oftentimes, a managed care program will send the reimbursement for ten codes total. From this it is possible to get an idea as to what is the rate of payment and whether you wish to continue the negotiation.

Many contracts are tied to the reimbursement rate for Medicare. Some managed care plans pay you based on "100% of regional managed care company's usual and customary fees." Oftentimes, this is less than Medicare rates, and it is imperative to ensure that you know exactly how you are being paid. Many managed care companies want you to take a fee reduction across the board for all radiation oncology CPT codes. Try to negotiate reduction in only a few codes (used less often), which may have a less deleterious effect on your practice. Some managed care companies will try to get you to contract for a case-rate structure. In this scenario, for any patient who requires radiation treatment, a certain dollar amount would be paid regardless of the complexity. Case-rate arrangements can sometimes be tiered, which allows two to three levels of complexity paid at a fixed rate. Case-rate reimbursements are difficult to manage and frequently do not increase year to year, while the complexity of treatment does increase. The physician is advised to use caution in accepting any case-rate structure.

There are a few managed care companies that reimburse based on a capitation basis. Under this scenario, a certain amount of money is paid monthly to the radiation oncology group to provide services regardless of the covered population's average age or need for radiation treatment. These contracts are extraordinarily difficult to negotiate and manage. Ultimately, to remain solvent, you would need to know the age of the population insured, as well as their cancer incidence, cancer screening availability, and so forth. Unfortunately, this information usually resides with the insurer, and likely they will not share this with the physician. Capitation rates can also be calculated from population-based data using the Surveillance, Epidemiology, and End Results (SEER) data (17). Nonetheless, these data underestimate the incidence of cancer and the volume of cancer treated with radiation.

Some managed care organizations bundle procedures together so that only one charge is paid rather than two separate services. For example, weekly physics management code 77336 may not be able to be billed with dose calculation code 77300 when both are rendered on the same day. Thus, the managed care plan finds that these two codes (which are mutually exclusive) are bundled together. Before signing a contract, a physician should understand which services are bundled together and which are not.

For hospital-based practices, it may be necessary for the managed care company to have a contract with the hospital for the technical component of radiation treatment and a contract with the radiation oncologist for professional services. Pitfalls to watch for include a provision that the codes with a professional/technical split must be billed on the same day by both the hospital and physician for either to obtain payment. This puts the physician in the position of auditing the hospital charge capture, a notoriously inefficient process (17).

A contract with the managed care company should spell out emergency care provisions. Many times emergency treatment for spinal cord compression or brain metastasis, and so forth, will be provided, and a managed care company will later indicate that this was a noncovered service on an emergency basis. Thus, an entire course of treatment may be denied in this way (17).

Economic Profiling: Insurance Companies Determine who Provides the Least Expensive Care

Economic profiling tracks physician care expenditures, including specialty referrals, laboratory testing, and utilization of other costly resources. Physicians are allowed to continue on the panel of certain insurance plans based on their level of utilization and cost to the insurance plan. Yet, expenditures to provide care to individual patients are variable (19). Patients who have complex cancers have a higher average cost of care, which may institute multiple inquiries from the insurance company about specialist referral, prescribing habits, and overall resource utilization. Higher average costs of care may lead to deselection from insurance plans for "outlier" utilization. When comprehensive care is provided in a single geographic setting, insurance companies know that patient compliance in the stated plan of disease management is enhanced, leading to fewer episodes of missed testing or treatment. This "dropout rate" is calculated as care prescribed by a physician but not undertaken by a patient (19). Physicians with high dropout rates reduce costs to the insurance company, but only temporarily.

Economic Credentialing

Economic credentialing is defined by the American Medical Association as the "use of economic criteria unrelated to the quality of care or professional competency to determine an individual physician's qualifications for granting or renewal of medical staff privileges" (19). The goal of economic credentialing in radiation oncology is to capture a revenue stream by denying hospital privileges to a group, or terminating hospital privileges and thereby limiting competition. Hospital bylaws are considered by many states to be a contract between a hospital and medical staff, serving as a guideline for actions against physicians, as well as outlining due process provisions for physicians (19). Hospitals may seek to institute differential credentialing to keep qualified physicians from becoming members of the medical staff, and thus limiting competition. One example is requiring radiation oncologists to complete 4 years of residency, whereas before 1994 radiation oncology residencies were only 3 years.

Contracts between physician groups and hospitals establish a business relationship to provide radiation oncology services. Traditionally, exclusive contracts assured patient access to care that would otherwise not be available. Because of increased access to cancer treatment in the United States, this is almost never the case today. Most hospitals enter into an exclusive contract strictly for financial reasons, which puts the physicians in the position of being controlled by the hospital master financial plan. Exclusive contracts may deprive patients of choices and limit the establishment of new physician practices. Some exclusive contracts contain "clean sweep" provisions that stipulate when a group loses an exclusive contract with a hospital, that each physician simultaneously forfeits clinical privileges without the benefit of due process afforded by the hospital bylaws.

The peer-review process may be misused to further a hospital's economic goals. Because in most states peer-review proceedings are protected from legal discovery, peer review affords an opportunity for physicians to evaluate their care and remediate their knowledge, if necessary. Protection from legal discovery also invites hospitals to target and eliminate physicians who are economic threats to their service lines. This is particularly true for hospital-based specialists, including radiation oncologists. Some radiation oncologists find themselves excluded from equipment or facilities when a health care institution changes radiation oncology from a hospital inpatient service to an outpatient service. This may occur with no change in location of building, equipment, or staffing. There is an entire consulting industry that teaches hospital personnel how to displace existing radiation oncologists and put their replacement physicians on salary. Fortunately, we are not the only target; physical medicine, diagnostic radiology, and cardiothoracic surgery physicians are also vulnerable to these tactics (19).

The American Medical Association has a long and continuous interest in fighting economic credentialing, and has a litigation department with years of accumulated information and experience and will assist physicians who challenge health care institutions about these issues.

Lobbying and Political Activity: the Role for Radiation Oncology

Americans place a high value on the quality and availability of medical care. In this country, we have massive government programs that provide the funds to pay for the health care of the poor, disabled, and elderly. Unfortunately, payment rules are created by the legislature for a large portion of all physicians' practices in the United States (13). The importance of interfacing with governmental payers, as well as in influencing the process that benefits our patients and brings them new technologies, cannot be underestimated. This can be accomplished through membership in and in financial support of organized medicine at all levels. Select the organizations that you support carefully and specifically with an eye toward those that provide lobbying power for you and for your patients (12,13,24,25). There are multiple organizations that interact with the Centers for Medicare and Medicaid Services. These include the American College of Radiation Oncology, the American Brachytherapy Society, the Association of Freestanding Radiation Oncology Centers, and the American Society for Therapeutic Radiology and Oncology (12–14,24,25).

Starting a Free-Standing Cancer Center

Starting a free-standing cancer center requires substantial time, effort, and diligence. The population area served by the free-standing center must be clearly defined by the radiation oncologist. In an area where there is no cancer program, the population data for the area can be gathered, complete with the age range of the population and the number of each potential patients within defined age ranges. The SEER data can then be applied using population-based numbers of cancer incidence. In 2002, the age-adjusted incidence of new cancers diagnosed was 4.7 cases per thousand of population (7). The raw cancer incidence provided by the SEER data does not tell us how many patients may undergo radiation treatment during the course of their illness. Take the number of estimated patients and then apply a yield ratio of approximately 50%, which should estimate the total number of patients that the new cancer center would serve. An additional 25% of patients will need to be retreated for other metastases or other new primary cancers (7). Model radiation oncology courses of treatment must be developed to estimate reimbursement per course of treatment (Table 98.1). A certain percentage of patients will receive a palliative treatment course, three-dimensional conformal treatment, and intensity-modulated radiation treatment. If an average length of treatment (including palliative treatment and definitive treatment) is approximately 5 weeks, to have 20 patients under continuous treatment per day will require 200 new patients per year.

A second way to estimate the population served is to count the number of occupied beds of hospitals serving the area. Each permanently filled hospital bed yields approximately one cancer patient per year, of which half will require radiation treatment.

For a cancer center in a competitive market, one must establish exactly how many patients would be treated in the new cancer center and specifically how the physicians plan to obtain these referrals. If a hospital-based group of physicians builds its own free-standing cancer center, some of the patients may follow because referring physicians will continue to refer. There are always surprises and changes in referral patterns when hospital-based radiation oncologists open a competing free-standing center.

Once the numbers of patients to be treated are established, along with their treatment length, the reimbursement for an "average course of treatment" can then be calculated. This average course of treatment should take into account intensity-modulated radiation treatment, palliative treatments, and three-dimensional conformal therapy. When one uses a conservative estimate and sets the total reimbursement at Medicare rates, this seems to be a reasonable approach to many lending institutions. Once total collections for the population to be served are established, the total expenses need to be established as well. This includes the costs of debt service, interest, principle, sales tax on equipment when installed, electric bills, costs of physics and dosimetry, costs of personnel including nursing and therapists, costs of water, building maintenance, professional liability, building insurance, employee benefits, physics equipment, accelerator maintenance, and so forth.

All of this can be packaged together as a pro forma to take to your financial institution. Generally, banks require a down payment of between 5% and 20% of the total amount borrowed. In addition, working capital will be needed for approximately 6 months of operation. The pro forma should be conservative. The goal should be to exceed the numbers that are projected, not just to meet them. This will give the bank a substantial amount of comfort as well. The carrying cost of maintaining a center, maintaining a competitive edge with equipment, and attracting and maintaining high-quality personnel is substantial. There is often underestimation of the cost of running a cancer center. If medical oncology is to be added, the costs of the monthly drug bill needs to be calculated.

Marketing a Practice

Marketing for radiation oncology is directed toward the referring physician. Determine the physicians most likely to refer to you and make a list. *Any* physician can be a referring physician. I have received two referrals from psychiatrists who had cancer patients who were unhappy with their care, underscoring this premise.

Presenting patient cases at a cancer conference at your local hospitals is a time-honored and useful form of individual marketing for your practice (7). Nursing staff usually attend, and they can be a referral source. Radiation oncology images can be rewarding to present at tumor boards. Outlines of isodose plans and other imaging studies, balloon brachytherapy depictions, high-dose-rate brachytherapy plans, and so forth, form an image in referring physicians' minds that medical oncologists cannot accomplish (7).

Making presentations to civic organizations and cancer support groups is also beneficial. Although I speak frequently to groups, there has never been an instance in which someone in the audience decided that to switch to me as a physician as the result of my presentation. Nonetheless, there have been multiple times when family members of new patients have said that they have heard me give a presentation. This underscored another physician's referral choice.

Advertising to the public generally does not yield new patients on its own. Advertising advanced technology may be helpful, but usually only bolsters the understanding and familiarity of the physicians and facility when another primary physician makes a referral.

If your hospital has a teaching program, it is often rewarding to give a lecture or two within this program (7). Physicians who attend such meetings will soon become your referring physicians, especially if they stay in the area.

Develop a telephone answering on-hold message that showcases your technology, as well as the talents of your physicians.

Thus, when patients and physicians call, they are given an explanation of exactly what your practice does while they are waiting for the receptionist.

Internet web site development can also be helpful. Again, this usually does not yield new patients, but rather reinforces the choice that other physicians have made to refer patients. Patients can find out about your practice on the Internet, as well as complete their intake forms, and so forth.

Some of these techniques may be helpful. However, none of these techniques will be useful unless outstanding patient care is delivered, both socially and medically.

Federal Stark Regulations Affecting Radiation Oncology

The second Stark law prohibiting self-referral was adopted in the 1993 Balanced Budget Bill (26). This law prohibited self-referral to designated health services, which included radiation oncology. Radiation oncologists who own their own facilities and equipment do not fall under violations of the Stark rule because it is not considered self-referral when the referring physician personally performs a designated health service.

There is also an in-office ancillary exemption that applies to ownership and investment interest for ancillary services. The in-office ancillary services must be provided in a building in which the referring physician also furnishes substantial physician services. The in-office ancillary exemption is the loophole exploited by some urologists who create a "group practice" with radiation oncologists and add a linear accelerator to their building. Curiously enough, the very radiation oncologists who join these ventures are often the displaced victims of hospital tactics of economic credentialing (see the preceding section).

Congress based some of their conclusions and wrote portions of the Stark law based on studies that examined the effects of ownership of free-standing radiation oncology facilities by referring physicians who are not radiation oncologists and who did not directly provide services. These "joint ventures" yielded a utilization rate 40% higher in these facilities in Florida than the rest of the United States, and cost of radiation treatment that was 60% higher than in the rest of the United States (10,26). In addition, these studies showed that there was less access to poorly served populations without any reduction in mortality among cancer patients that indicated improved quality of care (10,26). State laws may strengthen current existing federal laws, and it is important to understand the laws in your state concerning self-referral (26).

Economic Issues Specific to New Graduates of Residency Programs

Most new graduates are largely concerned about mastering the amount of medical knowledge necessary to become a specialist, as well as passing their radiation oncology boards. Few articles have been written on contracting that is specific to radiation oncology (16). A contract is simply a promise between two parties that the law recognizes as a duty. Five elements are required to create a valid contract: two competent parties, mutual consent, consideration, a legal purpose and duty, and a mutual obligation. When evaluating a first contract, obtaining legal advice from a health care attorney is essential.

The terms and conditions of the contract should set forth working conditions, provision of nursing service, transcription, ancillary help, on-call arrangements, vacation time, and coverage. Arrangements should be spelled out for professional liability insurance coverage, including term limits and a tail policy in the event that termination of employment occurs. Duties

should be specific to the practice of radiation oncology and not be vaguely worded so the new physician is expected to "perform all duties as the board of directors may assign" (16). The employer should also spell out the terms of potential termination. Reasonable terms of automatic contract termination include loss of your medical license, loss of hospital privileges for patient care issues, loss of a drug-enforcement agency license, loss of ability to prescribe controlled substances, conviction of a felony, and so forth. If there is a provision for termination of the contract prior to the end of the term, it should be clear and available to both parties. For example, "either party may terminate this agreement with 90 days' written notice with or without cause" (16). Written performance reviews should be given at least quarterly. This assists the employer and the employee to identify potential areas of conflict and allow resolution.

Restrictive covenants protect employers by placing limitations on the rights of the employee to compete with the employer. They should include the period of time the restriction shall remain in effect, as well as the geographic restriction. Because some of these restrictive covenants are not enforceable in certain states, liquidated damages for terminating employment and remaining in an area to compete has also been used by some practices (16). A liquidated damage clause provides a payment to the practice owner, negotiated in advance, that allows the employed physician to work in the area and compete after the contract is terminated (16).

Associates are invited to become partners after some period of time, which varies from region to region. Traditionally, this has meant financial parody with the senior partners. Many physicians are being offered positions without a partnership track. Partnership has also traditionally meant voting and decision-making parody. Some groups offer graduated financial parody: the first 2 years may be salaried, and during the next 3 years associates may gradually reach financial parody with senior partners in percentage increments. Formulas for buying into the practice are similarly variegated. In a hospital-based practice with an exclusive contract to provide professional services, the buy-in should be minimal, simply because the costs of maintaining the contract and capital equipment costs are minimal. One should only purchase assets that have real value or cover the cost of maintaining the contract over time. The accounts receivable are usually generated by the physician during the years of nonpartnership. One questions a "buy-in" for these accounts receivable that the new physician helped to generate. Good will is augmented by the employed physician as well. It is my opinion that these particular items are not worth a great deal financially.

Fewer than one third of radiation oncologists are still in their first postresidency job 5 years later (16). If negotiated into the contract, arbitration or mediation can be an effective and cost-efficient means to negotiate a dispute and avoid litigation between parties, should you decide to separate (16).

Economics of Medical Oncology

As a way to achieve the prescription drug coverage for our seniors, chemotherapy drug payment margins are the target for Medicare payment cuts. The target is huge: Medicare spends $70 billion each year for chemotherapy drugs and administration. Compare that to the amount spent on radiation oncology professional and technical fees, which totals 6 billion dollars per year, and our services appear very cost-effective (18,21). Outpatient drug reimbursement has changed from paying a percentage of the average wholesale price to paying a percentage of the average sales price. The average sales price is the sales price that is actually paid by outpatient practices with a tiny margin added. Medical oncologists argue appropriately that the administration of chemotherapy does not cover the cost of nursing time, waste disposal, and supplies. Medicare responded to this reality by increasing the fee for administration of the first hour of chemotherapy infusion by more than 270% between 2003 and 2004 (18). New drugs are still paid at an average of 95% of average wholesale price, and these are the most profitable drugs that a medical oncologist can administer. Once a new drug gets a permanent billing code, called a "J code," they are then paid at the average *sales* price plus 6% (a considerably lower profit). Because reimbursement for the first hour of chemotherapy has had the most dramatic increase in reimbursement for medical oncology, this makes any regimen that requires multiple days of therapy profitable for our medical oncology colleagues. These include daily or weekly chemoradiation protocols (18). There is a new drug update by Medicare every 12 weeks as the average sales price for chemotherapeutic drugs is recalculated by the Centers for Medicare and Medicaid.

Consulting groups are letting medical oncologists know that they can profit from incorporating positron emission tomography scanners and radiation oncology equipment into their practices. Perhaps more realistically, medical oncologists will be looking for reduction in their overhead through combining with radiation oncologists and being able to enhance patient care by giving daily chemotherapy sensitization protocols within a combined cancer center. Do not build a new cancer center without at least considering adding space for them.

Medicare's New Paradigm: Pay for Performance

The CMS is moving toward a system of Pay for Performance. Under this system, a physician practice meeting a certain benchmark of quality in patient care does not receive a reduction in Medicare payments. This movement, in its various combinations and permutations, started in 1999 when the Institute of Medicine released a report called *To Err is Human* (9). This report documented quality of care concerns in our health care system and pointed out that 98,000 people die each year as a result of preventable medical errors from all health care professionals. Subsequently, a Rand study found that many hospital deaths were preventable (8). In our legislators' minds, the findings of these studies sharpened their resolve to improve the quality of care delivered in our health care system. "Pay for Performance" has the objective of improving the quality of care by linking physician reimbursement to quality measures and outcomes. Pay for Performance was first tried in hospitals. Under the Deficit Reduction Act of 2005, hospitals receive a 2% reduction if they do not report to CMS on 10 quality measures and have acceptable performance targets. This pilot project with hospitals has been viewed by Congress to be successful. The results in quality of care measures for these areas are available on the CMS web site for any hospital that participates.

There has been substantial interest in adopting a Pay for Performance program for physician services rendered to Medicare beneficiaries. Congress and the American Medical Association have expressed support for this effort (1). To begin implementing this in January 2006, CMS started a limited pilot volunteer reporting program for physicians, which encourages physicians to voluntarily report quality of care data provided to Medicare beneficiaries. This initial objective was to gain experience with reporting from physician offices on quality of care delivered. Certain specialties lend themselves better to Pay for Performance measures than others. For example, diabetic patients should have retina examinations as a component part of their care, and not doing so would not be optimal care for them. The care of cancer patients is, however, quite variegated. As we all know, some patients with brain metastasis live only a few months, and others live for a year or more. Thus, outcome measures for patients who have cancer would probably not be appropriate. It is the physicians themselves within each specialty who should shape the compliance program linked to Pay for Performance. In this regard, it is likely that the better measure of quality of care would be practice accreditation. Practice accreditation is currently required in several states in the United States (5).

Professional Staffing Issues: Radiation Oncology Staffing in a Shortage Environment

Currently in the United States there is a critical manpower shortage in radiation therapy personnel. Regional shortage of therapists, dosimetrists, and physicists create a musical chair job market: the bell rings and everyone changes position. This situation is neither beneficial to patient care nor fiscally sound for our shrinking health care dollar. For those of us who have depended on temporary workers, we know that this is both an expensive proposition and seriously disruptive to employee morale (23).

In November 2001, the U.S. Bureau of Labor statistics predicted that by the year 2010, there would be a shortage of 7,000 radiation therapists (23). One way to stabilize your work force, create good will, and create excellence in our field is to start a scholarship program for radiation therapy professionals. Currently, most scholarship programs support radiographers to take an additional year of training to become radiation therapists. During the time of training, the student can receive a stipend, as well as have tuition and books paid for. In exchange, the candidate agrees to work for the cancer center for a period of time after graduation. One source of candidates can be a local radiography training program. Contact the director of the program and let them know that you are offering a scholarship program to qualified candidates. For students who receive monthly stipend support, the best way to ensure that they are serious about accepting the obligation is to have them sign a promissory note. If they fail to honor their contract or pass the registry within a specified period of time, the amount that the practice advanced them becomes due with interest (23).

Although many dosimetrists today are trained "on the job," there are 1-year programs that enroll therapists in full-time dosimetry training. If you have a candidate willing to relocate to one of the cities that has these programs, it is worth the investment to train them outside your facility and hopefully bring back some fresh ideas. For a radiation therapist who may have a baccalaureate degree in radiation therapy, and for the right individual who wishes to train in medical physics, this may be an opportunity to train a medical physicist for your program.

Opening your practice to scholarship programs and scholarship support creates a unique marketing opportunity for your facilities (23). This also augments cancer center morale in which the seasoned employees can teach the new graduates the tricks of the trade (23).

Practice Accreditation

Practice accreditation is a way to demonstrate the quality of radiation oncology practice to the public, as well as third-party payers. Practice accreditation may be one avenue whereby a practice that demonstrates quality does not receive payment reduction under Pay for Performance. Currently, the American College of Radiation Oncology and the American College of Radiology are the two practice accreditation bodies for radiation oncology practices. Some states (Alabama, New Jersey, and New York) require practice accreditation for state certification (5).

Most importantly, practice accreditation constitutes a mechanism to accomplish quality assurance and assess compliance with recognized standards for hospital or free-standing radiation oncology practices (4,5). Practice accreditation can also be a value-added qualification for third-party payers.

Standards for accreditation should include external review of randomly selected radiation oncology treatment courses, peer review, and quality assurance activities performed regularly, physics and dosimetry standards consistent with drafted standards for external-beam radiation treatment, brachytherapy, and medical physics quality assurance (4,23). An on-site verification visit by both physicists and physicians is essential to practice accreditation (4,23).

Economics of Radiation Oncology: Selected International Perspectives

Radiation oncologists from around the world were polled and asked questions about the economics of radiation oncology. This survey included questions about patient access to new technology, waiting times to start radiation treatment, and their country's system of medical care. This section represents a review of selected literature as well as the perspective and responses of those polled.

The rate of installation of megavoltage radiation therapy equipment was compared in Canada, Germany, and the United States (15). Rublee et al. (15) concluded that the higher proliferation of radiation equipment in the United States promoted rapid access to advanced medical services but was not necessarily associated with improved outcomes, more patient utilization, or efficient use of health care funds. They noted an average rate of growth of 10.3 radiation therapy units per million persons in the United States, 4.6 units per million persons in Germany, and 4.8 units per million persons in Canada.

Canada's socialized health care system creates some access problems for cancer patients. Currently, Canada has a scoring system that lists the severity of each curative cancer patient and urgency in starting radiation treatment. Curable head and neck cancers received the highest score, whereas curable prostate cancers were the lowest. This system sorts access to radiation treatment. Canadian physicians responding to our survey did not think that their health care system limited access to advanced technology but rather concentrated it into specific centers in geographic locations.

Radiation oncologists in China note that they have a single governmental payer system with socialized medicine and staggering cost increases. Patients in China who require chemotherapy are required to pay cash up front for their medication prior to its delivery. With respect to radiation oncology, radiation oncologists note a dearth of intensity-modulated radiation treatment, image-guided radiation treatment, and access to three-dimensional conformal radiation treatment as well. Perhaps the situation will be remedied in the future. On May 28, 2006, a linear accelerator manufacturer held a ground-breaking ceremony launching the construction of a new linear accelerator manufacturing facility for producing linear accelerators in China to serve the Chinese market.

Physician respondents from Western European countries did not specifically note that a socialized health care system impacted the delivery of radiation treatment nor the adoption of new technology. In contrast with this specific opinion, Calvo and Santos (2) describe monetary limits on the investment in innovative radiation treatment techniques. These authors note that the need for cost containment in the public health care system in Western European countries have slowed investment in stereotactic radiosurgery, conformal radiation treatment, high-dose-rate brachytherapy, and intraoperative radiation treatment. They reported on cost-benefit analysis of each of these technologies. Their conclusion was that Western Europe was not adopting new technology rapidly enough (4).

Radiation oncologists responding to our survey in England thought that access to curative radiation oncology was good. However, access to palliative radiation oncology was suboptimal.

Radiation oncologists in the Netherlands thought that their cancer programs limited neither access nor the development of new technology. Dutch radiation oncologists reported limited waiting times for patients to start radiation treatment.

Radiation oncologists in South America and Latin America cite too few radiation oncology installations, particularly in Mexico, Bolivia, and Venezuela. They also note a rapidly growing number of radiation oncology installations, especially in Argentina. The latter have tended to be for-profit centers. Latin American radiation oncologists also point with pride to the Organization of Radiation Oncologists, which currently serves their members needs and also seeks to engage more Latin American patients in cooperative prospective, randomized trials.

Radiation oncologists in Scandinavian countries of Denmark and Sweden point with pride to their innovative and large cancer centers. They do point out that they are geographically distant from each other, but there appears to be minimal to no limit in their access to new technology, nor long waiting times for patient treatment.

Practice accreditation is uncommon internationally. However, the American College of Radiation Oncology currently has accredited a number of international facilities, and practice accreditation in other countries continues to be in greater demand and is growing.

In general, countries with socialized medicine have certain defined limits on capital investment each year. As our technology grows ever more costly, these issues will need to be dealt with both at home as well as in the international community.

References

1. American Society of Therapeutic Radiology and Oncology Government Relations update: Pay for Performance and Quality of Care. 2006.
2. Calvo FA, Santos M. Innovative techniques in modern radiation oncology: the economic and organizational impact. *Rays* 1999;24:379–389.
3. Cancer prevention and early detection facts and figures, 2005. Washington DC: American Cancer Society 2005:14–26.
4. Cotter GW, Dobelbower RR. The American College of Radiation Oncology Practice Accreditation Program. *Crit Rev Oncol Hematol* 2005;55:93–102.
5. Dobelbower, RR, Cotter GW, Schilling PJ, et al. Radiation oncology practice accreditation. *Rays* 2002;26:191–198.
6. Gastrointestinal Study Group. Prolongation of the disease free interval in surgically treated rectal carcinoma. *N Engl J Med* 1985;312:1465–1472.
7. Gillette R. Marketing and Practice, *American College of Radiation Oncology Practice Management Guide*. Bethesda, MD: American College of Radiation Oncology; 2005:39–46.
8. Hayward RA, Hofer TP. Estimating hospital deaths due to medical errors. *JAMA* 1998;285:415–420.
9. Kohn LT, Corrigan JM, Donalson MS, et al. *To err is human: building a safer healthcare system*. Washington DC: National Academy Press; 1999.
10. Mitchell JM. Consequences of physician ownership of healthcare facilities: joint ventures in radiation therapy. N Engl J Med 1992;327:1497–1501. *Radiation Oncology Practice Management Guide*. Bethesda, MD: American College of Radiation Oncology; 2005.
11. Regaz J, Jackson SM, Le N: Adjuvant radiotherapy and chemotherapy in node-positive premenopausal woman with breast cancer. *N Engl J Med* 1997;337:956–962.
12. Rubenstein J. ACRO Responds to Proposed CMS Payment Cuts. Bethesda, MD: American College of Radiation Oncology; *ACRO Alert*. October 6, 2002.
13. Rubenstein J. Political activity, American College of Radiation Oncology practice management guide. Bethesda, MD: American College of Radiation Oncology 2004;2:87–88.
14. Rubinstein J. Political activity, *American College of Radiation Oncology practice management guide*. Bethesda, MD: American College of Radiation Oncology; 2004:87–88.
15. Rublee DA. Medical technology in Canada, Germany and the United States: an update. *Health Affairs* 1994;113–117.
16. Schilling PJ, Woods A. Anatomy of a Professional Services' Contract for Radiation Oncology. American College of Radiation Oncology. Available at: www.acro.org Accessed 1999.
17. Schilling PJ. Radiation Oncology Negotiation for Managed Care: *American College of*

Radiation Oncology Practice Management Guide. Bethesda, MD: American College of Radiation Oncology; 2008. In press.

18. Schilling PJ. AWP and ASP: what does the alphabet soup of medical oncology mean to the practicing radiation oncologist? Bethesda, MD: American College of Radiation Oncology; ACROGram, June 2004.

19. Schilling PJ. Economic profiling and economic credentialing: the increasing challenge for organized medicine. *Fla Med Assoc Q J* January 2003:33–35.

20. Schilling PJ. Managing the insurance denials and appeals process. *American College of Radiation Oncology Practice Management Guide*. Bethesda, MD: American College of Radiation Oncology; 2004: 67–69.

21. Schilling PJ. Radiation oncology and the prescription drug program: what does it mean to us? Bethesda, MD: American College of Radiation Oncology; ACROGram, September 18, 2003.

22. Schilling PJ. Tips on how to appeal denied medicare claims for radiation oncology. Bethesda, MD: American College of Radiation Oncology; *ACROGram* May 26, 2005.

23. Schilling PJ. Your cancer center can benefit from starting a scholarship program for radiation therapy professionals. *American College of*

24. Woods A. ACRO supports Quality Care Preservation Act. Bethesda, MD: American College of Radiation Oncology; *ACRO Alert*, April 23, 2003.

25. Woods A. The American College of Radiation Oncology Lobbies Washington: Our Specialty Succeeds in Reversing Payment Cuts. Bethesda, MD: American College of Radiation Oncology; *ACROGram*, December 1, 2003.

26. Woods A. The impact of federal Stark laws on radiation therapy. *American College of Radiation Oncology Practice Management Guide*. Bethesda, MD: American College of Radiation Oncology; 2004.

Index

Page numbers followed by "*f*" indicate figure and Page numbers followed by "*t*" indicate table.

A

A33 antigen, radioimmunotherapy with, 591
Abdominal compression method, radiation therapy, 10
Abdominal hysterectomy
    cervical cancer therapy, 1550, 1551*t*
    endometrial cancer, 1614–1615, 1622–1623
Abdominoperineal resection, rectal cancer therapy, 1374
Absolute survival criteria, end point selection, phase III clinical
      trials, 358
Absorbed dose, basic principles of, 157–160
Absorption rate distribution (ARD), electromagnetic heating,
      hyperthermia, 650, 650*f*–651*f*
Accelerated fractionation
    cervical cancer radiation therapy, 1556–1557
    chemoradiation/chemotherapy *vs.,* 315
    clinical trials, 310
    concomitant boost regimen, 312
    hybrid techniques, 308*t*–309*t*, 311–312
    non-small cell lung cancer radiation therapy, 1088–1089
    pure regimen, 307*t*, 310
    rationale for, 304, 306, 307*t*–309*t*
    regimens, 100–101
    split-course regimen, 308*t*–309*t*, 312
Accelerated partial breast irradiation (APBI)
    adjuvant brachytherapy, 500–502, 501*f*–503*f*
    breast cancer therapy, 1259–1264, 1261*t*
      intraoperative techniques, 1263–1264, 1264*f*
      MammoSite technique, 1262
      multicatheter interstitial techniques, 1260–1262, 1261*f*
Accelerated radiotherapy with carbogen and nicotinamide (ARCON),
      chemical modifiers of radiation therapy, 611–612
Accelerated repopulation
    chemoradiation therapy and repopulation inhibition, 672
    radiation therapy, 23, 24*f*–25*f*
Accounting systems, radiation therapy, 2023–2024, 2025*f*
Accreditation issues, radiation oncology, 2048–2049
Achillodynia, radiation therapy, 1949, 1950*f*, 1951*t*
Acoustic neuromas
    proton/α-particle radiotherapy, 415
    stereotactic radiosurgery, 384–385
Acquired immunodeficiency syndrome (AIDS)
    anal carcinoma, 711–712
    cervical carcinoma, 712–713
    Kaposi's sarcoma, 707–711
      combined treatment regimens, 708–710
      diagnostic workup, 708
      disease patterns, 707–708, 707*f*–711*f*
      pathology, 708
      radiation therapy, 710–711
    lymphomas, 703–707
      Hodgkin's lymphoma, 706–707
      non-Hodgkin's lymphoma, 703–706, 705*f*, 705*t*, 1739
    malignant neoplasms
      future research issues, 713
      HIV infection, 702–703
      pediatric malignancies, 713
    perianal cancer and, 1391
Actinium series, basic properties, 146

Active Breathing Coordinator (ABC), respiratory-gated radiotherapy,
      10, 10*t*
Activity-based costing (ABC), radiation therapy, 2023–2024, 2025*f*
Activity-exposure rate relationship, brachytherapy dosimetry, 434
Acupuncture, xerostomia management and, 2013
Acusticus neurinoma, diagnosis and management, 1937–1939
Acute acidification, hyperthermia, isoeffect dose modification, 639
Acute dermatities, in cancer patients, 2016–2017, 2016*f*
Acute esophagitis, late effects syndromes in esophagus and, 343–344
Acute lymphoblastic leukemia (ALL)
    central nervous system prophylaxis, 1781–1782
    classification and risk factors, 1778–1779
    hyperfractionated radiation therapy, 310
    meningeal leukemia, 1782
    testicular relapse, 1783
    treatment of, 1780–1783
Acute morbidity, brachytherapy, low-dose-rate irradiation, 517
Acute myelocytic leukemia (AML)
    classification and risk factors, 1777–1779, 1779*t*
    treatment, 1780
Acute pericarditis, as radiotherapy effect, 335–336, 335*f*
Acute responses
    ioffect formulae, time-dose effects, 97–98, 98*f*
    radiation therapy, mechanisms of, 79
Acute toxicity
    Hodgkin's lymphoma radiation therapy, pediatric patients,
      1899–1901
    intracranial tumor radiation therapy, 730
    ovarian cancer therapy, 1644
    rhabdomyoscarcoma radiation therapy, pediatric patients, 1882
    total body irradiation, 372
Acute urinary retention (AUR), prostate cancer brachytherapy,
      1472–1473, 1474*f*
Adaptive radiation therapy (ART)
    image-guided systems, 289–293, 290*f*–293*f*
    planned target volume in, 230
Adenocarcinoma
    bile duct, pediatric patients, 1917–1920, 1918*t*
    breast, pediatric patients, 1915–1916
    cervical cancer, 1540–1541
      survival rates, 1577, 1577*t*
    endometrial cancer, 1610, 1612, 1612*f*
    esophageal cancer, 1137
    gallbladder, 1359–1360
    pancreatic cancer, 1337, 1342*t*
    perianal cancer, 1391
    prostate cancer, 1441–1445
      pathology, 1453–1455, 1454*f*
    renal cell carcinoma, 1400
    stomach cancer, 1320–1321
    vaginal clear-cell adenocarcinoma, 1658
      epidemiology and risk factors, 1658
      management and treatment outcomes, 1672
      pathology, 1659
Adenocystic carcinomas
    breast cancer, 1197
    cervical cancer, 1541

Adenocystic carcinomas (*contd.*)
  esophageal cancer, 1137
  fast neutron radiotherapy, 409–410, 409*t*
  prostate tumors, 1455–1456
Adenoma malignum, cervical cancer, 1541
Adenomas
  adrenal gland tumors, 1719
  pituitary, nonmalignant disease, 1936–1937, 1937*t*, 1938*f*
  prolactin-secreting adenomas, 759–760, 760*t*
  thyrotropin-secreting adenomas, 760
Adenosarcomas, endometrial cancer, 1613
Adenosis, vaginal cancer, 1659
Adenosquamous carcinoma, vaginal cancers, 1660
Adipose tissue, mesenchymal tumors, 1122–1123
Adjacent field separation techniques
  electron beam therapy, 206, 206*f*–208*f*
  photon external-beam dosimetry, 184–185, 184*f*–187*f*
Adjuvant therapies. *See* Combined treatment modalities
Adnexa carcinomas
  epidemiology and management, 699–700
  orbital tumor radiation therapy, 794
Adrenal gland tumors
  anatomy, 1717
  clinical presentation, 1718, 1718*f*, 1718*t*
  cortical tumors, 1717
  diagnostic work-up, 1718–1719, 1718*t*
  epidemiology, 1717
  management, 1719–1720
  medulla tumors, 1717
  metastases, palliative therapy, 2001
  natural history, 1717–1718, 1718*t*
  pathologic classification, 1719, 1719*t*
  pediatric patients, 1921–1922
  radiation therapy, 1720
  staging, 1718–1719, 1718*t*
Adrenocorticotropic hormone (ACTH)
  late effects syndromes in neuroendocrine system and, 345
  pituitary adenoma, 1937
Africa, radiation therapy in, 606
Afterloading technology
  brachytherapy, 423
    cervical cancer, 1558–1566, 1560*f*
  esophageal cancer therapy, 1148, 1149*f*
  high-dose-rate brachytherapy, 540, 541*f*
  interstitial brachytherapy, 476–481
    iodine-125 plastic tube implants, 479–481
    iridium-192 wires or ribbons, 477–478, 477*f*–479*f*
    removable iridium-192 hairpin technique, 479, 480*f*
    suturing techniques, needles, guides, and plastic buttons,
      478–479, 479*f*
Age
  breast cancer risk and, 1176–1177, 1178*f*
    in elderly women, 1223–1224, 1224*f*, 1225*t*
    metastases, 1201
  cervical cancer prognosis and, 1541
  cutaneous T-cell lymphoma, 1768–1769
  ovarian cancer risk and, 1629–1631, 1630*f*
  prostate cancer risk and, 1441, 1443*t*
Age-related macular degeneration, diagnosis and management,
  1943, 1943*f*
Aggressive fibromatosis, soft tissue sarcomas, 1818
Air cavities
  electron-beam therapy, dosage calculations, 195, 197*f*
  photon external-beam dosimetry, 168–169, 169*f*, 173
Air-kerma strength, brachytherapy dosimetry, 433–435
Alcohol consumption, breast cancer risk and, 1180
Alignment systems, radiation therapy, 7
Allogeneic stem cell transplantation (ASCT)
  multiple myeloma, 1795
  radioimunoglobulin therapy with, 588
Allowed energy bands, thermoluminescence dosimetry, 159
Alloy block dosimetry, field shaping applications, 180–181, 180*f*
α-particle radiotherapy, 413–419
  acoustic neuromas, 415
  arteriovenous malformations, 417
  astrocytomas, 415
  breast cancer, 419
  gastrointestinal cancer, 418
  juxtaspinal cord tumors, 416–417, 416*f*
  lung cancer, 417–418
  optic pathway gliomas, 413

  pediatric malignancies, 418–419, 418*f*
  pituitary tumors, 414–415
  prostate cancer, 417
  skull-base tumors, 413–414, 414*t*, 415*f*
  uveal melanoma, 413, 414*f*
Alphafetoprotein (AFP) markers, hepatobiliary tract tumors,
      pediatric patients, 1918–1920
Alpha-particles, basic properties, 144–145, 144*t*
Altered fractionation schedules. *See also* Accelerated fractionation;
      Hyperfractionation
  bladder cancer radiation therapy, 1423
  clinical studies, 306, 310–317
  concurrent chemotherapy, 312, 313*t*–314*t*, 315
  dose escalations for therapeutic ratio improvement, 316–317
  dose size per fraction and interfraction interval length, 300–302,
      301*t*, 302*f*
  future research issues, 317
  isoeffect formulas, 303–304, 304*f*
  lowered biologically effective dose and cure probability, 316, 316*t*
  nasopharyngeal cancer radiation therapy, 836–837, 840, 841*f*,
      841*t*
  oral cavity tumor radiation therapy, 904
  overall treatment time, 303
  radiation therapy, 22–23, 23*f*, 23*t*
  radiobiology background, 300–304
  repair kinetics, 303
  simultaneous integrated boost (SIB) intensity-modulated
      radiation therapy, 245–246
  time-dose parameters, 300
Alveolar ridge
  anatomy, 891–892
  disease treatment and results, 909
American Association of Physicists in Medicine Task Group 43
      Report, brachytherapy dose calculations, 440–442,
      441*f*–442*f*, 441*t*
American College of Radiation Oncology Code of Ethics, 2038
American Medical Association Code of Ethics, 2037
Americium 241, brachytherapy applications, 428
Amifostine
  cervical cancer therapy, 1596
  chemical radioprotection, 614–615
  gastrointestinal mucositis, 2015–2016
  xerostomia management, 2012–2013
Aminolevulinic acid (ALA), photodynamic therapy, 599
Anal canal tumors. *See also* Rectal cancer
  acquired immunodeficiency syndrome, 711–712
  anatomy, 1383, 1384*f*
  brachytherapy, 524–525, 524*f*–525*f*
  clinical presentation, 1385
  combined chemoradiation therapy, 681*t*, 683
  diagnostic work-up, 1385
  epidemiology, 1383–1384
  metastases, 1384–1385, 1388, 1390
  natural history, 1384–1385
  pathologic classification, 1383
  perianal cancer, 1391–1394
  prognostic factors, 1385–1386
  risk factors, 1384
  staging, 1385, 1386*t*
  treatment, 13861394
    combined-modality therapy, 1386–1388 1387*t*, 1389*t*–1390*t*
    radiation therapy, 1390, 1391*t*, 1392–1394
    surgical management, 1390–1391
Anaplastic astrocytoma, 737
Anaplastic ependymomas, pediatric patients, 1834
Anaplastic ganglioma, pediatric patients, 1835
Anaplastic glioma
  chemotherapy, 735–736
  molecular genetics, 735
  radiosensitizers, 736–737
  treatment, 735
Anaplastic oligodendroma/oligoastrocytoma, 737
Anaplastic thyroid cancer
  classification, 1061
  management, 1067
  prognostic factors, 1062
  radiation therapy, 1068
Anaplastic Wilms' tumor, 1856
Anatomy-base optimization, interstitial brachytherapy, 454–456
Androgen response elements, prostate physiology, 1440
Androgens, prostate physiology, 1439–1440

Androgen suppression therapy, prostate cancer, 1488, 1489*t*, 1491–1495, 1492*t*–1493*t*, 1495*t*, 1499–1500
Anemia
    cervical cancer and, 1542–1543
    chemical modifiers of radiation therapy, 612
Anesthesia, implant brachytherapy, 486
Aneurysmatic bone cyst, radiation therapy, 1954
Angiogenesis
    cervical cancer, 1544
    chemoradiation therapy, molecular targeting and, 675–676
    induction and sustaining of, 113
    radiation oncology and, 47–48
    tumor molecular pathophysiology, vascular compartment, 126–127, 128*t*
Angiosarcoma, breast cancer radiation therapy and, 1276–1277
Anisotropy factor, brachytherapy dose calculation, 436–437, 441–442, 442*f*, 443*t*
Anoikis, radiation therapy and cell death, 78
Anthracycline, cardiomyopathy linked to, 334–335
Antibody-cytokine fusion proteins, cancer therapy, 586
Anticonvulsant therapy, brain metastases, 1978–1979
Antidepressants, pain management and, 2007
Antigen-processing, radioimmunoglobulins, 583
Antimetabolites, combined chemoradiation therapy, 677*t*, 678–679
Antioangiogenic therapies, tumor pathophysiology, 136–137, 137*f*
Aperture margins
    adaptive radiation therapy, 292–293, 293*f*
    intensity-modulated radiation therapy, 243–245, 246*f*
Apoptosis
    cervical cancer, 1544
    irradiation effects and, 35–36, 35*f*, 36*t*
    molecular radiation and, 115
    radiation oncology and, 43, 43*f*–44*f*
    radiation therapy and, 77–78
        characteristics of, 112*t*
        location variations, 78
        tumor cells, 84
    radioimmunoglobulins and, 583
    resistance to, 112–113, 112*t*
    in tumors, predictive assays, 84
Appendix, pediatric patients, 1917
Applicator systems, high-dose-rate brachytherapy safety, 548
Appropriateness criteria, radiation therapy, 2034
Arc therapy. *See* Electron arc therapy; Rotation therapy
Aromatase inhibitors, breast cancer therapy, 1306, 1306*t*
Arrhenius plots, hyperthermia isoeffect dose, 637–639, 638*f*–639*f*
Arteriovenous malformation (AVM). *See also* Vascular system
    hemangiomas, pediatric patients, 1925
    nonmalignant disease, 1939, 1939*t*
    proton and α-particle radiotherapy, 417
    spinal cord tumors, 769
    stereotactic radiosurgery, 383–384, 384*f*
    tumor molecular pathophysiology, 127–128
Aryepiglottic fold/arytenoid lesions, characteristics of, 978
Asia and Pacific region, radiation therapy in, 606–607, 607*t*
Astrocytomas
    pediatric patients, 1824–1832, 1824*t*
        high-grade tumors, 1828–1829
        low-grade tumors, 1824–1828, 1826*f*
        spinal cord, 1832
    proton/α-particle radiotherapy, 415
Asymmetric x-ray collimators, photon external-beam dosimetry, monitor unit calculations, 167
Atomic mass unit (amu), defined, 142
Atomic numer, defined, 142–143
Atomic structure
    basic principles, 142–143, 143*f*
    matter-particle interaction, 148–149
Attenuation coefficients, radioactivity, 146–147, 147*f*
Atypical teratoid/rhabdoid tumor, pediatric patients, 1841–1842
Auger electrons, defined, 144
Autologous stem cell transplantation, multiple myeloma, 1794–1795, 1795*f*
Autophagy
    molecular radiation and, 115
    radiation therapy and, 77–78
Avascular necrosis, late effects syndromes on bone and, 347–349, 349*f*, 349*t*
Avogadro's number, defined, 143
Axillary lymph nodes, breast cancer metasetases, 1183–1184, 1184*t*, 1198, 1198*f*

    in pediatric patients, 1915–1916
    posterior boost therapy, 1253–1254, 1254*f*
    radiation therapy, 1253, 1253*f*
    surgical management, 1205–1206
        radiation therapy *vs.*, 1224–1230
    unknown primary tumors, 1311

B
Back-projection techniques, intensity-modulated radiation therapy, 31
Backup batteries, high-dose-rate brachytherapy safety, 550
Balloon catheterization, vascular brachytherapy, 1960–1961, 1961*f*, 1962*t*
Bartholin's glands, vulvar cancer, 1694, 1697–1698
Basal cell carcinoma
    cervical cancer, 1541
    eyelid tumors, 792–793
    penile tumors, 1522
    skin cancer, epidemiology and etiology, 690, 691*f*
    staging and classification, 692
Basal cell nervous syndrome (BCNS), 1927–1928
Base excision repair (BER) mechanism, molecular radiation and, 116
Base of tongue (BOT) tumors
    oropharyngeal metastases, 924*t*–925*t*
    prognostic factors, 926–927, 928*t*
Bax protein, cervical cancer, 1544–1545
B-cell chronic lymphocytic leukemia, pathology and classification, 1741–1742
Bcl-2 oncogene, cervical cancer, 1544–1545
Beam orientation
    breast cancer radiation therapy, 1245–1246, 1247*f*–1250*f*, 1248
    cervical cancer radiation therapy, 1556, 1558*f*
    image-guided radiation therapy (IGRT), 288–289
    intensity-modulated radiation therapy, 242–243, 244*f*–245*f*
        oropharyngeal tumors, 949
    prostate cancer radiation therapy, 1459–1461, 1460*f*, 1460*t*
    three-dimensional conformal radiation therapy, 221, 222*f*
Beam-shaping blocks, radiation therapy, 8
Beam splitter techniques, photon external-beam dosimetry, adjacent field separation techniques, 184–185, 184*f*–185*f*
Beam uniformity verification, electron-beam therapy, water-based dose distribution, 193, 193*f*
Beaumont adaptive radiation therapy system, 289, 290*f*
Beckwith-Wiedemann syndrome, pediatric patients, 1917
Becquerel radiation
    defined, 145
    history of, 3–4
Belmont Report, 2038
Beneficence principle, medical ethics and, 2035–2036
Benign tumors. *See also* Nonmalignant disease
    stereotactic radiosurgery, 384
Benzydamine, chemical radioprotection, 617–618
β-catenin, growth control and, 111
β-radiation, in-stent restenosis, 1964–1965, 1965*t*–1966*t*
Betacath system, in-stent restenosis, 1962–1964, 1963*f*
Beta decay, radioactivity, 145
Beta-particles, basic properties, 144–145, 144*t*
Bexxar conjugate, leukemia and lymphoma therapy, 588–589
Bilateral salpingo-oophorectomy (, endometrial cancer, 1614–1615, 1622–1623
Biliary tract cancers
    cholangiocarcinoma, 1356–1360
        anatomy, 1356
        diagnosis, 1356–1357, 1356*t*
        distal bile duct, 1359
        epidemiology and risk factors, 1356
        future research, 1360
        intrahepatic, 1357–1358
        metastases, 1357
        pathology, 1357
        perihilar, 1358–1359
        radiation therapy, 1359–1360, 1360*f*
        staging, 1357, 1358*t*
    gallbladder adenocarcinoma, 1360–1361
    high-dose-rate brachytherapy, 572
    low-dose-rate brachytherapy, 504–506, 506*f*, 506*t*
    metastases, palliative therapy, 2000–2001
    pediatric patients, 1917–1920, 1918*t*
    sarcomas, 1361
    symptoms and etiology, 1349
Binding energy, atomic structure, 143

Bioethics, defined, 2035
Bioheat transfer, interstitial hyperthermia, 653–655, 654f–655f
Biologically-based optimization, radiation oncology, 68
Biologically equivalent dose (BED)
    altered fractionation radiotherapy, limits of, 316, 316t
    chemoradiation therapy, head and neck squamous-cell tumors, 815–816, 815t
    non-small cell lung cancer radiation therapy, 1086–1088
    radiation therapy, (α/β ratio), 27–28
Biologically targeted therapy, chemoradiation, head and neck squamous-cell tumors, 816–817
Biologic modifiers
    non-small cell lung cancer therapy, 1099
    radiation response, 614
Biology (radiobiology)
    brachytherapy, 464–466
    breast cancer, locally advanced and recurrent disease, 1296
    combined radiation and chemotherapy, 49–50, 50f
    high-dose-rate brachytherapy, 543
    Hodgkin's lymphoma, pediatric patients, 1892
    hyperthermia, 637–642
    of metastasis, 44–46
    molecular radiation, 114–121
    nonmalignant disease radiation and, 1933–1934
    particle beam radiotherapy, 407–408
    radiation oncology and, 12–13, 36–37, 37f
    radiation therapy and, 76–103
        cell cycle redistribution, 86–87
        dose fractionation patterns, 99–103
        fractional subunits, 80
        hypoxia and, 88–89
        linear quadratic formula, 91–92, 91f–92f, 93t, 98, 98f
        mammalian cell survival curves, 90–92, 91f
        molecular responses, normal tissue, 82
        multifraction survival curves, 93–94, 94f
        normal tissue cell death, 78
        normal tissue radiobiology, 77–78
        oxygen effect, 87–90, 89f
        pathobiology and kinetics, normal tissue injury, 78–80
        quality alterations, 103–104
        quantitative analysis and dose fractionation, 90–97
        random cell killing, 90, 91f
        regeneration/repopulation, normal tissue, 82–83, 83f, 98–99, 99f
        remembered dose, tolerance mechanisms and, 83–84, 84f
        survival model comparisons, 92–93, 93f–94f
        time-does isoeffect formulae and dose fractionation, 97–99, 98f
        tumor control probability, 95–97, 95f–97f
        tumor radiobiology, 84
        tumor regeneration, 85–86, 85f, 87f–88f
        tumor regression, 84–85
        tumor reoxygenation, 89–90, 89t
        tumor response and dose fractionation, 93t, 95
        two-component model, 92
        in vivo tumor response kinetics, 84
        volume effects, 80–82
    radioimmunoglobulins, 583–584, 584t
    stereotactic radiosurgery, 378
        body radiation therapy, 389–390
    three-dimensional conformal radiation therapy evaluation, 232–233
    total body irradiation, 364
    Wilms' tumor, 1850
Biopsies
    breast cancer, 1179–1180
        diagnosis, 1194
        sentinel lymph node biopsy, 1206
    cervical cancer screening, 1536
    nasal cavity and paranasal sinuses, 861
    neck metastases, unknown primary tumors, 1045–1046, 1048, 1050t
    prostate cancer classification and staging, 1455
    thyroid disease, 1059
Bisphosphonates, bone metastases palliative therapy, 1991–1992, 1996–1997
Bite block device, photon external-beam dosimetry, patient positioning and immobilization, 182–183, 182f
Bladder cancer
    anatomy, 1412
    brachytherapy, 521–522, 1429–1430

chemotherapy, 1432–1433
    combined chemoradiation therapy, 681t, 683
        organ preservation, 1430–1432, 1431t
        systemic and neoadjuvant techniques, 1432–1433, 1433t
    diagnostic work-up, 1413
    epidemiology, 1412, 1413t
    extravesical, lymph node-negative tumors, 1418
    hyperfractionation radiation therapy, clinical trials, 306
    hyperthermia therapy, 1430
    incidence and metastatic patterns, 1412–1413
    intraoperative radiotherapy for, 402
    metastases, 1418–1419, 1419t
    morbidity and mortality, 1415–1417, 1416t–1417t
    organ-confined, lymph node-negative tumors, 1417
    particle beam therapy, 1426
    pathology, 1414, 1417, 1418t
    radiation therapy, 1421–1426
        altered fractionation schedules, 1423
        elderly patients, 1424
        external beam radiation, 1421–1423, 1422t, 1427–1429, 1427f–1430f
        postoperative radiation, 1426
        preoperative radiation, 1424–1426
        salvage cystectomy and, 1423–1424
    recurrent disease, 1419–1420, 1420t
    rhabdomyosarcoma, pediatric patients, 1876
    staging, 1414, 1414t, 1417, 1418t
    superficial tumor therapy, 1414–1415
    surgical management, 1415–1417, 1416t–1417t, 1421
        bladder preservation, 1430–1432, 1431t
    symptoms and signs, 1413
    toxicity effects and quality of life issues, 1434–1435
    uncommon tumors, 1426
Blood flow
    hyperthermia manipulation of, 645–646
    spinal canal, 765–766
    tumor cells, 128–130, 129f–130f
B-mode acquisition and targeting (BAT), image-guided radiation therapy, 268–271, 270f
Body mass index, breast cancer risk and, 1180, 1202
Body radiation therapy, stereotactic (SBRT). See also Total body irradiation (TBI)
    biological and oncological rationale, 389–390
    future research issues, 394
    liver, 391–392, 393f
    lung, 392, 394t, 395f
    miscellaneous cancers, 394
    overview, 389
    physics and dosimetry principles, 390–391
    spine, 392, 394
Bohr atomic model, 143, 143f
Bolus properties
    electron arc therapy, 213–215, 214f–215f
    electron-beam therapy, 202–204, 203f–205f, 203t
    photon external-beam dosimetry, 182
Bone and bone marrow
    Ewing's sarcoma
        chemotherapy, 1886–1889
        clinical presentation, 1886
        diagnostic work-up, 1886
        epidemiology, 1886
        future research issues, 1890
        metastases, 1889
        outcome assessment, 1889
        prognostic factors, 1886, 1887t
        radiation therapy, 1887–1890, 1888t
        stem cell rescue, 1889–1890
    Gorham syndrome, pediatric patients, 1925
    hematologic malignancies, marrow ablation, 594–595
    interfaces
        electron-beam therapy, dosage calculations, 196, 199f
        photon external-beam dosimetry, 173
    late effects syndromes on normal tissue in, 347–349, 349f, 349t
    lymphomas of, 1758–1759
    metastases
        palliative therapy
            chemotherapy, 1991–1992
            combined system therapy, 1991–1992
            epidemiology, 1986, 1987f
            evaluation, 1987–1988, 1988f–1989f
            pain management, 1988–1989

pathophysiology, 1987–1988
  radiation therapy, 1992–1997, 1993f, 1994t–1995t
  radiopharmaceuticals, 1997–1998
  surgical management, 1989–1991, 1990f, 1990t
phosphorus-32 therapy, 595
radionuclide scanning, 624–625
rhenium-188, 594–595
samarium-153, 594
strontium-89 therapy, 592–593
nasal cavity and paranasal sinus therapy and, 871
non-Hodgkin's lymphoma, pediatric patients, 1908
nonmalignant disease, radiation therapy, 1954–1956
osteosarcoma
  chemotherapy, 1801–1803, 1803t
  clinical presentation, 1801
  diagnostic evaluation, 1801, 1802f
  epidemiology and risk factors, 1801
  pathology, 1801
  radiation therapy, 1803–1806, 1804t–1806t
  staging, 1801, 1802t
  surgical management, 1802–1803
radionuclide scanning, 624–625
Bone marrow transplant (BMT)
  delayed toxicity, lung, 372
  growth, gonadal, and endocrine effects, 373
  late effects syndromes on normal tissue
    bone and bone marrow, 348–349, 349f, 349t
    central nervous system, 325
    liver, 337–338, 337f, 338t
    lung, 330, 330f–331f
  neuroblastoma in pediatric patients, 1866–1869
  non-total-body irradiation, 365–366
  radioimunoglobulin therapy and, 588–589
Bone scans
  bone metastases, 1987–1988, 1987f–1989f
  breast cancer diagnosis and staging, 1193
  prostate cancer imaging, 1451
  stomach cancer diagnosis, 1320
Bony orbit, radiation injury to, 796
Bony tissue disease, 1954–1956
Boost regimens. *See also* Simultaneous integrated boost (SIB)
        intensity-modulated radiation therapy
  accelerated fractionation, 312
  altered fractionation, 245–246
  brain metastases, 1975, 1979t
  breast cancer radiation therapy, 1248
    electron boosts, 1250–1252
    electron *vs.* interstitial boosts, 1249–1250, 1252t
  cervical cancer radiation therapy, 1555, 1557–1558
  pediatric radiation therapy, medulloblastoma, 1839–1840, 1841f
  total body irradiation, 372
Boron neutron capture therapy (BNCT), principles and terminology,
        33–35, 33f
Borrowed-servant doctrine, radiation oncology, 64–65
Botho method, photon external-beam dosimetry, tissue
        inhomogeneity correction, 170
Bowen's disease
  penile tumors, 1522
  premalignant skin lesions, 691
Brachial plexopathy, 1271
  pain management, 2008
Brachytherapy. *See also* High-dose-rate brachytherapy
  accelerated treatments, 100–101
  acute morbidity, 517
  bladder cancer, 1429–1430
  cervical cancer, 508–515, 509f, 510–512, 511f–512f, 1558–1566,
        1560f–1562f
    applicators, 510–512
    carcinoma, 510, 511f–512f
    dose fractionation, 1565–1566
    dose rate impact on outcome, 1561
    Henschke applicator, 512, 513f
    high-dose-rate regimen, 1562–1564, 1563f–1564f,
        1563t–1565t, 1588–1589
    interstitial implants, 512–515, 513f–514f, 515t
    low-dose/high-dose comparisons, 1552–1553, 1553t,
        1577–1581, 1578f, 1579t–1580t
    low-dose-rate regimen, 1562
    minicolpostats, 512
    miscellaneous protocols, 515, 515t
    postoperative intracavitary protocols, 1583–1584, 1584t

pulse-pulse brachytherapy, 1566
  results, 1566–1573, 1567f
  three-dimensional treatment planning, 1564–1565
cesium 137 sources, 427–428, 428f
dose calculation formalism
  AAPM Task Group 43 report, 440–442
  one-dimensional source approximation, 442
  two-dimensional case, 440–442, 441f–442f
dose-rate effect, 29–30
endometrial cancer, 1616–1621, 1616t–1617t
esophageal cancer, 1142, 1148, 1149f, 1150t
future research issues, 470
glioblastoma multiforme dose escalation, 731–732
historical background, 4
interstitial implantation, 442–456, 442t–443t
  classical radium-substitute sources, 443–449
  dose specification, 449, 451–454
  Fletcher system, 450t
  Manchester system, 444–447, 444f, 445t–446t, 446f–448f
  modern developments, 454–456
  Paris system, 448–449, 449t
  Quimby system, 447–448
intracavitary techniques, 456–464
  dose specification, 458–464
  Fletcher-suit applicator systems, 456–458, 457f–458f
  image-guided systems, 464
  low-dose-rate sources, 426–428, 427f–428f
  Manchester systems, 456–458, 457f
isotropic point source dose calculation, 435–438
  anisotropy factor, 436–437
  Sievert integral model, 437–438, 437f
linear quadratic model, 465–470
  high-dose-rate cervical cancer effectiveness, 468–469, 469f
  low-dose-rate rational, 466
  nonuniform dose distribution, 467–468
  optimized dose protraction for prostate cancer, 469–470
  radioisotope effectiveness, 468
  redistribution and reoxygenation, 467
  treatment time modeling, 466, 467f
low-dose-rate applications
  anal canal and rectum, 524–525, 526f
  biliary tree, 504–506, 506f, 506t
  breast, 499–502, 501f
  endovascular system, 532
  esophagus, 502–504, 503f–505f
  eye targeting, 490–493, 491f–493f
  gynecologic malignancies, 517
  head and neck, 493–499
  implantation techniques, 486
  interstitial afterloading, 476–481
  interstitial brain implants, 487–490, 488f–489f
  low-dose-rate targeting, 487–532
  maxillary sinus, 494
  molds, 481–483
  nasal vestibule, 494
  nasopharynx, 495, 496t
  operating room safety, 486–487
  oral cavity, 495, 497
  overview, 476
  pancreas, 504
  penis and male urethra, 525–527, 526f
  permanent implant sources, 430
  prostate cancer, 527–531, 527t–528t, 528f–529f, 531f
  pterygium, 493
  quality assurance and safety issues, 532–534, 533f
  radioactive material selection, 476
  remote control afterloading, 483–486
  skin and lip, 494–495
  soft tissue sarcomas, 507–508, 507f
  templates, 481
  tongue and mouth, 497–498, 497f–499f
  tonsilar region/fauchal arch, 498–499, 500f
  uterine cervix, 508–517
  vagina, vulva, and female urethra, 517–524
nasal vestibule disease, 864
nasopharyngeal cancer, 836–837, 840, 841t
  persistent/recurrent disease, 846–848, 846t–847t, 848f
oral cavity tumors, 904–905, 905f
oropharyngeal cancer, 942f–943f, 943–944, 944t, 945f
penile cancer, 1526, 1528, 1529t
permanent interstitial sources, 429–432

Brachytherapy (*contd.*)
 posterior uvea melanoma, 784, 785*f*
 prostate cancer, 527–531, 527*t*–528*t*, 528*f*–529*f*, 531*f*
  intermediate/high-risk cancer, boost therapy with EBRT,
   1490–1491
  low-risk cancer, 1463–1465, 1464*f*, 1465*t*
   erectile dysfunction, 1474
   external beam radiation combined with, 1465, 1470,
    1474–1475
   outcomes assessment, 1469–1470, 1470*t*
   rectal tolerance, 1473–1474
   urinary toxicity, 1472–1473
 pulsed brachytherapy, 470
 quality assurance, 57, 532–534, 533*f*
 quantitative dosimetry, 438–440
  computational methods, 439–440
  experimental techniques, 438–439
 radioactive decay mathematics, 429–430, 430*f*, 430*t*
 radiobiology, 464–466
 radionuclide sources and properties, 423–426, 424*t*
  experimental intracavitary sources, 428
 retinoblastomas, 790
 source-strength specification, 432–435
  activity-exposure rate relationships, 434
  air-kerma strength, 433–435
  milligram-hours and integrated reference air-kerma, 435
  quantity activity measurement, 434
  source output quantities, 434–435
 temporary interstitial technique
  low-dose-rate sources, 428–429
  low-energy sources, 429
 terminology, 423
 tonsillar fossa and soft palate tumors, 926, 927*t*
 ultra-low-dose-rate permanent implant sources, 430–432
 vaginal cancer, 1669–1671, 1670*t*
Bragg-Gray cavity ionization measurement, absorbed dose
  calculation from, 159
Bragg peak
 charged particle radiotherapy, 412–413, 412*t*
 proton radiosurgery, 380
 protons and heavy ions, 148–149, 149*f*
Brain
 arteriovenous malformations, proton and α-particle
  radiotherapy, 417
 interstitial brachytherapy implants, 487–490, 488*f*–489*f*, 495*t*
 late effects syndromes on normal tissue, 323–326, 326*t*, 327*f*
 malignant tumors
  heavy ion therapies, 419–420, 419*t*
  intraoperative radiotherapy in, 404
  palliative therapy for metastases
   anticonvulsants, 1978–1979
   clinical presentation, diagnosis, and prognosis, 1974, 1975*t*
   concurrent radiosensitizers, 1977
   corticosteroids, 1974
   neurocognitive decline, 1977–1978
   postoperative radiation therapy, 1976
   radiosurgery boost trials, 1975, 1976*t*, 1979*t*
   surgical resection, 1974–1975, 1975*f*, 1978*t*
   whole-brain radiation therapy, 1974–1977, 1975*t*, 1977*f*,
    1980*t*
  partial brain irradiation, 726–727, 728*f*
  stereotactic radiosurgery, 386
  whole brain irradiation, 727, 729*f*, 1974–1977, 1975*t*, 1977*f*,
   1980*t*
 ovarian cancer metastases, 1644–1645
Brainstem
 encephalopathy, nasopharyngeal cancer therapy, 852
 gliomas
  adult patients, 739–740, 740*t*
  pediatric patients, 1830–1832, 1831*f*
 radiation imaging, 632–633
BRCA1/BRCA2 gene
 breast cancer risk and
  breast-conserving surgery in patients with, 1234–1237,
   1235*t*, 1236*f*–1237*f*
  male breast cancer, 1311–1312
  pediatric patients, 1915–1916
  screening protocols, 1181, 1181*t*
 ovarian cancer risk and, 1630
Breast augmentation, breast cancer surgery and irradiation after,
  1242

Breast cancer
 anatomical illustrations, 630–631, 631*t*
 bilateral carcinoma, 1242–1243
 brachytherapy, 499–502, 501*f*–503*f*
 clinical presentation, 1187
 combined treatment modalities
  breast-conserving surgery with, 1231*t*, 1231–1232
  sequencing protocols, 1229–1234, 1231*f*
  tamoxifen-radiation sequencing, 1232, 1233*t*, 1234
 contralateral breast cancer, 1257, 1274–1275, 1275*t*
 ductal carcinoma in situ, 1164–1172
  clinical presentation and epidemiology, 1184
  decision tree for, 1171–1172
  mammography, 1164, 1165*f*
  natural history, 1167
  pathology and biology, 1164–1167, 1166*f*–1167*f*
  treatment options, 1167–1171, 1168*f*–1169*f*, 1169*t*–1171*t*
 early stage
  anatomy, 1175, 1176*f*–1178*f*
  breast-conserving surgery, 1219–1224
   controversies and special circumstances, 1234–1243
   no radiation, 1219–1224
  chemotherapy, cosmetic effects, 1266–1268, 1267*t*
  cosmetic outcomes and sequelae, 1264–1269
   breast conservation surgery, 1268–1269
   cosmesis, 1264–1268, 1266*t*
   radiation therapy and, 1268
  cost issues in treatment of, 1277–1278
  diagnosis and work-up, 1189–1194
  epidemiology, 1175–1176, 1178*f*
  management of, 1202–1206
  multicentric disease patients, 1241, 1242*t*
  natural history and origins, 1183–1186
  pathologic classification, 1194, 1196–1197
  pathologic stage, 1194
  prevention and genetic screening, 1181–1183, 1181*t*–1182*t*
  prognostic factors, 1197–1202
  psychoemotional and quality of life issues, 1278–1279
  radiation therapy, 1206–1210
   accelerated partial breast irradiation, 1259–1260
   angiosarcoma, 1276–1277
   beam calculations, 1248, 1249*f*–1250*f*
   boost to tumor site, 1248
   brachial plexopathy, 1271
   cardiac sequelae, 1272–1274
   contralateral breast cancer, 1274–1275, 1275*t*
   cosmetic surgery following, 1268
   electron boosts, 1250–1252
   electron *vs.* interstitial boosts, 1249–1250, 1252*t*
   external beam radiation, 1262–1263
   in Hodgkin's patients, 1240–1241, 1240*t*
   intraoperative accelerated partial breast technique,
    1263–1264
   irradiation dose to contralateral breast, 1257
   lymphatics irradiation, 1252–1255
   lymphedema/breast edema following, 1269–1270
   MammoSite technique, 1262
   multicatheter interstitial techniques, 1260–1262
   patient positioning, 1243, 1245*f*
   pulmonary sequelae, 1271–1272, 1272*f*
   randomized data, 1248
   secondary malignancies, 1275–1276
   sequelae, 1269–1277
   skin/breast complications, 1270–1271
   stroke risk, supraclavicular radiation, 1274
   tangential beam alignment, 1245–1246, 1247*f*–1248*f*
   tangential field/supraclavicular field alignment,
    1255–1257, 1256*f*
   three-dimensional conformal *vs.* intensity-modulated
    therapies, 1257, 1259
   treatment volume, 1243–1244, 1246*f*
   whole breast dose, 1246, 1248
  recurrent disease prognosis, 1210–1219, 1212*t*
  regional lymphatics, radiation management, 1224–1230
  risk factors, 1176–1181, 1179*t*
  screening guidelines, 1187–1189, 1187*t*–1188*t*
  sequenced chemotherapy and hormonal therapy, 1230–1234
  staging systems, 1194, 1195*t*
  systemic management, 1206, 12152
 high-dose-rate brachytherapy, 558–559, 574–576, 575*t*
 hyperthermia therapy, 660–662, 661*f*

intensity-modulated radiation therapy, 258–259
intraoperative radiotherapy, 400*t*, 402–404
lobular carcinoma in situ, 1162–1163
locally advanced and recurrent disease
  breast conservation therapy, 1299–1300, 1299*f*
  chemotherapy, 1297–1298, 1297*t*
  clinical presentation, 1294–1296, 1295*f*
  epidemiology, 1292, 1293*t*, 1294*f*
  hormonal therapy, 1298–1299
  inflammatory breast cancer, 1293–1294
    management and treatment results, 1308–1309
  management of, 1296–1297, 1297*f*, 1297*t*
  mastectomy, 1300–1305, 1300*t*
    neoadjuvant chemotherapy and radiation therapy,
      1304–1305
    radiation therapy following, 1300–1302, 1301*f*, 1303*t*,
      1312–1315
    recurrence risk following, 1303–1304, 1303*t*
  natural history, 1292–1294, 1295*f*
  pathology and biology, 1296
  radiation therapy, 1300–1303, 1301*f*, 1303*t*, 1312–1315
  staging, 1296
  systemic therapies, 1305–1307, 1305*t*–1307*t*
  treatment algorithms for, 1307–1308, 1307*f*
  treatment results, 1308
male breast cancer, 1311
metastatic patterns, 1183–1186
  axillary spread, 1183–1184, 1184*t*
    unknown primary cancer, 1311
  bone metastases, palliative therapy, 1991–1992
  internal mammary spread, 1184, 1184*t*, 1228–1230, 1229*t*
  local control mechanisms, 1185, 1186*f*
  supraclavicular spread, 1184–1185, 1253, 1253*f*
  systemic spread, 1185
Paget's disease, 1163–1164
palliative therapy
  bone metastases, 1991–1992
pediatric patients, 1915–1916
photodynamic therapy, 601
proton and α-particle radiotherapy, 419
recurrent disease
  age as risk factor, 1210–1219, 1211*f*–1212*f*, 1211*t*
  breast conservation therapy and, 1309–1310
  managment and treatment results, 1309–1311
  margin status, 1212–1215
  mastectomy and risk of, 1309–1311
  regional nodal relapse, 1311
Breast conservation strategies
  combined treatment modalities, 1230*t*, 1231–1232
  ductal carcinoma in situ, 1168–1171, 1169*f*, 1169*t*–1171*t*
  early stage breast cancer, 1219–1224
    controversies and special circumstances, 1234–1243
    no radiation, 1219–1224
  locally advanced and recurrent disease, 1299–1300, 1299*f*
  recurrent disease, 1309–1310
Breastfeeding, breast cancer risk and, 1177
  lactation after breast-conservation therapy, 1240
Breath control devices, stereotactic body radiation therapy, 390–391
Bremsstrahlung radiation, defined, 144, 144*f*
Bronchogenic carcinoma, pediatric patients, 1915, 1915*f*
Bronchoscopy, tracheal tumor diagnosis, 1120
Buccal mucosa
  anatomy, 892
  disease treatment and results, 909–910
Buildup cap, radiation exposure measurement, 157
Bursitis, radiation therapy, 1948, 1948*f*

C
CA 15-3 marker, breast cancer prognosis and, 1202
CA 19-9 marker, fallopian tubes, 1651
CA 27-29 markers, breast cancer prognosis and, 1202
CA 125 markers
  cervical cancer, 1545
  fallopian tubes, 1651
  ovarian cancer screening, 1631–1632
Calcaneodynia, radiation therapy, 1949, 1950*f*, 1951*t*
Californium 252
  brachytherapy applications, 428
  cervical cancer radiation therapy, 1573
Calorimetry, absorbed dose measurements, 157–158
Cancer epidemiology, global trends, 604, 605*f*

Cancer management
  integrated multimodality and organ preservation, 50
  morbidity and mortality, 53*f*
  survival rates, 54*t*
Capacitive heating, hyperthermia, 650, 650*f*–651*f*
Capillary hemangioma, 779
Carbogen utilization, chemical modifiers of radiation therapy,
  611–612
Carboplatin, seminoma testis therapy, 1510–1512, 1511*t*
Carcinoembryonic antigen (CEA), cervical cancer, 1545
Carcinoma in situ. *See also* Ductal carcinoma in situ (breast)
  cervical cancer, 1546–1547
  vaginal cancer, brachytherapy, 520
  vaginal intraepithelial neoplasia, 1660–1661, 1664*t*
Carcinosarcoma
  bladder tumors, 1426
  prostate tumors, 1456
Cardiac pacemakers, photon external-beam dosimetry, 185, 187*t*
Cardiac sequelae, breast cancer therapy, 1272–1274
Cardiac tumors. *See also* Great vessel tumors
  anatomy of, 1154–1155
  clinical presentation, 1155–1156, 1156*t*
  diagnostic work-up, 1156–1157, 1157*f*
  incidence and epidemiology, 1154, 1155*t*
  management of, 1157–1158
  natural history, 1155
  radiation therapy, 1158–1159, 1159*f*
  staging system and pathologic classification, 1157, 1157*t*
Cardiomyopathy, late effects syndromes and, 332–336, 333*f*–335*f*,
  334*t*–335*t*
Cardiovascular effects, Hodgkin's lymphoma radiation therapy,
  pediatric patients, 1901
Carotid artery injury, nasopharyngeal cancer therapy, 853
Carotid body chemodectomas, 998, 1003*t*
Casuistry, medical ethics and, 2035
Cataracts, total body irradiation effects, 373
Catheter attachment lock, high-dose-rate brachytherapy safety, 548
Cause-specific survival, end point selection, phase III clinical trials,
  358
Cavity-gas calibration factor, absorbed dose calculation, 159
CD34 antigen, cervical cancer, 1545
CD109 protein, cervical cancer, 1545
Cell cycle
  chemoradiation therapy redistribution of, 671
  control of, 41–42
  hyperthermia, cytotoxicity mechanisms, 640, 641*f*
  irradiation effects on, 35–36, 35*f*, 36*t*
  loss of control in, 111–112
  radiation therapy and, 13
    delay in, 117
    redistribution mechanisms, 86–87, 87*f*
  tumor molecular pathophysiology, 126–127, 127*f*
Cell death. *See* Apoptosis
Cell injury, radiation therapy, pathology and kinetics, 78–80
Cell kill rate
  dose fractionation and, 90, 90*f*
  logarithmic, 13–14, 22*f*
  radiation dose and, 13, 18*f*
Cell proliferation, radiation therapy and, 13
Cell repair mechanisms, chemoradiation therapy inhibition of, 671
Cell survival
  dose-rate effect, radiation therapy, 29–30
  high-dose-rate brachytherapy, 544–545, 545*f*
  hyperthermia, 637, 638*f*
CEM 43° profile, hyperthermia isoeffect dose, 639, 639*f*
  clinical applications, 659–660
Central axis value, electron-beam therapy, water-based dose
  distribution, 193
Central-field depth dose, electron-beam therapy, 192
Central lung distance (CLD) alignment, breast cancer radiation
  therapy, 1245–1246, 1247*f*–1248*f*
Central nervous system (CNS) tumors. *See also* Intracranial tumors
  anatomy, 717–718, 718*f*–719*f*
  late effects syndromes on normal tissue in, 323–326, 325*f*, 325*t*
  lymphomas, 1759–1760
  malignant cysts, phosphorus-32 therapy, 595
  meningioma, 743–744
  natural history, 720
  non-Hodgkin's lymphoma, acquired immunodeficiency
    syndrome, 704–705
  pediatric patients

Central nervous system (CNS) tumors (*contd.*)
    astrocytic tumors, 1824–1832
    atypical teratoid/rhabdoid tumor, 1841–1842
    choroid plexus tumors, 1834–1835
    embryonal tumors, 1836–1842
    ependymal tumors, 1832–1834
    germ cell tumors, 1842–1844
    neuronal/mixed neuronal-glial tumors, 1835
    non-Hodgkin's lymphoma, 1908
    pineal parenchymal tumors, 1835–1836
    radiation therapy, 1822–1824, 1824*t*
    sellar region, 1844–1845
    supratentorial primitive neuroectodermal tumor, 1841, 1842*f*
  pediatric patients, epidemiology, 1822, 1826*f*
  primary lymphomas, 741–743
Central venous thrombosis, late effects syndromes on normal tissue
    in liver and, 336–338, 337*f*, 338*t*
c-erbB-2 oncogene, cervical cancer, 1544–1545
Cerebral edema
  intracranial tumor management, 724
  late effects syndromes on normal tissue, 326, 326*t*, 327*f*
Cerebrospinal fluid cytology, intracranial tumors, 723
Cervical cancer
  acquired immunodeficiency syndrome, 712–713
  anatomy, 1532, 1532*f*
  brachytherapy, 508–515, 509*f*, 510–512, 511*f*–512*f*, 1558–1566,
    1560*f*–1562*f*
    applicators, 510–512
    carcinoma, 510, 511*f*–512*f*
    dose fractionation, 1565–1566
    dose rate impact on outcome, 1561
    Henschke applicator, 512, 513*f*
    high-dose-rate regimen, 1562–1564, 1563*f*–1564*f*,
      1563*t*–1565*t*, 1588–1589
    interstitial implants, 512–515, 513*f*–514*f*, 515*t*
    low-dose/high-dose comparisons, 1577–1581, 1578*f*,
      1579*t*–1580*t*
    low-dose-rate regimen, 1562
    minicolpostats, 512
    miscellaneous protocols, 515, 515*t*
    postoperative intracavitary protocols, 1583–1584, 1584*t*
    pulse-pulse brachytherapy, 1566
    results, 1566–1573, 1567*f*
    three-dimensional treatment planning, 1564–1565
  cervical stump carcinoma, 1598–1599
  chemotherapy, 1591–1597, 1594*t*
    amifostine, 1596
    cisplatin and 5-fluorouracil, 1591–1592
    hyperfractionated radiation, 1596–1597
    intra-arterial, 1592
    mitomycin C/tirapazamine, 1592
    neoadjuvant therapy, 1596
  clinical presentation, 1535
  combined treatment modalities
    chemoradiation therapy, 681*t*, 682–683, 1591–1597,
      1594*f*–1595*f*, 1596*t*
      cisplatin, 1593
      hydroxyurea, 1592–1593
    chemotherapy regimens, 1591–1592
    hyperthermia and irradiation, 1597
    results, 1566–1584
    sequelae, 1589
    surgery and radiation, 1546–1550, 1551*t*
  cost issues in management of, 1599
  diagnostic work-up, 1535–1538, 1536*t*–1537*t*, 1538*f*
  elderly patients, 1572
  epidemiology, 1532, 1534
  high-dose-rate brachytherapy, 556–558, 557*f*–558*f*, 562–564,
    563*t*–565*t*
  hormone replacement therapy following treatment, 1589
  hyperbaric oxygen and hypoxic sensitizers, 1596–1597
  hyperthermia, 664–665, 664*f*
    radiation therapy and, 1597
  metastases, 1534–1535, 1534*t*–1536*t*, 1535*f*
    para-aortic lymph nodes, 1574–1576, 1576*t*
  natural history, 1534–1535, 1534*t*–1536*t*, 1535*f*
  oncological anatomy, 633
  pathologic classifications, 1540–1541
  pregnancy and, 1597–1598
  prognostic factors, 1541–1546
    age, 1541
    anemia and tumor hypoxia, 1542–1543
    angiogenesis and tumor vascularity, 1544
    apoptosis and radiation response markers, 1544
    carcinoembryonic antigen, 1545
    cyclooxygenases, 1546
    cytokeratin markers, 1545–1546
    cytokine markers, 1546
    flow cytometry studies and DNA and growth fraction, 1544
    histology, 1544
    HIV infection, 1546
    hormonal receptors, 1546
    molecular genetics, 1544–1545
    oncogenes, 1545
    race/socioeconomic status, 1541–1542
    tumor volume, 1543
  radiation therapy
    dose calculation, 1566
    elective para-aortic lymph node irradiation, 1576–1577, 1576*f*
    external beam irradiation, 1553–1556, 1554*f*–1555*f*
    hyperthermia and, 1597
    interstitial implants, 1573
    intraoperative irradiation, 1591
    palliative radiation, 1589
    postoperative, 1581–1583, 1582*f*, 1583*t*, 1589
    pretreatment laparotomy and nodal staging, 1551–1552,
      1552*t*
    prolonged treatment times, 1574, 1575*f*
    recurrent disease, 1590
    results, 1566–1584
    sequelae, 1584–1589, 1585*f*–1586*f*
    staging protocols and, 1547–1548
    surgery and, 1546–1550, 1551*t*
    techniques, 1552–1566
  recurrent disease, 1568–1591, 1574*t*
  secondary malignancies, 1599
  staging protocols, 1538–1540, 1539*t*, 1540*f*
    management based on, 1546–1548
    pretreatment laparotomy, 1551–1552, 1552*t*
    results analysis and, 1566–1573
  surgical management
    postoperative irradiation, 1581–1583, 1582*f*, 1583*t*
    radiation therapy and, 1546–1550, 1551*t*
    recurrent disease, 1590
    results, 1566–1584
    sequelae, 1589
    techniques, 1550–1552, 1551*t*–1552*t*
  treatment guidelines, 1540, 1544*t*
Cervical (neck) lymph nodes, neck metastases, unknown primary
    tumors, management of, 1041, 1043–1044, 1045*f*,
    1048, 1050*t*–1051*t*, 1051–1053, 1052*f*
Cervical stump carcinoma, 1598–1599
Cervicomedullary tumors, pediatric patients, 1831–1832
Cesium 137 sources
  brachytherapy, 427–428, 427*f*–428*f*
    nonafterloading sources, 428
  cervical cancer brachytherapy, 1558–1559
Charged particle radiotherapy
  pituitary tumor management, 754
  principles and applications, 412–413, 412*t*
Chemical modifiers, radiation therapy
  hypoxic cell sensitization, 612–613
  hypoxic cell targeting, 613–614
  mitigation, 615–617, 616*f*
  oxygen effect, 611
  radioprotection, 614–615
  treatment, 617–618
  tumor oxygenation augmentation, 611–612, 612*f*
Chemical radioprotection, 614–615
Chemodectomas
  classification, 998, 999*t*
  nonmalignant disease, 1940–1941, 1941*t*
  radiation therapy, 998, 1003*t*
Chemoprevention, for cancer, 53–54
Chemoradiation therapy. *See* Chemotherapy; Radiation therapy
Chemotherapy. *See also* Combined treatment modalities
  accelerated fractionation *vs.*, 315
  acute lymphoblastic leukemia, 1780–1783
  adrenal gland tumors, 1719–1720
  altered fractionation radiotherapy with, 312, 313*t*–314*t*, 315
  anal cancer, combined treatment modalities, 1386–1388, 1387*t*,
    1389*t*–1390*t*

anaplastic glioma, 736–737
bladder cancer, 1432–1433, 1433*t*
bone metastases, 1991–1992
breast cancer
    cosmesis and, 1266–1268, 1267*t*
    inflammatory breast cancer, 1308–1309
    locally advanced and recurrent disease, 1297–1300, 1297*t*, 1299*f*
        neoadjuvant chemotherapy and postmastectomy radiation, 1304–1305
        systemic therapy analysis, 1305–1307, 1305*t*–1307*t*
    sequencing protocols, 1230–1234, 1230*f*–1231*f*
    systemic therapy, 1206
cervical cancer, 1591–1597, 1594*t*
    amifostine, 1596
    cisplatin and 5-fluorouracil, 1591–1592
    hyperfractionated radiation, 1596–1597
    intra-arterial, 1592
    mitomycin C/tirapazamine, 1592
    neoadjuvant therapy, 1596
    staging protocols and, 1547–1548
colon cancer, 1368
    radiation and, 1368–1370, 1369*t*–1370*t*, 1370*f*
Cushing's disease, 758, 758*f*
cutaneous T-cell lymphoma, 1773
endometrial cancer, 1619, 1625
esophageal cancer, 1145
esthesioneuroblastoma, 1017–1018, 1914
Ewing's sarcoma, 1886–1889
fallopian tube malignancies, 1653–1654
germ-cell tumors, pediatric patients, 1925
glioblastoma multiforme, 733–734
head and neck sarcomas, 1031
hepatocellular carcinoma, 1353–1355
    pediatric patients, 1919–1920
Hodgkin's lymphoma, 1726, 1727*t*
    clinical trials, 1735
    pediatric patients, 1896, 1897*t*, 1898
    results, 1730–1733
    sequelae, 1733–1735
hyperfractionated radiotherapy concurrent with, 315
hyperthermia and, 648–649, 649*f*
hypopharyngeal cancers, 969–970
intracranial tumor management, 727–729
intraoperative radiotherapy with, 397–399, 400*t*
Kaposi's sarcoma, 708–710
Langerhans cell histiocytosis, 1921
medulloblastoma, 741
    pediatric patients, 1840–1841
meningiomas, nonmalignant disease, 1936
nasal cavity and paranasal sinuses, 862
nasopharyngeal cancer, 840–844, 842*t*, 843*f*, 844*t*
    pediatric patients, 1913
neuroblastoma, 1865–1869
non-Hodgkin's lymphoma, 1748–1750
    pediatric patients, 1905–1907, 1905*f*, 1906*t*, 1907*f*
nonpilocytic/diffusely infiltrating gliomas, 738–739
non-seminomatous germ cell tumors, 1512–1513, 1516
non-small cell lung cancer
    metastatic disease, 1098–1099
    postoperative, 1085
    preoperative, 1083–1084
oral cavity radiation therapy, 902
    radiation therapy combined with, 906
oropharyngeal cancer, 944–946
osteosarcoma, 1801–1803, 1803*t*
ovarian cancer, 1636–1637
pancreatic cancer, 1345–1346
pediatric patients
    germ-cell tumors, 1925
    hepatocellular carcinoma, 1919–1920
    Hodgkin's lymphoma, 1896, 1897*t*, 1898
    Langerhans cell histiocytosis, 1921
    medulloblastoma, 1840–1841
    nasopharyngeal cancer, 1913
    neuroblastoma, 1865–1869
    rhabdomyosarcoma, 1878
penis, cancer of, 1525
pituitary tumors, 754, 757

Cushing's disease, 758–759, 758*f*–759*f*
prostate cancer, 1495–1497
radiation therapy combined with, 48–50, 49*f*–50*f*
    anal cancer, 681*t*, 683
    antimetabolites, 677*t*, 678–679
    antitumor efficacy strategies, 674
    bladder cancer, 681*t*, 683
    cervical cancer, 681*t*, 682–683
    drug-radiation interaction, 670–672, 670*f*
    emerging strategies, 673–677
    esophageal cancer, 681*t*, 683–684
    future research, 684–685
    glioblastoma multiforme, 681*t*, 684
    head and neck cancers, 681–682, 681*t*, 807–818
        adjuvant postoperative irradiation, 813
        alternating radiation and chemotherapy, 810
        biologically target therapy, 816–817
        curative intent treatment, 810–813, 811*f*–814*f*, 814*t*
        efficacy of, 807–808
        future research issues, 817–818
        selection criteria, 813–816
        sequential chemoradiation, 816
        synchronous radiation and multiagent chemotherapy, 809–810
        synchronous radiation and single-agent chemotherapy, 808–809, 808*t*
        toxicity management strategies, 817
    long-term toxicity effects, 680*t*
    lung cancer, 679–681, 681*t*
    mitomycin C, 677*t*, 678
    molecular targeting strategies, 674–676, 674*t*, 675*f*
    normal tissue protection, 676–677
    overview, 669
    platinum-based drugs, 677, 677*t*
    rectal cancer, 681*t*, 684
    strategies in, 669–670
    taxanes, 677–678, 677*t*
    therapeutic index, 669
    timing protocols, 672–673, 673*t*
    topoisomerase I inhibitors, 677*t*, 679
    tumer cell repopulation inhibition, 672
retroperitoneal cancer, 1711, 1713
rhabdomyoscarcoma, pediatric patients, 1878
salivary gland tumors, 888
seminoma testis, 1510–1512, 1511*t*, 1516
small cell lung carcinoma, 1101–1102
soft tissue sarcomas, 1813–1814
spinal cord tumors, 771–772
stomach cancer
    basic principles, 1333
    surgery and, 1329–1332, 1329*t*–1330*t*
superior sulcus tumors, 1093
thymomas, 1115
thyroid disease, 1070
total body irradiation, 365–366
urethral cancer
    female, 1690
    male, 1529–1530
uterine sarcoma, 1624
vaginal cancer, 1667–1668
vulvar tumors, 1704–1705, 1705*t*
    sequelae, 1705–1706
Chiasmatic gliomas, pediatric patients, 1830
Childhood brainstem tumor, hyperfractionation radiation therapy, clinical trials, 306
Chloroma, diagnosis and management, 1012
Cholangiocarcinoma, 1356–1360
    anatomy, 1356
    diagnosis, 1356–1357, 1356*t*
    distal bile duct, 1359
    epidemiology and risk factors, 1356
    future research, 1360
    intrahepatic, 1357–1358
    metastases, 1357
    pathology, 1357
    pediatric patients, 1917–1920, 1918*t*
    perihilar, 1358–1359
    radiation therapy, 1359–1360, 1360*f*
    staging, 1357, 1358*t*
Cholecystectomy, gallbladder adenocarcinoma, 1360
Chondrosarcomas, nonmalignant disease, 1940, 1940*f*

Chordomas, 1005–1010
  anatomy, 1005
  clinical presentation, 1005–1006
  diagnostic work-up, 1006, 1006*t*
  epidemiology, 1005
  general management, 1006
  natural history, 1005
  nonmalignant disease, 1939–1940, 1940*f*, 1940*t*
  pathology, 1005
  photons, 1006–1009
  protons, 1009–1010
  radiation therapy, 1006, 1007*f*–1008*f*
  treatment sequelae, 1010
Choriocarcinoma, classification, 1505
Choroidal hemangiomas
  diagnosis and management, 779, 781*f*
  pediatric patients, 1925
  radiation therapy, 1942–1943
Choroidal melanoma
  diagnosis and management, 784, 785*f*
  episcleral plaque therapy, 490–493, 491*f*–492*f*
Choroid plexus tumors, pediatric patients, 1834–1835
Chromosome translocations, radiation oncology and, 37–39, 38*f*–40*f*
Chronic lymphocytic leukemia (CLL)
  staging, 1784*t*
  therapy, 1784–1785
Chronic myelogenous leukemia (CML)
  diagnosis, 1783
  treatment, 1783–1784
Chronic skin conditions, in cancer patients, 2016–2017, 2016*f*
Circumcision, penile cancer and, 1519
Cisplatin
  cervical cancer therapy, 1591–1594
  combined chemoradiation therapy, head and neck squamous-cell
    tumors, 809
  ovarian cancer therapy, 1637
Clear-cell carcinoma
  cervical cancer, 1541
  endometrial cancer, 1611–1612, 1612*t*
    uterine papillary serous and clear cell carcinoma, 1623–1624
  vaginal clear-cell adenocarcinoma, 1658
    epidemiology and risk factors, 1658
    management and treatment outcomes, 1672
    pathology, 1659
Clear-cell sarcoma, Wilms' tumor, 1856
Clinically detectable disease criteria, tumor control probability and,
    95–97, 96*f*
Clinical target volume (CTV)
  external beam radiation therapy, 7
  interstitial brachytherapy, 454–456
  lung cancer radiation therapy, 1095
  prostate cancer radiation therapy, 1459
  stereotactic body radiation therapy, liver, 391–392, 393*f*
  stomach cancer radiation therapy, 1324–1325, 1324*t*–1325*t*
  three-dimensional conformal radiation therapy
    applications, 227–230, 228*f*–230*f*
    specifications, 225
  treatment planning for radiation therapy, 30–31
Clinical trials
  breast cancer mastectomy, postmastectomy radiation,
    1300–1303, 1301*f*, 1303*t*, 1312–1315
  breast cancer systemic therapies, 1305–1307, 1305*t*–1307*t*
  cervical cancer therapies, 1567–1573
    chemotherapies, 1592–1597, 1594*t*
  combined chemoradiation therapy, head and neck squamous-cell
    tumors, 809–813, 811*f*–814*f*
  ethical issues in, 2040
  Ewing's sarcoma, pediatric patients, 1889–1890
  future research issues, 362
  meta-analysis, defined, 357
  methodology
    data collection, 360
    evolution of, 356
    final analysis, 361, 361*t*
    interim analysis, 360–361
    subset analyses, 362
    survival analyses, 361–362
  nonmalignant disease radiation therapy, 1933
  oropharyngeal cancer therapy, 945–946
  pancreatic cancer chemoradiation therapy, 1341–1346
  prospective studies

    defined, 356–357
    phase III trials, 358–360, 360*t*
    phase II trials, 357–358
    phase I trials, 357
  prostate cancer, whole-pelvic irradiation trial, 1488–1489
  radiation therapy, 2031–2032
  retrospective studies, defined, 356
  rhabdomyosarcoma, pediatric patients, 1880–1882, 1881*f*
  study design and classification, 356–357
  Wilms' tumor, 1854–1857, 1855*t*
Clonogenic cell proportion, radiosensitivity and, 15
Cluster of differentiation (CD) molecules, acute lymphoblastic
    leukemia (ALL), 1778–1779
c-myc oncogene, cervical cancer, 1545
Coaxial beam arrangements, photon external-beam dosimetry, 177,
    177*f*–178*f*
Cobalt-60 teletherapy, instrumentation, 150, 150*f*
Cognitive dysfunction
  brain metastases, 1977–1978
  leukemia radiation therapy, 1786–1787
Collagen vascular disease, breast cancer and, breast-conserving
    surgery in patients with, 1237–1238, 1237*t*
Collimator components, linear accelerator, 152, 152*f*
Colorectal cancer
  anatomy and metastatic patterns, 1366, 1367*f*
  epidemiology and risk factors, 1366
  intraoperative radiotherapy, 400–401, 402*f*
  late effects syndromes on normal tissue in, 342–344
  metastatic patterns, 1366–1367
  pathology, 1367
  pediatric patients, 1916–1917
  prevention and early detection, 1367
  radiation and chemotherapy, 1368–1370, 1369*f*, 1369*t*–1370*t*
    future research issues, 1371–1372
    locally advanced disease and palliation, 1370–1371
    techniques, 1371, 1372*f*
  staging and evaluation, 1367, 1368*t*
  surgical management, 1367–1368
Combined treatment modalities
  anal cancer, 1386–1388, 1387*t*, 1389*t*–1390*t*
  biological aspects, 49–50, 50*f*
  bladder cancer therapy, 1430–1435, 1431*t*
  bone metastases, 1991–1992, 1996–1997
  brain metastases, palliative therapy, 1974–1979, 1980*t*
  breast cancer chemoradiation
    breast-conserving surgery with, 1230*t*, 1231–1232
    sequencing protocols, 1230–1234, 1230*f*
    tamoxifen-radiation sequencing, 1232, 1233*t*, 1234
  cervical cancer, 1548–1550, 1549*f*
    chemotherapy and radiation, 1591–1597
    multicomponent chemotherapy, 1591–1592
    results, 1566–1573
    sequelae, 1589
  chemoradiation
    concurrent protocols, 673, 673*t*
  chemoradiation techniques, 48–50, 49*f*–50*f*
    anal cancer, 681*t*, 683
    antimetabolites, 677*t*, 678–679
    antitumor efficacy strategies, 674
    bladder cancer, 681*t*, 683
    cervical cancer, 681*t*, 682–683
    drug-radiation interaction, 670–672, 670*f*
    emerging strategies, 673–677
    esophageal cancer, 681*t*, 683–684
    future research, 684–685
    glioblastoma multiforme, 681*t*, 684
    head and neck cancers, 681–682, 681*t*, 807–818
      adjuvant postoperative irradiation, 813
      alternating radiation and chemotherapy, 810
      biologically target therapy, 816–817
      curative intent treatment, 810–813, 811*f*–814*f*, 814*t*
      efficacy of, 807–808
      future research issues, 817–818
      multiagent chemotherapy, 809–810
      selection criteria, 813–816
      sequential chemoradiation, 816
      single-agent chemotherapy, 808–809, 808*t*
      squamous-cell tumors, 809
      toxicity management strategies, 817
    lung cancer, 679–681, 681*t*
    mitomycin C, 677*t*, 678

molecular targeting strategies, 674–676, 674*t*, 675*f*
normal tissue protection, 676–677
overview, 669
platinum-based drugs, 677, 677*t*
rectal cancer, 681*t*, 684
strategies in, 669–670
taxanes, 677–678, 677*t*
therapeutic index, 669
timing protocols, 672–673, 673*t*
topoisomerase I inhibitors, 677*t*, 679
tumer cell repopulation inhibition, 672
colon cancer
palliative therapy, locally advanced disease, 1370–1371
radiation and chemotherapy, 1368–1370, 1369*t*–1370*t*, 1370*f*
surgery and chemotherapy, 1368
desmoplastic small round-cell tumor (DSCRT), 1927
esophageal cancer, 681*t*, 683–684, 1138–1139
postoperative regimen, 1145–1146, 1146*t*
radiation *vs.*, 1146–1147
surgery and, 1147, 1147*f*
hepatocellular carcinoma, transcatheter arterial
chemoembolization and radiation therapy, 1354,
1354*t*, 1355*f*
Hodgkin's lymphoma, 1726–1727, 1727*t*, 1730–1732, 1730*t*
pediatric patients, 1894–1896, 1899–1902, 1900*f*–1901*f*, 1900*t*
hypopharyngeal cancers, unresectable, nonmetastatic disease,
968, 971*t*
Kaposi's sarcoma, 708–710
late effects syndromes
central nervous system, 325–326
gastrointestinal tract, 343
heart, 334–336, 335*t*
kidney, 339–340
liver, 337–338, 337*f*, 338*t*
lung, 329–330, 330*f*–331*f*, 330*t*
skin and soft tissue, 332, 332*t*
medulloblastoma, pediatric patients, 1837–1841
metastatic spinal cord compression, 1981–1982, 1982*t*, 1983*f*
methotrexate/radiation therapy, late effects syndromes on
normal tissue, 325–326, 326*t*, 327*f*
nasopharyngeal cancer, 844–846, 845*f*, 845*t*
pediatric patients, 1913
non-Hodgkin's lymphoma, 1746–1747
non-small cell lung cancer
chemoradiation, 1089–1091, 1089*t*–1090*t*
nonplatinum chemotherapy combinations, 1099
postoperative, 1085
preoperative, 1084
oral cavity tumors, 906
ovarian cancer, 1640–1643
pain management, 2008–2009
pancreatic cancer
prospective trials, 1341–1343
quality of life issues, 1346
penile cancer, 1525
postoperative radiation, head and neck squamous-cell tumors,
813
prostate cancer
intermediate/high-risk cancer, androgen suppression and
radiation therapy, 1491–1495, 1492*t*–1493*t*, 1495*t*
low-risk cancer, external beam radiation and brachytherapy,
1465, 1470, 1474–1475
rectal cancer
neoadjuvant therapy, 1377–1378
postoperative adjuvant therapy, 1375–1377
side effects, 1376
renal cell carcinoma, 1403–1404
retroperitoneal cancer, 1709–1713, 1713*t*
small cell lung carcinoma, 1101
stomach cancer radiation therapy, 1329–1332, 1329*t*–1330*t*
superior sulcus tumor chemoradiation, 1092–1093
surgery and radiation therapy, 48, 48*f*
thymomas, 1115, 1116*t*
thyroid disease, 1070–1071
tracheal tumors, 1121–1122
urethral cancer, male, 1529–1530, 1529*t*
vaginal cancer, 1667–1668
vocal cord carcinomas, 990, 990*t*–992*t*
vulvar cancer, 1696–1697, 1699–1700, 1703–1704, 1704*t*
Communication equipment, high-dose-rate brachytherapy safety,
548

Compensating filter systems, photon external-beam dosimetry,
181–182, 182*f*
Complete response criteria, end point selection, phase III clinical
trials, 358
Complication probability, accelerated repopulation and, 23,
25*f*
Compton effect, basic principles, 147–148, 147*f*
Computational dosimetry, brachytherapy, 439
Computed tomography (CT)
adrenal gland tumors, 1718
bone metastases, 1987, 1993*f*
breast cancer diagnosis and staging, 1193
locally advanced and recurrent disease, 1294–1295, 1295*f*
cervical cancer screening, 1536–1537, 1537*t*
cone-beam computed tomography (CBCT)
gantry-mounted systems, 283, 284*f*
kilovoltage components, 282–283, 283*f*–284*f*
megavoltage components, 282, 283*f*
evolution of, 190
fallopian tube imaging, 1651
hypopharyngeal cancer imaging, 962, 962*f*
image-guided radiation therapy
in-room volumetric systems, 279–281, 280*f*–281*f*
on-rail systems, 280–281, 281*f*
intracranial tumors, 720–722, 722*f*, 723*t*
lung cancer diagnosis, 1080
oncologic imaging, 620–621, 621*f*
prostate cancer imaging, 1450–1451
radiation therapy, 1458–1459, 1462–1463
simulators
components and instrumentation, 155, 156*f*
three-dimensional conformal radiation therapy applications,
220–221, 220*f*–221*f*
spinal cord tumors, 768
stomach cancer diagnosis, 1320
supraglottic carcinoma diagnosis, 979–980, 980*t*
testicular cancer imaging, 1506
three-dimensional conformal radiation therapy, target volume
calculations, 227–230, 228*f*–230*f*
thyroid disease imaging, 1058, 1059*f*
vaginal cancer staging, 1661–1662, 1662*f*
Computer isodose calculations, interstitial brachytherapy, 454–456
Concomitant boost fractionation
accelerated treatment regimens, 100, 312
breast brachytherapy, 502
cervical cancer radiation therapy, 1557–1558
Cone-beam computed tomography (CBCT)
gantry-mounted systems, 283, 284*f*
kilovoltage components, 282–283, 283*f*–284*f*
megavoltage components, 282, 283*f*
oropharyngeal tumors, 951
prostate cancer radiation therapy, 1462–1463
Conference chart rounds
brachytherapy quality assurance, 57
external beam radiation therapy quality assurance, 56–57
Conformal therapy. *See also* Three-dimensional conformal radiation
therapy
data management, 233–234
historical development of, 218–219, 219*t*
overview, 218
quality assurance, 234–236
volume and dose specification, 224–230
dose reporting and prescription, 227
GTV, CTV, and PTV concepts, 227–230, 228*f*–230*f*
tumor/target volume definition, 224–226, 225*f*, 226*t*
Congestive heart failure, Wilms' tumor and, 1857
Conization, cervical cancer screening, 1536
Conjunctival tumors, 793, 793*f*
Connective tissue disease
desmoid (aggressive fibromatosis), 1949–1950, 1950*f*
induratio penis plastica, 1950–1951
keloids and hypertrophic scars, 1952–1954, 1953*f*
Morbus Dupuytren/Morbus Ledderhose, 1951–1952, 1951*t*,
1952*f*, 1953*t*
nonmalignant disease, 1949–1954
radiation effects on, 1934
Continence issues, prostate cancer therapy, 1471–1473
Continuous hyperfractionated accelerated radiation (CHA-RT),
accelerated treatment regimens, 100
Convection-enhanced chemotherapy delivery, intracranial tumor
management, 729

Convolution/superposition dose calculation algorithm
    photon external-beam dosimetry, tissue inhomogeneity
        correction, 170
    three-dimensional conformal radiation therapy, 231
Cordectomy techniques, vocal cord carcinoma, 983
Corneal injury, orbital tumor radiation therapy, 795
Coronary anatomy, vascular brachytherapy, 1960, 1960*f*
Coronary artery disease
    de novo coronary artery stenosis research, 1966–1967
    Hodgkin's lymphoma and, 1735
Corpus Hippocraticum, 2036
Corticosteroids
    bone metastases, 1991–1992
    brain metastases, 1974
    metastatic spinal cord compression, 1981
Cosmetic surgery (cosmesis), breast cancer therapy and, 1264–1268,
    1265*f,* 1266*t*
Cost issues. *See also* Economic analysis
    afterloading brachytherapy, 486
    breast cancer therapy, 1277–1278
    cervical cancer, 1599
    cost-benefit analysis, radiation therapy, 2026–2027
    high-dose-rate brachytherapy, 543
    oropharyngeal radiation therapy, 939*t*
    radiation therapy, 59–61
        activity-based costing *vs.* traditional accounting, 2023–2024,
            2025*f*
Cost utility analysis, radiation therapy, 2023, 2026–2027
Couch top, radiation therapy, 8
Coulomb force, atomic structure, 143
Cranial irradiation. *See also* Intracranial tumors
    acute lymphoblastic leukemia, 1781–1782
    high-risk acute lymphoblastic leukemia, 310
    leukemia therapy, 1785, 1785*f*
    small cell lung carcinoma radiation therapy and, 1102
    somnolence syndrome, 1786
Cranial nerves
    anatomical illustrations, 629–630, 629*t*
    neuropathy, nasopharyngeal cancer therapy, 852–853
    stereotactic radiosurgery tolerance, 382
Craniohypophysis xanthomatoses, 1920
Craniopharyngioma
    diagnosis and management, 744–745
    nonmalignant disease, 1937, 1939*f*
    pediatric patients, 1844–1845
Craniospinal irradiation
    electron-beam therapy, 210
    image-guided radiation therapy, Novalis system, 276–277, 276*f*
    leukemia therapy, 1785–1786
    orthogonal field junction separation, 185
    techniques for, 727
Critical organ tolerance, late effects syndromes on normal tissue, 323
Critical structure delineation, three-dimensional conformal radiation
    therapy, 221, 221*f*
Critical volume model, three-dimensional conformal radiation
    therapy evaluation, 232–233
Cross hairs, radiation therapy, 7
Cryosurgery/cryotherapy
    nonmelanoma skin cancer, 692–693
    prostate cancer therapy
        current techniques, 1456
        outcome assessment, 1466
        sequelae, 1471
Cumulative dose-volume histograms, three-dimensional conformal
    radiation therapy, 231, 232*f*
Cure probability, altered fractionation radiotherapy, limits of, 316,
    316*t*
Curie, Marie and Pierre, radiation oncology and, 3–4
Cushing's disease
    adrenal gland tumors, 1718, 1718*t*
    pituitary tumors, 758–759, 758*f*–759*f,* 1936–1937
    proton/α-particle radiotherapy, 415
    stereotactic radiosurgery, 385–386
Cutaneous lymphomas, 1757–1758, 1757*t*
    T-cell lymphoma
        diagnostic work-up, 1767, 1767*t*
        epidemiology, 1755
        etiology, 1755
        management, 1769–1770
        natural history, 1766–1767, 1767*f*
        pathologic classification, 1768

        prognostic factors, 1768–1769
        radiation therapy, 1769–1774, 1769*t*
        staging systems, 1767–1768, 1768*t*
Cutaneous melanoma, diagnosis and management, 1025
Cyberknife
    characteristics of, 154
    image-guided radiation therapy, 274, 274*f,* 275*t,* 276*f*
    oropharyngeal tumors, 951, 951*f*
Cyclo-oxygenase 2 molecules
    cervical cancer, 1546
    chemoradiation therapy, molecular targeting, 674–676, 674*t,*
        675*f*
    non-small cell lung cancer therapy, 1100
Cyclo-oxygenase-mediated signaling
    chemoradiation therapy, molecular targeting, 674–676, 674*t,* 675*f*
    mechanisms, 120
Cyclotrons, components and instrumentation, 154–155, 155*f*
Cystectomy. *See* Radical cystectomy; Salvage cystectomy
Cystosarcoma phylloides
    pathophysiology, 1197
    in pediatric patients, 1916
Cytokeratin markers, cervical cancer, 1545–1546
Cytokines
    late effects syndromes on normal tissue, central nervous system,
        325
    radiation effects on, 119
    radiation therapy, molecular responses, 82
    radiation therapy and, 78
    receptor tyrosine kinases, 111
    tumor cells, vessel wall movement, 131
Cytoplasmic nanoreceptor kinases, growth control and, 111
Cytoreductive surgery, ovarian cancer, 1636
Cytotoxic agents, modification of radiation response, 35
Cytotoxicity mechanisms, hyperthermia, 640, 641*f*
    pH modification, 645–646, 646*f*

D

Data collection and analyses
    clinical trials, 360
    high-dose-rate brachytherapy, 551–552
Data management, conformal therapy, 233–234
Daughter nuclides, basic properties, 146
DBS repair, molecular recognition of, 116–117
Death by neglect hypothesis, radiation therapy, 78
Decay constant, radioactivity and, 145
Decision trees
    ductal carcinoma in situ management, 1171–1172, 1172*t*
    radiation therapy, 48
Deep lesions, nonmalignant disease radiation, 1935
Degenerative osteoarthritis, radiation therapy, 1946–1947, 1947*f,*
    1947*t*
Delayed toxicity, total body irradiation, 372
Deletion-type chromosome lesions, radiation therapy and,
    mammalian cell survival curves, 90–92, 91*f*
Deliverable dose distributions, intensity-modulated radiation
    therapy, 240–241
Delta rays, basic properties, 148
"Demons" algorithm, adaptive radiation therapy, 291, 292*f*
Demyelination, central nervous system, late effects syndromes on
    normal tissue, 324–325
De novo coronary artery stenosis, clinical trials, 1966–1967
Dentition
    late effects syndromes in, 344
    oral cavity radiation therapy and dental care, 906–907,
        907*f*–908*f*
Deontology, medical ethics and, 2035
Depth dose
    electron-beam therapy
        patient uncertainties and, 194–196, 195*f*–199*f*
        water-based dose distribution, 190–192, 191*f*–192*f,* 191*t*
    photon external-beam dosimetry, 172, 172*f*–173*f,* 172*t*
Dermatofibrosarcoma protuberans
    epidemiology and management, 699
    soft tissue sarcomas, 1818
Dermoid tumors, 770
Desmoid (aggressive fibromatosis), diagnosis and management,
    1949–1950, 1950*f*
Desmoid tumors, retroperitoneal cancer, 1714
Desmoplastic small round-cell tumor (DSCRT), diagnosis and
    management, 1925, 1927
Developing countries, high-dose-rate brachytherapy, 577–578

Diarrhea, gastrointestinal mucositis, 2015–2016
Diet. *See also* Nutritional support, radiation therapy and
    breast cancer risk and, 1180
    gastrointestinal mucositis management and, 2015–2016
    prostate cancer risk and, 1441–1444, 1443*t*
    xerostomia management and, 2013
Differential dose-volume histograms, three-dimensional conformal
        radiation therapy, 231, 231*f*
Differentiated thyroid cancer
    chemotherapy, 1070
    classification, 1059
    external-beam radiation, 1064–1065, 1065*f*
    iodine therapy, 1063–1064, 1064*f*–1065*f*
    prognostic factors, 1061–1062
    surgical management, 1062–1063
    thyroglobulin therapy, 1066
    thyroid hormone therapy, 1065
    thyroid-stimulating hormone therapy, 1065–1066
Diffuse intrinsic brainstem tumors, pediatric patients, 1832
Diffuse large B-cell lymphoma (DLBCL)
    chemotherapy, 1748–1750
    clinical-histopathological correlates, 1744
    combined treatment modalities, 1746–1747, 1749–1751, 1751*f*
    gastric lymphoma, 1755
    head and neck lymphomas, 1756–1757
    pathology and classification, 1740–1741
    prognostic factors, 1743–1744
    radiation therapy, 1745–1748
    stem cell transplantation/chemotherapy, 1749–1750
Diffuse pontine gliomas, radiation imaging, 632–633
Diffusion-limited hypoxia, radiation therapy and, 13
Digitally reconstructed radiography (DRR)
    computed tomography simulators, 155
    evolution of, 218–219
    three-dimensional conformal radiation therapy, verification
        protocols, 224
Digital mammography, breast cancer screening, 1189
Digital tomosynthesis (DTS), image-guided radiation therapy, 283
Dilatation and curettage, cervical cancer screening, 1536
Disease-free survival, end point selection, phase III clinical trials, 358
Distal bile duct carcinoma, 1359
Distal urethra tumors, brachytherapy, 522–524, 523*f*–524*f*
Distribution rules, interstitial brachytherapy, 443
DNA damage
    biological basis for, 76–77
    cervical cancer, 1544
    chemoradiation therapy, 671
        molecular targeting and, 676
    ionizing radiation, 10, 11*f*, 11*t*–12*t*
    radiation-induced, recognition of, 115–116, 116*f*
    repair mechanisms, 116
DNA ploidy index, breast cancer metastases, 1200
Docetaxel, non-small cell lung cancer therapy, 1099
Documentation protocols, radiation therapy effects, 58
Door interlock systems, high-dose-rate brachytherapy, emergency
        procedures, 547
Dose-based objective functions, intensity-modulated radiation
        therapy, 247–248
Dose calculation methods. *See also* Dosimetry methods
    brachytherapy
        anisotropy factor, 436–437
        interstitial brachytherapy, 443–444
        isotropic point source, 435–438, 435*f*
        Sievert integral model, 437–438, 437*f*–438*f*
    breast cancer radiation therapy, 1246, 1248
        postmastectomy radiation, 1313–1314
    cervical cancer radiation therapy, 1566
    cholangiocarcinoma radiation therapy, 1359–1360
    electron-beam therapy
        algorithms for, 199–200, 201*f*
        standards for, 198–199
    esophageal cancer radiation therapy, 1141–1142
    glioblastoma multiforme, 731–732
    hepatocellular carcinoma radiation therapy, 1353, 1353*t*
    high-dose-rate brachytherapy, consistency quality and safety, 550
    interstitial brachytherapy, 449, 451–454
    intracavitary brachytherapy, 458–464
        point A dose and milligram-hours, 458–460, 459*f*
        prescription and reporting systems, 461–462, 463*t*–464*t*
        volumetric specification, 460–461, 461*f*
    intraoperative radiotherapy, 397

late effects syndromes in normal tissue and, 321–322, 322*f*
nasopharyngeal cancer radiation therapy, 831–832, 833*t*
nonmalignant disease radiation, 1934, 1934*t*
oral cavity radiation therapy, 903–904
oropharyngeal tumor radiation therapy, 935, 951
oropharyngeal tumors, 951
pancreatic radiation therapy, 1338–1341, 1339*f*–1340*f*
pediatric patients' radiation therapy, 1423
    astrocytomas, 1828
    Wilms' tumor, 1853–1854
photon external-beam dosimetry, 166–168
pituitary tumor radiation therapy, 761, 761*t*
prostate cancer radiation therapy, 1461
    brachytherapy techniques, 1464–1465
small cell lung carcinoma radiation therapy, 1102
soft tissue sarcoma radiation therapy, 1816–1817
solitary plasmacytoma radiation therapy, 1797–1798, 1797*f*
spine/spinal cord tumors, 774–775
three-dimensional conformal radiation therapy, 221–222
    algorithms for, 231
total-body irradiation, 366
Dose distribution techniques
    high-dose-rate brachytherapy, 555–556, 556*f*
    water-based dose distribution, electron-beam therapy, 190–193
        depth dose, 190–192, 191*f*–192*f*, 191*t*
        isodose plots, 193–194, 194*f*
        off-axis dose, 192–193, 193*f*
Dose escalation
    glioblastoma multiforme radiation therapy, 731–732
    nasopharyngeal cancer radiation therapy, 836–837, 840, 841*f*,
        841*t*
    non-small cell lung cancer radiation therapy, 1088–1089
    prostate cancer radiation therapy, 1466–1467
        intermediate/high-risk cancer, 1489–1491
Dose fractionation
    brain metastases, palliative radiation therapy, 1976*t*
    cell killing randomness and, 90, 90*f*
    chemoradiation therapy, head and neck squamous-cell tumors,
        815–816, 815*t*
    high-dose-rate brachytherapy, cervical cancer, 1565–1566
    hypoxia and, 90
    ioffect formulae, time-dose effects, 97–99, 98*f*
    mammalian cell survival curves, 90–92
    maxillary sinus radiation therapy, 865*t*, 868
    nasal cavity and ethmoid sinus radiation therapy, 865*t*, 866
    pattern modification, 99–103
    pediatric patients' radiation therapy, 1423
    tumor responses, 95, 95*f*
Dose heterogeneity, dose-volume histograms, 102, 103*f*
Dose homogeneity, total body irradiation, 370
Dose in free space, defined, 158
Dose-limiting issues, pancreatic radiation therapy, 1338
Dose painting technology, radiation oncology, 68
Dose perturbation factors (DPFs), photon external-beam dosimetry,
        bone interfaces, 173
Dose prescription
    fractionated stereotactic radio therapy, pituitary tumor
        management, 762
    radiation therapy, determination of, 6
Dose profiles, basic properties, 162–163, 164*f*
Dose rate
    cervical cancer brachytherapy and, 1561–1562
    clinical relevance, 29–30
    radiation therapy, 28–30, 28*f*–29*f*
    total body irradiation, 370
Dose reduction to normal tissue, high-dose-rate brachytherapy,
        542
Dose reporting/prescription, three-dimensional conformal radiation
        therapy, specifications, 227
Dose-specification criteria, interstitial brachytherapy, 443
Dose-time factors
    anal cancer radiation therapy, 1392–1393, 1393*f*
    radiation therapy, 22–28
        accelerated repopulation, 23, 24*f*–25*f*
        altered fractionation, 22–23, 23*f*, 23*t*
        isoeffect graphs, 24–25, 26*f*
        linear-quadratic equation, 26–28, 26*f*–27*f*, 27*t*
        nominal standard dose, 25–26
Dose-volume-based objective functions, intensity-modulated
        radiation therapy, 248–249, 248*f*–249*f*
Dose volume constraint, lung cancer radiation therapy, 1097

Dose-volume histograms (DVHs)
   adaptive radiation therapy, 292
   high-dose-rate brachytherapy, 555–556, 555f
   intensity-modulated radiation therapy, 248–249, 249f
   interstitial brachytherapy, 453–454, 453f
   prostate cancer radiation therapy, 1461f–1462f
   radiation therapy, 19–20
   stomach cancer radiation therapy, 1328–1329, 1329f
   three-dimensional conformal radiation therapy, 231–232,
        231f–232f
   tumor control probability and, 102, 102f
Dose-volume statistics, three-dimensional conformal radiation
        therapy, 231–232, 232f
Dosimetry methods
   absorbed dose calculation, 159–160
   brachytherapy, 432–435
      activity-exposure rate relationships, 434
      air-kerma strength, 433–435
      milligram-hours and integrated reference air-kerma, 435
      modern quantitative techniques, 438–440
      quantity activity measurement, 434
      source output quantities, 434–435
   breast cancer radiation therapy, postmastectomy radiation,
        1313–1314
   high-dose-rate brachytherapy, 543–546
      linear quadratic model, 543–545, 545f
      low-dose-rate conversion to, 545–546
      quality assurance and safety, 548–552, 551f
      treatment planning and, 552–556
   intensity-modulated radiation therapy, verification, 253–255
   isodose curves, 162, 163f
   oropharyngeal radiation therapy, intensity-modulated
        techniques, 948–949, 948f–949f
   output factor, 162, 162f
   percentage depth dose, 160–161, 160f
   photodynamic therapy, 600
   prostate cancer brachytherapy, 1464–1465
   scatter-air/scatter-maximum ratios, 161–162
   stereotactic body radiation therapy, 390–391
   thermal dosimetry, interstitial hyperthermia, 653
   tissue-air ratio, 161, 161f
   tissue-phantom/tissue-maximum ratios, 161, 161f
   total body irradiation, 368–369
   wedge filter, 163, 164f
Drug-eluting stents (DES)
   in-stent restenosis, 1965–1966
      vascular brachytherapy following, 1966
   vascular brachytherapy, overview, 1959
Drug-radiation interaction, combined chemoradiation therapy,
        670–672, 670f
Ductal adenocarcinoma, prostate cancer, 1455
Ductal carcinoma in situ (breast), 1164–1172
   clinical presentation and epidemiology, 1184
   decision tree for, 1171–1172
   mammography, 1164, 1165f
   natural history, 1167
   pathology and biology, 1164–1167, 1166f–1167f
   prognostic factors, 1167–1168, 1168f
   treatment options, 1167–1171, 1168f–1169f, 1169t–1171t
Dwell-weight optimization, interstitial brachytherapy, 454–456
Dynamic multileaf collimator (DMLC), image-guided radiation
        therapy
   beam tracking, 288–289
   respiratory motion management, 288
Dysgerminoma
   management of, 1645
   pediatric patients, 1924–1925
Dysphagia
   late effects syndromes in esophagus and, 343–344
   oropharyngeal radiation therapy, 941f–942f, 942–943

E
Ear
   anatomy, 800, 801f–802f
   skin tumors, radiation therapy, 695
   toxicity effects on, nasopharyngeal cancer therapy, 853
   tumors
      diagnostic workup and classification, 800–801, 801t, 802f
      epidemiology, 800
      external auditory canal, 801, 805f
      external ear, 800, 803, 803t
      management, 801–803, 804t
      middle ear and temporal bone, 803, 803f, 804t
      prognostic factors, 801
      radiation therapy, 803–804
      staging, 801, 803, 803t
Early-responding tissues, radiation therapy, 93t
Eastern Europe, radiation therapy in, 607f, 608
Economic analysis
   credentialing protocols, 2045–2046
   radiation oncology, 2043–2049
   radiation therapy, 2023–2024, 2025f
Economic profiling, radiation oncology and, 2045
Edema, cerebral, radiation-induced, late effects syndromes on
        normal tissue, 326, 326t, 327f
Edge restenosis, vascular brachytherapy, 1968–1969
Effective dose calculation, radiation therapy, multifraction survival
        curves, 94, 94f
Effective uniform dose (EUD), 103, 103f
Effective volume method, three-dimensional conformal radiation
        therapy evaluation, 232–233
Efficacy/toxicity profile, chemical modifiers of radiation therapy,
        611, 674
Elderly patients
   bladder cancer radiation therapy, 1424
   breast cancer metastatic risk, 1223–1224, 1224f, 1225t
   cervical cancer, 1572
   cervical cancer therapy in, 1752
   Hodgkin's lymphoma, 1732
Elective nodal irradiation
   lung cancer therapy, 1095, 1096f
   treatment planning and, 633–634, 634f
Electromagnetic heating, hyperthermia, 650, 650f–651f
Electromagnetic radiation, basic principles, 143–144
Electrometer, radiation exposure measurement, 157
Electron affinity, oxygen effect and, 88
Electron arc therapy, specialized techniques, 213–215, 214f–215f
Electron-beam radiation therapy (EBRT)
   bladder tumors, 1426–1427, 1427f–1429f
   brachytherapy with, interstitial brain implants, 489–490
   dose algorithms, 199–200, 201f
   dose prescription guidelines, 196–197
   future applications, 215
   intraoperative radiotherapy and, 397–404
   monitor unit calculations, 197–198, 199f
   overview, 190
   patient heterogeneity, dosage calculations, 194–196, 195f–199f
   specialized electron techniques, 209–215
      craniospinal irradiation, 210
      electron arc therapy, 213–215, 214f–215f
      intracavitary irradiation, 209–210, 209f–210f
      total-limb irradiation, 211–212, 212f
      total-scalp irradiation, 210–211, 211f
      total-skin irradiation, 212–213, 213f
   standard patient dose calculations, 198–199
   treatment planning principles, tools, and methods, 200–209, 201f
      bolus specifications, 202–204, 203f–205f
      electron collimation design, 201–202
      energy selection criteria, 200–201, 201f
      field abutment, 206, 206f–208f
      internal collimation, 204–205, 206f
      mixed-beam therapy, 206, 208f, 209
      multileaf collimation, 202
      skin collimation, 202, 202f
   treatment units, 150
   water-based dose distribution, 190–193
      depth dose, 190–192, 191f–192f, 191t
      isodose plots, 193–194, 194f
      off-axis dose, 192–193, 193f
Electron collimation, electron-beam therapy, 201–202
Electron conformal therapy, bolus design, 204, 205f
Electronic equilibrium, radiation exposure, 156–157
Electronic portal imaging devices (EPID)
   image-guided radiation therapy, 271, 272f, 273–274
   prostate cancer radiation therapy, 1462–1463
Electronic record-keeping and billing
   economic analysis, 2043, 2044t
   paperless electronic records, 952, 952f
   radiation oncology ethics and, 2039
Electrons, basic principles, 148
Electron-scattering foil, linear accelerator, 152
Electron volt (eV), defined, 142

Electrostatic (coulomb) force, basic principles, 145
Elekta Synergy Systems, image-guided radiation therapy, 279, 279*f*, 283, 284*f*
Elements, atomic structure, 142–143
Ellis technique, photon external-beam dosimetry, compensating filter systems, 181–182, 182*f*
Embryonal carcinoma
    classification, 1504*t*, 1505
    pediatric patients, 1836–1842
        medulloblastoma, 1836–1841, 1836*f*
Emergency procedures, high-dose-rate brachytherapy, 547
Empirical research methodology, radiation oncology, 10–12
Encapsulation technology
    brachytherapy, 424–426
    high-dose-rate brachytherapy, 543
    hyperthermia and, 648–649, 649*f*
Endobronchial irradiation, high-dose-rate brachytherapy, 567–569, 568*t*
Endodermal sinus tumor
    classification, 1504*t*, 1505
    ovarian cancer, 1633
    vaginal cancer, 1674–1675
End of exhale (EOE) phase, image-guided radiation therapy, respiratory motion management, 288
Endometrial cancer
    anatomy, 1610
    carcinomas, 1611–1612
    chemotherapy, 1619, 1625
    clinical presentation and diagnostic work-up, 1610
    diagnostic work-up, 1610–1611
    endometrial stromal sarcomas, classification, 1613
    epidemiology and risk factors, 1610
    high-dose-rate brachytherapy, 565–567, 566*t*–567*t*
    hyperplasia, 1611
    low-dose-rate brachytherapy, 516–517, 516*f*
    palliative therapy, 1623
    pathologic classification, 1611–1613, 1612*f*, 1612*t*
    prognostic factors, 1614
    radiation therapy, 1615–1624, 1616*t*–1618*t*
    recurrent disease, 1622–1623
    staging protocols, 1613–1614, 1613*t*–1614*t*
    surgical management, 1614–1615, 1622–1623
    uterine papillary serous and clear cell carcinoma, 1623–1624
    uterine sarcoma, 1624–1625
Endometroid tumors
    cervical cancer, 1540–1541
    classification, 1611–1612, 1612*t*
    prostate cancer, 1455
Endorectal magnetic resonance imaging, prostate cancer, 1451, 1452*f*
Endoscopic ultrasonography
    laryngeal cancers, 979
    oncologic imaging, 625, 625*t*
    rectal cancer imaging, 1373
    stomach cancer diagnosis, 1319–1320
Endothelial precursor cells (EPCs), tumor molecular pathophysiology, 126–127
Endovascular system
    brachytherapy, 532
        β-radiation in-stent coronary artery restenosis, 1964–1965, 1965*t*–1966*t*
        clinical trials, 1964–1967
        coronary anatomy, 1960, 1960*f*
        coronary in-stent restenosis, Betacath system, 1962–1964, 1963*f*
        de novo coronary artery restenosis, 1966–1967
        drug-eluting stents, coronary in-stent restenosis, 1965–1966
        edge restenosis, 1968–1969
        future research, 1969–1970
        γ-radiation in-stent coronary artery restenosis, 1964, 1965*t*
        historical perspective, 1959–1960
        in-stent restenosis following DES, 1966
        overview, 1959
        percutaneous coronary intervention, 1960–1961, 1961*f*, 1962*t*
        peripheral vascular brachytherapy trials, 1967–1968, 1968*t*
        physics and devices, 1962
        radioactive stents, 1967
        saphenous vein graft in-stent restenosis, 1966
        subacute thrombosis, 1969
        terminology, 1969

external-beam irradiation studies, 1961–1962
End point selection, phase III clinical trials, 358
Energy selection criteria
    electron-beam therapy, 200–201
    soft tissue sarcoma radiation therapy, 1816–1817
Environmental factors
    non-Hodgkin's lymphoma, 1739–1740
    ovarian cancer risk and, 1630–1631
Ep-CAM, radioimmunotherapy with, 590
Ependymoma
    diagnosis and management, 740
    pediatric patients, 1832–1834, 1833*f*
Epidermal growth factor receptors (EGFRs)
    chemoradiation therapy, molecular targeting, 674–676, 674*t*, 675*f*
    growth control and, 110
    non-small cell lung cancer therapy, 1099
    pancreatic cancer targeting, 1346
    signaling mechanisms, 119
    solid tumors, radioimmunoglobulin therapy, 589–590
Epidermoid tumors, 770
    vulvar cancer, 1693–1694
Episcleral plaque therapy, eye tumors, 490–493, 491*f*–492*f*
Episiotomy, vaginal cancer in, 1676
Epistaxis, nasopharyngeal cancer therapy, 853
Epithelial tumors
    ovarian cancer
        chemotherapy, 1636–1637
        consolidative therapy, 1640–1643
        management of, 1635–1638
        radiation therapy, 1637–1643, 1638*t*
        risk factors, 1630*t*
    vaginal intraepithelial neoplasia, 1658–1661
Epratuzumab, leukemia and lymphoma therapy, 589
Epstein-Barr virus (EBV)
    cervical cancer, 1546
    nasopharyngeal cancer, 1913, 1914*t*
Equilibrium conditions, basic properties, 146
Equivalent square table calculations, photon external-beam dosimetry, 167
Equivalent uniform dose (EUD), three-dimensional conformal radiation therapy evaluation, 233
Erectile dysfunction
    prostate cancer brachytherapy, 1474
    radiation-induced injury and, 2017
Error parameters
    error reduction, 576–577, 576*t*–577*t*
    high-dose-rate brachytherapy, 543
    phase III clinical trials, sample size criteria, 359, 360*t*–361*t*
Erythroplakia, oral cavity, 896, 896*f*
Erythroplasia of Queyrat, penile tumors, 1522
Esophageal cancer
    anatomy, 1131, 1132*f*
    brachytherapy, 1142, 1148, 1149*f*, 1150*t*
    chemotherapy, 1145
    clinical presentation, 1134
    combined chemoradiation therapy, 681*t*, 683–684, 1138–1139
        postoperative regimen, 1145–1146, 1146*t*
        radiation *vs.*, 1146–1147
        surgery and, 1147, 1147*f*
    diagnostic work-up, 1134–1136, 1136*f*
    epidemiology and risk factors, 1131–1133, 1133*f*
    failure patterns, 1134, 1135*t*–1136*t*
    future research issues, 1150–1151
    high-dose-rate brachytherapy, 569–570, 570*t*
    hyperthermia therapy, 663
    intraoperative radiotherapy and, 400
    late effects syndromes on normal tissue in, 342–344
    low-dose-rate brachytherapy, 502–504, 503*f*–505*f*
    lymphatic drainage, 1131, 1132*f*
    management, 1137–1139, 1138*f*
        palliative treatment, 1147
    natural history and metastases, 1133–1134, 1134*f*–1135*f*, 1134*t*
    pathologic classification, 1136–1137, 1137*t*
    pediatric patients, 1916
    photodynamic therapy, 602
    positron emission tomography, 624
    prognostic factors, 1137
    radiation therapy, 1139–1143, 1140*f*–1141*f*, 1143*t*
        chemoradiation *vs.*, 1146–1147
        iridium techniques, 1148, 1149*f*

Esophageal cancer (*contd.*)
  postoperative regimen, 1143–1144
  preoperative regimen, 1143–1144, 1144*t*
  sequelae, 1148, 1150
 staging systems, 1136, 1136*t*
 surgical management, 1138, 1142, 1143*t*, 1145–1146, 1146*t*
Esthesioneuroblastoma (ENB), 1012–1018
 diagnostic work-up and staging, 1013, 1014*f*, 1014*t*
 elective neck treatment, 1015
 epidemiology, 858–859, 1013
 management of, 1014–1015
 natural history, 859, 1013, 1013*f*
 pathologic features and prognostic factors, 1013–1014
 pediatric patients, 1914
 radiation therapy, 1016–1018, 1016*f*, 1017*t*
 treatment results, 869, 871*t*
Estrogen receptors
 breast cancer metastases, 1199
 cervical cancer, 1546
Etanidazole, chemical modifiers of radiation therapy, 613
Ethics in medicine
 clinical trials, 2040
 conceptual approaches, 2035
 formal oaths and codes of ethics, 2036–2038, 2036*f*–2037*f*
 medical errors and, 2040–2041
 principles, 2035–2036
 radiation oncology, 2038–2039
Ethmoid sinuses
 anatomy, 858
 clinical presentation, 860–861
 disease management, 862
 natural history, 859
 radiation therapy, 864–866, 865*f*
 treatment results, 869, 870*t*
Evidence-based medicine research
 quality of medical care and, 2032
 radiation therapy, 2027–2028, 2027*t*–2028*t*
Ewing's sarcoma
 desmoplastic small round-cell tumor (DSCRT), 1927
 pediatric patients
  chemotherapy, 1886–1889
  clinical presentation, 1886
  diagnostic work-up, 1886
  epidemiology, 1886
  future research issues, 1890
  metastases, 1889
  metastatic spinal cord compression, 1984
  outcome assessment, 1889
  prognostic factors, 1886, 1887*t*
  radiation therapy, 1887–1890, 1888*t*
  stem cell rescue, 1889–1890
Exercise
 breast cancer risk and, 1180
 fatigue management and, 2011–2012
Exposure calibration factor, radiation exposure measurement, 157
Extended pelvic lymph node dissection, prostate cancer, 1486–1487
Extended surgical staging (ESS), endometrial cancer, 1611,
  1614–1618, 1618*t*
External beam conformal radiation
 bladder cancer, 1421–1423, 1422*t*, 1427–1429, 1427*f*–1429*f*
 breast cancer therapy, 1262–1263, 1263*f*
External beam radiation therapy (EBRT)
 bladder cancer, 1426*f*–1429*f*, 1427–1429
  bladder-preservation therapy, 1430–1435
 bone metastases, 1992–1997
 cervical cancer, 514–515, 515*t*, 1553–1556, 1554*f*–1555*f*,
  1573–1574, 1574*t*
  sequelae, 1584–1588, 1585*f*–1586*f*
 cholangiocarcinoma, 1359–1360
 coronary balloon angioplasty and, 1961–1962
 differentiated thyroid cancer, 1064–1065, 1065*f*
 dose painting technology, 68
 endometrial cancer, 1615–1621
 high-dose-rate brachytherapy and, 560–562, 561*t*
  breast cancer, 575–576, 575*t*
  cervical carcinoma, 562–564, 563*t*–565*t*
  endobronchial irradiation, 567–569, 568*t*
  endometrial cancer, 566–567, 566*t*
  esophageal cancer, 569–570, 570*t*
  prostate cancer, 570–572, 571*t*–572*t*
 historical background, 3–4

intraoperative radiation/intraoperative electron irradiation
  therapy (IORT/IOERT) and, 397–398
multiple myeloma, 1796
nasal vestibule disease, 863–864, 863*f*
nasopharyngeal cancer, 836–837, 840, 841*f*, 841*t*
oropharyngeal tumors, 950–951
osteosarcoma, 1803–1804, 1804*t*
pancreatic cancer, 1339–1340, 1339*f*
  dose increases, 1344–1345
  locally advanced carcinoma, 1343
  prospective trials, 1341–1346, 1344*t*
pediatric patients, thyroid disease, 1923–1924
penile cancer, 1525–1526, 1526*f*–1527*f*, 1528, 1528*t*–1529*t*
pituitary tumor management, 756, 757*f*, 757*t*
prostate cancer
  intermediate/high-risk cancer
   brachytherapy boost, 1490–1491
   dose escalation, 1489–1490
  low-risk cancer
   brachytherapy combined with, 1465, 1470, 1474–1475
   current trends, 1456–1457
   dose escalation, 1466
   outcome assessment, 1466
   potency preservation, 1472, 1473*t*
   randomized control trials, 1466–1468, 1467*f*
   sequelae, 1471
   surgery *vs.*, 1468–1469
   techniques, 1457, 1458*f*
 quality assurance, 55–57
 retinoblastoma, 789–790
 retroperitoneal cancer, 1712, 1714*t*
 stomach cancer, 1329–1332, 1329*t*–1330*t*
 thyroid disease, pediatric patients, 1923–1924
 treatment planning, 6–7
 vaginal cancer, 1665–1666, 1668–1669, 1670*f*
 volume determination, 6–
External practice audit, quality assurance and, 58
External volume index, interstitial brachytherapy, 453–454
Extracapsular extension (ECE)
 breast cancer metastases, 1228
 prostate cancer recurrence, 1497–1498
Extracellular matrix (ECM)
 integrin-mediated signaling, 120–121, 120*f*
 tumor invasion and metastasis, 113–114
Extracranial meningiomas, diagnosis and management, 1024
Extradural tumors, spinal cord, 770
Extramedullary plasmacytomas, diagnosis and management,
  1018–1020
Extranodal non-Hodgkin's lymphoma
 central nervous system, 1758–1759
 cutaneous lymphomas, 1757–1758, 1757*t*
 gastrointestinal, 1754–1756
 head and neck, 1756–1757
 orbital lymphomas, 1758
 pathology and classification, 1742, 1742*t*
Extrapelvic metastases, anal cancer, 1384–1385, 1388, 1390
Extravascular compartment, solid tumor construction, 131–132
Extravasive intraductal carcinoma (breast), incidence and
  epidemiology, 1216–1217, 1216*t*
Extravesical lymph node-negative tumors, bladder cancer, 1418
Extremity sarcomas
 intraoperative radiotherapy, 401–402
 rhabdomyosarcoma, pediatric patients, 1877
Eye and orbit
 anatomy, 778, 779*f*
 benign ocular disease, 778–781
  capillary hemangiomas, 779
  choroidal hemangiomas, 779, 781*f*
  Graves' ophthalmopathy, 781
  prelymphoma, lymphoid hyperplasia and lymphoma,
   780–781
  pterygium, 778–779, 1941–1942, 1942*f*
 brachytherapy targeting, 490–493, 491*f*–493*f*
 lacrimal gland tumors, 794, 796, 796*f*
 late effects syndromes on normal tissue, 328
 malignant ocular disease, 781
  intraocular lymphomas, 791
  optic glioma, 791–792
  posterior uvea carcinoma, 781–782
  posterior uvea melanoma, 782–787, 783*t*–784*t*, 785*f*–786*f*
  retinal tumors, 787–791

nasal cavity and paranasal sinus therapy and, 871–872
nonmalignant disease, radiation therapy, 1941–1946
orbital and ocular tumor categories, 780*t*
orbital tumors, 792–794
    conjunctival tumors, 793, 793*f*
    eyelid basal and squamous cell carcinomas, 792–793
    lymphoma, 794, 795*f*
    metastatic tumors, 794
    rhabdomyosarcoma, 793–794
    sebaceous carcinoma, 793
radiation therapy sequelae, 794–796
    bony orbit, 796
    cornea, 795
    hypothalamus and pituitary dysfunction, 796
    lacrimal gland, 796
    lens, 795–796
    retina and choroid, 796
    skin and adnexa, 794
total body irradiation effects, 373
Eyelid tumors
    basal and squamous cell carcinomas, 792–793
    radiation therapy, 695

F
Facility design
    high-dose-rate brachytherapy, 547–548
    intensity-modulated radiation therapy, 257
Failure patterns in therapy, economic analysis of, 2043–2049
Fallopian tubes, tumors of
    anatomy, 1650
    chemotherapy, 1653–1654
    clinical presentation, 1650–1651
    diagnostic work-up, 1651, 1652*t*
    epidemiology, 1650
    future research issues, 1655
    molecular genetics, 1653
    natural history, 1650
    pathologic classification, 1652–1653
    prognostic factors, 1653, 1654*t*
    radiation therapy, 1654–1655
    second-look laparatomy, 1655
    staging, 1651–1652, 1652*t*
    surgical management, 1653
    treatment algorithm, 1655*t*
    treatment sequelae, 1655
False-positive rate, clinical trials, interim analyses, 360–361
False vocal cord lesions. *See also* Vocal cord carcinomas
    characteristics of, 978
Familial dysplastic nevi syndrome, 692
Family history
    breast cancer risk and, 1178–1179
        breast-conserving surgery in patients with, 1234–1237,
            1235*t*, 1236*f*–1237*f*
    colorectal cancer risk and, 1366–1367
    hereditary nonpolyposis colorectal cancer, 1366–1367
    ovarian cancer risk and, 1629–1631, 1630*f*
    prostate cancer risk and, 1444
Fast neutron radiotherapy, 408–412, 408*t*
    head and neck squamous-cell tumors, 410
    non-small-cell lung cancer, 410, 410*f*
    prostate cancer, 410–411, 411*f*
    salivary gland tumors, 408–410, 409*f*, 409*t*
    sarcomas, 411–412
Fatigue in cancer patients, supportive care for, 2011–2012
Fauchal arch tumors, brachytherapy, 498–499, 500*f*
Federal regulations, radiation oncology practices, 2047
Female gonadal function, late effects syndromes on normal tissue in,
    347
Fetal dose guidelines, photon external-beam dosimetry, 187, 188*t*
Few electron-leaf collimators (FELC), MERT therapy and, 215
f-factor, absorbed dose measurement, 158, 158*f*
Fibrous valvular endocardial thickening, as radiotherapy effect, 336
Field settings
    bladder cancer radiation therapy, 1427–1429, 1427*f*–1429*f*
    cervical cancer radiation therapy, 1553–1555, 1554*f*–1555*f*
    electron beam therapy, 206, 206*f*–208*f*
        water-based dose distribution, 191, 192*f*
    hepatocellular carcinoma radiation therapy, 1354
    Hodgkin's lymphoma radiation therapy, 1727–1730, 1729*f*
        pediatric patients, 1899, 1899*t*
    maxillary sinus radiation therapy, 867–868

nasal cavity and ethmoid sinus radiation therapy, 864–866
neuroblastoma, pediatric patients, 1867–1868, 1868*f*
non-Hodgkin's lymphoma radiation therapy, 1747–1748
photon external-beam dosimetry, separation techniques,
    184–185, 184*f*–187*f*
radiation therapy, 7
    stomach cancer, 1324–1329, 1324*t*–1326*t*, 1326*f*–1329*f*
skin cancer radiation therapy, 694
three-dimensional conformal radiation therapy, 221, 222*f*
total body irradiation, 367–368, 368*f*
Field shaping, photon external-beam dosimetry, 178–181
File transfer protocol (FTP), conformal therapy data, 233–234
Film dosimetry, absorbed dose calculation, 159
Final analyses, clinical trials, 360–361
Fine-needle aspiration biopsy
    breast cancer diagnosis, 1194
    thyroid disease, 1059
Fixed field settings
    intensity-modulated radiation therapy, 250–251, 250*f*
    photon external-beam dosimetry, monitor and dose unit
        calculations, 166–168
Fixed-gantry intensity-modulated fields
    intensity-modulated radiation therapy (IMRT), 255–256
    tomotherapy *vs.*, 256–257
Fletcher-Suit system
    brachytherapy, cervical carcinoma, 510–512, 511*f*–512*f*,
        1558–1566, 1560*f*
    interstitial brachytherapy, 450*t*
    intracavitary brachytherapy, 457–460, 457*f*–458*f*
Flow cytometry studies, cervical cancer, 1544
Fluorescence, thermoluminescence dosimetry, 159
18-Fluorodeoxyglucose-positron emission tomography ([18]FDG-PET)
    breast cancer diagnosis and staging, 1193
    cervical cancer screening, 1538, 1538*f*
    image-guided radiation therapy, 264–265, 264*f*–265*f*
Fluorodeoxyglucose-positron emission tomography (FDG-PET),
    hypopharyngeal cancer imaging, 962
5-Fluorouracil
    cervical cancer therapy, 1591–1592
    colon cancer therapy, 1368–1370, 1369*t*–1370*t*, 1370*f*
    pancreatic cancer, 1343–1344
    radiation combined with, head and neck squamous-cell tumors,
        809
FMSIO-PET imaging, tumor pathophysiology, prognostic
    implications, 136
Foam molds, photon external-beam dosimetry, patient positioning
    and immobilization, 183–184, 183*f*
FOCAL (fusion of computed tomography and linear accelerator)
    system, image-guided radiation therapy, in-room
    volumetric systems, 279, 280*f*
Focused biology, radiation oncology and, 16*f*
Follicular lymphoma
    clinical-histopathological correlates, 1744
    pathology and classification, 1741
    radiation therapy, 1751–1753
Follicular thyroid cancers
    classification, 1061
    pediatric patients, 1922–1924, 1923*t*
Forbidden energy bands, thermoluminescence dosimetry, 159
Four-dimensional imaging, image-guided radiation therapy,
    285–288, 286*f*–287*f*
Fractionated external-beam radiation therapy/surgery, pituitary
    tumors, 756, 757*t*
Fractionated radiation therapy. *See also* Accelerated fractionation;
    Altered fractionation; Hyperfractionation
    bone metastases, 1992–1997, 1994*t*–1995*t*
    breast cancer, 1246, 1248
    chemotherapy concurrent with, clinical trials, 315–316
    high-dose-rate brachytherapy, 560–562, 561*t*
        cervical cancer, 1564*t*
    intensity-modulated radiation therapy, 245–246
        critical regime issues, 316
    nasopharyngeal cancer, 831–832, 833*t*
    non-small cell lung cancer, 1088–1089, 1088*t*
    oral cavity tumors, 903–904
    oropharyngeal tumors, 935, 951
    pituitary tumors, 761
    radiosensitivity and, 15
    small cell lung carcinoma, 1101–1102
    total-body irradiation, 366–367
    vocal cord carcinoma, 984

Fractionated stereotactic radio therapy (FSRT)
craniopharyngiomas, 1937
defined, 378
pituitary tumors, 761–762
Fractionated steriotactic radiation therapy (FSRT)
glioblastoma multiforme radiation therapy dose escalation, 731
pituitary tumor management, 754, 755t
Fracture risk, bone metastases, 1989–1991, 1990t, 1993–1995, 1995t
Free-air ionization chamber
brachytherapy dosimetry, 433, 433f
radiation exposure measurement, 157
Free-standing radiation oncology centers, 2046
Fricke dosimetry, absorbed dose measurements, 157–158
Frontal sinus, anatomy, 858
Functional subunits (FSUs)
normal tissue effects, radiation therapy, 19–20
radiation therapy, 80–82, 81f
Function distribution and tissue organization, late effects syndromes on normal tissue, 320–321, 321f
Functioning pituitary tumors, 756

G
G1 phase, radiation damage and, 117, 118f
G2 phase, radiation damage and, 118
Gadd45 gene, cervical cancer, 1545
Gallbladder, adenocarcinoma, 1359–1360
γ-radiation, in-stent restenosis, 1964, 1965t
Gamma knife
acusticus neurinoma, 1938–1939
fast neutron radiotherapy with, salivary gland tumors, 409–410
hemangiomas in children, 1925
instrumentation, 150, 150f
stereotactic radiosurgery, 379–380
Gamma rays, basic properties, 144–145, 144t
Ganglioma, pediatric patients, 1835
paraganglioma, 1922
Ganglioneuroblastoma, pediatric patients, 1860–1861
Ganglioneuroma, pediatric patients, 1860–1861
Ganglion nodosum chemodectomas, 998, 1003t
Gantry-mounted systems
cone-beam computed tomography (CBCT), 283, 284f
planar imaging systems, 278–279, 278f–279f
Gastric artery, late effects syndromes in, 341–342, 342f
Gastric carcinoma
staging system, 1320, 1321t
surgical managment of, 1329–1332, 1329t–1330t
Gastrointestinal cancer
image-guided radiation therapy, Real-time Tumor Tracking, 277
intensity-modulated radiation therapy, 259
mucositic prevention, 2014–2016, 2015t
pediatric patients, 1916
photodynamic therapy, 602
stomach
anatomy, 1318
chemotherapy, 1333
clinical presentation, 1319
diagnostic work-up, 1319–1320
epidemiology, 1318
failure patterns for surgical resection, 1323, 1323t
future research issues, 1333–1334
metastatic patterns, 1318–1319, 1319f
pathology, 1320–1321
prognostic factors, 1321–1322, 1321t
radiation therapy, 1323–1329
indications for, 1323
palliative therapy, 1332
sequelae, 1332–1333, 1332t
techniques, 1323–1329, 1324t–1326t, 1326f–1329f
staging, 1320, 1320t–1321t
surgical management, 1322–1323, 1323t
results, 1329–1332, 1329t–1330t
Gastrointestinal tract, late effects syndromes in, 340–344, 342f–343f
Gemcitabine
non-small cell lung cancer therapy, 1099
pancreatic cancer therapy, 1345–1346
Gene expression. See also Molecular genetics
non-Hodgkin's lymphoma, 1743
radiation damage and, 118–119
salivary gland tumors, 888
Gene therapy

glioblastoma multiforme, 734–735
hyperthermia and, 649, 649f
Genetically significant dose data, photon external-beam dosimetry, 187
Genetic screening
breast cancer, 1181–1183, 1181t–1182t, 1201, 1201f
ovarian cancer risk and, 1630, 1630t
Geneva Declaration, 2037–2038
Genitourinary tract
photodynamic therapy, 602
radiation-induced injury, 2017
Genomics
mutagenesis and instability in, 121
radiation oncology, 67–68, 68f
Geographic overdosage, radiation therapy, 102–103
Geographic underdosage, intensity-modulated radiation therapy, 101–102, 102f
Germ-cell tumors. See also Germinoma; specific tumors, e.g. Dysgerminoma
extragonadal, retroperitoneal cancer, 1715, 1715t
mediastinum, 1117–1119
ovarian cancer, 1633–1634
management of, 1645
pediatric patients, 1842–1844
clinical presentation, 1924, 1925t
pathology and classification, 1924, 1924f
treatment, 1924–1925
testis (See also Intratubular germ-cell neoplasia)
classification, 1504, 1504t
non-seminomatous tumors, 1504t, 1505, 1512–1513
staging, 1506–1508, 1508f
Germinoma, pediatric patients, 1843, 1844f, 1924–1925
Given dose, electron-beam therapy, 196–197
Glasscock-Jackson glomus tumor classification, 998, 999t
Glassy cell carcinoma, cervical cancer, 1541
Gleason score, prostate cancer
clinical presentation and diagnosis, 1447–1449
epidemiology and risk factors, 1441
metastatic patterns, 1445–1446
prognostic classification, 1454–1455
prostate-specific antigen velocity, 1449
recurrent disease and, 1497–1498
treatment criteria and, 1456–1457
Glioblastoma multiforme (GBM)
chemotherapy, 733–734
combined chemoradiation therapy, 681t, 684
hyperthermia therapy, 663–664, 664f
magnetic resonance imaging, 622
molecular genetics, 723–724, 734
particle therapy, 734
radiation therapy, 730–735, 730t
brachytherapy techniques, 731–732
dose escalation
altered fractionation and, 731
FSRT and, 731
radiosensitizers, 733
radiotherapy dose, 730–731, 730t
radiotherapy target volume, 730
radioimmunotherapy, 734
recurrence therapy modalities, 735
stereotactic radiosurgery, 386
targeted therapies, 734–735
Gliomagenesis, intracranial tumors, 723–724
Gliomas
brainstem gliomas, 739–740, 740t
pediatric patients, 1830–1832, 1831f
diffuse pontine gliomas, 632–633
interstitial brachytherapy, 489–490
low-grade gliomas, 737–739
management of, 730
nonpilocytic/diffusely infiltrating gliomas, 737–738
optic glioma, 791–792
pediatric patients, 1829–1830
Gliomatosis cerebri, diagnosis and management, 739
Global agents, boron neutron capture therapy, 34
Global disease burden, radiation oncology, 604
Glomus tumors, 996–1002
anatomy, 996, 997f
clinical presentation, 996, 998, 998f, 998t
diagnostic workup, 996, 998, 998t
epidemiology, 996

nonmalignant disease, 1940–1941, 1941*t*
radiation management, 999–1002, 1000*f*–1003*f*, 1003*t*–1007*t*
staging, 998, 999*t*
surgical management, 998–999
Glottic larynx, lesions of, 978
radiation therapy, 989*t*–990*t*
treatment modalities, 990*t*
Gold radionuclides
brachytherapy, prostate cancer, 530, 1486–1489
low-dose-rate permanent implant brachytherapy, 430
Gonadal dose guidelines
Hodgkin's lymphoma radiation therapy, pediatric patients, 1901
photon external-beam dosimetry, 187
total-body irradiation, 373
Gonadal function, late effects syndromes on normal tissue in, 347
Gorham syndrome, 1925, 1926*f*–1927*f*
Gorlin-Goltz syndrome, 1927–1928
Graft *versus* leukemia effect, total body irradiation, 364–365
Gram-atomic mass, defined, 143
Granulocyte colony stimulating factor, accelerated fractionation *vs.*
chemoradiation/chemotherapy, 315
Granulosa cell tumors, ovarian germ cell tumors, 1646
Graves' disease, 781
radiation therapy, 1944–1945, 1944*t*–1945*t*, 1945*f*
Great vessel tumors, diagnosis and management, 1159–1160
Gross tumor volume (GTV)
external beam radiation therapy, 7
lung cancer radiation therapy, 1095
three-dimensional conformal radiation therapy
applications, 227–230, 228*f*–230*f*
specifications, 225
treatment planning for radiation therapy, 30–31
Growth control
molecular cancer biology and loss of, 110–114
self-sufficiency in, 110–111
total body irradiation and, 373
Growth factors
angiogenesis induction and, 113
radiation therapy, molecular responses, 82
signal transduction and, 42
Growth fraction, tumor regeneration after radiation, 85, 85*f*
Growth hormone (GH)
late effects syndromes in neuroendocrine system and, 345
pituitary tumor secretion, 757–758, 757*f*, 758*t*
Gynecologic cancer. *See also* specific organs, e.g. Cervical cancer
intensity-modulated radiation therapy, 259
interstitial brachytherapy, 517
intraoperative radiotherapy in, 404
metastases, palliative therapy, 2002, 2002*t*, 2003*f*
photodynamic therapy, 602
rhabdomyosarcoma, pediatric patients, 1877

H
Hadron beams, radiation therapy, 32
Half-life, radioactive nuclide, 145
Half-value layer (HVL)
brachytherapy radionuclides, 426
defined, 146–147
Hand-Schuller-Christian disease, 1920–1921
Hand tumors, radiation therapy, 695
Hard palate
anatomy, 891
treatment and results, 909
Head and neck tumors. *See also* Neck metastases; Salivary gland
tumors; specific regions, e.g. Hypopharyngeal cancer
accelerated fractionation radiotherapy, 307*t*, 310
hybrid techniques, 308*t*–309*t*, 311
brachytherapy, 493–499
feeding protocols, 487
chloroma, 1012
chordomas, 1005–1010
anatomy, 1005
clinical presentation, 1005–1006
diagnostic work-up, 1006, 1006*t*
epidemiology, 1005
general management, 1006
natural history, 1005
pathology, 1005
photons, 1006–1009
protons, 1009–1010

radiation therapy, 1006, 1007*f*–1008*f*
treatment sequelae, 1010
combined chemoradiation therapy, 681–682, 681*t*
esthesioneuroblastoma, 1012–1018
extracranial meningiomas, 1024
extramedullary plasmacytomas, 1019–1020
glomus tumors, 996–1002
anatomy, 996, 997*f*
clinical presentation, 993*f*, 996, 998, 998*t*
epidemiology, 996
radiation management, 999–1002, 1000*f*–1003*f*, 1003*t*–1007*t*
staging, 998, 999*t*
surgical management, 998–999
hemangiopericytoma, 1002–1005
high-dose-rate brachytherapy, 572, 573*t*
hyperfractionation radiation therapy, clinical trials, 306
intensity-modulated radiation therapy, 257–258
lentigo maligna melanoma, 1026–1027
lethal midline granuloma, 1010–1012
lymphomas, 1756–1757
nasopharyngeal angiofibroma, 1020–1024
nonlentiginous melanoma, 1024–1026
nonmalignant disease, radiation therapy, 1935–1941
oral cavity metastases, 822–823, 827*f*
osteosarcomas, 1805
pediatric patients, 1913–1915
nasohpharyngeal carcinoma, 1913
rhabdomyosarcoma, 1875–1876
photodynamic therapy, 601–602, 602*f*
rhabdomyosarcoma, pediatric patients, 1875–1876
sarcomas, 1027–1030
diagnosis and treatment, 1817
squamous-cell tumors
combined radiotherapy and chemotherapy, 807–818
adjuvant postoperative irradiation, 813
alternating radiation and chemotherapy, 810
biologically target therapy, 816–817
curative intent treatment, 810–813, 811*f*–814*f*, 814*t*
efficacy of, 807–808
future research issues, 817–818
selection criteria, 813–816
sequential chemoradiation, 816
synchronous radiation and multiagent chemotherapy, 809–810
synchronous radiation and single-agent chemotherapy, 808–809, 808*t*
toxicity management strategies, 817
fast neutron radiotherapy, 410
Health Insurance Portability and Accountabilty Act (HIPPA),
radiation oncology and, 65–66
Hearing loss. *See* Sensorineural hearing loss
nasopharyngeal cancer therapy, 853
Heart
late effects syndromes on normal tissue in, 332–336, 333*f*–335*f*,
334*t*–335*t*
tumors of
anatomy of, 1154–1155
clinical presentation, 1155–1156, 1156*t*
diagnostic work-up, 1156–1157, 1157*f*
incidence and epidemiology, 1154, 1155*t*
management of, 1157–1158
natural history, 1155
radiation therapy, 1158–1159, 1159*f*
staging system and pathologic classification, 1157, 1157*t*
Heat shock response, hyperthermia, 642
Heavy ion therapies
basic properties, 148–149
cervical cancer, 1573
charged particle radiotherapy, 412–413
principles and applications, 419–420, 419*t*
Heavy particle beams
components and instrumentation, 154–155, 155*f*
radiation therapy, 31–33
Helical tomotherapy
megavoltage components, 281–282, 282*f*
oropharyngeal tumors, 950–951
Hemangioblastoma, diagnosis and management, 746
Hemangiomas
liver, 1360
pediatric patients, 1925
vertebral, 1954–1955

Hemangiopericytoma, 1002–1005
  diagnosis and managment, 746
Hematagenous dissemination, nasopharyngeal cancer, 823
Hematologic malignancies, bone marrow ablation, 594–595
Hematometra, cervical cancer, 1540
Hematopoietic system, total body irradiation effects, 364
Hemibody irradiation (HBI)
  applications and complications, 374
  bone metastases, 1996–1997
  multiple myeloma, 1796
Henschke applicator, brachytherapy, cervical carcinoma, 512, 513*f*
Hepatitis B virus, hepatocellular carcinoma risk and, 1349–1350
Hepatitis C virus (HCV), hepatocellular carcinoma risk and, 1349–1350
Hepatobiliary tract tumors. *See* Biliary tract cancers; Liver cancer
Hepatoblastoma
  diagnosis and management, 1360
  pediatric patients, 1917–1920, 1918*t*
Hepatocellular carcinoma (HCC)
  anatomy, 1349, 1350*f*
  biliary tract cancer, 1355–1356
  clinical presentation, 1350–1351
  diagnostic work-up, 1351
  epidemiology, 1349
  future research on, 1355
  management, 1352–1355
  pathologic classification, 1351
  pediatric patients, 1917–1920, 1918*t*
  prevention, 1350
  risk factors, 1349–1350
  staging, 1351, 1352*t*
  surveillance, 1350
Hepatopathy, late effects syndromes in liver and, 338, 338*t*
Hereditary nonpolyposis colorectal cancer (HNPCC), clinical presentation and risk factors, 1366–1367
Heterotopic ossification, diagnosis and therapy, 1955–1956, 1955*f*, 1956*t*
High-dose-rate brachytherapy, 432, 432*t*, 540–559
  advantages and disadvantages, 541–543
  applicators, 540–541, 542*f*
  biliary cancers, 572
  breast cancer, 558–559, 574–576, 575*t*
  cervical cancer, 562–564, 563*t*–565*t*
    biology of, 1562–1563, 1563*f*, 1563*t*
    clinical experience, 1563–1564, 1564*f*, 1564*t*–1565*t*
    dose fractionation, 1565–1566
    dose specifications, 1564
    fractionation schedules, 1564*t*
    low-dose-rate comparisons, 1577–1581, 1578*f*, 1579*t*–1580*t*
    models, 468–469, 469*f*, 556–558, 557*f*
    sequelae, 1588–1589
  clinical applications, 556–559
    biliary cancers, 572
    breast cancer, 574–576, 575*t*
    cervical carcinoma, 562–564, 563*t*–565*t*
    in developing countries, 577–578
    endobronchial irradiation, 567–569, 568*t*
    endometrial carcinoma, 565, 566*t*–567*t*
    error reduction, 576–577, 577*t*
    esophageal cancer, 569–570, 570*t*
    head and neck cancers, 572, 573*t*
    image-based treatment planning, 564–567
    intraoperative techniques, 576–577, 576*t*
    limitations of, 578
    lung cancer, 567–569, 569*t*
    pediatric tumors, 573–574, 574*t*
    prostate cancer, 570–572, 571*t*–572*t*
    radiobiological principles, 560–562, 561*t*
    skin cancer, 576
    soft tissue sarcomas, 572–573, 574*t*
    vaginal cuff irradiation, 565–567, 567*t*
  in developing countries, 577–578
  dosimetry and treatment planning, 543–546, 552–556
  emergency procedures, 547
  endobronchial irradiation, 567–569, 568*t*
  endometrial carcinoma, 565, 566*t*–567*t*
  error reduction, 576–577, 577*t*
  esophageal cancer, 569–570, 570*t*
  facility design, 547–548
  head and neck cancers, 572, 573*t*

image-based treatment planning, 564–567
intraoperative techniques, 576–577, 576*t*
limitations of, 578
linear quadratic model, 543–545, 544*f*–545*f*
low-dose conversion to, 545–546
lung cancer, 567–569, 569*t*
normal procedures, 546–547
pediatric tumors, 573–574, 574*t*
personnel requirements, 546
physics and dosimetry, 540–559
  advantages and disadvantages, 541–543
  applications, 556–559
  applicators, 540–541, 542*f*
  dosimetry and treatment planning, 552–556
  emergency procedures, 547
  facility design, 547–548
  linear quadratic model, 543–545, 544*f*–545*f*
  low-dose conversion to, 545–546
  normal procedures, 546–547
  personnel requirements, 546
  pulsed brachytherapy, 546
  quality assurance, remote afterloading device, 548–552
  remote afterloaders, 540, 541*f*
  sources, 540, 542*f*
prostate cancer, 558, 570–572, 571*t*–572*t*, 1465, 1470, 1472
  morbidity, 1475
pulsed brachytherapy, 546
quality assurance, remote afterloading device, 548–552
radiobiological principles, 560–562, 561*t*
remote afterloaders, 540, 541*f*
retroperitoneal cancer, 1712
skin cancer, 576
soft tissue sarcomas, 572–573, 574*t*
sources, 432, 432*t*, 540, 542*f*
urethral cancer, female, 1688, 1688*f*
vaginal cancer, 1670–1671
vaginal cuff irradiation, 565–567, 567*t*
High-dose total-body irradiation, complications, 372
High-energy bent-beam linear accelerator, components and schematic, 151, 151*f*
Highly active antiretroviral therapy (HAART)
  Kaposi's sarcoma, 707–711
  malignant neoplasms and, HIV infection, 702–703, 713
Hinge angle, wedge filters, photon external-beam dosimetry, 175, 175*f*
Hippocratic oath, 2036, 2036*f*
Histiocytosis X, 1920–1921
Histologic diagnosis, intracranial tumors, 722, 723*t*
Hodgkin's lymphoma
  acquired immunodeficiency syndrome, 706–707
  anatomy, 1721
  chemotherapy, 1726, 1727*t*
    clinical trials, 1735
    results, 1730–1733
  combined treatment modalities, 1726, 1727*t*
  diagnostic work-up, 1722–1723, 1722*t*, 1723*f*
  elderly patients, 1732
  epidemiology and risk factors, 1721
  follow-up protocols, 1733
  hematopoietic cell transplantation, 1732–1733
  natural history and clinical presentation, 1721–1722
  oncological anatomy, 633
  pathologic classification, 1724–1725, 1724*t*–1725*t*
  pediatric patients, 1732, 1892–1903
    biology, 1892
    chemotherapy, 1896, 1897*t*, 1898
    clinical presentation, 1893
    combined treatment modalities, 1894, 1895*t*–1896*t*
    diagnostic work-up, 1893
    epidemiology, 1892
    future research issues, 1902
    long-term therapy effects, 1901–1902, 1902*f*
    pathologic classification, 1892–1893, 1893*t*
    prognostic factors, 1894
    radiation therapy, 1894–1896, 1899–1902, 1900*f*–1901*f*, 1900*t*
    recurrent/refractory disease, 1898–1899
    risk-adapted therapy, 1898
    staging, 1893
    therapy sequencing, 1898
positron emission tomography, 624, 624*f*

prognostic factors, 1725–1726, 1726t
radiation therapy, 1726–1730
  involved fields, 1729
  results, 1730–1733
  sequelae, 1733–1735
  subdiaphragmatic fields, 1728–1731, 1729f
  three-dimensional treatment planning, 1729–1730, 1730f
recurrent disease, 1732
secondary cancers, 1730–1731
staging, 1723–1724, 1723t–1724t, 1724f
surgical management, 1726
Holliday-functon, DBS repair, 116–117
Homologous recombination
chemoradiation therapy, molecular targeting and, 676
DBS repair, 116–117
Hormone receptors
breast cancer metastases, 1199
cervical cancer, 1546
prostate cancer risk and, 1441
Hormone-refractory prostate cancer (HRPC), chemotherapy, 1496
Hormone replacement therapy. *See also* Androgen suppression
       therapy
bone metastases, 1991–1992
breast cancer
  locally advanced and recurrent disease, 1298–1299
  recent advances in, 306–1307, 1306t
  risk factors, 1177–1178
  sequencing protocols, 1230–1234, 1230f
  systemic therapy, 1206
cervical cancer, post-therapy application, 1589
endometrial cancer, 1619
Hospital-physician relationships, radiation oncology ethics, 2039
Hot spots, radiation therapy, 102–103
Human epidermal growth factor receptor 2 (HER2/Neu)
breast cancer metastases, 1200
non-small cell lung cancer therapy, 1099
vaginal carcinoma, 1662–1663
Human immunodeficiency virus (HIV) infection. *See also* Acquired
       immunodeficiency syndrome (AIDS)
cervical cancer, 1534, 1546
malignant neoplams and, 702–703
perianal cancer and, 1391
Human lymphocyte antigen-1 (HLA-1), down-regulation, 583
Human papilloma virus (HPV)
cervical carcinoma epidemiology, 1534
hypopharyngeal cancer and, 959
penis, cancer of, 1524
Hybrid phantom planning, intensity-modulated radiation therapy,
       dosimetry verification, 254
Hydroxyurea, cervical cancer therapy, 1592–1593
Hyperbaric oxygen
cervical cancer therapy, 1596–1597
chemical modifiers of radiation therapy, 611–612
modification of radiation response, 35
Hyperfractionated radiation therapy
cervical cancer, 1556–1557
  chemotherapy and, 1595–1596
chemical modifiers of radiation therapy, 612
chemotherapy concurrent with, 315
concurrent chemotherapy with, head and neck squamous-cell
       tumors, 814, 814t
non-small cell lung cancer, 1088–1089, 1088t
radiation therapy, 100
  clinical trials, 305t, 306, 310
rationale for, 304, 305t
Hypertension, cervical cancer risk and, 1543
Hyperthermia
cell survival effects, 637, 638f
cervical cancer radiation therapy and, 1597
chemotherapy and, 648–649, 649f
clinical applications, 658–665
  breast cancer, 660–662, 661f
  cervical cancer, 664–665, 664f
  esophageal cancer, 663
  general considerations, 658–659
  glioblastoma multiforme, 663–664, 664f
  head and neck cancers, 663
  malignant melanoma, 663
  rectal cancer, 662
  sarcoma, 662–663

superficial tumors, 662
  thermal dosimetry principles, 659–660
cytotoxicity mechanisms, 640, 641f
  pH modification, 645–646, 646f
defined, 637
gene therapy and, 649, 649f
heat shock response, 642
interstitial brachytherapy and, 531
metastases, 646–647
modification of radiation response, 35
physics of, 649–658
  electromagnetic heating, 650, 650f–651f
  interstitial hyperthermia, 651–655, 652f–655f
  invasive thermometry, 655–657, 656f–657f
  noninvasive thermal dose measurements, 657–658,
    657f–659f
  ultrasound heating, 650–651, 651f–652f
physiology, 642–644, 643f–644f
quality assurance for, 57
radiation therapy with, 637
  rationale for, 647–648
thermal isoeffect dose
  Arrhenius relationship, 637–639, 638f–639f
  modifiers, 639–640
thermotolerance, 640–642, 641f
tissue damage, 644–645
Hyperthyroidism, late effects syndromes and, 345–346
Hypofractionation
accelerated treatment regimens, 100–101
metastatic spinal cord compression, contraindications,
    1983–1984
radiation therapy, 100
Hypopharyngeal cancer
anatomy, 957, 959f–960f
clinical presentation, 961–963, 962f–963f
epidemiology and etiology, 958–959
etiology, 958
future research issues, 973
metastastatic patterns, 960–961, 961f, 969–970
pretreatment evaluation, 963
prognostic factors, 959–960
recurrent disease management, 972–973
  quality of life, 973
staging protocols, 960, 960t, 963t
T1-T2 tumor management, 963–965, 964f–965f, 965t–966t,
  967f
T3-T4 resection
  radiation therapy, 966–968, 966t–967t, 967f–969f
  surgery, 965–966
therapy complications, 971
treatment results, 971–972
unresectable metastatic disease, 968, 971t
Hypothalamus, radiation injury and dysfunction, 796
Hypothyroidism
Hodgkin's lymphoma radiation therapy, 1734
late effects syndromes and, 345–346
Hypoxia
cell sensitization
  cervical cancer therapy, 1596–1597
  chemical modifiers of radiation therapy, 612–613
  pharmacologic targeting, 613–614
cervical cancer and, 1542–1543, 1596–1597
chemoradiation therapy and tumor radioresistance, 671–672
positron emmission tomography, image-guided radiation
    therapy, 265
radiation therapy and, 13, 88–89
radiosensitivity and, 15
tumor metabolism, 134–136, 135t
Hypoxia-inducing factor 1-a, tumor metabolism, 136
Hypoxic gain factor, neutron radiation quality, 104
Hypoxic sensitizers, modification of radiation response, 35
Hysterectomy
cervical cancer therapy, 1546–1548
  ovarian preservation, 1552
  para-aortic lymph node metastases, 1574–1576, 1576t
  postoperative radiation, 1581–1583, 1582f
  radiation therapy and, 1548–1550, 1549f, 1551t
  recurrent disease, 1590
  results, 1566–1573
  techniques for, 1550–1552
endometrial cancer, 1614–1615, 1622–1623

I

Illumination, photodynamic therapy, 599–600
Image-based planning systems
    high-dose-rate brachytherapy, 564–567, 565*t*
    pediatric patients, 1423
    photon external-beam dosimetry, compensating filter systems, 181–182, 182*f*
Image-guided intracavitary brachytherapy, 464
Image-guided radiation therapy (IGRT)
    adaptive radiotherapy, 289–293, 290*f*–293*f*
    beam tracking, 288–289
    cervical anatomy, 1532, 1533*f*
    evolution of, 218
    four-dimensional imaging, 285–288, 285*f*–287*f*
    future research, 293
    linear accelerators, 152, 153*f*
    overview of, 263
    planar imaging systems, 271–279
        cyberknife, 274, 274*f*, 275*t*, 276*f*
        electronic portal imaging devices, 271, 272*f*, 273–274
        gantry-mounted systems, 278–279, 278*f*–279*f*
        Novalis system, 274, 276–277, 276*f*
        real-time tumor tracking, 277, 277*f*
        University of Michigan system, 277
    respiratory motion management, 284–285, 284*f*–285*f*
        tumor treatment, 288
    stereotactic body radiation therapy and, 391
    target delineation, 263–268
        magnetic resonance imaging, 265–266, 267*f*
        positron emission tomography, 264–265, 264*f*–266*f*
        single photon emission computed tomography, 266, 268, 269*f*
    technology and clinical applications, 268–289
    tumors with respiratory motion, 288
    ultrasound systems, 268–271, 270*f*
    video systems, 271, 272*f*
    volumetric imaging systems, 279–284
        in-room CT systems, 279–281, 280*f*–281*f*
        kilovoltage systems, 282–283, 283*f*–284*f*
        megavoltage systems, 281–282, 282*f*
Imaging studies
    bone metastases, 1987–1988, 1987*f*–1989*f*
    brain metastases, 1974
    breast cancer diagnosis, 1190–1194, 1190*t*
    cervical cancer
        follow-up, 1540
        screening, 1536–1537
    fallopian tube disease, 1651
    glomus tumors, 996, 998*f*
    Hodgkin's lymphoma, 1722, 1723*f*
    laryngeal cancers, 979, 980*f*
    lung cancer, 1080
    metastatic spinal cord compression, 1981
    nasal cavity and paranasal sinuses, 861
    neck metastases, unknown primary tumors, 1036–1037, 1038*f*
    neuroblastoma, pediatric patients, 1860, 1861*f*
    non-Hodgkin's lymphoma, 1742–1743, 1742*t*
    pancreatic cancer, 1336–1337
    prostate cancer, 1450–1453
        intermediate/high risk cancer, 1487
        low-risk cancer, 1450–1453
    rectal cancer, 1373
    soft tissue sarcomas, 1809, 1811*f*
    spinal cord tumors, 768
    stomach cancer diagnosis, 1319–1320
    superior sulcus tumors, 1091–1093, 1092*f*
    testicular cancer, 1506
    thyroid disease, 1058–1059
Immobilization protocols. *See also* Organ motion; Patient positioning
    fractionated stereotactic radio therapy, pituitary tumors, 761–762
    high-dose-rate brachytherapy, 541–542
    intensity-modulated radiation therapy, 1098
    maxillary sinus radiation therapy, 867–868
    nasal cavity and ethmoid sinus radiation therapy, 864–866
    pediatric medulloblastoma radiation therapy, 1838
    photon external-beam dosimetry, 182–184, 183*f*
    prostate cancer radiation therapy, 1458–1459
    radiation therapy, 8–10, 9*t*
    stereotactic body radiation therapy, 390–391
    three-dimensional conformal radiation therapy, 220–221, 220*f*–221*f*
Immunobiology, non-Hodgkin's lymphoma, 1740

Immunodeficiency, Non-Hodgkin's lymphoma and, 1739
Immunohistochemical staining, soft tissue sarcoma classification, 1811
Immunoliposomes, cancer therapy, 585–586
Immunology
    hyperthermia effects, 642
    radioimmunoglobulins, 583–584, 584*t*
Immunotherapy, non-Hodgkin's lymphoma, 1750
Immunotoxins, cancer therapy, 585
Implantation techniques
    brachytherapy, 486
        cervical cancer, 1573
        prostate cancer, 527–530, 528*f*–529*f*
        removal protocols, 487
    radiation therapy, urethral cancer, female, 1685–1688, 1686*f*–1688*f*, 1689*t*, 1690
Implant-optimization criteria, interstitial brachytherapy, 443
    Manchester system, 444–447, 444*f*, 445*t*–446*t*, 446*f*–448*f*
In-air calibration, absorbed dose measurement, 158
Incessant ovulation hypothesis, ovarian cancer risk and, 1629–1631, 1630*f*
Induratio penis plastica, 1950–1951
Industrial relations, medical ethics and, 2040
Infectious agents, non-Hodgkin's lymphoma, 1739
Inflammatory breast cancer
    management and treatment results, 1308–1309
    natural history, 1293–1294
    in pediatric patients, 1916
Inflammatory response, radiation therapy, 82
Informed consent procedures, radiation oncology, 66–67, 67*t*
Infrahyoid epiglottis lesions, characteristics of, 977
Inguinal lymph nodes
    penis, cancer of, 1520, 1520*f*, 1521*t*, 1524–1525, 1524*t*, 1527*f*
    vulvar cancer metastases, 1692–1693, 1693*t*, 1699–1700
Inherited cancer syndromes, molecular biology, 109–114
In-stent restenosis
    β-radiation, 1964–1965, 1965*t*–1966*t*
    Betacath system, 1962–1964, 1963*f*
    drug-eluting stents, 1965–1966
        vascular brachytherapy following, 1966
    γ-radiation, 1964, 1965*t*
    saphenous vein graft, 1966
Institutional comparisons, total body irradiation, 370
Instrumentation, radiation therapy, 58–61
Insurance companies, economic profiling of, 2045
Integrated radiotherapy imaging system (IRIS), gantry-mounted systems, 278–279, 278*f*–279*f*
Integrated reference air-kerma (IRAK), brachytherapy dosimetry, 435
Integrated target volume (ITV), image-guided radiation therapy, four-dimensional imaging, 286–288, 286*f*–287*f*
Integrins
    cervical cancer, 1546
    signaling mechanisms, 120–121, 120*f*
Intensity-modulated arc therapy, 240
Intensity-modulated photon therapy (IMPT), charged particle radiotherapy and, 412–413, 412*t*
Intensity-modulated radiation therapy (IMRT)
    alternative techniques, 240, 241*f*
    aperture margins, 243–245, 246*f*
    beam configurations, 242–243, 244*f*–245*f*
    breast cancer, 258–259, 1257–1259, 1260*f*
    cervical cancer, 1558, 1559*f*–1560*f*
    coaxial beam arrangements, 177
    dose-based objective functions, 247–248
    dose-volume-based objective functions, 248–249, 248*f*–249*f*
    dosimetric verification, 253–255, 254*f*–255*f*
    electron arc therapy and, 215
    endometrial cancer, 1621, 1621*f*
    facility design requirements, 257
    fixed-gantry fields, 255–256
    fractionation, 245–246
    gastrointestinal cancer, 259
    geographic underdosage, 101–102, 102*f*
    gynecologic cancer, 259
    head and neck cancer, 257–258
    hypopharyngeal cancers, 965, 967*f*
        complications, 971
    imaging and volumes, 242
    intracranial malignancies, 259–260
    leaf sequence generatio, 250–252

limitations and risks, 239–240
lung cancer, 259, 1097–1098
map optimization, 246–247, 247f
nasopharyngeal cancer, 834–836, 836t, 837f–839f, 840t
objective function parameters, 249, 249f
oropharyngeal tumors, 946–950, 947t–948t, 948f–949f, 950t
  beam orientations, 949
  dosimetric quality assurance, 948–949, 948f–949f
  optimization and evaluation, 950
  patient setup verification, correction, and PTV regimens, 947–948, 948t
  simultaneous integrated boost, 949–950
  step-and-shoot and segmental techniques, 950
  treatment planning, 946–947, 947t
  treatment results, 950, 951t
ovarian cancer whole-abdominal radiation and, 1643
overview of, 239
pancreatic cancer, 1340–1341
pituitary tumor management, 756
process overview, 240–242, 242f–243f
prostate cancer, 258
  beam selection and planning, 1459–1461, 1460f–1461f, 1460t
  dose calculation methods, 1461
  intermediate/high-risk cancer treatment planning, 1489
  long-term results, 1468
  techniques, 1457–1458
quality assurance protocols, 253
rationale, 239–240
serial tomotherapy with, 256
tomotherapy vs. fixed-gantry techniques, 256–257
treatment planning for, 31, 242
  evaluation of, 249–250
treatment setup and delivery, 255–256
vocal cord carcinoma, 984
Interfollicular Hodgkin's lymphoma, 1725
Interim analyses, clinical trials, 360–361
Interleukins, radiation therapy, molecular responses, 82
Intermediate low-energy range, radionuclides, 425–426
Internal collimation, electron beam therapy, 204–205, 206f
Internal mammary chain (IMC) electron fields
  breast cancer management, 1228–1230, 1229t
  electron beam therapy, mixed-beam techniques, 206–207, 208f, 209
Internal mammary nodes
  anatomical illustrations, 630–631, 631t
  breast cancer metastases, 1184, 1184t, 1228–1230, 1229t
    radiation therapy, 1254–1255, 1258f–1259f
      tangential field alignment, 1256, 1258f–1259f
Internal margins, planning target volume, three-dimensional
    conformal radiation therapy, 226
International Commission on Radiation Units (ICRU)
  reference point, three-dimensional conformal radiation therapy, dose reporting/prescription, 227
  volumetric specifications, 224–226, 226t
    intracavitary brachytherapy, 460–461, 460f–461f
International economics, radiation oncology, 2049
International system (SI) units, radiation therapy, 145t
Interphase cell death, radiation therapy, 77–78
Interstitial hypertension, tumor cells, 134
Interstitial hyperthermia, physics principles for, 651–655, 652f–655f
Interstitial implant brachytherapy, 442–456, 442t–443t
  afterloading, 476–481
    iodine-125 plastic tube implants, 479–481
    iridium-192 wires or ribbons, 477–478, 477f–479f
    removable iridium-192 hairpin technique, 479, 480f
    suturing techniques, needles, guides, and plastic buttons, 478–479, 479f
  brain implants, 487–490, 488f–489f, 495t
  breast, 499–502, 501f–503f
  cervical cancer, 512–515, 513f–514f, 515t, 1558–1566, 1561f
    implants, 1573
  classical radium-substitute sources, 443–449
  dose specification, 449, 451–454
  Fletcher system, 450t
  gynecological malignancies, 517
  high-dose-rate regimens, 572, 572t
  hyperthermia with, 531
  iridium implants, prostate cancer, 530–531, 531f
  Manchester system, 444–447, 444f, 445t–446t, 446f–448f
  Martinez universal perineal interstitial template, 481
  modern developments, 454–456

Paris system, 448–449, 449t
Quimby system, 447–448
soft tissue sarcomas, 1817
vaginal cancer, 1671–1672
Interstitial transport, tumor cells, 132
Intestinal lymphomas, 1755–1756
Intra-arterial chemotherapy, cervical cancer, 1592
Intracavitary brachytherapy, 423, 456–464
  cervical cancer, 556–558, 557f, 1558–1566, 1560f
    postoperative protocols, 1583–1584
  dose specification, 458–464
  endometrial cancer, 1616–1621, 1616t–1617t, 1619–1622
  Fletcher-suit applicator systems, 457–458, 457f–458f
  high-dose rate model, cervical cancer, 468–469, 469f
  image-guided systems, 464
  low-dose-rate sources, 426–428, 427f–428f
  Manchester systems, 456–458, 457f
  vaginal cancer, 1669–1671
  vaginal carcinoma, 520, 520f
Intracavitary electron-beam therapy, 209–210, 209f–210f
Intracellular adhesion molecule (ICAM), radiation effects on, 1934
Intracranial tumors
  anaplastic glioma, 735–737
  anatomy, 717–718, 718f–719f
  brainstem glioma, 739–740
  chemotherapy and target agents, 727–729
  clinical presentation, 720
  craniopharyngioma, 744–746
  diagnostic work-up, 720–723, 721t
    histologic confirmation, 722–723
    imaging studies, 720–722, 721t, 722f, 723t
  differential dianosis, 723, 723t
  ependymoma, 740
  epidemiology, 718, 720
  follow-up, 729
  general management, 724
  glioblastoma multiforme, 731–735
  gliomatosis cerebri, 739
  hemangioblastoma/hemangiopericytoma, 746
  image-guided radiation therapy, Cyberknife system, 274, 274f, 275t, 276f
  intensity-modulated radiation therapy, 259–260
  low-grade glioma, 737–739
  malignant glioma, 730–731
  medulloblastoma, 740–741
  molecular genetics, 723–724
  natural history, 720
  nonmalignant disease radiation, 1935
  pathology, 723, 723t
  radiation therapy, 725–727
  seizures, 724
  stereotactic radiosurgery, 384
  surgery, 724–725
  treatment sequelae, 729–730
  vestibular schwannoma and neurofibroma, 745–746
Intradural-extramedullary tumors
  pathologic classification, 769–770
  surgical management, 771
Intrahepatic bile duct cancer, staging, 1351, 1352t
Intrahepatic cholangiocarcinoma, 1357–1358
Intramedullary tumors
  metastatic spinal cord compression, 1984
  pathologic classification, 768–769
  radiation therapy, 775
  surgical management, 771
Intraoperative high-dose-rate brachytherapy
  basic principles, 543
  prostate cancer, 1463, 1464f
Intraoperative radiation/intraoperative electron irradiation therapy (IORT/IOERT)
  bladder and kidney, 402
  bladder tumors, 1426
  breast, 400t, 402–404
  breast cancer therapy, 1263–1264, 1264f
  cervical cancer, 1591
  colon and rectum, 400–401, 402f
  colon cancer, 1370–1371
  doses and techniques, 397
  error reduction, 576–577, 576t–577t
  esophagus, 400
  extremity sarcomas, 401

Intraoperative radiation (*contd.*)
 gynecological cancer, 404
 lung, 400
 miscellaneous indications, 404
 modern trends in, 397, 398*f*
 osteosarcoma, 1804, 1804*t*
 ovarian cancer, 1643–1644
 pancreatic cancer, 399, 403*t*, 1343, 1345
 pediatric tumors, 402
 rationale for, 397, 399*f*
 retroperitoneal and pelvic soft tissue sarcomas, 401
 retroperitoneal cancer, 1712, 1714*t*
 stomach, 399–400
 stomach cancer, 1329–1332, 1329*t*–1330*t*
 tolerance and dose-limiting structures, 397–399
Intraoral cone radiation, oral cavity tumors, 905–906, 906*f*
Intraperitoneal phosphorus radiation therapy, ovarian cancer,
  1639–1644, 1639*t*, 1642*t*
Intratubular germ-cell neoplasia (IGCN)
 classification, 1504, 1504*t*
 treatment, 1512
Invasive (infiltrating) ductal carcinoma (IDC), pathological
  characteristics, 1196
Invasive lobular carcinoma (ILC)
 pathological characteristics, 1196–1197
 recurrent disease, 1217
Invasive micropapillary carcinoma, pathology, 1197
Invasive thermometry, hyperthermia, 655–657, 656*f*–657*f*
Inverse-square law, radionuclide properties, 425–426
In vivo kinetics, tumor responses, 84
Iodine therapy
 administrative procedures, 1072–1073
 differentiated thyroid cancer, 1063–1064, 1064*f*–1065*f*,
  1069–1070
 implants
  brachytherapy, 430–432, 431*f*
   line-source radial dose functions, 441–442, 443*t*
   retropubic prostate cancer implants, 527–530, 528*f*–529*f*,
    528*t*
  interstitial brachytherapy
   permanent implants, 480–481
   removable plastic tubes, 479–480
  nonsealed radionuclide therapy, 591
  posterior uvea melanoma, 784–787, 785*f*–786*f*
 medullary thyroid cancer, 1066–1067, 1067*f*, 1069–1070
 outpatient regimens, 1071–1072, 1072*f*
Ionizing radiation
 basic principles, 144
 biological effects, 115, 115*f*
 DNA damage, 10, 11*f*, 11*t*–12*t*
Ion recombination factor, absorbed dose calculation, 159
Iridium radionuclides
 esophageal cancer therapy, 1148, 1149*f*
 interstitial brachytherapy
  afterloading technology, 477–478, 478*f*–479*f*
  gynecological malignancies, 517
  hairpin technique, 479, 480*f*
  prostate cancer, 530–531, 531*f*
  ribbons and wires, 428–429
Irinotecan, non-small cell lung cancer therapy, 1099
Iris melanoma, 784, 785*f*
Iritis, nasal cavity and paranasal sinus therapy and, 871–872
Irradiated volume, three-dimensional conformal radiation therapy,
  225
Irregular fields, photon external-beam dosimetry, monitor unit
  calculations, 168, 168*f*
Ischemia-reperfusion injury, tumor metabolism, 134
Iseganan, chemical radioprotection, 617–618
Isocenter techniques, radiation therapy, 7
 breast cancer, supraclavicular and tangential field alignment,
  1256–1257, 1256*f*–1257*f*
Isodose shift method, photon external-beam dosimetry
 air gap corrections, 169, 169*f*
 tissue inhomogeneity correction, 169–170
Isoeffect dose
 basic properties, 162, 163*f*
 cervical cancer radiation therapy, 1556, 1558*f*
 electron-beam therapy
  treatment planning and, 200, 201*f*
  water-based dose distribution, 193–194, 194*f*
 episcleral plaque therapy, 492–493, 492*f*

graphs, radiation therapy, 24–25, 26*f*
hyperthermia
 Arrhenius relationship, 637–639, 638*f*–639*f*
 modifiers, 639–640
 photon external-beam dosimetry, clinical applications, 171–172,
  171*f*, 171*t*
 time-dose effects, dose fractionation and, 97–99
 wedge filter, 163, 164*f*
Isoflavones, prostate cancer risk and, 1443
Isotones, defined, 143
Isotopes
 bone metastases, palliative therapy with, 1997–1998
 defined, 143
 prostate cancer brachytherapy, 1464–1465
Isotropic point, brachytherapy dose calculation, 435–438, 435*f*, 442,
  443*t*

J

jun gene expression, radiation damage and, 118
Juvenile granulosa cell tumors, 1646
Juvenile nasopharyngeal angiofibroma (JNA), 1914–1915, 1914*t*,
  1941, 1942*t*
Juvenile secretory carcinoma of the breast, 1915–1916
Juxtaspinal tumors, proton and α-particle radiotherapy, 416–147,
  416*f*

K

Kantianism, medical ethics and, 2035
Kaposi's sarcoma, acquired immunodeficiency syndrome (AIDS),
  707–711
 combined treatment regimens, 708–710
 diagnostic workup, 708
 disease patterns, 707–708, 707*f*–711*f*
 epidemiology and risk factors, 707
 pathology, 708
 radiation therapy, 710–711
Kasabach-Merritt syndrome, 1925, 1926*f*
Keloids and hypertrophic scars, 1952–1954, 1953*f*
Keratitis, nasal cavity and paranasal sinus therapy and, 871–872
Keratoacanthoma, premalignant skin lesions, 691
Keratoses, premalignant skin lesions, 691
KERMA (kinetic energy released in the medium)
 absorbed dose calculation, 157–158, 158*f*
 brachytherapy dosimetry, 433–434
Khan scatter analysis, photon external-beam dosimetry, 167–168
Kidney. *See also* Renal cell carcinoma
 anatomy, 1397
 intraoperative radiotherapy in, 402
 late effects syndromes on normal tissue in, 338–340, 339*f*–341*f*,
  340*t*–341*t*
 rhabdoid tumor of, 1856
 total body irradiation and, 373
Kilovoltage systems, image-guided radiation therapy, 282–283,
  283*f*–284*f*
 prostate cancer, 1462–1463
Kilovoltage units, radiation therapy machines, 149–150, 149*f*–150*f*
Klystron, lnear accelerators, 151–152
K-means clustering, intensity-modulated radiation therapy, 251–252
"Knudson two hit" hypothesis, tumor-suppressor genes, 40–41, 41*f*,
  41*t*
Kyphosis, late effects syndromes on bone and, 347–349, 349*f*, 349*t*

L

Labetuzumab, radioimmunotherapy with, 590
Laboratory studies
 cervical cancer screening, 1536
 cutaneous T-cell lymphoma, 1769
 nasal cavity and paranasal sinuses, 861
 neuroblastoma, pediatric patients, 1860
 testicular cancer, 1506
Lacrimal gland
 radiation injury to, 796
 tumors, 794, 795*f*
Langerhans cell histiocytosis, pediatric patients, 1920–1921
Laparoscopy, stomach cancer diagnosis, 1320
Laparotomy
 cervical cancer pretreatment and nodal staging, 1551–1552, 1552*t*
 fallopian tubes, tumors of, 1655
 Hodgkin's lymphoma diagnosis, 1722–1723, 1723*t*
 ovarian cancer, secondary surgery, 1636
 ovarian cancer therapy, 1640, 1642*t*

Laryngeal cancer
 anatomy, 975, 976f–977f
 aryepiglottic fold/arytenoid lesions, 978
 clinical presentation, 979
 computed tomographic imaging, 620, 621f
 diagnostic work-up, 979–980, 980t
 epidemiology and risk factors, 975–976
 false cord carcinomas, 978
 follow-up policy, 993
 glottic larynx lesions, 978
 infrahyoid epiglottis lesions, 977
 lymphatic metastases, 978–979, 978f
 metastatic patterns, 976–979
 pathological classification, 981
 pediatric patients, 1913–1914
 prognostic factors, 981
 radiographic studies, 979, 980f
 staging, 980–981, 981t
 subglottic larynx lesions, 978
 supraglottic larynx lesions, 976–977
  diagnosis, 979–980, 980t
  radiation therapy, 987–988, 987f
  recurrent disease management, 988–989
  surgical treatment, 987
  treatment modalities, 985–988, 989t–990t
  treatment results, 990, 991t–992t
  treatment sequelae, 993
 suprahyoid epiglottis lesions, 976–977
 vocal cord carcinoma, 979
  radiation therapy, 983–984, 984f–986f
  recurrent disease management, 984–985
  surgical treatment, 983
  treatment modalities, 981–985
  treatment results, 988t–989t, 990
  treatment sequelae, 993
Laryngectomy techniques
 supracricoid laryngectomy, 987
 supraglotic lesions, 987
 vocal cord carcinoma, 983
 wide-field total laryngectomy, 987
Late effects morbidity scale, 321
Late effects on normal tissue (LENT) paradigm
 defined, 323
 intracranial tumor radiation therapy, 730
 stomach cancer radiation therapy, 1332–1333, 1332t
Late effects syndromes. See also Radiation necrosis
 bone and bone marrow, 347–349, 349f, 349t
 brain, 323–326, 326t, 327f
 central nervous system, 323–326, 325f, 325t
 cervical cancer therapy, 1585–1588, 1585f–1586f
 cholangiocarcinoma radiation therapy, 1360
 colorectum, 342–344
 critical organ tolerance, 323
 dentition, 344
 esophagus, 342–344
 eye, 328
 future research issues, 350
 gastrointestinal tract, 340–344, 343f
 hearing loss, 327–328
 heart, 332–336, 333f–335f, 334t–335t
 hepatocellular carcinoma radiation therapy, 1354
 Hodgkin's lymphoma radiation therapy, pediatric patients,
  1901–1902
 intraoperative radiotherapy, 397–399
 kidney, 338–340, 339f–341f, 340t–341t
 LENT paradigm, 323
 liver, 336–338, 337f, 338t
 lung, 328–330, 330f–331f, 330t
 nasopharyngeal cancer therapy, 851–853, 851t, 852f
  pediatric patients, 1913
 neuroblastoma in pediatric patients, 1869, 1869t
 neuroendocrine system, 345
 organ tolerance principles, 320–321, 321f
 osteosarcoma therapy, 1806
 overview of, 320
 pediatric patients
  Hodgkin's lymphoma radiation therapy, 1901–1902
  nasopharyngeal cancer therapy, 1913
  rhabdomyoscarcoma radiation therapy, 1882
  spinal cord, 776
  Wilms' tumor, 1857

 prostate cancer therapy, 1471–1473
 radiation effects, 321–323, 322f, 322t–323t
 radiation therapy, cell injury kinetics, 80
 reproductive systems, 346–347
 rhabdomyoscarcoma radiation therapy, pediatric patients, 1882
 salivary glands, 344–345
 second malignant neoplasms, 349–350
 skin and soft tissue, 330–332, 332t
 small intestine, 342–344
 spinal cord, 323–327, 328t
  in children, 776
 stomach, 342–344, 342f
 thyroid, 345–346
  iodine therapy, 1069–1070
 total body irradiation, 365
 Wilms' tumor, 1857
Late responses
 ioffect formulae, time-dose effects, 97–98, 98f
 radiation therapy, 79–80
Latin America, radiation therapy in, 607–608
Leaf sequences, intensity-modulated radiation therapy, 250–252,
  250f–252f
Legal issues
 medical ethics and, 2035–2036
 radiation oncology, 61–65
Leiomyosarcomas
 endometrial cancer, 1613
 esophageal cancer, 1137
Lens injury, orbital tumor radiation therapy, 795–796
Lentigo maligna, premalignant skin lesions, 691
Lentigo maligna melanoma, diagnosis and management, 1026–1027
Lentigo midline granuloma (LMG), diagnosis and treatment,
  1010–1012, 1011t
Lethal dose (LD50) principle, radiation therapy and, 13
Lethal-potentially lethal (LPL) model, stereotactic body radiation
  therapy, 389–390
Leukemia
 acute leukemias, 1777–1783
  classification, pathology and risk factors, 1777–1779, 1779t
  radiotherapeutic emergencies, 1779–1780, 1780f
  treatment, 1780–1783
 anatomic considerations, 1777, 1778f
 B-cell chronic lymphocytic leukemia, 1741–1742
 chronic leukemias, 1783–1785
 plasma cell, 1791
 radiation-induced, 1933
 radiation therapy, 1785–1787
 radioimmunotherapy, 588–589
 total body irradiation effects, 364–365
 vaginal cancers, 1660
Leukemic retinopathy, 791
Leukoencephalopathy, leukemia radiation therapy, 1787
Leukoplakia, oral cavity, 895, 895f
Lhermitte's syndrome
 Hodgkin's lymphoma and, 1734
 radiation-induced spinal cord transection, 323, 326–327,
  328t
Liability issues, radiation oncology, 64–65
Li-Fraumeni syndrome
 rhabdomyoscarcoma, 1872
 soft tissue sarcomas, 1808
Light-beam congruence, radiation therapy, 7
Linear accelerators
 image-guided radiation therapy
  stereotactic techniques, 380
  ultrasound therapy, 268–271, 270f
  volumetric imaging systems, 279–284, 280f–284f
 instrumentation and schematics, 150–151, 151f–152f
 stereotactic radiosurgery, 380
Linear energy transfer (LET)
 boron neutron capture therapy, 33–35, 33f
 modification of radiation response, 35–36
 particle beam radiotherapy, 407–408
 quality assurance, 103
 radiation-induced tumors, 54–55
Linear quadratic (LQ) formula
 brachytherapy modeling, 465–466
  high-dose-rate intracavitary therapy, cervical cancer,
   468–469, 469f
  low-dose-rate rationale, 466
  nonuniform dose distribution, 467–468

Linear quadratic (LQ) (*contd.*)
  permanent implants, 468
  prostate cancer dose optimization, 469–470
  radioisotope effectiveness, 468
  redistribution and reoxygenation, 467
  treatment time modeling, 466, 467*f*
  tumor shrinkage, 467
 dose fractionation, 91–92, 91*f*
  late effects syndromes in normal tissue and, 322
 high-dose-rate brachytherapy, 560–562
  dosimetry calculations, 543–545, 545*f*
 isoeffect relationships, 98, 98*f*
 radiation therapy, (α/β ratio), 26–28, 26*f*–27*f*, 27*t*
 stereotactic body radiation therapy, 389–390
Line-source radial dose functions, brachytherapy, 441–442, 443*t*
Lipomas, spinal cord, 770
Liposomally encapsulated drugs, hyperthermia and, 648–649, 649*f*
Lipowitz metal shielding block system, photon external-beam
    dosimetry, 179–180, 180*f*
Lip tissue
 anatomy, 891
 brachytherapy, 494, 495*f*
 carcinomas, treatment and results, 908
 skin tumors, radiation therapy, 695
Liver
 late effects syndromes on normal tissue in, 336–338, 337*f*, 338*t*
 stereotactic body radiation therapy, 391–392, 393*f*
 total-body irradiation, 372–373
Liver cancer
 cholangiocarcinoma, 1356–1360
  anatomy, 1356
  diagnosis, 1356–1357, 1356*t*
  distal bile duct, 1359
  epidemiology and risk factors, 1356
  future research, 1360
  intrahepatic, 1357–1358
  metastases, 1357
  pathology, 1357
  perihilar, 1358–1359
  radiation therapy, 1359–1360, 1360*f*
  staging, 1357, 1358*t*
 gallbladder adenocarcinoma, 1360–1361
 hepatocellular carcinoma
  anatomy, 1349, 1350*f*
  biliary tract cancer, 1355–1356
  clinical presentation, 1350–1351
  diagnostic work-up, 1351
  epidemiology, 1349
  future research on, 1355
  management, 1352–1355
  pathologic classification, 1351
  prevention, 1350
  risk factors, 1349–1350
  staging, 1351, 1352*t*
  surveillance, 1350
 metastases, palliative therapy, 2000, 2001*f*, 2001*t*
 pediatric patients, 1917–1920, 1918*t*
 sarcomas, 1361
 symptoms and etiology, 1349
Lobbying, for radiation oncology, 2046
Lobular carcinoma *in situ*
 diagnosis and treatment, 1162–1163
 invasive cancer and, 1218, 1218*t*
Local excision techniques, rectal cancer surgery, 1374–1375
Local tumor control
 breast cancer therapy and, 1215, 1215*t*
 hypopharyngeal cancer radiation therapy, 971, 972*t*
 intraoperative radiation/intraoperative electron irradiation
    therapy (IORT/IOERT), 397, 399*f*
 lung cancer metastases, 1079
 neuroblastoma in pediatric patients, 1867
 radiation therapy, survival probability and, 21
 soft tissue sarcoma metastases and, 1813
 temporal lobe chemodectomas, 998, 1004*t*
 vocal cord carcinomas, 989*t*
Location effects, stereotactic radiosurgery, 381, 381*f*
Logarithmic cell kill, radiation oncology and, 13–14, 15*t*, 22*f*
Loop excision, cervical cancer screening, 1536
Low anterior resection, rectal cancer therapy, 1374
Low-dose-rate irradiation
 advantages of, 101

brachytherapy
 acute morbidity, 517
 anal canal and rectum, 524–525, 524*f*–525*f*
 biliary tree, 504–506, 506*f*, 506*t*
 breast, 499–502, 501*f*–503*f*
 cervical cancer, 1552–1553, 1553*t*, 1562, 1563*t*
  high-dose-rate comparisons, 1577–1581, 1578*f*,
    1579*t*–1580*t*
 conversion to high-dose-rate brachytherapy, 545–546
 endometrium, 516–517, 516*f*
 endovascular, 532
 esophagus, 502–504, 503*f*–505*f*
 eye, 490–493, 491*f*–493*f*
 gynecologic malignancies, 517
 head and neck, 493–499
 interstitial brain implants, 487–490, 488*f*–489*f*, 490*t*
 intracavitary sources, 426–428, 427*f*–428*f*
 maxillary sinus, 494
 nasal vestibule, 494
 nasopharynx, 495, 496*t*
 oral cavity, 495, 497
 pancreas, 504
 penis and male urethra, 525–527, 526*f*
 prostate, 527–531, 527*t*–528*t*
  gold grain implants, 530
  interstitial irradiation and hyperthermia, 531
  iodine implants, 527–530, 528*f*–529*f*
  iridium interstitial implants, 530–531, 531*f*
  palladium implants, 530
 site targeting, 487–532
 skin and lip, 494–495, 495*f*
 soft-tissue sarcomas, 507–508, 507*f*
 temporary interstitial brachytherapy, 428
 tongue and mouth floor, 497–498, 497*f*–498*f*
 tonsillar/fauchal arch region, 498–499, 500*f*
 uterine cervix, 508–515, 509*f*
  applicators, 510–512
  carcinoma, 510, 511*f*–512*f*
  Henschke applicator, 512, 513*f*
  interstitial implants, 512–515, 513*f*–514*f*, 515*t*
  miscellaneous protocols, 515, 515*t*
 vagina, vulva, and female urethra, 517–524
  bladder/urethral lesions, 521–522
  carcinoma in situ, 520
  rectovaginal septum tumor, 521
  stage I, 520, 520*f*
  stage II, 520
  stages III and IV, 521, 521*f*
  vaginal cylinders, 518–520, 518*f*–519*f*, 524*f*
  vulva/distal urethra tumors, 522–524, 523*f*–524*f*
 vaginal cancer, 1669–1670
 total-body irradiation, complications, 372
Low-malignant potential (LMP) tumors, ovarian cancer, 1629, 1633
Low-melting alloy blocks, photon external-beam dosimetry, field
    shaping, 179–180, 180*f*
Lumpectomy, breast cancer management with, 1203–1204, 1203*f*,
    1223
 complications, 1270
Lung
 anatomy, 1076, 1077*f*
 breast cancer therapy sequelae in, 1271–1272, 1272*f*
 hepatobiliary tract cancer metaseases to, pediatric patients,
    1919–1920
 Hodgkin's lymphoma radiation therapy sequelae in, pediatric
    patients, 1901
 late effects syndromes in, 328–330, 330*f*–331*f*, 330*t*
 total body irradiation, delayed toxicity in, 372
 toxicity effects of therapy in, 1102–1104
Lung cancer
 chemoradiotherapy, 1089–1091, 1089*t*–1090*t*
 clinical presentation, 1078–1079
 combined chemoradiation therapy, 679–681, 681*t*
 diagnostic work-up and staging, 1079–1081, 1081*t*, 1082*f*
 epidemiology, 1076–1077
 high-dose-rate brachytherapy, 568–569, 569*t*
 Hodgkin's lymphoma and, 1735
 image-guided radiation therapy, Real-time Tumor Tracking, 277
 intensity-modulated radiation therapy, 259, 1097–1098
 lymphomas, 1759
 metastatic patterns, 1078, 1078*t*
 natural history, 1077–1078

non-small cell lung cancer, 1083–1091
    adjuvant therapy, 1084–1086
    chemotherapy rationale, 1098–1100
    inoperable staging, 1086–1089, 1086*t*
    neoadjuvant treatment, 1083–1084, 1084*t*
    operable tumor staging, 1083
    proton radiotherapy, 1098
oncologic imaging, 627*f*
pathologic classification, 1081–1082, 1082*t*
pediatric patients, 1915, 1915*f*
photodynamic therapy, 602
prognostic factors, 1082
proton and α-particle radiotherapy, 417–418
radiation therapy, 1094–1097, 1096*f*, 1097*t*
    normal tissue toxicity, 1102–1104, 1103*t*
small cell lung carcinoma, 1100–1102
stereotactic body radiation therapy (SBRT), 386–387, 392, 394*t*,
    395*f*
superior sulcus tumors, 1091–1093, 1094*f*
superior vena cava syndrome, 1093–1094
Lung interfaces
    electron-beam therapy, dosage calculations, 195, 198*f*
    photon external-beam dosimetry, 173, 174*f*
Lycopene, prostate cancer risk and, 1443–1444
Lyman NTCP model, three-dimensional conformal radiation therapy
    evaluation, 232–233
Lymphadenectomy
    bladder cancer treatment, morbidity and mortality, 1415, 1417
    cervical cancer, para-aortic lymph node metastases, 1575–1576,
        1576*t*
    vaginal cancer, 1663–1665
Lymphangiography, cervical cancer radiation therapy, 1553–1555,
    1554*f*–1555*f*
Lymphangioma, pediatric patients, 1925
Lymphatic metastases
    anal cancer, 1384–1385, 1388, 1390
    bladder cancer, 1418–1419, 1419*t*
    breast cancer, 1199
        radiation therapy, 1224–1230, 1252–1255, 1253*f*–1255*f*
    cervical cancer, 1534–1535, 1534*t*–1536*t*, 1535*f*
    esophageal cancer, 1131, 1132*f*
    gallbladder adenocarcinoma, 1360
    hypopharyngeal cancer, 961
    laryngeal cancers, 978–979, 978*f*
    nasopharyngeal cancer, 822–823, 827*f*
    to neck, unknown primary tumors
        anatomy, 1035, 1036*f*, 1036*t*
        biopsy procedures, 1045–1048, 1050*t*
        cervical lymph node metastasis, 1048, 1050*t*–1051*t*,
            1051–1053, 1052*f*
        clinically negative nodes, 1046–1047, 1046*t*
        clinically positive nodes, 1047–1048, 1047*f*, 1047*t*–1049*t*
        diagnostic work-up, 1035–1037
        dissection complications, 1039, 1040*t*, 1041*f*
        natural history, 1035, 1037*t*–1039*t*
        radiation therapy, 1039–1045, 1042*f*–1045*f*, 1046*t*
        radiographic studies, 1036–1037, 1038*f*
        staging, 1037, 1040*t*
        surgical management, 1037, 1039
    oral cavity tumors, 896–897, 897*t*
    oropharyngeal tumors, 916–919, 916*t*–918*t*, 918*f*–923*f*, 920*t*,
        926*t*
    pancreatic cancer, 1336, 1337*f*
    penis, cancer of, 1524–1525, 1524*t*, 1527*f*
    prostate cancer, 1446
        whole pelvic radiation and incidence of, 1486
    renal cell carcinoma, 1398
    renal pelvis and ureter carcinoma, 1398
    stomach cancer, 1318–1319, 1319*f*
    testicular cancer, 1503
    tumor cells, 132–134, 133*f*
    vulvar cancer, 1692–1693, 1693*t*, 1699–1700
Lymphedema, breast cancer radiation therapy and, 1269–1270
Lymph nodes
    anal cancer diagnosis, 1385
    bladder cancer metastases, 1418–1419, 1419*t*
    breast cancer recurrence and, 1218
    cervical anatomy, 1532, 1533*f*
        para-aortic lymph node irradiation, 1556, 1556*f*–1557*f*
    differentiated thyroid cancer involvement, 1062
    elective melanoma radiation therapy involving, 697

Hodgkin's lymphoma, 1721
melanoma radiation therapy involving, 697
mesenchymal tumors, 1122–1123
non-Hodgkin's lymphoma, pathology and classification, 1742,
    1742*t*
prostate cancer, extended pelvic lymph node dissection,
    1486–1487
Lymphocyte depletion Hodgkin's lymphoma, 1725
Lymphoid hyperplasia
    orbital tumors, 780–781
    radiation therapy, 1946
Lymphomas. *See also* Non-Hodgkin's lymphoma; specific
        lymphomas, e.g., Hodgkin's lymphoma
    acquired immunodeficiency syndrome, 703–707
        Hodgkin's lymphoma, 706–707
        non-Hodgkin's lymphoma, 703–706, 705*f*, 705*t*
    central nervous system, 741–743
    cervical cancer, 1541
    gastrointestinal, 1754–1756
    intraocular, 791
    mammary lymphoma, 1197
    orbital tumors, 780–781, 794
    penile tumors, 1523
    prostate tumors, 1456
    radioimmunotherapy, 588–589
    retroperitoneal cancer, 1713
    thyroid lymphoma, 1062, 1067–1069, 1069*f*
    vaginal cancer, 1660, 1674
Lymphotropic superparamagnetic particles, prostate cancer imaging,
    1487

M
Magnetic induction heating, hyperthermia, 650, 650*f*–651*f*
Magnetic resonance imaging (MRI)
    bladder cancer, 1413
    bone metastases, 1988, 1989*f*
    breast cancer
        diagnosis and work-up, 1191*f*, 1192–1193
        screening protocols, 1189
    cervical cancer screening, 1537–1538
    fallopian tubes, 1651
    image-guided radiation therapy, 265–266, 267*f*
    intracranial tumors, 721, 722*f*, 723*f*
    metastatic spinal cord compression, 1981
    oncologic imaging, 621–623, 622*f*–623*f*, 622*t*
        positron emission tomography, 623–624, 623*t*, 624*f*
    prostate cancer, 1451, 1452*f*
    rectal cancer imaging, 1373
    spinal cord tumors, 768, 769*f*
    thyroid disease, 1058, 1059*f*
Magnetic resonance spectroscopic imaging (MSRI)
    image-guided radiation therapy, 266
    prostate cancer, 1451–1453
Magnetron, linear accelerators, 151
Malabsorption syndrome, late effects in small intestine, 344
Male breast cancer, 1311–1312
Male gonadal function, late effects syndromes on normal tissue in,
        346–347
Malignant ascites, phosphorus-32 therapy, 595
Malignant fibrous histiocytoma, classification, 1811
Malignant melanoma, pediatric patients, 1928
Malignant mesenchymal tumors, endometrial cancer, 1610
Malignant mixed müllerian tumors, endometrial cancer, 1613
Malignant pleural mesothelioma, anatomical illustrations, 630
Malpractice issues, radiation oncology, 61–65
Mammalian cell survival curves, radiation therapy and, 90–92, 91*f*
Mammography
    breast cancer
        breast density measurement, 1181
        diagnosis and work-up, 1190–1192, 1190*t*, 1191*f*–1192*t*
        screening protocols, 1187–1189, 1187*t*–1189
    ductal carcinoma in situ, 1164, 1165*f*
    oncologic imaging, 625–626, 626*f*, 627*t*
Mammoplasty, breast cancer therapy and, 1242
MammoSite radiation therapy, breast cancer, 1262
Managed care, radiation oncology and
    ethics issues, 2039
    negotiations between, 2044–2045
Manchester system
    interstitial brachytherapy, 444–447, 444*f*, 445*t*–446*t*, 446*f*–448*f*
    intracavitary brachytherapy, 456–458, 457*f*

Mantle cell lymphoma
    pathology and classification, 1742
    treatment of, 1754
Mantle fields, Hodgkin's lymphoma radiation therapy, 1728, 1728*f*
Marginal zone lymphomas
    clinical-histopathological correlates, 1744–1745
    pathology and classification, 1741
    treatment of, 1753–1754
Margin status
    breast cancer recurrence and, 1212–1215
    prostate cancer recurrence, 1497–1498
    rectal cancer therapy, 1374
    stomach cancer, surgical management and, 1322–1323,
        1322*t*
Marketing issues, radiation oncology practices, 2046–2047
Martinez universal perineal interstitial template (MUPIT),
        brachytherapy, 481, 482*f*
Mass attenuation coefficient, basic principles, 146–147, 147*f*
Mass number, defined, 142–143
Mastectomy
    breast-conserving surgery *vs.*, 1208–1210, 1208*t*, 1209*f*
    ductal carcinoma in situ, 1168
    locally advanced and recurrent disease, 1300–1305, 1300*t*
        neoadjuvant chemotherapy and postmastectomy radiation
            and, 1304–1305
        neoadjuvant chemotherapy and radiation therapy, 1304–1305
        radiation therapy following, 1300–1303, 1301*f*, 1303*t*,
            1312–1315
        recurrence risk following, 1303–1304, 1303*t*, 1310–1311
    nipple-sparing, 1203
    in pediatric patients, 1915–1916
    radiation techniques following, 1312–1315
        breast reconstruction and, 1314–1315
    radiation *vs.*, 1204–1205, 1204*t*
    skin-sparing, 1203
Matrix proteasis, tumor invasion and metastasis, 113–114
Matter-particle interactions, radioactivity, 147–148, 148*f*
Maxillary sinuses
    anatomy, 858
    brachytherapy, 494
    clinical presentation, 861
    disease management, 862
    natural history, 859–860, 860*f*
    radiation therapy, 866–868, 866*f*–867*f*
    treatment results, 870–871, 872*t*
Maximal heart distance (MHD), breast cancer radiation therapy,
        1245–1246, 1247*f*–1248*f*
McCabe-Fletcher chemodectoma classification, 998, 999*t*
Mean central dose (MCD) calculation, interstitial brachytherapy
    calculation methods, 453
    Manchester system, 446–447, 447*f*
Mechanical uncertainties, radiation therapy, 7–8
Mediastinoscopy
    lung cancer diagnosis, 1080
    superior sulcus tumors, 1092
Mediastinum
    anatomy, 1109, 1110*f*, 1111*t*
    germ cell tumors, 1117–1119
    mesenchymal tumors, 1122–1123
    myasthenia gravis management, 1116
    neurogenic tumors, 1123–1124
    primary tumor incidence, 1109
    thymic carcinoid, 1117
    thymic carcinoma, 1116–1117
    thymoliposarcoma, 1117
    thymomas, 1109–1116
        chemotherapy, 1115
        combined treatment modalities, 1115, 1116*t*
        diagnosis, 1110
        epidemiology, 1109
        natural history, 1109–1110
        pathologic classification, 1110–1112, 1111*t*
        prognostic factors, 1112–1113, 1113*t*–1114*t*
        radiation therapy, 1114–1116
        recurrent disease, 1114
        staging, 1112, 1112*t*
        surgical management, 1113–1114
    tracheal carcinomas, 1119–1122
Medical errors, medical ethics and, 2040–2041
Medical ethics. *See* Ethics in medicine
Medicare claims

pay for performance paradigm, 2048
    radiation oncology and denial of, 2043
Medullary carcinoma
    breast cancer, 1196
    pediatric patients, 1922–1924, 1923*t*
    thyroid cancer
        chemotherapy, 1070
        classification, 1061
        management of, 1066–1068, 1067*f*
        prognostic factors, 1062
        radiation therapy, 1068
Medulloblastoma
    diagnosis and management, 740–741
    pediatric patients, 1836–1841, 1836*f*
        management, 1837–1841
        staging, 1837, 1837*t*
Megavoltage photon units
    electron beam radiation, 150
    image-guided radiation therapy, volumetric imaging systems,
        281–282, 282*f*
Melanomas
    hyperthermia therapy, 663
    nonlentiginous melanoma, 1025–1026
    pediatric patients, 1928
    posterior uvea, 782–784, 783*t*–784*t*
    skin lesions
        epidemiology, 695–696
        epidemiology and etiology, 690
        follow-up, 698
        management, 696–698
        staging, 696, 696*t*
    vaginal cancer, 1659, 1663, 1672–1673
    vulvar cancer, 1694, 1697
Meningeal leukemia, diagnosis and treatment, 1782–1783
Meningiomas
    diagnosis and management, 743–744
    extracranial, 1024
    intradural-extramedullary tumors, 769–770
    nonmalignant disease, radiation therapy, 1935–1936, 1935*t*,
        1936*f*
    stereotactic radiosurgery, 385
Merkel cell carcinoma
    epidemiology and etiology, 690, 698
    prognosis, 699
    treatment, 698–699
    vulvar cancer, 1694
MERT technique, electron arc therapy, 214–215
Mesenchymal tumors
    endometrial cancer, 1613
    mediastinum, 1122–1123
Meta-analysis
    defined, 357
    high-dose-rate *vs.* low-dose-rate brachytherapy, 563–564, 563*t*
Metal oxide semiconductor-field effect transistors (MOSFETs),
        semiconductor dosimetry, 160
Metaplastic carcinoma, breast cancer, 1197
Metastases. *See also* Recurrent disease; Secondary cancers
    adrenal, palliative therapy, 2001
    anal cancer, 1384–1385, 1388, 1390
    biliary tract, palliative therapy, 2000–2001
    biology of, 44–46, 45*f*–46*f*
    bladder cancer recurrence, 1419
    brain
        magnetic resonance imaging, 622, 622*f*
        palliative therapy
            anticonvulsants, 1978–1979
            clinical presentation, diagnosis, and prognosis, 1974, 1975*t*
            concurrent radiosensitizers, 1977
            corticosteroids, 1974
            neurocognitive decline, 1977–1978
            postoperative radiation therapy, 1976
            radiosurgery boost trials, 1975, 1976*t*, 1979*t*
            surgical resection, 1974–1975, 1975*f*, 1978*t*
            whole-brain radiation therapy, 1974–1977, 1975*t*, 1977*f*,
              1980*t*
        stereotactic radiosurgery, 386
    breast cancer, 1183–1186, 1197–1202
        age as factor, 1201
        axillary spread, 1183–1184, 1184*t*, 1198, 1199*f*
            unknown primary tumors, 1311
        DNA ploidy index, 1200

estrogen/progesterone hormone receptors, 1199
genetic cancer, 1201, 1201*f*
HER-2/neu activity, 1200
internal mammary spread, 1184, 1184*t*, 1228–1230, 1229*t*
local control and, 1185–1186, 1187*f*
lymphatic and vascular invasion, 1199
micrometastasis, 1198–1199
obesity/body mass index, 1202
p53 gene mutation, 1200–1201
pregnancy, 1202
proliferative indices/S-phase/thymidine labeling index, 1200
race as factor, 1201–1202
serum markers, 1202
smoking risk, 1202
supraclavicular spread, 1184–1185, 1253, 1253*f*
systemic spread, 1185
tumor grade, 1199
tumor location, 1202
tumor size, 1198, 1198*f*
tumor type, 1199
urokinase-type plasminogen activator/plasminogen activator
inhibitor type, 1201
cardiac tumors, 1155, 1155*t*, 1158
cervical cancer
para-aortic lymph nodes, 1574–1576, 1576*t*
patterns of, 1534–1535, 1534*t*–1536*t*, 1535*f*
small-cell carcinomas, 1548
tumor factors in, 1543–1544, 1544*t*
cholangiocarcinoma, 1357
colorectal cancer, 1366–1367
endometrial cancer, 1622–1623
esophageal cancer, 1133–1134, 1134*t*, 1135*f*
Ewing's sarcoma, 1886, 1889
gynecologic cancer, palliative therapy, 2002, 2002*t*, 2003*f*
Hodgkin's lymphoma, 1721–1722
hyperthermia and, 646–647
hypopharyngeal cancer and patterns of, 960–961, 961*f*, 969–970
intraocular tumors, 782–787, 783*t*–784*t*, 785*f*–786*f*
laryngeal cancer, 976–979
liver, palliative therapy, 2000, 2001*f*, 2001*t*
lung cancer, 1078, 1078*t*
nasopharyngeal cancer
hematogenous dissemination, 823
lymphatic spread, 822–823, 827*f*
oral cavity, 896–897, 897*t*
orbital tumors, 794
ovarian cancer, 1631, 1634
brain metastases, 1644–1645
pancreatic cancer, 1336, 1337*f*
penis, cancer of, 1520, 1523, 1524–1525, 1524*t*, 1527*f*
prostate cancer, 1445–1446
renal cell carcinoma, 1398
local therapy, 1405
renal pelvis and ureter carcinoma, 1398, 1405–1406
retroperitoneal cancer, 1708–1709
rhabdomyosarcoma, 1872, 1877
soft tissue sarcomas, 1808–1809, 1818
spinal cord compression (MSCC), palliative therapy
clinical presentation, diagnosis, and prognosis, 1979, 1981
corticosteroids, 1981
epidemiology, 1979
intramedullary metastases, 1984
pathophysiology, 1979
pediatric patients, 1984
radiation therapy, 1982–1984
surgical management, 1981–1982, 1982*t*, 1983*f*
spine, stereotactic radiosurgery, 386
splenic, 2001–2002
stomach cancer, 1318–1319, 1319*f*
thyroid cancer, pediatric patients, 1923–1924
tumor invasion and, 113–114
urethral cancer, female, 1682
vaginal cancers, 1660, 1661*t*
vulvar tumors, 1692–1693, 1693*t*
Wilms' tumor, 1851, 1856
Methotrexate
acute lymphoblastic leukemia, 1781–1782
radiation combined with
head and neck squamous-cell tumors, 809
late effects syndromes on normal tissue, 325–326, 326*t*, 327*f*
Microcirculation, tumor cells, 128–130, 129*f*–131*f*

Microinvasive breast cancer
classification, 1167
defined, 1196
Microinvasive cervical cancer, 1547–1548
Micrometastasis, breast cancer, 1198–1199
Microtrons, components and applications, 152, 154
Microwave power, lnear accelerators, 151
Middle East, radiation therapy in, 608
Milligram-hours, brachytherapy dosimetry, 435
intracavitary brachytherapy, 458–460, 459*f*
MIMIC collimator, tomotherapy, and, 240
Minicolpostats, brachytherapy, cervical carcinoma, 512
Minimum peripheral dose, interstitial brachytherapy, 451–454
Minority practice doctrine, radiation oncology, 62–65
Misonidazole, chemical modifiers of radiation therapy, 613
Mitigating compounds, chemical radioprotection, 615–617, 616*f*
Mitogenic signals, growth control and, 110–111
Mitomycin C (MMC)
cervical cancer therapy, 1592
combined chemoradiation therapy, 677*t*, 678
hypoxic cell targeting, 613–614
Mitotane, adrenal gland tumor therapy, 1719
Mitotic cell death, radiation therapy, 77–78
Mixed-beam techniques
electron beam therapy, 206–207, 208*f*, 209
fast neutron radiotherapy
prostate cancer, 411
salivary gland tumors, 409–410
Mixed cellularity Hodgkin's lymphoma, 1725
Mixed epithelial tumors, endometrial cancer, 1613
Mixed germ-cell tumors, testis, 1505
Mixed neuronal-glial tumors, pediatric patients, 1835
MLC and associated dosimetry, field shaping applications, 181,
181*f*
Mobile fluoroscopic C-arm systems, image-guided radiation therapy,
282–283, 283*f*
Modulation factor, tomotherapy, 154
Modulator instrumentation, lnear accelerators, 151
Mold techniques, brachytherapy, 481, 483
Molecular cascade, colorectal cancer, 1366–1367
Molecular forensics, radiation-induced tumors, 54–55
Molecular genetics
anaplastic glioma, 735–736, 736
breast cancer, recurrent disease, 1218–1219, 1219*t*
ductal carcinoma in situ, 1164–1167, 1166*f*–1167*f*
Ewing tumor, 1886
fallopian tube malignancies, 1653
intracranial tumors, 723–724
nonpilocytic/diffusely infiltrating gliomas, 737–738
oral cavity tumors, 895
principles of, 109–114
prostate cancer risk, 1444, 1445*t*
radiation oncology and, 36–37, 37*f*
soft tissue sarcomas, 1808, 1811*f*
Molecular imaging
altered fractionation radiotherapy and, 317
defined, 109
Molecular pathology, defined, 109
Molecular pathophysiology, defined, 109
Molecular radiation biology
base excision repair, 116
biological consequences, 115
cell cycle delay, 117
cell death, 115
DNA damage, 115–116
DNA repair, 116
DSB repair, 116–117
G1 phase, 117, 118*f*
G2 phase, 118, 118*f*
gene expression, 118–119
mutagenesis and genomic instability, 121
signaling mechanisms, 119–121
S phase, 117–118
target molecules, 114–115
Molecular targeting
altered fractionation radiotherapy and, 317
chemoradiation therapy, 674–676, 674*t*, 675*f*
defined, 109
non-small cell lung cancer therapy, 1099–1100
pancreatic cancer, 1346
renal cell carcinoma, 1404

Monitor unit (MU) calculations
electron-beam therapy, 197–198, 199f–200f
intensity-modulated radiation therapy, 252
verification, 254
photon external-beam dosimetry, 166–168, 167f–168f
Monoclonal antibodies
cancer targeting, 584–588
immunoliposomes and radioimmunoliposomes, 585–586
immunotoxins, 585
naked antibodies, 584–585, 585t
radioimmunoglobulins, 585
clinical results, 587–588
development of, 586
isotope selection, 586
leukemia and lymphoma therapy, 588–589
solid tumor therapy, 589–591
toxicity effects, 586–587
Monoclonal gammopathy, plasma cell myeloma/plasmacytoma,
1790, 1791t
Monte Carlo calculations
brachytherapy, photon transport simulation, 439–442, 439f, 441t
electron-beam therapy, dose algorithms, 199–200, 201f
evolution of, 190
MERT therapy and, 215
photon external-beam dosimetry, tissue inhomogeneity
correction, 170–171
three-dimensional conformal radiation therapy, 231
Mood dysfunction, supportive care for, 2011–2012
Morbidity rates
interstitial brachytherapy, 517
photodynamic therapy, 603
Morbus Dupuytren/Morbus Ledderhose, 1951–1952, 1951t, 1952f,
1953t
Morbus Peyronie, 1950–1951
Morning check protocol, high-dose-rate brachytherapy, 548
Motion artifacts
image-guided radiation therapy (IGRT), 268
radiation therapy, 8–10, 8f, 9t–10t
Motorized wedge filter, photon external-beam dosimetry, 175
Mouth floor tumors
anatomy, 891
brachytherapy, 497–498, 497f–498f
treatment and results, 909
MSKCC system, image-guided radiation therapy, 279–280
MUC-1 glycoprotein, radioimmunotherapy with, 590–591
Mucinous carcinoma
breast cancer, pathological characteristics, 1197
prostate tumors, 1455
Mucosal-associated lymphoid tissue (MALT) lymphomas
clinical-histopathological correlates, 1744–1745
gastric lymphomas, 1755
pathology and classification, 1741
treatment of, 1753–1754
Mucosal injury, supportive care for, 2013–2016
Mucosal melanomas, diagnosis and management, 1025
Mucositis
chemical radioprotection, 615–617, 616f
gastrointestinal, 2014–2016, 2015t
nasal cavity and paranasal sinus therapy and, 871–872
oral, supportive care for, 2013–2014, 2014f, 2014t
pain management, 2009
Multicentric disease
breast cancer in patients with, 1241, 1242t
prostate cancer, 1445–1446
Multifraction survival curves, radiation therapy, 92f–94f, 93–94
Multileaf collimator (MLC)
electron-beam therapy, 202
Hodgkin's lymphoma radiation therapy, 1727
image-guided radiation therapy, beam tracking technology, 289
intensity-modulated radiation therapy, 240
characteristics of, 252, 252f
fixed-field sequences, 250–251, 250f
quality assurance, 253–255
step-and-shoot/multisegment techniques, 251–252
linear accelerator, 152, 152f
photon external-beam dosimetry, monitor unit calculations, 167
Multiple-beam arrangements, photon external-beam dosimetry, 177,
177f–178f
Multiple endocrine neoplasia (MEN) syndrome
adrenal gland tumors, 1717–1718
pediatric patients, 1922

Multiple myeloma
asymptomatic, 1790, 1791t
clinical presentation, 1790
management, 1794, 1795f
prognostic factors, 1792–1793
radiation therapy, 1795–1796
staging, 1792t
Multisegment approach, intensity-modulated radiation therapy, 240
leaf sequence generation, 251–252
Multivariate analysis, cervical cancer therapy outcomes, 1572–1573
Muscle spasm, pain management, 2008–2009
Musculoskeletal effects, Hodgkin's lymphoma radiation therapy,
pediatric patients, 1901, 1901f
Mutagenesis, genomic instability and, 121
Myasthenia gravis
management of, 1116
natural history, 1109–1110
MYCN proto-oncogene, neuroblastoma, 1863
Mycosis fungoides, cutaneous T-cell lymphoma, 1766–1767, 1767f
radiation therapy, 1769–1774, 1771t
Myc transcription factors, molecular cancer biology and, 111
Myeloablative stem cell transplantation
multiple myeloma, 1795
neuroblastoma in pediatric patients, 1867
total body irradiation, 365
Myeloma, classification, 1790, 1791t
Myocardial tumors, 1155
Myxopapillary ependymoma, pediatric patients, 1834

N
Naked antibodies, cancer targeting, 584–585, 585t
Nasal cavity tumors
anatomy, 858
chemotherapy, 862
clinical presentation, 860
diagnostic work-up, 861, 861t
epdiemiology, 858–859
follow-up and recurrences, 868
lymphomas, 1757
management, 862
natural history, 858
palliative therapy, 862
pathologic classification, 861–862
prognostic factors, 862
radiation therapy, 695, 863–868
brachytherapy, 864
dose fractionation schedule, 865t, 866
external beam, 863–864, 863f
setup and field arrangement, 863f, 864–866, 865f, 865t
target volumes, 863–864
sequelae of treatment, 871–872, 872t
treatment results, 868–871, 870t
tumor staging, 861, 861t
Nasal vestibule
anatomy, 858
brachytherapy, 494
clinical presentation, 860
disease management, 862
natural history, 858, 858f, 859, 859f
pathologic classifications, 861–862
radiation therapy, 863–864, 863f
treatment results, 868–869, 869t
Nasopharyngeal cancer
accelerated fractionation radiotherapy, 310
α-particle radiotherapy, 416
anatomy, 820, 821f–822f, 822t
angiofibroma
clinical presentation and pathology, 1020–1021
diagnostic work-up, 1021, 1022f
epidemiology, 1020
juvenile nasopharyngeal angiofibroma, 1914–1915, 1914t
management, 1022–1023
radiation therapy, 1023–1024, 1023f
staging and prognostic factors, 1021–1022, 1022t
brachytherapy, 494–495, 496t
chemotherapy, 840–844, 842t, 843f, 844t
clinical presentation, 823, 827t
combined chemoradiation therapy, 844–846, 845f, 845t
diagnosis and staging, 823–825, 828t
dose escalation and altered fractionation, 836–837, 840, 841f,
841t

epidemiology, 820, 823f–824f, 824t
future research issues, 853–854
hematogenous dissemination, 823
local extension, 822, 825f–826f, 825t
lymphatic metastases, 822–823, 827f
magnetic resonance imaging, 622–623, 623f
oncological anatomy, 629–630, 629t
pathologic classification, 826, 830f, 830t
pediatric patients, 1913, 1914t
persistent/recurrent cancer, 846–848, 846t–847t, 848f
prognositic factors, 826–830, 831f
proton and α-particle radiotherapy, 416
radiation therapy, 831–840
    dose, time, and fractionation, 831–832, 833t
    intensity-modulated techniques, 834–836, 836t, 837f–839f, 840t
    three-dimensional conformal techniques, 833–834, 835f
    treatment preparation, 831, 831f–832f
    tumor target volumes, 832, 833t
    two-dimensional techniques, 832–833, 834f–835f
sequelae of treatment, 851–853, 851t, 852f
staging system, 825–826, 828f, 829t
treatment results, 848–850, 849f–850f, 849t–850t
treatment strategy, 831
National Electrical Manufacturers Association Code of Ethics, 2038
Natural killer (NK) cell suppression, radioimmunoglobulins, 583
Nausea and vomiting, gastrointestinal mucositis, 2015, 2015t
Near-surface lesions, nonmalignant disease radiation, 1935
Neck metastases
nasal cavitiy and paranasal sinus radiation therapy, 868
oropharyngal tumors, 916–919, 916t–918t, 918f–923f, 920t, 926t
unknown primary tumors
    anatomy, 1035, 1036f, 1036t
    biopsy procedures, 1045–1048, 1050t
    cervical lymph node metastasis, 1048, 1050t–1051t, 1051–1053, 1052f
    clinically negative nodes, 1046–1047, 1046t
    clinically positive nodes, 1047–1048, 1047f, 1047t–1049t
    diagnostic work-up, 1035–1037
    dissection complications, 1039, 1040t, 1041f
    natural history, 1035, 1037t–1039t
    radiation therapy, 1039–1045, 1042f–1045f, 1046t
    radiographic studies, 1036–1037, 1038f
    staging, 1037, 1040t
    surgical management, 1037, 1039
Necrotic cell death
molecular radiation and, 115
radiation therapy and, 77–78
Neoadjuvant therapy
bladder cancer, 1432–1433, 1433t
breast cancer, locally advanced and recurrent disease, 1297–1299, 1297t
cervical cancer, 1596
non-small cell lung cancer, 1083–1084, 1084t
oral cavity radiation therapy, 902
pancreatic cancer, 1342–1343
rectal cancer, 1377–1378
Neovagina, squamous cell carcinoma in, 1675–1676
Nephrectomy
renal cell carcinomas
    results and techniques, 1402–1403
    survival analyses, 1400–1402, 1401t, 1407–1409, 1408t
Wilms' tumor, 1853, 1856
Nephroureterectomy, renal pelvis and ureter carcinomas, 1405, 1409
Nerve sheath tumors, pathologic classification, 770
Nested isotherms, hyperthermia, 656, 656f
Neuraxis imaging, intracranial tumors, 722
Neuroablative pain management protocols, 2008
Neuroaxial pain management, 2008
Neuroblastoma
pediatric patients
    chemotherapy, 1865–1869
    clinical presentation, 1859–1860
    combined treatment modalities, 1863–1867, 1865t
    diagnostic work-up, 1860, 1861f–1863f
    epidemiology, 1859
    metastatic spinal cord compression, 1984
    natural history, 1859
    pathologic classification, 1860–1861
    prognostic factors, 1861, 1863, 1864t

radiation therapy, 1867–1869, 1868f
    staging, 1860, 1864t
    surgical management, 1863, 1865, 1865t, 1868–1869
retroperitoneal cancer, 1713
Neurocytoma, pediatric patients, 1835
Neuroendocrine system. See also specific organs
late effects syndromes in, 345
nasopharyngeal cancer therapy effects on, 853
pediatric patients, 1921–1927
prostate cancer, 1455
small cell carcinoma, breast cancer, 1197
total body irradiation and, 373
vaginal cancers, 1660
Neurofibroma, diagnosis and management, 745–746
Neurofibromatosis, pediatric patients
low-grade astrocytomas, 1824–1828
optic gliomas, 1829–1830
Neurogenic tumors, epidemiology and management, 1123–1124
Neurologic injury
photodynamic therapy, 601
stereotactic radiosurgery, 381, 381f
Neuronal tumors, pediatric patients, 1835
Neuropathy
intraoperative radiation therapy and, 398–399
pain management and, 2007
Neutron capture therapy. See Boron neutron capture therapy (BNCT)
Neutron radiation therapy. See also Fast neutron radiotherapy
beam units
    components and instrumentation, 154–155, 155f
    quality assurance for, 103–104
bladder tumors, 1426
cervical cancer, 1573
salivary gland tumors, 887–888
Neutrons, basic properties, 149
Neutropenia, late effects syndromes on bone and, 349
Nevi, premalignant skin lesions, 692
NFκB expression, radiation damage and, 118–119
Nimorazole, chemical modifiers of radiation therapy, 613
No action level (NAL) strategy, electronic portal imaging devices, 273
Nociceptive pain, defined, 2005
Nodular lymphocyte predominance Hodgkin's lymphoma, 1724–1725, 1731
Nodular sclerosis Hodgkin's lymphoma, 1725
Nominal standard dose (NSD), time-dose factor, radiation therapy, 25–26
Nonacoustic schwannomas, stereotactic radiosurgery, 385
Nonafterloading (preloaded) systems, temporary interstitial brachytherapy, 428
Noncoplanar directional availability, fixed-gantry intensity-modulated field protocols, 256–257
Nonendometroid tumors, classification, 1611–1612, 1612t
Nonepithelial tumors, vaginal cancer, 1659–1660, 1672–1673
Nonfunctioning pituitary tumors, management of, 756, 756f
Nongerminomatous germ cell tumors, pediatric patients, 1843–1844, 1844t
Non-Hodgkin's lymphoma (NHL). See also specific lymphomas
acquired immunodeficiency syndrome, 703–706, 705f, 705t
    central nervous system, 703–705
    diagnostic work-up, 704
    disease patterns, 703, 704f
    epidemiology and risk factors, 703
    general management, 704
    pathology and prognostic factors, 704
    radiation, 704–705, 705f, 705t
    systemic, 705–706
chemotherapy, 1748–1750
clinical features, 1742–1743
clinical-histopathologic correlates, 1744–1745
combined treatment modallities, 1747–1750
epidemiology, 1739
etiology, 1739–1740
immunotherapy, 1750
nodal vs. extra-nodal disease, 1742, 1742t
pathology and immunology, 1740–1742, 1740t, 1742t
pediatric patients
    chemotherapy, 1905–1907, 1905f, 1906t, 1907f
    clinical presentation, 1903–1904, 1903t
    diagnostic evaluation, 1904
    epidemiology, 1903
    future research issues, 1908–1909
    overt central nervous system disease, 1908

Non-Hodgkin's lymphoma (NHL) (*contd.*)
    pathologic classification, 1903*t*
    prognostic factors, 1905, 1905*f*, 1905*t*
    radiation therapy, 1907–1909, 1909*f*
    staging systems, 1904–1905, 1904*t*
  positron emission tomography, 624, 624*f*
  prognostic factors, 1743–1744, 1743*t*–1744*t*
  radiation therapy, 1745–1748, 1746*f*–1747*f*
  risk factors, 703
  staging, 1742–1743, 1742*t*–1743*t*
  stem cell transplantation, 1749–1750
  surgical management, 1745
Non-homologous end-joining (NHEJ), DBS repair, 116–117
Noninvasive thermal dose measurements, hyperthermia, 657–658, 657*f*–659*f*
Nonlentiginous melanoma, diagnosis and management, 1025–1026
Nonmaleficence principle, medical ethics and, 2035–2036
Nonmalignant disease, radiation therapy
  application principles, 1933, 1934*t*
  bony tissue, 1954–1956
  clinical trials, 1933
  connective tissue effects, 1934
  deep lesions, 1935
  disease classification, 1933
  dose principles, 1934, 1934*t*
  eye and orbit, 1941–1946
  head and neck tumors, 1935–1941
  inflammatory effects, 1934
  intracranial lesions, 1935
  joints and tendons, 1946–1949
  near-surface lesions, 1935
  pain and related symptoms, 1934
  radiobiological aspects, 1933–1934
  rationale, 1933
  skin and connective tissue disease, 1949–1954
  treatment planning, 1935
  tumor/leukemia induction risk, 1933
  vascular system effects, 1934
Nonmelanoma skin cancer (NMSC)
  epidemiology and etiology, 690, 691*f*
  follow-up and prevention, 693
  radiation therapy, 695
  staging and classification, 692, 692*t*
  surgical management, 692–693
Nonmyeloablative stem cell transplantation, total-body irradiation, 367
Non-nociceptive pain, defined, 2005
Nonoral adminstration routes, for pain management, 2007–2008
Nonpilocytic/diffusely infiltrating gliomas, 737–738
Nonsealed radionuclide therapy
  biophysical properties, 591–592
  bone metastases, 592–594, 593*t*
  clinical results, 592–594
  safety and quality assurance, 595–596
Non-small cell lung cancer (NSCLC), 1083–1091
  accelerated fractionation radiotherapy, 310
    hybrid techniques, 308*t*–309*t*, 311–312, 311*f*
  adjuvant therapy, 1084–1086
  anatomical illustrations, 631–632
  chemotherapy rationale, 1098–1100
  combined chemoradiation therapy, lung cancer, 680–681, 681*t*
  fast neutron radiotherapy, 410, 410*f*
  hyperfractionation radiation therapy, clinical trials, 306, 310
  inoperable staging, 1086–1089, 1086*t*
  neoadjuvant treatment, 1083–1084, 1084*t*
  operable tumor staging, 1083
  positron emission tomography, 623–624, 623*t*, 624*f*
  proton radiotherapy, 1098
Non-total body irradiation regimens, development of, 366
Nonuniform dose distribution, brachytherapy, 467–468
Normal tissue complication probability (NTCP)
  chemical modifiers of radiation therapy, 611
  hepatocellular carcinoma radiation therapy, 1353–1354, 1354*t*
  intensity-modulated radiation therapy, breast cancer, 258–259
  radiation therapy, 19–20
  stereotactic body radiation therapy, liver, 391–392, 393*f*
  three-dimensional conformal radiation therapy evaluation, 232–233
Normal tissue effects
  chemoradiation therapy, protection strategies, 676–677
  imaging, 626–627, 626–628, 627*f*, 627*t*

  intraoperative radiotherapy, 401*t*
  late effects of cancer treatment
    bone and bone marrow, 347–349, 349*f*, 349*t*
    brain, 326, 326*t*, 327*f*
    central nervous system, 323–326, 325*f*, 325*t*
    colorectum, 342–344
    critical organ tolerance, 323
    dentition, 344
    esophagus, 342–344
    eye, 328
    future research issues, 350
    gastrointestinal tract, 340–344, 343*f*
    hearing loss, 327–328
    heart, 332–336, 333*f*–335*f*, 334*t*–335*t*
    kidney, 338–340, 339*f*–341*f*, 340*t*–341*t*
    LENT paradigm, 323
    liver, 336–338, 337*f*, 338*t*
    lung, 328–330, 330*f*–331*f*, 330*t*
    neuroendocrine system, 345
    organ tolerance principles, 320–321, 321*f*
    overview of, 320
    radiation effects, 321–323, 322*f*, 322*t*–323*t*
    reproductive systems, 346–347
    salivary glands, 344–345
    second malignant neoplasms, 349–350
    skin and soft tissue, 330–332, 332*t*
    small intestine, 342–344
    spinal cord, 326–327, 328*t*
    stomach, 342–344, 342*f*
    thyroid, 345–346
  lung cancer therapy, 1102–1104, 1103*t*
  oropharyngeal tumor radiation therapy, 936–937
  prostate cancer radiation therapy, 1459
  radiotherapy, 18–20, 19*f*–20*f*
    cell death mechanisms, 77–78
    dose volume histograms, 103
    functional subunits (FSUs), 80
    injury pathobiology and kinetics, 78–80
    molecular responses, 82
    regeneration and repopulation, 82–83, 83*f*
    tumor control probability and, 95–97, 96*f*
  stereotactic body radiation therapy
    liver, 391–392, 393*f*
    lung, 392, 394*t*, 395*f*
  stereotactic radiosurgery, 381–382
Norton-Simon hypothesis, stereotactic body radiation therapy, 390
Novalis system, image-guided radiation therapy, 274, 276–277, 276*f*
Nuclear scan imaging
  fallopian tubes, 1651
  neuroblastoma, pediatric patients, 1860
Nuclear structure, basic principles, 142–143, 143*f*
Nuremberg Code, 2037–2038
Nutritional support, radiation therapy and, 2017–2018

O

Obesity, breast cancer metastatic risk and, 1202
Objective functions
  high-dose-rate brachytherapy, dosimetry and treatment planning, 552–555
  intensity-modulated radiation therapy, 247–249, 248*f*
Oblique filtration, radionuclides, 425–426
Occupational exposure, non-Hodgkin's lymphoma, 1739–1740
Odynophagia, late effects syndromes in esophagus and, 343–344
Off-axis ratios (OARs)
  electron-beam therapy
    total-skin irradiation, 212–213, 213*f*
    water-based dose distribution, 192–193, 193*f*
  photon external-beam dosimetry, 167–168
Oligometastases theory, stereotactic body radiation therapy, 390
Oncogenes
  cervical cancer, 1544–1545
  molecular cancer biology, 109, 110*t*
  radiation oncology and, 37–39, 38*f*–39*f*
Oncologic anatomy (onco-anatomy). *See also* Radiation oncology
  basic principles, 628–629, 628*t*
  breast cancer and internal mammary nodes, 630–631, 631*t*
  cervical cancer and uterosacral ligaments, 633
  elective nodal irradiation and modern treatment planning, 633
  Hodgkin's disease and spleen, 633
  malignant pleural mesothelioma and pleural recesses, 630, 630*f*
  nasopharynx and cranial nerves, 629–630, 629*t*

non-small-cell lung cancer and postoperative radiation therapy, 631–632, 632*f*

white matter tracts, brainstem, diffuse pontine gliomas, 632–633

Oncologic imaging
    computed tomography, 620–621, 621*f*
    endoscopic ultrasonography, 625, 625*t*
    intracranial tumors, 720–722, 721*t*, 722*f*, 723*t*
    magnetic resonance imaging, 621–623, 622*f*–623*f*, 622*t*
    mammography/ultrasonography, 625–626, 626*f*
    positron emission tomography, 623–624, 623*t*, 624*f*
    radionuclide bone scan and metastases, 624–625

Oncologist education, 633–634, 634*f*

Ophthalmic disease, photodynamic therapy, 601

Opiates
    adjuvant therapy and, 2007
    pain management and side effects of, 2006–2007, 2006*t*

Optical density, film dosimetry, 159

Optic glioma, 791–792
    pediatric patients, 1829–1830

Optic nerve tolerance
    radiation injury and, 796
    stereotactic radiosurgery, 381–382

Optic pathway
    gliomas, proton/α-particle radiotherapy, 413
    nasal cavity and paranasal sinus therapy and, 871–872

Optimal dose rate, low-dose rate irradiation, 101

Optimization
    high-dose-rate brachytherapy, 541
        dosimetry and treatment planning, 552–555, 554*f*
    intensity-modulated radiation therapy, 246–247, 247*f*
        oropharyngeal tumors, 950
    MERT therapy and, 215
    stomach cancer radiation therapy, 1324–1329, 1324*t*–1326*t*, 1326*f*–1329*f*

Oral cavity tumors
    anatomy, 891–892
    brachytherapy, 495, 497
    carcinoma distribution, 896*f*
    clinical presentation, 898, 898*f*–899*f*
    diagnostic evaluation, 898–900
    epidemiology, 893–895
    lymphatic metastases, 896–897, 897*t*
    management of, 900–901
    metastates, patterns of, 896–897, 896*f*
    molecular biology, 895–896, 895*f*–896*f*
    nasopharyngeal cancer therapy complications in, 853
    overview, 891, 892*f*–894*f*
    pathologic classification, 897–898, 898*f*
    premalignant lesions, 895
    radiation therapy, 901–907
        adjuvant protocols, 902
        altered fractionation, 904
        brachytherapy, 904–905, 905*f*
        chemotherapy and, 906
        dental care, 906–907, 907*f*–908*f*
        dose and fractionation, 903–904
        intraoral cone, 905–906, 906*f*
        neoadjuvant therapy, 902
        prognostic and predictive factors, 907–908
        techniques, 902–903, 902*f*–904*f*
    staging protocols, 900, 900*t*
    subsite-specific treatment and results, 908–910
    surgical management, 901

Oral hygiene
    mucositis prevention, 2013–2014
    xerostomia management and, 2013

Orbital lymphomas, 1758

Orbital rhabdomyosarcoma, pediatric patients, 1874–1875, 1875*f*

Orchiectomy, seminoma therapy, 1508–1510, 1509*t*–1510*t*

Organ boosting, total body irradiation, 372

Organ-confined, lymph-node negative tumors, bladder cancer, 1417

Organ motion
    prostate cancer radiation therapy, 1461–1463, 1484–1486
    radiation therapy, 8–10, 8*f*, 9*t*

Organ tolerance, late effects syndromes on normal tissue
    basic principles of, 320–321, 321*f*
    critical organ tolerance, 323

Oropharyngeal tumors
    anatomy, 913, 914*f*–915*f*
    base of tongue, 926–927, 928*t*
    brachytherapy, 943–944, 943*f*, 944*t*
    chemotherapy and altered fractionation regimes, 944–946, 945*f*
    clinical presentation, 919–920
    diagnostic work-up, 920–921
    epidemiology, 913
    lateral and posterior pharyngeal wall tumors, 927, 929–930, 931*t*
    lymphatics, 916–919, 916*t*–918*t*, 918*f*–923*f*, 920*t*, 926*t*
    management strategies, results and outcomes, 923–925
    natural history, 913, 915–916, 915*f*
    pathologic classification, 921–922
    pediatric patients, 1913–1914
    prognostic factors, 922–923
    radiation therapy, 933–938, 933*f*–936*f*
        clinical results, 950
        cone beam computed tomography, 951
        cyberknife, 951, 951*f*
        dose and fractionation sites, 935
        dose-calculation algorithms, 951
        external beam radiation therapy, 950–951
        helical tomography, 950
        intensity-modulated radiation therapy, 946–950, 947*t*–948*t*, 948*f*–949*f*, 950*t*
        nonrandomized studies, 945–946
        paperless electronic records, 952, 952*f*
        randomized trials, 946
        side effects, 936–938, 938*t*
        three-dimensional conformal therapy, 946–950
        xerostomia, 937–938, 939*f*
    socioeconomic outcomes and quality of life, 938–943, 939*f*–943*f*, 939*t*
    staging protocols, 921
    tonsillar fossa and/or soft palate tumors, 925–926, 925*f*–926*f*, 925*t*–927*t*
    treatment results, 929–932, 929*f*–930*f*, 932*f*–933*f*

Orthogonal field junctions, photon external-beam dosimetry, 185, 186*f*–187*f*

Orthovoltage (deep-therapy) units. *See also* Intraoperative radiation/intraoperative electron irradiation therapy (IORT/IOERT)
    radiation therapy machines, 149–150

Osteosarcoma
    chemotherapy, 1801–1803, 1803*t*
    clinical presentation, 1801
    diagnostic evaluation, 1801, 1802*f*
    epidemiology and risk factors, 1801
    pathology, 1801
    radiation therapy, 1803–1806, 1804*t*–1806*t*
    staging, 1801, 1802*t*
    surgical management, 1802–1803

Outcomes research
    breast cancer, 1264–1269
    cervical cancer, 1566–1572, 1568*t*, 1574
        radiation dose rates and, 1561
    lung cancer, 1085, 1086*t*
    oropharyngeal tumors, 923–925, 938–943, 939*f*–943*f*, 939*t*
    penile cancer, 1527–1528, 1527*t*–1529*t*, 1530, 1530*f*
    prostate cancer, 1469–1470, 1470*t*
    radiation therapy, 2028–2029, 2028*f*
    renal cell carcinoma, 1407–1409, 1408*t*
    rhabdomyosarcoma, pediatric patients, 1880–1882, 1881*f*
    testicular cancer, 1514–1515, 1515*f*
    urethral cancer, 1409, 1528–1530, 1529*f*
    vaginal cancer, 1672, 1675
    Wilms' tumor therapy, 1854–1857, 1855*t*

Outpatient treatment, high-dose-rate brachytherapy, 542

Output factor, basic properties, 162, 162*f*

Ovarian cancer
    adult granulosa cell tumors, 1645–1646
    advanced-stage disease, 1637
    anatomy, 1629
    chemotherapy, 1636–1637
    clinical presentation, 1631
    combined treatment modalities, 1640–1643
    cytoreductive surgery, 1636
    diagnostic work-up, 1631–1632
    early-stage disease, 1637
    epidemiology, 1629
    epithelial tumor management, 1635–1638, 1640–1643
    future research issues, 1646
    germ cell tumor management, 1645
    intraperitoneal chemotherapy, 1637
    metastatic patterns, 1631

Ovarian cancer (*contd.*)
  pathologic classification, 1632–1633, 1632*t*, 1633*t*–1635*t*
  pediatric patients, 1646
  radiation-induced injury and, 2017
  radiation therapy, 1637–1643
    consolidative therapy, 1640–1643
    epithelial ovarian carcinoma, 1637–1638
    intraoperative radiation, 1643–1644
    intraperitoneal phosphorus, 1639–1643, 1639*t*, 1642*t*
    palliative treatment, 1643
    stereotactic techniques, 1643
    whole-abdominal irradiation, 1638–1639, 1638*t*, 1641*t*,
        1643–1645
  recurrent disease, 1637
  risk factors, 1629–1631, 1630*f*
  screening, 1631
  sex cord-stromal tumors, 1646
  staging and survival factors, 1629, 1630*t*, 1635*t*
  surgical management, 1633–1637
  treatment, 1633, 1636*t*
    sequelae, 1644–1645
Ovarian function
  breast cancer risk and, 1177
  cervical cancer therapy and preservation of, 1552
Oxygenation (oxygen effect)
  chemical modifiers of radiation therapy, 611
  hyperthermia, 643–644, 644*f*
  radiation therapy, 13, 87–90, 88*f*–89*f*
Oxygen enhancement ratio (OER), particle beam radiotherapy,
    407–408
Oxygen fixation hypothesis, tumor metabolism, 135–136, 135*t*

P
p27/Kip1 gene, cervical cancer, 1545
p53 tumor suppressor gene
  apoptosis resistance and, 112–113
  breast cancer metastases, 1200–1201
  breast cancer screening, 1181
  cervical cancer, 1544–1545
Paclitaxel
  non-small cell lung cancer therapy, 1099
  pancreatic cancer therapy, 1345–1346
Paget's disease
  breast cancer
    diagnosis and treatment, 1163–1164
    pathophysiology, 1197
  vulvar cancer, 1694
Pain management
  adjuvant therapies, 2007, 2007*t*
  bone metastases, 1988–1989
    radiation therapy, 1992–1997
  complementary therapies, 2008
  interventional techniques, 2008
  medical guidelines, 2005–2006, 2006*f*, 2006*t*
  mucositis and proctitis, 2009, 2014
  muscle spasm, 2008–2009
  neuroaxial techniques, 2008
  neuroblative techniques, 2008
  nociceptive/non-nociceptive classification, 2005
  nonoral administration routes, 2007–2008
  opiate side effects, 2006–2007
  plexopathy, 2009
  radiation therapy, 1934
    interventional management during, 2008
Pair production, basic principles, 148, 148*f*
Palifermin, chemical radioprotection, 615–617, 616*f*
Palladium implants, brachytherapy, 430–432
  prostate cancer, 530
Palliative therapy. *See also* Supportive care
  adrenal metastases, 2001
  biliary tract metastases, 2000–2001
  bone metastases
    chemotherapy, 1991–1992
    combined system therapy, 1991–1992
    epidemiology, 1986, 1987*f*
    evaluation, 1987–1988, 1988*f*–1989*f*
    pain management, 1988–1989
    pathophysiology, 1987–1988
    radiation therapy, 1992–1997, 1993*f*, 1994*t*–1995*t*
    radiopharmaceuticals, 1997–1998
    surgical management, 1989–1991, 1990*f*, 1990*t*

brain metastases
  anticonvulsants, 1978–1979
  clinical presentation, diagnosis, and prognosis, 1974, 1975*t*
  concurrent radiosensitizers, 1977
  corticosteroids, 1974
  neurocognitive decline, 1977–1978
  postoperative radiation therapy, 1976
  radiosurgery boost trials, 1975, 1976*t*, 1979*t*
  surgical resection, 1974–1975, 1975*f*, 1978*t*
  whole-brain radiation therapy, 1974–1977, 1975*t*, 1977*f*,
      1980*t*
cervical cancer, 1589
colon cancer, 1370–1371
endometrial cancer, 1623
esophageal cancer, 1147
gynecologic malignancies, 2002, 2002*t*, 2003*f*
liver metastases, 2000, 2001*f*, 2001*t*
nasal cavity tumors, 862
ovarian cancer, 1639, 1643
rectal cancer recurrence, 2003
spinal cord compression
  clinical presentation, diagnosis, and prognosis, 1979, 1981
  corticosteroids, 1981
  epidemiology, 1979
  intramedullary metastases, 1984
  pathophysiology, 1979
  pediatric patients, 1984
  radiation therapy, 1982–1984
  surgical management, 1981–1982, 1982*t*, 1983*f*
splenic metastases, 2001–2002
stomach cancer, 1332
Pancarditis, as radiotherapy effect, 336
Pancreatic cancer
  anatomy and metastases, 1336, 1337*f*
  brachytherapy, 504
  chemotherapy clinical trials, 1341–1346, 1341*t*–1342*t*
  clinical presentation, 1336
  combined treatment modalities, 1342–1343, 1346
  computed tomographic imaging, 621, 621*f*
  epidemiology and risk factors, 1336
  future research issues, 1346
  imaging studies, 1336–1337
  intraoperative radiation/intraoperative electron irradiation
      therapy (IORT/IOERT), 399, 403*t*
  pathologic classification, 1337
  pediatric patients, 1917
  radiation therapy, 1338–1341, 1339*f*–1340*f*, 1345
  staging, 1337*t*
  stereotactic body radiation therapy, 394
  surgical management, 1337–1338, 1338*t*
  targeted therapies, 1346
Panhypopituitarism, craniopharyngioma and, 1937
Paperless electronic records, oropharyngeal tumor radiation
      therapy, 952, 952*f*
Papillary/mixed-papillary-follicular thyroid cancers, classification,
      1059, 1061
Pap smears, cervical cancer
  follow-up, 1540
  screening, 1535–1536
Para-aortic lymph nodes, cervical cancer radiation therapy, 1556,
      1556*f*–1557*f*
  elective irradiation, 1576–1577, 1576*f*
  metastases to, 1534, 1534*t*, 1574–1576, 1576*t*
  recurrent disease, 1590
  sequelae, 1587–1588
Paraganglioma
  nonmalignant disease, 1940–1941, 1941*t*
  pediatric patients, 1922
Parallel-opposed fields, photon external-beam dosimetry, 175–176,
      176*f*
Parameningeal sites, rhabdomyosarcoma, pediatric patients,
      1875–1876
Parametrium
  anatomy, 1532
  cervical cancer radiation therapy, boost regimen, 1555
Paranasal sinus tumors
  α-particle radiotherapy, 416
  anatomy, 858
  chemotherapy, 862
  epidemiology, 858–859
  general management, 862

lymphomas, 1757
natural history, 859–860, 860*f*
palliative therapy, 862
pathologic classifications, 861–862
pretreatment evaluation, 861, 861*t*
prognostic factors, 862
proton and α-particle radiotherapy, 416
staging, 861, 861*t*
Paraneoplastic syndromes, lung cancer metastases, 1079
Paris system, interstitial brachytherapy, 448–449, 449*t*, 452*f*
Parotid gland tumors
   anatomy, 874, 875*f*
   clinical presentation, 876
   diagnostic work-up and staging, 876–877, 877*f*, 878*t*, 879*f*
   epidemiology, 874–875
   late effects syndromes on normal tissue in, 345
   management of, 880–882
   pathologic classification, 876–877, 878*t*, 880*f*
   prognostic factors, 878–880, 881*f*
   radiation therapy, 882–883, 884*f*
Partial response criteria, end point selection, phase III clinical trials, 358
Particle beam radiotherapy
   biological models, 407–408
   bladder tumors, 1426–1429, 1427*f*–1429*f*
   charged particle radiotherapy, 412–413, 412*t*
   fast neutron techniques, 408–412, 408*t*
      head and neck squamous-cell tumors, 410
      non-small-cell lung cancer, 410, 410*f*
      prostate cancer, 410–411, 411*f*
      salivary gland tumors, 408–410, 409*f*, 409*t*
      sarcomas, 411–412
   future research issues, 420
   glioblastoma multiforme, 734
   heavy ion therapies, 419–420, 419*t*
   osteosarcoma, 1804–1805, 1805*t*
   overview, 407
   π-meson radiotherapy, 420
   posterior uvea melanoma, 786–787
   proton and α-particle radiotherapy, 413–419
      acoustic neuromas, 415
      arteriovenous malformations, 417
      astrocytomas, 415
      breast cancer, 419
      gastrointestinal cancer, 418
      juxtaspinal cord tumors, 416–417, 416*f*
      lung cancer, 417–418
      optic pathway gliomas, 413
      paranasal sinus and nasopharyngeal tumors, 416
      pediatric malignancies, 418–419, 418*f*
      pituitary tumors, 414–415
      prostate cancer, 417
      skull-base tumors, 413–414, 414*t*, 415*f*
      uveal melanoma, 413, 414*f*
Past-pointing technique, rotation therapy, photon external-beam dosimetry, 177–178
Paterson-Parker (P-P) system, interstitial brachytherapy, 444–447, 444*f*, 445*t*–446*t*, 446*f*–448*f*
Patient comfort issues
   high-dose-rate brachytherapy, 542–543
   oropharyngeal radiation therapy, intensity-modulated techniques, 947–948, 948*t*
Patient dose calculation standards, electron-beam therapy, 198–199
Patient evaluation
   intraoperative radiation/intraoperative electron irradiation therapy (IORT/IOERT), 397
   thyroid disease management, 1071
Patient positioning. *See also* Immobilization protocols
   breast cancer radiation therapy, 1243, 1244*f*–1245*f*
   pediatric medulloblastoma radiation therapy, 1838
   photon external-beam dosimetry, 182–184, 183*f*
   skin cancer radiation therapy, 694–695
   soft tissue sarcoma radiation therapy, 1815–1816, 1815*f*
   three-dimensional conformal radiation therapy, 220–221, 220*f*–221*f*
   total body irradiation, 370, 371*f*
Patient-related uncertainties
   electron-beam therapy, dosage calculations, 194–196, 195*f*–199*f*
   photon external-beam dosimetry, air gap correction, 168–169
   radiation therapy, 8
Patient selection and eligibility criteria

high-dose-rate brachytherapy, 543
intraoperative radiotherapy, 397
phase III clinical trials, 358
Patterns of care studies, radiation therapy, 2034
Patterns-of-failure model, stereotactic body radiation therapy, 390
Pauli Exclusion Principle, principles of, 142
Pay for performance paradigm in Medicare, radiation oncology and, 2048
Peacock tomotherapy system, 240, 241*f*
Peakscatter factor (PSF)
   photon external-beam dosimetry, 167–168
   tissue-air ratio, 161, 161*f*
Pedal lymphangiography, cervical cancer screening, 1536–1537
Pediatric patients
   acquired immunodeficiency syndrome, malignant neoplasms, 713
   adrenocortical carcinoma, 1921–1922
   appendix, 1917
   breast tumors, 1915–1916
   central nervous system (CNS) tumors
      astrocytic tumors, 1824–1832
      atypical teratoid/rhabdoid tumor, 1841–1842
      choroid plexus tumors, 1834–1835
      embryonal tumors, 1836–1842
      ependymal tumors, 1832–1834
      germ cell tumors, 1842–1844
      neuronal/mixed neuronal-glial tumors, 1835
      pineal parenchymal tumors, 1835–1836
      radiation therapy, 1822–1824, 1824*t*
      sellar region, 1844–1845
      supratentorial primitive neuroectodermal tumor, 1841, 1842*f*
   colorectal cancer, 1916–1917
   esophageal cancer, 1916
   Ewing's sarcoma
      chemotherapy, 1886–1889
      clinical presentation, 1886
      diagnostic work-up, 1886
      epidemiology, 1886
      future research issues, 1890
      metastases, 1889
      outcome assessment, 1889
      prognostic factors, 1886, 1887*t*
      radiation therapy, 1887–1890, 1888*t*
      stem cell rescue, 1889–1890
   gastrointestinal cancer, 1916
   hemangiomas, 1925
   hepatobiliary tract cancers, 1917–1920, 1918*t*
   high-dose-rate brachytherapy, 573–574, 574*t*
   Hodgkin's lymphoma, 1732, 1892–1903
      biology, 1892
      chemotherapy, 1896, 1897*t*, 1898
      clinical presentation, 1893
      combined treatment modalities, 1894, 1895*t*–1896*t*
      diagnostic work-up, 1893
      epidemiology, 1892
      future research issues, 1902
      long-term therapy effects, 1901–1902, 1902*f*
      pathologic classification, 1892–1893, 1893*t*
      prognostic factors, 1894
      radiation therapy, 1894–1896, 1899–1902, 1900*f*–1901*f*, 1900*t*
      recurrent/refractory disease, 1898–1899
      risk-adapted therapy, 1898
      staging, 1893
      therapy sequencing, 1898
   intraoperative radiotherapy for, 402
   juvenile nasopharyngeal angiofibroma, 1914–1915, 1914*t*
   Langerhans cell histiocytosis, 1920–1921
   late effects syndromes in neuroendocrine system of, 345
   lung cancer, 1915, 1915*f*
   lymphangiomas, 1925
   malignant melanoma, 1928
   metastatic spinal cord compression, 1984
   nasopharyngeal carcinoma, 1913, 1914*t*
   neuroblastoma
      chemotherapy, 1865–1869
      clinical presentation, 1859–1860
      combined treatment modalities, 1863–1867, 1865*t*
      diagnostic work-up, 1860, 1861*f*–1863*f*
      epidemiology, 1859
      natural history, 1859

Pediatric patients (*contd.*)
  pathologic classification, 1860–1861
  prognostic factors, 1861, 1863, 1864*t*
  radiation therapy, 1867–1869, 1868*f*
  staging, 1860, 1864*t*
  surgical management, 1863, 1865, 1865*t*, 1868–1869
 non-Hodgkin's lymphoma (NHL)
  chemotherapy, 1905–1907, 1905*f*, 1906*t*, 1907*f*
  clinical presentation, 1903–1904, 1903*t*
  diagnostic evaluation, 1904
  epidemiology, 1903
  future research issues, 1908–1909
  overt central nervous system disease, 1908
  pathologic classification, 1903*t*
  prognostic factors, 1905, 1905*f*, 1905*t*
  radiation therapy, 1907–1909, 1909*f*
  staging systems, 1904–1905, 1904*t*
 oropharyngeal and salivary gland cancers, 1913–1914
 ovarian cancer, 1646
 pancreatic cancer, 1917
 pheochromocytoma/paraganglioma, 1922
 proton and α-particle radiotherapy, 418–419, 418*f*
 rhabdomyosarcoma
  anatomy, 1872
  chemotherapy, 1878
  clinical presentation, 1872
  clinical trials, 1880–1882, 1881*f*
  diagnostic work-up, 1872–1873, 1873*t*
  epidemiology and risk factors, 1872
  extremities, 1877
  future research issues, 1882–1883
  head and neck, 1875–1876
  late effects, 1882
  metastases, 1872, 1877
  natural history and metastases, 1872
  orbital tumors, 1874–1875, 1875*f*
  outcomes, 1880–1882, 1881*f*
  pathologic classification, 1873–1874, 1874*t*
  pelvis, 1876–1877
  prognostic factors, 1874–1877, 1875*f*
  radiation therapy, 1878–1880, 1879*f*
  staging, 1873, 1873*t*–1874*t*
  surgical management, 1877–1878, 1882
 skin cancer, 1927–1928
 spine/spinal cord tumors, 772–773, 773*f*
 stomach cancer, 1916
 thyroid carcinoma, 1922–1924, 1923*t*
 Wilms' tumor
  anaplastic tumor, 1856
  biology, 1850
  clear cell sarcoma, 1856
  clinical presentation, 1851
  clinical trials and outcomes, 1854–1857, 1855*t*
  diagnostic work-up, 1851, 1851*f*, 1852*t*
  end stage renal disease, 1857
  epidemiology, 1850
  late effects of treatment, 1857
  natural history, 1851
  older patients, 1856
  pathologic classification, 1850–1851
  radiation therapy, 1853–1857, 1853*t*, 1854*f*
  rhabdoid tumor of kidney, 1856
  secondary cancer, 1857
  staging, 1851, 1852*t*–1853*t*
  surgical management, 1853
Pelvic disease
 bladder cancer recurrence, 1419
 cervical cancer metastases, 1534–1535, 1534*t*
 osteosarcomas, 1805
 rhabdomyosarcoma, pediatric patients, 1876–1877
Pelvic exenteration, cervical cancer therapy, 1550
Pencil-beam algorithm (PBA)
 electron-beam therapy
  standard for, 199–200, 201*f*
  water-based dose distribution, 193
 evolution of, 190
Pencil-beam redefinition algorithm (PBRA), electron-beam therapy, 199–200, 201*f*
Penectomy, 1524
Penis, cancer of
 anatomy, 1519, 1520*f*

 brachytherapy, 525–527, 526*t*
 chemotherapy, 1525
 clinical presentation, 1520–1521, 1520*f*
 diagnostic work-up, 1521, 1521*t*
 epidemiology, 1519
 inguinal lymph node involvement, 1524–1525, 1524*t*, 1527*f*
 natural history, 1519–1520
 pathologic classification, 1522–1523, 1522*t*–1523*f*
 prognostic factors, 1523–1524, 1523*f*
 radiation therapy, 1525–1526, 1526*t*
 staging, 1521–1522, 1521*t*–1522*t*
 surgical management, 1524
 treatment outcomes, 1527–1528, 1527*t*–1529*t*, 1530, 1530*f*
Percentage depth dose (PDD)
 basic principles, 160–161, 160*f*
 photon external-beam dosimetry, 166–168, 171–172, 171*f*, 171*t*
  wedge filters, 175
 total body irradiation, 369
Percival's medical ethics, 2036–2037, 2037*f*
Percutaneous ablation therapy, hepatocellular carcinoma, 1352–1353
Percutaneous coronary intervention, vascular brachytherapy, 1960–1961, 1961*f*, 1962*t*
Perfluorocarbons, modification of radiation response, 35
Performance status scale (PSS), oropharyngeal radiation therapy, 938–943, 940*f*
Perfusion-limited hypoxia
 radiation therapy and, 13
 tumor metabolism, 134
Perianal cancer, diagnosis and treatment, 1391–1394
Pericardial tumors
 inicidence and epidemiology, 1154, 1155*t*
 management of, 1157–1158
 natural history, 1155
Pericarditis, radiation-induced, Hodgkin's lymphoma, 1734
Perihilar cholangiocarcinoma, 1358–1359
Peripheral T-cell lymphomas (PTCL)
 clinical-histopathological correlates, 1745
 pathology and classification, 1741
 treatment of, 1754
Peripheral vascular brachytherapy, clinical trials, 1967–1968, 1968*t*
Periurethral duct carcinoma, histology, 1455
Permanent interstitial brachytherapy, 429–432, 430*t*
 implantation techniques, 455–456, 455*f*
 linear-quadratic model, 468
 low-dose-rate sources, 430
 radioactive decay mathematics, 429–430
 ultra low-dose-rate and permanent energy sources, 430–432
Persistent disease, nasopharyngeal cancer, 846–848, 846*t*–847*t*, 848*f*
Personnel roles, high-dose-rate brachytherapy, 546
Peyronie's disease
 induration penis plastica, 1950–1951
 penile tumors, 1523
Pharyngeal wall tumors
 prognostic factors and treatment, 927, 929–930, 931*t*
 radiation therapy, 971, 972*t*
Phase I clinical trials, defined, 357
Phase II clinical trials, defined, 357–358
Phase III clinical trials
 defined, 358–360, 360*t*
 eligibility criteria and patient selection, 358
Phenomenological model, stereotactic body radiation therapy, 390
Pheochromocytomas
 adrenal gland tumors, 1718–1720
 pediatric patients, 1922
pH levels
 hyperthermia modification of, 645–646, 646*f*
 tumor metabolism, 134
Phosphorescence, thermoluminescence dosimetry, 159
Phosphorus-32
 malignant ascites and pleural effusion, 595
 nonsealed radionuclide therapy, 592
 ovarian cancer therapy, 1639–1643, 1639*t*, 1642*t*
Photodynamic therapy
 breast, 601
 components, 599–600
 esophagus/gastrointestinal cancer, 602
 future research, 603
 genitourinary cancer, 602
 gynecological cancer, 602

head and neck, 601–602, 602f
lung cncer, 603
morbidity, 603
ophthalmic/neurologic conditions, 601
skin cancer, 600–601
Photoelectric effect, principles of, 147
Photon attenuation
  brachytherapy, 436, 436f
  chordoma radiation therapy, 1006–1009
Photon radiation therapy
  adjacent x-ray field separation, 184–185, 186f–187f
  bolus tissue equivalent, 182
  in cardiac pacemaker patients, 185, 187t
  chordomas, 1940, 1940t
  clinical applications, 171–175
  compensating filters, 181–182
  fetal dosage, 186, 187t
  field shaping, 178–181
  gonadal dosage, 186
  monitor unit and dose calculation methods, 166–168
  patient positioning, registration, and immobilization, 182–184, 183f
  patient topography corrections (air gaps), 168–169
  tissue inhomogeneities, correction for, 169–171
  treatment planning, 175–178
Photons
  electromagnetic radiation, 143–144, 143f–144f
  spectrum properties, brachytherapy, 423–426, 424f–427f, 424t
  transport simulation, brachytherapy, 439–440, 439f
Photosensitizers, photodynamic therapy, 599, 600t
Physical modifiers, radiation therapy, 35
Physics
  of hyperthermia, 649–658
    electromagnetic heating, 650, 650f–651f
    interstitial hyperthermia, 651–655, 652f–655f
    invasive thermometry, 655–657, 656f–657f
    noninvasive thermal dose measurements, 657–658, 657f–659f
    ultrasound heating, 650–651, 651f–652f
  radiation oncology and, 12–13
  stereotactic body radiation therapy and, 390–391
  vascular brachytherapy, 1962
Physiology
  of hyperthermia, 642–644, 643f–644f
  spinal cord tumors, 767–768, 767t
Pigmented villonodular synovitis (PVNS), diagnosis and therapy, 1954
Pilocarpine, xerostomia management and, 2013
Pilocytic astrocytoma, 737
Pineal parenchymal tumors, pediatric patients, 1835–1836
Pineoblastoma, pediatric patients, 1835
Pineocytoma, pediatric patients, 1835–1836
π-meson radiation therapy
  basic principles, 412
  principles and applications, 420
Pituitary gland
  leukemia radiation therapy, 1786
  radiation injury and dysfunction, 796
Pituitary tumors
  adenomas
    nonmalignant disease, 1936–1937, 1937t, 1938f
    pediatric patients, 1845
    stereotactic radiosurgery, 385–386
  anatomy and physiology, 751, 752f
  carcinomas, 760
  clinical presentation and diagnostic work-up, 751–752, 752f, 752t–753t
  Cushing's disease, 758–759, 758f–759f
  epidemiology, 751
  management, 753–756, 754f
    medical management, 754
    nonfunctioning tumors, 756, 756f
    posttherapy evaluations, 756
    radiation therapy, 754–756, 755t, 760–763
    results, 756–760
    surgical management, 754
    treatment sequelae, 762–763, 763t
  natural history, 751
  pathologic classification, 753, 754t
  prolactin-secreting hormones, 759–760, 761t

proton/α-particle radiotherapy, 414–415
staging, 752–753
Planar imaging systems, image-guided radiation therapy (IGRT), 271–279
  cyberknife, 274, 274f, 275t, 276f
  electronic portal imaging devices, 271, 272f, 273–274
  gantry-mounted systems, 278–279, 278f–279f
  Novalis system, 274, 276–277, 276f
  real-time tumor tracking, 277, 277f
Planning target volume (PTV)
  computed tomography and, 190
  electron arc therapy, 214–215
  electron-beam therapy
    energy selection, 200–201
    isodose contours, 200, 201f
    patient uncertainties and, 194–196, 195f–199f
    standard patient dose calculations, 198–199
  external beam radiation therapy
    Hodgkin's lymphoma radiation therapy, 1729–1730
    lung cancer radiation therapy, 1095–1096
    oropharyngeal radiation therapy, intensity-modulated techniques, 947–948, 948t
    prostate cancer radiation therapy, 1459
    stereotactic body radiation therapy, 391
  three-dimensional conformal radiation therapy
    applications, 227–230, 228f–230f
    specifications, 225–226
Plasma cell myeloma/plasmacytoma
  clinical presentations, 1791
  diagnostic work-up and staging, 1791–1792, 1791t–1792t
  epidemiology and etiology, 1790
  management, 1793–1798, 1793t
    assessment and follow-up, 1798
    autologous stem cell transplantation, 1794–1795
    multiple myeloma, 1794, 1795f
    novel therapies, 1795
    radiation therapy, 1795–1798
    radioimmuntherapy, 1796–1797
    solitary plasmacytoma, 1793–1794, 1793t–1794t, 1797
  monoclonal gammopathy, 1790
  natural history and genetics, 1790, 1791t
  pathophysiology, 1790
  prognostic factors, 1792–1793
Plaster casting, photon external-beam dosimetry, patient positioning and immobilization, 183, 183f
Platelet-derived growth factor (PDGF), signaling mechanisms, 119–120
Platinum-based drugs
  combined chemoradiation therapy, 677, 677t
  ovarian cancer therapy, 1637
Pleomorphic adenoma, radiation therapy, 882
Pleomorphic rhabdomyosarcoma, classification, 1811
Pleural effusion, phosphorus-32 therapy, 595
Pleural recesses, anatomical illustrations, 630, 630f
Pleuropulmonary blastoma (PPB), pediatric patients, 1915, 1915f
Plexopathy
  brachial, 1271
  pain management, 2009
Plummer-Vinson syndrome, oral cavity tumors, 894–895
Pneumonitis, radiation-induced
  breast cancer therapy, 1271–1272, 1272f
  Hodgkin's lymphoma, 1733–1734
  late effects syndromes on lung and, 329–330, 330f–331f, 330t
  total body irradiation, 365
    delayed toxicity, 372, 373f
Poikiloderma, late effects syndromes on normal tissue, 332, 332t
Point A dose specification, intracavitary brachytherapy, 458–460, 459f
Polarographic electrode, chemical modifiers of radiation therapy, 611–612
Political activity, radiation oncology and, 2046
Polymer delivery systems, chemotherapy, intracranial tumor management, 729
Polymer-gel dosimetry, absorbed dose calculation, 160
Polymorphic reticulosis (PMR), diagnosis and treatment, 1010–1012, 1011t
Population-based demographics, retroperitoneal cancer, 1709
Portal dose images (PDIs), intensity-modulated radiation therapy, 255

Positron emission tomography (PET)
  bone metastases, 1988
  breast cancer diagnosis and staging, 1193
  cervical cancer screening, 1538, 1538*f*
  intracranial tumors, 721–722, 722*f*
  oncologic imaging, 623–624, 623*t*, 624*f*
  prostate cancer imaging, 1487
  testicular cancer imaging, 1506
Posterior pelvis radiotherapy, anal cancer, 1392
Posterior uvea, metastatic carcinoma, 782–787, 783*t*–784*t*,
    785*f*–786*f*
Postoperative radiation therapy
  astrocytomas, pediatric patients, 1827, 1827*f*
  bladder cancer, 1426
  brain metastases, whole-brain radiation, 1976
  cervical cancer
    hysterectomy and, 1548–1550, 1549*f*, 1551*t*, 1581–1583,
        1582*f*
    sequelae, 1589
  endometrial cancer, 1620–1621
  esophageal cancer, 1144
  hypopharyngeal cancers, 966, 967*t*
  non-small-cell lung cancer, 631–632
  oropharyngeal tumors, 919, 924*f*
  pituitary adenoma, 1936–1937
  prostate cancer, 1499–1500
  rectal cancer, 1375–1377
  renal cell carcinoma, 1403–1404, 1407–1409, 1408*t*
  retroperitoneal cancer, 1712
  salivary gland tumors, 884–887, 886*t*–887*t*
  soft tissue sarcomas, 1814
  superior sulcus tumors, 1093
  supraglottic lesions, 987–988
  vulvar tumors, 1703–1704
Posttransplant lymphoproliferative disorder, non-Hodgkin's
    lymphoma, pediatric patients, 1908
Posttreatment evaluation
  implant brachytherapy, 486
  pituitary tumor radio therapy, 756
PSA doubling time (PSADT), prostate cancer therapy, 1475
Potency issues
  prostate cancer therapy, 1471–1473, 1473*t*
  radiation-induced injury and, 2017
Potential doubling time, tumor regeneration after radiation, 85
Potentially lethal damage repair (PLDR), radiation therapy, 78
Power law tissue-air ratio, photon external-beam dosimetry, tissue
    inhomogeneity correction, 170
Power sources, linear accelerator, 151–152
Practice guidelines
  radiation oncology marketing, 2046–2047
  radiation therapy, 2032–2034
Predictive assays
  radiation oncology, 68
  tumor cell death, 84
  tumor radiosensitivity, 16–17
Pregnancy
  breast cancer and
    disease management protocols, 1238–1239
    metastatic risk and, 1202
    post-therapy pregnancies, 1239–1240
    risk factors, 1177
  cervical cancer and, 1597–1598
  Hodgkin's lymphoma and, 1722
  Wilms' tumor and, 1857
Preoperative chemotherapy
  non-small cell lung cancer, 1083–1084, 1084*t*
  rectal cancer, 1378–1379, 1379*f*
  superior sulcus tumors, 1092
Preoperative radiation therapy
  bladder cancer, 1424–1426
  endometrial cancer, 1620
  esophageal cancer, 1143–1144, 1144*t*
  hepatocellular carcinoma, pediatric patients, 1919–1920
  implant brachytherapy, 486
  meningiomas, nonmalignant disease, 1936
  non-small cell lung cancer, 1083–1084, 1084*t*
  rectal cancer, 1378–1379, 1379*f*
  renal cell carcinoma, 1407–1409, 1408*t*
  retroperitoneal cancer, 1711–1713, 1713*t*–1714*t*
  soft tissue sarcomas, 1814
  stomach cancer, 1331–1332

supraglottic carcinomas, 987–988
  vulvar cancer, 1703
Prevention strategies
  breast cancer, 1181–1183, 1182*t*
  chemoprevention, 53–54
  colorectal cancer, 1367
  hepatocellular carcinoma, 1350
  mucositis, 2013–2014
  nonmelanoma skin cancer (NMSC), 693
  radiation oncology, 50–54, 51*f*–53*f*, 54*t*
  radiation oncology and, 50–54, 52*f*–53*f*, 54*t*
  xerostomia, 2012–2013
Primary chemotherapy, defined, 49
Primary prevention strategies, radiation oncology, 51–52
Primary standards, brachytherapy dosimetry, 433–434
Principal quantum number, defined, 142
Principlism, medical ethics and, 2035
Proctitis, pain management, 2009
Progesterone receptors, breast cancer metastases, 1199
Prognostic factors, tumor pathophysiology, 136
Programmed cell death type 1, radiation therapy and, 77
Programmed cell death type 2, radiation therapy and, 77–78
Progressive endarteritis, late effects syndromes in gastrointestinal
    tract and, 341–344, 342*f*
Prolactin-secreting adenomas, diagnosis and management, 759–760,
    760*t*
Proliferation indices, breast cancer metastases, 1200
Prophylactic surgery, breast cancer prevention, 1182–1183
Prospective studies
  defined, 356–357
  phase I trials, 357
  phase II trials, 357–358
  phase III trials, 358–360, 360*t*
Prostate cancer
  anatomy, 1439, 1440*f*–1441*f*
  brachytherapy, 527–531, 527*t*–528*t*
    gold grain implants, 530
    interstitial irradiation and hyperthermia, 531
    iodine implants, 527–530, 528*f*–529*f*, 528*t*
    iridium interstitial implants, 530–531, 531*f*
    palladium implants, 530
  brachytherapy, optimized dose protraction, 469–470
  fast neutron radiotherapy, 410–411, 411*f*
  high-dose-rate brachytherapy, 558, 570–572, 571*t*–572*t*
  image-guided radiation therapy
    Cyberknife system, 274, 274*f*, 275*t*, 276*f*
    electronic portal imaging devices, 273–274, 273*f*
    gantry-mounted systems, 278–279, 278*f*–279*f*
    ultrasound techniques, 268–271
  intensity-modulated radiation therapy, 258
  intermediate/high-risk cancer
    androgen-suppression therapy, 1488, 1489*t*, 1491–1495
    biochemical failure, 1497–1498
    chemotherapy, 1495–1497
    clinical presentation, 1483
    combined treatment modalities, 1491–1495
    epidemiology, 1483
    prognostic factors and risk classification, 1483–1484
    radiation therapy, 1484–1491
      adjuvant therapy, 1498–1500
      dose escalation, 1489–1491
      organ motion, 1484–1486
      prophylactic pelvic irradiation, 1486–1489
      prostate-specific antigen relapse, 1495
      whole pelvic irradiation, 1484, 1484*f*–1485*f*
    radical prostatectomy, biochemical failure following, 1497
  low-risk cancer
    brachytherapy, 1463–1465, 1469–1470, 1470*t*, 1472–1475
    combined brachytherapy/external beam radiation, 1470
    cryosurgery, 1457, 1466, 1471
    epidemiology and risk factors, 1441–1445, 1442*f*, 1443*t*,
        1445*t*, 1453, 1453*t*
    erectile dysfunction posttherapy, 1474
    imaging studies, 1450–1453, 1452*f*
    lymph node metastases, 1446–1447
    management trends, 1456–1457
    natural history, 1445–1446
    pathology and histology, 1453–1456
    potency preservation with external-beam radiation, 1472
    radiation therapy, 1457–1463, 1458*f*, 1460*f*–1462*f*, 1460*t*,
        1466–1469, 1467*f*, 1469*f*, 1471–1475, 1472*f*

radical prostatectomy, 1457, 1465–1466, 1471
rectal tolerance effects of therapy, 1473–1474
screening methods and markers, 1447–1449, 1448t
sequelae of therapy, 1471–1475
staging, 1449–1450, 1450t, 1453, 1453t
toxicity effects of therapy, 1472–1473, 1473t, 1474f
mortality studies, 1498
physiology, 1439–1440
proton and α-particle radiotherapy, 4r17
radiation-induced injury and, 2017
radioimmunotherapy, 591
rhabdomyosarcoma, pediatric patients, 1876
stereotactic body radiation therapy, 394
Prostatectomy. *See* Radical prostatectomy
Prostate-specific antigen (PSA)
density measurements, 1448
postirradiation increase in, 1475–1476
prostate cancer
metastatic patterns, 1445–1446
physiology, 1439–1440
screening methods with, 1447–1449, 1448t
staging work-up with, 1449–1450, 1450t
recurrent prostate disease and, 1495
reverse-transcriptase-polymerase chain reaction assay, 1449
serum tests for, 1449
velocity measurements, 1449
Prostatic acid phosphatase
prostate cancer screening, 1447–1449, 1448t
prostate physiology, 1439–1440
Prostheses (steel and silicone), photon external-beam dosimetry,
173–174
Proteomics, radiation oncology, 67–68, 68f
Protocol compliance, radiation therapy, quality assurance, 57–58
Proton radiation therapy, 413–419
acoustic neuromas, 415
arteriovenous malformations, 417
astrocytomas, 415
breast cancer, 419
chordoma radiation therapy, 1009–1010
components and instrumentation, 154–155, 155f
gastrointestinal cancer, 418
juxtaspinal cord tumors, 416–417, 416f
lung cancer, 417–418
non-small cell lung cancer, 1098
optic pathway gliomas, 413
paranasal sinus and nasopharyngeal tumors, 416
pediatric malignancies, 418–419, 418f
pituitary tumors, 414–415
prostate cancer, 417
radiation therapy, 32
skull-base tumors, 413–414, 414t, 415f
uveal melanoma, 413, 414f
Proton radiosurgery, techniques and applications, 380
Protons, basic properties, 148–149
Proto-oncogenes
normal and transformed cells, 39–40
radiation oncology and, 37–39, 38f–39f
Protracted radiation therapy
dose fractionation and, 100
human tumor regeneration, 86
Pseudosclerodermatosus panniculitis, breast cancer therapy
complications, 1270
Pseudotumor orbitae, radiation therapy, 1946, 1946t
Psychoemotional issues
breast cancer patients, 1278–1279
Hodgkin's lymphoma and, 1735
mood dysfunction, supportive care for, 2011–2012
Pterygium
brachytherapy and resection, 493, 493f
diagnosis and management, 778–779
radiation therapy, 1941–1942, 1942f
Pulsed brachytherapy
basic principles, 470
cervical cancer, 1566
high-dose-rate regimen, 546
Pulsed dose rate brachytherapy
cervical cancer, 1566
remote-control afterloading, 483, 484t, 485, 485f–486f
Pulse sequences, magnetic resonance imaging, 621–623, 622f–623f,
622t
Pyriform sinus tumors, radiation therapy, 971, 972t

Q
Quadratic objective function, intensity-modulated radiation therapy,
248
Quality assurance
brachytherapy, 57–58, 532–534, 533f
conformal therapy, 234–236
department committee structure for, 58
external beam radiation therapy, 55–57
external practice audit, 58
high-dose-rate brachytherapy
operation protocols, 546
remote afterloading device, 548–552
treatment plan evaluation, 555–556
intensity-modulated radiation therapy, 253
lung cancer, 1098
patient- and equipment-specific protocols, 253–255, 254f
medical care and evidence-based medicine, 2032
nonsealed radionuclide therapy, 595–596
oropharyngeal radiation therapy, intensity-modulated
techniques, 948–949, 948f–949f
prostate brachytherapy, 1464–1465, 1465t
protocol compliance, radiation therapy, 57–58
radiation oncology, 55–58
developing world, 608–609
radiation therapy, 103–104
three-dimensional conformal radiation therapy, verification
protocols, 222, 224, 224f
total body irradiation, 370–372
Quality conversion factor, absorbed dose calculation, 159
Quality of life issues. *See also* Supportive care
bladder cancer, 1434–1435
breast cancer patients, 1278–1279
hypopharyngeal cancer, 973
oropharyngeal radiation therapy, 939–943
pancreatic cancer chemoradiation, 1346
supportive care
basic principles, 2011
fatigue and mood dysfunction, 2011–2012
genitourinary tract injury, 2017
mucosal injury, 2013–2016
nutrition, 2017–2018
salivary gland injury, 2012–2013
skin injury, 2016–2017
Quantitative dosimetry
brachytherapy, 438–440
treatment planning for radiation therapy, 30–31
Quantity activity, brachytherapy dosimetry, 434
Quantum physics, electromagnetic radiation, 143–144, 143f–144f
Quimby system, interstitial brachytherapy, 447–448

R
Race
breast cancer metastatic risk and, 1201–1202
cervical cancer prognosis and, 1541–1542
Radiation exposure
absorbed dose calculation from, 157–158
basic principles, 156–157
breast cancer risk and, 1180
soft tissue sarcoma risk, 1808, 1811f
Radiation-induced tumors, 54–55
thyroid cancer, classification, 1061
Radiation myelitis, radiation therapy "remembered" dose tolerance,
83–84
Radiation necrosis
in brain, 326, 326t
chemoradiation therapy, 671
nasopharyngeal cancer therapy, 851–853, 851t, 852f
Radiation nephropathy, late effects syndromes on normal tissue and,
338–340, 339f–341f, 340t–341t
Radiation oncology. *See also* Oncologic anatomy (onco-anatomy)
accreditation issues, 2048–2049
Africa, 606
angiogenesis, 47–48
apoptosis, 43, 43f–44f
Asia and Pacific region, 606–607, 607t
cancer genetics and biology, 36–37, 37f
cancer prevention, 50–54, 51f–53f, 54t
cell-cycle control, 41–42, 42f
defined, 4–5
denied Medicare claims, 2043
in developing world

Radiation oncology (*contd.*)
    cancer epidemiology, 604, 605*f.*
    global disease burden, 604
    global status of radiation therapy, 604–605
    quality control and, 608–609
  DNA damage, 10
  Eastern Europe, 607*f,* 608
  economic analysis, 2043–2049
  empiricism *vs.* research-based oncology, 10–12
  ethical issues in, 2038–2040
  etymology of, 5
  evidence-based research on, 2029–2032, 2030*t*–2031*t,* 2031*f*
  federal regulations, 2047
  free-standing centers for, 2046
  future research issues, 67–68
  Health Insurance Portability and Accountability Act issues, 65–66
  historical perspective, 2–4
  international economics and, 2049
  irradiation effects on cells, 35–36, 35*f,* 36*t*
  Latin America, 607–608
  lobbying and political activity and, 2046
  logarithmic cell kill, 13–14, 22*f*
  malpractice issues, 61–65
  managed care negotiations and, 2044–2045
  marketing issues, 2046–2047
  metastasis biology, 44–46, 45*f*
  Middle East, 607*f,* 608
  molecular biology, 46–47
  oncogenesis, 37–39, 38*f*–40*f*
  patient management, 48–50, 48*f*–49*f*
  pay for performance paradigm in Medicare, 2048
  physics *vs.* biology in, 12–13
  prostate cancer, whole-pelvic irradiation trial, 1488
  proto-oncogenes, normal and transformed cells, 39–40, 40*f*–41*f,* 41*t*
  quality assurance, 55–58
  radiobiologic concepts in, 10
  radiosensitivity and radiocurability, 14–20, 15*t*
    normal tissue microenvironment, 17*f,* 18–20, 19*f*–20*f*
    tumor control probability, 17–18
    tumor sensitivity and predictive assays, 16–17
  residency program economics and, 2047
  risk management, 66–67, 67*t*
  staffing issues, 2048
  stereotactic radiosurgery, body radiation therapy, 389–390
  techniques of, 6
  telomeres, 42–43
  tumor markers, 44, 44*t*
  tumor-suppressor genes, 40–41, 41*f,* 41*t*
  work of suit principles, 14*t*
Radiation quality, systems for, 156
Radiation response markers
  biologic modifiers, 614
  cervical cancer, 1544
  chemical modifiers
    hypoxic cell sensitization, 612–613
    hypoxic cell targeting, 613–614
    mitigation, 615–617, 616*f*
    oxygen effect, 611
    radioprotection, 614–615
    treatment, 617–618
    tumor oxygenation augmentation, 611–612, 612*f*
Radiation therapy. *See also* Combined treatment modalities; specific therapies, e.g. External beam radiation therapy
  activity-based cost *vs.* traditional accounting, 2023–2024, 2025*f*
  acusticus neurinomas (schwannomas), 1937–1939
  acute and late ill effects, documentation, 58–61, 59*f,* 61*t*
  acute lymphoblastic leukemia, 1780–1783
  adrenal gland tumors, 1720
  age-related macular degeneration, 1943, 1943*f*
  anal cancer
    combined treatment modalities, 1386–1388, 1387*t,* 1389*t*–1390*t*
    sequelae, 1394
    techniques, 1390, 1391*t,* 1392–1394
  aneurysmatic bone cyst, 1954
  angiogenesis therapy, 47–48
  appropriateness criteria, 2033
  arteriovenous malformation, 1939, 1939*t*
  astrocytomas, pediatric patients, 1827–1832
  biological basis for, 76–103

    cell cycle redistribution, 86–87
    dose fractionation patterns, 99–103
    fractional subunits, 80
    hypoxia and, 88–89
    linear quadratic formula, 91–92, 91*f*–92*f,* 93*t,* 98, 98*f*
    mammalian cell survival curves, 90–92, 91*f*
    molecular responses, normal tissue, 82
    multifraction survival curves, 93–94, 94*f*
    normal tissue cell death, 78
    normal tissue radiobiology, 77–78
    oxygen effect, 87–90, 89*f*
    pathobiology and kinetics, normal tissue injury, 78–80
    quality alterations, 103–104
    quantitative analysis and dose fractionation, 90–97
    random cell killing, 90, 91*f*
    regeneration/repopulation, normal tissue, 82–83, 83*f,* 98–99, 99*f*
    remembered dose, tolerance mechanisms and, 83–84, 84*f*
    survival model comparisons, 92–93, 93*f*–94*f*
    time-does isoeffect formulae and dose fractionation, 97–99, 98*f*
    tumor control probability, 95–97, 95*f*–97*f*
    tumor radiobiology, 84
    tumor regeneration, 85–86, 85*f,* 87*f*–88*f*
    tumor regression, 84–85
    tumor reoxygenation, 89–90, 89*t*
    tumor response and dose fractionation, 93*t,* 95
    two-component model, 92
    in vivo tumor response kinetics, 84
    volume effects, 80–82
  bladder cancer, 1421–1426
    altered fractionation schedules, 1423
    elderly patients, 1424
    external beam radiation, 1421–1423, 1422*t,* 1427–1429, 1427*f*–1430*f*
    postoperative radiation, 1426
    preoperative radiation, 1424–1426
    salvage cystectomy and, 1423–1424
  bone metastases, palliative therapy, 1992–1997, 1993*f,* 1994*t*–1995*t*
  boron neutron capture therapy, 33–35
  box technique, cervical cancer radiation therapy, 1555
  brain metastases, 1974–1977
  breast cancer, 1206–1210
    accelerated partial breast irradiation, 1259–1260
    after breast augmentation, 1242
    angiosarcoma, 1276–1277
    beam calculations, 1248, 1249*f*–1250*f*
    boost to tumor site, 1248
    brachial plexopathy, 1271
    cardiac sequelae, 1272–1274
    contralateral breast cancer, 1257, 1274–1275, 1275*t*
    cosmetic surgery following, 1267*t,* 1268
    electron boosts, 1250–1252
      interstitial boosts *vs.,* 1249–1250, 1252*t*
    external beam radiation, 1262–1263
    Hodgkin's disease patients, 1240–1241, 1240*t*
    inflammatory breast cancer, 1309
    intraoperative accelerated partial breast technique, 1263–1264
    irradiation dose to contralateral breast, 1257
    lymphatics irradiation, 1224–1230, 1252–1255
    lymphedema/breast edema following, 1269–1270
    MammoSite technique, 1262
    multicatheter interstitial techniques, 1260–1262
    multicentric disease and, 1241, 1242*t*
    neoadjuvant chemotherapy and postmastectomy radiation, 1304–1305
    patient positioning, 1243, 1245*f*
    postmastectomy radiation, 1300–1303, 1301*f,* 1303*t,* 1312–1315
      breast reconstruction and, 1314–1315
      dosimetry and dose, 1313–1314
      target definitions, 1312
      technique, 1312–1313, 1313*f*–1314*f*
    pulmonary sequelae, 1271–1272, 1272*f*
    randomized data, 1248
    secondary malignancies, 1275–1276
    sequelae, 1269–1277
    skin/breast complications, 1270–1271
    stroke risk, supraclavicular radiation, 1274

tamoxifen-radiation sequencing, 1232, 1233*t*, 1234
tangential beam alignment, 1245–1246, 1247*f*–1248*f*
tangential field/supraclavicular field alignment, 1255–1257, 1256*f*
three-dimensional conformal *vs.* intensity-modulated therapies, 1257, 1259
treatment volume, 1243–1244, 1246*f*
whole breast dose, 1246, 1248
calcaneodynia/achillodynia, 1949, 1950*f*, 1951*t*
cardiac tumors, 1158–1159, 1159*f*
central nervous system lymphoma, 742
cervical cancer
chemoradiation, 1591–1597
combined treatment modalities, 1548–1550, 1549*f*, 1551*t*
dose calculation, 1566
elective para-aortic lymph node irradiation, 1576–1577, 1576*f*
external beam irradiation, 1553–1556, 1554*f*–1555*f*
hyperthermia and, 1597
interstitial implants, 1573
intraoperative irradiation, 1591
midline anteroposteror-posteroanterior portals, 1555
palliative radiation, 1589
postoperative, 1581–1583, 1582*f*, 1583*t*, 1589
pretreatment laparotomy and nodal staging, 1551–1552, 1552*t*
prolonged treatment times, 1574, 1575*f*
recurrent disease, 1590
results, 1566–1584
sequelae, 1584–1589, 1585*f*–1586*f*
staging protocols, 1547–1548
surgery and, 1546–1550, 1551*t*
techniques, 1552–1566, 1553*t*
chemodectoma, nonmalignant disease, 1940–1941, 1941*t*
chemoradiation therapy, 48–50, 49*f*–50*f*
anal cancer, 681*t*, 683
antimetabolites, 677*t*, 678–679
antitumor efficacy strategies, 674
bladder cancer, 681*t*, 683
cervical cancer, 681*t*, 682–683
drug-radiation interaction, 670–672, 670*f*
emerging strategies, 673–677
esophageal cancer, 681*t*, 683–684
future research, 684–685
glioblastoma multiforme, 681*t*, 684
head and neck cancers, 681–682, 681*t*, 807–818
adjuvant postoperative irradiation, 813
alternating radiation and chemotherapy, 810
biologically target therapy, 816–817
curative intent treatment, 810–813, 811*f*–814*f*, 814*t*
efficacy of, 807–808
future research issues, 817–818
multiagent chemotherapy, 809–810
selection criteria, 813–816
sequential chemoradiation, 816
single-agent chemotherapy, 808–809, 808*t*
toxicity management strategies, 817
long-term toxicity effects, 680*t*
lung cancer, 679–681, 681*t*
mitomycin C, 677*t*, 678
molecular targeting strategies, 674–676, 674*t*, 675*f*
normal tissue protection, 676–677
overview, 669
platinum-based drugs, 677, 677*t*
rectal cancer, 681*t*, 684
strategies in, 669–670
taxanes, 677–678, 677*t*
therapeutic index, 669
timing protocols, 672–673, 673*t*
topoisomerase I inhibitors, 677*t*, 679
tumer cell repopulation inhibition, 672
chloroma, 1012
cholangiocarcinoma, 1359–1360, 1360*f*
chordomas, 1006, 1007*f*–1008*f*
nonmalignant disease, 1939–1940, 1940*f*, 1940*t*
choroidal hemangioma, 1942–1943
clinical trials, 2031–2032
colon cancer
chemotherapy and, 1368–1370, 1369*t*–1370*t*, 1370*f*
techniques, 1371, 1372*f*
cost-benefit analysis, 2026–2027

course planning and administration, 5–6
craniopharyngioma
nonmalignant disease, 1937
pediatric patients, 1844–1845
current research overview, 2022
Cushing's disease, 759, 759*f*
cutaneous T-cell lymphoma, 1769–1774, 1769*t*
defined, 4–5
degenerative osteoarthritis, 1946–1947, 1947*f*, 1947*t*
desmoid (aggressive fibromatosis), 1949–1950
diffuse large B-cell lymphoma (DLBCL), 1745–1748
dose rate, 28–30, 28*f*–29*f*
dose-time factors, 22–28
accelerated repopulation, 23, 24*f*–25*f*
altered fractionation, 22–23, 23*f*, 23*t*
isoeffect graphs, 24–25, 26*f*
linear-quadratic equation, 26–28, 26*f*–27*f*, 27*t*
nominal standard dose, 25–26
economic analysis, 2023
endocrine orbitopathy (Graves disease), 1944–1945, 1944*t*–1945*t*, 1945*f*
endometrial cancer, 1615–1624, 1616*t*–1618*t*
ependymoma, 740
pediatric patients, 1833–1834, 1833*f*
esophageal cancer, 1139–1143, 1140*f*–1141*f*, 1143*t*
chemoradiation *vs.*, 1146–1147
iridium techniques, 1148, 1149*f*
postoperative regimen, 1143–1144
preoperative regimen, 1143–1144, 1144*t*
sequelae, 1148, 1150
esthesioneuroblastoma, 1016–1018, 1016*f*, 1017*t*
pediatric patients, 1914
evidence-based medicine and, 2027–2028, 2027*t*–2028*t*
quality assurance, 2032, 2032*f*
evidence-based oncology, 2029–2032, 2030*t*–2031*t*, 2031*f*
Ewing's sarcoma, pediatric patients, 1887–1890, 1888*t*
extramedullary plasmacytomas, 1019–1020
fallopian tubes, tumors of, 1654–1655
fatigue with, 2011–2012
follicular lymphoma, 1751–1753
glioblastoma multiforme, 730–735, 730*t*
brachytherapy techniques, 731–732
dose escalation
altered fractionation and, 731
FSRT and, 731
radiosensitizers, 733
radiotherapy dose, 730–731, 731*t*
radiotherapy target volume, 731
global status, 604–605, 605*f*
glomus tumors, 999–1002, 1000*f*–1003*f*, 1003*t*–1007*t*
nonmalignant disease, 1940–1941, 1941*t*
goals of, 5
heavy particle beams, 31–33
hemangiopericytoma, 1004–1005
hepatocellular carcinoma, 1353–1354, 1354*t*, 1355*f*
transcatheter arterial chemoembolization and, 1354, 1354*t*, 1355*f*
heterotopic ossification, 1955–1956, 1955*f*, 1956*t*
Hodgkin's lymphoma, 1726–1730
acquired immunodeficiency syndrome, 706–707
involved fields, 1729
mantle field, 1728, 1728*f*
pediatric patients, 1894–1896, 1899–1902, 1900*f*–1901*f*, 1900*t*
results, 1730–1733
sequelae, 1733–1735
subdiaphragmatic fields, 1728–1731, 1729*f*
three-dimensional treatment planning, 1729–1730, 1730*f*
hyperthermia with, 637
rationale for, 647–648
hypopharyngeal cancers
complications, 971
long-term follow-up, 972
outcome assessment, 971, 972*t*
postoperative treatment, 966, 967*t*
T1-2 tumors, 963–965, 964*f*–965*f*, 965*t*–966*t*, 967*f*
T3-4 tumors, 966, 968, 968*f*–969*f*
unresectable, nonmetastatic disease, 968, 971*t*
immobilization, 8–9
indications for, 5
induratio penis plastica (Morbus Peyronie), 1950–1951

Radiation therapy (*contd.*)
   instrumentation, 58–61
   international system of units (SI) for, 145*t*
   intracranial tumor management, 725–727
      anatomic landmarks, 726
      sequelae of, 730
   intratubular germ-cell neoplasia, 1512
   juvenile nasopharyngeal angiofibroma, 1914–1915, 1914*t*, 1941,
      1942*t*
   Kaposi's sarcoma, 710–711
   keloids and hypertrophic scars, 1952–1954, 1953*f*
   Langerhans cell histiocytosis, pediatric patients, 1921
   lentigo maligna melanoma, 1026–1027
   lentigo midline granuloma, 1010–1012, 1011*t*
   leukemia, radiotherapeutic emergencies, 1779–1780, 1780*f*
   lung cancer, 1094–1097, 1096*f*, 1097*t*
      non-small cell lung cancer
         definitive therapy, 1086–1089, 1086*t*
         outcomes, 1085, 1086*t*
         postoperative radiation, 1084–1085
      normal tissue toxicity, 1102–1104, 1103*t*
      small cell lung carcinoma, 1100–1102
      toxicity effects, 1102–1104, 1103*t*
   medulloblastoma, 741
      pediatric patients, 1837–1841, 1838*f*
   meningiomas, 743–744
   molecular cancer research and, 109
   Morbus Dupuytren/Morbus Ledderhose, 1951–1952, 1951*t*,
      1952*f*, 1953*t*
   multiple myeloma, 1795–1796
   myasthenia gravis, 1116
   nasopharyngeal cancer, 831–840
      angiofibroma, 1023–1024, 1023*f*
      dose, time, and fractionation, 831–832, 833*t*
      dose escalation and altered fractionation, 836–837, 840, 841*f*,
         841*t*
      intensity-modulated techniques, 834–836, 836*t*, 837*f*–839*f*,
         840*t*
      pediatric patients, 1913
      results of treatment, 848–850, 849*t*–850*t*, 849*f*–850*f*
      sequelae of, 851–853, 851*t*, 852*f*
      three-dimensional conformal techniques, 833–834, 835*f*
      treatment preparation, 831, 831*f*–832*f*
      tumor target volumes, 832, 833*t*
      two-dimensional techniques, 832–833, 834*f*–835*f*
   neck metastases, unknown primary tumors, 1039–1045,
      1042*f*–1045*f*, 1046*t*
      cervical lymph node involvement, 1041, 1043–1044, 1045*f*
      clinically negative nodes, 1046–1047, 1046*t*
      clinically positive nodes, 1047–1048, 1047*f*, 1047*t*–1049*t*
      complications, 1044–1045
   neuroblastoma, pediatric patients, 1867–1869, 1868*f*
   non-Hodgkin's lymphoma, 1745–1748, 1746*f*–1747*f*
      acquired immunodeficiency syndrome, 704–705, 705*f*, 705*t*
      pediatric patients, 1907–1909, 1909*f*
   nonmalignant disease
      application principles, 1933, 1934*t*
      bony tissue, 1954–1956
      clinical trials, 1933
      connective tissue effects, 1934
      craniopharyngioma, 1937
      deep lesions, 1935
      disease classification, 1933
      dose principles, 1934, 1934*t*
      eye and orbit, 1941–1946
      head and neck tumors, 1935–1941
      inflammatory effects, 1934
      intracranial lesions, 1935
      joints and tendons, 1946–1949
      meningioma, 1935–1936, 1935*t*, 1936*f*
      near-surface lesions, 1935
      pain and related symptoms, 1934
      radiobiological aspects, 1933–1934
      rationale, 1933
      skin and connective tissue disease, 1949–1954
      treatment planning, 1935
      tumor/leukemia induction risk, 1933
      vascular system effects, 1934
   nonpilocytic/diffusely infiltrating gliomas, 738
   nutritional support during, 2017–2018
   oral cavity tumors, 901–907
      adjuvant protocols, 902
      altered fractionation, 904
      brachytherapy, 904–905, 905*f*
      chemotherapy and, 906
      dental care, 906–907, 907*f*–908*f*
      dose and fractionation, 903–904
      intraoral cone, 905–906, 906*f*
      neoadjuvant therapy, 902
      prognostic and predictive factors, 907–908
      techniques, 902–903, 902*f*–904*f*
   oropharyngeal tumors, 933–938, 933*f*–936*f*
      clinical results, 950
      cone beam computed tomography, 951
      cyberknife, 951, 951*f*
      dose and fractionation sites, 935
      dose-calculation algorithms, 951
      external beam radiation therapy, 950–951
      helical tomography, 950
      intensity-modulated radiation therapy, 946–950, 947*t*–948*t*,
         948*f*–949*f*, 950*t*
      nonrandomized studies, 945–946
      paperless electronic records, 952, 952*f*
      randomized trials, 946
      side effects, 936–938, 938*t*
      three-dimensional conformal therapy, 946–950
      xerostomia, 937–938, 939*f*
  osteosarcoma, 1803–1806, 1804*t*–1806*t*
  outcomes research on, 2028–2029, 2028*f*
  ovarian cancer, 1637–1643
      consolidative therapy, 1640–1643
      epithelial ovarian carcinoma, 1637–1638
      intraoperative radiation, 1643–1644
      intraperitoneal phosphorus, 1639–1643, 1639*t*, 1642*t*
      palliative therapy, 1643
      palliative treatment, 1643
      stereotactic techniques, 1643
      whole-abdominal irradiation, 1638–1639, 1638*t*, 1641*t*,
         1643–1645
pain management during, 2008
pancreatic cancer, 1338–1341, 1339*f*–1340*f*, 1345
paragangliomas
  nonmalignant disease, 1940–1941, 1941*t*
  pediatric patients, 1922
patterns of care analysis, 2033
pediatric patients
  astrocytomas, 1827–1832
  craniopharyngioma, 1844–1845
  dose and dose-fractionation regimens, 1823
  ependymoma, 1833–1834, 1833*f*
  Ewing's sarcoma, 1887–1890, 1888*t*
  follow-up protocols, 1823–1824
  Hodgkin's lymphoma, 1894–1896, 1899–1902, 1900*f*–1901*f*,
    1900*t*
  Langerhans cell histiocytosis, 1921
  medulloblastoma, 1837–1841, 1838*f*
  nasopharyngeal cancer, 1913
  neuroblastoma, 1867–1869, 1868*f*
  rhabdomyoscarcoma, 1878–1880, 1879*f*
  sequelae, 1822–1824
  thyroid disease, 1923–1924
  Wilms' tumor, 1853–1857, 1853*t*, 1854*f*
penis, cancer of, 1525
perianal cancer, 1393–1394
personnel issues, 61*t*
pigmented villonodular synovitis, 1954
pituitary tumors, 754–756, 755*t*, 760–763
  conventional therapy, 760
  external-beam radiation therapy, 754
  nonmalignant disease, 1936–1937, 1937*t*, 1938*f*
  simulation techniques, 760–761, 761*f*
practice guidelines, 2032–2033, 2033*t*
prostate cancer
  intermediate/high-risk cancer, 1484–1491
    adjuvant therapy, 1498–1500
    androgen suppression therapy with, 1491–1495,
      1492*t*–1493*t*, 1495*t*
    chemotherapy and, 1496–1497
    dose escalation, 1489–1491
    extended lymph node dissection and, 1487
    organ motion, 1484–1486
    prophylactic pelvic irradiation, 1486–1489

prostate-specific antigen relapse, 1495
    salvage therapy, 1499–1500
    survival studies, 1499t
    whole pelvic irradiation, 1484, 1484f–1485f
  low-risk cancer
    beam selection and planning, 1459–1461, 1460f, 1460t
    current trends in, 1456–1457
    immobilization, simulation, and CT scanning, 1458–1459
    long-term results, 1468
    randomized dose-escalation trials, 1466–1468, 1467f
    target and normal tissue contouring, 1459
    techniques overview, 1457–1463
    treatment delivery and organ motion issues, 1461–1463
pterygium, 1941–1942, 1942f
quality assurance
  brachytherapy, 57–58
  evidence-based medicine and, 2032, 2032f
  external-beam therapy, 55–57
radiation-induced tumors, 54–55
reactive lymphoid hyperplasia/pseudotumor orbitae, 1946, 1946t
rectal cancer, 1375–1379
renal cell carcinoma, 1403–1404, 1407–1409, 1408t
renal pelvis and ureter carcinoma, 1409
resource utilization in, 2024
respiratory-dampened, respiratory-gated, and
      respiratory-synchronized therapy, 9–10
response modifiers, 36
retroperitoneal cancer, 1711–1713, 1713t–1714t
rhabdomyosarcoma, pediatric patients, 1878–1880, 1879f
rotator cuff syndrome, 1948, 1949t
salivary gland tumors, 882–888
  neutron therapy, 887–888
  primary radiotherapy, 887
  recurrent cancers, 888–889, 889f
  sequelae, 888
  surgery and, 884–887, 886t–887t
  systemic therapy, 888
  xerostomia management, 2012–2013
sarcomas, head and neck, 1029–1030, 1030t
seminoma testis, 1508, 1509t–1510t, 1510
skin cancer
  anatomical site specification, 695
  field size, 694
  melanoma, 696–698
  Merkel cell carcinoma, 698–699
  nonmelanoma, 693
  quality assurance, 693–694, 693t
  results, 695
  sequelae, 700
  time-dose fractionation, 694, 694t
skin injury from, 2016–2017, 2016f
soft tissue sarcomas, 1814–1819, 1818t
solitary plasmacytoma, 1797–1798, 1797f
spine/spinal cord tumors, 772–776, 773t, 774f
  dose calculation, 775–775
  metastatic spinal cord compression, 1982–1984
  results, 775
  sequelae, 775–776
  target volume, 773–774, 774f
stomach cancer, 1323–1329
  indications for, 1323
  palliative therapy, 1332
  sequelae, 1332–1333, 1332t
  techniques, 1323–1329, 1324t–1326t, 1326f–1329f
supraglottic lesions, 987–988, 987f
surgery combined wtih, 48, 48f
technology assessment, 2022–2023
tendonitis and bursitis, 1948, 1948f
tennis/golfer's elbow, 1948–1949
testicular cancer, 1513–1516, 1513f–1514f
thymomas, 1115–1116
thyroid disease
  management of, 1067–1069, 1068t, 1069f
  pediatric patients, 1923–1924
  radiation-induced cancer, 1055–1056, 1061
  sequelae, 1069–1070
time and effort analysis, 2024
toxicity quantitation, 20–21
tracheal tumors, 1120–1122, 1121t
treatment machines, 149–155
treatment planning, 30–31

tumor metabolism, 134–135
uncertainties, 7–8
urethral cancer
  female, 1685–1688, 1686f–1688f, 1689t, 1690
  male, 1526–1527, 1527f
uterine sarcoma, 1624
vaginal cancer, 1663–1669, 1668f–1669f, 1670t
  complications, 1676–1678
  external beam radiation, 1668–1669, 1670f, 1673–1675
  high-dose-rate intracavitary brachytherapy, 1670–1671
  interstitial brachytherapy, 1671–1672
  low-dose-rate intracavitary brachytherapy, 1669–1670
  salvage therapy, 1676
vertebral hemangiomas, 1954–1955
vocal cord carcinoma, 983–984, 984f–986f
  recurrent disease following, 984–985
  sequelae, 993
volumes in, 5–6, 5f
vulvar tumors, 1696–1697, 1700–1704, 1701f–1703f, 1704t
  sequelae, 1705–1706
whole-brain radiation, 1974–1977
Wilms' tumor, 1853–1857, 1853t, 1854f
Radiation Therapy Oncology Group (RTOG) Dose-Escalation Studies,
     stereotactic radiosurgery, 381, 382f
Radical cystectomy, bladder cancer
  chemotherapy following, 1432–1433, 1432t–1433t
  high-grade invasive bladder cancer, 1415, 1416t–1417t
  morbidity and mortality, 1415, 1416t–1417t, 1417
  organ preservation, 1430–1432, 1431t
  recurrent disease, 1419–1420
Radical hysterectomies
  cervical cancer therapy, 1550
  postoperative irradiation, 1581–1583, 1582f, 1583t
Radical prostatectomy
  current techniques, 1456
  external beam radiation therapy vs., 1468–1469
  outcome assessment, 1465–1466
  prostate cancer, 1471
Radioactive stents, clinical trials, 1967
Radioactivity
  basic principles, 144–146, 144t
  decay mathematics, permanent interstitial brachytherapy,
     429–430, 430f
Radiobiology. See Biology (radiobiology)
Radiochromic film dosimetry, absorbed dose calculation, 159–160
Radiocurability, principles of, 14–20
Radiodermatitis, late effects syndromes on normal tissue, 332, 332t
Radiofrequency phased array heating, hyperthermia, 650, 650f–651f
Radiographic studies. See Imaging studies
Radioimmunoglobulins, cancer therapy
  basic cancer biology and immunology, 583–584, 584t
  leukemia and lymphoma, 588–589
  monoclonal antibodies, 585
  solid tumors, 589–591
Radioimmunoliposomes, cancer therapy, 585–586
Radioimmunotherapy
  bone marrow ablation, 594–595
  bone mestastases, 592–595, 593t
  central nervous system malignancies, 595
  glioblastoma multiforme, 734
  iodine-131, 591–592
  leukemia and lymphoma, 588–589
  malignant ascites and pleural effusion, 595
  monoclonal antibodies
    cancer therapy, 584–588
    clinical results, 587–588
    development of, 586
    isotope selection, 586, 587f, 587t
    RIT toxicity, 586–587
  multiple myeloma, 1796–1797
  nonsealed radionuclide therapy, 591–594
  ovarian cancer, 1644
  phosphorus-32, 592, 595
  radioimmunoglobulins
    basic cancer biology and immunology, 583–584, 584t
    leukemia and lymphoma, 588–589
    solid tumors, 589–591
  radionuclide selection, 587t
  rhenium186/188, 592, 594–595
  safety and quality assurance, 595—596
  samarium-153, 592, 594

Radioimmunotherapy (*contd.*)
  strontium-89, 591–592
  thyroid malignancies, 592
Radioisotopes
  brachytherapy
    effectiveness, 468
    prostate cancer, 528*t*
    selection criteria, 476
  radioimmunotherapy and, 586, 587*f*, 587*t*
Radionuclides
  bone metastases, 1997–1998
  bone scan and metastases, 624–625
  brachytherapy
    experimental intracavitary radionuclides, 428
    sources, 423–426, 424*f*–426*f*, 424*t*
  neuroblastoma, pediatric patients, 1867–1869, 1868*f*
  nonsealed therapy, 591–594
  osteosarcoma radiation therapy, 1805, 1806*t*
  thyroid disease radiographic studies, 1058, 1058*t*
Radiopharmaceuticals. *See* Radionuclides
Radioprotectors, modification of radiation response, 35
Radiosensitivity, laws of, 12
  evolution of, 14–20
  oxygen effect and, 88, 89*f*
  stereotactic radiosurgery, 381
  tumor sensitivity, predictive assays, 16–17, 16*f*
Radiosensitizers
  anaplastic glioma, 737
  brain metastases, palliative therapy, 1977, 1980*t*
  combined chemoradiation therapy, head and neck squamous-cell
      tumors, 809
  glioblastoma multiforme radiation therapy, 732
  pancreatic cancer therapy, 1343
Radiosurgical techniques
  pituitary tumor management, 754, 757–758, 758*t*
  stereotactic radiosurgery, 379
Radium sources, brachytherapy
  activity-exposure rate, 434
  basic properties, 426
  interstitial substitutes, 443–449
  nonafterloading sources, 428
  radium 226, 426–427
Rad unit, absorbed dose measurements, 157
RAGE campaign (Radiation in Action Group Exposure), radiation
      oncology and, 65
Randomization, phase III clinical trials, 359–360
Range-straggling, defined, 147
ras oncogene, cervical cancer, 1545
Ras oncogene, signaling mechanisms, 119
Ratio of tissue-air ratio (RTAR), photon external-beam dosimetry,
      tissue inhomogeneity correction, 169
Real-time position management (RPM) system, image-guided
      radiation therapy, respiratory gating, 284–285, 285*f*,
      288
Real-Time Tumor-Tracking (RTRT) system, image-guided radiation
      therapy, 277, 277*f*
  respiratory gating with, 284–285, 285*f*
Receptor tyrosine kinases (RTKs), growth control and, 110–111
Recombinant human keratinocyte growth factor-1 (rhuKGF-1),
      mucositis prevention, 2013–2014
Rectal cancer. *See also* Colorectal cancer
  anatomy and tumor location, 1372, 1373*f*
  brachytherapy, 524–525, 524*f*–525*f*
  hyperthermia therapy, 662
  imaging studies, 1373
  locally advanced disease, 1379–1380
  neoadjuvant therapy, 1377–1378
  palliative therapy, 2003
  pediatric patients, 1916–1917
  postoperative adjuvant therapy, 1375–1377
  preoperative *vs.* postoperative radiation therapy, 1378–1379,
      1379*f*
  prognostic factors, 1372–1373
  recurrent disease, 1379
  reirradiation, 1380
  surgical management, 1373–1375
Rectal complications, prostate cancer
  brachytherapy, 1473–1474
  fast neutron radiotherapy, 411
Rectovaginal septum tumors, brachytherapy, 521
Recurrent disease. *See also* Metastases; Secondary cancers

acute lymphoblastic leukemia, 1782–1783
bladder cancer cystectomy, 1419–1420
breast cancer
    BRCA1/2 carriers, 1234–1237, 1235*t*, 1236*f*–1237*f*
    breast conservation therapy and risk of, 1309–1310
    ductal carcinoma in situ, 1171
    extravasive intraductal carcinoma, 1216–1217, 1216*t*
    histology, 1217–1218
    hyperthermia therapy, 660–662, 661*f*
    local control and systemic therapy, 1215, 1215*ti*
    lymphatic mestases, 1224–1230, 1226*t*
    mastectomy and systemic treatment, local-regional
        recurrence, 1303–1304, 1303*t*, 1310–1311
    molecular factors, 1218–1219
    nodal relapse, 1311
    postmastectomy radiation and, 1300–1303, 1301*f*, 1303*t*,
        1312–1315
    systemic therapies and, 1305–1307, 1305*t*–1307*t*
  cervical cancer, 1568–1591, 1571*t*, 1574*t*
    radiation therapy and, 1590
    tumor factors in, 1543–1544, 1544*t*
  colon cancer, 1371–1372
  endometrial cancer, 1622–1623
    high-dose-rate brachytherapy and, 566–567, 567*t*
  glioblastoma multiforme therapy, 735
  gynecologic malignancies, palliative therapy, 2002, 2002*t*, 2003*f*
  Hodgkin's lymphoma, 1732–1733
    pediatric patients, 1898
  hypopharyngeal cancers, 972–973
  intraoperative radiotherapy, 397–399
    colorectal cancer, 400–401, 402*f*
  intratubular germ-cell neoplasia, 1512
  lobular carcinoma *in situ*, 1218, 1218*t*
  meningiomas, 744
  nasal cavity and paranasal sinus disease, 868
  nasopharyngeal cancer, 846–848, 846*t*–847*t*, 848*f*
  oral cavity tumors, 910
  oropharyngeal tumors, 930, 932–933, 932*f*–933*f*
  ovarian cancer, 1637–1638
  pancreatic cancer, 1341, 1341*t*
  prostate cancer, 1495
    biochemical failure, 1497–1498
  rectal cancer, 1379
    palliative therapy, 2003
  renal pelvis and ureter carcinomas, 1405–1406
  retroperitoneal cancer, 1713, 1713*t*–1714*t*
  salivary gland tumors, 888–889
  seminoma testis, 1510–1512
  supraglottic carcinoma, 988
  testicular cancer, seminomas, 1508, 1509*t*–1510*t*, 1510
  thymomas, 1112–1114, 1113*t*–1114*t*
  time-to-tumor recurrence measurements, 86
  urethral cancer, female, 1685
  vaginal cancer, 1667*t*
  vocal cord carcinoma, 984–985
  Wilms' tumor, 1856
Redistribution modeling, brachytherapy, 467
Reduced intensity stem cell transplantation, total-body irradiation,
      367
Reed-Sternberg cells, Hodgkin's lymphoma pathology, 1724–1725
Reference dose, interstitial brachytherapy, 449, 451–454
Regeneration mechanisms
  human tumors, 86
  isoeffect formulae, 98–99
  radiation therapy
    normal tissue effects, 82–83, 83*f*
    tumor cells, 85–86, 85*f*
Regimen techniques, total-body irradiation, 366–367
Regression mechanisms, radiation therapy and, 84–85
Relative biological effectiveness (RBE) calculations
  altered fractionation, radiation therapy, 23
  particle beam radiotherapy, 407–408
  quality assurance and, 103–104
"Remembered" doses, radiation therapy retreatment tolerance,
      83–84
Remote afterloading system
  brachytherapy, 423, 483, 484*t*, 485–486, 485*f*
  high-dose-rate brachytherapy, 540, 541*f*
  quality assurance, 548–552
Renal cell carcinoma
  clinical presentation, 1398

diagnostic work-up, 1398–1399, 1399t
epidemiology and risk factors, 1397–1398
metastatic and recurrent disease, 1405
molecular targeting, 1404
natural history, 1398
pathologic classification, 1400
prognostic factors, 1400–1402, 1401t
radiation therapy, 1403–1404, 1406–1407, 1406f
 sequelae, 1409–1410
staging, 1399–1400, 1400t
stereotactic body radiation therapy, 394
surgical management, 1402–1403
therapy outcomes, 1407–1409, 1408t
Renal dysfunction, late effects syndromes in kidney and, 340, 340t–341t, 341f
Renal pelvis, tumors of
clinical presentation, 1398
diagnostic work-up, 1399, 1399t
epidemiology and risk factors, 1398
management and recurrence risk, 1405–1406
natural history, 1398
pathologic classification, 1400
prognostic factors, 1402
radiation therapy, 1407
radiation therapy sequelae, 1409–1410
staging, 1400, 1401t
therapy outcomes, 1409
Renal tolerance measurements, late effects syndromes in kidney and, 339–340, 340f
Reoxygenation mechanisms
brachytherapy, 467
radiation therapy and, 89–90, 89t
tumor metabolism, 134
Replication, cell death resistance and, 113
Repopulation mechanisms
isoeffect formulae, 98–99
radiation therapy, normal tissue effects, 82–83, 83f
Repositioning, radiation therapy, 8
Reproductive systems
Hodgkin's lymphoma therapy and, 1734
late effects syndromes on normal tissue in, 346–347
Research-based radiation oncology, empiricism *vs.*, 10–12
Resensitization, radiation therapy, (α/β ratio), 28
Residency program economics, in radiation oncology, 2047
Respiratory gating techniques, image-guided radiation therapy (IGRT), 284–285, 285f
Res ipsa loquitur doctrine, radiation oncology, 62–65
Resonant transformer x-ray machine, 150
Resource utilization analysis, radiation therapy, 2024
Respiration effects, radiation therapy, 9–10, 10t
Respiratory-dampened radiotherapy, 10
Respiratory-gated radiotherapy, 10, 10t
Respiratory motion management
image-guided radiation therapy (IGRT), 284–285, 284f–285f
 four-dimensional imaging, 285–288, 286f–287f
 tumor treatment, 288
stereotactic body radiation therapy, 390–391
Respondent superior doctrine, radiation oncology, 64–65
Retinal injury, orbital tumor radiation therapy, 796
Retinal tumors, 787–791
Retinoblastomas
brachytherapy, 790
characteristics and management, 787–791, 788f
classification, 788t
episcleral plaque therapy, 490–493, 491f–492f
external beam radiotherapy, 789–790
molecular genetics, 723–724
secondary cancers, 790–791
soft tissue sarcomas, 1808
staging, 789t
tree-dimensional conformal radiation therapy, 790
Retinoblastoma tumor suppressor protein (pRB)
cell cycle control loss and, 111
molecular genetics, 723–724
Retreatment doses, radiation therapy "remembered" dose tolerance, 83–84
Retromolar trigone
anatomy, 892
disease treatment and results, 909
Retroperitoneal cancer
anatomy, 1708, 1709f

chemotherapy, 1711, 1713
clinical presentation, 1709, 1711t
desmoid tumors, 1714
diagnostic work-up, 1709
epidemiology, 1708, 1710f
extragonadal germ cell tumors, 1715, 1715t
lymphomas, 1713
natural history, 1708–1709
neuroblastoma, 1713
radiation therapy, 1711–1713, 1713t–1714t
recurrent disease, 1713–1714
schwannomas, 1714
SEER system demographics, 1709, 1712t
surgical management, 1709–1713, 1713t
Wilms' tumor, 1713–1714
Retroperitoneal lymph node dissection, non-seminomatous germ cell tumors, 1512–1513
Retroperitoneal sarcomas, intraoperative radiotherapy, 401
Retrospective studies, defined, 356
Reverse-transcriptase-polymerase chain reaction (RT-PCR) assay, prostate-specific antigen, 1449
Rhabdoid tumor, Wilms' tumor, 1856
Rhabdomyoscarcoma
diagnosis and treatment, 793–794
group III pediatric patients, hyperfractionated radiation therapy, 310
late effects syndromes, 328
pediatric patients
 anatomy, 1872
 breast metaseases, 1916
 chemotherapy, 1878
 clinical presentation, 1872
 clinical trials, 1880–1882, 1881f
 diagnostic work-up, 1872–1873, 1873t
 epidemiology and risk factors, 1872
 extremities, 1877
 future research issues, 1882–1883
 head and neck, 1875–1876
 late effects, 1882
 metastases, 1872, 1877
 natural history and metastases, 1872
 orbital tumors, 1874–1875, 1875f
 outcomes, 1880–1882, 1881f
 pathologic classification, 1873–1874, 1874t
 pelvis, 1876–1877
 prognostic factors, 1874–1877, 1875f
 radiation therapy, 1878–1880, 1879f
 staging, 1873, 1873t–1874t
 surgical management, 1877–1878, 1882
Rhenium-186–188
bone metastases, 594–595
nonsealed radionuclide therapy, 592
Risk-adapted therapy, Hodgkin's lymphoma, pediatric patients, 1898
Risk factors
acute leukemias, 1777–1779, 1779t
anal cancer, 1384
breast cancer, 1176–1181, 1179t
cervical cancer, 1532, 1534
cholangiocarcinoma, 1356
colorectal cancer, 1366–1367
endometrial cancer, 1610, 1615t–1616t
esophageal cancer, 1131–1133, 1133f
hepatocellular carcinoma, 1349–1350
Hodgkin's lymphoma, 1721
Kaposi's sarcoma, 707
laryngeal cancer, 975–976
neck metastases, unknown primary tumors, 1035, 1037t
non-Hodgkin's lymphoma, 1739–1740
ovarian cancer, 1629–1631, 1630f
pancreatic cancer, 1336
penis and male urethral cancer, 1519
prostate cancer
 intermediate/high-risk cancer, 1483–1484
 low-risk cancer, 1441–1445, 1442f, 1443t, 1445t, 1453, 1453t
  diet influences, 1441–1444, 1443t
  familial risk factors, 1444
  genetic influences, 1444, 1445t
  hormonal influences, 1441
  stratification systems and staging classification, 1453, 1453t

Risk factors (*contd.*)
    radiation oncology, 66–67, 67*t*
    renal cell carcinoma, 1397–1398
    renal pelvis and ureter cancer, 1398
    rhabdomyoscarcoma, pediatric patients, 1872
    soft tissue sarcomas, 1808
    testicular cancer, 1503–1504, 1504*t*
    vaginal cancer, 1657–1658
    vulvar cancer, 1692
Risk management, radiation oncology, 66–67, 67*t*
Roentgen-to-rad conversion factor, absorbed dose measurement, 158, 158*f*
Roentgen unit, radiation exposure, 156–157
Röntgen, Wilhelm, history of radiation oncology and, 2–3, 3*f*
Room's-eye-view (REV) display, digitally reconstructed radiography, 218–219
Rotating gamma system, stereotactic radiosurgery, 380
Rotating slit tomotherapy, 243, 244*f*–245*f*
Rotational settings, radiation therapy, 7
Rotation therapy, photon external-beam dosimetry
    clinical applications, 177–178, 179*f*
    monitor unit calculations, 167–168
Rotator cuff syndrome, radiation therapy, 1948, 1949*t*

S

Safety issues
    brachytherapy
        implant removal, 487
        operating room protocols, 486–487
        U. S. regulations, 532–534, 533*f*
    high-dose-rate brachytherapy, 548–552
    iodine therapy administration, 1073
    nonsealed radionuclide therapy, 595–596
Salivary gland tumors
    anatomy, 874, 875*f*
    clinical presentation, 876
    diagnostic work-up and staging, 876–877, 877*f*, 878*t*, 879*f*
    epidemiology, 874–875
    fast neutron radiotherapy, 408–410, 409*f*, 409*t*
    injury, supportive care for, 2012–2013
    late effects syndromes on normal tissue, 344–345
    managment of, 880–882
    natural history, 875–876, 876*f*, 876*t*
    pathologic classification, 876–877, 878*t*, 880*f*
    pediatric patients, 1913–1914
    prognostic factors, 878–880, 881*t*
    radiation therapy, 882–888
        neutron therapy, 887–888
        primary radiotherapy, 887
        recurrent cancers, 888–889, 889*f*
        sequelae, 888
        surgery and, 884–887, 886*t*–887*t*
        systemic therapy, 888
Salvage surgery
    cystectomy, 1423–1424
    endometrial cancer, 1622–1623
    Ewing's sarcoma, 1887
    vaginal cancer, 1676
Samarium-153
    bone metastases, 594
    bone metastases, palliative therapy with, 1997–1998
    nonsealed radionuclide therapy, 592
Sample size criteria, phase III clinical trials, 358–359, 360*t*–361*t*
Saphenous vein graft, in-stent restenosis, 1966
Sarcomas. *See also* Soft tissue sarcomas
    breast cancer, 1197
    cardiac tumors, 1154, 1155*t*
    cervical cancer, 1541
    Ewing's sarcoma
        desmoplastic small round-cell tumor (DSCRT), 1927
        pediatric patients
            chemotherapy, 1886–1889
            clinical presentation, 1886
            diagnostic work-up, 1886
            epidemiology, 1886
            future research issues, 1890
            metastases, 1889
            metastatic spinal cord compression, 1984
            outcome assessment, 1889
            prognostic factors, 1886, 1887*t*
            radiation therapy, 1887–1890, 1888*t*

            stem cell rescue, 1889–1890
    fast neutron radiotherapy, 411–412
    head and neck, 1027–1030
        chemotherapy, 1030
        clinical presentation and diagnostic work-up, 1028
        general management, 1028–1029
        natural history, 1027–1028, 1027*t*
        prognostic work-up, 1028
        radiation therapy, 1029, 1030*t*
        tumor characteristics, 1030
    high-dose-rate brachytherapy, 5r72–573, 574*t*
    hyperthermia therapy, 662–663
    intraoperative radiotherapy, 401–402
    liver, 1360
    low-dose-rate brachytherapy, 507–508, 507*f*
    prostate tumors, 1456
    retroperitoneal cancer, 1709–1713, 1713*t*
    uterine, 1613
    vaginal cancer, 1673–1674
Sarcomatoid carcinoma, prostate tumors, 1455
Scatter-air/scatter-maximum ratios, basic principles, 161–162
Scatter factors, brachytherapy, 436, 436*f*
Scattergram analysis, human tumor regeneration, 86, 86*f*
Schiller-Duval bodies
    ovarian cancer, 1633
    yolk sac tumor, 1505
Schwannomas
    acusticus neurinoma, 1937–1939
    retroperitoneal cancer, 1714
Scoliosis
    late effects syndromes on bone and, 347–349, 349*f*, 349*t*
    Wilms' tumor and, 1857
Scoring system, late effects syndromes on normal tissue, 321
Screen film mammography, breast cancer screening, 1189
Screening protocols
    breast cancer, 1181–1183, 1181*t*–1182*t*, 1187–1189, 1187*t*
        digital *vs.* screen film mammography, 1189
        magnetic resonance imaging, 1189
        mammography, 1187–1189, 1187*t*–1188*t*
        physical examination, 1189
        ultrasound screening, 1189
        in under-50 women, 1188–1189
    cancer prevention and, 52–53
    cervical cancer, 1535–1538, 1536*t*–1537*t*
    genetic screening
        breast cancer, 1181–1183, 1181*t*–1182*t*, 1201, 1201*f*
        ovarian cancer risk and, 1630*t*, 1631
    neuroblastoma in pediatric patients, 1859
    ovarian cancer, 1631
    prostate cancer, 1447–1449, 1448*t*
"Seattle method," transperineal iodine implants, prostate cancer brachytherapy, 1463–1465, 1464*f*, 1465*t*
Sebaceous carcinoma, 700
    eyelids, 793
Secondary cancers
    breast cancer and, 1275–1276
    cervical cancer, 1599
    Ewing's sarcoma, 1890
    Hodgkin's lymphoma and, 1734–1735
    Hodgkin's lymphoma radiation therapy, pediatric patients, 1902
    intraoperative radiation therapy, 397–399
    as late effect on normal tissue, 349–350
    leukemia radiation therapy, 1787
    nasopharyngeal cancer therapy, 853
    prevention strategies, radiation oncology, 51–52
    retinoblastoma, 790–791
    total-body irradiation, 373–374
    Wilms' tumor and, 1857
Segmental techniques, intensity-modulated radiation therapy, oropharyngeal tumors, 950
Seizures, intracranial tumors, 724
Selenium, prostate cancer risk and, 1443
Sellar region tumors, pediatric patients, 1844–1845
Semiconductor dosimetry, absorbed dose calculation, 160
Seminomatous tumors
    mediastinum, 1118–1119
    surveillance protocols, 1508, 1510, 1510*t*
    testis
        chemotherapy, 1510–1512, 1511*t*
        classification, 1504, 1504*t*
        orchiectomy, 1508–1510, 1509*t*–1510*t*

radiation therapy, 1508, 1509*t*, 1510, 1514–1515, 1514*f*
  staging, 1505*t*, 1506, 1507*t*
Senescence, tissue damage and, 115
Sensorineural hearing loss (SNHL), late effects of radiation, 327–328
Sentinel lymph node biopsies, breast cancer, 1206
Sepsis, Hodgkin's lymphoma therapy and, 1734
Sequential chemoradiation, head and neck squamous-cell tumors, 816
Serous carcinoma, endometrial cancer, 1611–1612, 1612*t*
Serous papillary adenocarcinoma, fallopian tubes, 1652–1653
Serum markers
  breast cancer prognosis and, 1202
  cholangiocarcinoma, 1356–1357, 1356*t*
  fallopian tubes, 1651
  hepatobiliary tract tumors, pediatric patients, 1918–1920
  ovarian cancer screening, 1631
  ovarian germ cell tumors, 1645*t*
  prostate cancer screening, 1447–1449, 1448*t*
Sex cord-stromal tumors
  management of, 1645–1646
  pathologic classification, 1634
Sexuality, radiation-induced injury and, 2017
Sexually transmitted disease (STD), cervical carcinoma
      epidemiology, 1534
Sézary's syndrome, cutaneous T-cell lymphoma, 1766–1767
  radiation therapy, 1769–1774
Short tau inversion recovery (STIR) imaging, bone metastases, 1988
Shrinking action level (SAL) strategy, electronic portal imaging
      devices, 273
Shrinking field technique, external beam radiation therapy, volume
      determination, 6–7, 7*f*
Sievert integral model, brachytherapy dose calculation, 437–438,
      437*f*–438*f*
Signal transduction
  cell cycle control, 42
  growth factors and, 42
  molecular genetics, 723–724
  radiation effects, 119
  receptor tyrosine kinase initiation, 110–111
Simulators
  components and instrumentation, 155
  fractionated stereotactic radio therapy, pituitary tumor
      management, 762
  prostate cancer radiation therapy, 1458–1459
  radiation therapy, pituitary tumor management, 760–761, 761*f*
Simultaneous integrated boost (SIB) intensity-modulated radiation
      therapy
  fractionation, 245–246
  head and neck cancer, 257–258
  oropharyngeal tumors, 949–950
Simultaneous modulated accelerated-radiation therapy,
      nasopharyngeal cancer, 834–836, 836*t*
Single-field isodose charts, photon external-beam dosimetry,
      171–172, 171*f*, 171*t*
Single photon emission computed tomography (SPECT),
      image-guided radiation therapy, 266, 268, 269*f*
Single-stepping source remote afterloading, interstitial
      brachytherapy, 454–456
"Six hallmarks of cancer," 110*t*
Skin cancer
  anatomy, 690
  dermatofibrosarcoma protuberans, 699
  epidemiology and etiology, 690, 691*f*
  followup and prevention, 693
  high-dose-rate brachytherapy, 576
  malignant sweat gland carcinoma, 699–700
  melanoma
      epidemiology, 695–696
      follow-up, 698
      management, 696–698
      staging, 696, 696*t*
  Merkel cell carcinoma, 698–699
  nonmelanoma carcinomas, 692, 692*t*
      radiation therapy, 693
      surgical management, 692–693
  orbital tumor radiation therapy, 794
  pediatric patients, 1927–1928
  photodynamic therapy, 600–601
  premalignant lesions, 691–692
  radiation therapy, 693–695, 693*t*–694*t*
      anatomical site specification, 695
      sequelae, 700

sebaceous carcinoma, 700
Skin collimation, electron-beam therapy
  bolus selection and, 203–204, 203*f*–205*f*
  thickness measurements, 201–202, 202*f*
Skin injury
  brachytherapy, 494–495, 495*f*
  in cancer patients, 2016–2017, 2016*f*
  late effects syndromes in, 330–332, 332*t*
Skin marks, radiation therapy, 8
  breast cancer patients, 1270
Skin surface dose, total body irradiation, 370
Skull-base tumors, proton/α-particle radiotherapy, 413–414, 414*t*,
      415*f*
Sliding-window leaf sequence generation, intensity-modulated
      radiation therapy, 251, 251*f*
Small-cell carcinoma
  breast cancer, 1197
  cervical cancer, 1541
      treatment of, 1548
  lung, combined chemoradiation therapy, 679–680
  lung carcinoma, diagnosis and management, 1100–1102
  perianal cancer, 1391–1392
  prostate tumors, 1455–1456
Small intestine (small bowel)
  late effects syndromes, 342–344
  pediatric patients, 1916
      Hodgkin's lymphoma radiation therapy, 1901–1902
Small lymphocytic lymphoma (SLL)
  clinical-histopathological correlates, 1745
  pathology and classification, 1741–1742
  treatment of, 1754
Smart technology, radiation oncology, 67–68, 68*f*
Smoking, breast cancer risk and, 1180, 1202
Smoldering myeloma, 1790, 1791*t*
Socioeconomic status
  breast cancer metastatic risk and, 1201–1202
  cervical cancer prognosis and, 1541–1542
  oropharyngeal radiation therapy, 938–943
Soft palate tumors
  curative protocol, 930*f*
  oropharyngeal metastases, 924*t*–925*t*
  prognostic factors, 925–926, 925*f*–927*f*
Soft tissue sarcomas
  anatomy, 1808, 1809*t*, 1810*f*
  chemotherapy, 1813–1814
  clinical presentation and evaluation, 1809
  epidemiology, genetics, and risk factors, 1808, 1811*f*
  future research issues, 1819
  high-dose-rate brachytherapy, 572–573, 574*t*
  hyperthermia therapy, 662–663
  intraoperative radiotherapy, 401
  late effects syndromes in, 330–332, 332*t*
  low-dose-rate brachytherapy, 507 508, 507*f*
  nasal cavity and paranasal sinus therapy and, 871
  natural history, 1808–1809
  pathologic classification, 1811, 1812*t*, 1813
  penile tumors, 1522
  prognostic factors, 1813
  radiation therapy, 1814–1819, 1818*t*
  retroperitoneal cancer, 1709–1713, 1713*t*
  staging, 1809–1810, 1812*t*
  surgical management, 1813, 1817–1818
Solid tumors, radioimmunoglobulin therapy, 589–591
Solitary plasmacytoma
  clinical presentation, 1790
  management, 1793, 1793*t*–1794*t*
  prognostic factors, 1792, 1792*f*
  radiation therapy, 1797–1798, 1797*f*
Somnolence syndrome, 1786
SonArray, image-guided radiation therapy, 268–271
Source anisotropy, brachytherapy, 436–437
Source positioning accuracy, high-dose-rate brachytherapy, quality
      assurance and safety, 548–550, 549*f*–550*f*
Source-strength specification, brachytherapy, 432–435
  activity-exposure rate relationships, 434
  air-kerma strength, 433–435
  milligram-hours and integrated reference air-kerma,
      435
  quantity activity measurement, 434
  source output quantities, 434–435
Source strength value, high-dose-rate brachytherapy, 550

Source-to-axis distances (SADs), photon external-beam dosimetry
    air gap correction, 169, 169*f*
    clinical applications, 172
    monitor and dose unit calculations, 166–168
Source-to-surface distance (SSD)
    basic principles, 160–161, 160*f*
    electron-beam therapy
        dose algorithms, 199–200, 201*f*
        monitor unit calculations, 197–198, 199*f*
        water-based dose distribution, 191–192, 192*f*
    photon external-beam dosimetry
        air gap correction, 169, 169*f*
        monitor and dose unit calculations, 166–168
    total body irradiation, 367–368, 369*f*
Specific absorption rate (SAR), interstitial hyperthermia, 653–655,
    654*f*
    noninvasive dose measurements, 657–658, 657*f*–659*f*
Speech function, oropharyngeal radiation therapy, 942
Spermatocytic seminoma, classification, 1504–1505, 1504*t*
S phase
    breast cancer metastases, 1200
    cervical cancer, 1544
    radiation damage and, 117–118
Sphenoid sinus, anatomy, 858
Spindle cell carcinoma, breast cancer, 1197
Spin echo, magnetic resonance imaging, 621–623, 622*f*–623*f*, 622*t*
Spine/spinal cord tumors
    anatomy, 765, 766*f*
    astrocytomas, pediatric patients, 1832
    blood supply, 765–766
    chemotherapy, 771–772
    clinical manifestation, 767
    diagnosis and management, 765
    epidemiology, 766, 767*t*
    extradural tumors, 770
    history and physical findings, 767–768, 767*t*
    intradural-extramedullary tumors, 769–770
    intramedullary tumors, 768–770, 770*f*, 771
    juxtaspinal tumors, proton and α-particle radiotherapy, 416–147,
        416*f*
    late effects syndromes on normal tissue, 323–327, 328*t*
    miscellaneous neoplasms, 770
    myelopathy, nasopharyngeal cancer therapy, 852
    natural history, 766–767
    neuroblastoma in pediatric patients, 1865–1866
    osteosarcomas, 1805
    pathologic classifications, 768–770
    prognostic factors, 770–771
    radiation therapy, 772–776, 774*f*
        dose calculation, 775–775
        results, 775
        sequelae, 775–776
        target volume, 773–774, 774*f*
    radiographic studies, 768
    spinal canal anatomy, 765
    spinal cord compression, palliative therapy
        clinical presentation, diagnosis, and prognosis, 1979, 1981
        corticosteroids, 1981
        epidemiology, 1979
        intramedullary metastases, 1984
        pathophysiology, 1979
        pediatric patients, 1984
        radiation therapy, 1982–1984
        surgical management, 1981–1982, 1982*t*, 1983*f*
    stereotactic body radiation therapy (SBRT), 392, 394
    stereotactic radiosurgery effects, 382
    surgical management, 771
    tissue diagnosis, 768
    tumors, stereotactic radiosurgery, 386
    vascular malformations, 769
Spleen
    leukemia radiation therapy, 1786
    metastases, palliative therapy, 2001–2002
    oncological anatomy, 633
Split-course treatment regimens
    accelerated treatments, 100–101, 308*t*–309*t*, 312
    human tumor regeneration, 86
Sprouting angiogenesis, tumor molecular pathophysiology,
    126–127
Sputum cytology, lung cancer diagnosis, 1080
Squamous cell carcinoma (SCC)
    anal cancer, 1384–1385
    bladder tumors, 1426
    cervical cancer, 1540–1541
    epidemiology and etiology, 690, 691*f*
    eyelid tumors, 792–793, 793*f*
    head and neck tumors, combined chemoradiation therapy,
        807–818
        adjuvant postoperative irradiation, 813
        alternating radiation and chemotherapy, 810
        biologically target therapy, 816–817
        curative intent treatment, 810–813, 811*f*–814*f*, 814*t*
        efficacy of, 807–808
        future research issues, 817–818
        selection criteria, 813–816
        sequential chemoradiation, 816
        synchronous radiation and multiagent chemotherapy,
            809–810
        synchronous radiation and single-agent chemotherapy,
            808–809, 808*t*
        toxicity management strategies, 817
    hypopharyngeal cancers, 965, 966*t*
    neck metastases, unknown primary tumors, 1035, 1036*t*
    penile tumors, 1522, 1522*t*
    renal pelvis and ureter carcinoma, 1400
    staging and classification, 692
    vaginal cancer, 1657–1658
        management, treatment and outcome, 1663–1664
        neovagina, 1675–1676
        prognostic factors, 1662–1663
        surgical approach, 1665
        treatment options and outcome, 1664–1665
Square-root method, electron-beam therapy, monitor unit
    calculations, 197–198, 199*f*
Stabilization devices
    high-dose-rate brachytherapy, 541–542
    radiation therapy, 9, 9*t*
Staff and personnel issues
    radiation oncology, 2048
    radiation therapy, 61*t*
Stainless steel guides, interstitial brachytherapy, afterloading
    technology, 477–478, 478*f*–479*f*
Stallard episcleral plaque therapy, eye tumors, 490–493, 491*f*–492*f*
Standing wave design, lnear accelerators, 151, 151*f*
Stark regulations, radiation oncology, 2047
Stem cell rescue
    Ewing's sarcoma, pediatric patients, 1889–1890
    total body irradiation, 364
Stem cell transplantation
    Hodgkin's lymphoma, 1732–1733
    multiple myeloma, 1794–1795, 1795*f*
    non-Hodgkin's lymphoma, 1749–1750
    total body irradiation, 364
        nonmyeloablative/reduced intensity stem cell transplantation,
            367
Step-and-shoot leaf sequence generation, intensity-modulated
    radiation therapy, 251–252
    oropharyngeal tumors, 950
Step down heating, hyperthermia, isoeffect dose modification,
    639–640, 640*f*
Stereotactic radiosurgery/radiotherapy
    acusticus neurinoma, 1938–1939
    body radiation therapy (SBRT)
        biological and oncological rationale, 389–390
        future research issues, 394
        liver, 391–392, 393*f*
        lung, 392, 394*t*, 395*f*
        miscellaneous cancers, 394
        overview, 389
        physics and dosimetry principles, 390–391
        spine, 392, 394
    brain metastases, palliative therapy, 1975,
        1979*t*
    clinical applications, 382–387, 383*t*
        benign tumors, 384
        brain metastases, 386
        functional techniques, 382, 383*f*
        lung tumors, 386–387
        meningiomas, 385
        nonacoustic schwannomas, 385
        pituitary adenoma, 385–386
        spinal metastases, 386

vascular malformations, 383–384, 384f
vestibular schwannomas, 384–385
functional applications, 382, 383f
gamma knife techniques, 379–380
image-guided techniques, 380
intracranial tumor management, 724–725
key requirements, 379t
linear accelerator systems, 380
metastatic spinal cord compression, 1983–1984
nasopharyngeal cancer, persistent/recurrent disease, 847–848
non-small cell lung cancer, 1086
normal tissue tolerance, 381–382
ovarian cancer, 1643
overview, 378, 379f
radiobiologic considerations, 378–379
renal cell carcinoma, 1404
rotating gamma system, 380
terminology, 378, 379t
tomotherapy, 380
Steroid receptors, molecular cancer biology and, 111
Steroid therapy, Langerhans cell histiocytosis, 1921
Stockholm system, brachytherapy, cervical carcinoma, 510–512,
    511f–512f
Stomach cancer
    anatomy, 1318
    chemotherapy, 1333
    clinical presentation, 1319
    diagnostic work-up, 1319–1320
    epidemiology, 1318
    failure patterns for surgical resection, 1323, 1323t
    future research issues, 1333–1334
    intraoperative radiotherapy, 399–400
    late effects syndromes on normal tissue in, 342–344, 342f
    metastatic patterns, 1318–1319, 1319f
    pathology, 1320–1321
    pediatric patients, 1916
    prognostic factors, 1321–1322, 1321t
    radiation therapy, 1323–1329
        indications for, 1323
        palliative therapy, 1332
        sequelae, 1332–1333, 1332t
        techniques, 1323–1329, 1324t–1326t, 1326f–1329f
    staging, 1320, 1320t–1321t
    surgical management, 1322–1323, 1323t
        results, 1329–1332, 1329t–1330t
Strandqvist plots, tumor control probability, 17–18
Stratification, phase III clinical trials, 359–360
Stroke, breast cancer therapy and risk of, 1274
Strong nuclear force, radioactivity and, 145
Strontium-89
    bone metastases, 592–594, 593t
    bone metastases, palliative therapy with, 1997–1998
    nonsealed radionuclide therapy, 591–592
Subacute responses
    intracranial tumor radiation therapy, 730
    radiation therapy, 79
Subacute thrombosis, vascular brachytherapy, 1969
Subadditive effect, chemoradiation therapy, 670
Subclinical disease criteria, tumor control probability and, 96–97, 97f
Subdiaphragmatic field setting, Hodgkin's lymphoma, 1728–1729,
    1729f
Subglottic larynx, lesions of, 978
Sublinugual gland, anatomy, 874, 875f
Submandibular gland
    anatomy, 874, 875f
    radiation therapy, 883, 885f
Subset analyses, clinical trials, 362
Subvolumes, dose heterogeneity, 102, 103f
Sucralfate, chemical radioprotection, 617–618
Suit principles of radiation oncology, 13, 14t
Superadditive effect, chemoradiation therapy, 670
Superficial tumors, hyperthermia therapy, 662
Superficial units, radiation therapy machines, 149
Superior sulcus tumors, 1091–1093, 1094f
    magnetic resonance imaging, 623
Superior vena cava syndrome, diagnosis and management,
    1093–1094
Supervoltage units, electron beam radiation, 150
Supportive care. See also Quality of life issues
    basic principles, 2011
    fatigue and mood dysfunction, 2011–2012

genitourinary tract injury, 2017
mucosal injury, 2013–2016
nutrition, 2017–2018
salivary gland injury, 2012–2013
skin injury, 2016–2017
Supraclavicular fossa, breast cancer metastases, 1184–1185
    radiation therapy, 1253, 1253f, 1274
        tangential field alignment, 1255–1257, 1256f–1257f
Supracricoid laryngectomy, 987
Supraglottic carcinoma, 976–977
    diagnosis, 979–980, 980t
    radiation therapy, 987–988, 987f
        sequelae, 993
    recurrent disease management, 988–989
    surgical treatment, 987, 990t
    treatment modalities, 985–988, 989t–990t
    treatment results, 990, 991t–992t
    treatment sequelae, 993
Supraglottic larynx carcinomas, 976–977
    diagnosis, 979–980, 980t
    radiation therapy, 987–988, 987f
    recurrent disease management, 988–989
    surgical treatment, 987
    treatment modalities, 985–988, 989t–990t
    treatment results, 990, 991t–992t
    treatment sequelae, 993
Suprahyoid epiglottis lesions, characteristics of, 976–977
Supratentorial primitive neuroectodermal tumor, pediatric patients,
    1841, 1842f
Surface dose
    brachytherapy, 423
    electron-beam therapy, water-based dose distribution, 191
Surface irregularities, electron-beam therapy, dosage calculations,
    194–196, 195f–199f
Surgical management
    adrenal gland tumors, 1719–1720
    anal cancer, 1390–1391
    astrocytomas, pediatric patients, 1827, 1828f, 1829
    bladder cancer, 1421
    bone metastases, 1989–1991, 1990f, 1990t
    brain metastases, palliative therapy, 1974–1975, 1975f, 1978t
    brainstem gliomas, pediatric patients, 1830–1832, 1831f
    breast cancer
        after breast augmentation, 1242
        axillary lymph node dissection, 1205–1206
            radiation therapy vs., 1224–1230
        breast-conserving techniques, 1204–1205, 1204t,
            1207–1210, 1209f
            age as risk factor, 1210–1211
            clinical trials, 1220, 1222–1223, 1222t
            collagen vascular disease, 1237–1238, 1237t
            concurrent chemoradiation with, 1230t, 1231–1232
            cosmesis and, 1264–1268, 1265f, 1266t
            familial breast cancer and BRCA1-2 mutation patients,
                1234–1237, 1235t, 1236f–1237f
            lactation following, 1240
            locally advanced and recurrent disease, 1299–1300, 1299f
            mammoplasty and, 1242
            no radiation, 1219–1220, 1220f–1221f
            patient follow-up, 1268
            prognostic factors, 1210–1219, 1211f–1212f, 1211t
            radiographic studies, 1268–1269
            recurrence risk and, 1309–1310
        breast reconstruction, postmastectomy radiation and,
            1314–1315
        early stages, 1203–1206
        in elderly women, 1223–1224, 1224f, 1225t
        locally advanced and recurrent disease, 1297, 1297t
        lumpectomy, 1203–1204, 1203f, 1223
        mastectomy, 1300–1305, 1300t
        multicentric disease and, 1241, 1242t
        nipple-sparing mastectomy, 1203
        patient selection criteria, 1207–1208, 1207t
        prophylactic surgery, 1182–1183
        radiation therapy vs., 1204–1205, 1204t
        sentinel node biopsies, 1206
        skin-sparing mastectomy, 1203
    central nervous system lymphoma, 742
    cervical cancer, 1546–1548 (See also Hysterectomy)
        ovarian function preservation, 1552
        recurrent disease, 1590

Surgical management (*contd.*)
  staging protocols, 1539–1540, 1540*f*
  techniques for, 1550–1552
colon cancer, 1367–1368
Cushing's disease, 758
differentiated thyroid cancer, 1062–1063
endometrial cancer, 1614–1615, 1622–1623
ependymoma, 740
  pediatric patients, 1833–1834
esophageal cancer, 1138, 1142, 1143*t*, 1145–1146, 1146*t*
esthesioneuroblastoma, 1015–1017, 1914
Ewing's sarcoma, 1886–1887
fallopian tube malignancies, 1653
germ-cell tumors, pediatric patients, 1924–1925
glomus tumors, 998–999
hepatocellular carcinoma, 1352, 1352*t*
  pediatric patients, 1918–1920
hypopharyngeal cancers
  complications, 971
  T1-2 tumors, 963–964
  T3-4 resectable tumors, 965–966
intracranial tumor management, 724–725
  sequelae of, 729–730
Langerhans cell histiocytosis in children, 1921
medullary thyroid cancer, 1066–1067, 1067*f*
medulloblastoma, 741
  pediatric patients, 1837–1841
meningiomas, 743–744
  nonmalignant disease, 1935–1936, 1935*t*
metastatic spinal cord compression, 1981–1982, 1982*t*, 1983*f*
nasopharyngeal cancer, 848, 848*f*
neck metastases, unknown primary tumors, 1037, 1039
neuroblastoma in pediatric patients, 1863, 1865, 1865*t*, 1868–1869
non-Hodgkin's lymphoma, 1745
nonpilocytic/diffusely infiltrating gliomas, 738
oral cavity tumors, 901
osteosarcoma, 1802–1803
ovarian cancer
  cytoreductive surgery, 1636
  palliative surgery, 1637
  secondary surgery, 1636
  staging and debulking, 1634–1635
pancreatic cancer, 1337–1338, 1338*t*
  locally advanced disease resectioning, 1345
penis, cancer of, 1524, 1527–1528, 1527*t*
pituitary tumors, 754
  transphenoidal resection, 757
pretreatment laparotomy, 1551–1552, 1552*t*
prostate cancer
  current trends in, 1456–1457
  extended pelvic lymph node dissection, 1486–1487
  external beam radiation therapy *vs.*, 1468–1469
  radical prostatectomy, 1457
  sequelae, 1471
radiation therapy and, 48, 48*f*
rectal cancer, 1373–1374
renal cell carcinoma, 1402–1403
retroperitoneal cancer, 1709–1713, 1713*t*
rhabdomyosarcoma, pediatric patients, 1877–1878, 1882
salivary gland tumors, radiation therapy with, 884–887, 886*t*–887*t*
skin carcinoma
  melanoma, 696
  Merkel cell carcinoma, 698
  nonmelanoma skin cancer, 692–693
soft tissue sarcomas, 1813, 1817–1818
spinal cord tumors, 771
  spinal cord compression, 1981–1982, 1982*t*, 1983*f*
stomach cancer, 1322–1323, 1323*t*
  results, 1329–1332, 1329*t*–1330*t*
superior sulcus tumors, 1092–1093
thymomas, 1113–1114
tracheal tumors, 1120–1121, 1121*t*
urethral cancer
  female, 1684–1685, 1688, 1689*t*, 1690
  male, 1525
uterine sarcoma, 1624
vaginal cancer, 1663–1665, 1672–1673
  complications, 1676–1678
vocal cord carcinoma, 983, 993

recurrent disease following, 985
vulvar cancer, 1696–1697, 1699–1700
  lymph node metastases, 1694–1696
  sequelae, 1705–1706
Wilms' tumor, 1853, 1856
xerostomia, 2012–2013
Surveillance protocols, hepatocellular carcinoma, 1350
Survival analyses
bladder cancer, 1412–1413, 1413*t*
  recurrent disease, 1419–1420, 1420*t*
breast cancer, locally advanced and recurrent disease, 1296, 1297*f*
cervical cancer therapies, 1566–1573, 1568*t*, 1571*t*, 1572*f*, 1577*t*, 1583*t*–1584*t*
clinical trials, 361–362
colon cancer, 1368–1370, 1369*t*–1370*t*, 1370*f*
hepatocellular carcinoma, 1355
  pediatric patients, 1919–1920
Hodgkin's lymphoma radiation therapy, pediatric patients, 1899, 1900*t*
laryngeal cancer, 989*t*
neuroblastoma, pediatric patients, 1868–1869
pancreatic cancer, 1338, 1338*t*, 1342*t*
renal cell carcinomas, 1400–1402, 1401*t*
renal pelvis and ureter carcinoma, 1402
stomach cancer, 1321–1322, 1321*t*–1322*t*
thymomas, 1112–1113, 1113*t*–1114*t*
vaginal cancer, 1663–1664
Survival model comparisons, dose fractionation, 92–93, 93*f*–94*f*
Survival pathway signaling, radiation therapy and cell death, 78
Survival rates for cancer, 54*t*
Suturing techniques, interstitial brachytherapy, afterloading technology, 478–479, 479*f*
Sweat gland carcinoma, epidemiology and management, 699–700
Syed-Nedblett templates, brachytherapy, 481, 481*f*–482*f*
Synchronized moving aperture radiation therapy (SMART), beam tracking technology, 289
Synchrotrons, components and instrumentation, 155

T
T3N0 rectal cancer, 1376
TAG-72 antigen, radioimmunotherapy with, 590
Tamoxifen, breast cancer and
  complications with, 1270–1271
  ductal carcinoma in situ therapy, 1171, 1171*t*
  prevention, 1181–1183, 1182*t*
Tandem transplantation, multiple myeloma, 1795
Target molecules, radiation damage, 114–115, 114*f*
Target volume definition
  altered fractionation radiotherapy, dose escalation for improvement of, 316–317
  boron neutron capture therapy, 34–35
  breast cancer radiation therapy, postmastectomy radiation, 1312
  chemotherapy, intracranial tumor management, 729
  fractionated stereotactic radio therapy, pituitary tumor management, 762
  glioblastoma multiforme, 731, 731*t*, 734–735
  hypoxic cells, 613–614
  image-guided radiation therapy, 263–268
    four-dimensional imaging, 286–288, 286*f*–287*f*
    magnetic resonance imaging, 265–266, 267*f*
    positron emission tomography, 264–265, 264*f*–266*f*
    single photon emission computed tomography, 266, 268, 269*f*
  intracranial tumor radiation therapy, 726
  lung cancer radiation therapy, 1095–1097, 1096*f*, 1097*t*
    intensity-modulated radiation therapy, 1098
  maxillary sinus radiation therapy, 866–867, 866*f*–867*f*
  nasal cavity and ethmoid sinus radiation therapy, 864–866, 865*f*
  nasopharyngeal cancer, 832, 833*t*
  pediatric radiation therapy
    astrocytomas, 1827–1828, 1828*f*
    medulloblastoma, 1838–1841, 1839*f*
  radiation therapy, 8
  retroperitoneal cancer radiation therapy, 1711–1713
  soft tissue sarcoma radiation therapy, 1815
  spine/spinal cord tumors, 773
  three-dimensional conformal radiation therapy, 221, 221*f*
    volume and dose specification, 224–226, 225*f*, 226*t*
Taxanes
  breast cancer therapy, trials of, 1306, 1306*t*
  combined chemoradiation therapy, 677–678, 677*t*
  ovarian cancer therapy, 1637

Technetium-99m bone scintigraphy, bone metastases, 1987
Technology assessment
    ethical issues and, 2039–2040
    radiation therapy, 2022–2023
Teletherapy, radiation therapy using, 6
Telomeres, radiation oncology and, 42–43
Templates, brachytherapy, 481
Temporal lobe necrosis
    chemodectomas, 998, 1004t
    nasopharyngeal cancer therapy, 851–853, 851t, 852f
Tenascin-C, radioimmunotherapy with, 590
Tendonitis, radiation therapy, 1948, 1948f
Tennis/golfer's elbow, radiation therapy, 1948–1949
Teratoma, classification, 1505
Testicular cancer. See also specific tumors, e.g., Choriocarcinoma
    acute lymphoblastic leukemia, 1783
        radiation therapy, 1786–1787
    anatomy, 1503
    chemotherapy, 1516
    classification, 1504–1505, 1504t
    clinical presentation, 1505
    diagnostic work-up, 1505–1506, 1506t
    epidemiology, 1503–1504
    laboratory studies, 1506
    lymphomas, 1758
    management, 1508
    natural history and staging, 1505, 1505t
    non-Hodgkin's lymphoma, pediatric patients, 1908
    pathology, 1504
    radiation therapy, 1513–1514, 1513f–1514f
    radiographic studies, 1506
    rhabdomyosarcoma, pediatric patients, 1876–1877
    risk factors, 1503–1504, 1504t
    sequelae of therapy, 1515–1516
    staging and prognostic factors, 1505–1508, 1505t–1508t
    therapeutic outcomes, 1514–1515, 1515f
TG-21 protocol, total body irradiation, 369
TG-51 protocol
    absorbed dose calculation, 159
    total body irradiation, 369
Therapeutic factors, tumor pathophysiology, 136–137, 137f
Therapeutic index, chemoradiation therapy, 669
Therapeutic ratio (gain)
    altered fractionation radiotherapy, dose escalation for
        improvement of, 316–317
    chemical modifiers of radiation therapy, 611
    toxicity effects, radiation therapy, 20–21, 21f
Thermal dosimetry
    hyperthermia
        clinical applications, 659–660
        noninvasive thermal dose measurements, 657–658,
            657f–659f
    interstitial hyperthermia, 653
Thermal enhancement ratio (TER), hyperthermia/radiation therapy
    regimen, 647–648
Thermal isoeffect dose. See Isoeffect dose
Thermoluminescent detectors (TLD)
    absorbed dose calculation, 159
    brachytherapy, 438–440
Thermotolerance, hyperthermia, 640–642, 641f
    isoeffect dose modification, 639
Thimble chamber, radiation exposure measurement, 157
Thorium series, basic properties, 146
Three-dimensional brachytherapy, cervical cancer, 1564–1565
Three-dimensional conformal radiation therapy
    biological plan evaluation models, 232–233
    breast cancer, 1257–1259, 1260f
    cervical cancer, 1558, 1559f–1560f
    coaxial beam arrangements, 177
    data management, 233–234
    dose calculation algorithms, 231
    dose-volume histogram, 231–232, 231f–232f
    future research issues, 236
    historical development of, 218–219, 219t
    intensity-modulated radiation therapy comparison with, 239–240
    late effects syndromes on lung, 330, 331f
    lung cancer, 1094–1095, 1096f
    nasopharyngeal cancer, 833–834, 835f
    oropharyngeal cancer, 945f, 946–947
    overview, 218

pancreatic cancer, 1340–1341, 1340f
prostate cancer
    beam selection and planning, 1459
    dose calculation methods, 1461
    long-term results, 1468
    sequelae, 1471–1472, 1472f
    techniques, 1457–1458
quality assurance protocols, 234–236
retinoblastoma, 790
retroperitoneal cancer, 1711–1713, 1713t–1714t
treatment planning, 219–224, 219t
    beam arrangement and field apertures, 221, 222f
    dose calculation, 221–222
    patient positioning and immobilization, 220–221, 220f–221f
    plan evaluation and improvement, 222, 223f
    plan implementation and treatment verification, 222, 224,
        224f
    quality assurance protocols, 234–236
    tumor, target volume, critical structure delineation and dose,
        221, 221f
volume and dose specification, 224–230
    dose reporting and prescription, 227
    GTV, CTV, and PTV concepts, 227–230, 228f–230f
    tumor/target volume definition, 224–226, 225f, 226t
Three-dimensional external beam radiation therapy chart rounds, 57
Three-dimensional imaging, interstitial brachytherapy, 454–456
Three-dimensional treatment planning
    Hodgkin's lymphoma radiation therapy, 1729–1730, 1730f
    radiation therapy, 30–31, 30f
Through-and-through plastic tubing, interstitial brachytherapy,
    afterloading technology, 477–478, 479f
Thymic carcinoid, diagnosis and management, 1117
Thymic carcinoma, diagnosis and management, 1116–1117
Thymidine labeling index (TLI), breast cancer metastases, 1200
Thymoliposarcoma, diagnosis and management, 1117
Thymomas, 1109–1116
    chemotherapy, 1115
    combined treatment modalities, 1115, 1116t
    diagnosis, 1110
    epidemiology, 1109
    natural history, 1109–1110
    pathologic classification, 1110–1112, 1111t
    prognostic factors, 1112–1113, 1113t–1114t
    radiation therapy, 1114–1116
    recurrent disease, 1114
    staging, 1112, 1112t
    surgical management, 1113–1114
Thyroglobulin therapy, differentiated thyroid cancer, 1066
Thyroid cancer
    anaplastic cancer, 1061–1062, 1067–1068
    anatomy, 1055, 1056f
    chemotherapy, 1070
    clinical manifestations and diagnostic work-up, 1056–1059,
        1057t, 1059f
        fine-needle aspiration biopsy, 1059
        imaging studies, 1058–1059, 1058t
    combined treatment modalities, 1070–1071
    differentiated thyroid cancer, 1059, 1061–1066
    epidemiology, 1055–1056
    follicular cancers, 1061
    Hodgkin's lymphoma radiation therapy, pediatric patients,
        1901
    late effects syndromes, 345–346
    lymphoma, 1062, 1067–1068
    management, 1062–1067
    medullary thyroid cancer, 1061–1062, 1066–1068
    outpatient iodine therapy, 1071–1072
    papillary/mixed-papillary-follicular cancers, 1059, 1061
    pathologic classification, 1059, 1061
    patient surveillance, 1071
    pediatric patients, 1922–1924, 1923t
        Hodgkin's lymphoma and, 1901
    prognostic factors, 1061–1062
    radiation-induced cancer, 1055–1056, 1061
    radiation therapy, 1067–1069
    radioactive iodine therapy, 1069–1073
    staging, 1059, 1060t
Thyroidectomy
    differentiated thyroid cancer, 1062–1063
    medullary thyroid cancer, 1066–1067, 1067f
    pediatric patients, 1923

Thyroid hormone therapy
  differentiated thyroid cancer, 1065
  medullary thyroid cancer, 1067
  pediatric patients, 1923–1924
Thyroid-stimulating hormone (TSH), differentiated thyroid cancer, 1065–1066
Thyrotropin-releasing hormone (TRH), late effects syndromes in neuroendocrine system and, 345
Thyrotropin-secreting adenomas, diagnosis and management, 760
Time and effort analysis, radiation therapy, 2024
Time course of procedures
  high-dose-rate brachytherapy, 552–555
  nasopharyngeal cancer radiation therapy, 831–832, 833t
  Wilms' tumor radiation in pediatric patients, 1853
Time-dose fractionation
  melanoma radiation therapy, 698
  nominal standard dose and, 25–26
  normal tissue effects, radiation therapy, 19–20
  pediatric radiation therapy, medulloblastoma, 1840
  skin cancer radiation therapy, 694, 694t
Time to tumor recurrence, human tumor regeneration, 86
Tirapazamine, cervical cancer therapy, 1592
Tissue-air ratio
  basic principles, 161, 161f
  photon external-beam dosimetry, 167–168
    air gap correction, 168–169, 169f
    tissue inhomogeneity correction, 169–171
Tissue diagnosis, spinal cord tumors, 768
Tissue heterogeneity, intensity-modulated radiation therapy, lung cancer, 1098
Tissue inhomogeneities, photon external-beam dosimetry, correction for, 169–171
Tissue interface, photon external-beam dosimetry, 173–174, 174f
Tissue maximum ratio (TMR), total body irradiation, 369
Tissue-phantom/tissue-maximum ratios
  basic principles, 161, 161f
  photon external-beam dosimetry, air gap correction, 168–169, 169f
Tissue response mechanisms
  hyperthermia
    cytotoxicity effects, 640, 641f
    damage effects, 644–645
  invasion and metastasis, 113–114
  radiation therapy, biological basis for, 76–77
Tolerance doses
  intraoperative radiotherapy, 397–399
  late effects syndromes on normal tissue, 321–322, 322f
    central nervous system, 325, 325f, 325t
  radiation therapy, 19
  radiation therapy "remembered" doses, 83–84
  spinal cord tumor radiation therapy, 775–776
Tolerance volumes, late effects syndromes on normal tissue, 322–323, 323t
Tomotherapy
  components and instrumentation, 154, 154f
  development of, 240
  equipment, 240, 241f
  fixed-gantry technique vs., 256–257
  helical systems, 281–282, 282f
  rotating slit approach, 243, 244f–245f
  rotation therapy techniques, 178
  serial setup and IMRT delivery, 256
  stereotactic radiosurgery, 380
Tongue. See also Base of tongue (BOT) tumors
  anatomy, 891
  brachytherapy, 497–498, 497f–498f
  carcinomas, treatment and results, 908–909
Tonsillar fossa tumors
  brachytherapy, 498–499, 500f
  curative protocol, 930f
  oropharyngeal metastases, 924t
  prognostic factors, 925–926, 925f–927f
Topical mechlorethamine chemotherapy, cutaneous T-cell lymphoma, 1773
Topoisomerase I inhibitors, combined chemoradiation therapy, 677t, 679
Tort law, radiation oncology, 63–65
Total body irradiation (TBI)
  acute toxicity, 372
  advantages of, 366
  basic requirements, 367

chemotherapy with, 365–366
clinical myeloablative stem cell transplantation, 365
complications, 372–374
current techniques, 367–368
delayed toxicity, 372
dose and fractionation schedule, 366–367
dose homogeneity, 370
dose-limiting toxicity, 365
dose rate, 370
dosimetry, 368–369
eye lens effect, 373
graft versus leukemia/tumor effects, 365
growth, gonadal, and endocrine effects, 373
hematopoietic system effects, 364
high-dose complications, 372
Hodgkin's lymphoma, 1732–1733
institutional comparisons, 370
kidney effects, 373
late effects syndromes on normal tissue
  bone and bone marrow, 348–349, 349f, 349t
  central nervous system, 325
  liver, 337–338, 337f, 338t
  lung, 330, 330f–331f
leukemia radiologic effects, 364–365
liver effects, 372–373, 373f
low-dose complications, 372
low-dose rate regimens, 101
lung/organ dose attenuation, 371–372, 371f
multiple myeloma, 1795–1796
neuroblastoma in pediatric patients, 1866–1869
nonmyeloablative or reduced intensity stem cell transplantation, 367
overview, 364–367
patient positioning, 370, 371f
quality assurance, 370–372
secondary cancers, 373–374
selected organ boosting, 372
skin surface dose, 370
stem cell rescue, 364
stem cell transplantation, 364
Total energy released by primary photon interactions per unit mass (TERMA), photon external-beam dosimetry, tissue inhomogeneity correction, 170
Total-limb irradiation, electron-beam therapy, 211–212, 212f
Total mesorectal excision, rectal cancer therapy, 1374
Total reference air-kerma (TRAK), brachytherapy dosimetry, 435
Total-scalp irradiation, electron-beam therapy, 210–211, 211f
Total-skin electron-beam (TSEB) radiation
  basic principles, 212–213, 213f
  cutaneous T-cell lymphoma, 1769–1774, 1772f
Tourniquet techniques, modification of radiation response, 35
Toxicity effects
  androgen suppression therapy, prostate cancer, 1493–1494
  ovarian cancer therapy, 1644–1645
  radiation therapy
    bladder cancer, 1434–1435
    chemical radioprotection, 614–615
    combined chemoradiation therapy, head and neck squamous-cell tumors, 817
    lung cancer therapy, 1102–1104, 1103t
    oropharyngeal tumors, 936–937
    prostate cancer, 1471–1473
      intensity modulated photon therapy toxicity, 1489
    quantitation of, 20–21
    radioimmunotherapy, 586–587
    stereotactic body radiation therapy, spinal cord, 394
    total body irradiation, 365
      complications, 372
  rhabdomyoscarcoma radiation therapy, pediatric patients, 1882
  soft tissue sarcoma radiation therapy, 1819
TP53 tumor suppressor gene, cell cycle control loss and, 111
Tracheal carcinomas, diagnosis and management, 1119–1122, 1120f
Transcatheter arterial chemoembolization (TACE), hepatocellular carcinoma
  basic principles, 1353
  pediatric patients, 1920
  radiation therapy and, 1354, 1354t, 1355f
Transcription factors, growth control and, 111
Transforming growth factor family
  cervical cancer, 1546
  growth inhibitory signals and, 112
  radiation effects on, 119

Transfusion therapy, cervical cancer, 1543

Transient equilibrium, radioactivity, 146, 146*f*

Transient myelopathy syndrome, spinal, late effects of radiation on, 326–327, 328*t*

Transitional cell carcinomas
  bladder cancer, 1414
    systemic therapy, 1432
  prostate cancer, 1455
  renal pelvis and ureter carcinoma, 1400

Transition energy, radioactivity, 146

Transperineal iodine implants, prostate cancer, 527–530, 528*f* 529*f*
  brachytherapy, 1463–1465, 1464*f*, 1465*t*
  dosimetric evaluation, 1464–1465, 1465*t*

Transplantation protocols, hepatocellular carcinoma, 1352

Transrectal ultrasonography (TRUS), prostate cancer imaging, 1450

Transsphenoidal adenectomy, pituitary adenoma, 1936

Transurethral resection of the bladder (TURB)
  diagnosis, 1413
  disease progression and, 1412–1413
  superficial tumor treatment, 1413–1414
  technique, 1421
  toxicity and quality of life issues, 1434–1435

Transverse cervical liagments, anatomy, 1532

Trastuzumab, breast cancer therapy, 1307, 1307*t*

Traveling wave design, lnear accelerators, 151

Treatment algorithms
  breast cancer, locally advanced disease, 1307–1308, 1308*f*
  vulvar cancer, 1698*t*–1699*t*

Treatment head instrumentation, instrumentation and schematics, 151*f*, 152

Treatment planning
  cervical cancer brachytherapy, 1562*f*, 1564–1565
  elective nodal irradiation, 633–634, 634*f*
  electron arc therapy, 214–215
  electron-beam therapy, 200–209, 201*f*
    bolus specifications, 202–204, 203*f*–205*f*
    electron collimation design, 201–202
    energy selection criteria, 200–201, 201*f*
    field abutment, 206, 206*f*–208*f*
    internal collimation, 204–205, 206*f*
    mixed-beam therapy, 206–207, 208*f*, 209
    multileaf collimation, 202
    skin collimation, 202, 202*f*
  fractionated stereotactic radio therapy, pituitary tumor management, 762
  high-dose-rate brachytherapy
    dosimetry methods and, 552–556
    operation protocols, 546
  Hodgkin's lymphoma radiation therapy, 1729–1730, 1730*f*
  intensity-modulated radiation therapy, 31, 242, 242*f*–243*f*
    evaluation of, 249–250
    lung cancer, 1098
  intensity-modulated radiation therapy (IMRT), setup and delivery, 255–256
  nasopharyngeal cancer, 831, 831*f*–832*f*
  neuroblastoma, pediatric patients, 1867–1868, 1868*f*
  nonmalignant disease radiation, 1935
  oropharyngeal radiation therapy, intensity-modulated techniques, 946–947, 947*t*
  pediatric radiation therapy, medulloblastoma, 1839, 1840*t*, 1841*f*
  photon external-beam dosimetry, 175–178
  prostate cancer radiation therapy, 1461–1463
  radiation therapy, 30–31
    esophageal cancer, 1139, 1141
    volume definitions, 628*t*
  soft tissue sarcoma radiation therapy, 1816, 1816*f*
  spine/spinal cord tumors, 773–774, 774*f*
  stereotactic body radiation therapy, 390–391
  three-dimensional conformal radiation therapy, 219–224, 219*t*
    beam arrangement and field apertures, 221, 222*f*
    dose calculation, 221–222
    patient positioning and immobilization, 220–221, 220*f*–221*f*
    plan evaluation and improvement, 222, 223*f*
    plan implementation and treatment verification, 222, 224, 224*f*
    quality assurance protocols, 234–236
    tumor, target volume, critical structure delineation and dose, 221, 221*f*

Treatment time modeling, brachytherapy, 466, 467*f*

Treatment volume

breast cancer radiation therapy, 1243–1244, 1245*f*–1246*f*
cholangiocarcinoma radiation therapy, 1359–1360, 1360*f*
hepatocellular carcinoma radiation therapy, 1353–1354, 1354*t*
non-Hodgkin's lymphoma radiation therapy, 1747–1748
pancreatic radiation therapy, 1338–1339
three-dimensional conformal radiation therapy, 225
vulvar cancer radiation therapy, 1700–1702, 1701*f*–1702*f*

Trismus, oropharyngeal radiation therapy, 939–941

Truncal sarcomas, diagnosis and treatment, 1817

Tubular carcinoma, breast cancer, 1196

Tumor-associated antigens (TAAs), radioimmunoglobulin targeting, 584, 584*t*
  solid tumors, 589–590

Tumor cells
  antigenic targets, radioimmunoglobulins, 583–584, 584*t*
  basic structure, 126, 127*f*
  blood flow and circulation, 128–130, 129*f*–130*f*
  breast cancer, metastases and characteristics of, 1199
  cell-loss factors in, 84
  cervical cancer and characteristics of, 1543–1544, 1544*t*
  chemoradiation therapy and repopulation inhibition, 672
  extravascular compartment, 131–132
  hyperthermia and metabolism of, 643–644, 644*f*
  inherent radiosensitivity of, 15–16
  interstitial hypertension, 134
  interstitial transport, 132
  isoeffect formulae, 99, 99*f*
  lymphatic transport, 132–134, 133*f*
  metabolic environment, 134–136
  molecular pathophysiology, 126–137
    angiogenesis, 126–127, 128*t*
    prognostic implications, 136
    therapeutic implications, 136–137, 137*f*
    vascular architecture, 127–128
    vascular compartment, 126–131
  radiation therapy
    cell death prediction, 84
    regeneration following, 85–86
    regression mechanisms, 84–85
  radiosensitivity, predictive assays, 16–17, 16*f*
  vascular permeability, 130
  vessel wall movement, 130–131

Tumor control probability (TCP)
  accelerated repopulation and, 23, 24*f*
  chemical modifiers of radiation therapy, 611
  dose-volume histograms, 102, 102*f*
  external beam radiation therapy volume, 6–7
  radiation oncology and, 17–18
  radiation therapy, 95–97, 96*f*
  three-dimensional conformal radiation therapy evaluation, 233
  treatment planning and, 30–31, 30*f*

Tumor grade, breast cancer metastases, 1199

Tumorigenesis, replicative potential and, 113

Tumor location
  breast cancer metastases and, 1202
    recurrent disease, 1215–1216
  rectal cancer, 1372, 1373*f*

Tumor markers, radiation oncology and, 44, 44*t*

Tumor motion
  image-guided radiation therapy, respiratory motion management, 288
  intensity-modulated radiation therapy, lung cancer, 1098

Tumor necrosis factor (TNF) family, radiation therapy, 78
  molecular responses, 82

Tumor oxygenation, chemical modifiers of radiation therapy, 611–612

Tumor reoxygenation, radiation therapy, 89–90, 89*t*

Tumor responses, radiation therapy
  dose fractionation, 95, 95*f*
  in vivo kinetics, 84

Tumor selective agents, boron neutron capture therapy, 34, 34*f*

Tumor shrinkage effect, brachytherapy, 467

Tumor size
  breast cancer metasetases and, 1198
    recurrent disease, 1215, 1216*t*
  cervical cancer outcomes and, 1574

Tumor suppressor genes
  cell cycle control and, 111–112
  molecular cancer biology, 109, 110*t*
  radiation oncology and, 37–41, 38*f*–39*f*

Two-component (TC) model, dose fractionation, 91*f*, 92

Two-dimensional dose calculations
  brachytherapy, 440–441
  nasopharyngeal cancer radiation therapy, 832–833, 834f–835f
Two-dimensional fluence verification, intensity-modulated radiation therapy, 254–255
Tyrosine kinases, non-small cell lung cancer therapy, 1099

U

Ultra-low-dose-rate implants, brachytherapy, 430–431
Ultrasonography
  bladder cancer, 1413
  breast cancer
    diagnosis and work-up, 1192
    screening, 1189
  endoscopic ultrasonography, 625, 625t
  fallopian tube disease, 1651
  image-guided radiation therapy, 268–271, 270f
  mammography and, 625–626, 626f
  testicular cancer, 1506
  thyroid disease, 1058
Ultrasound heating, hyperthermia, 650–651, 651f–652f
Ultraviolet radiation
  lip carcinomas, 894
  skin cancer epidemiology and etiology, 690, 691f
Uncertainty, radiation therapy, 7–8
Unit Center Point (UCP), gamma knife systems, 150
University of Michigan system, image-guided radiation therapy, 277
Uranium series, basic properties, 146
Urethral cancer
  clinical presentation, 1398
  diagnostic work-up, 1399, 1399t
  epidemiology and risk factors, 1398
  female
    anatomy, 1682, 1683f
    anterior (distal), 1684–1685
    brachytherapy, 521–522
    chemotherapy, 1690
    clinical presentation, 1682, 1683f
    diagnostic workup, 1683, 1683f, 1683t
    epidemiology and etiology, 1682
    low-dose-rate brachytherapy, 517–524
      bladder/urethral lesions, 521–522
      carcinoma in situ, 520
      rectovaginal septum tumor, 521
      stage I, 520, 520f
      stage II, 520
      stages III and IV, 521, 521f
      vaginal cylinders, 518–520, 518f–519f, 524f
      vulva/distal urethra tumors, 522–524, 523f–524f
    metastatic patterns, 1682
    pathologic classification, 1683–1684
    posterior (proximal), 1685
    prognostic factors, 1684, 1685f
    radiation therapy, 1685–1688, 1686f–1688f, 1689t, 1690
    staging system, 1683, 1684t
    surgical management, 1684–1685, 1688, 1689t, 1690
  male
    anatomy, 1519, 1520f
    brachytherapy, 525–527, 526t
    clinical presentation, 1520–1521, 1520f
    diagnostic work-up, 1521, 1521t
    epidemiology, 1519
    natural history, 1519–1520
    pathologic classification, 1522–1523, 1522t–1523f
    prognostic factors, 1523–1524, 1523f
    radiation therapy, 1526–1527, 1527f
    staging, 1521–1522, 1521t–1522t
    surgical management, 1525
    therapy outcomes, 1528–1530, 1529t
  management and recurrence risk, 1405–1406
  natural history, 1398
  pathologic classification, 1400
  prognostic factors, 1402
  radiation therapy, 1407
    sequelae, 1409–1410
  recurrent disease, 1419–1420
  staging, 1400, 1401t
  therapy outcomes, 1409
Urinary toxicity
  prostate cancer brachytherapy, 1472–1473, 1474f
  radiation therapy and, 2017

Urinary tract tumors. *See* specific organs, e.g. Kidney, ureter, prostate
  radiation-induced injury and, 2017
Uterine cancers
  sarcomas, 1613
    chemotherapy, 1625
    radiation therapy, 1624
    surgical management, 1624
  uterine papillary serous and clear cell carcinoma, 1623–1624
  vaginal cancer risk and, 1675
Uterine cervix, cancer of. *See* Cervical cancer
Uterosacral ligaments, oncological anatomy, 633
Uterus, anatomy, 1532
Utilitarianism, medical ethics and, 2035
Uveal melanoma, proton/α-particle radiotherapy, 413, 414f

V

Vaginal cancer
  anatomy, 1657, 1658f
  clear-cell adenocarcinoma
    epidemiology and risk factors, 1658
    management and treatment outcomes, 1672
    pathology, 1659
  clinical presentation, 1660–1661, 1661t
  combinatorial treatment modalities, 1667–1668
  diagnostic work-up, 1661
  endodermal sinus (yolk sac) tumors, 1674–1675
  epidemiology and risk factors, 1657–1658
  episiotomy carcinoma, 1676
  histology, 1663
  leukemia, 1660
  low-dose-rate irradiation, brachytherapy, 517–524
    bladder/urethral lesions, 521–522
    carcinoma in situ, 520
    rectovaginal septum tumor, 521
    stage I, 520, 520f
    stage II, 520
    stages III and IV, 521, 521f
    vaginal cylinders, 518–520, 518f–519f, 524f
    vulva/distal urethra tumors, 522–524, 523f–524f
  lymphomas, 1660, 1674
  melanocytic tumors, 1659
  natural history, 1660, 1672–1673
  neuroendocrine small-cell carcinoma, 1660
  nonepithelial tumors, 1659–1660, 1672–1675
  pathology, 1658–1660
  prognostic factors, 1662–1663
  radiation-induced injury and, 2017
  radiation therapy, 1663–1669, 1668f–1669f, 1670t
    complications, 1676–1678
    external beam radiation, 1668–1669, 1670f, 1673–1675
    high-dose-rate intracavitary brachytherapy, 1670–1671
    interstitial brachytherapy, 1671–1672
    low-dose-rate intracavitary brachytherapy, 1669–1670
    salvage therapy, 1676
  recurrent disease, 1667t
  salvage therapy, 1676
  sarcomas, 1673–1674
  squamous cell carcinoma, 1657–1658
    management, treatment and outcome, 1663–1664
    neovagina, 1675–1676
    prognostic factors, 1662–1663
    surgical approach, 1665
    treatment options and outcome, 1664–1665
  staging, 1661–1662, 1662t
  treatment options and outcome, 1663–1667, 1666t
    complications, 1676–1678, 1677t
  uterine tumors and, 1675
  vaginal adenosis, 1659
  vaginal intraepithelial neoplasia
    clinical presentation, 1660–1661, 1661t
    epidemiology and risk factors, 1657–1658
    pathology, 1658–1659
    treatment options and outcome, 1664–1665, 1664t
Vaginal cuff irradiation
  cervical cancer radiation therapy, 1553–1555, 1554f–1555f
  high-dose-rate brachytherapy, 565–567, 567t
Vaginal cylinders
  brachytherapy, 518–520, 518f–519f, 524f
  cervical cancer radiation therapy, 1553–1555, 1554f–1555f
Valence electrons, atomic structure, 143

Van de Graaff generator, 150
Varian On-Board Imaging (OBI) system, image-guided radiation therapy, 278–279, 278*f*, 283, 284*f*
Vascular brachytherapy (VBT), 532
  β-radiation in-stent coronary artery restenosis, 1964–1965, 1965*t*–1966*t*
  clinical trials, 1964–1967
  coronary anatomy, 1960, 1960*f*
  coronary in-stent restenosis
    Betacath system, 1962–1964, 1963*f*
    drug-eluting stents, 1965–1966
  de novo coronary artery restenosis, 1966–1967
  edge restenosis, 1968–1969
  future research, 1969–1970
  γ-radiation in-stent coronary artery restenosis, 1964, 1965*t*
  historical perspective, 1959–1960
  in-stent restenosis following DES, 1966
  overview, 1959
  percutaneous coronary intervention, 1960–1961, 1961*f*, 1962*t*
  peripheral vascular brachytherapy trials, 1967–1968, 1968*t*
  physics and devices, 1962
  radioactive stents, 1967
  saphenous vein graft in-stent restenosis, 1966
  subacute thrombosis, 1969
  terminology, 1969
Vascular endothelial growth factor (VEGF)
  chemoradiation therapy, molecular targeting and, 675–676
  non-small cell lung cancer therapy, 1100
  pancreatic cancer targeting, 1346
  renal cell carcinoma targeting, 1404
  salivary gland tumors, 888
  signaling mechanisms, 120
  tumor molecular pathophysiology, 127
    lymphatic transport, 132–134, 133*f*
Vascular malformation. *See* Arteriovenous malformation (AVM)
Vascular occlusive disease (VOD)
  late effects syndromes on normal tissue in liver and, 336–338, 337*f*, 338*t*
  total-body irradiation, liver, 372–373
Vascular system. *See also* Arteriovenous malformation (AVM); Great vessel tumors
  breast cancer metastases, 1199
  cervical cancer, 1544
  mesenchymal tumors, 1122–1123
  radiation effects on, 1934
  tumor cells and permeability of, 130
  tumor molecular pathophysiology, 126–131
Verification protocols, three-dimensional conformal radiation therapy, 222, 224, 224*f*
  quality assurance protocols, 235–236
Verrucous carcinoma
  cervical cancer, 1540–1541
  vulvar cancer, 1694, 1698–1699
Vertebral hemangiomas, diagnosis and therapy, 1954–1955
Vertebroplasty, bone metastases palliation, 1991
Vestibular schwannomas
  diagnosis and management, 745–746
  stereotactic radiosurgery, 384–385
Video systems, image-guided radiation therapy (IGRT), 271, 272*f*
Vinorelbine, non-small cell lung cancer therapy, 1099
Virtual stimulation, computed tomography simulators, 155
Virtue theory, medical ethics and, 2035
Vocal cord carcinomas, 979
  radiation therapy, 983–984, 984*f*–986*f*
  recurrent disease management, 984–985
  surgical treatment, 983
  treatment modalities, 981–985
  treatment results, 988*t*–989*t*, 990
  treatment sequelae, 993
Volume effects
  cervical cancer radiation therapy, 1553–1555, 1554*f*–1555*f*
  late effects syndromes on normal tissue, 322–323, 323*t*
  pediatric patients' radiation therapy, Wilms' tumor, 1854, 1854*f*
  radiation therapy, 80–82
    prostate cancer, 1488–1489
    treatment planning, 628*t*
  small cell lung carcinoma radiation therapy, 1102
Volumetric imaging systems
  adaptive radiation therapy, 289–293, 290*f*–293*f*
  image-guided radiation therapy, 279–284
    in-room CT systems, 279–281, 280*f*–281*f*

    kilovoltage systems, 282–283, 283*f*–284*f*
    megavoltage systems, 281–282, 282*f*
Von Hippel-Lindau disease
  renal cell carcinoma risk and, 1397–1398
  vascular malformation, 769
Vulvar tumors
  anatomy, 1692, 1693*f*
  brachytherapy, 522–524, 523*f*–524*f*
  chemotherapy, 1704–1705, 1705*t*
    sequelae, 1705–1706
  clinical presentation, 1693
  epidemiology, 1692
  histologic variants, 1697–1698
  low-dose-rate irradiation, brachytherapy, 517–524
    bladder/urethral lesions, 521–522
    carcinoma in situ, 520
    rectovaginal septum tumor, 521
    stage I, 520, 520*f*
    stage II, 520
    stages III and IV, 521, 521*f*
    vaginal cylinders, 518–520, 518*f*–519*f*, 524*f*
    vulva/distal urethra tumors, 522–524, 523*f*–524*f*
  natural history and metastases, 1692–1693, 1693*t*
  pathology, 1693–1694
  prognostic factors, 1694–1695
  radiation therapy, 1696–1697, 1700–1704, 1701*f*–1703*f*, 1704*t*
    sequelae, 1705–1706
  staging, 1695–1696, 1696*t*
  surgical management, 1696–1697, 1699–1700
    lymph node metastases, 1694–1696
    sequelae, 1705–1706
  treatment algorithms, 1697*f*–1699*f*
  verrucous carcinoma, 1698–1699

W
Water-based dose distribution, electron-beam therapy, 190–193
  depth dose, 190–192, 191*f*–192*f*, 191*t*
  isodose plots, 193–194, 194*f*
  off-axis dose, 192–193, 193*f*
Waveguide instrumentation, linear accelerators, 151–152
Wave-particle duality, electromagnetic radiation, 143–144, 143*f*–144*f*
Wedge filter
  basic properties, 163, 164*f*
  photon external-beam dosimetry, 174–175, 175*f*–176*f*
Wegener's granulomatosis, diagnosis and treatment, 1010–1012, 1011*t*
Wet macular degeneration, photodynamic therapy, 601
White matter tracts, radiation imaging, 632–633
Whole abdominal irradiation
  endometrial cancer, 1621
  ovarian cancer, 1638–1639, 1638*t*, 1641*t*, 1643–1645
Whole-brain radiation therapy
  brain metastases, 1974–1977, 1975*t*, 1977*f*, 1980*t*
  skin injury from, 2016–2017, 2016*f*
Whole breast radiotherapy
  adjuvant brachytherapy, 499–502, 501*f*–503*f*
  protocols for, 1246, 1248
Whole-liver radiation, 2000, 2001*f*, 2001*t*
Whole-lung irradiation
  osteosarcoma, 1805, 1805*t*
  pediatric patients, 1919–1920
Whole pelvic radiation, prostate cancer
  intensity modulated photon therapy toxicity, 1489
  prophylactic rationale for, 1486–1489, 1487*f*, 1489*t*
  techniques, 1484, 1484*f*–1485*f*
Whole-pelvis radiation therapy, anal cancer, 1392, 1392*f*
WHO Pain Ladder, 2005, 2006*f*
Wilms' tumor
  anaplastic tumor, 1856
  bilateral, 1855
  biology, 1850
  clear cell sarcoma, 1856
  clinical presentation, 1851
  clinical trials and outcomes, 1854–1857, 1855*t*
  desmoplastic small round-cell tumor (DSCRT), 1927
  diagnostic work-up, 1851, 1851*f*, 1852*t*
  end stage renal disease, 1857
  epidemiology, 1850
  late effects of treatment, 1857
  late effects syndromes in kidney and, 340

Wilms' tumor (*contd.*)
  natural history, 1851
  older patients, 1856
  pathologic classification, 1850–1851
  radiation therapy, 1853–1857, 1853*t*, 1854*f*
  retroperitoneal cancer, 1713–1714
  rhabdoid tumor of kidney, 1856
  secondary cancer, 1857
  staging, 1851, 1852*t*–1853*t*
  surgical management, 1853
Wnt proteins, growth control and, 111

X

Xeroderma pigmentosum (XP), 1927–1928
Xerostomia
  Hodgkin's lymphoma, 1734
  hypopharyngeal cancer radiation, 971
  nasopharyngeal cancer radiation, 1913
  oropharyngeal tumors, 937–938, 939*f*
  salivary gland injury, supportive care, 2012–2013
X-rays
  basic principles, 144
  beam quality and penetration, 156
  stomach cancer diagnosis, 1319–1320

Y

Yolk sac tumor
  classification, 1504*t*, 1505
  ovarian cancer, 1633
  vaginal cancer, 1674–1675
Ytterbium 169, brachytherapy applications, 428

Z

Zevalin, leukemia and lymphoma therapy, 588–589